QUICK REFERENCE (QR) VIDEO ACCESS

The images below are QR codes. Each code corresponds to a video from the *Goldman-Cecil Medicine 25* collection. For fast and easy video access, right from your mobile device, follow these instructions. The videos are also available on Expertconsult.com.

What You Need

- **A mobile device, such as a smartphone or tablet, equipped with a camera and Internet access**
- **A QR code reader application (If you do not already have a reader installed on your mobile device, look for free versions in your app store.)**

How It Works

- **Open the QR code reader application on your mobile device.**
- **Point the device's camera at the code and scan.**
- **Each code opens an individual video player for instant viewing—no log-on required.**

Confusion Assessment Method (CAM)
Chapter 28, Video 28-1 – Marcos Mialnez, Jorge G. Ruiz, and Rosanne M. Leipzig

Standard Echocardiographic Views: Four-Chamber Image Plane
Chapter 55, Video 55-1D – Catherine M. Otto

Interlaminar Epidural Steroid Injection
Chapter 30, Video 30-1 – Ali Turabi

Dilated Cardiomyopathy: Long Axis View
Chapter 55, Video 55-2A – Catherine M. Otto

Standard Echocardiographic Views: Long Axis Image Plane
Chapter 55, Video 55-1A – Catherine M. Otto

Dilated Cardiomyopathy: Short Axis View
Chapter 55, Video 55-2B – Catherine M. Otto

Standard Echocardiographic Views: Short Axis Image Plane
Chapter 55, Video 55-1B – Catherine M. Otto

Dilated Cardiomyopathy: Apical Four-Chamber View
Chapter 55, Video 55-2C – Catherine M. Otto

Standard Echocardiographic Views: Short Axis Image Plane
Chapter 55, Video 55-1C – Catherine M. Otto

Three-Dimensional Echocardiography
Chapter 55, Video 55-3 – Catherine M. Otto

Stress Echocardiography: Normal Reaction
Chapter 55, Video 55-4A – Catherine M. Otto

Stress Echocardiography: Normal Reaction
Chapter 55, Video 55-4B – Catherine M. Otto

Stress Echocardiography: Proximal Stenosis of the Left Anterior Descending Coronary Artery
Chapter 55, Video 55-4C – Catherine M. Otto

Stress Echocardiography: Proximal Stenosis of the Left Anterior Descending Coronary Artery
Chapter 55, Video 55-4D – Catherine M. Otto

Pericardial Effusion: Parasternal Long Axis
Chapter 55, Video 55-5A – Catherine M. Otto

Pericardial Effusion: Parasternal Short Axis
Chapter 55, Video 55-5B – Catherine M. Otto

Pericardial Effusion: Apical Four-Chamber Views
Chapter 55, Video 55-5C – Catherine M. Otto

Secundum Atrial Septal Defect
Chapter 69, Video 69-1 – Ariane J. Marelli

Perimembranous Ventricular Septal Defect
Chapter 69, Video 69-2 – Ariane J. Marelli

Coronary Stent Placement
Chapter 74, Video 74-1 – Paul S. Teirstein

Guidewire Passage
Chapter 74, Video 74-2 – Paul S. Teirstein

Delivering the Stent
Chapter 74, Video 74-3 – Paul S. Teirstein

Inflating the Stent
Chapter 74, Video 74-4 – Paul S. Teirstein

Final Result
Chapter 74, Video 74-5 – Paul S. Teirstein

Superficial Femoral Artery (SFA) Stent Procedure
Chapter 79, Video 79-1 – Christopher J. White

Orthotopic Bicaval Cardiac Transplantation
Chapter 82, Video 82-1 – Y. Joseph Woo

Wheezing
Chapter 87, Video 87-1 – Jeffrey M. Drazen

Endoscopic Mucosal Resection Using Saline Lift Polypectomy of a Colon Adenoma Followed by Closure of the Mucosal Defect with Clips
Chapter 193, Video 193-3 – Douglas O. Faigel

VATS Wedge Resection
Chapter 101, Video 101-1 – Malcolm M. DeCamp

Endoscopic View of Rectal Cancer
Chapter 193, Video 193-4 – Douglas O. Faigel

Ventilation of an Ex Vivo Rat Lung
Chapter 105, Video 105-1 – Arthur S. Slutsky, George Volgyesi, and Tom Whitehead

Endoscopic Ultrasound
Chapter 193, Video 193-5 – Douglas O. Faigel

Renal Artery Stent
Chapter 125, Video 125-1 – Renato M. Santos and Thomas D. DuBose, Jr.

Laparoscopic Roux-en-Y Gastric Bypass
Chapter 220, Video 220-1 – James M. Swain

Interpretation of a Computed Tomographic Colonography
Chapter 133, Video 133-1 – David H. Kim

Pituitary Surgery
Chapter 224, Video 224-1 – Ivan Ciric

Donor Liver Transportation–Donor and Recipient
Chapter 154, Video 154-1 – Igal Kam, Thomas Bak, and Michael Wachs

Skin Testing
Chapter 251, Video 251-1 – Larry Borish

Snare Polypectomy of a Colon Adenoma
Chapter 193, Video 193-1 – Douglas O. Faigel

Nasal Endoscopy
Chapter 251, Video 251-2 – Larry Borish

Laparascopic-Assisted Double Balloon Enteroscopy with Polypectomy of a Jejunal Adenoma Followed by Surgical Oversew of the Polypectomy Site
Chapter 193, Video 193-2 – Douglas O. Faigel

Hip Arthroscopy Osteochondroplasty
Chapter 276, Video 276-1 – Bryan T. Kelly

Cervical Provocation
Chapter 400, Video 400-1 – Richard L. Barbano

Spurling Maneuver
Chapter 400, Video 400-2 – Richard L. Barbano

Cervical Distraction Test
Chapter 400, Video 400-3 – Richard L. Barbano

Straight Leg Raise
Chapter 400, Video 400-4 – Richard L. Barbano

Contralateral Straight Leg Raise
Chapter 400, Video 400-5 – Richard L. Barbano

Seated Straight Leg Raise
Chapter 400, Video 400-6 – Richard L. Barbano

Discectomy
Chapter 400, Video 400-7 – Jason H. Huang

Absence Seizure
Chapter 403, Video 403-1 – Samuel Wiebe

Left Rolandic Seizure
Chapter 403, Video 403-2 – Samuel Wiebe

Left Temporal Complex Partial Seizure
Chapter 403, Video 403-3 – Samuel Wiebe

Left Temporal Complex Partial Seizure Postictal Confusion
Chapter 403, Video 403-4 – Samuel Wiebe

Left Temporal Complex Partial Seizure
Chapter 403, Video 403-5 – Samuel Wiebe

Supplementary Sensory-Motor Seizure
Chapter 403, Video 403-6 – Samuel Wiebe

Right Posterior Temporal Seizure - Dramatic Frontal Semiology
Chapter 403, Video 403-7 – Samuel Wiebe

Right Mesial Frontal Seizure
Chapter 403, Video 403-8 – Samuel Wiebe

Nonconvulsive Status Epilepticus
Chapter 403, Video 403-9 – Samuel Wiebe

GTC Seizure Tonic Phase
Chapter 403, Video 403-10 – Samuel Wiebe

Minimally Conscious State
Chapter 404, Video 404-3 – James L. Bernat and Eelco F. M. Wijdicks

GTC Seizure Clonic Phase
Chapter 403, Video 403-11 – Samuel Wiebe

Akinetic Mutism
Chapter 404, Video 404-4 – James L. Bernat and Eelco F. M. Wijdicks

Myoclonic Facial Seizure
Chapter 403, Video 403-12 – Samuel Wiebe

Early Parkinson's Disease
Chapter 409, Video 409-1 – Anthony E. Lang

Tonic Seizure Lennox Gastaut
Chapter 403, Video 403-13 – Samuel Wiebe

Freezing of Gait in Parkinson's Disease
Chapter 409, Video 409-2 – Anthony E. Lang

Atonic Seizure Lennox Gastaut
Chapter 403, Video 403-14 – Samuel Wiebe

Gunslinger Gait in Progressive Supranuclear Palsy
Chapter 409, Video 409-3 – Anthony E. Lang

Reflex Auditory Seizure
Chapter 403, Video 403-15 – Samuel Wiebe

Supranuclear Gaze Palsy in Progressive Supranuclear Palsy
Chapter 409, Video 409-4 – Anthony E. Lang

Four Score
Chapter 404, Video 404-1 – James L. Bernat and Eelco F. M. Wijdicks

Applause Sign in Progressive Supranuclear Palsy
Chapter 409, Video 409-5 – Anthony E. Lang

Persistent Vegetative State
Chapter 404, Video 404-2 – James L. Bernat and Eelco F. M. Wijdicks

Apraxia of Eyelid Opening in Progressive Supranuclear Palsy
Chapter 409, Video 409-6 – Anthony E. Lang

Cranial Dystonia in Multiple System Atrophy
Chapter 409, Video 409-7 – Anthony E. Lang

Hemiballism
Chapter 410, Video 410-3 – Anthony E. Lang

Anterocollis in Multiple System Atrophy
Chapter 409, Video 409-8 – Anthony E. Lang

Blepharospasm
Chapter 410, Video 410-4 – Anthony E. Lang

Stridor in Multiple System Atrophy
Chapter 409, Video 409-9 – Anthony E. Lang

Oromandibular Dystonia
Chapter 410, Video 410-5 – Anthony E. Lang

Alien Limb Phenomenon in Corticobasal Syndrome
Chapter 409, Video 409-10 – Anthony E. Lang

Cervical Dystonia
Chapter 410, Video 410-6 – Anthony E. Lang

Myoclonus in Corticobasal Syndrome
Chapter 409, Video 409-11 – Anthony E. Lang

Writer's Cramp
Chapter 410, Video 410-7 – Anthony E. Lang

Levodopa-Induced Dyskinesia in Parkinson's Disease
Chapter 409, Video 409-12 – Anthony E. Lang

Embouchure Dystonia
Chapter 410, Video 410-8 – Anthony E. Lang

Essential Tremor
Chapter 410, Video 410-1 – Anthony E. Lang

Sensory Trick in Cervical Dystonia
Chapter 410, Video 410-9 – Anthony E. Lang

Huntington's Disease
Chapter 410, Video 410-2 – Anthony E. Lang

Generalized Dystonia
Chapter 410, Video 410-10 – Anthony E. Lang

Tics
Chapter 410, Video 410-11 – Anthony E. Lang

Limb Symptoms and Signs
Chapter 419, Video 419-1 – Pamela J. Shaw

Tardive Dyskinesia
Chapter 410, Video 410-12 – Anthony E. Lang

Bulbar Symptoms and Signs
Chapter 419, Video 419-2 – Pamela J. Shaw

Hemifacial Spasm
Chapter 410, Video 410-13 – Anthony E. Lang

Normal Swallowing
Chapter 419, Video 419-3 – Pamela J. Shaw

Wernickes Encephalopathy Eye Movements: Before Thiamine
Chapter 416, Video 416-1 – Barbara S. Koppel

Charcot-Marie-Tooth Disease Exam and Walk
Chapter 420, Video 420-1 – Michael E. Shy

Wernickes Encephalopathy Eye Movements: After Thiamine
Chapter 416, Video 416-2 – Barbara S. Koppel

GOLDMAN-CECIL MEDICINE

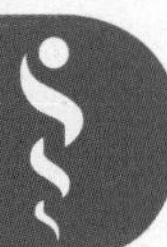

GOLDMAN-CECIL MEDICINE

25TH EDITION

Volume I

EDITED BY

LEE GOLDMAN, MD

Harold and Margaret Hatch Professor
Executive Vice President and Dean of the Faculties of Health Sciences and Medicine
Chief Executive, Columbia University Medical Center
Columbia University
New York, New York

ANDREW I. SCHAFER, MD

Professor of Medicine
Director, Richard T. Silver Center for Myeloproliferative Neoplasms
Weill Cornell Medical College
New York, New York

ELSEVIER
SAUNDERS

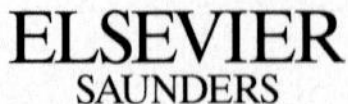

ELSEVIER
SAUNDERS

1600 John F. Kennedy Blvd.
Ste. 1800
Philadelphia, PA 19103-2899

GOLDMAN-CECIL MEDICINE, 25TH EDITION
ISBN: 978-1-4557-5017-7
Volume 1 Part Number: 9996096564
Volume 2 Part Number: 9996096629

International Edition (IE):
ISBN: 978-0-323-28800-2
IE Volume 1 Part Number: 9996118347
IE Volume 2 Part Number: 9996118282

Notices

Knowledge and best practice in this field are constantly changing. As new research and experience broaden our understanding, changes in research methods, professional practices, or medical treatment may become necessary.

Practitioners and researchers must always rely on their own experience and knowledge in evaluating and using any information, methods, compounds, or experiments described herein. In using such information or methods they should be mindful of their own safety and the safety of others, including parties for whom they have a professional responsibility.

With respect to any drug or pharmaceutical products identified, readers are advised to check the most current information provided (i) on procedures featured or (ii) by the manufacturer of each product to be administered, to verify the recommended dose or formula, the method and duration of administration, and contraindications. It is the responsibility of practitioners, relying on their own experience and knowledge of their patients, to make diagnoses, to determine dosages and the best treatment for each individual patient, and to take all appropriate safety precautions.

To the fullest extent of the law, neither the Publisher nor the authors, contributors, or editors assume any liability for any injury and/or damage to persons or property as a matter of products liability, negligence or otherwise, or from any use or operation of any methods, products, instructions, or ideas contained in the material herein.

Library of Congress Cataloging-in-Publication Data
Goldman's Cecil medicine.
Goldman-Cecil medicine / [edited by] Lee Goldman, Andrew I. Schafer.—25th edition.
p. ; cm.
Cecil medicine
Preceded by Goldman's Cecil medicine / [edited by] Lee Goldman, Andrew I. Schafer. 24th ed. c2012.
Includes bibliographical references.
ISBN 978-1-4557-5017-7 (hardcover, 2 vol set : alk. paper)—ISBN 978-0-323-28800-2 (international edition : alk. paper)—ISBN 978-9996096563 (volume 1 : alk. paper)—ISBN 9996096564 (volume 1 : alk. paper)—ISBN 978-9996096624 (volume 2 : alk. paper)—ISBN 9996096629 (volume 2 : alk. paper)
I. Goldman, Lee (Physician), editor. II. Schafer, Andrew I., editor. III. Title. IV. Title: Cecil medicine.
[DNLM: 1. Medicine. WB 100]
RC46
616—dc23

2014049904

Executive Content Strategist: Kate Dimock
Senior Content Development Manager: Maureen Iannuzzi
Publishing Services Manager: Anne Altepeter
Senior Project Manager: Cindy Thoms
Design Specialist: Paula Catalano

Printed in the United States of America

Last digit is the print number: 9 8 7 6 5 4 3 2 1

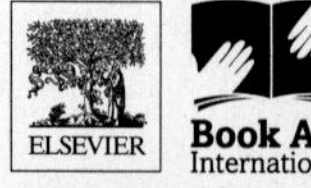
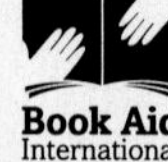

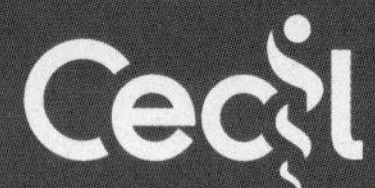

ASSOCIATE EDITORS

Mary K. Crow, MD
Joseph P. Routh Professor of Rheumatic Diseases in Medicine
Weill Cornell Medical College
Physician-in-Chief and Benjamin M. Rosen Chair in Immunology and Inflammation Research
Hospital for Special Surgery
New York, New York

James H. Doroshow, MD
Bethesda, Maryland

Jeffrey M. Drazen, MD
Distinguished Parker B. Francis Professor of Medicine
Harvard Medical School
Senior Physician
Brigham and Women's Hospital
Boston, Massachusetts

Robert C. Griggs, MD
Professor of Neurology, Medicine, Pediatrics, and Pathology and Laboratory Medicine
University of Rochester School of Medicine and Dentistry
Rochester, New York

Donald W. Landry, MD, PhD
Samuel Bard Professor of Medicine
Chair, Department of Medicine
Physician-in-Chief
Columbia University Medical Center
New York, New York

Wendy Levinson, MD
Professor of Medicine
Chair Emeritus
Department of Medicine
University of Toronto
Toronto, Ontario, Canada

Anil K. Rustgi, MD
T. Grier Miller Professor of Medicine and Genetics
Chief of Gastroenterology
American Cancer Society Professor
University of Pennsylvania Perelman School of Medicine
Philadelphia, Pennsylvania

W. Michael Scheld, MD
Bayer-Gerald L. Mandell Professor of Infectious Diseases
Professor of Medicine
Clinical Professor of Neurosurgery
Director, Pfizer Initiative in International Health
University of Virginia Health System
Charlottesville, Virginia

Allen M. Spiegel, MD
Dean
Albert Einstein College of Medicine
Bronx, New York

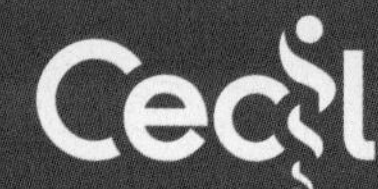

PREFACE

In the 90 years since the first edition of the *Cecil Textbook of Medicine* was published, almost everything we know about internal medicine has changed. Progress in medical science is now occurring at an ever-accelerating pace, and it is doing so within the framework of transformational changes in clinical practice and the delivery of health care at individual, social, and global levels. This textbook and its associated electronic products incorporate the latest medical knowledge in multiple formats that should appeal to students and seasoned practitioners regardless of how they prefer to access this rapidly changing information.

Even as *Cecil's* specific information has changed, however, we have remained true to the tradition of a comprehensive textbook of medicine that carefully explains the *why* (the underlying pathophysiology of disease) and the *how* (now expected to be evidence-based from randomized controlled trials and meta-analyses). Descriptions of physiology and pathophysiology include the latest genetic advances in a practical format that strives to be useful to the nonexpert. Medicine has entered an era when the acuity of illness and the limited time available to evaluate a patient have diminished the ability of physicians to satisfy their intellectual curiosity. As a result, the acquisition of information, quite easily achieved in this era, is often confused with knowledge. We have attempted to address this dilemma with a textbook that not only informs but also stimulates new questions and gives a glimpse of the future path to new knowledge. Grade A evidence is specifically highlighted in the text and referenced at the end of each chapter. In addition to the information provided in the textbook, the *Cecil* website supplies expanded content and functionality. In many cases, the full articles referenced in each chapter can be accessed from the *Cecil* website. The website is also continuously updated to incorporate subsequent Grade A information, other evidence, and new discoveries.

The sections for each organ system begin with a chapter that summarizes an approach to patients with key symptoms, signs, or laboratory abnormalities associated with dysfunction of that organ system. As summarized in E-Table 1-1, the text specifically provides clear, concise information regarding how a physician should approach more than 100 common symptoms, signs, and laboratory abnormalities, usually with a flow diagram, a table, or both for easy reference. In this way, *Cecil* remains a comprehensive text to guide diagnosis and therapy, not only for patients with suspected or known diseases but also for patients who may have undiagnosed abnormalities that require an initial evaluation.

Just as each edition brings new authors, it also reminds us of our gratitude to past editors and authors. Previous editors of *Cecil* include a short but remarkably distinguished group of leaders of American medicine: Russell Cecil, Paul Beeson, Walsh McDermott, James Wyngaarden, Lloyd H. Smith, Jr., Fred Plum, J. Claude Bennett, and Dennis Ausiello. As we welcome new associate editors—Mary K. Crow, James H. Doroshow, and Allen M. Spiegel—we also express our appreciation to William P. Arend, James O. Armitage, David R. Clemmons, and other associate editors from the previous editions on whose foundation we have built. Our returning associate editors—Jeffrey M. Drazen, Robert C. Griggs, Donald W. Landry, Wendy Levinson, Anil K. Rustgi, and W. Michael Scheld—continue to make critical contributions to the selection of authors and the review and approval of all manuscripts. The editors, however, are fully responsible for the book as well as the integration among chapters.

The tradition of *Cecil* is that all chapters are written by distinguished experts in each field. We are also most grateful for the editorial assistance in New York of Maribel Lim and Silva Sergenian. These individuals and others in our offices have shown extraordinary dedication and equanimity in working with authors and editors to manage the unending flow of manuscripts, figures, and permissions. We also thank Cassondra Andreychik, Ved Bhushan Arya, Cameron Harrison, Karen Krok, Robert J. Mentz, Gaétane Nocturne, Patrice Savard, Senthil Senniappan, Tejpratap Tiwari, and Sangeetha Venkatarajan, who contributed to various chapters, and we mourn the passing of Morton N. Swartz, MD, co-author of the chapter on "Meningitis: Bacterial, Viral, and Other" and Donald E. Low, MD, author of the chapter "Nonpneumococcal Streptococcal Infections, Rheumatic Fever." At Elsevier, we are most indebted to Kate Dimock and Maureen Iannuzzi, and also thank Maria Holman, Gabriela Benner, Cindy Thoms, Anne Altepeter, Linda McKinley, Paula Catalano, and Kristin Koehler, who have been critical to the planning and production process under the guidance of Mary Gatsch. Many of the clinical photographs were supplied by Charles D. Forbes and William F. Jackson, authors of *Color Atlas and Text of Clinical Medicine*, Third Edition, published in 2003 by Elsevier Science Ltd. We thank them for graciously permitting us to include their pictures in our book. We have been exposed to remarkable physicians in our lifetimes and would like to acknowledge the mentorship and support of several of those who exemplify this paradigm—Eugene Braunwald, Lloyd H. Smith, Jr., Frank Gardner, and William Castle. Finally, we would like to thank the Goldman family—Jill, Jeff, Abigail, Mira, Samuel, Daniel, Robyn, Tobin, and Dashel—and the Schafer family—Pauline, Eric, Melissa, Nathaniel, Pam, John, Evan, Samantha, Kate, and Sean, for their understanding of the time and focus required to edit a book that attempts to sustain the tradition of our predecessors and to meet the needs of today's physician.

LEE GOLDMAN, MD
ANDREW I. SCHAFER, MD

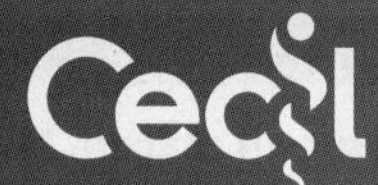

CONTRIBUTORS

Charles S. Abrams, MD
Professor of Medicine, Pathology, and Laboratory Medicine, University of Pennsylvania School of Medicine; Director, PENN-Chop Blood Center for Patient Care & Discovery, Hospital of the University of Pennsylvania, Philadelphia, Pennsylvania
Thrombocytopenia

Frank J. Accurso, MD
Professor of Pediatrics, University of Colorado School of Medicine; Attending Physician, Children's Hospital Colorado, Aurora, Colorado
Cystic Fibrosis

Ronald S. Adler, MD, PhD
Professor of Radiology, New York University School of Medicine; Department of Radiology, NYU Langone Medical Center, New York, New York
Imaging Studies in the Rheumatic Diseases

Cem Akin, MD, PhD
Associate Professor, Harvard Medical School; Attending Physician, Director, Mastocytosis Center, Brigham and Women's Hospital, Department of Medicine, Division of Rheumatology, Immunology, and Allergy, Boston, Massachusetts
Mastocytosis

Allen J. Aksamit, Jr., MD
Professor of Neurology, Mayo Clinic College of Medicine, Consultant in Neurology, Mayo Clinic, Rochester, Minnesota
Acute Viral Encephalitis

Qais Al-Awqati, MB ChB
Robert F. Loeb Professor of Medicine, Jay I. Meltzer Professor of Nephrology and Hypertension, Professor of Physiology and Cellular Biophysics, Division of Nephrology, Columbia University, College of Physicians and Surgeons, New York, New York
Structure and Function of the Kidneys

Ban Mishu Allos, MD
Associate Professor of Medicine, Division of Infectious Diseases, Associate Professor, Preventive Medicine, Vanderbilt University School of Medicine, Nashville, Tennessee
Campylobacter Infections

David Altshuler, MD, PhD
Professor of Genetics and of Medicine, Harvard Medical School, Massachusetts General Hospital; Professor of Biology (Adjunct), Massachusetts Institute of Technology, Boston and Cambridge, Massachusetts
The Inherited Basis of Common Diseases

Michael Aminoff, MD, DSc
Professor, Department of Neurology, University of California San Francisco, San Francisco, California
Approach to the Patient with Neurologic Disease

Jeffrey L. Anderson, MD
Professor of Internal Medicine, University of Utah School of Medicine; Vice-Chair for Research, Department of Internal Medicine, Associate Chief of Cardiology and Director of Cardiovascular Research, Intermountain Medical Center, Intermountain Healthcare, Salt Lake City, Utah
ST Segment Elevation Acute Myocardial Infarction and Complications of Myocardial Infarction

Larry J. Anderson, MD
Professor, Division of Infectious Disease, Department of Pediatrics, Emory University School of Medicine and Children's Healthcare of Atlanta, Atlanta, Georgia
Coronaviruses

Aśok C. Antony, MD
Chancellor's Professor of Medicine, Indiana University School of Medicine; Attending Physician, Indiana University Health Affiliated Hospitals and Richard L. Roudebush Veterans Affairs Medical Center, Indianapolis, Indiana
Megaloblastic Anemias

Gerald B. Appel, MD
Professor of Medicine, Division of Nephrology, Department of Medicine, Columbia University College of Physicians and Surgeons, New York, New York
Glomerular Disorders and Nephrotic Syndromes

Frederick R. Appelbaum, MD
Executive Vice President and Deputy Director, Fred Hutchinson Cancer Research Center; President, Seattle Cancer Care Alliance; Professor, Division of Medical Oncology, University of Washington School of Medicine, Seattle Washington
The Acute Leukemias

Suneel S. Apte, MBBS, DPhil
Staff, Cleveland Clinic Lerner College of Medicine at Case Western Reserve University, Cleveland, Ohio
Connective Tissue Structure and Function

James O. Armitage, MD
The Joe Shapiro Professor of Internal Medicine, University of Nebraska Medical Center, Omaha, Nebraska
Approach to the Patient with Lymphadenopathy and Splenomegaly; Non-Hodgkin Lymphomas

M. Amin Arnaout, MD
Professor of Medicine, Departments of Medicine and Developmental and Regenerative Biology, Harvard Medical School; Physician and Chief Emeritus, Division of Nephrology, Massachusetts General Hospital, Boston, Massachusetts
Cystic Kidney Diseases

Robert M. Arnold, MD
Leo H. Criep Professor of Clinical Care, Chief, Section of Palliative Care and Medical Ethics, University of Pittsburgh; Medical Director, UPMC Palliative and Supportive Care Institute, Pittsburgh, Pennsylvania
Care of Dying Patients and Their Families

David Atkins, MD, MPH
Director, Health Services Research and Development, Veterans Health Administration, Washington, D.C.
The Periodic Health Examination

John P. Atkinson, MD
Chief, Division of Rheumatology, Internal Medicine, Washington University School of Medicine in St. Louis, St. Louis, Missouri
Complement System in Disease

Bruce R. Bacon, MD
Endowed Chair in Gastroenterology, Professor of Internal Medicine, Co-Director, Saint Louis University Liver Center; Director, Saint Louis University Abdominal Transplant Center, Saint Louis University School of Medicine, St. Louis, Missouri
Iron Overload (Hemochromatosis)

Larry M. Baddour, MD
Professor of Medicine, Chair, Division of Infectious Diseases, Mayo Clinic, Rochester, Minnesota
Infective Endocarditis

Grover C. Bagby, MD
Professor of Medicine and Molecular and Medical Genetics, Knight Cancer Institute at Oregon Health and Science University and Portland VA Medical Center, Portland, Oregon
Aplastic Anemia and Related Bone Marrow Failure States

Barbara J. Bain, MBBS
Professor in Diagnostic Haematology, Imperial College London; Honorary Consultant Haematologist, St. Mary's Hospital, London, United Kingdom
The Peripheral Blood Smear

Dean F. Bajorin, MD
Attending Physician and Member, Medicine, Memorial Hospital, Memorial Sloan Kettering Cancer Center; Professor of Medicine, Weill Cornell Medical College, New York, New York
Tumors of the Kidney, Bladder, Ureters, and Renal Pelvis

Robert W. Baloh, MD
Professor of Neurology, University of California Los Angeles School of Medicine, Los Angeles, California
Neuro-Ophthalmology; Smell and Taste; Hearing and Equilibrium

Jonathan Barasch, MD, PhD
Professor of Medicine and Pathology and Cell Biology, Department of Medicine, Division of Nephrology, Columbia University College of Physicians & Surgeons, New York, New York
Structure and Function of the Kidneys

Richard L. Barbano, MD, PhD
Professor of Neurology, University of Rochester, Rochester, New York
Mechanical and Other Lesions of the Spine, Nerve Roots, and Spinal Cord

Elizabeth Barrett-Connor, MD
Professor of Community and Family Medicine, University of California San Diego, San Diego, California
Menopause

John R. Bartholomew, MD
Section Head, Vascular Medicine, Cardiovascular Medicine, Cleveland Clinic, Professor of Medicine, Cleveland Clinic Lerner College of Medicine of Case Western Reserve University, Cleveland, Ohio
Other Peripheral Arterial Diseases

Mary Barton, MD, MPP
Vice President, Performance Measurement, National Committee for Quality Assurance, Washington, D.C.
The Periodic Health Examination

Robert C. Basner, MD
Professor of Medicine, Columbia University Medical Center; Director, Columbia University Cardiopulmonary Sleep and Ventilatory Disorders Center, Columbia University College of Physicians and Surgeons, New York, New York
Obstructive Sleep Apnea

Stephen G. Baum, MD
Chairman of Medicine, Mount Sinai Beth Israel Hospital; Professor of Medicine and of Microbiology and Immunology, Albert Einstein College of Medicine, New York, New York
Mycoplasma Infections

Daniel G. Bausch, MD, MPH&TM
Associate Professor, Department of Tropical Medicine, Tulane University Health Sciences Center, New Orleans, Louisiana
Viral Hemorrhagic Fevers

Arnold S. Bayer, MD
Professor of Medicine, David Geffen School of Medicine at University of California Los Angeles; LA Biomedical Research Institute; Vice Chair for Academic Affairs, Department of Medicine, Harbor-UCLA Medical Center, Los Angeles, California
Infective Endocarditis

Hasan Bazari, MD
Associate Professor of Medicine, Harvard Medical School, Department of Medicine, Clinical Director, Nephrology, Program Director, Internal Medicine Residency Program, Massachusetts General Hospital, Boston, Massachusetts
Approach to the Patient with Renal Disease

John H. Beigel, MD
National Institute of Allergy and Infectious Diseases, National Institutes of Health, Bethesda, Maryland
Antiviral Therapy (Non-HIV)

George A. Beller, MD
Professor of Medicine, University of Virginia Health System, Charlottesville, Virginia
Noninvasive Cardiac Imaging

Robert M. Bennett, MD
Professor of Medicine, Oregon Health and Science University, Portland, Oregon
Fibromyalgia, Chronic Fatigue Syndrome, and Myofascial Pain

Joseph R. Berger, MD
Professor of Neurology, Chief of the Multiple Sclerosis Division, Department of Neurology, Perelman School of Medicine, University of Pennsylvania, Philadelphia, Pennsylvania
Cytomegalovirus, Epstein-Barr Virus, and Slow Virus Infections of the Central Nervous System; Neurologic Complications of Human Immunodeficiency Virus Infection; Brain Abscess and Parameningeal Infections

Paul D. Berk, MD
Professor of Medicine, Department of Medicine, Columbia University College of Physicians and Surgeons, New York, New York
Approach to the Patient with Jaundice or Abnormal Liver Tests

Nancy Berliner, MD
Professor of Medicine, Harvard Medical School; Chief, Division of Hematology, Brigham and Women's Hospital, Boston, Massachusetts
Leukocytosis and Leukopenia

James L. Bernat, MD
Louis and Ruth Frank Professor of Neuroscience, Professor of Neurology and Medicine, Geisel School of Medicine at Dartmouth, Hanover, New Hampshire; Department of Neurology, Dartmouth-Hitchcock Medical Center, Lebanon, New Hampshire
Coma, Vegetative State, and Brain Death

Philip J. Bierman, MD
Professor, Department of Internal Medicine, University of Nebraska Medical Center, Omaha, Nebraska
Approach to the Patient with Lymphadenopathy and Splenomegaly; Non-Hodgkin Lymphomas

Michael R. Bishop, MD
Professor of Medicine, Director, Hematopoietic Cellular Therapy Program, Section of Hematology and Oncology, Department of Medicine, University of Chicago, Chicago, Illinois
Hematopoietic Stem Cell Transplantation

Bruce R. Bistrian, MD, PhD, MPH
Professor of Medicine, Beth Israel Deaconess Medical Center; Professor of Medicine, Harvard Medical School, Boston, Massachusetts
Nutritional Assessment

Joseph J. Biundo, MD
Clinical Professor of Medicine, Tulane Medical Center, New Orleans, Louisiana
Bursitis, Tendinitis, and Other Periarticular Disorders and Sports Medicine

Adrian R. Black, PhD
Assistant Professor, Director of Tissue Sciences for the Eppley Institute, The Eppley Institute for Research in Cancer and Allied Diseases, University of Nebraska Medical Center, Omaha, Nebraska
Cancer Biology and Genetics

Charles D. Blanke, MD
Professor of Medicine, Oregon Health and Science University, Portland, Oregon
Neoplasms of the Small and Large Intestine

Joel N. Blankson, MD, PhD
Associate Professor, Johns Hopkins University School of Medicine, Baltimore, Maryland
Immunopathogenesis of Human Immunodeficiency Virus Infection

Martin J. Blaser, MD
Muriel and George Singer Professor of Medicine, Professor of Microbiology, Director, Human Microbiome Program, New York University Langone Medical Center, New York, New York
Acid Peptic Disease; Human Microbiome

William A. Blattner, MD
Professor and Associate Director, Institute of Human Virology, School of Medicine, University of Maryland; Professor of Medicine, School of Medicine, University of Maryland; Professor and Head, Division of Cancer Epidemiology, Department of Epidemiology and Public Health, School of Medicine, University of Maryland, Baltimore, Maryland
Retroviruses Other Than Human Immunodeficiency Virus

Thomas P. Bleck, MD
Professor of Neurological Sciences, Neurosurgery, Internal Medicine, and Anesthesiology, Associate Chief Medical Officer (Critical Care), Rush Medical College, Chicago, Illinois
Arboviruses Affecting the Central Nervous System

Joel A. Block, MD
The Willard L. Wood MD Professor and Director, Division of Rheumatology, Rush University Medical Center, Chicago, Illinois
Osteoarthritis

Henk Blom, MD
Laboratory of Clinical Biochemistry and Metabolism, Department of General Pediatrics, Adolescent Medicine and Neonatology, University Medical Centre Freiburg, Head of Laboratory/Clinical Biochemical Geneticist, Freiburg, Germany
Homocystinuria and Hyperhomocysteinemia

Olaf A. Bodamer, MD
Medical Genetics, University of Miami Hospital, Miami, Florida
Approach to Inborn Errors of Metabolism

William E. Boden, MD
Professor of Medicine, Albany Medical College; Chief of Medicine, Albany Stratton VA Medical Center; Vice-Chairman, Department of Medicine, Albany Medical Center, Albany, New York
Angina Pectoris and Stable Ischemic Heart Disease

Jean Bolognia, MD
Professor of Dermatology, Yale Medical School; Attending Physician, Yale-New Haven Hospital, New Haven, Connecticut
Infections, Hyperpigmentation and Hypopigmentation, Regional Dermatology, and Distinctive Lesions in Black Skin

Robert A. Bonomo, MD
Chief, Medical Service, Louis Stokes Cleveland VA Medical Center; Professor of Medicine, Pharmacology, Biochemistry, Molecular Biology, and Microbiology, Case Western Reserve University School of Medicine, Cleveland, Ohio
Diseases Caused by Acinetobacter and Stenotrophomonas Species

Larry Borish, MD
Professor of Medicine, Allergy, and Clinical Immunology, University of Virginia Health System, Charlottesville, Virgina
Allergic Rhinitis and Chronic Sinusitis

Patrick J. Bosque, MD
Associate Professor of Neurology, University of Colorado Denver School of Medicine; Neurologist, Denver Health Medical Center, Denver, Colorado
Prion Diseases

David J. Brenner, PhD, DSc
Higgins Professor of Radiation Biophysics, Center for Radiological Research, Columbia University Medical Center, New York, New York
Radiation Injury

Itzhak Brook, MD, MSc
Professor of Pediatrics and Medicine, Georgetown University, Georgetown University Medical Center, Washington, D.C.
Diseases Caused by Non–Spore-Forming Anaerobic Bacteria; Actinomycosis

Enrico Brunetti, MD
Assistant Professor of Infectious Diseases, University of Pavia; Attending Physician, Division of Infectious and Tropical Diseases, IRCCS San Matteo Hospital Foundation; Co-Director, WHO Collaborating Centre for Clinical Management of Cystic Echinococcosis, Pavia, Italy
Cestodes

David M. Buchner, MD, MPH
Shahid and Ann Carlson Khan Professor in Applied Health Sciences, Department of Kinesiology and Community Health, University of Illinois at Urbana-Champaign, Champaign, Illinois
Physical Activity

Pierre A. Buffet, MD, PhD
Research Unit Head, Erythrocyte Parasite Pathogenesis Research Team INSERM–University Paris 6, CIMI–Paris Research Center, University Pierre and Marie Curie; Associate Professor of Parasitology, Faculty of Medicine, University Pierre and Marie Curie, Pitié-Salpêtrière Hospital, Paris, France
Leishmaniasis

H. Franklin Bunn, MD
Professor of Medicine, Harvard Medical School; Physician, Brigham and Women's Hospital, Boston, Massachusetts
Approach to the Anemias

David A. Bushinsky, MD
John J. Kuiper Distinguished Professor of Medicine, Chief, Nephrology Division, University of Rochester School of Medicine; Associate Chair for Academic Affairs in Medicine, University of Rochester Medical Center, Rochester, New York
Nephrolithiasis

Vivian P. Bykerk, MD
Associate Professor of Medicine, Weill Cornell Medical College; Associate Attending Physician, Hospital for Special Surgery, New York, New York
Approach to the Patient with Rheumatic Disease

Peter A. Calabresi, MD
Professor of Neurology and Director of the Richard T. Johnson Division of Neuroimmunology and Neuroinfectious Diseases, Johns Hopkins University; Director of the Multiple Sclerosis Center, Johns Hopkins Hospital, Baltimore, Maryland
Multiple Sclerosis and Demyelinating Conditions of the Central Nervous System

David P. Calfee, MD, MS
Associate Professor of Medicine and Healthcare Policy and Research, Weill Cornell Medical College; Chief Hospital Epidemiologist, New York-Presbyterian Hospital/Weill Cornell Medical Center, New York, New York
Prevention and Control of Health Care–Associated Infections

Douglas Cameron, MD, MBA
Professor of Ophthalmology and Visual Neurosciences, University of Minnesota, Minneapolis, Minnesota
Diseases of the Visual System

Michael Camilleri, MD
Atherton and Winifred W. Bean Professor, Professor of Medicine, Pharmacology, and Physiology, College of Medicine, Mayo Clinic, Consultant, Division of Gastroenterology and Hepatology, Mayo Clinic, Rochester, Minnesota
Disorders of Gastrointestinal Motility

Grant W. Cannon, MD
Thomas E. and Rebecca D. Jeremy Presidential Endowed Chair for Arthritis Research, Associate Chief of Staff for Academic Affiliations, George E. Wahlen VA Medical Center, Salt Lake City, Utah
Immunosuppressing Drugs Including Corticosteroids

Maria Domenica Cappellini, MD
Professor of Internal Medicine, University of Milan, Fondazione IRCCS Ca' Granda Ospedale Maggiore Policlinico, University of Milan, Milan, Italy
The Thalassemias

Blase A. Carabello, MD
Professor of Medicine, Chairman, Department of Cardiology, Mount Sinai Beth Israel Heart Institute, New York, New York
Valvular Heart Disease

Edgar M. Carvalho, MD
Professor of Medicine and Clinical Immunology, Faculdade de Medicina da Bahia, Universidade Federal da Bahia and Escola Bahiana de Medicina e Saúde Pública, Salvador, Bahia, Brazil
Schistosomiasis (Bilharziasis)

William H. Catherino, MD, PhD
Professor and Research Head, Department of Obstetrics and Gynecology, Uniformed Services University of the Health Sciences Division of Reproductive Endocrinology and Infertility; Program in Reproductive and Adult Endocrinology, Eunice Kennedy Shriver National Institute of Child Health and Human Development, National Institutes of Health, Bethesda, Maryland
Ovaries and Development; Reproductive Endocrinology and Infertility

Jane A. Cauley, DrPH
Professor of Epidemiology, University of Pittsburgh Graduate School of Public Health, Vice Chair of the Department of Epidemiology, Pittsburgh, Pennsylvania
Epidemiology of Aging: Implications of the Aging of Society

Naga P. Chalasani, MD
David W. Crabb Professor and Director, Division of Gastroenterology and Hepatology, Indiana University School of Medicine, Indianapolis, Indiana
Alcoholic and Nonalcoholic Steatohepatitis

Henry F. Chambers, MD
Professor of Medicine, University of California San Francisco School of Medicine; Director, Clinical Research Services, Clinical and Translational Sciences Institute, San Francisco, California
Staphylococcal Infections

William P. Cheshire, Jr., MD
Professor of Neurology, Mayo Clinic, Jacksonville, Florida
Autonomic Disorders and Their Management

Ilseung Cho, MD, MS
Assistant Professor of Medicine, Division of Gastroenterology, Department of Medicine, New York University, New York, New York
Human Microbiome

Arun Chockalingam, PhD
Professor of Epidemiology and Global Health, Director, Office of Global Health Education and Training; Dalla Lana Faculty of Public Health, University of Toronto, Toronto, Ontario, Canada
Global Health

David C. Christiani, MD
Professor of Medicine, Harvard Medical School; Physician, Pulmonary and Critical Care, Massachusetts General Hospital; Elkan Blout Professor of Environmental Genetics, Environmental Health, Harvard School of Public Health, Boston, Massachusetts
Physical and Chemical Injuries of the Lung

David H. Chu, MD, PhD
Director, Contact Dermatitis, Division of Dermatology and Cutaneous Surgery, Scripps Clinic Medical Group, La Jolla, California
Structure and Function of the Skin

Theodore J. Cieslak, MD
Pediatric Infectious Diseases, Clinical Professor of Pediatrics, University of Texas Health Science Center at San Antonio; Department of Pediatrics, Fort Sam Houston, Texas
Bioterrorism

Carolyn Clancy, MD
Interim Under Secretary for Health, Veterans Administration, Washington, D.C.
Measuring Health and Health Care

David R. Clemmons, MD
Kenan Professor of Medicine, University of North Carolina School of Medicine; Attending Physician, Medicine, UNC Hospitals, Chapel Hill, North Carolina
Approach to the Patient with Endocrine Disease

David Cohen, MD
Professor of Medicine, Division of Nephrology; Medical Director, Kidney and Pancreas Transplantation, Columbia University Medical Center, New York, New York
Treatment of Irreversible Renal Failure

Jeffrey Cohen, MD
Chief, Laboratory of Infectious Diseases, National Institute of Allergy and Infectious Diseases, National Institutes of Health, Bethesda, Maryland
Varicella-Zoster Virus (Chickenpox, Shingles)

Myron S. Cohen, MD
Associate Vice Chancellor for Global Health, Director, UNC Institute for Global Health and Infectious Diseases, Chief, Division of Infectious Diseases, Yeargan-Bate Eminent Professor of Medicine, Microbiology, and Immunology and Epidemiology, Chapel Hill, North Carolina
Approach to the Patient with a Sexually Transmitted Infection; Prevention of Human Immunodeficiency Virus Infection

Steven P. Cohen, MD
Professor of Anesthesiology and Critical Care Medicine and Physical Medicine and Rehabilitation, Johns Hopkins School of Medicine, Baltimore, Maryland, and Uniformed Services University of the Health Sciences, Bethesda, Maryland; Director, Pain Research, Walter Reed National Military Medical Center, Bethesda, Maryland
Pain

Steven L. Cohn, MD
Professor of Clinical Medicine, University of Miami Miller School of Medicine; Medical Director, UHealth Preoperative Assessment Center; Director, Medical Consultation Service, University of Miami Hospital, Miami, Florida
Preoperative Evaluation

Robert Colebunders, MD
Emeritus Professor, Institute of Tropical Medicine, Antwerp, Belgium
Immune Reconstitution Inflammatory Syndrome in HIV/AIDS

Joseph M. Connors, MD
Clinical Professor, University of British Columbia; Clinical Director, BC Cancer Agency Centre for Lymphoid Cancer, Vancouver, British Columbia, Canada
Hodgkin Lymphoma

Deborah J. Cook, MD, MSc
Professor of Medicine, Clinical Epidemiology and Biostatistics, McMaster University, Hamilton, Ontario, Canada
Approach to the Patient in a Critical Care Setting

Kenneth H. Cowan, MD, PhD
Director, Fred & Pamela Buffett Cancer Center; Director, The Eppley Institute for Research in Cancer and Allied Diseases; Professor of Medicine, University of Nebraska Medical Center, Omaha, Nebraska
Cancer Biology and Genetics

Joseph Craft, MD
Paul B. Beeson Professor of Medicine and Immunobiology, Section Chief, Rheumatology, Program Director, Investigative Medicine, Department of Internal Medicine, Yale University School of Medicine, New Haven, Connecticut
The Adaptive Immune Systems

Jill Patricia Crandall, MD
Professor of Clinical Medicine, Division of Endocrinology and Diabetes Research Center, Albert Einstein College of Medicine, Bronx, New York
Diabetes Mellitus

Simon L. Croft, BSc, PhD
Professor of Parasitology, Faculty of Infectious and Tropical Diseases, London School of Hygiene and Tropical Medicine, London, United Kingdom
Leishmaniasis

Kristina Crothers, MD
Associate Professor, Department of Medicine, Division of Pulmonary and Critical Care, University of Washington School of Medicine, Seattle, Washington
Pulmonary Manifestations of Human Immunodeficiency Virus and Acquired Immunodeficiency Syndrome

Mary K. Crow, MD
Joseph P. Routh Professor of Rheumatic Diseases in Medicine, Weill Cornell Medical College; Physician in Chief and Benjamin M. Rosen Chair in Immunology and Inflammation Research, Hospital for Special Surgery, New York, New York
The Innate Immune Systems; Approach to the Patient with Rheumatic Disease; Systemic Lupus Erythematosus

John A. Crump, MB ChB, MD, DTM&H
McKinlay Professor of Global Health, Centre for International Health, University of Otago, Dunedin, New Zealand
Salmonella Infections (Including Enteric Fever)

Mark R. Cullen, MD
Professor of Medicine, Department of Medicine, Stanford University School of Medicine, Stanford, California
Principles of Occupational and Environmental Medicine

Charlotte Cunningham-Rundles, MD, PhD
Professor of Medicine and Pediatrics, Icahn School of Medicine at Mount Sinai, New York, New York
Primary Immunodeficiency Diseases

Inger K. Damon, MD, PhD
Director, Division of High Consequence Pathogens and Pathology, Centers for Disease Control and Prevention, Atlanta, Georgia
Smallpox, Monkeypox, and Other Poxvirus Infections

Troy E. Daniels, DDS, MS
Professor Emeritus of Oral Pathology and Pathology, University of California San Francisco, San Francisco, California
Diseases of the Mouth and Salivary Glands

Nancy E. Davidson, MD
Hillman Professor of Oncology, University of Pittsburgh; Director, University of Pittsburgh Cancer Institute and UPMC CancerCenter, Pittsburgh, Pennsylvania
Breast Cancer and Benign Breast Disorders

Lisa M. DeAngelis, MD
Chair, Department of Neurology, Memorial Sloan-Kettering Cancer Center; Professor of Neurology, Weill Cornell Medical College, New York, New York
Tumors of the Central Nervous System

Malcolm M. DeCamp, MD
Fowler McCormick Professor of Surgery, Feinberg School of Medicine, Northwestern University; Chief, Division of Thoracic Surgery, Northwestern Memorial Hospital, Chicago, Illinois
Interventional and Surgical Approaches to Lung Disease

Carlos del Rio, MD
Hubert Professor and Chair and Professor of Medicine, Hubert Department of Global Health, Rollins School of Public Health and Department of Medicine, Emory University School of Medicine, Atlanta, Georgia
Prevention of Human Immunodeficiency Virus Infection

Patricia A. Deuster, PhD, MPH
Professor and Director, Consortium for Health and Military Performance, Department of Military and Emergency Medicine, Uniformed Services University of the Health Sciences, Bethesda, Maryland
Rhabdomyolysis

Robert B. Diasio, MD
William J. and Charles H. Mayo Professor, Molecular Pharmacology and Experimental Therapeutics and Oncology, Mayo Clinic, Rochester, Minnesota
Principles of Drug Therapy

David J. Diemert, MD
Associate Professor, Department of Microbiology, Immunology, and Tropical Medicine, School of Medicine and Health Sciences, The George Washington University, Washington, D.C.
Intestinal Nematode Infections; Tissue Nematode Infections

Kathleen B. Digre, MD
Professor of Neurology, Ophthalmology, Director, Division of Headache and Neuro-Ophthalmology, University of Utah, Salt Lake City, Utah
Headaches and Other Head Pain

James H. Doroshow, MD
Bethesda, Maryland
Approach to the Patient with Cancer; Malignant Tumors of Bone, Sarcomas, and Other Soft Tissue Neoplasms

John M. Douglas, Jr., MD
Executive Director, Tri-County Health Department, Greenwood Village, Colorado
Papillomavirus

Jeffrey M. Drazen, MD
Distinguished Parker B. Francis Professor of Medicine, Harvard Medical School; Senior Physician, Brigham and Women's Hospital, Boston, Massachusetts
Asthma

Stephen C. Dreskin, MD, PhD
Professor of Medicine and Immunology, Division of Allergy and Clinical Immunology, Department of Medicine, University of Colorado Denver, School of Medicine, Aurora, Colorado
Urticaria and Angioedema

W. Lawrence Drew, MD, PhD
Professor Emeritus, Laboratory Medicine and Medicine, University of California San Francisco, San Francisco, California
Cytomegalovirus

George L. Drusano, MD
Professor and Director, Institute for Therapeutic Innovation, College of Medicine, University of Florida, Lake Nona, Florida
Antibacterial Chemotherapy

Thomas D. DuBose, Jr., MD
Emeritus Professor of Internal Medicine and Nephrology, Wake Forest School of Medicine, Winston-Salem, North Carolina
Vascular Disorders of the Kidney

F. Daniel Duffy, MD
Professor of Internal Medicine and Steve Landgarten Chair in Medical Leadership, School of Community Medicine, University of Oklahoma College of Medicine, Tulsa, Oklahoma
Counseling for Behavior Change

Herbert L. DuPont, MD, MACP
Mary W. Kelsey Chair and Director, Center for Infectious Diseases, University of Texas School of Public Health; H. Irving Schweppe Chair of Internal Medicine and Vice Chairman, Department of Medicine, Baylor College of Medicine; Chief of Internal Medicine, St. Luke's Hospital System, Houston, Texas
Approach to the Patient with Suspected Enteric Infection

Madeleine Duvic, MD
Professor and Deputy Chairman, Department of Dermatology, The University of Texas MD Anderson Cancer Center, Houston, Texas
Urticaria, Drug Hypersensitivity Rashes, Nodules and Tumors, and Atrophic Diseases

Kathryn M. Edwards, MD
Sarah H. Sell and Cornelius Vanderbilt Chair in Pediatrics, Vanderbilt University School of Medicine; Director, Vanderbilt Vaccine Research Program, Monroe Carrell Jr. Children's Hospital at Vanderbilt, Nashville, Tennessee
Parainfluenza Viral Disease

N. Lawrence Edwards, MD
Professor of Medicine, Vice Chairman, Department of Medicine, University of Florida; Chief, Section of Rheumatology, Medical Service, Malcom Randall Veterans Affairs Medical Center, Gainesville, Florida
Crystal Deposition Diseases

Lawrence H. Einhorn, MD
Distinguished Professor, Department of Medicine, Division of Hematology/Oncology, Livestrong Foundation Professor of Oncology, Indiana University School of Medicine, Indianapolis, Indiana
Testicular Cancer

Ronald J. Elin, MD, PhD
A.J. Miller Professor and Chairman, Department of Pathology and Laboratory Medicine, University of Louisville School of Medicine, Louisville, Kentucky
Reference Intervals and Laboratory Values

George M. Eliopoulos, MD
Professor of Medicine, Harvard Medical School; Physician, Division of Infectious Diseases, Beth Israel Deaconess Medical Center, Boston, Massachusetts
Principles of Anti-Infective Therapy

Perry Elliott, MD
Professor in Inherited Cardiovascular Disease, Institute of Cardiovascular Science, University College London, London, United Kingdom
Diseases of the Myocardium and Endocardium

Jerrold J. Ellner, MD
Professor of Medicine, Boston University School of Medicine; Chief, Section of Infectious Diseases, Boston Medical Center, Boston, Massachusetts
Tuberculosis

Dirk M. Elston, MD
Director, Ackerman Academy of Dermatopathology, New York, New York
Arthropods and Leeches

Ezekiel J. Emanuel, MD, PhD
Vice Provost for Global Initiatives, Diane V.S. Levy and Robert M. Levy University Professor, Chair, Department of Medical Ethics and Health Policy, University of Pennsylvania, Philadelphia, Pennsylvania
Bioethics in the Practice of Medicine

Joel D. Ernst, MD
Director, Division of Infectious Diseases and Immunology, Jeffrey Bergstein Professor of Medicine, Professor of Medicine, Pathology, and Microbiology, New York University School of Medicine; Attending Physician, New York University Langone Medical Center, New York, New York
Leprosy (Hansen Disease)

Gregory T. Everson, MD
Professor of Medicine, Director of Hepatology, University of Colorado School of Medicine, Aurora, Colorado
Hepatic Failure and Liver Transplantation

Amelia Evoli, MD
Associate Professor of Neurology, Catholic University, Agostino Gemelli University Hospital, Rome, Italy
Disorders of Neuromuscular Transmission

Douglas O. Faigel, MD
Professor of Medicine, Mayo Clinic, Chair, Division of Gastroenterology and Hepatology, Scottsdale, Arizona
Neoplasms of the Small and Large Intestine

Matthew E. Falagas, MD, MSc, DSc
Director, Alfa Institute of Biomedical Sciences, Athens, Greece; Adjunct Associate Professor of Medicine, Tufts University School of Medicine, Boston, Massachusetts; Chief, Department of Medicine and Infectious Diseases, Iaso General Hospital, Iaso Group, Athens, Greece
Pseudomonas and Related Gram-Negative Bacillary Infections

Gary W. Falk, MD, MS
Professor of Medicine, Division of Gastroenterology, University of Pennsylvania Perelman School of Medicine, Philadelphia, Pennsylvania
Diseases of the Esophagus

Gene Feder, MBBS, MD
Professor, Centre for Academic Primary Care, School of Social and Community Medicine, University of Bristol; General Practitioner, Helios Medical Centre, Bristol, United Kingdom
Intimate Partner Violence

David J. Feller-Kopman, MD
Director, Bronchoscopy and Interventional Pulmonology, Associate Professor of Medicine, The Johns Hopkins University, Baltimore, Maryland
Interventional and Surgical Approaches to Lung Disease

Gary S. Firestein, MD
Dean and Associate Vice Chancellor of Translational Medicine, University of California San Diego School of Medicine, La Jolla, California
Mechanisms of Inflammation and Tissue Repair

Glenn I. Fishman, MD
Director, Leon H. Charney Division of Cardiology, Vice-Chair for Research, Department of Medicine, William Goldring Professor of Medicine, New York University School of Medicine, New York, New York
Principles of Electrophysiology

Lee A. Fleisher, MD
Robert D. Dripps Professor and Chair, Anesthesiology and Critical Care, Professor of Medicine, University of Pennsylvania Perelman School of Medicine, Philadelphia, Pennsylvania
Overview of Anesthesia

Paul W. Flint, MD
Professor and Chair, Otolaryngology, Head and Neck Surgery, Oregon Health and Science University, Portland, Oregon
Throat Disorders

Evan L. Fogel, MD, MSc
Professor of Clinical Medicine, Indiana University School of Medicine, Indianapolis, Indiana
Diseases of the Gallbladder and Bile Ducts

Marsha D. Ford, MD
Adjunct Professor of Emergency Medicine, School of Medicine, University of North Carolina-Chapel Hill; Director, Carolinas Poison Center, Carolinas HealthCare System, Charlotte, North Carolina
Acute Poisoning

Chris E. Forsmark, MD
Professor of Medicine, Chief, Division of Gastroenterology, Hepatology, and Nutrition, University of Florida, Gainesville, Florida
Pancreatitis

Vance G. Fowler, Jr., MD, MHS
Professor of Medicine, Duke University Medical Center, Durham, North Carolina
Infective Endocarditis

Manuel A. Franco, MD, PhD
Director of Postgraduate Programs, School of Sciences, Pontificia Universidad Javeriana, Bogota, Colombia
Rotaviruses, Noroviruses, and Other Gastrointestinal Viruses

David O. Freedman, MD
Professor of Medicine and Microbiology, University of Alabama at Birmingham; Director, Gorgas Center for Geographic Medicine, Birmingham, Alabama
Approach to the Patient before and after Travel

Martyn A. French, MD
Professor in Clinical Immunology, School of Pathology and Laboratory Medicine, University of Western Australia, Perth, Australia
Immune Reconstitution Inflammatory Syndrome in HIV/AIDS

Karen Freund, MD, MPH
Professor of Medicine, Associate Director, Tufts Clinical and Translational Science Institute, Tufts University School of Medicine, Tufts Medical Center, Boston, Massachusetts
Approach to Women's Health

Cem Gabay, MD
Professor of Medicine, Head, Division of Rheumatology, University Hospitals of Geneva, Geneva, Switzerland
Biologic Agents

Kenneth L. Gage, PhD
Chief, Entomology and Ecology Activity, Centers for Disease Control and Prevention, Division of Vector-Borne Diseases, Bacterial Diseases Branch, Fort Collins, Colorado
Plague and Other Yersinia Infections

John N. Galgiani, MD
Professor of Medicine, Valley Fever Center for Excellence, University of Arizona, Tucson, Arizona
Coccidioidomycosis

Patrick G. Gallagher, MD
Professor of Pediatrics, Pathology, and Genetics, Yale University School of Medicine; Attending Physician, Yale–New Haven Hospital, New Haven, Connecticut
Hemolytic Anemias: Red Blood Cell Membrane and Metabolic Defects

Leonard Ganz, MD
Director of Cardiac Electrophysiology, Heritage Valley Health System, Beaver, Pennsylvania
Electrocardiography

Hasan Garan, MD
Director, Cardiac Electrophysiology, Dickinson W. Richards, Jr. Professor of Medicine, Columbia University Medical Center, New York, New York
Ventricular Arrhythmias

Guadalupe Garcia-Tsao, MD
Professor of Medicine, Yale University School of Medicine; Chief, Digestive Diseases, VA Connecticut Healthcare System, West Haven, Connecticut
Cirrhosis and Its Sequelae

William M. Geisler, MD, MPH
Professor of Medicine, University of Alabama at Birmingham, Birmingham, Alabama
Diseases Caused by Chlamydiae

Tony P. George, MD
Division of Brain and Therapeutics, Department of Psychiatry, University of Toronto; Schizophrenia Division, The Centre for Addiction and Mental Health, Toronto, Ontario, Canada
Nicotine and Tobacco

Lior Gepstein, MD, PhD
Edna and Jonathan Sohnis Professor in Medicine and Physiology, Rappaport Faculty of Medicine and Research Institute, Technion–Israel Institute of Technology, Rambam Health Care Campus, Haifa, Israel
Gene and Cell Therapy

Susan I. Gerber, MD
Team Lead, Respiratory Viruses/Picornaviruses, Division of Viral Diseases/Epidemiology Branch, National Center for Immunization and Respiratory Diseases, Centers for Disease Control and Prevention, Atlanta, Georgia
Coronaviruses

Dale N. Gerding, MD
Professor of Medicine, Loyola University Chicago Stritch School of Medicine, Research Physician, Edward Hines, Jr. VA Hospital, Hines, Illinois
Clostridial Infections

Morie A. Gertz, MD
Consultant, Division of Hematology, Mayo Clinic, Rochester, Minnesota; Roland Seidler, Jr. Professor of the Art of Medicine in Honor of Michael D. Brennan, MD, Professor of Medicine, Mayo Clinic, College of Medicine, Rochester, Minnesota
Amyloidosis

Gordon D. Ginder, MD
Professor, Internal Medicine, Director, Massey Cancer Center, Virginia Commonwealth University, Richmond, Virginia
Microcytic and Hypochromic Anemias

Jeffrey S. Ginsberg, MD
Professor of Medicine, McMaster University, Member of Thrombosis and Atherosclerosis Research Institute, St. Joseph's Healthcare Hamilton, Hamilton, Ontario, Canada
Peripheral Venous Disease

Geoffrey S. Ginsburg, MD, PhD
Director, Duke Center for Applied Genomics and Precision Medicine; Professor of Medicine, Pathology and Biomedical Engineering, Duke University, Durham, North Carolina
Applications of Molecular Technologies to Clinical Medicine

Michael Glogauer, DDS, PhD
Professor, Faculty of Dentistry, University of Toronto, Toronto, Ontario, Canada
Disorders of Phagocyte Function

John W. Gnann, Jr., MD
Professor of Medicine, Department of Medicine, Division of Infectious Diseases, Medical University of South Carolina, Charleston, South Carolina
Mumps

Matthew R. Golden, MD, MPH
Professor of Medicine, University of Washington, Director, HIV/STD Program, Public Health–Seattle & King County, Seattle, Washington
Neisseria Gonorrhoeae *Infections*

Lee Goldman, MD
Harold and Margaret Hatch Professor, Executive Vice President and Dean of the Faculties of Health Sciences and Medicine, Chief Executive, Columbia University Medical Center, Columbia University, New York, New York
Approach to Medicine, the Patient, and the Medical Profession: Medicine as a Learned and Humane Profession; Approach to the Patient with Possible Cardiovascular Disease

Ellie J.C. Goldstein, MD
Clinical Professor of Medicine, David Geffen School of Medicine at University of California Los Angeles, Los Angeles, California; Director, R.M. Alden Research Laboratory, Santa Monica, California
Diseases Caused by Non–Spore-Forming Anaerobic Bacteria

Larry B. Goldstein, MD
Professor of Neurology, Director, Duke Stroke Center, Neurology, Duke University; Staff Neurologist, Durham VA Medical Center, Durham, North Carolina
Approach to Cerebrovascular Diseases; Ischemic Cerebrovascular Disease

Lawrence T. Goodnough, MD
Professor of Pathology and Medicine, Stanford University; Director, Transfusion Service, Stanford University Medical Center, Stanford, California
Transfusion Medicine

Eduardo H. Gotuzzo, MD
Professor of Medicine, Director, Alexander von Humboldt Tropical Medicine Institute, Universidad Peruana Cayetano Heredia; Chief Physician, Department of Infectious, Tropical, and Dermatologic Diseases, National Hospital Cayetano Heredia, Lima, Peru
Cholera and Other Vibrio Infections; Liver, Intestinal, and Lung Fluke Infections

Deborah Grady, MD, MPH
Professor of Medicine, University of California San Francisco, San Francisco, California
Menopause

Leslie C. Grammer, MD
Professor of Medicine, Northwestern University Feinberg School of Medicine; Attending Physician, Northwestern Memorial Hospital, Chicago, Illinois
Drug Allergy

F. Anthony Greco, MD
Medical Director, Sarah Cannon Cancer Center, Nashville, Tennessee
Cancer of Unknown Primary Origin

Harry B. Greenberg, MD
Professor, Departments of Medicine and Microbiology and Immunology, Stanford University School of Medicine, Stanford, California
Rotaviruses, Noroviruses, and Other Gastrointestinal Viruses

Steven A. Greenberg, MD
Associate Professor of Neurology, Harvard Medical School; Associate Neurologist, Brigham and Women's Hospital, Boston, Massachusetts
Inflammatory Myopathies

Robert C. Griggs, MD
Professor of Neurology, Medicine, Pediatrics, and Pathology and Laboratory Medicine, University of Rochester School of Medicine and Dentistry, Rochester, New York
Approach to the Patient with Neurologic Disease

Lev M. Grinberg, MD, PhD
Professor, Chief, Department of Pathology, Ural Medical University; Chief Researcher of the Ural Scientific Research Institute of Phthisiopulmonology, Chief Pathologist of Ekaterinburg, Ekaterinburg, Russia
Anthrax

Daniel Grossman, MD
Vice President for Research, Ibis Reproductive Health, Oakland, California; Assistant Clinical Professor, Bixby Center for Global Reproductive Health, Department of Obstetrics, Gynecology and Reproductive Sciences, University of California San Francisco, San Francisco, California
Contraception

Lisa M. Guay-Woodford, MD
Hudson Professor of Pediatrics, The George Washington University; Director, Center for Translational Science, Director, Clinical and Translational Institute at Children's National, Children's National Health System, Washington, D.C.
Hereditary Nephropathies and Developmental Abnormalities of the Urinary Tract

Richard L. Guerrant, MD
Thomas H. Hunter Professor of International Medicine, Founding Director, Center for Global Health, Division of Infectious Diseases and International Health, University of Virginia School of Medicine, University of Virginia Health Sciences Center, Charlottesville, Virginia
Cryptosporidiosis

Roy M. Gulick, MD, MPH
Gladys and Roland Harrison Professor of Medicine, Medicine/Infectious Diseases, Weill Cornell Medical College; Attending Physician, New York–Presbyterian Hospital, New York, New York
Antiretrovial Therapy of HIV/AIDS

Klaus D. Hagspiel, MD
Professor of Radiology, Medicine, and Pediatrics, Chief, Noninvasive Cardiovascular Imaging, University of Virginia Health System, Charlottesville, Virginia
Noninvasive Cardiac Imaging

John D. Hainsworth, MD
Chief Scientific Officer, Sarah Cannon Research Institute, Nashville, Tennessee
Cancer of Unknown Primary Origin

Anders Hamsten, MD, PhD
Professor of Cardiovascular Diseases, Center for Molecular Medicine and Department of Cardiology, Karolinska University Hospital, Department of Medicine, Karolinska Institute, Stockholm, Sweden
Atherosclerosis, Thrombosis, and Vascular Biology

Kenneth R. Hande, MD
Professor of Medicine and Pharmacology, Vanderbilt/Ingram Cancer Center, Vanderbilt University School of Medicine, Nashville, Tennessee
Neuroendocrine Tumors and the Carcinoid Syndrome

H. Hunter Handsfield, MD
Professor Emeritus of Medicine, University of Washington Center for AIDS and STD, Seattle, Washington
Neisseria Gonorrhoeae *Infections*

Göran K. Hansson, MD, PhD
Professor of Cardiovascular Research, Center for Molecular Medicine at Karolinska University Hospital, Department of Medicine, Karolinska Institute, Stockholm, Sweden
Atherosclerosis, Thrombosis, and Vascular Biology

Raymond C. Harris, MD
Professor of Medicine, Ann and Roscoe R. Robinson Chair in Nephrology, Chief, Division of Nephrology, Vanderbilt University School of Medicine, Nashville, Tennessee
Diabetes and the Kidney

Stephen Crane Hauser, MD
Associate Professor of Medicine, Internal Medicine, Division of Gastroenterology and Hepatology, Mayo Clinic College of Medicine, Rochester, Minnesota
Vascular Diseases of the Gastrointestinal Tract

Frederick G. Hayden, MD
Stuart S. Richardson Professor of Clinical Virology and Professor of Medicine, University of Virginia School of Medicine; Staff Physician, University of Virginia Health System, Charlottesville, Virginia
Influenza

Douglas C. Heimburger, MD, MS
Professor of Medicine, Associate Director for Education and Training, Vanderbilt University School of Medicine, Vanderbilt Institute for Global Health, Nashville, Tennessee
Nutrition's Interface with Health and Disease

Erik L. Hewlett, MD
Professor of Medicine and of Microbiology, Immunology, and Cancer Biology, University of Virginia School of Medicine, University of Virginia Health System, Charlottesville, Virginia
Whooping Cough and Other Bordetella Infections

Richard J. Hift, PhD, MMed
School of Clinical Medicine, University of KwaZulu-Natal, Durban, South Africa
The Porphyrias

David R. Hill, MD, DTM&H
Professor of Medical Sciences, Director of Global Public Health, Frank H. Netter MD School of Medicine at Quinnipiac University, Hamden, Connecticut
Giardiasis

Nicholas S. Hill, MD
Professor of Medicine, Tufts University School of Medicine; Chief, Division of Pulmonary, Critical Care, and Sleep Medicine, Tufts Medical Center, Boston, Massachusetts
Respiratory Monitoring in Critical Care

L. David Hillis, MD
Professor and Chair, Department of Medicine, University of Texas Health Science Center at San Antonio, San Antonio, Texas
Acute Coronary Syndrome: Unstable Angina and Non-ST Elevation Myocardial Infarction

Jack Hirsh, CM, MD, DSc
Professor Emeritus, McMaster University, Hamilton, Ontario, Canada
Antithrombotic Therapy

Steven M. Holland, MD
Chief, Laboratory of Clinical Infectious Diseases, National Institute of Allergy and Infectious Diseases, National Institutes of Health, Bethesda, Maryland
The Nontuberculous Mycobacteria

Steven M. Hollenberg, MD
Professor of Medicine, Cooper Medical School of Rowan University; Director, Coronary Care Unit, Cooper University Hospital, Camden, New Jersey
Cardiogenic Shock

Edward W. Hook III, MD
Professor and Director, Division of Infectious Diseases, University of Alabama at Birmingham, Birmingham, Alabama
Granuloma Inguinale (Donovanosis); Syphilis; Nonsyphilitic Treponematoses

David J. Hunter, MBBS, MPH, ScD
Vincent L. Gregory Professor of Cancer Prevention, Harvard School of Public Health; Professor of Medicine, Harvard Medical School, Brigham and Women's Hospital, Boston, Massachusetts
The Epidemiology of Cancer

Khalid Hussain, MBChB, MD, MSc
Developmental Endocrinology Research Group, Clinical and Molecular Genetics Unit, Institute of Child Health, University College London, Department of Paediatric Endocrinology, Great Ormond Street Hospital for Children, London, United Kingdom
Hypoglycemia/Pancreatic Islet Cell Disorders

Steven E. Hyman, MD
Director, Stanley Center for Psychiatric Research, Broad Institute, Distinguished Service Professor of Stem Cell and Regenerative Biology, Harvard University, Cambridge, Massachusetts
Biology of Addiction

Michael C. Iannuzzi, MD, MBA
Chairman, Department of Internal Medicine, State University of New York Upstate Medical University, Syracuse, New York
Sarcoidosis

Robert D. Inman, MD
Professor of Medicine and Immunology, University of Toronto; Staff Rheumatologist, University Health Network, Toronto, Ontario, Canada
The Spondyloarthropathies

Sharon K. Inouye, MD, MPH
Professor of Medicine, Harvard Medical School; Director, Aging Brain Center, Institute for Aging Research, Hebrew SeniorLife, Boston, Massachusetts
Neuropsychiatric Aspects of Aging; Delirium or Acute Mental Status Change in the Older Patient

Geoffrey K. Isbister, MD, BSc
Associate Professor, Clinical Toxicologist, Calvary Mater Newcastle, Callaghan, Senior Research Academic, School of Medicine and Public Health, University of Newcastle, New South Wales, Australia
Envenomation

Michael G. Ison, MD, MS
Associate Professor in Medicine-Infectious Diseases and Surgery-Organ Transplantation, Northwestern University Feinberg School of Medicine, Chicago, Illinois
Adenovirus Diseases

Elias Jabbour, MD
Associate Professor, Department of Leukemia, Division of Medicine, The University of Texas MD Anderson Cancer Center, Houston, Texas
The Chronic Leukemias

Michael R. Jaff, DO
Professor of Medicine, Harvard Medical School, Chair, Institute for Heart, Vascular, and Stroke Care, Massachusetts General Hospital, Boston, Massachusetts
Other Peripheral Arterial Diseases

Joanna C. Jen, MD, PhD
Professor of Neurology, University of California Los Angeles School of Medicine, Los Angeles, California
Neuro-Ophthalmology; Smell and Taste; Hearing and Equilibrium

Dennis M. Jensen, MD
Professor of Medicine, David Geffen School of Medicine at University of California Los Angeles; Staff Physician, Medicine-GI, VA Greater Los Angeles Healthcare System; Key Investigator, Director, Human Studies Core & GI Hemostasis Research Unit, CURE Digestive Diseases Research Center, Los Angeles, California
Gastrointestinal Hemorrhage

Michael D. Jensen, MD
Professor of Medicine, Endocrine Research Unit, Director, Obesity Treatment Research Program, Mayo Clinic, Rochester, Minnesota
Obesity

Robert T. Jensen, MD
Chief, Cell Biology Section, Digestive Disease Branch, National Institute of Diabetes and Digestive and Kidney Diseases, National Institutes of Health, Clinical Center, Bethesda, Maryland
Pancreatic Neuroendocrine Tumors

Stuart Johnson, MD
Professor of Medicine, Loyola University Chicago Stritch School of Medicine; Associate Chief of Staff for Research, Edward Hines, Jr. VA Hospital, Hines, Illinois
Clostridial Infections

Richard C. Jordan, DDS, PhD
Professor of Oral Pathology, Pathology and Radiation Oncology, University of California San Francisco, San Francisco, California
Diseases of the Mouth and Salivary Glands

Ralph F. Józefowicz, MD
Professor, Neurology and Medicine, University of Rochester, Rochester, New York
Approach to the Patient with Neurologic Disease

Stephen G. Kaler, MD
Senior Investigator and Head, Section on Translational Neuroscience, Molecular Medicine Program, Eunice Kennedy Shriver National Institute of Child Health and Human Development, Bethesda, Maryland
Wilson Disease

Moses R. Kamya, MB ChB, MMed, MPH, PhD
Chairman, Department of Medicine, Makerere University College of Health Sciences, Kampala, Uganda
Malaria

Louise W. Kao, MD
Associate Professor of Emergency Medicine, Department of Emergency Medicine, Indiana University School of Medicine, Indianapolis, Indiana
Chronic Poisoning: Trace Metals and Others

Steven A. Kaplan, MD
E. Darracott Vaughan, Jr. Professor of Urology, Chief, Institute for Bladder and Prostate Health, Weill Cornell Medical College; Director, Iris Cantor Men's Health Center, NewYork–Presbyterian Hospital, New York, New York
Benign Prostatic Hyperplasia and Prostatitis

Daniel L. Kastner, MD, PhD
Scientific Director, National Human Genome Research Institute, National Institutes of Health, Bethesda, Maryland
The Systemic Autoinflammatory Diseases

Sekar Kathiresan, MD
Associate Professor in Medicine, Harvard Medical School; Director, Preventive Cardiology, Massachusetts General Hospital, Boston, Massachusetts
The Inherited Basis of Common Diseases

David A. Katzka, MD
Professor of and Consultant in Medicine, Gastroenterology, Mayo Clinic, Rochester, Minnesota
Diseases of the Esophagus

Debra K. Katzman, MD
Professor of Pediatrics, Senior Associate Scientist, The Research Institute, The Hospital for Sick Children and University of Toronto, Toronto, Ontario, Canada
Adolescent Medicine

Carol A. Kauffman, MD
Professor of Internal Medicine, University of Michigan Medical School; Chief, Infectious Diseases Section, Veterans Affairs Ann Arbor Healthcare System, Ann Arbor, Michigan
Histoplasmosis; Blastomycosis; Paracoccidioidomycosis; Cryptococcosis; Sporotrichosis; Candidiasis

Kenneth Kaushansky, MD
Senior Vice President for Health Sciences, Dean, School of Medicine, Stony Brook University, Stony Brook, New York
Hematopoiesis and Hematopoietic Growth Factors

Keith S. Kaye, MD, MPH
Professor of Medicine, Division of Infectious Diseases, Wayne State University School of Medicine, Detroit, Michigan
Diseases Caused by Acinetobacter and Stenotrophomonas Species

Armand Keating, MD
Professor of Medicine, Director, Division of Hematology, Epstein Chair in Cell Therapy and Transplantation, Professor, Institute of Biomaterials and Biomedical Engineering, University of Toronto, Toronto, Ontario, Canada
Hematopoietic Stem Cell Transplantation

Robin K. Kelley, MD
Assistant Professor of Medicine, University of California San Francisco, Helen Diller Family Comprehensive Cancer Center, San Francisco, California
Liver and Biliary Tract Cancers

Morton Kern, MD
Chief of Medicine, VA Long Beach Health Care System School of Medicine; Professor of Medicine, Associate Chief, Cardiology, University of California–Irvine, Irvine, California
Catheterization and Angiography

Gerald T. Keusch, MD
Professor of Medicine and International Health and Public Health, Boston University School of Medicine, Boston, Massachusetts
Shigellosis

Fadlo R. Khuri, MD
Professor and Chair, Hematology and Medical Oncology, Deputy Director, Winship Cancer Institute, Emory University, Atlanta, Georgia
Lung Cancer and Other Pulmonary Neoplasms

David H. Kim, MD
Vice Chair of Education, Professor of Radiology, Section of Abdominal Imaging, University of Wisconsin School of Medicine and Public Health, Madison, Wisconsin
Diagnostic Imaging Procedures in Gastroenterology

Matthew Kim, MD
Instructor of Medicine, Harvard Medical School; Associate Physician, Brigham and Women's Hospital, Boston, Massachusetts
Thyroid

Louis V. Kirchhoff, MD, MPH
Professor, Departments of Internal Medicine (Infectious Diseases) and Epidemiology, University of Iowa Health Care; Staff Physician, Medical Service, Department of Veterans Affairs Medical Center, Iowa City, Iowa
Chagas Disease

David S. Knopman, MD
Professor of Neurology, Mayo Clinic College of Medicine, Rochester, Minnesota
Regional Cerebral Dysfunction: Higher Mental Function; Alzheimer Disease and Other Dementias

Tamsin A. Knox, MD, MPH
Associate Professor of Medicine, Nutrition/Infection Unit, Tufts University School of Medicine, Boston, Massachusetts
Gastrointestinal Manifestions of HIV and AIDS

D.P. Kontoyiannis, MD, ScD
Professor, Department of Infectious Diseases, Infection Control and Employee Health, The University of Texas MD Anderson Cancer Center, Houston, Texas
Mucormycosis; Mycetoma

Barbara S. Koppel, MD
Professor of Clinical Neurology, New York Medical College, Chief of Neurology, Metropolitan Hospital Center, New York City Health and Hospital Corporation, New York, New York
Nutritional and Alcohol-Related Neurologic Disorders

Kevin M. Korenblat, MD
Associate Professor of Medicine, Department of Medicine, Washington University School of Medicine, St. Louis, Missouri
Approach to the Patient with Jaundice or Abnormal Liver Tests

Bruce R. Korf, MD, PhD
Wayne H. and Sara Crews Finley Chair in Medical Genetics, Professor and Chair, Department of Genetics, University of Alabama at Birmingham, Birmingham, Alabama
Principles of Genetics

Neil J. Korman, MD, PhD
Professor, Dermatology, Case Western Reserve University School of Medicine, University Hospitals Case Medical Center, Cleveland, Ohio
Macular, Papular, Vesiculobullous, and Pustular Diseases

Mark G. Kortepeter, MD, MPH
Associate Dean for Research, Associate Professor of Preventive Medicine and Medicine, Consultant to the Army Surgeon General for Biodefense; Office of the Dean, Edward Hébert School of Medicine, Uniformed Services University of the Health Sciences, Bethesda, Maryland
Bioterrorism

Joseph A. Kovacs, MD
Senior Investigator and Head, AIDS Section, Critical Care Medicine Department, National Institutes of Health, Bethesda, Maryland
Pneumocystis Pneumonia

Thomas O. Kovacs, MD
Professor of Medicine, Division of Digestive Diseases, David Geffen School of Medicine at University of California Los Angeles, Los Angeles, California
Gastrointestinal Hemorrhage

Monica Kraft, MD
Professor of Medicine, Duke University School of Medicine; Chief, Division of Pulmonary, Allergy, and Critical Care Medicine, Duke University Medical Center, Durham, North Carolina
Approach to the Patient with Respiratory Disease

Christopher M. Kramer, MD
Ruth C. Heede Professor of Cardiology, Professor of Radiology, Director, Cardiovascular Imaging Center, University of Virginia Health System, Charlottesville, Virginia
Noninvasive Cardiac Imaging

Donna M. Krasnewich, MD, PhD
Program Director, National Institute of General Medical Sciences, National Institutes of Health, Bethesda, Maryland
The Lysosomal Storage Diseases

Peter J. Krause, MD
Senior Research Scientist in Epidemiology, Medicine, and Pediatrics, Yale School of Public Health and Yale School of Medicine, New Haven, Connecticut
Babesiosis and Other Protozoan Diseases

John F. Kuemmerle, MD
Chair, Division of Gastroenterology, Hepatology, and Nutrition, Professor of Medicine, and Physiology and Biophysics, Center for Digestive Health, Virginia Commonwealth University, Richmond, Virginia
Inflammatory and Anatomic Diseases of the Intestine, Peritoneum, Mesentery, and Omentum

Ernst J. Kuipers, MD, PhD
Professor of Medicine, Department of Gastroenterology and Hepatology, Chief Executive Officer, Erasmus MC University Medical Center, Rotterdam, The Netherlands
Acid Peptic Disease

Paul W. Ladenson, MD
Professor of Medicine, Pathology, Oncology, and Radiology and Radiological Sciences, John Eager Howard Professor of Endocrinology and Metabolism, University Distinguished Service Professor, The Johns Hopkins University School of Medicine; Physician and Division Director, The Johns Hopkins Hospital, Baltimore, Maryland
Thyroid

Daniel Laheru, MD
Ian T. MacMillan Professorship in Clinical Pancreatic Research, Medical Oncology, Johns Hopkins University School of Medicine, Baltimore, Maryland
Pancreatic Cancer

Donald W. Landry, MD, PhD
Samuel Bard Professor of Medicine, Chair, Department of Medicine, Physician-in-Chief, NewYork-Presbyterian Hospital/Columbia University Medical Center, New York, New York
Approach to the Patient with Renal Disease

Anthony E. Lang, MD
Director, Division of Neurology, Jack Clark Chair for Research in Parkinson's Disease, University of Toronto; Director, Morton and Gloria Shulman Movement Disorders Clinic and the Edmond J. Safra Program in Parkinson's Disease and the Lily Safra Chair in Movement Disorders, Toronto Western Hospital, Toronto, Ontario, Canada
Parkinsonism; Other Movement Disorders

Richard A. Lange, MD, MBA
President and Dean, Paul L. Foster School of Medicine, Texas Tech University Health Sciences Center El Paso, El Paso, Texas
Acute Coronary Syndrome: Unstable Angina and Non-ST Elevation Myocardial Infarction

Frank A. Lederle, MD
Core Investigator, Center for Chronic Disease Outcomes Research, Minneapolis VA Medical Center; Professor of Medicine, University of Minnesota School of Medicine, Minneapolis, Minnesota
Diseases of the Aorta

Thomas H. Lee, MD, MSc
Senior Physician, Department of Medicine, Brigham and Women's Hospital; Chief Medical Officer, Press Ganey, Boston, Massachusetts
Using Data for Clinical Decisions

William M. Lee, MD
Professor of Internal Medicine, University of Texas Southwestern Medical Center, Dallas, Texas
Toxin- and Drug-Induced Liver Disease

James E. Leggett, MD
Associate Professor, Department of Medicine, Oregon Health and Science University; Infectious Diseases, Department of Medical Education, Providence Portland Medical Center, Portland, Oregon
Approach to Fever or Suspected Infection in the Normal Host

Stuart Levin, MD
Professor of Medicine, Emeritus Chairman, Department of Medicine, Rush University Medical Center, Chicago, Illinois
Zoonoses

Stephanie M. Levine, MD
Professor of Medicine, Division of Pulmonary Diseases and Critical Care Medicine, The University of Texas Health Science Center San Antonio, South Texas Veterans Health Care System, San Antonio, Texas
Alveolar Filling Disorders

Gary R. Lichtenstein, MD
Professor of Medicine, Perelman School of Medicine at the University of Pennsylvania, Director, Center for Inflammatory Bowel Disease, University of Pennsylvania, Philadelphia, Pennsylvania
Inflammatory Bowel Disease

Henry W. Lim, MD
Chairman and C.S. Livingood Chair, Department of Dermatology, Henry Ford Hospital; Senior Vice President for Academic Affairs, Henry Ford Health System, Detroit, Michigan
Eczemas, Photodermatoses, Papulosquamous (Including Fungal) Diseases, and Figurate Erythemas

Aldo A.M. Lima, MD, PhD
Professor of Medicine and Pharmacology, School of Medicine, Federal University of Ceará, Fortaleza, Ceará, Brazil
Cryptosporidiosis; Amebiasis

Geoffrey S.F. Ling, MD, PhD
Professor of Neurology, Uniformed Services University of the Health Sciences, Bethesda, Maryland
Traumatic Brain Injury and Spinal Cord Injury

William C. Little, MD
Patrick Lehan Professor of Cardiovascular Medicine, Chair, Department of Medicine, University of Mississippi Medical Center, Jackson, Mississippi
Pericardial Diseases

Donald M. Lloyd-Jones, MD, ScM
Senior Associate Dean, Chair, Department of Preventive Medicine, Eileen M. Foell Professor of Preventive Medicine and Medicine, Northwestern University Feinberg School of Medicine, Chicago, Illinois
Epidemiology of Cardiovascular Disease

Bennett Lorber, MD
Thomas M. Durant Professor of Medicine and Professor of Microbiology and Immunology, Temple University School of Medicine, Philadelphia, Pennsylvania
Listeriosis

Donald E. Low, MD†
Nonpneumococcal Streptococcal Infections, Rheumatic Fever

Daniel R. Lucey, MD, MPH
Adjunct Professor, Microbiology and Immunology, Georgetown University Medical Center, Washington, D.C.
Anthrax

James R. Lupski, MD, PhD
Cullen Professor of Molecular and Human Genetics, Professor of Pediatrics, Baylor College of Medicine and Texas Children's Hospital, Houston, Texas
Gene, Genomic, and Chromosomal Disorders

Jeffrey M. Lyness, MD
Senior Associate Dean for Academic Affairs, Professor of Psychiatry and Neurology, University of Rochester School of Medicine and Dentistry, Rochester, New York
Psychiatric Disorders in Medical Practice

Bruce W. Lytle, MD
Chair, Heart and Vascular Institute, Professor of Surgery, Thoracic and Cardiovascular Surgery, Cleveland Clinic, Cleveland, Ohio
Interventional and Surgical Treatment of Coronary Artery Disease

†Deceased.

C. Ronald MacKenzie, MD
Assistant Attending Physician, Department of Medicine-Rheumatology, C. Ronald MacKenzie Chair in Ethics and Medicine, Hospital for Special Surgery, Associate Professor of Clinical Medicine and Medical Ethics, Weill Cornell Medical College of Cornell University, New York, New York
Surgical Treatment of Joint Disease

Harriet L. MacMillan, MD, MSc
Professor, Departments of Psychiatry and Behavioural Neurosciences, and Pediatrics, Chedoke Health Chair in Child Psychiatry, Offord Centre for Child Studies, McMaster University, Hamilton, Ontario, Canada
Intimate Partner Violence

Robert D. Madoff, MD
Professor of Surgery, Stanley M. Goldberg, MD, Chair, Colon and Rectal Surgery, University of Minnesota, Minneapolis, Minnesota
Diseases of the Rectum and Anus

Frank Maldarelli, MD, PhD
Head, Clinical Retrovirology Section, HIV Drug Resistance Program, National Cancer Institute, National Institutes of Health, Bethesda, Maryland
Biology of Human Immunodeficiency Viruses

Atul Malhotra, MD
Chief of Pulmonary and Critical Care, Kenneth M. Moser Professor of Medicine, Director of Sleep Medicine, University of California San Diego, La Jolla, California
Disorders of Ventilatory Control

Mark J. Manary, MD
Helene B. Roberson Professor of Pediatrics, Washington University School of Medicine; Attending Physician, St. Louis Children's Hospital, St. Louis, Missouri; Adjunct Professor, Children's Nutrition Research Center, Baylor College of Medicine, Houston, Texas; Senior Lecturer in Community Health, University of Malawi College of Medicine, Blantyre, Malawi
Protein-Energy Malnutrition

Donna Mancini, MD
Professor of Medicine, Department of Medicine, Division of Cardiology, Columbia University College of Physicians and Surgeons, Center for Advanced Cardiac Care, Columbia University Medical Center, New York, New York
Cardiac Transplantation

Lionel A. Mandell, MD
Professor of Medicine, Faculty of Health Sciences, McMaster University, Hamilton, Ontario, Canada
Streptococcus Pneumoniae *Infections*

Peter Manu, MD
Professor of Medicine and Psychiatry, Hofstra North Shore–LIJ School of Medicine at Hofstra University, Hempstead, New York; Adjunct Professor of Clinical Medicine, Psychiatry and Behavioral Sciences, Albert Einstein College of Medicine, Bronx, New York; Director of Medical Services, Zucker Hillside Hospital, Glen Oaks, New York
Medical Consultation in Psychiatry

Ariane Marelli, MD, MPH
Professor of Medicine, McGill University, Director, McGill Adult Unit for Congenital Heart Disease, Associate Director, Academic Affairs and Research, Cardiology, McGill University Health Centre, Montreal, Québec, Canada
Congenital Heart Disease in Adults

Xavier Mariette, MD, PhD
Professor, Rheumatology, Université Paris-Sud, AP-HP, Le Kremlin Bicêtre, France
Sjögren Syndrome

Andrew R. Marks, MD
Wu Professor and Chair, Department of Physiology and Cellular Biophysics, Founding Director, Helen and Clyde Wu Center for Molecular Cardiology, Columbia University College of Physicians and Surgeons, New York, New York
Cardiac Function and Circulatory Control

Kieren A. Marr, MD
Professor of Medicine and Oncology, The Johns Hopkins University, Director, Transplant and Oncology Infectious Diseases, Baltimore, Maryland
Approach to Fever and Suspected Infection in the Compromised Host

Thomas J. Marrie, MD
Dean, Faculty of Medicine, Dalhousie University; Professor of Medicine, Capital District Health Authority, Halifax, Nova Scotia, Canada
Legionella Infections

Paul Martin, MD
Professor of Medicine and Chief, Division of Hepatology, Miller School of Medicine, University of Miami, Miami, Florida
Approach to the Patient with Liver Disease

Joel B. Mason, MD
Professor of Medicine and Nutrition, Tufts University; Staff Physician, Divisions of Gastroenterology and Clinical Nutrition, Tufts Medical Center, Boston, Massachusetts
Vitamins, Trace Minerals, and Other Micronutrients

Henry Masur, MD
Chief, Critical Care Medicine Department, Clinical Center, National Institutes of Health, Bethesda, Maryland
Infectious and Metabolic Complications of HIV and AIDS

Eric L. Matteson, MD, MPH
Professor of Medicine, Mayo Clinic College of Medicine, Consultant, Divisions of Rheumatology and Epidemiology, Mayo Clinic, Rochester, Minnesota
Infections of Bursae, Joints, and Bones

Michael A. Matthay, MD
Professor, Departments of Medicine and Anesthesia, University of California San Francisco, San Francisco, California
Acute Respiratory Failure

Toby A. Maurer, MD
Professor of Dermatology, University of California San Francisco; Chief of Dermatology, San Francisco General Hospital, San Francisco, California
Skin Manifestations in Patients with Human Immunodeficiency Virus Infection

Emeran A. Mayer, MD, PhD
Professor of Medicine, Physiology, and Psychiatry, Division of Digestive Diseases, Department of Medicine, University of California Los Angeles, Los Angeles, California
Functional Gastrointestinal Disorders: Irritable Bowel Syndrome, Dyspepsia, Chest Pain of Presumed Esophageal Origin, and Heartburn

Stephan A. Mayer, MD
Director, Institute for Critical Care Medicine, Icahn School of Medicine at Mount Sinai, New York, New York
Hemorrhagic Cerebrovascular Disease

Stephen A. McClave, MD
Professor of Medicine, Director of Clinical Nutrition, University of Louisville School of Medicine, Louisville, Kentucky
Enteral Nutrition

F. Dennis McCool, MD
Professor of Medicine, The Warren Alpert Medical School of Brown University; Medical Director of Sleep Center, Memorial Hospital of Rhode Island, Pawtucket, Rhode Island
Diseases of the Diaphragm, Chest Wall, Pleura, and Mediastinum

Charles E. McCulloch, PhD
Professor of Biostatistics, Department of Epidemiology and Biostatistics, University of California San Francisco, San Francisco, California
Statistical Interpretation of Data

William J. McKenna, MD
Professor of Cardiology, Institute of Cardiovascular Science, University College London, London, United Kingdom
Diseases of the Myocardium and Endocardium

Vallerie McLaughlin, MD
Kim A. Eagle, MD, Endowed Professor of Cardiovascular Medicine, Director, Pulmonary Hypertension Program, University of Michigan, Ann Arbor, Michigan
Pulmonary Hypertension

John J.V. McMurray, MB, MD
Professor of Cardiology, Institute of Cardiovascular and Medical Sciences, University of Glasgow, Glasgow, Scotland, United Kingdom
Heart Failure: Management and Prognosis

Kenneth R. McQuaid, MD
Professor of Clinical Medicine, Marvin H. Sleisenger Endowed Chair, Vice Chairman, University of California San Francisco; Chief, Medical Services and Gastroenterology, San Francisco VA Medical Center, San Francisco, California
Approach to the Patient with Gastrointestinal Disease

Marc Michel, MD
Professor of Internal Medicine, Head of the Unit of Internal Medicine at Henri Mondor University Hospital, National Referral Center for Adult's Immune Cytopenias, Creteil, France
Autoimmune and Intravascular Hemolytic Anemias

Jonathan W. Mink, MD, PhD
Frederick A. Horner, MD Endowed Professor in Pediatric Neurology, Professor of Neurology, Neurobiology & Anatomy, Brain & Cognitive Sciences, and Pediatrics, Chief, Division of Child Neurology, Vice Chair, Department of Neurology, University of Rochester, Rochester, New York
Congenital, Developmental, and Neurocutaneous Disorders

William E. Mitch, MD
Gordon A. Cain Chair in Nephrology, Director of Nephrology, Baylor College of Medicine, Houston, Texas
Chronic Kidney Disease

Mark E. Molitch, MD
Martha Leland Sherwin Professor of Endocrinology, Division of Endocrinology, Metabolism, and Molecular Medicine, Northwestern University Feinberg School of Medicine, Chicago, Illinois
Neuroendocrinology and the Neuroendocrine System; Anterior Pituitary

Bruce A. Molitoris, MD
Professor of Medicine, and Cellular and Integrative Physiology Director, Indiana Center for Biological Microscopy, Indiana University, Indianapolis, Indiana
Acute Kidney Injury

Jose G. Montoya, MD
Professor of Medicine, Division of Infectious Disease and Geographic Medicine, Stanford University School of Medicine, Stanford, California; Director, Palo Alto Medical Foundation Toxoplasma Serology Laboratory, National Reference Center for the Study and Diagnosis of Toxoplasmosis, Palo Alto, California
Toxoplasmosis

Alison Morris, MD, MS
Associate Professor of Medicine, Clinical Translational Science, and Immunology, Division of Pulmonary, Allergy, and Critical Care Medicine, University of Pittsburgh School of Medicine, Pittsburgh, Pennsylvania
Pulmonary Manifestations of Human Immunodeficiency Virus and Acquired Immunodeficiency Syndrome

Ernest Moy, MD, MPH
Medical Officer, Center for Quality Improvement and Patient Safety Agency for Healthcare Research and Quality, Rockville, Maryland
Measuring Health and Health Care

Atis Muehlenbachs, MD, PhD
Infectious Diseases Pathology Branch, Centers for Disease Control and Prevention, Atlanta, Georgia
Leptospirosis

Andrew H. Murr, MD
Professor and Chairman, Roger Boles, MD Endowed Chair in Otolaryngology Education, Department of Otolaryngology-Head and Neck Surgery, University of California San Francisco School of Medicine, San Francisco, California
Approach to the Patient with Nose, Sinus, and Ear Disorders

Daniel M. Musher, MD
Professor of Medicine, Molecular Virology, and Microbiology, Distinguished Service Professor, Baylor College of Medicine, Infectious Disease Section, Michael E. DeBakey Veterans Affairs Medical Center, Houston, Texas
Overview of Pneumonia

Robert J. Myerburg, MD
Professor of Medicine and Physiology, Division of Cardiology, Department of Medicine, American Heart Association Chair in Cardiovascular Research, University of Miami Miller School of Medicine, Miami, Florida
Approach to Cardiac Arrest and Life-Threatening Arrhythmias

Sandesh C.S. Nagamani, MD
Assistant Professor, Department of Molecular and Human Genetics, Director, Clinic for Metabolic and Genetic Disorders of Bone, Baylor College of Medicine and Texas Children's Hospital, Houston, Texas
Gene, Genomic, and Chromosomal Disorders

Stanley J. Naides, MD
Medical Director and Interim Scientific Director, Immunology, Quest Diagnostics Nichols Institute, San Juan Capistrano, California
Arboviruses Causing Fever and Rash Syndromes

Yoshifumi Naka, MD, PhD
Professor of Surgery, Department of Surgery, Columbia University College of Physicians and Surgeons, New York, New York
Cardiac Transplantation

Theodore E. Nash, MD
Principal Investigator, Clinical Parasitology Section, Laboratory of Parasitic Diseases, National Institute of Allergy and Infectious Diseases, National Institutes of Health, Bethesda, Maryland
Giardiasis

Avindra Nath, MD
Chief, Section of Infections of the Nervous System, National Institute of Neurological Disorders and Stroke, National Institutes of Health, Bethesda, Maryland
Cytomegalovirus, Epstein-Barr Virus, and Slow Virus Infections of the Central Nervous System; Neurologic Complications of Human Immunodeficiency Virus Infection; Meningitis: Bacterial, Viral, and Other; Brain Abscess and Parameningeal Infections

Eric G. Neilson, MD
Vice President for Medical Affairs and Lewis Landsberg Dean, Northwestern University Feinberg School of Medicine, Northwestern Memorial Hospital, Chicago, Illinois
Tubulointerstitial Nephritis

Lawrence S. Neinstein, MD
Professor of Pediatrics and Medicine, Keck School of Medicine of USC; Executive Director, Engemann Student Health Center, Division Head of College Health, Assistant Provost, Student Health and Wellness, University of Southern California, Los Angeles, California
Adolescent Medicine

Lewis S. Nelson, MD
Professor of Emergency Medicine, Director, Fellowship in Medical Toxicology, New York University School of Medicine; Attending Physician, New York University Langone Medical Center and Bellevue Hospital Center, New York, New York
Acute Poisoning

Eric J. Nestler, MD, PhD
Nash Family Professor and Chair, Department of Neuroscience, Director, The Friedman Brain Institute, Icahn School of Medicine at Mount Sinai, New York, New York
Biology of Addiction

Anne B. Newman, MD, MPH
Professor of Epidemiology, The University of Pittsburgh Graduate School of Public Health; Chair, Department of Epidemiology, Director, University of Pittsburgh Center for Aging and Population Health, Pittsburgh, Pennsylvania
Epidemiology of Aging: Implications of the Aging of Society

Thomas B. Newman, MD, MPH
Professor, Epidemiology & Biostatistics and Pediatrics, University of California San Francisco, San Francisco, California
Statistical Interpretation of Data

William L. Nichols, MD
Associate Professor, Medicine and Laboratory Medicine, Mayo Clinic College of Medicine; Staff Physician, Special Coagulation Laboratory, Comprehensive Hemophilia Center, and Coagulation Clinic, Mayo Clinic, Rochester, Minnesota
Von Willebrand Disease and Hemorrhagic Abnormalities of Platelet and Vascular Function

Lindsay E. Nicolle, MD
Professor of Internal Medicine and Medical Microbiology, University of Manitoba, Health Sciences Centre, Winnipeg, Manitoba, Canada
Approach to the Patient with Urinary Tract Infection

Lynnette K. Nieman, MD
Senior Investigator, Program on Reproductive and Adult Endocrinology, Eunice Kennedy Shriver National Institute of Child Health and Human Development, Bethesda, Maryland
Approach to the Patient with Endocrine Disease; Adrenal Cortex; Polyglandular Disorders

Dennis E. Niewoehner, MD
Professor of Medicine, University of Minnesota; Staff Physician, Minneapolis Veterans Affairs Health Care System, Minneapolis, Minnesota
Chronic Obstructive Pulmonary Disease

S. Ragnar Norrby, MD, PhD
Director General, Swedish Institute for Infectious Disease Control, Solna, Sweden
Approach to the Patient with Urinary Tract Infection

Susan O'Brien, MD
Professor, Department of Leukemia, Division of Medicine, The University of Texas MD Anderson Cancer Center, Houston, Texas
The Chronic Leukemias

Christopher M. O'Connor, MD
Professor of Medicine and Chief, Division of Cardiology, Director, Duke Heart Center, Durham, North Carolina
Heart Failure: Pathophysiology and Diagnosis

Francis G. O'Connor, MD, MPH
Professor and Chair, Military and Emergency Medicine, Medical Director, Uniformed Services University Consortium for Health and Military Performance, Bethesda, Maryland
Disorders Due to Heat and Cold; Rhabdomyolysis

Patrick G. O'Connor, MD, MPH
Professor and Chief, General Internal Medicine, Yale University School of Medicine, New Haven, Connecticut
Alcohol Abuse and Dependence

James R. O'Dell, MD
Bruce Professor and Vice Chair of Internal Medicine, Chief, Division of Rheumatology, University of Nebraska Medical Center and Omaha VA Nebraska–Western Iowa Health Care System, Omaha, Nebraska
Rheumatoid Arthritis

Anne E. O'Donnell, MD
Professor of Medicine, Chief, Division of Pulmonary, Critical Care, and Sleep Medicine, Georgetown University Medical Center, Washington, D.C.
Bronchiectasis, Atelectasis, Cysts, and Localized Lung Disorders

Jae K. Oh, MD
Professor of Medicine, Director, Echocardiography Core Laboratory and Pericardial Clinic, Division of Cardiovascular Diseases, Co-Director, Integrated Cardiac Imaging, Division of Cardiovascular Diseases, Mayo Clinic, Rochester, Minnesota
Pericardial Diseases

Jeffrey E. Olgin, MD
Gallo-Chatterjee Distinguished Professor of Medicine, Chief, Division of Cardiology, Co-Director, Heart and Vascular Center, University of California San Francisco, San Francisco, California
Approach to the Patient with Suspected Arrhythmia

Walter A. Orenstein, MD
Professor of Medicine, Pediatrics, and Global Health, Emory University School of Medicine, Atlanta, Georgia
Immunization

Douglas R. Osmon, MD, MPH
Professor of Medicine, Mayo Clinic College of Medicine; Consultant, Division of Infectious Diseases, Mayo Clinic, Rochester, Minnesota
Infections of Bursae, Joints, and Bones

Catherine M. Otto, MD
J. Ward Kennedy-Hamilton Endowed Chair in Cardiology, Professor of Medicine, University of Washington School of Medicine; Director, Heart Valve Clinic, University of Washington Medical Center, Seattle, Washington
Echocardiography

Mark Papania, MD, MPH
Medical Epidemiologist, Division of Viral Diseases, Measles, Mumps, Rubella, and Herpes Virus Laboratory Branch, Centers for Disease Control and Prevention, Atlanta, Georgia
Measles

Peter G. Pappas, MD
Professor of Medicine, University of Alabama at Birmingham, Birmingham, Alabama
Dematiaceous Fungal Infections

Pankaj Jay Pasricha, MD
Director, The Johns Hopkins Center for Neurogastroenterology; Professor of Medicine and Neurosciences, The Johns Hopkins School of Medicine; Professor of Innovation Management, Johns Hopkins Carey Business School, Baltimore, Maryland
Gastrointestinal Endoscopy

David L. Paterson, MD
Professor of Medicine, University of Queensland Centre for Clinical Research, Royal Brisbane and Women's Hospital Campus, Brisbane, Queensland, Australia
Infections Due to Other Members of the Enterobacteriaceae, Including Management of Multidrug Resistant Strains

Carlo Patrono, MD
Professor and Chair of Pharmacology, Department of Pharmacology, Catholic University School of Medicine, Rome, Italy
Prostaglandin, Aspirin, and Related Compounds

Jean-Michel Pawlotsky, MD, PhD
Professor of Medicine, The University of Paris-Est; Director, National Reference Center for Viral Hepatitis B, C, and Delta and Department of Virology, Henri Mondor University Hospital; Director, Department of Molecular Virology and Immunology, Institut Mondor de Recherche Biomédicale, Créteil, France
Acute Viral Hepatitis; Chronic Viral and Autoimmune Hepatitis

Richard D. Pearson, MD
Professor of Medicine and Pathology, University of Virginia School of Medicine and University of Virginia Health System, Charlottesville, Virginia
Antiparasitic Therapy

Trish M. Perl, MD, MSc
Professor of Medicine and Pathology, The Johns Hopkins School of Medicine; Professor of Epidemiology, Johns Hopkins Bloomberg School of Public Health; Infectious Diseases Specialist and Senior Epidemiologist, The Johns Hopkins Hospital and Health System, Baltimore, Maryland
Enterococcal Infections

Adam Perlman, MD, MPH
Associate Professor, Department of Medicine, Duke University Medical Center; Executive Director, Duke Integrative Medicine, Duke University Health System, Durham, North Carolina
Complementary and Alternative Medicine

William A. Petri, Jr., MD, PhD
Wade Hampton Frost Professor, Departments of Medicine, Pathology, Microbiology, Immunology, and Cancer Biology, School of Medicine, University of Virginia; Chief, Division of Infectious Diseases and International Health, University of Virginia Hospitals, Charlottesville, Virginia
Relapsing Fever and Other Borrelia Infections; African Sleeping Sickness; Amebiasis

Marc A. Pfeffer, MD, PhD
Dzau Professor of Medicine, Harvard Medical School; Senior Physician, Cardiovascular Division, Brigham and Women's Hospital, Boston, Massachusetts
Heart Failure: Management and Prognosis

Perry J. Pickhardt, MD
Professor of Radiology and Chief, Gastrointestinal Imaging, Section of Abdominal Imaging, University of Wisconsin School of Medicine and Public Health, Madison, Wisconsin
Diagnostic Imaging Procedures in Gastroenterology

David S. Pisetsky, MD, PhD
Chief of Rheumatology, Medical Research Service, Durham VA Medical Center; Professor of Medicine and Immunology, Department of Medicine, Duke University Medical Center, Durham, North Carolina
Laboratory Testing in the Rheumatic Diseases

Marshall R. Posner, MD
Professor of Medicine, Director of Head and Neck Medical Oncology, Director of the Office of Cancer Clinical Trials, The Tisch Cancer Institute, Icahn School of Medicine at Mount Sinai, New York, New York
Head and Neck Cancer

Frank Powell, PhD
Professor of Medicine, Chief of Physiology, University of California San Diego, La Jolla, California
Disorders of Ventilatory Control

Reed E. Pyeritz, MD, PhD
William Smilow Professor of Medicine and Genetics and Vice Chair for Academic Affairs, Perelman School of Medicine at the University of Pennsylvania, Philadelphia, Pennsylvania
Inherited Diseases of Connective Tissue

Thomas C. Quinn, MD, MSc
Associate Director for International Research, Head, Section of International HIV/AIDS Research, Division of Intramural Research, National Institute of Allergy and Infectious Diseases, National Institutes of Health; Professor of Medicine, Pathology, International Health, Molecular Microbiology and Immunology, and Epidemiology, The Johns Hopkins Medical Institutions, Baltimore, Maryland
Epidemiology and Diagnosis of Human Immunodeficiency Virus Infection and Acquired Immunodeficiency Syndrome

Jai Radhakrishnan, MD, MS
Professor of Medicine, Division of Nephrology, Department of Medicine, Columbia University Medical Center; Associate Division Chief for Clinical Affairs, Division of Nephrology, New York-Presbyterian Hospital, New York, New York
Glomerular Disorders and Nephrotic Syndromes

Petros I. Rafailidis, MD, PhD, MSc
Senior Researcher, Alfa Institute of Biomedical Sciences, Attending Physician, Department of Medicine and Hematology, Athens Medical Center, Athens Medical Group, Athens, Greece
Pseudomonas and Related Gram-Negative Bacillary Infections

Ganesh Raghu, MD
Adjunct Professor of Medicine and Laboratory Medicine, University of Washington, Director, CENTER for Interstitial Lung Diseases at the University of Washington; Co-Director, Scleroderma Clinic, University of Washington Medical Center, Seattle, Washington
Interstitial Lung Disease

Margaret Ragni, MD, MPH
Professor of Medicine and Clinical Translational Science, Department of Hematology/Oncology, University of Pittsburgh Medical Center; Director, Hemophilia Center of Western Pennsylvania, Pittsburgh, Pennsylvania
Hemorrhagic Disorders: Coagulation Factor Deficiencies

Srinivasa N. Raja, MD
Professor of Anesthesiology and Neurology, Director, Division of Pain Medicine, The Johns Hopkins University School of Medicine, Baltimore, Maryland
Pain

S. Vincent Rajkumar, MD
Professor of Medicine, Division of Hematology, Mayo Clinic, Rochester, Minnesota
Plasma Cell Disorders

Stuart H. Ralston, MB ChB, MD
Professor of Rheumatology, Institute of Genetics and Molecular Medicine, Western General Hospital, The University of Edinburgh, Edinburgh, United Kingdom
Paget Disease of Bone

Didier Raoult, MD, PhD
Professor, Aix Marseille Université, Faculté de Médecine; Chief, Hôpital de la Timone, Fédération de Microbiologie Clinique, Marseille, France
Bartonella Infections; Rickettsial Infections

Robert W. Rebar, MD
Professor, Department of Obstetrics and Gynecology, Western Michigan University Homer Stryker MD School of Medicine, Kalamazoo, Michigan
Ovaries and Development; Reproductive Endocrinology and Infertility

Annette C. Reboli, MD
Founding Vice Dean, Professor of Medicine, Cooper Medical School of Rowan University, Cooper University Healthcare, Department of Medicine, Division of Infectious Diseases, Camden, New Jersey
Erysipelothrix Infections

K. Rajender Reddy, MD
Professor of Medicine, Professor of Medicine in Surgery, Perelman School of Medicine at the University of Pennsylvania; Director of Hepatology, Director, Viral Hepatitis Center, Hospital of the University of Pennsylvania, Philadelphia, Pennsylvania
Bacterial, Parasitic, Fungal, and Granulomatous Liver Diseases

Donald A. Redelmeier, MD
Professor of Medicine, University of Toronto; Senior Scientist and Staff Physician, Sunnybrook Health Sciences Centre, Toronto, Ontario, Canada
Postoperative Care and Complications

Susan E. Reef, MD
Centers for Disease Control and Prevention, Atlanta, Georgia
Rubella (German Measles)

Neil M. Resnick, MD
Thomas P. Detre Endowed Chair in Gerontology and Geriatric Medicine, Professor of Medicine and Division Chief, Geriatrics, Associate Director, University of Pittsburgh Institute on Aging, University of Pittsburgh; Chief, Division of Geriatric Medicine and Gerontology, University of Pittsburgh Medical Center, Pittsburgh, Pennsylvania
Incontinence

David B. Reuben, MD
Director, Multicampus Program in Geriatric Medicine and Gerontology; Chief, Division of Geriatrics, Archstone Professor of Medicine, David Geffen School of Medicine at University of California Los Angeles, Los Angeles, California
Geriatric Assessment

Emanuel P. Rivers, MD, MPH
Professor and Vice Chairman of Emergency Medicine, Wayne State University; Senior Staff Attending, Critical Care and Emergency Medicine, Henry Ford Hospital, Detroit, Michigan
Approach to the Patient with Shock

Joseph G. Rogers, MD
Professor of Medicine, Senior Vice Chief for Clinical Affairs, Division of Cardiology, Durham, North Carolina
Heart Failure: Pathophysiology and Diagnosis

Jean-Marc Rolain, PharmD, PhD
Professor, Institut Hospitalo-Universitaire Méditerranée-Infection, Aix-Marseille Université, Marseille, France
Bartonella Infections

José R. Romero, MD
Professor of Pediatrics, University of Arkansas for Medical Sciences, Horace C. Cabe Professor of Infectious Diseases; Director, Section of Pediatric Infectious Diseases, Arkansas Children's Hospital, Little Rock, Arkansas
Enteroviruses

Karen Rosene-Montella, MD
Professor and Vice Chair of Medicine, Director of Obstetric Medicine, The Warren Alpert Medical School of Brown University; Senior Vice President, Women's Services and Clinical Integration, Lifespan Health System, Providence, Rhode Island
Common Medical Problems in Pregnancy

Philip J. Rosenthal, MD
Professor, Department of Medicine, University of California San Francisco, San Francisco, California
Malaria

Marc E. Rothenberg, MD, PhD
Director, Division of Allergy and Immunology, Director, Cincinnati Center for Eosinophilic Disorders; Professor of Pediatrics, Cincinnati Children's Hospital Medical Center, University of Cincinnati College of Medicine, Cincinnati, Ohio
Eosinophilic Syndromes

James A. Russell, MD
Professor of Medicine, University of British Columbia; Associate Director, Intensive Care Unit, St. Paul's Hospital, Vancouver, British Columbia, Canada
Shock Syndromes Related to Sepsis

Anil K. Rustgi, MD
T. Grier Miller Professor of Medicine and Genetics, Chief of Gastroenterology, American Cancer Society; Professor, Perelman School of Medicine at the University of Pennsylvania, Philadelphia, Pennsylvania
Neoplasms of the Esophagus and Stomach

Daniel E. Rusyniak, MD
Professor of Emergency Medicine, Adjunct Professor of Neurology and Pharmacology and Toxicology, Department of Emergency Medicine, Indiana University School of Medicine, Indianapolis, Indiana
Chronic Poisoning: Trace Metals and Others

Robert A. Salata, MD
Professor and Executive Vice Chair, Department of Medicine, Chief, Division of Infectious Diseases and HIV Medicine, Case Western Reserve University, University Hospitals Case Medical Center, Cleveland, Ohio
Brucellosis

Jane E. Salmon, MD
Collette Kean Research Chair, Hospital for Special Surgery, Professor of Medicine, Weill Cornell Medical College, New York, New York
Mechanisms of Immune-Mediated Tissue Injury

Edsel Maurice T. Salvana, MD, DTM&H
Associate Professor of Medicine, Section of Infectious Diseases, Department of Medicine, Philippine General Hospital; Director, Institute of Molecular Biology and Biotechnology, National Institutes of Health, University of the Philippines Manila, Manila, Philippines
Brucellosis

Renato M. Santos, MD
Associate Professor, Cardiology, Wake Forest School of Medicine, Winston-Salem, North Carolina
Vascular Disorders of the Kidney

Michael N. Sawka, PhD
Professor, School of Applied Physiology, Georgia Institute of Technology, Atlanta, Georgia
Disorders Due to Heat and Cold

Paul D. Scanlon, MD
Professor of Medicine, Division of Pulmonary and Critical Care Medicine, Mayo Clinic, Rochester, Minnesota
Respiratory Function: Mechanisms and Testing

Carla Scanzello, MD, PhD
Assistant Professor of Medicine, Division of Rheumatology, Perelman School of Medicine at the University of Pennsylvania and Translational Musculoskeletal Research Center, Philadelphia Veterans Affairs Medical Center, Philadelphia, Pennsylvania
Osteoarthritis

Andrew I. Schafer, MD
Professor of Medicine, Director, Richard T. Silver Center for Myeloproliferative Neoplasms, Weill Cornell Medical College, New York, New York
Approach to Medicine, the Patient, and the Medical Profession: Medicine as a Learned and Humane Profession; Approach to the Patient with Bleeding and Thrombosis; Hemorrhagic Disorders: Disseminated Intravascular Coagulation, Liver Failure, and Vitamin K Deficiency; Thrombotic Disorders: Hypercoagulable States

William Schaffner, MD
Professor and Chair, Department of Preventive Medicine, Department of Health Policy; Professor of Medicine (Infectious Diseases), Vanderbilt University School of Medicine, Nashville, Tennessee
Tularemia and Other Francisella Infections

W. Michael Scheld, MD
Bayer-Gerald L. Mandell Professor of Infectious Diseases, Professor of Medicine, Clinical Professor of Neurosurgery, Director, Pfizer Initiative in International Health, University of Virginia Health System, Charlottesville, Virginia
Introduction to Microbial Disease: Host-Pathogen Interactions

Manuel Schiff, MD
Professor, Université Paris 7 Denis Diderot, Sorbonne Paris Cité, Head of Metabolic Unit/Reference Center for Inborn Errors of Metabolism, Robert Debré University Hospital, APHP, Paris, France
Homocystinuria and Hyperhomocysteinemia

Michael L. Schilsky, MD
Associate Professor, Medicine and Surgery, Yale University School of Medicine, New Haven, Connecticut
Wilson Disease

Robert T. Schooley, MD
Professor and Head, Division of Infectious Diseases, Executive Vice Chair for Academic Affairs, Department of Medicine, University of California San Diego, La Jolla, California
Epstein-Barr Virus Infection

David L. Schriger, MD, MPH
Professor, Department of Emergency Medicine, University of California Los Angeles, Los Angeles, California
Approach to the Patient with Abnormal Vital Signs

Steven A. Schroeder, MD
Distinguished Professor of Health and Healthcare and of Medicine, University of California San Francisco, San Francisco, California
Socioeconomic Issues in Medicine

Lynn M. Schuchter, MD
Professor of Medicine, University of Pennsylvania; Chief, Hematology/Oncology Division, Program Leader, Melanoma and Cutaneous Malignancies Program, Abramson Cancer Center, Hospital of the University of Pennsylvania, Philadelphia, Pennsylvania
Melanoma and Nonmelanoma Skin Cancers

Sam Schulman, MD, PhD
Professor, Division of Hematology and Thromboembolism, Director of Clinical Thromboembolism Program, Department of Medicine, McMaster University, Hamilton, Ontario, Canada
Antithrombotic Therapy

Lawrence B. Schwartz, MD, PhD
Charles and Evelyn Thomas Professor of Medicine, Internal Medicine, Virginia Commonwealth University, Richmond, Virginia
Systemic Anaphylaxis, Food Allergy, and Insect Sting Allergy

Carlos Seas, MD
Associate Professor of Medicine, Vice Director, Alexander von Humboldt Tropical Medicine Institute, Universidad Peruana Cayetano Heredia; Attending Physician, Department of Infectious, Tropical, and Dermatologic Diseases, National Hospital Cayetano Heredia, Lima, Peru
Cholera and Other Vibrio Infections

Steven A. Seifert, MD
Professor of Emergency Medicine, University of New Mexico School of Medicine, Medical Director, New Mexico Poison and Drug Information Center, University of New Mexico Health Sciences Center, Albuquerque, New Mexico
Envenomation

Julian L. Seifter, MD
Associate Professor of Medicine, Harvard Medical School; Senior Physician, Brigham and Women's Hospital, Boston, Massachusetts
Potassium Disorders; Acid-Base Disorders

Duygu Selcen, MD
Associate Professor of Neurology and Pediatrics, Department of Neurology, Mayo Clinic, Rochester, Minnesota
Muscle Diseases

Clay F. Semenkovich, MD
Herbert S. Gasser Professor and Chief, Division of Endocrinology, Metabolism and Lipid Research, Washington University School of Medicine, St. Louis, Missouri
Disorders of Lipid Metabolism

Carol E. Semrad, MD
Professor of Medicine, The University of Chicago Medicine, GI Section, Chicago, Illinois
Approach to the Patient with Diarrhea and Malabsorption

Harry Shamoon, MD
Professor of Medicine and Associate Dean for Clinical and Translational Research, Albert Einstein College of Medicine; Director, Harold and Muriel Block Institute for Clinical and Translational Research at Einstein and Montefiore, Bronx, New York
Diabetes Mellitus

James C. Shaw, MD
Associate Professor, Department of Medicine, University of Toronto; Head, Division of Dermatology, Department of Medicine, Women's College Hospital, Toronto, Ontario, Canada
Examination of the Skin and an Approach to Diagnosing Skin Diseases

Pamela J. Shaw, DBE, MBBS, MD
Professor of Neurology, University of Sheffield, Consultant Neurologist, Royal Hallamshire Hospital, Sheffield, United Kingdom
Amyotrophic Lateral Sclerosis and Other Motor Neuron Diseases

Robert L. Sheridan, MD
Associate Professor of Surgery, Burn Service Medical Director, Boston Shriners Hospital for Children, Massachusetts General Hospital, Division of Burns, Harvard Medical School, Boston, Massachusetts
Medical Aspects of Injuries and Burns

Stuart Sherman, MD
Professor of Medicine and Radiology, Director of ERCP, Indiana University School of Medicine, Indianapolis, Indiana
Diseases of the Gallbladder and Bile Ducts

Michael E. Shy, MD
Professor of Neurology, Pediatrics, and Physiology, University of Iowa, Iowa City, Iowa
Peripheral Neuropathies

Ellen Sidransky, MD
Chief, Section on Molecular Neurogenetics, Medical Genetics Branch, National Human Genome Research Institute, National Institutes of Health, Bethesda, Maryland
The Lysosomal Storage Diseases

Richard M. Siegel, MD, PhD
Clinical Director, National Institute of Arthritis, Musculoskeletal, and Skin Diseases, National Institutes of Health, Bethesda, Maryland
The Systemic Autoinflammatory Diseases

Robert F. Siliciano, MD, PhD
Professor, The Johns Hopkins University School of Medicine, Howard Hughes Medical Institute, Baltimore, Maryland
Immunopathogenesis of Human Immunodeficiency Virus Infection

Michael S. Simberkoff, MD
Chief of Staff, VA New York Harbor Healthcare System; Professor of Medicine, NYU School of Medicine, New York, New York
Haemophilus and Moraxella Infections

David L. Simel, MD, MHS
Professor of Medicine, Duke University; Chief, Medical Service, Durham Veterans Affairs Medical Center, Durham, North Carolina
Approach to the Patient: History and Physical Examination

Kamaljit Singh, MD
Associate Professor of Medicine, Attending Physician, Infectious Diseases, Rush University Medical Center, Chicago, Illinois
Zoonoses

Karl Skorecki, MD
Annie Chutick Professor in Medicine, Rappaport Faculty of Medicine and Research Institute, Technion–Israel Institute of Technology; Director, Medical and Research Development, Rambam Health Care Campus, Haifa, Israel
Gene and Cell Therapy; Disorders of Sodium and Water Homeostasis

Itzchak Slotki, MD
Associate Professor of Medicine, Hebrew University, Hadassah Medical School; Director, Division of Adult Nephrology, Shaare Zedek Medical Center, Jerusalem, Israel
Disorders of Sodium and Water Homeostasis

Arthur S. Slutsky, MD
Professor of Medicine, Surgery, and Biomedical Engineering, University of Toronto; Vice President (Research), St. Michael's Hospital, Keenan Research Centre, Li Ka Shing Knowledge Institute, Toronto, Ontario, Canada
Acute Respiratory Failure; Mechanical Ventilation

Eric J. Small, MD
Professor of Medicine and Urology, Deputy Director and Director of Clinical Sciences, Helen Diller Family Comprehensive Cancer Center; Chief, Division of Hematology and Oncology, University of California San Francisco School of Medicine, San Francisco, California
Prostate Cancer

Gerald W. Smetana, MD
Professor of Medicine, Harvard Medical School; Division of General Medicine and Primary Care, Beth Israel Deaconess Medical Center, Boston, Massachusetts
Principles of Medical Consultation

Frederick S. Southwick, MD
Professor of Medicine, Division of Infectious Diseases, University of Florida and VF Health, Gainesville, Florida
Nocardiosis

Allen M. Spiegel, MD
Dean, Albert Einstein College of Medicine, Bronx, New York
Principles of Endocrinology; Polyglandular Disorders

Robert F. Spiera, MD
Professor of Clinical Medicine, Weill Cornell Medical College; Director, Scleroderma, Vasculitis, and Myositis Center, The Hospital for Special Surgery, New York, New York
Polymyalgia Rheumatica and Temporal Arteritis

Stanley M. Spinola, MD
Professor and Chair, Department of Microbiology and Immunology, Professor of Medicine, Microbiology and Immunology, and Pathology and Laboratory Medicine, Indiana University School of Medicine, Indianapolis, Indiana
Chancroid

David Spriggs, MD
Head, Division of Solid Tumor Oncology, Department of Medicine, Memorial Sloan Kettering Cancer Center; Professor of Medicine, Department of Medicine, Weill Cornell Medical College, New York, New York
Gynecologic Cancers

Paweł Stankiewicz, MD, PhD
Department of Molecular and Human Genetics, Baylor College of Medicine, Houston, Texas
Gene, Genomic, and Chromosomal Disorders

Paul Stark, MD
Professor Emeritus, University of California San Diego; Chief of Cardiothoracic Radiology, VA San Diego Healthcare System, San Diego, California
Imaging in Pulmonary Disease

David P. Steensma, MD
Professor of Medicine, Harvard Medical School, Adult Leukemia Program, Dana-Farber Cancer Institute, Boston, Massachusetts
Myelodysplastic Syndrome

Martin H. Steinberg, MD
Professor of Medicine, Pediatrics, and Pathology and Laboratory Medicine, Boston University School of Medicine; Director, Center of Excellence in Sickle Cell Disease, Boston Medical Center, Boston, Massachusetts
Sickle Cell Disease and Other Hemoglobinopathies

Theodore S. Steiner, MD
Associate Professor, University of British Columbia; Associate Head, Division of Infectious Diseases, Vancouver General Hospital, Vancouver, British Columbia, Canada
Escherichia Coli *Enteric Infections*

David S. Stephens, MD
Stephen W. Schwarzmann Distinguished Professor of Medicine, Emory University School of Medicine and Woodruff Health Sciences Center, Atlanta, Georgia
Neisseria Meningitidis *Infections*

David A. Stevens, MD
Professor of Medicine, Stanford University Medical School; President, Principal Investigator, Infectious Diseases Research Laboratory, California Institute for Medical Research, San Jose and Stanford, California
Systemic Antifungal Agents

James K. Stoller, MD, MS
Chairman, Education Institute, Jean Wall Bennett Professor of Medicine, Cleveland Clinic Lerner College of Medicine; Staff, Respiratory Institute, Cleveland Clinic, Cleveland, Ohio
Respiratory Monitoring in Critical Care

John H. Stone, MD, MPH
Professor of Medicine, Director, Clinical Rheumatology, Harvard Medical School, Massachusetts General Hospital, Boston, Massachusetts
The Systemic Vasculitides

Richard M. Stone, MD
Professor of Medicine, Harvard Medical School, Clinical Director, Adult Leukemia Program, Dana-Farber Cancer Institute, Boston, Massachusetts
Myelodysplastic Syndrome

Raymond A. Strikas, MD, MPH
Education Team Lead, Immunization Services Division, National Center for Immunization and Respiratory Diseases, Centers for Disease Control and Prevention, Atlanta, Georgia
Immunization

Edwin P. Su, MD
Associate Professor of Clinical Orthopaedics, Orthopaedic Surgery, Weill Cornell University Medical College; Associate Attending Orthopaedic Surgeon, Adult Reconstruction and Joint Replacement, Hospital for Special Surgery, New York, New York
Surgical Treatment of Joint Disease

Roland W. Sutter, MD, MPH&TM
Coordinator, Research, Policy and Product Development, Polio Operations and Research Department, World Health Organization, Geneva, Switzerland
Diphtheria and Other Corynebacteria Infections

Ronald S. Swerdloff, MD
Professor of Medicine, David Geffen School of Medicine at University of California Los Angeles; Chief, Division of Endocrinology, Department of Medicine, Harbor-UCLA Medical Center, Torrance, California
The Testis and Male Hypogonadism, Infertility, and Sexual Dysfunction

Heidi Swygard, MD, MPH
Associate Professor of Medicine, University of North Carolina at Chapel Hill, Chapel Hill, North Carolina
Approach to the Patient with a Sexually Transmitted Infection

Megan Sykes, MD
Michael J. Friedlander Professor of Medicine, Director, Columbia Center for Translational Immunology, Columbia University Medical Center, New York, New York
Transplantation Immunology

Marian Tanofsky-Kraff, PhD
Associate Professor, Department of Medical and Clinical Psychology, Uniformed Services University of Health Sciences, Bethesda, Maryland
Eating Disorders

Susan M. Tarlo, MBBS
Professor of Medicine, Department of Medicine and Dalla Lana School of Public Health, University of Toronto, Respiratory Physician, University Health Network, Toronto Western Hospital and St. Michael's Hospital, Toronto, Ontario, Canada
Occupational Lung Disease

Victoria M. Taylor, MD, MPH
Professor of Medicine, University of Washington, Fred Hutchinson Cancer Research Center, Seattle, Washington
Cultural Context of Medicine

Ayalew Tefferi, MD
Professor of Medicine, Department of Hematology, Mayo Clinic, Rochester, Minnesota
Polycythemia Vera, Essential Thrombocythemia, and Primary Myelofibrosis

Paul S. Teirstein, MD
Chief of Cardiology, Department of Medicine, Scripps Clinic, La Jolla, California
Interventional and Surgical Treatment of Coronary Artery Disease

Sam R. Telford III, ScD
Professor, Tufts University Cummings School of Veterinary Medicine, North Grafton, Massachusetts
Babesiosis and Other Protozoan Diseases

Rajesh V. Thakker, MD
May Professor of Medicine, University of Oxford; Radcliffe Department of Clinical Medicine, OCDEM, Churchill Hospital, Headington, Oxford, United Kingdom
The Parathyroid Glands, Hypercalcemia, and Hypocalcemia

Antonella Tosti, MD
Professor of Clinical Dermatology, Department of Dermatology and Cutaneous Surgery, University of Miami, Miami, Florida
Diseases of Hair and Nails

Indi Trehan, MD, MPH, DTM&H
Assistant Professor of Pediatrics, Washington University School of Medicine; Attending Physician, St. Louis Children's Hospital, Barnes-Jewish Hospital, St. Louis, Missouri; Visiting Honorary Lecturer in Paediatrics and Child Health, University of Malawi College of Medicine; Consultant Paediatrician, Queen Elizabeth Central Hospital, Blantyre, Malawi
Protein-Energy Malnutrition

Ronald B. Turner, MD
Professor of Pediatrics, University of Virginia School of Medicine, Charlottesville, Virginia
The Common Cold

Thomas S. Uldrick, MD
Staff Clinician, HIV and AIDS Malignancy Branch, National Cancer Institute, Bethesda, Maryland
Hematology and Oncology in Patients with Human Immunodeficiency Virus Infection

Anthony M. Valeri, MD
Professor of Medicine, Columbia University Medical Center; Director, Hemodialysis, Medical Director, Kidney and Pancreas Transplantation, New York-Presbyterian Hospital (CUMC); Director, Hemodialysis, Columbia University Dialysis Center, New York, New York
Treatment of Irreversible Renal Failure

John Varga, MD
John and Nancy Hughes Professor of Medicine, Northwestern University Feinberg School of Medicine, Chicago, Illinois
Systemic Sclerosis (Scleroderma)

Bradley V. Vaughn, MD
Professor of Neurology, Department of Neurology, University of North Carolina, Chapel Hill, North Carolina
Disorders of Sleep

Alan P. Venook, MD
Professor of Medicine, University of California San Francisco, Helen Diller Family Comprehensive Cancer Center, San Francisco, California
Liver and Biliary Tract Cancers

Joseph G. Verbalis, MD
Professor of Medicine, Georgetown University; Chief, Endocrinology and Metabolism, Georgetown University Hospital, Washington, D.C.
Posterior Pituitary

Ronald G. Victor, MD
Professor of Medicine, Burns and Allen Chair in Cardiology Research, Director, Hypertension Center, Associate Director, The Heart Institute, Cedars-Sinai Medical Center, Los Angeles, California
Arterial Hypertension

Angela Vincent, MBBS
Professor of Neuroimmunology, University of Oxford; Honorary Consultant in Immunology, Oxford University Hospital Trust, Oxford, United Kingdom
Disorders of Neuromuscular Transmission

Robert M. Wachter, MD
Professor and Associate Chairman, Department of Medicine, University of California San Francisco, San Francisco, California
Quality of Care and Patient Safety

Edward H. Wagner, MD, MPH
Director Emeritus, MacColl Center for Health Care Innovation, Group Health Research Institute, Seattle, Washington
Comprehensive Chronic Disease Management

Edward E. Walsh, MD
Professor of Medicine, University of Rochester School of Medicine and Dentistry; Head, Infectious Diseases, Rochester General Hospital, Rochester, New York
Respiratory Syncytial Virus

Thomas J. Walsh, MD
Director, Transplantation-Oncology Infectious Diseases Program, Chief, Infectious Diseases Translational Research Laboratory, Professor of Medicine, Pediatrics, and Microbiology and Immunology, Weill Cornell Medical Center; Henry Schueler Foundation Scholar, Sharp Family Foundation Scholar in Pediatric Infectious Diseases, Adjunct Professor of Pathology, The Johns Hopkins University School of Medicine; Adjunct Professor of Medicine, The University of Maryland School of Medicine, Baltimore, Maryland
Aspergillosis

Jeremy D. Walston, MD
Raymond and Anna Lublin Professor of Geriatric Medicine and Gerontology, The Johns Hopkins University School of Medicine, Baltimore, Maryland
Common Clinical Sequelae of Aging

Christina Wang, MD
Professor of Medicine, David Geffen School of Medicine at University of California Los Angeles; Associate Director, UCLA Clinical and Translational Research Institute, Harbor-UCLA Medical Center, Torrance, California
The Testis and Male Hypogonadism, Infertility, and Sexual Dysfunction

Christine Wanke, MD
Professor of Medicine and Public Health, Director, Division of Nutrition and Infection, Associate Chair, Department of Public Health, Tufts University School of Medicine, Boston, Massachusetts
Gastrointestinal Manifestions of HIV and AIDS

Stephen I. Wasserman, MD
Professor of Medicine, University of California San Diego, La Jolla, California
Approach to the Patient with Allergic or Immunologic Disease

Thomas J. Weber, MD
Associate Professor, Medicine/Endocrinology, Duke University, Durham, North Carolina
Approach to the Patient with Metabolic Bone Disease; Osteoporosis

Heiner Wedemeyer, MD
Professor, Department of Gastroenterology, Hepatology, and Endocrinology, Hannover Medical School, Hannover, Germany
Acute Viral Hepatitis

Geoffrey A. Weinberg, MD
Professor of Pediatrics, University of Rochester School of Medicine and Dentistry; Director, Pediatric HIV Program, Golisano Children's Hospital at University of Rochester Medical Center, Rochester, New York
Parainfluenza Viral Disease

David A. Weinstein, MD, MMSc
Professor of Pediatric Endocrinology, Director, Glycogen Storage Disease Program, Division of Pediatric Endocrinology, University of Florida College of Medicine, Gainesville, Florida
Glycogen Storage Diseases

Robert S. Weinstein, MD
Professor of Medicine, Department of Medicine, University of Arkansas for Medical Sciences; Staff Endocrinologist, Department of Medicine, Central Arkansas Veterans Health Care System, Little Rock, Arkansas
Osteomalacia and Rickets

Roger D. Weiss, MD
Professor of Psychiatry, Harvard Medical School, Boston, Massachusetts; Chief, Division of Alcohol and Drug Abuse, McLean Hospital, Belmont, Massachusetts
Drug Abuse and Dependence

Martin Weisse, MD
Chair, Pediatrics, Tripler Army Medical Center, Honolulu, Hawaii; Professor, Pediatrics, Uniformed Services University of the Health Sciences, Bethesda, Maryland
Measles

Jeffrey I. Weitz, MD
Professor of Medicine and Biochemistry, McMaster University; Executive Director, Thrombosis and Atherosclerosis Research Institute, Hamilton, Ontario, Canada
Pulmonary Embolism

Samuel A. Wells, Jr., MD
Medical Oncology Branch, National Cancer Institute, National Institutes of Health, Bethesda, Maryland
Medullary Thyroid Carcinoma

Richard P. Wenzel, MD, MSc
Professor and Former Chairman, Internal Medicine, Virginia Commonwealth University, Richmond, Virginia
Acute Bronchitis and Tracheitis

Victoria P. Werth, MD
Professor of Dermatology and Medicine, Hospital of the University of Pennsylvania and Philadelphia Veterans Administration Medical Center; Chief, Dermatology Division, Philadelphia Veterans Administration Medical Center, Philadelphia, Pennsylvania
Principles of Therapy of Skin Diseases

Sterling G. West, MD, MACP
Professor of Medicine, University of Colorado School of Medicine; Associate Division Head for Clinical and Educational Affairs, University of Colorado Division of Rheumatology, Aurora, Colorado
Systemic Diseases in Which Arthritis Is a Feature

A. Clinton White, Jr., MD
Paul R. Stalnaker Distinguished Professor and Director, Infectious Disease Division, Department of Internal Medicine, University of Texas Medical Branch, Galveston, Texas
Cestodes

Christopher J. White, MD
Professor of Medicine, Ochsner Clinical School, University of Queensland School of Medicine; System Chairman of Cardiovascular Diseases, Ochsner Medical Center, New Orleans, Louisiana
Atherosclerotic Peripheral Arterial Disease; Electrophysiologic Interventional Procedures and Surgery

Perrin C. White, MD
Professor of Pediatrics, The Audry Newman Rapoport Distinguished Chair in Pediatric Endocrinology, University of Texas Southwestern Medical Center, Chief of Endocrinology, Children's Medical Center Dallas, Dallas, Texas
Disorders of Sexual Development

Richard J. Whitley, MD
Distinguished Professor of Pediatrics, Loeb Eminent Scholar Chair in Pediatrics, Professor of Pediatrics, Microbiology, Medicine, and Neurosurgery, The University of Alabama at Birmingham, Birmingham, Alabama
Herpes Simplex Virus Infections

Michael P. Whyte, MD
Professor of Medicine, Pediatrics, and Genetics, Division of Bone and Mineral Diseases, Washington University School of Medicine; Medical-Scientific Director, Center for Metabolic Bone Disease and Molecular Research, Shriners Hospital for Children, St. Louis, Missouri
Osteonecrosis, Osteosclerosis/Hyperostosis, and Other Disorders of Bone

Samuel Wiebe, MD, MSc
Professor of Clinical Neurosciences, University of Calgary; Co-Director, Calgary Epilepsy Program, Alberta Health Services, Foothills Medical Centre, Calgary, Alberta, Canada
The Epilepsies

Jeanine P. Wiener-Kronish, MD
Henry Isaiah Dorr Professor of Research and Teaching in Anaesthesia and Anesthestist-in-Chief, Department of Anesthesia, Critical Care and Pain Medicine, Massachusetts General Hospital/Harvard Medical School, Boston, Massachusetts
Overview of Anesthesia

Eelco F.M. Wijdicks, MD, PhD
Professor of Neurology, Division of Critical Care Neurology, Department of Neurology, Mayo Clinic, Rochester, Minnesota
Coma, Vegetative State, and Brain Death

David J. Wilber, MD
George M. Eisenberg Professor of Medicine, Loyola Stritch School of Medicine; Director, Division of Cardiology, Director, Clinical Electrophysiology, Loyola University Medical Center, Maywood, Illinois
Electrophysiologic Interventional Procedures and Surgery

Beverly Winikoff, MD, MPH
President, Gynuity Health Projects; Professor of Clinical Population and Family Health, Mailman School of Public Health, Columbia University, New York, New York
Contraception

Gary P. Wormser, MD
Professor of Medicine and Chief, Division of Infectious Diseases, Department of Medicine, New York Medical College, Valhalla, New York
Lyme Disease

Myron Yanoff, MD
Professor and Chair, Ophthalmology, Drexel University College of Medicine, Philadelphia, Pennsylvania
Diseases of the Visual System

Robert Yarchoan, MD
Branch Chief, HIV and AIDS Malignancy Branch, National Cancer Institute, Bethesda, Maryland
Hematology and Oncology in Patients with Human Immunodeficiency Virus Infection

Neal S. Young, MD
Chief, Hematology Branch, NHLBI and Director, Trans-NIH Center for Human Immunology, Autoimmunity, and Inflammation, National Institutes of Health, Bethesda, Maryland
Parvovirus

William F. Young, Jr., MD, MSc
Professor of Medicine, Mayo Clinic College of Medicine; Chair, Division of Endocrinology, Diabetes, Metabolism, and Nutrition, Mayo Clinic, Rochester, Minnesota
Adrenal Medulla, Catecholamines, and Pheochromocytoma

Alan S.L. Yu, MB, BChir
Harry Statland and Solon Summerfield Professor of Medicine, Director, Division of Nephrology and Hypertension and the Kidney Institute, University of Kansas Medical Center, Kansas City, Kansas
Disorders of Magnesium and Phosphorus

Sherif R. Zaki, MD, PhD
Chief, Infectious Diseases Pathology Branch, Centers for Disease Control and Prevention, Atlanta, Georgia
Leptospirosis

Mark L. Zeidel, MD
Herman L. Blumgart Professor of Medicine, Harvard Medical School; Physician-in-Chief and Chairman, Department of Medicine, Beth Israel Deaconess Medical Center, Boston, Massachusetts
Obstructive Uropathy

Thomas R. Ziegler, MD
Professor, Department of Medicine, Division of Endocrinology, Metabolism, and Lipids, Emory University School of Medicine, Atlanta, Georgia
Malnutrition, Nutritional Assessment, and Nutritional Support in Adult Hospitalized Patients

Peter Zimetbaum, MD
Associate Professor of Medicine, Harvard Medical School; Director of Clinical Cardiology, Beth Israel Deaconess Medical Center, Boston, Massachusetts
Cardiac Arrhythmias with Supraventricular Origin

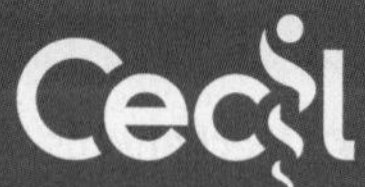

CONTENTS

VOLUME I

SECTION XI: RENAL AND GENITOURINARY DISEASES

SECTION XII: GASTROINTESTINAL DISEASES

SECTION XIII: DISEASES OF THE LIVER, GALLBLADDER, AND BILE DUCTS

SECTION XIV: HEMATOLOGIC DISEASES

SECTION XV: ONCOLOGY

VOLUME II

SECTION XVI: METABOLIC DISEASES

SECTION XVII: NUTRITIONAL DISEASES

SECTION XXIII: INFECTIOUS DISEASES

SECTION XXIV: HIV AND THE ACQUIRED IMMUNODEFICIENCY SYNDROME

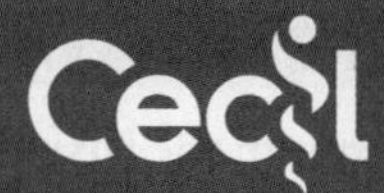

VIDEO CONTENTS

This icon appears throughout the book to indicate chapters with accompanying video available on ExpertConsult.com. For quick viewing, use your smartphone to scan the QR codes in the front of the book.

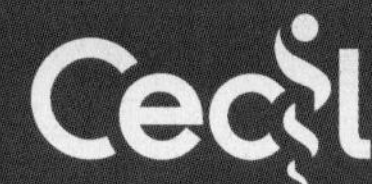

I SOCIAL AND ETHICAL ISSUES IN MEDICINE

1

APPROACH TO MEDICINE, THE PATIENT, AND THE MEDICAL PROFESSION: MEDICINE AS A LEARNED AND HUMANE PROFESSION

LEE GOLDMAN AND ANDREW I. SCHAFER

APPROACH TO MEDICINE

Medicine is a profession that incorporates science and the scientific method with the art of being a physician. The art of tending to the sick is as old as humanity itself. Even in modern times, the art of caring and comforting, guided by millennia of common sense as well as a more recent, systematic approach to medical ethics (Chapter 2), remains the cornerstone of medicine. Without these humanistic qualities, the application of the modern science of medicine is suboptimal, ineffective, or even detrimental.

The caregivers of ancient times and premodern cultures tried a variety of interventions to help the afflicted. Some of their potions contained what are now known to be active ingredients that form the basis for proven medications (Chapter 29). Others (Chapter 39) have persisted into the present era despite a lack of convincing evidence. Modern medicine should not dismiss the possibility that these unproven approaches may be helpful; instead, it should adopt a guiding principle that all interventions, whether traditional or newly developed, can be tested vigorously, with the expectation that any beneficial effects can be explored further to determine their scientific basis.

When compared with its long and generally distinguished history of caring and comforting, the scientific basis of medicine is remarkably recent. Other than an understanding of human anatomy and the later description, albeit widely contested at this time, of the normal physiology of the circulatory system, almost all of modern medicine is based on discoveries made within the past 150 years. Until the late 19th century, the paucity of medical knowledge was perhaps exemplified best by hospitals and hospital care. Although hospitals provided caring that all but well-to-do people might not be able to obtain elsewhere, there is little if any evidence that hospitals improved health outcomes. The term *hospitalism* referred not to expertise in hospital care but rather to the aggregate of iatrogenic afflictions that were induced by the hospital stay itself.

The essential humanistic qualities of caring and comforting can achieve full benefit only if they are coupled with an understanding of how medical science can and should be applied to patients with known or suspected diseases. Without this knowledge, comforting may be inappropriate or misleading, and caring may be ineffective or counterproductive if it inhibits a sick person from obtaining appropriate, scientific medical care. *Goldman-Cecil Medicine* focuses on the discipline of *internal medicine,* from which neurology and dermatology, which are also covered in substantial detail in this text, are relatively recent evolutionary branches. The term *internal medicine,* which is often misunderstood by the lay public, was developed in 19th-century Germany. *Inneren medizin* was to be distinguished from clinical medicine because it emphasized the physiology and chemistry of disease, not just the patterns or progression of clinical manifestations. *Goldman-Cecil Medicine* follows this tradition by showing how pathophysiologic abnormalities cause symptoms and signs and by emphasizing how therapies can modify the underlying pathophysiology and improve the patient's well-being.

Modern medicine has moved rapidly past organ physiology to an increasingly detailed understanding of cellular, subcellular, and genetic mechanisms. For example, the understanding of microbial pathogenesis and many inflammatory diseases (Chapter 256) is now guided by a detailed understanding of the human immune system and its response to foreign antigens (Chapters 45 to 49). Advances in our understanding of the human microbiome raise the possibility that our complex interactions with microbes, which outnumber our cells by a factor of 10, will help explain conditions ranging from inflammatory bowel disease (Chapter 141) to obesity (Chapter 220).[1]

Health, disease, and an individual's interaction with the environment are also substantially determined by genetics. In addition to many conditions that may be determined by a single gene (Chapter 41), medical science increasingly understands the complex interactions that underlie multigenic traits (Chapter 42). The decoding of the human genome holds the promise that personalized health care increasingly can be targeted according to an individual's genetic profile, in terms of screening and presymptomatic disease management, as well as in terms of specific medications and their adjusted dosing schedules.[2]

Although gene therapy has been approved for only one disease, lipoprotein lipase deficiency (Chapter 206), and only in Europe, it has shown promise in other conditions, such as Leber congenital amaurosis (Chapter 423). Cell therapy is now beginning to provide vehicles for the delivery of genes, gene products, and vaccines. It has also opened the way for "regenerative medicine" by facilitating the regeneration of injured or diseased organs and tissues. Such advances and others, such as nanomedicine, have already led to targeted and personalized therapies for a variety of cancers.[3] Knowledge of the structure and physical forms of proteins helps explain abnormalities as diverse as sickle cell anemia (Chapter 163) and prion-related diseases (Chapter 415). Proteomics, which is the normal and abnormal protein expression of genes, also holds extraordinary promise for developing drug targets for more specific and effective therapies.

Concurrent with these advances in fundamental human biology has been a dramatic shift in methods for evaluating the application of scientific advances to the individual patient and to populations. The randomized controlled trial, sometimes with thousands of patients at multiple institutions, has replaced anecdote as the preferred method for measuring the benefits and optimal uses of diagnostic and therapeutic interventions (Chapter 10). As studies progress from those that show biologic effect, to those that elucidate dosing schedules and toxicity, and finally to those that assess true clinical benefit, the metrics of measuring outcome has also improved from subjective impressions of physicians or patients to reliable and valid measures of morbidity, quality of life, functional status, and other patient-oriented outcomes (Chapter 11). These marked improvements in the scientific methodology of clinical investigation have expedited extraordinary changes in clinical practice, such as recanalization therapy for acute myocardial infarction (Chapter 73), and have shown that reliance on intermediate outcomes, such as a reduction in asymptomatic ventricular arrhythmias with certain drugs, may unexpectedly increase rather than decrease mortality. Just as physicians in the 21st century must understand advances in fundamental biology, similar understanding of the fundamentals of clinical study design as it applies to diagnostic and therapeutic interventions is needed. An understanding of human genetics will also help stratify and refine the approach to clinical trials by helping researchers select fewer patients with a more homogeneous disease pattern to study the efficacy of an intervention.

This explosion in medical knowledge has led to increasing specialization and subspecialization, defined initially by organ system and more recently by locus of principal activity (inpatient vs. outpatient), reliance on manual skills (proceduralist vs. nonproceduralist), or participation in research. Nevertheless, it is becoming increasingly clear that the same fundamental molecular and genetic mechanisms are broadly applicable across all organ systems and that the scientific methodologies of randomized trials and careful clinical observation span all aspects of medicine.

The advent of modern approaches to managing data now provides the rationale for the use of health information technology. Computerized health records, oftentimes shared with patients in a portable format, can avoid duplication of tests and assure that care is coordinated among the patient's various health care providers.

Extraordinary advances in the science and practice of medicine, which have continued to accelerate with each recent edition of this textbook, have transformed the global burden of disease.[4] Life expectancies for men and women are increasing, a greater proportion of deaths are occurring among people older than age 70 years, and far fewer children are dying before the age of 5 years. Nevertheless, huge regional disparities remain, and disability from conditions such as substance abuse, mental health disorders, injuries, diabetes, musculoskeletal disease, and chronic respiratory disease have become increasingly important issues for all health systems.

APPROACH TO THE PATIENT

Patients commonly have complaints (symptoms). These symptoms may or may not be accompanied by abnormalities on examination (signs) or on laboratory testing. Conversely, asymptomatic patients may have signs or laboratory abnormalities, and laboratory abnormalities can occur in the absence of symptoms or signs.

Symptoms and signs commonly define *syndromes,* which may be the common final pathway of a wide range of pathophysiologic alterations. The fundamental basis of internal medicine is that diagnosis should elucidate the pathophysiologic explanation for symptoms and signs so that therapy may improve the underlying abnormality, not just attempt to suppress the abnormal symptoms or signs.

When patients seek care from physicians, they may have manifestations or exacerbations of known conditions, or they may have symptoms and signs that suggest malfunction of a particular organ system. Sometimes the pattern of symptoms and signs is highly suggestive or even pathognomonic for a particular disease process. In these situations, in which the physician is focusing on a particular disease, *Goldman-Cecil Medicine* provides scholarly yet practical approaches to the epidemiology, pathobiology, clinical manifestations, diagnosis, treatment, prevention, and prognosis of entities such as acute myocardial infarction (Chapter 73), chronic obstructive lung disease (Chapter 88), obstructive uropathy (Chapter 123), inflammatory bowel disease (Chapter 141), gallstones (Chapter 155), rheumatoid arthritis (Chapter 264), hypothyroidism (Chapter 226), tuberculosis (Chapter 324), and virtually any known medical condition in adults.

Many patients, however, have undiagnosed symptoms, signs, or laboratory abnormalities that cannot be immediately ascribed to a particular disease or cause. Whether the initial manifestation is chest pain (Chapter 51), diarrhea (Chapter 140), neck or back pain (Chapter 400), or a variety of more than 100 common symptoms, signs, or laboratory abnormalities, *Goldman-Cecil Medicine* provides tables, figures, and entire chapters to guide the approach to diagnosis and therapy (see E-Table 1-1 or table on inside back cover). By virtue of this dual approach to known disease as well as to undiagnosed abnormalities, this textbook, similar to the modern practice of medicine, applies directly to patients regardless of their mode of manifestation or degree of previous evaluation.

The patient-physician interaction proceeds through many phases of clinical reasoning and decision making. The interaction begins with an elucidation of complaints or concerns, followed by inquiries or evaluations to address these concerns in increasingly precise ways. The process commonly requires a careful history or physical examination, ordering of diagnostic tests, integration of clinical findings with test results, understanding of the risks and benefits of the possible courses of action, and careful consultation with the patient and family to develop future plans. Physicians can increasingly call on a growing literature of evidence-based medicine to guide the process so that benefit is maximized while respecting individual variations in different patients. Throughout *Goldman-Cecil Medicine,* the best current evidence is highlighted with specific grade A references that can be accessed directly in the electronic version.

The increasing availability of evidence from randomized trials to guide the approach to diagnosis and therapy should not be equated with "cookbook" medicine. Evidence and the guidelines that are derived from it emphasize proven approaches for patients with specific characteristics. Substantial clinical judgment is required to determine whether the evidence and guidelines apply to individual patients and to recognize the occasional exceptions. Even more judgment is required in the many situations in which evidence is absent or inconclusive. Evidence must also be tempered by patients' preferences, although it is a physician's responsibility to emphasize evidence when presenting alternative options to the patient. The adherence of a patient to a specific regimen is likely to be enhanced if the patient also understands the rationale and evidence behind the recommended option.

To care for a patient as an individual, the physician must understand the patient as a person. This fundamental precept of doctoring includes an understanding of the patient's social situation, family issues, financial concerns, and preferences for different types of care and outcomes, ranging from maximum prolongation of life to the relief of pain and suffering (Chapters 2 and 3). If the physician does not appreciate and address these issues, the science of medicine cannot be applied appropriately, and even the most knowledgeable physician will fail to achieve the desired outcomes.

Even as physicians become increasingly aware of new discoveries, patients can obtain their own information from a variety of sources, some of which are of questionable reliability. The increasing use of alternative and complementary therapies (Chapter 39) is an example of patients' frequent dissatisfaction with prescribed medical therapy. Physicians should keep an open mind regarding unproven options but must advise their patients carefully if such options may carry any degree of potential risk, including the risk that they may be relied on to substitute for proven approaches. It is crucial for the physician to have an open dialogue with the patient and family regarding the full range of options that either may consider.

The physician does not exist in a vacuum, but rather as part of a complicated and extensive system of medical care and public health. In premodern times and even today in some developing countries, basic hygiene, clean water, and adequate nutrition have been the most important ways to promote health and reduce disease. In developed countries, adoption of healthy lifestyles, including better diet (Chapter 213) and appropriate exercise (Chapter 16), is the cornerstone to reducing the epidemics of obesity (Chapter 220), coronary disease (Chapter 52), and diabetes (Chapter 229). Public health interventions to provide immunizations (Chapter 18) and to reduce injuries and the use of tobacco (Chapter 32), illicit drugs (Chapter 34), and excess alcohol (Chapter 33) can collectively produce more health benefits than nearly any other imaginable health intervention.

APPROACH TO THE MEDICAL PROFESSION

In a profession, practitioners put the welfare of clients or patients above their own welfare.[5] Professionals have a duty that may be thought of as a contract with society. The American Board of Internal Medicine and the European Federation of Internal Medicine have jointly proposed that medical professionalism should emphasize three fundamental principles: the primacy of patient welfare, patient autonomy, and social justice.[6] As modern medicine brings a plethora of diagnostic and therapeutic options, the interactions of the physician with the patient and society become more complex and potentially fraught with ethical dilemmas (Chapter 2). To help provide a moral compass that is not only grounded in tradition but also adaptable to modern times, the primacy of patient welfare emphasizes the fundamental principle of a profession. The physician's altruism, which begets the patient's trust, must be impervious to the economic, bureaucratic, and political challenges that are faced by the physician and the patient (Chapter 5).

The principle of patient autonomy asserts that physicians make recommendations but patients make the final decisions. The physician is an expert advisor who must inform and empower the patient to base decisions on scientific data and how these data can and should be integrated with a patient's preferences.

The importance of social justice symbolizes that the patient-physician interaction does not exist in a vacuum. The physician has a responsibility to the individual patient and to broader society to promote access and to eliminate disparities in health and health care.

To promote these fundamental principles, a series of professional responsibilities has been suggested (Table 1-1). These specific responsibilities represent practical, daily traits that benefit the physician's own patients and society as a whole. Physicians who use these and other attributes to improve their patients' satisfaction with care are not only promoting professionalism but also reducing their own risk for liability and malpractice.

An interesting new aspect of professionalism is the increasing reliance on team approaches to medical care, as exemplified by physicians whose roles are defined by the location of their practice—historically in the intensive care unit or emergency department and more recently on the inpatient general hospital floor. Quality care requires coordination and effective communication across inpatient and outpatient sites among physicians who themselves now typically work defined hours.[7] This transition from reliance on a single, always available physician to a team, ideally with a designated coordinator, places new challenges on physicians, the medical care system, and the medical profession.

TABLE 1-1 PROFESSIONAL RESPONSIBILITIES

Commitment to:
Professional competence
Honesty with patients
Patient confidentiality
Maintaining appropriate relations with patients
Improving the quality of care
Improving access to care
Just distribution of finite resources
Scientific knowledge
Maintaining trust by managing conflicts of interest
Professional responsibilities

From Brennan T, Blank L, Cohen J, et al. Medical professionalism in the new millennium: a physician charter. *Ann Intern Med.* 2002;1136:243-246.

The changing medical care environment is placing increasing emphasis on standards, outcomes, and accountability. As purchasers of insurance become more cognizant of value rather than just cost (Chapter 12), outcomes ranging from rates of screening mammography (Chapter 198) to mortality rates with coronary artery bypass graft surgery (Chapter 74) become metrics by which rational choices can be made. Clinical guidelines and critical pathways derived from randomized controlled trials and evidence-based medicine can potentially lead to more cost-effective care and better outcomes.

These major changes in many Western health care systems bring with them many major risks and concerns. If the concept of limited choice among physicians and health care providers is based on objective measures of quality and outcome, channeling of patients to better providers is one reasonable definition of better selection and enlightened competition. If the limiting of options is based overwhelmingly on cost rather than measures of quality, outcomes, and patient satisfaction, it is likely that the historical relationship between the patient and the truly professional physician will be fundamentally compromised.

Another risk is that the same genetic information that could lead to more effective, personalized medicine will be used against the very people whom it is supposed to benefit—by creating a stigma, raising health insurance costs, or even making someone uninsurable. The ethical approach to medicine (Chapter 2), genetics (Chapter 40), and genetic counseling provides means to protect against this adverse effect of scientific progress.

In this new environment, the physician often has a dual responsibility: to the health care system as an expert who helps create standards, measures of outcome, clinical guidelines, and mechanisms to ensure high-quality, cost-effective care; and to individual patients who entrust their well-being to that physician to promote their best interests within the reasonable limits of the system. A health insurance system that emphasizes cost-effective care, that gives physicians and health care providers responsibility for the health of a population and the resources required to achieve these goals, that must exist in a competitive environment in which patients can choose alternatives if they are not satisfied with their care, and that places increasing emphasis on health education and prevention can have many positive effects. In this environment, however, physicians must beware of overt and subtle pressures that could entice them to underserve patients and abrogate their professional responsibilities by putting personal financial reward ahead of their patients' welfare. The physician's responsibility to represent the patient's best interests and avoid financial conflicts by doing too little in the newer systems of capitated care provides different specific challenges but an analogous moral dilemma to the historical American system in which the physician could be rewarded financially for doing too much.

In the current health care environment, all physicians and trainees must redouble their commitment to professionalism. At the same time, the challenge to the individual physician to retain and expand the scientific knowledge base and process the vast array of new information is daunting. In this spirit of a profession based on science and caring, *Goldman-Cecil Medicine* seeks to be a comprehensive approach to modern internal medicine.

GENERAL REFERENCES

For the General References and other additional features, please visit Expert Consult at https://expertconsult.inkling.com.

2

BIOETHICS IN THE PRACTICE OF MEDICINE

EZEKIEL J. EMANUEL

It commonly is argued that modern advances in medical technology, antibiotics, dialysis, transplantation, and intensive care units have created the bioethical dilemmas that confront physicians in the 21st century. In reality, however, concerns about ethical issues are as old as the practice of medicine itself. The Hippocratic Oath, composed sometime around 400 BC, attests to the need of ancient Greek physicians for advice on how to address the many bioethical dilemmas that they confronted. The Oath addresses issues of confidentiality, abortion, euthanasia, sexual relations between physician and patient, divided loyalties, and, at least implicitly, charity care and executions. Other Hippocratic works address issues such as termination of treatments to dying patients and telling the truth. Whether we agree with the advice dispensed or not, the important point is that many bioethical issues are not created by technology but instead are inherent in medical practice. Technology may make these issues more common and may change the context in which they arise, but many, if not most, bioethical issues that regularly confront physicians are timeless and inherent in the practice of medicine.

Many physicians have been educated that four main principles can be invoked to address bioethical dilemmas: autonomy, nonmaleficence, beneficence, and justice. Autonomy is the idea that people should have the right and freedom to choose, pursue, and revise their own life plans. Nonmaleficence is the idea that people should not be harmed or injured knowingly; this principle is encapsulated in the frequently repeated phrase that a physician has an obligation to "first do no harm"—*primum non nocere*. This phrase is not found either in the Hippocratic Oath or in other Hippocratic writing; the only related, but not identical, Hippocratic phrase is "at least, do not harm." Whereas nonmaleficence is about avoiding harm, beneficence is about the positive actions that the physician should undertake to promote the well-being of his or her patients. In clinical practice, this obligation usually arises from the implicit and explicit commitments and promises surrounding the physician-patient relationship. Finally, there is the principle of justice as the fair distribution of benefits and burdens.

Although helpful in providing an initial framework, these principles have limited value because they are broad and open to diverse and conflicting interpretations. In addition, as is clear with the principle of justice, they frequently are underdeveloped. In any difficult case, the principles are likely to conflict. Conflicting ethical principles are precisely why there are bioethical dilemmas. The principles themselves do not offer guidance on how they should be balanced or specified to resolve the dilemma. These principles, which are focused on the individual physician-patient context, are not particularly helpful when the bioethical issues are institutional and systemic, such as allocating scarce vaccines or organs for transplantation or balancing the risks and benefits of mammograms for women younger than 50 years. Finally, these four principles are not comprehensive. Other fundamental ethical principles and values, such as communal solidarity, duties to future generations, trust, and professional integrity, are important in bioethics but not encapsulated except by deformation in these four principles.

There is no formula or small set of ethical principles that mechanically or magically gives answers to bioethical dilemmas. Instead, medical practitioners should follow an orderly analytic process. First, practitioners need to obtain the facts relevant to the situation. Second, they must delineate the basic bioethical issue. Third, it is important to identify all the crucial principles and values that relate to the case and how they might conflict. Fourth, because many ethical dilemmas have been analyzed previously and subjected frequently to empirical study, practitioners should examine the relevant literature, whether it is commentaries or studies in medical journals, legal cases, or books. With these analyses, the particular dilemma should be reexamined; this process might lead to reformulation of the issue and identification of new values or new understandings of existing values. Fifth, with this information, it is important to distinguish clearly unethical practices from a range of ethically permissible actions. Finally, it is important not only to come to some resolution of the case but also to state clearly the reasons behind the decisions, that is, the interpretation of the principles used and how values were balanced. Although unanimity and consensus may be desirable ideals, reasonable people frequently disagree about how to resolve ethical dilemmas without being unethical or malevolent.

A multitude of bioethical dilemmas arise in medical practice, including issues of genetics, reproductive choices, and termination of care. In clinical practice, the most common issues revolve around informed consent, termination of life-sustaining treatments, euthanasia and physician-assisted suicide, and conflicts of interest.

PHYSICIAN-PATIENT RELATIONSHIP: INFORMED CONSENT

History

It commonly is thought that the requirement for informed consent is a relatively recent phenomenon. Suggestions about the need for a patient's informed consent can be found as far back as Plato, however. The first recorded legal case involving informed consent is the 1767 English case of *Slater v. Baker and Stapleton,* in which two surgeons refractured a patient's leg after it had healed improperly. The patient claimed they had not obtained consent. The court ruled:

> *[I]t appears from the evidence of the surgeon that it was improper to disunite the callous without consent; this is the usage and law of surgeons: then it was ignorance and unskillfulness in that very particular, to do contrary to the rule of the profession, what no surgeon ought to have done.*

Although there may be some skepticism about the extent of the information disclosed or the precise nature of the consent obtained, the notable fact is that an 18th-century court declared that obtaining prior consent of the patient is not only the usual practice but also the ethical and legal obligation of surgeons. Failure to obtain consent is incompetent and inexcusable. In contemporary times, the 1957 case of *Salgo v. Leland Stanford Junior University Board of Trustees* constitutes a landmark by stating that physicians have a positive legal obligation to disclose information about risks, benefits, and alternatives to patients; this decision popularized the term *informed consent.*

Definition and Justification

Informed consent is a person's autonomous authorization of a physician to undertake diagnostic or therapeutic interventions for himself or herself. In this view, the patient understands that he or she is taking responsibility for the decision while empowering someone else, the physician, to implement it. However, agreement to a course of medical treatment does not necessarily qualify as informed consent.

There are four fundamental requirements for valid informed consent: mental capacity, disclosure, understanding, and voluntariness. Informed consent assumes that people have the mental capacity to make decisions; disease, development, or medications can compromise patients' mental capacity to provide informed consent. Adults are presumed to have the legal competence to make medical decisions, and whether an adult is incompetent to make medical decisions is a legal determination. Practically, physicians usually decide whether patients are competent on the basis of whether patients can understand the information disclosed, appreciate its significance for their own situation, and use logical and consistent thought processes in decision making. Incompetence in medical decision making does not mean a person is incompetent in all types of decision making and vice versa. Crucial information relevant to the decision must be disclosed, usually by the physician, to the patient. The patient should understand the information and its implications for his or her interests and life goals. Finally, the patient must make a voluntary decision (i.e., one without coercion or manipulation by the physician). It is a mistake to view informed consent as an event, such as the signing of a form. Informed consent is viewed more accurately as a process that evolves during the course of diagnosis and treatment.

Typically, the patient's autonomy is the value invoked to justify informed consent. Other values, such as bodily integrity and beneficence, have also been cited, especially in early legal rulings.

Empirical Data

Fairly extensive research has been done on informed consent. In general, studies show that in clinical situations, physicians frequently do not communicate all relevant information for informed decision making. In a study of audiotapes from 1057 outpatient encounters, physicians mentioned alternatives in only 11.3% of cases, provided pros and cons of interventions in only 7.8% of situations, and assessed the patient's understanding of the information in only 1.5% of decisions. The more complex the medical decisions, the more likely it was that the elements of informed consent would be fulfilled. Importantly, data suggest that disclosure is better in research settings, both in the informed consent documents and in the discussions. For instance, in recorded interactions between researchers and prospective participants, the major elements of research, such as that the treatment was investigational and the risks and benefits of treatment, were disclosed in more than 80% of interactions. Greater disclosure in the research setting may be the consequence of requiring a written informed consent document that has been reviewed by an independent committee, such as an institutional review board or a research ethics committee. Some have suggested that for common medical interventions, such as elective surgery, standardized informed consent documents should include the risks and benefits as quantified in randomized controlled trials, relevant data on the surgeon, the institution's clinical outcomes for the procedure, and a list of acceptable alternatives.[1]

Patients frequently fail to recall crucial information disclosed, although they usually think they have sufficient information for decision making. Whether patients fail to recall key information because they are overwhelmed by the information or because they do not find much of it salient to their decision is unclear. The issue is what patients understand at the point of decision making, not what they recall later.

Studies aimed at improving informed consent in the clinical setting suggest that interactive media, such as videos and interactive computer software, can improve understanding by patients. Conversely, data on shared decision making show that interactive media do not improve participants' understanding, whereas more personal interaction, whether as an additional telephone call by a research nurse or as an additional face-to-face meeting, does enhance understanding.[2]

One of the most important results of empirical research on informed consent is the gap between information and decision making. Many studies show that most patients want information, but far fewer prefer decision-making authority. One study showed that most patients wanted information, but only about one third desired decision-making authority, and patients' decision-making preferences were not correlated with their information-seeking preferences. Several investigators found that patients' preference for decision-making authority increases with higher educational levels and declines with advancing age. Most important, the more serious the illness, the more likely patients are to prefer that physicians make the decisions. Several studies suggest that patients who have less of a desire to make their own decisions generally are more satisfied with how the decisions were made.

Practical Considerations

Implementing informed consent raises concerns about the extent of information to be disclosed and exceptions to the general requirement. A major area of ethical and legal disagreement has been what information to disclose and how to disclose it. As a practical matter, physicians should disclose at least six fundamental elements of information to patients: (1) diagnosis and prognosis; (2) nature of the proposed intervention; (3) alternative interventions, including no treatment; (4) risks associated with each alternative; (5) benefits of each alternative; and (6) likely outcomes of these alternatives (Table 2-1). Because risk is usually the key worry of physicians, it generally is recommended that physicians disclose (1) the nature of the risks, (2) their magnitude, (3) the probability that each risk will occur, and (4) when the consequence might occur.[3] Increasingly, these disclosures should include data both from clinical trials as well as the actual data from the institution and physician performing the test and treatments. Some argue that minor risks need not be disclosed. In general, all serious risks, such as death, paralysis, stroke, infections, or chronic pain, even if rare, should be disclosed, as should common risks.

The central problem is that the physician should provide this detailed information within reasonable time constraints and yet not overwhelm patients with complex information in technical language. The historical constraint of office time is no longer tenable. Interactive electronic media, which patients can view at home on their own time, can facilitate the transfer of information outside of the physician's office. Different states have adopted two contrasting legal standards defining how much information should be disclosed. The *physician* or *customary* standard, adapted from malpractice law, states that the physician should disclose information "which a reasonable medical practitioner would make under the same or similar circumstances." Conversely, the *reasonable person* or *lay-oriented* standard states that physicians should disclose all information that a "reasonable person in the patient's circumstances would find material to" the medical decision. The physician standard is factual and can be determined empirically, but the patient-oriented standard, which is meant to engage physicians with patients, is hypothetical. Currently, each standard is used by about half the states.

TABLE 2-1 FUNDAMENTAL ELEMENTS FOR DISCLOSURE TO PATIENTS

Diagnosis and prognosis
Nature of proposed intervention
Reasonable alternative interventions
Risks associated with each alternative intervention
Benefits associated with each alternative intervention
Probable outcomes of each alternative intervention

There are exceptions to the requirements of informed consent. In emergency situations, consent can be assumed because patients' interests concentrate on survival and retaining maximal mental and physical functioning; as a result, reasonable persons would want treatment. In some circumstances, physicians may believe the process of informed consent could pose a serious psychological threat. In rare cases, the "therapeutic privilege" promoting a patient's well-being trumps autonomy, but physicians should be wary of invoking this exception too readily.

If patients are deemed incompetent, family members—beginning with spouse, children, parents, siblings, then more distant relatives—usually are selected as surrogates or proxies, although there may be concerns about conflicting interests or knowledge of the patient's wishes. In the relatively rare circumstance in which a patient formally designated a proxy, that person has decision-making authority.

The *substituted judgment* standard states that the proxy should choose what the patient would choose if he or she were competent. The *best interests* standard states that the proxy should choose what is best for the patient. Frequently, it is not clear how the patient would have decided because the situation was not discussed with the patient and he or she left no living will. Similarly, what is best for a patient is controversial because there are usually tradeoffs between quality of life and survival. These problems are exacerbated because a proxy's predictions about a patient's quality of life are poor; proxies tend to underestimate patients' functional status and satisfaction. Similarly, proxy predictions are inaccurate regarding life-sustaining preferences when the patient is mentally incapacitated. Families tend to agree with patients about two thirds of the time in deciding whether to provide life-sustaining treatments if the patient became demented, when chance alone would generate agreement in 50% of the cases. Such confusion about how to decide for incapacitated patients can create conflicts among family members or between the family and medical providers. In such circumstances, an ethics consultation may be helpful.

TERMINATION OF MEDICAL INTERVENTIONS

History

Since the start of medicine, it has been viewed as ethical to withhold medical treatments from the terminally ill and "let nature take its course," while keeping the patient as comfortable as possible.[4] Hippocrates argued that physicians should "refuse to treat those [patients] who are overmastered by their disease." In the 19th century, prominent American physicians advocated withholding of cathartic and emetic "treatments" from the terminally ill and using ether to ease pain at the end of life. John Collins Warren, who wrote *Etherization: with Surgical Remarks* in 1848, included a chapter on using ether to ease the pain of a cancer patient's death. The editors of *The Lancet*, in 1900, argued that physicians should intervene to ease the pain of death and that they did not have an obligation to prolong a clearly terminal life. The contemporary debate on terminating care began in 1976 with the *Quinlan* case, in which the New Jersey Supreme Court ruled that patients had a right to refuse life-sustaining interventions on the basis of a right of privacy and that the family could exercise the right for a patient in a persistent vegetative state.

Definition and Justification

It generally is agreed that all patients have a right to refuse medical interventions. Ethically, this right is based on the patient's autonomy and is implied by the doctrine of informed consent. Legally, state courts have cited the right to privacy, right to bodily integrity, or common law to justify the right to refuse medical treatment. In the 1990 *Cruzan* case and in the subsequent physician-assisted suicide cases, the U.S. Supreme Court affirmed that there is a "constitutionally protected right to refuse lifesaving hydration and nutrition." The Court stated that "[A] liberty interest [based on the 14th Amendment] in refusing unwanted medical treatment may be inferred from our prior decisions." All patients have a constitutional and an ethical right to refuse medical interventions. These rulings were the basis of the consistent state and federal court rulings to permit the husband to terminate artificial nutrition and hydration in the *Schiavo* case.

Empirical Data

Data show that termination of medical treatments is now the norm, and the trend has been to stop medical interventions more frequently based on the preferences of patients and their surrogate decision makers.[5] More than 85% of Americans die without cardiopulmonary resuscitation, and more than 90% of decedents in intensive care units do not receive cardiopulmonary resuscitation. Of decedents in intensive care units, more than 85% die after the withholding or withdrawal of medical treatments, with an average of 2.6 interventions being withheld or withdrawn per decedent.

Despite extensive public support for use of advance care directives and the passage of the Patient Self-Determination Act mandating that health care institutions inform patients of their right to complete such documents, less than 30% of Americans have completed one.[6] Even among severely or terminally ill patients, less than 50% have an advance directive in their medical record. Data suggest that more than 40% of patients required active decision-making about terminating medical treatments in their final days, but more than 70% lacked decision-making capacity, thereby emphasizing the importance of advance directives. Efforts to improve completion of advance care directives have generated mixed results. In La Crosse County, Wisconsin, for example, after health care organizations in the county added an "Advance Directive" section to their electronic medical records, 90% of decedents had some type of advance directive. Unfortunately, even successful pilot efforts like La Crosse County's have not been adopted or easily scaled. A persistent problem has been that even when patients complete advance care directives, the documents frequently are not available, physicians do not know they exist, or they tend to be too general or vague to guide decisions. The increasing use of electronic health records should make it possible for advance directives to be available whenever and wherever the patient presents to a health care provider. Although electronic health records will help in making existing advance directives available, they will not solve the problem of actually having a conversation between the physician and the patient about advance care planning. Starting that conversation still seems to be a persistent barrier.

Just as proxies are poor at predicting patients' wishes, data show that physicians are probably even worse at determining patients' preferences for life-sustaining treatments. In many cases, life-sustaining treatments are continued even when patients or their proxies desire them to be stopped. Conversely, many physicians discontinue or never begin interventions unilaterally without the knowledge or consent of patients or their surrogate decision makers. These discrepancies emphasize the importance of engaging patients early in their care about treatment preferences.

Practical Considerations

There are many practical considerations in enacting this right (Table 2-2). First, patients have a right to refuse any and all medical interventions, from blood transfusions and antibiotics to respirators, artificial hydration, and nutrition. Although initiation of cardiopulmonary resuscitation was the focus of the early court cases, this issue is viewed best as addressing just one of the many medical interventions that can be stopped or withheld.

The question of what medical interventions can be terminated—or not started—is a recurrent topic of debate among physicians and other health care providers. The fact is that any treatment prescribed by a physician and administered by a health care provider can be stopped. The issue is not whether the treatment is ordinary, extraordinary, or heroic, or whether it is high technology or low technology. Treatments that can be stopped include not only ventilators, artificial nutrition, and hydration but also dialysis, pacemakers, ventricular assist devices, antibiotics, and any medications.

Second, there is no ethical or legal difference between withholding an intervention and withdrawing it. If a respirator or other treatment is started because physicians are uncertain whether a patient would have wanted it, they always can stop it later when information clarifies the patient's wishes. Although physicians and nurses might find stopping a treatment to be more difficult psychologically, withdrawal is ethically and legally permitted—and required—when it is consonant with the patient's wishes.

Third, competent patients have the exclusive right to decide about terminating their own care.[7] If there is a conflict between a competent patient and his or her family, the patient's wishes are to be followed. It is the patient's right to refuse treatment, not the family's right. For incompetent patients, the situation is more complex; if the patients left clear indications of their wishes, whether as explicit oral statements or as written advance care directives, these wishes should be followed. Physicians should not be overly concerned about the precise form patients use to express their wishes; because patients have a constitutional right to refuse treatment, the real concern is whether the wishes are clear and relevant to the situation. If an incompetent patient did not leave explicit indications of his or her wishes or designate a proxy decision maker, the physician should identify a surrogate decision maker and rely on the decision maker's wishes while being cognizant of the potential problems noted. There is a potential problem in terminating life-sustaining care to patients who are permanently incompetent but still conscious. Some state courts have restricted what treatments a proxy decision maker can terminate,

TABLE 2-2 PRACTICAL CONSIDERATIONS IN TERMINATION OF MEDICAL TREATMENTS

PRACTICAL QUESTION	ANSWER
Is there a legal right to refuse medical interventions?	Yes. The U.S. Supreme Court declared that competent people have a constitutionally protected right to refuse unwanted medical treatments based on the 14th Amendment.
What interventions can be legally and ethically terminated?	Any and all interventions (including respirators, antibiotics, pacemakers, ventricular assist devices, intravenous or enteral nutrition and hydration) can be legally and ethically terminated.
Is there a difference between withholding life-sustaining interventions and withdrawing them?	No. The consensus is that there is no important legal or ethical difference between withholding and withdrawing medical interventions. Stopping a treatment once begun is just as ethical as never having started it.
Whose view about terminating life-sustaining interventions prevails if there is a conflict between the patient and family?	The views of a competent adult patient prevail. It is the patient's body and life.
Who decides about terminating life-sustaining interventions if the patient is incompetent?	If the patient appointed a proxy or surrogate decision maker when competent, that person is legally empowered to make decisions about terminating care. If no proxy was appointed, there is a legally designated hierarchy, usually (1) spouse, (2) adult children, (3) parents, (4) siblings, and (5) available relatives.
Are advance care directives legally enforceable?	Yes. As a clear expression of the patient's wishes, they are a constitutionally protected method for patients to exercise their right to refuse medical treatments. In almost all states, clear and explicit oral statements are legally and ethically sufficient for decisions about withholding or withdrawing medical interventions.

thereby requiring the incompetent patient to have given very specific instructions about the particular treatments he or she does not want to receive and the conditions under which care should be withheld or withdrawn. This requirement severely limits the authority and power of proxy decision makers in these cases.

Fourth, the right to refuse medical treatment does not translate into a right to demand any treatment, especially treatments that have no pathophysiologic rationale, have already failed, or are known to be harmful. Futility has become a justification to permit physicians unilaterally to withhold or withdraw treatments despite the family's requests for treatment. Some states, such as Texas, have enacted futility laws, which prescribe procedures by which physicians can invoke futility either to transfer a patient or to terminate interventions. However, the principle of futility is not easy to implement in medical practice. Initially, some commentators advocated that an intervention was futile when the probability of success was 1% or lower. Although this threshold seems to be based on empirical data, it is a covert value judgment. Because the declaration of futility is meant to justify unilateral determinations by physicians, it generally has been viewed as an inappropriate assertion that undermines physician-patient communication and violates the principle of shared decision making. Similar to the distinction between ordinary and extraordinary, futility is viewed increasingly as more obfuscating than clarifying, and it is being invoked much less often.

ASSISTED SUICIDE AND EUTHANASIA

History

Since Hippocrates, euthanasia and physician-assisted suicide have been controversial issues. In 1905, a bill was introduced into the Ohio legislature to legalize euthanasia; it was defeated. In the mid-1930s, similar bills were introduced and defeated in the British Parliament and the Nebraska legislature. As of January 2014, physician-assisted suicide is legal in Oregon and Washington State, based on statewide public referenda, and in Vermont, based on legislation passed in May 2013. Both euthanasia and physician-assisted suicide are legal in the Netherlands, Belgium, and Luxembourg, and physician-assisted suicide is legal in Switzerland. The Montana Supreme Court did not recognize a constitutional right to physician-assisted suicide, but it ruled that the law permitting the termination of life-sustaining treatment protected physicians from prosecution if they helped hasten the death of a consenting, rational, terminally ill patient.

TABLE 2-3 DEFINITIONS OF ASSISTED SUICIDE AND EUTHANASIA

TERM	DEFINITION
Voluntary active euthanasia	Intentional administration of medications or other interventions to cause the patient's death with the patient's informed consent
Involuntary active euthanasia	Intentional administration of medications or other interventions to cause the patient's death when the patient was competent to consent but did not consent (e.g., the patient may not have been asked)
Nonvoluntary active euthanasia	Intentional administration of medications or other interventions to cause the patient's death when the patient was incompetent and was mentally incapable of consenting (e.g., the patient might have been in a coma)
Passive euthanasia	Withholding or withdrawal of life-sustaining medical treatments from a patient to let him or her die (termination of life-sustaining treatments)—a poor term that should not be used
Indirect euthanasia	Administration of narcotics or other medications to relieve pain with the incidental consequence of causing sufficient respiratory depression to result in the patient's death
Physician-assisted suicide	A physician provides prescription medications or other interventions to a patient with the understanding that the patient can use them to commit suicide

Definition and Justification

The terms *euthanasia* and *physician-assisted suicide*[8] require careful definition (Table 2-3). So-called passive and indirect euthanasia are misnomers and are not instances of euthanasia, and both are deemed ethical and legal.

There are four arguments against permitting euthanasia and physician-assisted suicide. First, Kant and Mill thought that autonomy did not permit the voluntary ending of the conditions necessary for autonomy, and as a result, both philosophers were against voluntary enslavement and suicide. Consequently, the exercise of autonomy cannot include the ending of life because that would mean ending the possibility of exercising autonomy. Second, many dying patients may have pain and suffering because they are not receiving appropriate care, and it is possible that adequate care would relieve much pain and suffering (Chapter 3). Although a few patients still may experience uncontrolled pain and suffering despite optimal end-of-life care, it is unwise to use the condition of these few patients as a justification to permit euthanasia or physician-assisted suicide for any dying patient. Third, there is a clear ethical distinction between intentional ending of a life and termination of life-sustaining treatments. The actual acts are different—injecting a life-ending medication, such as a muscle relaxant, or providing a prescription for one is not the same as removing or refraining from introducing an invasive medical intervention. Finally, adverse consequences of permitting euthanasia and physician-assisted suicide must be considered. There are disturbing reports of involuntary euthanasia in the Netherlands and Belgium, and many worry about coercion of expensive or burdensome patients to accept euthanasia or physician-assisted suicide. Permitting euthanasia and physician-assisted suicide is likely to lead to further intrusions of lawyers, courts, and legislatures into the physician-patient relationship.

There are four parallel arguments for permitting euthanasia and physician-assisted suicide. First, it is argued that autonomy justifies euthanasia and physician-assisted suicide. To respect autonomy requires permitting individuals to decide when it is better to end their lives by euthanasia or physician-assisted suicide. Second, beneficence—furthering the well-being of individuals—supports permitting euthanasia and physician-assisted suicide. In some cases, living can create more pain and suffering than death; ending a painful life relieves more suffering and produces more good. Just the reassurance of having the option of euthanasia or physician-assisted suicide, even if people do not use it, can provide "psychological insurance" and be beneficial to people. Third, euthanasia and physician-assisted suicide are no different from termination of life-sustaining treatments that are recognized as ethically justified. In both cases, the patient consents to die; in both cases, the physician intends to end the patient's life and takes some action to end the patient's life; and in both cases, the final result is the same: the patient's death. With no difference in the patient's consent, the physician's intention, or the final result, there can be no difference in the ethical justification. Fourth, the supposed slippery slope that would result from permitting euthanasia and physician-assisted suicide is not likely. The idea that permitting euthanasia and physician-assisted suicide would undermine the physician-patient relationship or lead to forced euthanasia is completely speculative and not borne out by the available data.

In its 1997 decisions, the U.S. Supreme Court stated that there is no constitutional right to euthanasia and physician-assisted suicide but that there also is no constitutional prohibition against states legalizing these interventions. Consequently, the legalization of physician-assisted suicide in Oregon, Vermont, and Washington State was constitutional.

Empirical Data

Attitudes and practices related to euthanasia and physician-assisted suicide have been studied extensively. First, surveys consistently indicate that between 50 and 80% of the American and British public support legalizing euthanasia and physician-assisted suicide for terminally ill patients who are suffering intractable pain.[9] However, public support declines significantly for euthanasia and physician-assisted suicide in other circumstances, such as for psychological reasons.[10] Physicians tend to be much less supportive of euthanasia and physician-assisted suicide, with oncologists, palliative care physicians, and geriatricians among the least supportive. Among American and British physicians, the majority opposes legalizing either practice. Second, approximately 25% of American physicians have received requests for euthanasia or physician-assisted suicide, including about 50% of oncologists. Third, multiple studies indicate that less than 5% of American physicians have performed euthanasia or physician-assisted suicide. Among oncologists, 4% have performed euthanasia and 11% have performed physician-assisted suicide during their careers. Fourth, in many cases, the safeguards are violated. One study found that in 54% of euthanasia cases, it was the family who made the request; in 39% of euthanasia and 19% of physician-assisted suicide cases, the patient was depressed; in only half of the cases was the request repeated.

In the Netherlands and Belgium, where euthanasia and physician-assisted suicide are legal, less than 2% of all deaths are by these measures, with 0.4 to 1.8% of all deaths as the result of euthanasia without the patient's consent.[11] Since the practice of assisted suicide was legalized in Oregon in 1997, a cumulative 0.2% of all deaths are by physician-assisted suicide.

Counterintuitively, data indicate that it is not pain that primarily motivates requests for euthanasia or physician-assisted suicide but rather psychological distress, especially depression and hopelessness. Interviews with physicians and with patients with amyotrophic lateral sclerosis, cancer, or infection with human immunodeficiency virus show that pain is not associated with interest in euthanasia or physician-assisted suicide; instead, depression and hopelessness are the strongest predictors of interest. Studies of patients in Australia and the Netherlands confirm the importance of depression in motivating requests for euthanasia. The desire to avoid dependence and loss of dignity are key motivations.

Finally, data from the Netherlands and the United States suggest that there are significant problems in performing euthanasia and physician-assisted suicide. Dutch researchers reported that physician-assisted suicide causes complications in 7% of cases, and in 15% of cases, the patients did not die, awoke from coma, or vomited up the medication. Ultimately, in nearly 20% of physician-assisted suicide cases, the physician ended up injecting the patient with life-ending medication, converting physician-assisted suicide to euthanasia. These data raise serious questions about how to address complications of physician-assisted suicide when euthanasia is illegal or unacceptable.

Practical Considerations

There is widespread agreement that if euthanasia and physician-assisted suicide are used, they should be considered only after all reasonable attempts at physical and psychological palliation have failed. A series of safeguards have been developed and embodied in the Oregon and the Dutch procedures, as follows: (1) the patient must be competent and must request euthanasia or physician-assisted suicide repeatedly and voluntarily; (2) the patient must have pain or other suffering that cannot be relieved by optimal palliative interventions; (3) there should be a waiting period to ensure that the patient's desire for euthanasia or physician-assisted suicide is stable and sincere; and (4) the physician should obtain a second opinion from an independent physician. Oregon and Washington State require patients to be terminally ill, whereas the Netherlands, Belgium, and Switzerland have no such requirement. Although there have been some prosecutions in the United States, there have been no convictions—except for Dr. Kevorkian—when physicians and others have participated in euthanasia and physician-assisted suicide.

FINANCIAL CONFLICTS OF INTEREST

History

Worrying about how payment and fees affect medical decisions is not new. In 1899, a physician reported that more than 60% of surgeons in Chicago were willing to provide a 50% commission to physicians for referring cases. He subsequently argued that in some cases, this fee splitting led to unnecessary surgical procedures. A 1912 study by the American Medical Association confirmed that fee splitting was a common practice. Selling patent medicines and patenting surgical instruments were other forms of financial conflicts of interest thought to discredit physicians a century ago. In the 1990s, the ethics of capitation for physician services and pharmaceutical prescriptions and payments by pharmaceutical and biotechnology companies to clinical researchers and practitioners raised the issue of financial conflicts of interest.

Definition and Justification

It commonly is argued that physicians have certain primary interests: (1) to promote the well-being of their patients, (2) to advance biomedical research, (3) to educate future physicians, and, more controversially, (4) to promote public health (Table 2-4). Physicians also have other, secondary interests, such as earning income, raising a family, contributing to the profession, and pursuing avocational interests, such as hobbies. These secondary interests are not evil; typically, they are legitimate, even admirable. A conflict of interest occurs when one of these secondary interests compromises pursuit of a primary interest, especially the patient's well-being.

Conflicts of interest are problematic because they can or appear to compromise the integrity of physicians' judgment, compromising the patient's well-being or research integrity. Conflict of interest can induce a physician to do something—perform a procedure, fail to order a test, or distort data—that would not be in a patient's best interest. These conflicts can undermine the trust of patients and the public, not only in an individual physician but also in the entire medical profession. Even the appearance of conflicts of interest can be damaging because it is difficult for patients and the public "to determine what motives have influenced a professional decision." The focus is on financial conflicts of interest, not because they are worse than other types of conflicts, but rather because they are more pervasive and more easily identified and regulated compared with other conflicts. Since ancient times, the ethical norm on conflicts has been clear: the physician's primary obligation is to patients' well-being, and a physician's personal financial well-being should not compromise this duty.

Empirical Data

Financial conflicts are not rare but are frequently under-reported.[12] The increased use of medical services and escalating health care spending, sometimes without clear benefit to patients, have been linked, at least statistically, to ownership of imaging facilities and referral to specialty hospitals owned by physicians. In Florida, it was estimated that nearly 40% of physicians were involved as owners of freestanding facilities to which they referred patients. In one study, 4 to 4.5 times more imaging examinations were ordered by self-referring physicians than by physicians who referred patients to radiologists. Similarly, patients referred to joint-venture physical therapy facilities have an average of 16 visits compared with 11 at non–joint-venture facilities. A recent study of urologists found that those who had integrated radiation

TABLE 2-4 PRIMARY INTERESTS OF PHYSICIANS
Promotion of the health and well-being of their patients
Advancement of biomedical knowledge through research
Education of future physicians and health care providers
Promotion of the public health

facilities into their practices increased their use of the radiation by 2.5 times compared with urologists who did not have financial relationships with radiation facilities.[13] There are no comparable data on the influence of capitation on physicians' judgment.

Similarly, multiple studies have shown that interaction with pharmaceutical representatives can lead to prescribing of new drugs, nonrational prescribing, and decreased use of generic drugs by physicians. Industry funding for continuing medical education payment for travel to educational symposia increases prescribing of the sponsor's drug.

Regarding researcher conflicts of interest, the available data suggest that corporate funding does not compromise the design and methodology of clinical research; in fact, commercially funded research may be methodologically more rigorous than government- or foundation-supported research. Conversely, data suggest that financial interests do distort researchers' interpretation of data. The most important impact of financial interests, however, appears to be on dissemination of research studies. Growing evidence suggests the suppression or selective publication of data unfavorable to corporate sponsors but the repeated publication of favorable results.

Practical Considerations

First, financial conflicts of interest are inherent in any profession when the professional earns income from rendering a service. Second, conflicts come in many different forms, from legitimate payment for services rendered to investments in medical laboratories and facilities, drug company dinners and payment for attendance at meetings, payment for enrolling patients in clinical research trials, and consultation with companies.

Third, in considering how to manage conflicts, it is important to note that people are poor judges of their own potential conflicts. Individuals often cannot distinguish the various influences that guide their judgments, do not think of themselves as bad, and do not imagine that payment shapes their judgments. Physicians tend to be defensive about charges of conflicts of interest. In addition, conflicts tend to act insidiously, subtly changing practice patterns so that they then become what appear to be justifiable norms.

Fourth, rules—whether laws, regulations, or professional standards—to regulate conflicts of interest are based on two considerations: (1) the likelihood that payment or other secondary interests would create a conflict and (2) the magnitude of the potential harm if there is compromised judgment. Rules tend to be of three types: (1) disclosure of conflicts, (2) management of conflicts, and (3) outright prohibition. Federal law bans certain types of self-referral of physicians in the Medicare program. The American Medical Association and the Pharmaceutical Research and Manufacturers of America have established joint rules that permit physicians to accept gifts of minimal value but "refuse substantial gifts from drug companies, such as the costs of travel, lodging, or other personal expenses . . . for attending conferences or meetings." Additionally, the Physician Payment Sunshine Act, which was passed in 2010 as part of the Affordable Care Act and went into effect in August 2013, requires that drug and device manufacturers report all payments and transfers of value given to physicians to the Centers for Medicare and Medicaid Services so that information can be published on a searchable public website.

Fifth, there is much emphasis on disclosure of conflicts, with the implicit idea being that sunshine is the best disinfectant. Disclosure may be useful in publications, but it is unclear whether this is a suitable safeguard in the clinical setting. Disclosure just may make patients worry more. Patients may have no context in which to place the disclosure or to evaluate the physician's clinical recommendation, and patients may have few other options in selecting a physician or getting care, especially in an acute situation. Furthermore, self-disclosure often is incomplete, even when required.

Finally, some conflicts can be avoided by a physician's own action. Physicians can refuse to engage in personal investments in medical facilities or to accept gifts from pharmaceutical companies at relatively little personal cost. In other circumstances, the conflicts may be institutionalized, and minimizing them can occur only by changing the way organizations structure reimbursement incentives. Capitation encourages physicians to limit medical services, and its potentially adverse effects are likely to be managed by institutional rules rather than by personal decisions.

FUTURE DIRECTIONS

In the near future, as genetics moves from the research to the clinical setting, practicing physicians are likely to encounter issues surrounding genetic testing, counseling, and treatment. The use of genetic tests without the extensive counseling so common in research studies would alter the nature of the bioethical issues. Because these tests have serious implications for the patient and others, scrupulous attention to informed consent must occur. The bioethical issues raised by genetic tests for somatic cell changes, such as tests that occur commonly in cancer diagnosis and risk stratification, are no different from the issues raised with the use of any laboratory or radiographic test.

In some cases, ethics consultation services may be of assistance in resolving bioethical dilemmas, although current data suggest that consultation services are used mainly for problems that arise in individual cases and are not used for more institutional or policy problems.

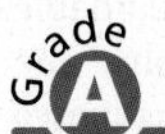

Grade A Reference

A1. Stacey D, Légaré F, Bennett CL, et al. Decision aids for people facing health treatment or screening decisions. *Cochrane Database Syst Rev.* 2014;1:CD001431.

GENERAL REFERENCES

For the General References and other additional features, please visit Expert Consult at https://expertconsult.inkling.com.

3 CARE OF DYING PATIENTS AND THEIR FAMILIES

ROBERT ARNOLD

By 2030, 20% of the U.S. population will be older than 65 years, and people older than 85 years constitute the fastest growing segment of the population. Owing to successes in public health and medicine, many of these people will live the last years of their lives with chronic medical conditions such as cirrhosis, end-stage kidney disease, heart failure, and dementia. Even human immunodeficiency virus (HIV) and many cancers, once considered terminal, have turned into chronic diseases.

The burden associated with these illnesses and their treatments is high. Chronically ill patients report multiple physical and psychological symptoms that lower their quality of life. The economic pressures associated with medical care adversely affect patients' socioeconomic status and cause family stress, especially among caregivers, who spend 20 or more hours a week helping their loved ones.

Palliative care, which was developed to decrease the burden associated with chronic illness, emphasizes patient- and family-centered care that optimizes quality of life by anticipating, preventing, and treating suffering. Palliative care throughout the continuum of illness addresses physical, intellectual, emotional, social, and spiritual needs while facilitating the patient's autonomy, access to information, and choice. Palliative care and services, which are coordinated by an interdisciplinary team, are available concurrently with or independent of curative or life-prolonging care. Palliative and nonpalliative health care providers should collaborate and communicate about care needs while focusing on peace and dignity throughout the course of illness, during the dying process, and after death.

Five points deserve special emphasis. First, palliative care can be delivered at any time during the course of an illness and is often provided concomitantly with disease-focused, life-prolonging therapy. Waiting until a patient is dying to provide palliative care is a serious error. For example, most elderly patients with chronic incurable illnesses, who might benefit from palliative care, are in the last 10 years of their lives but do not consider themselves to be dying. If palliative care is to have an impact on patients' lives, it should be provided earlier in a patient's illness, in tandem with other treatments.[A1] Second, prediction is an inexact science. Although many cancers have a predictable trajectory in the last 3 to 6 months of life, for most illnesses, doctors rarely can accurately predict whether a patient is in the last 6 months of life[1] (E-Fig. 3-1). Third, palliative care primarily focuses on the illness's burden rather than treating the illness itself. Because these burdens can be physical, psychological, spiritual, or social, good palliative care requires a multidisciplinary approach. Fourth, palliative care takes the family unit as the central focus of care. Treatment plans must be developed for both the patient and the family. Fifth, palliative care recognizes that medical treatments are not uniformly successful and that patients die. At some point in a patient's illness, the treatments may cause more burden than benefit. Palliative care recognizes this reality and starts with a discussion of the patient's goals and the development of an individualized treatment plan.

Many people confuse palliative care with hospice—an understandable confusion because hospices epitomize the palliative care philosophy. The two, however, are different. In the United States, hospice provides palliative care, primarily at home, for patients who have a life expectancy of 6 months or less and who are willing to forgo life-prolonging treatments. However, the requirement that patients must have a life expectancy of 6 months or less limits hospice's availability, as does the requirement that patients give up expensive and potentially life-prolonging treatments. Moreover, because doctors and patients often are unwilling to cease these treatments until very late in the disease course, so are most patients.

Palliative care is both a subspeciality and a domain of good internal medicine.[2] Given the need for palliative care, every clinician must be able to provide basic palliative care, and subspecialties such as oncology need special expertise.

PALLIATIVE CARE DOMAINS

Palliative care is a holistic discipline with physical, psychological, spiritual, existential, social, and ethical domains. When caring for patients with chronic life-limiting illness, good palliative care requires that the following questions be addressed:

Is the Patient Physically Comfortable?

Across many chronic conditions, patients have a large number of inadequately treated physical symptoms (Table 3-1). The reasons are multifactorial and range from inadequate physician education, to societal beliefs regarding the inevitability of suffering in chronic illness, to public concerns regarding opioids, to the lack of evidence-based treatments in noncancer patients.

The first step to improve symptom management is a thorough assessment. Standardized instruments such as the Brief Pain Inventory (Fig. 3-1) measure both the patient's symptoms and the effect of those symptoms on the patient's life. Use of standardized instruments assures that physicians will identify overlooked or underreported symptoms and, as a result, will enhance the satisfaction of both the patient and family.

The evidence for the treatment of end-stage symptoms continues to improve. The use of nonsteroidal anti-inflammatory agents and opioids[A2] can result in effective pain management in more than 75% of patients with cancer. Advances such as intrathecal pumps and neurolytic blocks are helpful in the remaining 25% (Chapter 30). The use of oxygen is not helpful for refractory dyspnea except when hypoxia has been documented[A3], whereas use of medications for depression often can be helpful[A4] (Chapter 397).

Is the Patient Psychologically Suffering?

Patients may be physically comfortable but still suffering. Psychological symptoms and syndromes such as depression, delirium, and anxiety are common in patients with life-limiting or chronic illnesses. It may be difficult to determine whether increased morbidity and mortality are caused by the physical effects of the illness or by the psychological effects of depression and anxiety on energy, appetite, or sleep. Screening questions focusing on mood (e.g., "Have you felt down, depressed, and hopeless most of the time for the past 2 weeks?") and anhedonism (e.g., "Have you found that little brings you pleasure or joy in the past 2 weeks?") have been shown to help in diagnosing depression in this population. Increasing data show that treatment of depression in chronic illness is possible and improves both morbidity and mortality.[A4-A6]

For patients and families facing mortality, existential and spiritual concerns are common. Progressive illness often raises questions of love, legacy, loss, and meaning. A physician's role is not to answer these questions or to provide reassurance, but rather to understand concerns of the patient and family, how they are coping, and what resources might help. Spirituality often is a source of comfort, and physicians can ascertain a patient's beliefs using a brief instrument such as the FICA Spiritual Assessment Tool (Table 3-2). A single screening question such as "Are you at peace?" may identify patients who are in spiritual distress and facilitate referrals to chaplains.

Is the Family Suffering?

Families, defined broadly as those individuals who care most for the patient, are an important source of support for most patients. Families provide informal caregiving, often at the expense of their own physical, economic, and psychological health. Good palliative care requires an understanding of how the family is coping and a search for ways to provide family members with the social or clinical resources they need to improve their well-being. Comprehensive and individually targeted interventions can reduce caregivers' burdens, although the absolute benefits are relatively small.

Because patients in palliative care often die, the palliative care team must address bereavement and postdeath family suffering. Good communication and informational brochures in an intensive care unit can decrease family members' adverse psychological outcomes after death.[A7] A letter of condolence or a follow-up phone call to the next of kin after a patient's death is respectful and offers the opportunity to clarify questions about the patient's care. Some family members suffer from complicated grief—a recently described syndrome associated with separation and traumatic distress, with symptoms persisting for more than 6 months. Primary care physicians, who have ongoing relationships with the loved one, and hospices, which provide bereavement services for a year after the patient's death, have the opportunity to assess whether the grief symptoms persist or worsen.

Is the Patient's Care Consistent with the Patient's Goals?

The sine qua non for palliative care is ensuring that the treatment plan is consistent with the patient's values. In one European cohort of elderly patients, most preferred longevity over quality of life, and half wanted resuscitation if necessary.[3] However, a large proportion of elderly, seriously ill patients are not focused on living as long as possible. Instead, they want to maintain a sense of control, relieve their symptoms, improve their quality of life, avoid being a burden on their families, and have a closer relationship with their loved ones.

Ensuring that treatment is consistent with a patient's goals requires good communication skills (Table 3-3). The approaches to giving bad news, discussing goals of care, and talking about forgoing life-sustaining treatment have similar structures (Table 3-4). First, the patient needs to understand the basic facts about the diagnosis, possible treatments, and prognosis. The communication skill that helps physicians communicate information is *Ask-Tell-Ask*—exploring what the patient knows or wants to know, then explaining or answering questions, and then providing an opportunity for the patient to ask more. In the hospital, where discontinuity of care is common and misunderstandings frequent, it is important to determine what the patient knows before providing information so as to keep everyone well coordinated. When giving bad news, knowing what the patient knows allows the physician to anticipate the patient's reaction. Finally, information must be titrated based on the patient's preferences. Although most patients want to hear everything about their disease, a minority do not. There is no foolproof way to ascertain what any patient wants to know other than by asking.

When giving patients information, it is important to give small pieces of information, not use jargon, and check the patient's understanding.[4] Giving information is like dosing a medication: one gives information, checks understanding, and then gives more information based on what the patient has heard.

After ensuring that the doctor and the patient have a shared understanding of the medical facts, the physician should engage in an open-ended conversation about the patient's goals as the disease progresses. This strategy requires that the patient be asked about both hopes and fears. One might ask: "What makes life worth living for you?" "If your time is limited, what are the things that are most important to achieve?" "What are your biggest fears or concerns?" "What would you consider to be a fate worse than death?" The clinician can use an understanding of these goals to make recommendations about which treatments to provide and which treatments would not be helpful. As a result, early palliative care can improve quality of life, mood, and even survival.

Physicians find talking about prognosis particularly difficult for two reasons: first, it is hard to foretell the future accurately; and second, they fear this information will "take away patients' hope." Thus, they often avoid talking to patients about these issues unless specifically asked. Although some patients do not want to hear prognostic information, for many patients, this

TABLE 3-1 APPROACHES TO THE MANAGEMENT OF PHYSICAL AND PSYCHOLOGICAL SYMPTOMS

SYMPTOM	ASSESSMENT	TREATMENT
Pain	How severe is the symptom (as assessed with the use of validated instruments) and how does it interfere with the patient's life? What is the etiology of the pain? Is the pain assumed to be neuropathic or somatic? What has the patient used in the past (calculate previous days' equal analgesic dose)?	Prescribe medications to be administered on a standing or regular basis if pain is frequent. For mild pain: use acetaminophen or a nonsteroidal anti-inflammatory agent (see Table 30-3). For moderate pain: titrate short-acting opioids (see Table 30-4). For severe pain: rapidly titrate short-acting opioids until pain is relieved or intolerable side effects develop; start long-acting opiates once pain is controlled. Rescue doses: prescribe immediate-release opioids—10% of the 24-hour total opiate every hour (orally) or every 30 minutes (parenterally) as needed. Concomitant analgesics (e.g., corticosteroids, anticonvulsants, tricyclic antidepressants, and bisphosphonates) should be used when applicable (particularly for neuropathic pain). Consider alternative medicine and interventional treatments for pain.
Constipation	Is the patient taking opioids? Does the patient have a fecal impaction?	Prescribe laxatives for all patients on opiates. If ineffective, add drugs from multiple classes (e.g., stimulant, osmotic laxatives, and enemas). Prescribe methylnaltrexone if still constipated.
Shortness of breath	Ask the patient to assess the severity of the shortness of breath. Does the symptom have reversible causes?	Prescribe oxygen to treat hypoxia-induced dyspnea, but *not* if the patient is not hypoxic. Opioids relieve breathlessness without measurable reductions in respiratory rate or oxygen saturation; effective doses are often lower than those used to treat pain. Aerosolized opiates do not work. Fans or cool air may work through a branch of the trigeminal nerve. Consider anxiolytics (e.g., low-dose benzodiazepines) and use reassurance, relaxation, distraction, and massage therapy.
Fatigue	Is the patient too tired to do activities of daily living? Is the fatigue secondary to depression? Is a disease process causing the symptom or is it secondary to reversible causes?	Provide cognitive education about conserving energy use. Treat underlying conditions appropriately.
Nausea	Which mechanism is causing the symptom (e.g., stimulation of the chemoreceptor trigger zone, gastric stimulation, delayed gastric emptying or "squashed stomach" syndrome, bowel obstruction, intracranial processes, or vestibular vertigo)? Is the patient constipated?	Prescribe an agent directed at the underlying cause (Chapter 132). If persistent, give antiemetic around the clock. Multiple agents directed at various receptors or mechanisms may be required.
Anorexia and cachexia	Is a disease process causing the symptom, or is it secondary to other symptoms (e.g., nausea and constipation) that can be treated? Is the patient troubled by the symptom or is the family worried about what not eating means?	A nutritionist may help find foods that are more appetizing (Chapter 213). Provide counseling about the prognostic implications of anorexia (Chapter 219).
Delirium	Is the confusion acute, over hours to days? Does consciousness wax and wane? Are there behavioral disturbances, marked by a reduced clarity in the patient's awareness of the environment, e.g., a problem of attention? Does the patient have disorganized thinking? Does the patient have an altered level of consciousness—either agitated or drowsy? Is there a reversible reason for the delirium? **D:** **D**rugs (opioids, anticholinergics, sedatives, benzodiazepines, steroids, chemotherapies and immunotherapies, some antibiotics) **E:** **E**yes and **E**ars (poor vision and hearing, isolation) **L:** **L**ow-flow states (hypoxia, myocardial infarction, congestive heart failure, chronic obstructive pulmonary disease, shock) **I:** **I**nfections **R:** **R**etention (urine/stool), **R**estraints **I:** **I**ntracranial (central nervous system metastases, seizures, subdural, cerebrovascular accident, hypertensive encephalopathy) **U:** **U**nderhydration, **U**ndernutrition, **U**ndersleep **M:** **M**etabolic disorders (sodium, glucose, thyroid, hepatic, deficiencies of vitamin B_{12}, folate, niacin, and thiamine) and toxic (lead, manganese, mercury, alcohol)	Identify underlying causes and manage symptoms (Chapter 28). Recommend behavioral therapies, including avoidance of excess stimulation, frequent reorientation, and reassurance. Ensure presence of family caregivers and explain delirium to them. Prescribe haloperidol, risperidone, or olanzapine.
Depression	Have you felt down, depressed, or hopeless most of the time during the past 2 weeks? Have you found that little brings you pleasure or joy during the past 2 weeks? (Somatic symptoms are not reliable indicators of depression in this population.)	Recommend supportive psychotherapy, cognitive approaches, behavioral techniques, pharmacologic therapies (see Table 397-5), or a combination of these interventions; prescribe psychostimulants for rapid treatment of symptoms (within days) or selective serotonin reuptake inhibitors, which may require 3 to 4 weeks to take effect; tricyclic antidepressants are relatively contraindicated because of their side effects.
Anxiety (applicable also for family members)	Does the patient exhibit restlessness, agitation, insomnia, hyperventilation, tachycardia, or excessive worry? Is the patient depressed? Is there a spiritual or existential concern underlying the anxiety?	Recommend supportive counseling and consider prescribing benzodiazepines.
Spiritual distress	Are you at peace?	Inquire about spiritual support.

Modified from Morrison RS, Meier DE. Palliative care. *N Engl J Med.* 2004;350:2582-2590.

information helps them plan their lives. Patients who are told that their disease is generally terminal are more likely to spend a longer period of time in hospice and to avoid aggressive technology at the end of life, without adverse psychological consequences. Furthermore, their families usually have fewer postdeath adverse psychological outcomes.

Given that one cannot guess how much information to provide, a physician can start these conversations by asking, "Are you the kind of person who wants to hear about what might happen in the future with your illness or would you rather take it day by day?" If the patient requests the latter, the physician can follow up by asking if there is someone else with whom he or she can talk about the prognosis. Second, before giving prognostic information, it is useful to inquire about the patient's concerns in order to provide information in the most useful manner. Finally, it is appropriate when discussing prognostic information to acknowledge uncertainty: "The course of this cancer can be quite unpredictable, and physicians don't have a crystal ball. I think you should be aware of the possibility that your health may

STUDY ID# ______ HOSPITAL ID# ______

DO NOT WRITE ABOVE THIS LINE

Brief Pain Inventory (Short Form)

Date: ___/___/___ Time: ____

Name: ______ Last ______ First ______ Middle Initial

1. Throughout our lives, most of us have had pain from time to time (such as minor headaches, sprains, and toothaches). Have you had pain other than these everyday kinds of pain today?

1. Yes 2. No

2. On the diagram, shade in the areas where you feel pain. Put an X on the area that hurts the most.

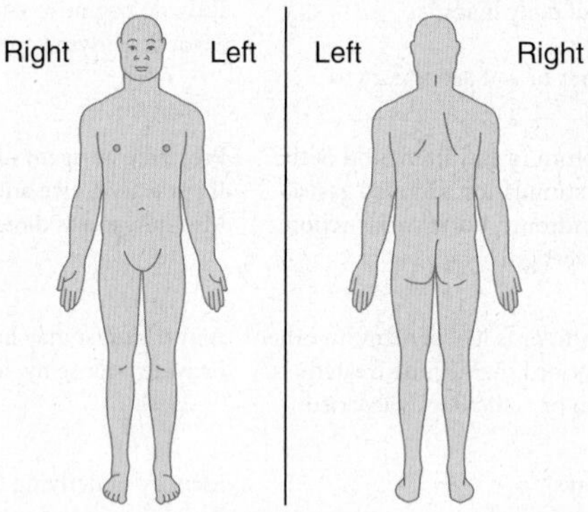

Right Left Left Right

3. Please rate your pain by circling the one number that best describes your pain at its worst in the last 24 hours.

0 No pain 1 2 3 4 5 6 7 8 9 10 Pain as bad as you can imagine

4. Please rate your pain by circling the one number that best describes your pain at its least in the last 24 hours.

0 No pain 1 2 3 4 5 6 7 8 9 10 Pain as bad as you can imagine

5. Please rate your pain by circling the one number that best describes your pain on the average.

0 No pain 1 2 3 4 5 6 7 8 9 10 Pain as bad as you can imagine

6. Please rate your pain by circling the one number that tells how much pain you have right now.

0 No pain 1 2 3 4 5 6 7 8 9 10 Pain as bad as you can imagine

FIGURE 3-1. Brief Pain Inventory (short form).

7. What treatments or medications are you receiving for your pain?

8. In the last 24 hours, how much relief have pain treatments or medications provided? Please circle the one percentage that shows how much relief you have received.

0% No pain	10%	20%	30%	40%	50%	60%	70%	80%	90%	100% Complete relief

9. Circle one number that describes how, during the past 24 hours, pain has interfered with your:

A. General Activity

0 Does not interfere	1	2	3	4	5	6	7	8	9	10 Completely interferes

B. Mood

0 Does not interfere	1	2	3	4	5	6	7	8	9	10 Completely interferes

C. Walking Ability

0 Does not interfere	1	2	3	4	5	6	7	8	9	10 Completely interferes

D. Normal Work (includes both work outside the home and housework)

0 Does not interfere	1	2	3	4	5	6	7	8	9	10 Completely interferes

E. Relations with Other People

0 Does not interfere	1	2	3	4	5	6	7	8	9	10 Completely interferes

F. Sleep

0 Does not interfere	1	2	3	4	5	6	7	8	9	10 Completely interferes

G. Enjoyment of Life

0 Does not interfere	1	2	3	4	5	6	7	8	9	10 Completely interferes

FIGURE 3-1, cont'd.

deteriorate quickly, and you should plan accordingly. We probably are dealing with weeks to months, although some patients do better, and some do worse. Over time, the course may become clearer, and if you wish, I may be able to be a little more precise about what we are facing."

The physician must discuss these topics in an empathic way. Palliative care conversations are as much about emotions as facts.[5] Talking about disease progression or death may elicit negative emotions such as anxiety, sadness, or frustration. These emotions decrease a patient's quality of life and interfere with the ability to hear factual information. Empathic responses strengthen the patient-physician relationship, increase the patient's satisfaction, and make the patient more likely to disclose other concerns. The first step is recognizing when the patient is expressing emotions. Once the physician recognizes the emotion being expressed, he or she can respond empathically.

It is also important for physicians to recognize their own emotional reactions to these conversations. The physician's emotional reactions color impressions of the patient's prognosis, thereby making it hard to listen to the patient, and may influence the physician to hedge bad news. The physician should become aware of her or his own emotional reactions to ensure that the conversation focuses on the patient rather than the health care provider's needs.

In addition to good communication skills, palliative care requires a basic knowledge of medical ethics and the law. For example, patients have the moral and legal right to refuse any treatment, even if refusal results in their death. There is no legal difference between withholding and withdrawing life-sustaining treatment. When confronted with areas of ambiguity, the physician should know how to obtain either a palliative care or ethics consultation.

TABLE 3-2 FICA SPIRITUAL ASSESSMENT TOOL

F—What is your **faith**/religion? Do you consider yourself a religious or spiritual person? What do you believe in that gives meaning/importance to life?
I—**Importance** and **influence** of faith. Is your faith/religion important to you? How do your beliefs influence how you take care of yourself? What are your most important hopes? What role do your beliefs play in regaining your health? What makes life most worth living for you? How might your disease affect this?
C—Are you part of a religious or spiritual **community**? Is this of support to you, and how? Is there a person you really love or is very important to you? How is your family handling your illness? What are their reactions/expectations?
A—How would you like me to **address** these issues in your health care? What might be left undone if you were to die today? Given the severity or chronicity of your illness, what is most important for you to achieve? Would you like me to talk to someone about religious/spiritual matters?

From Puchalski C, Romer A. Taking a spiritual history. *J Palliat Med.* 2000;3:129-137.

TABLE 3-3 CORE COMMUNICATION SKILLS

RECOMMENDED SKILL	EXAMPLE
A. IDENTIFYING CONCERNS AND RECOGNIZING CUES	
Elicit Concerns	
Open-ended questions	"Is there anything you wanted to talk to me about today?"
Active listening	Allowing patient to speak without interruption; allowing pauses to encourage patient to speak
Recognize Cues	
Informational concerns	Patient: "I'm not sure about the treatment options"
Emotional concerns	Patient: "I'm worried about that"
B. RESPONDING TO INFORMATIONAL CONCERNS	
"Ask-tell-ask"	Topic: communicating information about cancer stage
Ask	"Have any of the other doctors talked about what stage this cancer is?"
Tell	"That's right, this is a stage IV cancer, which is also called metastatic cancer…"
Ask	"Do you have questions about the staging?"
C. RESPONDING TO EMOTIONAL CONCERNS	
Nonverbal Empathy: S-O-L-E-R	
S	Face the patient **S**quarely
O	Adopt an **O**pen body posture
L	**L**ean toward the patient
E	Use **E**ye contact
R	Maintain a **R**elaxed body posture
Verbal Empathy: N-U-R-S-E	
N	**N**ame the emotion: "You seem worried"
U	**U**nderstand the emotion: "I see why you are concerned about this"
R	**R**espect the emotion: "You have shown a lot of strength"
S	**S**upport the patient: "I want you to know that I will still be your doctor whether you have chemotherapy or not"
E	**E**xplore the emotion: "Tell me more about what is worrying you"

From Back AL, Arnold RM, Tulsky JA. *Discussing Prognosis.* Alexandria, VA: American Society of Clinical Oncology; 2008.

During the past 10 years, there has been a societal push to encourage patients to designate health care proxies and to create advance care planning documents, typified by the use of living wills. These documents are meant to protect patients against unwanted treatments and to ensure that as they are dying, their wishes are followed.[6] Unfortunately, there are few empirical data showing that these documents actually change practice. Still, discussions of the documents with health professionals and family members generally provoke important conversations about end-of-life care decisions and may help families confronted with difficult situations know they are respecting their loved one's wishes.

TABLE 3-4 DISCUSSING PALLIATIVE CARE

GENERAL APPROACH
- Plan what to say. Create the right setting, allow adequate time, and determine who else should be present at the meeting.
- Listen carefully. Be prepared for strong emotions, respond empathetically, encourage description of feelings, and allow time for silence and response.

ESTABLISHING GOALS OF MEDICAL CARE
- Determine what the patient knows. Clarify any uncertainties or misconceptions.
- Understand what the patient is hoping to accomplish as well as any fears and worries.
- Repeat the goals back to the patient to make sure they are heard.
- Suggest treatments to meet these goals and clarify what will not be done because it will not help achieve the goals. Focus on the goals that you think you can achieve. Plan follow-up, review and revise plan as needed.

COMMUNICATING BAD NEWS
- Determine what the patient knows, wants to know, and can comprehend.
- Share information, recognizing that people handle information in different ways.
- Avoid jargon, pause frequently, check for understanding, and use silence.
- Recognize and support the patient's emotional reaction.
- Assess the patient's safety.
- Agree to a plan that enlists potential sources of support.

WITHDRAWING TREATMENT
- Discuss the context of the current discussion and what has changed to precipitate it.
- Review prior treatment goals and reassess their virtues.
- Discuss alternative treatments based on the new goals.
- Document a plan for forgoing treatment and share with the patient, the patient's family, and the health care team.

Adapted from Morrison RS, Meier DE. Clinical practice. Palliative care. *N Engl J Med.* 2004;350:2582-2590.

Is the Patient Going to Die in the Location of Choice?

Most patients say that they want to die at home. Unfortunately, most patients die in institutions—either hospitals or nursing homes. Burdensome transitions decrease quality in end-of-life care. Good palliative care requires establishing a regular system of communication to minimize transitional errors. A social worker who knows about community resources is important in the development of a dispositional plan that respects the patient's goals.

Hospice programs are an important way to allow patients to die at home. In the United States, *hospice* refers to a specific, government-regulated form of end-of-life care, available under Medicare since 1982 but subsequently adopted by Medicaid and many other third-party insurers. Hospice care typically is given at home, a nursing home, or specialized acute care unit. Care is provided by an interdisciplinary team, which usually includes a physician, nurse, social worker, chaplain, volunteers, bereavement coordinator, and home health aides, all of whom collaborate with the primary care physician, patient, and family. Bereavement services are offered to the family for a year after the death.

Hospices are paid on a per diem rate and are required to cover all the costs related to the patient's life-limiting illness. Because of this and the fact that their focus is on comfort rather than life prolongation, many hospices will not cover expensive treatments such as inotropic agents in heart failure or chemotherapy in cancer, even if they have a palliative effect. Many hospices are experimenting with different service models in an attempt to enroll patients earlier in the course of their illness and increase access to their services.

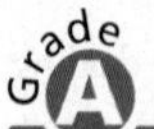

Grade A References

A1. Temel JS, Greer JA, Muzikansky A, et al. Early palliative care for patients with metastatic non-small-cell lung cancer. *N Engl J Med.* 2010;363:733-742.
A2. Michna E, Cheng WY, Korves C, et al. Systematic literature review and meta-analysis of the efficacy and safety of prescription opioids, including abuse-deterrent formulations, in non-cancer pain management. *Pain Med.* 2014;15:79-92.
A3. Abernethy AP, McDonald CF, Frith PA, et al. Effect of palliative oxygen versus room air in relief of breathlessness in patients with refractory dyspnoea: a double-blind, randomised controlled trial. *Lancet.* 2010;376:784-793.
A4. Laoutidis ZG, Mathiak K. Antidepressants in the treatment of depression/depressive symptoms in cancer patients: a systematic review and meta-analysis. *BMC Psychiatry.* 2013;13:140.
A5. Gallo JJ, Morales KH, Bogner HR, et al. Long term effect of depression care management on mortality in older adults: follow-up of cluster randomized clinical trial in primary care. *BMJ.* 2013;346:f2570.

A6. Jiang W, Krishnan R, Kuchibhatla M, et al. Characteristics of depression remission and its relation with cardiovascular outcome among patients with chronic heart failure (from the SADHART-CHF Study). *Am J Cardiol.* 2011;107:545-551.
A7. Lautrette A, Darmon M, Megarbane B, et al. A communication strategy and brochure for relatives of patients dying in the ICU. *N Engl J Med.* 2007;356:469-478.

GENERAL REFERENCES

For the General References and other additional features, please visit Expert Consult at https://expertconsult.inkling.com.

4

CULTURAL CONTEXT OF MEDICINE

VICTORIA M. TAYLOR

The 2010 U.S. Census counted about 39 million blacks or African Americans (13% of the population), nearly 15 million Asian Americans (5% of the population), about 3 million American Indians and Alaska Natives, and more than 500,000 Native Hawaiians and other Pacific Islanders. It also counted more than 50 million individuals of Hispanic or Latino origin (16% of the population). Approximately 40 million Americans (13% of the population) were foreign born. One in 2 immigrants to the United States have limited English proficiency (i.e., they do not speak English very well or fluently), and 1 in 10 immigrants do not speak English at all (Fig. 4-1).

During the past two decades, a large body of literature has documented substantial disparities in health status. Although some of these disparities are based on socioeconomic status, many are based on race, ethnicity, or other characteristics. Black men have a substantially higher age-adjusted incidence of prostate cancer than do white men (236 per 100,000 versus 147 per 100,000). American Indians/Alaska Natives are more than twice as likely as non-Latino whites of a similar age to have diabetes. More than half of the Americans who are living with chronic hepatitis B infection are Asians or Pacific Islanders. Lesbian, gay, bisexual, and transgender individuals have higher rates of suicidal behavior compared with heterosexual individuals. A major goal of Healthy People 2020 is to eliminate health disparities for preventable and treatable conditions such as cancer, diabetes, and human immunodeficiency virus infection.

Culture can be defined as a shared system of values, beliefs, and patterns of behavior, and it is not simply defined by race and ethnicity. Culture can also be shaped by factors such as country and region of origin, acculturation, language, religion, and sexual orientation. For instance, the black population of the northeastern United States includes individuals who moved from southern states decades ago as well as recent immigrants from Ethiopia. As the United States population becomes increasingly diverse and as pronounced differences in health status continue to be documented, consideration of the cultural context of medicine is becoming a national priority.

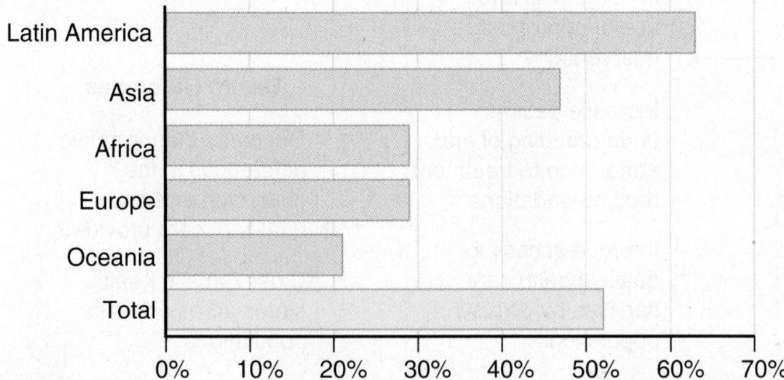

FIGURE 4-1. Proportion of immigrants aged 5 years and older with limited English proficiency by region of origin. (From Grieco EM, Acosta YD, de la Cruz P, et al. The foreign-born population in the United States: 2010. Washington DC: U.S. Department of Commerce; 2012.)

DISPARITIES IN HEALTH CARE ACCESS AND QUALITY

Components of health care access include the ability to get into the health care system as well as to obtain appropriate care once in the system. The availability of health care providers who meet an individual patient's needs is another key component of access to care. Quality care is based on scientific evidence (i.e., is effective), avoids injury to the patient (i.e., is safe), minimizes harmful delays (i.e., is timely), is responsive to the individual patient's needs (i.e., is patient centered), promotes communication among providers (i.e., is coordinated), does not vary because of personal characteristics (i.e., is equitable), and avoids waste (i.e., is efficient).

Access to Health Care

Racial and ethnic minority groups, particularly immigrants, disproportionately have problems accessing health care. Before the implementation of the Affordable Care Act, the proportions of Latinos and Native Americans/Alaska Natives who lacked health insurance was more than twice the proportion among non-Latino whites, and less than two thirds of Americans with limited English proficiency were insured. About 1 in 3 Korean American and Vietnamese American adults had no regular source of medical care compared with about 1 in 10 non-Latino white adults.

Blacks and Latinos are far less likely than are whites and Asians to have access to physicians of their own race and ethnicity. This imbalance is important because racial concordance between physicians and patients can improve the processes of care. For example, patients with race-concordant physicians are more likely to use needed health services, are less likely to postpone or delay seeking care, and are more satisfied with their care than are patients in race-discordant relationships. Whether these differences translate into different health outcomes, however, is less clear.[1]

Quality of Health Care

National surveys confirm population-level disparities in the quality of preventive care. Recent immigrants have far lower levels of interval screening for breast, cervical, and colorectal cancer than do individuals who were born in the United States (Fig. 4-2). The proportion of Native Hawaiians and other Pacific Islanders whose serum cholesterol levels are measured at least once every 5 years is significantly lower than among whites. In 2011, only 40% of Asians aged 65 years and older had ever received the pneumococcal vaccine compared with 67% of non-Latino whites.

Racial and ethnic disparities have been documented for a number of specific clinical situations. For example, Latino women with breast cancer are less likely to receive radiation therapy within a year of breast-conserving surgery than are white women, Native Americans and Alaska Natives are less likely than whites to receive recommended care such as initial antibiotics within 6 hours of hospital arrival, and blacks with end-stage renal disease

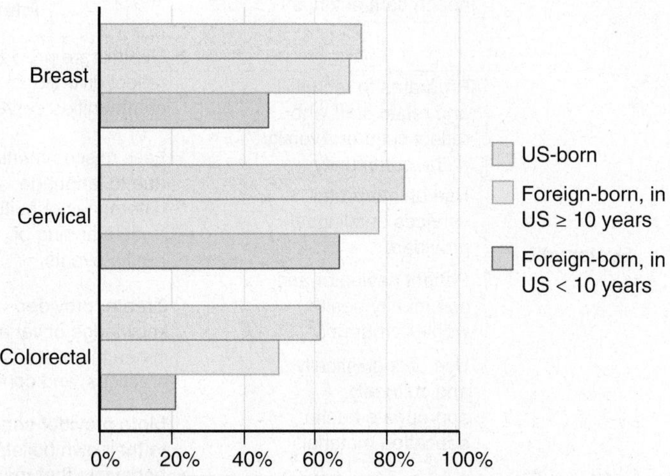

FIGURE 4-2. Adherence to cancer screening guidelines by immigration status. Breast = mammography during last 2 years among women aged 50 to 74 years. Cervical = Papanicolaou test during last 3 years among women aged 21 to 65 years. Colorectal = among individuals aged 50 to 75 years, fecal occult blood test last year; sigmoidoscopy last 5 years and fecal occult blood test last 3 years; or colonoscopy last 10 years. (From Centers for Disease Control and Prevention. Cancer screening—United States, 2010. *MMWR Morb Mortal Wkly Rep.* 2012; 61:41-45.)

are less likely to be entered to a transplant list than are whites. Moreover, disparities in the quality of care are found even when variations in insurance status, income, and comorbid conditions are taken into account.

Disparities in health care quality exist even in systems that are generally believed to provide equal access.[2] For example, in the Veterans Affairs Health System, disparities between blacks and whites have been documented for blood pressure control among patients with hypertension, cholesterol control among patients with coronary heart disease, and glucose control among patients with diabetes. Moreover, these disparities persist even after adjusting for location and socioeconomic status. Similar disparities have been documented in Medicare managed care programs between elderly blacks and whites with diabetes and cardiovascular disorders.

CULTURAL COMPETENCE IN HEALTH CARE

Health disparities can be reduced or perhaps even eliminated by maintaining culturally competent health care systems. Cultural competence may be defined as a set of congruent attitudes, behaviors, and policies that come together both among professionals and within systems to enable effective work in cross-cultural situations (Fig. 4-3). Ongoing efforts to improve cultural competence in the health care system target organizational, structural, and clinical barriers. These initiatives aim to close gaps in health status, to decrease differences in the quality of care, to enhance patients' satisfaction, and to increase patients' trust.

Organizational Barriers and Interventions

Diversity among health care professionals is associated with better access to care for disadvantaged populations. Black and Latino physicians are more likely than their white colleagues to work in medically underserved communities and to have a better understanding of barriers to health care. Because less than 10% of practicing physicians are black or Latino, and only about 15% of medical school students are from one of these groups, many U.S. medical schools have implemented comprehensive programs to infuse diversity among their students, resident physicians, and faculty.

About two thirds of the patients who receive care at federally funded community health centers in medically underserved areas are members of racial and ethnic minority groups. In these health centers, patients are three times more likely to have limited proficiency in English compared with the general population. The community health center model has proved effective not only in increasing access to care but also in improving continuity of care and health outcomes. For example, medically underserved communities with community health centers have fewer preventable hospitalizations and uninsured emergency department visits than do similar communities without health centers. Compared with national rates, community health centers report minimal racial and ethnic disparities in clinical outcomes such as the control of diabetes and hypertension.[3]

Structural Barriers and Interventions

Accumulating evidence suggests that trained professional interpreters can improve the clinical care received by individuals with limited English proficiency.[A1] However, interpreter services often remain ad hoc, with family members and untrained nonclinical employees acting as interpreters.[4] Use of ad hoc services has potentially negative clinical consequences, including breach of the patient's confidentiality and inaccurate communication. One major obstacle to the implementation of professional interpreter programs is a lack of reimbursement; Medicare and most private insurers do not pay for interpretation and related services, and most states do not pay for interpretation under Medicaid.

Assistance with navigation represents a promising model to enable racial and ethnic minority patients to move through the health system effectively and to be actively involved in decision making about their medical care.[5] Guides may be nurses, social workers, or volunteers who are familiar with the health care system. They help patients and their families navigate the treatment process, steering them around obstacles that may limit their access to quality care, choice of doctors, and access to treatment options. For example, an American Cancer Society navigation program is effective in reducing the time to diagnostic resolution after abnormal cancer screening tests in medically underserved patients.[A2]

Another option for closing the gap in health care among various minority populations is community health workers.[6] In general, community health workers live locally and share the language and culture of the patients being served. Lay community health workers provide cultural mediation between communities and the health care system; culturally appropriate and accessible health education and information; help in obtaining needed medical services, informal counseling, and social support; and advocacy within the health care system. The effectiveness of community health workers is documented by a study in which Mexican American women randomized to

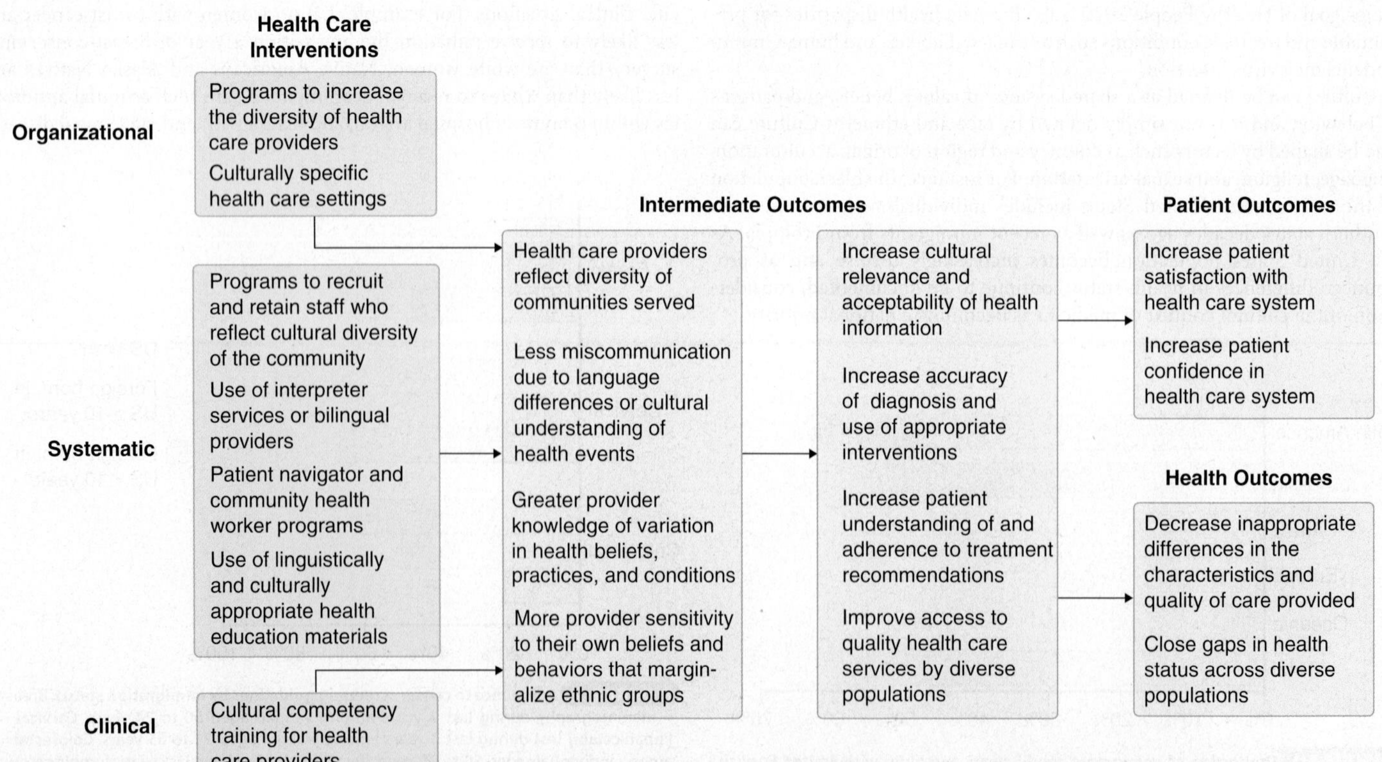

FIGURE 4-3. **Analytic framework for evaluating the effectiveness of health care interventions to increase cultural competence.** (From Anderson LM, Scrimshaw SC, Fullilove MT, et al., for the Task Force on Community Preventive Services. Culturally competent healthcare systems: a systemic review. *Am J Prev Med.* 2003; 24[suppl]:68-79.)

receive health worker education were significantly more likely to obtain Papanicolaou tests than were women randomized to receive usual care.[A3] The largest formal system of community health workers is the Indian Health Service, which currently has about 1400 community health representatives.

Clinical Barriers and Interventions

Patients who are members of racial and ethnic minority groups often understand health and disease (i.e., explanatory model) differently than the general population. For example, many Vietnamese people believe that disease is caused by an imbalance of the humoral forces of yin and yang. When ill, they commonly use Chinese herbal medicine as well as indigenous folk practices known as Southern medicine in an effort to restore the balance of humoral forces. In addition, Vietnamese patients may think that Western medicine is too strong and will upset the internal balance. Consequently, a hypertensive Vietnamese patient may, for example, use Chinese herbal medicines instead of prescribed antihypertensive medication. Alternatively, the patient may take a lower dose of medication than prescribed by his or her physician.

Cultural competency training for health care providers generally includes teaching cross-cultural knowledge and communication skills, while avoiding stereotypes.[7] Examples include the effect of prejudice on gays and lesbians and how this prejudice shapes their interactions with the health care system, and common spiritual practices that might interfere with prescribed therapies (such as Ramadan fasting practices, when observed by diabetic Muslim patients). Communication skills that can be addressed in cultural competence training include approaches to eliciting patients' explanatory models and use of traditional treatments, as well as methods for negotiating different styles of communication and levels of family participation in decision-making. Cultural competency training improves the attitudes and skills of health professionals as well as patient satisfaction, but there is less evidence that it improves clinical outcomes.[A4]

SUMMARY

Individual clinical practices should regularly assess their current organizational climate, policies, and training related to diversity. Practices can address health disparities by hiring clinical and office staff who are representative of the communities they serve, by routinely using professional interpreters during clinical encounters with patients who have limited proficiency with English, by offering cultural competency education and training to physicians and staff, and by providing educational and informational materials that are culturally and linguistically appropriate for their patient populations.[8]

National and state efforts to improve cultural competence in health care, whether used alone or in conjunction with socioeconomic initiatives, are likely to play a significant role in reducing health disparities across population subgroups. An important goal of the Affordable Care Act is to reduce health disparities by expanding health insurance coverage, addressing diversity in the health care workforce, increasing the capacity of community health centers, and promoting the use of patient navigators and community health workers.

Grade A References

A1. Bagchi AD, Dale S, Verbitsky-Savitz N, et al. Examining effectiveness of medical interpreters in emergency departments for Spanish-speaking patients with limited English proficiency: results of a randomized controlled trial. *Ann Emerg Med*. 2011;57:248-256.

A2. Paskett ED, Katz ML, Post DM, et al. The Ohio Patient Navigation Research Program: does the American Cancer Society patient navigation model improve time to resolution in patients with abnormal screening tests? *Cancer Epidemiol Biomarkers Prev*. 2012;21:1620-1628.

A3. Byrd TL, Wilson KM, Smith JL, et al. AMIGAS: a multicity, multicomponent cervical cancer prevention trial among Mexican American women. *Cancer*. 2013;119:1365-1372.

A4. Sequist TD, Fitzmaurice GM, Marshall R, et al. Cultural competency training and performance reports to improve diabetes care for black patients: a cluster randomized, controlled trial. *Ann Intern Med*. 2010;152:40-46.

GENERAL REFERENCES

For the General References and other additional features, please visit Expert Consult at https://expertconsult.inkling.com.

5 SOCIOECONOMIC ISSUES IN MEDICINE

STEVEN A. SCHROEDER

All nations—rich and poor—struggle with how to improve the health of the public, obtain the most value from medical services, and restrain rising health care expenditures. Many developed countries also wrestle with the paradox that their citizens have never been so healthy or so unhappy with their medical care. Despite the reality that only about 10% of premature deaths result from inadequate medical care, the bulk of professional and political attention focuses on how to obtain and pay for state-of-the-art medical care. By comparison, 40% of premature deaths stem from unhealthy behaviors—including smoking (about 44%; Chapter 32), excessive or unwise drinking (about 11%; Chapter 33), obesity and insufficient physical activity (about 15% but estimated to rise substantially in the years to come; Chapters 16 and 220), illicit drug use (about 2%; Chapter 34), and imprudent sexual behavior (about 3%; Chapter 285). Genetics (Chapter 40) account for an additional 30%; social factors—discussed next—account for 15%, and environmental factors (Chapter 19) account for 5%. Of the major behavioral causes of premature deaths, tobacco use (Chapter 32) is by far the most important, although recent increases in obesity (Chapter 220) and physical inactivity (Chapter 16) are also alarming. Health is influenced by genetic predisposition, behavioral patterns, environmental exposures, social circumstances, and health care.

SOCIAL STATUS INFLUENCES HEALTH

Socioeconomic status, or class, is a composite of many different factors, including income, net wealth, education, occupation, and neighborhood. In general, people in lower classes are less healthy and die earlier than people at higher socioeconomic levels, a pattern that holds true in a stepwise fashion from the poorest to the richest. In the United States, the association between health and class is usually discussed in terms of racial and ethnic disparities; but in fact, race and class are independently associated with health status, and it can be argued that class is the more important factor. For example, U.S. racial disparities in the prevalence of adult smoking are relatively small among whites, blacks, and Hispanic Americans, whereas there are huge differences among smoking rates by educational level (Fig. 5-1).[1] U.S. physicians have reduced their smoking prevalence to a record low of only 1%. Although both smoking rates and the numbers of cigarettes smoked by those who continue to smoke are gradually declining (Fig. 5-2), more than 43 million Americans and millions more elsewhere continue to smoke.[2] Because people of higher socioeconomic status adopt health-promoting behaviors at a faster rate than people of lower socioeconomic status, overall population health can increase while health disparities also widen (Fig. 5-3).

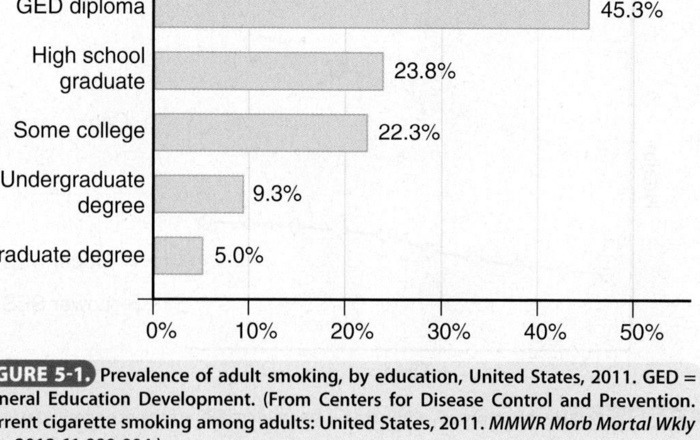

FIGURE 5-1. Prevalence of adult smoking, by education, United States, 2011. GED = General Education Development. (From Centers for Disease Control and Prevention. Current cigarette smoking among adults: United States, 2011. *MMWR Morb Mortal Wkly Rep*. 2012;61:889-894.)

In part, the relationship between class and health is mediated by higher rates of unhealthy behaviors among the poor, such as the inverse relationship between educational attainment and cigarette smoking, but unhealthy behaviors do not fully explain the poor health of those in the lower socioeconomic classes. Even when such behaviors are held constant, people in lower socioeconomic classes are much more likely to die prematurely than are people of higher classes. Of interest is that first-generation immigrants to the United States appear to be more protected from the adverse health consequences of low socioeconomic status than are subsequent generations.

It is unclear which of the components of class—education, wealth (either absolute wealth or the extent of the gap between rich and poor), occupation, or neighborhood—makes the greatest impact on a person's health. Most likely, it is a combination of all of them. For example, the constant stress of a lower class existence—lack of control over one's life circumstances, social isolation, and the anxiety derived from the feeling of having low status—is linked to poor health. This stress may trigger a variety of neuroendocrinologic responses that are useful for short-term adaptation but bring long-term adverse health consequences.

What can clinicians do with this knowledge? Clearly, it is difficult to write prescriptions for more income, a better education, good neighborhoods, or high-paying jobs. Physicians can, however, encourage healthy behavior. At key times of transition, such as during discharge planning for hospitalized patients, clinicians should be attentive to social circumstances. For patients who are likely to be socially isolated, clinicians should encourage or arrange interactions with family, neighbors, religious organizations, or community agencies to improve the likelihood of optimal outcomes. Access points to vital social services, such as child care, disability insurance, and food supplementation, can be provided in clinical settings.[3] In addition, physicians should seek to identify and eliminate any aspects of racism in health care institutions (Chapter 4). Finally, in their role as social advocates, physicians can promote such goals as safe neighborhoods, improved schools, and access to quality health care.

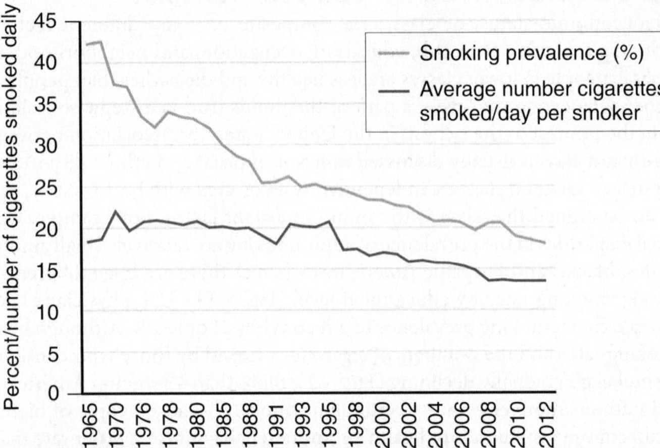

FIGURE 5-2. Smoking prevalence and average number of cigarettes smoked per day per current smoker. (Data based on Centers for Disease Control and Prevention (CDC). Smoking prevalence, 1965-2010. *MMWR Morb Mortal Wkly.* 2011;60:109-113; Current cigarette smoking in the United States: current estimate. CDC; http://www.cdc.gov/tobacco/data_statistics/fact_sheets/adult_data/cig_smoking. Accessed February 10, 2015; National Health Interview Survery. CDC; http://www.cdc.gov/nchs/nhis/quest_data_related_1997_forward.htm. Accessed February 10, 2015; Jamal A, Agaku IT, O'Connor E, et al. Current cigarette smoking among adults—United States, 2005-2013. *MMWR Morb Mortal Wkly.* 2014;63:1108-1112.)

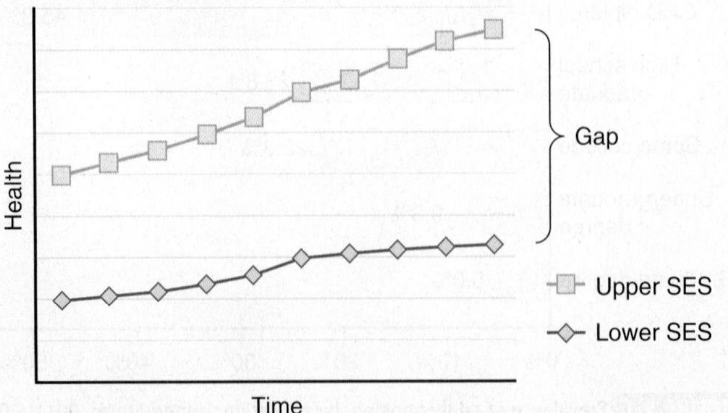

FIGURE 5-3. Health improves while disparities widen. SES = socioeconomic status.

ECONOMIC ISSUES IN MEDICAL CARE

Medical care today is on a collision course. On the one hand, an ever-expanding science base continuously generates new technologies and drugs that promise a longer and healthier life. Add a public eager to obtain the latest breakthroughs touted in the media and over the Internet, plus a well-stocked medical industry eager to meet that demand, and it is easy to understand why expenditures continue to soar. On the other hand, payers for medical care—health insurance companies, government (federal, state, and local), and employers—increasingly bridle at medical care costs.

The United States continues to lead the world in health care expenditures.[4] In 2011, it spent more than $2.7 trillion, amounting to 17.9% of the gross domestic product. Most policy analysts contend that this rate of increase in medical care expenditures is unsustainable, but this claim has been made for many years. A potent combination of supply and demand factors explains why the United States spends so much.[5] On the supply side, the United States far exceeds other countries in the availability and use of expensive diagnostic technologies, such as magnetic resonance imaging and computed tomography. For example, the United States has four times as many magnetic resonance imaging machines per capita as does Canada. Similar patterns exist for therapeutic technologies, whether coronary angioplasty, cancer chemotherapy, or joint prostheses. The differences are especially dramatic in older patients. Other supply factors that drive high medical expenditures in the United States include a fee-for-service payment system that compensates physicians much more when they use expensive technologies than when they do not[6]; a medical professional work force that earns much higher incomes relative to the population than in other nations and that emphasizes specialist rather than generalist practice; accelerated development of new and costly medications that are directly marketed to consumers; much higher administrative costs; higher rates of fraud and abuse; and a high rate of defensive medicine in response to pervasive fears about medical malpractice suits. Supply factors that do not appear to be unique to the United States are the number of physicians or hospitals. Many other developed countries have a much larger physician work force relative to their population, as well as a much higher ratio of primary care physicians to specialists. The number of hospitals and hospital beds, the frequency of hospitalizations, and the length of hospital stay are relatively low in the United States, although it does have a much greater proportion of intensive care beds. Finally, recent analyses suggest that a principal driver of high expenditures on health care in the United States is the much greater price charged per unit of service compared with other developed countries.

Demand factors also drive medical expenditures. The extent to which the media and the medical profession feature medical "breakthroughs" is extensive and one-sided. New promising treatments merit front-page stories and commercial advertisements, whereas subsequent disappointing results are buried or ignored. The cumulative result is to whet patients' appetite for more and to leave the impression that good health depends only on finding the right treatment. This same quest explains the popularity of alternative medicine, for which patients are willing to spend $34 billion annually out of their own pockets (Chapter 39). The cumulative impact of these supply and demand drivers is that there are incentives to do more at every step of the American medical system.[5]

It could be argued that rising expenditures for medical care are not a bad thing. What could be more important than ensuring maximal health? There are several rebuttals to that argument. First, it is not clear that money spent on medical care brings appropriate value in the United States, given that its health statistics are worse than those of virtually every other developed country. Second, there are substantial regional differences in the supply and use of medical care, such as a two-fold difference in the supply of acute hospital beds and a four-fold difference in the risk of being hospitalized in an intensive care unit at the end of life. Similar regional differences exist for procedures such as transurethral prostatectomy, hysterectomy, and coronary artery bypass surgery. Yet there is no evidence that "more is better" on a regional basis.

Consequently, rising health care expenditures are stressing public programs such as Medicare, Medicaid, the Veterans Administration health system, and municipal hospitals, with budget requests outstripping the tax base to pay for them. Medical debt is by far the most important cause of bankruptcy. Finally, as health care becomes less affordable for businesses and government, the number of people without health insurance will continue to increase.

Cost-Containment Strategies

Since the mid-1970s, a variety of strategies to contain rising medical expenditures have yielded limited success.[5] These attempts have tried to restrict the supply of costly medical technologies as well as the production of physicians, especially specialists; to promote health maintenance organizations that have incentives to spend less on medical care; to ration indirectly by limiting health insurance coverage; to institute prospective payment for hospital care; to use capitation payments or discounted fee schedules for physician reimbursement; to introduce gatekeeper mechanisms to reduce access to costly care; to put patients at more financial risk for their own medical care; to reform malpractice procedures; to reduce administrative costs; and to encourage less aggressive care at the end of life. The most recent suggestions—comparative effectiveness research to curtail the use of unnecessary technology, electronic medical records to avoid duplication of tests, payment for performance, accountable care organizations that change payment incentives—all hold promise to improve quality, but their potential for substantial cost reduction is only theoretical at present.

Recently, however, the rate of increase in health care expenditures has slowed relative to the gross domestic product.[7] Two basic hypotheses have been offered: the recession that began in 2008, and heightened cost consciousness among hospitals, health insurers, and some physician groups.

Payment for medical care varies by country. In the United States, health insurance coverage is an incomplete patchwork, consisting of government-sponsored programs for elderly people (Medicare), poor people (Medicaid), and veterans, plus employer-based coverage for workers and their families. Medicare covers acute care services in the hospital and in physicians' offices but has limited coverage for prescription drugs and long-term care. More than half of all Medicare subscribers also buy supplemental insurance. Medicaid covers more services than Medicare does, but Medicaid payments to physicians and hospitals are so low in many states that patients have restricted access to care. At any given time, more than 44 million Americans have lacked health insurance, and 70 million have been without insurance at some point during the year. In addition, millions of immigrant workers are also uninsured. The lack of health insurance contributes to poor health, such as delayed diagnosis and undertreatment of asthma, diabetes, hypertension, and cancer.

The 2010 Patient Protection and Affordable Care Act (ACA) contains numerous insurance reform features that took effect in 2010 and 2011, as well as coverage expansions that began in 2014.[8] The ACA was originally expected to cover 32 million previously uninsured Americans, with about half enrolling in subsidized private insurance plans and half in expanded state Medicaid programs. However, a 2012 Supreme Court decision gave states the choice of opting out of the Medicaid expansion. As a result, only 27 states plus the District of Columbia accepted that expansion. States that opted out of Medicaid expansion, such as Texas, tend to be those with the highest proportion of uninsured—mainly poor—people. In addition, various coverage components, especially regarding contraception, continue to be litigated. Revenue-generating provisions of the ACA are split about evenly between spending reductions and cost containment. In contrast to what happened after the passage of Medicare and Medicaid, the ACA continues to be highly controversial politically, and thus subject to potential changes, depending on election results.

Because medical care is both so valued and so expensive, physicians everywhere will inevitably become more involved in issues of medical economics. As cost-containment pressures force patients to assume more of their medical expenses, patients will become more aware of costs and more demanding about the price and value of care. In addition, knowledge will continue to accumulate about the real and potential harm from unnecessary or marginally useful medical services. Thus, informed clinical decision making will require that physicians have accurate information about the risks, benefits, and costs of medical care and better ways to communicate what is known and what is not.

GENERAL REFERENCES

For the General References and other additional features, please visit Expert Consult at https://expertconsult.inkling.com.

6

GLOBAL HEALTH

ARUN CHOCKALINGAM

Health is a human right, but more than 2 billion people live with a daily income of less than $2 and have no access to good health care. Health is determined by the context of people's lives. Individuals are unable to control many of the social determinants of health (Chapter 5), such as income and social status, education, physical environment, social support network, genetics, health services, and gender.[1]

In the process of modernization from a less developed to a more developed nation, the epidemiologic transition of modern sanitation, medications, and health care has drastically reduced infant and maternal mortality rates and extended average life expectancy. As a result, the world has progressed from the age of pestilence and famine, with a life expectancy between 20 and 40 years, to the age of receding pandemics, with a life expectancy of 30 to 50 years, and now to the current age of degenerative and man-made diseases, with a life expectancy of 60 years or more.

These trends, coupled with subsequent declines in fertility rates, have driven a demographic transition in which the major causes of death change from infectious diseases to chronic and degenerative diseases.[2] As many countries around the world have undergone globalization, owing to their internal urbanization, modernization, and economic development, an increased proportion of their burden of morbidity and mortality is now due to chronic noncommunicable diseases, including cardiovascular, cerebrovascular, and renovascular diseases as well as cancer, diabetes, chronic respiratory diseases, and mental disorders (Table 6-1).

WHAT IS GLOBAL HEALTH?

The term *global health* is sometimes confused with public health, international health, tropical medicine, and population health. Global health, which is defined as the health of populations in a global context, transcends the perspectives and concerns of individual nations and crosses national borders. Global health depends on the public health efforts and institutions of all countries, including their strategies for improving health, both population-wide and for individuals. Global health depends on multiple factors, including social, political, environmental, and economic determinants of health. Although global health often focuses on improving the health of people who live in low- and middle-income countries, it also includes the health of any marginalized population in any country.

Global health requires use of a wide range of institutions that collaborate in addressing all health issues. Global health also depends on the constructive use of evidence-based information to provide health and health equity, in part by strengthening primary health care and the health care delivery system.

Millennium Development Goals

In an attempt to address global inequity, the United Nations advanced eight millennium development goals with the objective of achieving these goals between 2000 and 2015. These eight goals incorporate 21 targets (Table 6-2), with a series of measurable health and economic indicators for each target.[3] Although many of the targets have not yet been achieved, substantial progress has been made toward all targets.

The millennium development goals emphasize that health and development are interconnected. To address global inequity, fundamental issues include reducing poverty, improving education, and empowering people. In addition to specific goals for reducing infant and child mortality, maternal mortality, and mortality due to infectious diseases such as human immunodeficiency virus infection/acquired immunodeficiency syndrome (HIV/AIDS), malaria, and tuberculosis, the millennium development goals strongly encourage environmental sustainability and global partnership.

GLOBAL BURDEN OF DISEASES

The global burden of disease is measured in terms of total and cause-specific mortality and morbidity as well as the national economic burden for health care. The Global Burden of Diseases, Injuries and Risk Factors Study 2010[4] shows that an estimated 53 million people died from all causes in 2010, with

TABLE 6-1 EPIDEMIOLOGIC TRANSITION IN CARDIOVASCULAR DISEASES

STAGES OF DEVELOPMENT	LIFE EXPECTANCY	BURDEN OF CARDIOVASCULAR DISEASE DEATHS, % OF TOTAL DEATHS	PREDOMINANT CARDIOVASCULAR DISEASES AND RISK FACTORS	MODERN REGIONAL EXAMPLES
1. Age of pestilence and famine	20-40 years	5-10	Infections, rheumatic heart disease, and nutritional cardiomyopathies	Rural India, sub-Saharan Africa, South America
2. Age of receding pandemics	30-50 years	10-35	As above plus hypertensive heart disease and hemorrhagic strokes	China
3. Age of degenerative and man-made diseases	50->60 years	35-65	All forms of strokes; ischemic heart disease at young ages; increasing obesity and diabetes	Aboriginal communities, urban India, former socialist economies
3A. Age of delayed degenerative diseases	>60 years	<50	Stroke and ischemic heart disease at old age	Western Europe, North America, Australia, New Zealand
3B. Age of health regression and social upheaval	50-60 years	35-55	Re-emergence of deaths from rheumatic heart disease, infections, increased alcoholism and violence; increase in ischemic and hypertensive diseases in the young	Russia

During stages 1 to 3A, life expectancy increases, whereas life expectancy decreases in stage 3B compared with stage 3A and even stage 3.
Modified from Omran AR. The epidemiological transition: a theory of the epidemiology of population change. *The Milbank Quarterly*. 2005;83:731-757. Reprinted from *The Milbank Memorial Fund Quarterly*. 1971;49:509-538; and Yusuf S, Reddy S, Ounpuu S, et al. Global burden of cardiovascular diseases: part I: general considerations, the epidemiologic transition, risk factors, and impact of urbanization. *Circulation*. 2001;104:2746-2753.

TABLE 6-2 MILLENNIUM DEVELOPMENT GOALS AND TARGETS (2000-2015)

GOAL 1: ERADICATE EXTREME POVERTY AND HUNGER

Target 1A: Halve, between 1990 and 2015, the proportion of people living on less than $1.25 a day.
Target 1B: Achieve decent employment for women, men, and young people.
Target 1C: Halve, between 1990 and 2015, the proportion of people who suffer from hunger.

GOAL 2: ACHIEVE UNIVERSAL PRIMARY EDUCATION

Target 2A: By 2015, all children (girls and boys) can complete a full course of primary schooling.

GOAL 3: PROMOTE GENDER EQUALITY AND EMPOWER WOMEN

Target 3A: Eliminate gender disparity in primary and secondary education preferably by 2005, and at all levels by 2015.

GOAL 4: REDUCE CHILD MORTALITY RATES

Target 4A: Reduce by two thirds, between 1990 and 2015, the under-five mortality rate.

GOAL 5: IMPROVE MATERNAL HEALTH

Target 5A: Reduce by three quarters, between 1990 and 2015, the maternal mortality ratio.
Target 5B: Achieve, by 2015, universal access to reproductive health.

GOAL 6: COMBAT HIV/AIDS, MALARIA, AND OTHER DISEASES

Target 6A: Have halted by 2015 and begun to reverse the spread of HIV/AIDS.
Target 6B: Achieve, by 2010, universal access to treatment for HIV/AIDS for all those who need it.
Target 6C: Have halted by 2015 and begun to reverse the incidence of malaria and other major diseases.

GOAL 7: ENSURE ENVIRONMENTAL SUSTAINABILITY

Target 7A: Integrate the principles of sustainable development into country policies and programs; reverse loss of environmental resources.
Target 7B: Reduce biodiversity loss, achieving, by 2010, a significant reduction in the rate of loss.
Target 7C: Halve, by 2015, the proportion of the population without sustainable access to safe drinking water and basic sanitation.
Target 7D: By 2020, to have achieved a significant improvement in the lives of at least 100 million slum-dwellers.

GOAL 8: DEVELOP A GLOBAL PARTNERSHIP FOR DEVELOPMENT

Target 8A: Develop further an open, rule-based, predictable, non-discriminatory trading and financial system.
Target 8B: Address the special needs of the least developed countries.
Target 8C: Address the special needs of landlocked developing countries and Small Island developing States.
Target 8D: Deal comprehensively with the debt problems of developing countries through national and international measures in order to make debt sustainable in the long term.
Target 8E: In cooperation with pharmaceutical companies, provide access to affordable, essential drugs in developing countries.
Target 8F: In cooperation with the private sector, make available the benefits of new technologies, especially information and communications.

From United Nations Millennium Development Goals. http://www.un.org/millenniumgoals/poverty.shtml. 2008. Accessed January 21, 2015.

13.2 million (25%) deaths due to communicable, maternal, neonatal, and nutritional disorders; 34.5 million (65%) due to noncommunicable diseases; and 5.1 million (10%) due to injuries (Table 6-3).[5] Although overall deaths between 1990 and 2010 increased by 13.5%, medical and public health advancements reduced deaths from communicable diseases by 17%, whereas deaths due to noncommunicable disease increased by 30% and deaths due to injury, including war-related deaths, increased by 24%.

CHANGING PATTERNS OF DISEASES

Despite the general trends of declining morbidity and mortality from communicable diseases, parts of Africa, Asia, and Latin America are still facing the challenges of infectious diseases, such as HIV infection, malaria, and tuberculosis, even as their prevalence of chronic noncommunicable diseases has risen—a so-called double burden. Concerted global health efforts and public awareness as well as investments by industrialized countries, multilateral agencies, and nongovernmental organizations have resulted in significant progress against HIV/AIDS (Chapter 384). Despite all of these efforts, however, the worldwide mortality due to HIV/AIDS and tuberculosis rose by 50% in 2010 compared with 1990 (Table 6-3). Although malaria deaths have fallen worldwide during the last decade, malaria is a rising threat in parts of Southeast Asia—especially Cambodia, Myanmar, Thailand, and Vietnam—where drug resistance to antimalaria medications is a problem.

TABLE 6-3 GLOBAL DEATHS IN 1990 AND 2010 FOR ALL AGES AND BOTH SEXES COMBINED

CAUSES OF DEATH	ALL AGES—DEATHS (THOUSANDS) 1990	2010	% CHANGE
All causes	46,511	52,769	+13
Communicable, maternal, neonatal, and nutritional disorders	15,859	13,156	−17
HIV/AIDS and tuberculosis	1770	2661	+50
Diarrhea, lower respiratory infection, and other common IDs	7772	5277	−32
Neglected tropical diseases and malaria	1211	1322	+ 9
Maternal disorders	359	255	−29
Neonatal disorders	3081	2236	−42
Nutritional deficiencies	977	684	−30
Other communicable, maternal, neonatal, and nutritional disorders	690	721	+5
Noncommunicable diseases	26,560	34,540	+30
Neoplasm	5779	7978	+38
Cardiovascular and circulatory diseases	11,903	15,616	+31
Chronic respiratory diseases	3986	3776	−5
Cirrhosis of the liver	778	1031	+33
Digestive diseases (except cirrhosis)	973	1112	+14
Neurologic disorders	595	1274	+14
Mental and behavioral disorders	138	231	+68
Diabetes, urogenital, blood, and endocrine diseases	1544	2726	+77
Musculoskeletal disorders	70	154	+121
Other noncommunicable diseases	794	642	−19
Injuries	4092	5073	+24
Transport injuries	958	1397	+46
Unintentional injuries other than transport injuries	2030	2123	+5
Self-harm and interpersonal violence	1009	1340	+33
Forces of nature, war, and legal intervention	95	214	+125

HIV/AIDS = human immunodeficiency virus infection/acquired immunodeficiency syndrome; ID = infectious diseases.
From Lozano R, Naghavi M, Foreman K, et al. Global and regional mortality from 235 causes of death for 20 age groups in 1990 and 2010: a systematic analysis for the Global Burden of Disease Study 2010. *Lancet.* 2012;380:2095-2128.

Noncommunicable diseases account for nearly two thirds of the global burden of disease. Nearly 80% of all noncommunicable diseases related to death and disability occur in the low- and middle-income countries, where they account for about 14 million deaths in people younger than 60 years. The prevention and control of noncommunicable diseases should involve both upstream and downstream approaches, such as social determinants; national and international policies regarding trade, agriculture, transportation, and environmental and other policies; health care, including accessibility, availability, and affordability; and settings, such as schools and worksites, where health promotion and disease prevention are targeted, as well as media by which health can be influenced.

Among noncommunicable diseases, cardiovascular diseases account for the largest burden of disease. One of the major worldwide risk factors for cardiovascular disease is hypertension (Chapter 67), which has an estimated prevalence of 35% to 45% of the global population—more than 2 billion people older than 25 years. The prevalence of hypertension is highest in Africa, where it is about 45% for both sexes, and lowest in the Americas, where it is about 35% for both sexes (Fig. 6-1). In all regions, men have a slightly higher prevalence of hypertension than do women. Despite significant efforts by global nongovernmental organizations and the World Health Organization, more than 50% of the world's population with hypertension does not even know their condition, and the percentage treated and controlled varies from less than 5% in Zambia to 66% in Canada.

As noncommunicable diseases have reached an epidemic proportion, all 192 United Nations Member States agreed to address their prevention and control worldwide, particularly in developing countries. The emphasis is on four major noncommunicable diseases (cardiovascular diseases, cancer, diabetes, and chronic respiratory diseases) and four key risk factors common to all four of these noncommunicable diseases (tobacco use, unhealthy diets, physical inactivity, and harmful use of alcohol). The World Health Organization developed a global monitoring framework to enable global tracking of progress in preventing and controlling these four major noncommunicable diseases and their key risk factors, aiming for a 25% reduction by 2025—with a slogan of *25 By 25*.[6]

Noncommunicable diseases represent a growing economic threat across the globe and are becoming an acute problem in low- and middle-income countries in which they are estimated to account for nearly $500 billion per year.[7] By contrast, worldwide adoption of best practices could substantially reduce that economic burden. For example, population-based interventions to reduce tobacco and harmful alcohol use as well as to improve unhealthy diets and to increase physical activity are estimated to cost less than $0.40 per person per year. These low-technology, population-wide interventions along with individual-based noncommunicable disease "best buy" interventions, such as individualized counseling and drug therapy, bring the total annual cost to $11.4 billion. Thus, on a per capita basis, the annual investment ranges from less than $1 in low-income countries to $3 in upper middle-income countries.

The growing epidemic of noncommunicable diseases, including mental health conditions, and the unfinished agenda of controlling infectious diseases (HIV/AIDS, malaria, tuberculosis, maternal and child health, and other infectious and parasitic diseases) pose a huge threat to the global population in terms of both human and fiscal losses. Although individual countries theoretically take responsibility for the health of their respective citizens, many low- and middle-income countries are unable to meet their domestic population's basic needs. The sum of public and private health care expenditure by countries based on their gross domestic product varies from 1.6% in South Sudan to 18% in the United States, with many high-income countries spending more than 10%. Thus, the worldwide solution requires a response of all of human society, including strategic domestic and international investments, both within countries and through multilateral agencies. This societal responsibility must be shared by the private sector, nongovernmental organizations, academia, professional societies, and the public themselves.

The modern global health agenda should move beyond false dichotomies—such as prevention versus treatment, infectious versus noncommunicable diseases, primary care versus specialized care, social determinants versus health services, life sciences versus social sciences—toward integration in the sense of common purpose. The approach to noncommunicable diseases should be integrated with the approach to communicable diseases. Health

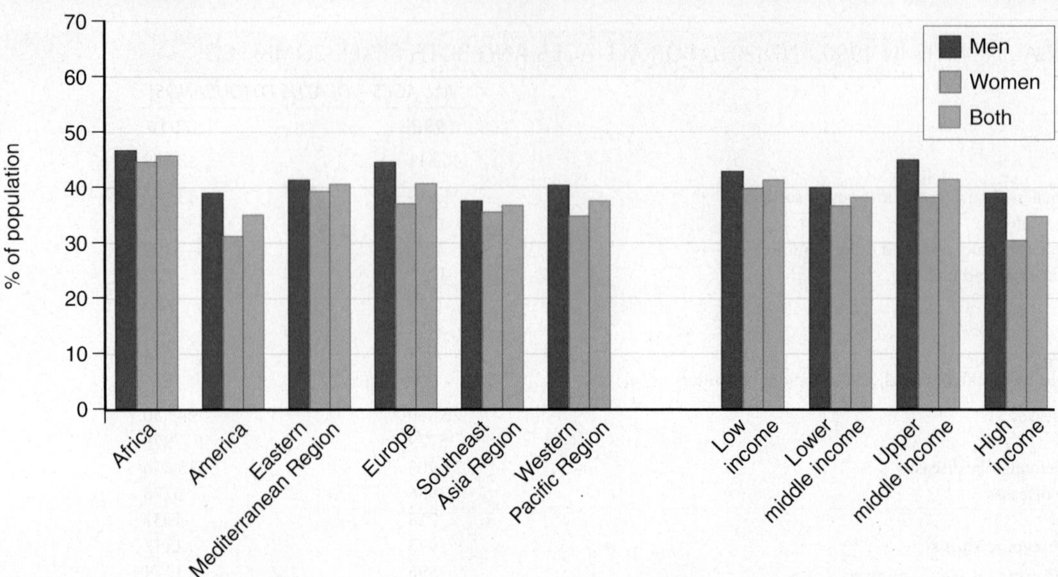

FIGURE 6-1. Global prevalence of hypertension. Age-standardized prevalence of hypertension, defined as systolic blood pressure ≥140 mm Hg or diastolic blood pressure ≥90 mm Hg or taking medications for lowering of blood pressure, in persons aged 25 years and older. (Data source: Noncommunicable Disease Global Monitoring Framework. World Health Organization. 2013. http://www.who.int/nmh/global_monitoring_framework/en/. Accessed January 21, 2015.)

targets should include noncommunicable diseases such as hypertension, diabetes, and cervical cancer, even in low- and middle-income countries. A critical component of health is a healthy lifestyle throughout life, from childhood to adolescence to adulthood, including risk factor reduction as well as treatment when it becomes necessary. Global health must integrate prevention and treatment in a cost-effective manner.

GENERAL REFERENCES

For the General References and other additional features, please visit Expert Consult at https://expertconsult.inkling.com.

II

PRINCIPLES OF EVALUATION AND MANAGEMENT

7

APPROACH TO THE PATIENT: HISTORY AND PHYSICAL EXAMINATION

DAVID L. SIMEL

OVERVIEW

Physicians may have multiple objectives with varying degrees of importance in their encounters with patients. These goals include, but are not limited to, the translation of symptoms and signs into diagnoses, the assessment of stability or change in known conditions, the provision of information and counseling for future prevention, and the reaffirmation or alteration of therapeutic interventions. A general health check will increase the number of diagnoses for a patient, but it may not affect overall morbidity and mortality.[1]

The interaction between the patient and physician represents not only a scientific encounter but also a social ritual centered on locus of control and meeting each other's expectations. Patients expect that their health care needs and concerns will be addressed competently. Physicians also have expectations: a need to feel that they have not missed something important in addressing diagnostic challenges, a need to put limits on the time available for each interaction, and a need to maintain objectivity so that their evaluation and recommendations are not clouded by their emotional feelings about the patient. The expertly performed rational clinical examination enhances the expected social ritual and the likelihood of acquiring relevant data. It also optimizes the physician's ability to understand the patient's symptoms and concerns, as well as to facilitate the healing process.[2]

Physical Examination Begins with the History

It is almost impossible to consider the history as distinct from the physical examination because the clinical examination begins as soon as the physician sees or hears the patient. From the patient's perspective, it matters little whether the physician determines the diagnosis from the history or the physical examination. The concept of deliberate practice, which has been demonstrated to be important in performing arts and in sports, can be applied to the performance of the clinical examination. This deliberate practice, which must be specifically designed to improve the ability to elicit symptoms and signs, requires appropriate training under observation, concentration, and commitment to ensure its consistent and accurate performance. The creation of simulation centers at many medical schools and hospitals provides new opportunities for this training.

Quantitative Principles of the Clinical Examination

The diagnostic accuracy of a symptom or sign is quantified by its sensitivity and specificity, often described as its likelihood ratio (LR) or predictive value (Chapter 10). Data on diagnostic accuracy can be obtained by a literature search for the evaluation of a disease-specific condition (e.g., melanoma) or a clinical finding (e.g., splenomegaly) (E-Tables 7-1 and 7-2). Each component of the history and physical examination has an associated sensitivity (the percentage of patients with a disorder who have an abnormal finding) and specificity (the percentage of patients without a disorder who have a normal finding). Measures of precision, such as the kappa (κ) statistic ($0 =$ random agreement; $+1 =$ perfect agreement), quantify the agreement between observers on a symptom or sign (Chapter 10). Current research on the clinical examination uses LRs that inform clinicians how likely they are to observe a particular finding in a patient with a given condition as opposed to a patient without the condition. A patient with an abnormal glabellar tap has an LR of 4.5 for Parkinson disease (Chapter 409), which means that the risk for Parkinsonism increases 4.5-fold compared with that in a patient who does not have the finding. Similarly, a patient who insists that he or she does not have "shaking in the arms" has an LR of 0.25 for Parkinson disease and is one fourth as likely (a reduced chance) to have the disease compared with the baseline risk.

MEDICAL HISTORY

The history begins by asking patients to describe, in their own words, the reason for seeking medical care (Table 7-1). Although patients may have many reasons for initiating a visit to the physician, they should be encouraged to select the one or two most important concerns they have. The physician should reassure the patient that other concerns will not be ignored, but that it is important to understand what is most concerning to the patient.

History of the Present Illness

Open-ended questions facilitate descriptions of problems in the patient's own words. Subsequently, specific questions fill in gaps and help clarify important points. These questions should be asked in an order dictated by the story the patient tells and targeted to suit the individual problem. When the patient is acutely ill, the physician should limit the amount of time spent in open-ended discussion and move promptly to the most important features that allow quick evaluation and management. In general, the history of the problem under consideration includes the following:

- Description of onset and chronology
- Location of symptoms
- Character (quality) of symptoms
- Intensity
- Precipitating, aggravating, and relieving factors
- Inquiry into whether the problem or similar problems occurred before and, if so, whether a diagnosis was established at that time

It is often helpful to ask patients to express what they believe is the cause of the problem or what concerns them the most. This approach often uncovers other pertinent factors and helps establish that the physician is trying to meet the patient's needs.

Past Medical and Surgical History

An astute clinician recognizes that patients may not report all their prior problems because they may forget, may assume that previous events are unrelated to their current problem, or simply may not want to discuss past events. Open-ended statements such as "Tell me about other medical illnesses that we did not discuss" and "Tell me about any operations you had" prompt the patient to consider other items. The physician should ask the patient about unexplained surgical or traumatic scars.

A list of current medications includes prescriptions, over-the-counter medications, vitamins, and herbal preparations. Patients who do not recall the names of medications should bring all medication bottles to the next visit. Patients may not consider topical medications (e.g., skin preparations or eyedrops) as important, so they may need prompting.

Information about allergies (Chapter 254) is particularly important, but challenging, to collect. Patients may attribute adverse reactions or intolerances to allergies, but many supposed allergic reactions are not truly drug allergies. For example, less than 20% of patients who claim a penicillin allergy are allergic on skin testing. Eliciting the patient's actual response to medications facilitates a determination of whether the response was a true allergic reaction.

Social and Occupational History and Risk Factors

The social history not only reveals important information but also improves understanding of the patient's unique values, support systems, and social situation. It can be helpful to ask the patient to describe what they would do during a typical day. Patients who lack confidence when filling out medical forms by themselves have an LR positive of 5.0 for problems with health care literacy.[3]

Data that may influence risk factors for disease should be gathered, including a nonjudgmental assessment of substance abuse. The tobacco history should include the use of snuff, chewing tobacco, and cigar and cigarette smoking (Chapter 32). Alcohol use should be determined quantitatively and by the effect that it has had on the patient's life (Chapter 33). Past or present use of illicit substances, prescription pain medications or sedatives, and intravenous drugs should be assessed (Chapter 34). The sexual history should address sexual orientation and gender identity, as well as current and past sexual activity. The physician can initiate this discussion with the question, "Do you have any concerns or questions about your sexuality, sexual orientation, or sexual desires?"[4] The employment history should include the current and past employment history, as well as any significant hobbies. All adult patients should be asked if they served in the military. Military veterans should be asked about their combat history, years of service, and areas of deployment (Table 7-2).[5]

The physician should also obtain information on socioeconomic status, insurance, the ability to afford or obtain medications, and past or current barriers to health care because of their impact on care of the patient (Chapter

TABLE 7-1 PATIENT'S MEDICAL HISTORY

Description of the patient
Age, gender, ethnic background, occupation
Chief reason for seeking medical care
State the purpose of the evaluation (usually in the patient's words)
Other physicians involved in the patient's care
Include the clinician that the patient identifies as his or her primary provider or the physician who referred the patient. Record contact information for all physicians who should receive information about the visit
History of the reason for seeking medical care
In chronologic fashion, determine the evolution of the indication for the visit and then each major symptom. It is best to address the patient's reason for seeking care first rather than what the physician ultimately believes is most important
Be careful to avoid "premature closure," in which a diagnosis is assumed before all the information is collected
Past medical and surgical history
List other illnesses and previous surgeries not related to the current problem
List all prescribed and over-the-counter medications with dose
Remember to ask about vitamin and herbal supplements
Allergies and adverse reactions
List allergic reactions to medications and food. Record the specific reaction (e.g., hives). Distinguish allergies from adverse reactions or intolerance to medication (e.g., dyspepsia from nonsteroidal anti-inflammatory agents)
Social, occupational, and military history (see Table 7-2)
Describe the patient's current family and a typical day for patient. The occupational history should focus on current and past employment as it might relate to the current problem
Risk factors
Include history of tobacco use, illegal drug use, and risk factors for sexually transmitted disease (including human immunodeficiency virus and hepatitis)
Family history
History of any diseases in first-degree relatives and a listing of family members with any conditions that could be risk factors for the patient (e.g., cardiovascular disease at a young age, malignancy, known genetic disorders, longevity)
Review of systems (see Table 7-3)

TABLE 7-2 BASIC MILITARY HISTORY

- Tell me about your military experience.
- When and where do you/did you serve?
- What do you/did you do while in the service?
- How has military service affected you?

If the patient answers "yes" to any of the questions below, ask the patient, "Can you tell me more about that?"

- Did you see combat, enemy fire, or casualties?
- Were you or a buddy wounded, injured, or hospitalized?
- Did you ever become ill while you were in the service?
- Were you a prisoner of war?

To screen for post-traumatic stress disorder, ask, "In your life, have you ever had an experience so horrible, frightening, or upsetting that, in the past month you …

- Have had nightmares about it or thought about it when you did not want to?"
- Tried hard not to think about it or went out of your way to avoid situations that reminded you of it?"
- Were constantly on guard, watchful, or easily startled?"
- Felt numb or detached from others, activities, or your surroundings?"

From Department of Veterans Affairs. Military Health History Pocket Card for Clinicians. http://www.va.gov/oaa/pocketcard/military-health-history-card-for-print.pdf. Accessed February 9, 2015.

5). Marital status and the living situation (i.e., whom the patient lives with, significant stressors for that patient) are important as risk factors for disease and to determine how best to care for the patient. A patient's culture (Chapter 4) and values should be known, including any prior advance directives or desire to overrule them (Chapter 3). The physician should explicitly elicit and record information regarding the next of kin; surrogate decision makers; emergency contacts; social support systems; and financial, emotional, and physical support available to the patient.

Family History

The family history is never diagnostic, but it allows risk stratification, which affects the pretest probability for an increasing number of disorders (e.g., heart disease, breast cancer, or Alzheimer disease). For common diseases such as heart disease, additional inquiry into the age of onset in first-degree relatives and death attributed to the disease should be obtained (Chapter 52). When a patient reports that a first-degree relative had a myocardial infarction,

TABLE 7-3 REVIEW OF SYSTEMS*

FOCUS all questions on a specific time frame (e.g., within the past "month" or "now") and on items not already addressed during the clinical examination:
Change in weight or appetite
Change in vision
Change in hearing
New or changing skin lesions
Chest discomfort or sensation of skipped beats
Shortness of breath, dyspnea on exertion
Abdominal discomfort, constipation, melena, hematochezia, diarrhea
Difficulty with urination
Change in menses
Joint or muscle discomfort not already mentioned
Problems with sleep
Difficulty with sexual function
Exposure to "street" drugs or medications not already mentioned
Depression (feeling "down, depressed, or hopeless"; loss of interest or pleasure in doing things)
A sensation of unsteadiness when walking, standing, or getting up from a chair

*Clinicians may start with this basic list and adapt the items to their specific patient population by considering factors such as age, gender, medications, and the problems identified during the examination. The process is facilitated by developing a routine personal approach to these questions, typically going through the systems from "head to toe."

the LR is 19 that the patient has a family history of myocardial infarction. Patients may lack appropriate information about the absence of disease, however, so a reported lack of a family history of myocardial infarction reduces the likelihood only by one third. In general, the specificity of the reported family history far exceeds its sensitivity; for example, only two thirds of patients with essential tremor (Chapter 410) report a family history, but 95% of such patients have first-degree relatives with tremor. The expansion of knowledge about genetic diseases (Chapter 40) requires clinicians not only to improve their skills in eliciting the family history but also to develop methods for confirming the information. For example, patients who report that a first-degree relative had carcinoma of the colon (LR 25), breast (LR 14), ovaries (LR 34), or prostate (LR 12) are usually providing accurate information.[6]

Review of Systems

The review of systems, which is the structural assessment of each of the major organ systems, elicits symptoms or signs that are not covered or may be overlooked in the history of the present illness (Table 7-3). Although a review of systems is required in many electronic records systems, it may only yield important diagnoses in less than 10% of patients, and the cost of pursuing false-positive findings is not known. In contrast to the open-ended nature of collecting the medical history, which allows the patient to "claim" or "deny" a variety of symptoms, the direct questioning technique of the review of systems leads the patient to "accept" or "reject" symptoms. The review of systems is more efficient if at least some questions are restricted to a specific time frame (e.g., "Has there been any recent change in your vision?" or "Have you recently had shortness of breath, wheezing, or coughing?") or by having the patient fill out a previsit questionnaire.

PHYSICAL EXAMINATION

Chaperones

Surveys suggest that most patients of either sex and all ages report a lack of preference for a chaperone, but it is not clear whether this response is their true feeling or a desire to give a "correct" response. Nevertheless, many adult women (29%) and adolescent girls (46%) do express a preference for a chaperone during a breast, pelvic, or rectal examination by a male physician (especially during their first examination). Examiners should offer patients the option of a chaperone, and a chaperone should be considered when the clinician and patient are of different genders. Many examiners prefer a chaperone to allay their own anxieties attributable to gender differences or to achieve a perceived need for protection should the patient become concerned during the procedure.

Vital Signs

Vital signs include the pulse rate and rhythm, blood pressure, respiratory rate, body temperature, and the patient's quantitative assessment of pain. Marked abnormalities require a rapid, focused evaluation that may take precedence over the typical structural approach to the remainder of the evaluation (Chapter 8).

When the blood pressure is abnormal (Chapter 67), the measurement should be repeated, assuring that the cuff size is appropriate. Many adults require a large adult cuff; using a narrow cuff can alter systolic/diastolic blood pressure by −8 to +10/+2 to +8 mm Hg. The appearance of repetitive sounds (Korotkoff sounds, phase 1) constitutes systolic pressure. (Record the value rounded upward to the nearest 2 mm Hg.) After the cuff is inflated about 20 to 30 mm Hg above the palpated pressure, the Korotkoff sounds muffle and disappear as the pressure is released (phase 5). The level at which the sounds disappear is the diastolic pressure.

Respirations should be assessed with the patient unaware that the rate is being observed. The examiner should decide whether patients have tachypnea (a rapid rate of breathing) or hypopnea (a slow or shallow rate of breathing). Tachypnea is not always associated with hyperventilation, which is defined by increased alveolar ventilation resulting in a lower arterial carbon dioxide level (Chapter 103). The subjective sensation of dyspnea (Chapter 83) is caused by an increased work of breathing.[7]

The body temperature of adults is measured with an oral electric thermometer. Rectal thermometers reliably record temperatures 0.4° C higher than oral thermometers. Tympanic thermometers vary too much in comparison with oral thermometers (−1.2° to +1.6° C vs. the oral temperature) to be reliable in hospitalized patients.

As a vital sign measure, patients should self-rate any pain on a scale of 0 to 10 (no pain to worst pain ever) (Chapter 30). However, the validity, usefulness, and value of this approach as a screening tool for clinical diagnosis are uncertain.

Head and Neck

Face

The examiner should note any asymmetrical facial features. Examples of asymmetry include skin lesions (Chapter 436), cranial nerve palsies (Chapter 396), parotid enlargement (Chapter 425), or the ptosis of Horner syndrome (Chapter 424). A variety of disorders may cause symmetrical, abnormal facies; examples include acromegaly (Chapter 224), Cushing syndrome (Chapter 227), and Parkinson disease (Chapter 409).

Ears

Physicians may not recognize their patient's hearing impairment (Chapter 428). The inability to appreciate the whispered voice increases the likelihood of hearing loss (LR 6).[8] Otoscopic evaluation of the tympanic membranes should reveal a translucent membrane and an obvious cone of light reflected where the eardrum meets the malleolus (see Fig. 426-7). Cerumen impaction is an easily treated cause of diminished hearing.

Nose

Patients with nasal symptoms often incorrectly self-diagnose bacterial sinusitis (Chapter 426). The nares should be examined for the presence of polyps, which can be seen as obstructing, glistening mucosal masses. Transillumination performed in a dark room is useful for diagnosing sinusitis, especially when combined with visualization of a purulent discharge, a patient's report of a poor response to decongestants or antihistamines, a maxillary toothache, and the presence of discolored rhinorrhea (Chapter 426). These patients have an LR greater than 6 for rhinosinusitis.

Mouth

The quality of the patient's dentition directly affects nutrition. Premalignant oral lesions (e.g., leukoplakia [see Fig. 190-1], nodules, ulcerations) found by generalist physicians are usually verified by dentists (LR > 6.5) (Chapter 425). Patients who use smokeless tobacco products are at significantly increased risk for premalignant and malignant oral lesions (Chapter 32). Bimanual palpation of the cheeks and floor of the mouth facilitates identification of potentially malignant lesions (Chapter 425).

Eyes

The eye examination begins with simple visual inspection to look for symmetry in the lids, extraocular movements, pupil size and reaction, and the presence of redness (Chapters 423 and 424). Abnormalities in extraocular movements should be grouped into nonparalytic (usually chronic with onset in childhood) or paralytic causes (third, fourth, or sixth cranial nerve palsy). Pupillary abnormalities may be symmetrical or asymmetrical (anisocoria). Red eyes should be categorized by the pattern of ciliary injection, presence of pain, effect on vision, and papillary abnormalities. When the eye examination is approached systematically, the generalist physician can evaluate the likelihood of conjunctivitis, episcleritis or scleritis, iritis, and acute glaucoma.

Routine determination of visual acuity can confirm a patient's report of diminished vision but does not replace the need for formal ophthalmologic evaluation in patients with visual complaints (Chapter 423). Aging patients often experience acute flashes and floaters, especially with posterior vitreal detachments. If acute flashes and floaters are associated with visual loss, the patient should be urgently referred for an ophthalmologic examination for the evaluation of a possible acute retinal detachment.[9] Cataracts can be detected with direct ophthalmoscopy, but the generalist's proficiency in this evaluation is uncertain.

After identifying the optic disc by ophthalmoscopy, the examiner should note the border of the disc for clarity, color, and the size of the central cup in relation to the total diameter (usually less than half the diameter of the disc). A careful observer usually can see spontaneous venous pulsations that indicate normal intracranial pressure, but about 10% of patients with normal intracranial pressure will not have spontaneous pulsations. Abnormalities of the optic disc include optic atrophy (a white disc), papilledema (see Fig. 423-27) (blurry margins with a pink, hyperemic disc), and glaucoma (a large, pale cup with retinal vessels that dive underneath and that may be displaced toward the nasal side). The generalist's examination inadequately detects early glaucomatous changes, so high-risk patients should undergo routine ophthalmologic examination for glaucoma.[10]

After inspecting the disc, the upper and lower nasal quadrants should be examined for the appearance of vessels and the presence of any retinal hemorrhages (see Fig. 423-24) or lesions. Proceeding from the nasal quadrants to the temporal quadrants decreases the risk for papillary constriction from the bright light focused on the fovea. Dilating the pupils leads to an improved examination. Patients with diabetes (Chapter 229) should undergo routine examination by eye care experts because the sensitivity of a generalist's examination is not adequate to exclude diabetic retinopathy or monitor it over time.

Neck

Carotid Pulses

The carotid pulses should be palpated for contour and timing in relation to the cardiac impulse. Abnormalities in the carotid pulse contour reflect underlying cardiac abnormalities (e.g., aortic stenosis) but are generally appreciated only after detecting an abnormal cardiac impulse or murmur (Chapter 51).

Many physicians listen for bruits over the carotid arteries because asymptomatic carotid bruits are associated with an increased incidence of cerebrovascular and cardiac events in older patients (Chapters 406 and 407). In asymptomatic patients, the presence of a carotid bruit increases the likelihood of a 70 to 90% stenotic lesion (LR 4 to 10), but the absence of a bruit is of uncertain value. Unfortunately, clinical data do not provide adequate data for judging the importance of detecting bruits in asymptomatic patients.

Jugular Veins

The examination of the neck veins is an interesting but often unreliable indicator of central venous pressure or fluid responsiveness in hospitalized sick patients (Chapter 51).[11] Inspection of the waveforms may facilitate the interpretation of the cardiac examination for right heart valvular lesions. The waves are seen best by shining a penlight obliquely on the vein while the examiner looks for the dynamic changes of the projected shadow on the bed linen.

Thyroid

The thyroid gland is felt best when standing behind the patient and using both hands to palpate the thyroid gland gently (Chapter 226). Palpation is enhanced when the patient swallows sips of water to allow the thyroid to glide underneath the fingers. When viewed from the side, lateral prominence of the thyroid between the cricoid cartilage and the suprasternal notch indicates thyromegaly. The generalist physician should estimate the size of the thyroid gland as normal or enlarged; the impression of an enlarged thyroid gland by a generalist physician has an LR of almost 4, whereas assessment of normal size makes thyromegaly less likely (LR 0.4). The volume of a normal thyroid gland is no greater than the volume of the patient's distal thumb phalanx.

Lymphatic System

While palpating the thyroid, the examiner may also identify enlarged cervical lymph nodes (Chapter 168). Lymph nodes can also be palpated in the supraclavicular area, axilla, epitrochlear area, and inguinofemoral region. Simple lymph node enlargement confined to one region is common and does not usually represent an important underlying disorder. Unexpected gross lymph node enlargement in a single area or diffuse lymph node enlargement is more important. Patients with febrile illnesses, underlying malignancy, or inflammatory diseases should routinely undergo an examination of each of the aforementioned areas for lymph node enlargement.

Chest

Inspection of the patient's posture may reveal lateral curves in the back (scoliosis) or kyphosis that may be associated with loss of vertebral height from osteoporosis (Chapter 243). When patients have back pain, the spine and paravertebral muscles should be palpated for spasm and tenderness (Chapter 400). The patient may be placed through maneuvers to assess loss of mobility associated with ankylosing spondylitis (Chapter 265), but a history of loss of lateral mobility may be just as efficient in the early stages of spondylitis.

Lungs

The incremental value of palpation and percussion of the chest to supplement the history, auscultation, and eventual chest radiograph is unknown. Normal vesicular sounds, which approximate a 3:1 inspiratory:expiratory ratio with no pause between phases, are heard throughout most of the normal posterior chest during quiet breathing. Auscultated wheezes are continuous adventitial sounds. Crackles (formerly called rales) are discontinuous sounds heard in conditions that stiffen the lung (heart failure, pulmonary fibrosis, and obstructive lung disease). The best piece of information for increasing the likelihood of chronic obstructive pulmonary disease is a history of more than 40 pack years of smoking (LR 19). The presence of wheezing or downward displacement of the larynx to within 4 cm of the sternum (distance between the top of the thyroid cartilage and the suprasternal notch) increases the likelihood of obstructive pulmonary disease (LR of 4 for either).

Heart

The patient should be examined in the sitting and lying positions (Chapter 51). Palpation of the apical impulse in the left lateral decubitus position helps detect a displaced apical impulse and can reveal a palpable S_3 gallop. When the apical impulse is lateral to the midclavicular line, radiographic cardiomegaly (LR 3.5) and an ejection fraction of less than 50% (LR 6) are more likely. Most examiners auscultate in sequence the second right then the second left intercostal spaces, the left sternal border, and then the apex. The examiner should concentrate on the timing, intensity, and splitting of sounds with respiration. The first and second heart sounds are heard best with the diaphragm, as are pericardial rubs. Gallops (S_3 and S_4) are heard best with the stethoscope bell. High-pitched versus low-pitched murmurs are detected by switching from the diaphragm to the bell. The location, timing, intensity, radiation patterns, and respiratory variation of murmurs should be noted. Special maneuvers during auscultation (e.g., Valsalva, auscultation during sudden squatting or standing) do not usually need to be performed if the results of routine precordial examination are entirely normal.

The presence of an S_3 gallop is useful for detecting left ventricular systolic dysfunction (LR > 4 for identifying patients with an ejection fraction of $<30\%$). The presence of a systolic thrill (palpable murmur, LR 12) or a holosystolic murmur increases the likelihood of moderate to severe aortic stenosis or mitral regurgitation. Quiet systolic murmurs (LR 0.08) are much less likely to herald important cardiac abnormalities. A loud, early diastolic murmur (LR 4) or a diastolic murmur associated with an S_3 suggests severe aortic regurgitation.

Breast

The most important determinants of the accuracy of the breast examination are the duration of the examination; the patient's position; careful evaluation of the breast boundaries; the pattern of the examination; and the position, movement, and pressure of the examiner's fingers (Chapter 198). To obtain the best sensitivity, the duration of the breast examination needs to be 5 to 10 minutes' total time, but few generalist physicians perform such a lengthy examination. Clinicians should recognize that the examination may make them (or their patient) feel uncomfortable—the presence of a chaperone may give the clinician the confidence to perform an intensive examination.

The patient should be examined with the pads of the fingers while she is supine, holding her hand first on her forehead (to flatten the lateral border of the breast) and then on her shoulder (to flatten the medial border). The examiner should make small circular motions with the fingers, moving up and down in parallel rows to span the entire breast-clavicle to the bra line. Cancerous breast lumps are difficult to distinguish from benign breast lumps on examination, but the presence of a fixed mass or a mass 2 cm in diameter has an LR of about 2 to 2.5 for cancer.

Abdomen

When patients have potential abdominal symptoms and the history suggests an acute problem, the examination should focus initially on identifying patients who require surgical evaluation. Palpation and percussion of the abdomen of patients with no symptoms or risk factors for an abdominal disorder seldom reveal important abnormalities (Chapter 132) except for asymptomatic widening of the abdominal aorta in older patients (LR of 16 for detecting aneurysms >4 cm in diameter). However, palpation misses a substantial proportion of small to medium aneurysms (Chapter 78).

The presence of bowel sounds in patients with acute symptoms can be falsely reassuring because the sounds can be present despite an ileus and may be increased early in an obstruction. For patients without gastrointestinal symptoms or abnormalities on palpation, auscultation for bruits is important primarily to detect renal bruits in patients with hypertension (Chapters 67 and 125). The presence of an abdominal bruit in a hypertensive patient, if heard in systole and diastole, strongly suggests renovascular hypertension (LR $\approx$ 40).

Liver

Detection of liver disease depends mostly on the history and laboratory evaluations (Chapter 146). By the time that signs are present on physical examination, the patient usually has advanced liver disease. The first abnormalities on physical examination associated with liver disease are extrahepatic. The clinician should assess the patient for ascites, peripheral edema, jaundice, or splenomegaly. In patients with an enlarged liver, palpation should begin at the liver edge, but palpation of the edge below the costal margin increases the likelihood of hepatomegaly only slightly (LR 1.7). The upper border of the liver may be detected by percussion, and a span of less than 12 cm reduces the likelihood of hepatomegaly. In the absence of a known diagnosis (e.g., a hepatoma, which may cause a hepatic bruit), auscultation of the liver rarely is helpful.

Spleen

Examination for splenomegaly in patients without findings suggestive of a disorder associated with splenomegaly almost always reveals nothing (Chapter 168). Approximately 3% of healthy teenagers may have a palpable spleen. The examination for an enlarged spleen begins first with percussion in the left upper quadrant to detect dullness. Palpation can be performed by any of the following three approaches ($\kappa \approx 0.2$ to 0.4): palpating with the right hand while providing counterpressure with the left hand behind the spleen, palpating with one hand without counterpressure (with the patient in the right lateral decubitus position for both techniques), or placing the patient supine with the left fist under the left costovertebral angle while the examiner tries to hook the spleen with the hands.

Musculoskeletal System

The musculoskeletal examination in adult patients is almost always driven by symptoms (Chapters 256 and 263). Most patients have back pain at some point during their life (Chapter 400). The patient's history helps assess the likelihood of an underlying systemic disease (age, history of systemic malignancy, unexplained weight loss, duration of pain, responsiveness to previous therapy, intravenous drug use, urinary infection, or fever). The most important physical examination findings for lumbar disc herniation in patients with sciatica all have excellent reliability, including ipsilateral straight leg raising causing pain, contralateral straight leg raising causing pain, and ankle or great toe dorsiflexion weakness.

The generalist physician should evaluate an adult patient with knee discomfort for torn menisci or ligaments. The best maneuver for demonstrating a tear in the anterior cruciate ligament is the anterior drawer or Lachman maneuver, in which the examiner detects the lack of a discrete end point as the tibia is pulled toward the examiner while the femur is stabilized. A variety of maneuvers that assess for pain, popping, or grinding along the joint line between the femur and tibia are used to evaluate for meniscal tears. As with many musculoskeletal disorders, no single finding has the accuracy of the orthopedist's examination, which factors in the history and a variety of clinical findings.

The shoulder examination is directed toward determining range of motion, maneuvers that cause discomfort, and assessment of functional disability.

Hip osteoarthritis is detected by evidence of restriction of internal rotation and abduction of the affected hip. Generalist physicians often rely on radiographs to determine the need for referral to orthopedic physicians, but routine radiographs are not needed early in the course of shoulder or hip disorders. The degree of pain and disability experienced by the patient may prompt confirmation of the diagnosis and referral.

The hands and feet may show evidence of osteoarthritis (local or as part of a systemic process) (Chapter 262), rheumatoid arthritis (Chapter 264), gout (Chapter 273), or other connective tissue diseases. In addition to regional musculoskeletal disorders, such as carpal tunnel syndrome, a variety of medical and neurologic conditions should prompt routine examination of the distal ends of the extremities to prevent complications (e.g., diabetes [neuropathy or ulcers] or hereditary sensorimotor neuropathy [claw toe deformity]).

Skin

The skin should be examined under good lighting (Chapter 436). It is best to ask the patient to point out any spots on the skin of concern. Examiner agreement on some of the most important features of melanoma (asymmetry, haphazard color, border irregularity) is fair to moderate (Chapter 203). A lesion that is symmetrical, has regular borders, is only one color, is 6 mm or smaller, or has not enlarged in size is unlikely to represent a melanoma (LR 0.07). However, an increasing number of findings greatly enhance the likelihood of melanoma (LR 2.6 for two or more findings and LR 98 for the presence of all five findings) (Chapter 203).

Basal cell carcinoma and squamous cell carcinoma occur more frequently than melanoma (Chapter 203). These lesions can be detected during routine examination by paying careful attention to sun-exposed areas of the nose, face, forearms, and hands.

Neurologic Examination

Full details of the neurologic examination are given in Chapter 396.

Psychiatric Evaluation

During the general examination, much of the psychiatric assessment (including cognition) is accomplished while eliciting the routine history and performing the review of systems (Chapter 397). Observation of the patient's mannerisms, affect, facial expression, and behavior may suggest underlying psychiatric disturbances. When a screening survey and review of systems are obtained by a questionnaire completed by the patient, the clinician should review the responses carefully to determine whether the patient exhibits symptoms of depression. Specific questioning for symptoms of depression is appropriate for all adult patients. Military veterans should be screened for post-traumatic stress disorder and possible prior traumatic brain injuries that may affect their behaviors. Delirium (Chapter 28) is common in both medical and surgical inpatients and is recognized by fluctuating mental status. Delirium should be suspected when the patient has trouble carrying on a normal conversation during bedside rounds; but the patient's nurse and visitors may detect delirium before the physician, so their report may contribute to diagnosis.[12]

Genitalia and Rectum

Pelvic Examination

A complete examination includes a description of the external genitalia, appearance of the vagina and cervix as seen through a speculum, and bimanual palpation of the uterus and ovaries (Chapters 199 and 237). About 10 to 15% of asymptomatic women have some abnormality on examination, and 1.5% have abnormal ovaries. However, screening for ovarian cancer is limited by the low sensitivity of the physical examination for detecting early-stage ovarian carcinoma (Chapter 199). In the emergency setting, all women of reproductive age with vaginal bleeding and pelvic pain should have a pregnancy test and an ultrasound to evaluate them for a possible ectopic pregnancy.[13]

Male Genitalia

Examination of the male genitalia should begin with a description of whether the penis is circumcised and whether there are any visible skin lesions (e.g., ulcers or warts). Palpation should confirm the presence of bilateral testes in the scrotum. The epididymis and testes should be palpated for nodules. The low incidence of testicular carcinoma means that most nodules are benign (Chapter 200).

The prostate should be examined in all quadrants, with attention focused on surface irregularities or differences in consistency throughout the prostate (Chapter 201). An estimate of prostate size may be confounded by the size of the examiner's fingers. It may be best to estimate the size of the prostate in centimeters of width and height.

Rectum

Patients can be examined while lying on their side, although this approach may place the examiner in an awkward stance (Chapters 132 and 145). The rectal examination in women can be performed as part of a bimanual examination, with the index finger in the vagina and the third finger in the rectum to permit palpation of the rectovaginal vault. Men may be asked to stand and lean over the examining table; alternatively, they may be examined while on their back with their hips and knees flexed. This latter maneuver is not used often, although it may facilitate examination of the prostate, which falls into the finger in this position.

The rectal examination begins with inspection of the perianal area for skin lesions. A well-lubricated, gloved finger is placed on the anus, and while applying gentle pressure, the examiner asks that the patient bear down as though having a bowel movement. This maneuver facilitates entry of the finger into the rectum. A normal rectal response includes tightening of the anal sphincter around the finger. The examiner should palpate circumferentially around the length of the fully inserted finger for masses. On withdrawing the gloved finger, the finger should be wiped on a stool guaiac card for fecal blood testing to assess for acute blood loss. As a screening test for colorectal carcinoma (Chapter 193), digital examination does not replace the need for testing stool samples collected by the patient (or using alternative screening strategies, such as flexible sigmoidoscopy or colonoscopy).

SUMMARIZING THE FINDINGS FOR THE PATIENT

The physician should summarize the pertinent positive and negative findings for the patient and be willing to express uncertainty to the patient, provided that it is accompanied by a plan of action (e.g., "I will reexamine you on your next visit"). The rationale for subsequent laboratory, imaging, or other tests should be explained. A plan should be established for providing further feedback and results to the patient, especially when there is a possibility that bad news may need to be delivered. Some physicians ask the patient if there is "anything else" to be covered. Patients who express additional new concerns at the end of the visit may have been fearful to address them earlier (e.g., "by the way, doctor, I'm getting a lot of chest pain"); when the problems seem non-urgent, it is acceptable to reassure the patient and offer the promise of evaluating the patient in a follow-up phone call or at the next visit.

FUTURE DIRECTIONS

The common assumption that physicians' diagnostic skills are deteriorating is not supported by evidence. There is considerable evidence that the scientific approach to understanding what is worthwhile and what is not worthwhile during the clinical examination identifies a core set of skills for clinical diagnosticians. Because good patient outcomes at good value are driven primarily by the quality of the information obtained during the clinical examination, continued application of scientific principles to the history and physical examination should improve diagnostic skills.

GENERAL REFERENCES

For the General References and other additional features, please visit Expert Consult at https://expertconsult.inkling.com.

8

APPROACH TO THE PATIENT WITH ABNORMAL VITAL SIGNS

DAVID L. SCHRIGER

Care of the patient is guided by integration of the chief complaint, history, vital signs, and physical examination findings (Chapter 7). Physicians should be keenly aware of a patient's vital signs but should seldom make them the centerpiece of the evaluation.

TABLE 8-1 NORMAL AND PANIC RANGES FOR KEY VITAL SIGNS IN ADULTS*

	NORMAL	PANIC
Temperature	36°-38° C (96.8°-100.4° F)	40° C (104° F)
Pulse	60-100 beats/min	<45 beats/min, >130 beats/min
Respirations	12-20 breaths/min	<10 breaths/min, >26 breaths/min
Oxygen saturation	95-100%	<90%
Systolic blood pressure	90-130 mm Hg	<80 mm Hg, >200 mm Hg
Diastolic blood pressure	60-90 mm Hg	<55 mm Hg, >120 mm Hg

*Normal values are for healthy adults. Values outside these ranges are common in patients who are ill or are anxious about their health care encounter. Panic values demand the health care provider's attention in any adult patient. These values are specific (rarely present in healthy patients) but not sensitive (most ill patients' vital signs will not include panic values). All vital signs must be interpreted in the context of the patient's presentation (see text).

THE IMPORTANCE OF VITAL SIGNS

The importance of vital signs in medical care is a conundrum for proponents of an evidence-based approach to the care of patients. No experienced physician would be willing to care for patients without them, yet a formal evaluation of the utility of vital signs for making specific diagnoses would conclude that they are not particularly useful because their likelihood ratios are too close to 1 to differentiate those who have a specific condition from those who do not (Chapter 7). For uncommon conditions, their predictive value is even worse. For example, the probability of tachycardia in a patient in thyroid storm is high, yet the probability of thyroid storm in a patient with isolated tachycardia is low. This application of Bayes theorem (Chapter 10) demonstrates why there is no justification for ordering thyroid tests for every tachycardic patient and why attempts to say "When vital sign *x* is high [low], do *y*" fail. Each vital sign can be normal or abnormal in almost every acute condition (Table 8-1), and vital signs can be transiently abnormal in healthy individuals. An algorithmic approach to testing and treatment in response to abnormal vital signs would be too vague and too complex to be of use.

Predictive Value

How can it be that vital signs are poor predictors of diagnoses but central to the practice of medicine? First, although vital signs are insufficiently predictive to be of use in rigid algorithms, these algorithms are but one of several heuristics used by physicians to diagnose and to treat patients. Pattern recognition and the hypothetical-deductive model are heuristics that are based not on average tendencies of a single factor (e.g., hypotension is present in *x*% of cases of septic shock) or a small number of factors (hypotension and tachycardia are present in *y*% of cases of septic shock) but on the complex interaction of multiple factors (e.g., because this patient is an ill-appearing elderly man with an enlarged prostate and a history of urinary tract infections, is tachycardic and hypotensive, has clear lungs and an enlarged but nontender prostate, and has an oxygen saturation of 97%, he should be treated for urosepsis [Chapter 284] while awaiting results of urinalysis and urine culture). Thus, vital signs can play an important function in medical decision making even though their likelihood ratios for specific conditions are unimpressive.

Despite their poor predictive value for any single diagnosis, abnormal vital signs help identify patients who are sicker.[1] For example, even one abnormal vital sign in the emergency department significantly increases the likelihood of adverse outcomes in elderly patients by about 50%,[2] and abnormal vital signs after admission carry a 20-fold increased risk for subsequent important deterioration.[3] Abnormal vital signs are also a key predictor of which patients are at risk of dying soon after being sent home from an emergency department.[4]

The usefulness of vital signs is also evidenced by the finding that more severe abnormalities are associated with an even worse prognosis. For example, among hospitalized patients, one critically abnormal vital sign carries about a 1% risk for inpatient death, whereas three simultaneously abnormal vital signs carry nearly a 25% risk for inpatient death.[5]

Vital Signs as Symptoms

Abnormal vital signs are seldom the fundamental pathophysiologic problem. In shock (Chapter 106), hypotension and tachycardia are manifestations of pathophysiologic processes occurring at cellular and molecular levels. Given the circuitous links from clinical disease to fundamental pathophysiology to abnormal vital signs, it is not surprising that the relationships between the disease states and vital signs are not strong. Until new technologies enable direct measurement of primary pathologic processes, vital signs remain an important, albeit imperfect, proxy.

The five key vital signs are temperature, pulse, blood pressure, respiratory rate, and oxygen saturation (pulse oximetry). Pulse oximetry is included because it has become widely available in acute care settings, is noninvasive and relatively inexpensive, and provides information unique from the respiratory rate. Advocates have suggested that pain, smoking status, and weight be considered routine vital signs; although a case can be made for each, they are not considered here. Clinicians should never forget that the most important vital sign is what the patient looks like; general appearance is a sign that guides the intensity and urgency of the evaluation.

MEASURING VITAL SIGNS

Although obtaining vital signs is generally straightforward, the validity and reliability of measurement depend on proper technique and, for blood pressure and pulse oximetry, well-maintained equipment. Rectal and oral temperatures are generally accurate (Chapter 280), although oral temperatures can be falsely depressed in patients who breathe through their mouths. Axillary temperature is unreliable and should not be used. There is wide variability in the validity and reliability of measurements performed with tympanic membrane thermometers. A hypothermia thermometer is preferred in patients with suspected hypothermia, and core temperature should be measured with an esophageal, bladder, or rectal temperature sensor in patients with severe hypothermia or hyperthermia (Chapter 109).

Blood pressure must be measured with an appropriately sized cuff (Chapter 67). Automated blood pressure machines occasionally provide spurious results, and questionable values should be confirmed by manual auscultation and by checking other limbs. Pulse is best obtained by palpation because this technique provides the opportunity to assess regularity and contour; the pulse should be counted for sufficient time for an accurate rate to be obtained (at least 15 seconds). High heart rates on the digital readout of a cardiac monitor must be confirmed by palpation because these monitors can spuriously count large P waves, T waves, or pacemaker spikes as R waves, thereby reporting a heart rate double the actual rate. Orthostatic vital signs—the comparison of blood pressure and pulse in the supine, sitting, and standing positions—are advocated by some but have proved to be insensitive and nonspecific for hypovolemia.

Because the typical respiratory rate is between 12 and 20 breaths per minute and because there is considerable breath-to-breath variation, the respiratory rate should be assessed for at least 30 seconds and preferably 1 minute. New technologies purporting to measure the respiratory rate have not proved clinically useful. Oxygen saturation is dependent on technology, so an understanding of the idiosyncrasies of the device being used is critical; valid measurements are unlikely unless there is good correlation of the machine's pulse reading and the patient's pulse. The probe should be placed on a part of the body that is warm and well perfused. Pulse oximeters compare the absorption of light at two wavelengths, so readings may be spuriously high under conditions that change the color of oxygenated or deoxygenated hemoglobin, including carbon monoxide poisoning (Chapter 94), methemoglobinemia (Chapter 161), and some of the less common hemoglobinopathies.

ROLE OF VITAL SIGNS IN MANAGEMENT OF THE PATIENT

Abnormal vital signs should be remeasured. Certain abnormalities require prompt evaluation (Table 8-2). Other vital sign abnormalities should be rechecked in the future unless they have been previously noted, in which case a work-up can be initiated, guided by the patient's past history and physical examination findings. It is critical that the physician always "treat the patient, not the vital signs."

Patients without Systemic Complaints

In patients presenting for a routine evaluation or nonsystemic complaint (e.g., knee injury), an abnormal vital sign will seldom be the harbinger of acute illness. Most commonly, it will be a false reading or a transient finding due to random variation or anxiety that requires no evaluation or treatment and can be rechecked in the future. On occasion, it will be the only or most apparent manifestation of a chronic condition or risk factor. The

TABLE 8-2 ABNORMALITIES REQUIRING RAPID EVALUATION IN THE ASYMPTOMATIC PATIENT

An irregularly irregular rapid pulse (if it is not known to be chronic) should trigger an evaluation of the patient's rhythm so that atrial fibrillation can be identified, evaluated, and treated (Chapter 64), thereby decreasing the patient's risk of stroke.
A heart rate above 130 beats per minute warrants an electrocardiogram to determine the patient's rhythm and a consideration of the differential diagnosis of tachycardia (hypovolemia, anemia, and thyroid disease in particular).
A markedly elevated diastolic blood pressure (e.g., >115 mm Hg) should stimulate an evaluation for hypertensive urgencies (Chapter 67). Note that hypertension in the absence of signs of acute end-organ damage does not require acute treatment, which can reduce intracranial perfusion pressure and cause stroke. Patients with elevated blood pressure should be offered standard evaluation and treatment for chronic hypertension (Chapter 67).
Markedly low pulse or blood pressure in patients receiving cardioactive medications should lead to a confirmation that the patient is truly asymptomatic, an inquiry into the dosing of these medications, and a reconsideration of the regimen.
Markedly low pulse in elderly patients who are not receiving rate-controlling drugs should trigger an evaluation of the patient's cardiac conduction system.
Oxygen saturation below 93% in the absence of known pulmonary problems should prompt an evaluation of the patient's pulmonary status.

measurement of an elevated blood pressure leading to a diagnosis of hypertension is the classic example of the value of vital signs in such patients.

Patients Who Complain of Systemic Illness but Do Not Appear to Be Very Ill

Vital signs serve two additional roles in symptomatic patients who do not appear particularly ill. First, abnormalities in vital signs provide information that may suggest or support a diagnosis. The presence of elevated temperature in a patient with productive cough, shortness of breath, and localized rales and egophony supports a diagnosis of infectious pneumonia. Vital signs may also play a role in defining therapy and triage. For example, guidelines for patients with community-acquired pneumonia (Chapter 97) formally incorporate vital signs.

The second role of vital signs in the stable symptomatic patient is to provide warning that the patient is sicker than he or she appears. For example, the presence of hypotension in a well-appearing patient thought to have pyelonephritis may be an indication of sepsis or hypovolemia. For vital signs to be of use, the physician must be aware of them and must incorporate them explicitly into a thought process that considers the dangerous diagnoses associated with the abnormal vital sign. The physician then must decide whether the likelihood of each potentially dangerous diagnosis is high enough to warrant specific evaluation. Unfortunately, no quick or easy rules differentiate spurious abnormalities that can be ignored from those that should trigger additional testing or treatment. What can be said is that the well-trained physician who is aware of abnormal vital signs and is willing to contemplate a change in treatment or disposition in response to them is less likely to make mistakes.

A few specific points bear mention. First, for most vital signs, "normal" is relative. Blood pressure must be interpreted in the context of the patient. For example, a blood pressure of 88/64 mm Hg may be reasonable for an otherwise healthy, young 50-kg woman but should cause concern in a 90-kg middle-aged man. Similarly, a blood pressure of 128/80 mm Hg would be fine in a 60-year-old man but worrisome in a 34-week pregnant woman. Second, because vital signs are insensitive measures of disease, normal vital signs should not dissuade the physician from pursuing potentially critical diagnoses. For example, young, well-conditioned adults may maintain normal vital signs well into the course of shock.

Use of Vital Signs in Patients Who Appear to Be Ill

For some patients, abnormal vital signs are expected on the basis of their appearance and their symptoms. For patients in extremis, care should proceed according to established guidelines such as Advanced Cardiac Life Support (Chapter 63), Advanced Trauma Life Support, and algorithms for the treatment of shock (Chapters 107 and 108). For other ill-appearing patients, two processes must occur. In one, the physician, armed with knowledge of the differential diagnosis of each abnormal vital sign and the ability to take a thorough history and to perform an appropriate physical examination, narrows the list of potential diagnoses and decides which are of sufficient probability to warrant evaluation. Simultaneously, the physician considers the list of treatment options for all diagnoses associated with the abnormal vital sign and, before establishing a diagnosis, initiates those treatments for which the potential benefit of prompt administration exceeds potential harms. For example, antibiotics for febrile patients at risk for bacterial infection, hydrocortisone for hypotensive patients at risk for hypoadrenalism, and thiamine for hypothermic patients at risk for Wernicke encephalopathy may improve outcome and are unlikely to cause harm even if the patient does not have the suspected condition. Although early presumptive treatment can be life-saving in selected patients, it should not be abused; physicians must avoid knee-jerk responses that can cause harm.

Differential Diagnosis and Treatment Options

Single Abnormal Vital Signs

Because vital signs can be abnormal in virtually any disease process, no differential diagnosis can be encyclopedic. The physician should focus initially on common diseases and diseases that require specific treatment. The thought process should begin with the chief complaint and history and then incorporate information about the vital signs and the remainder of the physical examination.

Multiple Abnormal Vital Signs

Patients who are acutely ill are likely to have several abnormal vital signs. Although certain patterns of abnormal vital signs predominate in specific conditions (e.g., hypotension, tachycardia, and hypothermia in profound sepsis), no pattern can be considered pathognomonic. The physician's goal is to work toward a diagnosis while simultaneously providing treatments whose benefits outweigh potential harms.

Fever is generally accompanied by tachycardia, with the general rule of thumb that the heart rate will increase by 10 beats per minute for every 1° C increase in temperature. The absence of tachycardia with fever is known as pulse-temperature dissociation and has been reported in typhoid fever (Chapter 308), legionnaires disease (Chapter 314), babesiosis (Chapter 353), Q fever (Chapter 327), infection with *Rickettsia* spp (Chapter 327), malaria (Chapter 345), leptospirosis (Chapter 323), pneumonia caused by *Chlamydia* spp (Chapter 318), and viral infections such as dengue fever (Chapter 382), yellow fever (Chapter 381), and other viral hemorrhagic fevers (Chapter 381), although the predictive value of this finding is unknown.

Much can be learned by comparing the respiratory rate with pulse oximetry. Hyperventilation in the presence of high oxygen saturation suggests a central nervous system process or metabolic acidosis rather than a cardiopulmonary process. Low respiratory rates in the presence of low levels of oxygen saturation suggest central hypoventilation, which may respond to narcotic antagonists.

Hypertension and bradycardia in the obtunded or comatose patient are known as the Cushing reflex, a relatively late sign of elevated intracranial pressure. Physicians should strive to diagnose and treat this condition before the Cushing reflex develops.

Approach to Abnormalities of Specific Vital Signs

Elevated Temperature

Normal temperature is often cited as 37° C (98.6° F), but there is considerable diurnal variation and variation among individuals, so 38° C is the most commonly cited threshold for fever. Fever thought to be due to infection should be treated with antipyretics and appropriate antimicrobials (Chapter 280). The importance of early administration of antibiotics to potentially septic patients cannot be overstated (Chapters 280 and 281). Hyperthermia (temperature above 40° C) should be treated with cooling measures such as ice packs, cool misting in front of fans, cold gastric lavage, and, for medication-related syndromes, medications such as dantrolene (Chapter 109). Most hospital anesthesia departments will have a designated kit for the treatment of malignant hyperthermia (Chapters 432 and 434).

Low Temperature

The treatment of hypothermia is guided by its cause (Chapter 109). The body's temperature decreases when heat loss exceeds heat production. Every logically possible mechanism for this phenomenon has been observed. Decreased heat production can result from endocrine hypofunction (e.g., Addison disease [Chapter 227], hypopituitarism [Chapter 224], hypothyroidism [Chapter 226]) and loss of the ability to shiver (e.g., drug-induced or neurologic paralysis or neuromuscular disorders). Malfunction of the hypothalamic regulatory system can be due to hypoglycemia (Chapter 229) and a variety of central nervous system disorders (Wernicke encephalopathy

[Chapter 416], stroke [Chapter 407], tumor [Chapter 189], and trauma [Chapter 399]). Resetting of the temperature set point can occur with sepsis. Increased heat loss can be due to exposure, behavioral and physical disorders that prevent the patient from sensing or responding to cold, skin disorders that decrease its ability to retain heat, and vasodilators (including ethanol). A careful history and physical examination should illuminate which of these possibilities is most likely.

Several considerations are worthy of emphasis. The spine of an obtunded hypothermic patient who is "found down" must be protected and evaluated because paralysis from a fall may have prevented the patient from seeking shelter and may have diminished the ability to produce heat. The physician should not forget to administer antibiotics to patients who may be septic (Chapter 108), thiamine to those who may have Wernicke encephalopathy (Chapter 416), hydrocortisone to those who may be hypoadrenal (Chapter 227), and thyroid hormone to those who may have myxedema coma (Chapter 226). Severely hypothermic patients (Chapter 109) should be treated gently because any stimulation may trigger ventricular dysrhythmias; even in the absence of pulses, cardiopulmonary resuscitation should be used only in patients with ventricular fibrillation or asystole.

Elevated Heart Rate

The rate, rhythm, and electrocardiogram differentiate sinus tachycardia from tachyarrhythmias (Chapters 62 to 65). Tachyarrhythmias can be instigated by conditions that may require specific treatment (e.g., sepsis [Chapter 108], electrolyte disorders [Chapters 116, 117, and 118], endocrine disorders [Chapter 221], and poisonings [Chapters 22 and 110]) before the arrhythmia is likely to resolve. For sinus tachycardia, treatment of the underlying cause is always paramount. Treatments may include antipyretics (for fever); anxiolytics; oral or intravenous fluids (for hypovolemia); nitrates, angiotensin-converting enzyme inhibitors, and diuretics (for heart failure and fluid overload [Chapter 59]); oxygen (for hypoxemia); α-blockers (for stimulant overdose); β-blockers (for acute coronary syndromes [Chapters 72 and 73] or thyroid storm [Chapter 226]); and anticoagulation (for pulmonary embolism [Chapter 98]). Tachycardia is often an appropriate response to a clinical condition and should not be treated routinely unless it is causing or is likely to cause secondary problems.

Low Pulse

Bradycardia can be physiologic (athletes and others with increased vagal tone), due to prescribed cardiac medications (e.g., β-blockers, calcium-channel blockers, digoxin), overdoses (e.g., cholinergics, negative chronotropic agents), disease of the cardiac conducting system, electrolyte abnormalities (severe hyperkalemia), and inferior wall myocardial infarction (Chapters 64 and 73). Asymptomatic patients do not require immediate treatment. The goal of therapy is to produce a heart rate sufficient to perfuse the tissues and alleviate the symptoms (Chapter 63). Overdoses should be treated with specific antidotes (Chapter 110). Endocrine disorders should be treated with replacement therapy. In patients with acute coronary syndrome (Chapter 72), the goal is to restore perfusion and alleviate the ischemia. Patients with profound bradycardia or hypotension may require chronotropic drugs to increase perfusion even if these agents increase myocardial oxygen demand. In normotensive patients with milder bradycardia, chronotropic agents should be used only if symptoms and ischemia cannot be resolved by other means. Atropine is the primary therapy for bradycardia; isoproterenol and cardiac pacing are reserved for those who do not respond (Chapter 63).

Elevated Blood Pressure

Elevated blood pressure does not require acute treatment in the absence of symptoms or signs of end-organ damage (Chapter 67). In patients whose blood pressure is markedly above their baseline, the history and physical examination should assess for the conditions that define "hypertensive emergency": evidence of encephalopathy, intracranial hemorrhage, ischemic stroke, heart failure, pulmonary edema, acute coronary syndrome, aortic dissection, renal failure, and preeclampsia. In the absence of these conditions, treatment should consist of restarting or adjusting the medications of patients with known hypertension and initiating a program of blood pressure checks and appropriate evaluation for those with no prior history of hypertension (Chapter 67).

The patient with a true hypertensive emergency should be treated with agents appropriate for the specific condition. Because rapid decreases in blood pressure can be as deleterious as the hypertensive state itself, intravenous agents with short half-lives, such as nitroprusside, labetalol, nitroglycerin, and esmolol, are preferred (Chapter 67).

Low Blood Pressure

Low blood pressure must be evaluated in the context of the patient's symptoms, general appearance, and physical examination findings. Treatment depends on context. The same blood pressure value may necessitate intravenous inotropic agents in one patient and no treatment in another.

In tachycardic hypotensive patients, the physician must rapidly integrate all available evidence to determine the patient's volume state, cardiac function, vascular capacitance, and primary etiology (Chapter 106). Not all patients with hypotension and tachycardia are in shock, and not all patients in shock will have hypotension and tachycardia. Patients in shock should be treated on the basis of the cause (Chapters 106 to 108).

Symptomatic hypotensive patients thought to be intravascularly volume depleted should receive intravenous fluid resuscitation with crystalloid or blood, depending on their hemoglobin level (Chapter 106). In patients with known heart disease, patients who are frail or elderly, and patients whose volume status is uncertain, small boluses of fluid (e.g., 250 mL of normal saline), each followed by reassessment, are preferred so that iatrogenic heart failure may be avoided. Inotropic support should be reserved for patients who do not respond to fluid resuscitation. High-output heart failure should be kept in mind in patients with possible thyroid storm or stimulant overdose.

Increased Respiratory Rate

Tachypnea is a normal response to hypoxemia (see later). Treatment of tachypnea in the absence of hypoxemia is directed at the underlying cause, which often is pain (Chapter 30). Anxiolytics (e.g., diazepam, 5 to 10 mg PO or IV; lorazepam, 1 to 2 mg PO, IM, or IV) or reassurance can calm patients with behavioral causes of hyperventilation. Breathing into a paper bag has been shown to be an ineffective treatment. Pulmonary embolism (Chapter 98) does not necessarily reduce the oxygen saturation or cause a low Po_2 and should always be considered in at-risk patients with unexplained tachypnea.

Decreased Respiratory Rate

Any perturbation of the respiratory center in the central nervous system can slow the respiratory drive (Chapter 86). Narcotics and other sedatives and neurologic conditions are common causes of a decreased respiratory rate. The primary treatment of apnea is mechanical ventilation (Chapter 105), but narcotic antagonists can be tried in patients with a history or physical examination findings (miosis, track marks, opiate patch) suggestive of narcotic use or abuse (Chapter 34). In nonapneic patients, mechanical ventilation is indicated for patients who are breathing too slowly to maintain an acceptable oxygen saturation and for patients who are retaining carbon dioxide in quantities sufficient to depress mental function. Patients who are unable to protect their airway should be intubated. Oxygen should be administered to all hypopneic patients who are hypoxemic (see earlier). Patients with chronic hypoventilation (Chapter 86) may have retained HCO_3^- to compensate for an elevated Pco_2 and so may depend on hypoxia to maintain respiratory drive; in these patients, overaggressive administration of oxygen can decrease the respiratory rate, increase the Pco_2, and increase obtundation (Chapter 104).

Decreased Oxygen Saturation

In hypopneic patients, initial efforts should try to increase the respiratory rate (see earlier) and tidal volume. Regardless of etiology, oxygen, in amounts adequate to restore adequate oxygen saturation ($Po_2 > 60$ mm Hg, oxygen saturation >90%), is the mainstay of therapy. When oxygen alone fails, noninvasive methods for improving ventilation or tracheal intubation are required (Chapter 104). Oxygen should increase the Po_2 in all patients except those who have severe right-to-left shunting (Chapter 69). Treatment of conditions that cause hypoxemia includes antibiotics (pneumonia), bronchodilators (asthma, chronic obstructive pulmonary disease), diuretics and vasodilators (pulmonary edema), anticoagulants (pulmonary embolism), hyperbaric oxygen (carbon monoxide poisoning), methylene blue (methemoglobinemia, sulfhemoglobinemia), and transfusion (anemia).

GENERAL REFERENCES

For the General References and other additional features, please visit Expert Consult at https://expertconsult.inkling.com.

9

STATISTICAL INTERPRETATION OF DATA

THOMAS B. NEWMAN AND CHARLES E. MCCULLOCH

ROLE AND LIMITATIONS OF STATISTICS

Much of medicine is inherently probabilistic. Not everyone with hypercholesterolemia who is treated with a statin is prevented from having a myocardial infarction, and not everyone not treated does have one, but statins reduce the *probability* of a myocardial infarction in such patients. Because so much of medicine is based on probabilities, studies must be performed on *groups* of people to estimate these probabilities. Three component tasks of statistics are: selecting a sample of subjects for study, describing the data from that sample, and drawing inferences from that sample to a larger population of interest.[1]

SAMPLING: SELECTING SUBJECTS FOR A STUDY

The goal of research is to produce generalizable knowledge, so that measurements made by researchers on samples of individuals will eventually help draw inferences to a larger group of people than was studied. The ability to draw such inferences depends on how the subjects for the study (the sample) were selected. To understand the process of selection, it is helpful to begin by identifying the group to which the results are to be generalized and then work backward to the sample of subjects to be studied.

Target Population

The *target population* is the population to which it is hoped the results of the study will be generalizable. For example, to study the efficacy of a new drug to treat obesity, the target population might be all people with a certain level of obesity (e.g., body mass index [BMI] of ≥30 kg/m^2) who might be candidates for the drug.

Sampling

The *intended sample* is the group of people who are eligible to be in the study based on meeting *inclusion criteria,* which specify the demographic, clinical, and temporal characteristics of the intended subjects, and not meeting *exclusion criteria,* which specify the characteristics of subjects whom the investigator does not wish to study. For example, for the study of a new obesity drug, the intended sample (inclusion criteria) might be men and women 18 years or older who live in one of four metropolitan areas, who have a BMI of 30 kg/m^2 or higher, and who have failed an attempt at weight loss with a standard diet. Exclusion criteria might include an inability to speak English or Spanish, known alcohol abuse, plans to leave the area in the next 6 months, and being pregnant or planning to become pregnant in the next 6 months.

In some cases, particularly large population health surveys such as the National Health and Nutrition Examination Survey (NHANES), the intended sample is a *random* sample of the target population. A *simple random sample* is a sample in which every member of the target population has an equal chance of being selected. Simple random samples are the easiest to handle statistically but are often impractical. For example, if the target population is the entire population of the United States (as is the case for NHANES), a simple random sample would include subjects from all over the country. Getting subjects from thousands of distinct geographic areas to examination sites would be logistically difficult. An alternative, used in NHANES, is *cluster* sampling, in which investigators take a random sample of "clusters" (e.g., specific census tracts or geographic areas) and then try to study all or a sample of the subjects in each cluster. Knowledge of the cluster sampling process must then be used during analysis of the study (see later) to draw inferences correctly back to the target population.

Regardless of the method used to select the intended sample, the *actual sample* will almost always differ in important ways because not all intended subjects will be willing to enroll in the study and not all who begin a study will complete it. In a study on treatment of obesity, for example, those who consent to be in the study probably differ in important, but difficult-to-quantify ways from those who do not (and may be more likely to do well with treatment). Furthermore, subjects who respond poorly to treatment may drop out, thus making the group that completes the study even less representative.

Statistical methods address only some of the issues involved in making inferences from a sample to a target population. Specifically, *most statistical methods address only the effect of random variation on the inference from the intended sample to the target population.* Estimating the effects of differences between the intended sample and the actual sample depends on the quantities being estimated and content knowledge about whether factors associated with being in the actual sample are related to those quantities. One rule of thumb about generalizability is that *associations between variables* are more often generalizable than measurements of single variables. For instance, subjects who consent to be in a study of obesity may be more motivated than average, but this motivation would be expected to have less effect on the *difference* in weight loss between groups than on the average weight loss in either group.

DESCRIBING THE SAMPLE

Types of Variables

A key use of statistics is to describe sample data. Methods of description depend on the *type of variable* (E-Table 9-1). *Numerical* variables include *continuous* variables (those that have a wide range of possible values), *count* variables (e.g., the number of times a woman has been pregnant), and *time-to-event* variables (e.g., the time from initial treatment to recurrence of breast cancer). Whereas *numerical* variables describe the data with numbers, *categorical* variables consist of named characteristics. Categorical variables can be further divided into *dichotomous* variables, which can take on only two possible values (e.g., alive/dead); *nominal* variables, which can take on more than two values but have no intrinsic ordering (e.g., race); and *ordinal* variables, which have more than two values and an intrinsic ordering of the values (e.g., tumor stage). Numerical variables are also ordinal by nature and can be made binary by breaking the values into two disjointed categories (e.g., systolic blood pressure >140 mm Hg or not), and thus sometimes methods designed for ordinal or binary data are used with numerical variable types, often for ease of interpretation.

Univariate Statistics for Numerical Variables: Mean, Standard Deviation, Median, and Percentiles

When describing data in a sample, it is a good idea to begin with *univariate* (one variable at a time) statistics. For numerical variables, univariate statistics typically measure *central tendency* and *variability.* The most common measures of central tendency are the *mean* (or average, i.e., the sum of the observations divided by the number of observations) and the *median* (the 50th percentile, i.e., the value that has equal numbers of observations above and below it).

One of the most commonly used measures of variability is the *standard deviation* (SD). The SD is defined as the square root of the *variance,* which is calculated by subtracting each value in the sample from the mean, squaring that difference, totaling all of the squared differences, and dividing by the number of observations minus 1. Although this definition is far from intuitive, the SD has some useful mathematical properties, namely, that if the distribution of the variable is the familiar bell-shaped, *normal,* or *Gaussian* distribution, about 68% of the observations will be within 1 SD of the mean, about 95% within 2 SD, and about 99.7% within 3 SD. Even when the distribution is not normal, these rules are often approximately true.

For variables that are not normally distributed, including most count and time-to-event variables, the mean and SD are not as useful for summarizing the data. In that case, the median may be a better measure of central tendency because it is not influenced by observations far below or far above the center. Similarly, the range and pairs of percentiles, such as the 25th and 75th percentiles or the 15th and 85th percentiles, will provide a better description of the spread of the data than the SD will. The 15th and 85th percentiles are particularly attractive because they correspond, in the Gaussian distribution, to about −1 and +1 SD from the mean, thus making reporting of the 50th, 15th, and 85th percentiles roughly equivalent to reporting the mean and SD.

Univariate Statistics for Categorical Variables: Proportions, Rates, and Ratios

For categorical variables, the main univariate statistic is the *proportion* of subjects with each value of the variable. For dichotomous variables, only one proportion is needed (e.g., the proportion female); for nominal variables and ordinal variables with few categories, the proportion in each group can be provided. Ordinal variables with many categories can be summarized by using proportions or by using medians and percentiles, as with continuous data that are not normally distributed.

It is worth distinguishing among *proportions, rates,* and *ratios* because these terms are often confused. *Proportions* are unitless, always between 0 and 1 inclusive, and express what fraction of the subjects have or develop a particular characteristic or outcome. Strictly speaking, *rates* have units of inverse time; they express the proportion of subjects in whom a particular characteristic or outcome develops over a specific time period. The term is frequently misused, however. For example, the term *false-positive rate* is widely used for the proportion of subjects without a disease who test positive, even though it is a proportion, not a rate. *Ratios* are the quotients of two numbers; they can range between zero and infinity. For example, the male-to-female ratio of people with a disease might be 3 : 1. As a rule, if a ratio can be expressed as a proportion instead (e.g., 75% male), it is more concise and easier to understand.

Incidence and Prevalence

Two terms commonly used (and misused) in medicine and public health are *incidence* and *prevalence. Incidence* describes the number of subjects who *contract* a disease *over time* divided by the population at risk. Incidence is usually expressed as a rate (e.g., 7 per 1000 per year), but it may sometimes be a proportion if the time variable is otherwise understood or clear, as in the lifetime incidence of breast cancer or the incidence of diabetes during pregnancy. *Prevalence* describes the number of subjects who *have* a disease at *one point in time* divided by the population at risk; it is always a proportion. At any point in time, the prevalence of disease depends on how many people contract it and how long it lasts: prevalence = incidence × duration.

Bivariate Statistics

Bivariate statistics summarize the relationship between two variables. In clinical research, it is often desirable to distinguish between *predictor* and *outcome variables.* Predictor variables include treatments received, demographic variables, and test results that are thought possibly to predict or cause the *outcome variable,* which is the disease or (generally bad) event or outcome that the test should predict or treatment prevent. For example, to see whether a bone mineral density measurement (the predictor) predicts time to vertebral fracture (the outcome), the choice of bivariate statistic to assess the association of outcome with predictor depends on the types of predictor and outcome variables being compared.

Dichotomous Predictor and Outcome Variables

A common and straightforward case is when both predictor and outcome variables are dichotomous, and the results can thus be summarized in a 2 × 2 table. Bivariate statistics are also called *measures of association* (E-Table 9-2).

Relative Risk

The *relative risk* or *risk ratio* (RR) is the ratio of the proportion of subjects in one group in whom the outcome develops divided by the proportion in the other group in whom it develops. It is a general (but not universal) convention to have the outcome be something bad and to have the numerator be the risk for those who have a particular factor or were exposed to an intervention. When this convention is followed, an RR greater than 1 means that exposure to the factor was (on average) bad for the study subjects (with respect to the outcome being studied), whereas an RR less than 1 means that it was good. That is, risk factors that cause diseases will have RR values greater than 1, and effective treatments will have an RR less than 1. For example, in the Women's Health Initiative (WHI) randomized trial, conjugated equine estrogen use was associated with an increased risk for stroke (RR = 1.37) and decreased risk for hip fracture (RR = 0.61).

Relative Risk Reduction

The *relative risk reduction* (RRR) is 1 − RR. The RRR is generally used only for effective interventions, that is, interventions in which the RR is less than 1, so the RRR is generally greater than 0. In the aforementioned WHI example, estrogen had an RR of 0.61 for hip fracture, so the RRR would be 1 − 0.61 = 0.39, or 39%. The RRR is commonly expressed as a percentage and used only when it is positive.

Absolute Risk Reduction

The *risk difference* or *absolute risk reduction* (ARR) is the difference in risk between the groups, defined as earlier. In the WHI, the risk for hip fracture was 0.11% per year with estrogen and 0.17% per year with placebo. Again, conventionally the risk is for something bad, and the risk in the group of interest is subtracted from the risk in a comparison group, so the ARR will be positive for effective interventions. In this case, the ARR = 0.06% per year, or 6 in 10,000 per year.

Number Needed to Treat

The *number needed to treat* (NNT) is 1/ARR. To see why this is the case, consider the WHI placebo group and imagine treating 10,000 patients for a year. All but 17 would not have had a hip fracture anyway because the fracture rate in the placebo group was 0.17% per year, and 11 subjects would sustain a fracture despite treatment because the fracture rate in the estrogen group was 0.11% per year. Thus, with treatment of 10,000 patients for a year, 17 − 11 = 6 fractures prevented, or 1 fracture prevented for each 1667 patients treated for 1 year. This calculation is equivalent to 1/0.06% per year.

Risk Difference

When the treatment *increases* the risk for a bad outcome, the difference in risk between treated and untreated patients should still be calculated, but it is usually just called the risk difference rather than an ARR (because the "reduction" would be negative). In that case, the NNT is sometimes called the number needed to harm. This term is a bit of a misnomer. The reciprocal of the risk difference is still a number needed to treat; it is just a number needed to treat per person harmed rather than a number needed to treat per person who benefits. In the WHI, treatment with estrogens was estimated to cause about 12 additional strokes per 10,000 women per year, so the number needed to be treated for 1 year to cause a stroke was about 10,000/12, or 833.

Odds Ratio

Another commonly used measure of association is the *odds ratio* (OR). The OR is the ratio of the *odds* of the outcome in the two groups, where the definition of the odds of an outcome is $p/(1 - p)$, with p being the probability of the outcome. From this definition it is apparent that when p is very small, $1 - p$ will be close to 1, so $p/(1 - p)$ will be close to p, and the OR will closely approximate the RR. In the WHI, the ORs for stroke (1.37) and fracture (0.61) were virtually identical to the RRs because both stroke and fracture were rare. When p is not small, however, the odds and probability will be quite different, and ORs and RRs will not be interchangeable.

Absolute versus Relative Measures

RRRs are usually more generalizable than ARRs. For example, the use of statin drugs is associated with about a 30% decrease in coronary events in a wide variety of patient populations (Chapter 206). The ARR, however, will usually vary with the baseline risk, that is, the risk for a coronary event in the absence of treatment. For high-risk men who have already had a myocardial infarction, the baseline 5-year risk might be 20%, which could be reduced to 14% with treatment, an ARR of 6%, and an NNT of about 17 for approximately 5 years. Conversely, for a 45-year-old woman with a high low-density lipoprotein cholesterol level but no history of heart disease, in whom the 5-year risk might be closer to 1%, the same RRR would give a 0.7% risk with treatment, a risk difference of 0.3%, and an NNT of 333 for 5 years.

The choice of *absolute* versus *relative measures* of association depends on the intended use of the measure. As noted earlier, RRs are more useful as summary measures of effect because they are more often generalizable across a wide variety of populations. RRs are also more helpful for understanding causality. However, absolute risks are more important for questions about clinical decision making because they relate directly to the tradeoffs between risks and benefits—specifically, the NNT, as well as the costs and side effects that need to be balanced against potential benefits. RRRs are often used in advertising because they are generally more impressive than ARRs. Unfortunately, the distinction between relative and absolute risks may not be appreciated by clinicians, thereby leading to higher estimates of the potential benefits of treatments when RRs or RRRs are used.

Risk Ratios versus Odds Ratios

The choice between RRs and ORs is easier: RRs are preferred because they are easier to understand. Because ORs that are not equal to 1 are always farther from 1 than the corresponding RR, they may falsely inflate the perceived importance of a factor. ORs are, however, typically used in two circumstances. First, in case-control studies (Chapter 11), in which subjects with and without the disease are sampled separately, the RR cannot be calculated directly. This situation does not usually cause a problem, however, because case-control studies are generally performed to assess rare outcomes, for which the OR will closely approximate the RR. Second, in observational studies that use a type of multivariate analysis called *logistic regression* (see later), use of the OR is convenient because it is the parameter that is modeled in the analysis.

Dichotomous Predictor Variable, Continuous Outcome Variable

Many outcome variables are naturally continuous rather than dichotomous. For example, in a study of a new treatment of obesity, the outcome might be change in weight or BMI. For a new diuretic, the outcome might be change in blood pressure. For a palliative treatment, the outcome might be a quality-of-life score calculated from a multi-item questionnaire. Because of the many possible values for the score, it may be analyzed as a continuous variable. In these cases, dichotomizing the outcome leads to loss of information. Instead, the *mean difference* between the two groups is an appropriate measure of the effect size. When the outcome is itself a difference (e.g., change in blood pressure over time), the effect is measured by the difference in the *within*-group differences *between* the groups.

Most measurements have units (e.g., kg, mm Hg), so differences between groups will have the same units and be meaningless without them. If the units of measurement are familiar (e.g., kg or mm Hg), the difference between groups will be meaningful without further manipulation. For measurements in unfamiliar units, such as a score on a new quality-of-life instrument, some benchmark is useful to help judge whether the difference between groups is large or small. In that case, authors typically express the difference in relation to the spread of values in the study by calculating the *standardized mean difference* (SMD), which is the difference between the two means divided by the SD of the measurement. It is thus expressed as the number of SDs by which the two groups are apart. To help provide a rough feel for this difference, a 1-SD difference between means (SMD = 1) would be a 15-point difference in IQ scores, a 600-g difference in birthweight, or a 40-mg/dL difference in total cholesterol levels.

Continuous Predictor Variable

When predictor variables are continuous, the investigator can either group the values into two or more categories and calculate mean differences or SMDs between the groups as discussed earlier or use a *model* to summarize the degree to which changes in the predictor variable are associated with changes in the outcome variable. Use of a model may more compactly describe the effects of interest but involves assumptions about the way the predictor and outcome variables are related. Perhaps the simplest model is to assume a linear relationship between the outcome and predictor. For example, one could assume that the relationship between systolic blood pressure (mm Hg) and salt intake (g/day) was linear over the range studied:

$$SBP_i = a + (b \times SALT_i) + \varepsilon_i$$

where SBP_i is the systolic blood pressure for study subject *i*, $SALT_i$ is that subject's salt intake, and ε_i is an error term that the model specifies must average out to zero across all of the subjects in the study. In this model, *a* is a constant, the *intercept,* and the strength of the relationship between the outcome and predictor can be summarized by the slope *b,* which has units equal to the units of SBP divided by the units of SALT, or mm Hg per gram of salt per day in this case.

Note that without the units, such a number is meaningless. For example, if salt intake were measured in grams per week instead of grams per day, the slope would only be one seventh as large. Thus, when reading an article in which the association between two variables is summarized, it is critical to note the units of the variables. As discussed earlier, when units are unfamiliar, they are sometimes standardized by dividing by the SDs of one or both variables.

It is important to keep in mind that use of a model to summarize a relationship between two variables may not be appropriate if the model does not fit. In the preceding example, the assumption is that salt intake and blood pressure have a linear relationship, with the slope equal to *b* mm Hg/g salt per day. The value of *b* is about 1 mm Hg/g salt per day for hypertensive patients. If the range of salt intake of interest is from 1 to 10 g/day, the model predicts that blood pressure will increase 1 mm Hg as a result of a 1-g/day increase in salt intake whether that increase is from 1 to 2 g/day or from 9 to 10 g/day. If the effect of a 1-g/day change in salt intake differed in subjects ingesting low- and high-salt diets, the model would not fit, and misleading conclusions could result.

When the outcome variable is dichotomous, the relationship between the probability of the outcome and a continuous predictor variable is often modeled with a *logistic* model:

$$\Pr\{Y_i = 1\} = \frac{1}{1 + e^{-(a + bx_i)}}$$

where the outcome Y_i is coded 0 or 1 for study subject *i*, and x_i is that subject's value of the predictor variable. Once again, *a* is a constant, in this case related to the probability of the disease when the predictor is equal to zero, and *b* summarizes the strength of the association; in this case, it is the natural logarithm of the OR rather than the slope. The OR is the OR *per unit change* in the predictor variable. For example, in a study of lung cancer, an OR of 1.06 for pack years of smoking would indicate that the odds of lung cancer increase by 6% for each pack year increase in smoking.

Because the outcome variable is dichotomous, it has no units, and "standardizing" it by dividing by its SD is unnecessary and counterproductive. On the other hand, continuous predictor variables do have units, and the OR for the logistic model will be per unit change in the predictor variable or, if standardized, per SD change in the predictor variable. Re-expressing predictors in standardized or at least more sensible units is often necessary. For example, suppose 10-year mortality risk decreases by 20% (i.e., RR = 0.8) for each increase in gross income of $10,000. The RR associated with an increase in gross income of $1 (which is what a computer program would report if the predictor were entered in dollars) would be 0.99998, apparently no effect at all because a change of $1 in gross income is negligible and associated with a negligible change in risk. To derive the coefficient associated with a $1 change, the coefficient for a $10,000 change is raised to the $^1/_{10{,}000}$ power: $0.8^{(1/10{,}000)} = 0.99998$.

Multivariable Statistics

In many cases, researchers are interested in the effects of multiple predictor variables on an outcome. Particularly in observational studies, in which investigators cannot assign values of a predictor variable experimentally, it will be of interest to estimate the effects of a predictor variable of interest *independent* of the effects of other variables. For example, in studying whether breastfeeding reduces the mother's risk for subsequent breast cancer, investigators would try to take differences in age, race, family history, and parity into account. Trying to stratify by all these variables would require a massive data set. Instead, models are used because they enable the information about individual predictors to be summarized by using the full data set. In this way, the estimated coefficients from the model are powerful descriptive statistics that allow a sense of the data in situations in which simpler methods fail. These models are similar to those described earlier but include terms for the additional variables.

Multiple Linear Regression

The multiple linear regression model for an outcome variable Y as function or predictor variables x_1, x_2, and so forth is as follows:

$$Y_i = a + (b_1 \times x_{1i}) + (b_2 \times x_{2i}) + \ldots + (b_k \times x_{ki}) + \varepsilon_i,$$

where the subscripts 1, 2, ..., k are for the first, second, ... k^{th} variables of the model, and the *i* subscripts are for each individual. As before, the relationships between each of these predictor variables and the outcome variable are summarized by coefficients, or slopes, which have units of Y divided by the units of the associated predictor. In addition, the linear combination of predictor variables adds a major simplifying constraint (and assumption) to the model: it specifies that the effects of each variable on the outcome variable are the same regardless of the values of other variables in the model. Thus, for example, if x_1 is the variable for salt intake and x_2 is a variable for sex (e.g., 0 for females and 1 for males), this model assumes that the average effect of a 1-g increase in daily salt intake on blood pressure is the same in men and women. If such is not believed to be the case, either based on previous information or from examining the data, the model should include *interaction* terms, or separate models should be used for men and women.

Multiple Logistic Regression

The logistic model expands to include multiple variables in much the same way as the linear model:

$$\Pr\{Y_i = 1\} = \frac{1}{1 + e^{-(a + b_1 x_{1i} + b_2 x_{2i} + \ldots + b_k x_{ki})}}$$

Again, the additional assumption when more than one predictor is included in the model is that in the absence of included interaction terms, the effect of each variable on the odds of the outcome is the same regardless of the values of other variables in the model. Because the logistic model is multiplicative, however, the effects of different predictors on the odds of the outcome are multiplied, not added. Thus, for example, if male sex is associated with a doubling of the odds for heart disease, this doubling will occur in both smokers and nonsmokers; if smoking triples the odds, this tripling will be true in both men and women, so smoking men would be predicted to have $2 \times 3 = 6$ times higher odds of heart disease than nonsmoking women.

Recursive Partitioning

Recursive partitioning, or *"classification and regression trees,"* is a prediction method often used with dichotomous outcomes that avoids the assumptions of linearity. This technique creates prediction rules by repeatedly dividing the sample into subgroups, with each subdivision being formed by further separating the sample on the value of one of the predictor variables. The optimal choice of variables and cut points may depend on the relative costs of false-positive and false-negative predictions, as set by the investigator. The end result is a set of branching questions that forms a treelike structure in which each final branch provides a yes/no prediction of the outcome. The methods of fitting the tree to data (e.g., cross-validation) help reduce overfitting (inclusion of unnecessary predictor variables), especially in cases with many potential predictors.

Proportional Hazards (Cox) Model

A multivariate model often used in studies in which subjects are monitored over time for development of the outcome is the *Cox* or *proportional hazards* model. Like the logistic model, the Cox model is used for continuous or dichotomous predictor variables, but in this case with a time-to-event outcome (e.g., time to a stroke). This approach models the *rate* at which the outcome occurs over time by taking into account the number of people still at risk at any given time. The coefficients in the Cox model are logarithms of *hazard ratios* rather than ORs, interpretable (when exponentiated) as the effect of a unit change in predictors on the *hazard* (risk in the next short time period) of the outcome developing. Like the logistic model, the Cox model is multiplicative; that is, it assumes that changes in risk factors multiply the hazard by a fixed amount regardless of the levels of other risk factors. A key feature of the Cox model and other *survival analysis* techniques is that they accommodate censored data (when the time to event is known only to exceed a certain value). For example, if the outcome is time to stroke, the study will end with many subjects who have not had a stroke, so their time to stroke is known only to exceed the time to their last follow-up visit.

INFERRING POPULATION VALUES FROM A SAMPLE

The next step after describing the data is drawing inferences from a sample to the population from which the sample was drawn. Statistics mainly quantify random error, which arises by chance because even a sample randomly selected from a population may not be exactly like the population from which it was drawn. Samples that were not randomly selected from populations may be unrepresentative because of *bias*, and statistics cannot help with this type of systematic (nonrandom) error.

Inferences from Sample Means: Standard Deviation versus Standard Error

The simplest case of inference from a sample to a population involves estimating a population mean from a sample mean. Intuitively, the larger the sample size, *N*, the more likely it will be that the sample mean will be close to the population mean, that is, close to the mean that would be calculated if every member of the population were studied. The more variability there is in the population (and hence the sample), the less accurate the sample estimate of the population mean is likely to be. Thus, the precision with which a population mean can be estimated is related to both the size of the sample and the SD of the sample. To make inferences about a population mean from a sample mean, the *standard error of the mean* (SEM), which takes both of these factors into account, is as follows:

$$\text{SEM} = \frac{\text{SD}}{\sqrt{N}}$$

To understand the meaning of the SEM, imagine that instead of taking a single sample of *N* subjects from the population, many such samples were taken. The mean of each sample could be calculated, as could the mean of those sample means and the SD of these means. The SEM is the best estimate from a single sample of what that SD of sample means would be.

Confidence Intervals

The SEM expresses variability of sample means in the same way that the SD expresses variability of individual observations. Just as about 95% of *observations* in a population are expected to be within ±1.96 SD of the mean, 95% of *sample means* are expected to be within 1.96 SEM of the population mean, thereby providing the 95% confidence interval (CI), which is the range of values for the population mean consistent with what was observed from the sample.

CIs can similarly be calculated for other quantities estimated from samples, including proportions, ORs, RRs, regression coefficients, and hazard ratios. In each case, they provide a range of values for the parameter in the target population consistent with what was observed in the study sample.

Significance Testing and *P* Values

Many papers in the medical literature include *P* values, but the meaning of *P* values is widely misunderstood and mistaught. *P* values start with calculation of a *test statistic* from the sample that has a known distribution under certain assumptions, most commonly the *null hypothesis,* which states that there is no association between variables. *P* values provide the answer to the question, "If the null hypothesis were true, what would be the probability of obtaining, by chance alone, a value of the test statistic this large or larger (suggesting an association between groups of this strength or stronger)?" When the *P* value is small, there are two possible explanations. First, something with a small possibility of occurring actually happened; or second, the null hypothesis is false, and there is a true association. Values of *P* less than 0.05 are customarily described as "statistically significant."

There are a number of common pitfalls in interpreting *P* values. The first is that because *P* values less than .05 are customarily described as being "statistically significant," the description of results with *P* values less than .05 sometimes gets shortened to "significant" when in fact the results may not be clinically significant (i.e., important) at all. A lack of congruence between clinical and statistical significance most commonly arises when studies have a large sample size and the measurement is of a continuous or frequently occurring outcome.

A second pitfall is concluding that no association exists simply because the *P* value is greater than .05. However, it is possible that a real association exists, but that it simply was not found in the study. This problem is particularly likely if the sample size is small because small studies have low *power,* defined as the probability of obtaining statistically significant results if there really is a given magnitude of difference between groups in the population. One approach to interpreting a study with a nonsignificant *P* value is to examine the power that the study had to find a difference. A better approach is to look at the 95% CI. If the 95% CI excludes all clinically significant levels of the strength of an association, the study probably had an adequate sample size to find an association if there had been one. If not, a clinically significant effect may have been missed. In "negative" studies, the use of CIs is more helpful than power analyses because CIs incorporate information from the study's results.

Finally, a common misconception about *P* values is that they indicate the probability that the null hypothesis is true (e.g., that there is no association between variables). Thus, it is not uncommon to hear or read that a *P* value less than .05 implies at least a 95% probability that the observed association is not due to chance. This statement represents a fundamental misunderstanding of *P* values. Calculation of *P* values is *based on the assumption* that the null hypothesis is true. The probability that an association is real depends not just on the probability of its occurrence under the null hypothesis but also on the probability of another basis for the association (see later)—an assessment that depends on information from outside the study, sometimes called the *prior probability* of an association (of a certain magnitude) estimated before the study results were known and requiring a different approach to statistical inference. Similarly, CIs do not take into account previous information on the probable range of the parameter being estimated. Bayesian methods, which explicitly combine prior knowledge with new information, are beginning to enter the mainstream medical literature.[2]

Appropriate test statistics and methods for calculating *P* values depend on the type of variable, just as with descriptive statistics (see E-Table 9-1). For example, to test the hypothesis that the mean values of a continuous variable are equal in two groups, a *t* test would be used; to compare the mean values across multiple groups, analysis of variance would be used. Because there are many different ways for the null hypothesis to be false (i.e., many different ways that two variables might be associated) and many test statistics that could be calculated, there are many different ways of calculating a *P* value for the association of the same two variables in a data set, and they may not all give the same answer.

Meta-analysis

Statistical techniques for inferring population values from a sample are not restricted to samples of individuals. *Meta-analysis* is a statistical method for drawing inferences from a sample of *studies* to derive a summary estimate and confidence interval for a parameter measured by the included studies, such as a risk ratio for a treatment effect.[3] Meta-analysis allows the formal combination of results while estimating and accommodating both the within-study and between-study variations. Meta-analysis is most often done when raw data from the studies are not available, as is typically the case when synthesizing information from multiple published results. For example, the previously cited estimate that a 1-g/day change in salt intake is associated with a 1-mm Hg change in blood pressure was obtained from a meta-analysis of randomized trials of low-salt diets in adults.

INFERRING CAUSALITY

In many cases, a goal of clinical research is not just to identify associations but also to determine whether they are *causal,* that is, whether the predictor causes the outcome. Thus, if people who take vitamin E live longer than those who do not, it is important to know whether it is *because* they took the vitamin or for some other reason.

Determination of causality is based on considering alternative explanations for an association between two variables and trying to exclude or confirm these alternative explanations. The alternatives to a causal relationship between predictor and outcome variables are *chance, bias, effect-cause,* and *confounding. P* values and CIs help assess the likelihood of *chance* as the basis for an association. *Bias* occurs when systematic errors in sampling or measurements can lead to distorted estimates of an association. For example, if those making measurements of the outcome variable are not blinded to values of the predictor variable, they may measure the outcome variable differently in subjects with different values of the predictor variable, thereby distorting the association between outcome and predictor.

Effect-cause is a particular problem in cross-sectional studies, in which (in contrast to longitudinal studies) all measurements are made at a single point in time, thereby precluding demonstration that the predictor variable preceded the outcome—an important part of demonstrating causality. Sometimes biology provides clear guidance about the direction of causality. For example, in a cross-sectional study relating levels of urinary cotinine (a measure of exposure to tobacco smoke) to decreases in pulmonary function, it is hard to imagine that poor pulmonary function caused people to be exposed to smoke. Conversely, sometimes inferring causality is more difficult: are people overweight because they exercise less, or do they exercise less because they are overweight (or both)?

Confounding

Confounding can occur when one or more extraneous variables are associated with both the predictor of interest and the outcome. For example, observational studies suggested that high doses of vitamin E might decrease the risk for heart disease. However, this association seems to have been largely due to confounding: people who took vitamin E were different in other ways from those who did not, including differences in factors causally related to coronary heart disease. If such factors are known and can be measured accurately, one way to reduce confounding is to *stratify* or *match* on these variables. The idea is to assemble groups of people who did and did not take vitamin E but who were similar in other ways. Multivariate analysis can accomplish the same goal—other measured variables are held constant statistically, and the effect of the variable of interest (in this case the use of vitamin E) can be examined. Multivariate analysis has the advantage that it can control simultaneously for more potentially confounding variables than can be considered with stratification or matching, but it has the disadvantage that a model must be created (see earlier), and this model may not fit the data well.

A new technique that is less dependent on model fit but still requires accurate measurements of confounding variables is the use of *propensity scores.* Propensity scores are used to assemble comparable groups in the same way as stratification or matching, but in this case the comparability is achieved on the basis of the *propensity* to be exposed to or be treated with the predictor variable of primary interest. Although propensity scores can adjust only for known confounders and are more subject to manipulation by investigators, systematic reviews suggest that they usually give answers that are generally similar to those of randomized trials addressing the same question.[4]

A major limitation of these methods of controlling for confounding is that the confounders must be known to the investigators and accurately measured. In the case of vitamin E, apparent favorable effects persisted after controlling for known confounding variables. It is for this reason that randomized trials provide the strongest evidence for causality. If the predictor variable of interest can be randomly assigned, confounding variables, both known and unknown, should be approximately equally distributed between the subjects who are and are not exposed to the predictor variable, and it is reasonable to infer that any significant differences in outcome that remain in these now comparable groups would be due to differences in the predictor variable of interest. In the case of vitamin E, a recent meta-analysis of randomized trials found no benefit and in fact suggested harm from high doses.

OTHER COMMON STATISTICAL PITFALLS

Missing Data

Research on human subjects is challenging. People drop out of studies, refuse to answer questions, miss study visits, and die of diseases that are not being studied directly in the protocol. Consequently, missing or incomplete data are a fact of medical research. When the particular data that are missing are unrelated to the outcome being studied (which might be true, for example, if the files storing the data got partially corrupted), analyses using only the data present (sometimes called a complete case analysis) are unlikely to be misleading. Unfortunately, such is rarely the case. Subjects refusing to divulge family income probably have atypical values, patients not coming for scheduled visits in a study of depression may be more or less depressed, and patients in an osteoporosis study who die of heart disease probably differ in many ways from those who do not.

Whenever a sizable fraction of the data is missing (certainly if it is above 10 or 15%), there is the danger of substantial bias from an analysis that uses only the complete data. This is the gap noted earlier between the intended and actual samples. Any study with substantial missing data should be clear about how many missing data there were and what was done to assess or alleviate the impact; otherwise, the critical consumer of such information should be suspicious. Multiple imputation is a technique of using observations with nonmissing data to estimate missing values; it can produce less biased estimates than simply excluding the observations with missing data.[5] In a randomized trial, the general rule is that the primary analysis should include all subjects who were randomized, regardless of whether they followed the study protocol, in an *intention-to-treat* analysis.

Clustered or Hierarchical Data

Data are often collected in a clustered (also called hierarchical) manner; for example, NHANES used a cluster sample survey, and a study of patient outcomes might be conducted at five hospitals, each with multiple admission teams. The cluster sample or the clustering of patients within teams within hospitals leads to correlated data. Said another way, and other things being equal, data collected on the same patient, by the same admission team, or in the same cluster are likely to be more similar than data from different patients, teams, or clusters. Failure to use statistical methods that accommodate correlated data can seriously misstate standard errors, widths of CIs, and *P* values, most often leading to overly optimistic estimates, that is, standard errors and *P* values that are incorrectly too small and CIs that are incorrectly too narrow. Statistical methods for dealing with correlated data include *generalized estimating equations* and the use of *robust standard errors* and *frailty models* (for time-to-event data). Studies with obvious hierarchical structure that fail to use such methods may be in serious error.

Multiple Hypothesis Testing

The "multiple hypothesis testing" or "multiple comparisons" issue refers to the idea that if multiple statistical tests are conducted, each at a significance level of .05, the chance that at least one of them will achieve a *P* value of less than .05 is considerably larger than .05, even when all the null hypotheses are true. For example, when comparing the mean value of a continuous variable across many different groups, analysis of variance is a time-tested method of performing an overall test of equality and avoiding making a large number of pairwise comparisons.

Because most medical studies collect data on a large number of predictor variables, performing a test on the association of each one with the outcome may generate false-positive results. The risk for falsely positive results is especially high with genomic studies, in which a researcher may test a million single-nucleotide polymorphisms for association with a disease.

A typical method for dealing with the problem of multiple testing is the *Bonferroni correction,* which specifies that the *P* value at which the null hypothesis will be rejected (e.g., .05) should be *divided by the number of hypothesis tests performed.* Although simple to use, a problem with this approach is that it is overly conservative. Studies with many listed or apparent outcomes or predictors (or both) are subject to inflation of the error rate to well above the nominal .05. Automated stepwise regression methods for choosing predictors in regression models typically *do not* alleviate and may exacerbate this problem. If no adjustment or method for dealing with multiple comparisons is used, the high probability of false-positive results should be kept in mind.

GENERAL REFERENCES

For the General References and other additional features, please visit Expert Consult at https://expertconsult.inkling.com.

10 USING DATA FOR CLINICAL DECISIONS

THOMAS H. LEE

Key functions in the professional lives of all physicians are the collection and analysis of clinical data. Decisions must be made on the basis of these data, including which therapeutic strategy is most appropriate for the patient and whether further information should be gathered before the best strategy can be chosen. This decision-making process is a blend of science and art in which the physician must synthesize a variety of concerns, including the patient's most likely outcome with various management strategies, the patient's worst possible outcome, and the patient's preferences among these strategies.

Only rarely does the physician enjoy true certainty regarding any of these issues, so a natural inclination for physicians is to seek as much information as possible before making a decision. This approach ignores the dangers inherent in the collection of information. Some of these dangers are immediate, such as the risk of cerebrovascular accident associated with coronary angiography. Some dangers are delayed, such as the risk of a malignant neoplasm due to radiation exposure from diagnostic tests. And some dangers are subtle, such as the risk of unnecessary anguish for patients due to delays, uncertainty, and confusion.

An additional concern is the cost of information gathering, including the direct costs of the tests themselves and the indirect costs that flow from decisions made on the basis of the test results. Substantial data demonstrate marked variation in use of tests among physicians located in different regions and even within the same group practice. Standards of medical professionalism endorse the need for physicians to exert their influence to minimize inefficiency, but this challenge grows increasingly complex as medical progress leads to proliferation of alternative testing strategies.

For the physician, there are three key questions in this sequence: Should I order a test to improve my assessment of diagnosis or prognosis? Which test is best? Which therapeutic strategy is most appropriate for this patient?

SHOULD I ORDER A TEST?

The decision of whether to order a test depends on the physician's and the patient's willingness to pursue a management strategy with the current degree of uncertainty.[1] This decision is influenced by several factors, including the patient's attitudes toward diagnostic and therapeutic interventions (e.g., a patient with claustrophobia might prefer an ultrasound to magnetic resonance imaging) and the information provided by the test itself. The personal tolerance of the patient and physician for uncertainty also frequently influences test-ordering approaches. A decision to watch and wait rather than to obtain a specific test also should be considered an information-gathering alternative because the information obtained while a patient is being observed often reduces uncertainty about the diagnosis and outcome. In other words, the "test of time" should be recognized as one of the most useful tests available when this tactic does not seem inappropriately risky.

TABLE 10-1 KEY DEFINITIONS*

Probability	A number between 0 and 1 that expresses an estimate of the likelihood of an event
Odds	The ratio of [the probability of an event] to [the probability of the event's not occurring]
TEST PERFORMANCE CHARACTERISTICS	
Sensitivity	Percentage of patients with disease who have an abnormal test result
Specificity	Percentage of patients without disease who have a normal test result
Positive predictive value	Percentage of patients with an abnormal test result who have disease
Negative predictive value	Percentage of patients with a normal test result who do not have disease
BAYESIAN ANALYSIS	
Pretest (or prior) probability	The probability of a disease before the information is acquired
Post-test (or posterior) probability	The probability of a disease after new information is acquired
Pretest (or prior) odds	(Pretest probability of disease)/(1 − pretest probability of disease)
Likelihood ratio	(Probability of result in diseased persons)/(Probability of result in nondiseased persons)

**Disease* can mean a condition, such as coronary artery disease, or an outcome, such as postoperative cardiac complications.

Most tests do not provide a definitive answer about diagnosis or prognosis but instead reduce uncertainty. Accordingly, the impact of information from tests often is expressed as *probabilities* (Table 10-1). A probability of 1.0 implies that an event is certain to occur, whereas a probability of 0 implies that the event is impossible. When all the possible events for a patient are assigned probabilities, these estimates should sum to 1.0.

It is often useful to use *odds* to quantify uncertainty instead of probability. Odds of 1 : 2 suggest that the likelihood of an event is only half the likelihood that the event will not occur, or a probability of 0.33. The relationship between odds and probability is expressed in the following formula:

$$\text{Odds} = P/(1-P)$$

where *P* is the probability of an event.

Performance Characteristics

Sensitivity and *specificity* are key terms for the description of test performance. These parameters describe the test and are in theory true regardless of the population of patients to which the test is applied. Research studies that describe test performance often are based, however, on highly selected populations of patients; test performance may deteriorate when tests are applied in clinical practice. The result of a test for coronary artery disease, such as an electron beam computed tomography scan, rarely may be abnormal if it is evaluated in a low-risk population, such as high-school students. False-positive abnormal results secondary to coronary calcification in the absence of obstructive coronary disease are common when the test is performed in middle-aged and elderly people. Another increasingly appreciated factor that can distort the performance of screening tests is the phenomenon of "overdiagnosis," in which the "disease" that is detected would not have led to clinical harm if it had not been found.[2]

Although researchers are interested in the performance of tests, the true focus of medical decision making is the patient. Physicians are more interested in the implications of a test result on the probability that a patient has a specific disease or outcome, that is, the predictive values of abnormal or normal test results. These predictive values are extremely sensitive to the population from which they are derived (Table 10-2; see also Table 10-1). An abnormal lung scan result in an asymptomatic patient has a much lower positive predictive value than that same test result in a patient with dyspnea and diminished oxygen saturation. Bayes theorem (see later) provides a

TABLE 10-2 EXAMPLE OF ODDS RATIO FORM OF BAYES THEOREM

Question: What is the probability of coronary disease for a patient with a 50% pretest probability of coronary disease who undergoes an exercise test if that patient develops (a) no ST segment changes, (b) 1 mm of ST segment depression, or (c) 2 mm of ST segment depression?

Step 1. Calculate the pretest odds of disease:

$$P/(1-P)=0.5/(1-0.5)$$
$$=0.5/0.5$$
$$=1$$

Step 2. Calculate the likelihood ratios for the various test results, using the formula LR = sensitivity/(1 − specificity). (Data from pooled literature.)

TEST RESULT	SENSITIVITY	SPECIFICITY	LIKELIHOOD RATIO
No ST segment changes	0.34	0.15	0.4
1-mm ST segment depression	0.66	0.85	4.4
2-mm ST segment depression	0.33	0.97	11

Step 3. Calculate the post-test odds of disease and convert those odds to post-test probabilities.

TEST RESULT	PRETEST ODDS	LIKELIHOOD RATIO	POST-TEST ODDS	POST-TEST PROBABILITY
No ST segment changes	1	0.4	0.4	0.29
1-mm ST segment depression	1	4.4	4.4	0.81
2-mm ST segment depression	1	11	11	0.92

framework for analyzing the interaction between test results and a patient's pretest probability of a disease.

As useful as the performance characteristics may be, they are limited by the fact that few tests truly provide dichotomous (i.e., positive or negative) results. Tests such as exercise tests have several parameters (e.g., ST segment deviation, exercise duration, hemodynamic response) that provide insight into the patient's condition, and the normal range for many blood tests (e.g., a serum troponin level) varies markedly according one's willingness to "miss" patients with disease. Tests that require human interpretation (e.g., radiologic studies) are particularly subject to variability in the reported results.

Bayes Theorem

The impact of a test result on a patient's probability of disease was first quantified by Bayes, an 18th century English clergyman who developed a formula that describes the probability of disease in the presence of an abnormal test result. The classic presentation of Bayes theorem is complex and difficult to use. A more simple form of this theorem is known as the *odds ratio* form, which describes the impact of a test result on the pretest odds (see Table 10-1) of a diagnosis or outcome for a specific patient.

To calculate the post-test odds of disease, the pretest odds are multiplied by the *likelihood ratio* (LR) for a specific test result. The mathematical presentation of this form of Bayes theorem is as follows:

$$\text{Post-test odds} = (\text{Pretest odds}) \times (\text{LR})$$

The LR is the probability of a particular test result in patients with the disease divided by the probability of that same test result in patients without disease. In other words, the LR is the test result's sensitivity divided by the false-positive rate. A test of no value (e.g., flipping a coin and calling "heads" an abnormal result) would have an LR of 1.0 because half of patients with disease would have abnormal test results, as would half of patients without disease. This test would have no impact on a patient's odds of disease. The further an LR is above 1.0, the more that test result raises a patient's probability of disease. For LRs less than 1.0, the closer the LR is to 0, the more it lowers a patient's probability of disease.

When it is displayed graphically (Fig. 10-1), a test of no value (*dotted line*) does not change the pretest probability, whereas an abnormal or normal result from a useful test moves the probability up or down. For a patient with a high pretest probability of disease, an abnormal test result changes the

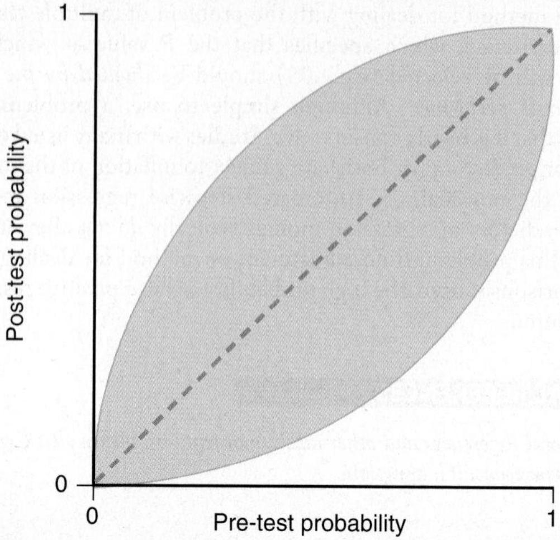

FIGURE 10-1. Impact of various test results on the patient's probability of disease. The *x*-axis depicts a patient's probability of disease before a test. If the test is of no value, the post-test probability (*dotted line*) is no different from the pretest probability. An abnormal test result raises the post-test probability of disease, as depicted by the concave downward arc, whereas a normal test result lowers the probability.

patient's probability only slightly, but a normal test result leads to a marked reduction in the probability of disease. Similarly, for a patient with a low pretest probability of disease, a normal test result has little impact, but an abnormal test result markedly raises the probability of disease.

Consider how various exercise test results influence a patient's probability of coronary disease (see Table 10-2). For a patient whose clinical history, physical examination, and electrocardiographic findings suggest a 50% probability of disease, the pretest odds of disease are 1.0. LRs for various test results are developed by pooling data from published literature. The sensitivity of an exercise test with any amount of ST segment changes is the rate of such test results in patients with coronary disease, and the specificity is the percentage of patients without coronary disease who do *not* have this test result. The LR for no ST change is less than 1, whereas the LRs for patients with ST changes are greater than 1 (see Table 10-2). Therefore, when the LRs for various test results are multiplied by the pretest odds to calculate post-test odds, the odds decrease for patients without ST segment changes but increase for patients with 1 or 2 mm of ST segment change. Post-test odds can be converted to post-test probabilities according to the following formula:

$$\text{Probability} = \text{Odds}/(1+\text{odds})$$

The calculations quantify how the absence of ST segment changes reduces a patient's probability of disease, whereas ST segment depression raises the probability of disease.

This form of Bayes theorem is useful for showing how the post-test probability of disease is influenced by the patient's pretest probability of disease. If a patient's clinical data suggest a *probability* of coronary disease of only 0.1, the *pretest odds* of disease would be only 0.11. For such a low-risk patient, an exercise test with no ST segment changes would lead to post-test probability of coronary disease of 4%, whereas 1-mm or 2-mm ST segment changes would lead to a post-test probability of disease of 33% or 55%, respectively.

Even if clinicians rarely perform the calculations that are described in Bayes theorem, there are important lessons from this theorem that are relevant to principles of test ordering (Table 10-3). The most crucial of these lessons is that the interpretation of test results must incorporate information about the patient. An abnormal test result in a low-risk patient may not be a true indicator of disease. Similarly, a normal test result in a high-risk patient should not be taken as evidence that disease is not present.

Figure 10-2 provides an example of the post-test probabilities for positive and negative results for a test with a sensitivity of 85% and a specificity of 90% (e.g., radionuclide scintigraphy for diagnosis of coronary artery disease). In a high-risk population with a 90% prevalence of disease, the positive predictive value of an abnormal result is 0.99 compared with 0.31 for the same test result obtained in a low-risk population with a 5% prevalence of disease. Similarly, the negative predictive value of a normal test result is greater in the low-risk population than in the high-risk population.

TABLE 10-3 PRINCIPLES OF TEST ORDERING AND INTERPRETATION

The interpretation of test results depends on what is already known about the patient.
No test is perfect; clinicians should be familiar with its diagnostic performance (see Table 10-1) and never believe that a test "forces" them to pursue a specific management strategy.
Tests should be ordered if they may provide *additional* information beyond that already available.
Tests should be ordered if there is a reasonable chance that the data will influence the patient's care.
Two tests that provide similar information should not be ordered.
In choosing between two tests that provide similar data, use the test that has lower costs or causes less discomfort and inconvenience to the patient.
Clinicians should seek all of the information provided by a test, not just an abnormal or normal result.
The cost-effectiveness of strategies using noninvasive tests should be considered in a manner similar to that of therapeutic strategies.

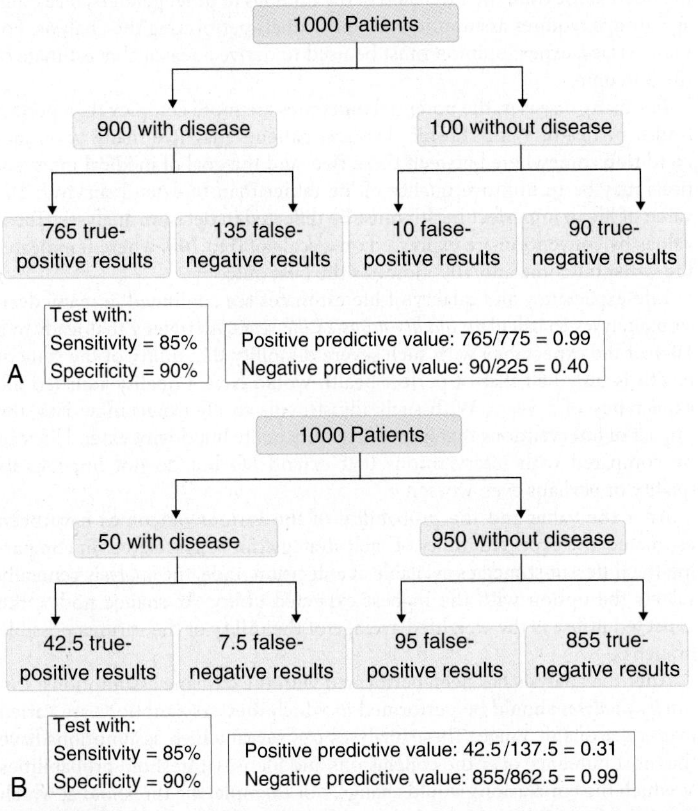

FIGURE 10-2. Interpretation of test results in high-risk and low-risk patients. **A,** High-risk population (90% prevalence of disease). **B,** Low-risk population (5% prevalence of disease).

Multiple Testing

Clinicians frequently obtain more than one test aimed at addressing the same issue and at times are confronted with conflicting results. If these tests are truly independent (i.e., the tests do not have the same basis in pathophysiology), it may be appropriate to use the post-test probability obtained through performance of one test as the pretest probability for the analysis of the impact of the second test result.

If the tests are not independent, this strategy for interpretation of serial test results can be misleading. Suppose a patient with chronic obstructive pulmonary disease and a history vaguely suggestive of pulmonary embolism is found to have an abnormal lung ventilation-perfusion scan. Obtaining that same test result over and over would not raise that patient's probability of pulmonary embolism further and further. In this extreme case, the tests are identical; serial testing adds no information. More commonly, clinicians are faced with results from tests with related but not identical bases in pathophysiology, such as ventilation-perfusion scintigraphy and pulmonary angiography.

Regardless of whether tests are independent, the performance of multiple tests increases the likelihood that an abnormal test result will be obtained in a patient without disease. If a chemistry battery includes 20 tests and the normal range for each test has been developed to include 95% of healthy individuals, the chance that a healthy patient will have a normal result for any specific test is 0.95. However, the probability that all 20 tests will be normal is $(0.95)^{20}$, or 0.36. Most healthy people can be expected to have at least one abnormal result. Unless screening test profiles are used thoughtfully, false-positive results can subject patients to unnecessary tests and procedures.

Threshold Approach to Decision Making

Even if a test provides information, that information may not change management for an individual patient. Lumbar spine radiographs of a patient who is not willing to undergo surgery may reveal the severity of disease but expose the patient to needless radiation. Similarly, a test that merely confirms a diagnosis that already is recognized is a waste of resources (see Table 10-3).

Before ordering a test, clinicians should consider whether that test result could change the choice of management strategies. This approach is called the *threshold approach to medical decision making*, and it requires the physician to be able to estimate the threshold probability at which one strategy will be chosen over another. The management of a clinically stable patient with a high probability of coronary disease might not be changed by any of the post-test probabilities shown in Table 10-2. If that patient had no ST segment changes, the post-test probability of 0.29 still would be too high for a clinician to consider that patient free of disease. An abnormal test result that strengthened the diagnosis of coronary disease might not change management unless it suggested a greater severity of disease that might warrant another management strategy.

Testing for Peace of Mind

Physicians frequently order tests even when there is little chance that the outcomes will provide qualitatively new insights into a patient's diagnosis or prognosis or alter a patient's management. In such cases, the cited goal for testing may be to improve a patient's peace of mind. Although a decrease in uncertainty can improve quality of life for many patients, individuals with hypochondriasis and somatization disorders rarely obtain comfort from normal test results; instead, their complaints shift to a new organ system, and their demands focus on other tests. For such patients, management strategies using frequent visits and cognitive tactics are recommended.

WHICH TEST IS BEST?

If the clinician decides that more information is needed to reduce uncertainty, and if it appears possible that tests might lead to a change in management strategies, the question arises as to which test is most appropriate. Note that just because guideline development committees have concluded that a specific test is "appropriate" in a given clinical context, it does not mean that this test is the *most* appropriate option. Several factors influence the choice among diagnostic strategies, including the patient's preferences, the costs and risks associated with the tests, and the diagnostic performance of alternative tests.

Diagnostic performance of a test often is summarized in terms of sensitivity and specificity,[3] but as shown in the example in Table 10-2, these parameters depend on which threshold (e.g., 1 mm vs. 2 mm of ST segment change) is used. A low threshold for calling a test result abnormal might lead to excellent sensitivity for detecting disease but at the expense of a high false-positive rate. Conversely, a threshold that led to few false-positive results might cause a clinician to miss many cases of true disease.

The receiver operating characteristic (ROC) curve is a graphic form of describing this tradeoff and providing a method for comparing test performance (Fig. 10-3). Each point on the ROC curve describes the sensitivity and the false-positive rate for a different threshold for abnormality for a test. A test of no value would lead to an ROC curve with the course of the dotted line, whereas a misleading test would be described by a curve that was concave upward (not shown).

The more accurate the test, the closer its ROC curve comes to the upper left corner of the graph, which would indicate a test threshold that has excellent sensitivity and a low false-positive rate. The closer an ROC curve comes to the upper left corner, the greater the area under the curve. The area under ROC curves can be used to compare the information provided by two tests.

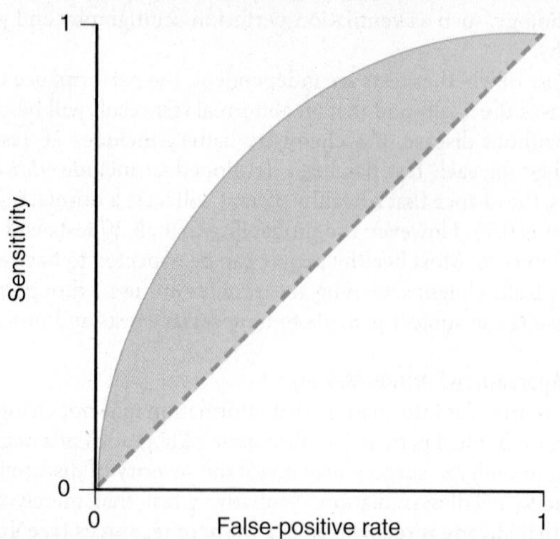

FIGURE 10-3. **Receiver operating characteristic curve. The points on the curve reflect the sensitivity and false-positive (1 − specificity) rates of a test at various thresholds. As the threshold is changed to yield greater sensitivity for detecting the outcome of interest, the false-positive rate rises. The better the test, the closer the curve comes to the upper left corner. A test of no value (e.g., flipping a coin) would lead to a curve with the course of the dotted line. The area under the curve is used often to compare alternative testing strategies.**

Even if one test is superior to another as shown by a greater area under its ROC curve, the question still remains as to what value of that test should be considered abnormal. The choice of threshold depends on the purpose of testing and on the consequences of a false-positive or false-negative diagnosis. If the goal is to screen the population for a disease that is potentially fatal and potentially curable, a threshold with excellent sensitivity is appropriate even if it leads to frequent false-positive results. In contrast, if a test is used to confirm a diagnosis that is likely to be treated with a high-risk invasive procedure, a threshold with high specificity is preferred. Only 1 mm of ST segment depression might be the appropriate threshold when exercise electrocardiography is used to evaluate the possibility of coronary disease in a patient with chest pain. If the question is whether to perform coronary angiography in a patient with stable angina in search of severe coronary disease that might benefit from revascularization, a threshold of 2 mm or more would be more appropriate.

CHOOSING A STRATEGY

Physicians and patients ultimately must use clinical information to make decisions. These choices usually are made after consideration of a variety of factors, including information from the clinical evaluation, patients' preferences, and expected outcomes with various management strategies. Insight into the impact of these considerations can be improved through the performance of decision analysis (Table 10-4).

The first step in a decision analysis is to define the problem clearly; this step often requires writing out a statement of the issue so that it can be scrutinized for any ambiguity. After the problem is defined, the next step is to define the alternative strategies.

Consider the question of which test is most appropriate to screen patients for breast cancer: mammography with or without breast magnetic resonance imaging—a technology that is highly sensitive for detecting breast cancer but is more costly and less specific. The expected outcomes for these strategies depend on each test's sensitivity and specificity for detecting breast cancer, which is influenced in turn by other factors, such as the frequency with which the test is performed. Patients' outcomes also are influenced by their underlying risk for breast cancer and the likelihood that earlier detection of tumors reduces the risk for death.

Each of these variables must be known or estimated for calculations to be made of each strategy's predicted life expectancy and direct medical costs. These outcomes differ for patients according to age, medical history, family history, and presence or absence of genetic markers such as *BRCA* mutations. Optimal strategies for an elderly patient with a short life expectancy and low clinical risk of cancer are unlikely to be the same as those for a younger patient with inherited mutations of the *BRCA1* or *BRCA2* gene, indicating a cumulative lifetime risk of breast cancer of 50 to 85% (Chapter 198).

TABLE 10-4 STEPS IN PERFORMANCE OF DECISION ANALYSIS

Frame the question.
Create the decision tree.
- Identify the alternative strategies.
- List the possible outcomes for each of the alternative strategies.
- Describe the sequence of events as a series of decision nodes and chance nodes.

Choose a time horizon for the analysis.
Determine the probability for each chance outcome.
Assign a value to each outcome.
Calculate the expected utility for each strategy.
Perform sensitivity analysis.

The credibility of the decision analysis depends on the credibility of these estimates. Published reports often do not provide information on the outcomes of interest for specific subsets of patients, or there may not have been sufficient statistical power within subsets of patients for the findings to be statistically significant. Randomized trial data are relevant to the populations included in the trial; the extension of the findings to other genders, races, and age groups requires assumptions by individuals performing the analysis. For many issues, expert opinion must be used to derive a reasonable estimate of the outcome.

For many diseases, the potential outcomes are more complex than perfect health or death. With chronic diseases, patients may live many years in a condition somewhere between these two, and the goal of medical interventions may be to improve quality of life rather than to extend survival. The value of life in imperfect health must be reflected in decision analyses. These values by convention are expressed on a scale of 0 to 100, where 0 indicates the worst outcome and 100 indicates the best outcome.

Life-expectancy and quality-of-life estimates are combined in many decision analyses to calculate *quality-adjusted life years.* A strategy that leads to a 10-year life expectancy with such severe disability that utility of the state of health is only half that of perfect health would have a quality-adjusted life expectancy of 5 years. With such adjustments to life-expectancy data, the impact of interventions that improve quality of life but do not extend life can be compared with interventions that extend life but do not improve its quality or perhaps even worsen it.[4]

After the value and the probability of the various outcomes have been estimated, the expected utility of each strategy can be calculated. In comparing the different strategies available at a decision node, the analysis generally selects the option with the highest expected utility. At chance nodes, the expected utility is the weighted average of the utility of the various possible branches.

After the analysis has been performed with the baseline assumptions, *sensitivity analyses* should be performed in which these assumptions are varied over a reasonable range. These analyses can reveal which assumptions have the most influence over the conclusions and identify threshold probabilities at which the conclusions would change. For example, the threshold at which breast magnetic resonance imaging should be added to mammography is likely to be influenced by the cost of the magnetic resonance imaging and the accuracy of the radiologists who interpret the images.

Cost-Benefit and Cost-Effectiveness Analyses

For clinicians and health care policymakers, the choices that must be addressed go beyond the choices within any single decision analysis. Because resources available for health care are limited, policymakers may have to choose among many competing options for "investments" in health. Although such decisions frequently are made on the basis of political considerations, cost-benefit and cost-effectiveness analyses can be informative in making the choices.

The methodology of these techniques is similar to that of decision analysis except that costs for the various possible outcomes and strategies also are calculated. *Discounting* is used to adjust the value of future benefits and costs because resources saved or spent currently are worth more than resources saved or expended in the future. In *cost-benefit* analyses, all benefits are expressed in terms of economic impact. Extensions in life expectancy are translated into dollars by estimating societal worth or economic productivity.

Because of the ethical discomfort associated with expressing health benefits in financial terms, *cost-effectiveness* analyses are used more commonly

TABLE 10-5 ESTIMATED COST-EFFECTIVENESS OF SELECTED HEALTH INTERVENTIONS

INTERVENTION	COST PER QUALITY-ADJUSTED LIFE YEAR (QALY) (2010 DOLLARS)
Treating rheumatoid arthritis with drugs that slow disease progression	Saves money and improves health
Using warfarin for 70-year-olds with atrial fibrillation	$3,000 per QALY
Daily dialysis for 60-year old critically ill men with kidney injury	$6,000 per QALY
Using an implantable cardioverter-defibrillator to prevent sudden cardiac death in high-risk patients	$38,000 per QALY
Treating spinal stenosis and leg pain with spine surgery	$90,000 per QALY
Screening 60-year-old heavy smokers with annual CT scans	$140,000 per QALY
Annual HIV screening for people with a low to moderate risk	Increases costs and makes health worse

Modified from the CEA Registry.[6]

than cost-benefit analyses. In these analyses, the ratio of costs to health benefits is calculated; one frequently used method for evaluating a strategy is calculation of cost per quality-adjusted life year.[5] These estimates can be used to identify strategies that are both cost-saving and health-improving, to compare strategies by which the health care system can "purchase" additional quality-adjusted life years, and even to caution about strategies that increase costs while worsening health (Table 10-5).[6]

Cost-effectiveness analyses can provide important insights into the relative attractiveness of different management strategies and can help guide policymakers in decisions about which technologies to make available on a routine basis. No medical intervention can have an attractive cost-effectiveness if its effectiveness has not been proved. The cost-effectiveness of an intervention depends heavily on the population of patients in which it is applied. An inexpensive intervention would have a poor cost-effectiveness ratio if it were used in a low-risk population unlikely to benefit from it. In contrast, an expensive technology can have an attractive cost-effectiveness ratio if it is used in patients with a high probability of benefiting from it. Table 10-5 shows cost-effectiveness estimates from published literature for some selected medical interventions. Such estimates should be used only with understanding of the population for which they are relevant.

GENERAL REFERENCES

For the General References and other additional features, please visit Expert Consult at https://expertconsult.inkling.com.

11 MEASURING HEALTH AND HEALTH CARE

CAROLYN M. CLANCY AND ERNEST MOY

Physicians routinely quantify a variety of health measures, including symptoms, vital signs, and findings on physical examination, to improve diagnosis, treatment, and prognostication. Similarly, the efficacy and quality of health care also can and should be measured for several reasons.

First, the quality of care delivered is often suboptimal.[1] Persistent variations in practice for patients with the same diagnosis reflect a combination of clinical uncertainty, individualized practice styles, patients' preferences and characteristics (age, race, ethnicity, education, income), and other factors. Both suboptimal care and varied care for the same condition undermine the historical assumption that a combination of highly trained health professionals and accredited facilities is sufficient to ensure consistent high-quality care.

A second major trend is attributable to the successes of biomedical science: the major challenge in health care today is the management of chronic disease for a population with increased life expectancy. For chronic conditions, health benefits are increasingly measured in improvements in functional status or quality of life, rather than simply using mortality rates or life expectancy.

A third trend relates directly to how the increasing costs of health care are now threatening public budgets and investments in other social goals, such as education. Although the United States spends more per capita on health care than any other developed nation (Chapter 5), the outcomes achieved lag far behind.

Finally, advances in communication and information technologies have inspired more people to play an active role in their health and health care. These innovations have accelerated demands for transparency and shared decision making.

As health insurance and health care regulation have expanded, requirements to track and justify health care services have grown. Intensifying urgency to improve the quality of health care, reduce disparities, control costs, and enhance transparency will likely lead patients and insurers to demand more data and to link quality measures to payments for services.

Fortunately, modern technology can help to meet the demand for data. Patients can record and submit their health parameters using hand-held devices connected to personal health records. Automated billing programs can track health care services, while electronic health records can assess the quality of physician care. Ultimately, fully integrated health information systems will allow patient information to be retrieved instantly and seamlessly wherever and whenever it is needed. In addition to assessing care quality today, these tools offer enormous promise for learning as a byproduct of care delivery.

HOW ARE HEALTH AND HEALTH CARE MEASURED?

Three types of measures typically assess health and health care. Measures of *health* quantify the sickness or well-being of a person. Measures of *health care quality* quantify the extent to which a patient receives needed care and does not receive unnecessary care. Health care quality is assessed using measures of *structure* (e.g., education and credentialing of clinicians), *process* (adherence to professional standards and evidence-based recommendations), and *outcomes* (or end results of care, including how patients experience their care and their self-reported health and function). Measures of *health care resources* quantify the resources used (e.g., radiographs, surgery, medication, intensive care) to improve the health of a patient.[2] All measures can be summed up across populations within a practice or community (Table 11-1).

Measures of health and health care often overlap (E-Fig. 11-1). Health measures that can be improved by health care, such as blood pressure or blood glucose levels, are often used as health care quality outcome measures. The delivery of quality health care requires the use of resources and the generation of direct health care costs, which may or may not improve health care at the margins of spending. Impaired health that reduces the ability to do work and earn wages but that could have been prevented by the delivery of health care contributes to the indirect costs of health care. At the intersection of health, health care quality, and health care resources are measures of health care value. These measures compare the health benefits of specific health care services with their costs.[2]

WHERE DO MEASURES OF HEALTH AND HEALTH CARE COME FROM?

Most researchers, provider groups, insurers, regulators, and credentialing organizations that develop measures consult with physicians to ensure that their metrics are consistent with professional standards. Insurers may create measures to allocate health care resources, to plan for future needs, and to identify efficient physicians for inclusion on panels or to be rewarded with performance bonuses. Regulators may develop measures to establish licensure requirements and to identify physicians who might benefit from remedial instruction. Credentialing organizations may construct measures to demonstrate the superior performance of physicians who meet their high standards. For example, the National Committee for Quality Assurance maintains the Healthcare Effectiveness Data and Information Set that is widely used to accredit health plans, and the American Board of Internal Medicine and other specialty boards include measures of practice performance as well as measures of medical knowledge for the maintenance of certification.

TABLE 11-1 MEASURES OF HEALTH AND HEALTH CARE

MEASURES OF HEALTH

- *Mortality:* rates of death typically adjusted for age and sex
- *Morbidity:* incidence and prevalence rates of diseases and their sequelae
- *Functional status:* assessments of a patient's ability to perform various actions such as activities of daily living or instrumental activities of daily living as observed by a provider or reported by the patient
- *Self-reported health status:* a patients' assessment of their health and well-being

MEASURES OF HEALTH CARE QUALITY

- *Health care outcomes:* the end results or health benefits derived from good health care or the health loss attributable to poor health care
- *Health care processes:* assessments of whether the right care was delivered at the right time and in the right way
- *Health care infrastructure:* the availability of resources needed to deliver good health care
- *Patient perceptions of health care:* a patient's assessment of health care received, usually emphasizing patient-provider communication and shared decision making
- *Access to health care:* the ability of patients to gain entry into health care and navigate to needed resources

MEASURES OF HEALTH CARE RESOURCES

- *Health care utilization:* the quantity of health care services that are used
- *Direct costs:* the costs of providers, supplies, and equipment needed to deliver health care
- *Indirect costs:* the costs of lost wages and decreased productivity due to illness or injury that could have been prevented by appropriate health care
- *Nonmedical costs:* the costs of health care not related to the delivery of services, such as administration, advertising, research, and profits earned by health industries

TYPE OF MEASURE	EXAMPLE
HEALTH	
Mortality	Deaths due to colorectal cancer per 100,000 population
Morbidity	New AIDS cases per 100,000 population
Functional status	% of people unable to perform one or more activities of daily living
Self-reported health status	% of people reporting that their overall health is excellent
HEALTH CARE QUALITY	
Health care outcomes	Death per 1000 hospitalizations with pneumonia
Intermediate outcomes	% of adults with diabetes whose blood pressure is <140/80 mm Hg
Health care processes	% of children who were given all recommended vaccinations
Health care infrastructure	% of office-based physicians with computerized systems for recording clinical notes
Patient perceptions of health care	% of patients who always reported good communication with their regular providers
Access to health care	% of patients who were unable or delayed in receiving medical care
HEALTH CARE RESOURCES	
Health care utilization	% of people with an emergency department visit in the past year
Direct costs	Expenditures for the treatment of depression
Indirect costs	Lost wages and productivity while caring for children with asthma
Nonmedical costs	Profits earned by pharmaceutical companies

WHY MEASURE HEALTH AND HEALTH CARE?

Measures of health and health care can be used for many purposes by different stakeholders (Table 11-2). Patients can use their own health information to track their progress, adjust their lifestyle, and plan for their future health care needs. Patient-level measures are important to physicians, hospitals, health plans, and policymakers, whether they are used to identify sentinel events that represent quality defects (e.g., amputating the wrong leg or giving a patient the wrong medication) or to initiate root cause analyses to improve health care quality.

Hospitals and health plans aggregate measures over their practices to identify opportunities for raising quality, improving efficiency, and reducing care disparities. For measures for which physicians are primarily accountable, these data can be used to acknowledge and reward high-performing physicians, select physicians for inclusion on a panel, and produce report cards to inform the public. Patients can use these report cards to select physicians and health plans that best match their health care needs. Measures that are aggregated to the community level can help policymakers allocate health care resources to locales with the greatest need and assess the success of any interventions.

WHAT ARE THE LIMITATIONS OF HEALTH AND HEALTH CARE MEASURES?

Historically, physicians recorded information on paper and had tremendous autonomy with respect to the level of detail and accuracy. Now, however, diverse stakeholders have a shared interest in standardizing measurements to facilitate fair comparisons. Detailed chart reviews largely have been replaced by data gathered for electronic medical records and by appropriately detailed registries composed of patients with a common condition or intervention. Examples of registries that have been used as platforms for assessing health care quality include the registry developed by the Society for Thoracic Surgeons to improve the quality of cardiothoracic surgery and the National Surgical Improvement Program registry, which was initially developed within the Veterans Health Administration, to assess processes and outcomes of major surgical procedures. Both registries rely on meticulous manual data, collected by trained nurses, that facilitate professional efforts to improve outcomes of care.

SELECTING MEASURES BASED ON EVIDENCE

Data used to measure the structure, process, and outcomes of health care can be gathered as part of rigorous hypothesis-driven research or from secondary sources of data initially collected for routine clinical care billing. The data's rigor and integrity are critical to the reliability of analyses performed on them.

In addition to the quality of the data themselves, however, the method of study design is also critical to the validity of reported findings. The most robust measures are supported by the concurrence of evidence derived from different research methodologies. In randomized controlled trials, random assignment of the intervention ensures that patients who do and do not receive it are as similar as possible. In double-blind studies, neither the patient nor the patient's physician knows the assigned treatment. For more complex interventions, such as the use of a team to manage depression, blinding is impractical. In all settings, controls typically receive the best standard care. In some situations, patients may serve as their own controls in a time-series randomized trial.

Although the randomized trial is a rigorous way to assess treatment effects, enrollment is often limited to selected individuals who meet strict entry criteria. This approach enhances a trial's internal validity but limits its generalizability. As a result, randomized trials are ideal for establishing an intervention's efficacy, which is its potential benefit under ideal conditions, but not necessarily its *effectiveness* in the real world. *Cluster randomized trials*, which randomize the level of the provider or system, represent a practical approach to determining effectiveness.

Although randomized trials are critical for assessing efficacy and effectiveness, *observational* and *case-control* studies are also important. In a *cohort study*, persons or patients are followed to determine their outcomes as a function of whether or not they possess a particular attribute or have been exposed to a particular condition or intervention. Cohort studies can provide a direct estimate of the absolute risk for an outcome in exposed patients but cannot guarantee whether such differences are related to interventions that were not randomly allocated.

In *case-control studies*, cases are defined based on having experienced an outcome not experienced by controls. Information that is gleaned from existing records or interviews can determine the proportion of case and control patients who experienced an exposure of interest. Case-control studies can achieve the same or higher statistical power as cohort studies despite enrolling fewer subjects, so they are especially attractive for investigating uncommon outcomes, such as serious adverse effects of medications when the events are too rare to study with clinical trials or cohort studies. Case-control studies are subject to the misclassification bias and recall bias, and they provide estimates of relative risk but not absolute risk.

TABLE 11-2 USES OF HEALTH AND HEALTH CARE MEASURES BY USER AND UNIT OF ANALYSIS

	USES BY PROVIDERS	USES BY POLICYMAKERS	USES BY PATIENTS
Patient-level measures	Diagnosis and prognosis Monitoring treatment response and compliance	Identifying sentinel events	Tracking health and health needs Retirement and estate planning
Provider practice or health plan–level measures	Improving quality Improving efficiency Reducing disparities	Public reporting Paying for performance Provider credentialing	Selecting providers and health plans
Community-level measures	Selecting practice location	Resource allocation Policy evaluation	Selecting place to live

TABLE 11-3 ATTRIBUTES OF MEASURES OF HEALTH AND HEALTH CARE

MEASURE ATTRIBUTES	CRITERIA FOR PROVIDERS	CRITERIA FOR POLICYMAKERS	CRITERIA FOR PATIENTS
Measure is scientifically sound			
Based on strong evidence	Based on high-quality studies?		
Valid	Measures what is intended and includes key elements?		
Reliable	Reproducible by different measurers and providers?		
Clearly specified	Numerator, denominator, exclusions, and risk adjustment defined?		
Endorsed by independent experts	Well accepted by scientific and medical communities?		
Condition is important Affects many people Causes high mortality or morbidity Costs a lot Is very unequal across populations	Important for my practice or the population I serve?	Important for population that will be affected by my policy?	Important to me?
Data collection is feasible Already available Could be collected at low cost relative to potential benefit Auditable	Available for my practice or the population I serve?	Available before and after policy implementation for affected population?	Available to me?
Findings are actionable Can be understood Can be improved Have been used successfully Have few unintended consequences	Do I know what actions I must change to improve quality? Used in practices like mine to improve quality with few unintended consequences?	Do I know what policies I must change to improve quality? Used for policies like mine to improve quality with few unintended consequences?	Do I know what actions I must take to improve my health? Used by patients like me to improve health with few unintended consequences?
When used as part of measure set, measures are: Balanced Able to be disaggregated	Represents multiple conditions, settings of care, populations, types of data (survey, administrative data, medical records), types of measures (structure, process, outcomes), and perspectives (patient, provider, system, society) as appropriate? Identifies individual measures that can be improved?		

Cross-sectional studies collect data at just one point in time. They can be used to estimate the prevalence of a condition or outcome but not to make valid inferences about whether a given outcome is related to any causal attribute or event.

There are additional methodologic issues beyond the credibility and quality of the source of data for quality measures. When presented with reports suggesting less-than-perfect performance, many physicians believe that their patients are sicker or are less likely to adhere to treatment recommendations. To address these concerns, risk adjustment for severity of illness, accurate identification of patient characteristics, and assessment of outcomes over time are all critical. Case-mix adjustment methods commonly use sophisticated statistical approaches in an attempt to adjust for such potential differences and to estimate whether observed differences result from differing patient populations rather than true differences in quality of care.

The precision of specific measures is also a challenge. Many stakeholders, especially payers and policymakers, are increasingly impatient and are generally more enthusiastic about use of measures that are only "pretty good" than are providers whose care is being judged.

SELECTING MEASURES: WHICH MEASURES ARE RIGHT FOR WHAT PURPOSE?

Creating measures is different from selecting which are most important and meaningful. Numerous publicly available sources provide a wealth of health and health care information (E-Table 11-1). The most prominent consensus-based organization that endorses measures is the National Quality Forum, which convenes panels of experts to assess the quality of a proposed measure based on criteria that include importance, scientific acceptability, feasibility, and usability. Endorsed measures are reassessed periodically to ensure they remain up to date and applicable.

The National Institutes of Health Patient Reported Outcomes Measurement Information System (http://www.nihpromis.org) is a repository of standardized patient-reported health status measures and collection instruments. Domains include physical, mental, and social well-being. The Agency for Healthcare Research and Quality National Quality Measures Clearinghouse (http://www.qualitymeasures.ahrq.gov) is an inventory of evidence-based measures of health care quality. Domains include clinical quality, efficiency, and population health. Also related are the National Guidelines Clearinghouse (http://www.guideline.gov) and the Health Care Innovations Exchange (http://www.innovations.ahrq.gov), collections of clinical guidelines and descriptions of successful uses of measures, respectively.

Potential users should examine the attributes of specific measures to ensure that they are appropriate for their intended application (Table 11-3). A number of organizations have developed scales or rating systems that summarize performance across multiple dimensions. Sometimes referred to as composite measures (e.g., a letter grade from the Leapfrog Group for hospital safety), these scales vary in comprehensiveness with little consensus regarding how components of a summary scale should be weighted. Indeed, it is not uncommon for a hospital to receive an "F" from one group and be rated a "top performer" by another. Thus, although appealing in their simplicity, the optimal use of these approaches remains unresolved.

GENERAL REFERENCES

For the General References and other additional features, please visit Expert Consult at https://expertconsult.inkling.com.

12 QUALITY OF CARE AND PATIENT SAFETY

ROBERT M. WACHTER

During the past two decades, scores of studies have demonstrated that the quality and safety of modern health care leave much to be desired, despite the fact that most physicians are well trained and work very hard. Yet the evidence is undeniable, with clear documentation of stunning variations in patterns of care that are neither supported by evidence nor justified by outcomes, major gaps between evidence-based best practices and current practice, and staggering numbers of serious medical errors. The recognition of these quality and safety problems has catalyzed a major transformation in thinking and practice, with new technologies, regulations, training models, incentive systems, and more.

To appreciate the problem and how to address it requires an understanding of quality measurement and improvement, the safety of patients, and value, which is the confluence of safety, quality, and cost.[1]

QUALITY

Definition

Quality of care has been defined by the Institute of Medicine as "the degree to which health services for individuals and populations increase the likelihood of desired health outcomes and are consistent with current professional knowledge." It includes six aims for a quality health care system, emphasizing that quality involves more than the delivery of evidence-based care (Table 12-1). Nevertheless, evidence-based medicine (Chapter 10) provides much of the scientific underpinning for quality measurement and improvement.[2] Previously, the lack of clinical evidence and the apprenticeship model of medical training promoted an idiosyncratic practice style by which a senior clinician or a marquee medical center determined the standard of care—a tradition now sometimes termed *eminence-based medicine*. Without discounting the value of experience and mature clinical judgment, the modern paradigm for determining optimal practice has changed, driven by the explosion in clinical research during the past 30 years; for example, the number of randomized clinical trials grew from 350 per year in 1970 to more than 27,000 per year in 2012. This research has helped define "best practices" in many areas of medicine, from preventive strategies for a healthy 62-year-old outpatient (Chapters 14 and 15) to the treatment of a patient with acute myocardial infarction and cardiogenic shock (Chapters 73 and 107).

Donabedian triad, which divides quality measures into *structure* (how care is organized), *process* (what is done), and *outcomes* (what happens to the patient), represents the most popular construct for quality measurement. Each element of the triad has important advantages and disadvantages as a quality measure (Table 12-2). Many of the widely used quality measures are process measures for which clinical research has established a link between such processes and improved outcomes. An example is the rate at which aspirin or a β-blocker is given to survivors of a myocardial infarction before hospital discharge (Chapter 73). However, when processes are less relevant and the science of case-mix adjustment is suitably advanced (e.g., cardiac bypass surgery; Chapter 74), outcome measurement (e.g., risk-adjusted mortality rate or 30-day readmission rate) is increasingly used. In other areas involving complex processes, structural measures are used as proxies for quality; examples here include the presence of intensivists to staff critical care units, a dedicated stroke service, and computerized physician order entry systems.

TABLE 12-1 THE INSTITUTE OF MEDICINE'S SIX QUALITY AIMS

Patient safety
Patient centeredness
Effectiveness
Efficiency
Timeliness
Equity

From Committee on Quality of Health Care in America, Institute of Medicine. Crossing the Quality Chasm: A New Health System for the 21st Century. Washington, DC: National Academy Press; 2001.

The Epidemiology of Quality-Related Problems

It is now well established that there are large and clinically indefensible variations in care from one city to another. Furthermore, U.S. practice adheres to the best evidence only slightly more than 50% of the time, even when adherence is known to correlate with ultimate clinical outcomes.

Levers for Change

For physicians, policymakers, administrators, and patients, evidence of major problems with quality has led to the recognition of structural problems that prevent the delivery of the highest quality of care. These problems include the lack of information regarding the performance of a provider or institution, the absence of incentives for quality improvement, the challenge for practicing physicians to stay abreast of modern evidence-based medicine, and the absence of an information technology support system for quality.

The first step in quality improvement is the creation of practice standards against which to measure quality. Scores of such measures have been promulgated by a variety of organizations, including payers (such as the Centers for Medicare and Medicaid Services), accreditors (such as the Joint Commission), and medical societies. These measures have identified many opportunities for improvement among individual physicians, practices, and hospitals.

Given the volume of new literature published each year, it is impossible for an individual physician to keep up with all the evidence-based advances in his or her field. *Practice guidelines*, such as those for the treatment of community-acquired pneumonia (Chapter 97) or the prophylaxis of deep venous thrombosis (Chapter 81), aim to synthesize evidence-based best practices into a set of summary recommendations.[3] Although concerns about "cookbook medicine" linger, there is a growing consensus that best practices should be "hard wired" if possible. The major challenges are to update guidelines as new knowledge accumulates and to recognize the complexity of guidelines when patients have multiple, potentially overlapping illnesses. *Clinical pathways* are similar to guidelines but attempt to codify a series of steps, usually temporally (on day 1, do the following; on day 2, do the

TABLE 12-2 COMPARISON OF THREE MEASURES OF CLINICAL QUALITY: THE DONABEDIAN TRIAD

MEASURE	SIMPLE DEFINITION	ADVANTAGES	DISADVANTAGES
Structure	How was care organized?	May be highly relevant in a complex health system	May fail to capture the quality of care by individual physicians Difficult to determine the "gold standard"
Process	What was done?	More easily measured and acted on than outcomes May not require case-mix adjustment No time lag—can be measured when care is provided May directly reflect quality (if carefully chosen)	A proxy for outcomes Not all may agree on "gold standard" processes May promote "cookbook" medicine, especially if physicians and health systems try to "game" their performance
Outcomes	What happened to the patient?	What we really care about	May take years to occur May not reflect quality of care Requires case-mix and other adjustment to prevent "apples-to-oranges" comparisons

Modified from Donabedian A. The quality of care. How can it be assessed? JAMA. 1988;270:1743-1748; and Shojania KG, Showstack J, Wachter R. Assessing hospital quality: A review for clinicians. Eff Clin Pract. 2001;4:82-90.

following; and so forth), making them more useful for stereotypical processes such as the postoperative management of patients after hip replacement. As more health care delivery organizations become computerized, pathways and guidelines are often translated into *order sets* or *clinical decision support systems* to guide clinicians at the point of care.

Although professionalism (Chapter 1) should be a sufficient incentive for physicians to provide high-quality care, reaching this goal typically depends on the existence of a system organized to translate research into practice and to deliver the right care every time. Such a system requires significant investments (in educating physicians, hiring case managers or clinical pharmacists, building information systems, and developing guidelines). The historical payment system, which compensates physicians and hospitals on the basis of volume rather than quality, provides no incentive to make the requisite investments, but this situation is changing rapidly.

The Changing Environment for Quality

The recent recognition of major gaps in quality and of the need for systemic change to improve quality has led to a variety of initiatives to catalyze quality improvement. Virtually all involve several steps: defining reasonable quality measures (evidence-based measures; capturing appropriate structures, process, or outcomes), measuring the performance of providers or systems, and using these results to promote change. This final imperative creates the greatest degree of uncertainty and experimentation.

Although one might hope that simply giving a physician information about prior performance would generate meaningful improvement, this strategy yields only modest change at best. Increasingly, a more aggressive and transparent strategy, such as disseminating the results of quality measurement to key stakeholders, is being adopted. In some cases, simple transparency is the main strategy—the rationale being that providers will find the exposure of their gaps in quality to be sufficiently concerning or embarrassing to motivate improvement. Although there is little evidence that patients use such data to choose among physicians or hospitals, transparency itself has frequently resulted in impressive improvements in some publicly reported quality measures.

The newest strategy in the United States is to tie payments for service to quality performance (pay for performance, or P4P). A number of P4P programs are under way, but early results indicate that differential payment leads to surprisingly modest gains beyond the improvements achieved by simple transparency.[4,5] P4P also raises a host of concerns, including whether presently captured quality data are accurate, whether payments should go to the best performers or those with the greatest improvements, whether existing measures adequately measure quality in patients with complex diseases, and whether P4P will create undue focus on certain measurable practices, leading to relative inattention to other important processes that are not being compensated. Another concern is that an overemphasis on "extrinsic" motivation (i.e., bonus payments) can actually extinguish "intrinsic" motivation (i.e., professionalism). One variation on the P4P theme is Medicare's "no pay for adverse events" program, in which hospital payments are withheld for certain "preventable" adverse events, such as injuries from falls or health care–associated infections.[A1] As with P4P more generally, the impact of such programs on quality and safety has been surprisingly modest.

Quality Improvement Strategies

Whether the motivation is professionalism, embarrassment, or economics, the next question is how actually to improve the quality of care. There is no simple answer; successful institutions and physicians have used a variety of strategies. In general, most use a variation of a "plan, do, study, act" (PDSA) cycle, recognizing that quality improvement activities must be carefully planned and implemented, that their impact needs to be measured, and that the results of these activities are often imperfect and require retooling.

In addition to the PDSA cycle, several other types of activities are useful. For quality improvement practices that require predictable repetition, efforts to "hard wire" the practice or to use alternative providers who focus on the activity are often beneficial. For example, the best strategy to increase the rate of pneumococcal vaccination (Chapter 18) among hospitalized patients with pneumonia is to embed it in a standard order set, either paper based or computerized. Another example is that having a nurse remove patients' shoes before the physician's entry can increase rates of diabetic foot examinations in an outpatient practice (Chapter 229).

In some areas, though, quality improvement involves much more complex and interdependent activities. In these circumstances, bringing teams together to examine their practices and to participate in a PDSA cycle is the most likely path to success. For example, a group of cardiac surgeons in the northeastern United States participated in an experiment in which they observed one another's practices, agreed on best practices, and measured one another's outcomes; the result was a 24% reduction in mortality with cardiac surgery. Many health care organizations are adopting one of the more sophisticated methodologies, such as Lean or Six Sigma, which involve mapping out all of the steps of a complex process (e.g., hospital admission) in an attempt to root out waste. For a hospital or clinic, the precise methodology chosen is probably less important than the decision to adopt a single way of approaching complex processes in need of improvement.

PATIENT SAFETY

Epidemiology

The concept of "first, do no harm" began more than 2 millennia ago, and many hospitals host periodic forums (e.g., morbidity and mortality conferences) to discuss errors. Until recently, however, there has been little teaching about the nature of medical mistakes, investment in safety research, regulation of safety standards, or emphasis on safety improvements, despite the fact that an estimated 44,000 to 98,000 Americans die each year of medical mistakes—the equivalent of a jumbo jet crashing each day. Such deaths may be related to medication errors, gaps in the discharge process, communication problems in intensive care units, or retained sponges in surgical patients—in short, virtually every aspect of modern medical care. Moreover, detailed clinical and statistical evidence of suboptimal safety has been reinforced by several high-profile and disquieting errors, sometimes apparently related to inadequate supervision and prolonged duty hours of trainees. These errors include the wrong patient getting a major procedure, the wrong limb being operated on, chemotherapy overdoses, mistaken mastectomies, and more. In the past few years, new classes of errors have emerged because of poorly designed health care information systems.[6] In addition, increasing attention is focusing on areas that were previously underemphasized, such as diagnostic errors.[7]

Because patients may be harmed despite receiving perfect care (i.e., from an accepted complication of surgery or a side effect of medication), it is important to separate *adverse events* from *errors*. The patient safety literature commonly defines an error as "an act or omission that leads to an unanticipated, undesirable outcome or to substantial potential for such an outcome." Adverse events, in contrast, are injuries due to medical management rather than the patient's underlying illness. This distinction is crucial. For example, when a patient who was appropriately prescribed warfarin for chronic atrial fibrillation develops a gastrointestinal bleed despite a therapeutic international normalized ratio, an adverse event, not a medical error, has occurred. Conversely, if the international normalized ratio was supratherapeutic because the physician prescribed a new medication without checking for possible drug interactions, a medical error would have occurred.

The Modern Approach to Patient Safety

The historical approach to medical errors often has been to blame the provider who was most proximate: whoever performed the surgery, hung the intravenous medication, or mixed the chemotherapy. It is now recognized that this approach fails to appreciate that most errors are committed by hard-working, well-trained individuals, and such errors are unlikely to be prevented by admonishing people to be more careful or by shaming and suing them. Instead, the modern approach, known as *systems thinking*, holds that humans will inevitably err and that safety depends on creating systems that anticipate errors and either prevent or catch them before they cause harm. Such an approach has been the cornerstone of safety improvements in other high-risk industries for some time.

The "Swiss cheese" model of accidents, drawn from innumerable investigations of accidents in commercial aviation and the nuclear power industry, for example, emphasizes that single errors by one individual working in an otherwise safety-conscious system rarely cause harm. Instead, such errors must penetrate multiple incomplete layers of protection ("layers of Swiss cheese") to cause terrible harm. The lesson is to focus not on the futile goal of trying to perfect human behavior but rather on creating multiple overlapping layers of protection to decrease the probability that the holes in the Swiss cheese will ever align, allowing an error to slip through.

How to Improve Patient Safety

Drawing on these models, modern thinking emphasizes efforts to design and implement systems to prevent or catch errors. For example, errors in routine behaviors can best be prevented by building in redundancies and crosschecks in the form of checklists, read-backs, and other standardized safety procedures, such as counting sponges in the operating room, signing a surgical site before an operation, or asking patients their names before administering a medication. In recent years, the use of checklists for the placement of central lines and to prepare patients for surgery has resulted in remarkable reductions in morbidity and mortality.[8] One way to decrease errors at the person-machine interface is by the use of "forcing functions," engineering solutions that decrease the probability of human error. The classic example outside of medicine is the modification of automobile braking systems to make it impossible to place a car in reverse when the driver's foot is off the brake. In health care, forcing functions include changing the gas nozzles and connectors so that anesthesiologists cannot mistakenly hook up the wrong gas, such as nitrogen instead of oxygen, and administer it to a patient. Given the ever-increasing complexity of modern medicine, building in such forcing functions in intravenous pumps, defibrillators, mechanical ventilators, and computerized order entry systems will be crucial to safety.

In addition to better systems, communication and teamwork must be improved. All commercial pilots must take "crew resource management" courses, in which they train for emergencies with other crew members, learn to flatten hierarchies that might stifle open communication, communicate clearly with standard language, and use checklists and other systematic approaches. The evidence that such interventions in medical care will improve the safety of patients is increasingly persuasive.[9] For example, better coordinated pharmacy practices can reduce medication errors after hospital discharge,[A2] and team-based approaches can reduce falls among hospital inpatients.[A3] The goal is a "culture of safety"—an environment in which teamwork, clear communication, and openness about errors, both with other health care professionals and with patients, is the norm.

Another key principle in ensuring the safety of patients is to learn from one's mistakes. Safe systems have a culture in which errors are openly discussed, often in morbidity and mortality conferences. To be most useful, these discussions should be interdisciplinary (involving physicians and other health professionals), identify when the errors occurred, and emphasize systems thinking and solutions; they should not be punitive. In addition to open discussions during conferences, safe organizations build in mechanisms to hear about errors from frontline staff, often through "incident reporting systems"; they also perform detailed "root cause" analyses of major errors or "sentinel events" in an effort to define all the layers of Swiss cheese that need improvement. The importance of open communication extends to patients as well. Disclosure of errors is now required by the Joint Commission. Patients and families value such openness, and reasonably strong evidence indicates that disclosure of errors might decrease the chance of a malpractice suit.[10]

Finally, there is increasing appreciation of the importance of a well-trained, well-staffed, and well-rested work force for the delivery of safe care. Lower nurse-to-patient ratios,[11] long work hours for residents, and lack of board certification are all linked to poor outcomes for patients. Safer systems cannot be created if the providers are overextended or poorly trained or supervised. In the United States, the Accreditation Council for Graduate Medical Education has limited duty hours for residents and has prohibited first-year residents from working 24-hour shifts. Evidence so far confirms that these standards have improved residents' quality of life but not patient safety, probably because of the concomitant increase in risky handoffs.[12]

In the absence of comparative evidence and in light of the high cost of interventions such as improved staffing, computerized order entry, and teamwork training, even institutions committed to safety must often make difficult choices. Given the natural tendency to focus on practices that are measured, publicly reported, and compensated, institutions and physicians tend to focus first on areas that are subject to regulation or on initiatives with multiple potential benefits, such as computerization. For example, computerization has been promoted in the United States by a federal incentive program, which provides billions of dollars to hospitals and physicians that implement computer systems meeting certain "Meaningful Use" standards.

Because improving culture is difficult to measure and to regulate, there is concern that it will not be as high a priority as it should be. Moreover, a safe culture depends on balancing the imperative to improve systems with the need to define and enforce accountability. The safety field is increasingly emphasizing more active enforcement of policies that address problems such as disruptive behavior by clinicians and failure to adhere to evidence-based safety practices.

VALUE: CONNECTING SAFETY AND QUALITY TO COST

Outside of health care, most purchasing decisions are based on perceived value: (quality + safety) ÷ cost. Health care decisions historically have not been made this way, in part because of the limited ability of patients and payers to make rational judgments about the quality and safety of a given provider or system, and in part because health care insurance insulates patients from the full cost of care. In the United States, which spends nearly 20% of its Gross Domestic Product on health care, policy pressures are increasingly being brought to bear on the entire value equation, that is, promoting value, not volume. For example, Medicare's Value-based Purchasing program modifies hospital reimbursement on the basis of quality, safety, and patient satisfaction scores. The organization's readmission initiative threatens substantial cuts in reimbursement to hospitals with higher-than-expected 30-day readmission rates.[13] Other federal programs seek to drive physicians and hospitals into arrangements in which they accept a fixed payment to manage a population of patients (Accountable Care Organizations) or for an episode of illness (bundled payments). Although such programs are controversial and of unproven value, they are part of a growing focus on quality, safety, the patient's experience, and the costs of care.

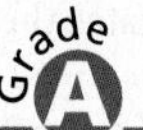

Grade A References

A1. Jack BW, Chetty VK, Anthony D, et al. A reengineered hospital discharge program to decrease rehospitalizations: A randomized trial. *Ann Intern Med.* 2009;150:178-187.

A2. Kripalani S, Roumie CL, Dalal AK, et al. Effect of a pharmacist intervention on clinically important medication errors after hospital discharge: a randomized trial. *Ann Intern Med.* 2012;157:1-10.

A3. Dykes PC, Carroll DL, Hurley A, et al. Fall prevention in acute care hospitals: a randomized trial. *JAMA.* 2010;304:1912-1918.

GENERAL REFERENCES

For the General References and other additional features, please visit Expert Consult at https://expertconsult.inkling.com.

13

COMPREHENSIVE CHRONIC DISEASE MANAGEMENT

EDWARD H. WAGNER

The World Health Organization defines chronic disease as "health problems that require ongoing management over a period of years or decades." This definition encompasses a broad array of physical, mental, and behavioral health problems. Regardless of cause or pathophysiology, chronic conditions require ongoing attention and adjustments by patients and their loved ones as well as care by professionals. Improving care for chronic illnesses has been facilitated by the realization that individuals with a wide variety of chronic health problems have similar needs to minimize morbidity and to optimize quality of life (Table 13-1). Because these needs are shared across conditions, clinical management of these seemingly disparate illnesses requires similar practice capacities and functions. The design and organization of care that leads to better outcomes are remarkably similar for conditions as clinically different as diabetes, depression, and substance abuse disorders.

To live effectively with their health conditions and to manage their treatments, patients must have access to essential information, skills, and encouragement. They must also receive evidence-based therapy and preventive care over time to improve disease control and to reduce the risk of complications and exacerbations. Because chronic illnesses are rarely cured and often change over time, effective care involves continuous monitoring and adjustments by patients and caregivers alike. When chronically ill patients experience periods of increased severity and risk, they often benefit from an intensification of management and support. Care for the chronically ill generally involves multiple health professionals and care settings, and it must be coordinated effectively.

TABLE 13-1 COMMON NEEDS OF PATIENTS WITH CHRONIC ILLNESS

Support and information that enables patients to be competent self-managers of their health and illness
Effective clinical and behavioral treatment that keeps the condition under control and optimizes health status
Effective preventive care to reduce the risk of complications and other morbidity
Ongoing monitoring of the patient's condition to detect and to respond to problems early in their course
Intensification of management and support during high-risk periods
Coordination of care to increase the efficiency and effectiveness of referrals and to prevent the mishaps that commonly occur during care transitions

THE GOALS OF CHRONIC CARE MANAGEMENT

The goals of chronic care management are to meet the aforementioned needs of patients with chronic illness routinely and efficiently. Chronic conditions, whether medical or psychiatric, present challenges for patients and their caregivers very different from those of acute illnesses or injuries. The decisions and behaviors undertaken by patients to deal with their illness, generally called self-management, influence the course and outcomes of most chronic diseases in major ways. Patients make decisions and take action in dealing with symptoms, coping with the social and emotional impacts of illness, monitoring their condition, taking medications, adjusting lifestyle, and interacting with the health care system. Most need training and ongoing support to become competent managers of their health and their illness. The competence and confidence with which patients self-manage have a major impact on outcomes. For example, participants in diabetes or hypertension self-management training programs generally experience clinically significant reductions in hemoglobin A_{1c} or blood pressure levels without major changes in drug therapy.[A1] Self-management can be enhanced in patients of all socioeconomic groups by empowering, training, and supporting them. Modern self-management support is a collaborative rather than a didactic process that seeks concordance between providers' and patients' perspectives on the goals of treatment and the actions needed to reach those goals.[1]

Whereas the primary goals of acute disease care are cure and recovery, cure is not an option for most chronic diseases, which are often characterized by slowly progressive deterioration, even with excellent care. Nevertheless, control of the metabolic or physiologic abnormalities or symptoms resulting from the underlying pathophysiologic processes (disease control) is now possible for most chronic conditions. Drugs and other therapies attempt to minimize morbidity, to limit further organ damage, to reduce the risk of exacerbations and complications, and to maintain quality of life and function. The metabolic or physiologic abnormalities or symptoms used to assess disease control often serve as clinical targets to guide therapy and as performance indicators to monitor the progress and quality of care for populations of patients (e.g., the percentage of diabetic patients with blood pressure <130/80 mm Hg). Disease control for many conditions requires the rigorous application of evidence-based treatment protocols that carefully step up or intensify treatment until clinical targets are reached.[A2]

Ongoing monitoring and assessment of chronically ill patients are essential to optimize treatment and to prevent losses to follow-up. Regular review of self-management activities reinforces their importance to the patient and to the overall management of the condition. Serious exacerbations and complications of common chronic illnesses are potentially preventable if they are identified early in their course and treated appropriately (e.g., recurrence of major depression, opportunistic infection in patients with HIV, foot ulcers among diabetic patients). The periodicity of assessments must change as the severity of illness waxes and wanes over time.

An increasingly important goal of effective chronic care management is to provide more intensive monitoring and management during periods of high risk, such as transitions from hospital to community or exacerbations. Clinical care or case management by nurses, pharmacists, or other nonphysician health professionals enables closer monitoring of patients, helps with medication adjustment, provides self-management support, and facilitates care coordination. Effective care management programs can reduce the likelihood of rehospitalization for chronically ill patients discharged from the hospital, reduce emergency department visits and hospitalizations among multiproblem ambulatory older adults, and improve disease control.

Chronically ill patients frequently receive medical and supportive services from multiple providers in different settings. Without good coordination, unnecessary hospital readmissions and emergency department visits, gaps and inefficiencies in care, and distress of the patient are all too common. Without assistance from their primary providers, patients or their loved ones must often assume responsibility for the onerous task of coordinating care.

MATCHING PATIENT NEEDS AND CARE DELIVERY

The percentage of chronically ill patients in good control varies widely from practice to practice, even after adjustment for patient differences. When individual practices are audited, failures to follow evidence-based guidelines or losses to follow-up appear almost randomly across different interventions and among patients within a practice, suggesting that they are related to flaws in care systems rather than to cognitive gaps. What, then, distinguishes practices that have high rates of control of major chronic conditions from the majority with much lower control rates?

Ambulatory care systems have for centuries been organized to react to acute problems, not to address the ongoing needs of the chronically ill. The focus on making a diagnosis and initiating treatment for the problem at hand leaves little time for addressing less urgent needs, such as medication adjustment, self-management support, and preventive care. Reimbursement systems that favor multiple short encounters aggravate the problem.

Failure to adhere to evidence-based guidelines and insufficient follow-up and attention to patient self-management are largely responsible for the poor control of chronic illness. The guidelines for most chronic conditions include recommendations to step up or to intensify therapy when clinical targets are not reached. Failure to intensify treatment in patients who have not achieved therapeutic targets, called clinical inertia, has been found in a large percentage of patients with uncontrolled diabetes, hypertension, depression, and other chronic illnesses. Clinicians have an understandable reluctance to increase drug doses or to add new drugs, but concerns about toxicity or nonadherence of the patient can be mitigated if practices have organized approaches to stepping up therapy and closely monitoring its impact.

Deficiencies in practice infrastructure and the professional environment compound the difficulties of meeting the needs of chronically ill patients. Despite electronic medical record systems, many practices still have difficulty in managing patient populations or measuring the quality of their care. Primary care physicians are increasingly uninvolved or even unaware when their patients are hospitalized. Efforts to improve the quality of chronic care must focus on improving the infrastructure and practice systems that busy clinicians require to meet the needs of their patients.

Interventions That Improve Care and Outcomes of Chronic Diseases

A wide array of systemic changes can improve the care and outcomes of major chronic diseases. These changes fall into four general categories. *Patient-directed interventions* try to enhance the knowledge of patients, increase their involvement in care, and alter their behavior. *Provider-directed interventions* give providers feedback about the quality of their care and try to change providers' knowledge and behavior through education and reminders. *Organizational changes* generally focus on the composition and functioning of the care team, the organization of patient encounters (e.g., planned visits), and the management of patients outside the office (e.g., follow-up, care management, and care coordination). *Information technology interventions* include the use of registries, computer reminders, and other decision support programs for management of populations and patients. Growing evidence suggests that the use of patient databases (registries) to measure performance, to identify individuals needing care, and to plan care of individual patients may be the information technology function that contributes the most to improving the care of the chronically ill.

Provider-directed interventions, especially educational programs, generally demonstrate weak effects. Conversely, interventions that promote the patient's self-management and change the composition or functioning of the practice team have the most salutary effects.[A3,A4] Across conditions, assigning responsibilities for care of patients to the nonphysician members of practice teams consistently leads to significant improvements in evidence-based care processes, disease control, and other outcomes. Better informed patients have better outcomes when they receive care from more informed providers who are supported by a well-organized clinical team and appropriate information technology.

The Chronic Care Model

Developed in the late 1990s, the chronic care model summarizes the basic elements for improving care of chronically ill individuals (Fig. 13-1). This

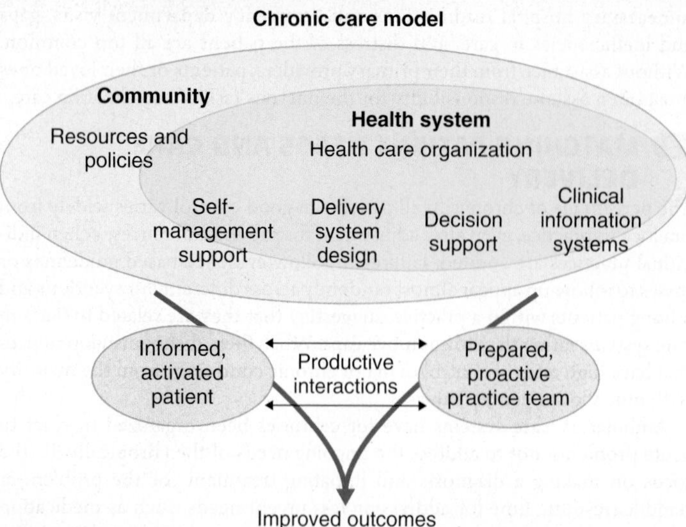

FIGURE 13-1. The chronic care model. (Modified from Wagner EH. Chronic disease management: what will it take to improve care for chronic illness? Eff Clin Pract. 1998;1:2-4. Chronic Care Model © American College of Physicians, Annals of Internal Medicine.)

model identifies six features of a health care system that facilitate high-quality chronic disease care: self-management support, delivery system design, decision support, clinical information systems, health care organization, and community resources. Evidence-based changes in these six areas foster productive interactions between informed patients who take an active part in their care and practice teams organized to meet their needs.

The chronic care model presumes that chronically ill patients have a primary care clinician, either a generalist or a specialist, who assumes responsibility for managing their care and coordinating the activities of other clinicians and institutions that provide advice and services. It posits that important patient outcomes, such as the prevention of morbidity, mortality, and avoidable emergency department visits and hospitalizations, can be affected by productive medical care. Accumulating evidence indicates that implementing the elements of the chronic care model is associated with improvements in the care and outcomes of chronic diseases.[A5-A7] Productive interactions are more likely when patients actively participate in their care. To do so, patients benefit from having the relevant information and skills needed to manage their illness as well as ongoing support and encouragement to overcome denial and passivity.

The other partner in productive interactions is the primary care clinician and the practice team. Before visits with chronically ill patients, practice teams should review accessible information to determine what services are needed, have clear assignments or standing orders for the delivery of those services, and include staff trained to perform them. Although all six elements of the chronic care model contribute to a delivery system that can effectively manage chronic illness, changes in two categories—delivery system design and self-management support—are essential to improve disease control and to reduce morbidity and mortality.

Self-Management Support

Didactic education of the patient alone has been demonstrated to have little if any impact on the patient's behavior or disease control. To change their lifestyle, to take medications as directed, to deal with symptoms and stress, and to address the other challenges of living with chronic illness, patients need to participate actively in their care, to understand and agree with the clinician's assessment of the problems and recommendations, and to learn the skills needed to carry out the recommendations. More active patients are more likely to engage in relevant self-management behaviors and to use health care more effectively,[2] so patients should be empowered to take an active role in their health care.

Group and individual interventions can help patients understand their illness and its treatment and give them the skills and confidence needed to be competent self-managers. In general, these programs share common features that include the teaching of critical skills (e.g., self-monitoring, use of medications), the collaborative development of realistic goals, and action plans for meeting these goals. Although self-management courses facilitated by peer or professional leaders improve disease control in diabetes, hypertension, and other chronic diseases, their effects diminish after termination of the program, so sustained follow-up and reinforcement are essential. Long-term self-management support is best accomplished by the primary care team in the context of ongoing chronic illness care. Although a physician's advice and encouragement are important, most primary care clinicians have neither the time nor the training to help patients set behavioral goals, to develop action plans, and then to follow up by telephone or e-mail. Clinical staff such as nurses or medical assistants with good communication skills and additional training in counseling methods can and should perform these functions.

Delivery System Design

Team Care

The goal of delivery system design is to match the organization of care delivery to the needs of the chronically ill. Without the help of a team, it is unlikely that physicians, in the course of a 15- to 20-minute visit, can effectively manage intercurrent problems, review and adjust treatment, provide recommended assessments and preventive care, discuss self-management goals and plans, and plan follow-up. Designing effective team care begins with a consideration of the various tasks required to meet the needs of the chronically ill and to ensure adherence to guidelines. Key tasks are allocated to the most appropriate members of the practice team. The team's routine involvement in patient visits is facilitated by protocols or standing orders that guide independent action by nonclinician staff. Brief meetings, often termed huddles, before clinic sessions allow practice teams to review key data (often from registries) of scheduled patients, to identify needed services, and to plan their delivery. The goal is to maximize the productivity of every patient interaction.

The specific practice change associated with the largest improvements in chronic disease outcomes is the increased involvement of the nonprovider members of practice teams in meeting the patient's clinical care needs.[A3,A4] For example, a recent trial showed that adding briefly trained lay "care guides" to primary care teams significantly increased the likelihood that patients would achieve disease-specific goals, such as diabetic retinal examinations and effective blood pressure control.[A8]

Planned Interactions

Much of chronic care management involves predictable preventive care or disease management activities, which are often postponed when chronically ill patients seek care for an acute problem. The availability of key patient data gives practice teams the opportunity to update chronic illness care even during visits for more urgent problems. Armed with information from an electronic medical record's reminder systems, nonphysician staff can provide flu shots, diabetic foot examinations, and other evidence-based actions. Practices also can initiate planned visits for patients who are noncompliant with guidelines, have failed to reach treatment targets, or have been lost to follow-up. Another format for the delivery of planned care is the group visit, in which patients receive their primary medical care together as a group. Group sessions generally include the same check-in activities that occur during an individual visit, followed by brief individual communications between the primary care provider and each patient, opportunities for private consultations, and an educational session with ample opportunity for peer-to-peer interaction. Approximately 30 to 50% of patients offered group visits attend them, and many prefer to receive much of their care in this setting.

Follow-up and Case Management

Follow-up tailored to a patient's needs and the clinical severity of the disease is a critical component of effective chronic care management. Traditionally, follow-up consisted of periodic in-person physician visits whose frequency is limited by cost and convenience. Ample evidence indicates that follow-up by telephone, e-mail, or telemedicine can be cost-effective and far more flexible than total reliance on repeated face-to-face return visits. Nonphysician team members, guided by protocols with clear referral criteria, can effectively manage much of electronic follow-up. Self-monitoring by patients is an important component of the follow-up plans for many chronic illnesses and is especially useful when patients use the results to adjust their therapy[A9] as well as to inform their practice team. Collecting self-monitoring data for the sole purpose of bringing them to the physician's office appears to be far less effective.

Chronically ill individuals at high risk of hospitalization, nursing home placement, major complications, or death often experience periods when more intensive monitoring and management would be helpful. Less severely ill patients also need closer follow-up during exacerbations or intercurrent illnesses, after hospital discharge, or when medications are being titrated or changed. Severely ill patients commonly have multiple chronic conditions, which often are complicated further by depression and other psychosocial problems. In response to these needs, nurse care management programs that regularly communicate with patients electronically or in person have proliferated. These programs assess a patient's status, review and support self-management goals and action plans, help coordinate care among providers and care settings, and may help manage medications. Case management is more likely to be effective if the case manager collaborates closely with the primary care clinician, has specific management goals (e.g., improve disease control or improve function), influences the medication regimen directly or indirectly, and reviews his or her caseload regularly with clinician experts.[3,4]

Decision Support

Efforts to educate health professionals have a limited impact on clinical performance. Inserting information and alerts directly into the flow of decision making is more helpful, although "alert fatigue" has become a serious problem. Even the most carefully developed evidence-based guidelines will have no impact on practice if they are not integrated into clinical management through computer templates, alerts, protocols, standing orders, and other efforts to standardize practice.

Many chronically ill patients who are cared for by generalists benefit from the advice and involvement of medical specialists. Truly shared care involving interactive communication between primary care clinicians and specialists can improve outcomes.[A10] Interactive communication channels between generalists and specialists (Chapter 430) can be improved by creating systems whereby consultants respond to questions by secure messaging within an electronic medical record system or through a web-based referral system.

Clinical Information Systems

Well-maintained registries that are either independent or incorporated in an electronic medical record enable practices to identify patients who need additional services, to produce rapid summaries of key clinical data and services for future patient encounters, and to measure clinical performance. Registries allow practices both to monitor and to manage their chronically ill populations. For example, individuals overdue for important preventive interventions or who fail to keep appointments can be efficiently identified and contacted.

Electronic two-way communication between patients and providers is playing an increasing role in the management of chronic disease. Telehealth, web portals, and mobile device applications enable providers to obtain and to respond to clinical data from patients, and they give patients efficient mechanisms for addressing their questions and concerns.

Community Resources

Programs and organizations in patients' local communities can most effectively meet many of their needs. Such needs include transportation, homemaker services, smoking cessation (Chapter 32), exercise (Chapter 16), weight control (Chapter 220), peer support, caregiver support and respite, self-management training, and financial counseling and assistance. For commonly needed services, practices should at least be able to provide specific information to advise patients on their best options.

TRANSFORMING PRACTICE

Measures of disease control and other indicators of the quality of chronic care begin to improve only when practices have made system-wide changes in most of the elements of the chronic care model, such that the routine care of all their chronically ill patients has been affected.[5] Practice routines and culture must change in ways that are initially foreign and uncomfortable for many practitioners. Team care means more meetings, new roles, and additional training for staff. To have useful registries and to provide proactive care, busy practices must define their population of patients and learn to manipulate software and data to obtain the information they need. Some of the changes may require additional financial investment. For all these reasons and more, improving chronic care management requires highly motivated physicians and practices that actively engage in continuous quality improvement. Practices must develop approaches that fit their population of patients, resources, and practice style, and they must refine and adapt them using rapid cycle improvement methods.

Health Care Organization

Many practices caring for chronically ill individuals are parts of larger health care organizations that can either encourage and promote the improvement of chronic care or undermine and obstruct it. Helpful organizations promote continuous quality improvement, incorporate a trusted performance measurement system, and provide financial or nonfinancial incentives for high quality.

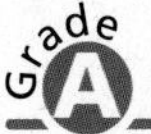

Grade A References

A1. Chodosh J, Morton SC, Mojica W, et al. Meta-analysis: chronic disease self-management programs for older adults. *Ann Intern Med.* 2005;143:427-438.
A2. McManus RJ, Mant J, Haque MS, et al. Effect of self-monitoring and medication self-titration on systolic blood pressure in hypertensive patients at high risk of cardiovascular disease: the TASMIN-SR randomized clinical trial. *JAMA.* 2014;312:799-808.
A3. Shaw RJ, McDuffie JR, Hendrix CC, et al. Effects of nurse-managed protocols in the outpatient management of adults with chronic conditions: a systematic review and meta-analysis. *Ann Intern Med.* 2014;161:113-121.
A4. Tricco AC, Ivers NM, Grimshaw JM, et al. Effectiveness of quality improvement strategies on the management of diabetes: a systematic review and meta-analysis. *Lancet.* 2012;379:2252-2261.
A5. Coleman K, Austin BT, Brach C, et al. Evidence on the Chronic Care Model in the new millennium. *Health Aff (Millwood).* 2009;28:75-85.
A6. Stellefson M, Dipnarine K, Stopka C. The chronic care model and diabetes management in US primary care settings: a systematic review. *Prev Chronic Dis.* 2013;10:E26.
A7. Miller CJ, Grogan-Kaylor A, Perron BE, et al. Collaborative chronic care models for mental health conditions: cumulative meta-analysis and metaregression to guide future research and implementation. *Med Care.* 2013;51:922-930.
A8. Adair R, Wholey DR, Christianson J, et al. Improving chronic disease care by adding laypersons to the primary care team: a parallel randomized trial. *Ann Intern Med.* 2013;159:176-184.
A9. Green BB, Cook AJ, Ralston JD, et al. Effectiveness of home blood pressure monitoring, Web communication, and pharmacist care on hypertension control: a randomized controlled trial. *JAMA.* 2008;299:2857-2867.
A10. Foy R, Hempel S, Rubenstein L, et al. Meta-analysis: effect of interactive communication between collaborating primary care physicians and specialists. *Ann Intern Med.* 2010;152:247-258.

GENERAL REFERENCES

For the General References and other additional features, please visit Expert Consult at https://expertconsult.inkling.com.

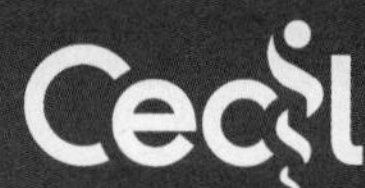

PREVENTIVE AND ENVIRONMENTAL ISSUES

14

COUNSELING FOR BEHAVIOR CHANGE

F. DANIEL DUFFY

Most medical care requires patients to change some behavior. For example, patients may need to keep appointments, stop an addictive behavior, eat different foods, take daily medications, monitor glucose levels, or increase their physical activity. The probability of effectuating change depends on the skills and language of the counselor, recognizing that clinicians typically see patients during brief and relatively infrequent visits for prevention and chronic care.

Behavior change counseling is talk therapy that engages patients in a partnership to execute a plan for change.[1] Behavior change counseling delivered by trained counselors is efficacious in sustaining healthy diets, increased physical activity, reduced alcohol and tobacco use, improved dental outcomes, reduced body weight, and self-care monitoring. Trained physicians who provide brief office-based counseling using patient-centered motivational methods can help patients successfully lose weight[A1] and improve diabetes self-care management.[A2] Modest success has been achieved with office-based counseling for medication adherence[A3] but not for heavy drinking[A4] or problem drug use.[A5]

MOTIVATIONAL INTERVIEWING

Motivational interviewing is an evidence-based therapy that has been adapted to the clinical setting to counsel patients about behavior change.[2] Using this approach, clinicians avoid giving advice and instead ask open-ended questions and then use "reflective listening" to uncover internal ambivalence that may restrain change. The verbal behaviors of trained clinicians include listening carefully and responding to patients' voiced desires, fears, and ambivalence about changing; using statements to affirm patients' autonomy and ability; summarizing patients' self-arguments for and against change; and helping patients intensify their motivation to make changes. With persistence, these conversations can convert patients' ambivalence into the belief and confidence that they can and will change. The overall advantage of motivational interviewing is about 50% greater than comparative counseling methods.[3]

Change counseling in medical care is based on the transtheoretical model of change (Fig. 14-1), which proposes that people change by moving through a cycle of five cognitive-experiential stages (Table 14-1): *precontemplation, contemplation, determination, action,* and *maintenance,*[4] often with a sixth stage (*relapse*). Many people cycle several times before adopting a new habit. By identifying a patient's stage along this continuum of change, a physician can select the most efficient counseling approach.

FITTING CHANGE COUNSELING INTO MEDICAL PRACTICE

The goal of change counseling is to help patients do what they need to do to achieve their own health goals. Physicians help but cannot make people change. Patients do the work, guided by clinicians who evoke their internal motivation to make the change.

To learn what behaviors patients need to change, the physician starts by taking a history of active problems, by performing an appropriate physical examination (Chapter 7), and by ordering any indicated diagnostic tests (Chapter 10). To optimize motivational interviewing, the history should rely primarily on open-ended questions so patients can tell their own stories. The physician's periodic reflections, expressions of empathy, and summaries of what patients say help patients believe they can and must change.

THE ASK-TELL-ASK APPROACH

The process of change counseling helps patients focus on their role in achieving their own health goals. In contrast to a paternalistic practice of making a diagnosis, ordering treatment, and giving expert advice, it promotes a patient's motivation, autonomy, and responsibility for making changes.

Iterative *ask-tell-ask* cycles remind clinicians first to *ask* patients to engage; second to *tell* information, answer questions, and correct misinformation; and third to *ask* patients to verbalize their understanding and intentions.

To use the ask-tell-ask strategy to initiate a conversation about the diagnosis and treatment, clinicians first ask permission to summarize their findings. Second, if patients agree, clinicians tell their diagnostic impressions and health assessments using clear and simple language. Third, clinicians ask an engaging follow-up question to clarify patients' understanding with a question such as, *What do you know about this situation?* The third ask may take the form of a reflective statement that invites patients to go deeper, affirm their courage, express empathy, or acknowledge nonverbal expressions of emotion. Usually, people know more than expected, thereby reducing the time needed for education of the patient.

To focus patients' attention on their role in making changes, clinicians might ask, *What ideas do you have about what you and I might do to improve your health?* Generating a list of hypothetical options may take several ask-tell-ask iterations. When a satisfactory list has been developed, the physician should summarize the patient's voiced health goals and the shared list of options for achieving them.

Clinicians then initiate change planning with a question such as, *What are you willing to do?* Patients' answers indicate their readiness to take action to change their behavior. Clinicians should guard against the "expert trap," in which patients skirt their own ambivalence for change and shift responsibility for change onto the clinician by stating, *You are the expert, and I'll do whatever you tell me to do.*

To avoid the trap, clinicians can estimate patients' motivational stages using a *conviction-confidence ruler* (Fig. 14-2). Clinicians show patients a ruler with markings from 1 to 10 and ask, *How convinced are you that it is important for you to do what is needed from 1 (not convinced at all) to 10 (totally convinced)?* They then ask, *Using the same scale, how confident are you that you will do it?*

Patients with low (0 to 2) scores are probably in the precontemplation stage. Midrange scores (3 to 7) suggest the contemplation stage. A high conviction score (8 to 10) implies determination to change, and moderate to high confidence scores (5 to 9) imply the preparation stage. High scores for conviction and confidence indicate action or maintenance stages. In the relapse stage, patients may have a low confidence score and, if very discouraged, a low conviction score as well. Scores of less than 7 on either question may indicate insufficient motivation for success.

The conviction-confidence scale can clarify patients' convictions about the importance of changing by asking, *Why four on conviction (or confidence) and not lower?* Or one might ask, *What would it take to raise your conviction (or confidence) score to a nine?* Voiced answers to these question help patients clarify their values and beliefs and see their strengths and resources to make needed changes.

STAGE-SPECIFIC CHANGE COUNSELING

A patient-centered change plan is far more comprehensive than a medical treatment plan, which forms only one part of a person's health plan. For example, filling a prescription is one step in a treatment plan, but remembering to take the medication several times a day, altering eating habits, monitoring medication effects, and quitting a self-destructive behavior are ongoing tasks in a change plan. The most common error in medical care is treating lifestyle changes as a simple prescription and being disappointed with the lack of patient adherence to recommendations. Nevertheless, physicians often must first focus the change plan on ensuring that patients take their medications before addressing more complex and time-consuming lifestyle changes.

Precontemplation stage counseling encourages patients to seek information from reading material and websites and to talk with family, friends, or others who have successfully made similar changes. This process highlights the conflict between the risks of the status quo and the benefits of new lifestyle behaviors. Precontemplation is not influenced by scare tactics, professional argument, or debate.

Contemplation stage counseling, which is more difficult, requires time and training. Trained physicians or counselors help patients explore and resolve the natural ambivalence that keeps them from doing the work needed to change. A *decisional balance table* (Table 14-2) can contrast a patient's reasons for sustaining current behaviors with the reasons for changing to healthier ones. Clinicians or counselors listen to what patients say and verbally reflect a patient's ambivalence to help patients begin to convince themselves to change. This approach helps patients "think out loud" about their conflicting desire to change and their simultaneous wish to sustain the status quo.

When momentum stalls or patients backslide from doing their part, physicians often blame patients for resisting change or label them noncompliant. More likely, the difficulty lies with insufficient resolution of the natural ambivalence about change and evolving discord in the physician-patient relationship. Physicians and patients begin talking at cross purposes, become

TABLE 14-1 STAGES OF CHANGE CHARACTERISTICS

STAGE OF CHANGE	PATIENT RESPONSE	PATIENT CHANGE TASKS	CLINICIAN COUNSELING TASKS	COUNSELING RESOURCES
Precontemplation	Surprise about problem Not thinking about changing Demoralized if in relapse	Learn about condition and change needed Develop self-awareness	Reflective listening Advise Inform	Information media Self-assessment logs or diary
Contemplation	Ambivalence Change talk—concern about health risks Sustain talk—prefers the status quo	Self–re-evaluation Raise conviction of importance of change Raise confidence in ability to change	Empathize with patient's ambivalence Open questions Affirm the positive Reflective listening Summarize patients' talking themselves into change	Conviction-confidence ruler Decisional balance Feedback logs Role models Referral for group training
Determination	I must change I can do it	Raise importance Raise confidence Develop action plan Pick start date Tell others	Support self-efficacy Facilitate action plan Anticipate problems Encourage social support	Menu of options Referral for formal counseling List of role models
Action	What will I do? Who or what might help? What problems might I have?	Take action steps to change Manage withdrawal from addiction	Manage cues to old behavior Be alert to positive effect of new behavior Reward self for change Manage withdrawal	Written plan Menu of cues Menu of consequences Menu of rewards Refer for counseling
Maintenance	Pleased with changed self Spontaneous talk about success and difficulties	Manage cues to go back to old behavior Manage bad effects of the new behavior Seek and use social support for change Become a role model to others	Discuss signs and times of danger for relapse Discuss "relapse thinking" Affirm new lifestyle habits	Role model for others Social support sources Referral for maintenance counseling
Relapse	Tells about thinking old behavior was no longer a concern Loss of control Demoralization	Learn the antecedents of relapse Recognize "relapse thinking" Keep open, do not hide Call for help	Reframe relapse to be a valuable lesson Evoke self-efficiency Move quickly back into action	Refer for formal relapse counseling Encourage finding role models who made change Frequent follow-up

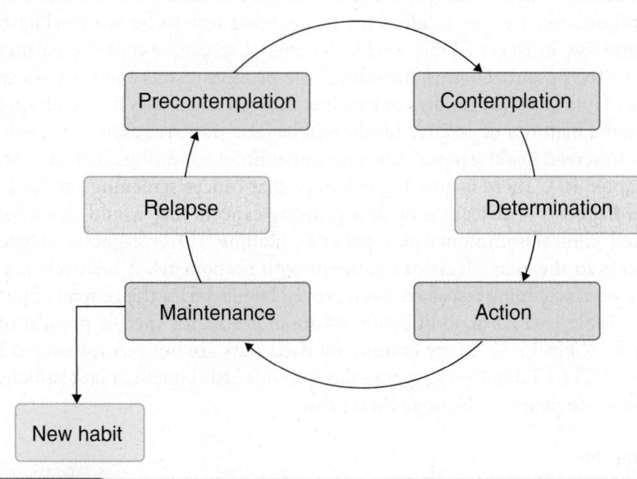

FIGURE 14-1. Cycle of change stages.

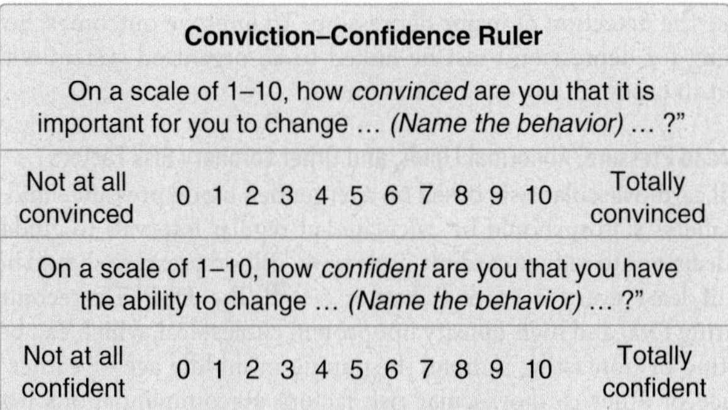

Conviction–Confidence Ruler
On a scale of 1–10, how *convinced* are you that it is important for you to change … *(Name the behavior)* … ?"
Not at all convinced
0 1 2 3 4 5 6 7 8 9 10
Totally convinced
On a scale of 1–10, how *confident* are you that you have the ability to change … *(Name the behavior)* … ?"
Not at all confident
0 1 2 3 4 5 6 7 8 9 10
Totally confident

FIGURE 14-2. Motivational counseling aid.

TABLE 14-2 DECISIONAL BALANCE

BEHAVIOR	REASONS NOT TO CHANGE	REASONS TO CHANGE
Unhealthy behavior	What do you like about it?	What are your concerns about it?
Healthy behavior	What are your concerns about it?	What do you like about it?

defensive, blame, interrupt, and disengage. Physicians might resolve the relational discord with an apology, by affirming patients' strengths, or by shifting the focus of counseling to empathy with the patient's ambivalence and encouragement to believe that she or he can change.

Determination and action stage counseling reinforces a patient's confidence. Counseling might begin with the question, *What are you going to do and when will you begin?* Picking a start date and committing to other people generates accountability and social support. Because it is difficult to change alone, asking *Who or what might help you?* encourages patients to solicit support from partners or others who are making similar changes. Patients may use reminders and rewards to reinforce the new behavior while avoiding situations that stir craving for the old behavior. To plan for relapse prevention and recovery and to handle problems and side effects, clinicians might ask, *What problems might arise and how might you handle them?* As with all change counseling, action plans work best when patients identify the people, resources, and coping strategies themselves. When the change involves quitting an addictive behavior, the plan also should include treatments to manage withdrawal and craving (Chapters 32, 33, and 34).

Maintenance stage counseling is frequently ignored on the assumption that once patients take action to change, the work is done. Moving from action to maintenance requires the new behavior to be internalized and to become routine, requiring little thought or effort. Counseling bolsters the new behavior when "change boredom" sets in, life stresses and competing priorities weaken commitment, or old behaviors become attractive and their consequences forgotten. Maintenance counseling keeps vigilance alive with questions such as, *What is working?* or *Most people have difficulty; how has this change gone for you?* Physicians can talk about relapse with questions like, *Many people begin to think that after a while it's safe to . . . [return to the old habit] just one more time; if you have had these thoughts, how have you handled them?* To engage patients in creative problem solving, physicians might ask, *Who or what has helped you sustain your new behavior?* Planning for recovery after a lapse can be initiated by asking, *Should you slip, what will you do, or who will you call?* A suggestion to call immediately tells patients that relapse is common and can be remediated; it should not be considered a sign of failure. By reframing relapse as a learning opportunity, physicians also help patients reflect on how to strengthen their action plan.

COUNSELING TEAMWORK AND REFERRAL

Behavior change counseling helps patients move from precontemplation to maintaining new habits. This counseling is not a single intervention but rather an ongoing process with long-term follow-up at frequent intervals. Longer counseling visits are appropriate in the first few months for the precontemplation and contemplation stages. Face-to-face or telephone follow-up visits every week or two are useful during the determination and action stages. For the maintenance stage, monthly brief follow-up counseling in the office combined with almost daily contact with supporting persons or role models works well. When intensive help is needed, physicians may refer the patient to education classes, behavioral counseling professionals, or self-help support groups to augment the medical treatment. Medical home primary care practices also can provide counseling for proactive prevention and chronic illness care using multidisciplinary teams of nurse educators, nutritionists, physical therapists, psychologists, and pharmacists. Changing of addictive behaviors usually requires referral to a behavioral change specialist.

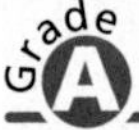

Grade A References

A1. Armstrong MJ, Mottershead TA, Ronksley PE, et al. Motivational interviewing to improve weight loss in overweight and/or obese patients: a systematic review and meta-analysis of randomized controlled trials. *Obes Rev.* 2011;12:709-723.

A2. Chen SM, Creedy D, Lin HS, et al. Effects of motivational interviewing intervention on self-management, psychological and glycemic outcomes in type 2 diabetes: a randomized controlled trial. *Int J Nurs Stud.* 2012;49:637-644.

A3. Easthall C, Song F, Bhattacharya D. A meta-analysis of cognitive-based behaviour change techniques as interventions to improve medication adherence. *BMJ Open.* 2013;3:e002749.

A4. Foxcroft DR, Coombes L, Wood S, et al. Motivational interviewing for alcohol misuse in young adults. *Cochrane Database Syst Rev.* 2014;8:CD007025.

A5. Roy-Byrne P, Bumgardner K, Krupski A, et al. Brief intervention for problem drug use in safety-net primary care settings: a randomized clinical trial. *JAMA.* 2014;312:492-501.

GENERAL REFERENCES

For the General References and other additional features, please visit Expert Consult at https://expertconsult.inkling.com.

15 THE PERIODIC HEALTH EXAMINATION

DAVID ATKINS AND MARY BARTON

Primary and secondary prevention is an essential part of primary care and the patient-centered medical home (Chapter 13). The appropriate services and their frequency vary with the age, gender, and individual risk factors of each patient. A periodic health examination focusing on prevention increases the delivery of appropriate screening and lifestyle counseling. The most comprehensive prevention recommendations are produced by the U.S. Preventive Services Task Force (USPSTF), an ongoing panel of experts supported by the federal Agency for Healthcare Research and Quality (http://www.uspreventiveservicestaskforce.org).

USPSTF recommendations are used by major primary care subspecialty groups, many health plans, and quality organizations, and their A and B recommendations guide preventive services that are covered under the Affordable Care Act. The USPSTF bases its recommendations on two factors: an estimate of the *net benefits* (benefits minus harms) of a service, and an assessment of the *certainty* of that estimate, based on the rigor of supporting studies. Grade A recommendations require high certainty of a substantial net benefit, most often from large, prospective, controlled studies that measure morbidity or mortality. Grade B recommendations have high certainty of moderate net benefit or have moderate certainty for substantial benefit. USPSTF recommendations are thus more conservative than those of some subspecialty organizations that may give more weight to indirect evidence, such as earlier detection of disease, and less weight to potential harms of interventions. Clinicians can draw several general conclusions from an evidence-based approach to prevention: we should be selective in our use of screening tests, especially in older patients, and involve patients in decisions about specific services for which a small chance of benefit must be balanced against possible harm.

HISTORY AND RISK ASSESSMENT

The history and risk assessment are important tools to identify individuals who may need additional screening tests or immunizations not generally recommended for their age group or who may benefit from specific counseling to address unhealthy behaviors. Formal health risk appraisals should be linked to a system to provide specific feedback and targeted interventions.[1] Risk assessment should address the following:

- Use of tobacco, alcohol, and other drugs (especially injection drugs) (Chapters 32, 33, and 34)
- Diet (Chapters 213 and 220)
- Physical activity (Chapter 16)
- Sexual behavior that may increase the risk for sexually transmitted diseases or unintended pregnancy (Chapters 285, 384, and 387)
- Family history of cancer and heart disease
- Birthplace and current residence (community risk for infectious diseases)
- Presence of chronic diseases, such as diabetes, and of other cardiovascular risk factors

SCREENING FOR EARLY DISEASE OR ASYMPTOMATIC RISK FACTORS

Every year, new screening tests are introduced and marketed on the basis of their ability to detect unrecognized diseases or risk factors for disease. Other conditions need to be fulfilled for a screening test to be worthwhile for routine use, however (Table 15-1). Benefits of screening must be balanced against the potential harms, including false-positive results and the risks and costs of follow-up procedures or treatments. Even when tests have high specificity, the majority of positive results will be false-positive results if the test is used to screen healthy populations for uncommon conditions such as cancer (Chapter 10). There is growing evidence that cancer screening can lead to "overdiagnosis"—detection of slow-growing cancers that would never have caused clinical symptoms in a patient's lifetime.[2] Overdiagnosis subjects patients to the side effects of treatment with no benefits. A relatively small number of screening tests have been proved beneficial for the general population (Table 15-2), but additional tests are indicated for specific populations at risk (Table 15-3). Many commonly used tests are not recommended by the USPSTF (Table 15-4) because they provide little benefit or lack sufficient evidence to prove or disprove their value.

Depression

Depression is common and frequently undetected in primary care (Chapter 397). Simple screening instruments, including the following two questions—During the past 2 weeks, have you felt down, depressed, or hopeless? During the past 2 weeks, have you felt little interest or pleasure in doing things?—increase the detection of major depression. To improve outcomes, however, screening for depression must be linked to an organized system with staff support to ensure follow-up and treatment.[3]

High Blood Pressure, Abnormal Lipids, and Other Coronary Risk Factors

Overall cardiovascular risk, based on age, gender, blood pressure, lipid levels, and diabetes status, should be calculated at regular intervals to guide treatment decisions to reduce cardiovascular risk.[4] Blood pressure should be measured at least every 2 years (Chapter 67).[A1] The USPSTF recommends measuring total and high-density lipoprotein cholesterol, which can be done on fasting or nonfasting samples, beginning in middle age or earlier in the presence of other cardiovascular risk factors. Recommendations from the American Heart Association and American College of Cardiology favor fasting lipoprotein analysis, which will identify patients with severe LDL-C

TABLE 15-1 REQUIREMENTS OF AN EFFECTIVE SCREENING TEST

The disease being screened for is an important cause of morbidity and mortality.
Screening can detect disease in an early, presymptomatic phase.
Screening and treatment of patients with early disease or risk factors produce better health outcomes than does treatment of patients when they present with symptoms.
Screening test is acceptable to patients and clinicians—safe, convenient, acceptable false-positive rate, acceptable costs.
Benefits of early detection and treatment are sufficient to justify potential harms and costs of screening.

TABLE 15-2 PREVENTION RECOMMENDATIONS FOR THE GENERAL POPULATION: FROM THE U.S. PREVENTIVE SERVICES TASK FORCE AND OTHER SOURCES

SCREENING

Height, weight, and body mass index (BMI) calculation: periodically
Blood pressure: at least every 2 yr
Screen for alcohol misuse
Brief screen for depression*
Total blood cholesterol and HDL cholesterol: every 5 yr for men and women ≥20 yr with CHD risk factors and men ≥35 yr without CHD risk factors
Colorectal cancer screening: age ≥50 yr (see text for options)
Mammogram: at least every 2 yr for women ≥50 yr; discuss with women 40–49 yr
Papanicolaou (Pap) test: at least every 3 yr for sexually active women aged 21–29 yr; every 5 yr when combined with HPV testing in women 30-65 yr; in absence of HPV testing, continue every 3 yr until age 65
HIV test: at least once in all adults; repeat based on high-risk sexual activity
Chlamydia and gonorrhea: sexually active women ≤24 yr and older women at risk
Bone mineral density test: women ≥65 yr and high-risk women <65 yr

COUNSELING

Substance use
- Tobacco cessation
- Reduction of risky or harmful alcohol use

Diet and exercise
- Limit saturated fat; maintain calorie balance; emphasize grains, fruits, and vegetables‡
- Regular physical activity†

Sexual behavior
- Unintended pregnancy: contraception
- STD prevention: avoid high-risk behavior, use condoms or female barrier with spermicide†

Injury prevention
- Lap and shoulder belts
- Motorcycle, bicycle, and ATV helmets†
- Smoke detector†

Dental health
- Regular visits to dental care provider†
- Floss, brush with fluoride toothpaste daily†

IMMUNIZATIONS

Pneumococcal vaccine (once, age ≥65 yr)
Influenza vaccine (annual)
Tetanus-diphtheria (Td) boosters (every 10 yr)
Measles, mumps, rubella (MMR) vaccine (susceptible adults aged 19–49 yr)§
Varicella (two doses, susceptible adults aged 30–49 yr)§
Human papillomavirus (HPV) vaccine (three doses, women ≤26 yr)

CHEMOPREVENTION

Multivitamin with folic acid (women planning or capable of pregnancy)
Discuss benefits and harms of aspirin to prevent cardiovascular disease in middle-aged adults and others at increased risk for vascular disease

*Depression screening is most effective where systems exist to improve its management.
†The ability of clinician counseling to influence this behavior is uncertain.
‡Diet counseling is most effective when it targets at-risk groups (overweight or with CHD risk factors).
§Immunity can be verified by serologic testing, documented history of illness, or vaccination.
Other sources for Tables 15-2 and 15-3 include U.S. Department of Health and Human Services (diet, physical activity) and Centers for Disease Control and Prevention (injury prevention, immunizations, PPD).
ATV = all-terrain vehicle; CHD = coronary heart disease; HDL = high-density lipoprotein; STD = sexually transmitted disease.

TABLE 15-3 RECOMMENDED SCREENING AND INTERVENTIONS FOR HIGH-RISK POPULATIONS

POTENTIAL INTERVENTION	POPULATION
Ultrasound examination for abdominal aortic aneurysm	Current or former male smokers aged 65-75 yr
Low-dose computed tomography for lung cancer	Smokers with at least 30 pack-year smoking history (current smokers and those who quit smoking within past 15 years)
Hepatitis C test	Born 1945 to 1965; history of injection drug use or other high risk behaviors
Syphilis (RPR/VDRL)	High-risk sexual behavior; consider local epidemiology*
Gonorrhea screen	High-risk sexual behavior; consider local epidemiology*
PPD	Specific immigrant groups, prisoners, HIV patients
Hepatitis B vaccine	Exposure to blood products; IV drug use; high-risk sexual behavior; travelers to high-risk areas
Hepatitis A vaccine	Persons living in or traveling to high-risk areas; institutionalized persons and workers in these institutions; those with certain chronic medical conditions
Meningococcal vaccine	First-year college students in dormitories; military recruits; those with asplenia; travelers to high-risk areas
Varicella vaccine	Adults born after 1980 without evidence of immunity
Breast cancer chemoprevention	Women at increased risk for breast cancer and with low risk for thromboembolic complications
Diabetes screen	Persons at increased risk of diabetes

*Routine screening may be indicated in communities or settings where infection is prevalent.
HIV = human immunodeficiency virus; IV = intravenous; PPD = purified protein derivative; RPR = rapid plasma reagin; VDRL = Venereal Disease Research Laboratory.

TABLE 15-4 INTERVENTIONS NOT RECOMMENDED FOR ROUTINE USE IN ASYMPTOMATIC AVERAGE-RISK ADULTS*

Resting or exercise electrocardiography (D) or helical computed tomography (CT) for asymptomatic coronary disease (I)
Ultrasound examination for asymptomatic carotid artery stenosis (D)
Chest radiograph for lung cancer
Oral examination for oral cancer (I)
Routine blood tests for anemia
Routine urine tests (to screen for infection, cancer, or chronic kidney disease) (I)
Blood tests or ultrasound examination for ovarian cancer (D)
Whole body CT
Brief tests of mental status to detect dementia (I)
Vitamin supplements (I, D)
Blood level of C-reactive protein to predict coronary risk (I)
Prostate-specific antigen for prostate cancer (D)

*These services have either insufficient evidence to support routine use (I) or at least fair evidence that they provide no benefit or that harms outweigh benefits (D).

elevations (>190 mg/dL) (Chapter 206). Either strategy is sufficient to calculate a 10-year cardiovascular risk and to identify patients who may benefit from statin therapy (Chapter 52), which should be considered whenever the 10-year risk exceeds 7.5%.[A2] Although factors such as C-reactive protein, homocysteine, and coronary calcification as assessed by computed tomography (CT) are associated with an increased risk for heart disease, the USPSTF found insufficient evidence to recommend their routine use.

Abdominal Aortic Aneurysm

Between 5 and 9% of men older than 65 years have an abdominal aortic aneurysm (Chapter 78). The risk for aneurysm is highest in smokers and is substantially lower in women (1%). The USPSTF recommends one-time screening with ultrasound examination in men aged 65 to 75 years who are current or former smokers,[5] based on trials demonstrating as much as a 40% lower death rate from abdominal aortic aneurysm rupture in screened men.

Colorectal Cancer

Screening can reduce both the incidence of and mortality from colorectal cancer. Options for screening men and women older than 50 years include an annual highly sensitive fecal occult blood test (FOBT) or fecal immunochemical test, flexible sigmoidoscopy every 5 years plus FOBT every 3 years, or colonoscopy every 10 years (Chapter 193).A3 Colonoscopy combines detection with the opportunity for biopsy and removal of lesions, so it is preferred in some guidelines. It carries higher costs and risks, however, and no single strategy has proved to be more effective or cost-effective than the alternatives. In a randomized trial, a single flexible sigmoidoscopy screening between 55 and 64 years of age reduced the colorectal cancer incidence by 33% and the colorectal cancer mortality by 43% after 11 years of follow-up in people who were screened.[6] In 2008, the USPSTF concluded that evidence was not yet sufficient to support newer technologies such as CT colonography or fecal tests for DNA markers of neoplasia. DNA tests were approved by FDA in 2014 and are more sensitive but less specific than FOBT.[7] The USPSTF recommends stopping routine screening at age 75 years.

Breast Cancer

In large trials, mammography screening (at intervals of 1 to 2 years, with or without clinical breast examination) reduces breast cancer mortality by 15 to 30% (Chapter 198). Most trials suggest that the benefits of screening extend to women in their 40s, but the benefits are smaller and the risks for false-positive results are higher than in women aged 50 to 70 years.[8] If a woman aged 40 to 49 years has a two-fold increased risk for breast cancer, she will have a similar benefit-to-harm ratio for biennial screening mammography as an average-risk woman aged 50 to 74 years.[9] No studies provide data on the benefits of screening women aged 75 and older. In a collaborative study, six independent models predicted that an average of 80% of the benefit of mammography could be achieved with biennial rather than annual mammography, whereas national mammography surveillance data indicate that false-positive results and other harms of screening would be reduced by about half if women were screened every other year instead of yearly. Although many cancers are discovered by patients, teaching women to perform breast self-examination increases the likelihood that a woman will undergo further evaluation for an unimportant finding, but it does not improve outcomes. Widespread screening for *BRCA1* or *BRCA2,* inherited mutations that increase the risk for breast cancer, is not recommended, but the USPSTF recommends that primary care providers screen women who have family members with breast, ovarian, tubal, or peritoneal cancer using one of several recommended family history screening tools designed to identify women at risk for potentially harmful mutations. Women with a positive family history should be referred for genetic counseling.[10]

Cervical Cancer

Papanicolaou (Pap) screening is highly effective in preventing invasive cervical cancer, but many low-risk women in the United States are screened more often than needed. The USPSTF and a multi-specialty-society collaborative[11] endorse delaying screening until age 21 and then screening women aged 21 to 30 years with previous normal test results only every 3 years instead of annually (Chapter 199).A4 In women ages 30 to 65 years, both groups recommend adding testing for the human papillomavirus (Chapters 18 and 373) to Pap testing (co-testing) and extending the interval between screens to 5 years. Women with adequate screening histories should be given the option of discontinuing screening after 65 years of age. Screening is not indicated in women who have undergone a hysterectomy for benign disease. Whether women who have received the human papillomavirus vaccine (Chapter 18) need less frequent screening is not yet known.

Prostate Cancer

Screening with prostate-specific antigen (PSA) can increase the detection of organ-confined prostate cancer, but two large trials provided conflicting results as to whether screening lowers morbidity or mortality from prostate cancer (Chapter 201). An American trial found no benefit of annual PSA testing, but it was hampered by a high rate of screening in the control group. A European study reported that men randomized to screening every 4 years had a 20% lower risk of dying from prostate cancer after 9 years; for each prostate cancer death prevented, 48 additional men were treated for prostate cancer, and 1068 men had to undergo screening. Because of the small benefit and significant morbidity associated with overdiagnosis and overtreatment, including incontinence and impotence, the USPSTF recommends against routine PSA screening,[12] but the American College of Physicians and some specialty groups recommend discussing PSA screening with men who have a life expectancy of at least 15 years.

Lung Cancer

The USPSTF now recommends annual screening with low-dose CT in adults aged 55 to 80 years who have at least a 30 pack-year smoking history and currently smoke or have quit within the last 15 years, based on a large trial in which such screening reduced deaths from lung cancer by 20% and all-cause mortality by 7%.[13] More than 10% of screened persons will have another clinically significant finding, such as a mass in the kidney or adrenal gland or an aortic aneurysm, and at least one false-positive test will occur in more than 40% of screened adults.

Osteoporosis

Tests of bone mineral density can identify men and women with a high risk for fracture due to osteoporosis and who may benefit from medications proved to lower the risk for fracture (Chapter 243). The USPSTF recommends screening for osteoporosis in women older than 65 years as well as in younger women who have risk factors that put them at comparable risk.[14] The most accurate predictor of risk for hip fracture is bone mineral density of the hip assessed with dual-energy x-ray absorptiometry. A tool developed by the World Health Organization (http://www.shef.ac.uk/FRAX/) incorporates bone mineral density and other risk factors, such as age and fracture history, to guide treatment decisions.

Thyroid Disease

Routine thyroid testing occasionally identifies patients with symptomatic but undiagnosed hypothyroidism (Chapter 226), but it more often detects subclinical hypothyroidism, a disorder marked by elevations in thyroid-stimulating hormone with normal levels of free thyroxine. Because the benefits of treating subclinical hypothyroidism remain uncertain, the USPSTF does not recommend routine thyroid testing in the absence of symptoms. Clinicians should be alert to subtle signs of thyroid disease and have a low threshold for testing patients in high-risk groups, including postpartum and postmenopausal women.

Diabetes

Routine screening for diabetes beginning at age 45 years is recommended by some groups, but the USPSTF recommends screening for abnormal blood glucose and type 2 diabetes only in patients at increased risk based on age, overweight, or family history. Although tight glucose control can reduce the incidence of microvascular disease, the benefit of early presymptomatic detection on clinically important retinopathy, neuropathy, and nephropathy is likely to be small. The benefits of early detection of diabetes are based primarily on the benefits of intensive lifestyle modifications.

HIV Infection

The USPSTF and Centers for Disease Control and Prevention (CDC) recommend screening for HIV infection (Chapters 387, 388, and 389) in all adolescents and adults aged 15 to 65 years, including pregnant women.A5 Whether to continue screening after age 65 years should consider risk factors such as new sexual partners. The optimal screening interval is unclear, but annual screening is reasonable in persons at very high risk, such as individuals who are actively engaged in risky sexual behaviors. Rescreening is not necessary in seronegative patients who have not been at increased risk since the last screen.

Hepatitis C Infection

Drugs for chronic hepatitis B and C infection (Chapter 149) have increased the ability to achieve viral suppression and prevent the complications of chronic liver disease in infected individuals. As a result, the USPSTF and CDC now recommend screening for hepatitis B and C in persons at high risk for infection, especially individuals with a history of past or current injection drug use.[15,16] Because persons born between 1945 and 1965 account for three fourths of Americans living with hepatitis C, one-time screening in this cohort is also recommended.

Sexually Transmitted Disease

Screening for chlamydia (Chapter 318) is recommended for all sexually active women aged 24 years and younger and for older women at risk.A6 Nucleic acid amplification tests can be performed on cervical or urine specimens. Early detection can reduce pelvic inflammatory disease (Chapter 285), a risk factor for infertility and ectopic pregnancy. Similar benefits are likely from screening women for gonorrhea (Chapter 299), but the risk for gonorrhea infection is more concentrated in high-risk urban and southeastern rural populations.

Vision and Hearing

Undetected but correctable vision (Chapter 423) and hearing (Chapter 428) problems are common in older adults and can be discovered by asking about problems and performing simple tests of visual acuity and hearing. Unfortunately, evidence is limited to show that regular screening leads to measureable benefits in function. Regular visual acuity testing is recommended for older adults by many organizations, but a large trial did not find any lasting benefits of screening, despite detecting many correctable causes of vision problems. The USPSTF concluded that evidence was insufficient to recommend routine vision or hearing screening.

BEHAVIORAL INTERVENTIONS

Lifestyle factors contribute to a large proportion of preventable deaths in the United States. Brief interventions are effective for some behaviors such as smoking and problem drinking, but changing other behaviors usually requires more intensive approaches. The 5 *As* framework—ask, assess, advise, assist, and arrange—which was developed from smoking cessation research, provides a useful framework for counseling (Chapter 14).

Tobacco Use

Brief interventions can produce small but clinically important increases in quit rates among smokers. Effects increase with more intensive counseling and support, including the use of medication (Chapter 33).

Alcohol Misuse

The USPSTF recommends screening all adults 18 years or older for alcohol misuse with one of three tools: the 10-question AUDIT instrument, its 3-question version AUDIT-C (http://www.integration.samhsa.gov/images/res/tool_auditc.pdf), or a single question: "How many times in the past year have you had five (for men) or four (for women and adults over 65 years old) or more drinks in a day?"[17] Brief multi-contact behavioral interventions can successfully reduce alcohol consumption in at-risk drinkers (Chapter 33).

Diet

Diet counseling can reduce the intake of saturated fat and increase the consumption of fruits and vegetables. Effects are most consistent with more intensive counseling (multiple sessions with trained counselors) and in higher risk patients, such as those with elevated lipid levels (Chapter 213).

Physical Activity

Moderate physical activity reduces the risk for obesity, diabetes, and coronary heart disease, among other benefits. Studies of counseling in the primary care setting, however, have reported inconsistent effects on long-term levels of physical activity (Chapter 16).

Injury Prevention

Motor vehicle injuries are the leading cause of years of potential life lost before age 65 years. In older persons, falls are a leading cause of unintentional injury and can be reduced with targeted interventions (Chapter 25). The USPSTF recommends targeted interventions for at-risk persons, such as exercise, physical therapy, and vitamin D supplementation (Chapter 25).[18] The USPSTF recommends that women of childbearing age be screened for intimate partner violence (Chapter 241)[19] but found insufficient evidence to recommend screening all elderly or other vulnerable adults for abuse and neglect.

IMMUNIZATIONS

Recommendations regarding immunization (Chapter 18) are regularly updated by the Advisory Committee on Immunization Practices of the Centers for Disease Control and Prevention (http://www.cdc.gov/vaccines).[20] Annual influenza immunization is recommended for all adults. Vaccination with pneumococcal polysaccharide (PPSV23) is recommended at least once at age 65 years or after for all adults and for younger adults with asplenia, chronic heart or lung disease, and other immune disorders. Revaccination is not generally recommended unless the initial immunization was before age 65 years or the patient has immune-related risk factors. Adults with immunocompromising conditions, including chronic renal failure, should also receive pneumococcal conjugate 13-valent vaccination (PCV13). Two doses of varicella vaccine are recommended for all adults born in the United States after 1980 without other evidence of immunity, and one dose of zoster vaccine is recommended for all adults at age 60 years. Adults should be revaccinated once with the Tdap vaccine (tetanus, diphtheria, acellular pertussis) and every 10 years with Td; if their vaccination history is uncertain, complete primary immunization with two additional doses of Td is recommended. A series of three doses of a vaccine against human papilloma virus (HPV) is recommended for young women up to age 26 years (with HPV4 or HPV2) to reduce the risk for cervical cancer and for men up to age 21 years (with HPV4) to reduce the risk for genital warts and the transmission of the virus.

CHEMOPREVENTION AND SUPPLEMENTS

Aspirin, postmenopausal hormone replacement therapy, breast cancer chemopreventive drugs, and supplements of vitamins or minerals can carry both benefits and risks. Decisions need to consider the likely benefits (which increase with the underlying risk of the disease being prevented), the probability of harm, and the individual preferences of each patient.

Aspirin

In men and women without known vascular disease, aspirin reduces the combined risk for myocardial infarction, stroke, and other serious cardiovascular events by 12%, but it also increases the risk for serious gastrointestinal bleeding and hemorrhagic stroke and does not significantly reduce cardiovascular mortality. For men ages 45 to 79 years and women ages 55 to 79 years, clinicians should assess whether the benefits, which increase with higher risk for vascular disease, outweigh the bleeding risks, which increase with age (Chapter 38).

Chemoprevention of Breast Cancer

Tamoxifen and raloxifene can reduce the incidence of invasive breast cancer by nearly 50% in women at increased risk, but both agents increase the risk for thromboembolic events and worsen menopausal symptoms; tamoxifen also increases the risk for endometrial cancer (Chapter 198). The USPSTF recommends clinicians discuss the balance of benefits and harms of these medications with women over age 35 years who are at increased risk for breast cancer. Women most likely to benefit are those who are younger than age 60 years and whose 5-year risk of invasive breast cancer is 3% or higher.[21] Online tools can be used to assess this risk (http://www.cancer.gov/bcrisktool/).

Postmenopausal Hormone Therapy

In long-term follow-up studies, estrogen-only therapy reduced the risk for fracture and invasive breast cancer but increased the risk for stroke, thromboembolism, gallbladder disease, and incontinence (Chapter 240). Combination therapy with estrogen and progestin generally has comparable benefits and risks, but it increases the risk for invasive breast cancer and also increases the risk for dementia.[22] Hormone therapy is a reasonable option for younger menopausal women with persistent, troublesome menopausal symptoms, but the USPSTF recommends against its routine use for preventive purposes.

Vitamin and Mineral Supplementation

The USPSTF does not recommend routine use of vitamin or mineral supplements because there is no convincing evidence that multivitamins or individual or paired supplements (e.g., vitamin A, C, D, or E; folic acid; beta-carotene; selenium; or calcium) reduce cardiovascular disease, cancer, or all-cause mortality in community-dwelling average-risk adults.[23] The USPSTF found insufficient evidence to support routine use of calcium and vitamin D supplements for the primary prevention of fractures in ambulatory adults, but primary prevention studies most commonly targeted healthy postmenopausal women. Vitamin D supplementation is recommended for individuals older than 65 years who are at risk for falls (see Injury Prevention), although the mechanism of action is uncertain.

FUTURE ISSUES

There is growing awareness that many older patients receive cancer screening well beyond the ages at which they are likely to benefit. Making clear recommendations for older patients is complicated by lack of good evidence, the difficulty assessing life expectancy, and differences in patients' preferences.[24] As the understanding of genetic factors that modify the risk for disease grows, clinicians may eventually be able to target screening, preventive treatments, or lifestyle interventions to those at greatest risk. The value of using currently available genomic tests to screen average-risk individuals is limited by an incomplete understanding of the predictive value of specific genotypes in the general population, the uncertain effect of such information on clinical decisions, and concerns about the possible adverse effects of screening (e.g., anxiety or "labeling," false reassurance, discrimination).

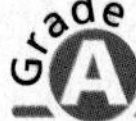

Grade A References

A1. James PA, Oparil S, Carter BL, et al. 2014 Evidence-based guideline for the management of high blood pressure in adults: report from the panel members appointed to the Eighth Joint National Committee (JNC 8). *JAMA*. 2014;311:507-520.

A2. Stone NJ, Robinson JG, Lichtenstein AH, et al. 2013 ACC/AHA guideline on the treatment of blood cholesterol to reduce atherosclerotic cardiovascular risk in adults: a report of the American College of Cardiology/American Heart Association Task Force on Practice Guidelines. *Circulation*. 2014;129:S1-S45.

A3. Whitlock EP, Lin JS, Liles E, et al. Screening for colorectal cancer: a targeted, updated systematic review for the U.S. Preventive Services Task Force. *Ann Intern Med*. 2008;149:638-658.

A4. Moyer VA. Screening for cervical cancer: U.S. Preventive Services Task Force recommendation statement. *Ann Intern Med*. 2012;156:880-891, W312.

A5. Moyer VA. Screening for HIV: U.S. Preventive Services Task Force recommendation statement. *Ann Intern Med*. 2013;159:51-60.

A6. LeFevre ML. Screening for chlamydia and gonorrhea: U.S. Preventive Services Task Force recommendation statement. *Ann Intern Med*. 2014;161:902-910.

A7. U.S. Preventive Services Task Force. Counseling and interventions to prevent tobacco use and tobacco-caused disease in adults and pregnant women: U.S. Preventive Services Task Force reaffirmation recommendation statement. *Ann Intern Med*. 2009;150:551-555.

A8. U.S. Preventive Services Task Force. Aspirin for the prevention of cardiovascular disease: U.S. Preventive Services Task Force recommendation statement. *Ann Intern Med*. 2009;150:396-404.

GENERAL REFERENCES

For the General References and other additional features, please visit Expert Consult at https://expertconsult.inkling.com.

16

PHYSICAL ACTIVITY

DAVID M. BUCHNER

DEFINITIONS

Physical activity can be broadly defined as body movement that is produced by skeletal muscles and expends energy. *Health-enhancing physical activity* is activity that, when added to light-intensity activities of daily life, produces health benefits and involves the large muscle groups of the body and substantial energy expenditure. Herein, *physical activity* refers to health-enhancing physical activity. *Exercise* refers to the subset of physical activity that involves a structured program to improve physical fitness.

Regular physical activity improves *health-related physical fitness*—the physiologic components of fitness that influence risk for disease, functional limitations, disability, and premature mortality. These components include cardiorespiratory endurance (aerobic capacity); skeletal muscle strength, power, and endurance; body composition and bone strength; and balance, flexibility, and reaction time.

The primary attributes of physical activity are *type* (mode), *frequency*, *duration*, and *intensity*. Types of physical activity (e.g., walking, swimming, lifting, stretching) are grouped according to their main physiologic effects into well-known categories: *aerobic* (or "cardio"), *muscle strengthening*, *flexibility*, and *balance*. Intensity is the level of effort during activity. For aerobic activity, the *absolute intensity* is measured in metabolic equivalents (METs), with 1 MET being the resting metabolic rate—an oxygen consumption of roughly 3.5 mL/kg/minute. *Absolute* intensity is commonly classified into: sedentary behavior (1.0 to 1.5 MET), light intensity (1.6 to 2.9 MET), moderate intensity (3.0 to 5.9 MET), and vigorous intensity (6.0 MET and higher). The *relative intensity*, which is the percentage of oxygen uptake (aerobic capacity) reserve required to perform an activity, ranges from 0 to 100%. In practice, the heart rate is used to monitor relative intensity because of the generally linear relationship between heart rate and percentage of oxygen uptake.

The *volume* (or amount) of activity is the product of frequency, duration, and intensity. Volume can be measured using self-report (questionnaires) as MET-minutes per week (a sum of the MET intensity of all activities multiplied by the minutes each activity is performed). Volume can also be assessed using objective measures of physical activity in either arbitrary units ("counts per day" from an accelerometer) or as activity-related energy expenditure (kcal/week). A commonly used objective measure is the accelerometer (usually worn at hip or wrist, for 1 week), which detects movement of the body and provides detailed information on the frequency, duration, and intensity of movement.

EPIDEMIOLOGY

Levels of Physical Activity

It is highly likely that Americans' total level of physical activity has declined since the 1950s. Occupational activity has probably declined the most, but activity around the home and as transportation for getting places has also declined. Trends in recreational physical activity are either stable or slightly improving.

Based on self-reported activity, about 60% of adults meet public health guidelines for physical activity,[1] but only about 10% to at most 45% of American adults meet these guidelines based on accelerometer data collected at the same time. Although one accelerometer reading is not a perfect measure of average physical activity levels, the magnitude of this discrepancy suggests that adults commonly over-report their activity levels and that physical inactivity is a larger public health problem than previously realized.

Physical activity levels decline with age, and men report more activity than women. Higher levels of income and education are associated with greater physical activity. Although white Americans self-report higher levels of physical activity than do other racial and ethnic groups, Mexican American adults are the most active group as judged by accelerometer data.[1]

Preventive Health Benefits in Adults

There is strong evidence that regular moderate or vigorous physical activity (Table 16-1) reduces the risk for premature mortality and coronary artery disease (Chapter 52), stroke (Chapter 406), high blood pressure (Chapter 67), adverse lipid profile (Chapter 206), type 2 diabetes mellitus (Chapter 229), metabolic syndrome, osteoporosis (Chapter 243), colon cancer (Chapter 193), breast cancer (Chapter 198), and obesity (Chapter 220).[2] Even 15 minutes per day or 90 minutes per week of moderately intensive exercise is associated with a 14% decrease in mortality.[3] Physical activity also reduces the risk for falls, cognitive impairment in older adults, age-related muscle loss, and depression (Chapters 25 and 397). There is moderate evidence that physical activity reduces the risk for hip fracture, lung cancer, endometrial cancer, and sleep disorders. Physical activity can delay age-related functional limitations and loss of independence.[A1] Some evidence also suggests that physical activity reduces the risk for anxiety disorders, osteoarthritis, and back pain.

The benefits of physical activity are independent of other risk factors. For example, a sedentary obese smoker achieves health benefits from exercise, even if smoking and obesity persist.

Epidemiologic studies report that low levels of activity are associated with an increased risk for adverse health outcomes,[4] including up to a 67% increase in overall mortality, a doubling of mortality from cardiovascular disease,[5] and an increased mortality from cancer. When a healthy diet, regular activity, and abstinence from smoking are considered simultaneously, the effect of lifestyle is even more dramatic.

The main determinant of the health benefits of physical activity is volume. Substantial health benefits begin to occur with a volume of 500 to 1000 MET-minutes/week. An adult can accumulate 500 MET-minutes by walking at 3.0 miles per hour (a 3.3-MET activity) on 3 days a week for 50 minutes (3.3 METs × 3 × 50 minutes =≈500 MET-minutes). When measured by caloric expenditure, this volume of walking in a 75-kg (165-lb) adult expends an extra 430 kcal above the 190 kcal that would have been expended under resting conditions.

The dose-response relationship between volume and health benefits is curvilinear, such that the marginal benefit of activity at lower levels is large, and the benefit decreases with higher activity levels.[5] Data from the Women's Health Initiative Observational Study (Table 16-2) provide an example of the dose-response effect. Compared with the least active women, the risk for cardiovascular disease was 19% less in women who averaged 600 MET-minutes/week, yet just 28% less in women who averaged 1968 MET-minutes/week. Dose-response effects are also found in intervention studies. For example, a randomized trial of two doses of exercise (doses equivalent to jogging 12 and 20 miles/week) found that the lower volume of exercise significantly improved plasma lipoproteins, but the higher volume had greater beneficial effects.[A2]

TABLE 16-1 EXAMPLES OF MODERATE-INTENSITY AND VIGOROUS-INTENSITY ACTIVITIES

MODERATE INTENSITY

Walking briskly (3 miles per hour or faster, but not race-walking)
Water aerobics
Bicycling slower than 10 miles per hour
Tennis (doubles)
Ballroom dancing
General gardening

VIGOROUS INTENSITY

Race-walking, jogging, or running
Swimming laps
Tennis (singles)
Bicycling 10 miles per hour or faster
Jumping rope
Heavy gardening (continuous digging or hoeing, with heart rate increases)
Hiking uphill or with a heavy backpack

From U.S. Department of Health and Human Services. *2008 Physical Activity Guidelines for Americans.* http://www.health.gov/paguidelines.

TABLE 16-2 RELATIVE RISK FOR CARDIOVASCULAR DISEASE IN THE WOMEN'S HEALTH INITIATIVE OBSERVATIONAL STUDY (*N* = 73,743)

MEDIAN MET-MINUTES PER WEEK	MULTIVARIATE ADJUSTED RELATIVE RISK FOR CARDIOVASCULAR DISEASE
0	1.0
252	0.89
600	0.81
1050	0.78
1968	0.72

Data from Manson JE, Greenland P, LaCroix AZ, et al. Walking compared with vigorous exercise for the prevention of cardiovascular events in women. *N Engl J Med.* 2002;347:716-725.

TREATMENT (Rx)

Therapeutic Health Benefits in Adults

Clinical practice guidelines assign a substantial therapeutic role to physical activity in patients with coronary heart disease (Chapter 52), high blood pressure (Chapter 67), type 2 diabetes (Chapter 229), obesity (Chapter 220), osteoporosis (Chapter 243), osteoarthritis (Chapter 262), claudication (Chapter 79), and chronic obstructive pulmonary disease (Chapter 88).

In individuals with impaired glucose tolerance and high cardiovascular risk, both baseline activity levels and changes in activity levels are associated with a reduction in subsequent cardiovascular events.[6] Physical activity also plays a role in the management of depression and anxiety disorders, elevated cholesterol levels, pain, heart failure, syncope, stroke, back pain, dementia, and constipation and in the prophylaxis of venous thromboembolism.

Although there is more evidence for the therapeutic effects of aerobic activity, muscle-strengthening exercise can also provide benefits. For example, a randomized trial of exercise in adults with diabetes reported that the combination of aerobic and muscle-strengthening exercise was superior to either by itself.[A3]

Physical activity effectively opposes age-related loss of fitness and functional limitations. In older adults, low fitness (exercise capacity of <85% of predicted value) is associated with doubled risk for mortality. Randomized controlled trials demonstrate that exercise by sedentary older adults improves health-related physical fitness (e.g., aerobic exercise improves aerobic capacity) and has beneficial effects on functional limitations, such as a slow gait speed.[A4] A systematic review of nine observational studies reported that slow gait speed is strongly related to mortality as well, with low-risk adults having gait speeds of 1.0 meter/second or higher.[7] Physical activity, especially balance training, prevents falls in older adults at increased risk for falling, such as those with impaired gait and balance.[A5] Because both low fitness and high body weight cause functional limitations, the question arises whether functional ability is best improved by weight loss, exercise, or both. With the doses of weight loss and exercise that are feasible in randomized trials, exercise alone appears more effective than weight loss alone, and combined exercise and weight loss is most effective.[A6]

Health Risks of Physical Activity

Physical activity and exercise have risks. Musculoskeletal injuries are by far the most common type of activity-related adverse event. The risk for injury depends on the type and volume of activity. Collision and contact sports have a much higher injury risk than noncontact activities such as walking, which is associated with about one musculoskeletal injury for every 1000 hours of walking for exercise.[8] The weekly volume of activity is directly related to the risk for musculoskeletal injuries, but when following public health guidelines, which involves participating in about 500 to 1000 MET-minutes/week, the risk for injury is low. The risk for injury is directly related to the rate of increase in the dose of activity, with more rapid increases having higher risk.[2] Previous musculoskeletal injuries and low fitness also increase the injury risk.

Overall, regular physical activity decreases the risk for sudden cardiac death and myocardial infarction; active adults have roughly a 70% lower risk for sudden death. However, relatively vigorous physical activity acutely increases the risk for these events in both active and inactive adults. About 5 to 10% of myocardial infarctions are associated with vigorous activity. Yet sudden death is a rare event during exercise, with published rates in the range of one death per year in 18,000 ostensibly healthy men and one death per 2.6 million workouts in fitness facilities.

Physical Activity Guidelines for Adults

In 2008, the U.S. Department of Health and Human Services issued the first national physical activity guidelines: the *2008 Physical Activity Guidelines for Americans*[2] (Table 16-3).

Recommended Amounts of Aerobic Activity for Prevention

To obtain substantial health benefits from physical activity, adults should do at least 150 minutes/week of moderate-intensity aerobic activity or 75 minutes/week of vigorous-intensity activity. Adults can do a combination of both moderate- and vigorous-intensity activity, using the rule of thumb that one vigorous-intensity minute of activity counts the same as two moderate-intensity minutes. Bouts of aerobic activity 10 or more minutes clearly have health benefits, and even short bouts of less than 10 minutes may also provide some health benefits.[9]

Recommended Amounts of Muscle-Strengthening Activity for Prevention

Adults should perform activities that strengthen the major muscle groups of the body at least 2 days each week. The major muscle groups are the legs, hips, back, chest, abdomen, shoulders, and arms.

Flexibility Activity

Flexibility activities are an acceptable part of a physical activity regimen, but there is insufficient evidence that flexibility activities have any health benefits, even for preventing injuries. Flexibility training does increase flexibility, and it may facilitate the types of physical activity that do have health benefits. If so, flexibility training is more important for people with reduced flexibility, such as older adults with age- and disease-related changes in range of motion.

Balance Activity

Balance training is currently recommended only for adults at increased risk for falls (Chapter 24), such as those older than 65 years with impaired gait or balance or frequent falls. Examples of balance exercises include sideways walking, backward walking, heel walking, and standing using a narrow base of support. Tai chi programs include exercises that improve balance, and tai chi exercise is an evidence-based approach to fall prevention. Preferably, adults at risk for falls should do balance training at least 3 days/week and follow an evidence-based program demonstrated to reduce the risk for falls.

Sedentary Behavior

Sedentary behavior can be defined as activities (not including sleeping) with energy expenditure of 1.0 to 1.5 METs; most of these behaviors involve sitting or lying down. Epidemiologic studies report that higher levels of sedentary time (or equivalently lower levels of light-intensity activity) have adverse health effects, independent of a person's volume of moderate- to vigorous-intensity activity. More sedentary time as assessed by accelerometers is associated with greater body weight, worse markers of metabolic health, and higher mortality. Currently, light-intensity activities expend calories and can be recommended as part of a plan to achieve and maintain a healthy weight. However, data are insufficient to issue guidelines on the amounts and patterns of sitting time that cause adverse health effects in adults.

Guidelines for Weight Management

The amount of activity required to maintain a healthy body weight varies widely among adults (Chapter 220). For some adults, the physical activity levels recommended in the guidelines will result in a stable, healthy body weight. Many adults, however, need higher levels of activity to achieve a healthy weight. These individuals should restrict their caloric intake and gradually increase their physical activity each week, to the point that is effective in achieving and maintaining a healthy body weight for them.

Additional Guidelines for Older Adults

In addition to balance training, the 2008 guidelines contain other recommendations specifically for older adults. Older adults who cannot do 150 minutes/week of moderate-intensity activity should be as active as their abilities and conditions allow. Progressive resistance strength training improves physical function in elderly people.[A7] Older adults should determine their level of physical activity using relative intensity, not absolute, intensity. This latter guideline seeks to avoid inappropriately high levels of effort in older adults with low fitness.

Recommending Physical Activity in Clinical Settings

Promoting physical activity in clinical settings involves essentially the same steps as the "5 As" of smoking cessation: ask, advise, assess, assist, arrange. (1) Ask about the amount of physical activity a patient typically engages in each week by questionnaire or interview. (2) Advise all patients to participate in at least a moderate amount of physical activity each week. Advise patients who do not meet the recommendations to increase their physical activity gradually to a specified minimal level, and tailor the recommendations according to their medical conditions. (3) Assess the next step or steps a patient needs to take to become more active. (4) Assist the patient in taking these steps. (5) Arrange an appointment to follow up on efforts to increase activity.

Health care providers should ask and advise patients about physical activity regularly. One quality-of-care measure assesses whether asking and advising are done at least once a year in older adults. Some recommend that physical activity should be a "vital sign" that is assessed at every visit. Studies consistently report that adults (especially older adults) identify their health care providers as an important source of advice on physical activity.

Nevertheless, the U.S. Preventive Services Task Force concluded that the benefit of routine counseling in the primary care setting is small.[10] The benefit is higher, however, if counseling is provided only when patients request it.

Exercise Prescription

For patients who want to exercise, a clinician can provide an exercise prescription. The prescription includes (1) the type, frequency, duration, and intensity of aerobic exercise; (2) the exercise movements (e.g., bench press), repetitions, and sets for resistance exercise; (3) other exercises such as stretching, balance exercises, warm-up, and cool-down; and (4) risk management strategies, such as increasing levels of activity gradually over time.

Lifestyle Prescription

A lifestyle prescription refers to approaches that integrate physical activity into daily life. For example, rather than walking specifically for exercise, a person walks to work or walks for pleasure as a recreational activity. Common ways to integrate physical activity into daily life are walking and biking for transportation and performing yard work and gardening.

Tailoring the Recommendation

Recommendations need to be tailored to individual abilities, individual preferences, medical conditions, and behavior techniques that improve adherence. Randomized trials show that home-based programs are superior to center-based programs in terms of long-term adherence.[A8] Although center-based programs are preferred by some, in most cases they serve a short-term purpose, such as assisting adults to initiate regular exercise.

A target level of physical activity below that of preventive recommendations is appropriate for adults with very low fitness, a large burden of chronic disease (e.g., severe chronic obstructive lung disease), or major functional limitations. An assessment of the nature of the activity limitation and the individual's capabilities and preferences can determine the target activity level and other details of the activity recommendation. Often, promoting physical activity in such adults relies on health care and community resources designed for people with preexisting limitations, such as cardiac rehabilitation, pulmonary rehabilitation, and exercise classes for adults with arthritis.

Risk Management

Strategies to reduce injury include increasing physical activity gradually over time, selecting activities in which collision or contact with people or objects is unusual, increasing physical fitness, using appropriate gear and sports equipment (e.g., bike helmets), engaging in activities in safe environments, and following basic safety rules and policies. Popular activities such as walking, biking, swimming, and gardening have a low risk for injury. When increasing the level of physical activity, the guidelines recommend using relative intensity to determine the level of effort, starting with relatively moderate-intensity activity, then increasing the duration and frequency first and the intensity last. In general, adding 5 to 15 minutes of moderate-intensity activity per session, two to three times a week, to a person's usual activities carries a low risk for musculoskeletal injury and no known risk for sudden cardiac death.[8]

TABLE 16-3 KEY PHYSICAL ACTIVITY GUIDELINES FOR ADULTS

All adults should avoid inactivity. Some physical activity is better than none, and adults who participate in any amount of physical activity gain some health benefits.

For substantial health benefits, adults should do at least 150 min (2.5 hr)/wk of moderate-intensity aerobic activity or 75 min (1.25 hr)/wk of vigorous-intensity aerobic activity, or an equivalent combination of moderate- and vigorous-intensity aerobic activity.

Aerobic activity should be performed in episodes lasting at least 10 min and should be spread throughout the week.

For additional and more extensive health benefits, adults should increase their aerobic physical activity to 300 min (5 hr)/wk of moderate-intensity or 150 min (2.5 hr)/wk of vigorous-intensity aerobic physical activity, or an equivalent combination of moderate- and vigorous-intensity activity. Additional health benefits are gained by engaging in physical activity beyond this amount.

Adults should also do muscle-strengthening activities that are moderate or high intensity and involve all major muscle groups on 2 or more days/wk because these activities provide additional health benefits.

From U.S. Department of Health and Human Services. *2008 Physical Activity Guidelines for Americans.* http://www.health.gov/paguidelines.

There is no evidence of the protective value of a medical consultation or of supervised exercise in healthy people of any age who seek to increase their level of physical activity. The U.S. Preventive Services Task Force recommended against routine screening for coronary disease in adults at low risk for it and concluded that in adults at high risk for coronary disease, there is insufficient evidence to recommend for or against screening with resting electrocardiography or an exercise treadmill test.[11]

Coordination between Medical Care and Community

Many factors affecting physical activity levels are difficult to influence in medical care settings, such as the characteristics of the communal environment (e.g., parks and recreational facilities) and the social environment (e.g., crime and social support). Community-level interventions that address such characteristics are essential to promoting physical activity. Effective community-based interventions include school physical education, social support interventions, community-wide campaigns, enhancement of access to places where physical activity is possible, and interventions that involve community design, such as improving the connectivity of streets and the walkability of neighborhoods.[12] Medical care and community efforts should be synergistic and mutually supportive. For example, health plans should be advocates for evidence-based community interventions. Community programs should serve as resources for evidence-based therapeutic activity for selected chronically ill adults, such as exercise classes designed to reduce the risk for falls.

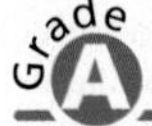

Grade A References

A1. Pahor M, Guralnik JM, Ambrosius WT, et al. Effect of structured physical activity on prevention of major mobility disability in older adults: the LIFE study randomized clinical trial. *JAMA.* 2014;311:2387-2396.

A2. Kraus WE, Houmard JA, Duscha BD, et al. Effects of the amount and intensity of exercise on plasma lipoproteins. *N Engl J Med.* 2002;347:1483-1492.

A3. Church TS, Blair SN, Cocreham S, et al. Effects of aerobic and resistance training on hemoglobin A_{1c} levels in patients with type 2 diabetes: a randomized controlled trial. *JAMA.* 2010;304:2253-2262.

A4. Pahor M, Blair SN, Espeland M, et al. Effects of a physical activity intervention on measures of physical performance: results of the Lifestyle Interventions and Independence for Elders Pilot (LIFE-P) study. *J Gerontol A Biol Sci Med Sci.* 2006;61:1157-1165.

A5. Gillespie LD, Robertson MC, Gillespie WJ, et al. Interventions for preventing falls in older people living in the community. *Cochrane Database Syst Rev.* 2012;9:CD007146.

A6. Villareal DT, Chode S, Parimi N, et al. Weight loss, exercise, or both and physical function in obese older adults. *N Engl J Med.* 2011;364:1218-1229.

A7. Liu CJ, Latham NK. Progressive resistance strength training for improving physical function in older adults. *Cochrane Database Syst Rev.* 2009;3:CD002759.

A8. Ashworth NL, Chad KE, Harrison EL, et al. Home versus center based physical activity programs in older adults. *Cochrane Database Syst Rev.* 2005;1:CD004017.

GENERAL REFERENCES

For the General References and other additional features, please visit Expert Consult at https://expertconsult.inkling.com.

17

ADOLESCENT MEDICINE

DEBRA K. KATZMAN AND LAWRENCE S. NEINSTEIN

Adolescence, a period of transition between childhood and adulthood, is marked by critical biologic, psychological, social, and cognitive changes. During this unique developmental period, patterns of behaviors and lifestyle choices are established that can influence current and future health, and unique medical and psychological problems can emerge.[1] Adult-oriented health care providers play a pivotal role in engaging youth in their health and in providing health care to adolescents and young adults.

NORMAL PHYSICAL GROWTH AND DEVELOPMENT

Biologic growth and development in adolescents are signified by the onset of puberty (Chapter 235), which varies temporally among adolescents and explains why adolescents of the same chronologic age can vary greatly in physical appearance. The first visible sign of puberty among girls is usually thelarche, or the development of breast buds, which occurs on average at 10.5 years in white girls and 1 year earlier in African American girls (Chapter 235).

Menarche occurs 2 to 4 years after the initial appearance of breast buds and pubic hair. The average age of menarche is 12.9 years for white girls and 12.2 years for African American girls. Menstrual periods are not always regular during the first 2 years after menarche. At menarche, only 20% of cycles are ovulatory; it may take up to another 4 years for 80% of cycles to be ovulatory. The average length for the completion of puberty in girls is 4 years (range, 1.5 to 8.0 years).

Puberty begins about 2 years later in boys than in girls. The first physical sign of puberty in boys, testicular enlargement and thinning of the scrotum, occurs at 11.5 years. Adrenarche occurs 6 months later at an average age of 12.0 to 12.5 years (Chapter 234). Facial hair starts to grow about 3 years after pubic hair. The completion of puberty in boys can take an average of 3 years (range, 2 to 5 years).

Pubertal weight gain accounts for about half of a person's ideal adult body weight. Peak weight gain follows the linear growth spurt by 3 to 6 months in adolescent girls and by about 3 months in adolescent boys. The average weight gain during puberty among adolescent girls is 15 to 55 lb or 7 to 25 kg (mean gain, 38.5 lb or 17.5 kg). Overall, adolescent boys gain 15 to 65 lb or 7 to 30 kg during puberty (mean gain, 52.2 lb or 23.7 kg).

Boys' body fat levels decrease during adolescence, dropping to 12% body fat by the end of puberty. On average, adolescent girls' lean body mass falls from 80 to 75%, whereas their average body fat levels increase from 16 to 27% by the end of adolescence. By the time adolescent girls are 16 years of age and adolescent boys are 18 years of age, they have accrued more than 90% of their adult skeletal mass.

Sexual maturity ratings (SMRs), also known as Tanner staging, are used to describe the progression of secondary sexual characteristics that occur in adolescents, irrespective of chronologic age. SMR is based on the development of breasts and the appearance of pubic hair among girls (Fig. 17-1) and on testicular and penile development and the appearance of pubic hair among boys (Fig. 17-2). SMR 1 corresponds to the prepubertal stage; puberty has not begun, and no sexual development has occurred. SMR 2 to SMR 5 indicate the progression of puberty to adulthood. Once young people reach SMR 5, they have fully developed secondary sexual characteristics. Sexual maturation correlates with linear growth, changes in weight and body composition, and hormonal changes. Sexual maturation provides important assurance of the normal progression of puberty or identification of abnormal pubertal development.[2]

NORMAL PSYCHOSOCIAL DEVELOPMENT

Adolescence is often divided into three psychosocial developmental phases: early adolescence (11 to 13 years), middle adolescence (14 to 16 years), and late adolescence (17 to 21 years). In early adolescence, adolescents begin to separate from their parents and establish an individual identity. As adolescents pull away from their parents in search of their own identity, their peer group takes on an important and special significance.

At the beginning of adolescence, cognitive abilities are dominated by concrete thinking. Young adolescents lack abstract reasoning capabilities, problem-solving skills needed to overcome barriers to behavioral changes, and the ability to appreciate how their current behaviors can affect their future health status.

Middle adolescence is characterized by growth in emotional autonomy and increasing separation from family. The adolescents' peer groups play a powerful role, and adolescents are increasingly involved in partnering relationships that include dating, sexual experimentation, and adverse health behaviors such as smoking cigarettes, drinking alcohol, using street drugs, and being truant. Abstract reasoning skills emerge but often regress to concrete thinking when adolescents are faced with stressful situations. These adolescents begin to understand the relationship between health behaviors and future health status, but peer pressure may make it challenging for them to make appropriate health-related choices.

During late adolescence, young people become increasingly more economically and emotionally independent. Peer group values become less important, and young people spend more time in a relationship with one person. The late stage of adolescence is characterized by the development of a strong personal identity. Abstract reasoning skills expand, and older adolescents have problem-solving skills that help them overcome challenges to behavioral change.

VITAL STATISTICS

Although adolescents and young adults are generally perceived to be healthy, their morbidity and mortality are often the result of risky behaviors and social forces (Table 17-1).[3] Unintentional injury, homicide, and suicide are the leading causes of death in 15- to 24-year-olds and account for more than 70% of all adolescent and young adult deaths. About 75% of these causes of death and injury are preventable.

Unintentional and Intentional Injuries

Unintentional injuries account for 44% of all injury deaths to children and adolescents. For every childhood death caused by injury, another 34 hospitalizations and 1000 emergency department visits occur. Major causes of unintentional injuries to adolescents include motor vehicle accidents, being struck by or against an object or person, cuts from sharp objects, and falls. Athletic injuries, which also are frequent, can be reduced by targeted prevention programs.A1 Factors that contribute to adolescent injuries include socioeconomic factors (poor adolescents are at greatest risk for injury), environmental factors (hazards such as all-terrain vehicles, backyard swimming pools, firearms, kerosene heaters, and gang activity), school environment, and developmental factors.

About 20% of all adolescents, especially adolescent girls in heterosexual relationships, report having experienced either psychological or physical violence from a dating partner. About 20 to 30% of students in grades 6 to 10 are involved in bullying, as a bully, victim, or bully-victim (those who are both aggressive to peers and victimized by peers). For younger adolescents, bullying can lead to a significantly higher risk of psychosomatic problems.

Suicide (Chapter 397) is the second leading cause of death among adolescents and young adults 15 to 24 years of age. Native Americans and white youth 15 to 24 years of age have the highest suicides rates, whereas African American youth 15 to 19 years of age and Asian youth 20 to 24 years of age have the lowest. The estimated ratio of attempted-to-completed suicides among adolescents ranges between 50 : 1 and 100 : 1. The most common methods used in suicide attempts are drugs and alcohol, whereas suffocation, hanging, or use of firearms is associated with completed suicides. Death rates caused by firearms are eight times higher in adolescent boys than in adolescent girls.

Homicide is the third leading cause of death in the 15- to 24-year-old U.S. population and the number one cause of death among African American males 15 to 24 years of age. About 75% of homicides in older adolescents and young adults involve firearms.

Clinicians should discuss the impact of alcohol and drugs on driving and stress the importance of routine use of seat belts when driving in a motor vehicle. Clinicians also should discuss safety during sports activities, such as use of bicycle helmets and sports-related protective gear.

Other Diseases

Excluding intentional and unintentional injuries, cancer is the leading cause of death in adolescents and is the leading cause of death by disease. Cancers with an increased incidence in adolescents include Hodgkin lymphoma

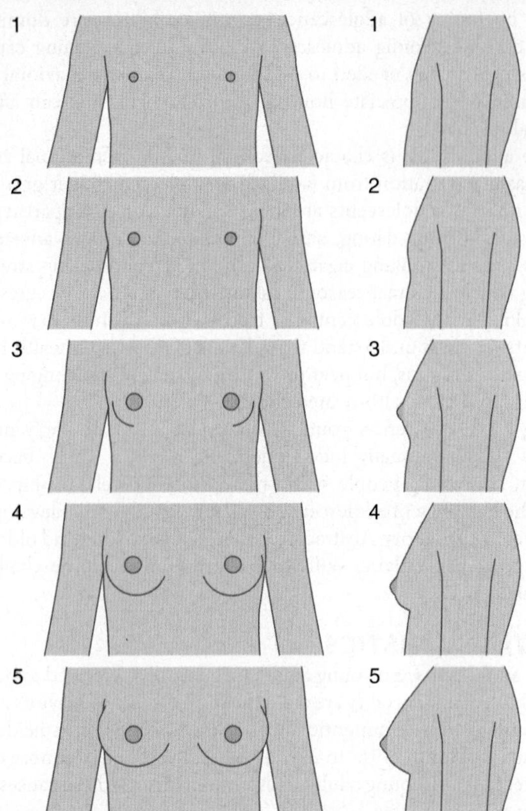

FIGURE 17-1. Female breast development. *Sexual maturity rating 1 (SMR 1):* Preadolescent; no glandular tissue. Areola and papilla: Areola conforms to general chest line. *SMR 2:* Breast buds appear; areola is slightly widened and projects as small mound. *SMR 3:* Enlargement of the entire breast with protrusion of the papilla or of the nipple. Breast and areola enlarge with no separation of their contours. *SMR 4:* Enlargement of the breast and projection of areola and papilla as a secondary mound. *SMR 5:* Adult configuration of the breast with protrusion of the nipple; areola no longer projects separately from remainder of breast. (Redrawn from Daniel WA, Paulshock BZ. A physician's guide to sexual maturity rating. Patient Care. 1979;30:122. Original illustration by Paul Singh-Roy.)

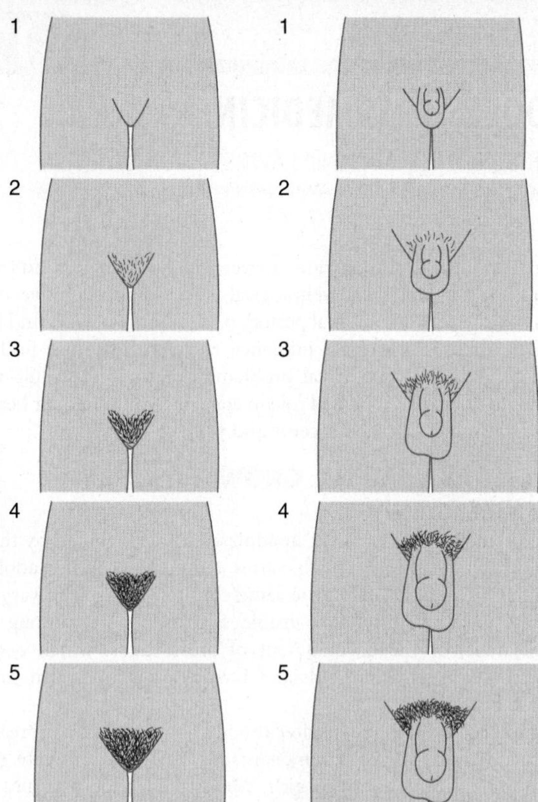

FIGURE 17-2. Female and male pubic hair development. *Sexual maturity rating 1 (SMR 1):* Prepubertal; no pubic hair. *SMR 2:* Small amount of scanty, long, slightly pigmented, along the base of the scrotum and phallus in the male and the medial border of the labia majora in females. *SMR 3:* Darker, coarser, starts to curl, small amount, extending laterally. *SMR 4:* Coarse, curly; resembles adult type but does not extend to the medial surface of the thighs. *SMR 5:* Abundant, adult-type pattern; hair extends onto the medial aspect of the thighs. ***Right,* Male genital development.** *SMR 1:* Penis preadolescent. Testicular volume <4 mL. *SMR 2:* Penis slight or no enlargement. Beginning enlargement of testes; testicular volume 4 to 8 mL; scrotal skin reddened, thinner. *SMR 3:* Penis increased in length. Testicular volume 10 to 15 mL. Further enlargement of scrotum. *SMR 4:* Penis larger in breadth, glans penis develops. Testes and scrotum nearly adult; testicular volume 12-20 mL. *SMR 5:* Penis adult size; testicular volume greater than 25 mL. (Redrawn from Daniel WA, Paulshock BZ. A physician's guide to sexual maturity rating. Patient Care. 1979;30:122. Original illustration by Paul Singh-Roy.)

(Chapter 186), germ cell tumors (Chapter 200), central nervous system tumors (Chapter 189), non-Hodgkin lymphoma (Chapter 185), thyroid cancer (Chapter 226), malignant melanoma (Chapter 203), and acute lymphoblastic leukemia (Chapter 183). HIV infection continues to be one of the 10 leading causes of death among people 15 to 24 years of age.

APPROACH TO THE ADOLESCENT PATIENT

When interviewing adolescent patients, the clinician should consider the adolescents' physical, cognitive, and psychosocial developmental stage; their growing autonomy and increasing role in taking responsibility for their own health and well-being; and their individual progression from childhood to adulthood. Chronologic age is not a guarantee that all adolescents will be at the same stage of physical, cognitive, and psychosocial development. The clinician should offer adolescent health care in a sensitive, flexible, and developmentally and culturally appropriate manner.

The clinician can meet with the adolescent alone at first to give the adolescent the message that she or he is the patient and the clinician is most eager to hear what the adolescent has to say. Conversely, the clinician can meet with the adolescent and her or his parents or guardians together for the initial part of the interview and then meet with the adolescent alone; this approach permits the clinician to develop an understanding of the reason for the visit from the perspective of the adolescent and his or her parents or guardians and to communicate that input from both the adolescent and the parents or guardians is highly valued. This approach also provides an opportunity for the clinician to observe the interaction between the adolescent and parents or guardians. The final approach to the interview is to greet the adolescent and family and request a meeting with the parents or guardians alone. This approach allows the parents or guardians to discuss concerns about the adolescent that they may not feel comfortable raising in the presence of the adolescent. Having this information may improve the focus of the visit. In this approach, the encounter with the parents or guardians is then followed by the clinician's meeting with the adolescent alone. With this interview structure, it is important that the adolescent be present from the time he or she meets with the clinician until the end of the visit, so that the adolescent does not perceive a breach of confidentiality.

TABLE 17-1 LEADING CAUSES OF DEATH IN U.S. ADOLESCENTS

CAUSE	PERCENTAGE OF DEATHS IN YOUTH AGED 15-24 YEARS
Unintentional injury	40.6
Suicide	15.8
Homicide	15.2
Malignant neoplasias	5.4
Diseases of the heart	3.2
Congenital anomalies	1.4
Cerebrovascular diseases	0.6
Pregnancy, childbirth, and the puerperium	0.6
All other causes	15.7

From Hoyert DL, Xu J. Deaths: preliminary data for 2011. National Vital Statistics Reports. Hyattsville, MD: National Center for Health Statistics; 2012.

Confidentiality

Issues of consent and confidentiality are central in the physician-adolescent interaction. Adolescents appreciate clinicians whom they trust and who can assure them of confidentiality. When guaranteed confidentiality, adolescents are more likely to seek necessary medical care, to disclose sensitive information, and to trust their clinician. Under these circumstances, most adolescents will involve their parents in their care. Parents appreciate education about the concept of confidentiality and recognize the importance of allowing the adolescent the opportunity to speak alone with the clinician. Confidentiality is also important for clinicians. To make an accurate diagnosis and to provide treatment, the clinician must obtain all relevant information from the adolescent. If the adolescent fears that such information will not be kept confidential, she or he may not provide all the necessary factual information.

Confidentiality and defining the limits of confidentiality should be discussed with the adolescent and his or her parents or guardians at the beginning of the interview. The adolescent and family need to know that the clinician will intervene if he or she believes that the adolescent's actions may cause him or her, or another person, significant harm. Examples of situations in which the clinician would not maintain confidentiality when dealing with young people include disclosure of current suicidal or homicidal intent.

Those who work with young people must have a clear understanding of consent and confidentiality and should make sure that adolescents are aware of confidentiality policies and practices. The duty of confidentiality does not preclude encouraging and empowering adolescents to talk to their parents or guardians about important health care issues and to include them in discussions of these issues. The legal definition of confidentiality varies, depending on geographic location, and clinicians should be familiar with the local laws.

Another goal of the interview is to build rapport with the adolescent and his or her parents or guardians. Clinicians can establish rapport with the adolescent at the start of the interview by creating an environment that is nonjudgmental, unintimidating, and supportive. The clinician's genuine interest in the adolescent is paramount. It is helpful to encourage the adolescent to talk about himself or herself—friends, hobbies, school. The clinician should listen carefully to the adolescent's statements and feelings. Sensitivity to and understanding of the adolescent's developmental stage and cultural background are important in interviewing an adolescent and interpreting answers accurately. The clinician should be respectful of the adolescent's growing need to be independent and desire to be treated as an individual person. Taking the time to build rapport is key to engaging the adolescent in a discussion of his or her personal health concerns with the clinician. It is the clinician's responsibility to familiarize himself or herself with the legal issues of confidentiality (as they relate to the adolescent patient and his or her parents or guardians) in his or her locality.

Preventive Health Care

Preventive health care for adolescents (Chapters 15 and 18) should promote physical and mental health and healthy physical, psychological, and social growth and development.[4] Positive behaviors such as exercise (Chapter 16) and nutritious eating (Chapter 213) should be encouraged, and health risk behaviors such as unsafe driving, use of tobacco (Chapter 32), unsafe sexual behaviors, and excess alcohol (Chapter 33) should be discouraged. Because lifelong health habits are established during adolescence, it is an important time to invest in health promotion and preventive services.

The U.S. Preventive Services Task Force recommends screening and counseling of all adolescents about depression and obesity and ensuring that all adolescents are up-to-date on their immunizations for tetanus, diphtheria, pertussis, varicella, measles, mumps, rubella, hepatitis B, meningococcus, polio, and human papillomavirus (HPV; Chapter 18). In addition, at-risk adolescents should be counseled about sexually transmitted diseases (e.g., HIV, chlamydia, gonorrhea, and syphilis) and advised about immunizations for influenza, pneumococcus, and hepatitis A.[5] Influenza immunization is recommended for all adolescents unless there is a vaccine shortage, in which case at-risk adolescents should be vaccinated first.

Components of the Adolescent Care Health Visit

History

Open-ended, nonjudgmental, developmentally appropriate, and gender-neutral questions help put the adolescent at ease and produce informative answers (Chapter 15). In addition to a standard medical history, the assessment should include a psychosocial history from the adolescent, either through a screening questionnaire or during the interview with the adolescent alone. The HEEADSSS assessment, which is a valuable screening tool for obtaining a comprehensive psychosocial history, covers the following topics:

- **H**ome: family members, living arrangements, and relationships
- **E**ducation/**E**mployment: academic or vocational success and future plans
- **E**ating: concerns about weight or body image or disordered eating attitudes and behaviors
- **A**ctivities: recreational activities, dating, and relationships
- **D**rugs: use of tobacco, alcohol, illicit drugs, anabolic steroids, and driving while intoxicated
- **S**exuality: sexual orientation, sexual activity, and sexual abuse
- **S**uicide (mental health): feelings of sadness, loneliness, depression; or suicidal ideation, attempts, and non-suicidal self-injury
- **S**afety: risk of unintentional injury or violence, fighting; or weapon carrying

Physical Examination

In general, the adolescent physical examination should occur without a parent or guardian present. In some situations, the adolescent is asked whether he or she would prefer to have a parent in the room during the physical examination. A male clinician should request that a female health care provider be present during the physical examination of a female patient, especially during the breast and genital examination. In theory, a female clinician should request a male health care provider be present during the genital examination of a male patient.

Care should be taken to ensure the adolescent's privacy. Providing an examination gown that covers the trunk and genital area is important. Talking with the adolescent during the examination also tends to increase comfort; explaining the procedures and commenting on the results are helpful. A comprehensive physical examination (Chapter 15) should include measuring the adolescent's weight and height, calculating his or her body mass index, plotting these measurements on standardized growth charts, and determining the adolescent's SMR.

The most recent American guidelines for cervical cancer screening recommend against screening women younger than 21 years.[6] These recommendations do not apply to young women with previously abnormal test results on cervical screening or to women who are immunosuppressed by HIV infection, organ transplantation, chemotherapy, or chronic use of corticosteroids. Indications for a pelvic examination in an adolescent include symptoms of vaginal or uterine infection, menstrual irregularities (e.g., amenorrhea, dysfunctional uterine bleeding, menorrhagia, and severe dysmenorrhea), undiagnosed abdominal or pelvic pain, tenderness, mass, trauma, sexual abuse, or assault. A careful history and a urine or patient-obtained specimen may be an alternative to the pelvic examination.

Conclusion of the Health Visit

At the conclusion of the adolescent health visit, the clinician should review the findings with the adolescent and talk about what happens next. The adolescent should have the opportunity to ask questions, get clarification, make comments, and respond to suggestions. The clinician should discuss with the adolescent what information will remain confidential. The clinician should then meet with the adolescent and the parents or guardians (if they have accompanied the adolescent to the health visit) to review the outcomes and to discuss the nonconfidential issues.

REPRODUCTIVE HEALTH

Reproductive health care includes issues of adolescent sexual development, adolescent sexual behaviors, adolescent pregnancy, and contraception. In the United States, nearly 50% of high-school boys and girls in grades 9 to 12 have had vaginal intercourse at least once. This number increases from 38% of boys and 28% of girls in grade 9 to about 63% of both boys and girls by their senior year. In addition, 3.4% of girls and 9% of boys in grades 9 to 12 started having sex before they were 13 years old, 15% of adolescents have had four or more sex partners during their lives, and 40% of sexually active high-school students did not use a condom when they last had sexual intercourse. About 60% of adolescent girls who are 13 years of age or younger when they first had sexual intercourse report having involuntary intercourse. Adolescents are more likely to report engaging in oral than in vaginal sex because they perceive oral sex as significantly less risky (fewer health, social, and emotional consequences) than vaginal sex, but adolescents who engage in oral sex also are more likely to engage in vaginal sex.[7]

Every year, about 750,000 pregnancies occur in girls 15 to 19 years of age in the United States. About 50% of these pregnancies result in a live birth, about 35% end with an abortion, and about 15% end with a miscarriage or stillbirth. During the past 20 years, teenage pregnancy rates in the United States have declined by 42%.[8] The birth rate for mothers 15 to 19 years of age decreased by about 50%, from about 62 per 100,000 to about 31 per 100,000.

Abortion rates also have decreased. Most of these decreases are because of increased use of effective contraception and decreased sexual activity. Adolescent pregnancy is more common among black and Hispanic girls as well as among girls from low-income families.

Positive outcomes of adolescent pregnancies are enhanced with good prenatal care, adequate initial and follow-up prenatal visits, nutritional counseling, assessment of psychosocial issues, and substance abuse counseling. Adolescents younger than 15 years are at increased risk for premature and low-birthweight infants; those older than 15 years who have adequate prenatal care do not have increased adverse outcomes.

Contraception

The most commonly used contraceptive methods in adolescents are oral contraceptive pills and condoms, although new hormonal delivery systems, such as transdermal patches, vaginal rings, and long-acting reversible contraceptives, are convenient and effective (Chapter 238). Long-acting reversible contraceptive methods (intrauterine devices and contraceptive implants) are increasingly popular in adolescents, who are at high risk of unintended pregnancy. Routine counseling about emergency contraception is an important part of the public health strategy to reduce teen pregnancy (Chapter 238).

Sexually Transmitted Diseases

Every year, about 4 million adolescents in the United States acquire a sexually transmitted disease (Chapter 285), representing 25% of the total cases of sexually transmitted disease diagnosed annually. *Chlamydia trachomatis,* which is the most commonly reported bacterial sexually transmitted disease, is reported annually in about 3.4% of female adolescents 15 to 19 years of age and 0.6% of male adolescents of the same age. The annual incidence of gonorrhea is about 0.6% for female adolescents 15 to 19 years of age and 0.25 % for adolescent males of the same age. In adolescents, HIV infection (Chapter 384) is contracted primarily as a sexually transmitted disease, and adolescents and young adults 15 to 24 years of age represent 14% of all new diagnoses of HIV infection in the United States. HPV (Chapter 373), which is the most prevalent of all sexually transmitted diseases in 15- to 24-year-olds, has a prevalence of about 20% in adolescent girls 14 to 17 years of age.

Adolescents are at greater risk of acquiring sexually transmitted diseases because they are more likely to engage in unprotected sexual intercourse with concurrent partners who have multiple other partners. Adolescent girls may have persistent vaginal columnar epithelium that is more susceptible than squamous epithelium to *Neisseria gonorrhoeae, C. trachomatis,* and HPV as well as lower levels of immunoglobulin A in their cervical mucus. Treatment may be delayed owing to an inability to access confidential health care services, lack of health care coverage, poverty, and drug trafficking and use.

Chlamydial infections (Chapter 318), often asymptomatic or minimally symptomatic in women, usually are manifested with a vaginal discharge in young adolescent girls. Otherwise, clinical presentations and treatments of sexually transmitted diseases (Chapter 285) in adolescents are similar to those in adults.

About 20% of adolescents given prescriptions for a sexually transmitted disease treatment fail to fill their prescriptions. Therefore, whenever it is available, an observed single-dose therapy is recommended.[9] In addition, expedited partner therapy, which is the treatment of sexual partners without requiring a prior clinical evaluation or prevention counseling, reduces the level of recurrent sexually transmitted diseases better than does standard management. Clinicians should consider the use of expedited partner therapy for partners exposed within 60 days to heterosexual males and females with chlamydia or gonorrhea infections when in-person evaluation and treatment are unlikely (Chapter 285).

ADOLESCENT OBESITY AND EATING DISORDERS

More than one third of children and adolescents are overweight or obese. Obese adolescents are significantly more likely to become severely obese in adulthood. Interventions should focus on changing behavior, increasing physical activity, and modifying the diet. Randomized trials also show that substituting sugar-free beverages for sugar-sweetened beverages can reduce short-term weight gain,[A2] but family-based behavioral treatment programs offer the best short- and long-term success for weight management.[A3] In extreme cases, pharmacotherapy and even bariatric surgery may be considered in the therapeutic plan (Chapter 220).

Eating disorders (Chapter 219) commonly begin during adolescence.[10] For adolescent-onset eating disorders, early recognition and aggressive treatment are critical to a successful outcome. The medical complications of eating disorders in adolescents include growth retardation, pubertal delay, low bone mineral density, and changes in brain structure and cognitive function. These complications, which occur early in the disease process, may not be completely reversible, thereby underscoring the need for early and aggressive treatment.

The goals of treatment are to restore physical health, normal eating behavior patterns, and mental health and to reduce the impact of the eating disorder on the quality of life. Adolescents should be treated at a facility where the health professionals understand eating disorders and have experience in treating adolescents. Successful management strategies for adolescents with eating disorders include early restoration of a normal nutritional and physiologic state, involvement of the family in the treatment, and incorporation of an interdisciplinary team in the treatment. Family-based therapy is an effective treatment for adolescents with eating disorders and helps protect against relapse.[A4]

SUBSTANCE ABUSE

Nearly half of adolescents try an illicit drug (Chapter 34) by the time they finish high school. About 75% of adolescents consume alcohol (Chapter 33) by the end of high school, and about half report having been drunk at least once in their life. Adolescents who begin using alcohol or drugs before 15 years of age are more than five times more likely to develop an addictive disorder later in life compared with those who first use alcohol at 21 years of age. About 45% of adolescents use marijuana, and 20% of 12th graders are current smokers.

Adolescents start using drugs or alcohol primarily because of social pressures but report continuing them to feel good or to cope with difficulties.[11] Boys tend to initiate drug and alcohol use at younger ages than girls do, but once girls begin to experiment, they are just as likely as boys to use drugs. Boys are more likely to consume marijuana, steroids, and smokeless tobacco, whereas girls are more likely to abuse amphetamines and methamphetamine.

Adolescents with poor self-esteem, low motivation, and poor academic achievement have a greater propensity for alcohol and drug abuse than those with positive self-esteem. Adolescents with a family member with a history of alcohol or other drug abuse are at greater risk. Adolescents are less likely to succumb to external pressures toward drug use if they have a strong sense of attachment to parents who clearly communicate their disapproval.

Signs and symptoms suggestive of substance abuse include changes in physical appearance, poor hygiene or dress, wearing long-sleeved shirts to hide scarring at injection sites, persistent cough or bronchitis, difficulty sleeping, sudden weight loss or weight gain, sudden changes in personality, aggressive behavior, irritability, nervousness, giddiness, changes in peer group, increased isolation from peers or family, depression, loss of interest in once favorite activities, decline in performance or attendance at school or work, forgetfulness, increased secretiveness, money or objects disappearing from the household, and prescription drugs that seem to be used up too quickly.

A validated screening tool for alcohol and substance abuse (Table 17-2) should be used in adolescents. Adolescents who answer yes to one of the six questions should receive advice on the adverse effects of substance abuse. Those who answer yes to two or more questions are at high risk and require further assessment or referral (Chapters 33 and 34). Urine drug testing has low sensitivity for detection of drug use, and there is no consensus about its role for screening of adolescents.

Alcohol and drug use contributes to more than 40% of adolescent deaths from motor vehicle crashes, to suicide attempts, and to an increased risk for subsequent use and its related problems in adulthood.

Historically, substance abuse treatment has been based on abstinence. More recently, a harm-reduction approach has gained acceptance. Adolescents discontinue drug and alcohol use mainly because of concern about their negative effects, and community-based interventions can be effective.[A5] To reduce alcohol abuse over time, individual interventions have a larger impact than family-based interventions.[A6]

CHRONIC ILLNESS AND TRANSITION

The prevalence of chronic diseases in adolescents has increased significantly because advances in medical technology and treatments have increased the survival of young people with childhood diseases formerly considered lethal.

TABLE 17-2 CRAFFT SCREENING TOOL FOR DRUG AND ALCOHOL USE IN ADOLESCENTS

The adolescent is instructed, "Please answer these next questions honestly. Your answers will be kept confidential. During the past 12 months, did you ..."
Drink any alcohol (more than a few sips)?
Smoke any marijuana or hashish?
Use anything else to get high?
If the adolescent answers no to the three opening questions, the provider only needs to ask the adolescent the first question—the CAR question. If the adolescent answers yes to any one or more of the three opening questions, the provider asks all six CRAFFT questions.
C—Have you ever ridden in a CAR driven by someone (including yourself) who was "high" or had been using alcohol or drugs?
R—Do you ever use alcohol or drugs to RELAX, feel better about yourself, or fit in?
A—Do you ever use alcohol/drugs while you are by yourself, ALONE?
F—Do you ever FORGET things you did while using alcohol or drugs?
F—Do your family or FRIENDS ever tell you that you should cut down on your drinking or drug use?
T—Have you gotten into TROUBLE while you were using alcohol or drugs?
CRAFFT is a mnemonic acronym of the first letters of key words in the six screening questions. The questions should be asked exactly as written.

About 18% of adolescents in the United States live with a chronic illness. Chronic illness may affect the adolescent's development, or the adolescent's development may affect the illness. For example, cystic fibrosis (Chapter 89) may delay puberty and hinder normal peer development. Puberty can exacerbate diabetes mellitus (Chapter 229). Increased risk-taking by adolescents with diabetes, asthma, or chronic renal failure can hinder their compliance with their medication regimen.

Adolescents in general, and those with special health care needs in particular, require a smooth, seamless, coordinated, and developmentally appropriate transition to the adult health care system. Barriers to a successful transition include a lack of adult physicians who can manage chronic childhood conditions (e.g., congenital heart disease; Chapter 69); patients, families, and pediatric subspecialists who are reluctant to terminate long-standing relationships; and patients and families who are poorly equipped to find their way in the adult health care system. As adolescents move closer to the age of transition, professionals should provide developmentally appropriate information and skills to support them and their families as they negotiate the adult health care system.

Adolescents benefit from an introductory visit with their adult-oriented care provider before leaving the pediatric health care system. This visit should give the adolescent a clearer idea about his or her new role as an adult patient, especially about expectations around decision making, giving consent, and the role of the family in his or her health care. The patient, family, and pediatric and adult health care systems should view the transition as a natural part of the developmental process of care for all adolescents.

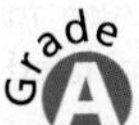

Grade A References

A1. Rossler R, Donath L, Verhagen E, et al. Exercise-based injury prevention in child and adolescent sport: a systematic review and meta-analysis. *Sports Med.* 2014;44:1733-1748.
A2. Ebbeling CB, Feldman HA, Chomitz VR, et al. A randomized trial of sugar-sweetened beverages and adolescent body weight. *N Engl J Med.* 2012;367:1407-1416.
A3. Sung-Chan P, Sung YW, Zhao X, et al. Family-based models for childhood-obesity intervention: a systematic review of randomized controlled trials. *Obes Rev.* 2013;14:265-278.
A4. Couturier J, Kimber M, Szatmari P. Efficacy of family-based treatment for adolescents with eating disorders: a systematic review and meta-analysis. *Int J Eat Disord.* 2013;46:3-11.
A5. Oesterle S, Hawkins JD, Fagan AA, et al. Testing the universality of the effects of the communities that care prevention system for preventing adolescent drug use and delinquency. *Prev Sci.* 2010;11:411-423.
A6. Tripodi SJ, Bender K, Litschge C, et al. Interventions for reducing adolescent alcohol abuse: a meta-analytic review. *Arch Pediatr Adolesc Med.* 2010;164:85-91.

GENERAL REFERENCES

For the General References and other additional features, please visit Expert Consult at https://expertconsult.inkling.com.

18

IMMUNIZATION

RAYMOND A. STRIKAS AND WALTER A. ORENSTEIN

Immunization is one of the most cost-effective means of preventing morbidity and mortality from infectious diseases. Routine immunization, particularly of children, has resulted in decreases of 90% or more in reported cases of measles, mumps, rubella, congenital rubella syndrome, poliomyelitis, tetanus, invasive *Haemophilus influenzae* type b, varicella, hepatitis A, and diphtheria. In many circumstances, immunization in children and adults not only prevents morbidity and mortality but also reduces health care costs in the long run.

GENERAL CHARACTERISTICS OF IMMUNIZATIONS

Immunization protects against disease or the sequelae of disease through the administration of an immunobiologic—a vaccine, toxoid, immune globulin preparation, or antitoxin. Protection induced by immunization can be active or passive.[1]

Active Immunization

Administration of a vaccine or toxoid causes the body to produce an immune response against the infectious agent or its toxins. Vaccines consist of suspensions of live (usually attenuated) or inactivated microorganisms or fractions thereof. Toxoids are modified bacterial toxins that retain immunogenic properties but lack toxicity. Active immunization generally results in long-term immunity, although the onset of protection may be delayed because it takes time for the body to respond. With live attenuated vaccines, small quantities of living organisms multiply within the recipient until an immune response cuts off replication. In most recipients, a single dose of a live vaccine generally induces a long-term immune response that closely parallels natural infection. In contrast, inactivated vaccines and toxoids contain large quantities of antigens. Killed (inactivated) vaccines often require multiple doses.

Passive Immunization

Passive immunization with use of immune globulins or antitoxins delivers preformed antibodies to provide temporary immunity. Immune globulins obtained from human blood may contain antibodies to a variety of agents, depending on the pool of human plasma from which they are prepared. Specific immune globulins are made from the plasma of donors with high levels of antibodies to specific antigens (such as tetanus immune globulin). Most immune globulins must be injected intramuscularly, although intravenous and subcutaneous preparations are also available. Antitoxins are solutions of antibodies derived from animals immunized with specific antigens (e.g., diphtheria antitoxin). Passive immunization usually is indicated to protect individuals immediately before anticipated exposure or shortly after known or suspected exposure to an infectious agent (Table 18-1), when active immunization either is not possible or has not been adequate.

Route and Timing of Vaccination

Each immunobiologic has a preferred site and route of administration. In adults, vaccines containing adjuvants should be injected intramuscularly, preferably in the deltoid muscle. For most adults, intramuscular injections should be administered with a 1- to 1½-inch, 22- to 25-gauge needle. Use of the buttocks is discouraged except when large volumes are required because of the potential for damage to the sciatic nerve and because of diminished immune response to some vaccines (such as hepatitis B), probably because vaccine is injected into fat rather than into muscle. Subcutaneous vaccines are usually administered in the triceps area. In general, inactivated vaccines and toxoids can be given at the same visit at different sites. Live and inactivated vaccines usually can be administered at the same time. For example, measles, mumps, and rubella (MMR) vaccine can be administered at the same time as inactivated poliovirus vaccine and live attenuated varicella vaccine. In general, injected and intranasally administered live vaccines not delivered on the same day should be separated by at least 4 weeks to avoid interference by the second vaccine of viral replication and immunity induced by the first vaccine. Orally administered live vaccines (such as oral typhoid vaccine) can be administered

TABLE 18-1 PASSIVE IMMUNIZATIONS FOR ADULTS

DISEASE	NAME OF MATERIAL	COMMENTS AND USE
Tetanus	Tetanus immune globulin, human	Management of tetanus-prone wounds in persons without adequate prior active immunization and treatment of tetanus
Cytomegalovirus	Cytomegalovirus immune globulin, intravenous	Prophylaxis for bone marrow and kidney transplant recipients
Diphtheria	Diphtheria antitoxin, equine	Treatment of established disease; high frequency of reactions to serum of nonhuman origin; in the United States, available only from CDC
Rabies	Rabies immune globulin, human	Postexposure prophylaxis of animal bites
Measles	Immune globulin, human	Prevention or modification of disease in exposed persons, not for control of outbreaks; particularly indicated for unvaccinated infants aged <12 months, pregnant women without evidence of measles immunity, and severely immunocompromised persons
Hepatitis A	Immune globulin, human	Pre-exposure and postexposure prophylaxis for travelers and others who need protection before immunity can be achieved with hepatitis A vaccine
Hepatitis B	Hepatitis B immune globulin, human	Prophylaxis for needle stick or mucous membrane contact with HBsAg-positive persons, for sexual partners with acute hepatitis B or carriers of hepatitis B, for infants born to mothers who are carriers of HBsAg, for infants whose mother or primary caregiver has acute hepatitis B
Varicella	Varicella-zoster immune globulin (VariZIG)	Persons with underlying disease and at risk for complications from chickenpox who have not had varicella or varicella vaccine and who are exposed to varicella; may be given up to 10 days after exposure to known susceptible adults, particularly if antibody negative; VariZIG is available under IND
Vaccinia	Vaccinia immune globulin	Treatment of eczema vaccinatum, vaccinia necrosum, and severe inadvertent inoculations such as ocular vaccinia after vaccinia (smallpox) vaccination; available only from CDC
Erythroblastosis fetalis	Rh immune globulin	Rh-negative women who give birth to Rh-positive infants or who abort
Hypogammaglobulinemia	Immune globulin, intravenous, subcutaneous	Maintenance therapy
Idiopathic thrombocytopenic purpura	Immune globulin, intravenous	Therapy for acute episodes
Botulism	Heptavalent A, B, C, D, E, F, E, G antitoxin, equine	Treatment of botulism; available through CDC
	Botulism immune globulin for infants	Treatment of botulism in infants
Snakebite	Antivenin, equine (North American coral snake antivenin)	Specific for North American coral snake, *Micrurus fulvius*
Crotalidae, polyvalent	Effective for viper and pit viper bites, including rattlesnakes, copperheads, moccasins	
Spider bite	Antivenin, equine	Specific for black widow spider, *Latrodectus mactans*, and other members of the genus
Scorpion	Fab fragments, equine	Specific for *Centruroides* genus scorpions

CDC = Centers for Disease Control and Prevention; HBsAg = hepatitis B surface antigen; IND = Investigational New Drug.

at any interval before or after live injected or intranasal vaccines. Immune globulin may interfere with the replication of injected live vaccine viruses; ideally, most live vaccines should be administered at least 2 weeks before or 3 to 11 months after immune globulin. Immune globulin does not interfere with the response to yellow fever vaccine and is not believed to interfere with orally or intranasally administered live virus vaccines.

Adverse Reactions

No vaccine is completely safe or completely effective. Adverse reactions fall into three general categories: local, systemic, and allergic. Local reactions are generally the most frequent but least severe. Systemic adverse reactions include fever, malaise, myalgias (muscle pain), headache, and loss of appetite. These symptoms, which are common and nonspecific, may occur in vaccinated persons because of the vaccine or because of something unrelated to the vaccine. Allergic reactions, which are the least frequent but most severe, may be caused by the vaccine antigen itself or by another component of the vaccine, such as the cell culture material, stabilizer, preservative, or antibiotic used to inhibit bacterial growth. Life-threatening allergic reactions occur at a rate of about one per million doses. The risk of an allergic reaction can be minimized by good screening before vaccination. All providers who administer vaccines must have an emergency protocol and supplies to treat anaphylaxis.

Antipyretics should not be administered routinely before or at the time of vaccination because they tend to reduce the immune response,[A1] but they can be used for the treatment of fever and local discomfort that might occur after vaccination. The egg protein contained in vaccines grown in chicken eggs (influenza and yellow fever vaccines) may cause reactions in persons severely allergic to eggs. In general, persons without anaphylactic-type allergies to eggs can be given these vaccines safely, but persons with anaphylactic reactions to eggs generally should not receive these vaccines except when it is absolutely necessary, and then only under established protocols by physicians who have expertise in such situations. Although measles and mumps vaccines are grown in chick embryo tissue culture, the risk of anaphylaxis even in persons with severe hypersensitivity to eggs is low, so they can be vaccinated without prior testing.

Suspected adverse events temporally related to vaccinations should be reported to the Vaccine Adverse Event Reporting System (at *www.vaers.hhs.gov*). The National Vaccine Injury Compensation Program was established in the 1980's to compensate individuals who experience certain health events after vaccination on a "no-fault" basis. No-fault means that persons filing claims are not required to prove negligence on the part of either the health care provider or manufacturer to receive compensation. The program covers all routinely recommended childhood vaccinations, although adults who receive a covered vaccine may also file a claim. Claims may be based on a Vaccine Injury Table (see *http://www.hrsa.gov/vaccinecompensation/vaccinetable.html*), which lists the adverse events associated with vaccines and is updated periodically.

General Considerations

The major group that makes comprehensive, detailed recommendations regarding immunization of adults is the Advisory Committee on Immunization Practices of the Centers for Disease Control and Prevention, which publishes its information in *Morbidity and Mortality Weekly Report* (also available at *http://www.cdc.gov/vaccines/schedules/hcp/adult.html*). Immunizations for adults depend on age, lifestyle, occupation, and medical conditions. Two adult immunization schedules are available, one based on age group (Fig. 18-1 and E-Table 18-1) and one based on underlying risk (Fig. 18-2 and Table 18-2).[1,2] All adults who have not received a primary series of diphtheria-tetanus-pertussis–containing vaccine as children should receive one dose of combined tetanus and diphtheria-pertussis vaccine (Tdap), followed by a second dose of tetanus and diphtheria toxoids (Td) 4 weeks later, a third Td dose 6 to 12 months later, and a Td booster every 10 years.[3] All adults (and especially health care personnel) who received a diphtheria-tetanus-pertussis (DTaP) vaccine series as children should have a one-time dose of Tdap, followed by Td every 10 years. Persons born in or after 1957 should have evidence of immunity to measles, mumps, and rubella (e.g., documentation of vaccination or presence of antibodies considered compatible with protection). Adults without evidence of immunity to varicella (documentation of age-appropriate vaccination with two doses of varicella vaccine; laboratory evidence of immunity or confirmation of disease; birth in the United States before 1980, except for health care personnel, pregnant women, or immunocompromised persons; or diagnosis or verification of a history of varicella or herpes zoster disease by a health care provider) should receive varicella vaccine.

Pneumococcal polysaccharide vaccine (PPSV23) is indicated for all adults 65 years and older and for younger adults with certain medical conditions that place them at high risk of complications (see Table 18-2). All adults aged 65 years and older and persons 19 years and older with immunocompromising conditions (including chronic renal failure and nephrotic syndrome), functional or anatomic asplenia, cerebrospinal fluid leaks, or cochlear implants should receive a single dose of pneumococcal conjugate vaccine, ideally before receiving pneumococcal polysaccharide vaccine. Adults 65 years and older should receive pneumococcal polysaccharide vaccine 6 to 12 months later. Adults with immunocompromising conditions should also receive a dose of PPSV23 at least 8 weeks later. Immunocompromised adults who already received PPSV23 should still receive pneumococcal conjugate vaccine 1 year or more after the PPSV23 dose; they should be revaccinated with PPSV23 once after pneumococcal conjugate vaccine when 5 years have passed since their first PPSV23 dose.

Influenza vaccination is recommended annually for all persons 6 months of age or older, including all health care personnel. Health care workers exposed to blood or blood products should receive hepatitis B vaccine. Health care workers should also be immune to measles, mumps, rubella, and varicella.

Text continued on page 73

Recommended Adult Immunization Schedule — United States–2014

Note: These recommendations *must* be read with the footnotes that follow containing number of doses, intervals between doses, and other important information.

Recommended adult immunization schedule, by vaccine and age group†

Vaccine ↓ Age Group →	19–21 years	22–26 years	27–49 years	50–59 years	60–64 years	≥65 years
Influenza †*	1 dose annually					
Tetanus, diphtheria, pertussis (Td/Tdap) †*	Substitute 1-time dose of Tdap for Td booster; then boost with Td every 10 yrs					
Varicella †*	2 doses					
Human papillomavirus (HPV) Female †*	3 doses					
Human papillomavirus (HPV) Male †*	3 doses	3 doses				
Zoster †					1 dose	
Measles, mumps, rubella (MMR) †*	1 or 2 doses					
Pneumococcal 13-valent conjugate (PCV13) †*	1 dose					
Pneumococcal polysaccharide (PPSV23) †	1 or 2 doses					1 dose
Meningococcal †*	1 or more doses					
Hepatitis A †*	2 doses					
Hepatitis B †*	3 doses					
Haemophilus influenzae type b (Hib) †*	1 or 3 doses					

For all persons in this category who meet the age requirements and who lack documentation of vaccination or have no evidence of previous infection; zoster vaccine recommended regardless of prior episode of zoster

Recommended if some other risk factor is present (e.g., on the basis of medical, occupational, lifestyle, or other indications)

No recommendation

*Covered by the Vaccine Injury Compensation Program

†See E-Table 18-1 for additional information.

Report all clinically significant postvaccination reactions to the Vaccine Adverse Event Reporting System (VAERS). Reporting forms and instructions on filing a VAERS report are available at http://www.vaers.hhs.gov or by telephone, 800-822-7967.

Information on how to file a Vaccine Injury Compensation Program claim is available at www.hrsa.gov/vaccinecompensation or by telephone, 800-338-2382. To file a claim for vaccine injury, contact the U.S. Court of Federal Claims, 717 Madison Place, N.W., Washington, D.C. 20005; telephone 202-357-6400.

Additional information about the vaccines in this schedule, extent of available data, and contraindications for vaccination are also available at http://www.cdc.gov/vaccines, or from the CDC-INFO Contact Center at 800-CDC-INFO (800-232-4636) in English or Spanish, 8:00 a.m. – 8:00 p.m. Eastern Time, Monday – Friday, excluding holidays.

Use of trade-names and commercial sources is for identification only and does not imply endorsement by the U.S. Department of Health and Human Services.

The recommendations in this schedule were approved by the Centers for Disease Control and Preventtion's (CDC) Advisory Committee on Immunization Practices (ACIP), the American Academy of Family Physicians (AAFP), the American College of Physicians (ACP), American College of Obstetricians and Gynecologist (ACOG) and American College of Nurse-Midwives (ACNM).

FIGURE 18-1. Recommended adult immunization schedule by vaccine and age group, United States, 2014. See E-Table 18-1 for footnotes. (Adapted from http://www.cdc.gov/vaccines/schedules/downloads/adult/adult-combined-schedule.pdf.)

Vaccines That Might Be Indicated for Adults Based on Medical and Other Indications†

Vaccine ↓ / Indication →	Pregnancy	Immuno-compromising conditions (excluding human immunodeficiency virus [HIV]) †	HIV infection CD4+ T lymphocyte count † < 200 cells/μL	HIV infection CD4+ T lymphocyte count † ≥ 200 cells/μL	Men who have sex with men (MSM)	Kidney failure, end-stage renal disease, receipt of hemodialysis	Heart disease, chronic lung disease, chronic alcoholism	Asplenia (including elective splenectomy and persistent complement component deficiencies) †	Chronic liver disease	Diabetes	Healthcare personnel
Influenza †*		1 dose IIV annually			1 dose IIV or LAIV annually			1 dose IIV annually			1 dose IIV or LAIV annually
Tetanus, diphtheria, pertussis (Td/Tdap) †*	1 dose Tdap each pregnancy				Substitute 1-time dose of Tdap for Td booster; then boost with Td every 10 yrs						
Varicella †*		Contraindicated						2 doses			
Human papillomavirus (HPV) Female †*		3 doses through age 26 yrs						3 doses through age 26 yrs			
Human papillomavirus (HPV) Male †*			3 doses through age 26 yrs					3 doses through age 21 yrs			
Zoster †		Contraindicated						1 dose			
Measles, mumps, rubella (MMR) †*		Contraindicated						1 or 2 doses			
Pneumococcal 13-valent conjugate (PCV13) †*						1 dose	1 dose				
Pneumococcal poly-saccharide (PPSV23) †						1 or 2 doses					
Meningococcal †*					1 or more doses						
Hepatitis A †*						2 doses					
Hepatitis B †*						3 doses					
Haemophilus influenzae type b (Hib) †*		post-HSCT recipients only				1 or 3 doses					

For all persons in this category who meet the age requirements and who lack documentation of vaccination or have no evidence of previous infection; zoster vaccine recommended regardless of prior episode of zoster

Recommended if some other risk factor is present (e.g., on the basis of medical, occupational, lifestyle, or other indications)

No recommendation

*Covered by the Vaccine Injury Compensation Program †For additional information please see http://www.cdc.gov/vaccines/schedules/downloads/adult/adult-schedule.pdf

These schedules indicate the recommended age groups and medical indications for which administration of currently licensed vaccines is commonly indicated for adults ages 19 years and older, as of Febuary 1, 2014. For all vaccines being recommended on the Adult Immunization Schedule: a vaccine series does not need to be restarted, regardless of the time that has elapsed between doses. Licensed combination vaccines may be used whenever any components of the combination are indicated and when the vaccine's other components are not contraindicated. For detailed recommendations on all vaccines, including those used primarily for travelers or that are issued during the year, consult the manufacturers' package inserts and the complete statements from the Advisory Committee on Immunization Practices (www.cdc.gov/vaccines/hcp/acip-recs/index.html). Use of trade names and commerical sources is for identification only and does not imply endorsement by the U.S. Department of Health and Human Services.

FIGURE 18-2. Recommended adult immunization schedule by vaccine and medical and other indications, United States, 2014. See E-Table 18-1 for footnotes. (Adapted from http://www.cdc.gov/vaccines/schedules/downloads/adult/adult-combined-schedule.pdf.)

TABLE 18-2 SELECTED IMMUNIZING AGENTS INDICATED FOR ADULTS*

DISEASE	IMMUNIZING AGENT	INDICATIONS	SCHEDULE	MAJOR CONTRAINDICATIONS AND PRECAUTIONS	COMMENTS
Anthrax	Anthrax vaccine, adsorbed, an inactivated vaccine	Pre-exposure prophylaxis of persons at high risk of exposure (e.g., military, certain laboratory workers) Consider with antibiotics for postexposure prophylaxis	0.5-mL dose IM at 0, 4, and 6 wk and boosters at 12 and 18 mo, then booster annually thereafter If used after exposure, three doses at 0, 2, and 4 wk with 60 days of antimicrobial therapy; antibiotics should be continued for 14 days after third dose	Severe allergic reaction to a vaccine component or after a prior dose Moderate or severe acute illness is a precaution to vaccination	Effectiveness against aerosol exposure inferred primarily from animal data Limited data on the benefits of postexposure use
Diphtheria	Tetanus and diphtheria toxoids combined	All adults	For incompletely immunized adults, three doses IM needed for primary series: two doses IM 4 wk apart, third dose 6-12 mo after second dose; one of these doses should be Tdap Booster every 10 yr No need to repeat if schedule is interrupted	History of neurologic reaction after a previous dose Severe allergic reaction to a vaccine component or after a prior dose	Tetanus and diphtheria toxoids combined with acellular pertussis vaccine (Tdap) preferred as one-time booster for all persons Moderate or severe acute illness is a precaution

TABLE 18-2 SELECTED IMMUNIZING AGENTS INDICATED FOR ADULTS—cont'd

DISEASE	IMMUNIZING AGENT	INDICATIONS	SCHEDULE	MAJOR CONTRAINDICATIONS AND PRECAUTIONS	COMMENTS
Hepatitis A	Inactivated hepatitis A vaccine	Travelers to highly or intermediately endemic countries Men who have sex with men Illegal drug users (injection and noninjection) Persons who work with hepatitis A virus–infected primates or who do research with the virus Persons with chronic liver disease Recipients of clotting factors	Two doses at least 6 mo apart for persons aged ≥1 yr	Severe allergic reaction to a vaccine component or after a prior dose Moderate or severe acute illness is a precaution to vaccination	Recommended for all children Should be considered for outbreak control
Hepatitis B	Inactivated hepatitis B virus subunit vaccine containing HBsAg	Adolescents Health care and public safety workers potentially exposed to blood Clients and staff of institutions for the developmentally disabled Hemodialysis patients Men who have sex with men Users of illicit injectable drugs Recipients of clotting factors Household and sexual contacts of HBV carriers Inmates of long-term correctional facilities Heterosexuals treated for sexually transmitted diseases or with multiple sexual partners Travelers with close contact for ≥6 mo with populations with high prevalence of HBV carriage Adults 19-59 yr with diabetes mellitus	Three doses IM at 0, 1, and 6 mo	Severe allergic reaction to a vaccine component or after a prior dose Moderate or severe acute illness is a precaution to vaccination	Pregnancy is not a contraindication. Health care workers who have contact with patients or blood, sexual contacts of persons with chronic HBV infection, hemodialysis patients, other immunosuppressed persons, and recipients of clotting factor concentrates should be tested 1-2 mo after vaccination to determine serologic response.
Human papillomavirus	Inactivated L1 capsid proteins of types 6, 11, 16, and 18 (quadrivalent) and types 16 and 18 (bivalent)	Females at 11-12 yr; catch-up vaccination of females through 26 yr Males 11-12 yr (quadrivalent vaccine only) and catch-up vaccination through 21 yr; consider catch-up through 26 yr to prevent anogenital and oropharyngeal cancers and genital warts	Three 0.5-mL doses IM at 0, 1 to 2, and 6 mo	Severe allergic reaction to a vaccine component or to a prior dose Vaccine is not recommended for pregnant women	The vaccine will not protect against existing infections. Because the types in the vaccine are not responsible for about 30% of infections associated with cervical cancer, screening for cancer should occur as for unvaccinated women.
Influenza	Inactivated virus vaccine	All persons ≥6 months of age, with greatest priority for those at higher risk for influenza complications (e.g., ≥65 yr old, persons with underlying medical conditions, pregnant women) or in contact with those at higher risk (e.g., health care workers, and persons with close contact with children <5 yr)	Annual vaccination; see annual ACIP recommendation	Severe allergic reaction to an influenza vaccine component (including eggs) or after a prior dose Recombinant vaccine (RIV) containing no egg protein may be given to persons 18-49 yr with severe egg allergies Moderate or severe acute illness is a precaution to vaccination GBS within 6 wk of prior dose of influenza vaccine	Optimum timing for vaccination is October. However, vaccination can occur throughout the influenza season, particularly for persons at high risk for complications and their contacts who were not vaccinated earlier. Only one dose of influenza vaccine per season is recommended for adults.

TABLE 18-2 SELECTED IMMUNIZING AGENTS INDICATED FOR ADULTS—cont'd

DISEASE	IMMUNIZING AGENT	INDICATIONS	SCHEDULE	MAJOR CONTRAINDICATIONS AND PRECAUTIONS	COMMENTS
Influenza (cont'd)	Live attenuated influenza virus	Persons 2 through 49 yr without underlying conditions that place them at high risk of complications from influenza	Annual vaccination; see annual ACIP statement Administered intranasally	Persons <2 yr or ≥50 yr Persons with underlying disorders that place them at high risk of influenza complications History of GBS within 6 wk of prior dose of influenza vaccine Pregnant women Hypersensitivity to eggs or components of vaccine	Can be used for household contacts and health care workers caring for patients without severe immunocompromise
Japanese encephalitis	Inactivated Japanese encephalitis virus vaccine	Travelers to Asia spending at least 1 mo in endemic areas during transmission season	Two 0.5-mL doses IM on days 0 and 28 for persons 18 yr and older	Pregnancy	
Measles	Live virus vaccine	All adults born after 1956 without history of live vaccine on or after first birthday or detectable measles antibody Persons born before 1957 generally can be considered immune	One dose sufficient for most adults; two doses at least 1 mo apart indicated for persons entering college or medical facility employment, traveling abroad, or at risk of measles during outbreaks	Altered immunity (e.g., leukemia, lymphoma, generalized malignant disease, congenital immunodeficiency, immunosuppressive therapy) Immune globulin or other blood products within prior 3-11 mo, depending on dose of immune globulin or blood product received Untreated tuberculosis Anaphylactic hypersensitivity to neomycin or gelatin Pregnancy Thrombocytopenia	Persons with anaphylactic allergies to eggs may be vaccinated (see text). Vaccine should be administered to persons with asymptomatic HIV infection and should be considered for patients except those with severe immunocompromise.
Meningococcal disease (two vaccines)	1. Meningococcal conjugate vaccines containing polysaccharide of serogroups A, C, W, and Y (age 2 mo–55 yr) 2. Polysaccharide vaccine containing tetravalent A, C, W, and Y (ages 56 yr and older, if never vaccinated and only one vaccination expected to be necessary)	All 11- to 18-yr-old persons and all persons with persistent complement component deficiencies or anatomic or functional asplenia Persons who will travel to areas with hyperendemic or epidemic diseases Certain laboratory workers May be useful during localized outbreaks	One dose with revaccination at age 16 yr of children who receive conjugate vaccine at 11-12 yr of age and every 5 yr for persons at high risk	Allergic reactions to a component of the vaccine, including diphtheria toxoid and latex	Conjugate vaccine is preferred to polysaccharide alone for persons aged 2 mo through 55 yr and for persons 56 yr and older previously vaccinated who continue to be at risk.
Mumps	Live virus vaccine	All adults born after 1956 without history of live vaccine on or after first birthday or detectable mumps antibody Persons born before 1957 generally can be considered immune	One dose sufficient for most adults Two doses at least 1 mo apart indicated for persons entering college or medical facility employment or traveling abroad	Altered immunity (e.g., leukemia, lymphoma, generalized malignant disease, congenital immunodeficiency, immunosuppressive therapy) Immune globulin or other blood products within prior 3-11 mo Anaphylactic hypersensitivity to neomycin or gelatin Pregnancy Thrombocytopenia if administered with measles vaccine	Although persons born after 1956 are generally immune, vaccine can be given to adults of all ages and may be particularly indicated for postpubertal males who are thought to be susceptible. Persons with anaphylactic allergies to eggs may be vaccinated.

TABLE 18-2 SELECTED IMMUNIZING AGENTS INDICATED FOR ADULTS—cont'd

DISEASE	IMMUNIZING AGENT	INDICATIONS	SCHEDULE	MAJOR CONTRAINDICATIONS AND PRECAUTIONS	COMMENTS
Pertussis	Adult preparation of pertussis antigens combined with tetanus and diphtheria toxoids (Tdap)	All 11- to 12-yr-olds Catch-up vaccination for all persons ≥13 yr	One dose Pregnant women: one dose during each pregnancy between 27 and 36 weeks of gestation	Severe allergic reaction to a vaccine component or after a prior dose Moderate or severe acute illness is a precaution to vaccination	Two preparations are available, one licensed for all persons ≥10 yr, one for 10- to 64-yr-olds.
Pneumococcal disease	23-Valent polysaccharide vaccine (PPSV23)	All adults with cardiovascular disease, pulmonary disease (including asthma), diabetes mellitus, alcoholism, cirrhosis, cerebrospinal fluid leaks, splenic dysfunction or anatomic asplenia, Hodgkin disease, lymphoma, multiple myeloma, chronic renal failure, nephrotic syndrome, immunosuppression, HIV infection, cigarette smokers 19 yr and older High-risk populations, such as certain Native Americans, and All adults ≥65 yr	One dose IM or SC; a second dose should be considered ≥5 yr later for adults at high risk of disease (e.g., asplenic patients) and those who lose antibody rapidly (e.g., nephrotic syndrome, renal failure, transplant recipients) Revaccinate adults who received a first dose when <65 yr who are now ≥65 yr and who received their vaccine at least 5 yr earlier	Severe allergic reaction to a vaccine component or after a prior dose Moderate or severe acute illness is a precaution to vaccination	
	Pneumococcal conjugate vaccine (PCV13)	One dose recommended for all adults age 65 years and older, for immunocompromised adults ≥19 yr, and those with functional/anatomic asplenia, cochlear implants, cerebrospinal fluid leaks	One dose if not previously vaccinated with PCV13) as an adult Give ≥1 year after PPSV23; or if PPSV23-naïve, if 65 years or older and not immunocompromised, give PPSV23 6-12 months after PCV13; if >19 yrs old and immunocompromised, give PPSV23 ≥8 wk after PCV13	Severe allergic reaction (e.g., anaphylaxis) to any component of PCV13 or any diphtheria toxoid-containing vaccine Moderate or severe acute illness is a precaution to vaccination	Although licensed for use in adults ≥50 yr, it is recommended only for adults ≥19 yr with the noted medical conditions.
Poliomyelitis	Inactivated poliovirus vaccine (IPV)	Certain adults who are at greater risk of exposure to wild poliovirus than the general population, including travelers to countries where poliomyelitis is epidemic or endemic or specific populations with disease caused by wild poliovirus	For unvaccinated adults, two doses IM or SC 4 wk apart and a third dose 6-12 mo after the second; if <4 wk available before protection is needed, a single dose of IPV For incompletely immunized adults, complete primary series of three doses of IPV or prior oral poliovirus vaccine (OPV); no need to restart interrupted series A single dose of IPV can be given to adults who previously received a primary series but now are at high risk, such as those traveling to an endemic area	On theoretical grounds, pregnant women should not receive IPV, but if immediate protection is needed, IPV can be used Severe allergic reaction to a vaccine component or after a prior dose Moderate or severe acute illness is a precaution to vaccination	
Rabies	Inactivated vaccine, HDCV or PCEC	High-risk persons, including animal handlers, selected laboratory and field workers, and persons traveling for ≥1 mo to areas with high risk of rabies	Pre-exposure prophylaxis: three doses of 1 mL IM on days 0, 7, and 21 or 28	History of severe hypersensitivity reaction	Further doses needed after exposure

TABLE 18-2 SELECTED IMMUNIZING AGENTS INDICATED FOR ADULTS—cont'd

DISEASE	IMMUNIZING AGENT	INDICATIONS	SCHEDULE	MAJOR CONTRAINDICATIONS AND PRECAUTIONS	COMMENTS
Rubella	Live virus vaccine	Adults, particularly women of childbearing age, who lack history of rubella vaccine and detectable rubella-specific antibodies in serum Males and females in institutions where rubella outbreaks may occur, such as hospitals, the military, and colleges Persons born before 1957, except women who can become pregnant, generally can be considered immune	One dose SC	Pregnancy, altered immunity (e.g., leukemia, lymphoma, generalized malignant disease, congenital immunodeficiency, immunosuppressive therapy) Immune globulin or other blood products within 3-11 mo before vaccination Anaphylactic hypersensitivity to neomycin Administration of blood products should not contraindicate postpartum vaccination Thrombocytopenia if administered with measles vaccine	Women should be counseled to avoid pregnancy for 1 mo after vaccination.
Smallpox	Live vaccinia virus	Persons working with orthopox viruses Members of public health and health care response teams	One dose intracutaneously with a bifurcated needle Boosters every 10 yr and perhaps every 3 yr for persons working with virulent orthopox viruses	History or presence of eczema or other acute, chronic, or exfoliative skin condition in patient or a close household or personal contact Immunosuppression or pregnancy in patient or a close household or personal contact History of heart disease Breast-feeding Age <1 yr Allergy to a vaccine component No contraindications if exposed to smallpox	Some complications of vaccination are treatable with vaccinia immune globulin. Vaccine is effective 3-4 days after exposure to variola and perhaps longer to prevent or to modify the illness. Serious adverse events are rare but significant, including eczema vaccinatum, progressive vaccinia, myopericarditis, autoinoculation, and encephalitis. Vaccinia is transmissible.
Tetanus	Tetanus and diphtheria toxoids combined	All adults	Three doses IM needed for primary series: two doses 4 wk apart, third dose 6-12 mo after second dose Booster every 10 yr; no need to repeat if schedule is interrupted	History of neurologic or severe allergic reaction after a prior dose	Special recommendations for wound treatment (see text) Persons with GBS within the first 6 wk after immunization, particularly adults who received a prior primary series, probably should not be revaccinated in most circumstances. Tetanus and diphtheria toxoids combined with acellular pertussis (Tdap) vaccine preferred for booster at age 11-12 yr One-time booster of Tdap for all adults
Typhoid fever	Vi capsular polysaccharide vaccine Live attenuated Ty21a oral vaccine	Travelers to areas where the risk of prolonged exposure to contaminated food and water is high May be considered for family and intimate contacts of carriers and laboratory workers who work with *Salmonella typhi*	Vi polysaccharide vaccine: one dose IM 0.5 mL; boosters every 2 yr Oral vaccine: four doses on alternate days; repeat series every 5 yr if risk continues	Severe local or systemic reaction to a prior dose Ty21a vaccine should not be administered to persons with altered immunity or those receiving antimicrobial agents	Efficacy only 50-77% Food and water precautions essential

TABLE 18-2 SELECTED IMMUNIZING AGENTS INDICATED FOR ADULTS—cont'd

DISEASE	IMMUNIZING AGENT	INDICATIONS	SCHEDULE	MAJOR CONTRAINDICATIONS AND PRECAUTIONS	COMMENTS
Varicella: chickenpox strain	Attenuated Oka strain of varicella virus	All persons without evidence of varicella immunity, especially health care personnel, childbearing-age women, and persons with household or other contact with persons at high risk of complications of varicella (e.g., susceptible immunosuppressed persons)	Two 0.5-mL doses SC 4-8 wk apart for persons ≥13 yr A second dose is recommended for all persons who previously received one dose	Immunocompromise Pregnancy Allergy to vaccine components	Adults with a history of prior clinician-diagnosed or verified varicella can be considered immune. Vaccine virus has rarely been transmitted to contacts from healthy vaccinees in whom rash developed. Women who receive vaccine should not become pregnant for 1 mo.
Varicella: zoster	Attenuated Oka strain of varicella virus, approximately 14 times more potent than varicella vaccine	Persons ≥60 years of age	One 0.65-mL dose SC	Immunocompromise Pregnancy Allergy to vaccine components	May be administered regardless of a prior history of shingles
Yellow fever	Live attenuated virus (17D strain)	Persons living or traveling in areas where yellow fever exists	One dose; booster every 10 yr	Immunocompromised persons History of anaphylactic allergies to eggs Pregnancy on theoretical grounds, although may be given if risk is high	Fever, jaundice, and multiple-organ system failure (viscerotropic disease) have been rarely reported in first-time recipients of 17D-derived yellow fever vaccinations. Vaccinate only persons traveling to areas endemic to yellow fever.

*See the text and package inserts for further details, particularly regarding indications, dosage, administration, side effects, and adverse reactions and contraindications.
ACIP = Advisory Committee on Immunization Practices; GBS = Guillain-Barré syndrome; HBsAg = hepatitis B surface antigen; HBV = hepatitis B virus; HDCV = human diploid cell vaccine for rabies; HIV = human immunodeficiency virus; IM = intramuscularly; IPV = inactivated poliovirus vaccine; MMR = measles, mumps, and rubella vaccine; OPV = live trivalent oral poliovirus vaccine; PCEC = purified chick embryo cell culture rabies vaccine; SC = subcutaneously.

Immunocompromised Persons

Patients with conditions that compromise their immune systems—immunodeficiency diseases, leukemia, lymphoma, and generalized malignant disease, and those who are immunosuppressed from therapy with corticosteroids, alkylating agents, antimetabolites, and radiation—generally should not receive live attenuated vaccines. An exception is infection with human immunodeficiency virus (HIV). Two doses of MMR vaccine are recommended for all persons aged 12 months and older who have HIV infection and do not have evidence of immunity to measles, rubella, and mumps and who are not severely immunosuppressed (i.e., a CD4 percentage ≥15% and $CD4^+$ lymphocyte counts ≥200 cells/μL for ≥6 months for persons aged >5 years). Varicella vaccination (two doses, 3 months apart) may be considered in HIV-infected persons with $CD4^+$ T-lymphocyte counts above 200 cells/μL. Patients with leukemia in remission who have not been receiving any chemotherapy for at least 3 months may receive live virus vaccines. Short-course therapy (<2 weeks) with corticosteroids, alternate-day regimens with low to moderate doses of short-acting corticosteroids, and topical applications or tendon injections are not ordinarily contraindications to the administration of live vaccines.

Immunocompromised patients can receive inactivated vaccines and toxoids, although the efficacy of such preparations may be diminished. Patients with known HIV infection should receive pneumococcal vaccine and annual influenza vaccination.

Pregnancy

In general, live vaccines should not be given to pregnant women because of the theoretical concern that the vaccines could adversely affect the fetus. No significant adverse events have been documented as attributable to vaccination of pregnant women with rubella-containing or varicella vaccines; nevertheless, pregnant women should not receive MMR or varicella vaccine, and women who do receive these vaccines should wait 1 month before becoming pregnant. Poliomyelitis and yellow fever vaccines usually should not be given to pregnant women unless the risk of disease is substantial. Tdap vaccination is indicated for pregnant women during each pregnancy, preferably between 27 and 36 weeks of gestation, to prevent pertussis in their infants and themselves. The safety of hepatitis A vaccination during pregnancy has not been determined, so the risk should be weighed against the benefit. All pregnant women should be screened for hepatitis B surface antigen (HBsAg). If HBsAg is positive, their children should receive hepatitis B vaccine and hepatitis B immune globulin within 12 hours of birth. All women who are or will be pregnant during the influenza season should receive inactivated influenza vaccine to protect themselves and their babies.

INDIVIDUAL IMMUNOBIOLOGICS

Hepatitis A

Two inactivated hepatitis A (Chapter 148) vaccines are available in the United States. Seroconversion rates after a single dose of either vaccine in persons older than 1 year exceed 95%, and protection is expected to persist for at least 25 years.

Indications

For adults, the vaccine is indicated primarily for persons traveling to countries (generally those in the developing world) with high or intermediate endemicity for hepatitis A, but it is also recommended for other groups at high risk for infection or for development of severe hepatitis. In addition, vaccine is routinely recommended for children 12 to 23 months of age. Vaccination also is recommended for persons aged 1 to 40 years for postexposure prophylaxis after close contact with an infected person or exposure to a contaminated food or water source. Health care workers have not been shown to be at higher risk than the general population for hepatitis A and do not need routine immunization. Although food handlers are not at increased risk for hepatitis A compared with the general population, the consequences of infection or suspected infection in this group, which can lead to extensive public health investigations, may make vaccination cost-effective in some settings. Doses vary by age and product. All schedules call for a second dose at least 6 months after the first dose.

Adverse Events

The most common adverse reaction after hepatitis A vaccination is tenderness and soreness at the injection site. Although rare and more serious adverse events have been reported in temporal association with vaccination, no causal relationships have been established.

Hepatitis B

Hepatitis B (Chapter 148) vaccine was the first vaccine known to prevent cancer. It also can prevent acute and chronic complications of hepatitis B, including an estimated 1800 deaths annually in the United States from liver cancer, cirrhosis, and fulminant hepatic disease. Currently produced vaccines are derived from insertion of the gene for HBsAg into *Saccharomyces cerevisiae.* When it is administered in a three-dose series, hepatitis B vaccine produces adequate antibody responses (anti-HBs ≥ 10 IU/L) in more than 90% of healthy adults younger than 40 years and in more than 95% of normal infants, children, and adolescents. By age 60 years, protective levels of antibody develop in only 75% of vaccinated persons. The duration of vaccine-conferred immunity is not known, although follow-up of vaccinees for more than 20 years indicates persistence of protection against clinically significant infections (i.e., detectable viremia and clinical disease). Booster doses are not currently recommended. Vaccine must be injected intramuscularly in the deltoid.

Indications

Hepatitis B vaccine is indicated for adults at increased risk of infection (see Fig. 18-1 and E-Table 18-1), including all persons 19 through 59 years of age with diabetes. Vaccination may be offered at the physician's discretion to persons 60 years of age or older with diabetes. Universal screening for HBsAg is recommended for all pregnant women; three doses of vaccine and one dose of hepatitis B immune globulin are recommended for infants of acutely or chronically infected mothers.

Adverse Events

The major adverse reaction is soreness at the injection site. Rare instances of Guillain-Barré syndrome, leukoencephalitis, optic neuritis, transverse myelitis, rheumatoid arthritis, type 1 diabetes, and autoimmune disease have been reported, but causal associations have not been confirmed with any systemic immune complications.

Human Papillomavirus

Two licensed human papillomavirus (HPV) vaccines contain the L1 capsid protein of types 16 and 18, which account for about 70% of cases of cervical cancer. The quadrivalent vaccine (HPV4), which also contains the L1 capsid protein of types 6 and 11 that are the most common causes of anogenital warts, is the only HPV vaccine licensed for boys and men.[4] Routine vaccination of 11- to 12-year-old girls and boys is recommended in a three-dose schedule at 0, 1 to 2, and 6 months. Catch-up vaccination should be undertaken for females through 26 years of age, all males through 21 years of age, and immunocompromised males and men who have sex with men through age 26 years. Catch-up vaccination may also be considered for other men 22 to 26 years of age. Women with a prior abnormal Papanicolaou smear and persons with genital warts should be vaccinated to prevent persistent infection with types of HPV they may not yet have acquired.

Adverse Events

The most commonly reported local symptoms are injection site pain, redness, and swelling. The most common generalized symptoms are dizziness, syncope, nausea, vomiting, fatigue, headache, fever, and urticaria. Anaphylaxis is very rare.

Influenza

Influenza vaccines for seasonal influenza include intramuscular and intradermal inactivated influenza vaccine, which may contain three or four influenza split or subvirion virus types—A(H3N2), A(H1N1), and one or two B strains—and intranasal live attenuated influenza vaccine. Live attenuated vaccine, which consists of four cold-adapted, temperature-sensitive attenuated viruses, one for each of the expected circulating strains, uses viruses that have been reassorted with circulating strains to contain six internal genes from the parent virus and genes for the surface hemagglutinin and neuraminidase of an A(H3N2), A(H1N1), and two B strains.

A recombinant inactivated influenza vaccine contains no egg protein and may be given to persons 18 to 49 years of age who experience hives after eating eggs; the alternative is to give the standard, egg-derived, inactivated vaccine followed by 30 minutes of observation. Persons with more severe symptoms after eating eggs may either receive the recombinant vaccine or be referred to a physician with expertise in management of allergic conditions.

Indications

Annual influenza (Chapter 364) vaccination is indicated for everyone 6 months of age and older, but especially persons at high risk of complications from the disease: all children aged 6 through 59 months; all persons aged 50 years and older; adults and children who have chronic pulmonary, cardiovascular, renal, hepatic, neurologic, hematologic, or metabolic disorders; persons who are immunosuppressed; women who are or will be pregnant during the influenza season; children and adolescents who are receiving long-term aspirin therapy and who might be at risk for experiencing Reye syndrome after influenza virus infection; residents of long-term care facilities; American Indians/Alaska Natives; and persons who are morbidly obese. To reduce transmission of influenza to high-risk patients, health care personnel[5] and household contacts of high-risk patients, including contacts of children younger than 5 years, also should be vaccinated annually.

The efficacy of inactivated influenza vaccine varies with the host's condition and the degree to which antigens in the vaccine match viruses that circulate during the following season. Provided the match is good, the vaccine's efficacy is usually 50% to 70% for healthy adults younger than 65 years. Effectiveness varies but averages about 60% in preventing laboratory-confirmed outpatient illness in persons 50 years and older but is only about 35% in the institutionalized elderly.[6] Live attenuated vaccine is licensed only for nonpregnant persons aged 2 through 49 years without underlying conditions that place them at high risk of complications from influenza. It also can be used for appropriately aged contacts of high-risk patients but is not recommended for contacts of severely immunosuppressed patients, such as patients with bone marrow transplants. Live attenuated vaccine is more than 85% effective in young children. In healthy adults, live attenuated vaccine and inactivated influenza vaccine are similarly effective.

Influenza vaccination also reduces cardiovascular events.[A2] Vaccination efforts should begin as soon as the vaccine becomes available, usually by October, and should continue throughout the season. Peak influenza activity usually recurs in January or February, and influenza season continues through March.

Adverse Events

The most common side effect of inactivated vaccine is soreness at the injection site. Fever, malaise, and myalgia may begin 6 to 12 hours after vaccination and persist for 1 or 2 days, although such reactions are most common in children exposed to vaccine for the first time. The most common adverse events after live attenuated influenza vaccine in adults are runny nose, headache, and sore throat. Severe allergic reactions are rare, including Guillain-Barré syndrome in about one case per 1 million doses.

Measles

Indications

Measles (Chapter 367) immunization is recommended for all persons born in or after 1957 without laboratory evidence of immunity, laboratory confirmation of prior disease, or prior appropriate vaccination. Children should routinely receive two doses of MMR vaccine—one at 12 to 15 months of age and one at 4 to 6 years of age. Most adults are considered to have been appropriately vaccinated if they received one dose of vaccine on or after their first birthday. However, adults who are at increased risk of exposure to measles or transmission of it (e.g., health care workers, college students, international travelers) should receive a second dose if they did not get a second dose as children, unless they have serologically documented immunity, have laboratory confirmation of disease, or were born before 1957. Persons embarking on foreign travel should have received two doses of MMR vaccine or have other evidence of measles immunity as defined before. Persons born before 1957 are usually immune as a result of natural infection and do not require vaccination, although vaccination is not contraindicated if they are believed to be susceptible.

During institutional outbreaks of measles, all persons who have not received two doses or who lack other evidence of measles immunity should be vaccinated. Although measles vaccine can be administered only with mumps and rubella as MMR, individuals already immune to one or more of the components may receive MMR without harm.

Measles vaccine is contraindicated for pregnant women on theoretical grounds, for persons with moderate to severe acute febrile illnesses, and for persons with altered immunocompetence, except those with HIV infection who are not severely immunocompromised. Patients with anaphylactic reactions to eggs can be vaccinated without prior skin testing.

Adverse Events

MMR vaccine can cause fever (<15%), rash (5%), transient lymphadenopathy (20% of adults), or parotitis (<1%). Febrile reactions, which usually are otherwise asymptomatic, generally occur 7 to 12 days after vaccination and persist for 1 or 2 days. MMR vaccination can rarely cause anaphylaxis, febrile seizures in children, thrombocytopenic purpura, transient arthralgia, and measles inclusion body encephalitis in persons with demonstrated immunodeficiencies.

Meningococcal Vaccines

Three quadrivalent meningococcal vaccines are available against disease caused by serogroups A, C, Y, and W135: meningococcal polysaccharide vaccine (MPSV4), which consists of 50 μg of polysaccharide of each of the four serogroups and is licensed for persons 2 years of age and older, and two meningococcal conjugate vaccines (MenACWY). A fourth vaccine, Hib-MenCY-TT, including *H. influenzae* type b plus meningococcal serotypes C and Y, was licensed in 2012 only for children ages 6 weeks through 18 months.

One conjugate vaccine consists of 4 μg of each polysaccharide covalently linked to 48 μg of diphtheria toxoid and licensed for persons 9 months to 55 years of age. The other conjugate vaccine consists of polysaccharide linked to CRM_{197} and is licensed for persons 2 months to 55 years of age. The four serogroups in each vaccine account for approximately two thirds of meningococcal disease in the United States and about 75% of the disease in persons 11 years of age or older (Chapter 298). Serogroup A and C polysaccharide vaccines are 85 to 100% efficacious in epidemic settings; vaccination with Y and W polysaccharides induces bactericidal antibodies and is presumed to be efficacious. In contrast to polysaccharide vaccines, conjugate vaccines induce immunologic memory, result in higher and more durable levels of high-avidity antibodies, and induce herd immunity. The duration of immunity for both MPSV4 and MenACWY is estimated at between 3 and 5 years.

Indications

Routine vaccination with MenACWY is recommended for all adolescents at 11 through 18 years of age, with a first dose administered at age 11 or 12 years and revaccination at age 16 years, or a first dose between 13 and 15 years and revaccination at age 16 to 18 years. Meningococcal vaccination once is also recommended for college freshmen who have not previously been vaccinated and will live in dormitories, military recruits, persons at risk during a community outbreak attributable to a vaccine serogroup, and persons who travel to or live in areas with hyperendemic or epidemic disease (e.g., the "meningitis belt" of sub-Saharan Africa, stretching from Mauritania to Ethiopia). For some persons at very high risk of meningococcal disease (e.g., microbiologists with frequent exposure to *Neisseria meningitidis* in culture and persons with persistent complement component deficiencies, splenic dysfunction, or asplenia), revaccination is recommended every 5 years.

MenACWY can be used for persons 2 months to 10 years of age with high-risk conditions but is not recommended routinely for this age group. For persons older than 55 years with an indication for vaccine, a single dose of MPSV4 is preferred. For persons now aged 56 years and older who were vaccinated previously with MenACWY and are recommended for revaccination or for whom multiple doses are anticipated (e.g., persons with asplenia and microbiologists), MenACWY is preferred.

Adverse Events

The major adverse reactions to MPSV4 are local reactions and systemic symptoms, such as headache and malaise, which generally persist for 1 or 2 days. The incidence of local reactions and low-grade fever is slightly higher after MenACWY than after MPSV4. An excess risk of Guillain-Barré syndrome was initially reported after MenACWY vaccines but has not been confirmed in subsequent studies.

Mumps

Indications

Mumps (Chapter 369) vaccine is indicated for all persons without evidence of immunity. For most adults, such evidence consists of a prior history of vaccination on or after the first birthday, laboratory evidence of immunity, or laboratory confirmation of disease. For adults at high risk, including health care workers, international travelers, and students at post-high school educational institutions, two doses of mumps vaccine constitute acceptable evidence of immunity. Most persons born before 1957 can be considered immune as a result of natural infection, although vaccination is not contraindicated if such persons are thought to be susceptible.

Adverse Events

Adverse events after the vaccine strain used in the United States are uncommon but include fever, parotitis, and allergic manifestations. Thrombocytopenic purpura has been reported rarely after MMR. Mumps vaccine is contraindicated for pregnant women on theoretical grounds, for persons with moderate to severe acute febrile illnesses, and for persons with altered immunocompetence. When it is combined with measles vaccine, it may be given to persons with asymptomatic HIV infection and considered for persons with symptomatic infection if they are not severely immunocompromised. Patients with anaphylactic reactions to eggs can be vaccinated without skin testing.

Pertussis Vaccine

Each of the two vaccines licensed for boosting immunity to pertussis in adults is combined with tetanus and diphtheria toxoids, and they have a lower content of pertussis antigens compared with the childhood pertussis-containing vaccines (Tdap). Boostrix (GlaxoSmithKline), which is licensed for adolescents and adults 10 years of age and older, contains three pertussis antigens—toxoid (PT), filamentous hemagglutinin (FHA), and pertactin (PRN). Adacel (Sanofi Pasteur), which is licensed for 10- through 64-year-olds, contains five pertussis antigens: PT, FHA, PRN, and two fimbriae. Both vaccines, when they are administered to previously vaccinated adolescents and adults, induce serologic responses that are comparable to those induced with effective childhood vaccination.

Indications

A single dose of Tdap is indicated for all adolescents at 11 to 12 years of age. Older adolescents and adults who have not received Tdap should get it instead of their next scheduled Td booster. Tdap can be given at any interval after a prior Td.[A3] All pregnant women should receive one dose of Tdap vaccine during each pregnancy, optimally between 27 and 36 weeks of gestation to maximize maternal antibody response and passive antibody transfer to the infant. If they have not been vaccinated during pregnancy, women should receive Tdap post partum if they have never previously been vaccinated with it. With the exception of pregnant women, booster doses of Tdap are not recommended.

Adverse Events

Adverse events, usually local reactions, are similar with the adult preparation of tetanus and diphtheria toxoids (Td) alone (see tetanus and diphtheria section later).

Pneumococcal Vaccines

Two pneumococcal vaccines are available for adults. Pneumococcal polysaccharide vaccine (PPSV23) consists of purified polysaccharide capsular antigens from the 23 types of *Streptococcus pneumoniae* that are responsible for 85 to 90% of the bacteremic disease in the United States (Chapter 289). Most adults, including elderly patients and those with alcoholic cirrhosis and diabetes mellitus, have a two-fold or greater rise in type-specific antibodies within 2 to 3 weeks of vaccination. Vaccination is approximately 60% effective against invasive pneumococcal disease, but its efficacy against pneumonia in high-risk populations, such as patients with alcoholic cirrhosis or Hodgkin disease, is not clear.[A4]

Pneumococcal conjugate vaccine (PCV13), licensed in 2011 for adults aged 50 years and older, should be administered once to eligible adults because it is expected to add protection to that offered by PPSV23. Ideally, PCV13 should precede PPSV23 by at least 8 weeks in immunocompromised persons over age 19 years and by at least 6 months in persons who are age 65 years or older and are not immunocompromised; if PPSV23 is administered first, an interval of 1 year should elapse before PCV13 is administered.

Indications

The preponderance of information supports the use of pneumococcal vaccines in high-risk populations, including all persons 65 years and older, persons 19 years or older who smoke cigarettes, and patients with asthma. Special efforts should target hospitalized patients. Approximately two thirds of patients who are admitted later with pneumococcal disease had been hospitalized for other reasons within the preceding 5 years. The newer PCV13 vaccine is recommended for all adults over age 65 years and for adults 19 years of age and older with immunocompromising conditions, functional or anatomic asplenia, cerebrospinal fluid leaks, or cochlear implants.

Because immunity may decrease 5 years or more after initial vaccination with PPSV23, a single booster dose of PPSV23 should be considered at that time for adults at highest risk of disease (such as asplenic patients) and for adults who lose antibody rapidly (such as patients with nephrotic syndrome or renal failure). Persons 65 years or older who received a dose more than 5 years earlier when they were younger than 65 years also should be revaccinated.

Adverse Events

Local reactions to PPSV23 are frequent, but less than 1% of vaccinees experience severe local reactions or systemic symptoms such as fever and malaise. Severe events, such as anaphylaxis or Arthus-like reactions at the site of injection, are rare. Because of the rarity of severe reactions in revaccinated patients, persons with indications for vaccination but with unknown histories of prior vaccination should be vaccinated. PCV13 reactions include pain, redness, and swelling at the injection site; limitation of movement of the injected arm; fatigue; and headache.

Poliomyelitis

Since 2000, inactivated poliovirus vaccine (IPV) has replaced the live attenuated oral poliovirus vaccine (OPV) in the United States because OPV vaccine caused about eight polio cases per year in the United States among recipients or their contacts (Chapter 379). OPV is still the vaccine used in most countries around the world.

Indications

Routine vaccination of persons 18 years of age or older is not recommended. If adults who are unvaccinated, are incompletely vaccinated, or have unknown vaccination status travel to areas where wild poliovirus is endemic or epidemic, they should receive a series of three doses: two doses of IPV administered at an interval of 4 to 8 weeks, with a third dose adminitered 6 to 12 months after the second. If three doses of IPV cannot be administered, alternatives include the following: three doses of IPV administered 4 weeks or more apart; if less than 8 weeks remain before protection is needed, two doses of IPV administered 4 weeks or more apart; and if less than 4 weeks remain before protection is needed, a single dose of IPV. If fewer than three doses are administered, the remaining doses needed to complete a three-dose series should be administered when feasible, at the intervals recommended, especially if the person remains at increased risk for poliovirus exposure.

As a precaution, adults (≥18 years of age) who are traveling to areas where poliomyelitis cases are occurring and who have received a routine series with either IPV or OPV in childhood should receive another dose of IPV before departure.[7] For adults, available data do not indicate the need for more than a single lifetime booster dose with IPV.

Adverse Events

Minor local reactions (pain, redness) commonly occur after IPV. Because IPV contains trace amounts of streptomycin, polymyxin B, and neomycin, allergic reactions may occur in persons allergic to these antibiotics.

Rabies

Two inactivated rabies vaccines are licensed in the United States.[8] Human diploid cell vaccine (HDCV), which is prepared from the Pitman-Moore strain of rabies virus, also contains small amounts of neomycin sulfate, albumin, and phenol red indicator. The purified chick embryo cell vaccine (PCECV), which is prepared from the Flury LEP rabies virus strain, also contains small amounts of polygeline, human serum albumin, potassium glutamate, and sodium EDTA. Both vaccines are given intramuscularly.

Indications

Rabies (Chapter 414) vaccine is indicated for pre-exposure prophylaxis of high-risk persons, including animal handlers, selected laboratory and field workers, and persons traveling for more than 1 month to areas where rabies is a constant threat. For both rabies vaccines, the pre-exposure regimen consists of three 1-mL intramuscular injections on days 0, 7, and 21 or 28. Post-exposure treatment depends on prior exposure to vaccine (Chapter 414). Persons being treated for the first time should be given human rabies immune globulin as well as four doses of vaccine at days 0, 3, 7, and 14.

Adverse Events

Local reactions (e.g., pain at the injection site, redness, swelling, and induration) are common after both rabies vaccine preparations. Hypersensitivity reactions can occur after booster doses.

Rubella

Indications

One dose of rubella vaccine (Chapter 368) is indicated for adults born in 1957 or later without evidence of immunity and for women of any age who lack evidence of immunity and who are considering becoming pregnant. Persons without a prior history of vaccination on or after the first birthday, laboratory evidence of immunity, or laboratory confirmation of disease should be considered as lacking evidence of immunity. A single dose of vaccine is 95% or more effective. Many persons receive two doses of rubella vaccine by the two-dose schedule of MMR.

Adverse Events

Follow-up of pregnant women who had no evidence of immunity and who received rubella vaccines within 3 months of the estimated date of conception show no evidence of defects compatible with congenital rubella syndrome in their offspring. Nevertheless, vaccine is contraindicated in pregnant women on theoretical grounds, and conception should be delayed for 1 month after rubella vaccination.

Arthralgia develops among about 25% of nonimmune postpubertal females after vaccination with rubella vaccine. Symptoms generally begin 1 to 3 weeks after vaccination, usually are mild, persist for about 2 days, and rarely recur. These symptoms are less common in postpubertal males compared with females. Other infrequent adverse events include transient peripheral neuritis and pain in the arms and legs. Thrombocytopenic purpura is rare when rubella vaccine is administered as MMR. Rubella vaccine is contraindicated for persons with moderate to severe acute illnesses and for persons with reduced immunocompetence. When it is given with measles vaccine, it may be administered to persons with asymptomatic HIV infection and considered for symptomatic persons who are not severely immunocompromised. Rubella vaccine is grown in human diploid cells and can be administered without problems to persons with allergy to eggs.

Tetanus and Diphtheria

Tetanus (Chapter 296) toxoid is one of the most effective immunizations, with more than 95% protection after a primary series of three doses. In persons aged 7 years or older, it should always be used in combination with diphtheria (Chapter 292) toxoid (Td), which is more than 85% effective in preventing disease. Combinations that also include pertussis antigens (Tdap) are preferred to Td for routine immunization of adolescents and adults who have yet to receive Tdap as well as for pregnant women (for whom Tdap is recommended during every pregnancy).[9] Doses need not be repeated if the schedule is interrupted. A booster dose of Td is recommended every 10 years.

Indications

After a wound, persons of unknown immunization status or persons who have received fewer than three doses of tetanus toxoid should receive a dose of Tdap or Td regardless of the severity of the wound. A3 Td also is indicated for persons who have previously received three or more doses if more than 10 years has elapsed since the last dose, in the case of clean and minor wounds, and if more than 5 years has elapsed for all other wounds. Persons who have never received a dose of Tdap should receive it instead of Td for wound management. Tetanus immune globulin should be administered simultaneously at a separate site to persons who have wounds that are not clean and minor if they have not previously received at least three doses of toxoid.

Adverse Events

Most reactions to Td consist of local inflammation and low-grade fever. Exaggerated local (Arthus-like) reactions, with extensive painful swelling, often from shoulder to elbow, are occasionally reported 2 to 8 hours after receipt of a diphtheria- or tetanus-containing vaccine, particularly in persons who have received frequent doses of diphtheria or tetanus toxoid. Severe systemic reactions, such as generalized urticaria, anaphylaxis, Guillain-Barré syndrome, and other neurologic complications, rarely have been reported after receipt of tetanus toxoid.

Varicella: Chickenpox

A single dose of live attenuated varicella vaccine (Oka strain), which can be combined with MMR vaccine, protects 70 to 90% of recipients against any disease and more than 95% of recipients against severe disease, but a two-dose schedule is recommended. Whether immunity wanes with increasing time after vaccination is unclear. Use of vaccine has been associated with dramatic decreases in the incidence of varicella.

Indications

Varicella vaccine is indicated routinely for all children without a contraindication. The two-dose schedule includes vaccination at 12 to 15 months of age and again at 4 to 6 years of age. For persons who previously received just a single dose, a catch-up second vaccination is recommended, preferably at least 3 months after the first dose. Persons 13 years or older without evidence of immunity to varicella should receive two doses at least 4 weeks apart. Evidence of immunity to varicella includes documentation of age-appropriate vaccination with two doses of varicella vaccine at least 28 days apart, laboratory evidence of immunity or laboratory confirmation of disease, birth in the United States before 1980, or diagnosis or verification of a history of varicella or herpes zoster disease by a health care provider. Serologic screening of adults in some situations may be cost-effective, provided that identified susceptible adults are vaccinated. Serologic testing is not indicated after vaccination. The vaccine is contraindicated in persons who are immunocompromised, persons with anaphylactic allergies to vaccine components, and pregnant women. Post-exposure vaccination within 3 days of exposure can reduce the likelihood of symptomatic infection by about two-thirds.[A5] Varicella vaccine is temperature sensitive, so it must be stored at −15° C or colder to retain potency and should be discarded if it is not used within 30 minutes of reconstitution.

Adverse Events

The most common side effect is soreness at the injection site, which is reported in 25 to 35% of recipients 13 years or older. Varicella-like rashes at the injection site (median of two lesions) have been reported in 3% of recipients in this age group after the first dose and in 1% after the second dose. Nonlocalized rashes with a median of five lesions have been reported in 5.5% of recipients after the first dose and in 0.9% after the second dose. Although the vaccine virus can cause herpes zoster (shingles), especially in children, the incidence is substantially lower than would be expected after natural varicella (Chapter 375). More severe events in temporal relation to the vaccine have been reported rarely, but a causal relationship has not been established. Transmission of vaccine virus to a contact is extremely rare and probably occurs only from vaccinees in whom a varicella-like rash developed.

Varicella: Zoster

The varicella-zoster virus vaccine, which is approximately 14 times more potent than the varicella vaccine used routinely in children, reduces zoster by about 50% and post-herpetic neuralgia by about two thirds in persons 60 years of age or older.[A6] The efficacy against zoster declines after age 70 years, but protection against post-herpetic neuralgia continues. As for the varicella-chickenpox vaccine, special freezer storage is required.

Indications

A single dose of zoster vaccine is recommended for persons 60 years of age or older, even if they have a prior history of zoster. It is not necessary to elicit a history of varicella or to test for varicella immunity before administering the vaccine. The vaccine is not recommended for immunocompromised persons or pregnant women.

Adverse Events

Local reactions (erythema, pain or tenderness, and swelling at the injection site) are common. Severe reactions were of similar incidence in vaccine and placebo recipients in clinical trials.

VACCINES INTENDED PRIMARILY FOR INTERNATIONAL TRAVELERS

Evaluation of people before travel should include a review and provision of routine vaccines recommended on the basis of age and other individual characteristics. Recommendations for specific vaccines related to travel will depend on itinerary, duration of travel, and host factors. Detailed recommendations are available at *www.cdc.gov/travel*.[10]

Japanese Encephalitis Vaccine

Indications

Japanese encephalitis (Chapter 383) vaccine is indicated primarily for travelers to Asia who will spend a month or longer in endemic areas during the transmission season, especially if travel will include rural areas. In all instances, travelers should be advised to take personal precautions to reduce exposure to mosquito bites. An older vaccine was reported to be 80 to 91% effective in preventing clinical disease, and the current whole virus inactivated vaccine (Ixiaro, Intercell Biomedical) was licensed on the basis of comparable immunogenicity. The primary series consists of two 0.5-mL doses given intramuscularly on days 0 and 28, with the second dose administered at least 1 week before travel (see Table 18-2). If the primary series was administered more than 1 year previously, a booster dose may be given before the next potential exposure to the virus.

Adverse Events

Headache and myalgia and local reactions (pain and tenderness) occur in more than 10% of vaccinees. However, the incidence rates of these events were similar to those in a comparison group that received a placebo with aluminum hydroxide.

Typhoid Vaccine

Indications

Two types of vaccines, a live attenuated Ty21a oral vaccine and a capsular polysaccharide vaccine (ViCPS), appear to be of comparable efficacy (50 to 77%). Typhoid (Chapter 308) vaccine is indicated primarily for travelers to areas where the risk of prolonged exposure to contaminated food and water is high. Because the vaccine is not always effective, food and water precautions are still essential. The vaccine also may be considered for family or other intimate contacts of typhoid carriers and laboratory workers who work with *Salmonella typhi*. For adults and children 6 years and older, either of the vaccines may be used. For Ty21a, one enteric-coated capsule is taken every other day for four doses. Alternatively, a single dose of the ViCPS vaccine may be given. The duration of protection with Ty21a is not known; repetition of the primary series is recommended every 5 years for persons at risk. Boosters are recommended every 2 years for the ViCPS vaccine if persons continue to be at risk. The ViCPS vaccine can be given to children as young as 2 years.

Adverse Events

Fever and headache may occur after receipt of typhoid vaccines. Stomach pain, nausea, and rash are rarely observed.

Yellow Fever Vaccine

Indications

Yellow fever (Chapter 381) occurs only in areas of South America and Africa. Vaccination with a single dose of the live attenuated 17D strain of virus confers protection to almost all recipients for at least 10 years. A booster dose is recommended every 10 years for persons at continued risk of exposure to yellow fever.

Adverse Events

Adverse reactions (fever, aches, and soreness, redness, or swelling where the injection was given) occur in up to 25% of vaccinees. Anaphylaxis has been reported in 0.8 to 1.8 persons per 100,000 doses of vaccine distributed. A rare syndrome (0.25 case per 100,000 doses distributed) of multiple organ system failure or viscerotropic disease with high rates of mortality has been reported, primarily among older adults and persons who have undergone thymectomy or have severe thymic dysfunction. Meningoencephalitis, Guillain-Barré syndrome, acute disseminated encephalomyelitis, and bulbar palsy have been reported in 1 to 2 persons per 100,000 doses and are more common in older vaccines. In patients 60 years and older who are going to spend time in yellow fever–endemic zones, yellow fever vaccine should be administered with caution and only after careful counseling. Yellow fever vaccine should not be given to immunocompromised persons or persons with anaphylactic allergies to eggs. The vaccine is contraindicated in pregnant women on theoretical grounds, although pregnant women who must travel to a high-risk area may be vaccinated.

VACCINES FOR POSSIBLE BIOTERRORISM AGENTS

Anthrax Vaccine

Anthrax (Chapter 294) vaccine adsorbed (AVA) is prepared from a cell-free filtrate of a nonencapsulated strain of anthrax and contains many cell products, including protective antigen. Protective antigen is responsible for binding to cells, allowing transport of lethal factor and edema factor into host cells. A recombinant protective antigen (rPA) vaccine is in clinical trials.

Indications

Pre-exposure prophylaxis consists of a three-dose primary intramuscular schedule at 0, 4 weeks, and 6 months, with booster doses at 12 and 18 months, followed by annual boosters. Protective efficacy of an earlier form of the vaccine against cutaneous anthrax was 92.5%. Animal models suggest efficacy against inhalation anthrax. Pre-exposure vaccination is recommended for persons engaged in work involving exposure to high concentrations of *Bacillus anthracis* or in activities with high potential for aerosol production. Vaccine is recommended in conjunction with antibiotics for postexposure prophylaxis after exposure to aerosolized *B. anthracis* spores. The recommended regimen is three doses of AVA administered at 0, 2, and 4 weeks, combined with at least 60 days of antibiotics, which should be continued for at least 14 days after the third dose of vaccine (Chapter 294).

Adverse Events

The most common adverse events are local reactions, including subcutaneous nodules, which are thought to be due to the deposition of the aluminum-containing adjuvant in subcutaneous tissue. These adverse events are less common with intramuscular injections than with subcutaneous injections.

Smallpox Vaccine

Smallpox vaccine uses vaccinia virus, an orthopox virus that is distinct from variola and cowpox viruses and that provides cross-protection from smallpox. Smallpox vaccine is close to 100% effective when it is administered properly with a bifurcated needle. Vaccination also prevents or modifies disease when it is administered within 3 to 4 days of exposure and perhaps even after greater delays. The skin usually does not need any special preparation. If alcohol is used for cleaning, the skin should be allowed to dry before vaccination to avoid inactivation of the vaccine. The needle is held perpendicular to the skin with 15 punctures for all vaccinees, made rapidly with enough vigor to ensure that a trace of blood appears within 15 to 20 seconds. With a primary take, the vaccination site should become reddened and pruritic within 3 or 4 days after vaccination; a large vesicle with a red areola forms and becomes pustular by 7 to 11 days. The lesion scabs by the third week.

Indications

The vaccine is indicated for persons who work with orthopox viruses. To increase preparedness for a smallpox attack, vaccination is often recommended for persons who will serve on public health or health care response teams. The duration of immunity is unclear. Revaccination is recommended at least every 10 years for persons who continue to be at risk. Contraindications include history or presence of eczema, other chronic or exfoliative skin conditions, and immunosuppression or pregnancy in the patient or a close household or other contact. Persons who are younger than 1 year, are breastfeeding, or have allergies to vaccine components should not be vaccinated. Because of reports of post-vaccination cardiac events, vaccination should be deferred in persons with ischemia or other severe heart diseases or persons at high risk for ischemic heart disease events (*http://emergency.cdc.gov/agent/smallpox/vaccination/index.asp*). In the event of exposure to variola, there are no contraindications. Should variola be introduced into a community, vaccination would be indicated for all exposed persons and their close contacts to prevent further spread, and recommendations for more widespread vaccination would have to be evaluated on a case-by-case basis.

Adverse Events

Fever is the most common adverse event. Other more serious complications include eczema vaccinatum, which is a local or disseminated vaccinia infection in persons with a history of eczema or other exfoliative dermatitis; vaccinia necrosum, which occurs in immunocompromised persons; autoinoculation, especially of the eye, which can cause keratitis and scarring; generalized vaccinia; myopericarditis; and encephalitis. The risk for death from vaccinia is about one case per 1 million primary vaccinations.

Other Agents

Other organisms or products that have been considered potential bioterrorism threats include plague (Chapter 312) and botulinum toxin (Chapter 296). Poisoning with botulinum toxin can be treated with a trivalent antitoxin available from the Centers for Disease Control and Prevention (see *http://www.cdc.gov/laboratory/drugservice/formulary.html*). An experimental heptavalent botulinum toxoid can be obtained from the Centers for Disease Control and Prevention for laboratory workers at high risk for exposure to toxin. Pre-exposure vaccination is not warranted or feasible for the general population.

OTHER VACCINES

A protein-conjugated vaccine for *H. influenzae* type b (Hib) should be considered for some adults at high risk for invasive Hib disease (e.g., asplenia, sickle cell disease, or recipient of a hematopoietic stem cell transplant) if they have not previously received Hib vaccine.

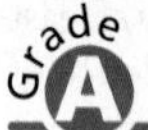

Grade A References

A1. Prymula R, Siegrist CA, Chlibek R, et al. Effect of prophylactic paracetamol administration at time of vaccination on febrile reactions and antibody responses in children: two open-label, randomised controlled trials. *Lancet.* 2009;374:1339-1350.
A2. Udell JA, Zawi R, Bhatt DL, et al. Association between influenza vaccination and cardiovascular outcomes in high-risk patients: a meta-analysis. *JAMA.* 2013;310:1711-1720.
A3. Thierry-Carstensen B, Jordan K, Uhlving HH, et al. A randomised, double-blind, non-inferiority clinical trial on the safety and immunogenicity of a tetanus, diphtheria and monocomponent acellular pertussis (TdaP) vaccine in comparison to a tetanus and diphtheria (Td) vaccine when given as booster vaccinations to healthy adults. *Vaccine.* 2012;30:5464-5471.
A4. Moberley S, Holden J, Tatham DP, et al. Vaccines for preventing pneumococcal infection in adults. *Cochrane Database Syst Rev.* 2013;1:CD000422.
A5. Macartney K, Heywood A, McIntyre P. Vaccines for post-exposure prophylaxis against varicella (chickenpox) in children and adults. *Cochrane Database Syst Rev.* 2014;6:CD001833.
A6. Gagliardi AM, Gomes Silva BN, Torloni MR, et al. Vaccines for preventing herpes zoster in older adults. *Cochrane Database Syst Rev.* 2012;10:CD008858.

GENERAL REFERENCES

For the General References and other additional features, please visit Expert Consult at https://expertconsult.inkling.com.

19

PRINCIPLES OF OCCUPATIONAL AND ENVIRONMENTAL MEDICINE

MARK R. CULLEN

In the first several decades after World War II, when many American workers came to enjoy coverage by health insurance—for everything *but* workplace injuries and illnesses—the myth grew that modern work is largely free of the risks of the industrial horrors of past eras. Starting in the 1970s, however, resurgence of societal and medical interest in these consequences of work found that diseases related to work are not truly extinct, just not well observed or studied. Occupational physicians, often cut off from mainstream medical practice, had difficulty in changing the perception, and most practicing internists were largely oblivious. It is now recognized that a substantial burden of ill health and disability is due to work-associated physical, chemical, and biologic hazards. Psychosocial aspects of work also may be injurious to health.

Although tens of thousands of toxic chemicals and other hazards can potentially cause or exacerbate a wide range of acute and chronic conditions, certain basic principles and clinical approaches apply broadly to general and specialty medical practice. This chapter outlines these basics, then briefly summarizes the most common occupational disorders seen by internists in developed countries, and finally reviews the effects of the environmental exposures most likely to be encountered.

PRINCIPLES OF OCCUPATIONAL AND ENVIRONMENTAL DISEASE

It is widely imagined that the major health effects of environmental and occupational exposures are unique disorders best recognized by their failure to fit easily into other diagnostic categories (e.g., arsenic poisoning). In reality, *the major consequences of chemical and physical exposures are, without further exploration of an environmental connection, indistinguishable in clinical presentations from disorders that make up the bulk of outpatient and inpatient medical practice:* common rashes (Chapter 438), nonspecific liver function abnormalities (Chapter 147), wheezing and irritative symptoms of the upper and lower respiratory tract (Chapter 87), various cancers (Chapter 180), peripheral neuropathies (Chapter 420), dysphoria (Chapter 397), and nonspecific cognitive dysfunction (Chapter 402). Although a handful of pathologically distinct disorders still occur, such as silicosis (Chapter 93) and lead poisoning (Chapter 22), when an environmental or workplace agent causes overt disease, physiologic and radiographic studies typically reveal manifestations completely consistent with common diagnoses such as asthma (Chapter 87), contact dermatitis (Chapter 438), fatty liver (Chapter 152), and lung cancer (Chapter 191).

The underlying cause of such conditions will inevitably remain obscure unless the clinician adheres to a disciplined approach designed to investigate and to exclude occupational or environmental causes whenever it is appropriate. The best approach is consistent use of the occupational and environmental history, a short series of questions that can be expanded on the basis of the responses (see later). The point is that the internist cannot "wait" to consider occupational or environmental issues until other diseases have been ruled out without running the risk of missing almost every occupational and environmental effect that he or she will encounter.

Whatever the pathway or time course, exposure dose is the major determinant of the risk for development of disease. As in pharmacology (Chapter 29), it is impossible to make any meaningful statement about cause and effect without appreciation of dose. Consider, for example, the difference in health effects of aspirin at 65 mg, 650 mg, and 6500 mg (Chapter 37). Over this two-order magnitude of change, the chemical goes from having one therapeutic target organ to having many to being lethal. It is no different with lead or organophosphate pesticides or solvents, except that there is rarely as simple a way to determine dose as in the drug situation, where pill bottles are labeled, drug prescriptions are recorded, and blood or urine levels are readily available in most laboratories. This limitation is exacerbated because, unlike with drugs, the range of toxic exposures may vary far more widely. For example, water in a contaminated drinking well or poor indoor air in an office could have toxins at a level that is two, three, or even four orders of magnitude (i.e., 10,000 times) lower than the level that may have been evaluated in epidemiologic studies of workers or tested in animals. Fortunately, it is much easier to "range find" than one might presuppose (see later discussion of history), and eagerness for precision—often unattainable—should not interfere with obtaining the great amount of information that *can* be readily gleaned from the patient and is often sufficient to act on. The key point is that no attempt to apply clinical information in relation to work or environment can be useful without some effort to characterize exposure dose.

Environmental hazards may affect preferentially vulnerable populations—those with underlying disease, those at the extremes of life, those with atopy, and those with other serious health risks such as smoking or diabetes. Genetic variability may underlie some of these differences, but few relevant genes have been sufficiently characterized for use in practice. Clinical studies of a host of common occupational diseases have identified behavioral and constitutional cofactors; for example, smoking dramatically increases the risk of lung cancer in asbestos-exposed workers (Chapter 191). This interaction creates a double demand on the clinician—the presence of smoking or atopy in a young woman with cough not only does not *preclude* the possibility of an occupational cause of her asthma but rather actually *increases* the likelihood that such an exposure may be important.

The Occupational and Environmental History and Exposure Assessment

Key to determining whether work and other environmental exposures may be causing or contributing to adverse health is the exposure history. The approach to obtaining this information and to the use of available resources to corroborate and complement it depends on the clinical context. In primary and much specialty medical care, where it is anticipated that a patient will be observed during a long period into the future, the most important step is to establish the hazards to which the patient may be exposed at work presently, the activities that may have resulted in past harmful exposures potentially relevant to future health (because of a latency with tobacco), and whether the present residential environment (including air and water and food sources) is thought to be contaminated by harmful materials. The recommended approach is to use a simple questionnaire, which can be self-administered or supervised by a medical extender (E-Fig. 19-1). These instruments can then be reviewed together by the patient and physician as time permits and updated over time. When jobs or materials are noted but the actual generic exposures are unknown, the patient and available reference sources can be enlisted to "translate" the history into specifics, such as which metals are being welded or what is actually contained in a cleaning agent or plastic. This information is obligatorily maintained and supplied on request by employers in most developed countries in the form of fact sheets termed Material Safety Data Sheets, many of which can be easily found online as well. In this way, the ongoing and former exposures, which may have an impact on health, can be noted and, where important, incorporated into routine preventive care or clinical surveillance for sequelae.

For patients with new clinical complaints or recently diagnosed conditions, the question of an environmental cause looms more urgently, so the approach must be more focused. If symptoms or signs of acute or subacute illness are suggested, the *timing* of recent or unusual environmental exposures in relation to the symptoms is key—more important than specific chemical detail. For example, if the patient develops shortness of breath shortly after the introduction of a new chemical or process at work or after a leak or spill, that fact should drive further questions, such as Did others get sick as well? For recurrent symptoms, such as cough or rash, cyclic changes are most often the strongest clue: Do symptoms get worse on workdays and improve on days off or holidays? For more insidious symptoms, such as weakness or numbness of the extremities or new-onset hepatic dysfunction, the appropriate question would be whether the onset of the abnormality has followed by weeks or months some demonstrable change in the work or home environment. Again, the coincidence of others similarly affected may be more valuable than detailed knowledge of the constituents of that environment. When such a temporal pattern is suggested, further efforts are warranted to establish what exposure may have occurred and what its dose may have been, often in conjunction with a specialty consultation.

In the elucidation of evidently more chronic conditions, such as pulmonary fibrosis, chronic renal insufficiency, or a malignant neoplasm, an alternative approach is suggested because the exposure, if relevant, is usually remote. In this situation, a detailed query about current work or ambient environments is *not* likely to be helpful in differential diagnosis, although knowledge of a past exposure to an important hazard (such as silica, asbestos, or cadmium) might, on the basis of the knowledge of its effects, influence the sequence of the evaluation. However, it is generally more efficient to explore past exposures *after* the pathophysiologic disturbance has been characterized, focusing inquiry on factors known to cause or suspected of causing that disorder—as easily found in suggested texts or literature searches.

In acute or chronic cases, information about *what* the exposure has been (generically) must be augmented by an estimation of exposure dose. A brief exposure to a fume containing a small percentage of lead will not, in general, cause acute lead poisoning (although hosts may differ in their responses), nor will trace contamination of a drinking well with benzene typically cause blood dyscrasias. The patient will rarely be able to supply detailed information about past or even current "dose" but often can provide valuable clues: Did the exposure continue during many years? Were fumes or fibers grossly visible in the air? Were respirators or other protective gear necessary or offered? Have episodes of unprotected exposure ever resulted in irritation or acute discomfort? A positive reply to any of these questions would suggest "high" exposure, where the reference point is the level at which the risk for development of a health effect becomes substantial. Conversely, if exposure has occurred in an otherwise typical office or around a home renovation, the levels of exposure are more likely "low." Nevertheless, such low-level exposure does not exclude a health effect, especially one caused by idiosyncratic mechanisms or occurring in hosts who are more "sensitive" to chemical exposures, a health characteristic found in 2 to 10% of the population. Although not to be condoned because of potential broader public health consequences, exposures to trace contaminants in food and drinking water are uncommon causes of *perceptible* clinical problems. When concern about the exposure is high, information from patients can be readily supplemented by information from employers (with the patient's consent!) and regulatory or health authorities or by consultation with specialists who should know the levels of most workplace hazards in the community. Finally, with an appropriate understanding of the limits of testing and awareness of "timing" issues in relation to exposure (as with measuring drug levels), an increasing number of hazardous chemicals can be biologically measured in blood or urine. Reliable testing is currently available for most metals and some pesticides, and testing may become available for a broad array of organic chemicals in the foreseeable future. Random sampling for "unknowns" is rarely helpful and most often leads to erroneous inferences because trace chemicals are ubiquitous, that is, almost everyone will have a higher than average level of "something."

OCCUPATIONAL AND ENVIRONMENTAL HEALTH DISORDERS COMMON IN PRACTICE

Although almost any medical complaint or condition could in theory have an occupational or environmental cause or contribution, certain conditions encountered in medical practice *commonly* do (Table 19-1). For these conditions, attention to the history is most important and most often rewarding.

Asthma

Atopic men and women with preexisting airways disease tolerate irritants in the workplace poorly and may experience exacerbations in temporal relation to one or more exposures. More important, numerous antigens are extant in the workplace, from large proteins, such as latex and animal danders, to small molecules, such as isocyanates needed to set polyurethane. More than 250 agents have been well characterized, and many others are suspect. Virtually no profession or work is immune, and up to 20% of all adult-onset asthma may have a work component. Presentation is often nonspecific; timing of symptoms during or slightly staggered from exposure is the clue to diagnosis, keeping in mind that there may be a lag of several hours between exposure and cough or other symptoms. The reward for early recognition of such causes is the likelihood that airway inflammation will abate when the noxious exposure is eliminated[1,2]; otherwise, lifelong, often generalized asthma is the rule (Chapter 87).

Chronic Interstitial, Parenchymal, and Inflammatory Lung Disorders

The rounded opacities of silicosis (Chapter 93) and coal workers' pneumoconiosis (Chapter 93) radiographically resemble sarcoid (Chapter 95); chronic beryllium disease (Chapter 93), a granulomatous disorder caused by sensitization to this widely used light metal, is clinically identical to sarcoid in almost all respects, but a reasonably specific test for blood and bronchoalveolar lavage fluid is now available to distinguish them. Asbestosis (Chapter 93) is identical to idiopathic pulmonary fibrosis (Chapter 92) in every clinical way except that benign pleural changes often accompany asbestosis, and asbestosis tends to be more indolent and usually stops progressing when exposure ceases or within a few years thereafter. Hypersensitivity pneumonitis (Chapter 93) is rarely suspected outside of agricultural settings but is occurring far more often; the causes are likely to be microbial contaminants of work materials, but some chemicals, such as the isocyanates, may also be causal. Occupational constrictive bronchiolitis, which can cause indolent or rapidly progressive dyspnea, is seen after exposure to a variety of noxious chemicals.[3] Recently, manufacturing and inorganic chemicals have been associated with outbreaks of allergic alveolitis, and synthetic fibers and food flavorings have precipitated severe and sometimes fatal airways responses. These observations support careful investigation of the environment in all cases of adult-onset lung disease.

TABLE 19-1 COMMON OCCUPATIONAL AND ENVIRONMENTAL HEALTH CONDITIONS IN GENERAL PRACTICE

CONDITION	EXPOSURE SETTINGS	COMMENT
Asthma	Virtually any indoor or outdoor workplace	New-onset, recrudescent, or exacerbated asthma
Interstitial, parenchymal, and inflammatory lung disorders	Dusts, metals, and organic materials	All parenchymal disorders have one or more environmental causes
Cancers of the respiratory tract	Asbestos, radon, silica, combustion fumes, tars, and some metals	Smokers are more likely to be affected
Sensorineural hearing loss	Noise, metals, and solvents	High-frequency loss, especially in younger workers
Musculoskeletal disorders of trunk and limbs	Heavy or repetitive activities or postures	Cold, vibration, and work stress contribute
Upper airway irritation	Dust and fumes	More common in smokers and atopic persons
Nonspecific building-related illness	Office work	Must exclude *specific* causes
Dermatitis, allergic or irritant	Repeated exposure to unprotected skin	Work and environmental exposures should be considered in every case
Multiple chemical sensitivities	Any	Complication of adverse environmental exposure

Cancers of the Respiratory Tract

Although most carcinomas of the lung and upper airway occur in smokers, occupational exposures to asbestos, silica, and the polyaromatic hydrocarbons in particulate air pollution, diesel exhaust, pitch, and asphalt contribute to the burden, as do radon and carcinogenic metals such as chromium and nickel found in most alloys (Chapter 191). Some organic materials, such as formaldehyde, are also likely culprits. Until there is an established strategy for secondary prevention, patients with these exposures should be observed expectantly; at a minimum, extraordinary efforts should be made to control smoking in these exposed individuals. Asbestos-exposed workers—smokers or otherwise—are additionally at risk for malignant mesothelioma (Chapters 99 and 191), but other than primary prevention, the only clinical implication is awareness for early diagnosis and compassionate care for this still largely incurable industrial disease.

Fatty Liver

With the widespread use of abdominal imaging, fatty liver has been recognized as more common than previously thought (Chapter 152). This disorder is common among individuals exposed regularly to organic solvents, a possibility that should be considered at the same time that infectious, metabolic, and pharmaceutical causes are considered. Once it is suspected, whether or not other factors are also present, chemical exposure should be reduced. Improvement tends to be slow, often during a period of many months, but the risk of progression is likely to have been averted or at least diminished.

Sensorineural Hearing Loss

Aside from aging, noise is the most important cause of high-frequency sensorineural hearing loss, recognizable as early as in adolescence (Chapter 426). Hobbies such as shooting and loud music may combine with industrial and agricultural noise to accelerate hearing loss. Although it is the responsibility of employers to conduct routine audiograms and to control exposure, clinicians should test noise-exposed patients periodically and reinforce whatever control strategies may be in place at work. Exposure to metals such as lead and organic solvents may compound the risk further.

Musculoskeletal Disorders of the Upper Extremity and Trunk

The most common cause of work disability, including permanent disability, is an injury to the back (Chapter 400) or upper extremity; the annual loss to the U.S. economy from disability and health care expenditures is estimated at a staggering 1 to 2% of the gross domestic product. Repetitive, heavy, awkward, and time-pressured activities are notorious contributors, as are cold and vibration.[4] A majority of cases, however, occur in workers without extremely physical jobs, such as health care or other service workers. Although an anatomically localized lesion may be identified and specifically treated in a small fraction of cases, as in carpal tunnel syndrome (Chapter 420) or thoracic outlet obstruction, the most important modalities of care in most cases are *early recognition* and *reduction of further insult*.[5] Physical therapy and medications may hasten recovery but cannot prevent recurrences and even progression unless the causal work and avocational activities are modified.[A1] Employers, who are increasingly familiar with these ergonomic issues, share an incentive to modify tasks or work stations.

Upper Airway Irritation

Virtually any smoke, fume, dust, or chemical has potential to irritate the upper respiratory tract (Chapter 93), causing acute or chronic symptoms indistinguishable from common allergic manifestations (Chapter 249) or upper respiratory infections (Chapter 96). Although the mucosae of the eyes, nose, sinuses, and throat tend to be forgiving, recurrent episodes are extremely nettlesome and cause substantial work disability. Atopic patients and patients with frequent infections are often the most sensitive to these ubiquitous environmental insults, which must ultimately be addressed along with the symptoms themselves and secondary infections.

Dermatitis

Erythematous rashes are a common consequence of topical exposures to workplace, avocational, and household materials, including latex, plastics, and many foods (Chapter 440). Although the keys to recognition are timing and the anatomic relation to clothing, allergenic and irritating chemicals can find their way into unlikely places, such as the groin and belt lines. Specialty consultation and patch testing are warranted in intractable cases but should not supplant careful observation and history taking in most situations. Acneiform lesions and folliculitis (Chapter 440) are also often caused by chemical irritation or physical factors at work, such as heat, pressure, or friction.

Sick Building Syndrome and Nonspecific Building-Related Illness

The effort to reduce the influx of "fresh" air into buildings to save heating and air-conditioning costs has resulted in upper airway and dermal irritation as well as vague central nervous system symptoms such as headache and fatigue, occurring shortly after beginning work and clearing minutes to hours after leaving the affected building. Many occupants are typically affected, especially those who spend the most time in one place. The cause is unknown, but recent evidence suggests that microbial materials may be the most common culprits. In every instance, a search for a specific allergen or irritant is worth undertaking (Chapter 249), but the most remedial sources are poor overall ventilation and dampness in which molds fester. When the cause is remedied, most building occupants typically experience symptomatic improvement. From a clinical perspective, the major consideration is whether any more serious problem, such as asthma, may have also developed.

Multiple Chemical Sensitivities

An environmental illness as transient as a single noxious inhalation or as persistent as a protracted course of nonspecific building-related illness can initiate a cycle of similar symptoms after exposures to odors or irritants at very low levels, thereby rendering everyday tasks such as shopping or driving problematic. A patient typically complains of feeling "allergic" to everything, although there is no evidence for allergic mechanisms (Chapter 249); the cause of this vexing complication, most prevalent in women and also seen in veterans of conflicts in the Middle East, is unknown and may involve psychological as well as physiologic factors. Despite the severity of complaints, which often include fatigue, muscle pain, stridor, chest tightness, and palpitations, laboratory test results are normal; many patients will meet clinical criteria for fibromyalgia (Chapter 274). Coexistent anxiety and depression often prompt psychiatric referral (Chapter 397), but the disorder has proved relatively refractory to all treatment modalities. Sympathetic support, environmental modification as needed to provide some symptomatic relief, and candor regarding the unknown nature of the disorder are appropriate; extensive clinical investigations often serve only to reinforce the patient's "sick" role and are best avoided. Despite all efforts, the most severely affected individuals will often seek the care of alternative practitioners (Chapter 39) with compelling if unproven theories and expensive, potentially harmful remedies.

COMMON HAZARDOUS EXPOSURES IN THE WORKPLACE AND AMBIENT ENVIRONMENT

Tens of thousands of chemicals in the workplace as well as important physical and biologic hazards may be encountered in the general environment (Table 19-2). Several of these hazards are of major current concern in industrialized countries.

TABLE 19-2 COMMON HAZARDS IN THE WORKPLACE AND AMBIENT ENVIRONMENT

HAZARD	HEALTH EFFECTS OF GREATEST CONCERN	COMMENTS
Metals	Neurotoxicity, cancer	Most can be measured in blood or urine to assess dose
Organic solvents	Respiratory and dermal irritation, neurotoxicity, hepatotoxicity	Benzene and a few others have unique effects
Organohalides (e.g., DDT, PCBs)	Cancer	Ubiquitous suspect carcinogens of high population concern
Herbicides and pesticides	Rare acute neurotoxicity, unknown long-term effects	Widespread hazards of high population concern
Electromagnetic radiation	Leukemia, glioblastoma	Ubiquitous exposures with unproven effects
Particulate matter	Acute and chronic atherosclerotic cardiovascular disease	Air pollution, workplace
Mold	Allergy	High population concern regarding putative chronic effects
Mineral dusts	Cancer	Old hazards still of high concern (e.g., asbestos, silica)

DDT = dichlorodiphenyltrichloroethane; PCBs = polychlorinated biphenyls.

Metals

Exposures to lead and arsenic (Chapter 22), once commonplace in industry, are now generally controlled; concern remains highest for environmental settings, especially for children. There is now greater concern for mercury—entrained in large ocean fish worldwide—and manganese, a potent neurotoxin that is found in welding fumes and various alloys and that affects extrapyramidal and autonomic function. For most metals—manganese being a notorious exception—blood or urine tests are available to quantify a patient's burden, but these tests must be mindful of timing, the form of metal, and possible "confounders," such as the largely benign form of arsenic excreted in urine for several days after even a single shellfish meal.

Organic Solvents

These petroleum derivatives remain ubiquitous in workplace and household products. All are irritating, potentially neurotoxic, and, to varying degrees, hepatotoxic (Chapter 110). Several more serious toxins, such as trichloroethylene and *n*-hexane, are no longer widely used. Benzene and the ethers of ethylene glycol are bone marrow toxins (Chapter 165).

Organohalides

Although these complex organic pesticides and industrial materials are no longer made and sold in developed countries, their remarkable biopersistence has resulted in entrainment into everyone's fat. Worse, the dread byproduct dioxin, once associated with herbicide manufacture, has now been recognized as a predictable consequence of combustion of any chlorine-containing materials. All are suspect carcinogens, although debate remains whether this effect is limited to soft tissue sarcomas (Chapter 202)—a relationship established for dioxin—or promotes cancers more globally. Some toxicologic and epidemiologic evidence links this class of agents to type 2 diabetes mellitus and dyslipidemias.

Herbicides and Pesticides

The acute neurotoxicity and irritant properties of most herbicides and pesticides have been well studied (Chapter 110). These agents are generally well controlled, although both occupational and residential overexposures occasionally occur. In developing countries, these substances remain a widespread vehicle for both suicide and homicide.

Nonionizing Electromagnetic Radiation

Electric wires, appliances, and, notoriously, cell phones emit low-frequency electromagnetic radiation at levels far below those that cause local thermal injuries (Chapter 20). These radiations are nonionizing, but there is some epidemiologic evidence of an increased risk of childhood leukemia with high-level exposure from household wiring and of excess brain tumors in adult workers with regular exposures. These data are difficult to interpret because study results differ according to how exposure is assessed; the only conclusion is that there is basis for concern and need for further study but not cause for widespread alarm or action other than precaution in the placement of new heavy power lines near schools and residences.

Particulate Matter

Evidence accumulated in the past decade points to the likelihood that ambient air pollution contributes measurably to the population risk of cardiovascular disease. Focus has turned from the well-established respiratory irritants—the gases sulfur dioxide and ozone—to the smallest particles, so-called $PM_{2.5}$. These particles may be laden with polyaromatic hydrocarbons from diesel exhaust, coal burning, and industrial sources, which are proinflammatory. This risk also accrues to more heavily exposed industrial workers, although it remains unclear if the risk is associated with particles of any origin or just those that evolve from combustion.

Mold

Molds are ubiquitous and long known for their unpleasant odors and potential for inducing allergic responses (Chapter 249), including asthma. Recently, concern has arisen over the potential for serious effects from various mycotoxins, long problems in veterinary medicine when domestic animals consume contaminated feed; however, a consensus panel concluded that there is no evidence of human risks beyond those well established from living or working in a moldy environment. Mold formation should be prevented wherever possible, especially in schools and offices, where molds contribute to problems with indoor air quality. Identification, with eradication of leaks and other sources of water accumulation, is key.

Mineral Dusts

Although asbestos has been largely abated, silica and human-made mineral fibers remain widely distributed in the environment. Silica (Chapter 93), present in virtually every form of "rock," is a potent cause of lung injury and cancer, so respiratory exposure should be carefully controlled in every setting. The evidence of serious risk from fibrous glass, mineral wool, and other human-made mineral fibers is less clear; probably only the finest fibers, such as slag wool, have cancer-causing potential, but many are potent dermal and upper respiratory irritants and should be well controlled for that reason alone.

SUMMARY

Occupational and environmental health problems remain prevalent, although their spectrum and nature have changed as rapidly as any in medicine and are likely to change even faster as technology, work, and knowledge continue to evolve. Physicians need not necessarily develop a large base of *facts*—themselves subject to revision frequently—but rather an *approach* that incorporates key elements and provides a foundation for efficient recognition and management of current and future clinical syndromes.

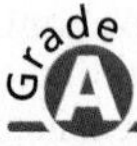

Grade A Reference

A1. Schaafsma FG, Whelan K, van der Beek AJ, et al. Physical conditioning as part of a return to work strategy to reduce sickness absence for workers with back pain. *Cochrane Database Syst Rev.* 2013;8:CD001822.

GENERAL REFERENCES

For the General References and other additional features, please visit Expert Consult at https://expertconsult.inkling.com.

20

RADIATION INJURY

DAVID J. BRENNER

IONIZING RADIATION

DEFINITION

Ionizing radiations include x-rays, gamma rays, beta particles, alpha particles, and neutrons. Unlike non-ionizing radiations, including radio waves, microwaves, infrared, visible light, and ultraviolet (UV) radiations, these radiations have enough energy to knock electrons out of atomic or molecular orbits, thereby breaking chemical bonds in biomolecules such as DNA.

A key difference among the various ionizing radiations is their ability to penetrate matter (Fig. 20-1). For example, alpha particles have very limited range, measured in micrometers. Because alpha particles cannot penetrate skin, their health significance is entirely in the context of internal exposure by inhalation or ingestion of alpha-emitting radioactive materials. Beta particles, which have intermediate ranges, can typically be stopped by a piece of paper. By contrast, x-rays, gamma rays, and neutrons are highly penetrating and are hard to shield.

Ionizing radiations are emitted by radioactive materials, which can either be naturally occurring or can be man-made, using machines such as nuclear reactors. The amount of ionizing radiation emitted by a radioactive material is determined by its activity, measured in becquerels (1 Bq = 1 radioactive disintegration/second) or Curies (Ci).

Radioactivity should be distinguished from absorbed dose, which is a measure of how much ionizing energy is actually absorbed by a structure of interest, such as a person or an organ. The basic measurement unit of absorbed dose, which is the energy deposited per unit mass, is the Gray (1 Gy = 1 J/kg). *Equivalent dose* takes into account the fact that not all types of radiation are equally effective, *effective dose* takes into account the fact that not all organs in the body are equally sensitive to ionizing radiation, and *collective dose* is a measure of the effective dose delivered summed over a whole exposed population (Table 20-1).

EPIDEMIOLOGY

Radiation exposure can come from natural sources, therapeutic or diagnostic medical exposures, or accidental exposures to individuals or to large populations. Natural sources and radiologic examinations are the major contributors to the overall collective radiation dose to the U.S. population (Fig. 20-2).[1]

Natural Sources of Ionizing Radiation

The largest naturally occurring source of radiation is from radon gas, which is an alpha-particle emitter. Radon is a constituent component of all rocks, particularly granite-type rocks. Radon is a member of a chain of radioactive elements that starts with naturally occurring uranium and radioactively decays from one element to the next; uniquely in this chain of elements, radon is a gas, which can emerge from the ground and result in high levels in the basement and higher floors of houses. Long-term exposure to radon gas can cause lung cancer because emitted alpha particles in the lung can damage cells in the bronchial epithelium. The three other main sources of naturally occurring radiation exposure are from terrestrial exposure (gamma rays emitted from naturally occurring radioactive materials in the ground), from space radiations (mainly intergalactic cosmic rays that penetrate through the atmosphere), and internal radiation (from naturally occurring radioactive elements in the body, such as potassium-40).

Medical Exposures

The single largest source of medical exposure is computed tomography (CT), which on average contributes about 25% of the collective dose to the U.S. population. This source of exposure is recent because CT has been commonly used only since the 1980s. Now, however, about 75 million CT scans are performed annually in the United States. In addition to CT, nuclear medicine, interventional fluoroscopy, and conventional radiography together constitute about 25% of the overall collective dose to the U.S. population.

Radiologic Accidents

Since the widespread introduction of nuclear power plants, major radiologic accidents have become an intermittent, although rare, source of radiation

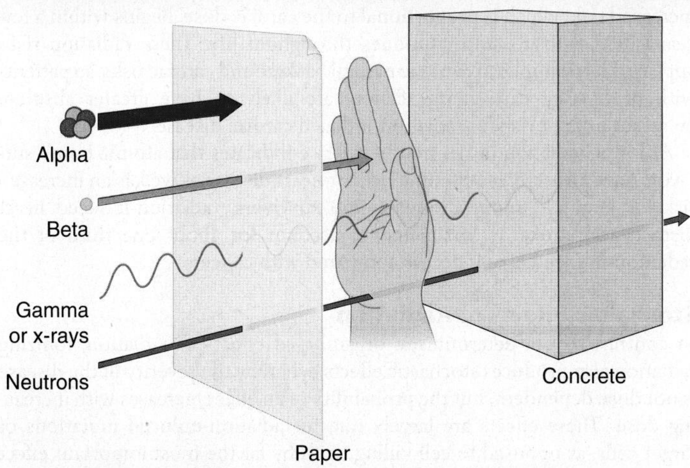

FIGURE 20-1. Schematic illustrating the relative ranges of alpha particles, beta rays, x-rays or gamma rays, and neutrons as they penetrate through matter.

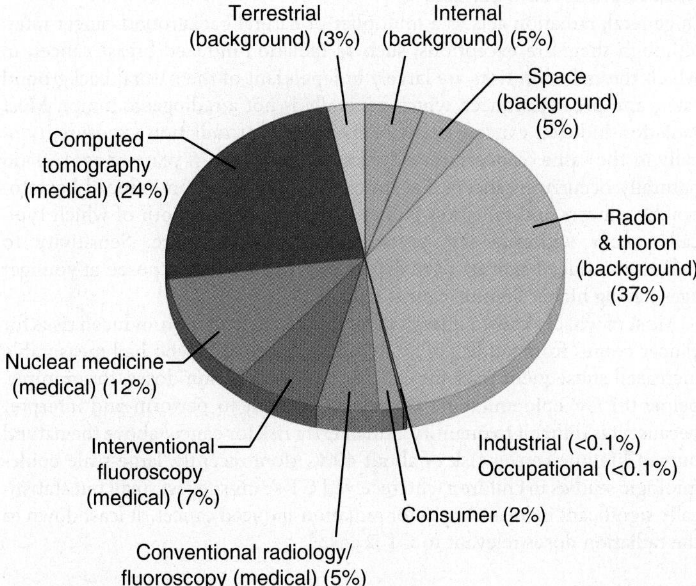

FIGURE 20-2. The major sources of radiation exposure to an average individual in the United States. (From Hall EJ. *Radiobiology for the Radiologist*. 7th ed. Philadelphia: Lippincott Williams & Wilkins; 2012.)

TABLE 20-1 STANDARD QUANTITIES AND UNITS ASSOCIATED WITH EXPOSURE TO IONIZING RADIATION

QUANTITY	DEFINITION	UNITS
Absorbed dose	Energy per unit mass	Gray (Gy)
Equivalent dose	Average dose × radiation-type-specific radiation weighting factor	Sievert (Sv)
Effective dose	Sum of equivalent doses to all exposed organs, each multiplied by an appropriate organ relative sensitivity factor	Sievert (Sv)
Collective dose	Sum of effective doses to a population of exposed individuals	Person-Sv

exposure. The accidents at Chernobyl in 1986 and at Fukushima in 2011 released far more radioactivity than any other accidents (Table 20-2).

Radiologic Terrorism

In the broadest of terms, two different types of such threats exist, one from an improvised nuclear device and the other from a radiologic dispersal device, sometimes called a *dirty bomb*.[2] The two are very different in terms of their potential consequences and also their likelihood of occurrence.

TABLE 20-2 ESTIMATED RELEASES OF RADIOACTIVE IODINE AND RADIOACTIVE CESIUM FROM THE FOUR HISTORICALLY BIGGEST NUCLEAR POWER PLANT ACCIDENTS

	^{131}I (TBq)	$^{137/134}$Cs (TBq)
Windscale, 1957	750	20
Three Mile Island, 1979	1	0.000001
Chernobyl, 1986	1,800,000	110,000
Fukushima, 2011	~500,000	~20,000

The consequences of exploding an improvised nuclear device, perhaps similar to those detonated at Hiroshima or Nagasaki, although more likely exploded at ground level, would be devastating in terms of loss of life and major injuries. For example, a 20-kT daytime surface improvised nuclear device explosion in midtown Manhattan might involve 2.2 million people exposed to high radiation doses, of whom perhaps only 1.6 million might survive.

By contrast, the consequences of exploding a radiologic dispersal device or dirty bomb, dispersing what could be very small or very large amounts of radioactive material, would likely involve a relatively small spatial area in which individuals are significantly exposed, as well as a much larger area in which individuals are exposed to very low levels of radioactivity. The significance of a dirty bomb depends on the amount of radioactivity in the device and the efficiency with which the explosion aerosolizes and disperses the radioactive material. Of course, the consequences of a radiologic dispersal device extend beyond health effects and could potentially involve large-scale social and economic disruption.[3]

PATHOBIOLOGY

Ionizing radiation can both mutate cells and kill them. The key initial damage site is a DNA double-strand break, although other types of damage are possible. This strand break is generally repaired by a variety of mechanisms, the most important of which is nonhomologous end rejoining. Imprecise nonhomologous end rejoining can lead to small mutations, whereas double-strand break misrepair (i.e., the wrong ends of breaks being rejoined to each other) can lead to chromosomal translocations, inversions, and telomere fusions.

Although chromosomal translocations, inversions, and point mutations are typically nonlethal lesions, such radiation-induced chromosomal aberrations can be the initial lesions associated with carcinogenesis. For example, the initial event in many hematopoietic cancers (Chapters 183 and 184) is often a recurrent translocation, which in turn results in the fusion of genes located at the translocation breakpoints. Radiation-induced point mutations and deletions also are often associated with loss of heterozygosity in tumor suppressor genes.

Misrepair of double-strand breaks can also induce dicentric chromosome aberrations and centric rings (Chapter 181), which are generally lethal lesions that cause reproductive cell death in which a cell loses its ability to divide. A second, quite different mechanism of radiation-induced cell death is apoptosis, or programmed cell death that, for example, is important after radiation exposure of hematopoietic cells and jejunal crypt cells.

CLINICAL MANIFESTATIONS

The consequences of radiation exposure are dose dependent and are also dependent on whether the exposure is to the whole body or only part of the body. After high doses of whole-body exposure, the major consequences are acute radiation syndromes, which may be fatal. After high doses of partial-body exposure, such as after radiotherapy, the consequences are highly organ specific. These high-dose tissue effects are deterministic, meaning that above a certain dose threshold, the probability of the effect rapidly increases to 100%, with the severity of the effect increasing with increasing dose. By contrast, the major concern at lower doses is with stochastic effects, in which there is no dose threshold, and it is the probability of the effect that increases with increasing dose. The major example here is radiation-induced cancer.

Acute Radiation Syndromes

The radiation dose needed to kill mitotically active dividing cells is far less than the dose needed to remove the functioning ability of differentiated cells. As a result, acute radiation syndromes generally relate to the failure of precursor cells to provide replacements for functional cells within an organ, when the latter need replacement. Acute radiation syndromes typically progress through four stages: prodromal, clinical latency, manifest illness, and recovery or death.

Prodromal Stage

Prodromal (early) symptoms occur shortly after irradiation, with the radiation dose determining the severity, duration, and onset. Typical prodromal symptoms include nausea, vomiting, anorexia, fatigue, diarrhea, abdominal cramping, and dehydration. At very high doses, these symptoms can appear within a few minutes of exposure; but at somewhat lower doses, they may not appear for many hours, if at all.

Latency Period

After the prodromal stage, a latency period typically precedes manifest illness. This delay occurs because the subsequent syndromes (hematopoietic and gastrointestinal) involve the failure of relevant tissues to self renew, and manifest illness does not occur until after the typical cellular turnover times in these tissues.

Manifest Illness

The *hematopoietic syndrome* results from whole-body or significant partial-body exposure to 3 to 9 Gy. At these doses, radiation kills some or all of the mitotically active hematopoietic precursor cells. Symptoms then result from lack of circulating blood elements some 4 to 8 weeks later as circulating cells die off and are not replaced. At this point, the hematopoietic syndrome may manifest as infections and possible hemorrhage, impairment of immune mechanisms, and potentially multiple-organ failure.

The *gastrointestinal syndrome* usually occurs after whole-body or significant partial-body exposure of about 8 Gy and above. These doses lead to death of intestinal stem cells in the regenerating crypts. Symptoms then result when differentiated cells of the villi are naturally sloughed off, but stem cells are unable to produce new cells, thereby leading to depopulation of the epithelial lining of the gastrointestinal tract. After a latency period of about 7 days, loss of, or significant shortening of, the villi on the intestinal epithelium leads to bacterial growth and increased risk for sepsis. Common symptoms include anorexia, nausea, vomiting, prolonged bloody diarrhea, abdominal cramps, dehydration, and weight loss. Should death occur, it is typically 7 to 10 days later.

At extremely high radiation doses, death is typically from the *cerebrovascular syndrome* within a few days after exposure. The cause of death is believed to be because changes in permeability of small blood vessels in the brain lead to cerebral edema.

Organ-Specific Late Effects after Radiotherapy

Iatrogenic organ-specific late effects follow quite predictably after targeted radiation therapy in which the organ in question is irradiated, although the severity of the response is less predictable. These tissue effects can be divided into global organ responses and focal responses, in which a particular part of the organ is differentially irradiated (Table 20-3).

As one example, significant radiation exposure to the heart increases the risk for subsequent major heart disease. These risks have been most notable in women who have had radiotherapy for left-sided breast cancer (Chapter 198),[4] patients treated with mantle radiation for Hodgkin lymphoma (Chapter 186), and some patients treated for lung tumors adjacent to the heart.[5] The effects to the heart can be wide ranging, including to the coronary arteries, the myocardium, the heart valves, and the pericardial sac. The increased risk, which is proportional to the cardiac dose, begins within a few years after exposure and continues throughout life. These radiation risks appear to be multiplicative of the natural background cardiac risks, so patients with preexisting cardiac risk factors are likely to have greater absolute increases in their risk for radiation-induced cardiac disease.

At lower radiation doses, good evidence indicates that atomic bomb survivors have an increased lifetime risk for heart disease as well as an increased risk for stroke.[6] Among atomic bomb survivors, radiation-induced heart disease and stroke are estimated to account for about one third of the radiation-induced excess deaths compared with cancers.

TABLE 20-3 TYPICAL ORGAN-SPECIFIC DETERMINISTIC LATE EFFECTS AFTER HIGH-DOSE RADIOTHERAPY

ORGAN	LOCALIZED END POINT	GLOBAL END POINT
Brain, cranial nerves	Focal weakness, vision loss	Neurocognitive deficit
Lung	Bronchial stricture	Shortness of breath
Heart	Coronary stenosis	Pericarditis, cardiomyopathy
Bladder	Bleeding	Urinary frequency, diarrhea
Bowel	Ischemia, bleeding	Enteritis

Adapted with changes from Rubin P, Constine LS, Marks LB, eds. *ALERT—Adverse Late Effects of Cancer Treatment. Vol. 1: General Concepts and Specific Precepts.* Heidelberg: Springer; 2014.

Stochastic Effects of Radiation

In contrast to the deterministic organ-based effects of radiation, ionizing radiation also produces stochastic effects, whereby the severity of the disease is not dose dependent, but the probability of an effect increases with increasing dose. These effects are largely due to radiation-induced mutations of target cells, as opposed to cell killing, with by far the most important effect being radiation carcinogenesis. Other potential radiation-induced stochastic health effects include deleterious radiation-induced genetic effects to subsequent generations.

Radiation Carcinogenesis

In general, radiation acts as a multiplier of natural background cancer rates, although there are exceptions, such as radiation-induced breast cancer, in which the radiation risks are largely independent of the natural background rates, and prostate cancer, which generally is not a radiogenic tumor. Most radiation-induced cancers occur many years after radiation exposure, typically in the same "cancer-prone" years (about 55 to 75 years of age), as do naturally occurring cancers. Exceptions include radiation-induced hematopoietic cancers and radiation-induced thyroid cancers, both of which typically occur within a few years of radiation exposure. Sensitivity to radiation-induced cancer is age dependent, with people exposed at younger ages having higher lifetime cancer risks.

Most of what is known quantitatively about the radiation-induced risks for cancer comes from studies of atomic bomb survivors, who had measurable increased subsequent risks for cancer.[6] At low radiation doses, for example, below 0.1 Gy, epidemiologic studies are difficult to perform and interpret because it is difficult to quantify a small extra risk for cancer above the natural human lifetime cancer risk of about 40%. More recently, large-scale epidemiologic studies in children who received CT scans suggest small but statistically significant increased risks for radiation-induced cancer, at least down to the radiation doses relevant to CT scans.[7,8]

Radiation Cataractogenesis

Ionizing radiation induces cataracts (Chapter 423) with a probability, severity, and latency related to the radiation dose.[9] Studies of atomic bomb survivors, Chernobyl cleanup workers, astronauts, and radiologic technicians have all shown increased incidence of cataracts, even at radiation doses below 1 Gy. Radiation cataractogenesis is a result of radiation damage or killing of dividing cells in the lens. Because there are essentially no mechanisms in the lens for removal of damaged cells, the resulting nontranslucent lens fibers migrate toward the posterior pole of the lens, where they represent the first stage of a cataract. Posterior subcapsular cataracts are less common than nuclear or cortical cataracts in the general population but are the type most commonly associated with ionizing radiation.

DIAGNOSIS

The diagnosis of radiation injury can be considered in two different contexts. The first context is when the radiation dose is not known, and the goal is to estimate the dose that was delivered in order to optimize treatment. Examples include accidents and radiologic terrorism scenarios. The second context is when the radiation dose is known, in particular after radiotherapy. Here the sequelae (see Table 20-3) are predictable, but the timing and the severity of the injury are less predictable.

Radiation Biodosimetry

For an individual exposed to a large whole-body radiation dose, the first critical task is to estimate the radiation dose that the individual received, because different syndromes (hematopoietic, gastrointestinal, cerebrovascular) are associated with different radiation dose ranges. The technique for estimating exposures to individuals is known as *radiation biodosimetry*. In this diagnostic process, a small amount of a body tissue, such as blood or urine, is analyzed, and dose-dependent end points in the sample are measured to provide an estimated dose. The most common end point, which is chromosomal aberrations in blood samples, can now be assessed by high-throughput technologies.[10] Other practical radiation-dose dependent assays include gene expression in blood or induction of metabolites in urine.

Post-Radiotherapy Sequelae

Deterministic radiation-induced organ syndromes are seen at reasonably predictable intervals after radiation therapy. For example, radiation pericarditis (Chapter 77) can develop during treatment or months to years later, initially with an effusion and progressing to pericardial constriction. Radiation enterocolitis (Chapter 140) can develop 6 to 12 months after radiation doses of 40 to 60 Gy for prostate cancer or gynecologic malignancies. Radiation-induced pulmonary injury can be detected in up to 50% of patients who receive thoracic radiation therapy, but only a minority of them will develop clinical symptoms (Chapter 94). In addition, the majority of all radiotherapy patients experience acute skin or mucosal toxicity, in particular radiation dermatitis, oral mucositis, and xerostomia.

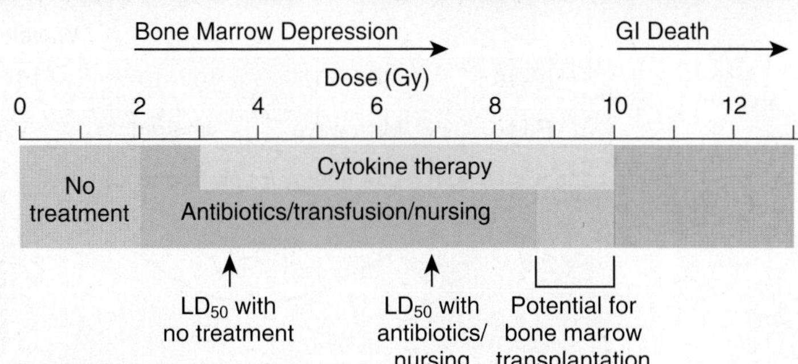

FIGURE 20-3. Schematic recommended treatment for acute radiation syndromes, as a function of the estimated dose that the individual received. Note the very narrow dose window for which bone marrow transplantations are potentially useful. (Adapted with changes from Hall EJ. *Radiobiology for the Radiologist*. 7th ed. Philadelphia: Lippincott Williams & Wilkins; 2012.)

TREATMENT Rx

Whole-Body Exposure Syndromes

For exposures below 2 Gy, no immediate treatment is needed (Fig. 20-3). For the hematopoietic syndrome, two primary treatment approaches are designed to reduce red blood cell depression, by using transfusions and cytokine therapy, and to minimize infection, by using antibiotics and possibly barrier nursing. Antibiotics and appropriate nursing care can raise the human LD_{50} (the dose at which 50% of exposed individuals die) from about 4 to 6 Gy, and the addition of human granulocyte colony-stimulating factor (e.g., filgrastim, 5 µg/kg daily for up to 2 weeks, subcutaneously or by IV infusion) may increase the LD_{50} to about 9 Gy.

The role of bone marrow transplantation in treating individuals with the hematopoietic syndrome is probably quite limited at doses less than about 9 Gy. In the aftermath of the Chernobyl accident, for example, 13 individuals underwent bone marrow transplantation, and three deaths were directly attributed to the sequelae of the procedure in patients in whom the transplantation was not indicated based on their exposure. Conservative treatment regimens, including antibiotics, cytokine therapy, transfusions, and nursing are clearly effective, but current treatment options are very limited at doses above about 10 Gy, when the gastrointestinal syndrome becomes the dominant cause of death.

Radiotherapy Sequelae

For radiotherapy-induced dermatitis, mucositis, and xerostomia, treatments include topical agents for dermatitis (Chapter 438), analgesics for mucositis, and saliva substitutes for xerostomia. Beyond dermatitis, mucositis, and xerostomia, radiation-induced deterministic tissue effects are typically treated in the same way as their non-radiation-induced counterparts. For example, the treatment of radiation-induced coronary artery disease is no different than the approach to coronary diseases in general (Chapters 71 to 74). However, the management of acute and chronic gastrointestinal symptoms after radiotherapy requires a more specialized approach because of the risk for local stricture (Chapter 142).[11]

PREVENTION

Countermeasures after Radiologic Accidents or Terrorism

Three FDA-approved pharmaceuticals can limit the radiation dose caused by exposures to specific radioisotopes: potassium iodide for radioactive iodine, Prussian blue for radioactive cesium or thallium, and diethylenetriamine pentaacetate (DTPA) for plutonium, americium, or curium. Although these pharmaceutical countermeasures can limit the organ doses and therefore the health consequences produced by these specific radioisotopes, they cannot be used to treat any of the adverse clinical effects caused by them.

The administration of potassium iodide (KI), which contains nonradioactive iodine, saturates the thyroid with nonradioactive iodine and thereby prevents radioactive iodine being absorbed into the thyroid, where it can cause thyroid cancer (Chapter 226). The protective effects of KI last about 24 hours, so it should be taken daily (130 mg for adults, 65 mg for children >3 years of age, 32 mg for children 1 to 3 years of age, 16 mg for infants) while there is a likelihood of exposure.

Prussian blue (ferric hexacyanoferrate [II]) binds cesium in the gastrointestinal tract and limits its reabsorption into the blood stream, thereby reducing the biologic half-life of cesium in the body from about 110 days to about 30 days and limiting the organ toxicities that it produces. The recommended dose of Prussian blue is 3 g orally three times daily for adults and 1 g orally three times daily for children 2 to 12 years of age, for a minimum of 30 days.

DTPA is a chelating agent that binds to radioactive plutonium, americium, and curium, thereby decreasing their persistence in the body. DTPA comes in two forms, Ca-DTPA and Zn-DTPA, with the calcium form considered more effective over the first 24 hours of exposure, and the zinc form preferable at later times, although both are effective over several weeks. They are administered intravenously (or with a nebulizer), with a daily intravenous dose of 1 g for adults and 14 mg/kg for children younger than 12 years.

Medical Imaging

Because CT is such a superb diagnostic tool and because individual CT risks are small, the nearly 90 million CT scans performed annually in the United States generally provide far more benefits than risks. However, organ doses from CT are typically far larger than those from conventional radiographic examinations, so CT should operate under the principle of using as low a dose as reasonably achievable. The first opportunity is to reduce the radiation dose per scan, so-called optimization, with improved technology. The second opportunity is justification—making sure that all CT scans are clinically justified. A substantial fraction of CT scans could potentially be replaced by other modalities, such as magnetic resonance imaging for some head examinations[12] and selective use of ultrasound for diagnosing appendicitis.[13] In addition, some CT scans could be avoided entirely by avoiding CT scans when imaging is not clinically necessary.

Radiation Therapy

Amifostine (200 mg/m^2 given intravenously daily, before each fraction of radiation therapy) has been approved by the U.S. Food and Drug Administration (FDA) for minimizing radiotherapy-associated xerostomia,[A1] but its use has been limited by significant toxicity. Several drugs have been designed to mitigate or treat the damage caused by radiation therapy, particularly to the mucosal barrier. Palifermin, which is a recombinant human keratinocyte growth factor, is FDA approved (60 µg/kg/day administered as an IV bolus injection for 3 consecutive days before therapy and 3 consecutive days after therapy for leukemia or lymphoma) to decrease the incidence or duration of severe oral mucositis.[A2]

NON-IONIZING RADIATION INJURY

Ionizing radiations uniquely have sufficient energy to cause DNA strand breaks, which in turn can lead to cell killing and mutations. By contrast, non-ionizing radiations, such as radio waves, microwaves, infrared radiation, and visible light, do not have sufficient energy to break DNA strands and have not been associated with health hazards. One exception is UV radiation, which is clearly a mutagen and a carcinogen. A second possible exception is radiofrequency radiation, although in this case the epidemiologic evidence and mechanistic considerations do not provide strong evidence of health risks.

Ultraviolet Radiation

UV radiations, which are part of the non-ionizing electromagnetic spectrum, cover a wavelength from about 150 to 400 nm (intermediate between visible light and x-rays). In turn, these UV wavelengths are subcategorized as UVA (400 to 320 nm), UVB (315 to 280 nm), and UVC (280 to 150 nm).

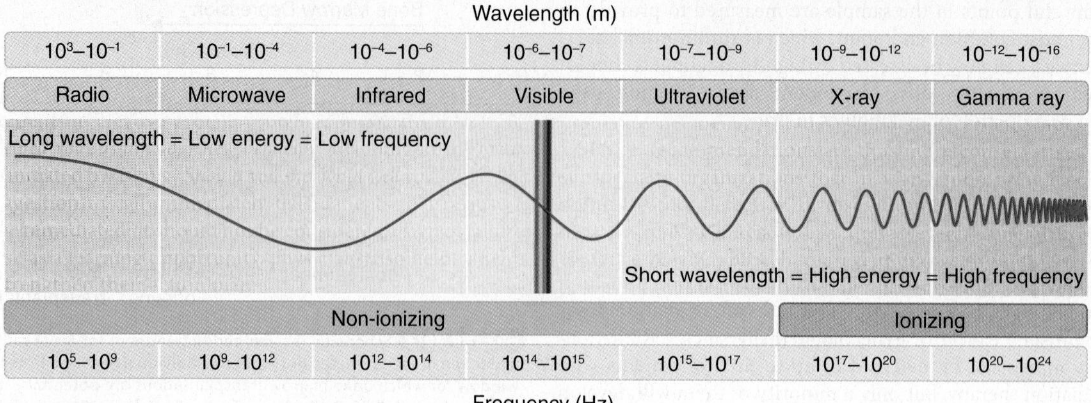

FIGURE 20-4. The electromagnetic spectrum.

Sunlight is by far the largest source of UV radiation to humans. Because of filtering in the atmosphere, about 95% of the UV spectrum that reaches the earth's surface is UVA, the remainder is nearly all UVB, and almost no UVC penetrates the ozone layer to reach the earth. Other sources of UV exposures include tanning beds and booths. Industrial exposures include welding arcs, plasma torches, germicidal and blacklight lamps, electric arc furnaces, hot-metal operations, mercury-vapor lamps, and some lasers.

PATHOBIOLOGY

UV radiations do not penetrate deeply into human tissues, so the injuries they cause are principally to the skin and eyes. The biologic effects of UV radiation are primarily attributable to its absorption in DNA, where pyrimidine dimers and their products are produced. These products are generally very efficiently removed, primarily through nucleotide excision repair but also through base excision repair, but errors in these repair processes ultimately can result in mutations. Although most UV radiation in sunlight is UVA, UVB is much more efficiently absorbed by nucleic acids, and most of the biologic effects of sunlight are associated with UVB.

The damaging effects of UV radiation are exacerbated in patients who have underlying defects in nucleotide excision repair. For example, studies of patients with xeroderma pigmentosum (Chapter 436) have provided key evidence of the link between UV light and skin cancer. In addition, the effects of UV are often enhanced in patients who are taking medications that contain photodynamic agents, such as tetracyclines, fluoroquinolones, nonsteroidal-anti-inflammatory drugs, diuretics, statins, phenothiazines, thioxanthenes, and antifungals. Such drug-related phototoxic reactions typically resolve after the drug is discontinued.

CLINICAL MANIFESTATIONS

The major acute effects of UVB exposure are sunburn and erythema, whereas UVA exposure is rarely the direct cause of sunburn. All ultraviolet radiations are well-established skin carcinogens (Chapter 203). Squamous cell carcinomas and basal carcinomas are typically associated with multiple or chronic exposures to sunlight, whereas melanoma is linked primarily to episodes of acute sunburn. Lighter skinned individuals, whose skin and eyes contain less melanin, are more prone to all UV effects because melanin acts as a photoprotector. Acute exposures of the eye to UVB (Chapter 423) can cause "welder flash" (photokeratitis), and chronic exposures are associated with cataracts as well as pterygium.

PREVENTION

Excessive exposure to sunlight or other sources of UV radiation should be avoided, especially in fair-skinned individuals. UV radiation–screening lotions or creams and UV radiation–blocking sunglasses should be used when appropriate.

During significant exposure to sunlight, it is important to use a broad-spectrum sunscreen that provides protection from UVB as well as UVA. Standard recommendations are use of sunscreen with a sun protection factor (SPF) of 30, with reapplication at least every 2 hours. Likewise, sunglasses should be rated to block 99% or 100% of UVB and UVA radiation.

Radiofrequency Radiation

Radiofrequency radiations are also part of the non-ionizing electromagnetic spectrum (Fig. 20-4). Examples are radiation emitted from mobile phones (800 MHz to 2 GHz) and radiation from electric power lines (50/60 Hz). Biologic studies of low-level radiofrequency exposure have shown slightly increased heating but no increase in DNA damage.[14]

Numerous epidemiologic studies have focused on the effects of electric power lines. Although some early studies showed an association between the proximity of residence to high-voltage power lines and the risk for childhood leukemia, these early studies have generally not proved repeatable.[15] Likewise, numerous studies of a possible relationship between cell phone use and head or neck tumors have not shown a convincing link. A recently launched prospective European study will follow 290,000 adult cell phone users over a 20-year period.

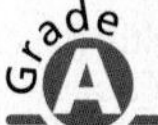

Grade A References

A1. Gu J, Zhu S, Li X, et al. Effect of amifostine in head and neck cancer patients treated with radiotherapy: a systematic review and meta-analysis based on randomized controlled trials. *PLoS ONE*. 2014;9:e95968.

A2. Le QT, Kim HE, Schneider CJ, et al. Palifermin reduces severe mucositis in definitive chemoradiotherapy of locally advanced head and neck cancer: a randomized, placebo-controlled study. *J Clin Oncol*. 2011;29:2808-2814.

GENERAL REFERENCES

For the General References and other additional features, please visit Expert Consult at https://expertconsult.inkling.com.

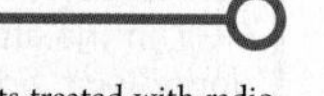

21 BIOTERRORISM

MARK G. KORTEPETER AND THEODORE J. CIESLAK

The likelihood that an individual physician would be called on to respond to a bioterror or biocrime incident is remote, but primary care physicians play critical roles as the point of entry into the medical system and as consultants for emergency services for any potential victims. Therefore, it is important for internal medicine physicians to be familiar with potential epidemiologic clues that an attack has occurred, general clinical aspects of agents considered to be the greatest threats, and how to alert the appropriate public health resources if they suspect an event.

HISTORY

Over centuries, biologic pathogens have repeatedly been used as weapons of warfare, ranging from tossing a dead animal carcass or feces into an adversary's water supply to releasing infectious agents by aerosol spraying.[1] Although biologic weapons can be used by governments as agents of warfare, a bigger concern now is their use by terrorists on civilian populations.

The opinions and assertions contained herein are the private views of the authors and are not to be construed as official or as necessarily reflecting the views of the Department of Defense, the United States Army, or the U.S. Government.

EPIDEMIOLOGIC CLUES

As with any other outbreak, the response to a potential act of bioterrorism relies on basic public health fundamentals. Although no single feature can be considered definitive, several features should raise the suspicion of an unnatural event (Table 21-1).

Victims of a chemical or conventional weapon release would likely become ill shortly after a release or explosion, whereas release of a biologic weapon would initially be silent because of its incubation period, with victims likely presenting for care in a delayed fashion to different care providers, dispersed in space and time. One way in which a bioterror attack might differ from a natural outbreak is in the unusual presentation of illness. For example, a disease that typically occurs on the skin or causes gastrointestinal illness might instead be manifested with respiratory features (e.g., anthrax, plague). Another clue could be illnesses that are unresponsive to standard therapies because of an unusual antibiotic sensitivity profile. Suspicion should also be raised by finding a disease outside the location or season in which it is typically found.

TABLE 21-1 EPIDEMIOLOGIC CLUES OF A BIOWEAPON ATTACK

A large outbreak with a similar disease or syndrome, especially in a discrete population
Many cases of unexplained diseases or deaths
More severe disease than expected for a specific pathogen or failure to respond to standard therapy
Unusual route of exposure for a pathogen, such as the inhalational route for diseases that normally occur through other exposures
A disease that is unusual for a given geographic area or transmission season, especially in the absence of a competent vector
Multiple simultaneous or serial epidemics
A single case of an uncommon agent (smallpox, some viral hemorrhagic fevers, inhalational anthrax, pneumonic plague)
Unusual strains or variants of organisms, or antimicrobial resistance patterns different from those known to be circulating
A similar or exact genetic type among agents isolated from distinct sources at different times or locations
Higher attack rates among those exposed in certain areas, such as inside a building after an indoor release, or lower rates in those inside a sealed building with an external release
Outbreaks of the same disease occurring simultaneously in noncontiguous areas
A zoonotic disease occurring in humans but not in animals
Direct evidence or intelligence of a release (equipment, munitions, tampering) or other potential vehicle of spread (spray device, contaminated letter)
A downwind pattern of casualty location

Modified from Dembek ZF, Alves DA, Cieslak TJ, et al. USAMRIID's Medical Management of Biological Casualties Handbook, 7th ed. September 2011. Found at www.usamriid.army.mil under reference materials tab. Accessed January 29, 2015.

AGENTS OF CONCERN

Among the myriad human infectious pathogens, a relatively small number possess the requisite properties to be considered potential weapons that could cause widespread disease, so-called weapons of mass destruction (Table 21-2). These agents typically remain stable in aerosol, which allows their relatively efficient spread, potentially over a large population.

ANTHRAX

EPIDEMIOLOGY

Anthrax, caused by infection with the gram-positive bacillus *Bacillus anthracis* (Chapter 294), is a worldwide scourge of herbivores. Most human cases have had direct contact with infected animals or their hides, hair, bone, or skins, although a recent outbreak occurred among injection drug users in the United Kingdom. Endemic areas tend to include underdeveloped parts of sub-Saharan Africa and Southeast Asia, where humans interact closely with animals that have not been vaccinated. Sporadic cases occur in the United States, typically along the trails of the historic cattle drives in the central plains. Animals are typically infected while grazing in areas contaminated with anthrax spores, which can survive in the soil for decades and are stable in a desiccated powder form. Although most cases worldwide are cutaneous, the spore form of the organism can be milled into the ideal particle size (2 to 6 μm) for infecting the lung and causing inhalational disease.

PATHOBIOLOGY AND CLINICAL MANIFESTATIONS

Exposure to spores can occur through a break in the skin, through the gastrointestinal tract, or by inhalation. Spores are taken up by macrophages and replicate in the local skin, or they can be transported to the regional lymph nodes in the gastrointestinal tract or lungs. While replicating, the bacilli secrete lethal toxin, which causes local necrosis, and edema toxin, which causes significant local edema. In untreated or unrecognized disease, the organism can cause bacteremia, systemic toxemia, and death.

Cutaneous anthrax can be readily recognized by the astute clinician on the basis of two clinical manifestations caused by its toxins: a black eschar, from which anthrax gets its name (from the Greek *anthrakis*, for coal), and surrounding edema that is out of proportion to the size of the lesion. The lesion starts as a papule that becomes a vesicle and eventually develops a central, black, necrotic area. Although this form of disease is readily treatable, it can lead to a 20% case-fatality rate if it is not recognized and treated appropriately. Gastrointestinal anthrax, which occurs after ingestion of infected, undercooked meat, is much more difficult to recognize and can have a case-fatality rate of 50% or more. Afflicted individuals develop fever, abdominal

TABLE 21-2 CENTERS FOR DISEASE CONTROL AND PREVENTION CATEGORY A BIOTERROR AGENTS

DISEASE (AND AGENT)	DIAGNOSTIC ASSOCIATIONS	WEAPONIZATION RATIONALE	TREATMENT (SEE TEXT FOR DETAIL)
Anthrax (*Bacillus anthracis*; Chapter 294)	Hemorrhagic mediastinitis	Highly lethal inhalational disease; stable spores survive desiccation; can be formulated as aerosol	Ciprofloxacin (400 mg IV q12h) or doxycycline (100 mg IV q12h) + clindamycin (600 mg IV q8h) + penicillin G (4 million units IV q4h)
Smallpox (variola virus; Chapter 372)	Synchronous exanthem	Virions stable in environment; population immunologically naïve	Supportive care; cidofovir and ST-246 are promising investigational drugs
Plague (*Yersinia pestis*; Chapter 312)	Hemoptysis	Contagious through respiratory droplets; "Black Death" conjures fear	Gentamicin (5 mg/kg IV qd) or ciprofloxacin (400 mg IV q12h) or doxycycline (100 mg IV q12h)
Tularemia (*Francisella tularensis*; Chapter 311)	Plague-like illness	Bacteria stable in environment; very low infectious dose	Same as for plague
Botulism (botulinum toxins; Chapter 296)	Descending, flaccid paralysis	Highly potent toxin; lends itself to food and water use; cases consume vast resources	Supportive care; ventilator support; botulinum antitoxin may halt (but will not reverse) symptom progression
Viral hemorrhagic fevers (Chapter 381; see Table 21-3)	Hemorrhagic diatheses	Fear factor is paramount; few countermeasures exist	Supportive care; ribavirin may be beneficial in select cases (e.g., Lassa fever, New World arenaviruses, Crimean-Congo hemorrhagic fever virus, hemorrhagic fever renal syndrome) when it is given under an experimental protocol: 30 mg/kg IV load, then 16 mg/kg q6h for 4 days, then 8 mg/kg q8h for 6 days

pain, diarrhea, hematochezia, hematemesis, and ascites. Paracentesis may yield hemorrhagic ascites.

Inhalational anthrax is of greatest concern after an aerosolized bioweapons attack. After an incubation period that averages 1 to 6 days but can be as long as 43 days, patients present with fever, profound drenching sweats, nausea, vomiting, diarrhea, shortness of breath, cough, and chest pain. Without prompt recognition and appropriate therapy, individuals can deteriorate rapidly with increasing dyspnea, stridor, cyanosis, and respiratory failure. Engorgement and hemorrhage of mediastinal lymph nodes with accompanying mediastinitis lead to the clinical hallmark of a widened mediastinum on the chest radiograph in about 60% of cases. Patients may also develop large hemorrhagic pleural effusions and infiltrates. Bacteremic dissemination can lead to widely metastatic infection in the gastrointestinal tract and meninges.

DIAGNOSIS

B. anthracis can be identified by Gram stain or culture of tissue or body fluids, including skin biopsy for cutaneous disease, peripheral blood, pleural effusions, and cerebrospinal fluid but not sputum. A chest radiograph may provide initial clues to inhalational disease with manifestations such as hilar or paratracheal fullness and pleural effusions. A chest computed tomography scan can confirm mediastinal adenopathy. Other techniques, such as fluorescent antibody staining or polymerase chain reaction (PCR), may provide more rapid diagnosis.

TREATMENT Rx

Antibiotics licensed for the treatment of inhalational anthrax include penicillin, ciprofloxacin, doxycycline, and levofloxacin, each for a total duration of 60 days (Table 21-2). After initial empirical therapy, antibiotic selection should be guided by sensitivity testing. In the 2001 outbreaks, patients who received more than one drug appeared to have better outcomes, so one of these drugs should be administered in combination with at least one other drug to which the organism is sensitive. Potential additional drugs include rifampin (300 to 600 mg orally once or twice daily), vancomycin (1 g or 15 mg/kg IV every 12 hours), ampicillin (2 g IV every 4 hours), chloramphenicol (500 mg IV or orally, every 6 hours), imipenem (1 g IV every 6 hours), clindamycin (600 mg IV every 8 hours), and clarithromycin (500 mg orally every 12 hours). Actual treatment doses and durations of combination therapy are based on clinical judgment or expert consultations.[2] A new monoclonal antibody, raxibacumab (single dose of 40 mg/kg IV during 2 hours and 15 minutes after premedicating with diphenhydramine 25 to 50 mg IV), is approved for additional therapy of inhalational anthrax along with antibiotics on the basis of animal efficacy data. Anthrax immune globulin remains an investigational product at this time.

PREVENTION

The anthrax vaccine, which is effective at preventing all forms of disease, has been reserved primarily for high-risk ranchers or veterinarians who have regular contact with herbivores, scientific personnel in research laboratories, and military personnel. The vaccine is now given as five doses intramuscularly during 18 months (day 0, followed by 1, 6, 12, and 18 months), with annual boosters if continued risk exists.

After a known exposure, chemoprophylaxis is recommended with ciprofloxacin (500 mg orally twice daily) or doxycycline (100 mg orally twice daily) for 60 days, although shorter durations are likely to be effective, especially if combined with vaccination. If the vaccine is available, three doses may be given concomitantly with antibiotics, but it is not licensed for this purpose and must be administered under an investigational protocol. Raxibacumab (dosed as before) is also approved for prophylaxis if antibiotics are not available.

PROGNOSIS

Factors associated with survival from anthrax include antibiotics or anthrax antiserum given during the prodromal phase, pleural fluid drainage, and a multiple drug regimen. Case-fatality rates in untreated patients approach 100%, although 55% of the victims of inhalation anthrax survived in a 2001 outbreak because of antibiotics and modern intensive care.

SMALLPOX

EPIDEMIOLOGY

Although smallpox was officially eradicated in 1980, concerns exist about undeclared stores outside approved repositories in the United States and Russia. The recent discoveries of unaccounted for vials of variola in the United States provide some credence to this concern. In addition to near-universal susceptibility, the environmental stability of smallpox viral particles makes it a formidable potential weapon.

Smallpox is caused by variola virus, an orthopoxvirus (Chapter 372) that is closely related to cowpox, vaccinia, and monkeypox. Variola generally spreads to household and other close contacts, but it can spread farther distances through aerosolized droplet nuclei as well as by direct contact with secretions of patients or fomites. Health care providers, who can be infected in the nosocomial setting, or unsuspecting individuals who have contact with contaminated objects are also at risk.

PATHOBIOLOGY AND CLINICAL MANIFESTATIONS

Infection initially occurs in the respiratory mucosa, followed by replication in the regional lymph nodes and then by an asymptomatic primary viremia that seeds the reticuloendothelial system. Approximately 1 week after infection (range, ~1 to 2 weeks), a secondary viremia seeds the skin. At this time, the sudden onset of illness includes fever, headache, backache, and vomiting. Within 2 or 3 days of this prodrome, and often as the temperature falls, the characteristic rash begins with small papules in a centrifugal pattern (more on the face and extremities than on the trunk) that progress in synchronous fashion during the next week to vesicles, umbilicated pustules, and finally scabs. Lesions are deep seated and can be intensely painful. Individuals are contagious at the onset of the rash and are considered to be free of contagion once the scabs have separated.

DIAGNOSIS

Chickenpox (varicella; Chapter 375), which can be confused with smallpox, occurs predominantly on the trunk rather than on the extremities (a centripetal pattern), and the lesions occur in successive crops, so macules, papules, pustules, and scabs can be seen simultaneously. In addition, varicella is transmissible before onset of the rash, but contagiousness abates when all the lesions are scabbed. Other diseases in the differential diagnosis of smallpox include monkeypox (Chapter 372), other poxviruses, disseminated vaccinia in a vaccine recipient or contact, disseminated herpes zoster (Chapter 375) or herpes simplex (Chapter 374), impetigo (Chapter 441), drug eruptions (Chapter 440), contact dermatitis (Chapter 438), erythema multiforme (Chapter 439), and rickettsialpox (Chapter 327).

Clinical recognition of the characteristic rash (Fig. 21-1) should raise suspicion of smallpox. Diagnosis would likely come from PCR or viral culture of skin or blood samples or from acute and convalescent serologies.

TREATMENT

The primary therapy for smallpox remains supportive care. Potential therapies include cidofovir (5 mg/kg IV; duration is determined on the basis of clinical response and potential side effects), a product licensed for treatment of cytomegalovirus retinitis in HIV-infected patients, and the investigational drug ST-246, which has been added to the strategic national stockpile for use in case of a smallpox outbreak.

PREVENTION

Vaccination uses vaccinia, an orthopoxvirus related to variola. In the event of an outbreak, postexposure vaccination within 4 days can prevent or ameliorate disease.[3] The U.S. government has stockpiled enough doses for the entire U.S. population of a newer, cell-cultured product for use in a national emergency. The surveillance and containment or ring vaccination method combines active case finding with vaccination of potential contacts within a certain radius around the cases. Health care providers would need to be vaccinated, and airborne and contact precautions (HEPA filter masks, negative-pressure rooms, gowns, gloves, eye protection) would be recommended in the hospital environment. Although there was an attempt to encourage health care providers to be vaccinated in the aftermath of the 2001 anthrax attacks, this effort was discontinued because of concerns about vaccine side effects, such as myocarditis, and skepticism about the true risk of an outbreak. Because the vaccine is a live agent, it is contraindicated in individuals with eczema or significant exfoliative skin conditions or immune compromise in the pre-exposure setting. Even in normal hosts, it can be associated with inoculation of other locations on the body, spread to close contacts, disseminated disease, postvaccine encephalitis, progressive vaccinia in individuals with defective cell-mediated immunity, eczema vaccinatum in people with prior eczema, and pericarditis or myocarditis. In the postexposure setting,

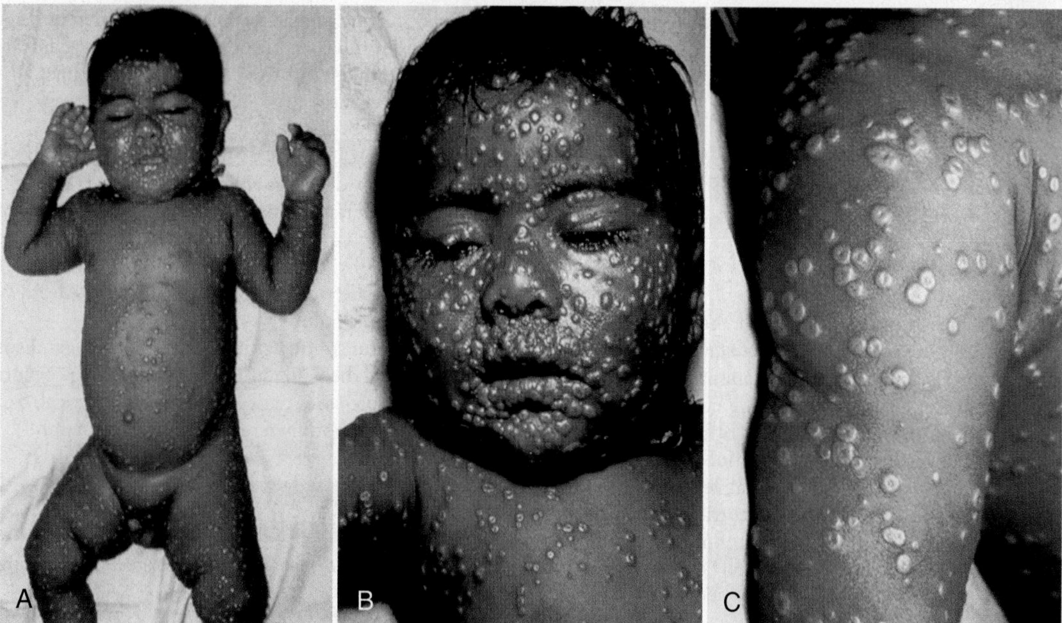

FIGURE 21-1. Smallpox. *A,* Demonstrates centrifugal nature of the rash. *B,* Demonstrates coalescences of some pustules. *C,* Demonstrates umbilicated pustules. (From Fenner F, Henderson DA, Arita A, et al. Smallpox and its eradication. Geneva: World Health Organization; 1988.)

risk benefits would have to be weighed regarding which individuals at risk for complications might receive vaccine and whether vaccinia immune globulin might be administered concomitantly. First-line therapy for significant vaccine reactions is vaccinia immune globulin.

PROGNOSIS

The case-fatality rate for the typical form of smallpox, known as variola major, is approximately 30%, but wide variations exist among races. In the minority of individuals who develop hemorrhagic smallpox or flat-type smallpox, the case-fatality rate approaches 100%. A different viral strain, variola minor, has case-fatality rates of only about 1%. Survivors of smallpox are often left with lifelong scarring from the lesions. Blindness and bone deformities, especially in children, are also known complications.

PLAGUE

EPIDEMIOLOGY

Plague was responsible for millions of deaths during three pandemics. Plague was used as a weapon by the Japanese before World War II when they released infected fleas in Chinese cities, and it was included in the former Soviet Union's biologic weapon arsenal. Plague is transmissible through the respiratory route, so an aerosol release could have devastating effects.

Plague is caused by the Gram-negative coccobacillus *Yersinia pestis* (Chapter 312). On light microscopy, the organism can have a bipolar appearance, making it look like a safety pin. In general, humans are infected during close proximity with rodents in areas where plague is enzootic or when their pets serve as vehicles for bringing infected fleas or the disease into their household. The "Black Death" of the 14th and 15th centuries owed much of its persistence to the ubiquitous presence of rats in homes and a lack of appreciation for their role in disease transmission.

Each year in the United States, several human cases are reported, usually in the Southwest. Most of these cases are bubonic, although occasional pneumonic plague is linked to infections in domestic cats.

PATHOBIOLOGY AND CLINICAL MANIFESTATIONS

Plague is manifested in three ways. Bubonic plague, which is the most common form, occurs after the bite of an infected flea. The organism spreads through the local lymphatics to the regional lymph nodes. As replication occurs, the lymph node or group of lymph nodes becomes swollen and extremely tender. As most flea bites occur on the lower extremities, the inguinal and femoral lymph nodes are most often affected. Untreated bubonic plague can progress to septicemic plague after organisms gain entry to the blood stream. In addition, patients can develop necrosis of cooler areas of the body, such as the tip of the nose, ears, or digits, as a result of a temperature-dependent coagulase produced by the organism. Septicemic plague may also occur in the absence of an antecedent bubo. Meningitis may occur from seeding through the blood stream. In pneumonic plague, the lungs are seeded secondarily by bacteremia from septicemic plague or primarily when a person inhales infected droplets. Although naturally occurring pneumonic plague is rare, this form of disease is the major concern after intentional aerosol release. In patients with pneumonic plague, viable organisms are found in the sputum, and the disease can then be spread to others. One of the hallmarks of the disease is the potential for purulent sputum to become hemorrhagic.

DIAGNOSIS

Plague bacilli are readily identified with Gram, Wright-Giemsa, or Wayson stains along with culture of the sputum or other infected body fluid, such as blood, fluid from a bubo, or cerebrospinal fluid. Other diagnostic methods include PCR for the F1 antigen, direct fluorescent antibody staining of body fluids, and serology by enzyme-linked immunosorbent assay or passive hemagglutination. However, serology is primarily useful in retrospect, because patients need to be treated empirically before a serologic response occurs.

TREATMENT

Rx

The historic drug of choice has been streptomycin (1 g IM twice daily for 7 to 10 days or for 3 days after the fever remits), but suitable alternatives include gentamicin (5 mg/kg IM or IV daily or a 2 mg/kg load followed by 1.7 mg IM or IV three times daily), doxycycline (200 mg IV load, then 100 mg IV every 12 hours), ciprofloxacin (400 mg IV every 12 hours), and levofloxacin (500 to 750 mg IV once daily) (Table 21-2). The drug of choice for plague meningitis is chloramphenicol (25 to 30 mg/kg IV load, followed by 50 to 60 mg/kg/day every 6 hours; on favorable clinical response, the dose can be reduced to 25 to 30 mg/kg/day every 6 hours).[4]

PREVENTION

Use of standard precautions is appropriate for bubonic plague. Droplet precautions should be applied for patients with pneumonic plague; this generally includes a private room where caregivers wear masks, gowns, gloves, and eye protection within 3 to 6 feet of the patients to minimize spread. These precautions should be continued until the patient demonstrates improvement and has been receiving effective antibiotics for 72 hours. Oral ciprofloxacin, levofloxacin, or doxycycline is recommended for postexposure prophylaxis of household contacts or individuals suspected of exposure in either the endemic or bioterrorism setting. Prophylaxis should continue for 7 days beyond the period of exposure.

No licensed vaccine for plague currently exists in the United States and a previously-licensed whole cell killed vaccine is no longer available. A new vaccine that uses the F1 and V antigens, which has demonstrated protection in animals against aerosol challenge, is being developed by the Department of Defense and is currently undergoing phase II testing.

PROGNOSIS

Case-fatality rates are 50% or more for untreated bubonic plague and nearly 100% for untreated septicemic and pneumonic plague. These fatality rates can be significantly reduced with prompt recognition and appropriate therapy.

TULAREMIA

Tularemia (Chapter 311) is caused by infection with the Gram-negative, aerobic nonmotile coccobacillary organism *Francisella tularensis*.[5] A zoonotic disease of rabbits, ground squirrels, and other small mammals, tularemia can be acquired by humans by skin or mucous membrane contact with body fluids or tissues of infected animals or from being bitten by infected deerflies, mosquitoes, or ticks. Disease can rarely occur by inhalation of contaminated dusts or ingestion of contaminated food or water. Relatively uncommon in the United States, fewer than 150 cases of naturally occurring human tularemia are typically reported each year. However, the environmental stability of *F. tularensis* as well as its very low infectious dose (as few as 10 organisms) makes it a potential weaponization threat.

CLINICAL MANIFESTATIONS AND DIAGNOSIS

Clinical manifestations of tularemia depend on the route of exposure. Although six different forms (glandular, oculoglandular, ulceroglandular, pharyngeal, pneumonic, and typhoidal) have been described, tularemia is perhaps more simplistically compared with plague, with glandular forms analogous to bubonic plague as well as pneumonic and typhoidal forms that present a clinical picture similar to what is seen in pneumonic and septicemic plague. A preponderance of these latter forms would be expected after an intentional release by aerosol. After an incubation period of 2 to 10 days, symptoms begin with fever and proceed to include severe exhaustion, substernal chest pain, nonproductive cough, and weight loss.

Diagnosis, which requires isolation of the organism in blood, sputum, skin, or mucus membrane lesions, may be difficult because of unusual growth requirements and overgrowth of commensal organisms. Therefore, serology is the mainstay of diagnosis, often in retrospect. Because of the risk of spread to microbiology laboratory personnel, it is important to notify the laboratory if infection with this organism is suspected.

TREATMENT AND PROGNOSIS Rx

Treatment of tularemia is similar to that of plague, with aminoglycosides for 10 to 14 days; streptomycin and gentamicin are considered the drugs of choice, although ciprofloxacin is a newer potential alternative (Table 21-2). Doxycycline/tetracycline and chloramphenicol are second-line choices because their use has been associated with relapses, and the recommended duration of therapy is 14 to 21 days.

Person-to-person spread is unusual, and standard precautions are adequate in caring for ill individuals. For known exposures, prophylaxis with tetracycline (500 mg orally four times a day for 2 weeks) is effective if it is begun within 24 hours of exposure; consensus recommendations in a bioterrorism setting are doxycycline 100 mg or ciprofloxacin 500 mg orally twice a day as postexposure prophylaxis.[6] A live attenuated vaccine has proven efficacy in preventing disease due to laboratory exposures and aerosol challenge in human volunteers, but it is not readily available to the public.

The case-fatality rate for untreated pneumonic and typhoidal tularemia is 35%, but this rate can be reduced to less than 5% with appropriate treatment.

BOTULISM

Botulism is caused by exposure to one of eight related neurotoxins (A to H) produced by certain strains of *Clostridium botulinum* (Chapter 296), a ubiquitous anaerobic spore-forming Gram-positive bacillus.[7] Botulinum toxins, which are among the most toxic substances known, can be lethal in doses as low as 0.001 μg/kg. These toxins, which act at presynaptic nerve terminals, block the release of acetylcholine, thereby resulting in a generalized flaccid paralysis with autonomic dysfunction. Although most toxins are unstable in the environment and thus constitute dubious weaponization threats, the potent nature of botulinum toxin, coupled with the ease with which it might be used to contaminate food and water, makes it an agent of concern. Naturally occurring human botulism is limited to types A, B, and E, although other toxin serotypes can produce an identical clinical syndrome. For this reason, a heptavalent antitoxin with activity against all seven serotypes has been licensed recently.

CLINICAL MANIFESTATIONS AND DIAGNOSIS

Botulism typically develops after a latent period ranging from hours to several days. Initial manifestations involve bulbar palsies, ptosis, photophobia, blurred vision, and other signs of cranial nerve dysfunction. Symptoms progress craniocaudally, leading to dysphonia, dysphagia, and, ultimately, a descending symmetrical paralysis. In fatal cases, death typically results from respiratory muscle failure.

Although botulism may mimic other neurologic disorders, such as myasthenia gravis and the Guillain-Barré syndrome, the occurrence of an outbreak involving multiple cases of descending, symmetrical, flaccid paralysis should make diagnosis of botulism relatively straightforward.

TREATMENT AND PROGNOSIS Rx

Supportive care measures plus antitoxin, including meticulous attention to ventilatory support, are the mainstay of botulism management. Patients may require such support for several months, so the management of a large-scale botulism outbreak would be especially problematic in terms of medical resources. Botulism is not contagious, so standard precautions are adequate in managing botulism victims. The first victims of an outbreak may have higher case-fatality rates because of delays in recognition. Those who recover can have long-term sequelae, such as dyspnea on exertion, fatigue, and weakness.

VIRAL HEMORRHAGIC FEVERS

EPIDEMIOLOGY

Viral hemorrhagic fever (Chapter 381) is a term used to describe the clinical syndrome caused by four families of RNA viruses: filoviruses (Ebola and Marburg), arenaviruses ("Old World" Lassa fever and "New World" South American viruses, Machupo, Junin, and others), bunyaviruses (hantaviruses, Crimean Congo hemorrhagic fever, and Rift Valley fever), and flaviviruses (yellow fever and dengue) (Table 21-3).[8] Agents of greatest concern from a bioterrorism perspective include the filoviruses and arenaviruses, which are infectious by the aerosol route and can replicate well in cell culture for large-scale production and whose clinical syndrome of hemorrhage and fever engenders fear. The massive outbreak of Ebola virus disease in West Africa in 2014 demonstrates the devastation that a hemorrhagic fever virus can have on a population, even in the absence of bioterrorism, especially when the medical infrastructure is sub-optimal.[9]

PATHOBIOLOGY AND CLINICAL MANIFESTATIONS

Once virus gains entry through the skin, mucous membranes, or respiratory tract, replication occurs in macrophages and dendritic cells. Organisms are then transported to regional lymph nodes and eventually through the lymphatics and blood stream to target organs, such as the liver and spleen, where local necrosis occurs. The body responds with activation of cytokines and chemokines, and massive depletion of lymphocytes disables the host's adaptive immune response. A sepsis-like picture ensues, with declining mean arterial pressure, increased vascular permeability, and a bleeding diathesis.

Clinical features of the hemorrhagic fevers include the acute onset of malaise, sore throat, fever, skin flushing, conjunctival injection, prostration, myalgias, and nonbloody diarrhea. These viruses have significant differences in the prominence of individual clinical findings. For example, dengue, the filoviruses, and Lassa more commonly cause a maculopapular rash in the first week. The filoviruses and South American viruses more typically cause obtundation and encephalitis. Although all of these produce modest elevations of aminotransferase levels, yellow fever and Rift Valley fever are known for causing significant hepatic dysfunction, thereby resulting in icterus and jaundice. Depending on a number of factors, including virulence, route of exposure, inoculum, and other host factors, illness can progress in the second week to overt signs of bleeding, including petechiae, purpura, ecchymoses, and oozing from venipuncture sites. If massive bleeding occurs, the source is usually the gastrointestinal tract. Severe cases will demonstrate a combination of neurologic and hematologic abnormalities.

TABLE 21-3 COMPARISON OF VIRAL HEMORRHAGIC FEVER AGENTS[4]

FAMILY	VIRUS	ENDEMIC AREA	FATALITY RATE	NOSOCOMIAL TRANSMISSION	COUNTERMEASURES
Filoviruses	Ebola	Africa, Philippines (Reston)	50-90% (Sudan/Zaire)	Yes	Anecdotal success with immune plasma; monoclonal antibodies demonstrate benefit after disease onset
	Marburg	Africa	23-70%	Yes	
Arenaviruses	Lassa	West Africa	1-2%	Yes	Ribavirin effective in a clinical trial with nonrandomized controls
	Junin	Argentine Pampas	30%	Rare	Immune plasma; reports of benefit with ribavirin; Candid 1 vaccine protective; not available in the United States
	Machupo	Bolivia	25-35%	Rare	Immune plasma; reports of benefit with ribavirin
Bunyaviruses	Crimean-Congo hemorrhagic fever	Africa, southeast Europe, Central Asia, India	30%	Yes	Anecdotal success with ribavirin treatment
	Rift Valley fever	Africa	<0.5%	No	Livestock vaccines in Africa; U.S. Department of Defense has two experimental vaccines
	Hantaviruses	Europe, Asia, South America (rare)	5% (Asian hemorrhagic fever with renal syndrome)	No*	Vaccines available in Asia; ribavirin effective in randomized trial but not licensed for that purpose
Flaviviruses	Yellow fever	Africa, South America	3-12%,(20-50% if second phase develops)	No	17D live attenuated vaccine
	Kyasanur Forest	Southern India	3-5%	No	Formalin-inactivated vaccine in India
	Omsk	Siberia	0.2-3%	No	Tick-borne encephalitis vaccines (not in United States) may offer some cross protection

*Exception is Andes, which causes hantavirus pulmonary syndrome (not addressed in this chapter).

DIAGNOSIS

Numerous more common diseases should be considered in the differential diagnosis of a viral hemorrhagic fever, including rickettsial infections (Rocky Mountain spotted fever, ehrlichia, anaplasma, and African tick typhus; Chapter 327), leptospirosis (Chapter 323), meningococcemia (Chapter 298), typhoid (Chapter 308), and falciparum malaria (Chapter 345). However, a viral hemorrhagic fever should be considered in patients who present with a clinically compatible syndrome, especially if a cluster of cases is seen. Laboratory features may include thrombocytopenia, elevated aminotransferase levels, leukopenia, anemia (although an elevated hematocrit may be seen in patients who have significant vascular leakage, as is sometimes seen with dengue and hantaviruses), hematuria, and proteinuria. PCR, viral culture, immunoglobulin M–specific enzyme-linked immunosorbent assay, acute and convalescent serology, or immunohistochemistry on autopsy specimens can establish the diagnosis. Routine clinical specimens and any attempt at viral isolation require a biosafety level 3 or 4 laboratory with expert consultation from the Centers for Disease Control and Prevention or the U.S. Army Medical Research Institute of Infectious Diseases.

TREATMENT Rx

No licensed therapies exist for the viral hemorrhagic fevers, so supportive care is the primary means of management with close attention to fluid status, avoidance of procedures that cause bleeding and medications that impair platelet function, use of blood products as necessary, use of vasopressors for hypotension, and dialysis for renal failure. Close attention to fluid status has significantly reduced mortality from dengue, and aggressive fluid repletion has been needed to address significant loss of fluid volume due to diarrhea, electrolyte abnormalities, and protein/nutritional depletion in Ebola infections.[10] Oral ribavirin or intravenous ribavirin (see Table 21-2) under an approved experimental protocol can reduce mortality in Lassa hemorrhagic fever, and it also appears to be beneficial against Argentine hemorrhagic fever (Junin virus) and hantaviruses that cause hemorrhagic fever with renal syndrome. It has no apparent efficacy against filoviruses (Ebola or Marburg) or flaviviruses (dengue, yellow fever). Monoclonal antibodies are a potentially promising option for Ebola virus.[11]

PREVENTION

Yellow fever vaccine is the only licensed vaccine against a viral hemorrhagic fever in the United States. Experimental vaccines exist against Junin virus and Rift Valley fever virus, but these vaccines have been used primarily to protect laboratory workers.

Certain viral hemorrhagic fevers (primarily Ebola, Marburg, Lassa, and Crimean-Congo hemorrhagic fever) produce high-level viremia during the period of greatest bleeding risk, thereby making them notorious for causing nosocomial outbreaks. In general, these outbreaks occur in environments, such as sub-Saharan Africa, where basic infection control practices are inadequate because of limited resources (e.g., lack of gowns, gloves, and eye protection as well as reuse of unsterilized needles and syringes). Spread of these viruses in the nosocomial environment can be significantly reduced with standard precautions that limit contact with blood and body fluids. In caring for patients at higher risk of spread (those who are coughing, vomiting, or hemorrhaging), enhanced precautions are recommended, using negative-pressure isolation and N-100 masks along with gowns, gloves, and eye protection. Even with these precautions, the infection of two nurses in Dallas in 2014 from a severely ill patient demonstrates the challenge of doing this right, as there is little room for error.

PROGNOSIS

Hemorrhagic viruses exhibit a wide range of mortality rates, ranging from less than 1% with Rift Valley fever to 80 to 90% with Ebola Zaire (Table 21-3). Despite the notoriety of these viruses for causing hemorrhage, the majority of individuals do not die of blood loss. Rather, death results from a sepsis-like picture, including a loss of vascular hemostasis, disseminated intravascular coagulation, hypotension, renal failure, shock, and death.

RESPONSE TO A BIOTERRORISM ATTACK

Even a relatively small bioterror event can have profound consequences. After the 2001 anthrax mailings, thousands of people were prescribed antibiotic prophylaxis, and government buildings were closed for decontamination. Since that event, significant improvements in future responses to a bioterrorism event include the licensure, manufacture, and storage of enough smallpox vaccine for everyone in the United States, production of anthrax and botulinum antitoxins for the strategic national stockpile, and development of protocols and authority for response. However, no country has yet achieved the ability to detect a pathogen release reliably in real time.[12] The 2014 Ebola outbreak also has identified shortcomings in preparedness in the U.S.

In any future bioterror attack, early warning signs might include clusters of patients with mediastinal adenopathy or widened mediastinum on the chest radiograph, a centrifugal pustular rash (smallpox), pneumonia and hemoptysis (plague), descending flaccid paralysis (botulism), or hemorrhagic manifestations and impaired clotting (viral hemorrhagic fever). Should such a cluster be identified or suspected, physicians should contact the local county or city health department, the state health department, and potentially the Centers for Disease Control and Prevention. Unlike a natural outbreak, a potential bioterror outbreak also requires a rapid dialogue between public health and law enforcement authorities, in part because patient and environmental samples constitute evidence against a perpetrator and must be handled under chain of custody. Physicians also must be prepared not only to protect themselves and their patients but also to serve as community resources, regardless of whether an outbreak is natural or terrorist in origin.

GENERAL REFERENCES

For the General References and other additional features, please visit Expert Consult at https://expertconsult.inkling.com.

22

CHRONIC POISONING: TRACE METALS AND OTHERS

LOUISE W. KAO AND DANIEL E. RUSYNIAK

About 80% of the elements in the periodic table are metals or metalloids, and various metals are in contact with humans in the home, workplace, and environment. Metals are part of a number of normal physiologic processes, such as iron in hemoglobin, but also can cause a number of toxic adverse effects.[1]

LEAD TOXICITY

EPIDEMIOLOGY

Lead (Pb) is a silver-gray, malleable metal that is resistant to corrosion. It has no known physiologic use, so any lead in the human body should be considered contamination.

The most common sources of lead poisoning are lead-based paints, lead-contaminated dust in older buildings, and lead-contaminated soil. Other sources include plumbing, solder, batteries, bullets, toys, curtain weights, necklace charms, food containers, and cosmetics, including Nigerian eyeliners. Adults in occupations such as battery manufacturing, welding, construction, mining, glass blowing, and shipbuilding have the highest lead exposures. Other less common but important routes of exposure include lead-contaminated moonshine and lead-containing ethnic folk remedies (e.g., greta and azarcon in Mexico).

Children in lower socioeconomic areas have the highest exposures to lead, and the majority of the scientific literature is biased toward pediatric studies. Much of what we have learned, however, is applicable to adults.

PATHOBIOLOGY

Lead's most devastating effects are on the central nervous system (CNS) of children. By disrupting the intracellular junction of capillary endothelium, lead impairs the blood-brain barrier, which further increases CNS absorption. Lead also increases capillary leak, which in severe cases can result in cerebral edema.

Lead inhibits several enzymes involved in heme synthesis: aminolevulinic acid synthetase, δ-aminolevulinic acid dehydratase, coproporphyrinogen decarboxylase, and ferrochelatase. Lead also inhibits the enzyme erythrocyte pyrimidine-5-nucleotidase, which impairs RNA degradation and contributes to red cell hemolysis. Collectively, the inhibition of these enzymes results in decreased concentrations of hemoglobin and a shorter life span of red blood cells.

By depositing lead-protein complexes in renal proximal tubular cells, lead interferes with normal mitochondrial function, thereby resulting in decreased reabsorption of glucose, amino acid, and phosphate. Chronically exposed persons can develop renal failure from tubular atrophy, interstitial fibrosis, and glomerular sclerosis.

Although lead has not been associated with specific bone-related disorders, the skeletal system serves as the main reservoir for lead; with chronic exposure, lead stores in bone can have a half-life of 5 to 19 years. As a result, soft tissues may be subjected to increased lead exposure during times of accelerated bone turnover, such as during childhood growth, after a long bone fracture, or during pregnancy.

CLINICAL MANIFESTATIONS

Lead poisoning can be subtle and difficult to diagnose because many of its historical clinical associations (e.g., neuropathy, gout, abdominal colic) are rarely seen today. In children, the most concerning long-term complications of environmental lead exposure are developmental cognitive deficits, especially when lead concentrations in young children exceed 100 μg/dL. Subacute neurologic problems include ataxia, lethargy, seizures, and coma. Adults can also experience severe neurologic symptoms (e.g., seizures and cerebral edema) with plumbism, but typically only when whole blood lead levels are higher than 150 μg/dL. More commonly, the neurologic problems caused by lead in adults are manifested as memory problems, insomnia, depression, and personality changes.

Other clinical effects of lead poisoning, in both children and adults, include a normocytic or microcytic anemia, abdominal pain, hepatotoxicity, and pancreatitis. The classic finding of peripheral neuropathy with footdrop and wristdrop is well described in adults but only occasionally seen in children. Nephrotoxicity most commonly is manifested as Fanconi syndrome (Chapter 128) with aminoaciduria, glycosuria, and phosphaturia. A consequence of this toxicity is impaired uric acid clearance and gout.[2] High lead levels also probably increase the risk of hypertension.

DIAGNOSIS

Diagnosis of lead intoxication involves a high level of suspicion. The best initial test is a whole blood lead level collected in a certified lead-free tube (Table 22-1). The blood lead level can be falsely elevated in individuals who have received chelation therapy, which mobilizes tissue lead stores, in the prior 7 days.

Radiographic imaging can support the diagnosis of lead poisoning and sometimes detect a lead-containing object or a retained bullet. Bone x-ray fluorescence technology can estimate bone lead levels, which can reflect chronic lead exposure, but this test is mostly a research tool and is not commonly available in clinical practice.

TREATMENT Rx

The first step in management of patients with elevated lead levels is prompt removal of the source, although the effectiveness of environmental cleanup and educational initiatives is disappointing.[A1] If lead comes from a work-related source, the Occupational Safety and Health Administration should be contacted. Chelation increases excretion of lead in a 24-hour urine sample and thereby decreases blood concentrations, but studies to date with the chelating agent succimer (2,3-dimercaptosuccinic acid, DMSA) in children have not shown improved neuropsychological function[3,4,A2] despite success in reducing blood lead levels. The current recommendation is that asymptomatic adults with blood lead levels of less than 70 μg/dL do not require chelation, patients with mild symptoms or blood lead levels between 70 and 100 μg/dL should receive only oral chelation, and patients with lead-induced encephalopathy or blood lead levels above 100 μg/dL should be considered for parenteral chelation. Although DMSA is approved by the Food and Drug Administration only for children, it also is commonly used in adults (Table 22-2).

Whole bowel irrigation with a polyethylene glycol–electrolyte solution should be considered if a patient has retained a gastrointestinal lead object. Patients who have lead-containing bullet fragments lodged in soft tissues or joint spaces may need to have them surgically removed.

PROGNOSIS

Despite controversy about long-term recovery from lead-associated cognitive deficits in children, adults with neurologic symptoms improve with removal of the exposure. The hematologic and nephrotoxic effects of lead also are reversible.

MERCURY TOXICITY

EPIDEMIOLOGY

Mercury (Hg) is a naturally occurring metal with three distinct forms. Although all forms are neurotoxic, elemental mercury (Hg^0) also causes pulmonary toxicity, inorganic mercury (Hg^+ or Hg^{++}) causes gastrointestinal and renal toxicity, and organic mercury (ethyl, methyl, alkyl, or phenyl) is a teratogen.

Elemental mercury is found in dental amalgams, thermometers, fluorescent lamps, batteries, and some paints. Occupational exposures may occur in dentists and dental hygienists, painters, gold extractors, bronzers, electroplaters, metallurgists, paper pulp manufacturers, miners, ceramic workers, and other workers who use mercury in processing. Mercury thermometers are becoming increasingly rare, and many countries have banned them because of potential mercury toxicity. Toxicity from elemental mercury is caused primarily from breathing its volatilized vapor.

Inorganic mercury has been used historically as a medicinal, cosmetic, and topical antiseptic in the forms of HgCl (calomel) and $HgCl_2$ (mercuric chloride). It is also used in the tanning industry, in taxidermy, in manufacturing of fireworks, and in dye manufacturing. Inorganic mercury may also be found in patent medicines, folk remedies (such as empacho among Mexican Americans), skin lightening creams, and Asian herbal remedies. Toxicity may occur from ingestion, inhalation, or dermal absorption.

Organic mercury compounds can be classified as short-chain alkyl (such as methylmercury), long-chain alkyl, and aryl compounds. The aryl compounds, such as thimerosal, behave like inorganic mercurial compounds. Methyl mercury has caused several large-scale human poisoning epidemics.

Soil and marine organisms methylate inorganic mercury from the air and industrial waste. Through a process known as bioamplification, methyl mercury concentrates in the tissues of marine life, reaching highest concentrations in large predatory fish such as tuna and swordfish. Fish consumption is now the largest route of organic mercury exposure in the general population. Organic mercury is also used as a fungicide, pesticide, wood preservative, and medicinal antiseptic or preservative (Mercurochrome and thimerosal). Toxicity is typically by ingestion.

TABLE 22-1 DIAGNOSTIC TESTING FOR METALS: REFERENCE RANGES

METAL	SERUM LEVEL	WHOLE BLOOD LEVEL	SPOT URINE	24-HOUR URINE
Lead		<10 µg/dL		
Mercury		<10 µg/L	<20 µg/L	<5 µg/g creatinine
Arsenic		<5 µg/L		<50 µg/L or <100 µg/g creatinine
Cadmium		<5 µg/L		<3 µg/g creatinine
Aluminum	<2 µg/L	<12 µg/L		4-12 µg/g creatinine
Bismuth	<1 µg/dL	<5 µg/dL	<20 µg/L	
Cobalt	0.1-1.2 µg/L		0.1-2.2 µg/L	
Manganese	0.9-2.9 µg/L	4-15 µg/L		<10 µg/L
Silver	<1 µg/L			<2 µg/L
Thallium		<2 µg/L		<5 µg/L
Zinc	109-130 µg/dL	600-1000 µg/dL		<500 µg/day

Modified from Nelson L, Goldfrank LR. Goldfrank's Toxicologic Emergencies. 9th ed. New York: McGraw-Hill Medical; 2011.

PATHOBIOLOGY

The pathophysiology of mercury poisoning is related to its disruption of cell physiology by binding to sulfhydryl, phosphoryl, carboxyl, and amide groups, thereby causing widespread dysfunction of normal cellular mechanisms. Each type of mercury causes differential effects depending on its route of exposure, solubility, and lipophilicity.

Elemental mercury is poorly absorbed by ingestion. If gastrointestinal motility or mucosal integrity is compromised, however, elemental mercury

TABLE 22-2 CHELATORS FOR ADULT HEAVY METAL POISONING

SYMPTOMS	CHELATOR	RECOMMENDED DOSE†	ADVERSE EFFECTS
LEAD			
Asymptomatic, BLL* < 70	None		
Mild-moderate, BLL 70-00	DMSA	10 mg/kg tid PO × 5 days, then bid for 14 days	Nausea, vomiting, diarrhea; mild elevations in aminotransferase levels
Encephalopathy, BLL > 100	BAL +	4 mg/kg deep IM q 4 h × 5days	Local injection site (pain, redness, sterile abscess); nausea, vomiting, diarrhea; anxiety, hypertension, tachycardia, fever; contraindicated in peanut allergy
	$CaNa_2EDTA$‡	1500 mg/m²/day (approximately 50-75 mg/kg/day) either continuous infusion or in 2-4 divided IV doses for 5 days	Renal toxicity (from metal chelate), constitutional symptoms, transient hypotension
MERCURY			
Acute (elemental or inorganic) with moderate/severe symptoms	BAL	5 mg/kg deep IM then 2.5 mg/kg every 12-24 hours for 10 days or until symptoms improve and patient is able to take PO	Local injection site (pain, redness, sterile abscess); nausea, vomiting, diarrhea; anxiety, hypertension, tachycardia, fever; contraindicated in peanut allergy
Chronic (elemental or inorganic) or organic with symptoms	DMSA	10 mg/kg tid PO × 5 days, then bid for 14 days	Nausea, vomiting, diarrhea, mild elevations in aminotransferase levels
ARSENIC			
Acute exposure with moderate to severe symptoms	BAL	3 mg/kg deep IM q 4 h × 2 days, then bid for 7 to 10 days	Local injection site (pain, redness, sterile abscess); nausea, vomiting, diarrhea; anxiety, hypertension, tachycardia, fever; contraindicated in peanut allergy
Chronic exposure with moderate symptoms§	DMSA	10 mg/kg tid PO × 5 days, then bid for 14 days	Nausea, vomiting, diarrhea, mild elevations in aminotransferase levels
ALUMINUM			
Acute or chronic exposure in dialysis patient with encephalopathy	Deferoxamine	See *http://www2.kidney.org/professionals/kdoqi/guidelines_bone/Guide12.htm*	Hypotension, increased risk of sepsis, acute lung injury
THALLIUM			
Acute thallium poisoning with moderate to severe symptoms	Prussian Blue	3 g tid PO until the urinary thallium excretion is less than 0.5 mg/day	Constipation, blue stool

*Adult recommendations.
†Chelation doses in general are not well studied or validated, with the exception of lead in children. Optimal dosing is not well established, particularly for BAL. Doses listed are author's suggestions.
‡Start 4 hours after first dose of BAL is administered.
§Benefit in this setting is not established.
BAL = British anti-Lewisite, dimercaprol; BLL = blood lead level; DMSA = 2,3-dimercaptosuccinic acid; succimer; EDTA = ethylenediaminetetraacetic acid.

may ionize into more readily absorbed forms. Elemental mercury toxicity occurs primarily by inhalation of the vapor into the alveoli, where it is well absorbed in the pulmonary circulation and readily crosses the blood-brain barrier. In the brain, it interferes with multiple cellular processes, including protein and nucleic acid synthesis. Mercury also inhibits catechol-*O*-methyltransferase, thereby elevating circulating catecholamine levels.

Inorganic mercury is absorbed after ingestion, initially binds the gastrointestinal mucosa, and accumulates in the kidneys, where it exerts direct oxidative damage. Although it does not readily cross the blood-brain barrier, CNS toxicity can be seen with chronic exposures because of the prolonged elimination rate. Mercuric ions do not appear to cross the placental barrier.

Organic mercury compounds are readily absorbed after ingestion and inhalation and are moderately absorbed after dermal exposure, particularly if skin is not intact. Owing to its high lipid solubility, organic mercury crosses the blood-brain barrier and concentrates in the CNS. It can also cross the placental barrier and concentrate in the fetus. Organic mercury concentrates in red blood cells, distributes throughout the body, and is primarily eliminated in the feces. Some forms of organic mercury are metabolized in the body to inorganic mercury compounds. Toxicity results from its inhibition of enzyme systems and interference with cellular maturity, microtubule function, and neurotransmitter synthesis and uptake.

CLINICAL MANIFESTATIONS

The manifestations of elemental mercury toxicity vary depending on the dose and chronicity of the exposure.[5] Inhalation of high concentrations of mercury vapor, as may occur in an industrial setting, may result in cough, chills, fever, and shortness of breath. Nausea, vomiting, and weakness may result. This syndrome may progress to a severe acute lung injury and respiratory as well as renal failure. Chronic exposure to lower concentrations of mercury vapor produces a classic triad of tremor, gingivostomatitis, and neuropsychiatric disturbances. The mercurial tremor may be both static and intentional. Sudden episodic bursts of tremor, also called tetanus mercurialis, have been described. Neuropsychiatric manifestations of mercury poisoning, also known as erethism, include fatigue, insomnia, memory dysfunction, social withdrawal, shyness, and depression.

Inorganic mercury poisoning can occur after dermal or mucosal absorption of mercury-containing cosmetics and teething powders as well as after accidental or intentional ingestion of mercuric chloride antiseptics. After acute ingestion, a hemorrhagic gastroenteritis is typically followed by renal failure from acute tubular necrosis. Chronic exposure is associated with erethism, renal dysfunction, and neurologic manifestations such as sensorimotor neuropathy, constriction of visual fields, tremor, and delirium. Acrodynia, or pink disease, has been described after elemental or inorganic mercury exposure, most notably in children after exposure to mercurial teething powder and diaper ointment. This syndrome is manifested as an erythematous, hyperkeratotic, often desquamating rash on the palms, soles, and face in conjunction with a papular rash. Acrodynia is also associated with an idiosyncratic hypersensitivity to mercury ions and mercury poisoning, which itself can increase circulating catecholamines and mimic pheochromocytoma (Chapter 228). Common findings include tremor, diaphoresis, tachycardia, and hypertension.

Human toxicity from organic mercury was first recognized when the dumping of mercury-containing waste into Minamata Bay in Japan led to a large-scale poisoning of the population, whose primary dietary staple was fish from the bay. In what is now called Minamata disease, patients presented with paresthesia, ataxia, dysarthria, tremor, and constriction of visual fields or "tunnel vision." These symptoms can be progressive and sometimes fatal. Children born to exposed mothers (congenital Minamata disease) suffer mental retardation, limb deformities, chorea, seizures, and microcephaly.

With organic mercury toxicity, symptoms are typically delayed for weeks to months. Other symptoms that follow organic mercury poisoning include mucous membrane irritation after ingestion and dermatitis after cutaneous exposure. However, no cardiovascular toxicities have been reported with up to moderate elevation in blood mercury levels.[6]

DIAGNOSIS

The diagnosis of mercury poisoning should be considered on recognition of the characteristic signs and symptoms coupled with a known or suspected exposure. Whole blood and urine mercury levels can confirm the exposure, but the correlation between levels and symptoms is inconsistent. In the setting of elemental mercury ingestion or injection, radiographs may also be useful. In a nonoccupationally exposed patient, whole blood mercury concentration should not exceed 10 μg/L, and a 24-hour urine mercury concentration should not exceed 20 μg/L (Table 22-1); urine must be collected in an acid-washed container. In general, urine concentrations are more reliable for monitoring of exposure and the response to therapy, but whole blood concentration is the preferred monitoring test for methyl mercury poisoning. The ratio of red blood cell to plasma mercury can differentiate organic mercury toxicity from inorganic mercury toxicity because organic mercury concentrates significantly in red blood cells. Hair analysis is unreliable because of the potential for external contamination. The practice of obtaining urine mercury levels after a chelation challenge is not recommended because levels obtained in this way are difficult to interpret.

TREATMENT Rx

Treatment is primarily symptomatic and supportive, with removal from the source of exposure. In cases of acute exposure, decontamination may be required. In cases of occupational or environmental exposure, environmental decontamination and surveillance by local or federal agencies may be necessary. After inhalation of elemental mercury vapor, support of respiratory function is crucial. After ingestion of inorganic mercury salts, fluid resuscitation, usually with normal saline, is needed to correct intravascular depletion, and renal replacement therapy may be required in cases of oliguric renal failure. Mercury compounds are poorly cleared by extracorporeal elimination measures, such as hemodialysis or peritoneal dialysis.

If dietary fish is the likely cause of an elevated mercury level, affected individuals should avoid eating any fish or shellfish for 1 month, after which blood or urine mercury levels should be reanalyzed. If mercury levels have declined into the normal range, as is usually the case, low-mercury fish (shrimp, canned light tuna, salmon, pollock, catfish) can be reintroduced into the diet at a frequency of no more than two meals per week.

Chelation therapy will increase urinary elimination of mercury (Table 22-2), and limited clinical data support its use early after acute poisonings. Oral DMSA, which is the chelator of choice, is generally well tolerated. If oral administration is not possible, dimercaprol (British anti-Lewisite, BAL) can be used except after methyl mercury exposure, in which it is contraindicated because it may shift mercury into the brain.

PROGNOSIS

The neurotoxicity that follows significant poisoning from all types of mercury may be irreversible, particularly in the setting of organic mercury poisoning, in which the diagnosis is often delayed. Nevertheless, 33 of 40 symptomatic children affected in the contaminated grain outbreak of 1971 in Iraq improved during a 2-year observation period. Acute renal failure after elemental or inorganic mercury poisoning can sometimes resolve. Patients with acrodynia have been reported to recover completely after chelation therapy and removal of the exposure.

ARSENIC TOXICITY

EPIDEMIOLOGY

Arsenic (As), which is found in soil, minerals, rocks, and metal ores, is present in all living organisms. It exists in several forms: elemental, inorganic (As^{3+} trivalent arsenite and As^{5+} pentavalent arsenate), gaseous (arsine, AsH^3), and organic. Elemental and organic arsenic have low toxicity, whereas gaseous arsine and inorganic arsenic are highly toxic. Arsenic's medicinal properties were recognized as early as 400 BC, and it has been used throughout history as a medicinal as well as a component of pigments, cosmetics, and famously as a poison.

Human exposure to arsenic may occur through contaminated air, groundwater, soil, and food, particularly seafood, rice, and produce. Marine organisms, especially shellfish, contain organic arsenicals arsenobetaine and arsenocholine, which are commonly reported in laboratory assays as elevated arsenic level but exert no known toxic effects.

In Bangladesh, ongoing epidemic arsenic poisoning from contaminated groundwater has affected millions of persons. Taiwan, Chile, the Cordoba province in Argentina, West Bengal, and other regions in the Ganga plain also have elevated levels of naturally occurring arsenic and cases of arsenic poisoning.

Occupational exposure to arsenic occurs in the microelectronics industry, where arsenide crystals are used to etch circuits on microchips. Arsine gas is liberated when inorganic arsenic contacts acid, as may occur in occupations such as metal smelting, galvanizing, and semiconductor manufacturing. Arsenic compounds are also used in the production of paint, fungicide, insecticide, pesticide, herbicide, wood preservatives, ceramics, and glass, and employees in these industries may also be potentially exposed.

Arsenic compounds may still be found in folk remedies and patent medicines. Modern medicinal uses of arsenic include arsenic trioxide (Trisenox) for the treatment of acute promyelocytic leukemia (Chapter 183) and melarsoprol, an organic arsenical, for the treatment of African trypanosomiasis (Chapter 346).

PATHOBIOLOGY

The toxicologically significant arsenic compounds are inorganic (trivalent and pentavalent). Arsine gas, which is also toxic, causes acute hemolysis. After absorption, inorganic arsenic binds to hemoglobin and is distributed to liver, kidney, heart, and lungs. In the liver, arsenic is methylated to form monomethylarsenoic and dimethylarsinic acid, both of which are less toxic. Arsenic concentrates in keratin-rich tissues, such as hair, skin, and nails. Much of an ingested dose of arsenic is eliminated in the urine. The mechanism of toxicity is by binding sulfhydryl groups of critical enzymes, including those of the Krebs cycle, thereby resulting in impaired gluconeogenesis, impaired oxidative phosphorylation, and ultimately depletion of cellular energy stores. Pentavalent arsenate may substitute for phosphate in biochemical reactions and disrupt normal oxidative phosphorylation. Arsenic also affects cardiac conduction by blocking cardiac potassium channels. Arsenic can alter gene expression through induction, downregulation, and upregulation of various genes involved in apoptosis, cell signaling, and growth factor response.

Arsine is a colorless, nonirritating gas. After inhalation, it is absorbed rapidly and binds to erythrocytes, where it exerts oxidative stress and causes severe Coombs-negative intravascular hemolysis. Renal failure is due to hemoglobin pigment deposition as well as to the direct toxic effects of arsine on renal tubular cells.

CLINICAL MANIFESTATIONS

The initial clinical features after ingestion of inorganic arsenic are nausea, vomiting, bloody diarrhea, and abdominal pain. Within several days, hematologic findings such as pancytopenia can be seen. QT prolongation, which can develop acutely or chronically, can lead to dysrhythmias such as torsades de pointes. After gastrointestinal symptoms improve, distal symmetrical peripheral neuropathy develops, potentially accompanied by weakness or encephalopathy.

Chronic exposures affect the bone marrow, skin, and peripheral nervous system.[7] Dermatologic effects include patchy or diffuse alopecia, hyperpigmentation, and melanosis as well as hyperkeratosis on the palms and soles. The pigmentation of chronic poisoning commonly appears in a finely freckled, "raindrop" pattern of symmetrical pigmentation or depigmentation that is particularly pronounced on the trunk and extremities. Nails may exhibit transverse white bands, which are known as Mees lines (Chapter 442) and reflect growth interruption during poisoning. Anemia, pancytopenia, neutropenia, thrombocytopenia, and eosinophilia can be seen. Neuropathy, which is a hallmark of arsenic poisoning, is described as a diffuse, symmetrical, ascending, painful sensorimotor neuropathy, most prominent in a stocking-glove distribution. In severe poisoning, ascending weakness and paralysis may result in respiratory failure that mimics the Guillain-Barré syndrome (Chapter 420). Arsenic exposure also causes a dose-dependent decline in lung function. Peripheral vascular disease, including peripheral vascular gangrene (black foot disease), can develop in chronically exposed patients. Even low to moderate chronic arsenic exposure increases the long-term risk of cardiovascular disease by about 30%.[8] Arsenic is a human carcinogen, and exposed populations have an increased risk of developing malignant neoplasms in the lung, skin, and bladder.

Arsine gas produces a clinical triad of abdominal pain, hemolysis, and hematuria, typically occurring hours after exposure. Patients may initially have headache, weakness, nausea, and vomiting. Several weeks after an acute exposure, peripheral neuropathy may develop.

DIAGNOSIS

Because arsenic clears from the blood quickly, an arsenic level above 100 μg/24 hours in urine collected in an acid-washed container requires further scrutiny (Table 22-1). Arsenic levels above 50 μg/L in a spot urine test warrant a 24-hour test. Patients who have recently ingested seafood may have urine arsenic levels exceeding 1500 μg/L, exclusively from organic arsenic, so differentiating inorganic from nontoxic organic arsenic is often critical. Total arsenic levels in hair or nails, where arsenic accumulates, are useful indicators of past exposures. Blood arsenic, urine arsenic, and urine arsenic metabolites can be used to confirm recent or ongoing exposure. In the unexposed individual, blood arsenic should be below 1 μg/L; hair and nail levels should be less than 1 ppm.

In patients with chronic arsenic exposure, a complete blood count may show anemia (normocytic, normochromic, or megaloblastic), leukopenia, and thrombocytopenia. A peripheral smear may show basophilic stippling (Fig. 157-14) or karyorrhexis. Renal dysfunction, hepatic enzyme elevation, and hyperbilirubinemia may be seen as well. The electrocardiogram may show QT prolongation and nonspecific ST-T wave changes. Nerve conduction studies typically show evidence of a distal symmetrical sensorimotor axonopathy. Conduction slowing may be seen in severe poisoning.

TREATMENT Rx

Initial treatment of arsenic toxicity includes supportive care, fluid repletion, decontamination if needed, and removal of the source of exposure. Hemodialysis may be required in patients who have significant renal dysfunction.

In cases of severe acute poisoning from inorganic arsenic, chelation is beneficial if it is instituted early. Dimercaprol (BAL; Table 22-2), which is the traditional chelating agent for arsenic, is effective in decreasing morbidity and mortality if it is administered within minutes to hours of acute exposure. In a small randomized trial, 2,3-dimercapto-1-propanesulfonate, which is not commercially available in the United States, significantly improved clinical symptoms, especially weakness, skin pigmentation, and lung disease, when given as 100 mg orally four times daily every other week for four cycles.[A3] The oral analogue of BAL, dimercaptosuccinic acid (DMSA, succimer) is also useful for subacute or chronic arsenic poisoning. In chronic inorganic arsenic intoxication, however, a clear benefit of chelation therapy has not been demonstrated.

Hemolysis caused by arsine gas poisoning should be treated with prompt exchange transfusion. Exchange transfusion can restore functional erythrocytes, remove hemoglobin pigments, remove arsenic itself, and remove toxic products formed in the arsine-hemoglobin reaction.

PROGNOSIS

Outcomes after arsenic poisoning are influenced by the dose, type of arsenic compound, and route and chronicity of exposure. Acute high-dose arsine gas inhalation with severe and rapid systemic toxicity can be fatal. With appropriate treatment, however, recovery has been reported. After acute inorganic arsenic ingestion, rapid diagnosis and treatment, including chelation, can reduce mortality from about 75% to about 45%. After acute or chronic arsenic poisoning, electrocardiographic abnormalities and bone marrow suppression are generally reversible after exposure ceases, but encephalopathy and neuropathy may be permanent. Skin changes, such as hyperpigmentation and hyperkeratoses, can progress to cancer but also can improve if exposure is reduced.

CADMIUM TOXICITY

EPIDEMIOLOGY

Cadmium (Cd) is primarily found in zinc ores as cadmium sulfide. Serious human exposures usually come from industrial use, including the production of nickel-cadmium batteries, electroplating, soldering, and welding. Workplace exposures occur through inhalation of dust containing oxides of cadmium or fumes from welding or smelting of metals containing cadmium. Depending on the particle size, more than 50% of cadmium can be absorbed through the lungs, but little cadmium is absorbed through the gastrointestinal tract. Many plants take up cadmium from the environment, but poor oral bioavailability and relatively low food concentrations make ingestion of food an unlikely source of significant cadmium, except when cadmium-containing industrial waste is dumped in agricultural regions, such as happened when cadmium-containing mining waste in waterways that irrigated rice fields caused a large outbreak of renal disease. Patients with renal disease often developed osteomalacia (Chapter 244), which can lead to painful fractures. Today, the most common source of environmental cadmium exposure is through smoking, because tobacco concentrates cadmium from the soil, and smoking exposes the lungs to these high levels of cadmium. Compared with nonsmokers, an average smoker has about double the concentration of total body cadmium.

PATHOBIOLOGY

Cadmium commonly exists as a divalent ion (Cd^{2+}) in salts such as cadmium sulfide and cadmium oxide. Like other divalent metals, it binds to and inhibits sulfhydryl-containing proteins and enzymes, thereby resulting in oxidative stress, cellular apoptosis, or necrosis. To survive in an environment where metals are ubiquitous, mammals have developed numerous antioxidant systems for protection. The one best studied in cadmium is the protein metallothionein, which is an intracellular, cysteine-rich protein especially found in the liver and kidney, where it is a potent protective antioxidant that binds to ionized cadmium.

CLINICAL MANIFESTATIONS

The most life-threatening manifestation of cadmium toxicity is acute chemical pneumonitis (Chapters 93 and 94). In persons who are exposed to high concentrations of cadmium fumes (e.g., smelter or welders), cadmium pneumonitis is manifested like metal fume fever with fever, malaise, myalgias, and elevated white blood cell counts that develop within 12 hours of exposure. Unlike metal fume fever, which typically resolves within a few days, cadmium pneumonitis can progress, with symptoms of dyspnea, hemoptysis, pulmonary edema, and respiratory distress as well as diffuse bilateral alveolar infiltrates on the chest radiograph.

The most problematic manifestation of chronic cadmium exposure is renal failure. Like lead, cadmium can damage the proximal tubules of the kidney and result in Fanconi syndrome (Chapter 128). Cadmium, bound to metallothionein, accumulates in the kidney, where its half-life is decades. Once metallothionein binding is saturated, toxicity can develop. Unlike the acute pulmonary manifestations, renal symptoms of cadmium toxicity may have a latency of 10 years of longer. Clinically, the signs of renal disease from cadmium are not different from those of other causes of proximal tubular disease. Patients will often manifest secondary symptoms of renal dysfunction, such as osteoporosis or ureteral stones, from impaired calcium metabolism. Hypertension and anemia from cadmium exposure are also likely secondary to its renal toxicity.

DIAGNOSIS

No laboratory tests can aid in the diagnosis of cadmium pneumonitis, so physicians must rely on their clinical suspicion or on alveolar infiltrates on a chest radiograph in a worker who presents with influenza-like symptoms.

Diagnosis of renal toxicity from chronic cadmium exposure relies predominantly on a 24-hour urine cadmium level standardized to grams of creatinine in a certified laboratory experienced in heavy metal testing (Table 22-1). In nonexposed nonsmokers, cadmium values should average about 0.08 μg per gram of creatinine. Levels of 7 μg cadmium per gram of creatinine and higher require removal from the workplace. For patients with levels above 3 μg cadmium per gram of creatinine, a medical evaluation and renal testing are indicated. Renal dysfunction has been reported in patients with lower levels, and the best test for evaluating renal function is urinary β_2-microglobulin levels, which serve as a useful early marker of toxicity; levels above 300 μg cadmium per gram of creatinine should raise concern for early kidney disease.

TREATMENT Rx

Because of the similarities between cadmium pneumonitis and metal fume fever, any patient presenting with influenza-like symptoms after working with heated cadmium should be admitted for observation. If the metal a patient was welding or cutting is not known, any clinical or radiographic sings of noncardiogenic pulmonary edema would also warrant hospital admission for supplemental oxygen and pulmonary support.

There are no effective treatments for renal toxicity caused by cadmium. Chelation therapy is not recommended.

PROGNOSIS

Patients with cadmium pneumonitis can survive with aggressive treatment, but severe cases can result in death, and survivors can have persistent restrictive lung disease. Because of its long half-life in the kidney, cadmium-induced renal damage is largely irreversible unless it is detected early when body burden is low (urinary cadmium < 10 μg per gram of creatinine).

SYNDROMES SPECIFIC TO OTHER TOXIC METALS

Aluminum (Dialysis Dementia)

In the 1970s, renal failure patients exposed to aluminum-containing phosphate binders or aluminum-contaminated dialysis fluid developed progressive neurologic impairment and multifocal seizures. Also known as dialysis dementia, this syndrome developed during weeks to years and was often fatal if undetected. Aluminum-containing phosphate binders and dialysis fluids are no longer used in patients with renal failure, and dialysis patients are routinely screened for aluminum toxicosis. However, occasional outbreaks continue to be reported, typically due to contamination of dialysis fluid with aluminum from electric pumps or drums.

Aluminum is found in air, soil, and water and is a component of metal alloys used in the home, such as cookware. Aluminum is also found in some antacids (sucralfate) and as aluminum potassium sulfate (Alum), which is used to treat hemorrhagic cystitis. Additional iatrogenic sources of aluminum include total parenteral nutrition solutions and vaccines. Ingested aluminum is not metabolized by the body and is excreted unchanged by the kidney. In patients with impaired renal function, aluminum is bound to transferrin and concentrates primarily in bone. Smaller amounts, however, are distributed to heart, liver, kidney, and brain. Ingested aluminum is thought to affect several biochemical functions, including neurotransmitter manufacture, uptake, and release. Aluminum also affects erythropoiesis and the normal function of bone, likely partially by interference with parathyroid function.

CLINICAL MANIFESTATIONS AND DIAGNOSIS

Clinical effects in patients with chronic exposures include anemia, osteomalacia, and neurologic effects including memory loss, tremor, dyspraxia, encephalopathy, and seizures. The relationship between aluminum and Alzheimer dementia has been debated, but the complex characteristics of aluminum bioavailability make it difficult to produce conclusive evidence.

Serum and urine aluminum levels can be obtained to estimate exposure. A serum aluminum concentration should not exceed 2 μg/L, and a 24-hour urine concentration is expected to be 4 to 12 μg per gram of creatinine in a patient with typical background aluminum exposure (Table 22-1).

TREATMENT AND PROGNOSIS Rx

Management of aluminum toxicity centers on removal from the source of exposure. The only chelator with proven benefit is deferoxamine (Table 22-2), which has a high affinity for aluminum and forms a dialyzable aluminum-deferoxamine complex.[9,10] If it is detected early, successful treatment with full recovery of neurologic function has been reported with deferoxamine.

Bismuth (Bismuth Encephalopathy)

Bismuth salts used to treat gastrointestinal disorders include bismuth subgallate, bismuth citrate, bismuth subnitrate, and bismuth subsalicylate (the active ingredient in Pepto-Bismol). Bismuth (Bi) is poorly absorbed from the gastrointestinal tract and is still used today to treat peptic ulcer disease and diarrhea. It also is used as an oral deodorant for patients with colostomies. Idiopathic bismuth toxicity is almost always associated with the chronic ingestion of over-the-counter preparations.

CLINICAL MANIFESTATIONS AND DIAGNOSIS

Bismuth toxicity is manifested primarily as a subacute encephalopathy with ataxia and incoordination followed by progressive memory loss, behavioral changes, insomnia, and muscle cramps. As symptoms progress, a prevalent feature is limb myoclonus when patients are startled or as they fall asleep. As symptoms worsen, myoclonus can progress to involve the whole body, including the tongue, and can occur without stimulus. Seizures can also develop.

The diagnosis of bismuth encephalopathy can be difficult. Blood and urine levels can indicate exposure to bismuth (Table 22-1) but do not correlate with symptoms. Furthermore, electroencephalographic findings, laboratory tests, and imaging studies are not specific. Because of its similarity in onset and symptoms, bismuth encephalopathy is often misdiagnosed as Creutzfeldt-Jakob disease (Chapter 415) or other progressive encephalopathies. Therefore, any patient in whom these diagnoses are being entertained should be screened for the use of bismuth products. As bismuth causes black stools, the finding of heme-negative black stool in a patient with a rapidly progressing encephalopathy should also warrant an investigation for bismuth toxicity.

Cobalt (Thyroid and Cardiac Toxicity)

Cobalt (Co) is an essential trace element that serves as the catalytic center of vitamin B_{12}. Toxicity is most commonly associated with chronic ingestion of

TREATMENT AND PROGNOSIS

Rx

The treatment of bismuth encephalopathy is to stop the use of the offending agent. Although there have been case reports purporting the benefits of metal chelators (e.g., DMSA, BAL, and 2,3-dimercapto-1-propansulfonic acid; Table 22-2) the rarity of the disorder makes a clinical trial impossible. Ethylenediaminetetraacetic acid (EDTA) may increase brain bismuth concentrations, and it should not be used. Although deaths have occurred from bismuth encephalopathy, full recovery is possible if the offending drug is stopped and the patient receives modern supportive care.

cobalt salts and more recently from cobalt-containing metal prostheses. One of the side effects of chronic ingestion is polycythemia. By stabilizing hypoxia-inducible transcription factors that normally respond to low concentrations of oxygen, cobalt mimics hypoxia and stimulates erythropoietin production. In the 1950s, cobalt chloride was used to treat iron deficiency anemia. Some of these patients developed hypothyroidism and goiter because of cobalt's ability to inhibit tyrosine iodinase. In addition, cobalt has caused dilated cardiomyopathy with pericardial effusions in adults who consumed large amounts of beer in which cobalt salts had been added as a foam stabilizer. Cobalt can also cause neurotoxicity with symptoms of hearing loss, visual impairment, and polyneuropathy.

Because cobalt is no longer used as a therapeutic or as an additive to beer, the concern for cobalt toxicity is now isolated to patients with cobalt-chromium prosthetic joints.[11] Cobalt liberated from a prosthesis has been linked to hypothyroidism, dilated cardiomyopathy, and neurotoxicity with metal-on-ceramics arthroplasty and metal-on-metal prosthetics. When it is viewed in the context of the millions of prosthetic joints placed each year and the few reported cases, this complication seems rare. The diagnosis in a patient with a cobalt-containing joint replacement requires symptoms of polycythemia, hypothyroidism, cardiomyopathy, and neurotoxicity. In these patients, a blood chromium level above 7 μg/L should stimulate a referral for a possible joint revision. There is little evidence that chelation improves outcomes in cobalt-poisoned patients.

Silver (Argyria)

Silver (Ag) is a precious metal long used in coinage and for its antibacterial properties. Silver is a broad-spectrum antimicrobial and commonly used as a topical antimicrobial in bandages, catheters, and medical devices. The ingestion of colloidal silver preparations as a "natural" supplement accounts for the majority of recent cases of significant toxicity.

When it is ingested continually, silver will be deposited in the skin and the liver.[12] The primary chronic toxicity of silver is argyria, which is a permanent blue-gray discoloration of the skin due to silver deposition over time (Fig. 22-1). Argyria can result from inhalation, ingestion, mucosal absorption, or dermal application or exposure. Argyria may be localized to the site of exposure, such as with corneal argyria, which was seen in the past from the use of colloidal silver-containing eye drops, or at the site of silver earrings and rings. Rarely, argyria has been reported after the implantation of silver-containing medical devices.

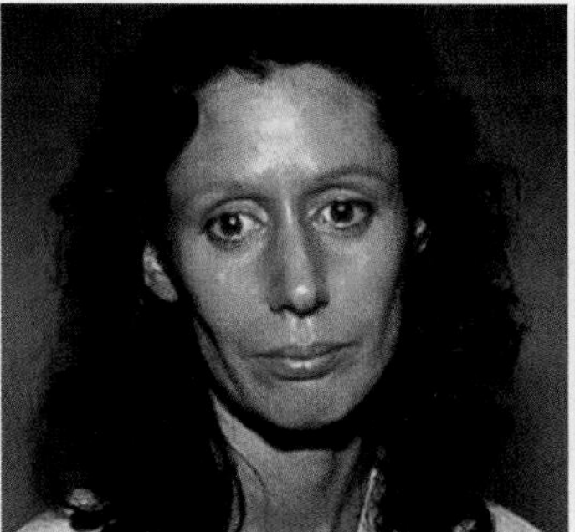
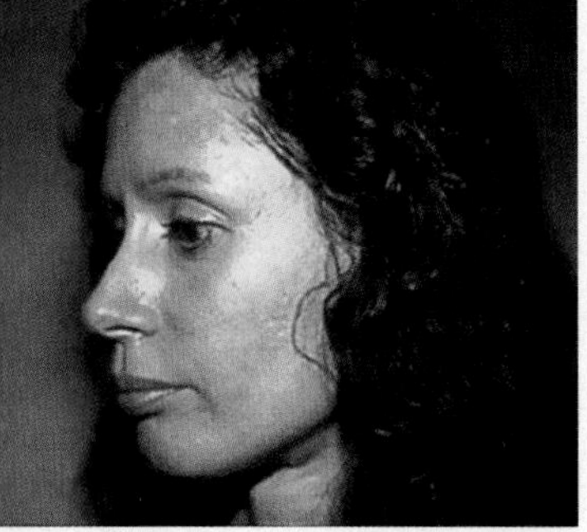

FIGURE 22-1. Frontal and side views of a 36-year-old woman with argyria show the gray discoloration of her face and neck. (From Jacobs R. "Argyria: my life story," *Clin Dermatol.* Elsevier, 2006;24:66-69. Figure 3).

The diagnosis of argyria is primarily based on history and physical examination. Localized skin biopsy, typically to differentiate argyria from malignant lesions, will show characteristic black-brown globules that are adherent to the dermal elastic fibers, blood vessels, basement membranes, hair follicles, and sweat glands on light microscopy; refractile particles on darkfield microscopy; and the presence of silver on scanning electron microscopy with energy dispersive radiography.

Chelation therapy is not effective for argyria, but successful laser treatment has been reported.[13]

Thallium (Neuropathy and Alopecia)

Thallium (Tl) has no beneficial role in the human body. Its salts are odorless, tasteless, well absorbed in the gastrointestinal tract, and very toxic. These characteristics make it a potential homicidal agent, and patients with thallium poisoning should always be considered victims of a crime. By interfering with potassium and sulfhydryl-containing enzymes, thallium interrupts normal energy production. Although it is toxic to all organs, the peripheral nervous system and integumentary system are the most sensitive.

The earliest clinical sign of thallium poisoning is a rapidly progressive, painful sensory polyneuropathy. Within 2 or 3 days of exposure, patients will describe painful burning paresthesias in their feet. These paresthesias can progress up the legs and, over time, can involve the hands. Motor nerves can also be affected, and profound weakness, including in respiratory muscles, can be misdiagnosed as Guillain-Barré syndrome (Chapter 420). Cranial neuropathies have also been reported. The best-known complication of thallium is painless hair loss, typically beginning 5 to 14 days after exposure and sometimes progressing to total body alopecia. Skin and nails can also be affected, with scaling of palms, acne-like lesions of the face, and Mees lines in the nails. Other neurologic symptoms of thallium poisoning include hallucinations, altered mental status, insomnia, psychosis, ataxia, and coma. Constipation, myalgias, pleuritic chest pain, arrhythmias, and hypotension can also occur.

Because systemic toxicities often develop before hair loss and because not all patients lose their hair, clinicians should consider thallium as a possible cause of any rapidly progressive painful neuropathy. In patients with thallium poisoning, a pulled hair will often have darkening of the hair root when it is visualized under a low-power light microscope. The definitive diagnosis of thallium poisoning requires the identification of elevated concentrations of thallium in a 24-hour urine sample (normal, <20 μg/specimen). As thallium undergoes enterohepatic circulation and is eliminated in the feces, treatment requires binding of thallium in the gut. The most effective antidote is Prussian Blue (a complex of potassium hexacyanoferrate), with recommended doses ranging from 3 g orally three times a day up to 250 mg/kg three times a day.[14]

Zinc (Myelopathy)

Zinc (Zn) is an essential mineral that is necessary for normal cellular functioning. It is involved in the catalytic activity of more than 100 enzymes and plays an important role in olfaction, taste, immune function, protein synthesis, and DNA synthesis. It is found naturally in a wide variety of foods and is absorbed in the jejunum, where it binds to metallothioneins. Zinc deficiency is manifested as a triad of dermatitis, diarrhea, and alopecia, which is reversible after zinc repletion.

In the setting of zinc overload, metallothioneins are upregulated; because copper has a higher affinity for metallothioneins, the result is increased copper binding and subsequent elimination of copper. Zinc-induced copper deficiency has been reported after overuse of zinc-containing supplements, with the improper use of zinc-containing denture adhesives, and from the presence of retained zinc-containing coins such as pennies.

The hematologic manifestations of zinc-induced copper deficiency include sideroblastic anemia, leukopenia, neutropenia, and myelodysplastic syndrome,[15] all of which are reversible with zinc cessation alone. In addition, a syndrome of myeloneuropathy, characterized by a spastic gait and sensory ataxia, is also associated with zinc overload/copper deficiency and may improve with copper supplementation and zinc cessation.

Diagnostic testing in patients suspected of zinc overload should include serum or urine zinc concentrations (Table 22-1), serum copper levels, and ceruloplasmin levels. In patients with myeloneuropathy, nerve conduction studies may show a sensory neuropathy, and magnetic resonance imaging (MRI) may show increased T2 signal in the cervical cord. Treatment of zinc overload–induced copper deficiency is primarily by cessation of zinc exposure and repletion of copper, such as with 6 mg/day of elemental copper orally daily for the first week, then 4 mg/day for the next week, and finally 2 mg/day after that until serum levels return to normal. Various chelation regimens have been reported, but data are insufficient to support their routine use in the setting of chronic toxicity.

Manganese (Parkinsonism)

Manganese (Mn) is an essential element necessary for the function of several enzymes, including superoxide dismutase and glutamine synthetase. Although there is no clear syndrome associated with manganese deficiency, a well-described constellation of symptoms and findings is associated with manganese toxicity. Associated primarily with chronic occupational exposure, manganese toxicity results from inhalation of high concentrations of either manganese dust (e.g., in miners) or manganese fumes (e.g., smelting, grinding, and rarely welding).[16] More recently, manganese toxicity has been reported in abusers of methcathinone, when this drug was illegally synthesized with potassium permanganate. Although the mechanism is not clear, manganese causes selective toxicity in the globus pallidus, striatum, and substantia nigra pars reticulata. In contrast to idiopathic Parkinson disease (Chapter 409), manganese does not affect the substantia nigra pars compacta.

The symptoms of manganism develop insidiously after years of exposure. Patients first develop changes in appetite, muscle weakness, and apathy. On occasion, patients will develop signs of central excitation and can have what is termed manganese psychosis. Symptoms often progress to difficulties with gait, speech, and facial expression. The gait abnormalities involve a slow and clumsy gait with the inability to walk backward. Patients often freeze while turning and frequently fall. Symptoms can progress to muscle hypertonia in extension and a peculiar gait in which patients walk on the balls of the feet with their ankles extended. Patients also develop stuttering speech, masked facies, sleep disturbances, and myalgias. Unlike with idiopathic Parkinson disease, manganese-exposed patients do not typically develop a resting tremor, and these symptoms are almost always symmetrical at onset.

Although there is no definitive test of manganese toxicity, a history of exposure, confirmatory laboratory testing (Table 22-1), radiographic studies, and clinical symptoms can support the diagnosis. The best laboratory test is a whole blood manganese level (normal, <15 μg/L), with elevated levels indicative of exposure but not necessarily correlating directly with symptoms. Because manganese can concentrate in the globus pallidus, MRI often will show an intense T1-weighted signal in the globus pallidus bilaterally. As with blood, however, MRI is indicative of manganese exposure but does not correlate with clinical symptoms. Because of the differences in the affected brain regions between manganese toxicity and Parkinson disease, fluorodopa positron emission tomography (PET) scanning can help differentiate between these disorders: patients with manganese toxicity will typically have normal PET scans, whereas patients with Parkinson disease have abnormal scans.

Manganism is not typically responsive to treatment. Although chelation with $CaNa_2EDTA$ has been associated with increased urinary elimination of manganese, there are no convincing data as to whether patient outcomes are improved.

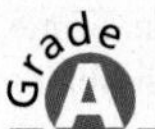

Grade A References

A1. Yeoh B, Woolfenden S, Lanphear B, et al. Household interventions for preventing domestic lead exposure in children. *Cochrane Database Syst Rev.* 2012;4:CD006047.

A2. Rogan WJ, Dietrich KN, Ware JH, et al. The effect of chelation therapy with succimer on neuropsychological development in children exposed to lead. *N Engl J Med.* 2001;344:1421-1426.

A3. Guha Mazumder DN, De BK, Santra A, et al. Randomized placebo-controlled trial of 2,3-dimercapto-1-propanesulfonate (DMPS) in therapy of chronic arsenicosis due to drinking arsenic-contaminated water. *J Toxicol Clin Toxicol.* 2001;39:665-674.

GENERAL REFERENCES

For the General References and other additional features, please visit Expert Consult at https://expertconsult.inkling.com.

IV

AGING AND GERIATRIC MEDICINE

23

EPIDEMIOLOGY OF AGING: IMPLICATIONS OF AN AGING SOCIETY

ANNE B. NEWMAN AND JANE A. CAULEY

DEMOGRAPHY: AGING OF SOCIETIES WORLDWIDE

More than 40 million adults older than 65 years are now living in the United States, and they account for 13% of the population. Even more notably, 5.5 million people (1.8% of the population) are older than 85 years, and more than 50,000 people (0.02% of the population) are older than 100 years. Although only 13% of the U.S. population is older than 65 years, they account for 36% of all medical expenditures.[1]

The trend toward an aging society has expanded to become a global health issue. The global population aged 65 years and older is more than 500 million people, about 7% of the world's population. By 2040, the world is projected to have 1.3 billion older people, accounting for 14% of the total population. In 2040, 28% of the population in western Europe will be 65 years and older, including about 9.3% older than 80 years. Japan is currently the oldest country in the world, with 22% of the population aged 65 years and older, compared with 18% in western Europe and 21% in North America (Table 23-1). Between 2005 and 2040, the overall world population is projected to increase by 35%, whereas the percentage aged 85 years or older will increase by 300% and the percentage aged 100 years or older will increase by 750%. The estimated number of centenarians was about 270,000 in 2005, but this number is projected to reach 2.3 million by 2040.[2]

Population aging, which has been accelerating in the United States and western Europe for more than 100 years, is now affecting countries such as India and China, where the population older than 65 years is projected to increase more than three-fold by 2040. The population aged 65 years and older was already 166 million in China and India in 2008, nearly one third of the world's total, and the absolute number will increase to 550 million by 2040. In the United States, increases in the elderly population are most prominent in minorities, especially Hispanics.

Life expectancy is also changing dramatically. Life expectancy is highest in Japan at 82 years and is in the 78- to 80-year range for other developed countries. Life expectancy has continued to increase at all ages and especially for people older than 85 years, except in some parts of the developing world, such as sub-Saharan Africa, where HIV/AIDS has had a major negative impact. In the United States, an average 65-year-old woman can expect to live for an additional 19.6 years, and the average 65-year-old man can expect to live for an additional 16.8 years. These changes have many important impacts on society because rates of illness and disability increase with age, and the relative proportion of younger adults who can help care for this older population is not increasing.

THE HEALTH OF OLDER ADULTS

Mortality

The current generation of older adults is healthier than previous generations because of the successful elimination of many infectious diseases and the prevention of injuries, but the population at risk for chronic diseases is increasing. In the United States in 1900, infectious diseases accounted for the largest share of deaths after 65 years of age, whereas heart disease, cancer, stroke, and lung disease account for more than half of all deaths today.

As people age, their mortality rate increases. Death rates are 1.8% per year in men and 1.2% per year in women between the ages of 65 and 70 years, increasing to 13% per year in women and 15% per year in men older than 85 years.[3] With increasing age, causes of death in older adults shift away from cancer and cardiovascular disease and toward stroke and dementia. Nevertheless, cardiovascular disease and cancer remain the top two causes of death in older adults into advanced old age (Table 23-2).

However, many factors contribute to mortality in old age, and death is usually multifactorial, with contributions from other chronic underlying conditions. Mortality in older adults is related to sociodemographic status and health habits; cardiovascular risk factors; and pulmonary, vascular, kidney, physical, and cognitive function. The inflammatory marker interleukin-6 is consistently associated with death from many different primary causes, thereby suggesting that inflammation is a common underlying pathway to death.[4]

Morbidity

The most common chronic conditions in older adults are hypertension, high cholesterol levels, and ischemic heart disease (Fig. 23-1). Prevalence varies by sex, with men having more heart disease than women and women having more arthritis than men. Because women live longer than men do, the prevalence of dementia is higher in women than in men, but incidence rates are more similar. Older African Americans and Hispanics have higher rates of hypertension, diabetes, and metabolic syndrome compared with older whites.[5]

The majority of older adults have one or more chronic health conditions, and 50% have two or more. Because of this high prevalence of multiple conditions, the care of older adults requires a balanced approach that considers the impact of treatment of one condition on the other conditions and the potential that some conditions may be masked by multiple overlapping symptoms. The presence of multiple conditions is commonly referred to as comorbidity, although multimorbidity may be a more accurate term.

Multimorbidity is strongly associated with disability, with a stepwise increase in the proportion of individuals who have self-reported difficulty in activities of daily living according to their number of medical conditions. Prospectively, the number of comorbid conditions predicts future disability. Multimorbidity also is associated with having a slower gait speed and poorer lower extremity strength and balance. Furthermore, disability and comorbidity provide distinct information and should not be considered equivalent constructs. The combined influence of multiple chronic diseases on physical functioning can be greater than the simple sum of their effects.

Subclinical Disease

Subclinical diseases are also common and increasingly recognized as important contributors to the risk of disability and mortality. With the advent of noninvasive functional testing and imaging, it is clear that many conditions can be advanced in older people, even if they are not symptomatic. Symptoms may also be nonspecific and attributed to aging rather than to underlying disease. For example, population studies of cardiovascular disease reveal that strokes are present on magnetic resonance imaging in about one third of older adults with no history of stroke, and advanced atherosclerosis is present also in one third of older adults with no history of a prior myocardial infarction. Ankle-brachial index screening documents that peripheral artery disease is 5 to 10 times more common than classic intermittent claudication. Other conditions, such as chronic obstructive pulmonary disease and osteoarthritis, are also more common when noninvasive testing is performed compared with clinically diagnosed disease. Importantly, subclinical disease burden is strongly related to mortality.

Obesity

Obesity (Chapter 220) is increasing in older adults at a rate faster than in any other age group. Obesity and disability disproportionately affect women and especially women of color. About one third of whites older than 60 years are obese, compared with about 50% of blacks and 40% of Hispanics. Obesity has a major impact on disability, including difficulty in walking or climbing steps. The epidemic of obesity is also contributing to the large increases in the incidence of diabetes in older adults. Increasing rates of obesity may halt or reverse increases in life expectancy, reduce quality of life, and increase disability.

Geriatric Syndromes

Many multifactorial conditions in older adults do not fall into a single disease category and are called geriatric syndromes. For example, urinary incontinence (Chapter 26) is a functional loss of bladder control that can be influenced by poor mobility, poor vision, loss of urinary concentrating ability, and certain medications as well as impaired bladder structure or function. Other important geriatric syndromes include impaired sleep (Chapter 405), delirium (Chapter 28), falling (Chapter 25), and weight loss. Rather than focusing on identification of a primary cause, all contributing factors need to be addressed in the evaluation and treatment of these syndromes.

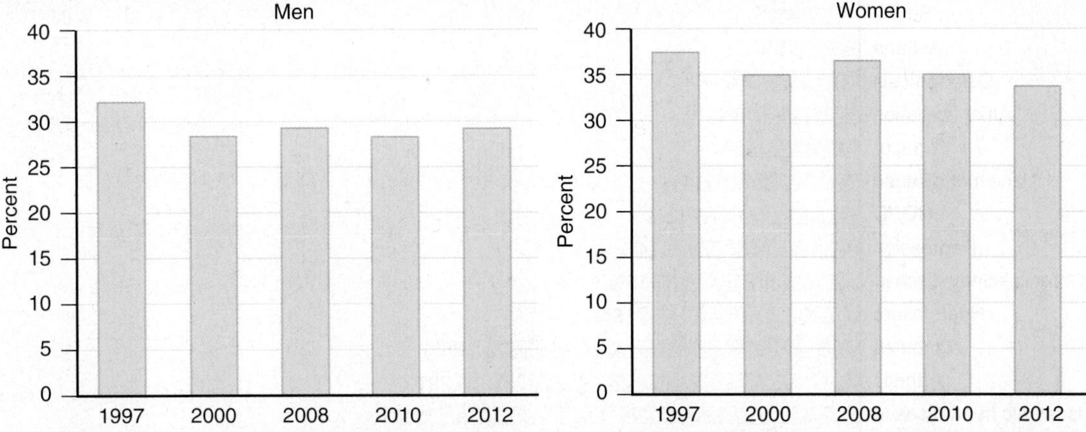

FIGURE 23-1. Prevalence of complex activity limitation among those 65 years and older in the United States. A complex activity limitation is defined as having one or more of the following limitations: self-care (activities of daily living or instrumental activities of daily living), social, or work. (Source: Centers for Disease Control and Prevention, National Center for Health Statistics: Health, United States, 2012, and Health, United States, 2010. Data from the National Health Interview Survey. http://www.cdc.gov/nchs/data/hus/hus12.pdf. Accessed January 29, 2015.)

TABLE 23-1 PERCENTAGE OF OLDER POPULATION BY REGION, 2014-2050

REGION	≥65 YEARS	≥75 YEARS	≥80 YEARS
NORTHERN AFRICA			
2014	4.9	1.7	0.8
2050	13.6	5.5	3.1
EASTERN AFRICA			
2014	2.8	0.9	0.4
2050	5.3	1.8	0.9
MIDDLE AFRICA			
2014	2.8	0.8	0.3
2050	5.4	1.7	0.8
SOUTHERN AFRICA			
2014	6	2.1	1
2050	11	4.9	3.1
WESTERN AFRICA			
2014	3.1	0.9	0.4
2050	5.3	1.8	0.8
ASIA (EXCLUDES NEAR EAST)			
2014	7.6	2.8	1.4
2050	18.8	9	5.2
WESTERN ASIA (NEAR EAST)			
2014	5.2	2	1
2050	14.2	6	3.4
EASTERN EUROPE			
2014	14.5	6.7	3.5
2050	27.9	13.7	8.5
WESTERN EUROPE			
2014	19.5	9.5	5.5
2050	27.5	16.6	11.6

Source: U.S. Census Bureau, International Data Base. http://www.census.gov/population/international/data/idb/informationGateway.php. Accessed January 29, 2015.

TABLE 23-2 LEADING CAUSES OF DEATH: U.S. POPULATION, 2011

CAUSE	RATE PER 100,000
Diseases of heart	173.7
Malignant neoplasms	168.6
Chronic lower respiratory diseases	42.7
Cerebrovascular diseases	37.9
Accidents (unintentional injuries)	38.0
Alzheimer disease	24.6
Diabetes mellitus	21.5
Influenza and pneumonia	15.7
Nephritis, nephrotic syndrome, and nephrosis	13.4
Intentional self-harm (suicide)	12.0
Septicemia	10.5
Chronic liver disease and cirrhosis	9.7
Essential hypertension and hypertensive renal disease	8.0
Parkinson disease	7.0
Pneumonitis due to solids and liquids	5.3

From Hoyert DL, Xu JQ. Deaths: preliminary data for 2011. *Natl Vital Stat Rep.* 2012;61:6.

Disability

In older adults, disability is usually related to multiple chronic conditions. Disability can be slowly progressive and chronic, or it can be sudden and catastrophic, as in the case of a stroke or hip fracture. Levels of disability include loss of basic self-care skills, such as bathing and toileting; loss of ability to live in the community for skills such as shopping and paying bills; loss of mobility; and loss of ability to function in high-level tasks. Classification schemes for disability in geriatrics are reviewed in Chapter 24.

The majority of older adults are not disabled. Data from the National Health Interview Survey show that disability levels declined in the 1980s and 1990s but have largely plateaued in recent years (Fig. 23-2). In 2012, about 28% of men and 34% of women older than 65 years reported difficulty with complex activities. Disability for activities of daily living appears to be declining worldwide, although evidence suggests that less severe levels of disability are becoming more common. It is possible, however, that the obesity epidemic will result in more years with disability.

Frailty versus Vigor

Frailty has been described as a state of decreased physiologic reserve and increased vulnerability to stress. Frailty is a wasting syndrome characterized by weakness, fatigue, low activity, slow movement, and weight loss. It has also been characterized by poor physical function alone or by a high burden of chronic disease. By the definition of a wasting syndrome, frailty is present in 7% of community-dwelling adults aged 65 years and older and 25% of adults aged 85 years and older. These estimates undoubtedly underestimate the prevalence of frailty because frail individuals are more likely to be temporarily in a medical care facility and unable to participate at any given time.

Loss of muscle mass, or sarcopenia, is an underlying component of frailty,[6] but excess fat, especially visceral fat and muscle fat, has a greater influence on physical function, inflammation, and metabolism than does low muscle mass. In the elderly, muscle strength, including contractile force, mitochondrial function, and speed of contraction or power, is more important to physical

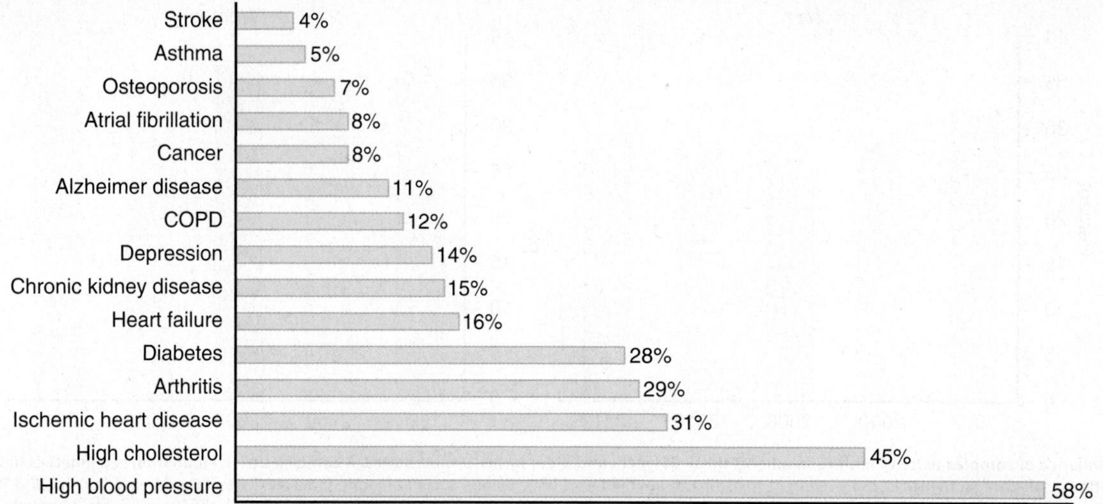

FIGURE 23-2. Percentage of Medicare fee-for-service beneficiaries with 15 selected chronic conditions: 2010. (Source: Centers for Medicare and Medicaid Services: Chronic Conditions among Medicare Beneficiaries, Chartbook: 2012 Edition. Based on 2010 Centers for Medicare and Medicaid Services administrative claims data for 100% of Medicare beneficiaries enrolled in the fee-for-service program.) COPD = chronic obstructive pulmonary disease.

function than muscle mass. Important weakness can be assessed in an office setting by measuring a grip strength (<30 kg in men and <20 kg in women).

Longevity and Healthy Aging

About 20 to 30% of longevity is heritable, similar to many complex chronic diseases.[7] Animal models of aging show that lifespan can be extended severalfold by altering genes, especially in the metabolic pathway. In lower organisms and mice, calorie restriction, achieved through long-term daily restriction of available calories, extends life, but this approach has mixed results in primates. Many hormonal factors are reduced with aging, but hormone replacement with estrogen, growth hormone, testosterone, and adrenal androgens is not beneficial for longevity and may be harmful. Among genetic factors, absence of the *ApoE4* allele remains the most robust predictor of longevity, and recent genome-wide association studies of centenarians also point to genes such as *FOX03A* in the pathway for metabolic control.

Many health conditions in late life may stem from early life exposures, including the health of the mother during pregnancy. For example, low birthweight or famine during pregnancy predicts early cardiovascular disease and diabetes when babies are later exposed to higher calorie intake. In Sweden, a lower lifetime exposure to infectious disease was associated with increased life expectancy. More research is needed to determine the critical periods for development and the optimal environmental exposures that can enhance healthy aging later in life.

PREVENTION

Osteoporosis treatment is effective in reducing fracture risk in advanced old age,[8] and treatment of hypertension is effective in decreasing mortality after 80 years of age.[A1] Statins are effective in reducing coronary heart disease in older adults.[A2] Physical activity significantly decreases the risk of disability[A3] and may reduce the risk of dementia, although the latter finding is primarily from observational studies that may be confounded by the fact that healthier people are more able to exercise. Ongoing research is evaluating the potential for aspirin to prolong active life in older adults and whether testosterone replacement in hypogonadal men will improve physical, cognitive, or sexual function in older men.

Grade A References

A1. Briasoulis A, Agarwal V, Tousoulis D, et al. Effects of antihypertensive treatment in patients over 65 years of age: a meta-analysis of randomised controlled studies. *Heart.* 2014;100:317-323.
A2. Savarese G, Gotto AM Jr, Paolillo S, et al. Benefits of statins in elderly subjects without established cardiovascular disease: a meta-analysis. *J Am Coll Cardiol.* 2013;62:2090-2099.
A3. Pahor M, Guralnik JM, Ambrosius WT, et al. Effect of structured physical activity on prevention of major mobility disability in older adults: the LIFE study randomized clinical trial. *JAMA.* 2014;311:2387-2396.

GENERAL REFERENCES

For the General References and other additional features, please visit Expert Consult at https://expertconsult.inkling.com.

24

GERIATRIC ASSESSMENT

DAVID B. REUBEN

Geriatric assessment is a broad term used to describe the evaluation of older patients, a process that recognizes the diverse medical and psychosocial conditions that influence the health status of older persons. In addition to the diseases that are common in the elderly population, these influences include social, psychological, and environmental factors. Geriatric assessment can range from brief screens by individual clinicians to an intensive interdisciplinary process that includes both evaluation and management.

Three fundamental concepts guide geriatric assessment and the resulting medical management. At the core of geriatric assessment is functional status, both as a dimension to be evaluated and as an outcome to be improved or maintained. A second overarching concept guiding geriatric assessment is prognosis, particularly life expectancy. Finally, geriatric assessment must be guided by the patient's goals.

FUNCTIONAL STATUS

Functional status can be viewed as a summary measure of the overall impact of health conditions in the context of an elderly person's environment and social support network. The underlying framework of functional status is a hierarchy of increasing complexity, beginning with specific physical movements (e.g., lifting, walking) that are integrated into higher level activities (e.g., fulfilling occupational and social roles). Impairment of functional status can be triggered by the onset of disease, deconditioning, changes in social support or environment, and advanced age.

Most commonly, older adults' functional status is assessed at two levels: activities of daily living (ADLs) and instrumental activities of daily living (IADLs). ADLs refer to self-care tasks such as bathing, dressing, toileting, maintaining continence, grooming, feeding, and transferring. Dependency in these tasks, which is present in up to 10% of older persons, usually requires full-time help at home or placement in a nursing home.

IADLs refer to tasks that are integral to maintaining an independent household, such as using the telephone, doing laundry, shopping for groceries, driving or using public transportation, preparing meals, taking medications, performing housework, and handling finances. Dependency in IADLs is more common, and almost 20% of persons aged 75 years or older are impaired in at least one task. With the progressive loss of multiple IADL functions, older persons find it more difficult to remain in their homes. Accordingly, many social services (e.g., Meals On Wheels, homemaker

TABLE 24-1 LIFE EXPECTANCY IN VARIOUS STATES OF FUNCTIONAL HEALTH ACCORDING TO AGE, GENDER, AND INITIAL FUNCTIONAL STATUS*

		LIFE EXPECTANCY IN YEARS IN EACH FUNCTIONAL STATUS							
		WOMEN				MEN			
AGE	INITIAL FUNCTIONAL CATEGORY	Independent Years	Mobility-Disabled Years	ADL-Disabled Years	Total Years	Independent Years	Mobility-Disabled Years	ADL-Disabled Years	Total Years
70 years	Independent	10.0	4.0	2.7	16.7	8.5	2.6	1.0	12.1
	Mobility disabled	7.3	5.6	2.8	15.7	5.6	4.1	1.1	10.7
	ADL disabled	3.0	2.9	5.6	11.5	1.6	1.5	3.4	6.5
75 years	Independent	7.0	3.6	2.6	13.2	6.0	2.4	1.0	9.4
	Mobility disabled	4.0	5.2	2.8	12.0	2.9	3.8	1.1	7.9
	ADL disabled	1.1	1.8	5.3	8.2	0.5	0.8	3.1	4.4
80 years	Independent	4.7	3.2	2.4	10.3	4.1	2.2	0.9	7.2
	Mobility disabled	2.0	4.4	2.7	9.0	1.4	3.3	1.0	5.7
	ADL disabled	0.4	1.0	4.7	6.0	0.2	0.4	2.6	3.1
85 years	Independent	3.3	2.9	1.8	8.0	2.9	2.1	0.7	5.8
	Mobility disabled	1.0	3.6	2.3	6.9	0.7	2.8	0.9	4.4
	ADL disabled	0.1	0.5	4.0	4.6	0.0	0.2	2.1	2.3

*Using 1988-1990 Established Populations for Epidemiologic Studies of the Elderly Data
ADL (activities of daily living) disabled = self-report of being unable to do or requiring human help to perform any of the following: bathing, transferring from bed to chair, dressing, eating, and using the toilet. Mobility disabled = self report of being unable to walk a half-mile or to walk up and down stairs to the second floor without help.

services, transportation services) are available to compensate for these deficiencies. A move to an assisted living facility can provide most IADL functions, but many facilities do not routinely provide assistance with ADLs except at an additional cost. In the United States, the costs of assisted living facilities are not covered by Medicare.

At a higher level of function, advanced activities of daily living (AADLs) refer to the ability to fulfill societal, community, and family roles as well as to participate in recreational or occupational tasks. These advanced activities vary considerably from individual to individual but may be valuable in monitoring functional status before the development of disability.

The choice of functional assessment tool depends on the characteristics of the population being assessed. For example, nursing home residents are almost always completely dependent in IADLs, so the focus should be on assessing ADLs and other basic dimensions of health. Hospitalized older persons should be assessed with regard to their prehospitalization functional status to provide insight into what may be achievable as well as their functional status at the time of discharge to identify any existing gap and to facilitate plans to close it.

Functional status is usually measured by self-report or proxy report. However, physical and occupational therapists often add objective information using structured clinical examinations or assessments. In addition, dimensions such as mobility and balance that contribute to function can be assessed by objective measures (described later).

Functional status should be assessed periodically: at the time of an initial visit; after a major illness; and at the time of social milestones, such as the illness of a spouse or a change in living or working situation. Changes in functional status should always prompt further diagnostic evaluation and intervention unless the change is expected and reflects a trajectory that is consistent with the patient's wishes. Measurement of functional status can be valuable in monitoring response to treatment (especially of chronic diseases) and can provide prognostic information that is useful in planning short- and long-term care.

PROGNOSIS

Life expectancy affects both the assessment process and the management decisions based on that assessment. For some older patients, comorbidities can worsen prognosis, such that screening tests (e.g., mammography) and treatments (e.g., for hypertension) with demonstrated effectiveness would not be beneficial within the expected survival period.

The probability that a patient will survive for a specified time (e.g., 5 years from the time of the assessment) or to a specified age (e.g., to age 100 years) can be estimated on the basis of age, gender, and race with government-generated life tables. Life expectancy also can be estimated with online calculators (see, for example, *eprognosis.org*) or by incorporating clinical characteristics. For example, better cognitive status and less comorbidity are the best predictors of 5-year survival in nonagenarians.[1] One simple approach is to incorporate functional status in addition to age and gender (Table 24-1).[2,3]

PATIENT GOALS

As people age, their current and future health may become a prominent factor in determining and achieving their life goals. Among very old patients, goals may be limited to achievement of a functional or health state (e.g., being able to walk independently), control of symptoms (e.g., pain, dyspnea), maintenance of their living situation (e.g., remaining at home), or short-term survival (e.g., living long enough to reach a personal milestone, such as an upcoming holiday). Sometimes the goals of patients and physicians differ. For example, a patient may want a cure, whereas the physician believes that only symptom management is possible. Conversely, the physician may believe that a better outcome is possible, but the patient declines to pursue the recommended path (e.g., hip replacement to restore mobility).[4] Physicians and patients alike must recognize that the elderly may receive less benefit from some interventions than younger do patients because of other adverse prognostic factors. For frail older persons with multiple chronic conditions or a short life expectancy, clinicians and patients should work together to identify the patient's personal goals within and across a variety of dimensions (e.g., symptoms, physical functional status, social and role functioning).[5] The care plan can then be developed and framed in the context of meeting these goals.

COMPONENTS OF GERIATRIC ASSESSMENT

Geriatric assessment begins with a medical evaluation. Some aspects (described later) that are rarely abnormal in younger adults (e.g., mobility, cognition) may cause substantial morbidity in older persons. In addition, some clusters of abnormal findings, such as muscle wasting, poor hygiene, bruises, pressure sores, and contractures, should raise the suspicion of elder mistreatment, neglect, or abuse. In such cases, patients should be questioned and examined without family members or caregivers present. Patients should then be queried as to whether anyone has threatened or hurt them, whether they have been receiving enough care, and whether anyone has taken their things. Answers to these questions may provide confirmatory information and prompt a report to adult protective services.

Nonmedical assessments are also important because they can identify problems that should be addressed and may be key to achieving the patient's goals. In addition to an assessment of functional status, older persons' environmental, financial, and nonfinancial support should be assessed. In some situations, particularly when older persons become acutely ill or experience caregiver stress or loss of a loved one, assessment of spiritual needs, with appropriate referral, may be valuable.

Advance Directives

Clinicians should discuss older patients' preferences for specific treatments while they still have the cognitive capacity to make these decisions. Patients should be asked to identify a spokesperson to make medical decisions for them if they cannot speak for themselves. This information should be conveyed through a durable power of attorney for health care, which also allows patients to specify treatments they do not want. Many states have allowed the use of Physician Orders for Life-Sustaining Treatment (POLST), a specific advance directive that documents a patient's end-of-life treatment preferences and serves as an order sheet. The standardized form, which is signed by both the physician and the patient, must be honored in all settings of care, including by emergency medical technicians responding to 911 calls.

Medical Assessment

The medical assessment includes vision; hearing; cognition; mood and affect; falls, mobility, and balance; medication review; nutrition; and urinary incontinence. Numerous screening instruments have been developed that assess many of these dimensions. Another important medical component of geriatric assessment includes[5] a determination of whether preventive services are up-to-date.

Vision

Each of the four major eye diseases—cataract, age-related macular degeneration, diabetic retinopathy, and glaucoma (Chapter 423)—increases in prevalence with age. Moreover, presbyopia is virtually universal, and most older persons require eyeglasses. Visual impairment has been associated with increased risk of falls, functional and cognitive decline, immobility, and depression.[6] Corrective lenses or other treatments may restore vision or prevent further decline of visual function.

A single question can be used to screen for visual impairment: Do you have difficulty driving, watching television or reading, or doing any of your daily activities because of your eyesight, even while wearing glasses?

The Snellen eye chart is the standard method of screening for visual acuity. The patient is asked to stand 20 feet from the chart and to read letters. Inability to read letters on or below the 20/40 line with the best-corrected vision (using glasses) indicates the need for further evaluation.

Hearing

Hearing loss (Chapter 428), which affects more than 60% of community-dwelling adults older than 70 years and 75% of residents living in nursing home settings, is associated with reduced cognitive, social, emotional, and physical functioning. When hearing loss is detected, amplification by hearing aids or assistive listening devices can improve quality of life and functional status.[7]

To identify hearing loss, simple questions (e.g., Would you say you have any difficulty hearing? Do you feel you have hearing loss?) can be asked, or the 10-item self-reported Hearing Handicap Inventory for the Elderly instrument can be administered. If either of these screens is positive or if the clinician suspects hearing loss, an objective test is the whisper voice test, which involves whispering three different random words in each ear at distances of 6, 12, and 24 inches from the patient's ear and then asking the patient to repeat the words. Patients who fail the test—that is, are unable to repeat half the whispered words correctly—should be referred to an audiologist for further evaluation.

A more accurate screening tool for hearing impairment is the Welch Allyn AudioScope. This handheld otoscope has a built-in audiometer that can be set at different levels of intensity. A pretone at 60 dB is delivered to the patient, and then four tones of 500, 1000, 2000, and 4000 Hz at 40 dB are presented. The inability to hear either the 1000- or 2000-Hz frequency in both ears or both the 1000- and 2000-Hz frequencies in one ear indicates a positive screen and identifies the need for formal audiometric testing.

Cognitive Assessment

The incidence of dementia (Chapters 27 and 402) increases with age, especially among those older than 85 years. Early detection of memory problems can lead to the identification of treatable conditions that contribute to cognitive impairment and the development of a proactive management plan with the patient's full participation.[8] Because the diagnosis of dementia has not been documented for as many as 80% of patients who meet diagnostic criteria for it, clinicians should routinely evaluate elderly patients using any of a variety of brief screening instruments (Chapter 27).[9]

Another component of cognitive assessment is decision-making capacity. In cognitively intact older persons, capacity is assumed. However, among those with cognitive impairment, decision making must be determined before many treatments are initiated. As a rule, capacity is specific to the decision the patient is being asked to make. Ask the following questions to determine a patient's decision-making capacity:

- Can the patient make and express personal preferences at all?
- Can the patient comprehend the risks and benefits?
- Does the patient comprehend the implications?
- Can the patient give reasons for the alternative selected?
- Are supporting reasons rational?

If the answer to all these questions is yes, the patient is competent to make the decision at hand. If not, a surrogate (the durable power of attorney for health care, if the patient has identified one) should make the decision. If a durable power of attorney for health care has not been identified, the decision can be made by a family member, friend, or caregiver who knows the patient well. The order of surrogates is determined by state law. If no one is available, the health care provider should make the decision on the basis of the patient's known value system or what the health care provider believes to be in the best interest of the patient.

Mood and Affect

Although major depression (Chapter 397) is no more common among the elderly than among the younger population, minor depression and other affective disorders are common and cause considerable morbidity. Moreover, the clinical manifestations of depression may be atypical, and depression may be masked in patients with cognitive impairment or other neurologic disorders such as Parkinson disease (Chapter 409).

A two-item version of the Patient Health Questionnaire can effectively screen for depression symptoms.[10] The screener asks the patient: Over the past 2 weeks, how often have you been bothered by any of the following problems?

- Little interest or pleasure in doing things
- Feeling down, depressed, or hopeless

Responses are scored as follows: 0, not at all; 1, several days; 2, more than half the days; 3, nearly every day. Persons who score a total of 3 points or higher on the two-item screen have a 75% probability of having a depressive disorder and should be evaluated in more detail (see Table 27-3 and Chapter 397).

Falls, Mobility, and Balance

Approximately one third of community-dwelling persons older than 65 years and half of those older than 80 years fall each year. Ten percent of these falls result in a serious injury. Patients who have fallen or have gait or balance problems are at higher risk of another fall. Performing a falls assessment (measuring orthostatic blood pressure; assessing vision; reviewing medications; and testing balance, gait, and lower extremity strength) and treating risk factors for falling can reduce falls by 30 to 40%.

All older patients should be asked at least annually if they have fallen,[11] and frail older persons should be asked about falls at every visit. In addition, asking about fear of falling can identify patients at risk of future falls.

Patients who have fallen or have a fear of falling should have their balance and gait assessed by direct observation of their ability to perform specific tasks. Tests of balance include the ability to maintain a side-by-side, semitandem, and full-tandem stance for 10 seconds; resistance to a nudge; and stability during a 360-degree turn. Quadriceps strength can be assessed by observing an older person rising from a hard armless chair without using his or her hands.

In addition, direct qualitative and quantitative observation of gait to determine stability is a quick and important component of assessment.[12] Qualitative aspects include evaluation of hesitancy; sway; step length, height, symmetry, and continuity; and path deviation. Gait speed is also a helpful marker for recurrent falls. Patients who take more than 13 seconds to walk 10 meters (0.8 meter per second) are more likely to have recurrent falls and to have a shorter life expectancy.[13]

The timed up-and-go test combines some features of strength and gait. It is a timed test of the patient's ability to rise from a standard armchair, walk 3 meters (10 feet), turn, walk back, and sit down again. Patients who take longer than 20 seconds to complete the test should receive further evaluation.

Medication Review

Older persons often see several different health care providers who prescribe multiple medications that increase the risk for drug-drug interactions and adverse drug events. At a minimum, the clinician should review the patient's updated and accurate medication list at each visit. A good method of detecting potential problems is to have patients bring in all their medications (prescription and nonprescription) in their bottles. Entering a patient's medication list into commercially available computer drug interaction programs can help prevent adverse events. Many electronic health records also alert clinicians to potential drug interactions.

Nutrition

Malnutrition in older adults includes obesity (Chapter 220), undernutrition (Chapter 214), and specific vitamin deficiencies (Chapter 218). Obesity in older adults is defined as a body mass index (BMI) of 30 kg/m^2 or greater. High BMI is associated with poorer function and more comorbidities, such as type 2 diabetes mellitus (Chapter 229), osteoarthritis (Chapter 262), hyperlipidemia (Chapter 206), coronary artery disease (Chapter 52), and sleep apnea (Chapter 100).

At the initial visit, patients should be weighed and asked about weight loss in the previous 12 months. They should be weighed at all follow-up visits. BMI should be calculated on the initial visit and periodically thereafter (e.g., yearly or when a change in weight suggests the need to recalculate). Serum markers, including serum albumin, prealbumin, and cholesterol levels, are nonspecific indicators of nutritional status and can be affected by inflammatory states, physiologic stress, and trauma.

Weight loss of 4% or more during 12 months predicts increased mortality and should prompt an evaluation of medical (e.g., malignant disease, gastrointestinal disorders, hyperthyroidism, diabetes), psychiatric (e.g., depression, dementia), dental, and social or functional (e.g., poverty, inability to shop or to prepare meals) causes. In community-based older adults, a serum 25-hydroxyvitamin D level below 50 nmol/L (20 ng/mL) is associated with an increased risk for relevant clinical disease events.[14]

Urinary Incontinence

Approximately one third of community-dwelling older adult women have some degree of urinary incontinence (Chapter 26), and 75% of older men have abnormal urinary tract symptoms. Complications of incontinence include skin irritation, pressure ulcers, urinary tract infections, sleep disruption, and falls. Identification of urinary incontinence is important because effective behavioral and pharmacologic treatments are available.

A simple screen for urinary incontinence asks the following question: Have you had urinary incontinence (do you "lose" your urine) to the extent that it is bothersome and you would like to know how it can be treated? This may be valuable in determining which patients want further evaluation and therapy. Patients who answer yes should be asked how much urine is leaked, how much it interferes with daily life, and when the leakage occurs. Further evaluation and treatment depend on whether the incontinence is overflow incontinence, urge incontinence, or stress incontinence (see Table 26-3).

PREVENTIVE SERVICES

Preventive services include lifestyle advice, screening tests to detect asymptomatic disease, and vaccinations. Recommended adult immunization schedules for older adults include annual influenza vaccination, one-time pneumonia vaccination, one-time pneumococcal vaccination, one-time herpes zoster vaccination (even if the patient reports a past episode of herpes zoster), and tetanus toxoid vaccination every 10 years after receiving one dose of tetanus, diphtheria, and pertussis vaccination (Tdap). (Chapter 18).

To help the clinician decide what is appropriate for a specific patient, the U.S. Preventive Services Task Force has created an interactive website (*http://epss.ahrq.gov/ePSS/search.jsp*) with recommendations based on the patient's age, gender, tobacco use, and current sexual activity (Chapter 14). For younger elderly persons, recommendations include screening for blood pressure, diabetes (if blood pressure >135/80 mm Hg), hyperlipidemia, obesity, alcohol misuse, colorectal cancer (to age 75 years), vitamin D supplementation, and osteoporosis as well as breast cancer in women (to age 75 years), with appropriate counseling and treatment if these disorders are detected. Exercise or physical therapy is recommended to prevent falls in patients who are at increased risk. Aspirin may be recommended to prevent cardiovascular disease in this population. Other recommendations depend on patient-specific risk factors.

With increasing age, fewer preventive services are recommended because of limited life expectancy and greater comorbidities. Accordingly, some preventive measures (e.g., aspirin to prevent cardiovascular disease) and cancer screenings are not recommended in the very elderly. When the evidence base for preventive services is sparse, decisions should be individualized, on the basis of the patient's personal values, goals, and preferences.

NONMEDICAL ASSESSMENTS

Environmental Assessment

Assessing a patient's environment includes evaluating three components: the person's ability to access community services (e.g., getting to the bank and stores if the patient cannot drive), the safety of the physical environment, and the appropriateness of the living situation for the person's functional ability and cognitive status. A brief screen for safety of the physical environment can be accomplished by using a checklist that is in the public domain (*http://www.cdc.gov/ncipc/pub-res/toolkit/Falls_ToolKit/DesktopPDF/English/booklet_Eng_desktop.pdf*). For home-bound older patients, a home safety evaluation by a home health agency is more appropriate.

Social Support Assessment

When older persons become frail, the adequacy of their social support network may be the determining factor in whether they can remain at home or need institutionalization. A brief screen of social support includes taking a social history, including asking who would be available to help if the patient becomes ill. For patients with functional impairment, the clinician should ascertain who can help the patient perform ADLs or IADLs. Early identification of problems with social support can help avoid crisis situations if the patient has a sudden medical or functional decline. Caregivers should be screened periodically for symptoms of depression or caregiver burnout and referred for counseling or support groups if necessary.

Financial Assessment

Although clinicians do not have the training or expertise to explore financial resources in detail, knowing the patient's insurance status may be helpful. For example, patients with Medicaid coverage may qualify for additional medical or social support benefits. Some may be eligible for other state or local benefits, depending on their income. Others may have long-term care insurance or veterans' benefits that can help pay for caregivers, obviating the need for institutionalization.

A STRATEGIC APPROACH TO GERIATRIC ASSESSMENT FOR THE PRACTICING CLINICIAN

Although assembling an interdisciplinary assessment team is beyond the capability of most practitioners, even small group practices can use teamwork and simple practice design to perform geriatric assessments efficiently and comprehensively. These assessments can lead to local implementation of or referral to comprehensive care models that can improve the outcomes of elderly individuals with a variety of chronic conditions.[A1][A2] Because of time constraints, screening is increasingly delegated to staff and to patients and their families by standing orders, forms, and questionnaires (Table 24-2). For example, previsit questionnaires can be used to gather information about past medical and surgical history; medications and allergies; social history, including available social support resources, preventive services, ability to perform functional tasks, and need for assistance; home safety; and advance directives. In addition, the previsit questionnaire can include specific questions that assess vision, hearing, falls, urinary incontinence, and depressive symptoms. A reasonable approach is to assess these issues annually beginning at age 75 years. Persons who are younger than 75 years but have multiple comorbidities should also be screened and reassessed annually. In addition, some elements of geriatrics assessment (assessing ADLs and IADLs; gait, balance, and falls; mood and affect; and cognition) should be performed after major illnesses, especially for those requiring hospitalization.

TABLE 24-2 APPROACHES TO ASSESSMENT OF FUNCTION IN ELDERLY INDIVIDUALS

ASPECT BEING ASSESSED	PREVISIT QUESTIONNAIRE		OFFICE STAFF ADMINISTERED	
	LENGTH OF SCREEN*	INSTRUMENTS	LENGTH OF SCREEN*	INSTRUMENTS
Functional status	D	Activities of daily living Instrumental activities of daily living		
Advance directives	B	Specific question about advance directives		
MEDICAL ASSESSMENT				
Visual impairment	B	Single-item question	B	Snellen eye chart (see Table 423-1)
Hearing impairment	B	Hearing Handicap Inventory for the Elderly	B (if needed)	Whisper test Audioscope
Cognitive problems	B		D	Mini-cog (see Chapter 27)
Mind, affective problems	D	PHQ	B	
Falls, mobility, balance	B	Simple questions	B	Timed up-and-go test
Medication review	D			Inspection of medication bottles
Malnutrition	D	Single question	B	Weight
Urinary incontinence	B	Single question	B	International Consultation on Incontinence Modular Questionnaire short form if single question is positive (see Chapter 26)
Preventive services	D	Specific questions		
OTHER DIMENSIONS				
Environment	D	Home safety checklist		
Social support	B	Single question		
Financial status			B	Insurance status

*B = brief screen (e.g., <2 minutes); D = detailed evaluation (usually ≥5 minutes); PHQ = Patient Health Questionnaire (see text).

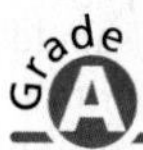

Grade A References

A1. Boult C, Green AF, Boult LB, et al. Successful models of comprehensive care for older adults with chronic conditions: evidence for the Institute of Medicine's "Retooling for an Aging America" report. *J Am Geriatr Soc.* 2009;57:2328-2337.

A2. Deschodt M, Flamaing J, Haentjens P, et al. Impact of geriatric consultation teams on clinical outcome in acute hospitals: a systematic review and meta-analysis. *BMC Med.* 2013;11:48.

GENERAL REFERENCES

For the General References and other additional features, please visit Expert Consult at https://expertconsult.inkling.com.

25 COMMON CLINICAL SEQUELAE OF AGING

JEREMY D. WALSTON

EPIDEMIOLOGY

Older adults make up the majority of patients actively treated in the health care system, in large part owing to their increased burden of chronic diseases but also because of their marked vulnerability to adverse health outcomes, such as functional and cognitive decline, falls, delirium (Chapter 28), and frailty. This age-related vulnerability is thought to have its basis in altered biology that results in tissue and physiologic system changes, which in turn may contribute to many of these conditions and to the chronic disease states commonly seen in older adults. Importantly, these biologic changes are likely to be heterogeneous and to occur at different chronologic ages and in different organs at different rates (Fig. 25-1). These complex age-related biologic changes represent a source of vulnerability that sets the stage for the marked increase in clinical sequelae observed in older adults.

PATHOBIOLOGY

Age-Related Cellular and Molecular Changes

The multiple biologic changes of aging affect important homeostatic functions and can lead to altered cellular function, declines in tissue resiliency, and cellular dropout. Several pathways become dysregulated with increasing age. First, autophagy, an intracellular process responsible for the recycling of damaged or redundant organelles or proteins, becomes less effective with age.[1] The result is an intracellular accumulation of dysfunctional mitochondria and proteins, which in turn can trigger cellular dysregulation through increased levels of free radicals, lower mitochondrial energy production, and programmed cell death or apoptosis. Second, senescent cell populations arise with increasing age and may lead to alterations in tissue and immune system function. For example, fibroblasts and fat cells evolve toward a phenotype whereby reproduction and cell death are less likely to take place, and survival persists in an altered, less functional state.[2] These senescent cells no longer function normally and often chronically secrete inflammatory cytokines and other bioactive molecules that alter surrounding tissues. Senescent T-cell populations also evolve with increasing age, perhaps related to early life viral infections. Although they are often normal in appearance and number, these T cells are less able to respond appropriately to immunogenic signals, thereby increasing vulnerability to infections. Third, some tissues become more sensitive to apoptosis, or programmed cell death. Although apoptosis is a normal cellular program that kills and disassembles damaged or redundant cells in all tissues, it accelerates with age and likely contributes to the vulnerability to chronic disease states, such as Parkinson disease, heart failure, and the generalized loss of cell number in many tissues. Fourth, evidence suggests that increased activity in transforming growth factor-β signaling may play an important role in the fibrotic changes that are observed in the heart, skeletal muscle, and lung tissue and that result in functional decrements with increasing age. Importantly, these aging-related molecular and cellular changes are heterogeneous and may affect individuals at different ages and in different tissues. However, the end result is increased susceptibility to chronic disease states, frailty, declines in function and cognition, and ultimately mortality.

Physiologic System Dysregulation and Its Consequences

Dysfunction in multiple physiologic stress response systems also plays a role in late-life vulnerability. Chronic diseases such as diabetes, vascular disease, chronic obstructive pulmonary disease, depression, and heart failure activate the innate immune system, the sympathetic nervous system, and the

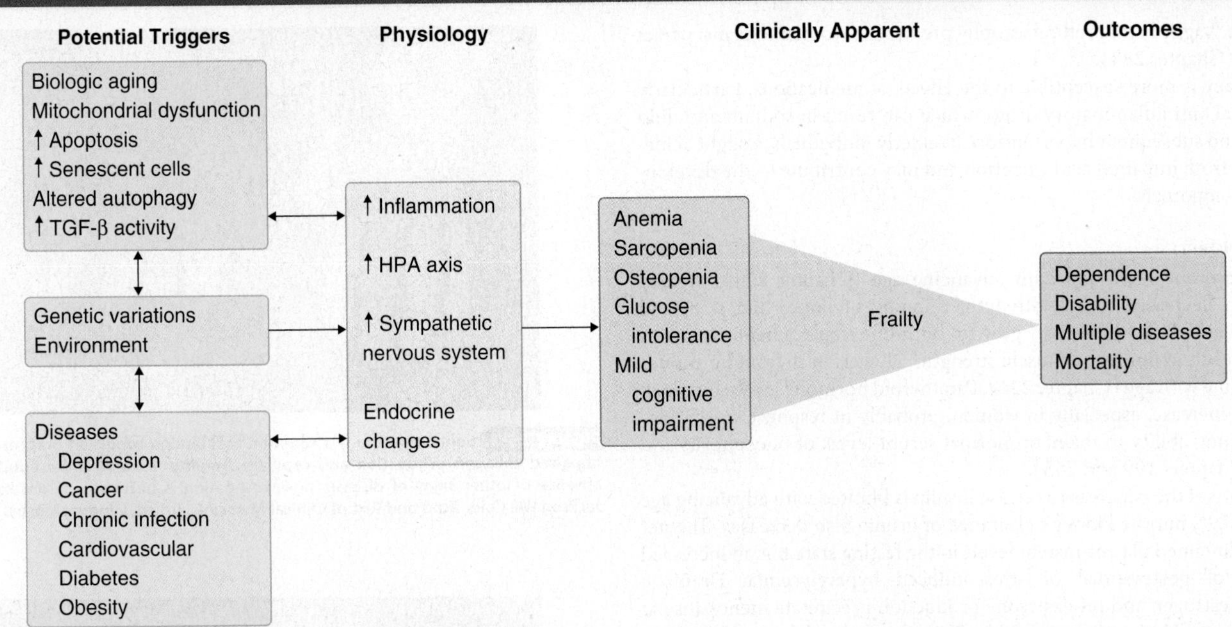

FIGURE 25-1. Comprehensive model pathway for biologic vulnerability to adverse outcomes in aging. HPA = hypothalamic-pituitary-adrenal; TGF-β = transforming growth factor-β.

hypothalamic-pituitary-adrenal axis, which in turn increase cortisol and the inflammatory cytokine interleukin-6 (IL-6).[3] These responses further exacerbate aging-related clinical conditions, such as osteoporosis and hypertension, and increase vulnerability to frailty, functional decline, accidental injury, and worsening chronic disease states[4] (E-Fig. 25-1).

CLINICAL MANIFESTATIONS

Some clinical manifestations are related not to physiologic aging but rather to cumulative exposures, such as with sun-related skin cancer (Chapter 203), or the delayed expression of genetic abnormalities, such as Huntington disease (Chapter 410) or polycystic kidney disease (Chapter 127). However, many organs and systems become less functional with age. For example, a healthy 70-year-old will have only about 50% of the lung function (Chapter 83) and renal function (Chapter 115) of a young adult. The resultant lack of physiologic reserve capacity does not affect day-to-day function but can greatly affect the ability to recover from a severe illness that exhausts the body's reserve capacity.

Despite normal baseline temperatures, older adults are more susceptible to hypothermia or hyperthermia (Chapter 109) after environmental exposure, even though they are less likely to develop fever with infections. For example, patients with pneumonia (Chapter 97) may present with confusion and dehydration rather than with fever and cough.

EFFECTS OF AGING ON SPECIFIC ORGANS AND SYSTEMS

Cardiovascular System

Between the ages of 20 and 80 years, left ventricular systolic function does not change, but the left ventricle gradually thickens. The result is that left ventricular filling in early diastole declines by 50%, and ventricular filling becomes more dependent on atrial contraction (Chapter 53). Although atherosclerosis is the most important cause of symptomatic cardiac disease in elderly people, the age-associated vascular stiffness results in an age-related increase in heart failure despite normal systolic function (Chapter 58). With the gradual loss of up to 90% of sinus node pacemaker cells by the age of 80 years, both the resting heart rate and the maximal heart rate with exercise decline. Conduction system dysfunction contributes to an increase in the prevalence of atrial fibrillation, which is seen in about 4% of community-dwelling older individuals (Chapter 64) and can develop in up to one third of the elderly after surgery (Chapter 433). Heart valves thicken and stiffen, and the prevalence of aortic stenosis and mitral annular calcifications rises (Chapter 75), often causing heart murmurs. Stiffening of the aorta causes an increase in systolic blood pressure, whereas diastolic blood pressure often stays stable or even declines (Chapter 67).

The combination of impaired ventricular filling and the inability to increase the heart rate with stress contributes to the postural hypotension that is seen in 20% of older individuals (Chapter 62) as well as their predisposition to syncope with stresses that younger individuals would tolerate. The reduced ability of the elderly to tolerate cardiovascular stress must be recognized and anticipated whenever they experience a major illness. In addition, coronary artery disease can limit cardiac reserve and increase the risk that hypotension will cause a secondary myocardial infarction.

Respiratory System

The chest wall stiffens with advancing age, and the lungs lose elastic recoil (Chapter 85). Maximal vital capacity declines by about 40%, but oxygen exchange declines by about 50% because of the additive effect of progressive ventilation-perfusion mismatching (Chapter 85). As a result, the arterial Po_2 of many 80-year-olds is about 70 to 75 mm Hg. The clinical manifestations are often progressive shortness of breath with exercise (Chapter 83) and an increased susceptibility to community-acquired pneumonia (Chapter 97) and even to aspiration pneumonia.

Gastrointestinal System

Taste and smell (Chapter 427) decline with advancing age. Food tends to taste less sweet and more bitter.

The esophageal sphincter can become lax (Chapter 138), thereby increasing reflux and even aspiration. Atrophic gastritis reduces the risk of duodenal ulcer but also the absorption of iron (Chapter 159) and vitamin B_{12} (Chapter 164). Delayed gastric emptying can lead to a sense of early satiety and decreased appetite.

A gradual decline in the number of hepatocytes decreases the weight of the liver by about one third by the age of 90 years and decreases the liver's ability to metabolize drugs (Chapter 29). Distal colonic motility from the rectosigmoid to the anal canal declines, and more than 60% of elderly individuals develop constipation (Chapter 136). Diverticula (Chapter 142) become more common with age and are seen in up to 50% of people older than age 80 years.

Urinary System

Glomerular filtration declines by about 1% per year, and kidney size declines by about one third in older adults (Chapter 115). Maximal concentrating capacity declines, and it becomes more difficult to excrete a salt load or to conserve water in the face of dehydration.

The bladder becomes more irritable with advancing age and may generate less power, which is especially a problem in men with prostatic hypertrophy (Chapter 129). By comparison, urinary incontinence (Chapter 26) is more prevalent in women. Residual bladder urine volume increases and nocturia is common. Vaginal and urethral atrophy predispose women to urinary tract infections (Chapter 284).[5]

The kidney is more susceptible to the effects of medications, particularly nonsteroidal anti-inflammatory drugs, which can result in sodium and fluid retention and subsequent hypertension. In elderly individuals, a slight acidemia results from impaired acid excretion and may contribute to the development of osteoporosis.

Endocrine System

Growth hormone levels fall with advancing age (Chapter 224), thereby resulting in decreased muscle strength, thinning of bones and skin, and increased central fat. However, growth hormone replacement does not appear to result in improved muscle strength.[A1] Levels of thyroid hormones do not decline with age (Chapter 226). Parathyroid hormone levels, however, commonly increase, especially in women, probably in response to the kidney's declining ability to maintain normal serum levels of phosphorus and calcium (Chapters 199 and 245).

The ability of the pancreas to release insulin is blunted with advancing age (Chapter 229), but the kidney's clearance of insulin also decreases. The net result is maintained plasma insulin levels in the fasting state but an increased likelihood of postprandial or stress-induced hyperglycemia. Dramatic declines in estrogen and progesterone production precipitate menopause at an average age of 51 years (Chapter 240). Testosterone levels begin to decrease in men by about 50 years of age, often with resulting declines in sexual function but not in the potency of semen (Chapter 234). Testosterone supplements reverse the muscle loss and sexual implications of declining testosterone levels but increase the risk of cardiovascular complications five-fold.[A2]

Immune System

Declines in the responsiveness of the immune system explain why the incidence of autoimmune conditions, such as systemic lupus erythematosus (Chapter 266) and multiple sclerosis (Chapter 411), declines in the elderly. However, this same decline explains increased morbidity and mortality with infectious diseases and the increased risk of reactivating infections such as tuberculosis (Chapter 324) and herpes zoster (Chapter 375). These risks emphasize the importance of vaccination against herpes zoster, influenza, pneumococcal pneumonia, and tetanus in the elderly (Chapter 18).

Hematopoietic System

Hematopoiesis (Chapter 156) is generally sustained with aging, except in response to marked stress. The one exception is that the hematocrit declines somewhat in elderly men, presumably owing to their lower testosterone levels.

Integumentary System

With aging, the epidermis and dermis adhere less tightly and the subcutaneous tissue thins, thereby making the skin feel looser and more likely to wrinkle and ulcerate. Clinical sequelae include senile purpura (Fig. 25-2) due to tears in small venules after bumps or abrasions (Chapter 440). Ultraviolet light exposure also predisposes to skin cancer (Chapter 203), rosacea (Chapter 439), xerosis, and hair loss (Chapter 442).

Wound healing is also compromised, and complete skin healing can take 5.5 weeks instead of 3.5 weeks in individuals older than 65 years. As a result, older adults are more prone to pressure sores when they are bedridden. Pressure sores, which are necrotic areas of muscle, subcutaneous fat, and skin, usually occur between underlying bone and a hard surface (or a soft surface during a prolonged time) as a result of compression and subsequent ischemia (Fig. 25-3). A continuous-pressure threshold of only 30 to 35 mm Hg is needed to cause pressure sores, and a standard mattress can generate pressures five times as high. In addition to pressure injury, other contributing factors include shear injury from rubbing constantly against underlying surfaces; burning injury from friction of the superficial skin layers; and moisture that softens the skin, makes it stick to underlying surfaces, and provides easy access for infection.

Safe positioning, regular turning, avoidance of direct pressure, pressure-reducing beds, deep foam mattresses, and air suspension beds can reduce the incidence of pressure sores. Pressure sores should be photographed to establish a baseline. The wound should be freed of any pressure to prevent additional pressure ulcers. Wet-to-dry dressings are a mainstay, and semiocclusive and occlusive dressings also can be helpful. Surgical or chemical débridement is often required. Topical or systemic antibiotics (Chapter 282) may be needed. Pressure ulcers usually heal within 6 months, but surgical repair is sometimes required.

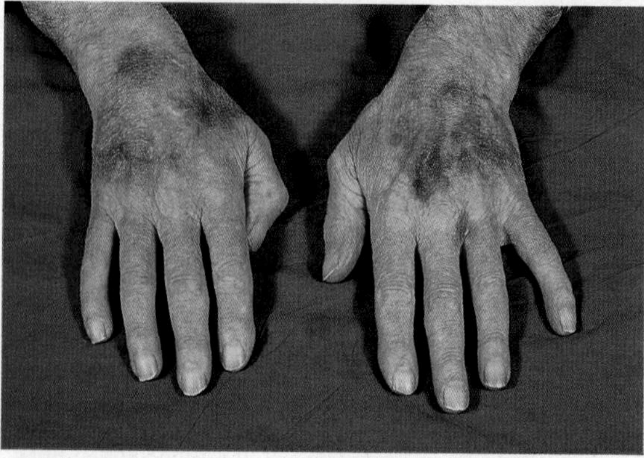

FIGURE 25-2. **Senile purpura is a common and benign condition that results from impaired collagen production and capillary fragility in some older adults. In the absence of other signs of disease, no investigation is necessary.** (From Forbes CD, Jackson WF. Color Atlas and Text of Clinical Medicine. 3rd ed. London: Mosby; 2003.)

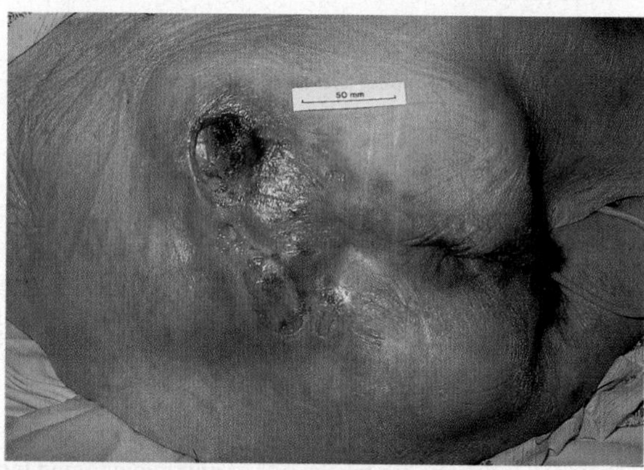

FIGURE 25-3. **Severe sacral pressure sore, one of the serious but preventable complications of immobility.** (From Forbes CD, Jackson WF. Color Atlas and Text of Clinical Medicine. 3rd ed. London: Mosby; 2003.)

Musculoskeletal System

Bone mass and density decrease by about 1% per year but by up to 2 to 3% per year in the first 5 to 10 years after menopause in women (Chapters 243 and 240). Tendons and ligaments become less elastic, thereby contributing to a higher incidence of rupture, especially of the Achilles tendon. Muscle mass declines by about 25% by the age of 70 years and by 30 to 40% by the age of 80 years unless it is offset by exercise.

Clinical Pharmacology

Older adults take a disproportionate share of all prescription (Chapter 29) and nonprescription medications (Chapter 39), and they are at increased risk of drug-drug interactions. Because the elderly have less muscle mass and more fat as a proportion of total body weight, they are more sensitive to the effects of water-soluble drugs and have prolonged effects from lipophilic drugs. Declines in renal and hepatic function reduce the clearance of most drugs, although drugs that are conjugated and glucuronidated are cleared relatively normally. Elderly people also are more likely to be nonadherent to prescribed regimens owing to the number of medications and their cost, mental impairment, and medication side effects.

Cancer and Cancer Screening

The incidence of most cancers rises with age, although many cancers may be less aggressive in the elderly than in younger persons. Some screening options, such as colonoscopy, are associated with their own intrinsic risks (Chapter 134), and all screening tests carry the potential side effects of false-positive results. All of these risks are greater in elderly persons, who also have fewer years of life to gain from early detection and treatment of cancer. As a result, screening recommendations should be adjusted in elderly persons. Examples include discontinuing colon cancer screening after the age of 75 years (Chapter 15), limiting screening mammography to women with at least a 10-year life expectancy,[6] advising any prostate cancer screening only to men with a 15-year life expectancy (Chapter 15), and often discontinuing Pap smear testing in women older than 65 years if prior active screening results have been negative.

Sensory and Sleep

In addition to age-related cognitive decline (Chapters 27 and 28), hearing loss develops in about 25% of individuals older than 65 years (Chapter 428), with decreased neural transmission leading to difficulty in discriminating important sounds from background noise. Presbycusis diminishes the ability to hear high-frequency sounds.

The thickening and stiffening of the lens diminish the ability to focus on nearby objects and increase glare (Chapter 423). Transmission of light through the lens may decline by 50% or more, so elderly individuals require more ambient light. Vitreal detachment causes floaters that also can interfere with vision. Decreased tear production causes dryness of the eyes. All of these conditions contribute to a decline in visual acuity to the extent that 40% of men and 60% of women older than 65 years have a visual acuity of 20/70 or worse.

Older adults tend to have difficulty in sleeping (Chapter 405) yet spend much more time in bed. Sleep apnea also becomes more common with advancing age (Chapter 100).

Frailty as a Clinical Marker of Vulnerability in Older Adults

Frailty, which is a late-life syndrome of weakness, slowness, and weight loss, is associated with high risk of adverse health outcomes and mortality. For example, diminished heart rate variability, which is a marker of dysregulated sympathetic nervous system activity, is associated with aging, frailty, and cardiac arrhythmias. Frail older adults have significantly higher levels of salivary cortisol during the afternoon nadir period, thereby suggesting chronically increased activity of the hypothalamic-pituitary-adrenal axis. Elevated levels of inflammatory cytokines, especially IL-6, tumor necrosis factor-α receptor 1 (TNFR1), and C-reactive protein, are strongly related to functional decline, frailty, chronic disease, and mortality in older adults,[7] probably owing to increased fat, more senescent cells, and free radical production from altered mitochondria. IL-6 is likely to have a negative impact on stem cells and satellite cells, which in turn may contribute to the chronic anemia and age-related declines in skeletal muscle (sarcopenia) and bone mass (osteopenia) commonly observed in frail, older adults. TNFR1 stimulates apoptosis and necroptosis, which are cell programs that lead to cell death and possibly tissue depletion and vulnerability later in life.

In addition to stress response systems, endocrine factors that normally maintain muscle mass also play a role in frailty. For example, the adrenal androgen dehydroepiandrosterone sulfate and insulin-like growth factor 1 are significantly lower in frail adults.

Frailty serves as a clinical indicator of which older adults are at high risk for adverse outcomes, including delirium (Chapter 28), falls, and mortality. Frailty is characterized by signs and symptoms of increasing weakness, fatigue, and declines in activity. Validated frailty screening tools (Table 25-1) enable physicians to identify patients at highest risk of adverse outcomes and mortality and to develop preventive interventions that will decrease risk and improve quality of life.

One approach is to measure physiologic parameters such as grip strength, walking speed, and weight loss as well as to gather information about activity and fatigue levels. With use of this approach, the prevalence of frailty rises with increasing age; approximately 10% of community-dwelling adults older than 65 years meet these frailty criteria and subsequently are at increased risk of functional decline, falling, hospitalization, and death, even after adjustment for age, socioeconomic and smoking status, and multiple common disease states.[8] The Fried or the Cardiovascular Health Study approach has been widely used to identify elders for whom interventions may be helpful.

Frailty increases the likelihood for development of influenza or influenza-like illness in the 6 months after vaccination; the likelihood of requiring care in a skilled nursing or long-term care facility after hospitalization for general surgery; poor renal transplant graft function and early hospital readmission after transplantation; falls, hospitalization, and mortality in patients on hemodialysis for chronic renal failure; and the risk of death in aging intravenous drug users. Biologic differences between frail and non-frail older adults (see Fig. 25-1) drive the marked vulnerability to adverse outcomes observed in the frail subjects.[9] Interventions should be targeted to the specific characteristics of a patient's frailty.[A3] Increasing physical exercise is the mainstay of most programs.[A4]

TABLE 25-1 FOUR COMMONLY USED INSTRUMENTS TO MEASURE FRAILTY IN OLDER ADULTS, WITH RELEVANT MEASUREMENT DOMAINS AND SCORING CRITERIA

INSTRUMENT	DOMAINS	SCORING
Fried frailty phenotype (biologic syndrome model)*	Physical function (slowness, low activity, weakness), nutritive (weight loss), and exhaustion	Score range: 0 to 5 Frail = ≥3 criteria present Intermediate/pre-frail = 1-2 criteria present Robust = 0 criteria present
Frailty index/accumulation of deficits (burden model)†	Diseases, ability in ADL, health attitudes/values, and symptoms/signs from the clinical and neurologic examinations	Number of deficits present and divided by the number of deficits taken into consideration Higher proportion equates to a higher level of frailty
Vulnerable Elders Survey (VES-13)‡	Physical function and ADL/IADL disability	Score range: 0 to 10 Frail = score ≥3
1994 Frailty measure (functional domains model)§	Physical function, nutritive function, cognitive function, sensory problems	Subject scoring a 3 or higher on at least one item in any domain is considered to have a problem or difficulty in that domain Frail = problems/difficulties in ≥2 domains

Details on the use and implementation of these tools can be found in the referenced articles.
ADL = activities of daily living; IADL = instrumental activities of daily living.
*Fried LP, Tangen CM, Walston J, et al. Frailty in older adults: evidence for a phenotype. *J Gerontol A Biol Sci Med Sci.* 2001;56:M146-M156.
†Rockwood K, Andrew M, Mitnitski A. A comparison of two approaches to measuring frailty in elderly people. *J Gerontol A Biol Sci Med Sci.* 2007;62:738-743.
‡Saliba D, Elliott M, Rubenstein LZ, et al. The Vulnerable Elders Survey: a tool for identifying vulnerable older people in the community. *J Am Geriatr Soc.* 2001;49:1691-1699.
§Strawbridge WJ, Shema SJ, Balfour JL, et al. Antecedents of frailty over three decades in an older cohort. *J Gerontol B Psychol Sci Soc Sci.* 1998;53:S9-S16.

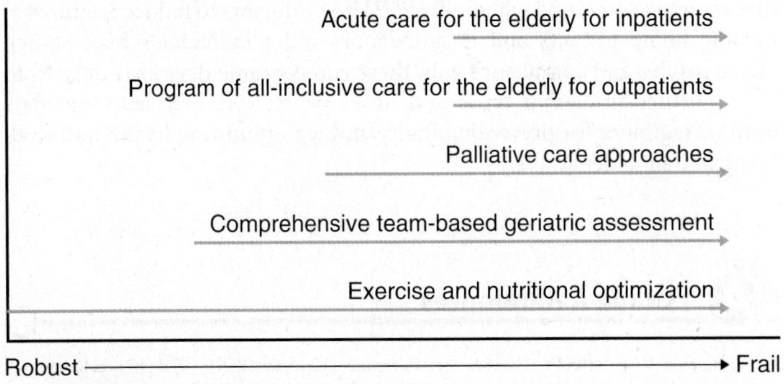

Acute care for the elderly for inpatients
Program of all-inclusive care for the elderly for outpatients
Palliative care approaches
Comprehensive team-based geriatric assessment
Exercise and nutritional optimization
Robust → Frail

FIGURE 25-4. Assessment and treatments in frail and vulnerable older adults.

The Care of Frail Older Patients in Clinical Settings

Focused prevention of iatrogenic injuries or recurrent hospitalizations and remediation of symptoms are often warranted for frail vulnerable older adults[10] (Fig. 25-4). Physical activity, exercise interventions, and nutritional supplementation can reduce disability and symptoms and improve quality of life across the spectrum of robust to frail older adults.[A5] In addition, exercise and weight loss together improve function in obese and frail older adults. Other options include a team-based approach that engages the patient, family members, caregivers, health care providers, and social workers. Classic palliative care, with appropriate pain management, less invasive treatment plans, limited hospital visits, and organized home care plans, can greatly improve quality of life. If the patient has frequently been admitted to an inpatient setting, a program for all-inclusive care or a medical daycare setting may help prevent recurrent admissions and improve quality of life. Once admitted to the hospital, frail older adults may benefit from being congregated in a unit that specializes in their care and can provide attention to their functionality, continence, sleep disturbances, delirium, and palliative care issues.

TABLE 25-2 EVALUATION OF A PATIENT WHO HAS FALLEN

Blood tests to exclude anemia, infection, and metabolic problems such as diabetes and thyroid disease
Electrocardiography to evaluate heart disease
24-Hour electrocardiographic recording or loop monitoring to evaluate arrhythmias (Chapter 62)
Echocardiography for patients with significant heart murmurs (Chapter 55)
Drug levels to determine whether a patient is being undertreated or overtreated with a particular drug
If focal neurologic signs or symptoms are present, a computed tomography scan of the brain
If suggestive symptoms are present, radiography of the neck or spine to look for spinal stenosis

Falls

Falls are a common manifestation of frailty. Contributing factors include cardiopulmonary disease, poor eyesight, hearing loss, balance disturbances, weakness, movement disorders, neuropathies, poor judgment, depression, osteoporosis, arthritis, and foot disorders. The risk of falling also increases in patients who take more prescription medications, especially hypnotics, muscle relaxants, antihypertensive agents, diuretics, and antidepressant medications. Environmental risks include stairs, loose objects, rugs, poor lighting, poorly fitting shoes, uneven pavements, and slippery surfaces.

The approach to a patient who has fallen must include a careful history of the circumstances surrounding the fall and all conditions that could contribute to it. The physical examination should test vision, gait, balance, muscle strength, neurologic function, and pulmonary function. Further testing is recommended whenever the history and physical examination do not reveal the cause of falling or if they reveal conditions that require further evaluation (Table 25-2). In general, this evaluation is similar to the evaluation for syncope (Chapter 62).

Given the strong relationship between vitamin D deficiency and frailty,[11] clinical trials are under way with some evidence that vitamin D_3 supplementation may reduce the mortality in elderly individuals.[A6] Exercise programs, including Tai Chi, improve strength and balance as well as help prevent falls that are often associated with frailty.[A7][A8] Hip protectors to reduce fractures in nursing home patients and in ambulatory older individuals have shown mixed results, and compliance with these cumbersome devices is only 25 to 70%. Further studies of types and doses of exercise may help elucidate optimal regimens for preventing frailty and for optimizing health and well-being of frail, older adults.

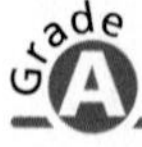

Grade A References

A1. Giannoulis MG, Martin FC, Nair KS, et al. Hormone replacement therapy and physical function in healthy older men. Time to talk hormones? *Endocr Rev.* 2012;33:314-377.

A2. Basaria S, Coviello AD, Travison TG, et al. Adverse events associated with testosterone administration. *N Engl J Med.* 2010;363:109-122.

A3. Cameron ID, Fairhall N, Langron C, et al. A multifactorial interdisciplinary intervention reduces frailty in older people: randomized trial. *BMC Med.* 2013;11:65.

A4. Gine-Garriga M, Roque-Figuls M, Coll-Planas L, et al. Physical exercise interventions for improving performance-based measures of physical function in community-dwelling, frail older adults: a systematic review and meta-analysis. *Arch Phys Med Rehabil.* 2014;95:753-769.

A5. Pahor M, Guralnik JM, Ambrosius WT, et al. Effect of structured physical activity on prevention of major mobility disability in older adults: the LIFE study randomized clinical trial. *JAMA.* 2014;311:2387-2396.

A6. Bjelakovic G, Gluud LL, Nikolova D, et al. Vitamin D supplementation for prevention of mortality in adults. *Cochrane Database Syst Rev.* 2014;1:CD007470.

A7. Moyer VA. Prevention of falls in community-dwelling older adults: U.S. Preventive Services Task Force recommendation statement. *Ann Intern Med.* 2012;157:197-204.

A8. El-Khoury F, Cassou B, Charles MA, et al. The effect of fall prevention exercise programmes on fall induced injuries in community dwelling older adults: systematic review and meta-analysis of randomised controlled trials. *BMJ.* 2013;347:f6234.

GENERAL REFERENCES

For the General References and other additional features, please visit Expert Consult at https://expertconsult.inkling.com.

26 INCONTINENCE

NEIL M. RESNICK

DEFINITION

Urinary incontinence is the involuntary leakage of urine sufficient to be a health or social problem.

EPIDEMIOLOGY

More than twice as common in women as in men, the prevalence of incontinence increases with age. Incontinence afflicts 15 to 30% of older adults living at home, one third of those in acute care settings, and half of those in nursing homes. It predisposes to perineal rashes, pressure ulcers, urinary tract infections, urosepsis, falls, and fractures, and it is associated with embarrassment, stigmatization, isolation, depression, anxiety, sexual dysfunction, and risk for institutionalization. Its cost in the United States exceeds $26 billion annually.

Despite these considerations, geriatric incontinence remains largely neglected, by patients and physicians alike. This is unfortunate because its increased prevalence with age relates more to age-associated diseases and functional impairments than to age itself. Most important, incontinence is usually treatable and often curable at all ages, even in frail elderly people, although the approach in older patients must be broader than that employed in younger patients.

PATHOBIOLOGY

At any age, continence depends not only on the integrity of lower urinary tract function but also on the presence of adequate mentation, mobility, motivation, and manual dexterity. Although incontinence in younger patients is rarely associated with deficits in these domains, such deficits occur commonly in older patients, in whom they can cause or exacerbate incontinence or influence therapeutic approaches.

With age, bladder capacity does not change, but bladder sensation and contractility decrease. At the cellular level, detrusor smooth muscle develops a "dense band pattern" characterized by dense sarcolemmal bands with depleted caveolae. This depletion may mediate the age-related decline in bladder contractility. In addition, an incomplete disjunction pattern characterized by scattered protrusion junctions develops and may underlie the high prevalence of involuntary bladder contractions (detrusor overactivity) in older adults of both sexes. Bladder ischemia and/or inflammation may also contribute.[1,2] Urethral length and sphincter strength decrease in women, whereas the prostate enlarges in most men and causes measurable obstruction in about half. The postvoid residual volume in the bladder also increases in both sexes but normally to less than 100 mL. In addition, elderly people often excrete most of their fluid intake at night, even in the absence of venous insufficiency, renal disease, heart failure, or prostatism. Because this shift in nocturnal fluid excretion is coupled with an age-associated increase in sleep disorders, most older adults have one or two episodes of nocturia per night.

None of these changes causes incontinence, but all predispose to it. This predisposition, combined with the increased likelihood that an older person will encounter an additional pathologic, physiologic, or pharmacologic insult, explains the increased prevalence of incontinence with age. Thus, the onset or exacerbation of incontinence in an older person is likely to be due to precipitants that are outside the lower urinary tract and that are amenable to medical intervention. Furthermore, treatment of the precipitants alone may be sufficient to restore continence, even if there is coexisting urinary tract dysfunction. For example, a flare of hip arthritis in a woman with age-related detrusor overactivity may decrease mobility sufficiently to convert her urinary urgency into incontinence. Treatment of the arthritis, rather than the involuntary detrusor contractions, will not only restore continence but also lessen pain and improve mobility. Because of their frequency, reversibility, and association with morbidity beyond incontinence, the transient precipitant causes should be addressed first.

Causes of Transient Incontinence

Incontinence is transient in up to one third of community-dwelling elderly people and in up to half of acutely hospitalized patients. Although most

TABLE 26-1 CAUSES OF TRANSIENT INCONTINENCE: DIAPERS MNEMONIC

Delirium	Result of underlying illness or medication; incontinence is secondary and abates once the cause of delirium is corrected	
Infection—*symptomatic* UTI	Acute, symptomatic UTI causes incontinence, but the far more common asymptomatic bacteriuria does not	
Atrophic urethritis/vaginitis	Characterized by vaginal erosions, telangiectasia, petechiae, and friability; may cause or contribute to incontinence. Although oral estrogen may worsen incontinence, a 3- to 12-month course of topical estrogen can be useful	
Pharmaceuticals	*Drug type:*	*Potential effects on continence:*
	Sedative-hypnotics (e.g., long-acting benzodiazepines; alcohol)	Sedation, delirium, decreased mobility
	Anticholinergics (dicyclomine, disopyramide, sedating antihistamines, antipsychotics, tricyclic antidepressants, anti-Parkinson, antidepressants) (*not* SSRIs)	Urinary retention, overflow incontinence, delirium, impaction; the antipsychotics also decrease mobility
	Opiates	Urinary retention, stool impaction, sedation, delirium
	α-Adrenergic antagonists	Relax sphincter; may induce stress incontinence in women
	α-Adrenergic agonists	Urinary retention in men (tighten sphincter, prostate)
	Calcium-channel blockers, especially the dihydropyridines	Urinary retention; nocturnal diuresis due to fluid retention
	"Loop" diuretics (thiazide-like agents only rarely cause it)	Polyuria, frequency, urgency
	NSAIDs	Nocturnal diuresis due to fluid retention
	Thiazolidinediones	Nocturnal diuresis due to fluid retention
	Some nociceptives (gabapentin, pregabalin)	Nocturnal diuresis due to fluid retention; sedation; delirium
	Dopamine receptor agonists (e.g., ropinirole, pramipexole)	Nocturnal diuresis due to fluid retention
	Angiotensin-converting enzyme inhibitors	Drug-induced cough leads to stress incontinence in women
	Vincristine	Urinary retention due to neuropathy
Excess urine output	From large intake, diuretic agents (theophylline, caffeinated beverages, alcohol), and metabolic disorders (hyperglycemia, hypercalcemia); nocturnal incontinence may result from mobilization of peripheral edema (heart failure, venous insufficiency, side effects of medications)	
Restricted mobility	Often results from overlooked, correctable conditions such as arthritis, pain, foot problems, postprandial hypotension, or fear of falling	
Stool impaction	May cause both fecal and urinary incontinence that remit with disimpaction	

NSAIDs = nonsteroidal anti-inflammatory drugs; SSRI = selective serotonin reuptake inhibitor; UTI = urinary tract infection.
Adapted from Resnick NM, Tadic SD, Yalla SV. Geriatric incontinence and voiding dysfunction. In: Wein AJ, Novick AC, Partin AW, et al, eds. *Campbell-Walsh Urology*, 10th ed. St. Louis: Elsevier; 2010.

transient causes are outside the lower urinary tract (Table 26-1), three points warrant emphasis. First, the risk for transient incontinence is increased if, in addition to physiologic changes of the lower urinary tract, there also are pathologic changes. Anticholinergic agents are more likely to cause overflow incontinence in individuals with a weak or obstructed bladder, whereas excess urine output is more likely to cause urge incontinence in people with detrusor overactivity or impaired mobility. Second, these transient causes may persist if left untreated and should not be dismissed merely because incontinence is long-standing. Third, identification of the most common cause is of little value because causes vary among individuals, and geriatric incontinence is rarely due to just one cause.

Causes of Established Incontinence Related to the Lower Urinary Tract

Detrusor overactivity, also called involuntary bladder contraction or *overactive bladder*, generally causes *urge incontinence* and is the most common type of lower urinary tract dysfunction in incontinent elderly people, in whom it accounts for about two thirds of cases. Histologically, detrusor overactivity is associated with the complete disjunction pattern, with widening of the intercellular space, reduction of normal (intermediate) muscle cell junctions, and emergence of novel protrusion junctions and ultraclose abutments that connect cells together in chains. These connections may mediate a change in cell coupling from a mechanical to an electrical mechanism that results in involuntary bladder contraction. Other potential causes include ischemia, abnormalities in suburothelial myofibroblasts, and changes in central nervous system structural and functional control mechanisms.

At any age, detrusor overactivity is usually idiopathic, but it can be associated with a variety of other causes that may affect prognosis and management. Such conditions include an upper motor neuron lesion (Chapters 400 and 419), urethral obstruction, stress incontinence, bladder calculus, and bladder carcinoma (Chapter 197).

Detrusor overactivity exists as two subsets in elderly people: one in which contractile function is preserved and one in which it is impaired. The latter condition, termed *detrusor hyperactivity with impaired contractility*, has several implications. First, because the bladder is weak, these patients commonly develop urinary retention, which is also seen in patients with outlet obstruction and detrusor underactivity. Second, even in the absence of retention, detrusor hyperactivity with impaired contractility mimics other lower urinary tract causes of incontinence. For instance, if the involuntary detrusor contraction occurs coincident with a stress maneuver and if the weak contraction is not detected, detrusor hyperactivity with impaired contractility will be misdiagnosed as stress incontinence. Alternatively, because detrusor hyperactivity with impaired contractility may be associated with urinary urgency, frequency, weak flow rate, elevated residual urine, and bladder trabeculation, in men it may mimic prostatic obstruction. Third, anticholinergic therapy of detrusor hyperactivity with impaired contractility may result in urinary retention owing to bladder weakness, thereby requiring alternative therapeutic approaches.

Stress incontinence, which is the second most common cause of incontinence in older women and the dominant cause in middle-aged women, usually reflects urethral hypermobility plus some degree of sphincter weakness. Stress incontinence is rare in men but can result from sphincter damage following radical but not transurethral prostatectomy.

Urethral obstruction is the second most common cause of established incontinence in older men, although most obstructed men are not incontinent. When obstruction is associated with incontinence, it usually presents as urge incontinence owing to the associated detrusor overactivity; overflow incontinence is uncommon. Outlet obstruction is rare in women but may result from a bladder neck suspension or from urethral kinking associated with a large cystocele.

Detrusor underactivity is usually idiopathic. When it causes incontinence, it is associated with overflow incontinence (<10% of incontinence).

Damage to lower urinary tract innervation can cause several types of dysfunction. A brain lesion may cause detrusor overactivity. A spinal cord lesion (Chapters 189 and 400) above the sacral level can cause both detrusor overactivity and detrusor-sphincter dyssynergia, a condition in which the sphincter contracts rather than relaxes during detrusor contraction; the result can be severe outlet obstruction and hydronephrosis. A spinal cord lesion below the sacral level can cause detrusor underactivity, sphincter weakness, or both. Peripheral and autonomic nerve damage can cause still additional problems. Because *neurogenic bladder* is such a nonspecific term, it is preferable to refer to the specific dysfunction that it causes.

Causes of Incontinence Unrelated to the Lower Urinary Tract (Functional Incontinence)

"Functional" incontinence, which is often cited as a distinct type of geriatric incontinence and attributed to deficits of cognition and mobility, implies that urinary tract function is normal. However, normal urinary tract function is the exception, even in continent elderly people, and is rarely observed in incontinent elderly people. Moreover, incontinence is not inevitable, even with dementia or immobility. Among the most severely demented institutionalized residents, nearly 20% are continent; among those who can transfer from a bed to a chair, nearly half are continent. Functionally impaired individuals also are the most likely to suffer from factors that cause transient incontinence, and a diagnosis of functional incontinence may result in failure to detect these reversible causes. Finally, if functionally impaired individuals also have urethral obstruction or stress incontinence, they may benefit from targeted therapy. Nonetheless, functional impairment often contributes to incontinence, and addressing its causes and those of transient incontinence may ameliorate incontinence sufficiently to obviate the need for further investigation.

CLINICAL MANIFESTATIONS

The manifestations of transient incontinence depend on the underlying condition. For established incontinence, detrusor overactivity usually manifests as *urge incontinence,* characterized by leakage that follows the *abrupt* onset or intensification of a desire to void, leakage of a moderate to large amount, urinary frequency (>8 voids/day), nocturia, and nocturnal incontinence. However, some patients with detrusor overactivity may present without the urge component. *Stress incontinence* causes leakage that coincides *instantaneously* with both the onset and cessation of a cough or other cause of increased abdominal pressure; nocturnal leakage is rare. Some patients report both types of incontinence, or *mixed incontinence,* but it is useful to determine which component is the most bothersome. In men with sphincter damage following radical prostatectomy, leakage resembles the intermittent drip of a leaky faucet. Occasionally, patients present with incontinence that is more difficult to characterize clinically without further testing.

DIAGNOSIS

In addition to a targeted clinical evaluation (Table 26-2), a bladder diary can provide diagnostic clues and guide therapy (Fig. 26-1). For example, incontinence occurring only between 8 AM and noon may be caused by a morning loop diuretic. Incontinence that occurs at night in a demented man with heart failure, but not during a 4-hour nap in his wheelchair, is likely due to nocturnal diuresis associated with his heart failure and not to dementia, impaired mobility, or prostatic obstruction. A woman with volume-dependent stress incontinence may leak only on the way to void after a full night's sleep, when

TABLE 26-2 CLINICAL EVALUATION OF THE INCONTINENT PATIENT

HISTORY

Type (urge, stress, overflow, or mixed)
Incontinence frequency, severity, duration
Pattern (diurnal, nocturnal, or both; also, e.g., after taking medications)
Associated symptoms (straining to void, incomplete emptying, dysuria, hematuria, suprapubic/perineal discomfort)
Alteration in bowel habit/sexual function (because of proximity to the bladder and shared innervation)
Other relevant factors (cancer, acute illness, neurologic disease, pelvic or lower urinary tract surgery/radiation therapy)
Medications, including nonprescription agents (see Table 26-1)
Brief assessment of cognitive and physical function

PHYSICAL EXAMINATION

Identify other relevant medical conditions (e.g., congestive heart failure, peripheral edema)
If stress incontinence suspected, determine whether leakage *coincides* with the onset *and* cessation of a single, forceful cough
Palpate for bladder distention after voiding
Pelvic examination to detect atrophic vaginitis, pelvic muscle laxity, pelvic mass
Rectal examination (skin irritation, resting tone and voluntary control of anal sphincter, prostate nodule; fecal impaction (*note:* prostate size correlates poorly with presence of urethral obstruction)
Neurologic examination (mental status and elemental examination, including sacral reflexes and perineal sensation)

INITIAL INVESTIGATION

Bladder diary (see Fig. 26-1)
Metabolic survey (electrolytes, calcium, glucose, and urea nitrogen as appropriate)
Measure postvoid residual volume, by portable ultrasound if available
Urinalysis to detect sterile hematuria or infection; culture if new-onset or worsening incontinence
Renal ultrasound to detect hydronephrosis in men whose postvoid residual volume urine exceeds about 200 mL
Urine cytology for patients with hematuria, pain, or unexplained new-onset or worsening incontinence
Uroflowmetry for men in whom urethral obstruction is suspected
Cystoscopy for patients with hematuria, suspicion of lower urinary tract pathology (e.g., bladder fistula, stone, or tumor; urethral diverticulum), or need for lower urinary tract surgery

Adapted from Resnick NM, Yalla SV. Management of urinary incontinence in the elderly. *N Engl J Med.* 1985;313:800-805.

Date	Time	Volume Voided (mL)	Are You Wet or Dry?	Approximate Volume of Incontinence	Comments
4/5	3:40 pm	240	Wet	Slight	
	6:05 pm	210	Dry		
	8:15 pm	150	Dry		Running water
	10:20 pm	150	Wet	15 mL	Bowel movement
	10:30 pm	30	Dry		
4/6	3:15 am	270	Wet	Slight	
	6:05 am	300	Wet	Slight	
	7:40 am	200	Dry		
	9:50 am	?	Dry		
	11:20 am	200	Dry		
	12:50 pm	180	Dry		
	1:40 pm	240	Dry		
	3:35 pm	160	Dry		
	6:00 pm	170	Dry		
	8:20 pm	215	Wet	Slight	Running water
	10:25 pm	130	Dry		

FIGURE 26-1. Sample bladder diary. Bladder diary of an incontinent 75-year-old man. Urodynamic evaluation excluded urethral obstruction and confirmed a diagnosis of detrusor hyperactivity with impaired contractility (detrusor hyperactivity with impaired contractility). Note the 24-hour urine output of nearly 3 liters due to the belief that drinking 10 glasses of fluid per day was "good for my health." (He did not mention this until queried about the voiding record.) Given the typical voided volume of 150 to 250 mL and a measured postvoid residual of 150 mL, excess fluid intake was overwhelming his usual bladder capacity of 400 mL (150 + 250 mL). Although involuntary bladder contractions were present, the easily reversible volume component of the problem, combined with the risk for precipitating urinary retention with an anticholinergic agent, prompted treatment with volume restriction alone. After daily urinary output dropped to 1500 mL, frequency abated, and incontinence resolved. (Adapted from DuBeau CE, Resnick NM. Evaluation of the causes and severity of geriatric incontinence: a critical appraisal. *Urol Clin North Am.* 1991;18:243-256.)

her bladder contains more than 400 mL—more than it ever does during her continent waking hours.

Because urinary retention is difficult to detect by examination and can affect diagnosis and therapy, the postvoid residual volume should be determined routinely, except possibly in middle-aged women with a classic presentation of stress incontinence. For example, in a randomized trial of women with uncomplicated, demonstrable stress urinary incontinence and a postvoid residual volume of less than 150 mL, preoperative office evaluation alone provided similar 1-year outcomes as did evaluation with urodynamic testing.[A1] Urodynamic testing is generally recommended only when diagnostic certainty is required, such as before most surgical repairs in older patients, or if there is evidence of a serious underlying cause of the incontinence, such as a brain or spinal cord lesion, carcinoma of the bladder or prostate, hydronephrosis, or bladder calculus.[3] Urodynamic evaluation comprises a battery of tests designed to assess the lower urinary tract during the filling and voiding phases of micturition. The selection among tests depends on the clinical setting and question to be answered; for instance, measuring detrusor pressure and urine flow during voiding can determine whether urethral obstruction is present, whereas monitoring bladder and urethral pressures during the filling phase and with coughing may be helpful for patients with an atypical presentation of mixed incontinence.

TREATMENT

Rx

Optimal therapy requires a multifactorial approach (Table 26-3), including treatment of transient causes, underlying medical conditions, functional impairments, and the urinary tract abnormality itself. Although pads and diapers have a role, they remain an adjunct to more specific therapy.

Behavioral Therapy

Behavioral therapy includes education, self-monitoring with a bladder diary, adjustment of the intake of fluid and caffeine,[3,4] weight loss for overweight women with stress incontinence,[A2] use of aids (e.g., a bedside urinal), and various types of bladder retraining and urethral sphincter exercises (e.g., progressively increasing voiding intervals, strategies to cope with urgency, and pelvic muscle exercises).[4,5][A3] The efficacy of behavioral therapy is equivalent to pharmacotherapy for urge incontinence. For stress incontinence, the efficacy of behavioral therapy is superior to drugs but inferior to surgery.[5][A3][A4] Moreover, combining behavioral and pharmacologic therapy may prove more beneficial than either treatment alone, especially for urge incontinence,[A3][A5] because neither therapy generally abolishes involuntary bladder contractions.[6] For institutionalized patients who are cognitively impaired but can state their name and are partly mobile, regular daytime reminders to void ("prompted voiding")

TABLE 26-3 STEPWISE APPROACH TO TREATMENT OF URINARY INCONTINENCE*

CONDITION	CLINICAL TYPE OF INCONTINENCE†	TREATMENT
Detrusor overactivity with normal contractility	Urge	1. Bladder retraining or prompted voiding regimens 2. ± Bladder relaxant medication if needed and not contraindicated (see drug list below). If treatment fails, consider posterior tibial neurostimulation, sacral neuromodulation, or intradetrusor injection of onabotulinumtoxinA 3. Indwelling catheterization alone is often unhelpful because detrusor spasms often increase, leading to leakage around the catheter 4. In selected cases, induce urinary retention pharmacologically and add intermittent or indwelling catheterization‡
Detrusor hyperactivity with impaired contractility	Urge§	1. If bladder empties adequately, behavioral methods (as above) ± bladder relaxant medication (low doses; especially feasible if sphincter incompetence coexists) 2. If residual urine >150 mL, augmented voiding techniques¶ or intermittent catheterization (± bladder relaxant medication). If neither feasible, undergarment or indwelling catheter‡ 3. In selected cases, induce urinary retention pharmacologically and add intermittent or indwelling catheterization‡
Stress incontinence	Stress	1. Conservative methods (weight loss if obese; treatment of cough or atrophic vaginitis; physical maneuvers to prevent leakage [e.g., tighten pelvic muscles before cough, cross legs]; occasionally, use of tampon or pessary is helpful) 2. If leakage threshold ≥150 mL identified, adjust fluid excretion and voiding intervals appropriately 3. Pelvic muscle exercises ± biofeedback/weighted intravaginal cones; must continue indefinitely 4. Surgery (sling, artificial sphincter, periurethral bulking injections)
Urethral obstruction	Urge/overflow‖	1. Conservative methods (including adjustment of fluid excretion, bladder retraining/prompted voiding) if hydronephrosis, recurrent symptomatic UTI, and hematuria have been excluded 2. α-Adrenergic antagonist 3. Also consider adding a bladder relaxant if detrusor overactivity coexists, postvoid residual volume is small, and surgery is not desired/feasible; *monitor postvoid residual volume!* 4. Finasteride, if not contraindicated and the patient either prefers it or is not a surgical candidate 5. Surgery (incision, prostatectomy) is an effective alternative before or after these steps
Underactive detrusor	Overflow	1. Decompress for at least several days (the larger the postvoid residual volume, the longer should be the decompression [up to a month]) and then perform a voiding trial 2. Exclude urethral obstruction if this has not already been done 3. If cannot void or if postvoid residual volume remains large, try augmented voiding techniques¶ ± α-adrenergic antagonist, but only if some voiding possible; bethanechol *rarely* useful 4. If fails, or voiding is not possible, intermittent or indwelling catheterization‡

BLADDER RELAXANT AGENTS FOR URGE INCONTINENCE

- Anticholinergic
  - Oxybutynin IR, 7.5-20 mg daily (2.5-5 mg tid-qid); oxybutynin XL, 5-30 mg once daily; oxybutynin patch (3.9 mg/day) twice weekly; oxybutynin 10% gel (1 g topically once per day)
  - Tolterodine, 1-2 mg twice daily; tolterodine LA, 4 mg once daily
  - Darifenacin, 7.5-15 mg once daily
  - Solifenacin, 5-10 mg once daily
  - Trospium, 20 mg daily to twice daily; 60 mg (extended release) once daily
  - Fesoterodine, 4-8 mg once daily
- β_3-Adrenergic agonist
  - Mirabegron, 25-50 mg once daily

*These treatments should be initiated only after adequate toilet access has been ensured, contributing conditions have been treated (e.g., atrophic vaginitis, UTI, fecal impaction, heart failure), fluid management has been optimized, and unnecessary or exacerbating medications have been addressed. For additional details, see text.

†*Urge:* leakage in the absence of stress maneuvers and urinary retention, usually preceded by *abrupt* onset or intensification of the need to void; *stress:* leakage that coincides *instantaneously* with stress maneuvers, in the absence of urinary retention or detrusor contraction; *overflow:* frequent leakage of small amounts associated with urinary retention.

‡UTI prophylaxis can be used for recurrent symptomatic UTIs, but only if catheter is not indwelling.

§May also mimic stress or overflow incontinence.

‖Also can cause postvoid "dribbling" alone, which is treated conservatively (e.g., by sitting to void and allowing more time, "double voiding," and in men by gently "milking" the urethra after voiding).

¶Augmented voiding techniques include Credé (application of suprapubic pressure) and Valsalva (straining) maneuvers, and double voiding. They should be performed only *after* voiding has begun.

UTI = urinary tract infection.

Adapted and updated in 2014 from Resnick NM. Voiding dysfunction and urinary incontinence. In: Beck JC, ed. *Geriatric Review Syllabus*. New York: American Geriatrics Society; 1991:141-154.

have proved effective for daytime incontinence; pads and diapers are appropriate for the others.[7]

Pharmacotherapy

Currently approved drugs have not proved effective for stress incontinence and overflow incontinence. For urge incontinence, however, several bladder relaxants have proved modestly and equally effective (see Table 26-3), even in trials that targeted older patients.[5] A3 A6 A7 All of the anticholinergics have antimuscarinic properties, such as dry mouth, constipation, visual blurring, and occasional confusion. Yet each is well tolerated even in cognitively impaired elderly patients when prescribed properly, although cognitive status should be monitored. A8 These drugs also can be well tolerated in patients taking cholinesterase inhibitors. The choice among these drugs often hinges on other considerations. For instance, immediate-release oxybutynin has the quickest onset of action, making it an inexpensive and effective choice for patients who need excellent control at predictable times. The other drugs, although more expensive, can be used less often and can be better tolerated for daily use. Mirabegron, a β_3-adrenergic agonist, is a newer drug with an efficacy similar to the anticholinergic agents.[8]

Regardless of the drug selected, the key is to begin with a low dose and increase it slowly, realizing that the full benefit is generally not apparent for about 2 months and that side effects may offset the benefit. With such titration, urge incontinence can be controlled in about one third of patients and substantially improved in another one third.

Surgical Procedures

Surgery for stress incontinence has proved effective for women of all ages, including elderly women, and is relatively durable. A4 Periurethral bulking injections can help frail women or those with mild stress incontinence, but it does not generally restore continence. However, urethral sling and mid-urethral tape suspension procedures can cure most women for at least 5 years. For women with more complex stress incontinence and for men with stress incontinence more than 1 year after radical prostatectomy, an artificial sphincter has proved effective and relatively durable. Experience with the "male sling" is still limited.

Surgical interventions for urge incontinence, including neuromodulation, A9 tibial nerve stimulation, A10 and injections of onabotulinum toxin, A11 A12 are third-line agents. However, these procedures have not yet been studied adequately in elderly people. In addition, the limited available data suggest that their efficacy may be only modestly better than that of pharmacotherapy, and that older patients may not fare as well as younger ones.

PREVENTION

There are scant data regarding the prevention of incontinence, but one randomized trial of an educational and behavioral modification program for women older than 55 years found that it reduced the risk for incontinence for 1 year. A13 A secondary analysis of the Diabetes Prevention Program found that, at the end of 3 years, an intensive lifestyle intervention was associated with reduced risk for self-reported incontinence, with most of the benefit explained by weight loss and a reduced risk for stress incontinence. A14

PROGNOSIS

Limited data suggest that incontinence progresses in about one third of patients and remits in about 10 to 15%, although it is unclear how much of the remission reflects intervention or improvement in functional or medical status.

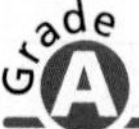

Grade A References

A1. Nager CW, Brubaker L, Litman HJ, et al. A randomized trial of urodynamic testing before stress-incontinence surgery. *N Engl J Med.* 2012;366:1987-1997.

A2. Subak LL, Wing R, West DS, et al. Weight loss to treat urinary incontinence in overweight and obese women. *N Engl J Med.* 2009;360:481-490.

A3. Shamliyan T, Wyman J, Kane RL. AHRQ Comparative Effectiveness Reviews. Nonsurgical treatments for urinary incontinence in adult women: diagnosis and comparative effectiveness. Rockville, MD: Agency for Healthcare Research and Quality; 2012;11(12):EHC074-EF.

A4. Labrie J, Berghmans BL, Fischer K, et al. Surgery versus physiotherapy for stress urinary incontinence. *N Engl J Med.* 2013;369:1124-1133.

A5. Rai BP, Cody JD, Alhasso A, et al. Anticholinergic drugs versus non-drug active therapies for non-neurogenic overactive bladder syndrome in adults. Cochrane Database System Review publications. 2012;12:CD003193.

A6. Myers DL. Female mixed urinary incontinence: a clinical review. *JAMA.* 2014;311:2007-2014.

A7. DuBeau CE, Kraus SR, Griebling TL, et al. Effect of fesoterodine in vulnerable elderly subjects with urgency incontinence: a double-blind, placebo controlled trial. *J Urol.* 2014;191:395-404.

A8. Wagg A, Dale M, Tretter R, et al. Randomised, multicentre, placebo-controlled, double-blind crossover study investigating the effect of solifenacin and oxybutynin in elderly people with mild cognitive impairment: the SENIOR study. *Eur Urol.* 2013;64:74-81.

A9. Herbison GP, Arnold EP. Sacral neuromodulation with implanted devices for urinary storage and voiding dysfunction in adults. Cochrane Database System Review publications. 2009;2:CD004202.

A10. Peters KM, Carrico DJ, Wooldridge LS, et al. Percutaneous tibial nerve stimulation for the long-term treatment of overactive bladder: 3-year results of the STEP study. *J Urol.* 2013;189:2194-2201.

A11. Visco AG, Brubaker L, Richter HE, et al. Anticholinergic therapy vs. onabotulinumtoxinA for urgency urinary incontinence. *N Engl J Med.* 2012;367:1803-1813.

A12. Nitti VW, Dmochowski R, Herschorn S, et al. OnabotulinumtoxinA for the treatment of patients with overactive bladder and urinary incontinence: results of a phase 3, randomized, placebo controlled trial. *J Urol.* 2013;189:2186-2193.

A13. Diokno AC, Sampselle CM, Herzog AR, et al. Prevention of urinary incontinence by behavioral modification program: a randomized, controlled trial among older women in the community. *J Urol.* 2004;171:1165-1171.

A14. Brown JS, Wing R, Barrett-Connor E, et al. Lifestyle intervention is associated with lower prevalence of urinary incontinence: the Diabetes Prevention Program. *Diabetes Care.* 2006;29:385-390.

GENERAL REFERENCES

For the General References and other additional features, please visit Expert Consult at https://expertconsult.inkling.com.

27

NEUROPSYCHIATRIC ASPECTS OF AGING

SHARON K. INOUYE

DEFINITION

The process of aging produces important physiologic changes in the central nervous system (Table 27-1), including neuroanatomic, neurotransmitter, and neurophysiologic changes. These processes result in age-related symptoms and manifestations (Table 27-2) for many older persons. These physiologic changes develop at dramatically variable rates among older persons, however, and the decline may be modified by factors such as diet, exercise, environment, lifestyle, genetic predisposition, disability, disease, and side effects of drugs. These changes can result in the common age-related symptoms of benign senescence, slowed reaction time, postural hypotension, vertigo or giddiness, presbyopia, presbycusis, stiffened gait, and sleep difficulties. In the absence of disease, these physiologic changes usually result in relatively modest symptoms and little restriction in activities of daily living. These changes decrease physiologic reserve, however, and increase the susceptibility to challenges posed by disease-related, pharmacologic, and environmental stressors. As a result, mild (relative risk, 1.2) and moderate (relative risk, 1.4) cognitive impairment are associated with increased mortality.[1]

EPIDEMIOLOGY

Neuropsychiatric disorders, the leading cause of disability in older persons, account for nearly 50% of functional incapacity. Severe neuropsychiatric conditions have been estimated to occur in 15 to 25% of older adults worldwide. These conditions are due to diseases that increase with age but are not part of the normal aging process. Alzheimer disease and related dementias occur in approximately 10% of adults aged 65 years and older and in 40% of

TABLE 27-1 AGE-RELATED PHYSIOLOGIC CHANGES IN THE CENTRAL NERVOUS SYSTEM

Neuroanatomic changes
Brain atrophy
Decreased neuron counts
Increased neuritic plaques
Increased lipofuscin and melanin
Neurotransmitter changes
Decline in cholinergic transmission
Decreased dopaminergic synthesis
Decreased catecholamine synthesis
Neurophysiologic changes
Decreased cerebral blood flow
Electrophysiologic changes (slowing of alpha rhythm, increased latencies in evoked responses)

TABLE 27-2 NEUROPSYCHIATRIC MANIFESTATIONS OF AGE-RELATED PHYSIOLOGIC CHANGES

SYSTEM	MANIFESTATION
Cognition	Forgetfulness Processing speed declines throughout adult life Neuropsychological declines: selective attention, verbal fluency, retrieval, complex visual perception, logical analysis
Reflexes	Stretch reflexes lose sensitivity Decreased or absent ankle reflexes Decreased autonomic and righting reflexes, postural instability
Sensory	Presbycusis (high-frequency hearing loss), tinnitus Deterioration of vestibular system, vertigo Presbyopia (decreased lens elasticity) Slowed pupil reactivity, decreased upgaze Olfactory system deterioration Decreased vibratory sensation
Gait and balance	Gait stiffer, slowed, forward flexed Increased body sway and mild unsteadiness
Sleep	Decreased sleep efficiency, fatigue Increased awakenings, insomnia Decrease in sleep stages 3 and 4 Sleep duration more variable, more naps

TABLE 27-3 GERIATRIC DEPRESSION SCALE—SHORT FORM

1. Are you basically satisfied with your life?	yes/NO
2. Have you dropped many of your activities and interests?	YES/no
3. Do you feel that your life is empty?	YES/no
4. Do you often get bored?	YES/no
5. Are you in good spirits most of the time?	yes/NO
6. Are you afraid that something bad is going to happen to you?	YES/no
7. Do you feel happy most of the time?	yes/NO
8. Do you feel helpless?	YES/no
9. Do you prefer to stay home rather than going out and doing new things?	YES/no
10. Do you feel you have more problems with memory than most?	YES/no
11. Do you think it is wonderful to be alive now?	yes/NO
12. Do you feel pretty worthless the way you are now?	YES/no
13. Do you feel full of energy?	yes/NO
14. Do you feel that your situation is hopeless?	YES/no
15. Do you think that most people are better off than you are?	YES/no

Scoring: Answers indicating depression are capitalized; six or more capitalized answers indicate depressive symptoms.
Modified with permission from Yesavage J, Brink T, Rowe T, et al. Development and validation of a geriatric depression screening scale: a preliminary report. *J Psychiatr Res.* 1983;17:37-49.

those older than 85 years (Chapter 402). Delirium occurs in 5 to 10% of all persons older than 65 years and in up to 80% of older persons during hospitalizations for acute illnesses (Chapter 28). Severe depression (Chapter 397) occurs in approximately 5% of older adults, with 15% having significant depressive symptoms. Anxiety disorders occur in 10% of older adults. Older individuals are also subject to substantial morbidity and functional disability from cerebrovascular disease (Chapters 406 through 408), Parkinson disease (Chapter 409), peripheral neuropathies (Chapter 420), degenerative myelopathies (Chapters 400 and 422), spinal stenosis and disc disease (Chapter 400), seizure disorders (Chapter 403), sleep apnea (Chapter 100), visual disturbances (Chapter 423), falls (Chapter 25), incontinence (Chapter 26), and impotence (Chapter 234).

DIAGNOSIS

To diagnose these neuropsychiatric conditions, physicians must understand and perform a mental status examination and an assessment of functional capacity and know the uses and side effects of psychoactive drugs in geriatric patients.

Mental Status Examination

In addition to a detailed neurologic examination, evaluation of neuropsychiatric disturbances in older persons requires a careful mental status examination, including an assessment of mood, affect, and cognition. Brief screening tests are available to evaluate these domains and to assist in the detection of potential problems requiring further evaluation and treatment (see Chapter 24). Scores of 6 or more on the 15-item short-form Geriatric Depression Scale (Table 27-3) indicate substantial depressive symptoms requiring further evaluation. For cognitively impaired patients, observer (proxy)–rated depression scales, such as the Hamilton Depression Scale or Cornell Scale, are recommended.

Early cognitive deficits can easily be missed during conversation because intellectual impairment can be masked with intact social skills. Given the high frequency of cognitive impairment, formal cognitive screening is reasonable but not required for all older persons.[2] Ideally, cognitive testing should evaluate at least the general domains of attention, orientation, language, memory, visuospatial ability, and conceptualization. To exclude delirium, attention should be assessed first by asking the patient to perform a task, such as repeating digits (normal span: more than five forward or more than three backward) or reciting the months backward (allow one error maximum); the remainder of cognitive testing would not be useful in an inattentive or delirious patient. For further cognitive testing, many brief, practical screening instruments are available. Historically, the most widely used instrument has been the Mini-Mental State Examination, a 19-item, 30-point scale that can be completed in 10 minutes. This copyrighted instrument now requires a per-use fee if the official version is used. Useful, brief alternative instruments include the Short Portable Mental Status Questionnaire (Table 27-4) and the Mini-Cog test (Table 27-5), both of which can be completed in less than 5 minutes. More detailed testing can be conducted with the Montreal Cognitive Assessment (Fig. 27-1), which requires 15 to 20 minutes; scores less than 26 indicate cognitive impairment. Questions to evaluate judgment and problem-solving ability in hypothetical situations, such as in a fire or when driving,

TABLE 27-4 SHORT PORTABLE MENTAL STATUS QUESTIONNAIRE

QUESTION	RESPONSE	ERROR?
What are the date, month, and year?*	Date Month Year	
What is the day of the week?		
What is the name of this place?		
What is your phone number?		
How old are you?		
When were you born?		
Who is the current president?		
Who was the president before him?		
What was your mother's maiden name?		
Can you count backward from 20 by 3s?		

*A mistake on *any* part of this question should be scored as an error.
Total possible errors: 10; more than three errors indicates cognitive impairment.
From Pfeiffer E. A short portable mental status questionnaire for the assessment of organic brain deficit in elderly patients. *J Am Geriatr Soc.* 1975;23:433-441. Copyright © E. Pfeiffer 1994. Reproduced with permission of the author.

TABLE 27-5 MINI-COG TEST

1. Instruct the patient to listen carefully to and remember three unrelated words and then to repeat the words: banana, sunrise, chair.
2. Instruct the patient to draw the face of a clock, either on a blank sheet of paper or on a sheet with a large circle already drawn on the page. After the patient puts the numbers on the clock face, ask him or her to draw the hands of the clock to read a specific time, such as 11:10. These instructions can be repeated, but no additional instructions should be given. Allow up to 3 minutes to complete the clock drawing.
3. Ask the patient to repeat the three previously presented words.
4. Give 1 point for each correct word and 2 points for a correctly drawn clock. Scores <3 suggest cognitive impairment.

Modified from Borson S, Scanlan J, Watanabe J, et al. Improving identification of cognitive impairment in primary care. *Int J Geriatr Psychiatry.* 2006;21:349-355. Reprinted by permission of the copyright holder (S. Borson).

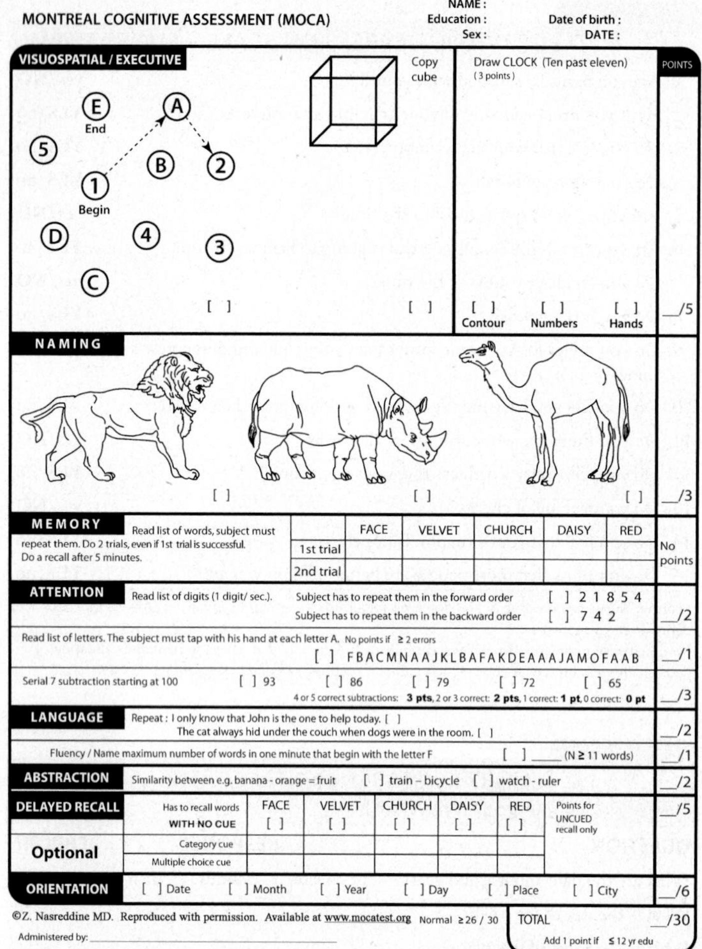

MONTREAL COGNITIVE ASSESSMENT (MOCA)

NAME :
Education :
Sex :
Date of birth :
DATE :

		POINTS
VISUOSPATIAL / EXECUTIVE	(E) End, (A), (5), (B), (2), (1) Begin, (D), (4), (3), (C) [ ] — Copy cube [ ] — Draw CLOCK (Ten past eleven) (3 points) [ ] Contour [ ] Numbers [ ] Hands	___/5
NAMING	[ ] [ ] [ ]	___/3
MEMORY	Read list of words, subject must repeat them. Do 2 trials, even if 1st trial is successful. Do a recall after 5 minutes. FACE VELVET CHURCH DAISY RED — 1st trial / 2nd trial	No points
ATTENTION	Read list of digits (1 digit/ sec.). Subject has to repeat them in the forward order [ ] 2 1 8 5 4. Subject has to repeat them in the backward order [ ] 7 4 2	___/2
	Read list of letters. The subject must tap with his hand at each letter A. No points if ≥ 2 errors [ ] FBACMNAAJKLBAFAKDEAAAJAMOFAAB	___/1
	Serial 7 subtraction starting at 100 [ ] 93 [ ] 86 [ ] 79 [ ] 72 [ ] 65 — 4 or 5 correct subtractions: **3 pts**, 2 or 3 correct: **2 pts**, 1 correct: **1 pt**, 0 correct: **0 pt**	___/3
LANGUAGE	Repeat : I only know that John is the one to help today. [ ] The cat always hid under the couch when dogs were in the room. [ ]	___/2
	Fluency / Name maximum number of words in one minute that begin with the letter F [ ] ___ (N ≥ 11 words)	___/1
ABSTRACTION	Similarity between e.g. banana - orange = fruit [ ] train - bicycle [ ] watch - ruler	___/2
DELAYED RECALL	Has to recall words WITH NO CUE: FACE [ ] VELVET [ ] CHURCH [ ] DAISY [ ] RED [ ] — Points for UNCUED recall only	___/5
Optional	Category cue; Multiple choice cue	
ORIENTATION	[ ] Date [ ] Month [ ] Year [ ] Day [ ] Place [ ] City	___/6

©Z. Nasreddine MD. Reproduced with permission. Available at www.mocatest.org Normal ≥26 / 30 TOTAL ___/30

Administered by: ______ Add 1 point if ≤ 12 yr edu

FIGURE 27-1. Montreal Cognitive Assessment. (Reproduced with permission from Nasreddine ZS, Phillips NA, Bedirian V, et al. The Montreal Cognitive Assessment, MoCA: A brief screening tool for mild cognitive impairment. *J Am Geriatr Soc.* 2005;53:695-699.)

can provide crucial insight into the patient's ability to function safely and independently.

Functional Assessment

Functional impairment, defined as difficulty in performing daily activities, is common among older persons. Although it is not routinely evaluated in the standard medical assessment, determination of the patient's degree of functional incapacity based on medical and neuropsychiatric conditions is crucial to diagnosis of mild cognitive impairment and dementia as well as to understanding of the burden of the disease and its impact on the individual's daily life. The important relationship between functional status and health in older persons is reflected by the finding that functional measures are stronger predictors of mortality after hospitalization than are admitting diagnoses. Functional measures strongly predict other important long-term outcomes in the elderly, such as future care needs, caregiver burden, risk for institutionalization, and long-term prognosis.[3] Functional independence is critical if patients are to remain living independently in the community, and functional decline represents the leading risk factor for nursing home placement.

The functional assessment should evaluate the patient's ability to perform basic self-care activities of daily living and instrumental activities of daily living, the higher level activities needed for independent living. Activities of daily living include basic self-care skills, such as feeding, grooming, bathing, dressing, toileting, transferring, and walking. Instrumental activities of daily living are more complex tasks, including shopping, preparing meals, managing finances, housekeeping, using the telephone, taking medications, and driving or using public transportation. The functional assessment is conducted with the patient, with corroboration from a family member or caregiver. Other related domains that should be assessed include vision, hearing, continence, nutritional status, safety, falls, living situation, availability of social support, and socioeconomic status.

The onset of acute cognitive or functional decline is often the first and sometimes the only sign of serious acute illness in older persons and warrants immediate medical attention. Similarly, the onset or worsening of related conditions, such as delirium, falls, incontinence, depression, frailty, or failure to thrive, heralds the need for prompt medical evaluation.

TREATMENT Rx

Psychoactive Effects of Drugs in Older Patients

Adverse Drug Events in the Elderly

Iatrogenic complications occur in 29 to 38% of older hospitalized patients, with a 3- to 5-fold increased risk in older compared with younger patients. Adverse drug events, the most common type of iatrogenic complication, account for 20 to 40% of all complications, and at least 27% of these are preventable.[4] The elderly are particularly vulnerable to adverse drug reactions because of multiple-drug regimens, multiple chronic diseases, relative renal and hepatic insufficiency, decreased physiologic reserve, and altered drug metabolism and receptor sensitivity with aging.[5] Inappropriate drug use has been reported in up to 40% of older patients who are hospitalized, with more than one quarter of these patients having absolute contraindications to the drug and the others being given a drug that was unnecessary. Among an estimated 100,000 annual drug-related emergency hospitalizations in patients older than 65 years, the most commonly implicated drugs are warfarin (33%), insulin (14%), oral antiplatelet agents (13%), and oral hypoglycemic agents (11%).[6] Because up to 50% of adverse drug events occur in patients receiving inappropriate drugs, the potential for reducing these adverse events is substantial.

Drugs with Psychoactive Effects

Nearly every class of drug has the potential to cause mental status changes in a vulnerable patient, but specific drugs are commonly implicated (Table 27-6) and should be used with caution in older patients.[6] Many cases of delirium or cognitive decline in older patients may be preventable through avoidance, substitution, or dose reduction of these psychoactive drugs. Long-acting benzodiazepines (e.g., diazepam, clonazepam, chlordiazepoxide) are particularly problematic medications for the elderly and should not be used to treat insomnia. If nonpharmacologic approaches to the management of insomnia are unsuccessful, short-term use of an intermediate-acting benzodiazepine without active metabolites (e.g., lorazepam 0.5 mg, half-life of 10 to 15 hours) is recommended. Drugs with anticholinergic effects (e.g., antihistamines, antidepressants, neuroleptics, antispasmodics) produce a panoply of poorly tolerated side effects in older patients, including delirium, postural hypotension, urinary retention, constipation, and dry mouth. Of the narcotics, meperidine causes delirium more frequently than other agents because of an active metabolite, normeperidine. Cardiac drugs, such as digitalis and antiarrhythmic agents, have prolonged half-lives, narrowed therapeutic windows, and decreased protein binding in older patients. The clinician should be aware that toxicity with these agents (e.g., digoxin) can occur even at therapeutic drug levels. The H_2-receptor antagonists (e.g., cimetidine, ranitidine, famotidine, nizatidine) are among the most common causes of drug-induced delirium in the elderly because of their frequent use; clinicians should strongly consider the use of less toxic alternatives (e.g., sucralfate, antacids) or dosage reductions for older patients, especially when the medication is being used for prophylaxis rather than treatment of active disease. Proton pump inhibitors have been associated with delirium in case reports but have less neuropsychiatric toxicity than H_2-receptor antagonists.

Psychoactive drugs account for nearly 50% of preventable adverse drug events, often in patients who have been prescribed three or more psychoactive drugs, frequently at inappropriately high doses in the elderly. Delirium and cognitive impairment are the most frequent adverse outcomes of psychoactive drugs. The use of any psychoactive drug is associated with a 4-fold increased risk of delirium or cognitive decline, but the outcomes of these conditions depend on the type or class of drug administered and the total number of drugs received. Sedative-hypnotic drugs are associated with a 3- to 12-fold increased risk for delirium or cognitive decline, narcotics are associated with a 2- to 3-fold increased risk, and anticholinergic drugs are associated with a 5- to 12-fold increased risk. Each drug carries its own individual risk for adverse outcomes, and when multiple drugs are used, the overall risk is compounded by the heightened potential for drug-drug and drug-disease interactions. If more than three drugs are added in a 24-hour period, the risk of delirium increases 4-fold. Similarly, the risk of cognitive decline increases directly with the number of drugs prescribed, from a 3-fold increased risk with two or three drugs to a 14-fold increased risk with six or more drugs.

Principles of Drug Therapy in the Elderly

Physicians always should consider whether nonpharmacologic approaches (Chapter 39) may be used as alternatives to medications in older persons. Relaxation techniques, massage, and music are highly effective for the treatment of insomnia and anxiety; localized pain can often be managed effectively

TABLE 27-6 DRUGS WITH PSYCHOACTIVE EFFECTS

Sedative-hypnotics
- Benzodiazepines (especially flurazepam, diazepam)
- Barbiturates
- Sleeping medications (chloral hydrate)

Narcotics (especially meperidine)

Anticholinergics
- Antihistamines (diphenhydramine, hydroxyzine)
- Antispasmodics (belladonna, Lomotil)
- Heterocyclic antidepressants (amitriptyline, imipramine, doxepin)
- Neuroleptics (chlorpromazine, haloperidol, thioridazine)
- Antiparkinson drugs (benztropine, trihexyphenidyl)
- Atropine, scopolamine

Cardiac drugs
- Digitalis glycosides
- Antiarrhythmics (quinidine, procainamide, lidocaine)
- Antihypertensives (β-blockers, methyldopa)

Gastrointestinal drugs
- H_2-receptor antagonists (cimetidine, ranitidine, famotidine, nizatidine)
- Proton pump inhibitors (esomeprazole, lansoprazole, omeprazole, pantoprazole)
- Metoclopramide (Reglan)

Miscellaneous drugs
- Nonsteroidal anti-inflammatory drugs
- Corticosteroids
- Anticonvulsants
- Levodopa
- Lithium

Over-the-counter drugs
- Cold and sinus preparations (antihistamines, pseudoephedrine)
- Sleep aids (diphenhydramine, alcohol-containing elixirs)
- Stay Awake (caffeine)
- Nausea, gastrointestinal relief (Donnagel, meclizine, H_2-receptor antagonists, loperamide)

TABLE 27-7 GUIDELINES FOR DRUG THERAPY IN THE ELDERLY

GENERAL PRINCIPLES

Remember that the elderly are highly sensitive to the psychoactive effects of all drugs.
Know the pharmacology of the drugs you prescribe. Know a few drugs well.

RECOMMENDED APPROACH

Use nonpharmacologic approaches whenever possible.
Avoid *routine* use of "as needed" drugs for sleep, anxiety, pain.
Choose the drug with the least toxic potential.
Substitute less toxic alternatives whenever possible (antacid or sucralfate for an H_2-blocker or proton pump inhibitors, Metamucil or Kaopectate for Imodium or Lomotil, scheduled acetaminophen regimen for pain management).
Reduce the dosage.
"Start low and go slow."
- Start with 25 to 50% of the standard dose of psychoactive drugs in the elderly.
- Titrate the drug slowly.
- Set realistic end points: titrate to improvement, not elimination of symptoms.

Keep the regimen simple.
Regularly reassess the medication list. Have the patient bring in all bottles and review what is being taken.
Reevaluate long-time drug use because the patient is changing.
Review over-the-counter medications, including herbal remedies.

with local measures such as injection, heat, ultrasound, and transcutaneous electrical stimulation.

When drug therapy is required in the elderly, physicians should choose the drug with the least toxic potential and emphasize drugs that have been well tested in older populations (Table 27-7). It is often wise to start with 25 to 50% of the standard adult dosage for a psychoactive drug and to increase the dose slowly. Drug regimens should be kept simple, with the fewest drugs and the fewest number of pills possible. Most important, the medication list should be reassessed frequently. Involving a clinical pharmacist in the care team can significantly improve healthcare outcomes.[A1] Systematic interventions involving geriatricians, clinical pharmacists, and computer-based monitoring systems also can significantly reduce the frequency of adverse drug reactions in older persons.[A2]

For persons with dementia or cognitive impairment, the following classes of drugs should be avoided or discontinued if possible: benzodiazepines, H_2-receptor antagonists, meperidine, sedative-hypnotics, and thioridazine.[4] Even long-standing medications should be reevaluated as the patient changes with age and illness. Long-term use does not justify continued use. The physician should review with the patient all prescribed and over-the-counter medications on a regular basis, preferably by having the patient bring in all medication bottles and indicate how each is being taken. Patients frequently underestimate the toxic potential of over-the-counter medications and herbal remedies, and they may be using a variety of such agents that could potentiate the side effects or directly counteract the desired effects of prescription medications (Chapter 29). For example, high-risk over-the-counter medications for older persons include nonsteroidal anti-inflammatory agents, H_2-blockers, and antihistamines. In addition, herbal remedies may interact with warfarin either to increase or to decrease its effect (St. John's wort decreases the effect and makes anticoagulation more difficult; gingko biloba increases the effect and may cause bleeding)[7]; others (such as kava kava, echinacea, and Chinese herbal preparations) have been associated with the risk of hepatotoxicity.

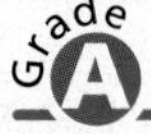

Grade A References

A1. Lee JK, Slack MK, Martin J, et al. Geriatric patient care by U.S. pharmacists in healthcare teams: systematic review and meta-analysis. *J Am Geriatr Soc*. 2013;61:1119-1127.
A2. Dalleur O, Boland B, Losseau C, et al. Reduction of potentially inappropriate medications using the STOPP criteria in frail older inpatients: a randomised controlled study. *Drugs Aging*. 2014; 31:291-298.

GENERAL REFERENCES

For the General References and other additional features, please visit Expert Consult at https://expertconsult.inkling.com.

28 DELIRIUM OR ACUTE MENTAL STATUS CHANGE IN THE OLDER PATIENT

SHARON K. INOUYE

Mental status change, one of the most common presenting symptoms in acutely ill elders, is estimated to account for 30% of emergency evaluations among older patients. Mental status often serves as a barometer of the underlying health of an elderly patient and is commonly the only symptom of serious underlying disease. A broad range of medical, neurologic, and psychiatric conditions can lead to mental status changes (Chapters 397 and 402). A systematic approach aids in the evaluation of suspected mental status change in an older patient (Fig. 28-1).

The first step in evaluating suspected altered mental status in an older patient is to obtain a detailed history from a reliable informant to establish the patient's baseline level of cognitive function and the clinical course of any cognitive changes. Chronic changes (those occurring during months to years) most likely represent an underlying dementing illness and should be evaluated accordingly (Chapter 402). Acute changes (those occurring during days to weeks)—even if superimposed on an underlying dementia—should be evaluated by a formal cognitive assessment to determine whether delirium is present. If features of delirium (e.g., inattention, disorganized thinking, altered level of consciousness, fluctuating symptoms) are not present, further evaluation for depression, acute nonorganic psychotic disorders, or other psychiatric conditions is indicated.

DELIRIUM

Delirium, a clinical syndrome characterized as an acute disorder of attention and cognitive function, is the most frequent complication of hospitalization for elders and is a potentially devastating problem. Delirium is often unrecognized despite sensitive methods for its detection, and its complications may be preventable.

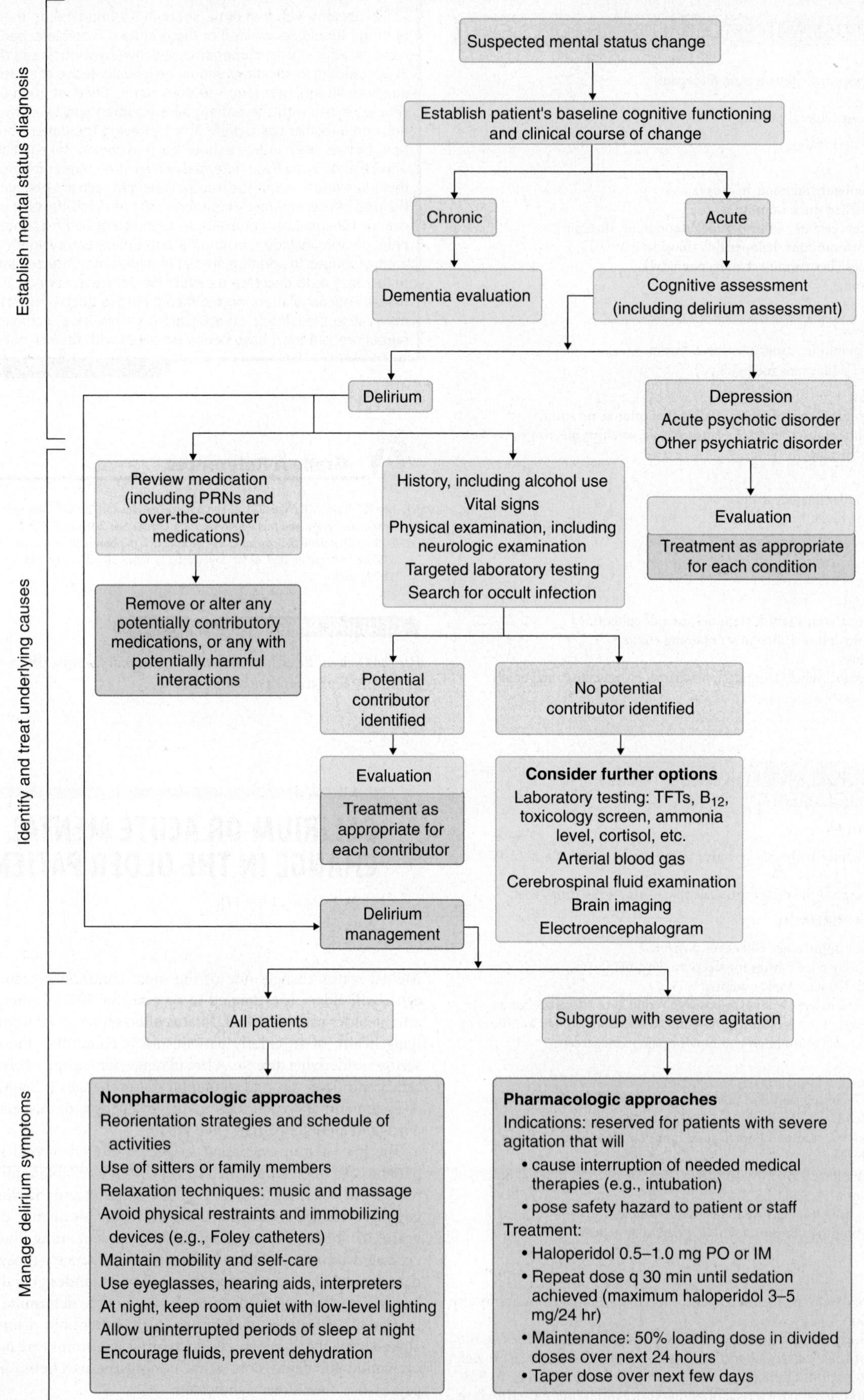

FIGURE 28-1. **Algorithm for the evaluation of suspected mental status change in older patients. PRN = as needed; TFTs = thyroid function tests.**

TABLE 28-1 DIAGNOSTIC CRITERIA FOR DELIRIUM

DSM-5 CRITERIA*

- Disturbed attention (i.e., reduced ability to direct, focus, sustain, and shift attention) and awareness (reduced orientation to the environment) that has developed in a short time (usually hours to a few days), represents a change from baseline attention and awareness, and tends to fluctuate in severity during the course of a day
- An additional disturbance in cognition (e.g., memory deficit, disorientation, language, visuospatial ability, or perception)
- Evidence from the history, physical examination, or laboratory findings that the disturbance is a direct physiologic consequence of another medical condition, substance intoxication or withdrawal, exposure to a toxin, or multiple causes
- No evidence for another preexisting, established, or evolving neurocognitive disorder to explain the inattention and cognitive disturbance
- No evidence for a reduced level of arousal, such as coma

CAM DIAGNOSTIC ALGORITHM†

Feature 1. Acute onset and fluctuating course. This information is usually obtained from a family member or nurse and is shown by positive responses to the following questions: Is there evidence of an acute change in mental status from the patient's baseline? Did the (abnormal) behavior fluctuate during the day—that is, tend to come and go or increase and decrease in severity?

Feature 2. Inattention. This feature is shown by a positive response to the following question: Did the patient have difficulty focusing attention—for example, was he or she easily distracted or did he or she have difficulty keeping track of what was being said?

Feature 3. Disorganized thinking. This feature is shown by a positive response to the following question: Was the patient's thinking disorganized or incoherent, such as rambling or irrelevant conversation, unclear or illogical flow of ideas, or unpredictable switching from subject to subject?

Feature 4. Altered level of consciousness. This feature is shown by any answer other than "alert" to the following question: Overall, how would you rate this patient's level of consciousness: alert (normal), vigilant (hyperalert), lethargic (drowsy, easily aroused), stupor (difficult to arouse), or coma (unable to arouse)?

*Modified with permission from American Psychiatric Association. Diagnostic and Statistical Manual of Mental Disorders. 5th ed. Washington, DC: American Psychiatric Association; 2013.
†The diagnosis of delirium requires the presence of features 1 and 2 and either 3 or 4. CAM = Confusion Assessment Method. From Inouye SK, van Dyck CH, Alessi CA, et al. Clarifying confusion: The Confusion Assessment Method. A new method for detection of delirium. *Ann Intern Med.* 1990;113:941-948. Copyright 2003, Hospital Elder Life Program, LLC. Not to be reproduced without permission.

DEFINITION

The diagnostic criteria for delirium are evolving (Table 28-1). The *Diagnostic and Statistical Manual of Mental Disorders* is based on expert consensus, but the diagnostic sensitivity and specificity of its criteria have not been tested. The Confusion Assessment Method provides a simple, operationalized diagnostic algorithm.[1] In studies of more than 1000 subjects, it had a sensitivity of 94%, a specificity of 89%, and a high interrater reliability.

EPIDEMIOLOGY

In persons older than 65 years admitted to general medical services, the prevalence of delirium at hospital admission is 18 to 35%. Delirium develops anew in an additional 11 to 14% of these patients during hospitalization. Higher rates are found when frequent surveillance is performed in older, surgical, and intensive care populations. Delirium occurs in 10 to 70% of postoperative patients, up to 80% of patients in medical intensive care units, up to 35% of nursing home patients, and at least 45% of patients at the end of life.[1]

The hospital mortality rates for delirium are 25 to 33%, as high as those associated with sepsis. The problem of delirium in hospitalized elderly patients has assumed particular prominence because patients aged 65 years and older currently account for more than 50% of all inpatient days of hospital care. Based on U.S. vital health statistics, delirium complicates hospital stays for at least 20% of the 12.5 million older persons hospitalized each year and increases hospital costs by more than $3000 per patient, amounting to more than $9 billion of Medicare expenditures yearly. Substantial additional costs are incurred after hospital discharge because of the increased need for rehabilitation services, nursing home placement, home care, and rehospitalization. Health care costs associated with delirium range from $50 billion to $200 billion per year. These extrapolations highlight the extensive economic and health policy implications of delirium.

PATHOBIOLOGY

Similar to other common geriatric syndromes (Chapter 25), delirium usually has multiple causes. A search for the innumerable potential underlying contributors requires clinical astuteness and a thorough medical evaluation, especially because many of these factors are treatable but may result in substantial morbidity and mortality if left untreated. The process is made more challenging by the frequently nonspecific, atypical, or muted features of the underlying illness in older persons. Delirium is commonly the only initial sign of an underlying life-threatening illness, such as pneumonia (Chapter 97), urosepsis (Chapter 284), or myocardial infarction (Chapter 73) in the older population.

The basic pathogenesis of delirium remains unclear. Recent evidence suggests that interacting biologic factors result in disruption of large-scale neuronal networks in the brain, thereby leading to acute cognitive disruption and delirium. Some of the leading proposed mechanisms include disruption in neurotransmitter systems, inflammation, physiologic stressors, metabolic derangements, electrolyte and acid-base disorders, and genetic factors. Many neurotransmitter systems are potentially involved, but relative cholinergic deficiency and dopamine excess are the most frequently linked. Inflammation may operate through both peripheral and central (brain) inflammatory cascades. Neuroimaging studies coupled with cognitive testing demonstrate a generalized disruption in higher cortical function, with dysfunction in the prefrontal cortex, frontal and temporoparietal cortex, fusiform cortex, lingual gyri, subcortical structures, thalamus, and basal ganglia.

The development of delirium usually involves a complex interrelationship between a vulnerable patient with pertinent predisposing factors and exposure to noxious insults or precipitating factors. Delirium may develop in vulnerable patients, such as cognitively impaired or severely ill patients, after a relatively benign insult, such as a single dose of sleeping medication. Conversely, in patients who are not vulnerable, delirium may develop only after exposure to multiple noxious insults. Previous studies have shown that the effects of these risk factors may be cumulative. Recognition of this multifactorial causation is important to the clinician because the removal or treatment of one factor in isolation usually is not sufficient to resolve the delirium. The full spectrum of vulnerability and precipitating factors should be addressed.

Factors that predispose patients to delirium include preexisting cognitive impairment or dementia, history of delirium, functional impairment, visual or hearing impairment, multiple comorbid conditions, severe underlying illness, depression, history of a stroke or transient ischemic attack, alcohol abuse, and advanced age. Dementia is an important and consistent risk factor for delirium; persons with dementia have a two-fold to five-fold increased risk for delirium, and 30 to 50% of delirious patients have underlying dementia.

Medications, the most common remediable causes of delirium, contribute to delirium in 40% of cases (Chapter 27). Insufficiency or failure of any major organ system, particularly renal or hepatic failure, can precipitate delirium. Surgical procedures are leading risk factors for delirium. Hypoxemia and hypercarbia have been associated with delirium. Clinicians must be attuned to occult respiratory failure, which in the elderly often lacks the usual signs and symptoms of dyspnea and tachypnea and can be missed by the measurement of oxygen saturation alone. Acute myocardial infarction or heart failure can be manifested as delirium in an elderly patient without the usual symptoms of chest pain or dyspnea. Occult infection is a particularly notable cause of delirium. Older patients frequently fail to mount the febrile or leukocytotic response to infection, and clinicians must assess them carefully for signs of pneumonia, urinary tract infection, endocarditis, abdominal abscess, or infected joints. A variety of metabolic disorders may contribute to delirium, including hypernatremia and hyponatremia, hypercalcemia, acid-base disorders, hypoglycemia and hyperglycemia, and thyroid or adrenal disorders. Immobilization and immobilizing devices (e.g., indwelling bladder catheters, physical restraints, bed alarms) are important factors in precipitating delirium. Dehydration and volume depletion and nutritional decline during hospitalization (e.g., weight loss, fall in serum albumin concentration) are well-documented factors contributing to delirium. Drug and alcohol withdrawal are important and often unsuspected causes of delirium in the elderly. Environmental factors, such as unfamiliar surroundings, sleep deprivation, deranged schedule, frequent room changes, sensory overload, and sensory deprivation, may aggravate delirium in the hospital. Psychosocial factors, such as depression, psychological stress, pain, and lack of social supports, also may precipitate delirium.

CLINICAL MANIFESTATIONS

The cardinal features of delirium include acute onset and inattention. Establishing the acuteness of onset requires accurate knowledge of the patient's baseline cognitive function. Patients with delirium are inattentive; that is, they have difficulty focusing, maintaining, and shifting attention. They appear easily distracted and have difficulty in maintaining conversation and following commands. Objectively, patients may have difficulty with simple repetitive tasks, digit spans, and recitation of months backward. Other key features include disorganized thought processes, which are usually a manifestation of underlying cognitive or perceptual disturbances; altered level of consciousness, which typically consists of lethargy with reduced awareness of the environment; and fluctuation of cognitive symptoms. Although not cardinal elements, other features that frequently occur during delirium include disorientation, cognitive deficits, psychomotor agitation or retardation, perceptual disturbances such as hallucinations and illusions, paranoid delusions, and sleep-wake cycle reversal.

DIAGNOSIS

The cornerstone of the evaluation of delirium is a comprehensive history and physical examination (Table 28-2). The first step is to establish the diagnosis of delirium through cognitive assessment and to determine whether the present condition represents an acute change from the patient's baseline cognitive function, such as from a family member. Because cognitive impairment may not be apparent during conversation, brief cognitive screening tests, such as the Short Portable Mental Status Questionnaire (Table 27-4) and the Confusion Assessment Method (CAM), should be used (Video 28-1). Attention should be assessed further with other simple tests, such as a forward digit span (inattention is indicated by an inability to repeat five digits forward) or recitation of the months backward (allow maximum of one error). A delirium assessment specifically for nonverbal (e.g., intubated) patients, called the CAM-ICU, has been developed. The history, which should be obtained from a reliable informant, is targeted to establish the patient's baseline cognitive function and the time course of any mental status change and to obtain clues about potential precipitating factors, such as recent medication changes, intercurrent infection, or medical illness. Physical examination should include a detailed neurologic examination for focal deficits and a careful search for signs of occult infection or an acute abdominal process.

Review of the patient's medication list, including over-the-counter medications and herbal remedies, is crucial, and the use of medications with psychoactive effects should be discontinued or minimized whenever possible.[2] In the elderly, these medications may cause psychoactive effects even at doses and measured drug levels within the "therapeutic range." Consideration should also be given to the possibility that withdrawal from alcohol or other medications is a contributor to delirium.

TABLE 28-2 EVALUATION OF DELIRIUM IN ELDERLY PATIENTS

Perform cognitive testing and determine baseline cognitive functioning: establish the diagnosis of delirium.
Obtain a comprehensive history and perform a physical examination, including a careful neurologic examination for focal deficits and a search for occult infection.
Review the patient's medication list: discontinue or minimize all psychoactive medications; check the side effects of all medications.
Perform a laboratory evaluation (tailored to the individual): complete blood count, electrolytes, blood urea nitrogen, creatinine, glucose, calcium, phosphate, liver enzymes, oxygen saturation.
Search for occult infection: physical examination, urinalysis, chest radiography, selected cultures (as indicated).
When no obvious cause is revealed after these steps, further targeted evaluation is considered in selected patients, as follows: Laboratory tests: magnesium, thyroid function, vitamin B_{12} level, drug levels, toxicology screen, ammonia level Arterial blood gas analysis: indicated in patients with dyspnea, tachypnea, any acute pulmonary process, or history of significant respiratory disease Electrocardiography: indicated in patients with chest or abdominal discomfort, shortness of breath, or cardiac history Cerebrospinal fluid examination: indicated when meningitis or encephalitis is suspected Brain imaging: indicated in patients with new focal neurologic signs or with a history or signs of head trauma Electroencephalography: useful in diagnosis of occult seizure disorder and in differentiating delirium from nonorganic psychiatric disorders

Laboratory Findings

Laboratory evaluation must be tailored to the individual situation (Table 28-2). In patients with preexisting cardiac or respiratory diseases or related symptoms, electrocardiography or arterial blood gas determination may be indicated. The need for cerebrospinal fluid examination is controversial except for the clear indication of the febrile delirious patient, in whom meningitis or encephalitis is suspected. Brain imaging should be reserved for patients with new focal neurologic signs, those with a history or signs of head trauma (e.g., upper body bruising), and those without another identifiable cause of the delirium. Electroencephalography, with a false-negative rate of 17% and a false-positive rate of 22% for distinguishing delirious from nondelirious patients, has a limited role and is most useful for detecting an occult seizure disorder and differentiating delirium from psychiatric disorders.

Differential Diagnosis

A crucial difficulty is distinguishing a long-standing confusional state (dementia) from delirium alone or delirium superimposed on dementia (see Fig. 28-1). These two conditions are differentiated by the acute onset of symptoms in delirium (dementia is much more insidious) and the impaired attention and altered level of consciousness associated with delirium. The differential diagnosis also includes depression and nonorganic psychotic disorders. Although paranoia, hallucinations, and affective changes can occur with delirium, the key features of acute onset, inattention, altered level of consciousness, and global cognitive impairment assist in the recognition of delirium. At times, the differential diagnosis can be difficult, particularly with an uncooperative patient or when an accurate history is unavailable. Because of the potentially life-threatening nature of delirium, it is prudent to manage the patient as if he or she has delirium and to search for and treat underlying precipitants (e.g., intercurrent illness, metabolic derangement, drug toxicity) until further information can be obtained.

TREATMENT Rx

Prevention

The most effective strategy to reduce delirium and its associated complications is primary prevention before delirium occurs. Preventive strategies should address important risk factors and target moderate- to high-risk patients at baseline (Table 28-3). Clinical trials document that multicomponent nonpharmacologic interventions targeted toward delirium risk factors can reduce the incidence of delirium by 30 to 40%. A1-A3 These components typically include strategies designed to improve orientation, to provide therapeutic activities, to increase mobilization and exercise, to enhance sleep with nonpharmacologic interventions, to optimize vision and hearing, and to manage dehydration. Preoperative geriatric consultation and lighter anesthesia also can reduce postoperative delirium. By comparison, no drug treatments, including antipsychotics or cholinesterase inhibitors, have been consistently effective in preventing delirium. Preventive efforts require system-wide changes to educate physicians and nurses, to improve their recognition of delirium and heighten their awareness of its clinical implications, to provide incentives to change practice patterns that lead to delirium (e.g., immobilization, sleep medications, bladder catheters, physical restraints), and to create systems that enhance high-quality geriatric care (e.g., geriatric expertise, case management, clinical pathways, quality monitoring).

Medical Therapy

In general, nonpharmacologic approaches should be used in all delirious patients, and these are usually successful in managing symptoms. Pharmacologic approaches should be reserved for patients whose symptoms may result in the interruption of needed medical therapies (e.g., intubation, intravenous lines) or may endanger the safety of the patient or other persons. No drug is ideal for the treatment of delirium, however; any drug can cloud the patient's mental status further and obscure efforts to monitor the course of the mental status change. The drug should be given at the lowest dose and for the shortest time possible. Neuroleptics are the preferred agents. Haloperidol, the most widely used agent, causes less orthostatic hypotension and fewer anticholinergic side effects than thioridazine and is available in parenteral form; however, it has a higher rate of extrapyramidal side effects and acute dystonias. Second-generation antipsychotics have not proved superior to haloperidol. If parenteral administration is required, intravenous haloperidol should be administered in a monitored setting because its use results in a rapid onset of action, short duration of effect, and risk of hypotension and torsades de pointes; oral and intramuscular administration has a more optimal duration of action, and these are the preferred routes. The recommended starting dose is 0.25 to 0.5 mg of haloperidol orally or intramuscularly, repeated every 30

TABLE 28-3 *NICE* GUIDELINES FOR PREVENTION OF DELIRIUM

CLINICAL FACTOR	RECOMMENDED PREVENTIVE INTERVENTIONS*
Cognitive impairment or disorientation	Provide orienting cues: calendars, clocks, photos. Reorient the patient to time, place, person, schedule. Provide cognitively stimulating activities, like reminiscence. Encourage regular visits from family and friends.
Dehydration or constipation	Encourage patients to drink fluids. Advise team about use of parenteral fluids if necessary. Carefully monitor fluid balance in patients with heart failure or renal disease.
Hypoxia	Assess for symptoms of hypoxia and monitor oxygen saturation levels.
Immobility or limited mobility	Encourage early mobilization and regular ambulation. Keep walking aids (canes, walkers) readily available at all times. Encourage all patients to conduct active range-of-motion exercises.
Infection	Look for and treat infection. Avoid unnecessary catheterization. Implement infection control procedures.
Multiple medications	Review medication for both the type and the number of medications. Monitor for potential interactions.
Pain	Assesses for pain, especially in those who have communication difficulties. Begin and monitor pain management in those with known or suspected pain.
Poor nutrition	Follow general nutrition guidelines and seek input from dietitian early on if needed. Ensure availability and proper fit of dentures.
Sensory impairment	Resolve reversible causes or contributors to impairment. Ensure that working hearing and visual aids are available and used by those who need them. Educate staff.
Sleep disturbance	Avoid medical/nursing procedures during sleep if possible. Schedule medications and procedures to avoid disturbing sleep. Reduce noise level at night unit-wide. Educate staff.

*Operationalized protocols for all recommended preventive interventions are available at www.hospitalelderlifeprogram.org.
Modified with permission from National Institute for Health and Care Excellence (NICE) Clinical Guideline 103. www.nice.org.uk/cg103.[A1]

minutes after the vital signs have been rechecked, until sedation has been achieved. The end point should be an awake but manageable patient. The average elderly patient who has not been treated previously with neuroleptics should receive no more than 3 to 5 mg of haloperidol in a 24-hour period. Subsequently, a maintenance dose consisting of half the loading dose should be administered in divided doses during the next 24 hours, with doses tapered during the next few days as the agitation resolves.

Benzodiazepines are not recommended as the first-line treatment of delirium because of their tendency to cause oversedation and to exacerbate the confusional state. They remain the drugs of choice, however, for the treatment of withdrawal syndromes from alcohol and sedative drugs (Chapters 33 and 34).

Nonpharmacologic Management

Multicomponent geriatric interventions may be effective in improving quality of life with the potential for significant cost savings.[1] Nonpharmacologic management techniques recommended for every delirious patient include encouraging the presence of family members, using "sitters" as orienting influences, and transferring a disruptive patient to a private room or closer to the nurses' station for increased supervision. Interpersonal contact and communication, including verbal reorientation strategies, simple instructions and explanations, and frequent eye contact, are vital. Patients should be involved in their own care and allowed to participate in decision making as much as possible. Eyeglasses and hearing aids may reduce sensory deficits. Mobility, self-care, and independence should be encouraged, and physical restraints and bed alarms should be avoided, if possible, because of their tendency to increase agitation, their lack of efficacy, and their potential to cause injury. Attention must be focused on minimizing the disruptive influences of the hospital environment. Clocks and calendars should be provided to assist with orientation. Room and staff changes should be kept to a minimum. A quiet environment with low-level lighting is optimal for delirious patients, and use of ear plugs may be helpful for management of delirium.[A4] Perhaps the most important intervention is to schedule the checking of vital signs, the administration of medications, and the performance of procedures to allow the patient's uninterrupted sleep at night.[3] Nonpharmacologic approaches to relaxation, including music, relaxation tapes, and massage, can be highly effective in managing agitation.

End-of-Life Care

Delirium occurs in at least 80% of patients at the end of life and is considered part of the dying process by many hospice care providers (Chapter 3). Establishing the goals for care in advance with the patient and family is critical to guide appropriate management. For example, some patients may prioritize the preservation of alertness and the ability to communicate with loved ones as long as possible; others may prioritize comfort above all else. Physicians must be aware that even in terminal patients, many causes of delirium are potentially reversible with simple interventions such as adjusting medications, providing oxygen, or treating dehydration; however, aggressive diagnostic evaluation is usually inappropriate in this population. Nonpharmacologic measures to treat agitation and delirium should be instituted in all patients (including massage, music, and relaxation therapies). Haloperidol remains the first-line therapy for delirium in terminally ill patients. If more sedation is indicated, a short-acting benzodiazepine such as lorazepam (starting dose, 0.5 to 1.0 mg PO, IM, or SL), which is easily titrated, is recommended in this setting. Because sedation may result in decreased interaction and communication, increased confusion, and respiratory depression, this choice should be made in conjunction with the family while honoring the patient's preferences.

PROGNOSIS

Delirium increases the risk of death about 2-fold, of institutionalization about 2.5-fold, and of dementia more than 12-fold[4] even after controlling for age, sex, severity of illness, comorbid conditions, and baseline dementia. Delirium also prolongs hospital stays and increases health care costs.

Delirium was previously considered a reversible, transient condition, but symptoms typically last for 30 days or more, only 20% of patients have complete resolution by 6 months, and its detrimental effects may persist at 1 year.[5] Delirium has even more pronounced effects in patients with underlying dementia. The rate of cognitive decline in patients with dementia more than doubles after an episode of delirium,[6] and about one in eight hospitalized patients with dementia who develop delirium will have at least one severe adverse outcome, including a five-fold increased risk of death and a nine-fold increased risk of institutionalization.[7] These studies suggest that strategies to prevent delirium in persons with dementia should be a priority to prevent future cognitive deterioration and adverse outcomes. The long-term detrimental effects are most likely related to the duration, severity, and underlying cause of the delirium and the vulnerability of the patients.

FUTURE DIRECTIONS

Because delirium is common, frequently iatrogenic, and linked to processes of care, it is a marker of the quality of care and safety of the patient in the hospital setting. Research is needed to elucidate the pathophysiologic mechanisms of delirium by the use of neuroimaging modalities, neuropsychological testing, and genetic and laboratory markers; to clarify the contribution of delirium to irreversible cognitive impairment and dementia; and to improve the evidence-based management of delirium.

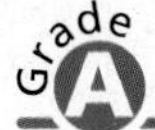

Grade A References

A1. O'Mahony R, Murthy L, Akunne A, et al. Synopsis of the National Institute for Health and Clinical Excellence guideline for prevention of delirium. *Ann Intern Med*. 2011;154:746-751.

A2. Deschodt M, Braes T, Flamaing J, et al. Preventing delirium in older adults with recent hip fracture through multidisciplinary geriatric consultation. *J Am Geriatr Soc*. 2012;60:733-739.

A3. Moyce Z, Rodseth RN, Biccard BM. The efficacy of peri-operative interventions to decrease post-operative delirium in non-cardiac surgery: a systematic review and meta-analysis. *Anaesthesia*. 2014;69:259-269.

A4. Van Rompaey B, Elseviers MM, Van Drom W, et al. The effect of earplugs during the night on the onset of delirium and sleep perception: a randomized controlled trial in intensive care patients. *Crit Care*. 2012;16:R73.

GENERAL REFERENCES

For the General References and other additional features, please visit Expert Consult at https://expertconsult.inkling.com.

V CLINICAL PHARMACOLOGY

29

PRINCIPLES OF DRUG THERAPY

ROBERT B. DIASIO

Under different conditions, a drug may produce diverse effects ranging from no effect to a desirable effect to an undesirable toxic effect. Physicians must learn how to choose the correct drug dosage for different conditions to ensure effective and safe therapy. This necessitates understanding the pharmacokinetics—the movement of a drug over time through the body—and the pharmacodynamics—the relationship between drug concentration and drug effect (Fig. 29-1). This chapter reviews the basic concepts of pharmacokinetics and pharmacodynamics, followed by guidelines on how to use this information to optimize therapeutic applications. Drug interactions and adverse drug responses are briefly discussed, with advice on how both can be recognized and minimized in clinical practice. Lastly, the increasing role of pharmacogenomics in individualizing therapy beyond preventing or predicting adverse drug responses is discussed.

PHARMACOKINETIC PRINCIPLES

Administration

The most efficient and straightforward means of administering a drug into the systemic circulation is by intravenous injection of the drug as a bolus. With this route, the full amount of a drug is delivered to the systemic circulation almost immediately. The same dose also may be administered as an intravenous infusion over a longer period, resulting in a decrease in the peak plasma concentration and an accompanying increase in the time the drug is present in the circulation. Many other routes of administration can be used, including sublingual, oral, transdermal, rectal, inhalational, subcutaneous, and intramuscular; each of these routes carries not only a potential delay in the time it takes the drug to enter the circulation but also the possibility that a large fraction of it will never reach the circulation.

Absorption

Absorption refers to the transfer of a drug from the site of administration to the systemic circulation. Many drugs cross a membrane barrier by passive diffusion and enter the systemic circulation. Because passive diffusion in this setting depends on the concentration of the solute at the membrane surface, the rate of drug absorption is affected by the concentration of free drug at the absorbing surface. Factors that influence the availability of free drug thus affect drug absorption from the administration site; this effect can be exploited to design medications that release a drug slowly into the circulation by prolonging drug absorption. With certain sustained-released oral preparations, the rate of dissolution of the drug in the gastrointestinal tract determines the rate at which the drug is absorbed (e.g., timed-release antihistamines). Similarly, a prolonged drug effect can be obtained by the use of transdermal medications (e.g., nitroglycerin) or intramuscular depot preparations (e.g., benzathine penicillin G).

First-Pass Effect

Some drugs that are administered orally are absorbed relatively efficiently into the portal circulation but are metabolized by the liver before they reach the systemic circulation. Because of this "first-pass" or "presystemic" effect, the oral route may be less suitable than other routes of administration for such drugs. A good example is nitroglycerin, which is well absorbed but efficiently metabolized during the first pass through the liver. However, the same drug can achieve adequate systemic levels when it is given sublingually or transdermally.

Bioavailability

The extent of absorption of a drug into the systemic circulation may be incomplete. The bioavailability of a particular drug is the fraction (F) of the total drug dose that ultimately reaches the systemic circulation from the site of administration. This fraction is calculated by dividing the amount of the drug dose that reaches the circulation from the administration site by the amount of the drug dose that would enter the systemic circulation after direct intravenous injection into the circulation (essentially the total dose). Bioavailability, or F, can range from 0, in which no drug reaches the systemic circulation, to 1.0, in which essentially all of the drug is absorbed. The bioavailability of a drug may vary in different formulations because the overall absorption differs. This variability has become a concern with the increasing use of generic preparations.

Distribution

After delivery of a drug into the systemic circulation either directly by intravenous injection or after absorption, the drug is transported throughout the body, initially to the well-perfused tissues and later to areas that are less perfused. The distribution phase can be assessed best by plotting the drug's plasma concentration on a log scale versus time on a linear scale (Fig. 29-2). For an intravenously administered drug, when absorption is not a factor, the initial phase—from immediately after administration through the rapid fall in concentration—represents the distribution phase, during which a drug rapidly disappears from the circulation and enters the tissues. This is followed by the elimination phase (see later), when drug in the plasma equilibrates with drug in the tissues. During this latter phase, the drug's plasma concentration is thought to be related to drug effect.

Volume of Distribution

The volume of distribution (VD) relates the amount of drug in the body to the concentration of drug in the plasma. It is calculated by dividing the dose that ultimately gets into the systemic circulation by the plasma concentration at time zero (C_{p0}):

$$VD = dose/C_{p0} \tag{1}$$

The C_{p0} can be calculated by extrapolating the elimination phase back to time zero (see Fig. 29-2). The VD is best considered the "apparent VD" because it represents the apparent volume needed to contain the entire amount of the drug, assuming it is distributed throughout the body at the same concentration as in the plasma. Table 29-1 lists pharmacokinetic data for commonly used drugs from several drug classes, showing the wide variation in VD. Digoxin, for example, has a large VD (>5 L), whereas glimepiride has a relatively small VD (0.18 L). As discussed later, VD is a useful pharmacokinetic tool for calculating the loading dose and appreciating how various changes can affect a drug's half-life.

Elimination

Drugs are removed from the body by two major mechanisms: hepatic elimination, in which drugs are metabolized in the liver and excreted through the biliary tract; and renal elimination, in which drugs are removed from the circulation by either glomerular filtration or tubular secretion. For most drugs, the rates of hepatic and renal elimination are proportional to the plasma concentration of the drug. This relationship is often described as a "first-order" process. Two measurements, clearance and half-life, are used to evaluate elimination.

Clearance

The efficiency of elimination can be assessed by quantifying how fast the drug is cleared from the circulation. Drug clearance is a measure of the volume of plasma cleared of drug per unit of time. It is similar to the clinical measurement used to assess renal function—creatinine clearance, which is the volume of plasma from which creatinine is removed per minute. Total drug clearance (Cl_{tot}) is the rate of elimination by all processes (El_{tot}) divided by the plasma concentration of the drug (C_p):

$$Cl_{tot} = El_{tot}/C_p \tag{2}$$

Drugs may be cleared by several organs, but as noted earlier, renal clearance and hepatic clearance are the two major mechanisms. Total drug clearance (Cl_{tot}) can best be described as the sum of clearances by each organ. For most drugs, this is essentially the sum of renal clearance and hepatic clearance:

$$Cl_{tot} = El_{Ren} + Cl_{Hep} \tag{3}$$

Table 29-1 shows the wide variation in clearance values among commonly used medications; some drugs (e.g., phenobarbital) have relatively low clearances (<5 mL/minute), and other drugs (e.g., aspirin) have relatively high clearances (>500 mL/minute). Tobramycin is cleared almost entirely by the kidneys, whereas aspirin, carbamazepine, and phenytoin are cleared less than 5% by the kidneys.

Drug clearance is affected by several factors, including blood flow through the organ of clearance, protein binding to the drug, and activity of the clearance processes in the organs of elimination (e.g., glomerular filtration rate and

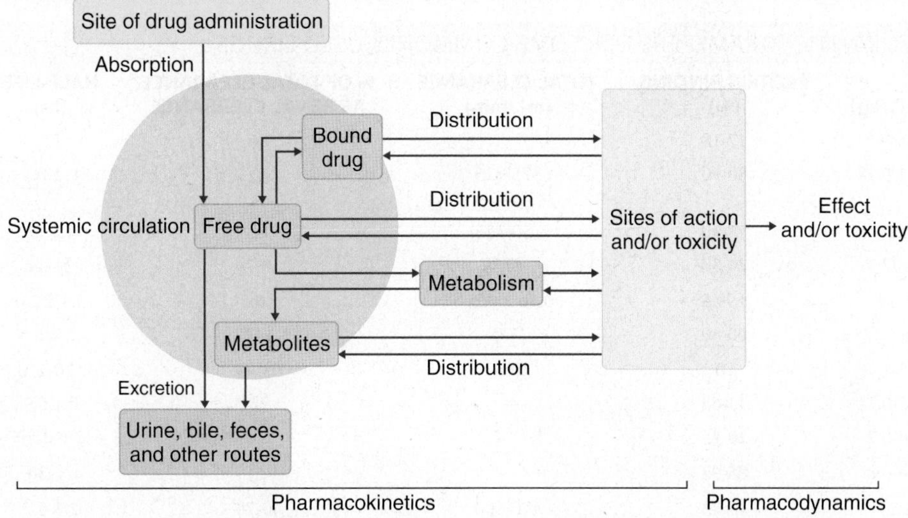

FIGURE 29-1. **Schematic of a drug's movement through the body, from the site of administration to production of a drug effect. The relationship between pharmacokinetics and pharmacodynamics is shown.**

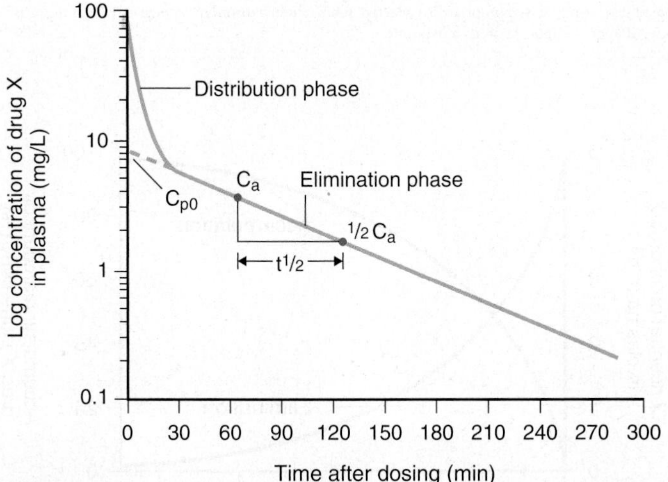

FIGURE 29-2. **Representative drug concentration versus time plot used in pharmacokinetic studies.** Concentration of drug is plotted with a logarithmic scale on the ordinate, and time is plotted with a linear scale on the abscissa. The resultant curve has two phases: the distribution phase, which is the initial portion of the plotted line when the concentration of drug decreases rapidly; and the later elimination phase, during which there is an exponential disappearance of drug from the plasma over time. The *dotted line* extrapolated from the elimination phase back to time zero is used to calculate plasma concentration at time zero (C_{p0}). During the elimination phase, the half-life ($t_{1/2}$) can be calculated as the time it takes to decrease the concentration by half (shown here as the time needed to decrease from concentration C_a to ½ C_a).

tubular secretion in the kidney, enzyme activity in the liver). Drug clearance is not affected by the distribution of drug throughout the body (VD) because clearance mechanisms act only on drug in the circulation.

Half-Life

The amount of time needed to eliminate a drug from the body depends on the clearance and the VD. The first-order elimination constant (K_e) represents the proportion of the apparent VD that is cleared of drug per unit of time during the drug's exponential disappearance from the plasma over time (elimination phase):

$$K_e = \mathrm{Cl/VD} \tag{4}$$

The value of this constant for a particular drug can be determined by plotting drug concentration versus time on a log-linear plot (see Fig. 29-2) and measuring the slope of the straight line obtained during the exponential (elimination) phase.

The time needed to eliminate the drug is best described by its half-life ($t_{1/2}$), which is the time required during the elimination phase (see Fig. 29-2) for the plasma concentration of the drug to be decreased by half. Mathematically, the half-life is equal to the natural logarithm of 2 (representing a reduction of drug concentration to half) divided by K_e. Substituting for K_e from Equation 4 and calculating the natural logarithm of 2, the half-life can be represented by the following equation:

$$t_{1/2} = 0.693\ \mathrm{VD/Cl} \tag{5}$$

From this equation, one can predict that at a given clearance, as the VD increases, the half-life increases. Similarly, at a given VD, as the clearance increases, the half-life decreases. Clinically, many disease states (see later) can affect VD and clearance. Because disease affects VD and clearance differently, the half-life may increase, decrease, or not change much at all. Therefore, the half-life by itself is not a good indicator of the extent of abnormality in elimination.

The half-life is useful to predict how long it takes for a drug to be eliminated from the body. For any drug that has a first-order elimination, one would expect that by the end of the first half-life, the drug would be reduced to 50%; by the end of the second half-life, to 25%; by the end of the third half-life, to 12.5%; by the end of the fourth half-life, to 6.25%; and by the end of the fifth half-life, to 3.125%. In general, a drug can be considered essentially eliminated after three to five half-lives, when less than 10% of the effective concentration remains. Table 29-1 shows the wide variation in half-life for several commonly used drugs.

CLINICAL APPLICATION OF PHARMACOKINETIC PRINCIPLES

Using a Loading Dose

To attain a desired therapeutic concentration rapidly, a loading dose is often used. In determining the amount of drug to be given, the clinician must consider the "volume" within the body into which the drug will be distributed. This volume is best described by the apparent VD. The loading dose can be calculated by multiplying the desired concentration by the VD:

$$\text{Loading dose} = \text{desired concentration} \times \mathrm{VD} \tag{6}$$

Rapid administration of the entire loading dose may produce an initially high peak concentration that results in toxicity. This problem can be avoided either by administering the loading dose as a divided dose or by varying the rate of access to the circulation, such as by administering the drug as an infusion (with an intravenous drug) or by taking advantage of the slower access to the circulation from various other routes (e.g., oral dosing). This approach is illustrated by phenytoin (see Table 29-1), which may need to be administered with a loading dose to achieve a therapeutic level (10 to 20 mg/L) rapidly. Because the VD for phenytoin is approximately 0.6 L/kg, the loading dose calculated from Equation 6 is 420 mg/L to attain a minimally

TABLE 29-1 PHARMACOKINETIC PARAMETERS FOR SOME COMMONLY USED DRUGS

DRUG	VD (L/kg)	PROTEIN BINDING (%)	TOTAL CLEARANCE (mL/min)	% OF TOTAL CLEARANCE AS RENAL CLEARANCE	HALF-LIFE (hr)	THERAPEUTIC RANGE (mg/L)
Amoxicillin	0.47	17-18		86	1.2	2-8
Aspirin (acetylsalicylic acid)	0.14-0.18	80-90	575-725	<2	0.2-0.3	20-250
Carbamazepine	1.2	75-90	50-125	1-3	12-17	4-12
Digoxin	5-7.3	20-30	75	50-70	34-44	0.5-2
Glimepiride	0.18	>99.5	0.62 ± 0.26	<0.5	3.4 ± 2.0	
Lidocaine	3	60-80	700	<10	1.5-2	1-5
Lithium carbonate	0.7-1	0	20-40	95-99	20-270	0.4-1.4*
Penicillin G	0.5-0.7	45-68	—	20	0.4-0.9	Variable
Phenobarbital	0.6-0.7	20-45	4	25	2-6 days	<10-40*
Phenytoin	0.4-0.8	88-93	—	<5	7-26	10-20
Procainamide	2.2	14-23	470-600	40-70	2.5-4.7	4-8
Theophylline	0.3-0.7	60	36-50	<10	4-16	5-20
Tobramycin	0.25-0.30	<10	70	>95	2-4	0.5-2 (TR) 4-8 (PK)
Vancomycin	0.4-1	52-60	65	85	4-6	5-10 (TR) 25-35 (PK)

*Therapeutic range varies according to the indication for the drug. For example, lithium carbonate in the range of 0.4-1.3 mg/L is appropriate for affective schizophrenia disorder; a range of 1.0-1.4 mg/L is appropriate for mania. Phenobarbital concentration below 10 mg/mL is appropriate for anticonvulsant therapy; 40 mg/L is appropriate as a hypnotic.
PK = peak value; TR = trough value; VD = volume of distribution.

therapeutic level of 10 mg/L in a 70-kg adult. However, administration of 420 mg of phenytoin by intravenous bolus carries the risk for cardiac arrest and death. By taking advantage of the reduced bioavailability (F = 0.8) and slow absorption of oral phenytoin, the loading dose can be administered safely as an oral dose of 500 mg.

The equation for the loading dose can also be used to calculate the dose needed to "boost" an inadequate blood level of drug to a desired therapeutic range. If therapeutic monitoring (see later under Drug Monitoring as a Guide to Therapy) shows that the phenytoin level is 5 mg/L and the desired level is 15 mg/L, it is necessary to multiply the difference needed to achieve the desired concentration (10 mg/L) by the VD (0.6 L/kg) to determine the dose (in mg/kg) necessary to achieve this drug level after distribution. In a 70-kg individual, 0.6 mg/kg is multiplied by 70 kg to obtain the calculated loading dose (420 mg) that can be administered safely. A 500-mg oral dose with a bioavailability of less than 1 (e.g., F = 0.8) would deliver to the systemic circulation the approximate amount needed and avoid the risks associated with rapid intravenous administration.

Determining Drug Accumulation

Continuing to administer a drug, either as a prolonged infusion or as repeated doses, results in accumulation until a steady state occurs. Steady state is the point at which the amount of drug being administered equals the amount being eliminated so that the plasma and tissue levels remain constant. The elimination half-life determines not only the time course of drug elimination but also the time course of drug accumulation. This mirror-image pattern of drug accumulation and elimination is illustrated in Figure 29-3. As with drug elimination, three to five half-lives determine the time it takes to reach steady state during drug accumulation. Whereas drugs with short half-lives accumulate rapidly, drugs with long half-lives require a longer time to accumulate, with a potential delay in achieving therapeutic levels. For drugs with long half-lives, a loading dose may be needed to obtain rapid drug accumulation and a more rapid therapeutic effect.

With each change in drug dose or rate of infusion, a change in steady state occurs. Although it is not obvious for drugs with short half-lives, the effects of dose adjustments for drugs with longer half-lives are delayed, and the time varies directly with the drug's half-life.

Using a Maintenance Dose

After steady state is reached in three to five half-lives with either a continuous infusion or intermittent doses, the rate of drug administered equals the rate of drug eliminated. For an intravenous drug, the administration rate is the infusion rate (I); for a drug administered by another route (e.g., orally), the administration rate is the dose per unit of time (D/t). Equation 7 shows that the rate of elimination (total) equals $Cl_{tot} \times C_p$. With an intravenously administered drug, because the infusion rate equals the elimination rate at steady state, it follows that

$$I = Cl_{tot} \times C_p \quad (7)$$

Similarly, with an orally administered drug, the dose administered per unit of time equals the elimination rate at steady state, with the result that

$$D/t = Cl_{tot} \times C_p \quad (8)$$

These equations show the direct relationship between the dose and the resultant plasma concentration at steady state. This relationship is independent of the distribution of the drug. By use of these equations, it is possible to determine the infusion rate or the interval and dose needed to achieve and maintain a specified drug concentration in the plasma.

When a drug is administered intermittently, it approaches steady-state concentration over time, with a pattern similar to that observed with continuous infusion (Fig. 29-4). With intermittent drug administration, such as with an

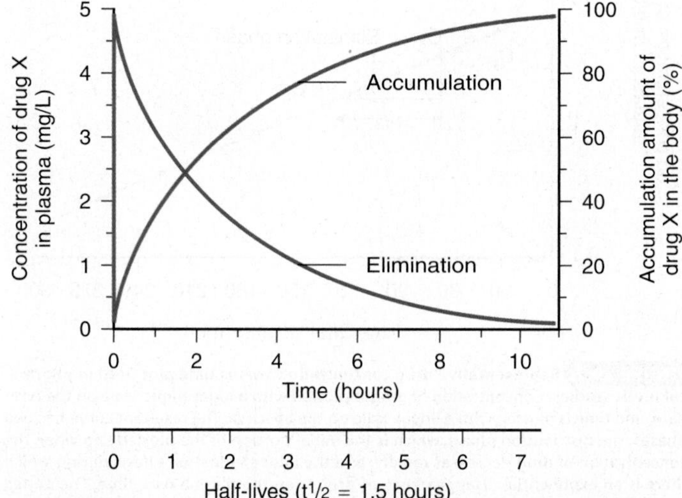

FIGURE 29-3. Representative plot of the mirror-image relationship between the elimination of drug (after drug is discontinued) and the accumulation of drug (during infusion). The plot shows the concentration on the left y-axis and time on the upper x-axis. The lower x-axis shows the time in half-lives, and the y-axis on the right shows the percentage of drug in the body. After three to five half-lives, elimination is essentially complete, and accumulation is essentially at a steady state.

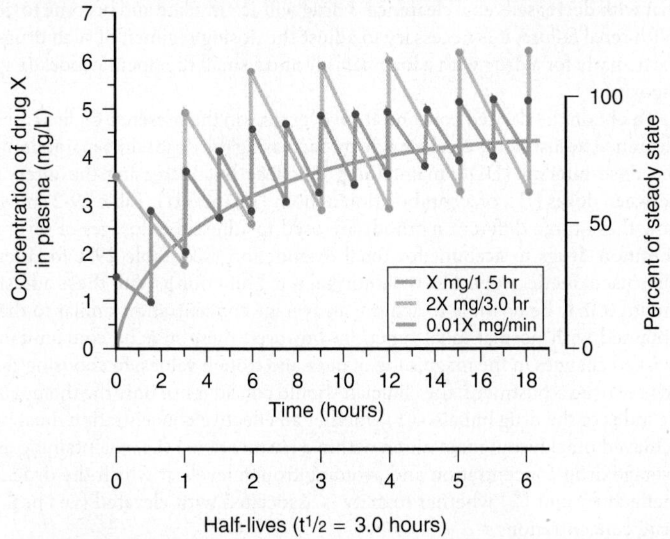

FIGURE 29-4. **Accumulation of drug over time, approaching a steady state. Time is depicted in hours (upper *x*-axis) and half-lives (lower *x*-axis, showing that steady state is reached in three to five half-lives). The *green line* depicts the pattern produced by an infusion of a hypothetical drug at a dose of 0.01X. The *orange line* shows the pattern resulting from oral administration of a 2X dose every 3 hours, and the *blue line* represents the pattern produced by oral administration of dose X every 1.5 hours.**

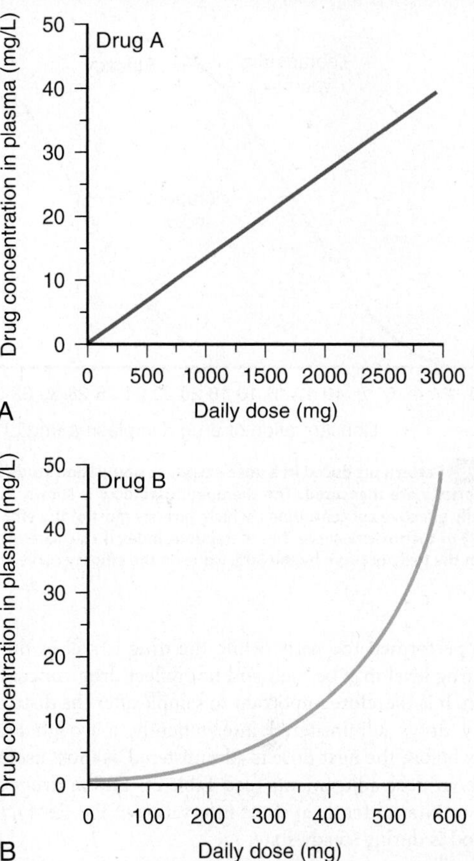

FIGURE 29-5. **Effect of increasing the dose of a drug on its serum concentration. A, Drug A follows first-order or linear kinetics. B, Drug B follows zero-order or nonlinear (or saturable) kinetics.**

oral dose, the drug concentration fluctuates; the magnitude of fluctuation between the peak and trough concentrations depends on the interval of administration, drug half-life, absorption characteristics, and site of administration. The effect of a change in the interval of administration for an oral drug is shown in Figure 29-4. As the intervals decrease below the half-life, the fluctuation decreases and approaches the curve produced by an intravenous infusion. Orally administered drugs may reach the blood stream more rapidly, attaining a higher peak concentration with one formulation, whereas the same drug administered as a timed-release formulation is absorbed more slowly, with a lower peak concentration but lasting longer in the plasma. Finally, the same drug administered by different routes may have different plasma profiles not only because of differing absorption characteristics but also because of other effects, such as first-pass metabolism.

Decreasing the Drug Level

At times, it may be necessary to decrease the plasma drug level while maintaining therapy (e.g., when signs of toxicity become apparent or a potentially dangerously high concentration of drug is noted; see later). The most effective and rapid response is to discontinue the drug; the length of time for which the drug is discontinued is determined by the estimated half-life of the drug in the specific patient. After discontinuation of the drug for a time based on its half-life, the total clearance (Cl_{tot}) of the drug can be used to determine what infusion rate (I, Equation 7) or dose and interval (D/t, Equation 8) must be used to achieve the new desired concentration (C_p).

Effect of Dose Increases on Elimination Kinetics

Although the previously discussed pharmacokinetic principles can be a guide to the dose of most drugs, not all drugs behave the same when the dose is increased. The elimination of most drugs follows first-order or linear kinetics; the amount of drug eliminated is directly proportional to the concentration of drug in the plasma (Fig. 29-5A). A few drugs have a different pattern of elimination. Three of the most commonly used drugs that exhibit this different pharmacokinetic pattern are ethanol, phenytoin, and salicylate. These drugs have dose-dependent, nonlinear saturation kinetics. As the dose of drug increases and the concentration of drug in the plasma rises, the relative amount of drug being eliminated falls (i.e., the clearance decreases) until the rate of drug metabolism is at its maximum. At this point, drug elimination is said to be zero order, and the drug concentration in plasma starts to increase much more (no longer linearly) with each subsequent increase in dose (Fig. 29-5B).

DRUG MONITORING AS A GUIDE TO THERAPY

Although published pharmacokinetic data (usually population averages) such as those in Table 29-1 are useful to determine initial drug dosing, modification of the dose may be needed in an individual patient. For some drugs (e.g., certain antihypertensives or anticoagulants), the therapeutic effects (e.g., blood pressure or coagulation) can be quantified easily over a range of concentrations, permitting adequate drug adjustment. For many other drugs (e.g., some antiarrhythmics or antiseizure medications), therapeutic effects over a range of concentrations are not readily detectable. With these drugs, the plasma concentration may provide further guidance in optimizing therapy if the plasma concentration of the drug is a reflection of its concentration at the site of action and the drug effects are reversible. A third, much smaller group of drugs produces irreversible effects (e.g., aspirin inhibition of platelet aggregation). With these drugs, plasma drug concentration does not correlate with drug effect, and drug monitoring is not useful.

To use drug concentration as a guide to therapy, it is necessary to establish a range of concentrations from minimally to maximally efficacious with tolerable toxicity. This range of concentrations, or the *therapeutic window*, is usually determined from a dose-response curve generated from a population of patients who have been examined closely for therapeutic and toxic effects (Fig. 29-6). This graph also may be used to determine the *therapeutic index*, a useful measure of drug toxicity calculated by dividing the 50% value from the toxicity curve by the 50% value from the efficacy curve. Because these curves are generated from population data, the values may not be applicable to all individuals.

Table 29-1, in addition to providing useful pharmacokinetic data, lists therapeutic ranges of several common drugs for which measuring the concentration and knowing the therapeutic range may be useful in clinical management. Many of these drugs are used to treat serious or life-threatening diseases. In these cases, it is essential to avoid inadequate doses because a therapeutic effect is often critical. Excessive doses must also be avoided because of the risk for toxicity with drugs that have a small therapeutic index. In contrast, it is not necessary to assay levels of drugs used to treat noncritical diseases (when inadequate treatment is not a serious problem) or for which the therapeutic index is large (when relative overtreatment is not likely to produce toxicity).

Problems with Interpreting Drug Concentration

The time of blood collection, perhaps more than any other factor, contributes to the misinterpretation of drug levels. As can be seen in Figure 29-2, if

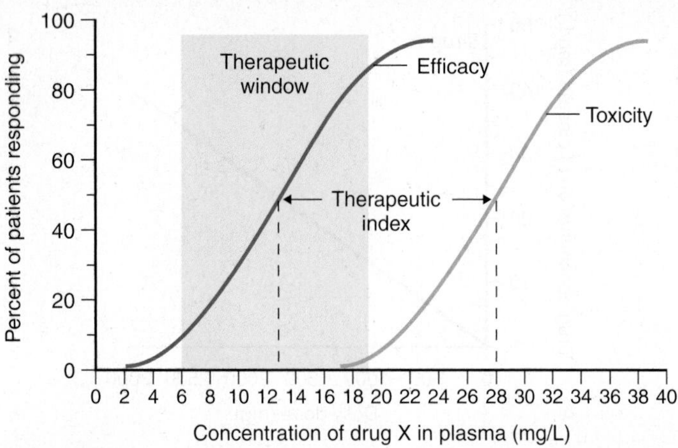

FIGURE 29-6. Pattern produced in a dose-response population study in which both effect and toxicity are measured. The therapeutic window is shown as the range of therapeutically effective concentrations, which includes most of the efficacy curve and less than 10% of the toxicity curve. The therapeutic index is calculated by dividing the 50% value on the toxicity curve by the 50% value on the efficacy curve.

sampling is performed too early, while the drug is still in the distribution phase, the drug level may be high and not reflect drug concentration at the site of action. It is therefore important to sample after the distribution phase.

For many drugs administered intermittently, a trough level, obtained immediately before the next dose is administered, is most useful for making decisions about dose adjustments (see Table 29-1). For drugs administered by infusion or intermittently at short intervals (see Fig. 29-4), the best time to draw blood is during steady state.

Protein binding is another major factor that contributes to the misinterpretation of drug levels. Free drug (not bound to protein and able to equilibrate with tissues and to interact with the site of action) is the critical drug concentration when therapeutic decisions are being made. Many drugs are tightly bound to plasma protein, however. Table 29-1 shows that many commonly used drugs, such as aspirin, carbamazepine, phenytoin, and glimepiride, have protein binding of more than 75%. Because many of the commonly used drug assays determine total drug concentration (which includes protein-bound drug and free drug), assessment of the "true" free drug concentration may be inaccurate, particularly if the fraction of drug bound to protein varies. In addition, the drug's binding may be decreased by disease or by other drugs, leading to increased unbound drug levels that alter the interpretation of the measured drug concentrations. Kidney and liver disease can change the binding of certain drugs (e.g., phenytoin) to protein because of a decrease in protein (e.g., decreased albumin, as in nephrotic syndrome or liver disease) or as a result of competition for protein binding by endogenously produced substances (e.g., uremia in kidney disease, hyperbilirubinemia in liver disease). Similarly, other drugs being administered may compete for binding to protein. A major problem secondary to these changes in protein binding is that free drug is not typically measured in many of the common drug assays used by clinical laboratories. Lastly, changes in drug binding to protein can affect the pharmacokinetics of the drug, the main effect being on the VD, which increases as protein binding decreases.

The usefulness of a drug assay is also limited by physiologic changes that may alter the response at a particular drug concentration. An example of this pharmacodynamic change is the response produced by a certain level of digoxin in the presence of altered electrolyte concentrations (e.g., potassium, calcium, and/or magnesium). Tolerance, a reduced response to a given concentration of drug with continued use, is another pharmacodynamic change that may alter how a drug concentration is interpreted. Tolerance is commonly observed with the continued use of narcotics (e.g., in terminal cancer patients); initially, adequate pain control is noted at a given drug concentration, but after long-term administration, the same drug concentration is no longer associated with pain relief.

ADJUSTMENTS OF DRUG DOSE WITH DISEASE

Kidney Disease

The major questions to be answered when determining whether a drug dosage needs to be adjusted in the setting of kidney disease are the following: Is the drug primarily excreted through the kidneys? Are increased drug levels likely to be associated with toxicity? If the answer to both is yes, it is likely that with decreased renal clearance, a drug will accumulate and become toxic. With renal failure, it is necessary to adjust the dosing regimen of such drugs, particularly for a drug with a long half-life and a small therapeutic index (e.g., digoxin).

To obtain the desired concentration over time in the presence of decreased clearance, adjustments can be made by decreasing the dose while maintaining the dose interval (DD), maintaining the dose but increasing the interval between doses (II), or a combination of both (DD and II). Table 29-2 shows how these three different methods are used to adjust the dosages of several common drugs to account for renal dysfunction (see Table 29-1 for their pharmacokinetic properties with normal renal function). With these adjustments, it may be possible to achieve an average concentration similar to that obtained with normal renal function; however, there may be concomitant marked changes in the magnitude of peak and trough values. In choosing the type of drug adjustment, the clinician should consider not only the therapeutic index of the drug but also (1) whether an effective concentration must be achieved quickly and maintained within a narrow range (i.e., maintaining an average drug concentration and avoiding trough levels at which the drug is ineffective) and (2) whether toxicity is associated with elevated (i.e., peak) drug concentrations.

Renal drug clearance correlates with creatinine clearance (whether the drug uses glomerular filtration or tubular secretion); therefore, any adjustment of drug dose in kidney disease can use the creatinine clearance to calculate the dose needed because renal drug clearance is proportional to creatinine clearance. The creatinine clearance (Cl_{cr}), which is used as an estimate of glomerular filtration rate, may be calculated directly from the serum creatinine concentration by the following equation:

$$Cl_{cr} = [(140 - \text{age}) \times \text{weight (kg)}]/[72 \times \text{serum creatinine (mg/dL)}] \quad (9)$$

The calculated creatinine clearance should be multiplied by 0.85 for females. (*Note:* This calculation applies only when the serum creatinine concentration is less than 5 mg/dL and renal function is not rapidly changing.)

Using Clearance for Dose Adjustment

The dose of a drug used in renal insufficiency ($dose_{D\text{-}RI}$) is proportional to the dose used with normal renal function ($dose_D$) in the same ratio as clearance of the drug in renal insufficiency ($Cl_{D\text{-}RI}$) to clearance with normal renal function (Cl_D). By rearranging, $dose_{D\text{-}RI}$ is defined as:

$$Dose_{D\text{-}RI} = dose_D \times [Cl_{D\text{-}RI}/Cl_D] \quad (10)$$

One can estimate the $Cl_{D\text{-}RI}$ by multiplying Cl_D by the ratio of the creatinine clearance in renal insufficiency ($Cl_{cr\text{-}RI}$) over Cl_{cr} with normal renal function:

$$Cl_{D\text{-}RI} = Cl_D \times [Cl_{cr\text{-}RI}/Cl_{cr}] \quad (11)$$

As shown in Equation 3, total clearance is the sum of clearance by renal and nonrenal (typically hepatic) mechanisms. Any nonrenal clearance is assumed to remain normal, and only the renal clearance is adjusted, with total clearance being reduced only to the extent that renal clearance is reduced. The dose may be calculated from the total (adjusted) clearance and the desired plasma concentration by either Equation 7 or Equation 8. The calculated dose is only an initial guide to the dose needed, however. By monitoring the drug response or the plasma drug concentration at various times after initial dosing, further dose adjustments can be made as necessary. From a practical perspective, most clinical dose adjustments in the presence of renal dysfunction can be guided by published tables based on changes in glomerular filtration rate (see Table 29-2) and the effectiveness of dialysis in removing the drug. Computerized decision support systems are particularly effective in guiding medication dosing for inpatients with renal insufficiency.

Loading Dose in Renal Insufficiency

For drugs typically administered with a loading dose in patients with normal renal function, the same approach can be used in those with renal insufficiency to ensure that the desired concentration is achieved rapidly. For drugs typically administered without a loading dose, the presence of a prolonged half-life resulting from renal insufficiency may delay drug accumulation to steady state. In this setting, a loading dose (equal to the amount needed to reach steady state with normal renal function) is required.

Additional Considerations in Renal Insufficiency

Because of individual differences among patients, the approaches outlined earlier should be considered only initial approximations to prevent ineffective

TABLE 29-2 ADJUSTMENT OF DRUG DOSAGE IN RENAL FAILURE

		HALF-LIFE (hr)			ADJUSTMENT FOR RENAL FAILURE			
DRUG	Type of Elimination	Normal	End-Stage Renal Disease	METHOD*	GFR > 50 mL/min	GFR 10-50 mL/min	GFR < 10 mL/min	Removed by Dialysis[†]
Amikacin	Renal	2-3	30	DD II	60-90% 12 hr	30-70% 12-18 hr	20-30% 24 hr	Yes
Aspirin	Hepatic (renal)	2-19	Unchanged	II	4 hr	4-6 hr	Avoid	Yes
Carbamazepine	Hepatic (renal)	35	?	DD	Unchanged	Unchanged	75%	No
Digoxin	Renal (nonrenal 15-40%)	36-44	80-120	DD II	Unchanged 24 hr	25-75% 36 hr	10-25% 48 hr	No
Lidocaine	Hepatic (renal < 20%)	1.2-2.2	1.3-3	DD	Unchanged	Unchanged	Unchanged	No
Lithium carbonate	Renal	14-28	Prolonged	DD	Unchanged	50-75%	25-50%	Yes
Penicillin G	Renal (hepatic)	0.5	6-20	DD	Unchanged 6-8 hr	75% 8-12 hr	25-50% 12-16 hr	Yes
Phenobarbital	Hepatic (renal 30%)	60-150	117-160	II	Unchanged	Unchanged	12-16 hr	Yes
Phenytoin	Hepatic (renal)	24	8	DD	Unchanged	Unchanged	Unchanged	No
Procainamide	Renal (hepatic 7-24%)	2.5-4.9	5.3-5.9	II	4 hr	6-12 hr	8-24 hr	Yes
Theophylline	Hepatic	3-12	?	DD	Unchanged	Unchanged	Unchanged	Yes
Tobramycin	Renal	2.5	56	DD II	60-90% 8-12 hr	30-70% 12 hr	20-30% 24 hr	Yes
Vancomycin	Renal	6-8	200-250	II	24-72 hr	72-240 hr	240 hr	No

*DD (alone) = decrease dose (maintain same interval); II (alone) = increase interval between doses (maintain dose); DD and II (together) = combination of both approaches.
[†]Dialysis refers to hemodialysis.
GFR = glomerular filtration rate.

(too low) or toxic (too high) doses. For maintenance therapy, it is desirable to monitor blood levels to guide dosing.

If a metabolite of the drug is responsible for its effect or toxicity and the metabolite accumulates in the setting of renal failure, the drug level alone may not provide sufficient guidance for planning therapy. For example, the major metabolite of procainamide is *N*-acetylprocainamide, which has a toxicity similar to that of the parent drug but only modest antiarrhythmic activity. In the setting of renal failure, *N*-acetylprocainamide may accumulate dramatically because it is more dependent on renal elimination. Measurement of procainamide levels alone does not accurately assess either the levels needed for antiarrhythmic effect or the risk for toxicity.

Liver Disease

Although many drugs are biotransformed in the liver, it is not possible to make any general recommendations for drug dose adjustments in liver disease. In contrast to renal disease, no useful laboratory test is available on which to base dose adjustments. It has been suggested that if the liver's capacity to produce protein (reflected by albumin concentration and prothrombin time) is reduced significantly, the clearance of drugs metabolized by the cytochrome P-450 enzymes is probably reduced as well.

One special situation that can develop with chronic liver disease and may require dose adjustment is the portacaval shunt. This condition produces not only a potential hemodynamic alteration, leading to decreased hepatic blood flow and accompanying decreased clearance, but also a possible bypassing of the first-pass effect, resulting in higher concentrations of drug reaching the systemic circulation. Drugs with a large hepatic extraction that are typically administered orally (e.g., propranolol) may appear in the systemic circulation at higher, potentially toxic concentrations.

Hemodynamic Diseases

Decreased cardiac output and hypotensive conditions lead to decreased perfusion of the organs, including those responsible for eliminating drugs. As noted earlier with regard to primary kidney disease, the dose can be adjusted for decreased renal perfusion by the use of creatinine clearance. The effect of decreased hepatic blood flow on pharmacokinetics is more difficult to assess. For drugs that have a high hepatic extraction (e.g., lidocaine), decreased hepatic blood flow suggests a need for dose reduction.

Altered hemodynamics also may affect the distribution of selected drugs. Drugs that have a relatively large VD (e.g., lidocaine, procainamide, quinidine) may be affected by conditions leading to hypotension, such as shock, resulting in a decrease in the apparent VD. With a reduced VD, the loading dose of a drug should be reduced to avoid potentially toxic drug levels.

In general, in the setting of severely compromised hemodynamics, it is advisable to be conservative, avoiding potentially toxic loading and maintenance doses of drugs. Drug levels and the clinical status should be monitored closely, and drug doses should be adjusted as necessary.

APPROACH TO DRUG OVERDOSE

The pharmacokinetic principles discussed earlier can be used to determine the best approach to drug removal in the setting of a drug overdose, particularly if hemodialysis or hemoperfusion is contemplated. The major goal is to increase the overall clearance of the drug, removing a substantial fraction of the total body load of drug. Examination of the VD and clearance values can provide some guidance. For drugs with a large VD (e.g., digoxin; see Table 29-1), only a small amount can be removed because clearance affects only the amount of drug present in the plasma, and a large portion of the drug is outside the plasma compartment. Similarly, for drugs with high clearance values, hemoperfusion may increase the overall clearance only minimally and is not indicated. Table 29-2 provides data for determining whether hemodialysis is likely to be useful to remove several commonly prescribed drugs.

DRUG USE IN ELDERLY PATIENTS

Administering drugs to elderly patients is perhaps the most challenging area of adult therapeutics because of several factors: the increasing likelihood of multiple illnesses, often with multisystemic involvement; the need for these patients to take multiple drugs (often prescribed by different physicians); and the increasing probability of altered pharmacokinetics and pharmacodynamics. These factors together contribute to a significantly increased frequency of drug interactions and adverse drug responses in this group of patients.

Pharmacokinetic Changes with Age

These changes can be secondary to the general physiologic effects of aging, such as alteration in body composition, or to specific changes in pharmacokinetically important organs (e.g., kidneys, liver). The distribution of drugs tends to change dramatically with age, mainly because of changes in body composition. Most typical is the increase in total body fat, with the accompanying decrease in lean body mass and total body water. The concentration of plasma proteins may also change; in particular, albumin decreases as the liver ages. Changes in drug distribution are manifested as a change in the apparent VD. For water-soluble drugs that are not bound to plasma proteins, the apparent VD is reduced; in contrast, for lipid-soluble drugs, the VD is increased. Minimal changes in metabolism accompany aging, but these alone cannot account for altered pharmacokinetics.

Excretion can be altered in the elderly, and the clearance of many drugs is decreased. Cardiac output and blood flow to the kidneys and liver also may be decreased. Glomerular filtration rate may be reduced by 50%. Hepatic elimination of drugs is less affected, except for drugs with a high hepatic clearance (e.g., lidocaine). The elimination half-life of many drugs is increased with aging as a consequence of a larger apparent VD and a decreased hepatic or renal clearance (see Equation 5).

Pharmacodynamic Changes with Age

These changes are a result of changes in the responsiveness of the target organ. They require the use of smaller drug doses in elderly patients, even if the pharmacokinetics are unchanged. This affects many drugs commonly used in elderly people; for example, antianxiety drugs and drugs from the sedative-hypnotic class may produce increased central nervous system depression in elderly patients at concentrations that are well tolerated in younger adults. Similarly, anticoagulants (e.g., warfarin) may produce hemorrhage in elderly people at concentrations that are well tolerated in younger adults.

General Recommendations for Drug Use in Elderly Patients

- Clearance of drugs eliminated by the kidneys may be reduced by 50%.
- Drugs eliminated primarily by the liver typically do not require dose adjustments for age, except for drugs with high hepatic clearances, which may be affected by the age-related decrease in hepatic blood flow.
- Because of the potential for increased target organ sensitivity in elderly people, only the lowest effective dose should be used.
- Frequent reviews of the patient's drug history should be conducted, including both prescription and over-the-counter medications, keeping in mind the increased potential risk for drug interactions and adverse drug responses.

INTERACTIONS BETWEEN DRUGS

Because patients are typically treated with multiple agents, even for a single disease, the possibilities for drug interactions are great. Many clinically important drug interactions typically involve a drug with a low therapeutic index (e.g., warfarin) and an easily detectable pharmacologic effect (e.g., bleeding), such that a small increase in the amount of drug produces a significant effect (toxicity).

It is difficult to accurately assess the prevalence of drug interactions in either the inpatient or the ambulatory setting, particularly because no formal and comprehensive surveillance mechanism is available. The risk for drug interactions seems to be increasing, particularly for critically ill, hospitalized patients, who are frequently taking more than 10 medications.[1]

There are basically two types of drug interaction: (1) pharmacokinetic drug interactions, caused by a change in the amount of drug or active metabolite at the site of action; and (2) pharmacodynamic drug interactions (without a change in pharmacokinetics), caused by a change in drug effect.

Pharmacokinetic Drug Interactions

Less Drug at the Site of Action

Decreased Absorption

The gastrointestinal lumen is perhaps the best example of an area where drug interactions can result in decreased drug absorption. Some commonly used drugs can illustrate this type of interaction. For many drugs, a physicochemical interaction prevents the drug from being absorbed. Drugs such as colestipol and cholestyramine (resins used to lower cholesterol and bind bile acids) can also bind other drugs present in the gastrointestinal lumen, including digoxin and warfarin. Because of the potential for many other drugs to be bound, it is generally recommended that other drugs not be administered within 2 hours of colestipol or cholestyramine. Another type of interaction occurs when metal ions (e.g., aluminum, calcium, and magnesium in antacids and iron in supplements to treat iron deficiency) form insoluble complexes with tetracyclines, which can act as chelating agents. Other commonly used medications that decrease absorption include kaolin-pectin suspensions to treat diarrhea. These medications can significantly inhibit the absorption of coadministered drugs (e.g., digoxin).

Drugs that are particularly susceptible to pH changes may have decreased absorption when they are administered with other drugs that either affect gastric acidity or alter the extent of exposure to low pH. Protein pump inhibitors or histamine-2 receptor antagonists may elevate gastric pH, which can inhibit the dissolution and subsequent absorption of drugs that are weak bases (e.g., ketoconazole). Medications that delay gastric emptying (e.g., belladonna alkaloids) can increase the degradation of a coadministered acid-labile drug (e.g., levodopa), resulting in decreased absorption.

Altered Distribution

Drugs that use the same active transport process to reach their site of action can compete at the level of transport, resulting in lower levels of drug reaching that site. The classic example of this type of interaction is the coadministration of guanidinium-type antihypertensives with tricyclic antidepressants, phenothiazines, and certain sympathomimetic amines (e.g., ephedrine), which block the effects of the antihypertensive drug.

Increased Metabolism

Many drugs (e.g., phenobarbital, phenytoin, ethanol, glutethimide, griseofulvin, rifampin) and toxic compounds (e.g., cigarette smoke, certain chlorinated hydrocarbons) can increase the hepatic metabolism of other drugs (e.g., corticosteroids, cyclophosphamide, cyclosporine, certain β-adrenergic blockers, theophylline, warfarin) by inducing the activity of the cytochrome P-450 super family of monooxygenase enzyme.

More Drug at the Site of Action

Increased Absorption

Any drug that increases the rate of gastric emptying (e.g., metoclopramide) can potentially increase the absorption of acid-unstable drugs. Also, drugs that decrease intestinal motility (e.g., anticholinergics) may increase the absorption of drugs that are relatively poorly absorbed (e.g., digoxin tablets) by increasing the drug's contact time with the absorbing surface.

Altered Distribution

Drugs bound to protein are limited in their distribution (particularly to the site of action) and are not available for metabolism or excretion. Drugs can compete with each other for binding to plasma proteins, resulting in drug interactions. Sulfonamides can displace barbiturates bound to serum albumin, leading to increased levels of free barbiturates and possible toxicity.

Decreased Metabolism

One of the most impressive drug interactions is produced when one drug inhibits the metabolism of another, leading to the second drug's accumulation and a significant risk for toxicity. This type of interaction results when 6-mercaptopurine, an antileukemic drug with a low therapeutic index, is used with allopurinol, often administered to control hyperuricemia. The interaction may result in potentially life-threatening toxicity.

Some drugs can inhibit the metabolism of many other drugs. For example, cimetidine can inhibit the metabolism of diazepam, imipramine, lidocaine, propranolol, quinidine, theophylline, and warfarin. Amiodarone inhibits the metabolism of calcium-channel blockers, phenytoin, quinidine, and warfarin. Of particular importance with amiodarone is its half-life of 1 to 2 months; it continues to inhibit drug metabolism for several months after it has been discontinued.

Other drugs are notable because their metabolism is inhibited by a variety of different drugs. The metabolism of the commonly used anticoagulant warfarin is inhibited not only by cimetidine and amiodarone but also by many other drugs, including alcohol, allopurinol, disulfiram, metronidazole, phenylbutazone, sulfinpyrazone, and trimethoprim-sulfamethoxazole. Similarly, the metabolism of phenytoin is inhibited by chloramphenicol, clofibrate, dicumarol, disulfiram, isoniazid (slow acetylators), phenylbutazone, and valproic acid.

Although most of these examples involve enzymes that metabolize the drug in the liver, drug-metabolizing enzymes outside the liver also may be affected by certain drugs. The best-known example is monoamine oxidase, which can be affected by nonspecific monoamine oxidase inhibitors, resulting in the accumulation of catecholamines at multiple sites after their release in response to the eating of tyramine-containing foods such as aged cheese, aged or cured meats, and any spoiled meat, poultry, or fish.

Decreased Excretion

Drugs can compete for the active transporters present in the kidney. Most of these interactions involve the acid transporters. The best-known interaction is probenecid's inhibition of penicillin transport, leading to decreased penicillin clearance and thus higher plasma levels, an interaction that was used in the past to maximize penicillin therapy. A similar inhibitory effect on the renal excretion of methotrexate can be produced by salicylates, phenylbutazone, and probenecid. The active transport of basic drugs (e.g., procainamide) can also be inhibited by other drugs (e.g., cimetidine, amiodarone).

Pharmacodynamic Drug Interactions

With pharmacodynamic interactions, drugs interact at the level of the receptor (target) or may produce additive effects by acting at separate sites on cells. An example of the first is the interaction of propranolol and epinephrine, which blocks β-adrenergic receptors; as a result, the α-adrenergic effects of epinephrine are unopposed. This undesirable interaction can result in severe hypertension.

Many examples exist of the additive effects of drugs. Aspirin, which can produce increased bleeding time by acting on platelets, can interact with warfarin, which affects clotting. The result is an increased risk for hemorrhage. Similarly, cardiac drugs, such as β-adrenergic blockers and calcium-channel blockers, have additive negative inotropic effects when they are coadministered, resulting in an increased risk for cardiac failure.

DIAGNOSIS AND PREVENTION OF DRUG INTERACTIONS

For a drug interaction to be recognized, the index of suspicion must be high whenever multiple drugs are used together. Because of the ever-increasing list of known and suspected drug interactions, it is impossible for a clinician to remember all or even many of the possible interactions.

Several clinical settings should raise concern about the possibility of drug interactions:

- The use of any drug with a low therapeutic index (Table 29-3) should be suspect.
- As the number of drugs being used concurrently increases, there is a disproportionately greater risk for drug interactions, particularly with more than 10 drugs.
- Critically ill patients who have multisystemic disease with compromised renal, hepatic, cardiac, or pulmonary function have an increased risk for drug interactions. This risk may be higher for patients with acquired immunodeficiency syndrome, who have an immunocompromised state and take a large number of drugs.
- Patients with various behavioral and psychiatric disorders (e.g., drug abusers taking a large number of prescription drugs as well as illicit drugs and alcohol) are at risk for drug interactions.

Another type of drug interaction that is becoming increasingly important is that between components of food (e.g., grapefruit juice) or natural products (e.g., herbs) and drugs. By inhibiting the intestinal cytochrome P-450 3A4 enzyme system, grapefruit juice can raise levels of drugs metabolized by this pathway (e.g., saquinavir, cyclosporine, verapamil) and result in toxicity or adverse drug effects.

Several steps can be taken to prevent drug interactions:

- When taking the medical history, it is important to document all drugs the patient is taking (and has recently taken), including prescription, over-the-counter, and other addictive drugs.
- It is desirable to minimize the number of drugs being taken by frequently reviewing the patient's drug list to ensure that each drug continues to be needed.

TABLE 29-3 DRUGS WITH LOW THERAPEUTIC INDICES AT HIGH RISK FOR ADVERSE DRUG RESPONSES AND DRUG INTERACTIONS

Anticoagulants
Antiarrhythmics
Anticonvulsants
Digoxin
Lithium carbonate
Oral hypoglycemics
Theophylline

- There should be a high degree of suspicion when medications with a low therapeutic index known to have a high risk for drug interactions (see Table 29-3) are used.
- High-risk clinical settings, such as occur with critically ill patients, should raise the suspicion of adverse drug interactions.
- Adverse drug interactions should be considered in the differential diagnosis whenever any change occurs in a patient's course.

ADVERSE REACTIONS TO DRUGS

An adverse drug response (ADR) is an undesired effect produced by a drug at standard doses, which typically necessitates reducing or stopping the suspected agent and may require treatment of the noxious effect produced. Further harm may occur with continued or future therapy with the drug.

EPIDEMIOLOGY

The financial impact of ADRs is estimated to be more than $100 billion per year. The actual incidence of ADRs is difficult to quantify because many cases are either not recognized or not reported. Several large studies have shown that the incidence may approach 20% for outpatients (even higher for patients taking more than 15 drugs) and 2 to 7% for inpatients. The incidence of ADRs increases exponentially with more than four drugs. Meta-analyses of several prospective studies suggest that ADRs are now the third leading cause of death in hospitalized patients. It is clear from more recent surveys that a relatively small group of drugs (see Table 29-3) continues to be implicated in most of the reported ADRs. Current trends suggest that the incidence of ADRs is likely to increase as a result of more prescribed and over-the-counter medications being used. Although still in an evolutionary phase, systems approaches have the potential to greatly advance the understanding of adverse drug events and the ability to predict them.[2]

PATHOBIOLOGY

Most ADRs are caused by an exaggerated (but predictable) pharmacologic effect of the drug or by a toxic or immunologic effect of the drug or a metabolite (not typically expected). Among an estimated 100,000 annual drug-related emergency hospitalizations in patients older than 65 years, the most commonly implicated drugs are warfarin (33%), insulin (14%), oral antiplatelet agents (13%), and oral hypoglycemic agents (11%).

Predictable Toxic Responses to Drugs

Exaggerated drug responses that cause adverse drug effects may be due to any condition that causes altered pharmacokinetics or pharmacodynamics (discussed earlier). There has been increasing interest in the discipline of pharmacogenomics, which explores the role of genetic factors in altered pharmacokinetics or pharmacodynamics and the resultant increased susceptibility to ADRs. Furthermore, a developing discipline of pharmacometabolomics should complement pharmacogenomics in personalized drug therapy by capturing environmental and microbiome-level influences on responses to drugs.[3] There is now ample evidence that molecular changes in the genes coding for drug-metabolizing enzymes can account for the variability in pharmacokinetics and drug effects observed in population studies. There are now many examples of the role of pharmacogenomics in altered drug response and effect. Three of the best-studied examples are genetic polymorphisms associated with debrisoquine-sparteine, *N*-acetylation, and mephenytoin. Each is associated with autosomal recessive inheritance, and together they are responsible for the metabolism of approximately 40 drugs (Table 29-4). Individuals with autosomal recessive genes are typically "poor metabolizers," with potentially altered pharmacokinetics that result in elevated plasma drug concentrations and can lead to toxicity. Recent studies have focused on genomic alterations associated with the variability in response to some commonly used drugs. Thus, the variability of response to warfarin (Chapter 38) is now understood to be due to single-nucleotide polymorphisms in the cytochrome P-450 2C9 (*CYP2C9*) and vitamin K epoxide reductase (*VKOR*) genes. These single-nucleotide polymorphisms have a significant effect on warfarin dose requirements. Similarly, polymorphisms in transporter genes can have profound effects on the pharmacokinetics of statins (Chapter 206). A common genetic variant of the organic anion-transporting polypeptide 1B1 can reduce the hepatic uptake of many statins, increasing the risk for statin-induced myopathy. Also, it is now appreciated that genetically impaired adenosine triphosphate (ATP)-binding cassette G2 transporter efflux activity can result in an increase in systemic exposure to various statins. Of particular importance to therapeutics is that the effects of these genetic polymorphisms differ, depending on the specific statin used.

TABLE 29-4 GENETIC POLYMORPHISMS OF DRUG-METABOLIZING ENZYMES

TYPE	PRIMARY DRUG EXAMPLES	OTHER DRUGS THAT ARE SUBSTRATES	INCIDENCE OF "POOR METABOLIZERS" IN WHITES (%)	ENZYME INVOLVED
Debrisoquine-sparteine polymorphism	Amitriptyline, codeine, tamoxifen	Antidepressants, antiarrhythmics, β-adrenergic receptor–blocking drugs, codeine, dextromethorphan, neuroleptics	5-10	Cytochrome P-450 IID6 (CYP2D6)
Mephenytoin polymorphism	Mephenytoin	Mephobarbital, hexobarbital, diazepam, omeprazole	4 (Japanese, Chinese, 15-20)	Cytochrome P-450 IIC (CYP2C)
N-acetylation polymorphism	Isoniazid, sulfadiazine	Hydralazine, phenelzine, procainamide, dapsone, sulfamethazine, sulfapyridine, aminoglutethimide, aminosalicylic acid, sulfasalazine	40-70 (Japanese, 10-20)	*N*-acetyltransferase (NAT2)
Methyl conjugation polymorphism	Catecholamines	L-Dopa, methyldopa	25-30	Catechol-*O* methyltransferase (COMT)

This provides a rational basis for an individualized approach to the use of lipid-lowering therapeutic agents.

A particularly impressive example occurs with certain cancer chemotherapy agents that have a relatively narrow therapeutic window and the potential to produce severe cytotoxicity (e.g., deficiency in dihydropyrimidine dehydrogenase activity can result in life-threatening toxicity after the administration of 5-fluorouracil). These defects typically are not recognized until the patient is given the drug. They are often described as "pharmacogenetic" syndromes.

Other genetic alterations do not affect metabolism specifically and do not produce a range of quantitative changes. These defects can produce "qualitative" defects and are often associated with structural defects. The classic example is glucose-6-phosphate dehydrogenase. Individuals who are deficient in this enzyme cannot tolerate the oxidative stress produced by some drugs, leading to hemolysis (Chapter 161). Drugs that can produce this clinical picture include aspirin, nitrofurantoin, primaquine, probenecid, quinidine, quinine, sulfonamides, sulfones, and vitamin K. Another similar defect is deficiency of methemoglobin reductase, which results in an inability to maintain iron in hemoglobin in the ferrous state, causing methemoglobinemia (Chapter 158) after exposure to oxidizing drugs such as nitrites, sulfonamides, and sulfones.

Unpredictable Toxic Responses to Drugs

Other toxic or immunologic ADRs are not predictable and are not obviously due to an increase in drug concentration (pharmacokinetic) or drug effect (pharmacodynamic). Unpredictable toxic responses include direct reactions between a drug and a specific organ (e.g., platinum-containing drugs, such as cisplatin, can produce direct toxicity in the kidney and the eighth cranial nerve). With other drugs, metabolism to an active intermediate must occur first. With a standard dose of acetaminophen, no untoward effects occur because the relatively small amount of reactive metabolite formed by oxidative metabolism is detoxified rapidly by reduced glutathione. In the presence of an overdose, the glutathione is depleted, and the remaining reactive metabolite can damage the liver. Understanding the mechanism of this toxicity has provided a rationale for treating acetaminophen overdose. Sulfhydryl-containing compounds (e.g., *N*-acetylcysteine), which can complex with the reactive metabolite, can be administered to reduce the amount of free toxic metabolite present, protecting the liver.

Immunologic reactions to drugs are generally not produced by the drug alone. Similar to other low-molecular-weight compounds (<1000 D), they are typically not antigenic themselves. When a drug or reactive metabolite combines with a protein to form a drug-protein complex, it can become antigenic, capable of eliciting an immune response.

Perhaps the most impressive form of drug allergy is anaphylaxis, which is due to an immunoglobulin E–mediated hypersensitivity. Many drugs from different classes have been shown to produce this type of drug allergy. The best-known example is the anaphylactic response produced by penicillin, which can occur after its administration by any route. Skin testing with penicillin G, penicilloic acid, or penicilloyl polylysine can identify patients at risk and should be performed in those with a suspected penicillin allergy who need treatment with penicillin. If the skin test result is positive, the patient must undergo desensitization before receiving penicillin. If the skin test result is negative, penicillin can be administered with caution.

DIAGNOSIS OF ADVERSE DRUG RESPONSES

Although many of the well-known adverse drug effects are due to a relatively small group of drugs, every drug has the potential to cause an ADR. A physician should always consider the possibility of an ADR in the differential diagnosis even if none has been reported previously for the particular drug. In earlier editions of this book, we provided a table listing many diverse clinical presentations associated with ADRs. The reader is now referred to the numerous websites providing more complete and up-to-date information on ADRs than can be detailed here. For example, *www.fdable.com* allows one to monitor drug safety with unlimited access to up-to-date information from the U.S. Food and Drug Administration (FDA) Adverse Event Reporting System (AERS).

In many instances, it is readily apparent that a specific drug has produced an ADR, such as the appearance of a rash in an otherwise healthy patient who was recently prescribed a single drug (e.g., penicillin). In other cases, the effect produced by the drug may be difficult to discern from other disease states. In still other cases, the adverse effect may mimic the illness being treated (e.g., development of an arrhythmia in a patient being treated with an antiarrhythmic drug).

From a public health perspective, it is highly desirable to have a mechanism available to detect, catalog, and track the incidence and severity of ADRs not only for drugs at various stages of development but also for drugs that were approved earlier. The FDA tracks adverse drug events through a voluntary reporting program, MedWatch. Health care professionals are encouraged to report any adverse events or product problems on a one-page form that can be sent by mail, fax, or electronically to the FDA. Nontraditional resources that are generated by patients via the Internet could supplement existing pharmacovigilance approaches.[4] Although various methods for surveying ADRs have been proposed, ultimately, the cooperation of alert clinicians, health care professionals, and patients must be encouraged.[4]

GENOMIC DATA PROVIDING GUIDANCE FOR CANCER THERAPEUTIC DECISION

In addition to genetic data being useful in understanding and increasingly predicting adverse drug effects (see earlier), it is becoming increasingly clear that genomic data (e.g., the presence of a specific genetic variant) can also help inform the clinician of the appropriate drug or dose of drug that should be used for the specific patient.[5,6] There is no therapeutic area in which this is more apparent than with oncologic drugs and particularly many of the new targeted therapy agents, for which the genomic profile of the tumor (vs. the host tissue) is critical.[7] A representative example is vemurafenib, a targeted agent that has recently been demonstrated to have therapeutic value in melanoma and potentially other malignancies as well. Vemurafenib is effective in tumors that have a specific mutation in their *BRAF* gene, a valine-to-glutamic acid mutation at residue 600 (V600E), that results in the oncogene protein product, BRAF(V600E) kinase, exhibiting a markedly elevated activity that overactivates the MAPK signaling pathway. Vemurafenib is an orally bioavailable, ATP-competitive, small-molecule inhibitor of BRAF(V600E) kinase with antineoplastic activity. It selectively binds to the ATP-binding site of BRAF(V600E) kinase and inhibits its activity, resulting in inhibition of an overactivated MAPK signaling pathway downstream in BRAF(V600E) kinase–expressing tumor cells, thereby reducing tumor cell proliferation. There are multiple other examples in oncology demonstrating that genomic data from the tumor of an individual patient can be useful in making a therapeutic decision.

GENERAL REFERENCES

For the General References and other additional features, please visit Expert Consult at https://expertconsult.inkling.com.

30 PAIN

STEVEN P. COHEN AND SRINIVASA N. RAJA

Pain is ubiquitous in life, usually serving as a warning sign of impending or actual injury to the organism. As such, pain is older than humans, dating back to our most primitive ancestors. Pain is also a vital diagnostic clue for physicians. Physicians should be intimately familiar with pain, for it is the most common symptom for which patients seek medical attention.

It is difficult to overestimate the impact that pain has on society. According to an Institute of Medicine report released in 2011, one in three Americans suffer from chronic pain, which is more than the total affected by heart disease, cancer, and diabetes combined. Among the various types of pain, back pain is the most common, followed by severe headaches, arthralgias, and neck pain. The estimated economic cost of chronic pain, to include medical costs and lost productivity, ranges between $560 and $635 billion (in 2010 dollars).[1] Spinal pain is the leading cause of disability in individuals younger than 45 years in industrialized nations, with the economic costs exceeding $100 billion annually in the United States by some estimates. Special populations at risk for chronic pain include the elderly, and individuals with physical and psychological morbidities. Several conditions characterized by chronic pain, such as headaches, irritable bowel syndrome, fibromyalgia, and complex regional pain syndrome, are more prevalent in women than in men.

DEFINITION

The International Association for the Study of Pain defines pain as "an unpleasant sensory and emotional experience associated with actual or potential tissue damage, or described in terms of such damage." This definition recognizes that pain may be experienced in some circumstances in the absence of ongoing tissue damage (e.g., phantom pain after a healed amputation). One implication of this construct is the assumption that pain is always subjective; hence, a patient's report of pain should always be accepted at face value in the absence of evidence to the contrary.

PATHOBIOLOGY

Classification of Pain States

Multiple classifications have been used to describe pain states on the basis of duration, anatomic source, and etiology. *Acute pain* usually results from injury or inflammation, has survival value, and may play a role in healing by promoting behaviors that minimize reinjury. In contrast, *chronic pain* is perhaps best construed as a "disease" that serves no useful purpose. Although there is no clear threshold at which acute pain transitions to a chronic state, it is generally accepted that pain persisting beyond the expected healing period is pathologic. In most cases, this period is between 3 and 6 months. The intensity of pain can be classified as mild (1 to 3), moderate (4 or 5), or severe (≥6 on a 0 to10 numerical rating scale).

Somatic and Visceral Pains

Pain can originate from somatic or visceral structures. *Somatic pain* is typically well localized and generally results from injury or disease of the skin, musculoskeletal structures, and joints. Different types of stimulation can evoke pain by binding to distinct receptors (also known as nociceptors), which can be broadly categorized as chemosensitive, thermosensitive, mechanosensitive, or polymodal. *Visceral pain* arises from internal organ dysfunction and can result from inflammation, ischemia, occlusion of flow resulting in capsular or organ distention (e.g., renal stones, bowel obstruction, cholecystitis), or functional disease (e.g., irritable bowel syndrome). In contrast to somatic pain, visceral pain is usually diffuse and poorly localized, is often referred to somatic regions (e.g., myocardial ischemia radiating into th and tends to be associated with exaggerated autonomic reflexes and gr emotional features. Some of the reasons for these differences betwee somatic and visceral pain include a lower density and different types (e.g., distention sensitive) of nociceptors in visceral structures and convergence with afferent pathways predominantly populated by somatic pain in the spinal cord.

Neuropathic, Nociceptive, and Mixed Pain

Pain can be etiologically classified as neuropathic, nociceptive, or mixed (Table 30-1). *Neuropathic pain* has been defined as pain arising as a direct consequence of a lesion or disease affecting the somatosensory system. Common peripheral neuropathic pain states include post-herpetic neuralgia, diabetic neuropathy, and radicular pain. One subtype of neuropathic pain is central pain, which is manifested as a constellation of symptoms requiring a primary lesion to the central nervous system as a necessary (but not sufficient) inciting event. Owing to its high prevalence, the most common overall cause of central pain is central post-stroke pain (occurring after approximately 8% of cerebrovascular accidents), although spinal cord lesions (e.g., syringomyelia or spinal cord injury) are associated with a higher incidence of central pain (>50%). Epidemiologic studies indicate that neuropathic pain is prevalent in 7% to 8% of the population, and that 20% to 25% of all chronic pain is neuropathic in nature. *Nociceptive pain* usually results from an injury or disease affecting somatic structures such as skin, muscle, tendons and ligaments, bone, and joints. Pain associated with cancer can result either from the tumor itself or as a consequence of therapy (e.g., surgery, chemotherapy, and radiation therapy). In light of the often multiple different causes, advanced cancer pain is a typical example of a mixed pain state.

Dysfunctional Pain

There is a group of pain syndromes that have been characterized by amplification of pain signaling in the absence of either inflammation or injury (as in nociceptive pain) or damage to the nervous system (as in neuropathic pain). These conditions include pain states such as fibromyalgia, irritable bowel syndrome and interstitial cystitis. The precise pathophysiologic mechanisms of pain in these disorders are still being elucidated, although they share some features of neuropathic pain such as augmented sensory perception and altered central neurotransmission.

Pain Mechanisms

Pain results from activation of specialized peripheral receptors (*nociceptors*) by a noxious event (stimulus). These receptors respond to various external stimuli: *mechanical* (e.g., pressure, tumor growth, incision), *thermal* (e.g., hot or cold), or *chemical* (e.g., ischemia or infection). In addition to distinct nociceptors that respond to each type of stimulus, there are also *polymodal* nociceptors that respond to multiple stimulus modalities. Once a stimulus is detected, it is converted into an electrical nerve signal (*transduction*), which is conveyed along the axons of thinly myelinated (A delta) or unmyelinated (C) nerve fibers through specific pathways (*transmission*). *Modulation* generally refers to the attenuation of pain signals through intrinsic inhibitory activity within the peripheral and the central nervous systems before being perceived as an unpleasant sensation (*perception*), though in some cases pain signals may be amplified during this process. *Pathologic pain* is the result of injury- or disease-induced changes in the peripheral or central nervous systems leading to alterations in pain signaling. One important example of pathologic pain from injury to the nervous system is *peripheral sensitization*. This form of pain is characterized by the development of spontaneous ectopic activity in injured nerves and dorsal root ganglion cells as well as enhanced sensitivity to mechanical, thermal, or chemical stimuli.

Prolonged and repeated activation of nociceptive afferent fibers produces *central sensitization*, a state of increased sensitivity of central pain signaling neurons. Activation of N-methyl-D-aspartate (NMDA) receptors by glutamate is thought to be an important mechanism for central sensitization. Studies indicate that in addition to functional changes in neurons, microglia and astrocytes may also play an important role in the central sensitization process. Other central neuroplastic changes that may contribute to neuropathic pain states include deafferentation hyperactivity that may occur after spinal cord or avulsion injuries, loss of large-fiber inhibition, reorganization of central connections of primary afferent fibers, and excitatory descending modulatory mechanisms. Central and peripheral sensitization are considered to be the prime culprits responsible for pain induced by innocuous stimuli (*allodynia*) and increased pain to normally noxious stimuli (*hyperalgesia*)

TABLE 30-1 CLASSIFICATION AND PREVALENCE OF COMMON PAIN CONDITIONS

NEUROPATHIC		NOCICEPTIVE		MIXED
*Peripheral**	*Central*	*Somatic*	*Visceral*	
Peripheral neuropathy (1-3%)	Central post-stroke pain (8%)	Arthritis (25-40% in people > 40 years)	Endometriosis (10% in women of reproductive age)	Headache (15% for migraine, 20-30% for tension type)
Post-herpetic neuralgia (annual incidence 0.1-0.2%)	Spinal cord injury (30-50%)	Myofascial pain (5-10%)	Irritable bowel syndrome (5-15%)	Cancer[§] (lifetime prevalence 30-40%)
Chronic postsurgical pain (5-20% after surgery)	Multiple sclerosis (25%)	Fibromyalgia[†] (2-4%)	Interstitial cystitis (0.2-1% of women)	Low back pain[‖] (point prevalence 10-30%)
Phantom limb pain (30-60%)	Parkinson disease (10%)	Connective tissue disorders (0.2-0.5%)	Ulcers, gastritis, esophagitis (3-9%)	Neck pain[‖] (annual incidence 20-30%)
Trigeminal neuralgia (0.01%)	Seizure disorder (1-3%)	Burn pain[‡] (annual incidence of burns requiring hospitalization 0.01%)	Cholecystitis, appendicitis	Ischemic pain[¶]
Radiculopathy, spinal stenosis (3%-10%)				
Complex regional pain syndrome (0.03%, 3-20% after orthopedic surgery)				
Nerve entrapment syndromes (e.g., carpal tunnel, thoracic outlet, meralgia paresthetica; 2-4%)				

*Prevalence rates represent proportion of patients with condition who develop pain.
[†]Some cases may represent a variant of central pain.
[‡]Third-degree burns are often associated with neuropathic pain.
[§]Neuropathic pain occurs in 20 to 50% of cases and may be secondary to tumor invasion, surgery, chemotherapy, and radiation treatment.
[‖]Neuropathic pain may accompany nociceptive pain in 10 to 35% of cases.
[¶]Typically nociceptive, but long-standing pain may result in ischemic neuropathy.

that are commonly observed in neuropathic pain states. Studies have shown an important role for neurotrophins, prostaglandins, cytokines such as tumor necrosis factor-α and interleukins, and glial cells in the sensitization processes.[2]

Genetics

Chronic pain is a prototypical example of the interplay between genes and environment. Although tissue or nerve injury is necessary for the development of most pain syndromes, by itself it is not sufficient, as only a small percentage of injuries result in chronic pain. There are many ways in which one's genetic makeup can influence pain to include differences in pain sensitivity, susceptibility to disease, immunomodulatory response to injury, psychological predisposition to pain persistence, interactions between genotype differences and environment, and response to analgesic therapy. Not only genetics but also epigenetics can affect how painful stimuli are perceived.

Heritability is estimated to account for between 30% and 60% of the variance in pain response and has been demonstrated to play a role in acute pain perception and the transition from acute injury to chronic pain.[3] Even when the variability associated with gender and racial differences is taken into consideration (i.e., women and African Americans are more likely to report pain than are men and whites, respectively), genetics continues to play a major role in explaining pain differences. Heritable pain conditions may occur through either dominant or recessive gene transmission, and involve an assortment of different phenotypes.

Although rare, examples of monogenic (single-gene mutation) pain conditions include hereditary sensory and autonomic neuropathies, familial hemiplegic migraine, and neurologic channelopathies such as primary erythromelalgia, which involves a mutation at the gene encoding the voltage-gated sodium channel Nav 1.7. This latter mutation causes increased excitability and ongoing activity in afferent sensory neurons.

More common are those conditions associated with multiple gene abnormalities and incomplete penetrance, with about a dozen genes accounting for more than half of the identified gene candidates. In most cases, genes may promote a predisposition to pain, which requires a subsequent environmental inciting event (e.g., an injury in the context of depression) for manifestation.

Compared with other specialties, the study of the genetic basis for pain variability is still in its infancy, with most research revolving around conditions containing pain as a major symptom (e.g., endometriosis, osteoarthritis) rather than pain itself as an independent measure. In the future, the translational application of genetic studies may involve the suppression of pain-facilitating alleles, increasing the expression of pain-protective alleles, and targeted analgesic therapies.

DIAGNOSIS

History

Similar to the work-up of any symptom, the evaluation of pain begins with a thorough history. One of the primary tenets of pain assessment is that subjective complaints should always be taken seriously. There is no diagnostic test that can measure pain or even ascertain its existence. The most promising techniques involve functional brain imaging that reflects cerebral metabolism. These research tools have helped us understand that the brains of chronic pain patients are different from those of normal individuals and undergo morphologic alterations such as a diminution in gray matter in the areas involved in pain perception. Studies have confirmed that these deleterious changes are a consequence, not a cause, of chronic pain and may be reversed by effective treatment.[4]

A comprehensive history should include the location of pain and its quality, exacerbating and relieving factors, temporal aspects, associated symptoms and signs (e.g., numbness or weakness), interference with activities of daily living, and response to prior treatments. The temporal aspects of pain can provide valuable clues to etiology. Most cases of acute pain develop subsequent to a specific inciting event (e.g., surgery, trauma), whereas chronic pain conditions are usually more insidious in onset. Because acute pain tends to be self-limited and the relationship to a precipitant event is more tangible, it is generally better tolerated and associated with fewer psychological sequelae.

The severity of pain can be measured by a variety of different rating scales. Some of the more common instruments include categorical scales, verbal and numerical rating scales (0 to 10), and the visual analog scale, in which a 10-cm line is anchored on each side by two points designated "no pain" and "worst possible pain." Because there are subtle differences between different scales, repeated assessments of response to therapy are ideally gauged by the same instrument. For young children and mentally incapacitated patients, the use of age-appropriate substitute scales or facial expressions has been validated.

Recent guidelines from experts across multiple specialties have concluded that pain scores represent only one component of pain management. Other important aspects of treatment include assessments of functional capacity (e.g., Oswestry disability index for back pain), psychological and emotional functioning, satisfaction ratings, adverse treatment effects and disposition (i.e., work status). It is therefore imperative that realistic goals be established and individually tailored treatment regimens be developed to achieve these ends.

Distinguishing between neuropathic and nociceptive pain can have important treatment implications (Table 30-2). Neuropathic pain is characterized by positive and negative symptoms. Negative symptoms, such as a loss of sensation, are usually the result of axon or neuron loss, whereas positive

TABLE 30-2 CATEGORIZATION OF NEUROPATHIC AND NOCICEPTIVE PAIN

CLINICAL CHARACTERISTIC	NEUROPATHIC PAIN	NOCICEPTIVE PAIN
Etiology	Nerve injury or peripheral or central sensitization	Tissue or potential tissue damage
Descriptors	Lancinating, shooting, electrical-like, stabbing	Throbbing, aching, pressure-like
Sensory deficits	Frequent (e.g., numbness, tingling, pricking)	Infrequent and, if present, in nondermatomal or non-nerve distribution
Motor deficits	Neurologic weakness may be present if motor nerve affected	May have pain-induced weakness
Hypersensitivity	Pain frequently evoked with nonpainful (allodynia) or painful (exaggerated response) stimuli	Uncommon except for hypersensitivity in the immediate area of an acute injury
Character	Distal radiation common	Distal radiation less common; proximal radiation frequent
Paroxysms	Exacerbations common and unpredictable	Exacerbations less common and associated with activity
Autonomic signs	Color changes, temperature changes, swelling, or sudomotor (sweating) activity occurs in one third to one half of patients	Autonomic signs uncommon in chronic nociceptive pain

symptoms reflect abnormal excitability of the nervous system. Numbness, tingling, and other symptoms suggestive of sensory dysfunction are strongly indicative of neuropathic pain, especially when they occur in a dermatomal or nerve distribution. Descriptors such as "burning," "shooting" and "electrical" are more likely to be associated with neuropathic pain, whereas adjectives such as "throbbing" and "aching" tend to be identified with nociceptive pain states such as arthralgias. Other positive symptoms observed in neuropathic pain states include pain evoked by normally innocuous stimuli (allodynia), and an exaggerated or prolonged pain response to noxious stimuli (hyperalgesia, hyperpathia). Although neuropathic pain tends to be more intermittent than nociceptive pain, mechanical spinal pain is classically exacerbated by movement. As alluded to earlier, some conditions, such as cancer, may be characterized by aspects of both nociceptive and neuropathic pain. There are several patient-report instruments available that may help distinguish neuropathic from nociceptive pain (e.g., painDETECT, s-LANSS, and DN4),[5] although determination by the physician through history, examination, and diagnostic testing remains the reference standard.[6]

A thorough history should evaluate sleep patterns. In epidemiologic studies, more than 50% of chronic pain patients exhibit some form of sleep disturbance, and sleep abnormalities are nearly ubiquitous in some conditions such as fibromyalgia. It is well known that pain can interfere with sleep, but what is not as commonly appreciated is that sleep deprivation may enhance pain sensitivity by lowering nociceptive thresholds and reduce response to analgesic therapy. Evidence also exists for a relationship between poor sleep and the development of chronic pain after an acute event. Although there is some evidence that improved sleep may lessen chronic pain, these studies are mostly correlational.

The proper evaluation of the patient in pain must include a psychosocial history. Between one half and two thirds of chronic pain patients exhibit varying degrees of psychopathology, with depression being the most common comorbidity, followed by anxiety disorders, somatoform disorders, and substance abuse. Many of these coexisting psychological conditions have been associated with poor treatment prognosis. People seeking chronic pain care may also be more likely to carry a concomitant axis II diagnosis (i.e., personality disorder), which can act as an additional barrier to effective treatment. Potential social factors that can have a negative impact on treatment should be identified, including low job satisfaction and secondary gain. A focused psychosocial history that includes prior psychiatric diagnoses, suicidal ideation, work history, legal history, and substance abuse is therefore essential in the formulation of a treatment plan.

Physical Examination

Examination of the patient in pain should encompass all body systems because pain is a frequent manifestation of systemic disease. A physical examination finding by itself is almost never pathognomonic but usually functions to confirm suspicions garnered from the history and to select patients for imaging studies or invasive diagnostic testing. Unlike acute pain, chronic pain is usually not associated with autonomic activation resulting in altered vital signs or facial grimacing.[7] Sensory symptoms can precede other neurologic findings by months or weeks. The most common forms of neuropathy are associated with sensory deficits in a glove-stocking distribution, but other patterns occur as well (Chapter 420). Numbness in the distribution of a nerve root or single nerve strongly suggests neuropathic pain, but nondermatomal sensory changes can accompany nociceptive pain (e.g., fibromyalgia) as well. Allodynia and hyperalgesia are hallmarks of neuropathic pain. Postural and gait abnormalities may be either causative factors for rheumatologic conditions (e.g., bursitis) or consequences of the underlying condition.

A careful evaluation of passive and active range of motion is useful because generalized and regional pain complaints are often accompanied by deconditioning. Distinctions should be drawn between pain-induced and neurologic weakness, with the latter often occurring in conjunction with muscle atrophy or asymmetry in reflexes. Sometimes reflex assessment is the only way to distinguish between a true neurologic condition and nonorganic causes.

Diagnostic Tests

Imaging has largely supplanted history and physical examination as the "gold standard" for diagnosis of disease but is not without drawbacks. There is a poor correlation between findings on magnetic resonance imaging (MRI) and the intensity of spinal pain, with more than 50% of asymptomatic individuals having abnormalities on lumbar, thoracic, and cervical films. Systematic reviews have found that early imaging for back pain does not improve outcomes or affect decision making and should be reserved for those patients with indications of a serious underlying condition.[A1] Absolute indications for MRI in patients with back pain are serious or progressive neurologic deficits, new-onset bowel and bladder dysfunction, suspected metastatic disease or infection, and referral of patients for procedural interventions. Yet, some have even questioned the utility of imaging as a prognostic tool before procedures. In a randomized trial evaluating whether MRI improved treatment outcomes in patients with sciatica who were referred for epidural steroid injections, preprocedure MRI was not shown to improve outcomes and only infrequently altered decision making.[A2] For back pain, the presence of "red flags" suggestive of more serious disease (e.g., trauma history, infection, history of intravenous drug abuse) should also alert the practitioner to seek further evaluation. For nonspinal pain conditions, MRI is ideal for discerning inflammation and soft tissue disease, whereas computed tomography scanning may be better for detecting bleeding and bone disease. The main advantage of ultrasound is that it is inexpensive and not associated with radiation. For chronic pain disorders, such as primary headaches and chronic abdominal or pelvic pain, imaging should be reserved for the evaluation of acute processes or a significant change in symptoms.

Electromyography and nerve conduction studies (Chapter 420) can be used to diagnose injury to large nerve fibers. However, because these studies are associated with significant false-negative and false-positive rates and are not sensitive in detecting impairment of small-fiber function, normal findings on a neurophysiologic study do not rule out neuropathic pain. For small-fiber neuropathies, a skin biopsy demonstrating decreased density of epidermal nerve fibers is a sensitive test.

TREATMENT

The goals of treatment should include elucidating the cause of pain and alleviating suffering. The biopsychosocial model posits that biologic, psychological, and social factors all play a role in chronic pain and should be addressed. Consequently, the goal of pain treatment should not be limited to pain reduction but also encompass improving function, psychological comorbidities, sleep, and social interaction. It has been argued that treatment should be mechanism based rather than etiology based, but at present, simple clinical tools to correlate symptoms and signs with mechanisms are lacking. The future development of diagnostic methods to identify mechanisms (e.g., intravenous

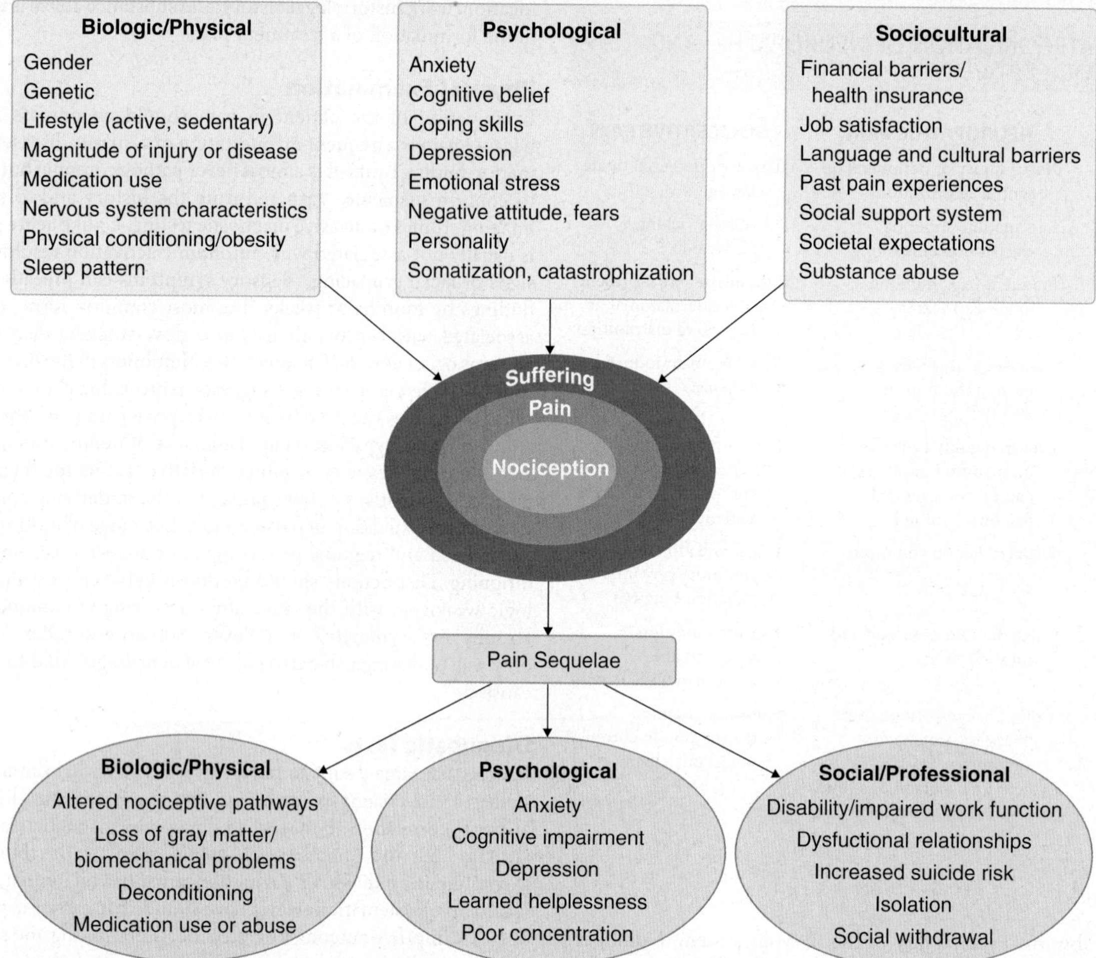

FIGURE 30-1. Schematic drawing of the biopsychosocial model of pain.

infusion tests) may help develop novel target-specific pharmacologic agents (Fig. 30-1).

Pain is a complex perceptual experience affected by a multitude of factors that include not only activation of nociceptors but also emotions, memory and cognition, social and cultural context, and expectations. Therefore, despite a paucity of studies evaluating a multidisciplinary approach to pain management, a strong consensus exists that this approach is beneficial.

Pharmacologic Therapies

Antipyretic Analgesics

Aspirin (Chapter 37) is the most widely used analgesic in the world. Along with its pharmacologic cousins nonsteroidal anti-inflammatory drugs (NSAIDs) and the antipyretic drugs acetaminophen and phenacetin, this group forms the backbone of pharmacologic pain treatment. Antipyretic analgesics exert their antinociceptive effects by the inhibition of cyclooxygenase, the rate-limiting enzyme in the production of prostaglandins, which sensitize nociceptors and regulate inflammation. There are several pharmacologic distinctions between NSAIDs and their counterparts, phenazone and acetaminophen. Whereas NSAIDs act both centrally and peripherally, making them effective topical agents for nociceptive inflammatory conditions, the primary site of enzyme inhibition for acetaminophen is in the central nervous system. Acetaminophen is also a weaker analgesic than NSAIDs and is largely devoid of anti-inflammatory effects.

The main drawback of nonopioid antipyretic analgesics is their ceiling effect, which can render them ineffective as stand-alone agents for severe pain. For cancer pain, the World Health Organization treatment paradigm advocates adding opioids to an analgesic regimen uncontrolled by NSAIDs, not replacing them. NSAIDs may act synergistically with opioids and have proven opioid-sparing effects. It is well acknowledged that aspirin, NSAIDs, and acetaminophen are more effective in treating nociceptive than neuropathic pain, although many neuropathic pain sufferers regularly take NSAIDs.

A major concern about nonopioid antipyretic agents is side effects. For NSAIDs, these include bleeding, gastrointestinal ulceration, renal toxicity, and increased risk of cardiovascular events (Chapter 37). Although the use of cyclooxygenase 2–selective inhibitors, such as celecoxib, or the addition of protein pump inhibitors to conventional NSAIDs may attenuate the risk of bleeding and ulcers, they do not affect the incidence of adverse renal or cardiovascular events. These risks are significantly increased in the elderly, in patients with multiple comorbidities, and with polypharmacy. In view of their considerable risks, NSAIDs should be prescribed in the lowest dose possible, for the shortest duration of time, and with periodic surveillance. Because it possesses a more favorable safety profile, acetaminophen is often considered a first-line therapy before NSAIDs, even for pain conditions associated with inflammation. Topical NSAIDs (e.g., diclofenac) have also been shown in randomized controlled studies to be beneficial for the treatment of rheumatologic disorders and have been touted as having comparable efficacy for regional pain conditions but with fewer adverse effects than systemic NSAIDs.[A3]

Adjuvant Analgesics

Multiple evidence-based guidelines for the treatment of chronic pain states, particularly neuropathic pain, have been published (Table 30-3). In general, these suggest that antidepressants and anticonvulsants should be the two first-line classes of medications for chronic neuropathic pain.[8,9] Depending on the particular drug and condition, these medications have been demonstrated to provide significant pain relief in carefully selected patients beyond that observed with placebo in 10 to 40% of ideal pharmacologic candidates. Whereas opioids have shown similar efficacy for neuropathic pain, anticonvulsants and antidepressants carry a lower risk of serious adverse events and long-term tolerance, rendering them preferable for long-standing noncancer pain (Table 30-4). In terms of efficacy, tricyclic antidepressants (TCAs) are superior to serotonin-norepinephrine reuptake inhibitors, which in turn are more efficacious than serotonin-specific reuptake inhibitors. However, because of their more favorable side effect profile, serotonin-norepinephrine reuptake inhibitors may be more effective than TCAs in some patients. Among the various TCAs, amitriptyline is the most studied but is probably comparable in efficacy to its metabolite nortriptyline and cousin imipramine. However, the last two drugs' more favorable side effect profiles (e.g., less sedation and anticholinergic activity) make them the preferred choices for neuropathic pain. In patients who cannot tolerate TCAs, serotonin-norepinephrine reuptake inhibitors such as duloxetine can be beneficial.[A4] In addition to neuropathic pain, antidepressants have also been shown to be effective in headache prophylaxis, abdominal and pelvic pain, fibromyalgia, and musculoskeletal pain.[A5]

Anticonvulsants are effective for neuropathic pain by virtue of their membrane-stabilizing properties. Although anticonvulsant drugs may be

TABLE 30-3 GUIDELINES FOR PHARMACOLOGIC TREATMENT OF CHRONIC NEUROPATHIC PAIN

NeuPSIG (IASP, 2010)*,[10]	CANADIAN PAIN SOCIETY (2007)*,[11]	EFNS (2010)[8]
First Line† TCA (nortriptyline, desipramine) Gabapentin Pregabalin Duloxetine Venlafaxine Topical 5% lidocaine	**First Line** TCA: amitriptyline, nortriptyline, imipramine, desipramine Anticonvulsants: gabapentin, pregabalin Carbamazepine for tic douloureux (idiopathic trigeminal neuralgia)	**DIABETIC NEUROPATHIC PAIN** **First Line** Duloxetine Gabapentin Pregabalin TCA Venlafaxine ER **Second or Third Line** Opioids Tramadol
Second Line Opioids Tramadol	**Second Line** SNRI: Duloxetine, venlafaxine Topical lidocaine 5%	**POST-HERPETIC NEURALGIA** **First Line** Gabapentin Pregabalin TCA Lidocaine plasters **Second or Third Line** Capsaicin Opioids
Third Line Antiepileptics Mexiletine Memantine Antidepressants Dextromethorphan Topical capsaicin	**Third Line** Tramadol Opioid analgesics	**TRIGEMINAL NEURALGIA** **First Line** Carbamazepine Oxcarbazepine **Second or Third Line** Surgery
	Fourth Line Cannabinoids Methadone SSRI: citalopram, paroxetine Other anticonvulsants: lamotrigine, topiramate, valproic acid Miscellaneous agents: mexiletine, clonidine	**CENTRAL PAIN** **First Line** Gabapentin Pregabalin TCA **Second or Third Line** Cannabinoids (multiple sclerosis) Lamotrigine Opioids Tramadol (spinal cord injury)

*Guidelines not disease specific, but for neuropathic pain in general.
†Consider lower starting dosages and slower titration in geriatric patients.
EFNS = European Federation of Neurological Societies; ER = extended release; NeuPSIG (IASP) = Neuropathic Pain Special Interest Group of the International Association for the Study of Pain; SNRI = serotonin norepinephrine reuptake inhibitors; SSRI = selective serotonin reuptake inhibitors; TCA = tricyclic antidepressant.

better than antidepressants for prototypical "lancinating-type" neuropathic pain, antidepressants are more versatile in that they have proven benefit in myriad other pain conditions. Owing to their high efficacy and favorable side effect profiles, gabapentin and pregabalin are first-line agents for most forms of neuropathic pain.[A6] In addition to independent pain-relieving properties, randomized controlled trials suggest that these drugs may act synergistically with opioids and antidepressants,[A7] provide anxiolysis, and exhibit preemptive analgesic effects when administered before surgery.[A8]

When gabapentinoid drugs are ineffective or intolerable, alternative anticonvulsants that act by different cellular mechanisms, such as lamotrigine and oxcarbazepine, may be employed. For trigeminal neuralgia, carbamazepine remains the treatment of choice, although adverse effects, such as the risk of agranulocytosis, limit its utility for other conditions. Other classes of adjuvants that may be effective in certain contexts include topical creams (e.g., capsaicin), *N*-methyl-D-aspartate antagonists (e.g., dextromethorphan), skeletal muscle relaxants (e.g., baclofen), cannabinoids, and antiarrhythmics (mexiletine). Topical lidocaine patches have been shown to reduce pain and allodynia in patients with post-herpetic neuralgia, and anecdotal evidence has suggested that they may be useful in the treatment of certain types of back pain. A high-concentration (8%) topical patch of capsaicin (the pungent chemical in chili pepper) has been demonstrated in clinical trials to provide significant pain relief compared with placebo for post-herpetic neuralgia and HIV neuropathy.[A9] A single 1-hour application can result in attenuation of pain for up to 12 weeks.

Opioid Analgesics

Opioid analgesics are the cornerstone of treatment for cancer pain (Table 30-5). Although randomized studies have found that opioids are effective in noncancer pain conditions, several reviews[12,13] and guidelines[A10] have concluded that they provide long-term improvement in only a minority of individuals, and that their superiority to other analgesics and ability to improve function are limited or inconclusive. Maximizing the therapeutic effects of opioid analgesics requires careful attention to balancing the beneficial effects with the undesirable adverse effects, including addiction. Understanding the clinical pharmacology of opioids, including their relative potency, duration of action, bioavailability, and pharmacokinetics, is essential for rational use. Their use for chronic pain management is limited primarily by myriad side effects that include nausea, constipation, sedation, itch, respiratory depression, and endocrine deficiency leading to sexual dysfunction and accelerated osteoporosis. Aggressive management with stool softeners and agents that enhance bowel motility, such as docusate and senna, can minimize constipation. Whereas most opioids are devoid of end-organ toxicity, an exception is meperidine. A metabolite, normeperidine, can accumulate after several days of treatment, causing myoclonus and anxiety; at higher concentrations, confusion, delirium, and seizures can ensue. Opioids that are predominantly renally eliminated, such as morphine, should be used with caution in patients with renal dysfunction. Two metabolites of morphine, morphine-6-glucuronide, which contains analgesic properties, and morphine-3-glucuronide, which may amplify pain in certain contexts, can accumulate in patients with renal dysfunction and contribute to the adverse effects of morphine. Alternative drugs include fentanyl and methadone.

For treatment of acute pain or an exacerbation of chronic pain in hospitalized patients (e.g., sickle cell crisis), patient-controlled analgesia (PCA) provides a convenient means of administering opioids. Intravenous morphine, fentanyl, or hydromorphone is commonly administered with an infusion device wherein a basal infusion, bolus dose, lockout interval, and maximum dose per hour can be programmed. PCA devices are safe and allow patients to control their pain management with less dependence on health care providers. Studies comparing PCA with conventional administration of opioids have generally found PCAs to be associated with better pain relief and higher satisfaction rates, albeit with larger amounts of medication consumed.

Critical steps in managing chronic pain patients with opioids include appropriate evaluation, clear and detailed documentation, a function-based treatment plan with well-defined patient goals that include an exit strategy, a written patient-physician agreement that includes informed consent and patient education, periodic review that focuses on progress toward functional goals, and specialist referrals in managing difficult patients. When considering a trial with opioids, health care providers need to consider the disease process, to assess traits such as compliance and responsibility, to perform risk stratification, and to monitor for predefined treatment goals and aberrant drug-related behaviors (Fig. 30-2).

The long-term use of opioids can be associated with tolerance and physical dependence. Cross-tolerance among opioids is not complete, and a strategy often used when tolerance is suspected is rotation to an alternative opioid, which may result in a 30 to 50% reduction in equianalgesic dose. Rates of addiction (Chapters 31 and 34) in reported studies vary widely, from less than 5% to 50%, which reflects differences in populations studied, definitions, and surveillance methods. A synthesis of evidence suggests that among chronic pain patients receiving opioid therapy, up to 40% will exhibit aberrant drug-related behaviors, 20% will abuse their drugs, and around 10% may become addicted.

Tramadol and tapentadol represent a newer class of analgesic drugs that have a dual mechanism of action. Tramadol is a weak agonist that inhibits the reuptake of norepinephrine and serotonin. Along with the usual side effects associated with opioids, seizures have been reported with tramadol, and adverse drug interactions can occur in patients taking coumadin and selective serotonin reuptake inhibitors. Tapentadol also has a dual mode of action as a μ-opioid agonist and a norepinephrine reuptake inhibitor and is slightly stronger than tramadol. Tramadol is presently approved for moderate to moderately severe severe pain. Tapentadol is approved for moderate to severe acute pain, while its extended-release formulation is approved for moderate to severe chronic pain and diabetic neuropathy.

Butorphanol, nalbuphine, and pentazocine are opioid agonist-antagonist drugs that can antagonize the actions of μ-opioid agonists and cause psychotomimetic effects due to their actions on the κ-opioid receptor. These drugs should be used with caution, particularly in patients receiving other μ-opioid agonists as they may precipitate withdrawal or reduce the effectiveness of pure opioid agonists. Buprenorphine, a partial agonist at the μ-opioid receptor and an antagonist at other opioid receptors, is available in various formulations, including a once per week transdermal patch for pain, and in combination with naloxone for the treatment of opioid addiction.

Combination Therapies

Most clinical trials have studied individual drugs in specific chronic pain states. Because no drug is universally effective and most provide only partial

TABLE 30-4 ADJUVANT ANALGESIC DRUGS FOR CHRONIC PAIN

DRUG	DOSAGE	INDICATIONS	ADVERSE EFFECTS	COMMENTS
TRICYCLIC ANTIDEPRESSANTS				
Amitriptyline, imipramine, desipramine, nortriptyline	10-150 mg/day	Peripheral neuropathy, post-herpetic neuralgia, other types of peripheral neuropathic pain, central pain, facial pain, fibromyalgia, headache prophylaxis, irritable bowel syndrome, and chronic low back pain with or without radiculopathy	Sedation, dry mouth, confusion, weight gain, constipation, urinary retention, ataxia, cardiac conduction delay (QTc prolongation)	First-line agents for neuropathic pain and headache prophylaxis Secondary amine drugs (e.g., nortriptyline) have fewer side effects than tertiary amines (e.g., amitriptyline) Contraindicated in glaucoma
SEROTONIN-NOREPINEPHRINE REUPTAKE INHIBITORS				
Venlafaxine	75-225 mg/day	Peripheral neuropathy, headache prophylaxis	Sedation, dry mouth, constipation, ataxia, hypertension, hyperhidrosis	Dose adjustment in patients with renal dysfunction
Duloxetine	60-120 mg/day	Peripheral neuropathy, fibromyalgia	Sedation, dry mouth, constipation, hyperhidrosis	U.S. Food and Drug Administration (FDA) approved for fibromyalgia and diabetic neuropathy Contraindicated in glaucoma
ANTICONVULSANTS				
Gabapentin	600-3600 mg/day	Peripheral neuropathy, post-herpetic neuralgia, other types of peripheral neuropathic pain, central pain, pelvic pain, headache prophylaxis, radiculopathy, chronic postsurgical pain	Sedation, weight gain, dry mouth, ataxia, edema	First-line agent for neuropathic pain FDA approved for post-herpetic neuralgia Effective preemptively for postoperative pain
Pregabalin	150-600 mg/day	Peripheral neuropathy, post-herpetic neuralgia, central pain, fibromyalgia	Sedation, weight gain, dry mouth, ataxia, edema	First-line agent for neuropathic pain FDA approved for diabetic neuropathy, post-herpetic neuralgia. and fibromyalgia Effective preemptively for postoperative pain. Same mechanism of action as gabapentin
Carbamazepine	200-1600 mg/day	Facial neuralgias, diabetic neuropathy	Sedation, ataxia, diplopia, hyponatremia, agranulocytosis, diarrhea, aplastic anemia, hepatotoxicity, Stevens-Johnson syndrome	First-line agent and FDA approved for trigeminal & glossopharyngeal neuralgia Contraindicated in patients with porphyria and atrioventricular conduction block
Topiramate	50-400 mg/day	Headache prophylaxis, chronic low back pain with or without radiculopathy	Sedation, ataxia, diplopia, weight loss, diarrhea, metabolic acidosis, kidney stones	First-line agent and FDA approved for migraine prophylaxis Often used as appetite suppressant
CORTICOSTEROIDS (SYSTEMIC)				
	5-60 mg/day (prednisone)	Inflammatory arthritis, other inflammatory pain conditions (e.g., inflammatory bowel disease), traumatic nerve injury, complex regional pain syndrome	Myriad psychiatric, gastrointestinal, neurologic, and cardiac side effects; immunosuppression, weakness, edema, weight gain, elevated glucose, poor wound healing, others	Stronger evidence supports local (i.e., injection) administration More effective for acute pain Strong anti-inflammatory effects
MISCELLANEOUS				
Muscle relaxants	Variable, depending on drug	Skeletal muscle spasm, acute spinal pain, temporomandibular disorder Baclofen effective for spasticity, dystonia, and trigeminal neuralgia	Sedation, ataxia, blurred vision, confusion, asthenia, xerostomia and other gastrointestinal effects, palpitations	First-line agents for acute back pain and skeletal muscle spasm
Lidocaine patch	1-3 patches every 12 hours	Post-herpetic neuropathy, peripheral neuropathy, other types of neuropathic and possibly myofascial pain associated with allodynia	Minimal systemic side effects when applied appropriately	Second-line agent and FDA approved for post-herpetic neuralgia
Capsaicin cream	0.025% applied 3 or 4 times per day	Post-herpetic neuralgia, peripheral neuropathy and other types of neuropathic pain, chronic postsurgical pain, arthritis and other musculoskeletal conditions	Burning on application Minimal systemic side effects when applied appropriately	FDA approved for arthritis Second-line agent for post-herpetic neuralgia and third-line agent for peripheral neuropathy
Cannabinoids	Variable, depending on drug and delivery route	Strongest evidence is for multiple sclerosis May be effective for peripheral neuropathy and other types of neuropathic pain and spasticity	Myriad psychiatric, neurologic and cardiac effects; xerostomia, abdominal pain, and other gastrointestinal effects	Fourth-line agent with narrow therapeutic index Modest analgesic effect comparable to codeine

pain relief, in clinical practice, two or more drugs are often used in combination. The rational use of polypharmacy should include drugs that act at different sites in the pain signaling process or modulate different neurotransmitter systems and ideally have antagonistic adverse effects (e.g., sedation and stimulation) (Fig. 30-3). For gabapentinoids, controlled trials suggest that combination therapy with either opioids or TCAs may be more effective than either drug alone.[A11][A12] For antidepressants, controlled studies have failed to establish a benefit for combination therapy with opioids. In a placebo-controlled crossover study performed in a population with chronic low back pain, treatment with pregabalin and celecoxib was found to be superior to monotherapy.[A13]

Psychological Treatment

The relationship between pain and psychopathology is complex. The lifetime prevalence of coexisting psychiatric illness in chronic pain patients

TABLE 30-5 FORMULATIONS, DOSAGES, AND PHARMACOLOGIC INFORMATION ON COMMONLY PRESCRIBED OPIOIDS

DRUG	EQUIANALGESIC DOSAGE (ORAL UNLESS SPECIFIED)	READILY AVAILABLE ROUTES OF ADMINISTRATION	DURATION OF ACTION	COMMENTS
PURE OPIOID AGONISTS				
Morphine	30 mg	IV, IM, PO, PR SR formulation	3-6 hr for short-acting 8-12 hr for SR	Reference standard for all opioids Renally excreted active metabolite
Oxycodone	20 mg	PO, PR SR formulation	3-6 hr for short-acting 8-12 hr for SR	Widely available in combination form with nonopioid analgesics Greater euphoric effects than morphine Both IR and SR forms popular among recreational users
Hydromorphone	3-6 mg	PO, PR, IV, IM SR formulation	3-6 hr 18-24 hr for SR	Higher PO : IV conversion ratio than other opioids SR form reserved for opioid-tolerant patients, and contraindicated in patients with recent monoamine oxidase inhibitor use
Hydrocodone	30-60 mg	PO SR formulation under development	3-6 hr 8-12 hr for SR	Wide variation in morphine-equivalent dose Most commonly prescribed opioid in the United States; typically used in combination form with nonopioid analgesic acetaminophen Formulations containing <15 mg hydrocodone are schedule III in the United States SR form being tested with and without acetaminophen
Oxymorphone	10mg	PO, IV, IM, Pr; SR formulation	4-8 hr, 12 hr for SR	Co-ingestion of alcohol with SR formulation can lead to "dose-dumping", or very high plasma levels and overdose. Very low (10%) oral bioavailability. Longer duration of action than morphine or oxycodone.
Methadone	2-20 mg	PO, PR, IV	6-12 hr for pain	Morphine:methadone conversion varies according to dose and length of opioid use, ranging from 2 : 1 to >20 : 1 in patients receiving very high doses Any physician with a schedule II DEA license may prescribe for pain May take 5-7 days to reach steady state because of extended half-life (i.e., accumulation) Electrocardiographic monitoring recommended with higher doses Other properties, such as NMDA receptor antagonism and reuptake inhibition of serotonin and norepinephrine, may slow the development of tolerance and increase efficacy for neuropathic pain
Fentanyl	12.5 μg/hr (TD) 800-1000 μg (TM) 200-400 μg (B)	TD, TM, B	72 hr for TD 1.5-3 hr for TM and B	TD, TM, and B formulations may be useful in patients with poor bowel function TD: Wide variation in conversion ratios; delivery system may be associated with fewer gastrointestinal side effects TM and B: delivery systems associated with more rapid (10 min) onset than IR oral opioids U.S. Food and Drug Administration approved for breakthrough cancer pain in opioid-tolerant patients
Codeine	200 mg	PO, PR, IM SR codeine combination products available as cough suppressant	3-6 hr 12 hr for SR	Often used in combination with nonopioid analgesics Efficacy and side effects may be affected by rate of metabolism to active metabolite morphine, which varies significantly Popular as cough suppressant
Propoxyphene	200 mg	PO, PR	3-6 hr	Wide variation in morphine-equivalent dose Often used in combination form with nonopioid analgesic Toxic metabolite may accumulate with excessive use, especially in elderly Weak antagonist at NMDA receptor
Meperidine	300 mg	PO, PR, IM, IV	2-4 hr	Toxic metabolite may accumulate with excessive use, especially in patients with renal insufficiency Associated with tachycardia and hypertension Concurrent use with monoamine oxidase inhibitors may result in fatal reactions May cause more "euphoria" than other opioids IM absorption erratic and injections painful
AGONIST-ANTAGONISTS, PARTIAL AGONISTS				
Buprenorphine Buprenorphine/Naloxone (Suboxone) (4 : 1 ratio of buprenorphine to naloxone)	0.3-24 mg SL 5-70 μg/hr (TD) 2-24 mg/day	SL, PR, IV, TD	6-8 hr 7 days for SR	Partial μ-agonist and κ-antagonist that may precipitate withdrawal in opioid-dependent patients receiving high doses Lower abuse potential and fewer psychomimetic effects than pure agonists Not readily reversed by naloxone Schedule III drug in the United States Primary use of SL preparation is to treat addiction Used in combination with naloxone (Suboxone, Subutex) for opioid dependence May prolong QT interval
Butorphanol	1 mg/ spray, repeat after 60-90 minutes (NS) 1-2 mg (IV or IM)	NS, IM, IV, PO	3-4 hr	Partial agonist and antagonist at μ-receptor and antagonist at κ-receptor Commonly used as nasal spray to treat migraine headache and less commonly for labor pain Significant abuse potential
Nalbuphine	1 : 1 parenteral ratio	SC, IM, IV	3-6 hr	Mixed agonist-antagonist, often used for labor and delivery Sometimes used to treat refractory opioid-induced pruritus
Levorphanol	4 mg	PO, IM, IV	4-8 hr	2 : 1 oral to IV conversion ratio Multiple mechanisms of action including inhibition of serotonin and norepinephrine reuptake, NDMA receptor antagonism, and σ-receptor agonism

TABLE 30-5 FORMULATIONS, DOSAGES, AND PHARMACOLOGIC INFORMATION ON COMMONLY PRESCRIBED OPIOIDS—cont'd

DRUG	EQUIANALGESIC DOSAGE (ORAL UNLESS SPECIFIED)	READILY AVAILABLE ROUTES OF ADMINISTRATION	DURATION OF ACTION	COMMENTS
Pentazocine Pentazocine/naloxone (Talwin) (100 : 1 ratio of pentazocine to naloxone)	90 mg	PO, SC, IM, IV	3-4 hr parenteral 8 hr PO	Mixed agonist-antagonist Naloxone added in 1970s to prevent abuse Also prescribed in preparation with acetaminophen
WEAK, DUAL-ACTION OPIOID AGONISTS				
Tramadol	150-300 mg	PO	4-6 hr 24 hr for SR	Dual action involves inhibition of serotonin and norepinephrine reuptake Affinity for μ-opioid receptor 6000× less than morphine Reduced side effects compared with morphine Analogue of codeine with active metabolite in which differences in metabolism may affect analgesia and side effects Available in combination form with acetaminophen Avoid concomitant use of serotonergic drugs Maximum recommended dose of 400 mg/day Not a federally controlled substance in the United States, although certain states have classified it as schedule IV
Tapentadol	75-110 mg	PO	4-6 hr 12 hr for SR	Dual action involves inhibition of norepinephrine reuptake May have fewer of certain side effects than morphine, such as gastrointestinal and respiratory depression Maximum dose 600 mg/day Avoid concurrent use of monoamine oxidase inhibitors

B = buccal; IM = intramuscular; IR = immediate release; IV = intravenous; NMDA = *N*-methyl-D-aspartate; NS = nasal spray; PO = oral; PR = rectal; SL = sublingual; SR = sustained release; TD = transdermal; TM = transmucosal.

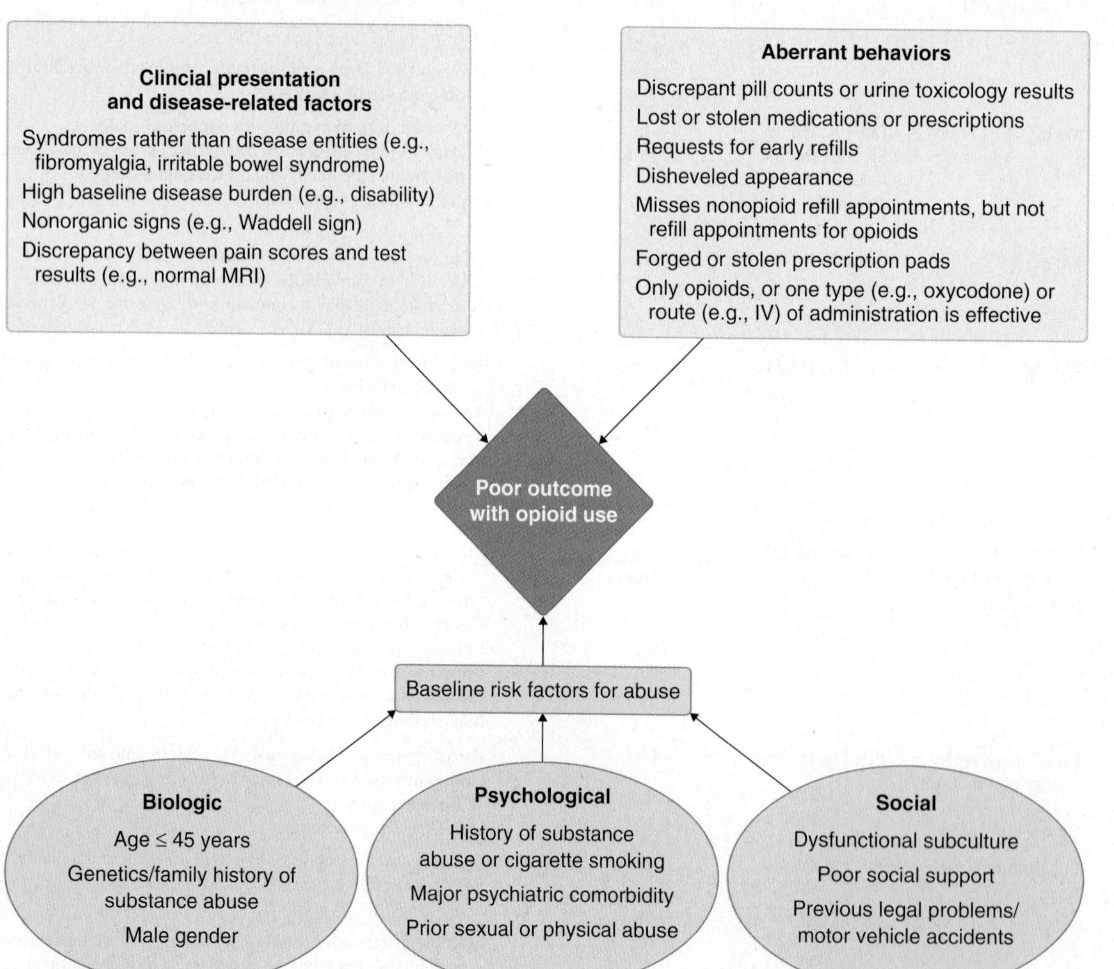

FIGURE 30-2. Factors associated with opioid abuse and treatment failure. IV = intravenous; MRI = magnetic resonance imaging.

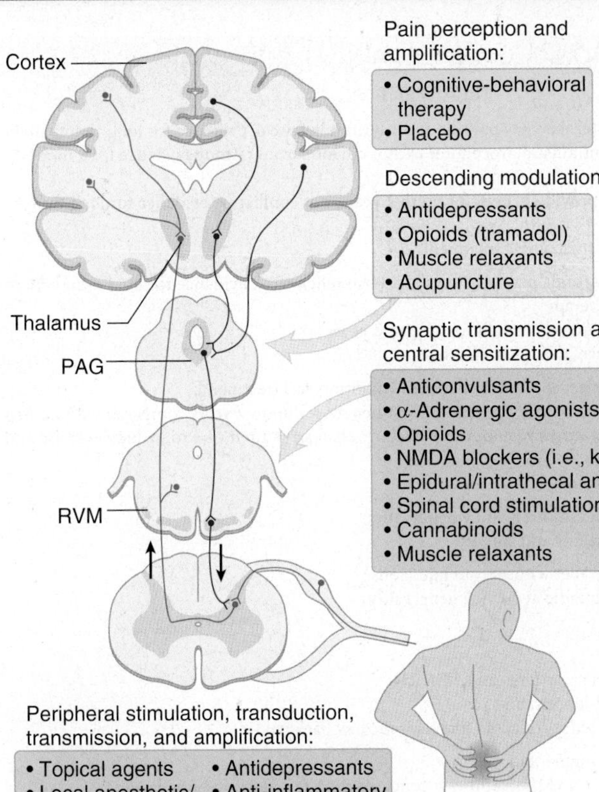

FIGURE 30-3. Rational choice of combination therapies for pain should be based on the mechanisms of drug actions. Combining drugs with disparate actions can have additive or synergistic analgesic effects and minimize adverse effects. NMDA = *N*-Methyl-D-aspartate; PAG = periaqueductal gray; RVM = rostral ventromedial medulla.

TABLE 30-6 PSYCHOSOCIAL FACTORS ASSOCIATED WITH CHRONIC PAIN

Multiple pain complaints
Poor job satisfaction, low pay
Inadequate coping skills
Fear-avoidance behavior
Manual labor, physically stressful job
Obesity
Somatization
Smoking
Low baseline activity levels
Ongoing litigation
Older age
Low education level
Higher presenting pain intensity, disability
Neurological symptoms
Anxiety
Depressed mood
Emotional distress

ranges from 50% to more than 80%. Between 30% and 60% of chronic pain sufferers experience symptoms of depression, making it the most common comorbidity. For anxiety disorders and substance abuse, co-prevalence rates are around 30% and 10 to 15%, respectively.

Viewed from a different perspective, the relationship is even more striking. More than 60% of patients with major depression and more than half of all patients with anxiety and substance abuse disorders experience chronic pain. Although it is widely acknowledged that chronic pain can predispose patients to depression, anxiety, and self-destructive behaviors such as substance abuse and suicide, what is less commonly appreciated is the effect that preexisting psychiatric conditions have on pain perception. There is a plethora of literature demonstrating that coexisting psychopathology is a strong predictor for the development of chronic pain after an acute, traumatic event (e.g., back pain episode, surgery) and is associated with poorer treatment outcomes.

It is incumbent on practitioners to screen all pain patients for psychological conditions that can adversely affect treatment (Table 30-6). Not only major psychiatric conditions, such as depression and generalized anxiety, but also maladaptive behaviors and secondary diagnoses, such as somatization disorder and poor coping skills, can negatively influence treatment.

Relaxation techniques such as biofeedback, self-hypnosis, and guided imagery have proved effective in a wide array of acute and chronic pain conditions but may be especially useful in those with high levels of anxiety. Cognitive-behavioral therapy is a highly structured form of psychotherapy predicated on the replacement of negative thought patterns and behaviors with more constructive ones. These therapies enhance modulation of pain signals and can also be effective for commonly associated symptoms such as fatigue and sleep abnormalities. Ideal candidates include educated, motivated patients in whom distorted thinking (e.g., catastrophization) and counterproductive behaviors serve to amplify pain behavior. In patients with personality disorders and ingrained maladaptive behaviors, long-term psychotherapy may be necessary.

Interventional Therapies: Nerve Blocks, Neuromodulation, and Surgery

Nerve Blocks

Injections may be performed for therapeutic, diagnostic, and sometimes prognostic purposes. Mechanistically, injections performed with local anesthetic may work by releasing entrapped nerves, enhancing blood flow, and interrupting processes involved in central sensitization (i.e., "breaking the cycle of pain"). Additional benefits of adding corticosteroid to local anesthetic include blocking the inflammatory cascade, suppressing ectopic discharges from injured nerves, and inhibiting the synthesis of prostaglandins, some of which serve to sensitize nociceptors.

Nerve blocks are almost never a panacea for noncancer pain but in appropriate candidates may provide intermediate-term pain relief, facilitate rehabilitative therapy, and improve quality of life for several weeks to months. Translating this relief into long-term improvement necessitates addressing the underlying causes and predisposing factors, which often entails psychotherapy and rehabilitation. Injections that can afford benefit in well-selected individuals include trigger point injections with local anesthetic for myofascial pain, intra-articular injection of steroids or viscosupplementation for chronic osteoarthritis, and nerve blocks with corticosteroid for entrapment syndromes (e.g., carpal tunnel syndrome). Among spinal injections, the strongest evidence is for epidural steroid injections in patients with radicular pain less than 6 months in duration, and radiofrequency denervation for facet joint pain. Neuroablative procedures such as celiac plexus neurolysis have been shown to provide significant pain relief lasting several months in patients with pain associated with upper abdominal cancers.

Electrical Stimulation

Electrical stimulation in various forms has been used for millennia to treat pain. The most commonly used type of electrical stimulation is transcutaneous electrical nerve stimulations (TENS), in which an electrical current is used to stimulate nerves for therapeutic purposes. The evidence supporting TENS to treat chronic pain is mixed, with one of the main criticisms being that any benefit is short-lasting. Spinal cord stimulation is a minimally invasive neuromodulatory technique for managing neuropathic pain states refractory to conservative measures in which an electrode(s) is inserted into the epidural space to stimulate the dorsal column. It was developed based on the gate-control theory, which postulates that activation of peripheral sensory A-fibers can attenuate pain signaling by slower-conducting pain C-fibers. Common indications include failed back surgery syndrome, complex regional pain syndrome, and outside of the United States, ischemic pain associated with peripheral vascular disease or angina. In patients with intractable chronic pain unresponsive to conservative measures, brain stimulation techniques have also shown promise. Deep brain stimulation has been demonstrated in uncontrolled studies to provide benefit for chronic neuropathic and nociceptive pain conditions, including phantom limb pain and cluster headache, whereas motor cortex stimulation has been successfully employed for trigeminal neuralgia and central pain.

Surgery

Surgical interventions are often advocated in chronic pain patients who have failed to respond to more conservative measures. A traumatic neuroma is an inexorable consequence of cutting or burning of a nerve, formed as a result of unregulated and disorganized nerve regeneration. Neuromas have been shown to fire ectopic pain signals and are often quite painful. Hence, neurolytic procedures are rarely successful in the long-term treatment of neuropathic

TABLE 30-7 EVIDENCE FOR TREATMENTS OF DIFFERENT CAUSES OF CHRONIC LOW BACK PAIN

CONDITION	PREVALENCE	TREATMENT
Lumbosacral radiculopathy from herniated disc	Annual prevalence 5-15%	Moderate evidence that epidural steroids may provide short-term relief, weak evidence for long-term benefit Weak evidence for percutaneous intradiscal procedures except chymopapain (strong evidence for a modest effect) Strong evidence that surgery may provide benefit for up to 2 years, but conflicting evidence for long-term benefit Negative or weak evidence for pharmacologic treatment
Spinal stenosis	5-10% of adults ≥ 65 years Rare in patients < 50 years	Moderate evidence that epidural steroids may provide short-term relief, weak evidence for long-term benefit Weak evidence for percutaneous therapy Strong evidence that surgery may provide benefit for at least 2 years Negative or weak evidence for pharmacologic treatment
Discogenic pain from degenerative disc disease	20-40% of patients with axial low back pain	Weak, conflicting evidence for modest short-term benefit with intradiscal treatments Weak, conflicting evidence that surgery may provide modest benefit for up to 2 years compared with no or unstructured treatment and that surgery is not more effective than structured care to include exercise and cognitive-behavioral treatment Negative evidence for epidural steroids
Facet arthropathy	10-15% of patients with axial low back pain, increasing with age	Moderate evidence for benefit with radiofrequency denervation Negative evidence for steroid injections and surgery
Sacroiliac joint pain	15-30% of patients with axial low back pain below L5 vertebra, increasing with age and inflammatory arthritis	Moderate evidence for short-term relief with steroid injections Moderate evidence for benefit with radiofrequency denervation Negative evidence for surgery
Myofascial pain	20%, but may be superimposed on a primary cause in more than 75% of patients	Strong evidence for exercise, muscle relaxants, and NSAIDs Weak, conflicting evidence for antidepressants Pharmacologic treatment more effective for acute than chronic low back pain
Vertebral fracture	6-18%, increasing with age and in certain ethnic groups (e.g., Asian women)	Conflicting evidence for vertebral augmentation Moderate extrapolated evidence for NSAIDs, although concerns exist for effect on bone healing Strong evidence for arthroses and bisphosphonates Anecdotal evidence for surgery, which may be necessary for stabilization Facet pain may play a role in pain after vertebral fracture

NSAIDs = nonsteroidal anti-inflammatory drugs.

pain. Part of the challenge in deciding when operative therapy is indicated revolves around the difficulty involved in establishing a causative relationship between the targeted pathologic process and pain. Roughly 10% of women of reproductive age have endometriosis (Chapter 236), but many patients with endometriosis have minimal symptoms, and pelvic pain is a frequent occurrence in young women with no detectable disease. With respect to inguinal hernia repair and spinal decompression, the incidence of chronic postsurgical pain is inversely correlated with the size of the bowel and disc herniation, respectively. This illustrates that in many individuals, the targeted disease may not be the primary cause of symptoms. On a similar note, scar tissue is a predictable sequela of surgical treatment, but lysis of adhesions is only infrequently associated with long-term symptom palliation because of the high recurrence rate and absence of any means to correlate the presence of adhesions with pain. Not surprisingly, surgery performed solely to remove a painful body part (e.g., hysterectomy, orchiectomy) rarely results in long-term benefit.

Back Pain

Back pain (Chapter 400) is the leading cause of disability in people younger than 45 years in the world. In patients who present with serious spinal disease (tumor, trauma), decompression, stabilization and fusion can be beneficial, but outcomes are strongly dependent on patient selection. Randomized studies have determined that decompression procedures done for radiculopathy and spinal stenosis are effective for short-term pain relief, but most demonstrate no long-term (>2 years) improvement compared with conservative treatment.[A14][A15] With respect to fusion or disc replacement performed for mechanical pain associated with common degenerative changes, randomized trials suggest that less than one third of patients can expect significant pain relief or a highly functional outcome, with the results diminishing over time[A16] (Table 30-7).

Physical Treatments

The use of "physical" therapies to provide pain relief and to enhance function is a cornerstone in the multimodal approach to the patient with pain. Physical therapists evaluate, educate, and provide minimally invasive procedural interventions to help prevent and alleviate pain and dysfunction. These include addressing causative mechanisms of pain (e.g., correcting gait abnormalities) and providing treatments (e.g., hot and cold packs, joint manipulation).

Exercise has been used for decades as a treatment for chronic pain and a means to prevent injury. Exercise works through a variety of mechanisms, including enhancing blood flow, releasing endorphins, exerting anti-inflammatory effects, activating inhibitory pathways, and improving sleep and mood. Whereas the largest body of research has been conducted for spinal pain, benefits have also been demonstrated in fibromyalgia, headaches, arthritis, neuropathic pain, and cancer.

Complementary and Alternative Therapies

Patients are seeking complementary and alternative medical (CAM) treatments (Chapter 39) with increasing frequency, with utilization rates around 40%. Pain is the most common indication for CAM therapies. Some of the most popular CAM modalities are acupuncture, chiropractic, and yoga, all of which have been shown to be beneficial in certain contexts. However, the effect size tends to be modest for these treatments,[A17] and there is little evidence to support one modality over another or against conventional medical treatments.

Pain Management in Older Persons

Older adults are more likely to report pain than are younger cohorts and often present with multiple comorbidities. The increased risk for drug-related adverse effects in this population is the basis for the popular recommendation "start low and go slow" in the titration of analgesic drugs. Age-related physiologic factors that can decrease the therapeutic dose of opioid and nonopioid analgesics include changes in volume of distribution and protein binding, decreased metabolism, decreased excretion, and increased pharmacologic sensitivity. For these reasons, nonpharmacologic interventions, such as ergonomic modifications, tailored physical therapy and exercise programs, nutritional consultation, psychobehavioral approaches, and injections, should be considered in appropriate patients.[14]

FUTURE DRUGS AND PREVENTION OF PAIN

Much research is being devoted to development of new routes of drug administration (e.g., transdermal, transmucosal), abuse-deterrent opioids, and novel nonopioid drug treatments, which can optimize outcomes and reduce risks and side effects. Two other areas receiving significant research attention involve the genotyping and phenotyping of chronic pain patients. The conceptual appeal of these endeavors is that pain treatment tailored to individuals may result in greater benefit and less harm than the shotgun approach.

Regenerative therapies, which seek to facilitate the body's ability to repair, replace, restore, or regenerate diseased or damaged tissue, are another frontier in pain medicine. Whereas many of these treatments are currently in preliminary stages of development, they may someday be used to treat central, joint, and spinal pain. Examples that are as yet unproven include stem cell therapy and the infusion of platelet-rich plasma, which involves stimulation of the body's natural healing processes.

Another area that has been underinvestigated is identifying patients at high risk for development of pain and employing strategies either to prevent pain or to minimize disease burden. In patients at high risk for chronic postsurgical pain (e.g., young patients with preexisting pain and psychological comorbidities), these measures might include the use of preemptive analgesics such as NSAIDs, anticonvulsants, and cytokine inhibitors and employing surgical techniques associated with less trauma. For patients with musculoskeletal complaints, this might entail educational initiatives and extensive rehabilitation.

Finally, the specialty of pain medicine must come to terms with the reality of spiraling health care costs by developing cost-effectiveness models by which to gauge benefit. Clinical trials evaluating new treatments should measure not only subjective outcomes such as pain scores but also objective ones that can result in societal cost savings, such as return to work or prevention of surgery. Proving that new treatments are more effective than existing or placebo treatments and result in cost-containment should be a cornerstone of future clinical research.

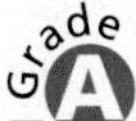

Grade A References

A1. Chou R, Fu R, Carrino JA, Deyo RA. Imaging strategies for low-back pain: systematic review and meta-analysis. *Lancet*. 2009;373:463-472.

A2. Cohen SP, Gupta A, Strassels SA, et al. Does MRI affect outcomes in patients with lumbosacral radiculopathy referred for epidural steroid injections? A randomized, double-blind, controlled study. *Arch Intern Med*. 2012;172:134-142.

A3. Derry S, Moore RA, Rabbie R. Topical NSAIDs for chronic musculoskeletal pain in adults. *Cochrane Database Syst Rev*. 2012;9:CD007400.

A4. Lunn MP, Hughes RA, Wiffen PJ. Duloxetine for treating painful neuropathy, chronic pain or fibromyalgia. *Cochrane Database Syst Rev*. 2014;1:CD007115.

A5. Moore RA, Derry S, Aldington D, et al. Amitriptyline for neuropathic pain and fibromyalgia in adults. *Cochrane Database Syst Rev*. 2012;12:CD008242.

A6. Moore A, Wiffen P, Kalso E. Antiepileptic drugs for neuropathic pain and fibromyalgia. *JAMA*. 2014;312:182-183.

A7. Chaparro LE, Wiffen PJ, Moore RA, Gilron I. Combination pharmacotherapy for the treatment of neuropathic pain in adults. *Cochrane Database Syst Rev*. 2012;7:CD008943.

A8. Clarke H, Bonin RP, Orser BA, et al. The prevention of chronic postsurgical pain using gabapentin and pregabalin: a combined systematic review and meta-analysis. *Anesth Analg*. 2012;115:428-442.

A9. Derry S, Sven-Rice A, Cole P, et al. Topical capsaicin (high concentration) for chronic neuropathic pain in adults. *Cochrane Database Syst Rev*. 2013;2:CD007393.

A10. Noble M, Treadwell JR, Tregear SJ, et al. Long-term opioid management for chronic noncancer pain. *Cochrane Database Syst Rev*. 2010;1:CD006605.

A11. Gilron I, Bailey JM, Tu D, et al. Morphine, gabapentin, or their combination for neuropathic pain. *N Engl J Med*. 2005;352:1324-1334.

A12. Gilron I, Bailey JM, Tu D, et al. Nortriptyline and gabapentin, alone and in combination for neuropathic pain: a double-blind, randomised controlled crossover trial. *Lancet*. 2009;374:1252-1261.

A13. Romano CL, Romano D, Bonora C, et al. Pregabalin, celecoxib, and their combination for treatment of chronic low-back pain. *J Orthop Traumatol*. 2009;10:185-191.

A14. Jacobs WC, van Tulder M, Arts M, et al. Surgery versus conservative management of sciatica due to a lumbar herniated disc: a systematic review. *Eur Spine J*. 2011;20:513-522.

A15. Kovacs FM, Urrútia G, Alarcón JD. Surgery versus conservative treatment for symptomatic lumbar spinal stenosis: a systematic review of randomized controlled trials. *Spine (Phila Pa 1976)*. 2011;36:E1335-E1351.

A16. Jacobs W, Van der Gaag NA, Tuschel A, et al. Total disc replacement for chronic back pain in the presence of disc degeneration. *Cochrane Database Syst Rev*. 2012;9:CD008326.

A17. Vickers AJ, Linde K. Acupuncture for chronic pain. *JAMA*. 2014;311:955-956.

GENERAL REFERENCES

For the General References and other additional features, please visit Expert Consult at https://expertconsult.inkling.com.

31 BIOLOGY OF ADDICTION

ERIC J. NESTLER AND STEVEN E. HYMAN

DEFINITION

Drug addiction is compulsive substance use despite serious negative consequences. Harmful drug use and addiction are significant contributors to medical morbidity and mortality both directly as a result of the toxic effects of abused drugs and indirectly through accidents, violence, nonsterile needle use, smoking, and other health hazards. By far the greatest contributors to illness and death are the widely used legal drugs, tobacco (Chapter 32), and alcohol (Chapter 33), although illegal addictive drugs and abused prescription drugs also exact a significant toll. In addition, addiction creates enormous burdens on society by impairing the function of the addicted person in multiple life roles, disrupting families and neighborhoods, and motivating crime. Globally, drug use is not distributed evenly and is not simply related to stringency of drug policy.[1]

Compulsive use, the cardinal feature of addiction, means that the affected person cannot control substance use for a significant time despite powerful reasons to do so, such as drug-related health problems, drug-associated arrests, or the threat of losing one's job or spouse. In the clinic, addiction can be remarkably frustrating to treat: drug seeking and administration are apparently voluntary behaviors that an otherwise sentient person seems unwilling to control. Even after significant efforts have been exerted to get an addicted patient into drug treatment, relapse is common, even long after the last withdrawal symptom has cleared. Relapses are often precipitated by stress or by reminders of drug use (cues) that may range from familiar drug use contexts (such as smoking after a meal) to interactions with drug-using friends, the smell of marijuana or tobacco smoke, and body feelings previously associated with drug seeking (so-called interoceptive cues). Molecular, cellular, and behavioral studies of drug action in animal models and noninvasive human neuroimaging studies are providing significant insights into the neurobiology underlying compulsive drug taking and its persistence. Other important frontiers of research include the human genetics of addiction risk and more recently, the neurobiology of what have been called behavioral addictions, such as compulsive gambling.

Drug users may repeatedly take drugs to gain pleasure or to escape from negative feelings, including the aversive feelings that may occur when drugs wear off. As a result of repeated drug administration over time, initial protein targets for the drugs and their downstream signaling pathways (Table 31-1) are excessively stimulated and may thus undergo homeostatic adaptations. These adaptations can produce tolerance (the need for increasing drug doses to achieve desired affects) or dependence (revealed by withdrawal symptoms between drug doses or with drug cessation). Both tolerance and dependence can contribute to ongoing drug use and to dosage increases; however, neither tolerance nor dependence alone explains compulsive use. First, tolerance and dependence occur not only with repeated use of many addictive drugs (e.g., heroin) but also with many nonaddictive drugs (e.g., β-adrenergic antagonists [propranolol], α_2-adrenergic agonist antihypertensive agents [clonidine], nitrates, selective serotonin reuptake inhibitor antidepressants). Second, some highly addictive drugs, such as cocaine, may produce little physical dependence and withdrawal in some individuals who nonetheless exhibit compulsive use. Finally, if dependence and withdrawal were necessary factors in addiction, the phenomenon of late, post-detoxification relapse would not be the major clinical problem that it is.[2] Although these forms of homeostatic adaptation play a role in addiction, as will be described, other types of plasticity within the nervous system are more significant.

RISK FACTORS FOR ADDICTION

Only a minority of individuals who use drugs go on to become addicted. The best-established risk factors for addiction are male sex and family history. Across countries and cultures, males have a greater risk for both heavy drug use and addiction, with risk ratios in the range of 1.4 : 1 to 2 : 1. In recent years, however, the sex ratios have narrowed in many countries, especially for tobacco use and alcohol. Moreover, females who succumb to addiction tend to do so more quickly after initial drug exposures, and drug use during pregnancy can have enormous deleterious effects on the fetus.

Genes play the preponderant role in familial risk as evidenced by twin and adoption studies.[3,4] Twin studies consistently show higher rates of concordance for heavy drug use and addiction within monozygotic twin pairs than within dizygotic twin pairs. Adoption studies that have been performed in several Scandinavian countries and in the United States have focused mostly on alcoholism. These studies demonstrate that individuals adopted early in life tend to resemble their biologic rather than their adoptive parents with respect to patterns of alcohol use. Large population genetic studies suggest that the heritable risk for addiction to any of several substances, including opiates, stimulants, nicotine, alcohol, and marijuana, is roughly the same and varies between 20 and 60%, depending on the study.

Although genes clearly play a significant role in vulnerability to addiction, few of the specific genetic variants that confer risk have been identified with certainty. Like all common neuropsychiatric disorders, addiction risk is highly

TABLE 31-1 PROPERTIES OF ADDICTIVE DRUGS

DRUG	NEUROTRANSMITTER	DRUG TARGET	EFFECT AFTER BINDING
Opiates (morphine, heroin, oxycodone)	Endorphins; enkephalins	μ and δ opioid receptor (agonist)	Activate G_i/G_o; activate K^+ channels
Psychostimulants (cocaine, amphetamines)	Dopamine (DA)	Dopamine transporter (DAT)* (antagonist)	Increase synaptic DA; stimulate presynaptic and postsynaptic DA receptors
Nicotine	Acetylcholine	Nicotinic acetylcholine receptor (nAChR) (agonist)	Stimulate cation channel (may desensitize)
Alcohol	γ-Aminobutyric acid (GABA) Glutamate	$GABA_A$ receptor (agonist) *N*-methyl-D-aspartate (NMDA) receptor (antagonist)	Activate Cl^- channel Inhibit Ca^{2+} entry
Marijuana (Δ^9-tetrahydrocannabinol)	Anandamide; 2-arachidonoylglycerol	Cannabinoid CB_1 (agonist)	Activate G_i/G_o; activate K^+ channels
Phencyclidine, ketamine		NMDA receptor (antagonist)	Inhibit Ca^{2+} entry

*The psychostimulants also interact with the norepinephrine and serotonin transporters, but under normal conditions, it is the DAT that is critical for rewarding and addictive properties. Unlike cocaine, amphetamines enter dopamine nerve terminals through the DAT and interact with a second target, the vesicular monoamine transporter (VMAT), to release DA into the cytoplasm and thence, through the DAT, to release it into the synapse.

Modified from Hyman SE, Malenka RC, Nestler EJ. Neural mechanisms of addiction: the role of reward-related learning and memory. *Annu Rev Neurosci.* 2006;29:565-598.

genetically complex; there is evidence from linkage and association studies for contributions by a large number of genetic variants of relatively small effect. Large genome-wide association studies and other applications of modern genomic methods are continuing. However, the task of gene identification is also complicated by the challenges of phenotype definition. There are no objective medical tests with which to make the diagnosis, and there may be independent genetic and nongenetic risk factors for different stages of substance use disorders, such as drug experimentation, addiction, and treatment responsiveness. Moreover, twin and family studies suggest that there may be both shared and unshared genetic risk factors underlying addictions to different drugs. As in other genetically complex disorders, it is hoped that with the identification of multiple risk-conferring variants, it will be possible to identify biochemical pathways involved in addiction pathogenesis, which will then suggest potential targets for new and more effective treatments.

REWARD CIRCUITRY: THE NEURAL SUBSTRATE OF ADDICTION

The survival and perpetuation of species require that animals, including humans, learn to predict threats and also learn the circumstances under which they can obtain "rewards," such as food, water, shelter, and opportunities for mating. A simple operational definition of reward is a stimulus that elicits approach and consummatory behaviors. Several interconnected neural circuits, highly conserved in evolution, control an individual's responses to rewarding and aversive stimuli (Fig. 31-1). Dopamine-releasing neurons in the ventral tegmental area (VTA) of the midbrain and their major target neurons in the nucleus accumbens (NAc) in the ventral striatum serve as a rheostat that detects and drives responses to rewards and threats, the amygdala and hippocampus are crucial for forming reward- and fear-related memories, the dorsal striatum (caudate and putamen) mediates well-learned behaviors and habits, and several regions of prefrontal cortex exert executive control over these subcortical systems. Addiction involves abnormal functioning of this entire circuit.[5]

The neurotransmitter dopamine, released from VTA nerve terminals in the NAc, plays the key (albeit not the only) role in binding rewards and reward-associated cues to adaptive reward-seeking responses. In animals, implanted electrodes can record firing of dopamine neurons; microdialysis catheters and electrochemical methods can be used to detect dopamine that has been released from presynaptic terminals. In humans, positron emission tomography permits indirect measures of dopamine release by observing the displacement of a positron-emitting D_2 dopamine receptor ligand previously bound to receptors after a stimulus or pharmacologic challenge. By use of such methods in multiple paradigms, it has been well established that natural rewards cause firing of VTA neurons and dopamine release in the NAc and other forebrain regions. When dopamine action is blocked, whether by lesioning of dopamine neurons, blocking of postsynaptic dopamine receptors, or inhibition of dopamine synthesis, rewards no longer motivate the behaviors necessary to obtain them.

New insights into the role of dopamine have emerged from studies of patients with Parkinson disease (Chapter 409). Parkinson disease results from the death of midbrain dopamine neurons; however, neurons within the substantia nigra, which project to the dorsal striatum, are more severely affected than neurons within the VTA. Patients are generally treated with

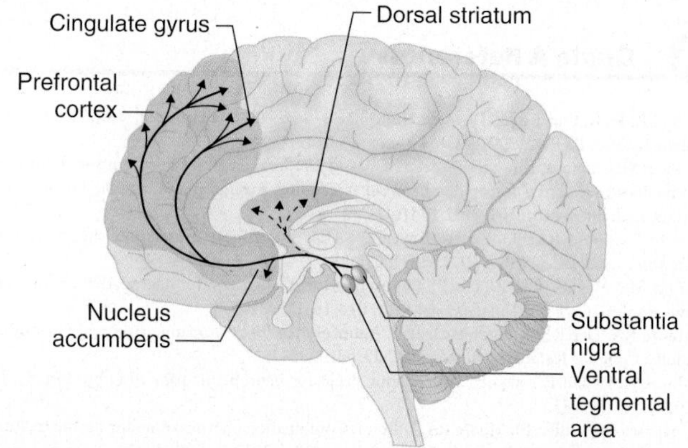

FIGURE 31-1. Brain reward circuits. The major dopaminergic projections to the forebrain that underlie brain reward are shown superimposed on a diagram of the human brain: projections from the ventral tegmental area to the nucleus accumbens, amygdala (not shown), hippocampus (not shown), and prefrontal cerebral cortex. Also shown are projections from the substantia nigra to the dorsal striatum (caudate and putamen and related structures) that play a role in habit formation and other deeply ingrained motor behaviors, including those related to drug consumption. (From Hyman SE, Malenka RC, Nestler EJ. Neural mechanisms of addiction: the role of reward-related learning and memory. *Annu Rev Neurosci.* 2006;29:565-598.)

L-dopa, a dopamine precursor, but as the disease progresses, other drugs may be needed, including selective D_2 dopamine receptor agonists. Relevant to this discussion is that a minority of patients treated with D_2 dopamine receptor agonists develop new risky, goal-directed behaviors, such as compulsive gambling or shopping. These behaviors generally cease when the drug is withdrawn. It is thought that whereas dopamine receptor agonists produce therapeutic effects on motor behavior in the more fully denervated dorsal striatum, they can combine with endogenous dopamine from preserved VTA neurons to overstimulate the NAc and other components of reward circuitry. These observations not only underscore the role of dopamine in motivation and reward seeking but also suggest that what have been called behavioral addictions share neural substrates with drug addiction.[6]

Much evidence suggests that the precise pattern of dopamine neuron firing and the resulting synaptic release of dopamine in forebrain circuits act to shape behavior so as to maximize future reward. In a basal state, dopamine neurons have a slow tonic pattern of firing. When a reward is encountered that is new, unexpected, or greater than expected, there is a phasic burst of firing of dopamine neurons causing a transient increase in synaptic dopamine. When a reward is predicted from known cues and is exactly as expected, there is little change from the tonic pattern of firing, that is, only small additional dopamine release. When a predicted reward is omitted or less than expected, dopamine neurons pause their firing to levels below their tonic rate. Phasic increases in synaptic dopamine signify that the world is better than expected, facilitate learning of new predictive information, and bind the newly learned predictive cues to action.

Dopamine is not the only neurotransmitter that signals reward. Others, including acetylcholine, endogenous opioid peptides (e.g., enkephalin and endorphin), and endogenous lipid substances called endocannabinoids (because cannabinoid drugs like marijuana are agonists at their receptors), are also released in the reward circuitry in response to natural rewards.

PROPERTIES OF ADDICTIVE DRUGS

Addictive drugs are chemically diverse and interact with different molecular targets in the nervous system (Table 31-1). They also exhibit significant differences from each other in many of their physiologic and behavioral effects. For example, cocaine and amphetamines are stimulants; they increase arousal, may cause anxiety, and at lower doses enhance cognitive performance. Alcohol is a depressant, is anxiolytic at low doses, and degrades cognitive performance. Heroin and other opiates are analgesic and cause drowsiness, constipation, and pupillary constriction. The shared behavioral effect of all addictive drugs is the liability, in vulnerable individuals, of causing compulsive use. The shared pharmacologic property that is required to cause addiction is the ability to increase levels of synaptic dopamine in the NAc and other forebrain regions. For example, cocaine blocks the dopamine uptake transporter that normally clears dopamine from synapses. Amphetamines cause reverse transport of dopamine into synapses through the dopamine uptake transporter. Opiates, nicotine, alcohol, and cannabinoids cause dopamine release, acting by different initial mechanisms to stimulate VTA dopamine neurons or to release them from resting inhibitory control. Each of these other drugs also induces reward through nondopamine mechanisms, that is, through activating cholinergic, opioid, or cannabinoid receptors within the reward circuitry (Table 31-1).

Natural rewards, such as food or sexual opportunities, regulate the firing of dopamine neurons through highly processed sensory information, both external and interoceptive. Addictive drugs short-circuit this kind of information processing by acting directly on proteins that control dopamine and other signals in the reward circuitry. Acting by such direct pharmacologic mechanisms, addictive drugs typically produce greater quantities of synaptic dopamine and other reward-related neurotransmitters over longer times than natural rewards do. In addition, addictive drugs provide a grossly pathologic learning signal by occluding pauses in dopamine and other neuron firing even when drug use proves less pleasurable than expected or even aversive. For example, when the inhalation of a smoker causes painful coughing, it might seem that the brain would signal an experience that is worse than expected with a resulting decrement in VTA neuron firing rate. However, because nicotine causes dopamine release pharmacologically, independent of the smoker's actual experience, reward circuits, unavailable to conscious introspection, still receive a positive message that reinforces nicotine seeking and nicotine use. In short, addictive drugs, by virtue of their effects on dopamine and related neurotransmitters, always signal "better than expected."

DRUG-INDUCED NEURAL PLASTICITY RELEVANT TO ADDICTION

Neurobiologic research on addiction has focused intensely on compulsive aspects of drug use, the ability of specific cues to activate drug seeking and craving, and the long persistence of stress and cue-dependent relapse risk. As described previously, compulsive drug use and the power of drug-associated cues reflect the usurpation of the brain's reward circuitry by drugs of abuse.[7] The persistence of addiction reflects long-term changes in neurons and synapses and their interacting circuits. Research during more than a decade has identified long-term changes in gene expression resulting from use of addictive drugs; recently, some long-lived alterations in gene expression have been attributed to drug-induced epigenetic mechanisms, such as modifications of chromatin.[8]

Long-term changes in gene expression may render the addicted person susceptible to stress and may also create persistent changes in hedonic state and mood regulation that may motivate drug taking. By themselves, however, changes in gene expression do not explain the ability of exquisitely specific cues to activate drug seeking or, if seeking is impeded, intense subjective drug craving. The ability of specific cues to activate drug seeking and wanting is based on long-term associative memories consolidated under the influence of dopamine and other reward signals. Long-term memory formation represents perhaps the most persistent changes in brain function that may occur in adult life. The neural substrates of memory are likely to include alterations in synaptic weights, such as long-term potentiation or long-term depression, and physical remodeling of dendritic spines. Processes of drug sensitization (or reverse tolerance), demonstrated in animal models and in humans, may contribute to these memory-related phenomena.[9]

The centrality of associative learning mechanisms for addiction was first recognized from clinical observation: much drug taking and, most notably, late relapses follow exposure to cues previously associated with drug use. Cues that can reinitiate drug use include environmental stimuli (e.g., persons with whom drugs have been used, drug paraphernalia) and body feelings. Because addictive drugs reliably increase synaptic dopamine and other reward-related neurotransmitters as a result of their direct pharmacologic actions—indeed, they produce excessive and grossly distorted reward signals—the brain receives a powerful impetus to connect the circumstances in which the drugs have been used with the motivation to take drugs again. Even if the drug is no longer pleasurable, the signals continue to reinforce drug wanting and seeking. Moreover, the certainty and magnitude of these signals give drugs a marked advantage over natural rewards and other learned goals, including prosocial activities.

In the laboratory, it has been possible to study the effects of drugs and drug cues on neural circuits, physiology, and subjective responding in addicted human subjects. For example, drug-associated cues have been shown to elicit drug urges and physiologic responses (such as sympathetic activation) as well as activation of reward circuits in addicted human subjects. By positron emission tomography, cocaine-related cues have been shown to elicit dopamine release in the dorsal striatum in addicted subjects.

Investigations at the cellular and molecular levels have begun to identify the physiologic and molecular changes that underlie the effects of addictive drugs on reward-related memory processes. Among psychotropic drugs that have been examined, only those drugs that can cause addiction produce long-term potentiation in brain reward circuits including the VTA. Addictive drugs also activate transcription factors, such as the cyclic adenosine monophosphate response element binding protein (CREB), and alter the composition of activator protein 1 (AP-1) complexes (composed of Fos and Jun families of transcription factors) in brain reward circuits. Cocaine, opiates, and other addictive drugs have been shown to regulate many genes downstream of CREB, AP-1, and other transcription factors. As well, it has been increasingly possible, through the use of genetically modified mice and virus-mediated gene transfer, to directly demonstrate the involvement of these transcriptional mechanisms in the range of behavioral abnormalities induced by repeated drug exposure in animal models. However, it is far more challenging to determine which drug-regulated proteins are causally involved in human addiction. Part of the challenge is that, whereas rodent models have provided many insights into drug action and behavior, it is difficult to model human compulsion in animals, that is, to model a free-living and independent person who loses control over drug use while experiencing the negative consequences of that use. That said, a growing body of knowledge is emerging about the neural and molecular processes that produce addiction, with the hope of translating these advances into medical diagnostic tests and more effective treatments of addictive disorders.

GENERAL REFERENCES

For the General References and other additional features, please visit Expert Consult at https://expertconsult.inkling.com.

32 NICOTINE AND TOBACCO

TONY P. GEORGE

DEFINITIONS

Cigarette smoking is the most common (>90%) method of tobacco use, although other forms of tobacco use, including pipe tobacco, cigars, and smokeless tobacco, are common. Nicotine is the active ingredient in tobacco that acts as a reinforcer for repeated use for all forms of tobacco.

EPIDEMIOLOGY

Cigarette smoking is the most preventable cause of morbidity and mortality in the Western world. In the United States, approximately 20% of the general population currently uses tobacco compared with 47% in 1965. Since the release of the U.S. Surgeon General's report in 1965, smoking prevalence has been substantially reduced, but this reduction appears to have slowed in recent years, likely because the remaining 20% of smokers are refractory to tobacco treatment. Approximately 450,000 people in the United States die each year as a result of smoking-attributable medical illnesses, including lung cancer, chronic obstructive pulmonary disease, cardiovascular disease, and stroke; and economic and health care costs of tobacco use exceed $400 billion annually. Smokeless tobacco (e.g., chewing tobacco) use has also increased, which has contributed to higher rates of oral pathologies, including precancerous oral lesions and cancers of the mouth and nasopharynx. Moreover, the health risks of environmental tobacco smoke (ETS) have become increasing clear, prompting the development of widespread tobacco bans in public settings.

Worldwide, it is estimated that approximately 1.1 billion people use tobacco on a regular basis, including approximately 65 million in the United States. Tobacco smoking is increasing rapidly throughout the developing world, and it is estimated that cigarette smoking will cause about 450 million deaths worldwide in the next 50 years.[1] In particular, the onset of smoking occurs at a younger age, the rates of smoking in women are increasing, and more smokers are of a lower socioeconomic status. Reducing smoking prevalence by 50% would prevent 20 to 30 million premature deaths in the first quarter of this century and 150 million in the second quarter.

For most smokers, quitting is the single most important thing they can do to improve their health.[2] A prospective cohort study in Norway suggests that even with sustained reductions (>25 to 75%) in daily smoking consumption, there is little if any decrease in cardiovascular disease and lung or other smoking-related cancer risk, further substantiating the merits of quitting versus reducing smoking.

PATHOBIOLOGY

Nicotine is the primary reinforcer in tobacco smoke, with contributions from more than 4000 components to the sensory (non-nicotine) aspects of cigarette smoking. The primary site of action of nicotine is the $\alpha_4\beta_2$ nicotinic acetylcholine receptor (nAChR), and the endogenous neurotransmitter acting on nAChRs is acetylcholine. nAChRs in the central nervous system (CNS) are pentameric ion channel complexes comprising two α- and three β-subunits; the seven α-subunits are designated α_2 to α_9 and the three β-subunits are designated β_2 to β_4. This produces considerable diversity in subunit combinations, which may explain the region-specific and functional selectivity of nicotinic effects in the CNS.[3] Activation of nAChRs leads to Na^+/Ca^{2+} ion channel fluxes and neuronal membrane depolarization. nAChRs are located presynaptically on several neurotransmitter-secreting neuron types in the CNS, including mesolimbic dopaminergic (DA) neurons that project from the ventral tegmental area (VTA) to the nucleus accumbens (NAc). Activation of nAChRs on mesolimbic DA neurons leads to DA secretion in the nucleus accumbens.

At low concentrations of nicotine, $\alpha_4\beta_2$ nAChR stimulation of afferent GABAergic projections onto mesoaccumbal DA neurons predominates, leading to reduced mesolimbic DA neuron firing and DA release. At higher nicotine concentrations, $\alpha_4\beta_2$ nAChRs desensitize, and predominant activation of α_7 nAChRs on glutamatergic projections occurs, leading to increased mesolimbic DA neuron firing and release. Within milliseconds of activation by nicotine, nAChRs desensitize. After overnight abstinence, nAChRs resensitize; this may explain why most smokers report that the first cigarette in the morning is the most satisfying. Interestingly, positron emission tomography (PET) neuroimaging studies have shown that smoking 2 or 3 puffs from a cigarette produces saturation of nAChRs in the brain reward system, suggesting that although binding to central nAChRs is an important first step in the effects of nicotine, it is not a complete explanation for continued smoking behaviors.

CLINICAL MANIFESTATIONS

Although there is a subset of cigarette smokers who do not smoke every day (e.g., "chippers"), most cigarette smokers are daily users and have some degree of physiologic dependence on nicotine. Smokers typically describe a "rush" and feelings of alertness, relaxation, and "satisfaction" when smoking, and it is well known that nicotine has both stimulating and anxiolytic effects depending on basal level of arousal. Airway stimulation is an important aspect of smoking behavior, and additives such as menthol enhance the experience by increasing the taste and reducing the harshness of smoked tobacco.

Interestingly, the positive effects of cigarette smoking (e.g., taste, satisfaction) appear to be mediated by non-nicotine components of tobacco such as tar. Besides positive reinforcement, withdrawal, and craving, there are several secondary effects of nicotine and tobacco use that may contribute to both maintenance of smoking and smoking relapse, including mood modulation (e.g., reduction of negative affect), stress reduction, and weight control. In addition, conditioned cues can elicit the urge to smoke even after prolonged periods of abstinence. Specific effects might be most relevant to smokers wishing to lose weight and to those with psychiatric presentations (mood modulation, cognitive enhancement, stress reduction). These secondary effects may present additional targets for pharmacologic intervention in certain subgroups of smokers (e.g., those with schizophrenia or depression, or those concerned about their weight).

DIAGNOSIS

The *Diagnostic and Statistical Manual*, 5th edition (DSM-5),[4] which was released in 2013 by the American Psychiatric Association, has changed the diagnostic terminology for nicotine and tobacco, eliminating the term *dependence* and instead using the term *tobacco use disorder*. Tobacco use disorder is established clinically by historical documentation of 2 of the following 11 criteria:

1. Tobacco often taken in larger amounts or over a longer period than was intended
2. Persistent desire or unsuccessful efforts to cut down or control tobacco use
3. A great deal of time spent in activities necessary to obtain or use tobacco
4. Presence of craving, or a strong desire or urge to use tobacco
5. Recurrent tobacco use resulting in failure to fulfill major obligations at work, school, or home
6. Continued tobacco use despite persistent or recurrent social or interpersonal problems caused or exacerbated by the effects of tobacco
7. Important social, occupational, or recreational activities given up or reduced because of tobacco use
8. Recurrent tobacco use in situations in which it is physically hazardous (e.g., smoking in bed)
9. Continued tobacco use despite persistent or recurrent physical or psychological problems that are caused or exacerbated by tobacco use
10. Tolerance, as defined by either a need for markedly increased amounts of tobacco to achieve desired effects, or markedly diminished effects with continued use of the same amount of tobacco
11. Withdrawal, manifested by the presence of the characteristic tobacco abstinence syndrome (e.g., four of the following: irritability, anxiety, difficulty concentrating, increased appetite, restlessness, dysphoric mood, insomnia), or tobacco (or nicotine) taken to relieve or avoid tobacco withdrawal symptoms.

For abstinent smokers, remission is classified as early (between 3 and 12 months of abstinence) or sustained (>12 months of abstinence). Moreover, current severity of tobacco use disorder is coded as mild (2 or 3 symptoms), moderate (4 or 5 symptoms) or severe (6 or more symptoms).

In addition, most physiologically dependent tobacco smokers state that they smoke their first cigarette of the day within the first 5 minutes of awakening (e.g., time to first cigarette <5 minutes after awakening). Timeline followback procedures and smoking diaries have been used successfully to monitor smoking consumption over time. Scales such as the Fagerstrom Test for Nicotine Dependence allow assessment of the level of nicotine dependence, with scores higher than 4 on a scale of 0 to 10 being consistent with physiologic dependence to nicotine. Nicotine craving and withdrawal can be reliably monitored using validated scales such as the Tiffany Questionnaire for Smoking Urges and the Minnesota Nicotine Withdrawal Scale. These scales have excellent test-retest reliability and internal consistency in smokers with schizophrenia compared with nonpsychiatric control smokers, suggesting that they can be used in psychiatric populations.

TREATMENT Rx

Psychosocial Treatments

Behavioral therapies are based on the theory that learning processes operate in the development, maintenance, and cessation of smoking (Table 32-1). Behavioral treatments for smoking can facilitate motivation to quit, provide an emphasis on the social and contextual aspects of smoking, and enhance overall success at smoking cessation.[5] In most reviews, 6-month quit rates with behavior therapies are 20% to 25%, and behavior therapy typically increases quit rates up to two-fold over standard medical advice. The primary goals of behavioral therapies in treatment of tobacco dependence include providing necessary skills to smokers to aid them in quitting smoking and teaching skills to avoid smoking in high-risk situations.

Brief Interventions

Brief advice has been found to increase smoking cessation rates and has been strongly endorsed in the latest U.S. Department of Health and Human Services Guidelines on Tobacco Dependence Treatment. Therefore, it is recommended that physicians use the "5 As" with all patients (*Ask* patients if they smoke, *Advise* patients to quit, *Assess* patients' motivation level for quitting, *Assist* with quit attempts, and *Arrange* follow-up contacts). Providing self-help material is a form of brief intervention used to increase motivation to quit and impart smoking cessation skills. Several recent studies have documented that minimal behavioral interventions such as community support groups, telephone counseling, and computer-generated tailored self-help materials can augment smoking cessation rates in controlled settings.

Motivational Interventions

The goal of motivational interviewing (MI) interventions is to elicit change through addressing ambivalence, increasing intrinsic motivation for change, and creating an atmosphere of acceptance in which patients take responsibility for making changes happen. Brief MI interventions have been developed for smoking cessation, and there is some evidence for increased smoking cessation using MI techniques.

TABLE 32-1 BEHAVIORAL TREATMENTS FOR TOBACCO DEPENDENCE

BEHAVIORAL TREATMENTS	MECHANISM OF ACTION	
Brief interventions	Increase motivation to quit and impart cessation skills (e.g., community support, telephone counseling)	2
Cognitive-behavioral and relapse-prevention therapies	Behavioral strategies are developed to manage triggers; cognitive coping strategies target maladaptive thoughts to prevent relapse	1
Motivational interviewing	Therapist promotes patient's self-motivational statements, and in turn, patient gains greater awareness of the problems with smoking; increases intention for smoking cessation	2

Effectiveness rating: 1 = strong evidence to support efficacy; 2 = moderate evidence to support efficacy; 3 = little evidence to support efficacy

Cognitive-Behavioral Therapies

In cognitive behavioral therapy (CBT), patients learn to anticipate situations in which they are likely to smoke and then plan to cope with these situations using behavioral (e.g., substitution of behavior) and cognitive (e.g., challenging thoughts) techniques. Some degree of efficacy of CBT in smokers has been observed for both individual and group counseling formats.

Relapse-Prevention (Coping Skills) Therapies

A large number of smokers relapse within 6 months of quitting. Focusing on relapse prevention skills, including recognizing high-risk situations and coping with lapses, can be included in initial smoking cessation treatment or following a quit attempt.

Pharmacologic Treatments

There are three U.S. Food and Drug Administration (FDA)-approved classes of smoking cessation pharmacotherapies: nicotine replacement therapy (NRT), sustained-release bupropion, and varenicline[6] (Table 32-2).

Nicotine Replacement Therapies

The goal of NRT is to alleviate tobacco withdrawal, which allows smokers to focus on habit and conditioning factors when attempting cessation. NRTs rely on systemic venous absorption and so do not produce the rapid high levels of arterial nicotine achieved when cigarette smoke is inhaled. Thus, individuals are unlikely to become addicted to NRT. Safety concerns regarding smoking while using an NRT patch appear to be less serious than previously thought. The most recent evidence suggests that treatment with a nicotine patch while concomitantly smoking is not hazardous, and that use of NRT *before* the quit date may actually facilitate smoking cessation compared with when given at the time of quitting smoking. All commercially available forms of NRT are effective and increase quit rates approximately 1.5- to 2.5-fold compared with placebo.[A1] The transdermal patch, gum, and lozenge are available over the counter (OTC), whereas the nasal spray is available by prescription.

Nicotine Gum

Nicotine ingested orally is extensively metabolized on first pass through the liver. Nicotine polacrilex gum avoids this problem through buccal absorption. Nicotine gum was approved as an OTC medication in the United States in 1996 and contains 2 or 4 mg of nicotine that can be released from a resin by chewing. Nicotine gum should be administered by scheduled dosing (e.g., 1 piece of 2-mg gum/hour). The original recommended duration of treatment was 3 months, although many experts believe longer treatment is more effective. Nicotine absorption from the gum peaks 30 minutes after beginning to use the gum. Venous nicotine levels from 2- and 4-mg gum are about one third and two thirds, respectively, of the steady-state (e.g., between cigarettes) levels of nicotine achieved with cigarette smoking. Nicotine delivered by cigarettes is absorbed directly into the pulmonary arterial circulation. Thus, arterial

TABLE 32-2 PHARMACOLOGIC TREATMENTS FOR TOBACCO DEPENDENCE

NICOTINE REPLACEMENT THERAPIES*		
Gum (OTC)	Slow nicotine absorption gradually reduces nicotine craving and withdrawal	1
Transdermal nicotine patch (OTC)	Slow nicotine absorption gradually reduces nicotine craving and withdrawal	1
Lozenge (OTC)	Slow nicotine absorption gradually reduces nicotine craving and withdrawal	1
Vapor inhaler (prescription) and e-cigarettes (nonprescription)	Fast nicotine absorption leads to stimulation of nAChR, which rapidly reduces nicotine craving and withdrawal. Electronic cigarettes (e-cigarettes) are not approved by the FDA and are under study to compare with other nicotine replacement therapies.	1
Nasal spray (prescription)	Fast nicotine absorption leads to stimulation of nAChR, which reduces craving and withdrawal	1
NON-NICOTINE PHARMACOTHERAPIES		
Bupropion SR*	Blocks reuptake of DA and NA; high-affinity, noncompetitive nAChR antagonism reduces nicotine reinforcement, withdrawal, and craving	1
Varenicline*	Acts as a partial agonist of $\alpha_4\beta_2$ nAChRs	1
Nortriptyline	Blocks reuptake of NA and 5-HT; probably reduces withdrawal symptoms and comorbid depressive symptoms; side effects limit utility.	1-2
Clonidine	α_2-Adrenoreceptor agonist reduces nicotine withdrawal symptoms	2
Mecamylamine	Noncompetitive, high-affinity nAChR antagonist combined with TNP reduces nicotine reinforcement, craving, and withdrawal and may increase smoking cessation rates versus TNP alone.	2-3
Naltrexone	Minimal evidence that this μ-opioid peptide receptor antagonist improves smoking cessation outcomes alone, or in combination with TNP. It may reduce alcohol use, and obviate cessation-induced weight gain.	3
Cytisine	Nicotinic partial agonist appears to be safe and efficacious for smoking cessation.[A8]	2
Nicotine vaccine	Limited evidence of efficacy for smoking cessation in early human trials, and recent phase III trials have been negative.	3

*Approved by the U.S. Food and Drug Administration (FDA).
Effectiveness rating: 1 = strong evidence to support efficacy; 2 = moderate evidence to support efficacy; 3 = little evidence to support efficacy.
5-HT = serotonin; DA = dopamine; NA = norepinephrine; nAChR= nicotine acetylcholine receptor; OTC = over the counter; TNP = transdermal nicotine patch.

levels from smoking are 5 to 10 times higher than those from the 2- and 4-mg gums. Absorption of nicotine in the buccal mucosa is decreased by an acidic environment, and patients should not drink beverages (e.g., coffee, soda, juice) immediately before, during, or after nicotine gum use.

Several placebo-controlled trials established the safety and efficacy of nicotine gum for smoking cessation.[6] There appears to be some evidence to support using higher doses of nicotine gum (4 mg pieces) in more highly dependent cigarette smokers (≥25 cigarettes per day [cpd]), which supports the idea of matching nicotine gum dose to dependence level of the smoker. Side effects from nicotine gum are rare and include those of mechanical origin (e.g., difficulty chewing, sore jaw) or of local pharmacologic origin (e.g., burning in mouth, throat irritation). Tolerance develops to most side effects over the first week, and education about proper use of the gum (e.g., do not chew too vigorously) decreases side effects.

Nicotine Lozenges

Nicotine lozenges that deliver nicotine (2 and 4 mg preparations) by buccal absorption were approved for OTC use in the United States in 2002. Lozenges offer further flexibility for nicotine replacement options for smokers and are known to allow greater absorption of nicotine compared with nicotine gum. Mild throat and mouth irritation have been reported in preliminary trials. Nicotine lozenges have shown their superiority to placebo lozenges, with significant reduction in nicotine craving and withdrawal. Furthermore, high lozenge doses may be more efficacious in more highly dependent smokers, suggesting that, similar to nicotine gum, lozenge dose can be matched with dependence level. Interestingly, the combination of nicotine lozenge and nicotine patch may lead to the higher long-term quit rates compared with both NRT monotherapies and bupropion.

Transdermal Nicotine Patch

Transdermal nicotine patch (TNP) formulations take advantage of ready absorption of nicotine across the skin. Three of the formulations are for 24-hour use, and one is for 16-hour use. Starting doses are 21 to 22 mg/24-hour patch and 15 mg/16-hour patch. Patches are applied daily each morning. Nicotine administered by patches is slowly absorbed so that, on the first day, venous nicotine levels peak 6 to 10 hours after administration. Thereafter, nicotine levels remain fairly steady, with a decline from peak to trough of 25% to 40% with 24-hour patches. Nicotine levels obtained with the use of patches are typically half those obtained by smoking. After 4 to 6 weeks on high-dose patch (21 or 22 mg/24 hours, and 15 mg/16 hours), smokers are tapered to a middle dose (e.g., 14 mg/24 hours or 10 mg/16 hours) and then to the lowest dose after an additional 2 to 4 weeks (7 mg/24 hours or 5 mg/16 hours). Most studies suggest that abrupt cessation of the use of patches often causes no significant withdrawal; thus, tapering does not appear to be necessary. The recommended total duration of treatment is usually 6 to 12 weeks.

The overall efficacy of the TNP for smoking cessation has been well documented.[6] The effects of active TNP are independent of patch type, treatment duration, tapering procedures, and behavioral therapy format or intensity, although it should be noted that behavioral treatment enhances outcomes with TNP compared with TNP alone. Severe adverse events with nicotine patches have not been found, with the most common minor side effects being skin reactions (50%), insomnia and increased or vivid dreams (15% with 24-hour patches), and nausea (5-10%). Tolerance to these side effects usually develops within a week. Rotation of patch sites decreases skin irritation. Insomnia reported in the first week after cessation appears to be mostly a result of nicotine withdrawal rather than the nicotine patch itself. A 24-hour patch can be removed before bedtime to determine whether the insomnia is caused by the nicotine patch. Without treatment, insomnia usually abates after 4 to 7 days. There is minimal dependence liability associated with patch use: only 2% of patch users continue to use it for an extended period after a cessation trial.

Nicotine Nasal Spray

Nicotine nasal spray is a nicotine solution in a nasal spray bottle similar to the type used with saline sprays. This NRT was approved for treatment of nicotine dependence in the United States in 1996. Nasal spray delivers about 1 mg nicotine per administration, and the patient administers the spray (10 mg/mL) to each nostril every 4 to 6 hours. This formulation produces a more rapid rise in nicotine levels than does nicotine gum, and the rise in nicotine levels produced by nicotine spray falls between the levels produced by nicotine gum and cigarettes. Peak nicotine levels occur within 10 minutes, and venous nicotine levels are about two thirds those of between-cigarette levels. Smokers may use the nasal spray as needed up to 30 times/day for 12 weeks.

Randomized, double-blind, placebo-controlled trials of nasal spray versus placebo spray[6] have established the safety and efficacy of the nasal spray for smoking cessation. Both trials employed treatment for 3 to 6 months, and active nasal spray led to a doubling of quit rates during active use. Differences were reduced or absent with extended follow-up, suggesting the need for maintenance use of this agent. However, such long-term studies to date have not been published. Major side effects from nicotine nasal spray are nasal and throat irritation, rhinitis, sneezing, coughing, and watering eyes. Nicotine nasal spray may have modest dependence liability; prolonged use occurs in about 10% of smokers using the nasal spray, so follow-up of smokers using nasal spray is recommended.

Nicotine Inhaler

Nicotine inhalers are cartridges (plugs) of nicotine (containing about 1 mg of nicotine each) placed inside hollow cigarette-like plastic rods. The cartridges produce a nicotine vapor when warm air is passed through them. Absorption from a nicotine inhaler is primarily buccal rather than respiratory. More recent versions of inhalers produce a rise in venous nicotine levels more rapidly than with nicotine gum but less rapidly than with nicotine nasal spray, with nicotine blood levels of about one third that of between-cigarette levels. Smokers are instructed to puff continuously on the inhaler (0.013 mg/puff) during the day, and recommended dosing is 6 to 16 cartridges daily. The inhaler is to be used as needed for about 12 weeks. No serious medical side effects have been reported with nicotine inhalers. Fifty percent of subjects report throat irritation or coughing. Double-blind, randomized controlled trials have demonstrated the superiority of inhaler to placebo inhalers for smoking cessation. Results revealed a two- to three-fold increase in quit rates (17 to 26%) at trial end point compared with placebo inhalers, and smaller differences at follow-up periods of 1 year or longer. These data support the short-term efficacy of the inhaler in cigarette smokers, but longer-term trials with the inhaler are needed, and there is some modest concern about abuse liability based on long-term use of the product in more than 10% of smokers.

Since their introduction in 2004, electronic cigarettes (e-cigarettes) to deliver nicotine have been purchased by millions (and rapidly increasing numbers) of people. Their role in tobacco control has been controversial, and there is a dearth of strong data to support or refute their efficacy in mitigating tobacco withdrawal and assisting quit attempts by smokers. One recent randomized controlled trial found that 13 weeks of nicotine e-cigarette use resulted in increased smoking abstinence at 6 months compared with use of patches or placebo e-cigarettes, although these differences were not statistically significant.[A2] Additional research will be required to determine their benefits and harms at both individual and population levels.[7]

Sustained-Release Bupropion

The phenylaminoketone, atypical antidepressant agent bupropion, in the sustained-release (SR) formulation (Zyban), is a non-nicotine first-line pharmacologic treatment approved by the FDA for nicotine dependent smokers who want to quit smoking.[A3] The mechanism of action of this antidepressant agent in the treatment of nicotine dependence likely involves dopamine and norepinephrine reuptake blockade, as well as antagonism of high-affinity nAChRs. The exact mechanism by which bupropion exerts antismoking effects is unclear. The goals of bupropion therapy are smoking cessation, reduction of nicotine craving and withdrawal symptoms, and prevention of cessation-induced weight gain.

The target dose of bupropion in nicotine dependence is 300 mg daily (150 mg bid), and it is typically started 7 days before the target quit date (TQD) at 150 mg daily, then increased to 150 mg twice daily after 3 or 4 days. Unlike with the NRTs, there is no absolute requirement that smokers completely cease smoking by the TQD, although many smokers report a significant reduction in urges to smoke and craving that facilitates cessation at the time of the TQD when drug levels reach steady-state plasma levels. Some smokers gradually reduce their cigarette smoking over several weeks before quitting.

A pivotal multicenter study established the efficacy and safety of bupropion SR for treatment of nicotine dependence, which led to its FDA approval in the United States in 1998. In a 7-week double-blind, placebo-controlled multicenter trial, four doses of bupropion SR (0, 100, 150, and 300 mg/day in twice-daily dosing), in combination with weekly individual cessation counseling, were prescribed to 615 cigarette smokers using at least 15 cpd. At 1-year follow-up, cessation rates were 12.4%, 19.6%, 22.9%, and 23.1%, respectively. Bupropion SR treatment dose-dependently reduced weight gain associated with smoking cessation and significantly reduced nicotine withdrawal symptoms at the 150- and 300-mg/day doses.

Subsequently, the efficacy of the combination of bupropion SR and TNP was studied in a double-blind, placebo-controlled, randomized multicenter trial. A total of 893 cigarette smokers, using at least 15 cpd, were randomized to one of four experimental groups: (1) placebo bupropion + placebo patch; (2) placebo bupropion + TNP; (3) bupropion (300 mg/day) + placebo patch; or (4) bupropion + TNP. Cessation rates at the 1-year follow-up assessment were 15.6%, 16.4%, 30.3%, and 35.5%, respectively. The bupropion groups were significantly better than the placebo-alone and TNP-alone conditions, but the combination of bupropion and TNP was not significantly better than bupropion alone. Weight suppression after cessation was most robust in the combination therapy group. Finally, a randomized controlled trial has demonstrated the efficacy of sustained-release bupropion in relapse prevention after smoking cessation. In individuals who quit smoking with 7 weeks of bupropion (300 mg/day) treatment, bupropion SR versus placebo for 12 months delayed smoking relapse and resulted in weight gain.

Common side effects reported with bupropion administration in cigarette smokers are headache, nausea and vomiting, dry mouth, insomnia, and activation, most of which occur during the first week of treatment. The main contraindication for the use of bupropion is a past history of seizures of any etiology. The rates of de novo seizures are low with this agent (<0.5%) at doses of 300 mg daily or less, and seizures have been observed when daily dosing exceeds 450 mg/day.

Varenicline

Varenicline tartrate (Chantix in the United States, Champix in Europe and Canada), an $\alpha_4\beta_2$ nAChR partial agonist, was approved as a first-line smoking cessation agent by the FDA in 2006 and in Canada and Europe in 2007. Varenicline (2 mg/day) is at least as good if not better than bupropion SR (300 mg/day) for providing long-term abstinence from cigarette smoking.[A4] Continuous abstinence over the follow-up period (weeks 9 to 52) were lower, and participants taking varenicline continued to show a higher rate of abstinence than participants taking bupropion and placebo. Varenicline has been also found to be effective in preventing smoking relapse compared with placebo.

Varenicline reduces tobacco cravings and smoking satisfaction and is generally well tolerated. The most common adverse events reported in the initial studies were nausea and insomnia. However, since approval of the drug, concerns have arisen over treatment-emergent neuropsychiatric events, including agitation, suicidal and homicidal ideation, mania, and psychosis. Thus, close monitoring of smokers, especially those with a history of psychiatric illness, has been strongly advised when prescribing this agent. In fact, there is recent evidence that vareniciline appears to be safe and efficacious in smokers with comorbid psychiatric disorders[8] and specifically disorders such as schizophrenia and bipolar disorder.

Combination Pharmacotherapies

There is substantial evidence to suggest that combining various formulations of NRTs, combining NRTs with bupropion SR or varenicline,[A5] or combining bupropion with varenicline[A6] may lead to enhanced smoking cessation outcomes compared with monotherapies. Although, less is known about how best to switch medications in the case of initial nonresponse, a recent study that used an adaptive trial design demonstrated that initial response to transdermal nicotine (e.g., a 50% reduction in smoking in the first 2 weeks after patch application) predicted success in subsequent smoking cessation.[A7] Moreover, those who failed to respond initially to transdermal nicotine responded to augmentation to bupropion SR or a switch to varenciline. Further studies of combination pharmacotherapies and strategies for switching among approved medications are warranted.

Off-Label Medications

Other medications (see Table 32-2) have demonstrated some evidence of efficacy for tobacco treatment, but are otherwise not approved for use for this indication and should be considered second-line treatments.

PREVENTION

Tobacco dependence remains one of the leading preventable causes of morbidity and mortality in the Western world. Nonetheless, smoking cessation therapies are amongst the most cost-effective and proven therapies in medicine. Yet, most health care providers do not identify tobacco use in their patients. Recent recommendations suggest that all smokers should be approached about quitting smoking. Moreover, effective tobacco policies such as state taxes and prevention efforts targeted to reducing the initiation of tobacco use by youth and adults are critical elements in the overall strategy to reduce the burden of tobacco-related disease and related social and health care costs.

PROGNOSIS

The prognosis for tobacco smokers who quit is excellent in terms of years of life and quality of life gained, and earlier quitting appears to be associated with increases in lifespan and quality of life.[9] Furthermore, although medication and behavioral treatments have documented efficacy in treating tobacco dependence, it is important that these therapies be used in combination to achieve the best overall results and ensure adequate skill acquisition and treatment adherence. The promise of novel treatment and prevention interventions and the employment of personalized medicine matching the right medications to smokers with preferential responses using pharmacogenetic (e.g. polymorphisms in genes for catecholamine-*O*-methyltransferase and the nicotinic receptor subunits CHRNA3 and CHRNA4) and neuroimaging biomarkers (e.g., positron emission tomography and functional magnetic resonance imaging) are of considerable excitement for the tobacco treatment field[10] and may be realized within the next decade. Furthermore, given the high rates of tobacco use and dependence in psychiatric populations and the lower rates of quitting in this subset of smokers compared with the general population, specific adaptation of tobacco treatments to mentally ill smokers will be of paramount importance to improving prognosis and outcomes in these hard-to-treat groups of smokers.[11] Additional future challenges include developing safer and more effective smoking cessation therapies and making these therapies available to all smokers who wish to quit.

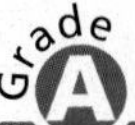

Grade A References

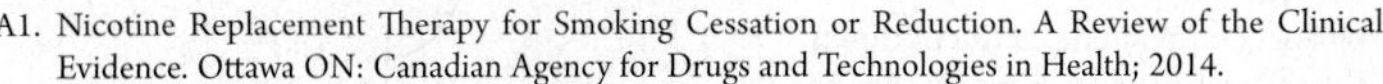

A1. Nicotine Replacement Therapy for Smoking Cessation or Reduction. A Review of the Clinical Evidence. Ottawa ON: Canadian Agency for Drugs and Technologies in Health; 2014.

A2. Bullen C, Howe C, Laugesen M, et al. Electronic cigarettes for smoking cessation: a randomized controlled trial. *Lancet*. 2013;382:1629-1637.

A3. Hughes JR, Stead LF, Hartmann-Boyce J, et al. Antidepressants for smoking cessation. *Cochrane Database Syst Rev*. 2014;1:CD000031.

A4. Hartmann-Boyce J, Stead LF, Cahill K, et al. Efficacy of interventions to combat tobacco addiction: Cochrane update of 2013 reviews. *Addiction*. 2014;109:1414-1425.

A5. Koegelenberg CF, Noor F, Bateman ED, et al. Efficacy of varenicline combined with nicotine replacement therapy vs varenicline alone for smoking cessation: a randomized clinical trial. *JAMA*. 2014;312:155-161.

A6. Rose JE, Behm FM. Combination treatment with varenicline and bupropion in an adaptive smoking cessation paradigm. *Am J Psychiatry*. 2014;171:1199-1205.

A7. Rose JE, Behm FM. Adaptive smoking cessation according to initial response to precessation nicotine patch. *Am J Psychiatry*. 2013;170:860-867.

A8. Cahill K, Stead LF, Lancaster T. Nicotine receptor partial agonists for smoking cessation. *Cochrane Database Syst Rev*. 2012;4:CD006103.

GENERAL REFERENCES

For the General References and other additional features, please visit Expert Consult at https://expertconsult.inkling.com.

33

ALCOHOL USE DISORDERS

PATRICK G. O'CONNOR

DEFINITION

A variety of terms have been used to describe the spectrum of medical, psychological, behavioral, and social problems associated with excessive consumption of alcohol (*alcohol problems*). *Alcoholism* is perhaps the most widely used term to describe patients with alcohol problems. In an attempt to define *alcoholism* more precisely, an expert panel of the National Council on Alcoholism and Drug Dependence and the American Society of Addiction Medicine developed a definition of alcoholism that included "a primary chronic disease with genetic, psychosocial and environmental factors ... often progressive and fatal ... characterized by impaired control over drinking, preoccupation with the drug alcohol, use of alcohol despite future consequences, and distortions of thinking, most notably denial." Because the term *alcoholism* is so broad, it also can be imprecise in defining the entire spectrum of alcohol problems.

Abstainers are individuals who consume no alcohol. *Moderate drinking* is defined by the National Institute on Alcohol Abuse and Alcoholism as the average number of drinks consumed daily that places an adult at low risk for alcohol problems. There is some epidemiologic evidence to suggest that moderate drinking may have some health benefits by reducing the risk for cardiovascular disease (Chapter 52). The scope of alcohol consumption that imparts this benefit may be low, however (e.g., less than one drink per day).

At-risk drinking is a level of alcohol consumption that imparts health risks (Table 33-1). This category of drinking behavior has been identified on the basis of epidemiologic evidence that certain threshold levels of alcohol consumption are associated with increased risk for specific health problems.

TABLE 33-1 TERMS AND CRITERIA FOR PATTERNS OF ALCOHOL USE

AT-RISK DRINKING
Men: >14 drinks/week or >4 drinks/day
Women: >7 drinks/week or >3 drinks/day
ALCOHOL USE DISORDER CRITERIA*
Tolerance
Withdrawal
More use than intended
Craving
Unsuccessful attempts to cut down
Excessive time acquiring alcohol
Activities given up because of use
Use despite negative effects
Failure to fulfill major role obligations
Recurrent use in hazardous situations
Continued use despite social or intrapersonal problems

*Mild = 2-3 criteria, moderate = 4-5 criteria, severe = 6 or more criteria.
(From American Psychiatric Association. *Diagnostic and Statistical Manual of Mental Disorders*. 5th ed. Arlington, VA: American Psychiatric Publishing; 2013.)

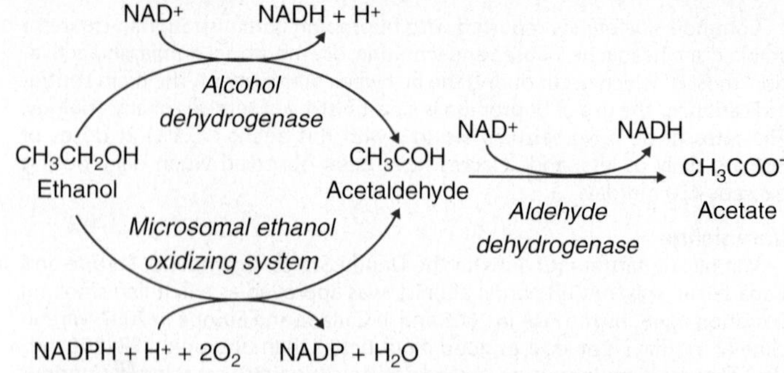

FIGURE 33-1. **Ethanol metabolism. Alcohol dehydrogenase predominates at low to moderate ethanol doses. The microsomal ethanol-oxidizing system is induced at high ethanol levels of chronic exposure and by certain drugs. Aldehyde dehydrogenase inhibition (genetic or drug induced) leads to acetaldehyde accumulation, particularly in the latter group.**

At-risk drinking is defined differently for men younger than 65 years than for women of all ages because of generally lower body weights and lower rates of metabolism of alcohol in women; the definition in men older than 65 years is the same as in women because of the age-related increased risk for alcohol problems, in part owing to changes in alcohol metabolism in older individuals. *Binge drinking* or *heavy drinking* is the episodic consumption of large amounts of alcohol, usually five or more drinks per occasion for men and four or more drinks per occasion for women. One standard drink contains 12 g of pure alcohol, an amount equivalent to that contained in 5 ounces of wine, 12 ounces of beer, or 1.5 ounces of 80-proof spirits.

The recently published *Diagnostic and Statistical Manual of Mental Disorders*, 5th edition (DSM-5) replaced the previous terminology of *alcohol abuse* and *alcohol dependence* with the term *alcohol use disorders* (see Table 33-1) in order to more clearly describe the spectrum of symptoms experienced by patients. Patients who meet 2 or 3 criteria are considered to have *mild*, 4 or 5 criteria *moderate*, and 6 to 11 criteria *severe* alcohol use disorder.[1]

EPIDEMIOLOGY

In national surveys, 52% of American adults reported that they use alcoholic beverages (liquor, wine, or beer), whereas 23% reported binge drinking, and 6.5% reported heavy drinking in the past 30 days.[2] Among individuals who use alcohol, many experience problems because of their drinking. It has been estimated that more than $100 billion is spent by American society each year to treat alcohol use disorders and to recover the costs of alcohol-related economic losses. Excessive alcohol consumption ranks as the third leading preventable cause of death in the United States after cigarette smoking and obesity. More than 100,000 deaths per year in the United States are attributed to alcohol use disorders.

Population-based epidemiologic studies have shown that alcohol use disorders are among the most prevalent medical, behavioral, or psychiatric disorders in the general population. An epidemiologic survey of the general population in the United States estimated a prevalence of alcohol abuse and dependence (using the older DSM-IV criteria) to be between 7.4 and 9.7%. The lifetime prevalence of abuse and dependence is estimated to be even higher. Despite higher thresholds and tolerance, men are at least twice as likely as women to meet criteria for alcohol abuse and dependence by standard diagnostic survey techniques. Although sociodemographic features, such as young age, low income, and low education level, have been associated with an increased risk for problem drinking, alcohol use disorders are prevalent throughout all sociodemographic groups, and all individuals should be screened carefully. The "skid row" stereotype of the alcohol-dependent patient is much more the exception than the rule.

The prevalence of alcohol use disorders is higher in most health care settings than it is in the general population because alcohol problems often result in treatment-seeking behaviors. The prevalence of problem drinking in general outpatient and inpatient medical settings has been estimated between 15 and 40%. These data strongly support the need for physicians to screen all patients for alcohol use disorders.

PATHOBIOLOGY

Beverage alcohol contains ethanol, which acts as a sedative-hypnotic drug. Alcohol is absorbed rapidly into the blood stream from the stomach and intestinal tract. Because women have lower levels of gastric alcohol dehydrogenase, the enzyme primarily responsible for metabolizing alcohol, they experience higher blood alcohol concentrations than do men who consume similar amounts of ethanol per kilogram of body weight. The absorption of alcohol can be affected by other factors, including the presence of food in the stomach and the rate of alcohol consumption. By means of metabolism in the liver, alcohol is converted to acetaldehyde and acetate (Fig. 33-1). Metabolism is proportional to an individual's body weight, but a variety of other factors can affect how alcohol is metabolized. A genetic variation in a significant proportion of the Asian population alters the structure of an aldehyde hydrogenase isoenzyme, resulting in the development of an alcohol flush reaction, which includes facial flushing, hot sensations, tachycardia, and hypotension.

In the brain, alcohol seems to affect a variety of receptors, including γ-aminobutyric acid (GABA), *N*-methyl-D-aspartate, and opioid receptors. Glycinuric and serotoninergic receptors also are thought to be involved in the interaction between alcohol and the brain. The phenomena of reinforcement and cellular adaptation are thought, at least in part, to influence alcohol-dependent behaviors. Alcohol is known to be reinforcing because withdrawal from ethanol and ingestion of ethanol itself are known to promote further alcohol consumption. After chronic exposure to alcohol, some brain neurons seem to adapt to this exposure by adjusting their response to normal stimuli. This adaptation is thought to be responsible for the phenomenon of tolerance, whereby increasing amounts of alcohol are needed over time to achieve desired effects. Although much has been learned about the variety of effects alcohol can have on various brain receptors, no single receptor site has been identified. A variety of neuropsychological disorders are seen in association with chronic ethanol use, including impaired short-term memory, cognitive dysfunction, and perceptual difficulties.

Although the brain is the primary target of alcohol's actions, a variety of other tissues have a major role in how alcohol affects the human body. Direct liver toxicity may be among the most important consequences of acute and chronic alcohol use (Chapter 152). A variety of histologic abnormalities ranging from inflammation to scarring and cirrhosis have been described. The pathophysiologic mechanism of these effects is thought to include the direct release of toxins and the formation of free radicals, which can interact negatively with liver proteins, lipids, and DNA. Alcohol also has substantial negative effects on the heart and cardiovascular system. Direct toxicity to myocardial cells frequently results in heart failure (Chapter 58), and chronic heavy alcohol consumption is considered to be a major contributor to hypertension (Chapter 67). Other organ systems that experience significant direct toxicity from alcohol include the gastrointestinal tract (esophagus, stomach), immune system (bone marrow, immune cell function), and endocrine system (pancreas, gonads).

CLINICAL MANIFESTATIONS

Alcohol has a variety of specific acute and chronic effects. The acute effects seen most commonly are alcohol intoxication and alcohol withdrawal. Chronic clinical effects of alcohol include almost every organ system.

Acute Effects

Alcohol Intoxication

After entering the blood stream, alcohol rapidly passes through the blood-brain barrier. The clinical manifestations of alcohol intoxication are related directly to the blood level of alcohol. Because of tolerance, individuals chronically exposed to alcohol generally experience less severe effects at a given blood alcohol level than do individuals who are not chronically exposed to alcohol.

The symptoms of mild alcohol intoxication in nontolerant individuals typically occur at blood alcohol levels of 20 to 100 mg/dL and include euphoria, mild muscle incoordination, and mild cognitive impairment. At higher blood alcohol levels (100 to 200 mg/dL), more substantial neurologic dysfunction occurs, including more severe mental impairment, ataxia, and prolonged reaction time. Individuals with blood alcohol levels in these ranges can be obviously intoxicated, with slurred speech and lack of coordination. These effects progress as the blood alcohol level rises to higher levels, to the point at which stupor, coma, and death can occur at levels equal to or greater than 300 to 400 mg/dL, especially in individuals who are not tolerant to the effects of alcohol. The usual cause of death in individuals with very high blood levels of alcohol is respiratory depression and hypotension.

Alcohol Withdrawal Syndrome

Alcohol withdrawal can occur when individuals decrease their alcohol use or stop using alcohol altogether. The severity of symptoms can vary greatly. Many individuals experience alcohol withdrawal without seeking medical attention, whereas others require hospitalization for severe illness. Because ethanol is a central nervous system depressant, the body's natural response to withdrawal of the substance is a hyperexcitable neurologic state. This state is thought to be the result of adaptive neurologic mechanisms being unrestrained by alcohol, with an ensuing release of a variety of neurohumoral substances, including norepinephrine. In addition, chronic exposure to alcohol results in a decrease in the number of GABA receptors and impairs their function.

The clinical manifestations of alcohol withdrawal include hyperactivity resulting in tachycardia and diaphoresis. Patients also experience tremulousness, anxiety, and insomnia. More severe alcohol withdrawal can result in nausea and vomiting, which can exacerbate metabolic disturbances. Perceptual abnormalities, including visual and auditory hallucinations and psychomotor agitation, are common manifestations of more moderate to severe alcohol withdrawal. Grand mal seizures commonly occur during alcohol withdrawal, although they do not generally require treatment beyond the acute withdrawal phase.

The time course of the alcohol withdrawal syndrome can vary within an individual and by symptom complex, and the overall duration of symptoms can be a few to several days (Fig. 33-2). Tremor is typically among the earliest symptoms and can occur within 8 hours of the last drink. Symptoms of tremulousness and motor hyperactivity typically peak within 24 to 48 hours. Although mild tremor typically involves the hands, more severe tremors can involve the entire body and greatly impair a variety of basic motor functions. Perceptual abnormalities typically begin within 24 to 36 hours after the last drink and resolve within a few days. When withdrawal seizures occur, they are typically generalized tonic-clonic seizures and most often occur within 12 to 24 hours after reduction of alcohol intake. Seizures can occur, however, at later time periods as well.

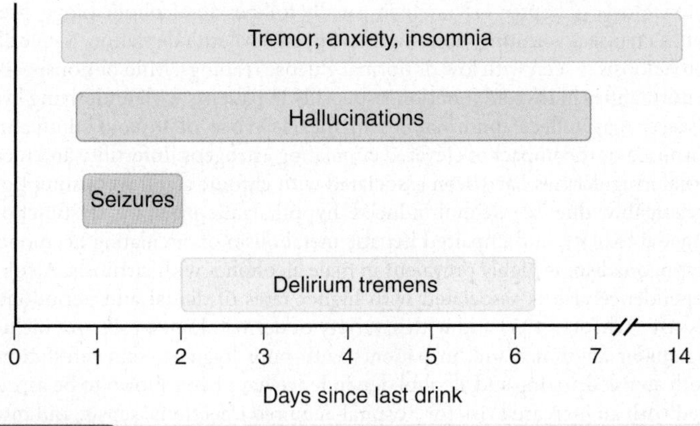

FIGURE 33-2. Time course of alcohol withdrawal.

The most severe manifestation of the alcohol withdrawal syndrome is delirium tremens. This symptom complex includes disorientation, confusion, hallucination, diaphoresis, fever, and tachycardia. Delirium tremens typically begins after 2 to 4 days of abstinence, and the most severe form can result in death.[3]

Chronic Effects

Acute manifestations, including intoxication and withdrawal, are generally stereotypical in their appearance and time course, but chronic manifestations tend to be more varied. Many patients with alcohol dependence may be without evidence of any chronic medical manifestations for many years. As time goes on, however, the likelihood that one or more of these manifestations will occur increases considerably. All major organ systems can be affected, but the primary organ systems involved are the nervous system, cardiovascular system, liver, gastrointestinal system, pancreas, hematopoietic system, and endocrine system (Table 33-2). Patients who drink are at risk for a variety of malignant neoplasms, such as head and neck, esophageal, colorectal, breast, and liver cancers (see individual chapters on those cancers). Excessive alcohol use often causes significant psychiatric and social morbidity that can be more common and more severe than the direct medical effects, especially earlier in the course of problem drinking.

Nervous System

In addition to the acute neurologic manifestations of intoxication and withdrawal, alcohol has major chronic neurologic effects. About 10 million Americans have identifiable nervous system impairment from chronic alcohol use. Individual predisposition to these disorders is highly variable and is related to genetics, environment, sociodemographic features, and gender; the relative contribution of these factors is unclear.

In the central nervous system, the major effect is cognitive impairment. Patients may present with mild to moderate short-term or long-term memory problems or may have severe dementia resembling Alzheimer disease (Chapter 402). The degree to which the direct toxic effect of alcohol is responsible for these problems or the impact of alcohol-related nutritional

TABLE 33-2 ALCOHOL-RELATED COMPLICATIONS

SYSTEM/REALM OF PROBLEM	COMPLICATIONS
Nervous system	Intoxication Withdrawal Cognitive impairment Cerebellar degeneration Peripheral neuropathy
Cardiovascular system	Cardiac arrhythmias Chronic cardiomyopathy Hypertension
Liver	Fatty liver Alcoholic hepatitis Cirrhosis
Gastrointestinal tract, esophagus	Chronic inflammation Malignant neoplasms Mallory-Weiss tears Esophageal varices
Stomach	Gastritis Peptic ulcer disease
Pancreas	Acute pancreatitis Chronic pancreatitis
Other medical problems	Cancers: mouth, oropharynx, esophagus, colorectal, breast, hepatocellular carcinoma Pneumonia Tuberculosis
Psychiatric	Depression Anxiety Suicide
Behavioral and psychosocial	Injuries Violence Crime Child or partner abuse Tobacco, other drug abuse Unemployment Legal problems

deficiencies is uncertain (Chapter 416). The deficiency of vitamins such as thiamine may plays a major role in promoting alcoholic dementia and severe cognitive dysfunction, as is seen in Wernicke encephalopathy and Korsakoff syndrome (Chapter 416). Alcohol also causes a polyneuropathy that can present with paresthesias, numbness, weakness, and chronic pain (Chapters 416 and 420). As with the central nervous system, peripheral nervous system effects are thought to be caused by a combination of the direct toxicity of alcohol and nutritional deficiencies. A small proportion (<1%) of patients with alcohol dependence may develop midline cerebellar degeneration, which presents as an unsteady gait.

Cardiovascular System

The most common cardiovascular complications of chronic alcohol consumption are cardiomyopathy, hypertension, and supraventricular arrhythmias. Alcoholic cardiomyopathy can present clinically in a manner similar to other causes of heart failure (Chapter 58). It is the most common cause of nonischemic cardiomyopathy in Western countries, accounting for about 45% of cases. Like these other causes, alcoholic cardiomyopathy also responds to conventional treatments of heart failure (Chapter 59). Abstinence from alcohol can result in significant improvement in cardiomyopathy in some patients. Increasing levels of alcohol consumption also are associated with increasing levels of systolic and diastolic hypertension (Chapter 67).

The most common arrhythmias associated with chronic alcohol use include atrial fibrillation and supraventricular tachycardia; these are seen commonly in the setting of acute intoxication and withdrawal (Chapter 64). The prevalence of alcohol-induced arrhythmias is unclear. Alcoholic cardiomyopathy also is associated with arrhythmias, in particular, ventricular arrhythmias (Chapter 65). Interestingly, the association between high levels of alcohol intake and increased cardiovascular mortality may be lessened in the presence of high physical activity.[4]

Liver

Alcohol abuse is the major cause of morbidity and mortality from liver disease in the United States. It has been estimated that there are more than 2 million people with known alcoholic liver disease in the United States. Factors that predispose to early liver disease include the quantity and duration of alcohol exposure, female gender, and malnutrition. The range of clinical manifestations includes acute fatty liver, alcoholic hepatitis, and cirrhosis (Chapter 153). Fatty liver associated with alcohol ingestion can be asymptomatic or associated with nonspecific abdominal discomfort; it generally improves with abstinence from alcohol. Alcoholic hepatitis can present as an asymptomatic condition identified through abnormalities in liver enzymes or as an acute episode with abdominal pain, nausea, vomiting, and fever. Patients with alcoholic hepatitis have particularly high levels of aspartate aminotransferase in the blood and elevated levels of γ-glutamyltransferase. Alcoholic hepatitis typically improves with abstinence from alcohol along with supportive care.

Alcohol-related cirrhosis is a major cause of death in the United States (Chapter 154). Although patients are often asymptomatic, patients with more advanced cirrhosis may present with a variety of symptoms and signs, including jaundice, ascites, and coagulopathy. Cirrhosis also is associated with gastrointestinal bleeding from esophageal varices (Chapter 138). Although there is some controversy about the use of liver transplantation to treat patients with alcoholic cirrhosis, many believe that patients in established recovery are good candidates for liver transplantation (Chapter 154). One randomized trial demonstrated that motivational enhancement therapy limited the quantity and frequency of pretransplantation alcohol consumption in patients with alcohol dependence.

Gastrointestinal Disease

Chronic alcohol use is associated with a variety of esophageal problems, including esophageal varices, Mallory-Weiss tears, and squamous cell carcinoma of the esophagus. The risk for squamous cell carcinoma is increased further in patients who smoke tobacco and drink alcohol (Chapter 192). Patients with these problems can present with difficulty swallowing, chest pain, gastrointestinal blood loss, and weight loss. Acute alcoholic gastritis typically presents with abdominal discomfort, nausea, and vomiting (Chapter 135).

Pancreas

The risk for pancreatitis in individuals with alcohol dependence is approximately four times that in the general population. Quantity and duration of alcohol exposure and a history of pancreatitis are predictive of future episodes. Acute alcoholic pancreatitis, which may present with severe abdominal pain, nausea, vomiting, fever, and hypotension, can be life-threatening (Chapter 144). Individuals who have recurrent acute pancreatitis may develop chronic pancreatitis, which typically presents with chronic abdominal pain, malabsorption, weight loss, and malnutrition.

Hematopoietic System

The anemia that commonly is seen in patients with chronic alcohol problems can be multifactorial (e.g., blood loss, nutrient deficiency, secondary to liver disease and hypersplenism). Studies of selected inpatients with alcohol dependence showed the prevalence of anemia to range from about 10 to 60%. Gastrointestinal blood loss due to Mallory-Weiss tears (Chapter 135), alcoholic gastritis (Chapter 132), or esophageal varices (Chapters 135 and 153) may be a key factor, and many patients develop subsequent iron deficiency. Dietary folate deficiency can be associated with megaloblastic anemias (Chapter 164). Alcohol also has a direct toxic effect on the bone marrow, which can lead to sideroblastic anemia that resolves after abstinence. Alcohol can suppress megakaryocyte production and cause thrombocytopenia, which may manifest as petechiae or bleeding (Chapter 172); the thrombocytopenia is particularly sensitive to abstinence, with platelet counts usually rebounding or returning to normal within 5 to 7 days after cessation of alcohol intake. Alcohol also appears to interfere directly with platelet function. Alcohol-related immune dysfunction, as evidenced by decreased production and function of white blood cells and derangement in humoral and cell-mediated immunity, partly explains why alcohol-dependent individuals are at higher risk for infectious diseases, such as pneumonia and tuberculosis.

Malignant Neoplasms

Alcohol intake has been associated with numerous cancers, including cancer of the upper digestive, respiratory, and liver malignant neoplasms. The amount of alcohol exposure that increases cancer risk may vary widely and may not correlate with what might be considered to be "safe" levels of alcohol consumption.[5] Concerning specific cancers, alcohol use is associated with squamous cell carcinomas of the esophagus (Chapter 192) and of the head and neck (Chapter 190). The co-occurrence of alcohol and tobacco abuse seems to be synergistic. Either heavy alcohol use or smoking individually increases the rate of oropharyngeal cancer by about six or seven times that of the general population, whereas the rate for people with both risk factors is about 40 times that of the general population. Patients with alcohol-induced liver disease who also have a history of hepatitis B or C are at particularly increased risk for hepatocellular carcinoma (Chapter 196).

Chronic alcohol use also has been associated with malignant neoplasms of the breast (Chapter 198), prostate (Chapter 201), pancreas (Chapter 194), cervix (Chapter 199), lung (Chapter 191), and colon (Chapter 193). Women who have more than one or two alcoholic drinks per day may increase their breast cancer risk 1.5-fold or more. Hormonal mechanisms and direct carcinogenic effects of alcohol have been postulated as causes of this association. The association of cervical cancer with alcohol dependence may be due to alcohol-associated high-risk sexual behaviors that are thought to increase the risk for cervical cancer.

Other Medical Issues

Gout has been associated with alcohol abuse, and flares can occur at lower serum urate levels than in nonalcoholic patients (Chapter 273). Alcoholic ketoacidosis (Chapter 118), which usually follows an alcoholic binge, presents as nausea, vomiting, abdominal pain, and volume depletion. Typically, ketoacidosis is seen with low or normal glucose readings. Mild or nonspecific abnormalities in thyroid function, especially in patients with underlying liver disease, may reflect abnormalities in the clearance of thyroid-stimulating hormone or the impact of elevated circulating estrogens. Infertility and menstrual irregularities have been associated with chronic alcohol consumption, presumably due to alcohol-induced hypothalamic-pituitary dysfunction, gonadal toxicity, and impaired hepatic metabolism of circulating hormones. Hypogonadism is highly prevalent in male alcoholics with cirrhosis. Alcohol dependence also is associated with higher rates of dental and periodontal disease (Chapter 425) and with a variety of dermatologic problems, including spider angiomas and, in patients with poor hygiene, skin infestations. Both at-risk drinking and alcohol dependence have been shown to be associated with an increased risk for hospital-acquired infections, sepsis, and mortality, especially in intensive care patients.

Psychiatric Issues

Psychiatric symptoms and illnesses are exceedingly common among individuals with alcohol problems. The prevalence of anxiety disorders is about 40%, and the prevalence of affective disorders is about 30%. Antisocial personality disorder is also more common in individuals with alcohol problems than in the general population. These psychiatric problems are more prevalent during periods of heavy drinking and withdrawal. All patients with alcohol use disorders require careful screening for psychiatric illnesses. Although alcohol dependence may be associated with worse outcomes in patients with common psychiatric problems such as depression and anxiety,[6] effective treatment of underlying psychiatric disorders may result in improved drinking behaviors.

Other Behavioral and Psychosocial Issues

Alcohol commonly is the underlying cause of domestic abuse, injuries, trauma, motor vehicle crashes, and burns. For example, of all substances of abuse, alcohol and cannabis appear to have the strongest association with intimate partner violence.[7] Patients presenting with injuries should be questioned carefully about their alcohol use. Tobacco use (Chapter 32) and other drug abuse (Chapter 34) are more prevalent in people with alcohol problems than in the general population.

DIAGNOSIS

Data from the history, physical examination, and laboratory generally are needed to provide a complete picture of the extent of alcohol problems in affected patients (Table 33-3).

Discussing the Diagnosis with Patients

In discussing alcohol problems, it is crucial that physicians be sensitive to the stigma and shame that may be felt by patients with alcohol problems and by their families. Alcohol-related diagnoses or problems should be discussed in a nonjudgmental manner, which forges a partnership and indicates commitment to helping with whatever problems the patients might have. Setting the stage for the discussion should include educating patients about the various levels of alcohol problems (e.g., at-risk drinking, alcohol use disorder) so that patients have an understanding of the spectrum of alcohol problems. Many patients may have a skewed view of what qualifies as problem drinking and may believe that only individuals with severe alcohol problems are truly problem drinkers. The history, physical examination, and laboratory studies should be provided as "proof" that a problem may or does exist.

TABLE 33-3 DIAGNOSIS OF ALCOHOL PROBLEMS

HISTORY

Step 1: Ask all patients about current and past use.
- Do you drink alcohol (ever or currently)?
- Do you have a family history of alcohol problems?

Step 2: Obtain detailed history regarding quantity and frequency of alcohol use.
- What types of alcohol do you consume?
- How often do you drink?
- How much do you usually drink?
- Do you ever drink more, and if so, how much?

Step 3: Standardized questionnaire
- CAGE questions:
  - Have you ever felt that you should ***c***ut down on your drinking?
  - Have people ***a***nnoyed you by criticizing your drinking?
  - Have you ever felt bad or ***g***uilty about drinking?
  - Have you ever taken a drink first thing in the morning (***e***ye opener) to steady your nerves or get rid of a hangover?

Step 4: Assess specific areas in suspected or known problem drinkers.
- Criteria for alcohol abuse and dependence
- Evidence of medical and psychiatric problems
- Evidence of behavioral or social problems
- Use of other substances
  - Tobacco
  - Mood-altering prescription drugs
  - Illicit drugs (e.g., heroin, cocaine)
  - Prior alcohol or substance abuse treatment

PHYSICAL EXAMINATION

Thorough and complete examination important in all patients
Focus attention to system with identified problems
In all patients, carefully examine:
- Central and peripheral nervous systems
- Cardiovascular system
- Liver
- Gastrointestinal tract

LABORATORY STUDIES (IN SELECTED PATIENTS)

Liver enzymes
Coagulation studies
Complete blood count
Carbohydrate-deficient transferrin

History

A four-step approach to the alcohol history includes comprehensive questions about alcohol use and a thorough evaluation for alcohol-related problems.

Step 1: Ask All Patients about Current and Past Alcohol Use

A single question—Do you currently or have you ever used alcohol?—can identify quickly patients who are not lifetime abstainers and require further screening. Patients who answer yes to this question should proceed through the subsequent three steps. Patients who answer no can be classified as lifetime abstainers from alcohol and require no further questioning unless their answer changes over time. It is crucial to ask about current and past alcohol use because many patients who meet lifetime criteria for alcohol use disorder but who are currently in recovery answer no to the question about current use; unless it is specifically asked about, important past use information may be missed.

Step 2: Obtain Detailed History Regarding Quantity and Frequency of Alcohol Use

A question to be asked routinely is, What type or types of alcoholic drinks (beer, wine, spirits) do you consume? Many patients do not consider the use of beer or wine "drinking." Quantity should be determined for typical use—How much do you usually drink on a typical drinking day?—and for range of use—Do you ever drink more than your usual amount, and if so, how much? This second question can be particularly important for identifying binge drinking. Quantity questions offer easy identification of at-risk drinking. Asking about the frequency of alcohol consumption—How often do you drink?—helps distinguish daily from nondaily alcohol users. Binge drinkers who drink only on weekends tend to have significant alcohol problems yet not be daily drinkers. A major goal of step 2 is to acquire a complete characterization of current alcohol use behaviors and the pattern of quantity and frequency of alcohol use during the patient's lifetime.

Step 3: Use Standardized Screening Instruments

Many standardized questionnaires have been developed to detect alcohol abuse and dependence. The two questionnaires that have been evaluated most extensively in medical settings are the CAGE (Cut down, Annoyed, Guilty, and Eye opener) questionnaire (see Table 33-3) and the Alcohol Use Disorder Identification Test (AUDIT). The CAGE questionnaire includes four questions and is scored by giving 1 point for each positive response. Given that the word *ever* is used in the CAGE questions, by definition this instrument is designed to detect lifetime alcohol problems and does not distinguish between lifetime problems and current problems. To screen for DSM-IV criteria alcohol abuse and dependence, the CAGE has a sensitivity of 43 to 94% and a specificity of 70 to 97% when a cutoff score of 2 is used to indicate a "positive" result. How this and other instruments relate to the new DSM-5 criteria for alcohol use disorder is the subject of ongoing inquiry.

The AUDIT's 10 questions cover the quantity and frequency of alcohol use, drinking behaviors, adverse psychological symptoms, and alcohol-related problems. The AUDIT was developed by the World Health Organization to identify hazardous (e.g., at-risk) drinking and harmful (e.g., alcohol use that results in physical or psychological harm) drinking. In contrast to the CAGE questionnaire, the AUDIT focuses on recent (current to past year) drinking behaviors. Each question is scored 0 to 4 (range for total score is 0 to 40), and a total score of 8 is considered to be a positive result.

Step 4: Assess Specific Areas in Suspected or Known Problem Drinkers

Questions asked in step 4 are based on the results of the questions asked in steps 2 and 3 to obtain more detailed information in patients with potential alcohol problems. Even patients who do not screen positive on the CAGE questionnaire may warrant detailed questioning about alcohol abuse and dependence (see Table 33-1), especially if they are drinking at or above at-risk levels or there is other evidence of possible alcohol problems. A detailed review for evidence of alcohol-related medical and psychiatric problems should occur, and the need for further medical and psychiatric evaluation should be determined. The physician should look for evidence of behavioral and social problems commonly associated with alcohol use and screen for family and occupational dysfunction and other problems, such as domestic violence. Patients should be asked about their use of tobacco, mood-altering prescription medications, and illicit drugs such as heroine and cocaine.

Finally, many patients with alcohol problems have prior treatment episodes that should be detailed. The inquiry should include questions not only about formal alcohol treatment (including number of episodes, duration of treatment, and inpatient versus outpatient treatment) but also about more informal treatments, such as attendance at self-help groups like Alcoholics Anonymous (AA). For patients who require a referral for treatment, knowledge of prior treatment experience is a crucial determinant of future referral recommendations.

The National Institute on Alcohol Abuse and Alcoholism has published *Helping Patients Who Drink Too Much: A Clinician's Guide,* which provides a similar approach to screening and evaluating patients for alcohol-related problems and includes an appendix of useful supporting materials.

Physical Examination

Patients with potential alcohol use disorders require a detailed physical examination to complement the history. In addition, attention should be focused on detecting common alcohol-related problems, including the nervous system, cardiovascular system, liver, and gastrointestinal system (see Table 33-2).

Laboratory Findings

A variety of laboratory tests have been proposed to aid screening for alcoholic abuse and dependence. Aminotransferase levels, red blood cell, mean corpuscular volume, and carbohydrate-deficient transferrin, alone or in combination, are not as effective as screening questionnaires, such as the CAGE and the AUDIT.

Laboratory tests do have a role in diagnosis and assessment of patients with potential alcohol problems. Routine laboratory testing, including liver enzymes (Chapter 147), bilirubin, complete blood count, and prothrombin time should be obtained in all patients with alcohol problems on a regular basis so that an appropriate and complete picture of the effects of alcohol on the individual can be obtained.

TABLE 33-4 ADVICE FOR PATIENTS WITH ALCOHOL PROBLEMS

State your medical concern:
Be specific about your patient's drinking patterns and related health risks.
Ask: How do you feel about your drinking?

Agree on a plan of action:
Ask: Are you ready to try to cut down or abstain?
Talk with patients who are ready to make a change in their drinking about a specific plan of action.

For patients who are not alcohol dependent:
Advise the patient to cut down if drinking is at or above at-risk drinking amounts (see Table 33-1) and there is no evidence of alcohol dependence.
Ask the patient to set a specific drinking goal: Are you ready to set a drinking goal? Some patients choose to abstain for a period of time or for good; others prefer to limit the amount they drink. What do you think will work best for you?
Provide patient education materials and tell the patient: It helps to think about your reasons for wanting to cut down and examine what situations trigger unhealthy drinking patterns. These materials will give you some useful tips on how to maintain your drinking goal.

For patients with evidence of alcohol dependence:
Advise to abstain if:
- Evidence of alcohol dependence
- History of repeated failed attempts to cut down
- Pregnant or trying to conceive
- Contraindicated medical condition or medication

Refer for additional diagnostic evaluation or treatment.
Procedures for patient in making referral decisions:
Involve your patient in making referral decisions.
Discuss available alcohol treatment services.
Schedule a referral appointment while the patient is in the office.

PREVENTION AND TREATMENT Rx

The relationship of change in alcohol use with prevention of subsequent problems has been well established. Treatment of alcohol use disorders should be based on the severity of potential or actual alcohol problems and tailored to meet the needs of individual patients. Separate advice and management approaches are suggested for nondependent at-risk or problem drinkers compared with individuals who are alcohol dependent (DSM-IV criteria) (Table 33-4). As with the screening instruments described previously, the manner in which the new DSM-5 criteria relate to specific treatment recommendations will become clearer in the near future.

Treatment of At-Risk Drinkers

Evidence confirms that generalist physicians, in a cost-effective manner, can help patients reduce their alcohol intake and prevent subsequent alcohol-related problems by using brief (5 to 20 minutes), focused counseling techniques (brief interventions) that are well suited for primary care and other medical settings.[8] More recent research has examined the use of brief interventions in more specialized settings, supporting their use in general medical inpatient settings and emergency departments.[A1] Newer approaches to decreasing alcohol use in heavy drinkers include providing personalized advice by computer[A2] and using text messaging and social media.

The brief counseling strategy includes four main components: motivational techniques, feedback about the problems with alcohol use, discussion of the adverse effects of alcohol, and setting recommended drinking limits. Motivational techniques are designed to motivate patients to change their alcohol use behavior by identifying potential or actual problems with which their alcohol use is associated. Feedback about these problems can make it clear to the patient that the problems exist. For at-risk and problem drinkers who do not meet criteria for alcohol dependence, setting recommended drinking limits below at-risk levels (e.g., less than one drink per day for women and less than two drinks per day for men) is a realistic and suitable goal. Epidemiologic evidence suggests that drinking below these levels is less likely to be associated with problems. Several randomized clinical trials confirm that patients who receive brief interventions significantly decrease their alcohol intake, often to "safe" levels, and can decrease health care use as well.

Treatment of Alcohol Use Disorders

Patients who meet criteria for an alcohol use disorder, in particular those who are dependent, usually require more intensive services than do patients who meet criteria for at-risk drinking. Most patients can be managed in outpatient treatment settings, whereas patients with a more severe alcohol use disorder or comorbid problems initially will likely require inpatient management, specific counseling programs, and pharmacologic therapy. Before entering a formal program to maintain remission, many patients first require medical management of alcohol withdrawal. Professional organizations have published practice guidelines that provide useful recommendations for how to select among treatment options for patients with alcohol dependence.

Management of Alcohol Withdrawal

Many patients may not present for medical management of alcohol withdrawal and deal with it on their own. However, a substantial subset do present for alcohol withdrawal treatment. Patients with mild to moderate withdrawal generally can be managed safely as outpatients with close follow-up. Patients with moderate to severe withdrawal, as manifested by hypertension, tremor, and any mental status changes, especially patients with significant comorbid medical or psychiatric illnesses, generally are treated best as inpatients. Patients who have a history of severe withdrawal in the past (e.g., delirium tremens) or who have a history of alcohol withdrawal seizures also generally should be managed as inpatients. The three major goals of medical management of alcohol withdrawal are to minimize the severity of withdrawal-related symptoms; to prevent specific withdrawal-related complications, such as seizures and delirium tremens; and to provide referral to relapse prevention treatment.

A wide variety of medications have been evaluated for their effectiveness in managing the alcohol withdrawal syndrome (Table 33-5). Longer-acting benzodiazepines are preferred because they provide a smoother withdrawal. Shorter-acting benzodiazepines, such as oxazepam, may be indicated in individuals with severe liver disease. The most common approach is to administer a standing dose of a benzodiazepine, with additional medication being given "as needed" on the basis of withdrawal symptoms. The specific benzodiazepine and dose often depend on the experience of the prescribing physician and the characteristics of the patient, including the severity of withdrawal (higher doses are used if withdrawal is more severe), the presence of liver disease (patients with severe liver disease should receive lower doses or shorter-acting medications), and the response to prior doses of medication (higher doses are given if symptom control is inadequate; lower doses are

TABLE 33-5 MEDICATIONS FOR THE TREATMENT OF ALCOHOL DEPENDENCE*

MEDICATION	DOSE AND ROUTE	FREQUENCY	EFFECTS	MAJOR COMMON ADVERSE EFFECTS
ALCOHOL WITHDRAWAL				
Benzodiazepines[‡]				
Chlordiazepoxide*	25-100 mg, PO/IV/IM[‡]	Every 4-6 hr	Decreased severity of withdrawal; stabilization of vital signs; prevention of seizures and delirium tremens	Confusion, oversedation, respiratory depression
Diazepam[†]	5-10 mg, PO/IV/IM[‡]	Every 6-8 hr		
Oxazepam[†]	15-30 mg, PO[‡]	Every 6-8 hr		
Lorazepam[†]	1-4 mg, PO/IV/IM[‡]	Every 4-8 hr		
β-Blockers				
Atenolol	25-50 mg, PO	Once a day	Improvement in vital signs	Bradycardia, hypotension
Propranolol	10-40 mg, PO	Every 6-8 hr	Reduction in craving	
α-Agonists				
Clonidine	0.1-0.2 mg, PO	Every 6 hr	Decreased withdrawal symptoms	Hypotension, fatigue
Antiepileptics				
Carbamazepine	200 mg, PO	Every 6-8 hr	Decreased severity of withdrawal; prevention of seizures	Dizziness, fatigue, red blood cell abnormalities
PREVENTION OF RELAPSE				
Disulfiram[†]	125-500 mg, PO	Daily	Decreased alcohol use among those who relapse	Disulfiram-alcohol reaction, rash, drowsiness, peripheral neuropathy
Naltrexone[†]	50 mg, PO 380 mg, IM	Daily Every 4 wk	Increased abstinence, decreased drinking days	Nausea, abdominal pain, myalgias-arthralgias
Acamprosate[†]	666 mg, PO	Three times a day	Increased abstinence	Diarrhea

*Most commonly used medications listed.
[†]Currently approved by U.S. Food and Drug Administration for the indication noted.
[‡]Dose and routes given for standard fixed-dose regimens, which include dose tapers over time.

given if adverse effects, such as oversedation, have occurred). In general, the amount of medication per dosing period is decreased gradually as the withdrawal syndrome abates. An individualized "symptom-triggered" dosing approach, in which benzodiazepines are administered on a dose-by-dose basis as guided by withdrawal symptoms, is safe and effective in certain patients and can reduce the total doses of benzodiazepines needed to treat withdrawal. β-Blockers (atenolol and propranolol), α-agonists (clonidine), and antiepileptics (carbamazepine) improve signs and symptoms of alcohol withdrawal but are viewed best as adjunctive medications to be used in addition to benzodiazepines.

Prevention of Relapse

Counseling Strategies Used by Alcohol Treatment Programs

Three commonly used psychotherapeutic techniques are motivational enhancement therapy, 12-step facilitation, and cognitive-behavioral coping skills. Two of these techniques are designed to give patients specific tools to help them avoid relapse to alcohol use. In motivational enhancement therapy, patients identify reasons for staying away from alcohol. The 12-step facilitation therapy uses the principles of AA to help patients focus their attention on abstinence. In cognitive-behavioral coping skills therapy, the patient identifies triggers to alcohol use and develops strategies to help deal with the triggers when they are present.

Project MATCH (Matching Alcohol Treatments to Client Heterogenicity) showed equivalence among three counseling approaches (cognitive-behavioral coping skills therapy, motivational enhancement therapy, or 12-step facilitation therapy) to treat alcohol dependence. At 1-year follow-up, most enrolled patients either remained abstinent or significantly decreased their alcohol use.

Self-Help Groups

Self-help groups such as AA and Rational Recovery are an important source of support and treatment for many patients with alcohol dependence. AA has the advantage of being widely available throughout the United States and is free of charge. The overall approach to treatment is based on the 12 steps for maintaining abstinence and dealing with the various effects of alcohol. AA meetings can be either "open" to anybody in the community or "closed" for active members only. The meetings vary in format, size, location, and demographic makeup. In counseling patients about attending AA, it is important for physicians to make them aware that variations in the nature of specific meetings, especially location and demographics of participants, require patients to be willing to attend more than one meeting site on a trial basis so that they find a comfortable setting.

Research on the effectiveness of AA has been limited, and there are no large controlled studies. Indirect evidence suggests, however, a significant improvement in alcohol use behaviors.

Pharmacotherapy to Prevent Relapse to Alcohol Use

The addition of medication to enhance the effectiveness of counseling therapies has been the subject of research for the past 40 years. As the neurobiology of alcohol use disorders has become more clearly understood, the potential to develop medications that may promote abstinence or decreased alcohol use has grown.[9,10] Three medications—disulfiram, naltrexone, and acamprosate—are approved for the treatment of alcohol dependence in the United States (see Table 33-5).

Disulfiram

Disulfiram is designed to prevent alcohol use by causing a severe adverse reaction when patients use alcohol. The disulfiram reaction, which includes flushing, nausea, vomiting, and diarrhea, is mediated by the inhibition of alcohol dehydrogenase and the resulting increase in serum levels of acetaldehyde and acetate after ingestion of alcohol (see Fig. 33-1). Disulfiram also affects monoamine metabolism, and the alcohol-disulfiram reaction may be related to changes in central monoamine functioning. Although disulfiram offers little benefit to most patients, it is effective in reducing alcohol intake in highly motivated patients who are supervised in an alcohol treatment program.

Naltrexone

Naltrexone is thought to decrease alcohol use by diminishing the euphorigenic effects of alcohol and by decreasing craving in alcohol-dependent patients. Randomized, placebo-controlled trials generally have shown that alcohol-dependent patients who receive naltrexone (50 mg/day) are more likely to decrease their alcohol use or remain abstinent compared with patients who receive placebo, and the effects persist after discontinuation of treatment, although one randomized trial did not show benefit in male veterans with severe alcohol dependence. Although most studies of naltrexone were performed in a specialty alcohol treatment setting and observed subjects for only 10 to 12 weeks, naltrexone also is effective in outpatient and primary care settings in patients who are followed for up to 34 weeks.[A3] Side effects of naltrexone are infrequent, most notably self-limited nausea in about 10% of patients. Dose-related hepatotoxicity has been reported in patients treated for obesity with high-dose naltrexone (300 mg/day). Mild liver enzyme abnormalities are not a contraindication to naltrexone, but patients should be followed with repeated liver enzyme studies. Patients with acute hepatitis or liver failure should not use naltrexone. In addition to the oral naltrexone, a newer long-acting injectable form of naltrexone was approved by the U.S. Food and Drug Administration (FDA) in 2006. Injectable naltrexone is typically administered at a dose of 380 mg intramuscularly every 4 weeks. Before beginning naltrexone, it is important to be sure that the patient is not opioid dependent in order to avoid a potentially severe opioid withdrawal reaction. Complete opioid abstinence for at least 7 to 10 days is recommended. Adverse reactions seen most commonly in patients who receive injectable naltrexone include injection site reactions (e.g., induration, itching) and symptoms such as nausea and headache, which are generally self-limited. This formulation of naltrexone may be particularly effective in those with more severe alcohol use disorders.[11]

Acamprosate

Approved by the FDA in 2004, acamprosate (calcium acetylhomotaurinate) has been identified as an effective agent for treatment of alcohol dependence. The precise mechanism of action of acamprosate is uncertain but may be related to its effects on neuroexcitatory amino acids and the inhibitory GABA system. In randomized, placebo-controlled clinical trials, subjects who received acamprosate were more likely to remain abstinent compared with subjects who received placebo.[A3] Side effects are minimal and typically include diarrhea. Like naltrexone, acamprosate is given as an adjunctive therapy to psychological treatments for alcohol dependence. Acamprosate appears to be effective in both men and women.

Other Pharmacologic Approaches to Prevent Relapse

There has been much interest in evaluation of the effectiveness of combinations of drug therapies to treat alcohol dependence. One study of 160 patients suggested that the combination of naltrexone and acamprosate was more effective than either medication alone. A larger federally funded study that enrolled 1383 subjects, Project COMBINE, examined naltrexone and acamprosate alone and in combination with two different psychological therapies to see which combination of pharmacologic and behavioral therapies is most effective. The behavioral therapies were medical management, which was designed to approximate counseling that can be provided in primary care and other medical settings, and combined behavioral intervention, which incorporated counseling techniques that are provided in alcohol treatment specialty settings. Results from this study demonstrated that patients receiving medical management with naltrexone, combined behavioral intervention, or both fared best, lending further support to the idea that alcohol-dependent patients can be effectively treated in primary care and other medical settings. Interestingly, acamprosate was not shown to be effective in this study. Gabapentin is effective as a single drug therapy for treating alcohol dependence and relapse-related symptoms, such as insomnia[A4], and the addition of gabapentin to naltrexone improves drinking outcomes in alcohol-dependent patients.[A5]

Topiramate, a fructopyranose derivative, is an effective treatment of alcohol dependence at a dose of up to 300 mg/day and is especially effective in patients with a *GRIK1* polymorphism.[12] Other medications that have shown promise include ondansetron, bromocriptine, and sodium valproate. Other drugs have shown possible benefits in patients with alcohol use disorders, perhaps more specifically those with concurrent depression (e.g., fluoxetine) or anxiety (e.g., buspirone).

PROGNOSIS

Alcohol abuse and dependence are chronic disorders that are characterized by exacerbations and remissions. The prognosis is better for patients who seek treatment and receive it in a systematic way (Table 33-6), but it can be poor for patients with advanced liver disease and continued alcohol use. In addition, the use of combinations of medications (e.g., naltrexone plus acamprosate) is under investigation.

FUTURE DIRECTIONS

To date, most studies have focused on shorter-term outcomes, from a few months to a year. It is important to understand more clearly what happens to these patients over time, especially the need for "booster sessions" to sustain improvements provided by brief interventions. Newer pharmacologic therapies may help many patients. More recently, there has been increased interest in expanding chronic care management approaches like those used in managing patients with diabetes or heart failure to patients with substance use disorders.[13] Although one large early trial failed to find a benefit, this approach may be beneficial in selected populations of patients with substance use disorders. Newer technology-based therapies, such as a smartphone application to support recovery in individuals with alcohol use disorders, hold promise for improving treatment outcomes in the future.[14]

TABLE 33-6 OVERVIEW OF TREATMENT APPROACH FOR PATIENTS WITH ALCOHOL PROBLEMS

Evaluate all patients
For patterns of problem alcohol use (Table 33-1)
For alcohol-related complications, if indicated (Table 33-2)
With use of data collected from history, physical examination, and laboratory testing (Table 33-3)
For at-risk and nondependent problem drinkers
Advise to decrease alcohol use to below at-risk levels (Table 33-4)
Advise patients who cannot decrease use to below at-risk levels to abstain
For patients who are alcohol dependent
Assess for need for withdrawal management medications (Table 33-5)
Refer to an alcohol treatment program
Consider medication to prevent relapse (Table 33-5)

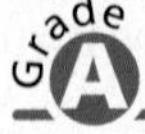

Grade A References

A1. D'Onofrio G, Fiellin DA, Pantalon MV, et al. A brief intervention reduces hazardous and harmful drinking in emergency department patients. *Ann Emerg Med*. 2012;60:181-192.

A2. Boon B, Risselada A, Huiberts A, et al. Curbing alcohol use in male adults through computer generated personalized advice: randomized controlled trial. *J Med Internet Res*. 2011;13:e43.

A3. Jonas DE, Amick HR, Feltner C, et al. Pharmacotherapy for adults with alcohol use disorders in outpatient settings: a systematic review and meta-analysis. *JAMA*. 2014;311:1889-1900.

A4. Mason BJ, Quello S, Goodell V, et al. Gabapentin treatment for alcohol dependence: a randomized clinical trial. *JAMA Intern Med*. 2014;174:70-77.

A5. Anton RF, Myrick H, Wright TM, et al. Gabapentin combined with naltrexone for the treatment of alcohol dependence. *Am J Psychiatry*. 2011;168:709-717.

GENERAL REFERENCES

For the General References and other additional features, please visit Expert Consult at https://expertconsult.inkling.com.

34 DRUGS OF ABUSE

ROGER D. WEISS

DEFINITION

The term *substance use disorder* has replaced *substance abuse* and *dependence* in the diagnostic lexicon; recent research has shown that the previous hierarchical distinction between abuse and dependence, with dependence representing a more severe form of the disorder, was problematic and not warranted. A substance use disorder is a clinical syndrome characterized by the following statement from the fifth edition of the American Psychiatric Association's *Diagnostic and Statistical Manual of Mental Disorders*: "The essential feature of a substance use disorder is a cluster of cognitive, behavioral, and physiological symptoms indicating that the individual continues using the substance despite significant substance-related problems."[1] There is no single pathognomonic symptom that is diagnostic of a substance use disorder. Rather, the syndrome is a series of 11 symptoms, of which the individual needs to meet two or more in the same 12-month period to warrant a diagnosis of a substance use disorder (Table 34-1). These 11 symptoms can be grouped into four general categories:

Impaired control: taking a substance in larger amounts or for a longer time than intended; persistent desire or unsuccessful attempts to stop or to reduce use; a great deal of time spent using a substance or recovering from the effects of its use; craving

Social impairment: failure to fulfill role obligations at home, work, or school as a result of repeated substance use; continued substance use despite experiencing interpersonal problems; or reducing or giving up important social, recreational, or occupational activities

Risky use: recurrent use in hazardous situations (e.g., driving) or despite knowledge that substance use is causing or exacerbating a physical or psychological problem

Pharmacological criteria: tolerance and physical dependence, when relevant; not all drugs cause these symptoms

For people who are prescribed medications that can cause tolerance and physical dependence, the diagnostic term *substance use disorder* should be used only with people whose medication use is problematic; tolerance and physical dependence are not considered criteria for a diagnosis of a substance use disorder in patients who are taking medications such as opioids or

TABLE 34-1 DSM-5 CRITERIA FOR SUBSTANCE USE DISORDERS

IMPAIRED CONTROL

1. Took larger amounts/for longer period of time than intended
2. Persistent desire or unsuccessful attempts to stop or reduce use
3. Much time spent using a substance or recovering from its effects
4. Craving

SOCIAL IMPAIRMENT

5. Failure to fulfill home, work, or school obligations because of repeated substance use
6. Continued use despite experiencing interpersonal problems
7. Reducing/giving up important social, recreational, or occupational activities

RISKY USE

8. Recurrent use in hazardous situations
9. Physical/psychological problems related to use

PHARMACOLOGICAL CRITERIA

10. Tolerance, when relevant*
11. Physical dependence, when relevant*

Substance use disorder is diagnosed if two or more of these 11 criteria are met within a 12-month period.

*"When relevant" indicates that these criteria are not counted, even if the symptoms are present, when an individual is using legitimately prescribed medications as intended and those medications are helping the person to function better.

From Hasin DS, O'Brien CP, Auriacombe M, et al. DSM-5 criteria for substance use disorders: recommendations and rationale. *Am J Psychiatry.* 2013;170:834-851.

sedative-hypnotics exclusively as part of appropriate medical care. If someone is using legitimately prescribed medications as intended (e.g., opioids for chronic pain or benzodiazepines for panic disorder) and those medications are helping the person to function better, that person will not meet criteria for a substance use disorder, even if the person is tolerant to the medication and is physically dependent.

EPIDEMIOLOGY

Use of illicit drugs and non-medical use of prescribed drugs are common. In 2011, approximately 22.5 million Americans reported using an illicit drug in the previous month, representing approximately 9% of the population. When asked about their substance use in the past month, 18 million people reported using marijuana, 6 million reported using potentially psychoactive prescription drugs nonmedically, 1.4 million people used cocaine, and 1 million people used hallucinogens; in fact, 10% of youths aged 12 to 17 years reported using an illicit drug in the past month. Illicit drug use is an important contributor to the global burden of disease, accounting for 20 million disability-adjusted life years in 2010. Worldwide, more people were dependent on opioids and amphetamines than other drugs.[2] Drug abuse produces substantial medical morbidity and mortality as well as tremendous social and economic costs.

PATHOBIOLOGY

Drug use disorders involve complex interactions between the pharmacology of a specific drug, an individual's genetic makeup, psychological strengths and weaknesses, environmental circumstances, and societal influences (such as physical and perceived drug availability, legal status and cost of the drug, religious and cultural mores, and presence of alternative rewarding activities). Thus, one can conceptualize the etiology of drug abuse by employing the public health model frequently cited in the study of infectious disease, that is, as an interaction among the host (i.e., the potential drug user), the agent (a specific drug in this case, as opposed to an infectious microorganism), and the environment (the person's family life and peer group and the social, cultural, and religious attitudes toward use of that substance).

The Host

A host factor that is well known to heighten vulnerability to drug abuse problems is a positive family history of a substance use disorder, which has been shown to increase the likelihood of development of both alcohol and drug dependence. Twin studies and adoption studies have shown that both genetic and environmental factors contribute to this vulnerability, although the precise nature by which this occurs is still unknown and a subject of active research. One area of great research interest relates to whether people can be vulnerable to drug dependence in general (e.g., as a result of a risk-taking temperament or poor decision making) or whether they are at high risk to abuse particular substances (perhaps because of a highly reinforcing response to a specific drug).

Psychiatric illness has been shown to influence the likelihood for development of drug abuse problems. For example, conduct disorder in childhood and adolescence and antisocial personality disorder in adulthood have both been found to predispose to subsequent drug abuse problems. Psychiatric disorders such as mood disorders are frequently noted in people with drug abuse problems. However, the presence of these two disorders in the same person does not necessarily imply causation, even if one of the disorders is manifested first.

In addition to the risk factors mentioned previously, certain individual protective factors may reduce the likelihood of a substance use disorder. Individuals who have positive familial relationships, success in academic activities, and meaningful religious affiliations have a lower likelihood for development of drug problems. The fact that many people have a mixture of risk and protective factors speaks to the complex etiologic nature of drug use disorders.

The Agent

Most drugs of abuse are inherently reinforcing; animals typically will self-administer most of the commonly abused drugs. Not all drugs are equally reinforcing in general, however, and there is a great deal of individual variation in drug preference. Some people like the stimulating effects of drugs such as cocaine and amphetamine, whereas others experience that level of stimulation as extremely uncomfortable. Some people like the relaxation induced by drugs such as marijuana and sedative-hypnotics, whereas others feel deadened and overly slowed down by these drugs. Although some people gravitate toward particular drugs of abuse because of their specific pharmacologic properties, other will use a variety of drugs indiscriminately, based on level of availability; some of these people are primarily seeking to alter their current emotional state, regardless of the direction in which it is changed. The reinforcing properties of many drugs of abuse appear to be mediated through dopaminergic pathways, although other neurotransmitters, including γ-aminobutyric acid, serotonin, and norepinephrine, are also involved in mediating drug-induced reinforcement.

The Environment

The third critical factor in the development, maintenance, and perhaps cessation of drug abuse is the environment in which the use occurs. Drug use does not occur in a vacuum. Rather, many societal factors, including legal status, availability, price, perception of dangerousness, social desirability, peer group, and religious beliefs, influence behavior relating to substance use. Drug availability is known to be a substantial influence on likelihood of substance use. For example, alcohol consumption has been shown to increase when the hours during which alcohol can be sold are extended. The restriction of alcohol availability by restricting hours of sale or by increasing its cost through taxation in turn reduces consumption. Illicit drugs are, of course, by definition less available than alcohol or tobacco. A major factor that influences use of these agents is the potential user's perception of the drug's safety, social cachet (or lack thereof), likelihood of incurring legal consequences, and peer group behavior. Treatment research has shown that environmental influences can have a powerful effect on drug use. Studies have shown, for example, that offering an alternative positive reward (e.g., a voucher that can be exchanged for desired goods and services such as movie tickets or clothes) in response to abstaining from drugs may help drug-dependent individuals overcome their severe craving and reduce their substance use. In fact, this type of treatment approach, based on the use of motivational incentives for abstinence, has been shown to be one of the most powerful treatment interventions available for the treatment of drug use disorders. The impact of environmental contingencies demonstrates the importance of appreciating the complexity of the interaction among the individual, the drug, and the environment in the determination of drug use.

CLINICAL MANIFESTATIONS

Medical Complications Related to Drug Use Disorders

Drug use disorders are associated with significant medical morbidity and sometimes with mortality. Medical complications are often directly related to the pharmacology of the abused agent, for example, the vasoconstrictor properties of cocaine; drug-specific complications are described later in the sections focusing on particular drugs of abuse.

In addition to these drug-specific sequelae, however, many medical complications incurred by patients with drug use disorders occur not as a result of the particular drug being abused. Rather, serious complications may occur as a result of three factors that cut across many of the drugs of abuse: paraphernalia, particularly unsterile needles; adulterants; and lifestyle issues.

Paraphernalia

Some of the most serious medical problems that occur in individuals with drug use disorders are a result of the route of administration rather than of the actual drug being used. The use of unsterile needles, particularly if they are shared with other drug users, can lead to a variety of localized and systemic infections, some of which can be life-threatening. Skin infections and cellulitis are relatively common among injection drug users. Systemic infections related to needle use are often serious; individuals who inject drugs may develop infective endocarditis (Chapter 76). Other relatively common infections among injection drug users include hepatitis B, hepatitis C, and HIV infection.

Adulterants

Drugs that are purchased and sold illicitly are often adulterated or "cut" with other similar-looking products, with the intention of increasing the dealer's profit margin. For example, other white powdery substances are typically added to cocaine and heroin during the dealing process to dilute their purity. Some of these adulterants can in turn cause medical problems.[3] At times, these complications occur because of the combined toxicity of the adulterant and the route of administration. Thus, for example, a patient may have granulomas in the lung or liver as a result of talc use; talc is commonly added to street heroin and can also cause difficulties in users who crush talc-containing pharmaceutical tablets (e.g., opioids) and then inject them. Other common adulterants in street drugs include quinine (frequently used with heroin) and lidocaine or levamisole (often added to cocaine), but such toxic materials as strychnine and ground glass have been found in samples of street drugs, leading to serious medical sequelae.

Lifestyle Issues

Many patients with drug use disorders expose themselves to multiple risks due to intoxication, participating in dangerous illegal activities, and associating with potentially violent people. As a result, these individuals experience a high rate of traumatic injuries and are at greater risk of being victims of assault, homicide, or suicide. Suicide is far more common among people with substance use disorders than among the general population; this may be related to a combination of the effects of acute intoxication, the high prevalence of depression among these individuals, and the higher rate of antisocial personality disorder in this population, which is associated with a propensity toward impulsiveness, risk taking, and violence. Although it is well known that intoxication can lead to motor vehicle crashes, intoxication can also serve as a risk factor for becoming a victim of someone else's vehicle; one study reported that one third of pedestrians who are killed by motor vehicles have alcohol in their blood, perhaps a reflection of the combination of risk taking, poor judgment, and impaired motor coordination that can occur during periods of intoxication.

TREATMENT Rx

General Treatment Principles

Drug use disorders represent a heterogeneous group of disorders. These are based on type of drug or drugs used; frequency and amount of use; severity of medical, behavioral, and social consequences; presence and severity of comorbid medical and psychiatric illness; and motivation to change. Treatment thus requires a careful medical and psychiatric assessment, including a detailed substance use history and laboratory testing. It is often helpful to enlist the help of a family member or significant other (with the patient's permission) in obtaining historical information. Intoxication and withdrawal syndromes need to be treated acutely; longer-term treatment involves helping the patient reduce or ideally abstain from substances of abuse and thus improve overall functioning.

Among the common drugs of abuse, medications with approval by the U.S. Food and Drug Administration (FDA) are available only for opioids and nicotine (nicotine is discussed in Chapter 32). However, researchers are actively studying a number of compounds for the treatment of other drugs of abuse, particularly stimulants and marijuana. Behavioral treatments are critically important in the treatment of substance use disorders. A number of behavioral treatments have a substantial evidence base supporting their efficacy; these include cognitive-behavioral therapy, motivational enhancement therapy, contingency management (also referred to as motivational incentive) therapy, 12-step facilitation therapy, and behavioral couples therapy. In addition to professional treatment, peer support groups such as the 12-step–oriented Alcoholics or Narcotics Anonymous and non–12-step groups such as SMART Recovery can be extremely helpful in facilitating recovery from drug abuse problems.

MAJOR DRUGS OF ABUSE

Opioids

For centuries, opioids have been a core part of the medical pharmacopoeia, primarily because of their capacity to treat pain but also because of their antitussive and antidiarrheal properties. Unfortunately, opioids are also powerful euphoriants and thus have substantial abuse liability. Although opium itself has been used for centuries, the isolation of morphine and codeine from opium in the 19th century along with the introduction of the hypodermic needle led to the increased prevalence of intravenous opioid use. Ironically, heroin was introduced near the end of the 19th century as a treatment for morphine addiction.

Opioids can be divided into four categories: natural opium alkaloids, including opium, morphine, and codeine; semisynthetic derivatives of morphine, including heroin and oxycodone; synthetic opioids that are not derived from morphine, including methadone and meperidine; and opioid-containing preparations, such as elixir of terpin hydrate.

EPIDEMIOLOGY

Opioid dependence represents a significant public health problem and accounts for more admissions for substance use disorder treatment than any substance other than alcohol. In the past two decades, there has been a shift in the epidemiology of opioid use disorders, however, with a reduction in heroin use and an increase in the abuse of opioid analgesic drugs; the latter has occurred as a result of either misuse of prescription opioids or illicit use of these agents. Approximately 620,000 people in the United States reported using heroin in 2011, with 178,000 trying the drug for the first time. During the same year, more than 11 million people either misused prescription opioids or used them illicitly, with 1.9 million doing so for the first time; opioids are currently the most commonly misused prescription drugs. Most people who use opioid analgesics in this way report that they initially obtained them from a friend or relative. It is thus likely that a portion of these people might, for example, have used a relative's opioid for the treatment of a temporary painful condition such as a migraine headache. However, the number of people seeking treatment as a result of an opioid analgesic use disorder has increased dramatically in the past decade.

PATHOBIOLOGY

Opioids are readily absorbed when they are taken orally, intranasally, or by smoking or injection. Heroin, which is almost immediately converted to morphine in the liver, is most commonly injected but may be smoked or used intranasally.

Opioids work by binding to specific opioid receptors and then exerting their activity. The major subtypes of opioid receptors have been identified and well described. Most of the commonly abused opioids bind as agonists to the μ-receptor and typically produce the effects most commonly associated with opioids: miosis, respiratory depression, analgesia, euphoria, and drowsiness. Opioids that bind to the κ-receptor, unlike μ-receptor agonists, often produce dysphoria rather than euphoria. The other two receptors, δ- and N/OFQ-receptors, do not appear to play a known significant role in opioid use disorders.

Opioid analgesics are ordinarily taken by the oral route, but they may be altered to be used through a different route of administration. This is particularly common with the extended- release preparations, which may be altered by chewing the pill (facilitating a rapid release of the opioid medication) or by crushing the pill, dissolving it in water, and then injecting it or using it intranasally.

CLINICAL MANIFESTATIONS

The initial response to the administration of heroin, particularly when it is used intravenously, is a "rush," often described as orgasmic, lasting 30 to

60 seconds. This sensation is generally followed by a profound sense of relaxation that is sometimes referred to as being "wrapped in warm cotton." During this period, the user generally feels drowsy and may be seen to be "nodding," with mental clouding and a sense of tranquility. A reduction in respiratory rate occurs, along with miosis, reduced contractility of smooth muscle, and reduced secretions in the stomach, pancreas, and biliary tract. Thus, constipation and urinary hesitancy may occur. Itching is commonly seen during opioid intoxication. Many people experience nausea and vomiting in their initial use of opioids, although tolerance tends to develop to this effect over time. Tolerance also occurs to some other effects rather quickly, particularly the analgesic, respiratory depressant, and euphoriant properties of opioids. In contrast, relatively little tolerance occurs to constipation or to pupillary constriction. It is important to be aware, then, that miosis is a manifestation of opioid use, but it is not diagnostic of opiate overuse or intoxication.[4]

Physical Dependence

Physical dependence on opioids leads to a characteristic withdrawal syndrome, the key signs of which include elevated heart rate and blood pressure, mydriasis, abdominal cramps, sweating, gooseflesh, rhinorrhea, lacrimation, and gastrointestinal distress, particularly diarrhea, nausea, and vomiting. Insomnia is common, particularly difficulty in falling asleep; this is often the most long-lasting complaint among people who experience opioid withdrawal. Yawning, muscle twitches, and difficulty with body temperature regulation are also commonly seen. The severity of withdrawal can be highly variable, depending on the dose of opioids taken, the length of time that they have been taken, and individual factors. For short-acting opioids such as heroin and hydrocodone, the earliest stages of withdrawal typically occur approximately 6 to 12 hours after the last use. Peak symptoms tend to occur 48 to 72 hours after the last dose, and most clinical symptoms usually resolve within 7 to 10 days. For longer-acting opioids such as methadone, each of these time periods associated with withdrawal from short-acting opioids should be approximately doubled or tripled.

Other Medical Complications

The most common serious medical complications that occur from opioid use are typically related to factors other than the opioids themselves, particularly needle use and adulterants; these were discussed previously. Common medical problems among heroin users include hepatitis B, hepatitis C, infective endocarditis, talc granulomatosis, HIV infection, cellulitis, and abscesses, all typically related to needle use.

An important noninfectious complication that has been reported with opioid use disorders is alteration of the cardiac conduction system, with a prolongation of the QT interval; this can lead to potentially serious arrhythmias, including torsades de pointes. This complication has been particularly noted with methadone.

Chronic pain is commonly seen among individuals with opioid use disorders, not just those who have received opioids for the treatment of pain. Pain can occur in these individuals for numerous reasons. In addition to the possibility that a chronic painful condition led to the use of opioids in the first place, those dependent on opioids are more likely to experience accidents, violence, and other forms of physical trauma that could produce chronic pain. There is also some evidence that chronic opioid use may lead to hyperalgesia, although there is some controversy regarding this issue. As with all substance use disorders, psychiatric illnesses (particularly mood disorders) are more common in those with opioid use disorders than in the general population. Moreover, the use of multiple drugs is common in patients with opioid use disorders, particularly among those using heroin. Indeed, the use of more than one drug is typically the rule rather than the exception in most substance use disorders.

TREATMENT Rx

Opioid Withdrawal

Opioid detoxification can be accomplished by switching patients from their current drug of abuse (e.g., heroin, hydrocodone) to methadone or buprenorphine and then tapering that medication. Although the details of accomplishing this vary, one method commonly used in hospital settings is to administer methadone 10 mg orally whenever a patient experiences objective signs of opioid withdrawal (e.g., mydriasis, tachycardia, hypertension, and sweating). This process can be repeated every 2 to 4 hours for 24 hours after the initial dose; the total amount of methadone given in that 24-hour period is the "stabilization dose," which should not ordinarily exceed 40 mg. The stabilization dose is then reduced by 5 mg a day until the detoxification is completed.

Buprenorphine can also be used successfully for opioid detoxification[A1]; patients who demonstrate objective signs of opioid withdrawal (often measured with a standardized withdrawal severity scale) can be stabilized with buprenorphine during a 1- to 2-day period; the subsequent taper from buprenorphine may occur either right away or after a period of stabilization with buprenorphine. The dose of buprenorphine will depend on whether the medication will be used for a brief, several-day detoxification or for longer-term stabilization or maintenance treatment.

Longer-Term Opioid Dependence Treatment

Three effective medications are approved by the FDA for the treatment of opioid dependence: methadone (a full opioid agonist), buprenorphine (a partial agonist), and naltrexone (an opioid antagonist). Methadone has been used successfully for both detoxification from opioids and maintenance treatment for many years.[A2] Unlike buprenorphine and naltrexone, which can be prescribed by physicians in their offices (although physicians wishing to prescribe buprenorphine for the treatment of opioid dependence must receive specialized training and certification to do so), methadone is available for the treatment of opioid dependence only in specially licensed treatment programs. Methadone is a long-acting μ-receptor agonist with a slow onset of peak effects (typically approximately 2 to 6 hours) and a slow offset of action, allowing for once-a-day administration. Methadone reduces opioid craving and induces cross-tolerance, thus blocking or attenuating the effects of other opioid use. Although the therapeutic dose of methadone for a particular individual may vary, doses of 60 mg or higher have typically been shown to be more effective than lower doses; there is some evidence that even higher doses (e.g., 80 mg a day or more) may be more effective than 60 mg. Methadone treatment has been shown to reduce opioid use, to increase employment, to decrease criminal behavior, and to reduce the rate of development of HIV infection.

When a patient enrolled in a methadone treatment program experiences pain (e.g., postoperatively) requiring opioid analgesia, the patient should continue to receive the baseline methadone maintenance treatment dose for the addiction and should receive a different opioid for treatment of the pain (Chapter 30); before administering methadone, it is a good idea to confirm the methadone dose with the patient's treatment program. The fact that the patient is receiving methadone every day does not obviate the need for opioid analgesia, however. In fact, many patients receiving methadone treatment for opioid dependence will require a dose of opioids that is relatively high as a result of cross-tolerance to other opioid drugs.

The Drug Addiction Act of 2000 revolutionized the treatment of opioid dependence by enabling the approval of the partial opioid agonist buprenorphine for the treatment of opioid dependence and allowing treatment with buprenorphine to be administered in physicians' offices rather than exclusively in specialized opioid treatment programs. To prescribe buprenorphine, physicians must apply to the Substance Abuse and Mental Health Services Administration for a waiver that allows them to prescribe buprenorphine, after taking an 8-hour training course on buprenorphine. At the time of this writing, physicians may treat up to 100 patients with buprenorphine in their office practice. Buprenorphine, a partial μ-agonist and κ-antagonist, has a more favorable safety profile than methadone because of its partial agonist properties. Respiratory depression, which can be induced by full agonists and is responsible for some overdose deaths, is far less likely to occur with buprenorphine because its partial agonist properties cause a plateau of opioid effects as the dose increases. Buprenorphine is administered sublingually, in either tablet or film form, for the treatment of opioid dependence either as buprenorphine alone (sometimes referred to as the "mono" product) or (more commonly, in the United States) as a combination product of buprenorphine and naloxone; the naloxone is added to discourage users from dissolving and injecting the medication because the naloxone in the combination product will precipitate withdrawal when it is injected. Buprenorphine has been shown to be effective for both opioid detoxification and maintenance treatment. Randomized trials have shown that extended treatment with buprenorphine-naloxone has produced far better outcomes compared with short-term detoxification in opioid-addicted youths aged 15 to 21 years.[A3] Typical doses of 12 to 16 mg of sublingual buprenorphine per day appear to be as effective as methadone in doses up to approximately 60 mg a day. Buprenorphine is also effective for maintenance therapy of heroin addiction[A4], but individuals who require much higher doses of methadone may respond better to that agent than to buprenorphine.[A5] To address problems with adherence, diversion, and nonmedical use, an implantable formulation of buprenorphine has been developed that provides a low, steady level of the drug during 6 months.[A6]

Naltrexone, a pure opioid antagonist, blocks the effects (including euphoria) of opioids. As a result, individuals taking naltrexone should have a reduced desire to use opioids because they will have no desired effect. When it is used orally (50 mg/day) or in its long-acting form (380 mg intramuscularly every 4 weeks), naltrexone is highly effective at suppressing illicit opioid use. A randomized clinical trial in prescription opioid-dependent outpatients has also demonstrated the effectiveness of naltrexone maintenance after buprenorphine taper.[A7] However, naltrexone has traditionally suffered from low acceptability; few patients have been interested in being treated with oral naltrexone. Moreover, among those who initially accept this treatment, the dropout rate is extremely high. An advantage of extended-release injectable naltrexone is that it can mitigate the traditionally poor adherence associated with the oral formulation[A8]; naltrexone can be a useful medication for patients who are willing (either as the result of external pressure or for internal motivation) to use it.

Methadone, buprenorphine, and naltrexone are not designed to be delivered alone but should be given in conjunction with counseling to be effective. It has been well demonstrated that the administration of methadone in the absence of counseling is an inadequate treatment approach; less is known about the optimal combination of buprenorphine and counseling. Two studies have demonstrated that counseling delivered within a medical office setting can be effective in conjunction with buprenorphine treatment, suggesting that general physicians who are trained to use buprenorphine can effectively treat at least a portion of patients with opioid dependence in their offices with a combination of buprenorphine and counseling.

Central Nervous System Stimulants: Cocaine and Amphetamines

The two most important central nervous system stimulants, cocaine and amphetamine (including methamphetamine[5]), are derived from different sources; cocaine is extracted from coca leaves, whereas amphetamine is a synthetic compound. However, both induce similar psychoactive activity when they are taken illicitly and can produce similar adverse consequences. Amphetamine has been used over the years to treat obesity and to combat fatigue and depression. Cocaine is still used as a topical anesthetic for otolaryngologic surgery. Ironically, its vasoconstrictor action, which is responsible for many of the cocaine-related medical complications described later, can be valuable for surgeons because of the resultant reduction of blood flow in the operating field. Although cocaine was not extracted from the coca leaf until the 19th century, coca leaves have been chewed for more than 1500 years for medicinal and religious purposes as well as to combat work-related fatigue. Sigmund Freud was one of the foremost advocates of cocaine, both extolling its psychoactive properties and discovering its ability to relieve pain, thus eventually leading to its discovery as the first local anesthetic. Cocaine was seen in the late 19th century as a "cure-all" and was included in numerous patent medicines as well as in Coca-Cola. The Harrison Narcotic Act of 1914 restricted the use of cocaine, and the drug was not widely used until the late 1970s, when there was a resurgence in cocaine use in the United States.

Like cocaine,[6] amphetamine was synthesized for the first time in the late 19th century. It was used for clinical purposes for the first time in the 1920s. Reports of amphetamine abuse first occurred in the 1930s, with intermittent epidemics since that time. In recent years, methamphetamine[5] abuse has been particularly prevalent and worrisome in the United States, with particularly high concentration of its use in the Midwestern and Western states, including Hawaii.

Cocaine can be used intranasally, by intravenous injection, or by smoking. Cocaine hydrochloride, which is the form of the drug used in medical therapeutics, is a water-soluble compound that can be used intranasally ("snorted") or injected. Adding an alkaline compound such as baking soda to an aqueous solution of cocaine hydrochloride produces a rocklike compound known as crack, which can be smoked. Smoking cocaine produces the most rapid onset of intoxication (6 to 10 seconds) and the shortest period of drug effect (10 to 15 minutes). Methamphetamine can also be used in multiple ways—orally, by smoking, or intravenously. Methamphetamine effects last much longer than those produced by cocaine; psychiatric symptoms such as paranoia that typically last only a matter of hours in cocaine users may persist for days to weeks after methamphetamine use and occasionally may result in a chronic psychotic state.

EPIDEMIOLOGY

Approximately 37 million Americans have used cocaine during their lifetime. In 2011, just less than 4 million people used cocaine; 1.4 million people, or 0.5% of the population, reported using cocaine in the past month. Of these past-month cocaine users, 17% (228,000) used crack, a decrease from 2010. Cocaine had the third highest rate of drug abuse or dependence in 2011 and was the third most common drug (behind opioids and cannabis) associated with a recent treatment episode; cocaine is also the drug of abuse most commonly involved in emergency department visits.

Other stimulant use is less common; approximately 20 million Americans have used stimulants nonmedically during their lifetime, with 12 million methamphetamine users. Methamphetamine use in the past month is reported by more than 400,000 people in the United States.

PATHOBIOLOGY

Both cocaine and amphetamine increase the accumulation and activity of specific neurotransmitters in the synaptic cleft, including dopamine, norepinephrine, and serotonin. Cocaine is believed to exert this effect by binding to the dopamine transporter. Increased dopaminergic activity, particularly in the nucleus accumbens, is thought to be responsible for the reinforcing effects of cocaine. Amphetamines appear to increase the level of dopamine in the synaptic cleft primarily by stimulating presynaptic dopamine release as opposed to reuptake blockade.

CLINICAL MANIFESTATIONS

Both cocaine and amphetamines reliably produce euphoria, wakefulness, a sense of initiative, increased self-confidence (sometimes to the point of grandiosity), and, in some instances, sexual stimulation. With higher doses, users may feel "wired," a syndrome characterized by anxiety, irritability, and perhaps paranoia. Withdrawal from either of these agents leads to opposite effects from those of intoxication: increased appetite, hypersomnia, and depression, which can occasionally be serious. Medical complications related to cocaine use[6] are related to a combination of cocaine's stimulant activity (increased heart rate and blood pressure) and its vasoconstrictor properties. Local complications that result from the drug's vasoconstrictor activity include ulcerations of the nasal mucosa, perforation of the nasal septum, and decreased pulmonary diffusion capacity. Systemic complications include myocardial infarction, intracranial hemorrhage, grand mal seizures (as a result of intoxication, not withdrawal), and ventricular tachyarrhythmias, which may be responsible for sudden death. Physicians seeing a patient in an emergency department for an unexplained seizure should consider drug abuse as a potential cause. (Not only cocaine but also phencyclidine and meperidine intoxication may lead to seizures, as can sedative-hypnotic or alcohol withdrawal). A serum or urine toxicology screen may thus be an important diagnostic tool in such a situation.

TREATMENT Rx

The treatment of stimulant use disorders primarily consists of behavioral therapies, including individual and group therapy, and self-help groups. Specific forms of treatment, such as cognitive-behavioral therapy, individual drug counseling by a 12-step–oriented disease model, and a behavioral treatment in which patients are reinforced for positive outcomes (e.g., drug-free urine screens), have been found to be successful. A great deal of research has been conducted in search of an effective pharmacotherapeutic treatment for stimulant dependence, but there is as yet no medication that has consistently been found to be effective enough to warrant approval by the FDA for this purpose.

Sedative-Hypnotic and Anxiolytic Drugs

Benzodiazepines and other sedative-hypnotic and anxiolytic medications such as barbiturates and zolpidem are frequently prescribed for the treatment of anxiety and sleep difficulties. Although different classifications of these drugs have very different chemical structures, they are grouped together according to their therapeutic applications. Most of these drugs act at the γ-aminobutyric acid type A receptor and can cause physical dependence and both dispositional and pharmacodynamic tolerance.

Because the benzodiazepines are far and away the most commonly prescribed sedative-hypnotics, they are also the most widely abused. There are two major patterns of benzodiazepine abuse. Many people who ultimately abuse these medications have initially received a legitimate benzodiazepine prescription for the treatment of anxiety or insomnia. However, a combination of tolerance and decreased effectiveness of the agent over time may lead some people to increase the dose on their own. In such circumstances, attempts by the physician to taper the person off of the medication can be very difficult.

A second pattern of benzodiazepine abuse occurs among individuals who are using other drugs of abuse, most commonly opioids or stimulants. For example, many individuals who are dependent on heroin or other opioids may use benzodiazepines as a means of either enhancing the opioid effect or buffering symptoms of opioid withdrawal. Such individuals typically use relatively large doses of benzodiazepines intermittently, and therefore many of these patients do not develop physical dependence on benzodiazepines, unlike the first category of patients, for whom physical dependence is common.

TREATMENT

Rx

The treatment of people who are abusing benzodiazepines depends to some extent on the pattern of abuse. For individuals who have an anxiety disorder and have been misusing a legitimately prescribed medication, a common approach would be to taper the benzodiazepine and to institute a different type of treatment, such as an antidepressant along with cognitive-behavioral therapy. Tapering a benzodiazepine that a person has been taking for an extended time (sometimes many years) is often a slow process, with careful monitoring of withdrawal symptoms (anxiety, agitation, insomnia, tachycardia, palpitations). Because benzodiazepine withdrawal, like alcohol withdrawal, can precipitate a seizure, gradual withdrawal is preferred. Most patients tolerate a benzodiazepine dose reduction initially with relatively little difficulty. However, as with most drug withdrawal regimens, people experience their greatest discomfort toward the end of the taper. One reason for this is that the percentage dose reduction at the low end of a taper regimen continues to increase over time; a reduction from 2 mg to 1.5 mg of clonazepam, for instance, is a 25% reduction, whereas the same half-milligram dose reduction from 1 mg to 0.5 mg represents a 50% drop.

For patients who are abusing benzodiazepines as part of a pattern of multiple substance use, medical detoxification from the benzodiazepine itself will often be unnecessary; for this population, psychosocial approaches that advocate abstinence from all substances of abuse, in conjunction with appropriate pharmacotherapy as needed (e.g., in the case of opioid dependence), are preferred. However, some deaths have been reported in France and elsewhere as a result of combinations of buprenorphine and benzodiazepines, usually used parenterally. Thus, physicians who are treating patients who are abusing both opioids and benzodiazepines need to be mindful of this issue when considering the use of buprenorphine.

Marijuana

Marijuana, which refers to the dried leaves and flowers of the plant *Cannabis sativa*, has been used for its psychoactive and medicinal properties for centuries. The major psychoactive substance in marijuana is Δ^9-tetrahydrocannabinol (THC); the concentration of THC has increased from 1 to 3% in 1970 to nearly 10% in recent years.

EPIDEMIOLOGY

Marijuana is the most commonly used illicit drug in the United States; more than 120 million Americans have used marijuana, and approximately 22 million report that they have used marijuana in the past month. With the recent trend toward legalization of medical marijuana and outright legalization of marijuana in some states, those numbers will likely continue to increase.

PATHOBIOLOGY

Marijuana and other cannabinoids such as hashish (dried cannabis resin) exert their effects by binding to the cannabinoid receptors, of which two are currently known. Binding to the CB1 receptor, which is located primarily in the brain, appears to be responsible for the psychoactive effects of THC, whereas the CB_2 receptor may be associated with immune system responses.

CLINICAL MANIFESTATIONS

When marijuana is smoked, its psychoactive effects occur almost immediately, with peak intensity approximately 30 minutes later; effects tend to disappear within 3 hours. Oral administration of marijuana leads to a delayed onset of action, but the effects of the drug persist for a longer time. Because THC is highly soluble in lipids, it can be stored in fat depots of regular users for several weeks, sometimes longer, with resultant positive urine test results for THC. Physiologic effects of marijuana intoxication include increased heart rate and conjunctival injection. Psychological effects include a sense of euphoria and well-being, friendliness, increased appetite, a distorted sense of time, impaired short-term memory, and sometimes a feeling of having achieved special insights. Cannabis has the capacity to cause tolerance in regular users, and some regular heavy users experience withdrawal symptoms on cessation of use, including irritability, difficulty in sleeping, and anxiety.[7]

TREATMENT

Rx

The most common acute adverse event that occurs in marijuana smokers is a sense of acute panic, most common in inexperienced smokers, when the user's level of intoxication is greater than expected and the individual feels out of control. This can be best managed with reassurance that the effects will go away as the drug wears off. Recent evidence has shown that cannabis use, particularly during adolescence, may increase the likelihood for development of a psychotic disorder such as schizophrenia later in life.

Compared with alcohol, opioids, and stimulants, it has been relatively uncommon for people to seek treatment of cannabis use disorder itself. However, that situation has gradually changed in recent years, and an increasing number of people have sought treatment because of difficulty in stopping marijuana use. There are no medications approved by the FDA for the treatment of cannabis use disorder. Psychosocial approaches similar to the treatment of other substance use disorders are currently the treatment of choice.

Hallucinogens

Hallucinogens are a group of plant-based and synthetic drugs that lead to primarily visual perceptual alterations, such as illusions and hallucinations, along with an alteration in the experience of external stimuli; ordinary events can appear profound to people while they are under the influence of these agents. The most common hallucinogens are lysergic acid diethylamide (LSD), mescaline, and psilocybin. Methylene dioxymethamphetamine (MDMA), also known as ecstasy, has both mild stimulant and potentially hallucinogenic properties and is thus sometimes categorized with the hallucinogens and sometimes as a stimulant.

EPIDEMIOLOGY

Approximately 1 million people in the United States report having used a hallucinogen in the previous month; approximately 36 million people have used these drugs during their lifetime. LSD is the most commonly used hallucinogen, with 23 million lifetime users in the United States; approximately 60% of that number have used MDMA.

PATHOBIOLOGY

LSD is thought to exert its action through serotonin agonist activity, particularly at the 5-HT_{2A} receptor. Other neurotransmitters may be involved in hallucinogenic activity as well. Hallucinogens can produce tolerance in a matter of days, but they do not produce physical dependence.

CLINICAL MANIFESTATIONS

In addition to their effects on perception and behavior, hallucinogens can produce sympathomimetic effects such as tachycardia, increased blood pressure and body temperature, and pupillary dilation. Hyperreflexia and muscle weakness can also be seen. The most commonly seen medical consequence of hallucinogen use is hyperthermia, which can occur most commonly in users of MDMA.

The most common acute psychological adverse event, similar to marijuana, is a feeling of panic over the sense of loss of control that a person may feel as a result of intoxication; as is the case with marijuana, this is most likely to occur in inexperienced users. Some hallucinogen users will develop psychotic symptoms that fail to remit after the drug has worn off. Some hallucinogen use can also lead to longer-term perceptual difficulties. When these occur, a spontaneous return of very brief hallucinogen-induced symptoms long after the drug has worn off is known as a flashback. People who have perceptual difficulties that are much more pervasive may be said to have *hallucinogen persisting perception disorder*, which can at times be quite disabling.

TREATMENT

Symptomatic treatment is focused on the specific adverse medical and psychiatric sequelae described previously. If a psychotic episode that occurs after use of a hallucinogen persisted over time, it would be treated like any other psychotic disorder. There is no specific treatment for hallucinogen use disorder, and it is uncommon for people to seek treatment specifically because they want to stop using hallucinogens.

Phencyclidine

Phencyclidine (PCP) was originally developed as a human general anesthetic, but its use for that purpose was stopped in the 1960s because it frequently led to psychosis and hallucinations in the postoperative period. Approximately 120,000 individuals report that they used PCP during 2011. Low doses of PCP can lead to symptoms that resemble alcohol intoxication, with slurred speech, ataxia, and a subjective feeling sometimes described as "feeling dead." PCP intoxication typically is accompanied by increased muscle tone, hyperreflexia, nystagmus, and ataxia.

When it is taken in high doses, PCP can have serious medical and psychiatric consequences. High-dose users may experience psychosis, catatonia, and extremely violent behavior. Medical sequelae of PCP intoxication can include muscle rigidity, seizures, hyperthermia, coma, and occasionally death.

Anabolic-Androgenic Steroids

Anabolic-androgenic steroids differ from other drugs described in this chapter because the motivation for use is typically related to the drug's physical rather than behavioral effects. Anabolic-androgenic steroids such as testosterone and its synthetic analogues have traditionally been used primarily to enhance strength and thus athletic performance, although in recent years, an increasing number of people have used these drugs primarily in an attempt to improve their physical appearance. Anabolic-androgenic steroids can have a legitimate medical purpose; they have most commonly been used to treat testosterone deficiency in men and more recently have been used to treat wasting syndromes in patients with AIDS.

Abuse of anabolic-androgenic steroids can cause a number of medical and psychiatric problems, including hypertension, elevated low-density lipoprotein cholesterol, cardiomyopathy, hepatotoxicity, acne, feminization (gynecomastia and reduced testicular size) in men, and masculinization (hirsutism, reduction in breast tissue, deeper voice) in women. Behavioral effects include aggressiveness (sometimes leading to violence) and an increased prevalence of mood disorders. There is no specific treatment to help people abusing anabolic steroids to stop. Rather, behavioral treatment approaches that are commonly used to treat other substance use disorders should be employed with this population.

CONCLUSIONS AND FUTURE DIRECTIONS

The ever-changing epidemiology of drug abuse means that the next decade will likely present new challenges as new drugs of abuse become increasingly popular. Recent research has focused on development and testing of effective pharmacologic and behavioral treatments for substance use disorders. Screening for these disorders in general medical practice and combining office-based interventions with referrals to specialty substance use disorder treatment as indicated can lead to successful outcomes for many of these patients.

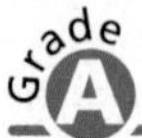

Grade A References

A1. Gowing L, Ali R, White JM. Buprenorphine for the management of opioid withdrawal. *Cochrane Database Syst Rev*. 2009;3:CD002025.

A2. Mattick RP, Breen C, Kimber J, et al. Methadone maintenance therapy versus no opioid replacement therapy for opioid dependence. *Cochrane Database Syst Rev*. 2009;3:CD002209.

A3. Minozzi S, Amato L, Bellisario C, et al. Maintenance treatments for opiate-dependent adolescents. *Cochrane Database Syst Rev*. 2014;6:CD007210.

A4. Mattick RP, Breen C, Kimber J, et al. Buprenorphine maintenance versus placebo or methadone maintenance for opioid dependence. *Cochrane Database Syst Rev*. 2014;2:CD002207.

A5. Weiss RD, Potter JS, Fiellin DA, et al. Adjunctive counseling during brief and extended buprenorphine-naloxone treatment for prescription opioid dependence a 2-phase randomized controlled trial. *Arch Gen Psychiatry*. 2011;68:1238-1246.

A6. Ling W, Casadonte P, Bigelow G, et al. Buprenorphine implants for treatment of opioid dependence: a randomized controlled trial. *JAMA*. 2010;304:1576-1583.

A7. Sigmon SC, Dunn KE, Saulsgiver K, et al. A randomized, double-blind evaluation of buprenorphine taper duration in primary prescription opioid abusers. *JAMA Psychiatry*. 2013;70:1347-1354.

A8. Krupitsky E, Nunes EV, Ling W, et al. Injectable extended-release naltrexone for opioid dependence: a double-blind, placebo-controlled, multicentre randomised trial. *Lancet*. 2011;377:1506-1513.

GENERAL REFERENCES

For the General References and other additional features, please visit Expert Consult at https://expertconsult.inkling.com.

35

IMMUNOSUPPRESSING DRUGS INCLUDING CORTICOSTEROIDS

GRANT W. CANNON

IMMUNOSUPPRESSIVE DRUGS

The immune response is an essential host defense mechanism to control and fight infection. The ability to suppress immune reactions is a critical component in autoimmune disease treatment and transplantation management. During autoimmune diseases, the basic immune physiology is altered, and one or more components of this process do not function properly. Current challenges with the selection, dosing, monitoring, and development of immunosuppressing drugs involve identifying the component of the immune system to be altered by the immunosuppressive therapy while at the same time maintaining a competent immune response to fight infection and perform other important immunoregulatory functions. After organ transplantation, most patients have an immune response to reject the organ that has been implanted. Immunosuppression during transplantation management, in contrast to autoimmune disease, involves the suppression of normal immune reactions rather than an effort to alter a pathologic process. In this latter case, immunosuppressive therapy is directed to act on the altered immune system. Suppression of natural host immune responses affects the ability of these protective mechanisms to fight infection. The general principles for selecting immunosuppressive therapy in transplantation patients involve specific monitoring for organ rejection with subsequent selection of immunosuppressive therapy proportionate to the degree of rejection or for maintaining tolerance to the implanted organ. The selection of the most effective therapy requires an individualized treatment program. These decisions require an understanding of the underlying pathophysiologic process, prognosis, and potential adverse events for the agents selected.

This chapter describes the mechanism of action—including the components of the immune response affected by the therapy, indications, and adverse events associated with commonly used immunosuppressive agents in autoimmune diseases and transplantation. Whereas each of these agents has an individual discussion, these drugs are frequently used in combination as their complementary effects are employed. The understanding of the principles and adverse events associated with immunosuppressive therapy is important for all physicians as the use of these drugs becomes more widespread; however, their specific management and initiation, particularly in patients with organ transplantation and severe autoimmune diseases, should generally be limited to specialists with specific training in immunosuppressive therapies.

Corticosteroids

Corticosteroids are highly effective immunosuppressive agents and have had a major impact on the treatment of autoimmune diseases and the effort to avoid rejection of transplants. Historically,[1] the initial enthusiasm for the marked clinical benefit of corticosteroids in the treatment of rheumatoid arthritis was dampened by the significant adverse events that developed after prolonged use. As opposed to many adverse events that may develop as allergic and idiosyncratic reactions to medications, most adverse events with corticosteroid therapy are a direct consequence of the physiologic effects of the drug. This observation sparked a determined effort to understand the mechanisms of actions of corticosteroids at physiologic levels and therapeutic doses. The objectives of these investigations have been to develop modifications of the naturally occurring hormones to exploit the clinical benefits provided by corticosteroids while avoiding the associated adverse effects.

Mechanism of Action

Corticosteroids affect multiple physiologic functions at the molecular, cellular, and organ level. The final result of corticosteroid treatment represents the composite effects of the drug on these multiple functions, which vary with the particular agent, dose, route, and duration of treatment[2] (Table 35-1).

TABLE 35-1 CLASSIFICATION OF IMMUNOSUPPRESSIVE AGENTS

CORTICOSTEROIDS

Binding to cytosol glucocorticoid receptor: results in suppression of pro-inflammatory cytokines (genomic effects)
Inhibition of arachidonic acid release and binding to surface receptor (nongenomic effects)
Results of corticosteroid actions
- Leukocyte numbers
  - Increase in circulating neutrophils
  - Decrease in circulating lymphocytes, monocytes, eosinophils, and basophils
- Leukocyte function
  - Neutrophils: decrease in trafficking
  - Lymphocytes: decrease in cellular immune functions and immunoglobulin production
- Cytokines
  - Decrease in pro-inflammatory cytokines: IL-1, IL-2, IL-6, and tumor necrosis factor-α
  - Increase in anti-inflammatory cytokines: IL-4, IL-10, and IL-13
- Prostaglandins and leukotrienes: decreased production

PURINE PATHWAY INHIBITORS

Azathioprine: inhibition of DNA synthesis and purine synthesis
Mycophenolate mofetil: inhibition of purine synthesis

PYRIMIDINE PATHWAY INHIBITORS

Leflunomide: inhibits pyrimidine synthesis by inhibiting dihydroorotate dehydrogenase

IMMUNOPHILIN-BINDING AGENTS

Calcineurin inhibition
- Cyclosporine: binds with cyclophilin to inhibit calcineurin, resulting in decreased T-cell activation
- Tacrolimus: binds with FKBP12 to inhibit calcineurin, resulting in decreased T-cell activation

Mammalian target of rapamycin (mTOR) inhibition
- Sirolimus: binds to FKBP12 to inhibit mTOR, resulting in decreased T-cell activation

ALKYLATING AGENTS

Cyclophosphamide: alkylation of nucleic acids with cytotoxic action

FKBP12 = 12-kD FK-binding protein; IL = interleukin.

Molecular Action

Genomic Effects

Corticosteroids are lipophilic and rapidly cross cell membranes into the cytosol, where they bind to the glucocorticoid receptor. The complex of glucocorticoid and its receptor then enters the nucleus and affects gene transcription by binding to glucocorticoid response elements. The complex may either stimulate or suppress gene transcription and subsequent protein production. This mechanism may have an impact on the function of 1% of all genes and suppresses the production of cytokines and other important inflammatory proteins. In addition to binding to glucocorticoid response elements, the glucocorticoid-glucocorticoid receptor complex also suppresses signal transduction pathways such as transcription factor activator protein-1 (AP-1), nuclear factor-κB (NF-κB), and nuclear factor of activator of T cells (NF-AT). Corticosteroids may also act to affect post-transcription and post-translation steps of protein synthesis. The anti-inflammatory actions of corticosteroids may be related to their action on the NF-κB and AP-1 pathways; the adverse events produced are related more to the activation or suppression of gene transcription. More recently, it has been recognized that corticosteroids can also regulate the mitochondrial genome. Glucocorticoid receptors are likewise present in mitochondria, and the mitochondrial genome contains glucocorticoid response elements.[3]

Nongenomic Effects

The genomic effects of corticosteroids require the diffusion of the drug into the cell, binding to the receptor, entry into the nucleus, and alteration of transcription. The ultimate effect on protein synthesis is not immediate, and it generally takes at least 30 minutes before any response is seen. The observation that some actions of corticosteroids are seen immediately has directed a search for nongenomic effects of corticosteroids. The glucocorticoid-glucocorticoid receptor complex can inhibit arachidonic acid release. In addition to the cytosol glucocorticoid receptor, membrane-bound receptors may be present that interact with cytoplasmic kinase–signaling molecules and G proteins and may mediate the rapid, nonclassic steroid effects and nongenomic functions.[2]

Systemic Effects

Impact on Leukocytes

Corticosteroids affect the activation, production, circulation, function, and survival of leukocytes. Whereas these impacts appear to be principally modulated by the genomic effects of corticosteroids on cytokines, corticosteroids also act on adhesion molecules and other mechanisms. The effects are on neutrophils, monocytes, macrophages, lymphocytes, eosinophils, and basophils. With corticosteroid therapy, neutrophils increase in the peripheral circulation (Chapter 167), primarily because of demargination, in contrast to a decrease in monocytes, lymphocytes, eosinophils, and basophils. Although the number of circulating neutrophils may increase, trafficking appears to be impaired. The impact on T cells is more pronounced than the effects on B cells, with the induction of apoptosis particularly in immature and activated T cells. Although function of B cells and neutrophils is not affected as strongly as that of T cells, high-dose prolonged use of corticosteroids can lead to suppression of antibody production.

Changes in Inflammatory Mediators

Corticosteroids result in a decrease in multiple pro-inflammatory cytokines and interleukins (ILs).[4] The cytokines affected include IL-1, IL-2, IL-6, and tumor necrosis factor-α, at the same time that there is an increase in anti-inflammatory cytokines—IL-4, IL-10, and IL-13. Corticosteroids have been associated with a reduction in the production of prostaglandins, leukotrienes, and other arachidonic acid metabolites, probably related to the reduced production of cyclooxygenase-2 and phospholipase A_2–related pro-inflammatory compounds (Chapter 37).

TREATMENT Rx

Specific Issues with Corticosteroid Therapy

Multiple corticosteroid compounds and preparations are available. Many of the commonly employed compounds are listed in Table 35-2. These compounds have differences in potency, half-life, and sodium-retaining properties. More recently, delayed-release prednisone has been licensed for clinical use and may have a special role in the treatment of inflammatory conditions with circadian features.[5] In many conditions, the local administration of corticosteroids will provide clinical benefit without the systemic toxicity associated with oral therapy. Local therapies include topical, ophthalmic, inhaled, and local injection, such as soft tissue and intra-articular injections. Although the potential for adverse events is generally reduced with local therapy, local toxicities can develop, as can systemic effects if large doses of topical corticosteroids are used.

Whereas most conditions can be treated with local or oral corticosteroids, intravenous administration can provide pulse doses if desired. Intravenous therapy may also be used in situations in which the patient cannot take oral medication or the absorption of oral agents is impaired. Pulse therapy is generally administered in high intravenous doses that are often given as divided treatments during 3 to 5 days. High-dose pulse therapy has particularly been advocated in acute organ transplantation rejection, severe systemic lupus erythematosus (SLE), aggressive vasculitis, and other acute and severe autoimmune disorders. The use of high-dose pulse corticosteroid therapy has been associated with the development of sudden cardiac arrhythmias and sudden death. Many of the patients described have had serious concurrent diseases that could in part be responsible for electrolyte abnormalities and other associated morbidities that could contribute to these observations. Despite the confusion about this association, close monitoring of patients receiving high-dose pulse corticosteroid therapy is warranted.

Indications

Corticosteroids are employed in a large range of autoimmune disorders and transplantation procedures. A listing of each indication for which corticosteroids have been employed and proven effective is beyond the scope of this chapter, but indications range from multiple rheumatologic disorders to transplantation and many other inflammatory conditions. For example, the demonstration that inflammation plays a significant role in reactive airway disease has dramatically increased the use of systemic and inhaled corticosteroids in asthma and chronic obstructive pulmonary disorders. The challenge is to determine the appropriate dose, route, and duration of therapy with these disorders. For severe autoimmune disorders, high doses of corticosteroids are employed. In many cases, oral administration of prednisone, 60 to 80 mg/day as single or divided doses, can be employed. If patients cannot take oral

TABLE 35-2 GLUCOCORTICOID PREPARATIONS

	ANTI-INFLAMMATORY POTENCY	EQUIVALENT DOSE (mg)	SODIUM-RETAINING POTENCY	PLASMA HALF-LIFE (min)	BIOLOGIC HALF-LIFE (hr)
Hydrocortisone	1	20	2+	90	8-12
Cortisone	0.8	25	2+	30	8-12
Prednisone	4	5	1+	60	12-36
Prednisolone	4	5	1+	200	12-36
Methylprednisolone	5	4	0	180	12-36
Triamcinolone	5	4	0	300	12-36
Betamethasone	20-30	0.6	0	100-300	36-54
Dexamethasone	20-30	0.75	0	100-300	36-54

From Garber EK, Targoff C, Paulus HE. Glucocorticoid preparations. In: Paulus HE, Furst DE, Droomgoole SH, eds. *Drugs for Rheumatic Diseases*. New York: Churchill Livingstone; 1987:446.

medication or high doses of corticosteroids are indicated, higher doses can be administered intravenously. Comparative data on the most appropriate doses and routes of administration are generally not available. Clinical judgment and empirical literature have formed the basis of these treatment regimens.

Adverse Effects

As noted previously, most adverse events associated with corticosteroid use are caused by the physiologic action of these drugs. Investigations are ongoing to determine whether separate mechanisms might be more associated with the therapeutic benefits whereas other pathways are more involved in the adverse events of corticosteroids. Currently available forms of corticosteroids do not selectively allow separation of the adverse events from the therapeutic effects. For example, the increase in infection associated with corticosteroids is the result of the impact of these drugs on leukocyte function and antibody production and is not an allergic reaction. The prevalence and severity of these adverse effects increase in proportion to the dose and duration of the therapy. The key to reducing adverse events with corticosteroids is to use the lowest needed dose and shortest possible duration for the required indication. Data also suggest that intermittent and every-other-day dosing may be associated with less toxicity than daily or divided daily doses.

Despite these limitations, corticosteroids are the only viable treatment option in many conditions, and efforts must be made to prevent, to detect development of, and to monitor for these adverse events. In most situations, education of the patient coupled with vigilant surveillance can detect these adverse events and often reduce their serious impact.

The following description of adverse events is not intended to be a comprehensive list of all reported adverse events associated with corticosteroids. The problems with infection, osteoporosis, metabolic abnormalities, and cardiovascular effects are highlighted because specific interventions can have an impact on these complications through proper education of the patient, monitoring, or prophylactic therapy.

Infections

Infections are increased in patients taking corticosteroids, particularly bacterial, fungal, and mycobacterial infections. The increased incidence and general severity of these infections are complicated by the anti-inflammatory actions of corticosteroids that can mask many of the cardinal signs of infection, such as fever, inflammation, and local discomfort. Patients taking corticosteroids should be alerted to the possibility of these "subclinical infections," and the provider must be vigilant in investigating signs and symptoms that may be less concerning in patients not taking corticosteroids. Management of infections in patients receiving corticosteroids requires close monitoring. Appropriate diagnostic procedures, antimicrobial therapy, and supportive measures are keys to successful management of infections in immunocompromised hosts. Patients with adrenal suppression may require "stress doses" of corticosteroids during the initial treatment of an infection. However, when possible, a reduction in corticosteroid dose may help restore a host immune response to the underlying infection, particularly with chronic infections.

Preventive measures to reduce infections include proper immunizations. If possible, for example, in a patient being evaluated for future transplantation, immunizations should be given before the immunosuppressive therapy. In many cases, a delay of immunosuppressive therapy is not possible to allow immunizations to be updated. However, in patients receiving chronic immunosuppressive therapy, routine immunizations should be offered when the disease is stable. Prophylactic antibiotics are generally not recommended to prevent infections in patients receiving corticosteroid therapy. However, two notable exceptions are the use of antituberculosis therapy in purified protein derivative–positive patients and trimethoprim-sulfamethoxazole therapy in patients receiving high-dose corticosteroid therapy for *Pneumocystis jirovecii* (previously named *Pneumocystis carinii*) prophylaxis.

Osteoporosis

Bone loss (Chapter 243) with corticosteroids affects multiple sites and has a greater impact on trabecular bone than on cortical bone. Common sites for involvement are the spine and femur, with associated fracture rates that may be as high as 20%, depending on the duration and dose of therapy. On initiation of long-term corticosteroid therapy, all patients should be evaluated for osteoporosis prophylactic therapy (Chapter 243). Unless it is contraindicated, patients should have adequate calcium and vitamin D through diet or supplements. In many patients, bisphosphonates will provide significant protection. Postmenopausal women should be evaluated for potential estrogen replacement therapy that may be helpful if benefits of therapy with corticosteroids are considered to outweigh the risks for cardiovascular disease and malignant disease. If osteoporosis develops in a patient receiving corticosteroids, efforts should be made to discontinue therapy or to reduce dose. Agents employed for treatment of osteoporosis should also be employed. Effective therapies include bisphosphonates, hormone replacement therapy, and anabolic agents such as parathyroid hormone preparations. These agents are generally used in association with calcium and vitamin D supplementation. An algorithm for prevention and treatment of glucocorticoid-induced osteoporosis is provided (Fig. 35-1).[6]

Metabolic Effects

The metabolic effects of corticosteroids may affect glucose metabolism, with results ranging from mild glucose intolerance to frank diabetes. Patients beginning corticosteroid therapy should be monitored for glucose intolerance and treated if significant hyperglycemia develops. The management of patients with existing diabetes is particularly challenging during corticosteroid therapy and requires close monitoring and adjustments of the diabetes management program. Other metabolic complications of corticosteroid treatment include weight gain with truncal obesity, electrolyte abnormalities including hypokalemia, and fluid retention.

Tapering Steroids

Exogenous corticosteroids will suppress the hypothalamic-pituitary-adrenal (HPA) axis. The likelihood of adrenal suppression increases with dose and duration of therapy. HPA axis suppression should be considered in patients receiving doses of 20 mg/day or more for 3 weeks or longer, although suppression can occur with lower doses. Formal evaluations can be performed to test the integrity of the HPA axis, but in most cases a scheduled taper of corticosteroid dose during several weeks will allow the return of HPA axis function without signs of adrenal insufficiency. The ideal rate for tapering corticosteroids has not been evaluated by clinical trials. The rate of reduction

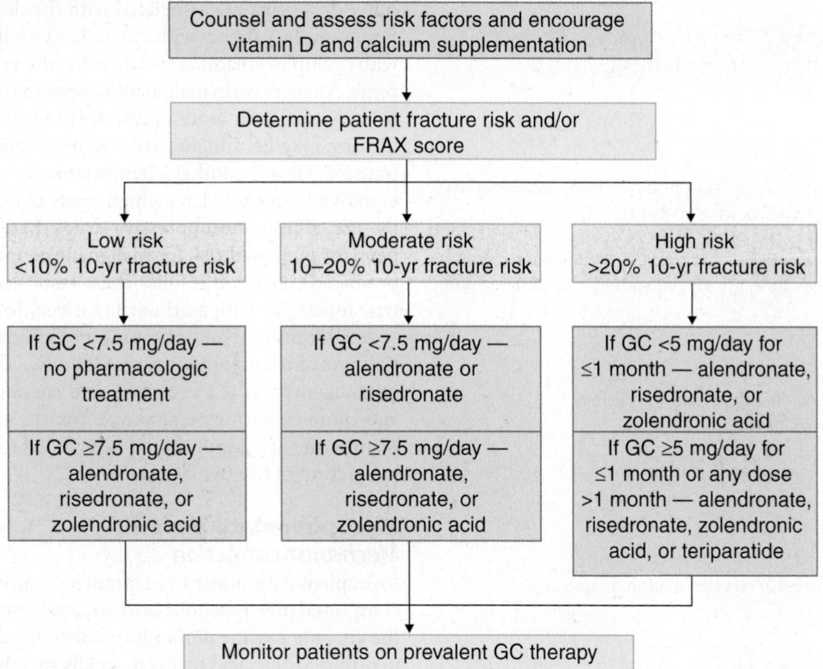

FIGURE 35-1. **Algorithm for prevention of steroid-induced osteoporosis on initiation of glucocorticoid (GC) therapy. FRAX = World Health Organization Fracture Risk Assessment Tool. (Modified from American College of Rheumatology 2010 recommendations for the prevention and treatment of glucocorticoid-induced osteoporosis. *Arthritis Rheum.* 2010;62:1515-1526.)**

in corticosteroid dose is often limited more by concerns over the potential relapses of disease activity than by the development of adrenal insufficiency. In general, if there is not a significant concern for a flare of the disease, a rapid reduction in dose to about 10 mg prednisone-equivalent per day is well tolerated. This dose replaces the normal physiologic production of cortisol. After this point, reductions in dose of 1 to 2.5 mg/day every 1 to 2 weeks will generally be well tolerated and may be accomplished by decreasing the dose of alternate-day treatment over 6 to 8 weeks. However, with acute medical illness, patients who have received corticosteroid doses in the past sufficient to cause HPA suppression should receive stress doses of steroids for a period of up to 1 year after the steroid treatment.

Cardiovascular Effects

Corticosteroids may induce or exacerbate cardiovascular risk factors, including hypertension, hyperlipidemia, and diabetes. Multiple mechanisms have been proposed for these effects, but the end result is that patients taking corticosteroids have an increased prevalence of atherosclerotic diseases and their associated complications. This problem is further complicated by the increased risk for cardiovascular disease in patients with inflammatory conditions, including rheumatoid arthritis and SLE, above that risk predicted by traditional risk factor assessment. These observations have emphasized the need to monitor corticosteroid-treated patients closely for cardiovascular risk factors with aggressive treatment of detected abnormalities.

Other Adverse Effects

Many other adverse events have been noted with corticosteroid therapy and are listed in Table 35-3. Osteonecrosis (avascular necrosis) is common during corticosteroid therapy and particularly involves the femoral head. Peptic ulcer disease is increased independently of concurrent nonsteroidal anti-inflammatory therapy. Cataracts and a variety of dermatologic abnormalities are more common. Muscle weakness or steroid myopathy, alteration of mood and behavior, and psychosis may develop. This broad spectrum of clinical complications requires the prescriber of corticosteroids to be aware of and alert to the development of these adverse events.

Purine Inhibition

Purines are critical components of nucleic acids and are particularly important in proliferating cells as part of cell growth and division. The inhibition of purines by competitive inhibitors (azathioprine and 6-mercaptopurine) or blocking critical enzymes (mycophenolate mofetil) in the purine pathway is an effective method of immunosuppression.

Azathioprine and 6-Mercaptopurine

Mechanism of Action

Azathioprine is an inactive compound that is metabolized to the active compound 6-mercaptopurine (6-MP). The exact mechanisms of action of 6-MP and its metabolites have not been fully established. At high doses, 6-MP may be incorporated into RNA and DNA, resulting in a cytotoxic effect; however, this effect is probably not the major action of the drug at the doses generally employed for immunosuppression. Most likely through feedback inhibition of de novo purine synthesis, 6-MP and its metabolites may reduce cell proliferation and thus produce immunosuppression. Genetically controlled differences in the activity of enzymes involved in the metabolism of 6-MP have been identified. The enzyme thiopurine *S*-methyltransferase is responsible for the metabolism of 6-MP to the metabolite methyl-6-MP. A rare homozygous (0.3%) and heterozygous (10%) defect in thiopurine *S*-methyltransferase is associated with increased toxicity, with severe hematologic toxicity in the homozygous patients.

The drug is metabolized eventually by xanthine oxidase. Because xanthine oxidase is inhibited by allopurinol, the concurrent use of allopurinol and azathioprine or 6-MP can result in a significant reduction in the metabolism of the active compounds and a significant increase in drug toxicity. For this reason, the combination of allopurinol and azathioprine should be avoided.

Indications

Azathioprine is approved by the U.S. Food and Drug Administration (FDA) for prevention of rejection of renal transplantation and treatment of rheumatoid arthritis. Clinical trials and reports have suggested that azathioprine also has efficacy during other types of organ transplantation and for autoimmune diseases. Azathioprine has been particularly effective at providing an adjunct to corticosteroid therapy, allowing a reduction in corticosteroid dose and avoiding the associated adverse events.

Adverse Effects

Serious infections are reported during treatment with azathioprine, similar to those seen with other immunosuppressive drugs. Opportunistic infections are a particular concern. Hematologic abnormalities include leukopenia, thrombocytopenia, and anemia. A complete blood count (CBC) is recommended on a regular basis, with increased frequency at the initiation of therapy. Current guidelines recommend a CBC weekly during the first month of azathioprine therapy, twice weekly during the second and third months, and monthly thereafter. Genotyping of the enzyme thiopurine *S*-methyltransferase may identify subjects with the highest risk for

TABLE 35-3 MAJOR ADVERSE EVENTS ASSOCIATED WITH IMMUNOSUPPRESSIVE THERAPIES*

CORTICOSTEROIDS

Serious and opportunistic infections
Osteoporosis
Metabolic disorders: hyperglycemia, adrenal suppression, hyperlipidemia, electrolyte abnormalities, fluid retention, hypertension, truncal obesity
Cardiovascular
Miscellaneous: osteonecrosis, peptic ulcer disease, cataracts, dermatologic abnormalities, steroid myopathy, psychosis, growth retardation, altered mood and behavior

AZATHIOPRINE

Serious and opportunistic infections
Hematologic abnormalities: leukopenia, thrombocytopenia, anemia
Gastrointestinal: nausea, vomiting, rare hepatitis
Reproductive: pregnancy class D
Miscellaneous: pancreatitis, interstitial pneumonitis, rashes

MYCOPHENOLATE MOFETIL

Serious and opportunistic infections
Leukopenia
Gastrointestinal: diarrhea, nausea, dyspepsia, elevated transaminases
Reproductive: pregnancy class C

CYCLOSPORINE

Serious and opportunistic infections
Renal disease and hypertension
Potential for increased malignant neoplasms
Reproductive: pregnancy class C
Miscellaneous: hirsutism, gingival hyperplasia, hyperuricemia, electrolyte abnormalities

TACROLIMUS

Serious and opportunistic infections
Renal disease and hypertension, perhaps lower than with cyclosporine
Potential for increased malignant neoplasms
Post-transplantation diabetes mellitus
Neurotoxicity: tremor, headaches, motor function abnormalities, mental status alteration, sensory changes
Reproductive: pregnancy class C
Miscellaneous: hirsutism, gingival hyperplasia, myocardial hypertrophy

SIROLIMUS

Serious and opportunistic infections
Renal disease and hypertension
Potential for increased malignant neoplasms
Reproductive: pregnancy class C
Miscellaneous: hyperlipidemia, pneumonitis, interstitial lung disease

CYCLOPHOSPHAMIDE

Serious and opportunistic infections
Increased incidence of malignant neoplasms
Hematologic toxicity: leukopenia, thrombocytopenia, anemia
Reproductive: pregnancy class D, premature ovarian failure, oligospermia, fetal abnormalities
Urologic: hemorrhagic cystitis, bladder cancer
Miscellaneous: nausea, vomiting, diarrhea, pulmonary fibrosis

*This list highlights the most serious and common adverse events but does not include all reported adverse events with these agents.

hematologic toxicity but does not substitute for monitoring of the CBC. Gastrointestinal toxicity is usually minor, but patients may have significant symptomatic complaints of nausea, vomiting, diarrhea, and epigastric pain that are often self-limited and reversible. A severe hepatic toxicity has been rarely reported, leading to a recommendation for regular monitoring of serum transaminases, alkaline phosphatase, and bilirubin, particularly during the first 6 months of therapy. Rare complications of azathioprine treatment include fever, arthralgia, rash, pancreatitis, and interstitial pneumonitis.

Azathioprine use in pregnancy is classified category D and has been associated with fetal abnormalities in animals. The use of azathioprine should be avoided, if possible, in pregnant women and nursing mothers, although patients with organ transplantation and autoimmune disease have had successful pregnancies while receiving azathioprine.

The association of azathioprine treatment with the development of malignant neoplasms has been controversial. In most clinical situations, azathioprine is used in conditions and in combination or temporal sequence with other drugs that are associated with the development of malignant diseases. For example, patients with systemic vasculitis or SLE may initially be treated with cyclophosphamide and then are often subsequently treated with azathioprine. An increase in malignant neoplasms in this population could be related to the concurrent azathioprine treatment, but the prior cyclophosphamide therapy may be a higher risk factor. In addition, patients with solid organ transplantation, another circumstance in which azathioprine is frequently employed, appear to have a higher rate of malignant neoplasms separate from the use of immunosuppressive drugs. Extensive efforts to identify an independent increased risk for malignant neoplasms with azathioprine have not produced consistent results. These results suggest that the risk for malignant transformation with azathioprine is very low if this risk exists at all.

Azathioprine is an important and effective therapy in organ transplantation and autoimmune disease. Often this drug is used in combination with other agents and as a corticosteroid-sparing drug. Surveillance for infection and monitoring for hematologic toxicity are important. Concurrent treatment with allopurinol should be avoided to prevent serious toxicity from an interaction of the two drugs.

Mycophenolate Mofetil

Mechanism of Action

Mycophenolate mofetil is a prodrug that is converted in vivo to the active compound mycophenolic acid. Mycophenolic acid acts through inhibition of the enzyme inosine monophosphate dehydrogenase, resulting in an increase in 6-thionosinic acid that is normally metabolized by this enzyme. The accumulation of 6-thionosinic acid acts through a negative feedback loop to suppress the de novo synthesis of purines and associated DNA production. Although it is not a cytotoxic agent, the actions of mycophenolic acid are most pronounced on proliferating cells, such as lymphocytes, to reduce cell division and associated functions of these critical cells in the immune response.

Indications

Mycophenolate mofetil is approved by the FDA for the prevention of allograft rejection in renal, hepatic, and cardiac transplantation. In addition to these approved indications, mycophenolate mofetil has been evaluated in SLE, for which its principal use has been in patients with lupus nephritis[A1], although the drug has been used for other manifestations. In the treatment of SLE, it can be used successfully in patients who no longer respond to azathioprine[7] and can be used as initial and maintenance therapy for lupus nephritis. Limited use has been reported in other autoimmune diseases such as rheumatoid arthritis, vasculitis, and polymyositis.

Adverse Effects and Monitoring

Common adverse events with mycophenolate mofetil include hematologic and gastrointestinal complications. Leukopenia is reported in 20 to 35% of patients receiving this drug for organ transplantation; however, severe neutropenia is seen in only 2 to 3% of subjects. Patients receiving mycophenolate mofetil have a higher susceptibility to infections, similar to that seen with other immunosuppressive agents, including opportunistic infections. Diarrhea, nausea, and dyspepsia are frequent. Abnormalities of liver enzymes are commonly noted and appear to be dose dependent. Rare complications include pulmonary fibrosis and malignant neoplasms. Mycophenolate mofetil is classified as category C by the FDA for use in pregnant women. Although the agent should be avoided in patients who are pregnant or not practicing adequate contraception, this drug appears to have less impact on the reproductive system than does cyclophosphamide. Patients with SLE who are concerned about a potential severe impact of cyclophosphamide on reproductive organs might elect to use mycophenolate mofetil instead.

Monitoring of patients receiving mycophenolate mofetil should include a monthly CBC and hepatic enzyme activities. Clinical monitoring for gastrointestinal and infectious complications should be conducted during regular clinical follow-up.

Mycophenolate mofetil is an important and effective agent in the management of transplantation patients. Ongoing work is studying the role of this drug in other autoimmune diseases. It is hoped that mycophenolate mofetil can provide effective therapy for rheumatic and autoimmune disorders with less toxicity than is seen with currently available agents, with a particular potential for use in lupus nephritis.

Immunophilin-Binding Agents

The development of immunophilin inhibitors has significantly advanced organ transplantation.[8] Each of these drugs—cyclosporine, tacrolimus (also known as FK506), and sirolimus (also known as rapamycin)—has significant immunosuppressive activity on T-cell-mediated functions. Whereas the mechanisms of action for each drug differ, they all have the common action of binding to a cytosolic protein. This binding results in a decrease in T-cell cytokine production and T-cell proliferation. These separate sites of action allow the use of these agents in combination in transplantation management. In addition, the differences in action and specific binding for each drug have resulted in unique adverse events profiles.

Cyclosporine

Mechanism of Action

Cyclosporine acts by binding to the cytosolic protein cyclophilin to form a cyclosporine-cyclophilin complex. The cyclosporine-cyclophilin complex inhibits the enzyme calcineurin. Calcineurin is an enzyme involved in multiple T-cell functions and is of particular importance in enhancing the transcription of genes for pro-inflammatory cytokines. The use of cyclosporine inhibits the production of IL-2 with a resulting decrease in T-cell activation. Cyclosporine also inhibits the production of other cytokines, including IL-3, IL-4, granulocyte-macrophage colony-simulating factor, tumor necrosis factor-α, and interferon-α. The overall impact of these actions is to reduce immune function and inflammation.

Indications

The use of cyclosporine and other calcineurin inhibitors has revolutionized solid organ transplantation. The specific FDA-approved indications include renal, liver, and heart transplantation. Most often the drug is used in conjunction with other immunosuppressive agents including corticosteroids and azathioprine. The critical clinical challenge is to balance the potent immunosuppressive effects of the drug against the adverse events produced by this agent, with particular attention to avoidance of infectious complications and monitoring for hypertension and renal toxicity. Because of these critical issues, prescribing information specifically limits this agent to physicians experienced with the use of immunosuppressive agents.

Oral cyclosporine is also approved for the treatment of rheumatoid arthritis as a disease-modifying antirheumatic drug (DMARD), either alone or in combination with methotrexate. Although it is effective in the treatment of rheumatoid arthritis and other rheumatic diseases, cyclosporine does not provide a substantially greater efficacy than the other DMARDs. Cyclosporine is also approved for the treatment of psoriasis. Because of the significant adverse event profile, cyclosporine is generally reserved for patients with autoimmune diseases whose therapy with more traditional and less toxic agents has failed.

Topical cyclosporine is effective and approved for treatment to increase tear production presumed to be suppressed secondary to inflammation in patients with keratoconjunctivitis sicca syndrome (Chapter 423). The topical treatment is associated with a much lower frequency of adverse drug events than is systemic cyclosporine therapy.

Adverse Effects

Close monitoring is required during cyclosporine therapy. Blood levels can be measured, which is useful in ensuring that the drug remains within a therapeutic range and below levels associated with increased toxicity. Because of multiple potential drug interactions that can both raise and lower cyclosporine levels, as well as food interactions, particularly increased levels with grapefruit and grapefruit juices, patients should be constantly monitored and blood levels obtained when indicated. These evaluations should ensure that when medical therapy is added, changed, or deleted, these adjustments will not have an impact on the effects of the cyclosporine, with its associated therapeutic and toxicity issues.

Infection

All infections have an increased potential for developing in patients receiving cyclosporine and other calcineurin inhibitors as with other immunosuppressive agents. Opportunistic infections associated with impaired cell-mediated immunity are particularly increased.

Renal Disease and Hypertension

Renal disease and hypertension are common adverse events during cyclosporine therapy and are increased in prevalence with increases in dose and duration of therapy. Close monitoring of blood pressure and serum creatinine concentration is critical during treatment with cyclosporine. In many cases, these conditions are reversible if they are detected early and appropriate dose adjustments are implemented. In many patients, a mild increase in serum creatinine concentration may be tolerated if the level remains stable. Whereas renal abnormalities and hypertension are commonly identified during treatment of patients with cyclosporine, most patients will not require discontinuation of the drug if adjustments in dose or other interventions are undertaken to avoid these complications.

Malignant Neoplasia

Malignant neoplasms, particularly lymphomas, have been noted to be more common in patients receiving solid organ transplantation with associated immunosuppressive therapy. However, the exact cause of these malignant neoplasms has not been determined. In vitro mutagenesis assays with cyclosporine have been negative. In vivo animal studies have yielded equivocal results, with some data suggesting a possible increased rate of malignant neoplasms in rats and mice.

Issues with Reproduction

Cyclosporine is a pregnancy class C drug. Data in animals have demonstrated toxicity to both the embryo and fetus. Patients should practice effective contraception while receiving this drug. Data from pregnant transplant patients are difficult to interpret because cyclosporine is generally not the only medical therapy received by these women and the impact of the disease associated with the organ transplantation is at times difficult to separate from the impact of therapy. Despite these limitations, normal pregnancies and early childhood development have been reported in many women receiving cyclosporine. Premature birth and low birth weight are more common in women receiving cyclosporine. Therefore, although the use of cyclosporine during pregnancy and breast-feeding should be avoided if at all possible, in patients who become pregnant, an assessment should determine whether the immunosuppressive therapy should be continued. In some cases, the risk for organ rejection with discontinuation of cyclosporine therapy may exceed the risk for exposure to the fetus during pregnancy.

Other Adverse Effects

Cyclosporine has also been associated with the development of hirsutism, gingival hyperplasia, hyperuricemia, and electrolyte abnormalities.

Tacrolimus

Mechanism of Action

Whereas cyclosporine binds to cyclophilin, tacrolimus binds to a different protein, the 12-kD FK-binding protein (FKBP12). The binding of FKBP12 and tacrolimus forms a complex that inhibits calcineurin in a fashion similar to cyclosporine. Through this mechanism, tacrolimus has similar inhibitory effects on T-cell function and cytokine production.

Indications

Tacrolimus is approved for the prophylactic treatment of organ rejection after kidney and liver transplantation. The efficacy and safety in rheumatoid arthritis is limited but encouraging. Experience with this agent is less extensive than the experience with cyclosporine.

Adverse Effects

The major adverse events with tacrolimus are similar to those of cyclosporine and include increased susceptibility to infection, renal disease, and hypertension. An increase in malignant neoplasia is also reported with a pattern similar to that reported in patients receiving cyclosporine.

Whereas many adverse events with tacrolimus are similar to those of other calcineurin inhibitors, some specific complications have been reported, including the development of post-transplantation diabetes mellitus. This adverse event was seen in 20% of subjects in phase III clinical trials of tacrolimus with an onset generally within the first 3 months of therapy. In many patients, post-transplantation diabetes mellitus will resolve after the drug is discontinued. Neurotoxicity is also reported, including tremor, headache, motor function abnormalities, mental status alterations, and sensory changes. Myocardial hypertrophy has been reported. Tacrolimus, like cyclosporine, is pregnancy class C. Patients receiving this drug should practice effective contraception.

Sirolimus

Mechanism of Action

Sirolimus (or rapamycin) in not a calcineurin inhibitor but has many actions and mechanisms similar to calcineurin inhibitors. The mechanism of action of sirolimus involves binding to FKBP12, the binding protein for tacrolimus, but the effect of this binding is different. Instead of acting on calcineurin, the sirolimus-FKBP12 complex binds to another protein, the mammalian target of rapamycin (mTOR), which is a key regulatory kinase. The inhibition of mTOR results in significant immunosuppression by decreasing T-cell proliferation and the progression from G_1 phase to S phase in the cell cycle. Because sirolimus works through a mechanism different from the mechanism of action for cyclosporine, the two drugs have been studied in combination. In renal transplantation patients, the use of these two agents in combination has a greater immunosuppressive effect than that of cyclosporine alone.

Indications

Sirolimus is approved for the prophylaxis of organ rejection in renal transplantation in combination with cyclosporine and corticosteroids for patients older than 12 years. Data with the use of sirolimus in other populations, including subjects with autoimmune diseases, are limited and generally are derived only from animal models.

Adverse Effects

The adverse event profile for infection and malignant neoplasms with sirolimus is similar to that with calcineurin inhibitors. Renal disease with cyclosporine and sirolimus in combination has been reported more frequently than in patients receiving cyclosporine alone. Adverse reactions specific for sirolimus include hyperlipidemia, interstitial lung disease, and the syndrome of calcineurin-induced hemolytic-uremic syndrome, thrombotic thrombocytopenic purpura, and thrombotic microangiopathy.

Alkylating Agents

Alkylating agents are an important component of immunosuppressive therapy in autoimmune diseases. The use of these agents is limited by their associated toxicity, particularly the potential for development of malignant neoplasia, reproductive toxicity, and increased incidence of infection. Patients considered candidates for alkylating therapy should be fully informed of the potential risks and benefits of these drugs and concur with the decision for their use. Regular monitoring of blood counts and urinalysis are important in observing patients receiving these drugs.

Cyclophosphamide

Cyclophosphamide has been used primarily as a cytotoxic drug for the treatment of malignant neoplasms; it is currently approved for this indication as well as for biopsy-proven minimal change nephrotic disease in children. Several severe autoimmune diseases have also been shown to be responsive to cyclophosphamide, often given in conjunction with initial high-dose corticosteroid therapy. Because of the significant toxicities associated with these drugs, a benefit-to-risk assessment and discussion should be undertaken with each patient as cyclophosphamide use is being considered. In most cases, the diseases warranting cyclophosphamide therapy will be life-threatening conditions with poor prognosis to justify the potential severe toxicity of this agent.

Mechanism of Action

Cyclophosphamide is an inactive compound that can be administered either orally or intravenously and is metabolized to the active drug by the cytochrome P-450 mixed function oxidase system. This process produces the active compounds phosphoramide mustard and the toxic metabolite acrolein. The cytotoxic effect of this drug results from the alkylation of various cellular constituents, especially nucleic acids. Changes in immune function with cyclophosphamide include depletion of lymphoid tissues, with decreases in both B and T cells, suppression of cellular immune function, and decreased antibody production.

Indications

Treatment of lupus nephritis and severe systemic vasculitis is the most well studied and common use of cyclophosphamide in the rheumatic diseases. Controlled clinical trials have demonstrated improved outcomes in these conditions, particularly with reduced progression to end-stage renal disease in patients with SLE and improved survival with systemic vasculitis such as granulomatosis with polyangiitis (GPA, formerly known as Wegener granulomatosis) and other forms of antineutrophil cytoplasmic autoantibody-associated vasculitis (AAV). However, there has been an increase use of rituximab (Chapter 36) in the treatment of AAV in place of cyclophosphamide with similar clinical benefit and less adverse events.[A2] The evaluation of cyclophosphamide in patients with SLE has demonstrated the benefit of intermittent, usually monthly, intravenous pulse therapy as a method to avoid some of the most severe toxic side effects while maintaining therapeutic efficacy. However, pulse intravenous cyclophosphamide has not been found to be as effective as continuous oral cyclophosphamide in all conditions, particularly GPA. Other conditions, such as polyarteritis nodosa, Takayasu arteritis, and Churg-Strauss syndrome, have been reported to benefit from cyclophosphamide; however, the low prevalence of these diseases has prohibited the conduct of controlled clinical trials to prove efficacy. Cyclophosphamide has also been demonstrated to be effective in the treatment of patients with rheumatoid arthritis, but it is generally not used in this condition because of the associated toxicity and availability of other effective agents. Although the use of cyclophosphamide has been a tremendous advance in the treatment of these life-threatening diseases, the use of less toxic medications, such as rituximab and mycophenolate mofetil, is under investigation to determine their relative clinical efficacy.

Adverse Effects

Before the initiation of cyclophosphamide therapy, a frank discussion with the patient about potential serious and even life-threatening adverse events should be undertaken and documented.

Malignant Neoplasia

Malignant neoplasms may develop in patients receiving cyclophosphamide for the treatment of both malignant and nonmalignant diseases. The risk for malignant change appears to increase with the duration and dose of cyclophosphamide. The most common malignant neoplasms are bladder, myeloproliferative, and lymphoproliferative disorders. The use of intravenous pulse cyclophosphamide may reduce but not eliminate the risk for bladder cancer. These malignant neoplasms may develop years after the discontinuation of the drug.

Reproductive Issues

Cyclophosphamide can be teratogenic, affect female reproduction, and reduce male fertility. Cyclophosphamide is pregnancy category D and should not be used in pregnant women unless life-threatening disease is present that warrants this treatment. Whereas successful pregnancies have been reported in patients receiving cyclophosphamide during pregnancy, fetal abnormalities are well documented secondary to chromosome damage in patients receiving cyclophosphamide. The use of cyclophosphamide in premenopausal women can induce premature ovarian failure. The use of gonadotropin-releasing hormone analogues during intravenous pulse cyclophosphamide therapy may reduce premature ovarian failure in patients with SLE; however, the risk of this complication is still present. In males, temporary and permanent decrease in sperm count may occur with cyclophosphamide. Because the recovery of fertility after cyclophosphamide is variable, sperm banking should be considered before therapy is begun.

Other Adverse Effects

As with other immunosuppressive agents, infections are more frequent and potentially more serious in patients receiving cyclophosphamide. Opportunistic infections are more likely to be seen in these subjects. Hematologic abnormalities can involve all cell lines. The CBC should be monitored regularly and cyclophosphamide discontinued or the dose reduced when cytopenias develop. Cyclophosphamide treatment may be complicated by hemorrhagic cystitis and bladder cancer, which are probably related to the toxic metabolite acrolein. Efforts to reduce the potential for hemorrhagic cystitis and bladder malignant neoplasms include the use of intravenous pulse therapy, hydration, frequent voiding, and treatment with agents containing sulfhydryl groups to scavenge acrolein. Regular urinalysis for blood is indicated to monitor for bladder toxicity. Patients may develop severe nausea, vomiting, and diarrhea with cyclophosphamide therapy.

Chlorambucil

Chlorambucil has not been evaluated as extensively as cyclophosphamide, but this agent appears to have properties and an adverse event profile similar to those of cyclophosphamide. Like cyclophosphamide, chlorambucil is associated with the development of malignant neoplasms and should be avoided during pregnancy.

Miscellaneous Agents

Although principally prescribed for other indications, methotrexate and leflunomide have been evaluated and used for their potential immunosuppressive effects. Leflunomide blocks the enzyme dihydroorotate dehydrogenase, resulting in an inhibition of pyrimidine synthesis and a reduction in

T-cell activation. Methotrexate has multiple mechanisms of action, but its major effect in autoimmune diseases is mediated by inhibition of the enzyme aminoimidazole-4-carboxamide ribonucleotide transformylase. This inhibition affects purine synthesis, increasing the intracellular concentration of aminoimidazole-4-carboxamide ribonucleotide, which stimulates the release of adenosine, a potent anti-inflammatory compound. Methotrexate has principally been advocated for its corticosteroid-sparing effects. Both methotrexate and leflunomide are effective DMARDs in the treatment of rheumatoid arthritis and are discussed in other chapters.

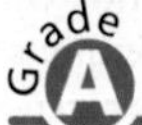

Grade A References

A1. Maneiro JR, Lopez-Canoa N, Salgado E, et al. Maintenance therapy of lupus nephritis with mycophenolate or azathioprine: systematic review and meta-analysis. *Rheumatology (Oxford)*. 2014; 53:834-838.

A2. Specks U, Merkel PA, Seo P, et al. Efficacy of remission-induction regimens for ANCA-associated vasculitis. *N Engl J Med*. 2013;369:417-427.

GENERAL REFERENCES

For the General References and other additional features, please visit Expert Consult at https://expertconsult.inkling.com.

36 BIOLOGIC AGENTS AND SIGNALING INHIBITORS

CEM GABAY

Biologic agents are a new class of therapeutic agents that target different mediators involved in the pathogenesis of human diseases. The development of these therapies has markedly improved the management of many diseases. In addition, their use has greatly increased our understanding regarding the pathophysiology of these diseases. One of the most compelling examples is the efficacy of tumor necrosis factor (TNF)-α inhibitors in rheumatoid arthritis and in inflammatory bowel diseases. In addition, new drugs targeting specifically intracellular enzymatic signaling pathways (kinases) have been developed. Most of these signaling inhibitors have been developed for the treatment of cancer. Recently, a kinase inhibitor was approved for the treatment of rheumatoid arthritis.

The United States Adopted Names Council has established a common classification of these different therapies (Table 36-1). The pharmaceutical company usually gives the prefix of the name, and the suffix defines whether this is a monoclonal antibody (mab), a soluble receptor (cept), or a kinase inhibitor (inib). Monoclonal antibodies, by far the largest group of biologic agents today, include also in their name the type of target (immune system, cancer, cardiovascular, system, and bone) as well as their origin (chimeric, humanized, and human).

TABLE 36-1 NOMENCLATURE OF MONOCLONAL ANTIBODIES

TARGET	ABBREVIATION	EXAMPLE
Immunology	li/l	ada**li**mumab
Cardiovascular	ci/c	beva**ci**zumab
Bone	os/s	den**os**umab
Interleukin	ki/k	cana**ki**numab
Miscellaneous tumors	tu/t	ofa**tu**mumab
SOURCE		
Chimeric	xi	ritu**xi**mab
Humanized	zu	trastu**zu**mab
Human	u	golim**u**mab

From the United States Adopted Names Council website (www.ama-assn.org).

To make mouse- or other animal-derived monoclonal antibodies less immunogenic, chemical and genetic engineering methods can replace two thirds of the mouse antibody with human antibody, creating "chimeric" monoclonal antibodies, or can replace 90 to 95% with human antibody to create "humanized" monoclonal antibodies. Chimeric and humanized monoclonal antibodies, being less immunogenic, elicit the production of less neutralizing human antimouse antibodies in the recipient present.

All biologic agents are large molecules that are administered by intravenous or subcutaneous routes, whereas kinase inhibitors are small chemicals that are prescribed as oral drugs. For safety reasons, combination of biologic agents or kinase inhibitors is not recommended. Rather than providing an exhaustive review of all tested approaches, this chapter aims to review the currently approved treatments.

TUMOR NECROSIS FACTOR-α INHIBITORS

The cytokine TNF-α binds to two different receptors, TNF-R55 and TNF-R75, and exerts important functions in the control of host responses against infections. However, uncontrolled TNF-α production may lead to chronic inflammation and subsequent tissue damage.

Types of Tumor Necrosis Factor-α Inhibitors

Different agents have been developed to inhibit the biologic activity of TNF-α, including monoclonal antibodies and soluble receptors. Monoclonal antibodies include infliximab (Remicade), adalimumab (Humira), and golimumab (Simponi). Infliximab is a chimeric antibody, whereas the two others are fully human antibodies. Certolizumab-pegol (Cimzia) is a pegylated humanized anti-TNF-α antibody Fab′ fragment. Etanercept (Enbrel) is a fusion protein that contains the extracellular portion of TNF-R75 coupled to the Fc domain of human immunoglobulin G1 (IgG1). All these agents bind to TNF-α and block its biologic activity. Etanercept binds also to lymphotoxin-α (previously termed TNF-β). Infliximab has been shown to exert cytotoxic effects on macrophages and T lymphocytes expressing TNF-α on their surface.

Indications

TNF-α antagonists are approved for the treatment of rheumatoid arthritis (Chapter 264). They exert marked anti-inflammatory effects and prevent the progression of structural joint damage. TNF-α inhibitors are efficacious in early rheumatoid arthritis and in long-standing disease refractory to conventional disease-modifying antirheumatic drugs (DMARDs) such as methotrexate. TNF-α inhibitors are more efficacious when administered in combination with methotrexate than alone. TNF-α inhibitors are also approved for the treatment of ankylosing spondylitis refractory to nonsteroidal anti-inflammatory drugs and psoriatic arthritis refractory to DMARDs (Chapter 265). Anti-TNF-α antibodies, but not etanercept, have proven efficacy in severe Crohn disease (Chapter 141) by reducing the disease activity score, inducing closure of draining fistulas, and allowing a decrease in the dose of chronic glucocorticoid medication. Infliximab, adalimumab, and golimumab are approved for the treatment of ulcerative colitis refractory to conventional therapy. Infliximab, adalimumab, and etanercept are also approved for the treatment of chronic plaque psoriasis (Chapter 438) refractory to phototherapy or systemic therapy.

Adverse Effects

TNF-α inhibitors can be associated with allergic reactions. Postmarketing data have shown that TNF- α inhibitors are associated with an increased risk for infections, including all types of bacterial and opportunistic infections. In particular, the use of TNF-α inhibitors has been associated with an increased risk for reactivation of latent tuberculosis. The results of cohort studies do not support an overall increased risk for cancer. Rare cases of demyelinating disorders, lupus-like manifestations, and cytopenia have been reported.

INTERLEUKIN-1 INHIBITORS

IL-1 (both IL-1α and IL-1β) binds to IL-1 receptors (type I IL-1R and IL-1R accessory protein) to induce a vast array of inflammatory signals. IL-1 receptor antagonist (IL-1Ra) competitively inhibits the interaction of IL-1 with its receptors.[1]

Types of Interleukin-1 Inhibitors

Anakinra (Kineret), recombinant human IL-1Ra, was the first IL-1 inhibitor used in clinical trials. Rilonacept (Arcalyst) is a fusion protein including the

IL-1 binding motifs of IL-1 receptors coupled to the Fc domain of human IgG1. Canakinumab (Ilaris) is a fully human monoclonal antibody against IL-1β.

Indications

Anakinra is approved for the treatment of rheumatoid arthritis refractory to conventional DMARDs but exhibits relatively modest efficacy. Anakinra, canakinumab, and rilonacept are approved for the treatment of cryopyrin-associated periodic syndromes, a set of hereditary systemic autoinflammatory diseases associated with *NLRP3* gene (encoding for cryopyrin) mutations (Chapter 261) and characterized by enhanced IL-1β release. Canakinumab is approved for the treatment of systemic-onset juvenile idiopathic arthritis in children aged 2 years and older. Anakinra is also effective in adult-onset Still disease and other autoinflammatory conditions. Clinical trials have reported encouraging results with IL-1 antagonists in crystal-induced arthritis such as gout and chondrocalcinosis. Promising results have also been reported from the use of gevokizumab, another fully human anti-IL-1β monoclonal antibody in Behçet uveitis.

Adverse Effects

Anakinra, canakinumab, and rilonacept have frequently been associated with injection site reactions and upper airway infections. A modest increase in serious infections has been reported with the three IL-1 antagonists. The combination of anakinra and etanercept (and probably also other TNF-α antagonists) increases the risk for infections and is not recommended.

INTERLEUKIN-6 INHIBITORS

IL-6 is a pro-inflammatory cytokine that binds to a heterodimeric receptor, including IL-6Rα and gp130. Tocilizumab (Actemra) is a humanized monoclonal antibody against IL-6Rα that inhibits its interaction with IL-6.

Indications

Tocilizumab is approved for the treatment of rheumatoid arthritis refractory to conventional DMARDs and TNF-α antagonists.[2] In clinical trials, tocilizumab prevented the progression of radiographic damage. Tocilizumab in monotherapy seems as effective as in combination with methotrexate and is superior to adalimumab (TNF-α inhibitor) in monotherapy. Tocilizumab is also approved for the treatment of systemic-onset juvenile idiopathic arthritis and polyarticular juvenile idiopathic arthritis in patients aged 2 years and older. In Japan, tocilizumab is approved for the management of Castelman disease. Tocilizumab is also effective for adult-onset Still disease. Clinical trials are in progress in other inflammatory rheumatic diseases. In addition, clinical trials examining the efficacy and safety of other monoclonal antibodies against IL-6R (sarilumab) or IL-6 (sirukumab, clazakizumab) in rheumatoid arthritis are in progress.[3]

Adverse Effects

Tocilizumab has been associated with an increased risk for serious infections. A transient increase in transaminase levels has been reported. Hypercholesterolemia and cytopenia may appear in some patients.

ANTIBODY AGAINST INTERLEUKIN-12 AND INTERLEUKIN-23

IL-12 and IL-23 are heterodimeric cytokines, including a common p40 subunit and a specific subunit—p35 for IL-12 and p19 for IL-23. IL-23 participates in the differentiation of T_H17 cells that produce IL-17. Experimental findings indicated that IL-23 and IL-17 are critical for the development of autoimmune pathologies. Ustekinumab (Stelara) is a human monoclonal antibody against p40 that targets both IL-12 and IL-23 and blocks their biologic activities.

Indications

Ustekinumab is approved for the treatment of psoriasis patients who have had prior exposure to phototherapy or use of other systemic therapies. In clinical trials, ustekinumab was associated with successful treatment of Crohn disease. In addition, ustekinumab alone or in combination with methotrexate is also approved for the treatment of active psoriatic arthritis. Anti-IL-17 and anti-IL-17R antibodies are in clinical trials for the treatment of psoriasis, psoriatic arthritis, ankylosing spondylitis, and rheumatoid arthritis.[4]

Side Effects

Ustekinumab has been associated with injection site reaction and allergic adverse events. Upper respiratory airway infections have been reported.

JANUS KINASE INHIBITOR

The janus kinase (JAK)-signal transducer and activator of transcription (STAT) signaling pathway transmits information from various receptors at the cell surface, including those of cytokines, interferons, and growth factors, to the DNA promoters in the nuclei, thus stimulating cell activation and gene expression. The JAK family comprises several members, such as JAK1, JAK2, JAK3, and Tyk2, that are associated as heterodimers or homodimers to the different receptors. Tofacitinib (Xeljanz) is a competitive inhibitor of JAK autophosphorylation, leading to the absence of STAT phosphorylation by JAK and the nuclear translocation of STAT. Tofacitinib preferentially inhibits the signaling associated with JAK3 and JAK1 activation, including the receptors involved in the immune and inflammatory responses.

Indications

Tofacitinib is approved for the oral treatment of moderate and severe rheumatoid arthritis refractory to conventional DMARDs and TNF antagonists.[5] Tofacitinib can be used alone or in combination with conventional DMARDs. Clinical trials in psoriasis, psoriatic arthritis, Crohn disease, and ulcerative colitis are ongoing. The JAK½ inhibitor ruxolitinib was recently approved for the treatment of myelofibrosis.[6]

Adverse Effects

Tofacitinib is associated with an increased rate of infectious events, including different types of bacterial infections, herpes zoster, and opportunistic infections. Increase in transaminase levels, hypercholesterolemia, and cytopenia has also been observed. Some of these adverse effects are potentially related to the inhibition of signals induced by IL-6 and hematopoietic growth factors.

INHIBITORS OF ANGIOGENESIS

Vascular endothelial growth factor (VEGF) is a family of growth factors involved in vasculogenesis and angiogenesis. VEGF-A binds to the tyrosine kinase receptors, VEGFR1 and VEGFR2. VEGF has been implicated in tumor growth and metastasis, in diabetic retinopathy, and in age-related macular retinopathy.

Types of Angiogenesis Inhibitors

Bevacizumab (Avastin) is a humanized monoclonal antibody against VEGF that acts as an angiogenesis inhibitor. Aflibercept (Zaltrap) is a fusion protein containing extracellular immunoglobulin motifs of VEGFR1 and VEGFR2 coupled to human IgG1. Several VEGF receptor–associated tyrosine kinase inhibitors have been approved for the treatment of cancer, including Sorafenib (Nexavar), Sunitinib (Sutent), Axitinib (Inlyta), Pazopanib (Votrient), Vandetanib (Caprelsa), and Sorafenib (Nexavar). Some of these tyrosine kinase inhibitors block not only VEGF receptors but also platelet-derived growth factor receptor-β, c-Kit, and Flt3 receptor.

Indications

Bevacizumab is approved for the treatment of glioblastoma (Chapter 189), and also for some patients with non–small cell lung cancer (Chapter 191), and metastatic colorectal cancer (Chapter 193). In Europe, bevacizumab is also approved for metastatic breast and ovarian cancer therapy. Intraocular injections of ranibizumab (Lucentis), an antibody fragment derived from bevacizumab, are effective in maintaining vision in most patients with wet macular degeneration (Chapter 423) and are approved for this indication. Aflibercept is approved for the treatment of metastatic colorectal cancer. Sunitinib is approved for the treatment of metastatic renal cell carcinoma (Chapter 197), gastrointestinal stromal tumor refractory to imatinib (Chapter 202), and unresectable pancreatic neuroendocrine tumors. Axitinib and pazopanib are approved for the treatment of renal cell carcinoma. Pazopanib is also approved for advanced soft tissue sarcoma. Vandetanib is approved for late-stage medullary thyroid cancer. Sorafenib is approved for advanced renal cell carcinoma, some cases of hepatocarcinoma (Chapter 196), and late-stage thyroid cancer.

Adverse Effects

Bevacizumab has been associated with a heightened risk for bleeding and gastrointestinal tract perforation. Delayed wound healing and hypertension have also been reported. Reported adverse events for kinase inhibitors include hypertension, fatigue, asthenia, diarrhea, and some abnormal laboratory tests, including transaminases, lipase, amylase, and leukocytes and platelets. Vandetanib is associated with prolonged QT, and more rarely with cases of torsades de pointes and sudden death.

INHIBITORS OF TUMOR GROWTH FACTORS

The epidermal growth factor receptor (EGFR), a member of the ErbB-1 (human epithelial growth factor receptor-1 [HER-1]) family of receptors, is a cell surface receptor for epidermal growth factor (EGF) and transforming growth factor-α. Binding of EGFR leads to tyrosine kinase activation. In tumor cells, EGFR overexpression or dysregulation due to *EGFR* gene mutations (exon 19 deletion or exon 21 [L858R] substitution) can lead to cell proliferation, apoptosis blockade, neovascularization, and tumor metastasis. HER-2 (also known as ErbB2) is a receptor with tyrosine kinase activity that is expressed at high levels in 20 to 30% of breast cancers and other types of cancers and may cause uncontrolled tumor cell proliferation.

Types of Inhibitors

Two types of strategies target the EGFR pathway: monoclonal antibodies to the extracellular domain of EGFR and orally available tyrosine kinase inhibitors. Cetuximab (Erbitux) is a chimeric monoclonal IgG1 anti-EGFR antibody that inhibits EGFR signaling and may also induce tumor cell death by antibody-dependent cellular cytotoxicity. Panitumumab (Vectibix) is a fully human monoclonal IgG2 antibody directed against EGFR. Erlotinib (Tarceva), gefitinib (Iressa), and afatinib (Gilotrif) are the three most commonly studied EGFR tyrosine kinase inhibitors. Trastuzumab (Herceptin) is a humanized monoclonal IgG1 antibody that binds to the extracellular domain of HER-2. Lapatinib (Tykerb) is a small molecule with inhibitory activity on EGFR and HER-2 tyrosine kinases.

Indications

Cetuximab is approved as second- and third-line treatment in colorectal and squamous cell carcinoma of the head and neck cancers. Panitumumab is approved for the treatment of metastatic colorectal cancer. Erlotinib and afatinib are approved for the treatment of metastatic non–small cell lung carcinoma with EGFR mutations, whereas gefitinib is approved for the same indication but with some additional limitations. Erlotinib is also approved for the treatment of pancreatic cancer. Trastuzumab and lapatinib are approved for the treatment of metastatic breast cancer expressing HER-2, and trastuzumab for metastatic stomach and gastroesophageal junction cancer expressing HER-2.

Adverse Effects

Cetuximab is sometimes associated with severe allergic reactions during infusion. Acne-like skin rash has been commonly reported. Erlotinib, gefitinib, and afatinib are associated with acne-like rash and mild gastrointestinal symptoms. Cardiotoxicity is a major problem in patients treated with trastuzumab. Approximately 10% of patients are unable to tolerate this drug because of pre-existing heart problems. The risk for cardiomyopathy is increased when combined with anthracycline (which itself is associated with cardiac toxicity). Lapatinib is in general well tolerated, but some cases of hepatotoxicity have been reported. Active research is in progress to develop more selective angiogenesis inhibitors in order to overcome acquired resistance to specific inhibitors of VEGF and VEGFR and to reduce their negative off-target effects.[7]

OTHER TYROSINE KINASE INHIBITORS

Imatinib mesylate (Gleevec or Glivec) works by binding to the adenosine triphosphate (ATP) binding site of BCR-ABL, resulting in competitive inhibition of its enzymatic activity. Imatinib inhibits also the tyrosine kinase activity of c-Kit and platelet-derived growth factor receptor.

Indications

Imatinib represents a major advance over conventional treatments for chronic myelogenous leukemia (Chapter 184), with more than 90% of patients obtaining complete hematologic response and 70 to 80% of patients achieving a complete cytogenetic response. Resistance to imatinib[8] represents a clinical challenge and is often a result of point mutations causing a conformation change in BCR-ABL, which impairs imatinib binding. Dasatinib (Sprycel) and Nilotinib (Tasigna), two other tyrosine kinase inhibitors, have been approved for the treatment of chronic myelogenous leukemia as first-line therapy or in patients who are not responsive or intolerant to imatinib. Bosutinib (Bosulif) and ponatinib (Iclusig) are second-generation tyrosine kinase inhibitors that are approved as second-line treatment for chronic myelogenous leukemia.

Imatinib is also approved for the treatment of patients with c-Kit-positive advanced gastrointestinal stromal tumor (Chapter 202). Early clinical trials also showed potential beneficial effect of imatinib in systemic mastocytosis, hypereosinophilic syndrome, and dermatofibrosarcoma protuberans.

Adverse Effects

Imatinib has been associated with the occurrence of cytopenia, edema, nausea, and rash, as well as rare cases of congestive heart failure. Cytopenia and congestive heart failure are also reported with all tyrosine kinase inhibitors. Nilotinib also carries a potential risk for severe cardiac arrhythmias. Ponatinib is associated with severe adverse events, including arterial and venous blood clots, leading to its approval only in patients refractory to all other tyrosine kinase inhibitors or in patients who carry a specific gene mutation (*T315I*).

BIOLOGIC AGENTS TARGETING T LYMPHOCYTES

T cells play a central role in immune responses and are thus important targets for therapies against graft rejection and autoimmune diseases.

Types of Agents Modulating T-Cell Activity

The agents targeting T cells include antibodies against T cells, soluble receptors inhibiting costimulation signals, and antibodies blocking T-cell migration. Therapies targeting CD3 were developed more than 30 years ago with a mouse monoclonal IgG2 antibody called OKT3. These antibodies were used in the treatment of kidney transplant rejection but were associated with limiting side effects due to the occurrence of a "cytokine release syndrome." Then, a series of non-Fc-binding humanized anti-CD3 monoclonal antibodies were developed to overcome this problem as well as the development of antimurine immunoglobulin antibodies.

Abatacept (Orencia) and belatacept (Nulojix) are fusion proteins containing the extracellular portion of cytotoxic T lymphocyte antigen-4 coupled to the Fc portion of human IgG1, and they inhibit costimulatory signals between CD28 and CD80/86. Alefacept (Amevive) is a recombinant fully human fusion protein, in which the extracellular domain of CD2 has been linked to the Fc portion of IgG1, and it inhibits costimulatory signals between CD2 and LFA-3.

Natalizumab (Tysabri), a humanized monoclonal antibody against α_4-integrin, inhibits the migration of T cells by blocking the interaction between α_4-integrin and adhesion molecules expressed on endothelial cells.

Indications

Different monoclonal anti-CD3 antibodies are used in clinical trials for the prevention of transplant rejection (Chapter 49) as well as for the treatment of acute graft-versus-host disease and type 1 diabetes mellitus.

Abatacept is approved for the treatment of patients with rheumatoid arthritis and polyarticular juvenile idiopathic arthritis aged 6 years and older refractory to conventional DMARDs and TNF-α inhibitors. Belatacept is approved for the prevention of acute kidney transplant rejection. Alefacept is approved for the treatment of chronic plaque psoriasis. Natalizumab is approved for the treatment of patients with highly active remitting-relapsing multiple sclerosis in monotherapy (Chapter 411) and for severe Crohn disease.

Adverse Effects

Abatacept is generally well tolerated, but serious infectious adverse events may occur. Belatacept has been associated with anemia, urinary tract infections, and post-transplant lymphoproliferative disorders in Epstein-Barr virus–unexposed patients. Lymphopenia may occur with alefacept, and infections, malignancies, and hepatotoxicity have been reported in clinical trials. Natalizumab can be associated with allergic reactions and hepatotoxicity. Some cases of multifocal progressive leucoencephalopathy (Chapter 370), a fatal neurologic complication of JC virus reactivation in immunosuppressed individuals, have been reported, thus limiting the use of natalizumab.

AGENTS TARGETING B LYMPHOCYTES

The B-cell lineage plays a critical role in immune responses through the production of immunoglobulins, the presentation of antigen to T cells, and production of cytokines. Therapies aiming to target B cells are used in B-cell lymphoma and in autoimmune diseases.

Mode of Action

B cells can be targeted either by the use of monoclonal antibodies depleting B cells or by inhibiting cytokines essential for their maturation and survival, such as B-cell-activating factor of the TNF family (BAFF). Rituximab

(Rituxan or MabThera), ofatumumab (Arzerra), and ocrelizumab are B-cell-depleting monoclonal antibodies by binding to CD20. Belimumab (Benlysta) is a fully human monoclonal antibody against BAFF.

Indications

Rituximab is approved for the treatment of non-Hodgkin B-cell lymphoma (Chapter 185), for rheumatoid arthritis patients with inadequate response to TNF-α inhibitors, and in antineutrophil cytoplasmic autoantibody–associated vasculitis, including granulomatosis with polyangiitis (formerly Wegener granulomatosis) and microscopic polyangiitis. Disappointing results were obtained in clinical trials with rituximab in systemic lupus erythematosus. Ofatumumab is approved for the treatment of chronic lymphocytic leukemia (Chapter 184). Ocrelizumab is currently in clinical trials in multiple sclerosis. Epratuzumab, a humanized monoclonal anti-CD22 B-cell-depleting antibody, is in clinical trials for non-Hodgkin B-cell lymphoma. Positive results were reported in systemic lupus erythematosus, suggesting that epratuzumab might be eventually approved for this indication. Belimumab is the first biologic agent approved for the treatment of systemic lupus erythematosus refractory to conventional therapy. However, phase III studies leading to the registration of belimumab in this indication did not include more severe cases with renal and central nervous system involvement. Belimumab did not show efficacy in rheumatoid arthritis, but encouraging results were reported in Sjögren syndrome. The efficacy of tabalumab, a monoclonal antibody targeting membrane-bound and soluble BAFF, is being tested in a clinical trial in systemic lupus erythematosus.

Adverse Effects

Rituximab is associated with allergic reaction during infusions, systemic reaction due to tumoral B-cell lysis, and an increased risk for infectious events. Rare cases of multifocal progressive leucoencephalopathy have been reported. Hypogammaglobulinemia may occur, particularly after several series of infusions. Belimumab is associated with allergic reaction during infusion and an increased risk for infections.

CONCLUSION

The use of biologic agents has led to major advances in the management of many severe diseases refractory to conventional therapies. These agents have also provided a unique way to confirm the role of basic mechanisms in human diseases. New developments in this field will follow different directions, including the refinement of existing strategies (using more selective inhibitors or human rather than chimeric antibodies), the extension to other indications than those for which the agents were primarily designed, the selection of novel targets, and the identification of biologic markers of response.

GENERAL REFERENCES

For the General References and other additional features, please visit Expert Consult at https://expertconsult.inkling.com.

37

PROSTANOIDS, ASPIRIN, AND RELATED COMPOUNDS

CARLO PATRONO

Arachidonic acid, or 5,8,11,14-eicosatetraenoic acid, is a 20-carbon polyunsaturated fatty acid esterified in the phospholipid domain of cell membranes. In response to chemical, physical, and hormonal stimuli, arachidonic acid is released from the glycerol backbone sn2 position by the action of various phospholipases A_2 and can be subjected to rapid enzymatic conversion to a series of oxygenated derivatives collectively called eicosanoids. The enzymes catalyzing various structural modifications of free arachidonic acid include prostaglandin H synthases, commonly known as cyclooxygenases (COX), lipoxygenases, and cytochrome P-450 isozymes. The resulting eicosanoids include prostanoids (prostaglandins and thromboxane A_2), leukotrienes, lipoxins, and epoxylins. Esterified arachidonic acid can also be subjected to in situ peroxidation, catalyzed by oxygen radicals, to form a series of corresponding isomers called isoeicosanoids.

Eicosanoids are not stored but are produced in response to diverse stimuli, with a pattern that reflects the cell-specific distribution of arachidonic acid–metabolizing enzymes and downstream isomerases and synthases. Eicosanoids are not circulating hormones but rather ubiquitous autacoids that modulate the intensity and duration of many important cellular responses in an autocrine (acting on the same cells that produced them) or paracrine (acting on nearby cells) fashion.

BIOSYNTHESIS AND ACTION OF PROSTANOIDS

Prostanoids include prostaglandins D_2, E_2, $F_{2\alpha}$, and I_2 (prostacyclin) and thromboxane A_2. They are formed through the sequential actions of phospholipase A_2 to release arachidonic acid from membrane phospholipids, prostaglandin H synthase to catalyze the cyclooxygenation of arachidonic acid to form the unstable intermediate prostaglandin G_2 and its reduction to prostaglandin H_2, and specific isomerases and synthases to catalyze the conversion of prostaglandin H_2 to different prostanoids (Fig. 37-1). Once formed, prostanoids interact with specific G protein–coupled receptors to evoke a variety of cellular responses, depending on the site of their biosynthesis (Fig. 37-1).

Two prostaglandin H synthases have been identified: prostaglandin H synthase 1 is expressed constitutively in all cells; prostaglandin H synthase 2 is constitutively expressed in some cells (e.g., neurons and renal cells) and is induced in other cell types in response to cytokines (e.g., in monocytes), tumor promoters (e.g., in intestinal epithelial cells), growth factors (e.g., in bone marrow–derived stem cells), and laminar shear stress (e.g., in endothelial cells). Because nonsteroidal anti-inflammatory drugs (NSAIDs) target the COX activity of these enzymes, they have become known colloquially as COX-1 and COX-2.[1] Both enzymes are homodimers that convert arachidonic acid, two oxygen molecules, and two electrons from one or more unknown reductants to prostaglandin H_2. COX-1 and COX-2 are found predominantly in the same cellular organelles, at the luminal surface of the endoplasmic reticulum and nuclear envelope of cells. Only one monomer of a dimer catalyzes arachidonic acid oxygenation at any given time. The cross-talk between monomers serves as a way for COX-2 to exhibit selectivity toward arachidonic acid, even when it is a minor component of the available fatty acid pool, and to sustain a "late phase" of prostanoid production. In contrast, COX-1 may efficiently oxygenate arachidonic acid in the early phase of prostanoid production, when this substrate represents a large fraction of free fatty acids, but may be inhibited by other competing fatty acids in the late phase.

Phenotypical analyses of COX-1–deficient and COX-2–deficient mice as well as studies with isoform-selective inhibitors suggest that there are processes in which each isozyme is uniquely involved (e.g., platelet aggregation for COX-1, ovulation and neonatal development for COX-2) and others in which both isozymes function coordinately (e.g., inflammation and its resolution, gastrointestinal ulceration and healing, and carcinogenesis). A way in which the two biosynthetic pathways may be dissociated metabolically is by a preferential coupling of the COX isozymes to various upstream phospholipases and downstream synthases, conditioning preferential formation of a particular prostanoid by a given cell type (e.g., COX-2–dependent prostacyclin by vascular endothelial cells).

Moreover, COX-2 oxygenation may play a unique role in a novel signaling pathway dependent on agonist-induced release of endocannabinoids.[2] Among the products of COX-2 oxygenation of endocannabinoids are glyceryl prostaglandins, some of which (e.g., glyceryl prostaglandin E_2 and glyceryl prostaglandin I_2) exhibit interesting biologic activities in inflammatory, neurologic, and vascular systems.

MEASUREMENTS OF THE PROSTAGLANDIN H SYNTHASE PATHWAY

Prostanoids are formed in vivo at a relatively low rate (e.g., 0.1 ng/kg per minute for both prostacyclin and thromboxane A_2) and are metabolized extensively by lung and liver enzymes to form chemically stable but biologically inactive derivatives that are excreted primarily through the kidney. Given the chemical instability and extremely low concentrations (1 to 2 pg/mL) of prostanoids in the systemic circulation, assessment of their production in humans is largely based on measurements of stable urinary metabolites (e.g., 11-dehydro-thromboxane B_2, a major enzymatic derivative of thromboxane A_2, and 2,3-dinor-6-keto-PGF$_{1\alpha}$, a major enzymatic derivative of prostacyclin). These analytical measurements have established that thromboxane metabolite excretion is primarily derived from platelet

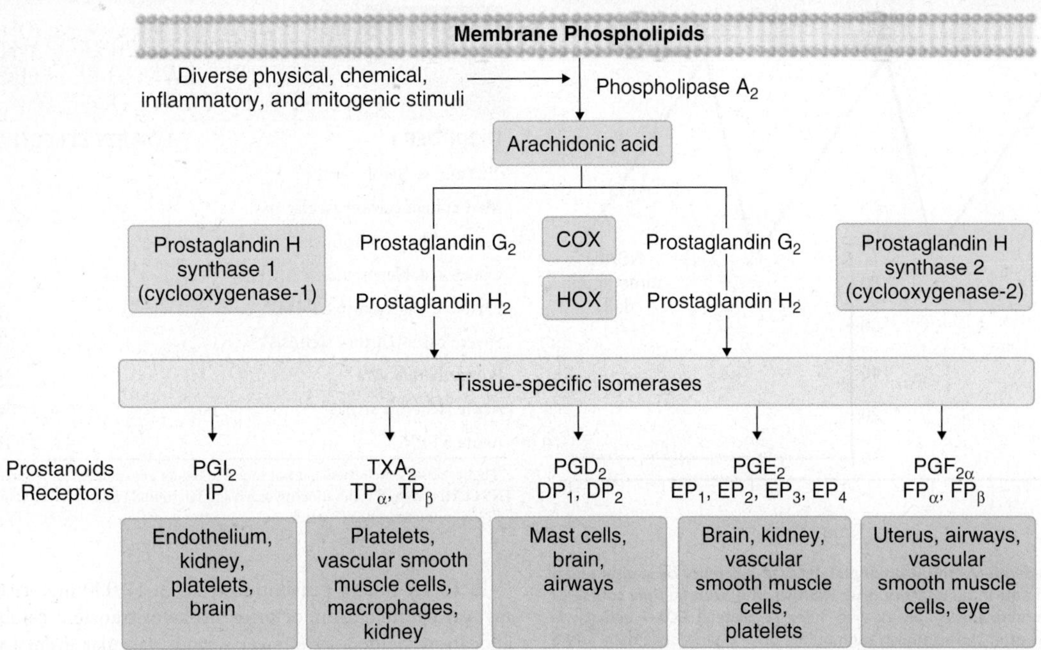

FIGURE 37-1. Production and actions of prostaglandins and thromboxane. Arachidonic acid, a 20-carbon fatty acid containing four double bonds, is liberated from the sn2 position in membrane phospholipids by phospholipase A_2, which is activated by diverse stimuli. Arachidonic acid is converted by prostaglandin H synthases, which have both cyclooxygenase (COX) and hydroperoxidase (HOX) activity, to the unstable intermediate prostaglandin H_2. The synthases are colloquially termed cyclooxygenases and exist in two forms, cyclooxygenase 1 and cyclooxygenase 2. Prostaglandin H_2 is converted by tissue-specific isomerases to multiple prostanoids. These bioactive lipids activate specific cell membrane receptors of the superfamily of G protein–coupled receptors. Some of the tissues in which individual prostanoids exert prominent effects are indicated. DP = prostaglandin D_2 receptor; EP = prostaglandin E_2 receptor; FP = prostaglandin $F_{2\alpha}$ receptor; IP = prostacyclin receptor; TP = thromboxane receptor.

thromboxane biosynthesis and largely reflects the rate of platelet activation in vivo. Similarly, prostacyclin metabolite excretion largely reflects the rate of vascular prostacyclin biosynthesis in vivo. Thromboxane biosynthesis is persistently enhanced in association with the major cardiovascular risk factors (e.g., diabetes mellitus). The biosynthesis of both thromboxane and prostacyclin is episodically increased in patients with acute coronary syndromes, perhaps reflecting a homeostatic response to accelerated platelet-vascular interactions.

Studies of the human pharmacology of COX inhibitors have largely relied on the development of whole blood assays of platelet COX-1 (based on serum thromboxane B_2 measurements) and monocyte COX-2 (based on lipopolysaccharide-induced prostaglandin E_2 production) activities. These assays have been useful in characterizing the variable potency of NSAIDs in inhibiting COX-1 and COX-2 in vitro (a measure of isozyme selectivity) and in determining ex vivo the dose and time dependence of their inhibitory effects in health and disease.

CLINICAL PHARMACOLOGY OF PROSTAGLANDIN H SYNTHASE INHIBITION

Most traditional NSAIDs inhibit COX-1 and COX-2 with similar potency (Fig. 37-2). Some traditional NSAIDs (e.g., nimesulide and diclofenac) and a class of COX-2 inhibitors called coxibs (e.g., celecoxib and etoricoxib) are more potent in inhibiting COX-2 than COX-1 (Fig. 37-2). These drugs fall into three general categories on the basis of their mechanism of action. One category of inhibitors includes freely reversible competitive inhibitors, such as ibuprofen and mefenamic acid. Binding of these inhibitors to the COX sites of both monomers composing a dimer is required for inhibition of COX-2 oxygenation of the substrate. A second group of inhibitors, including flurbiprofen, meclofenamate, diclofenac, and indomethacin, comprises time-dependent, noncovalent inhibitors. These NSAIDs are allosteric inhibitors that bind to one monomer of COX to inhibit its activity. Aspirin is unique to a third group of inhibitors that cause a time-dependent, covalent inhibition. Binding of aspirin to COX-1 or COX-2 leads to irreversible acetylation of a highly conserved serine residue (Ser-529 and Ser-516 in human COX-1 and COX-2, respectively). Aspirin acetylates only one monomer of a COX-1 dimer to cause complete loss of COX activity. Aspirin also maximally acetylates one monomer of human COX-2. The acetylated monomer of aspirin-treated COX-2 forms 15-hydroperoxyeicosatetraenoic acid from arachidonic acid, whereas the nonacetylated partner monomer forms mainly prostaglandin H_2 but only at 15 to 20% of the rate of native COX-2. Thus, the

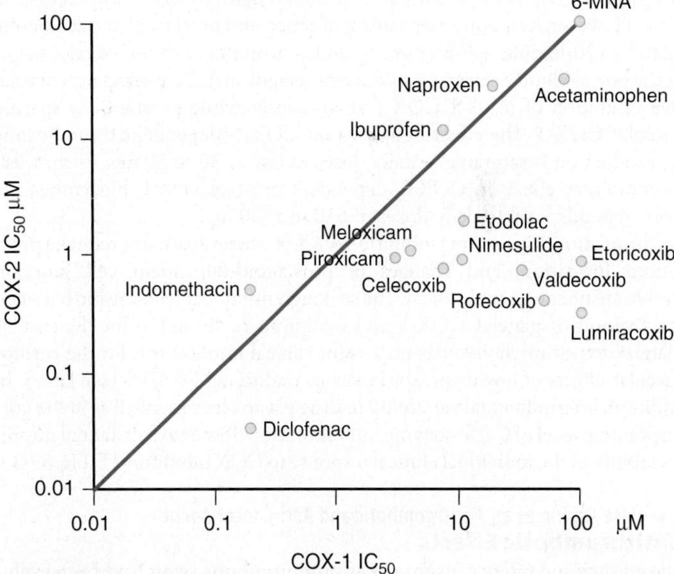

FIGURE 37-2. COX-2 selectivity as a continuous variable. Concentrations of various COX-2 inhibitors to inhibit the activity of platelet COX-1 and monocyte COX-2 by 50% (IC_{50}) are plotted on the abscissa and ordinate scales, respectively. The *solid line* describes equipotent inhibition of both COX-1 and COX-2. Symbols to the left of this line denote greater inhibition of COX-1 than of COX-2. Symbols to the right of this line indicate progressively greater inhibition of COX-2 than of COX-1, that is, increasing degrees of COX-2 selectivity. Aspirin is not shown on the figure because the long-term incubation required for monocyte COX-2 expression in human whole blood affects the chemical stability of the drug and underestimates its inhibitory potency. 6-MNA = 6-methoxy-2-naphthylacetic acid, the active metabolite of nabumetone.

effect of aspirin on COX-2 is an incomplete allosteric inhibition compared with that seen with COX-1.

Traditional NSAIDs typically inhibit platelet COX-1 and monocyte COX-2 by 50 to 90%, depending on dose; this effect is usually transient, depending on dose and half-life (Fig. 37-3). Coxibs inhibit monocyte COX-2 to the same extent as other NSAIDs while substantially sparing platelet (and presumably other cells) COX-1 in most patients exposed to therapeutic

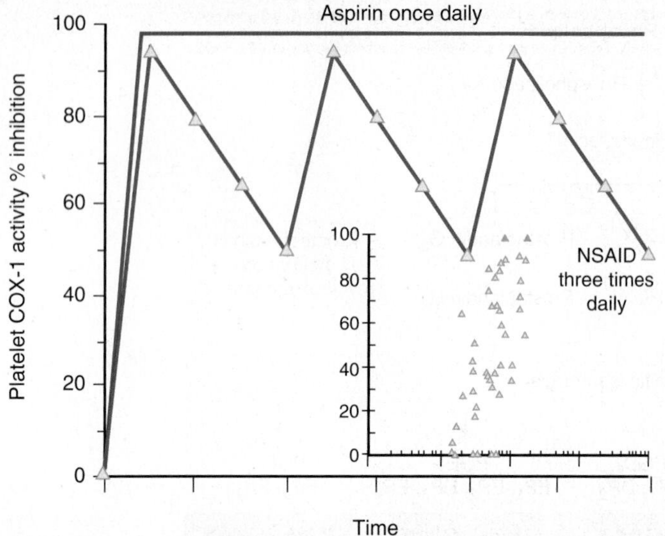

FIGURE 37-3. **Time-dependent inhibition of platelet COX-1 activity by aspirin and a traditional nonsteroidal anti-inflammatory drug (NSAID). The average time course of inhibition of serum thromboxane B_2, an ex vivo index of platelet COX-1 activity, is depicted during 24 hours after the administration of low-dose aspirin once daily and a traditional NSAID with short half-life given every 8 hours. The *inset* depicts the interindividual variability in the relationship between NSAID plasma levels plotted on the abscissa log scale and the corresponding level of inhibition of platelet COX-1 plotted on the ordinate.**

doses. In contrast, aspirin achieves virtually complete (i.e., >97%) and persistent (i.e., ≥24 hour) inactivation of platelet COX-1 by virtue of its irreversible mechanism of action and inability of anucleate platelets to resynthesize the enzyme. Aspirin is equally potent in acetylating COX-1 and COX-2 in vitro. However, its unique mechanism of action and unusual pharmacokinetic features (20-minute half-life; presystemic encounter with the platelet target in the portal blood before first-pass liver metabolism) allow selective, cumulative inhibition of platelet COX-1 at low doses while substantially sparing vascular COX-2. The effect of aspirin on COX-1–dependent thromboxane A_2 production is saturable at daily doses as low as 30 to 50 mg; in contrast, its inhibitory effect on COX-2–dependent prostaglandin I_2 biosynthesis is dose dependent up to daily doses of 650 to 1300 mg.

The relationships among inhibition of COX isozyme activity, reduced prostanoid formation, and changes in prostanoid-dependent cell function in vivo are not necessarily linear. The strikingly nonlinear relationship between inactivation of platelet COX-1 and inhibition of thromboxane-dependent platelet activation in vivo has important clinical implications for the cardiovascular effects of low-dose aspirin versus traditional NSAIDs (see later). In addition, interindividual variability in drug plasma levels as well as in the corresponding level of COX isozyme inhibition contributes to substantial unpredictability of the individual clinical response to COX inhibitors (E-Fig. 37-1).

Low-Dose Aspirin as an Antithrombotic and Anti-Cancer Agent

Antithrombotic Effects

The efficacy and safety of aspirin as an antithrombotic agent have been evaluated in several populations, ranging from apparently healthy persons at low risk of vascular complications (so-called primary prevention) to high-risk patients presenting with or surviving an acute myocardial infarction or an acute ischemic stroke (so-called secondary prevention). The clinical efficacy of aspirin was demonstrated at doses ranging from 50 to 162 mg given once daily (Table 37-1), consistent with the irreversible nature of its mechanism of action. Furthermore, higher doses (e.g., 300 to 325 mg) were not found to confer additional benefits, consistent with saturability of platelet COX-1 acetylation at low doses.[3,4]

In the six primary prevention trials among 95,000 low-risk individuals, aspirin allocation yielded a 12% relative risk reduction in serious vascular events (myocardial infarction, stroke, or vascular death).[A1] This protective effect was mainly due to a reduction in nonfatal myocardial infarction. The net effect on stroke was not significant, reflecting a small reduction in ischemic stroke and counterbalancing effects on hemorrhagic stroke. There was no significant reduction in vascular mortality. Aspirin increased gastrointestinal (or other extracranial) bleeds by approximately 50%.[A1] The balance of cardiovascular benefits and bleeding risk associated with low-dose aspirin in specifically primary prevention is uncertain.[5]

TABLE 37-1 VASCULAR DISORDERS FOR WHICH ASPIRIN HAS BEEN SHOWN TO BE EFFECTIVE AND THE LOWEST EFFECTIVE DOSE

DISORDER	LOWEST EFFECTIVE DAILY DOSE (mg)
TIA and ischemic stroke*	50
Men at high cardiovascular risk	75
Essential hypertension	75
Chronic stable angina	75
Unstable angina or NSTEMI*	75
Severe carotid artery stenosis*	75
Polycythemia vera	100
Acute ischemic stroke*	160
Acute STEMI	162

*Higher doses were tested and not found to confer any greater risk reduction.
NSTEMI = non–ST elevation myocardial infarction; STEMI = ST elevation myocardial infarction; TIA = transient ischemic attack.

In 16 secondary prevention trials in 17,000 high-risk patients with prior myocardial infarction, or prior stroke or transient cerebral ischemia, aspirin allocation yielded 19% fewer serious vascular events, with similar proportional reductions in coronary events (20% relative risk reduction) and ischemic stroke (22% relative risk reduction) but a nonsignificant increase in hemorrhagic stroke.[A1] The absolute benefit of aspirin was about 25 times larger in secondary than in primary prevention (15 vs. 0.6 fewer vascular events per 1000 per year). In both primary and secondary prevention trials, the proportional reductions in serious vascular events appeared similar for men and women and for older and younger people. The risks of serious vascular events and of major extracranial bleeds were predicted by the same independent risk factors (age, male gender, diabetes mellitus, current smoking, blood pressure, and body mass index), so those with high risk of vascular complications also had a high risk of bleeding. For secondary prevention of cardiovascular disease, the net benefits of adding aspirin to other preventive measures (e.g., statins) substantially exceed the bleeding hazards, irrespective of age and gender.

Anti-Cancer Effects

Aspirin, 75 mg daily or more for at least several years, reduces the incidence and mortality of colorectal cancer.[A2] Long-term follow-up of randomized vascular prevention trials of daily aspirin versus control showed that aspirin reduced not only the incidence of and mortality due to colorectal cancer but also death due to several other common cancers. Furthermore, meta-analysis has shown short-term reduction by daily aspirin in cancer incidence and mortality in women as well as in men and in non-smokers as well as in smokers.[A3] In a randomized trial of carriers of hereditary colorectal cancer genes, aspirin (600 mg daily) for a mean of 25 months substantially reduced the incidence of cancer after about 5 years.[A4] Low-dose aspirin also reduces the risk of metastases,[A5] especially for adenocarcinomas. The mechanism underlying the chemopreventive effect of low-dose aspirin might involve inhibition of platelet activation.[6] More recent evidence shows that the risk of major bleeding with aspirin diminishes with prolonged use, suggesting that the balance of risk and benefit favors the use of daily aspirin in primary prevention of colorectal and other cancers.[7] A regulatory review of the existing evidence as well as treatment guidelines are needed for this potential chemopreventive strategy.

Traditional Nonsteroidal Anti-inflammatory Drugs and Coxibs

NSAIDs constitute a chemically heterogeneous group of compounds that provide symptomatic relief of pain and inflammation associated with a variety of human disorders, including the rheumatic diseases. Their shared therapeutic actions (i.e., analgesic, anti-inflammatory, and antipyretic) are usually accompanied by mechanism-based adverse effects on gastrointestinal, cardiovascular, and renal functions. Prostanoids reproduce the main signs and symptoms of the inflammatory response and cause hyperalgesia and fever. Because of the redundancy of mediators of these responses, it is not surprising that NSAIDs exert only a moderate anti-inflammatory effect, are effective only against pain of low to moderate intensity, and reduce fever but do not interfere with the physiologic control of body temperature. The analgesic, anti-inflammatory, and antipyretic actions of traditional NSAIDs are largely reproduced by coxibs, a class of selective inhibitors of COX-2.

COX-2 selectivity is a continuous variable (see Fig. 37-2). Thus, one can pragmatically characterize three levels of COX-2 selectivity in terms of the probability of sparing COX-1 at therapeutic plasma levels: low (e.g., acetaminophen), intermediate (e.g., celecoxib, nimesulide, and diclofenac), and high (e.g., rofecoxib, etoricoxib, and lumiracoxib).

Drug Interactions

NSAIDs can modify the pharmacokinetics or pharmacodynamics of other drugs given concurrently, resulting in clinically important drug interactions. A pharmacodynamic interaction may occur between most NSAIDs and several classes of antihypertensive drugs. Reduced production of vasodilator prostacyclin and natriuretic prostaglandin E_2, as a consequence of renal COX-2 inhibition, results in vasoconstriction and sodium and water retention that in turn tend to elevate blood pressure, regardless of the mechanism of action of antihypertensive drugs. This pharmacodynamic interaction has been described with most traditional NSAIDs (including acetaminophen) and coxibs, but not with low-dose aspirin.

Some NSAIDs favoring COX-1 over COX-2 inhibition, such as ibuprofen and naproxen, may interfere with the antiplatelet effect of low-dose aspirin by competing with acetylsalicylic acid for a common docking site (arginine-120) within the COX-1 channel. Drugs favoring COX-2 versus COX-1 inhibition, such as acetaminophen and diclofenac, do not interfere with the pharmacodynamic effect of low-dose aspirin, similar to celecoxib and rofecoxib.

Gastrointestinal and Bleeding Complications

Upper gastrointestinal complications (bleeds, perforations, and obstructions)[8,9] occur in 1 to 2% of NSAID-treated patients (Chapter 139). The mortality rate associated with hospitalization due to major gastrointestinal events is 5 to 6% in recent studies. Mortality rates associated with upper or lower gastrointestinal complications due to NSAIDs are similar. The major risk factors for upper gastrointestinal bleeding are represented by age and a prior history of gastrointestinal disorders (E-Fig. 37-1). Male gender, cigarette smoking, and heavy alcohol intake increase this risk by less than two-fold, as do oral glucocorticoids. Oral anticoagulants, thienopyridines, and low-dose aspirin increase the risk of NSAID-induced bleeding complications by two- to three-fold. The excess of these complications due to traditional NSAIDs has been estimated to range between 3 and 30 events per 1000 patients treated per year, depending on the absence or presence of risk factors (E-Fig. 37-1).

Highly selective COX-2 inhibitors are associated with a statistically significant 50 to 66% relative risk reduction in ulcer complications compared with naproxen or ibuprofen. However, no such agent is currently available on the U.S. market.

Cardiovascular Complications

A meta-analysis of individual participant data from randomized trials of five different coxibs has revealed that in placebo comparisons, allocation to a coxib was associated with a 37% increased risk of major vascular events with no statistically significant heterogeneity among the different coxibs.[A6] This excess risk of vascular events was derived primarily from a two-fold increased risk of myocardial infarction. Overall, there was no significant difference in the incidence of vascular events between a coxib and any traditional NSAID, but there was evidence of significant heterogeneity between naproxen and the other traditional NSAIDs (largely represented by ibuprofen and diclofenac). The proportional effects on major vascular events were independent of baseline characteristics, including vascular risk. Therefore, the absolute excess of major vascular events caused by coxibs and some traditional NSAIDs varied between 2 and 9 for every 1000 patients allocated to a year of treatment, depending on the baseline level of cardiovascular risk.

Current evidence suggests that the risk of myocardial infarction depends on the extent of COX-2 inhibition and not on the variable COX-2 selectivity of the inhibitor.[10] This risk appears to be modulated by concomitant high-grade and persistent inhibition of platelet COX-1 activity, as suggested by the neutral cardiovascular phenotype associated with a high-dose regimen of naproxen.[A6] However, in patients at high cardiovascular risk, whose platelet COX-1 is completely and persistently inactivated by low-dose aspirin, the administration of any COX-2 inhibitor (including naproxen) is likely to produce detrimental cardiovascular consequences.

Given the nonlinear relationship between inhibition of platelet COX-1 activity and inhibition of platelet activation in vivo, it is perhaps not surprising that the cardiovascular safety profiles of coxibs and some traditional NSAIDs (e.g., diclofenac) appear similar because they both fail to inhibit platelet activation adequately irrespective of their COX-2 selectivity. Early appearance, dose dependence, and slow dissipation of risk are important features of COX-2-related cardiotoxicity.

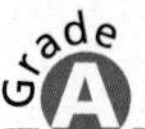

Grade A References

A1. Baigent C, Blackwell L, Collins R, et al. for the Antithrombotic Trialists' (ATT) Collaboration. Aspirin in the primary and secondary prevention of vascular disease: collaborative meta-analysis of individual participant data from randomised trials. *Lancet.* 2009;373:1849-1860.

A2. Rothwell PM, Wilson M, Elwin CE, et al. Long-term effect of aspirin on colorectal cancer incidence and mortality: 20-year follow-up of five randomised trials. *Lancet.* 2010;376:1741-1750.

A3. Rothwell PM, Price JF, Fowkes FG, et al. Short-term effects of daily aspirin on cancer incidence, mortality, and non-vascular death: analysis of the time course of risks and benefits in 51 randomised controlled trials. *Lancet.* 2012;379:1602-1612.

A4. Burn J, Gerdes AM, Macrae F, et al. Long-term effect of aspirin on cancer risk in carriers of hereditary colorectal cancer: an analysis from the CAPP2 randomised controlled trial. *Lancet.* 2011;378:2081-2087.

A5. Rothwell PM, Wilson M, Price JF, et al. Effect of daily aspirin on risk of cancer metastasis: a study of incident cancers during randomised controlled trials. *Lancet.* 2012;379:1591-1601.

A6. CNT Collaboration. Vascular and upper gastrointestinal effects of non-steroidal anti-inflammatory drugs: meta-analyses of individual participant data from randomised trials. *Lancet.* 2013;382:769-779.

GENERAL REFERENCES

For the General References and other additional features, please visit Expert Consult at https://expertconsult.inkling.com.

38

ANTITHROMBOTIC THERAPY

SAM SCHULMAN AND JACK HIRSH

Antithrombotic therapy suppresses the natural hemostatic mechanisms (Chapter 171) and is effective for preventing and treating venous, cardiac, and arterial thromboembolism. A variety of medications are now available that interfere with different steps in coagulation and platelet activation, sometimes with synergistic effects. Randomized clinical trials have produced a substantial body of evidence-based literature to guide the use of antithrombotic therapy for a wide range of clinical conditions. Updated recommendations have been published in the new 2012 American College of Chest Physicians (ACCP) evidence-based clinical practice guidelines, 9th edition (also accessible at http://journal.publications.chestnet.org/ss/guidelines.aspx). (See Grade A Recommendations for Antithrombotic Therapy at the end of the text in this chapter.)

PHARMACOLOGIC AGENTS

Vitamin K Antagonists

For more than 60 years, vitamin K antagonists have been the only oral anticoagulants available for clinical use. Now, with the development of new oral agents that target single coagulation enzymes (see later), the situation is changing. Coumarins are vitamin K antagonists, of which warfarin is the most widely used. Coumarins inhibit a vitamin K reductase that catalyzes the reduction of 2,3-epoxide (vitamin K epoxide), thereby leading to the depletion of vitamin KH_2, which is required for the production of functionally active (γ-carboxylated) coagulation proteins (factors II [prothrombin], VII, IX, and X) and anticoagulant proteins (protein C and protein S) (Chapter 175). Vitamin K_1 in food sources can reverse these effects of coumarins because it is reduced to vitamin KH_2 by a warfarin-insensitive vitamin K reductase (Fig. 38-1).

Warfarin is rapidly and almost completely absorbed from the gastrointestinal tract. It has a half-life of about 40 hours, a delayed onset of action (2 to 7 days, depending on dose), and a residual anticoagulant effect for up to 5 days after treatment is discontinued. The dose-response relationship of warfarin varies widely among individuals and is influenced by many factors, including age, body weight, liver disease, dietary vitamin K_1, genetic factors, concomitant drug use, compliance of the patient, and inappropriate dosage adjustments. Of these factors, inappropriate dosage adjustment and improved compliance through patient education are the most readily correctable.

The effect of warfarin must be monitored closely to prevent overdosing or underdosing. Laboratory monitoring is performed by measuring the

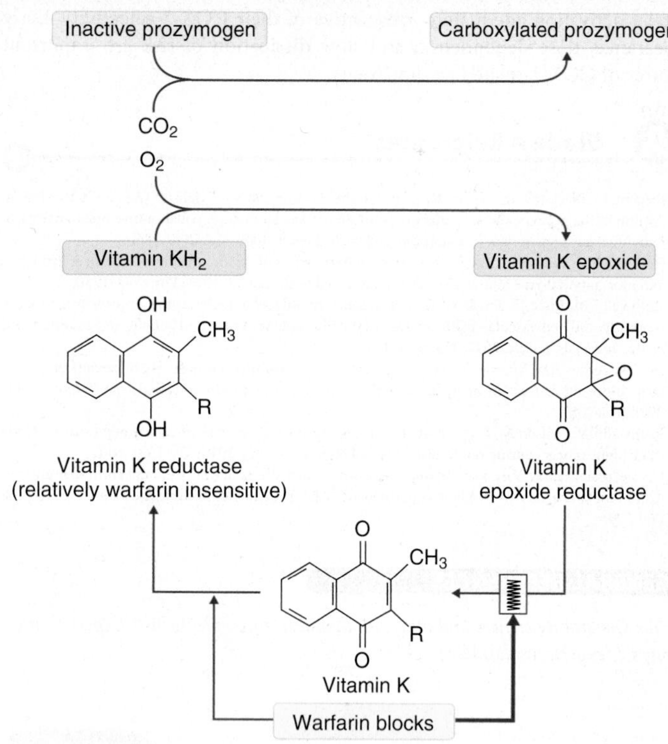

FIGURE 38-1. Warfarin inhibits vitamin K epoxide reductase and leads to the intracellular depletion (in the hepatocyte) of vitamin KH_2. Vitamin KH_2 is required for the conversion (by γ-carboxylation) of functionally inactive to active coagulation proteins. The anticoagulant effect of warfarin can be reversed by vitamin K_1 in food because it is reduced to vitamin KH_2 by a warfarin-insensitive vitamin K reductase.

prothrombin time and is reported as an international normalized ratio (INR). During initiation of warfarin therapy, the INR reflects primarily the depression of factor VII, which has a half-life of only 6 hours. The reliability of warfarin monitoring appears to be improved by using paper nomograms or computer-assisted algorithms. The convenience of monitoring is increased with a portable point-of-care instrument. Pharmacogenetic-guided dosing of warfarin has been evaluated in four randomized trials without producing evidence that the rate of major hemorrhage or thromboembolic complications is reduced, and the current cost is $100 to $200 per patient. The 2012 ACCP practice guidelines (http://journal.publications.chestnet.org/ss/guidelines.aspx) summarize published literature concerning the laboratory and clinical characteristics of vitamin K antagonists.

Indications for Warfarin

Warfarin is effective in the primary and secondary prevention of systemic embolism in patients with atrial fibrillation (Chapter 64),[A1] with rheumatic mitral valve complicated stenosis or by left atrial thrombus[A2]; with bioprosthetic or mechanical heart valves (Chapter 75); in the primary and secondary prevention of venous thromboembolism (VTE) (Chapters 81 and 98); in the prevention of acute myocardial infarction in high-risk patients (Chapters 72 and 73); and in the prevention of stroke (Chapter 407), recurrent infarction, and death in patients with acute myocardial infarction (Chapter 73). A target INR of 2.5 (range, 2.0 to 3.0) is recommended for almost all indications. Exceptions are mechanical prosthetic heart valve in the mitral position or caged-ball or caged-disk valve in the aortic position or any mechanical aortic valve in combination with atrial fibrillation, anterior myocardial infarction, left atrial enlargement, or low ejection fraction, when an INR of 3.0 (range, 2.5 to 3.5) is recommended.

Dosing and Monitoring

If a rapid anticoagulant effect is required, heparin and warfarin should be started at the same time and overlapped for at least 5 days. Warfarin is started with the estimated maintenance dose of about 5 mg/day, with the first INR measurement after 2 to 3 days, and patients usually reach an INR of 2.0 in 4 or 5 days. If there is no increase of the INR after two or three doses, the daily dose should be progressively increased until an INR response is observed. In patients with a low risk for bleeding, warfarin may be started at a dose of 10 mg and then adjusted according to daily INR results. Heparin treatment is discontinued when the INR has been in the therapeutic range for 2 days.

TABLE 38-1 RECOMMENDED MANAGEMENT OF ELEVATED INR WITH OR WITHOUT BLEEDING IN PATIENTS TREATED WITH WARFARIN

INR	BLEEDING	WARFARIN	VITAMIN K_1	FFP/PCC/rFVIIa
<5.0	Negligible	Hold 1 dose or reduce dose	No	No
5.0-9.9	Negligible	Hold 1-2 doses	Generally no*	No
≥10	Negligible	Hold	2.5-5 mg PO	No
Any	Serious or life threatening	Hold	10 mg IV† and repeat PRN	Yes

*1-2.5 mg PO for patients at increased risk for bleeding.
†Intravenous (IV) infusion should be given slowly.
FFP = fresh-frozen plasma; INR = international normalized ratio; PCC = prothrombin complex concentrate; PO = orally; PRN = as needed; rFVIIa, recombinant factor VIIa.

The INR is then performed two or three times weekly for 1 to 2 weeks and then weekly up to a maximal interval of 4 weeks, depending on the stability of INR results, and more frequently when a new drug is added to the treatment. Once the dose is stable, warfarin assessment up to every 12 weeks appears as safe and effective as every 4 weeks.[A3][A4]

Adjustments to the dose when the INR drifts out of the therapeutic range should be gradual and based on the weekly dose (e.g., 10 to 20% changes in weekly dose). Patients should be encouraged to keep a log of their dose and their INR response.

Adverse Effects

Warfarin-related bleeding is increased by the level of the INR. The risk for bleeding is also increased with concomitant aspirin use, in persons older than 65 years, in those with a history of stroke or gastrointestinal bleeding, and in those with serious comorbid conditions. Elderly patients are more sensitive to warfarin, requiring lower doses to reach the therapeutic range, and have an increased tendency to bleed, including intracranially, even when their INR is in the therapeutic range (Chapter 24).

Warfarin-induced skin necrosis (Fig. 176-1) occurs in 1 in 5000 patients, more frequently in women, and affects mainly breasts, buttocks, and thighs. An imbalance between moderately reduced procoagulant factors and severely depressed natural inhibitors may cause this hypercoagulable state in patients with congenital deficiency of protein C or protein S (Chapter 176), dietary deficiency of vitamin K, cancer, or heparin-induced thrombocytopenia with premature start of vitamin K antagonists (Chapter 172).

Reversing the Effect of Warfarin

The anticoagulant effect of warfarin can be reversed in one of three ways: by discontinuation of therapy, with the expectation that the INR will return to baseline in about 5 days; by administration of vitamin K_1, with the expectation that the anticoagulant effect will be reduced in 6 hours and reversed in 24 hours; and by infusion of fresh-frozen plasma (FFP), prothrombin complex concentrate (PCC), or recombinant coagulation factor VIIa (rFVIIa), which produce immediate reversal (Table 38-1).

Heparin and Low-Molecular-Weight Heparins

Heparin

Heparin binds to antithrombin (AT), thereby increasing the rate at which AT inactivates thrombin, activated factor X (factor Xa), and other coagulation enzymes. Heparin accelerates the inactivation of thrombin by AT by providing a template to which both the enzyme and the inhibitor bind to form a ternary complex (Fig. 38-2). In contrast, the inactivation of factor Xa by the AT-heparin complex does not require ternary complex formation and is achieved by binding of the heparin-bound AT to factor Xa. Heparin binds to a number of plasma, platelet, and endothelial cell–derived proteins that compete with AT for heparin binding. Binding of heparin to plasma proteins contributes to the variability of its anticoagulant response, whereas binding to hepatic macrophages is responsible for its dose-dependent clearance. Both properties contribute to the unpredictable anticoagulant effect of heparin and the need for laboratory monitoring. The plasma half-life is about 60 minutes at therapeutic concentrations.

Heparin is effective for the prevention and treatment of VTE,[A5] for the early treatment of patients with unstable angina and acute myocardial infarction,[A6] for patients who have cardiac surgery under cardiopulmonary bypass, for patients undergoing vascular surgery, and during and after coronary angioplasty and coronary stent placement.

The anticoagulant effects of heparin are usually monitored by the activated partial thromboplastin time (aPTT). A therapeutic effect is achieved when the aPTT ratio is equivalent to a heparin level of 0.3 to 0.7 anti–factor Xa units, which for many reagents is an aPTT ratio of 1.5 to 2.5. The risk for bleeding complications is increased with increasing heparin dosage, which in turn is related to the anticoagulant response. However, other clinical factors, such as recent surgery, trauma, and invasive procedures, are also important as predictors of bleeding during heparin treatment.

For the treatment of VTE, heparin is given in doses of 80 U/kg followed by 18 U/kg per hour by continuous infusion; the dose is adjusted according to the aPTT result at 6 hours by use of a validated nomogram. Lower doses (70 U/kg or 5000 U followed by 15 U/kg/h or 1000 U/hour) of heparin are used in patients with acute myocardial ischemia, who also receive aspirin and platelet glycoprotein IIb/IIIa complex (GPIIb-IIIa) antagonists or thrombolytic therapy.

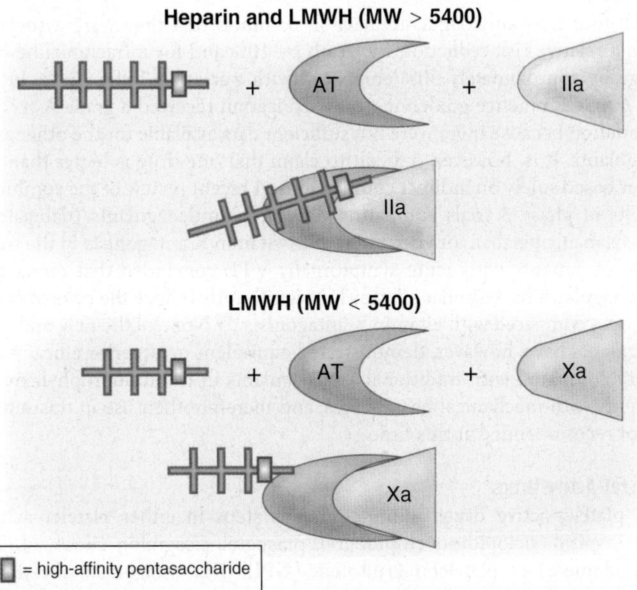

FIGURE 38-2. Only one third of high-affinity pentasaccharide-containing heparin molecules and one fifth of pentasaccharide-containing low-molecular-weight heparin (LMWH) molecules activate antithrombin (AT). Virtually all of the high-affinity heparin molecules are large enough to bridge between AT and factor IIa (thrombin). In contrast, only 25 to 50% of LMWH molecules have a molecular weight (MW) of 5400 or more, and although these smaller molecules inactivate factor Xa, they do not inactivate factor IIa. Although heparin has equal anti–factor IIa and anti–factor Xa activities, LMWH has reduced anti–factor IIa activity.

The main complications of heparin are bleeding and heparin-induced thrombocytopenia. Less common complications are heparin-induced osteoporosis and hyperkalemia. Heparin-related bleeding is dose related, and the risk is increased in patients who undergo an invasive procedure and if heparin is used in combination with a platelet GPIIb-IIIa antagonist or a thrombolytic agent.

If heparin-induced thrombocytopenia (Chapter 172) is suspected on clinical grounds and anticoagulant treatment is indicated, heparin should be stopped and replaced with a thrombin inhibitor: hirudin (lepirudin), argatroban, or danaparoid. Warfarin should not be used alone to treat acute heparin-induced thrombocytopenia because it can aggravate the thrombotic process, but it is safe in combination with a thrombin inhibitor after the platelet count has risen above 100×10^9/L.

Low-Molecular-Weight Heparins

Low-molecular-weight heparins (LMWHs) are fragments produced by either chemical or enzymatic depolymerization of heparin. LMWHs are approximately one third the size of heparin (Table 38-2). Depolymerization of heparin changes the anticoagulant profile. As a result, LMWHs have less protein and cellular binding and, as a consequence, have a more predictable dose response, better bioavailability, and a longer plasma half-life than regular heparin. LMWHs can therefore be administered subcutaneously once daily without laboratory monitoring.

Compared with heparin, which has a ratio of anti–factor Xa to anti–factor IIa activity of approximately 1 : 1, the various commercial LMWHs have ratios of anti–factor Xa to anti–factor IIa varying between 4 : 1 and 2 : 1, depending on their molecular size distribution. LMWHs are cleared principally by the renal route. They are associated with a lower incidence of heparin-induced thrombocytopenia and heparin-induced osteoporosis than is heparin.

LMWHs are effective in the prevention and treatment of VTE (Chapter 81),[A5] in the treatment of patients with unstable angina and non–ST elevation myocardial infarction (Chapters 72 and 73),[A6] and as an adjunct to fibrinolytic therapy in patients with acute ST elevation myocardial infarction (Chapter 73).

Pentasaccharides

On the basis of knowledge of the AT-binding sequence on heparin, a pentasaccharide, fondaparinux, with high affinity for AT has been synthesized. The structure of fondaparinux has been modified to increase its affinity to AT. Fondaparinux inactivates factor Xa through an AT-mediated mechanism. Because it is too short to bridge AT to thrombin, fondaparinux has no activity against thrombin.

After subcutaneous injection, fondaparinux is rapidly and completely absorbed and exhibits a bioavailability of 100%. The volume of distribution is similar to the blood volume. The drug is mainly excreted unchanged in the urine, with a terminal half-life of 17 hours in young volunteers and 21 hours in elderly volunteers.

TABLE 38-2 ANTICOAGULANT PROFILES, MOLECULAR WEIGHTS, PLASMA HALF-LIVES, AND RECOMMENDED DOSES OF COMMERCIAL LOW-MOLECULAR-WEIGHT HEPARINS AND HEPARINOID

				RECOMMENDED DOSE (INTERNATIONAL ANTI-XA UNITS)		
AGENT	**ANTI-X_a/ANTI-II_a RATIO**	**MOLECULAR WEIGHT**	**PLASMA HALF-LIFE (min)**	***General Surgery Prophylaxis***	***Orthopedic Surgery Prophylaxis***	**ACUTE TREATMENT**
Enoxaparin	2.7 : 1	4500	129-180	4000 U SC daily	4000 U SC daily or 3000 U SC bid	7000 U SC bid[*†] or 10,500 U SC daily[*]
Dalteparin	2 : 1	5000	119-139	2500 U SC daily	2500 U SC bid or 5000 U SC daily	8400 U SC bid[*†] or 14,000 U SC daily[*]
Nadroparin	3.2 : 1	4500	132-162	2850 U SC daily	2700 U SC daily,[*] 4000 U SC daily[*] from day 4	13,300 U SC daily[*]
Tinzaparin	1.9 : 1	4500	111	3500 U SC daily	3500 U SC daily[*] or 4500 U SC daily[*]	12,250 U daily[*]
Ardeparin	2 : 1	6000	200		50 U/kg SC bid	
Danaparoid[‡]	20 : 1	6500	1100	750 U SC daily	750 U SC bid	2500 U IV, then 4 hr each of 400 U/hr and 300 U/hr, then 200 U/hr; or 2000 U SC bid

*Weight-adjusted dose; stated dose for 70-kg patient.
†The higher daily dose is for acute coronary syndromes; the lower dose is for deep vein thrombosis.
‡Danaparoid sodium is a heparinoid.
IV = intravenously; SC = subcutaneously.

Fondaparinux circulates extensively bound to AT with minimal binding to other plasma proteins. Limited experimental and clinical studies suggest that fondaparinux has a lower risk for heparin-induced thrombocytopenia than that of heparin or LMWH as well as a lower risk for bone loss and of local skin reactions.

Fondaparinux is effective in the prevention and treatment of VTE[A5] and is also effective and safe in the treatment of acute coronary syndromes.

New Anticoagulants

The limitations of established anticoagulants have prompted the development of a variety of new anticoagulant agents that target various specific steps in the coagulation mechanism.[1,2]

Direct Thrombin Inhibitors

Direct thrombin inhibitors act independently of AT to inactivate both free thrombin and thrombin bound to fibrin. The direct thrombin inhibitors include hirudin, synthetic hirudin fragments (hirugen, lepirudin, and bivalirudin [Hirulog]), and low-molecular-weight inhibitors that react with the active site of thrombin (dabigatran and argatroban).[3]

Bivalirudin is approved for use in coronary angioplasty (Chapter 73) and reduces the risk for major bleeding in comparison with heparin.[A7] Argatroban and lepirudin are approved in patients with heparin-induced thrombocytopenia (Chapter 172). Data comparing argatroban with hirudin in heparin-induced thrombocytopenia are too limited for conclusions to be drawn about their relative efficacy and safety. Argatroban is metabolized in the liver and can be used in patients with renal failure, whereas the other direct thrombin inhibitors depend on elimination through renal excretion, and they may be used in patients with liver disease.

Dabigatran etexilate is administered orally and metabolized by ubiquitous esterases to dabigatran, a reversible, active-site thrombin inhibitor. The pharmacokinetic characteristics of dabigatran and the oral factor Xa inhibitors are summarized in Table 38-3. Dabigatran etexilate has been approved in Europe and several other countries for prophylaxis against VTE after hip or knee arthroplasty (first dose, 110 mg; then 220 mg once daily; for patients older than 70 years or with creatinine clearance of 30 to 50 mL/minute, first dose 75 mg and then 150 mg daily). The effect is similar to that of enoxaparin (40 mg subcutaneously daily). Dabigatran (150 mg twice daily) is more effective than warfarin for stroke prophylaxis in atrial fibrillation,[A1] whereas a lower dose (110 mg twice daily) is equally effective with lower risk for major bleeding. Both doses resulted in fewer intracranial hemorrhages than warfarin.[A8] The 110-mg regimen has not been approved in the United States, but for patients with a calculated creatinine clearance of 15 to 30 mL/minute, the dose of 75 mg twice daily is available. In the treatment of VTE, dabigatran (150 mg twice daily) has comparable effect to warfarin and is at least as safe regarding bleeding. In terms of periprocedural bleeding, dabigatran and warfarin are equivalently safe, and dabigatran facilitates a shorter interruption of oral anticoagulation.

Direct Factor Xa Inhibitors

A number of orally available low-molecular-weight active site-directed factor Xa inhibitors have been designed and are in various stages of clinical development (rivaroxaban, apixaban, betrixaban, edoxaban). Unlike heparins and pentasaccharide, direct inhibitors inactivate factor Xa without the need for AT as a cofactor.

Rivaroxaban, an oxazolidinone derivative (10 mg daily for 30 to 39 days), is more effective than enoxaparin in patients undergoing hip or knee arthroplasty but with a trend to more bleeding. For stroke prophylaxis in atrial fibrillation, rivaroxaban when compared with warfarin showed similar efficacy and safety.[A9] In patients with acute coronary syndromes, rivaroxaban, when added to standard antiplatelet therapy, reduced the risk for thromboembolic events at the cost of increased bleeding. In the treatment of VTE, rivaroxaban had similar efficacy to vitamin K antagonists, and in the trial with patients with pulmonary embolism, rivaroxaban reduced the risk for major bleeding.[A10]

Apixaban (2.5 mg twice daily) for prophylaxis against VTE after hip or knee arthroplasty has similar or better efficacy than LMWH and similar or lower risk for bleeding. In atrial fibrillation, apixaban (5 mg twice daily) reduces the risk for stroke and for major bleeding compared with warfarin,[A11] and it reduces the risk for stroke without any increase of major bleeding in comparison with aspirin.[A12] For patients with VTE, apixaban (5 mg twice daily) has similar effect as warfarin but with a reduced risk for major bleeding.[A13]

Edoxaban (60 mg daily after initial LMWH) for patients with VTE has similar effect and risk for major bleeding as warfarin.[A14] For patients with extensive pulmonary embolism, edoxaban appears to be more effective than warfarin. For patients with atrial fibrillation, edoxaban (60 mg daily) has similar risk for stroke and lower risk for major bleeding compared with warfarin.[A15]

All four new anticoagulants have in common that they were associated with a relative risk reduction for death by 10% and for intracranial hemorrhage by approximately 50% compared with warfarin (Table 38-4). In the 2012 ACCP practice guidelines, only dabigatran received a grade A recommendation because there were not sufficient data available for the other anticoagulants. It is, however, difficult to claim that one drug is better than the other based solely on indirect comparisons. A recent review of the combined results of phase 3 trials comparing direct oral anticoagulants (dabigatran, rivaroxaban, apixaban, or edoxaban) with vitamin K antagonists in the treatment of patients with acute symptomatic VTE concluded that direct oral anticoagulants have similar efficacy but significantly reduce the risks of major bleeding compared with vitamin K antagonists.[A16] None of the new oral anticoagulants have, however, demonstrated equivalent or superior efficacy and safety compared with traditional anticoagulants in thromboprophylaxis for patients with mechanical heart valves, and therefore their use in this setting is not recommended at this time.

Platelet-Active Drugs

The platelet-active drugs inhibit different steps in either platelet activation (aspirin, ticlopidine, clopidogrel, prasugrel, ticagrelor, cilostazol, and dipyridamole) or platelet recruitment (GPIIb-IIIa antagonists abciximab, tirofiban, and eptifibatide) (Fig. 38-3).

Aspirin and Other Cyclooxygenase Inhibitors

Mechanism of Action and Pharmacology

Aspirin permanently inactivates cyclooxygenase isoenzymes (COX-1 and COX-2) that catalyze the conversion of arachidonic acid to prostaglandin H_2, a precursor of a variety of eicosanoids, including thromboxane A_2 in platelets and prostacyclin (prostaglandin I_2) in vascular endothelial cells (Chapter 37).

Aspirin is rapidly absorbed in the stomach and upper intestine, attaining peak plasma levels about 30 minutes after ingestion; it has a half-life of about 15 minutes. Inhibition of platelet function is evident by 1 hour with uncoated aspirin but can be delayed after administration of enteric-coated aspirin. Therefore, if only enteric-coated tablets are available when a rapid effect is required, the tablets should be chewed.

Aspirin potentiates the antithrombotic effects of warfarin (in high-risk subjects), dipyridamole (in those with ischemic stroke), clopidogrel (in those

TABLE 38-3 PHARMACOKINETIC CHARACTERISTICS AND DRUG INTERACTIONS OF THE ORAL THROMBIN AND FACTOR Xa INHIBITORS

AGENT	BIOAVAILABILITY (%)	TIME TO PEAK PLASMA CONCENTRATION (hr)	PATHWAYS OF ELIMINATION	PLASMA HALF-LIFE (hr)	PLASMA PROTEIN BINDING (%)	MECHANISMS FOR DRUG INTERACTIONS
Dabigatran	6	2	80% renal excretion active	14-17	35	Induction or inhibition of P-gp
Rivaroxaban	80	2-3	⅓ renal excretion active ⅓ metabolized, renal excretion inactive ⅓ liver metabolism, fecal excretion	7-11	92-95	Induction or inhibition of P-gp Induction or inhibition of CYP3A4
Apixaban	50	3	Renal and fecal excretion, oxidative metabolism	8-14	87	Induction or inhibition of P-gp Induction or inhibition of CYP3A4
Edoxaban	50	1-2	⅓ renal excretion active, ⅔ fecal excretion	8-10	40-59	Induction or inhibition of P-gp

P-gp = P-glycoprotein.

TABLE 38-4 ABSOLUTE ANNUAL RISK REDUCTION* OF MAIN CLINICAL OUTCOMES WITH THE ORAL THROMBIN AND FACTOR Xa INHIBITORS COMPARED WITH WARFARIN IN PATIENTS WITH ATRIAL FIBRILLATION

AGENT	ISCHEMIC STROKE (%)	ALL-CAUSE MORTALITY (%)	MAJOR BLEEDING (%)	INTRACRANIAL BLEEDING (%)	GASTROINTESTINAL BLEEDING (%)
Warfarin	Reference	Reference	Reference	Reference	Reference
Dabigatran 110 mg	+0.14	−0.38	**−0.65**	**−0.26**	+0.10
Dabigatran 150 mg	**−0.28**	−0.47	−0.25	**−0.28**	**+0.49**
Rivaroxaban	−0.08	−0.4	+0.2	**−0.18**	**+0.61**
Apixaban	−0.08	**−0.42**	**−0.96**	**−0.47**	−0.10
Edoxaban 30 mg	**+0.52**	**−0.55**	**−1.82**	**−0.31**	**−0.41**
Edoxaban 60 mg	0.0	−0.36	**−0.68**	**−0.21**	**+0.28**

*Positive numbers correspond to absolute increase in risk. Statistically significant differences are in bold.

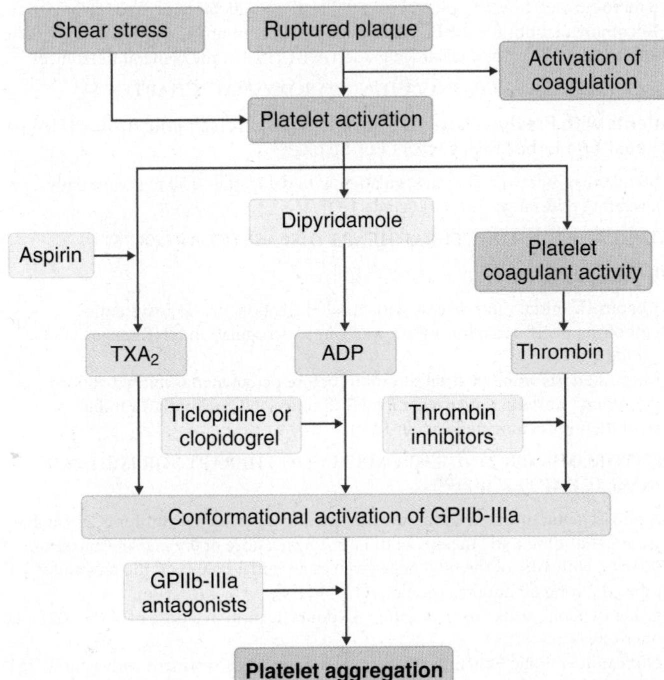

FIGURE 38-3. **Sites of action of platelet inhibitors. ADP = adenosine diphosphate; GPIIb-IIIa = glycoprotein IIb/IIIa complex; TXA_2 = thromboxane A_2.**

with coronary stents or acute myocardial ischemia), and heparin (in the prevention of recurrent miscarriages in pregnant women with antiphospholipid antibody syndrome and in patients with acute coronary ischemia). Aspirin produces a small increase in major bleeding and a very small increase in the risk for cerebral hemorrhage. It also potentiates bleeding when it is added to another antithrombotic agent.

Aspirin causes gastrointestinal side effects that are dose dependent. Aspirin is contraindicated in individuals with active peptic ulcer disease or aspirin-induced asthma or if gastrointestinal side effects are severe.

Clinical Uses

Based on the results of a meta-analysis, there is evidence that aspirin reduces vascular death by approximately 15% and nonfatal vascular events by about 30% in patients with cardiovascular disease.[A6] These effects are achieved in patients with silent myocardial ischemia or stable angina,[A6] unstable angina,[A6] non–ST elevation myocardial infarction,[A6] ST elevation myocardial infarction,[A6] noncardioembolic ischemic cerebrovascular disease,[A17] and peripheral arterial disease.[A18] Aspirin is also effective in patients after coronary angioplasty,[A6] coronary[A6] or peripheral artery stenting,[A18] angioplasty,[A18] or bypass graft,[A6] symptomatic carotid artery stenosis,[A17] or for 1 year after coronary artery bypass surgery[A6] and in preventing symptomatic coronary events in asymptomatic men and women older than 50 years.[A6] Aspirin has a favorable risk-to-benefit ratio for secondary prevention in patients with overt vascular disease, but the risk-to-benefit ratio is marginal when aspirin is used as primary prevention in asymptomatic individuals, even individuals with type 2 diabetes. Aspirin is less effective than oral anticoagulants in the prevention of recurrent stroke in atrial fibrillation.

Phosphodiesterase Inhibitors

Dipyridamole and cilostazol are phosphodiesterase inhibitors, which elevate platelet cyclic adenosine and guanine monophosphate (cAMP and cGMP) levels. They block platelet reactivity and also inhibit vasoconstriction. The most common side effect is headache.

Dipyridamole is a pyrimidopyrimidine derivative with a terminal half-life of 10 hours and elimination primarily by biliary excretion. Favorable results were obtained with a modified-release preparation in combination with aspirin in patients with carotid stenosis[A18] and in patients with prior noncardioembolic stroke or transient ischemic attack,[A17] in whom the risk for stroke was reduced by 16% with dipyridamole alone and by 37% with aspirin and dipyridamole in combination, compared with placebo.

In a meta-analysis, cilostazol (100 mg twice daily) was shown to reduce vascular events, driven by fewer cerebrovascular events,[A17] and in another meta-analysis to improve maximal and pain-free walking distance in patients with intermittent claudication.[A19] Cilostazol is contraindicated in patients with congestive heart failure, owing to reports of fatal events with similar drugs.

Thienopyridines

Ticlopidine, clopidogrel, and prasugrel are thienopyridines that inhibit adenosine diphosphate–induced platelet aggregation through the action of their active metabolites at the $P2Y_{12}$ receptor level. The drugs are administered orally, but their onset of action is delayed until their active metabolites are formed. Similarly, recovery of platelet function is delayed until the circulating affected platelets are replaced by newly formed, unaffected platelets.

Based on a better safety profile and equal efficacy, clopidogrel has replaced ticlopidine. Clopidogrel is rapidly absorbed and metabolized, producing inhibition of platelet aggregation as soon as 90 minutes after an oral loading dosing of 300 mg. With repeated daily administration of low doses (75 mg), there is cumulative inhibition of platelet function with a return to normal 7 days after the last dose of clopidogrel.

Clopidogrel is marginally more effective than aspirin in patients who have experienced a recent stroke[A17] or recent myocardial infarction[A6] and in patients presenting with symptomatic peripheral arterial disease.[A18] The additional benefit over aspirin is modest and similar to that observed with ticlopidine (about 10% relative risk reduction). Clopidogrel is also recommended for patients with symptomatic carotid artery stenosis[A18] or peripheral artery angioplasty.[A18] The combination of clopidogrel and aspirin is also more effective than aspirin alone in patients with unstable angina and non–ST elevation myocardial infarction (20% risk reduction) and in patients with atrial fibrillation, but at a cost of a modest increase in bleeding. The combination of clopidogrel and aspirin is also more effective than aspirin alone in patients who have percutaneous coronary intervention procedures and is recommended for 1 month after insertion of a bare metal stent, and for 3 to 6 months after a drug eluting stent.[A5][A6] Clopidogrel appears to be as well tolerated as aspirin.

Prasugrel is more potent and has a more rapid onset of action than clopidogrel. Given as a bolus dose of 60 mg, followed by 10 mg daily, when compared with clopidogrel, prasugrel reduces the absolute risk for cardiovascular death or nonfatal myocardial infarction or stroke by 2.2%, which is partly offset by an absolute increase of serious bleeding of 0.5%.

Ticagrelor, an oral direct and reversible $P2Y_{12}$ receptor inhibitor, provides a faster response than the thienopyridines.[A20] In a randomized trial in patients with acute coronary syndromes, ticagrelor was more effective than clopidogrel, providing an absolute risk reduction for cardiovascular death, myocardial infarction, or stroke of 1.9% without any significant increase of major bleeding.

Integrin $\alpha_{IIb}\beta_3$ (GPIIb-IIIa) Receptor Antagonists

The final common pathway of platelet aggregation is mediated by the binding of fibrinogen to the functionally active integrin $\alpha_{IIb}\beta_3$ (GPIIb-IIIa) on the platelet surface. Inhibitors of this process include monoclonal antibodies, synthetic peptides containing Arg-Gly-Asp (RGD) or Lys-Gly-Asp (KGD), and peptidomimetic and nonpeptide RGD mimetics. These compounds are administered intravenously, and they inhibit platelet function by competing with fibrinogen (and von Willebrand factor) for occupancy on the platelet integrin receptor.[A20] Abciximab (ReoPro), a mouse-human chimeric 7E3 Fab antibody, inhibits platelet aggregation in a concentration-dependent manner. Platelet function is impaired rapidly after an intravenous bolus of abciximab and gradually recovers over 24 to 48 hours. Tirofiban (MK-383, Aggrastat) is a nonpeptide derivative of tyrosine. It has a plasma half-life of 1.6 hours, and its effect on hemostasis is reversed within 4 hours of stopping treatment. Eptifibatide (Integrilin) is a synthetic disulfide-linked cyclic heptapeptide. It has a rapid onset and offset of action, and its effect on platelet function is reduced by more than 50% after 4 hours.

All three GPIIb-IIIa receptor antagonists are effective intravenous agents in patients undergoing percutaneous coronary interventions (Chapter 74), and tirofiban and eptifibatide are effective in patients with unstable angina or non–ST elevation myocardial infarction. The GPIIb-IIIa receptor antagonists are administered in combination with heparin and aspirin. Orally active nonpeptide GPIIb-IIIa inhibitors have been developed for long-term use, but the results of clinical trials have been disappointing.

Fibrinolytic Agents

Fibrinolytic agents convert plasminogen to the enzyme plasmin, which then degrades fibrin to soluble fragments, thereby lysing the thrombus. Of the available fibrinolytic agents, streptokinase and urokinase are not fibrin specific; in contrast, recombinant tissue-type plasminogen activator (rt-PA, alteplase) and the rt-PA variant tenecteplase are relatively fibrin specific (Chapter 73).

Streptokinase is an indirect fibrinolytic agent. It binds to plasminogen, converting it into a plasmin-like molecule that in turn converts plasminogen to plasmin. Streptokinase has a number of disadvantages. It is antigenic, rendering its repeated use problematic, and allergenic, producing chills, fever, and rigors in some patients and, in rare instances, anaphylaxis. Anistreplase (APSAC) is an acylated complex of streptokinase and Lys-plasminogen. Compared with streptokinase, it is more fibrin specific, has a longer plasma half-life, and is inactive until it is selectively activated by deacylation on the fibrin surface. Its side-effect profile, antigenicity, and efficacy are similar to those of streptokinase.

Urokinase is a naturally occurring plasminogen activator that differs from streptokinase in that it directly activates plasminogen and is not antigenic. Urokinase was used extensively to treat peripheral vascular occlusions, but production problems have curtailed its availability.

In its natural state, tissue plasminogen activator is produced by vascular endothelium; rt-PA (alteplase) is produced by recombinant DNA technology. Alteplase is not antigenic or allergenic, and it has greater fibrin specificity than streptokinase. It has a short half-life of about 3.5 minutes and therefore is given as a continuous intravenous infusion.

Truncated forms of rt-PA have been developed; the first was reteplase (r-PA), a single-chain deletion mutant that lacks certain domains. As a result, its half-life is about twice that of rt-PA, permitting double-bolus therapy 30 minutes apart. r-PA has lower affinity for fibrin than does rt-PA, but fibrinogen depletion with r-PA is less than that with streptokinase. No antigenicity has been reported with this compound.

Tenecteplase (TNK-tPA) is a mutant tissue plasminogen activator with amino acid substitution at three sites. Compared with rt-PA, it has a longer half-life, allowing single-bolus administration, increased fibrin specificity, and increased resistance to inhibition by plasminogen activator inhibitor 1.

Clinical Uses

Thrombolytic therapy reduces mortality in patients with ST-elevation myocardial infarction and for whom primary percutaneous coronary intervention is unavailable, as well as in patients with extensive pulmonary embolism and hypotension. Treatment with rt-PA intravenously within 3 hours from onset of symptoms of ischemic stroke increases the likelihood of good functional outcome despite a small increase in the risk for intracerebral hemorrhage.[A4] Thrombolysis can be justified for severe pulmonary embolism without contraindications, but thrombolysis in patients with moderate-risk pulmonary embolism does not improve outcomes despite better hemodynamics, because of increases in major bleeding and stroke.[A21]

SUMMARY OF GRADE A RECOMMENDATIONS FOR ANTITHROMBOTIC THERAPY

Grade 1A indicates that experts are certain that benefits do or do not outweigh risks, burdens, and costs. The reduction in number of grade A recommendations compared with previous editions is due to several changes in the development of the American College of Chest Physicians (ACCP) guidelines. In particular, (a) the GRADE methodology was strictly adhered to, (b) much less importance was paid to surrogate outcomes, and (c) intellectual conflicts were taken into account. Recommendations for the Prevention and Treatment of Venous Thromboembolic Disease that were not considered grade 1A are cited in the General References.[4-9]

ATRIAL FIBRILLATION, INCLUDING PAROXYSMAL (CHAPTER 64)

Patients with Previous Ischemic Stroke, Transient Ischemic Attack (TIA) or At Least Two Other Risk Factors For Stroke[A1]

- Standard approach: oral anticoagulation with dabigatran, 150 mg twice daily, or warfarin (INR range, 2.0-3.0) (grade 1A)

VALVULAR AND STRUCTURAL HEART DISEASE (CHAPTER 75)

Mitral Valve Disease[A2]

- Rheumatic mitral valve disease with atrial fibrillation, previous systemic embolism, or left atrial thrombus: warfarin anticoagulation (INR range, 2.0-3.0) (grade 1A)
- Mitral stenosis with left atrial thrombus before percutaneous mitral balloon valvotomy: warfarin anticoagulation (INR range, 2.0-3.0) until thrombus resolution is documented (grade 1A)

ANTITHROMBOTIC AND THROMBOLYTIC THERAPY FOR ISCHEMIC STROKE (CHAPTER 407)[A17]

- Acute ischemic stroke treatment within 3 hours of onset of symptoms, in eligible patients: thrombolytic therapy with IV rt-PA in a dose of 0.9 mg/kg (maximum of 90 mg), with 10% of the total dose given as an initial bolus and the remainder infused during 60 minutes (grade 1A)
- Acute ischemic stroke or TIA within 48 hours: aspirin in a dose of 160 to 325 mg once daily (grade 1A)
- Noncardioembolic ischemic stroke or TIA: long-term treatment with aspirin, 75 to 100 mg once daily, or clopidogrel, 75 mg once daily; or a combination of aspirin and extended-release dipyridamole, 25 mg/200 mg twice daily, or cilostazol, 100 mg twice daily (grade 1A)
- Cryptogenic stroke and patent foramen ovale or atrial septal aneurysm: long-term treatment with aspirin 50 to 100 mg once daily (grade 1A)
- Ischemic stroke or TIA and atrial fibrillation, including paroxysmal: long-term oral anticoagulation with dabigatran, 150 mg twice daily, or warfarin (INR range, 2.0-3.0) (grade 1A)

CORONARY ARTERY DISEASE (CHAPTER 72, 73, 74)[A6]

- Established coronary artery disease, including coronary artery stenoses >50% by coronary angiogram, cardiac ischemia on diagnostic testing, 1 year after acute coronary syndrome or after coronary artery bypass graft: long-term aspirin, 75 to 100 mg daily, or clopidogrel, 75 mg daily (grade 1A)
- Elective percutaneous coronary intervention with placement of bare metal stent: dual antiplatelet therapy for 1 month with aspirin, 75 to 325 mg daily, and clopidogrel, 75 mg daily (grade 1A)
- Elective percutaneous coronary intervention with placement of drug eluting stent: dual antiplatelet therapy for 3 to 6 months with aspirin, 75 to 325 mg daily, and clopidogrel, 75 mg daily (grade 1A)

PERIPHERAL ARTERIAL DISEASE (CHAPTER 79)[A18]

- Symptomatic peripheral arterial disease: long-term aspirin, 75 to 100 mg daily, or clopidogrel, 75 mg daily (grade 1A)
- Peripheral artery percutaneous transluminal angioplasty with or without stenting: long-term aspirin, 75 to 100 mg daily, or clopidogrel 75 mg daily (grade 1A)
- Peripheral artery bypass graft surgery: long-term aspirin, 75 to 100 mg daily, or clopidogrel, 75 mg daily (grade 1A)
- Symptomatic carotid artery stenosis, including recent carotid endarterectomy: long-term aspirin, 75 to 100 mg daily, or clopidogrel, 75 mg daily, or aspirin with extended-release dipyridamole, 25 mg/200 mg twice daily (grade 1A)

From: Antithrombotic therapy and prevention of thrombosis, 9th ed. American College of Chest Physicians Evidence-Based Clinical Practice Guidelines. *Chest* 2012.

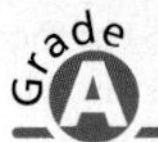

Grade A References

A1. You JJ, Singer DE, Howard PA, et al. Antithrombotic therapy for atrial fibrillation: antithrombotic therapy and prevention of thrombosis, 9th ed. American College of Chest Physicians Evidence-Based Clinical Practice Guidelines. *Chest.* 2012;141:e531S-e575S.

A2. Whitlock EP, Sun JC, Fremes SE, et al. Antithrombotic and thrombolytic therapy for valvular disease: antithrombotic therapy and prevention of thrombosis, 9th ed. American College of Chest Physicians Evidence-Based Clinical Practice Guidelines. *Chest.* 2012;141:e576S-e600S.

A3. Schulman S, Parpia S, Stewart C, et al. Warfarin dose assessment every 4 weeks versus every 12 weeks in patients with stable international normalized ratios: a randomized trial. *Ann Intern Med.* 2011;155:653-659.

A4. Holbrook A, Schulman S, Witt DM, et al. Evidence-based management of anticoagulant therapy: antithrombotic therapy and prevention of thrombosis, 9th ed. American College of Chest Physicians Evidence-Based Clinical Practice Guidelines. *Chest.* 2012;141:e89S-119S.

A5. Kearon C, Akl EA, Comerota AJ, et al. Antithrombotic therapy for VTE disease: antithrombotic therapy and prevention of thrombosis, 9th ed. American College of Chest Physicians Evidence-Based Clinical Practice Guidelines. *Chest.* 2012;141:e419S-94S.

A6. Vandvik PO, Lincoff AM, Gore JM, et al. Primary and secondary prevention of cardiovascular disease: antithrombotic therapy and prevention of thrombosis, 9th ed. American College of Chest Physicians Evidence-Based Clinical Practice Guidelines. *Chest.* 2012;141:e637S-e668S.

A7. Steg PG, van't Hof A, Hamm CW, et al. Bivalirudin started during emergency transport for primary PCI. *N Engl J Med.* 2013;369:2207-2217.

A8. Connolly SJ, Ezekowitz MD, Yusuf S, et al. Dabigatran versus warfarin in patients with atrial fibrillation. *N Engl J Med.* 2009;361:1139-1151.

A9. Patel MR, Mahaffey KW, Garg J, et al. Rivaroxaban versus warfarin in nonvalvular atrial fibrillation. *N Engl J Med.* 2011;365:883-891.

A10. Buller HR, Prins MH, Lensing AW, et al. Oral rivaroxaban for the treatment of symptomatic pulmonary embolism. *N Engl J Med.* 2012;366:1287-1297.

A11. Granger CB, Alexander JH, McMurray JJ, et al. Apixaban versus warfarin in patients with atrial fibrillation. *N Engl J Med.* 2011;365:981-992.

A12. Connolly SJ, Eikelboom J, Joyner C, et al. Apixaban in patients with atrial fibrillation. *N Engl J Med.* 2011;364:806-817.

A13. Agnelli G, Buller HR, Cohen A, et al. Oral apixaban for the treatment of acute venous thromboembolism. *N Engl J Med.* 2013;369:799-808.

A14. The Hokusai-VTE Investigators. Edoxaban versus warfarin for the treatment of symptomatic venous thromboembolism. *N Engl J Med.* 2013;369:1406-1415.

A15. Giugliano RP, Ruff CT, Braunwald E, et al. Edoxaban versus warfarin in patients with atrial fibrillation. *N Engl J Med.* 2013;369:2093-2104.

A16. van Es N, Coppens M, Schulman S, et al. Direct oral anticoagulants compared with vitamin K antagonists for acute venous thromboembolism: evidence from phase 3 trials. *Blood.* 2014;124:1968-1975.

A17. Lansberg MG, O'Donnell MJ, Khatri P, et al. Antithrombotic and thrombolytic therapy for ischemic stroke: antithrombotic therapy and prevention of thrombosis, 9th ed. American College of Chest Physicians Evidence-Based Clinical Practice Guidelines. *Chest.* 2012;141:e601S-636S.

A18. Alonso-Coello P, Bellmunt S, McGorrian C, et al. Antithrombotic therapy in peripheral artery disease: antithrombotic therapy and prevention of thrombosis, 9th ed. American College of Chest Physicians Evidence-Based Clinical Practice Guidelines. *Chest.* 2012;141:e669S-e690S.

A19. Robless P, Mikhailidis DP, Stansby GP. Cilostazol for peripheral arterial disease. *Cochrane Database Syst Rev.* 2008;1:CD003748.

A20. Eikelboom JW, Hirsh J, Spencer FA, et al. Antiplatelet drugs: antithrombotic therapy and prevention of thrombosis, 9th ed: American College of Chest Physicians Evidence-Based Clinical Practice Guidelines. *Chest.* 2012;141:e89S-119S.

A21. Meyer G, Vicaut E, Danays T, et al. Fibrinolysis for patients with intermediate-risk pulmonary embolism. *N Engl J Med.* 2014;370:1402-1411.

GENERAL REFERENCES

For the General References and other additional features, please visit Expert Consult at https://expertconsult.inkling.com.

39

COMPLEMENTARY AND ALTERNATIVE MEDICINE

ADAM PERLMAN

The National Institutes of Health's National Center for Complementary and Alternative Medicine (NCCAM) has defined complementary and alternative medicine (CAM) as " a group of diverse medical and health care systems, practices, and products that are not generally considered to be part of conventional medicine." The use of CAM by the general public has continued to grow. In the United States, approximately 12% of children and 38% of adults are using some form of CAM, and when the use of megavitamins as well as the use of prayer specifically for health reasons is added, the number increases to 62%. Use of CAM is higher in women and those with more education, but CAM use cuts across all socioeconomic levels, races, and ethnicities. In certain populations, such as patients with cancer or rheumatologic conditions, use of CAM can be significantly higher. In one study, 75% of cancer patients surveyed had used at least one CAM modality, and 58% of those using CAM initiated use after they were diagnosed.[1]

Perhaps motivated by growing patient interest in an era of increased consumerism in health care or frustration with the current evolution of health care, many conventional providers have developed interest and expertise in the integration of CAM into patient care. However, it is important to differentiate between integrating CAM and another growing field within health care, integrative medicine. Integrative medicine has been defined as "an approach to care that puts the patient at the center and addresses the full range of physical, emotional, mental, social, spiritual, and environmental influences that affect a person's health. Employing a personalized strategy that considers the patient's unique conditions, needs, and circumstances, it uses the most appropriate interventions from an array of scientific disciplines to heal illness and disease and help people regain and maintain optimum health."[2] Integrative medicine and integrative medicine programs are increasingly prevalent within the academic medical community. Formed in 1999, the Consortium of Academic Health Centers for Integrative Medicine now includes more than one third of all Academic Health Centers in North America.

Many of the principles as defined in Table 39-1 are not unique to integrative medicine, and interest in them has been increasing as a part of the evolving transformation of the U.S. health care system. This has led to a growing interest in integrative medicine as well as CAM and the need for physicians and all health care providers to have, at a minimum, a basic understanding of CAM. Health care providers must be comfortable engaging in a dialogue with patients about their potential use of CAM and the evidence base or lack thereof for the more popular CAM modalities as well as any potential safety concerns.

Most recently, NCCAM has used the term *complementary health approaches* to describe the practices and products that are studied as a part of NCCAM's research portfolio. In general, that portfolio can be separated into two main subgroups: natural products and mind and body practices.

NATURAL PRODUCTS

Natural products, often referred to as dietary supplements, include vitamins and minerals, herbs or botanicals, and a category referred to as nonvitamin, nonmineral natural products. After prayer, use of natural products was the most common complementary health approach among adults surveyed in 2007, with 17.7% of adults having reported using natural products during the previous 12 months. The 2007 National Health Interview Survey (NHIS) also revealed that 83 million U.S. adults spent almost $44 billion dollars out of pocket on visits to CAM practitioners and purchases of CAM products, classes, or materials. Of that out-of-pocked spending, $14.8 billion, or 43.7%, was for nonvitamin, nonmineral natural products (Table 39-2).

Commonly used natural products in adults include such substances as fish oil, glucosamine, and probiotics, and in children, fish oil, probiotics, and Echinacea. There is a growing body of research literature on numerous natural products with mixed conclusions regarding efficacy. As with any substance that has a physiologic effect on the body, many natural products, although typically safe, do have the potential for side effects as well as the potential to interact with medication. Many commonly used dietary supplements, such vitamin E, Ginkgo, and fish oil, can affect platelet function and therefore lead to an increased risk for bleeding. Patients are often unaware of these potential side effects or interactions with medications.

Currently, natural products are regulated under the Dietary Supplement Health and Education Act (DSHEA). Enacted by Congress in 1994, this act gives the U.S. Food and Drug Administration (FDA) the power to regulate both finished dietary supplement products and dietary ingredients. Dietary supplements are defined as products (other than tobacco) that are intended to supplement the diet and include one or more of the following ingredients: a vitamin, a mineral, an herb or other botanical, an amino acid, a substance for use by humans to supplement the diet by increasing the total dietary intake; or a concentrate, metabolite, constituent, extract, or combination of any of the aforementioned ingredients.

Manufacturers are responsible for ensuring that products are safe before bringing them to market, and the FDA is responsible for taking action against any unsafe product after it has reached the market. Although the FDA has a system in effect for the collection and review of adverse effects linked to dietary supplements, that system is voluntary, and concerns have been raised that the agency does not have adequate resources to ensure safety of products currently on the market in a timely and effective way.

TABLE 39-1 DEFINING PRINCIPLES OF INTEGRATIVE MEDICINE

The defining principles of integrative medicine are as follow:

- The patient and practitioner are partners in the healing process.
- All factors that influence health, wellness, and disease are taken into consideration.
- The care addresses the whole person, including body, mind, and spirit in the context of community.
- Practitioners use all appropriate healing sciences to facilitate the body's innate healing response.
- Effective interventions that are natural and less invasive are used whenever possible.
- Because good medicine is based in good science, integrative medicine is inquiry driven and open to new models of care.
- Alongside the concept of treatment, the broader concepts of health promotion and the prevention of illness are paramount.
- Care is individualized to best address the person's unique conditions, needs, and circumstances.
- Practitioners of integrative medicine exemplify its principles and commit themselves to self-exploration and self-development.

Data from Horrigan, B, Lewis, S, Abrams D, et al. *Integrative Medicine in America: How Integrative Medicine Is Being Practiced in Clinical Centers across the United States.* Encinitas, CA: The Bravewell Collaborative; 2012.

TABLE 39-2 USE OF COMPLEMENTARY OR ALTERNATIVE MEDICINE BY U.S. ADULTS IN 2007

MODALITY	PERCENTAGE OF ADULTS WHO USED IT
BIOLOGICALLY BASED THERAPIES	
Herbal or natural products	17.7
Dietary supplements	N/A
Diet-based therapy	3.5
BODY-BASED PRACTICES	
Chiropractic or osteopathic manipulation	8.6
Massage	8.3
Movement therapies*	1.5
MIND-BODY THERAPIES	
Biofeedback	0.2
Hypnosis	0.2
Meditation	9.4
Guided imagery	2.2
Progressive relaxation	2.9
Deep breathing	12.7
Yoga	6.1
Tai chi	1.0
Qi gong	0.3
ENERGY MEDICINE†	
Reiki, biofield, and other therapies	0.5
WHOLE MEDICAL SYSTEMS	
Naturopathy	0.3
Homeopathy	1.8
Ayurveda	0.1
Traditional Chinese medicine (acupuncture)	1.4
Traditional healers	0.4

*Pilates, Trager, Feldenkrais, and Alexander.
†Energy medicine is based on the theory that there are energy fields surrounding and penetrating the human body. Energy therapies are intended to manipulate these energy fields.

DSHEA also allowed for the enactment of regulations to ensure that manufacturers follow good manufacturing practices. In addition, the act clarified which claims are permissible for dietary supplement labels. It does not allow claims that a dietary supplement will "diagnose, prevent, mitigate, treat, or cure a specific disease" but does allow assertions that a dietary ingredient will affect the structure or function of the body. The Federal Trade Commission has responsibility and authority to regulate advertising for dietary supplements.

DSHEA also established the Office of Dietary Supplements (ODS) at the National Institutes of Health. This Mission of ODS is to "strengthen knowledge and understanding of dietary supplements by evaluating scientific information, stimulating and supporting research, disseminating research results, and educating the public to foster an enhanced quality of life and health for the U.S. population."

MIND AND BODY PRACTICES

As defined by NCCAM, mind and body practices "include a diverse group of procedures or techniques administered or taught by a trained practitioner or teacher." Mind and body practices include such therapies as meditation, acupuncture, massage therapy, movement therapy, relaxation techniques, spinal manipulation, tai chi, yoga, and various energy therapies, such as healing touch, Reiki, or qi gong. Mind and body practices as defined by NCCAM should not be confused with the commonly used term *mind-body medicine*. Mind-body medicine is typically used to describe techniques that are specifically designed to enhance the mind's ability to cause physiologic effects that will lead a positive therapeutic outcome, such as decreased pain or anxiety.

Meditation

Meditation, which involves various techniques to self-regulate attention, has been used for thousands of years by various religions and cultures, primarily in Asia, to increase awareness and ultimately improve self-understanding, inner peace, and enlightenment. In Western culture, meditation has gained in popularity since the 1960s and is often used without a religious context to help manage stress and improve overall health.

The physiologic effect of meditation has been extensively studied. Meditation has been shown to increase activity of the autonomic nervous system and bring about what Benson has termed "the relaxation response."[3] This response can lead not only to the subjective sense of decreased stress but also to measurable effects such as a lowering of blood pressure and heart rate. Other investigators have found evidence of increased blood flow in the brain and altered brain chemistry (see Relaxation Techniques, later). Regular meditation is associated with increased α-wave activity as well as decreased levels of hormones associated with stress, such as cortisol and epinephrine, and increased levels of melatonin.

Many meditation techniques exist, and meditation can be taught in individual or group sessions. Meditation has been shown to have potential benefits for managing conditions such as stress, anxiety, cognitive function in elderly people, gastrointestinal disorders, chronic pain, addictions, and even psoriasis.[A1] Although some techniques, such as transcendental meditation, have been more extensively studied, evidence comparing the potential effectiveness of various techniques is largely lacking.

Although safe for most patients, limited evidence suggests that meditation should be approached cautiously for anyone at risk for seizures, symptomatic low blood pressure, or psychotic illness. In one small study of meditators involved in an intensive meditation retreat, more than half of the participants experienced at least one adverse effect.

Acupuncture

Practiced in China for more than 5000 years, acupuncture involves the insertion of very fine needles at specific points in the body. These approximately 360 acupoints reside along 14 channels in the body called *meridians*. In Chinese medical theory, the insertion of the needles is intended to stimulate or improve the balance of the flow of "life energy" or *qi* (pronounced chi). Symptoms or disease are thought to be related to a blockage of flow or imbalance of *qi*. Although very different from a Western medical view of pathophysiology, acupuncture has been shown to have various physiologic effects on the body, including stimulation of endorphins and various brain centers.

There is a growing body of research investigating the potential benefits of acupuncture for a number of conditions. To date, there is evidence suggesting that acupuncture may be beneficial for pain from conditions such as dental pain, fibromyalgia, and headache,[4] as well as beneficial in stroke, analgesia during childbirth, and infertility treatment. A meta-analysis suggests that stimulation of the P6 acupuncture point at the wrist is a potentially effective intervention for reducing postoperative nausea and vomiting.[5] Randomized trials evaluating acupuncture for osteoarthritis of the knee show conflicting results, in part depending on study design[A2], but a recent carefully controlled, blinded trial showed no benefit.[A3]

It is important to explain to patients interested in a trying acupuncture, that the needles are typically ultra-fine and often not painful. An acupuncturist's assessment of the patient will determine the exact location of the needles to be placed. Repeat treatment most commonly occurs once a week, and it often requires 8 to 10 treatments to assess whether acupuncture will have a therapeutic effect.

Modern acupuncture using primarily sterile, disposable needles is generally safe. Risk for infection, although rare, does exist, and electro-acupuncture, which involves stimulation of the acupuncture point by passing a very weak electrical current along the needle, should be avoided in patients with electronic implantable devices such as pacemakers.

Massage Therapy

Massage therapy is perhaps one of the oldest healing modalities. Hippocrates is quoted as saying "the physician must be experienced in many things, but most assuredly in rubbing." Massage is most commonly used to relieve pain from musculoskeletal and other conditions as well as to improve function or relieve stress and aid in relaxation. However, there are more than 80 different types of therapeutic massage, and certain techniques may be more beneficial than others for specific conditions or complaints. Massage has a high use and acceptability in the United States, with approximately 18 million U.S. adults receiving massage in 2007.

The exact mechanism by which massage may exert a therapeutic effect is not clear. Massage is reported to improve local circulation, tone of supportive musculature, and joint flexibility. One commonly held belief was that lactic acid build-up led to delayed-onset muscle soreness and that massage removed lactic acid from muscle. Lactic acid is only present substantially during and immediately after high-intensity anaerobic exercise. It is metabolized within 60 minutes after such exercise ceases and converted back to pyruvate for processing in the Krebs cycle to produce further energy. Some research has suggested that massage may impair lactic acid removal from muscle after strenuous exercise by mechanically impeding blood flow. One study found that massage appeared to exert a clinical benefit by reducing inflammation and promoting mitochondrial biogenesis.[6] In a study of 11 young male athletes, massage was found to activate the mechanotransduction signaling pathways, focal adhesion kinase (FAK) and extracellular signal–regulated kinase 1/2 (ERK1/2), potentiate mitochondrial biogenesis signaling (nuclear peroxisome proliferator–activated receptor γ coactivator 1α [PGC-1α]), and mitigate an increase in nuclear factor κB (NFκB) (p65) nuclear accumulation caused by exercise-induced muscle trauma. Massage was also found to decrease the production of the inflammatory cytokines, tumor necrosis factor-α (TNF-α) and interleukin-6 (IL-6), and to reduce heat shock protein 27 (HSP27) phosphorylation, ultimately decreasing the cellular stress resulting from muscle fiber injury. Massage is also believed to decrease emotional stress through activation of the autonomic nervous system, leading to a variety of neuroendocrine effects.

Clinically, massage has been shown to be of potential benefit for a number of conditions, including neck pain, low back pain, constipation, high blood pressure, lymphedema, stress, and depression. A randomized controlled trial of massage for osteoarthritis of the knee found that an 8-week course of massage decreased pain and improved function, with many of the effects persisting for weeks after cessation of treatment.[A4] Massage appeared to be a viable option as an adjunct to more conventional treatment modalities.

Massage is safe in most settings. Although massage is not entirely risk free, serious adverse events are probably true rarities. Massage should be avoided over rashes, open wounds, fractures, blood clots, or a tumor and is controversial in patients with lymphatic malignancies. Massage can result in increased soreness or bruising and should done with caution in anyone with a bleeding disorder such as thrombocytopenia.

Movement Therapy

Movement therapy is a term used to describe a broad category of approaches that address health and disease by focusing on restoring balance to the body using physical movement. It includes such therapies as yoga, tai chi, Alexander Technique, Feldenkrais Method, and others. Although some therapies involve complex movements and require a trained instructor, others can be self-directed using instructional materials such as videos or books. Yoga and tai chi in particular have gained in popularity in the West and have a growing body of research suggesting positive health benefits.

Originating in India, yoga has been practiced for more than 5000 years. There are hundreds of different types of yoga, which typically involve principles of proper exercise, relaxation, breathing, diet, and meditation and were traditionally practiced to develop one physically, emotionally, and spiritually. In the West, yoga practices have focused on exercise or physical postures (asana), breathing exercises (pranayama), and meditation or relaxation (dharana). Popular forms of yoga in the West include Ashtanga, a vigorous style often taught in the United States as power yoga; Bikram, practiced in rooms heated to about 100° F; Iyengar, a slow form of yoga with strict attention to posture and alignment; Kundalini, a more spiritual form using postures combined with hand positions, breathing, and meditation; and Hatha, which has a focus on postures and breathing exercises to promote a balance of physical health and mental calmness.

Numerous studies have explored the potential health benefits of yoga. A study in the United Kingdom involving 313 adults with chronic low back pain found that yoga led to more improvement in function than usual care when offered once a week for 3 months.[A5] In a meta-analysis, yoga reduced low back pain and back-specific disability but did not improve overall health-related quality of life compared with usual care, educational programs, and exercise programs.[A6]

When guided by a well-trained instructor, yoga is generally safe for most healthy individuals. People with certain chronic conditions, such as glaucoma, hypertension, neck pain, or sciatica, should modify or avoid certain poses, as should women who are pregnant. Certain forms of yoga may be safer or more appropriate for people with particular conditions. For example, Bikram, or hot yoga, is best avoided in individuals with known heart disease, lung disease, or history of heat stroke. A review of comparison studies of yoga and exercise concluded that yoga may be as effective or superior to exercise in improving a number of health-related outcomes in both healthy and patient populations.[7]

Tai chi, also know as tai chi chuan, is an ancient Chinese practice involving a series of movements coordinated with breathing and practiced to strengthen the physical body, improve mental sharpness, and enhance the flow of energy or qi. The healthy flow of qi or this vital energy is thought to be a critical aspect of maintaining health in traditional Chinese medicine. A gentle form of movement that emphasizes continuous slow, often symmetrical flexion and extension of the upper and lower body, tai chi can often be practiced even by individuals with conditions such as heart disease or arthritis as well as by seniors at risk for falls.

Tai chi has been studied as an adjunct to conventional treatments for a number of conditions. A systematic review of the efficacy of tai chi for mostly healthy seniors found limited evidence that tai chi is effective in decreasing falls or blood pressure. A systemic review of tai chi for osteoarthritis came to a similar conclusion. There was some encouraging evidence to support efficacy, but future trials with larger patient samples and longer treatment periods were needed. However, a randomized trial in patients with fibromyalgia found that a 12-week course of tai chi compared with wellness education and stretching exercises led to significant improvement in pain as well as quality of life.[A7] Another randomized controlled trial in patients with mild to moderate Parkinson disease found that tai chi, compared with resistance training or stretching, reduced balance impairments, with additional benefits of improved functional capacity and reduced falls.[A8]

As with other movement therapies, tai chi is best practiced under the guidance of a trained instructor, although it can be learned from videos or books. Safe for most populations, guidelines for appropriate practice of tai chi are the same as those for other land-based exercise programs.

Relaxation Techniques

Relaxation techniques involve a broad range of therapies and techniques, including meditation, yoga, and tai chi, which have been practiced for thousands of years for their purported mental, physical, and spiritual benefits. In more modern times, a number of techniques have been developed with the intent of eliciting the "relaxation response." The relaxation response leads to decreased sympathetic nervous system activation and has been shown to increase α waves on electroencephalogram. Through an effect on the limbic system and its influence on the hypothalamic-pituitary-adrenal axis, there is a subsequent slowing of heart rate and respiratory rate, as well as numerous other neuroendocrine effects, including decreased plasma cortisol. Common techniques include progressive relaxation, breathing exercises, guided visualization, biofeedback, and autogenic training.

Although commonly used to control or manage stress, relaxation techniques have been studied for a number of medical conditions, including anxiety, pain, irritable bowel syndrome, diabetes, premenstrual syndrome, tension headaches, and smoking cessation. Relaxation techniques and meditation programs can provide small to moderate reductions in stress from a wide range of conditions. Relaxation techniques can lead to improvement in both acute and chronic pain, but little evidence exists that the improvement is sustained over time.[8]

Relaxation techniques are a safe, typically low-cost option for patients in need of managing stress more effectively or as a part of an overall plan to manage any of a myriad of stress-related conditions. Given the broad diversity of options, it is important for patients to find a technique that feels most comfortable to them based on goals, personality, beliefs, and lifestyle.

Spinal Manipulation

Spinal manipulation is a method based on the belief that misalignment of the spine can have deleterious effects on health. The technique typically involves correction of a subluxation of the spine by applying a sudden force to the vertebrae or other joint while the patient is lying in various positions on an examining table. Chiropractic manipulation is similar to osteopathic manual therapy practiced by osteopathic physicians. However, osteopaths are medical physicians who may or may not use manipulation as a part of their treatment options. Whereas chiropractors may use a range of modalities, their main focus is on manipulation and restoring of proper alignment of the spine. According to the 2007 NHIS study, more than 18 million adults and more than 2 million children had undergone chiropractic or osteopathic manipulation during the previous 12 months.

The efficacy of manipulation has been studied for a number of diverse conditions, with most studies focused on musculoskeletal disorders. A review of the evidence concluded that manipulation was effective for acute, subacute, and chronic low back pain; migraine and cervicogenic headache; cervicogenic dizziness; several extremity joint conditions; and acute or subacute neck pain.[9] The existing evidence was found to be inconclusive for cervical neck pain of any duration, and for mid-back pain, sciatica, tension-type headache, cocydynia, temporomandibular joint disorders, fibromyalgia, premenstrual syndrome, and pneumonia in older adults.

Although minor side effects such as soreness or light-headedness are not uncommon, overall the risk for a serious adverse event is very low. Concern has been raised that manipulation of the cervical spine may put patients at increased risk for vertebrobasilar artery stroke. However, any small increased risk for such a stroke associated with both chiropractic care and visits to primary care physicians may be because such patients were already having headaches or neck pain because of impending or ongoing vertebral artery dissection.

Energy Therapies

Energy therapies include a number of approaches in which the practitioner intends to channel healing energy (typically through the hands) into the person seeking help in order to restore balance of energy in the body and health. The core concept is that all humans have a subtle vital energy or biofield that flows through them and can be manipulated or used to influence health. Examples of therapies that use this concept are therapeutic touch, healing touch, Reiki, qi gong, and intercessory prayer (prayer for an individual that is specifically directed at that person's health).

NCCAM distinguishes two categories of energy therapies or energy medicine: the veritable and the putative. Veritable energy therapies involve energy that can be measured, such as light therapy or electromagnetic radiation (radiation therapy), and are not considered CAM. Putative energy therapies are not measurable in a reliable way and involve theoretical manipulation or modulation of the vital force or biofield as described previously.

Putative energy therapies have been challenged as being nonplausible biologically and as such are perhaps among the more controversial therapies categorized as CAM. Despite that, prayer for health was the most commonly used intervention in the 2007 NHIS report, with approximately 30% of respondents having had others pray for their health. Approximately 1% had used Reiki and 0.5% qi gong.

A review of the literature on energy healing and pain, focused on Reiki, therapeutic touch, and healing touch, concluded that despite interest in these modalities, particularly in the nursing practice literature, few well-conducted studies existed. A 2008 study funded by NCCAM assessed the efficacy of qi gong in the treatment of osteoarthritis of the knee. This randomized controlled trial comparing two qi gong masters and a "sham" master found that although qi gong may have benefit for patients with osteoarthritis of the knee, the two healers were not equivalent.[10] This study points out the challenge of determining the qualification and competency of energy therapy providers for those interested in pursuing energy therapies as a possible therapeutic modality. Despite the lack of definitive research, energy therapies remain popular with patients, and putative energy therapies are generally regarded as offering no measurable risk.

WHOLE MEDICAL SYSTEMS

It is important to recognize that many of the therapies and approaches described previously come from complete systems of healing, or *whole medical systems*. These systems, with their own particular paradigm or way of viewing disease and health, include systems such as traditional Chinese medicine, Ayurvedic medicine, homeopathy, Native American healing, and naturopathy.

CONCLUSION

Although still controversial, use of CAM by both patients and conventionally trained providers has continued to increase. As evidenced by the growth of the Consortium of Academic Health Centers for Integrative Medicine, as well as such events as the Institute of Medicine's 2009 Summit on Integrative Medicine and the Health of the Public, integration and acceptance of the concepts and principles of integrative medicine into the mainstream and academic medical settings has also grown. This is perhaps a result of a realization that many of the principles of integrative medicine, such as a partnering of patients and providers, care that addresses the whole person, and an emphasis on not only treatment but also the broader concepts of health promotion and illness prevention, offer at least part of the solution to the challenges of our evolving health care system. All health care providers, present and future, should be familiar with these concepts, including the safe and appropriate use of a broad range of healing sciences and providers to facilitate the body's innate healing response, relieve suffering, and optimize vitality.

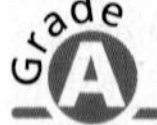

Grade A References

A1. Goyal M, Singh S, Sibinga EM, et al. Meditation programs for psychological stress and well-being: a systematic review and meta-analysis. *JAMA Intern Med.* 2014;174:357-368.

A2. Corbett MS, Rice SJ, Madurasinghe V, et al. Acupuncture and other physical treatments for the relief of pain due to osteoarthritis of the knee: network meta-analysis. *Osteoarthritis Cartilage.* 2013;21:1290-1298.

A3. Hinman RS, McCrory P, Pirotta M, et al. Acupuncture for chronic knee pain: a randomized clinical trial. *JAMA.* 2014;312:1313-1322.

A4. Perlman AI, Sabina A, Williams A, et al. Massage therapy for osteoarthritis of the knee: a randomized controlled trial. *Arch Intern Med.* 2006;166:2533-2538.

A5. Tilbrook HE, Cox H, Hewitt CE, et al. Yoga for chronic low back pain: a randomized trial. *Ann Intern Med.* 2011;155:569-578.

A6. Cramer H, Lauche R, Haller H, et al. A systematic review and meta-analysis of yoga for low back pain. *Clin J Pain.* 2013;29:450-460.

A7. Wang C, Schmid CH, Rones R, et al. A randomized trial of tai chi for fibromyalgia. *N Engl J Med.* 2010;363:743-754.

A8. Li F, Hammer P, Fitzgerald K, et al. Tai chi and postural stability in patients with Parkinson's disease. *N Engl J Med.* 2012;366:511-519.

GENERAL REFERENCES

For the General References and other additional features, please visit Expert Consult at https://expertconsult.inkling.com.

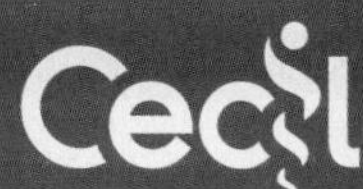

VI GENETICS

40

PRINCIPLES OF GENETICS

BRUCE R. KORF

The elucidation of the structure and function of the genome is one of the great scientific triumphs of the 20th century. The relevance of inheritance to health and disease probably has been recognized throughout history, but it is only during the last century that the rules governing inheritance and the mechanisms whereby genetic information is stored and used have come to light. The application of this knowledge to medical practice had long been focused on relatively rare monogenic and chromosomal disorders. Major contributions have been made in these areas in the form of approaches to genetic counseling, genetic testing, prenatal diagnosis, newborn screening, carrier screening, and, to a limited extent, treatment. As important as these contributions are, however, their impact has been limited by the rarity of these disorders. Powerful tools resulting from the sequencing of the human genome are changing this situation (Chapter 43).[1] Genetic factors that contribute to common and rare disorders are being identified, leading to new approaches to diagnosis, prevention, and treatment. Genetics and genomics are increasingly occupying center stage in medical practice, guiding treatment decisions and preventive strategies. This chapter reviews the paradigm whereby genetics is being integrated into the routine practice of medicine.

GENETIC CONTRIBUTION TO DISEASE

It may be argued that no disorder is either completely determined genetically or completely determined by non-genetic factors. Even monogenic conditions, such as phenylketonuria, are modified by the environment, in this case by dietary intake of phenylalanine. Genetically determined host factors are known to modify susceptibility to infection or other environmental agents. Even individuals who are victims of trauma may find themselves at risk in part because of genetic traits that affect behavior or ability to perceive or escape from danger.

Multifactorial Inheritance

Complex traits that are important for both health and disease are the result of an interaction of multiple genes with one another and with the environment (Fig. 40-1). In some cases, individual genes or environmental factors contribute overwhelmingly to the cause of a disorder, as with a genetic condition, such as neurofibromatosis or Marfan syndrome, or an acquired disorder, such as bacterial infection or trauma. Other times, there may be interplay among many factors, making it difficult to dissect out the specific genes or environmental exposures.

From a medical perspective, it is helpful to divide the genetic contribution to disease into three categories: (1) high-penetrance monogenic or chromosomal disorders; (2) monogenic versions of common disorders; and (3) complex, multifactorial disorders. Each of these has an impact on medical practice in distinctive ways.

High-Penetrance Monogenic or Chromosomal Disorders

High-penetrance monogenic or chromosomal disorders are the disorders that most clinicians think of as "genetic conditions" (Chapter 41). They include rare but familiar single-gene disorders, such as neurofibromatosis, Marfan syndrome, and cystic fibrosis, and chromosomal abnormalities, such as trisomy 21 (Down syndrome). Several thousand distinct human genetic disorders have been described and cataloged in *Mendelian Inheritance in Man* (available at www.omim.org). These include mendelian dominant or recessive disorders, sex-linked disorders, and conditions that are due to mutations within the 16.6-kilobase mitochondrial genome. They also include major chromosomal aneuploidy syndromes and syndromes associated with duplication or deletion of small regions of the genome that result in either reproducible syndromes, such as Williams syndrome (deletion of contiguous loci from a region of chromosome 7), or nonspecific intellectual disability or autism spectrum disorder.

ROLE OF THE NONSPECIALIST

Because of the rarity of many of these conditions, most practitioners have limited experience with a given disorder and are likely to need to refer the patient to an appropriate specialist for assistance with diagnosis and management. Nevertheless, the nonspecialist has many distinct roles in the care of these patients. These roles begin with recognition of the fact that the patient may have such a disorder and arrangement for appropriate diagnostic evaluation.[2] Many genetic disorders produce obvious signs or symptoms that at least prompt referral even if they are not immediately suggestive of a diagnosis. Others can be more subtle, with nevertheless significant consequences if the diagnosis is missed. An example is Marfan syndrome (Chapter 260). The physician needs to be alert to the physical characteristics of patients with Marfan syndrome because life-threatening aortic dissection can be avoided with appropriate monitoring and treatment. Table 40-1 lists examples of some adult-onset monogenic conditions with which the internist should be familiar.

Treatment of Patients with Genetic Disorders

The treatment of patients with genetic disorders may require the assistance of a specialist, but the nonspecialist is likely to be the first contact when an affected individual is ill. The primary care physician needs to be familiar with the disorder and major potential complications. For example, the patient with neurofibromatosis who experiences chronic back pain may be presenting with a malignant peripheral nerve sheath tumor, requiring more aggressive evaluation than would be typical for an unaffected individual with back pain. Formation of a good working relationship between the specialist and nonspecialist is crucial to ensure effective care.

The nonspecialist also has an important role in supporting the patient and helping to explain the difficult choices that may be offered for management. This includes providing support for patients who have disorders that cannot be treated and for the emotional impact that accompanies knowledge that a disorder may be transmitted to one's offspring or shared with other relatives. Most patients have little understanding of the mechanisms of genetics and genetic disease. Although the responsibility to explain these issues may reside with specialists and counselors, the primary care physician has an important supportive role.

ADVANCES IN GENETICS

Many of the disorders in this group have been known for a long time, but more recent advances in genetics have had a substantial impact on approaches to diagnosis and management. Genetic testing has been refined with the advent of molecular diagnostic tests that detect mutations within individual genes. Even rare disorders may be amenable to diagnostic testing; a database of testing laboratories can be found on the Internet (available at www.genetests.org or at www.ncbi.nlm.nih.gov/gtr/). Whole-genome scanning using cytogenomic microarrays is revealing small deletions or duplications in patients with disorders such as autism spectrum disorder, for whom standard chromosomal analysis had previously been unrevealing. Sequencing of the entire coding region of the genome ("*whole exome sequencing*") or the entire genome itself ("*whole genome sequencing*") is now being applied clinically.[3] (Actually, these tests do not detect every possible gene or DNA base, hence the use of the word "whole" is disputed, but the techniques do look across the entire genome, so the word "whole" distinguishes these from approaches that target specific genes.) Population screening for carrier status for autosomal recessive disorders has been offered for many years, with specific ethnic groups being offered testing for conditions of high prevalence in the group. Genomic approaches are now making it possible to vastly expand the scope of testing, increasing the numbers of conditions tested and making it possible to offer a similar comprehensive screen of dozens or even hundreds of genes regardless of ethnicity. Prenatal screening for trisomy can be offered noninvasively by sequencing of fetal DNA isolated from maternal blood. Newborn screening is being expanded beyond inborn errors of metabolism such as phenylketonuria and galactosemia, with the advent of tandem mass spectrometry and the availability of a standardized panel of tests.

Finally, treatment of some monogenic disorders is becoming feasible. Life expectancy for patients with cystic fibrosis has been increasing gradually with better treatments for chronic lung disease; dietary therapy is available for many inborn errors of metabolism; novel therapies that use either pharmaceuticals or gene or enzyme replacement strategies are in use or being tested for many conditions. The principles of management of genetic disorders are evolving rapidly, and care of patients increasingly requires active partnership of specialists and primary care physicians. Moreover, individuals with congenital disorders such as Down syndrome are routinely surviving to adulthood and require primary care physicians who are familiar with their special needs.

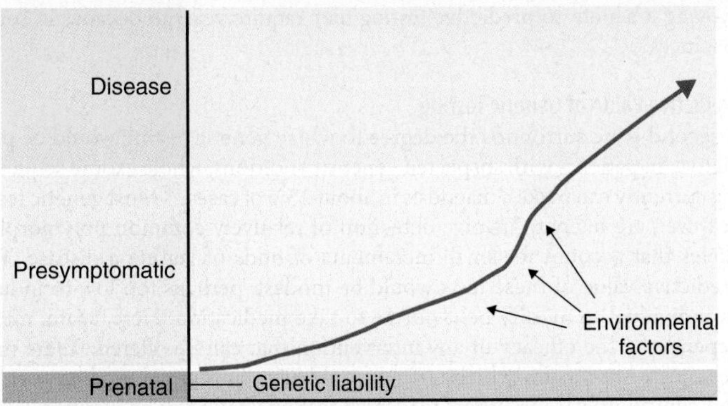

FIGURE 40-1. Multifactorial etiology of disease. An individual is born with a genetic liability but remains in a presymptomatic state for some time until additional events occur, including exposure to environmental factors, that result in crossing a threshold that is identified as *disease*. In instances of high-penetrance monogenic disorders, the genetic liability may be overwhelming. In other instances, genetic factors may contribute only slightly to disease risk.

TABLE 40-1 HIGH-PENETRANCE SINGLE-GENE DISORDERS THAT MAY PRESENT IN ADULTHOOD, WITH SOME MAJOR MEDICAL IMPLICATIONS*

DISORDER	INHERITANCE	MAJOR MEDICAL IMPLICATIONS
CARDIOVASCULAR		
Marfan syndrome	AD	Risk for aortic dissection; lens dislocation
Long QT syndrome	AD, AR	Arrhythmia, sudden death
RENAL		
Adult polycystic kidney disease	AD	Renal failure
PULMONARY		
α_1-Antitrypsin deficiency	AR	Emphysema, cirrhosis
NEUROLOGIC		
NF1	AD	Benign and malignant nerve sheath tumors, gliomas
NF2	AD	Schwannomas (especially vestibular), meningiomas
Von Hippel-Lindau	AD	Hemangioblastoma of cerebellum, brain stem, eye; pheochromocytoma; renal cell carcinoma
Huntington disease	AD	Movement disorder, psychiatric disorder, dementia
HEMATOLOGIC		
Globin disorders	AR	Stroke, iron overload
ENDOCRINE		
MEN syndromes	AD	Tumors of thyroid and parathyroid, pheochromocytoma

*See Table 40-2 for examples of lower penetrance disorders.
AD = autosomal dominant; AR = autosomal recessive; MEN = multiple endocrine neoplasia; NF = neurofibromatosis.

Monogenic Versions of Common Disorders

Not all monogenic disorders produce obscure phenotypes, and not all common disorders have complex multifactorial causes. Some common disorders occur in some families as single-gene traits (Table 40-2). This is usually true for only a proportion of affected individuals, but in some cases, it is a significant proportion and represents an important group of patients to be recognized.

Breast Cancer

An example is breast cancer (Chapter 198). Familial predisposition to breast and ovarian cancer in many cases is attributable to mutation of *BRCA1* or *BRCA2*. Women who inherit a mutation in one of these genes face a high risk for eventually developing breast or ovarian cancer—more than 80% by age 70 years for breast cancer. Women at risk because of mutation do not look different from women with sporadic breast cancer but can be distinguished by many features, including family history of breast or ovarian cancer in multiple relatives, early age at onset of cancer, and multifocality of the cancer (e.g., bilateral breast cancer or breast and ovarian cancer).

TABLE 40-2 SINGLE-GENE DISORDERS WITH INCOMPLETE PENETRANCE THAT MAY ACCOUNT FOR INHERITED FORMS OF SELECTED COMMON DISORDERS

DISORDER	INHERITANCE: GENES	MAJOR MEDICAL IMPLICATIONS
Hemochromatosis	AR: *HFE*	Cirrhosis, cardiomyopathy, diabetes mellitus
Thrombophilia	AD, AR: multiple genes	Deep vein thrombosis
Breast and ovarian cancers	AD: *BRCA1, BRCA2*	Breast and ovarian cancers
Familial adenomatous polyposis	AD: *APC*	Multiple colonic polyps, colon cancer
Lynch syndrome	AD: DNA mismatch repair genes	Colorectal cancer, endometrial cancer
Maturity-onset diabetes of the young	AD: multiple genes	Diabetes mellitus
Cardiomyopathy	AD: genes involved in cardiac contractile apparatus	Arrhythmia, heart failure

AD = autosomal dominant; AR = autosomal recessive.

COLON CANCER AND OTHER COMMON DISORDERS

Another example from cancer genetics is colon cancer (Chapter 193). Two syndromes, familial adenomatous polyposis and Lynch syndrome, are autosomal dominantly inherited and convey a high risk for colon cancer. Other noncancer examples are hemochromatosis (Chapter 212), in which cirrhosis, cardiomyopathy, diabetes, joint disease, and other problems ensue from excessive iron absorption; 10% of whites carry an allele that predisposes to this recessive disorder. Mutations in the factor V gene or the prothrombin gene occur commonly and predispose to deep vein thrombosis (Chapter 176). Rarer examples include inherited forms of cardiomyopathy, hypertension, and familial hypercholesterolemia.

MANAGEMENT

The physician may be called on to address these disorders in many ways. There is a compelling reason to make an early diagnosis of hemochromatosis because the complications can be prevented, but not reversed, by phlebotomy and subsequent monitoring of iron stores. Individuals at risk for colon cancer can be offered surveillance with colonoscopy or surgical resection of the colon to reduce the risk for cancer. Individuals at risk for breast and ovarian cancer likewise can be offered surveillance, chemoprevention, or surgery. The benefits of knowledge of genetic risks are less clear in some instances. Carriers of the factor V Leiden mutation would not be treated with anticoagulation until after an event of thrombosis, and the treatment may not be different for a carrier versus a noncarrier. In some cases, however, knowledge of carrier status may help ensure prompt diagnosis or avoid situations of high risk.

GENETIC TESTING

As with other medical tests, the physician should carefully consider risks, benefits, and clinical utility in deciding to use a genetic test. Some distinct ethical and legal risks may apply to some genetic tests. These may include anxiety, stigmatization, guilt, and possibly discrimination for insurance or employment. Some of these risks may be addressed by legislation to maintain privacy of genetic information, such as the Genetic Information Nondiscrimination Act of 2008, but the risks for anxiety, guilt, and stigmatization cannot be legislated away. To some extent, further research may improve the basis for surveillance or lead to effective treatments. For now, many of these disorders present a double-edged sword of potentially useful knowledge and potentially harmful information.

ROLE OF THE PHYSICIAN

The role of the physician in dealing with monogenic disorders includes recognition of individuals at risk and participation in formulation of a care plan.[4] Individuals at risk may not be identifiable by physical appearance and usually are not evident from medical history or physical examination findings. The most valuable screening tool is the family history. Directed questioning about a family history of major monogenic disorders, especially breast, ovarian, and colon cancer, as well as hypercholesterolemia, hypertension, deep vein thrombosis, cirrhosis, and diabetes, can identify the occasional patient with mendelian segregation of these common disorders. Even if the information is of uncertain reliability, eliciting a family history can prompt referral for further evaluation, documentation of the family history, and consideration for genetic testing. The physician's job is not simply to identify individuals at risk; some people believe they are at high risk even in the absence of well-documented risk factors. Addressing these misconceptions can bring peace of mind and usually does not require genetic testing.

Complex, Multifactorial Disorders

Understanding the genetics of common disorders is one of the great challenges of modern medicine, with the promise of major returns in terms of prevention, diagnosis, and treatment. The etiology of these disorders is complex in that they result from an interaction of multiple genes with one another and with environmental factors. The specific genes that are relevant may be different from one person to the next. Identification of these genes is difficult given this heterogeneity and the relatively small impact that any particular gene may have in a particular person.

POPULATION STUDIES

Dissection of the genetic contribution to common disease cannot be accomplished by the standard genetic approaches involving study of rare variants or family-based linkage studies. Most recent efforts have focused on study of large groups of patients, comparing the prevalence of particular genetic markers in case patients and control subjects. The availability of markers has been boosted by the identification of *single-nucleotide polymorphisms* (SNPs) (Chapter 43). These are differences in single DNA bases between individuals that occur every several hundred bases. Some of these account for common genetic differences between people, including differences that may contribute to disease. The catalog of SNPs currently includes several million variants; it has been found that the genome has evolved as blocks of clusters of genes, making it possible to use only a limited number of SNPs within a given region to determine whether there is a gene in that region that is associated with a disease. Since completion of the HapMap Project, there has been a dramatic increase in the number of SNPs found to be associated with common disorders. For most disorders, however, the total contribution to heritability of the condition has not been accounted for by SNP association studies.

GENETIC RISK ASSESSMENT

The goal of genetic risk assessment is the identification of individuals at risk for disease before the onset of signs or symptoms. In principle, the genetic factors could be identified at birth, or any time in life, by testing a DNA sample. Any individuals found to be at risk might be offered treatment in advance of onset of the disease to avoid complications or might be advised to modify their lifestyle to avoid exposure to environmental factors that might increase risk for disease. Genetic testing has been offered on a direct-to-consumer basis by some companies, although the clinical validity and clinical utility of such testing is a matter of debate.

Although the concept of genomic risk assessment would appear to be an attractive paradigm, many questions may be raised about its practicality and implementation. First, predictive testing is useful only insofar as it guides further management. This is likely to be a moving target because ability to test for risk can be developed more quickly than ability to modify that risk. The utility of interventions may be valued differently by different people. This already has been the case for testing of disorders such as breast cancer. Some women at risk choose not to know their *BRCA* status because the options, including surveillance or prophylactic surgery, are unacceptable to them. If there were a low-cost, safe, and effective treatment that would neutralize any risk the decision to test would be simple, but short of that, there are reasonable arguments on both sides of the issue of whether to test. For many disorders, it will take a long time to show the efficacy of any intervention because there may be a period of many years between the test and the onset of a disorder. Unless surrogate markers can be identified and followed, the task of proving a benefit to predictive testing may require years to decades in some instances.

Predictive Value of Genetic Testing

A second issue surrounds the degree to which genetic testing would be predictive. In patients with suspected genetic conditions, whole exome sequencing currently can make a diagnosis in about 25% of cases.[5,6] Most genetic tests, however, are likely to involve detection of relatively common polymorphic alleles that account for small increments of odds of getting a disease. The predictive value of these tests would be modest, perhaps too low to induce an individual to modify behavior or to take medication. Here, again, much depends on the efficacy of any intervention that can be offered. There may be some disorders for which testing would have substantial predictive value and clinical utility and others for which testing would not be justified.

Social and Ethical Issues

A third concern relates to social and ethical issues. Will people use test results as an excuse to pursue self-destructive behaviors, having received what may be false reassurance of "immunity"? Will people misinterpret results of testing in terms of a simplistic notion of genetic determinism, erroneously believing that their futures have been written, leaving them no recourse but to meet their fate? The rapid pace of technologic change is going to challenge the ability of the social and legal systems to keep pace.

Service Models

Finally, there are questions of the ideal context in which to offer such testing. The personal genomics companies provide their services directly to the consumer in most cases. This creates the obvious risk for incorrect interpretation of results by the patient, although it is not clear that the health care work force is otherwise prepared to deal with the challenges of interpretation of genome-wide studies. The challenges are increasing as the cost of genome sequencing continues to plummet. Genome sequencing also raises the complex question of how to handle incidental findings (i.e., discovery of an unexpected disease risk that may or may not be amenable to medical intervention).

DISEASE STRATIFICATION

A second application of genomics in medical practice entails stratification of disease. Even if genetic testing is not used to predict individuals at risk, it may well be used to determine the most appropriate treatment for a clinically diagnosed disorder. Most common disorders, such as hypertension and diabetes, are symptom complexes that probably result from a variety of causes. The particular combination of causes may differ in different individuals and may respond to different types of treatments. Choice of antihypertensive drug may come to depend on genetic testing to determine the specific cause of hypertension in a patient. The concept of disease stratification is particularly well developed in treatment of cancer, where targeted multigene tests and even genome sequencing is increasingly being used to guide therapy. It is likely that genetic tests eventually will accompany many if not most treatment decisions.

EFFECTS AND IDENTIFICATION OF DRUGS

Aside from helping to choose the most efficacious drug, genetic testing may play a role in avoidance of side effects and in appropriate dosing. Many drugs are known to be associated with rare side effects, some of which are sufficiently severe as to lead the drug to be withdrawn from use. Some of these side effects may occur only in individuals who are susceptible on the basis of having a particular allele at a polymorphic locus. An example is the association of polymorphisms in certain sodium or potassium channel genes with risk for arrhythmia on exposure to specific drugs.

Absorption and metabolism of drugs are largely under genetic control. Several polymorphisms are known to lead to particularly rapid or slow metabolism, accounting for individuals who experience dose-related side effects or lack of efficacy at standard dosages (Table 40-3). Detection of these polymorphisms would allow customization of drug dosage to an individual's pattern of metabolism, increasing the likelihood of efficacy without a prolonged period of trial-and-error dosing.[7]

The greatest gift of genetics and genomics to medicine may be in the ability to identify new drug targets and develop new approaches to treatment. Identification of genes that contribute to common disorders is revealing the cellular mechanisms that lead to disease. This knowledge offers the opportunity to develop new pharmaceutical agents that would target the physiologic mechanisms more precisely, leading to drugs that work better and cause fewer

TABLE 40-3 GENES IN WHICH COMMON POLYMORPHISMS AFFECT RATES OF DRUG METABOLISM OR ACTION

GENE	MEDICATIONS (EXAMPLES)
CYP2C9	Phenytoin, warfarin
CYP2D6	Debrisoquin, β-blockers, antidepressants
VKORC1	Warfarin
UGT1A1	Irinotecan
Thiopurine methyltransferase	Mercaptopurine, azathioprine
N-acetyltransferase	Isoniazid, hydralazine
CYP2C19	Clopidogrel

side effects. New approaches to gene replacement or insertion of genes into cells as localized drug delivery systems also may be developed. The treatment of common disorders likely would entail the use of approaches developed as a result of genomics even in cases in which genetic testing is not used to predict individuals who are at risk.

CONCLUSION

Most physicians in practice today trained before the elucidation of the sequence of the human genome. Nevertheless, physicians will be using the products of the genome project increasingly in their day-to-day practice during the coming years. Whether they are providing care for a patient with a rare genetic disorder or for a patient with a common condition not usually regarded as genetic, management choices increasingly will be informed by tests and treatments that in some way are based on information from the genome sequence.

The essence of the encounter between a physician and a patient can be distilled to two questions: Why this person? Why this time? A person who seeks medical care is doing so as the product of human evolution, having an ancestry associated with certain genetic vulnerabilities, because of inheritance of certain familial risk factors, because of exposure to some environmental factors, because of a particular physiologic process gone awry, because of behavioral traits that lead the person to seek medical care, because of prompting by family or friends to go to the doctor, because society makes medical services available, and because the person can afford to seek care. Genetics cannot answer all of these questions, but it is providing the key to addressing many of the biologic questions that underlie the medical mysteries that have puzzled humankind for generations.

GENERAL REFERENCES

For the General References and other additional features, please visit Expert Consult at https://expertconsult.inkling.com.

41 GENE, GENOMIC, AND CHROMOSOMAL DISORDERS

SANDESH C. S. NAGAMANI, PAWEŁ STANKIEWICZ, AND JAMES R. LUPSKI

THE HUMAN GENOME

Unprecedented technologic advances in molecular biology during the past two decades have enabled the determination of the entire DNA (deoxyribonucleic acid) sequence content of the human genome (Human Genome Project, HGP; http://web.ornl.gov/sci/techresources/Human_Genome/index.shtml) and establishment of a reference haploid genome.[1,2] Sequencing of other personal diploid human genomes and international collaborative efforts (http://www.1000genomes.org/) have generated DNA sequence data that have revolutionized our views on human history, evolution, and the genetic and genomic bases of disease.[3]

Human genomic DNA is packaged within the nucleus in 23 chromosome pairs, 22 autosomes, and 2 sex chromosomes, XX in females and XY in males. The diploid genome (2n) in each cell consists of two identical haploid copies of about 3×10^9 base pairs (bp), thus equaling in total 6 billion nucleotides. Most of the human genome consists of repetitive elements: tandem repeats (e.g., satellite sequences in centromeres), telomeric repeats, microsatellites, minisatellites, and short and long interspersed retrotransposable elements (e.g., *Alu* elements and LINE elements, respectively) (Table 41-1). These elements form constitutive heterochromatin, and their functional roles are not yet well elucidated. The unique "coding" DNA sequences comprise the minority of our genome and include about 23,000 protein-coding genes, conserved sequences that encode noncoding RNAs (i.e., not translated to protein), including microRNAs (miRNAs), small nucleolar RNAs (snoRNAs), and long noncoding RNAs (lncRNAs), as well as conserved regulatory elements. Although protein-coding sequences occupy only about 1 to 2% of the human genome, it has been demonstrated recently that most of our DNA may be transcribed into RNA.

Approximately 4 to 5% of the human genome, including both repetitive and unique sequences, is present in two or more copies in the haploid genome. DNA fragments larger than 1 kb and of DNA sequence identity greater than 90% have been termed *low-copy repeats* (LCRs) or *segmental duplications* (SDs). Most LCRs have arisen during primate speciation. A subset of LCRs with DNA sequence identity greater than 95% and longer than 10 kb can lead to local genome instability during both meiotic (constitutional) and mitotic (somatic) cell divisions, resulting in genomic rearrangements and conveying genomic disorders.

GENE

The concept of a gene can be traced back to 1865 when Gregor Mendel observed the inheritance of phenotypic traits in the garden pea, *Pisum sativum*. Mendel noted that two *factors* that we now know to be corresponding DNA loci (alleles) located on homologous chromosomes separate from each other during meiosis and segregate to two different gametes. This phenomenon of independent segregation is now known as *Mendel's first law. Mendel's second law* described the independent segregation of two different (nonallelic) loci during gamete formation. The *inheritance factors* or *units of heredity* encoding the genetic information were later defined as *genes*. We now define a *gene* as a fragment of DNA that carries the information used to transcribe it into a functional RNA (ribonucleic acid).

The DNA double helix is built of four nucleotides: two purine bases, adenine (A) and guanine (G), and two pyrimidine bases, thymine (T) and cytosine (C), all connected to deoxyribose sugars and linked by phosphodiester bonds at the 5′ and 3′ carbon of the sugar. (In RNA, thymine is replaced by uracil, U.) Three consecutive nucleotides (triplet codon) of the coding DNA encode an amino acid. There are 64 possible different codons (4^3 combinations) but only 20 amino acids; therefore, the genetic code has been termed *degenerate*. Most of the protein-coding genes in our genome comprise several coding regions or *exons* that are separated by noncoding *introns*. The entire gene (exons and introns) is transcribed into messenger RNA (mRNA) by RNA polymerase II starting from its 5′ end and continuing beyond the poly A recognition signal at the 3′ end. Typically, mRNA begins with a cap and terminates with a polyadenylated (polyA) tail at the 3′ end. In the subsequent process of splicing, the intervening noncoding introns are deleted, and the spliced, mature mRNA is translated into a polypeptide. The polypeptides start at the 5′ end (NH_2 terminus) with a methionine encoded by the AUG triplet. At the 3′ end (COOH terminus), the polypeptides are terminated by one of three terminating codons, UAA, UAG, or UGA (Fig. 41-1).

Micro-RNA (miRNA) (about 22 bp single-stranded RNA), *small nucleolar RNA* (snoRNA) (60 to 300 bp single-stranded RNA), and *long noncoding RNA* (lncRNA) (>200 bp RNA) are transcribed but are not translated. These noncoding RNAs are involved in many important biologic processes. There is evidence that dysregulation of noncoding RNA may have a role in cancer, cardiovascular, neurologic, and developmental disorders.

GENETIC AND GENOMIC VARIATION IN HUMANS

In addition to the Human Genome Project, the International HapMap (http://hapmap.ncbi.nlm.nih.gov), Human Genome Diversity (http://www.stanford.edu/group/morrinst/hgdp.html), ENCODE (http://www

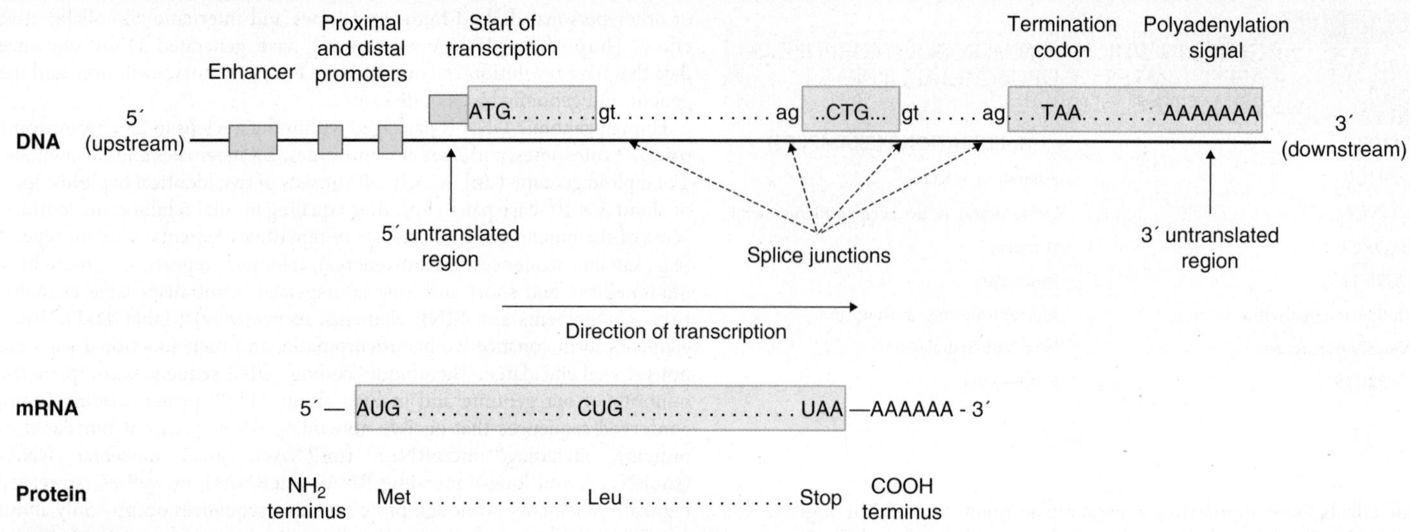

FIGURE 41-1. Gene structure. Schematic representation of the general structure of a typical human gene. Three exons are depicted as open rectangles. Note that the translation usually starts with an ATG triplet encoding methionine. The 5′ (upstream) portion of a gene corresponds to the NH_2 terminus, and the 3′ (downstream) segment encodes the COOH terminus of the polypeptide. Enhancers and promoters are shown as blue rectangles.

TABLE 41-1 STRUCTURE OF THE HUMAN GENOME

CHROMATIN FEATURE	SEQUENCE TYPE	HUMAN GENOME (HAPLOID)	% of Haploid Genome*
Euchromatin	Protein coding	20,000-25,000 genes	~2
	Noncoding	RNA genes	
		Regulatory elements	
		Pseudogenes	~38
		Gene fragments	
		Conserved sequences	
Heterochromatin	Repetitive		~60
		Tandem: satellite DNA, minisatellites, microsatellites	~14
		Interspersed (transposons):	~45
		Retrotransposons	~8
		LTR	
		Non-LTR	
		SINE (*Alu*)	~13
		LINE	~21
		DNA transposons	~3

*Estimated.
LINE = long interspersed nuclear elements; LTR = long-terminal repeat; SINE = short interspersed nuclear elements.

.genome.gov/10005107), 1000 Genomes project (http://www.1000genomes.org/), and other collaborative efforts, including personal genome sequencing projects, have revealed the tremendous and underappreciated extent of variation in the human genome.[3] Genetic variation consists of two major types: (1) nucleotide sequence changes, or single nucleotide variants (SNVs); and (2) genome structural changes, or copy-number variants (CNVs) (Fig. 41-2).

Single Nucleotide Variants

A genetic *polymorphism* is defined as a heterozygous DNA variation present in greater than 1% of the population (http://www.ncbi.nlm.nih.gov/SNP/, http://www.1000genomes.org/, http://evs.gs.washington.edu/EVS/). Genome-wide nucleotide variation uncovered in the early phase of DNA sequencing analyses showed that human genomes differ from the haploid reference genome mainly by single nucleotide changes. These differences have been termed *single nucleotide polymorphisms* (SNPs) and defined as a nucleotide change at a given position generated by substitution. Any two human beings differ on average by about 3.5 million SNPs (0.1% of the 3.0 $\times 10^9$ reference haploid genome). Whereas most of these SNPs map outside of the exons, on average about 20,000 SNPs occur in coding regions, and among these, about 7000 to 10,000 are nonsynonymous (i.e., change the encoded amino acid).[3] It is important to note that SNPs located outside of the protein-coding regions can still exert phenotypic effects, such as by modifying gene regulatory elements, transcription factor–binding sites, generating splicing mutations, or affecting noncoding RNAs.

A set of consecutive SNPs (or other markers) is defined as a *haplotype*. A nonrandom association of markers in a population not interrupted by meiotic recombination (*crossing over*) is described as *linkage disequilibrium*. (Note that linkage disequilibrium exemplifies the exception to Mendel's second law).

Copy-Number Variants

A more recently characterized group of major polymorphic genetic variation in the human genome is represented by *structural changes*. High-resolution genome-wide analysis of human genome sequences has revealed higher-order architectural features, with a potential to cause genomic instability and extensive submicroscopic structural variations.[4] These structural variations consist of unbalanced CNVs, including deletions, duplications, triplications, insertions, and translocations, that differ from the normal diploid state, as well as balanced rearrangements such as genomic inversions. Recent analyses have revealed that about 11,700 CNVs (size > 443 bp) cover more than 112 million base pairs (Mb) (3.7%) of the reference human genome. A validated subset of these CNVs overlap 13% of the Reference Sequence (RefSeq) (http://www.ncbi.nlm.nih.gov/projects/RefSeq/RSG) genes and 12% of the Online Mendelian Inheritance in Man (OMIM) (http://www.ncbi.nlm.nih.gov/sites/entrez?db=omim) genes and was predicted to alter the structure of 12.5% gene transcripts and 5.5% mRNAs. On average, each individual harbors about 1000 CNVs that range in size between 500 bp and 1.2 Mb; the frequency of smaller CNVs (<1 kb) and indels (insertion or deletion of bases < 100 bp) is much higher than the larger rearrangements. It is noteworthy that any two human genomes contain more base-pair differences due to CNVs than to SNVs.

Despite all these recent achievements, the total number, position, size, gene content, and population distribution of CNVs remain obscure because we still do not have accurate and reliable molecular methods to study smaller

CNVs on a genome-wide scale in different populations, particularly when copy-number changes are greater than $n = 4$ or 5.

CNVs have been shown to be responsible for Mendelian diseases, non-Mendelian traits such as complex diseases, and common traits (including neurobehavioral traits), or to represent benign polymorphic variants (Chapter 40).[5] CNVs can lead to abnormal phenotypes by disrupting the gene structure or changing the copy-number of dosage-sensitive genes. However, long-range effects of CNVs involving nongenic sequences, leaving a gene intact, have been also demonstrated. Furthermore, evidence suggests that a combination of two or more CNVs at the same or different loci may be responsible for phenotypic variation. The genome-wide scale of phenotypic effects exerted by CNVs (genomic load) is unknown and awaits further studies.

A summary of CNVs can be found in the Toronto Database of Genomic Variants (http://projects.tcag.ca/variation). Many clinically relevant CNVs can be found in the Database of Chromosomal Imbalance and Phenotype in Humans using Ensembl Resources (DECIPHER) (https://decipher.sanger.ac.uk/information).

Tandem Repeats

Variable number of tandem repeats (VNTR), or *minisatellites,* and short tandem repeats (STRs), such as unstable dinucleotides, trinucleotides, and tetranucleotides—$(GT)_n$, $(CAA)_n$, or $(GATA)_n$—referred to as *microsatellites,* are highly variable. Both minisatellites and microsatellites have been successfully used in linkage and association studies that enable the mapping of traits and the identification of genes and loci responsible for both Mendelian disorders and complex traits. These highly polymorphic sequence repeats are extremely variable in the copy number of their repeating subunits; this property enables the use of a number of such markers to derive a unique pattern of marker genotypes for each human individual. Thus, such markers have been useful in DNA fingerprinting for identity testing and DNA forensics.

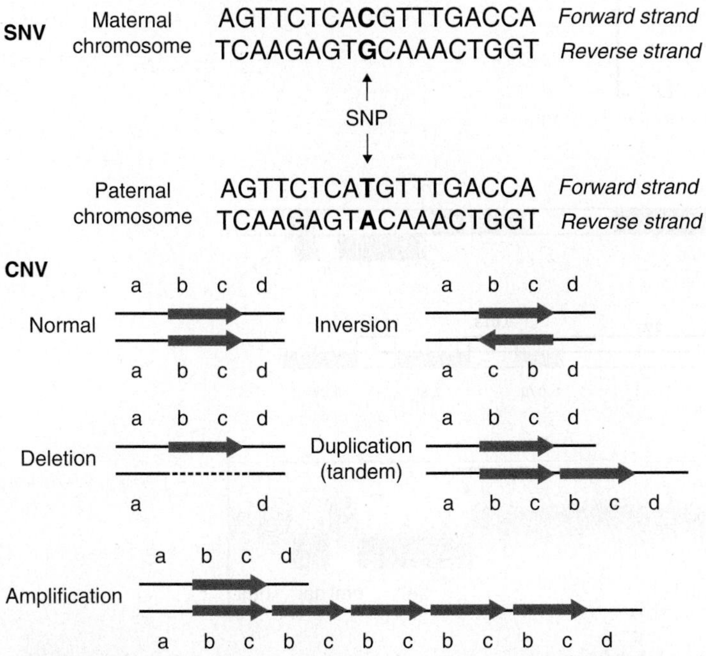

FIGURE 41-2. **Genetic variation.** (*Upper*) Heterozygous single nucleotide polymorphism (SNP, or single nucleotide variant, SNV) representing the most common transition C→T is shown. (*Bottom*) Structural genomic changes: a balanced inversion and the unbalanced copy-number variants (CNVs), deletion, duplication, and amplification are shown with *blue arrows* on two homologous chromosomes (*black lines*). The *dashed line* represents a deleted fragment of one chromosome.

Repetitive Elements

The other group of polymorphic elements in the human genome is represented by retrotransposons, long and short interspersed nuclear elements (LINEs and SINEs) (see Table 41-1). The most common *Alu* and L1 elements introduce recombinogenic genomic instability and insertional mutagenic activity; their positions within an individual human personal diploid genome can vary tremendously.[6] It has been recently estimated that repetitive elements may represent more than two thirds of the human genome.[7]

CHROMOSOMES

The recombined haploid (1n) human genome formed during meiosis is stored as chromosomes in female and male gametes. They merge at conception, and this diploid genome instructs the development of a zygote; the diploid human genome is subsequently transmitted to the mitotically dividing daughter cells. Human chromosomes can be distinguished from each other in a light microscope by differences in size and characteristic banding patterns after specific chemical staining (e.g., G-banding with Giemsa) when the chromosomes are arrested in a condensed phase (metaphase) of mitotic divisions.

Each human metaphase chromosome is composed of two chromatids that form short (p) and long (q) arms connected by a centromere built with α-satellite DNA. Based on the relative position of the centromere along the chromosome, chromosomes have been described as metacentric (similar-sized p and q arms), submetacentric (q arm significantly longer than p), and acrocentric (chromosomes 13, 14, 15, 21, and 22, with centromeres located close to the end of a chromosome) (Fig. 41-3).

Telomeres consist of repetitive DNA sequences (thousands of copies of TTAGGG repeats) located at the ends of both chromosome arms that are stabilized by a reverse transcriptase enzyme, *telomerase,* which adds TTAGGG sequence to the 3′ end of DNA strands. In contrast to germline and cancer cells, human somatic cells lacking telomerase gradually lose the telomeric sequences. As a result, cells reach the limit of their replicative capacity and fall into senescence.[8]

Chromosomal Aberrations

Microscopically visible chromosomal aberrations have been divided into numerical and structural aberrations and are found in about 1 in 160 live births.

Numerical Aberrations

The numerical aberrations typically result in lethality. Numerical aberrations are classified as either polyploidy (number of chromosomes are in multiples of haploid set of 23 chromosomes) or aneuploidy (with extra or missing chromosomes). Polyploidies such as triploidies (3n), 69,XXX, 69,XXY, and

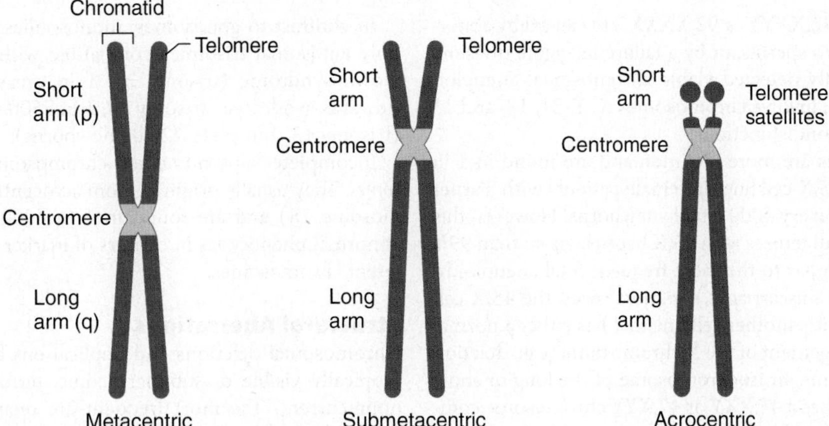

FIGURE 41-3. **Types of metaphase chromosomes. Metacentric, submetacentric, and acrocentric chromosomes are composed of two arms connected by a centromere. Each chromosome arm consists of two chromatids.**

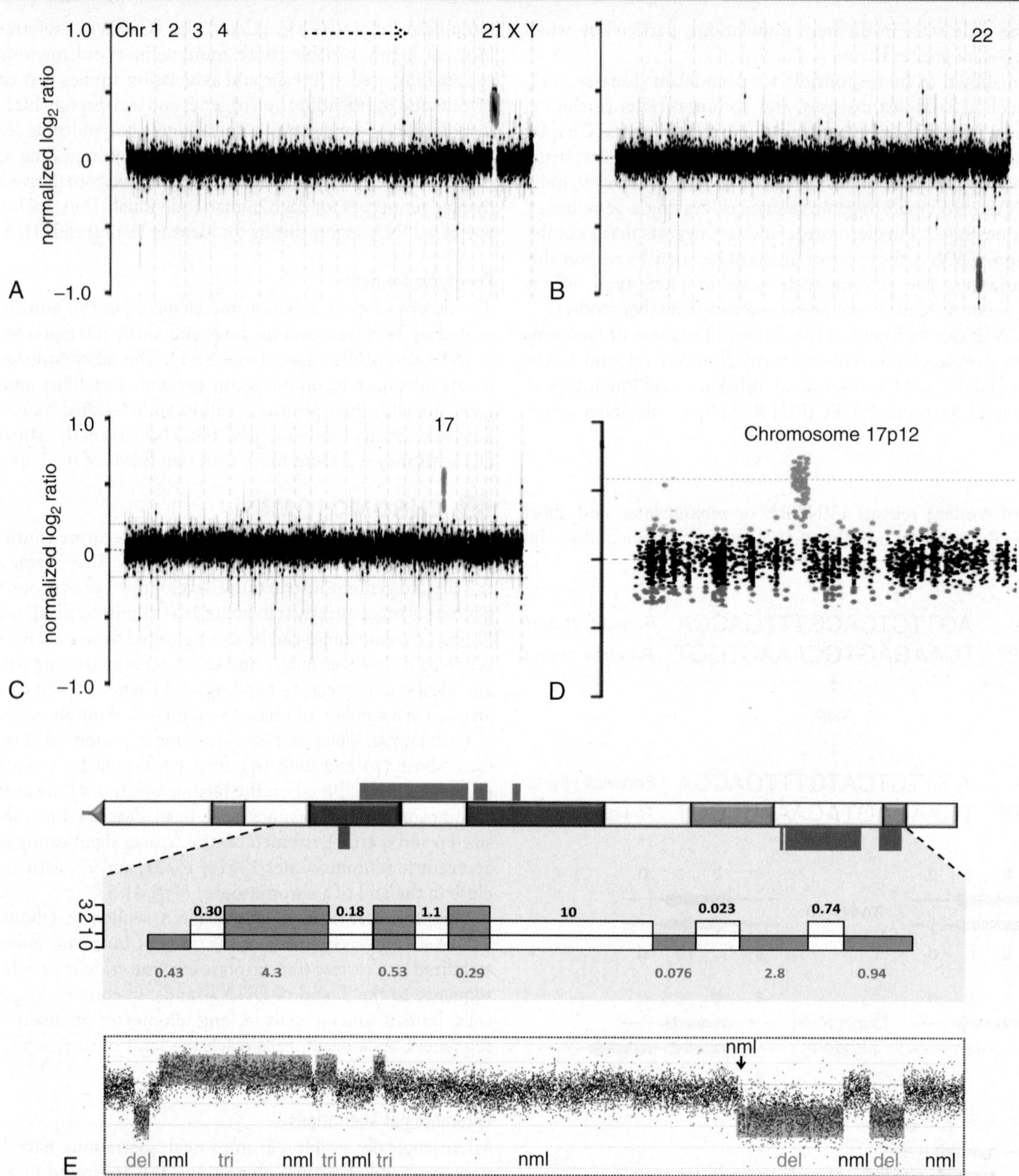

FIGURE 41-4. **Assaying copy-number variants (CNVs). Plots of array-based comparative genomic hybridization from patients with genomic rearrangements. Each "dot" on the plot represents an oligonucleotide that interrogates specific regions of the human genome from chromosome 1 (depicted on left) to the sex chromosomes depicted on the right). Gain of copy number is depicted in green, and loss of copy number is depicted in red. A, Patient with Down syndrome showing gain (three copies) of chromosome 21. B, Patient with congenital heart disease and velocardiofacial syndrome with a 3 Mb deletion of chromosome 22q11.2. C, Patient with autosomal dominant sensorimotor neuropathy (CMT1A) with a gain of copy number (duplication) on chromosome 17p12. D, Expanded view of the 17p12 duplication shown in C. E, Complex genomic rearrangement in a pediatric patient with epilepsy and hypotonia showing multiple breakpoints in a single chromosome. The rectangular boxes below the ideogram of the chromosome show copy-number of genomic segments, and the numbers depict the size of the CNVs in Mb. del = Deletion; nml = normal; tri = triplication.**

69,XYY, and tetraploidies (4n), 92,XXYY or 92,XXXX, are caused by abnormal fertilization of the egg by two sperms, or by a failure in zygote division, respectively. The most commonly detected viable chromosomal aneuploidies, trisomies and monosomies, involve chromosomes X, Y, 21, 18, and 13 and arise as a result of meiotic nondisjunctions.

Sex chromosome aneuploidies are more common and are found in 1 in 440 newborns. Monosomy X (45,X cell line) in female patients with Turner syndrome is identified in one in every 4000 female newborns. However, this birth rate represents only 1% of all fetuses with 45,X because more than 99% result in miscarriage. (This is similar to the most frequent fetal aneuploidy, trisomy 16, that results in 100% miscarriages.) In most cases, the 45,X cell line is found as a mosaic along with another cell line that has either a normal karyotype or a structural rearrangement of the X chromosome (e.g., deletion of the short arm, ring chromosome, or isochromosome of the long or short arms). One in every 1000 males has a 47,XXY or 47,XYY chromosome complement; the former results in Klinefelter syndrome, whereas the latter typically has mild if any manifestations.

In contrast to gonosomes, monosomies of all autosomes are lethal. The only autosomal trisomies compatible with life are found in patients with Down syndrome (trisomy 21, 1 in every 670 newborns) (Fig. 41-4A), Edwards syndrome (trisomy 18, 1 in 7500 newborns), and Patau syndrome (trisomy 13, 1 in every 22,700 newborns).

Incomplete supernumerary chromosomes are termed *marker chromosomes*. They usually originate from acrocentric autosomes (~50% from chromosome 15) and are found in 1 in 4000 newborns. The severity of the abnormal phenotypes in carriers of marker chromosomes varies among different chromosomes.

Structural Aberrations

Chromosomal deletions and duplications have been categorized as microscopically visible or submicroscopic, terminal or interstitial, recurrent or nonrecurrent. The most frequent are recurrent common-sized rearrangements flanked by directly oriented LCRs or SDs that mediate nonallelic homologous recombination (NAHR). For example, a 3 Mb microdeletion in chromosome 22q11.2 that results in DiGeorge (velocardiofacial) syndrome is found in 1 in 4000 newborns (Fig. 41-4B); a 1.4 Mb duplication of chromosome 17p12 accounts for greater than half of all adult-onset forms of inherited Charcot-Marie-Tooth (CMT) neuropathies (Fig. 41-4C and D). Evidence suggests that ectopic crossovers that lead to NAHR are preceded by an ectopic synapsis. Nonrecurrent rearrangements are of variable sizes with different breakpoint junctions in each patient reflecting distinct mechanisms of formation that include nonhomologous end joining (NHEJ) and replicative mechanisms such as FoSTeS (fork stalling and template switching) and MMBIR (microhomology-mediated break-induced replication). Whereas most recurrent rearrangements are typically "simple," a significant fraction of nonrecurrent genomic rearrangements with two or more breakpoint junctions referred to as *complex genomic rearrangements* (CGRs) have been implicated in causation of human disease phenotypes (Fig. 41-4E). These CGRs often occur as de novo events, vary in size from those involving a single exon to megabases of genomic sequence, and typically involve loss (i.e., deletion) and/or gain (i.e., duplication, triplication, etc.) in a single or multiple gene loci.[9] An extreme example of CGRs is a chromosome catastrophe wherein several copy-number changes and multiple breakpoints are concentrated on a single chromosome. This phenomenon, termed *chromothripsis*, has been noted in about 3% of all cancers and up to 25% of bone cancers and may portend a more severe disease.[10]

Balanced reciprocal translocations result from an exchange of the DNA material between two chromosomes and are found in about 1 in 600 individuals. During meiosis, the translocation chromosomes form a pachytene tetrad structure, and depending on the segregation type (alternate or adjacent, symmetrical or asymmetrical), either balanced or unbalanced products are transmitted to progeny. The unbalanced products often lead to either spontaneous miscarriage or birth of a child with significant clinical consequences. Recently, it has been shown by high-resolution genome analyses that up to 40% of apparently balanced translocations found in subjects with abnormal phenotypes are associated with additional imbalances at or near the translocation breakpoint or elsewhere in the genome.

Translocations involving short arms (or centromeres) of acrocentric chromosomes are described as *Robertsonian translocations*. Balanced Robertsonian translocations (45 chromosome complement) are present in 1 in 900 newborns and are thus the most common chromosome rearrangements in humans. The most frequent Robertsonian translocation, t(13;14), is found in 1 in 1300 individuals. The carriers of balanced Robertsonian translocations have a significantly increased risk for an unbalanced karyotype in progeny (e.g. trisomy 21 or trisomy 13) or uniparental disomy for chromosomes 14 and 15 that are known to contain imprinted genes.

Constitutional non-Robertsonian chromosomal translocations are nonrecurrent with the exception of three recurrent translocations: t(11;22)(q11.2;q23.3), which utilize AT-rich cruciforms, and t(4;8)(p16;p23) and t(4;11)(p16;p15.2), which are mediated by low-copy repeat gene clusters.

When a fragment of one chromosome is translocated into another chromosome's arm, the aberration is termed an *insertion* or *insertional translocation*. Insertional translocations have been recently shown by high-resolution human genome analyses to occur more than 100 times more frequently than recognized previously. The carrier of a balanced insertion has up to a 50% chance of an abnormal offspring.

An *inversion* is defined as a chromosome fragment that is reversed end to end. Inversions harboring the centromere are termed *pericentric*, and those with breakpoints mapping in the same chromosome arm are termed *paracentric*. Usually, only the products of pericentric inversions (unbalanced terminal deletion of one chromosome arm accompanied by a terminal duplication of the second arm) are found in a progeny. The acentric or dicentric products of paracentric inversions are unstable and thus not transmitted.

Other less common structural chromosomal abnormalities include ring chromosomes, isochromosomes, complex chromosome rearrangements, and heterochromatin variants. Rings arise when two broken ends of the same chromosome fuse. Usually, chromosome material telomeric to the breakpoints is lost and leads to an abnormal phenotype. Rings are commonly unstable mitotically and often form double ring structures. Isochromosomes arise when one part of the chromosome is duplicated and separated from the other. Isochromosomes can be monocentric (breakpoint in the centromere) or dicentric and thus unstable unless one of the centromeres becomes inactivated (pseudoisodicentric).

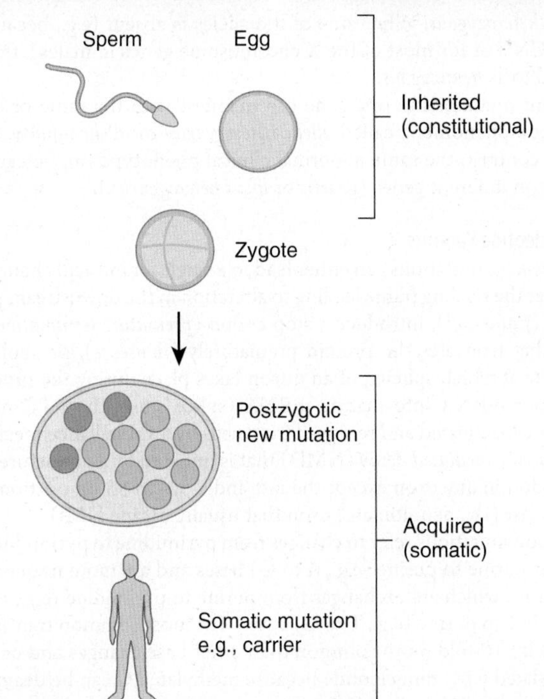

FIGURE 41-5. **Mutation. Constitutional mutations are inherited from one of the parents. They can be present in the somatic cells of a parent (carrier) or can arise during gametogenesis (de novo). Mutations that occur postzygotically (acquired, somatic) are usually found in a mosaic state.**

Mosaicism and Chimeras

The presence of two or more cell lines with different chromosome complements in one individual is termed *mosaicism* when they originate from the same zygote or *chimeras* when the cells originate from different zygotes. Chromosomal mosaicism is a common phenomenon and is observed in about 50% of embryos at the eight-cell stage and up to 75% of blastocysts. Somatic chromosomal mosaicism is found, for example, in patients with hypomelanosis of Ito and Pallister-Killian syndrome (tetrasomy 12p). Genome mosaicism in an organism may be more prevalent than appreciated and can be responsible for disease.[11]

MUTATIONS

Mutation is defined as a change in nucleotide sequence due to errors of DNA replication, recombination, repair, or radiation, chemical mutagens, viruses, or transposons. Gene mutations can be inherited from a parent (hereditary, constitutional, or *germline mutations*) and thus present in every cell or can be acquired in some tissues during development or any time throughout a person's life (*somatic mutations*) (Fig. 41-5). Whole genome sequencing of lung cancer tissue suggests one new point mutation for every pack of cigarettes smoked. Point mutations, usually involving only one or a few nucleotides, have been divided into substitutions, insertions, and deletions. Mutations mapping in protein-coding sequences and changing the protein structure have been termed *nonsynonymous*, whereas those that do not lead to protein change are known as *synonymous* or silent mutations. The latter mutations can still have functional consequences, for example, by generating a cryptic splice site, an exon splice enhancer, or affecting the regulatory elements.

Based on the functional consequences, mutations have been divided into loss-of-function and gain-of-function mutations. The former, also known as *hypomorphic* (partial loss) or *amorphic* or *null* (complete loss), affect the dosage-sensitive or haploinsufficient genes, in which a decreased amount of protein is not sufficient for normal function. Gain-of-function mutations increase or add a new function for the protein (*neomorphic*), whereas dominant negative mutations encode a protein that interacts antagonistically with the normal product from the other allele (*antimorphic*).

The situation in which one allele is mutated and the second is normal (wild-type) is referred to as *heterozygous*. A combination of the same two mutations in each of the alleles of the same locus (e.g., in consanguineous families) is defined as *homozygous*, or *compound heterozygous* when the two mutant alleles are distinct. Two mutant alleles at different loci are described as *double heterozygous*. When one of the alleles is absent (e.g., because of a deletion CNV or for most of the X chromosome genes in males), the locus is referred to as *hemizygous*.

Different mutations in one gene can manifest with the same or distinct phenotypes, phenomena called *allelic heterogeneity* or *allelic affinity*, respectively. By contrast, the same abnormal clinical phenotype can be caused by mutations in different genes (*genetic* or *locus heterogeneity*).

Single Nucleotide Variants

Nonsynonymous mutations can either lead to a single amino acid change (*missense*), alter the reading frame leading to alteration in the downstream protein structure (*frameshift*), introduce a stop codon (*premature termination codon* [PTC]) that truncates the protein prematurely (*nonsense*), or abolish the specific site at which splicing of an intron takes place during the processing of precursor mRNA into mature mRNA (splice site). The PTC mutated mRNAs are inactivated and removed from cells by a surveillance mechanism called *nonsense mediated decay* (NMD) that is initiated by a premature termination codon in any exon except the last and a 50- to 55-bp portion of the second to last (i.e., penultimate) exon that usually escape NMD.

Transition mutations refer to changes from pyrimidine to pyrimidine (e.g., C to T) or purine to purine (e.g., A to G) bases and are more frequent than transversions, which are exchanges from purine to pyrimidine (e.g., A to C) or pyrimidine to purine (e.g., T to G) bases. The most common transition, C to T, is about 10-fold more common than other base changes and occurs in the methylated CpG dinucleotide because methylated C can be deaminated and converted to T (see Fig. 41-2).

Unstable Repeat Expansions

Mutations that are unstable have been termed *dynamic*. Pathogenic dynamic expansion of trinucleotide, tetranucleotide, and pentanucleotide repeat sequences can be located in coding (e.g., CAG triplet in Huntington disease) or noncoding regions such as introns (e.g., GAA in Friedreich ataxia), or untranslated regions, either 5′ (e.g., CGG in fragile X syndrome) or 3′ (e.g., CTG in myotonic dystrophy). The mutations convey phenotypes that can be inherited as autosomal dominant (e.g., myotonic dystrophy), autosomal recessive (e.g., Friedreich ataxia), or X-linked (e.g., fragile X syndrome) traits due to gain or loss of function of the encoded protein. For each of the dynamic mutation diseases, there is a specific repeat number limit, above which the disease is manifested. The number of repeats below that threshold but greater than normal is referred to as a *premutation*. However, in some "disease genes," premutations are also associated with a milder, later onset, and sometimes distinct phenotype (e.g., ovarian failure in females and late-onset neurologic disorders in males with premutations in the fragile X syndrome *FMR1* gene). The number of repeats tends to expand in the next generations, a phenomenon called *anticipation*; this typically occurs in a sex-specific manner.

Copy-Number Variants

The Watson-Crick DNA base-pair changes are not the only mutational mechanism responsible for Mendelian monogenic diseases and complex traits. Higher order genomic architectural features can lead to a regional intrinsic instability of the human genome and susceptibility to DNA rearrangements, that is, CNVs that can be a frequent cause of diseases in humans. Such conditions that result from structural genome changes or CNVs have been referred to as *genomic disorders*.

A major mechanism by which rearrangements convey phenotypes is alteration of gene dosage because of a variation in gene copy-number. CNVs can lead to deletion, duplication, or disruption of the dosage-sensitive gene, generate gene fusions, exert position effects, or unmask mutations in the coding region or other functional SNPs in the second allele, as when a deletion CNV results in a hemizygous state.

Different calculations have shown that the de novo locus-specific mutation rates for genomic rearrangements are between 10^{-4} and 10^{-5}, at least 1000 to 10,000 fold more frequent than de novo point mutations. Thus, new-mutation CNV can contribute significantly to sporadic disease[12], including various common human neurodevelopmental conditions such as schizophrenia, autism, and intellectual disability, as well as sporadic cases of rare Mendelian disorders.[13]

Many genomic disorders occur sporadically and are often caused by de novo rearrangements. Recurrent rearrangements (deletions, duplications, or inversions) are caused by NAHR between low-copy repeats that are located less than 5 to 10 Mb from each other and have greater than 97% DNA sequence identity. The fixed position of these low-copy repeats or segmental duplications in the human genome result in recurrent rearrangements having a common size for a given region. NAHR between directly oriented low-copy repeats leads to deletions or reciprocal duplications of the genomic region located between them, whereas NAHR between the oppositely oriented low-copy repeats results in an inversion of the intervening genomic segment. Interestingly, the strand exchanges for NAHR sites are not scattered throughout the entire length of homology within low-copy repeats but instead cluster in recombination hotspots.

Most nonrecurrent CNVs appear to occur by nonhomologous recombination mechanisms, and one often observes microhomology at the breakpoints. The remainder of nonrecurrent different-sized rearrangements likely result from a NHEJ recombination mechanism. One prominent mechanism, particularly for complex (e.g., deletion/normal/duplication) rearrangements is the microhomology-mediated break-induced replication (MMBIR) mechanism.

Microduplication and Microdeletion Syndromes

Some of the microduplication and microdeletion syndromes are caused by a copy-number change of the dosage-sensitive or haploinsufficient gene. Among the best characterized genomic disorders are common autosomal dominant peripheral neuropathies, CMT1A and hereditary neuropathy with liability to pressure palsies (HNPP), that are caused by duplication and deletion CNV, respectively, of an about 1.4 Mb genomic interval within 17p12 harboring a dosage sensitive myelin gene *PMP22*. This genomic segment is flanked by two approximately 24 kb and 98.7% identical LCRs, termed the *proximal* CMT1A-REP and the *distal* CMT1A-REP, which serve as substrates for NAHR. Another example of common predominantly monogenic reciprocal microdeletion/microduplication syndromes is Potocki-Lupski syndrome, which can present clinically as autism and occurs due to dup(17)(p11.2p11.2), the recombination reciprocal to del(17)(p11.2p11.2) found in patients with Smith-Magenis syndrome. When two or more dosage-sensitive genes that are usually functionally unrelated are involved, these are referred to as contiguous gene deletion or duplication syndromes, for example, Potocki-Shaffer syndrome resulting from deletion del(11)(p11.2p11.2). LCR-mediated recurrent microdeletion and microduplication syndromes usually have similar prevalence in different populations; however, for a few genomic disorders, significant differences in incidences in different world populations have been observed, likely demonstrating that variation of genomic architecture is a significant factor for disease susceptibility (e.g., 17q21.31 microdeletion syndrome, Sotos syndrome, and 5q35). Examples of well-known and characterized microdeletion syndromes include Williams-Beuren syndrome (7q11.23), Prader-Willi and Angelman syndromes (15q11.2q12), DiGeorge syndrome (22q11.2), microdeletion 17q21.31 syndrome, microdeletion 1q21.1 syndrome, and Sotos syndrome. For all these microdeletions, the reciprocal microduplications predicted by the NAHR model have been reported, with phenotypes typically being milder. Whereas the role of CNVs in the causation of disorders like the aforementioned syndromes has been known for a while, recent studies have shown that a proportion of patients with neuropsychiatric manifestations including autism and schizophrenia harbor CNVs involving specific loci (e.g., 1q21.1, 15q13.3, and 16p11.2).[13] It is now becoming apparent that CNVs may be important for the some of the complex human traits.

PATTERNS OF INHERITANCE

Mendelian Inheritance

Most characterized disease-associated mutations in humans can be assigned to a single gene (monogenic) or locus and segregate as a Mendelian trait in an autosomal dominant, autosomal recessive, or X-linked fashion.

Autosomal dominant mutation is present in only one allele and thus is transmitted in meiosis to 50% of the gametes and is expected to manifest in half the offspring unless the trait is incompletely penetrant (e.g., in BRCA-related breast and ovarian cancer), represents variable expressivity (e.g., in Marfan syndrome), is age dependent (e.g., in Huntington disease), or is lethal (e.g., alveolar capillary dysplasia). In pedigree analysis, autosomal dominant inheritance is revealed as a vertical transmission of the trait.

In an autosomal recessive trait, the affected individuals carry two mutant alleles at a specific locus that are either the same (homozygous) or different (compound heterozygous). In general, both mutations are inherited from unaffected carrier parents (but note that occasionally heterozygous carriers of the mutated allele may manifest a mild phenotype or have an increased susceptibility to complex or multifactorial traits). Theoretically, affected probands represent 25% of the progeny; one half of the unaffected siblings carry one mutated allele, and the remaining one fourth of all progeny (one third of unaffected) have two wild-type (normal) alleles. In pedigree analysis, autosomal recessive inheritance is observed as horizontal transmission of the trait.

In X-linked (both dominant and recessive) diseases, no male-to-male transmission is observed, and all daughters of affected fathers are obligate carriers of the mutated allele. X-linked dominant diseases are more rare than X-linked recessive disorders and present both in males and in females. Usually, there are twice as many affected females as males; however, if the disease is lethal in males, only females are affected (e.g., Rett syndrome). Because of X inactivation, the phenotype in females is milder than in males in X-linked dominant diseases. In an X-linked recessive trait, only males are affected; in female carriers, the X chromosome harboring a mutated recessive allele is preferentially inactivated by nonrandom X inactivation. However, females with an incomplete or skewed X inactivation, females with only one X chromosome (Turner syndrome), or females carrying a balanced translocation between the X chromosome and an autosome (X material on the derivative chromosomes is not inactivated) can manifest the X-linked recessive disease.

Non-Mendelian Inheritance

The occurrence of sporadic cases of the disease can be explained by a classic Mendelian inheritance, such as de novo autosomal dominant, autosomal recessive, or X-linked mutation. However, one has to consider other possibilities, including non-Mendelian inheritance—genomic imprinting, uniparental disomy, mosaicism, mitochondrial DNA mutations, and digenic or triallelic inheritance.

Some genes acquire different activity status (usually methylation) after passage through spermatogenesis compared with oogenesis. As a result, a gene can be silenced (*imprinted*) depending on the parent of origin. This parent-of-origin effect is observed for the *UBE3A* gene on chromosome 15q12 that is imprinted during spermatogenesis, and only the maternal copy is active. When the active maternal copy of *UBE3A* is mutated, deleted, or inactivated in a different way, the offspring is affected with Angelman syndrome.

Sporadically, a chromosome pair may not be inherited from both parents. This distortion from biparental inheritance, termed *uniparental disomy* (UPD), may have clinical consequences when the uniparental chromosomes contain an autosomal recessive mutation or an imprinted gene. When both homologues are inherited from one parent, it is referred as *heterodisomy*. In *isodisomy*, both homologues in an offspring originate from only one of the parental homologues. The most frequent mechanism for UPD is trisomy rescue, in which an early postzygotic embryo is trisomic as a result of chromosome nondisjunction in meiosis I, and the extra chromosome is then lost during further development to restore disomy. Because this is a random event, in one third of cases, the disomic chromosomes remaining after trisomy to disomy rescue will represent UPD. Consequently, UPD is associated with advanced maternal age.

In some diseases, pathogenic mutations have been found in single alleles of two different genes with the other alleles at each given locus being normal. This double heterozygous phenomenon of two interacting genes has been reported, for example, for *ROM1* and *RDS* in retinitis pigmentosa and *GJB6* and *GJB2* in deafness.

In some patients, three abnormal alleles in two different genes have been identified. The phenomenon of triallelic (or oligogenic) inheritance has been observed, for example, in Bardet-Biedl syndrome, familial hypercholesterolemia, and cortisone reductase deficiency. Monogenic chromosomal microduplication syndromes (e.g., Charcot-Marie-Tooth type 1A) can also be categorized as triallelic given the presence of three alleles at a given locus because of duplication CNV.

Another distortion from Mendelian inheritance can be caused by mosaicism. Two or more cell lines can be present either in the gonads only (germline mosaicism) or in somatic cells. Mosaicism should be suspected when healthy parents have two or more children with a dominant disease. Mosaicism can be particularly relevant when mutational processes involve DNA replication errors and occur mitotically (e.g., point mutation and MMBIR).

Very rarely, a disease trait is transmitted to daughters and sons only from mothers. In such cases, one should consider a mitochondrial disease due to mutations in mitochondrial DNA (mtDNA). Multiple copies of mtDNA are present in the cell cytoplasm and are transmitted to progeny only through the oocytes. Initial clinical signs and symptoms typically originate from the most energy-dependent tissues (e.g., eyes, brain, skeletal muscle, and heart), and the phenotypic expression among family members varies and depends mainly on the proportion of mtDNA in the cytoplasm that carries the mutation, that is, *heteroplasmy*.

ASSAYING GENETIC VARIATION

Chromosome aberrations larger than about 5 Mb can be detected by light microscopy after specific staining that reveals characteristic banding patterns (e.g., G-banded karyotype analysis). Submicroscopic rearrangements, such as microdeletions or microduplications (30 kb to 5 Mb), have been analyzed previously using molecular cytogenetic techniques such as fluorescence in situ hybridization. In these routine clinical cytogenetic techniques, usually subpopulations of peripheral blood T lymphocytes stimulated by phytohemagglutinin are analyzed. Rearrangements of similar size (30 kb to 5 Mb) can be analyzed also using pulsed-field gel electrophoresis. However, both of these technologies are limited to the analysis of specific genomic regions, that is, locus-specific testing.

The development of array-based comparative genomic hybridization (array CGH) has enabled screening of the entire human genome for imbalances, with the level of genome resolution depending only on the number, size, and distance between the arrayed interrogating probes. These genome-wide imaging techniques are analogous to digital photography wherein the resolution observed is dependent on the pixels used. Initial clinical array CGH used large genomic clones, BACs and PACs (bacterial or P1 artificial chromosomes), as interrogating probes. These were rapidly replaced by oligonucleotides, of which millions can be synthesized on one glass slide. Oligonucleotide probes are also used on SNP arrays, which, in contrast to microarray-based CGH, enable association studies or detection of uniparental disomies. The widespread use of array CGH for diagnostic purposes not only has increased the sensitivity in detecting CNV associated with disease but also has led to the discovery of many new genomic disorders.

For detection of genomic imbalances, an alternative quantitative polymerase chain reaction–based technique, multiplex ligation-dependent probe amplification (MLPA), has been developed. MLPA is an inexpensive, simple, rapid, and sensitive tool to detect dosage alterations in selected genomic regions.

Most recently, several next-generation sequencing (NGS) technologies have been developed that enable simultaneous and massively parallel DNA sequencing. Such technologies have ushered in the era of "panel testing" (simultaneous assay of multiple genes implicated in a particular phenotype), whole exome sequencing (sequencing the entire coding regions of the genome), and whole genome sequencing (sequencing of the entire genome of an individual). In NGS, DNA sequencing uses chemistries other than the traditional Sanger dideoxy chain termination method. NGS methods generate far larger quantities of data at less expense; however, the individual raw sequence reads that are generated from individual amplified DNA template sequences have shorter read lengths and lower quality. Nevertheless, massive redundant sequencing of a personal diploid human genome (e.g., 30-fold coverage with respect to the haploid human reference genome sequence) provides robust and accurate personal genome sequencing. The NGS technologies have led to an explosion in gene discovery and understanding of the mechanistic bases of genetic disorders.[14] The use of whole exome sequencing alone for clinical diagnosis at the present time has resulted in a diagnostic yield of about 25%, a significant improvement over the currently available testing modalities.[15] NGS technologies have also made it possible to amplify cell-free DNA from maternal serum to facilitate prenatal screening for trisomies involving chromosomes 13, 18, or 21.

Recent advances and the relatively widespread use of array CGH and NGS technologies have transformed our understanding and diagnosis of human disease. With decreasing costs of sequencing and more extensive use of these methodologies, our understanding of the human history, evolution, disease, and treatment will inevitably advance to new levels of sophistication.

CONCLUSION

Mutations in humans are caused by SNVs and CNVs. New mutations can contribute to sporadic disease. The total genomic load can be important to clinical phenotype. Individual genetic variation is extensive. It is a sobering thought that for about 80 to 90% of the annotated genes in the reference human genome, a function remains to be elucidated for the potential clinical consequences of mutations. Furthermore, 98% of the human genome is noncoding, and the functional consequences of variation within it cannot be deciphered using the genetic code.

GENERAL REFERENCES

For the General References and other additional features, please visit Expert Consult at https://expertconsult.inkling.com.

42

THE INHERITED BASIS OF COMMON DISEASES

SEKAR KATHIRESAN AND DAVID ALTSHULER

A central question in medicine is to understand why some people get sick and others do not. We seek these answers for multiple reasons: to provide explanations to our patients, to predict disease risk early enough to prevent it, and most important, to understand pathophysiology so as to design rational approaches to prevention and therapy. In some cases, a single environmental exposure is found to play a major role in disease (e.g., smoking and lung cancer, or HIV infection and AIDS). In others, such as Huntington disease or cystic fibrosis, mutation of a single gene is both necessary and sufficient to cause illness. Of course, singular answers are the exception rather than the rule; in most cases, disease arises from the combined action of inborn and somatically acquired alterations in genome sequence, environmental and behavioral exposures, and bad luck. Such disorders, which explain most morbidity and mortality in human populations, are termed *complex traits*.[1]

As a tool for generating new hypotheses about the root causes of disease, human genetics has a number of unique features. First, it is now possible to systematically query the entire genome sequence of an individual in a manner unlimited by any prior assumption about underlying genes and pathophysiologic processes responsible. Second, because the constitutional genome sequence is established at conception and unaltered throughout life, associations between genome sequence and human phenotype can be interpreted as causal rather than reactive in their relationship to disease. However, although we have entered an era in which the specific genes and variants that contribute to risk for common human diseases can be identified, much work is needed to understand their functions and to learn whether and how this knowledge can improve the practice of medicine.[2]

HERITABILITY: INHERITED VARIATION IN DISEASE RISK

Susceptibility to disease varies within and across human populations. Studies of *familial aggregation* can determine the extent to which inherited difference in the genome sequence contributes to variation in disease risk. Such studies are simple in concept and ask whether members of the same family are more similar in disease risk compared with individuals chosen at random from the population. Of course, familial clustering can reflect not only shared genotype but also shared environment. The contribution of shared genotype can be dissected further by examining concordance of disease in proportion to the extent of genetic relatedness. The simplest such design involves comparing rates of disease concordance among dizygotic and monozygotic twin pairs. More sophisticated methods have now been developed in which the relatedness of individuals is estimated directly from genotype data (rather than based on pedigrees) and concordance compared with these empirically derived estimates of relatedness. With each of these approaches, common diseases such as types 1 and 2 diabetes mellitus, obesity, hypertension, coronary artery disease, autoimmune diseases, common cancers, schizophrenia, and bipolar disease show rates of disease concordance that rise with genetic similarity. However, many other traits of clinical interest (e.g., most drug responses) have not been studied with these methods, and thus the role of inheritance in these characteristics cannot be assumed. That is, variability in a clinical phenotype (such as drug response) cannot be assumed to be inherited in nature—family studies or molecular genetic studies are needed to draw any such conclusion.

Data about familial aggregation allow the calculation of *heritability*, defined as the fraction of interindividual variability in disease risk attributable to additive genetic influences. In this framework, the remaining variability among individuals is due to the sum of all other contributions to disease risk: environmental influences on disease, nonadditive (*epistatic*) genetic effects (e.g., gene-gene interactions or gene-environment interactions), error in the measurement of relatedness or disease, and random chance. For most clinically important traits (diseases and risk factors), empirical estimates of heritability range from 20 to 80% (see Online Mendelian Inheritance in Man, available at *www.ncbi.nlm.nih.gov:80/entrez/query.fcgi?db=OMIM*, for comprehensive information).

In interpreting estimates of heritability,[3] it is important to consider two crucial factors: the effect of measurement errors and the environmental context. *Measurement errors* decrease the estimate of the observed heritability of a trait. For example, a single measurement of blood pressure is much less heritable than a composite score based on serial measures of blood pressure over time. That is, estimates of heritability are lower bounds because day-to-day variability and imprecision in clinical measures can obscure the underlying biologic susceptibility entrained by inheritance. For the patient and physician, this means that although the blood pressure on a given day may not be particularly heritable, the blood pressure over time (which is the relevant risk factor for vascular disease) is heritable to a greater extent.

Second, estimates of heritability apply only to the context of the environment in which the study was performed. In the case in which environmental triggers of disease are relatively constant across a study population, inherited factors may explain much of the variation in rates of disease. In contrast, in the case in which exposure to environmental causes of disease is highly varied across the study population, nongenetic factors may outweigh the contribution of that same extent of variability in inborn susceptibility. For example, the rate and diversity of smoking behavior have a major impact on how much of the variability in rates of lung cancer (in any given study or patient cohort) is explained by inheritance. If smoking was absent from a given population (or ubiquitous), little of the variation in lung cancer risk would be due to smoking behavior; if, in contrast, half the population smoked multiple packs a day and the other half not at all, smoking behavior would dominate over inborn susceptibility.

For these reasons, heritability is not a fixed characteristic of a given disease but an assessment of a given population, a set of measurements, and the extent to which variability in genetic and environmental exposure explains disease risk. Thus, there is no contradiction between a disease's being highly heritable (in a given population) and yet having rates that vary dramatically across populations separated by time, geography, or socioeconomic status. In broad comparisons across groups, environmental exposure and methods of clinical ascertainment often vary substantially and contribute to secular changes in patterns of disease. Conversely, within a group exposed to a relatively uniform environment and studied in a standardized manner, genetic susceptibility may play a major role in determining individual risk.

HETEROZYGOSITY: INHERITED VARIATION IN GENOME SEQUENCE

Heritability expresses the inherited variation in rates of disease; *heterozygosity* expresses the rate of inherited variation in genome sequences (Table 42-1). Heterozygosity is defined as the proportion of sites on the chromosome at which two randomly chosen copies differ in DNA sequence. Because cells are *diploid* (carry two copies of the genome sequence) and because these two copies were selected in a semirandom manner from the population, heterozygosity is equivalent to the fraction of base pairs that vary between the two copies each of us inherited from our mother and our father. That is, heterozygosity is the rate of genetic variation in the individual.

Single-nucleotide polymorphisms (SNPs) are sites at which a single letter in the DNA code has been swapped for a single alternative letter. Such variants are observed at approximately 1 in 1000 positions in the human genome sequence. In the protein-coding regions of genes, rates of genetic variation are lower—less than 1 in every 2000 bases; the rate of variation that substantially alters the sequence of the encoded protein is lower still (see Table 42-1). The lower rate of variation in coding regions is due to natural selection against alteration in the amino acid sequence of encoded proteins.

Our genomes also contain other types of sequence variation: insertions and deletions of nucleotides; alteration in the number of copies of particular genes and sequences; and larger-scale alterations, such as inversions and translocations. All types of DNA sequence change can influence gene function and contribute to disease.

The genetic variation in each individual is largely attributable to variants that are common. Empirically, more than 98% of the heterozygous sites in each individual display frequency of greater than 1% in the worldwide human population. During the last 15 years, a public database has been built that

TABLE 42-1 CHARACTERISTICS OF HUMAN GENOME SEQUENCE VARIATION

Length of the human genome sequence (base pairs)	3,000,000,000
Number of human genes (estimated)	20,000
Fraction of base pairs that differ between the genome sequences of a human and a chimpanzee	1.3% (1 in 80)
Fraction of base pairs that vary between the genome sequences of any two humans	0.1% (1 in 1000)
Fraction of coding region base pairs that vary in a manner that substantially alters the sequence of the encoded protein	0.2% (1 in 5000)
Number of sequence variants present in each individual as heterozygous sites	3,000,000
Number of amino acid–altering variants present in each individual as heterozygous sites	12,000
Number of sequence variants in any given human population with frequency of >1%	10,000,000
Number of amino acid polymorphisms present in the human genome with a population frequency of >1%	75,000
Fraction of all human heterozygosity attributable to variants with a frequency of >1%	98%

contains essentially all common sequence variants in the human population (with frequency >1%). At the time of this writing, this public database contains more than 44 million human genetic variants (*www.ncbi.nlm.nih.gov:80/SNP/index.html*). Not all these entries represent common variants (some are rare), and a small fraction may represent technical false-positive findings.

The major contribution of common variation in human sequence diversity is explained by the unique demographic history of the human population. Despite the global distribution of the current human population, it is now clear that all humans are the descendants of a single population that lived in Africa only 10,000 to 40,000 years ago. The ancestral population was small (with an effective size of perhaps 10,000 individuals), lived a hunter-gatherer existence at low population densities (relative to other humans and later domesticated animals), and had evolved in Africa during millions of years. Most human genetic variation arose in this phase of human history, before the more recent migrations, expansions, and invention of technologies (e.g., farming) that resulted in widespread population of the globe. Most common human genetic variation predates the Diaspora and is shared by all populations on earth.

A second factor is the slow rate of change in human DNA. Mutation and recombination occur at very low rates, on the order of 10^{-8} per base pair per generation; and yet, any pair of human genes traces a lineage back to a shared ancestor who lived on the order of 10^3 to 10^4 generations ago (if a generation is 20 years, then 10^4 generations is 200,000 years). In other words, considering the typical nucleotide in two unrelated humans, it is more likely that they trace back to a shared ancestor without any mutation having occurred than it is that a mutation has arisen in the intervening time. This explains why 99.9% of base pairs are identical when any two copies of the human genome are compared.

Another aspect of human variation is explained by these simple mathematical and population genetic relationships: the extent of human DNA sequence diversity attributable to rare and common variants. Each of us inherits from our parents some 3 million common polymorphisms (classically defined as those with frequency of >1%). We inherit genetic variants that are shared by apparently unrelated individuals but are at frequencies less than 1%, and we inherit thousands of variants that are limited only to the individual and the individual's closest relatives.

The shared ancestry of human populations explains another aspect of human genetic variation: the correlations among nearby variants known as *linkage disequilibrium*. Empirically, individuals who carry a particular common variant at one site in the genome are observed to be more likely than chance to carry a particular set of variants at nearby positions along the chromosome. That is, not all combinations of nearby variants are observed in the population but rather only a small subset of the possible combinations. These correlations reflect the fact that most variants in our genomes arose once in human history (typically long ago) and did so on an arbitrary but unique copy carried by the individual in whom the mutation first arose. This unique ancestral copy can be recognized in the current population by the stretch of particular alleles (known as a *haplotype*). These ancestral haplotypes, passed down from shared prehistoric ancestors in Africa, offer a practical tool in association studies of human disease because it is not necessary to measure directly each nucleotide to capture much of the information.

THE SEARCH FOR GENES UNDERLYING MONOGENIC DISEASES

The *genetic architecture* of a disease refers to the number and magnitude of genetic risk factors that exist in each patient and their frequencies and interactions in the population. Diseases can be due to a single gene in each family (*monogenic*) or to multiple genes (*polygenic*). It is easiest to identify genetic risk factors when only a single gene is involved and this gene has a large impact on disease in that family. In cases in which a single gene is necessary and sufficient to cause disease, the condition is termed a *mendelian* disorder because the disease tracks perfectly with a mutation (in the family) that obeys Mendel's simple laws of inheritance.

Some single-gene disorders are caused by the same gene in all affected families; for example, cystic fibrosis is always caused by mutations in *CFTR*. Although many individuals with cystic fibrosis carry the same founder mutation (δ-508), others carry any pair of a wide variety of different mutations in *CFTR*. The existence of many different mutations at a given disease gene is known as *allelic heterogeneity*.

A mendelian disorder can be due to a single genetic lesion in any given family but in different families can be due to mutations in a variety of genes. This phenomenon, termed *locus heterogeneity*, is illustrated by retinitis pigmentosa. Although mutation in a single gene is typically necessary and sufficient to cause retinitis pigmentosa, there are dozens of different genes in which retinitis pigmentosa mutations have been found (Online Mendelian Inheritance in Man #268000). In each family, however, only one such gene is mutated to cause disease.

Most single-gene disorders are rare (present in <1% of the population) and are manifested early in life. Many are severe and cause death before reproduction in the absence of modern medical care. The fact that most monogenic disorders are severe in childhood and rare in the population is not a coincidence but reflects the impact of *natural selection*. The deleterious effect of these mutations results in a decrease in reproductive fitness (in individuals unlucky enough to inherit them), and the mutations and the disease are therefore unlikely to drift to high frequency in the population.

There are exceptions to this general idea: cases in which the mutation causing a severe monogenic disease (such as hemoglobin S, the cause of sickle cell anemia) is common in populations. Such cases appear to be the result of a different kind of selection, known as *balancing selection*—situations in which a gene mutation is beneficial in one circumstance (a genotype or environment) but deleterious in another. Heterozygous carriers of hemoglobin S are relatively protected against malaria, and this benefit balances the deleterious effect of sickle cell disease in homozygotes.

Starting in the 1980s, the advent of genome-wide linkage analysis led to rapid success at identifying the specific genetic mutations that cause mendelian disorders, and now thousands of genes have been identified for clinically important conditions (for comprehensive information, see *www.ncbi.nlm.nih.gov:80/entrez/query.fcgi?db=OMIM*). Progress was sparked by the development of a suite of powerful research techniques—*family-based linkage analysis* followed by *positional cloning*—in which a genome-wide search is undertaken for the causal gene, which is first localized to a chromosomal region. (The initial idea of genetic linkage mapping traces to Sturtevant in fruit flies in 1913 but did not become practical in humans until the 1980s.)

Once the search discovered linkage between a chromosomal region and a disease, that chromosomal neighborhood was scoured for the genetic culprit, which was recognized by the observation of mutations that altered the protein-coding sequence, enriched in cases of disease compared with unaffected relatives and population-based controls. The power of these approaches prompted and was fueled by the Human Genome Project, which provided the foundation of information on DNA structure, sequence, and genetic variation required to undertake such searches.

More recently, it has become possible to search for the mutations underlying mendelian diseases by skipping the step of family-based linkage, instead sequencing the genome of the individual and searching for mutations that might explain the disease. If the gene is already known and the mutation easily interpreted (e.g., truncating the protein), this approach is highly efficient and successful. If the gene is rarely mutated and not yet known to cause the disease, or if the mutations are in noncoding regions, direct sequencing still runs up against the analytical and clinical challenge of genome interpretation.

GENETIC INVESTIGATION OF COMMON DISEASES

Similar to mendelian disorders, most common diseases are influenced by inheritance. In contrast to mendelian disorders, the genetic contribution to common diseases is typically due to the action of many genes rather than a single gene in each family. Empirical evidence in favor of this model comes from classical family studies, which failed to observe classical mendelian ratios for common diseases. In the 1990s, the tools of family-based linkage analysis were applied to nearly all common disorders. Much of this work was done in isolated founder populations (such as Finland and Iceland) with the goal of simplifying the genetic architecture and accessing extended pedigrees. Excepting a few notable successes, these studies revealed few strong signals that localized the genes responsible for disease, indicating that few cases of common diseases are due to individual genes of large effect. If a single gene contained rare mutations of large effect that explained 20% or more of the inherited risk for type 2 diabetes, hypertension, or schizophrenia, it would long since have been found with linkage analysis.

The next shortcut to understanding the genetic determinants of common diseases was to identify and study rare families with early-onset forms of common diseases that clearly demonstrate mendelian patterns of inheritance. Important examples include the role of *BRCA1* and *BRCA2* in early-onset breast cancer, maturity-onset diabetes of the young as a form of type 2 diabetes, many monogenic disorders of blood pressure and electrolyte regulation, early-onset Alzheimer disease, and many others.

These successes provide diagnostic information for families burdened with severe, early-onset forms of disease and insight into the underlying pathways responsible for disease. For example, more than 20 genes have been identified that, when mutated, cause rare mendelian disorders of blood pressure and electrolyte regulation. So far, every one of these genes is active in the kidney, and most are involved in the renin-angiotensin-aldosterone pathway. This result is a compelling demonstration of the central importance of the kidney in human blood pressure regulation and has suggested new therapeutic targets of substantial promise.

It was hoped that the genes found to be responsible for early-onset, monogenic forms of common diseases would contribute to the more common forms of disease in the population. In this scenario, severe mutations might cause early-onset forms, and more prevalent but subtle alterations in the same genes might contribute to common forms of disease. A comprehensive test of this hypothesis awaited tools from the Human Genome Project and improved methods of genetic epidemiologic analysis.

ASSOCIATION STUDIES: FROM CANDIDATE GENES TO GENOME-WIDE ASSOCIATION STUDIES

Genome-wide association studies (GWAS) became possible in the mid-2000s on the basis of the sequencing of the human genome, cataloguing of common genetic variants, and high-throughput tools for measuring genetic variation. However, genetic association studies long predated genomic technologies and are simple in concept: the frequency of a common variant is measured in individuals with the disease of interest and compared with well-matched controls (drawn from the population at large or unaffected family members). Now, this process is routinely performed with hundreds of thousands or millions of genetic variants from the genome-wide collection.

Genetic association studies were pioneered in the context of the human leukocyte antigen (HLA) locus on chromosome 6. The HLA complex was discovered on the basis of its role in transplantation tolerance and is characterized by diverse allelic variation that can be measured by interactions of antibodies and antigens. By measurement of these protein-based (immunologic) readouts of the underlying genetic variation, HLA alleles were found to be a major determinant of susceptibility to infectious and autoimmune diseases. Starting in the 1960s, empirical data on human population genetics and genetic association studies were developed in the context of the HLA complex.

By the 1980s, tools of molecular biology made it possible to directly measure DNA variation (rather than using protein or phenotype measurements as surrogates for the underlying genetic variation), ushering in the modern era of human genetic research. In this pregenomic era, it was only practical to measure one or a small number of genetic variations in each study, limiting association studies to incomplete assessments of individual "candidate" genes selected on the basis of biologic criteria.

The study of candidate genes led to a modest number of robust and reproducible associations, such as the contribution of apolipoprotein E4 to Alzheimer disease; factor V Leiden to deep venous thrombosis; a 32-base deletion in the chemokine receptor CCR5 to HIV infection; common variants in the insulin gene to type 1 diabetes; and SNPs in the peroxisome proliferator–activated receptor γ and the β-cell potassium channel Kir6.2 to the risk for type 2 diabetes.

Early in the 2000s, comprehensive surveys of published genetic association studies showed that valid associations were few and far between, with many initial claims of association proving irreproducible, likely representing false-positive claims. One such analysis estimated that in the pre-GWAS era, only 10 to 20 bona fide associations had been documented of common genetic variants with common diseases.

A major reason for the state of this literature was the intrinsically low likelihood of finding a gene and variant contributing to any given disease. Each genome contains millions of genetic variants, and presumably only a small fraction of these influence disease. This is often described as a problem of "multiple hypothesis testing," with the investigative community searching for associations between multiple genes, multiple variants in each gene, and multiple diseases. An alternative (bayesian) statistical framework frames this issue on the basis of low prior probabilities of association. Regardless, it is conceptually clear that much more stringent statistical thresholds (than the traditional $P < .05$) are required for declaring association of genetic variants and disease.

As in linkage analysis for mendelian traits, a key to success in association studies was the advent of genome-wide search, unbiased by prior hypotheses about biologic mechanisms. With the sequencing of the human genome, development of large-scale SNP databases, and tools for genotyping up to one million SNPs per individual, by 2005 it became practical to perform GWAS to identify genomic loci harboring allelic variation. With a recognition that any given variant had a very low likelihood of truly being associated with disease, much more stringent statistical thresholds were deployed (typically requiring a P value of 10^{-7} or lower to declare "genome-wide significance").

Age-related macular degeneration (AMD) provided an early success of GWAS.[4] AMD is a typical common, polygenic disease (Chapter 423); siblings of affected patients are perhaps three to six times as likely as unrelated individuals to become afflicted, and yet family-based linkage analysis revealed only modestly significant (and modestly reproducible) linkage results. The pathophysiologic defects that underlie AMD were largely unknown until it was found that a common coding polymorphism in the gene for complement factor H is a major risk factor for AMD. The variant (*Y402H*) has a high population frequency (approximately 35% in European populations) and increases risk by 2.5- to 3-fold in heterozygotes and by 5- to 7-fold in homozygotes. Multiple other complement factors have since been found to harbor common genetic variation that influences the risk for AMD in a highly reproducible manner, providing unambiguous information about the primary role of complement in this common disease.

Since 2005, GWAS has been used to identify literally hundreds of novel genetic variants that show reproducible associations to a large variety of common human diseases. The field evolved a set of criteria and standards that largely eliminated the previous difficulties with irreproducible claims of association, making association studies a reliable method to identify genomic loci related to human diseases. The National Human Genome Research Institute of the National Institutes of Health maintains a catalogue of GWAS findings (*www.genome.gov/26525384*) that, at the time of this writing, included 12,987 such associations across 1871 publications. This represents dramatic progress compared with the two dozen or so such findings known at the start of the decade.

The results of GWAS support a number of conclusions about the role of common genetic variants in common disease. First, nearly all diseases investigated by GWAS have yielded novel findings, in many cases yielding dozens to more than 100 independent common variants associated with risk of disease. Second, only a small fraction of these findings were previously known, confirming that an unbiased genetic mapping approach can provide new clues about the etiology of common diseases. Third, most of the associations demonstrate modest odds ratios (on the order of 1.1-fold to 1.5-fold), indicating that the genetic nature of common disease is highly polygenic and that natural selection has likely purged alleles of large effect from the pool of common variants. Fourth, in only a few cases (perhaps 10%) does the associated haplotype carry a variant that alters protein structure; this suggests that much of the risk of common disease acts through effects on gene regulation rather than protein sequences. Fifth, in sum, the variants thus far identified explain only a modest fraction (ranging between 1% and 20%) of the estimated heritability of each disease, indicating that the rest of the inherited risk is due to some combination of common variants of more modest effect, rare variants not yet discovered, nonadditive interactions between genotypes and between genotype and the environment, or other (as yet unanticipated) factors.

Genome-wide approaches (not limited to candidate genes) can be thought of as testing the completeness of the sets of genes previously discovered for each disease by other approaches. For example, in the case of autoimmune diseases, many (perhaps half) of the findings from GWAS lie near a gene previously known to play a role in the immune system. Similarly, a substantial fraction of the genetic variants found to influence lipid levels lie near genes that were previously known to play a role in lipid biology (because they either carry rare mutations that contribute to mendelian forms of hyperlipidemia or were discovered on the basis of laboratory studies).[5] Examples such as autoimmune disease and lipids provide a reassuring alignment of mendelian genetics, biologic investigation, and the genes mapped by GWAS.

However, for the majority of diseases and of disease-associated genetic variants, the genomic regions showing association to disease are novel and do not contain any genes previously studied. One such case is type 2 diabetes, for which more than 80 independent genomic loci have been found to influence risk for disease, and yet only a handful were previously implicated by other methods. A second is myocardial infarction, for which perhaps one third of the SNPs lie near genes involved in low-density lipoprotein cholesterol, but the other two thirds do not contain any previously studied gene. These examples indicate that there are important gaps in our previous knowledge of pathophysiology and biologic mechanisms and that genome-wide approaches can point to high-priority candidates for study.

Although tantalizing, the results of GWAS have raised many more questions than they have answered. Each discovery implicates a particular genomic region, but it has proved challenging to establish which gene is responsible for the association. This is challenging in large part because so many of these common variants are noncoding, and methods to connect noncoding variation to the genes they regulate remain in their infancy. Even where novel genes are identified, much work is needed to discover their biologic and physiologic functions. Finally, GWAS findings explain only a fraction of the estimated heritability of most diseases, leaving open the question of which genes, and which types of variants and genetic effects, explain the remainder.

FROM COMMON VARIANTS TO INDIVIDUAL GENOMES

Although much of human genetic variation is due to common DNA variants (such as those tested through GWAS), each of us also inherits many thousands of variants that arose more recently and that tend to be lower in frequency and more population specific. To the extent that such variants have large effects on phenotype, they might have been previously identified on the basis of family-based linkage studies of mendelian disorders. However, there certainly exists a large universe of lower-frequency variations that have effects too modest to have been recognized and identified in family-based linkage analyses and are too rare to have been captured by the first generation of GWAS.

The study of lower-frequency and rare variants is now practical owing to advances in technology for DNA sequencing. With dramatic drops in price and increases in throughput, it is increasingly routine to sequence individual genomes in the context of medical research (and, in the future, clinical practice).[6] Such an approach will provide a much more complete assessment of genetic variation than was previously obtainable and will incorporate common as well as rare variants—and points to the major challenge of genome interpretation.[7]

For mendelian diseases, the sequencing of individual genomes has made it possible to bypass family-based linkage analysis and positional cloning and instead directly to sequence all protein-coding genes in the genome (so-called exome sequencing) among affected and unaffected individuals. Since 2009, the use of exome sequencing has led to the identification of numerous genes for mendelian disorders that had proved intractable with previous methods. For example, we studied a family in whom four siblings displayed extremely low blood low-density lipoprotein cholesterol, high-density lipoprotein cholesterol, and triglyceride levels—an apparently recessive disorder termed familial combined hypolipidemia. Previous linkage studies had identified a chromosomal region in which the causal gene lay, but because of the prohibitively large number of genes in the region, causal mutations had not been found. Exome sequencing of DNA samples from two of the siblings revealed only one gene, angiopoietin-like 3 (*ANGPTL3*), that harbored rare DNA variants in both alleles in both siblings.[8] Subsequent studies confirmed the presence of additional *ANGPTL3* mutations in unrelated individuals with the same disease.

For common diseases, elucidation of the role of low-frequency and rare variants is just beginning. At the time of this writing, initial genome sequencing studies of hundreds or a thousand cases of common diseases (compared with appropriate controls) have yielded few findings. This is likely due to some combination of (1) the causal rare variants being lower in frequency and more modest in effect size (that is, not deterministic) and thus requiring large samples to achieve statistical significance; (2) the current limitations in our ability to recognize functional mutations from the sea of benign DNA variants, which is needed to increase signal compared with noise; (3) the need for improved statistical methods for relating rare variants to disease; and (4) the natural selection during human evolution, which shaped the overall balance of rare and common variants that contribute to each disease.

CLINICAL IMPACT: PREDICTION, PREVENTION, AND DRUG TARGETS

Much has been written about the future use of genetic prediction in clinical medicine, but a sober appraisal requires consideration of the natural history of each disease, the available approaches for presymptomatic prevention, and the predictive nature of each test. Where genetic prediction is strong, disease outcomes are serious, and prevention exists, the combination can be of great clinical value. For example, in hemochromatosis, knowledge of genetic risk and measurement of iron stores allow presymptomatic phlebotomy, a safe and effective approach that reduces the development of end-organ damage and that would otherwise not be used. Similarly, testing for *BRCA* mutations in at-risk individuals provides valuable information about cancer risk, allowing women to choose between intensive monitoring and preventive surgery (mastectomy and oophorectomy) to reduce risk of cancer. What these examples share is that the disease is relatively rare, a robustly measured genetic risk factor dramatically increases risk, and an established prevention exists that otherwise (because of cost, convenience, or risk) would not be used.

For most common diseases, the role of genetic prediction remains unclear. This is because the disease is common, and genetic risk (as we understand it today) is probabilistic rather than deterministic in nature. Thus, the discrimination in risk due to genetics is much more limited. Moreover, in many cases, it is the characteristic of available interventions (rather than the genetic test per se) that limits utility. For example, some prevention strategies, such as diet and lifestyle modification for type 2 diabetes, are useful for everyone. In such settings, identification of a high-risk population is either of limited use or could even be counterproductive (if a focus on high-risk individuals ended up denying the rest of the population a worthwhile and safe prevention strategy). In other cases, we simply lack a proven preventive intervention, and thus risk estimation alone is not what limits progress. For example, the genetics of AMD has identified common variants with substantial effects on risk and a cumulative score of such variants that can stratify risk in the population by dozens-fold. However, at present, prevention for AMD involves smoking cessation, diet, and exercise, all of which are best deployed widely in the population rather than in a targeted manner.

To realize the value of genetic insights into disease, it will be necessary to develop new and more effective approaches to prevention that target causal mechanisms. One encouraging example involves the gene encoding proprotein convertase subtilisin/kexin type 9 (*PCSK9*) and risk of myocardial infarction. Mutations in *PCSK9* were first identified through genetic mapping studies of rare families with very high levels of low-density lipoprotein cholesterol. Soon, candidate gene association studies of *PCSK9* revealed the existence of common variants that reduced or eliminated the function of the *PCSK9* protein; in one study, 2.6% of African Americans carried nonsense mutations in *PCSK9*. These "loss of function" variants in *PCSK9*, being common, could be studied in large populations for impact on clinical phenotypes and were soon shown to reduce plasma low-density lipoprotein cholesterol and to protect against coronary heart disease. This indicated that reduction in *PSCK9* function would be expected to reduce risk of myocardial infarction through its effects on low-density lipoprotein cholesterol. Moreover, a small number of people were found to be homozygous for these loss-of-function *PCSK9* mutations and, despite lacking immunoreactive *PCSK9* protein, to be healthy and well. This indicated that even complete reduction in risk of *PSCK9* would likely be safe.

On the basis of these results, several companies have developed monoclonal antibody–based drugs targeting the *PCSK9* protein.[9] Preliminary data from clinical trials of these agents have demonstrated large reductions in blood low-density lipoprotein cholesterol levels, in some cases surpassing even the most potent statin drugs. A reduction in risk of myocardial infarction is predicted on the basis of the genetic data for loss-of-function *PCSK9* mutations as well as the experience with other drugs that lower low-density lipoprotein cholesterol. However, definitive outcomes trials remain important and, at the time of this writing, have not yet been completed.

IMPLICATIONS AND FUTURE DIRECTIONS

Inherited factors contribute substantially to common as well as to rare diseases. Mendelian disorders are typically caused by rare mutations in the protein-coding regions of genes. On the basis of the results of GWAS, it is clear that common variants play a role in common disease, with typically modest effects that often act through effects on gene regulation rather than on protein structure. Each person carries a deep reservoir of less common and rare genetic variations that will be tested in coming years for a role in disease. It seems reasonable to expect that in the coming decade, systematic and integrative analyses of millions of genome sequences will define lists of genes and variants (both common and rare) that contribute to each human disease. If this international effort incorporates large and epidemiologically valid samples and takes into account factors that could bias results, such as case ascertainment, it should provide reference information needed to annotate each individual genome sequence for disease risk.

However, success in identifying genes and mutations will prove of value only if it leads to improved prediction, diagnosis, understanding, and treatment. Biologic understanding requires bedside-to-bench research, in which genes found mutated in patients are studied in the laboratory. It will be necessary to place new genes into known (and as yet unrecognized) biologic pathways and to understand how dysfunction and dysregulation lead to disease. In some cases, such as the role of complement in AMD (see earlier), initial answers may come quickly; in others, in which the relevant pathobiology is as yet unknown, the information to be gleaned from following these clues is unpredictable. In the fullness of time, genetic insights gleaned from patients should lead to a new generation of therapies that more directly target the underlying root causes of risk in the population.

New approaches to "precision" medicine will require not only development of predictive models and new therapies but also a foundation of clinical trial evidence that demonstrates benefit. That is, it is not sufficient simply to hypothesize that a genetic test or targeted therapy benefits patients, but it will be necessary to test this hypothesis in controlled trials. Such clinical trials will involve measuring DNA variation in study participants and testing approaches to intervention (prevention or treatment) based on such information. Genetic tests may prove predictive without being useful, and only careful research can demonstrate value and justify society's investment in their use.

Whereas much remains uncertain, it is clear that genetic and genomic information is accumulating at a staggering rate and holds much potential as well as challenges for the future of medicine. Rather than leaping to deploy genomics in medicine before value has been shown, it is incumbent on us to carefully develop and critically evaluate the use of this new technology to inform and improve the understanding, prevention, and treatment of disease.

GENERAL REFERENCES

For the General References and other additional features, please visit Expert Consult at https://expertconsult.inkling.com.

43 APPLICATION OF MOLECULAR TECHNOLOGIES TO CLINICAL MEDICINE

GEOFFREY S. GINSBURG

The completion of the Human Genome Project more than a decade ago has become an enabler of the systematic exploration of the molecular underpinnings of disease and the expectation that these insights would lead to a transformation of medical practice. Until we were able to probe the molecular architecture of disease using genome technologies, most diseases were defined by anatomic location and clinical symptoms and treated with one-size-fits-all therapies that failed to account for the unique biologic background of the individual. The Human Genome Project laid the foundation for molecular medicine along with advances in genotyping and sequencing technologies, bioinformatics, systems biology, and computational biology. Today, molecular medicine aims to build on this foundation, translating these discoveries into clinical practice, with the ultimate goal of personalized and precision medicine.

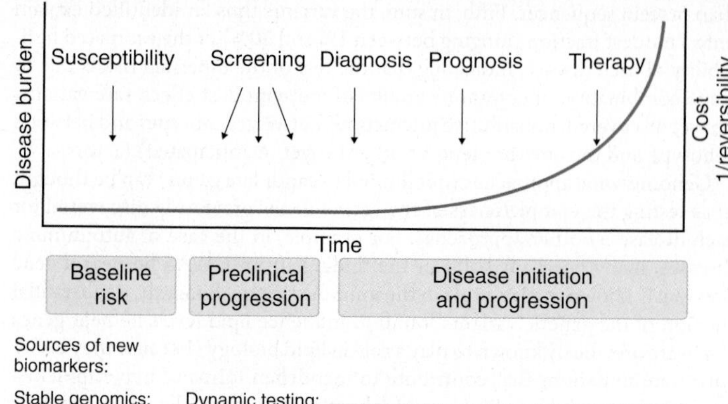

FIGURE 43-1. Use of molecular technologies across the continuum from health to disease. Various molecular technologies may be used to complement the traditional approach to evaluating at the time points indicated. (Adapted from Ginsburg GS, Willard HF. *Genomic and Personalized Medicine.* 2nd ed. Philadelphia, PA: Elsevier; 2013.)

MOLECULAR TECHNOLOGIES ALONG THE CONTINUUM FROM HEALTH TO DISEASE

Along the continuum from health to disease (as shown in Fig. 43-1), there are several important points where clinical decision making is now directly influenced and advantaged by molecular technologies (Table 43-1).[1,2] Risk estimates for developing some diseases can be defined during health and possibly even at birth using a variety of DNA analyses. Molecular signatures from technology platforms that measure the expressed genome (RNA, proteins, metabolites) can be used to define physiologic states in response to our environment and predict future clinical outcomes. These approaches also form the basis for a new molecular classification and taxonomy of disease and diagnosis. They can also provide more precise ways to screen for and detect disease at its earliest molecular manifestations, often preclinically. In addition, the selection of certain drugs may now be guided by a patient's underlying genetic makeup as well as the molecular makeup of the disease. Given that a disease's evolution from baseline risk often occurs over many years (see Fig. 43-1), periodic molecular profiling defines a novel form of health care monitoring that focuses on disease prevention and proactive management rather than the current paradigm of acute intervention and crisis response.

GENOMES, DISEASE, AND TREATMENT

A key question in medicine is to what extent genetic variation influences the likelihood of disease onset, affects the natural history of disease in combination with the environment, or provides clues relevant to the management of disease. In addition, it is not just the *human* genome that is relevant to an individual's state of health. The genomes of thousands of microorganisms that constitute *our microbiota* are also relevant to human phenotypes, and insights from *their* genomes are providing new approaches for the diagnosis, study, and treatment of disease (see later).

Sequencing: A Driver of Molecular Medicine

Genome-wide association study (GWAS) debuted in 2005 with the identification of variants in the complement factor H gene as a cause of age-related macular degeneration, (http://www.genome.gov/gwastudies). GWAS has been a transformative approach to identifying common genetic variation across the entire human genome in an unbiased fashion, offering an unprecedented opportunity to uncover new biologic pathways of disease. GWAS has been carried out on large cohorts of patients and controls across numer-

TABLE 43-1 APPLICATION OF MOLECULAR DIAGNOSTICS ALONG THE CONTINUUM FROM HEALTH TO DISEASE: EXAMPLES

TIME POINT IN CLINICAL DECISION MAKING	CANCER		CARDIOVASCULAR DISEASE	
	Test	**Indication**	**Test**	**Indication**
Risk/susceptibility	*BRCA1, BRCA2* *HNPCC* *TP53, PTEN*	Breast Colon Sarcomas	*KIF6, 9p21* Familion five-gene profile	CAD LQTS
Screening	HPV genotypes	Cervical	Corus CAD	CAD
Diagnosis	Cancer Type ID OVA1	Cancer of unknown primary Ovarian mass malignancy	Corus CAD	CAD
Prognosis	Oncotype DX (21-gene assay) MammaPrint (70-gene assay) HER2/neu, ER, PR	Breast	TnI, BNP, CRP	ACS
Pharmacogenomics	HER2/neu *UGT1A1* *KRAS* *EGFR* *ALK* *BRAF* NGS of somatic variation for targeted therapy AmpliChip; DMET *CYP2D6/CYP2C19*	Herceptin Irinotecan Cetuximab Erlotinib, gefitinib Crozotinib Vemurafenib Various (see E-Table 43-1)	*KIF6, SLCO1B1* AmpliChip; DMET *CYP2D6/CYP2C19* *VKORC1*	Statins Various (see E-Table 43-1) Warfarin
Monitoring	CTCs	Tumor recurrence or progression	AlloMap gene profile	Transplant rejection

ACS = acute coronary syndromes; BNP = brain natriuretic peptide; CAD = coronary artery disease; CRP = C-reactive protein; CTCs = circulating tumor cells; ER = estrogen receptor; HPV = human papillomavirus; LQTS = long QT syndrome; NGS = next-generation sequencing; PR = progesterone receptor; TnI = troponin I.
Data from Ginsburg GS, Willard H, eds. *Genomic and Personalized Medicine*. 2nd ed. New York, NY: Academic Press; 2012.

ous traits and diseases, revealing hundreds of common genetic variants associated with those traits.

Since 2001, the cost of sequencing a human genome dropped from \$3 billion to less than \$10,000. Next-generation sequencing (NGS) technology can now read approximately 250 billion bases in a week and allows direct measurement not just of common variants but also theoretically of *all* variations in a genome. It is estimated that the population frequency of germline variants is approximately 1 in every 1000 of the 3.2 billion nucleotide positions, giving rise to approximately 3 million variants in a given human genome. The challenge lies in figuring out the meaning of variants, many of which occur in noncoding regions (introns) of the genome whose function is largely unknown. Until the significance of the noncoding variants is understood, the focus clinically has been on exome sequencing (which examines variation in the coding sequence of exons that are translated into proteins), where mutations have predictable effects on downstream protein structure. Exome sequencing, which represents only about 1.5% of the 3 billion nucleotides that constitute the human genome, is still less expensive to perform than *whole-genome sequencing*. Individuals typically carry several hundred rare and potentially deleterious coding region variants. The first successful clinical applications of exome sequencing in 2009 revealed the diagnosis of patients with Freeman-Sheldon syndrome, and it is increasingly being explored for clinical applications, including the clinical diagnosis of rare genetic diseases,[3] the selection of cancer treatments based on molecular characterization of the tumor,[4] and the tracking of infectious disease outbreaks in real time[5] (see later).

Genetics of Common Complex Diseases

Despite strong statistical associations linking genetic variants with complex diseases, the low relative risk of the disease alleles (generally <2) limits their use for disease predisposition testing and risk assessment. There are notable exceptions, including genetic variation underlying breast cancer, Lynch syndrome, and celiac disease, where some variants have enabled preventive treatment or screening of family members. Despite these technologic advances in genomics, a simple family history continues to be among the best tools to identify risks for common diseases. In fact, for conditions with high heritability, such as cardiovascular disease, family history is a much stronger predictor of disease than any single or combination of genetic/genomic markers.[6] One model suggests that neither family history nor genetic testing should be used as a standalone but that the real power for disease prediction, risk assessment, and differential diagnosis comes from their combined use.

Clinical Sequencing for Diagnostic Dilemmas

More than 3500 mendelian disorders have a known molecular basis (http://omim.org/). However, there are nearly as many suspected mendelian traits for which the molecular basis remains to be identified. The potential for clinical sequencing to find the underlying cause and identify treatment options for these rare, sometimes debilitating diseases has led to the formation of various large national and international rare disease consortia. In some specialized clinical centers and through programs such as the National Human Genome Research Institute Undiagnosed Diseases Program (http://www.genome.gov/27544402), clinical sequencing is being offered to patients with suspected genetic diseases, the so-called diagnostic dilemmas. Early results from these clinical sequencing programs suggest that the success rate of disease gene identification is about 50%, offering hope for a diagnosis to thousands of individuals with previously undiagnosed or untreated rare disorders.[7]

Newborn Screening, Prenatal Diagnosis, and Preconception Carrier Testing

A natural outcome of identifying genes for rare mendelian disorders is the application of these findings to earlier detection, at birth (newborn screening), in utero (prenatal diagnosis) or before conception (carrier testing). Newborn screening—mandatory, state-supported public health programs meant to protect newborn children by screening them for rare, treatable (and thus preventable) disorders at birth—has been steadily increasing from an average of five conditions in 1995, to a panel of 31 core disorders and 26 secondary disorders currently recommended by the U.S. Department of Health and Human Services.[8] Rapid whole-genome sequencing (about 50 hours from test to result) was recently reported, and because the number of conditions considered for newborn screening will undoubtedly grow, rapid whole-genome sequencing can potentially broaden and foreshorten differential diagnoses, resulting in fewer empirical treatments and faster progression to genetic and prognostic counseling.

Cell-free fetal DNA circulating in maternal blood was isolated, amplified, and sequenced noninvasively through a sample of maternal plasma in 1997, In 2008, NGS technologies were used successfully to identify fetal aneuploidy from cell-free fetal DNA in maternal plasma. Clinical trials of the new method rapidly followed, and by late 2011, noninvasive prenatal testing of trisomy 21 by sequencing of maternal plasma DNA was being offered on a clinical and commercial basis in the United States and China. Noninvasive prenatal testing eliminates the need for invasive procedures, while also greatly expanding the number of genetic variants that have traditionally been detected in utero.[9]

Before conception, carrier screening enables couples to assess their risk for having a child with a recessive mendelian disorder and to use this information to guide their reproductive decisions. There are more than 1000 rare, *recessive* mendelian disorders for which the underlying genetic mutation is known. Although individually rare, these can have a sizable public health impact considering that each person is estimated to carry on average 2.8 mutations for known severe recessive disorders,[10] and the impact of screening could be substantial in terms of reduced disease morbidity and mortality in the population.

Pharmacogenomics: Germline Genetics Variants and Drug Response

Several genomic markers of efficacy, adverse events, and dosing of therapeutics have been discovered (E-Table 43-1), but their uptake into clinical practice has been variable, despite their clear actionability. In some cases, such as with the *HLA-B*5701* genotype for the HIV drug abacavir and *HLA-B*1502* for the antiseizure drug carbamazepine, carriers of these genotypes should avoid the drug entirely to eliminate a specific serious adverse event. In other cases, such as thiopurine *S*-methyltransferase (*TPMT*) for mercaptopurine or *CYP2C9/VKORC1* for warfarin, adjusting the dose of drug based on genotype can help to avoid toxicity and improve efficacy. *Actionability* is not enough to ensure diffusion of pharmacogenomics testing into clinical practice, as exemplified by the antiplatelet drug clopidogrel, for which despite having a U.S. Food and Drug Administration black box warning for efficacy in individuals carrying the *CYP2C19* genetic variant, there is no clear consensus among physicians on its use. In hepatitis C treatment, on the other hand, the *IL28B* genotype test not only has proved highly predictive of response to pegylated interferon/ribavirin used to treat chronic hepatitis C virus infection but also has seen rapid and widespread adoption in the clinic.[11] Genetic markers that predict reduced therapeutic efficacy may face a high hurdle for established drugs, unless evidence supporting clinical validity and utility of the test is indisputable.

Cancer Pharmacogenomics: Somatic Sequencing of Tumor DNA for Targeting Drug Therapies

Cancer arises as a result of somatic DNA mutations that confer a growth advantage on the cells in which they have occurred, giving rise to tumors. Comparison of the genetic profiles of tumors and the surrounding normal tissue (*gene expression profiling*) can reveal the acquired DNA variation that drives growth and that may reveal targets for treatment.

Targeted Therapies for Cancer

The idea of pairing medicines with specific tumor markers in a targeted fashion became a reality in the mid-1980s when detailed molecular studies of breast tumors led to the discovery of human epidermal growth factor receptor-2 (HER-2), a biomarker overexpressed in approximately 30% of breast tumors and associated with adverse outcomes. Subsequently, trastuzumab (Herceptin), a humanized monoclonal antibody targeting HER-2, was developed in 1998 and was shown to have increased efficacy in patients whose tumors tested positive. HER-2 testing of tumor is now part of the standard work-up and management of breast cancer. In the past decade, other examples of cancer therapies with companion diagnostics have emerged (Table 43-2). For example, *EGFR* mutation testing has markedly improved the efficacy of gefitinib and erlotinib, small molecule drugs for the treatment of non–small cell lung cancer that target *EGFR*. In metastatic colorectal cancer, tumors with mutated *KRAS* are usually resistant to treatment with cetuximab and panitumumab, leading the American Society of Clinical Oncology and the U.S. Food and Drug Administration (FDA) to recommend withholding the drugs in these patients. NGS now allows a comprehensive assessment of actionable tumor markers that indicate the potential for a specific therapeutic to have efficacy in a given tumor (see Table 43-1). In 2011, two cancer drugs received accelerated approval by the FDA for use with a companion diagnostic test: (1) crizotinib for the treatment of patients with locally advanced or metastatic non–small cell lung cancer with its companion diagnostic designed to detect the *EML4-ALK* fusion gene, and (2) vemurafenib for the treatment of patients with metastatic or unresectable melanoma positive for *BRAF* V600E mutations. The International Cancer Genome Consortium (https://www.icgc.org/icgc) and the Cancer Genome Atlas (http://cancergenome.nih.gov/) represent international collaborative efforts to define the spectrum of mutations found in tumors, mapping the genomic landscape of cancer. These efforts will provide a foundation from which to develop additional therapeutic strategies against new targets. However, even when successful, the results may be short-lived as therapeutic resistance evolves. Thus, although NGS is a promising new tool for surveying cancer genomes, it may not be a panacea for cancer genomic medicine.

Microbial Genomes: Friends or Foes?

We can now rapidly sequence the genomes of microorganisms—both the commensal bacteria that regularly inhabit our bodies (the *human microbiome*)[12] as well as the pathogenic infectious agents that cause acute and sometimes fatal diseases.[13] The Human Microbiome Project recently published a study of the microbial populations inhabiting various human body sites[14] and provided reference sequences for many taxa in health individuals as well as their correlation with host characteristics, including ethnicity, age, and body mass index. There are now emerging associations of human microbiota and diseases such as diabetes, asthma, psoriasis, atherosclerosis, and obesity.[15,16] Moreover, strategies to modify the gut microbiome are being explored as treatments for inflammatory bowel disease, including the use of fecal transplantation or engraftment of microbiota from a healthy donor into a recipient.[17] The human microbiome will play an important role in molecular medicine because microbial composition can be altered noninvasively through diet or the use of probiotics or antibiotics.

In infectious disease, diagnosis by NGS may supplant the need to first grow microorganisms in culture, previously a major impediment to pathogen identification. For example, in 2003, sequencing of samples from infected patients with the severe acute respiratory syndrome identified the causative agent as a coronavirus. Comparison of sequences of multiple isolates of an organism from a single epidemic gives a picture of the organism's evolution, allowing one to infer where the outbreak began and how the infection spread. Sequencing has been used to determine the origins of historical outbreaks of cholera, tuberculosis, and the 2009 H1N1 influenza. The clinical application of NGS to infectious disease was highlighted recently when the source of carbapenem-resistant *Klebsiella pneumoniae* in a hospital outbreak was identified by sequencing isolates of the bacteria—in real time—from infected individuals and examining the genetic differences.[18]

TABLE 43-2 MOLECULAR MARKER INFORMED CANCER THERAPIES (TARGETED THERAPEUTICS)

BIOMARKER	DRUG	CANCER TYPE	FDA DRUG LABELING RECOMMENDED OR REQUIRED
Estrogen receptor	Tamoxifen	Breast	Yes
Her2/neu	Trastuzumab	Breast	Yes
EGFR	Cetuximab	Colorectal	Yes
Kras	Cetuximab	Colorectal	Yes
EGFR	Panitumumab	Colorectal	Yes
Kras	Panitumumab	Colorectal	Yes
DPYD	5-FU	Breast/colorectal	No
EGFR	Erlotinib	Lung	No
EGFR	Gefitinib	Lung	No
BCR-ABL	Imatinib	CML	Yes
C-KIT	Imatinib	CML/ALL	Yes
ALK	Crozotinib	Lung	Yes
BRAF	Vemurafenib	Melanoma	Yes

5-FU = 5-flurouracil; ALL = acute lymphoblastic leukemia; CML = chronic myelogenous leukemia; FDA, U.S. Food and Drug Administration.

THE EXPRESSED GENOME

Complex Multimarker Genomic Tests for Disease Diagnosis and Prognosis

Beyond DNA sequence, measures of gene expression, proteins, metabolites, and epigenetic changes are being used to generate comprehensive profiles of biologic systems in health and disease. Many of the computational challenges of analyzing these large, complex data sets are being addressed to yield next-generation biomarkers that are multianalyte, diagnostic, prognostic, and predictive. A growing number of marketed tests now typically measure protein or RNA levels, often with complex algorithms, enabling diagnosis and prognosis (see Table 43-1). One example is Oncotype DX (Genomic Health Inc., Redwood City, CA), a test that examines expression of 21 genes in tumor tissue to determine the likelihood of disease recurrence in women with early-stage hormone estrogen receptor–positive breast cancer. The test, which is currently covered by many major insurance companies, analyzes expression levels and converts them to a recurrence risk score that has been shown to help guide treatment in patients, reduce overall health care costs, and improve outcomes.[19] Other examples include MammaPrint (Agendia Inc., Irvine, CA), which analyzes the expression of 70 genes to determine whether patients are at high or low risk for breast cancer recurrence; OVA1 (Vermillion, Inc., Austin, TX), a five-protein test that gauges whether a woman's ovarian mass is malignant and requires surgery; AlloMap (XDx Expression Diagnostics, Inc., Brisbane, CA), an 11 blood gene RNA signature for monitoring rejection after cardiac transplantation; and Corus CAD (CardioDx, Inc., Palo Alto, CA), a 23-gene blood RNA signature to screen for obstructive coronary artery disease.

Despite their complexity, in vitro diagnostic multianalyte index assays (IVDMIAs) like these are finding their way to the clinic. The 2007 draft guidance from the FDA suggested that IVDMIAs are used to make critical health care decisions and thus should be regulated by the FDA. Some of the marketed IVDMIAs have demonstrated analytical and clinical validity, but evidence of clinical utility is usually lagging. Moreover, the very nature of IVDMIAs presents challenges to insurers, who grapple not only with limited data on clinical utility but also with how to reimburse such tests that comprise both a laboratory component and an associated algorithm used to score risk, the latter part being integral to realizing the test's value.

The success of some IVDMIAs is evidence of the power of computational biology but also of the importance of advocacy and financial resources that the commercial developers of these tests must bring. Companies developing IVDMIAs are able to finance key studies aimed at demonstrating clinical validity, navigate regulatory hurdles, advocate for coverage by insurance companies, and disseminate their tests through marketing to health care providers. Their efforts offer valuable lessons on the effective translation of complex molecular tests to medicine.

Proteomics

The large-scale study of proteins, *proteomics*, allow for both protein identification and differential expression between two physiologic states (such as health and a specific disease). Quantitative proteomics, in which global differences in protein abundances are measured, continues to be a priority area for biomarker discovery and molecular medicine. This area has been dominated by stable isotope approaches, but recent label-free quantitative methods have been developed that rely on the measured intensity of a peptide ion and compares this to its intensity in other samples. Label-free methods have the advantage of higher throughput and fewer sample manipulation steps. Multiple—or selected-reaction monitoring of specific peptides within biofluids allows quantitation of absolute abundance of proteins in clinical samples. Although this technology is relatively immature in its applications to human health and disease, compared with RNA and metabolic profiling, it is anticipated that these methods, combined with the development of mass spectroscopy technology, will advance proteomics to more routine use in disease classification and diagnosis, prognosis, and pharmacogenomics within the next several years.

Metabolic Profiling

A metabolic profile is very similar to some of the traditional targeted profiles, such as a lipid profile, although it is more comprehensive. *Metabolomics* measures changes in the metabolic or chemical milieu that are downstream of genomic and proteomic alterations. It is estimated that humans contain approximately 5000 discrete small molecule metabolites, and the identification of metabolic fingerprints for specific diseases may have particular practical utility for the development of therapies because metabolic changes immediately suggest enzymatic drug targets. Similar to genomics and proteomics, metabolomics may be useful in disease diagnosis, prognosis, and drug development. In particular, metabolomics will likely be a valuable tool in assessing drug toxicity. Targeted mass-spectroscopy-based metabolic profiling has also been increasingly applied to studies of human diseases and conditions. These tools are being applied to diverse areas, such as diabetes, obesity, cardiovascular disease, cancer, and mental disorders.

CLINICAL IMPLEMENTATION OF MOLECULAR PROFILES

In order for molecular medicine to be practiced, it must be woven into current systems of health care delivery, with due consideration given not only to the providers of health care but also to the organizations in which they practice as well. Implementation scientists have outlined various aspects that need to be considered in order for molecular medicine to take hold in the clinical setting. Beyond the scientific soundness of the molecular or genomic test, measured by a strong evidentiary base and regard for potential benefits and harms, there is consideration of how the new test will integrate into the clinical workflow. Consideration should be given to aspects such as access to a laboratory certified by the Clinical Laboratory Improvement Amendments of 1988, methods for sample preparation and transport, test ordering, and receipt and delivery of results. Genomic test implementation is complicated by issues of privacy, complex interpretation of results, and the need to involve third parties for counseling in some cases; they may require the development of new systems to accommodate them.

A robust means of integrating genomic and molecular data into electronic health records will be required, with consideration of not only data storage formats and privacy issues but also appropriate decision support tools for prompting their use at the point of care and delivering results in an easily interpretable format. Currently, there are several examples of decision support tools, such as Warfarin Dosing (www.WarfarinDosing.org), but they are typically standalone tools and not part of routine clinical workflow. To maximize their effectiveness, such tools should be integrated into electronic health records. Tapping into the collective knowledge and experience of various institutions working in this space would greatly facilitate this effort. Ultimately, a national, standardized technical architecture for integrating clinical decision support into electronic health records will be required. Notable efforts in this space include those of Health Level 7 (http://www.hl7.org), an organization that provides interoperability standards for the exchange, integration, sharing, and retrieval of electronic health information. Through their Clinical Genomics Workgroup, this organization has developed a standards guide for genetic testing that includes document templates to support integration of genetic testing into electronic health records.[1] Appropriate clinical decision support, provided in the context of the electronic health record, will greatly facilitate the diffusion and uptake of genomic medicine.

GENERAL REFERENCES

For the General References and other additional features, please visit Expert Consult at https://expertconsult.inkling.com.

44

REGENERATIVE MEDICINE, CELL, AND GENE THERAPIES

LIOR GEPSTEIN AND KARL SKORECKI

CELL THERAPY

Introduction and Definitions

A remarkable clinical need exists for the development and clinical assessment of various methods to facilitate the regeneration of injured or diseased tissues and organs. This need derives from the unrelenting prevalence of trauma, congenital disorders, ischemia, and degenerative processes, which becomes increasingly urgent as the global population expands and ages. Cancer is tied to this field both directly (e.g., replacement of lost vital organ function as a result of cancer invasion or treatment modalities, cell-based delivery of cancer immune and gene therapies) and indirectly (e.g., role of stem cells in cancer pathogenesis, risk for tumorigenesis in stem cell–based therapies). The recent developments in stem cell biology, molecular interventions, biopolymers, and other related biologic and engineering disciplines have paved the way to the emerging research and clinical discipline of regenerative medicine.[1]

Regenerative Medicine

Regenerative medicine seeks to harness methods for the replacement or repair of dysfunctional cells, tissue, or organs in an attempt to restore normal function. It therefore draws on therapies from the three conventional pillars of medical therapeutics (pharmaceuticals, biologics, and medical devices) as well as from the newest platform technology, namely, cell therapy. The long-term goal of regenerative medicine is to cure disease by replacing the lost functions of tissues and organs, and thus it truly represents a paradigm shift from conventional therapies aiming to alter the natural course of disease or to provide symptomatic control. Consequently, regenerative medicine aims to develop curative strategies for unmet clinical needs such as diabetes, heart failure, and neurodegenerative disorders, among others.

Cell Therapy

Cell therapy involves the application of cells to achieve a therapeutic benefit, regardless of the cell type or clinical indication. Although achieving tissue and organ regeneration through cell replacement represents an important goal of cell therapy technology, its applications may reach far beyond the field of regenerative medicine. Hence, the spectrum of cell therapy approaches may range from permanent cell replacement strategies (attempting to replace lost or dysfunctional cells) to more transient cell therapies aiming to modulate disease progression or to protect tissues at risk, to achieve immunomodulatory effects (e.g., for prevention of graft-versus-host disease), to act as vehicles for the delivery of genes or gene products (cell-based gene therapy strategies), and even to act as cell-based cancer vaccines. This chapter focuses on the use of cell therapy for regenerative medicine and specifically concentrates on the potential role of different stem cell types to meet this challenge.

Stem Cells

Stem cells possess two defining properties: (1) the capacity for self-renewal and (2) the ability to differentiate into cell types with specialized cellular functions (Fig. 44-1). This may occur at the individual stem cell level through the process of asymmetrical cell division or at the cell population level wherein a subset of cells differentiate and the remaining stem cells remain dormant or replicate themselves as stem cells. After asymmetrical cell division, non–stem cell derivatives may either generate a pool of organ system–restricted, transit-amplifying cells with enhanced proliferative capacity or continue to differentiate by epigenetic and gene expression profile changes until reaching the terminally differentiated state. This conceptual framework was developed after the discovery of bone marrow cells that were capable of reconstituting the adult hematopoietic system. These hematopoietic stem cells constitute the basis for hematopoietic stem cell transplantation, the only form of stem cell therapy currently routinely well established in clinical practice (Chapter 178).

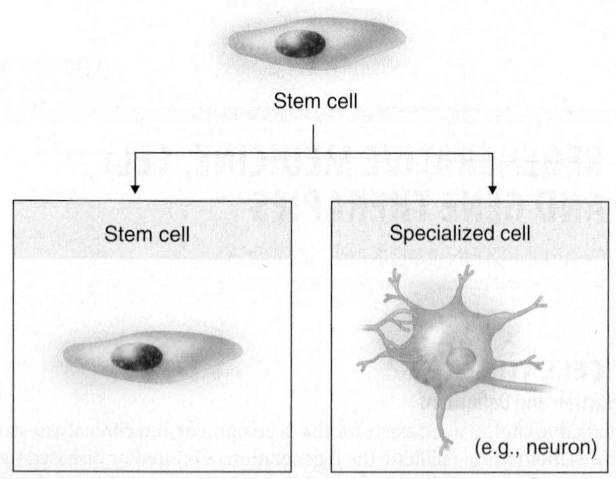

FIGURE 44-1. Asymmetrical cell division. Although this first characteristic was considered a required characteristic for stem cells based on their original description in the adult hematopoietic system, not all cell types currently named as stem cells necessarily display this property. For instance, human embryonic stem cells divide by symmetrical cell division.

The different stem cells types are routinely classified based on the protein or transcription factors they express, but also according to three basic additional attributes. These include replicative capacity (limited vs. unlimited), the scope or potency of differentiation (e.g., pluripotent, multipotent, oligopotent, unipotent), and their place in the life history of the organism (developmental or postdevelopmental). Thus, more recent terminology has broadened use of the term *stem cells* to cover a wider array of cell types that contribute to organ development or have the capacity to repopulate tissues and organ systems. The term *stem cells*, together with the formulations noted previously, has also recently been extrapolated to describe certain cellular subpopulations that may be principally responsible for the growth of malignant tumors. However, because cancer stem cells have no role in tissue regeneration, they are considered in Chapter 181.

Adult (Postnatal) Stem Cells

After birth, many tissues are thought to contain a subpopulation of cells with the capacity for extended self-renewal, combined with the ability to differentiate into more mature cell types with specialized functions (Fig. 44-2). Adult stem cells, thought to represent less than 0.01% of the total number of cells, are located in specialized supportive niche compartments at various sites within the hematopoietic system and elsewhere, and respond to cues in their local microenvironment. As a result of the success of hematopoietic stem cell transplantation in the treatment of bone marrow failure or in conjunction with myeloablative therapy in malignancy, scientists have been motivated to find adult stem cells in other organs. Adult tissues and organ systems reported to contain putative stem cells include bone marrow (hematopoietic and mesenchymal compartments) and peripheral blood, blood vessel endothelium, dental pulp, epithelia of the skin, adipose tissue, digestive system, cornea, retina, testis, and liver. Similar stem/progenitor cells were also reported in organs historically not thought to contain such cells, such as the central nervous system, the heart, and the kidney. Whether adult stem cells represent remnants of developmental stem cells that persist into adulthood for purposes of organ maintenance and repair or represent a distinct cell type dedicated for this latter purpose is not clear. Importantly, in many organs, despite the presence of such tissue-specific stem cells, their regenerative capacity is still inadequate to deal with massive cell loss such as occurs, for example, after a large myocardial infarction or after ischemic brain injury.

Embryonic and Induced Pluripotent Stem Cells

In contrast to adult stem cells that have relatively limited differentiation potency, cells in the developing preimplantation embryo still retain the capacity to differentiate into derivatives of all three germ layers (ectoderm, mesoderm, and endoderm), eventually contributing to all tissues in the body (Fig. 44-3). In normal development, however, such cells do not persist beyond the blastocyst stage. When isolated from unused preimplantation blastocysts generated for in vitro fertilization, the inner cell mass cells isolated can be used to generate human embryonic stem cell (hESC) lines (see Fig. 44-3). The generated hESCs exhibit unlimited self-renewal in cell culture in the undifferentiated state, while retaining the capacity to differentiate into cell derivatives of all three germ layers, essentially giving rise to any cell type in the body. Taking advantage of lessons learned from embryology, scientists were able to utilize the sequential application of different combinations of growth factors to achieve efficient differentiation systems from hESCs, yielding purified populations of different types of neurons, glial cells, cardiomyocytes, vascular endothelial and smooth muscle cells, pancreatic β cells, hepatocytes, different blood cells (platelets, red blood cells), and several other cell lineages.

One of the limitations of the hESC technology is the inability to derive such cells from an adult individual, preventing their utilization in a patient-specific manner. These limitations can be overcome with the introduction of induced pluripotent stem cell (iPSC) technology.[2] This approach allows adult somatic cells (e.g., fibroblasts) to be reprogrammed into pluripotent stem cells by introduction of a set of transcription factors linked to pluripotency (the originally reported combination of factors included OCT3/4, SOX2, c-MYC, and KLF4). The human iPSCs (hiPSCs) generated in this manner can then be coaxed to differentiate into a variety of cell types, using differentiation protocols similar to those already in place for hESC (Fig. 44-4). Importantly, because the hiPSCs can be generated in a patient-specific manner, this technology can potentially be used to develop autologous cell-replacement strategies that can evade the immune system, to generate patient- and disease-specific models of different genetic disorders, and to establish screens for drug testing and drug discovery.

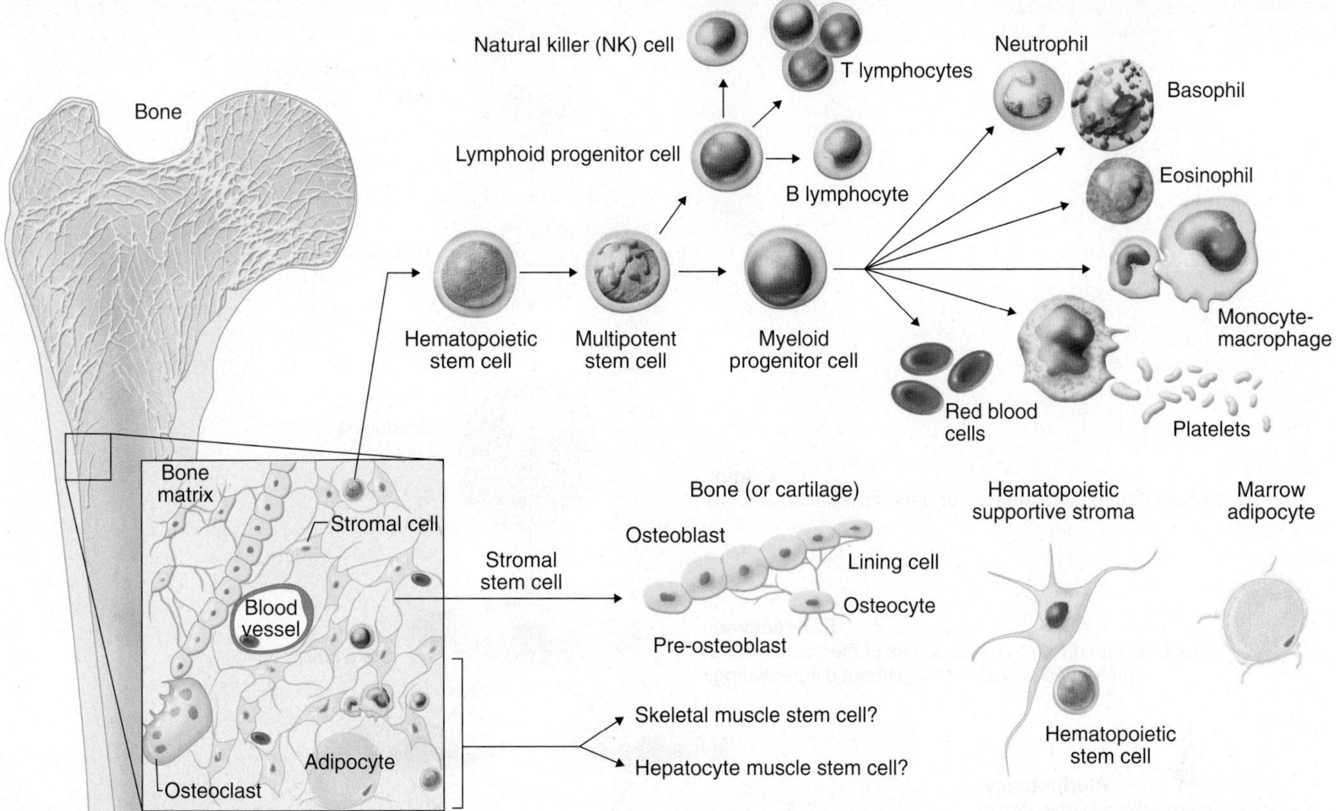

FIGURE 44-2. Adult stem cells. Adult stem cells can be multipotent and have the capacity to differentiate into a limited number of different cell types, often restricted to a given tissue or organ system, as in the case of adult hematopoietic or epidermal stem cells. Two stem cell types have been isolated from adult bone marrow—the hematopoietic stem cell and the mesenchymal stem cell. Adult mesenchymal stem cells of bone marrow origin, although their range of differentiation has been shown to be broader than that of any other adult stem cell type, do not reach pluripotency. It is thought that in some organ systems, such as the gastrointestinal epithelium, a unipotent pool of progenitors exists for repopulating a rapid population turnover of only one type of cell—although it is difficult to be certain whether such progenitors can be distinguished from the overall population of fully differentiated cells in tissues with high cellular turnover.

Cell Therapy Approaches to Regenerative Medicine

Historically, the field of cell therapy can be traced to the transfusion of blood and blood products (Chapter 177), solid organ transplantation (Chapter 49), in vitro fertilization, and bone marrow transplantation (Chapter 178). Nevertheless, beyond the aforementioned therapies, which have become the mainstay treatments in several medical fields, additional cell therapy approaches are considered highly experimental and are still at different stages of preclinical and clinical development. These ongoing efforts can be conceptually grouped into six different approaches (Fig. 44-5).

Delivery of Bone Marrow– and Blood-Derived Stem/Progenitor Cells

A flurry of studies during the past decade evaluated the ability of bone marrow–derived hematopoietic or mesenchymal stem cells to achieve tissue repair after delivery to a variety of organs. These studies were based initially on the assumption that these types of adult stem cells may display some degree of plasticity, allowing them to transdifferentiate into the relevant cell types (e.g., heart cells, nerve cells, and liver cells) after transplantation into the appropriate tissue environment. Although mounting evidence suggests that such transdifferentiation probably does not occur to a significant extent, many of these studies appeared to result in some degree of functional improvement after stem cell delivery to different organs. This clinical benefit may stem from the secretion of different growth factors by the engrafted cells ("paracrine hypothesis"); these factors in turn are thought to augment endogenous tissue repair mechanisms, improve tissue vascularization, modulate inflammation, and protect tissues at risk.

Delivery or Activation of Tissue-Specific Stem/Progenitor Cells or Induction of Cell Proliferation

In contrast to the conventional dogma, recent evidence suggests that a number of organs previously believed to lack any regenerative capacity (e.g., the brain, pancreas, kidney, and heart) in fact do possess such ability, albeit at a limited capacity. Whether this capability is due to the presence of tissue-specific stem/progenitor cells or due to some replication capability of terminally differentiated cells is still a matter of debate for each organ.

Significant efforts have been made in recent years to isolate such putative tissue-specific stem/progenitor cells based on the expression of general or specific stem cell markers or based on their unique culturing properties. These studies also highlighted the potential of such cells to be cultured in a clonal manner and to give rise to one or more cell types relevant to the organs from which they were isolated. Current efforts to utilize the aforementioned findings for regenerative medicine are focused either on the isolation, ex vivo expansion, and transplantation of such putative stem/progenitor cells back to their respective native organs or on the augmentation of their endogenous reparative potential in vivo. The former strategy can be exemplified in the central nervous system where progenitor cells are harvested, cultivated in culture (as neurospheres), and give rise to different types of neurons and supporting glial cells. Similar efforts have followed in other organs. In the heart, for example, such efforts have already reached early clinical trials, in which autologous cardiac stem cells were harvested from the heart, expanded ex vivo, and then engrafted back to the heart. The latter approach, in contrast, aims to influence putative stem cell niches within damaged organs to enhance the endogenous reparative properties of those stem/progenitor cells. Such an effect may underlie the potential therapeutic benefit of bone marrow–derived stem cells after their delivery to different organs.

The final strategy aims to boost endogenous organ repair through the replication of terminally differentiated tissue-specific cells. Such strategies can either augment the inherent physiologic capability of a given organ (e.g., insulin secretagogues for pancreatic β cells) or attempt to induce replication in cells that have already withdrawn from the cell cycle. Caution is warranted with respect to the latter approach because induction of uncontrolled proliferation (e.g., by genetic manipulation) may increase the risk for tumorigenesis.

Engraftment of Fetal Tissue

The most straightforward approach to organ repair would be to replace the missing cells with identical counterparts. Harvesting and expanding adult

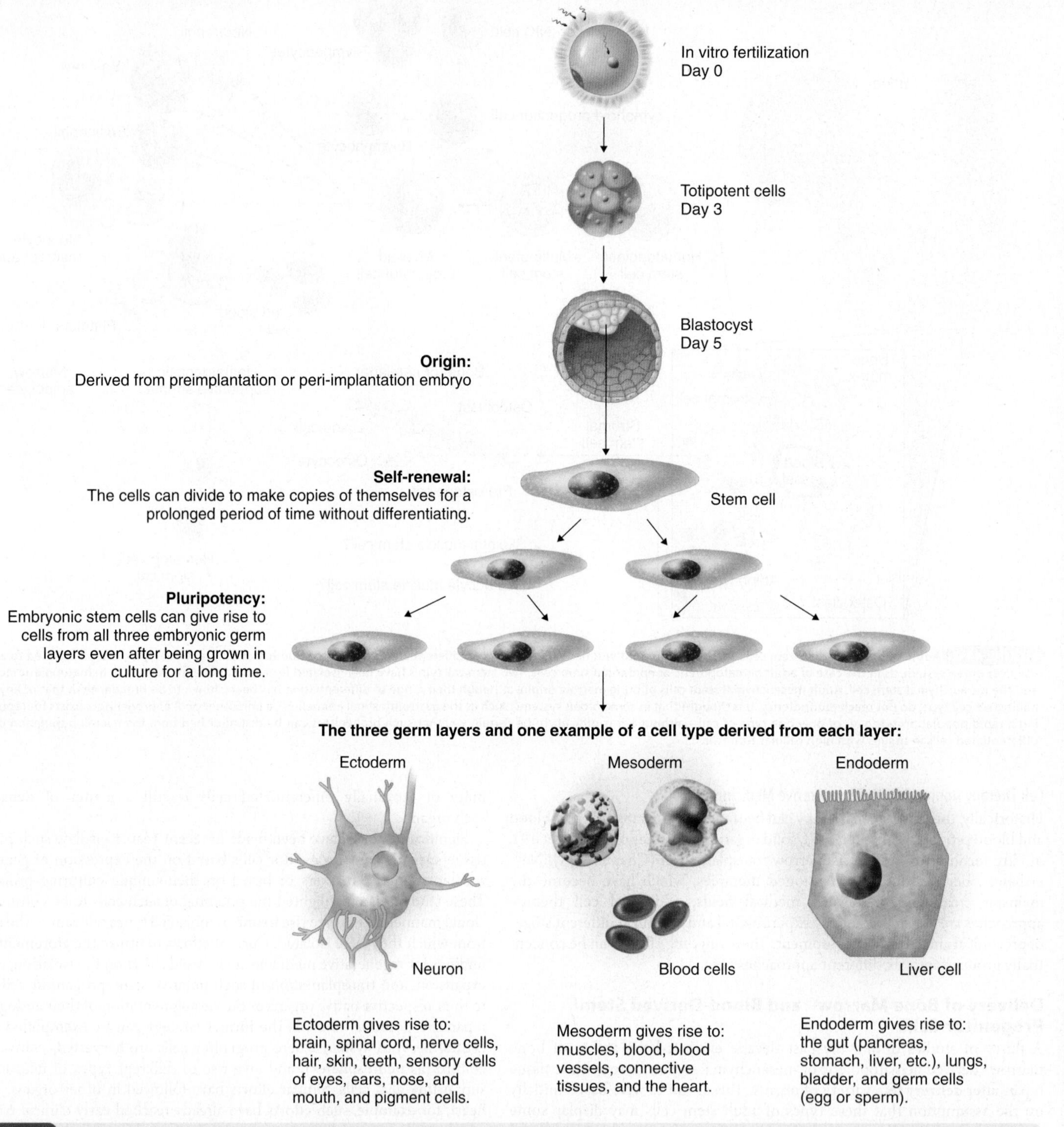

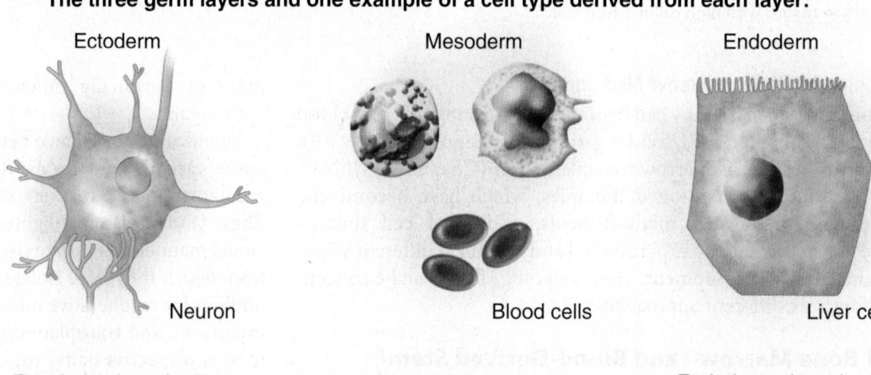
In vitro fertilization
Day 0
Totipotent cells
Day 3
Blastocyst
Day 5
Origin:
Derived from preimplantation or peri-implantation embryo
Self-renewal:
The cells can divide to make copies of themselves for a prolonged period of time without differentiating.
Stem cell
Pluripotency:
Embryonic stem cells can give rise to cells from all three embryonic germ layers even after being grown in culture for a long time.
The three germ layers and one example of a cell type derived from each layer:
Ectoderm
Mesoderm
Endoderm
Neuron
Blood cells
Liver cell
Ectoderm gives rise to: brain, spinal cord, nerve cells, hair, skin, teeth, sensory cells of eyes, ears, nose, and mouth, and pigment cells.
Mesoderm gives rise to: muscles, blood, blood vessels, connective tissues, and the heart.
Endoderm gives rise to: the gut (pancreas, stomach, liver, etc.), lungs, bladder, and germ cells (egg or sperm).

FIGURE 44-3. Embryonic stem cells. ***Totipotency*** **refers to the capacity to differentiate into all cell types in an organism, including extraembryonic tissues, placenta, and umbilical cord, a property confined to the fertilized egg itself, including the cells derived from the first few cell divisions after fertilization.** ***Pluripotency*** **refers to the capacity to differentiate into all the specialized cell types derived from the three germ layers (ectoderm, mesoderm, endoderm) of the developing embryo and is a hallmark feature of embryonic stem and germ cells.**

human cells for transplantation, however, may not be possible in the case of several organs with limited regenerative capacity. During prenatal human development, cells of fetal origin often show enhanced proliferative capacity as well as the ability to differentiate into more than one type of mature or specialized cell. Moreover, animal studies have demonstrated that transplantation of tissues harvested from developing organs (harvested within a specific time window during embryonic development) may give rise to entire functioning organs such as kidneys, lungs, and pancreas. Nevertheless, to date, the only fetal-derived cells that have been used in human clinical applications are the dopaminergic cells derived from the developing fetal nervous system for the treatment of Parkinson disease (Chapter 409). The broader use of fetal tissues for regenerative medicine may be hampered by the limited access to such cells for both technical and ethical reasons, the allogeneic nature of such procedures (requiring immune suppression), and the potential for tumor formation as already described in some case reports.

Transplantation of Ex Vivo Differentiation of Pluripotent Stem Cells

Unlike fetal tissues, hESCs are truly pluripotent (can give rise to advanced cell derivatives of all three germ layers). Importantly, hESCs can be propagated in the undifferentiated state and then coaxed to differentiate into a variety of cell types, giving rise to a potentially unlimited number of specialized cell types for transplantation. Consequentially, numerous preclinical studies have demonstrated the ability of hESC derivatives to engraft, survive,

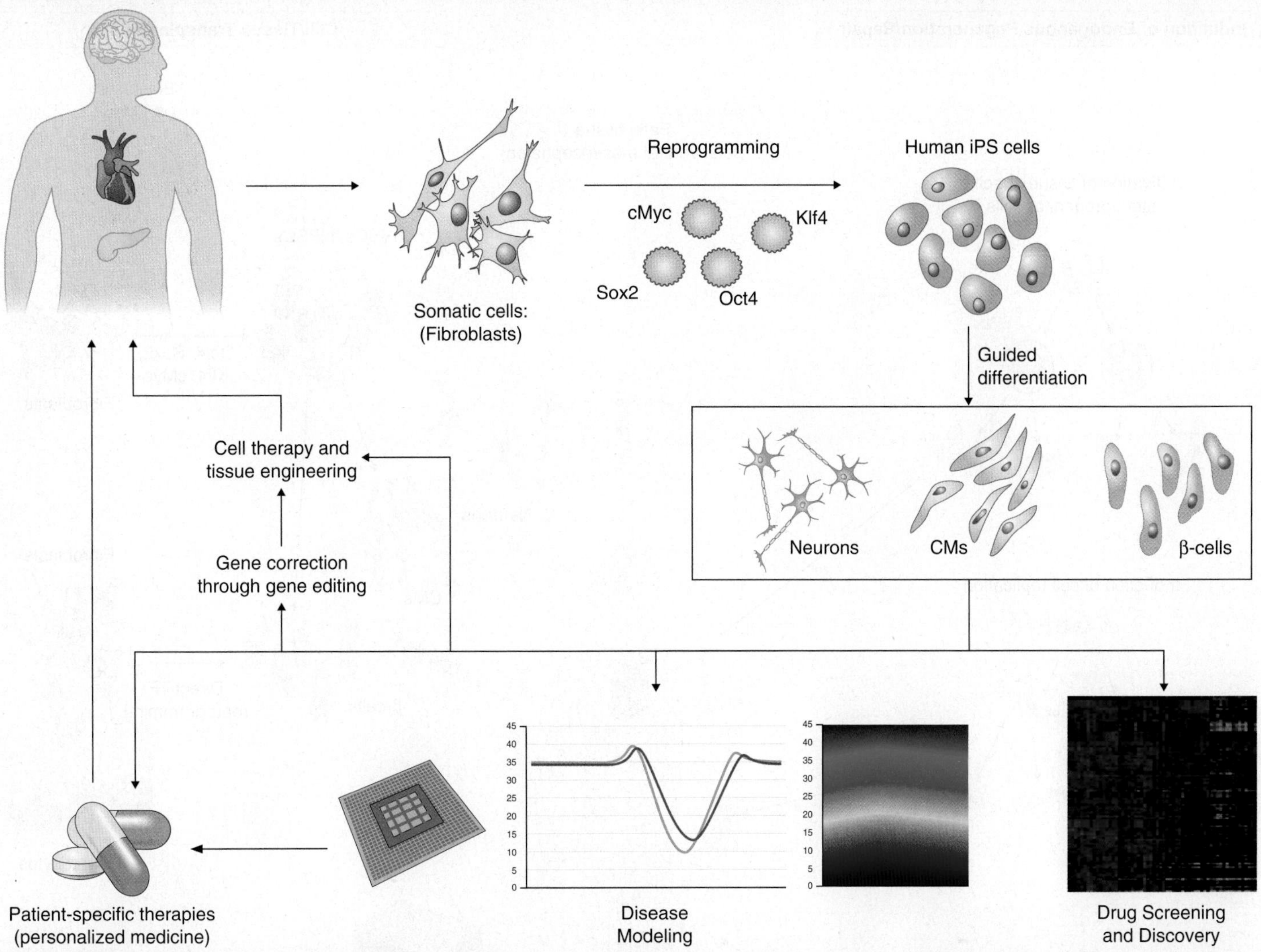

FIGURE 44-4. Application of the induced pluripotent stem cells (iPSC) technology. Patient-specific human iPSC can be generated by reprogramming of adult somatic cells (fibroblasts) with a set of transcription factors and then coaxed to differentiate into a variety of cell lineages. The patient-specific human iPSCs can then be transplanted back to the patient in an autologous manner for regenerative medicine applications. In a similar manner disease- and patient-specific human iPSC models of inherited disorders could be generated ("disease-in-a-dish models") and used for better understanding of genetic disorders, for drug development, and for optimizing patient-specific therapies. Gene editing techniques can be used for mutation correction and for transplantation of healthy cells. CM = cardiomyocytes; iPS = induced pluripotent stem cells.

and improve organ performance in a wide spectrum of relevant animal disease models (e.g., heart failure, Parkinson disease and other neurodegenerative disorders, diabetes). Early clinical studies using hESC derivatives are just emerging and have been focused so far on the retina (transplantation of retinal pigment epithelium [RPE] cells) and spinal cord injury (using oligodendrocyte progenitors).

Despite the significant achievements made with hESCs, the inability to create patient-specific hESCs from adult individuals, the ethical issues arising from destructive use of human embryos, and the anticipated immune rejection associated with such allogeneic cell transplantation impose important hurdles for their clinical utilization. The hiPSC technology provides a potential solution to these challenges. As noted, the patient's own somatic cells (fibroblasts, hair follicles, urine epithelial cells, or blood cells) could be reprogrammed by a set of transcription and chemical factors to yield pluripotent stem cells. The patient-specific hiPSCs could then be coaxed to differentiate to a variety of cell lineages, using protocols similar to those already in place for hESCs. In turn, these differentiated derivatives could then be transplanted either in an autologous or allogeneic manner. Clinical trials using hiPSC-derived cell lineages are expected to be initiated in the coming few years, with the initial targets being macular degeneration (RPE cells), Parkinson disease (dopaminergic neurons), blood product transfusion (hiPSC-derived platelets and red blood cells), and heart failure (cardiomyocytes).

One of the concerns in translating hESCs and hiPSCs into a therapeutic platform is the oncogenic risk. This concern stems from the potential for remaining undifferentiated cells within the cell grafts to form teratomas, from the use of oncogenic reprogramming factors, from the random integration of the viral vectors used in cellular reprogramming ("insertional oncogenesis"), and from genetic instability, potentially leading to both chromosomal aberrations and mutations. Progress to clinical trials requires definitive clarification of this key concern.

Direct Reprogramming

In contrast to the iPSC approach, which seeks to initially reprogram somatic cells to a pluripotent state followed by differentiation of the generated iPSCs to specific cell lineages, recently described direct reprogramming strategies aim to convert the phenotype of one mature cell type (fibroblasts) directly to another. The prototype for such a strategy was the demonstration that *MyoD*, a master regulator of skeletal muscle formation, can convert fibroblasts directly to skeletal muscle. Progress to derive other cell types after this report was delayed for many years because, unlike skeletal muscle, a single master developmental regulatory gene does not exist for most cell lineages.

Based on the experimental approach used to identify the combination of transcription factors that can reprogram somatic cells into iPSCs, researchers evaluated the ability to achieve analogous transcription factor reprogramming strategies to convert the cell fate of somatic cells directly. Consequentially, using a combination of lineage-specific developmental transcription factors, scientists were able to convert terminally differentiated fibroblasts or other somatic cells directly to neurons, β cells, different hematopoietic cell lineages, and cardiomyocyte-like cells. Recent studies have taken this concept a further step forward by demonstrating that transcription factor–based

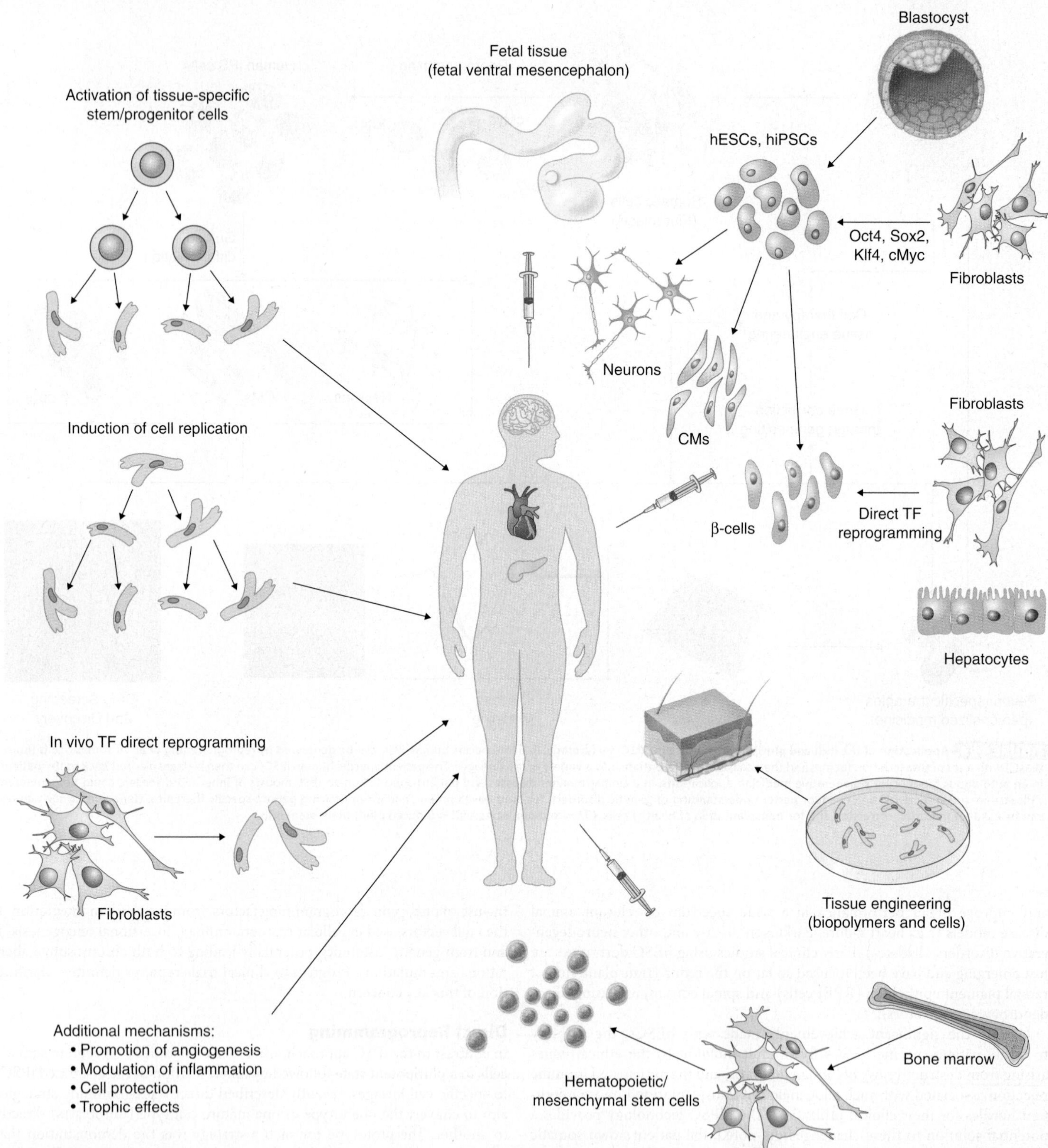

FIGURE 44-5. Conceptual framework for regenerative medicine approaches. These strategies can be divided into those attempting to augment endogenous regeneration *(left side)* and those focusing on transplantation of cells *(right side)*. The former could be achieved through the activation of putative tissue-specific stem/progenitor cells, through induction of cell replication, by in vivo transcription factor (TF)-based direct reprogramming (directly converting one somatic cell [fibroblast] into another), and by several other indirect means (e.g., modulation of inflammation, induction of angiogenesis, trophic effect, protection of tissue at risk). Cell sources that can be used for cell transplantation include fetal tissues (e.g., dopaminergic-rich fetal ventral mesencephalon for Parkinson disease), pluripotent stem cells (human embryonic stem cells [hESCs] and human induced pluripotent stem cells [hIPSCs]), derived cell-lineages, and somatic cells that can be generated ex vivo by direct transcription factor–based reprogramming of fibroblasts. CMs = cardiomyocytes.

transdifferentiation can also be achieved in vivo, suggesting a method whereby resident cells (fibroblasts, hepatic cells, or other cells) could be converted to the appropriate cell types for organ repair. Development of the latter approach for clinical application may be considered more analogous to gene therapy, with the associated advantages, shortcomings, and challenges of this discipline (see later).

Tissue Engineering

Tissue engineering is an interdisciplinary technology combining principles from life sciences and engineering with the goal of developing functional substitutes for damaged tissues and organs.[3,4] Rather than simply introducing cells into a diseased area, in tissue engineering, cells are embedded or seeded onto three-dimensional scaffolds (derived from different biomaterials) before transplantation. Regardless of the specific clinical application, tissue-engineering strategies usually involve the utilization of combinations of biomaterials, cells, and biologically active factors. The scaffold serves many purposes, including the control of the shape and size of the engrafted tissue, the delivery of biologic signals and adequate biomechanical support to the cells, the induction of vascularization of the graft, and the protection of the cells from physical damage. Scaffolds used in tissue engineering approaches are commonly divided into two general categories: (1) cellular scaffolds that are seeded ex vivo with cells before their in vivo transplantation; and (2) acellular scaffolds that depend on cells in the recipient to repopulate the scaffold with subsequent reconstitution after transplantation. Such tissue-engineered efforts have already reached proof-of-concept clinical trials. These efforts have mainly concentrated on the musculoskeletal system (bone and cartilage repair) but have also targeted other organs such as the heart and even complex organ structures such as the esophagus, trachea, and urinary bladder.

Specific Disease Applications in Cell Therapy

Although a growing number of experimental cell therapies have reached various stages of clinical trials, as yet none has become an established or approved treatment, with the aforementioned exception of hematopoietic stem cells and solid organ transplantation. Nonetheless, with the expectation of significant advances on the horizon, examples of some of the current cell therapy efforts being made in the fields of neurodegenerative disorders, heart failure, and diabetes are provided.

Neurodegenerative Disorders

The central nervous system has limited capacity for regenerating lost tissue both in slowly progressive degenerative neurologic conditions such as Parkinson disease, Alzheimer disease, and amyotrophic lateral sclerosis (ALS) and in acute injuries leading to rapid cell loss (ischemic stroke or traumatic spinal cord injury). Stem cell–based therapies are being explored as potential novel therapeutic paradigms for both acute and chronic neurodegenerative disorders.[5] Consistent with the spectrum of cell therapy–related mechanistic actions described above, these procedures could potentially act through the following mechanisms: (1) cell replacement, whereby cells (precommitted to specific neuronal or glial lineages) are transplanted to replace the specific subtypes of cells that were lost (i.e., dopaminergic neurons in Parkinson disease, motor neurons in ALS, or a mixture of different neuronal and glial subtypes in other disorders); (2) trophic support, whereby the engrafted cells are used to promote the survival of affected neurons or glia or stimulate endogenous repair of the diseased central nervous system through the secretion of neurotrophic factors; and (3) modulation of the inflammatory process thought to contribute to the pathogenesis of many neurodegenerative processes. Achieving the first mechanistic goal, despite being the most attractive, is probably also the most challenging because one would need not only to derive a clinically relevant number of the specific glial or neuronal subtypes or a combination of these cells but also to deliver them to the appropriate site (either focally or diffusely throughout the brain), as well as to assure cell-graft survival, its continuous and appropriate function, and importantly, its integration with the host neuronal network.

Parkinson disease (Chapter 409) involves loss of melanin-containing dopaminergic neurons within the substantia nigra pars compacta of the midbrain, coupled with accompanying depletion of striatal dopamine. This cellular loss is responsible for the major motor features of the disease. In the search for a more definitive therapy than pharmacology, early reports of cell replacement therapy suggested significant improvement in motor function after intrastriatal implantation of mesencephalic dopamine-rich tissue, obtained from aborted human fetuses aged 6 to 9 weeks. Long-term immunosuppressive treatment is essential to allow transplanted dopaminergic neurons to develop into their full functional potential despite the notion of an immunologic sanctuary within the brain. Clinical assessment standards have provided evidence of long-lived graft survival, morphologic and functional integration, and clinical benefit after therapy with cells of fetal origin that have now lasted up to 10 years or longer in some patients. Further progress, however, has been limited by lack of sufficient source tissue to treat a large number of affected patients, prohibitive variability in functional outcome, reports of serious dyskinesias in a subset of treated patients, and ethical considerations.

Given the aforementioned limitations of fetal tissue engraftment, stem cell derivatives could offer a viable alternative for the treatment of Parkinson disease by either replacing the dopaminergic neurons or slowing the degeneration process and restoring the integrity of the nigrostriatal pathway through the release of trophic factors. Importantly, dopaminergic neuroblast-like cells have been generated ex vivo from different stem cell sources, including pluripotent stem cells (hESCs and hiPSCs) by direct fibroblast reprogramming, neural stem cells and progenitors from the embryonic ventral mesencephalon, and adult neural stem cells from the subventricular zone. Preclinical engraftment studies demonstrated that such cells could survive in animal models of Parkinson disease and exert beneficial functional effects after cell maturation. Nevertheless, some properties that are fundamental for successful clinical translation have not been fully met in animal transplantation trials employing human stem cell–derived dopaminergic neurons. Additional challenges that should be addressed include development of methods to prevent the disease process from also destroying the grafted neurons (e.g., engineering the cells to secrete neurotrophic factors) and limiting graft-induced dyskinesia (e.g., by minimizing the number of serotonergic neuroblasts in the grafted tissue).

Investigations of stem cell–based approaches for the treatment of other neurodegenerative diseases, including ALS, Alzheimer disease, Batten disease, stroke, and brain and spinal cord injury, are now moving from experimental animal model studies to planning of clinical trials. Recent reports have shown a major clinical benefit in animal models of directed differentiation and transplantation of hESCs and hiPSCs toward retinal pigment epithelum. Human studies with these cells were recently initiated for patients suffering from macular degeneration.

Heart Disease

Although recent studies have challenged the dogma of the heart being a completely terminally differentiating organ, the endogenous repair mechanisms of the adult heart are usually inadequate in dealing with an extensive myocardial infarction. The resulting decrease in the contractile mass, which is associated with the loss of approximately 1 billion cardiomyocytes, may lead to the development of clinical heart failure (Chapters 58 and 59). With heart failure being the leading cause of hospitalization and with the paucity of donor organs limiting the number of heart transplantations worldwide, it is not surprising that the heart has become the focus of various regenerative medicine efforts.[6]

The first cells that reached clinical trials for heart failure were skeletal myoblasts. Such cells could be harvested (satellite cells) in an autologous manner, expanded ex vivo, and transplanted to the heart. However, skeletal myoblasts display different physiologic properties than cardiomyocytes and cannot form electromechanical connections with host cardiac tissue. Consequentially, these clinical efforts have largely been abandoned because of lack of efficacy as well as evidence suggesting increasing arrhythmogenicity in some patients.

The largest clinical experience in myocardial cell therapy comes from the use of bone marrow–derived stem cells (primarily hematopoietic stem cells and more recently also mesenchymal stem cells). The effects of delivery of such cells (mainly through the coronary circulation) were studied in thousands of patients, primarily in the setting of acute or recent myocardial infarction. These studies revealed either a neutral effect on myocardial performance or mild functional improvement. Although a recent meta-analysis of 33 randomized controlled trials studying transplantation of adult bone marrow–derived cells revealed a statistically significant improvement in left ventricular ejection fraction, this improvement was not associated with a change in mortality.[A1]

Bone marrow–derived stem cells are thought to exert their beneficial effects through the secretion of different growth factors rather than transforming to become new heart cells. Consequentially, a cell source that could truly re-muscularize the heart is direly needed. A potential candidate for such a task could be the recently described cardiac progenitor cells. Several reports have described cardiac progenitor cells as multipotent clonogenic cells that could be isolated based on different markers or culturing properties and potentially differentiate into cardiomyocytes and vascular cells. Such cells can be harvested from the heart (during surgery or a percutaneous cardiac catheterization biopsy approach), expanded ex vivo, and then transplanted back to the left ventricle in an autologous manner.

In contrast to the aforementioned cell types, human pluripotent stem cell lines (hESCs and hiPSCs) can undoubtedly become cardiomyocytes during ex vivo differentiation. Research efforts in recent years established efficient directed differentiation systems that could give rise to clinically relevant numbers of cardiomyocytes and demonstrated the ability of the generated cells to engraft, functionally integrate with host cardiac tissue, and improve myocardial performance in animal models of myocardial infarction. Nevertheless, issues related to ethics and the allogeneic nature of the graft (hESCs), to the inefficient and incomplete reprogramming process (iPSCs), to the heterogeneous and relatively immature properties of the generated cardiomyocytes, to the tumorigenic risk, and to the complex regulatory and financial issues have hindered clinical development of these cells to date.

Most recent efforts in the field have focused on attempting to induce mature cardiomyocytes to reenter the cell cycle (directly or after an initial dedifferentiation phase) or to convert the phenotype of nonmyocytes (fibroblasts) into cardiomyocytes. In the latter approach, recent studies have demonstrated the ability to convert the phenotype of murine fibroblasts both in vitro and in vivo into cardiomyocyte-like cells by the expression of a combination of cardiomyocyte-specific transcription factors (GATA-4, MEF-2C, and TBX-5 in one study). Although these and other efforts have the potential to augment the number of cardiomyocytes and consequentially improve contraction of the failing heart, they are still in the early phase of discovery.

Diabetes Mellitus

Successful pancreatic transplantation and improved glucocorticoid-free protocols for transplantation of islets of Langerhans have been shown not only to restore glucose control in patients with diabetes mellitus but also to prevent or even reverse some of the disease's complications (Chapters 229). However, whole organ or islet-based transplantation approaches are limited both by immunologic rejection and by limitation of an available source of transplantable tissues. This has motivated the search for cell types that can replace (type 1 diabetes mellitus) or augment (type 2 diabetes mellitus) deficient β-cell function.[7]

The development of hESCs and hiPSCs, coupled with improved understanding of β-cell development, has provided a potentially unique cell source to derive β cells for transplantation therapy. β cells make an especially attractive case for cell replacement strategies because only a single cell type is missing, cell replacement does not necessarily need to be performed in the native environment (pancreas), and, theoretically, such cells could even be engrafted subcutaneously. Harnessing lessons from embryology, efficient protocols were developed to promote differentiation of pluripotent cells in vitro into precursor or early-stage β-cell phenotype. More recent efforts have moved the field even closer to clinical application by tackling the challenge of creating more mature and functional β cells.

One of the problems with using β cells for cell replacement therapy is that the autoimmune destruction of endogenous β cells, which underlies the pathogenesis of type 1 diabetes, will probably also result in the destruction of the pluripotent cell–derived β cells, even when derived from an autologous (hiPSCs) source. Consequentially, significant efforts are being made to develop the biotechnologic means (encapsulation technologies) to deliver the cells in an immunoprotective environment that will prevent cell rejection but will retain the capacity of the engrafted β cells to sense glucose and to secrete insulin.

Beyond the derivation of new β cells from pluripotent stem cells, progress has also been made in reprogramming closely related cell types to β cells by the overexpressing of master regulatory transcription factors. Early studies focused on the conversion of hepatocytes to β-like cells through the overexpression of PDX1, the transcription factor MAFA, and NeuroD. In vivo transdifferentiation of mouse acinar cells to β cells has been achieved by transient viral overexpression of three transcription factors (PDX1, NGN3, and MAFA), whereas overexpression of a single transcription factor, PAX4, has successfully converted murine α cells to β cells.

Regenerative strategy focuses on increasing pancreatic β-cell mass by inducing the replication of existing β cells. This therapeutic approach would probably mainly target type 2 diabetic patients by decreasing the burden on existing overworked β cells but may also be beneficial for some patients with type 1 diabetes who still retain some β-cell mass. Whereas several tissues are regenerated by differentiation of tissue-specific stem cells, new pancreatic β cells are derived from the replication of existing β cells. Promising candidates for augmenting β-cell replication were recently identified and include the use of glucokinase activators or betatrophin, a protein secreted by the liver.

Stem Cell–Derived Platforms for Disease Modeling, Personalized Medicine, and Drug Discovery

In addition to the generation of cells for regenerative applications, the ability to grow a wide variety of different specialized cell types of human origin in culture provides unparalleled opportunities for gene and drug discovery and testing. For example, the ability to grow human cardiomyocytes in culture provides a preclinical human cellular-based experimental platform for screening newly developed drugs in terms of their potential to cause QT-interval prolongation and hence the risk for arrhythmia in the clinical setting. Other examples include the creation of an experimental tissue microenvironment of human origin for studying the stromal response to tumor growth and testing anticancer drugs that target tumorigenic responses such as angiogenesis.[8]

The hiPSC technology has further revolutionized this field because it allows for the first time the generation of disease/genotype- and patient-specific hiPSC models of a wide array of inherited disorders. Initial studies focused on diseases with monogenic inheritance, but more recent studies have included diseases with more complex inheritance patterns.[9] Consequently, different types of patient-specific hiPSC-derived neurons, cardiomyocytes, skeletal muscle, blood cells, hepatocytes, and other cell types were demonstrated to recapitulate in a culture dish the abnormal phenotype of a wide array of genetic disorders, including neurodegenerative disorders (e.g., spinal muscular atrophy, familial dysautonomia, ALS, schizophrenia, and even late-onset diseases such as Parkinson and Alzheimer disease), different cardiomyopathies and arrhythmogenic syndromes, a wide array of blood disorders, and several other genetic disorders. These models have already yielded important insights into the mechanisms underlying these disease states and have established unique experimental platforms that will enable the testing of existing therapies in a patient-specific manner (personalized medicine) to evaluate evolving therapies ("clinical studies in the culture dish") and to develop new therapeutic strategies.

GENE THERAPY

Gene therapy can be broadly defined as the transfer of genetic material into cells to restore or correct a cellular dysfunction or to provide a new cellular function in an attempt to cure a disease or at least to improve the clinical status of a patient. The use of genes as therapeutic platforms emerged during the mid-20th century, and in the 1990s, the first regulated registered studies were performed in the United States. In the first clinical study, a 4-year-old girl with adenosine deaminase (ADA) deficiency was treated by transfecting the ADA gene into her white blood cells, resulting in improvements in her immune system. Since then, more than 10,000 patients have been involved in more than 1700 gene therapy clinical studies performed throughout the world. The most common patient populations targeted in these studies have been cancer patients (more than 1000 studies), with another important category being monogenic inherited disorders (more than 100 studies). Although gene therapy initially was conceived as a way to treat life-threatening disorders (inborn errors, cancers) refractory to conventional treatment, it is now being explored for non-life-threatening conditions that adversely affect a patient's quality of life.

Although early clinical failures and a number of reported deaths (only two of which were actually attributed directly to gene therapy) and cases of gene therapy–related leukemic transformation led many to dismiss gene therapy as hazardous and premature, recent clinical successes have bolstered new optimism in the promise of this discipline. These include entirely novel initiatives in treating primary immunodeficiency syndromes, the improvement of vision in patients with the retinal disease (e.g., Leber congenital amaurosis), the successful treatment of X-linked adrenoleukodystrophy,[10] and the encouragement of experimental results in treating different forms of cancer.

Despite these success stories, only a few gene therapy agents are currently approved and available. Fomivirsen (Vitravene) is used for the treatment of cytomegalovirus retinitis in patients with AIDS. In 2012, Glybera became the first gene therapy treatment to be approved for clinical use in either Europe or the United States. Glybera uses a virus injected into a patient to deliver a working copy of a gene for producing lipoprotein lipase (LPL) to treat the rare inherited disorder of LPL deficiency. Finally, the *p53* tumor suppressor coding sequence in an adenovirus vector is used for the treatment of head and neck cancer but is registered only in China.

Classifications and Mechanisms of Action

In general, somatic gene therapy applications can be divided into those aiming to treat or correct various genetic disorders and those targeting nongenetic diseases by attempting to alter cell, tissue, and organ function in a favorable manner. According to the World Health Organization, there are more than 10,000 disorders with monogenic inheritance described in humans (http://www.who.int/genomics/public/geneticdiseases/en/index2.html), but only a small fraction of these may be amenable to gene therapy. Traditional gene therapy efforts for inherited disorders have mainly focused on the exogenous expression of genes encoding the missing or abnormal proteins and to a lesser extent also on altering the abnormal gene expression patterns. Future efforts are expected to shift the focus from uncontrolled overexpression of the missing protein to directly correcting the mutation at the DNA level (gene-editing strategies) in affected cells, using the newly emerging technologies known as the TALEN and CRISPR[11] approaches described in greater detail later under Gene Editing. With successful widespread use in research studies and proven applications in editing of gene sequence in stem cells, the transition to clinical application is sure to follow.

For nongenetic disorders, gene therapy efforts are aimed at overexpressing a specific protein in an attempt to alter cellular function favorably (e.g., to increase contractility in heart failure by overexpression of the sarcoplasmic reticulum calcium ATPase SERCA2a), protect tissue at risk (e.g., in acute kidney injury), exert paracrine effects through local secretion of specific proteins by the engineered cells (e.g., promote angiogenesis in ischemic tissues or induce neurotrophic effects in neurodegenerative disorders), and even secrete proteins systemically (e.g., in gene therapy trials attempting to correct bleeding disorders by secretion of coagulation factors or for systemic delivery of hormones such as erythropoietin for the treatment of anemia). Major efforts in the gene therapy arena to date have been in designing various methods to treat cancer (see later).

Progress in the field of gene therapy has developed into two different strategies: ex vivo and in vivo gene therapy. The ex vivo gene therapy approach (combined cell and gene therapy strategy) involves the initial harvesting of cells from a given patient followed by genetic modification of these cells in the laboratory. The genetically modified cells can then be selected, amplified in numbers, and returned to the same patient in an attempt to achieve the desired therapeutic effect. This strategy is particularly attractive for the genetic modification of stem cells that could reconstitute the relevant tissues, organs, and organ systems after transplantation. The most prominent example is using hematopoietic stem cell grafts in gene therapy trials for hematopoietic disorders.

The in vivo gene therapy approach, in contrast, involves the delivery of the relevant transgene (through the use of various vectors) directly to the targeted tissue, followed by the stable or transient expression of the transgene in the relevant cells. The expression of the transgene only in the relevant cells/tissues can be achieved by a combination of localized delivery (injection), a particular tropism of the vector used for the tissue of interest, and the expression of the transgene under the control of a cell/tissue-specific promoter.

Gene Therapy Delivery Methods

Gene therapy agents are often composed of two elements: the genetic material itself (i.e., the DNA expression cassette [the most common therapeutic payload used], short interfering RNA, or an antisense molecule) and the vector delivery system. The latter is usually the more complex and limiting component, and it is important to select the most efficient delivery method for any genetic therapy as well as to be aware of the potential adverse effects of each vector type, thus tailoring the therapy to specific clinical considerations. There are formidable barriers to successful gene transfer, such as crossing the cellular membrane, escaping from the endosome, moving through the nuclear membrane, and integrating into the host genome. Vectors that have been developed to try to overcome these obstacles fall into two broad categories: nonviral and viral vectors.

Gene therapy mediated by nonviral vectors is referred to as *transfection* and consists of the direct delivery of naked DNA by injection, the use of liposomes (cationic lipids mixed with nucleic acids), nanoparticles, and other means. Although nonviral vectors can be produced in relatively large amounts and are likely to present minimal toxic or immunologic problems, their major shortcoming is inefficient gene transfer. In addition, expression of the foreign gene tends to be transient, precluding the application of nonviral vectors to many disease states in which sustained and high-level expression of the transgene is required. The efficiency of nonviral vector delivery could be enhanced by the use of different physical methods that have evolved, such as electroporation (for well-circumscribed body compartments or masses such as muscle, skin, and tumors), gene gun (for DNA vaccination), and ultrasound delivery (for cardiovascular and tumor-related applications).

Gene therapy mediated by viral vectors is referred to as *transduction*, and this approach has been the main conduit for transferring genes to human cells in most gene therapy trials. The basic concept of viral vectors is to harness the innate ability of viruses to deliver genetic material into the infected cell. Viruses used in gene therapy have been modified to enhance safety, increase specific uptake, and improve efficiency. However, for each specific virus-based gene therapy vector, there have been major disadvantages that should be balanced against potential therapeutic benefits. For example, in cancer gene therapy, the immune response to the delivery vehicle carrying the anticancer genetic material can be used to advantage by serving as an adjuvant. In contrast, the system for delivery of a gene to be expressed for a prolonged period to replace or supplement a missing gene product in monogenic disease states should preferably be ignored by the immune system.

Viral vectors are derived from viruses with either RNA (retroviruses and lentiviruses) or DNA (adenovirus, adeno-associated virus [AAV], herpes simplex virus [HSV], and poxvirus [vaccine virus]) genomes. Viral vectors also fall into one of two main categories: integrating vectors, which insert themselves into the recipient's genome, and nonintegrating vectors, which often (although not always) form an extrachromosomal genetic element. Integrating vectors, such as γ-retroviral vectors and lentiviral vectors, are generally used to transfect actively dividing cells because they are stably inherited. Integrating vectors, however, may carry the risk for insertional mutagenesis (with clinical oncogenic transformations reported with the use of retroviruses). Nonintegrating vectors, such as adenoviral vectors and AAV vectors, can be used to transfect quiescent or slowly dividing cells, but they are quickly (in the case of adenoviral vectors) lost from cells that divide rapidly. Finally, efficient gene transduction can also be achieved using vectors that are maintained as episomes, especially in nondividing cells.

Adenoviral vectors and retroviral vectors based on Moloney murine leukemia virus featured prominently in early gene therapy trials. There has been a movement away from both, however, after the case of a fatality, which was linked to the toxicity of the adenoviral vector (used to introduce the ornithine transcarbamylase gene in that specific study) and the leukemia cases in SCID-X1 patients (which were linked with activation of *LMO2*, an oncogene on chromosome 11, due to insertional mutagenesis associated with the murine leukemia viral vector). Consequentially, these vectors have been largely been replaced with AAV and lentiviral vectors, respectively, which have become the most common vectors used in clinical trials today. Other viral vectors may have applications in specific settings. For example, in gene therapy applications being developed for pain management, a replication-defective HSV vector is being used because of its tropism for nerve tissues. Also, different oncolytic viruses with a preferential tropism to cancer cells are being used for gene therapy applications in cancer.

Diseases Treated by Gene Therapy

Inherited Immunodeficiency

More than 30 patients reported to date worldwide have undergone treatment with different retroviral vectors for inherited immunodeficiencies (Chapter 250). Patients with one of the following three diseases are included in this group: two types of severe combined immunodeficiency (SCID), both of which are characterized by dysregulation of lymphocyte development, and X-linked chronic granulomatous disease (X-CGD), an inherited immune deficiency with absent phagocyte reduced nicotinamide adenine diphosphate oxidase activity caused by mutations in the *gp91* (*phox*) gene. Individuals with adenosine deaminase (ADA) SCID suffer from premature death of T, B, and natural killer (NK) cells as a result of the accumulation of purine metabolites; patients with this condition have been treated with vectors expressing the *ADA* gene. In the first patients with ADA SCID, transduced T cells expressing transgenic *ADA* have been shown to persist for longer than 10 years; however, the therapeutic effect of gene therapy resulted in incomplete correction of the metabolic defect. More recently, an improved gene transfer protocol of bone marrow CD34-positive cells, combined with low-dose busulfan, resulted in multilineage, stable engraftment of transduced progenitors at substantial levels, restoration of immune function, correction of the *ADA* metabolic defect, and proven clinical benefit.[12] Overall, no adverse effect or toxicity has been observed in patients treated with *ADA* gene transfer in mature lymphocytes or hematopoietic progenitors.

The X-linked type (X-SCID group), in which there is defective cytokine-dependent survival signaling in T and NK cells, was shown to be corrected by introduction of the wild-type sequence of the common γ-C chain, which is an essential component of five cytokine receptors. In one clinical study, hematologic malignancies developed in four patients. One of the four died of this complication. Ten patients were successfully treated with a different viral transduction protocol, with one reported malignancy in up to 8 years of follow-up. Two adult X-CGD patients who suffered recurrent bacterial infections have been treated with CD34-positive cells transduced with a γ-retroviral vector expressing *gp91 phox*, with significant clinical improvement in the short term. However, in both these patients, there was an expansion of gene-transduced cells caused by the transcriptional activation of growth-promoting genes leading to myelodysplasia and gradual loss of efficacy. In summary, of the nearly 30 patients worldwide treated with gene therapy for immunodeficiency disorders, significant clinical improvement has been observed in many. However, severe and even life-endangering adverse consequences have been encountered with certain viral vectors and protocols. Additional clinical information from long-term observation and new clinical studies will be important for a clearer assessment of clinical benefit.[13]

Visual Loss

Both cell- and gene-based therapy approaches are leading areas for promising inroads in retinal disease. Although early trials of stem cell–based retinal cell therapy have not yet achieved proof of efficacy, at the level of gene therapy, clinical scientists have used gene augmentation therapy with direct subretinal injection of a recombinant AAV expressing *RPE65* complementary DNA in adults and children with Leber congenital amaurosis. This rare inherited eye disease destroys photoreceptors (Chapter 424), and the gene therapy results have shown medical evidence of visual preservation despite continued retinal degeneration.[14]

Cardiovascular and Pulmonary Conditions

Gene therapy efforts in the cardiovascular field have focused on achieving therapeutic angiogenesis in patients suffering from chronic ischemic heart disease[A2][A3] or from critical limb ischemia (CLI) and for improving cardiac function in heart failure patients. The use of genes to revascularize the ischemic myocardium due to coronary artery disease and CLI due to peripheral artery disease has been the focus of two decades of preclinical research with a variety of angiogenic mediators, including vascular endothelial growth factor, fibroblast growth factor, hepatocyte growth factor, and others, encoded by DNA plasmids or adenovirus vectors. Overall, these gene therapy studies in animal experimental models of ischemia were very encouraging, leading eventually to several clinical trials. Despite the established proof of concept and reasonable safety, however, results of the latest clinical trials on therapeutic angiogenesis for myocardial ischemia and CLI have provided inconsistent results, and the definite means of inducing clinically useful therapeutic angiogenesis remain elusive. These less than optimal results may stem from a number of reasons, including the application of a single growth factor that may not be sufficient to meet the multifaceted challenge for developing efficient induction of collateral vessels, the need for more sustained growth factor delivery in order to establish more stable vessels, and the need to target arteriogenesis rather than angiogenesis to achieve a more significant increase in perfusion. Therefore, efforts in the field are moving toward the use of different cell therapies for these ischemic conditions, as well as using combined cell and gene delivery strategies to achieve better outcomes. For example, a recent trial has used combined delivery of endothelial and smooth muscle cells (each cell type modified to secrete a different angiogenic growth factor) in CLI patients.

For heart failure, gene therapy trials have focused on restoring the abnormal calcium handling characteristic of failing human cardiomyocytes.[15] Because a reduction in levels of the sarcoplasmic reticulum calcium ATPase (SERCA2a), the sarcoplasmic reticulum calcium pump, was found to be a key factor in the alteration of calcium cycling in heart failure, this protein became an attractive clinical target for gene delivery purposes. Overexpression of SERCA2a levels by cardiomyocyte gene delivery has led to the restoration of previously abnormal calcium transients and to improved cardiac contractility, reduction of the frequency of arrhythmias, and improved oxygen utilization in animal models of heart failure. More recently, the clinical benefits of overexpressing SERCA2a have been demonstrated in phase I and II of the Calcium Upregulation by Percutaneous Administration of Gene Therapy in Cardiac Disease (CUPID) trials.[A4] These studies demonstrated that AAV delivery of the SERCA2a transgene by intracoronary delivery is feasible and safe, results in persistent expression of the transgene, and is associated with a significant improvement in associated biochemical alterations and clinical symptoms of heart failure in the treated patients.

Cystic Fibrosis

Experimental protocols for gene therapy for cystic fibrosis (CF) (Chapter 89) have been implemented since 1990. The cystic fibrosis transmembrane conductance regulator (CFTR) protein is mutated in patients with CF. Transducing the epithelium of the nasal and bronchial tree is potentially feasible through nonsystemic approaches. Nonviral gene therapy methods that deliver a copy of the *CFTR* gene to the airway of CF patients have been developed. Several placebo-controlled clinical trials of liposome-mediated *CFTR* gene transfer to the nasal epithelium have confirmed its safety and demonstrated variable degrees of functional correction. In addition, several clinical studies have assessed the potential of retrovectors, adenovectors, and AAV vectors for gene therapy for CF. With both nonviral and viral delivery systems, there were only mild side effects. However, the long-term clinical benefit has been marginal. Improved vectors are being assessed in preclinical studies.

Cancer

One of the most exciting opportunities for gene therapy lies in the cancer arena. Gene therapy strategies targeting cancer can be grouped according to their proposed mechanisms of action and include gene therapies aiming to directly induce cytotoxic effects in cancer cells (through the use of oncolytic viruses or by the delivery of apoptotic inducers and suicide genes), gene therapies aiming to boost the immune response to tumor antigens, and gene therapies targeting the tumor microenvironment.

Direct Cytotoxic Effects

An interesting approach for cancer gene therapy is to harness the action of oncolytic viruses.[16] Oncolytic viruses are therapeutically useful anticancer viruses that will selectively infect, amplify, and then damage cancerous tissues without causing harm to normal tissues. Cancer selectivity of the different oncolytic viruses takes advantage of defects commonly found across many tumor types, such as lack of antiviral responses, activation of Ras pathways, loss of tumor suppressors, and defective apoptosis. Oncolytic viruses can kill infected cancer cells in many different ways, ranging from direct virus-mediated cytotoxicity through a variety of cytotoxic immune effector mechanisms.

Several viruses such as the Newcastle disease virus (which activates the innate or adaptive immune response), reovirus (which activates host protein kinases to shut down protein production), and mumps virus have an inherent ability to specifically target cancer cells and, upon virus replication, cause significant cell death and tumor regression. Other viruses (HSV, adenovirus, vaccinia virus, vesicular stomatitis virus, and poliovirus) need to be genetically engineered to engender oncolytic activity. Genetically engineered viruses and inherently antitumor-selective viruses are being tested in early and late clinical conditions to determine their effectiveness in specific types of cancer (e.g., metastatic melanoma and different brain tumors).

Beyond the direct viral cytopathic effect, viral vectors can be used to deliver genes to cancer cells that will result in tumor cell death. The relevant transgenes encode for cellular proteins that are involved in apoptosis or prevent proliferation. The selectivity for the activation of such genes only in tumor cells is achieved either through the use of the aforementioned oncolytic viruses or by the expression of the transgenes under the control of promoters that are activated only in cancer cells, either as a general property of cancer (e.g., human telomerase or survivin) or in specific types of tumors (probasin in prostate cancer, ceruloplasmin in ovarian cancer, HER2 in breast cancer, and carcinoembryonic antigen in colon cancer). The most clinically advanced gene therapy drug against cancer is the replication-deficient adenovector expressing the human *p53* gene. This therapy (Gendicine) is approved in China for the treatment of patients with head and neck squamous cell carcinoma by direct administration into the tumor bed.

Another attractive approach is the use of suicide genes. Suicide gene therapy involves delivery of a pro-drug activating enzyme (suicide gene) that converts nontoxic pro-drugs to cytotoxic metabolites. The prototype for such a suicide gene/pro-drug combination is HSV thymidine kinase (TK)/ganciclovir (GCV). The TK gene is selectively expressed only in cancer cells (by one of the methods described previously), and after application of GCV, it converts it to the cytotoxic agent phosphorylated GCV. Interestingly, phosphorylated GCV is only toxic to dividing cells, further increasing the selectivity to the cancer cells. Other cytotoxic strategies are to express secreted pro-apoptotic proteins, such as tumor necrosis factor–related apoptosis-inducing ligand (TRAIL) or cytotoxins such as *Pseudomonas* exotoxin.

Immunomodulatory Cell and Gene Therapy for Cancer and Autoimmune Disease

In recent years, the focus of gene- and cell-based therapy for cancer has shifted away from directly manipulating or targeting the cancer cells toward modulation of the immune system itself. Cytotoxic T-lymphocyte antigen 4 (CTLA-4) and programmed death 1 (PD-1) are two T-lymphocyte proteins that have long been known to attenuate immune destruction of cancer cells. Blocking monoclonal antibodies to circumvent this attenuation have been shown to induce limited remissions in several forms of previously intractable metastatic tumors, including malignant melanoma. These partial successes have now revived still more sophisticated therapeutic approaches, based on the ex vivo personalized genetic engineering of cytotoxic T lymphocytes of cancer patients to enable the immune system to target tumor cells. Chimeric antigen receptor (CAR) therapy releases the encumbrance of major histocompatibility complex restriction in cancer antigen recognition by combining the antigen-binding site of a monoclonal antibody with the signal-activating machinery of the cytotoxic T lymphocytes. This enables combining a high level of target specificity typical of monoclonal antibodies with in vivo expansion and the potential for a durable response, as has been demonstrated in clinical treatment protocols in leukemia and other malignancies.[17] It can be anticipated that CAR-modified T lymphocytes might also prove useful as a combined genetic engineering/cell therapy approach to the management of autoimmune disease.

Disrupting Tumor Microenvironment

Targeting the tumor microenvironment is another attractive approach for cancer gene therapy because it consists of normal cells that should not develop resistance to the therapy. The most obvious target is the tumor neovascularization process. The use of antiangiogenic drugs such as bevacizumab (Avastin), an anti–vascular endothelial growth factor monoclonal antibody, has shown success in clinical trials for some cancer cell types, but the effect may be transient or negligible in others. This may be because the angiogenesis process is complex, and inhibiting just one aspect may not be sufficient. Developing alternative strategies such as combination therapies, including targeting multiple angiogenic pathways, might be a better strategy, especially because inhibiting angiogenesis is cytostatic and not cytotoxic. A number of antiangiogenic factors (e.g., angiostatin) have been expressed in viral vectors and have been used in preclinical studies but have not reached the clinic yet.

Other Forms of Molecular Therapies: RNA Interference and Gene Editing

RNA Interference

RNA interference (RNAi) regulates gene expression by a highly precise mechanism of sequence-directed gene silencing at the stage of translation by degrading specific messenger RNAs or by blocking their translation into protein. Research on the use of RNAi for therapeutic applications has gained considerable momentum. It has been suggested that many of the novel disease-associated targets that have been identified are amenable to conventional small molecule drug blockade and can potentially be targeted with RNAi. In the coming years, the concept of RNAi will be actively translated into a therapeutic option, with numerous early-phase trials already underway.

Gene Editing

The center of gravity for gene therapy may be shifting from gene restoration (where a whole new gene is pasted into the genome) to genome editing, whereby the pathogenic mutation is corrected in its natural gene location with zinc finger nucleases, transcription activator–like effector nucleases (TALENs), or clustered regulatory interspaced short palindromic repeats (CRISPRs).[18,19] These hybrid molecules act as highly specific "molecular scissors," which are engineered to target a specific location in the genome and introduce a double-strand break in the DNA proximal to the targeted mutation. The cleavage in the DNA is then resolved by homologous recombination between the endogenous genes and an exogenously introduced donor fragment containing the normal sequence. In this fashion, the pathogenic mutation is permanently changed back to the normal sequence. This also preserves the architecture of the genome and maintains gene control under the normal cellular regulatory elements.

Consequentially, gene editing represents a paradigm shift in the way gene therapy could be performed. To date, gene editing techniques have been used to correct the disease-causing mutations associated with X-linked SCID, hemophilia B, sickle cell disease,[20] and α_1-antitrypsin deficiency and to repair Parkinson disease–associated mutations (*SNCA* gene) in patient-derived hiPSCs or in preclinical mouse models. Targeted gene knockout through similar technologies promises to be a potentially powerful strategy for combating HIV/AIDs. Zinc finger nucleases have been used to confer HIV-1 resistance by disabling the HIV coreceptor C-C chemokine receptor type 5 (CCR5) in primary T cells and hematopoietic stem/progenitor cells. This approach is currently used in clinical trials. Additionally, zinc finger nucleases have been used to improve the performance of T-cell-based immunotherapies by inactivating the expression of endogenous T-cell-receptor genes, thereby enabling the generation of tumor-specific T cells with improved efficacy profiles.

Finally, site-specific nucleases may also bring a unique value to the conventional gene-adding approach by enabling insertion of therapeutic transgenes into specific "safe harbor" locations in the human genome, ensuring long-term expression of the transgene as well as reducing the potential for random insertional mutagenesis.

It is important to mention that the use of site-specific nuclease technology at its current state requires the presence of proliferating cells, and its utility is therefore still relatively limited for nonproliferating somatic cells and for direct in vivo applications. Continued progress in stem cell research, including the production and manipulation of hiPSCs cells, will ultimately open countless new directions for gene therapy, including treatments based on autologous stem cell transplantation.

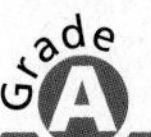

Grade A References

A1. Clifford DM, Fisher SA, Brunskill SJ, et al. Stem cell treatment for acute myocardial infarction. *Cochrane Database Syst Rev*. 2012;2:CD006536.

A2. Fisher SA, Brunskill SJ, Doree C, et al. Stem cell therapy for chronic ischaemic heart disease and congestive heart failure. *Cochrane Database Syst Rev*. 2014;4:CD007888.

A3. Wang ZX, Li D, Cao JX, et al. Efficacy of autologous bone marrow mononuclear cell therapy in patients with peripheral arterial disease. *J Atheroscler Thromb*. 2014;21:1183-1196.

A4. Zsebo K, Yaroshinsky A, Rudy JJ, et al. Long-term effects of AAV1/SERCA2a gene transfer in patients with severe heart failure: analysis of recurrent cardiovascular events and mortality. *Circ Res*. 2014;114:101-108.

GENERAL REFERENCES

For the General References and other additional features, please visit Expert Consult at https://expertconsult.inkling.com.

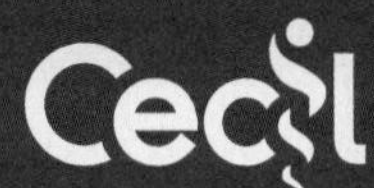

VII

PRINCIPLES OF IMMUNOLOGY AND INFLAMMATION

45

THE INNATE IMMUNE SYSTEM

MARY K. CROW

THE INNATE IMMUNE SYSTEM IN HOST DEFENSE AND DISEASE PATHOGENESIS

The immune system, comprising cells, the molecules they produce, and the organs that organize those components, evolved over millions of years in response to infections with pathogenic microorganisms.[1] Its essential role in maintaining health is based on its recognition and elimination or control of those foreign microbes. Central to the success of the protective role of the immune system is its capacity to distinguish foreign and dangerous invaders from self-components.[2,3] In addition to its contributions to host defense, the immune system is involved in the prevention of malignancy by surveying and recognizing self-cells that express novel antigens,[4] and it also plays a role in resolution and repair of tissue damage.

The immune system is generally described as including an *innate immune system* and an *adaptive immune system*. The former provides the first and rapid line of defense and cellular response to a foreign stimulus. The latter, dependent on activation by the innate immune response, develops a more specific response targeted to the offending organism and generates memory for that stimulus that can be elicited rapidly should that organism be encountered again on a later occasion.

Immune system cells derive from precursor cells of the hematopoietic lineage and populate discrete lymphoid organs, including lymph nodes, spleen, and thymus, as well as skin and intestine. Cells of the innate immune system serve as sentinels at locations that are likely to encounter foreign organisms, and after activation they will often travel to a local lymphoid organ. The induction of the adaptive immune response occurs in the context of structured aggregates of innate and adaptive immune cells in the lymphoid organs. Once activated and differentiated to produce effector molecules, immune system cells can be sampled in blood as they travel to sites of infection or tissue damage. There they can interact directly with target cells to mediate cell death or, alternatively, provide activating signals to expand or regulate a response, or secrete high local levels of immunomodulatory substances called cytokines. Cytokines are small soluble proteins that communicate among cells within the immune system or between immune system cells and cells in other tissues.[5] The cells and products of the immune system function as an exquisitely regulated complex system.[6] Inherited variations in hundreds of genes have evolved, under pressure of microbial challenge, to ensure adequate defense against pathogenic organisms across the human population.[1] However, in any one individual, the composite genetic profile can generate predisposition to infection or, alternatively, autoimmune or inflammatory disease.

The innate immune response was traditionally viewed as mediating nonspecific protection through the production of preformed effector molecules. However, important advances in characterization of the cell surface and intracellular pattern recognition receptors (PRR), particularly the toll-like receptor (TLR) family, and signaling pathways used by innate immune cells to implement a defensive response are now understood to have relative specificity for pathogen-associated molecular patterns (PAMPs) that are characteristic of categories of microbes.[7,8] In contrast to those receptor systems that initiate an innate immune response, the protein products that implement the response, whether to expand the reaction to additional cells, promote trafficking to the most relevant location, or shape the differentiation programs of adaptive immune system cells, do not show specificity based on the initial triggering stimulus. The products of the innate immune response can be highly effective at ablating or limiting the extent of infection and can generate a tissue repair program that establishes a satisfactory resolution of the episode of infection. However, when sustained or poorly regulated, they can represent an important pathophysiologic mechanism for many autoimmune and inflammatory diseases.

Cells of the Innate Immune System

Monocytes and Macrophages

Monocytes circulate in the peripheral blood with a half-life of 1 to 3 days. Macrophages arise from monocytes that have migrated out of the circulation and have proliferated and differentiated in tissue. Tissue macrophages include alveolar macrophages in the lung, Kupffer cells in the liver, osteoclasts in bone, microglia in the central nervous system, and type A synoviocytes in the synovial membrane. Macrophages secrete myriad products, including hydrolytic enzymes, reactive oxygen species, cytokines, and chemokines. Macrophages engulf microorganisms and foreign particles directly or are activated by protein complexes containing antibodies that bind to cell surface receptors for the Fc portion of immunoglobulin molecules (Fc receptors, or FcRs). These encounters activate intracellular signaling pathways that induce transcription of target genes, primarily those encoding mediators that promote inflammation or enzyme-mediated death of the microbe. Cytokines from other immune system cells, including interferon (IFN)-γ or interleukin (IL)-4, can drive macrophage differentiation toward the production of mediators that are primarily pro-inflammatory or to a wound healing functional profile. Researchers have characterized those functional phenotypes as M1 or M2, although it is recognized that the context of an innate immune response will determine the functional response, with composite profiles common.[9]

In addition to responding to foreign microbes, macrophages contribute to the elimination of senescent or apoptotic cells in a manner that avoids induction of an inflammatory response. Macrophages also interact with other cell types through complementary cell surface adhesion or costimulatory receptors. After capturing antigen, they can function as antigen-presenting cells for T lymphocytes, and they can interact with non–immune system cells such as endothelial cells or fibroblasts.

Dendritic Cells

Dendritic cells (DCs) comprise a complex family of cells that perform essential functions in the innate immune response and serve as a bridge to activation of an adaptive immune response. Myeloid dendritic cells can incorporate antigens derived from invading microbes, travel to nearby lymph nodes, and present processed antigenic peptides to T lymphocytes (T cells) in the form of peptide–major histocompatibility complex (MHC) molecule complexes. They are the most effective antigen-presenting cells based on expression of cell surface costimulatory molecules, and they produce cytokines, including IL-12 and IL-23, after interaction with PAMPs. They thereby contribute to the shaping of the T-cell differentiation program to generate effector cell functions. Plasmacytoid dendritic cells (pDCs) have been identified as highly effective producers of type I interferon, a key mediator of host defense against viral infections.

Natural Killer Cells

Natural killer (NK) and NK T cells provide early defense against viral infections and other intracellular pathogens while adaptive responses are developing.[10] NK cells are sensitized by cytokines, including type I interferons, released from pDCs and macrophages, and secrete abundant IFN-γ, which activates macrophages and other cells. They also are poised to kill virus-infected cells by injecting pore-forming enzymes and granzymes. Activation of NK cells is inhibited by interaction with self-MHC class I molecules on target cells. When those self-histocompatibility antigens are not present, NK cell–mediated killing is implemented. NK cells are important in tumor surveillance because they are able to kill MHC class I–deficient tumor cells that are no longer susceptible to adaptive immune responses. In addition to NK cells, a type of lymphocytes, so-called innate lymphoid cells, which participate early in innate immune responses but do not express rearranged receptors, is a focus of current study.[11]

Neutrophils

Neutrophils are the most abundant circulating white blood cells. They are recruited rapidly to inflammatory sites and can phagocytose and digest microbes (Chapters 167 and 169). Activation of neutrophils and phagocytosis is facilitated through the triggering of FcRs or complement receptors. Microbe-containing phagosomes fuse with lysosomes, which contain enzymes, proteins, and peptides that inactivate and digest microbes. Beyond their phagocytic capability, neutrophils produce a variety of toxic products. The release of toxic products is known as the respiratory burst because it is accompanied by an increase in oxygen consumption. During the respiratory burst, oxygen radicals are generated by nicotinamide adenine dinucleotide phosphate (NADPH) oxidases. Neutrophils also contribute to host defense through extrusion of DNA and associated proteins in the form of neutrophil extracellular traps, or NETs, to which bacteria can stick, facilitating their clearance. Despite their effective contributions to the innate immune response and microbial host defense, neutrophils can generate considerable collateral damage. NETs have the capacity to induce production of cytokines by pDCs and may damage vascular endothelial cells. Secretion of neutrophil granule contents, particularly their enzymes (myeloperoxidase, elastase, collagenase, and lysozyme), causes direct cellular injury and damages macromolecules at inflamed sites.

Eosinophils

In contrast to macrophages and neutrophils, eosinophils are only weakly phagocytic but are potent cytotoxic effector cells against parasites. Their major effector mechanism is the secretion of cationic proteins (major basic protein, eosinophil cationic protein, and eosinophil-derived neurotoxin). These proteins are released into the extracellular space, where they directly destroy the invading microorganism but can also damage host tissue (Chapter 170).

Basophils and Mast Cells

Basophils and tissue mast cells secrete inflammatory mediators such as histamine, prostaglandins, leukotrienes, and some cytokines.[12] Release of these substances is triggered when cell surface immunoglobulin E (IgE) receptors encounter monomeric IgE. They play a role in atopic allergies, in which allergens bind immunoglobulin (IgE) and cross-link FcεRs. Mast cells have been observed in rheumatoid arthritis synovial tissue and have been implicated in local inflammatory responses (Chapter 255). Like pDCs and macrophages, mast cells express TLRs and FcRs and produce cytokines after encountering immune complexes composed of TLR ligands.

Recognition Receptors and Triggers of an Innate Immune Response

Toll-like Receptors

The innate immune system utilizes both cell surface and intracellular PRRs to recognize conserved structures on microbes (PAMPs). Examples of PAMPs are bacterial lipopolysaccharides, peptidoglycans, mannans, bacterial DNA, double-stranded RNA, and glucans. The discovery and characterization of the TLR family of receptors and their relevant ligands has focused attention on the mechanisms that allow an innate immune response to shape the nature of the resulting inflammatory or repair programs, as well as the T-cell effector cell functions that follow recognition of antigens from the relevant pathogen. The TLRs have in common leucine-rich domains and bind PAMPs common to classes of pathogenic organisms.[7,8] For example, TLR-4, a cell surface–expressed PRR, binds lipopolysaccharide of gram-negative bacteria, and TLR-2 recognizes bacterial peptidoglycans and lipoproteins, often based on dimerization with other TLR family members. Important advances in understanding systemic autoimmune diseases have followed the characterization of endosomal TLRs with relative specificity for single-stranded RNA (TLR-7 and TLR-8), demethylated CpG-enriched DNA (TLR-9), and double-stranded RNA (TLR-3, which has both cell surface and endosomal forms). The distribution of particular TLRs among cells of the innate immune system varies, and additional members of the TLR family may still be discovered and characterized. The TLRs play central roles in alerting the immune system that a microbe, typically a bacteria in the case of TLR-2 and TLR-4 or a virus in the case of TLR-3, TLR-7, TLR-,8 and TLR-9, is threatening the host. But in some cases, when an immune complex with self-nucleic acid gains access to an endosomal TLR, a self-directed innate immune response can be initiated or amplified.

Cytoplasmic Nucleic Acid Sensors

Following the description of the TLR family and the capacity of the endosomal TLRs to recognize microbial and self-nucleic acids, a second category of intracellular innate immune system receptors was defined that recognize RNA or DNA from microbes, primarily viruses, that gain access to the cell cytoplasm. The DExD/H-box family of helicases include retinoic acid–inducible gene I (RIG-I) and melanoma differentiation–associated protein 5 (MDA5), described as members of the RIG-I-like receptor (RLR) family that recognizes viral RNAs with particular structural characteristics that distinguish the viral RNA from most host RNAs (Fig. 45-1).[13,14] Cytoplasmic DNA receptors have also been defined, with cyclic guanosine monophosphate–adenosine monophosphate synthase (cGAS) recently identified as an important sensor of cytoplasmic DNA that triggers an innate immune response after interacting with the stimulator of interferon genes (STING).[15] Whether RNA or DNA triggers these cytoplasmic sensors, the result is transcription and production of interferon-β and other proinflammatory cytokines that orchestrate the early phase of an antiviral immune response.

NOD Receptors

Another category of intracellular receptors is proving important in antimicrobial defense as well as contributing to activation of inflammatory states. The nucleotide-binding oligomerization domain (NOD)-like receptor (NLR) family comprises components of an intracellular structure called the inflammasome, a signaling platform that organizes innate immune system activation in response to some stimuli.[16] The inflammasome can activate caspase 1, an enzyme important for maturation of the pro-inflammatory cytokines IL-1β and IL-18. The NLRP3-containing inflammasome has been best studied and implicated in the inflammatory response to monosodium urate crystals, the triggers of gout attacks (Chapter 273). Mutations in the *NLRP3* gene are the basis of chronic autoinflammatory syndromes that are associated with exaggerated production of IL-1 (reviewed in Chapter 261).

C-Type Lectin Receptors

Members of the C-type lectin receptor family have a carbohydrate recognition domain and a calcium-binding domain that promotes signaling after interaction with carbohydrate-expressing microbes as well as self-molecules. DC-SIGN (DC-specific intracellular adhesion molecule-3 grabbing nonintegrin) is an example of a family member that recognizes high-mannose-containing structures on foreign antigens and supports DC activation. Mannose receptors on macrophages, dendritic cells, and other cell types, such as renal mesangial cells, participate in clearance of microbes as well as antigen trapping for presentation to adaptive immune system cells. The selectin family of proteins have a lectin domain, bind to carbohydrate ligands, and mediate the first steps of leukocyte migration. L-selectin is present on virtually all leukocytes; P-selectin and E-selectin are expressed on activated endothelial cells, and P-selectin is also stored in platelets. Selectins capture floating leukocytes and initiate their attachment and rolling on activated endothelial cells.

Scavenger Receptors

Scavenger receptors comprise a diverse family of receptors with the common functional role of binding various ligands and transporting or removing nonself or altered-self targets.[17] They can participate in clearance of microorganisms and cholesterol transport but can also contribute to disease pathology. For example, among the scavenger receptors is the receptor for oxidized low-density lipoproteins, which can promote generation of lipid-laden macrophages and atherosclerosis when accumulated in excess, and receptors for relatively inert substances such as silicon, which can drive an inflammatory response once taken into phagocytic cells. Scavenger receptors can also participate in activation of the inflammasome, as can occur after binding serum amyloid A protein.

Inhibitory Natural Killer Cell Receptors

The immunoglobulin-like killer inhibitory receptor (KIR) family of receptors participates in distinguishing self-cells from cells of foreign origin or tumor cells expressing modified-self-molecules. NK cells are ready to produce their toxic mediators, but they are held in check by inhibitory receptors that recognize MHC class I or MHC class I–like molecules.[10] Recognition of MHC class I molecules provides a negative signal that suppresses cell activity. The observation that NK cells kill target cells lacking MHC class I molecules recognized as self led to the missing-self hypothesis. By screening cell surfaces for the expression of MHC class I molecules, the innate immune system collects information about the intactness of tissues, emphasizing the crucial role of MHC class I molecules as markers of tissue integrity.

Fc and Complement Receptors

Most cells of the innate immune system possess receptors (FcRs) that specifically interact with the constant region (Fc portion) of immunoglobulins and can bind antibodies attached to antigens. The isotype of the antibody determines which cell type is activated in a given response. Triggering of most FcRs transmits activating signals; however, inhibitory FcRs on B lymphocytes (B cells) and macrophages can limit responses. Ligation of an FcγR on macrophages or neutrophils triggers phagocytosis of the antigen, activation of respiratory burst, and induction of cytotoxicity. On NK cells, FcγRs initiate antibody-dependent cell-mediated cytotoxicity. FcRs on pDCs are important for bringing immune complexes into intracellular compartments containing endosomal TLRs. FcRs on mast cells, basophils, and activated

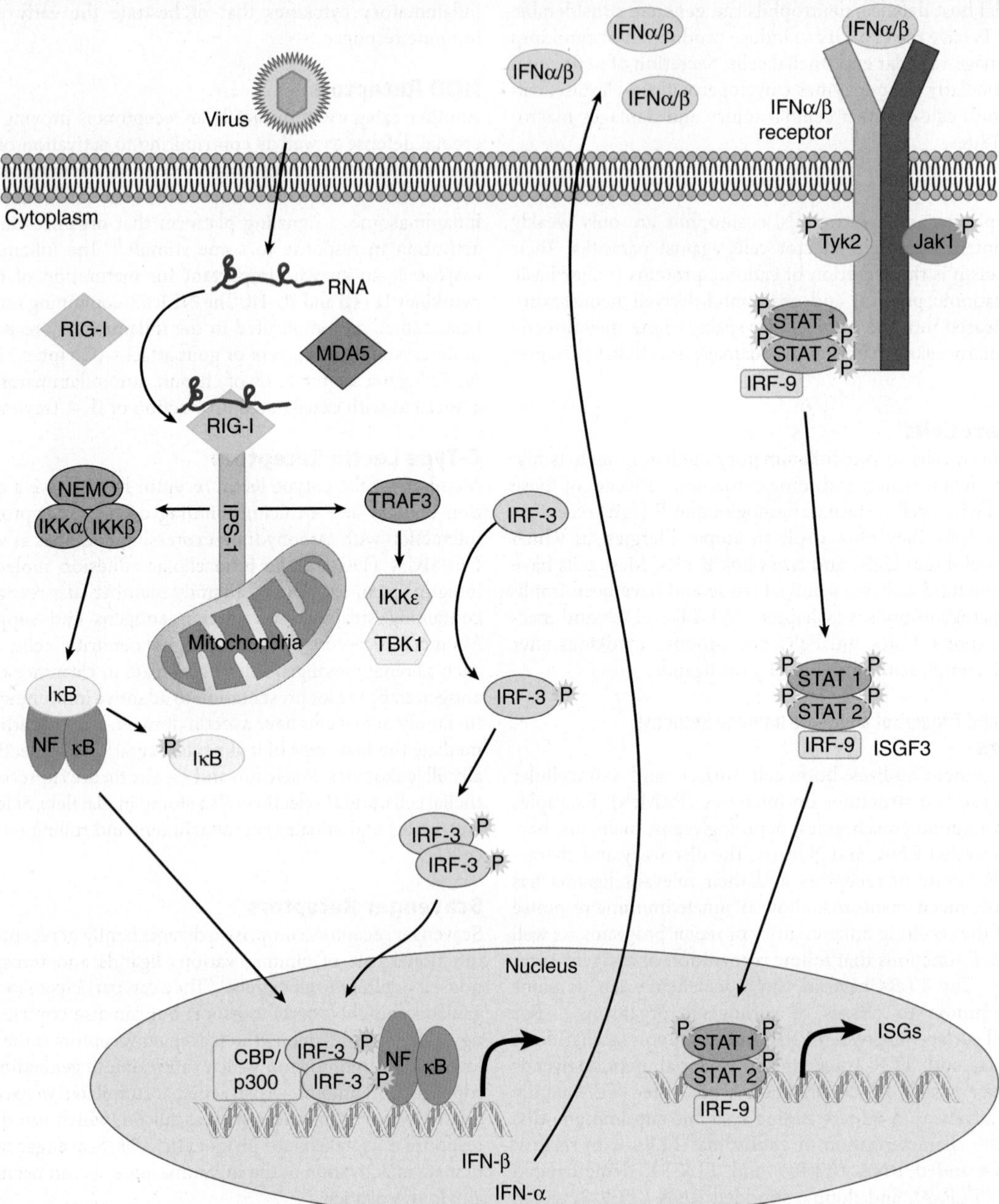

FIGURE 45-1. **Induction of antiviral type I interferon response. Cytoplasmic sensors of RNA, including RIG-I and MDA5, trigger a signaling cascade that results in translocation of IRF-3 to the nucleus and transcription of interferons. Those cytokines promote an antiviral immune response after binding to their receptor and activating the JAK-STAT pathway. CBP/p300 = CREB binding protein; NEMO = NF-κB essential modulator; IFN = interferon; IKK = inhibitor of nuclear factor κB kinase subunit; IPS-1 = interferon-β promoter stimulator-1; IRF = interferon response factor; ISG = interferon stimulated gene; ISGF3 = interferon-stimulated gene factor 3; JAK = Janus kinase; MDA5 = melanoma differentiation-associated protein 5; RIG-1 = retinoic acid–inducible gene 1; STAT = signal transducer and activator of transcription; TRAF3 = TNF (tumor necrosis factor) receptor–associated factor; Tyk = tyrosine kinase. (From Wilkins C, Gale M Jr. Recognition of viruses by cytoplasmic sensors. *Curr Opin Immunol.* 2010;22:41-47.)**

eosinophils bind monomeric IgE with extremely high affinity. Cross-linking of the constitutively cell surface–bound IgE induces cell activation and the release of cytoplasmic granules. Some immunoglobulin isotypes fix complement, and complement receptors on monocytes amplify cell activation induced by antigen-antibody-complement immune complexes[18] (Chapter 50). Complement receptor 1 (CR1) binds C3b and C4b, initial degradation products of complement activation, and when activated promotes phagocytosis of a complement-bearing immune complex. CR3 and CR4 are β_2-integrins and bind the degradation product iC3b.

Cytokine and Chemokine Receptors

Cells of the innate immune system express receptors for many cytokines, soluble, low-molecular-weight glycoproteins that derive from many cellular sources.[5] Binding of IFN-γ, produced by NK or type 1 helper T cells (T_H1 cells), by its receptor on monocytes activates a differentiation program that expands an inflammatory response. Receptors for IL-4 on monocytes induce a gene transcription program that is more supportive of a wound healing and repair program. Tumor necrosis factor-α (TNF-α) is a product of activated macrophages but also binds to those cells through its specific receptor, expanding an inflammatory response. Innate immune cells also express receptors for IL-6, which induces acute phase reactants and type I interferon, which orchestrates a broad host defense program in response to virus infection (see Fig. 45-1). Chemokine receptors include many family members that are differentially distributed among immune system cells and sense the gradient generated by soluble chemokines, resulting in attraction of cells to sites where they are needed to implement inflammatory or immune functions.

Signaling Pathways and Effector Mediators of the Innate Immune System

Each family of innate immune system receptors utilizes a complex network of molecules to transmit information from the cell surface or its cytoplasm to the nucleus, resulting in induction of a broad gene transcription and protein synthesis program that implements the next phase of the response. The contributions of each of the signal transduction pathways to the overall innate immune response will depend on the proteins produced and will determine whether the resulting cell products focus the overall immune function on ablating the damaging effects of virus infection on the host, limiting the inflammation and tissue damage that follow a bacterial or fungal infection, or healing a tissue wound through the production of scar tissue.

Receptor-Mediated Signaling Pathways

Certain common cell signaling systems are utilized by many cells and receptor systems.[6,7] Arguably the most important is the nuclear factor κ light-chain enhancer of activated B cells (NF-κB) pathway. NF-κB is a rapid-acting transcription factor because it is preformed in cells of the innate immune system and does not require new protein synthesis to take action. Its activity is induced by ligation of TLRs and many cytokine receptors. Its component transcription factors translocate to the cell nucleus after degradation of an inhibitory component, inhibitor of κB (IκB), and bind to promoter regions of genes encoding mediators of inflammation and cell proliferation. Another important pathway is mediated by the interferon regulatory factor (IRF) family, including transcription factors that are activated by endosomal TLRs in response to ligation by DNA or RNA, or by cytoplasmic nucleic acid sensors, usually from viral sources. IRF-3 is particularly important for promoting transcription of interferon-β, typically produced early in an antivirus innate immune response. IRF-7 is particularly supportive of interferon-α production induced by endosomal TLRs and is constitutively present in pDCs, the most active producers of IFN-α.

The Janus kinase (JAK)-signal transducer and activator of transcription (STAT) pathway is utilized by many cytokine receptors and involves sequential enzymatic reactions by kinases that eventuate in translocation of STAT proteins to the nucleus, where they bind to gene promoters and induce transcription and production of products important in implementing immunoregulation and inflammation.

TNF receptor family members activate a complex signaling pathway that involves proteins called TNF receptor–associated death domain (TRADD) proteins and TNF receptor–associated factors (TRAFs), ultimately activating the NF-κB and the mitogen-activated protein (MAP) kinase pathways.

The TGF-β receptor is a serine/threonine receptor kinase that phosphorylates cytoplasmic proteins of the SMAD family, which act as transcription factors after receptor engagement by TGF-β. TGF-β signaling can play an important role in terminating an innate immune response and initiating a wound healing or tissue repair program.

It is apparent that common intracellular signaling strategies are used by many of the receptor systems that activate and regulate the innate immune system, with ligand-receptor engagement triggering the activation of kinases that phosphorylate downstream pathway proteins, and result in translocation of important transcription factors from cytoplasm to nucleus where new gene transcription takes place.

Soluble Products of the Innate Immune Response

Cells of the innate immune system are the principal producers of many pro-inflammatory and regulatory cytokines already mentioned, and are also their targets. In addition to the cytokines described, cells of the innate immune system produce chemokines that attract immune system cells to sites of tissue damage or infection, and they produce cell survival and differentiation factors that help to develop an adaptive immune response. Macrophages and dendritic cells produce IL-12 and IL-23 to support development of effector T-cell programs, and they produce B-cell-activating factor (BAFF), a soluble mediator of the TNF family. BAFF supports B-cell survival and can provide costimulatory signals to B cells that have received antigen-specific activation signals through their surface B-cell antigen receptors, promoting differentiation to antibody-producing plasma cells.

A particularly important set of products includes components of the complement system, a group of plasma enzymes and regulatory proteins that are converted from inactive pro-enzymes to active enzymes in a controlled and systematic cascade, which is crucial in linking microbial recognition to cellular effector function (Chapter 50). Mannose-binding lectin circulates in the plasma, functioning as an opsonin, and is involved in activation of the complement pathway. C-reactive protein, an acute phase protein, participates in opsonization by binding to bacterial phospholipids. Macrophages and neutrophils are important in the initiation phase of an innate immune response through their production of antimicrobial defensins, cysteine-rich cationic proteins, and cathelicidin peptides, such as LL37.[19] Both categories of mediators can assist in killing of microbes in phagosomes. Neutrophils extrude stimulatory DNA in the form of NETs or release mitochondrial DNA, along with DNA-associated proteins like high mobility group box 1 (HMGB1) that amplifies TLR responses in pDCs or macrophages.

Role of the Innate Immune System in Localization, Extension, and Resolution of a Host Defense Reaction

Localization of Innate Immune System Cells

Most cells of the innate immune response are free agents, moving through blood or lymph in transit from one site to another. Mobility of the cellular constituents of the innate immune system is required for effective initiation of a response to invading microbes. Cells use a multistep process of adherence and activation. Initially, leukocytes roll on activated endothelial cells, activate chemokine receptors, increase adhesiveness, and eventually migrate through the endothelial layer across a chemokine gradient. The selectin family of proteins mediates the first steps of leukocyte migration. P-selectin and E-selectin are expressed on activated endothelial cells, and P-selectin is also stored in platelets. Selectins capture floating leukocytes and initiate their attachment and rolling on activated endothelial cells. To transform attachment and rolling into firm adhesion, the concerted action of chemokines, chemokine receptors, and integrins is necessary. Integrins are heterodimers formed of many different α chains and β chains; different α/β combinations are expressed on different cell subsets. Only after activation can integrins interact with ligands on endothelial cells. Activation involves modification of the cytoplasmic domain of the β chain, which leads to a structural change of the extracellular domains. This process is termed *inside-out signaling*. The last step of homing is transendothelial migration. Here, the firmly attached leukocytes migrate through the endothelial cell monolayer and the basement membrane of the vessel wall.

Transition to an Adaptive Immune Response

Movement of innate immune system cells is also required to transition a host response from primarily one depending on cells of the innate immune system to one that engages T and B lymphocytes. Dendritic cells resident in the skin and gut serve as sentinels and a first line of defense against invading organisms. When those cells are activated following sensing of PAMPs by PRRs and following uptake of microbial components by those cells, the DCs migrate to local lymph nodes where their contents, by now expressed on their surface in association with MHC class I or II molecules, can be sampled by T cells. As noted, activated macrophages, DCs, and pDCs produce cytokines that shape the differentiation program of T cells. In addition, cell surface costimulatory molecules induced after TLR-mediated activation, such as CD80 and CD86, provide essential accessory activation signals to T cells to ensure their effective activation. Macrophages and DCs also support the development of an adaptive immune response through their production of survival and differentiation factors. Chapter 46 provides a full description of the adaptive immune system and its implementation.

Role of Innate Immune System Cells in Resolution of an Immune Response and Wound Repair

Macrophages are particularly important in resolving an immune response and organizing the repair of damaged tissue. A classic paradigm describing pro-inflammatory/classically activated (M1) and anti-inflammatory/alternatively activated (M2) macrophages (see earlier under Monocytes and Macrophages) is likely to be overly simplistic. Yet it is clear that in the course of a chronic infection, macrophages can shift their functional profile from M1 to M2, in some cases promoted by the T-cell cytokines IL-4 and IL-13, to develop a gene expression program that includes production of TGF-β, supportive of a fibrotic response, and IL-10, a cytokine that inhibits antigen-presenting cell function.[9] Although an M1-like profile driven by IFN-γ is highly productive in achieving initial control over a pathogenic invading microbe, and M2-derived mediators promote wound healing, it should be recognized that either macrophage phenotype, and complex in-between profiles, can also be associated with pathologic states (Fig. 45-2). Current research is unraveling the innate immune mechanisms that account for such diverse diseases as atherosclerosis (Chapter 70), viewed as associated with M1 macrophages, and idiopathic pulmonary fibrosis (Chapter 92), possibly involving M2-like macrophages.

Contribution of the Innate Immune Response to Pathogenesis of Autoimmune Disease

Among the most significant insights of the past decade is the essential contribution of the innate immune system to the pathogenesis of autoimmune and inflammatory diseases. As described, the cells of the innate immune system are integral players in the early recognition of invading pathogenic microbes, and when the functions of this complex system are carefully

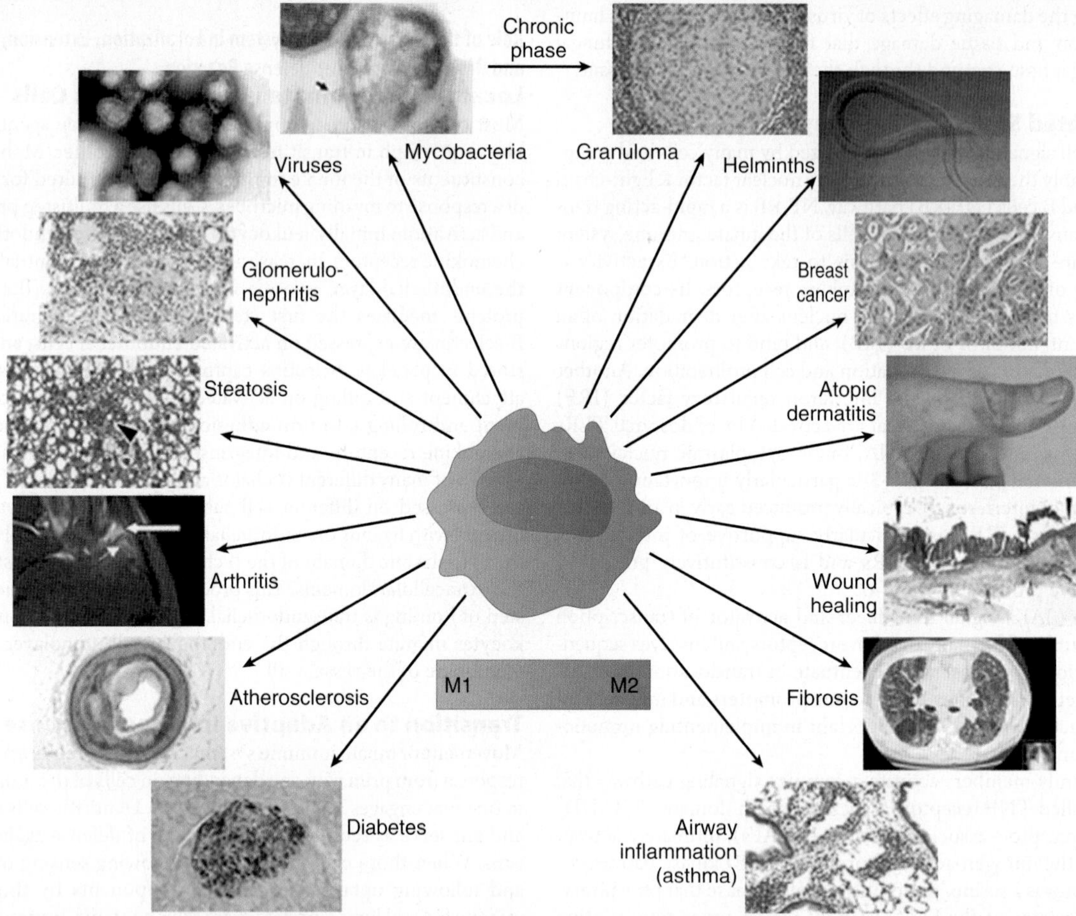

FIGURE 45-2. Schematic representation of macrophage plasticity and polarization in pathology. Dynamic changes occur over time with evolution of pathology: for instance, a switch from M1 to M2 macrophage polarization characterizes the transition from early to chronic phases of infection. Moreover, mixed phenotypes or populations with different phenotypes can coexist. (From Sica A, Mantovani A. Macrophage plasticity and polarization: in vivo veritas. *J Clin Invest.* 2012;122:787-795.)

orchestrated and balanced, the result is efficient ablation, or at least isolation, of the microbe. However, if the microbe is not effectively cleared from the system and persists, a chronic state of infection associated with immune activation and tissue damage is the result. Interestingly, many parallels can be seen between the immune alterations observed in the setting of chronic viral infection and the impaired immunoregulation characteristic of the prototypic autoimmune disease systemic lupus erythematosus. Excessive production of interferon-α is a feature of most patients with that disease, and it is now understood that activation of the endosomal TLRs by nucleic acid–containing immune complexes amplifies the activity of the innate immune response and drives production of interferon-α and other proinflammatory cytokines. Neutrophils are now recognized to contribute to the induction of that response through their production of HMGB1, cathelicidins, and extrusion of stimulatory DNA aggregates. TLR activation is proposed to contribute to many additional autoimmune and inflammatory diseases; as endogenous TLR ligands can act as effective TLR stimuli in the setting of a pro-inflammatory environment associated with oxidative cell damage. The inflammasome and its component proteins, including the NOD-like receptors, are recognized as mediators of inflammatory responses induced by urate crystals that result in gout attacks (Chapter 273), and they are targets of mutations that define dramatic autoinflammatory syndromes (Chapter 261), particularly seen in children.

Conclusion

The cells and products of the innate immune response, for many years viewed as less sophisticated and important than the highly specific T and B lymphocytes of the adaptive immune response, have taken their place as essential defenders against pathogenic microbes. Through the recognition of common molecular patterns characteristic of microbes by members of receptor families, some still being discovered, the cells of the innate immune response orchestrate the effector programs that are fine-tuned to target the vulnerabilities of each pathogen and kill, or at least limit the expansion of, that microbe. Advances in understanding the mechanisms utilized by the innate immune response and the clinical syndromes that result when components of that system are genetically altered, have elucidated the central role that receptors and products of the innate immune system play in the pathogenesis of autoimmune and inflammatory diseases. These insights are guiding efforts to develop targeted therapies that will leverage the new knowledge to control or even prevent human diseases in which the innate immune system plays an important pathogenic role.

GENERAL REFERENCES

For the General References and other additional features, please visit Expert Consult at https://expertconsult.inkling.com.

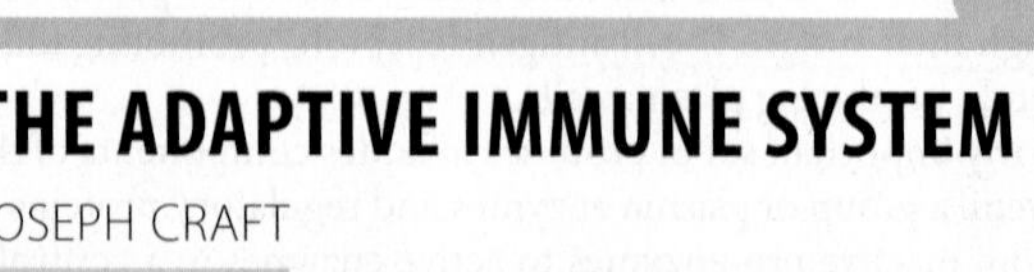

46 THE ADAPTIVE IMMUNE SYSTEM

JOSEPH CRAFT

PRINCIPLES OF ADAPTIVE IMMUNE SYSTEM ACTIVATION: RECOGNITION OF ANTIGEN

Structure of Antigen-Specific Receptors

The innate immune system recognizes structural patterns that are common in the microbial world, whereas the adaptive immune system is designed to respond to the entire continuum of antigens. This goal is achieved through two principal types of antigen recognition receptors: antibodies and T-cell receptors (TCRs). Antibodies, or immunoglobulins, are expressed as cell surface receptors on B cells or are secreted, both of which have the same specificity for antigen. They recognize conformational structures formed by the tertiary configuration of proteins. In contrast, α/β TCRs, the most abundant class of TCRs, fit specifically to epitopes formed by a small linear peptide embedded into major histocompatibility complex (MHC) molecules on the surface of antigen-presenting cells.

Antibodies

Antibodies consist of two identical heavy chains and two identical light chains, which are covalently linked by disulfide bonds. The amino (N)-terminal domain of each chain is variable and represents the recognition structure that interacts with the antigen. Each antibody has two binding arms of identical specificity. The carboxy (C)-terminal ends of the heavy and light chains form the constant region, which defines the subclass of the antibody (κ or λ for light chains; immunoglobulin M (IgM), IgA, IgD, IgE, or IgG for heavy chains). Additional subclasses can be distinguished for IgG and IgA. The constant region of antibodies includes the Fc region. Fc regions can polymerize (IgA) or pentamerize in the presence of a J (joining) chain (IgM). Fc regions are also the ligand for Fc receptors (FcRs) on cells of the innate immune system.

T-Cell Receptors

TCRs are dimers of α chains and β chains or of γ chains and δ chains, each of which contains three complementary-determining binding sites in the N-terminal domain. These complementary-determining sites define the specificity. α/β TCRs recognize peptide fragments in the context of MHC molecules, although certain ones bind glycolipid antigens, for example from mycobacteria, displayed by molecules with structural similarity to MHC. γ/δ TCRs are more variable and can recognize peptides or certain glycolipid antigens in the context of MHC-like molecules, or even unprocessed antigens, functioning similar to antibodies; the latter is a reflection of their structural similarity.

Specificities of Antibodies and T-Cell Receptors

The repertoires, or total number of specificities, of antibodies and TCRs are extremely diverse and have been estimated in the human to account for up to 10^{11} or higher, and 10^{18}, respectively, combinations. This enormous diversity reflects the anticipatory nature of adaptive immune receptors and must be acquired; it cannot be genetically encoded in contrast to that of innate receptors. Its foundation consists of fewer than 400 genes that are recombined and modified. Immunoglobulin heavy chains are formed from four gene segments—the variable, diversity, joining, and constant region gene segments. Also, TCR β chains and δ chains are assembled by the recombination of variable, diversity, joining, and constant region segments of TCR genes. Immunoglobulin light chains and TCR α chains and γ chains lack the diversity segment and are composed of three gene segments. During antibody or TCR rearrangement, gene segments are cut out by nucleases and recombined at the DNA level to form linear coding units for each receptor gene. Through the combination of several different mechanisms, an enormous diversity of receptors is generated. First, the genome contains multiple forms of gene segments; each receptor or antibody uses a different combination of these gene segments. Second, the splicing process is imprecise, introducing nucleotide variations at the variable-diversity, diversity-joining, and variable-joining junctions. These inaccuracies lead to frame shifts and result in completely different amino acid sequences. Finally, random nucleotides can be inserted at the junctional region by an enzyme, deoxyribonucleotidyl transferase.

Once generated, TCR sequences remain unchanged. This rule does not apply to immunoglobulins, which undergo modification. Immunoglobulin modification includes (1) replacement of an entire variable region, or receptor editing, typically occurring in the bone marrow during B-cell development to modify those immunoglobulin receptors that inadvertently bind self-antigens on initial recombination of gene segments; (2) class switching, in which the variable-diversity-joining unit combines with different constant region genes (isotype switching); or (3) somatic hypermutation, in which the antigen-contact areas of the antibody undergo mutations during an immune response to improve the affinity (affinity maturation). The latter two events occur in secondary lymphoid tissues, such as the spleen, lymph nodes, and mucosal lymphoid tissue, where immune responses to antigens are initiated.

Antigen Processing

T cells bearing α/β TCRs recognize peptide fragments that are displayed in the context of MHC class I and class II molecules through a process named *antigen presentation*. The two classes of MHC molecules are used as restriction elements by two different subsets of T cells. $CD4^+$ T cells recognize antigenic peptides embedded into MHC class II molecules, whereas $CD8^+$ T cells bind peptides complexed with MHC class I molecules. Generally, MHC class II molecules are expressed only on specialized, so-called professional, antigen-presenting cells, such as dendritic cells, monocytes, macrophages, and B cells, whereas class I proteins are displayed by virtually all nucleated cells, facilitating recognition by $CD8^+$ T cells of peptides from viruses that often have a broad range of target tissues. Peptides bound to MHC class II molecules typically derive from extracellular antigens that are captured and internalized into endosomes to be digested by proteinases, notably cathepsin. Occasionally, however, intracellular proteins or membrane proteins are also funneled into this pathway. MHC class II molecules are assembled in the endoplasmic reticulum in association with a protein called the *invariant chain* (Fig. 46-1). The molecules are transported to the endosome, where the invariant chain is removed from the peptide-binding cleft, making the cleft accessible to peptides derived from extracellular proteins. MHC class II molecules, stabilized by peptides of 10 to 30 amino acids in length, are displayed on the cell surface, where they are recognized by $CD4^+$ T cells.

MHC class I–associated peptides are produced in the cytosol by the proteasome, a large cytoplasmic multiprotein enzyme complex (see Fig. 46-1). Specialized transporter proteins, called *transporter in antigen processing* (TAP), facilitate translocation of peptides from the cytosolic proteasome to the endoplasmic reticulum. There, the peptides bind to newly formed MHC class I molecules and are transported to the cell surface, where they are recognized by antigen-specific $CD8^+$ T cells. MHC class I–associated peptides may also originate in the extracellular environment and be presented to T cells through the appropriately named *cross-presentation pathway*. This enables $CD8^+$ T cells to recognize foreign peptides, for example, from viruses, that

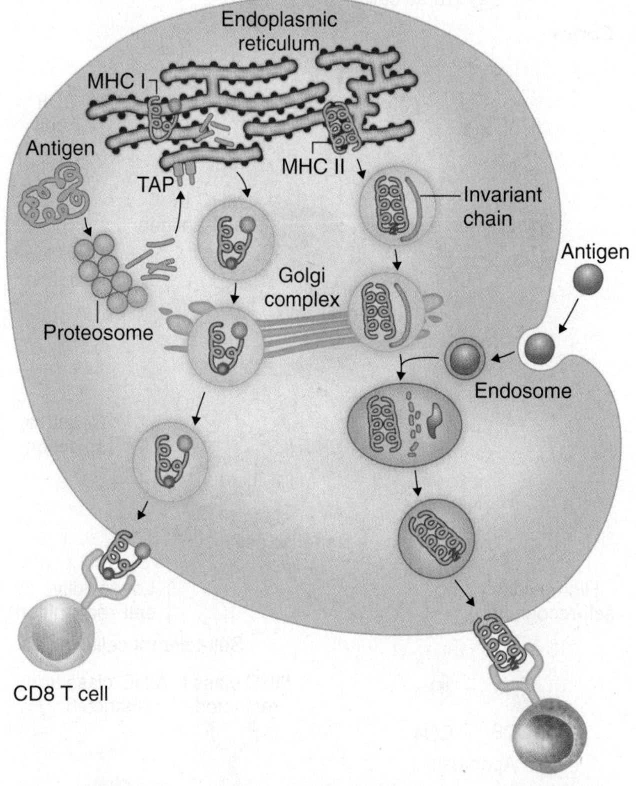

FIGURE 46-1. Pathways of antigen processing and delivery to major histocompatibility complex (MHC) molecules. Cytosolic proteins are broken down by the proteosome to generate peptide fragments, which are transported into the endoplasmic reticulum by specialized peptide transporters (TAP). After peptides are bound to MHC class I molecules, MHC-peptide complexes are released from the endoplasmic reticulum and travel to the cell surface, where they are ligands for $CD8^+$ T-cell receptors (TCRs). Extracellular foreign antigens are taken into intracellular vesicles, called *endosomes*. As the pH in the endosomes gradually decreases, proteases are activated that digest antigens into peptide fragments. After fusing with vesicles that contain MHC class II molecules, antigenic peptides are placed in the antigen-binding groove. Loaded MHC class II–peptide complexes are transported to the cell surface, where they are recognized by the TCRs of $CD4^+$ T cells.

are derived from infected and dying cells that are ingested by myeloid cells and then presented by MHC class I molecules.

The nature of the antigen-processing pathway determines the sequence of events in immune responses. Extracellular antigens, in general, enter the endosomal pool and associate with MHC class II molecules to stimulate CD4$^+$ T cells. Cytosolic antigens, including antigens from intracellular infectious agents, are degraded and displayed in the context of MHC class I molecules to initiate CD8$^+$ T-cell responses.

CELLULAR ELEMENTS OF THE ADAPTIVE IMMUNE SYSTEM

T Cells

T-Cell Development

T precursor cells are derived from hematopoietic stem cells that migrate to the thymus, a primary lymphoid tissue, where all the subsequent stages of T-cell maturation occur (Fig. 46-2). Pre-T cells express two enzymes, recombinase and terminal deoxynucleotidyl transferase, enabling them to recombine TCR genes. The β chain of the TCR is rearranged first and is expressed together with a pre-TCR α chain. Signals from the immature TCR complex inhibit rearrangement of the second β-chain allele and induce thymocyte proliferation and expression of both CD4 and CD8 molecules, so-called double positive thymocytes. Subsequently, the TCR α chain is recombined, with formation of a mature TCR. From here, the thymocyte undergoes many differentiation and selection steps modulated by the thymic microenvironment, with the end result being formation of a T cell that is ready to migrate to secondary lymphoid tissues and to be poised to recognize antigenic peptides. Early-stage thymocytes reside in the thymic cortex, where they mostly interact with epithelial cells. They then migrate toward the medulla, encountering dendritic cells and macrophages at the corticomedullary junction. Thymic stromal cells regulate T-cell proliferation by secreting lymphopoietic growth factors, such as interleukin-7 (IL-7). Interactions of the TCR with MHC molecules expressed on epithelial cells and on dendritic cells or macrophages determine the fate of the thymocyte.[1] Low-avidity recognition of peptide-MHC complexes on thymic epithelial cells by the TCR results in positive selection.[2] This recognition event rescues cells from apoptotic cell death and ensures that only T cells with functional receptors that can recognize MHC molecules, critical for T-cell activation on subsequent residence in the spleen and lymph nodes, survive. Thymocytes that express a receptor not fitting any MHC antigen complex die by neglect. High-affinity interaction between the TCR and peptide-MHC complex induces apoptotic death of the recognizing T cell. This process of negative selection eliminates T cells with specificity for self-antigens and is responsible for central tolerance to many autoantigens. It has been estimated that approximately 1% of thymocytes survive the stringent selection process. While undergoing selection, T cells continue to differentiate, with orderly expression of cell surface molecules. Double-positive thymocytes expressing both CD4 and CD8 molecules downregulate one or the other, developing into single-positive CD4$^+$ helper T cells that have been selected on MHC class II complexes or CD8$^+$ cytotoxic T cells that are restricted to MHC class I complexes. These single-positive cells are now mature T cells that are ready for exit and migration through the circulation to secondary lymphoid organs, including the spleen, lymph nodes, and mucosal lymphoid tissues, following chemokine cues and using adhesion molecules to enter. They exist in these tissues as inactivated, or naïve, cells until receiving the appropriate antigenic signal for activation and subsequent effector function.

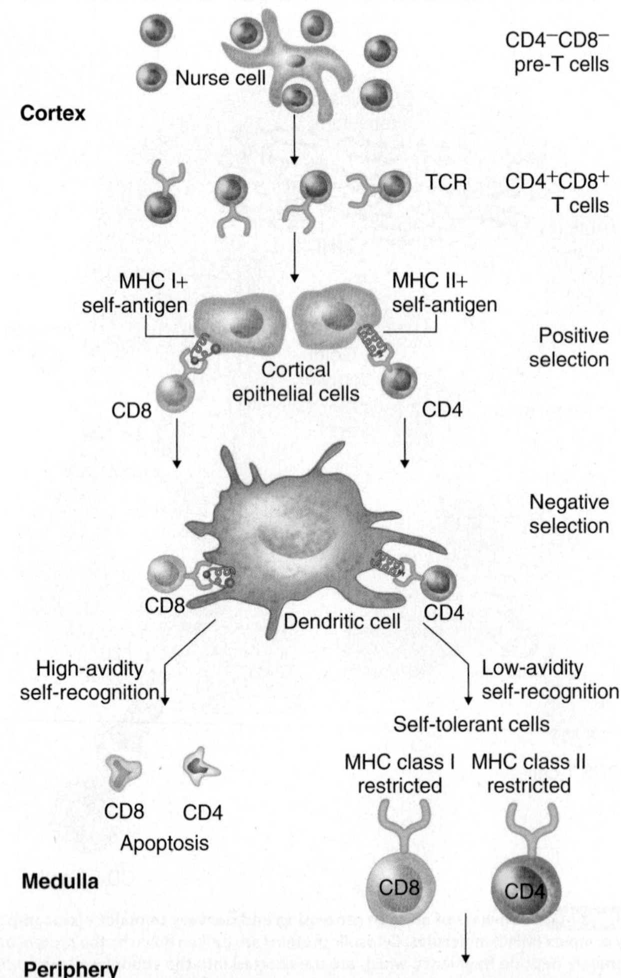

FIGURE 46-2. Maturation of T cells in the thymus. Precursors committed to the T-cell lineage arrive in the thymus and begin to rearrange their T-cell receptor (TCR) genes. Immature T cells with receptors binding to self–major histocompatibility complex (MHC) on cortical epithelial cells receive signals for survival (positive selection). At the corticomedullary junction, surviving T cells probe self-antigens presented by dendritic cells and macrophages. T cells reacting strongly to self-antigens are deleted by apoptosis (negative selection). T cells released into the periphery are tolerant toward self and recognize foreign antigens in the context of self-MHC.

T-Cell Stimulation and Accessory Molecules

T-cell activation is initiated when TCR complexes recognize antigenic peptides in the context of the appropriate MHC molecule on the surface of an antigen-presenting cell in secondary lymphoid organs. The principal antigen-presenting cells for activation of naïve T cells are dendritic cells. MHC-peptide recognition by the TCR, the first signal for T-cell activation, leads to receptor clustering and phosphorylation of the intracellular portion of the CD3 protein complex, the signaling component of the TCR, by receptor-associated tyrosine kinases. These events transmit signals to the nucleus of the T cell and initiate its activation. The coreceptors CD4 and CD8 are also critical for the initial events in T-cell activation, through their interaction with MHC class II and class I molecules, respectively, supporting CD3-mediated signals. Yet, this first activation signal delivered by the TCR and coreceptors is not alone sufficient for robust T-cell survival and differentiation. It needs to be complemented by the interaction of accessory molecules on the T cell and their ligands on the antigen-presenting cell. A spectrum of accessory molecules is known, of which the best known is CD28, which are engaged by CD80 and CD86 (also known as B7.1 and B7.2, respectively) on antigen-presenting cells (E-Table 46-1). Engagement of CD28 provides to the T cells a second, or costimulatory, signal to the T cell.[3] This second signal, delivered by the antigen-presenting dendritic cell, ensures T-cell survival and expansion. CD28-mediated signals are mandatory for the expression of many activation markers on the responding T cells and, in particular, for the secretion of IL-2. In the absence of such a second signal, T cells are rendered nonresponsive and anergic or undergo apoptosis. Finally, adhesion molecules (integrins) stabilize the interactions between T cells and antigen-presenting cells.

Signals from the TCR result in the activation of many genes and entry of the T cell into the cell cycle. The signals are transmitted by a cascade of cytoplasmic events. Cross-linking of the TCR and associated CD3 molecules results in the recruitment and activation of phosphotyrosine kinases and the phosphorylation of molecular constituents of the TCR and various adapter molecules. Signals mediated through the TCR then activate several biochemical pathways, which collectively lead to the activation of transcription factors that regulate gene expression

Three major variables determine the outcome of TCR stimulation: the duration and affinity of the TCR-antigen interaction, the maturation stage of the responding T cell, and the nature of the antigen-presenting cell. Antigen-presenting cells are gatekeepers in the initiation of T-cell responses. They can upregulate the expression of accessory molecules that provide costimulatory signals. MHC-peptide complexes are particularly dense on dendritic cells, enabling them to activate naïve T cells. In contrast, memory and effector cells have a lower threshold for activation and can react to antigens presented on peripheral tissue cells.

T-Cell Differentiation and Effector Functions

T-cell activation induces T-cell proliferation, with the goal of clonally selecting and expanding antigen-specific T cells. The extent of clonal proliferation is impressive. Antigen-specific $CD8^+$ T cells expand several thousand–fold; $CD4^+$ T cells expand somewhat less. During the phase of rapid growth, T cells differentiate from naïve T cells that are essentially devoid of effector functions into effector T cells that are needed for clearance of infectious organisms, or pathogens. The transition into effector cells is associated with a fundamental shift in functional profiles. First, effector T cells have a lower activation threshold; they do not require costimulation and can scan tissues that lack professional antigen-presenting cells. Second, they switch the expression of chemokine receptors and adhesion molecules to gain access to peripheral tissues. Finally, they gain effector functions.

The principal effector function of $CD8^+$ T cells is to lyse infected, antigen-bearing target cells. This commitment to eventual cytotoxic function is made during development in the thymus. Upon emigration from the thymus in the naïve, or inactivated, state, $CD8^+$ T cells circulate through secondary lymphoid tissues, surveying antigen-presenting dendritic cells for the appropriate MHC class I–peptide complex that can engage the TCR and that can supply costimulatory signals. On activation, $CD8^+$ T cells acquire cytotoxic functions and, using a variety of receptors and adhesion molecules, can emigrate from secondary lymphoid organs to peripheral tissue sites seeking cells infected by viruses or intracellular bacteria displaying pathogen-derived peptides on MHC class I molecules. On recognizing the appropriate MHC class I–peptide complex, $CD8^+$ T cells induce apoptosis of target cells. The T cell polarizes toward the area of antigen contact; specialized lytic granules are clustered in the contact area. A pore-forming protein, perforin, is released from the lytic granules and inserted into the target cell membrane. Proteases (granzymes) are injected into the target cells to initiate the apoptotic process by activating enzyme cascades. Mechanisms deployed by $CD8^+$ T cells are essentially identical to those of natural killer (NK) cells. $CD4^+$ T cells can also induce apoptosis but by a different mechanism than $CD8^+$ T cells. On activation, they express cell surface molecules such as Fas ligand (CD178) and TRAIL, which initiate the apoptotic cascade selectively in cells expressing the respective ligands Fas (CD95) or the death receptors DR4 and DR5.

Compared with $CD8^+$ T cells, the spectrum of options for $CD4^+$ T cells is larger. They are generally characterized as helper T, or T_H cells, because they produce cytokines and express cell surface molecules that promote the effector function of other lymphocytes and phagocytes. Like $CD8^+$ T cells, they are initially activated in secondary lymphoid tissues on contact with dendritic cells displaying the MHC–peptide complex (MHC class II, compared with MHC class I for $CD8^+$ T-cell activation) bound by a specific TCR along with the proper costimulatory signals. On activation, different subsets of $CD4^+$ effector T cells can be distinguished based on the preferential production of certain cytokines (see E-Table 46-1). T_H1 T cells predominantly produce interferon-γ (IFN-γ) and tumor necrosis factor-α (TNF-α) and are involved in cell-mediated immunity, such as delayed-type hypersensitivity reactions. These cytokines, among other actions, promote macrophage activation that is critical for protective responses against intracellular pathogens such as mycobacteria and listeria. T_H2 T cells preferentially produce IL-4, IL-5, and IL-13, cytokines that promote eosinophil maintenance, expansion, and tissue accumulation, as well as macrophage function; these are all important for host protection following infection with helminths, such as schistosomes and other worms. T_H17 T cells produce IL-17, critical for neutrophil expansion and function, with killing of extracellular bacteria, such as streptococci, and pathogenic fungi.[4] These cells may also produce IL-22 that promotes host-protective function at barrier surfaces, such as the skin and gut. Follicular helper T (T_{FH}) cells home to lymphoid follicles, where B cells congregate, where they express CD40 ligand (CD154) and other surface proteins along with cytokines, including IL-21, IL-4, and IFN-γ, that are critical for B-cell maturation to plasma cells and memory B cells. The decision as to which differentiation pathway to take is made during the early stages of naïve T-cell activation by antigen-presenting cells in secondary lymphoid organs. Pathway differentiation depends on several factors, including (1) the cytokines produced by the activating antigen-presenting cell and other innate cells in the microenvironment, (2) the nature of costimulatory signals, and (3) the avidity of the TCR–MHC antigen interaction. $CD4^+$ T-cell subset, or lineage, development is generally correlated with the expression of specific transcription factors (T-bet for T_H1, GATA3 for T_H2, RORγt for T_H17, and Bcl6 for T_{FH} cells). However, lineage commitment among differentiated $CD4^+$ T cells is not absolute and is not terminal, and transition between different effector types is possible.

Regulatory T Cells

Depending on their cytokine profile, $CD4^+$ T cells have the ability to cross-regulate each other, influence T-cell differentiation, and suppress T-cell effector activity. Classic examples of T cells with regulatory activity generated during the normal immune response are IL-10– and transforming growth factor-β (TGF-β)–producing cells. In addition, specialized subsets of regulatory T (Treg) cells are characterized by expression of the transcription factor forkhead box P3 (Foxp3). Naturally occurring $Foxp3^+$ Treg cells are generated during T-cell development in the thymus and recognize self-antigens. $Foxp3^+$ Treg cells can also arise from conventional $CD4^+$ T cells in the periphery. Natural and inducible Treg cells are in many ways indistinguishable, particularly because their development and function depend on Foxp3, and they are able to suppress T-cell expansion and constitutively express several cell surface markers, albeit markers that are not necessarily specific for Treg because activated T cells can also express them. Treg cells are important in peripheral tolerance, controlling the expansion of autoreactive T cells. They also play a role in immune responses to pathogens by virtue of their ability to suppress T-cell effector function and consequently downmodulate the inflammatory response incited by the former, a natural consequence of pathogen elimination. A principal difference between natural and induced Treg cells is that the latter largely survey mucosal and other environmentally exposed surfaces. Despite extensive studies in various models, the mechanism by which Treg cells function in vivo remains incompletely understood, although it is certainly a consequence of secretion of regulatory cytokines, like IL-10 and TGF-β, that can dampen inflammatory responses. Tregs may also express the T-cell molecule cytotoxic T-lymphocyte antigen (CTLA)-4 (CD152) that, like CD28, engages CD80 and CD86 on antigen-presenting cells. In contrast to CD28, which receives a positive signal from CD80 and CD86, leading to robust T-cell activation, engagement of these molecules on antigen-presenting cells by CTLA-4 on Tregs suppresses the ability of antigen-presenting cells to activate naïve T cells.

T-Cell Homeostasis

Effective immunity depends on the ability of the immune system to generate large numbers of antigen-specific T cells rapidly, yet the space in the T-cell compartment is limited. To avoid competition for space and resources and to prevent perturbation of T-cell diversity by lifelong exposure to antigens, the adaptive immune system employs several counterbalancing mechanisms. In the later stages of the activation process, a strong negative signal derives from interaction of CTLA-4 with CD80/CD86 on antigen-presenting cells. In addition, T cells undergo activation-induced cell death. Activated $CD4^+$ T cells begin to secrete Fas ligand and acquire sensitivity to Fas-mediated death, inducing apoptotic suicide and fratricide in neighboring T cells. These mechanisms impose constraints in the early stages of the T-cell antigen response. Other mechanisms control the rapid decline of expanded antigen-specific T cells when elimination of the antigen has been achieved. Removal of the driving antigen causes a deprivation of cytokines and costimulatory molecules, and growth factor–deprived T cells die from apoptosis. It has been estimated that only 5% of the antigen-expanded population survives after antigen clearance, becoming memory cells that are poised to respond if the host is again challenged by the same offending pathogen.

B Lymphocytes

B-Cell Development

B cells are generated in the bone marrow, like the thymus, a primary lymphoid organ. Lymphoid stem cells differentiate into distinctive B-lineage cells in the marrow, supported by a specialized microenvironment of nonlymphoid stromal cells supplying necessary chemokines, including stromal cell–derived factor 1 and cytokines (IL-7). Precursor B cells enter a process of tightly controlled sequential rearrangements of heavy chain and light chain immunoglobulin genes. On pre-B cells, the membrane μ chain is associated with a surrogate light chain to form a pre-B-cell receptor (BCR). Signals provided through this receptor induce proliferation of progeny that subsequently rearrange different light chain gene segments.

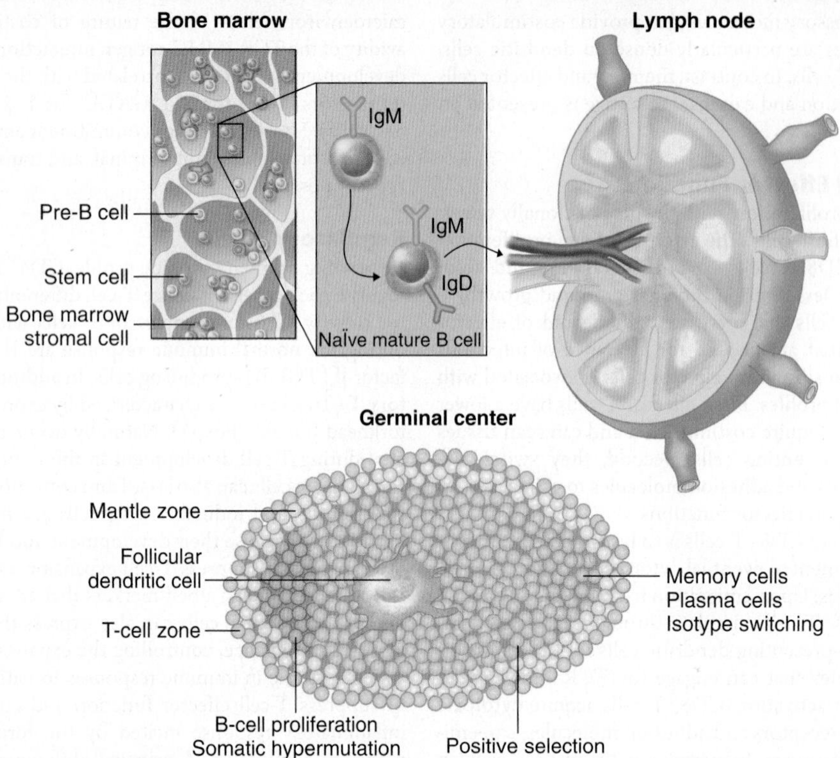

FIGURE 46-3. B-cell development and differentiation. The early stages of B-cell development occur in the bone marrow, with cells progressing through a developmental program determined by the rearrangement and expression of immunoglobulin (Ig) genes. Immature B cells with receptors for multivalent self-antigens die in the bone marrow. Surviving B cells coexpress IgD and IgM surface receptors. They are seeded into peripheral lymphoid organs, where they home to selected locations and receive signals to survive and become longer-lived naïve B cells. Antigen-binding B cells and antigen-presenting B cells that receive help from antigen-specific T cells are activated through membrane-bound and secreted molecules. Activated B cells migrate into the follicles, leading to the formation of germinal centers. B cells in germinal centers undergo somatic hypermutation of immunoglobulin genes; cells with high affinity for antigens presented on the surface of follicular dendritic cells are selected to differentiate into either memory B cells or plasma cells.

It is estimated that only 10% of B cells generated in the bone marrow reach the circulating pool. Losses are mostly due to negative selection and clonal deletion of immature B cells that express receptors directed against self-antigens. Cross-linking of surface IgM by multivalent self-antigens causes immature B cells to die. Such self-reactive B cells can be rescued from death by replacing the light chain with a newly rearranged light chain that is no longer self-reactive, a process named *receptor editing*.[5] On maturation, B cells begin to express surface IgD. B cells positive for IgD and IgM are exported from the bone marrow and migrate to peripheral lymphoid tissues following a chemokine gradient, in a process analogous to the migration of naïve T cells from the thymus to the same tissues (Fig. 46-3). There, colocalization of both types of lymphocytes facilitates their interaction following pathogen challenge. This enables B cells to receive T-cell help for the former's activation and subsequent function, including memory development and antibody secretion, required for responses to protein antigens.

B-Cell Stimulation

Mature, but naïve, B cells in secondary lymphoid organs are activated by soluble and cell-bound antigens to develop into antibody-secreting effector cells. B cells respond to a large variety of antigens, including proteins, polysaccharides, and lipids. Binding of antigen to cell surface IgM molecules induces BCR clustering, the initial step in B-cell activation. In addition to the antigen-binding immunoglobulin, the BCR comprises two proteins, Ig-α and Ig-β. The Ig-α/Ig-β heterodimer functions to transduce a signal and initiates the intracellular signaling cascade, analogous to the CD3 molecule of the TCR. Thus, the composition of the BCR, with ligand-binding and signal-transducing units, and the signaling events that lead to gene induction, are similar to those of the TCR. BCR triggering is enhanced by coreceptors, as for the TCR. The BCR-coreceptor complex is composed of CD81, CD19, and CD21, analogous to the TCR coreceptors CD4 and CD8. CD21 binds to complement fragments on opsonized antigens that are bound by the BCR, resulting in phosphorylation of the intracellular tail of CD19 by tyrosine kinases and augmentation of the BCR-mediated signal.

Like naïve T cells, naïve B cells require accessory signals in addition to triggering of their antigen-binding receptor. They receive second signals either from follicular helper T cells or from microbial components. Microbial constituents, such as bacterial polysaccharides, can induce antibody production in the absence of helper T cells, comprising thymus-independent, or T-independent, antigens.[6] In contrast, in the case of protein antigens, which are thymus- or T-dependent, the initial BCR stimulation prepares the cell for subsequent interaction with follicular helper T cells. These activated B cells start to enter the cell cycle; upregulate cell surface molecules, such as CD80 and CD86, that provide costimulatory signals to T cells; and upregulate certain cytokine receptors. As such, these B cells are prepared to activate helper T cells and to respond to cytokines secreted by those T cells, but they cannot differentiate into antibody-producing cells in the absence of T-cell help. Survival and differentiation factors produced by myeloid cells, such as B-cell-activating factor (BAFF), also stimulate B cells and help to maintain the B-cell pool.[7]

B-Cell Differentiation

Differentiation of B cells activated by protein antigens depends on interaction with helper T cells. B cells use their antigen receptor not only to recognize antigens but also to internalize them. After processing endocytosed antigens, MHC class II–peptide complexes appear on the cell surface, where antigen-specific CD4$^+$ T cells detect them. Also, B cells express costimulatory molecules and provide optimal conditions for T-cell activation. On activation, CD4$^+$ T cells express CD154, also known as CD40 ligand, on their surface and are able to stimulate the CD40 molecule on their B-cell partner. CD40-CD154 interaction is essential for subsequent B-cell proliferation and differentiation. Cytokines secreted by the helper T cells act in concert with CD154 to amplify B-cell differentiation and to determine the antibody type by controlling isotype switching. Isotypes greatly influence the versatility of antibodies as effector molecules, and cytokines drive isotype switching by stimulating the transcriptional activation of heavy chain constant region genes and enabling switching from transcription of the IgM heavy chain gene to that of IgG, IgA, or IgE.

T-cell-dependent B-cell differentiation and maturation take place in germinal centers, specialized areas in secondary lymphoid tissues where B cells rapidly proliferate, with mutation of the variable, or antigen-binding portion, of their immunoglobulin surface receptors (BCRs) (see Fig. 46-3). Those B cells bearing receptors with the highest affinity for antigen are selected for survival with the help of specific signals delivered by follicular helper T cells, whereas those with lesser affinity die by apoptosis. This process enables affinity maturation of B cells that most efficiently bind antigen and thereby facilitate its removal. As somatic hypermutation and affinity maturation proceed in the germinal center, isotype class switching of the immunoglobulin receptors is also occurring.[8]

Lymphocytes and Lymphoid Tissue

The initiation of adaptive immune responses depends on rare antigen-specific T cells and B cells meeting antigen-presenting cells and their relevant antigen. The recognition of a specific antigen in the tissue by uncommon T cells has a low probability, and it is unlikely that sufficient numbers of antigen-presenting cells and lymphocytes can be brought together to provide crucial momentum. The immune system uses specialized lymphoid microstructures to bring antigens to the site of lymphocyte traffic and accumulation. Secondary lymphoid organs include the spleen for blood-borne antigens, the lymph nodes for antigens encountered in peripheral tissues, and the mucosa-associated, bronchial-associated, and gut-associated lymphoid tissues, where antigens from epithelial surfaces are collected. Lymphocytes circulate through secondary lymphoid organs, constantly searching for their antigen. Their homing to lymph nodes is facilitated by specialized microvessels, called *high endothelial venules*, which provide the proper structure for them to leave the circulation and enter the tissue. Secondary lymphoid tissues have developed several strategies to sequester the relevant antigen. Antigens in peripheral tissue are encountered first by dendritic cells that, after activation, are mobilized to transport antigens into the local lymph nodes by the draining lymph. These antigen-bearing dendritic cells enter the lymph nodes through the afferent lymphatic vessel and settle in the T-cell-rich zones to present processed antigens to T cells. The net result of this process is an accumulation and concentration of the antigen in an environment that can be readily screened by infrequent antigen-specific T cells.

B cells are segregated from T cells in the lymph nodes and are localized in follicles. If, on antigen engagement, B cells find their cooperating (cognate) T cells at the borders of the T-cell-rich areas and the follicle, they receive cues to enter germinal centers along with their cognate follicular helper T cells. Germinal centers contain a network of follicular dendritic cells that capture particulate antigen or immune complexes on the cell surface. This unprocessed antigen is taken up by antigen-specific B cells, processed and presented, and recognized by antigen-specific T_{FH} cells. These T cells provide cytokines and cell-cell contact signals to support the germinal center reaction, a process that includes somatic hypermutation, affinity selection, and isotype switching (see Fig. 46-3). Germinal centers are essential for generating long-lived antibody-secreting plasma cells and memory B cells.

Lymphoid organ development is highly dependent on environmental cues. The symbiotic relationship between the host immune system and microorganisms is best exemplified in the gastrointestinal tract. Development of gut-associated lymphoid tissue is absolutely dependent on bacterial colonization. Increasing evidence suggests that host-symbiont interactions regulate adaptive immune functions throughout life. Disturbances in the bacterial microbiota and failure to maintain intestinal homeostasis are important in diverse diseases, including inflammatory bowel disease (Chapter 143) and HIV-associated immune defects.

Memory

An important consequence of adaptive immunity is the generation of immunologic memory, the basis for long-lived protection after a primary infection. Memory induction by vaccination is one of the landmark successes in medicine. Immunologic memory is defined as the ability to respond more rapidly and effectively to pathogens that have been encountered previously. The bases of immunologic memory are qualitative and quantitative changes in antigen-specific T cells and B cells. As a direct result of clonal expansion and selection in antigen-driven responses, the frequencies of antigen-specific memory B cells and memory T cells are increased 10-fold to 1000-fold compared with the naïve repertoires. The mechanisms through which memory T cells and B cells escape clonal downsizing in the terminal stages of the primary immune response are consequences of upregulation of a selected group of transcription factors that ensure survival. The enrichment of antigen-specific B cells and T cells enhances the sensitivity of the system to renewed challenges and provides a head start of 4 to 10 cell divisions. In addition to increased frequencies, memory T cells and B cells are functionally different from their naïve counterparts. Memory cells are long-lived and survive in the presence of certain cytokines without the need for continuous antigenic stimulation, guaranteeing immunologic memory for the life expectancy of the individual cell. Memory B cells produce predominantly IgG and IgA antibodies with evidence of somatic hypermutation and high affinity for the antigen. Cell surface expression of high-affinity antibodies allows more efficient antigen uptake, which enhances the crucial interaction with T cells. On antigen encounter, memory B cells change to antibody-secreting plasma cells, or re-enter the germinal center, where the high affinity of their immunoglobulin receptor gives them a competitive advantage over naïve B cells in antigen binding, leading to progressive affinity maturation of somatically mutated antibody molecules.

Because the TCR does not undergo isotype switching or affinity maturation, memory T cells are more difficult to distinguish from naïve or effector T cells. In contrast to effector cells, memory T cells lack activation markers and need antigen stimulation to resume effector functions. In contrast to naïve T cells, memory T cells have a lower activation threshold and are less dependent on costimulatory signals. In essence, their requirements for antigen stimulation are fewer, and their clonal size is larger, permitting fast, efficient responses to secondary antigen encounters. Also, memory T cells resume effector functions without having to undergo cell divisions.

Immunologic Tolerance and Autoimmunity

Unresponsiveness to self is a fundamental property of the immune system and is a condition, *sine qua non*, to maintain tissue integrity of the host. Self/nonself distinction is relatively straightforward for the innate immune system, in which receptors to nonself molecules are genetically encoded and evolutionarily selected. Self/nonself discrimination is much more complex for the adaptive immune system, in which antigen-specific receptors are generated randomly and the entire spectrum of antigens can be recognized. Thus, the adaptive immune system must acquire the ability to distinguish between self and nonself. Several different mechanisms are used, collectively called *tolerance*. Tolerance is antigen specific; its induction requires the recognition of antigen by lymphocytes in a defined setting. Failure of self-tolerance results in immune responses against self-antigens. Such reactions are called *autoimmunity* and may give rise to chronic inflammatory autoimmune disease.

Central and peripheral tolerance mechanisms can be distinguished. In central tolerance, self-reactive lymphocytes are deleted during development. This process of negative selection is particularly important for T cells. During thymic development, T cells that recognize antigen with high affinity, in particular antigens that are constitutively expressed on antigen-presenting cells, are deleted. Central tolerance for B cells follows the same principles. Recognition of antigen by developing B cells in the bone marrow induces apoptosis, or receptor editing that replaces the self-reactive receptor with one containing the product of a newly rearranged light chain gene. Negative selection is particularly important for B cells that recognize multivalent antigens because they do not depend on T-cell help and cannot be controlled peripherally.

Not all self-reactive T cells are centrally purged from the repertoire; certain antigens are not encountered at sufficient densities in the thymus. Also, all T cells have some degree of self-reactivity, which is necessary for positive selection in the thymus and for peripheral survival. Mechanisms of peripheral T-cell tolerance include (1) anergy, (2) peripheral deletion, (3) clonal ignorance, and (4) suppression of immune responses by regulatory T cells. T-cell anergy is transient and is actively maintained. It is induced if $CD4^+$ T cells recognize antigens presented by MHC class II molecules without receiving costimulatory signals. In general, costimulatory molecules such as CD80 and CD86 are restricted to antigen-presenting cells, and their expression is dependent on microbial recognition, leading to activation of the antigen-presenting cells. MHC-peptide presentation to T cells by immature or inactivated, resting antigen-presenting cells or on any cell other than peripheral antigen-presenting cells results in anergy because these cells typically lack expression of costimulatory molecules. Tissue-residing immature dendritic cells need to be activated by cytokines or recognition of pathogen-associated molecular patterns (PAMPs) to stimulate and not to anergize T cells. A second tolerance mechanism, peripheral deletion, is induced as a consequence of hyperstimulation. Hyperstimulation of T cells (e.g., by high doses of antigen and high concentrations of IL-2) preferentially activates pro-apoptotic pathways and causes elimination of the responding T-cell specificity. This mechanism may be responsible for the elimination of T cells specific for plentiful peripheral self-antigens and for foreign antigens abundantly present during infection. Whereas induction of anergy and activation-induced cell death are active consequences of antigen recognition, the third tolerance mechanism, clonal ignorance, is less well understood. Clonal ignorance is defined as the presence of self-reactive lymphocytes that fail to recognize or to respond to peripheral antigens. These cells remain responsive to antigenic challenge if given in the right setting. An example of clonal ignorance is nonresponsiveness to sequestered antigens that are not accessible to the immune system. Other mechanisms must exist, however, because clonal ignorance has also been shown for accessible antigens. Fourth, Treg cells play a pivotal role in maintaining peripheral tolerance. During an immune response, T cells can acquire the ability to produce regulatory cytokines, such as TGF-β, IL-10, or IL-4, that dampen or suppress immune responses. A dedicated subset of Treg cells, Foxp3 $CD4^+$ T cells, has been identified and characterized. Harnessing the frequencies and function of these cells may offer a promising approach to restoring peripheral tolerance in treating autoimmune diseases or facilitating transplantation tolerance; their elimination or functional suppression may potentiate cancer immunotherapy.

A critically important mechanism of peripheral tolerance of B cells is maintained through the absence of T-cell help. B cells require signals from T cells to differentiate into effector cells. B lymphocytes that recognize self-antigens in the periphery in the absence of T-cell help are rendered anergic or are unable to enter lymphoid follicles, where they could receive T-cell help, effectively excluding them from immune responses.

Generation and maintenance of self-tolerance can fail, in which case autoimmune responses are generated. Overall, chronic inflammatory diseases induced by tolerance failure occur in about 5% of the general population. Given the complexity of regulation, it is surprising that autoimmune diseases are not more frequent. It is thought that most autoimmune diseases result from dysfunction of the adaptive immune system, although activation of the innate immune system can set the stage for a self-reactive adaptive immune response. Many models of autoimmunity rely on the hypothesis that peripheral anergy is broken. Aberrant expression of costimulatory molecules on nonprofessional antigen-presenting cells or inappropriate activation of tissue-residing dendritic cells sets the stage for the induction of "forbidden" T-cell responses. Also, autoreactive B cells that recognize self-antigen complexed with foreign antigen may engulf this complex and receive help from T cells specific for the foreign antigen. Autoimmunity also may emerge if antigen ignorance is broken. This could happen if tissue barriers break down and antigens that are usually sequestered from the immune system, such as antigens from the central nervous system or the eye, become accessible. Tolerance mechanisms of anergy or clonal ignorance can also fail if a foreign antigen is sufficiently different from a self-antigen to initiate an immune response but sufficiently similar for activated T cells to elicit T-cell and B-cell effector functions (molecular mimicry).

GENERAL REFERENCES

For the General References and other additional features, please visit Expert Consult at https://expertconsult.inkling.com.

47 MECHANISMS OF IMMUNE-MEDIATED TISSUE INJURY

JANE E. SALMON

THE ADAPTIVE IMMUNE RESPONSE

Definition

The adaptive immune response is a crucial component of host defense against infection. Its distinguishing and unique feature is the ability to recognize pathogens specifically, based on clonal selection of lymphocytes bearing antigen-specific receptors. Antigens unassociated with infectious agents also may elicit adaptive immune responses. Many clinically important diseases are characterized by normal immune responses directed against an inappropriate antigen, typically in the absence of infection. Immune responses directed at noninfectious antigens occur in allergy, in which the antigen is an innocuous foreign substance, and in autoimmunity, in which the response is to a self-antigen.

Effector mechanisms that eliminate pathogens in adaptive immune responses are essentially identical to those of innate immunity. The specific antigen recognition feature of the adaptive immune response seems to have been appended to the preexisting innate defense system. As a result, the inflammatory cells and molecules of the innate immune system are essential for the effector functions of B and T lymphocytes. In addition to initiating protective responses, they mediate tissue injury in allergy, hypersensitivity, and autoimmunity.

Effector Mechanisms

Effector actions of antibodies depend on recruiting cells and molecules of the innate immune system. Antibodies are adapters that bind antigens to nonspecific inflammatory cells and direct their destructive effector responses. Antibodies also activate the complement system, which enhances opsonization of antigens, recruits phagocytic cells, and amplifies (or "complements") antibody-triggered damage. The isotype or class of antibodies produced determines which effector mechanisms are engaged.

Cell-bound receptors for immunoglobulin (Ig) constitute the link between humoral and cellular aspects of the immune cascade and play an integral part in the process by which foreign and endogenous opsonized material is identified and destroyed. These cell-based binding sites for antibodies, termed *Fc receptors,* interact with the constant region (Fc portion) of the immunoglobulin heavy chain of a particular antibody class regardless of its antigen specificity. Accessory cells that lack intrinsic specificity, such as neutrophils, macrophages, and mast cells, are recruited to participate in inflammatory responses through the interaction of their Fc receptors with antigen-specific antibodies. Distinct receptors for different immunoglobulin isotypes are expressed on different effector cells.

Receptors for IgG (FcγRs) are a diverse group of receptors expressed as hematopoietic cell surface molecules on phagocytes (macrophages, monocytes, neutrophils), platelets, mast cells, eosinophils, and natural killer (NK) cells. FcγRs often are expressed as stimulatory and inhibitory pairs.[1] Triggering of stimulatory FcγRs initiates a series of events, including phagocytosis; antibody-dependent, cell-mediated cytotoxicity; secretion of granules; and release of inflammatory mediators, such as cytokines, reactive oxidants, and proteases. Extensive structural diversity among FcγR family members leads to differences in binding capacity, signal transduction pathways, and cell type–specific expression patterns. This diversity allows IgG complexes to activate a broad program of cell functions relevant to inflammation, host defense, and autoimmunity. Phagocyte activation is triggered by stimulatory FcγRs, facilitating the recognition, uptake, and destruction of antibody-coated targets, whereas multivalent IgG binding to FcγRs on platelets leads to platelet aggregation and thrombosis, and binding to FcγRs on NK cells mediates cytotoxicity of antibody-coated targets.

IgE binds to high-affinity FcεRs on mast cells, basophils, and activated eosinophils.[2] In contrast to FcγRs, which are low affinity and bind to multivalent IgG rather than circulating individual IgG molecules, FcεRs can bind monomeric IgE. A single mast cell may be armed with IgE molecules specific for different antigens, all bound to surface FcεRs. Mast cells, localized beneath the mucosa of the gastrointestinal and respiratory tracts and the dermis of the skin, await exposure to multivalent antigens, which cross-link surface IgE bound to FcεRs and cause release of histamine-containing granules and generation of cytokines and other inflammatory mediators. IgE-mediated activation of eosinophils, cells normally present in the connective tissue of underlying respiratory, urogenital, and gut epithelium, leads to the release of highly toxic granule proteins, free radicals, and chemical mediators such as prostaglandins, cytokines, and chemokines. These amplify local inflammatory responses by activating endothelial cells and recruiting and activating more eosinophils and leukocytes. Prepackaged granules and high-affinity FcεRs that bind to free monomeric IgE enable an immediate response to pathogens or allergens at the first site of entry, a location where FcεR-bearing cells reside.

Inhibitory FcγRs, which modulate activation thresholds and terminate stimulating signals, are key elements in the regulation of effector function. Given that inhibitory and stimulatory Fc receptors are often coexpressed on the same cells, the effector response to a specific stimulus in a particular cell represents the balance between stimulatory and inhibitory signals. Inhibitory FcγRs can dampen responses triggered by FcεRs on mast cells and FcγR-mediated inflammation at sites of immune complex deposition.

Effector activities targeted by IgG and IgM also may be mediated by components of the complement system (Chapter 50). Antigen-bound multimeric immunoglobulin can initiate activation of the classic pathway of complement, causing enhanced phagocytosis of antigen-antibody complexes, increased local vascular permeability, and recruitment and activation of inflammatory cells. The target of injury is specified by the antibody, and the extent of damage is determined by the synergistic activities of immunoglobulin and complement.

Antigen-specific effector T cells also may initiate tissue injury. On exposure to an appropriate antigen, memory T cells are stimulated to release cytokines and chemokines that activate local endothelial cells and recruit and activate macrophages and other inflammatory cells. The effector cells directed by T-cell-derived cytokines, or cytolytic T cells themselves, mediate tissue damage. T helper 1 (T_H1) cells produce interferon-γ (IFN-γ) and activate macrophages to cause injury, whereas T_H2 cells produce interleukin-4 (IL-4), IL-5, and eotaxin (an eosinophil-specific chemokine) and trigger inflammatory responses in which eosinophils predominate. T_H17 cells secrete several effector molecules, including IL-17, which act on both immune and nonimmune cells to trigger differentiation; release of antimicrobial molecules, cytokines, and chemokines; and recruitment to sites of inflammation.[3] New T_H effector subsets have recently been identified, including follicular T helper cells (T_{FH}), which provide help to B cells in germinal centers and thus are key regulators of humoral responses and antibody production.

HYPERSENSITIVITY REACTIONS

In predisposed individuals, innocuous environmental antigens may stimulate an adaptive immune response, immunologic memory, and, on subsequent exposure to the antigen, inflammation. These "overreactions" of the immune system to harmless environmental antigens (allergens), called *hypersensitivity* or *allergic reactions,* produce tissue injury and can cause serious disease. Hypersensitivity reactions are grouped into four types according to the effector mechanisms by which they are produced (Table 47-1). The effectors for types I, II, and III hypersensitivity reactions are antibody molecules, whereas type IV reactions are mediated by antigen-specific effector T cells.[4]

Autoimmune disease is characterized by the presence of antibodies and T cells specific for self-antigens expressed on target tissues. The mechanisms of antigen recognition and effector function that lead to tissue damage in autoimmune disease are similar to the mechanisms elicited in response to pathogens and environmental antigens. These mechanisms resemble certain hypersensitivity reactions and may be classified accordingly (Table 47-2). Autoimmune disease caused by antibodies directed against cell surface or extracellular matrix antigens corresponds to type II hypersensitivity reactions; disease caused by formation of soluble immune complexes that subsequently are deposited in tissue corresponds to type III hypersensitivity; and disease caused by effector T cells corresponds to type IV hypersensitivity. Typically, several of these pathogenic mechanisms are operative in autoimmune disease. However, IgE responses are not associated with damage in autoimmunity.

Type I Hypersensitivity Reactions

Type I hypersensitivity reactions (Fig. 47-1) are triggered by the interaction of antigen with antigen-specific IgE bound to FcεRs on mast cells, which

TABLE 47-1 FOUR MAJOR TYPES OF IMMUNOLOGICALLY MEDIATED HYPERSENSITIVITY REACTIONS*

IMMUNOLOGIC SPECIFICITY	TYPE I (IgE ANTIBODY)	TYPE II (IgG ANTIBODY)	TYPE III (IgG ANTIBODY)	TYPE IV (T CELLS): T_H1 Cells	T_H2 Cells	T_H17 Cells	T Cells
Antigen	Soluble antigen allergen	Cell- or matrix-associated antigen	Soluble antigen	Soluble antigen	Soluble antigen	Soluble antigen	Cell-associated antigen
Effector mechanism	FcεRI- or FcγRIII-dependent mast cell activation, with release of mediators/cytokines	FcγR⁺ cells (phagocytes, NK cells), complement	FcγR⁺ cells, complement	Macrophage activation	Eosinophil activation	Macrophage activation Neutrophil activation	Direct cytotoxicity
Examples	Systemic anaphylaxis, asthma, allergic rhinitis, urticaria, angioedema	Certain drug reactions and reactions to incompatible blood transfusions	Arthus reaction and other immune complex–mediated reactions (e.g., serum sickness, subacute bacterial endocarditis)	Contact dermatitis, tuberculin reaction	Chronic allergic inflammation (e.g., chronic asthma, chronic allergic rhinitis)	Contact dermatitis, atopic dermatitis, asthma, rheumatoid arthritis	Contact dermatitis (e.g., poison ivy), reactions to certain virus-infected cells, some instances of graft rejection

*Hypersensitivity reactions were classified into four types by Coombs and Gell (1963) and modified by Janeway and colleagues (2001).
FcγR = Fc receptor for immunoglobulin G; FcεR = Fc receptor for immunoglobulin E; NK = natural killer.
From Coombs RRA, Gell PGH: Classification of allergic reactions responsible for clinical hypersensitivity and disease. In: Gell PGH, Coombs RA, eds. *Clinical Aspects of Immunology.* Oxford, UK: Blackwell; 1963; and Janeway C, Travers P, Walport M, Shlomchick M: *Immunobiology: The Immune System in Health and Disease.* 5th ed. New York: Garland Publishing; 2001.

TABLE 47-2 CLASSIFICATION OF AUTOIMMUNE DISEASES ACCORDING TO MECHANISM OF TISSUE INJURY

HYPERSENSITIVITY REACTION	AUTOIMMUNE DISEASE	AUTOANTIGEN
TYPE II		
Antibody against cell surface antigens	Autoimmune hemolytic anemia	Rh blood group antigens, I antigen
	Autoimmune thrombocytopenic purpura	Platelet integrin glycoprotein IIb/IIIa
Antibody against receptors	Graves disease	Thyroid-stimulating hormone receptor (agonistic antibodies)
	Myasthenia gravis	Acetylcholine receptor (antagonistic antibodies)
Antibody against matrix antigens	Goodpasture syndrome	Basement membrane collagen (α_3-chain of type IV collagen)
	Pemphigus vulgaris	Epidermal cadherin (desmoglein)
TYPE III		
Immune complex diseases	Mixed essential cryoglobulinemia	Rheumatoid factor IgG complexes (with or without hepatitis C antigens)
	Systemic lupus erythematosus	DNA, histones, ribosomes, binuclear proteins
TYPE IV		
T-cell-mediated diseases	Insulin-dependent diabetes mellitus	Pancreatic B-cell antigen
	Rheumatoid arthritis	Unknown synovial joint antigen
	Multiple sclerosis	Myelin basic protein, proteolipid protein

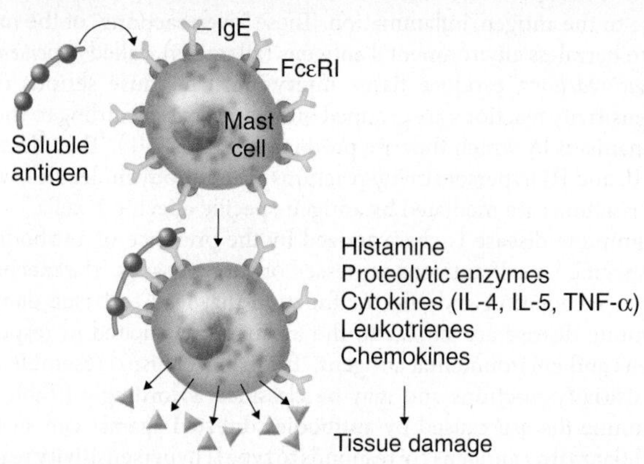

FIGURE 47-1. Type I hypersensitivity. Type I responses are mediated by immunoglobulin E (IgE), which induces mast cell activation. Cross-linking of the Fc receptor for IgE (FcεR) on mast cells, triggered by the interaction of multivalent antigen with antigen-specific IgE bound to FcεR, causes the release of preformed granules containing histamine and proteases. Cytokines, chemokines, and lipid mediators are synthesized after cell activation. IL = interleukin; TNF = tumor necrosis factor.

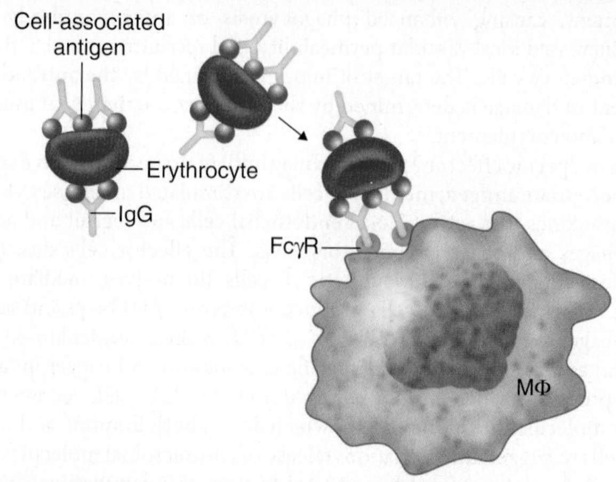

FIGURE 47-2. Type II hypersensitivity. Type II responses are mediated by immunoglobulin G (IgG) directed against cell surface or matrix antigens, which initiates effector responses through the Fc receptor for IgG (FcγR) and complement. The relative contributions of these pathways vary with the IgG subclass and the nature of the antigen. Only FcγR-mediated phagocytosis by macrophages (MΦ) is depicted in this figure. Activation of complement components would result in binding of C3b to the red blood cell membrane, rendering red blood cells susceptible to phagocytosis and leading to formation of the membrane attack complex and cell lysis.

causes mast cell activation. Proteolytic enzymes and toxic mediators, such as histamine, are released immediately from preformed granules, and chemokines, cytokines, and leukotrienes are synthesized after activation. Together, these mediators increase vascular permeability, break down tissue matrix proteins, promote eosinophil production and activation (IL-3, IL-5, and granulocyte-macrophage colony-stimulating factor [GM-CSF]), and cause influx of effector leukocytes (tumor necrosis factor-α [TNF-α], platelet-activating factor, and macrophage inflammatory protein [MIP-1]), constriction of smooth muscle, stimulation of mucus secretion, and amplification of T_H2 cell responses (IL-4 and IL-13). Eosinophils and basophils, activated through cell surface FcεRs, rapidly release highly toxic granular proteins (major basic protein, eosinophil peroxidase, and collagenase) and, over a longer period, produce cytokines (IL-3, IL-5, and GM-CSF), chemokines (IL-8), prostaglandins, and leukotrienes that activate epithelial cells, leukocytes, and eosinophils to augment local inflammation and tissue damage.

FcεR-bearing effectors act in a coordinated fashion. The immediate allergic inflammatory reaction initiated by mast cell products is followed by a late-phase response that involves recruitment and activation of eosinophils, basophils, and T_H2 lymphocytes.[5] The manifestations of IgE-mediated reactions depend on the site of mast cell activation. Mast cells reside in vascular and epithelial tissue throughout the body. In a sensitized host (an individual with IgE responses to antigens), re-exposure to antigen leads to type I hypersensitivity responses only in the mast cells exposed to the antigen. Inhalation of antigens produces bronchoconstriction and increased mucus secretion (asthma and allergic rhinitis); ingestion of antigens causes increased peristalsis and secretion (diarrhea and vomiting); and the presence of subcutaneous antigens initiates increased vascular permeability and swelling (urticaria and angioedema). Blood-borne antigens cause systemic mast cell activation, increased capillary permeability, hypotension, tissue swelling, and smooth muscle contraction—the characteristics of systemic anaphylaxis.

Type II Hypersensitivity Reactions

Type II hypersensitivity reactions (Fig. 47-2) are caused by chemical modification of cell surface or matrix-associated antigens that generates "foreign" epitopes to which the immune system is not tolerant. B cells respond to this antigenic challenge by producing IgG, which binds to these modified cells and renders them susceptible to destruction through complement activation, phagocytosis, and antibody-dependent cytotoxicity.

This phenomenon is seen clinically when drugs interact with blood constituents and alter their cellular antigens. Hemolytic anemia caused by immune-mediated destruction of erythrocytes (Chapter 160) and thrombocytopenia caused by destruction of platelets (Chapter 172), both type II hypersensitivity reactions, are adverse effects of certain drugs. Chemically reactive drug molecules bind covalently to the surface of red cells or platelets creating new epitopes that in a small subset of individuals are recognized as foreign antigens by the immune system and stimulate production of IgM and IgG antibodies reactive with the conjugate of drug and cell surface protein. Penicillin-specific IgG binds to penicillin-modified proteins on red blood cells and triggers activation of the complement cascade. Activation of complement components C1 through C3 results in covalent binding of C3b to the red cell membrane and renders circulating red cells susceptible to phagocytosis by FcγR and complement receptor–bearing macrophages in the spleen or liver. Activation of complement components C1 through C9 and formation of the membrane attack complex cause intravascular lysis of red cells. The factors that predispose only some people to drug-induced type II hypersensitivity reactions are unknown. Penicillin, quinidine, and methyldopa have been associated with hemolytic anemia and thrombocytopenia through this mechanism. Another example is heparin-induced thrombocytopenia or thrombosis, a severe, life-threatening complication that occurs in 1 to 3% of patients exposed to heparin (Chapter 172). Interactions among heparin, human platelet factor 4, antibodies to the human platelet factor 4–heparin complex, platelet FcγRIIA, and splenic FcγRs (which remove opsonized platelets) are involved in the pathogenesis of this disease.

Autoantibodies directed at antigens on the cell surface or extracellular matrix cause tissue damage by mechanisms similar to type II hypersensitivity reactions. IgG or IgM antibodies against erythrocytes lead to cell destruction in autoimmune hemolytic anemia because opsonized cells (coated with IgG or IgM and complement) are removed from the circulation by phagocytes in the liver and spleen or are lysed by formation of the membrane attack complex. Platelet destruction in autoimmune thrombocytopenic purpura occurs through a similar process. Because nucleated cells express membrane-bound complement regulatory proteins, they are less sensitive to lysis through the membrane attack complex, but when coated with antibody, they become targets for phagocytosis or antibody-dependent cytotoxicity. This mechanism is responsible for autoimmune and alloimmune neutropenia (Chapter 167).

IgM and IgG antibodies recognizing antigens within tissue or binding to extracellular antigens cause local inflammatory damage through FcγR and complement mechanisms. Pemphigus vulgaris (Chapter 439) is a serious blistering disease that results from a loss of adhesion between keratinocytes caused by autoantibodies against the extracellular portions of desmoglein 3, an intercellular adhesion structure of epidermal keratinocytes. Another example of a type II hypersensitivity reaction is Goodpasture disease (Chapter 121), in which antibodies against the α_3-chain of type IV collagen (the collagen in basement membranes) are deposited in glomerular and lung basement membrane. Tissue-bound autoantibodies activate monocytes, neutrophils, and basophils through FcγRs, initiating release of proteases, reactive oxidants, cytokines, and prostaglandins. Local activation of complement, particularly C5a, recruits and activates inflammatory cells and amplifies tissue injury. Neighboring cells are lysed by assembly of the membrane attack complex or by FcγR-initiated, antibody-dependent cytotoxicity.

Autoantibodies against cell surface receptors produce disease by stimulating or blocking receptor function. In myasthenia gravis (Chapter 422), autoantibodies against the acetylcholine receptors on skeletal muscle cells bind the receptor and induce its internalization and degradation in lysosomes, reducing the efficiency of neuromuscular transmission and causing progressive muscle weakness. In contrast, Graves disease (Chapter 226) is

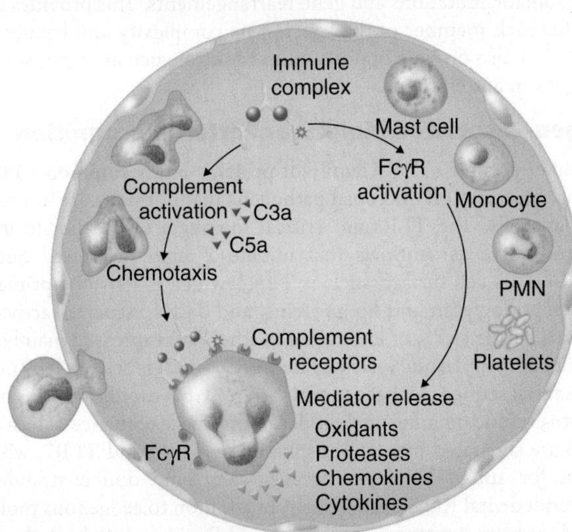

FIGURE 47-3. Type III hypersensitivity. Type III responses are mediated by immunoglobulin G (IgG) directed against soluble antigens. Localized deposition of immune complexes activates mast cells, monocytes, neutrophils, and platelets bearing the Fc receptor for IgG (FcγR), and initiates the complement cascade, all effectors of tissue damage. Generation of complement components C3a and C5a recruits and stimulates inflammatory cells and amplifies effector functions. PMN = polymorphonuclear leukocyte (also called *neutrophil*).

characterized by autoantibodies that act as agonists. Autoantibodies to thyroid-stimulating hormone receptors bind the receptor, mimicking the natural ligand, inducing thyroid hormone overproduction, disrupting feedback regulation, and causing hyperthyroidism.

Type III Hypersensitivity Reactions

Type III hypersensitivity reactions (Fig. 47-3) are caused by tissue deposition of small soluble immune complexes that contain antigens and high-affinity IgG antibodies directed at these antigens. Localized deposition of immune complexes activates FcγR-bearing mast cells and phagocytes and initiates the complement cascade, all effectors of tissue damage.[6]

Immune complexes are generated in all antibody responses. The formation and the fate of immune complexes depend on the biophysical and immunologic properties of the antigen and the antibody. These properties include the size, net charge, and valence of the antigen; the class and subclass of the antibody; the affinity of the antibody-antigen interaction; the net charge and concentration of antibody; the molar ratio of available antigen and antibody; and the ability of the immune complex to interact with the proteins of the complement system. The lattice size of the immune complex is influenced strongly by the physical size and valence of the antigen, the association constant of antibody for that antigen, the molar ratio of antigen and antibody, and the absolute concentrations of the reactants. Larger aggregates fix complement more efficiently, present a broader multivalent array of ligands for complement and FcγRs to bind, and are taken up more readily by mononuclear phagocytes in the liver and spleen and thereby removed from the circulation. Smaller immune complexes, which form in antigen excess—as occurs early in an immune response—circulate in the blood and are deposited in blood vessels, where they initiate inflammatory reactions and tissue damage through interactions with FcγRs and complement receptors.

Serum sickness is a systemic type III hypersensitivity reaction, historically described in patients injected with therapeutic horse antiserum for the treatment of bacterial infections. In general, serum sickness occurs after the injection of large quantities of a soluble antigen. Clinical features include chills, fever, rash, urticaria, arthritis, and glomerulonephritis. Disease manifestations become evident 7 to 10 days after exposure to the antigen, when antibodies are generated against the foreign protein and form immune complexes with these circulating antigens. Immune complexes are deposited in blood vessels, where they activate phagocytes and complement, producing widespread tissue injury and clinical symptoms. The effects are transient, however, and resolve after the antigen is cleared.

A syndrome similar to serum sickness occurs in chronic infections in which pathogens persist in the face of continued immune response. In subacute bacterial endocarditis (Chapter 76), antibody production continues

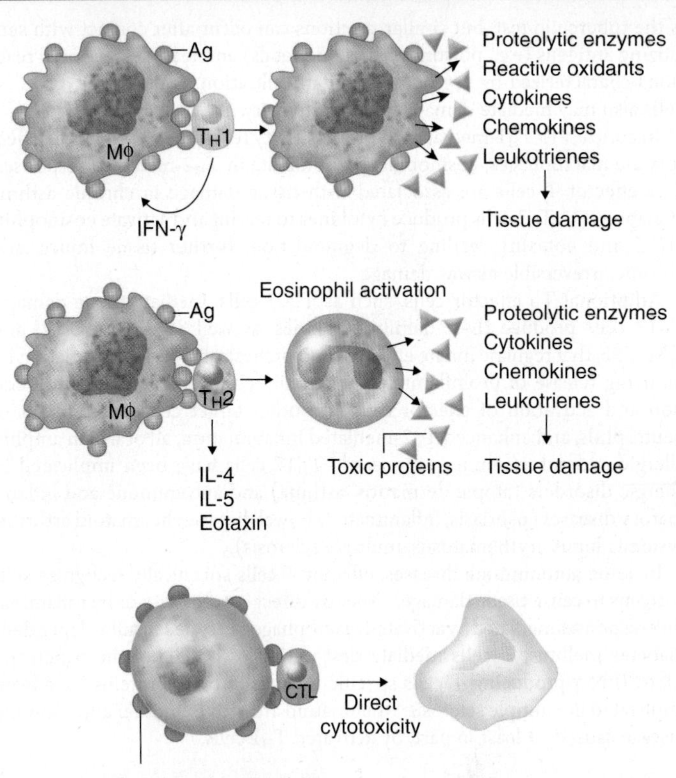

FIGURE 47-4. Type IV hypersensitivity. Type IV responses are mediated by T cells through three different pathways. In the first, type 1 helper T (T_H1) cells recognize soluble antigens (Ag) and release interferon-γ (IFN-γ) to activate effector cells, in this case macrophages (MΦ), and cause tissue injury. In T_H2-mediated responses, eosinophils predominate. T_H2 cells produce cytokines to recruit and activate eosinophils, leading to their degranulation and tissue injury. In the third pathway, damage is caused directly by cytolytic T lymphocytes (CTL). IL = interleukin.

but fails to eliminate the infecting microbes. As the pathogens multiply, generating new antigens, immune complexes form in the circulation and are deposited in small blood vessels, where they lead to inflammatory damage of skin, kidney, and nerve. Hepatitis B virus infection (Chapters 148 and 149) may be associated with immune complex deposition early in its course, during a period of antigen excess, because antibody production in response to hepatitis B surface antigen is as yet relatively insufficient; some anicteric patients may present with acute arthritis. Mixed essential cryoglobulinemia, which may be associated with hepatitis C viral infection, is an immune complex–mediated vasculitis in which deposition of complexes containing IgG, IgM, and hepatitis C antigens causes inflammation in peripheral nerves, kidneys, and skin. Serum sickness also can develop in transplant recipients who are treated with mouse monoclonal antibodies specific for human T cells to prevent rejection, and in patients with myocardial infarction who are treated with the bacterial enzyme streptokinase to effect thrombolysis.

Systemic lupus erythematosus (Chapter 266), the prototypical immune complex–mediated autoimmune disease, is characterized by circulating IgG directed against common cellular constituents, typically DNA and DNA-binding proteins. Small immune complexes are deposited in skin, joints, and glomeruli and initiate local tissue damage.

Type IV Hypersensitivity Reactions

Type IV hypersensitivity reactions (Fig. 47-4), also known as *delayed-type hypersensitivity reactions,* are mediated by antigen-specific effector T cells. They are distinguished from other hypersensitivity reactions by the lag time from exposure to the antigen until the response is evident (1 to 3 days). Antigen is taken up, processed, and presented by macrophages or dendritic cells. T_H1 effector cells that recognize the specific antigen (these are scarce and take time to arrive) are stimulated to release chemokines, which recruit macrophages to the site, release cytokines that mediate tissue injury and growth factors that stimulate monocyte production. IFN-γ activates macrophages and enhances their release of inflammatory mediators, whereas TNF-α and TNF-β activate endothelial cells, enhance vascular permeability, and damage local tissue. The prototypical type IV hypersensitivity reaction is the tuberculin test, but similar reactions can occur after contact with sensitizing antigens (e.g., poison ivy, certain metals) and lead to epidermal reactions characterized by erythema, cellular infiltration, and vesicles. $CD8^+$ T cells also may mediate damage by direct toxicity.

In contrast to T_H1-mediated hypersensitivity reactions, in which the effectors are macrophages, eosinophils predominate in T_H2-mediated responses. T_H2 effector T cells are associated with tissue damage in chronic asthma (Chapter 87). T_H2 cells produce cytokines to recruit and activate eosinophils (IL-5 and eotaxin), leading to degranulation, further tissue injury, and chronic, irreversible airway damage.

Additional T_H effector cells, such as T_H17 cells, mediate tissue damage. T_H17 cells produce IL-17 family cytokines, as well as IL-21, IL-22, and GM-CSF, that regulate innate effectors and orchestrate local inflammation by inducing release of proinflammatory cytokines and chemokines, proliferation and activation of effector cells and other target cells, recruitment of neutrophils, and enhanced T_H2-mediated inflammation, all of which amplify allergic and autoimmune responses.[3,7] T_H17 cells have been implicated in allergic disorders (atopic dermatitis, asthma) and autoimmune and inflammatory diseases (psoriasis, inflammatory bowel disease, rheumatoid arthritis, systemic lupus erythematosus, multiple sclerosis).

In some autoimmune diseases, effector T cells specifically recognize self-antigens to cause tissue damage, either by direct cytotoxicity or by inflammatory responses mediated by activated macrophages. In type 1 insulin-dependent diabetes mellitus, T cells mediate destruction of β cells of the pancreatic islets. IFN-γ-producing T cells specific for myelin basic proteins have been implicated in multiple sclerosis. Rheumatoid arthritis is another autoimmune disease caused, at least in part, by activated T_H1 cells.

GENERAL REFERENCES

For the General References and other additional features, please visit Expert Consult at https://expertconsult.inkling.com.

48 MECHANISMS OF INFLAMMATION AND TISSUE REPAIR

GARY S. FIRESTEIN

Host defense mechanisms have evolved to recognize pathogens rapidly, render them harmless, and repair the damaged tissue. This complex and highly regulated sequence of events can also be triggered by environmental stimuli such as noxious mechanical and chemical agents. Under normal circumstances, tightly controlled responses protect against further injury and clear damaged tissue. In disease states, however, pathologic inflammation can lead to marked destruction of the extracellular matrix (ECM) and organ dysfunction.

INITIATION OF THE INFLAMMATORY RESPONSE

When normal tissue encounters a pathogen, resident cells are stimulated by engagement of pattern recognition receptors that activate an ancient arm of host defense known as *innate immunity*. In contrast to *adaptive immunity*, which provides exquisite antigen specificity, innate immune responses recognize common motifs on pathogens (Chapter 45). Additional cytoplasmic receptors can sense "danger" signals from a toxic environment or cellular stress, such as urate or adenosine triphosphate (ATP). Innate mechanisms are designed for rapid responses (minutes to hours) compared with the more leisurely adaptive system that can take days to weeks to develop. In addition to orchestrating early events that are critical to host defense, cells of the innate system like dendritic cells orchestrate the subsequent adaptive cascade through the generation of chemokines that organize lymphoid tissue and presentation of antigens to lymphocytes. Innate immunity provides intergenerational continuity in that the receptors are encoded in the germline and are passed unchanged to progeny to protect the species. In contrast, each individual must generate his or her own adaptive immune system through complex somatic mutations and gene rearrangements. This provides defense tailored for each member of the species; its complexity and beauty permit specificity but also provide opportunities for error such as responses against self-antigens in autoimmunity.

Pathogen-Associated Molecular Pattern Recognition

The toll-like receptor (TLR) family of proteins binds common patterns of molecular structures on microbial pathogens that normally are not found in mammalian cells. The TLRs are critical members of the innate immune system and serve as sentinels that initiate a rapid response.[1] Some are expressed on the cell surface, such as TLR2, which is activated primarily by bacterial peptidoglycan and lipoproteins, and TLR4, which is activated by lipopolysaccharide (LPS, or endotoxin). Others are expressed mainly on the inner leaflet of cytoplasmic vesicles, like TLR9, which is activated by unmethylated bacterial sequences that are enriched for CpG motifs (regions of DNA where cytosine and guanine nucleotides in the linear sequence of bases along its length are separated by one phosphate), or TLR3 and TLR7, which are important for antiviral defense because they bind double-stranded and single-stranded viral RNA, respectively. In addition to exogenous molecules, some endogenous structures can bind to TLRs, including heat shock proteins and oxidized low-density lipoproteins (oxLDLs). The latter might be especially important in the pathogenesis of atherosclerosis, in which LDL activates TLR4 within vascular plaques. Local endothelial cell– and macrophage-derived chemotactic factors can then recruit activated T cells into the atheroma.

Signaling by TLR2 and TLR4 progresses through adaptor proteins and often converges on a kinase known as MyD88, which orchestrates several downstream cascades. By directing the phosphorylation of IκB kinase-β (IKKβ), MyD88 activates nuclear factor-κB (NF-κB), a master switch for inflammatory genes.[2] Translocation of NF-κB to the cell nucleus stimulates the production of cytokines (e.g., interleukin-6 [IL-6], IL-8, and tumor necrosis factor [TNF]), the machinery for prostaglandin release (e.g., cyclo-oxygenase 2 [COX2]), and genes that regulate the ECM (e.g., metalloproteinases). This rapid response is normally transient, although it can persist in pathogenic states. MyD88-independent pathways that stimulate innate immunity also exist. For instance, TLR3 stimulation by RNA viruses uses a separate pathway involving IKKε and interferon regulating factor-3 (IRF-3). IRF-3, in combination with several other transcription factors, induces the expression of genes such as interferon-β (IFN-β) to establish an antiviral state.

These genes primarily offer protection against pathogens by initiating key defense mechanisms. However, these same pathways can create a hazardous milieu that is toxic to normal cells through the production of oxygen radicals, nitric oxide, and other reactive intermediaries. These molecules can damage DNA and harm bystander cells, or even lead to neoplasia (E-Table 48-1). For instance, long-standing inflammation in the colon, as in ulcerative colitis, is associated with adenocarcinoma. Increased COX2 expression as a result of NF-κB translocation is another mechanism that contributes to the development of tumors at inflammatory sites. An unanticipated finding is that NF-κB itself can also directly augment carcinogenesis by serving as a survival signal for damaged cells that would normally be deleted by apoptosis.

The TLR signal transduction mechanisms integrate the environmental stimuli and generate a broadly antipathogen response. Fine-tuning of host defenses against unique pathogen structures to provide long-lived immunity requires the slower, more precise adaptive immune system. Although it is more cumbersome and primitive, innate immunity provides signals that activate adaptive responses. For instance, TLRs can direct dendritic cells (Chapter 45), which have internalized and processed antigen, to migrate from peripheral tissues to central lymphoid organs. The dendritic cells can also produce cytokines and, after maturation, present antigens to T cells in the context of class II major histocompatibility molecules and surface costimulatory proteins. The activated T cells can then migrate to the tissue to enhance and amplify the host response. T cells also provide help to B cells, thereby stimulating antibody production and activating other components of innate immunity (e.g., the complement system, Chapter 50).

Other non-TLR cytoplasmic sensors also serve a similar purpose in the environment. For instance, retinoic acid–inducible gene 1 (RIG-1) and melanoma differentiation–associated gene 5 (MDA5) can detect RNA viruses and initiate an inflammatory response. These are, in some cases, partially redundant with TLR3 and TLR7 and can activate similar signaling mechanisms, such as NF-κB through the IKKß and IRFs through a distinct pathway involving IKKε and TBK1.

Environmental Stress and Danger-Associated Molecular Patterns

Danger-associated molecular pattern molecules serve as a mechanism to detect and respond to damage to the microenvironment. Tissue injury due to direct trauma or a noxious stimulus initiates an inflammatory response and is associated with microvascular damage, extravasation of leukocytes through vascular walls, and leakage of plasma and proteins into the tissue. Endogenous proteins, including ATP receptors, S100, heat shock proteins, and high mobility-group box 1 (HMGB1), mediate release of molecules that reflect cellular toxicity and induce a cellular response. Acid-sensitive ion channels (ASICs) on the cell surface can also detect the environmental stress caused by a decrease in tissue pH. ASICs can mediate a variety of cellular functions, including cell death through apoptosis or pain responses that can lead to adaptive pain behaviors that limit further exposure to noxious stimuli.

Proteases, Coagulation, and Inflammation

Although the coagulation system's primary function is to maintain vascular integrity (Chapter 171), the proteases that regulate its functions also play an important role in the early responses to tissue damage and inflammation. For example, plasminogen is a circulating proenzyme that can be cleaved to plasmin by enzymes in the coagulation pathway, including factors XIa and XIIa. Tissue plasminogen activating factor and kallikrein also have this capacity. When activated, the serine protease plasmin can digest fibrin, fibronectin, thrombospondin, and laminin as well as activating pro-matrix metalloproteinases like collagenase (MMP1). By remodeling the extracellular matrix, this system can ultimately regulate cell recruitment and tissue damage.

Thrombus formation at the site of vascular damage can begin the inflammatory cascade through the release of vasoactive amines (e.g., serotonin), release of lysosomal proteases, and formation of eicosanoid products. The platelets can also later regulate healing with release of growth factors such as platelet-derived growth factor (PDGF) and transforming growth factor-β (TGFβ).

Inflammasome

The inflammasome[3] is among the best characterized mechanisms for sensing danger and includes the 22-member human Nod-like receptor (NLR) family of cytoplasmic proteins. The activated NLR proteins recruit additional proteins to form a complex with caspase-1 and adaptor molecule apoptosis-associated specklike protein (ASC). Activation of caspase-1 is a key function of inflammasomes, with resultant cleavage and activation of IL-1, IL-18, and IL-33. The latter molecule is also known as an "alarmin" because of its rapid release in the presence of tissue damage or a pathogen. Alarmins are often preformed in cells, such as mast cells, and can be either released directly into the microenvironment or quickly processed and secreted. Other alarmins include products of cell destruction, such as ATP or uric acid.

Disorders of the inflammasome are associated with a group of conditions known as autoinflammatory diseases (Chapter 261). The prototypic syndromes known as familial cold autoinflammatory disease, Muckle-Wells disease, and neonatal-onset multisystem inflammatory disease (NOMID) are due to nonconserved mutations in the *NLR* gene that encodes cryopyrin (also known as *NALP3*). These rare diseases are characterized by abnormal inflammasome activation with aberrant release of processed IL-1β. The clinical manifestations, including fever, rash, hearing impairment, and arthritis, depend on the specific amino acid substitution as well as other less well-defined genetic influences. The critical role of IL-1 has been proved by studies using treatment with IL-1 inhibitors, which prevent flares and can reverse end-organ damage. The inflammasome also participates in some common diseases, such as gout (Chapter 273), in which urate crystals can activate the inflammasome.

Immune Complexes and Complement

The complement system (Chapter 50) is another ancient defense mechanism that links innate immunity and the humoral arm of adaptive immunity. Both the classical complement pathway, activated by immunoglobulin G (IgG)- and IgM-containing immune complexes, and the alternative pathway, activated by bacterial products, converge at the third component of complement, C3, with proteolytic release of fragments that amplify the inflammatory response and mediate tissue injury. C3a and C5a directly increase vascular permeability and contraction of smooth muscle. C5a induces mast cell release of histamine, thereby indirectly mediating increased vascular permeability. C5a also activates leukocytes and enhances their chemotaxis, adhesion, and degranulation, with release of proteases and toxic metabolites. C5b attaches to the surface of cells and microorganisms and is the first component in the assembly of the C5b-9 membrane attack complex.

Individuals with abnormalities of the early complement components, especially C1q, C2, and C4, usually have a minimally increased incidence of infection but demonstrate an enhanced risk for developing autoimmune diseases such as systemic lupus erythematosus (SLE) (Chapter 266). The mechanism of increased disease susceptibility is probably related to inefficient clearance of immune complexes. Enhanced activation and consumption of complement proteins can also occur in SLE accompanied by low plasma C3 and C4 levels, especially in association with disease exacerbations. C3 or C5 deficiency increases susceptibility to bacterial infections, whereas defects in the late components that form the membrane attack complex result in an increased incidence of *Neisseria* sp bacteremia (Chapter 298).

SECOND WAVE OF THE INFLAMMATORY RESPONSE

Activation of innate immunity quickly leads to the robust influx of inflammatory cells. Resident cells, such as vascular endothelial cells, mast cells, dendritic cells, and interstitial fibroblasts, respond by releasing soluble mediators, including eicosanoids and pro-inflammatory cytokines (E-Table 48-2). These mediators amplify the inflammatory response and recruit additional leukocytes. Locally stimulated cells, along with the newly arrived inflammatory cells, release toxic reactive intermediates of nitrogen and oxygen as well as a myriad of proteases, principally matrix metalloproteinases (MMPs), serine proteases, and cysteine proteases. These molecules help destroy infectious agents and remove damaged cells, thus clearing the injured site for tissue repair. In most situations, the normal physiologic response is an exquisitely coordinated program that uses proteolytic enzymes to remodel the ECM and promote a supportive environment for wound healing rather than tissue damage.

Cellular Response

Inflammatory cell infiltration at the site of initial tissue damage typically begins with release of chemokines and soluble mediators from resident cells, including interstitial fibroblasts, mast cells, and vascular endothelial cells. Signaling from these events alters the local adhesion molecule profile and creates a chemotactic gradient that recruits cells from the blood stream. Mast cells, in particular, act as sentinels that degranulate within seconds after ligation of immunoreceptors and activation of the signaling molecule spleen tyrosine kinase (Syk) to release vasoactive amines. In most acute responses, polymorphonuclear leukocytes (PMNs) are the first inflammatory cells to arrive at the site of injury, followed later by mononuclear cells.

Most tissue fibroblasts and vascular endothelial cells are generally quiescent before migration of PMNs into the tissue. However, these resident cells can be triggered to proliferate and migrate toward the site of injury as well as to synthesize cytokines, proteases, and ECM components. Growth factors are released, such as basic fibroblast growth factor (bFGF) and vascular endothelial growth factor (VEGF), stimulating new blood vessel formation. Together with granulocyte-macrophage colony-stimulating factor (GM-CSF), these locally released growth factors contribute to cellular proliferation and amplification of the inflammatory response and also induce maturation of dendritic cells that process antigens. In addition, fibroblasts and endothelial cells secrete new ECM proteins, MMPs, and other ECM-digesting enzymes. Initially, the response favors proteolytic activity to clear damaged infrastructure. This is followed by a shift to increased production of new ECM to allow tissue repair and wound healing.

Increased vascular permeability, caused by disruption of endothelial cell tight junctions, allows blood-borne proteins such as fibrinogen, fibronectin, and vitronectin to extravasate into the perivascular ECM. Interaction with preexisting ECM allows the assembly of new ligands for a subset of adhesion molecules (e.g., integrins $\alpha_5\beta_1$ and $\alpha_v\beta_3$). This increased vascular permeability and change in the profiles of adhesion molecules and ligands, in conjunction with release of chemoattractant molecules, leads to the recruitment of leukocytes to sites of inflammation. Some of the chemokines involved are IL-8 (for neutrophils), macrophage chemoattractant protein-1 (MCP-1) for monocytes, RANTES (regulated on activation, T-cell expressed and secreted) for monocytes and eosinophils, and IL-16 (for $CD4^+$ T cells).

Chemokines have the capacity to recruit specific subsets of cells by binding to G protein–coupled chemokine receptors. Directly targeting chemokines, either with biologics or with small molecules, has met with limited success in clinical trials, perhaps because the system is quite complex and highly redundant. An alternative approach might be to target intracellular mechanisms distal to receptor ligation. Chemokine receptors generally signal through the phosphoinositide-3 kinase (PI3K) system, especially the gamma isoform. PI3Kγ is mainly expressed in bone marrow–derived cells and is the convergence point for multiple chemotactic factors. Preclinical studies suggest that blocking this pathway decreases inflammatory cell recruitment in models of lupus and rheumatoid arthritis.

The precise combination of chemokines and vascular adhesion molecules present in an inflammatory lesion determines the timing for recruitment of individual inflammatory cell types. Ligation of integrins on leukocytes also prolongs cell survival after they have moved into the tissue, by preventing apoptosis. The central role of certain specific adhesion molecule–ligand pairs has been confirmed in human diseases. For instance, $\alpha_4\beta_1$ plays a key role in the recruitment of lymphocytes to the central nervous system in multiple sclerosis, and blocking this interaction suppresses disease activity (Chapter 411). Eosinophils use the same adhesion receptors to migrate into the lung in allergen-induced asthma (Chapter 87).

Increased expression of intracellular adhesion molecule 1 (ICAM-1) and vascular cell adhesion molecule 1 (VCAM-1), as well as increased chemokine expression, is evident in other cell types, such as the airway epithelium after allergen challenge in asthma. Rapid transient influx of neutrophils occurs in allergic airway disease, along with activation of the local T cells and mast cells. These neutrophils produce lipid mediators, reactive oxygen intermediates, and proteases such as elastase, which may contribute to airflow obstruction, epithelial damage, and remodeling. Neutrophil elastase, together with chemokines released by both recruited and allergen-activated T cells and mast cells, serves to recruit eosinophils.

Soluble Mediators

PRO-INFLAMMATORY CYTOKINES

Pro-inflammatory cytokines, often derived from macrophages and fibroblasts, are mediators that activate the immune system. The pro-inflammatory members of the IL-1 family (e.g., IL-α, IL-1β, IL-18, and IL-33) and TNF have pleiotropic activities and can enhance adhesion molecule expression on endothelial cells, induce proliferation of endogenous cells, and stimulate antigen presentation. IL-1 and TNF also increase expression of matrix-degrading enzymes, such as collagenase and stromelysin. In addition, they stimulate synthesis of other inflammatory mediators such as prostaglandins from fibroblasts. TNF inhibitors (Chapter 36) are effective in inflammatory diseases such as psoriasis, rheumatoid arthritis, and inflammatory bowel disease, and IL-1 inhibitors (Chapter 36) are beneficial in genetic diseases such as Muckle-Wells syndrome and familial cold autoinflammatory syndrome.

IL-1 and TNF comprise only a small fraction of the acute cytokine response. Many other factors also participate, including IL-6 and its related cytokines (IL-11, osteopontin, and leukemia inhibitory factor), which can both induce acute phase reactants and bias an immune response toward a helper T type 1 (T_H1) or T_H2 phenotype (Chapter 47). GM-CSF can regulate dendritic cell maturation, increase expression of human leukocyte antigen (HLA-DR) on these cells, and enhance antigen presentation. The T_H1 lymphokine IFN-γ, although often considered part of the secondary wave that ensues after T-cell activation, can also induce expression of HLA-DR, increase expression of endothelial cell adhesion molecules, and inhibit collagen production. IL-1, IL-6, and IL-23 can coordinate differentiation toward T_H17 cells, a phenotype that is thought to play a major role in inflammation and autoimmunity owing to the production of IL-17 family members (IL-17A through F). Of these, IL-17A and perhaps IL-17F are especially important because they can synergize with IL-1 and TNF. The growth factor TGF-β biases cells toward the regulatory T cell (Treg) phenotype, which can suppress antigen-specific responses of other T cells (see later). The benefit of individual cytokine inhibitors varies depending on the disease. For instance, IL-6 blockade is effective in rheumatoid arthritis, whereas IL-12/23 and IL-17A inhibition suppresses skin inflammation in psoriasis. Clinical trials now clearly show that IL-17A antibodies are effective in psoriasis.[A1]

Many cytokines activate cells by ligating their receptors and engaging the Janus kinase (JAK) family of signaling molecules, including JAK1, JAK2, JAK3, and Tyk2. These kinases, in turn, phosphorylate the signal transducer and activator of transcription (STAT) proteins. The STATs serve as transcription factors that initiate expression of many other cytokines and mediators of the inflammation and amplify the response. JAK inhibition represents an alternative approach to abrogating the inflammatory response.

Cytokines play a key role in the establishment and perpetuation immune-mediated diseases. As noted earlier, autocrine and paracrine cytokine networks play a critical role in the perpetuation of inflammation in rheumatoid arthritis[4] (Chapter 264). MCP-1 recruits and activates macrophages into atheromas containing oxLDLs and foam cells. In allergic asthma (Chapter 87), IL-13 is emerging as a central inflammatory cytokine. IL-13 functions through binding to cell surface IL-4 receptors, and IL-4R–deficient mice are relatively resistant to the development of asthma.

EICOSANOIDS

In addition to cytokines and immune complexes, local inflammatory responses lead to the release of eicosanoids, which are lipid-derived molecules. Because lipids are present in the cell membrane, they are readily available substrates for the synthesis of mediators. These molecules are produced adjacent to sites of injury, and their half-lives range from seconds to minutes. Eicosanoids are not stored but are produced de novo from membrane lipids when cell activation by mechanical trauma, cytokines, growth factors, or other stimuli leads to release of arachidonic acid. Cytosolic phospholipase A_2 ($cPLA_2$) is the key enzyme in eicosanoid production. Cell-specific and agonist-dependent events coordinate the translocation of $cPLA_2$ to the nuclear envelope, endoplasmic reticulum, and Golgi apparatus, where interaction with COX (in the case of prostaglandin synthesis) or 5-lipoxygenase (in the case of leukotriene synthesis) can occur.

PROSTAGLANDINS

Prostanoids[5] are produced when arachidonic acid is released from the plasma membrane of injured cells by phospholipases and metabolized by cyclooxygenases and specific isomerases (Chapter 37). These molecules act both at peripheral sensory neurons and at central sites within the spinal cord and brain to evoke pain and hyperalgesia. Their production is increased in most acute inflammatory conditions, including arthritis and inflammatory bowel disease. In response to exogenous and endogenous pyrogens, prostaglandin E_2 (PGE_2) derived from COX2 mediates a central febrile response. In addition, prostaglandins synergize with bradykinin and histamine to enhance vascular permeability and edema. The levels of prostaglandins are usually very low in normal tissues and increase rapidly with acute inflammation, well before leukocyte recruitment. COX2 induction with inflammatory stimuli most likely accounts for the high levels of prostanoids in chronic inflammation.

COX2 also plays a key role in platelet–endothelial cell interactions by increasing the production of prostacyclin (PGI_2) in endothelial cells (Chapter 37). Increased risk for myocardial infarction associated with the use of selective COX2 inhibitors may be related to unopposed production of thromboxane A_2 by COX1 in platelets. Prostacyclin also protects against atherosclerosis in mice, and COX2 blockade abrogates this beneficial effect. Thus, COX inhibitors can potentially increase thrombotic events.

LEUKOTRIENES

A distinct set of enzymes direct arachidonic acid metabolites toward the synthesis of leukotrienes (Chapter 87). Their relative importance depends on the specific target organ of an inflammatory response. For instance, leukotriene receptor antagonists are effective in asthma, whereas similar approaches have been less impressive in rheumatoid arthritis. Unlike prostaglandins, leukotrienes are primarily produced by inflammatory cells such as neutrophils, macrophages, and mast cells. 5-Lipoxygenase is the key enzyme in this cascade, transforming released arachidonic acid to the epoxide leukotriene A_4 (LTA_4) in concert with 5-lipoxygenase-activating protein (FLAP). LTA_4 can be hydrolyzed by cytosolic LTA_4 hydrolase to LTB_4, a potent neutrophil chemoattractant and stimulator of leukocyte adhesion to endothelial cells. LTA_4 can also conjugate with glutathione to form LTC_4 by LTC_4 synthase at the nuclear envelope. LTC_4 can be metabolized extracellularly to LTD_4 and LTE_4. These three cysteinyl leukotrienes promote plasma leakage from postcapillary venules, upregulation of expression of cell surface adhesion molecules, and bronchoconstriction.

HISTAMINE

Histamine is a vasoactive amine produced by basophils and mast cells that markedly increases capillary leakage. In basophils, histamine is released in response to bacterial formylmethionyl-leucyl-phenylalanine (f-MLP) sequences, complement fragments C3a and C5a, and IgE. The resultant edema can be readily observed clinically in urticaria (Chapters 252 and 440) and allergic rhinitis (Chapter 251). The stimulus for release of histamine from mast cell granules is the same as in basophils, except for the absence of f-MLP receptors in this cell type. Histamine can also synergize with locally produced LTB_4 and LTC_4. In addition, histamine enhances leukocyte rolling and firm adhesion, and induces gaps in the endothelial cell lining, enhancing leukocyte extravasation.

Despite the production of histamine in asthma and in acute synovitis, currently available histamine blockers have minimal therapeutic effect in these conditions. Targeting the more recently described histamine type 4 receptor (HR4), which has a variety of immunomodulatory effects on bone marrow–derived cells, suggests that more precise inhibition of this novel histamine pathway might have greater success.[6]

KININS

Kinins induce vasodilation, edema, and smooth muscle contraction, as well as pain and hyperalgesia, through stimulation of C fibers. They are formed from high- and low-molecular-weight kininogens by the action of serine protease kallikreins in plasma and peripheral tissues. The primary products of kininogen digestion are bradykinin and lysyl-bradykinin. These products have high affinity for the B2 receptor, which is widely expressed and is responsible for the most common effects of kinins. The peptides desArg-BK and Lys-desArg-BK are generated by carboxypeptidases and bind the kinin B1 receptor subtype, which is not expressed in normal tissues but is rapidly upregulated by TLR ligands and cytokines. The kinin B2 receptor is internalized rapidly and desensitized, whereas the B1 receptor remains highly responsive. Kinin actions are associated with the secondary production of other mediators of inflammation, including nitric oxide, mast cell–derived products, and the pro-inflammatory cytokines IL-6 and IL-8. In addition, kinins can increase IL-1 production through initial stimulation of TNF and can increase prostanoid production through activation of phospholipase A_2 and release of arachidonic acid.

NEURAL NETWORKS

Neural outflow also can rapidly activate inflammatory mechanisms and alter vascular permeability at sites of tissue damage. Pain receptors can activate type δ fibers and carry information to the spinal cord about noxious stimuli where cytokines like IL-1 or TNF are produced. Spinal cytokines lead to phosphorylation of signal molecules in the central nervous system like mitogen activated protein kinases (MAPKs). Reflex neural loops, including sympathetic and parasympathetic nerves, release mediators like substance P, acetylcholine, epinephrine or norepinephrine into the immediate location as well as surrounding tissue. Vascular permeability and activation of resident cells like macrophages can help recruit additional cells to the affected region.

MECHANISMS OF TISSUE DAMAGE IN INFLAMMATION

Reactive Oxygen and Nitrogen

Macrophages, neutrophils, and other phagocytic cells can generate large amounts of toxic reactive oxygen intermediates (ROIs) and reactive nitrogen intermediates (RNIs) that can directly kill pathogens. ROIs and RNIs also serve as critical signal transduction molecules that regulate expression of inflammatory genes.

These molecules can also have deleterious effects on normal tissue by damaging DNA, oxidizing membrane lipids, and nitrosylating proteins. Release of reactive intermediates can be initiated by microbial products such as LPS and lipoproteins, by cytokines such as IFN-γ and IL-8, and by engagement of Fc receptors by IgG. These events cause translocation of several cytosolic proteins, including Rac2 and Rho-family guanosine triphosphatase (GTPase) to the membrane-bound complex carrying cytochrome *c*, with subsequent activation of reduced nicotinamide adenine dinucleotide phosphate (NADPH) oxidase. The reaction catalyzed by NADPH oxidase leads to superoxide production, which, in turn, increases hydrogen peroxide, hydroxyl radicals and anions, hypochlorous acid, and chloramines.

In some cases, ROIs can contribute directly to the initiation of chronic disease. Lipid oxidation produces aldehydes that substitute lysine residues in apolipoprotein B-100. This altered moiety either binds to TLR2 to induce cytokine production or is internalized by macrophages, leading to the production of foam cells and fatty streaks, the primary lesions of atherosclerosis (Chapter 70). Subsequently, altered epitopes in damaged host proteins can be presented to T cells to initiate an adaptive immune response that amplifies the inflammatory vascular lesion.

Nitric oxide synthases (NOS) convert L-arginine and molecular oxygen to L-citrulline and nitric oxide (NO). There are three known isoforms of NOS: neuronal NOS (ncNOS or NOS1) and endothelial cell NOS (ecNOS or NOS3) are both constitutively expressed, whereas macrophage NOS (macNOS, iNOS, or NOS2) is induced by inflammatory cytokines such as TNF and IFN-γ, as well as by products of viruses, bacteria, protozoa, and fungi and by low oxygen tension and low environmental pH.

Together with prostaglandins, the production of NO by NOS2 and ROIs by NADPH oxidase is a key mechanism by which macrophages paradoxically impair T-cell proliferation. This might control inflammatory processes or delete autoreactive T cells and partially accounts for the immunosuppression observed in certain infections and malignancies.

Proteases and Matrix Damage

Production of enzymes that degrade the ECM regulates tissue turnover in inflammation. Reconfiguring of the matrix remodels damaged tissue, releases matrix-bound growth factors and cytokines, prepares the tissue for the ingrowth of new blood vessels, and alters the local milieu to permit adherence and retention of newly recruited cells.

The MMPs are a family of more than 20 extracellular endopeptidases that participate in degradation and remodeling of the ECM matrix (Table 48-1). They are produced as pro-enzymes and require limited proteolysis or partial denaturation to expose the catalytic site. Their name is derived from their dependence on metal ions (zinc/metzincin superfamily) for activity and from their potent ability to degrade structural ECM proteins. MMPs can also cleave cell surface molecules and other pericellular nonmatrix proteins, thereby regulating cell behavior. For instance, MMPs can alter cell growth by digesting matrix proteins associated with growth factors. FGF and TGF-β have high affinities for matrix molecules that serve as depots for storage of these cytokines. Matrix proteolysis releases some growth factors and can make them available to cell surface receptors. In addition, MMPs can directly cleave and activate growth factors. MMPs affect cell migration by altering cell-matrix or cell-cell receptor sites. The adhesion molecule $β_4$ integrin is

TABLE 48-1 COMMON MATRIX METALLOPROTEINASES AND THEIR SUBSTRATES

MMP FAMILY	MATRIX SUBSTRATES	OTHER SUBSTRATES
Collagenases	Collagen I, II, III, VII, and X Aggrecan	Pro-MMP-1, -2, -8, -9, and -13 Pro-TNF
Entactin	$α_1$-Proteinase inhibitors Gelatin Tenascin	
Gelatinases	Aggrecan Denatured collagen Elastin Fibronectin Laminin Vitronectin	Pro-MMP-1, -2, and -13 Pro-TNF Pro-IL-1β Latent TGF-β
Matrilysins	Proteoglycans Denatured collagens Entactin Fibrin, fibrinogen Fibronectin Gelatin Laminin Tenascin Vitronectin	Pro-MMP-2 and -7 Pro-TNF Membrane-bound Fas ligand (FasL) Plasminogen $β_4$ Integrins
Stromelysins	Proteoglycans Aggrecan Collagen III, IV, V, IX, X, and XI Pro-IL-1β Entactin Fibrin, fibrinogen Fibronectin Gelatin Laminin Tenascin Vitronectin	Pro-MMP-1, -3, -7, -8, -9, -10, and -13 Pro-TNF Plasminogen $α_1$-Proteinase inhibitors

IL = interleukin; MMP = matrix metalloproteinase; TGF = transforming growth factor; TNF = tumor necrosis factor.

cleaved by MMP-7. MMP-3 and MMP-7 digest E-cadherin and not only disrupt endothelial cell junctions but also stimulate cell migration.

Degradation of the ECM is usually initiated by collagenases, which cleave native collagen. Denatured collagen is then recognized and further degraded by gelatinases and stromelysins. Unlike the collagenases, stromelysins demonstrate broad substrate specificity and act on many ECM proteins, such as proteoglycan, fibronectin, laminin, and many cartilage proteins. Stromelysins can also amplify the remodeling process by activating collagenase through limited proteolysis.

MMP gene expression can be induced by many pro-inflammatory cytokines, including TNF, IL-1, IL-17A, and IL-18. One common element in MMP promoters that regulates transcription is activator protein-1 (AP-1). AP-1 is a dimer that includes members of the Jun and Fos families. Cytokines can regulate the *MMP* gene by activating MAPKs, especially c-Jun amino terminal kinase (JNK), which, in turn, phosphorylates c-Jun and markedly enhances MMP production. NF-κB and NF-κB-like binding sites also can contribute to protease transcription.

Several other classes of proteases remodel the matrix, including serine proteases and cysteine proteases. High levels of active serine proteases, such as trypsin, chymotrypsin, and elastase, are released by infiltrating PMNs at sites of inflammation and can directly digest the ECM or activate the proenzyme forms of secreted MMPs. The ADAM (a disintegrin and metalloproteinase) family can cleave the extracellular domain of cytokine receptors. These ECM proteases include two members of the aggrecanase family. One of the aggrecanases (aggrecanase 2, or ADAMTS5) has been implicated in osteoarthritis because mice deficient in this enzyme have decreased cartilage destruction in models of osteoarthritis (Chapter 262).

TISSUE REPAIR AND RESOLUTION OF INFLAMMATION

Inflammation is a normal physiologic response but can cause serious host injury if allowed to persist. Additional mechanisms are required to reestablish homeostasis after this response is initiated. Suppression of acute inflammation by removal or deactivation of mediators and effector cells permits the host to repair damaged tissues through elaboration of appropriate growth factors and cytokines (Fig. 48-1). As in the initial generation of an inflammatory response, components of resolution include a cellular response (apoptosis and necrosis), formation of soluble mediators (such as anti-inflammatory cytokines and antioxidants), and production of direct effectors (such as protease inhibitors).

Deletion of Inflammatory Cells

Cells can be removed from an inflammatory site by several mechanisms. First, the influx of cells can be decreased by suppressing chemotactic factor production and vascular adhesion molecule expression. Second, cells, especially lymphocytes, can be released from the tissue and return to the circulation through lymphatics. Third, stressed cells can undergo necrosis with the release of their contents into the local environment. A fourth mechanism, known as autophagy,[7] can lead to digestion of internal organelles and ultimately to cell death. Perhaps the most critical and effective method for clearing cells from an inflammatory site is programmed cell death, or apoptosis.

Apoptosis is a highly regulated process in eukaryotic cells that leads to cell death and marks the surface membrane for rapid removal by phagocytes. This clearance process does not elicit an inflammatory response, in contrast to cell death by necrosis. PMN phagocytes have a very short half-life in the tissue, and the persistence or release of their contents into the microenvironment after death can be deleterious. In some pathologic conditions, such as leukocytoclastic vasculitis (Chapter 270), abundant neutrophil apoptosis is readily apparent on histopathologic examination. Other cells, including T lymphocytes, undergo postactivation apoptosis to prevent an overwhelming persistent host response. Defective apoptosis or even persistence of apoptotic cells that escape clearance may contribute to chronic inflammatory and autoimmune diseases. For instance, loss of tolerance to self-antigens might participate in autoimmune responses in SLE.

Commitment of a cell to apoptosis can be initiated by a number of factors, including the ROIs in the cellular microenvironment as well as signaling through several death receptor pathways (e.g., FasL/Fas and TNF-related apoptosis-inducing ligand [TRAIL]). The former can damage DNA, which is a common byproduct of the genotoxic environment created by inflammation. If DNA damage is excessive, repair by tightly regulated mismatch repair mechanisms is terminated, and programmed cell death can be initiated by genes such as the p53 tumor suppressor. The burden of mutations induced by ROIs or RNIs in chronic inflammation can potentially accumulate over time and eventually lead to amino acid substitutions in key regulatory proteins. Ultimately, as has been observed in ulcerative colitis, neoplastic disease can ensue.

Removal of apoptotic bodies, or the remnants of packaged apoptotic cells, is rapid and can be accomplished by macrophages, fibroblasts, epithelial and endothelial cells, muscle cells, and dendritic cells. The surface receptors used in recognition and engulfment of apoptotic cells include integrins (e.g., $\alpha_v\beta_3$), lectins, scavenger receptors, ATP-binding cassette transporter 1, LPS receptor, CD14, and complement receptors CR3 and CR4. However, some of these membrane molecules can be used in both pro-inflammatory and apoptotic pathways, the divergence of which may be based on differing ligands and accessory molecules. Apoptotic cells display a series of membrane-associated molecular patterns that interact with receptors on phagocytes. A general feature of apoptotic cells is loss of phospholipid asymmetry, with external presentation of phosphatidylserine. Externalized phosphatidylserine

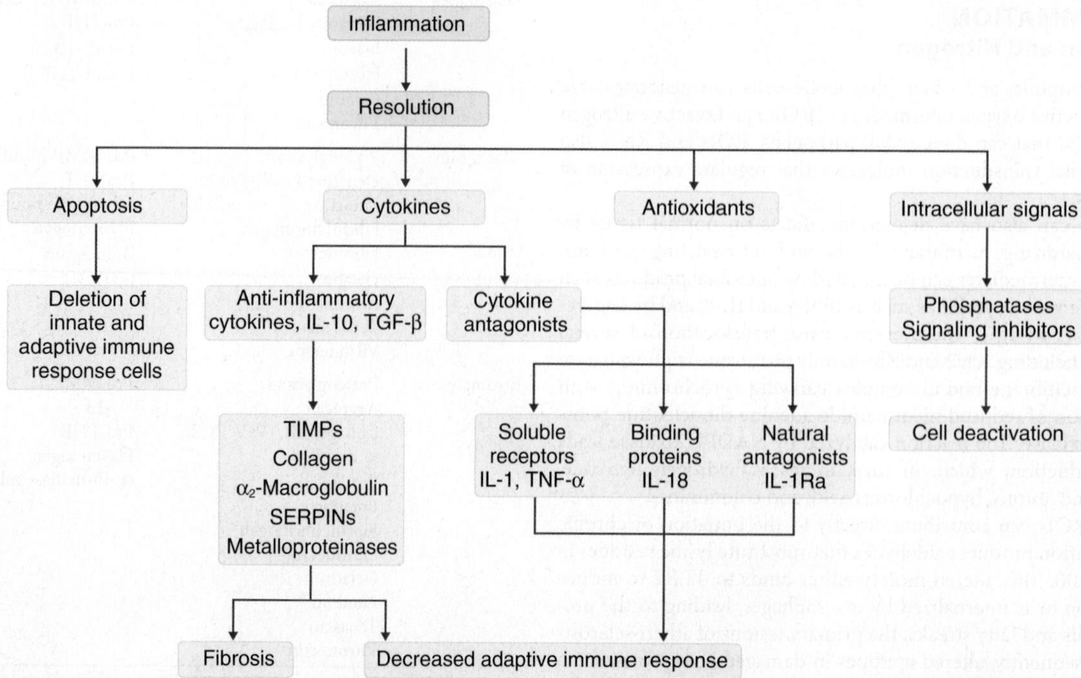

FIGURE 48-1. Anti-inflammatory mechanisms that resolve inflammation and lead to repair of the extracellular matrix. IL = interleukin; SERPINs = serine protease inhibitors; TGF = transforming growth factor; TIMPs = tissue inhibitor of metalloproteinases; TNF = tumor necrosis factor.

may be sufficient to trigger phagocytosis, but other apoptotic cell surface structures exist.

Although some inflammatory and immune cells are being deleted, other cell lineages expand during the resolution phase. Mesenchymal cells, especially fibroblasts, proliferate and produce new matrix that can contract to form a fibrotic scar. Locally produced growth factors such as PDGF induce DNA synthesis of these stromal cells through activation of PI3Ks. TGF-β[8] also stimulates fibroblast proliferation and converts cell phenotype to matrix formation rather than matrix destruction by increasing collagen production and suppressing MMP expression. In addition, mesenchymal stem cells that either reside in the tissue or migrate from the peripheral blood can differentiate into the appropriate organ-specific lineage. The pluripotential cells, in the presence of the appropriate milieu, can become adipocytes, chondrocytes, bone cells, or other terminally differentiated stromal cells.

Soluble Mediators

ANTI-INFLAMMATORY CYTOKINES

A variety of anti-inflammatory cytokines are released by resident and infiltrating cells. TGF-β and IL-10 are examples that are produced by macrophages, interstitial fibroblasts, or T cells. Some T-cell cytokines, including IL-4, IL-10, and IL-13, suppress the expression of MMP by cells stimulated by IL-1 or TNF. In addition to increasing fibroblast proliferation, TGF-β suppresses collagenase production, increases collagen deposition, and decreases MMP activity by inducing production of the tissue inhibitors of metalloproteinases (TIMPs). The repair phase is abnormal in diseases in which tissue fibrosis represents a major pathologic manifestation. For example, scleroderma (Chapter 267) is marked by diffuse fibrosis and is accompanied by high levels of TGF-β and increased production of ECM.

Cytokine decoy receptors can also downregulate the inflammatory response. Receptors can also be shed from the cell surface after proteolytic cleavage and can absorb cytokines, thereby preventing them from ligating functional receptors on cell membranes. These cytokine inhibitors can be released as a coordinated attempt to prevent unregulated inflammation, as in septic shock (Chapter 108), in which endotoxin induces production of soluble receptors after initial massive production of TNF and IL-1. Other types of cytokine-binding proteins are also produced as counter-regulatory mechanisms, including IL-18-binding protein (IL-18BP), which is an Ig superfamily–related receptor that captures IL-18. In bone remodeling (Chapter 243), interactions of receptor activator of NF-κB (RANK) with RANK ligand are required for osteoclast-mediated resorption. The competitive antagonist osteoprotegerin is a member of the TNF receptor family that binds to RANK ligand and inhibits osteoclast activation.

At least two distinct mechanisms contribute to natural IL-1 inhibition. An IL-1 decoy receptor (type II IL-1R) has both cell membrane and soluble forms that neutralize IL-1 activity. In addition, a natural IL-1 antagonist, IL-1Ra, can bind to functional IL-1 receptors and compete with IL-1α or IL-1β. However, IL-1Ra does not transduce a signal to the cell and blocks the biologic functions of ambient IL-1. The balance of IL-1 and IL-1Ra production depends on many influences. For instance, monocytes produce more IL-1, whereas mature macrophages produce IL-1Ra.

DEACTIVATION OF SIGNALING PATHWAYS

The signaling pathways described previously that initiate an inflammatory response have intracellular mechanisms to ensure that the process is self-limited. Many kinases, such as the MAPKs, require post-translational modification through phosphorylation to increase enzyme activity. A system of phosphatases that remove these phosphates can return the kinase to its resting form. For example, dual specificity phosphatase 1 (DUSP1) is an enzyme that dephosphorylates p38 MAPK as well as other MAPKs. DUSP1 expression is increased by p38 MAPK; thus, the very process of activating the cell through p38 is responsible for its own counter-regulatory mechanism. NF-κB activation is typically initiated by phosphorylation of the inhibitor of kB (IkB), which targets it for proteolysis. IkB expression later increases dramatically and stops the signaling through this pathway. JAK-STAT signaling is inhibited by the suppressor of cytokine stimulation (SOCS) proteins. Thus, cellular defense mechanisms have evolved to prevent persistent cell activation.

ANTI-INFLAMMATORY PROSTANOIDS AND CYCLOOXYGENASE

COX2 induced by pro-inflammatory mediators appears early and can contribute to inflammatory responses. However, COX2 expression late in the process has led to speculation that it also functions in the resolution of inflammation. This regulation might occur through formation of the cyclopentenone prostaglandins (CyPG). The prostanoids can serve as ligands for peroxisome proliferator-activated receptors (PPARs) (Chapter 206). There are three main classes of PPAR receptors—PPARα, PPARβ/δ, and PPARγ—all of which bind to DNA as heterodimers in association with the retinoid X receptor. Activation of PPARγ by CyPG is associated with the suppression of AP-1 and STAT transcriptional pathways in macrophages. A variety of natural and synthetic PPAR agonists have demonstrated efficacy in models of ischemia-reperfusion injury, arthritis, and inflammatory airway disease.

Inhibitors of Direct Effectors

ANTIOXIDANTS

Antioxidant enzymes that can inactivate the toxic intermediates and protect normal tissues include catalase and superoxide dismutase. Catalase is a peroxisomal enzyme that catalyzes the conversion of hydrogen peroxide to water and oxygen. Superoxide dismutases (SODs) catalyze the dismutation of superoxide to hydrogen peroxide, which is then removed by catalase or glutathione peroxidase. Glutathione peroxidases and glutathione reductase are additional mechanisms for maintaining redox balance and removal of toxic metabolites. Insufficient production of intracellular antioxidants such as glutathione can suppress lymphocyte responses and could account for defective T-cell receptor signaling and blunted immunity in T cells derived from rheumatoid arthritis synovium (Chapter 264).

Interactions of free radicals with surrounding molecules can generate secondary radical species in a self-propagating chain reaction. Chain-breaking antioxidants are small molecules that can receive or donate an electron and thereby form a stable byproduct with a radical. These antioxidant molecules are categorized as either aqueous phase (vitamin C, albumin, reduced glutathione) or lipid phase (vitamin E, ubiquinol-10, carotenoids, and flavonoids). In addition, transition metal-binding proteins (ceruloplasmin, ferritin, transferrin, and lactoferrin) can serve as antioxidants by sequestering cationic iron and copper and thereby inhibiting the propagation of hydroxyl radicals.

PROTEASE INHIBITORS

Protease inhibitors regulate the function of endogenous proteases and reduce the likelihood of collateral damage to tissues. These proteins form two functional classes, active site inhibitors and α_2-macroglobulin (α_2M). The latter class of protease inhibitors acts by covalently linking the protease to the α_2M chain and thereby blocking access to substrates. α_2M binds to all classes of proteases and, after forming a covalent bond, conveys them to cells through receptor-mediated endocytosis with subsequent enzymatic inactivation. The family of inhibitors of serine proteases (SERPINs) are the most abundant members of the former class of protease inhibitors and play a major role in regulation of blood clot resolution and inflammation, as indicated by many of their names: antithrombin III, plasminogen activator inhibitors 1 and 2, α_2-antiplasmin, α_1-antitrypsin, and kallistatin.

The TIMP family blocks the function of most MMPs. The TIMPs bind to activated MMPs and irreversibly block their catalytic sites. Examples of disease states with an unfavorable balance between TIMPs and MMPs include loss of cartilage in arthritis and regulation of tumor metastasis. TIMP-MMP imbalance in destructive forms of arthritis appears be caused by the limited production capacity for protease inhibitors, which is overwhelmed by the prodigious expression of MMPs. Whereas IL-1 and TNF induce MMPs, IL-6 and TGF-β suppress production of MMPs and increase levels of TIMPs. Therefore, the cytokine profile has a profound influence on the status of remodeling. When pro-inflammatory cytokines predominate, the balance favors matrix destruction; in the presence of pro-inflammatory cytokine inhibitors and growth factors, matrix protein production increases, and MMPs are inhibited by TIMPs.

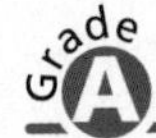

Grade A Reference

A1. Langley RG, Elewski BE, Lebwohl M, et al. Secukinumab in plaque psoriasis—results of two phase 3 trials. *N Engl J Med*. 2014;371:326-338.

GENERAL REFERENCES

For the General References and other additional features, please visit Expert Consult at https://expertconsult.inkling.com.

49

TRANSPLANTATION IMMUNOLOGY

MEGAN SYKES

DEFINITION

Clinical transplantation encompasses transplantation of organs and islets of Langerhans containing insulin-producing β cells, in which it is necessary to overcome the host-versus-graft (HVG) immune response to avoid rejection, as well as hematopoietic cell transplantation (HCT) (Chapter 178), in which it is necessary to contend with not only the HVG but also the graft-versus-host (GVH) immune response. Because preparations of bone marrow or mobilized peripheral blood stem cells (mPBSCs) contain mature T cells, their administration to conditioned and consequently immunoincompetent recipients is associated with the risk for GVH disease. Organs transplanted include corneas, kidneys, livers, hearts, lungs, small intestines, pancreases, and composite tissue allografts such as hands and faces. The list of transplanted allogeneic cells is likely to expand in the future to include other cell types, such as hepatocytes, myoblasts, and stem cell–derived replacement cells. Transplants originating from a member of the same species are referred to as *allotransplants.* However, transplants from other species, termed *xenografts,* are believed by many to be a promising solution to the severely inadequate supply of allogeneic organs and tissues, and such grafts may be used in the future. Transplants of tissues or cells originating from the recipient, either by processing of cells from the recipient's own organ (e.g., islets of Langerhans following pancreatectomy for chronic pancreatitis) or cell populations (e.g., CD34$^+$ hematopoietic progenitor and stem cells collected from leukapheresis products following mobilization from the bone marrow before high-dose radiation or chemotherapy to treat cancer) are referred to as *autologous.* In the future, these transplants may include stem cell–derived autologous cells used for therapeutic purposes.

ANTIGENS IN TRANSPLANTATION

The major antigens recognized during graft rejection and the cell types targeting them are summarized in Table 49-1.

Major Histocompatibility Antigens

The major histocompatibility complex (MHC; human leukocyte antigens [HLAs] in the human) controls adaptive and some innate immune responses and is of central importance in many immune-mediated diseases. The MHC also presents the strongest immunologic obstacle to all types of allografts. The HLA molecules include two major isoforms, termed class I and class II, and are all encoded in the MHC complex of chromosome 6. Although all HLA molecules have a similar general structure, class I and class II molecules show different expression patterns, with class I MHC expressed on most cells of the body, whereas class II antigens are expressed mainly on antigen-presenting cell (APC) populations, such as dendritic cells, macrophages, and B cells, as well as thymic epithelial cells involved in T-cell selection. Class II MHC can also be expressed on vascular endothelial cells and activated T cells of some species, including humans.

The specialized function of both classes of MHC molecules is the presentation of peptide antigens to T-cell receptors (TCRs), allowing adaptive immune responses to occur. In general terms, the peptides presented by class I molecules are 8- to 9-amino acid peptides derived from cytosolic proteins (e.g., viral proteins) that are transported into the endoplasmic reticulum, where they are processed and loaded onto class I molecules during their synthesis. CD8 molecules interact with the α_3 domain of the class I heavy chain, thereby strengthening the interaction of CD8$^+$ T cells that recognize class I–peptide complexes. Peptides presented by class II MHC molecules, on the other hand, are mostly 10 to 20mers derived from exogenous proteins (e.g., phagocytosed bacteria) that are processed through the endosomal processing pathway, and these are recognized by TCRs of T cells whose CD4 molecules strengthen the overall T cell–APC interaction. The class I presentation pathway is of particular importance in allowing destruction of virally infected cells, consistent with the expression of class I MHC on almost all cell types in the body. However, there are exceptions to this paradigm that account for the phenomenon of cross-priming and cross-presentation, wherein peptides from exogenous proteins are presented by class I molecules, a phenomenon that may have significance for transplantation. Class II MHC presentation of exogenous antigens takes place primarily on professional APCs and B cells, consistent with the role of CD4$^+$ T cells in initiating immune responses by activating APCs, providing direct and indirect (through activated APCs that also present peptides on class I molecules) "help" for CD8$^+$ cytotoxic T lymphocytes (CTLs), and providing help for antibody-producing B cells. B cells are able to focus the antigens recognized by their specific surface immunoglobulin receptors by binding and internalizing these antigens, which thereby predominate in the endosomal antigen-processing pathway and become presented by a high proportion of class II molecules on that B cell. This ability of B cells to preferentially present peptides derived from their cognate antigens to CD4 T cells recognizing those alloantigens is very important in driving alloantibody production.

A number of MHC molecules have been crystallized, both alone and with TCRs that recognize them. The TCR binding structure of class I and II MHC molecules is similar overall and includes both the peptide binding cleft formed by a β-pleated sheet and two α-helices forming the sides of the cleft (E-Fig. 49-1). However, class I and II MHC molecules also have significant structural differences, as summarized in E-Table 49-1. Although class I molecules are formed by the combination of a highly variable heavy (45-kD) chain (α chain) noncovalently linked to a nonpolymorphic, smaller (12-kD) light chain (β_2-microglobulin), class II molecules are heterodimers of two polymorphic chains, a 32-kD α chain and a noncovalently bound 28-kD β chain. TCRs interact physically with both the α-helices of the MHC molecules and side chains of the peptide that is bound in the groove, representing a trimolecular MHC-peptide-TCR interaction (see E-Fig. 49-1). It is the most variable ("hypervariable") portion of the TCR, produced by V-D-J somatic rearrangements and N insertions in the TCR α and β chains, known

TABLE 49-1 LYMPHOCYTES INVOLVED IN GRAFT REJECTION

CELL TYPE	ANTIGENS RECOGNIZED	FUNCTION	RELEVANCE
CD4$^+$ T cells	Allogeneic class II MHC (+ peptide) Self class II MHC + donor peptide	Antigen-presenting cell activation Help (cytokines and costimulation) Proinflammatory cytokine production Cytotoxicity Regulatory function	Organ allografts Cellular allografts Xenografts GVHD
CD8$^+$ T cells	Allogeneic class I MCH (+ peptide) Self class I MHC + donor peptide	Cytotoxicity Cytokine production Regulatory function	Organ allografts Cellular allografts Xenografts GVHD
NK cells	Class I MHC (activates or inhibits NK cell function) Other activating ligands	Cytotoxicity Cytokine production	? Organ allografts Cellular allografts Xenografts
B cells	Class I and class II MHC blood group antigens Xenogeneic carbohydrates	Antibody-mediated rejection (hyperacute, acute humoral, and chronic rejection)	Organ allografts Cellular allografts Xenografts

CTL = cytotoxic T lymphocyte; GVHD = graft-versus-host disease; MHC = major histocompatibility complex; NK = natural killer.

as complementarity-determining region 3 (CDR3), that recognizes specific MHC-peptide complexes.

The HLA molecules are all encoded within a 3.6-million base-pair region that encodes more than 200 genes, including complement and tumor necrosis factor (TNF) genes and many others in addition to MHC that have immunologic functions. The organization of the HLA region is illustrated in E-Figure 49-2, which shows that the heavy chains for "classic" class I HLA-A, B, and C and "nonclassic" class I molecules are encoded in a region that is telomeric to the "central MHC" region that includes complement and TNF genes among others, and lies between the class II and class I HLA regions. The class II region contains two α- and β-chain genes, only one of which is functional, for each of HLA-DQ and DP. However, the DR locus contains different numbers of β chains for different HLA alleles. Some of these DR β chains are pseudogenes, but various HLA-DR alleles contain either one or two functional β-chain genes.

One of the striking features of HLA molecules (and the MHC of most mammalian species) is their extensive polymorphism. There are thousands of defined HLA alleles in the class I and class II regions. Because the primary function of antigen presentation to T cells is to permit responsiveness to and clearance of pathogenic microorganisms, this polymorphism may have evolved to maintain the diversity of immune responsiveness to various pathogens within a population, avoiding annihilation of that population by a single microorganism that might not be presented well by a particular MHC. HLA alleles were originally distinguished by panels of highly sensitized human sera containing multiple alloantibodies. Although it effectively identified structurally related HLA alleles, this method failed to distinguish many allelic differences that are of functional importance for antigen binding and T-cell recognition. It was only with the development of molecular methods to distinguish alleles at the genomic level, eventually through specific genomic sequences, that the full extent of the polymorphism in this region was revealed. In association with this knowledge, it has been necessary to continually revise and refine the system of nomenclature defining these alleles. According to the most recently accepted nomenclature,[1] HLA alleles are identified by the locus (e.g., HLA-A), followed by an asterisk, and then a unique number with up to four sets of digits separated by colons. The first set describes the allele group (e.g., HLA-A*02), which usually corresponds to a serologically defined antigen, and the second set indicates the specific allele (e.g., HLA-A*02:101). The third and fourth set of digits are of less practical importance because they identify silent nucleotide substitutions in different alleles and variations in the nontranslated regions of the gene, respectively.

Within certain populations, however, the level of diversity within allele groups may be quite limited because of the common genetic origin of the allele. For example, for the originally serologically defined HLA-DR3 allele group, there is little diversity among Northern Europeans, such that most carry the DRB1*0301 allele. Thus, for this population, it is reasonable to refer to the serologic HLA-DR3 type as defining this allele. There are certain alleles that predominate within racial groups. For example, as few as five DRB1 alleles predominate among Northern Europeans, with each allele represented in 10 to 30% of this population. E-Table 49-2 summarizes the major DRB1 allelic groups defined initially at the serologic level and later at the level of genomic sequencing.

Most organ transplantations are performed across HLA disparities, and the strong immunosuppressive regimens used in transplant recipients are designed to prevent rejection by this exceptionally strong immune response. In contrast to T-cell responses to peptide antigens derived from foreign proteins, which are recognized by a very small fraction of naïve T cells (in the range of 1 in 10^5), a very high proportion, estimated at 1 to 10% of the T-cell repertoire, recognizes MHC alloantigens. The strong immunogenicity of allogeneic MHC molecules relates to the manner in which T cells are selected in the thymus; developing thymocytes do not survive unless they can weakly recognize a self MHC/peptide complex on a thymic stromal cell. This process is termed *positive selection*. Thymocytes whose receptors have high affinity for self/MHC complexes are deleted, however, so strongly autoreactive T cells rarely make it into the peripheral T-cell pool. Allogeneic antigens are not part of this *negative selection* process. The net result of these two selection steps is that the human T-cell "repertoire" is strongly biased to have cross-reactivity to allogeneic MHC molecules, providing a barrier to organ and hematopoietic cell transplantation. In the case of organ transplantation, in which long-term pharmacotherapy with powerful immunosuppressive drugs is used in an effort to prevent graft rejection, this can translate into improved results with matched organs in some situations. However, for unrelated, deceased donor transplantation, the benefits of HLA matching may be counterbalanced by the disadvantages associated with prolonged graft ischemia when attempts are made to transport organs to the most closely matched recipient.[2]

For hematopoietic cell transplantation (Chapter 178), the risks for GVH disease and marrow graft failure are so greatly amplified in the presence of extensive HLA mismatches that such transplantations have been avoided whenever possible; if a sufficiently matched, related donor cannot be found, a search is conducted through large registries containing millions of volunteer unrelated donors. Because of its extensive polymorphism, truly MHC-identical, unrelated donors can be difficult to find in the human population at large. For individuals with common HLA genotypes, the likelihood of finding a matched unrelated donor is markedly greater than that for individuals with rare genotypes. This situation relates in part to the phenomenon of *linkage disequilibrium*, wherein alleles at nearby loci are found together on the same chromosomal segment, or *haplotype*, more frequently than would be predicted by chance. The pattern of linkage disequilibrium is different in different racial groups, so the chance of finding a truly genotypically identical haplotype is greatest within the same population. For example, among whites, the DRB1*0301 allele is in linkage disequilibrium with DQB1*0201, which is located several hundred thousand base pairs away on chromosome 6; this complex, in addition to the DR4 alleles that are in linkage disequilibrium with DQB1*0302, confers the greatest genetic component of risk for the development of type 1 diabetes. Many autoimmune diseases demonstrate similarly strong HLA associations. Although there are data to indicate that HLA-specific autoantigen presentation plays a major role in determining disease susceptibility, non-HLA genes in linkage disequilibrium likely account for a significant component of these genetic risk factors.

The use of alternative donors has also increased the availability of hematopoietic cell transplantation (HCT) in individuals for whom an HLA-identical related or unrelated donor cannot be identified (Chapter 178). The use of cord blood transplantation, which has reduced GVH disease–inducing activity compared with adult stem cell products, as well as advances in avoiding GVH disease in haploidentical related donor HCT, has recently increased the safety and use of HLA-mismatched HCT.[3]

Minor Histocompatibility Antigens

"Minor" histocompatibility antigens are peptides derived from polymorphic peptides presented by an MHC molecule. Even genotypically HLA-identical siblings have different minor histocompatibility antigens. These are sufficient to induce graft rejection if immunosuppressive pharmacotherapy is not used. In the case of HCT, significant GVH disease frequently (about 30 to 50% of the time) complicates transplantation between HLA-identical siblings, even with the use of pharmacologic immunoprophylaxis.

Other Antigens

The major blood group (ABO) antigens can be the targets of a dramatic "hyperacute" rejection process that occurs when mismatched vascularized grafts are transplanted. Recognition of blood group antigens on the endothelial surface of the graft vessels by recipient "natural" antibodies (antibodies that are present without known sensitization to the antigens) activates the complement and coagulation cascades, resulting in rapid graft thrombosis and ischemia. A similar outcome can occur after transplantation to an individual with preformed anti–donor HLA antibodies resulting from presensitization by prior transplantations, transfusions, or pregnancies. Antibodies against other polymorphic antigens, such as MHC class I–related chain A (MICA), have been associated with graft rejection. In the past, transplantation could not be successfully performed in the presence of a positive anti-donor crossmatch. However, considerable success has been achieved in the transplantation of ABO-mismatched kidneys, livers, and hearts (the latter in the neonatal period only), and in transplantation of kidneys to highly presensitized patients.[4,5] In the case of kidney and liver transplantation, initial removal of the antibody and sometimes depletion of B cells, as well as the infusion of intravenous immunoglobulin (IVIG), has led to these successes. ABO-mismatched neonatal heart transplantation has succeeded because the transplantations are performed before the recipient has developed high levels of anti–blood group antigen antibodies, and the B cells seem to be rendered tolerant to the donor blood group antigen by the grafting process. Recognition of blood group antigens can also be of significance in HCT, in which ABO barriers are routinely crossed in both directions. This can cause hemolysis of recipient erythrocytes if the mismatch is in the GVH direction, but this complication can be avoided by washing the cellular product before infusion. Mismatches in the HVG direction can cause more persistent problems due to ongoing destruction of donor erythropoietic cells, resulting in pure red cell aplasia. More often, however, donor erythropoiesis is successfully established, and antidonor isohemagglutinins disappear from the circulation.

A and B blood group antigens are the consequence of the presence or absence of specific glycosylation enzymes in different individuals. Likewise, an antigenic specificity of the utmost importance in xenotransplantation is a carbohydrate epitope, Galα1–3Galβ1–4GlcNAc (αGal), which is produced by a specific galactosyl transferase. Humans and Old World monkeys lack a functional αGal transferase and produce high levels of natural antibodies against the ubiquitous αGal epitope. Because animals of interest as xenograft sources (e.g., pigs) express αGal at high levels on their vascular endothelium, transplantation of vascularized organs from pigs results in hyperacute rejection unless something is done to absorb the antibodies or inactivate complement. The development of αGal-knockout pigs, therefore, was an important milestone, and encouraging results have been obtained in pig-to-primate transplantation in initial studies.

In another type of transplant reaction, recognition as foreign results not from the presence of an antigen, but paradoxically from the absence of a self MHC molecule. Natural killer (NK) cells express a series of surface inhibitory and activating receptors that, collectively, determine whether the NK cell does or does not kill a potential target cell. The ligands for the inhibitory receptors are MHC class I molecules, and the receptors recognize specific groups of alleles. An NK cell may kill an allogeneic target that lacks a self MHC inhibitory ligand. This phenomenon has been shown in animal models to result in rapid bone marrow rejection when the donor marrow cells are not given in excess numbers or when a fraction of them are destroyed by an incompletely suppressed T-cell response. A similar phenomenon has not been clearly demonstrated in clinical HCT. The possibility that NK cells play a role in organ allograft rejection has long been an area of controversy. NK cells may be of particular importance in xenotransplantation, where they appear early in infiltrates of organ xenografts undergoing acute vascular rejection. NK cells clearly play a strong role in rejection of xenogeneic bone marrow, an observation that is relevant in one approach to inducing tolerance (see later discussion).

MECHANISMS OF REJECTION AND GRAFT-VERSUS-HOST DISEASE

Cellular Mediators

Many different cell types participate in rejection responses, and there is considerable redundancy. T cells are key players in most forms of rejection, with the exception of rejection that can be induced by antibodies in the absence of T-cell help. These include hyperacute and acute vascular rejection processes that may be induced by natural antibodies, as described earlier, or by antibodies that are present due to presensitization. The possible role of NK cells has already been discussed.

Direct and Indirect Allorecognition

T-cell responses are induced by APCs that present alloantigens. There are two forms of alloantigen recognition, termed *direct* and *indirect* (Fig. 49-1). Direct allorecognition denotes recognition of donor antigens on donor APCs provided by the graft. The extraordinarily high frequency of T cells with alloreactivity is caused by direct recognition of allogeneic MHC. Indirect recognition is the recognition of donor antigens that are picked up and presented on recipient MHC molecules on recipient APCs. The indirect response is more similar to "normal" T-cell responses, in which professional APCs present peptide antigens to T cells that are present at relatively low frequency in the naïve repertoire.

In organ transplantation, direct alloreactivity is particularly important in the early post-transplantation period, when APCs within the transplanted organ are still present; many of these cells migrate to the lymphoid tissues, where they initiate the alloresponse. However, the APC supply that comes with the donor graft is not renewable, so if the direct response is not maintained by recognition of donor antigens on endothelial cells or other cells in the graft, it may recede in importance. The indirect response, on the other hand, can be maintained by the constantly renewed pool of recipient APCs. The indirect response is of particular importance in inducing antibody responses.

Effector Mechanisms of Rejection

T cells can promote graft rejection through several effector mechanisms. One is the antibody-dependent processes that have already been discussed, which can be induced by $CD4^+$ helper T cells that promote differentiation and immunoglobulin (Ig) class switching of B cells that recognize other specificities on the same alloantigens. T cells provide cognate help to B cells when the TCRs recognize complexes of self MHC with donor MHC–derived peptide antigens (produced by B cells whose surface Ig receptors recognize and pick up the donor MHC antigen). If antidonor antibody is not present before transplantation but is induced afterward, the response can lead to the pathologic picture of acute humoral rejection. Antibodies may also participate in a slower, poorly understood process of chronic rejection, which, in the case of kidney and heart, is characterized by unique vascular lesions with intimal thickening and loss of the vessel space, and in the case of lung transplantation, by obliterative bronchiolitis. The mechanisms underlying these chronic rejection lesions are not well understood, and several different immune processes may in fact lead to similar lesions.

Direct Allorecognition

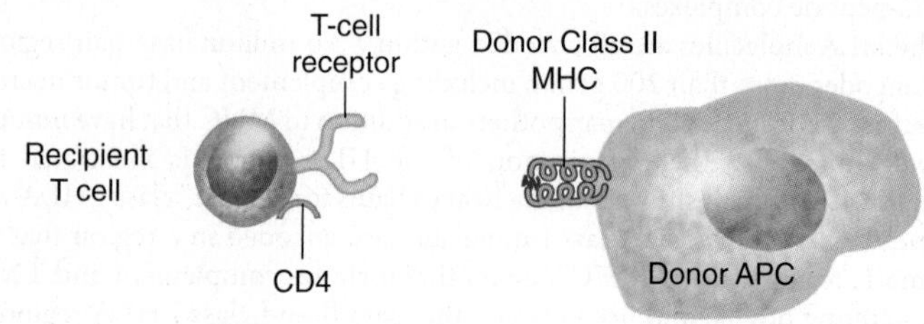

Indirect Allorecognition

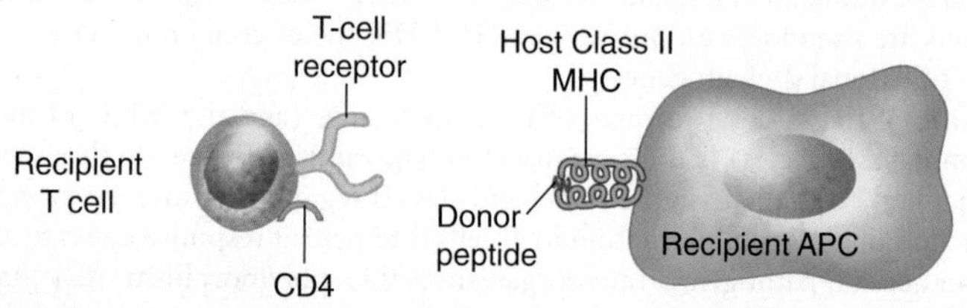

FIGURE 49-1 **Direct and indirect allorecognition. Direct allorecognition involves the recognition by a T-cell receptor of major histocompatibility complex (MHC) molecules (with or without a peptide) on a donor antigen-presenting cell (APC). Indirect allorecognition involves recognition by the T-cell receptor of a donor peptide presented on a recipient APC that has picked up and processed donor antigens.**

Another major effector pathway leading to graft rejection involves CTLs, which are predominantly members of the $CD8^+$ T-cell subset but also include $CD4^+$ T cells. Several effector mechanisms lead to killing of target cells by CTLs, and these include the granzyme/perforin-mediated pathway and the pathways involving Fas/Fas ligand (FasL) and other members of the TNF receptor family and their ligands (Chapter 47). Because $CD8^+$ cells recognize class I MHC molecules, which are widely expressed, it is not difficult to envision graft destruction by $CD8^+$ CTLs. $CD8^+$ CTLs may be activated through an APC that is stimulated initially through contact with an alloreactive $CD4^+$ cell. This is one form of CD4 "help" for $CD8^+$ cells. In addition, $CD8^+$ cells may be dependent on cytokines such as interleukin-2 (IL-2) from $CD4^+$ cells for their expansion and cytotoxic differentiation. However, there are also many examples of $CD8^+$ cell–mediated rejection that is independent of "help" from $CD4^+$ cells. Class II MHC, which is recognized by $CD4^+$ T cells, is less widely expressed on graft tissues than is class I MHC, although it may be induced on endothelial cells and graft parenchymal cells in the presence of inflammatory cytokines such as interferon-γ (IFN-γ).

In addition to cytotoxic mechanisms resulting from direct allorecognition, $CD4^+$ and $CD8^+$ T cells with indirect specificity seem also to be capable of causing graft destruction under some circumstances. Cytokines such as IFN-γ have been implicated in some instances, but in general, the pathways of indirect graft destruction are not well understood. A $CD8^+$ cell–mediated form of skin graft rejection that is dependent on donor antigens cross-presented on recipient MHC molecules (a form of indirect allorecognition for $CD8^+$ cells) has been described in an animal model. This form of graft rejection may be directed at antigen presented on endothelial cells of recipient vessels that revascularize the graft. This mechanism would not apply to primarily vascularized organ allografts.

The Role of T-Cell Trafficking

All the rejection processes described require trafficking of T cells into the graft. This process is made possible after the initial activation of naïve T cells in the lymphoid tissues. Naïve T cells can migrate into lymph nodes because of their expression of the CCR7 chemokine receptor and the adhesion molecule L-selectin. These T cells are activated by migratory graft APCs that also enter the lymph nodes. T-cell activation is associated with loss of CCR7 and L-selectin expression and acquisition of a new set of chemokine receptors and adhesion molecules that allow rolling and adhesion on the graft endothelium and entry into the graft parenchyma (Chapter 47). Inflammation in the graft, such as that induced by ischemia-reperfusion injury and the transplantation procedure, as well as that induced by initially responding T cells, is associated with upregulation of chemokines and adhesion ligands that promote entry of lymphocytes into the graft. Nevertheless, well healed-in grafts can be slowly rejected by adoptively transferred memory T cells, demonstrating that acute graft injury and inflammation are not essential for rejection in the presence of an established memory T-cell response. Rejection of hematopoietic cell grafts may involve many of the same mechanisms as those discussed for solid organs, although less detailed work has been done in this area.

Mechanisms of Graft-versus-Host Disease

Initiation of GVH disease (Chapter 178) requires that donor T cells recognize host alloantigens. The disease involves attacks on a variety of recipient epithelial tissues, namely skin, the intestine, and liver. Animal models have demonstrated clear roles for both $CD4^+$ and $CD8^+$ cells in initiating GVH disease, and each subset is able to do so independently of the other. The mechanisms of GVH disease include activation of alloreactive donor T cells by recipient APCs, leading to the differentiation of effector cells with direct cytotoxic activity and cytokine production in response to host antigens. A prominent role is played by TNF-α, whose production is induced in part by the translocation of bacteria across the intestinal wall, promoting innate immune system activation through toll-like receptors (Chapter 45). An intensely pro-inflammatory environment is produced by the combination of conditioning-induced tissue injury and disruption of mucosal barriers, bacterial activation of the innate immune system, and the GVH alloresponse. An important role is now appreciated for the inflamed microenvironment in target tissues in promoting the trafficking of GVH-reactive T cells into these tissues.[6]

STRATEGIES TO PREVENT GRAFT-VERSUS-HOST DISEASE

In view of the critical role of donor T cells in inducing GVH disease, an obvious strategy for preventing this complication is to remove mature T cells from the marrow graft. This approach has indeed been shown in both animal models and clinical studies to prevent GVH disease effectively. However, there are several disadvantages to this approach. One is that adult humans, particularly those who have undergone prior chemotherapy and radiotherapy, have little remaining thymic tissue and therefore demonstrate sluggish T-cell recovery, leading to serious opportunistic infections.

The second disadvantage applies to the most common indication for allogeneic HCT, namely the treatment of hematologic malignancies (Chapter 178). In this setting, T-cell depletion is often associated with an increased relapse rate due to loss of a graft-versus-tumor (GVT) effect, which is in large part mediated by GVH alloreactivity. Separation of GVH disease from GVT effects is a major goal of research in HCT, and some promising strategies are being explored (E-Table 49-3). These include control of T-cell trafficking so that the GVH alloresponse is confined to the lymphohematopoietic tissues where the tumor resides and a number of other approaches.[6,7]

The third disadvantage of donor T-cell depletion in HCT is that it increases the rate of engraftment failure. GVH alloreactivity and a "veto" effect of donor T cells help to overcome host resistance to donor engraftment. A veto cell, which may be a T cell or an NK cell, kills a CTL that attacks it. Although the phenomenon has been well established in animal models, its mechanisms are not clearly established, and its potential role in humans is uncertain. NK-cell recognition in the GVH direction resulting from the absence in the recipient of a class I MHC ligand (E-Fig. 49-3) that can trigger a donor NK-cell inhibitory receptor (KIR) may promote donor marrow engraftment and antitumor effects against acute myeloid leukemias in the setting of T-cell-depleted, HLA-mismatched HCT.

Clinically, pharmacologic immunosuppressive prophylaxis is usually used in at least the first 6 months after HCT to minimize the complication of GVH disease. Additionally, HLA-matched or closely matched donors are chosen whenever possible because GVH disease increases in frequency and severity as increased HLA barriers are transgressed. These measures, nevertheless, are insufficient, and GVH disease remains a major complication of HCT. Therefore, many of the new strategies being explored in organ transplantation and other fields are also being examined for the prevention of GVH disease in experimental models. It should be borne in mind, however, that tolerance of donor T cells to recipient alloantigens (see later discussion) might not be entirely beneficial in the HCT setting for the treatment of malignant disease because loss of GVH alloreactivity is likely to come with loss of antitumor effects.

STRATEGIES TO PREVENT ALLOGRAFT REJECTION

Nonspecific Immunosuppression

Immunosuppressive drugs are the mainstay of clinical organ transplantation, and improvements in these drugs following the discovery of cyclosporine have extended organ transplantation to include hearts, lungs, pancreases, livers, and other organs and tissues in the past 30 years. The mechanisms of action of these agents are discussed in Chapter 35. However, it is noteworthy that, despite these improvements and their enormous impact on early graft survival, these agents have been less effective in attenuating late graft loss. Because chronic immunologic rejection processes and side effects of the immunosuppressive drugs themselves are responsible for much of this late graft loss, improved immunosuppressive agents and induction of immune tolerance (see later discussion) are major research goals in transplantation.

Costimulatory Blockade

As understanding of immune responses has increased, recent years have seen the exploration of numerous biologic agents, including antibodies and small molecules targeting receptors of the immune system as well as cell-based therapies, in efforts to improve allograft survival. Because of the central role played by T cells in the immune response, considerable attention has been focused on blockers of T-cell costimulation. When a naïve T cell recognizes antigen through its unique TCR, additional "costimulatory" signals are required to allow full activation, expansion, and differentiation to occur. These signals are often provided by APCs in the form of ligands (e.g., B7-1, B7-2) for costimulatory receptors (e.g., CD28) on the T cell. Cross-talk between the T cell and the APC (e.g., due to CD40 activation by CD154 upregulation on the activated T cell) further amplifies the costimulatory activity of the APC, allowing it to effectively activate other T cells as well. The CD154 (T cell)–CD40 (B cell) interaction also promotes Ig class switching and functioning of B cells as APCs. Blockade of these processes (e.g., by CTLA4Ig and anti-CD154 monoclonal antibodies [mAbs]) has led to marked prolongation of allograft survival in stringent rodent and large-animal models. Robust, systemic tolerance to donor antigens has been achieved in rodents receiving bone marrow transplantation with costimulatory blockade and little or no additional conditioning. Some of these agents have joined the armamentarium of immunosuppressive agents in clinical trials in transplantation and autoimmune diseases.[8] Although anti-CD154 antibodies have been associated with thromboembolic complications, precluding further evaluation in transplantation trials, recently developed anti-CD40 antibodies have shown promise in animal studies. Numerous additional costimulatory and inhibitory pathways that affect T-cell responses have been described, and these all are potential targets for further manipulation of the alloresponse.

Immune Tolerance

Immune tolerance denotes a state in which the immune system is specifically unreactive to the donor graft (or recipient in the case of GVH reactivity) while remaining normally responsive to other antigens.[9-11] Tolerance is distinct from the state produced by nonspecific immunosuppressive agents, which increase risks for infection and malignancy. Numerous approaches to tolerance induction have been described in rodent models, largely owing to the strong tolerogenicity of primarily vascularized heart, liver, and kidney grafts in these animals. Because such grafts are less tolerogenic in humans, none of these strategies has been effectively applied clinically to date. Therefore, tolerance strategies that are appropriate for clinical evaluation must first be tested in "stringent" models, including relatively nontolerogenic grafts such as MHC-mismatched skin in rodents and vascularized organ graft models in large animals. In most of the models, only a superficial understanding of the mechanisms leading to tolerance is currently available.

The three major mechanisms of T-cell tolerance are deletion, anergy, and suppression (often referred to as "regulation"). *Deletion* denotes the destruction of T cells with receptors that recognize donor antigens; it can be achieved during T-cell development in the thymus, for example, by induction of mixed chimerism in T-cell-depleted hosts. Deletion can also be applied to mature T cells in the periphery, for example, by transplantation of a tolerogenic organ or marrow graft in combination with blockade of costimulatory molecules. *Anergy* denotes the inability of T cells to respond fully to antigens they recognize, and it can be induced by antigen presentation without costimulation. *Suppression* has attracted considerable interest since the discovery that constitutively $CD25^+$ T cells of the $CD4^+$ subset have suppressive activity that is dependent on expression of the transcription factor Forkhead Box Protein 3 (FoxP3). These and other types of suppressive T cells (e.g., NKT cells, regulatory $CD8^+$ cells and B cells, myeloid-derived suppressor cells) have been implicated in rodent transplantation tolerance models and in prevention of autoimmunity. The use of expanded regulatory cells has recently entered clinical trials, and both the ultimate practicality of the approach and the relative advantages of antigen-specific versus nonspecific regulatory cell therapy remain to be determined. There is also interest in strategies for activating or expanding regulatory T cells in vivo, thereby favoring the suppressive immune response over destructive alloimmunity.[12]

The developments in animal models and understanding of immune mechanisms described here have provided impetus for efforts to achieve immune tolerance in clinical transplantation. Every transplantation center has anecdotal cases of patients who have removed themselves from chronic immunosuppression without experiencing graft rejection. However, for every such patient, there are dozens more who have experienced rejection on dose reduction or removal of immunosuppressive drugs. Although trials of minimization and slow withdrawal of nonspecific immunosuppressive therapy are underway in organ transplant recipients, a major current limitation is the absence of good predictors of success. It remains to be seen whether recently identified molecular "tolerance signatures" will provide markers with sufficient predictive value to allow such withdrawal to be safely undertaken.

One approach developed in animal models has been successfully applied to the induction of immune tolerance in a small group of patients receiving renal allografts. This approach, involving bone marrow transplantation after nonmyeloablative conditioning, which is much less toxic than standard HCT conditioning, was shown to be effective in the most stringent rodent and large-animal models before being evaluated clinically. Initial success using combined kidney and bone marrow transplantation in patients with renal failure due to multiple myeloma led to pilot studies in patients with renal failure without malignant disease, with encouraging preliminary results. This approach and others that have emerged from ongoing investigations provide hope that, in the future, transplantation might be routinely performed without the need for chronic immunosuppressive therapy, with its attendant complications and limited ability to control chronic rejection.[11] Because autoimmune diseases are major contributors to end-stage renal disease, diabetes, and other types of organ failure, the potential for tolerance strategies to reverse autoimmunity while inducing allograft tolerance is also a source of hope. All these approaches must, however, be undertaken with the caution that successful regimens could also lead to immune tolerance to active infectious organisms.

GENERAL REFERENCES

For the General References and other additional features, please visit Expert Consult at https://expertconsult.inkling.com.

50 COMPLEMENT SYSTEM IN DISEASE

JOHN P. ATKINSON

The complement system consists of plasma and membrane proteins that participate in host defense against infections and in clearance of cellular and extracellular debris, as well as in a wide variety of autoimmune and inflammatory states (Fig. 50-1).[1,2] Complement is essential in innate immunity and a potent effector arm of adaptive (humoral) immunity. It is a *first* responder, especially in blood, to bacterial and viral invasion (Table 50-1). It helps to maintain sterility ("guardian of the intravascular space") by depositing within seconds its opsonic and membrane-perturbing fragments on a pathogen's surface. A second major activity of complement is to promote the inflammatory response via the release of soluble fragments *(anaphylatoxins)*. They bind to their receptors, leading to cellular activation, including chemokinesis and chemotaxis by phagocytic cells, and thereby enhance protection against infections. Furthermore, the deposition of complement fragments on immune complexes keeps them from precipitating and promotes their adherence to red blood cells (RBCs) for a hand-off to monocytes and dendritic cells in the liver and spleen.

Through these interactions, complement also instructs the adaptive immune response. Antigens decorated by complement proteins are taken up

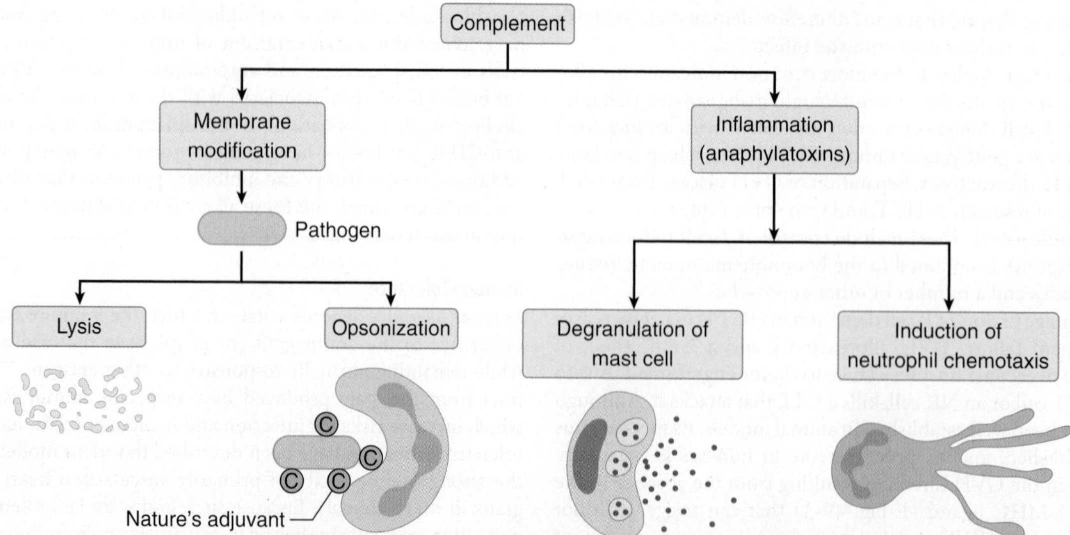

FIGURE 50-1. Function of the complement system. The most important function of the complement system is to alter the membrane of the pathogen by coating its surface with clusters of activation fragments. In one case, they facilitate the key process of opsonization in which C4b and C3b interact with complement receptors. In the other case, as with certain gram-negative bacteria and viruses, the membrane attack complex lyses the organism. The second critical function of complement is to activate cells and thus promote inflammatory and immune responses. The complement fragments C3a and C5a (known as anaphylatoxins) stimulate many cell types such as mast cells to release their contents and stimulate phagocytic cells to migrate to sites of inflammation (chemotaxis). Through these phenomena of opsonization and cell activation, complement serves as nature's adjuvant to prepare, facilitate, and instruct the host's adaptive immune response. Because complement activation occurs in a few seconds, this innate immune system initially engages most pathogens, especially those that try to enter the vascular space. As will be illustrated, these basic functions are also required to handle immune complexes and prevent autoimmunity. (Modified from Arthritis Foundation. *Primer on the Rheumatic Diseases*. 12th ed. Arthritis Foundation; Atlanta, Ga 2001.)

TABLE 50-1 COMPLEMENT SYSTEM IN HOST DEFENSE AGAINST BACTERIA AND VIRUSES

THE ACTIVITY	THE PLAYERS
Opsonization	(C3b > C4b, C1q, MBL)*
Membrane perturbation including lysis (the membrane attack complex)	(C5b-C9)
Proinflammatory via cellular activation (the anaphylatoxins and their receptors)	(C3a, C5a)

*C3b is the major opsonin of the complement system. C1q and MBL (mannose- or mannan-binding lectin) both participate in classical and lectin pathway activation, respectively, but also bind to their specific receptors upon attachment to a target.

TABLE 50-2 SALIENT FEATURES OF THE COMPLEMENT SYSTEM

Ancient innate system of immunity predominantly found in blood (the "guardian of the intravascular space")
Capable of rapidly opsonizing and lysing bacteria and viruses (millions of active fragments can be deposited on a target)
Works in seconds!
Most proteins are synthesized by the liver
Constantly turning over (AP protein C3 "ticks over" at a rate of 1% to 2% per hr)
The AP also features a feedback or amplification loop, which requires tight control
Effector arm of the humoral immune system (IgM and IgG)
Critical for clearance of self-debris (garbage removal)
After immunoglobulins and albumin, complement proteins are among the most abundant in blood
Nature's adjuvant (almost all foreign antigens are coated with complement fragments); instructs the adaptive immune response
A deficiency of an activator leads to bacterial infections or autoimmunity (SLE)
A deficiency of a regulator leads to undesirable cellular and tissue damage at sites of injury or degeneration (excessive activation)

AP = alternative pathway; SLE = systemic lupus erythematosus.

by monocytes, follicular-dendritic cells, B lymphocytes, and other antigen-presenting cells, resulting in an adaptive immune response. (The complement system is often called "nature's adjuvant.") Thus, complement activation is required for an optimal antibody response to most foreign antigens. Individuals lacking a functional complement system are predisposed to bacterial infections, predominantly by encapsulated organisms, including streptococcus, staphylococcus, *Haemophilus* spp., and *Neisseria* spp.[3] Surprisingly, a complete deficiency in an early component of the classical complement pathway predisposes to autoimmune diseases, particularly systemic lupus erythematosus (SLE).[4] This association suggests that complement is required not only for host defense against foreign agents but also to identify and safely clear self-materials (debris removal), particularly RNA and DNA species.

A remarkable feature of the complement system is that it reacts within seconds (Table 50-2). In less than 2 minutes, it can coat an encapsulated gram-positive bacterium with several million C3b opsonic fragments and lyse gram-negative bacteria by insertion of its terminal components (the membrane attack complex [MAC]). It works even more efficiently if driven by IgM or IgG binding to an antigen on a microbial membrane to activate the cascade. Antibodies and lectins direct the activation process to the pathogen's surface. Overall, the complement cascade is designed to become engaged on the surface of a pathogen, particularly bacteria. Plasma and membrane *regulators of complement activation* inhibit formation on normal "self" cells.

Much of the complement-mediated pathology revolves around the alternative pathway's (AP's) amplification loop. This feedback amplification loop is key in triggering activation early in an immune response; however, it must be rigorously regulated to prevent activation on normal self and excessive activation on injured self.[5] Approximately half of the proteins associated with the complement system are dedicated to the control of its activation and effector functions, especially to maintain homeostasis of the AP's amplification loop.

In clinical medicine (Table 50-3), the complement system participates in three pathologic processes (Table 50-4): (1) an inherited decrease in functional activity leading to increased susceptibility to bacterial infections and to autoimmunity, (2) mediating undesirable tissue damage upon activation by autoantibodies and immune complexes, and (3) excessive activation at sites of tissue injury in individuals carrying genetic variants in regulators.

Knowledge of how complement is activated and how it can be controlled points to opportunities for the development of therapeutic agents such as anti-C5 monoclonal antibody (mAb) therapy, which has been recently approved to treat several complement-dependent hemolytic disorders.

TABLE 50-3 PARTICIPATION OF THE COMPLEMENT SYSTEM IN HUMAN DISEASE

Activation by autoantibody (formation of immune complexes)

Engagement with modified self (clearance of debris or garbage)
- Degenerative processes (diseases of aging such as age-related macular degeneration)
- Cell and tissue damage (ischemia-reperfusion injury; atypical hemolytic uremic syndrome)

TABLE 50-4 PATHOLOGIC CONDITIONS ASSOCIATED WITH COMPLEMENT ACTIVATION

Examples of diseases in which complement activation contributes to the immunopathology:
Atypical hemolytic uremic syndrome*†
Paroxysmal nocturnal hemoglobinuria†
Age-related macular degeneration*†
Membranoproliferative glomerulonephritis (types 1, 2 and 3)†‡
Myasthenia gravis‡
Bullous pemphigoid‡
Systemic lupus erythematosus/antiphospholipid syndrome‡
Rheumatoid arthritis‡
Immune hemolytic anemias‡
Immune vasculitis (the ANCA-positive syndromes)‡
Ischemia reperfusion injury*†
Allotransplantation‡
Serum sickness‡
Exposures to foreign materials (e.g., membranes, nanoparticles)*

*Injury, ischemia, trauma, degeneration, or foreign body is the trigger (innate immune activation).
†Lack of adequate regulation contributes to disease pathogenesis.
‡Antibody dependent activation of the complement system (adaptive humoral immune activation).

ACTIVATION OF COMPLEMENT

Classical Pathway

The binding of IgM or IgG to a target antigen activates this exceptionally powerful and quick acting pathway to destroy microbes (Figs. 50-2 and 50-3). The classical pathway (CP) reaction cascade is designed to opsonize and perturb the surface membrane of microorganisms. Of course, autoantibodies also trigger this highly efficient CP. Complement action mediated by immune complexes may then lead to cellular and tissue damage. Instructive examples of autoantibodies and complement-mediated diseases are immune hemolytic anemias, myasthenia gravis, and bullous pemphigoid. The basic problem or pathologic defect in this type of human disease is, of course, the formation of the autoantibody. A misidentification of self that has occurred because of a breaking of tolerance. In this pathologic situation, the complement system is working at the behest of the autoantibody.

The CP is also activated by means other than the formation of IgM- and IgG-bearing immune complexes. β-Amyloid in the neuritic plaques of patients with Alzheimer disease directly engages the CP via an interaction with C1q. Likewise, C-reactive protein (CRP) and serum amyloid protein (SAP) bind to chromatin and other ribonucleoprotein complexes released from apoptotic cells, and these types of complexes activate the CP. As noted, the CP plays a key role in the opsonization and removal of nuclear debris. Approximately 80% of patients with hereditary absence of C1q or C4 develop SLE. Deposits of CRP and activated C1 have been demonstrated in ischemic tissue such as infarcted human myocardium. These observations indicate that CP activation via these antibody-independent means is critical in protecting against autoimmune responses by facilitating debris clearance.

Regulation of the CP activation occurs at two levels. First, the *ser*ine *pro*tease *in*hibitor (serpin) known as the C1-inhibitor (C1-INH) blocks the activity of many proteases, including factor XIIa, kallikrein, and factor XIa of

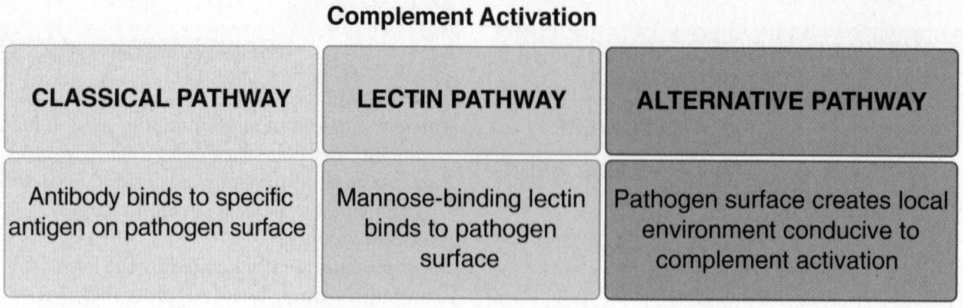

Complement Activation

CLASSICAL PATHWAY	LECTIN PATHWAY	ALTERNATIVE PATHWAY
Antibody binds to specific antigen on pathogen surface	Mannose-binding lectin binds to pathogen surface	Pathogen surface creates local environment conducive to complement activation

FIGURE 50-2. The three pathways of complement activation.

TABLE 50-5 TISSUE INJURY OR DEGENERATION AND COMPLEMENT ACTIVATION*

Age-related macular degeneration
Osteoarthritis (degenerative joint disease)
Ischemic stroke
Myocardial infarction
Traumatic brain injury (e.g., liver, kidney, gut)
Ischemia-reperfusion injury
Burns
Acute respiratory distress syndrome
Septic shock
Multiorgan failure syndromes
Alzheimer disease

*In these conditions, complement activation leads to deposition of fragments at the site of injury; however, how much of the tissue injury is attributable to complement system is unknown. In many cases, animal models support a pathologic role for the complement system. Only in age-related macular degeneration do we also have powerful genetic evidence in humans to indicate a key role for the complement system.

the clotting system as well as C1r, C1s, and MASP2 of the complement system. The importance of C1-INH is exemplified by its role in hereditary angioedema (Table 50-6). In this dominantly inherited disease, a deficiency of C1-INH allows uncontrolled proteolysis of C4 and C2 and generation of bradykinin, leading to recurrent swelling episodes. This serpin prevents chronic activation of the CP cascade and, after a few minutes, helps to shut down the system. CP activation is also regulated by multiple inhibitors at the key step of C3 activation. These plasma and membrane proteins inhibit C3 convertase formation on healthy self. Membrane regulators are highly expressed on most cell types, where they prevent activation on normal self and overexuberant activation on altered and nonself.

Lectin Pathway

The protein mannose-binding lectin (MBL) is a member of the collectin family that also includes pulmonary surfactants A and D.[6] MBL has a structure similar to C1q in that it consists of several subunits; namely, a globular recognition head domain for carbohydrates and a collagen-like tail that interacts with serine proteases. In the case of MBL, the globular domain is a lectin (protein) that binds to repeating mannose and *N*-acetylglucosamine residues on the surface of pathogens (see Figs. 50-2 and 50-3). Many microorganisms are recognized by MBL, including gram-positive and gram-negative bacteria, mycobacteria, fungi, parasites, and viruses (including human immunodeficiency virus 1 [HIV-1]). In general, as would be expected, mammalian glycoproteins and glycolipids are not readily recognized by MBL and the related lectins (ficolins and collectins) that activate the lectin pathway.

Three serine proteases, MASP-1, MASP-2, and MASP-3, associate with MBL (and the ficolins and collectins) through their collagen-like domain. This is analogous to the association of C1r and C1s with C1q. Activation of MASP-2, with some help from MASP-1, results in cleavage of C2 and C4, leading to formation of the classical/lectin pathway C3 convertase (C4b2a).

Genetic variations in the structural and regulatory portions of the MBL gene lead to wide differences in serum levels. A low level of MBL is associated with recurrent infections in children and adults and is a risk factor for the development of SLE. More striking is the association of low levels of MBL with infections in the setting of the treatment of SLE. For example, heterozygous MBL deficiency has been associated with a fourfold increase in the risk of bacterial pneumonia and homozygous deficiency with a more than 100-fold increase.

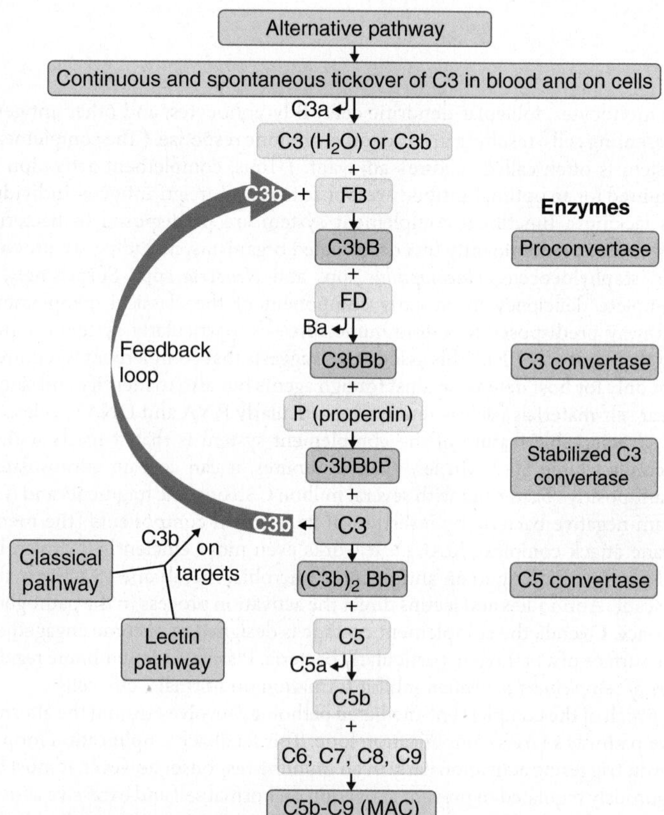

FIGURE 50-3. **Complement activation pathways.** In the reaction cascade shown, C3b or C3 (H_2O) binds the proenzyme factor B (FB), and the C36B complex then cleaved by the protease factor D (FD). The addition of properdin (P) to the enzyme complex increases the half-life of the enzyme complex approximately 10-fold. Although the source of the C3b can be from spontaneous turnover or via lectin pathway (LP) and classical pathway (CP) activation, the alternate pathway (AP) feedback loop commonly takes over to generate most of the C3b that binds to a target. The alternate pathway is continuously turning over. If activated C3b or C3 (H_2O) remains in the fluid phase, it is rapidly inhibited by the plasma regulator factor H. if activated C3 binds to normal or healthy self, it is prevented from forming a convertase by the ubiquitously expresses membrane cofactor protein (MCP [CD46]) and decay-accelerating factor (DAF [CD55]). DAF "kicks out" the catalytic Bb domain (a temporary stop), but MCP is a permanent stop because, upon its binding, the C3b is proteolytically cleaved to inactive C3b (iC3b) by a serine protease known as factor I. The feedback loop is a powerful amplification system. A single *Escherichia coli* organism in blood can be coated with several million C3bs in a couple of minutes!

Alternative Pathway

The AP takes advantage of the fact that C3 undergoes spontaneous, chronic, low-grade activation (Figs. 50-2 to 50-4). This C3b may covalently attach to any cell; however, on normal self, amplification of the cascade is blocked by inhibitors. In contrast, deposition on polysaccharides of bacterial membranes and to other targets, such as endotoxin and virally infected cells, leads to a rapid engagement of this pathway. These sites, similar to immune complexes and almost any type of biomaterial (cardiopulmonary bypass and hemodialysis membranes, nanoparticles, and so on), lack regulators, so rapid, massive activation may occur.

During spontaneous activation, called *tickover*, small amounts of activated C3 are continuously generated (C3 turns over in blood at 1% to 2%/hr). It can initiate a feedback loop and cleave more C3 to C3b. Also, the initial C3b

TABLE 50-6 SOLUBLE AND MEMBRANE FACTORS REGULATING COMPLEMENT

SOLUBLE FACTORS REGULATING COMPLEMENT			
NAME	**LIGAND OR BINDING FACTOR**	**FUNCTIONAL ACTIVITY**	**PATHOLOGY, IF DEFICIENT**
C1-INH	C1r, C1s, MASP-2	Binds to and displaces C1r and C1s from C1q and MASP-2 from MBL	HAE
C4bp* (C4 binding protein)	C4b, GAGs	Displaces C2a (DAA); cofactor for C4b cleavage by factor I (CA)	No clinical syndrome clearly defined
CPN-1 (carboxypeptidase-N)	C3a, C5a	Inactivates C3a and C5a	Urticaria and angioedema
Factor H*†	C3b, C3d, GAGs	Displaces Bb from AP C3 and C5 convertases (DAA) and is a cofactor for factor I to cleave C3b (CA)	AMD, aHUS, C3 glomerulopathies; bacterial infections secondary to low C3
Factor I†	C3b, C4b	Serine protease; cleaves C3b and C4b, requires a cofactor protein (CA)	AMD, aHUS; bacterial infections secondary to low C3
Protein S (vitronectin)	C5b67	Inhibits membrane attachment by C5b67	None defined
MEMBRANE-BOUND FACTORS REGULATING COMPLEMENT			
NAME	**LIGAND OR BINDING FACTOR**	**FUNCTIONAL ACTIVITY**	**DISEASE, IF DEFICIENT**
DAF (CD55)	C3 and C5 convertases	Displaces Bb from AP convertase and C2a from CP or LP convertases, respectively	PNH
Membrane cofactor protein (MCP, CD46)	C3b, C4b	Cofactor for factor I (CA)	aHUS
Protectin (CD59)	C8, C9	Inhibits MAC formation or insertion	PNH
CR1 (CD35) (immune adherence or C4b/C3b receptor)	C3b, C4b, C3, and C5 convertases	Cofactor for factor I to cleave C4b and C3b (CA); displaces Bb from C3b and C2a from C4b to inhibit convertases (DAA)	No complete deficiency described; decreased levels in immune complex–mediated diseases such as lupus
CRIg	C3b, iC3b, C3c	Inhibits activation of AP	None defined

*Factor H and C4bp also bind to surfaces, particularly at sites of tissue and cellular injury, where they also carry out regulatory activity.
†If heterozygous deficient, individual is predisposed to AMD and aHUS. If homozygous deficient, the AP turns over excessively, resulting in kidney disease (C3 glomerulopathies) and bacterial infections (secondary to the very low C3).
aHUS, atypical hemolytic uremic syndrome; AMD, age-related macular degeneration; AP, alternative pathway; $(C3b)_2$ Bb, alternative pathway C5 convertase; C3bC4bC2a, classical and lectin pathway C5 convertase; C4bC2a, classical and lectin pathway C3 convertase; CA, cofactor activity; CR1, complement receptor type 1; CRIg, complement receptor of the Ig superfamily; DAA, decay-accelerating activity; GAG, glycosaminoglycan; HAE, hereditary angioedema; MAC, membrane attack complex; MASP, mannan-binding lectin-associated serine protease; MBL, mannan or mannose binding lectin; PNH, paroxysmal nocturnal hemoglobinuria.

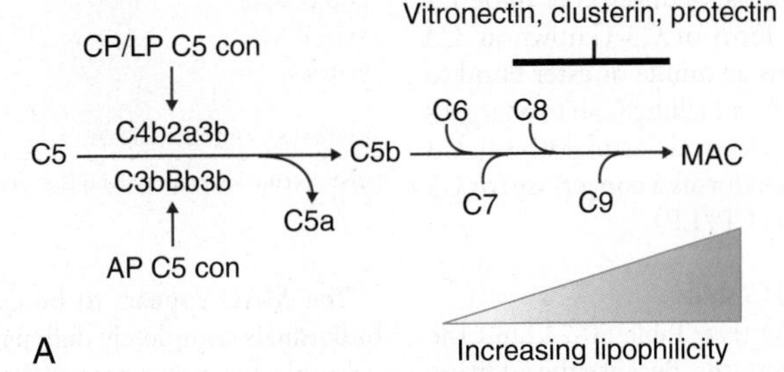

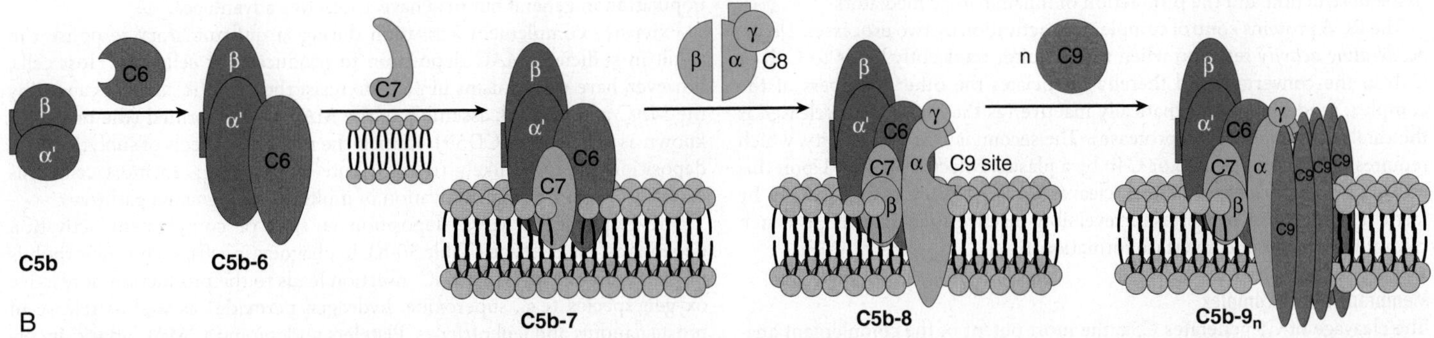

FIGURE 50-4. Activation of C5 and the membrane attack complex (MAC). A, The C5 convertases ("con") are the same as C3 convertases except a C3b has been attached to C4bC2a or a second C3b in the case of AP C5 convertase. B, Schematic representation of the assembly of the MAC on a cell membrane. C5b (composed of two chains) binds C6 and then C7. The C5b-7 complex can insert into a membrane and then bind C8 (composed of three chains) and multiple C9s to form a pore or channel in the membrane. (Modified from Liszewski MK, et al. *The Human Complement System in Health and Disease.* Marcel Dekker; New York, NY 1998.)

may be derived from either the classical or lectin pathway. Thus, activation of complement by any one of the three pathways has the potential to be rapidly magnified.[7] The AP C3 convertase is negatively controlled (to maintain homeostasis) both in the fluid phase and on host cells by two abundant plasma proteins and two widely expressed membrane proteins.[8]

The central role of the AP as an amplifier of complement activation is borne out by its association with a number of clinicopathologic states in the setting of deficient regulation (Tables 50-6 and 50-7). For example, multiple forms of membranoproliferative glomerulonephritis are associated with excessive C3 fragment deposition in the kidney because of either the

TABLE 50-7 COMPLEMENT SYSTEM MEDIATES THE DISEASE PROCESS AND ITS INHIBITION TREATS THE CONDITION

DISEASE	PATHOPHYSIOLOGY	ETIOLOGY	TREATMENT	FDA APPROVED
PNH	Lyse RBCs	Acquired hemopoietic somatic stem cell mutation in gene required for synthesis of GPI anchor	mAb to C5	Yes
aHUS	Damage to endothelial cells	Inherited loss of function variants in AP regulators or gain of function variants in AP activators	mAb to C5	Yes
HAE	Bradykinin generation	Autosomal dominant variants in the C1-inhibitor gene	C1 inhibitor replacement Bradykinin receptor blockage Kallikrein inhibitor	Yes Yes Yes
AMD	Degeneration of the retina	Inherited variants in a regulator (FH or FI) or gain of function in an alternative pathway component (C3 or FB)	Clinical trials in progress	No

aHUS= atypical hemolytic uremic syndrome; AMD = age-related macular degeneration; FDA = Food and Drug Administration; HAE= hereditary angioedema; GPI = glycosyl phosphatidylinositol; mAb = monoclonal antibody; PNH= paroxysmal nocturnal hemoglobinuria; RBC = red blood cell.

presence of autoantibodies (C3 or C4 nephritic factors) that stabilize C3 convertases or a genetic deficiency in complement regulatory protein (factor H or factor I).[9] Likewise, atypical hemolytic uremic syndrome (i.e., not associated with a preceding enteropathic infection featuring a *Shiga*-like toxin) occurs in individuals who harbor heterozygous missense mutations in factor H or I or have gain-of-function mutations in factor B or C3.[10] Genome-wide association and targeted deep sequencing studies have also linked age-related macular degeneration (AMD) to functional coding mutations in factor H and factor I and more uncommonly in factor B and C3.[11] Finally, rodent models of rheumatoid arthritis, SLE, and ANCA-positive vasculitic syndromes are ameliorated if the AP is disrupted.

C3 and C5 Convertases

The three activation pathways converge at C3. A remarkable feature of C3 is the presence of a thioester bond. Buried within the three-dimensional structure of the C3 protein lies a γ-carboxy group of a reactive glutamic acid residue linked to a cysteine in an "internal thioester." Upon its cleavage, for a few microseconds, a covalent attachment can occur via an ester or amide linkage to any nearby hydroxyl or amino group. Most of the cleaved thioester bonds are hydrolyzed by water to produce a form of C3 (known as C3 [H_2O]); however, a substantial percentage forms an amide or ester bond to amino groups or carbohydrates thereby covalently attaching C3b to a target's surface. Also, the addition of a C3b to C4b2a (classical/lectin pathway C3 convertase) or to C3bBb (AP C3 convertase) then forms a convertase for C5 (C3bBbC3b for the AP and C4bC2aC3b for the CP/LP).

TABLE 50-8 DISTRIBUTION OF ANAPHYLATOXIN RECEPTORS AND THEIR CELLULAR RESPONSES

CELL TYPE	RESPONSES
C5aR (CD88)	
Neutrophils	Chemotaxis
Eosinophils	Enzyme release
Basophils	Generation of reactive oxygen species
Mast cells	Upregulation of adhesion molecules
Monocytes	Increased synthesis of IL-1, IL-6, and IL-8
	Prostaglandin and leukotriene synthesis
Hepatocytes	Increased synthesis of acute phase reactants
Pulmonary epithelium	Increased IL-8
Neuronal cells	Cellular activation
Endothelial cells	Increased expression of P-selectin
Renal epithelial/mesangial cells	Proliferation
	Synthesis of growth factors
C3aR	
Eosinophils	Chemotaxis
Mast cells	Enzyme release
Platelets	Generation of reactive oxygen species
	Upregulation of adhesion molecules
Epithelial, endothelial, etc.	Cellular activation

CNS = central nervous system; IL = interleukin.

Regulators of Complement Activation at the C3 and C5 steps

The regulators of complement activation (RCA) (see Table 50-2) limit the production of C3b, primarily by the AP C3 convertases. Because the addition of C3b to a C3 convertase makes it a C5 convertase, regulation of the two enzyme complexes is linked. Modulation of their activity on host cells limits tissue destruction and the production of inflammatory mediators.

The RCA proteins control complement activation by two processes. *Decay-accelerating activity* refers to when the inhibitor transiently binds to C3b or C4b in the convertase and thereby dissociates the other members of the complex, rendering it enzymatically inactive (as the component released is the catalytic domain of the protease). The second is cofactor activity, which requires recognition of C3b or C4b by a plasma cofactor protein. Upon this interaction, the protease, factor I, cleaves C3b or C4b. Cleavage of C3b by factor I renders the convertase irreversibly inactive (generates iC3b which cannot participate in convertase formation).

Membrane Attack Complex

The cleavage of C5 generates C5a, the most potent of the complement anaphylatoxins, and C5b. C5b associates with C6 and C7 to create a lipophilic trimer as the initial part of the MAC (Fig. 50-4). The C5b67 trimer inserts into the lipid bilayer and serves as a binding site for C8 and C9. C9 self-polymerizes, leading to 12 to 18 C9 molecules that form a ring structure (completing the MAC). The MAC resembles a doughnut with a 10-nm pore running through the center. This pore allows water and ions to enter the cells, ultimately leading to osmotic lysis. Many pathogens such as gram-positive bacteria possess a capsule that makes them resistant to lysis.[12] Opsonization leading to phagocytosis is thus the major means of eliminating such organisms.

The MAC appears to be essential only for elimination of *Neisseria* spp. Individuals completely deficient in C5, C6, C7, C8, or C9 are at an increased risk only for meningococcal and gonococcal infections. C9 deficiency is a common immunodeficiency in Japan, with a heterozygote frequency of 3% to 5%. Thus, heterozygous deficiency seems to not be deleterious to the population in general but may have a selective advantage.

Extensive complement activation during an inflammatory response can result in sufficient MAC deposition to produce host cell lysis. Host cells, however, have mechanisms in place to resist the osmotic changes caused by the MAC and to block assembly of the MAC as it is formed (the protein is known as protectin or CD59). Rather, the nonlethal effects of sublytic MAC deposition are more likely to contribute to pathology. In most cells, this occurs through a general activation of multiple cell signaling pathways.

The response to MAC deposition at sites of complement activation depends on the cell type (Table 50-8). In phagocytic cells, such as neutrophils or macrophages, sublytic MAC insertion leads to the production of reactive oxygen species (e.g., superoxide, hydrogen peroxide) as well as release of prostaglandins and leukotrienes. Platelets undergoing a "MAC attack" incorporate phosphatidylserine on their outer membrane, facilitating formation of blood coagulation enzyme complexes with a potentially procoagulant effect. On endothelial cells, MAC deposition induces the synthesis of interleukin-1α (IL-1α), which leads to further autocrine and paracrine endothelial cell activation. It stimulates a procoagulant state by (1) altering the phospholipid composition of the endothelial membrane; (2) inducing the synthesis of tissue factor and upregulating the synthesis of plasminogen activator inhibitor; (3) upregulating the expression of adhesion molecules, including intercellular adhesion molecule 1 (ICAM-1) and E-selectin; and (4) stimulating endothelial cells to proliferate through growth factor production. In summary,

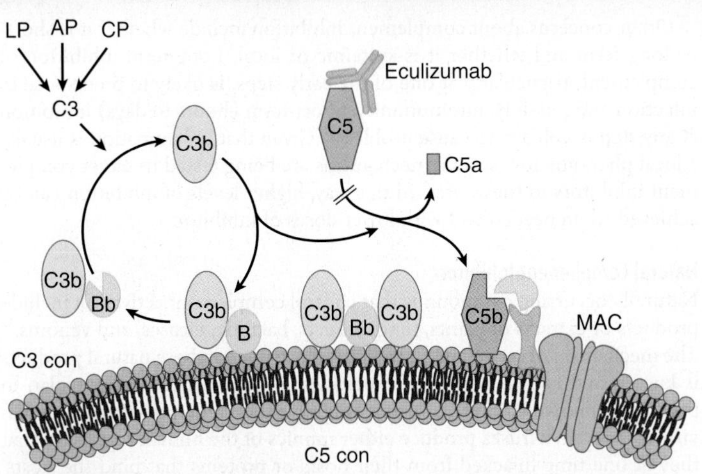

FIGURE 50-5. **Complement activation and the mechanism of action of eculizumab (monoclonal antibody [mAb] to C5). The alternate pathway (AP) constantly undergoes "tickover" but can also be primed by the classical pathway (CP) and lectin pathway (LP). The C3b that is formed interacts with factor B (B), which is then cleaved by factor D to form a C3 convertase (C3Bb). As more C3b is generated, some binds to the C3 convertase to form a C5 convertase. mAb to C5 (eculizumab) prevents the cleavage of C5 by the C5 convertase. Not shown is properdin that binds to both the C3 and C5 convertases to increase their half-lives approximately five- to 10-fold (from ≈30 seconds to several minutes).[7] (Modified from Wong EK, Goodship TH, Kavanagh D. Complement therapy in atypical haemolytic uraemic syndrome (aHUS).** ***Mol Immunol*****. 2013;56(3):199-212.)**

although cell death does not usually occur, deposition of the sublytic levels of MAC leads to a potentially dangerous situation, with increased inflammation, a procoagulant state, and cellular proliferation. Of course, part of this response is necessary at sites of injury to eliminate pathogens and debris and to facilitate wound repair. The short duration of complement activation and the presence of inhibitors help to maintain homeostasis.

Regulation of MAC formation is important clinically (Fig. 50-5). Two plasma proteins, clusterin and S-protein (vitronectin), bind the C5b-7 complex and prevent its association with the lipid membrane. C8 and multiple C9 molecules adhere to this soluble complex, termed *soluble C5b-9*, which is lytically inactive. CD59 (protectin) is a membrane-bound inhibitor of MAC formation. This small glycoprotein is attached to the cell membrane through a glycosyl phosphatidylinositol tail (GPI anchor). It binds to C5b-8, inserted in the cell membrane, to prevent binding to and polymerization of C9. The expression of CD59 is defective in patients with paroxysmal nocturnal hemoglobinuria (PNH), owing to the failure to synthesize the GPI anchor used by this and many other membrane proteins (including decay-accelerating factor [DAF]) to insert on the cell. The clinical features of PNH are primarily chronic hemolysis and intermittent thrombosis. Hemolysis is caused by complement activation on RBCs because of a lack of DAF and particularly CD59. Thrombosis is likely secondary to intravascular complement activation, leading to endothelial cell activation. The primary defect is an acquired hematopoietic stem cell mutation of a gene on the X chromosome responsible for encoding the first enzyme in the pathway to synthesize a GPI-anchor.

Anaphylatoxins

The anaphylatoxins serve a key early role in initiating a local inflammatory response as they trigger pathways to prepare a cell to face a pathogen or injury (Table 50-9). Similar to the MAC, anaphylatoxins are another major source of potential pathologic damage to self that results from complement activation. These peptides, C3a and C5a, are cleaved from their respective proteins during complement activation. They were named in 1910 to describe their toxic effects, including shock after the transfer of complement-activated serum into laboratory animals. They are 77 (C3a) or 74 (C5a) amino acids long and contain a key carboxy (C)-terminal arginine. They interact with the anaphylatoxin receptors. In plasma, the C-terminal arginine is removed by carboxypeptidase-N from anaphylatoxins not bound to their receptors. Depending on the response studied, this removal totally inactivates the anaphylatoxin or reduces its potency by about 1000-fold.

The C5a receptor (C5aR [CD88]) is a seven-transmembrane-spanning protein that couples ligand binding to G-protein signaling. Expressed on myeloid cells, particularly neutrophils and eosinophils, it mediates the potent

TABLE 50-9 RESPONSES TO SUBLYTIC MEMBRANE ATTACK COMPLEX ACTIVATION

CELL TYPE	EFFECTS
Most cells	Increased intracellular calcium flux Activation of G proteins Activation of protein kinases Activation of transcription factors Proliferation
Neutrophils and macrophages	Release of reactive oxygen species Activation of phospholipase A_2 Release of prostaglandins, thromboxane, and leukotrienes
Platelets	Release of ATP Increased P-selectin expression Procoagulant membrane changes
Endothelial cells	Increased synthesis of IL-1α Increased release of tissue factor Increased release of von Willebrand factor Increased synthesis of basic fibroblast and platelet-derived growth factors
Synoviocytes	Increased synthesis of prostaglandin Increased synthesis of IL-6 Increased production of matrix metalloproteinase
Glomerular epithelium	Activation of phospholipase A_2 Synthesis of prostaglandin Increased synthesis of collagen and fibronectin
Oligodendrocytes	Increased synthesis of myelin basic protein and proteolipids Increased proliferation

ATP = adenosine triphosphate; IL = interleukin.

chemoattractant property of C5a for both of these cell types. Signaling through CD88 leads to rapid secretion of all granule contents. These include lipases and proteases as well as lactoferrin from neutrophils, and peroxidase, major basic protein, and cationic protein from eosinophils. C5a also induces the release of cytokines, such as tumor necrosis factor (TNF), IL-1, IL-6, IL-8, and adhesion molecules, promoting the inflammatory response. The C5aR is expressed by numerous other tissues, including hepatocytes, bronchial and alveolar epithelium, vascular endothelium, renal mesangial and tubular epithelial cells, and brain neuronal cells. These cells are activated by receptor engagement, leading to production and release of cytokines, chemokines, and prostaglandins and to cellular proliferation.

The C3a receptor is also a seven-transmembrane-domain protein. It is expressed on almost all myeloid cells, including mast cells, where it mediates the release of allergic mediators. The C3aR also has been detected on many tissues, including in the brain and lung.

The anaphylatoxins have multiple biologic effects. In general, they cause smooth muscle contraction and recruitment of granulocytes, monocytes, and mast cells. In theory, they can contribute to the pathophysiology of any inflammatory condition. In disease models, C3a and C5a have been shown to play a role in diseases such as acute respiratory distress syndrome (ARDS), multisystem organ failure, septic shock, myocardial ischemia-reperfusion injury, asthma, rheumatoid arthritis, SLE, and inflammatory bowel disease. The anaphylatoxin peptides also are responsible for the "postpump" syndrome seen in patients undergoing cardiopulmonary bypass or hemodialysis. Exposure of blood to dialysis or perfusion membranes leads to complement activation. Within minutes of starting bypass, there is a sharp increase in the levels of C3a and C5a in the extracorporeal circuit being returned to the patient. This increase can be associated with respiratory distress, pulmonary hypertension, and pulmonary edema. It has been shown that the length of time that patients stay on the ventilator after bypass surgery correlates with the level of C3a generated during reperfusion.

C3a and C5a have been implicated in the initiation and prolongation of ARDS and multisystem organ failure. After severe trauma, levels of C3a have been measured that suggest activation of the entire circulating C3 pool. This activation leads to bronchoconstriction, increased vascular permeability, hypotension, and vascular plugging with leukocytes. The activation of white blood cells continues the cycle of tissue damage with further complement activation. Continued elevation of C3a in shock or ARDS is a poor prognostic sign. C3a and C5a also appear to play a major role in the pathogenesis of asthma.

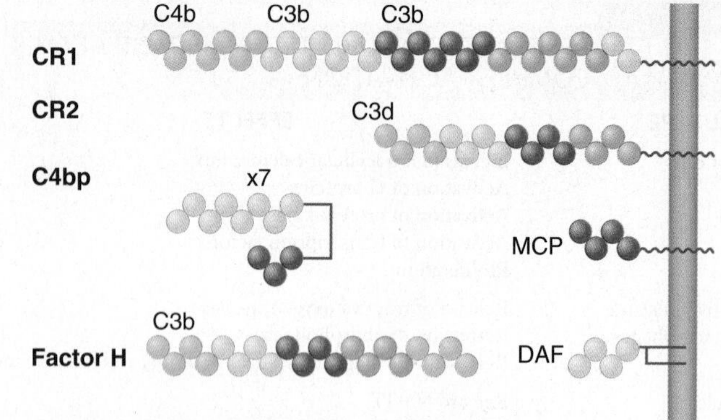

FIGURE 50-6. **Model of the complement regulators required to inhibit complement activation on self at the steps of C3 and C5 cleavage.** ***Circles*** **represent individual complement control repeats (~60 amino acids each), and** ***shading*** **indicates higher organizational units composed of several repeats. The approximate locations for binding of C3b and C4b fragments are indicated. Factor H and C4bp are plasma proteins. C4bp = C4-binding protein; CR = complement receptor; DAF = decay-accelerating factor; MCP = membrane cofactor protein.**

Complement Receptors

Opsonization of target by C4b and C3b is effective in preventing infections because these two complement fragments (and the further cleavage products in the case of C3b) are ligands for complement receptors (Fig. 50-6). After covalent attachment of C4b and C3b, immune adherence occurs between the opsonized microbe and immune cells, predominantly neutrophils, monocytes, and macrophages. Complement opsonins are highly effective mediators of immune adherence. On phagocytic cells, this is the prelude to the ingestion and destruction of the target antigen. On RBCs, immune adherence is followed by transfer of the C4b/C3b-coated cargo to monocytes and macrophages in the liver and spleen. CR1 is particularly efficient at immune adherence. Proteolytic modification of C3b leads to iC3b, which is a ligand for the highly phagocytic CR3 and CR4. A further degradation of iC3b to C3d leads to an interaction with CR2 to lower the threshold of B cell activation. Overall, the process is designed with two goals in mind: first is destruction by phagocytosis of the microbe and second is to coat microbial antigens for an adaptive immune response. For example, follicular dendritic cells and B lymphocytes express CR1, CR2, CR3, and CR4 that facilitate complement-coated antigens to be bound, internalized, and presented to other immune cells. CR3 and CR4 facilitate phagocytosis, and CR2 on follicular dendritic cells facilitates immunologic memory generation.

COMPLEMENT INHIBITORS

Given the many disease states in which complement is one of the central mediators of pathology, it is no surprise that complement inhibitors are in preclinical or clinical development for treatment of human diseases (see Table 50-2 and Fig. 50-6). These inhibitors take several different forms. Whereas some are variations of physiologic inhibitors, others are the products of molecular biologic searches for novel compounds.

It is important to consider where in the complement pathway to design an inhibitor to act. Inhibition of the activation pathways limits the production of biologically active peptides. Inhibiting the activation of C3 not only prevents the generation of the C3a anaphylatoxin but also may leave the patient susceptible to infection by limiting the deposition of C3b on targets as an opsonin. Inhibition of C3b deposition would decrease the patient's ability to clear immune complexes, potentially resulting in renal, pulmonary, and vascular damage. It also might promote the development of antibodies to self-antigens.

Inhibition of the C5 convertases is an attractive goal because it would prevent the generation of the C5a anaphylatoxin and the MAC (see Fig. 50-5). This strategy would inhibit complement activation without limiting C3b deposition. Inhibitors based on this concept have been successful; the mAb to C5 is approved by the Food and Drug Administration (FDA) to treat PNH and atypical hemolytic-uremic syndrome (aHUS).

Other concerns about complement inhibition include whether it is short- or long term and whether it is systemic or local. Long-term inhibition of complement, particularly at one of the early steps, is likely to predispose to infection and possibly autoimmunity. Short-term (hours to days) inhibition at any step is unlikely to cause problems. Given that inflammation is usually a local phenomenon, several mechanisms are being tested to target complement inhibitors to these sites. In this way, higher levels of inhibition can be achieved when needed and with lower doses of inhibitor.

Natural Complement Inhibitors

Naturally occurring compounds that control complement activation include products or extracts of plants, fungi, insects, bacteria, viruses, and venoms.[12] The mechanism of complement inhibition by some of these natural products is known and is of clinical and experimental importance. In particular, to protect themselves from the host's complement system, poxviruses, herpesviruses, and flaviviruses produce either mimics of the human regulators that they at one time hijacked from their hosts or proteins that bind the hosts' regulators such as the plasma protein factor H. Bacteria also express a wide variety of inhibitors of the human complement system. *Staphylococcus aureus,* for example, synthesizes up to 10 distinct proteins that inhibit at almost every key step of the complement cascade. Cobra venom factor (CVF) is a modified form of cobra C3b secreted by venom glands in the oral cavity. It is an 144,000-dalton glycoprotein that forms an AP convertase in association with host factor B. Upon injection, CVF leads to massive activation of the AP, leading to shock and pulmonary microvascular injury in experimental animals. It is resistant to the host's inhibitors because the site for that interaction is altered on CVF. Perhaps the most widely used natural inhibitor of complement activation is heparin. It decreases activation of the CP and AP. In clinical practice, the anticomplementary effect of heparin has been used to prevent complement activation during cardiopulmonary bypass. Measurement of complement activation products such as C3a or soluble C5b-9 after bypass showed decreases of 35% to 70% for adult and pediatric patients when heparin-coated extracorporeal circuits were used. Although numerous studies have looked at the decrease in complement activation by heparin-coated bypass circuits, there have been few attempts to correlate this with clinical outcome.

Anti-C5

The complement inhibitor that has achieved the widest attention as a therapeutic agent to stop complement activation is a mAb to C5 that prevents its cleavage to C5a (potent anaphylatoxin) and C5b (initiator of the MAC) (see Fig. 50-5). The generation of the C3b and C4b still occurs, allowing opsonization of pathogens and formation of immune complexes. Because activation of early complement components is also important for the maintenance of tolerance to self-antigens, inhibition of C5 activation is less worrisome than inhibition of C3 activation. The one consequence of C5 deficiency in humans is an increased risk of *Neisseria* infections that can largely be mitigated through vaccination. The anti-C5 mAb eculizumab has been approved for use in patients with PNH and aHUS.

The complement system is undergoing a renaissance. There are several reasons but probably the foremost is the discovery of mutations in complement regulators leading to aHUS and AMD. Second is the therapeutic success of a mAb to C5 in the treatment of aHUS and PNH. Third is the introduction of purified C1-Inhibitor, kallikrein inhibitors, and a bradykinin receptor antagonist to prevent and treat swelling attacks in hereditary angioedema. Last, intriguing recent data implicate the complement system in the pathophysiology of multiple disorders, including AMD, ischemia/reperfusion injury, organ regeneration, brain development (pruning of undesirable synapses), obesity, asthma, T-cell activation phenomena associated with allergic and rheumatic diseases,[13] and more.

GENERAL REFERENCES

For the General References and other additional features, please visit Expert Consult at https://expertconsult.inkling.com.

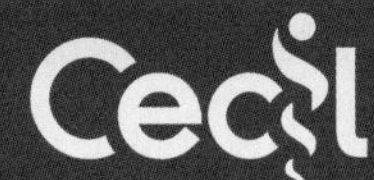

VIII

CARDIOVASCULAR DISEASE

51

APPROACH TO THE PATIENT WITH POSSIBLE CARDIOVASCULAR DISEASE

LEE GOLDMAN

Patients with cardiovascular disease may present with a wide range of symptoms and signs, each of which may be caused by noncardiovascular conditions. Conversely, patients with substantial cardiovascular disease may be asymptomatic. Because cardiovascular disease is a leading cause of death in the United States and other developed countries, it is crucial that patients be evaluated carefully to detect early cardiovascular disease, that symptoms or signs of cardiovascular disease be evaluated in detail, and that appropriate therapy be instituted. Improvements in diagnosis, therapy, and prevention have contributed to a 70% or so decline in age-adjusted cardiovascular death rates in the United States since the 1960s. Furthermore, among people age 65 years and older, regular visits to a primary care physician are associated with a 25 to 30% reduction in overall mortality. However, the absolute number of deaths from cardiovascular disease in the United States has not declined proportionately because of the increase in the population older than 40 years as well as the aging of the population in general.

In evaluating a patient with known or suspected heart disease, the physician must determine quickly whether a potentially life-threatening condition exists. In these situations, the evaluation must focus on the specific issue at hand and be accompanied by the rapid performance of appropriately directed additional tests. Examples of potentially life-threatening conditions include acute myocardial infarction (MI) (Chapter 73), unstable angina (Chapter 72), suspected aortic dissection (Chapter 78), pulmonary edema (Chapter 59), and pulmonary embolism (Chapter 98).

USING THE HISTORY TO DETECT CARDIOVASCULAR SYMPTOMS

Patients may complain spontaneously of a variety of cardiovascular symptoms (Table 51-1), but sometimes these symptoms are elicited only by obtaining a careful, complete medical history. In patients with known or suspected cardiovascular disease, questions about cardiovascular symptoms are key components of the history of present illness; in other patients, these issues are a fundamental part of the review of systems.

Chest Pain

Chest discomfort or pain is the cardinal manifestation of myocardial ischemia resulting from coronary artery disease or any condition that causes myocardial ischemia by an imbalance of myocardial oxygen demand compared with myocardial oxygen supply (Chapter 71). New, acute, often ongoing pain may indicate an acute MI, unstable angina, or aortic dissection; a pulmonary cause, such as acute pulmonary embolism or pleural irritation; a musculoskeletal condition of the chest wall, thorax, or shoulder; or a gastrointestinal abnormality, such as esophageal reflux or spasm, peptic ulcer disease, or cholecystitis (Table 51-2). The chest discomfort of MI commonly occurs without an immediate or obvious precipitating clinical cause and builds in intensity for at least several minutes; the sensation can range from annoying discomfort to severe pain (Chapter 73). Although a variety of adjectives may be used by patients to describe the sensation, physicians must be suspicious of any discomfort, especially if it radiates to the neck, shoulder, or arms. The probability of an acute MI can be estimated by integrating information from the history, physical examination, and electrocardiogram (Fig. 51-1).

The chest discomfort of unstable angina is clinically indistinguishable from that of MI except that the former may be precipitated more clearly by activity and may be more rapidly responsive to antianginal therapy (Chapter 72). Aortic dissection (Chapter 78) classically presents with the sudden onset of severe pain in the chest and radiating to the back; the location of the pain often provides clues to the location of the dissection. Ascending aortic dissections commonly present with chest discomfort radiating to the back, whereas dissections of the descending aorta commonly present with back pain radiating to the abdomen. The presence of back pain or a history of hypertension or other predisposing factors, such as Marfan syndrome, should prompt a careful assessment of peripheral pulses to determine whether the great vessels are affected by the dissection and of the chest radiograph to evaluate the size of the aorta. If this initial evaluation is suggestive, further testing with transesophageal echocardiography, computed tomography (CT), or magnetic resonance imaging (MRI) is indicated. The pain of pericarditis (Chapter 77) may simulate that of an acute MI, may be primarily pleuritic, or may be continuous; a key physical finding is a pericardial rub. The pain of pulmonary embolism (Chapter 98) is commonly pleuritic in nature and is associated with dyspnea; hemoptysis also may be present. Pulmonary hypertension (Chapter 68) of any cause may be associated with chest discomfort with exertion; it commonly is associated with severe dyspnea and often is associated with cyanosis.

Recurrent, episodic chest discomfort may be noted with angina pectoris and with many cardiac and noncardiac causes (Chapter 71). A variety of stress tests (Table 51-3) can be used to provoke reversible myocardial ischemia in susceptible individuals and to help determine whether ischemia is the pathophysiologic explanation for the chest discomfort (Chapter 71).

Dyspnea

Dyspnea, which is an uncomfortable awareness of breathing, is commonly caused by cardiovascular or pulmonary disease. A systematic approach (see Fig. 83-3) with selected tests nearly always reveals the cause. Acute dyspnea can be caused by myocardial ischemia, heart failure, severe hypertension, pericardial tamponade, pulmonary embolism, pneumothorax, upper airway obstruction, acute bronchitis or pneumonia, or some drug overdoses (e.g., salicylates). Subacute or chronic dyspnea is also a common presenting or accompanying symptom in patients with pulmonary disease (Chapter 83). Dyspnea also can be caused by severe anemia (Chapter 158) and can be confused with the fatigue that often is noted in patients with systemic and neurologic diseases (Chapters 256 and 396).

In heart failure, dyspnea typically is noted as a hunger for air and a need or an urge to breathe. The feeling that breathing requires increased work or effort is more typical of airway obstruction or neuromuscular disease. A feeling of chest tightness or constriction during breathing is typical of bronchoconstriction, which is commonly caused by obstructive airway disease (Chapters 87 and 88) but also may be seen in pulmonary edema. A feeling of heavy breathing, a feeling of rapid breathing, or a need to breathe more is classically associated with deconditioning.

In cardiovascular conditions, chronic dyspnea usually is caused by increases in pulmonary venous pressure as a result of left ventricular failure (Chapters 58 and 59) or valvular heart disease (Chapter 75). Orthopnea, which is an exacerbation of dyspnea when the patient is recumbent, is caused by increased work of breathing because of either increased venous return to the pulmonary vasculature or loss of gravitational assistance in diaphragmatic effort. Paroxysmal nocturnal dyspnea is severe dyspnea that awakens a patient at night and forces the assumption of a sitting or standing position to achieve gravitational redistribution of fluid.

Palpitations

Palpitations (Chapter 62) describe a subjective sensation of an irregular or abnormal heartbeat. Palpitations may be caused by any arrhythmia (Chapters 64 and 65) with or without important underlying structural heart disease. Palpitations should be defined in terms of the duration and frequency of the episodes; the precipitating and related factors; and any associated symptoms of chest pain, dyspnea, lightheadedness, or syncope. It is crucial to use the history to determine whether the palpitations are caused by an irregular or a regular heartbeat. The feeling associated with a premature atrial or ventricular contraction, often described as a "skipped beat" or a "flip-flopping of the heart," must be distinguished from the irregularly irregular rhythm of atrial fibrillation and the rapid but regular rhythm of supraventricular tachycardia. Associated symptoms of chest pain, dyspnea, lightheadedness, dizziness, or diaphoresis suggest an important effect on cardiac output and mandate further evaluation. In general, evaluation begins with ambulatory electrocardiography (ECG) (Table 51-4), which is indicated in patients who have palpitations in the presence of structural heart disease or substantial accompanying symptoms. Depending on the series, 9 to 43% of patients have important underlying heart disease. In such patients, more detailed evaluation is warranted (see Fig. 62-1).

Lightheadedness or *syncope* (Chapter 62) can be caused by any condition that decreases cardiac output (e.g., bradyarrhythmia, tachyarrhythmia, obstruction of the left ventricular or right ventricular inflow or outflow, cardiac tamponade, aortic dissection, or severe pump failure), by reflex-mediated vasomotor instability (e.g., vasovagal, situational, or carotid sinus syncope), or by orthostatic hypotension (see Table 62-1). Neurologic

TABLE 51-1 CARDINAL SYMPTOMS OF CARDIOVASCULAR DISEASE

Chest pain or discomfort
Dyspnea, orthopnea, paroxysmal nocturnal dyspnea, wheezing
Palpitations, dizziness, syncope
Cough, hemoptysis
Fatigue, weakness
Pain in extremities with exertion (claudication)

diseases (e.g., migraine headaches, transient ischemic attacks, or seizures) also can cause transient loss of consciousness. The history, physical examination, and ECG are often diagnostic of the cause of syncope (see Table 62-2). Syncope caused by a cardiac arrhythmia usually occurs with little warning. Syncope with exertion or just after conclusion of exertion is typical of aortic stenosis and hypertrophic obstructive cardiomyopathy. In many patients, additional testing is required to document central nervous system disease, the cause of reduced cardiac output, or carotid sinus syncope. When the history, physical examination, and ECG do not provide helpful diagnostic information that points toward a specific cause of syncope, it is imperative that patients with heart disease or an abnormal ECG be tested with continuous ambulatory ECG monitoring to diagnose a possible arrhythmia (see Fig. 62-1); in selected patients, formal electrophysiologic testing may be indicated

TABLE 51-2 CAUSES OF CHEST PAIN

CONDITION	LOCATION	QUALITY	DURATION	AGGRAVATING OR RELIEVING FACTORS	ASSOCIATED SYMPTOMS OR SIGNS
CARDIOVASCULAR CAUSES					
Angina	Retrosternal region; radiates to or occasionally isolated to neck, jaw, epigastrium, shoulder, or arms (left common)	Pressure, burning, squeezing, heaviness, indigestion	<2-10 min	Precipitated by exercise, cold weather, or emotional stress; relieved by rest or nitroglycerin; atypical (Prinzmetal) angina may be unrelated to activity, often early morning	S_3 or murmur of papillary muscle dysfunction during pain
Rest or unstable angina	Same as angina	Same as angina but may be more severe	Usually <20 min	Same as angina, with decreasing tolerance for exertion or at rest	Similar to stable angina but may be pronounced; transient heart failure can occur
Myocardial infarction	Substernal and may radiate like angina	Heaviness, pressure, burning, constriction	≥30 min but variable	Unrelieved by rest or nitroglycerin	Shortness of breath, sweating, weakness, nausea, vomiting
Pericarditis	Usually begins over sternum or toward cardiac apex and may radiate to neck or left shoulder; often more localized than the pain of myocardial ischemia	Sharp, stabbing, knifelike	Lasts many hours to days; may wax and wane	Aggravated by deep breathing, rotating chest, or supine position; relieved by sitting up and leaning forward	Pericardial friction rub
Aortic dissection	Anterior chest; may radiate to back	Excruciating, tearing, knifelike	Sudden onset, unrelenting	Usually occurs in setting of hypertension or predisposition, such as Marfan syndrome	Murmur of aortic insufficiency, pulse or blood pressure asymmetry; neurologic deficit
Pulmonary embolism (chest pain often not present)	Substernal or over region of pulmonary infarction	Pleuritic (with pulmonary infarction) or angina-like	Sudden onset; minutes to <1 hr	May be aggravated by breathing	Dyspnea, tachypnea, tachycardia; hypotension, signs of acute right ventricular failure, and pulmonary hypertension with large emboli; rales, pleural friction rub, hemoptysis with pulmonary infarction
Pulmonary hypertension	Substernal	Pressure; oppressive	Similar to angina	Aggravated by effort	Pain usually associated with dyspnea; signs of pulmonary hypertension
NONCARDIAC CAUSES					
Pneumonia with pleurisy	Localized over involved area	Pleuritic, localized	Brief or prolonged	Painful breathing	Dyspnea, cough, fever, dull to percussion, bronchial breath sounds, rales, occasional pleural friction rub
Spontaneous pneumothorax	Unilateral	Sharp, well localized	Sudden onset, lasts many hours	Painful breathing	Dyspnea; hyperresonance and decreased breath and voice sounds over involved lung
Musculoskeletal disorders	Variable	Aching	Short or long duration	Aggravated by movement; history of muscle exertion or injury	Tender to pressure or movement
Herpes zoster	Dermatomal in distribution	Burning, itching	Prolonged	None	Vesicular rash appears in area of discomfort
Esophageal reflux	Substernal, epigastric	Burning, visceral discomfort	10-60 min	Aggravated by large meal, postprandial recumbency; relief with antacid	Water brash
Peptic ulcer	Epigastric, substernal	Visceral burning, aching	Prolonged	Relief with food, antacid	
Gallbladder disease	Epigastric, right upper quadrant	Visceral	Prolonged	May be unprovoked or follow meals	Right upper quadrant tenderness may be present
Anxiety states	Often localized over precordium	Variable; location often moves from place to place	Varies; often fleeting	Situational	Sighing respirations, often chest wall tenderness

Modified from Andreoli TE, Carpenter CCJ, Griggs RC, et al. Evaluation of the patient with cardiovascular disease. In: *Cecil Essentials of Medicine*, 6th ed. Philadelphia: WB Saunders; 2004:34-35.

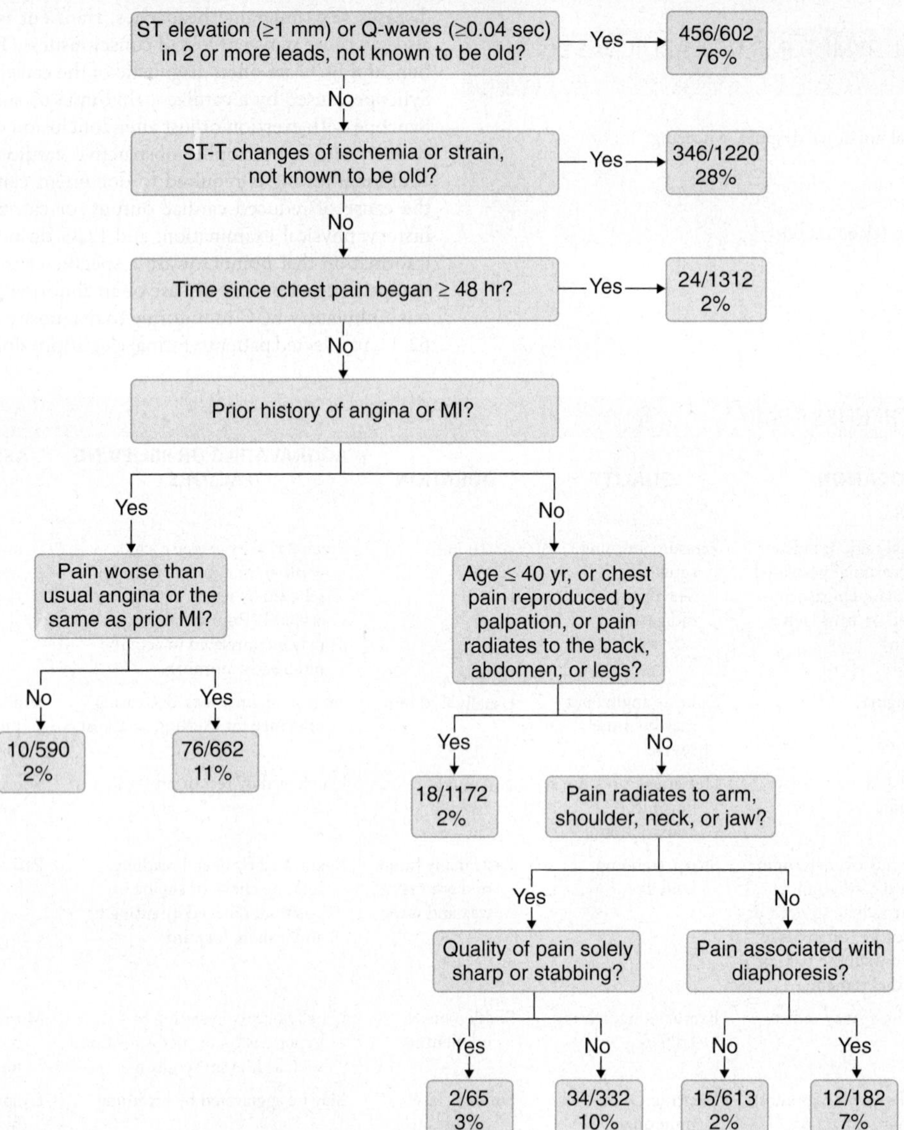

FIGURE 51-1. **Flow diagram to estimate the risk for acute myocardial infarction (MI) in emergency departments in patients with acute chest pain. For each clinical subset, the numerator is the number of patients with the set of presenting characteristics who had an MI; the denominator is the total number of patients presenting with that characteristic or set of characteristics. CHF = congestive heart failure; DVT = deep vein thrombosis. (Modified from Pearson SD, Goldman L, Garcia TB, et al. Physician response to a prediction rule for the triage of emergency department patients with chest pain. *J Gen Intern Med.* 1994;9:241-247.)**

TABLE 51-3 COMMON EXERCISE TEST PROTOCOLS*

PROTOCOL	STAGE	DURATION (min)	GRADE (%)	RATE (mph)	METABOLIC EQUIVALENTS AT COMPLETION	FUNCTIONAL CLASS
Modified Bruce protocol†	1	3	0	1.7	2.5	III
	2	3	10	1.7	5	II
	3	3	12	2.5	7	I
	4	3	14	3.4	10	I
	5	3	16	4.2	13	I
Naughton protocol‡	0	2	0	2	2	III
	1	2	3.5	2	3	III
	2	2	7	2	4	III
	3	2	10.5	2	5	II
	4	2	14	2	6	II
	5	2	17.5	2	7	I

*Ramp protocols in which the workload is gradually increased on the basis of the patient's estimated functional capacity to achieve maximal effort in approximately 10 minutes are also useful.
†Commonly used in ambulatory patients.
‡Commonly used in patients with recent myocardial infarction, unstable angina, or other conditions that are expected to limit exercise.
Modified from Braunwald E, Goldman L, eds. *Primary Cardiology*. 2nd ed. Philadelphia: WB Saunders; 2003.

TABLE 51-4 AMERICAN HEART ASSOCIATION/AMERICAN COLLEGE OF CARDIOLOGY GUIDELINES FOR USE OF DIAGNOSTIC TESTS IN PATIENTS WITH PALPITATIONS*

AMBULATORY ELECTROCARDIOGRAPHY	
Class I	Palpitations, syncope, dizziness
Class II	Shortness of breath, chest pain, or fatigue (not otherwise explained, episodic, and strongly suggestive of an arrhythmia as the cause because of a relation of the symptom with palpitation)
Class III	Symptoms not reasonably expected to be caused by arrhythmia
ELECTROPHYSIOLOGIC STUDY	
Class I	Patients with palpitations who have a pulse rate documented by medical personnel as inappropriately rapid and in whom electrocardiographic recordings fail to document the cause of the palpitations Patients with palpitations preceding a syncopal episode
Class II	Patients with clinically significant palpitations, suspected to be of cardiac origin, in whom symptoms are sporadic and cannot be documented; studies are performed to determine the mechanisms of arrhythmias, to direct or provide therapy or to assess prognosis
Class III	Patients with palpitations documented to have extracardiac causes (e.g., hyperthyroidism)
ECHOCARDIOGRAPHY	
Class I	Arrhythmias with evidence of heart disease Family history of genetic disorder associated with arrhythmias
Class II	Arrhythmias commonly associated with, but without evidence of, heart disease Atrial fibrillation or flutter
Class III	Palpitations without evidence of arrhythmias Minor arrhythmias without evidence of heart disease

*Class I, general agreement the test is useful and indicated; class II, frequently used, but there is a divergence of opinion with respect to its utility; class III, general agreement the test is not useful.
From Braunwald E, Goldman L, eds. *Primary Cardiology.* 2nd ed. Philadelphia: WB Saunders; 2003:132.

TABLE 51-5 A COMPARISON OF THREE METHODS OF ASSESSING CARDIOVASCULAR DISABILITY

CLASS	NEW YORK HEART ASSOCIATION FUNCTIONAL CLASSIFICATION	CANADIAN CARDIOVASCULAR SOCIETY FUNCTIONAL CLASSIFICATION	SPECIFIC ACTIVITY SCALE
I	Patients with cardiac disease but without resulting limitations of physical activity Ordinary physical activity does not cause undue fatigue, palpitation, dyspnea, or anginal pain.	Ordinary physical activity, such as walking and climbing stairs, does not cause angina. Angina with strenuous or rapid or prolonged exertion at work or recreation	Patients can perform to completion any activity requiring ≥7 metabolic equivalents, e.g., can carry 24 lb up 8 steps; carry objects that weigh 80 lb; do outdoor work (shovel snow, spade soil); do recreational activities (skiing, basketball, squash, handball, jog or walk 5 mph)
II	Patients with cardiac disease resulting in slight limitation of physical activity They are comfortable at rest. Ordinary physical activity results in fatigue, palpitations, dyspnea, or anginal pain.	Slight limitation of ordinary activity Walking or climbing stairs rapidly, walking uphill, walking or stair climbing after meals, in cold, in wind, or when under emotional stress, or only during the few hours after awakening Walking >2 blocks on the level and climbing >1 flight of ordinary stairs at a normal pace and in normal conditions	Patient can perform to completion any activity requiring ≥5 metabolic equivalents but cannot and does not perform to completion activities requiring ≥7 metabolic equivalents, e.g., have sexual intercourse without stopping, garden, rake, weed, roller skate, dance foxtrot, walk at 4 mph on level ground
III	Patients with cardiac disease resulting in marked limitation of physical activity They are comfortable at rest. Less than ordinary physical activity causes fatigue, palpitations, dyspnea, or anginal pain.	Marked limitation of ordinary physical activity Walking 1 or 2 blocks on the level and climbing >1 flight in normal conditions	Patient can perform to completion any activity requiring ≥2 metabolic equivalents but cannot and does not perform to completion any activities requiring ≥5 metabolic equivalents, e.g., shower without stopping, strip and make bed, clean windows, walk 2.5 mph, bowl, play golf, dress without stopping
IV	Patients with cardiac disease resulting in inability to carry on any physical activity without discomfort Symptoms of cardiac insufficiency or of the anginal syndrome may be present even at rest. If any physical activity is undertaken, discomfort is increased.	Inability to carry on any physical activity without discomfort—anginal syndrome may be present at rest	Patient cannot or does not perform to completion activities requiring ≥2 metabolic equivalents; cannot carry out activities listed above (Specific Activity Scale, class III)

From Goldman L, Hashimoto B, Cook EF, et al. Comparative reproducibility and validity of systems for assessing cardiovascular functional class: advantages of a new specific activity scale. *Circulation.* 1981;64:1227-1234. Reproduced by permission of the American Heart Association.

(Chapter 62). In patients with no evident heart disease, tilt testing (Chapter 62) can help detect reflex-mediated vasomotor instability.

Other Symptoms

Nonproductive *cough* (Chapter 83), especially a persistent cough (see Fig. 83-1), can be an early manifestation of elevated pulmonary venous pressure and otherwise unsuspected heart failure. *Fatigue* and *weakness* are common accompaniments of advanced cardiac disease and reflect an inability to perform normal activities. A variety of approaches have been used to classify the severity of cardiac limitations, ranging from class I (little or no limitation) to class IV (severe limitation) (Table 51-5). *Hemoptysis* (Chapter 83) is a classic presenting finding in patients with pulmonary embolism, but it is also common in patients with mitral stenosis, pulmonary edema, pulmonary infections, and malignant neoplasms (see Table 83-6). *Claudication,* which is pain in the extremities with exertion, should alert the physician to possible peripheral arterial disease (Chapters 79 and 80).

Complete Medical History

The complete medical history should include a thorough review of systems, family history, social history, and past medical history (Chapter 15). The review of systems may reveal other symptoms that suggest a systemic disease as the cause of any cardiovascular problems. The family history should focus on premature atherosclerosis or evidence of familial abnormalities, such as may be found with various causes of the long QT syndrome (Chapter 65) or hypertrophic cardiomyopathy (Chapter 60).

The social history should include specific questioning about cigarette smoking, alcohol intake, and use of illicit drugs. The past medical history may reveal prior conditions or medications that suggest systemic diseases, ranging from chronic obstructive pulmonary disease, which may explain a complaint of dyspnea, to hemochromatosis, which may be a cause of restrictive cardiomyopathy. A careful history to inquire about recent dental work or other procedures is crucial if bacterial endocarditis is part of the differential diagnosis.

PHYSICAL EXAMINATION FOR DETECTION OF SIGNS OF CARDIOVASCULAR DISEASE

The cardiovascular physical examination, which is a subset of the complete physical examination, provides important clues to the diagnosis of asymptomatic and symptomatic cardiac disease and may reveal cardiovascular manifestations of noncardiovascular diseases. The cardiovascular physical examination begins with careful measurement of the pulse and blood pressure (Chapter 8). If aortic dissection (Chapter 78) is a consideration, blood pressure should be measured in both arms and, preferably, in at least one leg. When coarctation of the aorta is suspected (Chapter 69), blood pressure must be measured in at least one leg and in the arms. Discrepancies in blood pressure between the two arms also can be caused by atherosclerotic disease of the great vessels. Pulsus paradoxus, which is more than the usual 10-mm Hg drop in systolic blood pressure during inspiration, is typical of pericardial tamponade (Chapter 77).

General Appearance

The respiratory rate may be increased in patients with heart failure. Patients with pulmonary edema are usually markedly tachypneic and may have labored breathing. Patients with advanced heart failure may have Cheyne-Stokes respirations.

Systemic diseases, such as hyperthyroidism (Chapter 226), hypothyroidism (Chapter 226), rheumatoid arthritis (Chapter 264), scleroderma (Chapter 267), and hemochromatosis (Chapter 212), may be suspected from the patient's general appearance. Marfan syndrome (Chapter 260), Turner syndrome (Chapter 235), Down syndrome (Chapter 41), and a variety of congenital anomalies also may be readily apparent.

Ophthalmologic Examination

Examination of the fundi may show diabetic (see Fig. 423-24) or hypertensive retinopathy (see Fig. 67-8) or Roth spots (see Fig. 423-28) typical of infectious endocarditis. Beading of the retinal arteries is typical of severe hypercholesterolemia. Osteogenesis imperfecta, which is associated with blue sclerae, also is associated with aortic dilation and mitral valve prolapse. Retinal artery occlusion (see Fig. 423-29) may be caused by an embolus from clot in the left atrium or left ventricle, a left atrial myxoma, or atherosclerotic debris from the great vessels. Hyperthyroidism may present with exophthalmos and typical stare (see Fig. 423-6), whereas myotonic dystrophy, which is associated with atrioventricular block and arrhythmia, often is associated with ptosis and an expressionless face (see Fig. 421-2).

Jugular Veins

The external jugular veins help in assessment of mean right atrial pressure, which normally varies between 5 and 10 cm H_2O; the height (in centimeters) of the central venous pressure is measured by adding 5 cm to the height of the observed jugular venous distention above the sternal angle of Louis (Fig. 51-2). The normal jugular venous pulse, best seen in the internal jugular vein (and not seen in the external jugular vein unless insufficiency of the jugular venous valves is present), includes an *a* wave, caused by right atrial contraction; a *c* wave, reflecting carotid artery pulsation; an *x* descent; a *v* wave, which corresponds to isovolumetric right ventricular contraction and is more marked in the presence of tricuspid insufficiency; and a *y* descent, which occurs as the tricuspid valve opens and ventricular filling begins (Fig. 51-3). Abnormalities of the jugular venous pressure (Fig. 51-4) are useful in detecting heart failure, and they correlate well with brain natriuretic peptide levels (Chapter 58) and echocardiographic evidence of an elevated pulmonary artery pressure (Chapter 55).[1] The jugular venous pressure also helps in the diagnosis of pericardial disease, tricuspid valve disease, and pulmonary hypertension (Table 51-6).

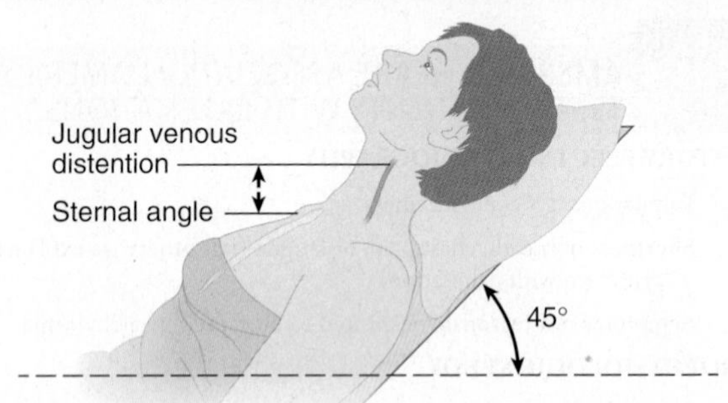

FIGURE 51-2. Jugular venous distention is defined by engorgement of the internal jugular vein more than 5 cm above the sternal angle at 45 degrees. The central venous pressure is the observed venous distention above the sternal angle plus 5 cm.

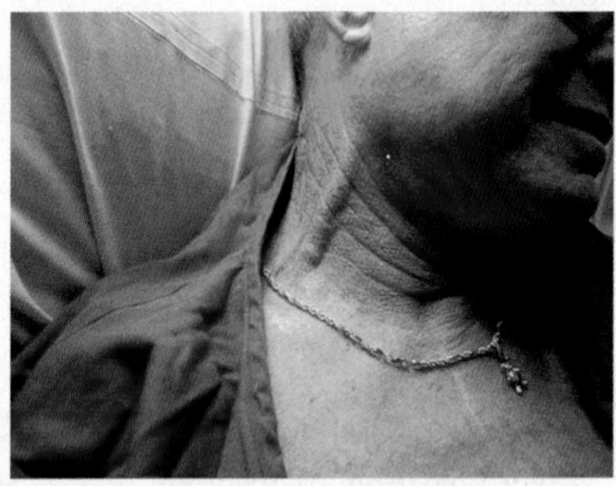

FIGURE 51-3. Typical distention of the internal jugular vein. (From http://courses.cvcc.vccs.edu/WisemanD/jugular_vein_distention.htm.)

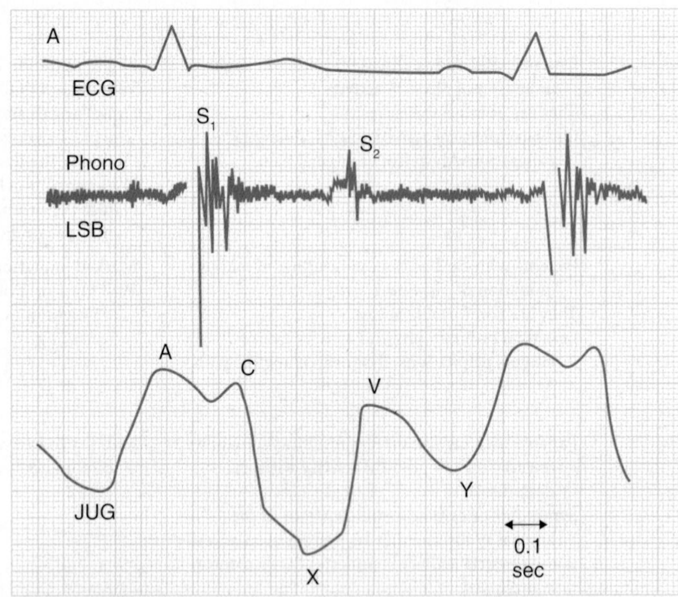

FIGURE 51-4. Normal jugular venous pulse. ECG = electrocardiogram; JUG = jugular vein; LSB = left sternal border; phono = phonocardiogram; S_1 = first heart sound; S_2 = second heart sound.

Carotid Pulse

The carotid pulse should be examined in terms of its volume and contour. The carotid pulse (Fig. 51-5) may be increased in frequency and may be more intense than normal in patients with a higher stroke volume secondary to aortic regurgitation, arteriovenous fistula, hyperthyroidism, fever, or anemia. In aortic regurgitation or arteriovenous fistula, the pulse may have a bisferious quality. The carotid upstroke is delayed in patients with valvular aortic stenosis (Chapter 75) and has a normal contour but diminished amplitude in any cause of reduced stroke volume.

Cardiac Inspection and Palpation

Inspection of the precordium may reveal the hyperinflation of obstructive lung disease or unilateral asymmetry of the left side of the chest because of right ventricular hypertrophy before puberty. Palpation may be performed with the patient either supine or in the left lateral decubitus position; the latter position moves the left ventricular apex closer to the chest wall and increases the ability to palpate the point of maximal impulse and other phenomena. Low-frequency phenomena, such as systolic heaves or lifts from the left ventricle (at the cardiac apex) or right ventricle (parasternal in the third or fourth intercostal space), are felt best with the heel of the palm. With the patient in the left lateral decubitus position, this technique also may allow palpation of an S_3 gallop in cases of advanced heart failure or an S_4 gallop in cases of poor left ventricular distensibility during diastole. The left ventricular apex is more diffuse and sometimes may be frankly dyskinetic in patients with advanced heart disease. The distal palm is best for feeling thrills, which are the tactile equivalent of cardiac murmurs. By definition, a thrill denotes a murmur of grade 4/6 or louder. Higher-frequency events may be felt best with the fingertips; examples include the opening snap of mitral stenosis or the loud pulmonic second sound of pulmonary hypertension.

TABLE 51-6 ABNORMALITIES OF VENOUS PRESSURE AND PULSE AND THEIR CLINICAL SIGNIFICANCE

Positive hepatojugular reflux	Suspect heart failure, particularly left ventricular systolic dysfunction (echocardiography recommended)
Elevated systemic venous pressure without obvious *x* or *y* descent, quiet precordium, and pulsus paradoxus	Suspect cardiac tamponade (echocardiography recommended)
Elevated systemic venous pressure with sharp *y* descent, Kussmaul sign, and quiet precordium	Suspect constrictive pericarditis (cardiac catheterization and MRI or CT recommended)
Elevated systemic venous pressure with a sharp brief *y* descent, Kussmaul sign, and evidence of pulmonary hypertension and tricuspid regurgitation	Suspect restrictive cardiomyopathy (cardiac catheterization and MRI or CT recommended)
A prominent *a* wave with or without elevation of mean systemic venous pressure	Exclude tricuspid stenosis, right ventricular hypertrophy caused by pulmonary stenosis, and pulmonary hypertension (echo-Doppler study recommended)
A prominent *v* wave with a sharp *y* descent	Suspect tricuspid regurgitation (echo-Doppler or cardiac catheterization to determine etiology)

CT = computed tomography; MRI = magnetic resonance imaging.
From Braunwald E, ed. *Heart Disease: A Textbook of Cardiovascular Medicine*. 5th ed. Philadelphia: WB Saunders; 1997.

Auscultation

The first heart sound (Fig. 51-6), which is largely produced by closure of the mitral and—to a lesser extent—the tricuspid valves, may be louder in patients with mitral valve stenosis and intact valve leaflet movement and less audible in patients with poor closure caused by mitral regurgitation (Chapter 75). The second heart sound is caused primarily by closure of the aortic valve, but closure of the pulmonic valve is also commonly audible. In normal individuals, the louder aortic closure sound occurs first, followed by pulmonic closure. With expiration, the two sounds are virtually superimposed. With inspiration, by comparison, the increased stroke volume of the right ventricle commonly leads to a discernible splitting of the second sound. This splitting may be fixed in patients with an atrial septal defect (Chapter 69) or a right bundle branch block. The split may be paradoxical in patients with left bundle branch block or other causes of delayed left ventricular emptying. The aortic component of the second sound is increased in intensity in the presence of systemic hypertension and decreased in intensity in patients with aortic stenosis. The pulmonic second sound is increased in the presence of pulmonary hypertension.

Early systolic ejection sounds are related to forceful opening of the aortic or pulmonic valve. These sounds are common in congenital aortic stenosis, with a mobile valve; in hypertension, with forceful opening of the aortic valve; and in healthy young individuals, especially when cardiac output is increased. Midsystolic or late systolic clicks are caused most commonly by mitral valve prolapse (Chapter 75). Clicks are relatively high-frequency sounds that are heard best with the diaphragm of the stethoscope.

An S_3 corresponds to rapid ventricular filling during early diastole. It may occur in normal children and young adults, especially if stroke volume is

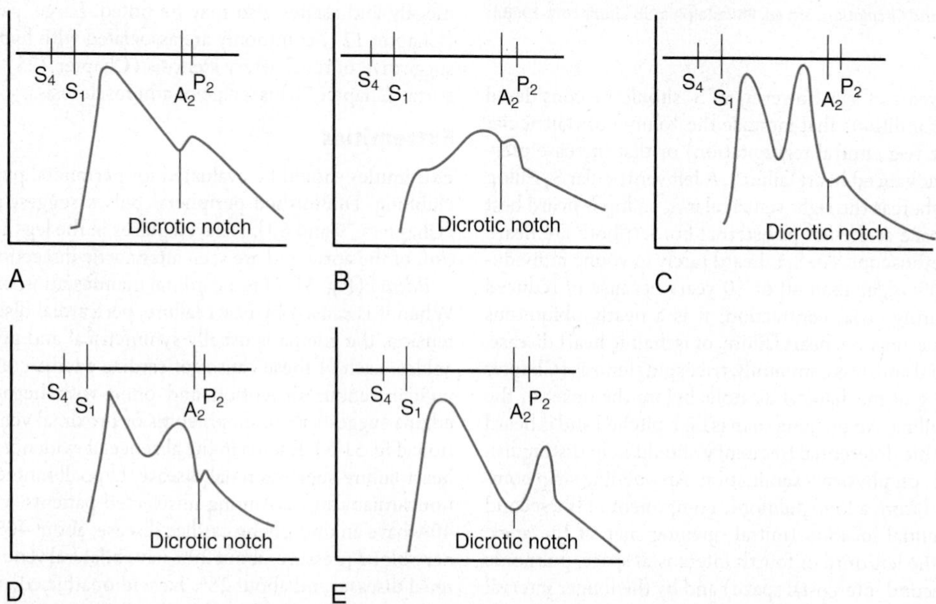

FIGURE 51-5. Schematic diagrams of the configurational changes in the carotid pulse and their differential diagnosis. Heart sounds also are illustrated. A, Normal. B, Anacrotic pulse with slow initial upstroke. The peak is close to the second heart sound. These features suggest fixed left ventricular outflow obstruction, such as valvular aortic stenosis. C, Pulsus bisferiens, with percussion and tidal waves occurring during systole. This type of carotid pulse contour is observed most frequently in patients with hemodynamically significant aortic regurgitation or combined aortic stenosis and regurgitation with dominant regurgitation. It rarely is observed in patients with mitral valve prolapse or in normal individuals. D, Pulsus bisferiens in hypertrophic obstructive cardiomyopathy. This finding rarely is appreciated at the bedside by palpation. E, Dicrotic pulse results from an accentuated dicrotic wave and tends to occur in sepsis, severe heart failure, hypovolemic shock, and cardiac tamponade and after aortic valve replacement. A_2 = aortic component of the second heart sound; P_2 = pulmonary component of the second heart sound); S_1 = first heart sound; S_4 = atrial sounds. (From Chatterjee K. Bedside evaluation of the heart: the physical examination. In: Chatterjee K, Chetlin MD, Karliner J, et al, eds. *Cardiology: An Illustrated Text/Reference*. Philadelphia: JB Lippincott; 1991:3.11-3.51.)

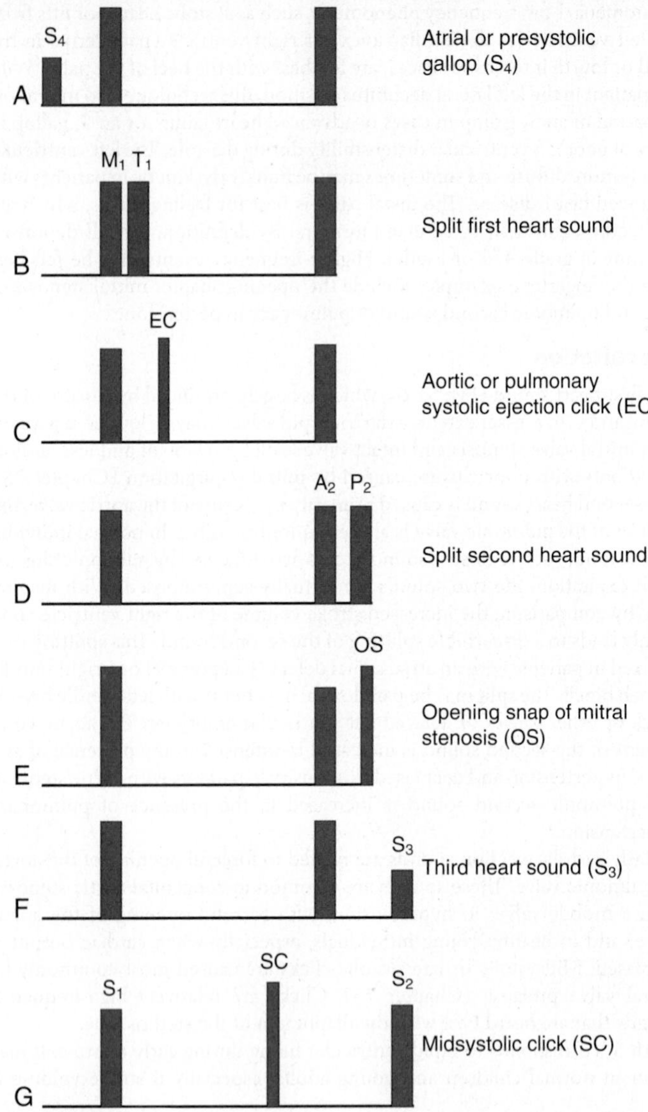

FIGURE 51-6. **Timing of the different heart sounds and added sounds. (Modified from Wood P. *Diseases of the Heart and Circulation*. 3rd ed. Philadelphia: JB Lippincott; 1968.)**

increased. After about 40 years of age, however, an S_3 should be considered abnormal; it is caused by conditions that increase the volume of ventricular filling during early diastole (e.g., mitral regurgitation) or that increase pressure in early diastole (e.g., advanced heart failure). A left ventricular S_3 gallop is heard best at the apex, whereas the right ventricular S_3 gallop is heard best at the fourth intercostal space at the left parasternal border; both are heard best with the bell of the stethoscope. An S_4 is heard rarely in young individuals but is common in adults older than 40 or 50 years because of reduced ventricular compliance during atrial contraction; it is a nearly ubiquitous finding in patients with hypertension, heart failure, or ischemic heart disease.

The opening snap of mitral and, less commonly, tricuspid stenosis (Chapter 75) occurs at the beginning of mechanical diastole, before the onset of the rapid phase of ventricular filling. An opening snap is high pitched and is heard best with the diaphragm; this differential frequency should help distinguish an opening snap from an S_3 on physical examination. An opening snap commonly can be distinguished from a loud pulmonic component of the second heart sound by the differential location (mitral opening snap at the apex, tricuspid opening snap at the left third or fourth intercostal space, pulmonic second sound at the left second intercostal space) and by the longer interval between S_2 and the opening snap.

Heart murmurs may be classified as systolic, diastolic, or continuous (Table 51-7). Murmurs are graded by intensity on a scale of 1 to 6. Grade 1 is faint and appreciated only by careful auscultation; grade 2, readily audible; grade 3, moderately loud; grade 4, loud and associated with a palpable thrill; grade 5, loud and audible with the stethoscope only partially placed on the chest; and grade 6, loud enough to be heard without the stethoscope on the chest. Systolic ejection murmurs usually peak in early to mid systole when left ventricular ejection is maximal; examples include fixed valvular, supravalvular, or infravalvular aortic stenosis and pulmonic stenosis. The murmur of hypertrophic obstructive cardiomyopathy has a similar ejection quality, although its peak may be later in systole when dynamic obstruction is maximal (Chapter 60). Pansystolic murmurs are characteristic of mitral or tricuspid regurgitation or with a left-to-right shunt from conditions such as a ventricular septal defect (left ventricle to right ventricle). A late systolic murmur is characteristic of mitral valve prolapse (Chapter 75) or ischemic papillary muscle dysfunction. Ejection quality murmurs also may be heard in patients with normal valves but increased flow, such as occurs with marked anemia, fever, or bradycardia secondary to congenital complete heart block; they also may be heard across a valve that is downstream from increased flow because of an intracardiac shunt. Maneuvers such as inspiration, expiration, standing, squatting, and hand gripping can be especially useful in the differential diagnosis of a murmur; however, echocardiography commonly is required to make a definitive diagnosis of cause and severity (Table 51-8).

High-frequency, early diastolic murmurs are typical of aortic regurgitation and pulmonic regurgitation from a variety of causes. The murmurs of mitral and tricuspid stenosis begin in early to mid diastole and tend to diminish in intensity later in diastole in the absence of effective atrial contraction, but they tend to increase in intensity in later diastole if effective atrial contraction is present.

Continuous murmurs may be caused by any abnormality that is associated with a pressure gradient in systole and diastole. Examples include a patent ductus arteriosus, ruptured sinus of Valsalva aneurysm, arteriovenous fistula (of the coronary artery, pulmonary artery, or thoracic artery), and a mammary soufflé. In some situations, murmurs of two coexistent conditions (e.g., aortic stenosis and regurgitation, atrial septal defect with a large shunt and resulting flow murmurs of relative mitral and pulmonic stenosis) may mimic a continuous murmur.

Unfortunately, the physical examination is limited for detecting meaningful valvular heart disease.[2] As a result, echocardiography (Chapter 55) is critical to the evaluation of patients with suspected structural heart disease.

Abdomen

The most common cause of hepatomegaly in patients with heart disease is hepatic engorgement from elevated right-sided pressures associated with right ventricular failure of any cause. Hepatojugular reflux is elicited by pressing on the liver and showing an increase in the jugular venous pressure; it indicates advanced right ventricular failure or obstruction to right ventricular filling. Evaluation of the abdomen also may reveal an enlarged liver caused by a systemic disease, such as hemochromatosis (Chapter 212) or sarcoidosis (Chapter 95), which also may affect the heart. In more severe cases, splenomegaly and ascites also may be noted. Large, palpable, polycystic kidneys (Chapter 127) commonly are associated with hypertension. A systolic bruit suggestive of renal artery stenosis (Chapter 125) or an enlarged abdominal aorta (Chapter 78) is a clue of atherosclerosis.

Extremities

Extremities should be evaluated for peripheral pulses, edema, cyanosis, and clubbing. Diminished peripheral pulses suggest peripheral arterial disease (Chapters 79 and 80). Delayed pulses in the legs are consistent with coarctation of the aorta and are seen after aortic dissection.

Edema (Fig. 51-7) is a cardinal manifestation of right-sided heart failure.[3] When it is caused by heart failure, pericardial disease, or pulmonary hypertension, the edema is usually symmetrical and progresses upward from the ankles; each of these causes of cardiac edema commonly is associated with jugular venous distention and often with hepatic congestion. Unilateral edema suggests thrombophlebitis or proximal venous or lymphatic obstruction (Fig. 51-8). Edema in the absence of evidence of right-sided or left-sided heart failure suggests renal disease, hypoalbuminemia, myxedema, or other noncardiac causes. Among unselected patients with bilateral edema, about 40% have an underlying cardiac disease, about 40% have an elevated pulmonary blood pressure, about 20% have bilateral venous disease, about 20% have renal disease, and about 25% have idiopathic edema.

Cyanosis (Fig. 51-9) is a bluish discoloration caused by reduced hemoglobin exceeding about 5 g/dL in the capillary bed. Central cyanosis is seen in patients with poor oxygen saturation resulting from a reduced inspired oxygen concentration or inability to oxygenate the blood in the lungs (e.g., as a result of advanced pulmonary disease, pulmonary edema, pulmonary arteriovenous fistula, or right-to-left shunting); it also may be seen in patients with marked erythrocytosis. Methemoglobinemia (Chapter 158) also can present with cyanosis. Peripheral cyanosis may be caused by reduced blood flow to the extremities secondary to vasoconstriction, heart failure, or shock.

TABLE 51-7 SOME COMMON CAUSES OF HEART MURMURS*

	USUAL LOCATION	COMMON ASSOCIATED FINDINGS
SYSTOLIC		
Holosystolic		
Mitral regurgitation	Apex → axilla	↑ with handgrip; S_3 if marked mitral regurgitation; left ventricular dilation common
Tricuspid regurgitation	LLSB	↑ with inspiration; right ventricular dilation common
Ventricular septal defect	LLSB → RLSB	Often with thrill
Early to mid systolic		
Aortic valvular stenosis	RUSB	
Fixed supravalvular or subvalvular	RUSB	Ejection click if mobile valve; soft or absent A_2 if valve immobile; later peak associated with more severe stenosis
Dynamic infravalvular	LLSB → apex + axilla	Hypertrophic obstructive cardiomyopathy; murmur louder if left ventricular volume lower or contractility increased, softer if left ventricular volume increased†; can be later in systole if obstruction delayed
Pulmonic valvular stenosis	LUSB	↑ with inspiration
Infravalvular (infundibular)	LUSB	↑ with inspiration
Supravalvular	LUSB	↑ with inspiration
"Flow murmurs"	LUSB	Anemia, fever, increased flow of any cause‡
Mid to late systolic		
Mitral valve prolapse	LLSB or apex → axilla	Preceded by click; murmur lengthens with maneuvers that decrease left ventricular volume†
Papillary muscle dysfunction	Apex → axilla	Ischemic heart disease
DIASTOLIC		
Early diastolic		
Aortic regurgitation	RUSB, LUSB	High-pitched, blowing quality; endocarditis, diseases of the aorta, associated aortic valvular stenosis; signs of low peripheral vascular resistance
Pulmonic valve regurgitation	LUSB	Pulmonary hypertension as a causative factor
Mid to late diastolic		
Mitral stenosis, tricuspid stenosis	Apex, LLSB	Low pitched; in rheumatic heart disease, opening snap commonly precedes murmur; can be caused by increased flow across normal valve‡
Atrial myxomas	Apex (L), LLSB (R)	"Tumor plop"
Continuous		
Venous hum	Over jugular or hepatic vein or breast	
Patent ductus arteriosus	LUSB	
Arteriovenous fistula		
Coronary	LUSB	
Pulmonary, bronchial, chest wall	Over fistula	
Ruptured sinus of Valsalva aneurysm	RUSB	Sudden onset

*See also Chapters 69 and 75.
†Left ventricular volume is decreased by standing or during prolonged, forced expiration against a closed glottis (Valsalva maneuver); it is increased by squatting or by elevation of the legs; contractility is increased by adrenergic stimulation or in the beat after an extrasystolic beat.
‡Including a left-to-right shunt through an atrial septal defect for tricuspid or pulmonic flow murmurs, and a ventricular septal defect for pulmonic or mitral flow murmurs.
LLSB = left lower sternal border (fourth intercostal space); LUSB = left upper sternal border (second and third intercostal spaces); RLSB = right lower sternal border (fourth intercostal space); RUSB = right upper sternal border (second and third intercostal spaces).

TABLE 51-8 SENSITIVITY AND SPECIFICITY OF BEDSIDE MANEUVERS IN THE IDENTIFICATION OF SYSTOLIC MURMURS

MANEUVER	RESPONSE	MURMUR	SENSITIVITY (%)	SPECIFICITY (%)
Inspiration	↑	RS	100	88
Expiration	↓	RS	100	88
Valsalva maneuver	↑	HC	65	96
Squat to stand	↑	HC	95	84
Stand to squat	↓	HC	95	85
Leg elevation	↓	HC	85	91
Handgrip	↓	HC	85	75
Handgrip	↑	MR and VSD	68	92
Transient arterial occlusion	↑	MR and VSD	78	100

HC = hypertrophic cardiomyopathy; MR = mitral regurgitation; RS = right sided; VSD = ventricular septal defect.
Modified with permission from Lembo NJ, Dell'Italia IJ, Crawford MH, et al. Bedside diagnosis of systolic murmurs. *N Engl J Med.* 1988;318:1572-1578. Copyright 1988 Massachusetts Medical Society. All rights reserved.

Clubbing (Fig. 51-10), which is loss of the normal concave configuration of the nail as it emerges from the distal phalanx, is seen in patients with pulmonary abnormalities such as lung cancer (Chapter 191) and in patients with cyanotic congenital heart disease (Chapter 69).[4]

Examination of the Skin

Examination of the skin may reveal bronze pigmentation typical of hemochromatosis (Chapter 212); jaundice (see Fig. 146-1) characteristic of severe right-sided heart failure or hemochromatosis; or capillary hemangiomas typical of Osler-Weber-Rendu disease (see Fig. 173-1), which also is associated with pulmonary arteriovenous fistulas and cyanosis. Infectious endocarditis may be associated with Osler nodes (see Fig. 76-2), Janeway lesions, or splinter hemorrhages (Fig. 51-11) (Chapter 76). Xanthomas (Fig. 51-12) are subcutaneous deposits of cholesterol seen on the extensor surfaces of the extremities or on the palms and digital creases; they are found in patients with severe hypercholesterolemia.

Laboratory Studies

All patients with known or suspected cardiac disease should have an ECG and chest radiograph. The ECG (Chapter 54) helps identify rate, rhythm, conduction abnormalities, and possible myocardial ischemia. The chest radiograph (Chapter 56) yields important information on chamber enlargement, pulmonary vasculature, and the great vessels.

Blood testing in patients with known or suspected cardiac disease should be targeted to the conditions in question. In general, a complete blood cell count, thyroid indices, and lipid levels are part of the standard evaluation. Point-of-care biomarker measurements in the emergency department can decrease unnecessary admissions and reduce median length-of-stay. For example, among patients who are being evaluated for an acute MI, an undetectable high-sensitivity troponin level at presentation reduces the probability of acute MI to less than 1%.[5] A protocol in which the ECG and troponin level are repeated in 2 hours is as good as longer observation periods for evaluating patients with acute chest pain and suspected MI.[A1] However, the advent of high-sensitivity troponin assays has also greatly increased the risk for a false-positive diagnosis of MI,[5] especially because of chronic troponin elevations in many cardiac conditions and in elderly patients (Chapter 72).[6]

Echocardiography (Chapter 55) is the most useful test to analyze valvular and ventricular function. By use of Doppler flow methods, stenotic and regurgitant lesions can be quantified. Hand-held ultrasonography performed by generalists can improve the assessment of left ventricular function, cardiomegaly, and pericardial effusion. Transesophageal echocardiography is the preferred method to evaluate possible aortic dissection and to identify clot in the cardiac chambers. Radionuclide studies (Chapter 56) can measure left ventricular function, assess myocardial ischemia, and determine whether ischemic myocardium is viable. CT can detect coronary calcium, which is a risk factor for symptomatic coronary disease (Chapter 56). In the setting

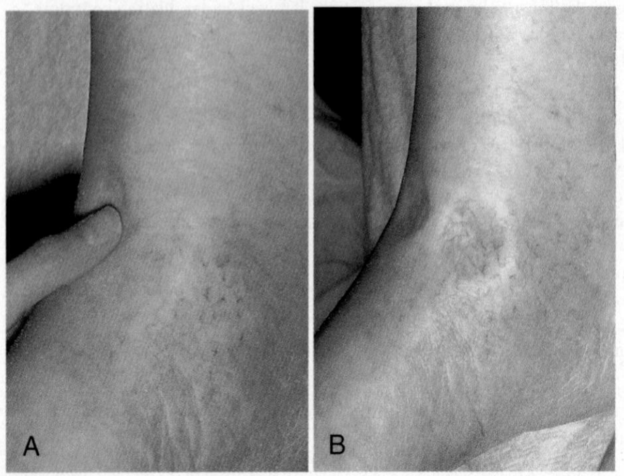

FIGURE 51-7. Pitting edema in a patient with cardiac failure. A depression ("pit") remains in the edema for some minutes after firm fingertip pressure is applied. (From Forbes CD, Jackson WD. *Color Atlas and Text of Clinical Medicine*. 3rd ed. London: Mosby; 2003.)

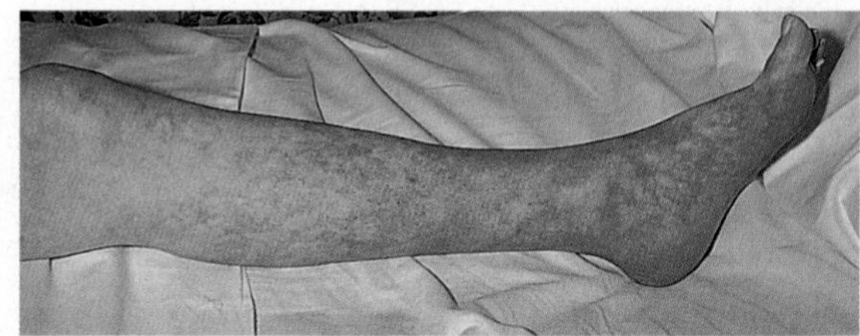

FIGURE 51-9. Arterial embolism causing acute ischemia and cyanosis of the leg. Initial pallor of the leg and foot was followed by cyanosis. (From Forbes CD, Jackson WD. *Color Atlas and Text of Clinical Medicine*. 3rd ed. London: Mosby; 2003.)

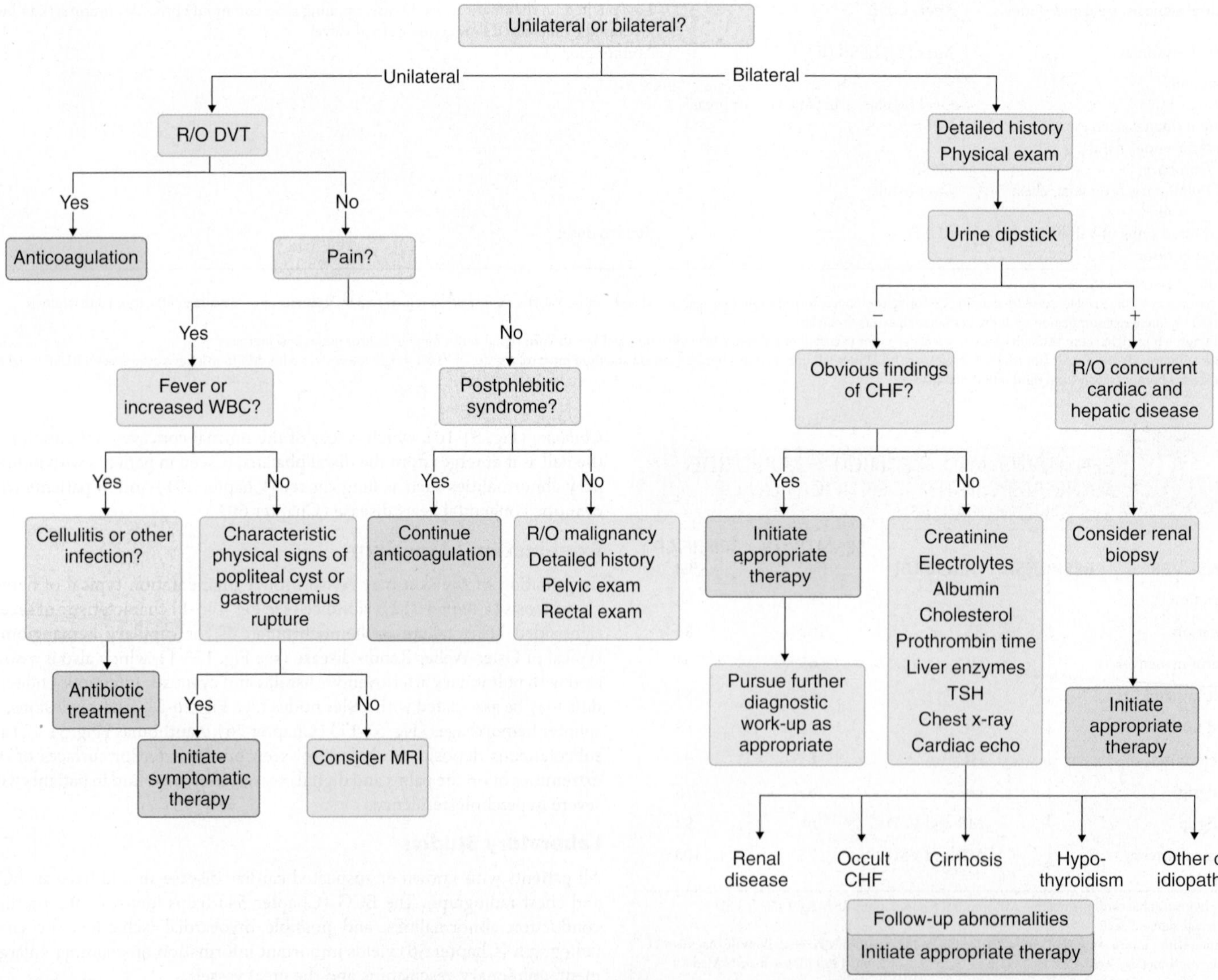

FIGURE 51-8. Diagnostic approach to patients with edema. CHF = congestive heart failure; DVT = deep vein thrombosis; MRI = magnetic resonance imaging; R/O = rule out; TSH = thyroid-stimulating hormone; WBC = white blood cell count. (From Chertow G. Approach to the patient with edema. In: Braunwald E, Goldman L, eds. *Primary Cardiology*. 2nd ed. Philadelphia: WB Saunders; 2003.)

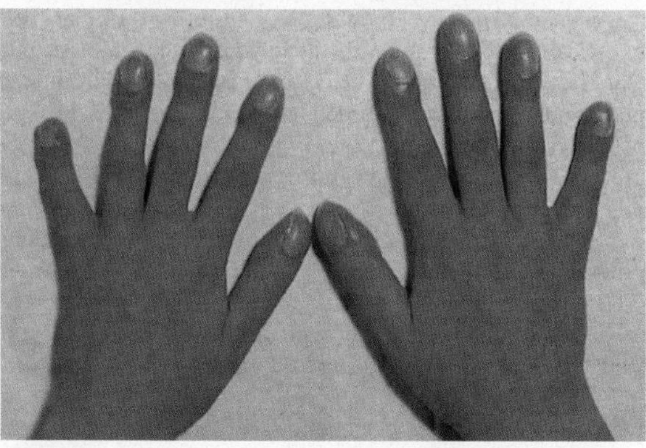

FIGURE 51-10. Severe finger clubbing in a patient with cyanotic congenital heart disease. (From Forbes CD, Jackson WD. *Color Atlas and Text of Clinical Medicine*. 3rd ed. London: Mosby; 2003.)

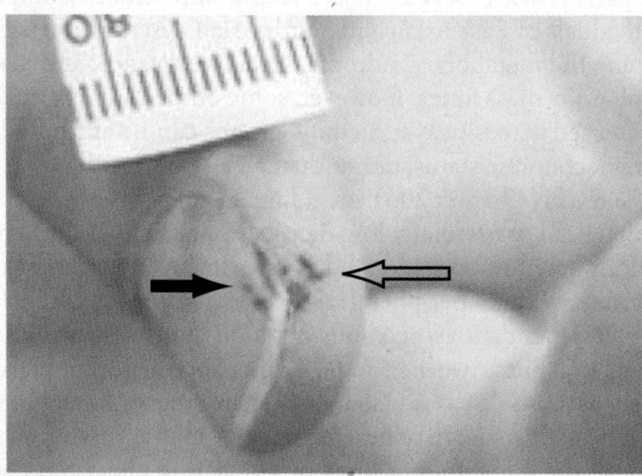

FIGURE 51-11. Splinter hemorrhage (*solid arrow*) and Janeway lesions (*open arrow*). These findings should stimulate a work-up for endocarditis. (Courtesy of Daniel L. Stulberg, MD.)

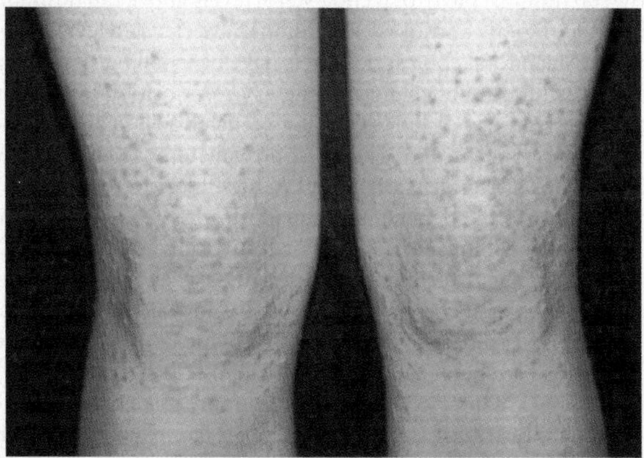

FIGURE 51-12. Eruptive xanthomas of the extensor surfaces of the lower extremities. This patient had marked hypertriglyceridemia. (From Massengale WT, Nesbitt LT Jr. Xanthomas. In: Bolognia JL, Jorizzo JL, Rapini RP, eds. *Dermatology*. Philadelphia: Mosby; 2003:1449.)

of acute chest pain, multislice CT is effective in diagnosing coronary disease.[A2] In a randomized trial of emergency department patients at low to intermediate risk for a possible acute coronary syndrome, coronary CT angiography resulted in a higher rate of discharge from the emergency department (50% vs. 23), a shorter length of stay (median, 18 vs. 24.8 hours), and a higher rate of detection of coronary disease (9% vs. 3.5%) without any change in the rate of serious adverse events.[A3] However, in a subsequent randomized trial of emergency department patients with symptoms suggestive of acute coronary syndromes but without ischemic ECG changes or an initially positive troponin test, incorporating coronary CT angiography into the triage strategy did not decrease overall costs of care.[A4]

Stress testing by exercise or pharmacologic stress is useful to precipitate myocardial ischemia that may be detected by ECG abnormalities, perfusion abnormalities on radionuclide studies, or transient wall motion abnormalities on echocardiography.[7,8] These tests are often crucial in diagnosis of possible myocardial ischemia (Chapter 71) and in establishment of prognosis in patients with known ischemic heart disease. However, they are not recommended for the screening of asymptomatic individuals[9] or prior to participation in sports.[10]

Cardiac catheterization (Chapter 57) can measure precise gradients across stenotic cardiac valves, judge the severity of intracardiac shunts, and determine intracardiac pressures. Coronary angiography provides a definitive diagnosis of coronary disease and is a necessary prelude to coronary revascularization with a percutaneous coronary intervention or coronary artery bypass graft surgery (Chapter 74).

Continuous ambulatory ECG monitoring can help diagnose arrhythmias. A variety of newer technologies allow longer-term monitoring in patients with important but infrequently occurring symptoms (Chapter 62). Formal invasive electrophysiologic testing can be useful in the diagnosis of ventricular or supraventricular wide-complex tachycardia, and it is crucial for guiding a wide array of new invasive electrophysiologic therapies (Chapter 66).

SUMMARY

The history, physical examination, and laboratory evaluation should help the physician establish the cause of any cardiovascular problem; identify and quantify any anatomic abnormalities; determine the physiologic status of the valves, myocardium, and conduction system; determine functional capacity; estimate prognosis; and provide primary or secondary prevention. Key preventive strategies, including diet modification, recognition and treatment of hyperlipidemia, cessation of cigarette smoking, and adequate physical exercise, should be part of the approach to every patient, with or without heart disease.

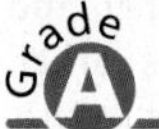

Grade A References

A1. Than M, Aldous S, Lord SJ, et al. A 2-hour diagnostic protocol for possible cardiac chest pain in the emergency department: a randomized clinical trial. *JAMA Intern Med*. 2014;174:51-58.

A2. Goodacre SW, Bradburn M, Cross E, et al. The randomised Assessment of Treatment using Panel Assay of Cardiac Markers (RATPAC) trial: a randomised controlled trial of point-of-care cardiac markers in the emergency department. *Heart*. 2011;97:190-196.

A3. Litt HI, Gatsonis C, Snyder B, et al. CT angiography for safe discharge of patients with possible acute coronary syndromes. *N Engl J Med*. 2012;366:1393-1403.

A4. Hoffmann U, Truong QA, Schoenfeld DA, et al. Coronary CT angiography versus standard evaluation in acute chest pain. *N Engl J Med*. 2012;367:299-308.

GENERAL REFERENCES

For the General References and other additional features, please visit Expert Consult at https://expertconsult.inkling.com.

52

EPIDEMIOLOGY OF CARDIOVASCULAR DISEASE

DONALD M. LLOYD-JONES

Cardiovascular diseases are the leading cause of death, disability, and medical costs in the world, and they are expected to remain so for the foreseeable future. Cardiovascular disease manifests in a number of different ways, including congenital heart and vascular malformations (Chapter 69); coronary heart disease (Chapters 70, 71, 72, 73, and 74); heart failure (Chapter 59); cardiomyopathies (Chapter 60); valvular heart disease (Chapter 75); dysrhythmias (Chapters 62, 63, 64, and 65); pericardial diseases (Chapter 77); aortic (Chapter 78), peripheral (Chapter 79), and cerebrovascular diseases (Chapter 406); systemic hypertension (Chapter 67); vasculitides (Chapter 270); venous thromboembolic disease (Chapter 81); and pulmonary vascular hypertension (Chapter 68). Of these, coronary heart disease, stroke, and heart failure, which share many common underlying risk factors, have by far the largest impact on the population in terms of incidence, prevalence, quality of life, and medical costs.

BURDEN IN THE UNITED STATES

Cardiovascular diseases have been the leading cause of death in the United States in every year of the 20th and 21st century except for 1918, when the influenza epidemic surpassed them. Cardiovascular diseases account for 1 in 3 deaths in America annually, or about 790,000 deaths, including about 400,000 in women and about 390,000 in men.[1] The overall rate of death due to cardiovascular disease in the United States is about 230 per 100,000 persons, with higher rates in men than in women and in blacks than in whites. Because of secular trends over the past 40 to 50 years, coronary heart disease alone may soon fall below all cancers combined, but all cardiovascular diseases combined are expected to remain the leading causes of death in the United States and globally for the foreseeable future.

Cardiovascular diseases also are the leading cause of hospitalizations and medical costs in the United States. Each year, about 5.8 million Americans are hospitalized for cardiovascular disease, more than 1.3 million cases of which are due to coronary heart disease and another 1 million or more due to heart failure. The United States currently spends more than $300 billion annually on direct and indirect costs for cardiovascular diseases, and these total costs are projected roughly to triple to more than $1 trillion annually by 2030.

In the United States, about 15.4 million adults have coronary heart disease, roughly half of whom have had a myocardial infarction. Each year, Americans suffer more than 900,000 new and recurrent myocardial infarctions, with about 380,000 deaths due to coronary heart disease, a large percentage of which are sudden cardiac deaths. There are about 6.8 million stroke survivors in the United States, with 800,000 new or recurrent strokes occurring every year. Strokes are especially prominent in the so-called "stroke belt" in the southeastern United States, where many African Americans live. With aging, the risks for stroke and heart failure tend to increase earlier in women and African Americans than in white men, whose coronary risk increases earlier. At present, more than 5 million Americans suffer from chronic heart failure, with approximately equal numbers of men and women affected. However, the prevalence of heart failure is about twice as high in blacks as in whites.

GLOBAL BURDEN

Cardiovascular diseases, including coronary heart disease and stroke, became the leading cause of death and disability globally in the early 21st century.[2] About 80% of cardiovascular deaths and events now occur in low- and middle-income countries, and the onset of cardiovascular disease tends to be at an earlier age in these countries. For example, about 50% of coronary deaths occur before age 70 years in India, whereas only 25% occur by that age in high-income countries. Unfavorable global trends in eating patterns, high rates of smoking, and increasing burdens of obesity, diabetes, and hypertension are driving the burden of cardiovascular disease.[3] Whereas stroke was the dominant cause of death and disability in East Asian countries for decades owing to high sodium intake and resulting hypertension, recent changes in diet, activity levels, and smoking have made coronary heart disease an equivalent or greater health burden in this area of the world.

RISK FACTORS FOR CARDIOVASCULAR DISEASE

Established Risk Factors

A number of factors have been established for cardiovascular disease based on their strength and consistency of associations, specificity, temporality, and biologic plausibility.[4,5] Furthermore, these established risk factors explain the vast majority of risk for incident myocardial infarction. Longitudinal cohort studies demonstrate that 90% of individuals who suffer a myocardial infarction have at least one established clinical risk factor before their first event, and adverse levels of nine risk factors and behaviors collectively account for 90% or more of the risk for myocardial infarction in men and women, in older and younger individuals, and in all regions of the world. These nine risk factors and behaviors include smoking (Chapter 32), elevated apolipoprotein B–to–apolipoprotein A1 ratio (Chapter 206), hypertension (Chapter 67), diabetes (Chapter 229), abdominal obesity (Chapter 220), psychosocial factors, lower consumption of fruits and vegetables (Chapter 213), alcohol intake (Chapter 33), and physical inactivity (Chapter 16). Many of the established risk factors tend to cluster in a *metabolic syndrome*, which is characterized by abdominal obesity, insulin resistance, hyperglycemia, elevated blood pressure, elevated triglyceride levels, and lower high-density lipoprotein (HDL) cholesterol levels.

Age is the most powerful risk factor for the development of most cardiovascular diseases, especially stroke (Chapter 407), heart failure (Chapters 58 and 59), and atrial fibrillation (Chapter 64). Chronologic age represents a person's aggregate exposure to multiple physiologic and environmental effects on the cardiovascular system. The incidence of cardiovascular disease at least doubles with each additional decade of age in adulthood until the oldest ages, when the heavy burden of competing causes of mortality (Chapter 23) limits further progression.

The impact of a person's *sex* on cardiovascular disease is important. More women than men die of cardiovascular diseases annually. However, women tend to develop risk factors later in life than do men, and women's incidence rates lag men's by approximately 10 years. The precise contributions of sex hormones to these age trends are uncertain, but many women develop worsening risk factor levels, particularly with regard to lipids, blood pressure, weight, and insulin resistance, during and after the menopausal transition (Chapter 240).

Race per se is not thought to be an independent risk factor for cardiovascular disease, and the established causal risk factors have broadly similar effects in all race and ethnic groups. Nevertheless, hypertension tends to be more prevalent in individuals of African ancestry, especially in environments with higher sodium intake, and to have a somewhat stronger association with cardiovascular events, especially heart failure and stroke. Compared with whites, individuals of East Asian and South Asian descent have a greater risk for developing the metabolic syndrome, insulin resistance, and diabetes at a lower overall body mass index. However, some of the cardiovascular risk differences observed across race and ethnic groups can be attributed to differences in socioeconomic status, rather than race or ethnicity.

Blood lipid levels (Chapter 206), including the total serum cholesterol level and its subfractions, particularly low-density lipoprotein (LDL) cholesterol, have significant, continuous, and graded associations with the risk for coronary heart disease and peripheral arterial atherothrombotic disease. By comparison, independent associations of blood lipids with stroke and heart failure events are much weaker, indicating a potentially lesser role in the pathogenesis of these diseases when they occur independently of their relationship to coexisting coronary heart disease. Apolipoprotein B–containing particles make up the subpopulation of circulating cholesterol-containing particles that represent the atherogenic lipoprotein fractions. These particles are considered to be the central actors in the initiation and promotion of atherogenesis on the basis of a substantial body of epidemiologic, clinical, and basic science evidence. Among U.S. adults aged 20 years and older, 43% (or nearly 100 million) have total cholesterol levels above the desirable range of less than 200 mg/dL, and 14% (31 million) have elevated levels of 240 mg/dL or higher. Mean total cholesterol levels have been falling sharply in recent decades, mostly because of changes in dietary composition but also because of more widespread use of lipid-lowering medications. In the 1970s, mean total cholesterol concentrations were approximately 220 mg/dL, whereas currently they are just under 200 mg/dL. These improvements have been a major contributor to the decline in coronary death rates over the same time period. Randomized clinical trials have unequivocally established LDL cholesterol as a causal agent for coronary heart disease, and statins are effective at reducing rates of both coronary heart disease and stroke, significantly and substantially.[A1] By comparison, niacin is of no apparent added value[A2] and other medications are being actively investigated (Chapter 206).

Blood pressure (Chapter 67) has a continuous, graded association with incident coronary heart disease, stroke, and heart failure events. In worldwide studies of nearly 1 million individuals, the risk at every age for all types of cardiovascular disease death doubled with each 20-mm Hg higher systolic blood pressure and each 10-mm Hg higher diastolic blood pressure, beginning at a blood pressure of 115/75 mm Hg.[6] Although the relationship with outcomes is linear, hypertension is typically defined by blood pressures of 140 mm Hg or higher systolic or 90 mm Hg diastolic (Chapter 67). Using this definition, hypertension is the most prevalent modifiable cardiovascular risk factor worldwide. Among people who are normotensive at age 55 years, the remaining lifetime risk for development of hypertension is 90%. Approximately one third of all American adults currently have hypertension, and its prevalence has been increasing owing to the obesity epidemic. Hypertension has stronger relative associations with stroke and heart failure than with coronary heart disease, in part because of its effects on myocardial and cerebrovascular remodeling. In the United States, rates of treatment and control for hypertension have been gradually increasing. The effective treatment of hypertension reduces the risk for stroke, heart failure, and coronary heart disease events.[A3]

Cigarette smoking (Chapter 32) is one of the strongest risk factors for cardiovascular disease events. After adjustment for other risk factors, smoking confers two- to three-fold higher risk for all manifestations of cardiovascular disease, especially coronary heart disease and peripheral arterial disease. Fortunately, consistent public health efforts have reduced the prevalence of smoking in the United States from about 45% in the 1960s to just under 20% currently. The prevalence of smoking remains higher in many European and Asian countries, and its continued increase in some parts of the world drives unfavorable trends in cardiovascular morbidity and mortality. A large body of evidence indicates that environmental exposure to tobacco smoke in nonsmokers ("second-hand" or "passive" smoking) also increases risk for cardiovascular events substantially (Chapter 32) and contributes to the population burden of disease. Substantial data also support the benefits of smoking cessation for reducing the risks for a subsequent coronary event and death.[7]

Overweight and obesity have been increasing in the United States and worldwide. Before 1985, fewer than 10% of Americans were obese, defined as having a body mass index of 30 kg/m^2 or higher. Now, however, about 35% of Americans are obese, and another 35% are overweight (Chapter 220). Major societal changes in the availability of food and in dietary content, coupled with reductions in physical activity, have produced this unprecedented epidemic. Although overweight and obesity themselves tend to be weak independent predictors of cardiovascular events in the short term, they are major drivers of elevated blood pressure, elevated blood glucose levels, and adverse lipid profiles that are themselves major contributors to the incidence of cardiovascular disease.[8]

Blood glucose and its surrogate marker, hemoglobin A1c, have a continuous and graded association with cardiovascular events. People with diabetes (Chapter 229), whether diagnosed or undiagnosed, have two- to three-fold higher adjusted risk for cardiovascular events compared with persons without diabetes, and they also have substantially higher risks for developing chronic renal disease (Chapter 130). Whereas diabetes was relatively uncommon before the 1980s, the obesity epidemic has led to a dramatic increase in the prevalence of type 2 diabetes and of impaired fasting glucose levels, termed *pre-diabetes*. At present in the United States, nearly 20 million people, representing more than 8% of all adults, have diagnosed diabetes, and another 8 million (about 3.5% of adults) have undiagnosed diabetes. Fully 87 million more adults, or about 38% of the adult U.S. population, currently have pre-diabetes. If current trends continue, an estimated 77% of men and 53% of women in the U.S. could have pre-diabetes by 2020. Diabetes affects non-white racial and ethnic groups, such as American Indians, African Americans, South Asians, East Asians, and Latinos, who appear to have greater sensitivity to insulin resistance at lower body mass index, in much greater proportions than whites. Unfortunately, tight control of glucose levels in persons with diabetes has not been associated with significant reductions in risk for macrovascular cardiovascular disease. A4 A5

Adverse diet (Chapter 213) is a major contributor to obesity, diabetes, hypertension, and hyperlipidemia. Healthy eating patterns emphasize a lower caloric intake and focus on fruits and vegetables, healthy fats from nuts and olive oil, lean sources of protein such as fish, whole grains, a reduced sodium intake, and limiting the intake of processed foods, unhealthy fats, and simple sugars. This eating pattern is typical of the "Mediterranean diet," which has been shown to be associated with a lower incidence of cardiovascular disease. A6 By comparison, no vitamin or mineral supplement has been shown conclusively to reduce cardiovascular risk.[9]

Alcohol (Chapter 33) has a complex association with cardiovascular events. Moderate intake of one serving of alcohol per day is associated with a modestly lower risk for cardiovascular disease. At higher levels of intake, however, risks for total mortality, hypertension, stroke, and heart failure tend to increase.

Physical inactivity (Chapter 16) *and a sedentary lifestyle* are also significant risk factors for cardiovascular disease. Individuals who participate in no physical activity are at highest risk for events. The risk is significantly lower for people who participate in even minimal physical activity, and risks decrease further with greater activity levels, particularly to the extent that they contribute to improvement in objective physical fitness. The biology and risks of sedentary time may be more than just the absence of physical activity because sedentary lifestyle, measured best by the hours of time spent in front of a television or computer screen, seems to have an adverse effect independent of time spent doing physical activity.

Family history is clearly an important cardiovascular risk factor, independent of other measurable risk factors. However, ideal levels of cardiovascular health do not appear to be genetically programmed nor inexorably compromised as a consequence of aging. Data indicate that the heritability of ideal cardiovascular health is less than 20%, thereby suggesting strong environmental and behavioral influences on this trait.

Novel Risk Markers

Blood markers of inflammation, thrombosis, and target organ damage also appear to characterize the atherosclerotic process (Chapter 70). Serum biomarkers such as C-reactive protein, fibrinogen, plasminogen activator inhibitor-1, interleukin-6, and lipoprotein-associated phospholipase A_2 have significant associations with incident cardiovascular events that are independent of established risk factors.[10] However, because of their lack of specificity and their relatively weak independent associations with incident disease, none of these markers has yet proved useful for routine screening or for incorporation into risk assessment algorithms in primary or secondary prevention. To date, none has provided meaningful reclassification of risk in individuals after quantitative assessment using traditional established risk factors. Newer biomarkers that indicate the presence of existing target organ damage, such as high-sensitivity troponin or natriuretic peptide levels, hold promise for screening and targeting of prevention efforts in older, asymptomatic individuals (Chapter 23).

Noninvasive cardiac testing and imaging holds the potential for detecting preclinical disease and potentially guiding early intervention. For example, electrocardiographic evidence of left ventricular hypertrophy confers significant excess risk for coronary heart disease over and above the presence of hypertension and other risk factors. High levels of coronary calcification on computed tomography (CT) imaging of the heart (Chapter 56) or greater carotid intima-media thickness measured by B-mode ultrasound of the carotid arteries portends a higher risk for future cardiovascular events. Because these imaging markers detect evidence of the actual underlying diseases of interest (i.e., left ventricular hypertrophy or atherosclerosis), rather than nonspecific risk factors, they are more effective at identifying individuals at high risk for incident clinical events, such as heart failure, stroke, and myocardial infarction. Of the available modalities, CT screening for coronary artery calcification appears to be the best widely available means for detecting individuals at near-term risk. For example, in the Multi-Ethnic Study of Atherosclerosis, asymptomatic individuals with coronary artery calcium scores of more than 100 Agatston units had relative hazards for a coronary event that were 7- to 10-fold higher than in individuals without any coronary calcification, even after adjustment for major established risk factors.[11] Coronary calcium scoring also has been shown to be the most effective and reliable means for reclassifying risk after a quantitative risk assessment using established risk factors, with the ability to identify otherwise low-risk individuals who nonetheless will have a cardiovascular event. Although noninvasive screening for cardiovascular disease holds much promise for the future, its precise role remains uncertain at the present time (Chapter 56).

Assessment of Risk for Cardiovascular Disease

Estimation of Short-Term Risk

Adverse levels of any single risk factor or risk marker are associated with elevated risk for incident cardiovascular events. However, combinations of adverse risk factors are additive and sometimes synergistic for increasing risk. To improve the prediction of cardiovascular events and provide quantitative risk assessment, a number of multivariable risk equations or scores, such as the Framingham equations (E-Tables 52-1 and 52-2), have been developed. The vast majority of risk scores available have focused on predicting 10-year absolute risk, and essentially all include age, sex, smoking status, cholesterol, and blood pressure, with some also including diabetes, family history, body mass index, socioeconomic status, or novel biomarkers. The end points of interest for diverse risk equations have varied widely, from the prediction of cardiovascular death alone to the prediction of fatal and nonfatal major coronary events, major atherosclerotic events (coronary disease and stroke), and a broader range of cardiovascular events (including heart failure, coronary revascularization, angina, or claudication). For example, the 10-year risk for incident atherosclerotic cardiovascular disease can be predicted in 50-year-old men and women according to sex, race, and different levels of risk factors (Fig. 52-1), and the risks are dramatically higher with a greater risk factor burden.

Lifetime Risk Estimation

Despite the widespread use of 10-year risk estimates to guide prevention strategies, this approach has important limitations. For example, one consequence of the substantial weighting of age in 10-year risk equations is that younger men and women, even those with substantial risk factor burden, do not tend to have a high short-term risk. When treatment thresholds are applied to quantitative risk estimates for clinical guidelines, men younger

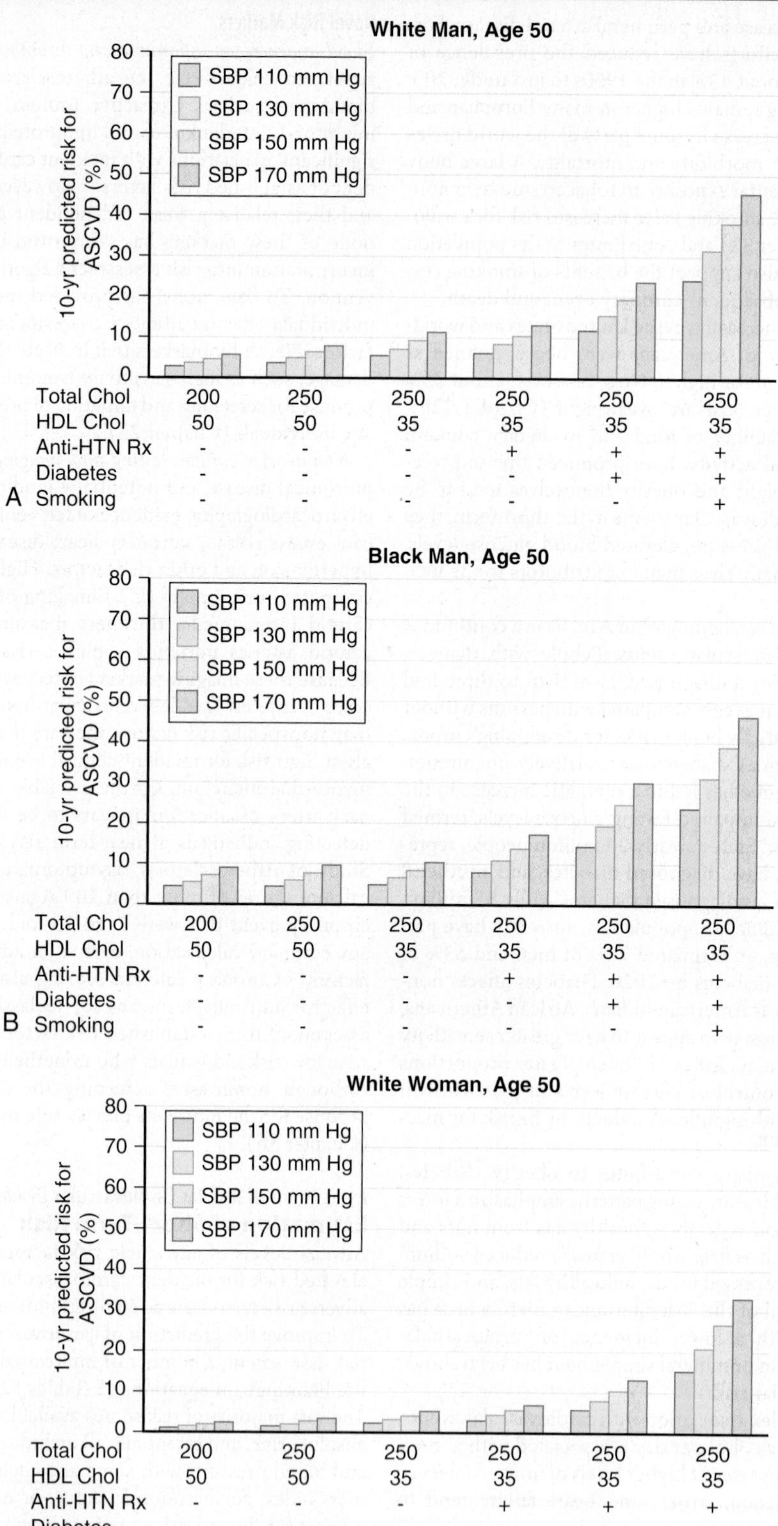

FIGURE 52-1. **Predicted 10-year risks for atherosclerotic cardiovascular disease (ASCVD), including fatal coronary heart disease, nonfatal myocardial infarction, and fatal or nonfatal stroke, as a function of selected risk factor levels in a 50-year-old black man (A), white man (B), white woman (C), or black woman (D). Chol = cholesterol; HDL = high-density lipoprotein; HTN = hypertension; Rx = medication. (Predicted risks are derived from the Pooled Cohort Equations from the 2013 American College of Cardiology/American Heart Association Guideline on the Assessment of Cardiovascular Risk. Goff DC Jr, Lloyd-Jones DM, Bennett G, et al. 2013 ACC/AHA guideline on the assessment of cardiovascular risk: a report of the American College of Cardiology/American Heart Association Task Force on Practice Guidelines.** ***J Am Coll Cardiol.*** **2014;63(25 Pt B):2935-2959.)**

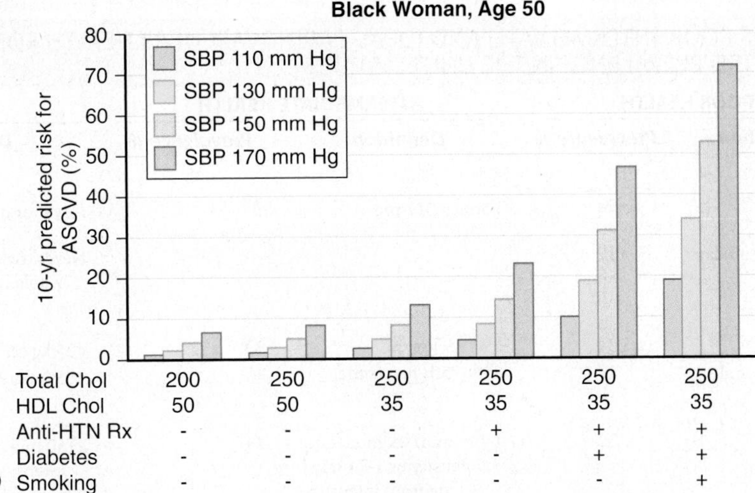

FIGURE 52-1, cont'd.

than 50 years and women younger than 60 years will infrequently exceed those thresholds. Therefore, recent guidelines have considered longer risk horizons, such as 30 years or the remaining lifespan.[12] The established risk factors are all associated with lifetime risks for cardiovascular disease, but the nature of the relationships sometimes differs from short-term associations because of competing risks. For example, smoking is a strong risk factor for near-term cardiovascular events but is a weaker predictor of lifetime risk for cardiovascular events because of the simultaneous and substantial risk for cancer death, which limits the lifetime risk for cardiovascular disease among smokers. As a result, lifetime risk estimates may enhance communication for individual patients, but how they should be used in decision making regarding the institution of preventive drug therapy is less certain.

Prevention of Cardiovascular Disease

Because patients with prevalent symptomatic cardiovascular disease are at the highest risk, preventive interventions such as lifestyle modifications and drug therapy to reduce risk are most effective and cost-effective when used as therapy for secondary prevention of recurrent events. Examples of intensive lifestyle modification and of proven therapies include aspirin,[A7] statins,[13][A1][A2] and antihypertensive medications,[14] as well as other medications and implantable devices that may prevent complications such as heart failure or fatal ventricular dysrhythmias.

For primary prevention, asymptomatic individuals may be at risk because of a heritable family history of premature cardiovascular disease, one or more markedly elevated risk factors, or multiple modestly elevated risk factors. The current primary prevention paradigm is to match the intensity of prevention efforts to the absolute risk of the patient. Appropriate lifestyle interventions (e.g., smoking cessation, weight loss, dietary modification) are recommended for all individuals, whereas drug therapy is recommended only for individuals in whom the absolute benefits can be expected to outweigh any potential adverse drug effects and to be cost-effective in doing so. Treatment that restores optimal risk factor levels does not always imply that the treated individual will now have the very low incidence rates observed in people who have maintained optimal risk factor levels throughout young adulthood and into middle age. As a result, another concept is *primordial prevention*, which is the prevention of the development of risk factors in the first place. Primordial prevention requires a focus on health behaviors that may prevent the development of dyslipidemia, diabetes, and hypertension, as well as population-level strategies that attempt to create an environment conducive to favorable health behaviors.

Cardiovascular Health: A New Paradigm

After decades of declining mortality rates from cardiovascular diseases and stroke in the United States, the new goal is to promote cardiovascular health in individuals and the population, monitor it over time, and improve it by concerted action. Central to the concept of cardiovascular health is the observation that optimal levels of seven health behaviors and health factors (Table 52-1) are associated with ideal cardiovascular health. Although about 40% of American adults believe they are in ideal cardiovascular health, fewer than 1% have all seven metrics at ideal levels, principally because of a poor-quality diet.[15] Persons who maintain high levels of cardiovascular health from young age to middle age have extremely favorable outcomes from middle to older ages, including a markedly increased longevity; a better quality of life; a substantially lower incidence of fatal and nonfatal cardiovascular disease events; a lower incidence of other chronic diseases of aging, including cancer and venous thromboembolism; a lower burden of subclinical atherosclerosis (e.g., carotid intima-media thickness, coronary artery calcification); higher levels of cognitive function in middle and older ages; and reduced medical care costs. These outcomes are observed in all segments of the population, as well as across all ages and both sexes.

People who pursue healthy lifestyles from young adulthood to middle age are far more likely to preserve ideal cardiovascular health than those who pursue none: 60% of the former group compared with only 3% of the latter group maintained ideal cardiovascular health factors into middle age. Cardiovascular health promotion thus represents a major paradigm shift and opportunity in public health efforts.

Future of Cardiovascular Epidemiology

Decades of success in observational epidemiology research continue to provide novel insights into trends and risk markers for cardiovascular disease, as well as the influence of in utero and early life exposures on the life course of cardiovascular diseases. New techniques to characterize environmental and behavioral exposures, physiology, health status, and precursors of disease include functional genomics, proteomics, metabolomics, and high-resolution imaging. With these tools, epidemiologic research has advanced to improve the characterization of the life course of cardiovascular diseases in living individuals and populations. For example, studies of the genotypes of individuals at the extremes of the distribution of LDL cholesterol levels have led to the discovery of polymorphisms in a novel gene termed proprotein convertase subtilisin/kexin type 9 (*PCSK9*). Although such polymorphisms are uncommon, specific missense and nonsense mutations in white and African American men and women are associated with substantially lower lifelong levels of LDL cholesterol. In turn, individuals with these polymorphisms have a 47 to 88% lower incidence of coronary heart disease over 15 years of follow-up through middle age compared with individuals without them. *PCSK9* has since become a novel potential therapeutic target.

A second emerging focus in cardiovascular epidemiologic research has been the study of effects of interventions in populations through public health and social policies. For example, studies have demonstrated marked reductions in hospitalizations for acute myocardial infarction occurring rapidly after the initiation of indoor smoking bans in diverse settings. Modeling studies have synthesized data from numerous epidemiologic sources to show that approximately 50 to 75% of the reductions in coronary death rates in Western countries may be attributable to population changes in risk factor levels, despite being offset by a recent worsening in obesity and diabetes prevalence, with the remainder likely attributable to advances in medical and surgical therapies.

TABLE 52-1 DEFINITIONS OF POOR, INTERMEDIATE, AND IDEAL CARDIOVASCULAR HEALTH FOR EACH OF SEVEN METRICS, AND UNADJUSTED PREVALENCE IN THE UNITED STATES

	POOR HEALTH		INTERMEDIATE HEALTH		IDEAL HEALTH	
Goal/Metric	***Definition***	***Prevalence %***	***Definition***	***Prevalence %***	***Definition***	***Prevalence %***
CURRENT SMOKING						
Adults >20 yr of age	Yes	24	Former ≤12 mo	3	Never or quit >12 mo	73 (51 never; 22 former >12 mo)
Children 12-19 yr of age	Tried prior 30 days	17			Never tried; never smoked whole cigarette	83
BODY MASS INDEX						
Adults >20 yr of age	≥30 kg/m²	34	25-29.9 km/m²	33	<25 kg/m²	33
Children 2-19 yr of age	>95th percentile	17	85th-95th percentile	15	<85th percentile	69
PHYSICAL ACTIVITY						
Adults >20 yr of age	None	32	1-149 min/wk moderate intensity or 1-74 min/wk vigorous intensity or 1-149 min/wk moderate + vigorous	24	≥150 min/wk moderate intensity or ≥ min/wk vigorous intensity or ≥150 min/wk moderate + vigorous	44
Children 2-19 yr of age	None	10	>0 and <60 min of moderate or vigorous activity every day	46	≥60 min of moderate of vigorous activity every day	44
HEALTHY DIET SCORE						
Adults >20 yr of age	0-1 components	76	2-3 components	24	4-5 components	<0.5
Children 5-19 yr of age	0-1 components	91	2-3 components	9	4-5 components	<0.5
TOTAL CHOLESTEROL						
Adults >20 yr of age	≥240 mg/dL	16	200-239 mg/dL or treated to goal	38 (27; 12 treated to goal)	<200 mg/dL	45
Children 6-19 yr of age	≥200 mg/dL	9	170-199 mg/dL	25	<170 mg/dL	67
BLOOD PRESSURE						
Adults >20 yr of age	SBP ≥140 or DBP ≥90 mm Hg	17	SBP 120-139 or DBP 80-89 mm Hg or treated to goal	41 (28; 13 treated to goal)	<120/<80 mm Hg	42
Children 8-19 yr of age	>95th percentile	5	90th-95th percentile or SBP ≥120 or DBP ≥80 mm Hg	13	<90th percentile	82
FASTING PLASMA GLUCOSE						
Adults >20 yr of age	≥126 mg/dL	8	100-125 mg/dL or treated to goal	34 (32; 3 treated to goal)	<100 mg/dL	58
Children 12-19 yr of age	≥126 mg/dL	0.5	100-125 mg/dL	18	<100 mg/dL	81

DBP = diastolic blood pressure; SBP = systolic blood pressure.
From National Health and Nutrition Examination Survey (NHANES) data and the American Heart Association. Reproduced from Lloyd-Jones DM, Hong Y, Labarthe D, et al. Defining and setting national goals for cardiovascular health promotion and disease reduction: the American Heart Association's strategic Impact Goal through 2020 and beyond. *Circulation.* 2010;121:586-613.

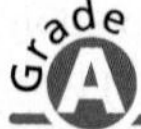

Grade A References

A1. Baigent C, Blackwell L, Emberson J, et al. Efficacy and safety of more intensive lowering of LDL cholesterol: a meta-analysis of data from 170,000 participants in 26 randomised trials. *Lancet.* 2010;376:1670-1681.

A2. Landray MJ, Haynes R, Hopewell JC, et al. Effects of extended-release niacin with laropiprant in high-risk patients. *N Engl J Med.* 2014;371:203-212.

A3. Thomopoulos C, Parati G, Zanchetti A. Effects of blood pressure lowering on outcome incidence in hypertension. 1. Overview, meta-analyses, and meta-regression analyses of randomized trials. *J Hypertens.* 2014;32:2285-2295.

A4. Fullerton B, Jeitler K, Seitz M, et al. Intensive glucose control versus conventional glucose control for type 1 diabetes mellitus. *Cochrane Database Syst Rev.* 2014;2:CD009122.

A5. Hemmingsen B, Lund SS, Gluud C, et al. Targeting intensive glycaemic control versus targeting conventional glycaemic control for type 2 diabetes mellitus. *Cochrane Database Syst Rev.* 2013; 11:CD008143.

A6. Estruch R, Ros E, Salas-Salvado J, et al. Primary prevention of cardiovascular disease with a Mediterranean diet. *N Engl J Med.* 2013;368:1279-1290.

A7. Sutcliffe P, Connock M, Gurung T, et al. Aspirin for prophylactic use in the primary prevention of cardiovascular disease and cancer: a systematic review and overview of reviews. *Health Technol Assess.* 2013;17:1-253.

GENERAL REFERENCES

For the General References and other additional features, please visit Expert Consult at https://expertconsult.inkling.com.

53

CARDIAC FUNCTION AND CIRCULATORY CONTROL

ANDREW R. MARKS

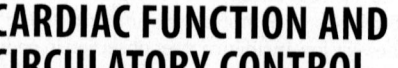

The heart has the daunting task of pumping sufficient amounts of blood to meet both its own metabolic demands and those of the other organs. Uniquely among all the organs, the heart's failure to perform its task for even a few minutes causes death. The heart continuously fulfills this physiologic role with a variety of electrical, contractile, and structural functions that control the flow of blood to the organs.

STRUCTURE OF THE HEART

Cardiac Development

In humans, the formation of a linear heart tube from the primary cardiac crescent occurs between days 21 and 23 of gestation. Looping of the heart

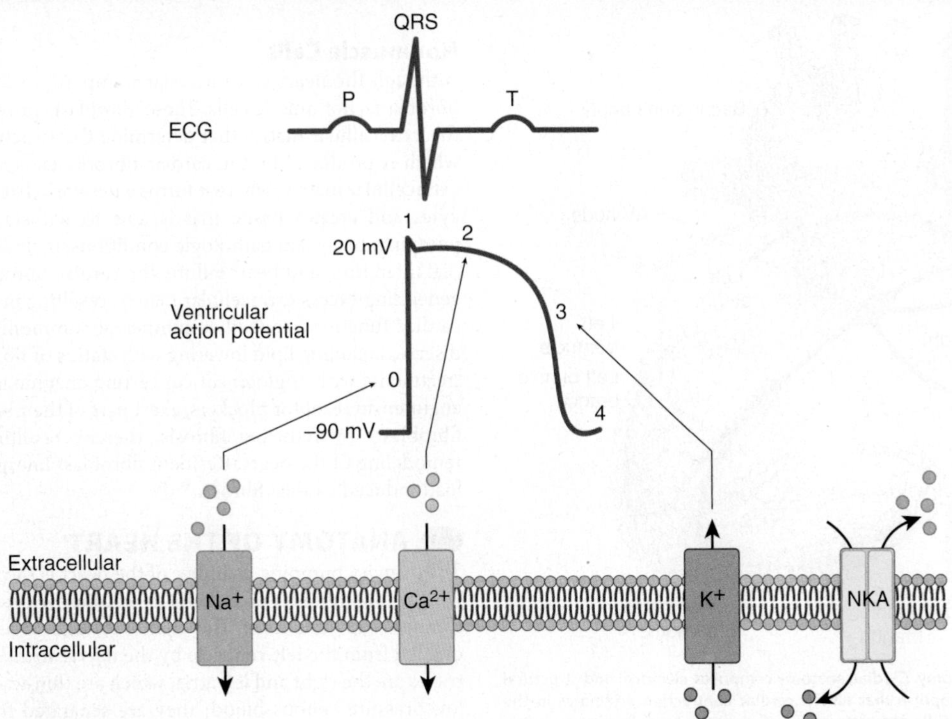

FIGURE 53-1. **Cardiac action potential and ion channels. Myocardial contraction begins when sodium channels open and positively charged sodium ions flow into the cell and cause membrane depolarization (phase 0). During phases 1, 2, and 3, calcium ions flow into the cell through L-type calcium channels, while potassium flows out of the cell through voltage-gated potassium channels. These three phases correspond to the myocardial contraction, which corresponds to the QRS complex on the surface electrocardiogram (ECG). The sodium-potassium adenosine triphosphatase (NKA) helps return the system to its resting state.**

tube and trabecular formation of the ventricle occur at 26 days of gestation (E-Fig. 53-1). At 6 weeks, the embryonic interventricular communication closes, followed by thickening and remodeling of the ventricular walls in the first trimester. By the end of week 7, heart development is essentially finished, although the heart continues to enlarge throughout gestation.[1,2]

Electrical Cells

The heart is a muscular pump controlled by regular electrical discharges from specialized muscle cells in the conduction system (Chapter 61). The molecular basis for the electrical activity of the heart is the activation of specific ion-conducting channels (Fig. 53-1). Coordinated activation and inactivation of cardiac ion channels regulate the membrane potential of the cardiac cells, thereby resulting in a rapid sequence of depolarization followed by repolarization. This electrical activity, which is manifested on the body surface as the electrocardiogram (ECG), is known as the action potential, and it is responsible for activating the contraction of the cardiac muscle. At a typical heart rate of 70 beats per minute, the heart beats about 100,000 times per day, or 37 million beats a year, corresponding to 3 billion beats during a lifespan of 80 years. Failure to propagate the signal throughout the heart (e.g., heart block) or abnormal rhythms (arrhythmias) that are either too slow (bradycardia) or too fast (tachycardia) can result in death (Chapter 62). Studies indicate that cardiac arrhythmias may be triggered by leak of calcium inside the cardiomyocytes, thereby suggesting a possible novel therapeutic target for a new generation of antiarrhythmic agents.

Ion Channels

Sodium, potassium, and calcium channels determine the electrical activity of the heart by opening and closing in a highly choreographed pattern that determines the action potential of the heart. The electrical regulation of the heart, which is reflected in the relative concentrations of ions inside and outside the heart muscle cells, determines the five phases of the action potential. The action potential is initiated when the opening of sodium channels results in a rapid influx of sodium (phase 0) down its concentration gradient (~145 mmol outside the heart muscle cell, ~10 mmol inside). After a brief early repolarization due to activation of potassium channels (phase 1), the rapid sodium influx depolarizes the cell, thereby activating calcium channels that allow calcium influx (phase 2) down its concentration gradient (~3 mmol outside, ~100 nmol inside). This calcium influx triggers excitation-contraction coupling that results in pumping by the heart. Potassium channels then open and cause repolarization (phase 3) as potassium fluxes out of the cell down its concentration gradient (~4 mmol outside, ~135 mmol inside). The membrane potential returns to the resting level of about −90 mV (phase 4).

Conduction System

Specialized pacemaker cells in the sinoatrial node (Fig. 53-2) have slightly higher (less negative) resting potentials and gradually depolarize during phase 5 owing to the activity of the potassium and calcium channels and the hyperpolarization-activated cyclic nucleotide–gated channels that are responsible for a small inward (depolarizing) current. In the normal heart, pacemaker cells are the first cells to depolarize, and they trigger the subsequent depolarization of the cells in specialized conducting fibers that propagate the electrical signal throughout the heart muscle in a highly regular and integrated fashion. Electrical activation (depolarization) spreading through the atria to the atrioventricular (AV) node is reflected as the P wave on the ECG (Chapter 54). The slowing of conduction in the AV node accounts for the PR interval on the ECG. After passing through the AV node, the depolarizing signal enters the bundle of His, where conduction is rapid. The bundle of His divides into the right and left bundle branches, which conduct the depolarizing signals into the ventricles and account for the QRS complex on the ECG. Repolarization is represented by the ST segment and the T and U waves of the ECG.

Contractile Cells

Heart muscle is composed of millions of individual cells known as cardiomyocytes, which contain an elaborate machinery required for coordinated contraction that pumps blood. Each cardiomyocyte is connected to its neighbors through specialized junctions that enable them to work as a single contractile unit.

The cardiomyocytes are filled with specialized contractile proteins arranged in highly regulated units, called sarcomeres, that give the muscles characteristic patterns known as striations (E-Fig. 53-2). Hence, like skeletal muscle, cardiac muscle is termed striated, as opposed to smooth muscles that form the vasculature and other organs such as the bladder, uterus, and stomach. Cardiomyocytes are also loaded with mitochondria that provide the energy (adenosine triphosphate [ATP]) required to fuel the heart's lifelong contractions (systole) and relaxations (diastole).

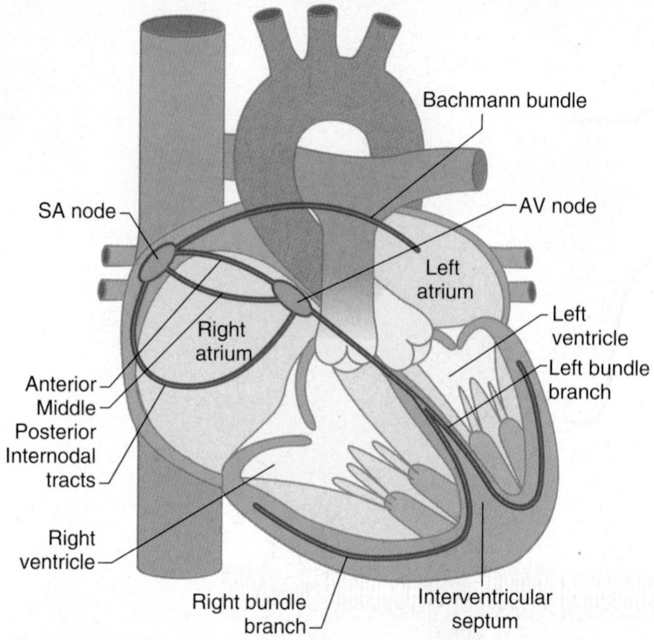

FIGURE 53-2. Cardiac anatomy. Cardiac anatomy comprises electrical and structural components. The electrical impulse that directs cardiac contraction originates in the sinoatrial (SA) node and is rapidly conducted through the atria by specialized conduction tracts. The impulses merge at the atrioventricular (AV) node, where, after a brief pause, they are rapidly conducted into the ventricles through the bundle of His, which is composed of specialized Purkinje cells. Blood moves from the atria into the ventricles through the tricuspid and mitral valves respectively, during diastole. During systole, blood from the ventricles is pumped into the pulmonary artery and aorta through the pulmonic and aortic valves, respectively.

Ultrastructure

The basic unit of the contractile system is the sarcomere, which is defined anatomically as the distance between two Z lines that anchor thin filaments composed of actin, tropomyosin, and troponin. Thin filaments slide past thick filaments (composed of myosin and titin) in a calcium-dependent manner to shorten the sarcomere length. The contractile proteins are surrounded by a calcium-filled membrane called the sarcoplasmic reticulum. The sarcoplasmic reticulum forms specialized associations with the transverse tubules, which are invaginations of the plasma membrane and contain voltage-gated calcium channels. When the muscle is activated by depolarization of its membrane, this electrical signal travels deep into the muscle through the transverse tubules. Inside the muscle, the electrical depolarizing signal activates the voltage-gated channels, which open to allow a small amount of calcium to enter the muscle cells. This influx of calcium in turn activates the type 2 ryanodine receptor (RyR2), calcium-release channels on the sarcoplasmic reticulum. The RyR channels open and release enough calcium from the sarcoplasmic reticulum to raise the calcium concentration in the myoplasm about 10-fold. As a result, calcium binds to troponin C in the thin filaments and causes a conformational change that enables cross-bridging between actin and myosin, thereby leading to sliding of the filaments, shortening of the sarcomere, and muscle contraction. Hydrolysis of ATP provides the energy required for the generation of force by the actin-myosin interaction. The conversion of electrical energy (depolarization of the cell membrane) to mechanical energy is known as excitation-contraction coupling. Relaxation of the heart muscle occurs when calcium is pumped back into the sarcoplasmic reticulum through the sarcoendoplasmic reticulum ATPase.

Signals That Regulate Contraction

Contractile force can be enhanced during stress by activation of the β-adrenergic pathway, which increases both the amount of calcium released and the rate of calcium uptake in the sarcoplasmic reticulum (E-Fig. 53-3). β-Agonists (e.g., epinephrine or norepinephrine) bind to β-adrenergic receptors to activate adenylyl cyclase, which generates cyclic adenosine monophosphate and activates protein kinase A. Protein kinase A phosphorylates phospholamban, the voltage-gated calcium channel, the ryanodine receptor, and sarcomeric regulatory proteins, thereby resulting in increased release of calcium from the sarcoplasmic reticulum and enhanced contractility of the heart.

Nonmuscle Cells

Although the heart is a muscular pump, 60 to 70% of its cells are cardiac fibroblasts, not muscle cells. These fibroblasts provide critical components of the extracellular matrix that determine the structure of the heart. Collagen, which is produced by the cardiac fibroblasts, is a major component of the extracellular matrix, where it forms a network that surrounds the cardiomyocytes and creates tissue that is able to withstand the stress of constant pumping. In certain pathologic conditions, including hypertension, myocardial infarction, and heart failure, the cardiac fibroblasts respond to stress by generating excess extracellular matrix, resulting in fibrosis, which can impair cardiac function.[3] Indeed, a number of commonly used therapies for heart disease, including lipid lowering with statins or fibrates and antihypertensive treatments with angiotensin-converting enzyme inhibitors, β-blockers, and angiotensin receptor blockers, exert part of their beneficial effects on cardiac fibroblasts by reducing fibrosis, thereby resulting in favorable "reverse" remodeling of the heart. Resident fibroblast lineages mediate pressure overload-induced cardiac fibrosis.[4]

ANATOMY OF THE HEART

The primary pumping chamber of the heart is the thick-walled left ventricle, which is composed of billions of cardiomyocytes connected end to end through gap junctions. The right ventricle is a thinner-walled chamber, divided from the left ventricle by the *interventricular septum*. Above the ventricles are the right and left atria, which are thin-walled chambers that receive low-pressure venous blood; they are separated from the ventricles by the *tricuspid valve* on the right side and the *mitral valve* on the left side. These valves are attached to *papillary muscles* that emerge from the ventricular walls through *chordae tendineae*. The pressure gradient between the ventricles and the atria opens the AV valves. The papillary muscles help establish the positions of the valve leaflets and prevent regurgitant flow during contraction. The *aortic and pulmonary valves* separate the left and right ventricles from their arterial connections and enable blood flow out of the ventricles.[5]

Coronary Blood Flow

The coronary arteries receive blood from the aorta, directly above the aortic valve, and travel through the epicardium that surrounds the heart to supply blood to the heart muscle (see Fig. 57-4). The diastolic blood pressure in the ascending aorta just above the aortic valve determines most of the flow of blood into the normal (nonstenosed) coronary arteries while the heart is relaxed. During systole, coronary flow is determined by the left ventricular intracavitary pressure, which equals the pressure within the inner myocardial wall, where coronary arteries are compressed during systole. Coronary blood flows to the epicardium during both systole and diastole but flows to the endocardium predominantly during diastole.

Metabolic Regulation of the Cardiovascular System

Cardiac muscle requires constant coronary perfusion to supply oxygen and other metabolites. Increased energy consumption due to enhanced contractility necessitated by increased pressures or higher heart rates (e.g., during exercise) can be met only by increased coronary blood flow. Signals that augment coronary blood flow (by up to six-fold) include nitric oxide, adenosine, bradykinins, prostaglandins, and carbon dioxide. The breakdown of ATP is the source of adenosine, whereas nitric oxide is produced by the action of nitric oxide synthases that metabolize the amino acid L-arginine. Autoregulatory mechanisms, including constriction in response to increased luminal pressures and dilation in response to reduced pressure, also play a role in determining coronary artery blood flow. Other metabolic factors that cause vasoconstriction include endothelin peptides, serotonin, 5-hydroxytryptamine, thromboxane, angiotensin II, and β_1-adrenergic stimulation.

Sympathetic and parasympathetic pathways of the autonomic nervous system and the renin-angiotensin system exert potent regulatory effects on cardiovascular function. The sympathetic nervous system plays the key role in the response to stress (e.g., the fight-or-flight response) by increasing heart rate and myocardial contractility and decreasing vascular tone. Regulation of cardiovascular function by the sympathetic nervous system is mediated by norepinephrine that is released at the nerve endings and by epinephrine from the adrenal gland. β-Adrenergic signaling is mediated by epinephrine, which increases the heart rate and vasodilates the central arterial bed, thereby resulting in reduced afterload, which in turn helps augment cardiac output.

The sinoatrial and AV nodes are regulated by parasympathetic innervation that slows the pacemaker's rate of firing and conduction through the AV node by the release of acetylcholine. Vasoconstriction of the venous system is mediated by the sympathetic nervous system, which limits fluid and blood loss after trauma.

The renin-angiotensin system also regulates blood pressure, peripheral vasoconstriction, and contractility in coordination with the sympathetic nervous system. Both the sympathetic nervous system and the renin-angiotensin system are chronically activated in heart failure (Chapter 58), in which the resulting maladaptive remodeling of the cardiovascular system promotes the progression of heart failure. Decreased perfusion to the kidney, decreased delivery of sodium to the macula densa, or increased sympathetic activity results in the release of the hormone renin from the macula densa cells within the juxtaglomerular apparatus of the kidney. Renin results in the production of angiotensin II, a potent constrictor of peripheral and coronary arteries. In turn, angiotensin II causes the release of the sodium-retaining hormone aldosterone from the adrenal gland (Chapter 227). Together, these signals result in sodium retention and increased arterial blood pressure.

PHYSIOLOGY OF THE HEART AND CIRCULATORY CONTROL

Cardiac Energetics

The major immediate source of energy in the heart is the oxidation of fatty acids and glucose. When oxygen supply is limited, glucose metabolism is favored because it generates more ATP per oxygen consumed. The heart has virtually no ability to conduct anaerobic metabolism (i.e., glycolysis) and therefore is dependent on oxygen for its function. For example, heart function deteriorates immediately under conditions of hypoxia, ischemia, and carbon monoxide poisoning.

Basal metabolism, total mechanical work performed by the heart, contractility, and heart rate determine the oxygen and energy consumption of the heart. During excitation-contraction coupling, two key steps require energy consumption (ATP hydrolysis): release of the myosin head–actin interaction and reuptake of calcium into the sarcoplasmic reticulum.

The mechanical work of the heart is determined by the total *pressure-volume area*, which is related to the number of actin-myosin cross-bridges formed during the contraction. It is the sum of the external work performed by the heart in pumping blood from the ventricle to the aorta (represented by the area inside the pressure-volume loop) plus energy stored in the myocardium at the end of contraction. Enhanced contractility requires increased oxygen consumption because an increased amount of calcium released from the sarcoplasmic reticulum requires increased ATP and oxygen consumption to pump the released calcium back into the sarcoplasmic reticulum through the sarcoplasmic reticular ATPase. On the basis of these principles, increasing the heart rate requires increased oxygen consumption. If the heart rate increases from 70 to 140 beats per minute during exercise or stress, oxygen consumption increases almost two-fold above the basal value.

Contractility and Relaxation

The Cardiac Cycle

In resting humans, the heart beats approximately once per second. With each beat, the heart cycles through a series of four hemodynamic events represented by changes in pressures and volumes (Fig. 53-3) as well as electrical activity as represented by the ECG. When the heart muscle is relaxed at end diastole, the ventricular pressure is at its resting level *(end-diastolic pressure)* and the ventricular volumes are at their maximal value *(end-diastolic volume)*. Aortic pressure declines as the blood ejected into the aorta during the previous ventricular contraction flows to the peripheral circulation. Atrial contraction provides a final boost to ventricular volume immediately before ventricular systole. Ventricular contraction increases the pressure in the ventricle; when this pressure exceeds the pressure in the atrium, the mitral valve closes. However, because ventricular pressure remains less than aortic pressure, the aortic valve remains closed, and no blood enters or leaves the ventricle during this first phase of the cardiac cycle, the *isovolumic contraction* phase. During systole, ventricular pressure eventually exceeds aortic pressure, at which time the aortic valve opens, blood is ejected into the aorta, and ventricular volume decreases during the *ejection* phase of the cycle. At the end of systole when contraction is maximum, ejection ends, and the ventricular volumes are at their lowest *(end-systolic volume)*. The volume of the ejected blood, which is termed the stroke volume (SV), is defined as the difference between the end-diastolic and end-systolic volumes. The ejection fraction

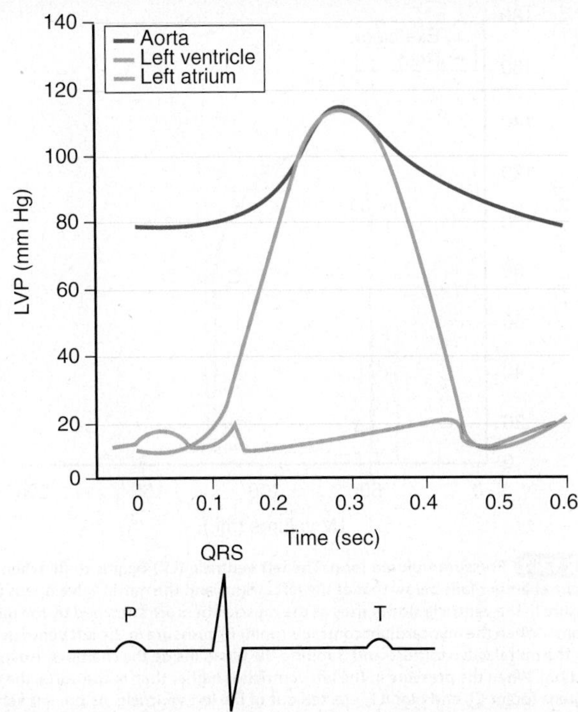

FIGURE 53-3. **Wiggers diagram. Changes in aortic, left ventricular, and left atrial pressures represented graphically as a function of time, with the corresponding electrocardiogram signal for each. LVP = left ventricular pressure.**

(EF), defined as the percentage of end-diastolic volume (EDV) ejected during a contraction (EF = 100 × SV/EDV), is an index of heart function. The next phase in the cycle occurs when the heart muscle relaxes, ventricular pressures are less than the aorta pressure, and the aortic valve closes. During this *isovolumic relaxation* phase, ventricular volumes remain constant because, once again, both the mitral and aortic valves are closed. When ventricular pressures fall below atrial pressures, the mitral and tricuspid valves open, and blood flows from the atria into the ventricles during the *filling* phase.

These four phases of the cardiac cycle can be represented by a *pressure-volume diagram* (Fig. 53-4), which plots the instantaneous ventricular pressure versus volume to calculate the *pressure-volume loop*. Similar effects occur on the left and right sides of the heart, but with higher pressures on the left side (Table 53-1).

Pressure-Volume Relationships

The volume of a ventricular chamber correlates with length of its muscles and sarcomeres. In the left ventricle, with its circular cross section, Laplace's law defines the relationship among pressure in the chamber (P), muscle tension (T, force/unit cross-sectional area of the muscle), chamber wall thickness (h), and internal radius of the chamber (R): $P \approx 2 \cdot T \cdot h/R$. Both calcium and the length of the heart muscle determine force (Fig. 53-5). Each muscle is composed of a linear array of sarcomere bundles. Maximal force is achieved at a sarcomere length of about 2.2 to 2.3 mm, which results in the optimal overlap of thick and thin filaments. When the sarcomere length is less than 2.0 mm, the ends of the thin filaments contact each other, thereby resulting in a reduction in force. Conversely, when sarcomeres are stretched beyond 2.3 mm, force decreases owing to reduced overlap between myosin heads and actin.

Force-length relationships, which are determined by measuring the force developed at different muscle lengths while preventing the muscle from shortening (isometric contractions), characterize the systolic and diastolic contractile properties of cardiac muscle. With increasing muscle length, end-systolic force increases to a greater degree than does end-diastolic force. The difference in force at end diastole versus end systole increases as muscle length increases as a result of the greater developed force of the stretched muscle. This relationship of force to length is referred to as the Frank-Starling law of the heart.

Work of the Heart

Cardiovascular performance is reflected in the arterial blood pressure and cardiac output (mean arterial blood flow), which in turn are dependent on four factors: preload, afterload, ventricular contractility, and heart rate.

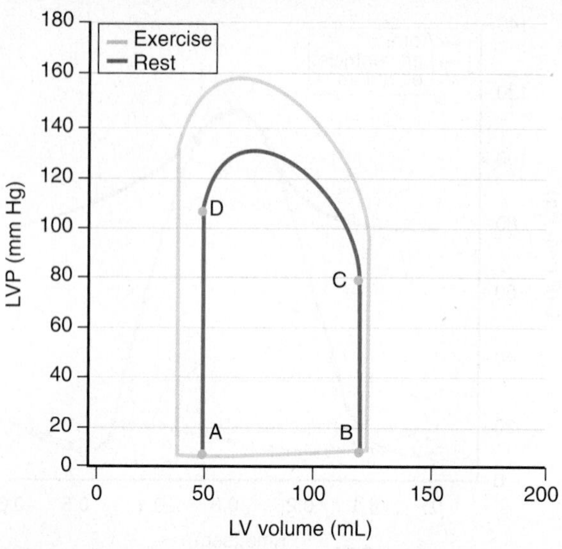

FIGURE 53-4. **Pressure-volume loop. The left ventricle (LV) begins to fill when pressure in the chamber falls below that of the left atrium, and the mitral valve opens (point A). Pressure in the ventricle slowly rises as the muscle fibers are stretched by the increasing volume. When the myocardium contracts (point B), pressure in the left ventricle rises, causing the mitral valve to close and trapping the blood inside the chamber (isovolumic contraction). When the pressure in the left ventricle is higher than in the aorta, the aortic valve opens (point C), and blood is ejected out of the left ventricle. As the left ventricle stops contracting, pressure in the aorta becomes higher than that in the left ventricle, and the aortic valve closes (point D). During this period of isovolumic relaxation, the ventricle rapidly relaxes until it starts filling again. During exercise, the release of norepinephrine from sympathetic nerve terminals leads to enhanced myocardial contractility. As a result, the left ventricle generates higher pressures and ejects a greater volume of blood during each beat. LVP = left ventricular pressure.**

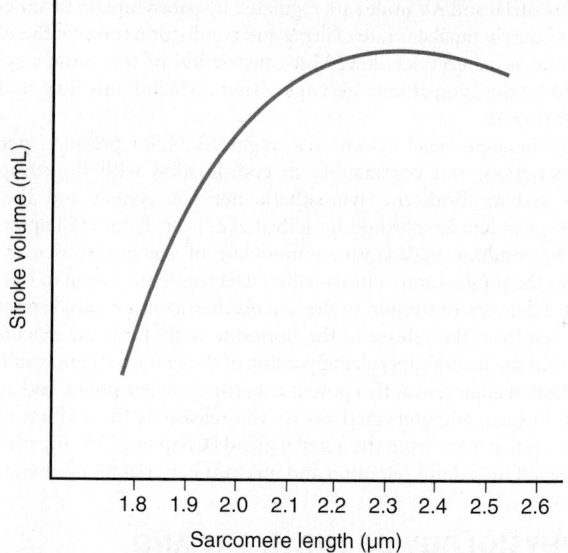

FIGURE 53-5. **Starling law. Cardiac output, represented as stroke volume (end-systolic volume minus end-diastolic volume), as a function of initial sarcomere stretch. The greater the initial stretch on the fibers during diastole, referred to as preload, the more force is generated during systole.**

TABLE 53-1 RANGE OF NORMAL RESTING HEMODYNAMIC VALUES

PRESSURE
Central venous (mean): 0-5 mm Hg
Right atrial (mean): 0-5 mm Hg
Right ventricular (systolic/diastolic): 20-30/0-5 mm Hg
Pulmonary artery (systolic/diastolic): 20-30/8-12 mm Hg
Left atrial (mean): 8-12 mm Hg
Left ventricular (systolic/diastolic): 100-150/8-12 mm Hg
Aortic (systolic/diastolic): 100-150/70-90 mm Hg
VOLUME-RELATED MEASURES
Right ventricular end-diastolic volume: 70-100 mL
Left ventricular end-diastolic volume: 70-100 mL
Stroke volume: 40-70 mL
Cardiac index: 2.5-4 L/min/m^2
Ejection fraction: 55-70%
ARTERIAL RESISTANCE
Systemic vascular resistance: 10-20 mm Hg · min/L
Pulmonary vascular resistance: 0.5-1.5 mm Hg · min/L

Preload, which refers to the degree to which sarcomeres are stretched just before systole, is defined as the end-diastolic pressure or volume. The Frank-Starling law of the heart dictates that ventricular pressure and output vary with preload, so a decrease in preload decreases end-diastolic volume and pressure, peak pressure, and stroke volume. Conversely, increased preload increases ventricular pressure and output, subject to the limits to which preload pressures can be increased. Left ventricular end-diastolic pressures of 20 to 25 mm Hg and greater cause exudation of fluid into the alveoli and pulmonary edema (Chapter 58).

Afterload refers to the stress that the ventricle must overcome to eject blood. Peak arterial pressure reflects the peak stress imposed on cardiomyocytes according to Laplace's law (described previously as $P \approx 2 \cdot T \cdot h/R$). As long as there is no left ventricular outflow obstruction, arterial pressure reflects myocyte afterload, as does *total peripheral resistance* (TPR), which corresponds to the tone of the resistance vessels. TPR is the ratio between the mean pressure decrease across the arterial system (mean arterial pressure [MAP] minus mean central venous pressure [CVP]) and cardiac output (CO): TPR = (MAP − CVP)/CO. When TPR is increased, the pressure-volume relationship shifts such that peak pressure is increased, whereas stroke volume and ejection fraction are decreased.

Contractility of cardiac muscle *(myocardial contractility)* or a ventricle *(ventricular contractility)* is the intrinsic ability to generate force independent of preload or afterload. When contractility is increased, the pressure-volume relationship shifts so that pressure, stroke volume, and ejection fraction are increased at constant preload volume and arterial resistance.

Cardiac output is measured in liters per minute and is equal to the amount of blood ejected at each heartbeat (stroke volume in liters per beat) multiplied by the number of beats per minute. As a result, *heart rate* is a powerful determinant of cardiac performance. Cardiac output and mean arterial pressure can be related to preload, afterload, contractility, and heart rate through the Frank-Starling curves, which plot end-diastolic pressure versus cardiac output or mean arterial pressure, to yield an overall picture of left ventricular function.

CARDIOVASCULAR RESPONSES TO STRESSORS

Exercise

Exercise requires dramatic increases in cardiac function combined with remodeling of the peripheral circulation to meet the enhanced metabolic demands of critical organs and to redirect blood flow to those organs. Indeed, the oxygen consumption during exercise can increase as much as 18-fold. About one third of the requirement for increased oxygen consumption is met by improved extraction of oxygen from the blood in the muscles (reducing venous saturation from about 75% to about 25%) and the remainder by increasing cardiac output as much as six-fold. Increased cardiac function is achieved largely through sympathetic stimulation and reduction in vagal tone, which combine to increase the heart rate, contractility, ejection fraction, filling rates, and systolic blood pressure and to decrease aortic impedance. In young healthy individuals, heart rate can increase from a baseline of 60 to 70 beats per minute at rest to as much as 170 to 200 beats per minute with exercise. To increase rather than to decrease cardiac output at these high heart rates, which can limit ventricular filling and stroke volume, contractility must also increase, through a phenomenon known as the positive force frequency relationship or Bowditch phenomenon. Along with increased cardiac contractility, arterial vasodilation in the aorta and other major arteries reduces the resistance to cardiac outflow. Both enhanced cardiac contractility and arterial vasodilation are triggered by the same sympathetic nervous system signals. With increased cardiac outflow, venous return also must increase so that preload can be maintained as well as possible to enhance cardiac function by the Frank-Starling mechanism. In response to the stress of repeated exercise (e.g., in trained athletes), the heart may undergo physiologic hypertrophy, which should be distinguished from the pathologic hypertrophy that is triggered by hypertension, myocardial infarction, and chronic activation of neurohormonal pathways (e.g., the renin-angiotensin system) (E-Fig 53-4).

Heart Failure

Heart failure can be defined as the inability of the heart to provide sufficient blood flow to meet the metabolic demands of the organs (Chapter 58). Heart failure can be due to systolic dysfunction with volume overload, most often as the consequence of ischemic heart disease (myocardial infarction) or as the end-stage consequence of hypertension.[6] Systolic heart failure is characterized by increases in the size of the various cardiac chambers (rightward shift of the end-diastolic pressure-volume relationship). In another form of heart failure, known as *diastolic heart failure,* the heart is not necessarily increased in size, and systolic function is preserved. Emerging data implicate altered regulation of calcium inside the cardiomyocyte in the pathogenesis of both the cardiac and skeletal muscle weakness that is seen in heart failure.

Aging

Prolongation of contraction and relaxation times, which are common abnormalities in older individuals, may be related to cardiac hypertrophy as a consequence of the high prevalence of hypertension with advancing age (Chapter 67). A progressive "stiffening" of the large arteries with advancing age increases resistance, although the mechanism underlying this change is not understood. The heart rate and contractile responses to sympathetic signals are reduced and lead to a diminished ability to respond to conditions of acute overload, such as increased blood pressure or an acute myocardial infarction.

Cardiac Regeneration

Some animals, such as zebrafish, can regenerate substantial portions of their hearts after injury, sometimes by recruiting atrial myocytes to replace damaged ventricular myocytes.[7] In mammals, however, cardiomyocytes stop proliferating right after birth. Any subsequent enlargement of the heart in response to stress (e.g., hypertension) or loss of myocardium (e.g., myocardial infarction) is limited to hypertrophy of existing cardiomyocytes. Studies, however, have shown that micro-RNAs (miRNAs) can activate cardiomyocyte proliferation and repair by enabling the terminally differentiated cardiomyocytes to re-enter the cell cycle and proliferate.[8] These miRNAs are short noncoding RNAs that downregulate target mRNAs by binding to partially complementary sequences and reducing the expression of the encoded proteins.[9] In mice, miRNAs can induce cardiac regeneration and prevent loss of heart function after myocardial infarction, thereby raising the possibility for a better understanding and potential treatment of cardiac diseases.

GENERAL REFERENCES

For the General References and other additional features, please visit Expert Consult at https://expertconsult.inkling.com.

54 ELECTROCARDIOGRAPHY

LEONARD GANZ

Electrocardiography, which has changed surprisingly little since initially introduced by Einthoven in the early 1900s, allows simultaneous recording of myocardial activation from several vantage points on the body's surface, thereby permitting analysis of electrical activation in different myocardial regions. Surface electrocardiography may be supplemented with intracardiac recordings, which are particularly helpful in the diagnosis and management of cardiac arrhythmias (Chapter 62).

NORMAL FUNCTION AND ELECTROCARDIOGRAM

Normal Cardiac Activation

Electrical activation of the heart depends on the spread of a depolarizing wave front from pacemaker cells through cardiac muscle as well as through specialized conducting tissues (Fig. 54-1). Under normal circumstances, cells in the sinoatrial nodal complex in the high lateral epicardial right atrium spontaneously depolarize at the highest rate and therefore constitute the dominant cardiac pacemaker (Chapter 61). This electrical wave front spreads throughout the right and left atria; specialized conducting tracts called Bachmann bundle speed the depolarizing wave front to the left atrium. Electrical atrial activation triggers atrial muscle contraction, which propels blood through the tricuspid and mitral valves into the right and left ventricles. Normally, the atrioventricular (AV) node, where conduction delay is physiologic, serves as the only electrical connection linking the atria and ventricles; the AV valve rings are insulated. The depolarizing wave front exits the AV node into the bundle of His, a specialized conducting tissue capable of rapid conduction. The bundle of His bifurcates into right and left bundle branches; the left bundle branch divides into the left anterior and left posterior fascicles. The bundle branches and their more distal ramifications of specialized conducting tissue are called the Purkinje system. From these specialized conducting tissues, the depolarizing wave front enters into and then moves through ventricular muscle. As in the atria, ventricular electrical activation begets muscle contraction, which pumps blood through the semilunar valves into the pulmonary and systemic circulations. After electrical activation, or depolarization, a period of electrical recovery, or repolarization, is necessary before repeated activation.

At the cellular level, a complex orchestration of ion channels opening and closing determines the membrane potential throughout this process. The flow of ions into and out of the myocardial cells inscribes an action potential that reflects depolarization and repolarization as well as the spontaneous depolarization of pacemaker cells (Chapter 61).

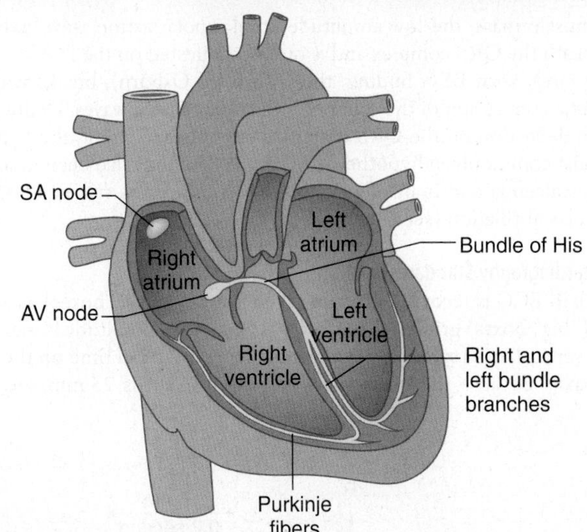

FIGURE 54-1. Cardiac conduction system. The normal conducting system consists of pacemaker cells in the sinoatrial (SA) nodal complex, specialized intra-atrial conducting tracts (including Bachmann bundle), the atrioventricular (AV) node, the His-Purkinje system, and working atrial and ventricular myocardium.

Electrocardiographic Waves

Labeled alphabetically, beginning with the P wave, the basic waves of the electrocardiogram (ECG) correspond to these electrical events (Fig. 54-2). The P wave represents atrial muscle depolarization; in severe hyperkalemia, atrial electrical activation may be unaccompanied by atrial muscle activation, and no P wave is inscribed. The QRS complex represents ventricular muscle depolarization; the disparity between ventricular and atrial muscle mass typically yields a QRS complex much larger in voltage amplitude than the P wave. Recorded from multiple vantage points, the QRS complex harbors tremendous information about the structure and function of ventricular tissue. Under normal circumstances, the PR interval, which is the segment from the onset of the P wave to the onset of the QRS complex, represents the delay between atrial and ventricular depolarization. The ST segment and T wave (and occasionally the U wave) reflect ventricular repolarization, a process of electrical recovery that must take place before the ventricle can be depolarized again. The J (junction) point denotes the end of the QRS complex and beginning of the ST segment. Atrial muscle also requires repolarization before the next depolarizing wave front. Because ventricular mass far exceeds atrial muscle mass, the low-amplitude atrial repolarization wave is buried underneath the QRS complex and is rarely manifested on the ECG.

One rarely seen ECG finding, the J wave (of Osborn), breaks with the alphabetic convention of the other electrocardiographic waves. Defined as a positive deflection on the QRS downstroke or at the J point, the J wave is seen most commonly in hypothermia (Fig. 54-3). It has also been described in hypercalcemia and brain injury and may increase the risk of idiopathic ventricular fibrillation (see later).

Electrocardiography Standards

A standard ECG is recorded on paper with 1-mm ("small" boxes) as well as 5-mm ("big" boxes) gridlines (see Fig. 54-2). Voltage amplitude is measured on the vertical axis (typically 10 mm equaling 1 mV) and time on the horizontal axis. Because the usual ECG recording speed is 25 mm/sec, each 1-mm gridline (small box) represents 0.04 second (40 msec), and each 5-mm gridline (big box) equals 0.2 second (200 msec). These standard calibrations can be modified in unusual circumstances, but such modifications are typically printed on the ECG.

A standard ECG is recorded during a 10-second period, although a rhythm or monitor strip can be recorded for substantially longer if necessary. Multiple leads are typically recorded simultaneously from the top to the bottom of the page. The usual groupings of leads include I, II, and III; aVR, aVL, and aVF; V_1, V_2, and V_3; and V_4, V_5, and V_6 (see later). Each group of leads is recorded for 2.5 seconds. A single lead (or multilead) rhythm strip is recorded below for the entire 10 seconds. Thus, as the ECG is scanned from left to right, one sees 10 seconds of cardiac activity, with each complex recorded simultaneously in multiple leads.

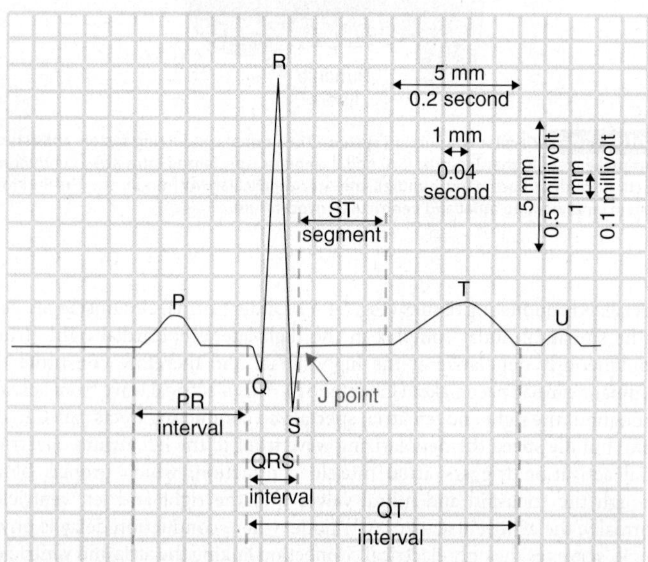

FIGURE 54-2. Inscription of a normal electrocardiogram (ECG). Sinoatrial nodal depolarization is not visible on the surface ECG; the P wave corresponds to atrial muscle depolarization. The PR interval denotes conduction through the atrial muscle, atrioventricular node, and His-Purkinje system. The QRS complex reflects ventricular muscle depolarization. The ST segment, T wave, and U wave (if present) represent ventricular repolarization. The J point lies at the junction of the end of the QRS complex and beginning of the ST segment. The QT interval is measured from the onset of the QRS to the end of the T wave. Note the gridlines. On the horizontal axis, each 1-mm line ("small" box) denotes 0.04 second (40 msec); a "big" box denotes 0.2 second (200 msec). On the vertical axis, 1 mm (small box) corresponds to 0.1 mV; 10 mm (two big boxes) therefore denotes 1 mV.

Normal Intervals

Each of the various ECG waves and intervals has normal ranges, defined from large numbers of electrocardiographic recordings in (presumably) healthy subjects (Table 54-1; see Fig. 54-2).

The RR interval (or PP interval), which is the measurement from R wave to R wave (or P wave to P wave), allows calculation of the heart rate. Because there are 60,000 msec in a minute, the heart rate (HR) in beats per minute can be easily calculated from the RR or PP interval in milliseconds:

$$HR = \frac{60{,}000}{RR}$$

Although the normal resting heart rate has traditionally been defined as being 60 to 100 beats per minute, a range of 50 to 90 at rest may actually be more reflective of normal physiology. When the heart rate is grossly irregular, as in atrial fibrillation (Chapter 64), the RR interval can be averaged over a number of cardiac cycles to estimate the heart rate. Because a standard ECG records 10 seconds in time, the heart rate (beats per minute) will equal the number of QRS complexes recorded on a standard ECG multiplied by 6. Alternatively, in a regular rhythm, the heart rate can be quickly estimated by

TABLE 54-1 NORMAL ELECTROCARDIOGRAPHIC INTERVALS

Heart rate	50-100 beats per minute
P wave duration	< 0.12 sec (120 msec)
PR interval	0.09-0.20 sec (90-200 msec)
QRS duration	0.075-0.11 sec (75-110 msec)
QTc	males: 0.39-0.45 sec (390-450 msec); females: 0.39-0.46 sec (390-460 msec)
QRS axis	−30 to +90 degrees

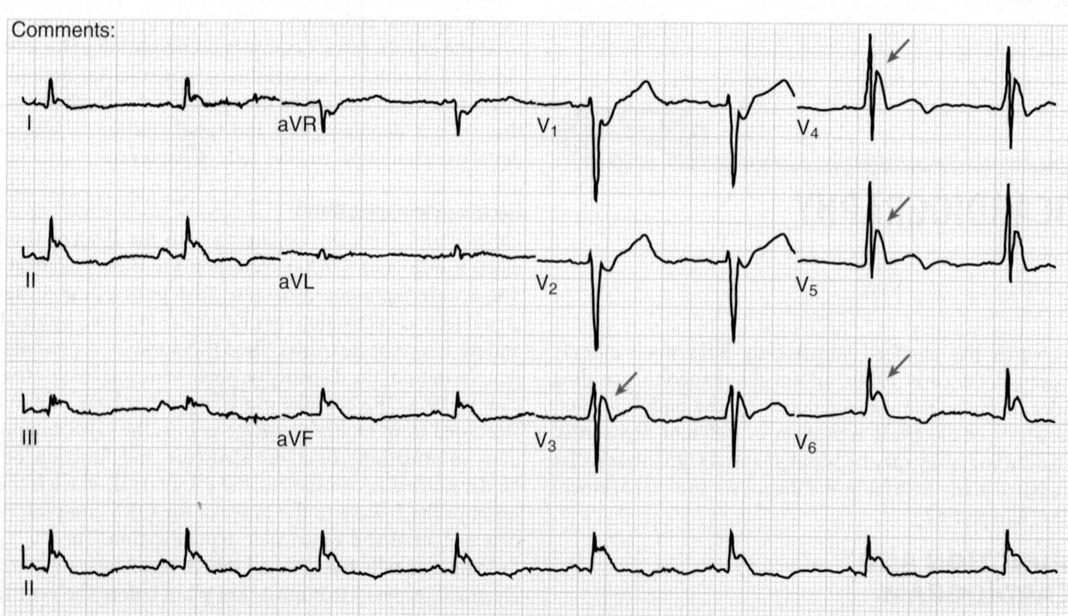

FIGURE 54-3. J wave (of Osborn). This ECG was recorded in a 40-year-old diabetic woman with profound hypothermia (26.6° C), diabetic ketoacidosis, and hypokalemia. Note the massive J waves in leads V_3 to V_6 (*arrows*) and smaller J waves in leads I, II, III, and aVF. Other notable findings include sinus bradycardia and QT prolongation.

counting the number of big boxes between consecutive QRS complexes or P waves (i.e., 2 large boxes = 150 beats per minute, 3 large boxes = 100 beats per minute, 4 large boxes = 75 beats per minute, 5 large boxes = 60 beats per minute, and so on).

P Wave Duration

The P wave duration, from the beginning to the end of a P wave, is typically less than 0.12 second (120 msec, three small boxes) in length. A broader P wave reflects an intra-atrial or interatrial conduction delay, or both. Abnormalities in P wave amplitude, morphology, and axis may reflect atrial enlargement.

PR Interval

The PR interval, measured from the onset of the P wave to the onset of the QRS complex, normally lasts between 0.09 and 0.2 second (90 to 200 msec). One-to-one AV conduction with a PR interval longer than 0.2 second has traditionally been called *first-degree AV block*, but *delayed AV conduction* may be a more appropriate term. Conduction through the atrial tissue, the AV node, and the His-Purkinje system contributes to the PR interval. When the PR interval is prolonged, delay is usually present in the AV node, although other sites of delay are possible. In the Framingham Heart Study, PR interval prolongation was associated with an increased risk of atrial fibrillation, a higher likelihood of later needing a pacemaker, and a higher overall mortality. A short PR interval may reflect ventricular preexcitation (Wolff-Parkinson-White syndrome), a junctional rhythm, or enhanced AV nodal conduction.

QRS Complex

The QRS complex, which reflects ventricular muscle electrical activation, carries important information in patients with coronary artery disease, cardiomyopathy, metabolic abnormalities, and other conditions. Capital letters (Q, R, S) denote large-amplitude deflections (≥5 mm or 0.5 mV), whereas lowercase letters (q, r, s) signify low-amplitude deflections (<5 mm or 0.5 mV). Q, q, S, and s waves are negative excursions from the isoelectric baseline, whereas R and r waves are positive deflections. Q and q waves are initial negative deflections, and S and s waves are negative deflections that follow a positive deflection (R or r wave); a QS complex is an entirely negative deflection. Q waves may reflect prior myocardial infarction (Chapter 73). An R′ or r′ wave refers to a second positive deflection after an S (or s) wave. The duration of the QRS complex reflects the time required for ventricular depolarization. Ventricular activation usually requires at least 0.075 second (75 msec, nearly two small boxes). There is some debate about the upper limit of the normal range for QRS duration; a consensus document specified 0.11 second (110 msec, nearly three small boxes). If the QRS duration is prolonged, an intraventricular or interventricular conduction delay (or both) is present. Particular patterns of interventricular conduction delay are termed bundle branch block (see later).

QT Interval

The QT interval, which reflects ventricular repolarization, is measured from the onset of the QRS complex to the end of the T wave. The QT interval is generally measured in leads II, V_5, and V_6 (see later) and reported as the longest interval among the three, averaged over three to five cycles. If the QT interval cannot be accurately measured in these leads, other leads may be used. The QT interval must be corrected to allow comparison of this interval at differing heart rates. Bazett's formula defines a corrected QT interval (QTc):

$$QTc = \frac{QT}{\sqrt{RR}}$$

Bazett's formula works reasonably well at heart rates in the normal range but overcorrects at high rates and undercorrects at low rates. Although more complex regression formulas have been developed to correct the QT interval at different heart rates, none has achieved widespread clinical use. Irregular rhythms (notably atrial fibrillation) complicate calculation of the QTc. Some investigators recommend measuring at least three QT intervals to get an average and then using an RR interval averaged over 10 cycles in Bazett's formula. The Fridericia formula,

$$QTc = \frac{QT}{\sqrt[3]{RR}}$$

may actually be more accurate than Bazett's formula in atrial fibrillation.[1]

The presence of a U wave complicates measurement of the QT (and therefore QTc) interval because it is not always clear where the T wave ends and whether the U wave should be included in a QTU interval. If the isoelectric baseline is reached between the T and U waves, the U wave is not generally included in the QT interval. If the T wave "merges" into the U wave without reaching the isoelectric baseline, the U wave is included in the QT (or QTU) interval. The QTc in a given patient may vary somewhat during the course of the day and tends to be slightly longer in young and middle-aged women than in men. The upper limit of a normal QTc is somewhat debatable, but a cutoff of 0.45 second (450 msec) in men and 0.46 second (460 msec) in women is generally used. The QT interval is sensitive to drug effects as well as to electrolyte and metabolic derangements. Patients with widened QRS complexes frequently have prolonged QT and QTc intervals. In these patients, the JT interval (from J point to the end of T wave) may be a more accurate index of repolarization, but normal standards have not been established.

Patients with a prolonged QTc, whether congenital or acquired, may be at risk for torsades de pointes ventricular tachycardia (Chapter 65). A short QTc interval (<390 msec) is unusual, and the rare patient with the short QT syndrome is at risk for malignant ventricular arrhythmias. Both short and longer QTc intervals are associated with a higher risk for development of atrial fibrillation, even in the absence of underlying structural heart disease.[2]

Electrocardiographic Leads

Recording a single ECG lead allows calculation of the heart rate and, frequently, accurate diagnosis of the heart rhythm. When the ECG is recorded from multiple skin leads simultaneously, the direction (or vector) of activation as the electrical wave front moves through the heart can be inferred. Although a number of different lead systems are possible (and some are actually used in research settings), standard electrocardiography uses 12 leads from 12 vantage points, recorded with 10 electrodes, six on the chest wall and four on the limbs. In reality, only three limb leads are actually used to generate recordings; the right leg lead serves as an electrical ground. The limb leads, called the frontal plane leads, generate bipolar and augmented unipolar lead recordings. The chest or precordial electrodes record unipolar recordings. Bipolar leads record the potential difference between two skin electrodes. In unipolar recordings, the lead of interest, the exploring electrode, is compared with a reference electrode. By convention, a positive deflection is recorded if the electrical wave front is moving toward the positive electrode in a bipolar pair or toward the exploring electrode in a unipolar lead.

The bipolar limb leads measure potential differences between electrodes on pairs of limb electrodes and closely resemble Einthoven original string galvanometer recordings. Lead I compares the right arm (negative) and left arm (positive); lead II, the right arm (negative) and left leg (positive); and lead III, the left arm (negative) and left leg (positive) (E-Fig. 54-1). Because the direction of both atrial and ventricular depolarization is away from the right arm and toward the left arm, a positive P wave and QRS complex are generally recorded in lead I. Similarly, the P wave and QRS complexes are positive in leads II and III in normal sinus rhythm because atrial and ventricular activation proceeds in a craniocaudal direction.

Leads aVR, aVL, and aVF are augmented unipolar leads in which the potential in each limb is compared with a reference electrode. For lead aVR, the potential of the right arm is compared with a reference composed of the left arm and left leg electrodes. Lead aVL compares the left arm potential with a reference combining the right arm and left leg; aVF compares the left leg with a right and left arm reference. Because atrial and ventricular activation normally moves from right to left and in a craniocaudal direction, the P wave and QRS complex are negative in lead aVR but positive in lead aVF. In lead aVL, P waves and QRS complexes are generally upright, although an rS complex may be recorded, particularly in young patients.

The precordial electrodes are positioned at specific points on the chest wall (E-Fig. 54-2A). These unipolar leads compare electrical potential between the chest electrode and a reference electrode called the Wilson central terminal. The Wilson central terminal combines the right arm, left arm, and left leg potentials through 5000-Ω resistors. The six precordial leads define atrial and ventricular activation with respect to a somewhat transverse plane through the chest wall (E-Fig. 54-2B). In this plane, atrial activation moves from right to left. Initial ventricular activation involving the septum is directed from left to right; left ventricular depolarization, which dominates right ventricular depolarization because of the differential in myocardial mass, then moves apically and laterally. In lead V_1, to the right of the sternum, the P wave is biphasic (reflecting right and then left atrial activation). Initial ventricular activation of the septum inscribes an r wave, whereas subsequent activation away from lead V_1 records a dominant S wave. In lead V_6, the P wave is positive, and initial ventricular septal depolarization inscribes a tiny "septal" q wave (usually ≤0.02 second). Subsequent ventricular depolarization records a dominant R wave.

Right-sided chest leads should be recorded when right ventricular abnormalities are suspected. RV_3, the mirror image of lead V_3, is routinely recorded in pediatric patients because of the possibility of congenital heart disease. In adults, ST elevation in lead RV_3 is specific for acute right ventricular infarction in those being evaluated for an acute inferior wall myocardial infarction.

Axis

An axis of electrical activation can be defined in the frontal plane axis by combining the bipolar and augmented unipolar limb leads (E-Fig. 54-3A). By convention, the axis parallel to lead I, toward the left, is called 0 degrees. A frontal plane axis between −30 and +90 degrees is normal, whereas other axes are abnormal (Fig. 54-4) in adults. Right axis deviation beyond +90 degrees is often a normal variant in children and adolescents. The frontal plane axis can be estimated by identifying the limb lead in which the QRS complex is most nearly isoelectric (similar positive and negative deflections); the axis is perpendicular to this lead (E-Fig. 54-3B). Because two lines pointing 180 degrees apart can be drawn perpendicular to any given line, examination of the other limb leads defines the direction in which the axis points. If the QRS complex is positive in any given limb lead, the axis will be oriented toward that limb lead, not away from it. Alternatively, the axis is in the normal range if the QRS complexes are primarily positive in both leads I and II.

An axis is not defined in the precordial leads. Rather, because the typical progression from leads V_1 to V_6 is from a predominantly negative to a positive QRS complex, the transition point is usually defined as the point at which the amplitude of the R wave first exceeds the amplitude of the S wave. Clockwise rotation (transition zone at V_4 or later) may portend a higher risk of future coronary events, and counterclockwise rotation (transition zone at V_3 or earlier) a lower risk of events.[3]

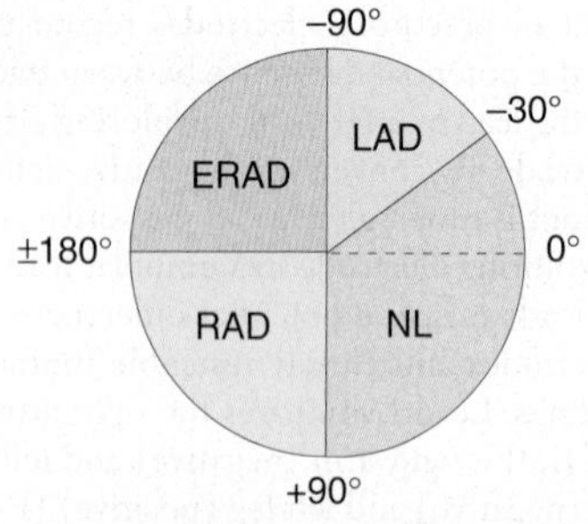

FIGURE 54-4. Chart of frontal plane axes. Normal (NL) = −30 to +90 degrees; left axis deviation (LAD) = −30 to −90 degrees (moderate, −30 to −45 degrees; marked, −45 to −90 degrees); right axis deviation (RAD) = +90 to +180 degrees (moderate, +90 to +120 degrees; marked, +120 to +180 degrees); extreme right axis deviation (ERAD) = −90 to ±180 degrees. Mild RAD is considered normal in children, adolescents, and young adults.

APPROACH TO INTERPRETING THE ELECTROCARDIOGRAM

A stepwise approach to interpreting the ECG ensures that no features of the tracing will be overlooked (Table 54-2).

Normal Electrocardiogram

Figure 54-5 is an example of a normal ECG. Sinus rhythm occurs at about 78 beats per minute, with minor variations in the RR intervals (sinus arrhythmia). The PR interval, QRS duration, and QTc are all normal. The QRS complex is most nearly isoelectric in lead aVL, so the QRS axis will be perpendicular to lead aVL. Because aVL points to −30 degrees, the QRS axis must be approximately −120 or +60 degrees. Because the QRS complex is positive in leads I and II (large R waves), the QRS axis is approximately +60 degrees. The transition in the precordial leads is typically at lead V_3 or V_4. The P wave is biphasic in lead V_1 and then positive in the other precordial leads. Septal q waves, reflecting not lateral infarction but rather normal early septal depolarization, are present in leads V_5 and V_6. Tiny q waves, a normal variant, are seen in the inferior leads.

Abnormal Electrocardiogram

Electrocardiography in patients with coronary artery disease is reviewed in Chapters 71 to 73.[4] Arrhythmias are reviewed in Chapters 61 to 66.

Conduction Abnormalities and Axis Deviation

Abnormalities of the specialized conduction system (i.e., His-Purkinje system) reflect slow or absent conduction in a particular structure (Table

TABLE 54-2 STEPWISE APPROACH TO INTERPRETING THE ELECTROCARDIOGRAM

Estimate the heart rate
Define the heart rhythm (regular vs. irregular; relationship of P waves to QRS complexes)
Measure intervals (PR, QRS duration, QT)
Calculate/estimate QTc
Estimate QRS axis
Examine P wave morphology, duration, and axis
Examine QRS progression and transition in precordial leads
Examine QRS complexes in regional groupings (septal leads [V_1,V_2], anterior leads [V_2, V_3, V_4], lateral leads [I, aVL, V_5, V_6], inferior and posterior leads [II, III, aVF, V_1,V_2])
Examine ST segments in regional groupings
Examine T waves in regional groupings

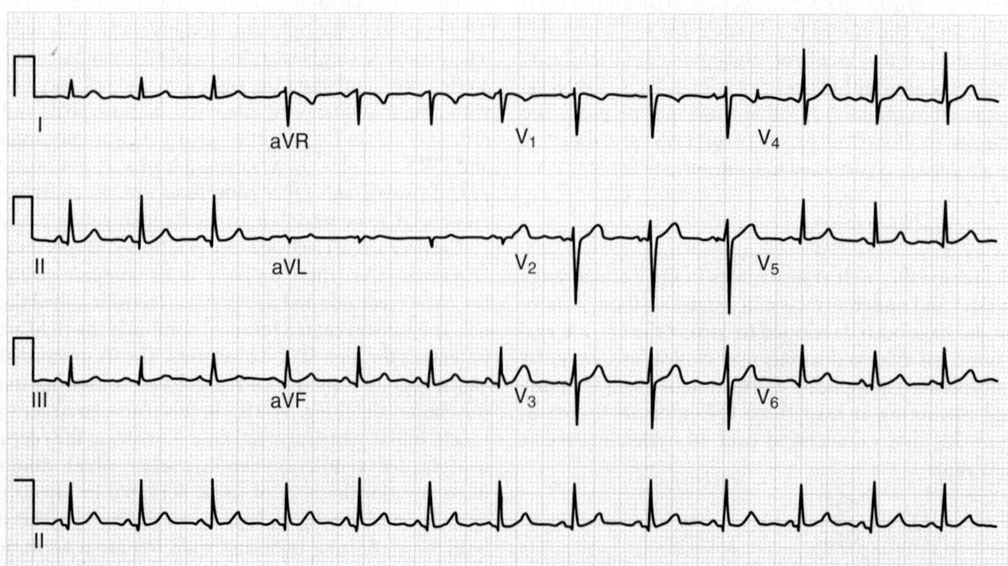

FIGURE 54-5. Normal electrocardiogram. The heart rate is approximately 78 beats per minute, with minor irregularity. Sinus arrhythmia is present. The axis is approximately +60 degrees. The PR, QRS, and QT intervals are approximately 140, 90, and 360 msec, respectively. P wave morphology, duration, and axis are normal. The transition is at lead V_4. No abnormal Q waves are present. ST segments are isoelectric, and T waves are concordant with QRS complexes.

54-3 and Fig. 54-6). Left anterior or posterior fascicular block does not prolong the QRS duration beyond 120 msec. Incomplete bundle branch refers to QRS patterns that are morphologically similar to left or right bundle branch block, but with a duration of less than 0.12 sec (120 msec). An interventricular conduction delay is generally defined as a QRS duration of more than 0.11 second (110 msec). When the QRS has a duration of at least 0.12 second (120 msec), it often has the configuration of a specific bundle branch block. An isolated left bundle branch block in an otherwise healthy person is associated with a two-fold higher risk for development of a cardiovascular event or dying of a cardiovascular cause. As a result, this finding should trigger an evaluation for possible cardiac disease. By comparison, a complete right bundle branch block generally has not been associated with an increased risk, although one study suggested up to a 30% increased risk in cardiovascular mortality.[5]

TABLE 54-3 FASCICULAR AND BUNDLE BRANCH BLOCKS

	QRS DURATION	AXIS	QRS MORPHOLOGY	ST SEGMENTS AND T WAVES
LAFB	<0.12 sec (120 msec)	−45 to −90 degrees	Delayed transition across the precordium qR aVL	Normal
LPFB	<0.12 sec (120 msec)	+90 to +180 degrees	Delayed transition across the precordium rS I, aVL qR in III, aVF	Normal
RBBB	≥0.12 sec (120 msec)	Normal	rsr′, rsR′, rSR′ in V_1 (and usually V_2); wide S in V_6 and I	Discordant in V_1 and V_2
RBBB with LAFB	≥0.12 sec (120 msec)	−45 to 90 degrees	rsr′, rsR′, rSR′ in V_1 (and usually V_2); wide S in V_6 and I	Discordant in V_1 and V_2
RBBB with LPFB	≥0.12 sec (120 msec)	+ 90 to +180 degrees	rsr′, rsR′, rSR′ in V_1 (and usually V_2); wide S in V_6 and I	Discordant in V_1 and V_2
LBBB	≥0.12 sec (120 msec)	Variable	rS or QS in V_1 (S wide and notched); wide notched R without q in V_5, V_6, and I Wide notched R with or without small q in aVL	Discordant in V_1 to V_6

LAD = left axis deviation; LAFB = left anterior fascicular block; LBBB = left bundle branch block; LPFB = left posterior fascicular block; RBBB = right bundle branch block.

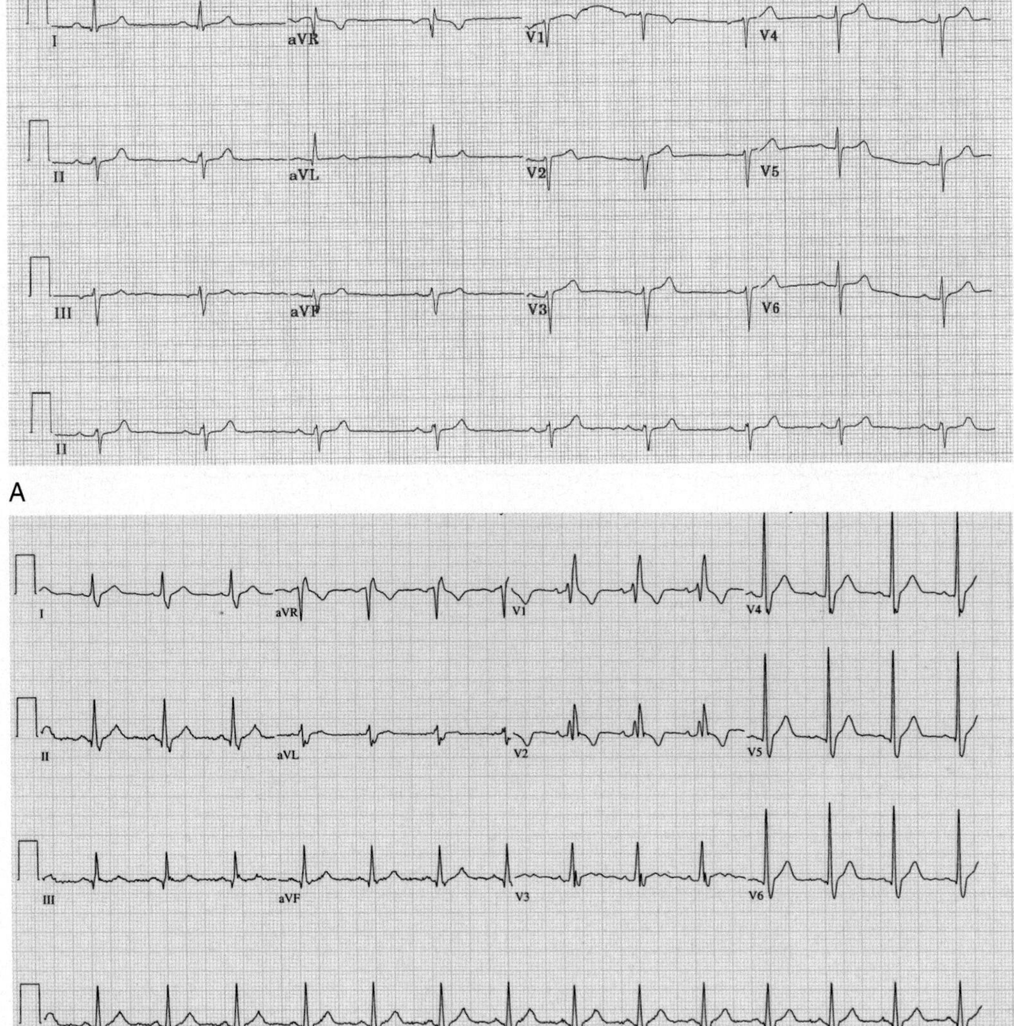

FIGURE 54-6. Fascicular and bundle branch blocks. A, Left anterior fascicular block (LAFB). Left axis deviation is present; the axis is approximately −60 degrees. The QRS duration is normal, and there is a delay in R wave progression across the precordial leads (late transition). Small q waves are present in leads I and aVL and small r waves in leads II, III, and aVF. **B,** Right bundle branch block (RBBB). The QRS is widened, with an rsR′ pattern in lead V_1 and a wide terminal S wave in lead V_6. ST segments are downsloping, and T waves are discordant with the QRS complex in the right precordial leads. The axis is normal, and signs of normal septal activation (q waves in lead V_6) are present.

Continued

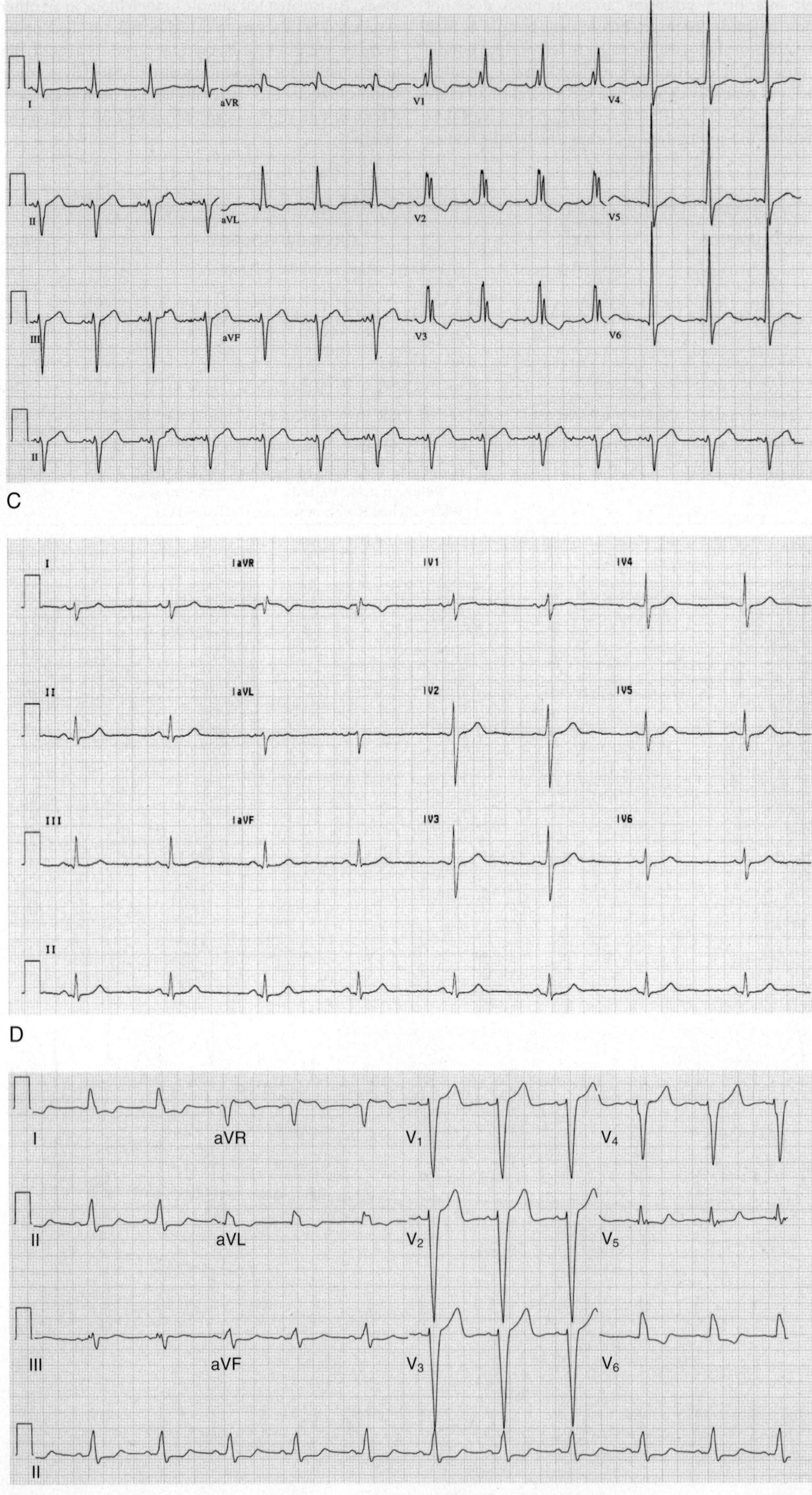

FIGURE 54-6, cont'd. **C,** RBBB and LAFB. In addition to features diagnostic of RBBB, an axis of −60 degrees is present. **D,** Left posterior fascicular block (LPFB). Right axis deviation (+120 degrees) is present. QRS duration is normal, and R wave progression across the precordial leads is delayed. Leads I and AVL have rS complexes, and the inferior leads have insignificant q waves. **E,** Left bundle branch block (LBBB). The QRS is widened, with a broad, notched complex in leads I and aVL and the left precordial leads. Small r waves and broad, deep S waves are present in the right precordial leads. With LBBB, the axis is usually normal or deviated to the left. ST segments and T waves are discordant with the QRS complex throughout the precordium.

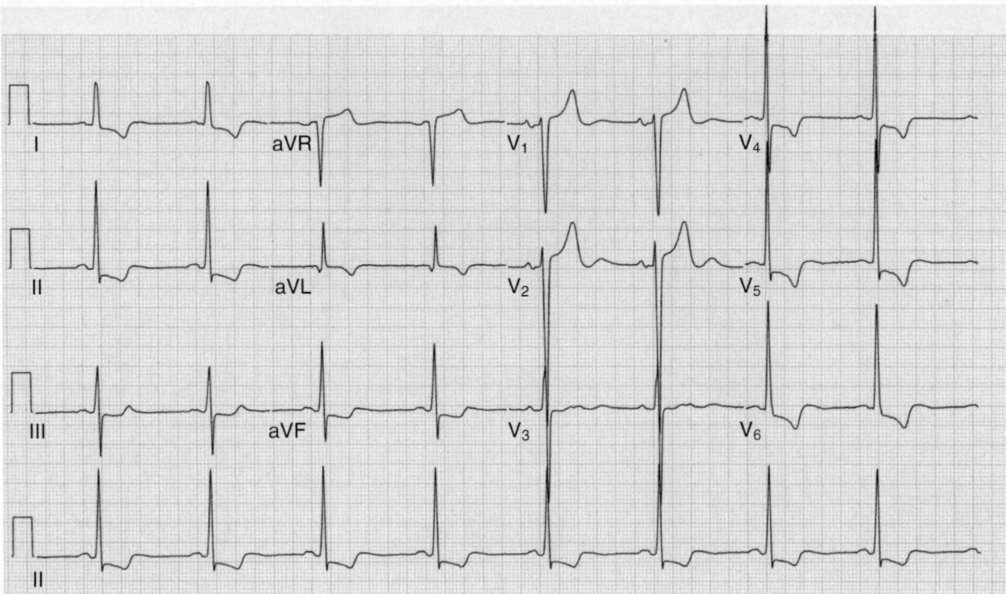

FIGURE 54-7. Left ventricular hypertrophy. Note the striking S wave amplitude in the right precordial leads and R wave amplitude in the left precordial leads. Repolarization abnormalities are present in the left precordial leads as well as in the limb leads. The S wave amplitude in V_3 (2.4 mV) plus the R wave amplitude in aVL (1.0 mV) totals 3.4 mV, easily satisfying the Cornell voltage criteria in this 76-year-old hypertensive man. Sinus bradycardia (50 beats per minute) is present as well.

Chamber Hypertrophy

A number of criteria for defining left ventricular hypertrophy (LVH; Fig. 54-7) and right ventricular hypertrophy (RVH) have been proposed. All of the LVH criteria suffer from poor sensitivity (ranging from 30 to 50%), although the specificity is good (85 to 95%). The Cornell voltage criterion, developed with an echocardiographic standard for LVH, simply adds the S wave amplitude in V_3 and the R wave amplitude in aVL; a total of more than 2.0 mV in women and 2.8 mV in men implies LVH. In many clinical settings, the Cornell criterion has replaced the more complicated Romhilt-Estes criteria, which assign points for QRS amplitude, repolarization abnormalities ("strain" pattern), left axis deviation, and other electrocardiographic features. RVH is much less common than LVH. Electrocardiographic criteria for diagnosis of RVH have even lower sensitivity (10 to 20%) than for LVH, although the specificity is similar. The Sokolow-Lyon criterion for RVH adds the R wave amplitude in lead V_1 to the S wave amplitude in lead V_5 or V_6; a sum of 1.05 mV or more implies RVH.

Low QRS Voltage

Low QRS voltage is defined as limb lead voltage of less than 5 mm (0.5 mV) in all leads or precordial voltage of less than 10 mm (1 mV) in all leads. The differential diagnosis is broad (Table 54-4), and many patients will not have a clinically apparent underlying explanation.

Repolarization Abnormalities

Abnormalities of the ST segment or T waves, or both, are extremely common (Table 54-5). T waves may be in the same direction (concordant) with the QRS complex or discordant. Electrolyte and other metabolic abnormalities, drug effects (particularly digoxin and antiarrhythmic drugs), and secondary effects caused by LVH, bundle branch block, or pacing are all commonly responsible. Furthermore, abnormal depolarization patterns frequently beget abnormal repolarization.

Early repolarization, a relatively common pattern of ST segment elevation, occurs more commonly in patients with idiopathic ventricular fibrillation compared with controls and has also been associated with an increased risk of cardiac mortality.[6] The risk is about 30% higher with 0.1 mV of ST elevation but three-fold higher with more than 0.2 mV of ST elevation. J waves in the absence of hypothermia also increase the risk of idiopathic ventricular fibrillation about four-fold.[7]

Pitfalls of Automated Computerized Electrocardiographic Readings

Automatic computerized ECG interpretations are generally accurate for calculating heart rates, axes, and intervals but have a sensitivity of only about 70% and a positive predictive value of only about 75% for diagnosis of acute myocardial infarction on the first electrocardiogram.[8] Computerized readings are not reliable for diagnosis of rhythm disturbances, a striking weakness of these programs. Over-reading by a physician, including comparison with previous tracings when available, remains mandatory. Formal over-reading by a cardiologist is also recommended, even though it may not alter clinical care very often compared with over-reading by an emergency physician or internist.[9]

TABLE 54-4 CAUSES OF LOW QRS VOLTAGE
Normal variant
Pericardial effusion
Myocardial infarction
Cardiomyopathy
Hypothyroidism
Obesity
Sarcoidosis
Amyloidosis
Chronic obstructive pulmonary disease
Anasarca

TABLE 54-5 CAUSES OF REPOLARIZATION ABNORMALITIES
Athlete's heart
Early repolarization (normal variant)
Myocardial ischemia/injury
Pericarditis
Electrolyte abnormalities
Left ventricular hypertrophy
Intraventricular conduction delay/bundle branch block
Drug effects (digitalis, antiarrhythmic drugs)
Long QT syndrome
Stroke/neurologic catastrophe

Electrocardiograms in Athletes

Extensive physical training leads to structural, electrophysiologic, and autonomic adaptations that can appear abnormal on an uninformed ECG reading.[10] Among the most important ECG findings are rhythms suggesting hypervagotonia, early repolarization, and increased chamber size (Table 54-6 and Fig. 54-8).[11] Differentiation between physiologic adaptations to exercise

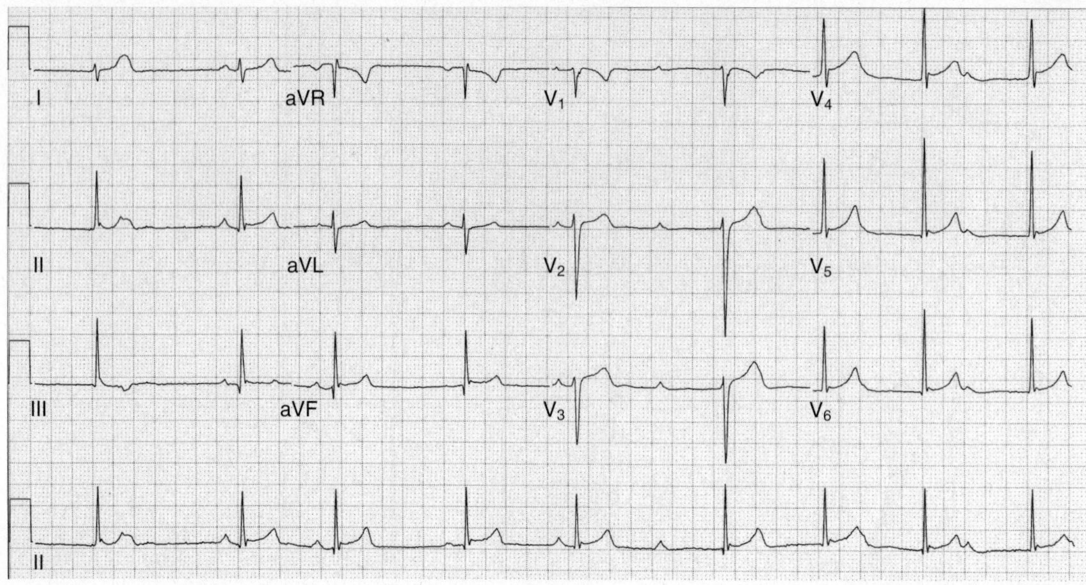

FIGURE 54-8. Athlete's heart. Bradycardia, variable P wave morphology, Mobitz I (Wenckebach) second-degree atrioventricular block, and junctional escape beats all reflect hypervagotonia in this thin, 18-year-old athlete. Mild right axis deviation is present, not uncommon in adolescents and young adults. Prominent S waves are present in leads V_2 and V_3, although formal voltage criteria for left ventricular hypertrophy are absent. Note blocked sinus P waves following junctional beats; this is not abnormal physiology.

TABLE 54-6 GENERALLY BENIGN FINDINGS IN AN ATHLETE'S ELECTROCARDIOGRAM

Sinus arrhythmia, sinus bradycardia, wandering atrial rhythm, junctional rhythm
First-degree atrioventricular block
Mobitz I (Wenckebach) second-degree atrioventricular block
Incomplete right bundle branch block
Isolated voltage criteria for left ventricular hypertrophy (e.g., without repolarization abnormalities, left axis deviation, left atrial abnormality, pathologic Q waves)
Early repolarization pattern

and potentially life-threatening abnormalities can be difficult and often requires expert consultation.

Screening Electrocardiograms

Although frequently recommended by cardiologists and primary care physicians, screening ECGs and exercise ECGs (i.e., exercise stress test) have not been shown to improve outcomes in asymptomatic adults. The U.S. Preventive Services Task Force recommends against screening resting or exercise ECG in asymptomatic adults who are at low risk of coronary heart disease events (Chapter 52).[12,13] For asymptomatic adults at intermediate or high risk, evidence is insufficient to make a recommendation.

GENERAL REFERENCES

For the General References and other additional features, please visit Expert Consult at https://expertconsult.inkling.com.

55 ECHOCARDIOGRAPHY

CATHERINE M. OTTO

Echocardiography is the clinical standard for evaluation of cardiac function in patients with known or suspected heart disease. This chapter reviews the basic principles of echocardiography, echocardiographic approaches, quantitative measurements, and clinical indications. The specific indications for echocardiography and additional echocardiographic images are presented in other chapters on individual types of cardiovascular diseases.

ECHOCARDIOGRAPHIC IMAGING

Principles

Echocardiography is based on the use of a piezoelectric crystal that converts electrical to mechanical energy, and vice versa, allowing both transmission and reception of an ultrasound signal. The frequency of ultrasound waves used for diagnostic imaging ranges from 2 to 10 MHz, with lower frequencies having greater tissue penetration and higher frequencies providing better image resolution. Each transducer consists of a complex array of piezoelectric crystals arranged to provide images in a fanlike two- or three-dimensional image, with the narrow top of this sector scan indicating the origin of the ultrasound signal. Transducers also include an acoustic lens that determines the focal depth, height, and width of the ultrasound beam.

Images are generated on the basis of the reflection of ultrasound from acoustic interfaces, for example, the boundary between the blood in the left ventricle and the myocardium. The time delay between transmission and reception is used to determine the depth of origin of the ultrasound reflection. The depths of the reflected signals from multiple ultrasound beams are combined to generate an image. The speed of signal analysis allows acquisition of two-dimensional ultrasound images at frame rates of 30 to 60 per second and of three-dimensional images at slower frame rates. Ultrasound is strongly attenuated by bone and air, so echocardiography relies on acoustic "windows," where, for example, ultrasound can penetrate to the heart while avoiding the ribs and lungs. With transthoracic imaging, the patient is positioned to bring the cardiac structures close to the chest wall, usually in a left lateral decubitus position, and the transducer is placed on the chest, with use of gel to provide acoustic coupling between the transducer and skin. Standard acoustic windows are parasternal, apical, subcostal, and suprasternal notch.[1]

Standard Image Planes

From the parasternal window, the image plane is adjusted manually by an experienced physician or sonographer to provide long and short axis views. Standard cardiac imaging planes are aligned relative to the axis of the heart, with the long axis defined as the plane that intersects the cardiac apex and the middle of the aortic valve. Short axis views are perpendicular to this long axis, with standard image planes at the cardiac base (aortic valve level), mitral valve, and midventricular levels. From the apical window, the transducer is rotated to provide three views oriented 60 degrees from each other, producing a four-chamber, a two-chamber, and a long axis view (Fig. 55-1; Video 55-1). These image planes also can be acquired with three-dimensional ultrasound transducers with standard two-dimensional plane reconstructed from the three-dimensional data set.

Measurements

Echocardiography provides accurate cardiac dimensions from three-dimensional, two-dimensional, or two-dimensional–guided linear depth

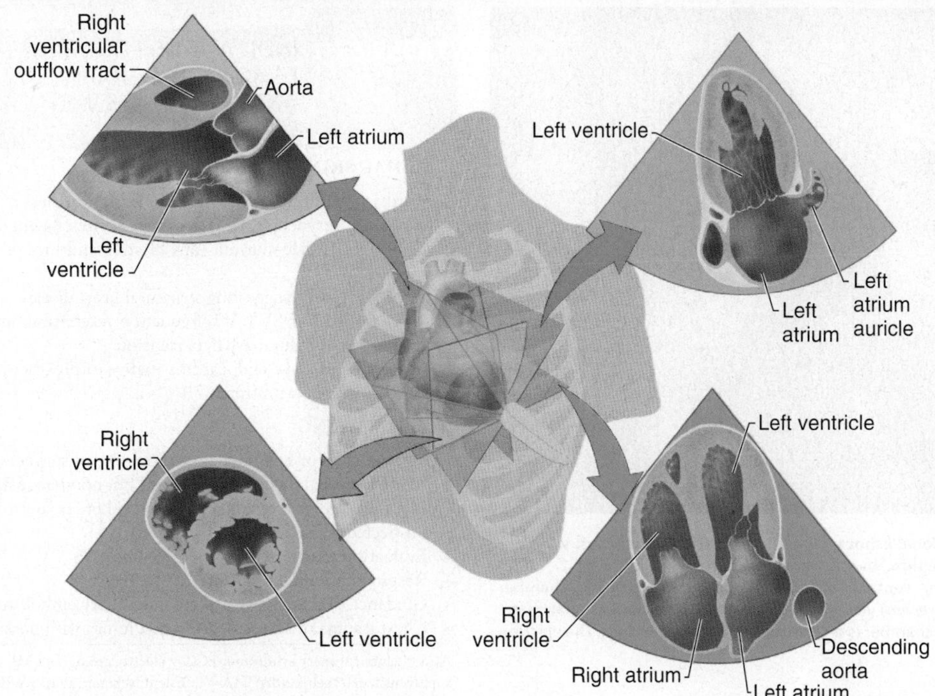

FIGURE 55-1. **The four basic image planes used in transthoracic echocardiography. A parasternal transducer position or "window" is used to obtain long and short axis views. The long axis view (*purple outline*) extends from the left ventricular apex through the aortic valve plane. The short axis view is perpendicular to the long axis view, resulting in a circular view of the left ventricle (*red outline*). The transducer is placed at the ventricular apex to obtain the two-chamber (*blue outline*) and four-chamber (*green outline*) views, each of which is about a 60-degree rotation from the long axis view and perpendicular to the short axis view. The four-chamber view includes both ventricles and both atria. The two-chamber view includes the left ventricle and left atrium; sometimes the atrial appendage is visualized. See Video 55-1. (From Otto CM. *Textbook of Clinical Echocardiography.* 5th ed. Philadelphia: Elsevier Saunders; 2013:32.)**

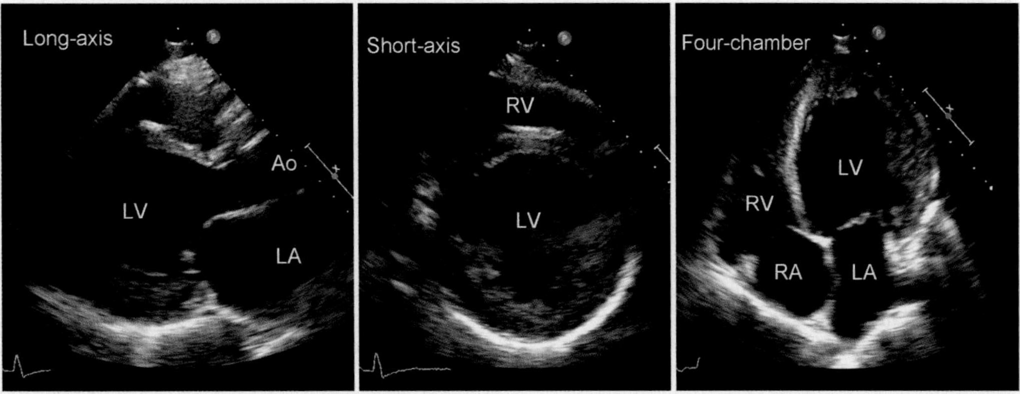

FIGURE 55-2. **Dilated cardiomyopathy on echocardiography. This example shows severe left ventricular dilation and systolic dysfunction in standard image planes of parasternal long axis (*left*), parasternal short axis (*center*), and apical four chamber (*right*). Ao = aorta; LA = left atrium; LV = left ventricle; RA = right atrium; RV = right ventricle. See Video 55-2.**

(M-mode) recordings. The measurements typically provided include left ventricular end-diastolic and end-systolic internal dimensions, left ventricular wall thickness, left atrial anterior-posterior diameter, and aortic sinus dimension. Left ventricular ejection fraction (EF) is determined by automated border detection from three-dimensional images or by tracing two-dimensional echocardiographic endocardial borders at end diastole and end systole in two orthogonal views (Figs. 55-2 and 55-3; Video 55-2).[2] End-diastolic and end-systolic ventricular volumes (EDV and ESV, respectively) are calculated by validated formulas, and the EF is determined as follows:

$$EF = (EDV - ESV)/EDV$$

Limitations

Echocardiography is an accurate, widely available, and widely used imaging approach. However, the quality of images can be suboptimal because of poor tissue penetration (e.g., excessive adipose tissue, position of the lungs relative to the heart), although images are nondiagnostic in less than 5% of patients with current instrumentation. Reflections are stronger when the interface is perpendicular to the ultrasound beam, so structures that are parallel to the beam may not be visible, an artifact called *echo dropout*. This potential limitation may be avoided by the use of appropriate imaging planes and the integration of data from multiple transducer positions. Ultrasound artifacts, such as beam width, shadowing, and reverberations, may be misinterpreted by inexperienced observers.

DOPPLER ECHOCARDIOGRAPHY

Principles

Ultrasound energy that is backscattered from moving red blood cells is shifted to a higher frequency when the blood is moving toward the transducer and a lower frequency when it is moving away. The magnitude of this Doppler shift corresponds to the velocity of blood flow.

Modalities

Pulsed Doppler allows measurement of flow velocity at a specific intracardiac site with the advantages of high spatial and temporal resolution. However, spatial localization is based on intermittent sampling at a time interval corresponding to the depth of interest. The sampling frequency, which is depth dependent, limits the maximum detectable velocity because

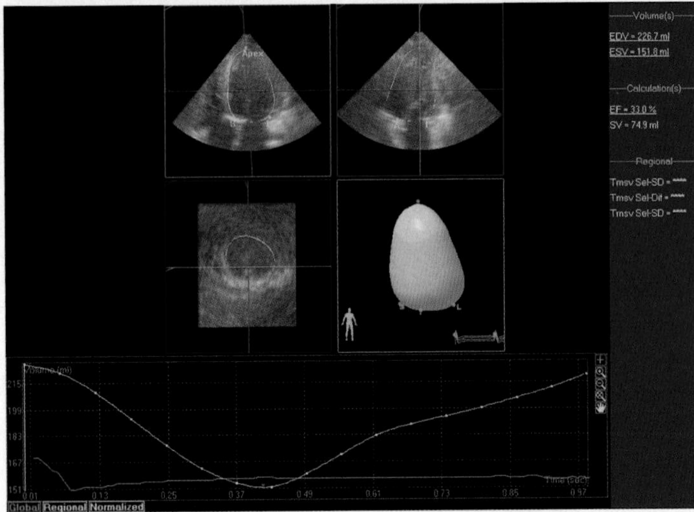

FIGURE 55-3. **Three-dimensional echocardiographic measurement of left ventricular volumes and ejection fraction. In the same patient as in Figure 55-2, three-dimensional imaging shows the ventricle in four-chamber (*upper left*), two-chamber (*upper right*), and short axis (*lower left*) views derived from the three-dimensional image acquisition. The left ventricular chamber is reconstructed in the lower right. The ejection fraction is 33%.**

of a phenomenon called *signal aliasing*. Normal intracardiac flow velocities are about 1 m/second, which can usually be recorded with pulsed Doppler.

Continuous-wave Doppler allows measurement of high velocities along the entire length of the ultrasound beam, but the origin of the high-velocity signal must be inferred from the two-dimensional images. With stenotic and regurgitant valves, blood flow velocities may be as high as 5 to 6 m/second, requiring the use of the continuous-wave Doppler mode. Both pulsed and continuous-wave Doppler velocities are displayed as a graph of velocity versus time, with the density of the spectral display corresponding to signal strength.

Color flow Doppler imaging is a modification of pulsed Doppler in which the flow velocity is displayed across a two-dimensional or three-dimensional image with a color scale to indicate direction and velocity. The advantage is a visually appealing display of intracardiac flow patterns. Disadvantages are low temporal resolution (frame rates of 10 to 30 per second) and poor velocity resolution due to signal aliasing.

Tissue Doppler uses the Doppler principle to record the velocity of motion of the myocardial wall. Tissue Doppler recordings of the myocardium adjacent to the mitral annulus are used to evaluate diastolic ventricular function. Speckle tracking strain imaging allows direct evaluation of myocardial mechanics (E-Fig. 55-1).[3]

Measurements

A standard echocardiographic study includes pulsed Doppler measurement of antegrade flow velocities (transmitral and transaortic) and evaluation for valve regurgitation by continuous-wave and color Doppler modalities. Other Doppler measurements depend on the specific clinical indication.

Quantitative measurements using Doppler data are derived from two basic concepts: volume flow rate and the pressure-velocity relationship. Stroke volume (SV, in cubic centimeters) can be calculated as the volume of a cylinder, where the base is the spatial cross-sectional area (CSA, in square centimeters) of flow, determined as the area of a circle from a two-dimensional diameter measurement. The height of the cylinder is the distance the average blood cell travels in one cardiac cycle, which is the velocity-time integral (VTI, in centimeters) of flow. Therefore,

$$SV\,(cm^3) = CSA\,(cm^2) \times VTI\,(cm)$$

This approach has been validated for measurement of transaortic, transmitral, and transpulmonic flow. Measurement of volume flow rate at two different intracardiac sites allows quantitation of intracardiac shunts and valvular regurgitation.

The relationship between the pressure gradient (ΔP) across a narrowing and the velocity (v) of blood flow is described by the simplified Bernoulli equation:

$$\Delta P = 4v^2$$

TABLE 55-1 INDICATIONS FOR TRANSTHORACIC ECHOCARDIOGRAPHY IN THE ACUTE SETTING AND IN PATIENTS WITH CARDIAC SIGNS OR SYMPTOMS

CARDIAC SIGNS AND SYMPTOMS

- Cardiac symptoms including chest pain, shortness of breath, palpitations, syncope/presyncope, TIA, stroke, or peripheral embolic event
- Abnormal cardiac murmur (any diastolic murmur or systolic murmur grade 3 or louder)
- Prior test results suggesting structural heart disease
- Atrial fibrillation, SVT, VT, frequent or exercise-induced VPCs
- Evaluation of pulmonary hypertension
- Suspected infective endocarditis (native or prosthetic valve) with positive blood cultures or a new murmur

ACUTE SETTING

- Hypotension or hemodynamic instability of suspected cardiac etiology
- Acute chest pain with suspected MI but nondiagnostic ECG
- Elevated cardiac biomarkers without other features of ACS
- Suspected complications of acute MI
- Evaluation of ventricular function after ACS
- Respiratory failure of uncertain etiology
- Guidance of therapy with acute pulmonary embolism
- Chest trauma or severe deceleration injury with possible cardiac consequences

ACS = acute coronary syndrome; ECG = electrocardiogram; MI = myocardial infarction; SVT = supraventricular tachycardia; TIA = transient ischemic attack; VPCs = ventricular premature contractions; VT = ventricular tachycardia.

Summarized from Douglas PS, Garcia MJ, Haines DE, et al. ACCF/ASE/AHA/ASNC/HFSA/HRS/SCAI/SCCM/SCCT/SCMR 2011 Appropriate Use Criteria for Echocardiography. A Report of the American College of Cardiology Foundation Appropriate Use Criteria Task Force, American Society of Echocardiography, American Heart Association, American Society of Nuclear Cardiology, Heart Failure Society of America, Heart Rhythm Society, Society for Cardiovascular Angiography and Interventions, Society of Critical Care Medicine, Society of Cardiovascular Computed Tomography, and Society for Cardiovascular Magnetic Resonance Endorsed by the American College of Chest Physicians. *J Am Coll Cardiol.* 2011;57:1126-1166. Reproduced from Otto CM. *Textbook of Clinical Echocardiography.* 5th ed. Philadelphia: Elsevier Saunders; 2013:119.

This equation allows calculation of maximum and mean gradients across stenotic valves, estimation of pulmonary systolic pressure, and detailed evaluation of intracardiac hemodynamics with regurgitant valves.

ECHOCARDIOGRAPHIC APPROACHES

Several echocardiographic modalities are in clinical use. If it is unclear which modality is optimum in a specific clinical setting, consultation with the echocardiographer is appropriate.

Transthoracic echocardiography is the standard clinical approach in most patients with suspected or known cardiac disease (Table 55-1). Advantages are that it is noninvasive, has no known adverse effects, and provides detailed data on cardiac anatomy and physiology. Limitations include poor image quality in some patients, limited visualization of structures distant from the transducer (e.g., atrial septum, left atrial appendage), and inability to visualize structures immediately distal to prosthetic heart valves (acoustic shadowing).[4]

Transesophageal echocardiography offers superior image quality because of a shorter distance between the transducer and the heart, the absence of interposed bone or lung, and the use of a higher-frequency transducer (Table 55-2). Transesophageal echocardiography usually is well tolerated, but intubation of the esophagus entails some risk, and most clinicians do this procedure with the patient under moderate sedation. Transesophageal echocardiography is much more sensitive than transthoracic echocardiography for detection of left atrial thrombus (95% vs. 50%), valvular vegetations (99% vs. 60%), and prosthetic mitral valve regurgitation (Fig. 55-4).

Point-of-care echocardiography refers to the use of smaller, less expensive ultrasound systems that can be carried by the physician, who can perform quick, limited examinations in the emergency department, at the inpatient bedside, or in the outpatient setting (Table 55-3). Point-of-care echocardiography units range from pocket sized to laptop sized. Some are very simple, with only two-dimensional imaging and limited controls; other systems provide high-quality imaging and all Doppler modalities. Point-of-care echocardiography does not replace a complete imaging study but can serve as an adjunct to the physical examination, particularly in the acute care setting, such as to distinguish ventricular dilation from a pericardial effusion, to estimate ventricular systolic performance (Table 55-4), or to screen for critical aortic stenosis.[5,6]

TABLE 55-2 INDICATIONS FOR USE OF TRANSESOPHAGEAL ECHOCARDIOGRAPHY AS THE INITIAL OR SUPPLEMENTAL TEST

- Patients with a high likelihood of nondiagnostic TTE due to patient characteristics or ability to visualize the structures of interest
- Suspected acute aortic disease including dissection and transection
- Suspected endocarditis with a moderate or high pretest probability (e.g., staphylococcal bacteremia, fungemia, prosthetic heart valve or intracardiac device)
- Evaluation of valve structure and function to evaluate suitability for surgical or transcatheter valve interventions
- Guidance of percutaneous noncoronary cardiac interventions, including but not limited to septal ablation, mitral valvuloplasty, PFO/ASD closure, radio frequency ablation
- Evaluation of patients with atrial fibrillation or flutter to facilitate clinical decision making with regard to anticoagulation, cardioversion, or radio frequency ablation
- Evaluation for cardiac source of embolus with no identified source on TTE
- Reevaluation for interval changes compared with prior TEE when a change in therapy is anticipated.
- Suspected complications of endocarditis (e.g., abscess, fistula)*
- Suspected prosthetic mitral valve dysfunction*
- Evaluation of posterior structure (e.g., atrial baffles) in congenital heart disease patients*

*Not considered in the appropriateness guidelines document but generally accepted as appropriate indications for transesophageal echocardiography as the initial approach.
PFO/ASD = patent foramen ovale/atrial septal defect; TEE = transesophageal echocardiography; TTE = transthoracic echocardiography.
Abstracted from Douglas PS, Garcia MJ, Haines DE, et al. ACCF/ASE/AHA/ASNC/HFSA/HRS/SCAI/SCCM/SCCT/SCMR 2011 Appropriate Use Criteria for Echocardiography. A Report of the American College of Cardiology Foundation Appropriate Use Criteria Task Force, American Society of Echocardiography, American Heart Association, American Society of Nuclear Cardiology, Heart Failure Society of America, Heart Rhythm Society, Society for Cardiovascular Angiography and Interventions, Society of Critical Care Medicine, Society of Cardiovascular Computed Tomography, and Society for Cardiovascular Magnetic Resonance Endorsed by the American College of Chest Physicians. *J Am Coll Cardiol.* 2011;57:1126-1166 with modification. Reproduced from Otto CM. *Textbook of Clinical Echocardiography.* 5th ed. Philadelphia: Elsevier Saunders; 2013:121.

Contrast echocardiography may be performed with intravenous injection of agitated saline to opacify the right-sided heart chambers. These microbubbles are relatively large and do not pass through pulmonary capillaries. Therefore, appearance of contrast material in the left side of the heart within one or two beats after right-sided heart opacification is consistent with an intracardiac shunt. Although most atrial-level shunts are predominantly left-to-right shunts, a small amount of right-to-left shunting occurs, which is the basis of this approach.

Contrast echocardiography also may be performed with commercially available microbubbles in the range of 1 to 5 μm. Because these microbubbles are smaller than the pulmonary capillaries, right-sided heart opacification is followed by left-sided heart opacification, which can enhance the evaluation of systolic function when image quality is suboptimal, especially during stress echocardiography (Fig. 55-5).

Three-dimensional echocardiography is increasingly available and is recommended for quantitation of left ventricular function, evaluation of complex structural heart disease, and guidance of transcatheter interventions (Fig. 55-6; Video 55-3).

Stress echocardiography is a standard approach for evaluating patients with known or suspected coronary artery disease; it has a sensitivity (85 to 95%) and a specificity (80 to 90%) similar to those of radionuclide stress imaging (Chapters 56 and 71). Myocardial infarction results in thinning and akinesis of the affected wall. However, in the absence of infarction, resting myocardial function is normal, even when severe epicardial coronary disease is present. The increased myocardial demand associated with exercise or pharmacologic stress leads to myocardial ischemia, which results in a regional wall motion abnormality, often before the onset of chest pain or electrocardiographic changes (Fig. 55-7; Video 55-4).

In patients who can exercise, standard views of the left ventricle are recorded at baseline and immediately after maximal treadmill or bicycle exercise. If endocardial definition is suboptimal, left-sided contrast is used. The rest and exercise images are compared in a side-by-side cine loop format. Myocardial ischemia is present if resting wall motion is normal but hypokinesis or akinesis is seen after exercise. The pattern of regional wall

TABLE 55-3 INDICATIONS FOR POINT-OF-CARE ECHOCARDIOGRAPHY

To complement a physical examination, especially in an intensive care unit
Rapid initial screening in an emergency setting or ambulance
Screening programs in schools, industry, and community activities
Triaging candidates for a complete echocardiographic examination
Teaching tool, especially to correlate with a cardiac examination

Modified from Sicari R, Galderisi M, Voigt JU, et al. The use of pocket-size imaging devices: a position statement of the European Association of Echocardiography. *Eur J Echocardiogr.* 2011;12:85-87.

TABLE 55-4 GOALS OF POINT-OF-CARE ECHOCARDIOGRAPHY IN THE SYMPTOMATIC EMERGENCY DEPARTMENT PATIENT

Assess possible pericardial effusion and guide pericardiocentesis
Assess global cardiac systolic function
Identify ventricular enlargement
Assess intravascular volume
Confirm potential positioning of a transvenous pacing wire

Modified from Labovitz AJ, Noble VE, Bierig M, et al. Focused cardiac ultrasound in the emergent setting: a consensus statement of the American Society of Echocardiography and American College of Emergency Physicians. *J Am Soc Echocardiogr.* 2010;23:1225-1230.

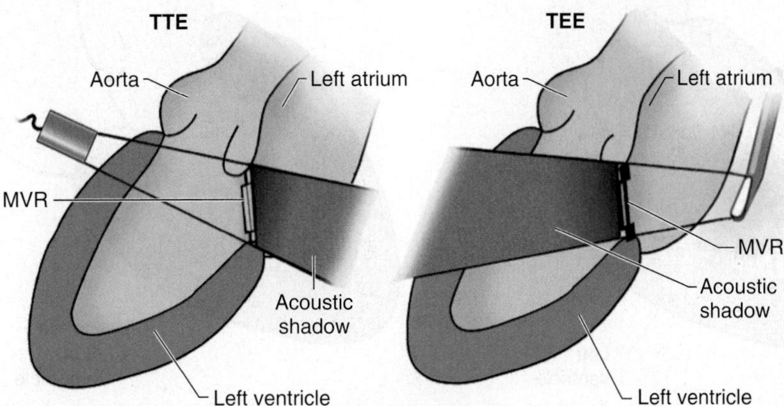

FIGURE 55-4. The problem of acoustic shadowing from a prosthetic mitral valve replacement (MVR). ***Left,*** **With transthoracic echocardiography (TTE), the acoustic shadow distal to the prosthetic valve obscures the left atrium, limiting assessment of valve regurgitation by Doppler techniques.** ***Right,*** **With transesophageal echocardiography (TEE), the left atrium now can be evaluated for valvular regurgitation. However, the acoustic shadow now obscures the left ventricle. (From Otto CM.** ***Textbook of Clinical Echocardiography.*** **5th ed. Philadelphia: Elsevier Saunders; 2013:121.)**

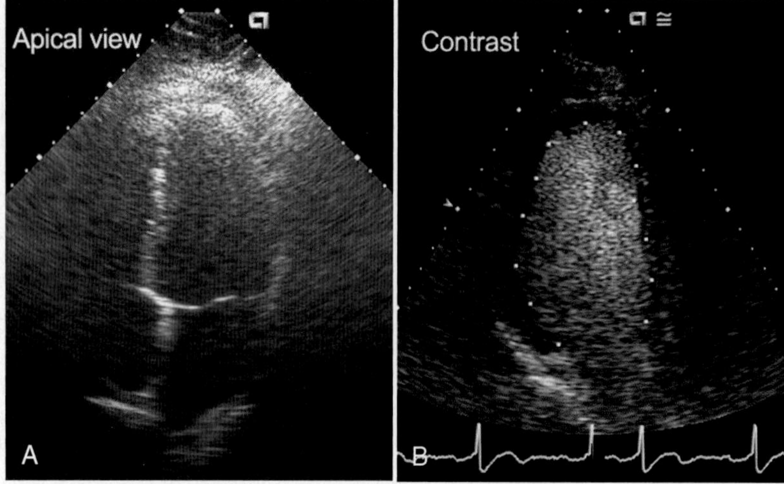

FIGURE 55-5. **Poor-quality apical view (A) with marked improvement in definition of the left ventricular cavity after opacification by contrast echocardiography (B). The *dots* indicate the left ventricular endocardial tracing for calculation of ejection fraction.**

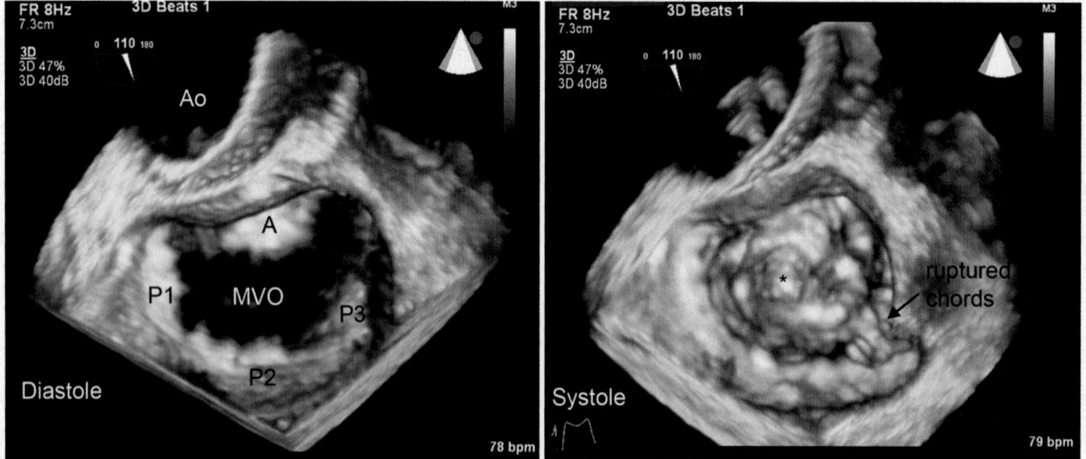

FIGURE 55-6. **The surgeon's three-dimensional view of the mitral valve from the left atrial side of the valve with the aortic valve at the top of the image.** In diastole, the anterior (A) leaflet and posterior leaflet (with P1, P2, and P3 scallops) are seen in the open position, with the normal mitral valve orifice (MVO). In systole, severe prolapse of the anterior leaflet is seen, particularly one bulging section (*asterisk*), and a flail segment with two small ruptured chords (*arrow*) is well visualized. These abnormalities cause severe, posteriorly directed mitral regurgitation. Ao = aorta. See Video 55-3. (From Otto CM. *Textbook of Clinical Echocardiography.* 5th ed. Philadelphia: Elsevier Saunders; 2013:327.)

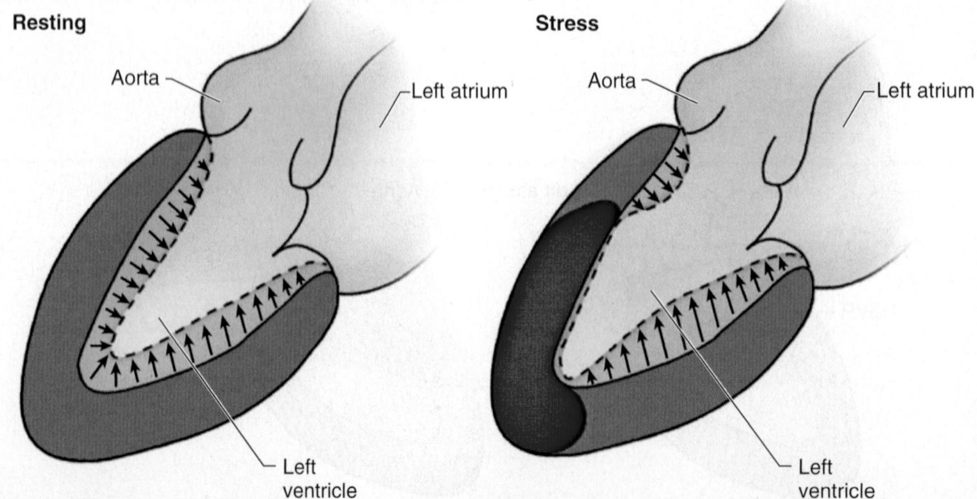

FIGURE 55-7. **The concept of stress echocardiography in a patient with 70% stenosis in the proximal third of the left anterior descending coronary artery.** At rest (*left*), endocardial motion and wall thickening are normal. After stress (*right*), either exercise or pharmacologic, the middle and apical segments of the anterior wall become ischemic, showing reduced endocardial wall motion and wall thickening. If the left anterior descending coronary artery extends around the apex, the apical segment of the posterior wall also will be affected, as shown here. The normal segment of the posterior wall shows compensatory hyperkinesis. See Video 55-4. (From Otto CM. *Textbook of Clinical Echocardiography.* 5th ed. Philadelphia: Elsevier Saunders; 2013:199.)

motion accurately identifies the area of myocardium at risk and is reasonably reliable for identification of the affected coronary artery. With three-vessel coronary disease, rather than a regional wall motion abnormality, the only clue on imaging may be an absence of the expected decrease in chamber size at peak exercise, caused by diffuse ischemia. Interpretation of an exercise echocardiogram includes exercise duration, hemodynamic response, symptoms, and electrocardiographic changes in addition to the echocardiographic images.

In patients who are unable to exercise, stress testing is performed with a graded intravenous infusion of dobutamine, beginning at 5 to 10 μg/kg/minute and increasing every 3 minutes to a maximum dose of 40 μg/kg/minute. If needed, atropine is used to achieve 85% of the maximum predicted heart rate. In addition to evaluation for myocardial ischemia, dobutamine stress echocardiography can assess myocardial viability in areas of stunning or hibernation, based on an improvement in endocardial motion from baseline to low-dose dobutamine, with subsequent worsening of function at higher doses—the "biphasic" response.

Intracardiac echocardiography is performed with an ultrasound probe on a catheter that is inserted into the right side of the heart through the femoral vein. Intracardiac echocardiography is used in the cardiac catheterization laboratory to guide percutaneous closure of a patent foramen ovale (PFO) and other procedures. In the electrophysiology laboratory, intracardiac echocardiography helps guide catheter positioning and identify complications.

CARDIAC FUNCTION MEASUREMENTS

In addition to qualitative descriptions of cardiac anatomy and physiology, echocardiography provides precise and accurate quantitation of cardiac function (including ventricular systolic and diastolic function), an estimate of the severity of valve stenosis and regurgitation, and a noninvasive estimate of pulmonary pressures.

Systolic Ventricular Function

Overall left ventricular systolic function is graded by visual estimation, with an approximate correspondence to EF as follows: normal (EF > 55%), mildly reduced (EF, 40 to 55%), moderately reduced (EF, 20 to 40%), and severely reduced (EF < 20%). More precise quantitation is performed when it is clinically indicated by calculation of a three-dimensional or biplane ejection fraction. Cardiac output calculations are not routine but may be helpful for noninvasive monitoring of therapy in patients with heart failure. Because EF measurements are affected by preload and afterload, measures that are less dependent on loading conditions, including the end-systolic dimension or volume, are generally preferred for clinical decision making in situations such as the timing of surgery for chronic valvular regurgitation.

Evaluation of right ventricular function by echocardiography is more challenging because of the complex shape of the chamber. Useful measurements include the basal diameter, the tricuspid annular plane systolic excursion, and the systolic Doppler tissue velocity at the annulus. Cardiac magnetic resonance imaging provides more accurate quantitation of right ventricular volumes and function when it is clinically needed.

Diastolic Ventricular Function

Evaluation of diastolic ventricular function is challenging because the patterns of ventricular filling are affected by preload, heart rate, and coexisting valvular regurgitation in addition to the diastolic properties of the ventricle. However, echocardiography can classify diastolic function on the basis of the combination of left ventricular inflow, pulmonary vein flow, tissue Doppler velocities, and isovolumic relaxation time. An estimate of left ventricular filling pressure (e.g., left ventricular end-diastolic pressure) also can be inferred by these approaches.

Valvular Stenosis

Echocardiography is the clinical standard for evaluation of aortic valvular heart disease (see Fig. 75-2). Cardiac catheterization is reserved for cases in which echocardiography is nondiagnostic, clinical data are discrepant with echocardiographic findings, or the coronary anatomy needs to be assessed (Chapter 75).

In patients with aortic stenosis, the most direct measure of stenosis severity is the antegrade velocity across the valve, indicating mild (<3 m/second), moderate (3 to 4 m/second), or severe (>4 m/second) valve obstruction. The maximum and mean transaortic pressure gradients also can be calculated by the Bernoulli equation. Accurate evaluation depends on a careful examination by an experienced echocardiographer.

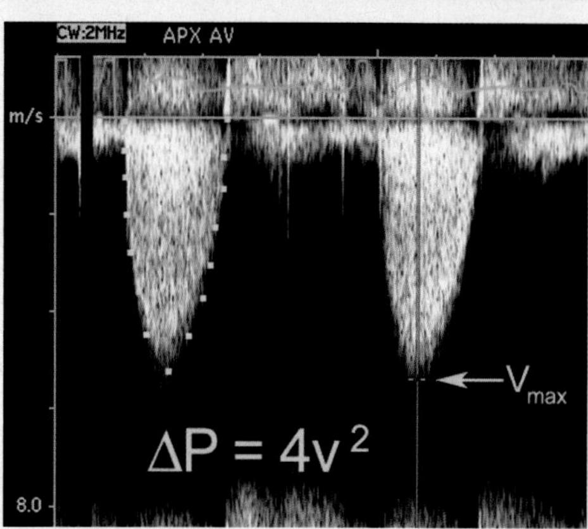

FIGURE 55-8. In a patient with aortic stenosis, the aortic jet velocity is recorded with continuous-wave Doppler from the window that yields the highest velocity signal. Maximum velocity (V_{max}) is used to calculate the maximum systolic gradient. The Doppler curve is traced, as shown, to calculate the mean systolic gradient with the Bernoulli equation, by which the pressure gradient (ΔP) equals four times the square of the velocity.

Aortic valve area (AVA) is calculated by the continuity equation, based on the concept that volume flow rates proximal to and within the narrowed orifice are equal:

$$AVA \times VTI_{AS} = CSA_{LVOT} \times VTI_{LVOT}$$

or

$$AVA = (CSA_{LVOT} \times VTI_{LVOT})/VTI_{AS}$$

where LVOT is left ventricular outflow tract, VTI is velocity-time integral, CSA is cross-sectional area, and AS is aortic stenosis (Fig. 55-8). It is especially important to calculate the AVA when left ventricular systolic dysfunction accompanies aortic valve disease. In some patients, low-dose dobutamine stress echocardiography is helpful in distinguishing ventricular dysfunction caused by severe aortic stenosis from primary myocardial disease with concurrent moderate stenosis.

The evaluation of mitral stenosis (see Fig. 75-4) includes measurement of the mean transmitral gradient from the velocity curve and calculation of the valve area, both from two-dimensional planimetry of a short axis image of the orifice and from the deceleration slope of the Doppler curve (pressure half-time method).

Valvular Regurgitation

The current approach to evaluating valvular regurgitation (see Fig. 75-8) is based on the proximal geometry of the regurgitant jet, with measurement of the narrowest jet width (vena contracta). When further quantitation is needed, regurgitant volume, regurgitant fraction, and regurgitant orifice area are calculated. Although color flow visualization of the flow disturbance may be helpful for detection of regurgitation and for understanding the mechanism of valve dysfunction, this approach should no longer be used to evaluate severity.

For aortic regurgitation, a narrow vena contracta (<3 mm) indicates mild regurgitation, whereas a wide vena contracta (>6 mm) indicates severe regurgitation. Additional evaluation of the severity of aortic regurgitation is based on the presence of holodiastolic flow reversal in the abdominal aorta and the density and slope of the continuous-wave Doppler velocity curve. The approach to evaluating mitral regurgitation (see Fig. 75-6) is similar, beginning with measurement of the vena contracta. In addition to calculation based on transmitral versus transaortic volume flow rates, the proximal acceleration of flow into the regurgitant orifice allows evaluation with central regurgitant jets. Color flow shows a proximal isovelocity surface area.

Pulmonary Pressures

Estimation of pulmonary artery systolic pressure (PAP) is a standard component of a complete examination.[7] The systolic pressure difference between the right ventricle and right atrium is calculated from the peak velocity in the tricuspid regurgitant (V_{TR}) jet, with use of the Bernoulli equation. Then, the right atrial pressure (RAP) is estimated from the size and appearance of the inferior vena cava. Because right ventricular and pulmonary artery systolic pressures are equal (in the absence of pulmonic stenosis),

$$PAP = 4(V_{TR})^2 + RAP$$

A small amount of tricuspid regurgitation is present in most patients, so pulmonary pressures can be estimated with this approach in more than 90% of patients. Because this approach measures only pulmonary systolic pressure, not pulmonary vascular resistance, invasive evaluation may still be needed in some clinical situations (Chapter 68).

THE ECHOCARDIOGRAPHIC EXAMINATION

Clinical Indications

Echocardiography is not useful for screening of the general population,[A1] but it is an effective approach to the initial evaluation of many cardiac signs and symptoms (Table 55-5).[8] Even when transesophageal imaging might be helpful, most clinicians begin with a transthoracic examination; exceptions are for the patient with a possible acute aortic dissection (Chapter 78), in whom transesophageal echocardiography should be performed as quickly as possible, and in the evaluation of possible left atrial thrombosis before cardioversion without anticoagulation (Chapter 64). Resting echocardiography is not helpful for diagnosis of coronary artery disease; stress imaging is needed if this diagnosis is suspected (Chapter 71). In patients with known cardiac disease, echocardiography is used to evaluate severity, to assess the results of medical and surgical interventions, and to guide procedures. Point-of-care ultrasound is useful for rapid screening to evaluate overall left ventricular function and to detect pericardial effusion (Fig. 55-9; Video 55-5).

Normal Findings

Trace to mild valve regurgitation is considered "physiologic" and is seen with 70 to 80% of mitral valves, 80 to 90% of tricuspid valves, and 70 to 80% of pulmonic valves in normal individuals. The prevalence of aortic regurgitation increases with age, but it is found in only 5% of young normal adults; the presence of aortic regurgitation raises the possibility of subtle aortic valve or root abnormalities.

A PFO (Chapter 69) is present in 25 to 35% of normal individuals and may be identified by color Doppler or by contrast echocardiography. Use of

TABLE 55-5 INDICATIONS FOR TRANSTHORACIC ECHOCARDIOGRAPHY (TTE) BY KNOWN DIAGNOSIS

CLINICAL DIAGNOSIS	KEY ECHOCARDIOGRAPHIC FINDINGS	LIMITATIONS OF ECHOCARDIOGRAPHY	ALTERNATIVE APPROACHES
VALVULAR HEART DISEASE (CHAPTER 75)			
Valve stenosis	Cause of stenosis, valve anatomy Transvalvular ΔP, valve area Chamber enlargement and hypertrophy LV and RV systolic function Associated valvular regurgitation	Possible underestimation of the stenosis severity Possible coexisting coronary artery disease	Cardiac catheterization; CMR
Valve regurgitation	Mechanism and cause of regurgitation Severity of regurgitation Chamber enlargement LV and RV systolic function PA pressure estimate	TEE may be needed to evaluate mitral regurgitant severity and valve anatomy (especially before MV repair)	Cardiac catheterization; CMR
Prosthetic valve function	Evidence for stenosis Detection of regurgitation Chamber enlargement Ventricular function PA pressure estimate	TTE is limited by shadowing and reverberations TEE is needed for suspected prosthetic MR due to "masking" of the LA on TTE	Cardiac catheterization; fluoroscopy
Endocarditis (Chapter 76)	Detection of vegetations (TTE sensitivity, 70-85%) Presence and degree of valve dysfunction Chamber enlargement and function Detection of abscess Possible prognostic implications	TEE more sensitive for detection of vegetations (>90%) A definite diagnosis of endocarditis also depends on bacteriologic criteria TEE more sensitive for detection abscess	Blood cultures and clinical findings also are diagnostic criteria for endocarditis
CORONARY ARTERY DISEASE			
Acute myocardial infarction (Chapters 72 and 73)	Segmental wall motion abnormality reflects "myocardium at risk" Global LV function (EF) Complications Acute MR vs. VSD Pericarditis LV thrombus, aneurysm, or rupture RV infarct	Coronary artery anatomy itself is not directly visualized	Coronary angiography (catheterization or CT) Radionuclide or PET imaging for myocardial perfusion
Angina (Chapter 71)	Global and segmental LV systolic function Exclude other causes of angina (e.g., AS, HCM)	Resting wall motion may be normal despite significant CAD Stress echocardiography is needed to induce ischemia and wall motion abnormality	Coronary angiography Radionuclide or PET imaging ETT
Pre-revascularization/ post-revascularization	Assess wall thickening and endocardial motion at baseline Improvement in segmental function after procedure	Dobutamine stress or contrast echocardiography is needed to detect viable but nonfunctioning myocardium	CMR Coronary angiography Radionuclide or PET imaging Contrast echocardiography
End-stage ischemic disease	Overall LV systolic function (EF) PA pressures Associated MR LV thrombus RV systolic function	—	Coronary angiography (Cath or CT) Radionuclide or PET imaging CMR for myocardial viability
CARDIOMYOPATHY (CHAPTERS 58-60)			
Dilated	Chamber dilation (all four) LV and RV systolic function (qualitative and EF) Coexisting atrioventricular valve regurgitation PA systolic pressure LV thrombus	Indirect measures of LVEDP Accurate EF may be difficult if image quality is poor	Radionuclide EF LV and RV angiography

TABLE 55-5 INDICATIONS FOR TRANSTHORACIC ECHOCARDIOGRAPHY (TTE) BY KNOWN DIAGNOSIS—cont'd

CLINICAL DIAGNOSIS	KEY ECHOCARDIOGRAPHIC FINDINGS	LIMITATIONS OF ECHOCARDIOGRAPHY	ALTERNATIVE APPROACHES
Restrictive	LV wall thickness LV systolic function LV diastolic function PA systolic pressure	Must be distinguished from constrictive pericarditis	Cardiac catheterization with direct, simultaneous RV and LV pressure measurement after volume loading CMR
Hypertrophic	Pattern and extent of LV hypertrophy Dynamic LVOT obstruction (imaging and Doppler) Coexisting MR Diastolic LV dysfunction	Exercise echo to detect inducible LV outflow tract obstruction	CMR Strain and strain rate imaging
HYPERTENSION (CHAPTER 67)			
	LV wall thickness and chamber dimensions LV mass LV systolic function Aortic root dilation	Diastolic dysfunction precedes systolic dysfunction, but detection is challenging because of age and other factors	Speckle tracking; strain and strain rate imaging LV twist and torsion
PERICARDIAL DISEASE (CHAPTER 77)			
	Pericardial thickening Detection, size, and location of PE Two-dimensional signs of tamponade physiology Doppler signs of tamponade physiology	Diagnosis of tamponade is a hemodynamic and clinical diagnosis Constrictive pericarditis is a difficult diagnosis Not all patients with pericarditis have an effusion	Intracardiac pressure measurements for tamponade or constriction CMR or CT to detect pericardial thickening
DISEASES OF THE AORTA (CHAPTER 78)			
Aortic root dilation	Cause of aortic dilation Accurate aortic root diameter measurements Anatomy of sinuses of Valsalva (especially Marfan syndrome) Associated aortic regurgitation	The ascending aorta is only partially visualized on TTE in most patients	CT CMR TEE
Aortic dissection	Two-dimensional images of ascending aorta, aortic arch, descending thoracic and proximal abdominal aorta Imaging of dissection "flap" Associated aortic regurgitation Ventricular function	TEE more sensitive (97%) and more specific (100%) Cannot assess distal vascular beds	Aortography CT CMR TEE
CARDIAC MASSES (CHAPTER 60)			
LV thrombus	High sensitivity and specificity for diagnosis of LV thrombus Suspect with apical wall motion abnormality or diffuse LV systolic dysfunction	Technical artifacts can be misleading 5-MHz or higher frequency transducer and angulated apical views needed	LV thrombus may not be recognized on radionuclide or contrast angiography
LA thrombus	Low sensitivity for detection of LA thrombus, although specificity is high Suspect with LA enlargement, MV disease	TEE needed to detect LA thrombus reliably	TEE
Cardiac tumors	Size, location, and physiologic consequences of tumor mass	Extracardiac involvement is not well seen Cannot distinguish benign from malignant tumor or tumor from thrombus	TEE CT CMR (with cardiac gating) Intracardiac echocardiography
PULMONARY HYPERTENSION (CHAPTER 68)			
	PA pressure estimate Evidence of left-sided heart disease to account for increased PA pressures RV size and systolic function (cor pulmonale) Associated TR	Indirect PA pressure measurement Cannot determine pulmonary vascular resistance accurately	Cardiac catheterization
CONGENITAL HEART DISEASE (CHAPTER 69)			
	Detection and assessment of anatomic abnormalities Quantitation of physiologic abnormalities Chamber enlargement Ventricular function	No direct intracardiac pressure measurements Complicated anatomy may be difficult to evaluate if image quality is poor (TEE is helpful)	CMR with three-dimensional reconstruction Cardiac catheterization TEE Three-dimensional echocardiography

AS = aortic stenosis; CAD = coronary artery disease; CMR = cardiac magnetic resonance; CT = computed tomography; EF = ejection fraction; ETT = exercise treadmill test; HCM = hypertrophic cardiomyopathy; LA = left atrium; LV = left ventricle; LVEDP = left ventricular end-diastolic pressure; LVOT = left ventricular outflow tract; MR = mitral regurgitation; MV = mitral valve; ΔP = pressure gradient; PA = pulmonary artery; PE = pericardial effusion; PET = positron emission tomography; RV = right ventricle; TEE = transesophageal echocardiography; TR = tricuspid regurgitation; TTE = transthoracic echocardiography; VSD = ventricular septal defect.

From Otto CM. *Textbook of Clinical Echocardiography.* 5th ed. Philadelphia: Elsevier Saunders; 2013:507-509.

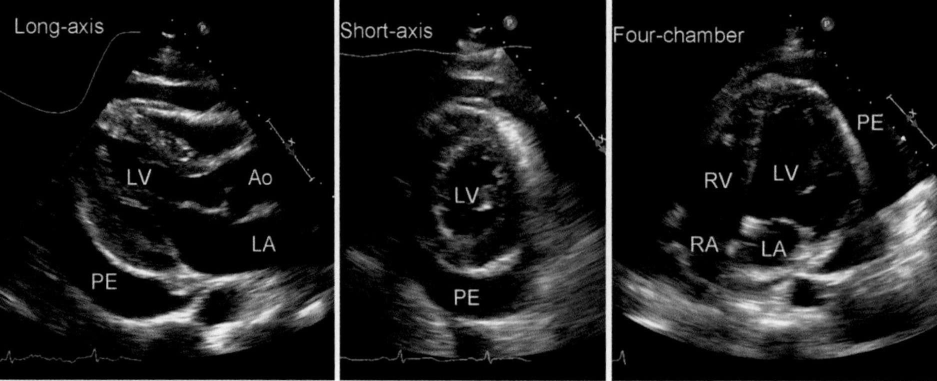

FIGURE 55-9. **Pericardial effusion.** A large echo-free space is seen anterior and posterior to the cardiac structure in the parasternal long axis view (*left*), short axis view (*center*), and apical four-chamber view (*right*) consistent with a pericardial effusion (PE). Ao = aorta; LA = left atrium; LV = left ventricle; RA = right atrium; RV = right ventricle. See Video 55-5.

the Valsalva maneuver enhances identification of a PFO because the slight elevation in right atrial pressure may lead to a brief right-to-left shunt. The significance of a PFO in patients without clinical events is unclear. Other common anatomic variants seen on echocardiography include aberrant chords (or "webs") in the left ventricle; small, linear, mobile echoes associated with the valves (Lambl's excrescences); and normal ridges in the left and right atria.

Unexpected abnormal findings also may be found on studies requested for other indications. A bicuspid aortic valve is present in 1 to 2% of the population; most of these patients are asymptomatic until late in life, so many cases are diagnosed "incidentally" by echocardiography. Aortic valve sclerosis, which is a frequent unexpected echocardiographic diagnosis, is a marker of cardiovascular disease and an increased risk of myocardial infarction even if valve function is normal.

INTEGRATING THE ECHOCARDIOGRAPHIC AND CLINICAL FINDINGS

The echocardiographic request should indicate the specific reason for the study and any relevant symptoms or signs. The echocardiographic examination then can be tailored to answer the clinical question. The echocardiographic results should be interpreted in conjunction with other clinical data.[8] If the echocardiographic data seem discrepant with the clinical data, the requesting physician should review the images with the echocardiographer to identify areas of uncertainty and to determine the next best diagnostic step.

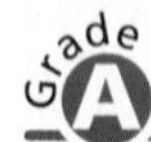

Grade A Reference

A1. Lindekleiv H, Lochen ML, Mathiesen EB, et al. Echocardiographic screening of the general population and long-term survival: a randomized clinical study. *JAMA Intern Med*. 2013;173:1592-1598.

GENERAL REFERENCES

For the General References and other additional features, please visit Expert Consult at https://expertconsult.inkling.com.

56

NONINVASIVE CARDIAC IMAGING

CHRISTOPHER M. KRAMER, GEORGE A. BELLER, AND KLAUS D. HAGSPIEL

RADIOGRAPHY OF THE HEART

Chest radiography is a widely available, relatively inexpensive, and rapid imaging modality, with an average effective radiation dose of 0.03 to 0.1 mSv. The heart is best evaluated on posteroanterior (PA) and lateral radiographs, with the heart closest to the image detector.

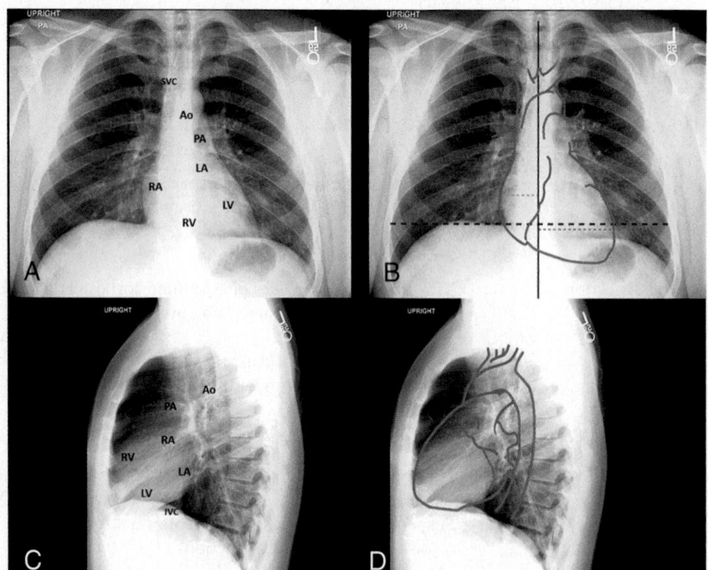

FIGURE 56-1. Normal anatomy. Posteroanterior (**A**) and lateral (**B**) chest radiograph projections in a healthy 28-year-old man. The cardiac chambers and the great vessels are marked on the corresponding drawings (**C, D**). The cardiothoracic ratio (**C**) is calculated by dividing the maximum transverse diameter of the cardiac silhouette (*blue line:* widest distance of the right heart border from the midpoint of the spine; *orange line:* widest distance from the left heart border to the midpoint of the spine) through the distance between the internal margin of the ribs at the top of the right diaphragm (*black line*). Ao = aorta; IVC = inferior vena cava; LA = left atrium; LV = left ventricle; RA = right atrium; RV= right ventricle; PA = pulmonary artery; SVC = superior vena cava.

On the chest radiograph, the heart appears as a homogeneous shadow surrounded by lung, so diagnostic assessment of the heart and great vessels is based on the size and shape of the cardiac silhouette, rather than on direct visualization of the heart's internal anatomy. Nevertheless, the size and shape of the heart and their changes over time, together with the appearance of the pulmonary vasculature, aid in the diagnosis of cardiac diseases. The radiographic appearance of the heart is also influenced by the radiographic technique, projection, body habitus, degree of inspiration, and whether the patient is supine or erect during the examination.

On the PA projection, the normal heart is located in the middle mediastinum, with approximately two thirds projecting to the left of the mid sternum (Fig. 56-1). The superior segment of the right heart border is a more or less straight line formed by the superior vena cava and right innominate vein. The inferior segment is convex and formed by the right atrium. The left heart border consists of three segments: the aortic arch superiorly, the main pulmonary artery in the middle, and the left ventricle (LV) in the longest segment inferiorly. The left atrial appendage is situated in the junction between the lower and middle segments; if enlarged, it can appear as a separate, prominent segment. The inferior border of the heart sometimes is not well differentiated from the diaphragm (see Fig. 56-1).

On lateral chest images, the right ventricle (RV) and the RV outflow tract form the anterior heart border, with the RV in contact with the lower third of the sternum. Lung between the sternum and the posteriorly curving RV and RV outflow tract forms the retrosternal clear space. The posterior heart border, which is seen between the carina and the diaphragm on lateral images, consists of the left atrium superiorly and the LV inferiorly. The inferior vena cava courses obliquely upward before it joins the right atrium. The ascending aorta, aortic arch, and proximal descending thoracic aorta are usually well seen on lateral images (see Fig. 56-1).

Alterations of the contour of the heart are generally caused by dilation of the atria, ventricles, or blood vessels. Chest images are not sensitive for detecting cardiac hypertrophy unless it is severe.

Comprehensive cardiovascular analysis of chest radiographs requires evaluation of the size and morphology of the heart and the great vessels, the pulmonary vasculature, and the presence and positioning of any calcifications or implanted devices such as valves, pacemakers, and defibrillators.

Radiographic Assessment of Heart Size

The cardiothoracic ratio (see Fig. 56-1) estimates the size of the heart. A value of less than 0.5 is considered normal on a radiograph taken during deep inspiration. Pectus excavatum deformities (Chapter 99) and epicardial fat pads can result in an abnormally large cardiothoracic ratio despite a normal-sized heart. Dilation of the LV, which increases the cardiothoracic ratio, appears as a concave mid left heart border and lengthening of the entire left heart border, with a downward pointing apex projecting below the diaphragm on PA views (Fig. 56-2). Extension of the posterior margin of the left ventricle more than 2 cm posterior to the inferior vena cava on the lateral film is considered a sign of left ventricular enlargement. Localized rather than global LV enlargement usually indicates the presence of ventricular aneurysms (Chapter 73). LV hypertrophy without dilation usually is not detectable on chest radiographs.

The most common cause of left atrial enlargement is secondary to LV dysfunction, especially LV dilation. Isolated enlargement of the left atrium is usually a sequela of mitral valve abnormalities or atrial fibrillation. Enlargement of the left atrium can also occur with LV hypertrophy without dilation in patients with aortic stenosis (Chapter 75) or hypertrophic cardiomyopathy (Chapter 60). Straightening of the left heart border between the main pulmonary artery and the LV just below the left main bronchus owing to enlargement of the left atrial appendage is one of the earliest signs of left atrial enlargement; with increasing size, this segment becomes convex. A double contour within the right cardiac border (double density sign), splaying of the carina, and elevation of the right main bronchus are less frequent signs (Fig. 56-3).

The RV normally does not form part of the heart's border on PA radiographs, but significant RV enlargement can lead to an abnormal convexity of the left heart border, with elevation and leftward displacement of the cardiac apex. The best radiographic indication of RV enlargement is obliteration of the retrosternal clear space in the lateral view owing to dilation of the RV outflow tract (Fig. 56-4).

Dilation of the right atrium causes the lower segment of the right heart border to become more prominent and increasingly round. In more severe cases, the entire right heart border is enlarged, and in extreme cases, the right atrium can become border-forming on the lateral view (see Fig. 56-3).

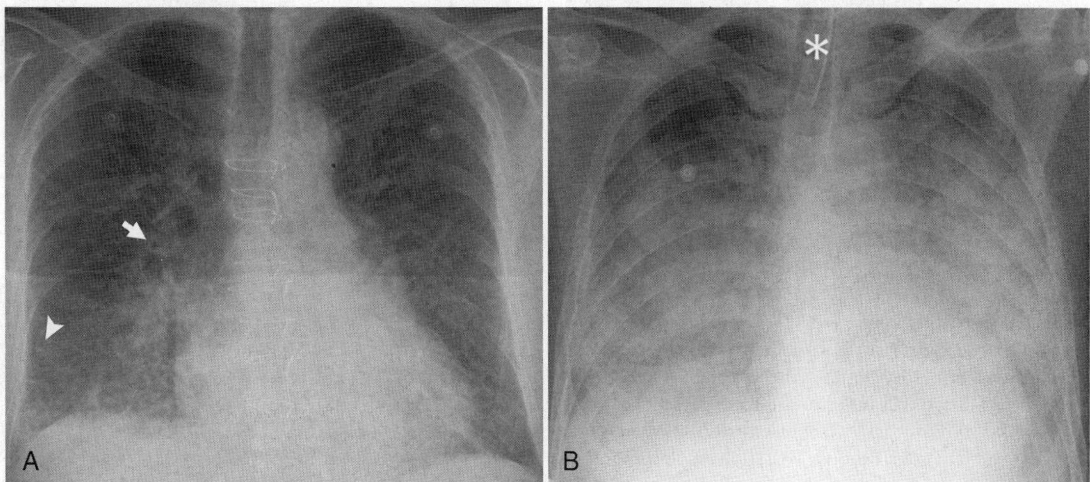

FIGURE 56-2. Left ventricular enlargement and pulmonary edema in two different patients. The image on the left (A) was obtained in a patient who had acute myocardial infarction and who had previously undergone aortic bypass grafting (sternotomy wires and bypass clips are seen). Interstitial edema is evidenced by the presence of vascular redistribution, Kerley B lines (*arrowhead*), and peribronchial cuffing (*arrow*). The image on the right (B) was obtained in a patient with cardiogenic alveolar edema. The left ventricle is significantly enlarged, and there is extensive bilateral air space consolidation with air bronchogram. Note normal position of an endotracheal tube (*asterisk*) and a nasogastric tube.

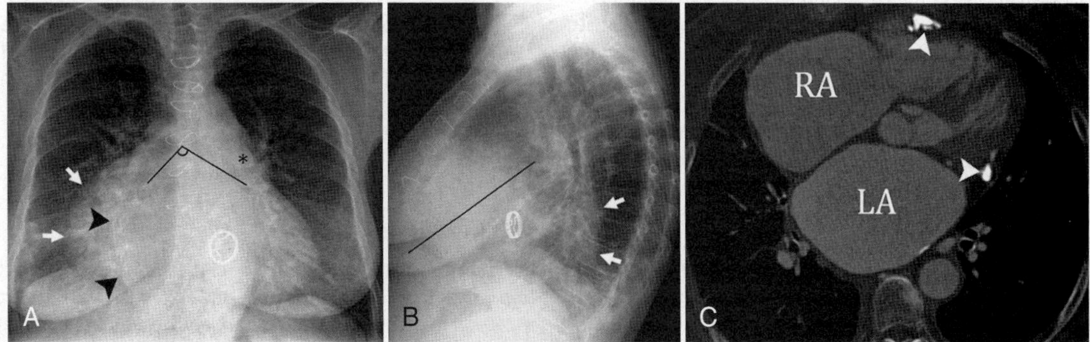

FIGURE 56-3. Biatrial enlargement in a patient who has undergone mitral valve repair. The posteroanterior (A) chest radiograph shows a prominent left atrial appendage (*asterisk*), the double density sign (*arrowheads*), and splaying of the carina. There is also enlargement of the right atrium, as evidenced by prominence and round shape of the right side border on the posteroanterior view (*arrows*). Posterior bulging of the heart (*arrows*) owing to biatrial enlargement is seen on the lateral view (B). Interstitial pulmonary edema is present. The location of the cardiac valves is best assessed on a lateral view (B) by drawing a line from the carina to the anterior costophrenic recess (*black line*). The pulmonic and aortic valves usually are positioned superior to this line, and the tricuspid and mitral valves are inferior to it. A computed tomographic image (C) also demonstrates biatrial enlargement as well as pericardial calcifications. LA = left atrium; RA = right atrium.

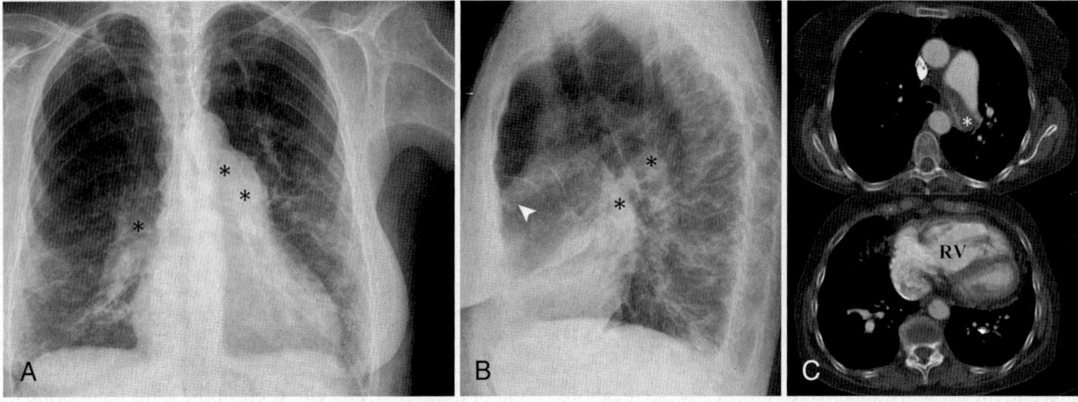

FIGURE 56-4. Pulmonary arterial hypertension in a patient with severe pulmonary emphysema and chronic pulmonary embolism. Enlarged central pulmonary arteries (*asterisks*) and the pruned-tree sign can be seen on the posteroanterior (**A**) and lateral (**B**) projections. Hyperlucency in both upper lobes is present owing to extensive pulmonary emphysema. Right ventricular enlargement has obliterated the retrosternal clear space on the lateral view (*arrowhead*) (**B**). The computed tomographic scan demonstrates dilated central pulmonary arteries with wall adherent chronic pulmonary embolus (*asterisk*) (**C**) as well as right ventricle (RV) dilation and hypertrophy.

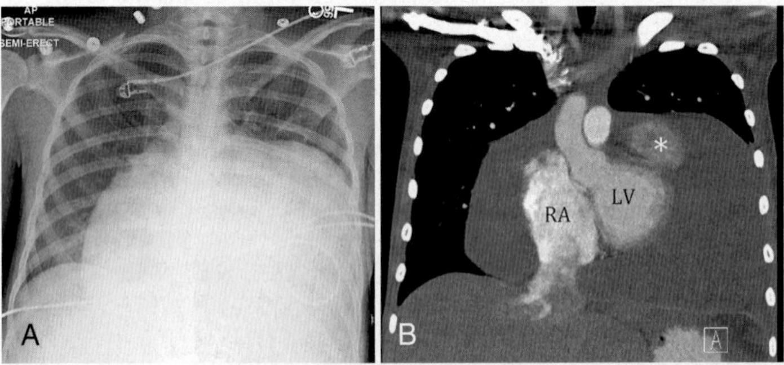

FIGURE 56-5. A 17-year-old girl presenting with massive pericardial effusion. The posteroanterior radiograph (**A**) shows the water-bottle sign; the hilar vessels are obscured. A coronal reformatted computed tomographic scan (**B**) shows the fluid in the pericardial sac as well as dilation of the right atrium and the left atrial appendage (*asterisk*). LV, left ventricle; RA, right atrium.

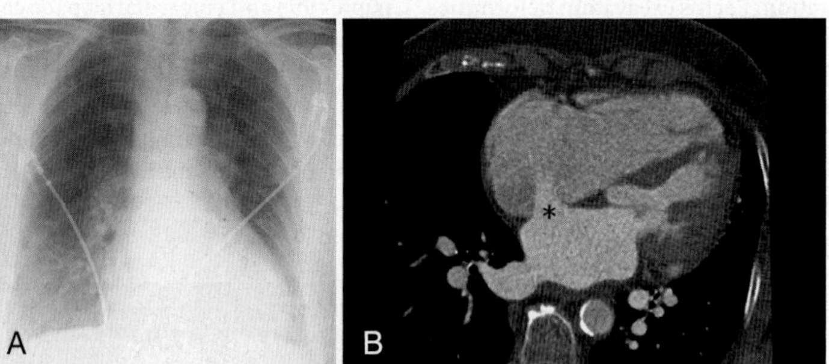

FIGURE 56-6. Female patient with known secundum type atrial septal defect. The posteroanterior radiograph (**A**) shows enlargement of the pulmonary arteries, shunt vascularity, and enlargement of the right heart border. A computed tomographic scan (**B**) shows the septal defect (*asterisk*) with left-to-right shunt. Enlargement of the right heart is also seen.

Pericardial Effusion

Large pericardial effusions cause significant enlargement of the cardiac silhouette despite a normal superior mediastinum—the so-called water-bottle sign. The fluid in the pericardial sac will obscure the hilar vessels on a PA chest film (Fig. 56-5), unlike cardiomegaly without effusion, in which the hilar structures often are relatively conspicuous. Posterior displacement of the pericardial fat line on lateral images is also a valuable finding for the detection of pericardial effusions.

Pulmonary Vasculature

The large and medium-sized pulmonary arteries and veins can be seen on the radiograph as linear shadows, and their size and appearance correlate with pulmonary blood flow and pulmonary venous pressure. The vessels in the lower lung zones are normally larger than in the upper zones as a result of the normal distribution of pulmonary blood flow (see Fig. 56-1). In patients with right-to-left shunts (Chapter 69), the pulmonary vasculature is decreased in caliber. In left-to-right shunts, the vascularity is increased, and the vessels are sharply outlined if the patient does not have heart failure (Fig. 56-6). With increasing pulmonary venous pressure, as is seen in heart failure (Chapters 58 and 59), the vessels in the upper zone enlarge on the chest radiograph. With further increases in pulmonary venous pressures, fluid extravasates into the pulmonary interstitium, and the pulmonary vessels lose their sharp demarcation. Horizontal lines in the periphery of the lungs (Kerley B) and vertical lines in the upper lobes (Kerley A) represent thickened interlobular septae. Fluid in the interstitium of the bronchial walls causes peribronchial thickening or cuffing (see Fig. 56-2). In more advanced cases, the lungs show a diffuse ground-glass appearance that masks the vascular structures, and pulmonary edema ultimately develops (see Fig. 56-2). Long-standing pulmonary arterial hypertension leads to dilation of the central pulmonary arteries with abrupt change in caliber instead of the normal tapering. The size and number of the peripheral arterial branches diminish, resulting in a pruned-tree appearance (see Fig. 56-4).

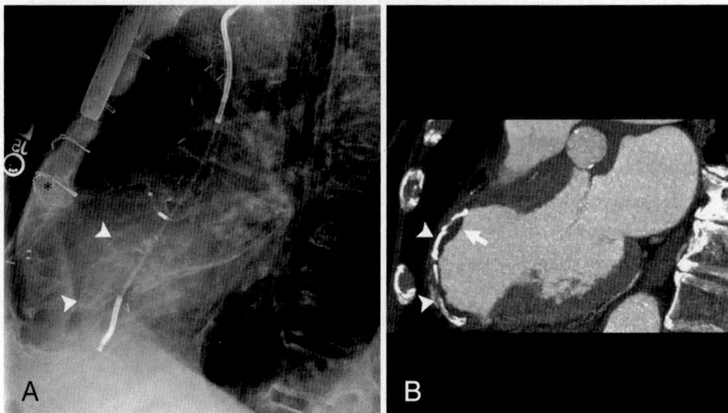

FIGURE 56-7. Calcified chronic myocardial infarction. Lateral radiograph (**A**) demonstrates thin curvilinear calcifications (*arrowheads*) in the region of the left ventricular apex. A reformatted cardiac computed tomographic scan (**B**) shows aneurysmal dilation and thinning of the apex, curvilinear calcifications, and thrombus (*arrow*). Dual-chamber pacer leads, aortocoronary bypass clips, and fracture of the most inferior sternotomy wire (*asterisk*) are also seen on the lateral radiograph (**A**).

Calcifications

Calcifications can often be seen on chest radiographs. In the heart, calcifications most frequently involve the valves and the mitral annulus (Chapter 75). Most aortic valvular calcifications are degenerative in nature and occur in otherwise normal valves, but their incidence is increased in bicuspid valves or in patients who have had rheumatic fever. Calcification of the mitral annulus is common and usually an asymptomatic finding. Coronary artery calcifications are frequent but are rarely seen on chest radiographs. Calcifications of the ventricles are most often seen in patients with prior myocardial infarction or ventricular aneurysms (Fig. 56-7). Pericardial calcifications tend to be thicker than calcifications in the myocardium and, in severe cases, can entirely surround the heart (see Fig. 56-3).

Implanted Devices

A great number of devices can be seen on a chest radiograph, and it is important to be familiar with their appearance to assess their correct position and integrity. However, accurate assessment of device position can occasionally require cross-sectional imaging because the radiographic projection, body habitus, degree of inspiration, and patient positioning (supine versus erect) greatly impact appearance of a device on the film (see Figs. 56-2, 56-3, and 56-7).

Characteristic Appearance of Cardiac Silhouette

Certain constellations of findings on chest radiographs can be characteristic of specific disorders. For example, in mitral stenosis, left atrial enlargement, pulmonary venous hypertension, a small aortic knob, and enlargement of the main pulmonary artery are typical findings. In aortic stenosis, LV enlargement, calcifications of the aortic valve, and dilation of the ascending aorta are often present. In pulmonic valve stenosis, enlargement of the pulmonary trunk is the most common radiographic sign, with or without signs of RV enlargement. In atrial septal defects, the heart is usually normal in size, with prominent pulmonary vasculature (shunt vascularity). In ventricular septal defects, the left atrium and LV are prominent, and shunt vascularity is present. A number of classic chest radiographic signs have been described for patients with more complex congenital heart disease (Chapter 69). These findings include the egg-on-a-string sign in transposition of the great arteries, the gooseneck sign in endocardial cushion defects, the boot-shaped heart in tetralogy of Fallot (Fig. 56-8), the figure-of-3 and reversed figure-of-3 signs in coarctation of the aorta, the box-shaped heart in Ebstein anomaly, the snowman sign in total anomalous pulmonary venous return, and the scimitar sign in partial anomalous pulmonary venous return (Fig. 56-8). Although these classic signs are useful when present, they are less frequently encountered than previously because congenital anomalies are diagnosed and treated earlier in life. As a result, chest radiography currently has a limited role in the diagnosis of congenital and acquired heart disease, but it remains a useful technique for monitoring the progression of disease and its response to treatment.

NUCLEAR CARDIOLOGY

The techniques of nuclear cardiology permit the noninvasive imaging of myocardial perfusion under stress and resting conditions and of resting regional and global function by use of radionuclide imaging agents and gamma or positron cameras with associated computer processing. All these techniques are based on acquiring images of radioactivity emanating from tracers localized in heart muscle or in the blood pools of the LV and RV. Myocardial perfusion imaging is the most commonly performed nuclear cardiology technique, most often in conjunction with either exercise or pharmacologic stress intended to produce flow heterogeneity between relatively hypoperfused and normally perfused myocardial regions. Single-photon emission computed tomography (SPECT) is one technique used to image uptake of tracers in the myocardium. Radionuclide angiography, in which technetium-99m (^{99m}Tc)-labeled red blood cells or other ^{99m}Tc-labeled agents are injected intravenously, is used for measurement of LV ejection fraction and assessment of regional wall motion, especially to monitor changes in global LV function in patients undergoing chemotherapy with cardiac toxic drugs. Positron emission tomography (PET) can assess regional myocardial metabolism to estimate myocardial viability, most often with fluorine-18-labeled 2-deoxyglucose (FDG), as well as myocardial perfusion by use of either nitrogen-13 (^{13}N) ammonia or rubidium-82 (^{82}Rb).

Myocardial Perfusion Imaging

IMAGING AGENTS

For the assessment of myocardial perfusion using SPECT technology, ^{99m}Tc-labeled perfusion agents, which provide higher-quality images more quickly, are used more commonly than thallium-201 (^{201}Tl) for exercise or pharmacologic stress perfusion imaging to evaluate patients with suspected or known coronary heart disease (CHD). Of the various ^{99m}Tc-labeled agents, ^{99m}Tc-sestamibi and ^{99m}Tc-tetrofosmin are the most common. These ^{99m}Tc agents permit simultaneous assessment of regional and global LV function and volumes with gated SPECT technology. Advantages of PET myocardial perfusion imaging compared with SPECT include higher sensitivity and specificity for the detection of coronary artery disease with a lower dose of radiation. By comparing stress blood flow to resting flow, PET also permits the quantification of absolute regional myocardial blood flow in mL/min/g and coronary flow reserve.

DETECTION OF CORONARY HEART DISEASE

The major indications for stress and rest myocardial perfusion imaging are to diagnose CHD, to assess prognosis, and to detect myocardial viability.[1] Exercise or pharmacologic stress myocardial perfusion imaging in patients with chest pain yields a sensitivity for detecting CHD of 88% for SPECT and 93% for PET.[2] The specificity for excluding CHD is 76% for SPECT and 81% for PET. Exercise or pharmacologic stress SPECT perfusion imaging has sensitivities and specificities that are superior to those of exercise electrocardiogram (ECG) testing alone. Specificity for SPECT myocardial perfusion imaging is enhanced by inspection of regional function on ECG-gated images and with computer algorithms, which correct for attenuation. Both the sensitivity and specificity for detecting CHD are enhanced by image quantitation.

Myocardial perfusion imaging is of particular value compared with exercise ECG testing alone in (1) patients with resting ECG abnormalities, such as those seen with LV hypertrophy, digitalis effect, Wolff-Parkinson-White syndrome, and intraventricular conduction abnormalities; and (2) patients who fail to achieve more than 85% of maximal predicted heart rate. The addition of stress perfusion imaging can assist in differentiating true-positive from false-positive ST depression. Detection of proximal left anterior descending stenoses and proximal multivessel CHD is enhanced by identifying regional systolic thickening or wall motion abnormalities on the gated SPECT images compared with assessment based on perfusion alone. If possible, drugs such as long-acting nitrates, β-blockers, and rate-lowering calcium blockers should be discontinued for 24 hours before exercise stress testing that is performed to diagnose or to exclude CHD as the cause of chest pain. Advances in gamma camera technology have yielded a new generation of high-speed gamma SPECT cameras that use cadmium zinc telluride semiconductor detectors.

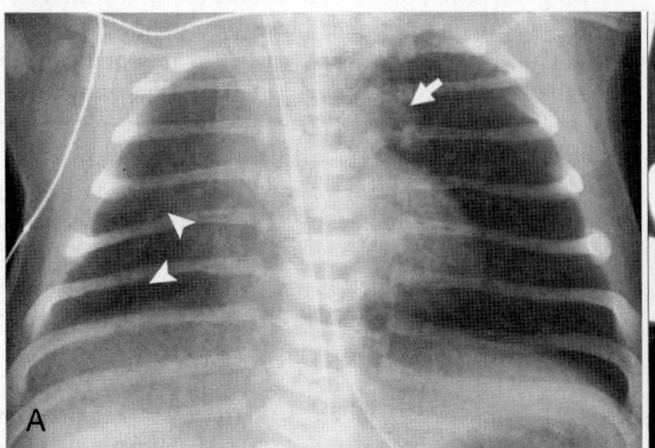

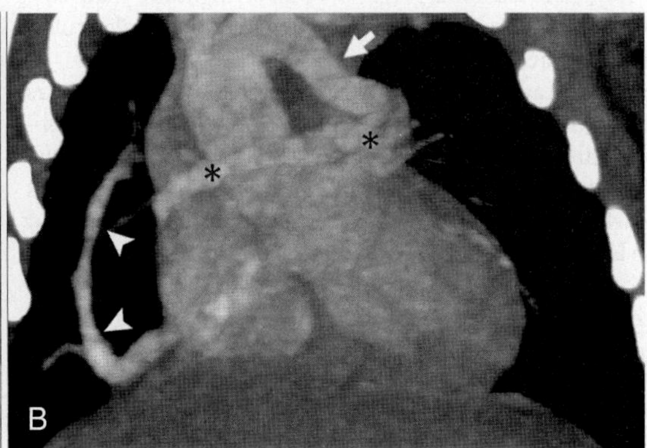

FIGURE 56-8. Infant with tetralogy of Fallot, pulmonary atresia, and partial anomalous pulmonary venous return. Anteroposterior radiograph (A) shows the classic boot-shaped heart seen with tetralogy of Fallot; the scimitar sign, owing to abnormal right pulmonary vein draining into the inferior vena cava (*arrowheads*); and abnormal superior parasternal left-sided mediastinal density caused by a left upper pulmonary vein draining into the left innominate vein (*arrow*). Coronal reformatted computed tomography (B) confirms these findings. The pulmonary arteries are diminutive (*asterisks*).

This technology has better spatial resolution, permits use of a lower effective dose of tracer for imaging, and requires less time compared with a conventional gamma camera (E-Fig. 56-1).

Employing a "stress-only" protocol for SPECT myocardial perfusion imaging in patients with a low or low-to-intermediate pretest probability of CHD based on clinical variables has reduced radiation exposure and imaging time. The conventional 1-day SPECT protocol entails performing a resting SPECT study first, followed by a stress study a few hours later using higher doses of the tracer. With the stress-only approach, the stress study is done first. If the stress study is normal, the resting study is not performed; but if the stress study is abnormal, then the patient is brought back the following day for the resting study to see if the perfusion defect in question is reversible and indicative of inducible ischemia. The two approaches are equally good for predicting future CHD event rates (E-Fig. 56-2).

Some gamma cameras are combined with a computed tomography (CT) scanner, which allows for multimodality hybrid imaging of anatomy and physiology. Myocardial perfusion imaging can be added to the coronary CT angiographic study if the latter shows an intermediate coronary stenosis of 50 to 70% in diameter. Conversely, the CT angiogram can be performed after an equivocal SPECT study to distinguish between true-positive and false-positive perfusion defects.

PHARMACOLOGIC STRESS IMAGING

In patients who are unable to exercise to 85% of their age-prediction maximum heart rate on exercise stress testing protocols, pharmacologic stress testing with use of vasodilators or dobutamine is an alternative to exercise for detecting physiologically significant coronary artery stenoses. Vasodilator stress SPECT myocardial perfusion imaging can use dipyridamole, adenosine, or regadenoson. The most commonly used vasodilator stress agent is now regadenoson, an A2A adenosine receptor agonist, administered as an intravenous bolus. The addition of limited exercise to adenosine or regadenoson imaging can attenuate the vasodilator-induced decrease in blood pressure and enhance image quality by increasing the heart-to-liver ratio of tracer uptake. Dobutamine stress is preferred in patients who have bronchospasm or a history of asthma or who have consumed caffeine, which is an adenosine receptor antagonist, within 12 hours before testing. Patients who experience side effects such as hypotension and chest pain during vasodilator infusion should be treated with intravenous aminophylline, an adenosine antagonist that immediately reverses these side effects. Regadenoson administration normally increases the heart rate, and its failure to do so is a bad prognostic sign.

ASSESSMENT OF PROGNOSIS

The extent of hypoperfusion on post-stress SPECT perfusion images provides important incremental prognostic information when added to clinical characteristics, the resting LV ejection fraction, exercise ECG stress test variables, and even coronary artery anatomy. Nondiabetic patients with chest pain and a normal myocardial perfusion scan at peak exercise or under vasodilator stress have a subsequent cardiac death or infarction rate of less than 1% per year and are generally appropriate candidates for medical therapy (Chapter 71) or require further diagnostic evaluation for a noncardiac cause of chest pain (Chapters 51 and 137). Conversely, patients with high-risk imaging results may benefit from early referral for invasive strategies, including coronary revascularization (Chapter 74), even if symptoms are mild. Patients who show inducible ischemia (Fig. 56-9) involving more than 10% of the LV myocardium may have a better outcome with coronary revascularization compared with medical therapy.

Transient ischemic LV cavity dilation, by which the LV cavity appears more dilated on stress images compared with rest images, occurs when subendocardial ischemia after stress causes a decrease in tracer uptake in the subendocardium. This finding is particularly predictive of poorer outcomes in diabetic patients who undergo SPECT myocardial perfusion imaging but is of limited value in low-risk patients whose scans are otherwise normal with no defects noted.

Assessment of regional LV function on post-stress gated SPECT images enhances the detection of multivessel CHD. LV ejection fraction and end-systolic and end-diastolic volumes can also be measured by gated SPECT imaging. Stress myocardial perfusion imaging does not appear to add any useful prognostic information over exercise ECG testing alone in patients who achieve 10 metabolic equivalents or more of workload without ischemic ST segment depression on the exercise ECG. Similarly, in low-risk women with good physical capacity, a diagnostic strategy using the exercise ECG alone is as good as exercise SPECT myocardial perfusion imaging for predicting 2-year outcomes at lower cost.[3] One significant limitation of SPECT myocardial perfusion imaging is failure to identify multivessel and left main coronary artery disease in some patients who have balanced ischemia, in which uptake of the imaging agent at peak stress is homogenously diminished throughout the LV myocardium because of diffusely reduced flow in regions supplied by all three major coronary arteries. Quantitative PET myocardial perfusion imaging will identify these patients by demonstrating global reduction in absolute coronary flow.

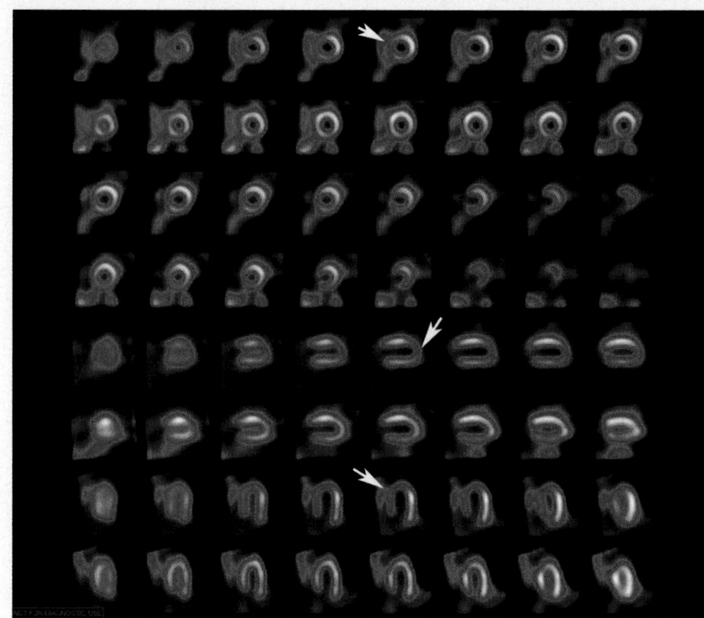

FIGURE 56-9. Exercise stress (rows 1 and 3 from top to bottom) and rest (rows 2 and 4) short axis, stress (row 5) and rest (row 6) vertical long axis, and stress (row 7) and rest (row 8) horizontal long axis single-photon emission computed tomography images showing reversible perfusion defects in the interventricular septum (*white arrows*) and the anteroapical region (*green arrows*). (Reproduced from Beller GA, Bateman TM. Provisional use of myocardial perfusion imaging in patients undergoing exercise stress testing. *J Nucl Cardiol.* 2013;20:711-714.)

DETERMINATION OF MYOCARDIAL VIABILITY WITH SINGLE-PHOTON EMISSION COMPUTED TOMOGRAPHY OR POSITRON EMISSION TOMOGRAPHY

SPECT perfusion imaging is performed in the resting state to identify residual myocardial viability in zones corresponding to severe regional wall motion abnormalities in patients with CHD and depressed LV function. When severe LV dysfunction is caused by "hibernation" (a state of chronic reduced contractility because of substantial ischemia), and not by irreversible myocardial necrosis, areas of resting hypoperfusion that are viable and contributing to hibernation show initial defects on early images but no or less severe defects on 3-hour delayed images. If uptake ultimately exceeds 50 or 60% of peak uptake in these regions, there is a high probability (65 to 75%) that regional myocardial function will improve after successful revascularization, compared with only a 10 to 20% probability for myocardial zones showing less than 50% of peak uptake on resting images.

Regional myocardial metabolism can be assessed noninvasively by PET with FDG and a flow tracer such as [^{13}N]ammonia or ^{82}Rb. FDG is a glucose analogue that is taken up initially in myocardial cells and is trapped by conversion to FDG-6-phosphate. FDG is cell membrane impermeable and remains within viable cells at high concentrations for more than 40 to 60 minutes. Increased FDG activity on clinical PET images in areas of diminished regional blood flow, as determined by [^{13}N]ammonia imaging, is characteristic of myocardial viability. These areas of blood flow–FDG mismatch usually show improved regional function after coronary revascularization. When the extent of viability (hibernation) by PET-FDG exceeds 10% of the LV, revascularization is associated with improved long-term survival compared with medical therapy.[4] Regions of the heart that show both diminished perfusion and FDG uptake (a "match" pattern) represent predominantly nonviable myocardium, with only a 10 to 15% probability of showing improved systolic function after revascularization. Patients who have an ischemic cardiomyopathy with poor viability on either resting SPECT or PET have a worse outcome after coronary revascularization compared with patients with predominantly viable myocardium.

Imaging of Ventricular Function

Global and segmental left and right ventricular function can be evaluated accurately by gated cardiac blood pool imaging to provide a radionuclide angiogram or ventriculogram. The equilibrium radionuclide angiographic approach is performed after thorough mixing of ^{99m}Tc-labeled blood cells within the intravascular compartment. Because ^{99m}Tc remains within the blood pool, serial imaging studies can be acquired during several hours. Acquisition of the images is synchronized with the QRS complex on the ECG through a multigated approach by which each cardiac cycle is divided into multiple frames. A uniform diminution of LV systolic function without segmental wall motion abnormalities suggests nonischemic dilated cardiomyopathy (Chapter 60), whereas depressed global LV function associated with segmental wall motion abnormalities suggests ischemic heart disease. LV function can also be assessed by gated SPECT myocardial perfusion imaging, and the LV ejection fraction and extent of wall motion abnormalities measured by this approach add prognostic information for risk stratification compared with perfusion alone.

CARDIAC COMPUTED TOMOGRAPHY

For CT, imaging with high spatial and temporal resolution and ECG gating during a breath-hold yields snapshots of the heart reconstructed from the same phase of the cardiac cycle. Coronary CT angiography can capture a three-dimensional image of the heart in one to two heartbeats on the latest generation scanners as well as provide coronary artery calcium scoring without the use of contrast and with little radiation.[5] Coronary CT angiography requires 60 to 100 mL of iodinated contrast and average radiation doses of less than 5 mSv. With latest generation scanners, radiation doses of less than 1 mSv are achievable. However, without careful planning of the imaging approach, radiation doses on the order of 5 to 20 mSv are typical on older 64-detector scanners. β-Blockade is often used to achieve a heart rate of 60 beats per minute or less to optimize imaging, and irregular rhythms such as atrial fibrillation may diminish image quality.

Coronary Artery Calcium Scoring

Coronary calcium is an indicator of the burden of atherosclerotic plaque, although there is no correlation of the amount of local coronary calcium with the physiologic or anatomic significance of an underlying coronary stenosis. Calcium scores are generally calculated as an Agatston score, which corresponds to each coronary lesion's calcium area multiplied by the maximal CT attenuation value of that lesion, and then summed for the entire coronary tree. Very high scores confer an increased risk for future cardiac events[6] (Fig. 56-10). Calcium scores are age, gender, and race dependent, and they must be normalized by these factors. Coronary calcium scores predict CHD events independently of standard risk factors, C-reactive protein levels, or the Framingham risk score. Calcium scores above 300 are especially associated with an increased risk for myocardial infarction and cardiac death. The utility of calcium scoring is highest in patients who are at intermediate risk for CHD, based on Framingham risk data (Chapter 52), and increasing scores over time portend a higher risk for a CHD event.[7] By comparison, a calcium score in otherwise low- or high-risk patients will rarely change management, although very high calcium scores may sometime encourage cardiac stress testing.

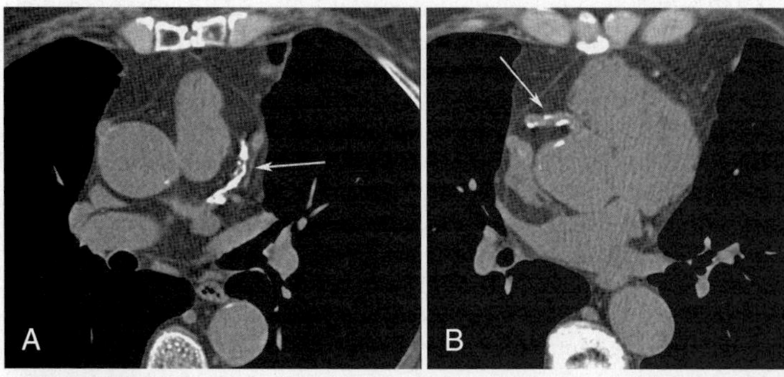

FIGURE 56-10. Non-contrast-enhanced computed tomography axial slices through the heart at two locations for coronary calcium scoring as risk assessment in an asymptomatic patient. **A,** The slice includes the left anterior descending artery with extensive calcification in its proximal portion *(arrow)*. **B,** The slice includes the right coronary artery with proximal spotty calcification *(arrow)*. This patient's calcium score was 457, putting him in a higher risk group regardless of his Framingham risk score.

Coronary Computed Tomographic Angiography

Coronary CT angiography is an excellent technique to diagnose anomalous coronary arterial anatomy in adults (Fig. 56-11). For detection of coronary artery disease, positive-predictive values are in the range of 64 to 91%, and negative-predictive values approach 99%. Thus, the technique is an excellent way to exclude (Fig. 56-12) significant coronary artery disease in the three major coronary vessels (Fig. 56-13). A limitation of the technique, however, is its lower specificity in heavily calcified vessels, which are more common in elderly patients. CT angiography tends to overestimate the percentage of stenosis compared with intravascular ultrasound. The accuracy for detecting stenoses in bypass grafts is quite high, although evaluation of native vessel coronary artery disease is limited in these patients owing to extensive calcification and smaller size vessels. Imaging within most coronary stents has proved difficult.

Coronary CT angiography is not recommended as a routine screening test, but it is useful in selected situations, such as in low- or low-intermediate-risk patients who present to the emergency department with chest pain but without ECG changes or elevations of cardiac biomarkers (Chapters 51 and 72). The high negative-predictive value of CT angiography often can exclude important CHD and avoid the need for other testing in this patient group, and randomized trials show that CT angiography in these patients allows earlier discharge from the emergency department without any increased risk. A1 A2

CT angiography also may be useful in patients with equivocal or nondiagnostic stress testing or new-onset heart failure. The extent and severity of coronary disease found at CT angiography correlate with subsequent all-cause mortality in a similar fashion to catheter-based coronary angiography. In asymptomatic patients, however, CT angiography does not improve risk stratification over calcium scoring.

Other Cardiac Applications

The same data acquired by coronary CT angiography can be reformatted and used for functional cardiac imaging, including measurement of LV volumes, ejection fraction, wall thickness, and global and segmental wall motion. In acute and chronic myocardial infarction, contrast-enhanced CT can demonstrate late enhancement in a manner similar to cardiovascular magnetic resonance imaging (CMR), albeit with a significantly lower signal and contrast-to-noise ratio. CT angiography can complement echocardiography to evaluate cardiac anatomy in patients with congenital heart disease, especially in patients with contraindications to CMR. CT can evaluate pericardial thickness and calcification in patients with suspected constrictive pericarditis (see Fig. 77-10) and can evaluate native and prosthetic valvular

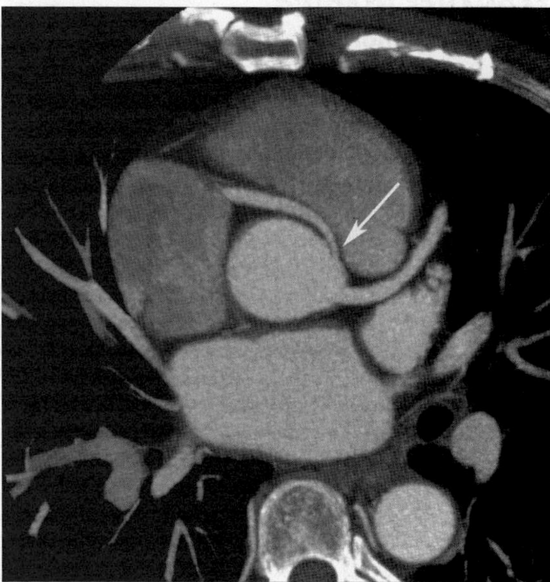

FIGURE 56-11. Contrast-enhanced computed tomographic angiogram in a young patient with chest pain and an anomalous right coronary artery (RCA). The RCA originates with a slitlike origin from the left coronary cusp *(arrow)* and passes anteriorly between the aorta and right ventricular outflow tract. The left main coronary artery originates normally from the left cusp.

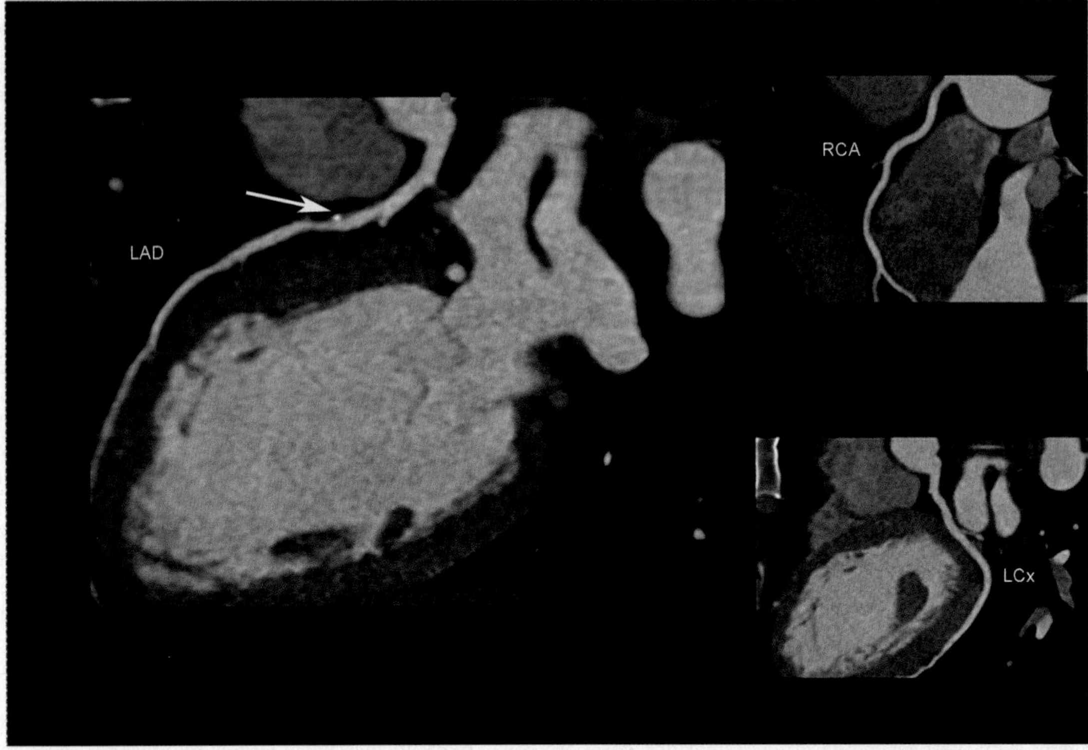

FIGURE 56-12. Contrast-enhanced computed tomographic coronary angiogram obtained on a dual-source 64-detector scanner in a patient with atypical chest pain. The left anterior descending (LAD) artery has a nonobstructive lesion *(arrow)* containing both noncalcified (soft) plaque, which appears dark, and a focal area of calcification. The right coronary artery (RCA) and left circumflex coronary artery (LCx) are normal.

structures (Fig. 56-14) and cardiac masses when imaging with other modalities is inadequate.

CT angiography is often used to image the left atrium and pulmonary venous anatomy for preprocedural planning for pulmonary vein ablation for atrial fibrillation (Chapter 66) or for post-procedural assessment of the possible complication of pulmonary vein stenosis (Fig. 56-15). Cardiac venous anatomy may be imaged to aid in the implantation of LV pacemakers in the cardiac venous system for biventricular pacing for heart failure (Chapters 59 and 66).

CARDIOVASCULAR MAGNETIC RESONANCE IMAGING

Indications, Contraindications, and Pulse Sequences

CMR is a versatile and flexible imaging modality that can be applied in diverse cardiovascular conditions,[8] especially using newer 1.5- or 3-Tesla (T) scanners. Advantages of CMR include the lack of ionizing radiation, the variety of tissues that can be characterized, and the ability to image the heart in any arbitrary plane. Images typically are obtained using ECG gating and breath-hold techniques.

In addition to general restrictions regarding magnetic resonance (e.g., certain intracranial aneurysm clips, transcutaneous electrical nerve stimulation units, intra-auricular implants), patients with cardiac pacemakers and implantable cardioverter-defibrillators generally should *not* undergo CMR because of safety concerns. Newer pacemaker systems under development may be compatible with magnetic resonance imaging. In addition, some non-pacemaker-dependent patients with newer pacemaker and defibrillator models have been scanned safely under controlled conditions, with close monitoring and then testing and reprogramming of the device after the procedure. CMR is safe for all prosthetic heart valves, although image distortions immediately around the prosthesis may obscure nearby pathology. CMR is safe for patients with intracoronary stents. Gadolinium-based contrast agents are contraindicated in patients with a glomerular filtration rate of less than 30 mL/minute/1.83 m^2, owing to their association with nephrogenic systemic fibrosis (Chapter 267).

A comprehensive CMR study includes evaluation of cardiac structure, function, tissue characteristics, perfusion, and scarring or fibrosis. CMR is highly accurate for the noninvasive quantitative assessment of LV and RV volumes and ejection fraction. The components of the examination are tailored to the particular diagnostic question at hand.

Specific Clinical Applications

CORONARY ARTERY DISEASE

For detection of myocardial ischemia, first-pass gadolinium perfusion imaging during vasodilator stress with adenosine or regadenoson shows defects, generally in the subendocardium, that persist for at least five heartbeats during the first pass of contrast (Fig. 56-16). Imaging is often repeated at rest after approximately 10 minutes to be sure any defect seen with stress was not either artifactual or caused by an infarct (the latter is excluded in combination with late gadolinium enhancement). Head-to-head comparisons of vasodilator stress perfusion CMR and dobutamine stress CMR suggest a higher sensitivity for contrast-enhanced perfusion imaging and higher specificity for dobutamine wall motion imaging. CMR stress testing is more accurate than SPECT[9] and is a strong predictor of cardiac events and survival. Coronary CT angiography has superior spatial resolution and accuracy compared with CMR for imaging of the coronary arteries, but CMR coronary imaging is useful for the diagnosis of anomalous coronary arteries.

CMR with late gadolinium enhancement is the gold standard technique for assessment of myocardial scar caused by myocardial infarction, with a better accuracy than nuclear imaging approaches, especially for smaller non–Q wave infarctions (Fig. 56-17). In acute myocardial infarction, CMR T2-weighted techniques can assess the myocardium at risk and estimate the amount of salvaged myocardium owing to reperfusion. Areas of low signal in the subendocardial core of the infarction represent regions of microvascular obstruction with severe capillary destruction and are a marker of subsequent adverse LV remodeling and poorer outcome. To assess myocardial viability in patients with chronic CHD, CMR with late gadolinium enhancement has the best sensitivity for recovery of function with revascularization, but low-dose dobutamine contractile reserve has better specificity.

CARDIOMYOPATHIES

CMR is often used to identify the underlying etiology of cardiomyopathies (Chapter 60). In patients who present in acute heart failure or with chest pain, elevated troponin levels, but a negative coronary arteriogram, CMR is ideally suited to identify myocarditis (Chapter 60) (Fig. 56-18). In patients

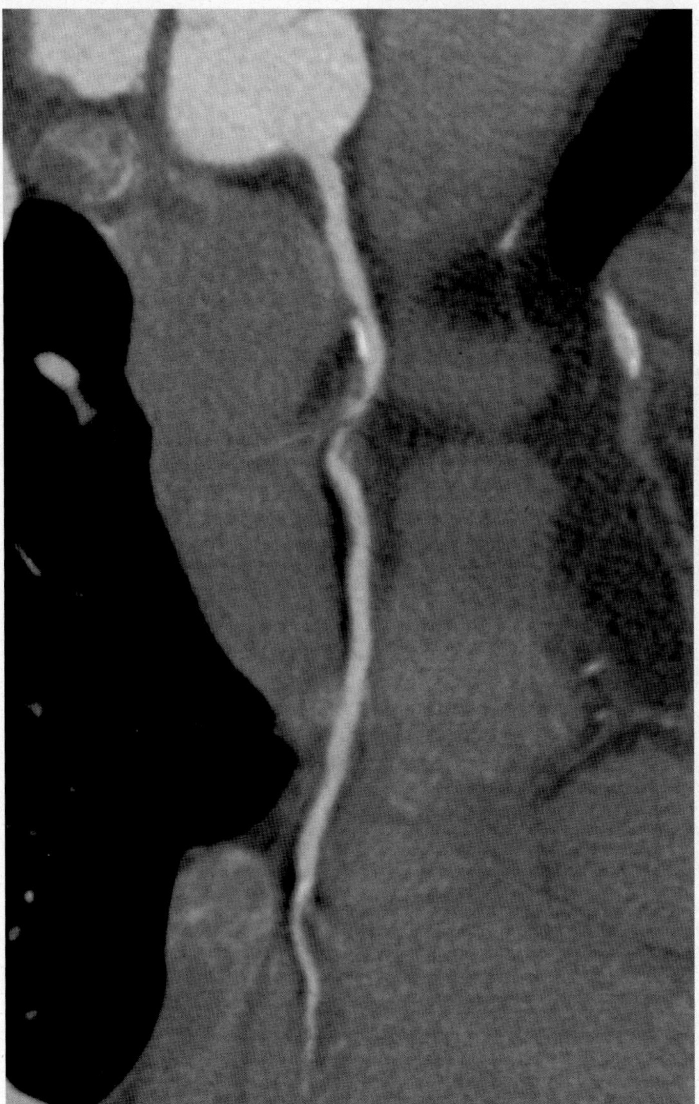

FIGURE 56-13. Contrast-enhanced computed tomographic coronary angiogram of the left anterior descending artery (LAD) in a 54-year-old man who presented to an emergency department with risk factors but atypical chest pain. The mid LAD demonstrates mixed obstructive plaque with calcified and noncalcified components.

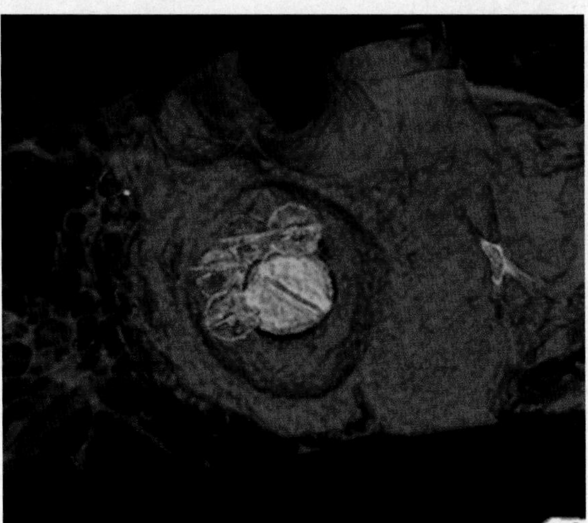

FIGURE 56-14. Three-dimensional reconstruction of a computed tomographic angiogram in a patient with a St. Jude's mechanical mitral valve with a paravalvular leak that has been closed with four Amplatzer devices.

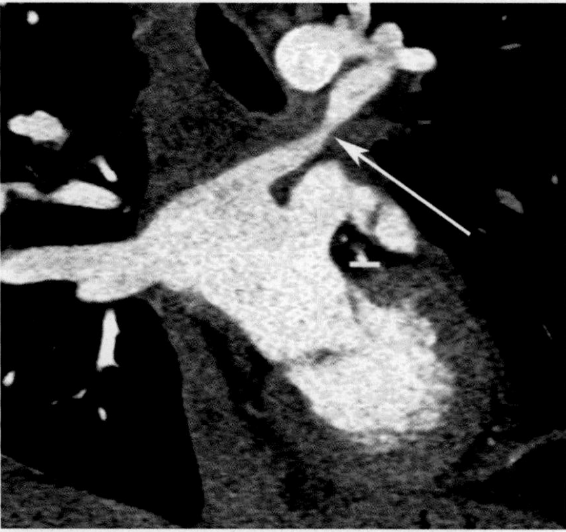

FIGURE 56-15. Contrast-enhanced computed tomographic coronary angiogram in a patient after pulmonary vein ablation for atrial fibrillation demonstrating stenosis of the left upper pulmonary vein toward its origin *(arrow)* relative to the more distal vessel.

with hypertrophic cardiomyopathy (Chapter 60), CMR is more sensitive than echocardiography for identifying increased regional wall thickness and can demonstrate late gadolinium enhancement (Fig. 56-19). Cardiac amyloidosis (Chapters 60 and 188) can be seen as diffuse subendocardial or patchy enhancement, or simply difficulty in nulling normal myocardium. A new noncontrast method entitled native T1 mapping can identify amyloidosis and other cardiomyopathies by measuring elevated T1 values in the myocardium. Patchy fibrosis is readily identified in cardiac sarcoidosis (Chapters 60 and 95) (Fig. 56-20) and is more sensitive than endomyocardial biopsy. The finding of fibrosis by late gadolinium enhancement in almost any form of heart disease is associated with adverse prognosis compared with those without fibrosis.[10]

CMR is often used in the diagnosis of arrhythmogenic right ventricular cardiomyopathy (Fig. 56-21; Chapters 60 and 65), which is characterized by global RV dilation and regional RV akinesis or dyskinesis. Late gadolinium enhancement sometimes may be seen but can be difficult to identify in the thin-walled right ventricle. Fat is a nonspecific finding. In iron overload conditions such as thalassemia (Chapter 162), multi-echo T1-weighted imaging of T2* can identify the extent of iron overload and can be used to follow effects of chelation therapy. Rarer causes of cardiomyopathy, such as ventricular noncompaction, Chagas disease (Chapters 60 and 347), and Takotsubo cardiomyopathy (Chapter 60), also have characteristic CMR findings.

AORTIC DISEASE, PERICARDIAL DISEASE, AND MASSES

CMR is an excellent test to image aneurysms but is a second-line test to detect acute aortic dissection (see Fig. 78-6) or intraluminal aortic hematoma (see Fig. 78-7) in stable patients. CMR is also an excellent test for the evaluation of chronic pericardial disease (Fig. 56-22) because it accurately identifies pericardial thickness as well as adherence of the pericardium to the epicardium in constrictive pericarditis. Real-time imaging can demonstrate ventricular interdependence, a hallmark of this disease. CMR is also an ideal tool to diagnose intracardiac (Fig. 56-23) and extracardiac masses such as myxomas, thrombus, and tumors (Chapter 60), owing to its high spatial resolution and ability to perform tissue characterization.

CONGENITAL HEART DISEASE

CMR is useful for the assessment of both simple and complex congenital heart disease and is often used as an adjunct to echocardiography (Chapter 69). For example, phase velocity CMR readily quantifies blood flow through the major blood vessels, thereby facilitating accurate assessment of the ratio of pulmonary to systemic blood flow in atrial or ventricular septal defects. CMR is particularly valuable for assessing abnormalities of the great vessels, such as aortic coarctation (Fig. 56-24), extracardiac anatomy, or anomalous pulmonary venous drainage, and in patients with complex congenital heart disease who have undergone prior corrective or palliative shunt surgery, such as in tetralogy of Fallot or hypoplastic left heart syndrome. CMR is uniquely

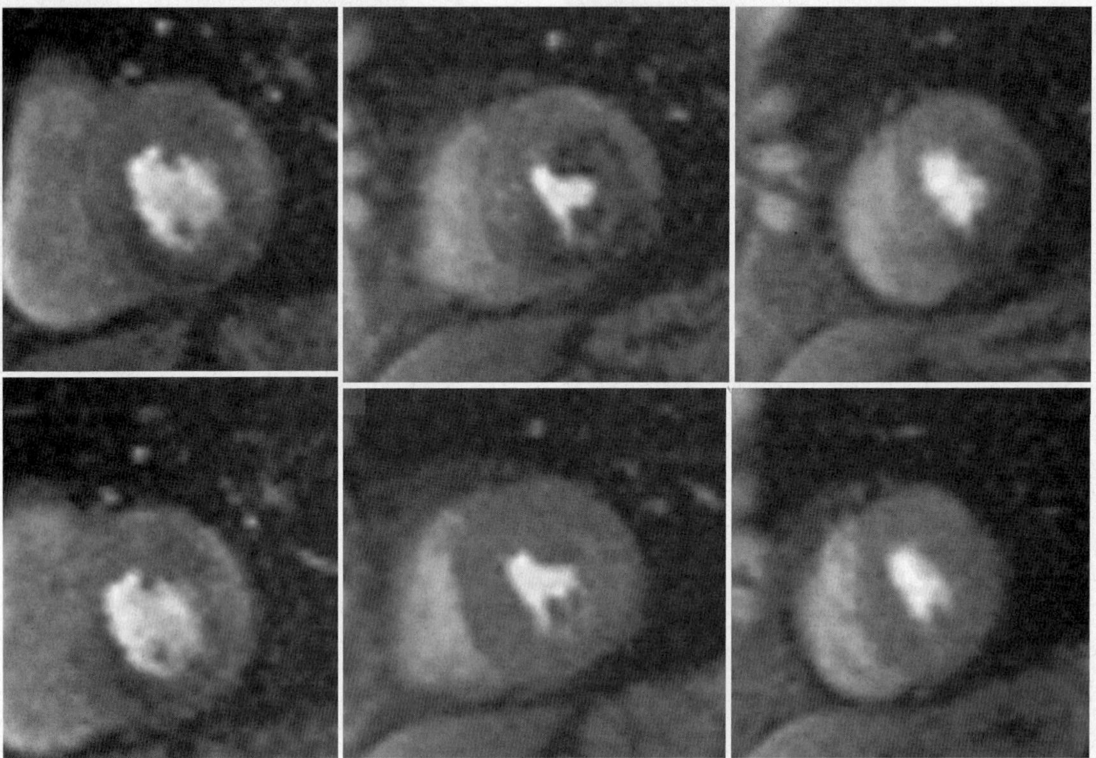

FIGURE 56-16. Set of first-pass gadolinium-enhanced magnetic resonance perfusion images during adenosine stress *(top row)* and at rest *(bottom row)* at the base *(left)*, mid ventricle *(center)*, and apex *(right)*. The stress images demonstrate a large perfusion deficit in the anterolateral and inferolateral walls (from 1 o'clock to 7 o'clock), especially in the mid ventricle and apex, whereas the same regions appear normal at rest.

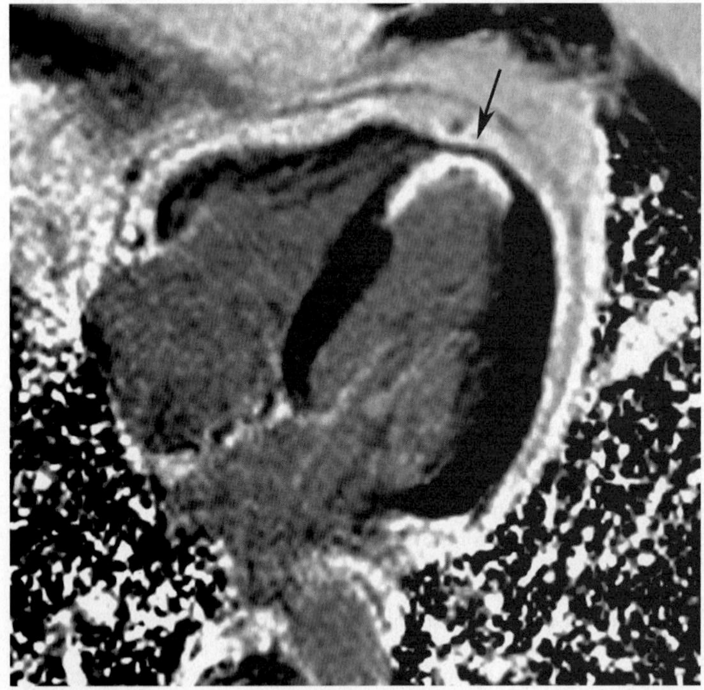

FIGURE 56-17. Late gadolinium-enhanced four-chamber long axis image in a patient with a scar *(arrow)* from a prior anterior myocardial infarction.

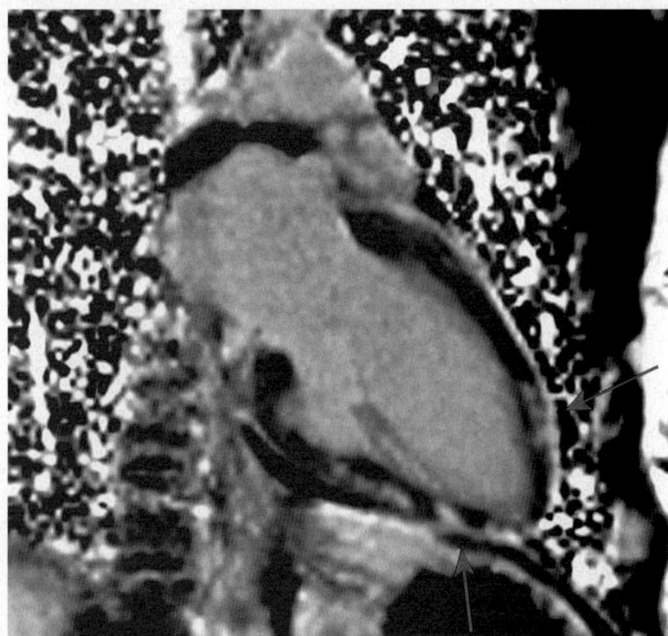

FIGURE 56-18. Gadolinium-enhanced image in a 22-year-old man shows patchy subepicardial enhancement *(arrows)*, characteristic of acute myocarditis.

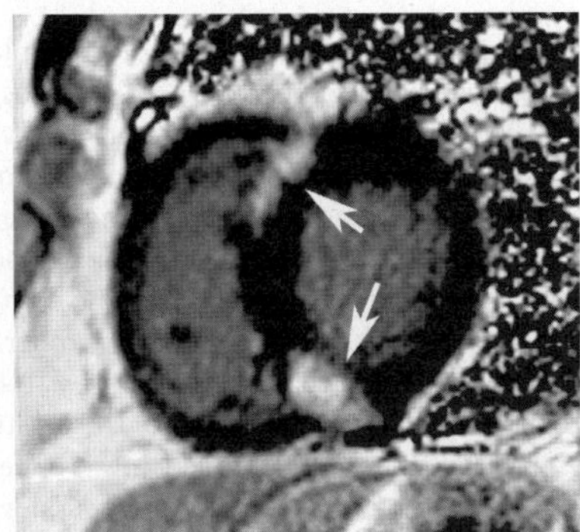

FIGURE 56-19. Late gadolinium-enhanced magnetic resonance short axis image of a 35-year-old man with hypertrophic cardiomyopathy demonstrates a classic pattern of enhancement, which identifies fibrosis *(arrows)*, in the right ventricular insertion sites.

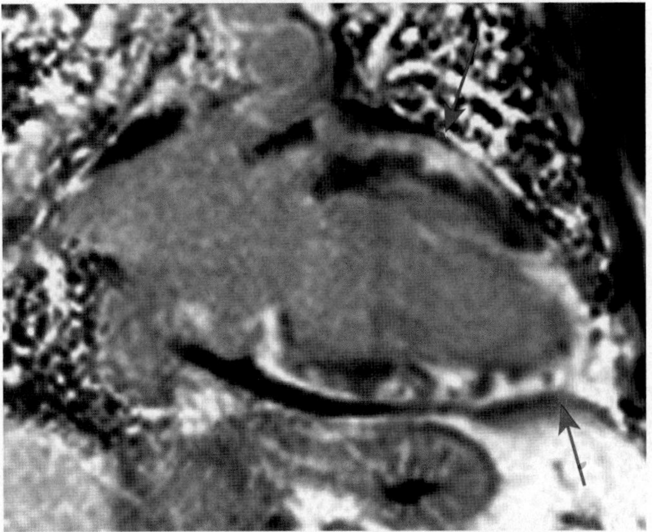

FIGURE 56-20. Late gadolinium-enhanced magnetic resonance image in a 47-year-old man with heart failure, heart block, and hilar lymphadenopathy shows patchy late gadolinium enhancement in a noncoronary distribution, including subepicardial anterior wall enhancement *(upper arrow)* and near transmural apical enhancement *(lower arrow)* consistent with myocardial sarcoidosis.

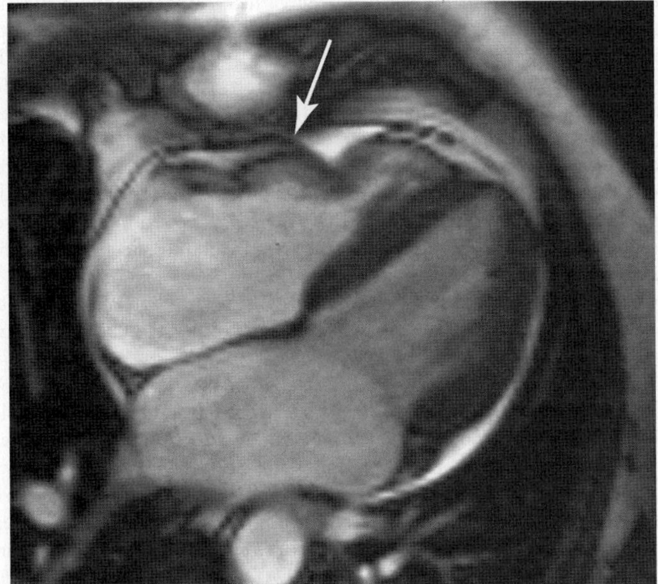

FIGURE 56-21. Magnetic resonance image in a 27-year-old woman with arrhythmogenic right ventricular cardiomyopathy demonstrates regional right ventricular (RV) systolic dysfunction, which is the hallmark of the disease. The *arrow* points to a region of RV dyskinesis at end systole, and the RV appears like an accordion at end systole.

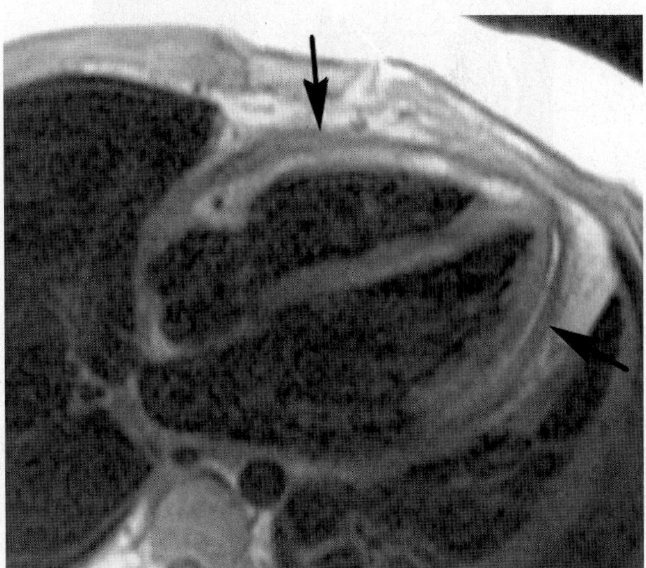

FIGURE 56-22. Magnetic resonance image of a 35-year-old man with dyspnea many years after mantle radiation for Hodgkin lymphoma shows a thickened pericardium *(arrows)* circumferentially around the left and right ventricles.

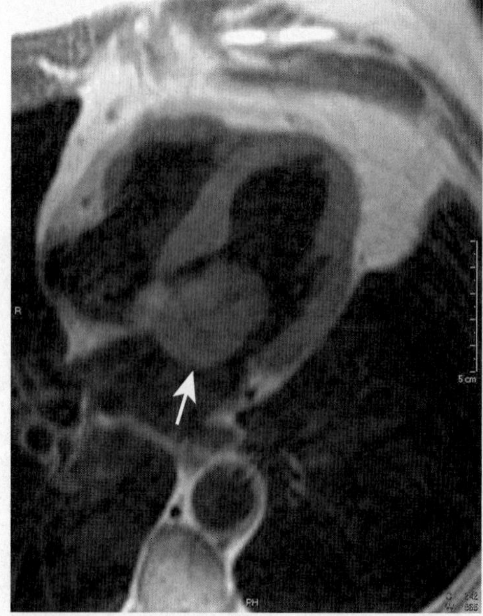

FIGURE 56-23. Diastolic magnetic resonance image of a large left atrial myxoma *(arrow)* showing that it is attached to the atrial septum and is prolapsing across the mitral valve.

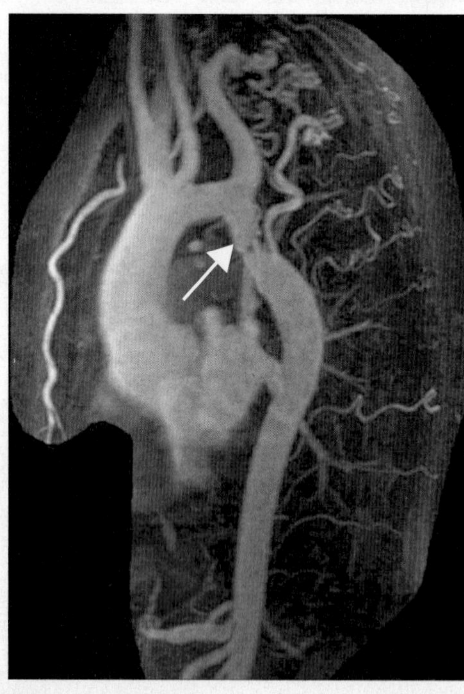

FIGURE 56-24. Three-dimensional contrast-enhanced magnetic resonance angiogram in a patient with an aortic coarctation *(arrow)*.

able to measure right ventricular volumes accurately, an often important determination in this setting.

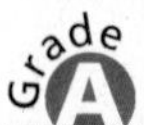

Grade A References

A1. Litt HI, Gatsonis C, Snyder B, et al. CT angiography for safe discharge of patients with possible acute coronary syndromes. *N Engl J Med.* 2012;366:1393-1403.

A2. Hoffmann U, Truong QA, Schoenfeld DA, et al. Coronary CT angiography versus standard evaluation in acute chest pain. *N Engl J Med.* 2012;367:299-308.

GENERAL REFERENCES

For the General References and other additional features, please visit Expert Consult at https://expertconsult.inkling.com.

57

CATHETERIZATION AND ANGIOGRAPHY

MORTON KERN

Cardiac catheterization is insertion and passage of small plastic tubes (catheters) into arteries and veins to the heart to obtain radiographic images of coronary arteries and cardiac chambers (angiography and ventriculography) and to measure pressures in the heart (hemodynamics). Coronary angiography defines the site, severity, and morphology of atherosclerotic lesions, and it identifies collateral blood supply beyond occluded vessel segments. Cardiac catheterization is used not only to diagnose coronary artery, valvular (Chapter 75), and myocardial diseases (Chapter 60) but also to perform therapeutic (interventional) procedures to relieve obstructing arterial stenoses (Chapter 74), to open or replace narrowed valves, or to close intracardiac defects (Chapter 69) through catheter-based, minimally invasive percutaneous techniques. These same diagnostic and therapeutic techniques are also used in the peripheral arterial circulation in a modified fashion to address carotid, renal, and peripheral vascular disease (Chapters 79 and 80), aortic aneurysms (Chapter 78), and vascular shunts (Table 57-1).

INDICATIONS FOR AND CONTRAINDICATIONS TO CARDIAC CATHETERIZATION

The indications to perform cardiac catheterization include the need to diagnose atherosclerotic coronary artery disease, abnormalities of cardiac muscle function, valvular abnormalities, and congenital heart disease (Table 57-2).[1] Contraindications to cardiac catheterization are few. Absolute contraindications involve only inadequate facilities or equipment for catheterization. Relative contraindications depend on the urgency of the procedure and conditions.

TECHNIQUE OF CATHETERIZATION

After the procedure and its indications, risks, and benefits are explained to the patient, the patient is placed on the cardiac catheterization table and centered under the C-arm of the radiographic gantry (E-Fig. 57-1). After sterile preparation and draping, local anesthetic is administered over the vascular access site—commonly the femoral artery but increasingly the radial artery, which is associated with better outcomes in patients with ST segment elevation myocardial infarction.[A1,A2] The artery is punctured, and a vascular sheath is inserted, through which the angiographic catheter is advanced over a soft spring-tipped 0.035-inch guidewire that permits safe, atraumatic passage of the catheter to the heart. The specially shaped catheters are seated and connected to a manifold to measure pressure and to inject radiographic contrast media.

Coronary arteriography records the images from multiple angles by rotation of the C-arm. The images are displayed and preserved on digital imaging systems.

After coronary angiography, the catheter is exchanged for a ventriculography catheter that is inserted into the left ventricle. After left ventricular (LV) pressure is measured, radiographic contrast medium (approximately 25 to 45 mL) is injected under high pressure (1000 psi) to assess LV wall motion, chamber size, presence of mitral valve regurgitation, and shape of the aortic root. The LV ejection fraction (normal is 50 to 70%), a measure of the heart function, is computed as a percentage of the diastolic volume ejected.

After diagnostic angiography is completed, the need for coronary revascularization (Chapter 74) is assessed. If suitable symptomatic coronary artery obstructions are present, percutaneous coronary intervention (PCI) may be performed at the same time if it was discussed with the patient and consented to in advance. Alternatively, the patient may be referred for later PCI or for coronary artery bypass graft surgery.

At the conclusion of the catheterization procedure, the catheters are removed. For the femoral artery, hemostasis is achieved either by manual compression, which requires the patient to remain stationary in bed for 4 hours, or by use of a vascular closure device while the patient remains in bed for 1 to 2 hours. For the radial approach, the arterial sheath is removed with the simple application of a specialized compression wrist band; the patient can ambulate immediately thereafter.

TABLE 57-1 PROCEDURES THAT MAY ACCOMPANY CORONARY ANGIOGRAPHY

PROCEDURE	COMMENTS
Central venous access: femoral, internal jugular, subclavian	Uses IV access for emergency medications or fluids, temporary pacemaker; pacemaker not mandatory for most coronary angiography
Hemodynamic assessment, left-sided heart pressures, aorta, and left ventricle	Routine for all studies
Right- and left-sided heart combined pressures	Not routine for coronary artery disease but mandatory for valvular heart disease and routine for heart failure, right ventricular dysfunction, pericardial disease, cardiomyopathy, intracardiac shunts, and congenital abnormalities
Left ventriculography	Routine for all studies; may be excluded with high-risk patients and those with left main coronary or aortic stenosis, severe congestive heart failure, or renal failure
Internal mammary and saphenous vein graft angiography	Routine for coronary bypass conduit
Pharmacologic studies: Assessment of coronary spasm (use of ergonovine or acetylcholine conducted in specialized centers for research only) Use of vasodilators	Conducted routinely for coronary angiography with nitroglycerin (for coronary spasm) Nitric oxide used for pulmonary hypertension
Aortography	Routine for aortic insufficiency, aortic dissection, and aneurysm and may be performed in patients with aortic stenosis; routine to locate bypass graft conduits not visualized by selective angiography
Cardiac pacing electrophysiologic studies	Arrhythmia evaluation
Interventional and special techniques	Percutaneous coronary intervention: includes balloon angioplasty, bare metal or drug-eluting stent, and rotational coronary atherectomy Assessment of fractional flow reserve to assess the functional severity of a coronary stenosis Balloon catheter valvuloplasty; transcatheter aortic valve replacement; myocardial biopsy; atrial septal defect or patent foramen ovale defect closure; transseptal puncture to assess valvular heart disease; electrophysiologic catheter ablation
Vascular closure devices	Routinely available for patients prone to femoral artery access bleeding

Modified from Kern MJ, ed. The Interventional Cardiac Catheterization Handbook. 3rd ed. Philadelphia: Elsevier; 2012.

COMPLICATIONS OF CARDIAC CATHETERIZATION

For diagnostic cardiac catheterization, risks are less than 0.2% for death, less than 0.5% for myocardial infarction, less than 0.07% for stroke, less than 0.5% for serious arrhythmia, and less than 1% for major vascular complications, including thrombosis and bleeding requiring transfusion or pseudoaneurysm (Table 57-3). Vascular complications occur more frequently with the femoral artery approach than with the radial artery approach; the brachial artery approach, which is used only when neither femoral nor radial access is possible, has the highest rate of vascular complications, and the radial artery has the lowest.

Patients are not routinely anticoagulated for a diagnostic catheterization, and special preparations must be made for patients who are receiving anticoagulants, patients who have diabetes or renal insufficiency, and patients who may have a potential allergy to radiographic contrast media. For the anticoagulated patient, provisions to withhold warfarin or heparin must be made to reduce the potential for femoral puncture site bleeding complications (e.g., retroperitoneal hematoma or pseudoaneurysm). For example, a patient taking warfarin after an aortic valve replacement would have the warfarin withheld for about 3 days before the catheterization, the international normalized ratio would be monitored, and the patient might be administered bridging heparin to the time of the procedure; warfarin would be restarted after the procedure.

For elective catheterizations in patients with insulin-dependent diabetes, half of the usual morning dose of insulin generally is given the morning of the procedure to provide reasonable diabetic coverage and to avoid hypoglycemia. Metformin should be withheld before the study. Medications for hypertension and other medical conditions are continued up to and including the morning of the procedure.

Contrast-induced nephropathy, which generally becomes clinically apparent 2 to 3 days after the catheterization, is uncommon. Patients with diabetes or renal insufficiency and patients who are dehydrated from any cause are at a three- to five-fold increased risk for contrast-induced renal failure. For

TABLE 57-2 INDICATIONS FOR AND CONTRAINDICATIONS TO CARDIAC CATHETERIZATION

INDICATIONS

Identification of the extent and severity of coronary artery disease and evaluation of left ventricular function
Assessment of the severity of valvular or myocardial disorders, such as aortic stenosis or insufficiency, mitral stenosis or insufficiency, and various cardiomyopathies, to determine the need for surgical correction
Collection of data to confirm and to complement noninvasive studies
Determination of the presence of coronary artery disease in patients with confusing clinical presentations or chest pain of uncertain origin

ABSOLUTE CONTRAINDICATIONS

Inadequate facilities
Patient refusal

RELATIVE CONTRAINDICATIONS

Severe uncontrolled hypertension
Ventricular arrhythmias
Recent acute stroke
Severe anemia
Active gastrointestinal bleeding
Allergy to radiographic contrast agents
Acute renal failure
Uncompensated congestive failure (patient cannot lie flat)
Unexplained febrile illness or untreated active infection
Electrolyte abnormalities (e.g., hypokalemia)
Severe coagulopathy
Pregnancy
Uncontrolled arrhythmias, hypertension
Uncooperative patient or patient refusal

TABLE 57-3 COMPLICATIONS OF CARDIAC CATHETERIZATION

MAJOR COMPLICATIONS

Death
Cerebrovascular accident
Myocardial infarction, shock
Ventricular tachycardia or fibrillation

RARE BUT SERIOUS COMPLICATIONS

Aortic dissection
Cardiac perforation
Tamponade
Heart failure
Reaction to contrast agents, anaphylaxis
Nephrotoxicity
Arrhythmias, including heart block, asystole, supraventricular tachyarrhythmias
Hemorrhage, including local or retroperitoneal
Infection
Protamine reaction
Vascular complications, including thrombosis, embolus, vascular injury, pseudoaneurysm

patients with renal insufficiency and those at high risk for contrast-induced renal failure because of diabetes or dehydration, hydration with sodium chloride is recommended to increase urine output.[A3] Treatment with *N*-acetylcysteine (Mucomyst) is no longer recommended to prevent contrast nephropathy.[A4] Recent data suggest a benefit from oral rosuvastatin, either 40 mg on admission followed by 20 mg per day for patients with an acute coronary syndrome[A5] or 10 mg for two days before and three days afterwards for patients with diabetes and chronic kidney disease.[A6]

Contrast media reactions are rare, with an overall incidence of 5% or less, but potentially serious. Adverse reactions occur in 10 to 12% of patients with a history of allergy and in 15% of patients with reported reaction on a previous contrast radiographic examination. There are three types of allergies to contrast media: cutaneous and mucosal manifestations, smooth muscle and minor anaphylactoid responses, and cardiovascular and major anaphylactoid responses involving laryngeal or pulmonary edema. Pretreatment with corticosteroids is helpful in reducing all types of reactions except urticaria. Patients reporting previous allergic reactions to contrast media should be premedicated with prednisone (60 mg orally the evening before and morning of the procedure) and diphenhydramine (25 to 50 mg orally the morning of the procedure). Patients with known prior anaphylactoid reactions should be pretreated with steroids in the same dose. Routine treatment with a histamine$_2$-receptor blocker (e.g., cimetidine) does not appear to have any benefit.

Hypotension during and after cardiac catheterization may occur from a vasovagal response, occult retroperitoneal bleeding, myocardial ischemia or infarction, or cardiac tamponade. Vasovagal hypotension is treated with volume and atropine (0.5 to 1.0 mg intravenously). Hypotension with back pain suggests retroperitoneal hematoma. Hypotension due to cardiac tamponade, which may occur during or after PCI, requires rapid diagnosis, reversal of anticoagulation, and urgent pericardiocentesis (Chapter 77).

Pulmonary congestion may develop in patients with marginal LV function or critical valvular heart disease. Congestion compromising respiratory and hemodynamic function is an emergency treated with oxygen, diuretics, nitroglycerin, inotropic agents, intubation, and intra-aortic balloon pumping as indicated (Chapter 107).

Chest pain during coronary angiography is unusual, but myocardial ischemia with pain and ST segment changes may occur during PCI (Chapter 74). Treatment with nitroglycerin, heparin, and antiplatelet medications usually controls myocardial ischemia before revascularization (Chapter 72). Minor arrhythmias (e.g., atrial or ventricular premature beats, brief episodes of supraventricular tachycardia) are common and usually resolve without treatment. Ventricular tachycardia or fibrillation is a rare occurrence but requires prompt defibrillation (Chapter 63).

HEMODYNAMIC DATA OBTAINED DURING CARDIAC CATHETERIZATION

Hemodynamic data are the recordings of the pressure and flow signals generated by the heart during the catheterization procedure.[2] A pressure wave is created by cardiac muscle contraction and is transmitted through the arterial circuit (Fig. 57-1). The pressure waves are measured by the fluid-filled catheters with a pressure transducer, which converts the mechanical pressure to an electrical signal that is displayed on a video monitor.

Simultaneous pressure measurements across the heart valves are used to diagnose valve function. In addition to pressure measurements, hemodynamic data also include analysis of multiple blood oxygen saturations sampled throughout the right and left sides of the heart to identify possible intracardiac shunting. Cardiac output is commonly measured by a thermodilution technique but can also be computed by knowing oxygen consumption and comparing systemic arterial oxygenation content to pulmonary arterial oxygen content by the Fick equation. Hemodynamic data permit calculation of vascular and pulmonary resistances and cardiac valve areas (see Table 53-1). Complete hemodynamic data requiring catheterization of the right and left sides of the heart are indicated to evaluate dyspnea of any cause; to confirm echocardiographic findings when data are not concordant with clinical or other testing results; and to determine the status of valvular heart disease, cardiomyopathy, and constrictive or restrictive cardiac physiology.

Complications of right-sided heart catheterization are rare. The most common problem is transient arrhythmia resulting from mechanical stimulation by the catheter as it passes through the right ventricular outflow tract. In patients with left bundle branch block, a temporary pacemaker may be needed if right bundle branch block occurs during right-sided heart catheterization.

Examples of Hemodynamics for Valvular Heart Disease

The severity of a valvular stenosis is based on the pressure gradient and flow across the valve. In patients with suspected aortic stenosis, a transvalvular pressure gradient should be obtained whenever there is conflicting clinical or echocardiographic data. Although the pressure recordings needed to assess the aortic valve gradient can be obtained with a catheter in the left ventricle and the side arm of the sheath in the femoral artery, more accurate recordings can be obtained with a dual-lumen pigtail catheter (Fig. 57-2). The normal aortic valve area is 2.5 to 3.5 cm^2 in adults. Severe aortic valve stenosis is associated with valve areas smaller than 1.0 cm^2.

In patients with mitral stenosis, the valve gradient often is measured with the LV and pulmonary capillary wedge pressures. The most accurate method to compute the mitral stenosis gradient uses the left atrial (obtained by transseptal puncture) and LV pressures (Fig. 57-3). The normal mitral valve area is 4 to 6 cm^2. Valve areas smaller than 1.0 to 1.2 cm^2 are considered severe mitral stenosis.

In patients with mitral regurgitation, the hemodynamics often show a characteristic large *v* wave on the pulmonary capillary wedge tracing

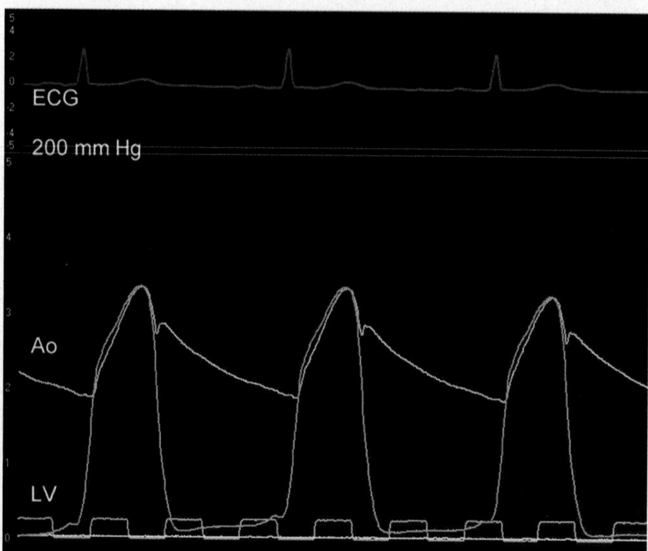

FIGURE 57-1. Normal left ventricular (LV) and aortic (Ao) pressures measured with a high-fidelity dual-transducer catheter.

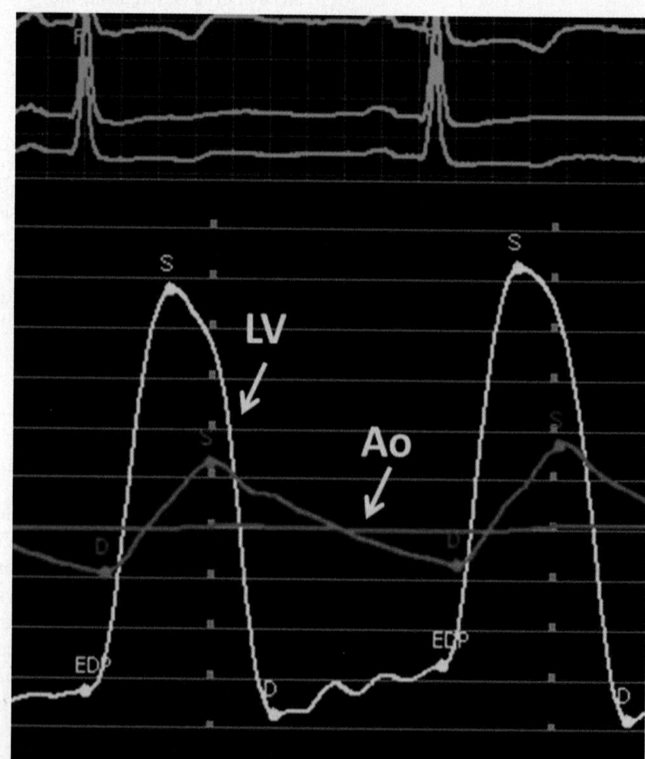

FIGURE 57-2. **Hemodynamics of aortic stenosis.** Aortic (Ao) and left ventricular (LV) pressure in patient with aortic stenosis measured with single dual-lumen catheter. Note delay in aortic pressure relative to left ventricular pressure. D = earliest point of diastolic LV pressure; EDP = end-diastolic pressure; S = peak LV pressure (systole).

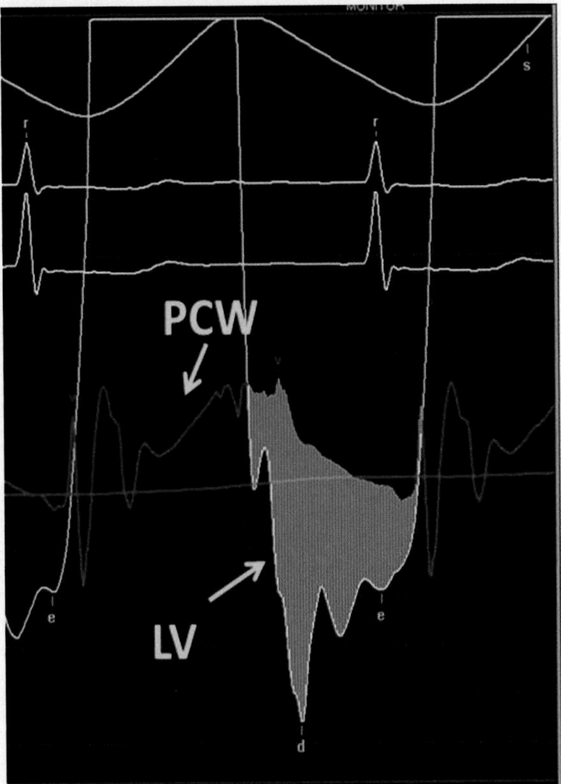

FIGURE 57-3. **Mitral stenosis. The difference between the pulmonary capillary wedge (PCW) pressure and the left ventricular (LV) pressure during diastole defines the gradient in mitral valve stenosis.**

(E-Fig. 57-2). During left ventriculography, the angiographic grading of mitral regurgitation is on a semiquantitative severity scale of 1 to 4 based on the amount of contrast material seen passing backward from the left ventricle through the incompetent mitral valve into the left atrium. Grade 1 angiographic mitral regurgitation demonstrates a brief puff of contrast material filling the left atrium and emptying immediately; grade 2 shows contrast material filling the left atrium on three beats with moderate density; grade 3 shows contrast material filling immediately and moderate density persisting for two or three beats; and grade 4 shows contrast material filling the entire left atrium, often including the appendage, with a density equal to that of the left ventricle for several beats after injection.

CORONARY ANGIOGRAPHY

Coronary angiography visualizes the epicardial arteries, branches, collaterals, and anomalies to diagnose and to treat patients with coronary artery disease (Fig. 57-4). In anticipation of PCI, the angiogram documents not only the presence and location of stenoses but also proximity to major and minor side branches, luminal abnormalities (e.g., thrombi), areas of calcification, and collateral supply, which will influence the decision and techniques used for revascularization. For the two-dimensional radiographic images to depict the three-dimensional coronary tree, multiple angulations of the radiographic imaging system are required.

Assessment of Coronary Stenoses

The degree of a stenosis is most often reported as the estimated percentage diameter luminal reduction of the most severely narrowed segment compared with the adjacent angiographically "normal" or unobstructed vessel segment, seen in the worst radiographic projection (Fig. 57-5). Because the operator uses visual estimations, an exact evaluation is impossible with less than 20% variation between readings of two or more experienced angiographers. The severity of a stenosis alone should not always be assumed to be associated with abnormal physiology (flow) and ischemia. Moreover, because coronary artery disease is a diffuse process, minimal luminal irregularities on angiography may represent significant, albeit nonobstructive, coronary artery disease at the time of angiography. The precise physiologic impact or morphologic detail of stenosis can be made with specialized catheters and sensor-tipped guidewires. For example, intermediately severe lesions (40 to 70% narrowed) without prior evidence of ischemia can be assessed with a pressure sensor guidewire to measure the translesional pressure during maximal blood flow (e.g., hyperemia induced by adenosine). The ratio of coronary to aortic pressure measured at maximal flow, called the fractional flow reserve (FFR), represents the percentage of normal flow across the stenosis. Lesions with FFR values higher than 0.80 are considered nonischemic and do not require revascularization. Conversely, PCI may be justified for a lesion with an FFR lower than 0.80. After PCI is undertaken, the lesion's length, true diameter, eccentricity, and degree of calcium involvement can be determined by intravascular ultrasound catheter-based imaging or with reflected light by optical coherence tomography to depict intravascular anatomy and to guide subsequent PCI (Fig. 57-6). However, neither intravascular ultrasound nor optical coherence tomography can substitute for a functional determination of ischemia by FFR calculation. The degree of collateralization detected on angiography is also important. For example, stable coronary artery disease patients with a high degree of collateral vessels have a 36% lower mortality compared with patients with low collateralization.[3]

Coronary Artery Anomalies

Coronary artery anomalies may be present in patients with chest pain syndromes or in young individuals who have survived sudden death. The angiographic appearance of coronary anomalies is not always straightforward, and computed tomographic angiography (Chapter 56) has become the diagnostic modality best suited to delineate the origin and course of the anomaly (Fig. 57-7).

At the time of coronary angiography, the misdiagnosis of an unsuspected anomalous origin of a coronary artery is a potential problem. Because the natural history of a patient with an anomalous origin of a coronary artery may depend on the anatomic pathway of the anomalous vessel, it is important to define accurately the origin and course of the vessel. Even experienced angiographers may have difficulty in delineating the true course of some anomalous vessels.

The most critical coronary anomaly is when the left main coronary artery arises from the right cusp and traverses a course between the aorta and pulmonary artery. The artery's initial course through the aortic wall creates a narrow oval opening; with aortic stretch during exercise, coronary blood flow is limited.

Ventriculography

The left ventriculogram, an integral part of nearly every coronary angiographic study, provides information on the motion of the walls of the heart (Fig. 57-8), LV volumes during systole and diastole, LV ejection fraction, rate of ejection, quality of contractility, presence of hypertrophic myopathy, and mitral valvular regurgitation. The normal pattern of LV contraction is a coordinated, uniform, almost concentric inward motion of all points along the ventricular inner surface during systole. Uncoordinated contractions are named according to their severity (e.g., moderate or severe hypokinesis, akinesis, and aneurysm-dyskinesis). Focal abnormal wall motion indicates the presence of ischemia, infarction, or aneurysm.

ADDITIONAL PROCEDURES PERFORMED IN THE CATHETERIZATION LABORATORY

Noncardiac Angiography

Other cardiovascular angiographic studies that may accompany coronary angiography and left ventriculography include aortography (Chapter 78), pulmonary angiography (Chapter 98), and peripheral vascular angiography of iliac and lower extremity arteries (Chapters 79 and 80) or renal arteries (Chapter 125).

Electrophysiologic Studies and Ablation Techniques

An electrophysiologic study (EPS) is an invasive procedure that involves the placement of multipolar catheter electrodes at various intracardiac sites (Chapter 62). The general purposes of an EPS are to characterize the electrophysiologic properties of the conduction system, to induce and analyze the mechanism of arrhythmias, and to evaluate the effects of therapeutic interventions. Electrode catheters are routinely placed in the right atrium, across the tricuspid valve annulus in the area of the atrioventricular node and His bundle, in the right ventricle, in the coronary sinus, and sometimes in the left ventricle. EPS is routinely used in the clinical management of patients who have supraventricular and ventricular arrhythmias (Chapters 64 and 65).

Transseptal Heart Catheterization

Transseptal access by use of a long catheter with a needle to puncture the thin atrial septal membrane at the fossa ovalis permits placement of a catheter into

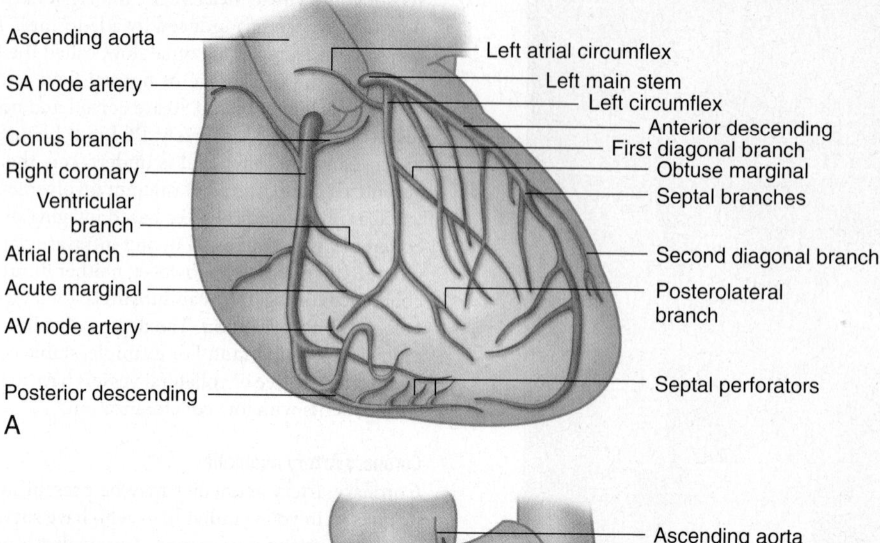

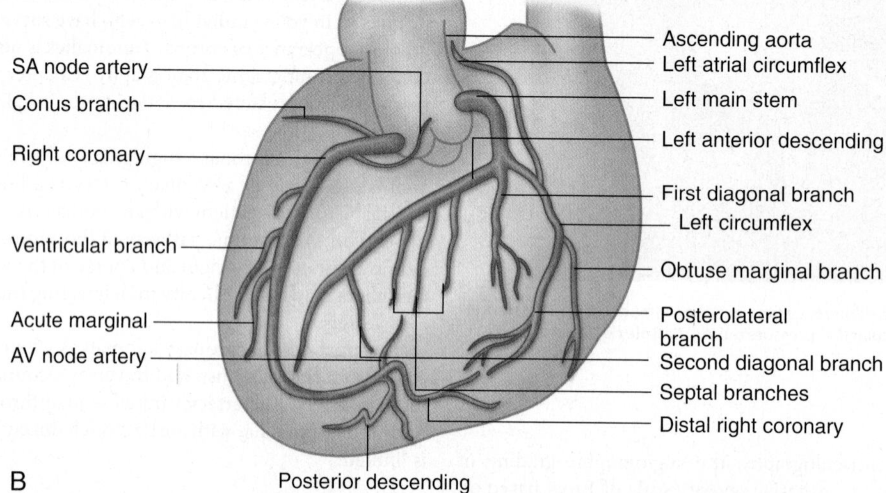

FIGURE 57-4. Coronary vessels. The right anterior oblique (A) and left anterior oblique (B) views are shown. The major arteries are the left main, left anterior descending, circumflex, and right coronary arteries. AV = atrioventricular; SA = sinoatrial. (Modified from Yang SS, Bentivoglio LG, Maranhao V, et al, eds. From Cardiac Catheterization Data to Hemodynamic Parameters. Philadelphia: Oxford University Press; 1988.)

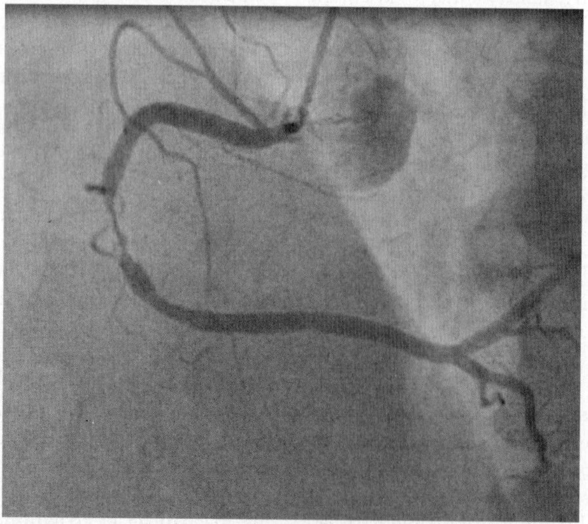

FIGURE 57-5. Example of a significant stenosis in the right coronary artery.

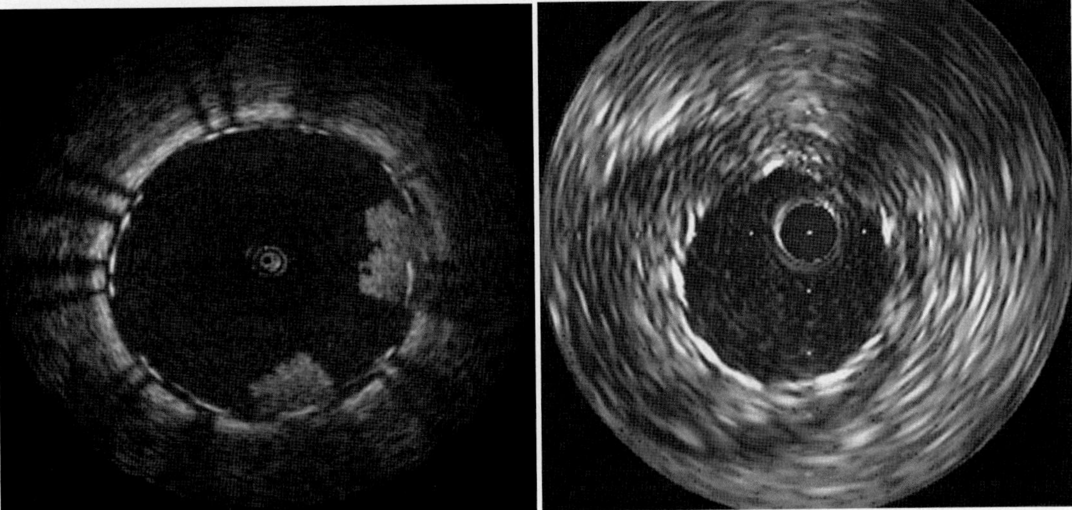

FIGURE 57-6. Cross-sectional image within a coronary artery by intravascular ultrasound (*right*) and optical coherence tomography (*left*).

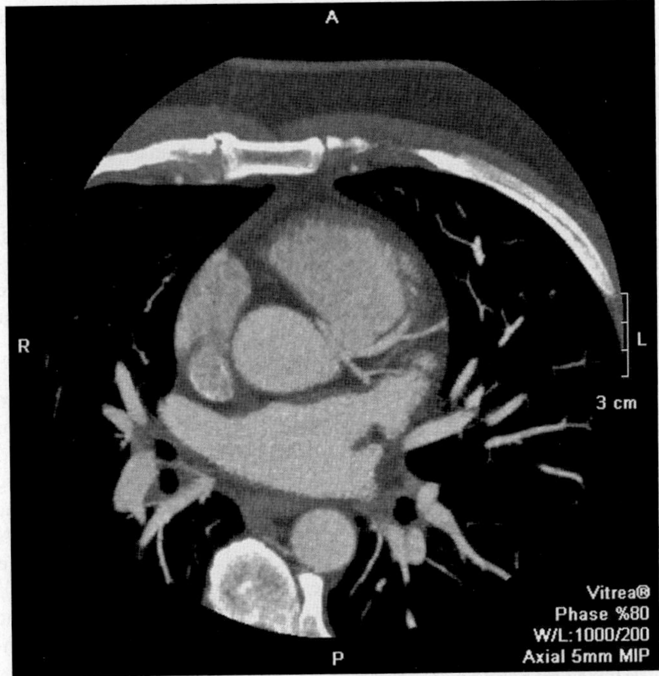

FIGURE 57-7. Frame from a computed tomographic angiographic study showing the origin of the left main coronary artery arising from the right sinus of Valsalva and coursing anteriorly between the aorta and pulmonary artery.

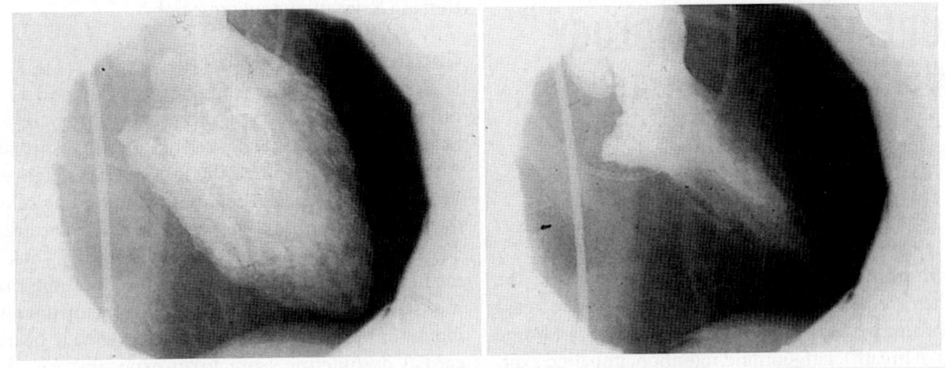

FIGURE 57-8. Example of left ventriculography. The ventricular contour is seen in diastole (*left*) and in systole (*right*).

the left atrium and then the left ventricle. It is an established technique used to acquire precise, high-quality hemodynamic data for patients with aortic stenosis, mitral valve disease (both stenosis and regurgitation), and hypertrophic cardiomyopathy (outflow tract obstructive gradient) and to provide access for valvuloplasty techniques (Chapter 75). The risks of transseptal catheterization, which include punctures of the aortic root, the coronary sinus, or the posterior free wall of the atrium, are potentially lethal problems.

Endomyocardial Biopsy

Endomyocardial biopsy procedures use venous access from the internal jugular vein or femoral vein to insert a flexible metal bioptome to obtain four to six 1-mm^3 pieces of right ventricular myocardium. There are two definitive indications for endomyocardial biopsy: monitoring for cardiac transplant rejection (Chapter 82) and detection of anthracycline cardiotoxicity (Chapter 60). Other indications in selected patients include diagnosis of cardiomyopathy and myocarditis and differentiation between restrictive and constrictive cardiomyopathies.

Other Procedures

Pericardiocentesis (Chapter 77) and PCI (Chapter 74) are performed in the catheterization laboratory for specific indications. Other procedures include balloon valvuloplasty and transcatheter aortic valve replacement for stenotic heart valves (Chapter 75),[4] and closure of an atrial septal defect or patent foramen ovale (Chapter 69), which is confirmed by typical oxygen saturations detected at catheterization.

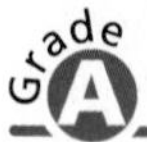

Grade A References

A1. Romagnoli E, Biondi-Zoccai G, Sciahbasi A, et al. Radial versus femoral randomized investigation in ST-segment elevation acute coronary syndrome: the RIFLE-STEACS (Radial Versus Femoral Randomized Investigation in ST-Elevation Acute Coronary Syndrome) study. *J Am Coll Cardiol.* 2012;60:2481-2489.

A2. Mehta SR, Jolly SS, Cairns J, et al. Effects of radial versus femoral artery access in patients with acute coronary syndromes with or without ST-segment elevation. *J Am Coll Cardiol.* 2012;60:2490-2499.

A3. Koc F, Ozdemir K, Altunkas F, et al. Sodium bicarbonate versus isotonic saline for the prevention of contrast-induced nephropathy in patients with diabetes mellitus undergoing coronary angiography and/or intervention: a multicenter prospective randomized study. *J Investig Med.* 2013;61:872-877.

A4. Acetylcysteine for prevention of renal outcomes in patients undergoing coronary and peripheral vascular angiography: main results from the randomized Acetylcysteine for Contrast-induced nephropathy Trial (ACT). *Circulation.* 2011;124:1250-1259.

A5. Leoncini M, Toso A, Maioli M, et al. Early high-dose rosuvastatin for contrast-induced nephropathy prevention in acute coronary syndrome: Results from the PRATO-ACS Study (Protective Effect of Rosuvastatin and Antiplatelet Therapy On contrast-induced acute kidney injury and myocardial damage in patients with Acute Coronary Syndrome). *J Am Coll Cardiol.* 2014;63:71-79.

A6. Han Y, Zhu G, Han L, et al. Short-term rosuvastatin therapy for prevention of contrast-induced acute kidney injury in patients with diabetes and chronic kidney disease. *J Am Coll Cardiol.* 2014;63:62-70.

GENERAL REFERENCES

For the General References and other additional features, please visit Expert Consult at https://expertconsult.inkling.com.

58 HEART FAILURE: PATHOPHYSIOLOGY AND DIAGNOSIS

CHRISTOPHER M. O'CONNOR AND JOSEPH G. ROGERS

DEFINITION

Heart failure is a clinical syndrome that results when abnormalities in the structure and function of the myocardium impair cardiac output or decrease filling of the ventricles. Characteristic features of the heart failure syndrome include dyspnea (shortness of breath), fatigue, fluid retention, impaired exercise performance, and edema. Pulmonary congestion is a common but not universal feature, so the term *congestive heart failure* is no longer used.

EPIDEMIOLOGY

The lifetime risk of heart failure is at least 20% for Americans and 25% for Europeans.[1] Although these cumulative incidences have remained stable during the past 30 years, the prevalence of heart failure has increased because of the improved long-term survival of patients with ischemic and other forms of heart disease as well as the strong association between heart failure and advancing age.[2] For example, more than 10% of the population older than 80 years has heart failure, and patients are living progressively longer with clinical heart failure. In the United States today, more than 5 million patients have clinical heart failure, and they generate more than one million hospitalizations for heart failure annually. Heart failure is the leading cause of hospitalization for patients older than 65 years. Once a patient is hospitalized for heart failure, the 30-day risk of rehospitalization is 25%, with a 10% risk of 30-day postdischarge mortality. Although survival has improved, the absolute mortality rates for heart failure remain approximately 50% within 5 years of diagnosis.

Approximately 40 to 50% of patients with heart failure have a preserved ejection fraction. Compared with patients who have heart failure with reduced ejection fraction, heart failure patients with a preserved ejection fraction tend to be older and are more likely to be women with a prior history of hypertension and diabetes. The mortality rate of patients with a preserved ejection fraction is somewhat lower than the rate for patients with reduced ejection fraction but is still higher than for an age-matched population.[3] Hospitalization and rehospitalization rates are comparable for heart failure patients regardless of their ejection fractions.

Disparities

African Americans are at increased risk for development of heart failure compared with white Americans and also have more frequent hospitalizations.[4] African Americans with heart failure have a similarly high mortality rate compared with white populations. The reasons for these disparities are multifactorial and include differences in heart failure etiology, prevalence of comorbidities, socioeconomic status, and response to therapies.

Hispanics represent a growing number of heart failure patients in the United States. Although large-scale studies are currently limited, preliminary data suggest this population is particularly vulnerable to heart failure.

Classification

The classification of heart failure considers the disease state and progression, degree of exercise intolerance (Chapter 51), measurement of heart function by ejection fraction, and its cause.[5] In the first approach, heart failure is classified by its progression through four stages from pre-disease to advanced symptoms (Fig. 58-1). The second approach evaluates functional states by classification systems such as the New York Heart Association classification, the Canadian Cardiovascular Society system, or other validated measures of exercise tolerance (see Table 51-5). Functional status is the most appropriate way to understand a patient's limitations and the impact of heart failure on quality of life. It also correlates with prognosis and is often used as a secondary end point in clinical trials. The third approach is to measure ejection fraction. This method, usually obtained by echocardiography (Chapter 55), dichotomizes the heart failure patient as either having a reduced (<50%) or preserved ejection fraction. This simple dichotomous classification helps in understanding the patient's underlying pathophysiologic process and in identifying appropriate treatment strategies. Classification based on cause, usually ischemic versus nonischemic (Chapter 60), is useful in guiding the diagnostic evaluation in tailoring treatment strategies. Deeper phenotypic characterization is a focus of ongoing research.[6]

Causes of Heart Failure

Heart failure has numerous causes (Table 58-1). In the United States and other developed countries, coronary artery disease causes about 70% of heart failure cases usually related to a myocardial infarction (Chapter 73). Although hypertension is the second leading cause of heart failure in Western developed countries, it represents the leading cause of heart failure in many developing countries. Diseases of the myocardium (Chapter 60), valves (Chapter 75), and pericardium (Chapter 77) as well as endocrinopathies, metabolic abnormalities, and genetic conditions may cause heart failure. Chemotherapy (e.g., anthracyclines and trastuzumab; Chapter 179) and chest radiation therapy (Chapter 20) may damage heart muscle. Reversible myocardial dysfunction from toxin exposure (e.g., cocaine [Chapter 34] and excessive alcohol intake [Chapter 33]), persistent tachycardia (Chapters 64 and 65), and severe mental/emotional stress (e.g., Takotsubo cardiomy-

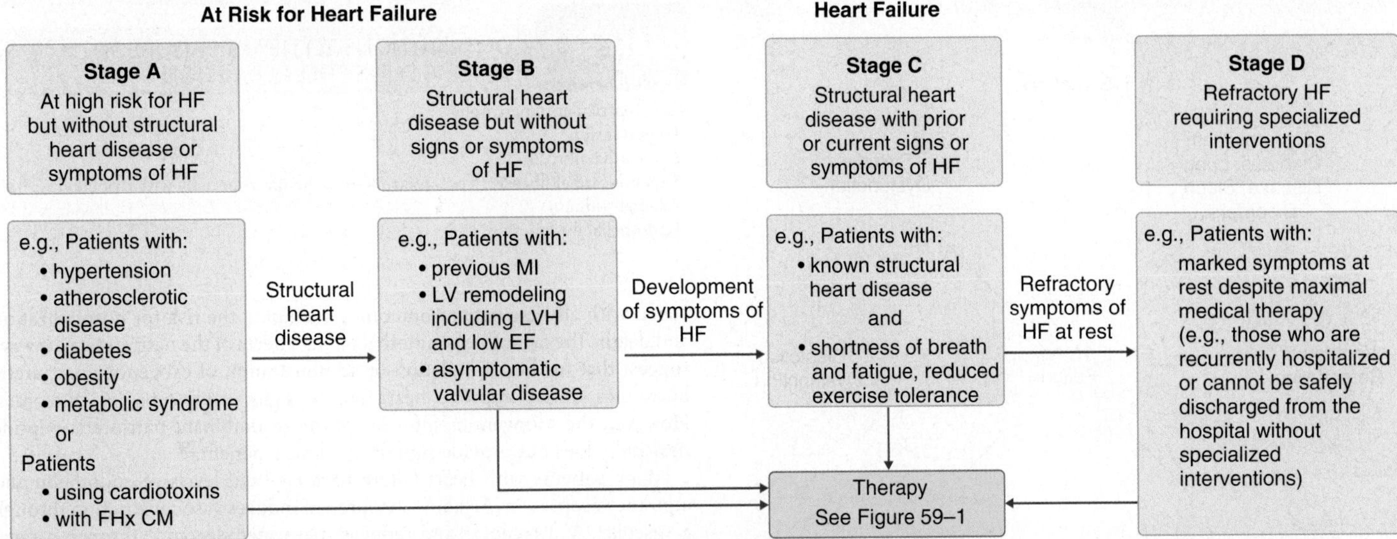

FIGURE 58-1. Stages of heart failure. EF = ejection fraction; FHx CM = family history of cardiomyopathy; HF = heart failure; LV = left ventricle; LVH = left ventricular hypertrophy; MI = myocardial infarction. (Modified from Hunt SA. ACC/AHA 2005 guideline update for the diagnosis and management of chronic heart failure in the adult: a report of the American College of Cardiology/American Heart Association Task Force on Practice Guidelines [Writing Committee to Update the 2001 Guidelines for the Evaluation and Management of Heart Failure]. *J Am Coll Cardiol.* 2005;46:e1-e82.)

TABLE 58-1 CAUSES OF HEART FAILURE
Coronary artery disease or prior myocardial infarction or ischemic injury
Hypertension
Familial and genetic disorders, including dilated cardiomyopathies, hypertrophic cardiomyopathies, storage diseases, and muscular dystrophies
Valvular disease: valvular stenosis or regurgitation
Toxic/drug-induced damage, including prior chemotherapy
Infiltrative processes, such as sarcoid, amyloid, and hemochromatosis (i.e., restrictive cardiomyopathy)
Arrhythmia-related dysfunction, including premature ventricular contraction–induced cardiomyopathy and atrial tachyarrhythmia–related dysfunction
Arrhythmogenic right ventricular cardiomyopathy
Pulmonary heart disease, including cor pulmonale
Infectious agents, including viral infections and Chagas disease
Immunologically mediated myocardial processes
Shunting: intracardiac or extracardiac, including arteriovenous fistulas
Constrictive pericarditis (i.e., nonmyocardial processes)
Age-related changes
Nutritional disorders, such as beriberi
High-output states, such as chronic anemia, thyrotoxicosis

opathy [Chapter 60]) may cause ventricular dysfunction that resolves following withdrawal of the inciting etiology.

The relative pathophysiologic mechanisms that contribute to the burden of heart failure vary by world region. For instance, infectious causes such as Chagas cardiomyopathy (Chapter 60) are prevalent in Central and South America. Rheumatic valvular disease is a common cause of heart failure in developing countries but is infrequent in developed countries.

Because of the large number of possible causes of heart failure, identification of the primary contributing factors may pose diagnostic challenges for the clinician. Furthermore, an acute decompensation of heart failure may be related to worsening of the primary cause, to a new cardiac or pulmonary problem, to the influence of cardiac conditions that demand increased cardiac output, or to poor adherence to otherwise successful therapies (Table 58-2). As a result, a systematic approach to the clinical evaluation is critical. Some patients will have decompensated heart failure that requires hospitalization, whereas others will have heart failure as an important comorbidity during hospitalization for another problem.

PATHOBIOLOGY

A number of factors contribute to the pathobiologic development and progression of heart failure (Table 58-3). The relative contribution of these different mechanisms to the overall pathophysiologic manifestations of heart failure (Fig. 58-2) varies in individual patients.

TABLE 58-2 FACTORS THAT MAY PRECIPITATE ACUTE DECOMPENSATION OF CHRONIC HEART FAILURE
Myocardial ischemia or infarction
Arrhythmias
Worsening hypertension
Worsening mitral or tricuspid regurgitation
Initiation of medications that worsen heart failure (calcium antagonists, β-blockers, nonsteroidal anti-inflammatory drugs, antiarrhythmic agents)
Discontinuation of therapy (patient noncompliance or physician initiated)
Dietary indiscretion
Iatrogenic volume overload (transfusion, fluid administration)
Alcohol consumption
Increased activity
Fever or infection
Anemia
Thyroid abnormalities
Exposure to high altitude
Pregnancy

TABLE 58-3 PATHOBIOLOGIC MECHANISMS OF HEART FAILURE
Hemodynamics
Neurohormones
Cardiorenal interactions
Abnormal calcium cycling
Cell death
Myocardial genetics

Heart Failure with a Reduced Ejection Fraction

A central tenet of the hemodynamic contribution to heart failure is that an abnormality of myocardial function is responsible for the failure of the heart to pump blood at a rate commensurate with the requirements of the metabolizing tissues or that it can do so only in the setting of elevated cardiac filling pressures.[7] In failing hearts, an increase in hemodynamic load causes maladaptive regulation of neurohormonal pathways that reduce intrinsic muscle

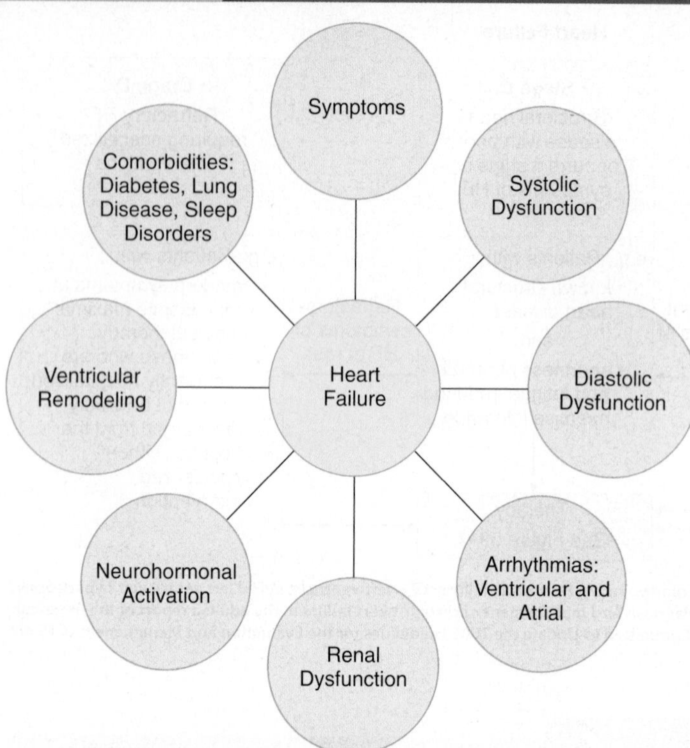

FIGURE 58-2. Pathophysiology of heart failure. The contributing and exacerbating factors to the pathophysiologic process of heart failure.

contractility (Chapter 53), in part because of ventricular remodeling. The structure of the extracellular matrix of the heart plays a pivotal role in ventricular scaffolding and overall pumping function. Replacement fibrosis after myocardial injury (e.g., myocardial infarction, toxin exposure, or chronic renin-angiotensin-aldosterone system activation) increases the connective tissue content and further impairs pump function (Chapter 53). Several neurohormonal pathways have been identified as regulators of myocardial fibrosis including aldosterone, matrix metalloproteinases, the tissue inhibitors of metaloproteinases (TIMPS), TNF-alpha and ST2.

Neurohumoral mechanisms emphasize the importance of adrenergic nervous system activation in the development and progression of left ventricular dysfunction. The initial activation of the sympathetic nervous system probably results from reduced pulse pressure, which activates arterial baroreceptors. Evidence for its activation comes from elevated levels of circulating norepinephrine, direct sympathetic nerve recordings showing increased activity, and increased release of norepinephrine by several organs, including the heart. Elements of the renin-angiotensin-aldosterone system are activated relatively early in heart failure. The presumptive mechanisms of induction include renal hypoperfusion, β-adrenergic system stimulation, and hyponatremia. Adrenergic and renin-angiotensin-aldosterone system activation stimulates the failing heart while also causing peripheral vasoconstriction and the retention of sodium and fluid. The initial result is improved circulation and perfusion of the vital organs. Over time, however, the prolonged activation of these systems causes maladaptive remodeling of the left ventricle and further dysfunction. Further, the sympathetic nervous system and renin-angiotensin-aldosterone system are co-regulated, such that increased activity of each pathway stimulates a simultaneous increase in the other. As cardiac function deteriorates, responsiveness to norepinephrine diminishes, as evidenced by baroreceptor desensitization and downregulation of cardiac adrenergic receptors. This desensitization may further stimulate sympathetic responses. When excessive vasoconstriction depresses left ventricular function, sodium retention increases already elevated ventricular filling pressures. As a result, heart failure is characterized by hypoperfusion associated with hypervolemia. The deleterious effects of vasoconstriction and volume retention are hallmarks of clinical heart failure syndromes.

Natriuretic peptides may counterbalance the vasoconstricting and sodium-retaining actions of the renin-angiotensin-aldosterone system and sympathetic nervous systems by causing both arterial and venous vasodilation as well as natriuresis and diuresis. Similar to other activated neurohormonal pathways in heart failure, the degree of natriuretic pathway activation is associated with adverse patient outcomes, including the risk for hospitalization and death. The favorable counterbalancing effects of the natriuretic pathways suggest that further stimulation or administration of exogenous natriuretic hormones might improve heart failure signs, symptoms, or outcomes. However, the intravenous infusion of the recombinant natriuretic peptide nesiritide does not provide significant clinical benefit.[A1]

TABLE 58-4 CONTRIBUTIONS TO HEART FAILURE WITH PRESERVED EJECTION FRACTION

Left ventricular hypertrophy
Hypertension
Myocardial fibrosis
Subendocardial fibrosis (from intermittent ischemia, especially with diabetes)
Arterial stiffness
Endothelial dysfunction

Many patients with heart failure have elevated levels of endothelin and arginine vasopressin. Arginine vasopressin induces vasoconstriction through a vascular (V_1) receptor and reduces free water clearance through a renal tubular (V_2) receptor. Endothelin causes prolonged vasoconstriction, reductions in glomerular filtration, and pulmonary arteriolar constriction. Although both endothelin and vasopressin are attractive targets for therapy, clinical trials with antagonists of these systems have been negative, thereby indicating that interdiction of neurohormonal activation is not uniformly beneficial.

Cardiorenal mechanisms emphasize the integral role of kidney dysfunction in the worsening of heart failure, with both organs contributing to the retention of sodium and water. In most patients with chronic heart failure, the kidneys are anatomically and structurally normal, but passive venous congestion and reduced renal perfusion lead to worsening renal function and a vicious circle of progressive dysfunction of both organ systems. Renal failure also compromises the ability to use inhibitors of the renin-angiotensin-aldosterone system to treat heart failure.

Abnormal calcium cycling reduces the calcium content in the cardiac sarcoplasmic reticulum owing to diastolic leak through altered ryanodine receptors. The reduced calcium content of the sarcoplasmic reticulum alters the contraction interactions between cardiac myosin and actin myofilaments. In addition, a loss of function of cardiac SERCA2a (sarcoendoplasmic reticulum calcium transport ATPase 2a) pumps, which are responsible for removal of cytoplasmic calcium, affects ventricular relaxation and causes diastolic dysfunction.

In all forms of heart failure, a variety of stressors (e.g., elevated neurohormone levels, adrenergic activation, inflammatory mechanisms, and toxin exposure) enhance cell death. Elevated serum levels of many proinflammatory cytokines (including tumor necrosis factor-α, interleukin-1β, and interleukin-6) may induce contractile dysfunction, myocardial fibrosis, and myocyte necrosis, perhaps by mediating some of the deleterious responses to catecholamines and angiotensin II. Cell death is also a cause of heart failure after myocardial infarction.

Persistent tachycardia (e.g., atrial fibrillation with rapid ventricular response) also can result in heart failure, presumably related to chronic hyperadrenergic stimulation. In some patients, the tachycardic response to heart failure may itself contribute to worsening heart failure. These forms of heart failure may be reversible, depending on the relative contribution of the tachycardia to the underlying myocardial dysfunction.

Genetic mutations are increasingly identified as important mediators of the cardiac structural and functional abnormalities linked to symptomatic heart failure (see Table 60-2). The majority of familial cardiomyopathies, most of which are inherited in an autosomal dominant fashion, are related to defects in the cytoskeleton or nuclear proteins. Inherited cardiomyopathy is also associated with muscular dystrophies, infiltrative diseases such as hemochromatosis, and mitochondrial disorders.

Heart Failure with a Preserved Ejection Fraction

The pathophysiologic mechanism of heart failure with a preserved ejection fraction is complex and includes alterations in cardiac structure and function, vascular abnormalities, end-organ dysfunction, and interrelated comorbidities (Table 58-4). In principle, diastolic dysfunction in heart failure with a preserved ejection fraction can result from increased left ventricular stiffness due to hypertrophy and interstitial fibrosis as well as from abnormal left ventricular relaxation due to dysfunctional calcium cycling. Although there are many potential causes of heart failure with a preserved ejection fraction,

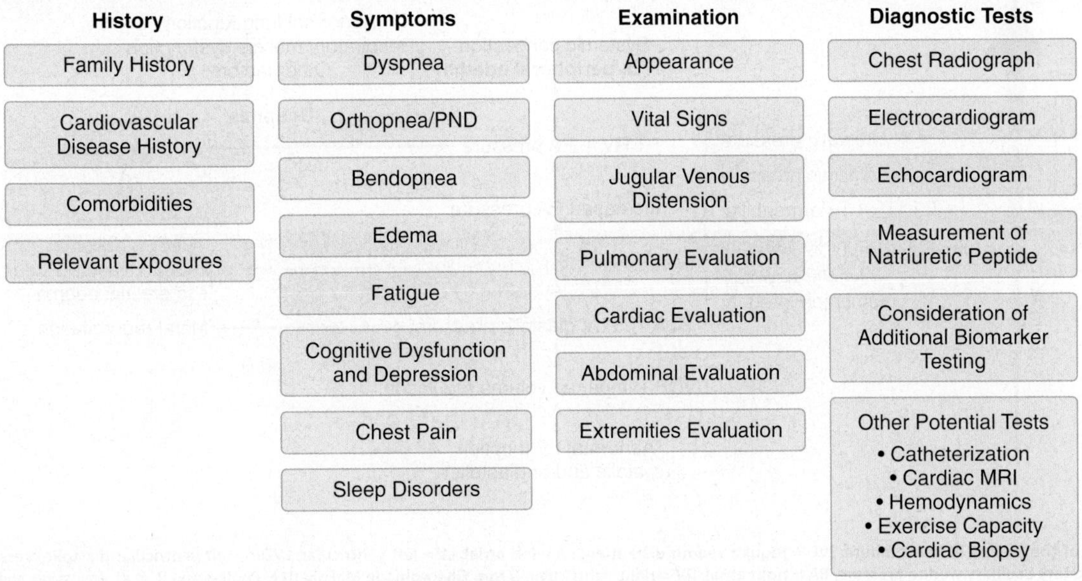

History	Symptoms	Examination	Diagnostic Tests
Family History	Dyspnea	Appearance	Chest Radiograph
Cardiovascular Disease History	Orthopnea/PND	Vital Signs	Electrocardiogram
Comorbidities	Bendopnea	Jugular Venous Distension	Echocardiogram
Relevant Exposures	Edema	Pulmonary Evaluation	Measurement of Natriuretic Peptide
	Fatigue	Cardiac Evaluation	Consideration of Additional Biomarker Testing
	Cognitive Dysfunction and Depression	Abdominal Evaluation	Other Potential Tests • Catheterization • Cardiac MRI • Hemodynamics • Exercise Capacity • Cardiac Biopsy
	Chest Pain	Extremities Evaluation	
	Sleep Disorders		

FIGURE 58-3. Diagnostic evaluation of heart failure. The various components of the diagnostic evaluation of heart failure patients are presented from the history, symptoms, and examination to diagnostic testing. MRI = magnetic resonance imaging; PND = paroxysmal nocturnal dyspnea.

most patients have current or prior hypertension; the resulting left ventricular hypertrophy and fibrosis are responsible for increased chamber stiffness. Ischemic heart disease also may contribute to heart failure with a preserved ejection fraction, by virtue of subendocardial fibrosis or as a result of intermittent ischemic dysfunction. Diabetes mellitus is often present, especially in women. Age itself is a crucial predisposing factor because it causes loss of myocytes (apoptosis), increased fibrosis with shifts to more rigid forms of collagen, and loss of vascular compliance.

Myocardial relaxation is an adenosine triphosphate–dependent process. Processes that interfere with myocardial energy metabolism (e.g., ischemia) compromise myocardial relaxation. These changes result in reduced ventricular compliance and elevated filling pressures. Elevated filling pressures increase the pulmonary capillary wedge pressure and contribute to the sensation of dyspnea. Diastolic dysfunction may remain asymptomatic for years, but increasing age, renal dysfunction, hypertension, and progressive left ventricular dysfunction are associated with the development of symptoms of heart failure. The resting hemodynamic profile in heart failure with preserved ejection fraction is frequently normal, but physiological perturbations such as tachycardia or exercise result in exaggerated increases in filling pressures. This phenomenon accounts for the marked exertional impairment seen in this syndrome. Furthermore, because atrial contraction is responsible for a disproportionately large percentage of the diastolic filling of a noncompliant ventricle, atrial fibrillation (i.e., loss of atrial contraction) can severely worsen patients' symptoms. Abnormalities in ventricular relaxation and myocardial stiffness limit ventricular filling, so patients may have a narrow window for optimal fluid volume. Modest volume overload can substantially exacerbate symptoms of dyspnea, and therapeutic diuresis may precipitate symptomatic hypotension owing to ventricular underfilling. Although diastolic dysfunction can occur alone as heart failure with a preserved ejection fraction, the majority of patients with significant diastolic dysfunction also have systolic dysfunction.[8] As a result, it is preferable to characterize patients as having heart failure with a preserved ejection fraction or heart failure with a reduced ejection fraction rather than as having systolic or diastolic heart failure.

CLINICAL MANIFESTATIONS

The diagnosis of heart failure may be apparent when patients present with classic symptoms of shortness of breath in combination with a clinical examination consistent with volume overload. A previous history of a myocardial infarction or poorly controlled hypertension should increase the clinician's suspicion for the diagnosis. In contrast, the diagnosis may be missed or delayed in patients who experience a more insidious course with vague symptoms, such as fatigue and exercise intolerance. The use of biomarkers such as natriuretic peptides has significantly improved the diagnostic yield in recent years.

The evaluation of a patient with suspected heart failure should proceed in an organized and focused manner (Fig. 58-3 and Table 58-5).

TABLE 58-5 APPROACH TO THE DIAGNOSIS OF HEART FAILURE

Obtain a history and physical examination to identify disorders or behaviors that might cause or exacerbate heart failure.
Obtain a family history to aid in diagnosis of familial causes of heart failure.
Assess volume status and vital signs at each encounter.
Patients with suspected new-onset or acute heart failure should undergo chest radiography to assess heart size and pulmonary congestion and to detect other diseases that may cause or contribute to the patient's symptoms.
A 12-lead electrocardiogram should be obtained for all patients presenting with heart failure.
Echocardiography should be performed during the initial evaluation of patients with heart failure to assess ventricular function and valve function.
Measurement of natriuretic peptides is recommended for the following indications: To support the diagnosis of heart failure in ambulatory patients with dyspnea as well as in those with possible acute heart failure, especially in the setting of an uncertain diagnosis. To establish prognosis or disease severity in heart failure.
The initial evaluation of patients presenting with heart failure should include a complete blood count, urinalysis and renal function, serum electrolytes, glucose and lipid profile, liver function tests, and thyroid-stimulating hormone.
Hemodynamic monitoring is recommended to guide therapy in patients who have respiratory distress or clinical evidence of impaired perfusion in whom the adequacy or excess of intracardiac filling pressures cannot be determined from clinical assessment.

Modified from Yancy CW, Jessup M, Bozkurt B, et al. 2013 ACCF/AHA guideline for the management of heart failure: a report of the American College of Cardiology Foundation/American Heart Association Task Force on Practice Guidelines. *J Am Coll Cardiol.* 2013;62:e147-e239.

Symptoms

Shortness of Breath

Dyspnea (Chapter 83) is the most common but nonspecific symptom of heart failure because patients with predominant lung disease or anemia may have similar symptoms. In most heart failure patients, dyspnea is present only with activity. It is the most common reason that patients seek care for heart failure, both during the chronic state and with acutely decompensated heart failure. The most important cause of dyspnea is pulmonary congestion that increases the accumulation of interstitial or intra-alveolar fluid, reduces lung compliance, and increases the work of breathing (Fig. 58-4). Dyspnea relief is a primary therapeutic target of heart failure treatment. Dyspnea can be quantified and monitored by a validated Likert dyspnea scale, which typically consists of 5- or 7-point demarcations that ask patients to rate their degree of improvement from baseline ranging from markedly better to markedly worse,

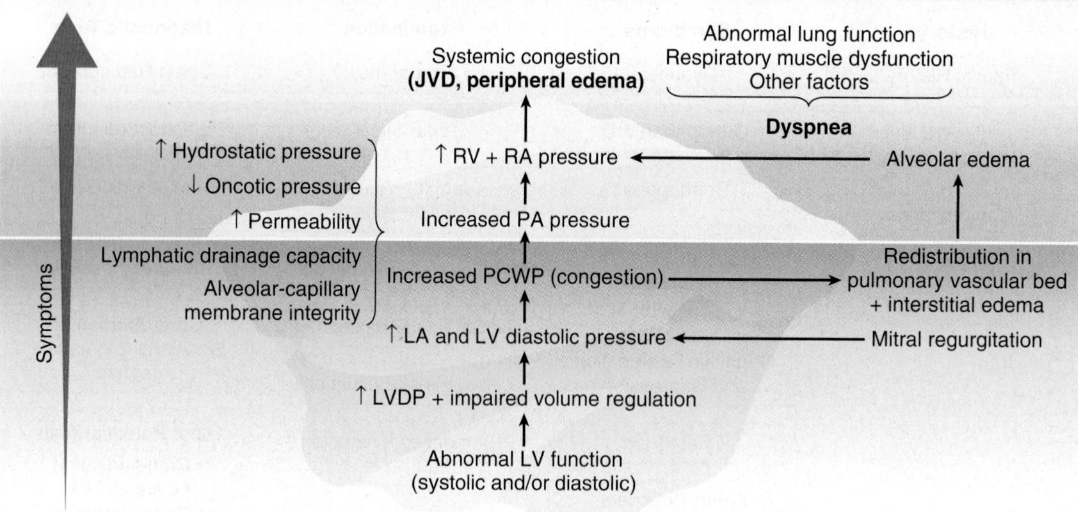

FIGURE 58-4. Role of congestion in heart failure. JVD = jugular venous distention; LA = left atrial; LV = left ventricular; LVDP = left ventricular diastolic pressure; PA = pulmonary artery; PCWP = pulmonary capillary wedge pressure; RA = right atrial; RV = right ventricular. (From Gheorghiade M, Follath F, Ponikowski P, et al. Assessing and grading congestion in acute heart failure: a scientific statement from the Acute Heart Failure Committee of the Heart Failure Association of the European Society of Cardiology and endorsed by the European Society of Intensive Care Medicine. *Eur J Heart Fail.* 2010;12:423-433.)

or a visual analog scale, which asks patients to rate their level of breathing difficulty on a vertical spectrum from 0 at the bottom to 100 at the top, with 100 being the best ability to breathe and 0 being the worst dyspnea. Improvement in dyspnea represents a major patient-reported outcome, and more severe dyspnea is associated with worse in-hospital and postdischarge outcomes.

When dyspnea occurs in the recumbent position, it is called *orthopnea*. This symptom is most commonly elicited by asking patients about their breathing while trying to lie flat during the night. Orthopnea results from the increase in venous return from the extremities and splanchnic circulation to the central circulation with changes in posture. The increase in ventricular preload raises pulmonary venous and pulmonary capillary hydrostatic pressures. Orthopnea is typically classified by an ordinal scale based on the number of pillows a patient requires to sleep comfortably without shortness of breath. Patients with prominent orthopnea may report an inability to sleep in a bed and instead may sleep in a recliner. Orthopnea is a specific symptom of heart failure, and it correlates well with the severity of pulmonary congestion.

Bendopnea is defined as severe dyspnea that occurs while bending over. The mechanism of bendopnea is poorly defined but appears to be related to increases in left ventricular filling pressures during bending in patients with a baseline elevation in pulmonary capillary wedge pressure.[9] There appears to be an association between bendopnea and baseline mismatch of left- and right-sided filling pressures (i.e., elevated wedge pressure out of proportion to right atrial pressure). The clinical spectrum of this symptom and its relationship to outcomes are not well understood, but recent data suggest that this symptom may be a more common than has previously been recognized.

Paroxysmal nocturnal dyspnea is acute, severe shortness of breath that wakes the patient from sleep. These symptoms should be distinguished from periods of apnea related to sleep-disordered breathing (Chapter 100). Paroxysmal nocturnal dyspnea usually is manifested about 1 hour after the patient goes to sleep and begins to subside shortly after awakening. Paroxysmal nocturnal dyspnea results from increased venous return and the mobilization of interstitial fluid from the splanchnic circulation and lower extremities, with accumulation of alveolar edema. Paroxysmal nocturnal dyspnea is relatively uncommon but almost always represents severe heart failure, and it appears to be associated with increased mortality.

Fatigue

Fatigue, which is one of the most common symptoms in heart failure, occurs in more than 90% of patients. Although fatigue is difficult to quantify and is not a specific symptom for heart failure, the severity of fatigue is associated with prognosis. As a result, clinicians should pay careful attention to this symptom as an occult manifestation of heart failure.

Chest Pain

Chest pain (Chapter 51) may be mediated by myocardial ischemia from underlying coronary artery disease, but also can occur in patients without obstructive coronary artery disease because of increased wall stress that is proportional to the degree of left ventricular dilation. Patients who have heart failure with a preserved ejection fraction and left ventricular hypertrophy may develop chest pain from a mismatch of oxygen supply and demand. Chest pain in amyloid heart disease results when deposition of amyloid protein in the medial layer of myocardial arterioles causes transient ischemia.

Cardiac Cachexia

Patients with heart failure can develop constitutional symptoms, including nausea, vomiting, anorexia, and diffuse abdominal pain. Muscle wasting is a frequent comorbidity among patients with advanced chronic heart failure.[10] In some patients, these symptoms can cause significant muscle mass and weight loss, termed cardiac cachexia, which is associated with a very poor prognosis. In many patients, these symptoms arise from prominent right-sided heart failure and resulting passive venous congestion in the abdominal vasculature or liver. In some patients, severe tricuspid regurgitation is a contributing factor. In patients with significant hepatic congestion, abdominal pain may be localized to the right upper quadrant, and jaundice may be observed. The group of patients most likely to experience these symptoms includes those with prominent right-sided heart failure. When patients present with this symptom complex including right upper quadrant tenderness due to hepatic congestion, these heart failure symptoms initially may be falsely attributed to gallbladder disease (Chapter 155) or other abdominal disease. In patients with advanced cardiogenic shock (Chapter 107), severe abdominal pain can be a particularly ominous sign of abdominal ischemia (Chapter 143).

Cognitive Dysfunction and Mood Disorders

Cognitive dysfunction (Chapter 402) is common, particularly in elderly heart failure patients. Confusion can be a manifestation of worsening heart failure related to relative hypotension precipitated by medications used to treat heart failure or of a specific complication of an individual drug, such as a β-blocker. Although intrinsic brain function itself is not affected in most patients with heart failure, cerebral hypoperfusion in advanced heart failure can cause memory impairment, limited attention span, and altered mentation.

Depressive symptoms (Chapter 397) occur in up to 25% of patients with heart failure. Depressive symptoms can be detected by simple questions such as the Patient Health Questionnaire depression module (see Chapter 24), which has an 80% predictive value for depression and is associated with worse outcomes in heart failure patients.

Sleep Disorders

Sleep-disordered breathing is observed in upward of 70% of heart failure patients and is associated with increased morbidity and mortality. Patterns of sleep-disordered breathing include obstructive sleep apnea (Chapter 100) and central sleep apnea/Cheyne-Stokes respiration (Chapter 86). Patients may have both types, and the relative proportion of each type varies with the severity of heart failure and its treatment. Nocturnal rostral fluid movement from the lower extremities of heart failure patients may worsen obstructive sleep apnea. Central sleep apnea is due in part to the instability of the ventilatory control systems in heart failure.

Chronic sleep-disordered breathing also causes a series of derangements that may precipitate or exacerbate heart failure. Sleep-disordered breathing increases blood pressure and the risk of arrhythmias.

Symptoms of sleep-disordered breathing include hypersomnolence, choking or gasping during sleep, recurrent awakenings, unrefreshing sleep, daytime fatigue, and impaired concentration or memory. The symptoms may be difficult to distinguish from other symptoms of heart failure, including unrefreshing sleep due to orthopnea and paroxysmal nocturnal dyspnea. Preliminary data suggest that attention to the diagnosis and management of sleep-disordered breathing with positive-pressure ventilation improves quality of life in some patients with heart failure.

Physical Examination

A carefully performed physical examination is critical to make an accurate diagnosis, to assess possible additional comorbid conditions, and to begin to estimate prognosis.

Global Observation and Vital Signs

The patient's general appearance may provide details related to the acuity and severity of the heart failure. Patients with severe symptoms may be pale or diaphoretic and unable to speak in complete sentences. In extreme circumstances, they may be unable to lie recumbent in bed because of severe dyspnea or pulmonary edema. The heart rate may be elevated (>100 beats per minute), and premature ventricular beats or atrial arrhythmias are common. Approximately 30% of heart failure patients have atrial fibrillation (Chapter 64). Pulsus alternans (alternating amplitude of successive beats) is an uncommon sign but is virtually diagnostic for advanced heart failure. Blood pressure is most commonly normal or high, but it may be low (systolic blood pressure <90 mm Hg) in advanced low-output heart failure. Blood pressure has historically been identified as an important prognostic marker (i.e., higher blood pressure is associated with improved long-term outcomes), but these associated data may not be applicable to all subgroups of patients, especially the elderly. A narrow pulse pressure (e.g., <30 to 35 mm Hg) also indicates more severe heart failure. Weight should be assessed and compared with the patient's known dry weight or recent weight trajectory. The assessment of weight not only helps the clinician to appreciate the severity of volume overload, but it may also assist with quantifying the degree of cardiac cachexia. The respiratory rate should be measured. Both low rates and high rates may be seen in heart failure. Likewise, both hypothermia and hyperthermia can be informative of impending shock or secondary causes of heart failure.

Jugular Veins

Examination of the jugular veins is a critical part of the heart failure physical examination (Chapter 51) both initially and serially.[11] The patient should be positioned in the partially recumbent position with his or her neck turned to the left. The patient's head should be rested on a pillow to limit tension in the neck muscles, which could obscure visualization of the venous pulsations (see Fig. 51-2). The ideal method for measurement is quantifying in centimeters of water (normal = 8 cm H_2O) and estimating the level of pulsations above the sternal angle (and adding 5 cm H_2O; see Fig. 51-3). To distinguish the venous pulsations from the carotid pulsations, clinicians should look for a double pulsation in the venous waveform and can compare the timing with the arterial pulsation in the wrist. If the top of the jugular venous pulsation cannot be appreciated in the initial position, it may be necessary to reposition the patient to see the peak of the pulsation. For instance, in some circumstances, it may be necessary to place the patient in the upright position to visualize the peak of the pulsation near the tragus. The presence of abdominal-jugular reflux should be assessed by putting sustained pressure on the abdomen for 30 seconds; a positive finding is at least a 1-cm rise in the jugular pressure, which then slowly declines when pressure is removed. These findings are a sign of abnormally elevated right ventricular filling pressures. Either an elevated jugular venous pressure or an abnormal abdominal jugular reflux has been reported in 80% of patients with advanced heart failure. No other simple sign is nearly as sensitive.

An additional important finding in the neck is evidence of tricuspid regurgitation, which is visualized as a large *cv* wave (see Fig. 51-4). This finding is confirmed by hepatic pulsations, which can be detected during the abdominal-jugular reflux determination. The carotid pulses should be evaluated for evidence of aortic stenosis (see Fig. 51-5), and thyroid abnormalities should be sought.

Pulmonary Examination

Despite having an elevated left ventricular filling pressure that is transmitted back into the left atrium and pulmonary vasculature, most patients with compensated heart failure do not have evidence of pulmonary congestion on their physical examination. The lungs of chronic heart failure patients undergo adaptive changes and have robust lymphatic drainage to compensate for elevated filling pressures. However, a subset of patients may develop alveolar fluid accumulation, which is appreciated as rales or "crackles" on the clinical examination (Chapter 83). These findings are more common in patients with acute pulmonary edema due to sudden decompensation from an inciting event, such as ischemia or worsening hypertension.

Fluid may also accumulate in the pleural space related to the increased transudation of fluid and impaired lymphatic drainage in the setting of elevated systemic venous pressures (Chapter 99). Pericardial effusions (Chapter 77) may also occur in the setting of heart failure, particularly in inflammatory cardiomyopathy, but this pattern of fluid accumulation is relatively uncommon overall. The clinician should listen and percuss for the possible presence of pleural effusions (Chapter 99), which tend to lateralize to the right side owing to the greater surface area of the lungs and the position of the diaphragm. The diagnosis of a moderate or large pleural effusion is critical because draining of the effusion may represent an important intervention to relieve dyspnea.

Cardiac Examination

The cardiac examination is the cornerstone of the evaluation of the patient with heart failure. Visual inspection may reveal a right ventricular heave, which provides information on right ventricular dysfunction and underlying pulmonary hypertension. Palpation of the location, size, and duration of the point of maximal impulse against the chest wall may provide details related to the degree of left ventricular dilation; the impulse is typically laterally displaced in the setting of ventricular enlargement and may be sustained in the setting of left ventricular hypertrophy.

Auscultation of the heart sounds provides important information related to the underlying rhythm and frequency of ectopic beats. Disorders such as pulmonary hypertension can be appreciated on the basis of an increase in the intensity of the second heart sound. The presence (or worsening) of valvular disorders (Chapter 75) can be characterized for their potential contribution to cardiac dysfunction. An apical S_3 gallop (see Fig. 51-6 in Chapter 51) is common in severe LV dysfunction, and its presence is correlated with an elevated left ventricular end-diastolic pressure and a poor prognosis. As patients are treated for volume overload, the intensity of and ability to detect an S_3 gallop may diminish. The S_4 gallop is common in patients who have ischemic heart disease and hypertension, and it is more likely indicative of diastolic dysfunction.

Abdomen

The physical examination should estimate the size of the liver and spleen and elicit the presence of ascites (Chapter 146). Intra-abdominal hypertension and abdominal venous congestion may cause renal venous hypertension and subsequent renal dysfunction. An enlarged and pulsatile liver is seen in individuals with markedly elevated right heart pressures and in patients with significant tricuspid insufficiency. Hepatic enlargement and dysfunction represent an important step in determining the most appropriate timing of intervention on a regurgitant tricuspid valve. In the setting of irreversible liver disease (i.e., cardiac cirrhosis), heart failure patients are at a substantially increased risk during surgical interventions. Thus, a thorough abdominal examination represents a critical component of the evaluation of heart failure patients.

Extremities

Edema (Chapter 51) results from the retention of sodium due to low cardiac output and reduced renal perfusion pressures, which ultimately result in elevated right-sided filling pressures, increased hydrostatic pressures in the venous circulation, and transudation of fluid into dependent interstitial spaces, especially in the ankles or lower extremities. Edema is commonly measured on a scale of 0 to 3+, but this system has marked interobserver variation. Peripheral edema is a nonspecific finding, and edema due to heart failure must be distinguished from edema related to medication use (e.g., calcium-channel blockers, thiazolidinediones, or nonsteroidal anti-inflammatory drugs), venous insufficiency, or hypoproteinemia.

The temperature of the extremities should also be assessed. Cool extremities suggest low cardiac output or concomitant peripheral arterial disease (Chapter 79).

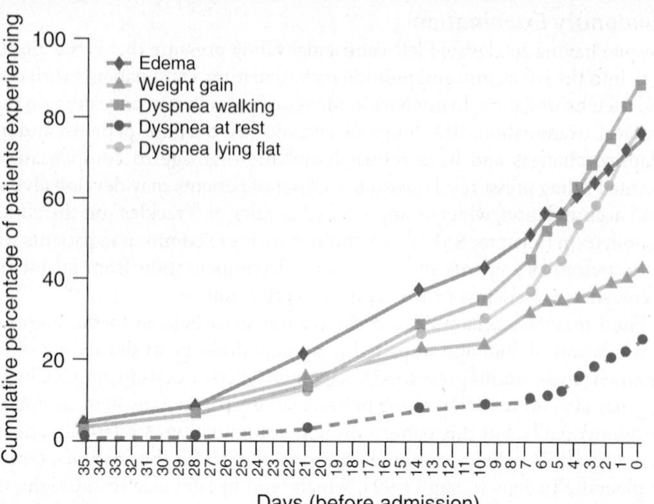

FIGURE 58-5. **Number of days from onset of worsening of selected symptoms of heart failure to admission to the hospital: cumulative percentage of patients.** (From Schiff GD, Fung S, Speroff T, et al. Decompensated heart failure: symptoms, patterns of onset, and contributing factors. *Am J Med.* 2003;114:625-630.)

DIAGNOSIS

Patterns of Presentation

The initial presentation ranges from subtle outpatient findings to acute decompensation that requires hospitalization. An initial presentation may represent the gradual progression of known but previously asymptomatic (stage A or B) heart failure or be the first indication of altered cardiac function. In patients who do not have an antecedent history of heart failure, precipitating factors, such as acute myocardial infarction (Chapter 73), tachyarrhythmias (Chapters 64 and 65), previously unrecognized or new valvular abnormalities (Chapter 75), toxic damage (including alcohol excess), or acute myocarditis (Chapter 60), should be considered.

When patients with stage C or D heart failure present with worsening symptoms, precipitating factors may also include myocardial ischemia, arrhythmias, or worsening of valvular function (see Table 58-2). Other conditions can include anemia, infection, hyperthyroidism, and any conditions that stimulate an increase in cardiac output. In many patients, however, the worsening may be gradual, augured by a sometimes subtle increase in outpatient signs and symptoms (Fig. 58-5).

Electrocardiography

A 12-lead electrocardiogram (Chapter 54) should be obtained for all patients who present with possible heart failure. The major importance of the electrocardiogram is to evaluate the cardiac rhythm, to identify current ischemia or prior myocardial infarction, and to detect evidence of left ventricular hypertrophy. Rhythm abnormalities may be responsible for the development or exacerbation of underlying cardiac dysfunction. For example, an underlying tachyarrhythmia can lead to the development of left ventricular systolic dysfunction that is reversible with appropriate intervention. Q waves suggest coronary artery disease as a likely contributor to ventricular dysfunction. The presence of voltage criteria for left ventricular hypertrophy supports a diagnosis of hypertensive heart disease, including heart failure with a preserved ejection fraction. Underlying conduction abnormalities, such as delayed ventricular conduction (i.e., bundle branch morphology), determine eligibility criteria for cardiac resynchronization therapy (Chapters 59 and 66) and have important prognostic implications. Holter monitoring sometimes may be helpful to determine the burden of ventricular arrhythmias or ectopic beats because tachycardia-mediated cardiomyopathies may be reversible with medical therapy or ablation therapy.

Chest Radiography

Patients with suspected new-onset or worsening heart failure should undergo chest radiography to assess heart size and pulmonary congestion as well as to detect other diseases that may cause or contribute to the patient's symptoms. Many patients with acute heart failure but only a minority of those with chronic heart failure have clear evidence of pulmonary venous hypertension (upper lobe redistribution, enlarged pulmonary veins) or pulmonary edema (perihilar or patchy peripheral infiltrates; see Fig. 56-2). Pleural effusions, usually on the right if unilateral but often bilateral, are also identified on the chest radiograph (see Fig. 99-3). Chest radiography may also play a role in identifying the location of the lead placement of intracardiac devices, such as biventricular pacemakers. Inappropriate lead placement may be observed in patients with worsening heart failure symptoms.

Laboratory Testing

The initial evaluation of patients presenting with heart failure should include a complete blood count to detect anemia and systemic diseases with hematologic manifestations; urinalysis and tests of renal function to assess renal states; serum electrolyte values to identify abnormalities needing treatment and to provide a baseline for subsequent therapy; glucose level and lipid profile to diagnose diabetes and dyslipidemia, which should be carefully managed in patients with heart failure; and thyroid-stimulating hormone level. Markers of hepatic congestion, such as elevated serum aminotransferase and bilirubin levels (Chapter 147), also should be measured because they are important prognostic signs in patients with heart failure. Screening for hemochromatosis (Chapter 212) or human immunodeficiency virus (HIV) infection is reasonable in selected patients with heart failure. Diagnostic tests for rheumatologic diseases (Chapter 256), amyloidosis (Chapter 188), or pheochromocytoma (Chapter 228) are not routinely indicated but rather should be targeted to patients with other ancillary findings suggestive of these conditions. Viral antibody titers yield relatively little incremental information and are rarely indicated in the evaluation of heart failure.

Natriuretic Peptides

Brain natriuretic peptide (BNP) and its amino-terminal fragment (NT-proBNP) provide incremental diagnostic and prognostic information above and beyond the history and physical examination in patients with heart failure. A BNP level should be measured to support the diagnosis of heart failure in ambulatory patients with dyspnea as well as in patients with possible acute heart failure, especially in the setting of an uncertain diagnosis. It also is useful to estimate the severity of heart failure and its prognosis.

Although BNP levels are relatively sensitive and specific markers for clinically confirmed heart failure, circulating levels are influenced by co-morbid processes. For example, obesity reduces BNP levels, whereas advancing age and renal dysfunction are associated with higher levels. Most heart failure therapies reduce BNP levels, but the usefulness of BNP-guided heart failure therapy is not well established.

Troponin

Owing to the increased sensitivity of currently available troponin assays, the majority of patients admitted with acute heart failure have elevations in circulating troponin even without any obvious myocardial ischemia. These elevations, which suggest ongoing myocyte injury or necrosis, are associated with worse clinical outcomes and mortality.[12]

Other Biomarkers: Galectin-3 and ST2

A number of additional biomarkers characterize inflammation, myocyte injury, neurohormonal upregulation, and extracellular matrix turnover in patients with heart failure (E-Table 58-1 and E-Fig. 58-1). For example, biomarkers of myocardial fibrosis, including soluble ST2 and galectin-3, are associated with hospitalization and death in patients with heart failure. In the future, strategies that combine multiple biomarkers into a risk stratification model may prove additive to clinical judgment.[13]

Echocardiography

An echocardiogram should be obtained during the initial evaluation of patients with heart failure to assess ventricular and valve function. Repeated echocardiograms are also indicated when patients have a significant change in their clinical status or receive treatment that may have had a significant effect on cardiac function. In contrast, routine repeated measurements of left ventricular function in the absence of a change in clinical status or treatment should not be performed.

Echocardiography (Chapter 55) allows the assessment of left ventricular systolic and diastolic function (see Figs. 55-2 and 55-3). Wall thickness, ventricular dilation, and regional wall motion abnormalities provide evidence of the underlying etiology and chronicity of heart failure. Right ventricular failure, which is associated with worse prognosis, can also be evaluated to assess the relative contribution of right-sided dysfunction. Echocardiography also evaluates valvular dysfunction (Chapter 75), which may be the result of or cause of worsening ventricular function. Quantitative measurements of pulmonary artery pressure and central venous pressure help characterize the degree of pulmonary hypertension and may guide diuretic therapies in circumstances in which the jugular veins are difficult to visualize. The presence of an atrial or ventricular thrombus requires anticoagulation. Novel methods using ventricular strain analysis and three-dimensional echocardiography can provide more detailed information about ventricular dyssynchrony and compliance and may, in the future, prove useful in patients with heart failure with a preserved ejection fraction.

Nuclear Cardiology and Coronary Angiography

When myocardial ischemia may be contributing to heart failure, coronary arteriography (Chapter 57) is reasonable to assess eligibility for revascularization. The most powerful predictors of prognosis for patients with ischemic cardiomyopathy are a history of prior myocardial infarction or revascularization, stenosis of 75% or greater of the left main or proximal left anterior descending artery, stenosis of 75% or greater of two or more epicardial vessels, and the severity of ventricular dysfunction. Coronary computed tomographic angiography (Chapter 56) may represent a non-invasive modality for assessing coronary disease in appropriately selected patients.

Noninvasive imaging (Chapter 56) to detect myocardial ischemia and viability is reasonable in patients who present with de novo heart failure and in patients who have known coronary artery disease and no angina, unless they are not eligible for revascularization. Viability assessment is reasonable in select situations in planning revascularization for patients who have heart failure and coronary artery disease. However, stress testing to assess myocardial viability so far has not been able to identify patients who will benefit from revascularization compared with medical therapy alone.[A2]

The single-photon emission computed tomography tracer *m*-iodobenzylguanidine (mIBG) has been widely used for studying causes and effects of cardiac sympathetic hyperactivity. Cardiac sympathetic imaging with mIBG is a noninvasive tool that may assist with the risk stratification of patients with heart failure. With mIBG imaging, the myocardial uptake and distribution can be visually assessed and quantified by calculating a heart-to-mediastinum ratio. This approach provides a highly reproducible index of cardiac sympathetic activity. Further study is required to determine the role of this imaging modality in heart failure risk stratification and clinical care.

Cardiac Magnetic Resonance Imaging

Cardiac magnetic resonance imaging (Chapter 56), which provides accurate data on left ventricular volume and ejection fraction, can be useful when echocardiography is inadequate. It is also helpful to assess for potential infiltrative cardiomyopathies when the cause of heart failure, especially heart failure with a preserved ejection fraction, is unclear. Late gadolinium enhancement adds important prognostic information related to ventricular arrhythmia and mortality risk (see Fig. 56-21).

Myocardial Biopsy

Guidelines indicate that endomyocardial biopsy should not be performed in the routine evaluation of patients with heart failure. However, endomyocardial biopsy may be useful in patients who present with heart failure when a specific suspected diagnosis would influence therapy. For example, in patients with acute myocarditis[14] or giant cell myocarditis and in patients with sarcoid or amyloid cardiomyopathy (Chapter 60), the appropriate pathologic diagnosis may inform treatment recommendations and prognosis. In certain circumstances, biopsy may be performed along with genetic testing (e.g., transthyretin gene mutation) to inform decisions on management and counseling of family members.

Assessment of Exercise Capacity

A heart failure patient's exercise capacity can be quantified by several testing modalities, including 6-minute walk distance and cardiopulmonary exercise testing (Chapter 85). Although these tests are not routinely recommended, they are helpful for determining the relative contribution of cardiac compared with pulmonary causes of functional limitation. The results of cardiopulmonary exercise testing are critical to determine the severity of disease in patients who are being considered for therapies such as heart transplantation or ventricular assist device placement (Chapter 82). A maximal oxygen consumption of less than 14 mL/kg/minute is associated with a poor enough prognosis that survival is probably better with transplantation or implantation of a left ventricular assist device compared with medical therapy. Serial cardiopulmonary exercise testing or 6-minute walk testing also can be useful to follow the disease course of specific patients objectively.

Invasive Diagnostics and Hemodynamic Monitoring

Invasive monitoring may be useful in selected patients who have acute heart failure, who have persistent symptoms despite adjustment of standard therapies, and whose fluid status or perfusion is uncertain. However, the routine use of pulmonary artery catheters should be discouraged.[A3]

Up to 30% of patients with heart failure with a reduced ejection fraction have an implantable device that detects arrhythmias and can provide hemodynamic assessment. Indirect measures, such as changes in impedance or heart rate variability, are precursors to worsening heart failure symptoms. Chronic hemodynamic monitors (i.e., direct measures of pulmonary pressures and right ventricular pressures) have been approved by the U.S. Food and Drug Administration and are now available for the serial measurement of left ventricular filling pressures. The interrogation of these devices may become part of the routine diagnostic follow-up to guide therapy in patients who have respiratory distress or clinical evidence of impaired perfusion in whom the adequacy or excess of intracardiac filling pressures cannot be determined from clinical assessment.

CONSEQUENCES OF MISDIAGNOSIS

The diagnosis of heart failure may be straightforward in a patient with dyspnea, signs of congestion, and elevated BNP level. Conversely, many patients have multiple comorbid conditions that make the assessment of shortness of breath more of a diagnostic dilemma. Pulmonary conditions such as chronic obstructive pulmonary disease (Chapter 88) represent the most common reason for misdiagnosis. The BNP level and echocardiogram results are useful in this situation. Other potential causes of edema or volume overload include renal failure (Chapter 131), venous thrombosis (Chapters 81 and 98), and venous insufficiency. If left ventricular systolic function is normal, it may be difficult to make a conclusive determination of the relative role of heart failure with preserved ejection fraction compared with other concomitant conditions, such as severe obesity, deconditioning, chronic anemia, or other systemic illnesses. BNP levels may be helpful in some circumstances. In other situations, exercise testing or invasive hemodynamic testing may be necessary to establish the appropriate diagnosis. Misdiagnosis can result in excessive and unnecessary diagnostic testing, higher costs, and increased morbidity and mortality because of the inappropriate use or nonuse of heart failure therapies.

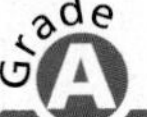

Grade A References

A1. O'Connor CM, Starling RC, Hernandez AF, et al. Effect of nesiritide in patients with acute decompensated heart failure. *N Engl J Med*. 2011;365:32-43.

A2. Bonow RO, Maurer G, Lee KL, et al. Myocardial viability and survival in ischemic left ventricular dysfunction. *N Engl J Med*. 2011;364:1617-1625.

A3. Binanay C, Califf RM, Hasselblad V, et al. Evaluation study of congestive heart failure and pulmonary artery catheterization effectiveness: the ESCAPE trial. *JAMA*. 2005;294:1625-1633.

GENERAL REFERENCES

For the General References and other additional features, please visit Expert Consult at https://expertconsult.inkling.com.

59

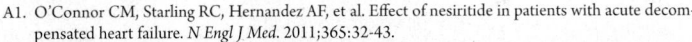

HEART FAILURE: MANAGEMENT AND PROGNOSIS

JOHN J. V. MCMURRAY AND MARC A. PFEFFER

EVALUATION AND MANAGEMENT OF HEART FAILURE

Heart failure is an overarching term for a syndrome (i.e., a constellation of signs and symptoms) that encompasses a vast spectrum of cardiovascular disorders and is associated with a greatly heightened risk for death and nonfatal adverse cardiovascular events (Chapter 58). Treatment is initially directed toward prevention of cardiac injury (e.g., due to hypertension or myocardial infarction) or toward limiting structural progression if cardiac damage has already occurred (e.g., left ventricular remodeling with declining left ventricular ejection fraction) and delaying the development of symptomatic heart failure. When symptoms develop, treatments are also directed at improving functional status as well as prognosis.

Approximately one in five adults will develop heart failure. In the United States, 5.8 million people have heart failure, and U.S. hospitals annually admit 1.0 million patients with a primary diagnosis of heart failure. The estimated cost of heart failure in the United States is about $24 billion per year. Randomized controlled clinical trials (RCTs) supply the framework for quantifying what different therapeutic approaches can offer. Even when they are definitive, RCTs only generate data about average risks and benefits of the tested therapeutic option in a selected cohort. Because an individual patient's responses can only be implied from the overall estimated group responses, RCTs cannot definitively direct the approach of every patient or answer the myriad questions that confront the practitioner regarding the specific circumstances of the patient. Another major limitation of RCTs is the relatively narrow time frame of observation, generally only months to several years, compared with epidemiologic experiences during decades. Despite these limitations, RCTs are the premier tool of evidence-based medicine, and the field of heart failure has fortunately been the focus of relatively high-quality RCTs that have provided robust evidence to improve clinical care and prognosis (Table 59-1 and E-Table 59-1). Indeed, the implementation of evidence from RCTs into clinical practice has resulted in impressive temporal improvements in survival after discharge from a first hospital admission for heart failure. Moreover, the age at which symptomatic heart failure first becomes evident has increased. Despite these tangible advances, heart failure continues to be a leading cause of morbidity and mortality in elderly people.

STAGES OF HEART FAILURE

The American Heart Association/American College of Cardiology Guidelines for the Evaluation and Management of Chronic Heart Failure in the Adult use a staging classification to underscore the evolution and progression of heart failure severity (Fig. 59-1).[1] This classification emphasizes the use of

TABLE 59-1 THERAPIES OF PROVEN BENEFIT IN HEART FAILURE*

Angiotensin-converting enzyme inhibitors
Angiotensin receptor blockers
β-Blockers
Mineralocorticoid receptor antagonists
Sacubitril-valsartan
Hydralazine-isosorbide dinitrate
Ivabradine
Digitalis
Cardiac resynchronization therapy
Cardioverter-defibrillator
Ventricular assist device
Exercise training

*See E-Table 59-1 for more details.

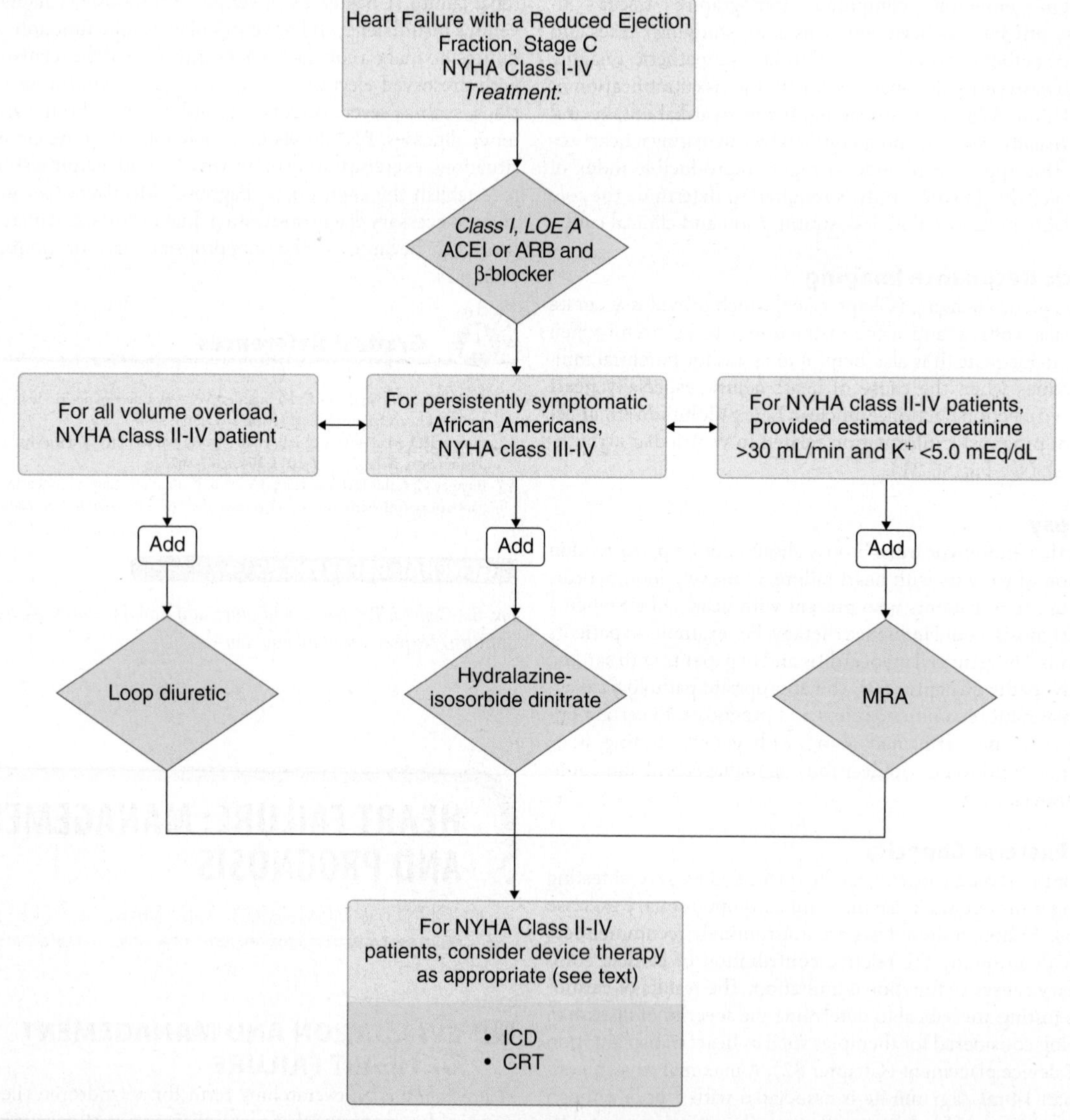

FIGURE 59-1. General approach to heart failure. Stage C heart failure with a reduced ejection fraction. Evidence-based, guideline-directed medical therapy. ACEI = angiotensin-converting enzyme inhibitor; ARB = angiotensin-receptor blocker; CRT = cardiac resynchronization therapy; ICD = implantable cardiovascular-defibrillator; MRA = mineralocorticoid receptor antagonist; NYHA = New York Heart Association. (Adapted from Yancy CW, Jessup M, Bozkurt B, et al. 2013 ACCF/AHA guideline for the management of heart failure: a report of the American College of Cardiology Foundation/American Heart Association Task Force on practice guidelines. *Circulation.* 2013;128:e240-327.)

different strategies and therapeutic options across the full spectrum of the syndrome, from prevention of heart failure to palliation of patients with end-stage disease.

Stage A: Individuals at Risk for Development of Heart Failure

Stage A designates patients at risk for development of heart failure based on concomitant cardiovascular diseases such as hypertension, coronary artery disease, and diabetes mellitus. Also included in stage A are individuals with prior exposure to cardiotoxic agents such as doxorubicin (Chapter 179) and those with a family history of a cardiomyopathy (Chapter 60). Although these predisposing factors do not by themselves technically constitute the syndrome of heart failure, the guidelines stress the importance of identifying individuals with modifiable factors because this represents an important opportunity to reduce the reservoir of patients at risk.

Population-based preventive approaches can reduce the incidence of heart failure. For example, public health programs targeting the eradication of the insect vector for *Trypanosoma cruzi* (Chapter 347) have reduced the incidence of Chagas cardiomyopathy (Chapter 60) in endemic regions of South and Central America.

Other population-based approaches to reduce the incidence of heart failure require specific screening efforts to identify individuals with modifiable risk factors. The most important although unfortunately nonmodifiable risk factor for the development of heart failure is advanced age; the incidence of heart failure rises sharply per decade after the age of 45 years (Chapter 58). For each decade of age after 45 years, the incidence of heart failure doubles, and heart failure is the leading hospital diagnosis for patients older than 65 years in the United States.

HYPERTENSION

Of the modifiable factors, hypertension (Chapter 67) undoubtedly contributes the greatest population attributable risk for heart failure. In other words, even though the increased risk for heart failure in an individual with hypertension is modest, the high prevalence of hypertension in the general population means that at a population level, hypertension is the major cause of heart failure.

The contribution of hypertension to the risk for heart failure was a consistent finding from all major cardiovascular epidemiologic studies, and the earliest RCTs of antihypertensive therapy showed unambiguous reductions in the risk for heart failure. Of the components of blood pressure, elevated systolic pressure has a greater influence on the incidence of heart failure than does diastolic pressure. In fact, aging is associated with a progressive rise in systolic blood pressure and fall in diastolic pressure as the compliance of the arterial tree diminishes (Chapter 67). In community-based studies, isolated systolic hypertension and elevated pulse pressure have been the most predictive blood pressure measurements for development of heart failure. In the Systolic Hypertension in the Elderly Program, antihypertensive treatment with chlorthalidone followed by atenolol reduced the incidence of new heart failure by about 50%, a treatment effect size recently exceeded (relative risk reduction 64%) with indapamide followed by perindopril in the Hypertension in Very Elderly Trial, probably the last placebo-controlled antihypertensive trial. In general, the actual extent of blood pressure lowering achieved, not the agent used, is the most important factor for preventing heart failure and reducing overall rates of major cardiovascular events.[A1] However, the greatest reduction in risk for heart failure seems to be seen when initial therapy is based on a diuretic and angiotensin-converting enzyme (ACE) inhibitor. By comparison, treatment with α-blockers increases the risk for heart failure compared with other antihypertensive drugs. Most important, it is estimated that effective treatment of hypertension (Chapter 67) will substantially reduce the age-adjusted incidence of heart failure by approximately 60% in women and 50% in men.

OTHER RISK FACTORS

Treatment of atherosclerotic risk factors, such as hypercholesterolemia (Chapter 206), and promotion of measures that encourage healthier lifestyles, such as smoking cessation (Chapter 32), weight control (Chapter 220), adoption of a Mediterranean diet (Chapter 213), and aerobic exercise (Chapter 16), should also reduce the number of individuals who progress from stage A to stage B (structural heart disease but without symptoms of heart failure). ACE inhibitors protect against the development of heart failure in patients with diabetes mellitus or with evidence of atherosclerosis. Although obesity is correlated with hypertension, lipid abnormalities, and glucose intolerance, an elevated body mass index is also an independent risk factor for the development of heart failure.

Stage B: Asymptomatic Structural or Functional Heart Disease

Stage B identifies asymptomatic (New York Heart Association or Canadian Cardiovascular Society class I; Chapter 58) patients who have a structural or functional cardiac disorder (e.g., left ventricular hypertrophy, enlargement, or dysfunction and valvar abnormalities) but do not have the signs and symptoms, such as dyspnea and fatigue, of the heart failure syndrome. In addition to history, physical examination, and electrocardiography (Chapter 54), more extensive screening with echocardiography (Chapter 55) or other imaging modalities (Chapter 56) is often required to detect patients with asymptomatic cardiac structural abnormalities.

A patient who has an acute myocardial infarction not complicated by early heart failure is an obvious example of someone who transitions from stage A to stage B. Rapid pharmacologic or mechanical coronary reperfusion is one of the immediate goals of therapy, with the aim of limiting the extent of myocardial injury and reducing the risk for death and future development of heart failure (Chapters 72 and 73). Survivors of the acute phase of myocardial infarction, a well-studied stage B cohort, are at particularly high risk for the future development of heart failure, with an overall annual incidence of 2% per year—but higher in patients who are older, have a lower left ventricular ejection fraction, do not routinely perform at least moderate exercise, or have concomitant hypertension or diabetes mellitus. For example, a clinically stable asymptomatic patient who has recovered from a myocardial infarction but who is older than 60 years with a left ventricular ejection fraction of less than 50% and a history of diabetes and hypertension has an estimated 30% 5-year likelihood of experiencing death or heart failure; without diabetes or hypertension, the 5-year estimated rate becomes 12%. By comparison, a younger myocardial infarction survivor who has a left ventricular ejection fraction over 50% and does not have hypertension or diabetes would be anticipated to have a 5-year rate for heart failure or death of only 3%. Data also suggest that an assessment of right ventricular function provides further independent incremental prediction for the risk for developing heart failure. With the continued improvements in care of patients with acute myocardial infarction (Chapters 72 and 73) and the use of implantable cardioverter-defibrillators (ICDs) after myocardial infarction in patients with reduced left ventricular ejection fraction, this pool of stage B patients, who represent a reservoir for new-onset heart failure, has been expanding. An ICD is recommended in patients who have a left ventricular ejection fraction of 35% or less and who survive at least 40 days after an acute myocardial infarction to reduce the risk for death (Chapter 73).

The impaired left ventricle, often due to a prior myocardial infarction, can undergo progressive chamber enlargement. This process, also termed left ventricular remodeling, describes the time-dependent and often insidious structural alterations of the impaired left ventricle, whereby the relationship of the left ventricular cavity volume increases out of proportion to mass, so the overall ventricular geometry becomes more distorted, usually more spherical. This distortion of left ventricular geometry often leads to mitral regurgitation. These structural changes produce regional and global increases in myocardial wall stress, which can promote further remodeling and contribute to the progressive deterioration of cardiac function and structure often associated with the later stages of symptomatic heart failure.

TREATMENT Rx

The treatment of heart failure is guided by the stage of symptoms and signs (see Fig. 59-1) as well as a robust literature of therapies proved to be beneficial by randomized trials (Fig. 59-2 and see E-Table 59-1).

Angiotensin-Converting Enzyme Inhibitors and Angiotensin Receptor Blockers

Mechanistic studies confirm that ACE inhibitors inhibit progressive left ventricular enlargement by reducing wall stress during the entire cardiac cycle as well as by more direct inhibition of the intracellular signaling pathways involved in myocardial hypertrophy and interstitial fibrosis. This attenuation of ventricular remodeling by ACE inhibitors reduces the development of symptomatic heart failure and death in stage B asymptomatic patients with left ventricular dysfunction by about 20%. In addition, deaths, often sudden and unexpected, attributed to cardiovascular causes, are reduced in stage B patients by ACE inhibitor therapy.

Therapy	Stage A	Stage B	Stage C	Stage D
	Trials			
Antihypertensive agents	✓	✓	✓	✓
Statins	✓	✓	(✓)	(✓)
β-Blockers		✓	✓	✓
ACE inhibitors	✓	✓	✓	✓
Angiotensin II receptor blockers (ARBs)		✓	✓	✓
Hydralazine/nitrates			✓	✓
Digoxin			✓	✓
Ivabradine			✓	✓
Mineralocorticoid antagonists			✓	✓
Implantable cardioverter-defibrillator (ICD)		✓	✓	(✓)
Cardiac resynchronization therapy (CRT)			✓	✓
Left ventricle assist device (LVAD)				✓

Stage A	Stage B	Stage C	Stage D
High risk for HF without structural heart disease or symptoms of HF	Structural heart disease but without signs or symptoms of HF	Structural heart disease with prior or current symptoms of HF	Refractory HF requiring specialized interventions
Patients with • Hypertension • Artherosclerotic disease • Diabetes • Obesity • Metabolic syndrome or Patients using • Cardiotoxins with family history of cardiomyopathy (FHx CM)	Patients with • Previous MI • LV remodeling including LVH and low EF • Asymptomatic valvular disease	Patients with • Known structural heart disease • Shortness of breath and fatigue, reduced exercise tolerance	Patients with marked symptoms at rest despite maximal medical therapy (e.g., those who are recurrently hospitalized or cannot be safely discharged from the hospital without specialized interventions)
↓ THERAPY	↓ THERAPY	↓ THERAPY	↓ THERAPY
Goals • Treat hypertension • Encourage smoking cessation • Treat lipid disorders • Encourage regular exercise • Discourage alcohol intake, illicit drug use • Control metabolic syndrome **Drugs** • ACEI or ARB as appropriate for patients with vascular disease or diabetes	**Goals** • Treat hypertension • Encourage smoking cessation • Treat lipid disorders • Encourage regular exercise • Discourage alcohol intake, illicit drug use • Control metabolic syndrome **Drugs** • ACEI or ARB as appropriate for patients with vascular disease or diabetes • β-Blockers in appropriate patients **Devices in selected patients** • Implantable defibrillators	**Goals** • Treat hypertension • Encourage smoking cessation • Treat lipid disorders • Encourage regular exercise • Discourage alcohol intake, illicit drug use • Control metabolic syndrome • Dietary salt restriction **Drugs for routine use** • Diuretics for fluid retention • ACEI • β-Blockers in appropriate patients • Mineralocorticoid antagonists **Drugs in selected patients** • ARBs • Digitalis • Hydralazine/nitrates • Ivabradine **Devices in selected patients** • Biventricular pacing • Implantable defibrillators	**Goals** • Appropriate measures under stages A, B, C • Decision re: appropriate level of care **Options** • Compassionate end-of-life care/hospice • Extraordinary measures • Heart transplantation • Chronic inotropes • Permanent mechanical support • Experimental surgery or drugs

FIGURE 59-2. **Stages of heart failure and therapies at various stages of heart failure (HF). Check marks indicate therapies proved by randomized trials to be beneficial; check marks in brackets indicate benefits uncertain. ACEI, angiotensin converting enzyme inhibitor; ARB, angiotensin receptor blocker; EF, ejection fraction; LV, left ventricle; LVH, left ventricular hypertrophy; MI, myocardial infarction.**

Several ACE inhibitors are effective as prophylactic therapy for high-risk stage B patients, and the target dose of each agent is established (Table 59-2). Therefore, patients with left ventricular systolic dysfunction, heart failure, or both complicating acute myocardial infarction should receive an ACE inhibitor to reduce the risk for chronic heart failure, reinfarction, stroke, and death.[1,2] The angiotensin receptor blocker (ARB) valsartan (Table 59-3) is as effective as captopril in reducing risk for cardiovascular death and other nonfatal cardiovascular outcomes, thereby providing an alternative pharmacologic class of agents for patients who cannot tolerate an ACE inhibitor because of cough or angioedema.[A2] Importantly, in patients with left ventricular dysfunction or acute heart failure in the context of a myocardial infarction, the combination of an ACE inhibitor and ARB is not better than either alone, so combination therapy is not recommended in this setting.

β-Blockers

β-Adrenergic receptor blockers (β-blockers) have long been known to reduce death and recurrent myocardial infarction when they are administered during the acute phase of myocardial infarction in patients without pulmonary congestion (Chapter 73). However, carvedilol (Table 59-4) also improves survival, reduces subsequent nonfatal myocardial infarctions, and has a favorable trend for reduced hospitalizations for heart failure in patients with a recent myocardial infarction and reduced left ventricular ejection fraction (≤40%) when it is added to an ACE inhibitor and should be considered in such patients.[A3] For stage B patients whose left ventricular dysfunction does not have an ischemic etiology, the evidence for β-blockers is less firm.

Treatment of Arrhythmias

Functional as well as structural problems may lead to the development of heart failure. For example, a persistently rapid ventricular rate in patients with atrial fibrillation can cause a rate-related (tachycardia-induced) cardiomyopathy (Chapter 64). Adequate pharmacologic control of the ventricular rate or interventions to restore sinus rhythm or to ablate re-entry pathways (Chapter 66) may reduce the risk for heart failure.

Other Therapies

Any treatments that control hypertension or reduce the risk for myocardial infarction will benefit stage B patients. Examples include statins, antiplatelet agents, and smoking cessation.

Stages C and D: Symptomatic Heart Failure

The development of symptoms and signs of the heart failure syndrome defines the transition from patients in the asymptomatic "at-risk" stages (A and B) to those who fulfill the clinical diagnosis of symptomatic heart failure (Chapter 58). This transition to the symptomatic phase underscores the progressive nature of heart failure and heralds a marked decline in prognosis. In one study, for example, the 2-year mortality rate was 27% in symptomatic patients compared with 10% in asymptomatic patients despite similarly reduced left ventricular ejection fractions and comorbidities.

TREATMENT Rx

The goals of treatment for patients with stage C and stage D heart failure are relief of symptoms, avoidance of hospital admission, and prevention of premature death. In general, the preventive measures that are of value during stages A and B should be sustained in patients with stages C and D heart failure.

Heart Failure with Reduced Left Ventricular Ejection Fraction

Pharmacologic Treatment

Drugs are the mainstay of the treatment of patients with symptomatic heart failure on the basis of the cumulative experiences from RCTs (see E-Table 59-1), particularly for patients with reduced left ventricular ejection fraction. However, devices and surgery have an important and increasing role in patients with advanced symptomatic heart failure (stages C and D; see Fig. 59-1). Exercise clearly improves well-being and clinical outcomes (see E-Table 59-1), but the evidence base for other lifestyle interventions is less robust. The organization and delivery of care can also have a substantial impact on outcomes.

Diuretics

Mechanism of Action

Diuretics act by blocking sodium reabsorption at specific sites in the renal tubule, thereby enhancing urinary excretion of sodium and water.

Clinical Benefits

Although not proven to improve mortality and morbidity in large trials, diuretics are required in nearly all patients with symptomatic heart failure (stages C and D) to relieve dyspnea and the signs of sodium and water retention ("congestion"), that is, peripheral and pulmonary edema. No other treatment relieves symptoms and the signs of sodium and water overload as rapidly and effectively. Once a patient needs a diuretic, treatment is usually necessary for the rest of the patient's life, although the dose and type of diuretic may vary.

Practical Use

The key principle is to prescribe the minimum dose of diuretic needed to maintain an edema-free state ("dry weight"). Excessive use can lead to electrolyte imbalances, such as hyponatremia, hypokalemia (and risk for digitalis toxicity), hyperuricemia (and risk for gout), and uremia. The risk for renal dysfunction is increased by concomitant use of nonsteroidal anti-inflammatory drugs (NSAIDs). Diuretic-induced hypovolemia may also cause symptomatic hypotension and prerenal azotemia. Restriction of dietary sodium intake may help reduce but does not eliminate the requirement for diuretics. Diuretic dosing should be flexible, with temporary increases for evidence of fluid retention (e.g., increasing symptoms, weight gain, edema) and decreases for evidence of hypovolemia (e.g., as a consequence of increased electrolyte loss due to gastroenteritis, decreased fluid intake, or both).

In some patients with milder symptoms of heart failure and preserved renal function (stage C), a thiazide diuretic such as chlorthalidone may suffice. In more advanced heart failure (stage D) or in patients with concomitant renal dysfunction, a loop diuretic such as furosemide is often needed. Loop diuretics cause a rapid onset of an intense but relatively short-lived diuresis compared with the longer lasting but gentler effect of a thiazide diuretic. The timing of administration of a loop diuretic, which need not be taken first thing every morning, can be adjusted according to the patient's social activities. The dose may be postponed or even temporarily omitted if the patient has to travel or has another activity that might be compromised by the prompt action of the diuretic. In severe heart failure (stage D), the effects of long-term administration of a loop diuretic may be diminished by increased sodium reabsorption at the distal tubule. This problem can be offset by use of the combination of a loop diuretic and a thiazide or thiazide-like diuretic (e.g., hydrochlorothiazide or metolazone), which act in synergy with a loop diuretic by blocking sodium reabsorption in different segments of the nephron. This combination requires more frequent monitoring of electrolytes and renal function for diuretic-induced hyponatremia, abnormalities of the serum potassium level, and prerenal azotemia.

A period of intravenous loop diuretic, given either as bolus injections or by continuous infusion, may be required in patients who become resistant to the action of oral diuretics. Why this resistance develops is uncertain, but factors thought to be important include impaired absorption of oral diuretics due to gut edema, hypotension, reduced renal blood flow, renal venous congestion, and adaptive changes in the nephron.

Patients with symptomatic heart failure (stages C and D) should be also considered for treatment with a mineralocorticoid receptor (aldosterone) antagonist, such as spironolactone, which increases excretion of sodium but not of potassium (see later). Patients receiving a combination of diuretics require careful monitoring of blood chemistry and clinical status. The use of a mineralocorticoid receptor (or, rarely, a potassium-sparing diuretic) along with an ACE inhibitor or ARB (treatment with all three is not recommended) requires particular care and surveillance for hyperkalemia.

Although they are highly effective in relieving symptoms and signs, diuretics alone are not sufficient for treatment of heart failure. In cases of severe resistant volume overload, mechanical removal of fluid by ultrafiltration may be considered. The addition of other disease-modifying treatments will better maintain clinical stability, slow structural progression, and reduce the risk for hospital admission and premature death.

ACE Inhibitors

Mechanism of Action

These drugs act by inhibiting the enzyme that converts the inactive decapeptide angiotensin I to the active octapeptide angiotensin II (and that also breaks down bradykinin). In patients with heart failure, excessive angiotensin II is thought to exert myriad harmful actions mediated through stimulation of the angiotensin II type 1 receptor subtype (AT1R), including vasoconstriction (which increases ventricular afterload), excessive growth of myocytes and the extracellular matrix (contributing to maladaptive left ventricular remodeling), activation of the sympathetic nervous system, prothrombotic actions, and augmentation of the release of arginine vasopressin and the retention of sodium (both directly and through stimulation of secretion of aldosterone, which activates the mineralocorticoid receptor).

ACE inhibitors also reduce the breakdown of bradykinin (because ACE is identical to kininase II), and the resultant accumulation of bradykinin is directly or indirectly responsible for two of the specific adverse effects of ACE inhibitors, cough, and angioedema. Bradykinin may, however, also have beneficial effects (vasodilation, inhibition of adverse cardiovascular remodeling, and

TABLE 59-2 PRACTICAL GUIDANCE ON THE USE OF ANGIOTENSIN-CONVERTING ENZYME INHIBITORS AND ANGIOTENSIN RECEPTOR BLOCKERS IN PATIENTS WITH HEART FAILURE DUE TO LEFT VENTRICULAR SYSTOLIC DYSFUNCTION

WHY?

Two major randomized trials (CONSENSUS I and SOLVD-T) and a meta-analysis of smaller trials have conclusively shown that angiotensin-converting enzyme (ACE) inhibitors increase survival, reduce hospital admissions, and improve New York Heart Association (NYHA) class and quality of life in patients with *all* grades of symptomatic heart failure. Other major randomized trials in patients with systolic dysfunction after acute myocardial infarction (SAVE, AIRE, TRACE) have shown that angiotensin-converting enzyme (ACE) inhibitors increase survival. In patients with heart failure (ATLAS), the composite end point of death or hospital admission was reduced by higher doses of ACE inhibitor compared with lower doses. ACE inhibitors have also been shown to delay or to prevent the development of symptomatic heart failure in patients with *asymptomatic* left ventricular systolic dysfunction.

In patients previously intolerant of an ACE inhibitor, candesartan has been shown to reduce the risk for the composite outcome of cardiovascular death or heart failure hospitalization, to reduce the risk for heart failure hospital admission, and to improve NYHA class. These findings in heart failure are supported by another randomized trial in patients with left ventricular systolic dysfunction, heart failure, or both complicating acute myocardial infarction (VALIANT) in which valsartan was as effective as the ACE inhibitor captopril in reducing mortality and cardiovascular morbidity.

Added to standard therapy, including an ACE inhibitor, in patients with all grades of symptomatic heart failure, the angiotensin receptor blockers (ARBs) valsartan and candesartan have been shown, in two major randomized trials (Val-HeFT and CHARM), to reduce heart failure hospital admissions, to improve NYHA class, and to maintain quality of life. The two CHARM low–left ventricular ejection fraction trials (CHARM-Alternative and CHARM-Added) also showed that candesartan reduced all-cause mortality.

IN WHOM AND WHEN?

ACE Inhibitors

Indications
- Potentially all patients with heart failure and a low ejection fraction
- First-line treatment (along with β-blockers) in patients with NYHA class II to IV heart failure; start as early as possible in course of disease. ACE inhibitors are also of benefit in patients with asymptomatic left ventricular systolic dysfunction (NYHA class I).

Contraindications
- History of angioedema
- Known bilateral renal artery stenosis

Cautions/seek specialist advice
- Significant hyperkalemia (K^+ > 5.0 mmol/L)
- Significant renal dysfunction (creatinine 221 μmol/L or >2.5 mg/dL)
- Symptomatic or severe asymptomatic hypotension (systolic blood pressure <90 mm Hg)

Drug interactions to look out for
- K^+ supplements/K^+-sparing diuretics, e.g., amiloride and triamterene (beware combination preparations with furosemide)
- Mineralocorticoid receptor antagonists (spironolactone, eplerenone), angiotensin receptor blockers, NSAIDs*
- "Low-salt" substitutes with a high K^+ content

Angiotensin Receptor Blockers

Indications
- First-line treatment (along with β-blockers) in patients with NYHA class II to IV heart failure intolerant of an ACE inhibitor because of cough or angioedema
- Second-line treatment (after optimization of ACE inhibitor and β-blocker*) in patients with NYHA class II–IV heart failure intolerant of a mineralocorticoid receptor antagonist

Contraindications
- Known bilateral renal artery stenosis

Cautions/seek specialist advice
- As for ACE inhibitors

Drug interactions to look out for
- As for ACE inhibitors

WHERE?

In the community for most patients

Exceptions—see Cautions/seek specialist advice

WHICH ACE INHIBITOR AND WHAT DOSE?

	STARTING DOSE	TARGET DOSE
Captopril	6.25 mg thrice daily	50 mg thrice daily
Enalapril	2.5 mg twice daily	10-20 mg twice daily
Lisinopril	2.5-5.0 mg once daily	20-35 mg once daily
Ramipril	2.5 mg once daily	5 mg twice daily or 10 mg once daily
Trandolapril	0.5 mg once daily	4 mg once daily

WHICH ARB AND WHAT DOSE?

	STARTING DOSE	TARGET DOSE
Candesartan	4 or 8 mg once daily	32 mg once daily
Valsartan	40 mg twice daily	160 mg twice daily
Losartan	50 mg once daily	150 mg daily

HOW TO USE?

Start with a low dose (see above).

Double dose at not less than 2-week intervals.

Aim for target dose (see above) or, failing that, the highest tolerated dose.

Remember: *some* ACE inhibitor/ARB is better than *no* ACE inhibitor/ARB.

Monitor blood pressure and blood chemistry (urea/blood urea nitrogen, creatinine, K^+).

Check blood chemistry 1-2 weeks after initiation and 1-2 weeks after final dose titration.

When to stop up-titration, reduce dose, stop treatment—see Problem Solving.

A specialist heart failure nurse may assist with education of the patient, follow-up (in person or by telephone), biochemical monitoring, and dose up-titration.

ADVICE TO PATIENT

Explain expected benefits (see Why?).

Treatment is given to improve symptoms, to prevent worsening of heart failure leading to hospital admission, and to increase survival.

Symptoms improve within a few weeks to a few months of starting treatment.

Advise patients to report principal adverse effects, (i.e., dizziness/symptomatic hypotension, cough)—see Problem Solving.

Advise patients to avoid NSAIDs* not prescribed by a physician (self-purchased over-the-counter) and salt substitutes high in K^+—see Problem Solving.

PROBLEM SOLVING

Asymptomatic low blood pressure
- Does not usually require any change in therapy

Symptomatic hypotension
- If dizziness, lightheadedness, or confusion and a low blood pressure, reconsider need for nitrates, calcium-channel blockers,† and other vasodilators.
- If no signs or symptoms of congestion, consider reducing diuretic dose.
- If these measures do not solve problem, seek specialist advice.

Cough
- Cough is common in patients with heart failure, many of whom have smoking-related lung disease.
- Cough is also a symptom of pulmonary edema, which should be excluded when a new or worsening cough develops.
- ACE inhibitor–induced cough rarely requires treatment discontinuation.
- When a troublesome cough does develop (e.g., one stopping the patient from sleeping) and can be proved to be due to ACE inhibition (i.e., recurs after ACE inhibitor withdrawal and rechallenge), substitution of an ARB can be considered

Worsening renal function
- Some rise in urea (blood urea nitrogen), creatinine, and potassium is to be expected after initiation of an ACE inhibitor/ARB; if an increase is small and asymptomatic, no action is necessary.
- An increase in creatinine of up to 50% above baseline, or 266 μmol/L (3 mg/dL), whichever is the smaller, is acceptable.
- An increase in potassium to ≤5.5 mmol/L is acceptable.
- If urea, creatinine, or potassium does rise excessively, consider stopping concomitant nephrotoxic drugs (e.g., NSAIDs*) and other potassium supplements or retaining agents (triamterene, amiloride, spironolactone-eplerenone‡) and, if no signs of congestion, reducing the dose of diuretic.
- If greater rises in creatinine or potassium than those outlined above persist despite adjustment of concomitant medications, the dose of the ACE inhibitor should be halved and blood chemistry rechecked within 1 to 2 weeks; if there is still an unsatisfactory response, specialist advice should be sought.
- If potassium rises to >5.5 mmol/L or creatinine increases by >100% or to above 310 μmol/L (3.5 mg/dL), the ACE inhibitor/ARB should be stopped and specialist advice sought.
- Blood chemistry should be monitored frequently and serially until potassium and creatinine have plateaued.

Note: It is rarely necessary to stop an ACE inhibitor/ARB, and clinical deterioration is likely if treatment is withdrawn. Ideally, specialist advice should be sought before treatment discontinuation.

*Avoid nonsteroidal anti-inflammatory drugs (NSAIDs) unless essential.

†Calcium-channel blockers should be discontinued unless absolutely essential (e.g., for angina or hypertension).

‡The safety and efficacy of an ACE inhibitor used with an angiotensin receptor blocker and spironolactone (as well as β-blocker) are uncertain, and the use of all three inhibitors of the renin-angiotensin-aldosterone system together is not recommended.

Modified from McMurray J, Cohen-Solal A, Dietz R, et al. Practical recommendations for the use of ACE inhibitors, β-blockers, mineralocorticoid receptor antagonists and angiotensin receptor blockers in heart failure: putting guidelines into practice. *Eur J Heart Fail.* 2005;7:710-721.

TABLE 59-3 PRACTICAL GUIDANCE ON THE USE OF Β-BLOCKERS IN PATIENTS WITH HEART FAILURE DUE TO LEFT VENTRICULAR SYSTOLIC DYSFUNCTION

WHY?

Several major randomized controlled trials (i.e., USCP, CIBIS II, MERIT-HF, COPERNICUS) have shown, conclusively, that certain β-blockers increase survival, reduce hospital admissions, and improve New York Heart Association (NYHA) class and quality of life when added to standard therapy (diuretics, digoxin, and angiotensin-converting enzyme [ACE] inhibitors) in patients with *stable* mild and moderate heart failure and in some patients with severe heart failure. In the SENIORS trial, which differed substantially in design from the aforementioned studies (older patients, some patients with preserved left ventricular systolic function, longer follow-up), nebivolol appeared to have a smaller treatment effect, although direct comparison is difficult. One other trial (BEST) did not show a reduction in all-cause mortality but did report a reduction in cardiovascular mortality and is otherwise broadly consistent with the aforementioned studies. The COMET trial showed that carvedilol was substantially more effective than a low dose of short-acting metoprolol tartrate* (long-acting metoprolol succinate was used in MERIT-HF).

IN WHOM AND WHEN?

Indications
- Potentially *all* patients with *stable* mild and moderate heart failure; patients with severe heart failure should be referred for specialist advice.
- First-line treatment (along with ACE inhibitors) in patients with *stable* NYHA class II to III heart failure; start as early as possible in course of disease.

Contraindications
- Asthma
- Second- or third-degree atrioventricular block

Cautions/seek specialist advice
- Severe (NYHA class IV) heart failure
- Current or recent (<4 weeks) exacerbation of heart failure (e.g., hospital admission with worsening heart failure, heart block, or heart rate <60 beats/minute).
- Persisting signs of congestion, hypotension/low blood pressure (systolic < 90 mm Hg), raised jugular venous pressure, ascites, marked peripheral edema

Drug interactions to look out for
- Verapamil, diltiazem (should be discontinued)†
- Digoxin, amiodarone

WHERE?

In the community in stable patients (NYHA class IV/severe heart failure patients should be referred for specialist advice)
Not in unstable patients hospitalized with worsening heart failure
Other exceptions—see Cautions/seek specialist advice

WHICH β-BLOCKER AND WHAT DOSE?

	STARTING DOSE	TARGET DOSE
Bisoprolol	1.25 mg once daily	10 mg once daily
Carvedilol	3.125 mg twice daily	25-50 mg twice daily
Metoprolol CR/XL	12.5-25 mg once daily	200 mg once daily*
Nebivolol	1.25 mg once daily	10 mg once daily

HOW TO USE?

Start with a low dose (see above).
Double dose at *not less than* 2-week intervals.
Aim for target dose (see above) or, failing that, the highest tolerated dose.
Remember: *some* β-blocker is better than *no* β-blocker.
Monitor heart rate, blood pressure, and clinical status (symptoms, signs—especially signs of congestion, body weight).
Check blood chemistry 1 to 2 weeks after initiation and 1 to 2 weeks after final dose titration.
When to stop up-titration, reduce dose, stop treatment—see Problem Solving.
A specialist heart failure nurse may assist with education of the patient, follow-up (in person or by telephone), and dose up-titration.

ADVICE TO PATIENT

Explain expected benefits (see Why?).
Treatment is given to improve symptoms, to prevent worsening of heart failure leading to hospital admission, and to increase survival.
Symptomatic improvement may develop slowly after starting treatment, taking 3 to 6 months or longer.
Temporary symptomatic deterioration *may* occur during initiation or up-titration phase; in the long term, β-blockers improve well-being.
Advise patient to report deterioration (see Problem Solving) and that deterioration (tiredness, fatigue, breathlessness) can usually be easily managed by adjustment of other medication; patients should be advised not to stop β-blocker therapy without consulting the physician.
To detect and to treat deterioration early, patients should be encouraged to weigh themselves daily (after waking, before dressing, after voiding, before eating) and to increase their diuretic dose should their weight increase, persistently (>2 days), by >1.5–2.0 kg.‡

PROBLEM SOLVING

Worsening symptoms or signs (e.g., increasing dyspnea, fatigue, edema, weight gain)
- If increasing congestion, increase dose of diuretic or halve dose of β-blocker (if increasing diuretic does not work).
- If marked fatigue (or bradycardia—see below), halve dose of β-blocker (rarely necessary); review patient in 1 to 2 weeks; if not improved, seek specialist advice.
- If serious deterioration, halve dose of β-blocker or stop this treatment (rarely necessary); seek specialist advice.

Low heart rate
- If <50 beats/minute and worsening symptoms, halve dose of β-blocker or, if severe deterioration, stop β-blocker (rarely necessary).
- Review need for other heart rate–slowing drugs (e.g., digoxin, amiodarone, diltiazem, or verapamil†).
- Arrange electrocardiogram to exclude heart block.
- Seek specialist advice.

Asymptomatic low blood pressure
- Does not usually require any change in therapy.

Symptomatic hypotension
- If dizziness, lightheadedness, or confusion and a low blood pressure, reconsider need for nitrates, calcium-channel blockers,† and other vasodilators.
- If no signs or symptoms of congestion, consider reducing diuretic dose or ACE inhibitor.
- If these measures do not solve problem, seek specialist advice.

Note: β-Blockers should not be stopped suddenly unless absolutely necessary (there is a risk for a "rebound" increase in myocardial ischemia or infarction and arrhythmias). Ideally, specialist advice should be sought before treatment discontinuation.
*Metoprolol tartrate should not be used in preference to an evidence-based β-blocker in heart failure.
†Calcium-channel blockers should be discontinued unless absolutely necessary, and diltiazem and verapamil are generally contraindicated in heart failure.
‡This is generally good advice for all patients with heart failure.
Modified from McMurray J, Cohen-Solal A, Dietz R, et al. Practical recommendations for the use of ACE inhibitors, β-blockers, mineralocorticoid receptor antagonists and angiotensin receptor blockers in heart failure: putting guidelines into practice. *Eur J Heart Fail.* 2005;7:710-721.

TABLE 59-4 PRACTICAL GUIDANCE ON THE USE OF MINERALOCORTICORTICOID RECEPTOR ANTAGONISTS IN PATIENTS WITH HEART FAILURE DUE TO LEFT VENTRICULAR SYSTOLIC DYSFUNCTION

WHY?

The RALES study showed that low-dose spironolactone increased survival, reduced hospital admissions, and improved New York Heart Association (NYHA) class when added to standard therapy (diuretic, digoxin, angiotensin-converting enzyme [ACE] inhibitor, and, in a minority of cases, β-blocker) in patients with severe (NYHA class III or IV) heart failure symptoms. The findings of RALES are supported by another randomized trial in patients with heart failure, reduced ejection fraction, and mild symptoms (NYHA class II) in which another mineralocorticoid receptor (MRA), antagonist, eplerenone, increased survival and reduced hospital admissions for heart failure when added to an ACE inhibitor (or angiotensin receptor blocker [ARB]) and β-blocker (EMPHASIS-HF). These findings in heart failure are supported by another randomized trial in patients with left ventricular systolic dysfunction and heart failure (or diabetes) complicating *acute* myocardial infarction (EPHESUS), in which eplerenone increased survival and reduced hospital admission for cardiac causes.

IN WHOM AND WHEN?

Indications
- Potentially all patients with symptomatic heart failure (class II to IV NYHA)
- Second-line therapy (after ACE inhibitors and β-blockers*) in patients with symptomatic heart failure (NYHA class II to IV); second-line therapy (after ACE inhibitors and β-blockers) in patients with a LVEF ≤ 40%

Cautions/seek specialist advice
- Significant hyperkalemia ($K^+ > 5.0$ mmol/L)[†]
- Significant renal dysfunction (creatinine > 221 μmol/L or 2.5 mg/dL)[†]

Drug interactions to look out for
- K^+ supplements/K^+-sparing diuretics (e.g., amiloride and triamterene; beware combination preparations with furosemide)
- ACE inhibitors, angiotensin receptor blockers, NSAIDs[‡]
- "Low-salt" substitutes with a high K^+ content

WHERE?

In the community or in the hospital
Exceptions—see Cautions/seek specialist advice

WHICH DOSE?[†]

	STARTING DOSE	TARGET DOSE
Spironolactone	25 mg once daily or on alternate days	25-50 mg once daily
Eplerenone	25 mg once daily	50 mg once daily

HOW TO USE?

Start with a low dose (see above).
Check blood chemistry at 1, 4, 8, and 12 weeks; 6, 9, and 12 months; 6-monthly thereafter.
If K^+ rises above 5.5 mmol/L or creatinine rises to 221 μmol/L (2.5 mg/dL), reduce dose to 25 mg on alternate days and monitor blood chemistry closely.
If K^+ rises to >6.0 mmol/L or creatinine to >310 μmol/L (3.5 mg/dL), stop spironolactone immediately and seek specialist advice.
A specialist heart failure nurse may assist with education of the patient, follow-up (in person or by telephone), biochemical monitoring, and dose up-titration.

ADVICE TO PATIENT

Explain expected benefits (see Why?).
Treatment is given to improve symptoms, to prevent worsening of heart failure leading to hospital admission, and to increase survival.
Symptom improvement occurs within a few weeks to a few months of starting treatment.
Avoid NSAIDs[‡] not prescribed by a physician (self-purchased over-the-counter agent) and salt substitutes high in K^+.
If diarrhea or vomiting occurs, patients should stop the mineralocorticoid receptor and contact the physician.

PROBLEM SOLVING

Worsening renal function/hyperkalemia
- See How to Use? section.

Major concern is hyperkalemia (>6.0 mmol/L); although this was uncommon in RALES and EMPHASIS-HF, it has been seen more commonly in clinical practice.
- Conversely, a high-normal potassium level may be desirable in patients with heart failure, especially if they are taking digoxin.

It is important to avoid other K^+-retaining drugs (e.g., K^+-sparing diuretics such as amiloride and triamterene) and nephrotoxic agents (e.g., NSAIDs[‡])
The risk for hyperkalemia and renal dysfunction when a mineralocorticoid receptor antagonist is given to patients already taking an ACE inhibitor and ARB is higher than when a mineralocorticoid receptor antagonist is added to just an ACE inhibitor or ARB given singly; close and careful monitoring is mandatory.*
Some "low-salt" substitutes have a high K^+ content.
Male patients treated with spironolactone may develop breast discomfort or gynecomastia (these problems are significantly less common with eplerenone).

Modified from McMurray J, Cohen-Solal A, Dietz R, et al. Practical recommendations for the use of ACE inhibitors, β-blockers, aldosterone antagonists and angiotensin receptor blockers in heart failure: putting guidelines into practice. *Eur J Heart Fail.* 2005;7:710-721.
*The safety and efficacy of spironolactone used with an ACE inhibitor and an ARB (as well as a β-blocker) are uncertain, and the use of all three inhibitors of the renin-angiotensin-aldosterone system together is not recommended.
[†]It is extremely important to adhere to these cautions and doses in light of recent evidence of serious hyperkalemia with spironolactone in usual clinical practice in Ontario.
[‡]Avoid nonsteroidal anti-inflammatory drugs (NSAIDs) unless essential.

antithrombotic actions), although the importance of these bradykinin-mediated actions to the clinical benefits of ACE inhibition is uncertain.

Clinical Benefits

Clinical trials have shown that treatment with an ACE inhibitor, when it is used alone or added to diuretics and digoxin, decreases left ventricular size, improves ejection fraction, reduces symptoms and hospital admissions, and prolongs survival (see E-Table 59-1). These agents also reduce the risk for development of myocardial infarction and possibly diabetes, and atrial fibrillation. Consequently, treatment with an ACE inhibitor is recommended for all patients with left ventricular systolic dysfunction, irrespective of symptoms or etiology. ACE inhibitors are not a substitute for a diuretic but mitigate diuretic-induced hypokalemia.

Practical Use

ACE inhibitors should be introduced as early as possible in a patient's treatment. The only contraindications are current symptomatic hypotension and bilateral renal artery stenosis (Chapter 125); the latter is often associated with a prompt and marked increase in serum levels of blood urea nitrogen and creatinine when renal perfusion is reduced precipitously by inhibiting the production and actions of angiotensin II. Treatment should be started in a low dose (see Table 59-2), with the dose gradually increased toward a target dose of proven benefit in a clinical trial. The patient should be evaluated for symptomatic hypotension, uremia, and hyperkalemia after each dose increment; these adverse effects are uncommon and can usually be resolved by reduction in the dose of diuretic (if the patient is edema free) or concomitant hypotensive or nephrotoxic medications (e.g., nitrates, calcium-channel blockers, or NSAIDs). A dry, nonproductive cough occurs in approximately 15% of patients treated with an ACE inhibitor, and if it is troublesome, substitution of an ARB is recommended. In the rare cases of angioedema (Chapter 252), the ACE inhibitor should be stopped and not used again; an ARB can be cautiously substituted (see later).

β-Blockers

Mechanism of Action

Heart failure is characterized by excessive activation of the sympathetic nervous system, which causes vasoconstriction and sodium retention, thereby increasing cardiac preload and afterload and often inducing myocardial ischemia or arrhythmias. In addition, norepinephrine can cause hypertrophy of myocytes and augment their apoptosis. β-Blockers counteract many of these harmful effects of the hyperactivity of the sympathetic nervous system. A rapid heart rate is an important prognostic factor in heart failure among patients in sinus rhythm, and β-blockers reduce heart rate.

Clinical Benefits

The long-term addition of a β-blocker to an ACE inhibitor (and diuretic, digoxin, and mineralocorticoid receptor antagonist) further improves left ventricular function and symptoms, reduces hospital admissions, and strikingly improves survival. Consequently, a β-blocker is recommended for all patients with symptomatic systolic dysfunction, irrespective of etiology and severity, and the combination of a β-blocker with an ACE inhibitor is now the cornerstone of the treatment of symptomatic heart failure (see Fig. 59-1). Treatment with a β-blocker, added to an ACE inhibitor, is recommended for all patients with symptoms (NYHA classes II to IV) and left ventricular systolic dysfunction, irrespective of etiology.

Practical Use

The major contraindications to use of a β-blocker in heart failure are asthma (although it is important to note that the dyspnea caused by pulmonary congestion can be confused with reactive airway disease) and second- or third-degree atrioventricular block. Initiation of treatment during an episode of acute decompensated heart failure should also be avoided until the patient is stabilized. In addition, caution is advised in patients with a heart rate below 60 beats per minute or a systolic blood pressure below 90 mm Hg. It is recommended that a β-blocker shown to produce benefits in a randomized trial be used (see E-Table 59-1).

Like ACE inhibitors, β-blockers should be introduced as early as possible in a patient's treatment, started in a low dose (see Table 59-3), and increased gradually toward a target dose used in a clinical trial (the "start low–go slow" approach). The patient should be checked for symptomatic hypotension and excessive bradycardia after each dose increment, but both of these side effects are uncommon, and hypotension can often be resolved by reduction in the dose of other nonessential blood pressure–lowering medications (e.g., nitrates and calcium-channel blockers). Bradycardia is more likely in patients who are also taking digoxin or amiodarone, and the simultaneous use of these agents should be reviewed if excessive bradycardia occurs. On occasion, symptomatic worsening and fluid retention (e.g., weight gain or edema) may occur after initiation of a β-blocker or during dose up-titration; these side effects usually can be resolved by a temporary increase in the diuretic dose without necessitating discontinuation of the β-blocker.

Treatment with a β-blocker should be given for life, although the dose may need to be decreased (or, rarely, treatment discontinued) temporarily during episodes of acute decompensation if the patient shows signs of circulatory underperfusion or refractory congestion.

Mineralocorticoid Receptor (Aldosterone) Antagonists

Mechanism of Action

Aldosterone, which is the second effector hormone in the renin-angiotensin-aldosterone cascade, has detrimental vascular, renal, autonomic, and cardiac actions when it is produced in excess in patients with heart failure. Excessive aldosterone promotes sodium retention and hypokalemia, and it is believed to contribute to myocardial fibrosis, all of which predispose to arrhythmias. Aldosterone mediates its effects by activating the mineralocorticoid receptor, which is also stimulated by other endogenous corticosteroids. Mineralocorticoid receptor antagonists block these undesirable actions and, at high doses, also act as potassium-sparing diuretics.

Clinical Benefits

The mineralocorticoid receptor antagonist spironolactone (see E-Table 59-1) improves symptoms, reduces hospital admissions, and increases survival when it is added to an ACE inhibitor (and diuretics and digoxin) in patients with a reduced left ventricular ejection fraction and severely symptomatic heart failure. Eplerenone, another mineralocorticoid receptor antagonist, reduces mortality and morbidity when it is added to both an ACE inhibitor and β-blocker in patients with a reduced left ventricular ejection fraction and heart failure with mild symptoms (NYHA class II) (see E-Table 59-1). Consequently, a mineralocorticoid receptor antagonist should be considered in all patients who remain symptomatic (class II to IV) despite treatment with a diuretic, ACE inhibitor (or ARB), and β-blocker.[2,A4] Addition of a mineralocorticoid receptor antagonist to an ACE inhibitor (and diuretic, digoxin, and β-blocker) is preferred to the addition of an ARB because of the greater benefit of a mineralocorticoid receptor antagonist, particularly in reducing all-cause mortality. When begun, a mineralocorticoid receptor antagonist should be given indefinitely. The combination of an ACE inhibitor, an ARB, and a mineralocorticoid receptor antagonist has not been adequately evaluated and is not recommended.

Practical Use

Treatment with a mineralocorticoid receptor antagonist should be initiated with a low dose (see Table 59-4) with careful monitoring of serum electrolytes and renal function. Hyperkalemia and uremia are the adverse effects of greatest concern (as with ACE inhibitors and ARBs), and a mineralocorticoid receptor antagonist should not be given to patients with a serum potassium concentration of more than 5.0 mmol/L, serum creatinine concentration above 2.5 mg/dL (>221 µmol/L), or other evidence of markedly impaired renal function. The importance of selection of patients and dose is underscored by reports of a worrisome incidence of serious hyperkalemia in community practice settings. Spironolactone can have antiandrogenic effects, especially painful gynecomastia, in men; because eplerenone has less of an action on the androgen receptor, it is a reasonable substitute in patients who experience this adverse effect.

Angiotensin Receptor Blockers

Mechanism of Action

Instead of inhibiting the production of angiotensin II through ACE, ARBs block the binding of angiotensin II to the AT1R. This pharmacologically distinct mechanism of action may be important because angiotensin II is also believed to be produced by other enzymes, such as chymase. ARBs do not inhibit kininase II or the breakdown of bradykinin, so they do not cause cough and cause less angioedema than do ACE inhibitors.

Clinical Benefits

When they are used as the sole agent in heart failure, ARBs produce benefits similar to those of ACE inhibitors. An ARB may be used as a substitute in patients who have cough or angioedema with an ACE inhibitor. When they are used in clinically effective doses, other adverse effects such as hypotension, renal dysfunction, and hyperkalemia are encountered as frequently as with an ACE inhibitor. As with an ACE inhibitor, the specific agents, dosing regimens, and target doses that were of demonstrable benefit in clinical trials are recommended (see E-Table 59-1).

In the broader population of patients with persistent heart failure symptoms (stage C or stage D, functional class II to IV) that can be treated with an ACE inhibitor, an ARB in combination with an ACE inhibitor (and β-blocker) further improves the left ventricular ejection fraction, relieves symptoms, reduces the risk for hospital admission for worsening heart failure, and can also reduce the risk for cardiovascular death (see Table 59-2), but the incremental benefits are not as great as adding a mineralocorticoid receptor antagonist (see later). Although a mineralocorticoid receptor antagonist is the preferred additional therapy because of its greater benefits (see above), an ARB is an alternative as the third disease-modifying drug (in addition to an ACE inhibitor and β-blocker) in patients who have persistent symptoms (stages C and D) and who do not tolerate a mineralocorticoid receptor antagonist. The efficacy and safety of the four-drug combination of an ACE inhibitor, β-blocker, ARB, and mineralocorticoid receptor antagonist are uncertain. Consequently, either a mineralocorticoid receptor antagonist or an ARB, but not both, should be added to an ACE inhibitor and a β-blocker in such patients.

The approach to initiation, titration, and monitoring of an ARB is similar to that of an ACE inhibitor (see Table 59-2). The adverse effects, with the exception of cough and angioedema, are similar. Use of multiple inhibitors of the renin-angiotensin-aldosterone system requires even more diligent monitoring, especially in patients at higher risk for uremia, hypotension, or hyperkalemia (i.e., patients 75 years of age and older or with a systolic blood pressure below 100 mm Hg, diabetes, or renal impairment) because combined treatment with an ACE inhibitor and an ARB significantly increases the risks for worsening renal function, hyperkalemia, and symptomatic hypotension. As with ACE inhibitors, β-blockers, and mineralocorticoid receptor antagonists, treatment with ARBs should be indefinite unless there is intolerance.

Neprilysin is an enzyme that breaks down natriuretic peptides and other vasoactive substances, including adrenomedullin and bradykinin. Inhibiting neprilysin augments the concentrations of these substances, which have vasodilator and natriuretic actions. Because neprilysin also degrades angiotensin II, a neprilysin inhibitor must be combined with an agent that blocks the renin-angiotensin system. Since ACE and neprilysin each breakdown bradykinin, inhibiting both enzymes leads to a significant increase in the risk of angioedema. For that reason, the angiotensin receptor neprilysin inhibitor (ARNI) sacubitril-valsartan (LCZ696) was developed. When 200 mg twice daily of sacubitril-valsartan was compared with enalapril 10 mg twice daily, the ARNI reduced cardiovascular mortality and heart failure hospitalization, as well as reducing other measures of progressive worsening of heart failure, including symptom deterioration.[A5] Sacubitril-valsartan causes more hypotension and slightly more angioedema than enalapril. Sacubitril-valsartan is currently undergoing regulatory review in the US and Europe.

Ivabradine

Mechanism of Action

Ivabradine is the first of a new class of drugs developed to inhibit the mixed sodium-potassium channel or current (also known as the funny channel, abbreviated as I_f or I_{Kf}) in the sinoatrial node and, in so doing, reduce heart rate. Reduction in heart rate is the only known cardiac action of ivabradine, which has this effect only in patients in sinus rhythm.

Clinical Benefits

Only one large RCT has examined the effect of ivabradine on mortality and morbidity in patients with symptomatic heart failure (NYHA class II to IV), a reduced ejection fraction (≤35%), and sinus rhythm with a rate of 70 beats per minute or greater. That trial showed that ivabradine improved symptoms and ejection fraction and reduced the risk for hospitalization for heart failure (but not mortality) when added to an ACE inhibitor (or ARB), a β-blocker, and a mineralocorticoid receptor antagonist.[A6]

Practical Use

Although not approved for use in the United States, ivabradine should be considered where it is available in patients who have persistent symptoms (NYHA class II to IV) despite treatment with other disease-modifying therapies, that is, an ACE inhibitor (or ARB), β-blocker, and mineralocorticoid receptor antagonist, and who are in sinus rhythm with a heart rate of 70 beats per minute or greater. Treatment should be started at 5 mg twice daily, increased to 7.5 mg twice daily after 14 days unless the heart rate is 60 beats per minute or less, and reduced usually to 2.5 mg twice daily if the rate is less than 50 beats per minute. Symptomatic bradycardia and visual disturbance (phosphenes) are uncommon but require the dose be reduced or ivabradine be discontinued. Ivabradine also may increase the risk for atrial fibrillation, which should prompt discontinuation of the drug. Ivabradine should not be used in combination with agents that prolong the QT interval (e.g., amiodarone) and must be used cautiously with inhibitors (including grapefruit juice) or inducers of CYP3A4.

Digoxin

Mechanism of Action

Digitalis glycosides inhibit the cell membrane Na^+, K^+-ATPase pump, thereby increasing intracellular calcium and myocardial contractility. In addition, digoxin is thought to enhance parasympathetic and reduce sympathetic nervous activity as well as to inhibit renin release.

Clinical Benefits

Only one large RCT has examined the effects of starting (as opposed to withdrawing) digoxin on mortality and morbidity in patients with heart failure in sinus rhythm. In that trial, digoxin did not reduce mortality but did decrease the risk for admission to hospital for worsening heart failure when it was added to a diuretic and an ACE inhibitor. In patients in sinus rhythm, addition of digoxin is recommended only for those whose heart failure remains symptomatic despite standard treatment with a diuretic and three disease-modifying drugs, that is, an ACE inhibitor (or ARB), a β-blocker, and a mineralocorticoid receptor antagonist (or ARB). In patients with atrial fibrillation, digoxin may be used at an earlier stage if a β-blocker fails to control the ventricular rate during exercise; Chapter 64). Digoxin can also be used to control the ventricular rate when β-blocker treatment is being initiated or up-titrated.

If the effect of digoxin is needed urgently, loading with 10 to 15 μg/kg lean body weight, given in three divided doses 6 hours apart, may be used. The maintenance dose should be one third of the loading dose. Smaller maintenance doses (e.g., one fourth of the loading dose and not more than 62.5 μg/day) should be used in elderly patients and in patients with reduced renal function as well as in patients with a low body mass. Monitoring of the serum digoxin concentration is recommended because of the narrow therapeutic window. A steady state is reached 7 to 10 days after treatment is started; blood should be collected at least 6 hours (and ideally 8 to 24 hours) after the last dose. The currently recommended therapeutic range is 0.5 to 1.0 ng/mL).

Digoxin can cause anorexia, nausea, arrhythmias, confusion, and visual disturbances, especially if the serum concentration is above 2.0 ng/mL. Hypokalemia increases susceptibility to the adverse effects. The dose of digoxin should be reduced in elderly patients and in patients with renal dysfunction. Certain drugs increase serum digoxin concentration, including amiodarone.

Hydralazine and Isosorbide Dinitrate

Mechanism of Action

Hydralazine is a powerful direct-acting arterial vasodilator. Its mechanism of action is not understood, although it may inhibit enzymatic production of superoxide, which neutralizes nitric oxide and may induce nitrate tolerance. Nitrates dilate both veins and arteries, thereby reducing preload and afterload by stimulating the nitric oxide pathway and increasing cyclic guanosine monophosphate in vascular smooth muscle. Neither drug on its own nor any other direct-acting vasodilator has been demonstrated to be beneficial in heart failure.

Clinical Benefits

Although this combination has been known for some time to improve systolic function and probably to reduce death in class II to IV heart failure compared with placebo, head-to-head comparison showed that an ACE inhibitor is superior for improving survival. Nevertheless, on the basis of subgroup analyses suggesting that African Americans responded better to hydralazine and isosorbide dinitrate, a subsequent RCT showed that the addition of hydralazine and isosorbide dinitrate in African Americans, most of whom were receiving an ACE inhibitor and β-blocker and many of whom were taking spironolactone, further reduced mortality and hospital admissions for heart failure and improved quality of life.[A7] The combination of hydralazine and isosorbide dinitrate is recommended in African American patients with NYHA class III or IV symptoms and an ejection fraction of 45% or less despite treatment with standard disease-modifying drugs, that is, an ACE inhibitor, β-blocker, and mineralocorticoid receptor antagonist.

A fixed combination of 37.5 mg of hydralazine and 20 mg of isosorbide dinitrate was used in the trial; one tablet was given, and if tolerated, a second was given 12 hours later. One tablet was then prescribed three times daily for 3 to 5 days, at which point the dose was increased to the target maintenance of two tablets three times daily, that is, a daily dose of 225 mg hydralazine and 120 mg isosorbide dinitrate. Because of the limited inclusion criteria of this RCT, however, it is uncertain whether this combination of vasodilators is an effective addition in other populations of patients.

Practical Use

Other than for African Americans, the main indication for hydralazine and isosorbide dinitrate is as a substitute in patients with intolerance to an ACE inhibitor and an ARB. Hydralazine and isosorbide dinitrate should be used as additional treatment in African Americans and considered for other patients who remain symptomatic with other proven therapies. The main dose-limiting adverse effects of hydralazine and isosorbide dinitrate are headache and dizziness. A rare adverse effect of higher doses of hydralazine, especially in slow acetylators, is a systemic lupus erythematosus–like syndrome (Chapter 266).

Omega-3 Polyunsaturated Fatty Acids

In one trial, 1 gram of n-3 PUFA (850 to 852 mg eicosapentaenoic acid and docosahexaenoic acid as ethyl esters in the average ratio of 1 : 1.2) per day led to a small reduction in cardiovascular morbidity and mortality in patients with heart failure. Although this agent may have beneficial anti-inflammatory and antiarrhythmic effects, its current role in the treatment of heart failure is uncertain, especially because trials in survivors of acute myocardial infarction have not shown benefit (Chapter 73).[A8]

The aforementioned treatments are the only pharmacologic therapies shown to be of benefit in patients with heart failure and a reduced left ventricular ejection fraction. Other treatments have been tested in randomized trials and shown to have a neutral (e.g., amlodipine) or uncertain (e.g., bosentan and etanercept) effect on mortality and morbidity or to increase mortality (e.g., dronedarone, milrinone, flosequinan, vesnarinone, and moxonidine).

Other Pharmacologic Issues

Some therapies that are of proven value for cardiovascular conditions that underlie or are associated with heart failure are of uncertain benefit (antiplatelet treatment, Chapter 38) or do not improve outcomes (statins, Chapter 206) in patients with persistent, symptomatic heart failure. Vitamin K antagonists such as warfarin and other non–vitamin K oral anticoagulants that inhibit factor Xa or thrombin are indicated in patients with atrial fibrillation to reduce the risk for thromboembolism, provided patients have no contraindications to their use (Chapter 64). Anticoagulants may also be used in patients with evidence of intracardiac thrombus (e.g., detected during echocardiographic examination) or systemic thromboembolism. The many interactions of warfarin with other drugs, including some statins and amiodarone (Chapter 38), must always be considered. The non–vitamin K oral anticoagulants are contraindicated in patients with severe renal impairment and should be given at a reduced dose in patients with less severe impairment (Chapter 38), keeping in mind that no therapy is available to reverse the actions of these agents.[A9][A10] Heparin prophylaxis (Chapter 38) against deep vein thrombosis is indicated when patients with heart failure are bed bound, such as during hospital admission. Vaccination against influenza and pneumococcal infection is advised (Chapter 18) in all patients with heart failure because these infections can lead to severe clinical deterioration.

Drugs to Use with Caution in Heart Failure

Patients with heart failure, especially if it is severe, often have renal and hepatic dysfunction, so any drug excreted predominantly by the kidneys or metabolized by the liver may accumulate (Chapter 29). Similarly, because of their extensive comorbidity, patients with heart failure are inevitably treated with multiple drugs, thereby increasing the risk for drug interactions.

Drugs that should be avoided, if possible, in heart failure include thiazolidinediones (because of the risk for fluid retention), most antiarrhythmic drugs (including dronedarone, although amiodarone and dofetilide may be used), most calcium-channel blockers (with the possible exception of amlodipine, although this drug may increase the risk for pulmonary edema), corticosteroids, NSAIDs, cyclooxygenase-2 inhibitors, many antipsychotics (e.g., clozapine), and antihistamines. The U.S. Food and Drug Administration recently raised the concern that the dopamine agonist pramipexole used to treat Parkinson disease (Chapter 409) also might increase the risk for developing heart failure. Metformin (because of the risk for lactic acidosis) should be used with caution. In a recent trial, saxagliptin was shown to increase the risk for developing heart failure in patients with diabetes.[A11] Some salt substitutes contain substantial amounts of potassium and must be used cautiously. Other dietary constituents (e.g., grapefruit and cranberry juice) and supplements such as St. John's wort can interact with drugs taken by patients with heart failure, especially warfarin and digoxin.

Organization of Care

Several studies have shown that organized, nurse-led, multidisciplinary care can improve outcomes in patients with heart failure, particularly by reducing recurrent hospital admissions. Thus it is recommended that all patients with heart failure be enrolled in a disease management program.[A12] The most successful disease management approach seems to involve education of the patients, their families, and caregivers about heart failure and its treatment (including flexible diuretic dosing and reinforcing the importance of adherence), recognizing (and acting on) early deterioration (dyspnea, sudden weight gain, edema), and optimizing proven pharmacologic treatments. A home-based rather than clinic-based approach may be best, although trials are needed to compare these types of interventions directly. Even telephone follow-up is of value.[A13] New technology enabling noninvasive home telemonitoring of physiologic measures (e.g., heart rate and rhythm, blood pressure, temperature, respiratory rate, weight, and estimated body water content) and implanted devices, which collect similar data and may be interrogated remotely, are also being tested as aids to monitoring and management, but studies to date have not given consistent results. However, in one moderate-sized trial, use of an implanted sensor for the noninvasive measurement of pulmonary artery pressure resulted in a 30% reduction in the number of heart failure hospitalizations.[A14] Despite the usefulness of brain-type natriuretic peptide (BNP) in the diagnosis of heart failure and as a prognostic measure, treatment guided by BNP levels has not been shown in randomized trials to be consistently better than standard, evidence-based care.

Education

Education of the patient, family, and caregivers is invaluable (Table 59-5). Self-detection of early signs and symptoms of deterioration provides for earlier intervention. Counseling on the proper use of therapies, with an emphasis on adherence, is critical.

Useful patient-oriented material is available from several reliable sources the Heart Failure Society of America (http://www.hfsa.org/hfsa-wp/wp/patient/education-modules/), American Heart Association (http://www.americanheart.org/presenter.jhtml?identifier=1486), National Heart, Lung and Blood Institute (http://www.nhlbi.nih.gov/health/dci/Diseases/Hf/HF_WhatIs.html), and the Heart Failure Association of the European Society of Cardiology (http://www.heartfailurematters.org/EN/Pages/index.aspx), and other organizations.

Medication Use Counseling

When appropriate, a patient should be taught how to adjust the dose of diuretic within individualized limits. The dose should be increased (or a supplementary diuretic added) if there is evidence of fluid retention (symptoms of congestion) and decreased if there is evidence of hypovolemia (e.g., increased thirst associated with weight loss or postural dizziness, especially during hot weather or an illness causing decreased fluid intake or sodium and water loss). If hypovolemia is more marked, the doses of other medications also will have to be reduced.

The expected effects, beneficial and adverse, of other drugs should also be explained in detail (e.g., possible association of cough with ACE inhibitor). It is useful to inform patients that improvement with many drugs is gradual and may become fully apparent only after several weeks or even months of treatment. It is also important to explain the need for gradual titration with ACE inhibitors, ARBs, and β-blocking drugs to a desired dose level, which again may take weeks or even months to achieve. Patients should be advised not to use NSAIDs without consultation and to be cautious about using herbal or other nonproprietary preparations (Chapter 39).

Adherence

Education and counseling of the patient, caregiver, and family promotes adherence, which is associated with better outcomes. Drug adherence can also be helped by home visits, specialized follow-up programs[3], and certain pharmacy aids, such as dose allocation (pill-organizing) boxes.

Lifestyle Modification

Exercise

Tailored, structured, supervised aerobic exercise is safe and improves functional capacity and quality of life in patients with heart failure (see E-Table 59-1). An appropriate exercise prescription may also reduce hospitalizations and mortality in patients with heart failure. Regular physical activity or exercise training if available is recommended for all patients with heart failure who are able to participate.[4]

Diet, Nutrition, and Alcohol

Most guidelines advocate avoidance of foods containing relatively high salt content in the belief that doing so may reduce the need for diuretic therapy. This recommendation is based on clinical experience, which suggests that excess sodium intake can be a precipitant of clinical decompensation. Some salt substitutes have a high potassium content, which can lead to hyperkalemia.

Restriction of fluid intake is indicated only during episodes of decompensation associated with peripheral edema or hyponatremia. In these situations, daily intake should be restricted to 1.5 to 2.0 L to help facilitate reduction in extracellular fluid volume and to avoid hyponatremia.

Reducing excessive weight will reduce the work of the heart and may lower blood pressure (Chapter 67). Conversely, malnutrition is common in severe heart failure, and the development of cardiac cachexia is an ominous sign. Reduced food intake is sometimes caused by nausea (e.g., related to digoxin use or hepatosplenic congestion) or abdominal bloating (e.g., due to ascites). In these cases, small frequent meals and high-protein and high-calorie liquids may be helpful. In severe decompensated heart failure, eating and bending may be difficult because of dyspnea.

Moderate alcohol intake is not thought to be harmful in heart failure, although excessive intake can cause cardiomyopathy and atrial arrhythmias in susceptible individuals. In patients with suspected alcoholic cardiomyopathy, abstinence from alcohol may improve cardiac function.

Smoking

Smoking causes peripheral vasoconstriction, which is detrimental in heart failure. Nicotine replacement therapy (Chapter 32) is believed to be safe in heart failure. The safety of bupropion in heart failure is uncertain, especially because it is known to increase blood pressure, and varenicline may increase cardiovascular risk.

Sexual Activity

Sexual activity need not be restricted in patients with compensated heart failure, although dyspnea may be limiting. In men with erectile dysfunction (Chapter 234), treatment with a cyclic guanine monophosphate phosphodiesterase type 5 inhibitor can be useful, but these drugs must not be taken within 24 hours of prior nitrate use, and nitrates must not be restarted for at least 24 hours afterward.

Driving

Patients with heart failure can continue to drive, provided their condition does not induce undue dyspnea, fatigue, or other incapacitating symptoms. Patients with recent syncope, cardiac surgery, percutaneous coronary intervention, or device placement may be restricted from driving, at least

TABLE 59-5 TOPICS THAT SHOULD BE DISCUSSED WITH A PATIENT WITH HEART FAILURE AND WITH HIS OR HER FAMILY AND CAREGIVERS

GENERAL ADVICE

Explain what heart failure is and why symptoms occur
- Causes of heart failure
- How to recognize symptoms
- What to do if symptoms occur
- Self-weighing (to identify fluid retention)

RATIONALE FOR TREATMENTS

Importance of adhering to pharmacologic and nonpharmacologic (e.g., dietary) treatments
Smoking advice
Prognosis

DRUG COUNSELING

Rationale (i.e., benefits of individual drugs)
Dose and time of administration
Potential adverse affects (and what, if any, action to take)
What to do in case of missed or skipped doses
Self-management (e.g., flexible diuretic dosing)

REST AND EXERCISE

Rest
Exercise and activities related to work
Daily physical activity
Sexual activity
Rehabilitation

PSYCHOSOCIAL ASPECTS

Depression
Cognitive function
Social support

VACCINATIONS AND IMMUNIZATIONS

Travel
Driving
Dietary and social habits
- Control sodium intake when necessary (e.g., some patients with severe heart failure)
- Avoid excessive fluids in severe heart failure
- Avoid excessive alcohol intake and illicit drugs

Modified from McMurray JJ, Adamopoulos S, Anker SD, et al. ESC Guidelines for the diagnosis and treatment of acute and chronic heart failure 2012: the Task Force for the Diagnosis and Treatment of Acute and Chronic Heart Failure 2012 of the European Society of Cardiology. Developed in collaboration with the Heart Failure Association (HFA) of the ESC. *Eur Heart J.* 2012;33:1787-1847.

temporarily, according to local regulations. Patients holding an occupational or commercial license may also be subject to additional restrictions.

Traveling

Short flights are unlikely to cause problems for a patient with compensated heart failure. Cabin pressure is generally maintained to provide an oxygen level no lower than equivalent to 6000 feet above sea level, which should be well tolerated in patients without severe pulmonary disease or pulmonary hypertension. Longer journeys may cause limb edema and dehydration, thereby predisposing to venous thrombosis. Adjustment of the dose of diuretics and other treatments should be discussed with the patient wishing to travel to a warm climate or a country where the risk for gastroenteritis is high. It is also advisable for heart failure patients to carry a list of medications and contact information for their health care provider.

Comorbidity

Comorbid conditions, which are common and important in patients with heart failure, may be due to the underlying cardiovascular disease that caused or contributed to heart failure (e.g., hypertension, coronary artery disease, diabetes mellitus), may arise as a complication of heart failure (e.g., arrhythmias), or can result from an adverse effect of treatment given for heart failure (e.g., gout). The exact causes of other comorbidities in heart failure, such as diabetes (Chapter 229), depression (Chapter 397), sleep apnea (Chapter 100), renal dysfunction (Chapter 130), and anemia (Chapter 158), are complex and uncertain. These and other comorbid conditions, such as chronic obstructive pulmonary disease and asthma, are important because they are a major determinant of prognosis and may limit the use of certain treatments for heart failure (e.g., renal dysfunction limiting use of ACE inhibitors or asthma limiting β-blockers) and because treatment of comorbidities may affect the stability of heart failure (e.g., NSAIDs needed for rheumatic conditions can cause salt and water retention and renal dysfunction). Both prevention (e.g., diabetes mellitus) and treatment (e.g., anemia) of comorbidities are being evaluated as a potential new therapeutic goal in heart failure.

Angina

β-Blockers are of benefit in both angina (Chapter 71) and heart failure. Similarly, ivabradine, which reduces heart rate by inhibiting the I_f current in the sinus node, is also beneficial in both angina and heart failure. Nitrates relieve angina but on their own are not of proven value in chronic heart failure. Calcium-channel blockers should generally be avoided in heart failure because they have a negative inotropic action and cause peripheral edema; only amlodipine has been shown to have no adverse effect on survival, but it may increase the risk for pulmonary edema. Trimetazidine, ranolazine, and nicorandil are antianginal drugs that are available in certain countries; their safety in patients with heart failure is uncertain. Percutaneous and surgical (Chapter 74) revascularization is also of value in relieving angina in selected patients with heart failure (see later). Coronary artery bypass grafting may reduce the risk for death from cardiovascular causes and cardiovascular hospitalization (including heart failure hospitalization) in selected heart failure patients with angina and a reduced ejection fraction (see later).

Atrial Fibrillation

Atrial fibrillation (Chapter 64) may be the cause of or a consequence of heart failure in a patient presenting with atrial fibrillation and a rapid ventricular rate, and the distinction can be difficult, especially because prolonged atrial fibrillation may lead to a rate-related cardiomyopathy. Thyrotoxicosis (Chapter 226) and mitral valve disease (Chapter 75), especially stenosis, must be excluded. Alcohol abuse should also be considered. β-Blockers and digoxin are given to control the ventricular rate. The patient should be supervised closely after the initiation of these treatments because underlying sinus node dysfunction may raise the risk for bradycardia. Unless the patient presents emergently with symptoms or signs of heart failure, myocardial ischemia, or hypertension, there is little or no evidence to support a strategy of restoring sinus rhythm rather than controlling the ventricular rate in most patients with heart failure (Chapter 64).[5] Atrioventricular node ablation and pacing may be required to control ventricular rate (Chapter 66). Catheter ablation can cure atrial fibrillation in some patients with heart failure, but the rate of success and its long-term benefits remain uncertain (Chapter 66). There is a strong indication for thromboembolism prophylaxis with warfarin in patients with heart failure and atrial fibrillation (Chapter 64).

Asthma and Reversible Airways Obstruction

Asthma is a contraindication for use of a β-blocker, but most patients with chronic obstructive pulmonary disease (Chapter 88) can tolerate a β-blocker. Pulmonary congestion can mimic chronic obstructive pulmonary disease. Systemic administration of a corticosteroid to treat reversible airways obstruction may cause sodium and water retention and exacerbate heart failure, whereas inhalation therapy is better tolerated.

Diabetes Mellitus

Diabetes mellitus is discussed in detail elsewhere (Chapter 229). The prevalence and incidence of diabetes mellitus are high in heart failure, and the risk for development of type 2 diabetes may be reduced by ACE inhibitors and ARBs. β-Blocker treatment is not contraindicated and is of benefit in patients with diabetes and heart failure. Thiazolidinediones cause sodium and water retention, may lead to decompensation, and are not recommended in patients with or at risk for heart failure. Metformin may cause lactic acidosis and is not recommended in patients with severe heart failure. Saxagliptin increases the risk for developing heart failure in patients with diabetes.

Abnormal Thyroid Function

Both thyrotoxicosis and hypothyroidism can cause heart failure (and thyrotoxicosis can cause atrial fibrillation, which may precipitate heart failure). Amiodarone can also induce both hypothyroidism and hyperthyroidism, the latter being particularly difficult to diagnose. The risk for thyroid dysfunction may be less with the related antiarrhythmic agent dronedarone, but dronedarone increases mortality in severe heart failure and should be avoided in patients with stage C or D heart failure or recently decompensated heart failure.

Gout

Hyperuricemia and gout (Chapter 273) are common in heart failure and can be caused or aggravated by diuretic treatment. Allopurinol may prevent gout, and acute attacks are better treated with colchicine, oral steroids, or intra-articular steroids rather than by an NSAID.

Renal Dysfunction

Most patients with heart failure have a reduced glomerular filtration rate. ACE inhibitors, ARBs, and mineralocorticoid receptor antagonists often cause a further small reduction in glomerular filtration rate and rise in serum blood urea nitrogen and creatinine levels, which, if limited, should not lead to discontinuation of treatment. Marked increases in blood urea nitrogen and creatinine, however, should prompt consideration of underlying renal artery stenosis (Chapter 125). Renal dysfunction may also be caused by sodium and water depletion, leading to relative hypovolemia (e.g., due to excessive diuresis, diarrhea, and vomiting) or hypotension. Nephrotoxic agents such as NSAIDs are also a common cause of renal dysfunction in heart failure.

Prostatic Obstruction

For prostatic disease (Chapter 129), a 5α-reductase inhibitor may be preferable to an α-adrenoceptor antagonist, which can cause hypotension and salt and water retention. A cyclic guanine monophosphate phosphodiesterase type 5 inhibitor is an alternative, but it cannot be used in patients taking nitrates. Prostatic obstruction should also be considered in male patients with deteriorating renal function.

Anemia

A normocytic, normochromic anemia (Chapter 158) is also common in heart failure, in part because of the high prevalence of renal dysfunction. Malnutrition and blood loss may also contribute. Intravenous iron treatment with 200 mg of ferric carboxymaltose improves quality of life and reduces symptoms in patients with NYHA class II to III heart failure, a reduced ejection fraction, and iron deficiency without adverse effects.[A15] By comparison, erythropoiesis-stimulating agent darbepoetin is not of benefit.[A16]

Depression

Depression (Chapter 397) is common in patients with heart failure, perhaps partly owing to disturbance of the hypothalamic-pituitary axis and other neurochemical pathways but also as a result of social isolation and the adjustment to chronic disease. Depression is associated with worse functional status, reduced adherence to treatment, and poor clinical outcomes. Both psychosocial interventions and pharmacologic treatment are helpful. Selective serotonin reuptake inhibitors are believed to be the best tolerated pharmacologic agents, whereas tricyclic antidepressants should be avoided because of their anticholinergic actions and potential to cause arrhythmias.

Cancer

Many anticancer drugs, particularly anthracyclines, cyclophosphamide, and trastuzumab (Herceptin), can cause myocardial damage and heart failure, as can mediastinal radiotherapy. Pericardial constriction can be a result of previous radiotherapy, and malignant pericardial involvement can cause effusion and tamponade (Chapter 77).

Devices and Surgery

Implantable Cardioverter-Defibrillators

About half of patients with heart failure die suddenly, mainly as the result of a ventricular arrhythmia. The relative risk for sudden death, as opposed to death from progressive heart failure, is greatest in patients with milder symptoms. In patients with more advanced heart failure, progressive pump failure deaths are relatively more common. Antiarrhythmic drugs have not been shown to improve survival in heart failure, but ICDs (Chapter 66) reduce the risk for death in selected patients after myocardial infarction (Chapter 73) and improve survival in patients with class II to III heart failure and systolic dysfunction who were otherwise treated with optimal medical therapy. All patients with class II or III heart failure, irrespective of etiology, and a left ventricular ejection fraction remaining at 35% or less despite at least 3 months of treatment with disease-modifying therapy (i.e., an ACE inhibitor [or ARB], β-blocker, and mineralocorticoid receptor antagonist [or ARB]) should be considered for an ICD provided they have no other conditions greatly limiting life expectancy (i.e., have an anticipated survival of at least a year) or quality of life.

Cardiac Resynchronization Therapy

About 30% of patients with heart failure have substantial prolongation of the QRS duration on the surface electrocardiogram, which is a marker of abnormal electrical activation of the left ventricle causing dyssynchronous contraction, less efficient ventricular emptying, and, often, mitral regurgitation. Atrioventricular coupling may also be abnormal, as reflected by a prolonged PR interval, as may interventricular synchrony. Cardiac resynchronization therapy (CRT) with atrial-biventricular or multisite pacing optimizes atrioventricular timing and improves synchronization of cardiac contraction. In symptomatic patients (NYHA class II to IV) who are in sinus rhythm, have marked systolic dysfunction (left ventricular ejection fraction ≤35%), and have a wide QRS, the addition of CRT to optimal medical therapy and an ICD improves pump function, reduces mitral regurgitation, relieves symptoms, and significantly prolongs exercise capacity. CRT also substantially reduces the risk for death and for hospital admission for worsening heart failure in such patients (see E-Table 59-1).[A17,A18] Many other outcome measures, including quality of life, are also improved. The greatest benefit appears to be in patients with a left bundle branch block (LBBB) morphology and in patients with mild symptoms (NYHA class II).[A19] Whether CRT is beneficial in patients in atrial fibrillation or with non-LBBB QRS widening is uncertain. All patients in sinus rhythm with persistent symptoms (NYHA class II to IV) and an ejection fraction of 35% or less despite optimal disease-modifying medical therapy (ACE inhibitor, β-blocker, and mineralocorticoid receptor antagonist) should be considered for CRT if they have a QRS duration of 130 msec or longer, especially if they have LBBB.[6]

Surgery

With the exception of cardiac transplantation and ventricular assist devices, there are no generally accepted criteria for surgical intervention. Use of operative procedures is variable among centers and greatly dependent on local experience and expertise. Expert imaging and detailed hemodynamic and functional assessments are usually required when any patient with heart failure is considered for surgery, and close liaison between the relevant experts in these fields is essential. The collective expertise in surgical centers is often used to make highly individualized decisions about whether to operate and what procedures will be attempted. "Established" operative treatments for patients with heart failure include coronary artery bypass grafting, surgery for mitral valve incompetence, surgery or percutaneous interventions for aortic valve stenosis (Chapter 75), implantation of ventricular assist devices, and heart transplantation.

A recent trial showed no benefit (in symptoms or rates of death or hospitalization for cardiac causes) of surgical ventricular reconstruction. Cardiomyoplasty and partial left ventriculectomy are other operations for heart failure now thought to be without benefit.

Percutaneous Coronary Intervention or Coronary Artery Bypass Grafting

Percutaneous coronary intervention or coronary artery bypass grafting (Chapter 74), as appropriate, is indicated for relief of angina. The extent of ischemia and residual myocardial viability can be determined by noninvasive assessments such as dobutamine echocardiography (Chapter 55), magnetic resonance imaging (Chapter 56), and positron emission tomographic scanning (Chapter 56) in patients with impaired left ventricular ejection fraction. Coronary artery bypass grafting may reduce the risk for cardiovascular death and hospitalization (including heart failure hospitalization) in selected heart failure patients with angina, a reduced ejection fraction, and two-vessel or three-vessel coronary disease.[A20] Coronary artery bypass grafting is therefore recommended in patients who have symptomatic heart failure (NYHA class II to III), angina pectoris, and suitable coronary anatomy and who are otherwise fit for surgery.

Whether coronary artery bypass grafting is beneficial in patients who have coronary artery disease but who do not have angina is less certain. Many physicians and surgeons consider revascularization in such asymptomatic patients only if ischemia affects a substantial area of myocardium as documented by noninvasive imaging. However, the hypothesis that improvement of coronary blood flow to viable but noncontracting ("hibernating") myocardium can improve ventricular function and clinical outcomes remains to be proved.

Cardiac Transplantation

Cardiac transplantation (Chapter 82) remains the most accepted surgical intervention in end-stage heart failure. Selection criteria usually focus on patients with refractory heart failure, that is, those with severe symptoms and functional limitations (peak oxygen consumption of less than 12 mL/kg per minute), as well as a particularly worrisome clinical course and prognosis attributed to their cardiac condition. These patients are often dependent on intravenous inotropic agents and mechanical support.

Mechanical Circulatory Support

Given the scarcity of organ donors, mechanical circulatory support using a left ventricular (or biventricular) assist device may be used as a "bridge to transplantation" or even as a permanent, definitive, procedure ("destination therapy") for some patients with advanced or end-stage heart failure. A pulsatile volume-displacement left ventricular assist device can provide a short but significant prolongation of survival in patients who have end-stage heart failure and are ineligible for transplantation (see E-Table 59-1), but the rates of bleeding, infective and thrombotic complications, and mechanical dysfunction necessitating repeat surgery were high with this older device. In patients with end-stage heart failure ineligible for transplantation, a newer continuous-flow device is significantly better than this older device in terms of 2-year survival without repeat device surgery or disabling stroke (46% versus 11%).[A21] Because not every hospital could or should be expected to offer all these levels of support for patients with advanced heart failure, there is a general recognition that such services should be concentrated in a limited number of tertiary centers.[7] Centers implanting these devices use criteria such as persistent (>2 months) severe symptoms despite optimal drug and device therapy and other features placing patients at high-risk for death (e.g., left ventricular ejection fraction <25%, three or more heart failure hospitalizations in the prior 12 months, peak oxygen consumption <12 mL/kg per minute, dependence on intravenous inotropic therapy, progressive end-organ dysfunction, and deteriorating right ventricular function) to decide who should considered for mechanical circulatory support.

Heart Failure with Preserved Left Ventricular Ejection Fraction (Diastolic Dysfunction)

Although all patients with symptomatic heart failure share a constellation of signs and symptoms, impaired physical capacity, and reduced quality of life, some have a preserved left ventricular ejection fraction (generally >40 or 50%), and many are thought to have diastolic dysfunction (Chapter 58).[8] Diastolic heart failure often has a cause different from that of systolic heart failure and a better survival rate (Chapters 53, 58, and 60), but sometimes it is an early manifestation of what will evolve into heart failure with a reduced left ventricular ejection fraction. The distinction is important, however, because most of the RCTs that generated the evidence for treatment of heart failure included only patients with reduced left ventricular ejection fractions (see E-Table 59-1). Treatment of the underlying cardiovascular and other disorders that contribute to symptomatic stage C and stage D of heart failure with preserved left ventricular ejection fraction, such as hypertension, myocardial ischemia, and diabetes, is critical and is as for stages A and B (see earlier). In patients with atrial fibrillation, control of the ventricular rate with a β-blocker or a rate-limiting calcium-channel blocker (or restoration of sinus rhythm) may be particularly important (Chapter 64). Diuretics are used empirically to treat sodium and water retention, according to the same principles as in heart failure with reduced left ventricular ejection fraction. In one trial of patients with a left ventricular ejection fraction greater than 40% (mean 54%), treatment with the ARB candesartan decreased the risk for hospital admission for heart failure but did not improve survival or the composite outcome of cardiovascular death or hospital admission for worsening heart failure. In a subsequent study of patients with a left ventricular ejection fraction of 45% or greater (mean 60%), the ARB irbesartan had no beneficial effect, raising the possibility that the benefit of candesartan in the earlier trial was largely in patients with borderline systolic dysfunction (i.e., a left ventricular ejection fraction of 40 to 50%). In a more recent study of patients with a left ventricular ejection fraction or 45% or greater (mean 56%), treatment with the mineralocorticoid receptor antagonist spironolactone decreased the risk for hospital admission for heart failure but did not improve survival or the composite outcome of cardiovascular death or hospital admission for worsening heart failure.[A22] Smaller studies in patients in sinus rhythm have shown that the calcium-channel blocker verapamil may improve symptoms and exercise capacity in patients with heart failure and preserved left ventricular ejection fraction, possibly by reducing heart rate and thereby increasing the duration of diastolic left ventricular filling as well as by directly enhancing myocardial relaxation. There are, however, no current RCTs in which this drug decisively reduced mortality or morbidity in patients with heart failure and preserved left ventricular ejection fraction, so treatment currently is aimed at relieving symptoms.

Heart Failure Due to Valvular Heart Disease

Heart failure also can arise as a result of regurgitant and stenotic valve disease (Chapter 75). It can sometimes be difficult to determine whether mitral regurgitation is primary or secondary in a patient with heart failure and left ventricular dilation, although a prior history of known valve disease or rheumatic fever may suggest a primary valve problem. The objective of treatment of primary valve disease is the prevention of heart failure by surgical repair or replacement of the diseased valve or valves (Chapter 75). The development of overt heart failure is an ominous sign, sometimes requiring emergent valve replacement (e.g., aortic stenosis) but sometimes indicating that valve replacement may not be possible (e.g., because of severe pulmonary hypertension).

Aortic Stenosis

Evaluation of the aortic valve (Chapter 75) can be difficult in patients with poor left ventricular systolic function. Such patients may have insufficient cardiac output to generate a high gradient across even a severely stenotic valve. Conversely, a calcified and degenerate but nonstenotic aortic valve may appear stenosed simply because it does not open normally in patients with very low cardiac output. A calculated valve area provides a better assessment of the severity of aortic stenosis in these patients. Stress echocardiography (Chapter 55) may help assess the potential for ventricular recovery after relief of aortic stenosis. Consideration should be given as to whether concomitant myocardial ischemia from coronary artery disease may also be contributing to a reversible depression of systolic function. Transcatheter valve replacement is a valuable technique for patients who have aortic stenosis but are at very high risk for open valve replacement.

Mitral Regurgitation

Mitral regurgitation can be a primary cause or a secondary manifestation in a patient with heart failure and left ventricular dilation (Chapter 75). Surgery sometimes will result in clinical improvement, but some patients with advanced left ventricular dysfunction will not achieve substantial benefit (e.g., mitral valve surgery in a patient with long-standing severe mitral regurgitation). Valve repair or annuloplasty may, however, be beneficial in carefully selected patients with secondary mitral regurgitation caused by or exacerbated by left ventricular dilation. It is not known whether valve repair is preferable to valve replacement.[A23] The role of percutaneous mitral valve repair is still uncertain and is under investigation.

Heart Failure Due to Nonischemic Dilated Cardiomyopathy

Patients with heart failure and normal coronary arteries should be evaluated for possible reversible causes. Untreated hypertension is now an unusual cause of dilated cardiomyopathy in the United States, but hypertension was once a leading cause in the United States and still remains a major consideration in many parts of the world. Infiltrative cardiomyopathies (e.g., hemochromatosis, amyloid, sarcoid) and arteritides sometimes have specific recommended therapies (Chapters 60, 95, 188, and 212). Chagas disease (Chapter 347) must be considered in patients from endemic areas. Alcohol and other toxins (e.g., chemotherapeutic agents) are other recognized causes of dilated cardiomyopathy. Dilated cardiomyopathy can also develop in the peripartum period. Most cases of nonischemic dilated cardiomyopathy are usually labeled "idiopathic" (i.e., no specific etiology can be determined), although many may have a genetic origin, especially if there is a positive family history. Irrespective of etiology, nonischemic dilated cardiomyopathy should be treated in the same way as dilated ischemic cardiomyopathy.

Heart Failure Due to Hypertrophic Cardiomyopathy

Heart failure can arise in patients with hypertrophic cardiomyopathy because of predominant diastolic dysfunction, associated mitral incompetence, or the development of systolic dysfunction. The management of hypertrophic cardiomyopathy and its complications is often very different from the management of dilated cardiomyopathy (Chapter 60), thereby underscoring the value of echocardiography in the evaluation of the patient with heart failure.

Acute Decompensated Heart Failure and Pulmonary Edema

Patients presenting with acute heart failure include those who develop heart failure de novo as a consequence of another cardiac event, usually a myocardial infarction, and those who present for the first time with decompensation of previously asymptomatic and often unrecognized cardiac dysfunction (patients previously in stage B, a transition with profound prognostic implications).[9] However, because of frequent recurrences, most episodes of acute decompensation occur in patients with established, chronic heart failure that has worsened as a result of the unavoidable natural progression of the syndrome, with an intercurrent cardiac (e.g., arrhythmia) or noncardiac (e.g., pneumonia) event, or as a consequence of an avoidable reason, such as nonadherence with treatment or use of an agent that can alter renal function. Although it is not always identified, searching for a reversible precipitant is an important aspect of the initial therapy plan (Table 59-6).

Most patients with acute heart failure require admission to the hospital, especially if pulmonary edema is present. In contrast to chronic heart failure, data from RCTs generally are not available to guide effective therapy for patients with acute decompensated heart failure. The principal goals of management of this heterogeneous group of patients are to relieve symptoms, the most important of which is extreme dyspnea, and to maintain or to restore vital organ perfusion. An intravenous bolus or infusion of a loop diuretic and, in hypoxemic patients, oxygen are the key first-line treatments.

TABLE 59-6 SOME COMMON PRECIPITATING CAUSES OF HEART FAILURE

Myocardial ischemia or infarction
Atrial fibrillation or other supraventricular tachycardias
Uncontrolled hypertension
Valvar disease
Ventricular tachycardia
Pulmonary embolism
Pericardial disease
Sepsis
Anemia
Poor dietary or medical adherence
Adverse drug effects
Hyperthyroidism or hypothyroidism

From Kimmelstiel CD, DeNofrio D, Konstam MA. Heart failure. In: Wachter RM, Goldman L, Hollander H, eds. *Hospital Medicine.* 2nd ed. Philadelphia: Lippincott Williams & Wilkins; 2005:360.

A small RCT suggested that high-dose diuretic (more than 2.5 times previous oral dose) resulted in greater relief of dyspnea and congestion compared with low-dose diuretic (same intravenous dose as prior oral dose), but at the expense of more, albeit transient, renal dysfunction.[A24] An intravenous opiate may also be given in selected patients to relieve anxiety and distress. Noninvasive ventilation using a tight-fitting mask to provide positive-pressure ventilation reduces respiratory distress and metabolic disturbances more rapidly than standard oxygen therapy but has not reduced short-term mortality. Intravenous infusion of a nitrate (e.g., continuous intravenous infusion of 20 to 200 μg/mm of nitroglycerin, titrated according to the symptomatic response and hemodynamic measurements, particularly arterial blood pressure) may also be valuable in patients with hypertension or myocardial ischemia (Fig. 59-3). Intravenous nesiritide (human B-type natriuretic peptide as a 2.0-μg/kg intravenous bolus followed by a continuous intravenous infusion of 0.01 to 0.03 μg/kg/mm titrated according to the symptomatic response and hemodynamic measurements, particularly arterial blood pressure) can reduce the pulmonary capillary wedge pressure more promptly than intravenous nitroglycerin but has minimal effect on dyspnea and does not improve other clinical outcomes.[A25] In volume-overloaded patients with severe heart failure unresponsive to diuretics, ultrafiltration is an option at specialized centers, although it was not superior to intensified pharmacologic therapy in a recent trial.

In patients with marked hypotension or other evidence of organ hypoperfusion, an inotropic agent such as dobutamine (continuous intravenous infusion of 2.5 to 25 μg/kg/min, titrated according to hemodynamic and heart rate response and induction of arrhythmias or myocardial ischemia) or a phosphodiesterase inhibitor (e.g., milrinone) should be considered, although neither treatment has ever been shown to reduce in-hospital deaths. In some countries, the calcium sensitizer levosimendan is also available for use in these patients. In general, potent inotropic agents should be used in a cardiac monitored setting at the lowest clinically effective dose and for the shortest duration possible (Chapter 107). Although low-dose dopamine (intravenous infusion of 2.5 μg/kg/mm) is often administered in an attempt to improve diuresis and renal function, such benefits were not confirmed in a recent RCT.[A26] In one trial of patients admitted to the hospital for acute heart failure and systolic blood pressure of 125 mm Hg or greater, serelaxin (recombinant human relaxin-2, at 30 μg/kg per day intravenously for 48 hours) improved dyspnea and reduced death at 6 months by one third, but this therapy has not been approved for use in the United States or the European Union. Patients with severe hyponatremia may benefit from the arginine vasopressin antagonist tolvapan (15 to 60 mg orally once daily).

In more critically ill patients, mechanical circulatory support (e.g., with an intra-aortic balloon pump) may also be considered (Chapter 107). The aim of treatment is to support the patient's circulation and vital organ function until either the patient's own heart recovers or a definitive operative procedure can be performed (e.g., transplantation or implantation of a long-term ventricular assist device).

In patients admitted to the hospital, discharge planning and subsequent management to reduce the risk for readmission are important.[10,11] Ideally, an effective oral diuretic regimen should have been identified, and fluid-volume and biochemical stability should have been achieved. This optimization of volume status and development of a stable oral regimen before discharge is thought to reduce the risk for early readmission. Treatment with an ACE inhibitor (or ARB), β-blocker, and mineralocorticoid receptor antagonist (or ARB), as appropriate, should also be started and titrated in the stabilized patient before discharge. Outpatient follow-up should be arranged to ensure that any of those treatments that have not been started before discharge are initiated

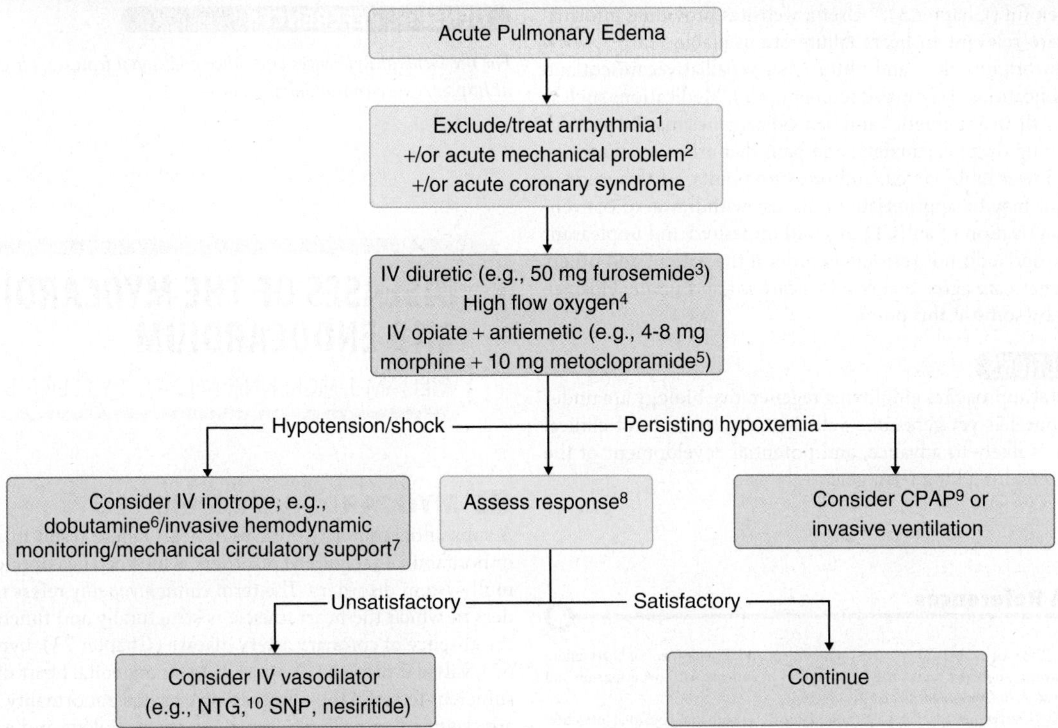

1 Causal arrhythmia (e.g., ventricular tachycardia). It can be difficult to determine whether atrial fibrillation is a primary cause of acute pulmonary edema or secondary to it. An ECG is an essential investigation.

2 Acute mechanical problems include ventricular septal rupture and mitral valve papillary muscle rupture. Mechanical support (e.g., an intra-aortic balloon pump) and urgent surgery should be considered. An echocardiogram should be performed as soon as possible, especially in a patient without a prior diagnosis of heart failure/other relevant heart disease (e.g., prior myocardial infarction or valve disease).

3 Dose of diuretic depends on prior diuretic use and renal function—a lower dose may suffice if preserved renal function and no prior diuretic use.

4 Oxygen causes an increase in systemic vascular resistance and a reduction in heart rate and cardiac output and should only be administered to patients with hypoxemia.

5 Consider if patient agitated/distressed/in pain; may cause respiratory depression and dose should be reduced in very elderly.

6 An intravenous infusion of dobutamine may be started at a dose of 2.5 μg/kg/min, doubling every 15 minutes according to response and tolerability (dose titration usually limited by excessive tachycardia, arrhythmias, or ischemia). A dose above 20 μg/kg/min is rarely needed.

7 E.g., an intra-aortic balloon pump

8 Improvement in symptoms and peripheral perfusion and adequate urine output—patient should be monitored closely, and usually a response will occur within 30 minutes. Bladder catheterization may help in monitoring urine output.

9 Continuous positive airways pressure (CPAP) is valuable in severe pulmonary edema, especially if associated with hypoxemia. Endotracheal intubation and invasive mechanical ventilation should be considered in patients with persisting hypoxemia and physical ventilatory exhaustion.

10 If systolic blood pressure is adequate (>100 mm Hg), an intravenous infusion of nitroglycerin (NTG) can be considered. Start at a dose of 10 μg/min and double every 10 minutes according to response and tolerability (usually dose up-titration is limited by hypotension). A dose of more than 100 μg/min is rarely needed.

FIGURE 59-3. **Approach to the patient with acute pulmonary edema.** SNP = sodium nitroprusside.

after discharge and that the dose of each drug is increased, as tolerated, to the appropriate target.

Outpatient Follow-Up

The key to successful follow-up is the careful tracking of clinical symptoms and the patient's weight, which often involves interviewing not only the patient but also family members, who may be more aware of changes in status than the patient is (see previous section, Organization of Care). Continuity of care and seamless transitions from the inpatient to the outpatient setting are crucial aspects of optimal management. Patients with advanced heart failure and patients requiring frequent hospitalization require special attention. Programs that provide telephone-based tracking of daily weights and symptoms can detect deterioration in time to intervene before the need for hospitalization. Although these programs may be costly, several evaluations have found them to be cost effective. Because the care of these patients requires considerable experience and expertise, specialized disease management programs and clinics have been developed and may provide additional benefit compared with traditional care.

PROGNOSIS

The prognosis of patients with heart failure is poor despite advances in therapy. Of patients who survive the acute onset of heart failure, only 35% of men and 50% of women are alive after 5 years. Although it is difficult to predict prognosis in individual patients, patients with symptoms at rest (class IV) have a 30 to 50% annual mortality rate, patients who are symptomatic with mild activity (class III) have mortality rates of 10 to 20% annually, and patients with symptoms only with moderate activity (class II) have a 5 to 10% annual mortality rate. Mortality rates are higher in older patients, men, and patients with a reduced left ventricular ejection fraction or underlying coronary heart disease.

End-of-Life Considerations

Although predicting the trajectory of illness in patients with advanced heart failure is notoriously difficult, it is often apparent when a patient has progressed to end-stage heart failure, commonly associated with concomitant renal failure. In these circumstances, the expertise of the palliative care team may be especially helpful (Chapter 3).[12] Useful websites providing information on palliative care relevant to heart failure are available (http://www.goldstandardsframework.nhs.uk/ and http://www.palliativecarescotland.org.uk/content/publications/HF-final-document.pdf). Medications such as parenteral opiates (with an antiemetic) and benzodiazepines may be particularly helpful in relieving dyspnea, anxiety, and pain that arises from ascites, hepatic congestion, lower limb edema, and pressure points. At this stage in the patient's illness, it may be appropriate to discuss withdrawal of conventional treatment, deactivation of an ICD to avoid undesired and unpleasant electrical discharges, and a do-not-resuscitate order if the patient and others involved in the patient's care agree that comfort care is appropriate. Hospice care may be chosen by some at this point.

FUTURE DIRECTIONS

Multiple experimental approaches employing regenerative biology are under investigation, but none has yet generated sufficient data to warrant clinical use. Device therapy is likely to advance, and potential development of the total artificial heart remains a long-term goal.

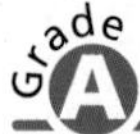

Grade A References

A1. Sciarretta S, Palano F, Tocci G, et al. Antihypertensive treatment and development of heart failure in hypertension: a Bayesian network meta-analysis of studies in patients with hypertension and high cardiovascular risk. *Arch Intern Med.* 2011;171:384-394.

A2. Pfeffer MA, McMurray JJ, Velazquez EJ, et al. Valsartan, captopril, or both in myocardial infarction complicated by heart failure, left ventricular dysfunction, or both. *N Engl J Med.* 2003;349:1893-1906.

A3. Dargie HJ. Effect of carvedilol on outcome after myocardial infarction in patients with left-ventricular dysfunction: the CAPRICORN randomised trial. *Lancet.* 2001;357:1385-1390.

A4. Zannad F, McMurray JJ, Krum H, et al. Eplerenone in patients with systolic heart failure and mild symptoms. *N Engl J Med.* 2011;364:11-21.

A5. McMurray JJ, Packer M, Desai AS, et al. Angiotensin-neprilysin inhibition versus enalapril in heart failure. *N Engl J Med.* 2014;371:993-1004.

A6. Swedberg K, Komajda M, Bohm M, et al. Ivabradine and outcomes in chronic heart failure (SHIFT): a randomised placebo-controlled study. *Lancet.* 2010;376:875-885.

A7. Taylor AL, Ziesche S, Yancy C, et al. Combination of isosorbide dinitrate and hydralazine in blacks with heart failure. *N Engl J Med.* 2004;351:2049-2057.

A8. Rizos EC, Ntzani EE, Bika E, et al. Association between omega-3 fatty acid supplementation and risk of major cardiovascular disease events: a systematic review and meta-analysis. *JAMA.* 2012;308:1024-1033.

A9. Anderson JL, Halperin JL, Albert NM, et al. Management of patients with atrial fibrillation compilation of 2006 ACCF/AHA/ESC and 2011 ACCF/AHA/HRS recommendations: a report of the American College of Cardiology/American Heart Association Task Force on Practice Guidelines. *J Am Coll Cardiol.* 2013;61:1935-1944.

A10. Camm AJ, Lip GY, De Caterina R, et al. 2012 Focused update of the ESC guidelines for the management of atrial fibrillation: an update of the 2010 ESC guidelines for the management of atrial fibrillation. Developed with the special contribution of the European Heart Rhythm Association. *Eur Heart J.* 2012;33:2719-2747.

A11. Scirica BM, Bhatt DL, Braunwald E, et al. Saxagliptin and cardiovascular outcomes in patients with type 2 diabetes mellitus. *N Engl J Med.* 2013;369:1317-1326.

A12. Konstam MA. Home monitoring should be the central element in an effective program of heart failure disease management. *Circulation.* 2012;125:820-827.

A13. Desai AS. Home monitoring heart failure care does not improve patient outcomes: looking beyond telephone-based disease management. *Circulation.* 2012;125:828-836.

A14. Abraham WT, Adamson PB, Bourge RC, et al. Wireless pulmonary artery haemodynamic monitoring in chronic heart failure: a randomised controlled trial. *Lancet.* 2011;377:658-666.

A15. Ponikowski P, van Veldhuisen DJ, Comin-Colet J, et al. Beneficial effects of long-term intravenous iron therapy with ferric carboxymaltose in patients with symptomatic heart failure and iron deficiency. *Eur Heart J.* 2014; [Epub ahead of print].

A16. Swedberg K, Young JB, Anand IS, et al. Treatment of anemia with darbepoetin alfa in systolic heart failure. *N Engl J Med.* 2013;368:1210-1219.

A17. Cleland JG, Abraham WT, Linde C, et al. An individual patient meta-analysis of five randomized trials assessing the effects of cardiac resynchronization therapy on morbidity and mortality in patients with symptomatic heart failure. *Eur Heart J.* 2013;34:3547-3556.

A18. Goldenberg I, Kutyifa V, Klein HU, et al. Survival with cardiac-resynchronization therapy in mild heart failure. *N Engl J Med.* 2014;370:1694-1701.

A19. Ruschitzka F, Abraham WT, Singh JP, et al. Cardiac-resynchronization therapy in heart failure with a narrow QRS complex. *N Engl J Med.* 2013;369:1395-1405.

A20. Velazquez EJ, Lee KL, Deja MA, et al. Coronary-artery bypass surgery in patients with left ventricular dysfunction. *N Engl J Med.* 2011;364:1607-1616.

A21. Slaughter MS, Rogers JG, Milano CA, et al. Advanced heart failure treated with continuous-flow left ventricular assist device. *N Engl J Med.* 2009;361:2241-2251.

A22. Pitt B, Pfeffer MA, Assmann SF, et al. Spironolactone for heart failure with preserved ejection fraction. *N Engl J Med.* 2014;370:1383-1392.

A23. Acker MA, Parides MK, Perrault LP, et al. Mitral-valve repair versus replacement for severe ischemic mitral regurgitation. *N Engl J Med.* 2014;370:23-32.

A24. Felker GM, Lee KL, Bull DA, et al. Diuretic strategies in patients with acute decompensated heart failure. *N Engl J Med.* 2011;364:797-805.

A25. O'Connor CM, Starling RC, Hernandez AF, et al. Effect of nesiritide in patients with acute decompensated heart failure. *N Engl J Med.* 2011;365:32-43.

A26. Chen HH, Anstrom KJ, Givertz MM, et al. Low-dose dopamine or low-dose nesiritide in acute heart failure with renal dysfunction: the ROSE acute heart failure randomized trial. *JAMA.* 2013;310:2533-2543.

GENERAL REFERENCES

For the General References and other additional features, please visit Expert Consult at https://expertconsult.inkling.com.

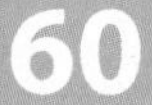

60 DISEASES OF THE MYOCARDIUM AND ENDOCARDIUM

WILLIAM J. MCKENNA AND PERRY ELLIOTT

MYOCARDIAL DISEASE

A substantial minority of cases of heart failure result from familial (genetic) or nonfamilial (acquired) disorders, which can be confined to the heart or be multisystem disorders. The term *cardiomyopathy* refers to myocardial disorders in which the heart muscle is structurally and functionally abnormal in the absence of coronary artery disease (Chapter 73), hypertension (Chapter 67), valvular disease (Chapter 75), or congenital heart disease (Chapter 69) sufficient to cause the observed myocardial abnormality.[1] Cardiomyopathies are classified according to ventricular morphology and pathophysiology into four major types: dilated cardiomyopathy, hypertrophic cardiomyopathy, restrictive cardiomyopathy, and arrhythmogenic right ventricular cardiomyopathy (ARVC) (Table 60-1 and Fig. 60-1). Diseases that do not fit into these groups (such as endocardial fibroelastosis and left ventricular noncompaction) are termed unclassified cardiomyopathies. Mixed phenotypes can exist; for example, patients with hypertrophic and dilated cardiomyopathies frequently have a restrictive left ventricular physiology or develop ventricular dilation.

Hypertrophic Cardiomyopathy

DEFINITION AND EPIDEMIOLOGY

Hypertrophic cardiomyopathy is defined as unexplained left ventricular hypertrophy in the absence of abnormal loading conditions (valve disease, hypertension, congenital heart defects) sufficient to explain the degree of hypertrophy.[2] The disease occurs in all racial groups, with a prevalence of between 0.2 and 0.5%.

PATHOBIOLOGY

Hypertrophic cardiomyopathy is usually familial with autosomal dominant inheritance. Mutations in sarcomeric contractile protein genes (Table 60-2) account for approximately 50 to 60% of cases. More than 1400 different mutations have been identified, with marked variation in disease penetrance and clinical expression. A similar clinical phenotype is seen in association with other uncommon genetic disorders, including Noonan syndrome (Chapter 69), Friedreich ataxia (Chapter 421), neurofibromatosis (Chapter 417), hereditary spherocytosis (Chapter 161), respiratory chain disorders, glycogen storage diseases (Chapter 207), and lysosomal storage disorders (Chapter 208) (see Table 60-2).

Pathology

In the common form of autosomal dominant hypertrophic cardiomyopathy, myocardial hypertrophy usually affects the interventricular septum more than other regions of the left ventricle. Other patterns, including concentric, mid-ventricular (sometimes associated with a left ventricular apical diverticulum), and apical, also occur. Coexistent right ventricular hypertrophy is present in up to 44% of cases. The papillary muscles are often poorly developed and may be displaced anteriorly, thereby contributing to systolic anterior motion of the anterior mitral valve leaflet in 25% of patients and of the posterior leaflets in 10% of cases in the resting state. Often, the mitral valve is structurally abnormal, with elongation of the anterior leaflet and occasional direct insertion of the papillary muscle into the anterior leaflet. The histologic hallmark of hypertrophic cardiomyopathy is a triad of myocyte hypertrophy, myocyte disarray, and interstitial fibrosis. Myocyte disarray refers to architectural disorganization of the myocardium, with adjacent myocytes aligned obliquely or perpendicular to each other in association with increased inter-

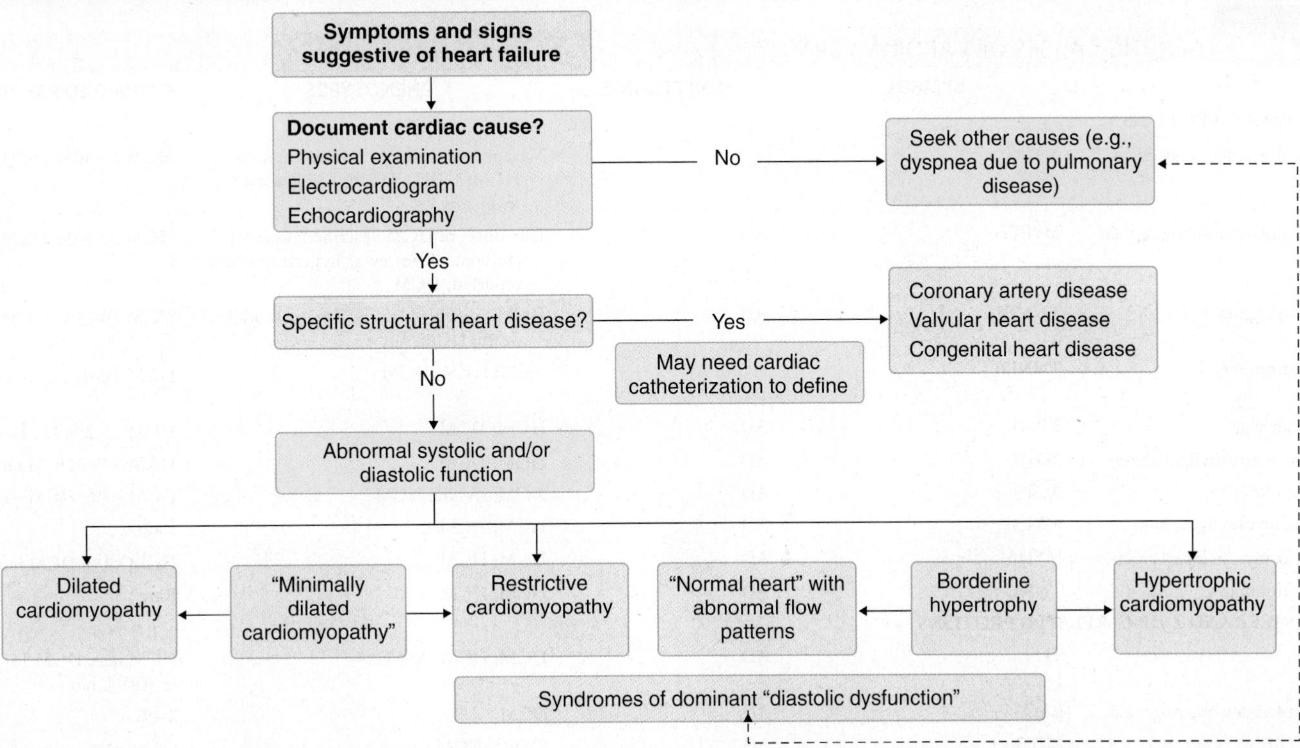

FIGURE 60-1. Initial approach to classification of cardiomyopathy. The evaluation of symptoms or signs consistent with heart failure first includes confirmation that they can be attributed to a cardiac cause. Although this conclusion is often apparent from routine physical examination and electrocardiography, echocardiography serves to confirm cardiac disease and provides clues to the presence of other cardiac diseases, such as focal abnormalities suggesting primary valve disease or congenital heart disease. Having excluded these conditions, cardiomyopathy is generally considered to be dilated, restrictive, or hypertrophic, as shown in Table 60-1. Patients with apparently normal cardiac structure and contraction are occasionally found to demonstrate abnormal intracardiac flow patterns consistent with diastolic dysfunction but should also be evaluated carefully for other causes of their symptoms. Most patients with so-called diastolic dysfunction also demonstrate at least borderline criteria for left ventricular hypertrophy, frequently in the setting of chronic hypertension and diabetes. A moderately decreased ejection fraction without marked dilation or a pattern of restrictive cardiomyopathy is sometimes referred to as minimally dilated cardiomyopathy, which may represent either a distinct entity or a transition between acute and chronic disease.

TABLE 60-1 PROFILES OF MYOCARDIAL DISEASE

	HYPERTROPHIC	DILATED	RESTRICTIVE	ARVC
Causes	Genetic (see Table 60-2)	Myocarditis (see Table 60-4) Metabolic/endocrine Genetic (see Table 60-2)	Infiltrative or storage diseases (see Table 60-8) Endomyocardial (e.g., Löffler, carcinoid) Genetic (see Table 60-2)	Genetic (see Table 60-2)
Ejection fraction	Increased	Reduced	25-50%	Normal until end stage 30% regional LV disease
LV end-diastolic dimension	Usually decreased	Increased	Normal	Normal until end stage Right ventricle dilated
LV wall thickness	Increased	Normal	Normal or mildly increased	Normal
Atrial size	Increased	Increased	Increased; may be massive	Left atrium normal; right dilated in severe disease
Valvular disease	Mitral regurgitation (SAM)	Mitral (functional); tricuspid regurgitation in late stages	Mitral and tricuspid regurgitation, rarely severe	Tricuspid regurgitation in severe disease
Common symptoms	Dyspnea; chest pain, syncope Late: orthopnea, PND	Dyspnea, fatigue Late: orthopnea, PND	Dyspnea Late: orthopnea, PND, right-sided heart failure	Palpitations, syncope Late: right-sided heart failure
Arrhythmia	Atrial fibrillation, ventricular tachycardia; conduction block in *PRKAG2*, mitochondrial; Fabry disease	Ventricular tachyarrhythmias; heart block in Chagas disease, giant cell myocarditis, laminopathies	Atrial fibrillation; conduction block in sarcoid, amyloidosis, desminopathy	Ventricular ectopy and tachycardia

ARVC = arrhythmogenic right ventricular cardiomyopathy; LV = left ventricular; PRKAG2 = protein kinase, AMP-activated, gamma 2 non-catalytic subunit mutation; SAM = systolic anterior motion of mitral valve; PND = paroxysmal nocturnal dyspnea.

stitial collagen. The myofibrillar architecture within the myocyte is also disorganized. Although myocyte disarray occurs in aortic stenosis, longstanding hypertension, and some forms of congenital heart disease, the presence of extensive disarray (more than 10% of ventricular septal myocytes) is thought to be a highly specific marker for hypertrophic cardiomyopathy. Small intramural coronary arteries are often dysplastic and narrowed because of wall thickening by smooth muscle cell hyperplasia.

PATHOPHYSIOLOGY

Abnormal ventricular geometry, wall thickening, myocyte hypertrophy, myocyte and myofibrillar disarray, and myocardial fibrosis all contribute to impairment of left ventricular diastolic function. The net result is elevation of left ventricular end-diastolic pressures, symptoms of heart failure, and reduced exercise tolerance. Global measures of left ventricular systolic

TABLE 60-2 GENETIC CAUSES OF CARDIOMYOPATHY

GENE	SYMBOL	INHERITANCE	PHENOTYPES	ESTIMATED FREQUENCY
SARCOMERIC PROTEINS				
Cardiac β-myosin heavy chain	MYH7	AD	Variable: moderate to severe prognosis; HCM; LVNC; DCM; Laing distal myopathy	HCM 30-40%; DCM 4-6%
Cardiac myosin-binding protein C	MYBPC3	AD	Late onset of HCM described; cases of children with a severe hypertrophy also reported; DCM	HCM 30-40%; DCM ~1%
Cardiac troponin T	TNNT2	AD	HCM: possible high incidence of sudden death; DCM	HCM 10-15%; DCM 3-5%
Cardiac troponin I	TNNI3	HCM: AD DCM: AD, AR	RCM; HCM; DCM	HCM 2-5%; DCM <1%
α-Tropomyosin	TPM1	AD	HCM; DCM	HCM ~1-2%; DCM <1%
Regulatory myosin light chain	MYL2	AD	HCM; DCM	HCM ~1%; DCM rare
Cardiac actin	ACTC	AD	DCM; LVNC; HCM	DCM ~1%; HCM ~1%
Essential myosin light chain	MYL3	AD	HCM; DCM	Rare
Cardiac α-myosin heavy chain	MYH6	AD	DCM; HCM	HCM <1%; DCM rare
Cardiac troponin C	TNNC	AD	HCM; DCM	Rare
SARCOMERE AND Z-DISC–RELATED PROTEINS				
Titin	TTN	AD	DCM; HCM; ARVC	HCM rare; DCM 15-25%; ARVC rare
BCL2-associated athanogene 3	BAG3	AD	DCM	2-4%
Cypher/ZASP	LDB3	AD	LVNC; DCM	DCM <1%
Titin-cap or telethonin	TCAP	AD	HCM; DCM	HCM <1%; DCM rare
α-Actinin-2	ACTN2	AD	HCM; DCM	Rare
Ankyrin repeat domain-containing protein 1	ANKRD1	AD	DCM	Rare
Cysteine and glycine-rich protein 3 (cardiac LIM protein)	CSRP3	AD	DCM; HCM	Rare
Four-and-a-half LIM protein 1	FHL1	AD	DCM	Rare
Four-and-a-half LIM protein 2	FHL2	AD	DCM	Rare
Myozenin 2	MYOZ2	AD	HCM	Rare
Myopalladin	MYPN	AD	DCM	Rare
Nexilin	NEXN	AD	HCM; DCM	Rare
Nebulette	NEBL	AD	DCM	Rare
PDZ and LIM domain protein 3	PDLIM3	AD	DCM; HCM	Rare
Metavinculin	VCL	AD	DCM; HCM	Rare
CYTOSKELETAL PROTEINS				
Desmin	DES	AD, AR	DCM; desminopathies; DCM with clinical features usually associated with ARVC	DCM <1%
Dystrophin	DMD	XL	DCM in Duchenne muscular dystrophy (DMD); Becker muscular dystrophy (BMD)	DCM <1%
Caveolin-3	CAV3	AD	HCM	Rare
α-B crystallin	CRYAB	AD	DCM; myofibrillar myopathies	Rare
α-, β-, γ-, and δ-sarcoglycans	SGCA, SGCB, SGCG, SGCD	SGCD: AD	DCM	Rare
NUCLEAR PROTEINS				
Lamin A/C	LMNA	LVNC, DCM: AD EMD2: AD EMD3: AR LGMD1B: AD ARVC: AD	LVNC; DCM; DCM in Emery-Dreifuss muscular dystrophy types 2 and 3 (EMD2 and EMD3); DCM in limb girdle muscular dystrophy; DCM with clinical features usually associated with ARVC	DCM 4-8%
Dystrobrevin	α-DTNA	AD	DCM; LVNC	Rare
Emerin	EMD	XL	DCM, Emery-Dreifuss muscular dystrophy	Rare
PR domain-containing protein 16	PRDM16	AD	LVNC; DCM	Rare
Syntrophin	SNTA1	AD	DCM	Rare
Spectrin repeat containing, nuclear envelope 1	SYNE1	AD	DCM	Rare
Spectrin repeat containing, nuclear envelope 2	SYNE2	AD	DCM	Rare
Transmembrane protein 43	TMEM43	AD	ARVC	Rare
Thymopoietin	TMPO	AD	DCM	Rare

TABLE 60-2 GENETIC CAUSES OF CARDIOMYOPATHY—cont'd

GENE	SYMBOL	INHERITANCE	PHENOTYPES	ESTIMATED FREQUENCY
ION CHANNEL AND ION CHANNEL RELATED				
Cardiac sodium channel	SCN5A	AD	DCM; LVNC	DCM 1-2%
Regulatory SUR2A subunit of the cardiac K(ATP) channel	ABCC9	AD	DCM	Rare
DESMOSOMAL PROTEINS				
Plakophilin 2	PKP2	AD, AR	ARVC	AD 30-40%; AR rare
Desmoglein 2	DSG2	AD	ARVC	12-40%
Desmoplakin	DSP	ARVC: AD Carvajal syndrome: AR	ARVC; DCM in Carvajal syndrome	ARVC 6-16%
Desmocollin 2	DSC2	AD	ARVC	Rare
Plakoglobin	JUP	ARVC: AD Naxos disease: AR	ARVC; Naxos disease	Rare
CALCIUM-HANDLING PROTEINS				
Phospholamban	PLN	AD	DCM; HCM; ARVC	DCM <1%; HCM rare; ARVC rare
Calsequestrin 2 (cardiac muscle)	CASQ2	AD	LVNC; CPVT	Rare
Junctophilin 2	JPH2	AD	HCM	Rare
Cardiac ryanodine receptor	RYR2	AD	ARVC; CPVT	Rare
METABOLIC PROTEINS				
Amylo-1,6-glucosidase	AGL	AR	Cardiomyopathy in Forbes disease	?
Acid α-1,4-glucosidase	GAA	AR	Cardiomyopathy in Pompe disease	?
α-Galactosidase A	GLA	XL	HCM in Anderson-Fabry disease	?
Lysosomal-associated membrane protein 2	LAMP2	XL	HCM in Danon disease	?
Protein kinase, AMP-activated, γ_2 noncatalytic subunit	PRKAG2	AD	HCM in Wolff-Parkinson-White syndrome	?
Frataxin	FRDA	AR	HCM in Friedreich ataxia	?
OTHERS				
RNA-binding protein 20	RBM20	AD	DCM	3-5%
M_2 muscarinic receptor	CHRM2	AD	DCM	Rare
Cardiotrophin 1	CTF1	AD	DCM	Rare
αT-catenin	CTNNA3	AD	ARVC	Rare
Dolichol kinase	DOLK	AD	DCM	Rare
Eyes absent 4	EYA4	AD	DCM	Rare
Fukutin-related protein	FKRP	AD, AR	DCM as part of limb-girdle muscular dystrophy 2I	Rare
Fukutin	FKTN	AD, AR	DCM; Limb-girdle muscular dystrophy	Rare
GATA zinc finger domain-containing protein 1	GATAD1	AR	DCM	Rare
Hereditary hemochromatosis	HFE	AR	DCM and RCM in hereditary hemochromatosis	Rare
Laminin α2	LAMA2	AD	DCM	Rare
Laminin α4	LAMA4	AD	DCM	Rare
Integrin-linked kinase	ILK	AD	DCM	Rare
Genes encoding mitochondrial components	MTTG, MTTY, MTND5, others	AD, maternal	HCM in MELAS, MERRF, LHON syndromes	?
Muscle-related coiled-coil protein	MURC	AD	DCM	Rare
Myosin light chain kinase 2	MYLK2	AD	HCM	Rare
Myomesin 1	MYOM1	AD	HCM	Rare
Myomesin 2	MYOM2	AD	HCM	Rare
Myotilin	MYOT	AD	DCM	Rare
Presenilin 1	PSEN1	AD	DCM	Rare
Presenilin 2	PSEN2	AD	DCM	Rare
RAS-MAPK pathway genes	PTPN11, RAF1, SOS1, KRAS, HRAS, BRAF, MEK1-2, others	AD	HCM in Noonan syndrome and LEOPARD syndrome	?
Tafazzin	TAZ	XL	DCM; LVNC; Barth syndrome	Rare
Transcription factor TBX20	TBX20	AD	DCM with developmental anomalies	Rare
Transforming growth factor β3	TGFB3	AD	ARVC	Rare
Muscle RING Finger 1 (MuRF1)	TRIM63	AD	HCM	Rare
Hereditary amyloidosis	TTR	AD	HCM and RCM in hereditary amyloidosis	Rare

AD = autosomal dominant; AR = autosomal recessive; ARVC = arrhythmogenic right ventricular cardiomyopathy; CPVT = catecholaminergic polymorphic ventricular tachycardia; DCM = dilated cardiomyopathy; HCM = hypertrophic cardiomyopathy; LVNC = left ventricular noncompaction; RCM = restrictive cardiomyopathy; XL = X-linked.

function are often normal, but regional myocardial dysfunction and progressive systolic impairment are relatively common.

Approximately 25% of patients have left ventricular outflow tract obstruction at rest caused by contact between the anterior leaflet of the mitral valve and the interventricular septum during ventricular systole. Many patients without outflow obstruction at rest develop it during physiologic and pharmacologic interventions that reduce left ventricular end-diastolic volume or increase left ventricular contractility.

CLINICAL MANIFESTATIONS

Most patients are asymptomatic or have only mild or intermittent symptoms. Symptomatic progression is usually slow, age related, and associated with a gradual deterioration in left ventricular function during decades. Less than 5% of patients may have rapid, symptomatic deterioration. Symptoms can develop at any age, even many years after the appearance of electrocardiographic (ECG) or echocardiographic manifestations of left ventricular hypertrophy. On occasion, sudden death may be the initial presentation. However, most individuals with hypertrophic cardiomyopathy have few if any symptoms, and the diagnosis is often made as a result of family screening or the incidental detection of a heart murmur or ECG abnormality.

Approximately 20 to 30% of adults develop chest pain (Chapters 51 and 71), which may occur on exertion, at rest, or nocturnally. Postprandial angina associated with mild exertion is typical. Mild to moderate dyspnea on exertion is relatively common, and some patients develop paroxysmal nocturnal dyspnea that may be caused by transient myocardial ischemia or arrhythmia. Approximately 20% of patients experience syncope (Chapters 51 and 62), and a similar proportion complain of presyncope. Palpitations (Chapter 62) are frequent and are usually attributable to supraventricular or ventricular ectopy or to forceful cardiac contraction. Sustained palpitations are usually caused by supraventricular tachyarrhythmias, but initial presentation with a symptomatic arrhythmia is uncommon. Patients with distal or apical hypertrophy have fewer symptoms and arrhythmias, better exercise capacity, and good prognosis. On occasion, however, patients with distal or apical hypertrophy may have severe refractory chest pain or may present with troublesome supraventricular arrhythmias.

DIAGNOSIS

A three- to four-generation family history, which should be obtained in all patients with a new diagnosis of cardiomyopathy, helps determine the probability of familial disease and its mode of inheritance. The initial diagnostic evaluation includes a family history focusing on premature cardiac disease or death, a comprehensive medical history focusing on cardiovascular symptoms, a careful physical examination, a 12-lead electrocardiogram, and a two-dimensional echocardiogram.

The general evaluation may provide diagnostic clues in patients whose hypertrophic cardiomyopathy is associated with syndromes or metabolic disorders. For example, Noonan syndrome is characterized by short stature, developmental delay, cutaneous abnormalities (cafe au lait spots), hypertelorism, ptosis, low-set posteriorly rotated ears, and webbed neck. These features are shared with the less common LEOPARD syndrome. Angiokeratomas, anhidrosis, Raynaud-like symptoms with neuropathy, cornea verticillata, retinal vascular dilation, tinnitus, diarrhea, and proteinuria are typical features of Fabry disease (Chapter 208).

Clinical examination of the cardiovascular system is often normal. In the presence of left ventricular outflow tract obstruction, the arterial pulse has a rapid upstroke and downstroke (sometimes with a bisferiens character), the apex beat is sustained or double (reflecting a palpable atrial impulse followed by left ventricular contraction), and auscultation will demonstrate a systolic ejection murmur that is heard loudest at the left sternal edge and that radiates to the right upper sternal edge and apex (Chapter 51). Most patients with left ventricular outflow tract obstruction also have the murmur of mitral regurgitation, which results from failure of the mitral valve leaflets to coapt due to the systolic anterior motion of the mitral valve. Physiologic and pharmacologic maneuvers that decrease afterload or venous return (e.g., standing, Valsalva maneuver, inhalation of amyl nitrite) or increase contractility (e.g., a post-extrasystole beat) will increase the intensity of the murmur, whereas interventions that increase afterload and venous return (e.g., squatting or handgrip) will reduce it (see Table 51-8). In contrast, physical signs in most patients who do not have left ventricular outflow tract obstruction are subtle and are limited to features that reflect the hyperdynamic contraction (rapid upstroke pulse) and poorly compliant right (prominent *a* wave in jugular venous pressure) and left (S_4 gallop, double-apex beat) ventricles (Chapter 51).

Diagnostic Testing

More than 95% of patients have abnormal ECG findings, but no changes are disease specific. The most common abnormalities are increased QRS voltage consistent with left ventricular hypertrophy, left axis deviation (15 to 20%), abnormal Q waves (25 to 30%, most commonly in inferolateral leads), and ST segment or T wave changes (>50%). An isolated increase in the QRS voltage without ST segment changes or T wave inversion is rare in hypertrophic cardiomyopathy. The presence of predominantly distal or apical thickening is associated with giant negative T wave inversion, which is maximal in leads V_3 and V_4.

Two-dimensional echocardiography (Chapter 55) is the mainstay of diagnostic imaging, but magnetic resonance imaging (Chapter 56) and computed tomography (Chapter 56) provide alternatives if the echocardiogram is of poor quality. In most patients, the hypertrophy is asymmetrical and involves the anterior and posterior intraventricular septum (Fig. 60-2). The hypertrophy, however, may be more generalized and involve the free wall of the left ventricle, or it may be localized and confined to areas other than the septum, such as the lateral or posterior wall of the left ventricle. The echocardiogram

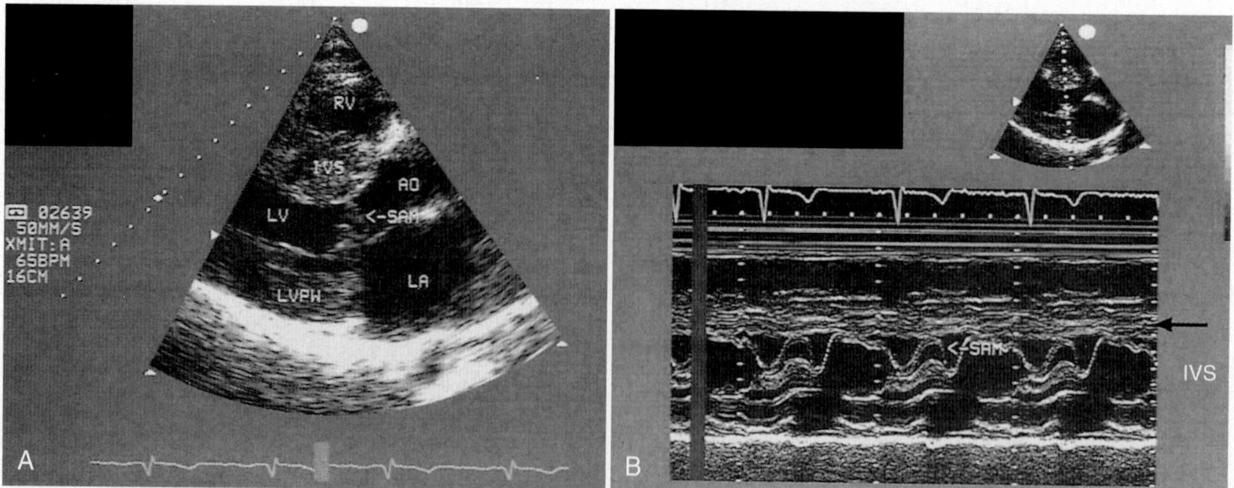

FIGURE 60-2. Hypertrophic obstructive cardiomyopathy. A, The two-dimensional long axis parasternal view shows the chambers of the heart. The left ventricle posterior wall (LVPW) is thickened, and the most striking abnormality is the hypertrophy of the interventricular septum (IVS). Another characteristic feature is a Venturi effect: as blood leaves the left ventricle (LV), it sucks the anterior leaflet of the mitral valve forward, a phenomenon called systolic anterior motion (SAM). **B,** This phenomenon is more clearly shown in the parasternal long axis M-mode echocardiogram. The massive thickening of the septum is also obvious in the M-mode image (IVS). AO = aorta; LA = left atrium; RV = right ventricle. (From Forbes CD, Jackson WF. Color Atlas and Text of Clinical Medicine. 3rd ed. London: Mosby; 2003.)

can measure left ventricular outflow tract obstruction, both at rest and after provocative maneuvers. Patients with an outflow tract gradient of 30 mm Hg or more typically have systolic anterior motion of the mitral valve, with contact of either the anterior or (less commonly) the posterior mitral leaflet with the intraventricular septum during systole, in association with a posteriorly directed jet of mitral regurgitation, the severity of which is proportionate to the severity of the obstruction. Most patients with hypertrophic cardiomyopathy have left atrial enlargement as well as echocardiographic evidence of diastolic dysfunction. Magnetic resonance imaging, although not needed for the diagnosis, readily demonstrates the characteristic abnormalities (E-Figs. 60-1 to 60-4).

When it is available, cardiopulmonary exercise testing with metabolic gas exchange measurements provides an accurate and reproducible assessment of exercise capacity, which can be followed serially. Cardiac catheterization is rarely required for diagnosis or management, but it may be indicated when measurement of intracardiac pressures is required to guide therapeutic decisions (e.g., in patients with severe mitral regurgitation) and for the exclusion of coexistent coronary artery disease in patients with chest pain.

Diagnostic Criteria

A wall thickness of more than 2 standard deviations above the mean, corrected for age, gender, and height, is generally accepted as diagnostic. In adults, this value is typically 1.5 cm or more in men and 1.3 cm or more in women. In the presence of other causes of left ventricular hypertrophy, such as long-standing systemic hypertension or aortic stenosis, the diagnosis of hypertrophic cardiomyopathy may be problematic. However, secondary hypertrophy from other causes rarely exceeds 1.8 cm. Hypertrophy in the highly trained athlete is usually less than 1.6 cm in men and 1.4 cm in women and typically occurs in association with an increased left ventricular end-diastolic dimension and stroke volume. An ECG tracing showing Q waves or inferolateral repolarization changes in an athlete favors the diagnosis of hypertrophic cardiomyopathy.

Given the 50% probability of disease in first-degree relatives of a patient with hypertrophic cardiomyopathy, modified diagnostic criteria (Table 60-3) consider the high probability that their otherwise unexplained ECG and echocardiographic findings reflect incomplete disease expression, with the corresponding risks for complications and for passing the gene to their children.

TABLE 60-3 DIAGNOSTIC CRITERIA FOR HYPERTROPHIC CARDIOMYOPATHY IN FIRST-DEGREE RELATIVES OF AFFECTED PATIENTS*

MAJOR CRITERIA	MINOR CRITERIA
ECHOCARDIOGRAPHY	
Left ventricular wall thickness ≥13 mm in the anterior septum or posterior wall or ≥15 mm in the posterior septum or free wall	Left ventricular wall thickness of 12 mm in the anterior septum or posterior wall or of 14 mm in the posterior septum or free wall
Severe SAM of the mitral valve (septal-leaflet contact)	Moderate SAM of the mitral valve (no mitral leaflet–septal contact)
	Redundant mitral valve leaflets
ELECTROCARDIOGRAPHY	
Left ventricular hypertrophy with repolarization changes (Romhilt and Estes)	Complete bundle branch block or (minor) interventricular conduction defects (in left ventricular leads)
T wave inversion in leads I and aVL (≥3 mm with QRS-T wave axis difference ≥30 degrees), V_3-V_6 (≥3 mm), or II and III and aVF (≥5 mm)	Minor repolarization changes in left ventricular leads
	Deep S wave in lead V_2 (>25 mm)
Abnormal Q waves (>40 msec or >25% R wave) in at least two leads from II, III, aVF (in absence of left anterior hemiblock), and V_1-V_4; or I, aVL, V_5-V_6	Unexplained chest pain, dyspnea, or syncope

*The diagnosis of hypertrophic cardiomyopathy in first-degree relatives of patients with the disease is based on the presence of one major criterion, two minor echocardiographic criteria, or one minor echocardiographic criterion and two minor electrocardiographic criteria.

aVF = augmented voltage unipolar left foot lead; aVL = augmented voltage unipolar left arm lead; SAM = systolic anterior motion.

Modified from McKenna WJ, Spirito P, Desnos M, et al. Experience in clinical genetics in hypertrophic cardiomyopathy. *Heart*. 1997;77:130-132.

TREATMENT

Clinical management is based mainly on symptoms (Fig. 60-3).[3,4] Exceptions include specific therapies for lysosomal storage diseases, such as Pompe disease (Chapter 207) and Fabry disease (E-Fig. 60-5; Chapter 208), and for Friedreich ataxia (Chapter 421). The treatment of the remaining patients with hypertrophic cardiomyopathy focuses on the counseling of family members, the management of symptoms, and the prevention of disease-related complications.

Family Evaluation

All patients with hypertrophic cardiomyopathy should be counseled on the implications of the diagnosis for their families. Careful pedigree analysis can reassure relatives who are not at risk for inheriting the disease. For those who are at risk, current guidelines recommend screening with a 12-lead electrocardiogram and echocardiogram at intervals of 12 to 18 months, usually starting at the age of 12 years (unless there is a "malignant" family history of premature sudden death, the child is symptomatic or a competitive athlete, or there is a clinical suspicion of left ventricular hypertrophy) until full growth and maturation are achieved (usually by the age of 18 to 21 years). Thereafter, if there are no signs of disease expression, screening approximately every 5 years is advised because the onset of left ventricular hypertrophy may be delayed until well into adulthood in some families. Modified diagnostic criteria (see Table 60-3) consider the high probability that otherwise unexplained ECG and echocardiographic findings in first-degree relatives reflect incomplete disease expression.

When it is available, genetic testing can identify a disease-causing mutation in an index case and thereby provide presymptomatic diagnosis of family members. Whenever genetic testing is considered, individuals should be informed about the purpose of the test, the most probable mode of inheritance, and the potential hazards and limitations of genetic testing.

Symptom Management

Medical Therapy

Therapeutic options in patients *without* left ventricular outflow gradients are limited predominantly to pharmacologic therapy. β-Blockade may improve chest pain and dyspnea. The dose (starting at a dose equivalent to propranolol 120 mg/day) should be titrated to achieve a target heart rate of 50 to 70 beats per minute at rest and 130 to 140 beats per minute at peak exercise. Calcium antagonists such as verapamil (starting at a dose of 120 mg/day) and diltiazem (starting at a dose of 180 mg/day) are useful alternatives, particularly in patients with refractory chest pain, but high doses (e.g., verapamil >480 mg/day, diltiazem >360 mg/day) may be required. In patients with paroxysmal nocturnal dyspnea and no evidence of ventricular outflow obstruction, a transient mechanism such as myocardial ischemia or arrhythmia may be implicated, although investigations usually fail to identify the precise cause. Such patients as well as those with chronically raised pulmonary pressures may require diuretics (e.g., furosemide, 20 to 40 mg orally as needed, followed by 20 mg/day if required). The dose and duration of diuretic therapy should be minimized because injudicious use of these drugs can be dangerous, particularly in patients with severe diastolic impairment or labile obstruction.

In patients with symptoms caused by left ventricular outflow tract obstruction, the main aim of treatment is to reduce the outflow tract gradient. Options include negative inotropic drugs, surgery,[5] atrioventricular sequential pacing, and percutaneous alcohol ablation of the interventricular septum. Approximately 60 to 70% of patients improve with β-blockers, although high doses (equivalent to propranolol at 480 mg/day) are frequently required, and side effects are often limiting. When β-blockade alone is ineffective, disopyramide, titrated to the maximal tolerated dose (usually between 400 and 600 mg/day), may be effective in up to two thirds of patients, but side effects related to the anticholinergic effects (e.g., dry eyes and mouth, urinary retention) limit its use. Disopyramide should be given concomitantly with a small to medium dose of a β-blocker (e.g., propranolol, 120 to 240 mg/day), which will slow the heart rate and also blunt rapid atrioventricular nodal conduction should supraventricular arrhythmias develop. In patients who have left ventricular outflow tract obstruction and are taking a β-blocker and disopyramide, other antiarrhythmic drugs that alter repolarization (e.g., sotalol or amiodarone) must be avoided because of the potential proarrhythmic effect. In patients with outflow tract gradients, verapamil can be effective, but caution is required in patients with severe obstruction or elevated pulmonary pressures.

Interventional Therapy

Surgery should be considered for significant outflow obstruction (gradient >50 mm Hg) in patients who have symptoms refractory to medical therapy. The most commonly performed surgical procedure, ventricular septal myectomy, either abolishes or substantially reduces the gradient in 95% of cases, reduces mitral regurgitation, and improves exercise capacity and symptoms. Surgery should be performed in an experienced center, where mortality rates should be less than 1% for isolated myomectomy. The main complications (atrioventricular block, ventricular septal defects) are uncommon (2 to 5%).

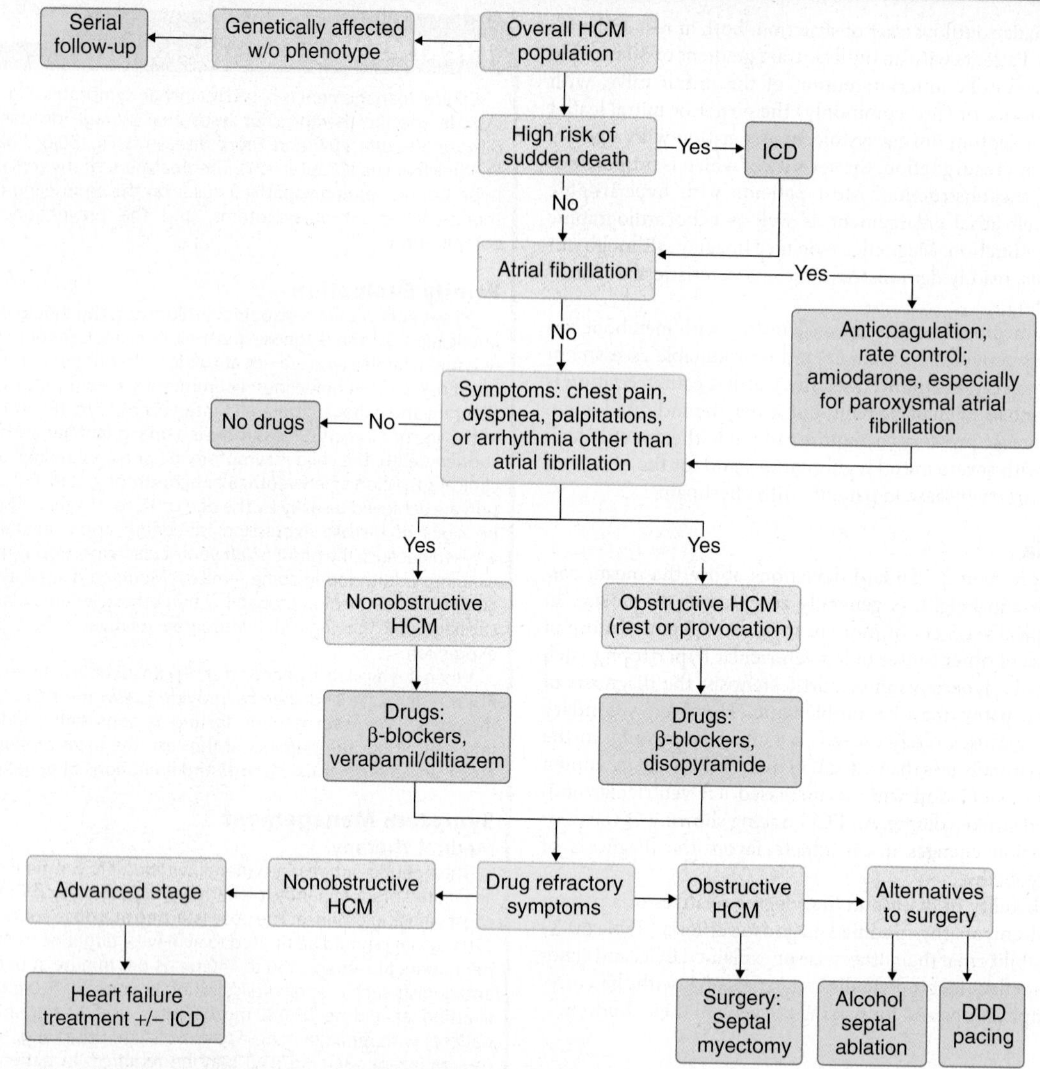

FIGURE 60-3. **Approach to the management of hypertrophic cardiomyopathy (HCM). DDD = dual chamber, ICD = implantable cardioverter-defibrillator. (Modified from Maron BJ, McKenna WJ, Danielson GK, et al. American College of Cardiology/European Society of Cardiology clinical expert consensus document on hypertrophic cardiomyopathy. *J Am Coll Cardiol*. 2003;42:1687-1713.)**

When concomitant procedures (e.g., mitral valve repair or replacement, coronary artery bypass grafting) are required or when other significant comorbidities are present, perioperative mortality rates are higher (4 to 5%).

In experienced centers, the selective injection of alcohol into a septal perforator branch of the left anterior descending coronary artery to create a localized septal scar yields outcomes similar to surgery. The main nonfatal complication is atrioventricular block requiring a pacemaker in 5 to 20% of patients.

Dual-chamber pacing with a short programmed atrial ventricular delay to produce maximal preexcitation while maintaining effective atrial transport can reduce the outflow gradient by 30 to 50% but provides little objective improvement in exercise capacity in most patients. Outcomes (gradient reduction, improved symptoms) are best in older patients with angulated septa and localized upper septal hypertrophy.

Supraventricular Arrhythmia

Atrial fibrillation in hypertrophic cardiomyopathy is associated with a high risk for systemic embolization, so anticoagulation (international normalized ratio in the range of 2.0 to 3.0) should be considered in all patients with sustained or paroxysmal atrial fibrillation (Chapter 64). Treatment with low-dose amiodarone, 1000 to 1400 mg/week, is effective in maintaining sinus rhythm and in controlling the ventricular response during breakthrough episodes. The addition of a low-dose β-blocker, verapamil, or diltiazem may be required for rate control. Serious side effects with low-dose amiodarone are uncommon. β-Blockers, particularly those with class III action (e.g., sotalol), are less effective alternatives. In general, the principles of managing atrial fibrillation in patients with hypertrophic cardiomyopathy are similar to those in other conditions (Chapter 64), with the provision that the threshold to use anticoagulation should be low because of the significant embolic risk.

Prevention of Sudden Death

The overall risk for sudden death in children and adults with hypertrophic cardiomyopathy is approximately 0.5 to 1% per year, but a minority of individuals have a much greater risk for ventricular arrhythmia and sudden death. The most powerful predictor of sudden cardiac death in hypertrophic cardiomyopathy is a history of previous cardiac arrest. In patients without such a history, the most useful markers of risk are a family history of premature (<40 years of age) sudden cardiac death, unexplained syncope (unrelated to neurocardiogenic mechanisms), flat or hypotensive blood pressure response to upright exercise, nonsustained ventricular tachycardia on ambulatory ECG monitoring or during exercise, and severe left ventricular hypertrophy on echocardiography (defined as a maximal left ventricular wall thickness of 30 mm or more). A clinical risk prediction model for sudden death (available online at http://www.hcmrisk.org/) can estimate an individual patient's absolute 5-year risk of sudden death.[5] Patients with an annual mortality rate of 4 to 6% based on the online risk predictor or on the presence of two or more of these markers should be considered for an implantable cardioverter-defibrillator (ICD) (Chapter 66). All patients with hypertrophic cardiomyopathy should be advised to avoid competitive sports and intense physical exertion. Patients without any risk factors do not warrant an ICD. For patients with one risk factor, decisions about an ICD should be individualized on the basis of the patient's age and severity of disease and level of risk that is acceptable to the patient.

PROGNOSIS

Most patients with hypertrophic cardiomyopathy follow a stable and benign course with a low risk for adverse events and a survival similar to that of age- and gender-matched normal populations, but many experience progressive symptoms caused by atrial arrhythmia and gradual deterioration in left ventricular systolic and diastolic function. Between 0.5 and 1% of affected individuals die suddenly each year. The annual incidence of stroke varies from 0.56 to 0.8% per year, rising to 1.9% in patients older than 60 years, and 23% of strokes are fatal. The development of severe systolic heart failure is associated with a poor prognosis, with an overall mortality rate of up to 11% per year. The incidence of infective endocarditis is 1.4 per 1000 person-years overall but 3.8 per 1000 person-years in patients with obstruction.

Myocarditis

DEFINITION AND EPIDEMIOLOGY

Myocarditis, which is an inflammatory process involving the myocardium, can be caused by infections, immune-mediated damage, or toxins (Table 60-4). The incidence and prevalence of myocarditis are difficult to estimate because the clinical presentation varies from asymptomatic ECG abnormalities to hemodynamic collapse and sudden death. Population estimates of the prevalence of myocarditis range from 1 in 100,000 to 1 in 10,000, whereas postmortem studies report myocarditis in up to 12% of young victims of sudden cardiac death.

Worldwide, the most common infective myocarditis is Chagas disease, caused by *Trypanosoma cruzi*, a protozoan organism endemic in rural areas of South and Central America (Chapter 347). In the Western world, viral myocarditis is the most common cause of inflammatory heart disease. Human immunodeficiency virus (HIV) infection (Chapter 384) is associated with lymphocytic myocarditis and is a strong predictor of poor prognosis. Smallpox vaccination (Chapter 18) causes myopericarditis with a reported incidence of 7.8 cases per 100,000 vaccine administrations. Other rare myocarditides include giant cell myocarditis, myocarditis complicating autoimmune disorders such as systemic lupus erythematosus (Chapter 266), and cocaine abuse (Chapter 34).

TABLE 60-4 CAUSES OF MYOCARDITIS

INFECTION
Viral
Coxsackievirus, human immunodeficiency virus, echovirus, adenovirus, influenza, measles, mumps, parvovirus, poliovirus, rubella, varicella-zoster virus, herpes simplex virus, cytomegalovirus, hepatitis C virus, rabies virus, respiratory syncytial virus, vaccine virus, dengue virus, yellow fever virus
Protozoal
Trypanosoma cruzi, Toxoplasma gondii
Bacterial
Brucella, Corynebacterium diphtheriae, Salmonella, Haemophilus influenzae, Mycoplasma pneumoniae, Neisseria meningitidis (meningococcus), *Streptococcus pneumoniae, Staphylococcus, Mycobacterium, Neisseria gonorrhoeae* (gonococcus), *Vibrio cholerae*
Spirochetal
Treponema pallidum, Borrelia, Leptospira
Fungal
Aspergillus, Candida, Cryptococcus, Actinomyces, Blastomyces, Histoplasma, Coccidioides
Rickettsial
Coxiella burnetii, Rickettsia rickettsii, Rickettsia tsutsugamushi
Parasitic
Trichinella spiralis, Echinococcus granulosus, Taenia solium
IMMUNE-MEDIATED DISORDERS
Alloantigens
Heart transplant rejection
Autoantigens
Churg-Strauss syndrome, celiac disease, Whipple disease, giant cell myocarditis, Kawasaki disease, systemic lupus erythematosus, systemic sclerosis, sarcoidosis, scleroderma, polymyositis, thrombocytopenic purpura
Allergens (Drugs)
Penicillin, sulfonamides, tetracycline, methyldopa, streptomycin, tricyclic antidepressants, thiazide diuretics, dobutamine, indomethacin
TOXIC CAUSES
Drugs
Anthracyclines, catecholamines, amphetamines, cocaine, cyclophosphamide, 5-fluorouracil, trastuzumab, interferon, interleukin-2
Physical Agents
Electric shock, radiation, hyperpyrexia
Heavy Metals
Copper, iron, lead
Others
Arsenic, snake bite, scorpion bite, wasp and spider stings, phosphorus, carbon monoxide
GENETIC DISORDERS
Inherited cardiomyopathies with immune-mediated pathogenesis (dilated and right ventricular cardiomyopathy)

PATHOBIOLOGY

Myocarditis is defined histologically by the presence of myocyte injury, with degeneration or necrosis, and an inflammatory infiltrate not due to ischemia. Four patterns are recognized: *active myocarditis*, with myocyte degeneration or necrosis and definite cellular infiltrate with or without fibrosis; *borderline myocarditis*, with a definite cellular infiltrate without evidence of myocardial cellular injury; *persistent myocarditis*, with continued active myocarditis on repeated biopsy; and *resolving or resolved myocarditis*, characterized by a diminished or absent infiltrate with evidence of connective tissue healing on repeated biopsy. Despite their widespread use, the so-called Dallas criteria have low specificity and sensitivity, with a diagnostic yield as low as 10 to 20% in some series. Therefore, newer virology techniques used in conjunction with conventional light microscopy include nested polymerase chain reaction or reverse transcription polymerase chain reaction on RNA and DNA extracted from endomyocardial biopsy specimens and immunohistochemical staining for subtypes of infiltrating lymphocytes and abnormal expression of cellular adhesion molecules on interstitial or endothelial cells.

Viral Myocarditis

Most data on the pathology of viral myocarditis come from murine models. Initially, there is direct invasion of the myocardium by cardiotropic viruses, which enter the cardiomyocyte through receptor-mediated endocytosis. The viral genome, which translated intracellularly to produce viral protein or is incorporated into the host cell genome, may contribute to myocyte dysfunction by cleaving dystrophin. In the second phase, activation of the host immune system, including recruitment of natural killer cells and macrophages, increases the expression of proinflammatory cytokines such as interleukin-1 and tumor necrosis factor. Activation of $CD4^+$ T lymphocytes promotes clonal expansion of B lymphocytes, thereby resulting in further myocardial cell damage, inflammation, and the production of circulating antiheart antibodies directed against contractile, structural, and mitochondrial proteins. This autoimmune response may result in long-term ventricular remodeling by direct effects on myocardial structural components or alterations in the extracellular matrix.

CLINICAL MANIFESTATIONS

Some patients report prodromal symptoms of viremia, including fever, myalgia, coryzal symptoms, and gastroenteritis, but many individuals with myocarditis are asymptomatic and manifest only transient ECG abnormalities, such as nonspecific ST segment and T wave abnormalities, pathologic Q waves, and low QRS voltages. Less common presentations include acute myocardial infarction with angiographically normal coronary arteries (Chapter 73), atrioventricular block (Chapter 64), and ventricular arrhythmias (Chapter 65). Patients with impairment of left ventricular function may present with symptoms and signs of fulminant cardiogenic shock (Chapter 107) with acute cardiovascular collapse. In some cases, sudden cardiac death is the first presentation.

DIAGNOSIS

The diagnosis of myocarditis requires a high index of suspicion because it may mimic other common conditions. There are no typical features on echocardiography, but impaired left or right ventricular systolic performance (with or without ventricular dilation), regional wall motion abnormalities, left (or right) ventricular thrombus, diastolic impairment, and pericardial effusions may be present. Cardiac magnetic resonance imaging can detect myocardial inflammation and myocyte injury, with pericellular and cellular edema.

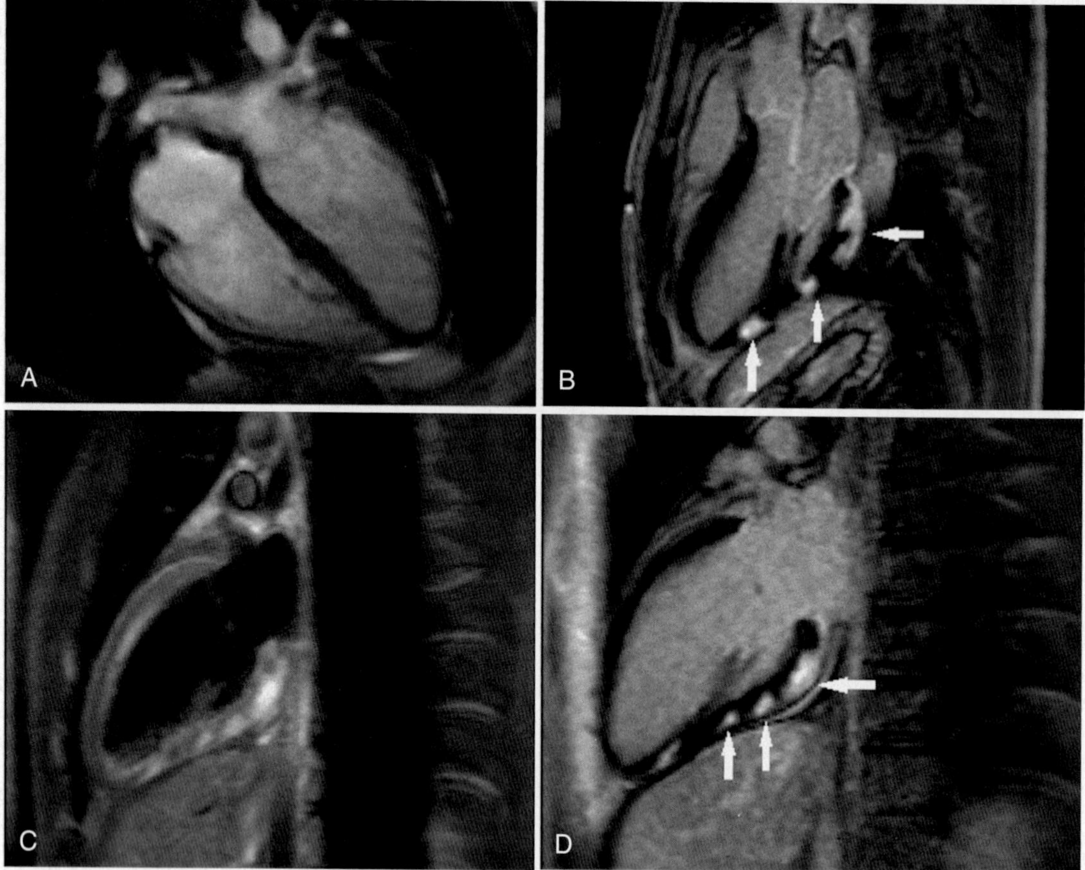

FIGURE 60-4. **A 17-year-old man presenting with apparent acute myopericarditis. The four-chamber end-diastolic view (A) presents a mildly dilated left ventricle. There is patchy late gadolinium enhancement involving the inferior and lateral walls (B, D, *arrows*). Edema is seen on T1 imaging (C), and there is extensive late enhancement. The differential diagnosis of this appearance also includes sarcoid and giant cell myocarditis.**

Routine blood tests, such as full blood count and erythrocyte sedimentation rate, are usually unhelpful. Serum markers of myocardial injury, such as troponins T and I, may be elevated, but myocarditis may be proven by biopsy even in the absence of elevated serum troponin levels. Creatine kinase and its cardiac isoform CK-MB are less sensitive and specific than troponin. Increased levels of autoantibodies against myocardial proteins (such as myosin and the adenine nucleotide translocator protein) are biomarkers of autoimmune myocarditis and correlate with progressive worsening of ventricular function.

Cardiac magnetic resonance imaging with gadolinium enhancement can show evidence of myocarditis (Fig. 60-4), but cardiac catheterization with right ventricular endomyocardial biopsy remains the "gold standard" diagnostic test. In the United States, biopsy has generally been reserved for patients with heart failure refractory to standard management, features suggestive of systemic disease (e.g., connective tissue disease [Chapter 260], amyloidosis [Chapter 188], hemochromatosis [Chapter 212], sarcoidosis [Chapter 95]), or suspicion of giant cell myocarditis because of new-onset heart failure associated with tachyarrhythmias or conduction disease. By comparison, a European consensus statement recommends endomyocardial biopsy to achieve an etiologic diagnosis and to guide potential novel treatment options in patients with "clinically suspected myocarditis,"[6] despite the absence of definitive outcome data to support this recommendation.

Specific Causes

Viral myocarditis may be suspected from the clinical picture of recent febrile illness, often with prominent myalgias, followed by angina-like chest pain, dyspnea, or arrhythmias. Elevated troponin levels support the diagnosis, and increasing viral titers (to coxsackievirus, echovirus, adenovirus, or influenza virus) are consistent with recent infection. The correlation with biopsy-proven myocarditis is strongest with HIV and Lyme disease. Clinical cardiomyopathy occurs in 10 to 40% of patients infected with HIV due to the HIV infection itself or to coinfection with cytomegalovirus.

Giant cell myocarditis, which accounts for 10 to 20% of biopsy-positive cases of myocarditis, is manifested with the rapid onset of chest pain, fever, and hemodynamic compromise, often with ventricular tachycardia or atrioventricular block. When ventricular tachyarrhythmias or progressive heart failure are major features of clinically suspected myocarditis, particularly in a young person, endomyocardial biopsy is recommended to determine whether giant cell myocarditis is present.

Toxoplasmosis (Chapter 349) *myocarditis,* due to intermittent rupture of cysts in the myocardium, can cause atypical chest pain, arrhythmias, pericarditis, and symptomatic heart failure. Diagnosis is made from antibody titers. Lyme carditis (Chapter 321) is classically manifested with conduction system abnormalities resulting from infection with *Borrelia burgdorferi,* which is diagnosed serologically.

Immune-mediated myocarditis can be associated with polymyositis (Chapter 269) or systemic lupus erythematosus (Chapter 266), although pericarditis and coronary artery vasculitis are more common. Hypersensitivity reactions, especially to drugs (Chapter 254), can cause myocarditis that is often associated with peripheral eosinophilia and can be confirmed by endomyocardial biopsy.

TREATMENT

The first-line treatment of myocarditis is supportive with afterload reduction and diuresis (Chapter 59). Patients with fulminant acute myocarditis may require inotropic support, mechanical assist devices, or extracorporeal membrane oxygenation (Chapter 107). After initial stabilization, patients with symptoms and signs of heart failure should receive angiotensin-converting enzyme inhibitors, diuretics, β-blockers, and anticoagulants in accordance with standard guidelines (Chapter 59). Patients with intractable and deteriorating heart failure may require cardiac transplantation (Chapter 82).

The role of immunosuppression is uncertain. In one randomized, placebo-controlled trial of 111 adults with biopsy-proven myocarditis, there was no difference in mortality or improvement in left ventricular function in patients treated with prednisolone plus either cyclosporine or azathioprine.[A1] Conversely, in a randomized trial of patients who had major histocompatibility complex expression on endomyocardial biopsy samples and who were randomized to prednisolone (1 mg/kg/day tapering to a maintenance dose of 0.2 mg/kg/day for a total of 90 days) and azathioprine (1 mg/kg/day for a total of 100 days) versus placebo, left ventricular ejection fraction improved in the immunosuppressed group, but no difference was observed in mortality or rates of transplantation or rehospitalization during a 2-year follow-up period.[A2] Immunosuppression has been reserved for patients with giant cell myocarditis,[A3] but recent recommendations now extend immunosuppression to other biopsy-proven, infection-negative immune-mediated forms of myocarditis including eosinophilic myocarditis, cardiac sarcoidosis, and lymphocytic myocarditis that is refractory to conventional heart failure therapy. The optimal regimens remain to be determined, and intravenous immune globulin therapy is not helpful.

PROGNOSIS

Patients with acute myocarditis with mild heart failure or symptoms suggestive of myocardial ischemia or infarction typically improve within weeks without sequelae. An acute presentation of myocarditis with advanced heart failure (ejection fraction <35%) may resolve but can lead to chronic left ventricular dysfunction (dilated cardiomyopathy) or progress to death or cardiac transplantation. Patients who present with acute fulminant myocarditis, however, may have an excellent prognosis, with survival rates of more than 90%. Overall, however, biopsy-proven viral myocarditis is associated with a long-term mortality of almost 20% at 4.7 years, and the presence of biventricular dysfunction at presentation is the best predictor of all-cause mortality. Giant cell myocarditis is usually fatal without heart transplantation, but it can be stabilized by early diagnosis and prompt introduction of immunosuppression.[7]

Dilated Cardiomyopathy

DEFINITION AND EPIDEMIOLOGY

Dilated cardiomyopathy is a heart muscle disorder defined by dilation and impaired systolic function of the left ventricle or both ventricles, in the absence of coronary artery disease, valvular abnormalities, or pericardial disease. In adults, prevalence estimates range from 14 to 36 per 100,000. In children, dilated cardiomyopathy is the most common cardiomyopathy, accounting for up to 58% of cases. Overall, males and females are approximately equally affected, except for dilated cardiomyopathy associated with neuromuscular disorders or inborn errors of metabolism, for which there is male predominance because some of these conditions have an X-linked inheritance.

PATHOBIOLOGY

A number of conditions are associated with dilated cardiomyopathy, including neuromuscular disorders, inborn errors of metabolism, and malformation syndromes. In most patients, no identifiable cause is found, and the disease is termed idiopathic dilated cardiomyopathy.

Genetic Dilated Cardiomyopathy

Between 20 and 50% of individuals with dilated cardiomyopathy have evidence of familial disease (see Table 60-2).[8] Autosomal dominant inheritance, which accounts for 68% of familial cases, has two major forms: isolated dilated cardiomyopathy, which is manifested with a clinical picture of heart failure; and dilated cardiomyopathy, in which an associated arrhythmia (i.e., conduction system disease, ventricular tachycardia or fibrillation) is usually the initial manifestation. The latter patients may also have an associated skeletal myopathy. Genes implicated in isolated dilated cardiomyopathy include cytoskeletal and sarcomeric protein genes. Truncating mutations in *TTN*, the gene encoding the sarcomere protein titin, occur in approximately 25% of familial cases of idiopathic dilated cardiomyopathy and in 18% of sporadic cases. Mutations in the lamin A/C gene, which encodes a nuclear envelope protein, cause atrial and ventricular arrhythmia and progressive atrioventricular conduction disease, which may precede the development of dilated cardiomyopathy.

X-linked inheritance accounts for between 2 and 5% of familial cases of dilated cardiomyopathy. Neuromuscular disorders account for 26% of cases, 90% of which are Duchenne, Becker, and Emery-Dreifuss muscular dystrophies (Chapter 421). Isolated X-linked dilated cardiomyopathy, also caused by mutations in the dystrophin gene, is characterized by raised serum creatine kinase muscle isoforms but does not result in clinical signs or symptoms of skeletal muscular dystrophy.

Acquired Dilated Cardiomyopathy

Common acquired causes of dilated cardiomyopathy include infectious myocarditis, chemotherapy (Chapter 179), radiation therapy (Chapter 20), alcohol (Chapter 33), cocaine (Chapter 34), nutritional deficiencies (Chapter 215), iron overload (Chapter 212), inflammatory and autoimmune disorders (Chapters 266 and 270), endocrinopathies (Chapter 226), and pregnancy (Chapter 239). Tachycardia-mediated cardiomyopathy (tachycardiomyopathy) is rare and usually reverses once the tachycardia is controlled.

CLINICAL MANIFESTATIONS

The symptoms and signs associated with dilated cardiomyopathy depend on the age of the patient and the degree of left ventricular dysfunction. Although the first presentation may be with sudden death or a thromboembolic event, most patients present with symptoms of high pulmonary venous pressure or low cardiac output (Chapter 58), which can be acute, sometimes precipitated by intercurrent illness or arrhythmia, or chronic. Increasingly, dilated cardiomyopathy is diagnosed incidentally in asymptomatic individuals during family screening.

Adults initially present with reduced exercise tolerance and dyspnea on exertion. With worsening left ventricular function, patients may develop dyspnea at rest, orthopnea, paroxysmal nocturnal dyspnea, peripheral edema, and ascites. Symptoms related to mesenteric ischemia, such as abdominal pain after meals, nausea, vomiting, and anorexia, may dominate, especially in children. Arrhythmia symptoms, such as palpitations, presyncope, and syncope, can occur at any age.

In advanced disease, features of low cardiac output include sinus tachycardia, weak peripheral pulses, and hypotension. The jugular venous pressure may be elevated, and the apical impulse is displaced. Peripheral edema, hepatomegaly, and ascites are common in patients with heart failure. Auscultation of the chest typically reveals basal crackles. Auscultation of the heart may reveal the presence of a third (and sometimes also a fourth) heart sound. In patients with functional mitral regurgitation, a pansystolic murmur may be heard at the apex and radiate to the axilla, but frequently no murmurs are heard, even in the presence of mitral incompetence, especially if cardiac output is very low.

DIAGNOSIS

The electrocardiogram may be normal but more typically shows sinus tachycardia, nonspecific ST segment and T wave changes (most commonly in the inferior and lateral leads), atrial enlargement, and voltage criteria for ventricular hypertrophy. Atrioventricular block raises the possibility of mutations in the lamin A/C gene. Supraventricular and ventricular arrhythmias are common. The chest radiograph is usually abnormal, with an increased cardiothoracic ratio (>0.5) reflecting left ventricular and left atrial dilation. Patients with pulmonary edema have increased pulmonary vascular markings and pleural effusion.

On echocardiography, the presence of ventricular end-diastolic dimensions greater than 2 standard deviations above body surface area–corrected means (or greater than 112% of predicted dimension) and fractional shortening less than 25% are sufficient to make the diagnosis. Other common features include functional mitral and tricuspid regurgitation and abnormalities of diastolic left ventricular function. Cardiac magnetic resonance imaging may show areas of myocardial fibrosis (E-Fig. 60-6).

Other recommended tests (Table 60-5) include a complete blood count and tests of renal, thyroid, and hepatic function. Levels of serum creatine kinase should be measured in all patients with dilated cardiomyopathy because this may provide important clues to the etiology. For example, dystrophin-linked dilated cardiomyopathy has been diagnosed in up to 8% of men with dilated cardiomyopathy and should be considered in men with increased serum creatine kinase levels and an X-linked family history. Other cardiac biomarkers, such as troponin I and troponin T, can be elevated. Plasma B-type natriuretic peptide levels predict survival, hospitalization rates, and listing for cardiac transplantation. Symptom-limited exercise testing, combined with respiratory gas analysis, is a useful technique to assess functional limitation and disease progression in patients with stable dilated cardiomyopathy.

Cardiac catheterization is rarely needed except perhaps to exclude severe coronary artery disease or to provide more precise information about possible valvular heart disease. Endomyocardial biopsy may be diagnostic for myocarditis and for some metabolic or mitochondrial disorders but is rarely advised. Hemodynamic assessment of left ventricular end-diastolic and pulmonary artery pressures may be necessary before transplantation.

TABLE 60-5 LABORATORY EVALUATION OF CARDIOMYOPATHY

CLINICAL EVALUATION

History and physical examination to identify cardiac and noncardiac disorders*
Assessment of ability to perform routine and desired activities*
Assessment of volume status*

LABORATORY EVALUATION

Electrocardiogram*
Chest radiograph*
Two-dimensional and Doppler echocardiogram*
Chemistry
  Serum sodium,* potassium,* glucose, creatinine,* blood urea nitrogen,* calcium,* magnesium*
  Albumin,* total protein,* liver function tests,* serum iron, ferritin
  Urinalysis
  Creatine kinase
  Thyroid-stimulating hormone*
Hematology
  Hemoglobin/hematocrit*
  White blood cell count with differential,* including eosinophils
  Erythrocyte sedimentation rate

INITIAL EVALUATION IN SELECTED PATIENTS ONLY

Titers for suspected infection
  Acute viral (coxsackievirus, echovirus, influenza virus)
  Human immunodeficiency virus, Epstein-Barr virus
  Lyme disease, toxoplasmosis
  Chagas disease
Catheterization with coronary angiography in patients with angina who are candidates for intervention*
Serologic studies for active rheumatologic disease
Endomyocardial biopsy

*Level I recommendations from Hunt SA, Abraham WT, Chin MH, et al. ACC/AHA 2005 Guideline Update for the Diagnosis and Management of Chronic Heart Failure in the Adult. *Circulation.* 2005;112:e154-e235.

TREATMENT

Rx

Supportive therapy includes sodium and fluid restriction, avoidance of alcohol and other toxins, and use of established heart failure medications (Chapter 59). Although older recommendations emphasized rest and avoidance of exercise, this advice should be limited to patients with myocarditis or peripartum cardiomyopathy; for other patients, a submaximal exercise regimen is desirable to sustain mobility, to avoid deconditioning, and to maintain physical and psychological health. Patients with atrial fibrillation or with echocardiographic evidence of a left atrial or left ventricular mural thrombosis should be anticoagulated to an international normalized ratio of 2.0 to 3.0. An ICD is preferred to medication for ventricular arrhythmias,[A4] and some patients require management for advanced heart failure (Chapter 59) with biventricular pacing, inotropic medications, ventricular assist devices, and cardiac transplantation (Chapter 82).

Family Screening

Familial evaluation of first-degree relatives by history and physical examination and with 12-lead ECG and two-dimensional echocardiographic studies is warranted at the time of diagnosis and serially thereafter. Precise algorithms to guide the interval of evaluation remain to be determined; because disease progression is usually slow, evaluation about every 5 years until the age of 50 years appears appropriate. The detection of early disease in a family member offers an opportunity to initiate treatment, usually with an angiotensin-converting enzyme inhibitor or β-blocker, but the efficacy of such therapy remains to be proved.

PROGNOSIS

The prognosis of idiopathic and genetically determined dilated cardiomyopathy is related to the severity of disease at the time of presentation and the response to treatment. Most patients improve with treatment, but 5-year survival is less than 50% in patients who present with severe disease (e.g., ejection fraction <25%, left ventricular end-diastolic dimension >65 mm, peak oxygen consumption <12 mL/kg/minute).[9]

Specific Causes of Dilated Cardiomyopathy

Alcoholic Cardiomyopathy

In the United States, excess alcohol consumption (Chapter 33) contributes to more than 10% of cases of heart failure. Alcohol and its metabolite, acetaldehyde, are cardiotoxins. Myocardial depression is initially reversible but, if alcohol consumption is sustained, can lead to myocyte vacuolization, mitochondrial abnormalities, and myocardial fibrosis. Even in chronic stages, however, the heart failure represents a sum of both reversible and irreversible myocardial dysfunction. The amount of alcohol necessary to produce symptomatic cardiomyopathy in susceptible individuals is not known but has been estimated to be six drinks (~4 oz of pure ethanol) a day for 5 to 10 years. Frequent binging without heavy daily consumption may also be sufficient. Alcoholic cardiomyopathy can develop in patients without social evidence of an alcohol problem. Abstinence leads to improvement in at least 50% of patients with severe symptoms, some of whom normalize their left ventricular ejection fractions. Patients with other causes of heart failure also should limit alcohol consumption.

Chemotherapy

Anthracycline (doxorubicin, daunorubicin, epirubicin) cardiotoxicity (Chapter 179) causes characteristic histologic changes on endomyocardial biopsy with overt heart failure in 5 to 10% of patients who receive doses of 450 mg/m^2 of body surface area or more. In adults who receive these drugs, combined treatment with enalapril (starting at 1.25 mg or 2.5 mg twice daily, increasing to 10 mg twice daily as tolerated with systolic blood pressure ≥90 mm Hg) and carvedilol (starting at 6.25 mg twice daily and increasing to 25 mg twice daily if there is no heart failure, bradycardia, or atrioventricular block) can significantly reduce the risk of left ventricular dilation and heart failure.[A5] Patients who have received anthracyclines in the prepubertal period without apparent cardiotoxicity may develop cardiac failure in young adulthood. The risk is higher in patients who have lower baseline ejection fractions, concomitant radiation therapy, or higher doses of anthracycline. *Cyclophosphamide* and *ifosfamide* can cause acute severe heart failure and malignant ventricular arrhythmias. Some *tyrosine kinase inhibitors* (e.g., sunitinib) cause a reduction in systolic function, especially in the presence of coronary artery disease, but there is good response to withdrawal and conventional medical therapy (Chapter 184). *5-Fluorouracil* can cause coronary artery spasm and depressed left ventricular contractility. Up to 11% of patients who receive *trastuzumab* (Chapter 198), a recombinant monoclonal antibody that binds to human epidermal growth factor type 2, develop dilated cardiomyopathy, which is reversible after withdrawal and conventional drug treatment. The risk for cardiotoxicity increases with previous anthracycline and radiation treatment. *Interferon alfa* may be associated with hypotension and arrhythmias in up to 10% of patients, and *interleukin-2* rarely has been associated with cardiotoxicity.

Metabolic and Endocrine Disease

Excess catecholamines, as in *pheochromocytoma* (Chapter 228), may injure the heart by compromising the coronary microcirculation or by direct toxic effects on myocytes. *Cocaine* (Chapter 34) increases synaptic concentrations of catecholamines by inhibiting reuptake at nerve terminals; the result may be an acute coronary syndrome or chronic cardiomyopathy.

Thiamine deficiency from poor nutrition or alcoholism (Chapter 218) can cause beriberi heart disease, with vasodilation and high cardiac output followed by low output. *Calcium deficiency* resulting from hypoparathyroidism, gastrointestinal abnormalities, or chelation directly compromises myocardial contractility.

Hypophosphatemia (Chapter 119), which may occur in alcoholism, during recovery from malnutrition, and in hyperalimentation, also reduces myocardial contractility. Patients with *magnesium depletion* due to impaired absorption or increased renal excretion (Chapter 119) also may present with left ventricular dysfunction.

Hypothyroidism (Chapter 226) depresses contractility and conduction and may cause pericardial effusions, whereas *hyperthyroidism* increases cardiac output, can worsen underlying heart failure, and may rarely be the sole cause of heart failure.

The presenting sign of *diabetes* (Chapter 229) can be cardiomyopathy, especially with diastolic dysfunction, independent of epicardial coronary atherosclerosis, for which it is a major risk factor.

Obesity (Chapter 220) can cause cardiomyopathy with increased ventricular mass and decreased contractility, which improve after weight loss, or it can aggravate underlying heart failure from other causes.

Peripartum Cardiomyopathy

Peripartum cardiomyopathy appears in the last month of pregnancy or in the first 5 months after delivery in the absence of preexisting cardiac disease (Chapter 239). The incidence is between 1 in 3000 and 1 in 15,000 deliveries, with increased risk in older mothers or in the setting of twins, malnutrition, tocolytic therapy, toxemia, or hypertension. Lymphocytic myocarditis, found in 30 to 50% of biopsy specimens, suggests an immune component, perhaps cross-reactivity between uterine and cardiac myocyte proteins or an enhanced susceptibility to viral myocarditis. More recently, it has been suggested that enhanced oxidative stress triggers activation of cathepsin D, an ubiquitous lysosomal enzyme that cleaves serum prolactin in its antiangiogenic and pro-apoptotic 16-kD form, which appears to promote endothelial inflammation and impair cardiomyocyte metabolism and contraction. Presentation is usually with orthopnea and dyspnea on minimal exertion, most often within the first weeks after delivery when the excess volume of pregnancy would normally be mobilized. Preexisting cardiac disease must be excluded. Diuretics facilitate postpartum diuresis, and angiotensin-converting enzyme inhibitors improve symptoms (Chapter 59). In a small randomized trial, oral bromocriptine (2.5 mg twice daily for 2 weeks, then daily for 6 weeks) significantly improved recovery of left ventricular function and may reduce deaths.[A6] The prognosis is improvement to normal or near-normal ejection fraction during the next 6 months in more than 50% of patients. About 4% require heart transplantation, and about 9% die suddenly or from complications of heart transplantation.

Overlap with Restrictive Cardiomyopathy

Diseases causing primarily restrictive cardiomyopathies can occasionally overlap to cause a picture consistent with dilated cardiomyopathy. For example, *hemochromatosis* (Chapter 212) and *sarcoidosis* (Chapter 95) should be considered in evaluating any patient with a cardiomyopathy, although these conditions are more often considered with the restrictive diseases. *Amyloidosis* (Chapter 188) is less commonly confused with dilated than with hypertrophic cardiomyopathy but should be considered in a patient with a thick-walled ventricle with moderately depressed contractile function.

Arrhythmogenic Right Ventricular Cardiomyopathy

DEFINITION AND EPIDEMIOLOGY

ARVC (Chapter 65) is a genetically determined heart muscle disorder characterized histologically by loss of cardiomyocytes with replacement by fibrous or fibrofatty tissue in the right ventricular myocardium; clinically by ventricular arrhythmias, heart failure, and sudden death; and histologically by cardiomyocyte loss and replacement. The disease is seen in patients of European, African, and Asian descent, with an estimated prevalence between 1 in 1000 and 1 in 5000 adults.

PATHOBIOLOGY

ARVC is inherited as an autosomal dominant disease with incomplete penetrance, although recessive forms with cutaneous manifestations are recognized (see Table 60-2). Most cases are caused by heterozygous mutations in genes encoding components of the desmosomal junction of cardiomyocytes. The most common occur in plakophilin 2, desmocollin 2, desmoplakin, and desmoglein 2. Homozygous mutations in plakoglobin and desmoplakin are responsible for the rare autosomal recessive forms (i.e., Naxos disease and Carvajal syndrome). A highly penetrant and lethal mutation in the transmembrane cytoplasmic protein 43 (TMEM43) has been described in families from Newfoundland. Two other nondesmosomal genes, the cardiac ryanodine receptor and transforming growth factor-β3, have been linked with ARVC but are probably not important in most patients.

Pathology

The main pathologic feature is progressive loss of right ventricular myocardium, which is replaced by adipose and fibrous tissue. These changes begin in the inflow, outflow, and apical regions of the right ventricle. Aneurysm formation in these areas is typical. Progressive myocardial involvement may lead to global right ventricular dilation. Severe right ventricular disease is often associated with fibrofatty substitution of the left ventricular myocardium, with the posterolateral wall preferentially affected.

Mutations in desmosomal protein genes may increase the susceptibility of the myocardium to the damaging effects of mechanical stress, thereby predisposing to cardiomyocyte detachment, death, and eventual replacement with fibrofatty tissue. The acute phase of myocardial injury may be accompanied by inflammation. The predilection for the right ventricle has been explained by its thin wall and greater distensibility. As desmosomal proteins interact with many other proteins, including components of the cellular cytoskeleton and intermediate filaments, it is possible that ventricular dysfunction occurs as the result of reduced cytoskeletal integrity and impaired force transduction. Some desmosomal proteins, in particular plakoglobin, are also important signaling molecules that regulate the transcription of many other genes. Finally, a reduction in the number and size of gap junctions may result in a electrical coupling defect, thereby increasing the propensity to arrhythmia without significant morphologic changes.

CLINICAL MANIFESTATIONS

By convention, the natural history of ARVC is divided into phases, but it is not inevitable that patients will progress through all phases. In the early phase, patients are usually asymptomatic, but resuscitated cardiac arrest and sudden death may be the initial manifestations, particularly in adolescents and young adults. The overt arrhythmic phase usually begins in adolescents and young adults, when patients note palpitations or syncope. Symptomatic sustained arrhythmias are usually accompanied by ECG, morphologic, and functional abnormalities of the right ventricle sufficient to fulfill diagnostic criteria for ARVC. A small proportion of patients progress to a more advanced phase, which is characterized by diffuse right or left ventricular impairment that requires conventional treatment for heart failure (Chapter 59).

DIAGNOSIS

Clinical evaluation includes inquiry for symptoms of arrhythmia (syncope, presyncope, sustained palpitation); a family history of premature cardiac symptoms or sudden death; 12-lead, 24-hour, and maximal exercise ECG testing; and two-dimensional echocardiography with specific right ventricular views. Contrast echocardiography may be required to obtain better endocardial definition of the right ventricular myocardium and apex of the left ventricle. Magnetic resonance imaging (Chapter 56) may provide accurate assessment of ventricular volumes as well as noninvasive characterization of the characteristic fibrous tissue and fat that establishes the diagnosis and provides prognostic information (Fig. 60-5).[10]

Ventricular arrhythmias with a left bundle branch block morphology, consistent with a right ventricular origin, are characteristic. However, the ECG and arrhythmic manifestations are not specific to ARVC and overlap with many other disease states, so standard criteria are recommended for diagnosis (Table 60-6). Because these criteria are highly specific but lack sensitivity for detection of early disease, more sensitive criteria are recommended for first-degree relatives of known cases (Table 60-7). The diagnosis of ARVC in a proband also raises the possibility of mutation analysis in the family to identify those at risk and in need of serial evaluation as well as those who need no specific follow-up.

Differential Diagnosis

The differential diagnosis includes other inherited cardiomyopathies, the inherited arrhythmia syndromes (long QT syndrome, Brugada syndrome, and catecholaminergic polymorphic ventricular tachycardia; Chapter 65), cardiac sarcoidosis, myocarditis, and causes of right ventricular dilation such as intracardiac or extracardiac shunts (Chapter 69). The differentiation from so-called benign right ventricular outflow tract tachycardia may be problematic, although the 12-lead ECG and right ventricular imaging studies are typically normal, and no familial disease is present. Some patients with desmosomal protein gene mutations demonstrate left ventricular involvement early in the disease, and a minority may have a predominant left ventricular dilated cardiomyopathy phenotype.

TREATMENT Rx

Pharmacologic treatment is the first-line therapy for patients with well-tolerated, non–life-threatening ventricular arrhythmias, such as frequent ventricular extrasystoles. Treatment of patients with symptomatic ventricular arrhythmias is with an ICD, with supplemental sotalol (160 to 240 mg/day) or even amiodarone (maintenance dose of 200 mg/day). Catheter ablation (Chapter 66) may be required in patients with drug-refractory incessant ventricular arrhythmia or frequent recurrences of ventricular tachycardia after implantation of an ICD, although recurrence is common.

Retrospective analyses of clinical and pathologic series have identified a number of possible predictors of adverse outcome in probands, including an early age at onset of symptoms, competitive sporting activity, severe right ventricular dilation, left ventricular involvement, syncope, episodes of complex

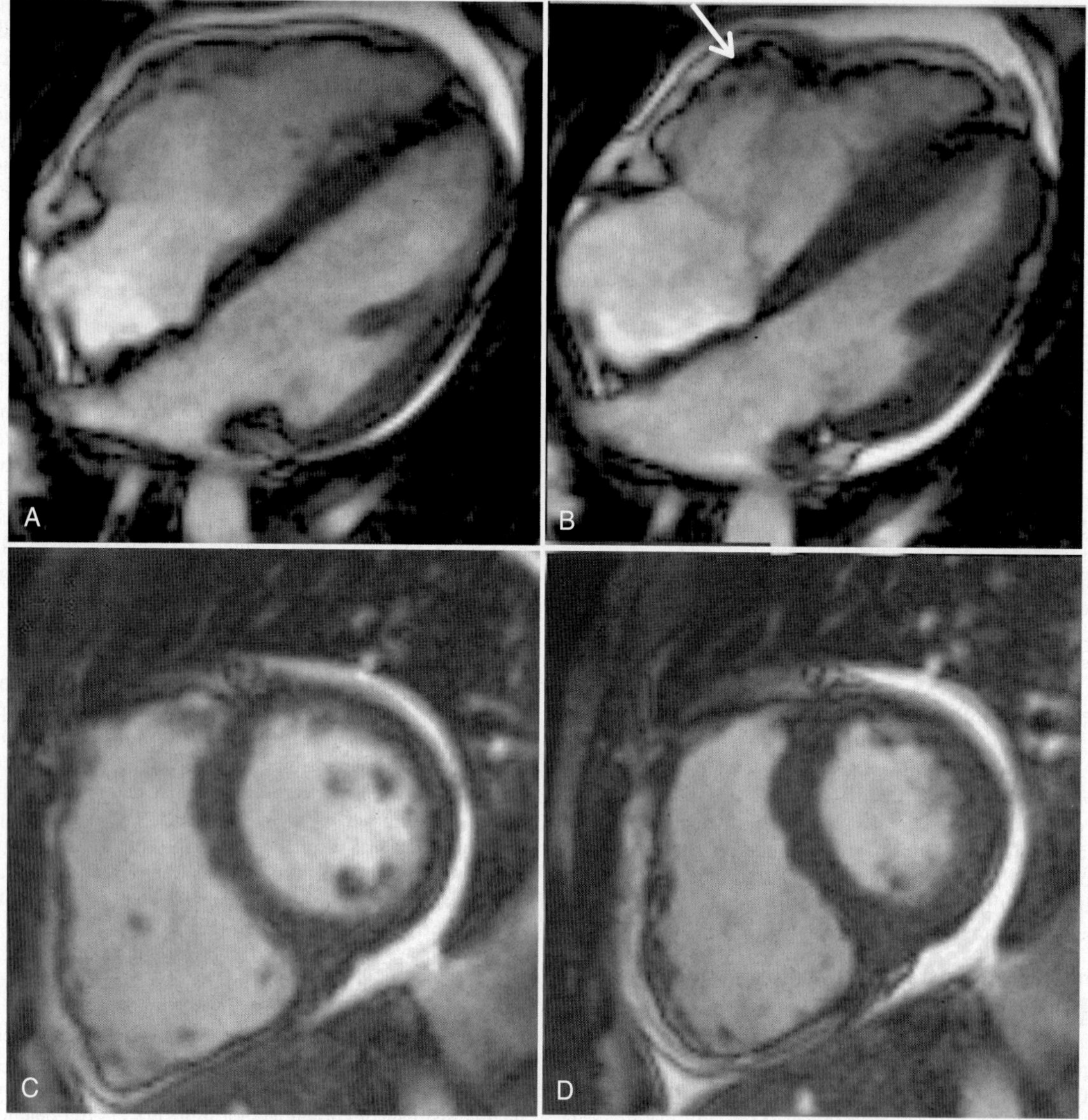

FIGURE 60-5. A 21-year-old man with arrhythmogenic right ventricular cardiomyopathy. End-diastolic (A) and end-systolic (B) frames from a four-chamber view, with a dilated and impaired right ventricle with a basal wall motion abnormality (*arrow*), confirmed on end-diastolic (C) and end-systolic (D) short axis views. This individual had no scar in the left ventricle with well preserved systolic function; scar imaging in the thin right ventricle (with adjacent fat and small effusion) was equivocal.

ventricular arrhythmias or VT, and increased QRS dispersion on the 12-lead electrocardiogram. ICD implantation is recommended for the prevention of sudden cardiac death in patients with documented sustained ventricular tachycardia or ventricular fibrillation and a reasonable expectation of survival with a good functional status for longer than 1 year. ICD implantation may also be appropriate in patients with extensive disease, including those with left ventricular involvement, or undiagnosed syncope when ventricular tachycardia or ventricular fibrillation has not been excluded as the cause.

Standard heart failure therapy, including diuretics, angiotensin-converting enzyme inhibitors, and β-blockers, is indicated in patients in whom ARVC has progressed to severe heart failure or biventricular systolic dysfunction (Chapter 59). Anticoagulation should be considered in the presence of atrial fibrillation (Chapter 64), marked ventricular dilation, or ventricular aneurysms. In patients in whom heart failure is refractory, cardiac transplantation (Chapter 82) should be considered.

PROGNOSIS

Most data on prognosis in ARVC are derived from small, high-risk populations. By the age of 40 years, event-free survival is 50 to 60% in patients with Naxos disease and some autosomal dominant forms. In patients who have syncope or sustained ventricular arrhythmias and are treated with an ICD, freedom from appropriate shock therapy is about 75% at 48 months after implantation, with 96% of patients alive. Risk factors for sudden cardiac death include severe right ventricular disease, left ventricular involvement, and a history of unexplained syncope.

Restrictive Cardiomyopathy

DEFINITION AND EPIDEMIOLOGY

The incidence and prevalence of restrictive cardiomyopathy in adults are unknown. Restrictive cardiomyopathies (Table 60-8) are characterized by stiffness, impaired filling, elevated left ventricular diastolic pressures, and reduced diastolic volume of the left or right ventricle despite normal or near-normal systolic function and wall thickness. Primary forms are uncommon, whereas secondary forms, in which the heart is affected as part of a multisystem disorder, usually present at the advanced stage of an infiltrative disease (e.g., amyloidosis or sarcoidosis) or a systemic storage disease (e.g., hemochromatosis). Idiopathic restrictive cardiomyopathy affects both male and female patients and may be manifested in children and young adults.

PATHOBIOLOGY

Approximately 30% of patients with idiopathic restrictive cardiomyopathy have familial disease, and most of these patients will have mutations in the cardiac sarcomere protein genes, particularly troponin I and β-myosin heavy chain. Mutations in the gene encoding desmin (an intermediate filament) cause restrictive cardiomyopathy associated with skeletal myopathy and cardiac conduction system abnormalities.

The macroscopic features of restrictive cardiomyopathy include biatrial dilation and small ventricular cavities. In many hearts, there is thrombus in the atrial appendages and patchy endocardial fibrosis. The histologic features of idiopathic restrictive cardiomyopathy are typically nonspecific with patchy interstitial fibrosis, but myocyte disarray is not uncommon in patients with

TABLE 60-6 REVISED TASK FORCE CRITERIA FOR ARRHYTHMOGENIC RIGHT VENTRICULAR CARDIOMYOPATHY IN PROBANDS*

CRITERIA	
MAJOR	**MINOR**
I. GLOBAL OR REGIONAL DYSFUNCTION AND STRUCTURAL ALTERATIONS*	
By Two-Dimensional Echo • Regional RV akinesia, dyskinesia, or aneurysm • *and* 1 of the following (end diastole): PLAX RVOT ≥32 mm (corrected for body size [PLAX/BSA] ≥19 mm/m^2) PSAX RVOT ≥36 mm (corrected for body size [PLAX/BSA] ≥21 mm/m^2) *or* fractional area change ≤33%	**By Two-Dimensional Echo** • Regional RV akinesia or dyskinesia • *and* 1 of the following (end diastole): PLAX RVOT ≥29 to <32 mm (corrected for body size [PLAX/BSA] ≥16 to <19 mm/m^2) PSAX RVOT ≥32 to <36 mm (corrected for body size [PSAX/BSA] ≥18 to <21 mm/m^2) *or* fractional area change >33% to ≤40%
By MRI • Regional RV akinesia or dyskinesia or dyssynchronous RV contraction • *and* 1 of the following: RV end-diastolic volume indexed to BSA ≥110 mL/m^2 (male) or ≥100 mL/m^2 (female) *or* RV ejection fraction ≤40%	**By MRI** • Regional RV akinesia or dyskinesia or dyssynchronous RV contraction • *and* 1 of the following: RV end-diastolic volume indexed to BSA ≥100 to <110 mL/m^2 (male) or ≥90 to <100 mL/m^2 (female) *or* RV ejection fraction >40% to ≤45%
By RV angiography • Regional RV akinesia, dyskinesia, or aneurysm	
II. TISSUE CHARACTERIZATION OF WALL	
• Residual myocytes <60% by morphometric analysis (or <50% if estimated), with fibrous replacement of the RV free wall myocardium in ≥1 sample, with or without fatty replacement of tissue on endomyocardial biopsy	• Residual myocytes 60% to 75% by morphometric analysis (or 50% to 65% if estimated), with fibrous replacement of the RV free wall myocardium in ≥1 sample, with or without fatty replacement of tissue on endomyocardial biopsy
III. REPOLARIZATION ABNORMALITIES	
• Inverted T waves in right precordial leads (V_1,V_2, and V_3) or beyond in individuals >14 years of age (in the absence of complete right bundle branch block QRS ≥120 msec)	• Inverted T waves in leads V_1 and V_2 in individuals >14 years of age (in the absence of complete right bundle branch block) or in V_4, V_5, or V_6 • Inverted T waves in leads V_1, V_2, V_3, and V_4 in individuals >14 years
IV. DEPOLARIZATION/CONDUCTION ABNORMALITIES	
• Epsilon wave (reproducible low-amplitude signals between end of QRS complex to onset of the T wave) in the right precordial leads (V_1 to V_3)	• Late potentials by SAECG in ≥1 of 3 parameters in the absence of a QRS duration ≥110 msec on the standard ECG • Filtered QRS duration (fQRS) ≥114 msec • Duration of terminal QRS <40 µV (low-amplitude signal duration) ≥38 msec • Root-mean-square voltage of terminal 40 msec ≤20 µV • Terminal activation duration of QRS ≥55 msec measured to the end of the QRS, including R′, in V_1, V_2, or V_3, in the absence of complete right bundle branch block
V. ARRHYTHMIAS	
• Nonsustained or sustained ventricular tachycardia of left bundle branch morphology with superior axis (negative or indeterminate QRS in leads II, III, and aVF and positive in lead aVL)	• Nonsustained or sustained ventricular tachycardia of RV outflow configuration, left bundle branch block morphology with inferior axis (positive QRS in leads II, III, and aVF and negative in lead aVL) or of unknown axis • >500 ventricular extrasystoles per 24 hours (Holter)
VI. FAMILY HISTORY	
• ARVC confirmed in a first-degree relative who meets current Task Force criteria • ARVC confirmed pathologically at autopsy or surgery in a first-degree relative • Identification of a pathogenic mutation[†] categorized as associated or probably associated with ARVC in the patient under evaluation	• History of ARVC in a first-degree relative in whom it is not possible or practical to determine whether the family member meets current Task Force criteria • Premature sudden death (<35 years of age) due to suspected ARVC in a first-degree relative

*Hypokinesis is not included in this or subsequent definitions of right ventricular (RV) regional wall motion abnormalities for the proposed modified criteria.
†A pathogenic mutation is a DNA alteration associated with ARVC that alters or is expected to alter the encoded protein, is unobserved or rare in a large non-ARVC control population, and either alters or is predicted to alter the structure or function of the protein or has demonstrated linkage to the disease phenotype in a conclusive pedigree.
ARVC = arrhythmogenic right ventricular cardiomyopathy; aVF = augmented voltage unipolar left foot lead; aVL = augmented voltage unipolar left arm lead; BSA = body surface area; ECG = electrocardiogram; MRI = magnetic resonance imaging; PLAX = parasternal long axis view; PSAX = parasternal short axis view; RVOT = right ventricular outflow tract; SAECG = signal-averaged electrocardiogram.
Diagnostic terminology for original criteria: this diagnosis is fulfilled by the presence of 2 major, 1 major plus 2 minor, or 4 minor criteria from different groups.
Diagnostic terminology for revised criteria: definite diagnosis: 2 major, 1 major and 2 minor, or 4 minor criteria from different categories; borderline: 1 major and 1 minor or 3 minor criteria from different categories; possible: 1 major or 2 minor criteria from different categories.
From Marcus FI, McKenna WJ, Sherrill D, et al. Diagnosis of arrhythmogenic right ventricular cardiomyopathy/dysplasia: proposed modification of the task force criteria. *Circulation.* 2010;121:1533-1541.

pure restrictive cardiomyopathy. Amyloidosis, hemochromatosis, and sarcoidosis are among the systemic diseases that cause restrictive cardiomyopathy (see later).

CLINICAL MANIFESTATIONS

Most patients present with symptoms and signs of heart failure and arrhythmia. Common symptoms include dyspnea on exertion, recurrent respiratory tract infections, general fatigue, and weakness. Symptoms may progress rapidly to dyspnea at rest, orthopnea, paroxysmal nocturnal dyspnea, and abdominal discomfort due to hepatic engorgement. Many patients complain of chest pain and palpitation. Syncope is a presenting symptom in 10% of children. Rarely, sudden death is the initial manifestation of the disease.

Physical examination typically reveals an elevated jugular venous pressure, which has a prominent *y* descent and fails to fall (or rises) during inspiration (Kussmaul sign). On cardiac auscultation, the pulmonary component of the second heart sound may be loud if pulmonary vascular resistance is high. A third heart sound and occasionally a fourth heart sound commonly produce a gallop rhythm. Peripheral edema, ascites, and hepatomegaly are common.

DIAGNOSIS

The most frequent ECG abnormalities include P mitrale and P pulmonale, nonspecific ST segment and T wave abnormalities, ST segment depression, and T wave inversion, usually in the inferolateral leads. Voltage criteria for left and right ventricular hypertrophy may be present, although patients with

TABLE 60-7 ARRHYTHMOGENIC RIGHT VENTRICULAR CARDIOMYOPATHY: CRITERIA FOR DIAGNOSIS OF FIRST-DEGREE RELATIVES WHO DO NOT FULFILL CRITERIA AS PROBANDS*

ARVC in a first-degree relative plus one of the following:	
ECG	T wave inversion in right precordial leads (V_2 and V_3)
Signal-averaged ECG	Late potentials seen on signal-averaged ECG
Arrhythmia	Left bundle branch block–type ventricular tachycardia on ECG, on Holter monitoring, or during exercise testing; >200 extrasystoles during a 24-hour period
Structural or functional abnormality of the right ventricle	Mild global right ventricular dilation or reduction in ejection fraction with normal left ventricle; mild segmental dilation of the right ventricle; regional right ventricular hypokinesia

*Any one criterion is adequate for the diagnosis.
ARVC = arrhythmogenic right ventricular cardiomyopathy; ECG = electrocardiogram.
From Hamid MS, Norman M, Quraishi A, et al: Prospective evaluation of relatives for familial arrhythmogenic right ventricular cardiomyopathy reveals a need to broaden diagnostic criteria. *J Am Coll Cardiol.* 2002;40:1445-1450.

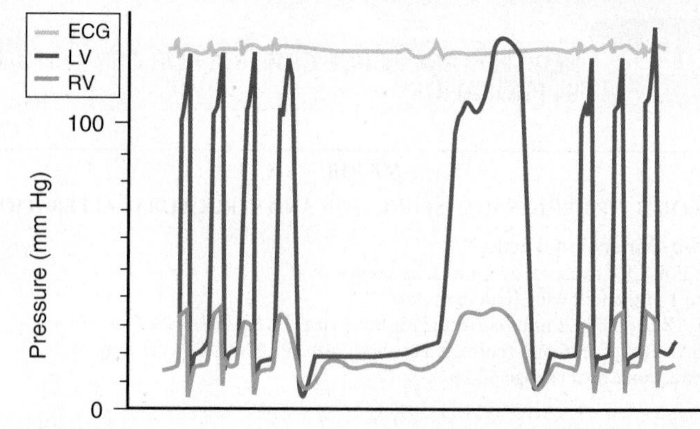

FIGURE 60-6. Idiopathic restrictive cardiomyopathy. Right ventricular (RV) and left ventricular (LV) pressure electrocardiographic (ECG) tracings in a patient with idiopathic restrictive cardiomyopathy. A dip-and-plateau pattern is seen in both ventricles, and diastolic filling pressures are elevated. The plateaus occur at different pressures, approximately 16 mm Hg for the RV tracing compared with 20 mm Hg for the LV tracing. The diagnosis of restrictive disease was confirmed by thoracotomy. (Redrawn from Benofti JR, Grossman W, Cohn PF. The clinical profile of restrictive cardiomyopathy. *Circulation.* 1980;61:1206.)

TABLE 60-8 CAUSES OF RESTRICTIVE CARDIOMYOPATHIES

INFILTRATIVE DISORDERS
Amyloidosis
Sarcoidosis
STORAGE DISORDERS
Hemochromatosis
Fabry disease
Glycogen storage diseases
FIBROTIC DISORDERS
Radiation
Scleroderma
Drugs (e.g., doxorubicin, serotonin, ergotamine)
METABOLIC DISORDERS
Carnitine deficiency
Defects in fatty acid metabolism
ENDOMYOCARDIAL DISORDERS
Endomyocardial fibrosis
Hypereosinophilic syndrome (Löffler endocarditis)
MISCELLANEOUS CAUSES
Carcinoid syndrome

amyloidosis have low-voltage QRS complexes. Conduction abnormalities include intraventricular conduction delay and abnormal Q waves.

On cardiac imaging, both atria are markedly dilated and can dwarf the size of the ventricles in patients with normal global systolic function and a nonhypertrophied, nondilated left ventricle. Pulsed-wave Doppler velocities typically show increased early diastolic filling velocity, decreased atrial filling velocity, increased ratio of early diastolic filling to atrial filling, decreased E wave deceleration time, and decreased isovolumic relaxation time. Pulmonary vein and hepatic vein pulsed-wave Doppler velocities demonstrate higher diastolic than systolic velocities, increased atrial reversal velocities, and atrial reversal duration greater than mitral atrial filling duration. Tissue Doppler imaging usually shows reduced diastolic annular velocities and an increased ratio of early diastolic tissue Doppler annular velocity to mitral early diastolic filling velocity, reflecting elevated left ventricular end-diastolic pressures.

The characteristic hemodynamic feature on cardiac catheterization is a deep and rapid early decline in ventricular pressure at the onset of diastole, with a rapid rise to a plateau in early diastole ("dip-and-plateau" or "square root sign") (Fig. 60-6). Left ventricular end-diastolic, left atrial, and pulmonary capillary wedge pressures are markedly elevated, usually 5 mm Hg or more above right atrial and right ventricular end-diastolic pressures. Volume loading and exercise accentuate the difference between left-sided and right-sided pressures.

The diagnostic evaluation aims to exclude potentially reversible conditions. In such cases, the cardiac manifestations may provide the clues, but definitive diagnosis relies on the demonstration of disease-specific features, such as amyloid protein in amyloidosis (Chapter 188), noncaseating granulomas in sarcoidosis (Chapter 95), abnormal iron studies in hemochromatosis (Chapter 212), or reduced α-galactosidase A levels in Fabry disease (Chapter 208). Endomyocardial biopsy is rarely required to make these diagnoses.

TREATMENT Rx

Diuretics are the main therapy for heart failure symptoms (Chapter 59), but they must be carefully administered so as not to reduce left ventricular filling pressures to the point of hypotension. Angiotensin-converting enzyme inhibitors and β-blockers are commonly recommended despite few data on their benefit. In patients with secondary restrictive cardiomyopathies, specific treatment of the underlying systemic disease is often appropriate (see later). Referral for transplant assessment should be considered early because pulmonary hypertension may develop and necessitate heart and lung transplantation.

PROGNOSIS

In adults with restrictive cardiomyopathy, the clinical course is usually slow and protracted. Survival from the time of diagnosis is often 10 years or more, except for AL amyloidosis, which progresses much more rapidly. Symptoms of heart failure are generally progressive and respond poorly to treatments for heart failure.

Specific Clinical Syndromes

SARCOIDOSIS

The frequency of myocardial involvement in patients with sarcoidosis (Chapter 95) is difficult to determine because it is frequently subclinical and patchy in nature. Postmortem studies suggest that the heart is involved in at least 25% of patients, but clinical cardiac involvement occurs in less than 10% of patients. Clinical manifestations of sarcoid include heart failure, conduction abnormalities, atrial and ventricular arrhythmias, pericardial effusion, valvular dysfunction, and, rarely, sudden cardiac death.[11] Right-sided heart failure secondary to pulmonary hypertension may occur in patients with extensive fibrotic lung disease. Myocardial infiltration by sarcoid granulomas results in restrictive or dilated cardiomyopathy. The most common site is in the lateral wall of the left ventricle. Papillary muscle involvement is responsible for the most common valvulopathy, mitral regurgitation. Granuloma formation in the basal interventricular septum may cause conduction abnormalities. Ventricular arrhythmias are also frequent. Biopsy of extracardiac sites is usually adequate for the diagnosis, but imaging with a gallium scan, T2 magnetic resonance imaging, or positron emission tomography/computed tomography often demonstrates cardiac inflammation. A myocardial biopsy may show granulomas but, because of the focal distribution of the lesions, may be nondiagnostic. Corticosteroid therapy may improve arrhythmias, but heart failure may worsen despite such therapy. An ICD is generally indicated for ventricular arrhythmias.

AMYLOIDOSIS

EPIDEMIOLOGY AND PATHOBIOLOGY

Amyloidosis can result in deposition of amyloid protein in the atria, ventricles, coronary vessels, conduction system, and valves. The degree of cardiac involvement varies among subtypes.[12] Hematologic disorders (Chapter 187) associated with excessive light chain (AL) immunoglobulin production are the most common cause of cardiac amyloid. Familial forms caused by the accumulation of mutant proteins (transthyretin or apolipoprotein A) (Chapter 188) have variable cardiac involvement. Secondary amyloidosis, due to deposition of serum amyloid A protein in chronic inflammatory diseases, rarely affects the heart. In senile systemic amyloidosis, cardiomyopathy is caused by deposition of normal wild-type transthyretin; this disease nearly always affects elderly persons (>70 years), with a clinical course that is considerably slower than with other types of amyloid.

DIAGNOSIS

The ECG tracing in most forms of cardiac amyloid characteristically shows decreased voltage despite increased wall thickness on echocardiography. Characteristic two-dimensional echocardiographic findings in advanced cardiac amyloidosis are biventricular hypertrophy, thickened valves and interatrial septum, dilated atria, and a small pericardial effusion. The myocardium has a hyperreflective granular texture (Fig. 60-7), best seen on digital image analysis. Echo Doppler in advanced disease demonstrates a restrictive left ventricular filling pattern. Cardiac magnetic resonance imaging may show subendocardial late gadolinium enhancement with abnormal gadolinium kinetics (Fig. 60-8). Nuclear scans with ^{123}I-labeled serum amyloid P component are highly specific. In hereditary transthyretin-related amyloidosis, abnormalities usually can be detected on ^{99m}Tc-DPD scintigraphy before the appearance of echocardiographic changes.

A definitive diagnosis of amyloidosis requires a tissue biopsy specimen, which can be obtained from other sites. For example, fine-needle aspiration of abdominal fat is positive for amyloid deposits in more than 70% of patients with AL amyloidosis. If the result is negative, endomyocardial biopsy has a very high sensitivity.

TREATMENT AND PROGNOSIS Rx

Specific therapies to impede precursor protein production and fibril formation should be implemented whenever possible (Chapter 188). Diuretics, often in high doses (e.g., furosemide, 40 to 80 mg daily), are the mainstay of the palliative heart failure regimen. Angiotensin-converting enzyme or angiotensin II inhibitors should be used cautiously because they are often poorly tolerated and of unproven efficacy in cardiac amyloid. Aldosterone inhibitors might be helpful in advanced cases. Patients may be hypersensitive to digoxin because of enhanced drug binding with amyloid fibrils. Patients with atrial fibrillation in AL amyloidosis should receive anticoagulation with warfarin (Chapter 38) because of a high rate of thromboembolism. Cardiac transplantation remains controversial, but heart transplantation (Chapter 82) with high-dose chemotherapy and with stem cell transplantation (Chapter 178) has been used in patients with AL amyloidosis.

Patients with amyloidosis with heart failure have a median survival time of less than 1 year and a 5-year survival rate of less than 5%. Most deaths occur suddenly. Patients with familial amyloidosis have a slower course than that of patients with a monoclonal gammopathy.

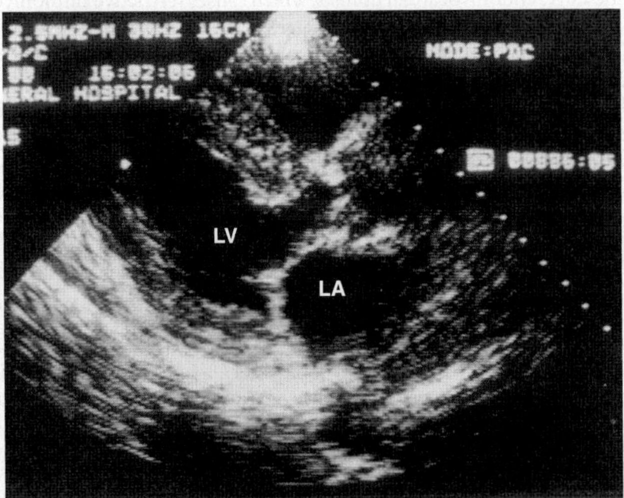

FIGURE 60-7. **Amyloidosis.** An apical four-chamber echocardiographic image demonstrates biventricular hypertrophy in a patient with biopsy-proven amyloidosis. LA = left atrium; LV = left ventricle. (From Levine RA. Echocardiographic assessment of the cardiomyopathies. In: Weyman AE, ed. Principles and Practice of Echocardiography. 2nd ed. Philadelphia: Lea & Febiger; 1994:810.)

HEREDITARY HEMOCHROMATOSIS

Hereditary hemochromatosis (Chapter 212) is an autosomal recessive disorder caused by excessive iron deposition in various organs, including the liver, spleen, pancreas, endocrine glands, and heart. In whites, its prevalence is between 1 in 200 and 1 in 500, with an even higher prevalence in the Irish population. The most common form is caused by mutations in the *HFE* gene, with two missense mutations accounting for most cases (C282Y and H63D).

Most patients with classic disease present between the ages of 40 and 60 years with hyperpigmentation, diabetes mellitus, and hepatomegaly. Up to 35% of patients with hemochromatosis experience heart failure, and 36% develop arrhythmias. Restrictive physiologic features dominate early in the disease, followed by ventricular dilation. The diagnosis is generally made from the clinical picture, an elevated serum iron level, and a high transferrin saturation. Genetic testing is helpful, and the diagnosis can be confirmed by endomyocardial biopsy. Phlebotomy and iron chelation therapy with deferoxamine (Chapter 212) may improve cardiac function before cell injury becomes irreversible. Standard heart failure treatment (Chapter 59) is generally recommended. Death from hemochromatosis results more often from cirrhosis and liver carcinoma than from cardiac disease.

Unclassified Cardiomyopathies

LEFT VENTRICULAR NONCOMPACTION

Failure of the trabecular or spongiform layer of the myocardium to compact may occur with congenital heart disease, including atrial and ventricular septal defects and coarctation of the aorta (Chapter 69), and with the rare X-linked multisystem disorder Barth syndrome.[13] With recent improvements in imaging technology, it has also been recognized in patients with hypertrophic and dilated cardiomyopathy. The prevalence of localized areas of noncompaction is unknown, but clinically significant isolated left ventricular noncompaction in the absence of other cardiac abnormalities is uncommon.

Areas of noncompacted myocardium may be best delineated from normal myocardium by the demonstration of flow within the myocardium by Doppler or contrast echocardiography or cardiac magnetic resonance imaging (Fig. 60-9). When extensive areas are involved, systolic performance may be impaired, and there is a risk of ventricular arrhythmias and systemic emboli. Treatment, when necessary, is for associated heart failure (Chapter 59), arrhythmias (Chapters 64 and 65), and the risk of emboli (Chapter 59). Natural history and prognosis are not well established.

TAKOTSUBO CARDIOMYOPATHY

Takotsubo cardiomyopathy is a syndrome of transient apical left ventricular dysfunction that mimics myocardial infarction (Chapter 73).[14] Postulated mechanisms include coronary artery spasm, myocarditis, a hyperadrenergic syndrome, and dynamic mid-cavity obstruction.

The clinical syndrome classically includes chest pain, ST segment elevation, and raised cardiac biomarkers in association with emotional or physical stress. Coronary arteriography reveals normal epicardial vessels. Conservative treatment with rehydration and removal of the determinants of stress usually results in rapid resolution within hours of the symptoms, ECG changes, and wall motion abnormalities. Of the approximately 12,000 patients who develop takotsubo cardiomyopathy each year in the United States, in-hospital mortality is 4.2%, mostly in people who have another underlying critical illness.

DISEASES OF THE ENDOCARDIUM

Endocardial fibrosis, fibroelastosis, and thrombosis are subclassified into endomyocardial diseases with hypereosinophilia (hypereosinophilic syndromes) and endomyocardial disease without hypereosinophilia (e.g., endomyocardial fibrosis) (see Table 60-8).

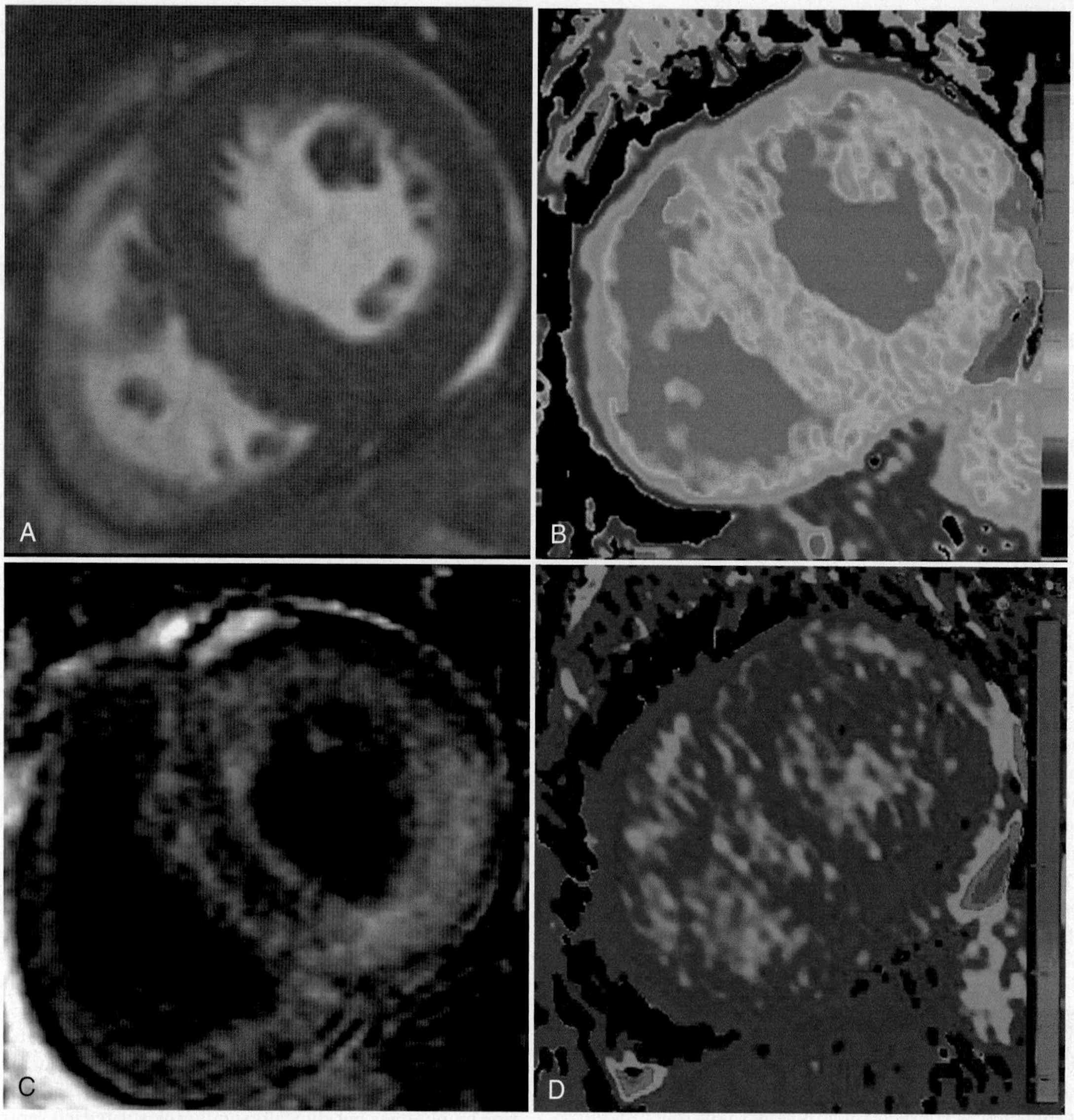

FIGURE 60-8. **A 66-year-old woman with AL amyloidosis and cardiac involvement.** Note the concentric hypertrophy in the short axis (A) and the presence of red signal in the myocardium suggestive of high "native" T1 (B). There is a transmural and circumferential late gadolinium pattern (C) that is typical of cardiac amyloidosis. On the postcontrast image (D), the dark blue areas inside the myocardium are characterized by presence of gadolinium and lower T1 than in the other parts of the myocardium and the blood (green). These findings suggest high extracellular volume (amyloid fibrils substitution) inside the myocardium.

Hypereosinophilic Syndrome

Hypereosinophilic syndromes are a rare and heterogeneous group of disorders defined as persistent blood eosinophilia ($>1.5 \times 10^9$/L) for more than 6 consecutive months, associated with evidence of eosinophil-induced organ damage in the absence of causes of hypereosinophilia, such as allergic, parasitic, and malignant disorders (Chapter 170). Pathogenic mechanisms include stem cell mutations that lead to expression of PDGFRA-containing fusion genes, mainly the *FIP1L1-PDGFRA* fusion gene, with constitutive tyrosine kinase activity and sustained overproduction of interleukin-5 by activated T-cell subsets. Clinically, hypereosinophilic syndrome can be classified into chronic eosinophilic leukemia, lymphocytic hypereosinophilic syndrome, myeloproliferative hypereosinophilic syndrome, and idiopathic hypereosinophilic syndrome. The term *organ-restricted eosinophilic disease*, such as eosinophilic gastroenteritis, dermatitis, or pneumonia, is used when a specific organ or tissue is the exclusive target of eosinophilic infiltration and damage. The term *Löffler fibroplastic endocarditis* with eosinophilia has been used to describe cardiac damage caused by direct toxicity of circulating eosinophils in patients with persistent hypereosinophilia, but its use is now discouraged.

CLINICAL MANIFESTATIONS AND DIAGNOSIS

Hypereosinophilic syndrome is a rare disorder that tends to occur in patients 20 to 50 years of age, but all age groups are affected. Cardiac involvement generally evolves in three phases: an early necrotic stage that involves the endomyocardium, which is usually asymptomatic but can be manifested as acute heart failure; a thrombotic stage, in which thrombi develop on the ventricular endocardium, sometimes causing peripheral emboli; and the final fibrotic stage, endomyocardial fibrosis, which causes restrictive cardiomyopathy and damage to atrioventricular valves. Chest pain, cough, dyspnea or orthopnea, and edema of the lower extremities are typical symptoms. Some patients may develop arrhythmias.

The characteristic two-dimensional echocardiographic findings include endocardial thickening, apical obliteration of one or both ventricles by an echogenic material, hyperdynamic contraction of the spared ventricular walls with bilateral atrial enlargement, and a restrictive pattern on echo Doppler.

TREATMENT

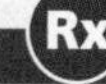

Patients with the F/P fusion gene chromosomal rearrangement should be treated with the tyrosine kinase inhibitor imatinib (100 mg daily for 1 week, increasing by 100 mg each week to 400 mg as guided by toxicity and hematologic response); the duration of therapy is still under investigation. Because some patients develop severe congestive heart failure within days after initiation of therapy, pretreatment with corticosteroids is recommended by some authorities. For patients without the F/P fusion gene, corticosteroids (median maximal daily dose of prednisone of 40 mg [range, 5 to 60 mg] for a duration of 2 months to 20 years; median maintenance dose of 10 mg daily [range, 1 to 40 mg/day]) are the most common first-line therapy. Steroid-sparing and second-line drugs include hydroxyurea (median maximal daily dose of 1000 mg [range, 500 to 2000 mg], adjusted to response), interferon alfa (median maximal dose of 14 million units per week [range, 3 to 40 million units per week], adjusted to response), and imatinib (as before).

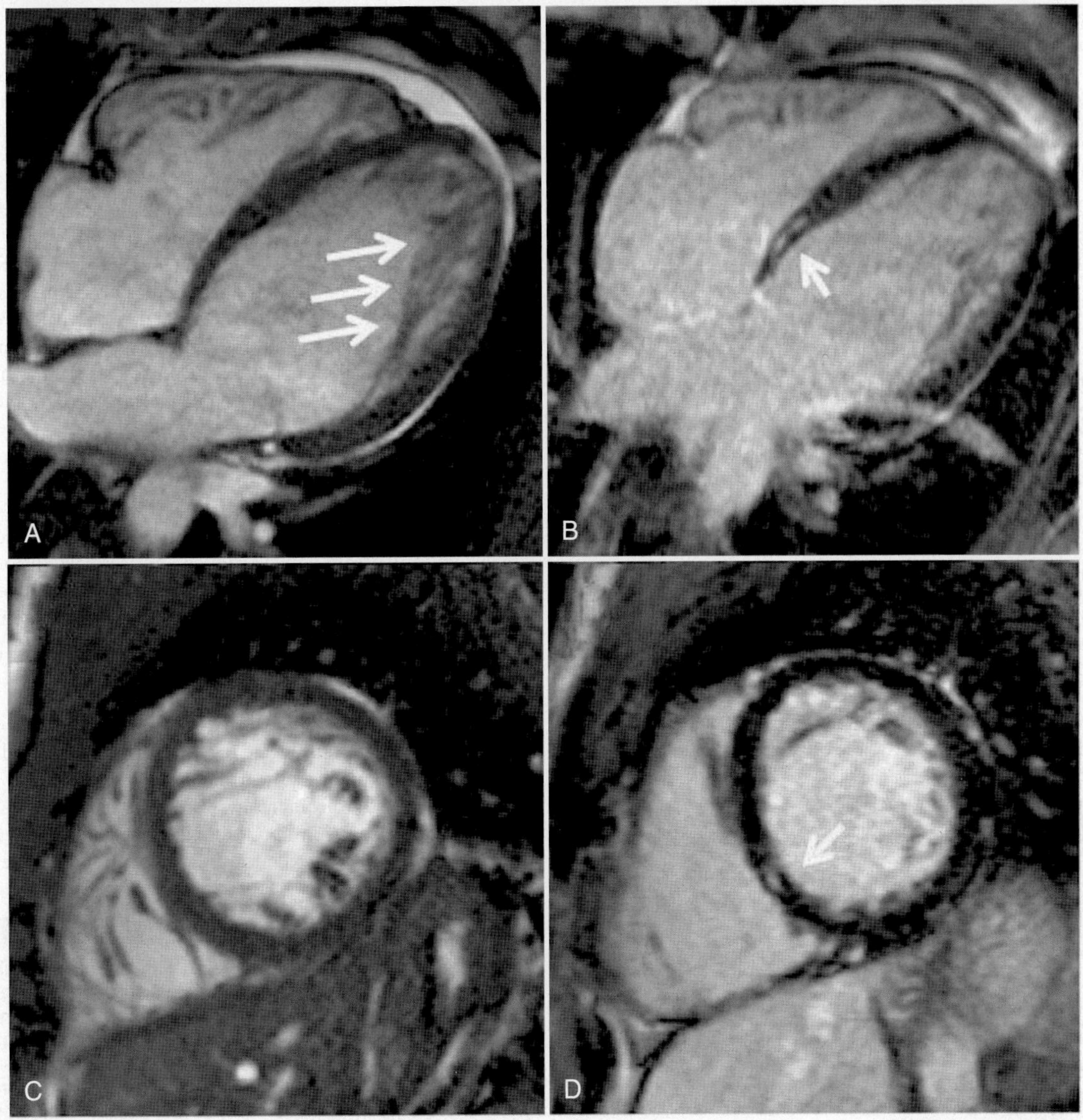

FIGURE 60-9. A 23-year-old white man with left ventricular noncompaction. Four-chamber end-diastolic (A) and short axis (C) views show left ventricular dilation, prominent trabeculae (*long arrows*), and poorly formed papillary muscles. The ejection fraction was 55%. There is limited mid-myocardial septal late gadolinium enhancement (B, D, *short arrows*).

Tropical Endomyocardial Fibrosis

Tropical endomyocardial fibrosis is probably the most common type of restrictive cardiomyopathy worldwide. The disease occurs predominantly within the tropics and affects mostly children and adolescents, usually from low socioeconomic backgrounds. Its cause is unknown, but potential contributors include infection, autoimmunity, genetic predisposition, ethnicity, diet, climate, and poverty.

Severe hypereosinophilia is found in some patients early in the initial stage of the illness; it is characterized by febrile illness, pancarditis, facial and periorbital swelling, pruritus, urticaria, and neurologic symptoms. This phase is followed by ventricular thrombosis that affects the apices and the subvalvular apparatus and then evolves to endocardial fibrosis. The final stage is characterized by restrictive physiology, atrioventricular valve regurgitation, and marked atrial dilation. Death results from complications of chronic heart failure but can occur suddenly from thromboembolism or arrhythmia.

Atrial fibrillation is common at presentation. In advanced disease, the electrocardiogram shows low-voltage QRS complexes, nonspecific ST-T wave changes, and conduction abnormalities. Echocardiography demonstrates apical obliteration, reduction of ventricular cavity size, and tethering or retraction of mitral or tricuspid leaflets or both. There is no specific laboratory test, and hypereosinophilia is present only early in the disease.

There is no specific treatment for endomyocardial fibrosis. Medical treatment is used to control the heart failure (Chapter 59) and arrhythmias (Chapters 64 and 65). Surgical endocardial resection, combined with valve repair or replacement, has an early postoperative mortality between 15 and 30%. The overall prognosis is poor, with a 44% mortality rate at 1 year, increasing to nearly 90% at 3 years.

Carcinoid Syndrome

EPIDEMIOLOGY AND PATHOBIOLOGY

Carcinoid tumors are rare (1 in 100,000) neuroendocrine malignant neoplasms originating mostly from enterochromaffin cells in the gastrointestinal tract (Chapter 232). Carcinoid syndrome, with flushing, diarrhea, and bronchospasm, occurs after tumor cells metastasize to the liver and the vasoactive substances produced by the tumors enter the systemic circulation through the hepatic vein. Carcinoid heart disease occurs in up to 70% of cases of carcinoid syndrome.

The typical cardiac lesion is the carcinoid plaque, which is composed of smooth muscle cells, myofibroblasts, and elastic tissue that forms a fibrous layer on the endocardial surface of the right ventricle and atrium, the valve leaflets, and the subvalvular apparatus, including the chordae and papillary muscles. The tricuspid valve plaques tend to develop on the ventricular side of the leaflets, where they adhere to the mural endocardium and cause valvular regurgitation. On the pulmonary valve, the predominant lesion is stenosis. In patients with a patent foramen ovale, left-sided valvular involvement can occur. Occasional patients may have concomitant myocardial metastases and pericardial effusions from direct tumor invasion.

The most common presentation is dyspnea with signs and symptoms of right-sided heart failure. The electrocardiogram and radiograph are nonspecific. Echocardiography shows thickening of the tricuspid valve, the subvalvular apparatus, and the pulmonary valve. In severe disease, the tricuspid leaflets are retracted and fixed, with loss of normal coaptation. Similar findings can be seen on cardiac magnetic resonance imaging.

TREATMENT AND PROGNOSIS

Treatment of the underlying carcinoid with a somatostatin analogue can improve systemic symptoms (Chapter 232). Valve replacement now has an operative mortality of less than 10% (Chapter 232). Without treatment, patients with carcinoid heart disease have a mean life expectancy of 1.6 years. In one series, cardiac surgery for valve disease was associated with about a 50% risk reduction.

Nonbacterial Thrombotic (Marantic) Endocarditis

EPIDEMIOLOGY AND PATHOBIOLOGY

Platelet-fiber masses that are adherent to the mitral or aortic valves are seen in about 20% of patients with malignant tumors, especially mucin-producing adenocarcinomas, melanomas, leukemias, and lymphomas. The lesions are sterile, commonly verruciform, and without accompanying inflammation.

CLINICAL MANIFESTATIONS AND DIAGNOSIS

Nonbacterial thrombotic endocarditis is virtually always asymptomatic but occasionally is a source of systemic emboli. Because of the small size of many of the emboli, the first presentation is often with cerebral symptoms. Larger lesions are detectable by echocardiography, but even transesophageal echocardiography is not sufficiently sensitive to identify lesions that may be found at autopsy and that may have been the source of systemic emboli.

TREATMENT

No treatment has been proved efficacious. However, systemic anticoagulation similar to that used in patients with tumor-associated deep venous thrombosis is often tried (Chapters 81 and 179).

CARDIAC TUMORS

Myocardial Tumors

Most primary cardiac tumors (Table 60-9) are benign. However, all tumors that extend from other tissues into the heart are malignant, as are metastatic lesions.

TABLE 60-9 CARDIAC TUMORS

PRIMARY
Benign
Myxoma
Lipoma
Fibroma
Rhabdomyoma
Fibroelastoma
Malignant
Sarcoma
Mesothelioma
Lymphoma
SECONDARY
Direct Extension
Lung cancer
Breast cancer
Mediastinal tumors
Metastatic Tumors
Malignant melanoma
Leukemia
Lymphoma
Venous Extension
Renal cell cancer
Adrenal cancer
Liver cancer

EPIDEMIOLOGY AND PATHOBIOLOGY

Primary tumors of the heart are unusual, with a prevalence of 1 in 2000 to 1 in 4000 in autopsy series. Nearly all these primary tumors are benign myxomas, although fibromas, lipomas, and fibroelastomas also occur. Rhabdomyomas are seen in children, especially with tuberous sclerosis (Chapter 417). The rare primary malignant tumors include sarcomas, especially angiosarcomas (see Table 60-9). Rarely, a primary mesothelioma or lymphoma may originate in the heart.

Up to 20% of advanced cancers may involve the pericardium, epicardium, or cardiac chambers either by direct extension of the primary tumor or by metastatic disease. Direct extension occurs principally from cancers of the lung, breast, esophagus, and mediastinum. Extension through the inferior vena cava to the right atrium and even to the right ventricle occurs with cancers of the kidney, adrenal gland, and liver. Metastatic spread is most common with melanomas or lymphomas.

Pericardial Tumors

CLINICAL MANIFESTATIONS

Pericardial tumors almost always result from direct extension of tumors, principally lung and breast, which produce a pericardial effusion that can progress to cardiac tamponade (Chapter 77). Patients typically are asymptomatic or minimally symptomatic in terms of the cardiac involvement until the effusion is large, although they often may be very ill because of progressive tumor elsewhere.

DIAGNOSIS

The diagnosis is often suspected in a patient with advanced malignant disease on the basis of evidence of heart failure, hypertension, or arrhythmia and is confirmed by echocardiography. The differentiation between pericardial involvement by tumor and postradiation pericarditis depends on pericardiocentesis, often guided by echocardiography, and cytologic examination.

TREATMENT

Cardiac tamponade must be treated with urgent pericardiocentesis, preferably under echocardiographic or radiologic guidance (Chapter 77). Although such a procedure can be life-saving and provide short-term to intermediate-term palliation, control of the effusion often requires prolonged drainage, administration of intrapericardial chemotherapeutic agents, or limited or full pericardiectomy (Chapter 77). Some patients with pericardial tumors may respond to aggressive systemic chemotherapy, but recurrent accumulation of fluid is sufficiently likely that creation of a pericardial window should be considered before hospital discharge.

PROGNOSIS

In many cases, a tumor that is causing pericarditis has extended or will eventually extend through the pericardial space and into the myocardium, so no therapy is likely to be successful. The prognosis is very poor, except in unusual cases in which the tumor responds dramatically to systemic therapy.

Intracavitary Tumors

MYXOMA

DEFINITION AND EPIDEMIOLOGY

A myxoma is a benign polypoid neoplasm that originates from endocardial cells and is attached to the interatrial septum, usually protruding into the left atrium but occasionally into the right atrium and rarely into the ventricles. Myxomas are more common in women, especially between the ages of 30 and 60 years, than in men. These tumors can be familial and are rarely associated with other systemic abnormalities.

CLINICAL MANIFESTATIONS

Myxomas are slow growing and usually do not produce symptoms or signs until they enlarge. The typical presentation is with a tumor embolus, whereby usually small portions of the myxoma break loose and cause a single embolism or a shower of emboli.[15] However, a large embolism from a myxoma can be of sufficient size to obstruct a medium-sized artery. Some patients have systemic symptoms, including fever, malaise, and arthralgias, as part of a clinical syndrome that may be confused with bacterial endocarditis (Chapter 76) or a collagen vascular disease. Large myxomas can prolapse into the mitral valve orifice during diastole, or they may obstruct blood flow from the left atrium to the left ventricle and mimic rheumatic mitral stenosis.

DIAGNOSIS

A myxoma large enough to obstruct the mitral orifice can produce an audible "tumor plop" when the myxoma prolapses and obstructs blood flow during diastole, at the same time that the opening snap of mitral stenosis would typically be heard. If obstruction is incomplete, the tumor plop may be followed by a diastolic rumble. As obstruction becomes more severe, cardiac output may fall precipitously. Echocardiography (Chapter 55) is usually definitive; transesophageal echocardiography provides a higher sensitivity than does transthoracic echocardiography, and magnetic resonance imaging can be helpful.

TREATMENT Rx

Surgical removal is generally curative, although myxomas can be multiple or recur in about 5% of cases. Follow-up postoperative echocardiography is generally recommended. However, the optimal frequency and duration for follow-up screening are uncertain.

OTHER PRIMARY INTRACAVITARY TUMORS

Papillary fibroelastomas are rare, typically frondlike tumors that may arise from a cardiac valve, often the mitral valve, and are generally detected incidentally by echocardiography. However, like myxomas, they can be manifested with systemic or even coronary emboli. Surgical excision is usually successful.

Angiosarcomas, which are more frequent in men than in women, typically involve the pericardium and right atrium. They cause obstruction with clinical signs and symptoms of right-sided heart failure. These sarcomas are generally not amenable to therapy.

EXTENSION OF TUMOR INTO THE CARDIAC CAVITIES

Direct extension of tumor up the inferior vena cava into the right atrium can be seen with renal cell carcinomas and less commonly with liver and adrenal cancers. In some cases, tumor extension is accompanied by adherent clot, and either the tumor or the clot may cause obstruction or pulmonary emboli (Chapter 98). No treatments are generally successful, and the prognosis is grim.

Intramyocardial Tumors

Benign tumors in the myocardium include lipomas, fibromas, and rhabdomyomas. Primary malignant tumors include sarcomas, lymphomas, and mesotheliomas. Metastatic tumors include melanomas, lymphomas, and leukemias. The tumors may be clinically silent, or they may produce arrhythmias or even impinge on coronary arteries, thereby causing ischemic syndromes. Large tumors may protrude into the cardiac chamber and cause obstruction. Therapies are not successful, except for occasional patients whose metastatic tumors may respond to systemic chemotherapy or whose primary tumors have been cured by heart transplantation.

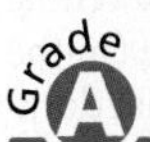

Grade A References

A1. Mason JW, O'Connell JB, Herskowitz A, et al. A clinical trial of immunosuppressive therapy for myocarditis: the Myocarditis Treatment Trial Investigators. *N Engl J Med.* 1995;333:269-275.

A2. Wojnicz R, Nowalany-Kozielska E, Wojciechowska C, et al. Randomized, placebo-controlled study for immunosuppressive treatment of inflammatory dilated cardiomyopathy: two-year follow-up results. *Circulation.* 2001;104:39-45.

A3. Cooper LT Jr, Hare JM, Tazelaar HD, et al. Usefulness of immunosuppression for giant cell myocarditis. *Am J Cardiol.* 2008;102:1535-1539.

A4. Kadish A, Dyer A, Daubert JP, et al. Prophylactic defibrillator implantation in patients with nonischemic dilated cardiomyopathy. *N Engl J Med.* 2004;350:2151-2158.

A5. Bosch X, Rovira M, Sitges M, et al. Enalapril and carvedilol for preventing chemotherapy-induced left ventricular systolic dysfunction in patients with malignant hemopathies: the OVERCOME trial (preventiOn of left Ventricular dysfunction with Enalapril and caRvedilol in patients submitted to intensive ChemOtherapy for the treatment of Malignant hEmopathies). *J Am Coll Cardiol.* 2013;61:2355-2362.

A6. Sliwa K, Blauwet L, Tibazarwa K, et al. Evaluation of bromocriptine in the treatment of acute severe peripartum cardiomyopathy: a proof-of-concept pilot study. *Circulation.* 2010;121:1465-1473.

GENERAL REFERENCES

For the General References and other additional features, please visit Expert Consult at https://expertconsult.inkling.com.

61

PRINCIPLES OF ELECTROPHYSIOLOGY

GLENN I. FISHMAN

The rhythmic beating of the heart reflects the tightly regulated and exquisitely integrated activity of numerous protein complexes that control the flow of ions across cell membranes, including channels, transporters, exchangers, and gap junction channels.[1] The human heart beats almost 3 billion times during a normal lifespan, and even brief periods of dysfunction may lead to life-threatening consequences. Thus, the failure rate of cardiac rhythmicity is exceptionally low. Nonetheless, inherited syndromes, as well as acquired heart disease, may affect cardiac rhythmicity, and these disorders lead to substantial morbidity and mortality, including sudden cardiac death (Chapter 63). This chapter reviews the molecular, cellular, and organ-level determinants of cardiac rhythmicity and relates these principles to fundamental mechanisms responsible for clinically important arrhythmias.

BASIC CONCEPTS

The function of the heart as a highly dynamic pump is intricately entwined with the tightly regulated electrical activation of its constituent cardiomyocytes. During each cardiac cycle, an electrical impulse known as an *action potential* is spontaneously generated by a relatively small number of pacemaker cells in the sinoatrial node and then propagated to neighboring cardiac myocytes through arrays of intercellular channels known as gap junctions. Subpopulations of myocytes within the heart have unique electrical properties that reflect regional specialization. Myocytes within the sinoatrial and atrioventricular nodes produce spontaneous action potentials that reflect their pace-making function. Cells within the His-Purkinje network are optimized to rapidly deliver excitatory current to the large mass of ventricular myocardium, whereas ventricular myocytes display action potentials optimized to facilitate excitation-contraction coupling, that is, to trigger the release of calcium ions from the sarcoplasmic reticulum and to promote the actomyosin cross-bridge formation that underlies cardiac contraction (Chapter 53). Abnormalities in cardiac electrophysiology, whether the result of congenital syndromes or acquired heart disease, can lead to disturbances in the initiation, propagation, or conduction of electrical impulses and, as a result, to a wide variety of arrhythmic syndromes.

IONIC BASIS OF CARDIAC ELECTROPHYSIOLOGY

The Cardiac Action Potential

The cardiac action potential (Fig. 61-1) is a recording of a cell's membrane potential, V_m, versus time. During each cardiac cycle, ions move back and forth across the cardiomyocyte cell membrane, thereby changing V_m. The cardiac action potential, which reflects the integrated behavior of numerous individual ionic currents, is largely dominated by the movement of Na^+, Ca^{+2}, and K^+ ions. These ions traverse the cell membrane through ion-selective pores formed by assemblies of integral membrane-spanning proteins and accessory proteins. The behavior of these ionic pathways is highly regulated, and permeation of specific ions is influenced by multiple factors, the most prominent of which are changes in membrane potential (i.e., voltage gating), ligand binding, second messengers such as cyclic adenosine monophosphate, and post-translational modification. Channel function and, by extension, action potential behavior are dynamically tuned in response to normal physiologic factors, especially heart rate. However, a number of pathologic stressors influence channel activity, including acquired syndromes that are associated with cardiac hypertrophy and failure, as well as an ever-growing number of congenital diseases. Regardless of the underlying pathology, the effects on action potential behavior may trigger arrhythmic activity.

The cardiac action potential is divided into phases, each reflecting the major ionic movements that take place. In working cardiomyocytes, such as ventricular or atrial myocytes, the *resting membrane potential* during diastole, or phase 4 of the cardiac action potential, is determined by the baseline ionic and charge gradients that exist across the sarcolemmal membrane. These gradients are generated by pumps and transporters, the most important of which is the Na^+, K^+-ATPase. This energy-requiring electrogenic pump, which is the major target of ouabain-like compounds such as digoxin, extrudes three Na^+ ions from the intracellular compartment in exchange for two K^+ ions,

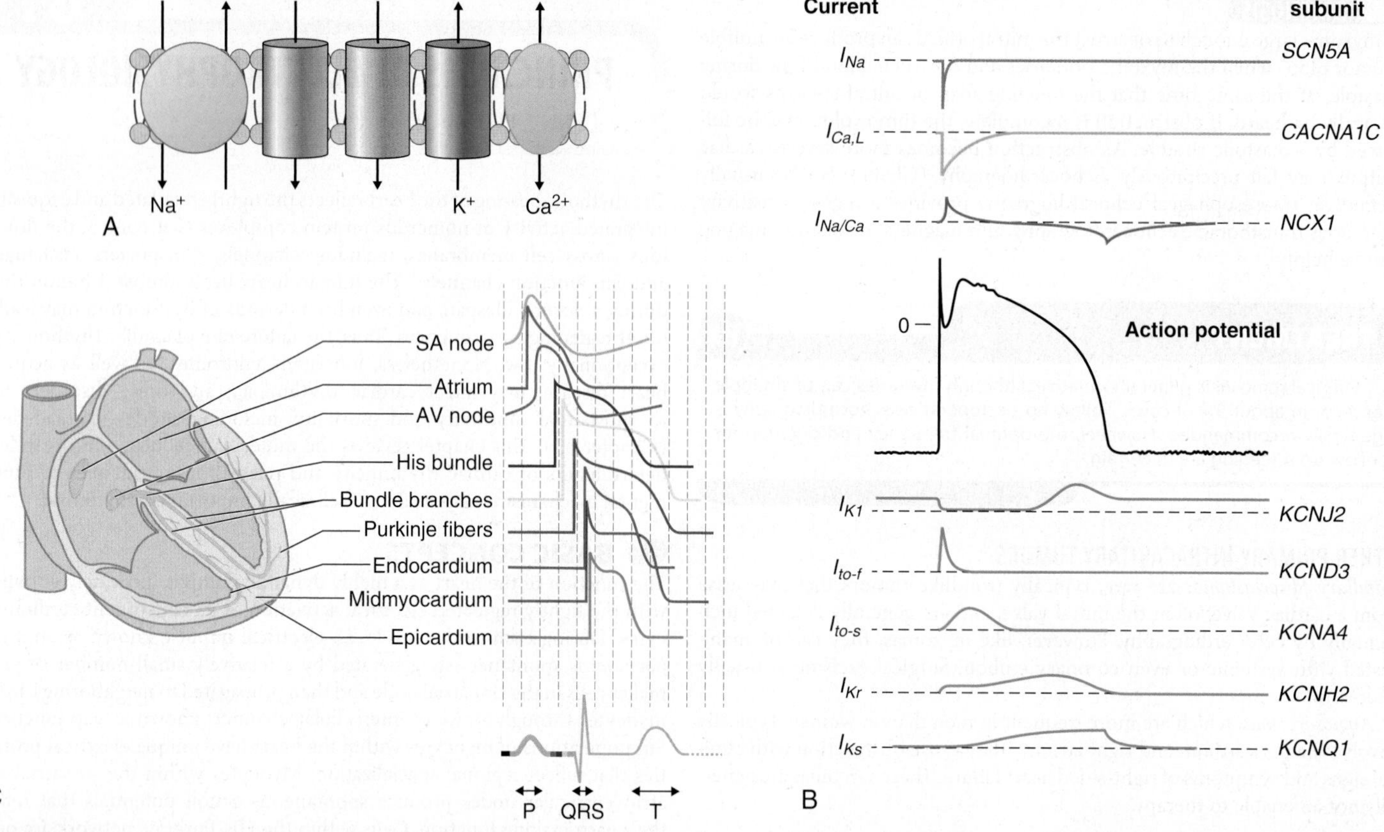

FIGURE 61-1. Ion channels and the cardiac action potential. A, Key channels involved in cardiac excitability and generation of the cardiac action potential. Inward currents are carried by Na^+ channels *(purple)* and Ca^{2+} channels *(red).* Repolarizing currents are primarily carried by K^+ channels *(blue).* The Na^+, K^+-ATPase is an energy-requiring exchanger that pumps K^+ out of the cell in exchange for Na^+ and is essential for establishing resting ionic gradients and the resting membrane potential. **B,** Time course and relative magnitude of ionic currents active during the cardiac action potential. Inward currents are represented by downward deflections and outward currents by upward deflections. **C,** Action potentials from different regions of the heart and their relationship to the surface electrocardiogram are indicated. AV = atrioventricular. (Adapted from Marbán E. Cardiac channelopathies. *Nature.* 2002;415:213-218.)

thereby resulting in directionally opposite gradients of Na^+ ions (outside > inside) and K^+ ions (inside > outside). Under resting conditions, a subset of membrane channels highly permeable to K^+ is open, but those that allow for the passage of other ions such as Na^+ or Ca^{2+} are only minimally permeable. As a consequence, the concentration gradient promotes the movement of potassium ions from inside to outside of the cell, until the resulting excess of negative charge within the cell balances the diffusional forces and an electrochemical equilibrium is established. The equilibrium potential for a given ion is calculated by the *Nernst equation,* where E_{eq} is the equilibrium potential, R is the universal gas constant, T is the absolute temperature, z is the valence of the ionic species, and F is Faraday constant:

$$E_{eq} = \frac{RT}{zF} ln\left(\frac{[X]_{out}}{[X]_{in}}\right)$$

If the cell membrane were *only* permeable to K^+ ions, at the measured concentrations of intracellular and extracellular K^+, the resting membrane potential would be approximately −100 mV. However, because of the slight but measurable permeability to other ionic species, which have Nerst potentials that are less negative than that for K^+, the actual resting membrane potential in a typical ventricular cardiac myocyte is closer to −85 mV.

When the cardiac cell is depolarized to its excitatory threshold, an action potential is triggered through a series of highly regulated time-dependent changes in ionic conductances (see Fig. 61-1B). The fast sodium current is activated and very rapidly depolarizes the membrane during phase 0 of the action potential. The sodium current is inactivated at the peak of depolarization, which is approximately +40 mV. The increase in V_m during phase 0 activates several additional voltage-gated currents. A transient outward potassium current, or I_{to}, partially *re*polarizes the cell, thereby producing a small notch in the action potential, denoted as phase 1. The increase in V_m during phase 0 also activates, albeit more slowly, the inward L-type calcium current, $I_{Ca\text{-}L}$. It is this trigger for Ca^{2+} that is responsible for Ca^{2+}-induced release from the sarcoplasmic reticulum and is integral to the process of excitation-contraction coupling (Chapter 53). The inward Ca^{2+} current is balanced by several outward repolarizing currents, including the rapid component of the delayed rectifier potassium current I_{Kr}, the slow component of the delayed rectifier potassium current I_{Ks}, and the electrogenic Na^+-Ca^{+2} exchanger, thereby resulting in a plateau in the action potential known as phase 2. When the outward potassium currents increase and the calcium current decreases at the end of phase 2, the action potential progresses to phase 3, which is the phase of rapid repolarization. The inward rectifier potassium current I_{K1} contributes significantly to this final phase of repolarization and brings the action potential back to its resting membrane potential, or phase 4, at which point the cell is primed for another action potential.

Action potential recordings from atrial cardiomyocytes and from cells of the His-Purkinje system are qualitatively similar to those described previously, but with some notable differences that primarily reflect the differential expression of repolarizing potassium currents that tend to abbreviate (in the case of atrial cells) or lengthen (for Purkinje cells) the action potential duration (see Fig. 61-1C).

The relatively small populations of cells in the sinoatrial node (SAN) and atrioventricular node (AVN) express unique complements of ionic currents that are responsible for spontaneous depolarization during phase 4 and the triggering of action potentials. Pacemaker cells express substantially less I_{K1} compared with ventricular myocytes, and as a consequence, their minimum V_m is −65 mV, and they do not repolarize to the same extent as working ventricular cardiomyocytes. In addition, pacemaker cells display what is known as the funny current, I_f, which is activated by *hyper*polarization and carried by sodium. Activation of I_f during phase 4 slowly depolarizes the cell membrane. In addition, a subsarcolemmal calcium clock contributes to diastolic depolarization through the spontaneous, rhythmic release of Ca^{2+} from the sarcoplasmic reticulum, a process that is linked to the voltage clock through the activity of the sodium-calcium exhange current, I_{NCX}. Inasmuch as there is minimal fast inward I_{Na} expressed in nodal cells, the action potential triggered by this spontaneous phase 4 depolarization is due to activation of calcium currents carried by $I_{Ca,L}$ and $I_{Ca,T}$. The magnitude of I_f and I_{Ca}, and hence the slope of phase 4 depolarization as well as the upstroke velocity of the action potential in pacemaker cells, is augmented by adrenergic stimulation, which produces a chronotropic response.

Owing to considerable regional heterogeneity in the density of individual ionic currents, even within distinct compartments of the heart such as the ventricular myocardium, not all ventricular action potentials are identical (see Fig. 61-1C). Much of this heterogeneity is due to differences in the magnitude of various repolarizing K^+ currents. For example, although electrotonic coupling through gap junction channels mitigates this intrinsic heterogeneity, action potentials recorded from epicardial, mid-myocardial, and endocardial cells show substantial differences in morphology, both at rest and especially in response to provocative stimuli such as changes in rate or pharmacologic agents. Moreover, action potential morphology is not static; it varies in response to changes in physiologic state. *Action potential duration adaption*, which reflects the normal shortening of the action potential observed during increased heart rate, provides a mechanism to preserve adequate time for ventricular filling during diastole. Action potential duration shortening in this setting is due to a net increase in repolarizing currents, primarily from increased I_{Ks} and reverse-mode I_{NaCa}. This adaptation is regulated, at least in part, by the kinetics of activation and inactivation of the channels that are responsible for these currents, as well as their modulation by various signaling cascades, such as those regulated by the autonomic nervous system. However, maladaptive regulation of ionic currents is a frequent manifestation of acquired forms of heart disease,[2] and this *pathologic electrical remodeling* may amplify intrinsic heterogeneities in cardiac electrophysiology and form a substrate that promotes arrhythmic behavior.

Impulse Propagation

In the intact heart, action potentials not only must be generated but also must propagate from cell to cell as a wave of excitation throughout the atrial and ventricular myocardium. For successful propagation, the upstream excited cell must provide sufficient charge to bring the membrane potential, V_m, of downstream cells up to their excitation threshold potential. Gap junctions, which comprise arrays of intercellular channels, provide the structural basis for this electrotonic flow of current from cell to cell. For propagation to be successful, the ratio of the charge generated to charge consumed during the excitation cycle, known as the *safety factor*, must be greater than 1.

Unlike nerves, the action potential duration of human cardiomyocytes is quite long, on the order of 200 msec. This longer action potential duration is required so that each myocyte has sufficient time for contraction and relaxation before the next heartbeat. Impulses that arrive too early in the cardiac cycle will not produce normal action potentials. If the impulse occurs during the upstroke or plateau phase (phases 0 to 2), the sodium channels will not have had sufficient time to recover from fast inactivation, and the cell displays *absolute refractoriness*. If the impulse occurs somewhat later, during phase 3 of the action potential, a supranormal stimulus is required to overcome the potassium currents that remain active during the terminal portion of the action potential, a phenomenon known as *relative refractoriness*. Moreover, because not all of the sodium channels will have recovered from inactivation, the rate of rise of voltage during phase 0 of the premature beat may be diminished.

MOLECULAR BASIS OF CARDIAC ELECTROPHYSIOLOGY

The individual currents that are responsible for cardiac excitability reflect the integrated behavior of various protein complexes that are assembled into ion-specific channels, transporters, and exchangers.[3] At the molecular level, ion channels comprise multi-subunit glycoproteins, including a pore-forming major, or α-subunit, and one or several accessory proteins (E-Figure 61-1). The latter influence a range of channel properties including trafficking of the major subunit to the sarcolemmal membrane as well as regulation of channel biophysical properties, that is, the opening and closing of the channel in response to various factors such as membrane voltage, ligands, mechanical stimuli, second messengers, or post-translational modification.

Sodium Channels

Voltage-gated sodium channels are responsible for the activation and propagation of the cardiac action potential. Not surprisingly, acquired and inherited syndromes that affect the function of voltage-gated sodium channels in the heart are responsible for a broad range of arrhythmic phenotypes. Cardiac sodium channels activate extremely rapidly, within 1 msec, and begin to inactivate almost completely within several milliseconds. The very small proportion of channels that remain active for several hundred milliseconds results in the persistent or late Na^+ current, I_{NaL}.

The most abundant cardiac sodium channel comprises a pore-forming α-subunit known as $Na_v1.5$ and several smaller accessory subunits, or β-subunits, designated $Na_v\beta1$ to 4. The α-subunit is an approximately 260-kD protein that consists of four homologous domains, each comprising six transmembrane segments. Substantial experimental work has identified the key regions of the protein that regulate channel properties, including voltage dependence, activation, and inactivation, as well as the binding sites for pharmacologic agents such as local anesthetics, antiarrhythmic drugs, and neurotoxins. The β-subunits are single-membrane-spanning proteins that associate with $Na_v1.5$ through their extracellular immunoglobulin-fold domains. They serve to increase the delivery of the α-subunit to the sarcolemmal membrane and to influence channel function. The β-subunits also enhance the subcellular localization of the channel and its interactions with various adaptors, signaling molecules, and cytoskeletal proteins. In addition to $Na_v1.5$, several "neuronal" α-subunits are expressed at low levels in the heart and likely contribute to regional heterogeneity in sodium channel function. Mutations in $Na_v1.5$, in specific β-subunits, and in several interacting regulatory and scaffolding proteins all may influence the behavior of the sodium current in the heart and thereby produce a range of arrhythmic syndromes, including long QT syndrome type 3 (LQT3) and Brugada syndrome (Chapter 65).[4]

The I_f current contributes to phase 4 depolarization in pacemaker cells and is a reflection of the activity of hyperpolarization-activated cyclic nucleotide gated, or *HCN* channels. The full channels are composed of dimers of *HCN* proteins, each of which has six transmembrane domains. *HCN4* and *HCN1* are the predominant isoforms found in the nodes, whereas *HCN2* is found throughout the conduction system. Binding of cyclic adenosine monophosphate, a key second messenger in the adrenergic signaling cascade, to the carboxy terminus of the channel shifts activation positively, thereby increasing the slope of phase 4 depolarization and linking autonomic tone to heart rate.

Calcium Channels

Voltage-gated calcium channels are important for generating the action potential in the sinoatrial and atrioventricular nodes and for excitation-contraction coupling in virtually all contractile cardiomyocytes. The dominant forms expressed in the heart are the L-type (large and long-lasting) and the T-type (tiny and transient) calcium channels, both of which include pore-forming α-subunits, similar in overall structure to that of voltage-gated sodium channels.

L-type Ca^{2+} channels comprise an α_1 subunit, a noncovalently bound β accessory subunit ($Ca_v\beta1$-4), and an alternatively spliced α_2-δ-subunit that is post-translationally processed through cleavage and disulfide bond formation. The dominant α_1-subunit in the heart is $Ca_v1.2$, whereas $Ca_v1.3$ is restricted primarily to nodal and atrial cells. Both α_1-subunits are alternatively spliced to produce variants that are uniquely regulated.

The related T-type calcium channels are also found in the heart but display distinct biophysical properties compared with L-type Ca^{2+} channels; they activate at more negative voltages (−70 mV) and inactivate more rapidly. The major isoform expressed in the heart is heart is $Ca_v3.1$ and, to a lesser extent, $Ca_v3.2$. These channels are normally restricted to the nodes, Purkinje cells, and atrial myocytes. In pace-making cells, the T-type currents contribute to phase 4 depolarization. Mutations in Ca^{2+} channel subunits are also responsible for a number of arrhythmic syndromes, including Timothy syndrome (LQT8) and a subset of individuals with Brugada syndrome.

Potassium Channels

Numerous classes of potassium channels are expressed in the heart, where they contribute to repolarization and maintenance of the resting membrane potential. The heterogeneous expression of potassium channels in different regions and cell types is largely responsible for the variable action potential morphologies that are observed. As with sodium and calcium channels, potassium channels are formed from the assembly of pore-forming subunits along with various accessory β-subunits. However, α-subunits of potassium channels include between two and six transmembrane domains, and the full channel is formed as a dimer or tetramer, depending on the specific subfamily. Dysregulation of expression and function of potassium channels is quite common in many acquired forms of heart disease. The resulting loss of repolarizing currents leads to action potential duration prolongation and acquired long QT syndrome. In addition, heritable mutations that diminish potassium currents are responsible for several forms of inherited long QT syndrome.

Voltage-gated potassium channels, or *Kv* channels, are activated by membrane depolarization. Numerous classes of *Kv* channels have been identified in the heart. The α-subunits are six transmembrane domain proteins. Unlike sodium and calcium channels, functional potassium channels are formed by the assembly of four such subunits and various β-subunits. The transient outward current is composed of two components, $I_{to,fast}$ and $I_{to,slow}$; both are rapidly activated and contribute to phase 1 of the cardiac action potential, but their recovery kinetics differ. $I_{to,fast}$ is particularly prominent in the epicardial layer of the ventricles, especially in the right ventricle. This differential expression is thought to contribute to the pathology of J wave syndromes, including Brugada syndrome.

The other major class of voltage-gated potassium channels in the heart is responsible for the delayed rectifier currents, broadly classified as I_K currents. These channels include the ultra-rapidly activating I_{Kur}, which is restricted to atrial myocytes, and the delayed rectifier currents, I_{Kr} and I_{Ks}, both of which contribute to phase 3 repolarization of the cardiac action potential. I_{Kr} activates and inactivates rapidly and shows strong inward rectification; that is, current moves more easily (but not exclusively) in the inward direction than in the outward direction, although it is the outward current that is physiologically relevant. I_{Ks} activates slowly and does not display inward rectification. Both currents also show marked regional heterogeneity. Numerous cardiac and noncardiac medications, as well as heritable syndromes that reduce the magnitude of these currents (particularly I_{Kr}), result in action potential duration prolongation and acquired or heritable long QT syndrome.

The second major class of potassium currents in the heart are the *Kir* currents carried by inwardly rectifying potassium channels. I_{K1} is observed in both atrial and ventricular cardiomyocytes. Conductance through these channels is high at negative membrane potentials, so this current is critical for terminal repolarization (phase 3) and for setting the resting membrane potential (phase 4). Another inwardly rectifying potassium current is carried by I_{KATP} channels. The full channels include not only the pore-forming subunit but also auxiliary *SUR* subunits, which are targets for channel inhibition by the sulfonylurea class of drugs. Because I_{KATP} currents are inhibited by intracellular adenosine triphosphate, they are activated in the setting of ischemia. The augmented outward current shortens action potential duration and abbreviates systole, thereby diminishing energetic requirements. Thus I_{KATP} channels provide a link between metabolic state and membrane excitability. Importantly, the resulting action potential duration shortening diminishes refractoriness, which may enhance the risk for re-entrant arrhythmias. The last major class of inward rectifiers includes the acetylcholine- and adenosine-activated potassium channels, which are encoded by $K_{ir}3.1$ and $K_{ir}3.4$. These channels, which are enriched in nodal and atrial cardiac myocytes, are activated when ligands bind to muscarinic or purinergic G protein–coupled receptors, which facilitate the uncoupling of $G_{\beta\gamma}$ from G_α and the activation of the K_{ir} channels by the released $G_{\beta\gamma}$.

Gap Junction Channels

Gap junction channels, which are responsible for the electrotonic coupling of cardiac myocytes, are essential for normal impulse propagation throughout the myocardium. The channels are formed by the hexameric assembly of connexin monomers, each of which is a tetramembrane spanning protein. Connexin 43 is the dominant isoform expressed in ventricular and atrial myocardium, whereas connexin 40 is also abundantly expressed in the atrium. The nodes express variable amounts of connexin 45 and connexin 30.2, and the bundle branches and Purkinje fibers express significant levels of connexin 40. Gap junctions in the node integrate the intrinsic beating rate of each nodal cell into a single functional unit. Abnormalities in connexin expression and function, a process known as pathologic gap junction remodeling, are observed in atrial and ventricular myocardium in many acquired forms of heart disease. The remodeling contributes to aberrant impulse propagation and predisposes to arrhythmic behavior. In addition, germline or somatic mutations in cardiac connexin genes are associated with arrhythmic syndromes, especially atrial fibrillation.

MECHANISMS OF ARRYHTHMOGENESIS

Cardiac arrhythmias, which are disturbances in the rate or rhythm of the heartbeat, are a reflection of abnormal impulse formation or conduction. Inasmuch as cardiac myocytes reside within a complex multicellular environment and are electrotonically coupled by gap junction channels, arrhythmic syndromes almost always reflect a complex interplay of individual, or *cell autonomous*, properties within a multicellular network.[5] Most clinically important arrhythmias arise in the setting of acquired heart disease, in which pathologic *electrical remodeling*, resulting from dysregulation of ion channel expression or function, accompanies *structural remodeling*. However, many arrhythmic syndromes result from, or are exacerbated by, genetic variations, including disease-causing alterations in coding regions that directly affect the function of proteins, which regulate cardiac electrophysiology, as well as sequence variants in regulatory or other noncoding genome regions, which appear to regulate transcriptional and post-transcriptional behavior.

Disorders of Impulse Formation

In the healthy heart, the sinus node, which is located at the junction of the right atrium and the superior vena cava, is the predominant pacemaker. Secondary pacemakers with intrinsically slower pacing rates are found further downstream in the specialized conduction system within the atrioventricular node and the His-Purkinje system. The firing rate of pacemaker cells is regulated primarily by autonomic tone: sympathetic stimulation increases the slope of phase 4 depolarization, whereas parasympathetic stimulation decreases the slope by augmenting repolarizing currents. Nodal suppression may result from pharmacologic agents, such as β-adrenergic blockers, calcium channel blockers, or digitalis, as well as from fibrotic diseases. Moreover, mutations in several genes that affect the voltage clock (*SCN5A* and *HCN4*), the calcium clock (*RYR2* and *CASQ2*), or both (*ANKB*) may cause familial sinus node dysfunction.

Conversely, under pathologic conditions, myocardial cells outside the specialized conduction system may exhibit spontaneous activity, a phenomenon termed *abnormal automaticity*. Abnormal automaticity is most often seen with ischemia or reperfusion, in which maximum diastolic potentials are reduced to approximately −60 mV to −50 mV, a level at which Na^+ or Ca^{2+} channels may reach their activation threshold and trigger action potentials.

Afterdepolarizations and Triggered Activity

During cardiac repolarization, a number of inward and outward currents are active, and small changes in conductance of individual channels can markedly affect the trajectory of repolarization. *Afterdepolarizations*, which are abnormal oscillations in membrane potential, occur either during (early afterdepolarizations) or after (delayed afterdepolarizations) an action potential. Afterdepolarizations of sufficient magnitude to evoke an action potential produce triggered activity. Early afterdepolarizations are almost always observed in the setting of abnormal action potential duration prolongation, which provides sufficient time for *re*-activation of L-type Ca^{2+} channels during the plateau phase of the action potential. Thus, congenital syndromes, as well as bradycardia, hypokalemia, hypomagnesemia, antiarrhythmic medications, and many noncardiac drugs, are associated with QT prolongation and promote early afterdepolarizations. Conversely, rapid pacing and drugs that shorten the action potential duration tend to suppress early afterdepolarizations. Early afterdepolarizations in the setting of action potential duration prolongation often trigger *torsades de pointes* (Chapter 65), a polymorphic ventricular tachycardia, especially when there is increased dispersion of repolarization. Delayed afterdepolarizations, in contrast, are usually the result of intracellular Ca^{2+} overload and are typically seen in the setting of catecholamine excess, ischemia, toxic concentrations of digitalis-like agents, and some congenital syndromes, including catecholaminergic polymorphic ventricular tachycardia. The excessive Ca^{2+} load activates the electrogenic Na^+-Ca^{2+} exchanger, producing a depolarizing transient inward current, I_{TI}.

Disorders of Impulse Conduction

During each cardiac cycle, impulses must be generated in pacemaker cells within the sinus node, and a wave of excitation must propagate throughout the atria, travel down the specialized conduction system (including the atrioventricular node and His-Purkinje network), and then activate the ventricular myocardium. Processes that diminish intercellular coupling, such as fibrosis or calcification of the specialized conduction system, can diminish the safety factor for conduction and produce varying degrees of heart block. Inherited defects in conduction have been observed with mutations in sodium channel subunits *SCN5A* and *SCN1B*, which affect phase 0 of the cardiac action potential; in *KCNJ2*, which affects terminal repolarization and the resting membrane potential; and in a number of developmental disorders that affect the cardiac conduction system, such as Holt-Oram syndrome, Emery-Dreifuss muscular dystrophy, and myotonic dystrophy type 1. Conduction block may also be seen with the secondary electrical remodeling that is associated with structural heart disease and with many cardioactive drugs.

Re-entry

Re-entry is considered the most common mechanism responsible for clinically significant cardiac arrhythmias, including both supraventricular and ventricular disorders. Fundamentally, re-entry involves self-perpetuating waves of excitation that circulate around an inexcitable obstacle. Depending on the number of re-entrant waves within a tissue (one or multiple), their size, and their spatial stability, the surface electrocardiogram may reveal a relatively organized rhythm, such as atrial flutter or monomorphic ventricular tachycardia, or a seemingly disorganized rhythm, such as atrial fibrillation or polymorphic ventricular tachycardia. Re-entry normally requires the presence of unidirectional block within a "fast" conducting pathway around an obstacle, combined with recirculation of the impulse from a second "slow" pathway in the retrograde direction, as might be the case at a bifurcating Purkinje-ventricular junction or around scar tissue of a healed myocardial infarction (Fig. 61-2). However, the "obstacle" may also be viable myocardium that is inexcitable owing to its intrinsic electrophysiologic properties, such as cellular uncoupling or refractoriness, a phenomenon referred to as *functional block*. Because refractoriness is critically dependent on the action potential duration, areas of myocardium with prolongation of the action potential duration may form a suitable substrate for functional re-entry.

Heterogeneity in action potential duration and the concomitant *dispersion of refractoriness* also play critical roles in the maintenance of arrhythmic behavior, especially through a phenomenon known as *phase 2 re-entry*. This term refers to the flow of current during phase 2 of the cardiac action potential from a depolarized cell to neighboring cells that are more fully repolarized and not refractory to reexcitation. This principle is best characterized in the J wave syndromes, especially Brugada syndrome, in which loss of function of inward currents (I_{Na} or I_{Ca}) or gain of function of outward currents (I_{to}, $I_{K\text{-}ATP}$) causes loss of the action potential dome during phase 2 and an abbreviated action potential duration in a subset of cardiac myocytes. Current can then flow into these cells from neighboring cells in which the action potential dome is maintained, thereby causing local reexcitation, a closely coupled extrasystole, and the initiation of re-entry. In Brugada syndrome, this process is thought to arise in the right ventricular outflow tract, where the transient outward current density is significantly greater in the epicardium compared with the endocardium (Fig. 61-3).

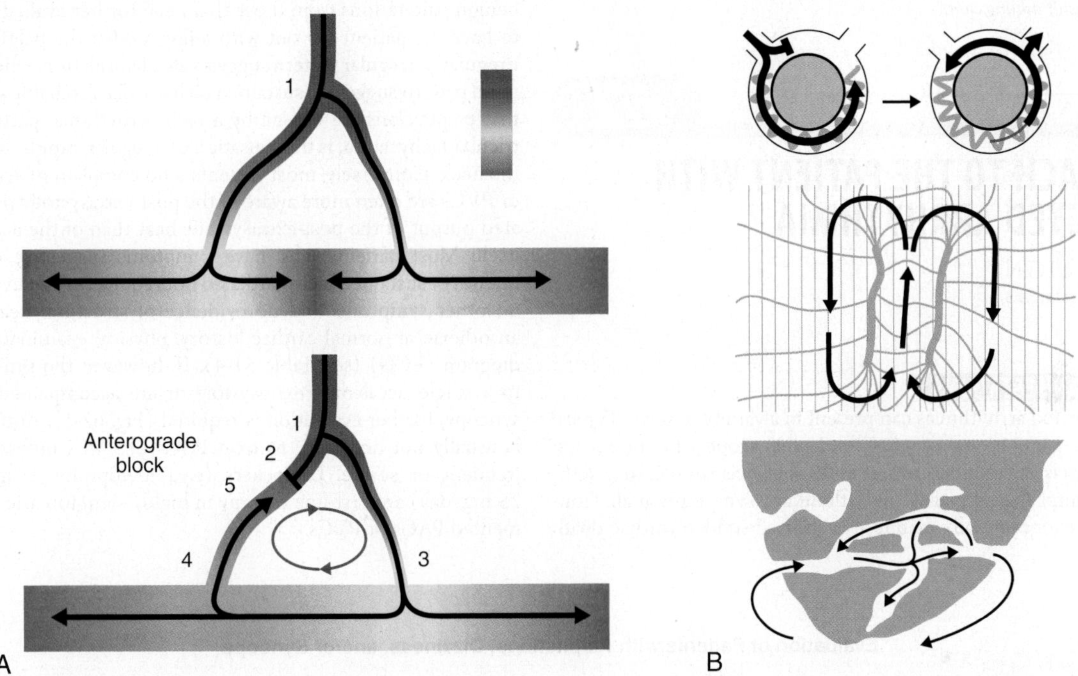

FIGURE 61-2. **Re-entrant cardiac arrhythmias. A,** Re-entry at the Purkinje-ventricular junction. *Upper panel:* Normally an impulse propagates along a Purkinje fiber and divides into two pathways (1), and together they activate the underlying ventricular myocardium. *Lower panel:* The impulse propagates along the right pathway (3) but is blocked within the left pathway (2). The original impulse travels within the ventricular myocardium, reenters the left pathway in the retrograde direction (4), and successfully propagates through the area with block (5). Continued propagation throughout this circuit *(red circle)* would produce re-entrant ventricular tachycardia. **B,** Re-entry associated with myocardium scar. *Upper panel:* Diagram representing a single circuit of re-entry that initiates with unidirectional block. The circuit length must be longer than the longest refractory period in the circuit. *Middle panel:* A figure 8, in which re-entry is established due to dispersion of refractoriness during tachycardia. *Lower panel:* Anatomic labyrinth circuit, created by strands of viable myocardium within the scar, with potential for multiple re-entry circuits. (The image to the right is reproduced from Benito B, Josephson ME. Ventricular tachycardia in coronary artery disease. *Rev Esp Cardiol [Engl Ed].* 2012;65:939-955.)

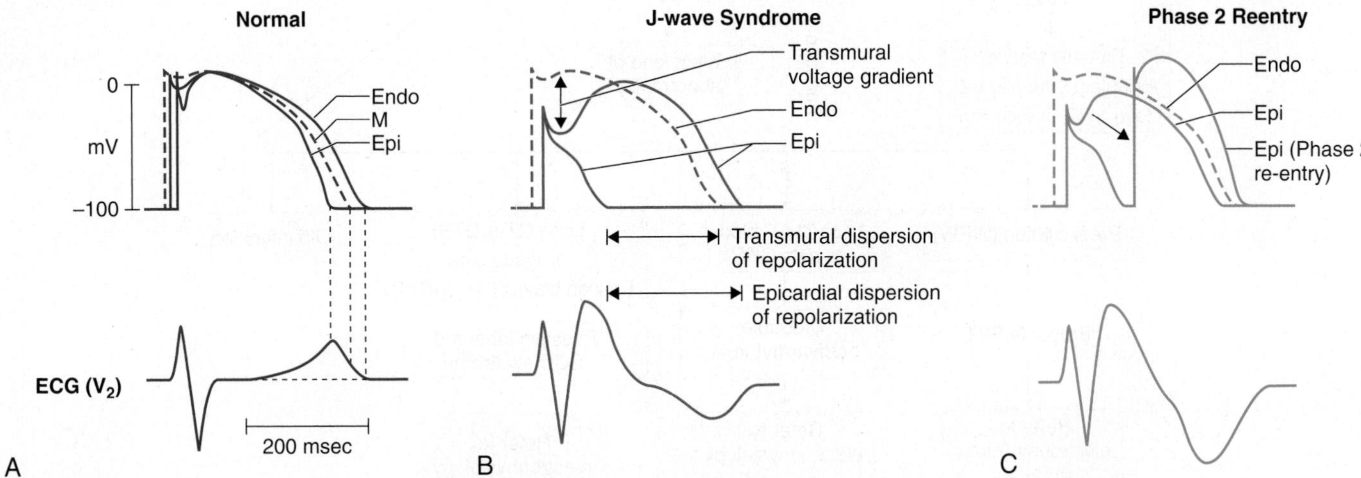

FIGURE 61-3. **Cellular basis for J wave syndromes and phase 2 re-entry.** Under normal conditions, the ST segment is isoelectric because of the absence of transmural voltage gradients at the level of the action potential plateau. Accentuation of the phase I notch under pathophysiologic conditions, such as loss of function of I_{Na} or gain of function of I_{to}, leads to loss of the action potential dome at some epicardial sites but not others, producing ST and T wave changes typically observed in Brugada syndrome. Loss of the action potential dome in epicardium but not endocardium results in the development of a marked transmural dispersion of repolarization and conduction of the action potential dome, from sites at which it is maintained to sites at which it is lost, thereby causing local reexcitation through a phase 2 re-entry mechanism. (Modified from Antzelevitch C, Brugada P, Brugada J, et al. Brugada syndrome: from cell to bedside. *Curr Probl Cardiol.* 2005;30:9-54.)

SUMMARY

The concepts of cardiac electrophysiology, including the genesis of the action potential, the molecular basis of cardiac excitability, and the mechanisms that are responsible for abnormal cardiac rhythms, provide a foundation for understanding and identifying clinically relevant arrhythmias. Insights into the biophysical basis of congenital arrhythmic syndromes and into the pathologic remodeling observed in acquired arrhythmic syndromes have already resulted in several targeted new therapies informed by the expression, function, and regulation of ion channels.

GENERAL REFERENCES

For the General References and other additional features, please visit Expert Consult at https://expertconsult.inkling.com.

62 APPROACH TO THE PATIENT WITH SUSPECTED ARRHYTHMIA

JEFFREY E. OLGIN

CLINICAL MANIFESTATIONS

Patients with suspected arrhythmias can present in a variety of ways. Typical symptoms include palpitations, syncope, and presyncope (dizziness). On occasion, arrhythmias can manifest more subtly as exercise intolerance, lethargy, and vague complaints of malaise or without any symptoms at all. Conversely, arrhythmias occasionally manifest as aborted sudden cardiac death (cardiac arrest) (Chapter 63). The specific differential diagnosis, prognosis, and treatment of these symptoms are determined by the severity of the symptom (i.e., whether it results in syncope) and whether the patient has underlying structural heart disease. In general, the likelihood of a life-threatening arrhythmia, such as ventricular tachycardia or ventricular fibrillation, in a patient with symptoms of palpitations or syncope is significantly greater in a patient who has structural heart disease. Therefore, the determination of whether structural heart disease is present is a key step in the diagnosis and prognosis of patients with suspected arrhythmias.

Palpitations

Palpitations, defined as an awareness of an irregular or rapid heartbeat, are most commonly due to ectopic beats—namely, premature atrial contractions (PACs; Chapter 64) and premature ventricular contractions (PVCs; Chapter 65)—or to tachyarrhythmias. A careful history can often distinguish benign palpitations from those that need further evaluation. It can be useful to have the patient tap out with a finger what the palpitations feel like. An irregularly irregular pattern suggests atrial fibrillation, whereas a more regular, rapid pattern suggests a sustained tachycardia. A reliable symptom suggesting that palpitations are caused by a tachyarrhythmia, particularly a supraventricular tachycardia, is the sensation of a regular, rapid-pounding sensation in the neck. Conversely, most patients who complain of symptoms from PACs or PVCs are often more aware of the post-extrasystolic pause or the accentuated output of the post-extrasystolic beat than of the actual premature beat itself. Most patients who have symptoms suggestive of premature beats but not of sustained tachycardia do not require further evaluation if they have no other symptoms and no evidence of structural heart disease—that is, an otherwise normal cardiac history, physical examination, and electrocardiogram (ECG) (see Table 51-4). If, however, the symptoms are not due to a single occasional extrasystole or are accompanied by presyncope or syncope, further evaluation is required (Fig. 62-1). Antiarrhythmic therapy is usually not necessary to treat PACs or PVCs unless the symptoms are frequent or severe. β-Blockers (e.g., metoprolol 25 mg/day or atenolol 25 mg/day) are first-line therapy in highly symptomatic patients with documented PACs or PVCs.

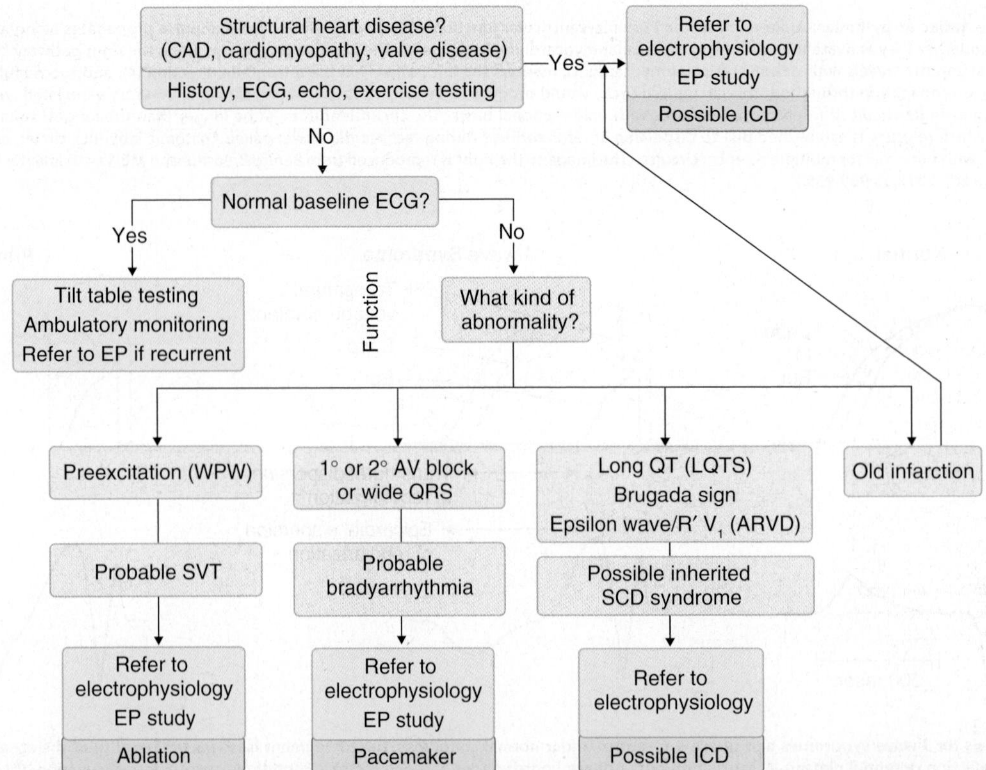

FIGURE 62-1. Algorithm for evaluating patients with symptoms of palpitation, dizziness, or syncope. ARVD = arrhythmogenic right ventricular dysplasia; AV = atrioventricular; CAD = coronary artery disease; ECG = electrocardiogram; echo = echocardiogram; EP = electrophysiology; ICD = implantable cardioverter-defibrillator; LQTS = long QT syndrome; SCD = sudden cardiac death; SVT = supraventricular tachycardia; WPW = Wolff-Parkinson-White syndrome.

Palpitations are the most common presentation of tachyarrhythmias. Most tachyarrhythmias in patients without structural heart disease are due to supraventricular tachycardias (Chapter 64) that resolve spontaneously within several seconds. When the tachyarrhythmia is more prolonged, it often resolves with simple interventions. Patients themselves can cough several times, perform the Valsalva maneuver, exhale forcefully against a closed glottis for several seconds, or even rub gently on their eyeballs. A physician can use carotid sinus massage (Chapter 64), performed by pressing and rubbing the carotid pulse just below the angle of the mandible for 5 to 15 seconds. This maneuver should be avoided in elderly patients and in patients with a history of cerebrovascular accident, known carotid artery stenosis, or carotid bruit on auscultation. In patients with structural heart disease, palpitations may signify ventricular tachycardia (Chapter 65), particularly if they occur with syncope or presyncope. Rarely do bradyarrhythmias manifest as palpitations.

Presyncope and Syncope

Syncope, defined as a sudden loss of consciousness, and presyncope, or lightheadedness, are caused by global impairment of blood flow to the brain (Table 62-1). Syncope can be a manifestation of tachyarrhythmias, bradyarrhythmias, or neurocardiogenic syncope, or it can be unrelated to any arrhythmia. A careful history and physical examination are necessary to exclude other cardiac causes (e.g., acute ischemia, aortic stenosis) or neurologic causes. Important historical features that suggest an arrhythmic cause are an association with palpitations and the lack of any neurologic deficits preceding or following the event. Important differential diagnoses include conditions other than lightheadedness that may be termed dizziness by the patient. Vertigo (Chapter 428), a sense of imbalance or of the "room spinning," and ataxia (Chapter 410) can usually be distinguished by the history and physical examination. The possibility of seizures (Chapter 403) must also be evaluated; syncope from an arrhythmia or neurocardiogenic syncope occasionally results in seizure-like activity, and seizures can sometimes be confused with syncope. The most important distinguishing feature is that postictal symptoms, a key feature of seizure disorders, are absent when syncope is the result of an arrhythmia. Patients with syncope from an arrhythmia usually awaken without any neurologic residual, unless the patient experienced a cardiac arrest with prolonged hypoxia and required resuscitation.

Because most spells of episodic loss of consciousness occur outside medical observation, the history is the most critical part of the evaluation (Table 62-2). Each syncopal episode should be reviewed in detail, with special attention to symptoms preceding the episode, events during unconsciousness, and the symptoms and time course of regaining orientation after consciousness is restored. Information from a witness can be essential to the evaluation.

The patient's presymptomatic activity and positioning, as well as symptoms when the syncopal episode began, are important clues to diagnosis. Seizures or cardiac arrhythmias can occur in any body position, but recumbent patients rarely develop neurocardiogenic (vasovagal) syncope and never have orthostatic hypotension. Prodromal lightheadedness, dizziness (but uncommonly vertigo), bilateral tinnitus, nausea, diffuse weakness, and dimming of vision are symptoms of cerebral hypoperfusion and support the diagnosis of syncope, which may be from a cardiac, orthostatic, or neurocardiogenic cause. Loss of consciousness so rapid that a prodrome is absent may occur with seizures and with some cardiac arrhythmias such as asystole, which typically causes loss of consciousness within 4 to 8 seconds in the upright position but usually requires 12 to 15 seconds in the recumbent position. Palpitations during the prodrome suggest a tachyarrhythmia. The activity of the patient immediately before the onset of symptoms may also provide clues. Syncope associated with the cessation of exertion or with anxiety or pain suggests neurocardiogenic syncope, whereas symptoms during exertion suggest an arrhythmia. Syncope associated with a change in posture suggests orthostatic causes, whereas syncope while straining at urination suggests situational neurocardiogenic syncope.

A witness's description of the events during the episode of unconsciousness is very helpful. Although body stiffening and limb jerking occur with generalized seizures, similar movements can result from cerebral hypoperfusion, especially if perfusion is not restored rapidly. Such muscle jerking is often

TABLE 62-1 CAUSES OF SYNCOPE AND THEIR PREVALENCE

NEUROCARDIOGENIC CAUSES
Vasovagal (8-41% of patients)
Situational (1-8% of patients)
Micturition
Defecation
Swallow
Cough
Carotid sinus syncope (0.4% of patients)
Neuralgias
Psychiatric disorders
Medications, exercise
ORTHOSTATIC HYPOTENSION (4-10% OF PATIENTS)
DECREASED CARDIAC OUTPUT
Obstruction to flow (1-8% of patients)
Obstruction to left ventricular outflow or inflow: aortic stenosis, hypertrophic obstructive cardiomyopathy, mitral stenosis, myxoma
Obstruction to right ventricular outflow or inflow: pulmonic stenosis, pulmonary embolism, pulmonary hypertension, myxoma
Other heart disease
Pump failure, myocardial infarction, coronary artery disease, coronary spasm, tamponade, aortic dissection
ARRHYTHMIAS (4-38% OF PATIENTS)
Bradyarrhythmias: sinus node disease, second- and third-degree atrioventricular block, pacemaker malfunction, drug-induced bradyarrhythmias
Tachyarrhythmias: ventricular tachycardia, torsades de pointes (e.g., associated with congenital long QT syndrome or acquired QT prolongation), supraventricular tachycardia
NEUROLOGIC AND PSYCHIATRIC DISEASES (3-32% OF PATIENTS)
Migraine
Transient ischemic attacks
UNKNOWN (13-41% OF PATIENTS)

Adapted from Kapoor W. Approach to the patient with syncope. In: Braunwald E, Goldman L, eds. *Primary Cardiology*, 2nd ed. Philadelphia: Saunders; 2003.

TABLE 62-2 CLINICAL FEATURES SUGGESTING SPECIFIC CAUSES

DIAGNOSTIC CONSIDERATION
Neurocardiogenic
Symptoms after prolonged motionless standing, sudden unexpected pain, fear, or unpleasant sight, sound, or smell
Syncope in a well-trained athlete after exertion (without heart disease)
Situational syncope during or immediately after micturition, cough, swallowing, or defecation
Syncope with throat or facial pain (glossopharyngeal or trigeminal neuralgia)
Organic Heart Disease (e.g., coronary artery disease, aortic stenosis, primary arrhythmia, obstructive hypertrophic cardiomyopathy, pulmonary hypertension)
Brief loss of consciousness, no prodrome, history of heart disease
Syncope with exertion
Family history of sudden death
Neurological
Seizures: confusion for >5 min after regaining consciousness
Transient ischemic attack, subclavian steal, basilar migraine: syncope associated with vertigo, dysarthria, diplopia, arm exercise
Migraine: syncope associated with antecedent headaches
Other Vascular
Carotid sinus: syncope with head rotation or pressure on the carotid sinus (as in tumors, shaving, tight collars)
Orthostatic hypotension: syncope immediately on standing
Subclavian steal or aortic dissection: differences in blood pressure or pulse between the two arms
Drug-Induced
Patient is taking a medication that may lead to long QT syndrome, orthostasis, or bradycardia
Psychiatric Illness
Frequent syncope, somatic complaints, no heart disease

Adapted from Kapoor WN. Syncope. *N Engl J Med.* 2000;343:1856-1862.

multifocal and can be synchronous or asynchronous. In contrast to epileptic seizures, which generally produce tonic-clonic activity for at least 1 to 2 minutes, muscle jerking in syncope rarely persists for longer than 30 seconds. If an arrhythmia continues or the patient is physically maintained upright, tonic stiffening of the body followed by jerking movements of the limbs can occur. Occasionally, motor movements identical to a tonic-clonic seizure occur, and a mistaken diagnosis of epilepsy can be made. Urinary incontinence during the spell is frequently used to support or refute a diagnosis of epilepsy; however, fainting with a full bladder can result in incontinence, whereas seizures with an empty bladder will not. Tongue biting favors seizures.

The time frame over which consciousness and orientation are regained is perhaps the most important clue in differentiating seizures from syncope. Recovery of orientation after neurocardiogenic syncope occurs within seconds of regaining consciousness. Recovery of orientation after self-reversible arrhythmia-associated syncope is usually proportional to the duration of the unconsciousness and is usually rapid (0 to 10 seconds). Life-threatening arrhythmias (e.g., prolonged asystole or ventricular fibrillation) usually do not resolve without resuscitation, and the confusion after regaining consciousness may be permanent owing to ischemic brain injury (Chapter 63). By comparison, the period of confusion after seizures, often accompanied by agitation, continues for 2 to 20 minutes after recovery of consciousness.

DIAGNOSIS

Arrhythmias are generally categorized as bradyarrhythmias (slow heart rates), tachyarrhythmias (fast heart rates), or premature beats (single extrasystoles from the atrium or the ventricle—PACs [see Fig. 64-10] or PVCs [see Fig. 65-1], respectively) (see Table 62-1). Although not a primary arrhythmia, neurocardiogenic syncope is a related diagnostic and management issue because its symptoms are frequently similar to those of arrhythmias and because neurocardiogenic syncope secondarily results in bradycardia (see later).[1] A systematic approach can optimize the likelihood of identifying the cause of transient loss of consciousness (Table 62-3).

TABLE 62-3 SUMMARY OF CLINICAL RECOMMENDATIONS FOR TRANSIENT LOSS OF CONSCIOUSNESS

TOPIC	RECOMMENDATIONS
Initial assessment	Detailed history, especially from witnesses Full clinical examination 12-lead ECG
Uncomplicated faints	Suggestive features include: Posture: occurrence during prolonged standing or similar previous episodes avoided by lying down Provoking factors, such as pain or a medical procedure Prodromal symptoms, such as sweating or feeling warm or hot before TLoC Further investigation and specialist referral are not needed.
Epilepsy	Suggestive features are a bitten tongue; head turning to one side during TLoC; no memory of abnormal behavior that occurred before, during, or after TLoC; unusual posturing; prolonged limb jerking (brief seizure-like activity often occurs during syncope, including uncomplicated faints); confusion after the event; or prodromal déjà vu or jamais vu. If features of epilepsy are present, arrange for early review by an epilepsy specialist. Do not arrange for EEG before neurologic assessment. Note that brief seizure-like activity often occurs during syncope, including uncomplicated faints. Do not suspect epilepsy unless suggestive features are present. Arrange for cardiovascular assessment if the cause of TLoC is unclear.
Urgent specialist referral	Give immediate treatment for clinically urgent problems (such as complete AV block or severe bleeding). Arrange for urgent specialist cardiovascular assessment for patients at risk for a severe adverse event (such as those with long QT interval, cardiac arrhythmia, or structural heart disease).
Further cardiovascular assessment	Focus on specific disorders that may cause TLoC, such as orthostatic hypotension, the carotid sinus syndrome, structural heart disease, or cardiac arrhythmia. Assessment should include repeated history, clinical examination, and 12-lead ECG. For suspected cardiac arrhythmia or unexplained TLoC, use ambulatory ECG for further assessment: Very frequent episodes: use 24- to 48-hour Holter monitoring. Moderately frequent episodes: use external event monitoring. Infrequent episodes: use an implantable event recorder.

AV = atrioventricular; ECG = electrocardiography; EEG = electroencephalogram; TLoC = transient loss of consciousness.

Adapted from Cooper PN, et al. Synopsis of the National Institute for Health and Clinical Excellence Guideline for management of transient loss of consciousness. *Ann Intern Med.* 2011;155:543-549.

Bradyarrhythmias

Bradyarrhythmias (Chapter 64) can be due to dysfunction in the sinoatrial node, atrioventricular (AV) node, or His-Purkinje system (below the AV node). Sinus bradycardia manifests as a slow atrial (sinus) rate and can occur at rest or as an inappropriately slow rate during exercise (chronotropic incompetence). Sinus arrest can be intermittent, when transient loss of sinus activity (loss of the P wave on the ECG) causes brief sinus pauses, or persistent, with prolonged loss of atrial activation. The sinus rate and even the presence of sinus pauses are influenced by autonomic tone. Therefore, healthy individuals—particularly younger patients and well-trained athletes (with high vagal tone)—have occasional sinus slowing, often during sleep. A sinus pause of more than 3 seconds is considered pathologic if it is associated with symptoms while a patient is awake. Sinus bradycardia and sinus arrest can also be the result of medications, typically β-blockers and calcium-channel blockers. When not "physiologic" or due to medications, sinus bradycardia and sinus arrest are the result of intrinsic conduction system disease. Sinus bradycardia, especially if it is intermittent, can also signify disease of the right coronary artery.

Bradyarrhythmias from AV nodal disease result from the failure of impulse conduction from the atrium to the ventricle. Like the sinus node, the AV node is dramatically affected by autonomic tone. Mobitz type I second-degree AV block (Wenckebach block; see Fig. 64-6) can be seen during periods of high vagal tone (such as while sleeping) and is not necessarily pathologic; for example, it does not progress to complete heart block and is not associated with a widened QRS. Many drugs, such as β-blockers and calcium-channel blockers, commonly cause first-degree AV block and should be considered a potential cause of any degree of AV block. Mobitz type II block (see Fig. 64-7) signifies that the level of AV block is below the AV node in the His-Purkinje system, which is not sensitive to autonomic tone; the resulting QRS is widened, and there is a high likelihood of progression to complete heart block (third-degree AV block; see Figs. 64-8 and 64-9). Idiopathic paroxysmal atrioventricular block, detected by continuous ECG monitoring, can also cause syncope. Intermittent complete heart block, which can result in drop attacks or Stokes-Adams attacks, is usually preceded by abnormal baseline findings on the ECG, such as a bundle branch block or second-degree AV block. The treatment of choice for patients with symptomatic bradyarrhythmias or those likely to progress to complete heart block is implantation of a permanent pacemaker (Chapter 66).

Tachyarrhythmias

Tachyarrhythmias can arise from the atrium or AV node (supraventricular tachycardia) or from the ventricle (ventricular tachycardia). Supraventricular tachyarrhythmias that may be associated with palpitations, presyncope, or syncope include atrial tachycardia (see Fig. 64-16), AV nodal re-entrant tachycardia (see Fig. 64-15), AV junctional tachycardia (see Fig. 64-18), atrial flutter (see Fig. 64-21), and atrial fibrillation (see Fig. 64-22), sometimes in association with accessory conduction pathways that facilitate the re-entry needed to sustain the arrhythmia. Ventricular tachyarrhythmias include the various forms of ventricular tachycardia (see Figs. 65-2 through 65-4). Treatment is guided by the specific tachyarrhythmia and its underlying cause (Table 62-4; see Tables 64-5 and 64-6) (Chapters 63 through 66).

Neurocardiogenic Syncope and Related Syndromes

Neurocardiogenic syncope is the sudden onset of lightheadedness or loss of consciousness as a result of autonomic reflexes and is more common in younger patients (teenage to third decade of life). It is sometimes called a vasovagal episode, a common faint, or situational syncope if it is clearly induced by a particular activity (e.g., micturition syncope). Some families have autosomal dominant vasovagal syncope, which is genetically heterogeneous but seems to be linked to chromosome 15q26.[2]

In this form of neurocardiogenic syncope, heightened parasympathetic output, either due to direct stimulation (e.g., micturition, defecation,

TABLE 62-4 INDICATIONS FOR INITIAL OBSERVATION AND RAPID EVALUATION OF SYNCOPE

EUROPEAN SOCIETY OF CARDIOLOGY*	CANADIAN CARDIOVASCULAR SOCIETY†
Known coronary or structural heart disease, heart failure, or prior arrhythmia	Heart failure or history of ischemic, arrhythmic, obstructive, or valvular heart disease
ECG showing nonsustained ventricular tachycardia, bifascicular block, sinus bradycardia <50 beats/min, sinoatrial block, preexcitation, or evidence of an inherited disease	Abnormal ECG: arrhythmia, conduction disease, new ischemia, or evidence of prior myocardial infarction
Syncope during exertion or when supine, palpitations preceding syncope, family history of sudden cardiac death	Systolic blood pressure <90 mm Hg
Important comorbidities (e.g., severe anemia, electrolyte disturbance)	Comorbid conditions: age >60 years, dyspnea, hematocrit <30%, hypertension, cerebrovascular disease, family history of sudden death before age 50 years, syncope while supine, syncope during exercise, syncope with no prodromal symptoms

ECG = electrocardiogram.
*Moya A, Sutton R, Ammirati F, et al. Guidelines for the diagnosis and management of syncope (version 2009): the Task Force for the Diagnosis and Management of Syncope of the European Society of Cardiology (ESC). *Eur Heart J.* 2009;30:2631-2671.
†Sheldon RS, Morillo CA, Krahn AD, et al. Standardized approaches to the investigation of syncope: Canadian Cardiovascular Society position paper. *Can J Cardiol.* 2011;27:246-253.

abdominal pain, or other gastrointestinal conditions) or as a reflex in response to sympathetic stimulation (e.g., seeing blood, abrupt cessation of exercise), results in arterial dilation (called the vasodilatory response) and an inhibition of sinus and AV node activity (the cardioinhibitory response). The result is a transient decrease in blood pressure, often manifested as lightheadedness or syncope. Because they are associated with parasympathetic (vagal) output, episodes are frequently accompanied by nausea, diaphoresis, and salivation. Twin analyses provide strong evidence for genetic factors in vasovagal syncope.

Treatment of this form of syncope can be challenging. The most effective therapies are behavioral (avoidance of triggers), wearing of compression stockings, and maintenance of adequate hydration and salt intake. Lying down with the feet elevated and performing isometric hand exercises may abort an acute episode. Medical therapy, including β-blockers (pindolol 5 to 15 mg twice daily), mineralocorticoids (fludrocortisone 0.1 mg/day), paroxetine (10 to 20 mg/day), and midodrine (an α-adrenergic agonist and vasoconstrictor; 5 to 10 mg three times daily), has shown some efficacy in reducing recurrence rates, although the efficacy of β-blockers for reducing syncopal episodes has been inconsistent.

Rarely, situational syncope is associated with swallowing or coughing. Swallowing can trigger brain stem reflexes that lead to vagally induced bradyarrhythmias, with resultant syncope. This phenomenon may or may not be associated with severe pain in the tonsillar pillar, which may radiate to the ear (i.e., glossopharyngeal neuralgia; Chapter 398). The pain can usually be prevented by carbamazepine (400 to 1000 mg/day total in divided doses of 2-3 times per day orally); in refractory cases, 300 mg/day in divided doses of 1-4 times per day of phenytoin can be added. Cough-related syncope can occur with severe, repeated coughing, which may increase thoracic pressure and result in increased vagal tone or a transient reduction in outflow from the intracranial veins, followed by a transient increase in intracranial pressure and impaired blood flow.

A related cause of syncope is carotid body hypersensitivity, in which vagal tone is increased by direct stimulation of the carotid body. This condition is frequently seen in older patients (particularly men older than 60 years), in whom episodes are associated with mechanical stimulation of the neck (e.g., turning the head, shaving, wearing a tight collar or necktie). Use of β-blockers, calcium-channel blockers, and digitalis can exacerbate or predispose to this condition. This form of syncope is diagnosed by documenting pauses longer than 3 seconds in response to carotid sinus massage and is curable with a pacemaker because carotid body stimulation does not cause significant vasodilation.

Postural or orthostatic hypotension can result in recurrent syncope. The history confirms that the patient is in the upright posture during spells, that the prodromal symptoms are those of cerebral hypoperfusion, and that the symptoms are relieved with recumbency. The diagnosis is supported by detecting a decrease of 30 mm Hg or greater in systolic blood pressure or a decrease of 10 mm Hg or greater in diastolic blood pressure between recumbent and upright postures. The many causes include drugs, polyneuropathies (Chapter 420), and neurodegenerative disorders (Chapter 409).

Cerebrovascular syncope results from cerebral hypoperfusion due to vascular phenomena, as opposed to generalized hypotension caused by arrhythmias or neurocardiogenic reflexes. Loss of consciousness can be a component of a basilar artery transient ischemic attack, but other brain stem symptoms nearly always precede or accompany the unconsciousness. Vertigo is most frequent, but diplopia or visual field disturbances, hemifacial or perioral numbness, and dysarthria or ataxia are also common. Recovery of consciousness may require 30 to 60 minutes. Although the diagnosis is suggested by the history and clinical presentation, imaging studies can be useful to confirm the diagnosis. Carotid Doppler studies may show various degrees of stenosis, especially in older patients. However, unconsciousness requires bihemispheric dysfunction; thus, unilateral carotid stenosis alone does not cause syncope. Transcranial Doppler studies or magnetic resonance angiography of the basilar artery is indicated only if brain stem ischemic symptoms are present in addition to loss of consciousness; false-positive tests are common, especially with increasing age. These patients, who are at risk for basilar artery stroke, should be treated with aspirin and should be considered for other treatments (e.g., surgery, stent placement) appropriate for their symptoms and anatomy (Chapter 407).

Other syndromes that can cause syncope include subclavian artery stenosis, which may result in retrograde blood flow from the vertebral artery to one arm, with resultant brain stem hypoperfusion (i.e., subclavian steal syndrome). Asymmetry in upper extremity systolic blood pressure, typically averaging 45 mm Hg, is nearly always present. Brain stem symptoms are similar to those in basilar transient ischemic attacks, including loss of consciousness, but a subsequent stroke from subclavian steal is rare. Repair of the stenosis is the treatment of choice. Syncope may also occur in up to 10% of patients with basilar artery migraine (Chapter 398). It can have a postural (orthostatic) manifestation or be associated with other basilar artery symptoms.

Neuropsychiatric syncope is a diagnosis of exclusion but is suggested by young age, frequent spells, multiple symptoms (e.g., dizziness, vertigo, lightheadedness, numbness), and duplication of the patient's symptoms by hyperventilation with the mouth open for 2 to 3 minutes. Whereas syncope and seizures occur with the eyes open, often with gaze deviation, psychogenic events frequently begin with eye closing.

Seizures (Chapter 403) can cause loss of consciousness and occasionally present clinically as syncope. However, seizures usually have a characteristic presentation and include a postictal phase, whereas most patients experiencing a syncopal episode quickly regain consciousness, except when cerebral perfusion is so compromised as to cause a secondary seizure or persistent anoxia and brain damage.

Diagnostic Tests

Electrocardiography

The baseline ECG is critical in the evaluation of a patient with palpitations or syncope. The presence of ventricular preexcitation, as manifested by a short PR interval and a delta wave (see Fig. 64-19), establishes the likely diagnosis of Wolff-Parkinson-White syndrome in a patient with palpitations and AV reciprocating tachycardia (Chapter 64); it can also be used to determine the location of the responsible accessory pathway. The baseline ECG provides useful predictive information about the likelihood of conduction system abnormalities being responsible for bradyarrhythmias (e.g., sinus bradycardia suggests sinus node dysfunction, a prolonged PR interval suggests AV nodal disease, and a widened QRS suggests disease below the AV node). The ECG is also useful in diagnosing prior myocardial infarction (i.e., pathologic Q waves), which raises the likelihood of ventricular tachycardia as a potential cause of syncope or palpitations. Abnormalities such as a prolonged QT interval in a patient with syncope and a family history of syncope or sudden death suggest one of the congenital long QT syndromes (Chapter 65). An incomplete right bundle branch block with coved ST segment elevation in ECG lead V_1 or V_2 in a patient with syncope or palpitations suggests Brugada syndrome, whereas an epsilon wave, incomplete right bundle branch block, and inverted T waves in V_1 are suggestive of right ventricular dysplasia (Chapter 65). All these syndromes carry an increased risk for recurrent syncope and sudden death if untreated (Chapters 63 through 65). The short QT syndrome also predisposes to ventricular arrhythmias, but currently there is no clear definition of a pathologically short QT duration.

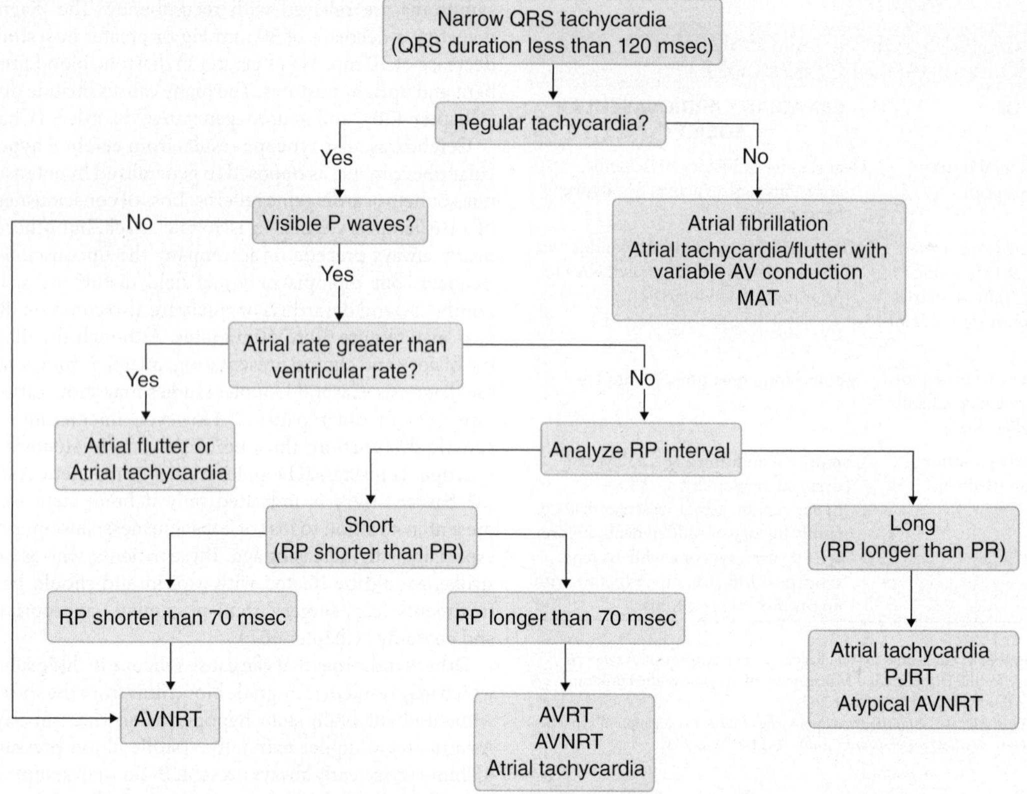

FIGURE 62-2. **ECG algorithm for diagnosis of narrow-complex tachycardias. AVNRT = atrioventricular nodal reciprocating tachycardia; AVRT = atrioventricular reciprocating tachycardia; MAT = multifocal atrial tachycardia; PJRT = permanent form of junctional reciprocating tachycardia. (From Blomstrom-Lundqvist C, Scheinman MM, Aliot EM, et al. ACC/AHA/ESC guidelines for the management of patients with supraventricular arrhythmias—executive summary. *Circulation*. 2003;108:1871-1909.)**

Performing an ECG during an episode of palpitations is extremely useful in making a definitive diagnosis. For narrow–QRS complex tachycardias, the specific supraventricular tachycardia can often be surmised from the 12-lead ECG obtained during symptoms (Fig. 62-2). Moreover, for wide–QRS complex tachycardias, the 12-lead ECG is useful in distinguishing a supraventricular tachycardia (with aberrancy) from a ventricular tachycardia (Fig. 62-3). The presence of fusion beats or AV dissociation during a wide–QRS complex tachycardia leads to the diagnosis of ventricular tachycardia. For ventricular tachycardias, the morphology of the QRS complex is useful in determining the location of the ventricular tachycardia focus and in identifying idiopathic ventricular tachycardia (right ventricular outflow tract or fascicular), which has a much more benign course than ventricular tachycardia in the setting of coronary disease (Chapter 65).

The effect of carotid sinus massage, vagal maneuvers, or adenosine (given as a rapid intravenous bolus of 6 mg and repeated at a dose of 12 mg if the initial dose is ineffective) is also useful in narrowing the differential diagnosis of a tachycardia. These maneuvers slow conduction through the AV node. Therefore, tachycardias that terminate with either maneuver are likely to involve the AV node as a critical component of the re-entrant circuit (AV nodal re-entrant tachycardia or AV re-entrant tachycardia). If the maneuver induces AV block but does not terminate the arrhythmia, likely causes are atrial fibrillation, atrial flutter, and atrial tachycardias (or occasionally ventricular tachycardia if the QRS is wide). On rare occasions, atrial tachycardias and some idiopathic ventricular tachycardias terminate in response to adenosine. Important clues to the specific mechanism can be obtained at the onset or termination of tachycardia, so obtaining a continuous 12-lead ECG during carotid sinus massage or the administration of adenosine is very useful.

During bradycardias, the ECG is useful in determining the level of the conduction system (sinus node, AV node, or His bundle) responsible for the bradycardia. Sinus bradycardia is diagnosed when a slow (<50/minute at rest) atrial rate (P wave) conducts to the ventricle. Sinus arrest or sinus pauses are diagnosed by absent or dropped P waves. First-degree AV block (see Fig. 64-5) is defined as a prolonged PR interval (>200 msec), and second-degree AV block is defined by P waves that occasionally do not conduct to the ventricle (P wave without an ensuing QRS); Mobitz type I second-degree AV block (also known as Wenckebach block; see Fig. 64-6) is characterized by progressive lengthening of the PR interval until one P wave does not conduct to the ventricle. This form of AV block is often seen in younger patients, is usually benign, and rarely progresses to complete AV (third-degree) block. Mobitz type II second-degree AV block (see Fig. 64-7), which is characterized by the sudden, unexpected loss of conduction of a P wave to the ventricle (dropped QRS), signifies disease of the His-Purkinje system and often progresses to complete heart block. Complete heart block or third-degree AV block (see Figs. 64-8 and 64-9) is diagnosed by the dissociation of P waves from QRS complexes, with an atrial rate faster than the ventricular rate.

Ambulatory Monitoring

For intermittent symptoms such as palpitations, dizziness, or syncope, it is often difficult to obtain a 12-lead ECG while the symptoms are occurring. Therefore, ambulatory monitoring, which allows ECG monitoring over long periods, is a vital diagnostic tool. There are currently three types of ambulatory monitors: Holter monitors, which continuously record the ECG for 24 to 48 hours; event recorders, which are wearable loop recorders that record only during specific events (when the patient activates the recorder because of symptoms or the recorder detects a heart rate above or below a specified threshold) and can be worn for 1 month or more; and implantable loop recorders, which function similarly to event recorders but can be used for up to 14 months. In addition, home telemetry units can allow patients to undergo prolonged continuous remote monitoring by wireless or Internet connections. The choice of ambulatory monitoring method is largely determined by the frequency of the symptoms and the likelihood of capturing an episode during a given monitoring period.

Ambulatory monitoring is diagnostic only if abnormalities occur during symptoms or if the patient has typical symptoms without any concurrent abnormalities. A "normal" monitoring record is nondiagnostic if the patient does not have symptoms during the period.

Holter Monitors

Holter monitors use either a tape (in older devices) or digital media (in newer devices) to record a 3-, 5-, or 12-lead surface ECG continuously, usually for 24 to 48 hours but for 3 weeks or more when indicated. Processing, printing, and analysis of the recordings are performed offline with commercial systems.

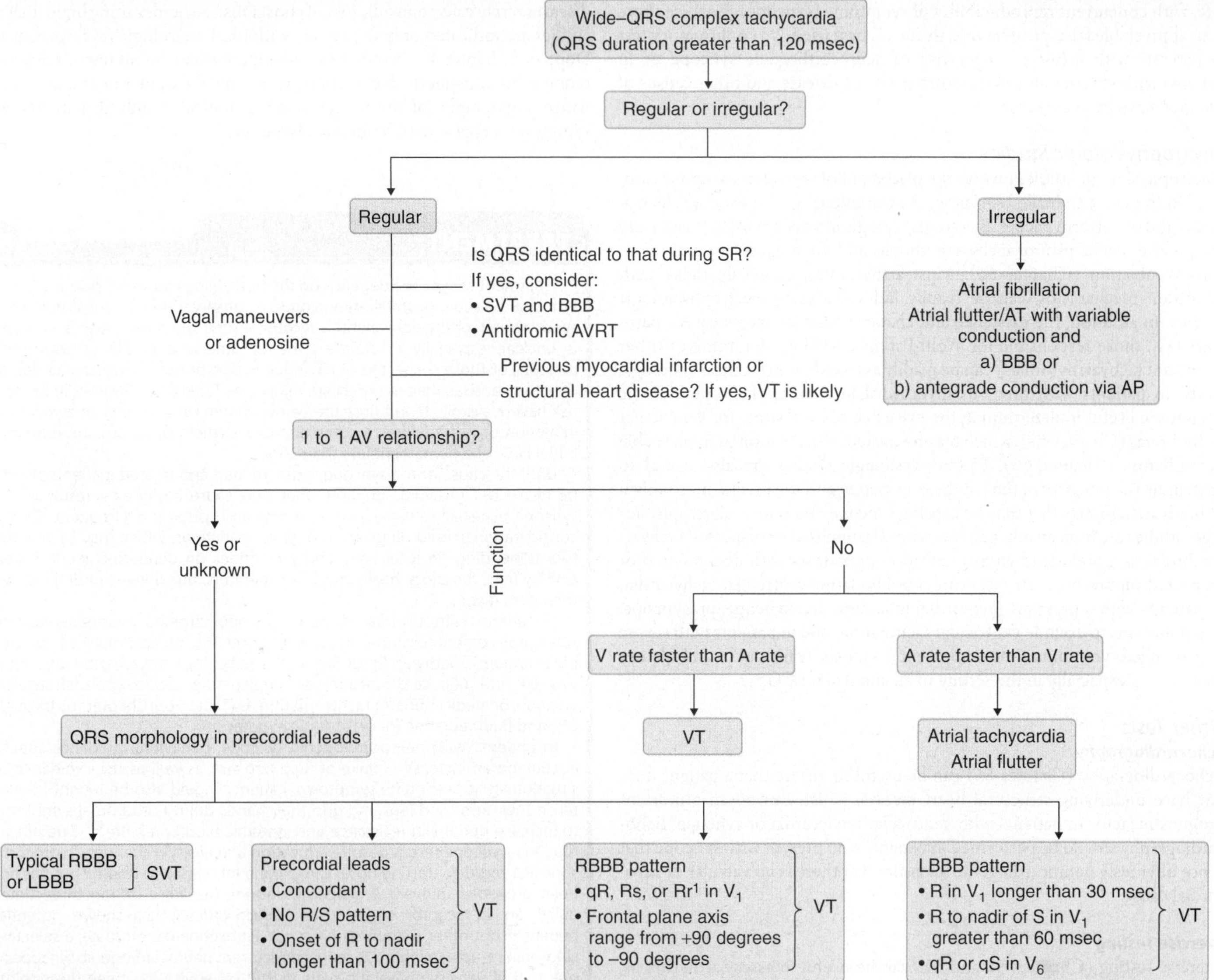

FIGURE 62-3. **ECG algorithm for diagnosis of wide-complex tachycardias. A = atrial; AP = accessory pathway; AT = atrial tachycardia; AV = atrioventricular; AVRT = atrioventricular reciprocating tachycardia; BBB = bundle branch block; LBBB = left bundle branch block; RBBB = right bundle branch block; SR = sinus rhythm; SVT = supraventricular tachycardia; V = ventricular; VT = ventricular tachycardia. (From Blomstrom-Lundqvist C, Scheinman MM, Aliot EM, et al. ACC/AHA/ESC guidelines for the management of patients with supraventricular arrhythmias—executive summary. *Circulation.* 2003;108:1871-1909.)**

In addition to recording the rhythm, analyses of heart rate variability and ST segment changes and accurate counts of PACs and PVCs can be automated. Some systems allow extrapolation to produce a "virtual" 12-lead recording at any time during the monitoring period. Holter monitoring is useful for detecting symptoms that are frequent (multiple times daily) and for diagnosing sinus node dysfunction (sinus node arrest, sick sinus syndrome) or intermittent AV block. It can also be useful to assess the adequacy of ventricular rate control in a patient with atrial fibrillation.

Event Monitors

Event monitors, also known as loop recorders, are designed to record intermittent episodes during long periods (weeks to months) and are thus useful for patients with less frequent symptoms. The system records the ECG into a loop buffer that is continuously updated and overwritten. The duration of memory varies from a few seconds to a few minutes and is usually programmable. When activated, the information is "locked" into memory and continues to record forward for a preprogrammed amount of time. Newer systems allow both patient-activated (when symptoms occur) and event-triggered (when the heart rate is above or below a preset threshold) recording. Some recorders have algorithms to detect and record atrial fibrillation automatically, regardless of the heart rate. After episodes have been recorded, the patient transmits the recording over the telephone to centralized receivers. Newer systems use cell-phone technology to transmit the data automatically. Some event monitors require leads similar to Holter monitors, whereas others are worn on the wrist or are put into small credit card–sized devices that are placed on the chest during symptoms. The latter type is useful only in patients whose symptoms last for several minutes and who do not have syncope.

Implantable Loop Recorders

Implantable loop recorders are small devices with integrated leads that are implanted in a small subcutaneous pocket during a simple surgery, usually performed in the electrophysiology laboratory. They function similarly to event recorders in terms of recording ECGs. Patients can activate the device with a small transmitter, or the device can be autotriggered on the basis of preprogrammed heart rates. The device can be interrogated by a computer, similar to the way pacemakers are interrogated to program the device's parameters and to retrieve ECGs that have been recorded. In patients with recurrent, difficult-to-diagnose syncope, an implantable loop recorder is better than the combination of tilt testing, an external loop recorder, and electrophysiologic testing.[A1]

Tilt Table Testing

Tilt table testing is used to confirm the diagnosis of neurocardiogenic syncope. The test involves continuous heart rate and blood pressure monitoring during head-up tilting. After baseline measurements in the supine position, the patient is tilted head-up at 60 to 80 degrees for 60 minutes. Some laboratories use isoproterenol or nitroglycerin as additional provocation. A positive result is a sudden and precipitous fall in blood pressure and heart rate, with concurrent reproducibility of symptoms (syncope). Because there is an appreciable false-positive rate, the test is best used as a confirmatory test in patients with a history suggestive of neurocardiogenic syncope or in patients with syncope in whom structural heart disease and other causes of syncope have been excluded.

Electrophysiologic Studies

Electrophysiologic studies involve the placement of several transvenous catheters in the heart to make temporary measurements of intracardiac electrograms and to perform pacing. Electrophysiologic studies are useful to identify the precise mechanism of tachyarrhythmias and are a necessary prelude to curative ablation (Chapter 66). Most arrhythmias, especially those with re-entrant mechanisms, can be readily induced during electrophysiologic studies. In addition, the existence and characteristics of accessory AV pathways (i.e., those responsible for Wolff-Parkinson-White syndrome or other re-entrant tachyarrhythmias) can be readily assessed by an electrophysiologic study. In patients with previous myocardial infarction, electrophysiologic studies are useful in determining the existence of a substrate for ventricular arrhythmias (Chapter 65), which may be treated with ablation or implantable defibrillators (Chapter 66). Electrophysiologic studies are also useful to determine the integrity of the conduction system and the precise mechanism of bradyarrhythmias that may be causing syncope. Therefore, electrophysiologic studies are indicated in patients with documented or suspected tachyarrhythmias as a prelude to curative ablation in patients with documented or suspected supraventricular tachycardia or idiopathic ventricular tachycardia; in patients with a previous myocardial infarction and syncope, presyncope, or palpitations to exclude ventricular tachycardia; and in patients with severe or prolonged symptoms and no apparent diagnosis by history or ambulatory monitoring, especially in the setting of an abnormal ECG.

Other Tests

Echocardiography

Echocardiography (Chapter 55) can be useful to ensure that a patient does not have underlying structural heart disease, which can be an important prognostic factor in patients with ventricular tachycardia or syncope. Echocardiography should be performed in patients who present with syncope that is not obviously neurocardiogenic to ensure that there is no valvular or myocardial cause.

Exercise Testing

Exercise testing (Chapters 51 and 71) can be useful to assess arrhythmias, particularly in patients whose symptoms are exercise related. Exercise testing can also be useful in the evaluation of patients with bradyarrhythmias to diagnose chronotropic incompetence, and it can differentiate AV block due to autonomic tone (improves with exercise) from intrinsic conduction disease (generally worsens with an increasing rate).

Neurologic Testing

Routine electroencephalography (Chapter 396) is not helpful because a single study may be normal, even in epileptic patients. Structural brain diseases rarely cause episodic loss of consciousness, and routine brain imaging studies are indicated only in patients with focal neurologic findings. Carotid Doppler (Chapter 407) studies can document stenosis, but unconsciousness requires bihemispheric dysfunction. Transcranial Doppler or magnetic resonance angiography of the basilar artery is indicated only in patients with symptoms suggestive of brain stem ischemia.

TREATMENT

Treatment of syncope depends on the underlying cause.[3,4] Proximate to the syncopal episode, hospital admission (e.g., observation in a chest pain unit, syncope unit, or the equivalent) is recommended when the cause of syncope is unclear, especially in elderly patients, otherwise fragile or worrisome patients, or those suspected of having a cardiac or cerebrovascular cause, or if the syncope resulted in significant injury (see Table 62-4). Patients at highest risk have a systolic blood pressure below 90 mm Hg, a history of myocardial infarction or heart failure, a complaint of shortness of breath, an abnormal initial ECG, or a hematocrit less than 30%.

Until the cause of the syncope is determined and treated, patients should be instructed to avoid situations that may cause injury as a result of the syncope, especially if there is no prodrome and episodes are frequent. Careful consideration should be given to driving restrictions, which may be mandatory depending on local laws, and restrictions on dangerous work-related activity (e.g., for pilots, heavy machine operators, bus drivers) until definitive therapy is given.

In patients with a cardiac cause of syncope, targeted treatments include valve replacement for aortic stenosis (Chapter 75); medications for hypertrophic cardiomyopathy (Chapter 60); a pacemaker for bradyarrhythmias (Chapters 64 and 66); cardioversion, an implantable cardioverter-defibrillator, ablation, or medications for tachyarrhythmias (Table 62-5; Chapters 63 through 65); and fluid repletion for orthostatic hypotension.

In patients with neurocardiogenic syncope, behavioral guidance should encourage an increased intake of fluid and salt, as well as the avoidance of situations that precipitate symptoms. Patients should also be taught how to tense their arms and legs and grip their hands during prodromal symptoms to increase peripheral resistance and systemic blood pressure.[A2] If neurocardiogenic syncope recurs despite education and lifestyle changes, fludrocortisone (0.1 mg/day, starting dose) can expand intravascular volume but has not been proved to prevent syncope. Midodrine (usually 5-10 mg three times daily), an α_1-receptor agonist and vasoconstrictor, has shown potential benefit,[A3] but other α-agonists have not. Paroxetine (20 mg/day), a selective serotonin re-uptake inhibitor, reduced recurrent neurocardiogenic syncope in one trial of very symptomatic patients but otherwise has been disappointing.[A4] In randomized trials, β-blockers have not been useful. Pacemakers reduce recurrent neurocardiogenic syncope in select patients with primarily a cardioinhibitory component or severely asystolic neutrally mediated syncope.[A5][A6] For example, in patients older than 40 years with frequent syncopal episodes (at least three episodes in 2 years) and demonstrated bradycardia (asystole or AV block) during an event (≥3 seconds during a syncopal episode or ≥6 seconds during a presyncopal episode), dual-chamber pacing reduces syncope by 32%.

TABLE 62-5 ARRHYTHMIC CAUSES OF PALPITATIONS AND SYNCOPE

ETIOLOGY	SPECIFIC ARRHYTHMIA	SYMPTOMS: *Palpitations*	SYMPTOMS: *Dizziness*	SYMPTOMS: *Syncope*	*Treatment*	*Comments*
BRADYARRHYTHMIAS						
Sinus node dysfunction	Sinus bradycardia	No	Occasional	Rare	Pacemaker (if symptoms)	Can be seen in association with neurocardiogenic syncope
	Sinus arrest	Occasional	Yes	Occasional	Pacemaker	Pause >3 sec
	Sick sinus syndrome	Occasional	Yes	Occasional	Pacemaker	
AV nodal disease	First-degree AV block	No	No	No	None	
	Type I second-degree AV block	Occasional	No	No	None	Can be seen in association with neurocardiogenic syncope
	Type II second-degree AV block	Occasional	Rare	No	Pacemaker if severe	Can progress to complete heart block
	Third-degree AV block	Yes	Yes	Yes	Pacemaker	
Tachy-brady syndrome		Yes	Yes	Occasional	Treat tachycardia if possible Pacemaker	Can also be manifestation of sick sinus syndrome

TABLE 62-5 ARRHYTHMIC CAUSES OF PALPITATIONS AND SYNCOPE—cont'd

		SYMPTOMS				
ETIOLOGY	SPECIFIC ARRHYTHMIA	Palpitations	Dizziness	Syncope	Treatment	Comments
TACHYARRHYTHMIAS						
SVT	Atrial tachycardia	Yes	Occasional	Rare	Ablation β-Blockers (e.g., metoprolol, atenolol)* Calcium-channel blockers (e.g., diltiazem)*	
	Atrial flutter	Yes	Occasional	Rare	Ablation Antiarrhythmic drugs (e.g., amiodarone)* Cardioversion (acute episode)	Often difficult to control rate
	Atrial fibrillation	Yes	Occasional	Rare	Ventricular rate control Warfarin Antiarrhythmic drugs (e.g., amiodarone)* Cardioversion (acute episode) Ablation	
	AV nodal re-entrant tachycardia	Yes	Yes	Rare	Ablation β-Blockers (e.g., metoprolol, atenolol)* Calcium-channel blockers (e.g., diltiazem)*	
	AV re-entrant tachycardia (WPW)	Yes	Yes	Rare	Ablation Antiarrhythmic drugs*	
VT	Idiopathic (RV outflow tract, fascicular)	Yes	Yes	Occasional	Ablation	Absence of structural heart disease Low risk for sudden death
	VT secondary to CAD, cardiomyopathy	Yes	Yes	Yes	ICD Amiodarone (400 mg qd)* Ablation	Increased incidence of sudden death
	Bundle branch re-entry	Yes	Yes	Yes	Ablation	Usually in the setting of LV dysfunction and baseline intraventricular conduction delay
	Genetic syndromes (e.g., long QT syndrome, Brugada, arrhythmic right ventricular dysplasia)	Occasional	Yes	Yes	ICD	Not always a clear family history Increased incidence of sudden death
Ectopy	PACs	Occasional	No	No	None β-Blockers (e.g., atenolol, metoprolol) if symptomatic*	
	PVCs	Occasional	No	No	None β-Blockers (e.g., atenolol, metoprolol) if symptomatic*	Benign in absence of structural heart disease
NEUROCARDIOGENIC SYNCOPE		No	Yes	Yes	Behavioral (hydration, avoid triggers, abort episodes) Midodrine (10 mg tid)	

*See Table 64-5 for drug doses.
AV = atrioventricular; CAD = coronary artery disease; ICD = implantable cardioverter-defibrillator; LV = left ventricle; PACs = premature atrial contractions; PVCs = premature ventricular contractions; RV = right ventricle; SVT = supraventricular tachycardia; VT = ventricular tachycardia; WPW = Wolff-Parkinson-White syndrome.

PROGNOSIS

One syncopal event predicts a substantial risk for recurrent syncope. Although syncope itself does not appear to increase the risk for death, patients with cardiac or cerebrovascular causes have higher mortality rates than patients with definable noncardiac causes or those without a definable cause. For otherwise healthy individuals discharged with a primary diagnosis of syncope, the subsequent risk for all-cause mortality is increased by 6%, with stroke increased by 35% and a cardiovascular hospitalization by 75%.[5] Among patients who come to an emergency department, the overall death rate is about 7.5% at 1 year. In patients with inherited arrhythmias, such as the long QT syndrome (Chapter 65), syncope worsens prognosis. Compared with other patients with supraventricular tachycardia, syncope per se does not increase mortality but does increase the likelihood of needing medical or ablation therapy (Chapter 66).

In patients with arrhythmias, a key issue is whether they should be allowed to drive a motor vehicle. Consensus recommendations vary depending on the arrhythmia and its treatment (Table 62-6).[6]

TABLE 62-6 DRIVING IN PATIENTS WITH ARRHYTHMIAS

CARDIOVASCULAR DISORDER	DRIVING RESTRICTION
SVT: atrial fibrillation, atrial flutter, narrow complex SVT, wide complex SVT	No driving if symptomatic Can drive if asymptomatic for 1 month (3-6 months for wide complex SVT)
VT, VF	No driving for 6 months
Bradyarrhythmias	No restriction if asymptomatic; no driving if syncope occurs
After successful catheter ablation	Can drive after recovery from procedure
After pacemaker implantation	No driving for 1 week (4 weeks for commercial drivers)
After ICD implantation	No driving for 6 months (barred from commercial driving)

ICD = implantable cardioverter-defibrillator; SVT = supraventricular tachycardia; VF = ventricular fibrillator; VT = ventricular tachycardia.
Adapted from Banning AS, Ng GA. Driving and arrhythmia: a review of scientific basis for international guidelines. *Eur Heart J.* 2013;34:236-244.

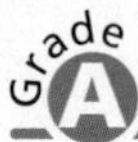

Grade A References

A1. Krahn AD, Klein GJ, Yee R, et al. Randomized assessment of syncope trial: conventional diagnostic testing versus a prolonged monitoring strategy. *Circulation*. 2001;104:46-54.

A2. van Dijk N, Quartieri F, Blanc JJ, et al. Effectiveness of physical counterpressure maneuvers in preventing vasovagal syncope: the Physical Counterpressure Manoeuvres Trial (PC-Trial). *J Am Coll Cardiol*. 2006;48:1652-1657.

A3. Izcovich A, Gonzalez Malla C, Manzotti M, et al. Midodrine for orthostatic hypotension and recurrent reflex syncope: A systematic review. *Neurology*. 2014;83:1170-1177.

A4. Moya A, Sutton R, Ammirati F, et al. Guidelines for the diagnosis and management of syncope (version 2009): the Task Force for the Diagnosis and Management of Syncope of the European Society of Cardiology (ESC). *Eur Heart J*. 2009;30:2631-2671.

A5. Brignole M, Menozzi C, Moya A, et al. Pacemaker therapy in patients with neurally mediated syncope and documented asystole. Third International Study on Syncope of Uncertain Etiology (ISSUE-3): a randomized trial. *Circulation*. 2012;125:2566-2571.

A6. Connelly SJ, Sheldon R, Thorpe KE, et al. Pacemaker therapy for prevention of syncope in patients with recurrent severe vasovagal syncope. Second Vasovagal Pacemaker Study (VPS II): a randomized trial. *JAMA*. 2003;289:2224-2229.

GENERAL REFERENCES

For the General References and other additional features, please visit Expert Consult at https://expertconsult.inkling.com.

63 APPROACH TO CARDIAC ARREST AND LIFE-THREATENING ARRHYTHMIAS

ROBERT J. MYERBURG

Sudden cardiac arrest is characterized by an abrupt loss of consciousness because of absence of blood flow owing to loss of cardiac pumping action. If not treated promptly, it will lead to central nervous system injury or death within minutes. Sudden cardiac arrest is often forewarned by a change in cardiovascular status, as indicated by the onset or worsening of symptoms related to transient arrhythmias, such as palpitations, lightheadedness, or near-syncope or syncope (Chapter 62). Other forewarnings may include new or worsening chest pain, dyspnea, or weakness. In individual patients, however, these warning symptoms have limited sensitivity and predictive power for sudden cardiac arrest because they also predict the acute coronary syndrome (Chapter 72) and acute myocardial infarction (MI) (Chapter 73).

EPIDEMIOLOGY

Patients with advanced ischemic and nonischemic cardiomyopathies (Chapter 60), heart failure (Chapters 58 and 59), and certain acquired and inherited arrhythmia syndromes (Chapters 64 and 65) have an increased risk for sudden cardiac arrest. However, most sudden cardiac arrests occur either as a first cardiac event in an apparently healthy individual with unrecognized disease or in patients known to be low risk. The incidence in the general population over the age of 35 years ranges from 1 to 2 per 1000 per year. Among adolescents and young adults, it is 1 per 100,000 per year. In addition, competitive and high-intensity recreational athletes have a low but finite increase in risk for sudden cardiac arrest during training or competition,[1] with estimates ranging from 1 in 75,000 to 1 in 200,000. These risks are higher in males and in association with specific sports, such as basketball and football in the United States and cycling, jogging, and soccer in Europe. In adolescents and younger adults in the United States, hypertrophic cardiomyopathy (Chapter 60) is the most commonly identified structural cause in competitive athletes;[2] but beyond the age of 30 to 35 years, coronary artery disease is more common (Chapter 73).[3] Offspring in families in which sudden cardiac arrest was the initial manifestation of heart disease are themselves at high risk for sudden cardiac arrest as the initial manifestation of heart disease, thereby emphasizing the importance of a careful family history for assessing risk.[4]

PATHOBIOLOGY

In the past, ventricular fibrillation (VF) and pulseless ventricular tachycardia (VT) were the most common electrical mechanisms of sudden cardiac arrest (Chapter 65), largely in association with acute MI and with chronic ischemic and nonischemic cardiomyopathies. Over the past two decades, however, asystole and pulseless electrical activity have now become the first recorded rhythm in the majority of both in-hospital and out-of-hospital cases. These rhythms may also follow deterioration or active termination of prolonged VF by electrical cardioversion. Pulseless electrical activity is defined as primary when it is the initial rhythm noted in patients with predisposing cardiac disorders and as secondary when it occurs in the setting of noncardiac predisposing factors, such as hypoxia, metabolic disorders, massive pulmonary embolism, or blood loss.[5]

Premature ventricular contractions (PVCs) and short runs of nonsustained ventricular tachycardia may forewarn a long-term risk for sudden cardiac arrest, primarily when associated with advanced structural heart disease, but there is no evidence that suppression of chronic PVCs is protective. In contrast, sustained wide QRS tachycardias are of greater concern and should be considered of ventricular origin, because of their potentially high immediate risk, until determined otherwise (Chapter 62). Most wide-QRS tachycardias are initially approached as a medical urgency or emergency, whereas most narrow-QRS tachycardias of supraventricular origin are approached with less urgency (Chapters 64 and 65).

CLINICAL MANIFESTATIONS

The absence of a pulse in conjunction with no respiratory efforts or only gasping or agonal respirations is diagnostic of cardiac arrest. Although the absence of a carotid or femoral pulse is a primary diagnostic criterion for the health care professional, palpation for a pulse is no longer recommended for lay responders. The absence of respiratory efforts or severe stridor with *persistence of a pulse* suggests a primary respiratory arrest that may lead to cardiac arrest in a short time; skin color may be pale or intensely cyanotic. In the latter circumstance, initial efforts should include oropharyngeal exploration in search of a foreign body and the Heimlich maneuver, which entails wrapping the arms around the victim from the back and delivering a sharp thrust to the upper part of the abdomen with a closed fist, particularly in a setting in which aspiration is likely (e.g., collapse in a restaurant).

DIAGNOSIS

Distinguishing Supraventricular from Ventricular Tachycardias

Differentiating supraventricular tachycardia (SVT) (Chapter 64) with either narrow or wide QRS complexes from VT is an important clinical challenge for both risk prediction and therapy. Although it is generally assumed that narrow-QRS tachycardias are SVTs, VT occasionally has a narrow QRS complex on a one- or two-lead rhythm strip, thereby mimicking SVT. Whenever possible, the classification of a tachycardia as SVT or VT should be based on a 12-lead electrocardiogram (ECG). However, a standard ECG will not always suffice because patients with intraventricular conduction abnormalities (such as a left or right bundle branch block) will have wide-complex tachycardias during SVTs, usually with a QRS vector similar to that seen in normal sinus rhythm. In addition, when an SVT is very rapid, a functional bundle branch block may transiently prolong the QRS duration and shift the QRS axis. In both examples, the wide QRS may mimic VT, and it may be necessary to perform an electrophysiologic study to determine the diagnosis (Chapter 62).

When wide-complex SVT is suspected clinically, transient vagal stimulation by carotid sinus massage or an atrioventricular nodal blocking agent, such as intravenous adenosine (see Table 64-5), may be useful for transiently slowing the ventricular rate or terminating an SVT. A continuous rhythm strip should be recorded during administration of adenosine or performance of vagal maneuvers because characterizing transient changes on a monitor screen may be unreliable. Intravenous calcium-blocking agents generally should not be used for the diagnosis or treatment of wide-QRS tachycardias, especially in the presence of structural heart disease, because of their myocardial depressant effects. The exception is when it is known with certainty that the tachycardia is an SVT in a patient with normal or near-normal left ventricular function.

Sustained VT occurs most commonly in the presence of structural heart disease and must be interpreted as a forewarning of fatal arrhythmia in that setting. It is characterized by QRS complexes that are usually longer than 0.12 second, with a mean vector that is markedly different from the QRS vector of normally conducted impulses. The rate of most VTs is between 140 and 200 impulses per minute, but rates may be slower or faster. VT may be electrically stable (such as monomorphic VT patterns at relatively slow rates; Fig. 63-1A) or unstable (such as polymorphic VTs or monomorphic VTs at rates exceeding 190 to 200 per minute; see Fig. 63-1B) (Chapter 65).

Monomorphic Nonsustained Ventricular Tachycardia

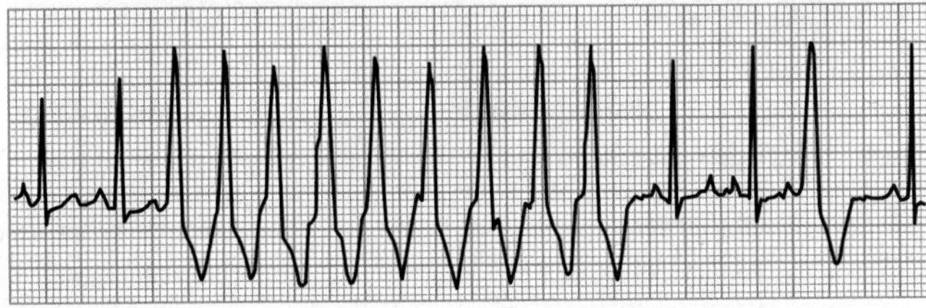

A

Polymorphic Nonsustained Ventricular Tachycardia

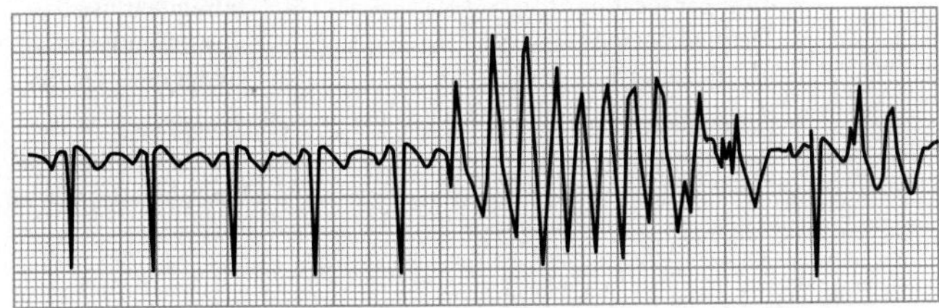

B

FIGURE 63-1. **Nonsustained ventricular tachycardia. Monomorphic patterns (A) are characterized by a slower and more stable electrical pattern than polymorphic patterns (B). Both have long-term prognostic implications in patients with advanced structural heart disease, but monomorphic patterns tend to be more stable over the short term.**

TREATMENT

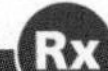

The management of a patient in cardiac arrest involves artificial maintenance of blood flow to preserve viability of the central nervous system, heart, and other vital organs, while striving to restore spontaneous circulation as quickly as possible. These goals are accomplished by assessing the patient and contacting an emergency response team; initiating basic life support (BLS); early defibrillation for those with VF or pulseless VT; advanced life support (ACLS) as needed; and post–cardiac arrest care, the latter now formally incorporated into the concept of the post–cardiac arrest syndrome. In a randomized trial, allowing family presence during cardiopulmonary resuscitation (CPR) was associated with better psychological health among family members and did not interfere with medical efforts, increase stress in the health care team, or result in medicolegal conflicts.[A1]

Basic Life Support

The first action in BLS is to confirm that the collapse is the result of a cardiac arrest. After an initial evaluation for response to voice or tactile stimulation, observation for respiratory movements and skin color, and simultaneous palpation of major arteries for the presence of a pulse, the determination that a life-threatening incident is in progress should immediately prompt a call to an emergency medical rescue system (911).

After confirming the cardiac arrest, the goal of BLS is to re-establish perfusion as quickly as possible using CPR or the newly proposed concept of cardiocerebral resuscitation (see later). The previous "ABC" algorithm of basic life support (airway-breathing-compression) has been changed to "CAB" (compression-airway-breathing), based on the recognition that compression alone is the primary maneuver because the patient is better perfused by minimizing interruptions between compressions and can be harmed by excessive ventilation.[5]

A precordial thump may be attempted by a properly trained rescuer as part of an initial response, although its added benefit is questionable. The technique involves one or two blows delivered firmly to the junction of the middle and lower thirds of the sternum from a height of 8 to 10 inches. A thump should not be used in an unmonitored patient with a perceptible rapid tachycardia or without complete loss of consciousness because of concern about converting cardiac electrical activity into VF, and the effort should be abandoned if a spontaneous pulse does not appear immediately.

Prompt initiation of CPR, which can be performed by professional and paraprofessional personnel, by experienced emergency medical technicians, and by trained laypersons, is the key element for successful resuscitation. The delay between diagnosis and preparatory efforts in the initial response and institution of CPR should be minimal. If only one witness is present, the only activity that should precede BLS is telephone contact (911) of emergency personnel.

Clearing the airway includes tilting the head backward and lifting the chin, in addition to exploring the airway for foreign bodies—including dentures—and removing them. The Heimlich maneuver should be performed if there is reason to suspect a foreign body lodged in the oropharynx, as suggested by severe respiratory stridor rather than by slow agonal respirations or apnea. When the person at the scene has insufficient physical strength to perform the maneuver, mechanical dislodgement of a foreign body can sometimes be achieved by abdominal thrusts with the unconscious patient in a supine position. If there is suspicion that respiratory arrest precipitated the cardiac arrest, particularly in the presence of a mechanical airway obstruction, a second precordial thump should be delivered after the airway has been cleared.

With the head properly positioned and the oropharynx clear, mouth-to-mouth respiration can be initiated, but bystander compression-only CPR is as good as, if not better than, compression plus rescue breathing.[A2] With the exception of Heimlich maneuvers, ventilation strategies are now reserved for emergency medical responders and medical professionals, rather than bystander responders. Devices available for establishing ventilation include plastic oropharyngeal airways, esophageal obturators for establishing ventilation, a masked Ambu bag, and endotracheal tubes. Intubation is the preferred procedure, but time should not be sacrificed, even in the in-hospital setting, while awaiting an endotracheal tube or a person trained to insert it quickly and properly. Temporary support with Ambu bag ventilation is the usual method in the hospital until endotracheal intubation can be accomplished. When ventilatory support is provided by emergency responders in the out-of-hospital setting, the lungs should be inflated twice in succession after every 30 chest compressions.[5]

Circulatory support, which is the primary element of BLS, is intended to maintain blood flow until definitive steps can be taken. The rationale is based on the hypothesis that chest compression maintains an externally driven pump function by sequential emptying and filling of its chambers, with competent valves favoring the forward direction of flow. The palm of one hand is placed over the lower part of the sternum while the heel of the other rests on the dorsum of the lower hand. The sternum is then depressed with the resuscitator's arms straight at the elbows to provide a less tiring and more forceful fulcrum at the junction of the shoulders and back. With this technique, sufficient force is applied to depress the sternum at least 2 inches (>5 cm), with abrupt relaxation. The cycle is carried out at a rate of about 100 compressions per minute. In current guidelines for emergency cardiac care, the integration of respiratory and compression actions was changed to a compression-ventilation ratio of 30 : 2 for single responders to victims from infancy (excluding newborns) through adulthood, and for two responders to adult victims.[6] For two-rescuer CPR for infants and children, the compression-ventilation ratio is 15 : 2. Another recently suggested modification is the "hands-only" (cardiac-only, compression-only) technique,[5] which uses 200 successive compressions without interruption.[7] This variation, which may be more effective than compression-ventilation sequences, encourages more bystander CPR by untrained or remotely trained bystanders who lack confidence and also allays concerns about mouth-to-mouth ventilation of unknown victims in the absence of mechanical airway devices.

Intermediate Life Support: Automated External Defibrillators

Despite the temporizing benefit of BLS, time to defibrillation is the major determinant of survival. Because ACLS strategies are generally implemented by in-hospital personnel or out-of-hospital emergency medical rescue system responders, an intermediate strategy is for nonconventional first responders to use automated external defibrillators (AEDs). Referred to as public access defibrillation or lay first-responder systems, the strategy relies on devices that prompt the user to deliver a defibrillation shock when deemed appropriate by a computerized rhythm detection system in the device. The operators can be trained police officers, security guards, airline personnel, or trained (or even untrained) lay responders (Table 63-1). A number of studies have suggested improved survival rates when such strategies are deployed in public sites,[8] but an initial study of a home deployment strategy was disappointing. Further study is warranted because most out-of-hospital cardiac arrests occur at home. AED programs are not a replacement for ACLS (see later), but rather are an intermediate supplement to the BLS-ACLS sequence that is intended to attempt earlier defibrillation while awaiting the arrival of ACLS-trained emergency rescue personnel.

Advanced Cardiac Life Support

ACLS methods, other than those directly related to control of tachyarrhythmias, are guided by comprehensive protocols to aid responders over a broad expanse of clinical circumstances and mechanisms of cardiac arrest ranging from transient clinical events to end-stage multisystem disease. The general goals of ACLS are to restore a hemodynamically effective cardiac rhythm, optimize ventilation, and maintain and support the restored circulation. During ACLS, the patient's cardiac rhythm is promptly cardioverted or defibrillated as the first priority, if appropriate equipment is immediately available. If cardiac arrest has lasted for 4 to 5 minutes before the availability of a defibrillator, a short period of closed-chest cardiac compression immediately before defibrillation increases the probability of survival.[A3]

After the initial attempt to restore a hemodynamically effective rhythm, the patient is intubated and oxygenated, if needed. Electrical pacing of the heart

TABLE 63-1 AUTOMATED EXTERNAL DEFIBRILLATOR STRATEGIES FOR RAPID RESPONSE TO CARDIAC ARRESTS CAUSED BY VENTRICULAR FIBRILLATION

DEPLOYMENT	EXAMPLES	RESCUERS	ADVANTAGES	LIMITATIONS
Emergency vehicles	Police cars Fire engines Ambulances	Trained emergency personnel	Experienced users Broad deployment Objectivity	Deployment time Arrival delays Community variations
Public access sites	Public buildings Stadiums, malls Airports Airliners	Security personnel Designated rescuers Random laypersons	Population density Shorter delays Lay and emergency personnel access	Low event rates Inexperienced users Panic and confusion
Multifamily dwellings	Apartments Condominiums Hotels	Security personnel Designated rescuers Family members	Familiar locations Defined personnel Shorter delays	Infrequent use Low event rates Geographic factors
Single-family dwellings	Private homes Apartments Neighborhood "Heart Watch"	Family members	Immediate access Familiar setting	Acceptance Victim may be alone One-time user; panic

should be attempted if a severe bradyarrhythmia or asystole is present (Chapter 66). An intravenous line is established to deliver medications. After intubation, the goal of ventilation is to reverse hypoxemia and not merely to achieve a high alveolar Po_2. When available, oxygen rather than room air should be used to ventilate the patient, and arterial O_2 saturation should be monitored, when possible. In the out-of-hospital setting, a face mask or an Ambu bag by means of an endotracheal tube is generally used.

Approach to Specific Arrhythmias

Tachyarrhythmic Cardiac Arrest

Slow, well-tolerated monomorphic VTs, especially in the absence of structural heart disease, can usually be treated with antiarrhythmic drugs or β-adrenergic blocking agents in some circumstances (see Table 64-5). In contrast, when rapid VT or VF is identified on a monitor or by telemetry, defibrillation should be performed immediately (Fig. 63-2).[5,6] When a reversible cause, such as an acute ischemic syndrome or electrolyte disturbance, is the mechanism, normal rhythm can be successfully restored in up to 90% of VF victims weighing up to 90 kg with a DC monophasic shock of up to 360 J, or a with a biphasic shock of up to 200 J, delivered within 2 to 3 minutes. Failure of the initial shock to restore an effective rhythm is a poor prognostic sign. Although some previous algorithms suggested a succession of monophasic shock energies from 200 to 360 J, or biphasic waveforms from 100 to 200 Joules, during a sequence of attempts to defibrillate, there is little to be gained from beginning with energies less than 300 J monophasic or less than 150 J biphasic during a cardiac arrest response.

After a single shock using a 150 or 200 J biphasic waveform or a 300 or 360 J monophasic waveform, the patient should be checked immediately for restoration of a spontaneous pulse; CPR should be continued for five cycles if a pulse remains absent. Subsequently, a second shock should be delivered, followed by epinephrine, 1 mg intravenously (IV). If a pulse is still absent, CPR is repeated for five cycles before the next shock. Epinephrine may be repeated at 3- to 5-minute intervals with defibrillator shocks in between, but high-dose epinephrine does not appear to provide added benefit. Vasopressin, 40 U given IV once, is an equally good alternative to epinephrine,[A4] but the combination does not appear to be better than either one alone.[A5]

SVTs can precipitate cardiac arrest in two circumstances. One is in patients with high-grade coronary artery stenoses, in whom rapid heart rates can cause myocardial ischemia because of the dependence of coronary blood flow on the diastolic interval. In this setting, the arrhythmia should be treated urgently by restoring sinus rhythm or slowing the heart rate, either by medical therapy (e.g., intravenous adenosine, β-blockers, or Ca^{2+} blockers) (Chapter 64) or by electrical direct current (DC) cardioversion (Chapter 66). The second mechanism of concern is atrial fibrillation in patients with Wolff-Parkinson-White syndrome, who may have ventricular rates greater than 300 beats per minute when the accessory pathway has a short refractory period (see Fig. 64-19). This pathophysiology can cause hypotensive VT or VF and requires prompt therapy (Chapter 64).

Pharmacotherapy for Resistant Arrhythmias

For a patient who continues in VF or pulseless VT despite multiple attempts at DC cardioversion after epinephrine, or who has recurrent episodes of VF or VT after cardioversion, electrical stability may be achieved by administering intravenous antiarrhythmic agents while continuing resuscitative efforts (see Fig. 63-2). Amiodarone (150 mg IV over a 10-minute period, followed by 1 mg/minute for up to 6 hours and 0.5 mg/minute thereafter) is the initial treatment of choice.[A6] Additional bolus dosing, to a maximum of 500 mg, can be tried if the initial bolus is unsuccessful. Amiodarone need not be given as a routine to individuals who respond to initial defibrillation with a persistently stable

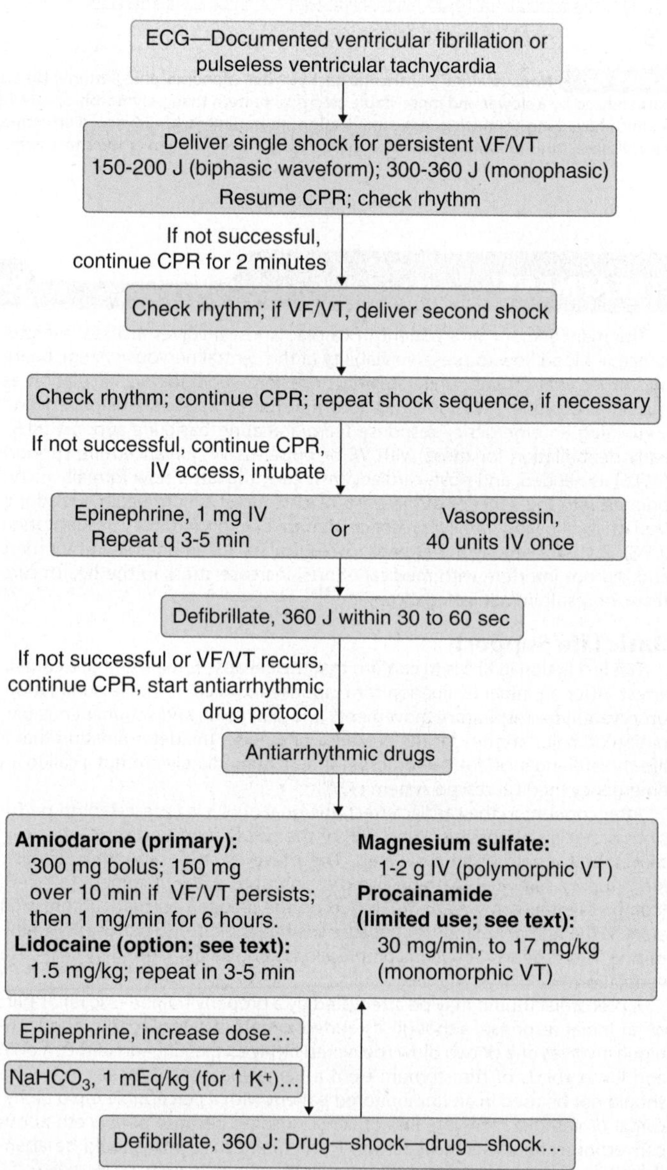

FIGURE 63-2. General algorithm for advanced cardiac life support (ACLS) response to ventricular fibrillation (VF) or pulseless ventricular tachycardia (VT). For more detail, see the ACLS guidelines in the Grade A References. *Note:* In a 2008 advisory, 200 compression-only sequences were suggested as an alternative to standard CPR cycles between shocks, and this approach is under consideration for future guidelines. CPR = cardiopulmonary resuscitation; ECG = electrocardiogram.

rhythm, but it is preferred for those who have recurrent episodes of VT or VF after initial defibrillation and oxygenation.

If there is sufficient clinical evidence that the cardiac arrest was heralded by the onset of an acute coronary syndrome, lidocaine (1.0- to 1.5-mg/kg bolus given IV, with the dose repeated in 2 minutes) may be used instead of amiodarone, or if amiodarone has failed. When acute or intermittent ischemia is not thought to be the mechanism, intravenous amiodarone is the preferred initial drug, but lidocaine may be tried if amiodarone fails. Intravenous procainamide (loading infusion of 100 mg/5 minutes to a total dose of 500 to 800 mg, followed by a continuous infusion at 2 to 5 mg/minute) is now rarely used but may be tried in those with persisting, hemodynamically unstable arrhythmias.

In patients with acute hyperkalemia as the triggering event for resistant VF, hypocalcemia, or arrest potentially caused by excess doses of calcium-blocking drugs, 10% calcium gluconate (5 to 20 mL infused at a rate of 2 to 4 mL/minute) may be helpful. Otherwise, calcium should not be used routinely during resuscitation, even though ionized Ca^{2+} levels may be low during resuscitation from cardiac arrest.

Resistant forms of polymorphic VT (torsades de pointes), rapid monomorphic VT, ventricular flutter (rate > 260/minute), or resistant VF may respond to $MgSO_4$ (1 to 2 g given IV over a 1- to 2-minute period) or to β-blocker therapy (propranolol, 1-mg boluses IV to a total dose of up to 15 to 20 mg; or metoprolol, 5 mg IV, up to 20 mg). $MgSO_4$ is specifically indicated for polymorphic VTs due to inherited or acquired (drug-induced) long QT patterns (Chapter 65). This VT pattern also occurs with marked hypokalemia, so 20 mEq/hour of intravenous potassium chloride should be included in the treatment of patients who have a serum K^+ of less than 3 mEq/L and whose polymorphic VT is resistant to other therapies. However, hypokalemia also may follow the acid-base and electrolyte shifts associated with prolonged arrests and should not be considered a primary cause of the cardiac arrest in that circumstance.

Asystole, Bradyarrhythmias, and Pulseless Electrical Activity

The approach to a patient with bradyarrhythmia, asystolic arrest, or pulseless electrical activity differs from the approach to patients with tachyarrhythmic events (VT/VF).[9] Effective CPR is critical because no electrical strategies are effective for restoring circulation. As soon as this form of cardiac arrest is recognized, efforts should focus on continuing CPR, intubation, and establishing intravenous access. Possible reversible causes, including hypovolemia, hypoxia, cardiac tamponade, tension pneumothorax, preexisting acidosis, drug overdose, hypothermia, and hyperkalemia, must be identified and treated immediately (Fig. 63-3). Respiratory causes of pulseless electrical activity or asystole may respond promptly to appropriate interventions, as do tamponade and hypovolemic causes. Epinephrine (1.0 mg IV every 3 to 5 minutes) or isoproterenol (up to 15 to 20 μg/minute IV), which are commonly used in an attempt to elicit spontaneous electrical activity or increase the rate of a bradycardia, have only limited success. In one observational study, prehospital epinephrine increased the chance of return of spontaneous circulation before hospital arrival but decreased the chance of survival and good functional outcomes 1 month after the event.[10] In a randomized trial of patients with cardiac arrest requiring vasopressors, combined vasopressin-epinephrine and methylprednisolone during CPR and stress-dose hydrocortisone in post-resuscitation shock improved survival to hospital discharge with favorable neurologic status compared with epinephrine/saline placebo.[A7] In the absence of an intravenous line, epinephrine (1 mg, i.e., 10 mL of a 1 : 10,000 solution) may be given by the intracardiac route, but there is danger of coronary or myocardial laceration. Sodium bicarbonate, 1 mEq/kg, may be tried for known or strongly suspected preexisting hyperkalemia or bicarbonate-responsive acidosis but is no longer recommended for routine use. Atropine is no longer recommended for initial management of bradyarrhythmic cardiac arrests because of lack of efficacy.

External pacing (Chapter 66) should be tried for out-of-hospital bradycardic or asystolic arrest, although existing data suggest little influence on outcome. In the hospital setting, external pacing is generally used during the initial response to a bradycardic or asystolic arrest, but it should be superseded by transvenous pacing if the arrest is prolonged, if continuous pacing is needed, or if the external device fails to pace. Unfortunately, an *asystolic* patient continues to have a very poor prognosis despite available techniques.

Post-Resuscitation Care

After return of spontaneous circulation, particularly after a prolonged resuscitation, attention shifts to the elements of injury caused by cardiac arrest. The four components of the post–cardiac arrest syndrome include brain injury, myocardial dysfunction, systemic ischemia-reperfusion responses, and control of persistent precipitating factors.[4] The therapeutic goal is to maintain a stable electrical, hemodynamic, and central nervous system status. Specific therapy is determined by the clinical circumstances.[11] The most pressing issue is the presence of anoxic encephalopathy, which is a strong predictor of in-hospital death and post-arrest disability.[12] To prevent post-arrest encephalopathy, therapeutic hypothermia to 33°C or 34°C is no better than cooling to 36°C.[A8,A9]

During or after therapy targeted to restoration of an electrically stable cardiac rhythm, the patient's general metabolic state should be addressed by improving oxygenation and reversing acidosis. Intravenous sodium bicarbonate (1 mEq/kg), with up to 50% of this dose repeated every 10 to 15 minutes during the course of CPR, is recommended for patients with known or suspected preexisting bicarbonate-responsive causes of acidosis, for certain drug overdoses (Chapter 110), and after prolonged and unsuccessful attempts at resuscitation. Caution must be exercised, however, because excessive quantities of sodium bicarbonate can be deleterious by causing alkalosis, hypernatremia, and hyperosmolality. When possible, arterial pH, Po_2, and Pco_2 should be monitored during the resuscitation. Myocardial injury (Chapter 73) and hemodynamic dysfunction (Chapter 107) are managed by standard techniques.

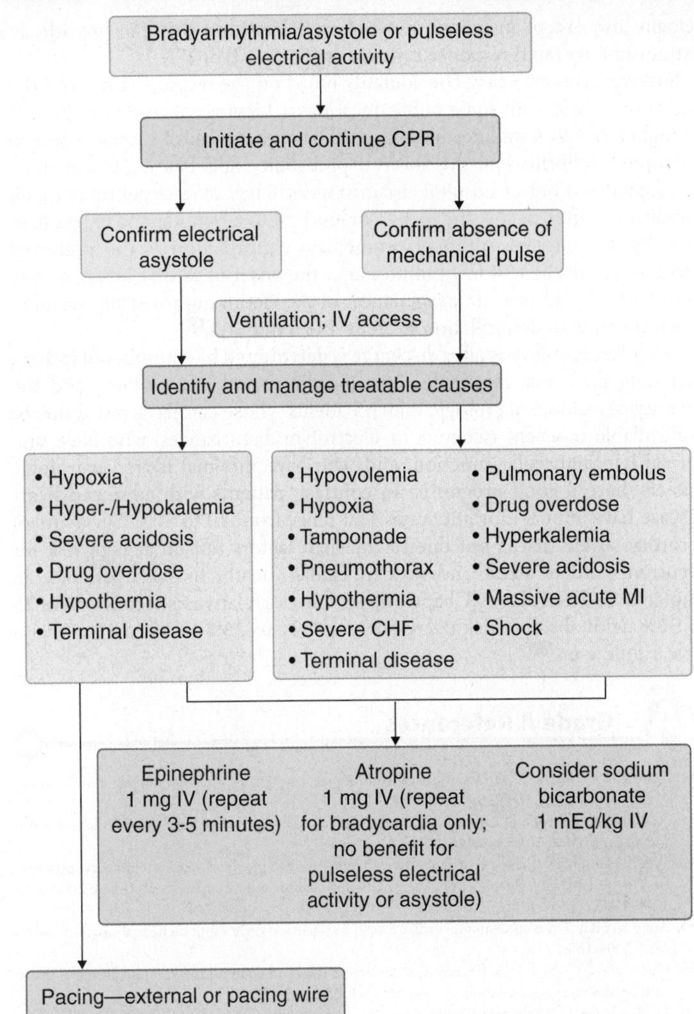

FIGURE 63-3. General algorithm for advanced cardiac life support response to bradycardic or asystolic cardiac arrest or pulseless electrical activity. For more detail, see the Grade A References. CHF = congestive heart failure; CPR = cardiopulmonary resuscitation; MI = myocardial infarction.

PROGNOSIS

The probability of survival after a prompt intervention is about 25% to 30% for VF/VT compared with about 15% for pulseless electrical activity and less than 5% for asystole.[13,14] In the hospital, the probability of survival is determined by the specific patient category (acute syndromes better than end-stage diseases), the mechanism of cardiac arrest (better for tachyarrhythmias than for bradyarrhythmias, asystole, or pulseless electrical activity), and the hospital site (better in intensive care units or other monitored settings than on an unmonitored general care unit). Immediate defibrillation in highly protected settings, such as a cardiac catheterization laboratory where response times of less than 60 seconds are the norm, is associated with greater than a 90% survival rate for VF in the absence of pathophysiologic conditions that tend to perpetuate the potentially fatal arrhythmia. In many acute care settings, including patients with acute coronary syndromes (Chapters 72 and 73), outcomes also can be excellent. For other in-hospital settings and most out-of-hospital settings, the absolute number and proportion of survivors remain low, except in unique out-of-hospital settings that can provide an extraordinarily rapid response time to victims in VF or VT.

Survival rates also vary considerably based on the response time and the site of the arrest, with some public locations achieving survival rates of 50% or higher. If 3 to 4 minutes have elapsed from the onset of cardiac arrest to attempted defibrillation, the survival probability falls below 50% in most in-hospital and out-of-hospital circumstances. Survival rates continue to fall rapidly thereafter, decreasing to 25% or less by 4 to 6 minutes and to less than 10% by 10 minutes. Although immediate defibrillation is the preferred method within the first few minutes after the onset of cardiac arrest, a brief period of CPR to provide oxygenation of the victim improves survivability when the time to defibrillation exceeds 4 to 5 minutes.[A3]

Long-term prognosis after discharge is determined by a number of factors, including pre-event ventricular function, history of heart failure, and the severity of residual neurologic injury. Patients whose cardiac arrest is due to controllable transient ischemia or electrolyte disturbances, who have preserved left ventricular function, and who have minimal if any neurologic defects, have a good prognosis. In contrast, patients with advanced heart disease have annual mortality rates that range from 10 to 50%. Survivors of a cardiac arrest that is not due to transient factors remain at high risk for recurrent cardiac arrest and sudden cardiac death. In such patients, an implantable defibrillator (Chapter 66) achieves a relative risk reduction of 25 to 30%, with absolute risk decreasing from 21 to 25% to 15 to 18% over a 2-year follow-up.[A10]

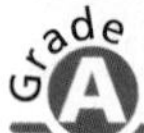

Grade A References

A1. Jabre P, Belpomme V, Azoulay E, et al. Family presence during cardiopulmonary resuscitation. *N Engl J Med*. 2013;368:1008-1018.

A2. Rea TD, Fahrenbruch C, Culley L, et al. CPR with chest compression alone or with rescue breathing. *N Engl J Med*. 2010;363:426-433.

A3. Wik L, Hansen TB, Fylling F, et al. Delaying defibrillation to give basic cardiopulmonary resuscitation to patients with out-of-hospital ventricular fibrillation: a randomized trial. *JAMA*. 2003;289:1389-1395.

A4. Aung K, Htay T. Vasopressin for cardiac arrest: a systematic review and meta-analysis. *Arch Intern Med*. 2005;165:17-24.

A5. Gueugniaud PY, David JS, Chanzy E, et al. Vasopressin and epinephrine vs. epinephrine alone in cardiopulmonary resuscitation. *N Engl J Med*. 2008;359:21-30.

A6. Dorian P, Cass D, Schwartz B, et al. Amiodarone as compared with lidocaine for shock-resistant ventricular fibrillation. *N Engl J Med*. 2002;346:884-890.

A7. Mentzelopoulos SD, Malachias S, Chamos C, et al. Vasopressin, steroids, and epinephrine and neurologically favorable survival after in-hospital cardiac arrest: a randomized clinical trial. *JAMA*. 2013;310:270-279.

A8. Nielsen N, Wetterslev J, Cronberg T, et al. Targeted temperature management at 33 degrees C versus 36 degrees C after cardiac arrest. *N Engl J Med*. 2013;369:2197-2206.

A9. Kim F, Nichol G, Maynard C, et al. Effect of prehospital induction of mild hypothermia on survival and neurological status among adults with cardiac arrest: a randomized clinical trial. *JAMA*. 2014;311:45-52.

A10. Connolly SJ, Hallstrom AP, Cappato R, et al. Meta-analysis of the implantable cardioverter defibrillator secondary prevention trials. AVID, CASH and CIDS studies. Antiarrhythmics vs Implantable Defibrillator study. Cardiac Arrest Study Hamburg. Canadian Implantable Defibrillator study. *Eur Heart J*. 2000;21:2071-2078.

GENERAL REFERENCES

For the General References and other additional features, please visit Expert Consult at https://expertconsult.inkling.com.

64 CARDIAC ARRHYTHMIAS WITH SUPRAVENTRICULAR ORIGIN

PETER ZIMETBAUM

Supraventricular arrhythmias are divided into bradyarrhythmias and tachyarrhythmias. Any rhythm that originates above where the His bundle bifurcates into the right and left bundle branches is considered to be supraventricular in origin.

ANATOMY AND NORMAL ELECTROPHYSIOLOGY

The normal cardiac impulse begins in the sinus node complex, which is located at the junction of the right atrium and the superior vena cava. It then travels through the right atrium and primarily activates the left atrium through the coronary sinus. The time it takes to activate the atria is represented by the P wave on the electrocardiogram (ECG). After depolarizing the atria, the impulse enters the atrioventricular (AV) node, which is located in the inferior septal region of the right atrium, where a delay occurs. This delay allows time for the atria to contract and fill the ventricles. In most individuals, the impulse travels through the AV node over a uniform functional pathway or route. Some people have two or more functional pathways called dual AV nodal pathways (fast and slow pathways). The delay in the AV node represents most of the isoelectric portion of the PR interval on the ECG (E-Fig. 64-1). The usual duration of atrial activation including delay in the AV node is up to 140 msec and can be measured directly as the atrial-His interval. The impulse then travels into the specialized infranodal conducting system, that is, through the His bundle, then right and left bundle branches, and into the Purkinje network. The Purkinje network extends or fans out throughout the ventricular endocardium. Impulses conduct rapidly through the Purkinje network, thereby allowing nearly simultaneous activation of the ventricles. A small portion of the isoelectric segment of the PR interval represents infranodal conduction. This infranodal conduction through the His-Purkinje system can also be measured directly (His-ventricle interval) and should take between 40 and 60 msec. Once out of the Purkinje network, the impulse proceeds relatively slowly from the endocardial to epicardial surface of the ventricles. The QRS complex on ECG represents depolarization of the bundle branches and ventricular myocardium. Patients who have ventricular preexcitation activate the ventricles through an alternative route to the normal ventricular conduction system. These patients have bypass tracts or accessory pathways over which the ventricular myocardium can be activated directly rather than traveling over the AV node and His-Purkinje network. These pathways, which develop as a failure of the normal fibrous separation of the atria and ventricles, are located in proximity to the tricuspid and mitral valves. Direct activation of the ventricular myocardium without the usual delay in the AV node results in a slurred upstroke of the QRS complex called a delta (δ) wave (E-Fig. 64-2).

The normal heart rate is generated by tissues or pacemaker cells with intrinsic automaticity. The sinus node cells produce the greatest rate (60 to 100 beats per minute) of automaticity and suppress other potentially automatic (AV junctional, 40 to 55 beats per minute; His-Purkinje cells, 15 to 40 beats per minute) tissues with slower rates of depolarization. The sinus node and AV node are heavily influenced by the parasympathetic (vagal) and sympathetic (adrenergic) nervous system. At rest, the parasympathetic system controls sinus node automaticity. With exertion or emotional or physical stress, a withdrawal of parasympathetic tone and an increase in heart rate, which is then perpetuated by sympathetic tone, further increase heart rate. Sinus arrhythmia refers to the normal variation in heart rate with inspiration and expiration. With inspiration, a withdrawal of vagal tone increases heart rate; by comparison, expiration is associated with a drop in heart rate (Fig. 64-1). During sleep, a dominance of vagal tone slows heart rate.

BRADYARRHYTHMIAS

Bradyarrhythmias may be caused by sinus node, AV node, or His-Purkinje dysfunction (Table 64-1).

Sinus Bradycardia and Sinus Node Dysfunction

Sinus bradycardia (Fig. 64-2) is generally defined as a sinus rate of less than 60 beats per minute. It should be noted, however, that sinus rates as low as 45 to 50 beats per minute, particularly at rest, can be physiologically normal. Sinus node dysfunction encompasses a group of disorders including sinus bradycardia, sinoatrial (SA) exit block, sinus arrest (pause of >2 to 3 seconds) during sinus rhythm, chronotropic incompetence, and tachycardia-bradycardia (tachy-brady) syndrome. Sinus node dysfunction in combination with symptoms such as fatigue, dizziness, near or complete syncope (Chapters 51 and 62), or worsening of heart failure (Chapter 58) is called sick sinus syndrome. The tachy-brady syndrome is often identified by a prolonged delay in sinus node recovery following the termination of atrial fibrillation (AF) (Fig. 64-3). SA exit block refers to the electrophysiologic phenomenon of sinus node firing with delay or block of the impulse as it travels from the sinus node to the surrounding atrial tissue (Fig. 64-4). SA exit block can be first degree, second degree (type 1 or 2), and third degree. First-degree SA block is difficult to diagnose from the surface ECG. Second-degree SA exit block type 1 is manifest by progressive PP shortening preceding the sinus pause. The PP interval following the pause must be greater than twice the PP interval that preceded the pause. Second-degree SA exit block type 2 is characterized by a pause equaling an exact multiple of the sinus rate

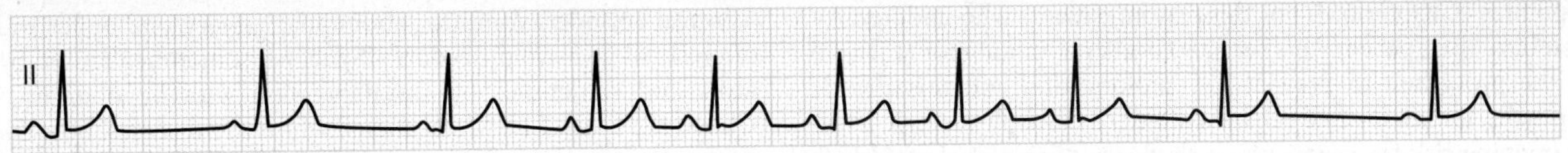

FIGURE 64-1. **Sinus arrhythmia.** Note the variation in sinus rates, which fluctuate with normal variations in autonomic tone.

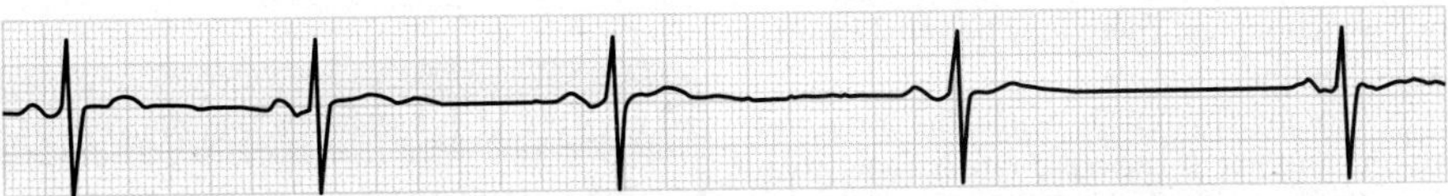

FIGURE 64-2. **Sinus bradycardia.** Progressive sinus bradycardia—in this case related to heightened vagal tone while sleeping.

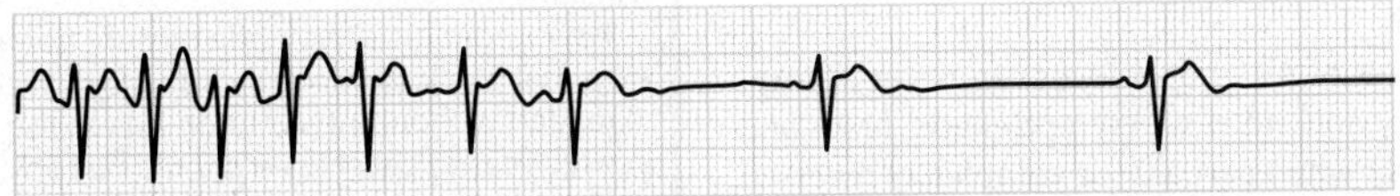

FIGURE 64-3. **Electrocardiographic evidence of tachy-brady syndrome.** Atrial fibrillation with a tachycardic ventricular response followed by conversion to sinus bradycardia.

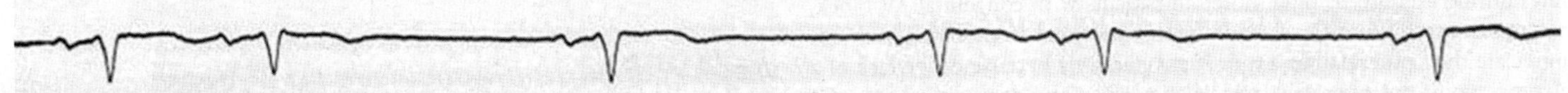

FIGURE 64-4. **Sinoatrial block.** Sinoatrial exit block, probably type 2, is characterized by a pause equaling an exact multiple of the sinus rate.

TABLE 64-1 BRADYCARDIAS

SINUS NODE DYSFUNCTION
Sinus bradycardia < 45 beats/min
Sinoatrial exit block
First-degree
Second-degree
Third-degree
Sinus arrest
Bradycardia-tachycardia syndrome
ATRIOVENTRICULAR BLOCK
First-degree
Second-degree
Mobitz type I (Wenckebach phenomenon)
Mobitz type II
Higher degree (e.g., 2 : 1, 3 : 1)
Third-degree
Atrioventricular node
His-Purkinje system

(i.e., constant PP interval before and after the pause). High-degree SA exit block refers to the absence of multiple P waves with a pause still corresponding to an absolute multiple of the underlying PP intervals, and third-degree AV block results in a complete absence of sinus P waves.

Chronotropic incompetence refers to the inability to increase the sinus rate appropriately in response to exercise or other physiologic demand. In most patients, chronotropic incompetence is manifest by a maximal heart rate of less than 100 beats per minute.

ATRIOVENTRICULAR CONDUCTION DISTURBANCES

AV conduction disturbances refer to abnormal conduction in the AV node or in the His-Purkinje system (HPS) below the AV node. Electrical transmission through the AV conduction system is primarily limited by the AV node, which conducts in a decremental fashion to prevent excessively rapid conduction to the ventricles. The normal AV node rarely conducts faster than 200 beats per minute and slows with aging. The AV node is heavily influenced by autonomic tone and may conduct more than 200 beats per minute in the presence of heightened sympathetic and withdrawal of parasympathetic tone. Conduction through the HPS system is faster and nondecremental.

The AV blocks are classified as first, second, high, and third degree. First-degree AV block is a misnomer because nothing is actually blocked—rather,

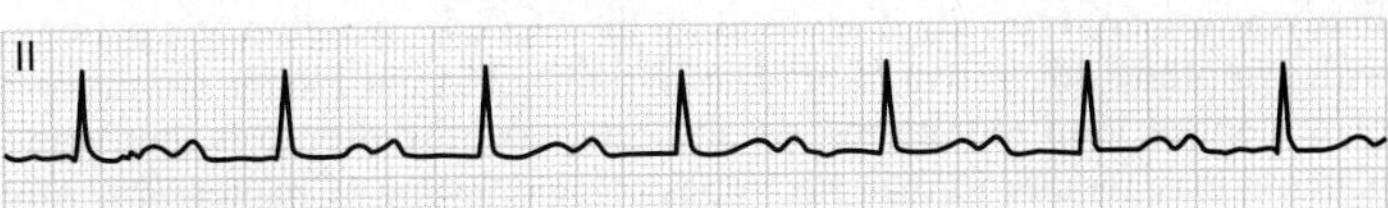

FIGURE 64-5. **First-degree atrioventricular (AV) block.** Note the prolonged (>200 msec) AV conduction.

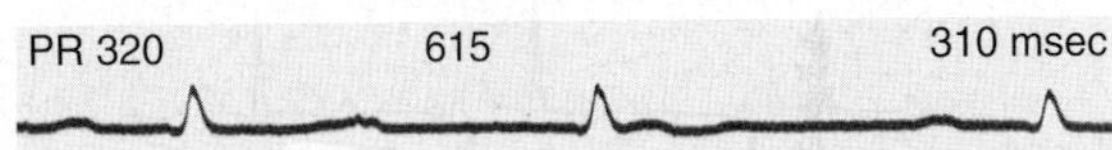

FIGURE 64-6. **Mobitz I block.** Progressive PR prolongation from 320 to 615 msec, followed by a blocked P wave. The subsequent conducted PR interval is less than the PR interval before the dropped P wave.

there is delay, usually in the AV node, manifest by a prolonged PR interval (Fig. 64-5). Second-degree AV block is divided into Mobitz type I (Wenckebach) or Mobitz type II. Mobitz type I is defined by progressive PR prolongation with eventual block after a P wave (Fig. 64-6). The initial PR prolongation is longest, the subsequent RR intervals shorten, and the PR interval following the blocked P wave is shorter than the last conducted PR interval before the blocked P wave. Mobitz type I usually occurs in the AV node. Mobitz type II, which is characterized by the abrupt failure of conduction after a P wave without preceding PR prolongation, usually represents conduction disease below the AV node. In patients with 2 : 1 block (two P waves for every QRS), it can be difficult to determine whether the block is Mobitz I in the AV node or Mobitz II below the AV node. Clues to conduction disease in the AV node include a prolonged PR interval (i.e., more than 300 msec) and a narrow QRS duration. Clues to conduction disease below the node include a normal PR interval but with bundle branch block (Fig. 64-7).

High-degree or advanced AV block, which is a form of second-degree block with multiple or successive nonconducted P waves, or both (Fig. 64-8), frequently recurs or persists. Third-degree block (or complete heart block) refers to a rhythm in which the atrial and ventricular activity occur independently, and the atrial rate usually exceeds the ventricular rate. Third-degree heart block can be seen with sinus rhythm or any atrial tachyarrhythmia with a regular escape rhythm in the AV junction or below (Fig. 64-9). Sometimes there is no escape rhythm, and heart block results in asystole. Complete heart block, particularly when it is acute and accompanied by an escape rhythm, can be associated with marked QT prolongation, which signifies a risk for torsades de pointes (Chapter 65). For this reason, patients who undergo AV node ablation have their pacemakers set at 80 beats per minute for at least 6 weeks after the procedure to prevent QT prolongation and torsades de pointes. Eventually, the pacing rate can be reduced to more physiologic levels without the ongoing risk for ventricular arrhythmia. Complete heart block and other types of severe bradyarrhythmia may present with syncope if there is a prolonged pause before an escape rhythm develops. More often, these rhythms present with fatigue and dyspnea. The blood pressure is often elevated owing to peripheral vasoconstriction, and there may be renal insufficiency secondary to reduced cardiac output.

The term AV dissociation refers to any rhythm in which the atria and ventricles beat independently of one another. If the atrial rate is faster than the ventricular rate, it is called complete heart block or third-degree AV block. AV dissociation with an atrial rate slower than the subsidiary pacemaker is usually seen with junctional or ventricular tachycardias.

CLINICAL MANIFESTATIONS

Sinus bradycardia and various degrees of AV nodal blocks can occur asymptomatically during sleep in healthy individuals. Asymptomatic first- and second-degree AV block, particularly when partially or completely reversed by exercise, is usually benign. Persistent second-degree and third-degree AV nodal block is abnormal and is often associated with dizziness, fatigue, exertional dyspnea, worsening of heart failure, near-syncope, or syncope. Third-degree AV block with a good junctional escape mechanism that accelerates during exercise, as often noted in patients with congenital AV block, may remain asymptomatic. Patients with congenital heart block may not appreciate their potential for a more active lifestyle because of the lack of a reference point but often feel much better when an appropriate heart rate acceleration can be achieved after pacemaker therapy.

DIAGNOSIS

Bradycardias are typically diagnosed by the ECG. In symptomatic patients with symptoms suggestive of bradyarrhythmia, 24-hour Holter monitoring or prolonged loop monitoring usually can make the diagnosis, but some patients may require formal electrophysiologic testing (Chapter 62). Any bradycardias, including sinus node dysfunction (Table 64-2) and AV nodal block (Table 64-3), can be caused at least in part by vagal influences, such as vasovagal episodes, vomiting, abdominal surgery, and upper and lower gastrointestinal invasive procedures. Syncope, sometimes caused by the bradycardia and sometimes by vasodepression with hypotension, may result (Chapters 51 and 62). Medications, infiltrative diseases, fibrocalcific degeneration, and a variety of other causes must be considered. Lyme disease also is a common cause of reversible complete heart block, usually localized to the AV node.

TREATMENT

The treatment of sinus node dysfunction and AV blocks consists of first removing any medications that may precipitate dysfunction (see Table 64-2). Although some patients will recover normal conduction, the susceptibility to medications usually indicates an underlying conduction abnormality that may worsen over time.

Asymptomatic sinus node dysfunction requires no therapy. Asymptomatic AV nodal block, particularly if the QRS escape complex is narrow, can also be managed without intervention unless the QT interval is markedly prolonged, in which case a pacemaker should be considered. For symptomatic sinus node dysfunction and second- and third-degree AV block, acute management includes intravenous atropine (1 mg) or isoproterenol (usually 1 to 2 µg/minute infusion) to increase the heart rate. Temporary cardiac pacing (Chapter 66) may be required. If sinus node dysfunction or AV block is due to transient

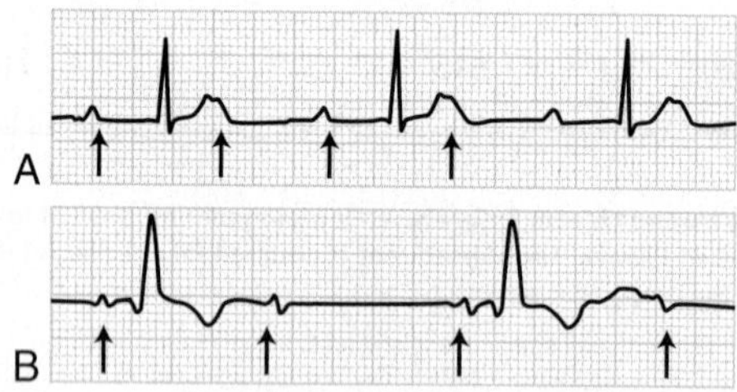

FIGURE 64-7. Two-to-one conduction in the atrioventricular (AV) node and below the AV node. A, Two-to-one conduction, with the conducted beats demonstrating a prolonged PR interval (>300 msec) and a narrow QRS, indicating Mobitz I block in the AV node. B, Normal-duration conducted PR interval and a wide QRS duration favoring Mobitz II block into an infranodal site of block.

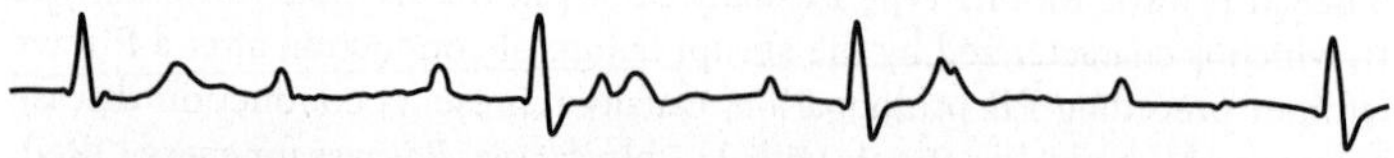

FIGURE 64-8. High-degree atrioventricular block. Periods of complete heart block with three nonconducted P waves (the first of which is buried in the first QRS complex) followed by two P waves, the second of which is conducted to the ventricle with a long PR interval. The subsequent three P waves are once again nonconducted, with the last P wave buried in the last QRS complex.

TABLE 64-2 CAUSES OF SINUS NODE DYSFUNCTION

INTRINSIC
Hypothyroidism
Fibrocalcific degeneration
Increased vagal tone, especially in sleep apnea
Congenital mutations
Scleroderma
Amyloidosis
Chagas disease
EXTRINSIC
Trauma, including cardiac surgery
Drugs
Calcium-channel blockers
β-Blockers
Digoxin
Antiarrhythmic medications (amiodarone, dronedarone, sotalol, flecainide, propafenone)
Lithium

TABLE 64-3 CAUSES OF ATRIOVENTRICULAR BLOCK

All causes of sinus node dysfunction listed in Table 64-2 and also:
Lyme disease
Bacterial endocarditis with abscess formation
Cardiac sarcoidosis with granuloma
Inferior myocardial infarction
Anterior myocardial infarction (less common and often associated with cardiogenic shock)
Congenital mutations (possibly associated with maternal lupus erythematosus and transmission of anti-Ro and La antibodies)
Corrected transposition of the great vessels
Chagas disease
Some neurologic conditions (especially myotonic dystrophy)
Drugs as in Table 64-2

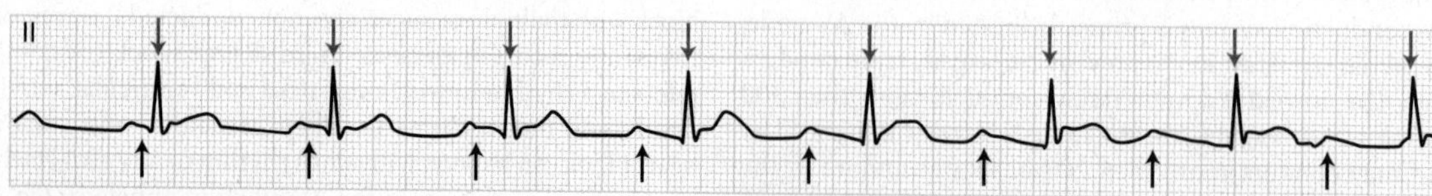

FIGURE 64-9. Complete heart block with the atrial beats *(black arrows)* dissociated from the ventricular beats *(red arrows)*. Note the ST elevation in leads III and aVF indicating acute inferior myocardial infarction as the cause of complete heart block.

abnormalities, such as drug-induced, acute ischemic syndromes, temporary pacing is usually sufficient; however, when intra-His or infra-His block is suspected (e.g., exercise-induced AV block or asymptomatic Mobitz type II block) and the site can be documented with His bundle recording, permanent pacing (see Tables 66-1 and 66-2) is the only effective chronic therapy, and consensus recommendations for pacemaker implantation should guide its use. For all forms of persistent symptomatic sinus node dysfunction or second- or third-degree AV block, permanent pacing is the therapy of choice (Chapter 66).[1,2] In patients with atrioventricular block and systolic dysfunction, biventricular pacing is preferred.[A1] The only exception is Lyme disease, in which most cases of heart block resolve within a week of antibiotic therapy (Chapter 321).

Supraventricular Rhythms with a Normal Rate

Atrial premature beats (APBs) can arise from the right or left atrium or the pulmonary veins. The P wave, which differs from the P wave of sinus rhythm unless the APB originates near the sinus node, always precedes the QRS complex (Fig. 64-10). If the P wave is blocked, however, it is not followed by a QRS complex. A blocked premature atrial contraction may be confused with second-degree AV block, unless its prematurity is recognized, or with sinus node dysfunction, if it is inconspicuous. Altered appearance of the ST-T segment is often a clue to the presence of a P wave. A premature QRS complex with the morphology of the underlying sinus rhythm in the absence of a premature P wave represents an AV junctional beat (Fig. 64-11).

An ectopic atrial rhythm refers to a nonsinus atrial rhythm from a single focus with a single P wave morphology (Fig. 64-12). Wandering atrial pacemaker refers to an ectopic atrial rhythm with at least three distinct P wave morphologies at rates between 50 and 100 beats per minute (Fig. 64-13).

CLINICAL MANIFESTATIONS

APBs are most often asymptomatic but can occasionally be experienced as palpitations (Chapter 62). Similarly, ectopic atrial rhythms, including a wandering atrial pacemaker, are virtually always asymptomatic. Rarely, ectopic atrial rhythm can be very slow and associated with symptoms of fatigue.

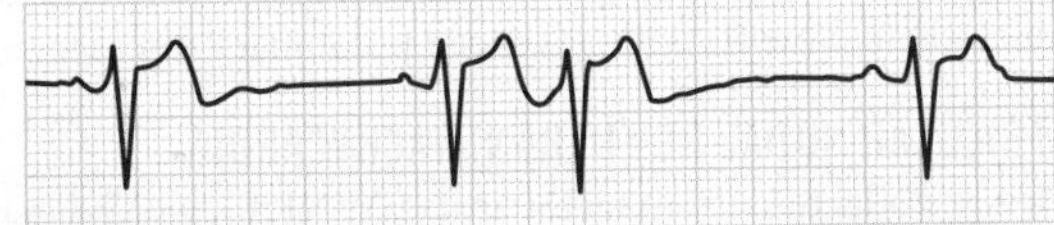

FIGURE 64-10. Atrial premature beat. Sinus rhythm with an atrial premature beat as the third complex in the rhythm strip. The P wave is buried in the preceding T wave.

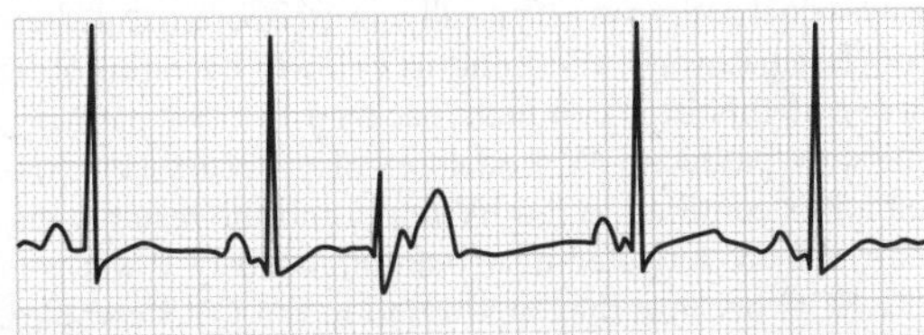

FIGURE 64-11. Junctional premature beat. The premature beat is narrow but slightly different in morphology compared with the surrounding sinus beats. This premature beat is from the atrioventricular junction or slightly more distal in the fascicles. The inverted P wave following the QRS represents retrograde activation of the atria.

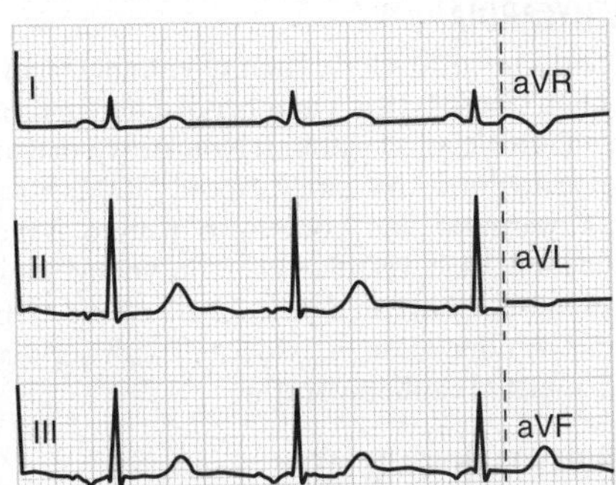

FIGURE 64-12. Ectopic atrial rhythm. The inverted P waves in leads II, III, and aVF indicate a nonsinus P wave originating in the low right atrium.

DIAGNOSIS

The diagnoses of atrial premature beats, ectopic atrial rhythms, and wandering atrial pacemakers are all made by ECG or on an ambulatory Holter monitor or loop event recorder (Chapter 62).

TREATMENT

Rx

Premature atrial contractions do not generally require treatment unless they are associated with significant symptoms. Treatment consists primarily of β-blockers (e.g., atenolol, 25 to 100 mg daily) or calcium-channel blockers (e.g., long-acting diltiazem, 180 to 300 mg daily). Ectopic atrial rhythms and wandering atrial pacemakers are rarely symptomatic and are not treated with medications. Rarely, a slow ectopic rhythm associated with fatigue can be treated with atrial pacing at a rate faster than the ectopic atrial rhythm.

Supraventricular Tachyarrhythmias

The supraventricular tachycardias (SVTs) are defined as arrhythmias with three or more beats at a rate of greater than 100 beats per minute (Table 64-4). The beats, which can be regular or irregular, are usually narrow complex but can be wide complex when associated with bundle branch block (aberration) or conduction over an accessory pathway. Atrial dilation, acute myocardial infarction, pulmonary embolism, acute or chronic inflammatory states, or scars from prior surgery involving atrial myocardium or pericardium are among the causes of atrial tachyarrhythmias.

The most important diagnostic clues for diagnosing the type of SVT include the ventricular response rate, regularity, and, if known, the suddenness of the onset of tachycardia. The QRS is regular during sinus tachycardia, atrial flutter, AV nodal re-entrant tachycardia, atrioventricular reciprocating tachycardia, and atrial tachycardia; it is irregular with atrial AF, atrial flutter with variable AV block, multiple atrial premature contractions, and multifocal atrial tachycardia. Sudden onset and termination suggest acute AF, atrial flutter, AV nodal re-entrant tachycardia, atrioventricular reciprocating tachycardia, and atrial tachycardia. Gradual onset and recession suggest sinus tachycardia, chronic AF, atrial premature contractions and multifocal atrial tachycardia.

SINUS TACHYCARDIA

Sinus tachycardia (Fig. 64-14) is an arrhythmia that is almost always a physiologic response to an emotional or physical stress such as anxiety, exercise, anemia, hypotension, hypoxemia, fever, thyrotoxicosis, or heart failure. It is characterized by a gradual increase and decrease in heart rate and rarely exceeds 180 beats per minute. In rare cases, it may be a nonphysiologic condition called inappropriate sinus tachycardia, which is characterized by sinus tachycardia that develops in response to minimal stress and that continues beyond the time when the normal response would have slowed.

Sinus node re-entry is a rare form of SVT caused by re-entry in the sinus node. As opposed to physiologic ST, it begins abruptly, is often triggered by a premature atrial beat, and ends abruptly. The P wave morphology is identical to sinus rhythm, and β-blockers are the treatment of choice if required for symptoms.

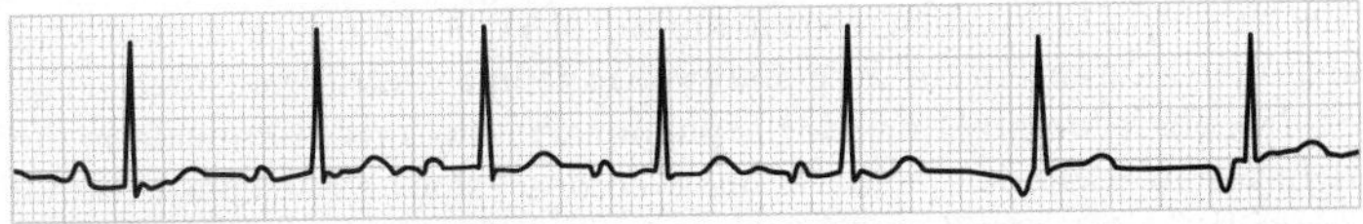

FIGURE 64-13. Wandering atrial pacemaker. Rhythm with three distinct P wave morphologies.

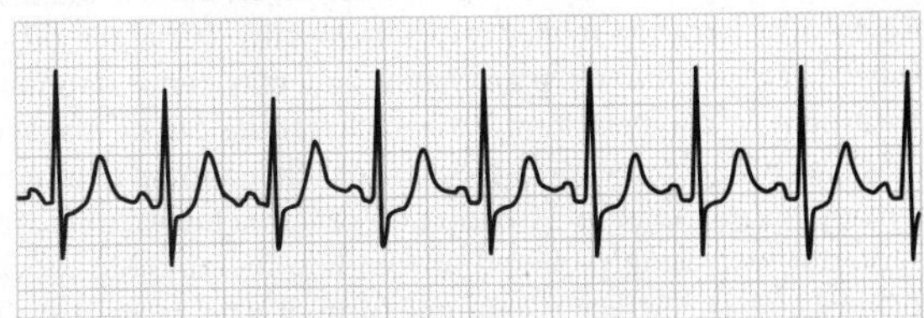

FIGURE 64-14. Sinus tachycardia at 120 beats/minute.

TABLE 64-4 SUPRAVENTRICULAR TACHYCARDIAS

	R-R REGULARITY	P WAVE MORPHOLOGY
ATRIAL TACHYCARDIAS		
Sinus tachycardia	Regular	Positive in II, III, aVF; negative in aVR
Sinus node re-entry	Regular	Positive in II, III, aVF; negative in aVR
Atrial tachycardia, unifocal	Regular	P different from sinus
Atrial tachycardia, multifocal	Irregular	Three or more different P wave morphologies
Atrial flutter, common: counterclockwise	Regular; irregular if variable AV block	Sawtooth flutter waves; regular waveform; negative in II, III, aVF, positive in V_1, negative in V_6
clockwise		Positive in II, III, aVF; negative in V_1; positive in V_6
Atrial flutter: uncommon	Regular; irregular if variable AV block	Pattern different than common atrial flutter (counterclockwise or clockwise)
Atrial fibrillation	Irregularly irregular	Irregular fibrillation waves
AV JUNCTIONAL TACHYCARDIAS		
AV re-entry (using accessory pathways)		
Orthodromic	Regular	Retrograde P in ST-T wave
Antidromic	Regular preexcited, except in irregular preexcited atrial fibrillation	Retrograde P, short RP
Slow conducting	Regular	Retrograde P at end of T wave or later (long RP)
Atriofascicular (antidromic)	Regular preexcited	Retrograde P, short RP
AV nodal re-entry		
Common (slow-fast)	Regular	Retrograde P obscured by QRS or alters the end of QRS (short RP)
Uncommon (fast-slow)	Regular	Retrograde P at end of T wave or later (long RP)
Others (slow-slow)	Regular	PR-RP approximately equal
Nonparoxysmal junctional tachycardia*	Regular, slow rate	AV dissociation
Automatic junctional tachycardia*	Regular	AV dissociation

AV = atrioventricular.
*Site of origin is usually infranodal.

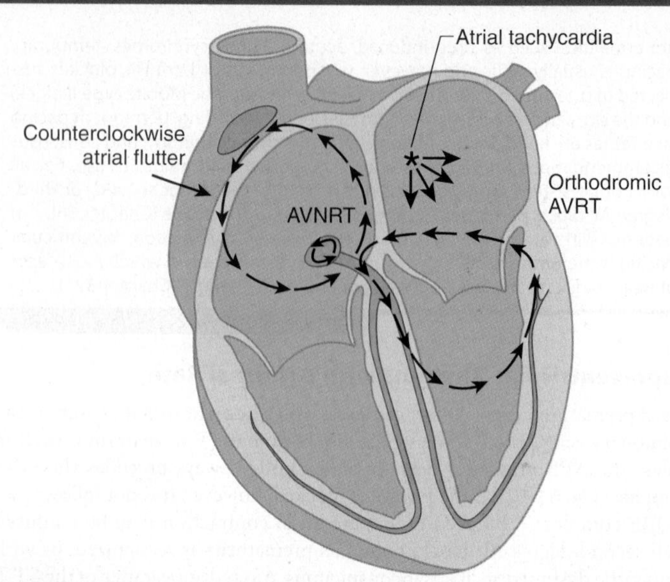

FIGURE 64-15. Diagram of the site and mechanism of common forms of supraventricular tachycardia. AVNRT = atrioventricular nodal re-entrant tachycardia; AVRT = atrioventricular re-entrant tachycardia.

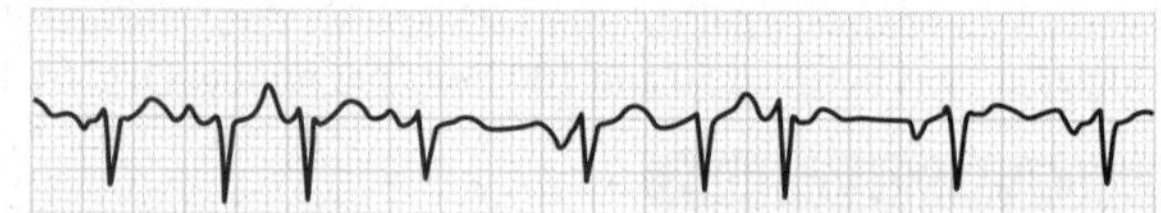

FIGURE 64-16. Multifocal atrial tachycardia. An atrial tachycardia with three different P wave morphologies.

ATRIAL TACHYCARDIA

The term atrial tachycardia refers to a group of SVTs that originate from focal anatomic locations in the atria and propagate in a centrifugal pattern (Fig. 64-15). These locations include the pulmonary veins, crista terminalis in the right atrium, tricuspid or mitral annulus, coronary sinus, atrial septa, left atrial appendage, aortomitral continuity, or regions of scar tissue from previous cardiac surgery. Atrial tachycardias, which are usually regular rhythms that rarely exceed 200 beats per minute, may present in young age but more often develop later in life. Atrial tachycardias can be re-entrant, triggered, or automatic in mechanism. Some forms of atrial tachycardia are incessant and can predispose to a tachycardia-related cardiomyopathy (Chapter 60). Other forms of atrial tachycardia are paroxysmal and may remit spontaneously without treatment. When persistent, atrial tachycardias can be managed with medications (calcium-channel or β-blockers or other antiarrhythmic drugs). Electrical mapping and ablation (Chapter 66) of atrial tachycardia are highly effective and are increasingly offered as first-line therapy. Multifocal atrial tachycardia (Fig. 64-16), which is a unique form of atrial tachycardia characterized by three or more P wave morphologies, is distinguished from wandering atrial pacemaker when the rate is 100 beats per minute or more rather than less than 100 beats per minute. It is an irregular rhythm and occurs almost exclusively in patients with advanced pulmonary disease.

ATRIOVENTRICULAR NODAL RE-ENTRANT TACHYCARDIA

Atrioventricular nodal re-entrant tachycardia (AVNRT), which is a common form of SVT in all age groups, presents most often in young adulthood and frequently occurs after a change in position. It is more common in women than men and may develop or be exacerbated by pregnancy or certain phases of the menstrual cycle. Patients with AVNRT have two functional AV nodal pathways (dual pathways). Typically, an atrial premature beat blocks in one pathway (fast pathway) and conducts slowly over the other pathway (slow pathway). If this beat conducts back up the fast pathway and then re-enters the slow pathway, AV nodal re-entry occurs (Fig. 64-17). This re-entrant circuit is confined to the AV node, and the result is that both the atria and ventricles are activated nearly simultaneously. P waves may not be visible on the ECG because they are buried in the QRS complex. When P waves are present, they usually are seen just after the QRS and have a negative or superior axis (negative in leads II, III, and aVF; short RP tachycardia) (see Fig. 64-15). Atypical AVNRT is rare and occurs with conduction down the fast pathway and up the slow pathway, with a long interval between the preceding R wave and subsequent negative P wave (e.g., long RP tachycardia).

JUNCTIONAL TACHYCARDIA

Junctional tachycardia refers to a focal (non-re-entrant) tachycardia originating in the AV junction (Fig. 64-18). A number of different forms of junctional tachycardia have differing clinical patterns. Nonparoxysmal junctional tachycardia is a benign arrhythmia that rarely exceeds 120 beats per minute and typically exhibits a "warm-up" and "cool-down" pattern. A more rapid paroxysmal form of junctional tachycardia occurs in young adults and is often associated with exercise. Congenital junctional ectopic tachycardia, which occurs in the pediatric population, is associated with very rapid rates and a risk for tachycardia-related cardiomyopathy.

ACCESSORY PATHWAY TACHYCARDIAS

Tachycardias associated with an accessory pathway or bypass tract are called atrioventricular re-entrant tachycardia (AVRT). These tachycardias most often conduct down the normal AV conducting system and back up

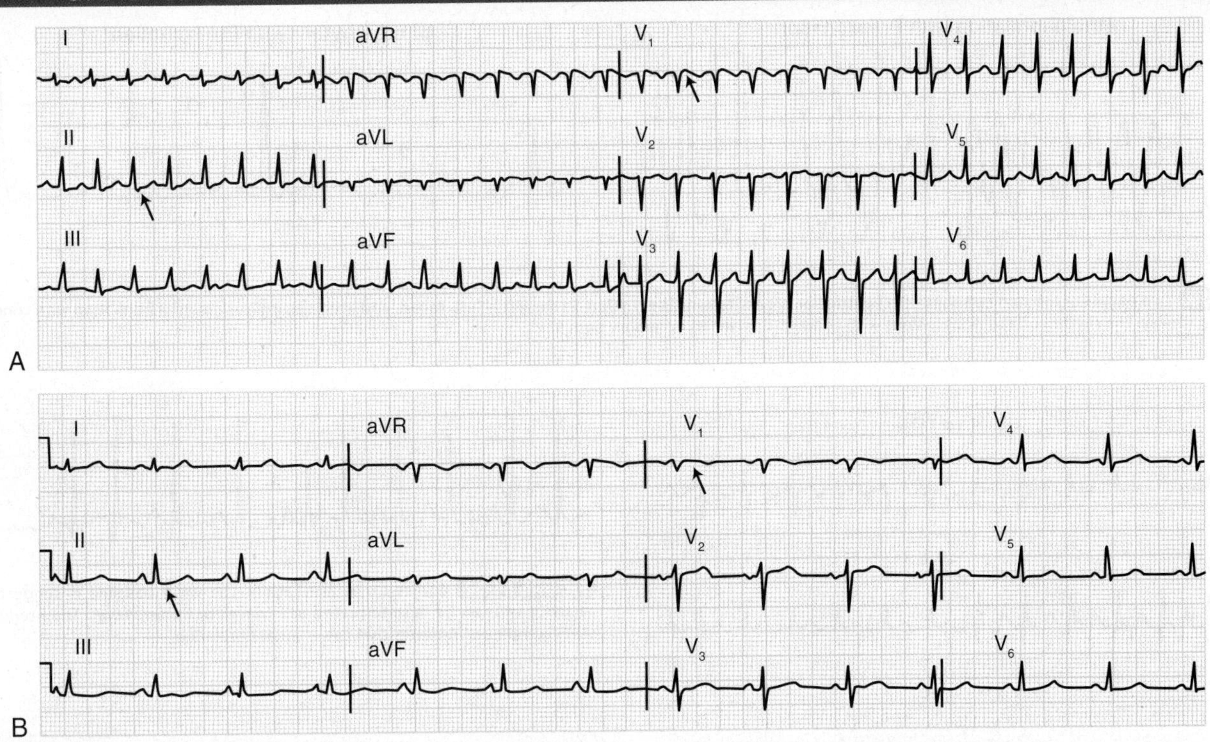

FIGURE 64-17. **Electrocardiograms demonstrating different rhythms in the same patient. A, Atrioventricular nodal re-entrant tachycardia, with *arrows* indicating retrograde P waves (negative in lead II, positive in V_1). B, Same patient in sinus rhythm. The absence of a negative deflection at the end of the QRS in lead II and positive deflection in V_1 confirms that those findings in panel A were retrograde P waves.**

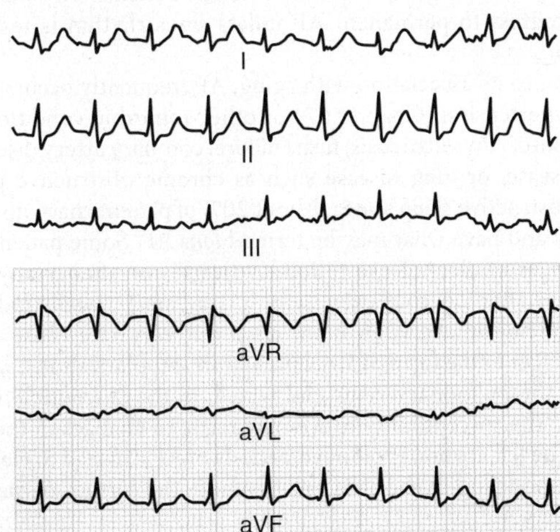

FIGURE 64-18. **Junctional tachycardia. A tachycardia without evident P waves. The negative deflections at the end of leads II, III, and aVF represent retrograde P waves. This rhythm is impossible to distinguish from atrioventricular nodal re-entrant tachycardia on the surface electrocardiogram.**

the accessory pathway (orthodromic AVRT) (see Fig. 64-15). Antidromic tachycardia is rare and represents conduction down the accessory pathway and back up the normal conducting system or, less commonly, a second accessory pathway. Wolff-Parkinson-White syndrome is defined by the presence of delta waves or preexcitation on the ECG in sinus rhythm (Fig. 64-19), in combination with a history of AVRT. It is important to recognize, however, that many patients with ventricular preexcitation never get AVRT. In addition, up to 40% of patients with accessory pathways have AF. Because accessory pathway tissue, unlike the AV node, is usually nondecremental, a rapidly conducting accessory pathway may allow AF to conduct to the ventricles at excessive rates and precipitate ventricular fibrillation. Drugs like digoxin, which accelerate accessory pathway conduction, should be avoided in these patients.

The ECG during orthodromic AVRT can have a narrow complex, but a wide QRS complex will be seen if there is aberration from a bundle branch block, especially at more rapid rates. The retrograde P wave is negative in leads I and aVL if it conducts over a left lateral accessory pathway and negative in leads II, III, and aVF if it conducts over a septal or posteroseptal accessory pathway (Fig. 64-20). The P wave occurs later (after the preceding R wave) compared with AVNRT because in AVRT, the impulse must conduct beyond the AV node and into the ventricle before returning to the atria over an accessory pathway. In antidromic AVRT, the QRS complex is wide with a slurred upstroke and resembles that seen with ventricular tachycardia as opposed to a bundle branch block. Antidromic conduction with AF is often fast, broad, and irregular (see Fig. 64-19).

ATRIAL FLUTTER

Atrial flutter is an arrhythmia with an atrial rate of approximately 300 beats per minute and a ventricular response of 150 (2 : 1), 100 (3 : 1), or slower multiples. Typical atrial flutter is a macro-re-entrant circuit that circulates in the right atrium in a clockwise or counterclockwise loop (Fig. 64-21). The inferior portion of typical flutter uses the narrow region between the inferior vena cava and tricuspid annulus as a critical isthmus of conduction. Typical atrial flutter almost always occurs in patients with underlying cardiovascular or pulmonary disease. It can also develop in patients who receive antiarrhythmic drugs (e.g., sodium-channel blocking drugs) for AF.[3] Atypical atrial flutter refers to macro-re-entrant atrial circuits that do not use this critical cavotricuspid isthmus of tissue. These atypical forms of atrial flutter often occur in the left atrium after mitral valve surgery or catheter ablation of AF. Typical atrial flutter can be recognized by a "sawtooth" P wave morphology, which is predominantly negative in leads II, III, and aVF and positive in V_1 (counterclockwise atrial flutter) or positive in leads II, III, and aVF and negative in V_1 (clockwise atrial flutter).

ATRIAL FIBRILLATION

AF is identified by the absence of P waves and the presence of an irregularly irregular ventricular rate. Coarse AF, which describes the presence of residual atrial activity on the ECG, is generally best seen in lead V_1 with the absence of P wave–like activity in other leads (Fig. 64-22). AF can be present with a regular ventricular rate when there is concomitant AV dissociation (e.g., complete heart block or ventricular tachycardia).

AF, which is the most common arrhythmia in clinical practice, afflicts more than 2 million Americans. The likelihood of developing AF increases with aging, with an anticipated three-fold increase in prevalence as the U.S. population ages in the next 20 years. AF is almost always a recurrent

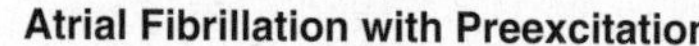

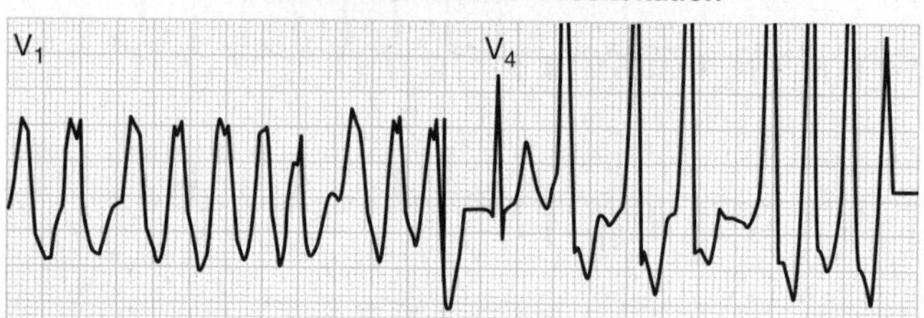

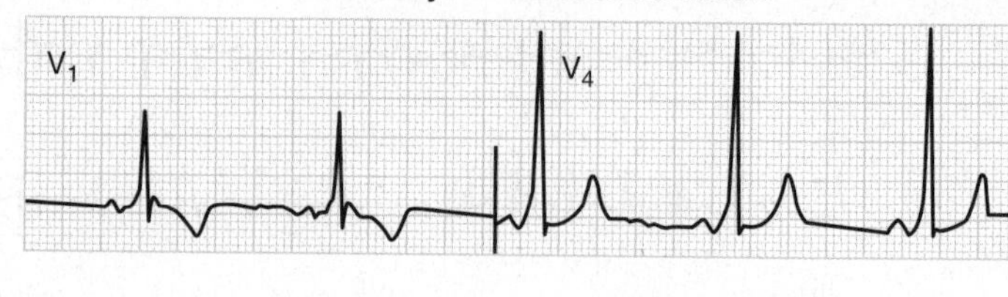

FIGURE 64-19. Two panels of the same patient with ventricular preexcitation. The rhythm on the left is fast, broad, and irregular, indicating atrial fibrillation with conduction over an accessory pathway. The rhythm on the right is sinus with conduction over an accessory pathway.

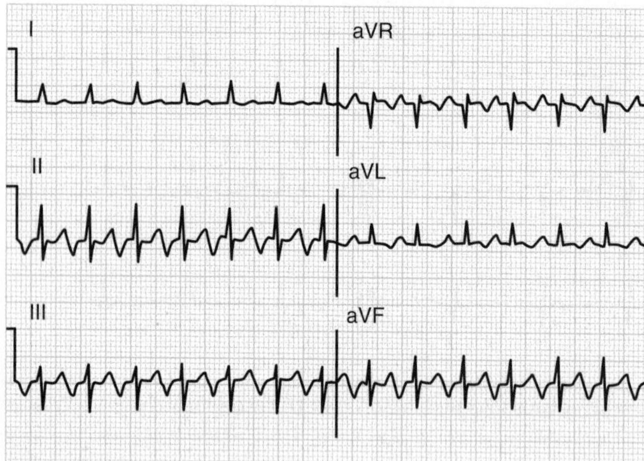

FIGURE 64-20. Atrioventricular re-entrant tachycardia. Negative P waves are seen in leads II, III, and aVF indicative of retrograde conduction to the atria over a septal accessory pathway.

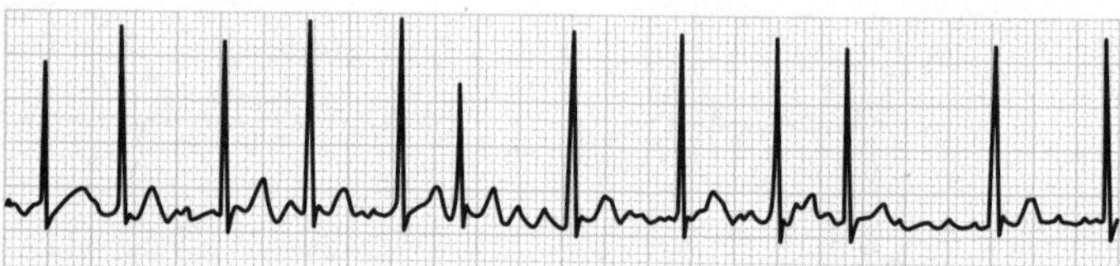

FIGURE 64-22. Coarse atrial fibrillation. The wavy baseline is suggestive of atrial activity and can be misinterpreted as P waves or flutter waves. The irregularity of the QRS complexes indicates that this is atrial fibrillation.

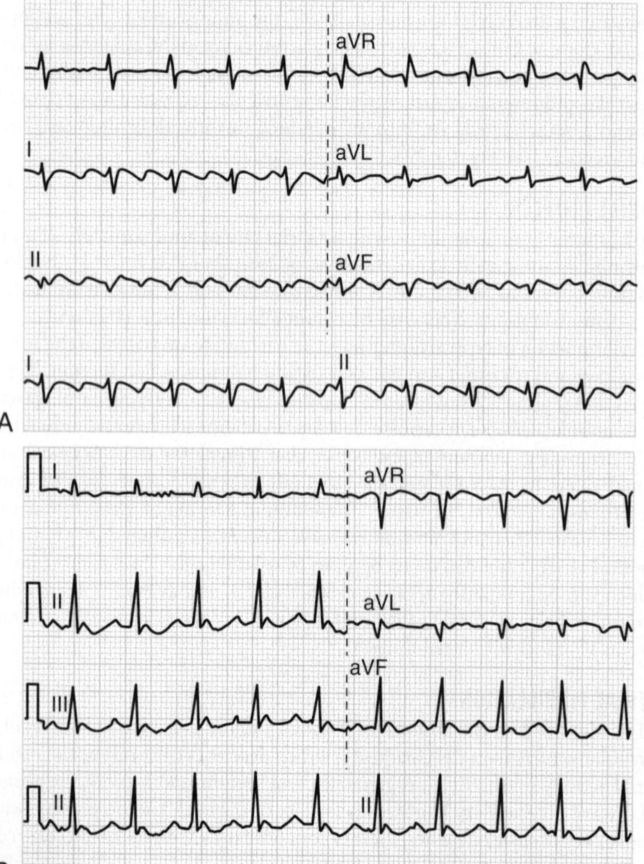

FIGURE 64-21. Two examples of atrial flutter. A, Typical counterclockwise right atrial flutter with classic sawtooth flutter waves seen in leads II, III, and aVF. B, Clockwise right atrial flutter.

disorder, with the possible exception of AF that develops in association with hyperthyroidism (Chapter 226) and surgery (Chapter 433). AF can be paroxysmal (terminates spontaneously) or persistent (persists for at least 7 days or until cardioverted). Paroxysmal AF can occur as self-remitting arrhythmia for decades or can progress to permanent AF. Patients with persistent AF generally progress to permanent AF unless sinus rhythm is restored with cardioversion.

In addition to its association with aging, AF frequently occurs in association with hypertension (Chapter 67) or other comorbid conditions such as diabetes mellitus, thyrotoxicosis, heart failure, coronary artery disease, valvular heart disease, or lung disease such as chronic obstructive pulmonary disease or obstructive sleep apnea. About 20% of patients have no associated comorbidity and have what may be termed *lone AF*. Some patients develop AF after binges of alcohol use ("holiday heart") or after parasympathetic surges such as after vigorous exercise or a large meal (vagally induced AF). Excessive caffeine intake is an often cited but very rare cause of AF. AF requires a trigger in the form of atrial premature depolarizations, which often originate in the pulmonary veins and which, in the susceptible individual, result in AF. The susceptibility to AF may relate to changes in the electrical function of the left atrium. Prolonged periods of AF can lead to electrical and structural remodeling of the atria and promote the further perpetuation of AF ("AF begets AF").

AF results in the loss of the atrial contribution to ventricular filling. This so-called loss of atrial kick is generally well tolerated in normal individuals, in whom only about 15% of ventricular filling is the result of atrial contraction. In patients who have stiff, noncompliant ventricles (e.g., patients with aortic stenosis, hypertrophic or restrictive cardiomyopathy, or long-standing hypertension), however, up to 40% of ventricular filling may be related to atrial contraction, so stroke volume may fall noticeably in such patients.

The primary morbidity associated with AF is thromboembolism. Thromboembolism in patients with nonvalvular AF typically results from thrombus formation in and dislodgement from the left atrial appendage. The risk for thromboembolism is related to the presence of underlying vascular disease but not to the pattern of AF (paroxysmal or persistent).[4] For example, even subclinical AF is associated with a 2.5-fold increased risk for ischemic stroke or systemic embolism. However, the risk for embolization is further increased in the first 3 to 4 weeks after cardioversion, when the gradual return of atrial mechanical function can result in a particularly high risk for thromboembolism. The risk for thromboembolism in AF increases with age, diabetes mellitus, hypertension, previous embolic episodes, vascular disease, and heart failure. The lowest incidence (<1% annually) is in patients younger than 65 years with lone AF. AF is associated with about a 1.4-fold higher risk for cognitive impairment and dementia, with or without a history of clinical stroke.

CLINICAL MANIFESTATIONS

SVTs can produce symptoms specifically related to the rhythm itself, including fatigue, palpitations (Chapter 62), dizziness, shortness of breath, chest discomfort, presyncope, and syncope. These symptoms are mostly related to the rapidity of the ventricular response and are most prevalent at the onset of the arrhythmia. In contrast to other forms of SVT, asymptomatic episodes of AF are common in patients who also have symptomatic AF.

Incessant SVT and uncontrolled ventricular rates can cause tachycardia-related cardiomyopathy, which is reversible with control of these arrhythmias. In some situations, however, the clinical presentation may be dominated by the underlying condition that precipitates the arrhythmia, such as fever, physical stress, hypovolemia, heart failure (Chapter 58), hypoxia, sympathomimetic or parasympatholytic medications, thyrotoxicosis (Chapter 226), and pheochromocytoma (Chapter 228).

Re-entrant tachycardias begin and end abruptly, whether without treatment or when terminated with vagal maneuvers or intravenous medications. An accessory pathway with ventricular preexcitation can be undiagnosed into adulthood, when it can mimic myocardial infarction or right ventricular hypertrophy on the electrocardiogram.

DIAGNOSIS

The first key to diagnosis is the 12-lead ECG. A Holter monitor is useful if the arrhythmia is likely to be detected by 24 to 48 hours of monitoring, whereas a continuous loop event recorder, which can be worn for up to a month and activated by the patient for symptoms, is preferred if the arrhythmia is less frequent (Chapter 62). Another alternative is a device that records data continuously and transmits to a central station, capturing both symptomatic and asymptomatic arrhythmias over a period of up to 1 month.

On physical examination, patients with a blocked atrial beat or AVNRT may have large (cannon) "a" waves detected in their jugular veins (see Fig. 51-4). Carotid sinus massage, which has a vagal effect on the AV node, can terminate SVTs that depend on the AV node as part of the circuit (AVNRT and AVRT). Carotid sinus massage also can occasionally terminate atrial tachycardia but more often will slow the pulse by reducing the number of atrial inputs conducted through the AV node. Similarly, carotid sinus massage will slow but not terminate atrial flutter and AF.

Adenosine (6 mg rapidly intravenously in 1 to 3 seconds) slows the heart rate in sinus tachycardia, atrial tachycardia, AF, or atrial flutter, and can terminate AV nodal re-entrant tachycardia, AV reciprocating tachycardia, and some atrial tachycardias. It should not be used in patients with wide, irregular QRS because it may exacerbate the AF of Wolff-Parkinson-White syndrome.

Electrophysiologic testing (Chapter 66) is the definitive way to distinguish SVT from ventricular tachycardia (see Table 65-2). The SVT can often be initiated by paced premature beats, after which the mechanism and location of the arrhythmia can be determined.

TREATMENT Rx

Acute Therapy

Sinus, Atrial, Atrioventricular Nodal Re-entrant, and Junctional Tachycardias

Sinus tachycardia rarely should be treated directly. Instead, treatment should focus on identifying and treating any precipitating underlying conditions, especially heart failure, pulmonary disease, fever, anemia, and thyroid disease. In the occasional patients who require treatment for symptoms associated with inappropriate sinus tachycardia, ivabradine 5 mg twice daily provides significant improvement and completely eliminates symptoms in approximately half of the patients.[A2]

Multifocal atrial tachycardia is relatively unresponsive to medical therapy, is very difficult to ablate, and is best treated by management of the underlying pulmonary disorder. Nondihydropyridine calcium-channel blocking drugs (diltiazem, verapamil; Table 64-5) are most often used if a therapy is absolutely required.

Sustained or repeated episodes of nonsustained SVT, however, generally require effective therapy. If rapid control is desired (e.g., in patients with myocardial ischemia or hypotension), cardioversion is the best solution (Chapter 66). Atrial tachycardias, including atrial flutter or AF, may also convert spontaneously or convert after treatment of an underlying cause, such as hypoxia or heart failure, or after cessation of precipitating medications.

TABLE 64-5 ANTIARRHYTHMIC DRUGS: DOSES AND SIDE EFFECTS

ANTIARRHYTHMIC DRUG AND COMMON USE	DOSE/METABOLISM	SIDE EFFECTS AND REQUIRED MONITORING	SELECTED DRUG INTERACTIONS
Ivabradine (not available in the U.S.)	2.5 mg starting dose, 5 mg bid for 1 month followed by increase to 7.5 bid if needed	Sinus bradycardia Headaches Visual brightness	Azole antifungals, macrolide antibiotics, nefazadone, nelfinavir, ritonavir
Quinidine	Hepatic CYP 3A4 (70%), renal (30%) Dose: sulfate—600 mg tid, gluconate—324 to 648 mg q8h Dose reduced for renal failure	Thrombocytopenia Cinchonism Pruritus, rash QT prolongation/torsades de pointes	↑ Digoxin and amiodarone concentrations Quinidine inhibits CYP 2D6 and may increase drugs metabolized by this enzyme, e.g., ↑ effect of tricyclic antidepressants, haloperidol, some β-blockers, fluoxetine, narcotics Quinidine metabolism inhibited by cimetidine Quinidine metabolism increased by phenobarbital, phenytoin, and rifampicin
Procainamide	Mostly hepatic—rapid acetylators produce more NAPA; NAPA renally cleared PO dose: 50 mg/kg/24 hr IV dose: 1 g over 25 min, then 20-60 μg/kg/min infusion Reduce dose for renal dysfunction or low cardiac output	Rash, fever, arthralgias, drug-induced lupus, particularly in slow acetylators Agranulocytosis QT prolongation/torsades de pointes	Procainamide clearance reduced by trimethoprim, cimetidine, and ranitidine
Disopyramide	Renal, hepatic (CYP 3A4) Dose: 100-400 mg q8-12h; max dose, 800 mg/24 hr Reduce dose for renal or hepatic dysfunction	Anticholinergic (contraindicated for narrow-angle glaucoma): dry mouth, urinary retention, constipation, blurry vision QT prolongation/torsades de pointes	None
Propafenone	Hepatic: 150-300 mg q8h or sustained release 225-425 mg bid	Metallic taste, dizziness, SIADH Atrial flutter, ventricular tachycardia	May decrease the metabolism of warfarin Increase digoxin levels
Flecainide	Renal, hepatic CYP 2D6 50-100 mg bid; max dose, 300-400 mg/day	Dizziness, headache, visual blurring Atrial flutter, ventricular tachycardia	May increase digoxin levels Flecainide levels increased by amiodarone, haloperidol, quinidine, cimetidine, and fluoxetine

TABLE 64-5 ANTIARRHYTHMIC DRUGS: DOSES AND SIDE EFFECTS—cont'd

ANTIARRHYTHMIC DRUG AND COMMON USE	DOSE/METABOLISM	SIDE EFFECTS AND REQUIRED MONITORING	SELECTED DRUG INTERACTIONS
β-Blockers (selected)	Hepatic, renal Only renal (atenolol, nadolol) IV esmolol: 250-500 μg over 1 min, then 50-300 μg/kg/min over 4 min Acebutolol, 200-600 mg bid; atenolol, 25-100 mg qd; carvedilol, 3.125-50 mg bid; metoprolol, 25-150 mg bid; nadolol, 20-120 mg qd; nebivolol, 5-40 mg qd; propranolol, 10-120 mg bid	Fatigue, depression, bronchospasm, impotence	Minimal, except for carvedilol and metoprolol, whose levels may be increased by amiodarone, propafenone, quinidine, fluoxetine, haloperidol, paroxetine, and cimetidine
Sotalol	Renal: 80-120 mg bid Max dose, 240 mg bid	Bronchospasm QT prolongation/torsades de pointes	No significant interactions
Dofetilide	Renal, hepatic CYP 3A4 CrCl > 60 (500 μg bid), CrCl 40-60 (250 μg bid), CrCl 20-39 (125 μg bid)	QT prolongation and torsades de pointes Three days of in-hospital monitoring is required during drug initiation	Contraindicated with verapamil, ketoconazole, cimetidine, megestrol, prochlorperazine, and trimethoprim Hydrochlorothiazide increases dofetilide levels Must discontinue amiodarone at least 3 mo before dofetilide initiation
Ibutilide	Hepatic CYP 3A4 1 mg IV over 10 min, repeat after 10 min if necessary	Nausea QT prolongation and torsades de pointes Must monitor for 4 hr after drug initiation	None
Amiodarone	Hepatic half-life 50 days PO load 10 g over 7-10 days, then 400 mg for 3 wk, then 200 mg/day for atrial fibrillation Maintenance dose of 400 mg/day for VT Dose reduce load for bradycardia or QT prolongation IV: 150-300 mg bolus, then 1 mg/min infusion for 6 hr, followed by 0.5 mg/min thereafter	Pulmonary (acute hypersensitivity pneumonitis, chronic interstitial infiltrates), hepatitis Thyroid (hypo- or hyperthyroidism) Photosensitivity, blue-gray discoloration with chronic high dose, nausea, ataxia, tremor, alopecia Avoid if identified thyroid nodule LFTs two to three times a year, TFTs twice yearly, PFTs and CXR at initiation and CXR yearly thereafter. QT prolongation expected; reduce dose if exceeds 500 msec	Inhibits CYP 450 enzymes—increases concentrations of warfarin, digoxin, cyclosporine, alprazolam, carbamazepine, HMG-CoA inhibitors, phenytoin, and quinidine
Dronedarone	Hepatic CYP 3A4 half-life 30 hr PO 400 mg bid Improved absorption with food	Reduces the secretion of creatinine without a reduction in GFR Hepatic failure Avoid in heart failure	Increases digoxin levels (dose reduce digoxin by half) May increase myositis with simvastatin Avoid grapefruit
Calcium-channel blocker (nondihydropyridine)	Hepatic Inhibit CYP 3A4 IV diltiazem, 20 mg bolus over 2 min, then 5-15 mg per hour maintenance infusion Verapamil long-acting 120-480 mg qd Diltiazem long-acting 180-300 mg qd	Constipation, rash, peripheral edema	Inhibits CYP 3A4—will increase levels of alprazolam, carbamazepine, dihydropyridine, cyclosporine, HMG-CoA inhibitors. Verapamil (but not diltiazem) increases digoxin levels
Adenosine	Erythrocyte, endothelial cell 6-mg IV push, followed if necessary by 12 mg after 1-2 min	Nausea, headache, flushing, chest pain, bronchospasm (contraindicated if asthma)	Methylxanthines compete for adenosine receptors with adenosine Dipyridamole decreases the metabolism of adenosine
Digoxin	Renal, hepatic, gastrointestinal, 0.125-375 mg/day	Anorexia, nausea, fatigue, confusion, altered vision with green-yellow halos	Levels of or sensitivity to digoxin increased by hypokalemia, quinidine, verapamil, amiodarone, propafenone, renal failure, hypoxia, decreased muscle mass Levels of or sensitivity to digoxin decreased by malabsorption, hyperkalemia, hypocalcemia

CXR = chest x-ray; CYP = cytochrome P-450; GFR = glomerular filtration rate; HMG-CoA = 3-hydroxy-3-methylglutaryl coenzyme A; IV = intravenous administration; LFT = liver function test; NAPA = *N*-acetyl procainamide; PFT = pulmonary function test; PO = oral administration; SIADH = syndrome of inappropriate diuretic hormone; TFT = thyroid function test; VT = ventricular tachycardia.

An acute episode of AVNRT can often be terminated with vagal maneuvers, such as carotid massage. In most atrial tachycardias, adenosine or vagal stimulation (or both) produces enough AV block to unmask the atrial origin of the tachycardia. However, some atrial tachycardias and most episodes of AVNRT terminate after administration of adenosine. Intravenous β-blockers or calcium-channel blockers (see Table 64-5) can be used for the same purpose. For sustained control of the ventricular rate during atrial tachycardia, intravenous esmolol and diltiazem are effective.

Accessory Pathway Tachycardia

The acute management of SVTs that use an accessory pathway (AVRT) depends on the mechanism of the rhythm. If the tachycardia uses the AV node as one limb of the circuit, it may terminate with vagal maneuvers such as carotid sinus massage. If the tachycardia uses an accessory pathway as the antegrade limb (antidromic AVRT), it is important to avoid measures that may accelerate the conduction properties of the accessory pathway. For example, digoxin and epinephrine will increase conduction over the accessory pathway and potentially accelerate the tachycardia. Patients may have an adrenergic response to a drop in blood pressure induced by the vasodilating properties of β-blockers and calcium-channel blockers, particularly when AF conducts over an accessory pathway. As a result of these potential complications, adenosine (see Table 64-5) is the drug of choice for the acute termination of antidromic AVRT, but a true antiarrhythmic drug, such as intravenous amiodarone, or cardioversion should be considered for antidromically conducted AF. In orthodromic AVRT, in which the AV node is the antegrade limb of the tachycardia, β-blockers or calcium-channel blockers can be used as well as adenosine.

Atrial Flutter

It can be very difficult to control the rate of acute atrial flutter, which generally must be treated by restoring sinus rhythm. Intravenous ibutilide is approximately 60% effective for converting atrial flutter to sinus rhythm. Direct current electrical cardioversion, which is highly (>95%) effective for restoring sinus rhythm, should not be performed unless the episode of atrial flutter is believed to be less than 48 hours in duration, or transesophageal echocardiogram has excluded clot in the left atrial appendage, or until the risk for stroke has been minimized by achieving a therapeutic international normalized ratio (INR) of 2 to 3 with warfarin or administration of a therapeutic dose of dabigatran, rivaroxaban, or apixaban (Chapter 38) for the prior 4 weeks.

Atrial Fibrillation

For acute AF without hypotension, rate control is crucial and can be accomplished with esmolol, metoprolol, verapamil, or diltiazem (see Table 64-5); digoxin is usually a third-line agent (Fig. 64-23). Most patients who have new-onset AF who are considered good candidates for cardioversion should be anticoagulated with heparin, warfarin, or a therapeutic dose of dabigatran, rivaroxaban, or apixaban (Chapter 38).[5,6] One half of patients with acute-onset AF will spontaneously revert to sinus rhythm within for the first 48 to 96 hours. The decision of whether to restore and maintain sinus rhythm or allow recurrences or progression to permanent AF is a fundamental component of AF management. Trials of a strategy of rate control compared with a strategy of rhythm control with antiarrhythmic drugs have demonstrated no difference in total or arrhythmic mortality associated with these two approaches,[A3] even in patients with a reduced ejection fraction.[A4] Because a significant component of the adverse events experienced in the rhythm control arms of these studies was due to stroke in un-anticoagulated patients and toxicity from antiarrhythmic drugs, advances in antiarrhythmic and anticoagulant medications as well as the advent of reliable ablative therapies for AF may necessitate a reevaluation of this question.

If a strategy of rate control is chosen, it is important to confirm a heart rate of 80 to 110 beats per minute at rest and less than 140 beats per minute with exercise, preferably by monitoring the heart rate during exercise on an exercise treadmill test or with an ambulatory monitor. More strict rate control is not beneficial.[A5] Failure to confirm rate control can result in the development of tachycardia-induced cardiomyopathy. First-line therapy for rate control includes β-blockers or calcium-channel blockers; digoxin can also be used but is generally less effective. Patients commonly require a combination of medications to achieve goal heart rates.[7]

If a strategy of rhythm control is chosen, many patients will first require cardioversion, either pharmacologic or electrical (Chapter 66). The risk for clot formation must be mitigated before cardioversion in all patients with AF of more than 48 hours' duration. The first step generally is to perform transesophageal echocardiography (TEE) (Chapter 55). If TEE shows no evidence of a left atrial clot, cardioversion can be undertaken without systemic anticoagulation; if the patient has risk factors for stroke in association with AF, however, most clinicians administer anticoagulation during the cardioversion and for the subsequent 4 weeks. If the TEE shows evidence of clot, 4 consecutive weeks of warfarin anticoagulation with an INR of at least 2, or equivalent anticoagulation with therapeutic doses of dabigatran, rivaroxaban, or apixaban is required; anticoagulation must be maintained for at least 3 to 4 weeks after cardioversion. Electrical cardioversion, which should be performed with a minimum of 200 joules, is successful in more than 90% of cases. Pharmacologic cardioversion can be performed with intravenous drugs such as ibutilide, which is more successful for atrial flutter (60% efficacy) than AF (50%). Oral medications can also be used as a "pill in the pocket" strategy. Patients can take a single dose of propafenone (600 mg) or flecainide (300 mg) with a conversion rate for recent-onset AF (<48 hours' duration) of approximately 50% without the need for a screening TEE. Oral amiodarone (typically loaded with 10 g over the first week, followed by 400 to 600 mg a day for the next 3

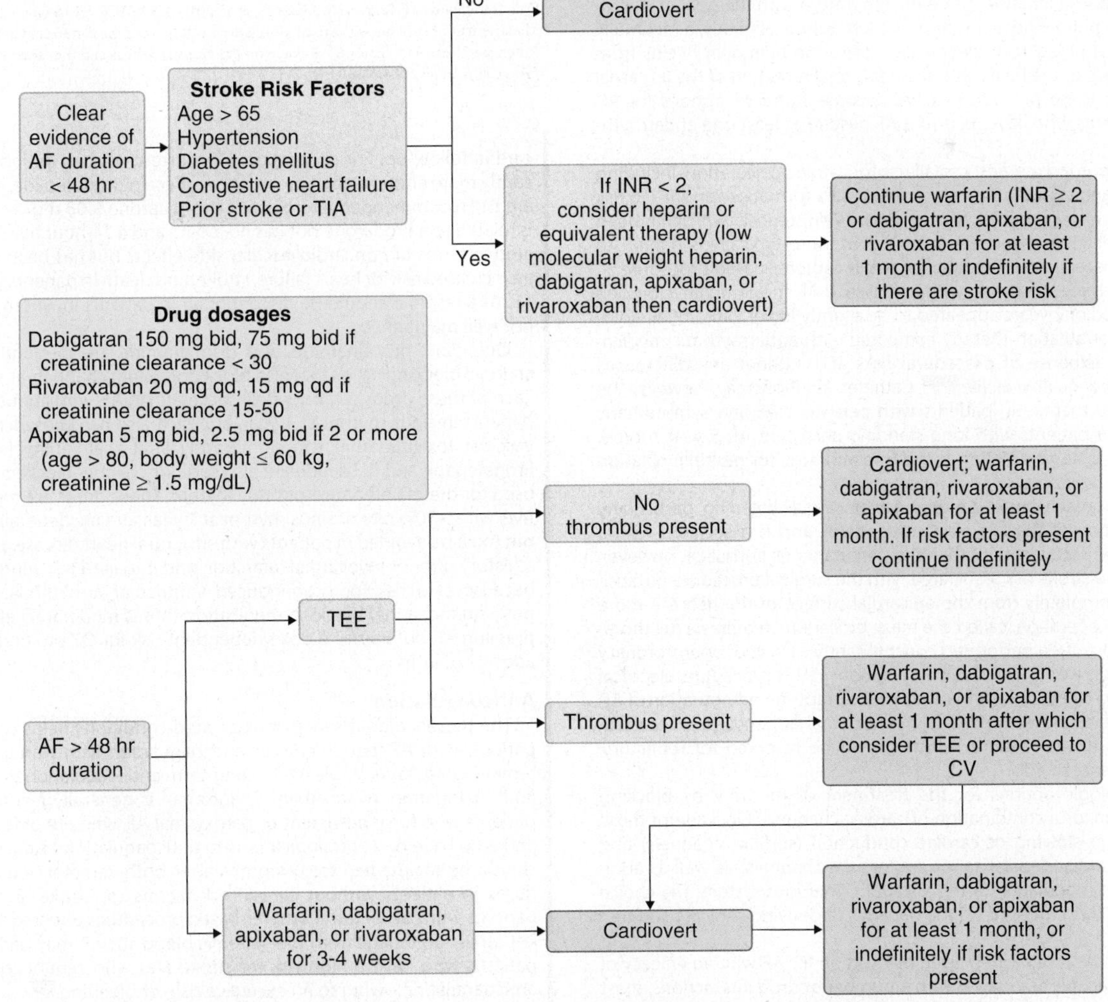

FIGURE 64-23. Management of recent-onset atrial fibrillation (AF). CV = cardioversion; INR = international normalized ratio; TEE = transesophageal echocardiography; TIA, transient ischemic attack.

weeks) can also be used for cardioversion and is successful in approximately 50% of patients with both recent and more prolonged AF.

Long-Term Management

AVNRT, AVRT, Atrial Tachycardias, and Atrial Flutter

Chronic therapy for AVNRT is guided by the frequency and severity of symptoms.[8] Many patients are able to live with this rhythm with infrequent recurrences, which terminate spontaneously or with adenosine. If chronic therapy is required, β-blockers or calcium-channel blockers and less commonly digoxin are used. Ablation of AVNRT (Chapter 66) is highly effective and should be considered before using sodium- or potassium-channel blocking drugs.

Most patients with symptomatic AVRT are treated with catheter ablation (Chapter 66). Ablation of an accessory pathway located near the AV node or His bundle carries a 1% risk for complete heart block, whereas ablation of accessory pathways on the left side of the heart and distant from the AV node and His bundle region is not associated with a risk for heart block but carries a small risk for stroke. At present, it is not standard of care to ablate accessory pathways in patients without symptomatic arrhythmias.[9,10]

The long-term management of atrial tachycardia depends on symptoms. If the rhythm is highly symptomatic, it is generally managed with a β-blocker or calcium-channel blocker. If these medications are unsuccessful or not tolerated, ablation is frequently recommended, but antiarrhythmic medications are an alternative.

In patients with atrial flutter, ventricular rate control is possible by achieving AV nodal block with β-blockers, calcium-channel blockers, and digitalis. However, radiofrequency ablation, which is curative, is now the preferred choice for most patients with atrial flutter (Chapter 66), especially recurrent atrial flutter. Because atrial flutter carries a 3% per year risk for thromboembolism, patients with atrial flutter should also receive long-term anticoagulation similar to what is recommended for AF (see later). If atrial flutter is successful, the risk for recurrence is very small, and long-term anticoagulation is not necessary.

Atrial Fibrillation

Therapies for the chronic maintenance of sinus rhythm in patients with AF include pharmacologic and procedural approaches. The procedural approaches include catheter-based ablation inside the left atrium with the goal of electrically isolating the pulmonary veins from the left atrium. Similarly, a minimally invasive surgical approach can electrically isolate the pulmonary veins from the external surface of the heart with the additional resection of the left atrial appendage. Both these procedures have become standard options for AF, especially in patients who have recurrent AF despite at least one antiarrhythmic drug.[A6]

The catheter approach carries a small risk for cardiac perforation, including pericardial tamponade and atrioesophageal fistula formation, and a 1% risk for stroke. There is also a small risk for pulmonary vein stenosis, which has been reduced by newer technologies. A second procedure typically is offered to patients who have recurrent AF following a first catheter-based procedure.

In randomized trials of patients with paroxysmal AF, the cumulative burden of AF over a period of 2 years appeared to be slightly lower with initial radiofrequency catheter ablation therapy compared with antiarrhythmic medications, but at the expense of procedural risks and without any differences in patient-reported quality of life.[A7][A8] Catheter ablation may, however, be preferred as initial therapy in patients with persistent AF and symptomatic heart failure.[A9] For patients with long-standing persistent AF, 5-year success rates are 20% for a single ablation procedure and 45% for multiple ablation procedures.

The surgical approach carries a higher risk for cardiac bleeding, particularly during the resection of the left atrial appendage, and is associated with a significantly longer recovery time than the percutaneous approach. However, there should be no stroke risk associated with the surgical procedure because it is performed completely from the epicardial surface of the heart. A more extensive surgical operation, called the maze procedure, requires a full thoracotomy and is most often performed concomitantly as part of open coronary artery bypass surgery or an open valve operation. In this procedure, electrical lines of block are created in the left atrium to interrupt the perpetuation of AF, the pulmonary veins are isolated, and the left atrial appendage is resected. Success rates for this procedure, which should be reserved for refractory, symptomatic AF, exceed 80%.

The pharmacologic options for the treatment of AF work by blocking sodium, potassium, or a combination of cardiac channels. Blockade of these channels results in slowing of cardiac conduction (sodium channels) and prolongation in cardiac repolarization (potassium channels) as well as additional effects from modulation of the autonomic nervous system. The choice of antiarrhythmic drug is based on the patient's underlying clinical condition (Table 64-6).

Amiodarone is the most widely used medication for AF with an efficacy of 60 to 70% at 1 year. It is associated with a number of drug interactions, most notably with warfarin and digoxin. Its associated risk for thyroid, liver, and lung toxicities, related in part to the iodine moieties on this compound, necessitate careful follow-up. For prevention of recurrent AF, oral amiodarone is significantly more effective than propafenone, flecainide, dofetilide, or sotalol, which are the recommended alternatives. Dronedarone (400 mg twice daily), which is related to amiodarone but has no iodine and a 24-hour half-life, is well tolerated in terms of noncardiovascular side effects but has been associated with an increased risk for heart failure, stroke, and death in patients with permanent AF. As a result, it should be discontinued in patients in whom sinus rhythm is not well maintained.

Quinidine, procainamide, and disopyramide are predominantly sodium-channel blocking drugs that also block potassium channels at slow heart rates. Each of these drugs is moderately successful in AF, with about 50% of treated patients in sinus rhythm at 1 year, but each also has idiosyncratic noncardiovascular toxicities that can significantly limit their utility (see Table 64-5). Propafenone and flecainide are also sodium-channel blockers that are widely used for the maintenance of sinus rhythm. These drugs are moderately effective, with a 50% rate of sinus rhythm at 1 year, and are generally well tolerated but must be avoided in patients with structural heart disease, particularly with a history of prior myocardial infarction and impaired left ventricular function, because of a risk for drug-induced ventricular arrhythmia. Dofetilide is a potassium-channel blocking medication that is moderately effective for suppressing AF but carries a dose-dependent risk for QT prolongation and torsades de pointes.

Anticoagulation

The presence or absence of associated conditions helps determine which patients with AF require chronic anticoagulation with warfarin or other systematic coagulants (Table 64-7). Long-term anticoagulation therapy with warfarin, dabigatran, rivaroxaban, or apixaban is generally recommended in all patients who have persistent or paroxysmal AF, who are older than 65 years, and who have no contraindications to anticoagulation.[4] Anticoagulation also should be maintained for 6 months after both catheter and surgical procedures in patients without clinical risk factors for stroke and chronically in patients with risk factors. Catheter-based procedures directed at excluding the left atrial appendage from the systemic blood stream may become options in patients who have a high risk for stroke and who cannot tolerate systemic anticoagulation owing to an excessive risk for bleeding.[A10]

Warfarin alone is superior to aspirin or the combination of clopidogrel and aspirin, with meta-analysis showing that adjusted-dose warfarin and

TABLE 64-6 SELECTION OF ANTIARRHYTHMIC DRUGS

PATIENT CHARACTERISTICS	ANTIARRHYTHMIC DRUG CHOICES
No structural heart disease	*First line:* flecainide, propafenone, dronedarone, sotalol *Second line:* amiodarone, dofetilide
Depressed left ventricular ejection fraction with heart failure	*First line:* amiodarone, dofetilide *Avoid:* dronedarone, flecainide, propafenone
Coronary artery disease without congestive heart failure	*First line:* sotalol, dronedarone, dofetilide, amiodarone *Avoid:* flecainide, propafenone
Hypertrophic cardiomyopathy	*First line:* amiodarone, sotalol, dronedarone *Second line:* disopyramide

TABLE 64-7 CURRENT RECOMMENDATIONS FOR THROMBOEMBOLIC PROPHYLAXIS FOR PATIENTS WITH ATRIAL FIBRILLATION BASED ON RISK FACTORS FOR STROKE

RISK FACTORS*	RECOMMENDATIONS
Heart failure (1 point) Hypertension (1 point) Age ≥65 (1 point), ≥75 (2 points) Diabetes (1 point) Stroke/TIA (2 points) Vascular disease (1 point) Female gender (1 point)	2 or more points: anticoagulation with warfarin or a new oral anticoagulant 1 point: anticoagulation or no therapy depending on the preference of the patient and treating physician 0 points: no therapy

*Based on the CHA_2DS_2-VASc risk stratification scoring system.
TIA = transient ischemic attack.
Data from January CT, Wann S, Alpert JS, et al. 2014 AHA/ACC/HRS Guideline for the Management of Patients with Atrial Fibrillation: A Report of the American College of Cardiology/American Heart Association Task Force on Practice Guidelines and the Heart Rhythm Society. *J Am Coll Cardiol* 2014;64:e1-e76.

antiplatelet agents reduce stroke by approximately 60% and 20%, respectively.[A11] Although there is some protective effect at an INR as low as 1.8, the target INR for chronic anticoagulation with warfarin should be 2 to 3 to avoid INRs less than 1.8. Guidelines no longer recommend aspirin or other antiplatelet agents in patients without an indication for warfarin or the newer anticoagulants.

New oral anticoagulant medications have the potential to replace warfarin as more effective and safer (except for gastrointestinal bleeding)[A12] primary therapy to prevent systemic emboli in patients with AF. In a randomized trial of patients with nonvalvular atrial fibrillation, rivaroxaban (an oral factor Xa inhibitor at 20 mg per day) was better than warfarin at preventing stroke or systemic embolization, with significantly less intracranial and fatal bleeding.[A13] In another randomized trial of patients with atrial fibrillation, apixaban (an oral factor Xa inhibitor at 5 mg twice daily) prevented more strokes and systemic emboli than warfarin, with less bleeding from all causes and fewer deaths.[A14] Dabigatran, a direct thrombin inhibitor (150 mg twice daily), is superior to warfarin for preventing thromboembolism, with a lower risk for intracranial bleeding but a slightly higher risk for extracranial bleeding.[A15] All three drugs are eliminated by the kidney (apixaban 25%, rivaroxaban 65%, and dabigatran 85%), so they are not recommended in patients with substantial renal dysfunction, and the doses should be reduced in patients with moderate renal dysfunction (Chapter 38). A reasonable approach is to use apixaban in patients at the highest risk for bleeding, to use rivaroxaban in patients who prefer once-daily dosing, and to avoid dabigatran in patients older than 80 years because of increased bleeding risk. The addition of aspirin to moderate-intensity warfarin (INR 2 to 3) or to dabigatran, rivaroxaban, or apixaban can decrease vascular events and is recommended, despite its increased risk of causing bleeding, in some AF patients with concomitant risk factors, such as coronary artery disease or a prior stroke that is attributed to vascular disease rather than to AF.

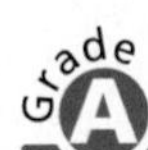

Grade A References

A1. Curtis AB, Worley SJ, Adamson PB, et al. Biventricular pacing for atrioventricular block and systolic dysfunction. *N Engl J Med.* 2013;368:1585-1593.

A2. Cappato R, Castelvecchio S, Ricci C, et al. Clinical efficacy of ivabradine in patients with inappropriate sinus tachycardia: a prospective, randomized, placebo-controlled, double-blind, crossover evaluation. *J Am Coll Cardiol.* 2012;60:1323-1329.

A3. Al-Khatib SM, Allen LaPointe NM, Chatterjee R, et al. Rate- and rhythm-control therapies in patients with atrial fibrillation: a systematic review. *Ann Intern Med.* 2014;160:760-773.

A4. Roy D, Talajic M, Nattel S, et al. Rhythm control versus rate control for atrial fibrillation and heart failure. *N Engl J Med.* 2008;358:2667-2677.

A5. Van Gelder I, Groenveld H, Crijns H. Lenient versus strict rate control in patients with atrial fibrillation. *N Engl J Med.* 2010;362:1363-1373.

A6. Wilber DJ, Pappone C, Neuzil P, et al. Comparison of antiarrhythmic drug therapy and radiofrequency catheter ablation in patients with paroxysmal atrial fibrillation: a randomized controlled trial. *JAMA.* 2010;303:333-340.

A7. Morillo CA, Verma A, Connolly SJ, et al. Radiofrequency ablation vs antiarrhythmic drugs as first-line treatment of paroxysmal atrial fibrillation (RAAFT-2): a randomized trial. *JAMA.* 2014;311:692-700.

A8. Cosedis Nielsen J, Johannessen A, Raatikainen P, et al. Radiofrequency ablation as initial therapy in paroxysmal atrial fibrillation. *N Engl J Med.* 2012;367:1587-1595.

A9. Jones DG, Haldar SK, Hussain W, et al. A randomized trial to assess catheter ablation versus rate control in the management of persistent atrial fibrillation in heart failure. *J Am Coll Cardiol.* 2013;61:1894-1903.

A10. Reddy VY, Möbius-Winkler S, Miller MA, et al. Left atrial appendage closure with the Watchman device in patients with a contraindication for oral anticoagulation: the ASAP study (ASA Plavix Feasibility Study With Watchman Left Atrial Appendage Closure Technology). *J Am Coll Cardiol.* 2013;61:2551-2556.

A11. Hart RG, Pearce LA, Aguilar MI, et al. Meta-analysis: antithrombotic therapy to prevent stroke in patients who have nonvalvular atrial fibrillation. *Ann Intern Med.* 2007;146:857-867.

A12. Ruff CT, Giugliano RP, Braunwald E, et al. Comparison of the efficacy and safety of new oral anticoagulants with warfarin in patients with atrial fibrillation: a meta-analysis of randomised trials. *Lancet.* 2014;383:955-962.

A13. Patel MR, Mahaffey KW, Garg J, et al. Rivaroxaban versus warfarin in nonvalvular atrial fibrillation. *N Engl J Med.* 2011;365:883-891.

A14. Granger CB, Alexander JH, McMurray JJ, et al. Apixaban versus warfarin in patients with atrial fibrillation. *N Engl J Med.* 2011;365:981-992.

A15. Connolly SJ, Ezekowitz MD, Yusuf S, et al. Dabigatran versus warfarin in patients with atrial fibrillation. *N Engl J Med.* 2009;361:1139-1151.

GENERAL REFERENCES

For the General References and other additional features, please visit Expert Consult at https://expertconsult.inkling.com.

65

VENTRICULAR ARRHYTHMIAS

HASAN GARAN

DEFINITIONS

Ventricular arrhythmias are cardiac rhythms that originate in the ventricular myocardium or in the His-Purkinje tissue. They include a wide spectrum of arrhythmias, from the most innocuous isolated premature ventricular contraction (PVC) to the most malignant and life-threatening ventricular arrhythmia (Fig. 65-1).

Two consecutive PVCs are termed a *couplet*, whereas *ventricular tachycardia* (VT) is arbitrarily defined as three or more ventricular contractions in a row at a rate faster than 100 beats per minute. The definition of *sustained* VT—a continuous ventricular rhythm, at a rate faster than 100 beats per minute, with no interruption for 30 seconds or longer—is equally arbitrary. However, most if not all sustained VTs are much faster than 100 beats per minute, persist for more than 30 seconds, and cause a substantial decrease in ventricular function and cardiac output, especially in patients with underlying organic heart disease. These abrupt physiologic changes may result in acute heart failure, hypotension, syncope, or even circulatory collapse within several seconds to minutes after the onset of VT.

Monomorphic VT is electrocardiographically defined as a wide-complex tachycardia with no change in QRS configuration, frontal axis, or horizontal axis from one beat to the next (see Fig. 65-1C). Monomorphic ventricular tachycardia (Fig. 65-2A) at a very rapid (>250 beats per minute) rate is sometimes called ventricular flutter, but there is no consensus for a definite rate cutoff, and it is not possible to separate the QRS clearly from the T waves when the rate exceeds 250 beats per minute. Polymorphic VT is characterized by beat-to-beat changes in the QRS morphology and axis, and very fast polymorphic VT may be difficult to distinguish from *ventricular fibrillation* (VF) (Fig. 65-2B). VF is a grossly irregular ventricular rhythm, usually at a rate faster than 300 beats per minute and with markedly variable low amplitude in the QRS morphology, during which there is no cardiac output. Torsades de pointes and bidirectional polymorphic VT are two distinct subtypes of polymorphic VT. To avoid confusion, the term *pleomorphic* VT should be used rather than the term *polymorphic* VT to describe the phenomenon of multiple clinical monomorphic VTs, each with distinct QRS configurations and axis observed at different times in the same patient.

EPIDEMIOLOGY

The prevalence of PVCs is a function of sampling method and duration, and PVCs may be seen in 50% of apparently healthy individuals if the monitoring time is 24 hours or longer. Nonsustained VT may be recorded in up to 3% of apparently healthy individuals with no identifiable heart disease. The prevalence of PVCs and nonsustained VT increases with age, but also with the presence and severity of an underlying heart disease. Therefore, the finding of nonsustained VT often leads to a cardiac evaluation to exclude organic heart disease, even if it is incidentally discovered in an asymptomatic patient. The prevalence of nonsustained VT rises to 7 to 12% in the late phase of myocardial infarction (MI) and may be as high as 80% in patients with heart failure owing to dilated cardiomyopathy (Chapter 60).

Approximately 10% of patients with documented sustained VT have no identifiable heart disease, in which case idiopathic VT is diagnosed. Idiopathic VF is exceedingly rare. Sudden cardiac death (Chapter 63) owing to ventricular arrhythmias accounts for an estimated 50% of all annual cardiovascular deaths in the United States.[1]

The nature of the underlying heart disease in patients dying of VT or VF is age dependent. Before 30 years of age, the organic heart disease most commonly associated with VT and VF is genetic cardiomyopathy (Chapter 60), whereas acute MI and chronic ischemic cardiomyopathy are the most common underlying heart diseases in individuals older than 40 years. In about one third of cases of sudden cardiac death without obvious underlying organic heart disease at autopsy, post-mortem genetic analysis may identify a deleterious mutation in an ion channel—a so-called channelopathy that predisposes to VT and VF.

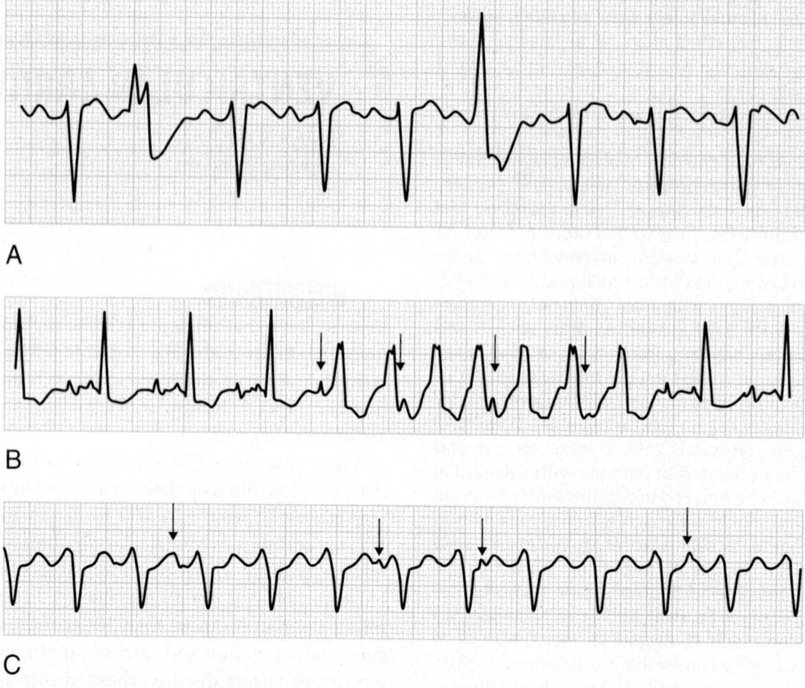

FIGURE 65-1. Ventricular arrhythmias. A, Multifocal premature ventricular beats. B, Nonsustained monomorphic ventricular tachycardia. Note dissociated P waves indicated by *arrows*. C, Sustained monomorphic ventricular tachycardia. Dissociated P waves are indicated by *arrows*.

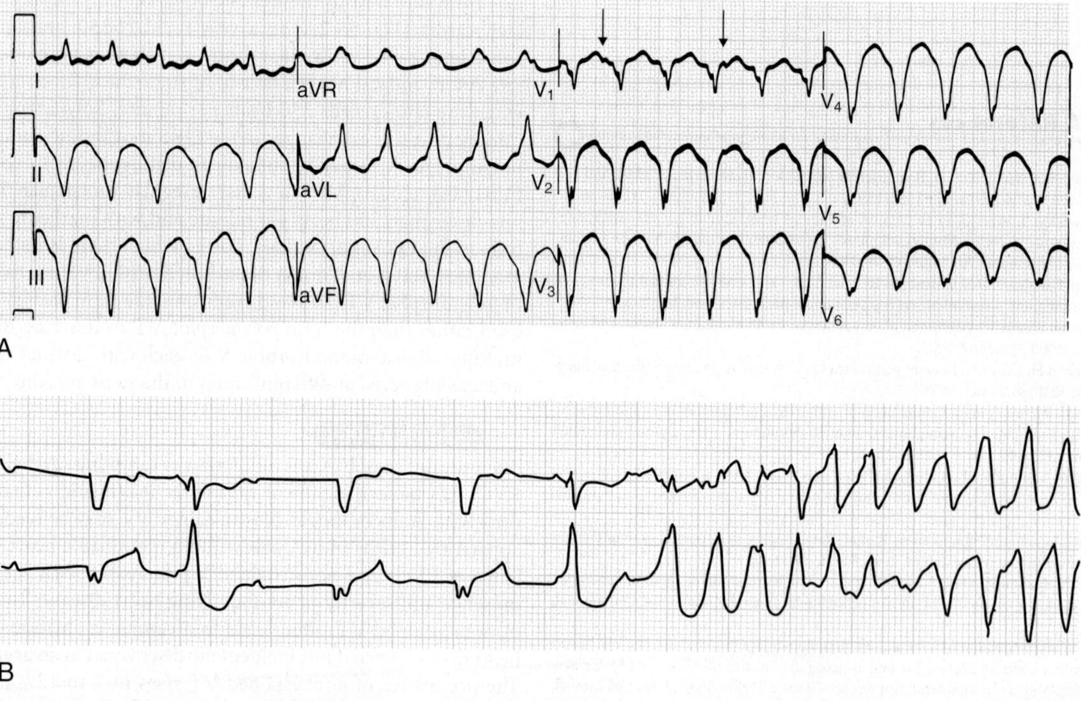

FIGURE 65-2. A, Monomorphic ventricular tachycardia (VT) in a patient with chronic myocardial infarction. The *arrows* identify P waves in lead V_1, showing atrioventricular dissociation. No R wave is recorded in any of the precordial leads V_1 to V_6 during VT. B, Polymorphic VT in a patient with chronic ischemic cardiomyopathy and marked first-degree atrioventricular block. There is no QT prolongation before the onset of the polymorphic VT.

PATHOBIOLOGY

Based on their underlying mechanisms, ventricular arrhythmias are classified as re-entrant, triggered, or automatic (Chapter 61). Re-entry, which results from activation in pathways sharing a common isthmus, is initiated by the simultaneous presence of conduction block in one limb and abnormally slow conduction in an adjacent limb, thereby allowing recovery of excitability in the former (E-Fig. 65-1A). One type of triggered activity results from early afterdepolarizations, which are oscillatory depolarizations occurring during the late phase of the action potential (E-Fig. 65-1B). Another type of triggered activity results from delayed afterdepolarizations, which are transient depolarizations that occur immediately after the termination of the action potential and may reach activation threshold. Automatic arrhythmias arise from accelerated pacemaker activity (E-Fig. 65-1C).

Sustained re-entrant activation in the myocardium, which is the most common cause of monomorphic VT, usually arises from subendocardial scarring, which is the result of prior ischemic injury and which creates an electrophysiologically abnormal substrate that results in re-entry. Other pathologic conditions capable of creating a substrate for re-entry include inflammation, granuloma (e.g., cardiac sarcoidosis), fibrofatty infiltration (e.g. arrhythmogenic right ventricular cardiomyopathy [ARVC]), genetically caused sarcomeric disarray (e.g., hypertrophic cardiomyopathy), and iatrogenic scar or patch (e.g., surgical repair of tetralogy of Fallot). These substrates may also result in polymorphic VT and VF by more than one mechanism.

The mechanism of ventricular arrhythmias in Brugada syndrome is not completely understood. One proposed mechanism is based on intraventricular phase 2 re-entry owing to an exaggerated endocardial-to-epicardial gradient in membrane potential due to differences in transient outward current. Other evidence suggests abnormal conduction in the epicardium of the right ventricular outflow tract.

Triggered activity, which results from adenosine-sensitive delayed afterdepolarizations rather than re-entry, is thought to be the underlying mechanism for idiopathic monomorphic VT of outflow tract origin. Idiopathic VT from re-entry in the fascicles of the left bundle branch has a relatively narrow QRS complex that always manifests right bundle branch block mimicry, most commonly with left, but rarely with right, frontal axis deviation.

Torsades de pointes is caused by early afterdepolarizations that arise during an abnormally prolonged action potential owing to a delayed repolarization process in the setting of genetic long QT syndromes or acquired long QT during therapy with QT-prolonging drugs. The cause may be either diminished outflowing potassium currents or enhanced inflowing sodium or calcium currents. Although many episodes terminate spontaneously, the rates are usually very fast, and a torsade episode, if long enough, can transform into VF.

Bundle branch re-entry, which results from re-entrant activation incorporating the right and the left bundle branches distally joined by the slowly conducting septal myocardium, may cause one or two nonsustained ventricular beats in a normal heart. However, sustained bundle branch re-entry occurs when myocardial disease causes chamber enlargement and bundle branch elongation and/or disease in the conduction system causes abnormal slow conduction, thereby creating the scenario for sustained bundle branch re-entry. The common type of bundle branch re-entry has anterograde activation over the right bundle and uses the left bundle retrogradely, thereby resulting in a left bunch branch block (LBBB) pattern on surface electrocardiogram (ECG), but the reverse direction with right bundle branch block (RBBB) may also occur rarely.

Accelerated pacemaker activity in an ectopic location, with rates exceeding the underlying sinus rhythm rate, may arise in settings such as transient inflammation, excess digoxin levels, intracellular calcium loading, electrolyte imbalance, and coronary reperfusion following thrombotic occlusion. Bidirectional VT is thought to result from calcium overload of the myocytes owing to congenitally acquired abnormal calcium release from the ryanodine receptor or digitalis toxicity.

Finally, there is no consensus regarding the mechanisms underlying VF. Theoretically, VF may be initiated when early or delayed afterdepolarizations fall in the vulnerable period of the action potential, thereby precipitating a re-entrant wave that breaks into sister wavelets and results in high-frequency electrical activity. In fact, VF may be regarded as an end stage for a variety of severe electrophysiologic abnormalities that result in chaotic activation.

TABLE 65-1 VENTRICULAR TACHYCARDIA AND CARDIAC DIAGNOSIS

STRUCTURAL HEART DISEASE
Acquired heart disease
Acute myocardial infarction
Chronic myocardial infarction, ischemic heart disease
Nonischemic dilated cardiomyopathy
Hypertensive heart disease
Valvar heart disease
Cardiac sarcoidosis
Cardiac amyloidosis
Other infiltrative diseases (e.g., Chagas disease)
Cardiac tumors
Congenital heart disease
Arrhythmogenic right ventricular cardiomyopathy
Hypertrophic cardiomyopathy
Genetic dilated cardiomyopathies
Iatrogenic
Surgically repaired congenital heart disease
Left ventricular assist devices
NO STRUCTURAL HEART DISEASE
Idiopathic ventricular tachycardia
Right and left ventricular outflow tract tachycardias
Left intrafascicular re-entry
Papillary muscle tachycardias
Idiopathic ventricular fibrillation
Ion channel mutations
Long QT syndromes
Catecholaminergic polymorphic ventricular tachycardia
Short QT syndrome
Mixed etiology
Brugada syndrome

CLINICAL MANIFESTATIONS

Ventricular arrhythmias can present in a variety of clinical settings (Table 65-1). Often, ventricular arrhythmias are asymptomatic and are detected by an irregular pulse on a physical examination, on a routine ECG, on an exercise test, or on routine inpatient monitoring. In other patients, symptomatic ventricular arrhythmias can present as palpitations, dizziness, syncope (Chapters 51 and 62), shortness of breath, or sudden cardiac arrest (Chapter 63). The diagnosis usually can be confirmed on an ECG, but ambulatory monitoring (Chapter 62) is often needed because the arrhythmia may be intermittent. Ambulatory monitoring can also help correlate arrhythmias with any potentially related symptoms. In some patients, exercise testing can be helpful, especially in patients with exercise-induced symptoms.

On the ECG, the QRS complex duration will typically be more than 0.12 seconds. In monomorphic VT (Fig. 65-3), the QRS complexes are the same from beat to beat, whereas polymorphic VT has multiple and changing QRS morphologies (Fig. 65-4). In VF, the ECG shows continuous irregular activation without any discrete QRS complexes (Fig. 65-5). Although underlying structural heart disease is usually present, these arrhythmias do not require a fixed structural substrate.

Acute Myocardial Infarction

VT and VF may arise as early as minutes to hours after the onset of symptoms during acute myocardial infarction (MI), and prehospital VT and VF during acute MI are responsible for a large proportion of out-of-hospital sudden cardiac deaths (Chapter 63). The incidence of peri-infarction VF has declined over the past two decades, presumably related to the widespread practice of coronary revascularization (Chapter 74) during acute MI. Among patients with ST elevation MI who now reach the hospital, about 3 to 4% develop VT, mostly during the acute phase. The incidence of VT in patients with non-ST elevation MI (Chapter 72) is lower, about 1%. Accelerated idioventricular rhythm (AIVR) is an automatic ventricular rhythm that is faster than the sinus rate but usually less than 120 beats per minute. It may occur in the setting of acute MI and is commonly observed immediately after coronary reperfusion. AIVR rates are slower than those of the fast and malignant VT and VF of acute MI, and this arrhythmia typically terminates spontaneously without causing hemodynamic instability.

DIAGNOSIS

Not every wide-complex tachycardia is VT. The diagnosis is straightforward from the His bundle electrogram recorded at the time of a wide-complex tachycardia during a cardiac electrophysiology study, but diagnosis on a standard 12-lead ECG may be challenging (Table 65-2). The differential diagnosis of a sustained regular-rate wide-complex tachycardia includes any type of supraventricular tachycardia with aberrant conduction (Chapter 64), supraventricular tachycardia with ventricular preexcitation, bundle branch re-entry (which is a specific type of VT), and myocardial VT. The clinical setting and the patient's background (e.g., history of previous MI or cardiomyopathy) play a major role in making an accurate diagnosis. New-onset wide-complex tachycardia in a young and otherwise healthy individual with no structural heart disease is most likely supraventricular tachycardia (SVT) with aberration, an SVT with preexcitation, or idiopathic VT.

The most reliable observation in favor of VT is evidence of AV dissociation, that is, absence of any relationship between the atrial and ventricular rate, with the ventricular rate faster than the atrial (see Fig. 65-2A), or a regular wide-complex tachycardia with the atria fibrillating. However, the absence of atrioventricular (AV) dissociation does not exclude VT because ventriculoatrial conduction is present in about 25% of VTs. Fusion beats (which occur when an occasional sinus beat conducts through the AV node and reaches the His-Purkinje system at the same time as the VT source activates the myocardium, thereby resulting in a beat with a morphology that is the hybrid of a conducted QRS complex and the VT complex) confirm AV

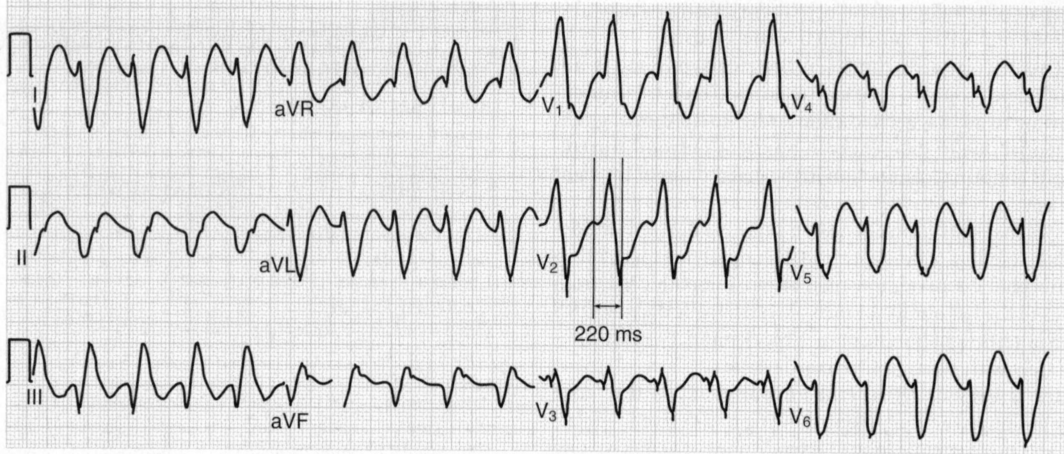

FIGURE 65-3. **Monomorphic ventricular tachycardia in a patient with chronic ischemic cardiomyopathy. In lead V_2, the duration from the onset of the R wave to the nadir of the S wave is more than 200 msec. See text for further explanation.**

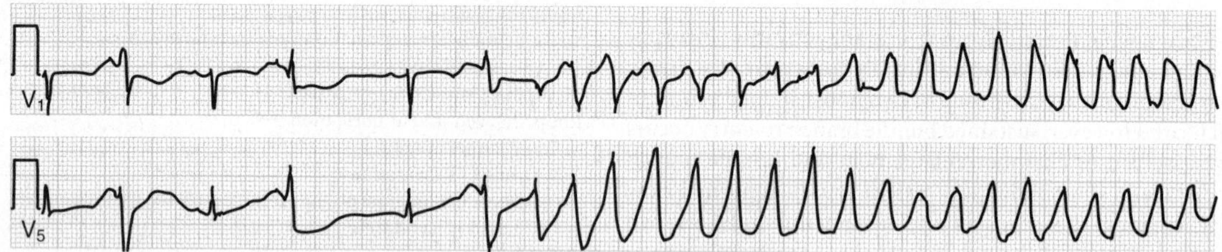

FIGURE 65-4. **Torsades de pointes (TdP) in a patient with a markedly prolonged QT interval. A premature ventricular beat just after the peak of the T wave initiates TdP. As the tachycardia progresses, the rotation or the "twist" in the QRS axis is clearly observed in lead V_1, with the polarity of the signal changing gradually from negative to positive.**

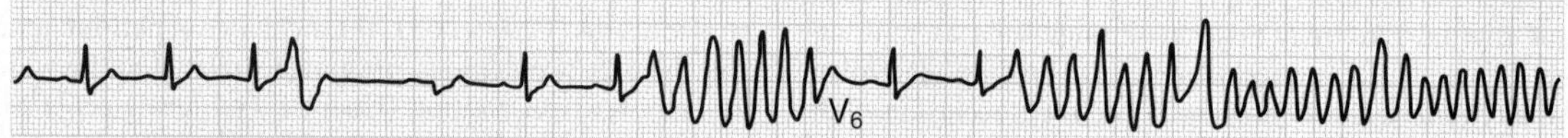

FIGURE 65-5. **This electrocardiogram in a patient with idiopathic ventricular fibrillation (VF) shows recurrent closely coupled premature ventricular contractions (PVCs) and the initiation of VF by one of these closely coupled PVCs.**

TABLE 65-2 DISTINGUISHING VENTRICULAR TACHYCARDIA FROM SUPRAVENTRICULAR TACHYCARDIA WITH ABERRANT CONDUCTION

VENTRICULAR TACHYCARDIA	SUPRAVENTRICULAR TACHYCARDIA
AV dissociation	Same QRS morphology as preexisting bundle branch block in sinus rhythm
aVR: initial R > S or initial R or Q > 40 msec	V_1: rsR′
Absence of any R wave in V_1 to V_6	
V_1 to V_6: onset of R to S > 100 msec in any lead	
QRS duration >160 msec	
Initial R wave in aVR	

AV = atrioventricular.

dissociation but are observed only when VT rates are relatively slow. Other findings that favor VT include a QRS duration longer than 160 msec, or longer than 140 msec with an RBBB pattern. One approach, based on the QRS configuration on the ECG, uses the absence of RS complex in all precordial leads or an interval of more than 100 msec from the onset of R to the nadir of S wave as observations strongly favoring VT (see Figs. 65-2A and 65-3). The absence of any R waves in the QRS complexes recorded from all six precordial leads, described as negative concordance, strongly suggests VT, but unfortunately is not a common finding. Prominent R waves observed in all six precordial ECG leads, termed *positive concordance,* may be seen in SVT with left ventricular preexcitation but otherwise also suggests VT with a basal site of origin. In the absence of preexcitation, a slow rate of rise in the voltage during the first 40 to 60 msec of the QRS onset suggests VT, as does the presence of initial R wave in lead aVR. A wide-complex tachycardia with a QRS morphology identical to that of aberrantly conducted beats manifesting bundle branch block (BBB) on a previously recorded ECG in the same patient should raise suspicion of bundle branch re-entry VT if AV dissociation is present.

If AV dissociation is not present, the differential diagnosis includes SVT with aberrant conduction, but the rare condition of preexcitation with an atriofascicular accessory pathway should also be considered in a patient with LBBB aberration. A monomorphic wide-complex tachycardia with an irregular rate, manifested by more than 60-msec difference in cycle length from one beat to the next, is likely to be atrial fibrillation (AF) or atrial flutter, with variable AV block and aberrant conduction or with preexcitation. It is important to emphasize that electrolyte imbalances or the use of antiarrhythmic drugs diminishes the predictive accuracy of all of these diagnostic clues.

Sustained polymorphic wide-complex tachycardia with marked beat-to-beat changes in the QRS morphology is always ventricular and either terminates spontaneously or transforms into VF. Torsades de pointes, a specific type of polymorphic VT, derives its name from the "twisting" or rotating of the QRS axis as the tachycardia progresses. It occurs in genetic or acquired long QT syndrome and is frequently pause dependent—typically starting when a premature beat falls on the prolonged T wave of the beat following a long RR interval (see Fig. 65-4). Finally, bidirectional VT manifesting a unique feature of beat-by-beat axis alternans may occur with digitalis toxicity or in the congenital catecholaminergic polymorphic ventricular tachycardia syndrome.

Several different algorithms based on the configurations of the QRS complexes have high sensitivity, high specificity, and acceptable predictive accuracy for distinguishing epicardial VT from endocardial VT (Table 65-3).[2] All

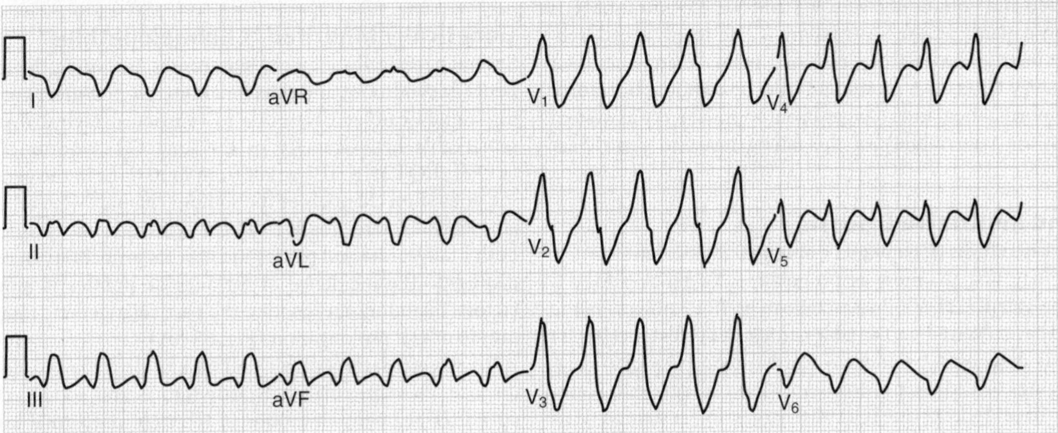

FIGURE 65-6. Monomorphic epicardial ventricular tachycardia in a patient with nonischemic dilated cardiomyopathy. The positive polarity pseudo-delta wave is prominent in the right precordial leads and the negative polarity pseudo-delta wave is prominent in the inferior limb leads.

TABLE 65-3 ELECTROCARDIOGRAPHIC PARAMETERS USED TO PREDICT AN EPICARDIAL ORIGIN OF VENTRICULAR TACHYCARDIA

PARAMETER	CRITERIA
Pseudo-delta wave	>75 msec favors epicardial site
Intrinsicoid deflection time	>85 msec favors epicardial site
Onset of R to nadir of S in precordial leads	>120 msec favors epicardial site
QRS duration	Epicardial longer
Q waves during VT in lead I	Favors epicardial site
Q waves during VT in II-III-aVF	Favors endocardial site
aVR/aVL amplitude ratio	Epicardial higher

VT = ventricular tachycardia.

are based on ECG criteria for whether the initial activation likely starts at an epicardial site. If so, the rapidly conducting His-Purkinje system is not available immediately, and the intramyocardial conduction delay produces a slurred initial component of the QRS complex, often called a *pseudo-delta wave*, which is manifested as a slow rate of rise of voltage before it reaches the intrinsicoid deflection (Fig. 65-6). Early recognition of ECG findings suggesting an epicardial origin of VT is important in planning and preparing a patient before a catheter ablation procedure (Chapter 66) because the epicardial approach requires a special technique in the cardiac electrophysiology laboratory.

Cardiac electrophysiology testing (Chapter 62) may be indicated in patients who have organic heart disease and recurrent syncope but in whom the history, physical examination, ECG, echocardiogram, and ambulatory cardiac rhythm monitoring fail to clarify the cause, especially if the patient has a history of myocardial infarction or cardiomyopathy, either of which increases the probability that VT may be the cause of syncope. A second diagnostic indication is to identify the mechanism underlying a documented wide-complex tachycardia before the consideration of catheter ablation therapy (Chapter 66).

Identifying the Underlying Cause of Ventricular Arrhythmias

In patients with a diagnosed ventricular arrhythmia, the next step is to conduct a careful evaluation to exclude any underlying structural heart disease. This evaluation must include a comprehensive history and physical examination (Chapter 51), echocardiography (Chapter 55), and stress testing (Chapter 71). The family history may provide clues to guide genetic testing for an inherited cardiomyopathy (Chapter 60). Cardiac magnetic resonance imaging (Chapter 56) is indicated in selected patients to exclude conditions such as sarcoidosis and ARVC.

Despite a comprehensive evaluation, about 10 to 15% of patients will have PVCs or VT with no identifiable structural or genetically identifiable cause. Most of the idiopathic monomorphic VTs are in one of two categories, defined by ECG morphology. VTs that arise in the right or left ventricular outflow tract typically manifest an inferiorly directed frontal axis and are markedly positive in inferior leads (E-Fig. 65-2); the QRS configuration observed in the right precordial leads may further discriminate the sites of origin as the right or the left ventricular outflow tract or one of the sinuses of Valsalva. By comparison, idiopathic left ventricular tachycardia usually manifests RBBB mimicry and left axis deviation, but there may also be right axis deviation. The QRS complexes typically are not very wide because the involved region is His-Purkinje tissue adjacent to the interventricular septum. The differential diagnosis includes idiopathic VT arising in one of the left ventricular papillary muscles (E-Fig. 65-3). When either of these typical patterns is observed in a patient with no structural heart disease, the physician should suspect idiopathic VT. Conversely, sustained VT that does not fall into either of these two broad categories should always raise a high index of suspicion that organic heart disease may be present.

Chronic Ischemic Heart Disease and Post–Myocardial Infarction Ventricular Tachycardia

In survivors of ST elevation MI, the prevalence of sustained VT by 6 weeks is about 1%, and VT may occur as late as 15 to 20 years after the acute MI without any intervening event. VT commonly, but not invariably, reflects poor left ventricular function, especially a dyskinetic left ventricular wall segment. The electrophysiologic substrate is the surviving but electrophysiologically abnormal tissue embedded in the infarcted zone, which creates the conditions for re-entry. The areas that harbor pathways underlying re-entry can be identified by low-amplitude fractionated local electrograms recorded from the endocardium. Up to 16% of the patients have VT of epicardial origin. The same substrate may cause polymorphic VT and VF, which do not depend on a long QT interval and are different than torsades de pointes seen with repolarization abnormalities.

Nonischemic Dilated Cardiomyopathy

The most common cause of sustained monomorphic VT in nonischemic cardiomyopathy (Chapter 60) is also re-entry within the myocardium, but it differs from the post-infarction VT of chronic ischemic heart disease. The pathologic substrate, such as fibrosis, may be hard to identify. The abnormal, low-voltage, fractionated local electrograms tend to be located in basal, lateral, and often perivalvar left ventricular areas, which may correlate with the location of intramyocardial or subepicardial scarring identified by cardiac magnetic resonance imaging. The proportion of monomorphic VTs due to bundle branch re-entry is higher in nonischemic dilated cardiomyopathy compared with chronic ischemic heart disease, and VT with a focal rather than re-entrant mechanism rarely may be observed. Also, VT of nonischemic dilated cardiomyopathy is more likely to have an epicardial origin—as high as 22 to 35% in many series—and reaching 70% in Chagas disease.[3] Ventricular tachycardia resulting from bundle branch re-entry also is more common in nonischemic dilated cardiomyopathy.

Heart Failure

The failing heart from any underlying cause (Chapter 58) is highly vulnerable to ventricular arrhythmias, and 40 to 60% of the deaths in patients with heart failure are sudden and commonly from VT and VF. Re-entrant VT is common especially in patients whose heart failure is due to advanced ischemic heart disease, but triggered activity resulting from derangements of calcium homeostasis may also play a prominent role. In addition, hormonal factors, electrolyte abnormalities, and changes in autonomic nervous system activity also increase the vulnerability of the failing heart to ventricular arrhythmias.

Inflammatory and Infiltrative Disease

Among patients with sarcoidosis (Chapter 95), about 40 to 50% have cardiac involvement, which may first manifest as progressive AV block and VT. Although the true prevalence of VT in sarcoidosis is not known, in the selected patients who have received implantable cardiac defibrillators (ICDs) for cardiac sarcoidosis diagnosed by endomyocardial biopsy, cardiac magnetic resonance imaging, or cardiac positron emission tomographic scans, about 15% per year have appropriate ICD discharges for sustained VT.[4] Patients with other infiltrative heart diseases such as amyloidosis (Chapter 188) also have an elevated risk for VT and life-threatening ventricular arrhythmias.[5]

Adult Congenital Heart Disease

VT may occur in the setting of any adult congenital heart disease when there is a ventricular surgical scar or patch, as is seen after repair of tetralogy of Fallot or a ventricular septal defect closure, or a failing ventricle such as after a Mustard or Senning procedure to palliate transposition of great arteries (Chapter 69). In patients with surgically repaired tetralogy of Fallot, the prevalence of VT is about 5%, and about 2% have sudden cardiac death.

Genetically Inherited Cardiomyopathies

Hypertrophic cardiomyopathy (Chapter 60) is responsible for more than one third of sudden cardiac deaths in patients younger than age 25 years (Chapter 63), and mortality in young hypertrophic cardiomyopathy patients is almost exclusively due to VT and VF. Neither genetic testing nor a cardiac EP study can definitively identify patients at high risk for VT and VF, and the risk is determined based on findings such as a history of syncope, documented nonsustained VT especially in a young patient, a markedly thickened (>3 cm) interventricular septum, and a paradoxical decrease in blood pressure during exercise.[6]

ARVC is a congenital cardiomyopathy (Chapter 60), usually with an autosomal dominant inheritance. The fibrofatty infiltration of the right ventricular myocardium, which may also involve the interventricular septum and the left ventricle, results in progressive histologic change and marked electrophysiologic abnormalities, which may be manifest on the surface ECG as an epsilon wave (Fig. 65-7). The markedly altered conduction characteristics are conducive to re-entry. The incidence of VT in ARVC is related to the severity of the pathologic myocardial changes and ranges from 25 to 100%, depending on the penetrance and the expressivity of the disease. VT typically is initiated by exercise and demonstrates LBBB mimicry in the precordial ECG leads. However, unlike idiopathic right ventricular outflow tract VT, the frontal axis may be variable and not always inferiorly directed, and the site of origin may be epicardial in about 40% of cases.

Genetically Inherited "Channelopathies"

Several genetically acquired syndromes, including the long QT syndromes, Brugada syndrome, and catecholaminergic polymorphic VT increase the risk for sudden cardiac death due to ventricular tachyarrhythmias. Despite the remarkable heterogeneity of the long QT syndrome, most of the cases (LQT1, LQT2, LQT3) result from mutations in the genes coding for one of the potassium channels or the sodium channel.[7] The other genetic mutations are extremely rare. The VT of long QT syndrome is torsades de pointes, and both bradycardia and pauses increase its probability in patients who are predisposed. The incidence of torsades de pointes is influenced by multiple factors, including age, gender, the particular genetic mutation, and the magnitude of QT prolongation (Fig. 65-8A).

The electrocardiographic hallmark of Brugada syndrome, which also predisposes to ventricular tachyarrhythmias and sudden cardiac death, is the coved ST segment elevations in the right precordial leads (Fig. 65-8B). In some cases, this pattern may not be present except when the patient is febrile. The inheritance is autosomal dominant, a sodium channel mutation is present in 20 to 30% of the cases, but the genetics are heterogenous. Catecholaminergic polymorphic VT is a rare genetic condition resulting from abnormal calcium homeostasis. It is characterized by exercise-induced, wide-complex tachycardia manifesting alternating ECG axes from one beat to the next. This condition also predisposes the patient to exercise-induced VF. In addition, a chromosomal haplotype causing overexpression of dipeptidyl peptidase-like protein-6 has been described in one type of familial idiopathic VF, a rare but challenging subset of inheritable arrhythmia syndromes causing sudden cardiac death.

Iatrogenic Ventricular Tachycardia and Ventricular Fibrillation

QT-prolonging drugs, including class III antiarrhythmic drugs (see www.sads.org.uk), may precipitate torsades de pointes and VF in genetically predisposed individuals even if the baseline QTc is normal or borderline. Class IC antiarrhythmic drugs may cause life-threatening VT in patients with ischemic or any other organic heart disease and in patients with Brugada syndrome. Ventricular scarring owing to aneurysmectomy, tetralogy of Fallot repair, ventricular septal defect repair, alcohol ablation of the interventricular septum to relieve dynamic outflow tract obstruction in hypertrophic cardiomyopathy, or implantation of a left ventricular assist device may create a substrate for re-entry and VT.

TREATMENT Rx

Premature Ventricular Contractions and Nonsustained Ventricular Tachycardia

In the absence of structural heart disease, there is no convincing evidence that ventricular ectopic activity influences survival. Therefore PVCs do not need treatment in asymptomatic patients. If ventricular ectopy results in symptoms that substantially decrease quality of life, a cardioselective β-blocker (e.g., metoprolol 50 mg twice daily or atenolol 50 mg once daily) is safe but

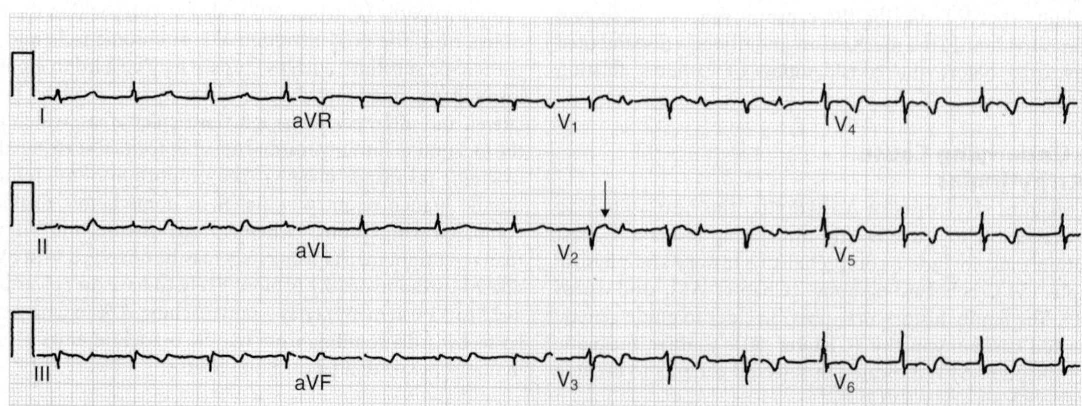

FIGURE 65-7. This electrocardiogram was recorded in a patient with arrhythmogenic right ventricular cardiomyopathy, marked first-degree heart block, and recurrent ventricular tachycardia. Epsilon waves, marked by the *arrow*, are visible in the right precordial leads.

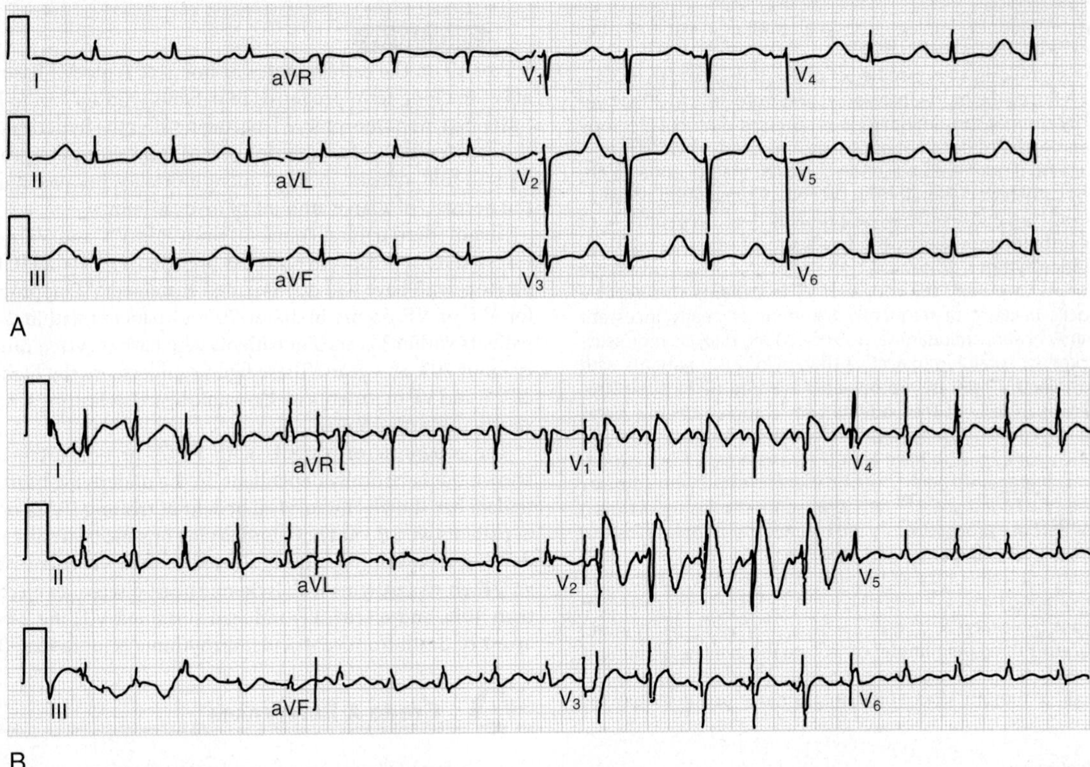

FIGURE 65-8. A, Electrocardiogram showing a QT interval of 640 msec in a woman with LQT1 syndrome, with the terminal portion of the T wave merging with the P wave. B, Electrocardiogram of a man with Brugada syndrome, showing the typical "coved" ST elevation in lead V_1.

not a very effective first-choice therapy to eradicate PVCs. PVCs may be more effectively suppressed using class IC antiarrhythmic agents such as flecainide (50 to 100 mg twice daily) or propafenone (150 to 225 three times daily), which are safe in the absence of organic heart disease but are contraindicated in organic heart disease, especially ischemic heart disease.[8]

In some patients, the frequency of PVCs and nonsustained VT reaches a critical level that results in decreased systolic ventricular function. These patients should be treated aggressively, including catheter mapping and ablation (Chapter 66) to avoid the potential adverse effects of antiarrhythmic drugs.

Acute Management of Ventricular Tachycardia and Ventricular Fibrillation

The management of VT with hemodynamic instability and VF should conform to the guidelines for advanced cardiac life support (Chapter 63), with an emphasis on defibrillation. For patients who have sustained VT with modest hypotension and normal mental status, intravenous drug therapy with lidocaine (given as a 50-mg bolus) or amiodarone (150 mg infused intravenously over 10 minutes) may be tried. Lidocaine, which works best at rapid heart rates, is an effective drug to terminate VT, which invariably occurs at a high rate, but not to prevent recurrences, except in the setting of acute ischemia. By comparison, amiodarone is more effective at slower heart rates and therefore is better for preventing recurrent VT after sinus rhythm is restored. Intravenous calcium channel blocker therapy should not be given unless the mechanism is known with certainty to be verapamil-sensitive idiopathic left ventricular tachycardia.

The most important factor in preventing early recurrence is the prompt identification and reversal of any precipitating causes. Examples include hypokalemia and other electrolyte imbalances, low oxygen saturation, intravenous β-agonist agents, and acute heart failure (Chapter 59) or myocardial ischemia (Chapter 72 and 73). Heart failure should be rigorously treated (Chapter 59). VF suggests the presence of residual ischemia; the feasibility of coronary revascularization (Chapter 74) should be addressed, but even then recurrences are common.

Treatment of Electrical Storm

Electrical storm is a term used to describe frequently recurrent VT or VF requiring repeated defibrillations. Electrical storm rarely occurs in nonischemic cardiomyopathy or in genetically acquired ventricular arrhythmias. When this condition is encountered in the early phase of acute MI, relief of ischemia is of paramount importance. If the electrical storm continues even after coronary reperfusion, insertion of an intra-aortic balloon pump and use of an intravenous β-blocker therapy, preferably with a short half-life drug (e.g., esmolol 50 to 300 μg/kg per minute by intravenous infusion) should be considered. Intravenous lidocaine (2 to 4 mg per minute) or intravenous amiodarone (0.5 to 1.0 mg per minute) may also be used if esmolol is ineffective.

Idiopathic Ventricular Tachycardia and Ventricular Fibrillation

Although cardiac arrest resulting from transformation of idiopathic VT to VF is exceedingly rare, sustained VT at a rate faster than 200 beats per minute commonly causes cardiopulmonary symptoms and even syncope (Chapter 62). Idiopathic VTs of outflow tract origin may respond to β-blocker therapy (e.g., metoprolol 50 mg every 12 hours, or atenolol 50 mg daily), and a few may respond to an empirical trial of calcium-channel blockers (e.g., sustained-release diltiazem 120 to 240 mg daily, or sustained-release verapamil 120 to 240 mg daily). The so-called idiopathic left ventricular tachycardia resulting from left fascicular re-entry frequently responds to verapamil (e.g., sustained-release 180 to 360 mg daily), but papillary muscle VT may not.

Catheter ablation therapy (Chapter 66), which may be curative for idiopathic VTs because of their focal origin in sites such as the right or left ventricular outflow tracts, epicardium, or papillary muscle, should be considered as a preferred alternative to long-term antiarrhythmic drug therapy.[9] The long-term success rate of catheter ablation for these focal sites can be about 85% or even higher. Studies with smaller groups of patients have reported even higher rates of success for idiopathic VT arising in the sinuses of Valsalva.

By comparison to the relatively benign prognosis of idiopathic sustained VT, idiopathic VF accounts for 5 to 10% of all cases of sudden cardiac death (Chapter 63). The appropriate treatment for survivors of idiopathic VF is no different than for any other survivor of VF (i.e., ICD therapy). The ECG may show recurrent PVCs with short coupling intervals. If these PVCs are monomorphic, they may be amenable to catheter ablation. Catheter ablation may decrease the risk for recurrence but still does not obviate the need for ICD protection.

Ventricular Tachycardia and Ventricular Fibrillation with Structural Heart Disease

Sustained VT and VF in patients with organic heart disease have become a common indication for ICD therapy. Three randomized trials comparing ICD therapy to antiarrhythmic drug therapy all showed significant survival benefit with ICD over drug therapy. After an acute MI, an ICD reduces mortality in patients who have survived more than 40 days and have a left ventricular ejection fraction of 30% or less or who have symptomatic heart failure and an ejection fraction of less than 0.35%; and patients more than 5 days after MI who have a reduced ejection fraction, nonsustained VT, and inducible sustained VT or VF on electrophysiologic testing.[A1] By comparison, ICDs do not reduce mortality when routinely implanted soon after MI or in patients after recent coronary artery revascularization.[A2]

In patients with a chronically depressed ejection fraction of less than 30%, insertion of an ICD reduces the mortality rate by 20%, from 36% to 29%, over the next 5 years.[A3] By comparison, amiodarone suppresses ventricular ectopy and reduces sudden death but does not appear to improve survival.[A3,A4]

However, there are no randomized placebo-controlled trials of antiarrhythmic drug therapy or catheter ablation for the secondary prevention of recurrent VT in patients with organic heart disease, probably because treatment of a potentially lethal arrhythmia with placebo has been considered unacceptable. As a result, antiarrhythmic drugs and catheter ablation currently serve as palliative treatments to modify the course of VT in patients who receive too many ICD shocks because of frequently recurrent or nearly incessant VT. If medications are chosen, amiodarone (100 to 400 mg daily) is more successful than β-blockers or sotalol for palliative therapy of VT in patients with ICD.[A5] However, sustained VT can be reproducibly initiated by focal electrophysiologic stimulation in 65% of the patients with chronic ischemic heart disease, and the identified site is usually amenable to treatment with catheter ablation. Among such patients who have an ICD for ischemic VT but experience recurrent VT, an average of about 50% of patients treated with catheter ablation will be free of VT for 2 years,[A6] although some studies report even higher success rates.[A7] These procedures should be undertaken only at institutions with the highest level of expertise and experience.

In patients who are clinically unstable because of incessant VT despite an ICD, reversible precipitating factors should be sought and, if present, corrected promptly. Intravenous β-blockers (e.g., esmolol 50 to 300 μg/kg per minute) and amiodarone (0.5 to 1.0 mg per minute) constitute the first line of therapy. Intravenous lidocaine (e.g., 2 to 4 mg per minute) can be added, especially if myocardial ischemia is present, and emergent catheter ablation may be considered.

Torsades de Pointes

The first line of therapy for torsades de pointes in patients with long QT syndrome is β-blocker therapy (e.g., metoprolol 50 to 100 mg daily, atenolol 50 mg daily, or nadolol 40 mg daily, and titrated as tolerated), but its success is influenced by gender and the magnitude of QT prolongation, as well as by the specific genotype.[10] In an acute setting with frequently recurrent torsades de pointes, magnesium sulfate (1 to 2 g intravenous infusion over 10 to 30 minutes) may be effective. An ICD is recommended if patients who are on β-blocker therapy develop recurrent syncope or documented torsades de pointes. Whether nonpharmacologic therapy, such as sympathetic ganglionic denervation, will prove effective in some cases is uncertain. β-Blockers are also the drugs of choice for catecholaminergic polymorphic VT, with ICD therapy recommended for patients with recurrent syncope or documented VT while on β-blocker therapy. Whether oral flecainide can obviate the need for ICD protection in such patients is uncertain.

Treatment of Genetically Acquired Ventricular Tachycardia and Ventricular Fibrillation

Most of the VTs observed in patients with ARVC may be reproducibly induced by programmed electrophysiologic stimulation and are amenable to catheter ablation. Recent clinical studies suggest that nearly half of these VTs have an epicardial site of origin, and simultaneous endocardial and epicardial catheter mapping and ablation may be the most effective method of treatment.[11] However, catheter ablation cannot substitute for ICD therapy. In patients with hypertrophic cardiomyopathy, ICD therapy is routinely recommended in high-risk patients (Chapter 60). Case reports suggest a benefit of catheter ablation in highly selected patients, and amiodarone may sometimes be useful.

For Brugada syndrome, catheter ablation of the electrophysiologically abnormal substrate in the right ventricular outflow tract epicardium can lead to eventual disappearance of the pathognomonic ST elevation on the ECG.[12] Quinidine (600 to 900 mg daily in three or four divided doses) is the only antiarrhythmic drug that appears to be useful to treat this syndrome, but whether catheter ablation or quinidine will be a substitute for an ICD in the highest risk patients, who have unprovoked Brugada pattern in their resting ECG and have a history of syncope, is unproved.

Iatrogenic Ventricular Tachycardia

For sustained monomorphic VT in patients with surgically repaired congenital heart disease, catheter mapping and ablation are recommended. The techniques are similar to those used for catheter ablation of ischemic VT.

Although sustained VT or VF during the course of LVAD therapy is usually well tolerated acutely, recurrent intractable VT or VF can result in right heart failure and in frequent ICD shocks, both of which may carry significant morbidity. Amiodarone (200 to 400 mg daily) and β-blocker therapy (e.g., metoprolol 100 to 200 mg daily) may be effective in at least rendering VT no longer incessant, and catheter ablation therapy has occasionally been tried in refractory VT with modest success.

PROGNOSIS

VT or VF in the early minutes or hours of acute MI has not been shown to affect the long-term prognosis in patients who survive to hospital discharge. Sustained monomorphic VT occurring after the hyperacute phase but within the next few days of an anterior wall MI portends poor prognosis, with about a seven-fold increase in subsequent mortality, because it usually occurs after the necrosis of a large amount of myocardium.

The modern natural course of untreated VT and VF perhaps can best be assessed from prospective studies of patients receiving ICD therapy. Among patients who have had documented sustained VT, appropriate ICD therapy for VT or VF occurs in about 70% of patients within 2 years and 85% of patients within 3 years. For patients who have survived cardiac arrest, the rate is about 70% at 3 years. These figures underscore the high rate of recurrence of VT and VF in patients with organic heart disease presenting with sustained ventricular arrhythmias.

The prognosis of patients with PVCs or nonsustained VT is less well known but is critically dependent on the underlying heart disease. No study to date has shown any survival benefit of treating PVCs or nonsustained VT in patients who do not have underlying organic heart disease and who do not develop a cardiomyopathy as a result of their ventricular ectopic activity. In very high-risk patients with ischemic heart disease, an ejection fraction of less than 40%, and electrically induced sustained VT, the 2-year rate of cardiac arrest or death from ventricular arrhythmia is more than 30%.

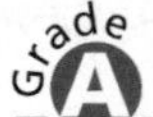

Grade A References

A1. Goldenberg I, Gillespie J, Moss AJ, et al. Long-term benefit of primary prevention with an implantable cardioverter-defibrillator: an extended 8-year follow-up study of the Multicenter Automatic Defibrillator Implantation Trial II. *Circulation.* 2010;122:1265-1271.

A2. Steinbeck G, Andresen D, Seidl K, et al. Defibrillator implantation early after myocardial infarction. *N Engl J Med.* 2009;361:1427-1436.

A3. Piccini JP, Berger JS, O'Connor CM. Amiodarone for the prevention of sudden cardiac death: a meta-analysis of randomized controlled trials. *Eur Heart J.* 2009;30:1245-1253.

A4. Bardy GH, Lee KL, Mark DB, et al. Amiodarone or an implantable cardioverter-defibrillator for congestive heart failure. *N Engl J Med.* 2005;352:225-237.

A5. Connolly SJ, Dorian P, Roberts RS, et al. Comparison of beta-blockers, amiodarone plus beta-blockers, or sotalol for prevention of shocks from implantable cardioverter defibrillators: the OPTIC Study: a randomized trial. *JAMA.* 2006;295:165-171.

A6. Kuck KH, Schaumann A, Eckardt L, et al. Catheter ablation of stable ventricular tachycardia before defibrillator implantation in patients with coronary heart disease (VTACH): a multicentre randomised controlled trial. *Lancet.* 2010;375:31-40.

A7. Reddy VY, Reynolds MR, Neuzil P, et al. Prophylactic catheter ablation for the prevention of defibrillator therapy. *N Engl J Med.* 2007;357:2657-2665.

GENERAL REFERENCES

For the General References and other additional features, please visit Expert Consult at https://expertconsult.inkling.com.

66

ELECTROPHYSIOLOGIC INTERVENTIONAL PROCEDURES AND SURGERY

DAVID J. WILBER

PACEMAKERS

Temporary Pacemaking

In emergencies such as asystolic cardiac arrest (Chapter 63), transcutaneous pacing with electrode pads applied to the chest wall occasionally can be lifesaving. Usually, however, time allows for temporary pacemaker leads to be inserted percutaneously, through an internal jugular or subclavian vein, and to be positioned and gently embedded in the right ventricular apex under fluoroscopic guidance. The lead is then attached to an external generator. A temporary pacemaker is often required as urgent therapy in a patient who has an indication for a permanent pacemaker and is awaiting that definitive procedure. Another indication for temporary pacing is the treatment of a

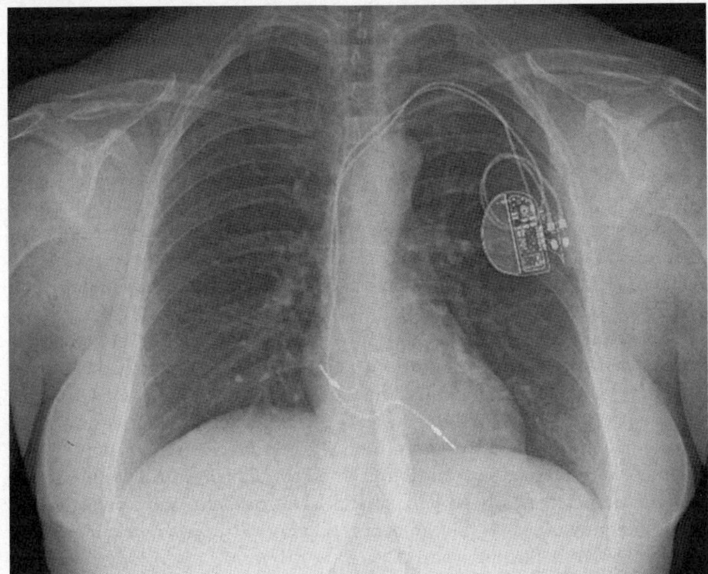

FIGURE 66-1. Typical lead placement for a dual-chamber permanent pacemaker.

transient symptomatic bradycardia, such as may be caused by drug toxicity or a metabolic perturbation, or to maintain a rate of 85 to 100 beats per minute in order to suppress torsades de pointes (Chapter 65) until the causative factor, especially an offending drug, has been eliminated. Prophylactic temporary pacing is used in patients who have high-degree atrioventricular (AV) block in the setting of an acute myocardial infarction (Chapter 73) and for patients who are at a high risk for developing symptomatic bradycardia during an interventional or surgical cardiac procedure.

The most common complication of temporary pacing is infection owing to inadequate sterile techniques at the time of implantation or to suboptimal antisepsis afterward. The risk can be minimized by limiting temporary pacing to 48 hours or by replacing the lead at that time under optimal sterile conditions.

Permanent Pacing

Permanent pacemaker leads can be inserted during cardiac surgery, but they much more frequently are inserted percutaneously through the subclavian vein or by cutdown through a cephalic vein. Ventricular leads are typically positioned in the right ventricular apex or, alternatively, higher on the right ventricular septum or outflow tract, and then are secured in place with a screw mechanism. Atrial leads are usually placed in the right atrial appendage (Fig. 66-1).

Lithium iodide pacemaker batteries, which have a 7- to 8-year lifespan and weigh less than 30 g, typically are implanted subcutaneously in the infraclavicular region (E-Fig. 66-1). The programmability of many different parameters has become standard, as has the ability of the pacemaker to provide diagnostic and telemetric data.

Indications for Permanent Pacemaking

Pacemakers are implanted either to alleviate symptoms caused by bradycardia or to prevent severe symptoms in patients in whom symptomatic bradycardia is likely to develop (Tables 66-1 and 66-2).[1-3] The most common bradycardia-induced symptoms are dizziness or lightheadedness, syncope or near-syncope (Chapters 51 and 62), exercise intolerance, and heart failure. Because these symptoms are nonspecific, documentation of an association between symptoms and bradycardia should be obtained before a pacemaker is recommended. If the bradycardia is persistent, such as in a patient with a complete AV block, a simple electrocardiogram may be sufficient to document the need for a pacemaker. If the bradycardia is intermittent, other diagnostic testing, such as 24-hour ambulatory monitoring, a continuous loop recorder, an implantable event monitor, or an electrophysiology test (Chapter 62), may be needed to document a relationship between symptoms and bradycardia.

Even after a symptomatic bradycardia has been documented, however, a correctable cause for the bradycardia (Chapter 64) should be excluded before a pacemaker is implanted. Correctable causes of symptomatic bradycardia include hypothyroidism (Chapter 226), an overdose with drugs such as

TABLE 66-1 CLASS I INDICATIONS* FOR IMPLANTATION OF A PERMANENT PACEMAKER

SINUS NODE DYSFUNCTION
Symptomatic sinus bradycardia
Symptomatic chronotropic incompetence
Symptomatic sinus bradycardia resulting from required drug therapy
ATRIOVENTRICULAR (AV) BLOCK
Third-degree and advanced second-degree AV block associated with symptomatic bradycardia
Third-degree and advanced second-degree AV block in an awake patient with asystole of >3 seconds or an escape rate of <40 beats per minute or with an infranodal escape rhythm
Atrial fibrillation with a pause of ≥5 seconds
Third-degree and advanced second-degree AV block due to postoperative AV block that is not expected to resolve
Third-degree and advanced second-degree AV block with neuromuscular diseases such as myotonic muscular dystrophy, Kearns-Sayre syndrome, and Erb dystrophy
Asymptomatic third-degree AV block if cardiomegaly or left ventricular dysfunction is present, or if the block is below the AV node
CHRONIC BIFASCICULAR BLOCK
Advanced second-degree or intermittent third-degree AV block
Type II second-degree AV block
Alternating bundle branch block
AFTER ACUTE PHASE OF MYOCARDIAL INFARCTION
Second-degree infranodal AV block with alternating bundle branch block
Third-degree infranodal AV block
Transient advanced second-degree or third-degree infranodal AV block and associated bundle branch block
Persistent symptomatic second-degree or third-degree AV block
CAROTID SINUS SYNDROME
Recurrent syncope caused by spontaneous carotid sinus stimulation or carotid sinus pressure that induces asystole of >3 seconds in duration

*Class I indications are conditions for which a pacemaker is indicated.
Adapted from Gillis AM, Russo AM, Ellenbogen KA, et al. HRS/ACCF expert consensus statement on pacemaker device and mode selection. *J Am Coll Cardiol.* 2012;60:682-703.

TABLE 66-2 CLASS IIA INDICATIONS* FOR IMPLANTATION OF A PERMANENT PACEMAKER

SINUS NODE DYSFUNCTION
Heart rate of <40 beats per minute when a clear association between symptoms consistent with bradycardia and the actual presence of bradycardia has not been demonstrated
Syncope of unclear etiology when sinus node dysfunction is demonstrated by electrophysiologic testing
ATRIOVENTRICULAR (AV) BLOCK
Persistent third-degree AV block with an escape rate of >40 beats per minute in an asymptomatic adult without cardiomegaly
Asymptomatic second-degree infranodal AV block
First-degree or second-degree AV block associated with symptoms similar to pacemaker syndrome
Asymptomatic type II second-degree AV block with a narrow QRS
CHRONIC BIFASCICULAR BLOCK
Syncope, when other potential causes of syncope have been excluded
An HV interval of ≥100 msec
Pathologic pacing-induced infranodal AV block during electrophysiologic testing
CAROTID SINUS SYNDROME
Syncope without clear provocative events and with asystole of >3 seconds during carotid sinus pressure

HIV = His-ventricle.
*Class IIA indications are conditions for which a pacemaker is reasonable.
Adapted from Tracy CM, Epstein AE, Darbar D, et al. 2012 ACCF/AHA/HRS focused update of the 2008 guidelines for device-based therapy of cardiac rhythm abnormalities: a report of the American College of Cardiology Foundation/American Heart Association Task Force on Practice Guidelines. *J Am Coll Cardiol.* 2012;60:1297-1313.

digitalis, electrolyte disturbances, and medications such as β-adrenergic blocking agents (administered either orally or in the form of eye-drops for glaucoma), calcium-channel blocking agents, and antiarrhythmic medications (Chapter 64). At times, a pacemaker is necessary to allow continued treatment with a medication that is responsible for the bradycardia, such as in a patient in whom symptomatic sinus bradycardia develops after initiation of therapy with a β-adrenergic blocking agent for paroxysmal atrial fibrillation (AF) associated with a rapid ventricular response.

Pacing Modes

Pacing modes are described by a simple code. The first letter represents the chamber being paced (A for atrium, V for ventricle, D for dual chamber). The second letter identifies the chamber whose depolarizations are being sensed by the pacemaker (A, V, D, or O for no sensing). The third letter indicates whether the pacemaker is functioning in an inhibited (I) mode, a tracking (T) mode, in both modes (D), or asynchronously (O). The fourth letter designates whether the pacemaker can modulate the heart rate on its own, independent of the patient's intrinsic atrial activity. An additional fifth letter may be used to define the pacemaker's ability to provide antitachycardia pacing (P), to deliver shocks (S), or both (D).

The most appropriate pacing mode must be determined for each individual. By far the most common permanent pacing modes now used in the United States are DDD (pacing and sensing of the atrium and ventricle in both inhibited and tracking fashion) and DDDR (with the additional ability to adjust the atrial rate independently in patients with a poor intrinsic heart rate response to exercise).

In patients with sinus node dysfunction, atrial or dual-chamber pacing significantly reduces the risk for AF[A1] and improves quality of life[A2] compared with ventricular pacing. Although atrial pacing alone is an option for younger active patients with normal AV conduction, the high risk that these patients will develop symptomatic AV block makes initial dual-chamber pacing attractive. In patients with AV block, dual-chamber pacing improves quality of life, reduces the risk for developing AF, and avoids the 25% risk for developing the pacemaker syndrome, which consists of symptoms of weakness, lightheadedness, exercise intolerance, or palpitations owing to the absence of AV synchrony during ventricular pacing. This syndrome is treated by restoring AV synchrony with atrial-based pacing modes, which would require an additional procedure to implant an atrial lead if a dual-chamber pacemaker were not originally placed. For these reasons, current consensus guidelines recommend dual-chamber pacing for most patients with sinus node dysfunction or AV block.

In patients who have paroxysmal AF and dual-chamber pacemakers, the ventricular rate will attempt to track the rapid atrial rates during the arrhythmia. Mode-switching pacemakers can pace in the DDD mode during sinus rhythm and automatically switch to rate-responsive ventricular pacing during AF or other supraventricular arrhythmias (Fig. 66-2). In patients who have long-standing persistent AF and in whom further attempts to restore sinus rhythm are not planned, there is no indication for atrial pacing or for the placement of an atrial lead.

An exception to the recommendation for dual-chamber pacing is in patients who have chronic AF with occasional symptomatic pauses. VVIR pacing is recommended to protect against the pauses and to provide a normal rate response to exercise if needed.

Another option for patients with AV block is biventricular pacing. In patients with AV block, class I to III heart failure, and left ventricular systolic dysfunction, biventricular pacing is superior to conventional right ventricular pacing with an insignificant 17% reduction in death but a larger reduction in severe heart failure.[A3]

Complications of Pacemakers

About 1 to 2% of patients develop complications from the implantation procedure itself, including pocket hematoma, pneumothorax, perforation of the atrium or ventricle, lead dislodgement, subclavian vein thrombosis, and infection. A strategy of continued warfarin treatment at the time of implantation of a pacemaker or an implantable cardioverter-defibrillator (ICD) markedly reduces the incidence of clinically significant device-pocket hematoma compared with bridging therapy with heparin.[A4] The subcutaneous pocket may develop a hematoma or local infection.[4] Pacemaker infections typically involve primarily the subcutaneous pacemaker pocket, but long-term resolution of infection generally requires removal of both the pulse generator and leads as well as long-term antibiotic therapy (Chapter 76). If the device becomes infected, nearly 40% of patients have coexisting valve involvement, predominantly tricuspid valve infection (Chapter 76), with mortality rates as high as 15% in the hospital and 20 to 25% at 1 year.[4]

During long-term follow-up after pacemaker implantation, potential problems include failure to pace, failure to capture, and changes in the pacing rate. These problems may be a manifestation of suboptimal programming, fracture of a lead or a break in its insulation, generator malfunction, or battery depletion.

Ventricular pacing, particularly from the right ventricular apex, is associated with a delayed and abnormal activation sequence, and interventricular and intraventricular mechanical dyssynchrony. When more than 40% of heart beats are the result of ventricular pacing, even in dual-chamber pacing modes, patients can develop adverse ventricular remodeling with ventricular dilation, systolic dysfunction, altered myocardial metabolism, and functional mitral regurgitation. Clinically, such patients are at greater risk for developing AF and heart failure. To avoid those complications, every attempt should be made to minimize the amount of ventricular pacing, including programming longer AV delays (220 to 250 msec) or implanting pacemakers with algorithms that minimize the cumulative percentage of ventricular pacing. In patients with bradycardia and a left ventricular ejection fraction of 35% or less, cardiac resynchronization therapy should be considered if significant right ventricular pacing (>40% of heart beats) is anticipated.

TRANSTHORACIC CARDIOVERSION AND DEFIBRILLATION

Techniques

Defibrillators generate and then discharge an electrical current across two paddle electrodes. The resulting shock simultaneously depolarizes large portions of the atria or ventricles, thereby terminating re-entrant circuits and extinguishing re-entrant arrhythmias that rely on such circuitry (Chapters 61, 64, and 65). Synchronization with the QRS complex (*cardioversion*) is always advised in patients with either a supraventricular tachycardia (SVT) or ventricular tachycardia (VT) because a nonsynchronized shock coincident with the T wave may precipitate ventricular fibrillation (VF). If a shock is needed

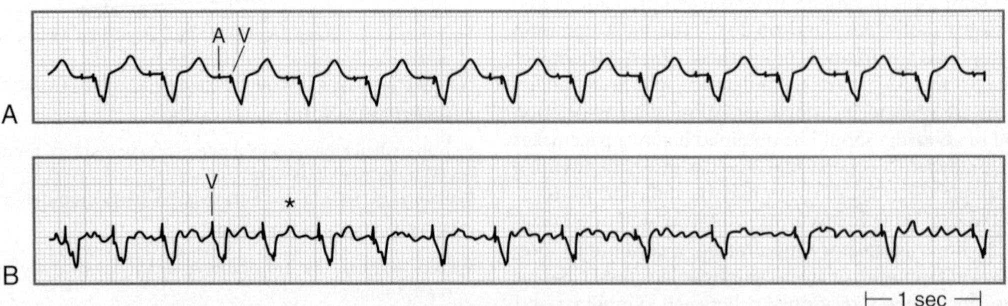

FIGURE 66-2. Rhythm strips from a Holter monitor in a patient with complete atrioventricular block, sinus bradycardia, paroxysmal atrial fibrillation, and a rate-responsive dual-chamber pacemaker with mode-switching capability. A, When the patient is in sinus rhythm, the pacemaker functions in a DDDR mode, with synchronized atrial and ventricular pacing at 105 beats per minute while the patient is walking. **B,** At the onset of an episode of atrial fibrillation, there is tracking of the atrium that results in ventricular pacing at 140 beats per minute, which is the upper rate limit of the pacemaker. Within 2 seconds *(asterisk)*, the mode-switch feature results in VVIR pacing, and the ventricular pacing rate gradually falls to 70 beats per minute, which is the lowest rate limit of the pacemaker. A = atrial stimulus; V = ventricular stimulus. (Courtesy of Dr. Fred Morady.)

to terminate VF, however, this *defibrillation* does not require synchronization to the QRS complex.

The success of cardioversion or defibrillation is affected by the shock waveform and shock strength. Biphasic shock waveforms are recommended because they are significantly more effective than monophasic waveforms at equivalent energies. Other technique-dependent variables that maximize the energy delivered to the heart include increasing paddle pressure, delivery of the shock during expiration, and repetitive shocks. Patient-related factors that may decrease the probability of successful cardioversion and defibrillation include metabolic disturbances, a longer duration of arrhythmia, and higher body weight.

Indications and Technique

The most common arrhythmias treated by cardioversion and defibrillation are VF, VT, AF, and atrial flutter (Chapters 63, 64, and 65). Treatment of VF is always an emergency: a 200-J defibrillation shock should be delivered emergently, followed by one or more 360-J shocks if necessary. Cardioversion of VT may be a life-saving emergency procedure, similar to defibrillation for VF, or an urgent but controlled procedure with an initial shock strength of 50 to 100 J followed by higher energy shocks if needed. For AF, cardioversion is usually an elective procedure, with an initial shock of 200 J in adults, followed by shocks of 300 to 360 J if necessary. For cardioversion of atrial flutter, an initial shock of 50 to 100 J is appropriate. Regardless of the underlying arrhythmia, the energy required is a probability function and not a discrete value, so subsequent shocks may be effective for successful cardioversion or defibrillation even if the first 360-J shock is not effective.

Elective cardioversion requires fasting for at least 8 hours, a reliable catheter in a peripheral vein, oxygen, suction, and equipment for potential emergency airway management. Patients are premedicated (Chapter 432), usually with propofol. In the anteroposterior configuration, which may be more effective for initial cardioversion of AF, one electrode is positioned to the left of the sternum at the fourth intercostal space, with the second electrode placed posteriorly, to the left of the spine, at the same level as the anterior electrode. In the anteroapical configuration, one electrode is placed to the right of the sternum at the level of the second intercostal space, and the second electrode is placed at the mid-axillary line, lateral to the apical impulse.

Precautions and Complications

Cardioversion of AF (Chapter 64) may be complicated by thromboembolism. If no atrial thrombi are seen on a transesophageal echocardiogram, preprocedure anticoagulation is not necessary. Otherwise, anticoagulation is necessary for 3 weeks before elective cardioversion. All patients should be anticoagulated for 1 month after cardioversion if AF has been present for 48 hours or longer.[5]

VF may rarely occur even when shocks are synchronized to the QRS complex. The risk for post-shock ventricular arrhythmias is increased in patients with electrolyte disturbances and digitalis toxicity, so elective cardioversion should be delayed in such patients. Many patients develop elevations of serum troponin levels, sometimes with transient ST segment elevation, after cardioversion, especially if higher energies were delivered in a short period of time, but clinical myocardial dysfunction is rare.

Post-shock bradycardia or asystole, which may occur because of vagal discharge or an underlying sick sinus syndrome, sometimes can require atropine or emergency transcutaneous pacing. If a patient has a pacemaker or ICD, the shocking electrodes should be placed as far away from the generator as possible, and both the generator and pacing threshold should be checked after the procedure.

OTHER IMPLANTABLE DEVICES: CARDIOVERTER-DEFIBRILLATORS AND CARDIAC RESYNCHRONIZATION THERAPY

Implantable Cardioverter-Defibrillators

ICD Pulse Generators and Leads

The procedures for implanting ICDs are analogous to those used for permanent pacemakers. The 60-g pulse generators are similarly implanted subcutaneously in the infraclavicular area. ICDs deliver biphasic shocks at strengths of less than 1 to 42 J while recording the electrogram during the arrhythmia and its treatment. They also can provide antitachycardia overdrive pacing as well as dual-chamber antibradycardia pacing.

A developing alternative is the totally subcutaneous, implantable ICD.[6] With this device, defibrillation is achieved by current flowing between a pulse

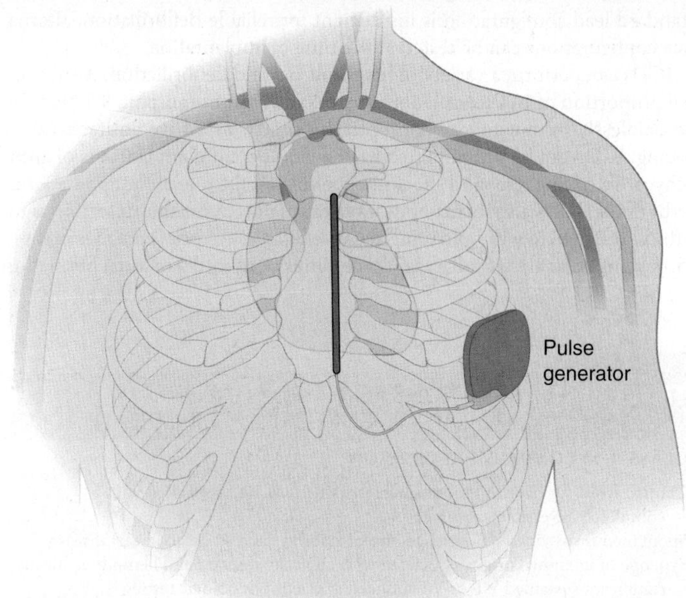

FIGURE 66-3. Schematic of pulse generator and lead position for the subcutaneous defibrillator.

generator implanted in the axilla and a subcutaneous coil implanted parallel and just lateral to the sternum (Fig. 66-3). The pulse generator must deliver higher stored energy (80 J) compared with transvenous defibrillation to ensure an adequate margin of safety for defibrillation, but initial data suggest that the device's effectiveness for sensing and terminating VF is comparable to transvenous systems. The device is not suitable for patients with concomitant bradycardia, in those with indications for cardiac resynchronization therapy, or in patients in whom frequent antitachycardia pacing is needed or anticipated. However, it is likely to become an attractive option for patients who have had prior complications from transvenous systems (e.g., vein thrombosis, infection) and for primary prevention in patients in whom frequent shocks are not anticipated.

Indications

ICD therapy initially evolved as secondary prevention to treat patients who had survived an episode of ventricular fibrillation or hemodynamically unstable ventricular tachycardia and were at high risk for subsequent death owing to recurrent ventricular arrhythmias.[6] Based on multiple randomized trials and careful risk-to-benefit analyses, ICDs now are also implanted as primary prevention in individuals at high risk for a first cardiac arrest (Table 66-3), including patients who have idiopathic dilated cardiomyopathy (Chapter 60) and unexplained episodes of syncope; patients who have dilated ischemic or nonischemic cardiomyopathy with an ejection fraction of 35% or less and class II or III heart failure; patients who have coronary artery disease, an ejection fraction or 35% or less, spontaneous episodes of nonsustained VT, and inducible sustained VT in the electrophysiology laboratory (Chapter 65); patients who have had a previous myocardial infarction and now have an ejection fraction of less than 30% (Chapter 73); and selected patients with conditions such as hypertrophic cardiomyopathy, Brugada syndrome, and long-QT syndrome (Chapters 60 and 65).[7,8] Further refinements in these criteria are to be expected over the coming years as data from ongoing and planned trials become available.

Programming of ICDs

A fundamental goal of ICD implantation and lead configuration is to deliver sufficient energy to the ventricular myocardium to ensure reliable defibrillation. The most common pathway for this energy is from the implanted pectoral pulse generator to a coil electrode on the distal portion of the transvenous lead that is positioned in the right ventricle. The energy required for successful defibrillation is probabilistic, and the relationship between successful defibrillation and energy of the shock is a sigmoidal curve, with an intermediate zone in which the success rate of any single defibrillation attempt is variable. Most transvenous ICD pulse generators can store and deliver 30 to 40 J, which exceeds the typical defibrillation energy threshold of 10 to 15 J, thereby allowing a substantial margin of safety for defibrillation. If the standard lead configuration is insufficient for reliable defibrillation, alternative configurations can be tested at the time of implantation.

ICDs can perform a variety of functions beyond defibrillation. A substantial proportion of ICD recipients have sustained monomorphic VT that can be painlessly terminated by appropriately timed, overdrive antitachycardia pacing. ICDs can be programmed to deliver different combinations of antitachycardia pacing rates and shocks depending on the rate of the spontaneous arrhythmia. ICDs also incorporate a variety of programmable detection algorithms designed to withhold unnecessary therapies for brief episodes of rapid supraventricular arrhythmias, especially sinus tachycardia or atrial fibrillation (Fig. 66-4). In addition, many ventricular arrhythmias, particularly at lower rates, will self-terminate within seconds, so algorithms designed to delay cardioversion for a few seconds can reduce unnecessary shocks. Optimal programming reduces the patient's discomfort, maximizes the life of the pulse generator battery, and reduces the potential adverse effects of unneeded shocks on left ventricular function. For example, optimized programming (incorporating higher rate cutoffs, detection delay, rhythm discriminators, and antitachycardia overdrive pacing can reduce inappropriate device shocks by 50% and mortality by 30% compared with standard ICD programming, without increasing the risk for syncope.[A5,A6] Many athletes with ICDs can engage in vigorous and competitive sports without physical injury or failure to terminate the arrhythmia.[9]

TABLE 66-3 INDICATIONS FOR IMPLANTABLE CARDIOVERTER-DEFIBRILLATOR IMPLANTATION

CLASS I*: SECONDARY PREVENTION
Cardiac arrest survivor (VF or unstable sustained VT not associated with a completely reversible cause)
Spontaneous sustained VT (irrespective of stability) and structural heart disease
Syncope of unknown origin associated with clinically relevant and hemodynamically significant sustained VT or VT induced at electrophysiologic testing
CLASS I*: PRIMARY PREVENTION
Prior myocardial infarction (≥40 days), LVEF < 35%, NYHA class II or III
Prior myocardial infarction (≥40 days), LVEF < 30%, NYHA class I
Nonischemic dilated cardiomyopathy, LVEF ≤ 35%, NYHA class II or III
Prior myocardial infarction, LVEF < 40%, spontaneous NSVT, inducible sustained VT or VF at electrophysiologic testing
CLASS IIA†
Nonischemic dilated cardiomyopathy, significant LV dysfunction, and syncope
Sustained VT and normal or near-normal ventricular function
Hypertrophic cardiomyopathy and one or more risk factors for sudden death
Arrhythmogenic right ventricular cardiomyopathy and one or more risk factors for sudden death
Long QT syndrome with syncope or VT despite β-blocker therapy
Nonhospitalized patients awaiting cardiac transplantation
Brugada syndrome and syncope or VT
Catecholaminergic polymorphic VT and syncope or VT on β-blocker therapy
Cardiac sarcoidosis, giant cell myocarditis, or Chagas disease

*Class I indications are conditions for which an implantable cardioverter-defibrillator is indicated.
†Class IIA indications are conditions for which an implantable cardioverter-defibrillator is reasonable.
LVEF = left ventricular ejection fraction; NSVT = nonsustained ventricular tachycardia, VF = ventricular fibrillation; VT = ventricular tachycardia.
Adapted from Tracy CM, Epstein AE, Darbar D, et al. 2012 ACCF/AHA/HRS focused update of the 2008 guidelines for device-based therapy of cardiac rhythm abnormalities: a report of the American College of Cardiology Foundation/American Heart Association Task Force on Practice Guidelines. *J Am Coll Cardiol.* 2012;60:1297-1313.

Cardiac Resynchronization Therapy

Cardiac resynchronization therapy (CRT) requires the transvenous placement of electrodes into the right ventricle and into the coronary venous system for synchronous pacing of both ventricles (Fig. 66-5).

Indications for CRT

Abnormal and prolonged ventricular activation, as indicated by QRS prolongation of more than 120 msec on the electrocardiogram (ECG), contributes to poorly coordinated dyschronous activation of the left ventricle, thereby resulting in spontaneously reduced systolic function as would occur iatrogenically with right ventricular pacing. Over time, these abnormal electrical patterns can lead to progressive ventricular remodeling with dilation, further impairment of systolic function, and new or worsening heart failure (Chapter 58). Implantation of an additional ventricular lead, typically into a posterolateral coronary vein, permits pacing of the region of latest left ventricular activation. Synchronizing the timing between pacing of the right ventricular septum and the left ventricular free wall promotes more synchronous ventricular contraction and results in "reverse remodeling" with a reduction in ventricular volumes, improved systolic function, and clinical improvement in heart failure (Chapter 59).[10] In clinical trials of patients with reduced systolic function, prolonged QRS duration, and class III or ambulatory class IV heart failure, the addition of CRT to guideline-directed medical therapy is associated with an approximately 30% reduction in hospitalizations and a 24 to 36% reduction in total mortality.[A7] Functional improvement in heart failure symptoms and quality of life is seen in a majority of patients, but 30 to 40% of patients may not improve symptomatically. Superior outcomes are associated with longer QRS delays and a left bundle branch block QRS configuration.[2] Although a prolonged QRS duration is typically associated with mechanical dyssynchrony as demonstrated by cardiac imaging, there is no evidence that imaging-identified mechanical dyssynchrony alone, in the absence of QRS prolongation, identifies patients who will improve with CRT.

Clinical trials have also established that the benefit of CRT extends to patients with less severe heart failure symptoms (class I or II), in whom CRT

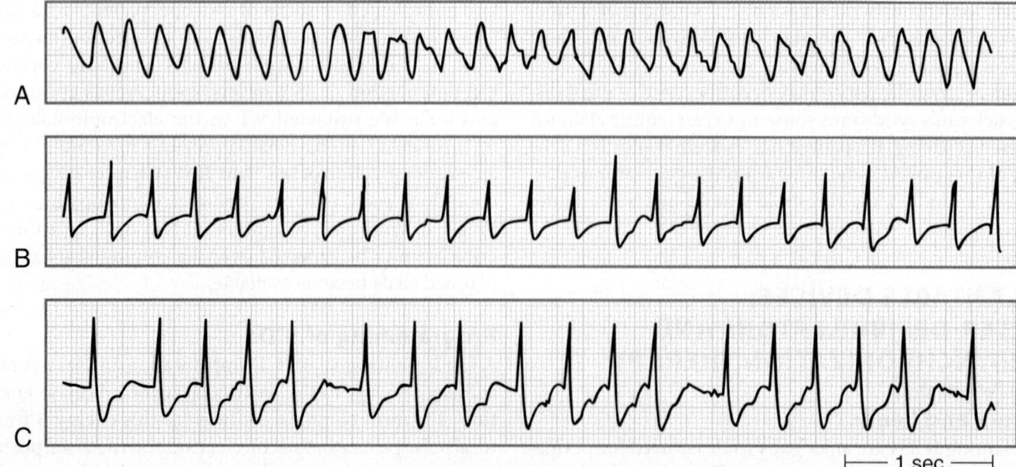

FIGURE 66-4. Examples of stored electrograms obtained several hours after three different patients had experienced a flurry of shocks from an implantable cardioverter-defibrillator and showing the rhythm recorded by the device immediately before a shock was delivered. **A,** In this patient, the stored electrogram demonstrates ventricular tachycardia at a rate of 300 beats per minute, thus indicating that the shock was appropriate. He was treated with amiodarone to reduce the frequency of episodes of ventricular tachycardia. **B,** This patient received shocks because of paroxysmal supraventricular tachycardia at a rate of 206 beats per minute, which exceeded the programmed rate cutoff of 170 beats per minute. He underwent radio frequency ablation of the paroxysmal supraventricular tachycardia and received no further inappropriate shocks. **C,** The stored electrograms in this patient indicate that the patient received inappropriate shocks that were triggered by atrial fibrillation at a rate of 180 beats per minute. The rate cutoff of the device in this patient was 150 beats per minute. This patient was treated with a β-blocker to keep the ventricular rate less than 150 beats per minute during atrial fibrillation. (Courtesy of Dr. Fred Morady.)

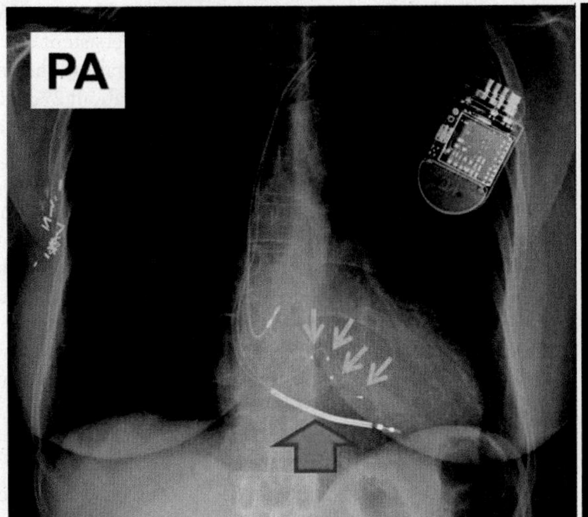

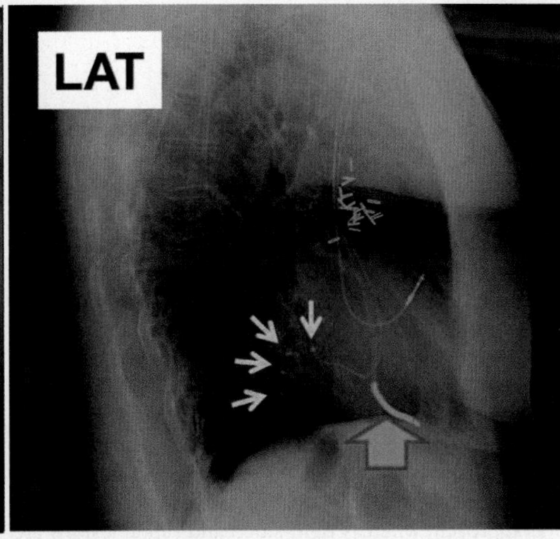

FIGURE 66-5. Typical position of the left ventricular pacing lead in a posterolateral branch of the coronary sinus in a patient with a cardiac resynchronization device. Note the presence of a defibrillator coil on the distal right ventricular lead, indicating that the device is also capable of defibrillation (CRT-D).

appears to delay the onset of symptomatic heart failure and significantly reduce heart failure events over the next 1 to 7 years if the ejection fraction is 30% or less and the QRS duration is more than 130 msec, especially in patients with left bundle branch block.[A8] Current indications for CRT therapy (Table 66-4) likely will continue to evolve as additional evidence accrues. In patients who meet criteria for both CRT and ICD implantation, some evidence suggests that implantation of devices with both functions (CRT-D) may provide additional mortality benefit.[3] However, CRT alone may be appropriate for some patients with more advanced heart failure, extensive comorbidity, and limited life expectancy, in whom the primary objective is symptomatic improvement.

Complications

Many of the complications related to ICD and CRT implantation procedures are somewhat more frequent but are similar to those associated with pacemakers. Major procedure-related complications include pneumothorax, myocardial perforation, and infection, all of which should have an incidence of less than 1%. The approach to infection is similar as for permanent pacemakers. Overall, major complications occur in 2 to 3% of new ICD implants and are more common during pulse generator replacement (5 to 6%). Long-term complications are primarily related to infection and lead failure. Given their larger size and complexity, ICD leads are more likely to fail (1 to 4% annually) than are pacemaker leads (<0.5% annually). Lead failure is most often due to insulation failure or fracture of the conductor wires. Survival of contemporary ICD leads has been estimated at 80 to 98% at 5 years, with lead failure rates accelerating thereafter. Lead failure is highly dependent on the lead's design and on the materials used. CRT devices have the highest likelihood of procedure-related complications, predominantly owing to dislodgement of the coronary sinus lead, and reoperation is required in 4 to 8% of patients.

Although an occasional therapeutic ICD discharge is common, flurries of discharges require urgent evaluation to determine the cause (see Fig. 66-3). Such causes can range from flurries of VT or VF, which may have a correctable precipitant (e.g., an electrolyte imbalance, drug toxicity), to AF or another SVT with a rapid ventricular response, lead fracture, or insulation failure. In some cases, antiarrhythmic drug therapy (see Tables 64-5 and 64-6), catheter ablation, or both may reduce or eliminate the arrhythmias associated with frequent shocks.

TABLE 66-4 INDICATIONS FOR IMPLANTATION OF CRT DEVICE

CLASS I INDICATIONS*
LVEF ≤ 35%, sinus rhythm, LBBB (≥150 msec), NYHA class II, III, or ambulatory class IV on guideline-directed medical therapy
CLASS IIA INDICATIONS†
LVEF ≤ 35%, sinus rhythm, LBBB (120-149 msec), NYHA class II, III, or ambulatory class IV on guideline-directed medical therapy
LVEF < 35%, sinus rhythm, non-LBBB (≥150 msec), NYHA class III or ambulatory class IV on guideline-directed medical therapy
LVEF ≤ 35, atrial fibrillation, on guideline-directed medical therapy, and both: • Requires ventricular pacing or otherwise meets CRT criteria • Near 100% pacing with CRT can be achieved by either atrioventricular node ablation or pharmacologic rate control
LVEF ≤ 35% on guideline-directed medical therapy and are undergoing new or replacement device implantation with anticipated requirement for significant (>40%) ventricular pacing

*Class I indications are conditions for which CRT is indicated.
†Class IIA indications are conditions for which CRT is reasonable.
CRT = cardiac resychronization therapy; LBBB = left bundle branch block; LVEF = left ventricular ejection fraction; NYHA=New York Heart Association (functional class).
Adapted from Brignole M, Auricchio A, Baron-Esquivias G, et al. 2013 ESC Guidelines on cardiac pacing and cardiac resynchronization therapy: the Task Force on cardiac pacing and resynchronization therapy of the European Society of Cardiology (ESC). Developed in collaboration with the European Heart Rhythm Association (EHRA). *Eur Heart J.* 2013;34:2281-2329; and Tracy CM, Epstein AE, Darbar D, et al. 2012 ACCF/AHA/HRS focused update of the 2008 guidelines for device-based therapy of cardiac rhythm abnormalities: a report of the American College of Cardiology Foundation/American Heart Association Task Force on Practice Guidelines. *J Am Coll Cardiol.* 2012;60:1297-1313.

CATHETER ABLATION

Catheter-based ablation techniques are based on the concept that each arrhythmia requires a critical anatomic region or regions to initiate and maintain the formation and propagation of the abnormal impulse. Selective destruction of myocardial tissue in these areas can eliminate the arrhythmia. Depending on the type of arrhythmia, target sites for ablation are selected by recording the electrical activation sequence during an episode of sustained tachycardia, with a goal of identifying a discrete site of origin or a critical component of a larger reentrant circuit. For these arrhythmias, reproduction of the clinical arrhythmia during diagnostic electrophysiologic testing (Chapter 62) is critical and can be facilitated by careful selection of pacing sites, judicious use of sedation, and intravenous infusion of catecholamines. Alternatively, the target site can sometimes be selected based on specific anatomic landmarks or tissue characteristics identified during sinus rhythm.

Tissue Effects of Applied Energy

Radio frequency current, typically in the range of 300 to 750 kHz, is the most common form of energy used in catheter ablation. The energy is applied in a unipolar fashion between a small electrode in contact with the targeted myocardium and a large dispersive cutaneous patch electrode placed on the back. The small electrode area at the myocardial interface results in a high-density current and rapid resistive heating in the myocardium that is immediately subjacent to the electrode, with slower conductive heating of deeper myocardial layers. A tissue temperature greater than 60° C is required for irreversible myocyte injury. Saline irrigation of the electrode reduces heating at the tissue-electrode interface, moves the zone of maximal heating deeper into the tissue, and results in larger, deeper lesions. Among other energy sources, cryoablation is the most widely used, whereas microwave, laser, and ultrasound have limited applications at present.

Radio Frequency Ablation of Supraventricular Tachycardias

Radio frequency ablation is the recommended first-line treatment for paroxysmal SVT, Wolff-Parkinson-White (WPW) syndrome, or type 1 (typical) atrial flutter that is symptomatic enough to warrant therapy (Chapter 64). For atrial flutter other than type 1 and for inappropriate sinus tachycardia, an ablation procedure is recommended only in patients who have significant symptoms and recurrences despite antiarrhythmic medications. AV nodal re-entrant tachycardia (Chapter 64), which is the most common type of paroxysmal SVT, is successfully eliminated in 98% of cases (with a <1% risk for high-degree AV block) by radio frequency ablation of the "slow" limb of the re-entry circuit, usually at the posteroseptal aspect of the right atrium, near the ostium of the coronary sinus. Cryoablation, which is associated with a lower risk for AV block but also a lower long-term success rate, may be considered for patients at higher risk for AV block, such as small children.

Left-sided accessory pathways are ablated by using either a retrograde aortic or a transseptal approach, whereas right-sided and septal lesions are ablated with a venous approach. Detailed mapping is essential to identify the optimal site for ablation, usually on either the atrial or the ventricular aspect of the mitral or tricuspid annulus. For the ablation of an accessory pathway, the success rate is 90 to 98%, with an overall complication rate of 2 to 3% and a less than 0.1% risk for a fatal complication. The most common serious complications are cardiac tamponade, owing to mechanical perforation of the heart by an electrode catheter, and high-degree AV block when the accessory pathway is near the AV node. Cryoablation is a reasonable alternative when the accessory pathway is near the AV node.

Most atrial tachycardias arise in the right atrium and are mapped using a venous approach, but left atrial tachycardias require a transseptal approach. Approximately 10 to 20% of patients with atrial tachycardia have more than one focus, and this rhythm may also be observed in association with other forms of SVT, particularly AV nodal re-entrant tachycardia. If the atrial tachycardia originates from a single site, ablation has about a 90% success rate, and complications are rare. For patients with multiple sources of atrial tachycardia, long-term success rates are lower.

Type 1 atrial flutter (Chapter 64), which arises in the right atrium, can be eliminated by ablation directed at a critical isthmus located in the low right atrium, between the tricuspid annulus and the inferior vena cava. The long-term success rate is more than 90%, with a less than 1% risk for serious complications.

Ablation of Atrial Fibrillation

Strategies for catheter ablation of AF (Chapter 64) are evolving.[11] At present, the primary aim of AF ablation is to reduce symptoms caused by recurrent episodes and thereby to improve quality of life. For patients with recurrent paroxysmal AF, a primary driver of the arrhythmia is from focal sources in the regions surrounding the proximal portions of the pulmonary vein and other thoracic veins as they insert into atrial myocardium. However, focally triggered arrhythmias may arise from other right and left atrial sites in 10 to 20% of patients.

For patients with recurrent symptomatic paroxysmal AF despite at least one antiarrhythmic drug trial, radio frequency or cryoballon catheter ablation reduces the risk for recurrent atrial arrhythmias by 50 to 70% and significantly improves quality of life compared with continued attempts to control the arrhythmia with alternative drug therapy.[12,13] Clinical trial data also demonstrate improved outcomes for reducing recurrent AF in selected patients with paroxysmal AF in whom catheter ablation is used as first-line treatment,[A9,A10] although rates of recurrence remain in the 50% range at 2 years even in patients who underwent ablation. Because AF is a progressive disease, however, the window of opportunity for intervention to prevent progression from paroxysmal to permanent AF or to prevent stroke, heart failure, or death may be limited. Ongoing large clinical trials are likely to provide more definitive information on long-term outcomes.

For patients with continuous persistent AF of greater than 1-year duration, catheter ablation is less successful. In patients with symptomatic heart failure, a left ventricular ejection fraction of 35% or less, and persistent AF, ablation can improve symptoms and neurohormonal status compared with rate control therapy.[A11] However, isolation of the pulmonary veins alone may be insufficient to maintain sinus rhythm. Adjunctive or alternative strategies, guided by anatomic considerations or mapping during AF, are the subject of ongoing investigation, and their long-term success is unclear.

Overall, the 1-year success rate of catheter ablation is 75 to 85% for paroxysmal AF and 60 to 75% for longstanding persistent AF. The most serious complications of AF ablation are atrial perforation, thromboembolism, and atrioesophageal fistula, with an overall risk of about 2%. Other complications are phrenic nerve injury or vascular access issues. Pulmonary vein stenosis is a potentially serious complication that can be avoided by not delivering energy within the tubular portion of the pulmonary veins.

In patients with refractory AF associated with an uncontrolled ventricular rate despite pharmacologic AV node blockade, ablation of the AV node can improve symptoms, functional capacity, and left ventricular function. In AV node ablation, third-degree AV block is intentionally induced with a success rate that approaches 100%. When the ablation lesions are placed sufficiently proximal in the AV junction, a junctional escape rhythm usually can be preserved. All patients require a permanent pacemaker to provide adequate rate response to physical activity.

Ablation of Ventricular Arrhythmias

Radio frequency ablation has an 85 to 100% success rate for the treatment of focal idiopathic VT (Chapter 65), whether it arises in the outflow tract of the right ventricle with a left bundle branch block configuration and superior axis, or arises from other sites, including the AV valve annuli, the sinuses of Valsalva, the left ventricular septum, or the papillary muscles. Given these outcomes, ablation is recommended in symptomatic patients, either after failure of initial drug therapy or as first-line therapy depending on a patient's preference.[14] Complications have been rare, and patients can avoid medications or an ICD.

By comparison, VT in patients with coronary artery disease usually arises in diseased tissue adjacent to an area of previous infarction in the left ventricle. Radio frequency ablation is not usually curative because the disease process is diffuse and the VT may originate from multiple sites. However, radio frequency ablation can be used as adjunctive therapy to reduce the number of ICD discharges, with a success rate of 65 to 95% and serious complications in about 5% of patients.

ARRHYTHMIA SURGERY

Ventricular Tachycardia

Subendocardial resection or cryoablation of the scar tissue that triggers monomorphic VT (Chapter 65) in patients with a prior myocardial infarction can eliminate VT in selected patients, with a success rate of 85 to 90% but an operative mortality rate of 5 to 15% even in experienced centers. Because of this high mortality rate, the procedure is limited to patients who have recurrent VT and other indications for cardiac surgery, such as large aneurysms associated with heart failure or the need to implant a left ventricular assist device.

Atrial Fibrillation

In the Maze procedure, a series of incisions or linear lesions or both are created by cryoablation or radio frequency ablation in the specific regions of the left and right atria to subdivide the atria into parts too small to sustain AF.[15] The success rate for eliminating AF is about 90%, and the operative mortality rate is less than 2%. The most common indication for the Maze procedure currently is for treatment of symptomatic AF in patients undergoing other cardiac surgical procedures, such as coronary revascularization or valve replacement or repair. A variety of simpler and even minimally invasive operative procedures have been developed for AF, but their long-term efficacy and their role in the treatment of AF remain unclear.

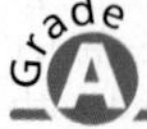

Grade A References

A1. Sweeney MO, Bank AJ, Nsah E, et al. Minimizing ventricular pacing to reduce atrial fibrillation in sinus-node disease. *N Engl J Med.* 2007;357:1000-1008.

A2. Lamas GA, Lee KL, Sweeney MO, et al. Ventricular pacing or dual-chamber pacing for sinus-node dysfunction. *N Engl J Med.* 2002;346:1854-1862.

A3. Curtis AB, Worley SJ, Adamson PB, et al. Biventricular pacing for atrioventricular block and systolic dysfunction. *N Engl J Med.* 2013;368:1585-1593.

A4. Birnie DH, Healey JS, Wells GA, et al. Pacemaker or defibrillator surgery without interruption of anticoagulation. *N Engl J Med.* 2013;368:2084-2093.

A5. Moss AJ, Schuger C, Beck CA, et al. Reduction in inappropriate therapy and mortality through ICD programming. *N Engl J Med.* 2012;367:2275-2283.

A6. Tan VH, Wilton SB, Kuriachan V, et al. Impact of programming strategies aimed at reducing nonessential implantable cardioverter defibrillator therapies on mortality: a systematic review and meta-analysis. *Circ Arrhythm Electrophysiol.* 2014;7:164-170.

A7. Cleland JG, Abraham WT, Linde C, et al. An individual patient meta-analysis of five randomized trials assessing the effects of cardiac resynchronization therapy on morbidity and mortality in patients with symptomatic heart failure. *Eur Heart J*. 2013;34:3547-3556.
A8. Goldenberg I, Kutyifa V, Klein HU, et al. Survival with cardiac-resynchronization therapy in mild heart failure. *N Engl J Med*. 2014;370:1694-1701.
A9. Cosedis Nielsen J, Johannessen A, Raatikainen P, et al. Radiofrequency ablation as initial therapy in paroxysmal atrial fibrillation. *N Engl J Med*. 2012;367:1587-1595.
A10. Morillo CA, Verma A, Connolly SJ, et al. Radiofrequency ablation vs antiarrhythmic drugs as first-line treatment of paroxysmal atrial fibrillation (RAAFT-2): a randomized trial. *JAMA*. 2014;311:692-700.
A11. Jones DG, Haldar SK, Hussain W, et al. A randomized trial to assess catheter ablation versus rate control in the management of persistent atrial fibrillation in heart failure. *J Am Coll Cardiol*. 2013;61:1894-1903.

GENERAL REFERENCES

For the General References and other additional features, please visit Expert Consult at https://expertconsult.inkling.com.

67

ARTERIAL HYPERTENSION

RONALD G. VICTOR

DEFINITION

Hypertension is defined as a usual office blood pressure of 140/90 mm Hg or higher (Table 67-1), blood pressure levels for which the benefits of drug treatment have been shown in randomized controlled trials. However, epidemiologic data show continuous positive relationships between the risk for death from coronary artery disease (CAD) and stroke with systolic or diastolic blood pressure values as low as 115/75 mm Hg (Fig. 67-1). The artificial dichotomy between "hypertension" and "normotension" may delay medical treatment until vascular health has been irreversibly compromised by elevated blood pressure values that were previously considered normal. As a result, guideline committees continue to debate how far to lower blood pressure with antihypertensive medication and whether to recommend drug therapy for high-risk patients with blood pressure in the "prehypertensive" range of 120 to 139/80 to 89 mm Hg.[1-4]

EPIDEMIOLOGY

Affecting one fourth of the adult population (78 million adults in the United States and more than 1 billion people worldwide), arterial hypertension is the leading cause of death in the world and the most common cause for an outpatient visit to a physician; it is the most easily recognized treatable risk factor for stroke (Chapters 406, 407, and 408), myocardial infarction (Chapters 72 and 73), heart failure (Chapters 58 and 59), peripheral vascular disease (Chapter 79), aortic dissection (Chapter 78), atrial fibrillation (Chapter 64), and end-stage kidney disease (Chapter 130). Because of increasing rates of obesity and aging of the population, hypertension is projected to affect 1.5 billion persons, one third of the world's population, by the year 2025. Presently, about 54% of strokes and 47% of ischemic heart disease worldwide is attributable to high blood pressure. Half of this disease burden is in people who meet the definition of hypertension, and the remainder is in people with lesser degrees of high blood pressure (*prehypertension*).

The asymptomatic nature of hypertension and the inherent variability in blood pressure delay diagnosis. Effective treatment requires frequent medical checkups and continuity of care by a knowledgeable clinician, both of which are less common in men and in members of low-income minority groups. Most cases of hypertension are multifactorial, and management remains empirical, often requiring three or more drugs with complementary mechanisms of action, in addition to any other medications that may be needed for concomitant medical conditions. Pill burden, prescription drug costs, medication side effects, and insufficient time for patient education contribute to nonadherence with medications. Busy primary care physicians often undertreat hypertension. Lifestyle modification (particularly diet and exercise) can lower blood pressure somewhat, but the reduction rarely is enough to eliminate the need for medication. For all these reasons, blood pressure remains elevated—140/90 mm Hg or higher—in more than half of affected individuals in the United States, with marked racial, ethnic, and gender disparities.[5] The resultant annual cost to the U.S. health care system exceeds $73 billion.

TABLE 67-1 STAGING OF OFFICE BLOOD PRESSURE*

BLOOD PRESSURE STAGE	SYSTOLIC BLOOD PRESSURE (mm Hg)	DIASTOLIC BLOOD PRESSURE (mm Hg)
Normal	<120	<80
Prehypertension	120-139	80-89
Stage 1 hypertension	140-159	90-99
Stage 2 hypertension	≥160	≥100

*Calculation of seated blood pressure is based on the mean of two or more readings on two separate office visits.
From Chobanian A, Bakris G, Black H, et al. The Seventh Report of the Joint National Committee on the Prevention, Evaluation, and Treatment of High Blood Pressure: the JNC 7 report. *JAMA*. 2003;289:2560-2572.

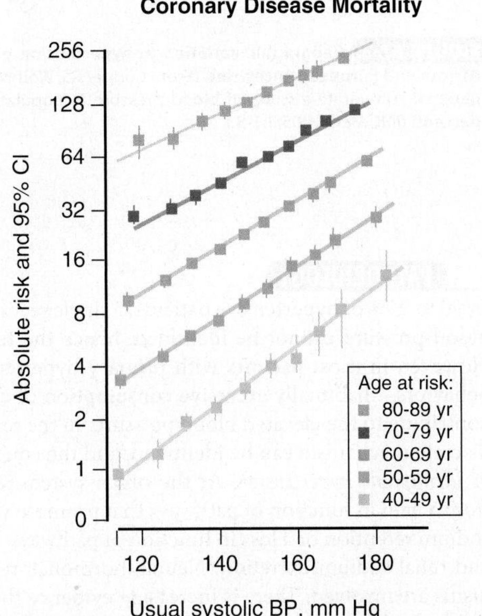

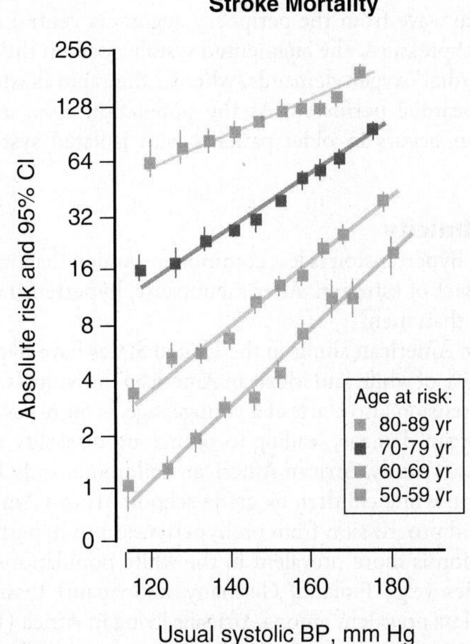

FIGURE 67-1. Absolute risk for coronary artery disease and stroke mortality by usual systolic blood pressure (BP) levels. CI = confidence interval. (From Lewington S, Clarke R, Qizilbash N, et al, for the Prospective Studies Collaboration. Age-specific relevance of usual blood pressure to vascular mortality: a meta-analysis of individual data for one million adults in 61 prospective studies. *Lancet*. 2002;360:1903-1913.)

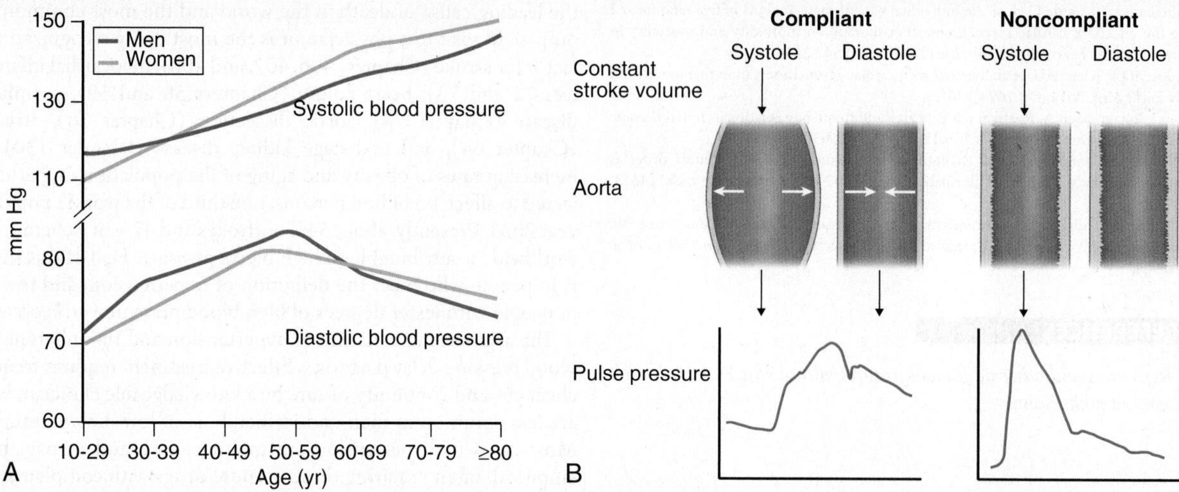

FIGURE 67-2. Aging and pulse pressure. **A,** Age-dependent changes in systolic and diastolic blood pressure in the United States. **B,** Schematic diagram showing the relation between aortic compliance and pulse pressure. (**A,** From Burt V, Whelton P, Rocella EJ, et al. Prevalence of hypertension in the U.S. adult population: results from the Third National Health and Nutrition Examination Survey, 1988-1991. *Hypertension.* 1995;25:305-313; **B,** Courtesy of Dr. Stanley Franklin, University of California at Irvine.)

Aging and Pulse Pressure

Patients often ask: is systolic or diastolic blood pressure more important? The answer is: both. In industrialized societies, systolic pressure rises progressively with age; if individuals live long enough, almost all (>90%) will develop hypertension. This age-dependent rise in blood pressure is not an essential part of human biology. In less developed countries where consumption of calories and salt is low, blood pressures remain low and do not rise with age. In developed countries, diastolic pressure rises until the age of 50 years and decreases thereafter, producing a progressive rise in pulse pressure (systolic pressure minus diastolic pressure) (Fig. 67-2).

Different hemodynamic faults underlie hypertension in younger and older persons. Patients who develop hypertension before the age of 50 years typically have *combined systolic and diastolic hypertension:* systolic pressure above 140 mm Hg *and* diastolic pressure above 90 mm Hg. The main hemodynamic fault is vasoconstriction at the level of the resistance arterioles. In contrast, most patients who develop hypertension after the age of 50 years have *isolated systolic hypertension:* systolic pressure above 140 mm Hg but diastolic pressure below 90 mm Hg (often below 80 mm Hg). In isolated systolic hypertension, the primary hemodynamic fault is decreased distensibility of the large conduit arteries. Collagen replaces elastin in the elastic lamina of the aorta, a process that is accelerated by both aging and hypertension. When pulse wave velocity increases sufficiently, the rapid return of the arterial pulse wave from the periphery augments central systolic (rather than diastolic) pressure. The augmented systolic load on the left ventricle increases myocardial oxygen demands, whereas the rapid diastolic runoff compromises myocardial perfusion. As the population ages, most uncontrolled hypertension occurs in older patients with isolated systolic hypertension.

Gender and Race/Ethnicity

Before the age of 50 years, hypertension is less common in women than men, suggesting a protective effect of estrogen. After menopause, hypertension is more common in women than men.

Forty percent of African American adults in the United States have hypertension, compared with 25% of white and Mexican American individuals.[5] In African Americans, hypertension also starts at a younger age, is more severe, and causes more target organ damage, leading to premature disability and death. In the Bogalusa Heart Study, African American children already had higher blood pressures than white children by grade school. African Americans also have a more rapid progression from prehypertension to hypertension. However, hypertension is more prevalent in the white populations of several European countries (e.g., Finland, Germany, and Spain) than in African Americans and is less prevalent among Africans living in Africa (Fig. 67-3), although hypertension is increasing in developing countries undergoing Westernization. These international data emphasize the importance of environmental factors.

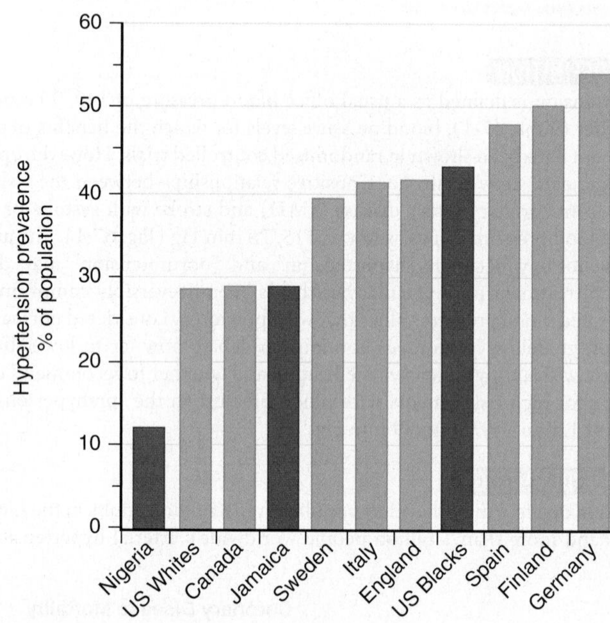

FIGURE 67-3. Geographic variation in hypertension prevalence in populations of African and European ancestries. (From Cooper RS, Wolf-Maier K, Luke A, et al. An international comparative study of blood pressure in populations of European vs. African descent. *BMC Med.* 2005;3:1-8.)

PATHOBIOLOGY

In 90 to 95% of hypertensive patients, a single reversible cause of the elevated blood pressure cannot be identified, hence the term *primary hypertension.* However, in most patients with primary hypertension, readily identifiable behaviors—habitually excessive consumption of calories, salt, or alcohol—contribute to the elevated blood pressure. In the remaining 5 to 10%, a more discrete mechanism can be identified, and the condition is termed *secondary or identifiable hypertension.* At the organ-system level, hypertension results from a gain in function of pathways that promote vasoconstriction and renal sodium retention or a loss in function of pathways that promote vasodilation and renal sodium excretion. Neural, hormonal, renal, and vascular mechanisms are involved. There is increasing evidence that neurohormonal activation contributes to the early pathogenesis by compromising vascular function (e.g., endothelium-dependent vasodilation) and structure (e.g., inward remodeling) that precede hypertension.

Behavioral Determinants of Human Blood Pressure Variation

The most important behavioral determinants of blood pressure are related to dietary consumption of calories and salt. Across populations, the prevalence of hypertension increases linearly with average body mass index. With the obesity epidemic in both developed and developing societies, increasing attention is being paid to the *metabolic syndrome* (Chapter 229) that often accompanies hypertension. The metabolic syndrome refers to the frequent clustering of elevated blood pressure with abdominal ("male pattern") adiposity, insulin resistance with glucose intolerance, and a dyslipidemic pattern consisting typically of elevated plasma triglyceride and low high-density lipoprotein cholesterol levels. In the Framingham Heart Study, obesity has been estimated to account for as much as 60% of the new cases of hypertension. The underlying mechanisms by which weight gain leads to hypertension are incompletely understood, but there is mounting evidence for an expanded plasma volume plus sympathetic overactivity. The sympathetic overactivity is thought to be a compensatory attempt to burn fat but at the expense of peripheral vasoconstriction, renal salt and water retention, and hypertension. In some obese individuals, sleep apnea (Chapter 100) is an important cause of hypertension. Repeated arterial desaturation sensitizes the carotid body chemoreceptors, causing sustained sympathetic overactivity even during waking hours.

Dietary sodium intake is another key behavioral determinant of human hypertension. In the INTERSALT study of 52 locations around the world, the risk for development of hypertension during three decades of adult life was linearly and tightly related to dietary sodium intake. Interindividual variability in blood pressure responses to dietary sodium loading and sodium restriction indicates an important genetic underpinning.

Genetic Determinants of Human Blood Pressure Variation

Concordance of blood pressures is greater within families than in unrelated individuals, greater between monozygotic twins than between dizygotic twins, and greater between biologic siblings than between adoptive siblings living in the same household. As much as 70% of the familial aggregation of blood pressure is attributed to shared genes rather than to shared environment.

The complex regulation of blood pressure has thwarted the genetic dissection of primary human hypertension, with the first positive genome-wide association studies suggesting multiple risk alleles, each having very small effects. Mutations in 20 salt-handling genes cause ultra-rare syndromes of severe, early-onset hypotension (salt-wasting syndromes) or hypertension (all inherited as mendelian traits). The clinical relevance of these mutations to common primary hypertension has been limited, although recent data indicate that heterozygous mutations in genes underlying the pediatric salt-wasting syndromes (Bartter and Gitelman) are present in 1 to 2% of the general adult population and confer resistance against primary hypertension.

CLINICAL MANIFESTATIONS

Hypertension is called the silent killer—an asymptomatic chronic disorder that silently damages the blood vessels, heart, brain, and kidneys if it is undetected and untreated. Although headaches (Chapter 398) are common in patients with mild to moderate hypertension, episodes of headaches do not correlate with fluctuations in blood pressure. Rather, they correlate with a person's awareness of his or her diagnosis.

DIAGNOSIS

Initial Evaluation for Hypertension

The initial evaluation for hypertension should accomplish three goals: (1) stage the blood pressure, (2) assess the patient's additional cardiovascular risk factors, and (3) detect clues of secondary hypertension that require further evaluation.

Goal 1: Accurate Assessment of Blood Pressure

Office Blood Pressure

Traditionally, blood pressure has been staged as normal, prehypertension, or hypertension based on the average of two or more readings taken at two or more office visits (see Table 67-1). The blood pressure should be measured at least twice after 5 minutes of rest with the patient seated, the back supported, and the arm bare and at heart level. A large adult-sized cuff should be used to measure blood pressure in overweight adults because the standard-sized cuff will cause falsely elevated readings. Tobacco and caffeine should be avoided for at least 30 minutes. Blood pressure should be measured in both arms, to exclude coarctation of the aorta, and after 5 minutes of standing, to exclude a significant postural fall, particularly in older patients and patients with diabetes or other conditions (e.g., Parkinson disease) that predispose to autonomic insufficiency.

Home and Ambulatory Blood Pressure Monitoring

A person's blood pressure varies so much throughout a 24-hour period that it is impossible to characterize it accurately except by repeated measurements under various conditions. Out-of-office readings are the only way to obtain a clear picture of a person's usual blood pressure for accurate diagnosis and management. These readings are more predictive of cardiovascular events than office readings and overcome many of the pitfalls of office measurement, including physician errors and "white coat" reactions. Home blood pressure monitoring can improve medication adherence by actively involving patients in their own medical care.

New recommendations include the following: (1) home blood pressure monitoring should become a routine part of the clinical management of patients with known or suspected hypertension the same way that home blood glucose monitoring is essential to the management of patients with diabetes; (2) two or three readings should be taken in the morning and at night for 4 days; the first day's readings should be discarded as being artificially high, and all the other readings should be averaged; and (3) the target treatment goal is an average home blood pressure of less than 135/85 mm Hg for most patients and less than 130/80 mm Hg for patients with proteinuric chronic kidney disease and possibly for some other high-risk patients.

A validated electronic oscillometric monitor with an arm cuff should be chosen from the dabl Educational Web site (www.dableducational.org). Each patient's monitor should be checked in the physician's office for its accuracy and appropriate cuff size. Patients must be taught correct measurement techniques and to avoid reporting bias. Wrist monitors are inaccurate and not recommended. The oscillometric method may not work well in patients with atrial fibrillation or frequent extrasystoles, for whom manual sphygmomanometry is required. Some patients will become obsessed about taking their blood pressure and need to stop.

Ambulatory blood pressure monitoring (Table 67-2) provides automated measurements of blood pressure during a 24-hour period while patients are engaged in their usual activities, including sleep (Fig. 67-4). Ambulatory blood pressure measurement is superior to standard office measurement in predicting fatal and nonfatal myocardial infarction and stroke. Recommended normal values are an average daytime blood pressure below 135/85 mm Hg, nighttime blood pressure below 120/70 mm Hg, and 24-hour blood pressure below 130/80 mm Hg (Table 67-3) Some experts have recommended a lower cutoff value of 130/80 mm Hg as a more stringent definition of normal daytime blood pressure.

TABLE 67-2 RECOMMENDED CLINICAL INDICATIONS FOR AMBULATORY BLOOD PRESSURE MONITORING

- Suspicion of white-coat hypertension
  - High office blood pressure in untreated patients with no target organ damage and low cardiovascular risk
- Suspicion of masked hypertension
  - Normal office blood pressure in untreated or treated patients with target organ damage or high cardiovascular risk
- Differentiation of pseudoresistant from truly resistant hypertension
- Labile blood pressure
  - Suspicion of dysautonomia: orthostatic hypotension ± supine hypertension, postprandial hypotension, baroreflex failure
  - Suspicion of drug-induced hypotension
- Suspicion of nocturnal hypertension in patients with sleep apnea, chronic kidney disease, or diabetes
- Assessment of hypertension in elderly people, children, and adolescents, and pregnant women.

Adapted from O'Brien E, Parati G, Stergiou G, et al. European society of hypertension position paper on ambulatory blood pressure monitoring. *J Hypertens.* 2013;31:1731-1768; and Mancia G, Fagard R, Narkiewicz K, et al. 2013 ESH/ESC Guidelines for the management of arterial hypertension: the Task Force for the management of arterial hypertension of the European Society of Hypertension (ESH) and of the European Society of Cardiology (ESC). *J Hypertens.* 2013;31:1281-1357.

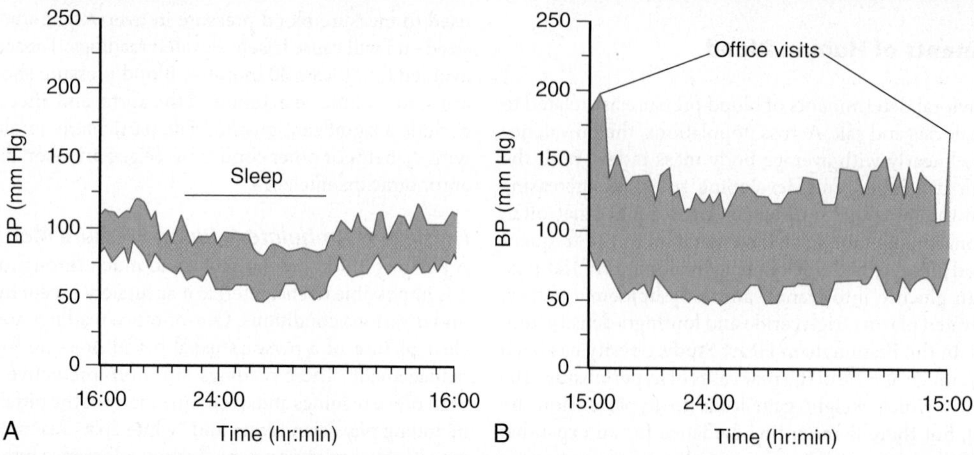

FIGURE 67-4. **The 24-hour ambulatory blood pressure (BP) monitor tracings of two different patients. A, Optimal blood pressure in a healthy 37-year-old woman. Note the normal variability in blood pressure, the nocturnal dip in blood pressure during sleep, and the sharp increase in blood pressure on awakening. B, Pronounced white coat effect in an 80-year-old woman referred for evaluation of medically refractory hypertension. Documentation of the white coat effect prevented overtreatment of the patient's isolated systolic hypertension. (A, Provided by Ronald G. Victor, MD, Hypertension Center, Cedars-Sinai Heart Institute, Los Angeles, California; B, Courtesy of Wanpen Vongpatanasin, MD, Hypertension Division, Department of Internal Medicine, University of Texas Southwestern Medical Center, Dallas, Texas.)**

TABLE 67-3 DEFINITIONS OF HYPERTENSION BY OFFICE AND OUT-OF-OFFICE BLOOD PRESSURE LEVELS

CATEGORY	SYSTOLIC (mm Hg)		DIASTOLIC (mm Hg)
Office blood pressure	≥140	and/or	≥90
Home blood pressure	≥135	and/or	≥85
Ambulatory blood pressure			
• Daytime (or awake)	≥135	and/or	≥85
• Nighttime (or sleep)	≥120	and/or	≥70
• 24 hour	≥130	and/or	≥80

Adapted from Mancia G, Fagard R, Narkiewicz K, et al. 2013 ESH/ESC Guidelines for the management of arterial hypertension: the Task Force for the management of arterial hypertension of the European Society of Hypertension (ESH) and of the European Society of Cardiology (ESC). *J Hypertens.* 2013;31:1281-1357.

About 20% of patients with elevated office blood pressures have normal home or ambulatory blood pressures. If the daytime blood pressure is below 135/85 mm Hg (or preferably below 130/80 mm Hg) and there is no target organ damage despite consistently elevated office readings, the patient has "office-only" or "white coat" hypertension, caused by a transient adrenergic response to the measurement of blood pressure in the physician's office. If there are no other risk factors (such as metabolic syndrome), the cardiovascular risk is similar to that in persons with consistently normal blood pressure. Many patients do not have pure white coat hypertension but rather white coat aggravation, a white coat reaction superimposed on a milder level of out-of-office hypertension that nevertheless needs treatment. For example, up to 30% of treated patients who have persistently elevated office blood pressure readings will be shown by ambulatory monitoring to have adequate or even excessive control of their hypertension, thereby eliminating overtreatment (see Fig. 67-4). In other patients, office readings underestimate ambulatory blood pressures, presumably because of sympathetic overactivity (e.g., owing to job stress, home stress, or tobacco smoke) that dissipates when the patient comes to the office. Such "masked hypertension" carries the same increased cardiovascular risk as sustained office and home hypertension and is particularly common in men, elderly patients, and patients with diabetes or chronic kidney disease (E-Fig. 67-1). Both white coat and masked hypertension are so common in elderly patients that office blood pressure measurement alone, without home or ambulatory monitoring, would lead to either overtreatment or undertreatment in three out of every four patients.[6] Current U.K. and European guidelines place far greater emphasis than U.S. guidelines on home and ambulatory blood pressure monitoring for clinical decision making.

Ambulatory monitoring is the only way to detect hypertension during sleep. Blood pressure normally dips during sleep and increases sharply when a person awakens and becomes active. Nocturnal hypertension increases the aggregate blood pressure burden on the cardiovascular system and is a stronger predictor of cardiovascular outcomes than daytime ambulatory blood pressure or office measurements. Nocturnal hypertension is particularly common in patients with chronic kidney disease (Chapter 130), presumably because of their sustained sympathetic overactivity, which does not shut down during sleep, and centralization of blood volume with nocturnal recumbence. Nocturnal hypertension also is prevalent in African Americans, in whom the normal nocturnal dipping of blood pressure is often impaired.

Goal 2: Cardiovascular Risk Stratification

Although cardiovascular risk increases with increasing blood pressure, it also increases if the patient has hypertensive target organ damage or additional cardiovascular risk factors (Table 67-4). More than 75% of hypertensive patients will benefit from lipid-lowering statins (Chapter 206), and 25% have diabetes. Thus, the minimal laboratory testing required for the initial evaluation of hypertension is determination of blood electrolyte, fasting glucose, and serum creatinine levels (with calculated glomerular filtration rate [GFR]), a fasting lipid panel, hematocrit, spot urinalysis (including urine albumin-to-creatinine ratio), and a resting 12-lead electrocardiogram (ECG).

The gradient of increasing levels of blood pressure with cardiovascular risk steepens as additional risk factors are added. The patient's global cardiovascular risk should be estimated from the 2013 ACC/AHA pooled atherosclerotic cardiovascular disease (ASCVD) risk calculator (http://www.cardiosource.org/Science-And-Quality/Practice-Guidelines-and-Quality-Standards/2013-Prevention-Guideline-Tools.aspx). Decisions regarding treatment thresholds and treatment targets, however, still depend largely on specific blood pressure values rather than on an individual's global cardiovascular risk. Higher risk hypertensive patients are more likely to be treated with blood pressure medications but less likely to have their office blood pressure controlled to less than 140/90 mm Hg.

Goal 3: Identification and Treatment of Secondary (Identifiable) Causes of Hypertension

The third goal of the initial evaluation is to screen for identifiable causes of hypertension (Table 67-5), in the hope of finding a surgical cure. A thorough search for secondary causes, which is not cost effective in most patients with hypertension, becomes critically important in two circumstances: (1) when there is a compelling finding on the initial evaluation and (2) when the hypertensive process is so severe that it either is refractory to intensive multiple-drug therapy or requires hospitalization.

RENAL PARENCHYMAL HYPERTENSION

Chronic kidney disease (Chapter 130) is the most common cause of secondary hypertension. Hypertension is present in more than 85% of patients with chronic kidney disease and is a major factor causing their increased cardiovascular morbidity and mortality. The mechanisms causing the hypertension include an expanded plasma volume and peripheral vasoconstriction; the peripheral vasoconstriction is caused by both activation of vasoconstrictor pathways (renin-angiotensin and sympathetic nervous systems) and inhibition of vasodilator pathways (nitric oxide).

Measurement of serum creatinine alone is an inadequate screening test for renal insufficiency. A spot urine specimen should be obtained to screen for microalbuminuria, which is defined as a urine albumin-to-urine creatinine ratio of 30 to 300 mg/g (equivalent to excretion of 30 to 300 mg of albumin per 24 hours); higher levels of albuminuria indicate more advanced kidney disease. Using the spot urine specimen, creatinine clearance should be calculated (www.nephron.com) (Chapter 114) to screen for an estimated GFR below 60 mL/minute per 1.73 m^2.

TABLE 67-4 FACTORS OTHER THAN BLOOD PRESSURE LEVEL THAT INFLUENCE GLOBAL CARDIOVASCULAR RISK IN PATIENTS WITH HYPERTENSION

RISK FACTORS

- Male
- Age (men ≥55 yr, women ≥65 yr)
- Smoking
- Dyslipidemia
- Impaired fasting glucose (100-125 mg/dL)
- Obesity (BMI ≥ 30 kg/m^2 or waist circumference: men, ≥102 cm, women, ≥88 cm)
- Family history or premature cardiovascular disease (men aged < 55 yr, women aged < 65 yr)

ASYMPTOMATIC TARGET ORGAN DAMAGE

- Left ventricular hypertrophy by ECG or transthoracic echocardiography
- Chronic kidney disease (eGFR ≤ 60 mL/min/1.73 m^2)
- Microalbuminuria (albumin-to-creatinine ratio, 30-300 mg/g)
- Ankle-brachial index < 0.9
- Pulse wave velocity > 10 m/sec

DIABETES MELLITUS

(fasting plasma glucose ≥126 mg/dL × 2; or hemoglobin A_{1C} ≥ 7%; or postload plasma glucose > 198 mg/dL)

ESTABLISHED CARDIOVASCULAR OR RENAL DISEASE

- Stroke or TIA
- CAD: myocardial infarction, angina, myocardial revascularization
- Heart failure (with decreased or preserved ejection fraction)
- Intermittent claudication (symptomatic peripheral artery disease)
- Chronic kidney disease with eGFR < 30 mL/min/1.73m^2
- Advanced retinopathy: hemorrhages or exudates, papilledema

BMI = body mass index; CAD = coronary artery disease; ECG = electrocardiogram; eGFR = estimated glomerular filtration rate; TIA = transient ischemic attack.
Adapted from Mancia G, Fagard R, Narkiewicz K, et al. 2013 ESH/ESC Guidelines for the management of arterial hypertension: the Task Force for the management of arterial hypertension of the European Society of Hypertension (ESH) and of the European Society of Cardiology (ESC). *J Hypertens.* 2013;31:1281-1357.

In patients with mild (stage 2: GFR of 60 to 90 mL/minute per 1.73 m^2) or moderate (stage 3: GFR of 30 to 60 mL/minute per 1.73 m^2) proteinuric chronic kidney disease, stringent blood pressure control is important both to slow the progression to end-stage renal disease and to reduce the excessive cardiovascular risk. In patients with severe chronic kidney disease, hypertension often becomes difficult to treat and may require either (1) intensive medical treatment with loop diuretics, potent vasodilators (e.g., minoxidil), high-dose β-adrenergic blockers, and central sympatholytics; or (2) initiation of chronic hemodialysis as the only effective way to reduce plasma volume. In chronic hemodialysis patients, the challenge is to control interdialytic hypertension without exacerbating dialysis-induced hypotension. The annual mortality rate in the hemodialysis population is 25%; half of this excessive mortality is caused by cardiovascular events that are related, at least in part, to hypertension.

RENOVASCULAR HYPERTENSION

PATHOBIOLOGY AND CLINICAL MANIFESTATIONS

The two main causes of renal artery stenosis (Chapter 125) are atherosclerosis (85% of cases), typically in older persons with other clinical manifestations of systemic atherosclerosis, and fibromuscular dysplasia (15% of cases), typically in young women who are otherwise healthy. Although renal artery stenosis and hypertension frequently coexist, the presence of a renal artery stenosis proves neither that the patient's hypertension is renovascular in origin nor that revascularization will improve renal perfusion and blood pressure.

Unilateral renal artery stenosis can lead to underperfusion of the juxtaglomerular cells, thereby causing renin-dependent hypertension even though the contralateral kidney is able to maintain normal blood volume. In contrast, bilateral renal artery stenosis (or unilateral stenosis with a solitary kidney) constitutes a potentially reversible cause of progressive renal failure and volume-dependent hypertension. The following clinical clues increase the suspicion of renovascular hypertension: any hospitalization for urgent or emergent hypertension; recurrent "flash" pulmonary edema; recent worsening of long-standing, previously well-controlled hypertension; severe hypertension in a young adult or after the age of 50 years; precipitous and progressive worsening of renal function in response to angiotensin-converting enzyme (ACE) inhibition or angiotensin II receptor blockade; unilateral small kidney by any radiographic study; extensive peripheral arteriosclerosis; and a flank bruit.

DIAGNOSIS

Contrast-enhanced computed tomography (CT) and magnetic resonance angiography are the preferred screening tests for renal artery stenosis, but gadolinium-enhanced magnetic resonance imaging (MRI) is contraindicated in patients with advanced chronic kidney disease to avoid potentially fatal gadolinium-induced nephrogenic systemic fibrosis (Chapter 267). Fibromuscular dysplasia classically causes a "string of beads" lesion in the midportion of a renal artery (Fig. 67-5A), whereas atherosclerotic renal artery lesions

TABLE 67-5 GUIDE TO EVALUATION OF IDENTIFIABLE CAUSES OF HYPERTENSION

SUSPECTED DIAGNOSIS	CLINICAL CLUES	DIAGNOSTIC TESTING
Chronic kidney disease	Estimated GFR < 60 mL/min/1.73 m^2 Urine albumin-to-creatinine ratio ≥ 30 mg/g	Renal sonography
Renovascular disease	New elevation in serum creatinine, marked elevation in serum creatinine with ACE inhibitor or ARB, drug-resistant hypertension, flash pulmonary edema, abdominal or flank bruit	Renal sonography (atrophic kidney), CT or MR angiography, invasive angiography
Coarctation of the aorta	Arm pulses > leg pulses, arm BP > leg BP, chest bruits, rib notching on chest radiography	MR angiography, TEE, invasive angiography
Primary aldosteronism	Hypokalemia, drug-resistant hypertension	Plasma renin and aldosterone, 24-hour urine aldosterone and potassium after oral salt loading, adrenal vein sampling
Cushing syndrome	Truncal obesity, wide and blanching purple striae, muscle weakness	1 mg dexamethasone-suppression test, urinary cortisol after dexamethasone, adrenal CT
Pheochromocytoma	Paroxysms of hypertension, palpitations, perspiration, and pallor; diabetes	Plasma metanephrines, 24-hour urinary metanephrines and catecholamines, abdominal CT or MR imaging
Obstructive sleep apnea	Loud snoring, large neck, obesity, somnolence	Polysonography

ACE = angiotensin-converting enzyme; ARB = angiotensin receptor blocker; BP = blood pressure; CT = computed tomography; GFR = glomerular filtration rate; MR, magnetic resonance; TEE = transesophageal echocardiography.

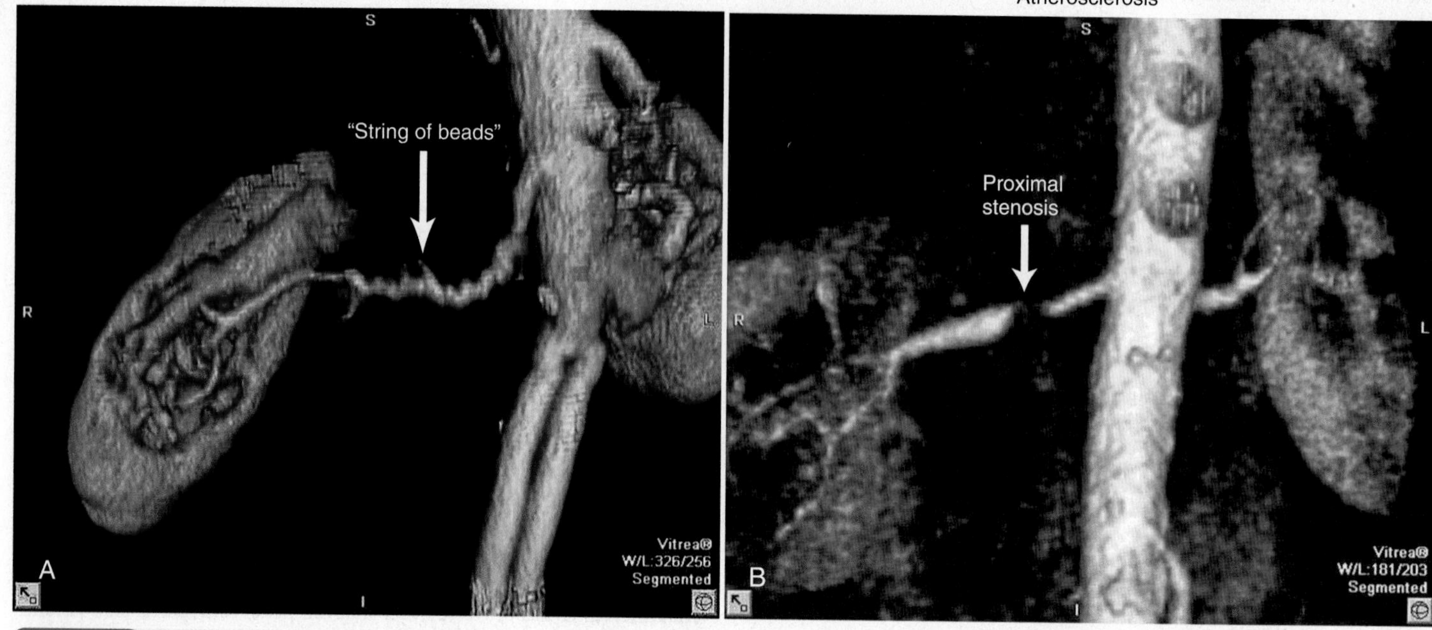

FIGURE 67-5. Computed tomographic angiogram with three-dimensional reconstruction. A, The classic "string of beads" lesion of fibromuscular dysplasia (bilateral in this patient). **B,** A severe proximal atherosclerotic stenosis of the right renal artery and mild stenosis of the left renal artery. (Images courtesy of Bart Domatch, MD, Radiology Department, University of Texas Southwestern Medical Center, Dallas, Texas.)

are proximal and discrete (Fig. 67-5B). Invasive renal angiography is the gold standard for confirming the diagnosis of renal artery stenosis.

TREATMENT Rx

Balloon angioplasty is the treatment of choice for fibromuscular dysplasia, with overall favorable outcomes and at least one third of patients no longer needing any antihypertensive medications.[7] In contrast, most atherosclerotic renal artery lesions do not cause hypertension or progressive renal failure, and most patients will not benefit from revascularization (balloon angioplasty or stenting), which carries substantial risks for serious complications.[A1,A2] As a result, medical management of hypertension (with a regimen that includes a renin-angiotensin system inhibitor) and the associated atherosclerotic risk factors is first-line treatment for atherosclerotic renal artery stenosis, except that patients with truly drug-resistant hypertension, a progressive decline in renal function (ischemic nephropathy), or recurrent acute ("flash") pulmonary edema may benefit from stent-based revascularization (Chapter 125).

MINERALOCORTICOID-INDUCED HYPERTENSION DUE TO PRIMARY ALDOSTERONISM

PATHOBIOLOGY

The most common causes of primary aldosteronism (Chapter 227) are a unilateral aldosterone-producing adenoma and bilateral adrenal hyperplasia. Because aldosterone is the principal ligand for the mineralocorticoid receptor in the distal nephron, excessive aldosterone production causes excessive renal Na^+-K^+ exchange, often resulting in hypokalemia.

CLINICAL MANIFESTATIONS AND DIAGNOSIS

The diagnosis should always be suspected when hypertension is accompanied by either unprovoked hypokalemia (serum potassium concentration below 3.5 mmol/L in the absence of diuretic therapy) or a tendency to develop excessive hypokalemia during diuretic therapy (serum potassium concentration below 3.0 mmol/L). However, more than one third of patients do not have hypokalemia on initial presentation, and the diagnosis should also be considered in any patient with resistant hypertension.

Screening for hyperaldosteronism should be restricted to the small fraction of hypertensive patients with hypokalemia or severe drug-resistant hypertension. If such patients have a positive screening test—a high serum aldosterone level and a suppressed plasma renin activity level—and want to consider laparoscopic adrenalectomy, the patient should be referred to an experienced center for further evaluation: salt-loading to test for nonsuppressible aldosteronism and, if present, adrenal vein sampling to test for lateralization.

TREATMENT Rx

Both CT and MRI have too many false-positive and false-negative results to be used as a noninvasive alternative to invasive adrenal vein sampling. Laparoscopic adrenalectomy and mineralocorticoid receptor blockade with eplerenone (50 to 100 mg per day) constitute highly effective therapeutic options that target the disease-causing mechanism with a favorable risk-to-benefit ratio.

MENDELIAN FORMS OF MINERALOCORTICOID-INDUCED HYPERTENSION

Almost all the rare mendelian forms of hypertension are mineralocorticoid induced and involve excessive activation of the epithelial Na^+ channel (ENaC), the final common pathway for reabsorption of sodium from the distal nephron (E-Fig. 67-2). Thus, salt-dependent hypertension can be caused both by gain-of-function mutations of ENaC or the mineralocorticoid receptor and by increased production or decreased clearance of mineralocorticoid receptor ligands, which are aldosterone, deoxycorticosterone, and cortisol.

PHEOCHROMOCYTOMAS AND PARAGANGLIOMAS

Pheochromocytomas are rare catecholamine-producing tumors of the adrenal chromaffin cells, whereas paragangliomas are even rarer tumors of the extra-adrenal chromaffin cells (Chapter 228). The diagnosis should be suspected when hypertension is drug resistant or paroxysmal, particularly when accompanied by paroxysms of headache, palpitations, pallor, or diaphoresis. In some patients, pheochromocytoma is misdiagnosed as panic disorder. A family history of early-onset hypertension may suggest pheochromocytoma as part of the multiple endocrine neoplasia syndromes (Chapter 231). An increasing number of pheochromocytomas are being detected incidentally on abdominal imaging studies for nonadrenal indications. If the diagnosis is missed, outpouring of catecholamines from the tumor can cause unsuspected hypertensive crisis during unrelated surgical procedures, in which case mortality rates exceed 80%.

OTHER NEUROGENIC CAUSES

Other causes of neurogenic hypertension that can be confused with pheochromocytoma include sympathomimetic agents (cocaine, methamphetamine; Chapter 34), baroreflex failure, and obstructive sleep apnea (Chapter 100). A history of surgery and radiation therapy for head and neck tumors (Chapter 190) raises suspicion of baroreceptor damage. Snoring and somnolence suggest sleep apnea, but continuous positive airway pressure to treat the sleep apnea rarely improves blood pressure substantially (Chapter 100).

OTHER CAUSES OF SECONDARY HYPERTENSION

Coarctation of the aorta typically occurs just distal to the origin of the left subclavian artery, so the blood pressure is lower in the legs than in the arms (opposite of the normal situation) (see Fig. 69-7). The clue is that the pulses are weaker in the lower than in the upper extremities, indicating the need to measure blood pressure in the legs as well as in both arms. Intercostal collaterals can produce bruits on examination and rib notching on the chest radiograph. Coarctations can be cured with surgery or angioplasty.

Hyperthyroidism tends to cause systolic hypertension with a wide pulse pressure, whereas hypothyroidism tends to cause mainly diastolic hypertension. Treatment is for the underlying disease. Hyperparathyroidism (Chapter 245) also has been associated with hypertension. Cyclosporine and tacrolimus are important causes of secondary hypertension in transplant recipients, apparently by inhibition of calcineurin, the calcium-dependent phosphatase that is expressed not only in lymphoid tissue but also in neural, vascular, and renal tissue. In the absence of outcomes data, nondihydropyridine calcium-channel blockers (CCBs) have become the drugs of first choice, but they increase cyclosporine blood levels. Combination therapy with diuretics, CCBs, and central sympatholytics often is required.

TABLE 67-6 LIFESTYLE RECOMMENDATIONS TO LOWER BLOOD PRESSURE IN ADULTS WITH HYPERTENSION OR PRE-HYPERTENSION

DIET

1. Adopt a diet that is:
   - *High* in vegetables, nuts, fruits, grains, low-fat dairy products, fish, poultry, etc.
   - *Low* in sweets, sugar-sweetened beverages, and red meats

   Adapt this dietary pattern to calorie requirements, personal/cultural food preferences, and medical conditions such as diabetes.
2. Lower sodium intake

PHYSICAL ACTIVITY

1. Engage in three to four 40-minute sessions of moderate-to-intense aerobic physical activity per week.

Adapted from Eckel RH, Jakicic JM, Ard JD, et al. 2013 AHA/ACC guideline on lifestyle management to reduce cardiovascular risk: a report of the American College of Cardiology/American Heart Association Task Force on Practice Guidelines. *J Am Coll Cardiol.* 2014;63:2960-2984.

PREVENTION AND TREATMENT OF HYPERTENSION

At the population level, the primary prevention of hypertension requires large-scale societal changes, including further efforts to influence the food industry to reduce salt in processed foods, efforts to increase exercise, and the availability of fresh fruits and vegetables. After a person's blood pressure rises to hypertensive or even prehypertensive levels, lifestyle modifications alone are almost never enough to return blood pressure to normal, and recidivism is typical.

Although short-term pharmacologic therapy with a low-dose angiotensin receptor blocker (ARB) may prevent the conversion from prehypertension to full-blown hypertension, blood pressure quickly rises again if the ARB is discontinued. Thus, lifelong prescription medication is the cornerstone of effective therapy for primary hypertension, with lifestyle modification serving as a very important adjunct but not as an alternative. The objective is to reduce the blood pressure and associated metabolic abnormalities sufficiently to reduce the risk for cardiovascular events and end-stage renal disease without compromising the patient's quality of life.

Randomized trials have proved beyond any doubt that antihypertensive drug therapy reduces cardiovascular risk, with benefits that are proportional to the reduction in blood pressure achieved (E-Fig. 67-3).A3 However, in practice, most treated patients do not achieve the same low risk levels of truly normotensive persons because their blood pressures remain higher than optimal owing to the threshold levels of guidelines, hesitation of practicing physicians to start and intensify drug treatment, costs of medications, and medication noncompliance despite the declining costs of generic medications. This residual risk also may be attributable to the cardiovascular damage sustained before starting drug therapy.

Multidrug regimens with two, three, or even more medications of different drug classes are almost always required to achieve currently recommended blood pressure goals. Low-dose drug combinations exert synergistic effects on blood pressure while minimizing dose-dependent side effects. For most patients with hypertension, lipid-lowering therapy (Chapter 206) is indicated as part of a comprehensive cardiovascular risk-reduction strategy (Chapter 52).

Lifestyle Modification

Lifestyle modification (Table 67-6) should be part of every antihypertensive regimen.A4 However, dietary and exercise interventions are difficult to sustain long term. For example, short-term trials have proved that individuals with prehypertension or stage 1 hypertension can lower their blood pressures on average by 6/3 mm Hg even without restricting calorie or sodium intake if they adhere to a diet rich in fresh fruits and vegetables and low-fat dairy products (www.nhlbi.nih.gov/files/docs/public/heart/dash_brief.pdf). Modest dietary sodium restriction produces a further reduction in blood pressure and decreases cardiovascular disease risk.[8] Sodium reduction is particularly effective in black hypertensive patients. Most dietary sodium comes from processed foods, and patients should be taught to read food labels (6 g of NaCl = 2.4 g of sodium = 100 mmol of sodium).

Moderately intense aerobic exercise programs can lower blood pressure by 2 to 5/1 to 2 mm Hg. The larger reductions in blood pressure are seen immediately after a bout of aerobic exercise (Chapter 16), but smaller reductions can persist for several hours.

Relaxation and stress management techniques (e.g., meditation, biofeedback, breathing exercises) can decrease blood pressure transiently but generally produce little if any demonstrable effect on ambulatory blood pressure (Chapter 39). However, some individuals with overwhelming home or job strain or anger can benefit from cognitive behavior therapy and anxiolytics (Chapter 397).

Blood pressure increases transiently by 10 to 15 mm Hg after each cigarette, so smokers of more than 20 cigarettes per day often have higher blood pressures out of the office than in the smoke-free medical office. Smokers should be counseled to quit tobacco (Chapter 32) not only because it raises blood pressure but also because it is such a potent risk factor for coronary heart disease, stroke, and the progression of hypertensive kidney disease.

Blood pressure increases by up to 10 to 15 mm Hg with the first morning cup of coffee, but the pressor response to caffeine often habituates throughout the day. Thus, caffeine consumption need not be totally eliminated but may need to be reduced.

Moderate alcohol (Chapter 33) consumption (one or two drinks per day) does not seem to increase the risk for hypertension in Western populations; but in Japanese populations, hypertension is more common in men who are moderate drinkers than in men who cannot drink because of a loss-of-function mutation in the alcohol dehydrogenase gene. In all populations, heavy drinking (three or more standard-sized drinks per day) and especially binge drinking activate the sympathetic nervous system the next day during withdrawal and are associated with an increased incidence and severity of hypertension, which is reversible if alcohol consumption decreases.

Antihypertensive Drugs

Although every hypertensive patient should adopt sensible lifestyle modifications, almost all will require medication to optimize outcomes. Lowering blood pressure with medication reduces but does not eliminate the risks for cardiovascular events, renal failure, and death.

Classes of Oral Antihypertensive Drugs

Multiple classes of oral antihypertensive drugs are approved by the U.S. Food and Drug Administration, although all have specific contraindications (Tables 67-7 and 67-8).

First-Line Drugs for Hypertension

Multiple practice guidelines[1-4] recommend initiating drug treatment with one or more of three classes of first-line drugs (Fig. 67-6), which have additive or synergistic effects when used in combination: (1) CCBs, (2) renin-angiotensin system blockers—either ACE inhibitors or ARBs, and (3) thiazide-like diuretics.

Calcium-Channel Blockers

Mechanism of Action. The CCBs block the opening of voltage-gated (L-type) Ca^{2+} channels in cardiac myocytes and vascular smooth muscle cells. The resultant decrease in the cytosolic Ca^{2+} signal decreases heart rate and ventricular contractility and relaxes vascular smooth muscle. Blood pressure lowering is related mainly to peripheral arterial vasodilation, with the rank

TABLE 67-7 SELECTED ORAL ANTIHYPERTENSIVE AGENTS

DRUG	DOSE RANGE, TOTAL, MG/DAY (DOSES PER DAY)	USUAL STARTING DOSE, MG/DAY (DOSES PER DAY)
DIURETICS		
Thiazide and Thiazide-Like Diuretics		
Chlorthalidone	6.25-50 (1)	6.25 (1)
HCTZ	6.25-50 (1)	12.5 (1)
Indapamide	1.25-5 (1)	1.25 (1)
Metolazone	2.5-5 (1)	2.5 (1)
Loop Diuretics		
Bumetanide	0.5-2 (2)	1 (2)
Ethacrynic acid	25-100 (2)	25 (2)
Furosemide	20-160 (2)	20 (2)
Torsemide	2.5-20 (1-2)	5 (2)
Potassium Sparing		
Amiloride	5-20 (1)	10 (2)
Eplerenone	25-100 (1-2)	25 (1)
Spironolactone	6.25-400 (1-2)	12.5 (1)
Triamterene	25-100 (1)	37.5 (1)
β-BLOCKERS		
Acebutolol	200-800 (2)	200 (2)
Atenolol	25-100 (1)	25 (1)
Betaxolol	5-20 (1)	5 (1)
Bisoprolol	2.5-20 (1)	2.5 (1)
Carteolol	2.5-10 (1)	2.5 (1)
Metoprolol	50-450 (2)	50 (2)
Metoprolol XL	50-200 (1-2)	50 (1)
Nadolol	20-320 (1)	40 (1)
Penbutolol	10-80 (1)	10 (1)
Pindolol	10-60 (2)	10 (1)
Propranolol	40-180 (2)	40 (2)
Propranolol LA	60-180 (1-2)	60 (1)
Timolol	20-60 (2)	20 (2)
VASODILATING β-BLOCKERS		
Carvedilol	6.25-50 (2)	6.25 (2)
Carvedilol CR	10-80 (1)	20 (1)
Labetalol	100-2400 (2)	200 (2)
Nebivolol	2.5-40 (1)	5 (1)
CALCIUM-CHANNEL BLOCKERS		
Dihydropyridines		
Amlodipine	2.5-10 (1)	2.5 (1)
Felodipine	2.5-20 (1-2)	2.5 (2)
Isradipine CR	2.5-20 (2)	2.5 (2)
Nicardipine SR	30-120 (2)	30 (2)
Nifedipine XL	30-120 (1)	30 (1)
Nisoldipine	10-40 (1-2)	10 (2)
Nondihydropyridines		
Diltiazem CD	120-540 (1-2)	180 (1)
Verapamil HS	120-480 (1)	180 (1)
ANGIOTENSIN-CONVERTING ENZYME INHIBITORS		
Benazepril	10-80 (1-2)	20 (1)
Captopril	25-150 (2)	25 (2)
Enalapril	2.5-40 (2)	5 (2)
Fosinopril	10-80 (1-2)	20 (2)
Lisinopril	5-80 (1-2)	40 (2)
Moexipril	7.5-30 (1)	7.5 (1)
Perindopril	4-16 (1)	4 (1)
Quinapril	5-80 (1-2)	40 (2)
Ramipril	2.5-20 (1)	2.5 (1)
Trandolapril	1-8 (1)	2 (1)
ANGIOTENSIN RECEPTOR BLOCKERS		
Candesartan	8-32 (1)	8 (1)
Eprosartan	400-800 (1-2)	400 (1)
Irbesartan	150-300 (1)	150 (1)
Losartan	25-100 (2)	50 (1)
Olmesartan	5-40 (1)	20 (1)
Telmisartan	20-80 (1)	40 (1)
Valsartan	80-320 (1-2)	160 (2)
DIRECT RENIN INHIBITOR		
Aliskiren	150-300 (1)	150 (1)
α-BLOCKERS		
Doxazosin	1-16 (1)	1 (1)
Prazosin	1-40 (2-3)	1 (2)
Terazosin	1-20 (1)	1 (1)
Phenoxybenzamine for pheochromocytoma	20-120 (2)	20 (2)
CENTRAL SYMPATHOLYTICS		
Clonidine	0.3-1.2 (3)	0.3 (3)
Clonidine patch	0.1-0.6 (weekly)	0.1 (weekly)
Guanabenz	2-32 (2)	2 (2)
Guanfacine	1-3 (1) (qhs)	1 (1)
Methyldopa	250-1000 (2)	250 (2)
Reserpine	0.05-0.25 (1)	0.05 (1)
DIRECT VASODILATORS		
Hydralazine	10-200 (2)	20 (2)
Minoxidil	2.5-100 (1)	2.5 (1)
FIXED-DOSE COMBINATIONS		
Aliskiren/HCTZ	150/12.5-300/25 (1)	150/12.5 (1)
Amiloride/HCTZ	5/50 (1)	5/50 (1)
Amlodipine/benazepril	2.5-5/10-20 (1)	2.5/10 (1)
Amlodipine/olmesartan	5-10/20-40 (1)	5/20 (1)
Amlodipine/telmisartan	5/20-10/80 (1)	5/20 (1)
Amlodipine/valsartan	5/160-10/320 (1)	5/160 (1)
Atenolol/chlorthalidone	50-100/25 (1)	50/25 (1)
Benazepril/HCTZ	5-20/6.25-25 (1)	20/6.25 (1)
Bisoprolol/HCTZ	2.5-10/6.25 (1)	2.5/6.25 (1)
Candesartan/HCTZ	16-32/12.5-25 (1)	16/12.5 (1)
Enalapril/HCTZ	5-10/25 (1-2)	5/25 (1)
Eprosartan/HCTZ	600/12.5-25 (1)	600/12.5 (1)
Fosinopril/HCTZ	10-20/12.5 (1)	10/12.5 (1)
Irbesartan/HCTZ	150-300/12.5-25 (1)	150/12.5 (1)
Losartan/HCTZ	50-100/12.5-25 (1)	50/12.5 (1)
Olmesartan/HCTZ	20-40/12.5 (1)	20/12.5 (1)
Spironolactone/HCTZ	25/25 (½-1)	25/25 (1/2)
Telmisartan/HCTZ	40-80/12.5-25 (1)	40/12.5 (1)
Trandolapril/verapamil	2-4/180-240 (1)	2/180 (1)
Triamterene/HCTZ	37.5/25 (½-1)	37.5/25 (1/2)
Valsartan/HCTZ	80-160/12.5-25 (1)	160/12.5 (1)
Valsartan/Amlodipine/HCTZ	80-160/5-10/12.5-25 (1)	160/5/12.5 (1)

HCTZ = hydrochlorothiazide.

TABLE 67-8 MAJOR CONTRAINDICATIONS AND SIDE EFFECTS OF ANTIHYPERTENSIVE DRUGS

DRUG CLASS	MAJOR CONTRAINDICATIONS	SIDE EFFECTS
Diuretics		
Thiazides	Gout	Insulin resistance, new-onset type 2 diabetes Hypokalemia, hyponatremia Hypertriglyceridemia Hyperuricemia, precipitation of gout Erectile dysfunction (more than other drug classes) Potentiate nondepolarizing muscle relaxants Photosensitivity dermatitis
Loop diuretics	Hepatic coma	Interstitial nephritis Hypokalemia Potentiate succinylcholine Potentiate aminoglycoside ototoxicity
Potassium-sparing diuretics	Serum potassium concentration > 5.5 mEq/L GFR < 30 mg/mL/1.73 m^2	Hyperkalemia
ACE inhibitors	Pregnancy Bilateral renal artery stenosis Hyperkalemia	Cough Hyperkalemia Angioedema Leukopenia Fetal toxicity Cholestatic jaundice (rare fulminant hepatic necrosis if the drug is not discontinued)
Dihydropyridine CCBs	As monotherapy in chronic kidney disease with proteinuria	Headaches Flushing Ankle edema Heart failure Gingival hyperplasia Esophageal reflux
Nondihydropyridine CCBs	Heart block Systolic heart failure	Bradycardia, AV block (especially with verapamil) Constipation (often severe with verapamil) Worsening of systolic function, heart failure Gingival edema or hypertrophy Increase cyclosporine blood levels Esophageal reflux
ARBs, DRI	Pregnancy Bilateral renal artery stenosis Hyperkalemia	Hyperkalemia Angioedema (very rare) Fetal toxicity
β-Adrenergic blockers	Heart block Asthma Depression Cocaine and methamphetamine abuse	New-onset type 2 diabetes (especially in combination with a thiazide) Heart block, acute decompensated heart failure Bronchospasm Depression, nightmares, fatigue Cold extremities, claudication (β_2 effect) Stevens-Johnson syndrome Agranulocytosis
α-Adrenergic blockers	Orthostatic hypotension Systolic heart failure Left ventricular dysfunction	Orthostatic hypotension Drug tolerance (in the absence of diuretic therapy) Ankle edema Heart failure First-dose effect (acute hypotension) Potentiate hypotension with PDE-5 inhibitors (e.g., sildenafil)
Central sympatholytics	Orthostatic hypotension	Depression, dry mouth, lethargy Erectile dysfunction (dose dependent) Rebound hypertension with clonidine withdrawal Coombs test–positive hemolytic anemia and elevated liver enzymes with α-methyldopa
Direct vasodilators	Orthostatic hypotension	Reflex tachycardia Fluid retention Hirsutism, pericardial effusion with minoxidil Lupus with hydralazine

ACE = angiotensin-converting enzyme; ARBs = angiotensin receptor blockers; AV = atrioventricular; CCBs = calcium-channel blockers; DRI = direct renin inhibitor; GFR = glomerular filtration rate; NSAIDs = nonsteroidal anti-inflammatory drugs; PDE-5 = phosphodiesterase-5.

order of potency being dihydropyridines > diltiazem ≫ verapamil. In contrast, for negative chronotropic and inotropic effects, the rank order of potency is verapamil ≫ diltiazem > dihydropyridines.

Therapeutic Principles. The most recommended CCBs are amlodipine followed by diltiazem. Amlodipine's long half-life permits once-daily dosing, and its costs are low since it became generic. Amlodipine is equivalent to a potent diuretic or lisinopril in protecting against nonfatal coronary events, stroke, and death, but it provides less protection against heart failure.[A5] Unlike diuretics, ARBs, and ACE inhibitors, a high-salt diet or concurrent nonsteroidal anti-inflammatory drug (NSAID) therapy does not compromise the effectiveness of dihydropyridine CCBs. The CCBs have some diuretic action because they dilate the afferent renal arteriole and may reduce requirements for additional diuretic therapy in mild hypertension. Amlodipine and other dihydropyridine CCBs are less renoprotective than ACE inhibitors or ARBs in patients with proteinuric chronic kidney disease. Such patients should not receive amlodipine as first-line therapy, but it may be useful as adjunctive therapy after initiation of appropriate first-line therapy with either an ACE inhibitor or ARB, as well as a diuretic.

Diltiazem is a usually well-tolerated alternative in patients who cannot tolerate amlodipine or would benefit from its other effects. Verapamil is not recommended because it is a weak antihypertensive medication and causes constipation.

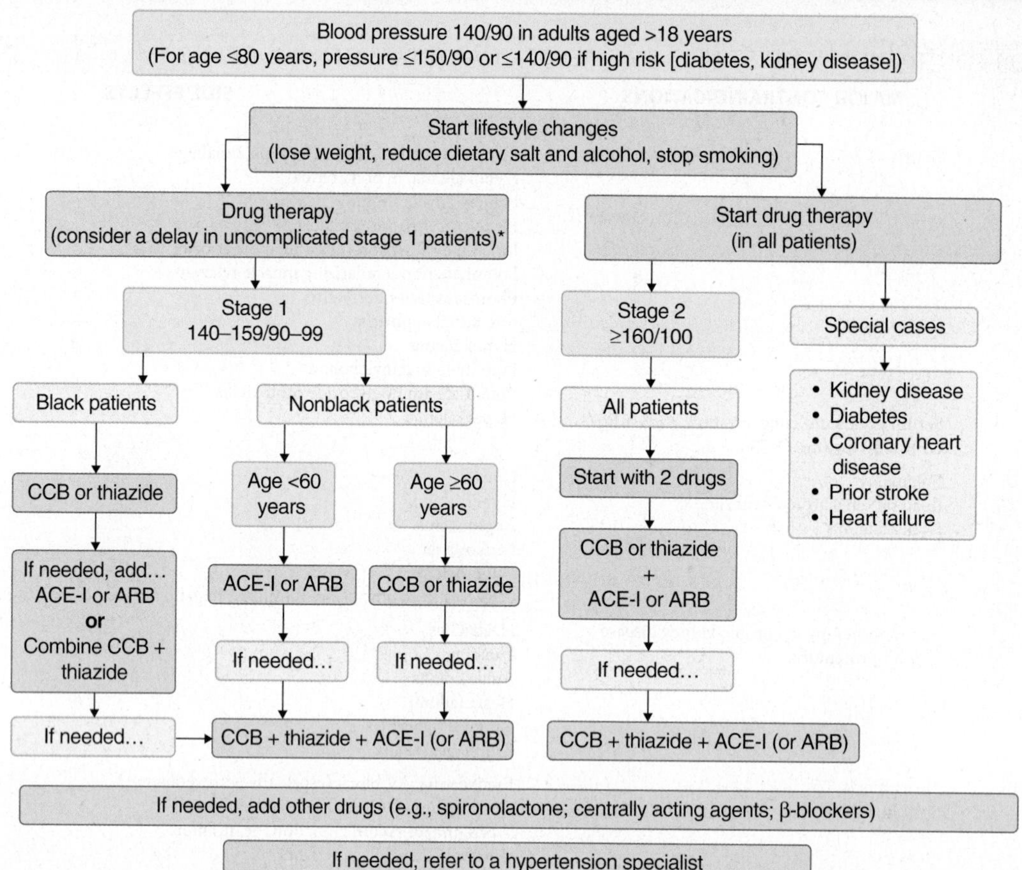

FIGURE 67-6. **2014 Hypertension Management Algorithm Recommended by the American Society of Hypertension and the International Society of Hypertension.** At any stage, it is entirely appropriate to seek help from a hypertension expert if treatment is proving difficult. *In patients with stage 1 hypertension and no history of a prior cardiovascular, stroke, or renal event, no evidence of end organ damage, and no diabetes or other major risk factors, drug therapy can be delayed for a short trial of lifestyle modification; however, most patients will require medication to achieve recommended blood pressure targets. In all other patients (including those with stage 2 hypertension), drug therapy should be started as soon as the diagnosis of hypertension is made. ACE-I = angiotensin-converting enzyme inhibitors; ARB = angiotensin receptor blocker; CCB = calcium channel blocker; thiazide = thiazide or thiazide-like diuretics. Blood pressure values are in mm Hg. (From Weber MA, Schiffrin EL, White WB, et al. Clinical practice guidelines for the management of hypertension in the community: a statement by the American Society of Hypertension and the International Society of Hypertension. *J Clin Hypertens.* 2014;16:14-26.)

Side Effects. *Short-acting dihydropyridines should not be used to treat hypertension.* By triggering an abrupt fall in blood pressure with reflex sympathetic activation, these rapidly acting arterial vasodilators can precipitate myocardial ischemia/infarction and death. The principal side effect of long-acting dihydropyridines is dose-dependent ankle edema, which is far more common with 10 mg of amlodipine than with lower doses. Because this vasogenic edema is caused by selective arterial dilation, it may be improved by adding an ACE inhibitor or ARB that produces balanced arterial and venous dilation. The long-acting dihydropyridines rarely cause flushing and headache. All CCBs can cause gingival hyperplasia, a rare side effect that is reversible if detected early but can otherwise lead to several dental problems. Dihydropyridines relax the smooth muscle of the distal esophagus and can exacerbate gastroesophageal reflux disease. Diltiazem can impair cardiac conduction, especially in older patients also receiving digoxin, β-blockers, or central sympatholytic agents.

Renin-Angiotensin System Inhibitors: ACE Inhibitors, ARBs, and Direct Renin Inhibitors

Mechanisms of Action. ACE inhibitors block conversion of the inactive precursor angiotensin I (AT1) to angiotensin 2 (AT2). ARBs block the action of AT2 on the type 1 angiotensin receptor. The direct renin inhibitor aliskiren blocks the conversion of pro-renin to renin, thereby blocking renin-angiotensin system activation at its origin. High levels of circulating pro-renin may stimulate AT1 receptor-independent signaling pathways that are both potentially beneficial and potentially harmful.

Clinical Use. ACE inhibitors are easy to use and have a rather flat dose-response curve. Lisinopril monotherapy is equivalent to amlodipine or chlorthalidone monotherapy except for producing a smaller reduction in blood pressure and thus less stroke protection for black hypertensive patients[A5] and older patients with low-renin hypertension. Even in these patients, however, ACE inhibitors are quite effective when combined with a diuretic or CCB. The ARBs confer the same benefits as ACE inhibitors in treating hypertension, while avoiding the ACE inhibitor cough (see later). There are no randomized trials of aliskiren monotherapy.

ACE inhibitors and ARBs are standard first-line therapy for patients with chronic kidney disease, especially if they have proteinuria. ACE inhibitors and ARBs have comparable effects on renal function, but ARBs produce more regression of left ventricular hypertrophy than do other antihypertensives.

Side Effects. All renin-angiotensin system inhibitors are contraindicated in pregnancy because they cause fetal renal agenesis and other birth defects. ACE inhibitors block the degradation of bradykinin, which activates nociceptive sensory fibers in the lungs that trigger a dry cough, which is more common in black patients and even more common in Asian patients. Bradykinin also may underlie the much less common ACE inhibitor-induced angioedema. If a cough develops in a patient who is on an ACE inhibitor and who needs renin-angiotensin system blockade, an ARB should be substituted.

The ACE inhibitors and ARBs can provoke hyperkalemia in the setting of chronic kidney disease or diabetes with type 4 renal tubular acidosis (Chapter 118). Serum potassium and creatinine levels must be monitored closely in all patients. In patients with stage 3 chronic kidney disease with proteinuria, initiation of ACE inhibitor or ARB therapy often causes a small transient increase in the serum creatinine level, but these drugs should be decreased in dose or temporarily discontinued only if the elevation is more than 30%.

Diuretics

Mechanism of Action. With initiation of diuretic therapy, contraction of blood volume causes the initial fall in blood pressure. With continued therapy, blood volume is partially restored, and vasodilator mechanisms (e.g., opening of adenosine triphosphate [ATP]-sensitive K^+ channels) sustain the antihypertensive action. Loop diuretics block Na^+-K^+-$2Cl^-$ transport in the thick ascending loop of Henle, where a large portion of the filtered sodium is reabsorbed. Thiazide diuretics and the indoline derivative indapamide block Na^+-Cl^- cotransporter in the distal convoluted tubule, where a smaller portion of the filtered sodium is reabsorbed.

Therapeutic Principles. Diuretics are still among the most effective antihypertensive medications. The thiazide-type diuretic chlorthalidone is at least as effective as (and in some circumstances more effective than) lisinopril or amlodipine in lowering blood pressure and preventing the attendant cardiovascular complications in all subgroups of patients.[A5] Combined with other classes of antihypertensive medications, diuretics exert a synergistic effect on blood pressure.

Despite the long-standing popularity of hydrochlorothiazide in clinical practice, chlorthalidone has a much longer duration of action and appears to be more efficacious in lowering blood pressure. A 25-mg dose of chlorthalidone is roughly equivalent in potency to a 50-mg dose of hydrochlorothiazide.

Loop diuretics are less effective blood pressure–lowering agents and should be reserved for treating hypertension in the setting of advanced chronic kidney disease (stage 3 or higher). Chlorthalidone also may be effective in stage 3 chronic kidney disease.

Side Effects. Thiazides and thiazide-like diuretics can aggravate glucose intolerance (particularly in higher doses and when used in combination with a β-blocker), cause hypokalemia and hypomagnesemia, precipitate gout, and elevate serum lipid levels, especially triglyceride levels. They sometimes cause photosensitive dermatitis and are more likely than any other antihypertensive drugs to cause erectile dysfunction. Though less well recognized than thiazide-induced hypokalemia, thiazide-induced hyponatremia (Chapter 116) is a common reason that some elderly hypertensive patients simply cannot tolerate even low-dose thiazides. In hypertensive patients with chronic kidney disease, high doses of loop diuretics may precipitate acute renal decompensation, especially if combined with a high-dose ACE inhibitor or ARB; the medications can be restarted carefully at low doses after the GFR has returned to baseline.

Add-on Drug for Difficult Hypertension

Mineralocorticoid Receptor Antagonists and ENaC Antagonists ("Potassium-Sparing Diuretics")

Mechanism of Action. Eplerenone and spironolactone prevent circulating aldosterone and other mineralocorticoids from activating the mineralocorticoid receptor in the distal nephron, thereby inhibiting the downstream activation of ENaC. By comparison, triamterene and amiloride block ENaC directly. Because less sodium is presented to the Na^+, K^+-ATPase on the vascular side of the collecting duct cells, less potassium is excreted in the urine than with thiazide or loop diuretics.

Therapeutic Principles. Eplerenone (25-100 mg daily) or low-dose spironolactone (12.5-100 mg daily) is widely recommended as a highly effective add-on drug for difficult cases of hypertension. Eplerenone is a much more specific antagonist that avoids the infrequent sexual side effects of low-dose spironolactone (painful gynecomastia, erectile dysfunction, nonmenstrual uterine bleeding). Hyperkalemia must be avoided when using these agents in patients with kidney disease.

β-Adrenergic Blockers

Vasodilating β-blockers (labetalol, carvedilol, and nebivolol) also are highly effective add-on drugs for difficult hypertension. Standard β-blockers (e.g., metoprolol, atenolol) are not.

Mechanism of Action. With the initiation of standard β-blocker therapy, blood pressure changes little at first because a compensatory increase in peripheral resistance offsets the fall in cardiac output. Over time, blood pressure falls progressively as the peripheral vasculature relaxes. Thus, the antihypertensive effect of β-blockade involves decreases in cardiac output (β_1-receptors), renin release (β_1-receptors), and norepinephrine release (prejunctional β_2-receptors). The prototype β-blocker propranolol nonselectively blocks both β_1- and β_2-receptors. Other standard β-blockers (metoprolol, atenolol, acebutolol, and bisoprolol) are relatively cardioselective. In low doses, they exert a greater inhibitory effect on β_1- than on β_2-receptors, but selectivity is lost at high doses. Vasodilating β-blockers such as labetalol or carvedilol also block α-adrenergic receptors, whereas nebivolol stimulates endogenous production of nitric oxide.

Therapeutic Principles and Side Effects. Although standard β-blockers are first-line medical therapy for ischemic heart disease (Chapters 72 and 73) and heart failure (Chapter 59), they are no longer first-line or even second-line agents for uncomplicated hypertension. They predispose to diabetes, particularly when combined with a thiazide, and offer less stroke protection than other antihypertensive drugs; they provide modest protection against cardiovascular events but do not reduce all-cause mortality. In addition to being rather weak antihypertensives, they are less effective than other agents in lowering central aortic blood pressure because bradycardia allows more time for wave reflection and thus central pressure augmentation.

By contrast, vasodilating β-blockers are much more potent antihypertensive agents and do not adversely affect glucose tolerance, but they have not been studied in large randomized trials. Labetalol is effective treatment for hypertensive urgencies but is too short acting to be recommended for chronic hypertension management. Common side effects such as fatigability cause high discontinuation rates for all β-blockers. β-Blockers also can impair cardiac conduction, precipitate acute bronchospasm, and promote weight gain.

α-Adrenergic Blockers

Mechanism of Action. By blocking the interaction of norepinephrine on vascular α-adrenergic receptors, these drugs cause peripheral vasodilation, thereby lowering blood pressure. By increasing skeletal muscle blood flow, they increase insulin sensitivity. By dilating urethral smooth muscle, they improve symptoms of prostatism. Prazosin, doxazosin, terazosin, and intravenous phentolamine selectively block α_1-adrenoreceptors; phenoxybenzamine blocks both α_1- and α_2-receptors.

Therapeutic Principles and Side Effects. Phenoxybenzamine is the drug of choice for preoperative management of pheochromocytoma (Chapter 228); after α-blockade is achieved, a β-blocker should be added to block an otherwise excessive reflex tachycardia. The selective α_1-blockers are not first-line agents and should not be used as monotherapy because their propensity to cause fluid retention can lead to tachyphylaxis and unmask or exacerbate heart failure. When used in a combination regimen that includes a diuretic, however, they are effective add-on therapy for difficult hypertension and are particularly useful in older men with prostatism. Although marketed specifically for prostatism and not as an antihypertensive agent, the selective α_{1A}-blocker tamsulosin lowers blood pressure in some men.

Central Sympatholytics

Mechanism of Action. Stimulation of postsynaptic α_2-adrenergic receptors and imidazoline receptors in the central nervous system lowers central sympathetic outflow, while stimulation of presynaptic α_2-receptors causes feedback inhibition of norepinephrine release from peripheral sympathetic nerve terminals. These combined actions reduce adrenergic drive to the heart and peripheral circulation.

Therapeutic Principles and Side Effects. The central sympatholytics are best reserved for short-term oral treatment of hypertensive urgency. They are potent antihypertensive agents that may be needed as add-on therapy for very difficult hypertension, but their troublesome central nervous system side effects reduce quality of life. To avoid rebound hypertension between doses, short-acting clonidine must be given every 6 to 8 hours or, whenever possible, discontinued using a gradual tapering schedule. Rebound hypertension is less of a problem with longer acting preparations (guanfacine, clonidine patch). α-Methyldopa remains a useful drug for management of hypertension in pregnancy (Chapter 239) but is no longer first-line therapy.

Direct Vasodilators

Mechanism of Action. Minoxidil and hydralazine are potent hyperpolarizing arterial vasodilators that work by opening vascular ATP-sensitive K^+ channels.

Therapeutic Principles and Side Effects. By causing selective and rapid arterial dilation, both drugs cause profound reflex sympathetic activation and tachycardia. Hydralazine is useful for the treatment of preeclampsia (Chapter 239). A combination of hydralazine plus nitrates is useful for the treatment of heart failure specifically in African American patients, in whom hypertensive heart disease causes heart failure most commonly (Chapter 59) Severe hypertension accompanying advanced chronic kidney disease is the main indication for minoxidil, which must be combined with aβ-blocker to prevent excessive reflex tachycardia and with a loop diuretic to prevent excessive fluid retention. Institution of hemodialysis is usually a more effective means of controlling hypertension in this setting.

Antihypertensive Drug Interactions

By inhibiting the kidney's ability to excrete sodium, NSAIDs can negate the antihypertensive action of diuretics and renin-angiotensin system inhibitors, but they do not interfere with CCBs. The risk for increased blood pressure and associated cardiovascular events is lowest with acetaminophen and low-dose aspirin (81 mg daily), intermediate with non-COX-2 selective NSAIDs including high-dose aspirin, and highest with COX-2-selective NSAIDs. Even a single glass of grapefruit juice increases the bioavailability of dihydropyridine CCBs by inhibiting the intestinal cytochrome P-450 3A4 (CYP34A) system, which is responsible for the first-pass metabolism of many oral medications. Diltiazem and verapamil, which are potent CYP3A4 inhibitors, should be avoided in patients undergoing anti-VEGF cancer chemotherapy with either sunitinib or sorafenib and should be used with caution in patients receiving digoxin or immunosuppressive therapy with either cyclosporine or tacrolimus because blood levels will increase and must be monitored. Carvedilol should be taken after meals to optimize its absorption, whereas a high-fat meal will impair the absorption of aliskiren.

Which Blood Pressure Goals and Which Drugs for Which Patients?

Despite the large evidence base for the medical treatment of hypertension, important gaps remain on (1) how far to lower blood pressure and (2) with which drugs for which patients. Current guidelines[1-4] recommend blood pressure goals of less than 150/90 mm Hg for "elderly" patients and less than 140/90 mm Hg for essentially all other patients. However, some experts recommend the goal of less than 140/90 mm Hg in patients older than 60 years if they are not frail (Chapter 25) and are able to tolerate such treatment without side effects.[9] The new guidelines place more emphasis on combination therapy with any two or all three of the first-line drug classes (CCBs, renin-angiotensin system blockers, thiazide diuretics; Tables 67-9 and 67-10). However, the preferred antihypertensive drug classes differ for specific types of patients (Table 67-11).

TABLE 67-9 BLOOD PRESSURE TREATMENT RECOMMENDATIONS SHAPED BY ALL OF OUR CURRENT MAJOR GUIDELINES

	2011-2014 GUIDELINES
Blood pressure treatment goals	<150/90 mm Hg for "elderly" patients <140/90 mm Hg for "nonelderly" patients and patients with diabetes or chronic kidney disease
Preferred first-line treatment	Three choices: calcium-channel blocker, ACE inhibitor or ARB, or thiazide diuretic (chlorthalidone preferred)
Combination treatment	Good option for stage 1 hypertension ACE inhibitor + calcium-channel blocker preferred over an ACE inhibitor + thiazide-type diuretic

Adapted from James PA, Oparil S, Carter BL, et al. 2014 Evidence-based guideline for the management of high blood pressure in adults: report from the panel members appointed to the Eighth Joint National Committee (JNC 8). *JAMA*. 2014;311:507-520; Weber MA, Schiffrin EL, White WB, et al. Clinical practice guidelines for the management of hypertension in the community: a statement by the American Society of Hypertension and the International Society of Hypertension. *J Hypertens*. 2014;32:3-15; Mancia G, Fagard R, Narkiewicz K, et al. 2013 ESH/ESC Guidelines for the management of arterial hypertension: the Task Force for the management of arterial hypertension of the European Society of Hypertension (ESH) and of the European Society of Cardiology (ESC). *J Hypertens*. 2013;31:1281-1357; National Institute for Health and Clinical Excellence (NICE). Clinical guideline 127. Hypertension: clinical management of primary hypertension in adults. 2011. www.nice.org.uk/guidance/cg127.
ACE = angiotensin-converting enzyme; ARB = angiotensin receptor blocker.

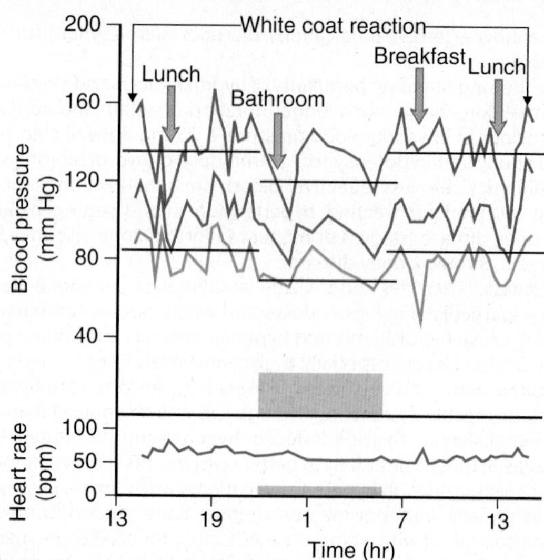

FIGURE 67-7. **The 24-hour blood pressure monitor tracing of a patient with postprandial and orthostatic hypotension. This frail 70-year-old woman was referred for evaluation of labile hypertension and dizziness. *Blue arrows* show repeated episodes of postprandial hypotension. The *red arrow* shows an episode of orthostatic hypotension when the patient walked to the bathroom 90 minutes after going to sleep. White coat reactions are also seen when the patient came to clinic both to have the monitor placed and then to have it removed. (Provided by Ronald G. Victor, MD, Hypertension Center, Cedars-Sinai Heart Institute, Los Angeles, California.)**

Hypertensive Patients in General

Current recommendations are based on hypertension trials, in which the active treatment group achieved a final mean systolic blood pressure below 140 mm Hg but never below 130 mm Hg. By comparison, some data indicate benefits of lowering blood pressure to less than 140/90 mm Hg for older as well as younger patients (see E-Fig. 67-3), and meta-regression analysis suggests—but does not prove—that additional lowering of blood pressure will provide additional cardiovascular protection even when the baseline blood pressure is 140/90 mm Hg or lower.

In randomized trials, differences in systolic blood pressure reduction rather than drug class explain the benefits of treatment with three caveats. First, β-blockers provide less stroke protection and CCBs more stroke protection than other drugs. Second, the combination of an ACE inhibitor and CCB may be an excellent initial option because it prevents more cardiovascular events than either the combination of a β-blocker with a thiazide diuretic or an ACE inhibitor with a thiazide diuretic (E-Fig. 67-4).[A6] CCBs also are better tolerated than diuretics and avoid their metabolic side effects. Third, dual renin-angiotensin system blockade with both an ACE inhibitor and an ARB has no advantage over monotherapy with either drug but results in much more symptomatic hypotension and more renal impairment (E-Fig. 67-5).[A7]

Systolic Hypertension in Elderly Patients

Most hypertensive patients are now older than 65 years, and most have isolated systolic hypertension. Placebo-controlled trials provide unequivocal proof that any blood pressure–lowering regimen reduces coronary events, strokes, heart failure events, and deaths in elderly hypertensive patients, even patients older than 80 years.[1] Although antihypertensive drugs are just as effective in preventing cardiovascular events in older patients, the intensity of their blood pressure reduction must be weighed against increased risks for hypotension, which can precipitate falls and ischemic cardiac events. The lowest mean systolic blood pressure reached in these trials in elderly patients is 145 mm Hg, so evidence supports an office systolic blood pressure treatment target below 150 mm Hg. Whether there are additional benefits to reducing office systolic blood pressure in active otherwise healthy elderly patients to below 140 mm Hg remains uncertain at this time.

Ambulatory monitoring is key for detecting postprandial hypotension and orthostatic hypotension, which are common in hypertensive elderly patients (Fig. 67-7). Although the management of postprandial hypotension is challenging, useful strategies include frequent small low-carbohydrate meals, caffeine with meals, and liberalized salt intake. If these nondrug strategies prove insufficient, fludrocortisone (0.1 to 0.2 mg daily) can be added; it often worsens supine hypertension, which can be managed with elevation of the head of the bed (with 6-inch cinder blocks producing a 30-degree head-up tilt) and a low-dose short-acting ARB (e.g., losartan 25-50 mg) at bedtime.[10]

Although most elderly patients will require combination therapy with two or three drugs to manage their hypertension, it is important to titrate medications more slowly in elderly patients and to check frequently for orthostatic hypotension and adverse drug reactions, such as thiazide-induced hyponatremia. Nonadherence and potential drug-drug interactions are key concerns. Therapy should be simplified and individualized, based more on the patient's overall health or frailty than on chronologic age. For example, a seated home blood pressure of 155 mm Hg may be an appropriate treatment target for a frail 70-year-old patient with marked orthostatic and postprandial hypotension, whereas a home seated blood pressure of 130 mm Hg may be an appropriate treatment target for a vigorous healthy 85-year-old patient whose chief concern is to avoid a disabling stroke.

Hypertension with Left Ventricular Hypertrophy

More than one third of hypertensive patients have electrocardiographic left ventricular hypertrophy by the time of diagnosis, a finding that places them at increased risk for hypertensive complications including heart failure, stroke, and atrial fibrillation. Meta-analyses consistently show the superiority of ARBs for the regression of left ventricular hypertrophy.[A8] In patients with stage 2 hypertension and left ventricular hypertrophy on their ECG, an ARB-based regimen is more effective than a β-blocker-based regimen for reducing cardiovascular events, especially stroke.

Hypertension in Patients with Diabetic Nephropathy or Nondiabetic Chronic Kidney Disease

Diabetic nephropathy (Chapter 124) is accompanied by proteinuria, loss of renal autoregulation, hypertension, progression to end-stage renal disease, and a high incidence of cardiovascular events. Because the addition of an ARB but not amlodipine to background antihypertensive therapy slows progression of nephropathy in patients with type 2 diabetes, type 2 diabetes with nephropathy is an indication for an ARB.[A9] Evidence suggests an office blood pressure goal of less than 140/90 mm Hg for patients with type 2 diabetic nephropathy and even a goal of less than 130/80 mm Hg in patients with significant proteinuria (urine plasma albumin-to-creatinine ratio of more than 30 mg/g (corresponding to >30 mg of urinary albumin excretion in 24 hours).[A9]

Similar goals are recommended for patients with proteinuric nondiabetic chronic kidney disease, in whom ramipil appears to be more renoprotective than either amlodipine or metoprolol. Aliskiren should not be added to background therapy with an ACE-I or ARB because such dual renin-angiotensin system blockade produces hyperkalemia and hypotension while producing no added cardiovascular benefit.

Blood Pressure Reduction in Patients with Prior Coronary Events or Strokes

Evidence from randomized trials is insufficient to determine an optimal blood pressure treatment target for the secondary prevention of coronary events in patients with preexisting coronary disease. Current recommendations include goal office blood pressure of less than 140/90 mm Hg and using two or more medications if this office goal is not achieved. β-Blockers and CCBs are preferred drugs because they are both antihypertensive and antianginal. Overtreatment of diastolic blood pressure can theoretically impair coronary perfusion, worsen myocardial ischemia, and provoke coronary events in patients with underlying coronary disease, but prospective data have not yet defined a critical lower limit of on-treatment diastolic blood pressure. Nevertheless, it is probably prudent not to treat a diastolic blood pressure below 60 mm Hg.

TABLE 67-10 DIFFERENCES AMONG CURRENT TREATMENT GUIDELINES FOR ADULTS WITH HYPERTENSION

GUIDELINE	POPULATION	GOAL BLOOD PRESSURE (mm Hg)	INITIAL DRUG TREATMENT OPTIONS
2014 JNC 8 Committee[1]	General ≥60 yr	<150/90	Nonblack: thiazide, ACE-I or ARB, CCB
	General <60 yr	<140/90	Black: thiazide, CCB
	Diabetes	<140/90	Thiazide, ACE-I or ARB, CCB
	CKD	<140/90	ACE-I or ARB
2014 ASH/ISH[2]	General ≥80 yr	<150/90	Nonblack/stage 1: thiazide, ACE-I or ARB, CCB
	General <80 yr	<140/90	Black/stage 1: thiazide, CCB Stage 2: CCB or thiazide *plus* ACE-I or ARB
	Diabetes	<140/90	ACE-I or ARB
	CKD	<140/90	ACE-I or ARB
2013 AHA/ACC/CDC[3]	General	<140/90	Stage 1: thiazide for most or ACE-I or ARB, CCB Stage 2: thiazide *plus* ACE-I or ARB *or* thiazide *plus* CCB *or* ACE-I or ARB *plus* CCB
2013 ESH/ESC[4]	General ≥80 yr	<150/90	BB, thiazide, CCB, ACE-I or ARB
	General 60-79 yr	<150/90 *or* <140/90	ARB
	General ≤60 yr	<140/90	ARB
	Diabetes	<140/85	ACE-I or ARB
	CKD no proteinuria	<140/90	ACE-I or ARB
	CKD + proteinuria	<130/90	ACE-I or ARB
2013 CHEP[5]	General ≥80 yr	<150/90	Thiazide, BB (<60 yr), ACE-I or ARB (nonblack)
	General <80 yr	<140/90	Thiazide, BB (<60 yr), ACE-I or ARB (nonblack)
	Diabetes	<130/80	ACE-I or ARB (+ additional CVD risk); ACE-I or ARB, thiazide, CCB (− additional CVD risk)
	CKD	<140/90	ACE-I or ARB
2013 ADA[6]	Diabetes	<140/80	ACE-I or ARB
2012 KDIGO[7]	CKD no proteinuria	≤140/90	ACE-I or ARB
	CKD + proteinuria	≤130/80	ACE-I or ARB
2011 UK NICE[8]	General ≥80 yr	<150/90	≥55 yr or black: CCB, thiazide
	General <80 yr	<140/90	<55 yr: ACE-I or ARB
2011ACCF/AHA: Elderly hypertensives[9]	General ≥80 yr	SBP ≤140 or 145	ACE-I or ARB, CCB, thiazide
	General <80 yr	SBP ≤140	
2010 ISHIB[10]	Black	<135/85	Thiazide, CCB
	Black + target organ disease or CVD risk	<130/80	

ACE-I = angiotensin-converting enzyme inhibitor; ARB = angiotensin receptor blocker; CCB = calcium-channel blocker; CVD = cardiovascular disease.

[1]James PA, Oparil S, Carter BL, et al. 2014 evidence-based guideline for the management of high blood pressure in adults: report from the panel members appointed to the Eighth Joint National Committee (JNC 8). *JAMA.* 2014;311:507-520.

[2]Weber MA, Schiffrin EL, White WB, et al. Clinical practice guidelines for the management of hypertension in the community a statement by the American Society of Hypertension and the International Society of Hypertension. *J Hypertens.* 2014;32:3-15.

[3]Go AS, Bauman M, Coleman King SM, et al. An effective approach to high blood pressure control: a science advisory from the American Heart Association, the American College of Cardiology, and the Centers for Disease Control and Prevention. *Hypertension.* 2014;63:1230-1238.

[4]Mancia G, Fagard R, Narkiewicz K, et al. 2013 ESH/ESC Guidelines for the management of arterial hypertension: the Task Force for the management of arterial hypertension of the European Society of Hypertension (ESH) and of the European Society of Cardiology (ESC). *J Hypertens.* 2013;31:1281-1357.

[5]Canadian Hypertension Education Program (CHEP) 2013 Recommendations. Retrieved August 4, 2014 from http://www.hypertension.ca/chep.

[6]American Diabetes Association. Standards of medical care in diabetes: 2013. *Diabetes Care.* 2013;36(Suppl 1):S11-66.

[7]Kidney Disease: Improving Global Outcomes (KDIGO) Blood Pressure Work Group. KDIGO clinical practice guideline for the management of blood pressure in chronic kidney disease. *Kidney Int Suppl.* 2012;2:337-414.

[8]National Institute for Health and Clinical Excellence (NICE). Clinical guideline 127. Hypertension: clinical management of primary hypertension in adults. 2011. www.nice.org.uk/guidance/cg127.

[9]Aronow WS, Fleg JL, Pepine CJ, et al. ACCF/AHA 2011 expert consensus document on hypertension in the elderly: a report of the American College of Cardiology Foundation Task Force on Clinical Expert Consensus Documents. *Circulation.* 2011;123:2434-2506.

[10]Flack JM, Sica DA, Bakris G, et al. Management of high blood pressure in blacks: an update of the International Society on Hypertension in Blacks consensus statement. *Hypertension.* 2010;56:780-800.

Stroke survivors are at high risk for recurrent stroke, further disability, and death. Reduction in systolic blood pressure to below 130 mm Hg with thiazide and ACE inhibitor combination therapy can reduce these risks.[11]

Hypertension in Minority Populations

Mexican Americans have the lowest rate of control of hypertension of all U.S. racial/ethnic groups but also have the highest risk for diabetes. Thus, antihypertensive regimens should be tailored to avoid causing more new cases of diabetes (e.g., by avoiding high-dose chlorthalidone). In African Americans, hypertension not only is more prevalent than in the general population but also starts at a younger age, is less well controlled, and causes disproportionate and premature disability and death.[5] African Americans commonly have lower plasma renin levels and have less response to monotherapy with an ACE inhibitor or ARB than do white hypertensive patients. African American participants have a higher risk for fatal stroke when taking an ACE inhibitor alone than when taking a diuretic alone, but racial/ethnic differences disappear when high doses of an ACE inhibitor or ARB are used in combination with a diuretic or CCB. ACE inhibitors or ARBs can help achieve excellent control of hypertension in African American patients when used as part of an appropriate multidrug regimen.

Hypertension Associated with Oral Contraceptives and Estrogen Replacement

Oral contraceptives, particularly current low-dose estrogen preparations, cause a small increase in blood pressure in most women but rarely cause a large increase into the hypertensive range. The mechanism is unknown, but women older than 35 years and those who smoke or are overweight appear to be at increased risk. If hypertension develops, oral contraceptive therapy

TABLE 67-11 PREFERRED ORAL ANTIHYPERTENSIVE DRUG CLASSES IN SPECIFIC CONDITIONS

CONDITION	DRUG CLASS(ES)
Prehypertension	ARB
Hypertension in general	CCB, ACE-I or ARB, D
Hypertension in elderly patients	CCB, ACE-I or ARB, D
Hypertension with left ventricular hypertrophy	ARB, D, CCB
Hypertension in patients with diabetes mellitus	CCB, ACE-I or ARB, D
Hypertension in patients with diabetic nephropathy	ARB, D
Hypertension in nondiabetic chronic kidney disease	ACE-I or ARB, BB, D
BP reduction for secondary prevention of coronary events	ACE-I, CCB, BB, D
BP reduction for secondary prevention of stroke	ACE-I + D, CCB
BP management for patient with heart failure	D, BB, ACE-I or ARB, aldosterone antagonist
Gestational hypertension (stage 2, without preeclampsia)	Labetalol, nifedipine, methyldopa
Thoracic aortic aneurysm	BB, ACE-I or ARB, D
Atrial fibrillation (ventricular rate control)	BB, nondihydropyridine CCB

ACE-I = angiotensin-converting enzyme inhibitor; ARB = angiotensin receptor blocker; BB = β-blocker; CCB = calcium-channel blocker; D, diuretic (thiazide-like such as chlorthalidone is preferred).

Adapted from Mancia G, Fagard R, Narkiewicz K, et al. 2013 ESH/ESC Guidelines for the management of arterial hypertension: the Task Force for the management of arterial hypertension of the European Society of Hypertension (ESH) and of the European Society of Cardiology (ESC). *J Hypertens.* 2013;31:1281-1357.

TABLE 67-12 CAUSES OF PSEUDORESISTANT AND TRULY RESISTANT HYPERTENSION

PSEUDORESISTANT HYPERTENSION	TRULY RESISTANT HYPERTENSION
Inadequate medical regimen Pressor substances (e.g., nonsteroidal anti-inflammatory drugs [NSAIDs], calcineurin inhibitors such as cyclosporine or tacrolimus, or sympathomimetics such as cocaine or methamphetamine) White coat reaction, improper blood pressure measurement Medication nonadherence	Chronic kidney disease Primary aldosteronism Other secondary hypertension (e.g., pheochromocytoma, Cushing syndrome, atherosclerotic renal artery stenosis, fibromuscular renal artery stenosis, Takayasu arteritis, coarctation of the aorta, hyperthyroidism, hypothyroidism, hyperparathyroidism) Difficult primary hypertension

should be discontinued in favor of other methods of contraception. Oral estrogen replacement therapy after menopause appears to cause a small increase in blood pressure, whereas transdermal estrogen (which bypasses first-pass hepatic metabolism) appears to cause a small decrease in blood pressure.

Hypertension in Pregnancy

Hypertension, the most common nonobstetric complication of pregnancy, is present in about 10% of all pregnancies (Chapter 239). About one third of cases are caused by chronic hypertension and two thirds by gestational hypertension or preeclampsia, the latter defined as an increase in blood pressure to 160/110 mm Hg or higher after the 20th week of gestation, accompanied by proteinuria and pathologic edema. Preeclampsia sometimes also is accompanied by seizures (eclampsia) and the multisystem HELLP syndrome (Chapter 239) of hemolysis, elevated liver enzymes, and low platelets. Preeclampsia is the most common cause of maternal mortality and perinatal mortality.

Current guidelines recommend low-dose aspirin, beginning in the first trimester, to reduce the risk for recurrent preeclampsia in women with a past history of preeclampsia.[12] Women with gestational hypertension or chronic hypertension should be monitored twice weekly with measurements of blood pressure and weekly assessment of platelet counts, liver enzymes, and proteinuria.

Antihypertensive medication of mild maternal hypertension does not improve perinatal outcome and may be associated with fetal growth retardation, so medications are not recommended for uncomplicated stage 1 gestational hypertension but rather are reserved for stage 2 hypertension (blood pressure > 160/110 mm Hg). For pregnant women with stage 2 hypertension but without severe preeclampsia/eclampsia, oral drug therapy should be initiated with any one of three preferred drugs: labetalol (400 to 2400 mg daily), nifedipine XL (30 to 120 mg daily), or methyldopa (500 to 3000 mg daily). Combination therapy is rarely needed, and excessive reductions in blood pressure must be avoided. All renin-angiotensin system blockers must be discontinued. The definitive cure of preeclampsia is termination of pregnancy.

Intravenous labetalol (0.5 to 2 mg/minute up to a cumulative dose of 300 mg) has replaced hydralazine as the drug of choice to treat severe preeclampsia/eclampsia. Intravenous magnesium sulfate is not a reliable antihypertensive agent but is effective in treating or preventing seizures (eclampsia). Delivery soon after maternal stabilization is recommended irrespective of gestational age for women with superimposed preeclampsia and any of the following: uncontrollable severe hypertension, eclampsia, pulmonary edema, abruptio placentae, disseminated intravascular coagulation, or fetal distress. Intravenous nitroglycerin (10 to 100 μg/minute) is the treatment of choice when pulmonary edema accompanies preeclampsia.

For women with preeclampsia or even gestational hypertension, blood pressure should be monitored closely in the hospital for 72 hours postpartum and again as an outpatient 7 to 10 days after delivery. All blood pressure drugs are secreted into human breast milk, but only propranolol and nifedipine are secreted in high enough concentrations that they should be avoided in mothers who are breast-feeding. Women whose preeclampsia caused preterm delivery have an almost 10-fold increased risk for cardiovascular disease in later life and are candidates for aggressive risk factor modification.

Drug-Resistant Hypertension

Up to one in five hypertensive patients has *resistant hypertension*, defined as high blood pressure uncontrolled with three antihypertensive drugs, including a diuretic, or controlled on four or more drugs.[13] More than half of such patients have *pseudoresistance* because of improper blood pressure measurement techniques, white coat reactions, medication nonadherence, intake of drugs that raise blood pressure (e.g., NSAIDs, excessive alcohol, psychiatric drugs), or an inadequate blood pressure regimen (Table 67-12). Common correctable issues are clonidine rebound (especially with as-needed dosing), inadequate diuretic therapy, inappropriate use of a loop diuretic in a patient with normal renal function, infrequent dosing with a short-acting loop diuretic (e.g., once-daily furosemide), and use of a low-dose thiazide in a patient with chronic kidney disease.

Truly drug-resistant patients are at high risk because of their severe hypertension and target organ damage. Patients should be screened for secondary hypertension, especially chronic kidney disease, obstructive sleep apnea (Chapter 100), primary aldosteronism (Chapter 227), and pheochromocytoma (Chapter 228). In the absence of an identifiable cause for the hypertension, a mineralocorticoid receptor antagonist or a vasodilating β-blocker can serve as highly effective add-on therapies. Low-dose eplerenone or spironolactone can be remarkably effective for resistant hypertension—even when the serum aldosterone is within the normal range.

Despite maximally tolerated doses of five or more different antihypertensive medications, some patients still have uncontrolled hypertension. Unfortunately, neither catheter-based renal denervation[A10,14] nor an implantable carotid baroreceptor pacemaker have been shown to be reliably beneficial in such patients.

Acute Severe Hypertension

Twenty-five percent of all emergency department patients present with an elevated blood pressure (Chapter 8). *Hypertensive emergencies* are acute, often severe elevations in blood pressure, accompanied by rapidly progressive target organ dysfunction, such as myocardial or cerebral ischemia or infarction, pulmonary edema, or renal failure. The blood pressure typically is 220/130 mm Hg or higher, but it may be much lower in women who have preeclampsia in the absence of preexisting hypertension. The full-blown clinical picture of a hypertensive emergency is a critically ill patient who presents with a blood pressure typically above 220/130 mm Hg, headaches, confusion, blurred vision, nausea and vomiting, seizures, pulmonary edema, oliguria, and grade 3 or grade 4 hypertensive retinopathy (Fig. 67-8). *Hypertensive emergencies* require immediate reduction of blood pressure with intravenous medication (Table 67-13) and intra-arterial monitoring in an intensive care unit (ICU). In contrast, *hypertensive urgency* denotes severe uncontrolled hypertension sometimes with vague symptoms (such as headache, malaise, anxiety) but without objective evidence of acute target organ damage. In the absence of acute target organ damage, a patient with a blood pressure of 220/130 mm Hg or higher should be treated with short-acting oral medication. *Severe hypertension,* defined as a blood pressure between 180/110 and 219/129 mm Hg without symptoms or acute target organ damage, almost always occurs in patients who have chronic hypertension and who ran out of or stopped taking their blood pressure medication. Long-acting oral medication simply can be restarted. Patients with a hypertensive urgency or severe hypertension require outpatient follow-up within 24 to 72 hours with either a primary care physician or hypertension specialist.

The most common hypertensive cardiac emergencies include acute aortic dissection (Chapter 78), hypertension after cardiac surgery (Chapter 74), acute

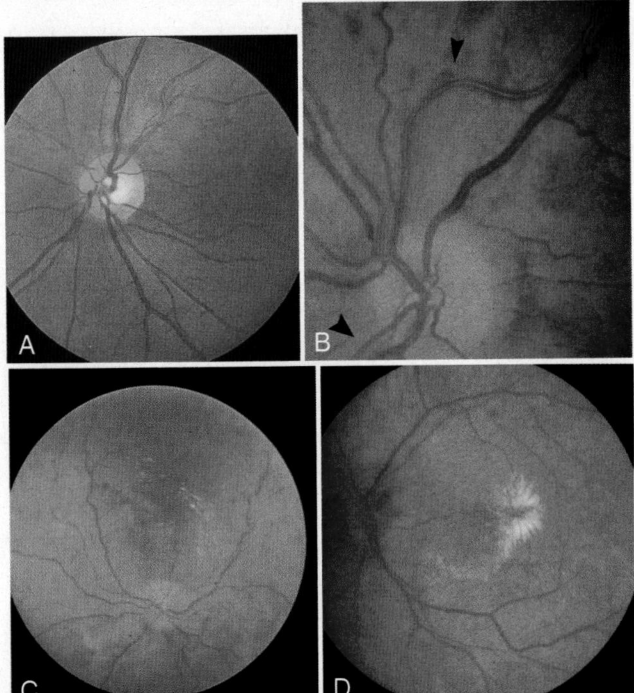

FIGURE 67-8. Hypertensive retinopathy is traditionally divided into four grades. A, Grade 1 shows early and minor changes in a young patient. Increased tortuosity of a retinal vessel and increased reflectiveness (silver wiring) of a retinal artery are seen at 1 o'clock in this view. Otherwise, the fundus is completely normal. B, Grade 2 also shows increased tortuosity and silver wiring *(arrowheads)*. In addition, there is "nipping" of the venules at arteriovenous crossings. C, Grade 3 shows the same changes as grade 2 plus flame-shaped retinal hemorrhages and soft "cotton-wool" exudates. D, In grade 4, there is swelling of the optic disc (papilledema), retinal edema is present, and hard exudates may collect around the fovea, producing a typical "macular star." (From Forbes CD, Jackson WF. *Color Atlas and Text of Clinical Medicine.* 3rd ed. London: Mosby; 2003.)

myocardial infarction (Chapter 73), and unstable angina (Chapter 72). Other hypertensive emergencies include cocaine-induced sympathetic crisis, eclampsia (Chapter 239), head trauma (Chapter 399), severe body burns (Chapter 111), postoperative bleeding from vascular suture lines, and epistaxis that cannot be controlled with anterior and posterior nasal packing. Neurologic emergencies—acute ischemic stroke, hemorrhagic stroke, subarachnoid hemorrhage, and hypertensive encephalopathy—can be difficult to distinguish from one another (Chapters 406 to 408). Hypertensive encephalopathy (Chapter 408) is characterized by severe hypertensive retinopathy (retinal hemorrhages and exudates, with or without papilledema) and a posterior leukoencephalopathy (affecting mainly the white matter of the parieto-occipital regions) seen on cerebral MRI or CT. A new focal neurologic deficit suggests a stroke in evolution, which demands a much more conservative approach to the elevated blood pressure (Chapter 407).

In most other hypertensive emergencies, the goal of parenteral therapy is to achieve a controlled and gradual lowering of blood pressure. A good rule of thumb is to lower the initially elevated arterial pressure by 10% in the first hour and by an additional 15% during the next 3 to 12 hours to a blood pressure of no less than 160/110 mm Hg. Blood pressure can be reduced further during the next 48 hours. Exceptions to this rule are aortic dissection (Chapter 78) and postoperative bleeding from vascular suture lines, two situations that demand much more rapid normalization of blood pressure. In most other cases, unnecessarily rapid correction of the elevated blood pressure to completely normal values places the patient at high risk for worsening cerebral, cardiac, and renal ischemia. In chronic hypertension, cerebral autoregulation is reset to higher than normal blood pressures. This compensatory adjustment prevents tissue overperfusion (increased intracranial pressure) at very high blood pressures, but it also predisposes to tissue underperfusion (cerebral ischemia) when an elevated blood pressure is lowered too quickly (Chapter 407). In patients with coronary disease, overly rapid or excessive reduction in diastolic blood pressure in the ICU can precipitate an acute myocardial ischemia or infarction.

Intravenous Drugs for Hypertensive Emergencies

First-line drug options for hypertensive emergencies (Table 67-14) are intravenous labetalol (a combined α- and β-blocker), nitroprusside, nicardipine (a dihydropyridine CCB), or urapadil (a new central sympatholytic that acts on central serotonergic pathways and also selectively blocks peripheral α_1-adrenergic receptors). In patients with impaired cerebral autoregulation (see

TABLE 67-13 RECOMMENDED TREATMENT OF HYPERTENSIVE EMERGENCIES BY END ORGAN INVOLVED

TYPE OF EMERGENCY	TIME-LINE, TARGET BP	FIRST-LINE THERAPY	ALTERNATIVE THERAPY
Hypertensive crisis with retinopathy, microangiopathy, or acute renal insufficiency	Several hours, MAP −20 to −25%	Labetalol	Nitroprusside Nicardipine Urapadil
Hypertensive encephalopathy	Immediate, MAP −20 to −25%	Labetalol	Nicardipine Nitroprusside
Acute aortic dissection	Immediate, Systolic BP < 110 mm Hg	Nitroprusside plus metoprolol	Labetalol
Acute pulmonary edema	Immediate, MAP 60 to 100 mm Hg	Nitroprusside with loop diuretic	Nitroglycerine Urapadil with loop diuretic
Acute coronary syndrome	Immediate, MAP 60 to 100 mm Hg	Nitroglycerine	Labetalol
Acute ischemic stroke and BP > 220/120 mm Hg	1 hr, MAP −15%	Labetalol	Nicardipine Nitroprusside
Cerebral hemorrhage and Systolic BP > 180 mm Hg or MAP > 130 mm Hg	1 hr, Systolic BP < 180 mm Hg and MAP < 130 mm Hg	Labetalol	Nicardipine Nitroprusside
Acute ischemic stroke with indication for thrombolytic therapy and BP > 185/110 mm Hg	1 hr, MAP < −15%	Labetalol	Nicardipine Nitroprusside
Cocaine/XTC intoxication	Several hours, Systolic BP < 140 mm Hg	Phentolamine (after benzodiazepines)	Nitroprusside
Pheochromocytoma crisis	Immediate	Phentolamine	Nitroprusside Urapadil
Perioperative hypertension during or after CABG	Immediate	Nicardipine	Urapadil Nitroglycerine
During or after craniotomy	Immediate	Nicardipine	Labetalol
Severe preeclampsia/eclampsia	Immediate, BP < 160/105 mm Hg	Labetalol (plus $MgSO_4$ and oral antihypertensive medication such as nifedipine with or without methyldopa)	Ketanserin Nicardipine

Adapted from van den Born BJ, Beutler JJ, Gaillard CA, et al. Dutch guideline for the management of hypertensive crisis: 2010 revision. *Neth J Med.* 2011;69:248-255.
BP = blood pressure; CABG = coronary artery bypass grafting; MAP = mean arterial pressure; MgSO4 = magnesium sulfate; XTC = ecstasy.

TABLE 67-14 INTRAVENOUS DRUGS FOR HYPERTENSIVE EMERGENCIES

DRUG	ONSET OF ACTION	HALF-LIFE	DOSE	CONTRAINDICATIONS AND SIDE EFFECTS
Labetalol	5-10 min	3-6 hr	0.25-0.5 mg/kg; 2-4 mg/min until goal BP is reached, thereafter 5-20 mg/hr	Second- or third-degree AV block; systolic heart failure, COPD (relative); bradycardia
Nicardipine	5-15 min	30-40 min	5-15 mg/hr as continuous infusion, starting dose 5 mg/hr, increase every 15-30 min with 2.5 mg until goal BP, thereafter decrease to 3 mg/hr	Liver failure
Nitroprusside	Immediate	1-2 min	0.3-10 µg/kg/min, increase by 0.5 µg/kg/min every 5 min until goal BP	Liver/kidney failure (relative), cyanide toxicity
Nitroglycerine	1-5 min	3-5 min	5-200 µg/min, 5 µg/min increase every 5 min	
Urapadil	3-5 min	4-6 hr	12.5-25 mg as bolus injections; 5-40 mg/hr as continuous infusion	
Esmolol	1-2 min	10-30 min	0.5-1.0 mg/kg as bolus; 50-300 µg/kg/min as continuous infusion	Second- or third-degree AV block, systolic heart failure, COPD (relative); bradycardia
Phentolamine	1-2 min	3-5 min	1-5 mg, repeat after 5-15 min until goal BP is reached; 0.5-1 mg/hr as continuous infusion	Tachyarrhythmia, angina pectoris

AV = atrioventricular; BP = blood pressure; COPD = chronic obstructive pulmonary disease.
Adapted from van den Born BJ, Beutler JJ, Gaillard CA, et al. Dutch guideline for the management of hypertensive crisis: 2010 revision. *Neth J Med.* 2011;69:248-255.

later), labetalol causes a smaller adverse fall in cerebral blood flow than nitroprusside but has a longer half-life, thereby leading to more adverse episodes of systemic hypotension.[15] Intravenous nicardipine appears to produce a more predictable and consistent reduction in blood pressure than labetalol with a similar safety profile; however, physicians and hospital pharmacies are less familiar with nicardipine.[16]

After the blood pressure has been brought under acute control, oral labetalol and dihydropyridine CCBs are particularly useful agents in weaning patients from parenteral therapy so that they can be transferred from the ICU. A few doses of intravenous furosemide are often needed to overcome drug resistance due to secondary volume expansion resulting from parenteral vasodilator therapy.

Secondary hypertension should be suspected in patients admitted to the ICU with hypertensive crisis. Normal 24-hour urinary catecholamine values or normal plasma normetanephrine and metanephrine values collected when the blood pressure is the highest (first 24 hours in ICU) effectively rule out pheochromocytoma (Chapter 228). Bilateral renal artery stenosis (Chapter 125) and other secondary causes should be excluded after the patient has been transferred out of the ICU but before discharge from the hospital.

Oral Medications for Hypertensive Urgencies

Labetalol is effective in a dose of 200 to 300 mg, which can be repeated in 2 to 3 hours and then prescribed in twice-daily dosing. If a β-blocker is contraindicated, clonidine is effective in an initial dose of 0.1 or 0.2 mg followed by additional hourly doses of 0.1 mg. Captopril, a short-acting ACE inhibitor, lowers blood pressure within 15 to 30 minutes of oral dosing. A small test dose of 6.25 mg should be used to avoid an excessive fall in blood pressure in hypovolemic patients; then, the full oral dose is 25 mg, which can be repeated in 1 to 2 hours and prescribed as 25 to 75 mg twice daily.

Incidental Blood Pressure Elevation in the Emergency Department

Blood pressures above 160/110 mm Hg are a common incidental finding among patients who present to emergency departments and other acute care settings for urgent medical or surgical care of symptoms that are unrelated to blood pressure (e.g., musculoskeletal pain, orthopedic injury). The elevated blood pressure more often is the first indication of chronic hypertension than a simple physiologic stress reaction, so there is an important opportunity to initiate primary care referral for formal evaluation of possible chronic hypertension. Home or ambulatory blood pressure monitoring is indicated to determine whether the patient's blood pressure normalizes completely after the acute illness has resolved.

PROGNOSIS

The prognosis of the patient with hypertension is related both to the severity of the blood pressure elevation and the presence of additional cardiovascular risk factors. Undertreatment of hypertension and underuse of combination drug therapy, both of which are common in busy outpatient practices,[17] worsens outcomes, whereas management protocols with fixed-dose/once-daily combination pills, proactive follow-up, and access to walk-in blood pressure checks can improve hypertension control rates to as high as 80% (Table 67-15). In many states, pharmacists can work with patients and can implement a preset medication intensification protocol under a collaborative practice agreement with physician oversight. Long-term continuation rates are best for the ARBs, intermediate for ACE inhibitors and CCBs, and worst for diuretics and β-blockers.[18] Patients with drug-resistant hypertension should be referred to a hypertension specialist (www.ash-us.org/HTN-Specialist.aspx).

TABLE 67-15 STRATEGIES TO OPTIMIZE HYPERTENSION MANAGEMENT

HEALTH SYSTEM
- Standardized medication intensification protocol
- Team-based approach involving clinical pharmacists
- Pay providers for performance

DRUG TREATMENT
- Low-dose combination therapy
- Best-tolerated drug classes
- Fixed-dose single pill combinations
- Long-acting once daily drugs
- Low-cost generics

PATIENT ENGAGEMENT
- Shared goals
- Medication reconciliation/education
- Out-of-office blood pressure monitoring
- Social support from family and peers

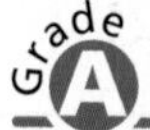

Grade A References

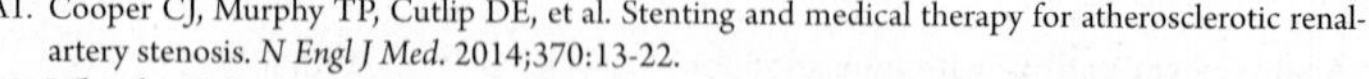

A1. Cooper CJ, Murphy TP, Cutlip DE, et al. Stenting and medical therapy for atherosclerotic renal-artery stenosis. *N Engl J Med.* 2014;370:13-22.

A2. Wheatley K, Ives N, Gray R, et al. Revascularization versus medical therapy for renal-artery stenosis. *N Engl J Med.* 2009;361:1953-1962.

A3. Sundstrom J, Arima H, Woodward M, et al. Blood pressure-lowering treatment based on cardiovascular risk: a meta-analysis of individual patient data. *Lancet.* 2014;384:591-598.

A4. Eckel RH, Jakicic JM, Ard JD, et al. 2013 AHA/ACC Guideline on Lifestyle Management to Reduce Cardiovascular Risk: A Report of the American College of Cardiology/American Heart Association Task Force on Practice Guidelines. *J Am Coll Cardiol.* 2014;63:2960-2984.

A5. ALLHAT Officers and Coordinators. Major outcomes in high-risk hypertensive patients randomized to angiotensin-converting enzyme inhibitor or calcium channel blocker vs diuretic: the Antihypertensive and Lipid-Lowering Treatment to Prevent Heart Attack Trial (ALLHAT). *JAMA.* 2002;288:2981-2997.

A6. Jamerson K, Weber MA, Bakris GL, et al. Benazepril plus amlodipine or hydrochlorothiazide for hypertension in high-risk patients. *N Engl J Med.* 2008;359:2417-2428.

A7. Mann JF, Schmieder RE, McQueen M, et al. Renal outcomes with telmisartan, ramipril, or both, in people at high vascular risk (the ONTARGET study): a multicentre, randomised, double-blind, controlled trial. *Lancet.* 2008;372:547-553.

A8. Fagard RH, Celis H, Thijs L, et al. Regression of left ventricular mass by antihypertensive treatment: a meta-analysis of randomized comparative studies. *Hypertension.* 2009;54:1084-1091.

A9. Kidney Disease: Improving Global Outcomes (KDIGO) Blood Pressure Work Group. KDIGO clinical practice guideline for the management of blood pressure in chronic kidney disease. *Kidney Int Suppl*. 2012;2:337-414.

A10. Bhatt DL, Kandzari DE, O'Neill WW, et al. A controlled trial of renal denervation for resistant hypertension. *N Engl J Med*. 2014;370:1393-1401.

GENERAL REFERENCES

For the General References and other additional features, please visit Expert Consult at https://expertconsult.inkling.com.

68 PULMONARY HYPERTENSION

VALLERIE MCLAUGHLIN

DEFINITION

The normal pulmonary vasculature is a low-pressure system, with less than one tenth the resistance to flow observed in the systemic vasculature. Pulmonary hypertension refers to the hemodynamic state in which the pressure in the pulmonary artery is elevated above a mean of 25 mm Hg. A specific type of pulmonary hypertension, pulmonary arterial hypertension, also requires that the left-sided heart filling pressure (pulmonary capillary wedge pressure, left ventricular end-diastolic pressure, or left atrial pressure) be 15 mm Hg or less and that the calculated pulmonary vascular resistance be greater than 3 Wood units (Wood unit = [pulmonary artery pressure minus mean pulmonary capillary wedge pressure] divided by cardiac output).[1] The syndrome of pulmonary arterial hypertension (Table 68-1)[2] results when blood flow through the pulmonary circulation is restricted, thereby leading to pathologic increases in pulmonary vascular resistance and, ultimately, to right ventricular failure. Pulmonary hypertension may also be a consequence of many other chronic diseases, including left-sided heart failure (Chapter 58), a variety of parenchymal lung diseases, and thromboembolic disease (Chapter 98).

EPIDEMIOLOGY

Normal pulmonary blood pressure is 20/10 (mean, 15) mm Hg at rest at sea level, rising to 30/13 (mean, 20) mm Hg with mild exercise. Pressures rise with altitude, and at an altitude of about 15,000 feet, normal resting pulmonary artery pressures are about 38/14 (mean, 20) mm Hg. Pulmonary arterial systolic pressure rises gradually with age, and each increase of 10 mm Hg is associated with a 2.7-fold greater risk for mortality.

Idiopathic pulmonary arterial hypertension, formerly called primary pulmonary hypertension, is the prototype of group 1 pulmonary arterial hypertension. This disease affects women more than men in a 2 : 1 ratio. It may be manifested at any age, with a mean age at onset of 37 years. The prevalence of pulmonary arterial hypertension is between 15 and 26 per million persons. Heritable pulmonary arterial hypertension occurs in a familial context, most often (70%) due to a mutation in the bone morphogenetic protein receptor type 2. (See Pathobiology.)

Drug- and toxin-induced pulmonary arterial hypertension has been most clearly linked to anorexigens, including aminorex, fenfluramine, and dexfenfluramine. Although these agents are no longer used, observational studies link amphetamines, methamphetamines, and L-tryptophan to pulmonary arterial hypertension. The tyrosine kinase inhibitor dasatinib also has been associated with the development of pulmonary arterial hypertension.

One of the most common types of group 1 pulmonary arterial hypertension occurs in the setting of connective tissue diseases. For example, the prevalence of pulmonary arterial hypertension in patients with scleroderma (Chapter 267) is in the range of 7 to 12%. It is less common in systemic lupus erythematosus (Chapter 266), rheumatoid arthritis (Chapter 264), and other systemic vasculitides (Chapter 270). Pulmonary arterial hypertension is a rare but well-established complication of human immunodeficiency virus (HIV) infection (Chapter 391), and its prevalence of 0.5% in such patients has not changed with the widespread use of highly active antiretroviral therapy. Prospective hemodynamic studies show that 2 to 6% of patients with portal hypertension (Chapter 153) develop pulmonary arterial hypertension, although the reason for the association is not clear.

TABLE 68-1 CLINICAL CLASSIFICATION OF PULMONARY HYPERTENSION

GROUP 1

Pulmonary arterial hypertension
- Idiopathic pulmonary arterial hypertension
- Heritable pulmonary arterial hypertension
  - BMPR2
  - ALK1, endoglin, SMAD9, CAV1, KCNK3
  - Unknown
- Drug- and toxin-induced pulmonary hypertension
- Associated with
  - Connective tissue diseases
  - HIV infection
  - Portal hypertension
  - Congenital heart diseases
  - Schistosomiasis

Pulmonary veno-occlusive disease and/or pulmonary capillary hemangiomatosis

Persistent pulmonary hypertension of the newborn

GROUP 2

Pulmonary hypertension due to left heart disease
- Systolic dysfunction
- Diastolic dysfunction
- Valvular disease
- Congenital or acquired left heart inflow or outflow tract obstruction

GROUP 3

Pulmonary hypertension due to lung diseases and/or hypoxia
- Chronic obstructive pulmonary disease
- Interstitial lung disease
- Other pulmonary diseases with mixed restrictive and obstructive pattern
- Sleep-disordered breathing
- Alveolar hypoventilation disorders
- Chronic exposure to high altitude
- Developmental lung diseases
  - Congenital diaphragmatic hernia
  - Bronchopulmonary dysplasia

GROUP 4

Chronic thromboembolic pulmonary hypertension

GROUP 5

Pulmonary hypertension with unclear multifactorial mechanisms
- Hematologic disorders: chronic hemolytic anemias, myeloproliferative disorders, splenectomy
- Systemic disorders: sarcoidosis, pulmonary Langerhans cell histiocytosis, lymphangioleiomyomatosis, neurofibromatosis, vasculitis
- Metabolic disorders: glycogen storage disease, Gaucher disease, thyroid disorders
- Others: segmental pulmonary arterial hypertension, tumoral obstruction, fibrosing mediastinitis, chronic renal failure

ALK1 = activin receptor-like kinase type 1; BMPR2 = bone morphogenetic protein receptor type 2; HIV = human immunodeficiency virus.

From Simonneau G, Gatzoulis MA, Adatia I, et al. Updated clinical classification of pulmonary hypertension. *J Am Coll Cardiol*. 2013;62:D34-D41.

A significant proportion of patients with untreated systemic-to-pulmonary shunts, commonly due to congenital heart disease (Chapter 69), develop pulmonary arterial hypertension. Persistent exposure of the pulmonary vasculature to increased blood flow and pressure leads to an elevated pulmonary vascular resistance. In some cases, Eisenmenger syndrome (Chapter 69), with a reversal of flow across the defect, results in right-to-left shunting. Pulmonary veno-occlusive disease (Chapter 98) and pulmonary capillary hemangiomatosis are rare disorders that directly affect the pulmonary vasculature. The presentation of each is often similar to pulmonary arterial hypertension, but the prognosis is particularly poor.

Pulmonary hypertension due to left-sided heart disease probably represents the most frequent cause of pulmonary hypertension seen in practice (group 2 patients). Left-sided ventricular (Chapter 58) or valvular (Chapter 75) disease may increase left atrial pressure, which then is transmitted back to the pulmonary vasculature. Often, the transpulmonary gradient and pulmonary vascular resistance are normal. In such cases, optimal treatment of the left-sided heart disease results in reduction of the left-sided heart filling pressures and, consequently, a reduction in the pulmonary artery pressures. On occasion, patients with left-sided heart disease have an elevation of pulmonary artery pressure greater than expected on the basis of the elevation of left-sided heart filling pressures, with a transpulmonary gradient of more than 12 mm Hg and a pulmonary vascular resistance of more than 3 Wood units. This difference may be due to an increase in pulmonary artery vasomotor tone or pulmonary vascular remodeling in the setting of persistently elevated left-sided heart filling pressures.

Group 3 patients have pulmonary hypertension due to lung diseases or hypoxia. Any disorder that results in hypoxemia (e.g., chronic obstructive lung disease [Chapter 88], interstitial lung disease [Chapter 92], sleep-disordered breathing [Chapter 100]) may result in pulmonary hypertension, although the pressure elevation tends to be modest, with a mean pulmonary artery pressure of 25 to 35 mm Hg. Echocardiography-based observations have suggested that up to 80% of patients with chronic obstructive lung disease and idiopathic pulmonary fibrosis have elevated pulmonary artery pressures. In patients who have more advanced parenchymal lung disease and undergo evaluation for lung volume reduction surgery or lung transplantation, 40 to 50% have pulmonary hypertension at the time of right-sided heart catheterization. Most often, the elevations in pulmonary artery pressures are modest, but a small proportion of patients have more substantial elevations.

Group 4 patients have chronic thromboembolic pulmonary hypertension (Chapter 98), which must be differentiated from the other groups because the treatment is different. Approximately 4% of patients who have suffered an acute pulmonary embolism progress to development of chronic thromboembolic pulmonary hypertension. Approximately half of those ultimately diagnosed with chronic thromboembolic pulmonary hypertension do not have a known history of an acute pulmonary embolism. Chronic thromboembolic pulmonary hypertension occurs equally in both genders. All age groups can be affected, with a median age of 63 years.

PATHOBIOLOGY

The pathobiology of pulmonary arterial hypertension is complex and incompletely elucidated (E-Fig. 68-1). The pulmonary arterial hypertension phenotype is characterized by endothelial dysfunction, a decreased ratio of apoptosis to proliferation in pulmonary artery smooth muscle cells, and a thickened, disordered adventitia in which adventitial metalloproteases are excessively activated. The evolution of pulmonary vascular disease frequently originates with the interaction of a predisposing state and one or more inciting stimuli, a concept referred to as the multiple-hit hypothesis.

In group 1 pulmonary arterial hypertension, patients have a panvasculopathy predominantly affecting the small pulmonary arterioles. It is characterized by a variety of arterial abnormalities, including intimal hyperplasia, medial hypertrophy, adventitial proliferation, thrombosis in situ, varying degrees of inflammation, and plexiform lesions. An individual patient may manifest all or some of these lesions, and the distribution of the lesions may be diffuse or focal.

The genetic defect best characterized in heritable pulmonary arterial hypertension is that of the bone morphogenetic protein receptor type 2, a member of the transforming growth factor-β (TGF-β) signaling family. Mutations in activin receptor–like kinase type 1, or endoglin, have also been identified, usually in families with coexistent hereditary hemorrhagic telangiectasia. Less commonly, mutations in activin receptor–like kinase type 1, or endoglin, have been identified in patients with pulmonary arterial hypertension, predominantly with coexistent hereditary hemorrhagic telangiectasia (Chapter 173). Mutations in other genes (i.e., BMPR1B, caveolin-1, and SMAD9), all of which are involved in the TGF-β signaling pathway, are considerably less common. A novel channelopathy of KCNK3, which has been identified in familial and idiopathic cases of pulmonary arterial hypertension, is the first indication that the disease may involve factors apparently independent of the TGF-β signaling pathway.

The imbalance in the production or metabolism of vasoactive mediators in the pulmonary vasculature includes a reduction in prostacyclin and nitric oxide, which have vasodilator and antiproliferative properties, and an increase in thromboxane and endothelin, which are vasoconstrictors as well as mitogens. The reduction in nitric oxide synthase in pulmonary arterial hypertension diminishes nitric oxide and, subsequently, cyclic guanosine monophosphate production. Endothelin-1 is a potent vasoconstrictor and smooth muscle mitogen that may contribute to the development of pulmonary arterial hypertension. Prostacyclin synthase is reduced in pulmonary arterial hypertension, resulting in an inadequate production of prostacyclin, which is a vasodilator with potent antiproliferative effects. Other aberrations include those of the voltage-dependent potassium channels and serotonin pathways. Disorders of inflammatory and coagulation pathways have also been described.

Chronic changes in the pulmonary vasculature also occur as a result of other types of pulmonary hypertension. Chronic elevation of left-sided heart filling pressures causes a backward transmission of pressure to the pulmonary venous system and triggers vasoconstriction in the pulmonary arterial bed. On histologic evaluation, the veins are thickened abnormally, and a neointima is formed. As secondary features, medial hypertrophy and thickening of the neointima on the arterial side of the pulmonary circulation occur. These changes can be reversed with therapies that result in chronic reduction of left-sided heart filling pressures.

In parenchymal lung disease, changes in the distal pulmonary arterial vessels are related to hypoxia. Hypoxia induces muscularization of the distal vessels and medial hypertrophy of the more proximal vessels. Neither neointima formation nor the development of plexiform lesions is observed.

The pathologic process of chronic thromboembolic pulmonary hypertension is often distinct from idiopathic pulmonary arterial hypertension. The lesions are frequently more variable, with some arterial pathways that appear relatively unaffected and others that show recanalized vascular thromboses. However, the involvement of distal microvessels, particularly when thromboses have occurred in subsegmental arteries, can resemble idiopathic pulmonary arterial hypertension with the formation of plexiform lesions.

Pathophysiology

The normal pulmonary vasculature bed has a remarkable capacity to dilate and recruit unused vasculature to accommodate increases in pulmonary blood flow. In pulmonary hypertension, the pulmonary artery pressure and pulmonary vascular resistance are increased at rest and further increase with exertion. In response to this increased afterload, the normally very thin right ventricle hypertrophies and eventually dilates. Early in the process, the right ventricle may be capable of maintaining normal cardiac output at rest, although it may fail to augment cardiac output with exercise, thereby leading to exertional dyspnea. As the disease progresses, the right ventricular dysfunction may progress to the point that resting cardiac output is impaired. Right ventricular function is a major determinant of functional capacity and prognosis in pulmonary arterial hypertension. Although the left ventricle is not affected by pulmonary vascular disease itself, progressive right ventricular dilation can impair left ventricular filling and lead to mildly increased left-sided heart filling pressure. The pathophysiologic mechanism of pulmonary hypertension related to left-sided heart and lung disease is further complicated by those underlying disorders.

The two most frequent mechanisms of death are progressive right ventricular failure and sudden death. Right ventricular failure, as evidenced by elevated jugular venous pressure, lower extremity edema, and occasionally ascites, may also be accompanied by evidence of poor forward flow due to inadequate filling of the left ventricle. Hypotension, hypoperfusion, and renal insufficiency may result. Other potential causes of death include pneumonia, sepsis, and pulmonary embolism.

CLINICAL MANIFESTATIONS

History

Dyspnea, which is the most common symptom of pulmonary hypertension, initially may be attributed to underlying disorders such as heart failure or obstructive lung disease, but the dyspnea of pulmonary hypertension typically is insidious in progression and reproducible. Dyspnea is classified by the World Health Organization (WHO) system, which is similar to the New York Heart Association classification system for angina and heart failure (see Table 51-5), and may progress to dyspnea at rest.

Other common symptoms of pulmonary hypertension include fatigue, lightheadedness, chest pain (Chapter 51), and palpitations (Chapters 51 and 62). Syncope (Chapter 62), which is an ominous finding, is often exertional in nature; it signifies the inability of the right ventricle to augment cardiac output as needed for physical activity. Symptoms of right-sided heart failure, including edema and ascites, signify advanced disease.

The nonspecific symptoms of pulmonary hypertension often explain its delayed recognition. In various reviews, the delay from onset of symptoms to diagnosis can be as long as 2 years.[3]

Patients often have symptoms associated with their underlying disease, which typically is far advanced by the time pulmonary arterial hypertension develops. For example, patients with pulmonary hypertension associated with left-sided heart disease (group 2) often have paroxysmal nocturnal dyspnea and orthopnea. Patients with pulmonary hypertension related to hypoxic lung disease (group 3) may have cough, sputum production, or wheezing. Clinical symptoms of chronic thromboembolic pulmonary

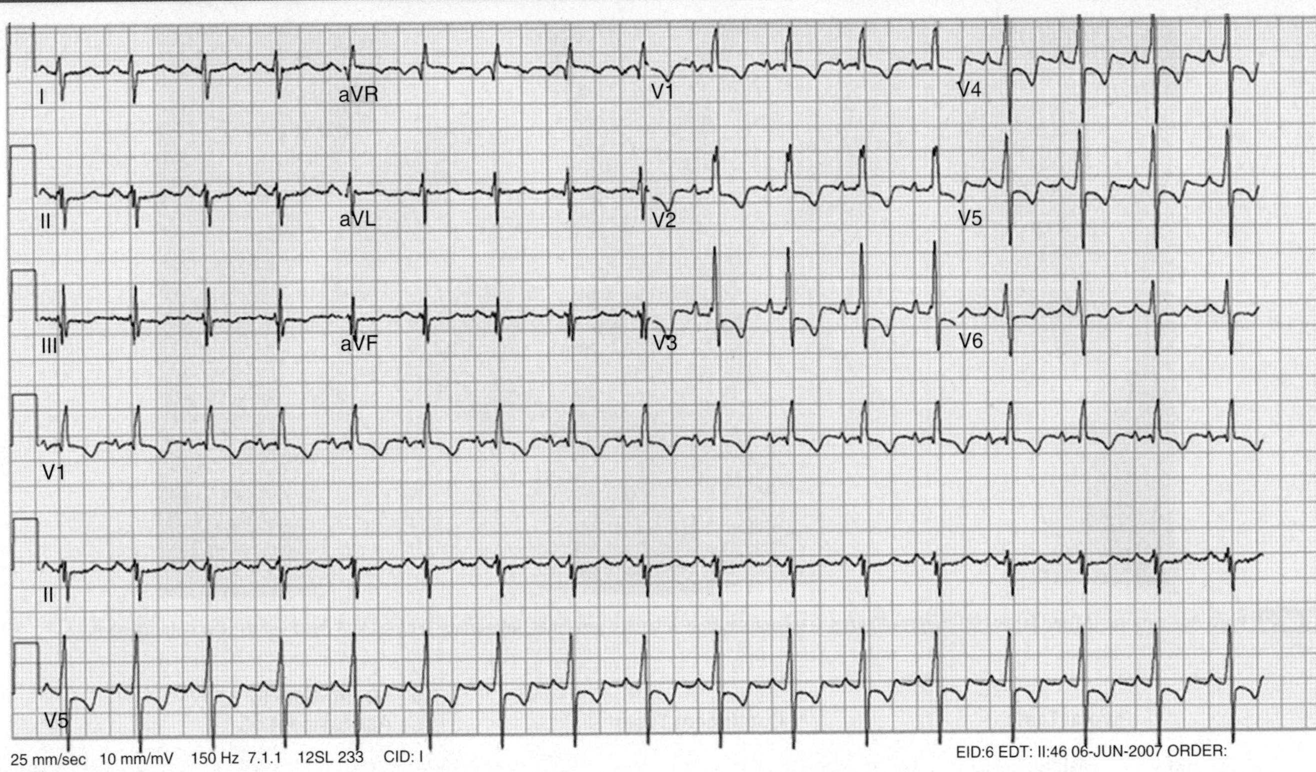

FIGURE 68-1. Electrocardiogram demonstrating sinus rhythm, right axis deviation, and right ventricular hypertrophy with a strain pattern.

hypertension resemble those of idiopathic pulmonary arterial hypertension, except that edema and hemoptysis occur more often in chronic thromboembolic pulmonary hypertension, whereas syncope is more common in idiopathic pulmonary arterial hypertension.

Physical Examination

Distention of jugular veins (see Fig. 51-3) may signify right ventricular failure, and prominent *v* waves (see Fig. 51-4) may be a result of tricuspid regurgitation. The amplitude of the carotid upstroke may give some insight into the cardiac output. The classic physical examination finding in pulmonary hypertension is a loud pulmonic component to the second heart sound, which reflects high pulmonary pressures that increase the force of the pulmonic valve closure. Palpation of the sternum often reveals a parasternal lift as the hypertrophied, pressure-overloaded right ventricle obliterates the retrosternal air space. A right ventricular fourth heart sound reflects diastolic filling of the hypertrophied, noncompliant right ventricle, akin to the left-sided fourth heart sound in a patient with systemic hypertension and left ventricular hypertrophy. The murmur of tricuspid regurgitation, which is holosystolic, located at the left lower sternal border, and augments with inspiration, is common in patients with moderate to severe pulmonary hypertension. Other findings on auscultation may include an early systolic click and the murmur of pulmonic regurgitation. A right ventricular third heart sound often signifies advanced disease and right-sided heart failure. Other signs consistent with right ventricular failure include hepatomegaly, peripheral edema (see Fig. 51-7), ascites, hypotension, diminished pulse pressure, and cool extremities.

Other physical examination findings may give some insight into the etiology of the pulmonary hypertension. For example, central cyanosis and clubbing may suggest an intracardiac shunt and Eisenmenger physiology. Sclerodactyly, telangiectasias (see Fig. 267-3), arthritis, Raynaud phenomenon (see Fig. 80-7), and rashes may increase the suspicion of an underlying connective tissue disease. Splenomegaly, spider angioma, palmar erythema (see Fig. 146-2), icterus (see Fig. 146-1), and caput medusae may suggest portal hypertension as an etiology. Signs of left-sided heart disease, such as pulmonary congestion, left-sided third heart sound, or findings of mitral or aortic valve disease on auscultation, may signify pulmonary hypertension as a result of left-sided heart disease. Fine rales, accessory muscle use, wheezing, protracted expiration, and productive cough may denote group 3 pulmonary hypertension as a result of hypoxic lung disease. Pulmonary vascular bruits suggest chronic thromboembolic pulmonary hypertension.

DIAGNOSIS

Initial assessments include an electrocardiogram and chest radiograph.[4] The electrocardiogram may show right axis deviation, right ventricular enlargement, right atrial enlargement, and ST and T wave changes across the anterior precordium that reflect right ventricular strain (Fig. 68-1). The chest radiograph may demonstrate enlarged proximal pulmonary arteries (see Fig. 56-6) with peripheral tapering or pruning of the pulmonary vasculature (Fig. 68-2A). The lateral radiograph may reveal the reduction in retrosternal air space as a result of right ventricular enlargement (Fig. 68-2B).

If, on the basis of history, physical examination, electrocardiogram, and chest radiograph, there is a reasonable suspicion for pulmonary hypertension, a series of diagnostic evaluations should follow (Fig. 68-3), usually beginning with an echocardiogram and with further testing guided by the patient's subtype. The echocardiogram gives insight not only into the presence of pulmonary hypertension but also into the presence of common disorders of the left side of the heart that may result in pulmonary hypertension. Two-dimensional echocardiographic findings reflective of elevated pulmonary artery pressures include right atrial enlargement, right ventricular enlargement, flattening of the intraventricular septum, and underfilled left ventricle (Fig. 68-4). The right ventricular systolic pressure may be estimated on the basis of the velocity of the tricuspid regurgitant jet by the modified Bernoulli equation (Chapter 55) (Fig. 68-5), although a reliable estimate of right ventricular systolic pressure is not always obtainable, and this measurement is prone to error, particularly in patients with parenchymal lung disease.

The echocardiogram is also useful to assess for left-sided heart causes of pulmonary hypertension, such as systolic dysfunction, diastolic dysfunction, and valvular heart disease. On occasion, a previously unknown congenital heart defect is discovered during this evaluation. In approximately 25% of patients, a previously trivial patent foramen ovale may shunt blood from the right atrium to the left atrium because of the high pulmonary vascular resistance and thereby worsen systemic oxygenation.

In a patient with unexplained dyspnea and evidence of pulmonary hypertension on echocardiography, chronic thromboembolic pulmonary hypertension must be excluded.[5] The study of choice for this assessment is the ventilation-perfusion (V/Q) scan (see Fig. 98-4), which often shows multiple perfusion defects that are not matched on ventilation. Although spiral computed tomography is excellent for the assessment of acute pulmonary embolus, it sometimes fails to detect surgically accessible chronic thromboembolic disease. If either of these studies detects an abnormality, further evaluation with pulmonary angiography may be required to determine

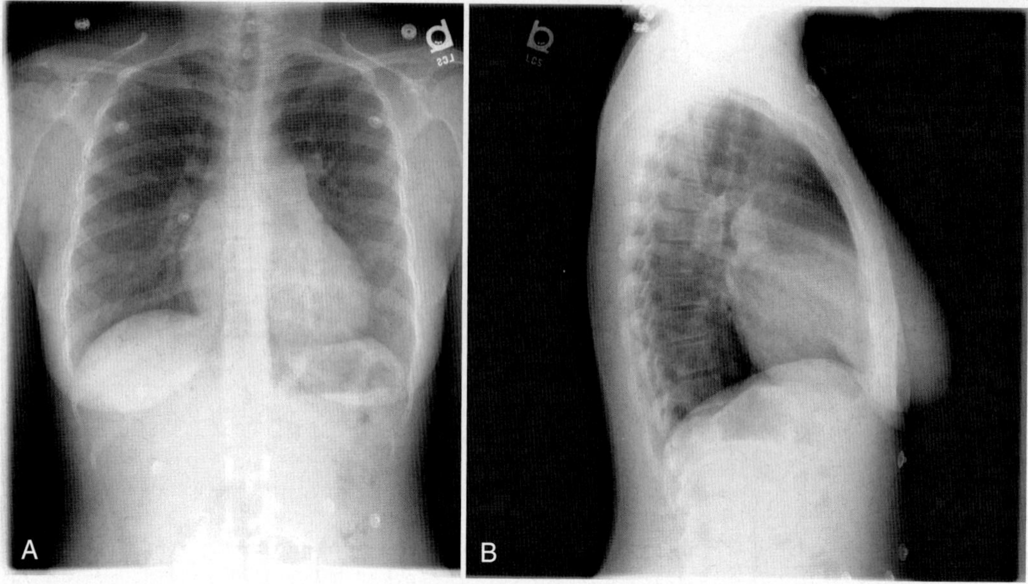

FIGURE 68-2. **Posterior-anterior (A) and lateral (B) chest radiographs demonstrating enlarged proximal pulmonary arteries and right ventricular enlargement.**

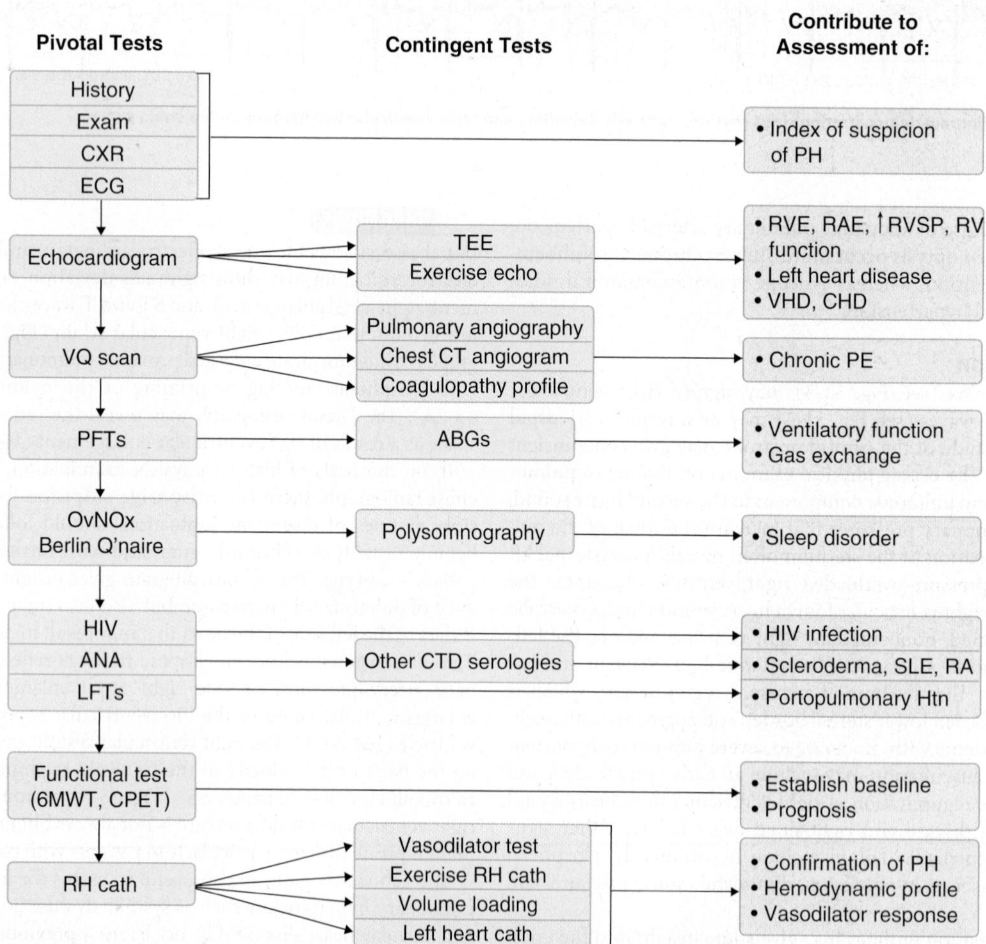

FIGURE 68-3. **Diagnostic approach to pulmonary arterial hypertension.** Because the suspicion of pulmonary arterial hypertension (PH) may arise in various ways, the sequence of tests may vary. However, the diagnosis of PH requires that certain data support a specific diagnosis. In addition, the diagnosis of idiopathic pulmonary arterial hypertension (IPAH) is one of excluding all other reasonable possibilities. *Pivotal tests* are those that are essential to establishing a diagnosis of any type of PH by either identification of criteria of associated disease or exclusion of diagnoses other than IPAH. All pivotal tests are required for a definitive diagnosis and baseline characterization. An abnormality of one assessment (such as obstructive pulmonary disease on pulmonary function tests) does not preclude that another abnormality (chronic thromboembolic disease on V/Q scan and pulmonary angiogram) is contributing or predominant. *Contingent tests* are recommended to elucidate or to confirm results of the pivotal tests and need be performed only in the appropriate clinical context. The *combination* of pivotal and appropriate contingent tests contributes to assessment of the differential diagnoses in the right-hand column. Definitive diagnosis may require additional specific evaluations not necessarily included in this general guideline. ABGs = arterial blood gases; ANA = antinuclear antibody serology; CHD = congenital heart disease; CPET = cardiopulmonary exercise test; CT = computed tomography; CTD = connective tissue disease; CXR = chest x-ray; ECG = electrocardiogram; HIV = human immunodeficiency virus screening; Htn = hypertension; LFTs = liver function tests; 6MWT = 6-minute walk test; OvNOx = overnight oximetry; PE = pulmonary embolism; PFTs = pulmonary function tests; RA = rheumatoid arthritis; RAE = right atrial enlargement; RH cath = right-sided heart catheterization; RV, right ventricle; RVE = right ventricular enlargement; RVSP = right ventricular systolic pressure; SLE = systemic lupus erythematosus; TEE = transesophageal echocardiography; VHD = valvular heart disease; V/Q scan = lung ventilation-perfusion scintigram. (From McLaughlin VV, Archer SL, Badesch DB, et al. ACCF/AHA 2009 expert consensus document on pulmonary hypertension: a report of the American College of Cardiology Foundation Task Force on Expert Consensus Documents and the American Heart Association developed in collaboration with the American College of Chest Physicians; American Thoracic Society, Inc.; and the Pulmonary Hypertension Association. *J Am Coll Cardiol.* 2009;53:1573-1619.)

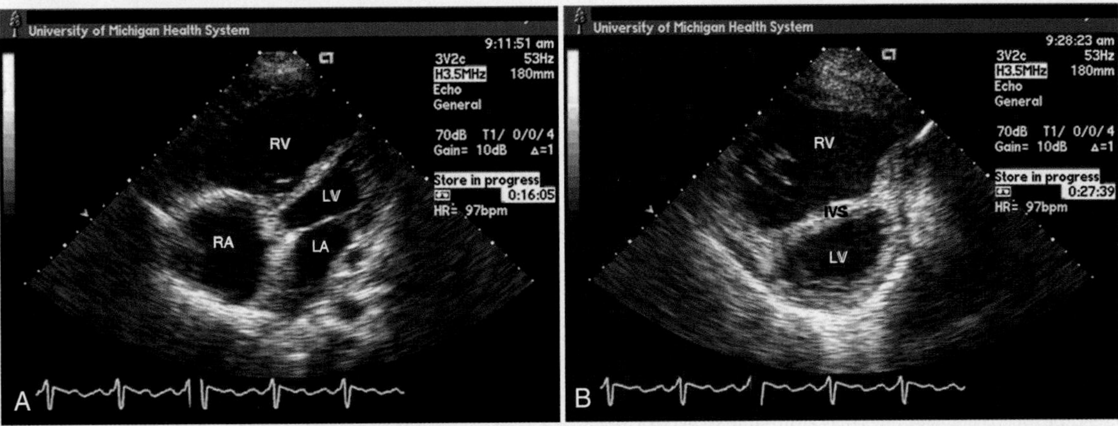

FIGURE 68-4. Echocardiographic images of the heart. A, Four-chamber view. Right atrial (RA) enlargement, right ventricular (RV) enlargement. The left atrium (LA) and left ventricle (LV) are small and underfilled. B, Short axis view. RV enlargement is present. Flattening of the intraventricular septum (IVS) results from pressure and volume overload of the RV.

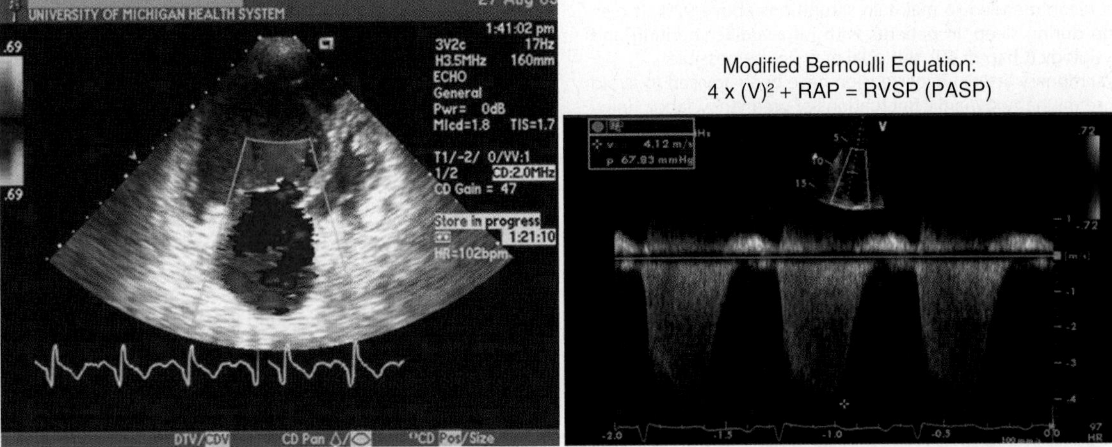

FIGURE 68-5. Calculation of estimated pulmonary artery pressure based on the velocity of the tricuspid regurgitant jet. RAP = right atrial pressure; RVSP = right ventricular systolic pressure; PASP = pulmonary artery systolic pressure; V = tricuspid jet velocity (m/sec).

whether chronic thrombolic disease is the diagnosis and, if so, whether it is surgically accessible.

Pulmonary function tests in patients with pulmonary arterial hypertension may show mild restrictive disease and a mildly reduced diffusing capacity for carbon monoxide. Patients with the scleroderma spectrum of diseases tend to have more substantial reductions in the diffusing capacity for carbon monoxide, which may even precede the development of pulmonary hypertension. Pulmonary function tests may disclose evidence of obstructive or restrictive lung disease; further evaluation with chest computed tomography may be necessary. Overnight oximetry is useful to screen for obstructive sleep apnea (Chapter 100). If indicated, formal polysomnography may be required.

Recommended serologic testing, given the known associations, includes an antinuclear antibody test and HIV serology in addition to liver function tests to assess for chronic liver disease. A study of functional capacity, most commonly the 6-minute walk test, is useful to assess the severity of disease, to determine the potential need for oxygen, and to establish a baseline against which to assess subsequent changes in exercise capacity as a result of medical interventions. The high prevalence of pulmonary arterial hypertension in patients with scleroderma serves as an opportunity for screening of this high-risk population with echocardiography to make an early diagnosis.[6]

If pulmonary arterial hypertension is suspected on the basis of the noninvasive evaluation, the diagnosis must be confirmed with a right-sided heart catheterization that measures right atrial pressure, right ventricular pressure, pulmonary artery (systolic, diastolic, and mean) pressures, pulmonary arterial wedge pressure (reflective of left ventricular end-diastolic pressure or left atrial pressure), cardiac output and index, heart rate, systemic blood pressure, and oxygen saturations in the superior vena cava, inferior vena cava, pulmonary artery, and a systemic artery. From this information, pulmonary vascular resistance and systemic vascular resistance may be calculated, right ventricular performance can be ensured, and an intracardiac or intrapulmonary shunt can be confirmed or excluded.

In patients with left-sided heart or parenchymal lung disease, however, optimal management of the underlying condition is often undertaken before right-sided heart catheterization is considered. Patients with suspected chronic thromboembolic disease often undergo both right-sided heart catheterization and pulmonary angiography (Chapter 98) to assess surgical candidacy and operative risk.

Measurement of the wedge pressure, a surrogate for left atrial pressure in the absence of pulmonary vein obstruction, is useful to exclude pulmonary hypertension caused by left-sided heart disease or, in rare cases, pulmonary veno-occlusive disease. If an optimal wedge pressure tracing cannot be obtained, or if there is any question about the accuracy of the wedge pressure tracing, a left ventricular end-diastolic pressure should be obtained.

Acute vasodilator testing is often performed at the time of the initial right-sided heart catheterization, not only for its prognostic implications but also to identify patients who might be candidates for therapy with calcium-channel blockers. Although the data regarding vasodilator testing and treatment with calcium-channel blockers are largely restricted to patients with idiopathic pulmonary arterial hypertension, vasodilator testing is often performed in patients with other types of pulmonary arterial hypertension. However, acute vasodilator testing is not indicated and may be harmful in patients with significantly elevated left-sided heart filling pressures because pulmonary edema may ensue.

The three agents most commonly used for acute vasodilator testing in the cardiac catheterization laboratory are inhaled nitric oxide, intravenous epoprostenol, and intravenous adenosine. A positive response to an acute vasodilator is a decrease in mean pulmonary artery pressure by at least 10 mm Hg to a mean pulmonary artery pressure of less than 40 mm Hg, without a decrease in cardiac output. If a patient meets these criteria, it is reasonable to administer a trial of oral calcium-channel blockers.

Unfortunately, adherence to the published algorithms for the diagnosis of pulmonary arterial hypertension is dismal. Studies that mistakenly remain unperformed include the V/Q scan (57%), HIV serology (29%), and serologies for connective tissue diseases (50%).[7] Ten percent of patients are given the diagnosis of pulmonary arterial hypertension without a right-sided heart catheterization confirmation, and only a minority of patients treated with calcium-channel blockers fulfilled the criteria for likely being an acute responder.

TREATMENT Rx

General Measures

Basic counseling and education are important components in the care of patients with pulmonary arterial hypertension. Patients are encouraged to engage in low-level graded aerobic exercise, such as walking, as tolerated, and to enroll in an intensive pulmonary rehabilitation program. Patients should avoid heavy physical exertion or isometric exercise, both of which may provoke exertional syncope. Exposure to high altitudes may contribute to hypoxic pulmonary vasoconstriction and may not be well tolerated. A sodium-restricted diet (<2400 mg/day) is advised and is particularly important to manage volume status in patients with right ventricular failure. Routine immunizations, such as those against influenza and pneumococcal pneumonia (Chapter 18), are advised. Because hypoxia is a potent pulmonary vasoconstrictor, supplemental oxygen is recommended to maintain saturations above 92% at rest, with exertion, and during sleep. In patients with intracardiac shunting and Eisenmenger physiology (Chapter 69), this goal may not be possible.

Women with pulmonary arterial hypertension have been advised to avoid pregnancy because the hemodynamic fluctuations of pregnancy, labor, delivery, and the postpartum period are potentially life-threatening. In a recent series of 26 women whose pulmonary arterial hypertension was well controlled and whose pregnancies were managed at highly specialized centers, three died, another developed refractory right-sided heart failure that required heart-lung transplantation, two had spontaneous abortions, and six had induced abortions.[8] Overall, 62% of the pregnancies resulted in a healthy baby without maternal complications. Current guidelines continue to recommend that pregnancy be avoided or terminated early in women with pulmonary arterial hypertension, although referral to a specialized center can be considered before termination. Women of childbearing potential should be counseled on contraception options at the time of diagnosis.

Background Therapy

On the basis of uncontrolled observational series in patients with primarily idiopathic pulmonary arterial hypertension, consensus recommendations advocate the use of warfarin titrated to an international normalized ratio of 1.5 to 2.5 in patients with idiopathic pulmonary arterial hypertension. Diuretics (e.g., furosemide, initiated at 20 mg and titrated as needed) are indicated to manage right ventricular volume overload; in some patients, intravenous diuretics may be necessary. Serum electrolytes and renal function must be closely monitored. Digoxin, 0.125 to 0.25 mg/day, is rarely used in patients with right ventricular failure and a low cardiac output and in patients with atrial arrhythmias, despite the paucity of data; if the patient experiences any evidence of digoxin toxicity, the drug should be discontinued because of the unfavorable risk-to-benefit ratio.

Vasodilator Therapy

Treatment of pulmonary arterial hypertension has evolved considerably, in part because of advances in understanding of the disease process and the availability of agents that target known pathobiologic derangements (Fig. 68-6).[A1]

Calcium-Channel Blockers

Approximately 7% of adult patients with idiopathic pulmonary arterial hypertension have a favorable response to acute vasodilator testing and excellent prognosis with calcium-channel blockers. Long-acting nifedipine (90 to 180 mg daily), diltiazem (360 to 720 mg daily), and amlodipine (10 to 20 mg daily) are the most commonly used calcium-channel blockers. Because of its potential negative inotropic effects, verapamil should be avoided. Patients must be observed closely for both the safety and efficacy of this therapy. If a patient who meets the definition of an acute response does not improve to WHO functional class I or II with calcium-channel blocker therapy, the patient should not be considered a chronic responder; alternative or additional pulmonary arterial hypertension–specific therapy should be instituted.

Targeted Therapies

In clinical trials, intravenous epoprostenol improves functional class, exercise endurance, hemodynamics, and survival in patients with idiopathic pulmonary arterial hypertension, and it also improves exercise tolerance and hemodynamics in patients with pulmonary arterial hypertension related to the scleroderma spectrum of diseases. Uncontrolled studies have also reported favorable effects with intravenous epoprostenol in patients with numerous forms of associated pulmonary arterial hypertension. Observational series suggest a long-term survival benefit with intravenous epoprostenol compared with historical controls. Epoprostenol must be delivered by continuous intravenous infusion, commonly initiated in the hospital at a dose of 2 ng/kg/minute, with the dose titrated up on the basis of symptoms of pulmonary arterial hypertension and side effects of the therapy. Each patient must learn the techniques of sterile preparation of the medication, operation of the ambulatory infusion pump, and care of the central venous catheter. Although dosing must be highly individualized, maintenance doses in the range of 25 to 40 ng/kg/minute are typically needed for patients receiving monotherapy. Common side effects include headache, jaw pain, flushing, nausea, diarrhea, rash, and musculoskeletal pain. Infections and infusion interruption can be life-threatening.

Subcutaneous treprostinil can provide a modest but statistically significant improvement in exercise tolerance. The main limitation of this therapy is pain and erythema at the site of the subcutaneous infusion, a complication that occurs in 85% of patients. Oral treprostinil (starting at 0.25 mg with meals twice daily and increased to as high as 12 mg twice daily as tolerated) also is modestly effective as monotherapy.[A2] For subcutaneous or oral therapy, other prostanoid-type side effects, including headache, diarrhea, rash, and nausea, also occur. Subcutaneous treprostinil is often started in the home, with the dose titrated up on the basis of symptoms of pulmonary arterial hypertension and drug side effects. Treprostinil is less potent than epoprostenol, and higher doses are required to achieve the desired efficacy. Inhaled treprostinil four times daily and inhaled iloprost six to nine times daily also are effective for improving exercise capacity. However, cough is an additional side effect with this method of administration.

The endothelin receptor antagonist bosentan (initiated orally at 62.5 mg twice daily and titrated up to 125 mg twice daily after 1 month) improves hemodynamics, exercise capacity, and the clinical course of pulmonary arterial hypertension.[A3] Liver enzymes must be monitored on a monthly basis; the dose should be reduced if liver enzymes rise to more than three to five times the upper limits of normal and discontinued if they rise to five times the upper limit of normal. Ambrisentan (administered orally at doses of either 5 mg or 10 mg once daily) has similar benefits.[A4] Other side effects include lower extremity edema, headache, and nasal congestion. Macitentan, a dual endothelin-receptor antagonist, significantly reduces the composite end point of death, atrial septostomy, lung transplantation, initiation of treatment with parenteral prostanoids, or worsening pulmonary arterial hypertension by 30% when it is given as 3 mg daily and by 46% if it is given as 10 mg daily.[A5] The most frequent adverse events are headache, nasopharyngitis, and anemia, without any increased rate of peripheral edema or elevated liver enzymes.

Riociguat is a first in class soluble guanylate cyclase stimulator, which directly stimulates soluble guanylate cyclase independent of nitric oxide and increases the sensitivity of soluble guanylate cyclase to nitric oxide. In a randomized controlled trial that included some patients who previously had been treated with endothelin receptor antagonists or nonparenteral prostanoids, riociguat (at a dose of 1.0 mg up to 2.5 mg three times daily) significantly improved the primary end point of 6-minute walking distance as well as pulmonary vascular resistance, brain natriuretic peptide levels, functional class, and time to clinical worsening.[A6] The most common adverse events included headache, dyspepsia, peripheral edema, and hypotension. Riociguat should not be used concurrently with phosphodiesterase type 5 inhibitors.

The chronic administration of inhaled nitric oxide is cumbersome and not clinically useful. However, the phosphodiesterase type 5 antagonists sildenafil and tadalafil are effective and useful for pulmonary arterial hypertension.[A7] Sildenafil is approved at a dose of 20 mg three times daily and tadalafil at a dose of 40 mg once daily. The most common side effects of the inhibitors are headache, flushing, dyspepsia, and epistaxis.

Given the availability of therapies that target different pathologic processes, combination therapy is an attractive theoretical option in pulmonary arterial hypertension. Emerging data support the incremental benefit of combining more than one targeted therapy under careful observation, usually in a specialized center.

Invasive Therapies

Despite advances in medical therapies for pulmonary arterial hypertension, many patients experience progressive functional decline, largely related to worsening right-sided heart failure. In carefully selected patients, atrial septostomy may improve symptoms. Atrial septostomy creates a right-to-left interatrial shunt, thereby decreasing right-sided heart filling pressures and improving right-sided heart function and left-sided heart filling. Although the right-to-left shunting decreases systemic arterial oxygen saturation, it is anticipated that the improvement in cardiac output will result in overall augmentation in systemic oxygen delivery. Contraindications to performing atrial septostomy include severe right ventricular failure on cardiorespiratory support, mean right atrial pressure of more than 20 mm Hg, pulmonary vascular resistance index of more than 55 U/m^2, resting oxygen saturation of less than 90% on room air, and left ventricular end-diastolic pressure of more than 18 mm Hg. Because of the high morbidity and mortality associated with this procedure, it should be performed only by experienced operators in specialized centers.

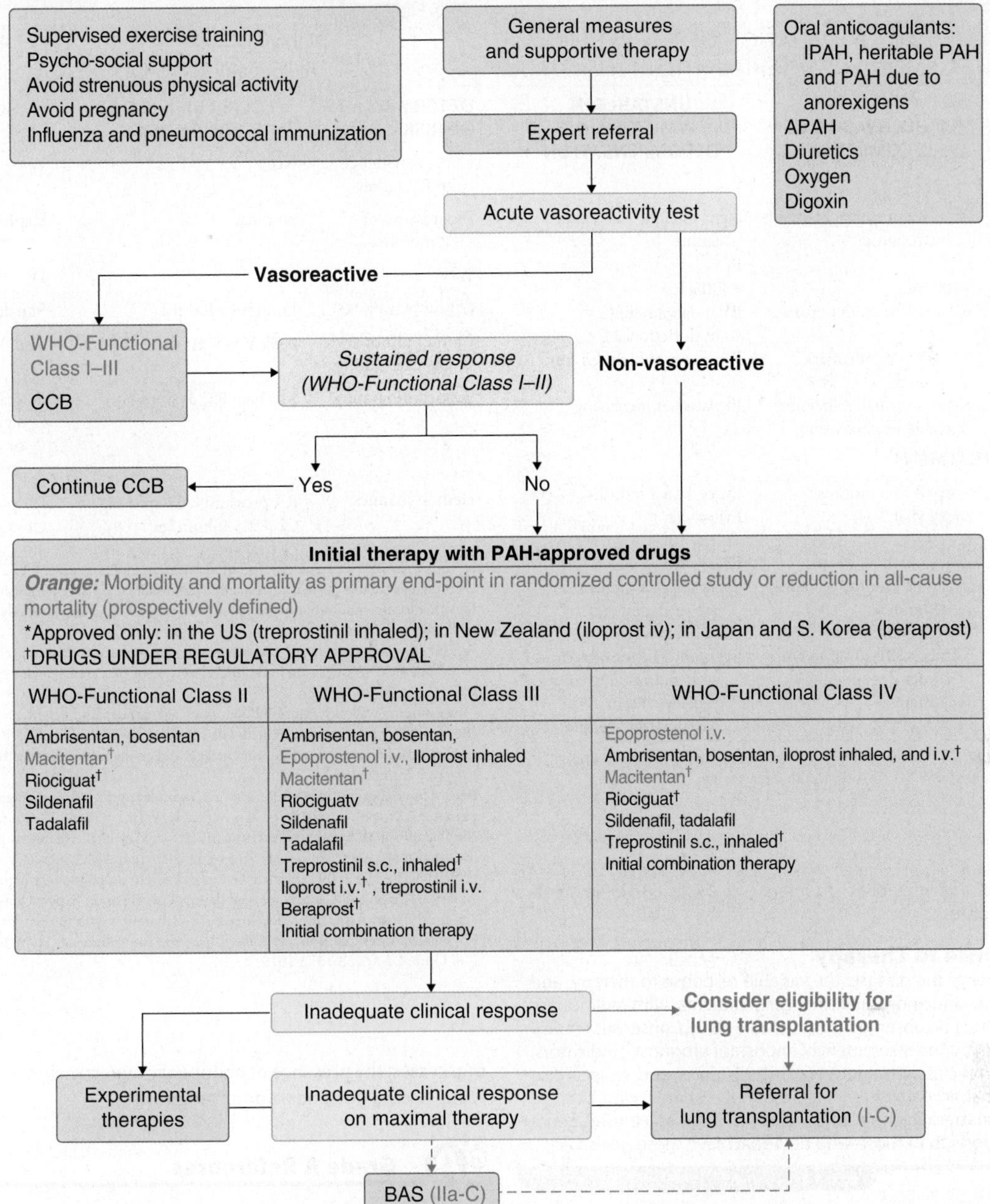

FIGURE 68-6. **Pulmonary hypertension evidence-based treatment algorithm. APAH = associated pulmonary arterial hypertension; BAS = balloon atrial septostomy; CCB = calcium-channel blockers; IPAH = idiopathic pulmonary arterial hypertension; i.v. = intravenous; PAH = pulmonary arterial hypertension; s.c. = subcutaneous; WHO = World Health Organization. (Modified from Galie N, Corris PA, Frost A, et al. Updated treatment algorithm of pulmonary arterial hypertension. *J Am Coll Cardiol.* 2013;62:D60-D72.)**

Bilateral lung (Chapter 101) or heart-lung (Chapter 82) transplantation is the final option for selected patients with pulmonary arterial hypertension when medical therapy fails. The 1-, 3-, 5-, and 10-year survival rates are 66%, 57%, 47%, and 27%, respectively, in patients with idiopathic pulmonary arterial hypertension who undergo transplantation. Transplantation as a potential therapeutic option should be discussed with selected patients at the time of diagnosis, although timing of referral is challenging. The International Society for Heart and Lung Transplantation recommends that patients with pulmonary arterial hypertension be referred for transplantation evaluation if they have persistent functional class III or IV symptoms despite treatment with pulmonary arterial hypertension–specific therapies, including prostanoids. Patients who are otherwise good transplant candidates should be referred when they have an unacceptable response to medical therapies.

Special Populations

Group 2: Pulmonary Venous Hypertension

No specific therapy is currently approved for the treatment of pulmonary venous hypertension that causes secondary pulmonary arterial hypertension. For example, a multicenter randomized controlled trial found no difference in peak oxygen consumption or secondary clinical end points when patients with stable heart failure and a preserved ejection fraction were treated with sildenafil compared with placebo.[A8]

Group 3: Primary Lung Disease

For these disorders, treatment of underlying lung disease is indicated.

Group 4: Chronic Thromboembolic Hypertension

For patients with chronic thromboembolic pulmonary hypertension and a significant clot burden, pulmonary endarterectomy (E-Fig. 68-2) is the treatment of choice and is a potentially curative procedure. Riociguat (a soluble guanylate cyclase stimulator at a dose of 1.0 up to 2.5 mg three times daily) improves 6-minute walking distance, pulmonary vascular resistance, NT-pro-brain natriuretic peptide level, and functional class[A9] in patients with either inoperable chronic thromboembolic pulmonary hypertension or persistent pulmonary hypertension after pulmonary endarterectomy. Warfarin anticoagulation is also recommended.

Group 5: Other Causes

Pulmonary hypertension also consists of several forms for which the etiology is unclear or multifactorial. Among these conditions are a number of

TABLE 68-2 LONGITUDINAL EVALUATION OF THE PATIENT WITH PULMONARY ARTERIAL HYPERTENSION

CLINICAL PARAMETER	STABLE SYMPTOMS, WELL COMPENSATED	UNSTABLE IN SYMPTOMS OR DECOMPENSATION
DEFINITION		
Physical examination	No evidence of right-sided heart failure	Signs of right-sided heart failure
WHO functional class	I/II	IV
6-minute walk distance	>400 m	<300 m
Echocardiography	RV size/function normal	RV enlargement/ dysfunction
Hemodynamics	RA pressure normal; CI normal	RA pressure high; CI low
BNP	Nearly normal, remaining stable or decreasing	Elevated or increasing
EVALUATION AND TREATMENT		
Frequency of visits	Every 3 to 6 months	Every 1 to 3 months
Functional class assessment	Every visit	Every visit
6-minute walk test	Every visit	Every visit
Echocardiography	Every 12 months or center dependent	Every 6 to 12 months or center dependent
BNP	Center dependent	Center dependent
RHC	Clinical deterioration and center dependent	Every 6 to 12 months or with clinical deterioration
Oral therapy	Treatment	IV prostacyclin or combination treatment

BNP = brain natriuretic peptide; CI = cardiac index; RA = right atrial; RHC = right-sided heart catheterization; RV = right ventricle; WHO = World Health Organization.

TABLE 68-3 PULMONARY ARTERIAL HYPERTENSION: DETERMINANTS OF PROGNOSIS*

DETERMINANTS OF RISK	LOWER RISK (GOOD PROGNOSIS)	HIGHER RISK (POOR PROGNOSIS)
Clinical evidence of RV failure	No	Yes
Progression of symptoms	Gradual	Rapid
WHO class[†]	II, III	IV
6-minute walk test[‡]	Longer (>400 m)	Shorter (<300 m)
Cardiopulmonary exercise testing	Peak V_{O_2} > 10.4 mL/kg/min	Peak V_{O_2} < 10.4 mL/kg/min
Echocardiography	Minimal RV dysfunction	Pericardial effusion, significant RV enlargement or dysfunction, right atrial enlargement
Hemodynamics	RA pressure < 10 mm Hg CI > 2.5 L/min/m^2	RA pressure > 20 mm Hg CI < 2.0 L/min/m^2
BNP level[§]	Minimally elevated	Significantly elevated

*Most data available pertain to idiopathic pulmonary arterial hypertension. Few data are available for other forms of pulmonary arterial hypertension. One should not rely on any single factor to make risk predictions.
[†]WHO class is the functional classification for pulmonary arterial hypertension and is similar to the New York Heart Association functional class, except that patients with syncope are defined as class IV.
[‡]The 6-minute walk test is also influenced by age, gender, and height.
[§]Because there are currently limited data regarding the influence of BNP on prognosis, and many factors including renal function, weight, age, and gender may influence BNP, absolute numbers are not given for this variable.
BNP = brain natriuretic peptide; CI = cardiac index; peak V_{O_2} = average peak oxygen uptake during exercise; RA = right atrial; RV = right ventricle; WHO = World Health Organization.
Modified from McLaughlin VV, Gaine SP, Howard LS, et al. Treatment goals of pulmonary hypertension. *J Am Coll Cardiol.* 2013;62:D73-D81; and McLaughlin VV, Archer SL, Badesch DB, et al. ACCF/AHA 2009 expert consensus document on pulmonary hypertension: a report of the American College of Cardiology Foundation Task Force on Expert Consensus Documents and the American Heart Association developed in collaboration with the American College of Chest Physicians; American Thoracic Society, Inc.; and the Pulmonary Hypertension Association. *J Am Coll Cardiol.* 2009;53:1573-1619.

hematologic, systemic, and metabolic disorders (see Table 68-1). No treatments are of proven value.

Assessing Response to Therapy

Given the complexity of the disease, the variable response to therapy, and the goal of optimizing and individualizing care, patients with pulmonary arterial hypertension must be observed closely (Table 68-2). Consensus recommendations rely on the routine assessment of important prognostic indicators, such as WHO functional class, 6-minute walking distance, and echocardiographic and hemodynamic parameters (Table 68-3).[9] Patients who achieve these parameters, no matter which specific therapy or approach is used, seem to have a better prognosis than those who do not achieve these goals.

PROGNOSIS

Several clinical factors are correlated with prognosis (see Table 68-3). The natural history of symptomatic idiopathic pulmonary arterial hypertension is a median survival of 2.8 years with 1-, 3-, and 5-year survival rates of 68%, 48%, and 34%, respectively. In the era of targeted therapies, survival has improved but still remains suboptimal, with 1-, 2-, and 3-year survival of 86%, 70%, and 55% for incident cases.[10] Pulmonary hypertension itself is the direct cause of death in about 50% of patients and contributes to but does not directly cause death in the other 50%.[11]

Patients with pulmonary arterial hypertension related to the scleroderma spectrum of diseases tend to have a poorer prognosis than that of those with idiopathic pulmonary arterial hypertension, whereas patients with pulmonary arterial hypertension related to congenital heart disease tend to have a better prognosis, perhaps because they have better right ventricular function. Two large registries have shed light on the prognosis of patients with pulmonary arterial hypertension. Important predictors of poorer survival include male gender, worse functional class, reduced exercise tolerance as measured by the 6-minute walking distance, elevated right atrial pressures, and lower cardiac output. The natural history of patients with groups 2, 3, and 4 pulmonary hypertension is influenced by their left-sided heart and lung disease. In most cases, the presence of pulmonary hypertension in addition to the underlying disease portends a poor prognosis.

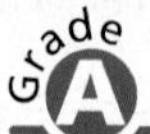

Grade A References

A1. Galie N, Corris PA, Frost A, et al. Updated treatment algorithm of pulmonary arterial hypertension. *J Am Coll Cardiol.* 2013;62:D60-D72.
A2. Jing ZC, Parikh K, Pulido T, et al. Efficacy and safety of oral treprostinil monotherapy for the treatment of pulmonary arterial hypertension: a randomized, controlled trial. *Circulation.* 2013;127:624-633.
A3. Rubin LJ, Badesch DB, Barst RJ, et al. Bosentan therapy for pulmonary arterial hypertension. *N Engl J Med.* 2002;346:896-903.
A4. Galie N, Olschewski H, Oudiz RJ, et al. Ambrisentan for the treatment of pulmonary arterial hypertension: results of the ambrisentan in pulmonary arterial hypertension, randomized, double-blind, placebo-controlled, multicenter, efficacy (ARIES) study 1 and 2. *Circulation.* 2008;117:3010-3019.
A5. Pulido T, Adzerikho I, Channick RN, et al. Macitentan and morbidity and mortality in pulmonary arterial hypertension. *N Engl J Med.* 2013;369:809-818.
A6. Ghofrani HA, Galie N, Grimminger F, et al. Riociguat for the treatment of pulmonary arterial hypertension. *N Engl J Med.* 2013;369:330-340.
A7. Galie N, Brundage BH, Ghofrani HA, et al. Tadalafil therapy for pulmonary arterial hypertension. *Circulation.* 2009;119:2894-2903.
A8. Redfield MM, Chen HH, Borlaug BA, et al. Effect of phosphodiesterase-5 inhibition on exercise capacity and clinical status in heart failure with preserved ejection fraction: a randomized clinical trial. *JAMA.* 2013;309:1268-1277.
A9. Ghofrani HA, D'Armini AM, Grimminger F, et al. Riociguat for the treatment of chronic thromboembolic pulmonary hypertension. *N Engl J Med.* 2013;369:319-329.

GENERAL REFERENCES

For the General References and other additional features, please visit Expert Consult at https://expertconsult.inkling.com.

69

CONGENITAL HEART DISEASE IN ADULTS

ARIANE J. MARELLI

The convergence of major progress in medicine, pediatrics, and cardiovascular surgery has resulted in the survival of an increasingly large number of adult patients with congenital heart disease. Adult physicians are becoming increasingly responsible for these patients, commonly in concert with a cardiologist and a tertiary care facility.

DEFINITIONS

Patients can be divided into three categories according to the surgical status: unoperated, surgically palliated, or physiologically repaired. Congenital heart lesions can be classified as *acyanotic* or *cyanotic*. *Cyanosis* refers to a blue discoloration of the mucous membranes resulting from an increased amount of reduced hemoglobin. Central cyanosis occurs when the circulation is mixed because of a right-to-left shunt.

A *native lesion* refers to an anatomic lesion present at birth. Acquired lesions, naturally occurring or as a result of surgery, are superimposed on the native anatomy. *Palliative* interventions are performed in patients with cyanotic lesions and are defined as operations that either increase or decrease pulmonary blood flow while allowing a mixed circulation and cyanosis to persist (Table 69-1). *Physiologic repair* applies to procedures that provide total or nearly total anatomic and physiologic separation of the pulmonary and systemic circulations in complex cyanotic lesions and results in patients who are acyanotic.

Eisenmenger complex refers to flow reversal across a ventricular septal defect (VSD) when pulmonary vascular resistance exceeds systemic levels. *Eisenmenger physiology* designates the physiologic response in a broader category of shunt lesions in which a right-to-left shunt occurs in response to an elevation in pulmonary vascular resistance. *Eisenmenger syndrome* is a term applied to common clinical features shared by patients with Eisenmenger physiology.

Each congenital lesion can influence the course of another. For example, the physiologic consequences of a VSD are different if it occurs in isolation or in combination with pulmonary stenosis. A *simple lesion* is defined as either a shunt lesion or an obstructive lesion of the right or left side of the heart occurring in isolation. A *complex lesion* is a combination of two or more abnormalities.

EPIDEMIOLOGY

Genetic Determinants

About 20% of congenital heart defects are associated with a syndrome or chromosomal anomaly, and the most common such chromosomal anomaly is Down syndrome (trisomy 21), in which about 50% of patients have defects of the endocardial cushions and the ventricular septum. VSDs also occur in 90% of patients with trisomy 13 and trisomy 18. The most frequently observed defects in patients with Turner syndrome (45,X) are aortic coarctation, aortic stenosis, and atrial septal defect (ASD). About 15% of patients with tetralogy of Fallot have a deletion on chromosome 22q11; prevalence is higher in those with a right aortic arch. Abnormalities involving the chromosomal band 22q11 can also result in a group of syndromes, the most common of which is DiGeorge syndrome. The shared phenotypic features are designated CATCH-22 syndromes, that is, a combination of *c*ardiac defects, *a*bnormal facies, *t*hymic hypoplasia, *c*left palate, and *h*ypocalcemia. For families with a child who carries a congenital cardiac malformation due to a chromosomal anomaly, the risk of the cardiac malformation in future children is related to the risk of recurrence of the chromosomal anomaly itself.

Typically, single mutant genes are also associated with syndromes of cardiovascular malformations, although not every patient with the syndrome has the characteristic cardiac anomaly. Examples include osteogenesis imperfecta (autosomal recessive; Chapter 260), associated with aortic valve disease; Jervell and Lange-Nielsen syndrome (autosomal recessive) and Romano-Ward syndrome (autosomal dominant), associated with a prolonged QT interval and sudden death; and Holt-Oram syndrome (autosomal dominant), in which an ASD occurs with a range of other skeletal anomalies. Osler-Weber-Rendu telangiectasias (Chapter 173) are associated with pulmonary arteriovenous fistulas. Williams syndrome (Chapters 40 and 41) occurs with supravalvular aortic stenosis in most cases. Noonan syndrome is associated with pulmonary stenosis, ASD, and hypertrophic cardiomyopathy. Although autosomal dominant inheritance has been implicated for both, most cases are sporadic. Deletion at chromosome 7q11.23 has been identified in patients with Williams syndrome, and a gene defect has been mapped to 12q22-qter in patients with Noonan syndrome (Chapter 60).

The risk for recurrence when the mother carries a sporadically occurring congenital lesion varies from 2.5 to 18%, depending on the lesion. Obstructive lesions of the left ventricular outflow tract have the highest recurrence rates in offspring. When the father carries the lesion, 1.5 to 3% of the offspring are affected. When a sibling has a congenital cardiac anomaly, the risk for recurrence in another sibling varies from 1 to 3%.

PREVENTION

Genetic screening for the 22q11.2 microdeletion should be considered if patients with tetralogy of Fallot plan to have children. Without the 22q11 deletion, the risk of congenital heart disease in the fetus is 4 to 6%.

Incidence and Prevalence

Congenital heart defects are diagnosed in approximately 1% of births in the United States. The prevalence of congenital heart disease has increased in the general population, with the steepest rise observed in adults with severe or complex lesions. An overall prevalence of 6 per 1000 adults has been documented. The median age of patients with severe lesions has increased from childhood to late adolescence. Currently, more than 1 million adults are expected to be alive in the United States with congenital heart disease.[1] Advances in medical and surgical therapy have increased the survival of patients with congenital heart defects, thereby emphasizing that congenital heart disease is a lifelong condition that influences health care utilization and costs across the lifespan.

Bicuspid aortic valve occurs in about 2% of the general population, is the most common congenital cardiac anomaly encountered in adult populations, and accounts for up to half of surgical cases of aortic stenosis in adults (Chapter 75). ASDs constitute 30 to 40% of cases of congenital heart disease in adults, with ostium secundum ASD accounting for 7% of all congenital lesions. A solitary VSD represents 15 to 20% of all congenital lesions and is the most common congenital cardiac lesion observed in children; its high spontaneous closure rates explain the lesser prevalence in adults. Patent ductus arteriosus (PDA) accounts for 5 to 10% of all congenital cardiac lesions in infants with a normal birthweight. Pulmonary stenosis and coarctation of the aorta represent 3 to 10% of all congenital lesions.

Tetralogy of Fallot is the most common cyanotic congenital anomaly observed in adults. Together with complete transposition of the great arteries, these lesions account for 5 to 12% of congenital heart disease in infants. More complex lesions, such as tricuspid atresia, univentricular heart, congenitally corrected transposition of the great arteries, Ebstein anomaly, and double-outlet right ventricle, account for 2.5% or less of all congenital heart disease.

TABLE 69-1 PALLIATIVE SURGICAL SHUNTS FOR CONGENITAL HEART LESIONS

PALLIATIVE SHUNT	ANASTOMOSIS
SYSTEMIC ARTERIAL TO PULMONARY ARTERY SHUNTS	
Classic Blalock-Taussig	Subclavian artery to PA
Modified Blalock-Taussig	Subclavian artery to PA (prosthetic graft)
Potts anastomosis	Descending aorta to left PA
Waterston shunt	Ascending aorta to right PA
SYSTEMIC VENOUS TO PULMONARY ARTERY SHUNTS	
Classic Glenn	SVC to right PA
Bidirectional Glenn	SVC to right and left PA
Bilateral Glenn	Right and left SVC to right and left PA

PA = pulmonary artery; SVC = superior vena cava.
From Marelli A, Mullen M. Palliative surgical shunts for congenital heart lesions. *Clin Paediatr.* 1996;4:189.

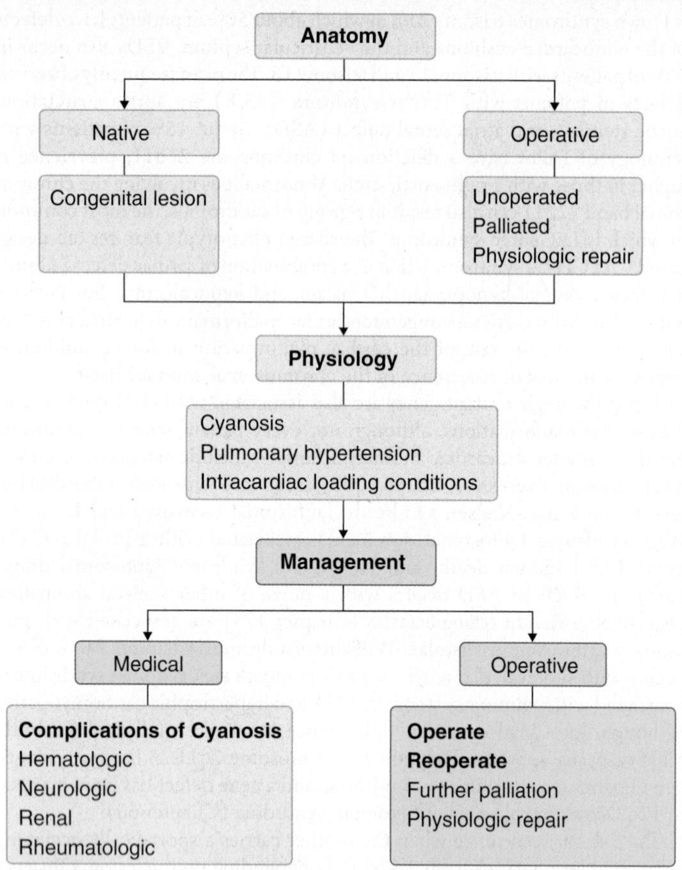

FIGURE 69-1. The goals of complete clinical assessment in congenital heart disease are to define the anatomy and physiology to determine appropriate management.

CLINICAL MANIFESTATIONS

Congenital heart disease is a lifelong condition during which the patient and the lesion evolve concurrently. A patient may have been monitored for many years because of an erroneous diagnosis made in infancy or childhood when diagnostic techniques were more limited. The differential diagnosis of native and surgical anatomy in the adult with an unknown diagnosis depends on whether the patient is cyanotic or acyanotic. On completion of the evaluation, the following questions should be answered (Fig. 69-1): What is the native anatomy? Has this patient undergone surgery for the condition? What is the physiology? What can and should be done for this patient both medically and surgically, and importantly, who should do it?

If the patient has not undergone surgery, the question is, Why not? If the patient is palliated, has the degree of cyanosis progressed as evidenced by a drop in systemic saturation or a rise in hemoglobin? If the patient has undergone a physiologic repair, what procedure was performed? Are residual lesions present, and have new lesions developed as a consequence of surgery? The patient's physiology is determined by the presence or absence of cyanosis, pulmonary hypertension, adequate filling of the cardiac chambers, and any resulting medical complications.

A clinical assessment, 12-lead electrocardiogram (ECG), chest radiograph, and baseline oxygen saturation should be part of every initial assessment. Two-dimensional transthoracic echocardiography (Chapter 55) and Doppler and color flow imaging are used to establish the diagnosis and to monitor the evolution of documented hemodynamic complications. Transesophageal echocardiographic examination is particularly useful in adults and is increasingly important during interventional catheter-guided therapy and surgery. Magnetic resonance imaging (Chapter 56) and computed tomography (Chapter 56) are useful adjuncts. Cardiac catheterization for congenital heart disease has shifted from pure diagnosis to include intervention. Coronary arteriography is recommended for adults older than 40 years in whom surgical intervention is contemplated.

Pulmonary Hypertension and Its Complications

Pulmonary hypertension secondary to structural disease of the heart or circulation can occur with or without an increase in pulmonary vascular resistance. Pulmonary vascular obstructive disease occurs when pulmonary vascular resistance rises and becomes fixed and irreversible. In the most common congenital anomalies, pulmonary hypertension is a result of increased pulmonary blood flow because of a native left-to-right shunt. Examples include ASD, a moderately sized VSD, PDA, and a variety of complex lesions. The rate at which pulmonary hypertension progresses to become pulmonary vascular obstructive disease varies from one lesion to another and depends at least in part on the source of pulmonary blood flow. Pulmonary hypertension typically develops in patients with an ASD after the fourth decade; Eisenmenger syndrome is a late complication seen in only 5 to 10% of cases. In contrast, in patients with a large VSD or persistent PDA, progressive elevation in pulmonary vascular resistance occurs rapidly because the pulmonary vascular bed is exposed not only to the excess volume of the left-to-right shunt but also to systemic arterial pressures. As a result, Eisenmenger complex develops in approximately 10% of patients with a large VSD during the first decade. Surgical pulmonary artery banding is a palliative measure aimed at decreasing pulmonary blood flow and protecting the pulmonary vascular bed against the development of early pulmonary vascular obstructive disease.

If forward flow from the right side of the heart is insufficient, native collaterals or surgical shunts provide an alternative source of pulmonary blood flow (see Table 69-1). With large surgical shunts, however, direct exposure of the pulmonary vascular bed to the high pressures of the systemic circulation causes pulmonary vascular obstructive disease. As a result, systemic to pulmonary arterial shunts are currently less favored in neonates and infants, in whom systemic venous to pulmonary arterial shunts are now preferred.

The term *Eisenmenger's syndrome* should be reserved for patients in whom pulmonary vascular obstructive disease is present and pulmonary vascular resistance is fixed and irreversible. These findings, in combination with the absence of left-to-right shunting, render the patient inoperable.

The clinical manifestations of Eisenmenger's syndrome include dyspnea on exertion, syncope, chest pain, congestive heart failure, and symptoms related to erythrocytosis and hyperviscosity. On physical examination, central cyanosis and digital clubbing are hallmark findings. Systemic oxygen saturations typically vary between 75 and 85%. The pulse pressure narrows as the cardiac output falls. Examination of jugular venous pressure can reveal a dominant *a* wave reflecting a noncompliant right ventricle until tricuspid insufficiency is severe enough to generate a large *v* wave. A prominent right ventricular impulse is felt in the left parasternal border in end expiration or in the subcostal area in end inspiration. A palpable pulmonary artery is commonly felt. The pulmonary component of the second heart sound is increased and can be felt in most cases. Pulmonary ejection sounds are common when the pulmonary artery is dilated with a structurally normal valve. Right atrial gallop is heard more frequently when the *a* wave is dominant. A murmur of tricuspid insufficiency is common, but the inspiratory increase in the murmur (Carvallo's sign) disappears when right ventricular failure occurs. In diastole, a pulmonary insufficiency murmur is often heard. The 12-lead ECG shows evidence of right atrial enlargement, right ventricular hypertrophy, and right axis deviation. Chest radiographic findings include a dilated pulmonary artery segment, cardiac enlargement, and diminished pulmonary vascular markings. Echocardiography confirms the right-sided pressure overload and pulmonary artery enlargement as well as the tricuspid and pulmonary insufficiency. Cardiac catheterization is indicated if doubt exists about the potential reversibility of the elevated pulmonary vascular resistance in a patient who might otherwise benefit from surgery.

Cyanosis occurs when persistent venous to arterial mixing results in hypoxemia. Adaptive mechanisms to increase oxygen delivery include an increase in oxygen content, a rightward shift in the oxyhemoglobin dissociation curve, a higher hematocrit, and an increase in cardiac output. When cyanosis is not relieved, chronic hypoxemia and erythrocytosis result in hematologic, neurologic, renal, and rheumatic complications.

Hematologic complications of chronic hypoxemia include erythrocytosis, iron deficiency, and bleeding diathesis. Hemoglobin and hematocrit levels as well as red blood cell indices should be checked regularly and correlated with systemic oxygen saturation levels. Symptoms of hyperviscosity include headaches, faintness, dizziness, fatigue, altered mentation, visual disturbances, paresthesias, tinnitus, and myalgia. Symptoms are classified as mild to moderate when they interfere with only some activities, or they can be marked to severe and interfere with most or all activities. Patients with compensated erythrocytosis establish an equilibrium hematocrit at higher levels in an iron-replete state with minimal symptoms. Patients with decompensated erythrocytosis manifest unstable, rising hematocrit levels and experience severe hyperviscosity symptoms.

Hemostatic abnormalities can occur in up to 20% of cyanotic patients with erythrocytosis. Bleeding is usually mild and superficial and leads to easy bruising, skin petechiae, or mucosal bleeding, but epistaxis, hemoptysis, or even life-threatening postoperative bleeding can occur. A variety of clotting factor deficiencies and qualitative and quantitative platelet disorders have been described.

Neurologic complications, including cerebral hemorrhage, can be caused by hemostatic defects and are most often seen after inappropriate use of anticoagulant therapy. Patients with right-to-left shunts may be at risk for paradoxical cerebral emboli. Focal brain injury may provide a nidus for brain abscess if bacteremia supervenes. Attention should be paid to the use of air filters in peripheral intravenous lines to avoid paradoxical emboli through a right-to-left shunt.

Prophylactic phlebotomy has no place in the prevention of cerebral arterial thrombosis. Indications for phlebotomy are the occurrence of symptomatic hyperviscosity in an iron-replete patient and prevention of excessive bleeding perioperatively.

Pulmonary complications include massive pulmonary hemorrhage and in situ arterial thrombosis. A rapid clinical deterioration associated with progressive hypoxemia often marks the terminal stage of disease. No clear benefits are observed with the use of anticoagulants (systemic or intrapulmonary) because of the risk for prolonged bleeding due to the underlying coagulopathy. The chronic disease process and high mortality prohibit pulmonary endarterectomy.

Renal dysfunction can be manifested as proteinuria, hyperuricemia, or renal failure. Focal interstitial fibrosis, tubular atrophy, and hyalinization of afferent and efferent arterioles can be seen on renal biopsy. Increased blood viscosity and arteriolar vasoconstriction can lead to renal hypoperfusion with progressive glomerulosclerosis. Hyperuricemia is commonly seen in patients with cyanotic congenital heart disease and is thought to be due mainly to the decreased reabsorption of uric acid rather than to overproduction from erythrocytosis. Asymptomatic hyperuricemia need not be treated because lowering of uric acid levels has not been shown to prevent renal disease or gout.

Rheumatologic complications include gout and hypertrophic osteoarthropathy, which is thought to be responsible for the arthralgias affecting up to one third of patients with cyanotic congenital heart disease. In patients with right-to-left shunting, megakaryocytes released from the bone marrow bypass the lung and are entrapped in systemic arterioles and capillaries, where they release platelet-derived growth factor, which promotes local cell proliferation. Digital clubbing and new osseous formation with periostitis occur and cause the symptoms of arthralgia. Symptomatic hyperuricemia and gouty arthritis can be treated as necessary with colchicine, probenecid, or allopurinol; nonsteroidal anti-inflammatory drugs are best avoided, given the baseline hemostatic anomalies in these patients.

TREATMENT Rx

In patients with Eisenmenger syndrome, bosentan (e.g., 62.5 mg twice daily for 4 weeks, then 125 mg twice daily) may improve hemodynamics and exercise capacity after 4 months of use.[A1] Chronic oxygen therapy is unlikely to benefit hypoxemia caused by right-to-left shunting in the setting of a fixed pulmonary vascular resistance. Oxygen therapy may be considered for cyanotic patients during long-distance flights.

In the iron-replete state, moderate to severe hyperviscosity symptoms typically occur when hematocrit levels exceed 65%. If no evidence of dehydration is present, removal of 500 mL of blood during a 30- to 45-minute period should be followed by quantitative volume replacement with normal saline or dextran (Fig. 69-2). The procedure may be repeated every 24 hours until symptomatic improvement occurs.

Treatment of spontaneous bleeding is dictated by its severity and the abnormal hemostatic parameters (Fig. 69-3). For severe bleeding, platelet transfusions, fresh-frozen plasma, vitamin K, cryoprecipitate, and desmopressin have been used. Reduction in erythrocyte mass also improves hemostasis, so cyanotic patients undergoing surgery should have prophylactic phlebotomy if the hematocrit is greater than 65%.

Iron deficiency is common in cyanotic adult patients because of excessive bleeding or phlebotomy. In contrast to normocytic erythrocytosis, which is rarely symptomatic at hematocrit levels less than 65%, iron deficiency may be manifested with hyperviscosity symptoms at hematocrit levels well below 65%. The treatment of choice is not phlebotomy but oral iron repletion until a rise in hematocrit is detected, typically within 1 week.

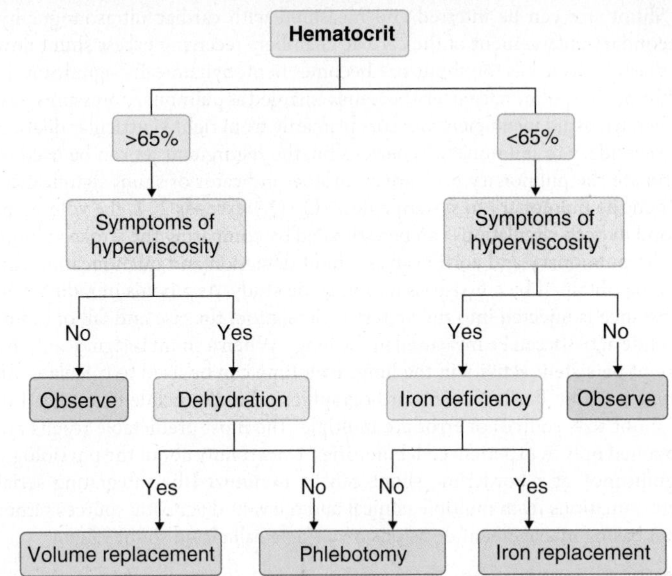

FIGURE 69-2. Treatment algorithm for erythrocytosis of cyanotic congenital heart disease.

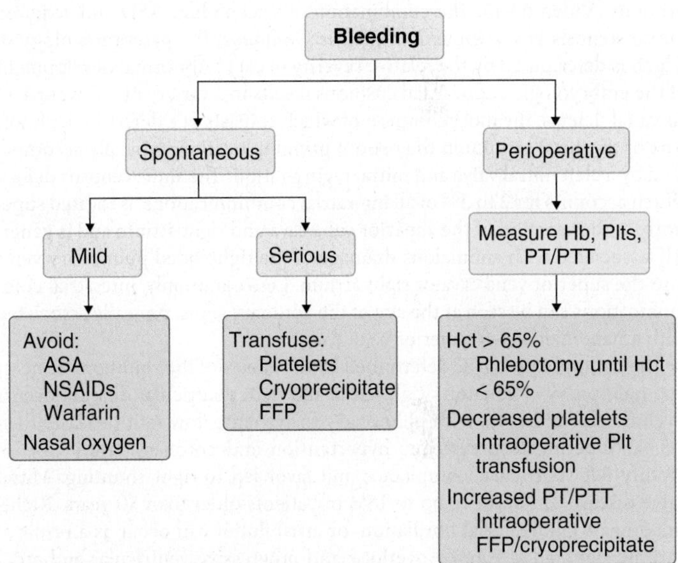

FIGURE 69-3. Treatment algorithm for bleeding diathesis of cyanotic congenital heart disease. ASA = acetylsalicylic acid; FFP = fresh-frozen plasma; Hb = hemoglobin; Hct = hematocrit; NSAIDs = nonsteroidal anti-inflammatory drugs; Plts = platelets; PT = prothrombin time; PTT = partial thromboplastin time.

SIMPLE LESIONS

Isolated Shunt Lesions

Hemodynamic complications of significant shunts relate to volume overload and chamber dilation of the primary chamber receiving the excess left-to-right shunt and to secondary complications of valvular dysfunction and damage to the pulmonary vascular bed. The size and duration of the shunt determine the clinical course and therefore the indications for closure. The degree of shunting is a function of both the size of the communication and, depending on its location, biventricular compliance or pulmonary and systemic vascular resistance. Clinically apparent hemodynamic sequelae of shunts are typically apparent or can be expected to occur when pulmonary to systemic flow ratios exceed 1.5 : 1.

Shunt size can be inferred and measured with cardiac ultrasonography. Secondary enlargement of the cardiac chambers receiving excess shunt flow in diastole occurs as the shunt size becomes hemodynamically significant; in addition, the pulmonary artery becomes enlarged as pulmonary pressure rises. When tricuspid insufficiency occurs primarily from right ventricular dilation or secondary to pulmonary hypertension, the regurgitant jet can be used to estimate the pulmonary pressure as another indicator of shunt significance. When the pulmonary to systemic flow ($\dot{Q}:\dot{Q}$) exceeds 2 : 1, the volume of blood in both circulations can be estimated by comparing the stroke volume at the pulmonary and aortic valves. Shunt detection and quantification can also be obtained by a first-pass radionuclide study. As a bolus of radioactive substance is injected into the systemic circulation, the rise and fall of radionuclide activity can be measured in the lungs. When a shunt is significant, the rate of persistent activity in the lungs over time can be used to calculate the shunt fraction. For both echocardiographic and radionuclide quantification of shunt size, sources of error are multiple. The most predictable results are obtained only in experienced laboratories. Uncertainty about the physiologic significance of a borderline shunt can be minimized by integrating serial determinations from multiple clinical and relevant diagnostic sources rather than basing management decisions on a single calculated shunt value.

Atrial Septal Defect

Classification of ASDs is based on anatomic location. Most commonly, an ostium secundum ASD occurs in the central portion of the interatrial septum as a result of an enlarged foramen ovale or excessive resorption of the septum primum (Video 69-1). The combination of a secundum ASD and acquired mitral stenosis is known as *Lutembacher syndrome*, the pathophysiology of which is determined by the relative severity of each. Abnormal development of the embryologic endocardial cushions results in a variety of atrioventricular canal defects, the most common of which consists of a defect in the lower part of the atrial septum in the ostium primum location, typically accompanied by a cleft mitral valve and mitral regurgitation. The sinus venosus defect, which accounts for 2 to 3% of all interatrial communications, is located superiorly at the junction of the superior vena cava and right atrium and is generally associated with anomalous drainage of the right-sided pulmonary veins into the superior vena cava or right atrium. Less commonly, interatrial communications can be seen at the site of the coronary sinus, typically associated with an anomalous left superior vena cava.

The pathophysiology is determined by the effects of the shunt on the heart and pulmonary circulation. Right atrial and right ventricular dilation occurs as shunt size increases with pulmonary to systemic flow ratios greater than 1.5 : 1. Superimposed systemic hypertension and coronary artery disease modify left ventricular compliance and favor left-to-right shunting. Mitral valve disease can occur in up to 15% of patients older than 50 years. Right-sided heart failure, atrial fibrillation, or atrial flutter can occur as a result of chronic right-sided volume overload and progressive ventricular and atrial dilation. Stroke can result from paradoxical emboli, atrial arrhythmias, or both. A rise in pulmonary pressure occurs because of the increased pulmonary blood flow. Pulmonary hypertension is unusual before 20 years of age but is seen in 50% of patients older than 40 years. The overall incidence of pulmonary vascular obstructive disease is 15 to 20% in patients with ASD. Eisenmenger disease with reverse shunting, a late and rare complication of isolated secundum ASD, is reported in 5 to 10% of patients.

DIAGNOSIS

Although most patients are minimally symptomatic in the first three decades, more than 70% become impaired by the fifth decade. Initial symptoms include exercise intolerance, dyspnea on exertion, and fatigue caused most commonly by right-sided heart failure and pulmonary hypertension.[2] Palpitations, syncope, and stroke can occur with the development of atrial arrhythmias.

On physical examination, most adults have a normal general physical appearance. When Holt-Oram syndrome is present, the thumb may have a third phalanx or may be rudimentary or absent. With an uncomplicated nonrestrictive communication between both atria, the *a* and *v* waves are equal in amplitude. Precordial palpation typically discloses a normal left ventricular impulse unless mitral valve disease occurs. Characteristically, if the shunt is significant, a right ventricular impulse can be felt in the left parasternal area in end expiration or in the subxiphoid area in end inspiration. A dilated pulmonary artery can sometimes be felt in the second left intercostal space. On auscultation, the hallmark of an ASD is the wide and fixed splitting of the second heart sound. Pulmonary valve closure, as reflected by P_2, is delayed

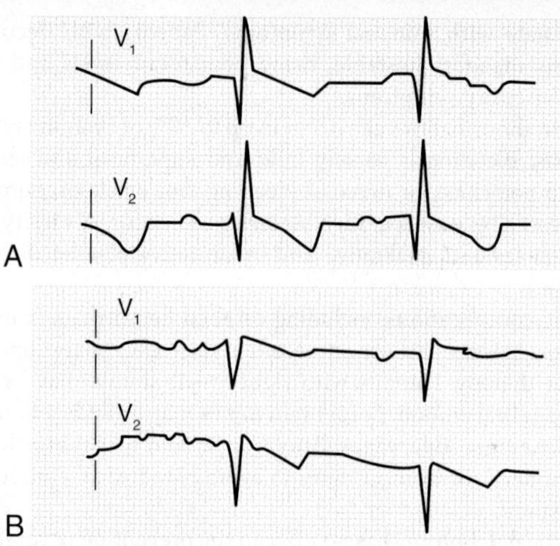

FIGURE 69-4. Electrocardiographic hallmark in atrial septal defect. Right precordial leads V_1 and V_2 illustrate two variants of an incomplete right bundle branch block pattern, the rSrT pattern (A) and the rsR′ pattern (B).

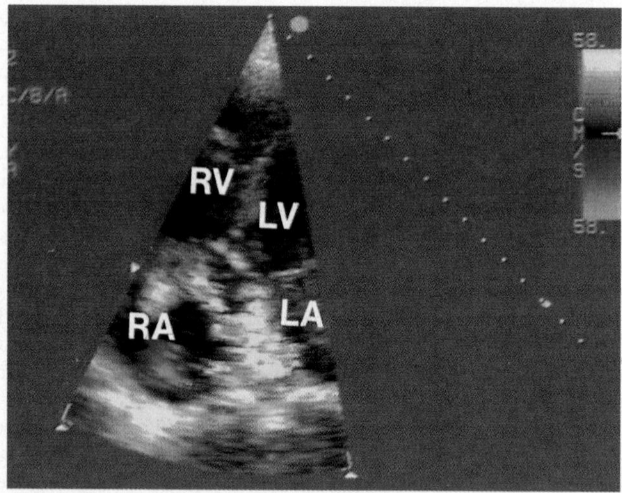

FIGURE 69-5. Color flow Doppler apical four-chamber view showing blood flow from the left atrium (LA) to the right atrium (RA) through a moderately sized atrial septal defect. LV = left ventricle; RV = right ventricle. (From Forbes CD, Jackson WF. Color Atlas and Text of Clinical Medicine. 3rd ed. London: Mosby; 2003.)

because of right ventricular overload and the increased capacitance of the pulmonary vascular bed. The A_2-P_2 interval is fixed because the increase in venous return elevates the right atrial pressure during inspiration, thereby decreasing the degree of left-to-right shunting and offsetting the usual phasic respiratory changes. In addition, compliance of the pulmonary circulation is reduced from the high flow, thus making the vascular compartment less susceptible to any further increase in blood flow. A soft midsystolic murmur generated by the increased flow across the pulmonary valve is usually heard in the second left interspace. In the presence of a high left-to-right shunt volume, increased flow across the tricuspid valve is heard as a mid-diastolic murmur at the lower left sternal border. With advanced right-sided heart failure, evidence of systemic venous congestion is present.

The ECG characteristically shows an incomplete right bundle branch block pattern (Fig. 69-4). Right axis deviation and atrial abnormalities, including a prolonged PR interval, atrial fibrillation, and flutter, are also seen. Typically, the chest radiograph shows pulmonary vascular plethora with increased markings in both lung fields consistent with increased pulmonary blood flow (see Fig. 56-6). The main pulmonary artery and both its branches are dilated. Right atrial and right ventricular dilation can be seen. Cardiac ultrasonography is diagnostic and provides important prognostic information (Fig. 69-5). Ostium primum and secundum ASDs are easily identifiable with transthoracic imaging, but a sinus venosus ASD can be missed unless it is specifically sought. For more accurate visualization of the superior interatrial septum and localization of the pulmonary veins, transesophageal echocardiography is useful. With Doppler study, pulmonary artery pressures can be quantified, and the $\dot{Q}:\dot{Q}$ can be measured.

TREATMENT Rx

Closure of an ASD either percutaneously or surgically is indicated in the presence of right-sided heart enlargement, with or without symptoms. Centrally located defects measuring up to 3.5 cm can be occluded by transcatheter techniques in a cardiac catheterization laboratory. Advantages of this approach include the avoidance of sternotomy and cardiopulmonary bypass. Uncomplicated secundum ASDs may be closed surgically in children and adults with minimal operative mortality, although surgical closure is usually reserved for patients in whom concomitant repair of associated valvular anomalies is required, anomalous pulmonary veins are present, or device closure is not technically feasible.

In patients older than 40 years with symptoms and significant shunts, closure improves functional status and survival.[A2] In the presence of a significant shunt, closure of an ASD before 25 years of age without evidence of pulmonary hypertension results in a long-term outcome that is similar to that of age- and sex-matched controls. Advanced age (60 years) is not a contraindication to ASD closure in the presence of a significant shunt because a significant number of patients will show evidence of symptomatic improvement. Preoperative pulmonary artery pressure and the presence or absence of pulmonary vascular disease are important predictors of successful interventional outcome.

Patent Foramen Ovale

Integrity of the fetal circulation depends on the patency of the foramen ovale. In most cases, the fall in pulmonary vascular resistance at birth induces the foramen to become sealed. Necropsy studies have revealed that the foramen ovale remains patent beyond the first year of life in about 30% of individuals, and clinical studies have demonstrated that the prevalence of patent foramen ovale is three times higher in patients with cryptogenic stroke (Chapter 407), particularly before the age of 55 years, because of right-to-left shunting and paradoxical embolization of material from the venous circulation. Cardiac investigation of the patient with cryptogenic stroke includes transesophageal echocardiography with agitated saline injection to visualize the presence of a right-to-left shunt (Chapter 55). Patent foramen ovale most likely to result in future paradoxical embolization is found in patients younger than 55 years with a prior cryptogenic stroke, in association with a hypermobile septum with aneurysm formation, and when a significant amount of right-to-left shunting is present at rest without provocative maneuvers.

TREATMENT Rx

Current information does not support closure of a patent foramen ovale for primary prevention of a first stroke in a patient in whom it is fortuitously diagnosed on routine echocardiography.[3] Among patients with a prior cryptogenic stroke, however, randomized trials provide some guidance. In one randomized trial of patients with cryptogenic stroke or transient ischemic attack and a patent foramen ovale, device closure was no better than medical therapy alone for preventing a recurrent stroke or transient ischemic attack.[A3] In a second trial, closure of a patent foramen ovale for secondary prevention of cryptogenic embolism did not significantly reduce recurrent embolic events or death (3.4%) after 4 years compared with medical therapy (5.2%).[A4] In a third randomized trial of adults who had had a cryptogenic ischemic stroke, there also was no significant benefit from closure of a patent foramen ovale, but closure was superior to medical therapy alone in prespecified analyses limited to patients who actually received and adhered to the original treatment (0.66 vs. 1.39 events per 100 person-years).[A5] These findings together suggest a probable small benefit of closure compared with medical therapy, which is warfarin to an international normalized ratio of 2.0 to 3.0.[4] Primary closure of a patent foramen ovale is clearly indicated when a patient has contraindications to medical therapy, if medical therapy has failed, or in the presence of a hypercoagulable state not treatable by medical therapy.

Ventricular Septal Defect

For anatomic classification of VSDs, the interventricular septum can be divided into four regions. Defects of the membranous septum, or infracristal VSDs, are located in a small translucent area beneath the aortic valve and account for up to 80% of VSDs. These VSDs typically show a variable degree of extension into the inlet or outlet septum, hence their designation as perimembranous (Video 69-2). Infundibular defects or supracristal outlet VSDs occur in the conal septum above the crista supraventricularis and below the pulmonary valve. Inlet defects are identified at the crux of the heart between the tricuspid and mitral valves and are usually associated with other anomalies of the atrioventricular canal. Defects of the trabecular or muscular septum can be multiple and occur distal to the septal attachment of the tricuspid valve and toward the apex.

The pathophysiology and clinical course of VSDs depend on the size of the defect, the status of the pulmonary vascular bed, and the effects of shunt size on intracardiac hemodynamics. Unlike ASDs, a VSD may decrease in size with time. Approximately half of all native VSDs are small, and more than half of them close spontaneously; moderate or even large VSDs may also close in 10% or less of cases. The highest closure rates are observed in the first decade of life; spontaneous closure in adult life is unusual.[5]

Patients who have a small defect with trivial or mild shunts are defined as those with a $\dot{Q}:\dot{Q}$ of less than 1.5 and normal pulmonary artery pressure and vascular resistance. Patients with moderate defects have a $\dot{Q}:\dot{Q}$ ratio of greater than 1.2 and elevated pulmonary artery pressure but not elevated pulmonary vascular resistance. Patients with a large and severe defect have an elevated $\dot{Q}:\dot{Q}$ ratio with high pulmonary pressure and elevated pulmonary vascular resistance. Eisenmenger complex develops in about 10% of patients with VSDs, usually when there is no resistance to flow at the level of the defect, which can be as large as the aorta. When a systolic pressure gradient is present between the ventricles, the physiologic severity may be trivial or mild but can also be moderate or severe.

Minimal or mild defects usually cause no significant hemodynamic or physiologic abnormality. A moderate or severe defect causes left atrial and ventricular dilation consistent with the degree of left-to-right shunting. Shunting across the ventricular septum occurs predominantly during systole when left ventricular pressure exceeds that on the right; diastolic filling abnormalities occur in the left atrium. With moderate or severe defects, the right side of the heart becomes affected as a function of the rise in pulmonary pressure and pulmonary blood flow.

DIAGNOSIS

An adult with a VSD most commonly has a small restrictive lesion that either was small at birth or has undergone some degree of spontaneous closure. A second group of patients consists of those with large, nonrestrictive VSDs that have not been operated on; these patients have had Eisenmenger complex for most of their lives. Patients with a moderately sized defect are typically symptomatic as children and are therefore more likely to have repair at a young age.

Patients with a trivial or mild shunt across a small, restrictive VSD are usually asymptomatic. Physical examination discloses no evidence of systemic or pulmonary venous congestion, and jugular venous pressure is normal. A thrill may be palpable at the left sternal border. Auscultation reveals normal S_1 and S_2 without gallops. A grade 4 or louder, widely radiating, high-frequency, pansystolic murmur is heard maximally in the third or fourth intercostal space and reflects the high-pressure gradient between the left and right ventricles throughout systole. The striking contrast between a loud murmur and otherwise normal findings on cardiac examination is an important diagnostic clue. The ECG and chest radiograph are also normal in patients with small VSDs.

At the other end of the spectrum are patients with Eisenmenger complex (see earlier). Between these two extremes are patients with a moderate defect, whose pathologic process reflects a combination of pulmonary hypertension and left-sided volume overload resulting from a significant left-to-right shunt. In adults, shortness of breath on exertion can be the result of both pulmonary venous congestion and elevated pulmonary pressure. On physical examination, a diffuse palpable left ventricular impulse occurs with a variable degree of right ventricular hypertrophy and an accentuated second heart sound. A systolic murmur persists as long as pulmonary vascular resistance is below systemic resistance. The ECG commonly shows left atrial enlargement and left ventricular hypertrophy. The chest radiograph shows shunt vascularity with an enlarged left atrium and ventricle. The degree of pulmonary hypertension determines the size of the pulmonary artery trunk.

Echocardiography can identify the defect and determine the significance of the shunt by assessing left atrial and ventricular size, pulmonary artery pressure, and presence or absence of right ventricular hypertrophy. Cardiac catheterization is reserved for those in whom surgery is considered. Adults with a small defect of no physiologic significance need not be studied invasively. Those with Eisenmenger complex have severe pulmonary vascular disease and are not surgical candidates. Patients who have a moderately sized shunt that appears hemodynamically significant and in whom pulmonary pressures are elevated are most likely to benefit from direct measurements of pulmonary vascular resistance and reactivity.

TREATMENT Rx

Patients with Eisenmenger complex have pulmonary vascular resistance that is prohibitive to surgery. For this group of patients, management centers on the medical complications of cyanosis (see earlier). In a few patients with small defects, complications can relate to progressive tricuspid insufficiency caused by septal aneurysm formation or to acquired aortic insufficiency when an aortic cusp becomes engaged in the high-velocity jet flow generated by the defect. The intermediate group of patients with a defect of moderate physiologic significance should have their VSDs closed unless closure is contraindicated by high pulmonary vascular resistance. For a perimembranous VSD, transcatheter closure is as effective as open surgical closure and has a lower rate of minor adverse events.[A6]

Late results after operative closure of isolated VSDs include residual patency in up to 20% of patients, only about 5% of whom need a reoperation. Rhythm disturbances after surgical closure of VSDs include tachyarrhythmias and conduction disturbances. Right bundle branch block occurs in one third to two thirds of patients, whereas first-degree atrioventricular block and complete heart block occur in less than 10%. Sudden cardiac death after surgical repair of VSD occurs in 2% of patients.

Patent Ductus Arteriosus

The ductus arteriosus connects the descending aorta to the main pulmonary trunk near the origin of the left subclavian artery (Fig. 69-6). Normal postnatal closure results in fibrosis and degenerative changes in the ductal lumen, leaving in its place the residual ligamentum arteriosum, which rarely can become part of an abnormal vascular ring. When the duct persists, significant calcification of the aortic ductal end is observed.

The physiologic consequences of a PDA are determined by its size and length as well as by the ratio of pressure and resistance of the pulmonary and aortic circulations on either end of the duct. If systolic and diastolic pressure in the aorta exceeds that in the pulmonary artery, aortic blood flows continuously down a pressure gradient into the pulmonary artery and then returns to the left atrium. The left atrium and subsequently the left ventricle dilate, whereas the right side of the heart becomes progressively affected as pulmonary hypertension develops.

A small PDA has continuous flow throughout the entire cardiac cycle without left-sided heart dilation, pulmonary hypertension, or symptoms. Patients with a small PDA, although protected from hemodynamic complications of a significant left-to-right shunt, remain at risk for infectious endarteritis, which usually develops on the pulmonary side of the duct and occurs at a rate of about 0.45% per year after the second decade. Because endarteritis accounts for up to one third of the total mortality in patients with PDA, ductal closure should be considered even when the PDA is small.

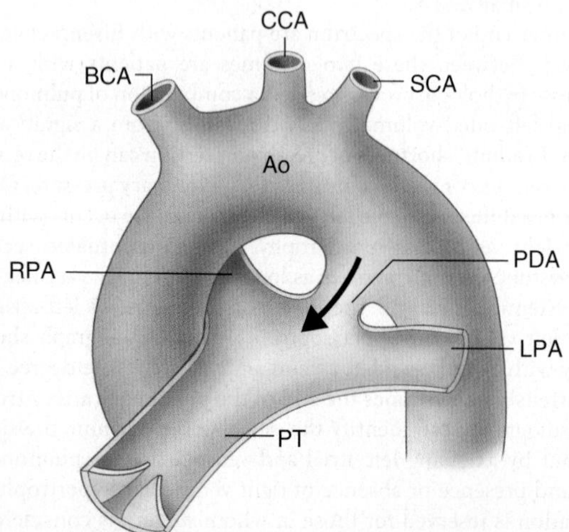

FIGURE 69-6. Anatomy of a patent ductus arteriosus. Note the relationships of the position of the ductus, left subclavian artery, and pulmonary artery bifurcation. Ao = aorta; BCA = brachiocephalic; CCA = common carotid artery; LPA = left pulmonary artery; PDA = patent ductus arteriosus; PT = pulmonary trunk; RPA = right pulmonary artery; SCA = subclavian artery. (From Perloff JK, ed. Clinical Recognition of Congenital Heart Disease. 4th ed. Philadelphia: WB Saunders; 1994:510.)

A PDA is of moderate or large size but still restrictive when a left-to-right shunt occurs throughout systole and diastole is of variable duration. Left atrial or ventricular dilation and pulmonary hypertension will vary with the quantity of left-to-right shunting as well as with the secondary effects on the pulmonary vascular bed. Symptoms generally increase by the second and third decades and include dyspnea, palpitations, and exercise intolerance. As heart failure, pulmonary hypertension, or endarteritis develops, mortality rises to 3 to 4% per year by the fourth decade, and two thirds of patients die by 60 years of age. Eisenmenger physiology with systemic or suprasystemic pulmonary pressure and a right-to-left shunt develops in 5% of patients with an isolated PDA.

DIAGNOSIS

In patients with Eisenmenger physiology, a right-to-left shunt from the pulmonary artery to the descending aorta results in decreased oxygen saturation in the lower extremities compared with the upper extremities. This difference in cyanosis and clubbing is most prominent in the toes; the left arm is variably affected through the left subclavian artery, and the right arm is typically spared. With a large left-to-right shunt, the pulse pressure widens as diastolic flow into the pulmonary artery lowers systemic diastolic pressure. The arterial pulse becomes bounding as a result of increased stroke volume. Precordial palpation discloses variable left and right ventricular impulses as determined by the relative degree of left-sided volume overload and pulmonary hypertension. In the presence of a continuous aortopulmonary gradient, the classic "machinery" murmur of a PDA can be heard at the first or second left intercostal space below the left clavicle. As the pulmonary pressure rises, the diastolic component of the murmur becomes progressively shorter. With the development of Eisenmenger physiology and equalization of aortic and pulmonary pressure, the entire murmur may disappear, and the clinical findings are dominated by pulmonary hypertension.

In adult patients with a significant left-to-right shunt, the ECG shows a bifid P wave in at least one limb lead consistent with left atrial enlargement and a variable degree of left ventricular hypertrophy. The PR interval is prolonged in about 20% of patients. In older patients, the chest radiograph shows calcification at the location of the PDA. Characteristically, the ascending aorta and pulmonary artery are dilated, and the left-sided chambers are enlarged. Echocardiography may not directly visualize the PDA but can accurately identify it by a Doppler signal that often parallels the length of the murmur. Left-sided heart dilation and pulmonary hypertension can be quantified and monitored. Cardiac catheterization to assess pulmonary vascular resistance is commonly indicated before closure.

TREATMENT Rx

After ligation of a PDA in infancy or early childhood, cardiac function is commonly normal, and no special follow-up is required. If pulmonary artery pressure and pulmonary vascular resistance are substantially elevated, preoperative evaluation should assess the degree of reversibility. With Eisenmenger disease, closure is contraindicated. Closure of a PDA either percutaneously or surgically is indicated in the presence of left-sided heart enlargement or if prior endarteritis has occurred. Reported operative mortality rates vary from less than 1 to 8%, depending on the presence of calcification and the degree of pulmonary hypertension. Transcatheter or coil occlusion is an accepted procedure in adults. Residual shunt rates vary from 0.5 to 8%, depending on the device used. Small residual defects that are detected by echocardiography but are not associated with an audible murmur or hemodynamic findings do not appear to carry a significant risk for endarteritis.

Aortopulmonary Window

An aortopulmonary window is typically a large defect across the adjacent segments of both great vessels above their respective valves and below the pulmonary artery bifurcation. The pathophysiologic mechanism is similar to that of a PDA. The shunt is usually large, so pulmonary vascular resistance rises rapidly and abolishes the aortopulmonary gradient in diastole. The murmur is usually best heard at the third left intercostal space. With a right-to-left shunt, differential cyanosis never occurs because the shunt is proximal to the brachiocephalic vessels. Differentiation of an aortopulmonary window from a PDA can usually be confirmed with echocardiography; the left-to-right shunt is seen in the main pulmonary artery in the aortopulmonary window compared with the left pulmonary artery bifurcation in PDA. Cardiac catheterization confirms the diagnosis and hemodynamics. Surgical repair is necessary unless pulmonary vascular obstructive disease precludes closure.

Pulmonary Arteriovenous Fistulas

Pulmonary arteriovenous fistulas can occur as isolated congenital disorders or as part of generalized hereditary hemorrhagic telangiectasia (Osler-Weber-Rendu syndrome; Chapter 173). These fistulas typically occur in the lower lobes or the right middle lobe and can be small or large, single or multiple. The arterial supply usually comes from a dilated, tortuous branch of the pulmonary artery.

The most common finding is that of abnormal opacity on a chest radiograph in a patient with buccal ruby patches or in an otherwise healthy adult who has mild cyanosis. Shunting between deoxygenated pulmonary arterial blood and the oxygenated pulmonary venous blood results in a physiologic right-to-left shunt. The degree of shunting is typically small and not significant enough to result in dilation of the left atrium and ventricle. Heart failure is unusual. Hemoptysis can result if a fistula ruptures into a bronchus. In patients with hereditary hemorrhagic telangiectasia, angiomas occur on the lips and mouth as well as in the gastrointestinal tract and on pleural, liver, and vaginal surfaces. Epistaxis is most common, but cerebrovascular accidents can also occur. Patients with hereditary hemorrhagic telangiectasia can have symptoms that resemble those of a transient ischemic attack even in the absence of right-to-left shunting. On physical examination, cyanosis and clubbing can be notable or barely detectable. Auscultation can disclose soft systolic or continuous noncardiac murmurs on the chest wall adjacent to the fistula. The murmur typically increases with inspiration. The ECG is usually normal. The chest radiograph shows one or more densities, typically in the lower lobes or in the right middle lobe. An echocardiogram can confirm the presence of the fistula by showing early opacification of the left atrium in the absence of any other intracardiac communication when saline is injected into a peripheral vein. The absence of a hemodynamically significant shunt can be confirmed by documenting normal cardiac chamber size.

If the hypoxemia is progressive or if a neurologic complication is documented to have occurred because of paradoxical emboli, fistula closure should be considered. Options include percutaneous catheter techniques if the fistula is small and accessible or a pulmonary wedge resection or lobectomy if the fistula is large. Multiple or recurrent fistulas create a major therapeutic challenge.

Isolated Obstructive Lesions of the Right and Left Ventricular Outflow Tract

Complications of obstructive lesions of the outflow tract relate to the secondary effects of exposure to pressure overload in the chamber proximal to the obstruction. The inability to increase systemic or pulmonary blood flow in the face of a fixed obstruction can cause exercise intolerance, inadequate myocardial perfusion, ventricular arrhythmias, and sudden death.

RIGHT VENTRICULAR OUTFLOW TRACT OBSTRUCTION

Obstruction of the right ventricular outflow tract can occur at the level of the pulmonary valve (see later), above it in the main pulmonary artery or its branches, or below it in the right ventricle itself. Supravalvular and branch pulmonary artery stenoses are important and common complications in patients with tetralogy of Fallot (see later). Residual supravalvular pulmonary stenosis is sometimes seen after palliative pulmonary artery banding to decrease pulmonary blood flow in patients with large left-to-right shunts. Congenital branch pulmonary artery stenosis can occur in isolation or with valvular pulmonary stenosis, shunt lesions, or a variety of syndromes. Patients with Noonan syndrome have a characteristic phenotypic facial appearance, short stature, and webbed neck; cardiac lesions may include a dysplastic pulmonary valve, left ventricular hypertrophic cardiomyopathy, and peripheral pulmonary artery stenosis. Supravalvular pulmonary stenosis can be seen with supravalvular aortic stenosis in Williams (elfin facies) syndrome.

Pulmonary atresia refers to an absent, imperforate, or closed pulmonary valve, which typically occurs in conjunction with other malformations. Pulmonary atresia with a nonrestrictive VSD is a complex cyanotic malformation that is discussed later.

Primary infundibular stenosis with an intact ventricular septum can result from a fibrous band just below the infundibulum. In a double-chambered right ventricle, obstruction is caused by anomalous muscle bundles that divide the right ventricle into a high-pressure chamber below the hypertrophied muscle bundles and a low-pressure chamber above the bundles and below the valve. The clinical features vary according to the presence or absence of other lesions, such as pulmonary valvular stenosis or VSD.

VALVULAR PULMONARY STENOSIS

Isolated congenital valvular pulmonary stenosis (Chapter 75) is a common lesion due to a bicuspid valve in 20% of cases, a dysplastic valve caused by myxomatous changes and severe thickening in 10% of cases, and an abnormal trileaflet valve in most of the remaining cases. Fusion of the leaflets results in a variable degree of thickening and calcification in older patients.

The 25-year survival of patients with valvular pulmonary stenosis is greater than 95% but is worse in those with severe stenosis and peak systolic gradients greater than 80 mm Hg. For patients with mild (<50 mm Hg gradients) and moderate (50 to 80 mm Hg gradients) pulmonary stenosis, bacterial endocarditis, complex ventricular arrhythmias, and progression of the stenosis are uncommon.

DIAGNOSIS

A patient with moderate or even severe pulmonary stenosis may be asymptomatic. With severe stenosis, exercise intolerance can be associated with presyncope and ventricular arrhythmias. Progressive right-sided heart failure is the most common cause of death. On physical examination of patients with significant pulmonary stenosis, jugular venous pressure has a dominant *a* wave, reflecting a noncompliant right ventricle. Palpation discloses a sustained parasternal lift of right ventricular hypertrophy. An expiratory systolic ejection click is characteristic if the leaflets are still mobile. In moderate or severe stenosis, a grade 3 or louder systolic murmur can be heard and felt in the second left interspace. The length of the murmur increases as it peaks progressively later in systole with an increasing degree of obstruction. If right-sided heart failure occurs, tricuspid insufficiency and systemic venous congestion develop. The ECG can show right axis deviation and tall, peaked right atrial P waves in lead II. With more than mild stenosis, the R wave exceeds the S wave in lead V_1. On chest radiography, the main pulmonary artery can be dilated even if the stenosis is mild. Characteristically, the left pulmonary artery is more dilated than the right because of the leftward direction of the high-velocity jet. A variable degree of right ventricular hypertrophy is manifested as right-sided chamber enlargement. Echocardiography can establish the diagnosis and determine the severity by Doppler ultrasound examination. Patients with valvular pulmonary stenosis do not require cardiac catheterization. The mean gradient at echocardiography correlates well with the gradient measured at cardiac catheterization and should be used for therapeutic decisions because peak instantaneous Doppler gradients tend to overestimate the severity of disease.

TREATMENT Rx

Depending on symptoms, percutaneous balloon valvotomy should be considered for patients with isolated valvular pulmonary stenosis and mean Doppler gradients of 30 mm Hg or greater unless there is moderate or severe pulmonary regurgitation. In the presence of a doming valve, pulmonary angioplasty is the procedure of choice for adults, who achieve persistently good results at 10-year follow-up. For patients with hypoplastic pulmonary arteries or subvalvular stenosis (double-chambered right ventricle), surgical resection of right ventricular muscle bands can be performed.

LEFT VENTRICULAR OUTFLOW TRACT OBSTRUCTION

Stenosis of the left ventricular outflow tract can occur at, below, or above the aortic valve. Discrete subaortic stenosis, most commonly caused by a fibromuscular ring just below the valve, accounts for 15 to 20% of all cases of congenital obstruction of the left ventricular outflow tract. Concomitant aortic insufficiency occurs in 50% of cases. Supravalvular aortic stenosis results from thickened media and intima above the aortic sinuses; early coronary atherosclerosis or even ostial coronary obstruction can occur.

CONGENITAL VALVULAR AORTIC STENOSIS

The normal aortic valve has three cusps and commissures. A unicuspid aortic valve accounts for most cases of severe aortic stenosis in infants (Chapter 75). A bicuspid aortic valve, which is the most common congenital cardiac malformation, functions normally at birth but often becomes gradually obstructed as calcific and fibrous changes occur; prolapse of one or both cusps can cause aortic insufficiency.

The pathophysiologic mechanism of aortic stenosis depends not only on its severity but also on the age at diagnosis. When a bicuspid aortic valve becomes stenotic in adulthood because of degenerative changes, criteria for diagnosis and intervention parallel those for other forms of acquired aortic stenosis (Chapter 75). The estimated overall 25-year survival rate for patients with congenital valvular aortic stenosis diagnosed in childhood is 85%. Children with initial peak cardiac catheterization gradients of less than 50 mm Hg have long-term survival rates of higher than 90%, as opposed to survival rates of 80% in those with gradients of 50 mm Hg or greater.

DIAGNOSIS

Symptoms include angina, exertional dyspnea, presyncope, and syncope and may progress to heart failure. The auscultatory hallmark of a bicuspid aortic valve is an audible systolic ejection click that is typically of a higher pitch than the first heart sound and is best heard not at the cardiac base but at the apex. The sound is caused by sudden movement of the stenotic valve as it moves superiorly in systole and is followed by the typical aortic stenosis murmur (Chapter 75). When significant calcification of the valve results in reduced mobility, the ejection sound is no longer heard. The diagnosis is easily confirmed by two-dimensional echocardiography, with which the number and orientation of aortic cusps can readily be identified.

TREATMENT Rx

Conservative management is generally indicated for mild stenosis with a peak gradient of less than 25 mm Hg, but close supervision is required because 20% of these patients require an intervention during long-term follow-up. Unlimited athletic participation is allowed only for asymptomatic patients with peak gradients of less than 20 to 25 mm Hg, a normal ECG, and a normal exercise test result. For children who are symptomatic or have gradients greater than 30 mm Hg but do not have significant aortic insufficiency, transcatheter aortic valvotomy is preferred. Aortic valvuloplasty can be considered in young adults, but calcification limits its success, and valve replacement is usually required (Chapter 75). For adults, treatment decisions are similar to those for aortic stenosis from other causes. For patients with subvalvular aortic stenosis, surgical intervention is indicated in the presence of peak gradients above 50 mm Hg, symptoms, or progressive aortic insufficiency.

COARCTATION OF THE AORTA

Aortic coarctation typically occurs just distal to the left subclavian artery at the site of the aortic ductal attachment or its residual ligamentum arteriosum. Less commonly, the coarctation ridge lies proximal to the left subclavian. A bicuspid aortic valve is the most common coexisting anomaly, but VSDs and PDAs are also seen. Pseudocoarctation refers to buckling or kinking of the aortic arch without the presence of a significant gradient.

The most common complications of aortic coarctation are systemic hypertension (Chapter 67) and secondary left ventricular hypertrophy with heart failure. Systemic hypertension is caused by decreased vascular compliance in the proximal aorta and activation of the renin-angiotensin system in response to renal artery hypoperfusion below the obstruction. Left ventricular hypertrophy occurs in response to chronic pressure overload. Congestive heart failure occurs most commonly in infants and then after 40 years of age. The high pressure proximal to the obstruction stimulates the growth of collateral vessels from the internal mammary, scapular, and superior intercostal arteries to the intercostals of the descending aorta. Collateral circulation increases with age and contributes to perfusion of the lower extremities and the spinal cord. This mechanism, although adaptive in a patient who has not undergone surgery, accounts for significant morbidity during surgery when the motor impairment results from inadequate protection of spinal perfusion. Aneurysms occur most notably in the ascending aorta and in the circle of Willis. Premature coronary disease is thought to be related to the resulting hypertension. Complications, including bacterial endarteritis at the coarctation site or, more commonly, endocarditis at the site of a bicuspid aortic valve, cerebrovascular complications, myocardial infarction, heart failure, and aortic dissection, occur in 2 to 6% of patients, more frequently in those with advancing age who have not undergone surgery.

DIAGNOSIS

Young adults may be asymptomatic with incidental systemic hypertension and decreased lower extremity pulses. Coarctation should always be considered in adolescents and young adult men with unexplained upper extremity hypertension. The pressure differential can cause epistaxis, headaches, leg fatigue, or claudication. Older patients have angina, symptoms of heart failure, and vascular complications.

On physical examination, the lower half of the body is typically slightly less developed than the upper half. The hips are narrow and the legs are short, in contrast to broad shoulders and long arms. Blood pressure measurements should be obtained in each arm and one leg; an abnormal measurement is an increase of less than 10 mm Hg in popliteal systolic blood pressure compared with arm systolic blood pressure. The diastolic pressure should be the same in the upper and lower extremities. A pressure differential of more than 30 mm Hg between the right and the left arms is consistent with compromised flow in the left subclavian artery. Right brachial palpation characteristically reveals a strong or even bounding pulse compared with a slowly rising or absent femoral, popliteal, or pedal pulse. Examination of the eyegrounds can reveal tortuous or corkscrew retinal arteries. Precordial palpation is consistent with left ventricular pressure overload. On auscultation, a systolic ejection sound reflecting the presence of a bicuspid aortic valve should be sought. The coarctation itself generates a systolic murmur heard posteriorly, in the midthoracic region, the length of which correlates with the severity of the coarctation. Over the anterior of the chest, systolic murmurs reflecting increased collateral flow can be heard in the infraclavicular areas and the sternal edge or in the axillae.

In adult coarctation, the most common finding on the ECG is left ventricular hypertrophy. Chest radiographic findings are diagnostic. Location of the coarctation segment between the dilated left subclavian artery above and the leftward convexity of the descending aorta below results in the "3 sign" (Fig. 69-7). Bilateral rib notching as a result of dilation of the posterior intercostal arteries is seen on the posterior of the third to eighth ribs when the coarctation is below the left subclavian. Unilateral rib notching sparing the left ribs is observed when the coarctation occurs proximal to the left subclavian artery. Transthoracic echocardiography documents the gradient in the descending aorta and determines the presence of left ventricular hypertrophy. Magnetic resonance imaging (Chapter 56) is the best modality for visualizing the anatomy of the descending aorta. Cardiac catheterization should measure pressures and assess collaterals when surgery is contemplated.

TREATMENT 

Intervention is recommended in patients who have gradients of 20 mm Hg or more on cardiac catheterization (Chapter 57) or who have evidence of significant collateral flow on imaging studies. The choice between catheter intervention and surgical intervention, which should be made in conjunction with a specialist, depends on the associated anomalies and the anatomy of the coarctation segment. Fifty percent of patients repaired when they are older

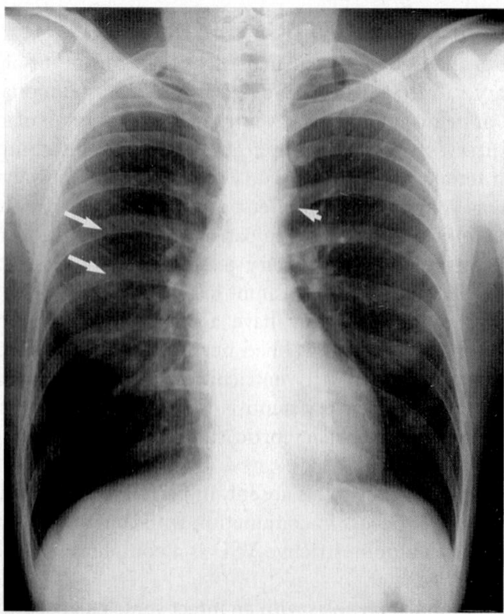

FIGURE 69-7. Chest radiograph of a patient with coarctation of the aorta. The radiographic *3* formed by the dilated subclavian artery above and the dilated aorta below (*short arrow*) is shown. Note the notching, best seen at the level of the seventh and eighth ribs (*long arrows*). The dilated ascending aortic segment can also be seen.

than 40 years have residual hypertension, whereas those who have undergone surgery between the ages of 1 and 5 years have a less than 10% prevalence of hypertension on long-term follow-up. Actuarial survival rates are 94%, 86%, and 74% at 10, 20, and 30 years, respectively, after initial surgical repair.[6]

Balloon angioplasty is the treatment of choice for focal recoarctation in patients who have previously been operated on. The incidence of incomplete relief and restenosis is decreased in adults by endovascular stent placement. Focal complications include aortic aneurysms and, rarely, aortic rupture.

Anomalies of the Sinuses of Valsalva and Coronary Arteries

SINUS OF VALSALVA ANEURYSMS

At the base of the aortic root, the aortic valve cusps are attached to the aortic wall, above which three small pouches, or sinuses, are seated. The right coronary artery originates from one sinus and the left main coronary artery from a second; the third is called the *noncoronary sinus*. A weakness in the wall of the sinus can result in aneurysm formation with or without rupture. In more than 90% of cases, the aneurysm involves the right or noncoronary cusp. Rupture typically occurs into the right side of the heart at the right atrial or ventricular level with a resulting large left-to-right shunt driven by the high aortic pressure.

A previously asymptomatic young man typically has chest pain and rapidly progressing shortness of breath sometimes after physical strain. The physical examination is consistent with significant heart failure. Even if the communication is between the aorta and the right side of the heart, biventricular failure is not unusual. The classic murmur is loud and continuous, often with a thrill. A murmur of aortic insufficiency secondary to damage to the adjacent aortic valve may be superimposed. The chest radiograph shows volume overload of both ventricles with evidence of shunt vascularity and pulmonary venous congestion. The echocardiogram is diagnostic. Cardiac catheterization can verify the integrity of the coronary artery adjacent to the ruptured aneurysm.

Even though symptoms may abate as the heart dilates, progressive cardiac decompensation typically results in death within 1 year of the rupture. A ruptured sinus of Valsalva aneurysm therefore requires urgent surgical repair.

CORONARY ARTERY FISTULAS

Fistulas arise from the right or left coronary arteries and in 90% of cases drain into the right ventricle, the right atrium, or the pulmonary artery in order of decreasing frequency. Typically, young patients are asymptomatic, but supraventricular arrhythmias are seen with progressive dilation of the intracardiac chambers. Angina can occur as the fistula creates a coronary steal by diverting blood away from the myocardium. Heart failure is seen with large fistulas. A continuous murmur heard in a young, otherwise normal acyanotic, asymptomatic patient should suggest the diagnosis. Most fistulas are associated with a small shunt, and hence the murmur is often less than grade 3 and is heard in the precordial area. Unless the shunt is large, the ECG is normal, as is the chest radiograph. The echocardiogram, especially the transesophageal echocardiogram, is diagnostic. Percutaneous transcatheter closure with coil embolization is preferred, but surgical ligation is also an alternative.

ANOMALOUS ORIGIN OF THE CORONARY ARTERIES

The left main coronary artery normally arises from the left sinus of Valsalva and courses leftward, posterior to the right ventricular outflow tract. The right coronary artery arises from the right sinus of Valsalva and courses rightward to the right ventricle. Isolated ectopic or anomalous origins of the coronary arteries (see Fig. 57-7) are seen in 0.6 to 1.5% of patients undergoing coronary angiography.

The most common anomaly is ectopic origin of the left circumflex artery from the right sinus of Valsalva, followed by anomalous origin of the right coronary artery from the left sinus and anomalous origin of the left main coronary artery from the right sinus. If the anomalous coronary artery does not course between the pulmonary artery and aorta, the prognosis is favorable. Risks of ischemia, myocardial infarction, and death are greatest when the left main coronary artery courses between both great vessels.

Coronary arteries can also originate from the pulmonary trunk. If both the right and left arteries originate from the pulmonary trunk, death usually occurs in the neonatal period. If only the left anterior descending coronary artery originates from the pulmonary trunk, the rate of survival to adulthood is approximately 10%, depending on the development of collateral retrograde flow to the anomalous artery from a normal coronary artery. This collateral flow may cause a continuous murmur along the left sternal border, congestive heart failure from the large shunt, and a coronary steal syndrome as blood is diverted away from the normal artery.

A single coronary ostium can provide a single coronary artery that branches into right and left coronary arteries, the left then giving rise to the circumflex and the anterior descending arteries. The ostium can originate from the right or left aortic sinus. The coronary circulation is functionally normal unless one of the branches passes between the aorta and the pulmonary artery.

Diagnostic procedures include angiography, magnetic resonance imaging, and transesophageal echocardiography. For an anomalous coronary artery that originates from the pulmonary artery, surgical reimplantation into the aorta is preferred. For an anomalous artery that courses between the pulmonary artery and aorta, a bypass graft to the distal vessel is preferred.

SPECIFIC COMPLEX LESIONS

Tetralogy of Fallot

Tetralogy of Fallot, the most common cyanotic malformation, is characterized by superior and anterior displacement of the subpulmonary infundibular septum, which causes the tetrad of pulmonary stenosis, VSD, aortic override, and right ventricular hypertrophy. The VSD is perimembranous in 80% of cases. Additional cardiac anomalies include a right-sided aortic arch in up to 25% of patients. An anomalous left anterior descending artery originating from the right coronary cusp and crossing over the right ventricular outflow tract is seen in 10% of cases. Other associated anomalies include ASD, left superior vena cava, defects of the atrioventricular canal, and aortic insufficiency. With pulmonary atresia, pulmonary blood flow occurs through aortic to pulmonary collaterals. Life expectancy is limited unless staged reconstructive surgery is performed.

The physiology in unrepaired tetralogy of Fallot is determined by the severity and location of the pulmonic outflow obstruction and by the interaction of pulmonary and systemic vascular resistance across a nonrestrictive VSD. Because the pulmonary stenosis results in a relatively fixed pulmonary resistance, a drop in systemic vascular resistance as occurs with exercise is associated with increased right-to-left shunting and increasing cyanosis. A child who squats after running is attempting to reverse the process by increasing systemic vascular resistance by crouching with bent knees. Native pulmonary blood flow is typically insufficient. Unless a PDA has remained open, a cyanotic adult will typically have undergone a palliative procedure to increase pulmonary blood flow.

Examination of unrepaired patients reveals central cyanosis and clubbing. The right ventricular impulse is prominent. The second heart sound is single and represents the aortic closure sound with an absent or inconspicuous P_2. Typically, little or no systolic murmur is heard across the pulmonary valve because the more severe the obstruction, the more right-to-left shunting occurs and the less blood flows across a diminutive right ventricular outflow tract. A diastolic murmur of aortic insufficiency is often heard in adults. In the presence of a palliative systemic arterial to pulmonary artery shunt, the high-pressure gradient generates a loud continuous murmur. In a patient who has not undergone surgery, progressive infundibular stenosis and cyanosis occur. Before the advent of palliative surgery, mortality rates were 50% in the first few years of life, and survival past the third decade was unusual.

Complete surgical repair consists of patch closure of the VSD and relief of the right ventricular outflow tract obstruction. Adequate pulmonary blood flow is ensured by reconstruction of the distal pulmonary artery bed. Previous palliative shunts are usually taken down. Complete repair in childhood yields a 90 to 95% 10-year survival rate with good functional results, and 30-year survival rates may be as high as 85%. Total correction with low mortality and a favorable long-term follow-up is possible even in adulthood.

After repair, residual pulmonary stenosis, proximal or distal, with a right ventricular pressure greater than 50% of systemic occurs in up to 25% of patients. Some degree of pulmonary insufficiency is common, particularly if a patch has been inserted at the level of the pulmonary valve or if a pulmonary valvotomy has been performed. Residual VSDs can be found in up to 20% of patients. Patients may be asymptomatic or may have symptoms related to long-term complications after surgical repair. Symptoms can reflect residual right ventricular pressure or volume overload or arrhythmias at rest or with exercise. Angina can occur in a young patient if surgical repair has damaged an anomalous left anterior descending artery as it courses across the right ventricular outflow tract. In acyanotic adults, clubbing commonly regresses.

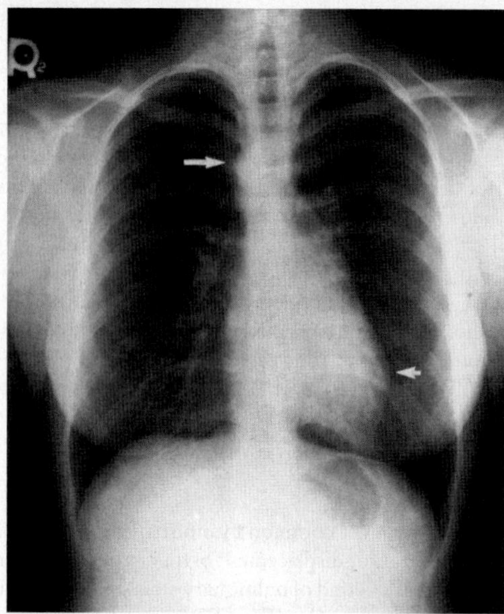

FIGURE 69-8. Chest radiograph of an adult after tetralogy of Fallot repair. A right aortic arch with rightward indentation of the trachea (*long arrow*) can be seen. The right ventricular apex remains upturned (*short arrow*). Note the sternal wires consistent with intracardiac repair, clarifying the fullness of the pulmonary artery segment often seen after extensive enlargement of the right ventricular outflow tract.

A right ventricular impulse is often felt as a result of residual pulmonary insufficiency or stenosis. A systolic murmur can represent residual pulmonary stenosis, residual VSD, or tricuspid insufficiency. A diastolic murmur can reflect aortic or pulmonary insufficiency. Ventricular arrhythmias are common after repair, with an incidence of sudden death as high as 5%.

The ECG in unrepaired tetralogy of Fallot shows right axis deviation, right atrial enlargement, and dominant right ventricular forces over the precordial leads. The most common finding after repair is complete right bundle branch block, which is seen in 80 to 90% of patients. The chest radiograph typically shows an upturned apex with a concave pulmonary artery segment giving the classic appearance of a boot-shaped heart. Figure 69-8 demonstrates the findings in an adult after repair. The apex is persistently upturned, although the pulmonary artery segment is no longer concave. Echocardiography can confirm the diagnosis and document intracardiac complications in repaired and unrepaired patients. Shunt patency can be determined by Doppler examination. Magnetic resonance imaging can accurately document stenosis in the distal pulmonary artery bed. Cardiac catheterization is reserved for patients in whom operative or reoperative treatment is contemplated or in whom the integrity of the coronary circulation needs to be verified.

Patients with a change in exercise tolerance, angina, or evidence of heart failure and those with symptomatic arrhythmias or syncope should be referred for complete evaluation. Surgical reintervention is generally considered when right ventricular pressure is more than two thirds as high as systemic pressure because of residual right ventricular outflow tract obstruction, free pulmonary regurgitation occurs with right ventricular dysfunction or sustained arrhythmias, or a residual VSD causes a significant shunt.

Patients should be seen yearly by an adult congenital heart specialist for assessment of right ventricular function, pulmonary valve dysfunction, and arrhythmia. Surveillance should include a history, physical examination, and 12-lead ECG. Sudden cardiac death can occur in 3 to 6% of patients observed between 20 and 30 years, sometimes despite favorable hemodynamics.[7]

Complete Transposition of the Great Arteries

Complete transposition of the great arteries is the second most common cyanotic lesion, and surgically corrected adults are increasingly common. In simple transposition of the great arteries, the atria and ventricles are in their normal positions, but the aorta arises from the right ventricle, and the pulmonary artery arises from the left ventricle. When the aorta is anterior and rightward with respect to the pulmonary artery, as is most common, D-transposition is present. The native anatomy has the pulmonary and systemic circulations in parallel, with deoxygenated blood recirculating between the right side of the heart and the systemic circulation, whereas oxygenated blood recirculates from the left side of the heart to the lungs. The condition is incompatible with life unless a VSD, PDA, or ASD is present or an ASD is created; a hemodynamically significant VSD is present in 15% of cases. Subpulmonary obstruction of the left ventricular outflow tract occurs in 10 to 25% of cases.

The Senning or Mustard atrial baffle repairs, which were the first corrective procedures, redirect oxygenated blood from the left atrium to the right ventricle so that it may be ejected into the aorta while deoxygenated blood detours the right atrium and heads for the left ventricle and into the pulmonary artery. Although this operation results in acyanotic physiology, the right ventricle assumes a permanent position under the aorta and pumps against systemic pressures, a lifelong task for which it was not designed. When the subpulmonary obstruction is significant, the Rastelli procedure reroutes blood at the ventricular level by tunneling the left ventricle to the aorta inside the heart through a VSD. A conduit is then inserted outside the heart between the left ventricle and aorta. The best current option, which is the arterial switch operation, transects the aorta and pulmonary artery above their respective valves and switches them to become realigned with their physiologic outflow tracts and appropriate ventricles. The proximal coronary arteries are translocated from the sinuses of the native aorta to the neoaorta (native pulmonary artery). In this operation, each ventricle reassumes the role that it was embryologically destined to fulfill. Long-term complications include neoaortic regurgitation, supravalvular stenosis, and chronotropic incompetence. In addition, surveillance is required for possible coronary artery complications.[8]

At present, adults with transposition of the great arteries most commonly have undergone an atrial baffle repair, with an expected 15-year survival rate of 75% and a 20-year survival rate of 70%. For patients with an atrial baffle procedure, symptoms include exercise intolerance, palpitations caused by bradyarrhythmias or atrial flutter, and right ventricular failure. The patient is typically acyanotic unless a baffle leak exists. Reoperation is required in approximately 20% of patients for baffle-related complications, progressive left ventricular outflow tract stenosis, or severe tricuspid regurgitation.

If an adult patient is cyanotic and has a native intracardiac shunt or a palliative shunt, referral to an appropriate facility should be undertaken to explore the possibility of intracardiac repair. Comprehensive echocardiographic imaging should be performed in a specialized adult congenital center. Echocardiography can confirm the diagnosis and explore related abnormalities.

Congenitally Corrected Transposition of the Great Arteries

In congenitally corrected transposition of the great arteries, the great arteries are transposed, the ventricles are inverted, but the atria remain in their normal position. The systemic circulation (left atrium, morphologic right ventricle, and aorta) and pulmonary circulation (right atrium, morphologic left ventricle, and pulmonary artery) are in series. The patient is therefore acyanotic unless an intracardiac shunt is also present. The right ventricle is aligned with the aorta and performs lifelong systemic work, which accounts in part for its eventual failure. Associated lesions include a VSD, pulmonary stenosis, and Ebstein malformation of the left-sided tricuspid valve. Complete heart block develops at a rate of 2% per year. Patients with congenitally corrected transposition of the great arteries and no other associated defects can remain free of symptoms until the sixth decade, at which time significant atrioventricular valve regurgitation, failure of the right (systemic) ventricle, supraventricular arrhythmias, and heart block occur.

Right-Sided Ebstein Anomaly

The septal and posterior cusps of the tricuspid valve are largely derived from the right ventricle as it liberates a layer of muscle that skirts away from the cavity to become valve tissue. When this process occurs abnormally, the posterior and septal cusps of the tricuspid valve remain tethered to the muscle and adhere to the right ventricular surface—hence the diagnostic hallmark of Ebstein anomaly, apical displacement of the septal tricuspid leaflet.

In right-sided Ebstein anomaly of the tricuspid valve, the right side of the heart consists of three anatomic components: the right atrium proper, the true right ventricle, and the atrialized portion of the right ventricle between the two. The displaced septal and posterior tricuspid leaflets lie between the atrialized right ventricle and the true right ventricle. In mild Ebstein anomaly, the degree of tricuspid leaflet tethering is only mild, the anterior leaflet retains mobility, and the size of the true right ventricle is only mildly reduced. Severe Ebstein anomaly is associated with severe tethering of the tricuspid leaflet tissue and a diminutive, hypocontractile true right ventricle. Functionally, the valve is regurgitant because it is unable to appose its three leaflets during ventricular contraction. Valvular regurgitation and asynchronous, abnormal right ventricular function cause the dilation and right-sided heart failure observed in the more severe forms of the lesion. The wide spectrum of severity of the anomaly is based on the degree of tricuspid leaflet tethering and the relative proportion of atrialized and true right ventricle. The most common associated cardiac defect, a secundum ASD or patent foramen ovale, is reported in more than 50% of patients. On physical examination, a clicking "sail sound" is heard as the second component of S_1 when tricuspid valve closure becomes loud and delayed.

The 12-lead ECG typically shows highly peaked P waves with a wide, often bizarre-looking QRS complex. Preexcitation occurs in 20% of patients; supraventricular tachyarrhythmias, atrial fibrillation, and atrial flutter occur in 30 to 40% of patients and constitute the most common findings in adolescents and adults with right-sided Ebstein anomaly.

When patients of all ages are taken together, the predicted mortality is approximately 50% by the fourth or fifth decade. Complications include atrial arrhythmias due to severe right atrial enlargement and cyanosis caused by a right-to-left atrial shunt as tricuspid insufficiency increases and the right ventricle fails. Atrial arrhythmias, cyanosis, and the presence of an intra-atrial communication also increase the risk for stroke.

Intervention is considered when functional status or cyanosis worsens, significant atrial arrhythmias are documented, or a cerebrovascular accident occurs. Surgical options include replacement or repair of the tricuspid valve and closure of the ASD. The feasibility of tricuspid valvuloplasty depends on the size and mobility of the anterior tricuspid leaflet, which is used to construct a unicuspid right-sided valve.

Atrioventricular Canal Defect

Embryologic septation of the atrioventricular canal results in closure of the inferior portion of the interatrial septum and the superior portion of the interventricular septum. Septation is achieved with the growth of endocardial cushions, which also contribute to development of the mitral and tricuspid valves. Hence, the nomenclature *atrioventricular canal defect* or *endocardial cushion defect* is used to designate this group of anomalies.

A partial atrioventricular canal defect refers to an ostium primum ASD with a cleft mitral valve. The anomaly is manifested as a hemodynamic combination of an ASD with a variable degree of mitral regurgitation. The 12-lead ECG shows the typical findings of left axis deviation with a Q wave in leads I and aVL and a prolonged PR interval. The echocardiogram shows a defect in the inferior portion of the interatrial septum and a cleft mitral valve.

A complete atrioventricular canal defect is an uncommon defect consisting of a primum ASD, an inlet VSD that usually extends to the membranous interventricular septum, and a common atrioventricular valve. Adults who have not been operated on usually have Eisenmenger syndrome unless concomitant pulmonary stenosis has protected the pulmonary vascular bed or the VSD has undergone spontaneous closure, in which case the physiologic consequences are similar to those of a partial atrioventricular canal.

Surgical repair of an atrioventricular defect consists of closing the interatrial or interventricular communication with reconstruction of the common atrioventricular valve or closure of the cleft in the mitral valve. An adult who has undergone repair may have significant residual regurgitation of the mitral or tricuspid valve. Even after surgery, acquired subaortic obstruction can occur in the long left ventricular outflow tract, which has a classic gooseneck deformity on cardiac angiography.

Univentricular Heart and Tricuspid Atresia

The terms *single ventricle, common ventricle,* and *univentricular heart* have been used interchangeably to describe the double-inlet ventricle, in which one ventricular chamber receives flow from both the tricuspid and mitral valves. In 75 to 90% of cases, the single ventricle is a morphologic left ventricle. Obstruction of one of the great arteries is common, and life expectancy is short without an operation. The patients most likely to survive to adulthood palliated or, rarely, without surgery have a single ventricle of the left morphologic type, with pulmonary stenosis protecting the pulmonary vascular bed.

In tricuspid atresia, no orifice is found between the right atrium and right ventricle, and an underdeveloped or hypoplastic right ventricle is present. The morphologic left ventricle is consistently normally developed and therefore becomes the single functional ventricle. Typically, blood flows into the right atrium, then through an obligatory ASD and to the left atrium, where it then proceeds to the left ventricle. Variable features include a VSD, the abnormal position of the great arteries, and the relative degree of pulmonary stenosis, all of which are used to classify tricuspid atresia. Without surgery, 50% of patients die in the first 6 months and 90% in the first decade.

Adult patients rarely have not been operated on. They may be acyanotic after the Fontan operation; if cyanotic and palliated, the patient may benefit from further palliation or may be eligible for the Fontan operation. With the Glenn shunt or the Fontan operation, a direct anastomosis is created between the systemic venous and pulmonary circulations. Venous blood flows passively from the systemic veins to the pulmonary circulation and returns oxygenated to a left-sided atrium and into the single functional ventricle, which then pumps oxygenated blood into the systemic circulation. The Glenn anastomosis diverts part of the systemic venous return to the lungs, whereas the Fontan procedure makes the patient acyanotic by diverting the entire systemic venous circulation to the pulmonary vascular bed. For optimal results, a successful Fontan operation requires low pulmonary vascular resistance, preserved single ventricular function, and unobstructed anastomosis between the systemic veins and the pulmonary arteries. At 5-year follow-up, 80% or more of Fontan survivors are in New York Heart Association functional class I or II, with successful pregnancy reported in a small number of patients. When patients of all ages are considered together, 10-year survival rates vary from 60 to 70%. Late deaths are due to reoperation, arrhythmia, ventricular failure, protein-losing enteropathy, and liver dysfunction. Yearly follow-up with specialized imaging is recommended.

Vascular Malformations

AORTIC ARCH ANOMALIES

Vascular Rings and Other Arch Anomalies

One of the most frequent developmental errors of the aortic arch is an aberrant right subclavian artery originating distal to the left subclavian and coursing rightward behind the esophagus at the level of the third thoracic vertebra. Although the finding is frequent, symptoms are uncommon. When symptoms occur, the term *dysphagia lusoria* has been used in reference to swallowing difficulties that result from esophageal compression. Abnormal development of the brachial arches and dorsal aorta can result in a variety of anomalies that lead to the formation of vascular rings around the trachea and esophagus. The outcome is often benign, but symptoms of respiratory compromise or dysphagia warrant surgery. When the left pulmonary artery arises from the right and passes leftward between the trachea and esophagus, a pulmonary artery sling occurs. Symptoms of tracheal compression warrant correction.

A right aortic arch occurs when the aortic arch courses toward the right instead of the left. Mirror-image branching is the most common anatomic variant. In most cases, this anomaly coexists with other congenital lesions, notably tetralogy of Fallot.

ANOMALOUS VENOUS CONNECTIONS

Anomalies of Systemic Venous Return

A persistent left superior vena cava can be fortuitously diagnosed on chest radiography or on echocardiography. Its clinical relevance depends on development of the coronary sinus. If the coronary sinus is normally formed, typically the left superior vena cava drains into the right atrium through the coronary sinus. If the coronary sinus is not normally developed, the persistent left superior vena cava drains into the left atrium, and cyanosis results from the obligatory right-to-left shunt; this commonly occurs with an ASD or a complex cardiac anomaly.

Venous return above the renal veins can be abnormal with inferior vena cava interruption and azygos or hemiazygos continuation. In the former, inferior vena cava flow above the renal veins continues into the azygos vein, which courses normally up the right of the spine to empty into the junction between the superior vena cava and right atrium. In a less common anatomic arrangement, the caval flow empties into a hemiazygos vein, which empties into a persistent left superior vena cava. The finding rarely occurs in isolation but can be seen in patients with associated simple or complex malformations.

Anomalies of Pulmonary Venous Return

In partial anomalous pulmonary venous return, one or more but not all four pulmonary veins are not connected to the left atrium. The most common pattern has the right pulmonary veins connected to the superior vena cava, usually with a sinus venosus ASD. Anomalous connection of the right pulmonary veins to the inferior vena cava results in a chest radiographic shadow that resembles a Turkish sword, hence the designation *scimitar syndrome.* Associated anomalies include hypoplasia of the right lung, anomalies of the bronchial system, hypoplasia of the right pulmonary artery, and dextroposition of the heart. Partial anomalous pulmonary venous return results in a left-to-right shunt physiology similar to that of an ASD.

In total anomalous pulmonary venous return, all the pulmonary veins connect abnormally to either the right atrium or one of the systemic veins above or below the diaphragm. Concurrent obstruction of the pulmonary veins is present when drainage occurs below the diaphragm and variable when drainage occurs above it. An ASD is essential to sustain life. One third of cases occur with major complex cardiac malformations.

In cor triatriatum, the pulmonary veins drain into an accessory chamber that is usually connected to the left atrium through an opening of variable size. The hemodynamic consequences are determined by the size of this opening and are similar to those of mitral stenosis. If symptoms of pulmonary venous hypertension occur, surgical treatment is indicated.

CARDIAC MALPOSITIONS

The normal heart is left sided and hence the designation *levocardia*. Cardiac malpositions are defined in terms of the intrathoracic position of the heart in relation to the position of the viscera (visceral situs), which are usually concordant with the position of the atria. That is, when the liver is on the right and the stomach is on the left, the atrium receiving systemic venous blood (right atrium) is right sided and the atrium receiving pulmonary venous blood (left atrium) is left sided. Asplenia and polysplenia syndromes are associated with a variety of complex cardiovascular malformations.

Dextrocardia and Mesocardia

In dextrocardia, the heart is on the right side of the thorax with or without situs inversus. When the heart is right sided with inverted atria, the stomach is right sided, and the liver is left sided, the combination is dextrocardia with situs inversus. In this arrangement, also called *mirror-image dextrocardia*, the ventricles are inverted, but so are the viscera and therefore the atria. The heart usually functions normally, and the diagnosis is often fortuitous. The heart sounds are louder on the right side of the chest, and the liver is palpable on the left. The chest radiograph shows a right-sided cardiac apex with a lower left hemidiaphragm and a right-sided stomach bubble. The ECG shows an inverted P and T wave in lead I with a negative QRS deflection and a reverse pattern between aVR and aVL. A mirror-image progression is seen from V_1 to a right-sided V_6 lead. An echocardiogram should be performed to ensure that intracardiac anatomy is normal.

When dextrocardia with situs solitus occurs, the ventricles are inverted but not the viscera and therefore not the atria. Associated severe cardiac malformations are typical.

In mesocardia, the heart is centrally located in the chest with normal atrial and visceral anatomy. The apex is central or rightward displaced on the chest radiograph. Typically, no associated cardiac malformations are present.

SPECIALIZED ISSUES

Endocarditis Prophylaxis

Prolonged survival of patients with complex congenital heart disease has resulted in a population at increased risk for infective endocarditis (Chapter 76). Adults with congenital heart disease should be informed about the risks of endocarditis. Any unexplained fever requires blood cultures to be drawn before antibiotics are initiated. Thorough transthoracic and transesophageal echocardiograms should be performed to assess the presence of vegetations. If infection of prosthetic material is suspected, early consultation with a specialist who has access to a congenital heart surgeon should be initiated because of the potential for rapid deterioration. The risk of endocarditis is highest in patients with cyanotic congenital heart disease and next highest in patients with endocardial cushion defects.[9]

Antibiotic prophylaxis before dental procedures that involve manipulation of the gingiva, periapical regions of the teeth, or mucosal tissue is indicated in patients with previous infective endocarditis, unrepaired cyanotic lesions, palliative shunts or conduits, prosthetic valves or prosthetic materials used for valve repair, repaired congenital heart disease with prosthetic material or transcatheter device within 6 months of intervention, and repaired congenital heart disease with residual lesions at or adjacent to the site of a prosthetic patch or device (Chapter 76). It is also reasonable to consider prophylaxis against endocarditis before vaginal delivery at the time of membrane rupture in such patients. Prophylaxis is not indicated for nondental procedures in the absence of active infection.

Exercise

The goal of exercise evaluation is to assess the functional results of therapeutic interventions and to provide guidelines for exercise prescriptions.[10]

TABLE 69-2 EXERCISE RECOMMENDATIONS IN ADULTS WITH CONGENITAL HEART DISEASE

CONDITION	UNRESTRICTED	LOW-MODERATE INTENSITY*	PROHIBITED
ASD†	No PHT; no arrhythmia; normal ventricular function	PA pressure >40 mm Hg *with* normal ETT; no arrhythmia	Eisenmenger
VSD†	Small; no PHT; no arrhythmia; normal ventricular function	Moderate VSD	Eisenmenger
PDA†	Small; no PHT; no arrhythmia; normal ventricular function	PA pressure >40 mm Hg *with* normal ETT; no arrhythmia	Eisenmenger
Coarctation‡	Gradient ≤20 mm Hg arm to leg; normal BP at rest and exercise	Gradient ≥20 mm Hg arm to leg *with* normal BP and normal ETT	Gradient ≥50 mm Hg arm to leg *or* aortic aneurysm
PS	Gradient <40 mm Hg; no arrhythmia; normal ventricular function	Gradient 40-60 mm Hg	Gradient ≥70 mm Hg *or* ventricular arrhythmia
AS	Gradient, <30 mm Hg; normal ECG; normal ETT; asymptomatic	Gradient 30-50 mm Hg *with* normal ECG, normal ETT; asymptomatic	Gradient >50 mm Hg *or* ventricular arrhythmia
TOF after repair	Normal RV pressure; no shunt; no arrhythmia	Increased RV pressure *or* moderate PR *or* SVT	RV pressure ≥65% systemic *or* ventricular arrhythmia on ETT *or* severe PR
Mustard or Senning		No cardiomegaly, arrhythmia, or syncope; normal ETT	Cardiomegaly *or* arrhythmia at rest or exercise
c-TGA unoperated	No cardiomegaly; mild TR; no arrhythmia; normal ETT	Moderate RV dysfunction, moderate TR; no arrhythmia	Severe TR *or* uncontrolled arrhythmia
Ebstein anomaly	Mild Ebstein; no arrhythmia; operated with mild TR	Moderate TR *with* no arrhythmia	Severe Ebstein *or* uncontrolled arrhythmia
Fontan		Normal O_2 saturation *with* near-normal ETT and ventricular function	Moderate-severe MR or TR *or* uncontrolled arrhythmia

*Based on peak dynamic and static components of exercise during competition for individual sports (see credit line).
†Unoperated or 6 months after surgery.
‡Unoperated or 1 year after surgery.
AS = aortic stenosis; ASD = atrial septal defect; BP = blood pressure; c-TGA = corrected transposition of the great arteries; ECG = electrocardiogram; ETT = exercise tolerance test; MR = mitral regurgitation; PA = pulmonary artery; PDA = patent ductus arteriosus; PHT = pulmonary hypertension; PR = pulmonary regurgitation; PS = pulmonary stenosis; RV = right ventricle; SVT = supraventricular tachyarrhythmia; TOF = tetralogy of Fallot; TR = tricuspid regurgitation; VSD = ventricular septal defect.
Based on guidelines recommended in Graham TP, Driscoll DJ, Gersony WM, et al. Task Force 2: Congenital heart disease. *J Am Coll Cardiol.* 2005;45:1326-1333.

Patients with residual hemodynamic lesions or unrepaired congenital cardiac anomalies should be evaluated on an annual basis with a physical examination, an ECG, and a cardiac ultrasonographic examination if indicated. Pertinent additional tests may include Holter monitoring and exercise testing. Attention should be directed to the detection of pulmonary hypertension, arrhythmias, myocardial dysfunction, and symptoms such as exercise-induced dizziness, syncope, dyspnea, or chest pain.

A series of exercise guidelines have been proposed for major groups of congenital heart defects (Table 69-2). Patients beyond 6 months after repair of a single shunt lesion without pulmonary hypertension, arrhythmias, or evidence of myocardial dysfunction can participate in all sports. With residual shunts, if the peak pulmonary artery pressure is less than 40 mm Hg in the absence of ventricular dysfunction or significant arrhythmias, patients can enjoy a free range of activity. Patients with elevated pulmonary vascular resistance are at risk of sudden death during intense exercise; although most self-limit their activity, participation in competitive sports is contraindicated. Patients with aortic and pulmonary stenosis should be counseled as recommended earlier, according to gradient severity. For patients with uncomplicated aortic coarctation, athletic participation is permitted if the arm-leg blood pressure gradient is 20 mm Hg or less at rest and the peak systolic blood pressure during exercise is normal. For patients after tetralogy of Fallot repair, repair of transposition of the great arteries, and the Fontan operation, exercise recommendations vary according to residual ventricular function and the presence or absence of arrhythmias. For such complex patients, care in a specialized center is associated with better outcomes.[11]

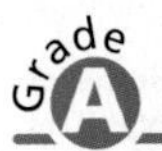

Grade A References

A1. Gatzoulis MA, Beghetti M, Galiè N, et al. Longer-term bosentan therapy improves functional capacity in Eisenmenger syndrome: results of the BREATHE-5 open-label extension study. *Int J Cardiol.* 2008;127:27-32.

A2. Attie F, Rosas M, Granados N, et al. Surgical treatment for secundum atrial septal defects in patients >40 years old: a randomized clinical trial. *J Am Coll Cardiol.* 2001;38:2035-2042.

A3. Furlan AJ, Reisman M, Massaro J, et al. Closure or medical therapy for cryptogenic stroke with patent foramen ovale. *N Engl J Med.* 2012;366:991-999.

A4. Meier B, Kalesan B, Mattle HP, et al. Percutaneous closure of patent foramen ovale in cryptogenic embolism. *N Engl J Med.* 2013;368:1083-1091.

A5. Carroll JD, Saver JL, Thaler DE, et al. Closure of patent foramen ovale versus medical therapy after cryptogenic stroke. *N Engl J Med.* 2013;368:1092-1100.

A6. Yang J, Yang L, Yu S, et al. Transcatheter versus surgical closure of perimembranous ventricular septal defects in children: a randomized controlled trial. *J Am Coll Cardiol.* 2014;63:1159-1168.

GENERAL REFERENCES

For the General References and other additional features, please visit Expert Consult at https://expertconsult.inkling.com.

70

ATHEROSCLEROSIS, THROMBOSIS, AND VASCULAR BIOLOGY

GÖRAN K. HANSSON AND ANDERS HAMSTEN

Atherosclerosis is the underlying cause of most cases of myocardial infarction, ischemic stroke, and peripheral arterial disease.[1] It is also a major cause of chronic heart failure and vascular dementia. Atherosclerosis, which is a chronic inflammatory response to the accumulation of lipid in the artery wall, is characterized by clinically silent intimal plaques that develop in arteries for years and even decades.[2] Fissuring or erosion of atherosclerotic plaques triggers the formation of a thrombus that accumulates during seconds to minutes to cause acute ischemia of the end organ. This ischemia, in turn, results in the dramatic clinical manifestations. It is estimated that approximately 90% of cases of myocardial infarction (Chapter 73), 60% of strokes (Chapter 407), most cases of heart failure (Chapter 58), and up to one third of all cases of dementia (Chapter 402) are due to atherosclerosis.

RISK FACTORS FOR ATHEROSCLEROSIS

The major risk factors that promote the development of atherosclerosis are an elevated low-density lipoprotein (LDL) cholesterol level, cigarette smoking, type 2 diabetes (Chapter 229), hypertension (Chapter 67), and a family history of coronary heart disease, ischemic stroke, or peripheral arterial disease. Other conditions that increase the risk of atherosclerotic disease or events include a low high-density lipoprotein (HDL) level (Chapter 206), abdominal obesity, hypertriglyceridemia, high plasma levels of lipoprotein (a), hyperfibrinogenemia, the inflammatory marker C-reactive protein, and physical inactivity (Chapter 52). Other emerging risk factors, including uric acid, psychosocial stress encompassing external stressors (e.g., job stress, life events, and financial problems), and reactions to stress (e.g., depression [Chapter 397], anxiety, psychosocial distress, and sleep disturbances [Chapters 100 and 405]), also appear to contribute. Elevation of plasma total homocysteine is also associated with increased cardiovascular risk, but it is possible that chronic renal dysfunction accounts for at least some of the vascular disease seen in hyperhomocysteinemia.

An atherogenic lipoprotein phenotype has been defined as the presence of a predominance of small, dense LDL particles, hypertriglyceridemia, and low plasma HDL cholesterol concentration. This lipoprotein phenotype, which is strongly linked to obesity, insulin resistance, hypertension, and abnormalities in postprandial lipoprotein metabolism, is similar to the so-called metabolic syndrome in that both are associated with a cluster of atherogenic and thrombotic risk factors—raised plasma levels of fibrinogen, plasminogen activator inhibitor-1, and coagulation factor VII as well as platelet hyperactivity. The inflammatory biomarker C-reactive protein, which is a predictor of cardiovascular events, is not causatively related to atherosclerosis but reflects ongoing inflammation, in atherosclerotic lesions or elsewhere in the body, that may accelerate the atherosclerotic process.

FORMATION OF ATHEROSCLEROTIC LESIONS

Atherosclerosis is thought to be initiated when apolipoprotein B–containing lipoproteins, predominantly LDL, accumulate in the vascular intima, the innermost layer of the artery (Fig. 70-1). Small, dense LDL particles are particularly prone to accumulate in the intima, where they associate with proteoglycans of the extracellular matrix. Lipoprotein lipase produced locally in the artery can bridge LDL to the extracellular matrix, and phospholipase and sphingomyelinase actions may contribute to the entrapment of LDL. Once trapped in the artery wall, LDL particles can be attacked by enzymes such as myeloperoxidase and NADPH oxidases; they may also be modified by nonenzymatic oxidation. During oxidative modification of LDL, certain biologically active oxidized phospholipid species are released and activate endothelial cells and macrophages. Such activation leads to production of chemokines and expression of leukocyte adhesion molecules that together instigate recruitment of monocytes and T cells to the intima. Local growth factors induce recruited monocytes to develop into macrophages.

In the intima, macrophages take up oxidized LDL through their scavenger receptors, start to accumulate cholesterol, and are gradually transformed into cholesterol-laden foam cells.[3] Some macrophages in the intima produce proinflammatory mediators, including tumor necrosis factor (TNF), interleukin-1, proinflammatory eicosanoids, radical oxygen and nitrogen species, and prothrombotic factors. At least some of this inflammatory activity may be instigated when intracellular cholesterol microcrystals in the macrophage activate the inflammasome machinery that generates the inflammatory mediator interleukin-1β.

T cells that are stimulated to enter the intima may recognize antigens presented by macrophages.[4] These antigens include components of LDL, other endogenous proteins, and possibly microbial antigens. Activated intimal T cells produce T_H1-type cytokines, such as interferon-γ, TNF, and lymphotoxin, all of which are strongly proatherogenic. For example, interferon-γ release also inhibits collagen fiber formation and smooth muscle proliferation. With the entry and activation of T cells and macrophages, the accumulation of lipid in the intima leads to the chronic inflammatory disease process of atherosclerosis.

Although adaptive immunity is believed to exert a net proatherogenic effect, antiatherogenic immune responses against LDL involve activation of regulatory T cells, secretion of the anti-inflammatory cytokines interleukin-10 and transforming growth factor-β, and production of anti-LDL antibodies.[5] In addition to T cells and macrophages, atheroma formation is also stimulated by dendritic cells that take up and present antigen and by mast cells that secrete enzymes and bioactive mediators.

Triglyceride-rich lipoprotein remnant particles, which have adverse effects on endothelial function, penetrate into the subendothelial space of normal intima and atherosclerotic plaques, where they are retained. Inflammation

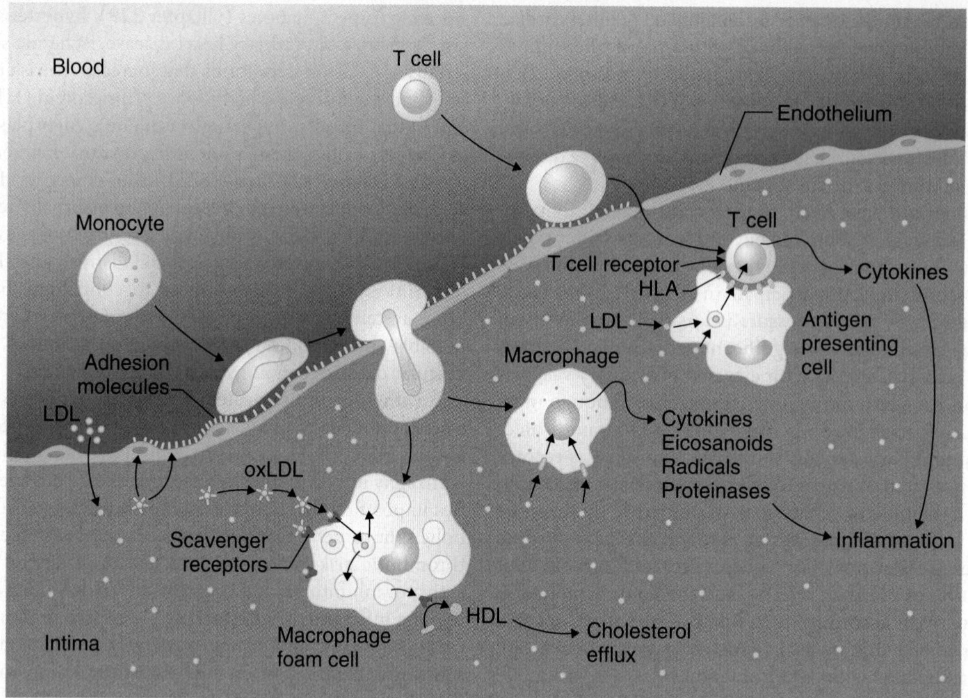

FIGURE 70-1. **Formation of atherosclerotic plaques. Low-density lipoproteins (LDL) transit from the blood stream to the arterial intima and accumulate under the endothelial cell layer. LDL particles undergo oxidative modification in the intima (denoted by spikes on LDL particles), thereby leading to their binding to scavenger receptors and uptake by macrophages, which accumulate cholesterol and develop into foam cells. Cholesterol efflux to high-density lipoprotein (HDL) counteracts the tendency to foam cell formation. Molecules released from oxidatively modified LDL (oxLDL) activate endothelial cells to express leukocyte adhesion molecules that promote binding of monocytes and T cells to the surface of the artery. Chemokines stimulate monocytes and T cells to migrate into the intima, where the monocytes differentiate into macrophages. Although many macrophages develop into foam cells, some are activated, thereby leading to release of proinflammatory cytokines, eicosanoids, radicals, and proteases. T cells entering through mechanisms similar to those of monocytes can recognize local antigens, such as LDL components, which are presented to them by antigen-presenting cells (dendritic cells and macrophages) that express human leukocyte antigen (HLA) molecules. T cells whose receptors can recognize local antigens are activated, thereby leading to release of a host of cytokines that can activate macrophages and enhance vascular inflammation. (Modified from Hansson GK. Inflammation, atherosclerosis, and coronary artery disease. *N Engl J Med.* 2005;352: 1685-1695.)**

may increase the levels of such lipoprotein particles in blood by inhibiting their clearance. The LDL-like lipoprotein (a) particle exerts both proatherogenic and prothrombotic actions.

Conversely, antiatherogenic HDL particles counteract the formation of atherosclerotic lesions in model systems.[6] These particles mediate cholesterol efflux from cells by acting as acceptors of cholesterol delivered from specific transport proteins termed adenosine triphosphate–binding cassette (ABC) A1 and G1. In addition, HDL particles carry anti-inflammatory and antioxidant proteins.

GROWTH, DEATH, AND THE PROGRESSION OF DISEASE

Early atherosclerotic lesions grow by the accumulation of cholesterol; the infiltration of inflammatory cells; the activation, proliferation, and death of such cells; and the gradual development of a core that contains cellular debris and lipids. As a tissue response to this process, smooth muscle cells form a subendothelial cap structure dominated by collagen fibers that are produced by these cells. The collagen cap mechanically stabilizes the plaque and creates a barrier between the hemostatic components of the blood and the thrombogenic material of the plaque. Until the plaque is far advanced, compensatory enlargement ("remodeling") of the arterial wall prevents it from significantly protruding into the arterial lumen. However, after the plaque has enlarged to a sufficient size, the lumen narrows as the plaque grows, and the artery remodels inward, often accompanied by exaggerated or paradoxical vasoconstriction.

PLAQUE ACTIVATION, THROMBOSIS, AND INFARCTION

The atherosclerotic process typically is silent for months, years, and even decades, and it may never result in clinical manifestations. However, if the plaque's surface is damaged, thrombotic occlusion of the artery may ensue.[7] Surface continuity may be damaged by fissuring (so-called plaque rupture, observed in 60 to 80% of cases of acute coronary syndrome) or surface erosion (present in 20 to 40% of cases with coronary thrombosis, especially in women and young victims of sudden coronary death). Recent studies suggest that the proportion of infarctions caused by rupture vs erosion is changing, with more cases due to erosion and fewer to overt plaque rupture.[8] Fissures and erosions trigger atherothrombosis by exposing thrombogenic material inside the plaque, such as phospholipids, tissue factor, and matrix molecules, to platelets and coagulation factors (Fig. 70-2). Platelet aggregates that form on these exposed surfaces are stabilized by a fibrin network. Tissue factor, expressed in vascular smooth muscle cells and macrophages of the atherosclerotic plaque, is the primary cellular initiator of the blood coagulation cascade that leads to fibrin formation. Atherothrombi expand rapidly and can fill the lumen within minutes, thereby leading to ischemia and infarction.

A range of factors may contribute to atherothrombosis.[9,10] Disturbance of the balance between prothrombotic and fibrinolytic activity on the plaque surface probably plays an important role for precipitating the thrombotic event, but the precise sequence of events that operate in vivo is not yet known.

The cause of plaque rupture also remains unclear. Clinical studies have associated ischemic atherothrombotic events such as myocardial infarction (Chapter 73) and stroke (Chapter 407) with infections and stressful events. Histopathologic analysis shows increased inflammation with infiltration of macrophages, activated T cells, dendritic cells, and mast cells as well as reduced thickness of the fibrous cap and increased neovascularity at sites of plaque rupture and thrombosis. Matrix metalloproteinases and cysteine proteinases, which are produced by macrophages, are found at sites of plaque rupture and have been implicated in rupture, but their effects on the composition and size of lesions are complex. Cell death alone may be an important trigger of plaque rupture. Apoptotic cells contained in the plaque are usually removed by efferocytosis. If this process fails, secondary necrosis ensues, thereby leading to reduced mechanical integrity and accumulation of prothrombotic material from dead cells.

Ruptured plaques also tend to have a large necrotic lipid core. In contrast, plaques underlying erosions do not have a large lipid core and show less inflammation compared with ruptured plaques. Plaque rupture frequently occurs without clinical manifestations, possibly reflecting variation in the

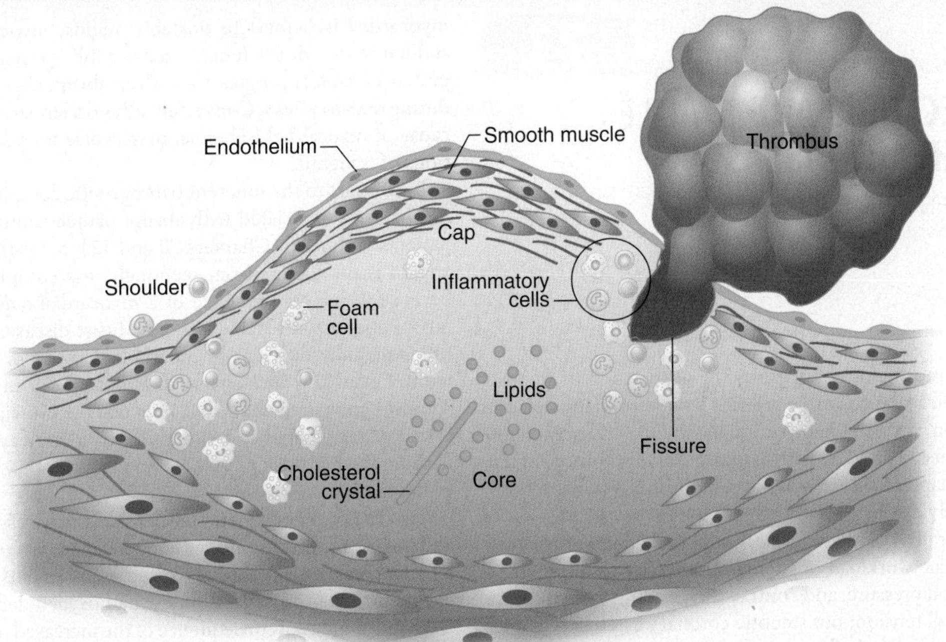

FIGURE 70-2. **Plaque rupture and atherothrombosis. The advanced atherosclerotic plaque has a central core with lipids (especially cholesterol), live and dead cells, necrotic material from dead foam cells, and calcium salts. The plaque is overlaid by a fibrous cap that consists of smooth muscle cells and collagen (produced by the muscle cells) and covered by an intact layer of endothelial cells. Inflammatory cells (macrophages, T cells, mast cells, dendritic cells, and occasional B cells) are interspersed with these components and are particularly abundant in the shoulder regions of plaques, where fissures (also called ruptures) may expose thrombogenic core material (e.g., lipids, collagen, tissue factor) to blood components. This event triggers platelet aggregation and humoral coagulation, thereby leading to thrombus formation at the site of fissuring. Thrombi may expand locally to obstruct blood flow or they may detach to cause embolization. (Modified from Hansson GK. Inflammation, atherosclerosis, and coronary artery disease. *N Engl J Med.* 2005;352:1685-1695.)**

thrombotic response depending on the thrombogenicity of exposed plaque constituents, local hemorrheology, shear-induced platelet activation, systemic clotting activity, fibrinolytic function, and sensitivity of the end organ to ischemia.

PRINCIPLES OF ANTIATHEROSCLEROTIC THERAPY

Current treatment of atherosclerosis aims to control risk factors and to maintain or to restore perfusion in affected arteries. However, progress in understanding the pathogenesis of atherosclerosis is expected to result in more direct approaches. To date, firmly established interventions include smoking cessation, dietary and pharmacologic reduction of LDL cholesterol (Chapter 206), and management of blood pressure (Chapter 67). Available data also strongly support intervention directed toward hyperglycemia (Chapter 229), hypertriglyceridemia (Chapter 206), obesity (Chapter 220), and physical inactivity (Chapter 16).

Cholesterol-lowering statins clearly reduce atherosclerotic lesions and inhibit their progression.[A1] Statins also prevent nitroglycerin-induced endothelial dysfunction and nitrate tolerance, and they inhibit immune activity and inflammation.[A2,A3] Aspirin and other inhibitors of platelet aggregation, β-adrenergic receptor blockers, and angiotensin-converting enzyme inhibitors or angiotensin II antagonists are also part of the routine secondary prevention of coronary heart disease (Chapters 71, 72, and 73). Inhibitors of platelet aggregation are widely used for secondary prevention of atherosclerotic cardiovascular disease. Aspirin inhibits formation of proaggregatory prostaglandins, whereas other inhibitors of platelet aggregation modulate expression of platelet adhesion molecules. Nitroglycerin and similar compounds that mimic the action of endogenous nitric oxide remain the most important vasodilators used in secondary prevention (Chapter 71). Eicosapentaenoic acid treatment has also shown promising results in secondary prevention.

FUTURE DIRECTIONS

Novel therapeutic approaches include new lipid-lowering treatment, immunosuppressive and anti-inflammatory compounds, and vaccination with disease-related antigens. Investigational agents targeting atherogenic lipoproteins include proprotein convertase subtilisin kexin type 9 (PCSK9),[A4] inhibitors of squalene synthase, microsomal triglyceride transfer protein, and antisense oligonucleotides to apolipoprotein B. In contrast, therapies to raise HDL levels have been disappointing (Chapter 206). Peroxisome proliferator-activated receptor agonists (Chapter 229), besides their beneficial effects on lipid and blood glucose levels, have shown direct antiatherosclerotic effects in experimental studies. However, inhibitors of secreted and lipoprotein-associated phospholipase A_2 have not reduced cardiovascular events in clinical trials.[A5,A6]

Members of the interleukin-1 and TNF families of proinflammatory proteins, eicosanoids, and cell surface proteins promoting antigen-specific T-cell activation are particularly promising targets of anti-inflammatory therapy, whereas stimulation of anti-inflammatory signaling pathways represents a different potential antiatherosclerotic therapy. Patients whose asthma is treated with the leukotriene receptor blocker montelukast have a reduced risk for ischemic stroke and myocardial infarction, but whether it or other anti-inflammatory agents will be clinically useful for reducing cardiovascular events is uncertain.

Vaccination against immunogenic epitopes in the protein and lipid moieties of LDL may induce anti-inflammatory regulatory immunity and also reduce LDL uptake in cells of the atherosclerotic lesion. Identification of genes that increase the risk of coronary artery disease by genome-wide association studies is likely to generate a new set of potential targets.[11]

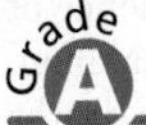

Grade A References

A1. Taylor F, Huffman MD, Macedo AF, et al. Statins for the primary prevention of cardiovascular disease. *Cochrane Database Syst Rev.* 2013;1:CD004816.

A2. Liuni A, Luca MC, Di Stolfo G, et al. Coadministration of atorvastatin prevents nitroglycerin-induced endothelial dysfunction and nitrate tolerance in healthy humans. *J Am Coll Cardiol.* 2011;57:93-98.

A3. Ridker PM, Danielson E, Fonseca FA, et al. Rosuvastatin to prevent vascular events in men and women with elevated C-reactive protein. *N Engl J Med.* 2008;359:2195-2207.

A4. Blom DJ, Hala T, Bolognese M, et al. A 52-week placebo-controlled trial of evolocumab in hyperlipidemia. *N Engl J Med.* 2014;370:1809-1819.

A5. White HD, Held C, Stewart R, et al. Darapladib for preventing ischemic events in stable coronary heart disease. *N Engl J Med.* 2014;370:1702-1711.

A6. Nicholls SJ, Kastelein JJ, Schwartz GG, et al. Varespladib and cardiovascular events in patients with an acute coronary syndrome: the VISTA-16 randomized clinical trial. *JAMA.* 2014;311:252-262.

GENERAL REFERENCES

For the General References and other additional features, please visit Expert Consult at https://expertconsult.inkling.com.

71

ANGINA PECTORIS AND STABLE ISCHEMIC HEART DISEASE

WILLIAM E. BODEN

DEFINITION

Ischemic heart disease is most commonly caused by obstruction or stenosis of one or more of the epicardial coronary arteries by atheromatous plaque (Chapter 70). Obstruction can result in myocardial ischemia and may culminate in infarction (Chapters 72 and 73) with associated symptoms of angina, dyspnea, heart failure (Chapter 58), arrhythmic complications (Chapters 63, 64, and 65), and ultimately death.

Angina pectoris is generally a consequence of a supply-demand imbalance: an activity increases cardiac workload or "demand," thereby resulting in an increase in heart rate, blood pressure, and contractility, leading to an increase in left ventricular (LV) wall tension; but stenotic coronary arteries (Chapter 57) are unable to augment antegrade flow or "supply" adequately in response to this increase in demand. Such an imbalance classically results in chest discomfort (Chapter 51) of varying intensity and duration. Angina pectoris is generally defined as a discomfort in the chest or adjacent areas caused by myocardial ischemia. Often, angina is described incorrectly as "chest pain." The term *angina*, however, derives from a neologism of two Latin words, *angor animi*, which literally translates into "fear of life being extinguished ('from the breast')," according to Heberden original description in 1768. Had Heberden been trying to convey the literal term for chest pain, he would more likely have used the Latin term *dolor pectoris*.

Grading of Angina Pectoris

The Canadian Cardiovascular Society (CCS) angina grading scale is a widely used four-point ordinal scale that classifies angina pectoris from mild (class I: angina occurring only during strenuous or prolonged physical activity) to severe (class IV: inability to perform any activity without angina, or angina at rest) and includes the full spectrum of angina from chronic stable to unstable (see Table 51-5). Operationally, the CCS angina scale permits clinicians to categorize patients as mild or stable (generally CCS classes I and II) versus severe or unstable (typically CCS classes III and IV). For classification purposes, subjects with stable ischemic heart disease generally exhibit CCS class I-II symptoms, which are typically provoked by exertion. Other grading systems include a specific activity scale, which is based on the metabolic cost of specific activities, and an anginal score, which integrates the clinical features and tempo of angina with electrocardiographic changes and offers independent prognostic information beyond that provided by age, gender, ventricular function, and coronary anatomy.

EPIDEMIOLOGY

An estimated 15 million Americans currently have coronary heart disease (Chapter 51).[1] Among individuals aged 45 years and older, the incidence of stable angina pectoris is about 500,000 per year, of whom about 65% are men. Nearly 8 million Americans have prevalent angina pectoris. Although deaths attributable to coronary disease have declined in the United States during the past several decades, ischemic heart disease is now the leading cause of death worldwide, and it is expected that this rate of rise will continue to accelerate in the coming decade as a consequence of the epidemic rise in obesity (Chapter 220), type 2 diabetes (Chapter 229), and the metabolic syndrome, which may give rise to an increasing risk for development of premature coronary artery disease in younger generations. An estimated 7 million patients went to emergency departments in 2010 for chest pain, and approximately 1.5 million of them were hospitalized with the acute coronary syndrome (ACS; Chapter 72).[2]

PATHOBIOLOGY

Angina is the most frequent clinical expression of myocardial ischemia. Ischemia, which rapidly develops when a mismatch arises between myocardial oxygen needs and myocardial oxygen supply, can be manifested clinically in many different ways besides angina, from no symptoms (e.g., silent myocardial ischemia) to unstable angina, myocardial infarction (MI), or sudden cardiac death. It may remain stable for many years in selected patients or may be rapidly progressive with an abrupt change in frequency and tempo during days to weeks. Conversely, atherosclerosis, which is the most common cause of myocardial ischemia, may evolve for years without any manifestations of ischemia.

In contrast to the inherent pathogenetic complexity mediated by differing mechanisms associated with abrupt plaque rupture, fissuring, or erosion in patients with ACS (Chapters 70 and 72), the pathogenesis of chronic stable angina is, by comparison, seemingly less complicated and heterogeneous because it is a consequence of a myocardial supply-demand mismatch. In most patients with stable ischemic heart disease, atherosclerosis involves a fundamentally different histopathologic process (small necrotic lipid core with an overlying thick or very thick fibrous cap and a low proclivity to plaque rupture) compared with ACS, in which the principal histopathologic picture is that of a large lipid core subtended by a thin-capped fibroatheroma, which harbors the high-risk or vulnerable plaque with a high proclivity for rupture (Chapter 70).

Two major pathogenetic mechanisms may result in myocardial ischemia and angina in the chronic setting: so-called *demand angina*, which is caused by an increase in myocardial oxygen requirements and workload; and *supply angina*, which is caused by diminished oxygen delivery to myocardial tissue. Demand angina is a consequence of the increased myocardial oxygen requirements that occur with increased physical activity, emotion, or stress. In a patient with chronic, restricted oxygen delivery due to atherosclerotic narrowing of a coronary artery, this increased demand may precipitate angina. Other extracardiac precipitants of angina include the excessive metabolic demands imposed by fever, thyrotoxicosis (Chapter 226), severe anemia (Chapter 158) from blood loss, tachycardia from any cause (Chapters 62, 63, and 64), hypoglycemia (Chapter 230), and pain.

By contrast, supply angina may occur in patients with either unstable angina (Chapter 72) or chronic stable angina by transient reductions in myocardial oxygen delivery as a consequence of coronary vasoconstriction with resulting dynamic coronary stenosis. In the presence of coronary luminal narrowing due to atherosclerosis, superimposed platelet thrombi and leukocytes may elaborate vasoconstrictor substances, such as serotonin and thromboxane A_2, whereas endothelial damage in diseased coronary arteries may decrease production of vasodilator substances such as nitric oxide and adenosine. The result is an abnormal physiologic vasoconstrictor response to exercise and other stimuli, such as exogenously administered adenosine, or the paradoxical vasoconstrictor response to the typical flow-mediated reactive hyperemia associated with brachial artery compression. In some clinical settings, patients who have normal coronary arteries or non–flow-limiting stenoses may exhibit dynamic obstruction alone, which can cause myocardial ischemia and result in angina at rest (Prinzmetal's [variant] angina). Conversely, in patients with severe fixed obstruction to coronary blood flow, only a minor increase in dynamic obstruction can reduce blood flow below a critical level and cause myocardial ischemia.

The pathophysiologic basis for angina and ischemia in patients with stable ischemic heart disease has important implications for the selection of anti-ischemic agents. The greater the contribution from increased myocardial oxygen requirements to the imbalance between supply and demand, the greater the likelihood that agents that reduce heart rate and wall tension, such as β-blockers or non-dihydropyridine calcium antagonists, will provide clinical benefit, whereas nitrates and calcium antagonists with more potent vasodilatory properties (particularly the dihydropyridines) will be more beneficial to alleviate angina and ischemia mediated by coronary vasoconstriction.

Although the most common cause of ischemic heart disease is atherosclerotic narrowing of the coronary arteries resulting in flow-limiting obstruction to epicardial blood flow, obstructive coronary artery disease may also have nonatherosclerotic causes, such as congenital abnormalities of the coronary arteries (Chapter 69), vasospasm, myocardial bridging, coronary arteritis in association with systemic vasculitides (Chapter 270), and radiation-induced coronary disease (Chapter 20). Radiation therapy for thoracic or mediastinal malignant neoplasms, particularly breast cancer and Hodgkin lymphoma, can cause long-term coronary microangiopathy and macroangiopathy. There is a four- to seven-fold increase in clinically significant, high-grade coronary artery stenosis of the mid and distal left anterior descending coronary artery in women with irradiated left-sided breast cancer compared with those treated with radiation for right-sided breast cancer. Myocardial ischemia and angina pectoris may also occur in the absence of obstructive coronary artery disease, as in the case of aortic valve disease (Chapter 75), hypertrophic cardiomyopathy (Chapter 60), and dilated cardiomyopathy. Moreover, ischemic heart disease may coexist with these other forms of heart disease.

CLINICAL MANIFESTATIONS

History

It is important to recognize that there are many causes of chest discomfort (see Table 51-2), that angina-like chest pain may not represent ischemic heart disease (Table 71-1), that ischemic heart disease causes symptoms other than anginal pain (Table 71-2), and that nonatherosclerotic coronary artery abnormalities may cause ischemic chest pain (Table 71-3).

Angina pectoris has four cardinal clinical features: the character of the discomfort, its site and distribution, its provocation, and its duration. The character of anginal discomfort is typically described as a pressure sensation that conveys a feeling of strangling and anxiety (Chapter 51), but patients may also use descriptors such as heaviness, squeezing, constricting, viselike, suffocating, and crushing. In some patients, especially women and the elderly, the quality of the sensation is more vague and atypical. Some patients may describe the discomfort as a burning sensation in the mid-epigastrium or as an uncomfortable, numb sensation. *Anginal equivalents* (i.e., symptoms of myocardial ischemia other than angina), such as dyspnea, fatigue, lightheadedness or dizziness, and gastric eructations, also may be manifestations of ischemic heart disease.

TABLE 71-1 PROBABILITY (%) OF CORONARY ARTERY DISEASE BY AGE, GENDER, AND SYMPTOMS

GENDER	AGE (yr)	DEFINITE ANGINA	ATYPICAL ANGINA	NONCARDIAC CHEST PAIN
Men	30-39	83	46	3
	40-49	88	57	12
	50-59	94	71	18
	60-69	95	78	31
	≥70	97	94	63
Women	30-39	—	20	4
	40-49	56	31	4
	50-59	68	30	6
	60-69	81	48	10
	≥70	96	56	—

From Chaitman BR, Bourassa MG, Davis K, et al. Angiographic prevalence of high-risk coronary artery disease in patient subsets (CASS). *Circulation.* 1981;64:360-367.

TABLE 71-2 NON–CHEST PAIN SYMPTOMS OF CHRONIC ISCHEMIC HEART DISEASE

DYSPNEA

Dyspnea on exertion
Dyspnea at rest
Paroxysmal nocturnal dyspnea
Temporal change of increasing exertional dyspnea with declining effort tolerance

NON–CHEST LOCATIONS OF DISCOMFORT (EITHER EXERTIONAL OR AT REST)

Neck or mandibular discomfort or pain
Throat tightness
Shoulder discomfort
Upper arm or forearm discomfort (more often left-sided)
Interscapular or infrascapular discomfort

MID-EPIGASTRIC OR ABDOMINAL

Mid-epigastric burning, often postprandially
Sharp abdominal pain (atypical, but more common in women)
Right upper quadrant discomfort (may mimic gallbladder disease or pancreatitis)
Nausea or vomiting (often associated with increased vagal tone secondary to inferior myocardial ischemia or infarction)

DIAPHORESIS

EXCESSIVE FATIGUE AND WEAKNESS

Often a discernible prodrome of increasing fatigue with declining effort tolerance

DIZZINESS AND SYNCOPE

Uncommon, unless precipitated or exacerbated by alterations in heart rate or rhythm (e.g., bradyarrhythmia, tachyarrhythmia, heart block), blood pressure (e.g., hypotension), or cardiac output (e.g., decreased cerebral perfusion)

The site and distribution of anginal discomfort are predominantly midsternal or retrosternal but can be precordial. Radiation is common, usually to the left side of the neck and shoulder and down the ulnar surface of the left arm; radiation to the right arm is less common. Discomfort radiating to the jaw is common and must be distinguished from dental pain. Epigastric discomfort alone or in association with chest pressure may occur. Provocation of angina is classically caused by physical exertion or activity, emotional stress, exposure to the cold, sexual intercourse, or eating a large meal. Angina that occurs at rest or nocturnally often heralds a change in the pattern from stable to unstable and may indicate that there is an incipient plaque rupture leading to ACS. Vasospastic (or Prinzmetal's) angina may occur spontaneously at rest or nocturnally without provocation.

The typical duration of an episode of angina pectoris is brief. An episode usually begins gradually and reaches its maximal intensity during a period of minutes before abating. It is unusual for angina pectoris to peak and trough in less than a minute, and it is common that patients with exertional angina usually prefer to rest, to sit, or to stop walking during episodes that may be precipitated by the offending activity. Chest discomfort that persists for more than 15 to 20 minutes, especially at rest or nocturnally, is likely to represent ACS or MI. By contrast, features that suggest a noncardiac etiology of angina pectoris include pleuritic pain, pain reproduced by movement or palpation of the chest wall or arms, sharp or constant pain lasting for many hours, pain or discomfort that a patient can localize to the chest wall with the tip of one finger, and very brief episodes of pain lasting seconds (Chapter 51). Typical angina pectoris is generally relieved within minutes by rest or the use of sublingual, oral, or cutaneous nitroglycerin. The response to sublingual nitroglycerin is often a helpful diagnostic tool, although some noncardiac pain (e.g., esophageal spasm) may also respond to nitroglycerin.

Although chest discomfort is usually the predominant symptom in ischemic heart disease, chest discomfort may be absent, atypical, or not prominent in some patients. Patients with stable ischemic heart disease may complain predominantly or exclusively of dyspnea, diminishing exercise tolerance, fatigue, or weakness. Others will first present with an abnormal exercise test result or other evidence of myocardial ischemia without any symptoms. Some patients may present with cardiac arrhythmias or even sudden cardiac death.

Physical Examination

Many patients with stable ischemic heart disease present with normal physical findings, but a diligent physical examination may reveal findings that represent either the consequences of myocardial ischemia or evidence of risk factors for coronary artery disease. Inspection of the eyes may reveal a corneal arcus, and examination of the skin may show xanthomas (see Fig. 51-12). Retinal arteriolar changes are common in patients with coronary artery disease who have hypertension or diabetes mellitus (see Figs. 423-26 and 423-24).

The cardiac examination is generally of limited benefit in evaluating patients with chest pain or establishing a diagnosis of ischemic heart disease.

TABLE 71-3 NONATHEROSCLEROTIC CAUSES OF ISCHEMIC CHEST PAIN

PRIMARY CARDIAC CAUSE

Coronary artery abnormalities
- Coronary spasm
- Coronary arteritis
- Coronary dissection
- Coronary artery anomalies
- Radiation-induced coronary disease

Myocardial bridging
Aortic stenosis
Hypertrophic cardiomyopathy
Dilated cardiomyopathy
Tachycardia

PRIMARY NONCARDIAC CAUSE

Anemia
Sickle cell disease
Hypoxemia
Carbon monoxide poisoning
Hyperviscosity (e.g., polycythemia)
Hyperthyroidism
Pheochromocytoma

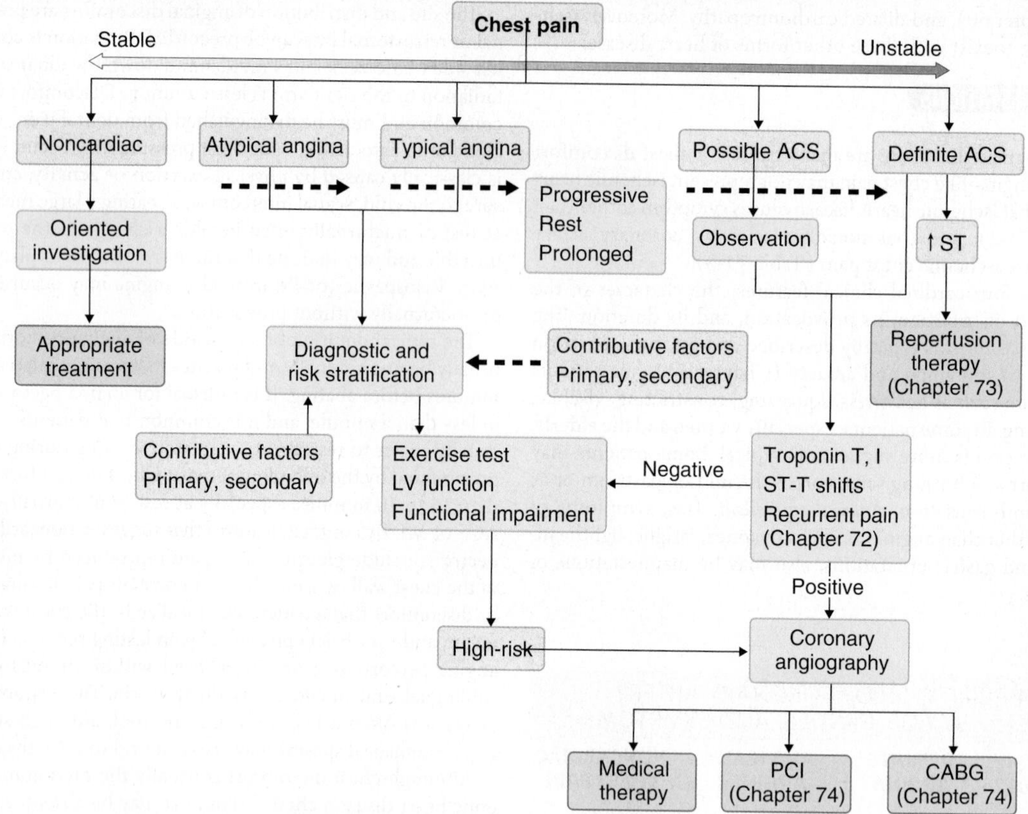

FIGURE 71-1. Evaluation of chest pain. ACS = acute coronary syndrome; CABG = coronary artery bypass graft; LV = left ventricular; PCI = percutaneous coronary intervention. (Modified from Théroux P. Angina pectoris. In: Goldman L, Ausiello DA, eds. Cecil Textbook of Medicine. 23rd ed. Philadelphia: Saunders Elsevier; 2008.)

During an episode of chest discomfort, myocardial ischemia may produce either a third or fourth heart sound.

Myocardial ischemia also can cause a transient holosystolic or mid-late systolic apical murmur due to reversible papillary muscle dysfunction that results in mitral regurgitation. These murmurs are more prevalent in patients with extensive coronary artery disease, especially with inferior or inferoposterior ischemia due to right coronary artery disease. It is important to distinguish such a murmur from the murmur of aortic stenosis or obstructive hypertrophic cardiomyopathy (see Tables 51-7 and 51-8). A displaced LV apical impulse, particularly if dyskinetic, is a sign of significant LV systolic dysfunction.

If patients have coexisting heart failure, an elevated jugular venous pressure, pulmonary rales, and peripheral edema may be present (Chapter 58). The physical examination may reveal other implicating or contributing conditions, such as thyroid enlargement (Chapter 226) or severe anemia (Chapter 158).

DIAGNOSIS

In addition to a careful history and physical examination, assessment of patients with stable ischemic heart disease includes the 12-lead electrocardiogram (ECG), measurement of biochemical and inflammatory markers, and noninvasive diagnostic testing.[3,4] The first goal is to assess the patient's probability of ischemia so that an appropriate evaluation can expedite effective therapy (Fig. 71-1).

Resting Electrocardiogram

Although there may be focal, diagnostic findings of ST segment depression or T wave inversions (Fig. 71-2) on the resting ECG in chronic ischemic heart disease, even patients with extensive anatomic coronary artery disease may have a normal tracing at rest. In addition to myocardial ischemia, other conditions that can produce ST-T wave abnormalities include LV hypertrophy and dilation due to long-standing hypertension and valvular heart disease (e.g., aortic stenosis, hypertrophic cardiomyopathy), electrolyte abnormalities, neurogenic effects, and antiarrhythmic drugs. The presence of new ST-T wave abnormalities on the resting ECG, however, can be helpful in the diagnosis of coronary artery disease and may correlate with the severity of the underlying heart disease.

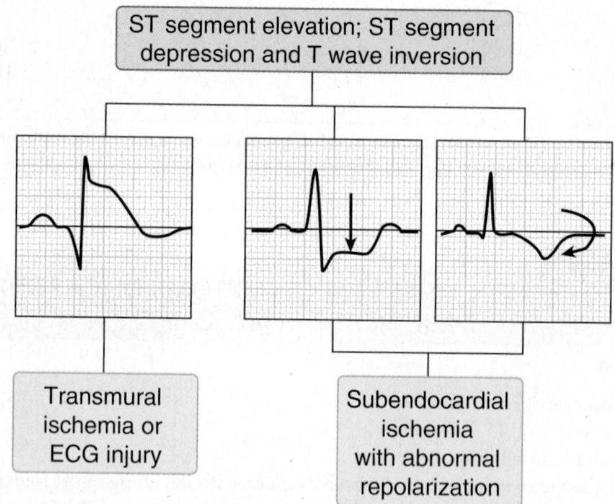

FIGURE 71-2. Ischemic ST segment shifts and repolarization changes on electrocardiogram (ECG).

In addition to focal ST-T wave abnormalities, the ECG may reveal various conduction disturbances, most frequently left bundle branch block and left anterior fascicular block (Chapter 54). The finding of abnormal Q waves is relatively specific for the presence of previous MI but may not help determine when such an event occurred. Arrhythmias, especially ventricular premature beats (Chapter 65), may be present on the ECG but have a low sensitivity and specificity for coronary artery disease.

During a spontaneous episode of angina pectoris or during exertion or stress, the ECG becomes abnormal in 50% or more of patients with normal resting ECGs. The most common abnormality observed is focal ST segment depression, usually in one or more ECG lead groups, which signifies the presence of subendocardial ischemia. On occasion, transient but diminutive ST segment elevation and normalization of previous resting ST-T wave depression or inversion (pseudonormalization) may develop during chronic angina and ischemia, although ST segment elevation is far more commonly observed in ACS patients with plaque rupture.

TABLE 71-4 BLOOD TESTS TO OBTAIN ROUTINELY (OR SELECTIVELY*) IN PATIENTS WITH CHRONIC STABLE ISCHEMIC HEART DISEASE

LIPID LEVELS
Low-density lipoprotein (LDL) and high-density lipoprotein (HDL) cholesterol
Triglyceride level
*LDL electrophoresis (especially apolipoprotein B and small dense LDL)
*Lipoprotein (a)
*Lipoprotein-associated phospholipase A_2
METABOLIC EVALUATION
Fasting plasma glucose concentration
Serum creatinine level
Thyroxine level
*Hemoglobin A_{1c} in patients with known or suspected diabetes
MARKERS OF INFLAMMATION OR CARDIAC FUNCTION
*High-sensitivity C-reactive protein
*Brain natriuretic peptide
PROTHROMBOTIC ASSESSMENT
Plasma fibrinogen
Platelet count
*Factor V Leiden
*D-dimer
*Plasminogen activator inhibitor type 1
TO ASSESS OTHER POTENTIAL CARDIAC RISK FACTORS
*Serum homocysteine level

Laboratory Testing

In patients with new-onset or worsening symptoms, serial troponin measurements can distinguish MI and ACS from stable ischemic heart disease (Chapters 72 and 73). The plasma level of brain natriuretic peptide, which increases in response to spontaneous or provoked ischemia, does not reliably distinguish stable from unstable ischemic heart disease but is associated with the risk of future cardiovascular events in patients who are at risk for coronary disease. High-sensitivity C-reactive protein, an acute phase reactant of inflammation, has a strong and consistent relationship to the risk of future cardiovascular events, and an elevated level may warrant more aggressive diagnostic evaluation and therapy.

All patients with chronic angina should have biochemical evaluation of total cholesterol, low-density lipoprotein (LDL) cholesterol, high-density lipoprotein (HDL) cholesterol, triglyceride, serum creatinine (estimated glomerular filtration), and fasting blood glucose levels (Table 71-4). Other biochemical markers that are not routinely recommended but are associated with higher risk of future cardiovascular events include lipoprotein (a), apolipoprotein B, small dense LDL cholesterol, and lipoprotein-associated phospholipase A_2. Homocysteine levels correlate with the risk for development of coronary heart disease, but randomized trials have failed to demonstrate a reduction of clinical events when elevated homocysteine levels are reduced; as a result, routine screening for an elevated homocysteine level is not recommended.

Noninvasive Testing

Noninvasive stress testing with a standard electrocardiographic treadmill or bicycle exercise, radionuclide imaging (Chapter 56), stress echocardiography (Chapter 55), or newer diagnostic modalities such as cardiac magnetic resonance (CMR; Chapter 56) and positron emission tomography (PET; Chapter 56) is a useful and clinically important approach to establishing the diagnosis and prognosis in patients with stable ischemic heart disease (Fig. 71-3). The predictive accuracy of these tests is defined not only by their sensitivity and specificity but also by the prevalence of disease (or pretest probability) in the population under study. Noninvasive testing should be performed only if the incremental information is likely to alter the planned management strategy. Thus, the value of noninvasive stress testing is greatest when the pretest likelihood is intermediate because the test result is likely to have the greatest effect on the post-test probability of coronary artery disease and, hence, on clinical decision making.

Each noninvasive test has a sensitivity and specificity (Table 71-5) that, when combined with a patient's pretest probability (see Table 71-1), can yield a post-test probability for coronary artery disease (Fig. 71-4). The choice among tests depends on the patient's characteristics (Table 71-6).

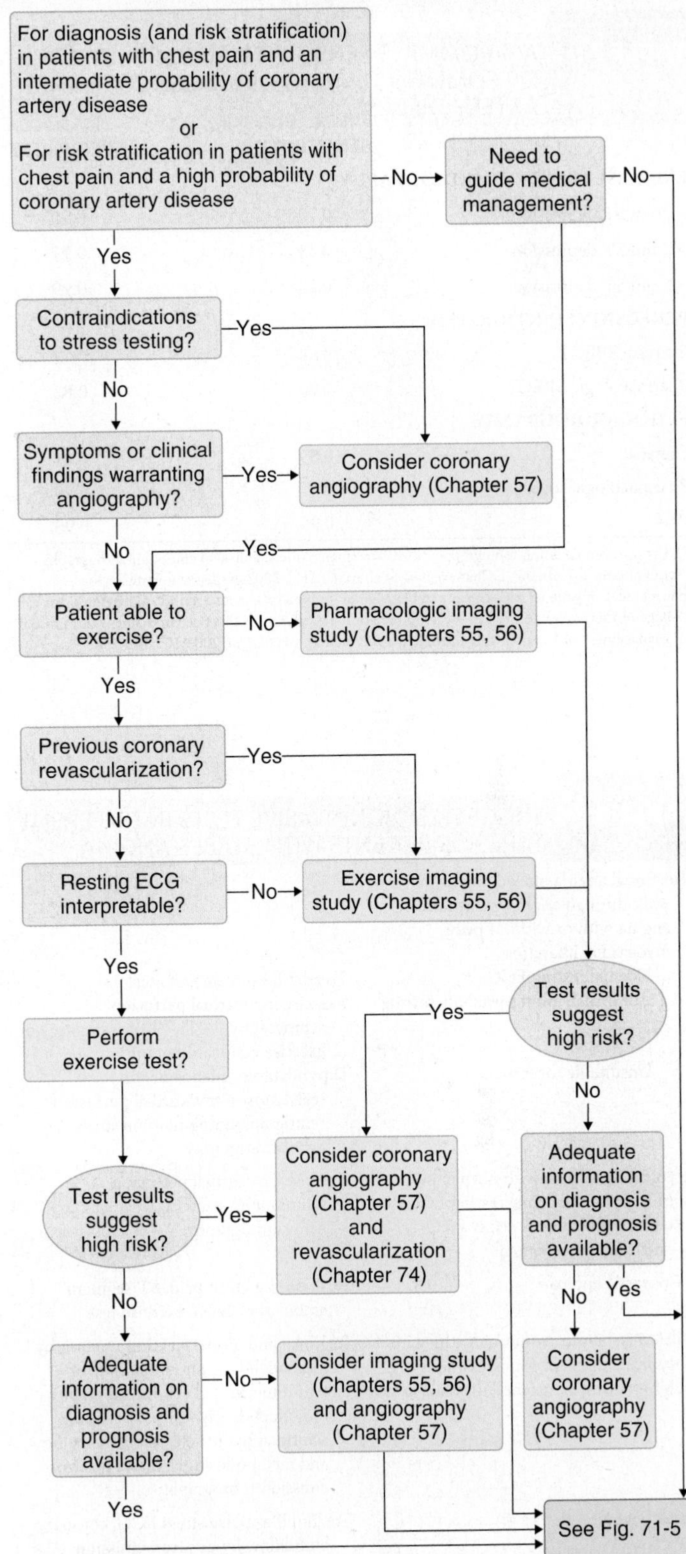

FIGURE 71-3. Approach to the use of stress testing and angiography for the evaluation of chronic stable angina. ECG = electrocardiogram. (Modified from American College of Cardiology/American Heart Association Task Force on Practice Guidelines. Management of Patients with Chronic Stable Angina. ACC/AHA/ACP-ASIM Pocket Guidelines. Philadelphia: Elsevier Science; 2000.)

Exercise Electrocardiography

An exercise ECG is the preferred test in patients who have suspected angina pectoris and are considered to have a moderate probability of coronary artery disease if the resting ECG is normal (i.e., ST segments are not obscured by structural heart disease or medication), provided subjects are capable of achieving an adequate workload. Interpretation of the exercise ECG should include the exercise capacity achieved (duration and metabolic equivalents of the external workload; see Table 51-3), the magnitude and extent of ST

TABLE 71-5 APPROXIMATE SENSITIVITY AND SPECIFICITY OF COMMON TESTS TO DIAGNOSE CORONARY ARTERY DISEASE

	SENSITIVITY	SPECIFICITY
EXERCISE ELECTROCARDIOGRAPHY		
>1 mm ST depression	0.70	0.75
>2 mm ST depression	0.33	0.97
>3 mm ST depression	0.20	0.99
PERFUSION SCINTIGRAPHY		
Exercise SPECT	0.88	0.72
Pharmacologic SPECT	0.90	0.82
ECHOCARDIOGRAPHY		
Exercise	0.85	0.81
Pharmacologic stress	0.81	0.79
PET	0.95	0.95

PET = positron emission tomography; SPECT = single-photon emission computed tomography.
From Gibbons RJ, Abrams J, Chatterjee K, et al. ACC/AHA 2002 guideline update for the management of patients with chronic stable angina—summary article: a report of the American College of Cardiology/American Heart Association Task Force on Practice Guidelines (Committee on Management of Patients with Chronic Stable Angina). *Circulation.* 2003;107:149-158.

TABLE 71-6 SUGGESTED NONINVASIVE TESTS IN DIFFERENT TYPES OF PATIENTS WITH STABLE ANGINA

Exertional angina, mixed angina, walk-through angina, postprandial angina with or without prior myocardial infarction	
Normal resting ECG	Treadmill exercise ECG test
Abnormal, uninterpretable resting ECG	Exercise myocardial perfusion scintigraphy (^{201}Tl, ^{99m}Tc-sestamibi) or exercise echocardiography
Unsuitable for exercise	Dipyridamole, adenosine, or regadenoson myocardial perfusion scintigraphy; dobutamine stress echocardiography
Atypical chest pain with normal or borderline abnormal resting ECG or with nondiagnostic stress ECG, particularly in women	Exercise myocardial perfusion scintigraphy, exercise echocardiography
Vasospastic angina	ECG during chest pain, ST segment ambulatory ECG, exercise test
Dilated ischemic cardiomyopathy with typical angina or for assessment of hibernating or stunned myocardium	Regional and global ejection fraction by radionuclide ventriculography or two-dimensional echocardiography, radionuclide myocardial perfusion scintigraphy; in selected patients, flow and metabolic studies with positron emission tomography
Syndrome X	Treadmill exercise stress ECG, coronary blood flow by positron emission tomography, Doppler probe
Known severe aortic stenosis or severe hypertrophic cardiomyopathy with stable angina	Exercise stress tests contraindicated; dipyridamole, adenosine, or regadenoson myocardial perfusion scintigraphy in selected patients; coronary angiography preferred
Mild aortic valvular disease or hypertrophic cardiomyopathy with typical exertional angina	"Prudent" treadmill myocardial perfusion scintigraphy; dipyridamole, adenosine, or regadenoson myocardial perfusion scintigraphy

ECG = 12-lead electrocardiogram.
Modified from Braunwald E, Goldman L, eds. Primary Care Cardiology. 2nd ed. Philadelphia: WB Saunders; 2003.

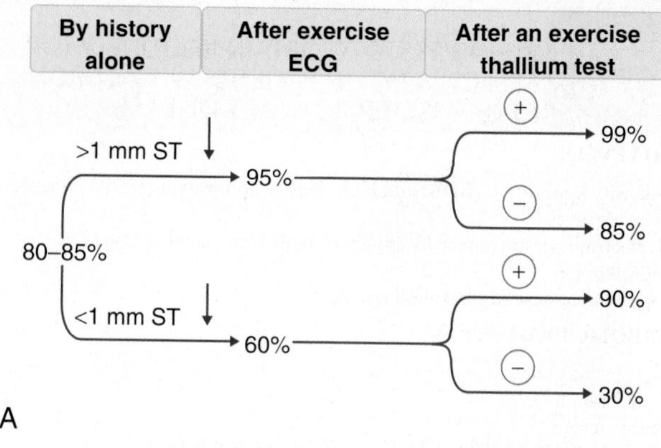

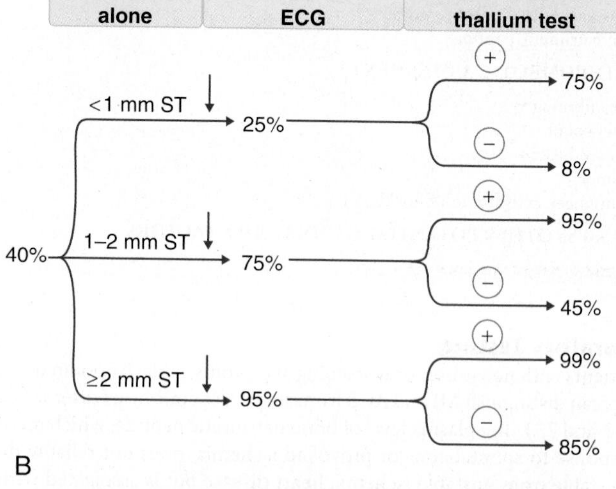

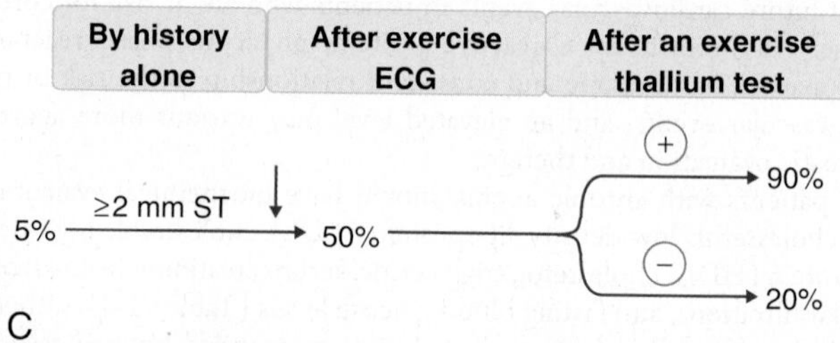

FIGURE 71-4. Approximate probabilities of coronary artery disease in different patient groups. A, Approximate probability of coronary artery disease before and after noninvasive testing in a patient with typical angina pectoris. These percentages demonstrate how the sequential use of an electrocardiogram (ECG) and an exercise thallium test may affect the probability of coronary artery disease in a patient with typical angina pectoris. B, Approximate probability of coronary artery disease before and after noninvasive testing in a patient with atypical angina symptoms. C, Approximate probability of coronary artery disease before and after noninvasive testing in an asymptomatic subject in the coronary artery disease age range. (Redrawn from Branch WB Jr, ed. Office Practice of Medicine. 3rd ed. Philadelphia: WB Saunders; 1994:45.)

segment deviation, the clinical and hemodynamic responses to exercise, and the rapidity with which the heart rate returns to normal after exercise.

The exercise test protocol is usually adjusted to a patient's tolerance, aiming for 6 to 12 minutes of exercise time (i.e., Bruce protocol stages II to IV) to achieve maximal oxygen consumption and to elicit objective evidence of inducible ischemia, if present. Exercise stress testing is generally safe, with death or MI occurring in less than one case per 2500 tests, when such provocative testing is avoided in patients with ACS, severe aortic stenosis, severe hypertension, or uncontrolled heart failure. Other contraindications are acute MI, symptomatic arrhythmias, acute pulmonary embolism, and suspected acute aortic dissection. Relative contraindications are hypertension above 200 mm Hg systolic or 110 mm Hg diastolic, hypertrophic cardiomyopathy, and high-degree atrioventricular block.

Concomitant antianginal therapy (notably the use of β-blockers) reduces the sensitivity of exercise testing as a screening tool. If the purpose of the exercise test is to diagnose ischemia, it should be performed, whenever possible, before β-blockers are initiated or 2 to 3 days after their discontinuation.

Nuclear Cardiology Imaging

Stress myocardial perfusion imaging (Chapter 56) with single-photon emission computed tomography (SPECT) with simultaneous electrocardiographic testing (see Fig. 56-9) is particularly helpful in the diagnosis of coronary artery disease in patients with abnormal resting ECGs and among those in whom ST segment responses cannot be interpreted accurately, such as patients with repolarization abnormalities caused by LV hypertrophy, those with left bundle branch block, and those receiving digitalis. Its sensitivity and specificity are superior to exercise electrocardiography alone in detecting coronary artery disease (especially multivessel disease), in identifying regional perfusion defects that may localize to and correlate with diseased vessels, and in delineating the magnitude and extent of ischemic and infarcted myocardium. Treadmill testing is preferred for patients who are capable of performing such physical activity because of the additional diagnostic and prognostic information achieved with graded exercise. In the 40 to 50% of patients who are unable to exercise adequately, however, pharmacologic vasodilator stress with dipyridamole, adenosine, or regadenoson may be the preferred approach to noninvasive testing.

Stress Echocardiography (Chapter 55)

Stress two-dimensional echocardiography with exercise or pharmacologic stress can detect regional ischemia by identifying new wall motion abnormalities (see Fig. 55-7). Additional clinical information about associated structural heart disease, chamber dimensions, and valve function can be readily obtained. Exercise echocardiography can detect the presence of coronary artery disease with an accuracy similar to that achieved with stress myocardial perfusion imaging and is useful for localizing and quantifying ischemic myocardial segments. Pharmacologic stress is usually performed with dobutamine in patients who are unable to exercise and in those unable to achieve adequate heart rates with exercise.

Ambulatory Ischemic Monitoring

Patients with symptomatic myocardial ischemia have episodes of silent ischemia that occur with the activities of daily living and are detectable on ambulatory monitoring but go unrecognized clinically because of the absence of angina or anginal equivalents. Although 24-hour ambulatory electrocardiography may detect such "silent myocardial ischemia" and may provide a quantitative estimate of the frequency and duration of ischemic episodes, its sensitivity for detection of coronary artery disease is much less reliable than that of exercise electrocardiography.

Stress Cardiac Magnetic Resonance Imaging (Chapter 56)

Pharmacologic stress perfusion with CMR imaging is becoming increasingly available in many centers and may provide additional diagnostic capability in detecting the presence of structural heart disease, in addition to suspected coronary artery disease. CMR with gadolinium enhancement is the most accurate way to diagnose a scar from a prior MI (see Fig. 56-17).

Chest Radiography

Unless there is a history of prior MI, heart failure, or structural heart disease, the chest radiograph (Chapter 56) is usually normal in patients with chronic angina or stable ischemic heart disease. If an enlarged cardiac silhouette is present, it is generally indicative of a previous MI with LV dilation and cardiac remodeling. Other causes of cardiomegaly include long-standing hypertension, concomitant valvular heart disease, pericardial effusion, and nonischemic cardiomyopathy.

Cardiac Computed Tomographic Angiography

Cardiac computed tomographic angiography (CCTA; Chapter 56) is a highly sensitive method to detect coronary calcification (see Fig. 56-10), which is strongly associated with coronary atherosclerosis, and can also provide noninvasive angiography of the proximal coronary arteries. Although coronary calcification is a highly sensitive (approximately 90%) finding in patients with coronary artery disease, the specificity for identifying patients with obstructive coronary artery disease is much lower (approximately 50%). Because of the potential unnecessary testing from false-positive results, CCTA is currently not recommended as a routine screening approach for suspected obstructive coronary artery disease in individuals at low risk (<10% 10-year estimated risk of coronary events). By contrast, selective screening of intermediate-risk patients may be reasonable because a high calcium score may reclassify such individuals at higher risk and thereby lead to more intense risk factor modification.[5] CCTA can also be coupled with PET imaging in a hybrid PET and computed tomography scanner, which can provide a quantitative assessment of coronary anatomy along with regional myocardial blood flow and cardiac metabolism.

Diagnostic Coronary Angiography

Despite the continued evolution of noninvasive diagnostic testing, invasive coronary angiography (Chapter 57) remains the "gold standard" for anatomic definition of coronary artery disease. Among patients with the clinical diagnosis of stable ischemic heart disease referred for coronary angiography, a 70% or more luminal diameter narrowing is found in one (about 25%), two (about 25%), or all three (about 25%) epicardial coronary arteries in about 75% of cases; another 5 to 10% of patients have obstruction of the left main coronary artery; and the remaining 15 to 20% have no flow-limiting coronary obstructions. These data emphasize the persisting role of coronary angiography for diagnostic purposes (Table 71-7), but angiography is also helpful for

TABLE 71-7 CORONARY ANGIOGRAPHY FOR DIAGNOSIS AND RISK STRATIFICATION IN PATIENTS WITH CHRONIC ANGINA AND STABLE ISCHEMIC HEART DISEASE

FOR INITIAL DIAGNOSTIC INDICATION
Recommended on the Basis of Evidence or General Consensus
Patients with suspected angina and evidence of intermediate-high risk, moderate-severe ischemia on noninvasive testing, or a changing angina pattern who have survived sudden cardiac death or serious ventricular arrhythmia
Weight of Evidence or Opinion is in Favor
Uncertain diagnosis after noninvasive testing, and the benefit of a more certain diagnosis outweighs the risk and cost of coronary angiography
Inability to undergo noninvasive testing because of disability, illness, or morbid obesity
Occupational requirement for a definitive diagnosis
Suspected nonatherosclerotic cause of myocardial ischemia
Suspicion of a coronary spasm
High pretest probability of left main or three-vessel disease
Recurrent hospitalization for chest pain in the absence of definitive diagnosis
Overriding desire for a definitive diagnosis and a greater than low probability of CAD
Not Recommended
Significant comorbidity in patients in whom the risk of coronary arteriography outweighs the benefit of the procedure
Overriding personal desire for a definitive diagnosis and a low probability of CAD
FOR INITIAL RISK STRATIFICATION OR TREATMENT INDICATION
Recommended on the Basis of Evidence or General Consensus
With disabling (CCS class III and class IV) chronic stable angina despite medical therapy
With high-risk criteria on noninvasive testing regardless of anginal severity
Patients with angina who have survived sudden cardiac death or serious ventricular arrhythmia
Angina and symptoms and signs of congestive heart failure
Clinical characteristics that indicate a high likelihood of severe CAD
Weight of Evidence or Opinion is in Favor
Significant left ventricular dysfunction (EF < 45%), CCS class I or class II angina, and demonstrable ischemia but less than high-risk criteria on noninvasive testing
High-risk criteria suggesting ischemia on noninvasive testing
Inadequate prognostic information after noninvasive testing
Clinical characteristics that indicate a high likelihood of severe CAD
CCS class I or class II angina, preserved left ventricular function (EF > 45%), and less than high-risk criteria on noninvasive testing
CCS class III or class IV angina that improves to class I or class II with medical therapy
CCS class I or class II angina but intolerance (unacceptable side effects) to adequate medical therapy
Not Recommended
CCS class I or class II angina in patients who respond to medical therapy and who have no evidence of ischemia on noninvasive testing
Patients who prefer to avoid revascularization after adequate explanation

CAD = coronary artery disease; CCS = Canadian Cardiovascular Society; EF = ejection fraction.
Modified from Gibbons RJ, Abrams J, Chatterjee K, et al. ACC/AHA 2002 guideline update for the management of patients with chronic stable angina—summary article: a report of the American College of Cardiology/American Heart Association Task Force on Practice Guidelines (Committee on Management of Patients with Chronic Stable Angina). *Circulation*. 2003;107:149-158.

risk stratification in patients with clear-cut angina and ischemic heart disease. In patients with less severe coronary stenoses (i.e., 50 to 70% on angiography), coronary intravascular ultrasonography (see Fig. 57-6) can substantially enhance the quantification of obstruction and vulnerability of the coronary atheroma to future instability. Alternatively, an invasive physiologic approach with use of a pressure wire positioned proximal and distal to a coronary stenosis can measure the severity of the stenosis and determine whether functionally significant flow reduction (i.e., a decreased fractional flow reserve [FFR] < 0.8) is present. This technique may be useful when there is a borderline (50 to 60%) visual coronary stenosis at angiography, particularly if such a stenosis subtends an ischemic myocardial segment observed on noninvasive testing. An FFR below 0.8 is generally considered to represent a sufficiently important reduction in coronary flow to justify proceeding to percutaneous coronary intervention (Chapter 74) to reduce symptoms and the subsequent need for urgent revascularization.A1 A2 By contrast, an FFR of 0.8 or higher would indicate that myocardial revascularization of the stenotic coronary artery would be of little benefit clinically.

Differential Diagnosis of Angina

Many common noncardiac disorders may be manifested with clinical features that can be confused with angina pectoris (see Table 51-2). In some instances, symptoms may be indistinguishable from ischemic heart disease. For example, many patients with angina have coexisting esophageal disorders (Chapter 138), and both angina and esophageal discomfort may be relieved by nitroglycerin (Chapter 51). A distinguishing feature from angina is that esophageal discomfort is often relieved by antacids, proton pump inhibitors, or food.

Costochondritis can mimic angina but can typically be distinguished by the presence of well-localized pain on palpation. However, pressure, if it is applied too firmly to the anterior chest wall during examination of a patient with suspected angina pectoris, may elicit symptoms of discomfort even in normal subjects. Cervical radiculopathy may cause pain radiating to the shoulders, neck, or upper arms and can be confused with angina. However, this condition typically causes a constant ache that is often exacerbated by neck movement or rotation and may be accompanied by a focal sensory deficit or radiculopathy.

Pulmonary hypertension (Chapter 68) can cause exertional chest discomfort that may share many of the characteristics of angina pectoris. It is believed that right ventricular ischemia during physical exertion may cause this discomfort along with associated symptoms of exertional dyspnea, dizziness, and syncope. Findings on physical examination typically include a parasternal lift, a loud (and sometimes palpable) pulmonary component of the second heart sound, and findings of right ventricular hypertrophy on electrocardiography.

Chest pain may also be an important presenting clinical feature of pulmonary embolism (Chapter 98). Physical findings typically include tachycardia and tachypnea, an accentuated pulmonic component of the second heart sound, and occasionally a right-sided S_4 gallop. Pleuritic discomfort suggests pulmonary infarction, whereas a history of pain exacerbated by inspiration or deep breathing, along with a pleural friction rub, usually helps distinguish it from angina pectoris.

Acute pericarditis (Chapter 77) may be confused with the discomfort of angina pectoris, but pericarditis tends to cause chest pain that is generally sharp, is not relieved by rest or nitroglycerin, is exacerbated by movement or deep breathing, and is associated with a pericardial friction rub that may be evanescent. Aortic dissection (Chapter 78), which may be manifested with acute, severe chest pain, may be confused with an acute MI but generally not with angina.

Risk Stratification

Clinical and noninvasive criteria can be used in a complementary fashion to refine the estimate of risk for the individual patient with stable ischemic heart disease (Table 71-8). Clinical characteristics that include age, male sex, diabetes mellitus, previous MI, and symptoms typical of angina are predictive of the presence of coronary artery disease. Heart failure and LV dysfunction (generally defined by an ejection fraction < 50%), the severity and extent of angina, and associated symptoms such as dyspnea are also important predictors of outcome in patients with stable ischemic heart disease.

The simple classification of disease into single-, double-, or triple-vessel or left main coronary artery disease remains the most widely used approach (Table 71-9). Additional prognostic information is provided by the severity and extent of coronary luminal narrowing and its location. For example,

TABLE 71-8 USING THE RESULTS OF NONINVASIVE RISK STRATIFICATION TO GUIDE CLINICAL DECISION MAKING

HIGH RISK (>3% ANNUAL MORTALITY RATE)
Severe resting left ventricular dysfunction (LVEF < 35%)
High-risk treadmill score (≤−11)*
Severe exercise left ventricular dysfunction (exercise LVEF < 35%)
Stress-induced large perfusion defect (particularly if anterior)
Stress-induced multiple perfusion defects of moderate size
Large, fixed perfusion defect with left ventricular dilation or increased lung uptake (^{201}Tl)
Stress-induced moderate perfusion defect with left ventricular dilation or increased lung uptake (^{201}Tl)
Echocardiographic wall motion abnormality (involving more than two segments) developing at low dose of dobutamine or at a low heart rate (<120 beats/min)
Stress echocardiographic evidence of extensive ischemia
INTERMEDIATE RISK (1-3% ANNUAL MORTALITY RATE)
Mild to moderate resting left ventricular dysfunction (LVEF = 35-49%)
Intermediate-risk treadmill score (−11 < score < 5)*
Stress-induced moderate perfusion defect without left ventricular dilation or increased lung intake (^{201}Tl)
Limited stress echocardiographic ischemia with a wall motion abnormality only at higher doses of dobutamine involving two segments or less
LOW RISK (<1% ANNUAL MORTALITY RATE)
Low-risk treadmill score (≥ 5)*
Normal or small myocardial perfusion defect at rest or with stress†
Normal stress echocardiographic wall motion or no change of limited resting wall motion abnormalities during stress†

*Score = (duration of exercise in minutes) − (5 × mm of ST segment depression) − (4 × angina score), where 0 = no angina, 1 = nonlimiting angina, and 2 = angina that causes discontinuation of the test.

†Although the published data are limited, patients with these findings will probably not be at low risk in the presence of either a high-risk treadmill score or severe resting left ventricular dysfunction (LVEF < 35%).

LVEF = left ventricular ejection fraction.

From Gibbons RJ, Abrams J, Chatterjee K, et al. ACC/AHA 2002 guideline update for the management of patients with chronic stable angina—summary article: a report of the American College of Cardiology/American Heart Association Task Force on practice guidelines (Committee on the Management of Patients with Chronic Stable Angina). *J Am Coll Cardiol.* 2003;41:159-168.

TABLE 71-9 CORONARY ARTERY DISEASE PROGNOSTIC INDEX

EXTENT OF CORONARY ARTERY DISEASE	5-YEAR MORTALITY RATE (%)*
1-vessel disease, 75%	7
>1-vessel disease, 50-74%	7
1-vessel disease, ≥95%	9
2-vessel disease	12
2-vessel disease, both ≥95%	14
1-vessel disease, ≥95% proximal LAD	17
2-vessel disease, ≥95% LAD	17
2-vessel disease, ≥95% proximal LAD	21
3-vessel disease	21
3-vessel disease, ≥95% in at least 1	27
3-vessel disease, 75% proximal LAD	33
3-vessel disease, ≥95% proximal LAD	41

*Assuming medical treatment only.

LAD = left anterior descending coronary artery.

From Califf RM, Armstrong PW, Carver JR, et al. Task Force 5: stratification of patients into high, medium and low risk subgroups for purposes of risk factor management. *J Am Coll Cardiol.* 1996;27:1007-1019.

high-grade lesions of the left main coronary artery or its equivalent, as defined by severe proximal left anterior descending and proximal left circumflex coronary artery disease, are particularly life-threatening. The SYNTAX trial has permitted the identification of subsets of coronary artery disease patients into three tertiles of low-, moderate-, and high-risk anatomic findings based on multiple lesional characteristics (see Tables 71-8 and 71-9). However, the plaque causing the most severe chronic stenosis is not necessarily the one that will subsequently rupture to cause ACS or acute MI.

TREATMENT Rx

Comprehensive management of angina and stable ischemic heart disease (Fig. 71-5) entails multiple therapeutic approaches to the identification and treatment of associated diseases that can precipitate or worsen angina and ischemia (Table 71-10): cardiac risk factor identification and intervention; application of pharmacologic and nonpharmacologic interventions for secondary prevention; pharmacologic and symptomatic management of angina and ischemia; and myocardial revascularization with percutaneous coronary intervention (PCI) or coronary artery bypass graft (CABG) surgery, when indicated (Table 71-11). A multidimensional management approach integrates all of these considerations, often simultaneously, in each patient. Among pharmacotherapies, three drug classes are classified as being "disease modifying" in that they have been demonstrated to reduce mortality and morbidity in patients with stable ischemic heart disease and preserved LV function: antiplatelet agents such as aspirin; inhibitors of the renin-angiotensin-aldosterone system, especially angiotensin-converting enzyme (ACE) inhibitors; and effective lipid-lowering agents, principally statins. Other therapies, such as nitrates, β-blockers, calcium antagonists, and ranolazine, can reduce myocardial ischemia,

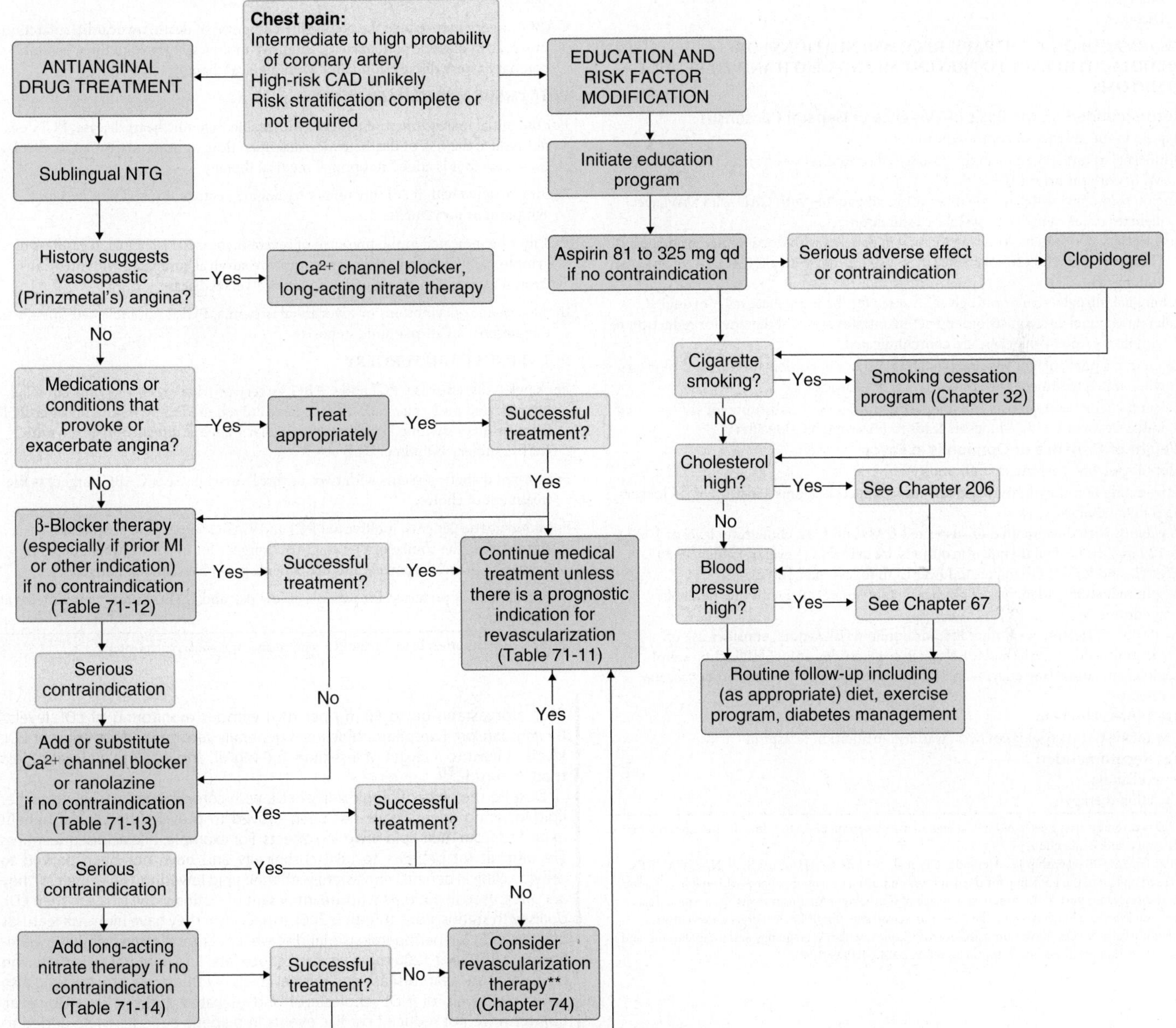

FIGURE 71-5 Algorithm for the treatment of stable angina. AS = aortic stenosis; CABG = coronary artery bypass graft; CAD = coronary artery disease; MI = myocardial infarction; NTG = nitroglycerin; PTCA = percutaneous transluminal coronary angioplasty. (Modified from American College of Cardiology/American Heart Association Task Force on Practice Guidelines. Management of Patients with Chronic Stable Angina. ACC/AHA/ACP-ASIM Pocket Guidelines. Philadelphia: Elsevier Science; 2000.)

TABLE 71-10 TREATMENT OF PATIENTS WITH STABLE ANGINA

GENERAL MEASURES
Rule out and control aggravating conditions
Associated noncardiac diseases
Associated cardiac disease
Use of drugs aggravating angina
Smoking cessation
Dietary counseling for body weight and lipid control
Exercise prescription
Treat to targets
Hypertension
Blood lipids
Diabetes
PHARMACOLOGIC THERAPY: RECOMMENDATIONS FOR PHARMACOTHERAPY TO PREVENT MI AND DEATH AND TO REDUCE SYMPTOMS
Recommended on the Basis of Evidence or General Consensus
Aspirin in the absence of contraindications
β-Blockers as initial therapy in the absence of contraindications in patients with prior MI or without prior MI
Angiotensin-converting enzyme inhibitor in all patients with CAD who also have diabetes or left ventricular systolic dysfunction
Low-density lipoprotein–lowering therapy in patients with documented or suspected CAD and LDL cholesterol greater than 130 mg/dL, with a target LDL of less than 100 mg/dL
Sublingual nitroglycerin or nitroglycerin spray for the immediate relief of angina
Calcium-channel antagonists or long-acting nitrates as initial therapy for reduction of symptoms when β-blockers are contraindicated
Calcium-channel antagonists or long-acting nitrates in combination with β-blockers when initial treatment with β-blockers is not successful
Calcium-channel antagonists and long-acting nitrates as a substitute for β-blockers if initial treatment with β-blockers leads to unacceptable side effects
Weight of Evidence or Opinion is in Favor
Clopidogrel when aspirin is contraindicated
Long-acting non-dihydropyridine calcium-channel antagonists instead of β-blockers as initial therapy
In patients with documented or suspected CAD and LDL cholesterol level of 100 to 129 mg/dL, several therapeutic options are available (Level of Evidence: B)
Lifestyle and/or drug therapies to lower LDL to less than 100 mg/dL
Weight reduction and increased physical activity in persons with the metabolic syndrome
Institution of treatment of other lipid or nonlipid risk factors; consider use of nicotinic acid or fibric acid for elevated triglycerides or low HDL cholesterol
Angiotensin-converting enzyme inhibitor in patients with CAD or other vascular disease
Usefulness Unclear
Low-intensity anticoagulation with warfarin in addition to aspirin
Not Recommended
Dipyridamole
Chelation therapy

CAD = coronary artery disease; HDL = high-density lipoprotein; LDL = low-density lipoprotein; MI = myocardial infarction.

From Fihn SD, Blankenship JC, Alexander KP, et al. 2014 ACC/AHA/AATS/PCNA/SCAI/STS focused update of the guideline for the diagnosis and management of patients with stable ischemic heart disease: a report of the American College of Cardiology/American Heart Association Task Force on Practice Guidelines, and the American Association for Thoracic Surgery, Preventive Cardiovascular Nurses Association, Society for Cardiovascular Angiography and Interventions, and Society of Thoracic Surgeons. *J Am Coll Cardiol.* 2014;64:1929-1949.

ameliorate or prevent angina, and improve exercise performance, but they have not been shown to reduce mortality in patients with stable ischemic heart disease.

Disease-Modifying Therapies

Careful attention to lifestyle and the management of coronary risk factors is essential (Fig. 71-6). Such secondary prevention strategies can reduce the risk of progressive coronary disease, morbidity, and mortality.

Drugs That Alter Lipid Metabolism

Each 1% increase in the LDL cholesterol level results in a 2 to 3% increase in risk for coronary events (Chapter 52). Large, randomized clinical trials in patients with ischemic heart disease have shown a consistent and significant reduction in mortality and cardiac events with statin therapy (Chapter 206). Patients with stable angina should routinely be treated with statins[3,6-8] (see Table 206-5). Recent U.S. guidelines recommend high-dose statin therapy (e.g., atorvastatin up to 80 mg per day) without monitoring of LDL levels.[8] By comparison, European guidelines[7] generally recommend lowering of LDL levels at least to a target of less than 100 mg/dL and often to a target of less than 70 mg/dL.[A3]

Despite the epidemiologic link of LDL with coronary disease events, other lipid-lowering agents have not been proved to provide the clinical benefit expected from their lipid-lowering effects. For example, bile acid sequestrants are difficult for patients to take chronically and have not been proved to provide clinical benefits consistent with their lipid lowering. Nevertheless, they are often used in patients who are intolerant of statins or fail to reach their LDL goals with statins alone (Chapter 206), especially if they have high-risk features of prior ACS, MI, peripheral arterial disease, or cerebral arterial disease. Gemfibrozil, a fibrate at 1200 mg daily, can reduce fatal and nonfatal MI in men who have coronary heart disease and normal levels of LDL cholesterol but who also have low levels of HDL cholesterol and elevated triglycerides. However, fibrates have not reduced cardiac events in diabetic patients when added to statins[A4] and have not been shown to reduce overall mortality despite about a 10% reduction in major cardiovascular events.[A5] Similarly, ezetimibe lowers LDL cholesterol levels but has not been shown to reduce cardiac events or mortality.

Epidemiologically, each decline of 1 mg/dL in HDL cholesterol is associated with a 2 to 3% increase in the risk of MI and death from cardiac causes. However, drug therapy that elevates HDL levels with either niacin or cholesteryl ester transfer protein inhibitors has been universally disappointing.[A6][A7]

TABLE 71-11 CURRENT RECOMMENDATIONS FOR MYOCARDIAL REVASCULARIZATION IN PATIENTS WITH CHRONIC STABLE ANGINA

CABG SURGERY VERSUS MEDICAL THERAPY
Among patients with medically refractory angina pectoris, CABG surgery is indicated for symptom improvement.
Among patients with medically stable angina pectoris, CABG surgery is indicated to prolong life in left main coronary artery disease or three-vessel disease (regardless of left ventricular function) and, possibly, to help symptoms.
CABG surgery may be indicated for prolongation of life if the proximal left anterior descending coronary artery is involved (regardless of the number of diseased vessels).
CABG surgery may reduce the composite end point of death, myocardial infarction, or stroke in diabetic patients with extensive multivessel (two- to three-vessel) coronary artery disease compared with medical therapy.
PCI VERSUS MEDICAL THERAPY
For the initial management of patients with stable ischemic heart disease, PCI does not reduce the risk of death, myocardial infarction, or other major cardiovascular events when it is added to optimal medical therapy.
Among patients with medically refractory angina pectoris, PCI is indicated for symptom improvement.
PCI may be indicated in the presence of severe myocardial ischemia, regardless of symptoms. PCI does not appear to improve survival compared with medical treatment among patients with one- or two-vessel disease.
In the absence of symptoms or myocardial ischemia, PCI is not indicated (merely for the presence of an anatomic stenosis).
PCI VERSUS CABG SURGERY
For single-vessel disease, PCI and CABG surgery provide excellent symptom relief, but repeated revascularization procedures are required more frequently after PCI. Intracoronary stenting is preferred to regular PCI, but direct comparison with CABG surgery is limited.
For treated diabetic patients with two- or three-vessel disease, CABG surgery is the treatment of choice.
For nondiabetic patients, multivessel PCI and CABG surgery are acceptable alternatives. The choice of PCI or CABG surgery for initial treatment depends primarily on local expertise and the patient's and physician's preferences.
In general, PCI is preferred for patients at low risk and CABG surgery for patients at high risk.

CABG = coronary artery bypass graft; PCI = percutaneous coronary intervention.

Angiotensin-Converting Enzyme Inhibitors

ACE inhibitor administration (see Table 67-7) reduces cardiac events, cardiovascular mortality, and all-cause mortality in patients with risk factors for or with previously diagnosed coronary artery disease,[A8] including high-risk patients with vascular disease or diabetes and patients with stable coronary artery disease and no clinical evidence of heart failure. By contrast, ACE inhibitors do not appear to prevent future cardiac events in post-MI patients with

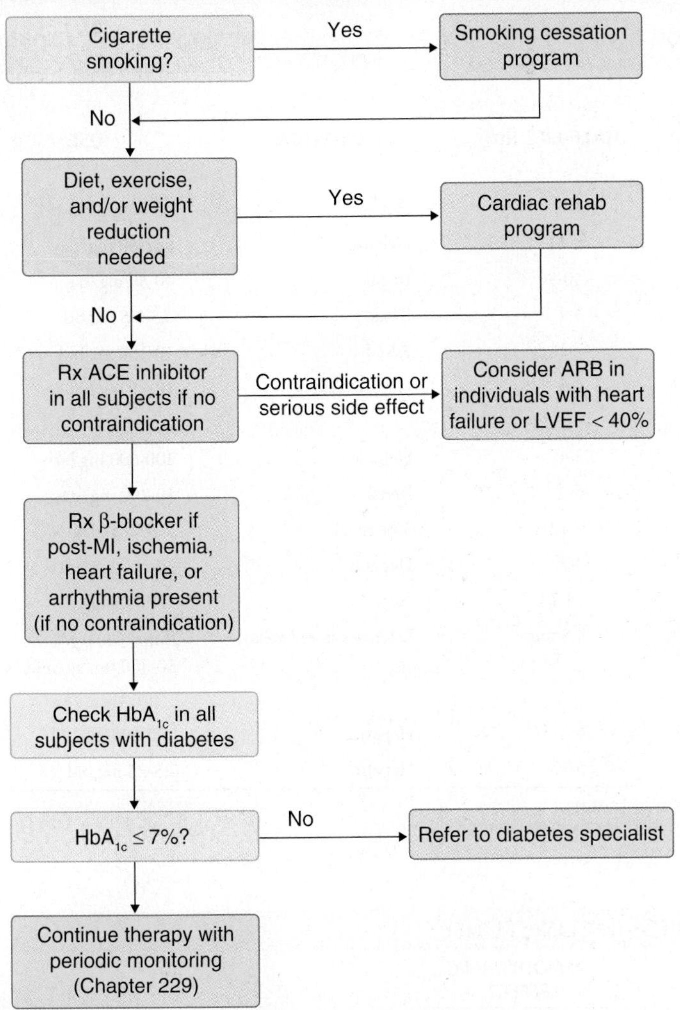

FIGURE 71-6. **Approach to lifestyle interventions and pharmacotherapy.** ACE = angiotensin-converting enzyme; ARB = angiotensin receptor blocker; HbA_{1c} = hemoglobin A_{1c}; LVEF = left ventricular ejection fraction; MI = myocardial infarction; Rx = prescribe.

preserved LV function. Whether angiotensin receptor blockers have similar benefits in patients with chronic angina and stable ischemic heart disease is not yet known.

Antiplatelet Agents and Anticoagulants

Aspirin reduces the risk of adverse cardiovascular events by 33% in patients with stable angina. The reduction in vascular events is comparable for doses of 75 to 150 mg daily and 160 to 325 mg daily, but daily doses of less than 75 mg have less benefit.[A9] Therefore, in the absence of contraindications, aspirin, 75 to 325 mg once daily, should be administered routinely in all patients with angina and stable ischemic heart disease.

Clopidogrel (Chapter 38), which is the most widely used thienopyridine in the treatment of patients with coronary artery disease, is of proven benefit when it is combined with aspirin to reduce the composite end point of death, MI, or stroke in ACS patients and in patients who undergo PCI, especially with drug-eluting stents (Chapters 72 and 74). The standard regimen is an initial loading dose of 300 to 600 mg orally, followed by a maintenance dose of 75 mg daily. In patients with angina and stable ischemic heart disease, however, adding clopidogrel to low-dose (75 to 162 mg/day) aspirin does not reduce the primary composite end point of MI, stroke, or death from cardiovascular causes,[A10] so clopidogrel should be reserved for patients who cannot tolerate aspirin or who have had an acute coronary event (Chapter 72) or a stent implantation (Chapter 74). Both prasugrel and ticagrelor are approved in patients with ACS and in those who undergo PCI with stent placement, but neither agent has yet been studied in the medical management of patients with chronic angina and stable coronary artery disease.

Warfarin is generally as effective as aspirin for preventing coronary events in patients with angina and is preferred to aspirin for patients with concomitant atrial fibrillation (Chapter 64), but it is associated with a higher risk of bleeding. Combination therapy with warfarin plus aspirin is superior to aspirin alone if the international normalized ratio is maintained above 2.0, but the benefit of the combination must be weighed against a 1 per 100 patient-years risk of bleeding.[A11] Factor Xa inhibitors (dabigatran, rivaroxaban, and apixaban) approved for the treatment of venous thromboembolic disease and for the prevention of systemic embolism (Chapter 38) in patients with nonvalvular atrial fibrillation have not yet been tested in patients with stable ischemic heart disease.

Therapeutic Agents to Reduce Angina and Ischemia

The goal of antianginal therapy is to reduce symptoms of cardiac ischemia and to improve quality of life. β-Blockers, which prevent the binding of catecholamines to the β-adrenergic receptor, lower heart rate and myocardial contractility, thereby reducing myocardial workload, myocardial oxygen demand, and ischemia and anginal symptoms. β-Blockers raise the ischemic threshold and delay or prevent the onset of angina with exercise. β-Blockers also reduce the rate of secondary cardiac events and sudden cardiac death in post-MI patients, but there have been no placebo-controlled outcome trials in angina patients. All β-blockers appear to be equally effective in patients with chronic stable angina (Table 71-12). The β-blocker dose should be titrated to a target resting heart rate of 50 to 60 beats per minute as tolerated by the patient.

Calcium-channel blockers (Table 71-13) reduce afterload by their peripheral vasodilatory effects and thus lower myocardial workload and myocardial oxygen demand. Calcium-channel blockers also reduce coronary vascular resistance and inhibit coronary vasospasm by preventing coronary arterial smooth muscle contraction. This favorable reduction in myocardial oxygen demand, coupled with an increase in myocardial oxygen supply, results in a reduction in angina and ischemia. Non-dihydropyridine calcium-channel blockers, such as verapamil and diltiazem, also reduce heart rate. Conversely, dihydropyridine calcium-channel antagonists, such as amlodipine, have greater effect on vascular smooth muscle, are better peripheral and coronary vasodilators, and hence may have advantages for use in the hypertensive patient with angina. In randomized clinical trials, calcium-channel blockers and β-blockers are generally equally effective in relieving angina, improving time to onset of angina, and improving time to ischemic ST depression during exercise. Because calcium-channel blockers have not been shown to reduce death or MI in patients with stable or previously unstable ischemic heart disease, these agents are usually used in patients who cannot tolerate β-blockers or who require additional pharmacotherapy to control their symptoms. When calcium-channel blockers are used with β-blockers, care must be taken not to cause symptomatic bradycardia with verapamil and diltiazem. When calcium-channel blockers are used alone, diltiazem is often preferred because the dihydropyridine calcium-channel blockers can increase the heart rate.

Nitrates (Table 71-14) continue to be widely prescribed for antianginal treatment and are effective when they are administered sublingually, orally, or topically. They act as vasodilators by entering vascular smooth muscle, where they are metabolized to nitric oxide, which relaxes vascular smooth muscle, including in coronary arteries. These effects reduce angina by improving coronary blood flow. Nitrates also lower preload because of their venodilatory effects, with a resulting reduction in LV end-diastolic pressure and wall tension, which in turn lowers subendocardial oxygen demand. When nitrates are used in patients with stable angina, they improve exercise tolerance, time to onset of angina, and ST segment depression during treadmill exercise testing. Long-acting nitrates, which are frequently combined with β-blockers and calcium-channel blockers, have additive antianginal and anti-ischemic effects in patients with stable ischemic heart disease. Sublingual nitroglycerin or oral spray can terminate an angina attack and can be used as prophylaxis to prevent exertional angina. Long-acting nitrates administered orally or transdermally are used to prevent angina and to improve exercise tolerance. For avoidance of nitrate tolerance or tachyphylaxis, an 8- to 12-hour nitrate-free interval daily is recommended. Nitroglycerin and nitrates can cause vasodilation-induced headache, a decrease in blood pressure, and, more rarely, severe hypotension with bradycardia due to activation of the vagal Bezold-Jarisch reflex. Because the vasodilation by nitroglycerin is markedly exaggerated and prolonged in the presence of the phosphodiesterase inhibitors sildenafil (Viagra), vardenafil (Levitra), and tadalafil (Cialis), these agents and nitrates should not be used concurrently.

Ranolazine (initiated at a dose of 500 mg twice daily and titrated up to a maximal dose of 1000 mg twice daily) acts by reducing intracellular calcium overload in ischemic myocytes by inhibiting late inward sodium current entry. The net effect of reduced late inward sodium current is a reduction in LV wall tension and myocardial oxygen demand, thereby reducing angina and ischemia. Ranolazine increases exercise tolerance in patients with stable angina, reduces episodes of recurrent ischemia, and provides additional antianginal benefit in patients who are already receiving intensive antianginal therapy with β-blockers and calcium-channel blockers.[A12] Whether ranolazine can reduce death, MI, or recurrent ischemia compared with placebo in patients with chronic angina is unproven.[2,6,9]

Nonpharmacologic Treatment

Enhanced external counterpulsation (EECP) is an alternative treatment for patients with refractory angina. EECP is generally administered as 35 sequential treatments (1 hour daily; 5 days/week) during 7 weeks. EECP does not reduce ischemia on myocardial perfusion imaging, and the mechanisms

TABLE 71-12 CLINICAL USE OF B-BLOCKERS

COMPOUND BY RECEPTOR ACTIVITY	INTRINSIC SYMPATHOMIMETIC ACTIVITY*	MEMBRANE STABILITY EFFECT	HALF-LIFE (hr)	EXCRETION	USE
β_1 AND β_2					
Propranolol	–	++	1-6	Hepatic	20-80 mg bid-tid
Propranolol long-acting	–	++	8-11	Hepatic	80-360 mg/day
Nadolol	–	–	40-80	Renal	40-80 mg/day
Pindolol	+	+	3-4	Renal	2.5-7.5 mg tid
Sotalol	–	–	7-18	Renal	40-160 mg bid
Timolol	–	–	4-5	Hepatic-renal	10-15 mg bid
β_1 SELECTIVE					
Acebutolol	+	+	3-4	Hepatic	200-600 mg bid
Atenolol	–	–	6-9	Renal	50-200 mg/day
Bisoprolol	–	–	9-12	50% renal	5-20 mg/day
Metoprolol	–	–	3-7	Hepatic	50-200 mg bid
Metoprolol long-acting	–	–	14-25	Hepatic	100-400 mg
Esmolol	–	–	4.5 min	Esterases in red cells	Bolus 500 μg/kg 50-300 μg/kg/min IV
β_1, β_2, α_2					
Labetalol	+	–	6	Hepatic	200-600 mg bid
Carvedilol	–	+	6-10	Hepatic	2.5-25 mg bid

*Presence commonly associated with maintenance of or increase in heart rate; absence associated with decrease in heart rate.
From Théroux P. Angina pectoris. In: Goldman L, Ausiello DA, eds. Cecil Textbook of Medicine. 23rd ed. Philadelphia: Saunders Elsevier; 2008.

TABLE 71-13 PROPERTIES OF CALCIUM-CHANNEL BLOCKING DRUGS IN CLINICAL USE

DRUGS	USUAL DOSE	ELIMINATION HALF-LIFE (hr)	HEMODYNAMIC EFFECT: HR	HEMODYNAMIC EFFECT: PVR	SIDE EFFECTS
DIHYDROPYRIDINES					
Nifedipine PA*	10-40 mg bid	10	↑↑	↓↓↓	Hypotension, dizziness, flushing, edema, constipation
Nifedipine XL*	30-120 mg/day	24	↑	↓↓	
Amlodipine	2.5-10 mg/day	30-50	=	↓↓↓	Headache, edema
Felodipine	2.5-10 mg/day	11-16	↑	↓↓↓	Headache, dizziness
Isradipine	2.5-10 mg bid	8	=	↓↓↓	Headache, fatigue
Nicardipine	20-40 mg tid	2-4	↑	↓↓↓	
Nicardipine SR*	30-60 mg bid	8-10	↑	↓↓	Headache, dizziness, flushing, edema
Nisoldipine	10-40 mg/day	7-12	=	↓↓↓	As for nifedipine
Nitrendipine	20 mg/day or bid	5-12	↑	↓↓↓	As for nifedipine
OTHERS					
Bepridil	200-400 mg/day	24-40	↓	↓	Arrhythmias, dizziness, nausea
Diltiazem	30-90 mg tid	4-6	↓	↓	Hypotension, dizziness, bradycardia, edema
Diltiazem CD*	120-540 mg/day	—	↓	↓	
Verapamil	80-160 mg tid	3-8	↓	↓↓	
Verapamil SR*	120-480 mg/day	—	↓	↓↓	Hypotension, heart failure, edema, bradycardia

*PA, XL, SR, CD: long acting.
HR = heart rate; PVR = peripheral vascular resistance.
From Théroux P. Angina pectoris. In: Goldman L, Ausiello DA, eds. Cecil Textbook of Medicine. 23rd ed. Philadelphia: Saunders Elsevier; 2008.

underlying its effects are poorly understood. Possible mechanisms include durable hemodynamic changes that reduce myocardial oxygen demand, improvement in myocardial perfusion by diastolic augmentation of retrograde coronary flow, and improved endothelial function. Although EECP increased the time to ST segment depression during exercise testing, reduced angina, and improved health-related quality of life for at least 1 year in one randomized, double-blind study of patients with chronic stable angina, its role in the treatment of angina remains unclear.[A13]

Myocardial Revascularization

Coronary revascularization with either PCI or CABG (Chapter 74) prolongs life, reduces major cardiovascular events, and improves health status, quality

TABLE 71-14 CLINICAL USE OF NITROGLYCERIN AND NITRATES

	DOSE	DURATION OF ACTION	INDICATION
NITROGLYCERIN			
Sublingual or buccal spray	0.15-1.5 mg	Relief of angina	Before or at onset of pain
Ointment	7.5-40 mg	8-12 hr	Prophylaxis of angina
Transdermal	0.2-0.8 mg/hr	8-16 hr	Prophylaxis of angina
Intravenous	5-400 μg/hr	Ongoing; increasing doses as needed	Recurrent chest pain, systemic hypertension, left-sided heart failure
ISOSORBIDE DINITRATE			
Oral	5-40 mg tid	6-8 hr	Prophylaxis of angina
ISOSORBIDE-5-MONONITRATE			
Oral	20 mg bid	8-12 hr	Prophylaxis of angina
Oral, slow release	30-240 mg/day	12-20 hr	Prophylaxis of angina

From Théroux P. Angina pectoris. In: Goldman L, Ausiello DA, eds. Cecil Textbook of Medicine. 23rd ed. Philadelphia: Saunders Elsevier; 2008.

of life, and functional capacity in selected patients with chronic, stable ischemic heart disease who meet certain anatomic criteria: the presence of significant left main coronary artery disease, three-vessel coronary artery disease, or multivessel coronary artery disease with an LV ejection fraction below 50%. For other patients, however, the data are more mixed.

Comparisons of PCI with Optimal Medical Therapy

Numerous randomized clinical trials have compared PCI with medical therapy in patients who have stable coronary heart disease and do have anatomic criteria as noted before. In these patients, PCI improves angina symptoms but does not reduce the risk of death, MI, or other major cardiovascular events when it is added to optimal medical therapy as an initial management strategy in patients with stable ischemic heart disease.[A14-A17] As a result, a trial of optimal medical therapy to control symptoms is justifiable and more cost-effective[10] for patients whose stable coronary disease is not associated with anatomic features for which revascularization has been shown to prolong life. For patients with stable angina and coronary lesions with reduced FFR below 0.8 in one or more visually stenotic arteries (≥50% stenosis), initial PCI significantly reduces the need for hospitalization for urgent revascularization but has not been shown to reduce the composite end point of MI or death.[A1] Because PCI as an initial management strategy does not reduce long-term death, MI, or other major cardiovascular events when it is added to optimal medical therapy in patients with stable coronary artery disease but without specific anatomic criteria, preventive pharmacotherapy and lifestyle modification for secondary prevention of major cardiovascular events must be paramount in such patients.

Comparisons of CABG with Medical Therapy

Randomized trials comparing CABG with medical therapy indicate that a greater severity of ischemia, a greater extent of disease, and the presence of LV dysfunction favor a greater magnitude of survival benefit of CABG over medical therapy. CABG prolongs survival in patients with significant left main coronary artery disease irrespective of symptoms, in patients with multivessel coronary artery disease and impaired LV function (ejection fraction < 50%), and in patients with three-vessel coronary artery disease that includes the proximal left anterior descending coronary artery. Patients with extensive multivessel coronary artery disease appear to benefit more from CABG surgery, particularly if they also have diabetes, whereas PCI is most appropriate for patients with one- or two-vessel coronary artery disease. Of note is that these randomized trials found little difference in mortality between CABG surgery and medical therapy at 1 year, but the benefits of CABG surgery over medical therapy steadily emerged during the next 3 to 5 years. Few patients in these early trials received arterial grafts (which would likely improve the long-term results of CABG surgery), aspirin to prevent graft occlusion, lipid-lowering drugs to mitigate late graft disease progression, or inhibitors of the renin-angiotensin-aldosterone system. With improvements in operative techniques, more common use of antiplatelet agents, more widespread use of disease-modifying therapies, and more aggressive risk factor management during the past decade, the benefits of modern-day CABG surgery compared with contemporary medical therapy have likely changed.

Comparisons of PCI with CABG Surgery for Multivessel Coronary Artery Disease

In randomized trials that have compared PCI with CABG in patients with multivessel coronary artery disease, most excluded patients with significant left main coronary artery disease and were conducted in an era before the advent of stents and other advances in PCI technology, including newer adjunctive medical therapies that are increasingly in widespread clinical use. In patients with severe three-vessel disease or left main disease randomized to either CABG surgery or PCI with a paclitaxel drug-eluting stent, CABG significantly reduced the end point of cardiac death, recurrent MI, and repeated revascularization in the CABG-treated patients with multivessel disease, especially in patients with diabetes.[A18] In a large randomized trial of diabetic patients with multivessel but stable ischemic heart disease, CABG significantly reduced both death and MI compared with PCI.[A19]

In summary, among patients who remain symptomatic despite intensive treatment or who have substantial ischemia or extensive coronary artery disease, revascularization with either PCI or CABG is appropriate, depending on the anatomic complexity of disease (see Table 71-11; Chapter 73). CABG surgery is clearly superior to PCI in symptomatic patients with three-vessel or left main coronary artery disease and in diabetic patients with stable ischemic heart disease. Although PCI appears to provide equivalent survival outcomes in lower risk patients and in patients with one- or two-vessel disease, repeated procedures are more often needed.

OTHER ANGINAL SYNDROMES

Variant Angina or Prinzmetal's Angina

The diagnosis of variant or Prinzmetal's angina is based on the documentation of transient ST segment elevation during an episode of chest pain in the absence of a severe, fixed coronary stenosis. Prinzmetal's variant angina typically is caused by an occlusive spasm superimposed on a coronary artery stenosis that otherwise does not limit blood flow significantly. In some patients, however, no underlying stenoses are seen. Associated Raynaud phenomenon and migraine headache have been described in some patients, suggesting that the syndrome may be part of a more generalized vasospastic disorder.

The chest discomfort occurs predominantly at rest, although approximately one third of patients may also experience pain during exercise. There is a predilection for the pain to wake the patient in the early morning hours when sympathetic activity is increasing. The syndrome is often cyclical; periods of exacerbation with repetitive episodes of chest pain may persist only for seconds or be more prolonged and severe, alternating with periods with few or no symptoms. The symptoms are typically relieved by nitroglycerin. The ST segment elevation accompanying the pain signifies transmural ischemia due to total abrupt occlusion of a nonsignificant stenosis in the absence of adequate collateral circulation. The subsequent rapid reperfusion may explain the high prevalence of severe life-threatening arrhythmias.

Coronary angiography, with a provocative test for spasm such as injection of acetylcholine into the affected coronary artery, usually precipitates the syndrome. Such testing is useful to establish the diagnosis and to assess the response to therapy, especially in patients with normal or nearly normal coronary angiograms, in whom the diagnosis is otherwise unclear. Dihydropyridine calcium-channel blockers (e.g., amlodipine, 5 to 10 mg orally per day) are preferred in patients with Prinzmetal's angina.

Microvascular Angina with Normal Coronary Angiography

Angina can occur despite normal coronary arteries, even after an acetylcholine challenge. More detailed testing may reveal increased coronary resistance and an inability to increase coronary resistance and to increase coronary flow in response to stimuli such as exercise, adenosine, dipyridamole, and atrial pacing.

Symptoms occur most frequently at rest and often in relation to emotional stress. Periods of exacerbation commonly alternate with symptom-free periods. The syndrome is more frequent in women, and some patients have an altered perception of pain or hypersensitivity to certain stimuli.

The diagnosis requires objective documentation of ischemia based on ST-T segment changes, a metabolic abnormality, a transient regional perfusion defect or new wall motion abnormality on echocardiography, or endothelial dysfunction that limits blood flow reserve. Abnormal endothelium-dependent vasoreactivity can be associated with regional myocardial perfusion defects on SPECT and PET imaging.

β-Blockers may be useful, particularly when a relative tachycardia, hypertension, or decreased heart rate variability on Holter monitoring is present. Nitroglycerin can relieve symptoms in approximately 50% of patients, and long-acting nitrates or calcium antagonists are sometimes helpful.

The prognosis is generally favorable and not different from that of a general age-matched population in the absence of coronary artery disease. However, some studies have indicated that an ischemic response to exercise is associated with increased mortality.

Silent Myocardial Ischemia

Up to 20% of patients with ischemic heart disease may not present with angina. Such patients are often described as having silent myocardial ischemia. Some patients are totally asymptomatic despite obstructive coronary artery disease, which may be severe. Others have silent ischemia after a prior documented MI. The third and most common form occurs in patients who may also exhibit the usual forms of chronic stable angina, unstable angina, and Prinzmetal's angina. When monitored, these patients, who typically have silent ischemia episodes in addition to symptomatic ischemia, are sometimes referred to as having *mixed angina*. This mixed angina is estimated to be present in approximately one third of all treated patients with angina, although an even higher prevalence has been reported in diabetic patients. In these patients, about 85% of ambulant ischemic episodes occur without chest pain, and 66% of angina episodes are not accompanied by ST segment depression, suggesting that overt angina pectoris is merely the "tip of the ischemic iceberg." Pharmacologic agents that reduce or abolish episodes of symptomatic ischemia also reduce or abolish episodes of silent ischemia.

PROGNOSIS WITH OPTIMAL MANAGEMENT

Modern treatments have improved the prognosis of patients with stable ischemic heart disease to an annual mortality rate of 1 to 3% and a 1 to 2% rate of major ischemic events. The 1-year rate of cardiovascular death is now 1.9% (95% confidence interval [CI], 1.7 to 2.1), with a 2.9% (95% CI, 2.6 to 3.2) rate of all-cause mortality and a 4.5% (95% CI, 4.2 to 4.8) rate of the combined outcome of cardiovascular death, MI, or stroke. Even in patients who have refractory angina and are not candidates for revascularization, modern medical treatment is associated with a 1-year mortality of only 4% and a 9-year mortality of 30%.[11]

Recurrent angina is a common subsequent complaint in many patients with stable ischemic heart disease, even those who were initially treated successfully with PCI. About 30% of patients continue to experience angina one or more times per week, with associated greater physical limitation and worse quality of life, and almost 80% of patients who underwent initially successful PCI for chronic angina still take one or more antianginal agents at 1 year.

Selection of optimal treatment requires a full understanding of the potential risks and benefits of each treatment approach. In patients with stable symptoms who have not had an adequate trial of medical therapy (e.g., 8 to 12 weeks of multifaceted medical therapy and lifestyle intervention), such an initial approach of aggressive medical therapy is recommended. For patients whose angina or quality of life is not adequately controlled with optimal medical therapy, revascularization with either PCI or CABG surgery should be considered. Recent clinical trials data now show convincing benefit of CABG surgery over PCI for patients with left main or three-vessel coronary artery disease and for diabetic patients with multivessel disease. Although the results of randomized trials must be individualized for specific patients, a multidisciplinary approach to clinical decision making can ensure that all therapeutic options are fully and transparently discussed so that patients are offered the most appropriate evidence-based treatment recommendations that are tailored to the level of ischemic risk and coronary anatomic findings.

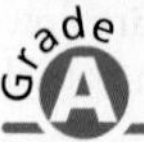

Grade A References

A1. De Bruyne B, Pijls NH, Kalesan B, et al. Fractional flow reserve–guided PCI versus medical therapy in stable coronary disease. *N Engl J Med*. 2012;367:991-1001.

A2. De Bruyne B, Fearon WF, Pijls NH, et al. Fractional flow reserve-guided PCI for stable coronary artery disease. *N Engl J Med*. 2014;371:1208-1217.

A3. Cannon CP, Braunwald E, McCabe CH, et al. Intensive versus moderate lipid lowering with statins after acute coronary syndromes. *N Engl J Med*. 2004;350:1495-1504.

A4. Ginsberg HN, Elam MB, Lovato LC, et al. Effects of combination lipid therapy in type 2 diabetes mellitus. *N Engl J Med*. 2010;362:1563-1574.

A5. Jun M, Foote C, Lv J, et al. Effects of fibrates on cardiovascular outcomes: a systematic review and meta-analysis. *Lancet*. 2010;375:1875-1884.

A6. Boden WE, Probstfield JL, Anderson T, et al. Niacin in patients with low HDL cholesterol levels receiving intensive statin therapy. *N Engl J Med*. 2011;365:2255-2267.

A7. Landray MJ, Haynes R, Hopewell JC, et al. Effects of extended-release niacin with laropiprant in high-risk patients. *N Engl J Med*. 2014;371:203-212.

A8. Dagenais GR, Pogue J, Fox K, et al. Angiotensin-converting enzyme inhibitors in stable vascular disease without left ventricular systolic dysfunction or heart failure: a combined analysis of three trials. *Lancet*. 2006;368:581-588.

A9. Lièvre M, Cucherat M. Aspirin in the secondary prevention of cardiovascular disease: an update of the APTC meta-analysis. *Fundam Clin Pharmacol*. 2010;24:385-391.

A10. Bhatt DC, Fox KA, Hacke W, et al. Clopidogrel and aspirin versus aspirin alone for the prevention of atherothrombotic events. *N Engl J Med*. 2006;354:1706-1717.

A11. Anand SS, Yusuf S. Oral anticoagulants in patients with coronary artery disease. *J Am Coll Cardiol*. 2003;41:62S-69S.

A12. Kosiborod M, Arnold SV, Spertus JA, et al. Evaluation of ranolazine in patients with type 2 diabetes mellitus and chronic stable angina: results from the TERISA randomized clinical trial (Type 2 Diabetes Evaluation of Ranolazine in Subjects With Chronic Stable Angina). *J Am Coll Cardiol*. 2013;61:2038-2045.

A13. McKenna C, McDaid C, Suekarran S, et al. Enhanced external counterpulsation for the treatment of stable angina and heart failure: a systematic review and economic analysis. *Health Technol Assess*. 2009;13:1-90.

A14. Stergiopoulos K, Boden WE, Hartigan P, et al. Percutaneous coronary intervention outcomes in patients with stable obstructive coronary artery disease and myocardial ischemia: a collaborative meta-analysis of contemporary randomized clinical trials. *JAMA Intern Med*. 2014;174:232-240.

A15. Boden WE, O'Rourke RA, Teo KK, et al. Optimal medical therapy with or without PCI for stable coronary disease. *N Engl J Med*. 2007;356:1503-1516.

A16. BARI Investigators. The final 10-year follow-up results from the BARI randomized trial. *J Am Coll Cardiol*. 2007;49:1600-1606.

A17. Frye R, August P, Brooks M, et al. BARI 2D: a randomized clinical trial of treatment strategies for type 2 diabetes and coronary artery disease. *N Engl J Med*. 2009;360:2503-2515.

A18. Mohr FW, Morice MC, Kappetein AP, et al. Coronary artery bypass graft surgery versus percutaneous coronary intervention in patients with three-vessel disease and left main coronary disease: 5-year follow-up of the randomised, clinical SYNTAX trial. *Lancet*. 2013;381:629-638.

A19. Farkouh ME, Domanski M, Sleeper LA, et al. Strategies for multivessel revascularization in patients with diabetes. *N Engl J Med*. 2012;367:2375-2384.

GENERAL REFERENCES

For the General References and other additional features, please visit Expert Consult at https://expertconsult.inkling.com.

72 ACUTE CORONARY SYNDROME: UNSTABLE ANGINA AND NON-ST ELEVATION MYOCARDIAL INFARCTION

RICHARD A. LANGE AND L. DAVID HILLIS

DEFINITION

The term *acute coronary syndrome* (ACS) is used to describe the continuum of myocardial ischemia (unstable angina pectoris) or infarction (with or without concomitant ST segment elevation). The patient with *unstable angina* has cardiac chest pain that is new, worsening (i.e., more severe, prolonged, or frequent than previous episodes of angina), or occurring at rest, *without* serologic evidence of myocyte necrosis—that is, no elevation of serum concentrations of troponin or the MB isoenzyme of creatine kinase (CK-MB). The patient with cardiac chest pain *with* serologic evidence of myonecrosis and without ST segment elevation is said to have a *non–ST segment elevation myocardial infarction* (MI). Because unstable angina and non–ST segment elevation MI are characterized by the absence of ST segment elevation, they are collectively termed *non–ST segment elevation ACS*, or NSTE ACS (Fig. 72-1). The patient with acute-onset cardiac chest pain, serologic evidence of myonecrosis, and persistent (>20 minutes) ST segment elevation is said to have an *ST segment elevation MI* (Chapter 73).

EPIDEMIOLOGY

Almost 1.2 million individuals in the United States are hospitalized annually with ACS, of whom approximately two thirds have NSTE ACS. More than

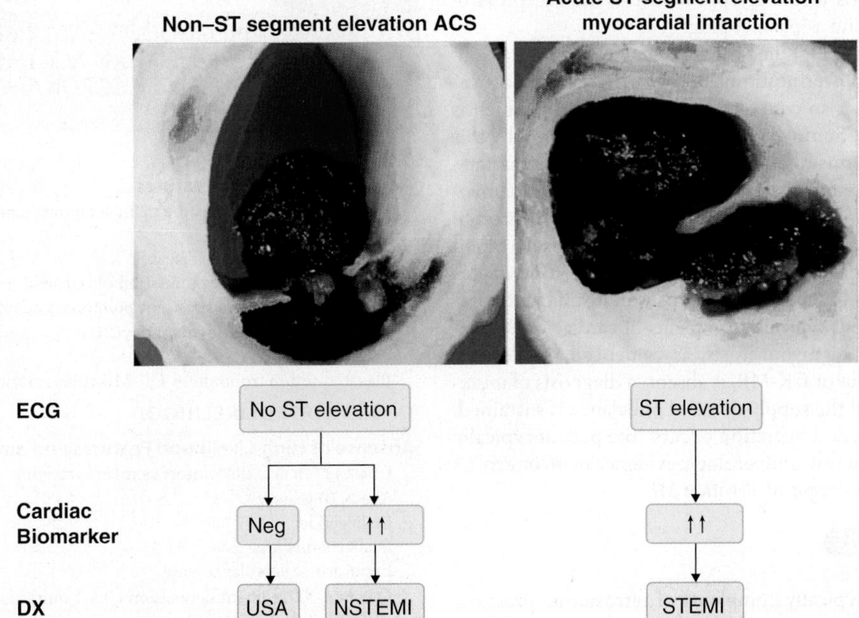

FIGURE 72-1. Acute coronary syndrome (ACS). Symptomatic, morphologic, electrocardiographic, and serologic findings in patients with various kinds of ACS. Subjects with ACS usually complain of chest pain. If the involved coronary artery is totally occluded by fresh thrombus (shown on the *right*), the patient's electrocardiogram (ECG) reveals ST segment elevation, cardiac biomarkers subsequently are elevated, and the patient is diagnosed with an ST segment elevation myocardial infarction (STEMI). If the involved coronary artery is partially occluded by fresh thrombus (shown on the *left*), the patient's ECG does not show ST segment elevation. If cardiac biomarkers are not elevated, the patient is diagnosed with unstable angina (USA). If cardiac biomarkers are elevated, the patient is diagnosed with a non–ST segment elevation MI (NSTEMI). Dx = diagnosis.

half of those with NSTE ACS are older than 65 years, and almost half are women. NSTE ACS is more common in individuals with one or more risk factors for atherosclerosis (Chapter 52), peripheral vascular disease, or a chronic inflammatory disorder, such as rheumatoid arthritis, psoriasis, or infection.

Most subjects with ACS have so-called primary ACS, which is precipitated by rupture of a coronary arterial atherosclerotic plaque, with subsequent platelet aggregation and thrombus formation, leading in turn to diminished blood flow in the involved artery. An occasional individual has so-called secondary ACS, which is caused by a transient or sustained marked imbalance between myocardial oxygen supply and demand. Substantial reductions in oxygen supply, for example, can be caused by severe systemic arterial hypotension, anemia, or hypoxemia; dramatic increases in oxygen demand can be caused by tachycardia, severe systemic arterial hypertension, or thyrotoxicosis. In the subject thought to have secondary ACS, therapy should be directed at the underlying cause.

PATHOBIOLOGY

The precipitating event in almost all subjects with NSTE ACS is coronary arterial atherosclerotic plaque rupture or erosion, with subsequent platelet aggregation and thrombus formation, leading to subtotal occlusion of the involved artery.[1] In an occasional patient, total thrombotic occlusion of the artery leads to NSTE ACS rather than to ST segment elevation MI when extensive collateral blood supply perfuses the region of myocardium that is distal to the occluded artery.

Rarely, intense vasospasm of a segment of an epicardial coronary artery, due to focal endothelial dysfunction (i.e., Prinzmetal's angina) or drug ingestion (caused, for example, by cocaine, chemotherapeutic agents, or one of the serotonin receptor agonist "triptans"), causes a transient or sustained compromise of coronary arterial blood flow, with resultant NSTE ACS. Spontaneous coronary arterial dissection, which occurs most often in peripartum women and patients with vasculitis, may result in NSTE ACS.

Plaque Rupture

Coronary arterial atherosclerotic plaque rupture (Chapter 70) or erosion is the initiating event in most patients with NSTE ACS. Several factors may play a role in the deterioration of the protective fibrous cap that separates the atheroma in the vessel wall from the coronary arterial lumen. Local and systemic inflammation, mechanical features, and anatomic changes contribute to the transformation of a stable atherosclerotic plaque to a so-called vulnerable plaque, the rupture of which triggers platelet adherence, activation, and aggregation, with subsequent thrombus formation.

The deposition of oxidized low-density lipoprotein in the coronary arterial wall stimulates an inflammatory response, which results in the accumulation of macrophages and T lymphocytes at the plaque border. These inflammatory cells secrete cytokines (e.g., tissue necrosis factor, interleukin-1, interferon-γ), which inhibit collagen synthesis and deposition, as well as enzymes (e.g., matrix metalloproteinases and cathepsins), which promote collagen and elastin degradation, thereby rendering the overlying fibrous cap vulnerable to rupture.

Systemic inflammation may play a role in plaque rupture, as evidenced by the predisposition to development of ACS in individuals with chronic gingivitis, rheumatoid arthritis, and chronic or acute infection. Angiographic and angioscopic studies of the coronary arteries of ACS patients often demonstrate plaque ulceration and thrombosis at more than one site, thereby suggesting that a systemic and diffuse inflammatory process is present.

The mechanical characteristics and location of coronary arterial plaques appear to influence their stability. For example, thin fibrous caps are more likely to erode or to rupture than are thick ones. Sites of low shear stress, such as vessel bifurcations, have reduced production of endothelial vasodilator substances (i.e., nitric oxide and prostacyclin), accelerated accumulation of lipids and inflammatory cells, increased degradation of the extracellular matrix, and thinning of the fibrous cap, all of which contribute to plaque instability.

Detailed histologic examination of evolving atherosclerotic plaques reveals a rich neovascularization that is the result of angiogenic peptides, such as fibroblast growth factors, vascular endothelial growth factor, placental growth factor, oncostatin M, and hypoxia-inducible factor, which are secreted by smooth muscle cells, inflammatory cells, and platelets. This neovascularization contributes to the growth of atheroma and to leukocyte trafficking, plaque hemorrhage, and destabilization.

Thrombus Formation

Platelets play a pivotal role in the pathobiology of ACS. After erosion or rupture of a vulnerable plaque, circulating platelets *adhere* to the exposed subendothelial proteins, after which they are *activated*. With activation, the platelets change shape from discoid to stellate, thereby increasing the surface area on which thrombin formation can occur. The platelets then release the contents of their intracellular granules (i.e., thromboxane, serotonin, adenosine diphosphate [ADP], von Willebrand factor, fibrinogen) into the immediate environment and promote focal vasoconstriction of the adjacent arterial segment and activation of nearby platelets. Platelets also increase the number of glycoprotein IIb/IIIa receptors on their surface and the affinity of these receptors to bind circulating fibrinogen. The result is platelet *aggregation*, which occurs as fibrinogen binds to the glycoprotein IIb/IIIa receptors of adjacent platelets, thereby creating a "platelet plug."

With formation of the platelet plug, the coagulation system activates and generates thrombin, which is a powerful stimulator of further platelet activation and aggregation. Thrombin also converts fibrinogen to fibrin, which is incorporated into the thrombus. Subtotal coronary arterial occlusion by this platelet-rich thrombus compromises blood flow in the involved artery, thereby resulting in an imbalance of oxygen supply and demand of the myocytes perfused by the artery. Distal embolization of platelet-rich thrombi from the site of a ruptured plaque may contribute to the compromise in blood flow. If the supply-demand imbalance is transient, the involved myocytes become ischemic but do not die because the ischemia is of insufficient duration to cause necrosis. The patient typically complains of cardiac chest pain at rest, but serologic evidence of myonecrosis, as evidenced by elevated serum concentrations of troponin or CK-MB, is absent; a diagnosis of *unstable angina* is made. In contrast, if the supply-demand imbalance is sustained, ischemic myocytes begin to die, and infarction occurs. The patient typically complains of cardiac chest pain at rest, and serologic evidence of myonecrosis confirms the diagnosis of *non–ST segment elevation MI.*

CLINICAL MANIFESTATIONS

Symptoms

The patient with NSTE ACS typically complains of retrosternal pressure, squeezing, or heaviness that may be intermittent and recurrent or persistent (Chapter 51). If the episodes are intermittent and recurrent, the duration of each episode may range from only a few minutes to several hours. The chest pain may radiate to the left arm, neck, or jaw, and it may be accompanied by diaphoresis, nausea, abdominal pain, dyspnea, or syncope.

Atypical presentations of NSTE ACS are not uncommon and may include aching or vague chest discomfort, epigastric pain, acute-onset indigestion, unexplained fatigue, or dyspnea. Such atypical complaints are often observed in younger (25 to 40 years of age) and older (>75 years of age) patients, women, and patients with diabetes mellitus, chronic renal insufficiency, or dementia.

Physical Examination

The patient with NSTE ACS often has normal findings on physical examination. On occasion, evidence of left ventricular dysfunction (Chapter 58), such as basilar rales or a ventricular gallop, hypotension, or peripheral hypoperfusion, may accompany an episode of NSTE ACS or appear shortly thereafter. An important goal of the physical examination is to exclude other potential causes of the patient's symptoms, including both noncardiac causes (i.e., costochondritis, pneumothorax, pulmonary embolism, pneumonia) and other cardiac disorders not attributable to myocardial ischemia (i.e., aortic dissection, pericarditis, severe systemic arterial hypertension, arrhythmias; Chapter 51). Accordingly, differences in blood pressure between the upper and lower limbs, decreased lung sounds, friction rubs, and pain on sternal palpation suggest a diagnosis other than NSTE ACS. Other findings on physical examination—such as an elevated blood pressure, tachycardia, pallor, or increased sweating or tremor—point toward precipitating conditions, such as uncontrolled hypertension (Chapter 67), arrhythmias (Chapters 64 and 65), anemia (Chapter 158), or thyrotoxicosis (Chapter 226).

DIAGNOSIS

The patient with suspected ACS should be evaluated promptly because an expedient and accurate diagnosis permits the timely initiation of appropriate therapy, which can reduce the rate of complications. The initial assessment should be directed at determining whether the subject's symptoms are likely to be caused by myocardial ischemia, MI, or some other disorder. The likelihood of ACS can be estimated from the history, physical examination, and electrocardiogram (ECG) (Table 72-1). In the acute setting, the presence or absence of traditional risk factors for atherosclerosis is less important for determining the presence or absence of ACS than are the patient's symptoms, ECG findings, and serologic evidence of myonecrosis. As a result, these long-term risk factors are not integral in determining whether an individual should be evaluated, hospitalized, or treated for ACS.

Conditions that increase the likelihood that the symptomatic patient is experiencing myocardial ischemia or MI include older age, male gender, diabetes mellitus, extracardiac vascular disease, and chest pain radiating to the left arm, neck, or jaw as the presenting symptom. Myocardial ischemia is highly likely if anginal symptoms are accompanied by ECG abnormalities (i.e., Q waves, ST segment depression or elevation ≥1 mm in magnitude, or T wave inversion in multiple precordial leads) or elevated serum concentrations of troponin or CK-MB.

TABLE 72-1 LIKELIHOOD THAT SYMPTOMS AND SIGNS REPRESENT AN ACUTE CORONARY SYNDROME CAUSED BY CORONARY ARTERIAL PLAQUE RUPTURE

HIGH LIKELIHOOD
Any of the Following Features
Chest or left arm pain as the main symptom, similar in nature to previously noted angina
Known coronary artery disease
Evidence on physical examination of transient murmur of mitral regurgitation, hypotension, diaphoresis, or pulmonary edema
New or transient ST segment deviation (≥1 mm) or T wave inversion in multiple precordial leads
Elevated serum troponin or CK-MB concentration
INTERMEDIATE LIKELIHOOD
Absence of High-Likelihood Features and any of the Following
Chest or left arm discomfort as main symptom
Age > 70 years
Male gender
Diabetes mellitus
Extracardiac vascular disease
Q waves, ST segment depression (0.5-1 mm), or T wave inversion (>1 mm) in leads with dominant R waves
Normal cardiac troponin or CK-MB
LOW LIKELIHOOD
Absence of High- or Intermediate-Likelihood Features, but May Have
Probable ischemic symptoms in the absence of any of the intermediate likelihood characteristics
Recent cocaine use
Chest discomfort reproduced by palpation
T wave flattening or inversion < 1 mm in leads with dominant R waves
Normal electrocardiogram
Normal serum troponin or CK-MB concentration

Modified from Anderson JL, Adams CD, Antman EM, et al. ACC/AHA 2007 guidelines for the management of patients with unstable angina/non-ST-elevation myocardial infarction. *Circulation.* 2007;116:e148-e304.

In a patient with known coronary artery disease, typical symptoms are likely to be caused by myocardial ischemia or MI rather than by another condition, particularly if the patient confirms that the symptoms are similar to previous anginal episodes. Conversely, a young individual who has a normal ECG and no risk factors for atherosclerosis is unlikely to be having ACS even when complaining of chest pain with features consistent with ischemia or infarction.

It is important to inquire about the use of cocaine and methamphetamines in the patient with suspected ACS, especially in those who are younger than 40 years or have few traditional risk factors for atherosclerosis. These drugs can increase myocardial oxygen demand and concomitantly decrease oxygen supply by causing vasospasm and thrombosis. A urine toxicologic analysis should be considered when substance abuse is suspected as a cause of ACS.

Electrocardiogram

An ECG, which should be obtained and examined promptly in the patient with suspected ACS, is particularly valuable if it is obtained during a symptomatic episode. If the patient has persistent (>20 minutes) ST segment elevation, prompt reperfusion therapy should be initiated (Chapter 73). Transient ST segment abnormalities that develop during a symptomatic episode at rest and resolve when the patient is asymptomatic strongly suggest NSTE ACS. ST segment depression (or transient ST segment elevation) and T wave abnormalities occur in up to 50% of NSTE ACS patients.

A completely normal ECG does not exclude the possibility of NSTE ACS; in fact, about 5% of patients who are discharged from the emergency department and ultimately diagnosed with ACS have a normal ECG. Ischemia or infarction in the territory of the left circumflex coronary artery often escapes detection with a standard 12-lead ECG, but it may be detected with right-sided leads (V_4R and V_3R) or posterior leads (V_7 to V_9). In the patient whose initial ECG is normal, subsequent ECGs should be obtained in the first 24 hours and during symptomatic episodes, and they should be compared with previous tracings to identify new ST segment or T wave abnormalities. Deep

(>2 mm), symmetrical T wave inversion in the anterior chest leads is often associated with a hemodynamically significant stenosis of the left main or proximal left anterior descending coronary artery.

Serum Biomarkers

With modern high-sensitivity assays, troponin (Chapter 73) is detectable in the blood within 2 hours of the onset of symptoms in patients with non–ST segment elevation MI.[2] An undetectable high-sensitivity troponin level at presentation to the hospital reduces the probability of acute MI to less than 1%.[3] With conventional assays, troponin elevations are generally detectable within 4 hours of the onset of myonecrosis, but detection may be delayed for up to 8 hours in some individuals. Because a single normal serum troponin measurement is insufficient to exclude MI in a patient with recent symptoms, patients with suspected MI are generally observed, either in the emergency department or in a chest pain evaluation unit, with a repeated troponin measurement (and a repeated ECG) 2 to 6 hours later or whenever chest pain recurs.[4] Serum troponin levels also help in acute risk stratification of all ACS patients at the time of the patient's arrival to the hospital.

Serum troponin concentrations can be measured with point-of-care instruments at the patient's bedside by desktop devices or handheld rapid qualitative assays. The advantage of point-of-care systems for avoiding delays must be weighed against their higher costs and the need for stringent quality control. In addition, point-of-care assays are qualitative or semiquantitative and observer dependent, whereas the central laboratory provides more accurate quantitative information concerning biomarker concentrations.

Up to one third of ACS patients whose serum CK-MB concentrations are normal have detectable serum concentrations of troponin T and I, indicating that myonecrosis has occurred and establishing the diagnosis of non–ST segment elevation MI. Current recommendations call for the use of the serum troponin concentration for acute risk stratification at the time of the patient's arrival to the hospital.

Noninvasive Testing

The patient considered to have a low likelihood for ACS (on the basis of the history, physical examination, ECG, and serum biomarkers) should undergo timely stress testing (Chapter 51). Although stress testing does not absolutely establish or exclude the presence of coronary artery disease, it has the advantage of also defining a patient's exercise tolerance, which helps tailor therapeutic decisions. Alternatively, multidetector coronary computed tomographic angiography, which has a high (>98%) negative predictive value to exclude coronary artery disease when it is performed and interpreted at experienced centers, can help reduce hospital stay when the findings are normal in emergency department patients at low to intermediate risk of possible ACS.[A1] Conversely, the patient who is believed to be at higher risk for ACS or who continues to have typical ischemic chest pain with ECG abnormalities or elevated cardiac biomarkers should not undergo stress testing or coronary computed tomographic angiography but rather should either undergo coronary angiography or be rendered symptom free with medical therapy before stress testing.

An echocardiogram may be helpful in the patient with chest pain if the ECG is nondiagnostic (i.e., minimal ST segment or T wave abnormalities). If left ventricular hypokinesis or akinesis is observed during an episode of chest pain and then improves when symptoms resolve, myocardial ischemia is likely. In the patient with anterior T wave inversion of uncertain etiology, hypokinesis of the left ventricular anterior wall suggests that the observed T wave abnormality is due to a severe stenosis of the left anterior descending coronary artery. Because echocardiography can help evaluate and identify alternative causes for the patient's chest pain (i.e., myocarditis [Chapter 60], aortic dissection [Chapter 78], or pulmonary embolism [Chapter 98]), it is recommended in patients whose diagnosis is uncertain.

Coronary Angiography

Coronary angiography (Chapter 57) should be performed in patients who are thought to be at high risk for death, MI, or recurrent ischemia in the ensuing days, weeks, and months (see later); in patients who have spontaneous or inducible myocardial ischemia despite appropriate medical therapy; and in patients who have a confusing or difficult clinical presentation and a subsequent inconclusive noninvasive evaluation. The results of angiography help determine whether revascularization is appropriate and, if so, whether it should be attempted by coronary artery bypass grafting or percutaneous coronary intervention (PCI) (Chapter 74).

In patients with NSTE ACS, coronary angiography demonstrates significant stenosis of the left main coronary artery in about 15% of patients, of all three major epicardial coronary arteries in about 30 to 35% of patients, of two of the three epicardial arteries in about 20 to 30% of patients, and of one major epicardial artery in 20 to 30% of patients. About 15% of patients have no coronary arterial narrowing of hemodynamic significance. Women with NSTE ACS are likely to have less extensive coronary artery disease than men have, and patients with non–ST segment elevation MI usually have more extensive disease than those with unstable angina.

On angiography, the coronary arterial lesion responsible for NSTE ACS (the so-called culprit lesion) typically is asymmetrical or eccentric, with scalloped or overhanging edges and a narrow base or neck, features that reflect underlying plaque disruption and thrombus formation. Although obvious thrombus is visible by angiography in only one third of patients with NSTE ACS, coronary angioscopy shows plaque rupture with overlying thrombus in the majority. Interestingly, the lesion that is the nidus for ACS often is not severely stenotic when it is assessed on recently performed angiograms; in fact, two thirds of culprit lesions previously had less than 50% luminal diameter narrowing (and therefore would not have been considered appropriate for revascularization).

Risk Assessment and Triage

The initial evaluation of the patient with possible or suspected ACS should focus on an assessment of the patient's risk of acutely sustaining a cardiac ischemic event (death, MI, or recurrent ischemia). Patients considered to be at low risk for a cardiac ischemic event may be observed in a chest pain evaluation unit for several hours, with repeated troponin level and ECG. If the findings of that brief evaluation are normal, the patient should be discharged home, with further evaluation performed on an outpatient basis. Conversely, patients not at low risk should be hospitalized for further evaluation and treatment (Fig. 72-2; see Fig. 51-1).

After the initial triage decision is made, therapeutic interventions are based on the risk of adverse events in the ensuing hours, days, weeks, and months—estimated by either the Thrombolysis in Myocardial Infarction (TIMI) or Global Registry of Acute Coronary Events (GRACE) risk algorithm—balanced against the risk of a bleeding complication from intensive medical therapy (Table 72-2) or an adverse event from an invasive cardiac procedure. On the basis of this initial assessment, the patient's therapy should be tailored to minimize the likelihood of adverse events.

Although serum markers of myonecrosis represent only one of the TIMI or GRACE risk variables, the presence of this variable alone identifies the patient as being at high risk. However, although elevated serum markers indicate myonecrosis, they provide no insight into its cause because myonecrosis can occur with disease entities other than coronary artery disease (e.g., pulmonary embolism, decompensated heart failure, severe hypertension or tachycardia, anemia, sepsis). Thus, in evaluation of the patient with possible ACS, the presence of elevated serum markers should be assessed in conjunction with other variables.

Increasing age is associated with a higher incidence of both ACS-related cardiac ischemic events and complications from intensive medical therapy and invasive cardiac procedures. Even though elderly individuals are at increased risk of treatment-related complications, they nonetheless derive a greater absolute and relative benefit from such intensive therapy compared with younger individuals. Apart from this initial risk assessment, the ACS patient's general medical and cognitive status, anticipated life expectancy, and, most important, personal preferences should be evaluated and considered.

Once the risk status of the ACS patient is established, therapy is initiated and tailored to the patient's risk of sustaining a subsequent ischemic cardiac event or a treatment-related complication (Table 72-3).[5] For example, the patient considered to be at low risk of a subsequent ischemic event does not benefit from intensive antithrombotic therapy or routine coronary angiography and revascularization. Conversely, in patients considered to be at high risk of sustaining an ischemic event, optimal therapy—including coronary angiography and revascularization (if appropriate)—results in a 20 to 40% decrease in the risk of recurrent ischemia and MI and an approximately 10% reduction in mortality.[A2][A3]

Differential Diagnoses

Several cardiac and noncardiac conditions, some of which are potentially life-threatening, may mimic NSTE ACS. The patient with a pulmonary embolism (Chapter 98) will often complain of chest pain and dyspnea and may have ECG abnormalities and an elevated serum troponin concentration. Aortic dissection (Chapter 78) should be considered and excluded because the therapies for NSTE ACS are contraindicated in patients with this

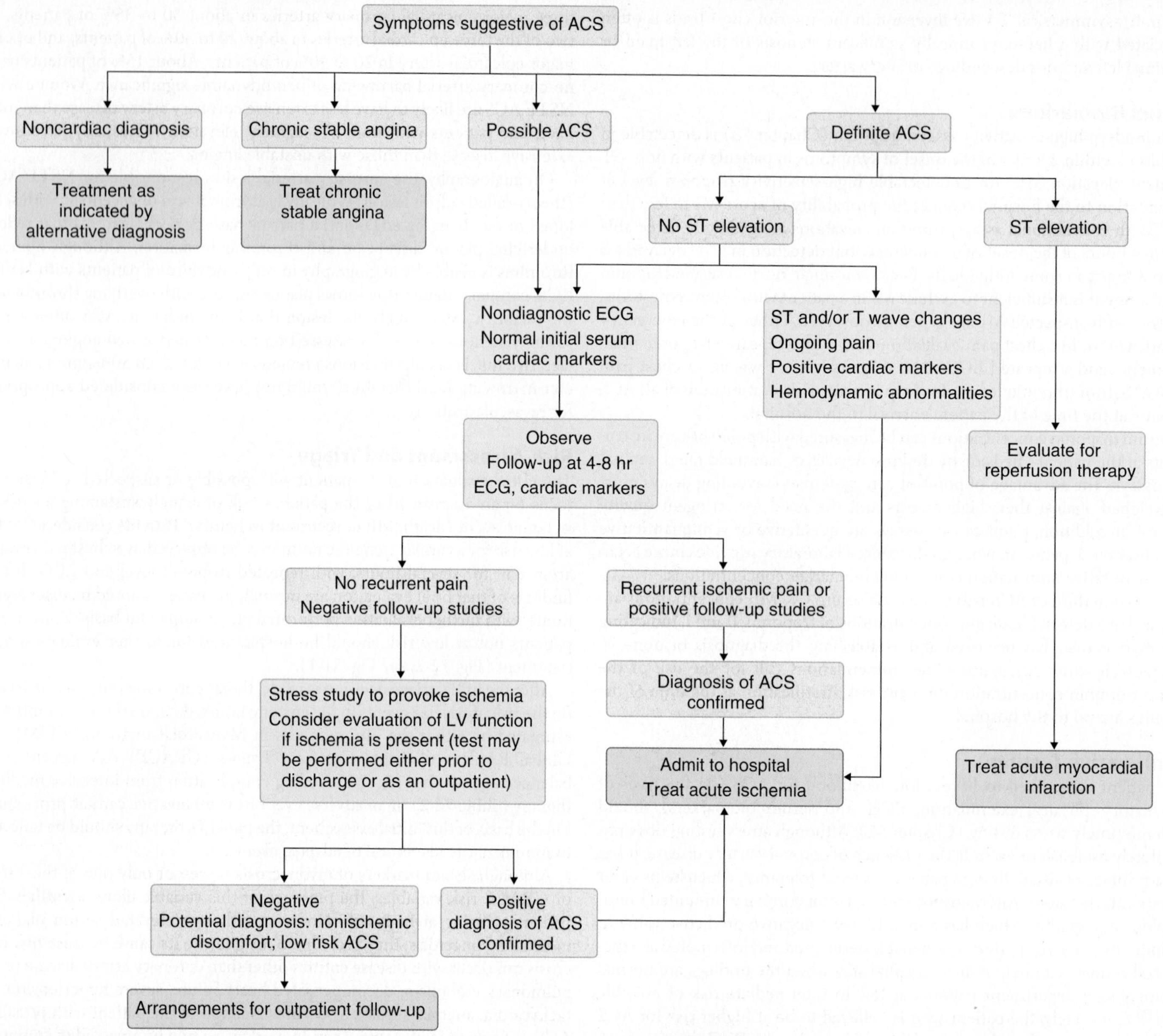

FIGURE 72-2. **Initial triage for patients with symptoms suggestive of an acute coronary syndrome (ACS). ECG = electrocardiogram; LV = left ventricular. (Modified from Anderson JL, Adams CD, Antman EM, et al. ACC/AHA 2007 guidelines for the management of patients with unstable angina and non-ST-segment elevation myocardial infarction. A report of the American College of Cardiology/American Heart Association Task Force on Practice Guidelines. *Circulation.* 2007;116:e148-e304.)**

condition. Stroke (Chapter 407) and subarachnoid hemorrhage (Chapter 408) may be accompanied by ECG abnormalities, left ventricular segmental wall motion abnormalities, and elevated serum biomarker concentrations. Underlying chronic cardiac conditions, such as valvular heart disease (i.e., aortic stenosis, aortic regurgitation) and hypertrophic cardiomyopathy (Chapter 60), may be associated with symptoms similar to those of NSTE ACS, elevated serum biomarker concentrations, and ECG abnormalities. Myocarditis (Chapter 60), pericarditis (Chapter 77), and myopericarditis often cause chest pain that resembles angina, ECG abnormalities, and elevated serum biomarker concentrations; an influenza-like or upper respiratory tract infection often precedes or accompanies these conditions. Patients with "stress cardiomyopathy" (takotsubo syndrome) typically have chest pain, ST segment abnormalities and deeply inverted T waves, and mildly elevated serum biomarker concentrations (Chapter 60).

TREATMENT Rx

The goals of treatment of the subject with NSTE ACS are to prevent recurrent ischemia (by correcting the imbalance between myocardial oxygen supply and demand), to prevent thrombus propagation, and to stabilize the vulnerable plaque. Antianginal medications, such as nitroglycerin (see Table 71-14), β-adrenergic blockers (see Table 71-12), and calcium-channel blockers (see Table 71-13), favorably affect myocardial oxygen supply and demand, thereby preventing recurrent ischemia. Antiplatelet and antithrombotic agents retard thrombus propagation, and statins promote plaque stabilization. Once the risk status of the ACS patient is established, treatment is initiated (see Table 72-3).

Every NSTE ACS patient, regardless of the level of risk, should promptly receive antianginal medications, antiplatelet therapy, and a statin, unless contraindicated. A patient considered to be at low risk may receive unfractionated heparin, but more intensive anticoagulant therapy is not necessary because such therapy increases the risk of bleeding without further reducing the risk of an ischemic cardiac event. Routine coronary angiography and revascularization are not beneficial and should be reserved for the patient with recurrent ischemia despite intensive medical therapy.

Conversely, the high-risk patient should receive antianginal medications, antiplatelet therapy, a statin, intensive anticoagulant therapy, and coronary angiography followed by revascularization (if indicated). In the patient whose coronary anatomy is suitable, revascularization reduces the incidence of ischemia and recurrent MI, and it also improves survival in certain patients (see later).

Antianginal Therapy

Nitroglycerin

Nitroglycerin (see Table 71-14), which is a venodilator at low doses and an arteriolar dilator at higher doses, may prevent recurrent ischemia in patients with unstable angina, but no studies of sufficient statistical power have

TABLE 72-2 RISK VARIABLES FOR ISCHEMIC EVENTS AND BLEEDING COMPLICATIONS

RISK VARIABLES PREDICTIVE OF DEATH, MYOCARDIAL INFARCTION, OR RECURRENT ISCHEMIA

Thrombolysis in Myocardial Infarction (TIMI) Score*

Age > 65 years
Three or more risk factors for atherosclerosis
Known coronary artery disease (previous coronary arteriography or myocardial infarction)
Two or more episodes of anginal chest pain at rest in the 24 hours before hospitalization
Use of aspirin in the 7 days before hospitalization
ST segment deviation ≥ 0.5 mV
Elevated serum concentrations of troponin or CK-MB

Global Registry of Acute Coronary Events (GRACE)†

Age
Heart failure class
Heart rate
Systolic blood pressure
ST segment deviation
Cardiac arrest during presentation
Serum creatinine concentration
Elevated serum markers of myonecrosis

RISK FACTORS FOR BLEEDING COMPLICATIONS WITH INTENSIVE THERAPY‡

Female gender
Older age
Renal insufficiency
Low body weight
Tachycardia
Systolic arterial pressure (high or low)
Anemia
Diabetes mellitus

*Individuals with three or more of these variables are considered to be at high risk, whereas those with none, one, or two are considered to be at low risk. (From Diez JG, Cohen M. Balancing myocardial ischemic and bleeding risks in patients with non-ST-segment elevation myocardial infarction. *Am J Cardiol.* 2009;103:1396-1402.)
†Each variable is assigned a numerical score on the basis of its specific value, and the eight scores are summed to yield a total score, which is applied to a reference nomogram to determine the patient's risk. The GRACE application tool is available online at www.outcomes-umassmed.org/grace. (From Brieger D, Fox KA, Fitzgerald G, et al. Predicting freedom from clinical events in non-ST-elevation acute coronary syndromes: the Global Registry of Acute Coronary Events. *Heart.* 2009;95:888-894.)
‡The patient's bleeding risk can be estimated with the tool available at www.crusadebleedingscore.org. (From Subherwal S, Bach RG, Chen AY, et al. Baseline risk of major bleeding in non-ST-segment-elevation myocardial infarction: the CRUSADE [Can Rapid risk stratification of Unstable angina patients Suppress ADverse outcomes with Early implementation of the ACC/AHA Guidelines] Bleeding Score. *Circulation.* 2009;119:1873-1882.)

determined whether it reduces the risk of MI in this population of patients. In patients who complain of recurrent symptoms, nitroglycerin should be given sublingually or by buccal spray (0.3 to 0.6 mg). Patients with ongoing or recurrent chest pain should receive intravenous nitroglycerin (5 to 10 μg/minute with use of nonabsorbable tubing), with escalation of the dose in increments of 10 μg/minute until symptoms resolve or adverse effects develop. Nitroglycerin's most common adverse effects are headache, nausea, dizziness, hypotension, and reflex tachycardia.

Nitrate tolerance can be avoided by periodically providing the patient with a nitrate-free period (i.e., a brief cessation of drug administration). Nitroglycerin should not be given to patients who have received a phosphodiesterase-5 inhibitor (i.e., sildenafil, tadalafil, or vardenafil) within the previous 24 to 48 hours as severe hypotension may ensue.

β-Adrenergic Blockers

β-Adrenergic blockers diminish symptoms and the risk of MI in ACS patients who are not already taking a β-blocker at the time of hospitalization. In the normotensive patient without ongoing chest pain or tachycardia, metoprolol should be initiated at 50 mg orally every 6 to 8 hours, with the dose increased (to 100 mg twice daily) as necessary to control heart rate, blood pressure, and symptoms. In high-risk patients and in patients with tachycardia or elevated systemic arterial pressure, metoprolol should be administered intravenously (three boluses of 5 mg each given 5 minutes apart) initially, after which an oral dose should be initiated. A reasonable target heart rate is 50 to 60 beats per minute at rest.

β-Blockers should not be administered to patients with decompensated heart failure, hypotension, hemodynamic instability, or advanced atrioventricular block. Because most patients with chronic obstructive pulmonary disease or peripheral vascular disease tolerate β-blockers without difficulty, these conditions should not preclude their use.

Calcium-Channel Blockers

Calcium-channel blockers, which cause arterial vasodilation, increase coronary arterial blood flow and lower systemic arterial pressure. The non-dihydropyridine calcium-channel blockers diltiazem and verapamil slow heart rate and are recommended for the patient with a contraindication to a β-adrenergic blocker or persistent or recurrent symptoms despite treatment with nitroglycerin or a β-blocker. Oral diltiazem (30 to 90 mg four times daily of the short-acting preparation or up to 360 mg once daily of the long-acting preparation) is the preferred calcium-channel blocker because it reduces the incidence of myocardial ischemia and recurrent MI in patients with NSTE ACS. Diltiazem is contraindicated in patients with left ventricular systolic dysfunction or pulmonary vascular congestion. Caution should be exercised when combining a β-blocker with diltiazem because the two drugs may act synergistically to depress left ventricular systolic function as well as sinus and atrioventricular nodal conduction. Patients with ACS should not be prescribed short-acting nifedipine unless they are already receiving a β-blocker because it may increase the risk of death. The risks and benefits of long-acting dihydropyridines in patients with NSTE ACS are undefined.

Antiplatelet Agents

ACS patients should receive dual antiplatelet therapy (aspirin and an ADP receptor inhibitor) acutely and for at least 1 year unless the patient has an aspirin allergy or active bleeding. In patients with NSTE ACS, aspirin (Chapter 37) reduces the risk of death or MI by about 50%.A4 The recommended dose is 75 to 162 mg daily, continued indefinitely. The choice of which ADP receptor antagonist to use in combination with aspirin is determined by each patient's characteristics (i.e., risk of bleeding), medication costs, and pharmacologic properties of the agent (see following details). The patient who is allergic to or intolerant of aspirin should be treated with an ADP receptor inhibitor (clopidogrel, ticagrelor, or prasugrel [if PCI treated]) alone.[5]

Clopidogrel (Chapter 38) is a thienopyridine that blocks the $P2Y_{12}$ ADP receptor, thereby diminishing ADP-mediated platelet activation. Its antiplatelet activity is synergistic with aspirin because the two agents inhibit different platelet-activating pathways. Clopidogrel is a prodrug that must be metabolized by the cytochrome P-450 system to the active form. Polymorphisms in the cytochrome P-450 isoform CYP2C19, which are present in 15 to 20% of individuals, slow metabolism of the prodrug to the active form, thereby reducing the magnitude of platelet inhibition. Drugs that are potent inhibitors of the CYP2C19 enzyme (e.g., omeprazole, esomeprazole, cimetidine, fluconazole, ketoconazole, voriconazole, etravirine, felbamate, fluoxetine, and fluvoxamine) should not be administered with clopidogrel because they affect the metabolism to its active form and reduce its antiplatelet effects.

In subjects with NSTE ACS, the addition of clopidogrel (a loading dose of 300 to 600 mg, then 75 mg daily for at least 1 year) to aspirin reduces the composite end point of cardiovascular death, nonfatal MI, or stroke by 20% (2.1% reduction in absolute risk) compared with treatment with aspirin alone.A5 The benefit of an aspirin-clopidogrel combination is seen as early as 24 hours after drug initiation and persisted for the 12 months of the study, despite an increase in minor bleeding.

Prasugrel (Chapter 38), another thienopyridine, has a greater antiplatelet effect and a more rapid onset of action than clopidogrel. In patients with ACS who are referred for PCI, prasugrel in combination with aspirin reduces ischemic events (i.e., a combination of cardiovascular death, nonfatal MI, and stroke) by 20% compared with concomitant clopidogrel and aspirin (2.2% absolute risk reduction) therapy.A6 However, this benefit is obtained at a 0.5% increased risk of life-threatening bleeding and a 0.3% increased risk of fatal bleeding. At present, prasugrel is approved for use in the ACS patient who is referred for PCI. In combination with aspirin, it is administered as a 60-mg oral loading dose followed by a 10-mg daily maintenance dose. Because prasugrel-associated bleeding complications are highest in patients with a previous stroke or transient ischemic attack, age older than 75 years, or a body weight of less than 60 kg, it should not be used in patients with any of these features.

Ticagrelor (Chapter 38), a thienopyridine that does not require hepatic activation, has more rapid onset and more pronounced platelet inhibition than clopidogrel. It is a reversible inhibitor of the $P2Y_{12}$ receptor, so platelet function returns more rapidly after discontinuation than with clopidogrel. In a randomized trial in NSTE ACS patients, the addition of ticagrelor to aspirin reduced the composite end point of vascular death, nonfatal MI, or stroke by about 15% compared with treatment with clopidogrel and aspirin but increased non–procedure-related bleeding by an absolute 0.7%.A7 In combination with aspirin, ticagrelor is administered as a 180-mg oral loading dose, followed by a 90-mg twice-daily maintenance dose. In patients who receive ticagrelor, the daily aspirin maintenance dose should be 100 mg or less, and ticagrelor should not be used in patients with a history of intracranial hemorrhage.

Glycoprotein IIb/IIIa inhibitors (Chapter 38) block platelet aggregation in response to all potential agonists, so they are the most potent antiplatelet agents available. Three glycoprotein IIb/IIIa inhibitors, each of which must be

TABLE 72-3 MANAGEMENT STRATEGIES FOR PATIENTS WITH ACUTE CORONARY SYNDROME

THERAPY	INITIATION	DURATION	DOSE, ROUTE, AND DURATION	BENEFIT VS. PLACEBO (REDUCED INCIDENCE OF . . .)
LOW-RISK PATIENT				
Antianginal				
β-Blocker[*]	Immediately	Hospitalization ± indefinitely	Metoprolol, 5-mg IV boluses (three given 2 to 5 minutes apart), then 50 mg orally twice daily, titrated up to 100 mg twice daily; or atenolol, 5 to 10 mg IV bolus, then 100 mg orally daily	Recurrent ischemia
Nitroglycerin	Immediately	Hospitalization ± indefinitely	0.3-0.6 mg sublingually or 5-10 μg/min IV initially and increased by 10 μg/min every 5 minutes	Not studied
Diltiazem or verapamil[*]	Immediately	Hospitalization ± indefinitely	30-90 mg orally four times daily or up to 360 mg of long-acting preparation orally daily	MI, recurrent ischemia
Lipid Lowering				
Statin	Before hospital discharge	Indefinitely	Atorvastatin, up to 80 mg orally daily	Recurrent ischemia
Antiplatelet				
Aspirin	Immediately	Indefinitely	162-325 mg orally initial dose, then 81 mg orally daily	Death, MI
Clopidogrel	Immediately	1-12 months	300 mg orally initial dose, then 75 mg orally daily	MI, recurrent ischemia
Anticoagulant				
Unfractionated heparin	Immediately	2 to 5 days	IV bolus of 60 U/kg, then 12 U/kg IV adjusted to achieve an aPTT of 50 to 70 seconds	Death or MI (combined)
HIGH-RISK PATIENT				
Antianginal				
β-Blocker[*]	Immediately	Hospitalization ± indefinitely	Metoprolol, 5-mg IV boluses (three given 2 to 5 minutes apart), then 50 mg orally twice daily titrated up to 100 mg twice daily; or atenolol, 5- to 10-mg IV bolus, then 100 mg orally daily	Death, MI, recurrent ischemia
Nitroglycerin	Immediately	Hospitalization ± indefinitely	0.3-0.6 mg sublingually or 5-10 μg/min IV initially and increased by 10 μg/min every 5 minutes	Not studied
Diltiazem or verapamil[*]	Immediately	Hospitalization ± indefinitely	30-90 mg orally four times daily or up to 360 mg of long-acting preparation orally daily	MI, recurrent ischemia
Lipid Lowering				
Statin	Before hospital discharge	Indefinitely	Atorvastatin, up to 80 mg orally daily	Recurrent ischemia
Antiplatelet				
Aspirin *and*	Immediately	Indefinitely	162-325 mg orally initial dose, then 81 mg orally	Death, MI
Clopidogrel *or*	Immediately	≥12 months	300 mg orally initial dose, then 75 mg orally daily	MI, recurrent ischemia
Prasugrel *or*	At time of PCI	15 months	60 mg orally initial dose, then 10 mg orally daily	Cardiovascular death, MI or stroke (combined)[†]
Ticagrelor	At time of PCI	12 months	180 mg orally initially, then 90 mg twice daily	Vascular death, MI or stroke (combined)[†]
Glycoprotein IIb/IIIa inhibitor (eptifibatide, tirofiban, or abciximab)	At time of PCI	12-24 hours after PCI	Abciximab, IV bolus of 0.25 mg/kg, then 0.125 μg/kg/min IV (max. 10 μg/min) for 12 hours; or eptifibatide, IV bolus of 180 μg/kg, then 2.0 μg/kg/min IV for 18-24 hours; or tirofiban, 0.4 μg/kg/min IV for 30 minutes, then 0.1 μg/kg/min IV for 12 to 24 hours	MI
Anticoagulants				
Unfractionated heparin *or*	Immediately	2 to 5 days; discontinue after successful PCI	IV bolus of 60 U/kg, then 12 U/kg IV adjusted to achieve an aPTT of 50 to 70 seconds	Death or MI (combined)
Enoxaparin *or*	Immediately	Duration of hospitalization (up to 8 days); discontinue after successful PCI	1 mg/kg subcutaneously twice daily	MI, recurrent ischemia[‡]
Bivalirudin *or*	Immediately	Up to 72 hours; discontinue 4 hours after PCI	IV bolus of 0.75 mg/kg, then 1.75 mg/kg/hr IV	Bleeding[§]
Fondaparinux	Immediately	Duration of hospitalization (up to 8 days); if used during PCI, it must be coadministered with another anticoagulant with factor IIa activity	2.5-mg subcutaneous injection once daily	Bleeding[¶]

TABLE 72-3 MANAGEMENT STRATEGIES FOR PATIENTS WITH ACUTE CORONARY SYNDROME—cont'd

THERAPY	INITIATION	DURATION	DOSE, ROUTE, AND DURATION	BENEFIT VS. PLACEBO (REDUCED INCIDENCE OF ...)
Invasive Management				
Coronary angiography followed by revascularization (if appropriate)	Up to 36-80 hours after hospitalization; within 24 hours in "very high risk" patients			MI, recurrent ischemia

*Avoid in the patient with decompensated heart failure, hypotension, or hemodynamic instability.
†Compared with clopidogrel.
‡Compared with unfractionated heparin.
§As monotherapy compared with heparin and glycoprotein IIb/IIIa inhibitor combination.
¶Compared with enoxaparin.
aPTT = activated partial thromboplastin time; MI = myocardial infarction; PCI = percutaneous coronary intervention.
Modified from Lange RA, Hillis LD. Optimal management of acute coronary syndromes. *N Engl J Med.* 2009;260:2237-2240.

administered parenterally, are available: abciximab is the Fab fragment of a monoclonal antibody to the receptor; eptifibatide is a peptide; and tirofiban is a peptidomimetic molecule.

Glycoprotein IIb/IIIa inhibitors reduce the incidence of recurrent ischemic events in patients with NSTE ACS who undergo PCI but not in patients who are managed with medical therapy alone. When a glycoprotein IIb/IIIa inhibitor is administered to PCI patients, it should be initiated at the time of angiography because its routine administration beforehand carries an increased bleeding risk and no improvement in outcomes. The glycoprotein IIb/IIIa inhibitor infusion (see Table 72-3) typically is continued for 12 to 24 hours after PCI.

Anticoagulants

Anticoagulant therapy should be administered to all patients with ACS unless a contraindication, such as active bleeding, is present. For the patient in whom a noninvasive, ischemia-guided management strategy is selected, treatment with unfractionated heparin, low-molecular-weight heparin (LMWH), or fondaparinux is appropriate, with fondaparinux recommended for the patient at increased risk of bleeding. For the patient in whom an invasive management strategy is selected, unfractionated heparin and LMWH are the agents of choice. Although bivalirudin may be preferred in patients undergoing PCI, it is not used in the initial management of the patient with ACS.

Heparin

Unfractionated heparin (Chapter 38) exerts its anticoagulant effect by accelerating the action of circulating antithrombin; it prevents thrombus propagation but does not lyse existing thrombi. In the patient with NSTE ACS, the addition of heparin to aspirin reduces the rate of in-hospital ischemic events (i.e., death or MI) by 33%.[A8]

Unfractionated heparin should be initiated with an intravenous bolus of 60 U/kg, followed by a continuous infusion of approximately 12 U/kg/hour (maximum, 1000 U/hour), adjusted to maintain the activated partial thromboplastin time (aPTT) at 1.5 to 2.5 times control (i.e., 50 to 70 seconds) or a heparin concentration at 0.3 to 0.7 U/mL (by anti–factor Xa determinations). The infusion should be continued for 48 hours or until revascularization is performed, whichever occurs sooner. Frequent monitoring of the aPTT or heparin concentration is necessary because the anticoagulant response to a standard dose of unfractionated heparin varies widely among individuals; even when a weight-based nomogram (see Table 81-4) is followed, the aPTT is outside the therapeutic range more than one third of the time.

Mild thrombocytopenia occurs in 10 to 20% of patients treated with unfractionated heparin. In 1 to 5% of patients, a more severe form of thrombocytopenia develops. This antibody-mediated response usually occurs 4 to 14 days after the initiation of treatment (although it may appear more quickly in patients who received heparin within the preceding 6 months) and is associated with thromboembolic sequelae in 30 to 80% of subjects (Chapter 172).

Low-Molecular-Weight Heparin

LMWHs (Chapter 38), which are fragments of unfractionated heparin, exert a more predictable anticoagulant effect, have a longer half-life, and are less likely to cause thrombocytopenia compared with unfractionated heparin. Because they provide predictable and sustained anticoagulation with once- or twice-daily subcutaneous administration, monitoring of their anticoagulant effect is not required.

LMWH is superior to unfractionated heparin in preventing MI or death during hospitalization in NSTE ACS patients who have elevated serum cardiac biomarkers as well as in those considered to be at high risk for recurrent ischemia (see Table 72-2). In the low-risk subject, unfractionated heparin and LMWH have similar efficacy.

Two LMWHs, enoxaparin and dalteparin, are approved for the treatment of the patient with NSTE ACS. The dose of enoxaparin is 1 mg/kg subcutaneously twice daily, and the dose of dalteparin is 120 IU/kg (maximum, 10,000 IU) subcutaneously twice daily. Therapy should be continued for the duration of the hospitalization, up to 8 days, or until revascularization is performed (whichever occurs first). In obese (>120 kg), thin (<60 kg), or renally impaired (creatinine clearance < 30 mL/minute) patients, the LMWH dose should be adjusted to achieve an anti–factor Xa concentration of 0.5 to 1.5 IU/mL 4 to 6 hours after drug administration. LMWH should be avoided in the patient with a history of heparin-induced thrombocytopenia. In the patient with renal failure, treatment with LMWH has been associated with the development of hyperkalemia.

Fondaparinux

Fondaparinux (Chapter 38), which is a selective factor Xa inhibitor, does not require dose adjustment and monitoring. Fondaparinux does not cause thrombocytopenia. Fondaparinux is as effective as enoxaparin in preventing ischemic cardiac events but with 50% fewer major bleeding episodes (2.2% vs 4.1%).[A9] Because an increased incidence of catheter-related thrombosis has been reported after fondaparinux treatment, it is not recommended for patients who are likely to undergo coronary angiography. Fondaparinux is a desirable anticoagulant for the ACS patients who are managed in an ischemia-guided fashion, especially patients at higher risk of a bleeding complication with anticoagulant therapy, but not for other patients.

For the patient with ACS, fondaparinux is administered as a 2.5-mg subcutaneous injection once daily for up to 5 days or until hospital discharge. Its use is contraindicated in patients with severe renal impairment and in those who weigh 50 kg or less, and it should not be used as the sole anticoagulant during a PCI.

Bivalirudin

Bivalirudin, a direct thrombin inhibitor, is currently recommended as an alternative anticoagulant for patients undergoing PCI. Because it has not been tested in patients whose ACS is managed with an ischemia-guided strategy, its administration in a setting other than the cardiac catheterization laboratory is not recommended. In the patient undergoing PCI, bivalirudin (0.75 mg/kg intravenous bolus followed by an infusion of 1.75 mg/kg/hour for up to 4 hours after the PCI) is as effective as combination heparin and glycoprotein IIb/IIIa inhibitor therapy in preventing ischemic events, but it causes fewer major bleeding episodes. Bivalirudin is the anticoagulant of choice for the patient with ACS who has heparin-induced thrombocytopenia.

Statins

Prompt initiation of statin therapy is recommended in all patients with NSTE ACS to promote plaque stabilization and to restore endothelial function. Moreover, when statin therapy is initiated during the patient's hospitalization (rather than at hospital discharge), long-term medical compliance is substantially improved. In the absence of contraindications, high-dose atorvastatin (80 mg daily) should be given orally to the patient with NSTE ACS, regardless of the baseline serum low-density lipoprotein cholesterol concentration; a lower dose is not as effective in reducing ischemic events.[A10]

Recurrent or Refractory Unstable Angina

In most patients hospitalized with NSTE ACS, symptoms do not recur after the institution of appropriate antianginal therapy. The occasional patient with continued or recurrent chest pain despite optimal medical therapy is at high risk for an MI. For the patient with refractory myocardial ischemia or hemodynamic instability despite optimal medical therapy, intra-aortic balloon counterpulsation can reduce the incidence of ischemic episodes until revascularization can be performed. Intra-aortic balloon function is synchronized with the patient's ECG so that it inflates during diastole and deflates during systole, thereby augmenting coronary arterial blood flow and reducing myocardial oxygen demand by decreasing afterload. Intra-aortic balloon counterpulsation causes lower limb ischemia in approximately 3% of patients in whom the device is placed, but this complication usually resolves with its removal.

Coronary Revascularization

Coronary revascularization is performed to relieve angina that is persistent or recurrent despite optimal medical therapy, to prevent recurrent ischemia or MI in patients at high risk for a subsequent ischemic event, and to improve survival in patients with suitable coronary arterial anatomy.

Coronary revascularization is successful in relieving symptoms in 90% of the patients with angina refractory to medical therapy. Whether coronary bypass surgery or PCI is the more appropriate method of revascularization is determined by the location and severity of coronary arterial stenoses and the presence of comorbid medical conditions that may affect the performance or safety of the revascularization procedure.[6,7]

The patient who has been rendered symptom free with optimal medical therapy should undergo an assessment to determine whether he or she is at high risk or relatively low risk of sustaining a cardiac ischemic event (death, MI, or recurrent ischemia) in the ensuing days, weeks, and months and a bleeding complication from intensive medical therapy or an invasive cardiac procedure. Patients who are at low risk of having a subsequent ischemic event (those with a normal serum troponin concentration, age younger than 75 years, and zero, one, or two TIMI risk variables) should be evaluated noninvasively for inducible ischemia before hospital discharge. If the patient has spontaneous or provocable ischemia, coronary angiography and, if appropriate, revascularization should be performed.

The ACS patient with a detectable serum troponin concentration, age older than 75 years, or three or more TIMI risk variables is considered to be at high risk for a subsequent event and should be referred for routine coronary angiography and revascularization (if appropriate) during the hospitalization because this management strategy reduces the incidence of subsequent ischemic cardiac events.[A11] In most subjects, early (within 24 hours of hospitalization) invasive therapy is no better at preventing death, MI, or stroke than somewhat delayed (median, 50 hours) invasive management, although it is associated with a modest decrease in the occurrence of recurrent ischemia. In contrast, in the one third of subjects considered to be at very high risk (GRACE risk score of >140, corresponding to an incidence of in-hospital death or MI of >20%), an early invasive management strategy is superior to a delayed strategy in reducing the incidence of death, MI, or stroke.

The patient with clinical features or noninvasive test results suggestive of severe coronary artery disease (i.e., left ventricular dysfunction, hemodynamic instability, life-threatening ventricular arrhythmias, or extensive inducible ischemia) should be referred for coronary angiography (Table 72-4) to determine if left main or three-vessel coronary arterial disease is present because patients with these coronary anatomic findings derive a survival benefit with coronary revascularization compared with medical therapy (Chapter 74). In patients who are taking an ADP receptor inhibitor and in whom coronary artery bypass grafting can be delayed, the drug should be discontinued (5 days for clopidogrel or ticagrelor and at least 7 days for prasugrel) to allow dissipation of the antiplatelet effect.

Complications

Patients with NSTE ACS can develop recurrent ischemic events or any of the complications associated with ST segment elevation MI, including arrhythmias, heart failure, and mechanical complications (Chapter 73). However, the acute complications other than recurrent ischemia occur less often in subjects with NSTE ACS because the amount of myocardial damage usually is less.

Because intensive medical therapy in conjunction with invasive management can lead to life-threatening bleeding complications, the patient's risk of such should be assessed before these therapies are instituted. Female gender, older age, renal insufficiency, low body weight, tachycardia, systolic arterial pressure, hematocrit, and diabetes mellitus predict an increased risk of major bleeding, often due to excessive dosing of antiplatelet or anticoagulant agents. The bleeding risk can be estimated with the tool available at www.crusadebleedingscore.org.

Integrated Approach to Treatment

Although the treatment of the subject with NSTE ACS should be individualized, taking into account the specific features of the disease and the particular circumstances of the patient, algorithms nonetheless provide a useful framework (Fig. 72-3). Smoking cessation (Chapter 32), cholesterol lowering (Chapter 206), and control of blood pressure (Chapter 67), obesity, and diabetes mellitus (Chapter 229) are important long-term prevention strategies.[8-11] Maintaining compliance long term with medical therapy appears to reduce the risk of a future ischemic event by up to 80%.

TABLE 72-4 SELECTION OF INITIAL TREATMENT STRATEGY: INVASIVE VERSUS CONSERVATIVE

GENERALLY PREFERRED STRATEGY	PATIENT CHARACTERISTICS
Invasive	Recurrent angina or ischemia at rest or with low-level activities despite intensive medical therapy Elevated cardiac biomarkers (troponin) New or presumably new ST segment depression Signs or symptoms of heart failure or new or worsening mitral regurgitation High-risk findings from noninvasive testing Hemodynamic instability Sustained ventricular tachycardia PCI within 6 months Previous CABG High-risk score (e.g., TIMI, GRACE) Mild to moderate renal dysfunction Diabetes mellitus Reduced left ventricular systolic function (EF < 40%)
Conservative	Low-risk score (e.g., TIMI, GRACE) Patient or physician preference in the absence of high-risk features

CABG = coronary artery bypass grafting; EF = left ventricular ejection fraction; GRACE = Global Registry of Acute Coronary Events; HF = heart failure; PCI = percutaneous coronary intervention; TIMI = Thrombolysis in Myocardial Infarction.

PROGNOSIS

Because the number of ECG leads demonstrating ST segment depression and the magnitude of such depression are indicative of the extent and severity of myocardial ischemia and MI, it is not surprising that ST segment depression correlates with the patient's prognosis. Compared with subjects without ST segment depression, the patient with NSTE ACS who has ST segment depression of 1 mm or greater in two or more leads is almost four times as likely to die within 1 year, and the patient with ST segment depression of 2 mm or greater in magnitude is almost six times as likely to die within 1 year. If ST segment depression of 2 mm or greater is present in more than one region of the ECG, the mortality is increased 10-fold. Even the 20% of patients with ACS who have only 0.5 to 1 mm of ST segment depression have an adverse prognosis. Patients with ST segment depression also have a higher risk for subsequent cardiac events compared with patients with only T wave inversions (>1 mm).

The magnitude of the serum troponin concentration predicts short-term (30 days) and long-term (1 year) risks of recurrent MI and death, independent of ECG abnormalities or markers of inflammatory activity. C-reactive protein measured with a highly sensitive assay, which is a widely used marker of inflammation, has no role in the diagnosis of ACS but is predictive of long-term (6 months) mortality among patients with troponin-negative NSTE ACS. Elevated serum concentrations of natriuretic peptides (B-type natriuretic peptide [BNP] or its N-terminal prohormone [NT-pro-BNP]) are associated with a three- to five-fold increased mortality in patients with NSTE ACS, although they have limited value for diagnosis, initial risk stratification, and selection of an initial management strategy. Natriuretic peptide concentrations measured a few days after the onset of symptoms have better predictive value than those measured at the time of hospitalization. In patients with NSTE ACS, a simultaneous assessment of troponin, high-sensitivity C-reactive protein, and BNP is superior to a single biomarker assessment at predicting short-term outcome.

In contrast to patients with ST segment elevation MI, in whom most events occur before or shortly after presentation to the hospital, patients with NSTE ACS continue to be at high risk for such events during the ensuing days, weeks, and months. Although in-hospital mortality is higher in patients with ST segment elevation MI than among those with NSTE ACS (7 vs. 5%, respectively), the mortality rates at 6 months are similar for the two conditions (12 vs. 13%, respectively). During long-term follow-up of patients hospitalized with ACS, rates of death are actually higher in those with NSTE ACS than in those with ST segment elevation MI, with a two-fold difference after 4 years. As a result, treatment strategies for NSTE ACS should address the issues related to both the acute event and longer-term treatment.

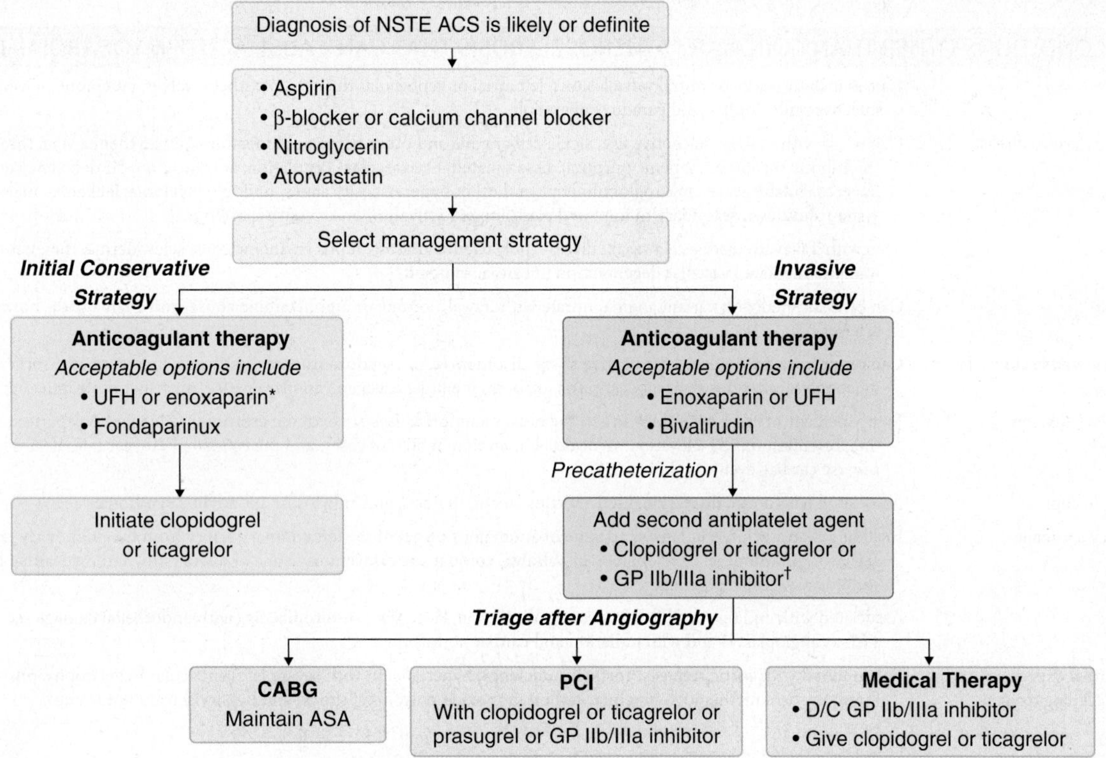

FIGURE 72-3. Approach to the patient with non–ST segment elevation acute coronary syndrome (NSTE ACS). *Enoxaparin or fondaparinux is preferred to unfractionated heparin (UFH). †Intravenous eptifibatide or tirofiban is preferred. ASA = aspirin; CABG = coronary artery bypass grafting; D/C = discontinue; GP = glycoprotein; PCI = percutaneous coronary intervention.

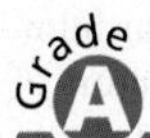

Grade A References

A1. Litt HI, Gatsonis C, Snyder B, et al. CT angiography for safe discharge of patients with possible acute coronary syndromes. *N Engl J Med.* 2012;366:1393-1403.

A2. Mehta SR, Granger CB, Boden WE, et al. Early versus delayed invasive intervention in acute coronary syndromes. *N Engl J Med.* 2009;360:2165-2175.

A3. O'Donoghue ML, Vaidya A, Afsal R, et al. An invasive or conservative strategy in patients with diabetes mellitus and non-ST-segment elevation acute coronary syndromes: a collaborative meta-analysis of randomized trials. *J Am Coll Cardiol.* 2012;60:106-111.

A4. Antithrombotic Trialists' Collaboration. Collaborative meta-analysis of randomised trials of antiplatelet therapy for prevention of death, myocardial infarction, and stroke in high risk patients. *BMJ.* 2002;324:71-86.

A5. Yusuf S, Zhao F, Mehta SR, et al. Effects of clopidogrel in addition to aspirin in patients with acute coronary syndromes without ST-segment elevation. *N Engl J Med.* 2001;345:494-502.

A6. Wiviott SD, Braunwald E, McCabe CH, et al. Prasugrel versus clopidogrel in patients with acute coronary syndromes. *N Engl J Med.* 2007;357:2001-2015.

A7. Kohli P, Wallentin L, Reyes E, et al. Reduction in first and recurrent cardiovascular events with ticagrelor compared with clopidogrel in the PLATO Study. *Circulation.* 2013;127:673-680.

A8. Eikelboom JW, Anand SS, Malmberg K, et al. Unfractionated heparin and low-molecular-weight heparin in acute coronary syndrome without ST elevation: a meta-analysis. *Lancet.* 2000;355:1936-1942.

A9. Yusuf S, Mehta SR, Chrolavicius S, et al. Comparison of fondaparinux and enoxaparin in acute coronary syndromes. *N Engl J Med.* 2006;354:1464-1476.

A10. Cannon CP, Braunwald E, McCabe CH, et al. Intensive versus moderate lipid lowering with statins after acute coronary syndromes. *N Engl J Med.* 2004;350:1495-1504.

A11. O'Donoghue M, Boden WE, Braunwald E, et al. Early invasive vs conservative treatment strategies in women and men with unstable angina and non-ST-segment elevation myocardial infarction: a meta-analysis. *JAMA.* 2008;300:71-80.

GENERAL REFERENCES

For the General References and other additional features, please visit Expert Consult at https://expertconsult.inkling.com.

73

ST SEGMENT ELEVATION ACUTE MYOCARDIAL INFARCTION AND COMPLICATIONS OF MYOCARDIAL INFARCTION

JEFFREY L. ANDERSON

DEFINITION

Conceptually, myocardial infarction (MI) is myocardial necrosis caused by ischemia. Practically, MI can be diagnosed and evaluated by clinical, electrocardiographic, biochemical, radiologic, and pathologic methods. Technologic advances in detecting much smaller amounts of myocardial necrosis than previously possible (e.g., by high-sensitivity troponin determinations) have required a redefinition of MI. Given these developments, MI now also should be qualified with regard to size, precipitating circumstance, and timing. This chapter focuses on acute MI associated with ST segment elevation on the electrocardiogram (ECG). This category of acute MI is characterized by profound ("transmural") acute myocardial ischemia affecting relatively large areas of myocardium. The underlying cause is essentially *complete* interruption of regional myocardial blood flow (resulting from coronary occlusion, usually atherothrombotic; Chapter 70). This clinical syndrome should be distinguished from non–ST segment elevation MI, in which the blockage of coronary flow is incomplete and for which different acute therapies are appropriate (Chapter 72).

EPIDEMIOLOGY

The risk of cardiovascular disease and MI has declined in recent years in the United States and the Western world, but the burden of disease remains high. Cardiovascular disease is responsible for almost half of all noncommunicable deaths worldwide (Chapter 52), and coronary heart disease causes about 1 of every 6 deaths in the United States or about 380,000 deaths per year. Each

TABLE 73-1 CONDITIONS OTHER THAN CORONARY ATHEROSCLEROSIS THAT CAN CAUSE ACUTE MYOCARDIAL INFARCTION

Coronary emboli	Causes include aortic or mitral valve lesions, left atrial or ventricular thrombi, prosthetic valves, fat emboli, intracardiac neoplasms, infective endocarditis, and paradoxical emboli
Thrombotic coronary artery disease	Can occur with oral contraceptive use, sickle cell anemia and other hemoglobinopathies, polycythemia vera, thrombocytosis, thrombotic thrombocytopenic purpura, disseminated intravascular coagulation, antithrombin III deficiency and other hypercoagulable states, macroglobulinemia and other hyperviscosity states, multiple myeloma, leukemia, malaria, and fibrinolytic system shutdown secondary to impaired plasminogen activation or excessive inhibition
Coronary vasculitis	Seen with Takayasu disease, Kawasaki disease, polyarteritis nodosa, lupus erythematosus, scleroderma, rheumatoid arthritis, and immune-mediated vascular degeneration in cardiac allografts
Coronary vasospasm	Can be associated with variant angina, nitrate withdrawal, cocaine or amphetamine abuse, and angina with "normal" coronary arteries
Infiltrative and degenerative coronary vascular disease	Can result from amyloidosis, connective tissue disorders (e.g., pseudoxanthoma elasticum), lipid storage disorders and mucopolysaccharidoses, homocystinuria, diabetes mellitus, collagen vascular disease, muscular dystrophies, and Friedreich ataxia
Spontaneous coronary dissection	Eighty percent of cases occur in women; the most common causes are extreme exertion in men and postpartum status in women; the presentation is ST elevation myocardial infarction in 50% of cases, and the estimated 10-year rate of subsequent major adverse cardiac events is about 50%
Coronary ostial occlusion	Associated with aortic dissection, luetic aortitis, aortic stenosis, and ankylosing spondylitis syndromes
Congenital coronary anomalies	Including Bland-White-Garland syndrome of anomalous origin of the left coronary artery from the pulmonary artery, left coronary artery origin from the anterior sinus of Valsalva, coronary arteriovenous fistula or aneurysms, and myocardial bridging with secondary vascular degeneration
Trauma	Associated with and responsible for coronary dissection, laceration, or thrombosis (with endothelial damage secondary to trauma such as angioplasty) and with radiation and cardiac contusion
Augmented myocardial oxygen requirements exceeding oxygen delivery	Encountered with aortic stenosis, aortic insufficiency, hypertension with severe left ventricular hypertrophy, pheochromocytoma, thyrotoxicosis, methemoglobinemia, carbon monoxide poisoning, shock, and hyperviscosity syndromes

year, about 635,000 Americans are diagnosed with a first MI, about 230,000 have a recurrent MI, and about 150,000 more have a silent first MI.[1] An American suffers a coronary event approximately every 30 seconds, and one dies from one every minute.

More than 5 million people visit emergency departments in the United States each year for evaluation of chest pain and related symptoms (Chapter 51), about 680,000 of whom are diagnosed with an acute coronary syndrome (non–ST segment elevation MI/unstable angina; Chapter 72). The presence of ST segment elevation or new left bundle branch block (LBBB) on the ECG distinguishes patients with acute MI who require consideration of immediate reperfusion (recanalization) therapy from other patients with an acute coronary syndrome. Changing demographics, lifestyles, and medical therapies have led to a decrease in the ratio of ST segment elevation MI (STEMI) to non–ST segment elevation acute coronary syndromes during the past 15 to 20 years, so STEMI now accounts for about 30% of all MIs.

PATHOBIOLOGY

Erosion, fissuring, or rupture of vulnerable atherosclerotic plaques has been determined to be the initiating mechanism of coronary thrombotic occlusion, thereby precipitating intraplaque hemorrhage, coronary spasm, and occlusive luminal thrombosis (Chapter 70). Plaque rupture most frequently occurs in lipid-laden plaques with an endothelial cap weakened by internal collagenase (metalloproteinase) activity derived primarily from macrophages. These macrophages are recruited to the plaque from blood monocytes responding to inflammatory mediators and adhesion molecules.

With plaque rupture, elements of the blood stream are exposed to the highly thrombogenic plaque core and matrix containing lipid, tissue factor, and collagen. Platelets adhere, become activated, and aggregate; vasoconstrictive and thrombogenic mediators are secreted; vasospasm occurs; thrombin is generated and fibrin formed; and a partially or totally occlusive platelet- and fibrin-rich thrombus is generated. When coronary flow is occluded, electrocardiographic ST segment elevation occurs, resulting in STEMI. Partial occlusion, occlusion in the presence of collateral circulation, and distal coronary embolization result in unstable angina or non–ST segment elevation MI (Chapter 72). Ischemia from impaired myocardial perfusion causes myocardial cell injury or death, ventricular dysfunction, and cardiac arrhythmias.

Although most MIs are caused by atherosclerosis, occasional patients can develop complete coronary occlusions due to coronary dissections,[2] emboli, in situ thrombosis, vasculitis, primary vasospasm, infiltrative or degenerative diseases, diseases of the aorta, congenital anomalies of a coronary artery, or trauma (Table 73-1). In a canine model of coronary occlusion and reperfusion, myocardial cell death begins within 15 minutes of occlusion and proceeds rapidly in a wave front from endocardium to epicardium. Partial myocardial salvage can be achieved by releasing the occlusion within 3 to 6 hours; the degree of salvage is inversely proportional to the duration of ischemia and occurs in a reverse wave front from epicardium to endocardium. The extent of myocardial necrosis can also be altered by modification of metabolic demands and collateral blood supply. The temporal dynamic of infarction in human disease, although more complex, is generally similar.

Susceptibility to coronary artery disease and subsequent MI is estimated to be 40% genetic, with the balance being environmental. A large international collaborative meta-analysis identified or validated 23 common genetic susceptibility loci for coronary artery disease, many unrelated to traditional risk factors, but these loci account for only 10% of genetic variance. Interestingly, among patients with coronary artery disease, only a variant in the glycosyltransferase gene associated with the ABO blood group O phenotype has been shown to protect against MI.

CLINICAL MANIFESTATIONS

The diagnosis of acute MI has traditionally rested on the triad of ischemic-type chest discomfort, electrocardiographic abnormalities, and elevated serum cardiac biomarkers of necrosis. Acute MI was considered present when at least two of the three were present. With their increasing sensitivity and specificity, serum cardiac biomarkers (i.e., troponin I [TnI] and troponin T [TnT]) have assumed a dominant role in confirming the diagnosis of acute MI in patients with suggestive clinical or electrocardiographic features.

History

Ischemic-type chest discomfort is the most prominent clinical symptom in most patients with acute MI (see Table 51-1). The discomfort is characterized by its quality, location, duration, radiation, and precipitating and relieving factors. The discomfort associated with acute MI is qualitatively similar to that of angina pectoris but more severe. It often is perceived as heavy, pressing, crushing, squeezing, bandlike, viselike, strangling, constricting, aching, or burning; it rarely is perceived as sharp pain and generally not as stabbing pain (Chapters 51 and 71).

The primary location of typical ischemic pain is most consistently retrosternal, but it also can present left parasternally, left precordially, or across the anterior chest (Chapter 51). On occasion, discomfort is predominantly perceived in the anterior neck, jaw, arms, or epigastrium. It generally is somewhat diffuse; highly localized pain (finger point) is rarely angina or acute MI. The most characteristic pattern of radiation is to the left arm, but the right arm or both arms can be involved. The shoulders, neck, jaw, teeth, epigastrium, and interscapular areas also are sites of radiation. Discomfort above the jaws or below the umbilicus is not typical of acute MI. Associated symptoms often include nausea, vomiting, diaphoresis, weakness, dyspnea, restlessness, and apprehension.

The discomfort of acute MI is more severe and lasts longer (typically 20 minutes to several hours) than angina, and it is not reliably relieved by rest or nitroglycerin. The onset of acute MI usually is unrelated to exercise or other apparent precipitating factors. Nevertheless, acute MI begins during physical or emotional stress and within a few hours of arising more frequently than is explained by chance.

It is estimated that at least 20% of acute MIs are painless ("silent") or atypical (unrecognized). Elderly patients, especially women, and patients with diabetes are particularly prone to painless or atypical MI, which is the presentation of MI in as many as one third to one half of such patients. Because the prognosis is worse in elderly patients and in those patients with diabetes, diagnostic vigilance is required. In these patients, acute MI can be manifested as sudden dyspnea (which can progress to pulmonary edema), weakness, lightheadedness, nausea, and vomiting. Confusional states, sudden loss of consciousness, a new rhythm disorder, and an unexplained fall in blood pressure are other uncommon presentations. The differential diagnosis of ischemic chest discomfort also should include gastrointestinal disorders (e.g., reflux esophagitis; Chapter 138), musculoskeletal pain (e.g., costochondritis), anxiety or panic attacks, pleurisy or pulmonary embolism (Chapter 98), and acute aortic dissection (see Table 51-2 and Chapter 78).

Physical Examination

No physical findings are diagnostic or pathognomonic of acute MI. The physical examination findings can be entirely normal or may reveal only nonspecific abnormalities. An S_4 gallop frequently is found if it is carefully sought. Blood pressure often is initially elevated, but it may be normal or low. Signs of sympathetic hyperactivity (tachycardia, hypertension, or both) often accompany anterior wall MI, whereas parasympathetic hyperactivity (bradycardia, hypotension, or both) is more common with inferior wall MI.

The examination is best focused on an overall assessment of cardiac function. Adequacy of vital signs and peripheral perfusion should be noted. Signs of cardiac failure, both left and right sided (e.g., S_3 gallop, pulmonary congestion, elevated neck veins) should be sought, and observation for arrhythmias and mechanical complications (e.g., new murmurs) is essential. If hypoperfusion is present, determination of its primary cause (e.g., hypovolemia, right-sided heart failure, left-sided heart failure) is critical to management.

DIAGNOSIS

Electrocardiogram

In patients with a possible acute MI, an ECG must be obtained immediately. Although the initial ECG is neither perfectly specific nor perfectly sensitive in all patients who develop acute STEMI, it plays a critical role in initial stratification, triage, and management (Chapter 51). In an appropriate clinical setting, a pattern of ST segment elevation of 2 mm (0.2 mV) or more at the J point in V_2 to V_3 in men or 1.5 mm (0.15 mV) or more in women in the absence of left ventricular (LV) hypertrophy or 1 mm (0.1 mV) or more in two or more other contiguous chest or limb leads suggests coronary occlusion causing marked myocardial ischemia.[1] In such patients, emergency reperfusion (primary angioplasty or fibrinolysis) should be performed unless it is contraindicated. Hyperacute T wave changes may suggest the diagnosis in the early phase of STEMI before the onset of ST elevation. A new or presumably new LBBB, which may obscure ST elevation analysis, may suggest a STEMI equivalent in the appropriate clinical setting. ST depression in two or more precordial leads V_1 to V_4 may indicate transmural posterior injury due to occlusion of the left circumflex coronary artery; extending ECG analysis to leads V_7 to V_9 can help confirm this diagnosis. Other ECG patterns (ST segment depression, T wave inversion, nonspecific changes, normal ECG) in association with ischemic chest discomfort are consistent with a non–ST segment elevation acute coronary syndrome and are treated with different triage and initial management strategies (Chapter 72).

Electrocardiographic Evolution

Serial ECG tracings improve the sensitivity and specificity of the ECG for the diagnosis of acute MI and assist in assessing the outcomes of therapy. When typical ST segment elevation persists for hours and is followed within hours to days by T wave inversions and Q waves, the diagnosis of acute MI can be made with virtual certainty. The ECG changes in acute STEMI evolve through three overlapping phases: hyperacute or early acute, evolved acute, and chronic (stabilized).

Early Acute Phase

This earliest phase begins within minutes, persists, and evolves during hours. T waves increase in amplitude and widen over the area of injury (hyperacute pattern). ST segments evolve from concave to a straightened to a convex upward pattern (acute pattern). When prominent, the acute injury pattern of blended ST-T waves can take on a tombstone appearance (Figs. 73-1 and 73-2). ST segment depressions that occur in leads opposite those with ST segment elevation are known as reciprocal changes and are associated with larger areas of injury and a worse prognosis but also with greater benefits from reperfusion therapy.

Other causes of ST segment elevation must be considered and excluded. These conditions include pericarditis (Chapter 77), LV hypertrophy with J point elevation, and normal variant early repolarization (Chapter 54). Pericarditis (or perimyocarditis) is of particular concern because it can mimic acute MI clinically, but fibrinolytic therapy is *not* indicated and can be hazardous.

Evolved Acute Phase

During the second phase, ST segment elevation begins to regress, T waves in leads with ST segment elevation become inverted, and pathologic Q or QS waves become fully developed (>0.03-second duration or depth >30% of R wave amplitude, or both).

Chronic Phase

Resolution of ST segment elevation is variable. Resolution is usually complete within 2 weeks of inferior MI, but it can be delayed further after anterior MI. Persistent ST segment elevation, often seen with a large anterior MI, is indicative of a large area of akinesis, dyskinesis, or ventricular aneurysm. Symmetrical T wave inversions can resolve during weeks to months or can persist for an indefinite period; hence, the age of an MI in the presence of T wave inversions is often termed indeterminate. Q waves usually do not resolve after anterior MI but often disappear after inferior wall MI.

Early reperfusion therapy accelerates the time course of ECG changes to minutes or hours instead of days to weeks. ST segments recede rapidly, T wave inversions and loss of R waves occur earlier, and Q waves may not develop or progress and occasionally may regress. Indeed, failure of ST segment elevation to resolve by more than 50 to 70% within 1 to 2 hours

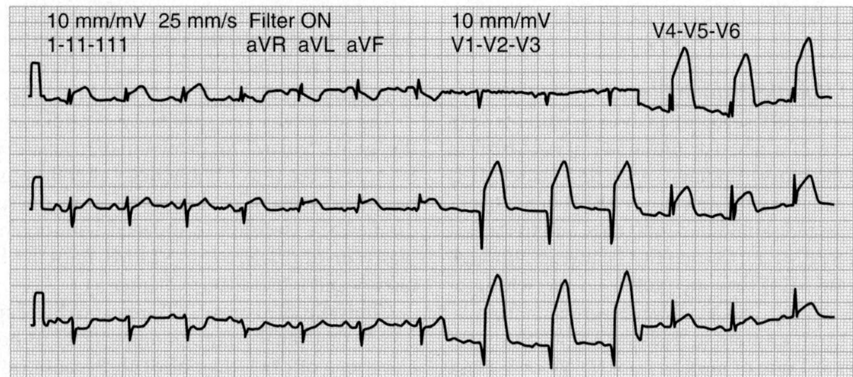

FIGURE 73-1. Electrocardiographic tracing shows an acute anterolateral myocardial infarction. Note ST segment elevation in leads I, aVL, and V_1 to V_6 with Q waves in V_1 to V_4.

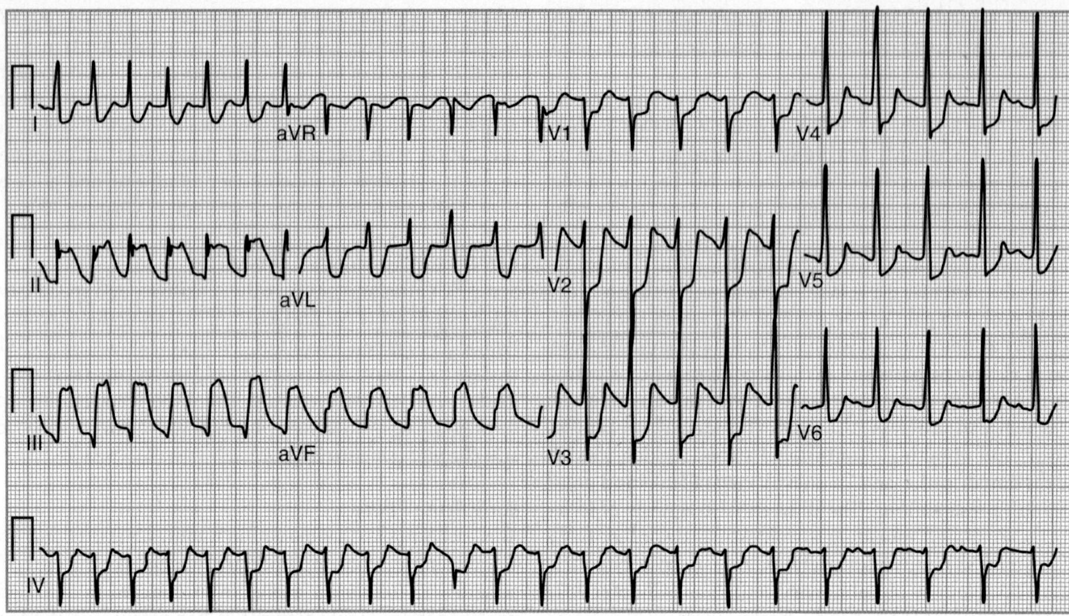

FIGURE 73-2. Electrocardiographic tracing shows an acute inferoposterior myocardial infarction.

suggests failure of fibrinolysis and should prompt referral for urgent angiography and consideration of "rescue angioplasty."

True Posterior Myocardial Infarction and Left Circumflex Myocardial Infarction Patterns

"True posterior" MI presents a mirror-image pattern of ECG injury in leads V_1 to V_2 to V_4 (Fig. 73-2). The location of injury of true posterior MI by magnetic resonance imaging actually involves portions of the *lateral* LV wall and is typically caused by occlusion of a nondominant left circumflex artery. In the precordial leads, the acute phase is characterized by ST segment depression rather than by ST segment elevation. The evolved and chronic phases show increased R wave amplitude and widening instead of Q waves. Recognition of a true posterior acute MI pattern is challenging but important because the diagnosis should lead to an immediate reperfusion strategy. Extending the ECG to measure left posterior leads V_7 to V_9 increases sensitivity for detection of acute left circumflex–related injury patterns (i.e., ST segment elevation) with excellent specificity (Chapter 54). Other causes of prominent upright anteroseptal forces include right ventricular (RV) hypertrophy, ventricular preexcitation variants (Wolff-Parkinson-White syndrome; Chapter 64), and normal variants with early R wave progression. New appearance of these changes or the association with an acute or evolving inferior MI usually allows the diagnosis to be made.

Right Ventricular Infarction

Proximal occlusion of the right coronary artery before the acute marginal branch can cause RV infarction as well as acute inferior MI in about 30% of cases. Because the prognosis and treatment of acute inferior MI differ in the presence of RV infarction, it is important to make this diagnosis. The diagnosis is assisted by obtaining right precordial ECG leads, which are routinely indicated for inferior acute MI (Chapter 54). Acute ST segment elevation of at least 1 mm (0.1 mV) in one or more leads V_4R to V_6R is both sensitive and specific (>90%) for identifying acute RV injury, and Q or QS waves effectively identify RV infarction.

Diagnosis in the Presence of Bundle Branch Block

The presence of LBBB often obscures ST segment analysis in patients with suspected acute MI. The presence of a new (or presumed new) LBBB in association with clinical (and laboratory) findings suggesting acute MI is associated with high mortality; patients with new-onset LBBB benefit substantially from reperfusion therapy and should undergo triage and treatment in the same way as patients with STEMI do. Certain ECG patterns, although relatively insensitive, suggest acute MI if they are present in the setting of LBBB: Q waves in two of leads I, aVL, V_5, and V_6; R wave regression from V_1 to V_4; ST segment elevation of 1 mm or more in leads with a positive QRS complex; ST segment depression of 1 mm or more in leads V_1, V_2, or V_3; and ST segment elevation of 5 mm or more associated with a negative QRS complex. The presence of right bundle branch block (RBBB) usually does not mask typical ST-T wave or Q wave changes except in rare cases of isolated true posterior acute MI, which are characterized by tall right precordial R waves and ST segment depressions.

TABLE 73-2 CONDITIONS THAT CAN MIMIC ST SEGMENT ELEVATION MYOCARDIAL INFARCTION

Early repolarization with noncoronary chest pain
Myocarditis
Pericarditis
Takotsubo ("stress") cardiomyopathy

Differential Diagnosis

Although STEMI is often an easy diagnosis to make on the basis of the presentation and test results (see later), other considerations include acute pericarditis (Chapter 77), acute myocarditis (Chapter 60), stress-induced (takotsubo) syndrome (Chapter 60), and early repolarization (Table 73-2). All but early repolarization can be associated with abnormal biomarkers, but none are associated with a coronary occlusion. Early coronary angiography is advised when the cause of ST segment elevation is unclear (see Table 73-1).

Serum Cardiac Biomarkers of Necrosis

Cardiac-derived TnI (cTnI) and TnT (cTnT), which are proteins of the sarcomere, are not normally present in the blood with standard sensitivity assays and have amino acid sequences distinct from their skeletal muscle isoforms. The troponins generally are first detectable 1 to 4 hours after the onset of acute MI,[3] are maximally sensitive at 8 to 12 hours, peak at 10 to 24 hours, and persist for 5 to 14 days. Their long persistence has allowed them to replace other markers for the diagnosis of acute MI in patients presenting late (>1 to 2 days) after symptoms. However, this persistence can obscure the diagnosis of an early recurrent MI, for which more rapidly cleared markers (i.e., the MB isoenzyme of creatine kinase [CK-MB]) may be selectively useful.

The sensitivity and specificity of cardiac-specific TnI and TnT make them the "gold standard" for detection of myocardial necrosis (see later). However, because of the 1- to 12-hour delay after the onset of symptoms before markers become detectable or diagnostic across the spectrum of acute coronary syndromes, the decision to proceed with urgent reperfusion (primary angioplasty or fibrinolysis) in STEMI must be based on the patient's clinical history and initial ECG (Chapter 51).

Clinically, cTnI and cTnT appear to be of approximately equivalent utility, except that renal failure is more likely to be associated with false-positive elevations of cTnT than of cTnI. Because troponins also may be present in low concentration in a number of nonischemic cardiovascular conditions, the

TABLE 73-3 NON–MYOCARDIAL INFARCTION CAUSES OF AN ELEVATED TROPONIN LEVEL

OTHER CARDIAC CAUSES
Myocardial injury: cardiac contusion, surgery, ablation, shocks
Myocardial inflammation: myocarditis, pericarditis
Heart failure
Cardiomyopathies: infiltrative, stress, hypertensive, hypertrophic
Aortic dissection
Severe aortic stenosis
Tachycardias
PULMONARY CAUSES
Pulmonary embolism
Pulmonary hypertension
Respiratory failure
NEUROLOGIC CAUSES
Stroke
Intracranial hemorrhage
OTHER
Shock: septic, hypovolemic, cardiogenic
Renal failure

Modified from Thygesen K, Alpert JS, Jaffe AS, et al. Third universal definition of myocardial infarction. *Circulation.* 2012;126:2020-2035.

clinician also must consider the clinical context and the temporal rise and fall of troponin levels (Table 73-3).

Other Laboratory Tests

On admission, routine assessment of complete blood count and platelet count, standard blood chemistry studies, a lipid panel, and coagulation tests (prothrombin time, partial thromboplastin time) is useful. Results assist in assessing comorbid conditions and prognosis and in guiding therapy. Hematologic tests provide a useful baseline before initiation of antiplatelet, anticoagulant, and fibrinolytic therapy or coronary angiography or angioplasty. Myocardial injury precipitates polymorphonuclear leukocytosis, commonly resulting in an elevation of white blood cell count of up to 12,000 to 15,000/μL, which appears within a few hours and peaks at 2 to 4 days. The metabolic panel provides a useful check on electrolytes, glucose, and renal function. On hospital admission or the next morning, a fasting lipid panel is recommended as a baseline for lipid-lowering (statin) therapy (Chapter 206). Unless carbon dioxide retention is suspected, finger oximetry is adequate to titrate oxygen therapy. The C-reactive protein level increases with acute MI, but its incremental prognostic value in the acute setting has not been established. B-type natriuretic peptide, which increases with ventricular wall stress and relative circulatory fluid overload, may provide useful incremental prognostic information in the setting of acute MI.

Imaging

A chest radiograph is the only imaging test *routinely* obtained on admission for acute MI. Although the chest radiograph is often normal, findings of pulmonary venous congestion, cardiomegaly, or widened mediastinum can contribute importantly to diagnosis and management decisions. For example, a history of severe, "tearing" chest and back pain in association with a widened mediastinum should raise the question of a dissecting aortic aneurysm (Chapter 78). In such cases, fibrinolytic therapy must be withheld pending more definitive diagnostic imaging of the aorta. Other noninvasive imaging (e.g., echocardiography [Chapter 55], cardiac nuclear scanning [Chapter 56], and other testing) is performed for evaluation of specific clinical issues, including suspected complications of acute MI. Coronary angiography (Chapter 57) is performed urgently as part of an interventional strategy for acute MI or later for risk stratification in higher-risk patients who are managed medically.

Echocardiography

Two-dimensional transthoracic echocardiography with color flow Doppler imaging is the most generally useful noninvasive test obtained on admission or early in the hospital course (Chapter 55). Echocardiography efficiently assesses global and regional cardiac function and enables the clinician to evaluate suspected complications of acute MI. The sensitivity and specificity of echocardiography for regional wall motion assessment are high (>90%), although the age of the abnormality (new vs. old) must be distinguished clinically or by electrocardiography. Echocardiography is helpful in determining the cause of circulatory failure with hypotension (relative hypovolemia, LV failure, RV failure, or mechanical complication of acute MI). Echocardiography also can assist in differentiating pericarditis and perimyocarditis from acute MI. Doppler echocardiography is indicated to evaluate a new murmur and other suspected mechanical complications of acute MI (papillary muscle dysfunction or rupture, acute ventricular septal defect, LV free wall rupture with tamponade or pseudoaneurysm). Later in the course of acute MI, echocardiography may be used to assess the degree of recovery of stunned myocardium after reperfusion therapy, the degree of residual cardiac dysfunction and indications for angiotensin-converting enzyme (ACE) inhibitors and other therapies for heart failure, and the presence of LV aneurysm and mural thrombus (requiring oral anticoagulants).

Radionuclide, Magnetic Resonance, and Other Imaging Studies

Radionuclide techniques generally are too time-consuming and cumbersome for routine use in the acute setting of definite or probable acute MI. More commonly, they are used in risk stratification before or after hospital discharge to augment exercise or pharmacologic stress testing (Chapter 56). Thallium Tl 201 or technetium Tc 99m sestamibi nuclear scans or rubidium Rb 82 positron emission tomography scans can assess myocardial perfusion and viability as well as infarct size. Cardiac magnetic resonance imaging (Chapter 56) with late gadolinium enhancement also can assess infarct size as well as myocardial function during the convalescent phase. Computed tomography and magnetic resonance imaging also can be useful to evaluate patients with a suspected dissecting aortic aneurysm (Chapter 78). When a nonatherosclerotic cause of myocardial necrosis is raised (e.g., perimyocarditis simulating acute MI), contemporary multislice (e.g., 64-slice) coronary computed tomography can assess coronary artery disease qualitatively and semiquantitatively as well as distinguish other causes of chest pain syndromes (Chapters 51 and 56).

TREATMENT Rx

Assessment and Management

Prehospital Phase

More than half of deaths related to acute MI occur within 1 hour of onset of symptoms and before the patient reaches a hospital emergency department. Most of these deaths are caused by ischemia-related ventricular fibrillation (VF) and can be reversed by defibrillation (Chapters 63 and 66). Rapid defibrillation allows resuscitation in 60% of patients when treatment is delivered by a bystander using an on-site automatic external defibrillator or by a first-responding medical rescuer (Chapter 63). Moreover, the first hour represents the best opportunity for myocardial salvage with reperfusion therapy. Thus, the three goals of prehospital care are to recognize symptoms promptly and seek medical attention; to deploy an emergency medical system team capable of cardiac monitoring, defibrillation and resuscitation, and emergency medical therapy; and to transport the patient expeditiously to a medical care facility staffed with personnel capable of providing expert coronary care, including reperfusion therapy (primary angioplasty or fibrinolysis).

The greatest time lag to reperfusion therapy is the patient's delay in calling for help. Public education efforts have yielded mixed results, and innovative approaches are needed. Emergency medical personnel should perform a 12-lead ECG at the site of first medical contact in patients with symptoms consistent with STEMI.[1,4] In coordinated systems and when transportation delays are substantial (i.e., >90 to 120 minutes), fibrinolytic and other antithrombotic therapy ideally is administered in the field, thereby shortening the time to reperfusion.

Hospital Phases

Emergency Department

The goals of emergency department care are to identify patients with acute myocardial ischemia rapidly, to stratify them into acute STEMI compared with other acute coronary syndromes (see Fig. 72-1 and Fig. 73-1), to initiate a reperfusion strategy and other appropriate medical care in qualifying patients with acute STEMI, and to prioritize by triage rapidly to inpatient care (cardiac intensive care unit, step-down unit, observation unit) or outpatient care (patients without suspected ischemia) (see Fig. 72-2).

The evaluation of patients with chest pain and other suspected acute coronary syndromes begins with a 12-lead ECG even as the physician is beginning a focused history, including contraindications to fibrinolysis and angiography, and a targeted physical examination. Continuous ECG monitoring should be started, an intravenous line should be established, and admission blood tests should be performed (including cardiac biomarkers such as cTnI or cTnT). As

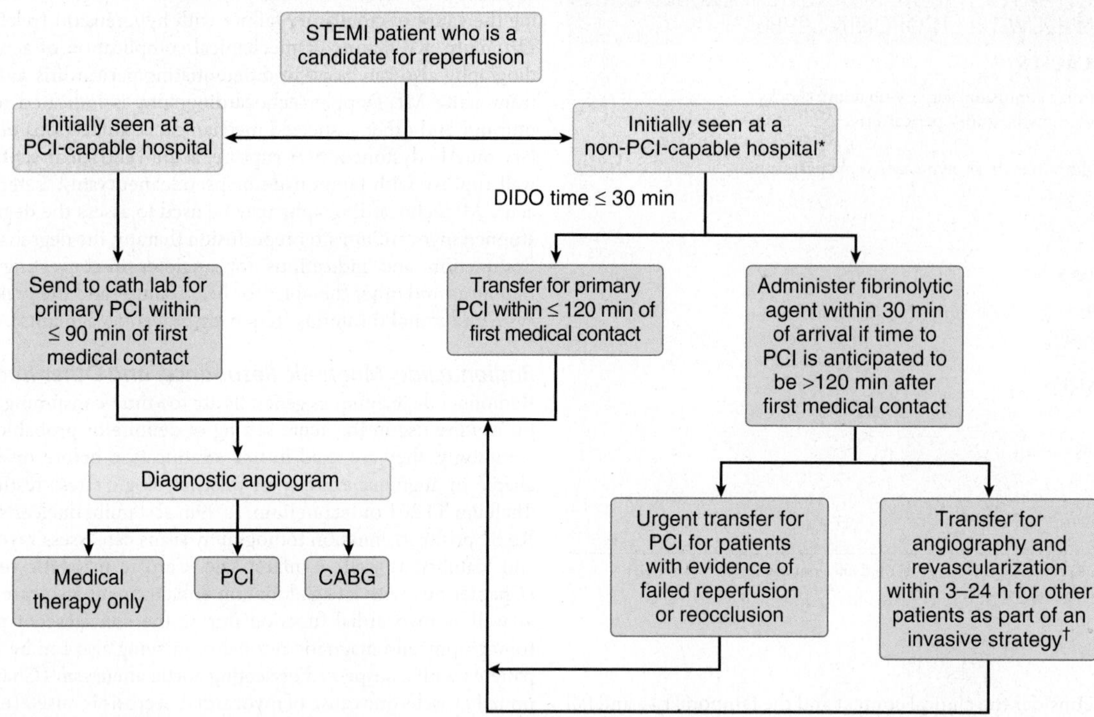

FIGURE 73-3. **Reperfusion therapy for patients with ST segment elevation myocardial infarction (STEMI). *Patients with cardiogenic shock or severe heart failure initially seen at a non–PCI-capable hospital should be transferred for cardiac catheterization and revascularization as soon as possible, irrespective of time delay from MI onset (Class I, Level of Evidence: B). †Angiography and revascularization should not be performed within the first 2 to 3 hours after administration of fibrinolytic therapy. CABG = coronary artery bypass grafting; DIDO = door in–door out; PCI = percutaneous coronary intervention. (Modified from O'Gara PT, Kushner FG, Ascheim DD, et al. 2013 ACCF/AHA guideline for the management of ST-elevation myocardial infarction: a report of the American College of Cardiology/American Heart Association Task Force on Practice Guidelines. *Circulation.* 2013;127:e362-e425.)**

rapidly as possible, the patient should be stratified as having a probable acute STEMI, a non–ST segment elevation acute MI, probable or possible unstable angina, or likely noncardiac chest pain.

In patients with acute STEMI by clinical and electrocardiographic criteria, a reperfusion strategy must be selected. Alternative choices are primary percutaneous coronary intervention (primary PCI; the patient is transferred directly to the cardiac catheterization laboratory with a systems goal of first medical contact to device time of less than 90 minutes) and fibrinolysis (begun immediately in the emergency department with a goal of door to needle time of less than 30 minutes)[1] (Fig. 73-3). In patients who present to a non–PCI-capable hospital, the goal is a first medical contact to device time of 120 minutes or less; otherwise, fibrinolytic therapy is indicated.

Specific Therapeutic Measures

Reperfusion Therapy

Early reperfusion of ischemic, infarcting myocardium represents the most important conceptual and practical advance for acute STEMI and is the primary therapeutic goal. Coronary reperfusion is accomplished by primary PCI with angioplasty and stenting or by fibrinolytic (thrombolytic) therapy. During the past decade, the application of reperfusion therapy has remained relatively constant in the United States and other Western countries at 70 to 75% of eligible patients with acute MI. The percentage of patients undergoing primary PCI has increased substantially over time, although fibrinolytic therapy continues to be commonly applied in developing countries.[5]

With broad application of reperfusion therapy, 30-day mortality rates from acute STEMI have progressively declined during the past three decades (from 20 to 30% to 5 to 10%). Each community should develop and follow an optimal STEMI system of care within the resources available (Fig. 73-3).

Primary Percutaneous Coronary Intervention

Prompt PCI by the femoral or, increasingly, the radial artery approach[A1] is the reperfusion strategy of choice in patients with STEMI and ischemic symptoms of less than 12 hours in duration at PCI-capable hospitals (Table 73-4). The relative benefits of primary PCI over fibrinolysis include a significantly lower acute mortality rate, lower rates of nonfatal reinfarction, and lower risks of intracerebral hemorrhage.[A2] PCI generally includes a bare metal or drug-eluting (e.g., sirolimus, paclitaxel, everolimus, zotarolimus) stent (Chapter 74).

Currently, a primary PCI strategy begins with initiation of a $P2Y_{12}$ inhibitor in the emergency department, together with aspirin and an anticoagulant (e.g., heparin or bivalirudin), followed by rapid PCI with stenting. Augmented antiplatelet therapy with a glycoprotein IIb/IIIa (GPIIb-IIIa) inhibitor may be given in selected patients, generally at the time of catheterization. The addition of a reduced dose of a plasminogen activator to GPIIb-IIIa therapy in the field or emergency department may further improve outcomes in selected patients who undergo early PCI, but this approach is generally not recommended. Pharmacologically facilitated PCI, whereby patients at hospitals without PCI capabilities are given adjusted doses of fibrinolytic or GPIIb-IIIa inhibitors, or both, and then are transferred to other hospitals for emergent (i.e., within 1 to 2 hours) PCI, overall appears to be no better than rapid transfer for primary PCI within 1 to 2 hours.[A3]

Primary PCI also is recommended in patients with STEMI and cardiogenic shock or acute, severe heart failure emergently and irrespective of time delay

TABLE 73-4 INDICATIONS FOR PRIMARY ANGIOPLASTY AND COMPARISON WITH FIBRINOLYTIC THERAPY

INDICATIONS
A preferred reperfusion strategy for ST segment elevation or LBBB acute MI within 12 hours of symptom onset (or >12 hours if symptoms persist)
Cardiogenic shock developing within 36 hours of ST segment elevation/Q wave acute MI or LBBB acute MI in patients <75 years old who can be revascularized within 18 hours of shock onset
Recommended only at centers performing >200 PCIs/year with backup cardiac surgery and for operators performing >75 PCIs/year
ADVANTAGES OF PRIMARY PCI
Higher initial reperfusion rates
Reduced risk of intracerebral hemorrhage
Less residual stenosis; less recurrent ischemia or infarction
Usefulness when fibrinolysis is contraindicated
Improvement in outcomes with cardiogenic shock
DISADVANTAGES OF PRIMARY PCI (COMPARED WITH FIBRINOLYTIC THERAPY)
Access, advantages restricted to high-volume centers and operators
Longer average time to treatment
Greater dependence on operators for results
Higher system complexity and costs

LBBB = left bundle branch block; MI = myocardial infarction; PCI = percutaneous coronary intervention (includes balloon angioplasty, stenting).

TABLE 73-5 CHARACTERISTICS OF INTRAVENOUS FIBRINOLYTIC AGENTS APPROVED BY THE U.S. FOOD AND DRUG ADMINISTRATION

	STREPTOKINASE (SK)	ALTEPLASE (t-PA)	RETEPLASE (r-PA)	TENECTEPLASE (TNK–t-PA)
Dose	1.5 MU in 30-60 minutes	100 mg in 90 minutes*	10 U + 10 U, 30 minutes apart	30-50 mg† during 5 seconds
Circulating half-life (minutes)	≅20	≅4	≅18	≅20
Antigenic	Yes	No	No	No
Allergic reactions	Yes	No	No	No
Systemic fibrinogen depletion	Severe	Mild to moderate	Moderate	Minimal
Intracerebral hemorrhage	≅0.4%	≅0.7%	≅0.8%	≅0.7%
Patency (TIMI 2/3) rate, 90 minutes‡	≅51%	≅73-84%	≅83%	≅77-88%
Lives saved per 100 treated	≅3§	≅4‖	≅4	≅4
Cost per dose (approximate U.S. dollars)	300	1800	2200	2200

*Accelerated t-PA given as follows: 15-mg bolus, then 0.75 mg/kg during 30 minutes (maximum, 50 mg), then 0.50 mg/kg during 60 minutes (maximum, 35 mg).

†TNK–t-PA is dosed by weight (supplied in 5-mg/mL vials): <60 kg = 6 mL; 61-70 kg = 7 mL; 71-80 kg = 8 mL; 81-90 kg = 9 mL; >90 kg = 10 mL.

‡TIMI = Thrombolysis in Myocardial Infarction. Data from Granger CB, Califf RM, Topol EJ. Thrombolytic therapy for acute myocardial infarction: a review. *Drugs.* 1992;44:293-325; and Bode C, Smalling RW, Berg G, et al. Randomized comparison of coronary thrombolysis achieved with double-bolus reteplase (recombinant plasminogen activator) and front-loaded, accelerated alteplase (recombinant tissue plasminogen activator) in patients with acute myocardial infarction: the RAPID II Investigators. *Circulation.* 1996;94:891-898.

§Patients with ST segment elevation or bundle branch block, treated <6 hours.

‖Based on the finding from the GUSTO trial that t-PA saves one more additional life per 100 treated than does SK. Data from The GUSTO Investigators. An international randomized trial comparing four thrombolytic strategies for acute myocardial infarction. *N Engl J Med.* 1993;329:673-682; and Simes RJ, Topol EJ, Holmes DR Jr, et al. Link between the angiographic substudy and mortality outcomes in a large randomized trial of myocardial reperfusion: importance of early and complete infarct artery reperfusion. GUSTO-I Investigators. *Circulation.* 1995;91:1923-1928.

from onset of MI symptoms[A4] (Chapter 107). Primary PCI also is reasonable in patients with STEMI who have clinical or electrocardiographic evidence of ongoing ischemia between 12 and 24 hours after the onset of symptoms. However, delayed PCI of a totally occluded infarct-related artery after 24 hours is not recommended in asymptomatic, stable patients with one- or two-vessel disease.[A5] PCI performed in a stenotic but noninfarcted artery at the time of primary PCI in STEMI patients who otherwise are hemodynamically stable has recently been shown to be superior to medical therapy alone[A6]; staged PCI of such arteries (i.e., at a somewhat delayed time after primary PCI) is a common current practice whose safety is supported by registry data. Increasing positive experience with PCI of the left main coronary artery with stents, especially drug-eluting stents, suggests that it may be an alternative to coronary artery bypass grafting (CABG) in STEMI patients with a culprit left main coronary artery with compromised flow when PCI can be performed more rapidly and safely than CABG. Routine application of mechanical thrombus aspiration at the time of angiography probably does not provide additional benefit over PCI alone, but selected use may be beneficial in patients with a large burden of thrombus.

Fibrinolytic Therapy

Various fibrinolytic agents (Table 73-5) are useful in patients with STEMI or new or presumed new LBBB who present for treatment within 12 hours of the onset of symptoms and who have no contraindications to their use (Table 73-6). Benefit declines from about 40 lives or more saved per 1000 within the first hour, to 20 to 30 lives saved per 1000 for hours 2 to 12, to a nonsignificant 7 lives saved per 1000 for hours 13 to 24. An accelerated regimen of tissue plasminogen activator (t-PA plus intravenous heparin) is preferred to streptokinase because the patency rate of the infarct-related artery at 90 minutes is higher and mortality is lower. Longer-acting variants of t-PA, given by single-bolus (tenecteplase) or double-bolus (reteplase) injections, are now in widespread clinical use because they are more convenient to give, but they have not led to further improvements in survival. A nonimmunogenic fibrinolytic agent is preferred for patients with a history of prior streptokinase use.

The major risk of fibrinolytic therapy is bleeding. Intracranial hemorrhage is the most serious and frequently fatal complication; its incidence rate is 0.5 to 1% with currently approved regimens. Older age (>70 to 75 years), female gender, hypertension, and higher relative doses of t-PA and heparin increase the risk for intracranial hemorrhage. The risk-to-benefit ratio should be assessed in each patient when fibrinolysis is considered and specific regimens are selected.

For failed fibrinolysis, rescue PCI is more effective than repeated fibrinolysis.[A7] After fibrinolysis, regardless of its apparent success, a preferred strategy is to transfer all STEMI patients with high-risk features rapidly to a hospital with PCI facilities to undergo angiography rather than to transfer only selected patients in whom fibrinolysis has failed or recurrent ischemia has developed.[A8] This early transfer and angiography strategy at a median of 3 hours after fibrinolysis reduces the risk for recurrent ischemia, reinfarction, heart failure, cardiogenic shock, or death by 36%.

Selecting a Reperfusion Regimen

Whether to use PCI or fibrinolytic therapy depends on local resources and experience as well as on patient factors. Primary PCI is feasible in community hospitals without surgical capability, but operator and team experience as well as organizational and transfer issues are critical to success.[A9] In general, primary PCI with stenting is preferred in experienced facilities that are able to mobilize and to treat patients quickly (<90 minutes door to device system time). PCI is particularly preferred for patients at higher risk for mortality (including shock), for later presentations (>3 hours), and for patients with greater risk of intracranial hemorrhage (age >70 years, female gender, therapy with hypertensive agents).

In non–PCI-capable hospitals and in other situations in which PCI is not feasible or would be significantly delayed (e.g., by a long transfer time to a PCI-capable facility) to more than 120 minutes after first medical contact, fibrinolytic therapy should be given to patients with STEMI within 12 hours of the onset of symptoms unless it is contraindicated. Fibrinolytic therapy is reasonable within 12 to 24 hours of the onset of symptoms in the setting of a large MI or hemodynamic instability. Prehospital fibrinolysis followed by a routine *emergent* (i.e., within 1 to 2 hours) invasive strategy on hospital arrival causes a *higher* rate of in-hospital mortality, cardiac ischemic events, and strokes compared with primary PCI alone or by a more delayed invasive approach after fibrinolysis in stabilized patients and cannot be recommended.

TABLE 73-6 INDICATIONS FOR AND CONTRAINDICATIONS TO FIBRINOLYTIC THERAPY

INDICATIONS

Ischemic-type chest discomfort or equivalent for 30 minutes–12 hours with new or presumed new ST segment elevation in two contiguous leads of ≥2 mm (≥0.2 mV) in leads V_1, V_2, or V_3 or ≥1 mm in other leads
New or presumed new left bundle branch block with symptoms consistent with myocardial infarction
Absence of contraindications

CONTRAINDICATIONS, ABSOLUTE

Active bleeding or bleeding diathesis (menses excluded)
Prior hemorrhagic stroke, ischemic stroke within 3 months, except acute ischemic stroke within 3-4.5 hours
Intracranial or spinal cord neoplasm or arteriovenous malformation
Suspected or known aortic dissection
Closed head or facial trauma within 3 months

CONTRAINDICATIONS, RELATIVE

Severe, uncontrolled hypertension by history or on presentation (>180/110 mm Hg)
Anticoagulation with therapeutic or elevated international normalized ratio (>2-3)
Old ischemic stroke (>3 months ago); intracerebral disease other than above
Recent (<3 weeks) major trauma/surgery or prolonged (>10 minutes) cardiopulmonary resuscitation or internal bleeding
Active peptic ulcer
Recent noncompressible vascular punctures
Pregnancy
For streptokinase/anistreplase: prior exposure (especially if >5 days ago) or allergic reaction

Modified from Kushner FG, Hand M, Smith SC Jr, et al. 2009 Focused updates: ACC/AHA guidelines for the management of patients with ST-elevation myocardial infarction and the ACC/AHA/SCAI guidelines on percutaneous coronary intervention. *Circulation.* 2009;120:2271-2306.

However, immediate transfer to a PCI-capable hospital for coronary angiography is recommended if such patients develop cardiogenic shock or severe heart failure and is reasonable in patients with suspected failed reperfusion or reocclusion after fibrinolytic therapy and even in hemodynamically stable patients with apparently successful reperfusion, provided angiography is delayed for at least 2 to 3 hours after fibrinolytic therapy.

Ancillary and Other Therapies

Initial Medical Management

Aspirin (162 to 325 mg) should be given on presentation to all patients unless it is contraindicated (Fig. 73-4). A loading dose of an adenosine diphosphate receptor ($P2Y_{12}$) inhibitor (i.e., clopidogrel, 600 mg, or prasugrel, 60 mg, or ticagrelor, 180 mg) also should be given as early as possible or at the time of primary PCI to STEMI patients for whom an invasive approach is planned. In addition, it is reasonable to start treatment with a GPIIb-IIIa receptor antagonist—abciximab (IV bolus of 0.25 mg/kg, then 0.125 μg/kg/minute [maximum, 10 μg/minute] for up to 12 hours), tirofiban (IV bolus of 25 μg/kg, then 0.15 μg/kg/minute for up to 12 to 18 hours; reduce infusion rate by 50% for estimated creatinine clearance < 30 mL/minute), or eptifibatide (IV bolus of 180 μg/kg, second bolus after 10 minutes, then 2.0 μg/kg/minute for up to 18 hours; reduce infusion by 50% for estimated creatinine clearance < 50 mL/minute)—at the time of primary PCI for STEMI in selected patients, such as those with a large burden of thrombus or those who have not received an adequate loading dose of a $P2Y_{12}$ inhibitor. The value of starting a GPIIb-IIIa receptor antagonist before arrival in the catheterization laboratory is less certain.

Anticoagulant therapy should be initiated on presentation. Options include intravenous heparin (initial bolus of 60 IU/kg [maximum, 4000 IU], then 12 IU/kg/hour [maximum, 1000 IU/hour] for patients >70 kg, adjusted to maintain activated partial thromboplastin time 1.5 to 2 times the control value), low-molecular-weight heparin (LMWH; e.g., enoxaparin, IV bolus of 30 mg, then 1 mg/kg subcutaneously twice daily for patients <75 years old without renal insufficiency with fibrinolysis or IV bolus of 0.5 mg/kg with primary PCI), and bivalirudin (with a primary PCI strategy, bolus of 0.75 mg/kg, then infusion of 1.75 mg/kg/hour). In STEMI patients who are undergoing PCI and who are at higher risk for bleeding, evidence supports use of bivalirudin anticoagulation with a $P2Y_{12}$ inhibitor but without a GPIIb-IIIa receptor antagonist. Fondaparinux may be used as adjunctive anticoagulant therapy with fibrinolysis but not as the sole anticoagulant with primary PCI.

Patients with chest pain should be given sublingual nitroglycerin (0.4 mg every 5 minutes for up to three doses), after which an assessment should be made of the need for intravenous nitroglycerin. Persistent ischemic pain may be treated with titrated intravenous doses of morphine (i.e., 2 to 4 mg intravenously, repeated every 5 to 15 minutes to relieve pain). Initiation of β-blocker therapy is usually indicated, especially in patients with hypertension, tachycardia, and ongoing pain; however, decompensated heart failure is a contraindication to the acute initiation of β-blocker therapy, particularly by the intravenous route. Oxygen should be used, if needed, in doses sufficient to avoid hypoxemia (e.g., initially at 2 to 4 L/minute by nasal cannula; fingertip oximetry may be used to monitor effect). The ideal systolic blood pressure is 100 to 140 mm Hg. Excessive hypertension usually responds to titrated nitroglycerin, β-blocker therapy, and morphine (also given for pain). Relative hypotension could require discontinuation of these medications, fluid administration, or other measures as appropriate to the hemodynamic subset (Table 73-7). Atropine (0.5 to 1.5 mg intravenously) should be available to treat symptomatic bradycardia and hypotension related to excessive vagotonia. Direct transfer to the catheterization laboratory or fibrinolysis followed by transfer to the cardiac intensive care unit should occur as expeditiously as possible.

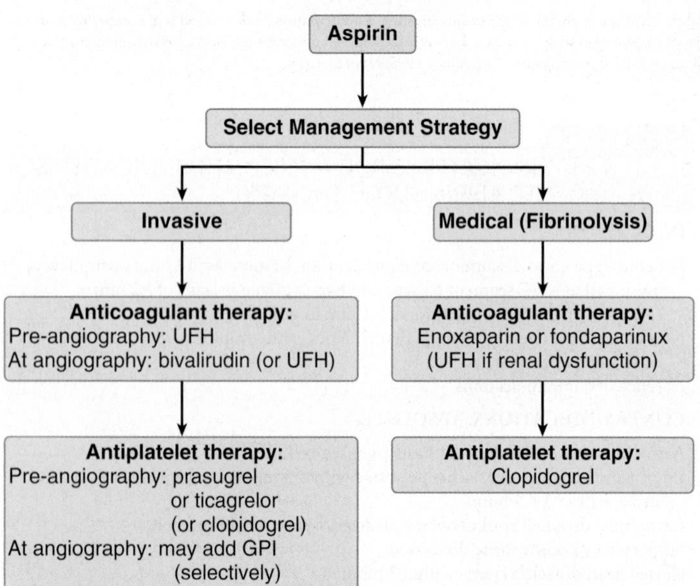

FIGURE 73-4. **Recommendations for antiplatelet and anticoagulant therapy for ST segment elevation myocardial infarction (STEMI). See text for doses. GPI = glycoprotein IIb/IIIa inhibitor; UFH = unfractionated heparin.**

Early Hospital Phase: Coronary Intensive Care

Coronary intensive care for early hospital management of acute MI has reduced in-hospital mortality by more than 50%. The goals of such care include continuous electrocardiographic monitoring and antiarrhythmic therapy for serious arrhythmias (i.e., rapid defibrillation of VF), initiation or continuation of a coronary reperfusion strategy to achieve myocardial reperfusion, initiation or continuation of other acute medical therapies, hemodynamic monitoring and appropriate medical interventions for different hemodynamic subsets of patients, and diagnosis and treatment of mechanical and physiologic complications of acute MI (Table 73-8).

TABLE 73-7 HEMODYNAMIC SUBSETS OF ACUTE MYOCARDIAL INFARCTION

	BLOOD PRESSURE (RELATIVE)	TYPICAL PHYSICAL FINDINGS	CARDIAC INDEX (L/min/m^2)	PA WEDGE PRESSURE (mm Hg)	SUGGESTED INTERVENTIONS
Normal	Normal	$\pm S_4$	>2.5	≤12	None required
Hyperdynamic	Normal or high	Anxious	>3	<12	Control pain, anxiety; β-blocker; treat SBP to <140 mm Hg
Hypovolemia	Low	Dry	≤2.7	≤9	Add fluids to maintain normal pressure; can develop pulmonary edema if hypotension caused by unrecognized LV failure
Mild LV failure	Low to high	Rales, $\pm S_3$	2-2.5	>15	Diuresis; nitrates, ACE inhibitor; consider low-dose β-blocker
Severe LV failure	Low to normal	Above $+S_3$, ± ↑ JVP, ± edema	<2	>20	Diuresis; nitrates; low-dose ACE inhibitor; avoid β-blockers; consider inotropes, urgent revascularization
Cardiogenic shock	Very low	Above + cool, clammy; ↓ mental or renal function	≤1.5	>25	Avoid hypotensive agents; place intra-aortic balloon pump; urgent revascularization if possible
RV infarct	Very low	↑ JVP with clear lungs	<2.5	≤12	Give IV fluids; avoid nitrates and hypotensive agents; dobutamine if refractory to fluids

↑ = increased; ↓ = decreased; ACE = angiotensin-converting enzyme; IV = intravenous; JVP = jugular venous pressure; LV = left ventricle; PA = pulmonary artery; RV = right ventricle; SBP = systolic blood pressure.
Modified from Forrester JS, Diamond G, Chatterjee K, et al. Medical therapy of acute myocardial infarction by application of hemodynamic subsets (second of two parts). *N Engl J Med.* 1976;295:1404-1413.

TABLE 73-8 SAMPLE ADMISSION ORDERS FOR ST SEGMENT ELEVATION ACUTE MYOCARDIAL INFARCTION

Diagnosis	Acute ST segment elevation myocardial infarction
Admit	Coronary care unit with telemetry
Condition	Serious
Vital signs	q ½h until stable, then q1-4h and PRN; pulse oximetry × 24 hr; notify if heart rate <50 or >100; respiratory rate <8 or >20; SBP <90 or >150 mm Hg; O_2 saturation <90%
Activity	Bedrest × 12 hr with bedside commode; thereafter, light activity if stable
Diet	NPO except for sips of water until pain free and stable; then 2 g sodium, heart-healthy diet as tolerated, unless on call for catheterization (or other test requiring NPO)
Laboratory tests*	Troponin I or T at 2 hours, then q8h × 3; comprehensive blood chemistry, magnesium, CBC with platelets; PT/INR, aPTT; BNP; lipid profile (fasting in morning); portable CXR
IV therapy	D_5W or NS to keep vein open (increase fluids for relative hypovolemia); second IV if IV medication given
Reperfusion therapy*	Emergency primary coronary angioplasty or fibrinolysis (if appropriate) 1. Primary angioplasty (preferred if available within 90 minutes) 2. Tenecteplase, alteplase, reteplase, or streptokinase (see Table 73-5 for doses), if primary PCI is unavailable within 90-120 minutes
Medications	1. Nasal O_2 at 2 L/min with or at risk of hypoxemia, titrated to keep O_2 saturation >90% 2. Aspirin 162-325 mg chewed on admission, then 81-162 mg PO daily 3. IV heparin, 60-U/kg bolus (maximum, 4000 U) and 12 U/kg/hr (maximum, 1000 U/hr), titrate to target aPTT 1.5-2.0 × control (about 50-70 seconds); *or* enoxaparin (preferred with fibrinolytic), 30 mg IV, then 1 mg/kg SC q12h (maximum SC doses, 100 mg on day 1; reduce to 0.75 mg/kg for age ≥75 years, increase interval to q24h for CrCl <30 mL/min); *or* bivalirudin (with primary PCI), 0.75-mg/kg IV bolus, then 1.75 mg/kg/hr (delay 30 minutes if heparin given) 4. Metoprolol, 12.5 PO q6h, incremented to 25-50 mg q6h as tolerated (hold for SBP < 100 mm Hg, pulse < 50 beats/min, asthma, heart failure); may consider IV metoprolol if immediate effect required (tachyarrhythmia, severe hypertension, unrelieved pain) in the absence of heart failure 5. Consider IV nitroglycerin drip × 24-48 hr (titrated to SBP 100-140 mm Hg) 6. Morphine sulfate, 2-4 mg IV and increment at 5-15 minutes PRN for unrelieved pain 7. Stool softener 8. Anxiolytic or hypnotic if needed 9. ACE inhibitor for hypertension, anterior acute MI, or LV dysfunction, in low oral dose (e.g., captopril, 6.25 mg q8h), begun within 24 hours or when stable (SBP > 100 mm Hg) and adjusted upward 10. Lipid-lowering therapy (i.e., high-intensity statin) regardless of LDL: target LDL reduction of ≥50%; give atorvastatin 80 mg PO on admission (pre-cath) and continue daily 11. Antiplatelet therapy: clopidogrel, 600 mg PO on admission for invasive strategy, 300 mg PO with fibrinolytic, then 75 mg PO daily; *or* ticagrelor, 180 mg PO on admission, then 90 mg bid (with primary PCI strategy); *or* prasugrel, 60 mg PO on admission, then 10 mg PO daily (with primary PCI strategy). For specific treatments for hemodynamic subgroups, see Table 73-7.

*If not ordered in the emergency department.
ACE = angiotensin-converting enzyme; aPTT = activated partial thromboplastin time; BNP = brain natriuretic peptide; CABG = coronary artery bypass graft surgery; CBC = complete blood count; CrCl = creatinine clearance; CXR = chest radiograph; D_5W = 5% dextrose in water; INR = international normalized ratio; IV = intravenous; LDL = low-density lipoprotein; LV = left ventricle; MI = myocardial infarction; NPO = nothing by mouth; NS = normal saline; PCI = percutaneous coronary intervention; PO = orally; PRN = as needed; PT = prothrombin time; daily = once daily; SBP = systolic blood pressure; SC = subcutaneous.
Modified from Kushner FG, Hand M, Smith SC Jr, et al. 2009 Focused updates: ACC/AHA guidelines for the management of patients with ST-elevation myocardial infarction and the ACC/AHA/SCAI guidelines on percutaneous coronary intervention. *Circulation.* 2009;120:2271-306.

General care measures include attention to activity, diet and bowels, education, reassurance, and sedation. Bedrest is encouraged for the first 12 hours. In the absence of complications, dangling, bed-to-chair, and self-care activities can begin within 24 hours or earlier after successful reperfusion therapy. When stabilization has occurred, usually within 1 to 3 days, patients may be transferred to a step-down unit where progressive reambulation occurs. The risk for emesis and aspiration or the anticipation of angiography or other procedures usually dictates nothing by mouth or clear liquids for the first 4 to 12 hours. Thereafter, a heart-healthy diet in small portions is recommended. In patients at high risk for bleeding gastric stress ulcers, a proton pump inhibitor or an H_2-receptor antagonist is recommended. Many patients benefit from an analgesic (e.g., morphine sulfate, in 2- to 4-mg increments) to relieve ongoing pain and an anxiolytic or sedative during the acute phase. A benzodiazepine is frequently selected, but routine use of anxiolytics is neither necessary nor recommended. Sedatives should not substitute for education and reassurance from concerned caregivers to relieve emotional distress and improve behavior. Constipation often occurs with bedrest and narcotics; stool softeners and a bedside commode are advised.

The ECG should be monitored continuously during the entire hospital course to detect serious arrhythmias and to guide therapy. Measures to limit infarct size (i.e., coronary reperfusion) and to optimize hemodynamics also stabilize the heart electrically. Routine antiarrhythmic prophylaxis (e.g., with lidocaine or amiodarone) is not indicated, but specific arrhythmias require treatment (see later text).

Hemodynamic evaluation is helpful in assessing prognosis and in guiding therapy (see Table 73-7). Clinical and noninvasive evaluation of vital signs is adequate for normotensive patients without pulmonary congestion. Patients with pulmonary venous congestion alone can usually be managed conservatively. Invasive monitoring is appropriate when the cause of circulatory failure is uncertain and when titration of intravenous therapies depends on hemodynamic measurements (e.g., pulmonary capillary wedge pressure and cardiac output). Similarly, an arterial line is not necessary in all patients and may be associated with local bleeding after fibrinolysis or potent antiplatelet and anticoagulant therapy. Arterial catheters are appropriate and useful in clinically unstable, hypotensive patients who do not respond to intravenous fluids to replete or to expand intravascular volume (see the later discussion of complications).

Later Hospital Phase

Transfer from intensive care to the step-down unit usually occurs within 1 to 3 days, when the cardiac rhythm and hemodynamics are stable. The duration of this late phase of hospital care is usually an additional 1 to 3 days in uncomplicated cases. Activity levels should be increased progressively under continuous electrocardiographic monitoring. Medical therapy should progress from parenteral and short-acting agents to oral medications appropriate and convenient for long-term outpatient use.

Risk stratification and functional evaluations are critical to assess prognosis and to guide therapy as the time for discharge approaches. Functional evaluation also can be extended to the early period after hospital discharge. Education must be provided about diet, activity, smoking, and other risk factors (e.g., lipids, hypertension, and diabetes).

Antiplatelet Therapy

Aspirin

Aspirin (Chapters 37 and 38) reduces the relative risk of vascular death in patients with acute MI and is strongly recommended at a dose of 162 to 325 mg, preferably chewed, both before primary PCI and with fibrinolytic therapy. Aspirin should be continued throughout hospitalization and then indefinitely on an outpatient basis at 81 mg/day; 325 mg/day may be preferable for the first month after PCI in patients who are taking clopidogrel.

Adenosine Diphosphate ($P2Y_{12}$) Receptor Antagonists

In addition to aspirin, *clopidogrel* (300 mg followed by 75 mg/day) is recommended in STEMI patients 75 years of age or younger who are treated with a fibrinolytic, in whom it reduces predischarge occlusion rates of infarct-related arteries (by 41%) and reduces ischemic complications at 30 days (by 20%) without increasing rates of intracerebral hemorrhage.A10 It is also recommended without a loading dose in STEMI patients older than 75 years who receive fibrinolytic therapy.A11 Clopidogrel also is indicated in STEMI patients undergoing primary PCI with stenting (loading dose, 600 mg); it is less effective but has a lower bleeding risk than prasugrel and ticagrelor (see later). Clopidogrel increases the risk of bleeding and blood transfusions with CABG; if CABG is planned, clopidogrel should be withheld for at least 5 days unless the urgency of surgery outweighs the risk of excessive bleeding. Common genetic variants (i.e., in CYP2C19) may reduce activation of clopidogrel, but dosing guided by genetic testing has not been shown to improve clinical outcomes. Similarly, proton pump inhibitors, especially omeprazole, impair clopidogrel's antiplatelet activity, but coadministration has not been associated with any adverse clinical consequences.

Prasugrel, a more potent thienopyridine, is indicated as adjunctive therapy (60 mg loading dose, 10 mg/day maintenance dose), on admission or at the time of angiography, in patients who receive primary PCI but not in patients who receive fibrinolytic therapy.A12 However, prasugrel is contraindicated in patients with a prior history of stroke or transient ischemia attack, should be used with caution (or in reduced doses) in older (≥75 years) and smaller (<60 kg) patients, and should be withheld for at least 7 days before nonemergent CABG.

Ticagrelor, a direct-acting and non-thienopyridine $P2Y_{12}$ inhibitor, also is more effective than clopidogrel and is indicated for adjunctive therapy (loading dose of 180 mg, maintenance dose of 90 mg twice daily) on admission or at angiography with primary PCI but not with fibrinolytic therapy.A13 Ticagrelor is contraindicated in patients with a history of intracranial hemorrhage.

The recommended duration of $P2Y_{12}$ inhibitor therapy is 1 year after PCI for STEMI with stenting to prevent stent thrombosis and recurrent ischemic events. Platelet function testing can be used to guide dosing of $P2Y_{12}$ inhibitors, but studies to date have not demonstrated sufficient benefit to warrant their routine use. Platelet function testing can be used to document adherence and may prove useful in high-risk patients with drug-eluting stents.

Glycoprotein IIb/IIIa Receptor Antagonists

High-risk patients with non–ST segment elevation acute coronary syndrome benefit from antagonists of the platelet membrane GPIIb-IIIa receptor, either on admission or after PCI (Chapters 38 and 72). The benefit is smaller in STEMI with routine stenting, but it is reasonable to administer a GPIIb-IIIa receptor antagonist at the time of primary PCI in STEMI patients who have a large burden of thrombus or who have not received adequate loading with a $P2Y_{12}$ inhibitor. If early CABG is a possibility after angiography, a shorter-acting inhibitor (eptifibatide, tirofiban) may impart a lower perioperative risk for bleeding than abciximab. Earlier ("upstream") glycoprotein inhibition before hospital admission or in the emergency department (precatheterization) can improve coronary patency at the time of emergency angiography, but incremental benefit on clinical outcomes has not been established.

Anticoagulant Therapy

Low-Molecular-Weight Heparins

In patients with acute STEMI who are treated with fibrinolytic therapy, LMWH can reduce reinfarction rates by 25% and mortality by about 10% compared with unfractionated heparin.A14 Enoxaparin is dosed according to age and weight (i.e., age <75 years: IV bolus of 30 mg, then 1 mg/kg SC every 12 hours [maximum, 100 mg for first two doses]; age ≥75 years: no bolus, 0.75 mg/kg SC every12 hours [maximum, 75 mg, first two doses]) as well as by creatinine clearance (if the creatinine clearance is <30 mL/minute: 1 mg/kg SC every 24 hours) until hospital discharge or up to 8 days. Enoxaparin is more complicated to use with a primary PCI strategy; it is an option in this setting in current European[6] but not in American[1] guidelines.

Unfractionated Heparin

Unfractionated heparin can benefit patients treated with primary PCI or fibrinolytic agents (see Fig. 73-3). When it is given with a fibrin-specific fibrinolytic agent, intravenous heparin is begun concurrently and continued for 48 hours, beginning with a bolus of 60 U/kg (maximum, 4000 U), followed initially by an infusion of 12 U/kg/hour (maximum, 1000 U/hour), with adjustment after 3 hours based on the activated partial thromboplastin time (target of 50 to 70 seconds, 1.5 to 2 times control). Experimental regimens including a GPIIb-IIIa inhibitor and a fibrinolytic agent have used even lower heparin doses. During primary PCI, high-dose heparin (bolus of 70 to 100 U/kg) is used to achieve an activated clotting time of 250 to 300 seconds. Given together with a GPIIb-IIIa inhibitor during PCI, the dose of heparin is adjusted (bolus of 50 to 70 U/kg) to achieve a lower activated clotting time range (200 to 250 seconds). Additional boluses are given as needed to maintain therapeutic activated time levels.

Factor Xa Inhibitors

Selective factor Xa inhibition (i.e., with fondaparinux, 2.5 mg, initial dose intravenously, then subcutaneously once daily for up to 8 days during index hospitalization) may reduce death or reinfarction at 30 days by 18 to 23% independent of heparin use in patients who receive fibrinolysis or no reperfusion therapy, but it is not of benefit in patients who have undergone PCI. As a result, it may be a preferred alternative to unfractionated heparin or no heparin (e.g., in patients who present later and in patients treated with streptokinase) in patients with STEMI who are not undergoing a primary PCI strategy. Fondaparinux is contraindicated if the creatinine clearance is less than 30 mL/minute.

Direct Antithrombins

Bivalirudin, a synthetic hirudin analogue with direct antithrombin activity (Chapter 38), combined with early administration of high-dose clopidogrel is better than the combination of heparin plus a GPIIb-IIIa inhibitor for STEMI patients who undergo primary PCI.A15 The recommended dose is an IV bolus of 0.75 mg/kg, followed by an infusion of 1.75 mg/kg/hour; an additional bolus of 0.3 mg/kg can be given if needed. Bivalirudin has not been tested and is not indicated in patients receiving fibrinolytic therapy.

Other Pharmacologic Therapies

Nitrates

Nitroglycerin and other organic nitrates (isosorbide dinitrate and isosorbide mononitrate) reduce excessive cardiac preload and afterload, increase coronary caliber in responsive areas of stenosis, reverse distal small coronary arterial vasoconstriction, improve coronary collateral flow to ischemic myocardium, and inhibit platelet aggregation in acute MI (Chapter 71). The results are improved oxygen delivery and reduced oxygen consumption.

Nitroglycerin is useful for the first 24 to 48 hours for patients with acute MI and pulmonary congestion, large anterior MI, persistent ischemia, or hypertension. In patients treated with fibrinolytic therapy and aspirin, nitrates provide a modest relative survival benefit of about 4 lives saved per 1000 patients treated. In patients undergoing primary PCI, however, no such benefit has been shown.

When it is used in the setting of an acute MI, intravenous nitroglycerin should begin with a bolus injection of 12.5 to 25 μg followed by an infusion of 10 to 20 μg/minute. The infusion rate is increased by 5 to 10 μg/minute every 5 to 10 minutes up to about 200 μg/minute during hemodynamic monitoring until clinical symptoms are controlled or blood pressure targets are reached (blood pressure decreased by 10% in normotensive patients or by 30% in hypertensive patients but not to less than 80 mm Hg mean or 90 mm Hg systolic). Nitrates should be avoided in patients with hypotension, marked bradycardia or tachycardia, or RV infarction, and they are not indicated routinely during the convalescent phase of STEMI.

β-Blockers

β-Adrenoceptor blockers reduce heart rate, blood pressure, and myocardial contractility, and they stabilize the heart electrically. These actions provide clinical benefit to most patients with acute MI by limiting myocardial oxygen consumption, relieving ischemia, reducing infarct size, and preventing serious arrhythmias.

Early (first-day) β-blockade is generally recommended for STEMI patients who do not have signs of heart failure, evidence of a low-output state or increased risk for cardiogenic shock, or other contraindications, such as heart block, severe bradycardia, and active reactive airways disease, regardless of concomitant fibrinolysis or PCI. Oral β-blocker therapy may be titrated to tolerance or goal (e.g., metoprolol, 25 to 100 mg twice daily; atenolol, 50 to 100 mg/day; or carvedilol, 6.25 to 25 mg twice daily). Intravenous β-blockade has been reserved for STEMI patients who have no contraindications to its use and who are hypertensive or have ongoing ischemia. β-Blocker therapy should be continued after hospitalization for all STEMI patients without contraindications, but it also may benefit patients with anterior STEMI if given before reperfusion.A16

Renin-Angiotensin-Aldosterone System Inhibitors

The renin-angiotensin-aldosterone system is activated in acute MI and heart failure. Use of an ACE inhibitor has been shown to improve remodeling after acute MI (especially after large anterior MI). ACE inhibitors also have demonstrated efficacy in heart failure, wherein they prevent disease progression, hospitalization, and death (Chapter 59). A meta-analysis of three major trials and 11 smaller ones involving more than 100,000 patients showed an overall mortality reduction of 6.5%, representing about 5 lives saved per 1000 patients treated. Benefit is concentrated and greater in higher-risk patients with large or anterior MI and with LV dysfunction or heart failure, although patients with lesser degrees of LV dysfunction and only moderate cardiovascular risk can also benefit in the long term.

Oral *ACE inhibitor therapy* should begin within the first 24 hours in patients with anterior infarction, heart failure, or low ejection fraction (≤0.40) in the absence of hypotension (systolic pressure <100 mm Hg or >30 mm Hg less than usual baseline) or other contraindications. An *angiotensin receptor blocker* (ARB) should be given to otherwise qualifying patients who are intolerant of ACE inhibitors.A17 An ACE inhibitor or an ARB also is reasonable for other patients with STEMI, especially those with a relative indication (e.g., hypertension, diabetes, or mild renal insufficiency), and in those with the expectation of a smaller but worthwhile benefit.

All patients without contraindications or intolerance to initial ACE inhibitor or ARB therapy also should receive these drugs during the in-hospital convalescent phase. ACE inhibitor therapy should begin with low oral doses and should be progressively advanced to a full or maximally tolerated dose. For example, the short-acting agent captopril may be started in a dose of 6.25 mg or less and adjusted during 1 to 2 days to 50 mg twice daily. Before discharge, a transition may be made in graded dose schedules to longer-acting agents such as ramipril (2.5 mg titrated to 10 mg/day), lisinopril (2.5 to 5 mg titrated to 10 mg/day), or enalapril (2.5 mg titrated to up to 20 mg twice daily). In patients who cannot tolerate ACE inhibitors (e.g., because of cough), graded doses of an ARB may be substituted (e.g., valsartan, 80 to 160 mg twice daily, or losartan, 50 to 100 mg/day).

Selective *aldosterone receptor blockade* with eplerenone (25 to 50 mg/day) reduces total and cardiovascular mortality (including sudden death) as well as cardiovascular hospitalizations in post-MI patients with an ejection fraction of 0.40 or less and heart failure or diabetes and who are already receiving other optimal therapies, including ACE inhibitors.[A18] Spironolactone also benefits patients with advanced heart failure, including those in whom it is caused by a remote MI. Hence, aldosterone receptor blockade should be added to other standard therapies (i.e., ACE inhibitors and β-blockers) during convalescence in STEMI patients with an ejection fraction of 0.40 or less and either symptomatic heart failure or diabetes mellitus. Hyperkalemia, the most common side effect, requires monitoring (Chapter 59).

Antiarrhythmic Agents and Implantable Cardioverter-Defibrillators

Antiarrhythmic therapy is reserved for treatment of or short-term prevention after symptomatic or life-threatening atrial fibrillation (AF) or ventricular arrhythmias, together with other appropriate measures (cardioversion, treatment of ischemia and metabolic disturbances). When medications are indicated, amiodarone usually is the most appropriate agent.

An implantable cardioverter-defibrillator (ICD) is indicated in patients with VF or hemodynamically significant sustained ventricular tachycardia (VT) occurring more than 2 days after STEMI and not due to a transient or reversible cause (e.g., ischemia, reinfarction, metabolic abnormalities). An ICD also may be considered for patients with severe LV dysfunction (ejection fraction ≤0.30) at least 40 days after STEMI and 3 months after CABG without spontaneous or induced VT or VF. These differences reflect an apparent time dependence, in which the benefit of an ICD appears to be delayed until the early post-MI and post-revascularization periods (Chapter 66). By comparison, early ICD implantation is not beneficial in a broader group of patients because its usefulness in preventing similar deaths is offset by the high rate of nonsudden deaths.[A19]

Inotropes

Digitalis and intravenous inotropes can increase oxygen demand, provoke serious arrhythmias, and extend infarction. Current opinion supports the use of digoxin in selected patients recovering from acute MI who develop supraventricular tachyarrhythmias (e.g., AF) or heart failure refractory to ACE inhibitors and diuretics. Intravenous inotropes (e.g., dobutamine, dopamine, milrinone, and norepinephrine) are reserved for temporary support of patients with hypotension and circulatory failure that is unresponsive to volume replacement (Chapters 59 and 107).

Lipid-Lowering Therapy

Lipid lowering, particularly with statins, reduces event rates in patients with coronary disease (Chapter 206). Initiation and continuation of high-intensity statin therapy (e.g., atorvastatin, 80 mg daily) is recommended in the setting of MI,[7,A20] independent of fasting lipid levels, although it is reasonable to obtain a fasting lipid profile within 24 hours of admission.

Other Medical Therapies

Calcium-channel blockers, although anti-ischemic, also are negatively inotropic and have not been shown to reduce mortality after acute STEMI. Furthermore, certain agents may cause harm in some patients. Verapamil or diltiazem (heart rate–slowing drugs) may be given to patients in whom β-blockers are ineffective or contraindicated for control of rapid ventricular response with AF or relief of ongoing ischemia in the absence of heart failure, LV dysfunction, or atrioventricular (AV) block (Chapter 64).

In comatose STEMI patients resuscitated from out-of-hospital cardiac arrest due to VF or pulseless VT, *therapeutic hypothermia* to a targeted temperature of 36°C is beneficial and should be started as soon as possible after hospital arrival (Chapter 63). Prehospital cooling does not provide incremental benefit.

Glucose-insulin-potassium affords no benefit on mortality, cardiac arrest, or cardiogenic shock when this combination is added to usual care in patients with acute STEMI. However, *glucose control*, by an insulin-based regimen to achieve and to maintain glucose levels of less than 180 mg/dL while avoiding hypoglycemia, is recommended in the acute phase of STEMI. After the acute phase, individualized treatment is indicated with agents or combinations of agents that best achieve glycemic control and are well tolerated (Chapter 229).

Magnesium is of no benefit in patients with acute MI who are treated with fibrinolysis. Supplementation is recommended if the magnesium level is below normal or in patients with torsades de pointes–type VT associated with a prolonged QT interval. Intracoronary infusion of *autologous bone marrow mononuclear cells* is not effective.

Management of Complications

Recurrent Chest Pain

When chest pain recurs after acute MI, the diagnostic possibilities include post-infarction ischemia, pericarditis, infarct extension, and infarct expansion. Characterization of the pain, physical examination, electrocardiography, echocardiography, and cardiac marker determinations assist in the differential diagnosis. CK-MB may discriminate reinfarction better than cTnI or cTnT.

Post-infarction angina developing spontaneously during hospitalization for acute MI despite medical therapy usually merits coronary angiography. β-Blockers (intravenously, then orally) and nitroglycerin (intravenously, then orally or topically) are recommended medical therapies. Pain with recurrent ST segment elevation or recurrent elevation of cardiac markers may be treated with readministration of t-PA or, possibly, a GPIIb-IIIa inhibitor, together with nitroglycerin, β-blockade, and heparin. Streptokinase, which induces neutralizing antibodies, generally should not be readministered after the first few days. If facilities for angiography, PCI, and surgery are available, an invasive approach is recommended to relieve discomfort occurring hours to days after an acute MI that is associated with objective signs of ischemia. Radionuclide perfusion stress testing can be helpful in patients with discomfort that is transient or of uncertain ischemic origin. For lesions with questionable degrees of stenosis at angiography, coronary pressure (fractional flow reserve) or Doppler velocimetry or intracoronary ultrasound can determine whether PCI is warranted.

Infarct expansion implies circumferential slippage with thinning of the infarcted myocardium. Infarct expansion can be associated with chest pain but without recurrent elevation of cardiac markers. Expansive remodeling can lead to an LV aneurysm. The risk for remodeling is reduced with early reperfusion therapy and administration of ACE inhibitors.

Acute pericarditis most commonly is manifested on days 2 to 4 in association with large, transmural infarctions causing pericardial inflammation. On occasion, hemorrhagic effusion with tamponade develops; thus, excessive anticoagulation should be avoided. Pericarditis developing later (2 to 10 weeks) after acute MI could represent Dressler syndrome, which is believed to be immune mediated. The incidence of this post-MI syndrome has decreased dramatically in the modern reperfusion era. Pericardial pain after STEMI is treated with aspirin, but colchicine, acetaminophen, or narcotic analgesics are reasonable if aspirin (even in high doses) is not effective. Glucocorticoids and nonsteroidal anti-inflammatory drugs are potentially harmful after STEMI and should be avoided.

Rhythm Disturbances

Ventricular Arrhythmias

Acute MI is associated with a proarrhythmic environment that includes heterogeneous myocardial ischemia, heightened adrenergic tone, intracellular electrolyte disturbance, lipolysis and free fatty acid production, and oxygen free radical production on reperfusion. Arrhythmias thus are common early during acute MI. Micro-re-entry is likely the most common electrophysiologic mechanism of early-phase arrhythmias, although enhanced automaticity and triggered activity also are observed in experimental models.

Primary VF, the most serious MI-related arrhythmia, contributes importantly to mortality within the first 24 hours. It occurs with an incidence of 3 to 5% during the first 4 hours and then declines rapidly during 24 to 48 hours. Polymorphic VT and, less commonly, monomorphic VT are associated life-threatening arrhythmias that can occur in this setting. Clinical features (including warning arrhythmias) are not adequately specific or sensitive to identify patients at risk for sustained ventricular tachyarrhythmias, so all patients should be continuously monitored. Prophylactic lidocaine, which reduces primary VF but does not decrease (and may increase) mortality, is not recommended. Primary VF is associated with a higher rate of in-hospital and short-term mortality, but longer-term risk of recurrent VT or VF and mortality is largely unaffected in survivors.

Accelerated idioventricular rhythm (60 to 100 beats per minute) frequently occurs within the first 12 hours and is generally benign (i.e., is not a risk factor for VF). Indeed, accelerated idioventricular rhythm frequently heralds reperfusion after fibrinolytic therapy. Antiarrhythmic therapy is not indicated except for sustained, hemodynamically compromising accelerated idioventricular rhythm.

Late VF, which is defined as VF developing more than 48 hours after the onset of acute MI, often occurs in patients with larger MIs or heart failure, portends a worse prognosis for survival, and is an indication for aggressive measures (e.g., consideration of an ICD). Monomorphic VT resulting from re-entry in the context of a recent or old MI also can appear late after MI, and patients may require long-term therapy (e.g., an ICD, see earlier).

Electrical cardioversion is required for VF and sustained polymorphic VT (unsynchronized shock) and for sustained monomorphic VT that causes hemodynamic compromise (synchronized shock) (Chapters 65 and 66). Brief intravenous sedation is given to conscious, "stable" patients. For slower, stable VT and nonsustained VT requiring therapy, intravenous amiodarone or intravenous lidocaine is commonly considered. After episodes of VT or VF, infusions of antiarrhythmic drugs may be given for 6 to 24 hours; the ongoing risk for arrhythmia then is reassessed. Electrolyte and acid-base imbalance and hypoxia should be corrected. β-Blockade is useful in patients with frequent polymorphic VT associated with adrenergic activation ("electrical storm"). Additional, aggressive measures should be considered to reduce cardiac ischemia (e.g., emergency PCI or CABG) and to address LV dysfunction (e.g., intra-aortic balloon pump) in patients with recurrent polymorphic VT despite the use of β-blockers or amiodarone, or both.

Patients with sustained VT or VF occurring late in the hospital course should be considered for long-term prevention and therapy. When indicated, an ICD provides greater survival benefit than antiarrhythmic drugs in patients with ventricular tachyarrhythmias and can improve survival after convalescence from acute MI for patients with an ejection fraction of 30% or less, regardless of their rhythm status (see earlier).

Atrial Fibrillation and Other Supraventricular Tachyarrhythmias

AF now occurs in 5 to 10% of patients with an acute MI, usually within the first 24 hours (Chapter 64). The incidence of atrial flutter or another supraventricular tachycardia is much lower. The risk for AF increases with age, larger MIs, heart failure, pericarditis, atrial infarction, hypokalemia, hypomagnesemia, hypoxia, pulmonary disease, and hyperadrenergic states. The incidence of AF is reduced by effective early reperfusion. Hemodynamic compromise with rapid rates and systemic embolism (in ~2%) are adverse consequences of AF. Systemic embolism can occur on the first day, so prompt anticoagulation with heparin is indicated.

Recommendations for management of AF include electrical cardioversion for patients with hemodynamic compromise or ischemia; rate control with intravenous digoxin for patients with ventricular dysfunction (i.e., give 1.0 mg, half initially and half in 4 hours), with an intravenous β-blocker (e.g., metoprolol, 5 mg during 2 minutes to a total of 15 mg during 10 to 15 minutes) in those without clinical ventricular dysfunction, or with intravenous diltiazem or verapamil in hemodynamically compensated patients with a contraindication to β-blockers; and anticoagulation with heparin (or LMWH). Amiodarone, which is generally reserved for patients with or at high risk for recurrence, may be started and continued for 6 weeks if sinus rhythm is restored and maintained.

Bradycardias, Conduction Delays, and Heart Block

Sinus and AV nodal dysfunction is common during acute MI. Sinus bradycardia, a result of increased parasympathetic tone often in association with inferior acute MI, occurs in 30 to 40% of patients. Sinus bradycardia is particularly common during the first hour of acute MI and with reperfusion of the right coronary artery (Bezold-Jarisch reflex). Vagally mediated AV block also can occur in this setting. Anticholinergic therapy (atropine, 0.5 to 1.5 mg IV) is indicated for *symptomatic* sinus bradycardia (heart rate generally <50 beats per minute associated with hypotension, ischemia, or escape ventricular arrhythmia), including ventricular asystole, and *symptomatic* second-degree (Wenckebach) or third-degree block at the AV nodal level (narrow QRS complex escape rhythm). Atropine is not indicated and can worsen infranodal AV block (anterior MI, wide-complex escape rhythm).

New-onset infranodal AV block and intraventricular conduction delays or bundle branch blocks predict substantially increased in-hospital mortality. Fortunately, their incidence has declined in the reperfusion era (from 10 to 20% to ~4%). Mortality is related more to extensive myocardial damage than to heart block itself, so cardiac pacing only modestly improves survival. Prophylactic placement of multifunctional patch electrodes, which allow immediate transcutaneous pacing (and defibrillation) if needed, is indicated for symptomatic sinus bradycardia refractory to drug therapy, infranodal second-degree (Mobitz II) or third-degree AV block, and new or indeterminate-age bifascicular block (LBBB; RBBB with left anterior or left posterior fascicular block) or trifascicular block (bilateral or alternating bundle branch block [any age], bundle branch block with first-degree AV block). Transcutaneous pacing is uncomfortable and is intended for prophylactic and temporary use only. Temporary pacing is indicated in the setting of STEMI for *symptomatic* bradyarrhythmias unresponsive to medical therapy. Patients who require a pacemaker to maintain an adequate heart rate or who are at very high risk (>30%) of requiring pacing (including patients with alternating, bilateral bundle branch block, with new or indeterminate-age bifascicular block with first-degree AV block, and with infranodal second-degree AV block) should have a transvenous pacing electrode inserted as soon as possible for temporary pacing.

Indications for permanent pacing after acute MI depend on the prognosis of the AV block and not solely on symptoms. Indications include even transient second- or third-degree AV block in association with bundle branch block and ongoing *symptomatic* AV block at any level. However, block at the AV nodal level (Wenckebach) rarely is persistent or symptomatic enough to warrant permanent pacing.

Heart Failure and Other Low-Output States

Cardiac pump failure is the leading cause of circulatory failure and in-hospital death from acute MI. Manifestations of circulatory failure can include a weak pulse, low blood pressure, cool extremities, a third heart sound, pulmonary congestion, oliguria, and obtundation. However, several distinct mechanisms, hemodynamic patterns, and clinical syndromes characterize the spectrum of circulatory failure in acute MI. Each requires a specific approach to diagnosis, monitoring, and therapy (see Table 73-7).

Left Ventricular Dysfunction

The degree of LV dysfunction correlates well with the extent of acute ischemia and infarction. Hemodynamic compromise becomes evident when impairment involves 20 to 25% of the left ventricle, and cardiogenic shock or death occurs with involvement of 40% or more (Chapter 107). Pulmonary congestion and S_3 and S_4 gallops are the most common physical findings. Early reperfusion (with fibrinolytic agents, PCI, or CABG) is the most effective therapy to reduce infarct size, ventricular dysfunction, and associated heart failure. Medical treatment of heart failure related to the ventricular dysfunction of acute MI is otherwise generally similar to that of heart failure in other settings (Chapter 59) and includes adequate oxygenation and diuresis (begun early, blood pressure permitting, and continued on a long-term basis if needed). Morphine sulfate (i.e., 2 to 4 mg intravenously, with increments as needed after 5 to 15 minutes or more) is useful for patients with pulmonary congestion. Nitroglycerin also reduces preload and effectively relieves congestive symptoms. Titrated oral ACE inhibitor therapy (e.g., captopril, incremented from 3.125 to 6.25 mg three times daily to 50 mg twice daily as tolerated, or lisinopril, 1.25 to 2.5 mg one or twice daily, titrated as tolerated up to 10 to 20 mg twice daily) also is indicated for heart failure and pulmonary edema unless excessive hypotension (systolic blood pressure <100 mm Hg) is present. Treatment can be begun sublingually (0.4 mg every 5 minutes three times), and then the transition can be made to intravenous therapy (initially 5 to 10 μg/minute, incrementing by 5 to 20 μg/minute until symptoms are relieved or until mean arterial pressure falls by 10% in normotensive patients or 30% in hypertensive patients but not <90 mm Hg or >30 mm Hg lower than baseline).

Intravenous vasodilator therapy to reduce preload and afterload (as blood pressure permits), inotropic support, intra-aortic balloon counterpulsation (IABP), and LV assist devices, together with urgent reperfusion, are indicated in cardiogenic shock (see later and Chapter 107).

Volume Depletion

Relative or absolute hypovolemia is a frequent cause of hypotension and circulatory failure and is easily corrected if it is recognized and treated promptly. Poor hydration, vomiting, diuresis, and disease- or drug-induced peripheral vasodilation can contribute to this condition. Hypovolemia should be identified and corrected with intravenous fluids before more aggressive therapies are considered. An empirical fluid challenge may be tried in the appropriate clinical setting (e.g., for hypotension in the absence of congestion, for inferior or RV infarction, and for hypervagotonia). If filling pressures are measured, cautious fluid administration to a pulmonary capillary wedge pressure of up to about 18 mm Hg may optimize cardiac output and blood pressure without impairing oxygenation.

Right Ventricular Infarction

RV ischemia and infarction occur with proximal occlusion of the right coronary artery (before the take-off of the RV branches). Ten percent to 15% of inferior acute STEMIs show classic hemodynamic features, and these patients form the highest-risk inferior MI subgroup for morbidity and mortality (25 to 30% vs. <6% hospital mortality). Improvement in RV function commonly occurs over time, a finding suggesting reversal of ischemic stunning and other favorable accommodations if short-term management is successful.

Hypotension in patients with clear lung fields and elevated jugular venous pressure in the setting of inferior or inferoposterior acute MI should raise the suspicion of RV infarction. Kussmaul sign (distention of the jugular vein on inspiration) is relatively specific and sensitive in this setting. ST segment elevation in lead V_1 and in right precordial lead V_4R (Chapter 54), particularly in the first 24 hours, is the most sensitive electrocardiographic marker of RV infarction. Echocardiography is helpful in confirming the diagnosis (RV dilation and dysfunction are observed). When right-sided heart pressures are measured, a right atrial pressure of 10 mm Hg or greater and 80% or more of the pulmonary capillary wedge pressure are relatively sensitive and specific for RV ischemic dysfunction.

Management of RV infarction consists of early maintenance of RV preload with intravenous fluids, reduction of RV afterload (i.e., afterload-only reducing drugs as for LV dysfunction; consider intra-aortic balloon pump), early reperfusion, short-term inotropic support if needed, and avoidance of venodilators (e.g., nitrates) and diuretics used for LV failure (they may cause marked hypotension). Volume loading with normal saline solution alone is often effective. If the cardiac output fails to improve after 0.5 to 1 L of fluid, inotropic support with intravenous dobutamine (starting at 2 μg/kg/minute and titrating to hemodynamic effect or tolerance, up to 20 μg/kg/minute) is recommended. High-grade AV block is common, and restoration of AV synchrony with temporary AV sequential pacing can lead to substantial improvement in cardiac output. Because the onset of AF (in up to one third of RV infarcts) can cause severe hemodynamic compromise, it requires prompt cardioversion. Early coronary reperfusion with fibrinolysis or PCI markedly improves outcomes.

Cardiogenic Shock

Cardiogenic shock (Chapter 107) is a form of severe LV failure characterized by marked hypotension (systolic pressures <80 mm Hg) and reductions in cardiac index (to <1.8 L/minute/m^2) despite high LV filling pressure (pulmonary capillary wedge pressure >18 mm Hg). The cause is loss of a critical functional mass (>40%) of the left ventricle. Cardiogenic shock is associated historically with mortality rates of more than 70 to 80% despite aggressive medical therapy. Risk factors include age, large (usually anterior) acute MI, previous MI, and diabetes. In patients with suspected shock, hemodynamic monitoring and IABP are indicated. Intubation often is necessary. Vasopressors are often needed.

Emergency revascularization with either PCI or CABG is recommended in STEMI patients with cardiogenic shock irrespective of the time delay from MI onset (Chapter 107). *IABP* and LV assist devices can be useful for patients with medically refractory unstable ischemic syndromes and cardiogenic shock. Primary IABP therapy for cardiogenic shock associated with acute MI provides temporary stabilization but does not reduce mortality.[A21] IABP is currently recommended in the setting of acute MI as a stabilizing measure for patients undergoing angiography and subsequent PCI or surgery for cardiogenic shock, mechanical complications (acute mitral regurgitation, acute ventricular septal defect), refractory post-MI ischemia, or recurrent intractable VT or VF associated with hemodynamic instability. In patients with acute anterior MI without shock, however, IABP plus PCI is no better than PCI alone for reducing infarct size. IABP also is not useful in patients with significant aortic insufficiency or severe peripheral vascular disease. LV assist devices may provide superior hemodynamic support, but clinical trials evidence is still limited.

Mechanical Complications

Mechanical complications usually occur within the first days to weeks and account for approximately 15% of MI-related deaths. Such complications include acute mitral valve regurgitation, ventricular septal defect, free wall rupture, and LV aneurysm. Suspicion and investigation of a mechanical defect should be prompted by a new murmur or sudden, progressive hemodynamic deterioration with pulmonary edema or a low-output state. Transthoracic or transesophageal Doppler echocardiography usually establishes the diagnosis. A balloon flotation catheter can be helpful in confirming the diagnosis. Arteriography to identify correctable coronary artery disease is usually warranted, and interim support with IABP may be useful. However, surgical consultation should be requested promptly, and urgent repair is usually indicated.

Acute mitral valve regurgitation (Chapter 75) results from infarct-related rupture or dysfunction of a papillary muscle. Total rupture leads to death in 75% of patients within 24 hours. Medical therapy is initiated with nitroprusside (beginning with 0.1 μg/kg/minute and titrating upward every 3 to 5 minutes to the desired effect, as tolerated by blood pressure response, up to 5 μg/kg/minute), to lower preload and to improve peripheral perfusion, and inotropic support (e.g., dobutamine, titrated from 2 up to 20 μg/kg/minute in normotensive patients; dopamine, titrated from 2 up to 20 μg/kg/minute in hypotensive patients; or combined dobutamine and dopamine). IABP is used to maintain hemodynamic stability. For papillary muscle rupture, emergency surgical repair (if possible) or replacement (more commonly) is then undertaken. Surgery is associated with high mortality (≥20%), but it leads to better functional and survival outcomes than medical therapy alone. For patients with ischemic (functional) mitral regurgitation but intact anatomy, key interventions include early reperfusion, diuretics, and afterload reduction. If residual mitral regurgitation is severe, however, surgery with mitral valve repair, mitral ring annuloplasty, or often mitral valve replacement may be needed.

Post-infarction septal rupture with *ventricular septal defect*, which occurs with increased frequency in elderly patients, in patients with hypertension, and possibly after fibrinolysis, also warrants urgent surgical repair. Because a small post-MI ventricular septal defect can suddenly enlarge and cause rapid hemodynamic collapse, all septal perforations should be repaired. On diagnosis, invasive monitoring is recommended, together with vasodilators (e.g., nitroprusside, initially 0.1 μg/kg/minute, titrated upward every 3 to 5 minutes to desired effect, as tolerated by blood pressure response, up to 5 μg/kg/minute) and, if needed, judicious use of inotropic agents (e.g., dobutamine, titrated from 2 up to 20 μg/kg/minute in normotensive patients; dopamine, titrated from 2 up to 20 μg/kg/minute in hypotensive patients; or combined dobutamine and dopamine). An intra-aortic balloon pump should be inserted, a surgical consultation promptly obtained, and the surgical repair undertaken as soon as feasible. Percutaneous closure is an appealing,[8] less invasive option for initial emergent treatment, but experience is limited and residual shunts are common.

LV free wall rupture usually causes acute cardiac tamponade with sudden death. In a small percentage of cases, however, resealing or localized containment ("pseudoaneurysm") can allow medical stabilization, usually with inotropic support or IABP, followed by emergency surgical repair.

An *LV aneurysm* can develop after a large, most commonly anterior, acute MI. If refractory heart failure, VT, or systemic embolization occurs despite medical therapy and PCI, aneurysmectomy with CABG is indicated.

Thromboembolic Complications

The risk of thromboembolism has declined markedly with contemporary therapy for STEMI. Systemic arterial emboli (including cerebrovascular emboli) typically arise from an LV mural thrombus, whereas pulmonary emboli commonly arise from thrombi in leg veins. Arterial embolism can cause dramatic clinical events, such as hemiparesis, loss of a pulse, ischemic bowel, or sudden hypertension, depending on the regional circulation involved.

Mural thrombosis with embolism typically occurs in the setting of a large (especially anterior) acute STEMI and heart failure. The risk for embolism is particularly high when a mural thrombus is detected by echocardiography. Thus, in patients with anterior acute STEMI and in other high-risk patients, echocardiography should be performed during hospitalization; if results are positive, anticoagulation should be started (with an anticoagulant), if not already initiated, and continued (with warfarin) for 6 months.

Deep venous thrombosis can be prevented by lower extremity compression therapy, by limiting the duration of bedrest, and by the use of subcutaneous unfractionated heparin or LMWH (in patients at risk not receiving intravenous heparin) until patients are fully ambulatory (Chapter 81). Patients with pulmonary embolism are treated with intravenous heparin and then oral anticoagulation for 6 months (Chapter 98).

Adding an anticoagulant (e.g., warfarin) to aspirin and a $P2Y_{12}$ receptor inhibitor for the prevention of venous thromboembolic disease (Chapters 176 and 98) or the prevention of systemic embolization in patients with AF (Chapter 64) should be restricted to situations in which the benefit of preventing a thromboembolic event exceeds that of the increased risk of bleeding. Anticoagulant therapy is indicated in STEMI patients with AF and a high risk of systemic emboli, mechanical heart valves, recent venous thromboembolism, or a hypercoagulable disorder.[1] The duration of triple antithrombotic therapy should be limited to the shortest time possible to minimize the risk of bleeding. Anticoagulant therapy also is reasonable for patients with STEMI and an asymptomatic LV mural thrombus and might be considered for at-risk patients with anterior akinesis or dyskinesis, with the duration of anticoagulation being limited to 3 months. In the absence of data on the new anti–factor Xa agents, warfarin, usually to an international normalized ratio of 2.0 to 2.5, is recommended. To minimize bleeding in at-risk patients, the physician must pay careful attention to the appropriate selection of antithrombotic regimens and to their doses based on age, weight, renal function, and other comorbidities.

Risk Stratification after Myocardial Infarction

Risk stratification is a continuous process that begins on admission and continues through hospital discharge. The goals of risk stratification before and early after discharge for acute MI are to assess ventricular and clinical function, latent ischemia, and arrhythmic risk; to use this information for patient education and prognostic assessment; and to guide therapeutic strategies. Formal risk stratification tools (e.g., Thrombolysis in Myocardial Infarction, Global Registry of Acute Coronary Events) have been developed and validated for acute coronary syndrome patients for use on admission and at discharge (E-Fig. 73-1).

Cardiac Catheterization and Noninvasive Stress Testing

Risk stratification generally involves functional assessment by one of three strategies: cardiac catheterization, submaximal exercise stress electrocardiography before discharge (at 4 to 6 days), or symptom-limited stress testing at 2 to 6 weeks after discharge. Many or most patients with acute STEMI undergo invasive evaluation for primary PCI or after fibrinolytic therapy. Catheterization generally is performed during hospitalization for patients at high risk. In others, predischarge submaximal exercise testing (to peak heart rate of 120 to 130 beats per minute or 70% of the predicted maximum) appears safe when it is performed in patients who are ambulating without symptoms; it should be avoided within 2 to 3 days of acute MI and in patients with unstable post-MI angina, uncompensated heart failure, or serious cardiac arrhythmias. Alternatively or in addition, patients may undergo symptom-limited stress testing at 2 to 6 weeks before they return to work or resume other increased physical activities. Abnormal test results include not only ST segment depression but also low functional capacity, exertional hypotension, and serious arrhythmias. Patients with positive test results should be considered for coronary angiography.

The sensitivity of stress testing can be augmented with radionuclide perfusion imaging (Chapter 56) or echocardiography (Chapter 55). Supplemental imaging also can quantify the LV ejection fraction and size the area of infarction or ischemia (e.g., by cardiac magnetic resonance imaging; Chapter 56). For patients with ST segment or QRS changes that preclude accurate interpretation of the ECG, an imaging study is recommended with initial stress testing. In others, an imaging study may be performed selectively for those in whom the exercise electrocardiography test result is positive or equivocal. For patients unable to exercise, pharmacologic stress testing can be performed with adenosine, a long-acting bolus analogue of adenosine (e.g., regadenoson), or dipyridamole scintigraphy or by dobutamine echocardiography.

To assess LV function, ejection fraction should be measured in all patients with STEMI before discharge. Patients who initially have a reduced LV ejection fraction and who are possible candidates for ICD therapy should have the LV ejection fraction reevaluated 40 days or more after discharge.

Electrocardiographic Monitoring

Modern telemetry systems capture complete rhythm information during hospital observations and allow identification of patients with serious arrhythmias, so routine 24- to 48-hour ambulatory electrocardiographic (Holter) monitoring before or after hospital discharge is not recommended. Patients with sustained VT or VF occurring late during hospitalization or provoked during electrophysiologic study with nonsustained VT on monitoring are candidates for an ICD, especially if the ejection fraction is less than 40% (Fig. 73-5) (Chapters 65 and 66). Prophylactic ICD placement at least 1 month after acute MI prevents sudden death for patients with severely depressed function (ejection fraction ≤ 0.30) regardless of the rhythm status.

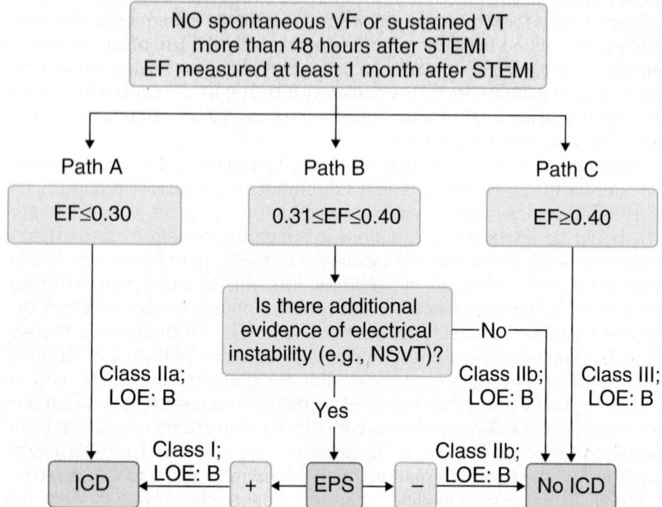

FIGURE 73-5. Algorithm to aid in selection of implantable cardioverter-defibrillator (ICD) in patients with ST segment elevation myocardial infarction (STEMI) and diminished ejection fraction (EF). The appropriate management path is selected on the basis of left ventricular EF measured at least 1 month after STEMI. All patients, whether an ICD is implanted or not, should receive medical therapy. EPS = electrophysiologic studies; LOE = level of evidence; NSVT = nonsustained ventricular tachycardia; VF = ventricular fibrillation; VT = ventricular tachycardia. (Modified from Antman EM, Anbe DT, Armstrong PW, et al. 2004 Update: ACC/AHA guidelines for the management of patients with ST-elevation myocardial infarction—executive summary. A Report of the American College of Cardiology/American Heart Association Task Force on Practice Guidelines [Writing Committee to Revise the 1999 Guidelines for the Management of Patients with Acute Myocardial Infarction]. ***Circulation.*** **2004;110:588-636.)**

Post-Hospital Care: Secondary Prevention, Patient Education, and Rehabilitation

Before discharge, a detailed, evidence-based plan of care should emphasize the importance of a healthy lifestyle, including diet, exercise, smoking cessation, and compliance with medications. Timely outpatient health care follow-up should be scheduled and a rehabilitation program referral provided.

Secondary Prevention

Advances in secondary prevention have resulted in increasingly effective measures to reduce recurrent MI and cardiovascular death. Secondary prevention should be conscientiously applied after acute MI (Table 73-9).

A fasting *lipid profile* is recommended within 24 hours of admission, and high-intensity *lipid-lowering therapy* with a statin should start in the hospital, preferably on admission, and be continued as outpatient therapy in all patients with STEMI and no contraindication to its use (e.g., atorvastatin, 80 mg daily; Chapter 206).

Continued smoking doubles the subsequent mortality risk after acute MI, and *smoking cessation* reduces the risk for reinfarction and death within 1 year (Chapter 32). An individualized smoking cessation plan should be formulated, including pharmacologic aids (nicotine gum and patches, bupropion, or varenicline).

Antiplatelet therapy (Chapter 38; Fig. 73-6) should consist of aspirin, given on a long-term basis to all patients without contraindications (recommended maintenance dose, 81 mg/day). Clopidogrel (75 mg/day) or prasugrel (10 mg/day) or ticagrelor (90 mg twice daily) is given to patients who received PCI with stenting, and clopidogrel is also appropriate for other patients at higher risk for recurrent vascular events. Therapy should continue for 1 year after stent placement, although a shorter duration may be considered for patients experiencing or at high risk of major bleeding, especially if they have a bare metal stent or a second-generation drug-eluting stent.

Anticoagulant therapy (i.e., warfarin, with an international normalized ratio goal of 2.0 to 3.0) is indicated after acute MI for patients unable to take antiplatelet therapy, for patients with persistent or paroxysmal AF, for patients with LV thrombus, and for patients who have suffered a systemic or pulmonary embolism. Anticoagulants also may be considered for patients with extensive wall motion abnormalities and markedly depressed ejection fraction with or without heart failure. Data on the benefits and risks of warfarin added to antiplatelet therapy (Fig. 73-6) are sparse.

ACE inhibitor therapy can prevent adverse myocardial remodeling after acute MI and can reduce heart failure and death; it is clearly indicated for long-term use in patients with anterior acute MI or an LV ejection fraction of less

TABLE 73-9 DISCHARGE MEDICATION CHECKLIST AFTER MYOCARDIAL INFARCTION*

MEDICATION	DOSES	REASONS NOT TO USE	COMMENTS
Aspirin	Initial: 162-325 mg Maintenance: 75-162 mg daily	High bleeding risk	Reduces mortality, reinfarction, and stroke
Clopidogrel *or*	Initial dose: 300-600 mg (75-150 mg after fibrinolysis in patients >75 years) Maintenance: 75 mg daily	High bleeding risk; suboptimal antiplatelet response	Indicated after PCI for at least 1 year (shorter time for BMS if high bleeding risk); also reduces vascular events when added to aspirin in non–ST segment elevation acute MI (also useful on the basis of clinical trials after ST segment elevation acute MI) Genetic variants (CYP2C19) may reduce response Controversial interaction with proton pump inhibitors (e.g., omeprazole)
Prasugrel *or*	Initial dose: 60 mg Maintenance: 10 mg daily	High bleeding risk	Avoid with history of prior stroke or TIA
Ticagrelor	Initial dose: 180 mg Maintenance: 90 mg bid		Consider 5 mg daily in patients >75 years or <60 kg Avoid if history of intracranial bleed Limit daily aspirin dose to 81 mg
β-Blocker (e.g., metoprolol, carvedilol)	Metoprolol: 25-200 mg daily Carvedilol: 6.25-25 mg bid	Asthma, bradycardia, heart failure	Reduces mortality, reinfarction, sudden death, arrhythmia, hypertension, angina, atherosclerosis progression
ACE inhibitor (e.g., ramipril, lisinopril) or ARB (e.g., valsartan, losartan)	Ramipril: 2.5-10 mg daily Lisinopril: 5-10 mg daily Valsartan: 80-160 mg daily-bid Losartan: 50-100 mg daily	Hypotension, allergy, hyperkalemia	Reduces mortality, reinfarction, stroke, heart failure, diabetes, atherosclerosis progression
Lipid-lowering agent (i.e., a high-intensity statin; e.g., atorvastatin, rosuvastatin)	Atorvastatin: 80 mg daily Rosuvastatin: 20-40 mg daily	Myopathy, rhabdomyolysis, hepatitis	Goal = LDL ≥50% reduction (statins also can benefit patients with lower LDL†)
Nitroglycerin sublingual	0.4 mg SL PRN for angina	Aortic stenosis; sildenafil (Viagra) use	Instruct on PRN use and appropriate need for medical attention

*Medications given at hospital discharge improve long-term compliance.
†Heart Protection Study (*Lancet.* 2002;360:7); and PROVE-IT study (*N Engl J Med.* 2004;350:1495).
ACE = angiotensin-converting enzyme; ARB = angiotensin receptor blocker; BMS = bare metal stent; LDL = low-density lipoprotein; MI = myocardial infarction; PCI = percutaneous coronary intervention; PRN = as needed; daily = once daily; SL = sublingual; TIA = transient ischemic attack.
Modified from Kushner FG, Hand M, Antman EM, et al. 2009 Focused updates: ACC/AHA guidelines for the management of patients with ST-elevation myocardial infarction and the ACC/AHA/SCAI guidelines on percutaneous coronary intervention. *Circulation.* 2009;120:2271-2306.

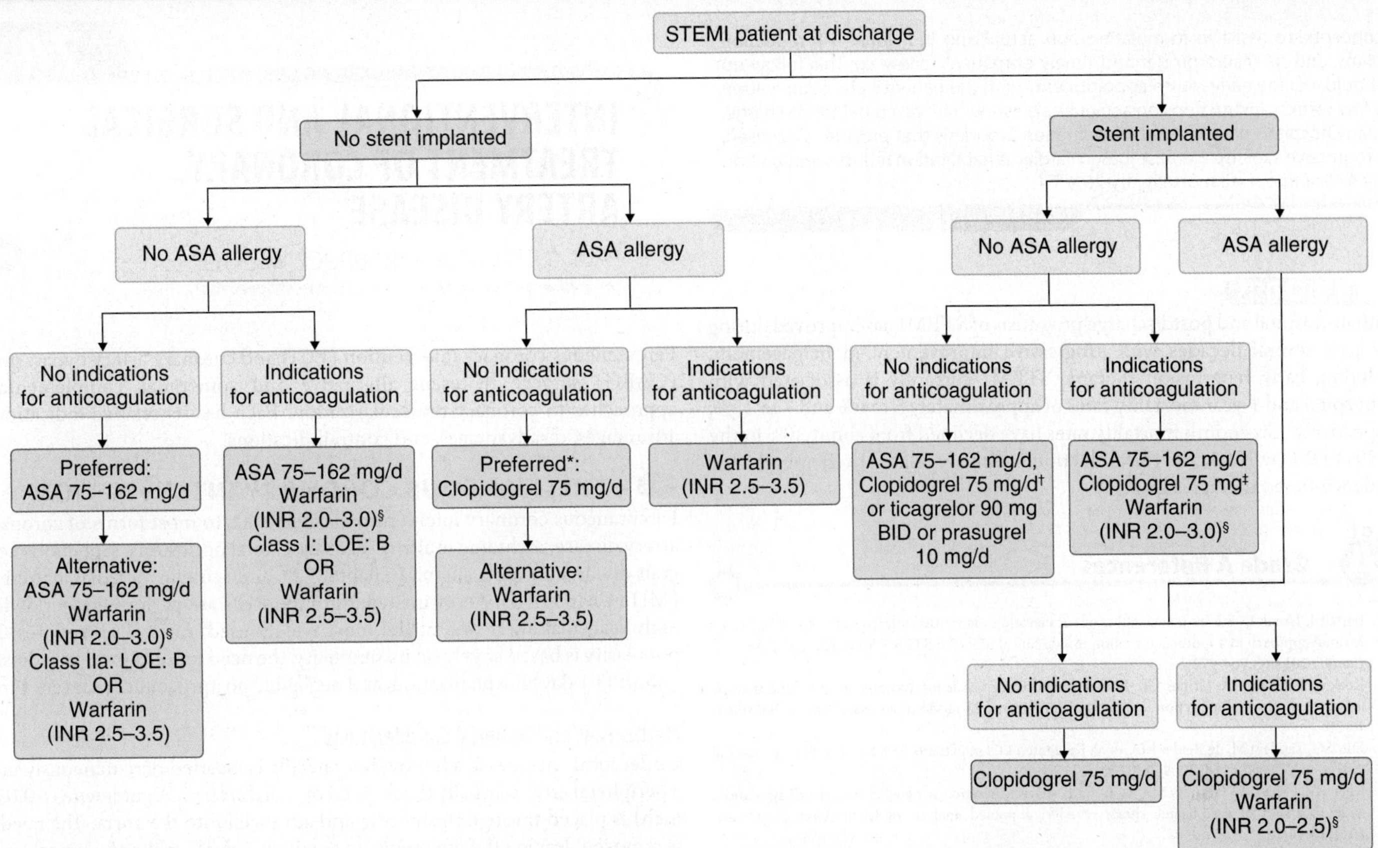

FIGURE 73-6. Long-term antithrombotic therapy at hospital discharge after ST segment elevation myocardial infarction (STEMI). *Clopidogrel is preferred to warfarin because of increased risk of bleeding and low patient compliance in warfarin trials. †For 12 months. ‡Discontinue clopidogrel 1 month after implantation of a bare metal stent or several months after implantation of a drug-eluting stent (3 months after sirolimus and 6 months after paclitaxel) because of the potentially increased risk of bleeding with warfarin and two antiplatelet agents. Continue aspirin (ASA) and warfarin on a long-term basis if warfarin is indicated for other reasons, such as atrial fibrillation, left ventricular thrombus, cerebral emboli, or extensive regional wall motion abnormality. §An international normalized ratio (INR) of 2.0 to 3.0 is acceptable with tight control, but the lower end of this range is preferable. The combination of antiplatelet therapy and warfarin may be considered in patients younger than 75 years who have a low bleeding risk and who can be monitored reliably. LOE = level of evidence. (Modified from Antman EM, Anbe DT, Armstrong PW, et al. ACC/AHA guidelines for the management of patients with ST-elevation myocardial infarction—executive summary. A report of the American College of Cardiology/American Heart Association Task Force on Practice Guidelines [Writing Committee to Revise the 1999 Guidelines for the Management of Patients with Acute Myocardial Infarction]. *Circulation.* 2004;110:588-636.)

than 40%. ACE inhibitors also reduce recurrent MI in higher-risk patients with an ejection fraction greater than 40%. In contrast, ACE inhibition, when added to other contemporary therapies, provides little additional benefit in reducing cardiovascular events in patients who have stable coronary disease and a low risk (<5%/year) for a coronary event. These data suggest a rationale for the long-term use of ACE inhibitors (e.g., ramipril, 2.5 mg titrated to 10 mg/day, or lisinopril, 2.5 to 5 mg titrated to 10 mg/day) in most patients after MI, except perhaps those at lowest risk (i.e., without heart failure, hypertension, glucose intolerance, or reduced ejection fraction).A22 An ARB (e.g., valsartan, 80 to 160 mg twice daily, or losartan, 50 to 100 mg/day) should be substituted in patients who cannot tolerate an ACE inhibitor; in patients with advanced heart failure, both an ACE inhibitor and an ARB may be complementary (Chapter 59).A17 An aldosterone receptor blocker (e.g., eplerenone, 25 mg/day orally, increased to 50 mg/day after 4 weeks if tolerated, with monitoring of serum potassium levels) also should be added to the ACE inhibitor or ARB (but not both) regimen on a long-term basis in patients with depressed ejection fraction (≤0.40) and clinical heart failure or diabetes, unless this approach is contraindicated.A18

Long-term β-blocker therapy is strongly recommended for all MI survivors without uncompensated heart failure or other contraindications. Options include metoprolol, 20 to 200 mg/day, and carvedilol, 6.25 to 25 mg twice daily. Long-term therapy in patients at low risk (normal ventricular function, successful reperfusion, absence of arrhythmias) is reasonable but not mandatory.

Nitroglycerin (0.4 mg) is prescribed routinely for sublingual or buccal administration for acute anginal attacks. Longer-acting oral therapy (isosorbide mononitrate, 30 to 60 mg orally every morning, or dinitrate, 10 to 40 mg orally two or three times daily) or topical nitroglycerin (e.g., start with 0.5 inch; can be titrated up to 2 inches, every 6 hours for 2 days) may be added to treatment regimens for angina or heart failure in selected patients.

Calcium-channel blockers are negatively inotropic and are *not* routinely given on a long-term basis. However, they may be given to selected patients without LV dysfunction (ejection fraction >0.40) who are intolerant of β-blockers and who require these drugs for antianginal therapy (e.g., amlodipine, 5 to 10 mg/day orally, or diltiazem, 120 to 480 mg/day orally, as sustained release or in divided doses) or for control of heart rate in AF (e.g., diltiazem, 120 to 480 mg/day orally, or verapamil, 180 to 480 mg/day orally, as sustained release or in divided doses). Short-acting nifedipine should be avoided.

Hormone therapy with estrogen with or without progestin is not begun after an acute MI because it increases thromboembolic risk and does not prevent reinfarction. For women already receiving hormone replacement, therapy should be discontinued unless it is being given for a compelling indication.

Hypertension (Chapter 67) and diabetes mellitus (Chapter 229) must be assessed and tightly controlled in patients after acute MI. ACE inhibitors or β-blockers as described earlier are usually the first-choice therapies for hypertension, with ARBs indicated when ACE inhibitors are not tolerated. ACE inhibitors and ARBs also can reduce the long-term complications of diabetes.

Antioxidant supplementation (e.g., vitamin E, vitamin C) does not benefit patients after acute MI and is *not* recommended. Folate therapy reduces homocyst(e)ine levels but does not reduce clinical events. Routine fish oil supplements also are not supported by accumulating evidence.

Antiarrhythmic drugs are *not* generally recommended after acute MI, and class I antiarrhythmic agents can increase the risk for sudden death. Class III drugs (amiodarone, sotalol, dofetilide) may be used as part of the management strategy for specific arrhythmias (e.g., AF, VT) (Chapters 64 and 65).

Patient Education and Rehabilitation

The hospital stay provides an important opportunity to educate patients about their MI and its treatment, coronary risk factors, and behavioral modification. Education should begin on admission and should continue after discharge. However, the time before hospital discharge is particularly opportune. Many hospitals use case managers and prevention specialists to augment physicians and nurses, to provide educational materials, to review important concepts, to assist in formulating and actualizing individual risk reduction plans, and to ensure proper and timely outpatient follow-up. This follow-up should include early return appointments with the patient's physician (within a few weeks). Instructions on activities also should be given before discharge. Many hospitals have cardiac rehabilitation programs that provide supervised, progressive exercise. Exercise-based cardiac rehabilitation reduces reinfarction by 47% and overall mortality by 26%.[A23]

PROGNOSIS

Both in-hospital and postdischarge prognosis of STEMI has improved during the past several decades with progressive improvement in management, including early reperfusion therapy. STEMI currently is associated with in-hospital and 1-year mortality rates of approximately 5 to 6% and 7 to 18%, respectively.[1] Six-month mortality rates have declined from about 30% in the 1970s to 9% by 2005, and this reduction is directly related to the number of evidence-based therapies given.

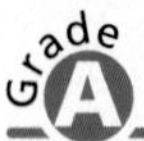

Grade A References

A1. Bernat I, Horak D, Stasek J, et al. ST-segment elevation myocardial infarction treated by radial or femoral approach in a multicenter randomized clinical trial: the STEMI-RADIAL trial. *J Am Coll Cardiol.* 2014;63:964-972.

A2. Keeley EC, Boura JA, Grines CL. Primary angioplasty versus intravenous thrombolytic therapy for acute myocardial infarction: a quantitative review of 23 randomised trials. *Lancet.* 2003;361:13-20.

A3. Ellis SG, Tendera M, de Belder MA, et al. Facilitated PCI in patients with ST-elevation myocardial infarction. *N Engl J Med.* 2008;358:2205-2217.

A4. Jeger RV, Urban P, Harkness SM, et al. Early revascularization is beneficial across all ages and a wide spectrum of cardiogenic shock severity: a pooled analysis of trials. *Acute Card Care.* 2011;13:14-20.

A5. Hochman JS, Reynolds HR, Dzavik V, et al. Long-term effects of percutaneous coronary intervention of the totally occluded infarct-related artery in the subacute phase after myocardial infarction. *Circulation.* 2011;124:2320-2328.

A6. Wald DS, Morris JK, Wald NJ, et al. Randomized trial of preventive angioplasty in myocardial infarction. *N Engl J Med.* 2013;369:1115-1123.

A7. Wijeysundera HC, Vijayaraghavan R, Nallamothu BK, et al. Rescue angioplasty or repeat fibrinolysis after failed fibrinolytic therapy for ST-segment myocardial infarction: a meta-analysis of randomized trials. *J Am Coll Cardiol.* 2007;49:422-430.

A8. Cantor WJ, Fitchett D, Borgundvaag B, et al. Routine early angioplasty after fibrinolysis for acute myocardial infarction. *N Engl J Med.* 2009;360:2705-2718.

A9. Aversano T, Lemmon CC, Liu L. Outcomes of PCI at hospitals with or without on-site cardiac surgery. *N Engl J Med.* 2012;366:1792-1802.

A10. Sabatine MS, Cannon CP, Gibson CM, et al. Addition of clopidogrel to aspirin and fibrinolytic therapy for myocardial infarction with ST-segment elevation. *N Engl J Med.* 2005;352:1179-1189.

A11. Chen ZM, Jiang LX, Chen YP, et al. Addition of clopidogrel to aspirin in 45,852 patients with acute myocardial infarction: randomised placebo-controlled trial. *Lancet.* 2005;366:1607-1621.

A12. Wiviott SD, Braunwald E, McCabe CH, et al. Prasugrel versus clopidogrel in patients with acute coronary syndromes. *N Engl J Med.* 2007;357:2001-2015.

A13. Wallentin L, Becker RC, Budaj A, et al. Ticagrelor versus clopidogrel in patients with acute coronary syndromes. *N Engl J Med.* 2009;361:1045-1057.

A14. Antman EM, Morrow DA, McCabe CH, et al. Enoxaparin versus unfractionated heparin with fibrinolysis for ST-elevation myocardial infarction. *N Engl J Med.* 2006;354:1477-1488.

A15. Mehran R, Lansky AJ, Witzenbichler B, et al. Bivalirudin in patients undergoing primary angioplasty for acute myocardial infarction (HORIZONS-AMI): 1-year results of a randomised controlled trial. *Lancet.* 2009;374:1149-1159.

A16. Pizarro G, Fernandez-Friera L, Fuster V, et al. Long-term benefit of early pre-reperfusion metoprolol administration in patients with acute myocardial infarction: results from the METOCARD-CNIC trial (Effect of Metoprolol in Cardioprotection During an Acute Myocardial Infarction). *J Am Coll Cardiol.* 2014;63:2356-2362.

A17. Pfeffer MA, McMurray JJ, Velazquez EJ, et al. Valsartan, captopril, or both in myocardial infarction complicated by heart failure, left ventricular dysfunction, or both. *N Engl J Med.* 2003;349:1893-1906.

A18. Pitt B, Remme W, Zannad F, et al. Eplerenone, a selective aldosterone blocker, in patients with left ventricular dysfunction after myocardial infarction. *N Engl J Med.* 2003;348:1309-1321.

A19. Steinbeck G, Andresen D, Seidl K, et al. Defibrillator implantation early after myocardial infarction. *N Engl J Med.* 2009;361:1427-1436.

A20. Cannon CP, Steinberg BA, Murphy SA, et al. Meta-analysis of cardiovascular outcomes trials comparing intensive versus moderate statin therapy. *J Am Coll Cardiol.* 2006;48:438-445.

A21. Thiele H, Zeymer U, Neumann FJ, et al. Intraaortic balloon support for myocardial infarction with cardiogenic shock. *N Engl J Med.* 2012;367:1287-1296.

A22. Braunwald E, Domanski MJ, Fowler SE, et al. Angiotensin-converting-enzyme inhibition in stable coronary artery disease. *N Engl J Med.* 2004;351:2058-2068.

A23. Lawler PR, Filion KB, Eisenberg MJ. Efficacy of exercise-based cardiac rehabilitation post-myocardial infarction: a systematic review and meta-analysis of randomized controlled trials. *Am Heart J.* 2011;162:571-584.e2.

GENERAL REFERENCES

For the General References and other additional features, please visit Expert Consult at https://expertconsult.inkling.com.

74

INTERVENTIONAL AND SURGICAL TREATMENT OF CORONARY ARTERY DISEASE

PAUL S. TEIRSTEIN AND BRUCE W. LYTLE

Percutaneous coronary intervention (PCI) and coronary artery bypass graft (CABG) surgery represent alternative and sometimes complementary approaches to coronary revascularization. Each has its relative indications, advantages, disadvantages, and contraindications.

PERCUTANEOUS CORONARY INTERVENTION

Percutaneous coronary intervention is applicable to most forms of coronary artery disease, including multivessel disease, total occlusions, saphenous vein graft disease, unstable angina (Chapter 72), and acute myocardial infarction (MI) (Chapter 73). An estimated 2 million PCIs are performed worldwide each year, making it one of the most widely used medical procedures. Its popularity is based largely on its simplicity, the need for only local anesthesia, a short (≈1 day) hospitalization, and negligible postprocedure recovery time.

Mechanisms and Technical Considerations

Under local anesthesia, a hollow-bore needle is inserted percutaneously into a peripheral artery (usually the femoral or radial artery). A guidewire (≈0.038 inch) is placed through this needle and advanced into the aorta. The needle is removed, leaving the guidewire, over which a small-caliber (≈3 mm), specially shaped catheter (called a guiding catheter) is advanced under fluoroscope guidance into the ostium of the obstructed coronary artery. By use of radiographic contrast injections that provide fluoroscopic visualization of the coronary artery lumen, a thin (≈0.014 inch), highly steerable guidewire is directed down the coronary artery and across the stenotic lesion. This guidewire becomes a "rail" over which therapeutic tools such as inflatable balloons, stents, and atherectomy catheters are passed to the diseased segment (Fig. 74-1).

Balloon catheters (Fig. 74-2) typically have two lumens, one to allow passage over the guidewire and another to carry a mixture of saline and radiographic contrast material to inflate a balloon at the distal catheter tip. Under fluoroscopy, the balloon is centered across the lesion and inflated to 3 to 20 atmospheres of pressure. Balloon inflation widens the narrowed lumen by stretching the vessel and, in most cases, causing a tear (a therapeutic dissection) at the edges of the plaque, where the atheroma meets the nondiseased media. Atherectomy catheters, which also are passed over a guidewire to the

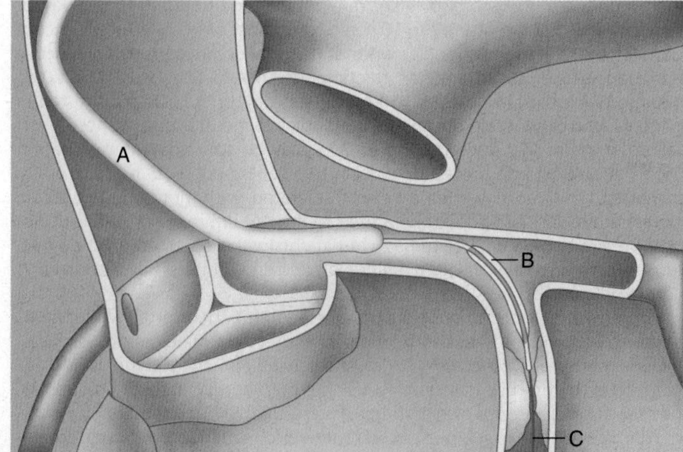

FIGURE 74-1. **Schematic view of coronary angioplasty technique. A guide catheter (A) is inserted into the orifice of the coronary artery (in this figure, the left main artery), and a balloon catheter (B) is advanced over a thin guidewire (C) into the lesion. Balloon inflation dilates the stenotic region. (Modified from Baim DS. Percutaneous balloon angioplasty and general coronary intervention. In: Baim DS, ed. *Grossman's Cardiac Catheterization, Angiography, and Intervention.* 7th ed. Philadelphia: Lippincott Williams & Wilkins; 2005.)**

diseased segment, remove plaque by a shaving, grinding, slicing, or suction mechanism. Coronary stents are metallic or polymeric scaffolding devices that are crimped onto a deflated balloon catheter before insertion into the diseased vessel (Videos 74-1 to 74-3). During balloon inflation, the collapsed stent expands to support the vessel lumen (Fig. 74-3 and Video 74-4). While balloons and atherectomy devices create an adequate, albeit rough channel through diseased arteries, the supporting structure of the stent can widen the lumen to near its predisease dimensions. With a stent, tissue flaps are "pinned" against the wall, and recoil is limited (Video 74-5). Most stents are designed so that the metallic struts comprise only about 20% of the surface area to allow endothelialization to reduce the risk of thrombosis. Drug-eluting stents release local medications that further reduce the risk of restenosis.[1]

Filters deployed within a coronary vessel beyond the target lesion to limit distal embolization of plaque, platelet aggregates, and other "debris" can further reduce ischemic complications in selected, high-risk patients. Stents composed of polymers or metals that provide a temporary scaffolding and then biodegrade (usually over several years) are currently undergoing intense clinical study.

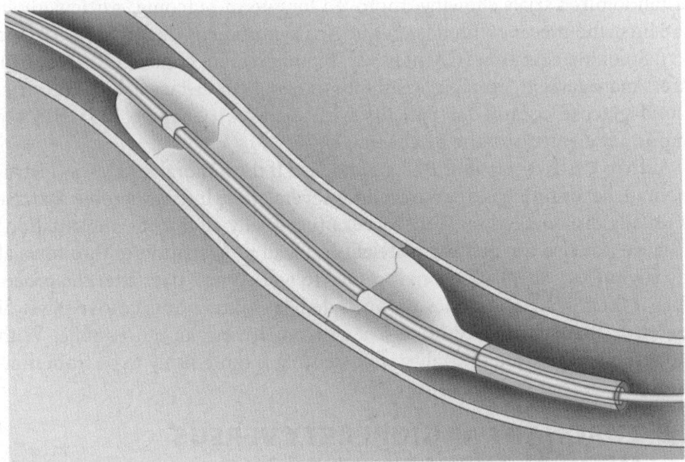

FIGURE 74-2. Balloon angioplasty catheter. The catheter consists of two lumens, an inflation lumen and a guidewire lumen. Two radiopaque markers, indicating the lateral balloon margins, aid in positioning of the balloon before inflation.

During the PCI procedure, the interventional cardiologist is able to assess the target vessel fluoroscopically by injections of contrast material through the guiding catheter (Fig. 74-4). When the coronary artery has been opened successfully, all catheters are withdrawn, and the arterial access site is sealed by mechanical pressure, an absorbable plug, or a remote suturing device. Patients without comorbidity ambulate in 3 to 6 hours. Discharge from the hospital usually occurs on the morning after the procedure after stability of the arterial access site, cardiac biomarkers, and electrocardiogram is confirmed. Increasingly, selected patients are treated as outpatients and released 6 to 12 hours after the procedure without an overnight stay.

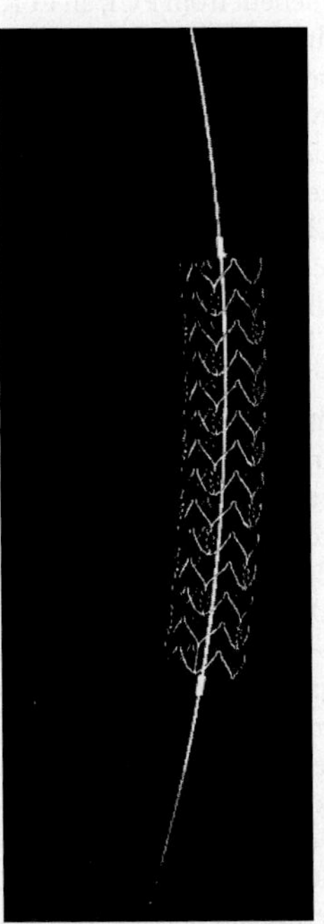

FIGURE 74-3. Balloon-expandable coronary stent. The stainless steel stent is crimped onto a balloon catheter to allow low-profile passage through the coronary artery. When it is positioned across the lesion, the balloon is inflated, expanding the stent. After balloon deflation and removal, the stent remains, providing a scaffold that supports the vessel lumen.

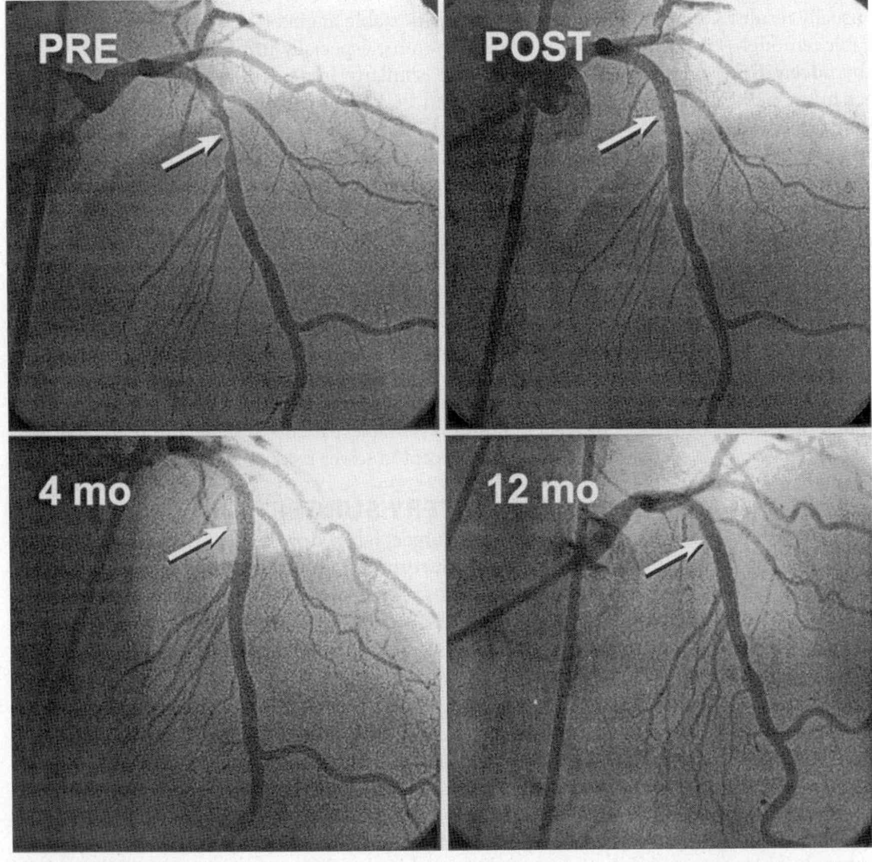

FIGURE 74-4. Angiographic images before, after, and at late follow-up after placement of a sirolimus-eluting stent. The left anterior descending artery contains a tight stenosis *(arrow, upper left panel)*. After stent implantation *(upper right panel)*, the stenosis is abolished *(arrow)*. Follow-up at 4 and 12 months *(bottom panels)* reveals a completely open lumen with no evidence of restenosis *(arrows)*.

Selection of Patients for Percutaneous Coronary Intervention

Any decision to perform PCI must include a review of the coronary angiogram (Chapter 57) by an experienced interventional cardiologist to assess the lesion's technical suitability for the procedure. The disease must narrow the coronary artery lumen by at least 60%, and the quantity of myocardium subtended by the vessel should not be trivial. The pressure drop across a stenosis, called the *fractional flow reserve* (FFR), during maximum hyperemia (usually induced by intravenous adenosine) reflects its hemodynamic severity. Whereas a pressure drop of more than 20% (which corresponds to a FFR <0.80) predicts a clinical benefit from PCI, an FFR greater than 0.80 has been correlated with clinical harm.[A1,A2] High-risk lesion characteristics, such as longer lesion length, vessel tortuosity, lesion calcification, or the presence of thrombus, must be taken into consideration. Subtle angiographic findings, such as the presence of collateral vessels that supply a different myocardial territory and that originate distal to the target, should be appreciated. For each patient, the benefits of PCI must be weighed against the procedural risk. Characteristics of the patient conveying increased risk include advanced age (i.e., >75 years), diabetes, smaller vessels that are often found in women, prior MI, significant impairment of left ventricular function, and renal insufficiency.

Procedural Success and Complications

With use of modern techniques in appropriately selected patients, most PCI procedures have a greater than 95% success rate. The single exception is a chronic total coronary occlusion (100% obstruction of the lumen), in which the interventional cardiologist's ability to negotiate a guidewire through the blockage is only about 50% to 90% and varies substantially with the operator's expertise. With the increased use of coronary stents and adjunctive antiplatelet agents (thienopyridines and platelet glycoprotein IIb/IIIa inhibitors), abrupt coronary artery closure is rarely encountered. When PCI is performed by an experienced interventional cardiologist in appropriately selected patients, the risk of in-hospital death is less than 1%; MI (usually small, non–ST segment elevation MI) is approximately 5%, the need for urgent or emergent CABG surgery is less than 1%, the risk of stroke is less than 0.1%, the chance of coronary perforation is less than 1%, and morbidity at the arterial access site (i.e., hematoma, pseudoaneurysm, or arteriovenous fistula) occurs in fewer than 5% of patients. As a result of these low complication rates, PCI without the availability of onsite surgery is not associated with higher mortality or rate of emergency CABG surgery.[A3,A4]

Restenosis and Thrombosis

Restenosis is a renarrowing of an artery after a PCI procedure, usually resulting from one of two mechanisms. The first mechanism, unfavorable remodeling and elastic recoil, is a mechanical renarrowing caused by adventitial constriction and shrinkage of the vessel lumen. The second mechanism, neointimal hyperplasia, is caused by the proliferation of smooth muscle cells and matrix in response to the injury caused by balloons, stents, or atherectomy devices. Restenosis occurs in 10% to 50% of PCI patients after balloon angioplasty without stenting, usually within the first 6 months after the procedure. Characteristics associated with higher risk of restenosis include longer lesions, small-diameter vessels, diabetes, and multivessel disease. Treatment with either balloon angioplasty or atherectomy devices results in similar rates of restenosis. Coronary stents, which provide a semirigid scaffolding within the lumen and reduce restenosis by eliminating the mechanical renarrowing caused by unfavorable remodeling and elastic recoil, reduce restenosis by about one third compared with balloon angioplasty alone.[1]

Although bare metal stents eliminate the mechanical component of restenosis, the proliferative component is enhanced. Smooth muscle cell division and matrix formation can migrate through the stent struts to renarrow the vessel lumen. Drug-eluting stents, which contain and release antiproliferative drugs (e.g., sirolimus, everolimus, zotarolimus, and paclitaxel) reduce the need for early repeat PCI to less than 5%.[A5,A6] However, drug-eluting stents may carry a slightly higher risk of thrombosis later (>1 year), especially if patients cannot or do not continue aspirin plus a thienopyridine.

Choices Related to Stenting

Based on long-term follow-up data, the choice between a bare metal stent and a drug-eluting stent remains controversial. Patients receiving drug-eluting stents must continue dual antiplatelet therapy with aspirin and a thienopyridine for a minimum of 12 months. If a patient is unlikely to be able to adhere to such therapy because of bleeding risks or the need for an invasive or surgical procedure, a bare metal stent is preferable. Biodegradable scaffolds, which completely dissolve over 2 to 3 years,[2] are approved in some countries but not currently in the U.S. Atherectomy is rarely used, with the exception of the Rotablator (Boston Scientific, Maple Grove, MN), which pulverizes plaque into microparticles that pass through the coronary microcirculation and is particularly helpful for the treatment of heavily calcified lesions. After plaque debulking with the Rotablator, a drug-eluting stent is usually implanted.

Discharge Issues

Discharge planning after PCI represents an important opportunity to emphasize evidence-based medical treatment of atherothrombotic disease and coronary risk factor modification. All patients should receive aspirin (81-325 mg/day) indefinitely. For patients receiving bare metal stents, a minimum 2-week course of a thienopyridine (e.g., clopidogrel 75 mg/day, prasugrel 10 mg/day, or ticagrelor 90 mg/day) is mandatory. If a drug-eluting stent is deployed, this dual antiplatelet therapy generally should be extended for at least 12 months, but aspirin alone may be sufficient in some lower-risk patients.[3] Extending dual antiplatelet therapy to 36 months reduces cardiovascular events, increases bleeding, and probably has no benefit for overall survival.[A7] Prolonged use of aspirin, clopidogrel, angiotensin-converting enzyme inhibitors, β-blockers, and lipid-lowering agents should be considered on the basis of randomized trials showing improved long-term outcome, particularly in patients who present with unstable angina syndromes (Chapters 71, 72, and 73). Smoking cessation (Chapter 32), blood pressure control (Chapter 67), stress management, exercise, weight loss, changes in dietary habits, and strict blood glucose control for patients with diabetes (Chapter 229) also are important elements of the discharge plan.

Activity restrictions after PCI are modest. If the femoral artery was instrumented, heavy lifting is discouraged for several days. Intense aerobic exercise is usually discouraged for 2 to 4 weeks (especially after stent implantation) because exercise can activate platelets and lead to formation of thrombus at the angioplasty site. Patients may return to work 1 or 2 days after the procedure if their occupation does not include heavy lifting or excessive physical exercise. There is usually no restriction on driving an automobile. With modern management, mortality after stenting is more likely to be from noncardiac than from cardiac causes.[4]

CORONARY ANGIOPLASTY VERSUS MEDICAL THERAPY

Percutaneous coronary intervention reduces angina and commonly leads to better treadmill exercise performance and improved quality-of-life measurements. However, PCI has not been shown to reduce the risks of death, MI, or other major cardiovascular events compared with modern optimal medical therapy in patients with stable angina (Chapter 71).[A8] PCI reduces symptoms for the first 24 months, especially in patients with more severe angina, but symptoms were similarly improved over baseline with both intensive medical therapy and PCI at 36 months.[A9] In truly asymptomatic patients, significant ischemia first should be documented by functional testing, or a large quantity of myocardium should be supplied by the stenotic coronary artery. Patients experiencing acute ST segment elevation MI (Chapter 73) represent an important subgroup in whom PCI has proved beneficial compared with medical therapy (Fig. 74-5). In ST segment elevation MI, randomized trials consistently have reported a reduction in mortality, stroke, subsequent MI, and recurrent ischemia with immediate PCI compared with thrombolytic therapy[A10] or with initial thrombolytic therapy followed by rescue PCI as needed[A11] even if immediate PCI requires transfer to another hospital. For non–ST segment elevation MI and many patients with unstable angina, an early aggressive approach that includes either PCI or CABG in angiographically suitable patients is generally preferable to a conservative strategy[A12,A13] except in lower risk patients (Chapter 72).

CORONARY ARTERY SURGERY

Coronary artery bypass graft surgery is based on the premise that the morbidity and mortality associated with coronary atherosclerosis are largely related to atherosclerotic coronary stenoses that can be demonstrated by coronary angiography (Chapter 57) and that if grafts are constructed to route blood flow around these stenoses, myocardial blood supply can be improved or preserved, cardiac symptoms relieved, cardiac events diminished, and survival prolonged. Over time, the fundamentals of that concept have been shown to be correct.

The most common types of grafts for coronary artery bypass have been reversed segments of saphenous vein and the internal thoracic arteries. Saphenous vein grafts are anastomosed to the aorta (proximal anastomosis) and to the coronary artery distal to the major obstruction (Fig. 74-6). Saphenous vein grafts have the advantages of availability, larger size than most coronary arteries, and favorable handling characteristics. With time,

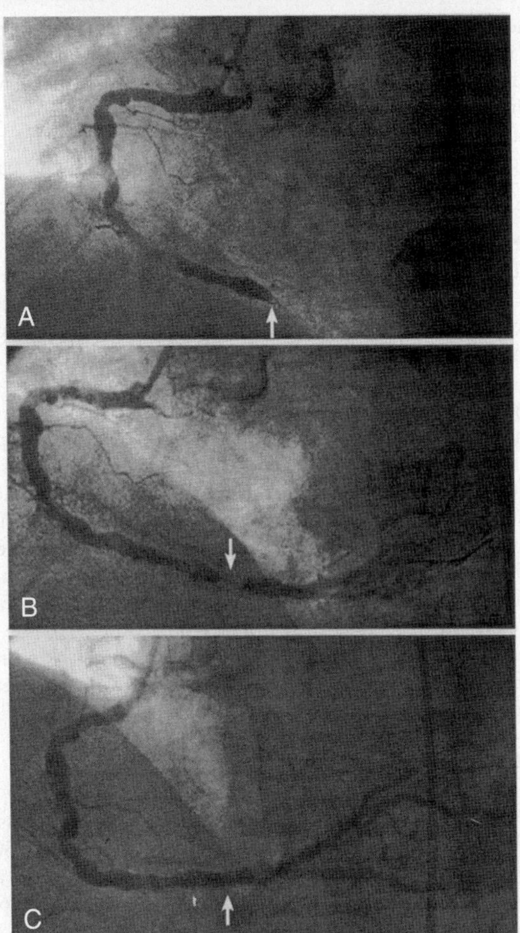

FIGURE 74-5. **Primary coronary angioplasty for acute myocardial infarction. This 50-year-old man presented at midnight with 70 minutes of crushing substernal chest pressure accompanied by inferior ST segment elevation. Emergency angiography performed 45 minutes after arrival found 100% occlusion of the right coronary artery (A, *arrow*). Within 10 minutes, a guidewire was negotiated through the obstruction (presumably caused by fresh thrombus), allowing perfusion into the distal vessel and uncovering a high-grade stenotic lesion (B, *arrow*). After deployment of a coronary stent (C, *arrow*), the stenosis was abolished and significant myocardial damage aborted.**

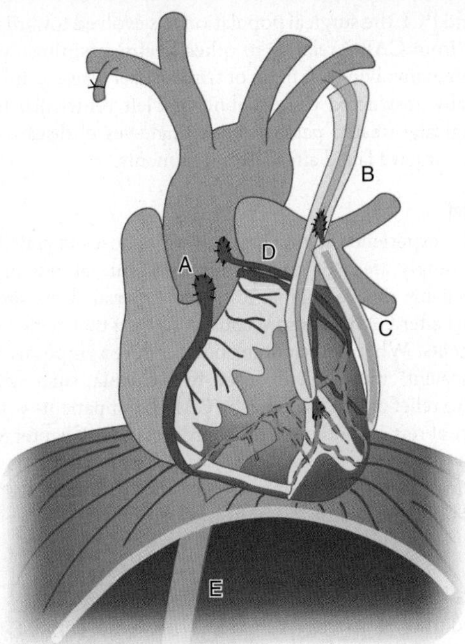

FIGURE 74-6. **Types of bypass grafts. Bypass grafts include reversed saphenous vein graft from the aorta to the right coronary artery (A), in situ left internal mammary artery graft to the anterior descending coronary artery (B), Y graft of the right internal mammary artery from the left internal mammary artery to the circumflex coronary artery (C), radial artery graft from the aorta to the circumflex coronary artery (D), and in situ gastroepiploic graft to the posterior descending branch of the right coronary artery (E).**

however, saphenous vein grafts may develop intrinsic pathologic changes, intimal fibroplasia, and vein graft atherosclerosis, each of which may lead to narrowing or occlusions. Modern treatment with platelet inhibitors and statins (Chapter 206) decreases the risk of vein graft failure but cannot eliminate it. Internal thoracic artery grafts, on the other hand, are resistant to the development of late atherosclerosis. When used as an in situ (subclavian origin intact) graft to the left anterior descending (LAD) coronary artery, the left internal thoracic artery graft has a more than 90% patency rate up to 20 years after operation. As a result, patients who receive a left internal thoracic artery to LAD graft, with or without saphenous vein grafts, have a better long-term survival rate, fewer reoperations, and fewer cardiac events compared with patients receiving only saphenous vein grafts. The right internal thoracic artery may also be used for revascularization as an in situ graft, as an aorta to coronary artery graft, or as a composite arterial graft from the left internal thoracic artery to a coronary artery. Use of both internal thoracic arteries as grafts provides incremental benefit over a single internal thoracic artery graft strategy and produces an improved survival with a lower risk for reoperation.[5] Although the experience is more limited, radial artery grafts also appear to function better than saphenous vein grafts.[A14]

Most CABG operations are performed with a full median sternotomy incision, historically with the aid of cardiopulmonary bypass, aortic cross-clamping, and cardioplegic solution—techniques that allow exposure and arrest of the heart such that detailed microsurgical anastomoses can be constructed while myocardial function is effectively protected. By comparison, operations performed through smaller incisions (minimally invasive surgery) have had limited application for coronary revascularizations. In randomized trials, beating heart ("off-pump") surgery without cardiopulmonary bypass has not consistently reduced morbidity and has often been associated with a lower rate of long-term graft patency[A15]; as a result, it is usually reserved for carefully selected patients.

Perioperative Risks

The risk of mortality associated with CABG correlates with ischemia at the time of operation, left ventricular function, extent of coronary stenoses, noncardiac atherosclerosis, and comorbid conditions, as well as with the experience, skill, and judgment of the surgeon. Effective myocardial protection has diminished much of the incremental risk based on the severity of cardiac disease. For patients younger than 70 years without serious comorbid conditions, the mortality risk of primary CABG surgery is less than 1% in experienced hands. Nevertheless, CABG surgery in the presence of ongoing myocardial ischemia caused by acute MI, unstable angina, or acute vessel closure after PCI is still associated with increased risk. Noncardiac comorbid conditions (aortic atherosclerosis, renal function, chronic obstructive pulmonary disease, and coagulation system disorders) increase perioperative risk when these conditions are severe.

The most serious postoperative morbidity after CABG is stroke, often related to aortic or cerebrovascular atherosclerosis and atherosclerotic embolization. Heightened awareness of the importance of aortic and carotid atherosclerosis and improved management strategies appear to have decreased the risk of focal stroke in patients previously at high risk. Serious wound complications of median sternotomy are uncommon (1%-2%).

Late Outcomes

The late outcomes after CABG are related to age, severity of cardiac disease before operation, noncardiac comorbid conditions, progression of atherosclerosis, and the operation itself. CABG tends to diminish but not eliminate long-term survival differences based on the number of diseased coronary vessels, left main stenosis, and left ventricular function. The achievement of complete revascularization (bypass grafts to all stenotic coronary vessels) and the use of internal thoracic artery grafts improve long-term survival rates and symptomatic status.

For subgroups of patients with severe coronary artery disease, CABG prolongs life expectancy (see later discussion). More than 80% of patients are alive more than 10 years after operation. Over the long term, control of the progression of atherosclerosis by lifestyle modifications, pharmacologic treatment of hypertension (Chapter 67) and lipids (Chapter 206), and platelet inhibitors (Chapter 38) appear to extend the benefits of CABG.

INDICATIONS FOR BYPASS SURGERY

The goals of CABG are to relieve symptoms and to prolong life expectancy. On the basis of randomized trials and the emergence of alternative medical treatments and PCI, the surgical population has evolved toward patients who benefit most from CABG relative to other treatments: those with complex conditions, often involving left main or triple-vessel disease, diffuse coronary stenoses, totally obstructed vessels, abnormal left ventricular function, and diabetes. Surgically treated patients with single-vessel disease usually have LAD stenoses or have failed alternative treatments.

Symptom Relief

If patients who experience angina have severe stenoses in graftable coronary arteries that supply areas of myocardium ischemic at rest or with stress, CABG will reliably relieve angina. Randomized trials have shown that the relief of angina after CABG is more consistent than that achieved with alternative treatments. When intermittent heart failure symptoms represent an "anginal equivalent" that is also caused by ischemia, such symptoms also respond well to relief of that ischemia by CABG. For patients with symptoms of heart failure at rest, dobutamine echocardiography (Chapter 55) and positron emission tomography (Chapter 56) can identify segments of viable but hibernating myocardium (ischemic at rest) that may improve with bypass grafting, thus reducing symptoms of heart failure.

Survival

Chronic Stable Angina

In randomized trials of patients with mild to moderate chronic stable angina, an improved survival rate has been documented for patients treated with initial CABG compared with those treated with initial medical treatment in the presence of a left main stenosis of more than 50% of the diameter, triple-vessel disease, double-vessel disease with a proximal LAD lesion, abnormal left ventricular function, or a strongly positive exercise test result (Chapter 71). Meta-analysis of these randomized trials also suggests a survival benefit of CABG for any patient with a proximal LAD lesion and myocardial ischemia. These are subgroups of patients for whom bypass surgery should be strongly considered even in the absence of severe symptoms. During these trials, patients with severe angina were not randomized but were included in observational studies that noted improved survival rates with CABG for patients with double- and triple-vessel disease and normal or abnormal left ventricular function.[A16] Medical, interventional, and surgical treatments have all advanced substantially since these trials were completed.

Unstable Angina or Non–ST Segment Elevation Myocardial Infarction

Current data suggest an aggressive strategy, including CABG when indicated, in patients with unstable angina or non–ST segment elevation acute MI (Chapter 72).[A12][A13]

Ischemic Syndromes without Randomized Trials

ST Segment Elevation Acute Myocardial Infarction

For patients with ST segment elevation acute MI, CABG may be indicated in the acute setting when thrombolytic therapy or PCI has not been effective, ischemia is ongoing, and large areas of myocardium remain jeopardized. CABG after a completed MI may be indicated in patients in whom persistent ischemia in noninfarcted areas of myocardium produces postinfarction angina or hemodynamic instability. Mechanical complications of myocardial necrosis, including papillary muscle rupture, ventricular septal rupture, and myocardial free wall rupture, are acute life-threatening situations that usually require urgent operation for repair of the defect, often combined with CABG (Chapter 73).

Failed Percutaneous Coronary Intervention

The availability of intracoronary stents has decreased the need for emergency CABG to treat acute failure of PCIs. Current indications for emergency CABG include closure or threatened closure of a vessel supplying a significant amount of myocardium.

Coronary Bypass Reoperations

Patients in whom new stenoses develop in native arteries or in bypass grafts may have recurrent ischemic syndromes. Severe vein graft atherosclerosis is an unstable lesion that often leads to serious cardiac events, particularly if the LAD or multiple vessels are jeopardized; reoperation appears to improve the survival rate of these patients. Conversely, if the LAD coronary artery is supplied by a patent internal thoracic artery graft, reoperation does not appear to improve survival, although it may improve symptoms. Reoperations are more difficult and dangerous than primary procedures, but the risk now approaches that for primary procedures in institutions performing a large number of reoperations. PCI is sometimes an alternative for the treatment of vein graft disease.

Coexisting Cardiac Disease

During cardiac operations performed for valvular (Chapter 75) or aortic (Chapter 78) disease, the standard treatment is to perform bypass grafts to major coronary arteries with angiographic stenoses of more than 50% of the luminal diameter. No randomized trials have addressed this issue, and these indications, although logical given the natural history of atherosclerosis, remain practice patterns based on consensus but not on definitive data.

PERCUTANEOUS CORONARY INTERVENTION VERSUS CORONARY ARTERY BYPASS GRAFTING

The decision between PCI and CABG surgery is largely determined by clinical status and anatomic features, but some areas remain controversial. For patients with acute coronary syndromes, PCI is the preferred initial approach and is known to improve the survival rate of patients with ST segment elevation MI. CABG is reserved for patients with failed acute PCI or residual myocardial ischemia. For patients with chronic coronary syndromes, there are currently no data to confirm that PCI prolongs life regardless of anatomy, but randomized trials, albeit older trials, demonstrate that CABG prolongs the life expectancy of patients with severe coronary artery disease, particularly patients with left ventricular dysfunction or severe ischemia. Surgery, therefore, is often the initial approach to these patient subsets.

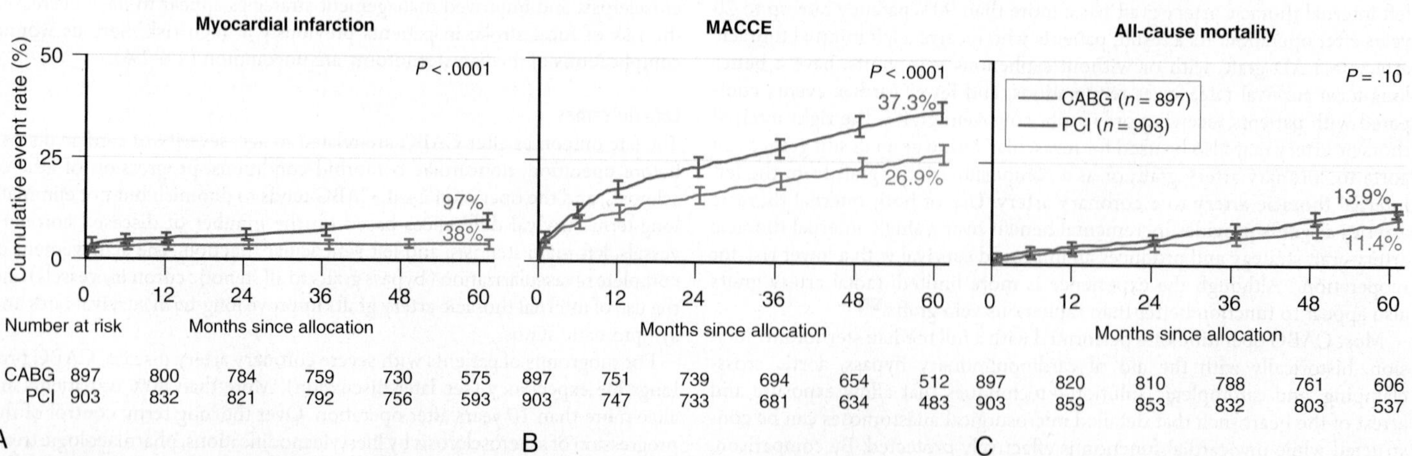

FIGURE 74-7. The SYNTAX trial randomized patients with left main vessel or three-vessel coronary artery disease to coronary artery bypass grafting (CABG) versus percutaneous coronary intervention (PCI). At 5 years, patients randomized to CABG surgery had fewer myocardial infarctions, fewer major acute coronary or cerebrovascular events (MACCE = death, myocardial infarction, stroke, and repeat revascularization), and a trend toward lower mortality. (Data from More F, Morice M, Serruys P, et al. Coronary artery bypass graft surgery versus percutaneous coronary intervention with three vessel disease and left main coronary disease: 5-year follow-up of the randomized, clinical SYNTAX Trial. *Lancet.* 2013;381:629-638.)

Randomized trials have provided information aiding in the selection of therapy. The SYNTAX trial randomized patients with triple vessel or left main disease to PCI or CABG and grouped patients based on scores reflecting the anatomic complexity and extent of coronary disease into low-, medium-, and high-risk subgroups. At 5-year follow-up, the entire group of patients randomized to bypass surgery had fewer MIs (9.7% vs. 3.8%; $P < .001$), fewer repeat revascularization (25.9% vs. 13.7%; $P < .001$), and a trend toward lower mortality rates (13.9% vs. 11.4%; $P = 0.10$)[A17] (Fig. 74-7). Patients with more complex coronary artery disease benefitted most from CABG, including a clear improvement in survival rate, but patients with more limited coronary disease had equivalent survival outcomes with PCI. Randomized trials also show that diabetic patients with multivessel coronary artery disease have better survival rates with CABG compared with PCI.[A16,A18]

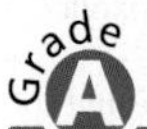

Grade A References

A1. De Bruyne B, Pijls N, Fearon W, et al. Fractional flow reserve-guided PCI versus medical therapy in stable coronary artery disease. *N Engl J Med.* 2012;367:991-1001.

A2. De Bruyne B, Fearon WF, Pijls NH, et al. Fractional flow reserve-guided PCI for stable coronary artery disease. *N Engl J Med.* 2014;371:1208-1217.

A3. Jacobs AK, Normand SL, Massaro JM, et al. Nonemergency PCI at hospitals with or without on-site cardiac surgery. *N Engl J Med.* 2013;368:1498-1508.

A4. Aversano T, Lemmon CC, Liu L, Atlantic CPORT Investigators. Outcomes of PCI at hospitals with or without on-site cardiac surgery. *N Engl J Med.* 2012;366:1792-1802.

A5. Palmerini T, Biondi-Zoccai G, Della Riva D, et al. Clinical outcomes with drug-eluting and bare-metal stents in patients with ST-segment elevation myocardial infarction: evidence from a comprehensive network meta-analysis. *J Am Coll Cardiol.* 2013;62:496-504.

A6. Bangalore S, Kumar S, Fusaro M, et al. Short- and long-term outcomes with drug-eluting and bare-metal coronary stents: a mixed-treatment comparison analysis of 117 762 patient-years of follow-up from randomized trials. *Circulation.* 2012;125:2873-2891.

A7. Mauri L, Kereiakes DJ, Yeh RW, et al. Twelve or 30 months of dual antiplatelet therapy after drug-eluting stents. *N Engl J Med.* 2014;371:2155-2166.

A8. Stergiopoulos K, Boden WE, Hartigan P, et al. Percutaneous coronary intervention outcomes in patients with stable obstructive coronary artery disease and myocardial ischemia: a collaborative meta-analysis of contemporary randomized clinical trials. *JAMA Intern Med.* 2014;174:232-240.

A9. Weintraub WS, Spertus JA, Kolm P, et al. Effect of PCI on quality of life in patients with stable coronary artery disease. *N Engl J Med.* 2008;359:677-687.

A10. Keeley EC, Boura JA, Grines CL. Primary angioplasty versus intravenous thrombolytic therapy for acute myocardial infarction: a quantitative review of 23 randomised trials. *Lancet.* 2003;361:13-20.

A11. Di Mario C, Dudek D, Piscione F, et al. Immediate angioplasty versus standard therapy with rescue angioplasty after thrombolysis in the Combined Abciximab REteplase Stent Study in Acute Myocardial Infarction (CARESS-in-AMI): an open, prospective, randomised, multicentre trial. *Lancet.* 2008;371:559-568.

A12. Mehta SR, Granger CB, Boden WE, et al., for the TIMACS Investigators. Early versus delayed invasive intervention in acute coronary syndromes. *N Engl J Med.* 2009;360:2165-2175.

A13. O'Donoghue M, Boden WE, Braunwald E, et al. Early invasive vs. conservative treatment strategies in women and men with unstable angina and non-ST-segment elevation myocardial infarction: a meta-analysis. *JAMA.* 2008;300:71-80.

A14. Deb S, Cohen EA, Singh SK, et al. Radial artery and saphenous vein patency more than 5 years after coronary artery bypass surgery: results from RAPS (Radial Artery Patency Study). *J Am Coll Cardiol.* 2012;60:28-35.

A15. Houlind K, Kjeldsen BJ, Madsen SN, et al. On-pump versus off-pump coronary artery bypass surgery in elderly patients: results from the Danish On-Pump Versus Off-Pump Randomization Study. *Circulation.* 2012;125:2431-2439.

A16. Frye RL, August P, Brooks MM, et al. A randomized trial of therapies for type 2 diabetes and coronary artery disease. *N Engl J Med.* 2009;360:2503-2515.

A17. Mohr F, Morice M, Serruys P, et al. Coronary artery bypass graft surgery versus percutaneous coronary intervention with three vessel disease and left main coronary disease: 5-year follow-up of the randomized, clinical SYNTAX Trial. *Lancet.* 2013;381:629-638.

A18. Deb S, Wijeysundera HC, Ko DT, et al. Coronary artery bypass graft surgery vs percutaneous interventions in coronary revascularization: a systematic review. *JAMA.* 2013;310:2086-2095.

GENERAL REFERENCES

For the General References and other additional features, please visit Expert Consult at https://expertconsult.inkling.com.

75

VALVULAR HEART DISEASE

BLASE A. CARABELLO

The cardiac valves permit unobstructed forward blood flow through the heart when they are open while preventing backward flow when they are closed. Most valvular heart diseases cause either valvular stenosis with obstruction to forward flow or valvular regurgitation with backward flow. Valvular stenosis imparts a pressure overload on the left or right ventricle (RV) because these chambers must generate higher than normal pressure to overcome the obstruction to pump blood forward. Valvular regurgitation imparts a volume overload on the heart, which now must pump additional volume to compensate for what is regurgitated. When valve disease is severe, these hemodynamic burdens can lead to ventricular dysfunction, heart failure, and sudden death (Table 75-1). In almost every instance, definitive therapy for severe valvular heart disease is mechanical restoration of valve function.

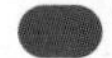

AORTIC STENOSIS

EPIDEMIOLOGY

Bicuspid and Other Congenitally Abnormal Aortic Valves

Approximately 1% of the population is born with a bicuspid aortic valve, with a male preponderance (Chapter 69). Although this abnormality does not usually cause a hemodynamic disturbance at birth, bicuspid aortic valves tend to deteriorate with age. Approximately one third of these valves become stenotic, another third become regurgitant, and the remainder cause only minor hemodynamic abnormalities. When stenosis develops, it usually occurs when patients are in their 40s, 50s, and 60s.

Sometimes congenital aortic stenosis from a unicuspid, bicuspid, or even abnormal tricuspid valve causes symptoms during childhood and requires correction by adolescence. Occasionally, these congenitally stenotic aortic valves escape detection until adulthood.

Tricuspid Aortic Valve Stenosis

In some patients born with apparently normal tricuspid aortic valves, thickening and calcification develop similar to what occurs in bicuspid valves. When aortic stenosis develops in previously normal tricuspid aortic valves, it usually does so in the 60s to 80s. Although stenosis and calcifications of bicuspid and tricuspid aortic valves were formerly considered to be degenerative processes, it is clear that this type of aortic stenosis arises from an active inflammatory process similar to that of coronary heart disease. This concept is supported by many pieces of evidence. First, the initial lesion of aortic stenosis is similar to the plaque of coronary disease. Second, both diseases have hypertension and hyperlipidemia, including elevated levels of lipoprotein(a), as risk factors. Third, there is excellent correlation between calcification of the aortic valve and calcification of the coronary arteries. Fourth, patients with the most severe aortic stenosis have the highest levels of C-reactive protein. However, many diseased aortic valves demonstrate actual bone formation, not merely calcification. Future targets for controlling or preventing the disease likely will aim at bone-forming pathways.

Rheumatic Valvular Heart Disease

Rheumatic valve disease is now a rare cause of aortic stenosis in developed countries, but rheumatic fever and its sequelae remain an important issue in many developing countries (Chapter 290). In virtually every case, the mitral valve is also detectably abnormal.

PATHOBIOLOGY

The normal aortic valve area is 3 to 4 cm^2, and little hemodynamic disturbance occurs until the orifice is reduced to about one third of normal, at which point a systolic gradient develops between the left ventricle (LV) and aorta.[1] LV and aortic pressures are normally nearly equal during systole. In aortic stenosis, intracavitary LV pressure must increase above aortic pressure, however, to produce forward flow across the stenotic valve and to achieve acceptable downstream pressure (see Fig. 57-2 in Chapter 57). Each of the processes that cause aortic stenosis has a typical pathoanatomic configuration (Fig. 75-1). There is a geometric progression in the magnitude of the gradient as the valve area narrows. Given a normal cardiac output, the gradient rises rapidly from 10 to 15 mm Hg at valve areas of 1.5 to 1.3 cm^2 to about 25 mm Hg at 1.0 cm^2, 50 mm Hg at 0.8 cm^2, 70 mm Hg at 0.6 cm^2, and 100 mm Hg at 0.5 cm^2. The rate of progression of aortic stenosis varies widely from patient to patient; it may remain stable for many years or increase by more than 15 mm Hg per year. A major compensatory response to the increased LV pressure associated with aortic stenosis is the development of concentric LV hypertrophy (LVH). The Laplace equation—tress (s) = Pressure (p) × Radius (r)/2 Thickness (th)—indicates that the systolic force on any unit of LV myocardium (afterload) varies directly with ventricular pressure and radius and inversely with wall thickness. As pressure increases, it can be offset by increased LV wall thickness (concentric hypertrophy). The

TABLE 75-1 SUMMARY OF SEVERE VALVAR HEART DISEASE

	AORTIC STENOSIS	MITRAL STENOSIS	MITRAL REGURGITATION	AORTIC REGURGITATION
Etiology	Idiopathic calcification of a bicuspid or tricuspid valve Congenital Rheumatic	Rheumatic fever Annular calcification	Mitral valve prolapse Ruptured chordae Endocarditis Ischemic papillary muscle dysfunction or rupture Collagen vascular diseases and syndromes Secondary to LV myocardial diseases	Annuloaortic ectasia Hypertension Endocarditis Marfan syndrome Ankylosing spondylitis Aortic dissection Syphilis Collagen vascular disease
Pathophysiology	Pressure overload on the LV with compensation by LVH As disease advances, reduced coronary flow reserve causes angina. Hypertrophy and afterload excess lead to systolic and diastolic LV dysfunction.	Obstruction to LV inflow increases LA pressure and limits cardiac output, thus mimicking LV failure. Mitral valve obstruction increases the pressure work of the RV Right ventricular pressure overload is augmented further when pulmonary hypertension develops.	Places volume overload on the LV. Ventricle responds with eccentric hypertrophy and dilation, which allow increased ventricular stroke volume. Eventually, however, LV dysfunction develops if volume overload is uncorrected.	*Chronic:* Total stroke volume causes hyperdynamic circulation, induces systolic hypertension, and causes pressure and volume overload. Compensation is by concentric and eccentric hypertrophy. *Acute:* Because cardiac dilation has not developed, hyperdynamic findings are absent. High diastolic LV pressure causes mitral valve preclosure and potentiates LV ischemia and failure.
Symptoms	Angina Syncope Heart failure	Dyspnea Orthopnea PND Hemoptysis Hoarseness Edema Ascites	Dyspnea Orthopnea PND	Dyspnea Orthopnea PND Angina Syncope
Signs	Systolic ejection murmur radiating to the neck Delayed carotid upstroke S_4, soft or paradoxical S_2	Diastolic rumble after an opening snap Loud S_1 RV lift Loud P_2	Holosystolic apical murmur radiating to the axilla, S_3 Displaced PMI	*Chronic:* Diastolic blowing murmur Hyperdynamic circulation Displaced PMI Quincke pulse de Musset sign Austin Flint murmur *Acute:* Short diastolic blowing murmur Soft S_1
Electrocardiogram	LAA LVH	LAA RVH	LAA LVH	LAA LVH
Chest radiograph	Boot-shaped heart Aortic valve calcification on lateral view	Straightening of left heart border Double density at right heart border Kerley B lines Enlarged pulmonary arteries	Cardiac enlargement	*Chronic:* Cardiac enlargement Uncoiling of the aorta *Acute:* Pulmonary congestion with normal heart size
Echocardiographic findings	Concentric LVH Reduced aortic valve cusp separation Doppler shows mean gradient ≥40 mm Hg in most severe cases	Restricted mitral leaflet motion Valve area ≤1.5 cm^2 in most severe cases Tricuspid Doppler may reveal pulmonary hypertension	LV and LAA in chronic severe disease Doppler: large regurgitant jet	*Chronic:* LV enlargement Large Doppler jet PHT <400 msec *Acute:* Small LV Mitral valve preclosure
Catheterization findings	Increased LVEDP Transaortic gradient 40 mm Hg AVA ≤0.8 in most severe cases	Elevated pulmonary capillary wedge pressure Transmitral gradient usually >5 mm Hg in severe cases MVA <1.5 cm^2	Elevated pulmonary capillary wedge pressure Ventriculography shows regurgitation of dye into LV	Wide pulse pressure Aortography shows regurgitation of dye into LV Usually unnecessary
Medical therapy	Avoid vasodilators Digitalis, diuretics, and nitroglycerin in inoperable cases	Diuretics for mild symptoms Anticoagulation in atrial fibrillation Digitalis, β-blockers, verapamil, or diltiazem for rate control	Vasodilators in acute disease No proven therapy in chronic disease	*Chronic:* Vasodilators in chronic asymptomatic disease with hypertension even if LV function is normal. *Acute:* Vasodilators
Indications for surgery	Appearance of symptoms in patients with severe disease (see text)	Appearance of more than mild symptoms Development of pulmonary hypertension Appearance of persistent atrial fibrillation	Appearance of symptoms EF <0.60 ESD ≥40 mm	*Chronic:* Appearance of symptoms EF <0.50 ESD ≥50 mm *Acute:* Even mild heart failure Mitral valve preclosure

AVA = aortic valve area; EF = ejection fraction; ESD = end-systolic diameter; LA = left atrium; LAA = left atrial enlargement; LV = left ventricle; LVEDP = left ventricular end-diastolic pressure; LVH = left ventricular hypertrophy; MVA = mitral valve area; PHT = pressure half-time; PMI = point of maximal impulse; PND = paroxysmal nocturnal dyspnea; RV = right ventricle; RVH = right ventricular hypertrophy.

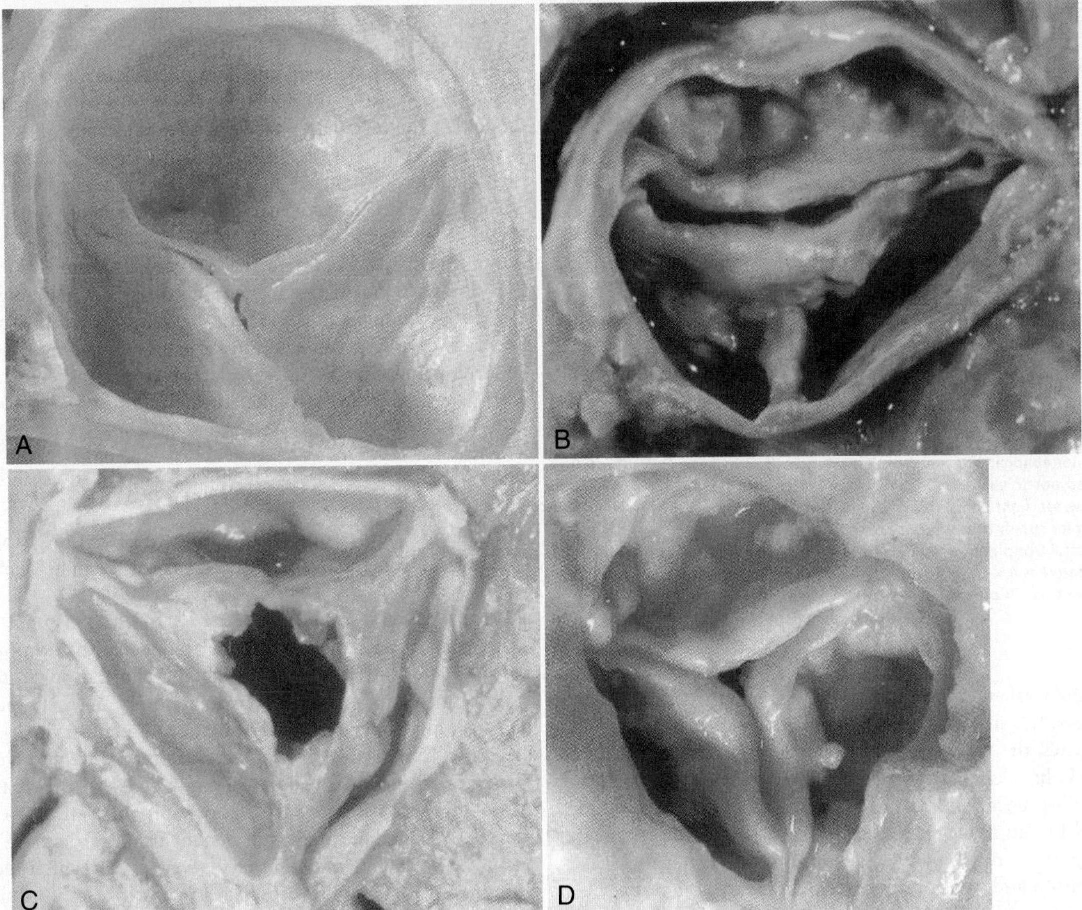

FIGURE 75-1. **Pathology of aortic stenosis. A, A normal aortic valve. B, A stenotic congenital bicuspid valve. C, Rheumatic aortic stenosis. D, A stenotic calcified tricuspid aortic valve. (From Bonow RO, Braunwald E. Valvular heart disease. In: Zipes DP, Libby P, Bonow RO, Braunwald E, eds. *Heart Disease: A Textbook of Cardiovascular Medicine.* 7th ed. Philadelphia: WB Saunders; 2005:1583.)**

determinants of LV ejection fraction are contractility, preload, and afterload. By normalizing afterload, the development of concentric hypertrophy helps preserve ejection fraction and cardiac output despite the pressure overload. Although hypertrophy clearly serves a compensatory function, it also has a pathologic role and is in part responsible for the classic symptoms and the poor outcome of untreated symptomatic aortic stenosis.

Angina

In general, angina (Chapter 71) results from myocardial ischemia when LV oxygen (and other nutrient) demand exceeds supply, which is predicated on coronary blood flow. In normal subjects, coronary blood flow can increase five- to eightfold under maximum metabolic demand, but in patients with aortic stenosis, this reserve is limited. Reduced coronary blood flow reserve may be caused by a relative diminution in capillary ingrowth to serve the needs of the hypertrophied LV or by a reduced transcoronary gradient for coronary blood flow because of the elevated LV end-diastolic pressure. Restricted coronary blood flow reserve is in part responsible for angina in many patients who have aortic stenosis despite normal epicardial coronary arteries, but many patients with restricted flow do not develop angina. In other patients, angina is caused by increased oxygen demand when inadequate hypertrophy allows wall stress, a key determinant of myocardial oxygen consumption, to increase.

Syncope

Syncope (Chapters 51 and 62) generally occurs because of inadequate cerebral perfusion. In aortic stenosis, syncope is usually related to exertion. It may result when exertion causes a fall in total peripheral resistance that cannot be compensated for by increased cardiac output because output is limited by the obstruction to LV outflow; this combination reduces systemic blood pressure and cerebral perfusion. In addition, high LV pressure during exercise may trigger a systemic vasodepressor response that lowers blood pressure and produces syncope. Cardiac arrhythmias, possibly caused by exertional ischemia, also cause hypotension and syncope.

Heart Failure

In aortic stenosis, contractile dysfunction (systolic failure) and failure of normal relaxation (diastolic failure) occur and cause symptoms (Chapter 58). The extent of ventricular contraction is governed by contractility and afterload. In aortic stenosis, contractility (the ability to generate force) is often reduced. The mechanisms of contractile dysfunction may include abnormal calcium handling, microtubular hyperpolymerization causing an internal viscous load on the myocyte, and myocardial ischemia. In some cases, contractile function is normal, but the hypertrophy is inadequate to normalize wall stress and excessive afterload results. Excessive afterload inhibits ejection, reduces forward output, and leads to heart failure.

The increased wall thickness that helps normalize stress increases diastolic stiffness. Even if muscle properties remain normal, higher filling pressure is required to distend a thicker ventricle. As aortic stenosis advances, collagen deposition also stiffens the myocardium and adds to the diastolic dysfunction.

CLINICAL MANIFESTATIONS

The diagnosis of aortic stenosis is usually first suspected when the classic systolic ejection murmur is heard during physical examination (Chapter 51). The murmur is loudest in the aortic area and radiates to the neck. In some cases, the murmur may disappear over the sternum and reappear over the LV apex, thereby giving the false impression that a murmur of mitral regurgitation is also present (Gallavardin phenomenon). The intensity of the murmur increases with cycle length because longer cycles are associated with greater aortic flow. In mild disease, the murmur peaks in intensity in early systole or midsystole. As the severity of stenosis worsens, the murmur peaks progressively later in systole. Perhaps the most helpful clue to the severity of aortic stenosis by physical examination is the characteristic delay in the carotid pulse with a diminution in its volume (see Fig. 51-5 in Chapter 51); in elderly patients, however, increasing carotid stiffness may pseudonormalize the carotid upstrokes. The LV apical impulse in aortic stenosis is not displaced but is enlarged and forceful. The simultaneous palpation of a forceful LV apex

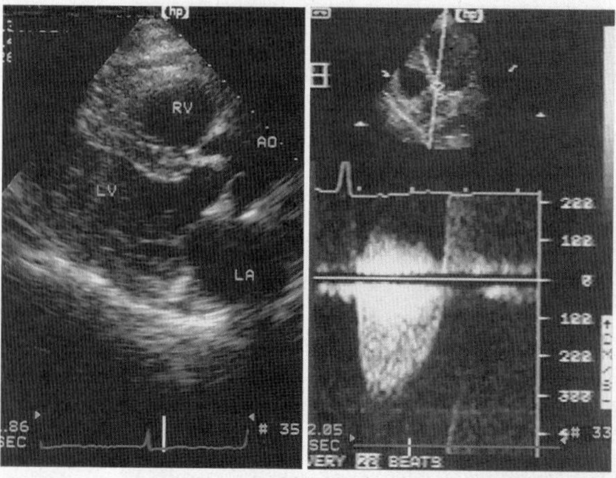

FIGURE 75-2. **Doppler echocardiogram from a patient with aortic stenosis. The *left panel* shows thickened aortic valve leaflets that dome into the aorta with restricted opening in systole. The *top right panel* shows a miniaturized apical four-chamber view at the top with a Doppler cursor through the aorta, and the *bottom right panel* shows a continuous-wave spectral Doppler signal with a peak velocity of 3 m/sec. The peak valve gradient can be calculated as 4×3^2, or 36 mm Hg. AO = aorta; LA = left atrium; LV = left ventricle; RV = right ventricle. (Courtesy of Dr. Anthony DeMaria.)**

beat and a delayed and weakened carotid pulse is a persuasive clue that severe aortic stenosis is present. S_1 in aortic stenosis is generally normal. In congenital aortic stenosis when the valve is not calcified, S_1 may be followed by a systolic ejection click. In calcific disease, S_2 may be single and soft when the aortic component is lost because the valve neither opens nor closes well. In some cases, delayed LV emptying secondary to LV dysfunction may create paradoxical splitting of S_2. An S_4 gallop is common. In advanced disease, pulmonary hypertension and signs of right-sided failure are common.

Because of the dire consequences of missing the diagnosis of aortic stenosis, the physician must have a low threshold for obtaining an echocardiogram whenever aortic stenosis cannot be excluded by physical examination, especially in patients with a history of angina, syncope, or heart failure. In asymptomatic patients with suspicious murmurs, early diagnosis allows the patient and physician to be more vigilant regarding possible early signs and symptoms.

DIAGNOSIS

The electrocardiogram (ECG) in patients with aortic stenosis usually shows LVH (Chapter 54). In some cases of even severe aortic stenosis, however, LVH is absent on the ECG, possibly because of the lack of LV dilation. Left atrial (LA) abnormality is common because the stiff LV increases LA afterload and causes the LA to dilate.

The chest radiograph in aortic stenosis is generally nondiagnostic. The cardiac silhouette is not usually enlarged but may assume a boot-shaped configuration. In advanced cases, there may be signs of cardiomegaly and pulmonary congestion; aortic valve calcification may be seen in the lateral view.

Echocardiography (Chapter 55) is indispensable to assess the extent of LVH, systolic ejection performance, and aortic valve anatomy (Fig. 75-2). Doppler interrogation of the aortic valve makes use of the modified Bernoulli equation (Gradient = $4 \times \text{Velocity}^2$) to assess the severity of the stenosis (Chapter 55). As blood flows from the body of the LV across the stenotic valve, the flow rate must accelerate for the volume to remain constant. Doppler interrogation of the valve can be performed to detect this increase in velocity for estimation of the valve gradient and valve area. The peak aortic flow velocity in patients with preserved LV systolic function is a useful clinical guide to prognosis. In patients with a flow velocity of 3.0 m/second or less, symptoms are unlikely to develop in the next 5 years; by comparison, in patients with a flow velocity of 4.0 m/second or greater, symptoms usually develop within 2 years; and when the velocity exceeds 5 m/second, symptoms are likely to develop within 1 year.

Although exercise testing is contraindicated in symptomatic patients with aortic stenosis because of the high risk for complications, cautious exercise testing is gaining favor in asymptomatic patients. Such testing often reveals latent symptoms or hemodynamic instability that has gone unrecognized during the patient's normal daily activities. Exercise-induced hypotension or symptoms are indications for aortic valve replacement in patients with severe aortic stenosis; in patients with mild to moderate aortic stenosis, another source of exercise limitation should be sought.

Brain natriuretic peptide (BNP) levels may be higher in patients who will become symptomatic in a short time span. Levels exceeding 550 pg/mL portend a poor prognosis, and rising BNP levels on repeated measurements should be a cause for concern. However, it is still premature to rely on this biomarker to indicate the need for valve replacement.

Cardiac catheterization for performance of coronary arteriography is usually undertaken before surgery because most patients with aortic stenosis are of the age at which coronary disease is common. When echocardiography shows severe aortic stenosis and the patient has one or more of the classic symptoms of the disease, formal invasive documentation of the severity of the stenosis is not necessary, and coronary angiography need not be performed in young adults. When the hemodynamic diagnosis is unclear, however, right- and left-sided heart catheterization should be performed to determine the transaortic valvular pressure gradient and cardiac output, which are used to calculate the aortic valve area by the Gorlin formula:

$$A = \frac{CO/SEP \times HR}{44.3\sqrt{h}}$$

where CO is cardiac output (mL/min), SEP is the systolic ejection period (seconds), HR is the heart rate, and *h* is the mean gradient.

Low Flow, Low Gradient Aortic Stenosis

Two types of pathophysiology can reduce cardiac output and reduce the aortic gradient, thereby misleading the clinician into underestimating the severity and clinical gravity of aortic stenosis.[2] The first type occurs in patients who have developed systolic dysfunction, either from long-standing neglected disease or from a coexisting myocardial infarction. In such patients, the ejection fraction and stroke volume are reduced, as is the transvalvular gradient. Although these patients have a poorer prognosis than do patients with preserved LV function, many still benefit from aortic valve replacement. The second type is patients who have severe LVH, which reduces LV volume. Although the ejection fraction is normal, stroke volume and the valve gradient are reduced. Such patients also usually benefit from valve replacement.

TREATMENT Rx

Medical Therapy

In asymptomatic patients, close follow-up is very important,[3] but no treatment is indicated, nor is any known to be beneficial. Even statins are not useful[A1] despite the similar pathobiology between aortic stenosis and coronary disease.

There also is no accepted effective medical therapy for symptomatic aortic stenosis. In patients with heart failure awaiting surgery, diuretics can be used cautiously to relieve pulmonary congestion. Nitrates may also be used cautiously to treat angina pectoris. Although vasodilators, especially angiotensin-converting enzyme (ACE) inhibitors, have become a cornerstone of therapy for heart failure, they are not recommended for aortic stenosis. With fixed valvular obstruction to outflow, vasodilation reduces pressure distal to the obstruction without increasing cardiac output and may cause syncope. When surgery and valvuloplasty are unsuccessful or impossible, diuretics can be used to improve symptoms with the understanding that they will not improve life expectancy.

Invasive Therapy

Valve Replacement Surgery

The only proven effective therapy for aortic stenosis is aortic valve replacement.[4-6] Even octogenarians benefit from valve replacement unless other comorbid factors preclude surgery, so aortic valve replacement should not be denied simply on the basis of age. Valve replacement should also not be denied because the ejection fraction is reduced; the excess afterload imposed by the stenotic valve is relieved with valve replacement, and a depressed ejection fraction usually improves dramatically after surgery. The exception to this rule is a severely reduced ejection fraction in the face of only a small aortic valve gradient; in this case, the severity of the aortic stenosis may be overestimated because the failing LV has difficulty opening a mildly to moderately stenotic valve. In such patients, LV muscle dysfunction either has another cause or is often so severe that it does not recover after valve replacement. Evidence indicates, however, that even some well-selected patients in this category, such as patients who demonstrate increased cardiac output during dobutamine infusion, may benefit from aortic valve replacement.

Percutaneous Aortic Valve Replacement

Percutaneous transcatheter aortic valve implantation reduces the 1-year mortality rate by 45% (from 51% to 31%) in patients who have severe aortic stenosis and are too ill to undergo surgery.[A2,A3] This 1-year survival advantage

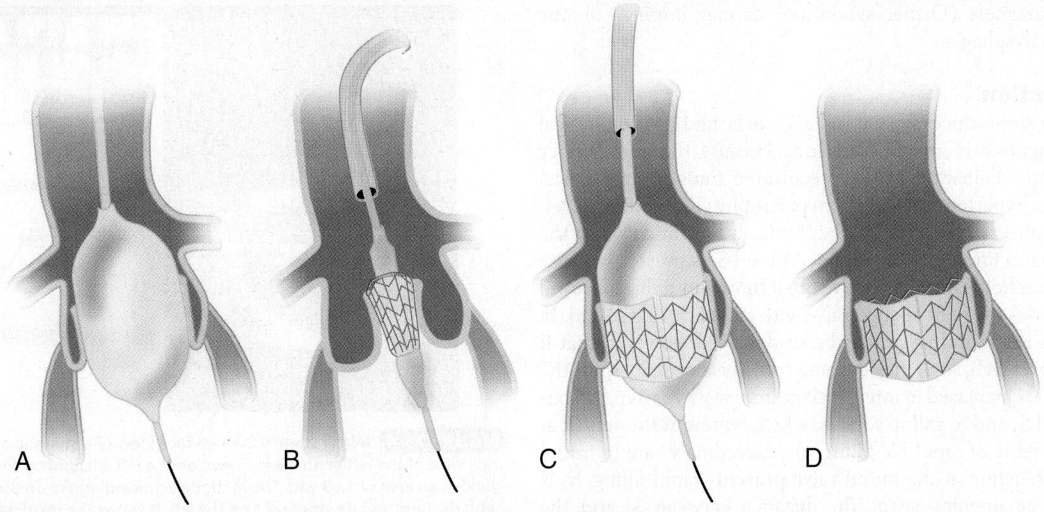

FIGURE 75-3. Steps for transcatheter aortic valve replacement. A, Dilation of the native stenotic valve. B, A crimped stented valve has been inserted over a guidewire into the aortic annulus. C, Inflation of the balloon deploys the valve. D, The balloon is deflated and removed with the aortic valve replaced. (Modified from Cleveland Clinic. Heart valve disease—percutaneous interventions. http://my.clevelandclinic.org/heart/percutaneous/percutaneousValve.aspx.)

remains significant (a subsequent 42% reduction in mortality) among patients who survive beyond the first year, but the mortality benefit may be limited to patients who do not have extensive coexisting conditions. Percutaneous valve implantation also is as good as standard valve replacement in high-risk adults[A4] and may be even better with the newer self-expanding prosthesis.[A5] Even in the high-risk patients who undergo the procedure, national statistics show a 5.5% in-hospital mortality rate and a 2% stroke rate.[7] Percutaneous valve implantation also benefits patients with severe low-flow aortic stenosis.[8]

Two types of valves are available throughout much of the world, including the United States. One is balloon expandable, and the other uses a self-expanding platform. In the first type, the native valve is dilated, and then a stented valve is inserted over a balloon into the aortic annulus (Fig. 75-3). The balloon is expanded to secure the valve and its stent, which is intended to help prevent restenosis. In the second type, the bimetallic frame expands when it contacts body heat. Paravalvular regurgitation, seen in more than 60% of patients, is associated with late morbidity in proportion to its severity, and engineering efforts are underway to limit paravalvular leak.

Balloon Aortic Valvotomy

In acquired calcific aortic stenosis, leaflet restriction results from heavy calcium deposition in the leaflets themselves and is not caused by commissural fusion. Balloon aortic valvotomy is relatively ineffective in improving aortic stenosis; it generally results in a residual gradient of 30 to 50 mm Hg and a valve area of 1.0 cm^2. The mortality rate after this procedure is similar to that in untreated patients. Balloon aortic valvotomy has generally been abandoned in centers that can perform percutaneous aortic valve replacement but still may be used in other settings when immediate temporary relief is required, either because of the demands of other noncardiac conditions or to improve cardiac status temporarily as a bridge to definitive aortic valve replacement.

PROGNOSIS

In asymptomatic patients with normally functioning or minimally dysfunctional bicuspid aortic valves, the survival rate is similar to age-matched control participants, and sudden death is rare, occurring in fewer than 1% of asymptomatic patients. However, 27% of patients require surgery by 20 years after diagnosis. In adults with asymptomatic but hemodynamically significant aortic stenosis, symptoms typically develop within 5 years.[9] A higher peak aortic jet velocity, heavy valve calcification, a positive exercise test result, severe LV dysfunction, and high β-type natriuretic peptide levels predict a worse prognosis and may warrant consideration of valve replacement in asymptomatic patients with severe disease.

The progression of mild to moderate aortic stenosis to severe disease is the key to the natural history of the disease and is quite variable.[10] Aortic stenosis may remain mild for a decade or more in some patients, but in others, it may progress to severe disease in as little as 5 years.

When symptoms develop, survival declines precipitously. Approximately 35% of patients with aortic stenosis are initially evaluated for angina. Of these, 50% are dead in 5 years unless aortic valve replacement is performed. Approximately 15% have syncope; of these, 50% are dead in only 3 years unless the aortic valve is replaced. Of the 50% with symptoms of heart failure, 50% are dead in 2 years without aortic valve replacement. In all, only 25% of patients with symptomatic aortic stenosis survive 3 years in the absence of valve replacement, and the annual risk for sudden death ranges from 10% in patients with angina to 15% with syncope to 25% with heart failure. After valve replacement surgery, prognosis improves to near normal, especially for patients older than 65 years at the time of valve implantation, presumably because older patients have fewer years at risk for valve-related complications.

MITRAL STENOSIS

EPIDEMIOLOGY

In almost all cases of acquired mitral stenosis, the cause is rheumatic heart disease. As the population ages, however, severe calcification of the mitral annulus is increasingly causing mitral stenosis in elderly adults in the absence of rheumatic involvement. Rheumatic mitral stenosis is three times more common in women and usually develops in the 40s and 50s. Although the disease has become rare in developed countries because of the waning incidence of rheumatic fever, mitral stenosis is still prevalent in developing nations, where rheumatic fever is common (Chapter 290).

PATHOBIOLOGY

At the beginning of diastole, a transient gradient between the LA and LV normally initiates LV filling. After early filling, LA and LV pressures equilibrate. In mitral stenosis, obstruction to LV filling increases LA pressure and produces a persistent gradient between the LA and the LV (see Fig. 57-2 in Chapter 57). The combination of elevated LA pressure (and pulmonary venous pressure) and restriction of inflow into the LV limits cardiac output. Although myocardial involvement from the rheumatic process occasionally affects LV muscle function, the muscle itself is normal in most patients with mitral stenosis. However, in approximately one third of patients with mitral stenosis, LV ejection performance is reduced despite normal muscle function because of reduced preload (from inflow obstruction) and increased afterload as a result of reflex vasoconstriction caused by reduced cardiac output.

Because the RV generates most of the force that propels blood across the mitral valve, the RV incurs the pressure overload of the transmitral gradient. In addition, secondary but reversible pulmonary vasoconstriction develops, thus further increasing pulmonary artery pressure and the burden on the RV. As mitral stenosis worsens, RV failure develops.

CLINICAL MANIFESTATIONS

Patients with mitral stenosis usually remain asymptomatic until the valve area is reduced to about one third its normal size of 4 to 5 cm^2. Then the symptoms typical of left-sided failure—dyspnea on exertion, orthopnea, and paroxysmal nocturnal dyspnea—develop. As the disease progresses and RV failure occurs, ascites and edema are common. Hemoptysis, which is common in mitral stenosis but uncommon in other causes of LA hypertension, develops when high LA pressure ruptures the anastomoses of small bronchial veins. In some cases, a large LA may impinge on the left recurrent laryngeal nerve and cause hoarseness (Ortner syndrome) or may impinge on the esophagus and cause dysphagia.

Physical Examination

Although mitral stenosis produces typical and diagnostic findings on physical examination, the diagnosis is missed frequently because the auscultatory findings may be subtle. Palpation of the precordium finds a quiet apical impulse. If pulmonary hypertension and RV hypertrophy (RVH) have developed, the examiner notes a parasternal lift. S_1 is typically loud and may be the most prominent physical finding of the disease. A loud S_1 is present because the transmitral gradient holds the mitral valve open throughout diastole until ventricular systole closes the fully opened valve with a loud closing sound. In far-advanced disease, the mitral valve may be so damaged, however, that it neither opens nor closes well, so S_1 may become soft. S_2 is normally split; the pulmonic component is increased in intensity if pulmonary hypertension has developed. Left-sided S_3 and S_4 gallop sounds, which represent the ventricular and atrial components of rapid LV filling, are exceedingly rare in mitral stenosis because obstruction at the mitral valve prevents rapid filling. S_2 is usually followed by an opening snap. The distance between S_2 and the opening snap provides a reasonable estimation of LA pressure and the severity of the mitral stenosis. The higher the LA pressure, the sooner the LA pressure and the falling LV pressure of early ventricular relaxation equilibrate. At this equilibration point, the mitral valve opens, and the opening snap occurs. When LA pressure is high, the opening snap closely (0.06 second) follows S_2. Conversely, when LA pressure is relatively normal, the snap occurs later (0.12 second) and may mimic the cadence of an S_3 gallop. The opening snap is followed by the classic low-pitched early diastolic mitral stenosis rumble, which increases in length as the mitral stenosis worsens. This murmur may be inaudible if the patient has a relatively low resting cardiac output. Modest exercise, such as isometric handgrip, may accentuate the murmur's intensity. If the patient is in sinus rhythm, atrial systole may produce a presystolic accentuation of the murmur. If pulmonary hypertension has developed, the pulmonic component of S_2 increases in intensity to become as loud or louder than the aortic component. With pulmonary hypertension, a diastolic blowing murmur of pulmonary insufficiency (Graham Steell murmur) is often heard, although in many cases, a coexistent murmur of mild aortic insufficiency is mistaken for this murmur. Neck vein elevation, ascites, and edema are present if RV failure has developed.

DIAGNOSIS

Atrial fibrillation is common, but LA abnormality is generally present on the ECG if the patient is in sinus rhythm. If pulmonary hypertension has developed, there is often evidence of RVH.

On the chest radiograph, LA enlargement produces straightening of the left heart border and a double density at the right heart border as a result of the combined silhouettes of the RA and LA. Pulmonary venous hypertension produces increased vascularity. Kerley B lines, which represent thickening of the pulmonary septa secondary to chronic venous engorgement, may also be seen.

The echocardiogram produces excellent images of the mitral valve and is the most important diagnostic tool in confirming the diagnosis (Fig. 75-4). Transthoracic echocardiography or, if necessary, transesophageal echocardiography makes the diagnosis in nearly 100% of cases and accurately assesses severity. Mitral stenosis, similar to aortic stenosis, can be quantified by assessing the transvalvular gradient with the modified Bernoulli principle. The stenosis is considered severe when the area is smaller than 1.5 cm^2 and very severe when valve area is smaller than 1.0 cm^2.

During echocardiography, the suitability of the valve for balloon valvotomy can also be assessed (see later). If even mild tricuspid regurgitation is present, the systolic gradient across the tricuspid valve can be used to gauge pulmonary artery pressure, which is an important prognostic factor in mitral stenosis because the prognosis worsens as pulmonary pressure increases.

Invasive Evaluation

Cardiac Catheterization

Cardiac catheterization is usually unnecessary to assess the severity of mitral stenosis. Because many patients with mitral stenosis are of an age when coronary disease might be present, however, coronary arteriography is generally performed if cardiac surgery is anticipated or if the patient has coexistent angina. In these cases, it is common to perform left- and right-sided heart catheterization to confirm the transmitral gradient and to calculate the valve area from the Gorlin formula (see earlier).

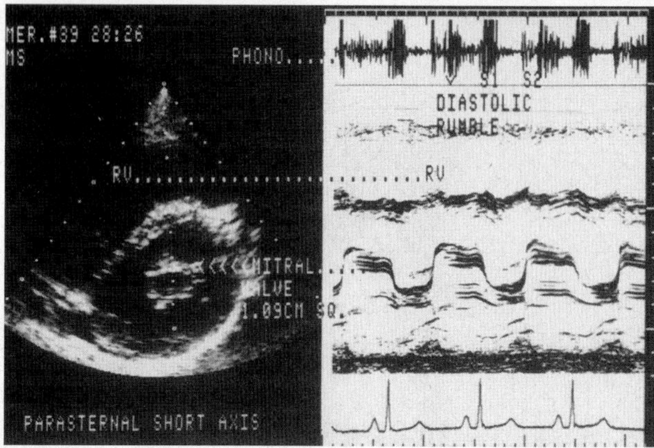

FIGURE 75-4. Mitral stenosis. An en face view of a stenotic mitral valve in the short-axis view of the left ventricle is shown on the *left*. Planimetry for the mitral valve orifice yielded an area of 1.09 cm^2. The M-mode echocardiogram on the *right* has been aligned with the appropriate structures on the *left*. It shows the restricted opening of the mitral valve in diastole associated with the classic diastolic rumbling murmur. RV = right ventricle. (From Assey ME, Usher BW, Carabello BA. The patient with valvular heart disease. In: Pepine CJ, Hill JA, Lambert CR, eds. *Diagnostic and Therapeutic Cardiac Catheterization*. 3rd ed. Baltimore: Williams & Wilkins; 1998:709.)

PREVENTION, TREATMENT, AND PROGNOSIS

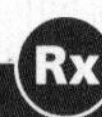

Mitral stenosis can be prevented by appropriate antibiotic treatment of β-hemolytic streptococcal infections (Chapter 290).

Medical Therapy

Asymptomatic patients with mitral stenosis and sinus rhythm require no therapy. Symptoms of mild dyspnea and orthopnea can be treated with diuretics alone. When symptoms worsen to more than mild or if pulmonary hypertension develops, mechanical correction of the stenosis is preferable to medical therapy because it improves longevity in severely symptomatic patients.[11]

Patients with mitral stenosis in whom atrial fibrillation develops usually decompensate because the rapid heart rate reduces diastolic filling time, increases LA pressure, and decreases cardiac output. The heart rate must be controlled promptly, preferably with an infusion of diltiazem, amiodarone, or esmolol for acute atrial fibrillation or with a β-blocker, a calcium channel blocker, or oral digoxin in chronic atrial fibrillation (Chapter 64).

Conversion to sinus rhythm is routinely recommended either pharmacologically or with direct-current countershock (Chapter 64) after anticoagulation is therapeutic. It should be noted that patients with rheumatic atrial fibrillation have been excluded from trials of echocardiogram-guided cardioversion without anticoagulation and trials of rate control versus rhythm control for the chronic management of atrial fibrillation. If sinus rhythm cannot be maintained, mechanical therapy for the mitral stenosis is generally recommended in the hope that sinus rhythm can be restored after the obstruction to atrial outflow is corrected. However, the cause of atrial fibrillation in patients with mitral stenosis probably includes atrial rheumatic inflammation, so restoration of sinus rhythm is unpredictable even after mechanical intervention.

Because patients with concomitant mitral stenosis and atrial fibrillation have an extraordinarily high risk for systemic embolism, they should undergo chronic anticoagulation with warfarin at an international normalized ratio (INR) target of 2.5 to 3.5. Anticoagulation is warranted in all patients unless there is a serious contraindication to its use.

Mechanical Therapy

When symptoms progress past early functional class II, that is, symptoms with more than ordinary activity, or if pulmonary hypertension develops, the prognosis is worse unless the mitral stenosis is relieved. In most instances, an excellent result can be achieved with percutaneous balloon valvotomy. In contrast to aortic stenosis, in mitral stenosis, there is fusion of the valve leaflets at the commissures. Balloon dilation produces a commissurotomy and a substantial increase in valve area that appears to persist for at least a decade and provides improvement comparable to that of closed or open commissurotomy in suitable patients. Nonrheumatic mitral stenosis caused by mitral annular calcification does not respond to balloon valvotomy. The only effective mechanical therapy for this condition is surgical debridement of the mitral annulus followed by mitral valve replacement. Suitability for balloon valvotomy is determined partially during echocardiography. Patients with pliable valves, little valvular calcification, little involvement of the subvalvular apparatus, and less than moderate mitral regurgitation are ideal candidates. Even when valve anatomy is not ideal, however, valvotomy may be attempted in patients with advanced age or in situations in which comorbid risk factors increase surgical risk. In otherwise healthy patients with unfavorable valve anatomy, surgery to perform an open commissurotomy or valve replacement is undertaken. Even at 20 years, 30% of patients have durable functional benefit after a percutaneous mitral commissurotomy.[12]

PRIMARY (ORGANIC) MITRAL REGURGITATION

EPIDEMIOLOGY

The mitral valve is composed of the mitral annulus, the leaflets, the chordae tendineae, and the papillary muscles. Abnormalities in any of these structures may lead to mitral regurgitation. In primary mitral regurgitation, valvular abnormalities cause the valve to leak; the resulting hemodynamic overload, if prolonged and severe, causes LV damage, heart failure, and eventual death if untreated. This condition must be distinguished from secondary or functional mitral regurgitation, wherein disease of the LV causes the valve to leak; this secondary mitral regurgitation is discussed later in this chapter.

The most common cause of primary mitral regurgitation in the United States is mitral valve prolapse, which is responsible for approximately 90% of all cases and comprises many diseases, including myxomatous degeneration of the valve (E-Fig. 75-E1). Annular calcification, endocarditis, papillary muscle dysfunction or infarction, collagen vascular disease, and rheumatic heart disease are less common causes. Use of the weight loss agents dexfenfluramine and fenfluramine has been implicated in causing valve damage in a few patients who received these drugs.

Primary mitral regurgitation can be subdivided on the basis of chronicity. Common causes of severe acute mitral regurgitation include ruptured chordae tendineae and infective endocarditis. Chronic severe mitral regurgitation is more likely to be caused by myxomatous degeneration of the valve, rheumatic heart disease, or annular calcification.

PATHOBIOLOGY

The pathophysiology of mitral regurgitation can be divided into three phases (Fig. 75-5). In acute mitral regurgitation of any cause, the sudden option for ejection of blood into the LA "wastes" a portion of the LV stroke volume as backward rather than forward flow. The combined regurgitant and forward flow causes volume overload of the LV and stretches the existing sarcomeres toward their maximum length. Use of the Frank-Starling mechanism is maximized, and end-diastolic volume increases concomitantly. The regurgitant pathway unloads the LV in systole because it allows ejection into the relatively low-impedance LA and thereby reduces end-systolic volume. Although increased end-diastolic volume and decreased end-systolic volume act in concert to increase total stroke volume, forward stroke volume is subnormal because a large portion of the total stroke volume is regurgitated into the LA. This regurgitant volume increases LA pressure, and the patient experiences heart failure with low cardiac output and pulmonary congestion despite normal LV contractile function.

In many cases, severe acute mitral regurgitation necessitates emergency surgical correction. By comparison, patients who can be managed through the acute phase or in whom the valve abnormalities develop more slowly may enter the phase of hemodynamic compensation. In this phase, eccentric LVH and increased end-diastolic volume, combined with normal contractile function, allow ejection of a sufficiently large total stroke volume to permit forward stroke volume to return toward normal. LA enlargement allows accommodation of the regurgitant volume at a lower filling pressure. In this phase, the patient may be relatively asymptomatic even during strenuous exercise.

Although severe mitral regurgitation may be tolerated for many years, the lesion often causes LV dysfunction, atrial fibrillation, or heart failure within 5 years of the detection of severe mitral regurgitation. The now damaged ventricle has impaired ejection performance, and end-systolic volume increases. Greater LV residual volume at end systole increases end-diastolic volume and end-diastolic pressure, and the symptoms of pulmonary congestion may reappear. Additional LV dilation may worsen the amount of regurgitation by causing further enlargement of the mitral annulus and malalignment of the papillary muscles. Although there is substantial contractile dysfunction, the increased preload and the presence of the regurgitant pathway, which tends to normalize afterload despite ventricular enlargement, augment the ejection fraction and may maintain it in a relatively normal range.

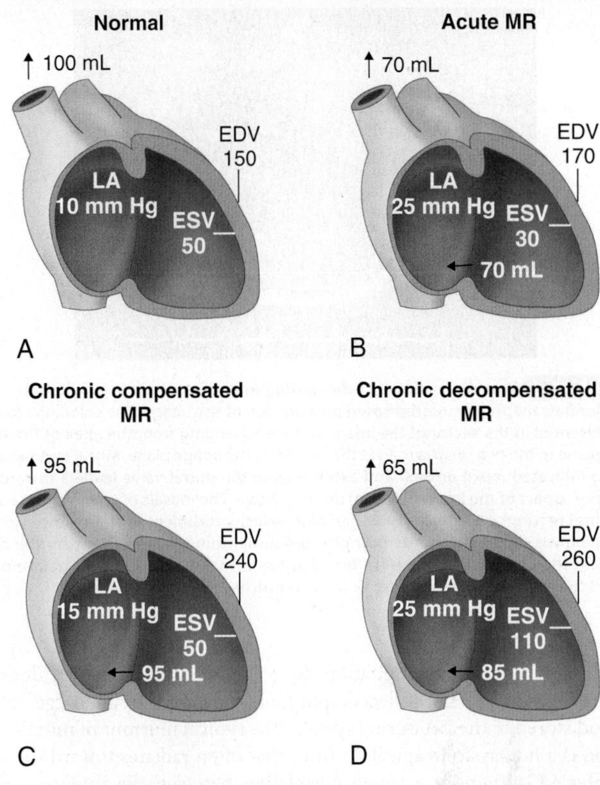

	Preload SL (μ)	Afterload ESS (kdyne/cm²)	CF	EF	RF	FSV (mL)
N	2.07	90	N	.67	.0	100
AMR	2.25	60	N	.82	.50	70
CCMR	2.19	90	N	.79	.5	95
CDMR	2.19	120	↓	.58	.57	65

FIGURE 75-5. Mitral regurgitation. Normal physiology (N) (**A**) is compared with the physiology of acute mitral regurgitation (AMR) (**B**). Acutely, the volume overload increases preload (sarcomere length [SL]), and end-diastolic volume (EDV) increases from 150 to 170 mL. Unloading of the left ventricle by the presence of the regurgitant pathway decreases afterload (end-systolic stress [ESS]), and end-systolic volume (ESV) falls from 50 to 30 mL. These changes result in an increase in the ejection fraction (EF). Because 50% of the total left ventricular (LV) stroke volume (regurgitant fraction [RF]) is ejected into the left atrium (LA), however, forward stroke volume (FSV) falls from 100 to 70 mL. At this stage, contractile function (CF) is normal. **C,** Chronic compensated mitral regurgitation (CCMR). In CCMR, eccentric cardiac hypertrophy has developed, and EDV has increased substantially. Increased EDV, combined with normal contractile function, permits ejection of a larger total stroke volume and a larger forward stroke volume than in the acute phase. Left atrial enlargement permits lower left atrial pressure. Because the radius term in the Laplace equation has increased with increasing LV volume, afterload and ESV return to normal. **D,** Chronic decompensated mitral regurgitation (CDMR). In this stage, contractile dysfunction causes a large increase in ESV with a fall in total and forward stroke volume. Additional LV enlargement leads to worsening mitral regurgitation. The relatively favorable loading conditions in this phase still permit a normal EF, however, despite contractile dysfunction. (From Carabello BA. Mitral regurgitation: basic pathophysiologic principles. *Mod Concepts Cardiovasc Dis.* 1988;57:53-57.)

The causes of LV contractile dysfunction in patients with mitral regurgitation may relate to loss of contractile proteins and abnormalities in calcium handling. In at least some cases, contractile dysfunction is reversible by timely mitral valve surgery

CLINICAL MANIFESTATIONS

In the medical history, the standard symptoms of left-sided heart failure should be sought (Chapter 58). An attempt to discover potential causes should be made by questioning for a prior history of a heart murmur or abnormal findings on cardiac examination (Chapter 51), rheumatic heart disease, endocarditis (Chapter 76), or the use of anorexigenic drugs.

Volume overload of the LV displaces the apical impulse downward and to the left. S_1 may be reduced in intensity, whereas S_2 is usually physiologically

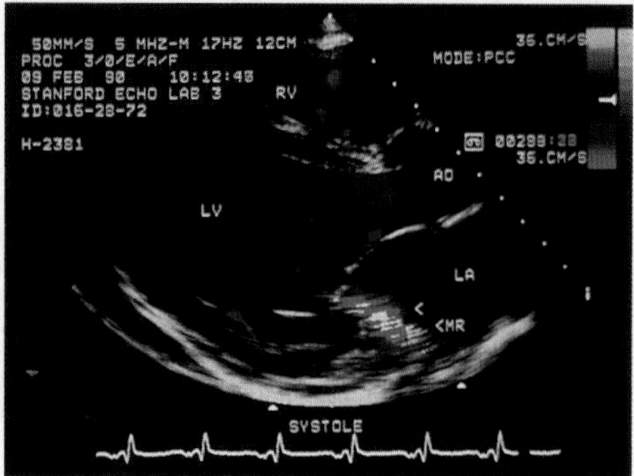

FIGURE 75-6. **Two-dimensional echocardiogram of mitral regurgitation with Doppler flow mapping superimposed on a portion of the image. The color information is represented in the sector of the imaging plane extending from the apex of the triangular plane to the *two small arrows* at the *bottom* of the image plane. Mitral regurgitation (MR) is indicated *(open arrows)* and extends from the mitral valve leaflets toward the posterior aspect of the left atrium (LA) during systole. The mosaic of colors representing the mitral regurgitant signal is typical of high-velocity turbulent flow. The low-intensity *orange-brown* signal represents flow directed away from the transducer on the chest wall, and the *blue* shades represent blood in the left ventricular outflow tract moving toward the transducer. AO = aorta; LV = left ventricle; RV = right ventricle.**

split. In severe mitral regurgitation, S_2 is followed by S_3, which does not indicate heart failure but reflects rapid filling of the LV by the large volume of blood stored in the LA during systole. The typical murmur of mitral regurgitation is a holosystolic apical murmur that often radiates toward the axilla (Chapter 51). There is a rough correlation between the intensity of the murmur and the severity of the disease, but this correlation is too weak to use in clinical decision making because the murmur may be soft when cardiac output is low. In contrast to aortic stenosis, murmur intensity does not usually vary with the RR interval. In acute mitral regurgitation, the presence of a large v wave may produce rapid equilibration of LA and LV pressure, thereby reducing the driving gradient and shortening the murmur. Pulmonary hypertension may develop and produce right-sided signs; including an RV lift, an increased P_2; and if RV dysfunction has developed, signs of right-sided heart failure.

DIAGNOSIS

The ECG usually shows LVH and LA abnormality. The chest radiograph typically shows cardiomegaly; the absence of cardiomegaly indicates either that the mitral regurgitation is mild or that it has not been chronic enough to allow cardiac dilation to occur.

Echocardiography shows the extent of LA and LV enlargement (Chapter 55). Ultrasonic imaging of the mitral valve is excellent and offers clues to the mitral valve abnormalities responsible for the regurgitation. In some patients, three-dimensional echocardiography can add pathoanatomic information of potential use in aiding surgical repair of the valve. Color-flow Doppler interrogation of the valve (Fig. 75-6) helps assess the severity of regurgitation, but because this technique images flow velocity rather than actual flow, it is subject to errors in interpretation. The Doppler technique is excellent for excluding the presence of mitral regurgitation and for distinguishing between mild and severe degrees. Newer techniques may quantify regurgitation more precisely but are not applicable in every patient, and standard color-flow Doppler examination may not be sufficient for exact quantification of mitral regurgitation or to determine whether the severity of the lesion is sufficient to cause eventual LV dysfunction. Cardiac magnetic resonance imaging (MRI) (Chapter 56), when available, can more precisely quantify the severity of the regurgitation. When the severity of mitral regurgitation is in doubt or if mitral valve surgery is being contemplated, cardiac catheterization (Chapter 57) is helpful in resolving the severity of the lesion; coronary arteriography should be included in patients older than 40 years or with symptoms suggesting coronary disease (Chapter 71).

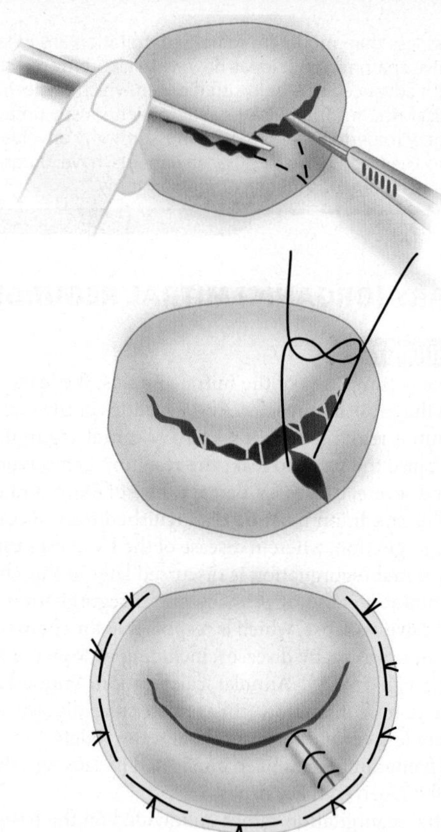

FIGURE 75-7. **The stages of mitral valve repair. (Modified from Cleveland Clinic. Mitral valve repair. http://my.clevelandclinic.org/heart/disorders/valve/mvrepair.aspx.)**

TREATMENT AND PROGNOSIS Rx

Medical Therapy

Severe Acute Mitral Regurgitation

In severe acute mitral regurgitation, the patient is usually symptomatic with heart failure or even shock. The goal of medical therapy is to increase forward cardiac output while concomitantly reducing regurgitant volume (Chapter 59). Arterial vasodilators reduce systemic resistance to flow and preferentially increase aortic outflow and simultaneously decrease the amount of mitral regurgitation and LA hypertension. If hypotension already exists, vasodilators such as nitroprusside lower blood pressure further and cannot be used. In these cases, intraaortic balloon counterpulsation (Chapter 107) is preferred if the aortic valve is competent. Counterpulsation increases forward cardiac output by lowering ventricular afterload while augmenting systemic diastolic pressure.

Chronic Symptomatic Mitral Regurgitation

In patients with *symptomatic* mitral regurgitation, ACE inhibitors (e.g., lisinopril, 20 mg/day) reduce LV volume and improve symptoms. Observational evidence suggests that such patients may also benefit from administration of β-blockers. Mitral valve surgery rather than medical therapy is generally preferred, however, in most symptomatic patients with mitral regurgitation. When atrial fibrillation is present, long-term anticoagulation should achieve the same INR goal as for mitral stenosis.

Chronic Asymptomatic Mitral Regurgitation

Vasodilators have had little effect in reducing LV volume or improving normal exercise tolerance in patients with mitral regurgitation, perhaps because afterload is not usually increased in those with chronic asymptomatic mitral regurgitation. There is no definitive indication to begin afterload reduction before symptoms appear because no large randomized trials have been performed, and smaller trials have generally shown no benefit from these therapies.

Surgical Therapy

The timing of mitral valve surgery must weigh the risks of the operation and placement of a prosthesis, if one is inserted, against the risk for irreversible LV dysfunction if surgery is delayed unwisely.[13] For most other types of valve diseases, surgical correction usually requires placement of a prosthetic valve, but in patients with mitral regurgitation, the native valve can often be repaired. Because conservation of the native valve obviates the risks associated with a prosthesis, the option of mitral valve repair should influence the patient and physician toward earlier surgery.

Types of Mitral Valve Surgery

Mitral Valve Repair

When feasible, mitral valve repair (Fig. 75-7) is the preferred operation. Repair restores valve competence, maintains the functional aspects of the apparatus, and avoids the insertion of a prosthesis. Repair is most applicable in cases of posterior chordal rupture; anterior involvement and rheumatic involvement make repair more difficult. Currently, the percentage of mitral valve surgeries that are valve repair varies from 0% to 95% at different hospital centers, averaging about 70% across the United States overall. For severe ischemic mitral regurgitation, mitral valve repair and chordal-sparing mitral valve replacement provide equivalent clinical outcomes at 1 year, although replacement results in less residual mitral regurgitation.[A6] For moderate ischemic mitral regurgitation, mitral valve repair does not clearly add benefit above and beyond the benefits of coronary artery bypass surgery.[A7]

Percutaneous mitral valve repair with implantation of a clip device is less invasive than conventional mitral valve repair but is also substantially less effective than open surgery for reducing the amount of mitral regurgitation.[A8] It is approved in the United States for use in symptomatic inoperable patients. In all cases, the feasibility of repair depends on the pathoanatomy that is causing the mitral regurgitation and the skill and experience of the operating surgeon.

Mitral Valve Replacement with Preservation of the Mitral Apparatus

In this procedure, a prosthetic valve is inserted, but continuity between the native leaflets and the papillary muscles is maintained. This procedure has the advantage of ensuring mitral valve competence while preserving the LV functional aspects of the mitral apparatus. Even if only the posterior leaflets and chordae are preserved, the patient benefits from improved postoperative ventricular function and possibly better survival. In many cases, it is possible to preserve the anterior and posterior chordal attachments, although anterior continuity can be associated with LV outflow tract obstruction. Although the patient benefits from restored mitral valve competence and maintenance of LV function, insertion of a prosthesis still carries all prosthesis-associated risks. Operative mortality with all mitral valve replacement operations is at least twice as high as with mitral valve repair.

Mitral Valve Replacement without Preservation of the Mitral Apparatus

When the native valve cannot be repaired or the chordae preserved, such as in severe rheumatic deformity, the mitral valve leaflets and its apparatus are removed, and a prosthetic valve is inserted. Although this operation almost guarantees mitral valve competence, the mitral valve apparatus is responsible for coordinating LV contraction and for helping maintain the efficient prolate ellipsoid shape of the LV. Destruction of the apparatus leads to a sudden fall in LV function and a decline in postoperative ejection fraction that is often permanent.

Timing of Surgery

Symptomatic Patients

Most patients with symptoms of dyspnea, orthopnea, or fatigue should undergo surgery regardless of which operation is performed because they already have lifestyle limitations from their disease. The mere presence of symptoms worsens the prognosis despite relatively well-preserved LV function. The onset or worsening of symptoms is a summary of the patient's pathophysiology and may give a broader view of cardiovascular integrity than possible with any single measurement of pressure or function. For patients with acute mitral regurgitation owing to flail mitral valve leaflets, earlier surgery appears to be better than prolonged medical management, but randomized trials have not been performed.[14]

Asymptomatic Patients with Normal Left Ventricular Function

Surgery has increasingly been considered in asymptomatic patients who have normal LV function but echocardiographic findings indicating that valve *repair* is likely to be successful. Although these patients are at low risk without surgery, the risk associated with valve repair is less than 1%, and this approach reduces the risks of subsequent LV dysfunction or atrial fibrillation, which may occur if the valvular disease progresses. Furthermore, life span can be normal after successful repair before LV dysfunction has developed. Valve repair obviates the need for protracted, expensive follow-up and provides a durable correction of the lesion. This approach is sensible, however, only if it is certain that valve repair can be performed because insertion of a prosthesis carries unacceptable risk in this low-risk group.

Asymptomatic Patients with Left Ventricular Dysfunction

The onset of LV dysfunction in patients with mitral regurgitation may occur without causing symptoms. Early surgery is warranted to prevent the muscle dysfunction from becoming severe or irreversible. Regardless of whether valve repair or replacement is eventually performed, survival is prolonged if surgery is performed before the ejection fraction declines to less than 0.60 or before the LV is unable to contract to an end-systolic dimension of 40 mm. Patients with severe mitral regurgitation should be monitored yearly with a history, physical examination, and echocardiographic evaluation of LV function. When the patient reports symptoms or echocardiography shows the onset of LV dysfunction, surgery should be undertaken.

Asymptomatic Elderly Patients

Among Medicare recipients, the operative mortality rate is 4% for patients undergoing mitral valve repair and 9% for patients undergoing replacement. The 1-, 5-, and 10-year survival estimates are 91%, 77%, and 54%, respectively, for patients undergoing repair compared with 83%, 65%, and 37% for patients undergoing replacement, respectively.[15] Patients older than 75 years of age may have poorer surgical results than younger patients, especially if coronary disease is present or if mitral valve replacement rather than repair must be performed. However, results of surgery in older patients with mitral regurgitation have steadily improved during the past decade, and elderly patients with symptoms refractory to medical therapy may benefit from surgery. Nevertheless, there is little compelling reason to commit elderly *asymptomatic* patients to a mitral valve operation.

MITRAL VALVE PROLAPSE

DEFINITION

Mitral valve prolapse occurs when one or both of the mitral valve leaflets prolapse into the LA superior to the mitral valve annular plane during systole.[16] The importance of mitral valve prolapse varies from patient to patient. In some cases, prolapse is simply a consequence of normal LV physiology without significant medical impact, such as in situations that produce a small LV (e.g., the Valsalva maneuver or an atrial septal defect), in which reduction of ventricular volume causes relative lengthening of the chordae tendineae and subsequent mitral valve prolapse. At the other end of the spectrum, severe redundancy and deformity of the valve, which occurs in myxomatous valve degeneration, increases the risk for stroke, arrhythmia, endocarditis, and progression to severe mitral regurgitation.

DIAGNOSIS

History

Most patients with mitral valve prolapse are asymptomatic. In some cases, however, mitral valve prolapse is associated with symptoms, including palpitations, syncope, and chest pain. In some cases, chest pain is associated with a positive thallium scintigram indicating the presence of true ischemia despite normal epicardial coronary arteries, perhaps because excessive tension on the papillary muscles increases oxygen consumption and causes ischemia. Palpitations, syncope, and presyncope, when present, are linked to autonomic dysfunction (Chapters 51, 62, and 418), which appears to be more prevalent in patients with mitral valve prolapse.

Physical Examination

On physical examination, the mitral valve prolapse syndrome produces the characteristic findings of a midsystolic click and a late systolic murmur. The click occurs when the chordae tendineae are stretched taut by the prolapsing mitral valve in midsystole. As this occurs, the mitral leaflets move past their coaptation point, permit mitral regurgitation, and cause the late systolic murmur (see Table 51-7 in Chapter 51). Maneuvers that make the LV smaller, such as the Valsalva maneuver, cause the click to appear earlier and the murmur to be more holosystolic and often louder (see Table 51-8 in Chapter 51). In some cases of echocardiographically proven mitral valve prolapse, neither the click nor the murmur is present; in other cases, only one of these findings is present.

Noninvasive Evaluation

Echocardiography is useful to prove that prolapse is present, to image the amount of regurgitation and its physiologic effects, and to discern the pathoanatomy of the mitral valve. Although an echocardiogram is not necessary to diagnose prolapse in patients with the classic physical findings, the echocardiogram adds significant prognostic information because it can detect patients who have specifically abnormal valve morphology and in whom most of the complications of the disease occur. Prolapse shown in the four-chamber echocardiographic view should be confirmed in the parasternal long-axis view.

TREATMENT Rx

Because most cases of mitral valve prolapse are asymptomatic, therapy is usually unnecessary. Although prophylaxis against infective endocarditis was previously recommended in these patients, guidelines no longer recommend antibiotic prophylaxis based on available data (Chapter 76). In patients with palpitations and autonomic dysfunction, β-blockers are often effective in relieving symptoms. Low-dose aspirin therapy has been recommended for patients with redundant leaflets because these patients have a slightly increased risk for stroke. No data from large studies are available to support this contention, however. If severe mitral regurgitation or a flail mitral leaflet develops, however, the therapy is the same as for other causes of mitral regurgitation.

PROGNOSIS

Most patients with mitral valve prolapse have a benign clinical course; even for complication-prone patients with redundant and misshapen mitral leaflets, complications are relatively rare. Approximately 10% of patients with thickened leaflets experience infective endocarditis, stroke, progression to severe mitral regurgitation, or sudden death. The progression to severe mitral regurgitation varies with gender and age, and men are approximately twice as likely to progress as women. By 50 years of age, only approximately one in 200 men requires surgery to correct mitral regurgitation. By the age of 70 years, the risk increases to approximately 3%.

SECONDARY (FUNCTIONAL) MITRAL REGURGITATION

DEFINITION

Secondary or functional mitral regurgitation is a very different disease than is primary mitral regurgitation. In primary mitral regurgitation, treating the mitral regurgitation cures the patient. Conversely, secondary mitral regurgitation is a consequence of LV myocardial dysfunction caused either by myocardial infarction or dilated cardiomyopathy. Because treating secondary mitral regurgitation cannot reverse those entities, the role of valve therapy is often unclear.

EPIDEMIOLOGY

An estimated 5 million Americans have heart failure (Chapters 58 and 59), and about half of them have heart failure with a reduced ejection fraction. About 75% of these latter patients also have some degree of secondary mitral regurgitation, which is severe in about 20% of them.

PATHOBIOLOGY

In secondary mitral regurgitation, the valve itself is normal. Regurgitation occurs because ventricular damage leads to dilation, which causes displacement of the papillary muscles, which in turn prevents a normal valve from reaching its coaptation point. Mitral closing is further impaired by mitral annular dilation and reduced closing force from the weakened myocardium.

CLINICAL MANIFESTATIONS

Because virtually all patients with secondary mitral regurgitation have heart failure, almost all complain of the symptoms of heart failure. Some may note a worsening of symptoms when more than mild secondary mitral regurgitation develops. Probably because the mitral valve itself is normal, as well as because of the weakened force of contraction, the murmur of functional mitral regurgitation may be unimpressive or even inaudible.

DIAGNOSIS

Echocardiography is the mainstay of the diagnosis. In addition to evaluating the severity of the mitral regurgitation itself, the echocardiogram is helpful in establishing the extent of the dilated cardiomyopathy or of the prior myocardial infarction that is responsible for causing the secondary mitral regurgitation.

THERAPY AND PROGNOSIS Rx

The presence of mitral regurgitation in patients with systolic dysfunction is associated with worsened prognosis, which in turn probably reflects both poorer LV function as well as the imposition of an extra volume overload on an already weakened LV.

Because all patients with secondary mitral regurgitation have heart failure, they should receive standard treatment for heart failure (Chapter 59). Many patients with secondary mitral regurgitation also have conducting system abnormalities, and patients with left bundle branch block may benefit from cardiac resynchronization therapy (Chapters 59 and 66), which improves systolic function while often reducing secondary mitral regurgitation, sometimes even eliminating it. When the above therapies fail to relieve symptoms, surgical treatment can be considered. Unlike in primary mitral regurgitation, it is unclear whether valve repair is superior to valve replacement, and it is also unclear whether mitral surgery prolongs life. Indeed, recent data from a randomized trial found no difference in overall outcome between repair and replacement for secondary mitral regurgitation. The average survival rate at 5 years is about 50%, and this figure has not changed much over the past several decades.

AORTIC REGURGITATION

DEFINITION

Aortic regurgitation is caused either by abnormalities of the aortic leaflets or by abnormalities of the proximal aortic root. Leaflet abnormalities causing aortic regurgitation include a bicuspid aortic valve,[17] infective endocarditis, and rheumatic heart disease; anorexigenic drugs have also been implicated. Common aortic root abnormalities that cause aortic regurgitation include Marfan syndrome (Chapter 260), hypertension-induced annuloaortic ectasia, aortic dissection (Chapter 78), syphilis (Chapter 319), ankylosing spondylitis (Chapter 265), and psoriatic arthritis (Chapter 265). Acute aortic regurgitation is usually caused by infective endocarditis (Chapter 76) or aortic dissection.

PATHOBIOLOGY

As with mitral regurgitation, aortic regurgitation imparts a volume overload on the LV because the LV must pump the forward flow entering from the LA and the regurgitant volume returning through the incompetent aortic valve. Also as with mitral regurgitation, the volume overload is compensated for by the development of eccentric cardiac hypertrophy, which increases chamber size and allows the ventricle to pump a greater total stroke volume and a greater forward stroke volume. Ventricular enlargement also allows the LV to accommodate the volume overload at a lower filling pressure. In contrast to mitral regurgitation, the entire stroke volume is ejected into the aorta in aortic regurgitation. Because pulse pressure is proportional to stroke volume and elastance of the aorta, the increased stroke volume increases systolic pressure. Systolic hypertension leads to afterload excess, which does not generally occur in mitral regurgitation. Accordingly, ventricular geometry also differs between mitral and aortic regurgitation because the afterload excess in aortic regurgitation causes a modest element of concentric hypertrophy, as well as severe eccentric hypertrophy.

In acute aortic insufficiency, such as might occur in infective endocarditis, severe volume overload of the previously unprepared LV results in a sudden fall in forward output while precipitously increasing LV filling pressure. It is probably this combination of pathophysiologic factors that leads to rapid decompensation, presumably because the severely diminished gradient for coronary blood flow causes ischemia and progressive deterioration in LV function. In acute aortic insufficiency, reflex vasoconstriction increases peripheral vascular resistance. In compensated chronic aortic insufficiency, vasoconstriction is absent, and vascular resistance may be reduced and contribute to the hyperdynamic circulation observed in these patients.

CLINICAL MANIFESTATIONS

The most common symptoms from chronic aortic regurgitation are those of left-sided heart failure, that is, dyspnea on exertion, orthopnea, and fatigue. In acute aortic regurgitation, cardiac output and shock may develop rapidly. The onset of symptoms in patients with chronic aortic regurgitation usually heralds the onset of LV systolic dysfunction. Some patients with symptoms have apparently normal systolic function, however, and the symptoms may be attributed to diastolic dysfunction. Other patients may have ventricular dysfunction yet remain asymptomatic.

Angina may also occur in patients with aortic insufficiency but less commonly than in those with aortic stenosis. The cause of angina in aortic regurgitation is probably multifactorial. Coronary blood flow reserve is reduced in some patients because diastolic runoff into the LV lowers aortic diastolic pressure while increasing LV diastolic pressure; these two influences lower the driving pressure gradient for flow across the coronary bed. When angina occurs in aortic regurgitation, it may be accompanied by flushing. Other symptoms include carotid artery pain and an unpleasant awareness of the heartbeat.

DIAGNOSIS

Physical Examination

Aortic regurgitation produces a myriad of signs because a hyperdynamic, enlarged LV ejects a large stroke volume at high pressure into the systemic

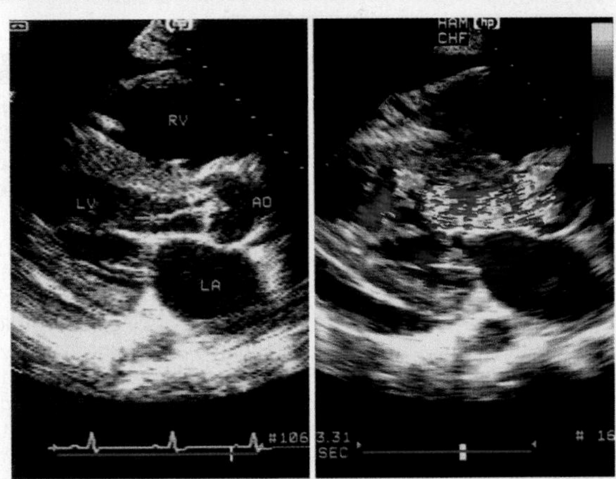

FIGURE 75-8. Echocardiogram of a patient with aortic regurgitation caused by infective endocarditis. The *left panel* shows a linear vegetation *(arrow)* prolapsing into the left ventricular (LV) outflow tract from the aortic valve leaflet in diastole. The *right panel* is a color-flow Doppler image exhibiting turbulent blood flow filling the LV tract during diastole. AO = aorta; LA = left atrium; RV = right ventricle. (Courtesy of Dr. Anthony DeMaria.)

circulation. Palpation of the precordium finds a hyperactive apical impulse displaced downward and to the left. S_1 and S_2 are usually normal. S_2 is followed by a diastolic blowing murmur heard best along the left sternal border with the patient sitting upright. In mild disease, the murmur may be short and heard only in the beginning of diastole when the gradient between the aorta and the LV is highest. As the disease worsens, the murmur may persist throughout diastole. A second murmur, a mitral valve rumble, is heard at the LV apex in patients with severe aortic insufficiency. Although the cause is still debated, this Austin Flint murmur is probably produced as the regurgitant jet impinges on the mitral valve and causes it to vibrate.

In chronic aortic regurgitation, the high stroke volume and reduced systemic arterial resistance result in a wide pulse pressure, which may generate a number of signs, including Corrigan pulse (sharp upstroke and rapid decline of the carotid pulse), de Musset sign (head bobbing), Duroziez sign (combined systolic and diastolic bruits created by compression of the femoral artery with the stethoscope), and Quincke pulse (systolic plethora and diastolic blanching in the nail bed when gentle traction is placed on the nail). Perhaps the most reliable of physical signs indicating severe aortic regurgitation is Hill sign, an increase in femoral systolic pressure of 40 mm Hg or more compared with systolic pressure in the brachial artery.

In contrast to chronic aortic insufficiency with its myriad clinical signs, acute aortic insufficiency may have a subtle manifestation. The eccentric hypertrophy, which compensates for chronic aortic insufficiency, has not yet had time to develop, and the large total stroke volume responsible for most of the signs of chronic aortic insufficiency is absent. The only clues to the presence of acute aortic insufficiency may be a short diastolic blowing murmur and reduced intensity of S_1. This latter sign occurs because high diastolic LV pressure closes the mitral valve early in diastole (mitral valve preclosure) so that when ventricular systole occurs, only the tricuspid component of S_1 is heard.

Noninvasive Evaluation

The ECG in patients with aortic insufficiency is nonspecific but almost always demonstrates LVH. The chest radiograph shows an enlarged heart, often with uncoiling and enlargement of the aortic root.

Echocardiography (Chapter 55) is the most important noninvasive tool for assessing the severity of aortic insufficiency and its impact on LV geometry and function (Fig. 75-8). During echocardiography, the LV end-diastolic dimension, end-systolic dimension, and fractional shortening are determined. Aortic valve anatomy and aortic root anatomy can be assessed and the cause of the aortic regurgitation can often be determined. Color-flow Doppler examination of the aortic valve helps quantify the severity of aortic regurgitation by assessing the depth and width to which the diastolic jet penetrates the LV. Another way to assess the severity of aortic regurgitation is the pressure half-time method: continuous-wave Doppler interrogation of the aortic valve displays the decay of the velocity of retrograde flow across the valve. In mild aortic insufficiency, the gradient across the valve is high throughout diastole, and its rate of decay is slow, with production of a long Doppler half-time (the time that it takes the velocity to decay from its peak to that value divided by the square root of 2). In severe aortic regurgitation, there is rapid equilibration between pressure in the aorta and pressure in the LV, and the Doppler half-time is short. If mitral valve preclosure is detected in acute aortic insufficiency, urgent surgery is necessary. In cases in which the severity of aortic insufficiency is in doubt, MRI can quantify regurgitant flow or catheterization with aortography can visualize regurgitant flow to resolve the issue.

TREATMENT AND PROGNOSIS Rx

Medical Therapy

Asymptomatic Patients with Normal Left Ventricular Function

Because aortic regurgitation increases LV afterload, which decreases cardiac efficiency, afterload reduction with nifedipine and other vasodilators, including ACE inhibitors and hydralazine, improves hemodynamics in the short term. Although initial data suggested that such therapy could delay or reduce the need for aortic valve surgery without any adverse effects when surgery is finally performed, more recent data suggest no benefit from such therapy. These discrepant results from relatively small trials preclude firm recommendations. When hypertension accompanies aortic regurgitation, it should be treated according to standard guidelines (Chapter 67).

Symptomatic Patients or Patients with Left Ventricular Dysfunction

Patients who have symptoms or manifest LV dysfunction should not be treated medically, except for short-term stabilization, but should undergo aortic valve surgery as soon as feasible.

Surgical Therapy

Acute Aortic Regurgitation

When any of the symptoms or signs of heart failure develop, even if mild, the medical mortality rate is high and approaches 75%. Echocardiographic evidence of preclosure of the mitral valve from high diastolic intracavitary LV pressure is an especially ominous sign. Therapy with vasodilators, such as nitroprusside, may temporarily improve the patient's condition before surgery but is never a substitute for surgery. In patients with acute aortic regurgitation caused by bacterial endocarditis (Chapter 76), surgery may be delayed to permit a full or partial course of antibiotics, but persistent, severe aortic regurgitation requires emergency valve replacement. Even when blood cultures have been positive recently and antibiotic therapy has been of brief duration, the valve reinfection rate is low, 0% to 10%, with valve replacement or valve repair. Emergency surgery should not be withheld simply because the duration of antibiotic therapy has been brief.

Chronic Aortic Regurgitation

Asymptomatic patients who manifest evidence of LV dysfunction benefit from surgery. Because loading conditions differ between aortic and mitral regurgitation, the objective markers for the presence of LV dysfunction also differ. In aortic regurgitation, when the ejection fraction is less than 0.50 or the end-systolic dimension is greater than 50 mm, postoperative outcome is impaired, presumably because these markers indicate that LV dysfunction has developed. Surgery should be performed before these benchmarks are reached. A calculated regurgitant orifice above 30 mm^2 portends a poorer prognosis and may warrant surgery.

Patients with advanced symptoms are at increased risk for a suboptimal surgical outcome regardless of whether they have evidence of LV dysfunction. Patients should undergo aortic valve replacement before symptoms impair lifestyle.

Although some patients may be able to undergo successful aortic valve repair to restore aortic valve competence, most patients require insertion of an aortic valve prosthesis.

TRICUSPID REGURGITATION

DEFINITION

Tricuspid regurgitation is usually secondary to a hemodynamic load on the RV rather than a structural valve deformity. Diseases that cause pulmonary hypertension, such as chronic obstructive airway disease or intracardiac shunts, lead to RV dilation and subsequent tricuspid regurgitation. Because most of the force that is needed to fill the LV is provided by the RV, LV dysfunction leading to elevated LV filling pressure also places the RV under a hemodynamic load and can eventually lead to RV failure and tricuspid regurgitation. In some instances, tricuspid regurgitation may be caused by pathology of the valve itself. The most common cause of primary tricuspid regurgitation is infective endocarditis, usually stemming from drug abuse and unsterile injections. Other causes include trauma (especially from hitting the steering wheel or dashboard in motor vehicle accidents), carcinoid syndrome, rheumatic involvement of the tricuspid valve, myxomatous degeneration, RV infarction, and mishaps during endomyocardial biopsy.

DIAGNOSIS

The symptoms of tricuspid regurgitation are those of right-sided heart failure and include ascites, edema, and occasionally right upper quadrant pain. On physical examination, tricuspid regurgitation produces jugular venous distention accentuated by a large v wave as blood is regurgitated into the RA during systole. Regurgitation into the hepatic veins causes hepatic enlargement and liver pulsation. RV enlargement is detected as a parasternal lift. Ascites and edema are common. The murmur of tricuspid regurgitation is a holosystolic murmur heard along the left sternal border, often increasing with inspiration. The murmur may be faint, and it usually can be heard only under the best auscultatory conditions.

The definitive diagnosis of tricuspid regurgitation is made during echocardiography. Doppler interrogation of the tricuspid valve shows systolic disturbance of the right atrial blood pool. Echocardiography (Chapter 55) can also be used to determine the severity of pulmonary hypertension, measure RV dilation, and assess whether the valve itself is intrinsically normal or abnormal.

TREATMENT AND PROGNOSIS Rx

Therapy for secondary tricuspid regurgitation is generally aimed at the cause of the lesion. If LV failure has been responsible for RV failure and tricuspid regurgitation, the standard therapy for improving LV failure (Chapter 59) lowers LV filling pressure, reduces secondary pulmonary hypertension, relieves some of the hemodynamic burden of the RV, and partially restores tricuspid valve competence. If pulmonary disease is the primary cause, therapy is directed toward improving lung function. Medical therapy directed at tricuspid regurgitation is usually limited to diuretics because the vasodilators that are so useful in the treatment of left-sided heart failure are often ineffective in treating pulmonary hypertension. However, a number of options can improve late-stage symptoms that are primarily caused by the pulmonary hypertension itself (Chapter 68).

Surgical intervention for the tricuspid valve is rarely entertained in isolation. However, if other cardiac surgery is planned in a patient with severe tricuspid regurgitation, concomitant ring annuloplasty or tricuspid valve repair is frequently attempted to ensure postoperative tricuspid competence. Because a second operation to address residual tricuspid regurgitation after successful left-sided valve surgery carries an unacceptably high mortality rate, concomitant tricuspid annuloplasty is now entertained for even mild to moderate tricuspid regurgitation during left-sided valve surgery. Tricuspid valve replacement is often not well tolerated and is rarely performed except when severe deformity, as is often seen in endocarditis or carcinoid disease, precludes valve repair.

PULMONIC STENOSIS

DEFINITION

Pulmonic stenosis is a congenital disease resulting from fusion of the pulmonic valve cusps (Chapter 69). It is usually detected and corrected during childhood, but occasionally cases are diagnosed for the first time in adulthood. Symptoms of pulmonic stenosis include angina and syncope. Occasionally, symptoms of right-sided heart failure develop. During physical examination, the uncalcified valve in pulmonic stenosis produces an early systolic ejection click on opening. During inspiration, the click diminishes or disappears because increased flow into the right side of the heart during inspiration partially opens the pulmonic valve in diastole so that systole causes less of an opening sound. The click is followed by a systolic ejection murmur that radiates to the base of the heart. If the transvalvular gradient is severe, RVH develops and produces a parasternal lift.

The diagnosis of pulmonic stenosis is confirmed by echocardiography, which quantifies the transvalvular gradient and the degree of RVH and dysfunction.

TREATMENT AND PROGNOSIS Rx

In asymptomatic patients with a gradient less than 25 mm Hg, no therapy is required. If symptoms develop or the gradient exceeds 50 mm Hg, balloon commissurotomy is effective in reducing the gradient and relieving symptoms. Although long-term prognosis is not yet established, 90% of patients do not require reintervention 10 years after balloon therapy.

Postoperative Care of Patients with Substitute Heart Valves

After a prosthetic valve has been inserted, a baseline echocardiogram should be obtained to provide a reference point in the event that valve dysfunction is suspected at a later date. Echocardiography does not need to be repeated unless there is a change in clinical status or physical findings. The major causes of mechanical valve dysfunction are infective endocarditis and thrombus formation. For bioprostheses, endocarditis is also a risk, but valve degeneration, which can cause either stenosis or regurgitation, is a major concern.

Whenever a patient with a prosthetic heart valve has a temperature higher than 100° F, endocarditis must be excluded by blood culture; for fever with signs of sepsis, broad-spectrum antibiotics must be begun while awaiting culture results. For patients with bioprosthetic valves, mechanical prostheses, and homografts, endocarditis prophylaxis should be instituted at the time of procedures that are associated with a high risk for bacteremia (Chapter 76). Whether prophylaxis is necessary for pulmonary autografts is currently unclear, but physicians usually prescribe prophylaxis for these patients.

All patients with a mechanical heart valve require anticoagulation.[18] Recommended INR values range from 2.0 for a young normotensive patient in sinus rhythm with an aortic valve prosthesis to 3.5 for a patient with atrial fibrillation and a mitral valve prosthesis. Aspirin, 325 mg, is recommended in addition to warfarin to reduce the risk for valve thrombosis in patients who have mechanical prosthetic valves that are at higher risk for thromboembolic complications. Newer anticoagulants such as dabigatran are associated with more thrombosis and bleeding in patients with mechanical prosthetic valves[A9] and should not be used. When thrombosis occurs on a prosthetic valve, about 60% of patients can have restored valve function after intravenous infusion of a thrombolytic agent.[19] In patients with periprosthetic paravalvular leaks, a percutaneous procedure can successfully close about 85% of the leaks.[20]

Choices among Prosthetic Valves

Different types of prosthetic valves (Fig. 75-9) have different advantages and disadvantages (Table 75-2). At long-term follow-up, primary valve failure with resulting need for reoperation is much more common with bioprosthetic valves,[A10][A11] and bleeding is generally more common with mechanical valves. For mitral valves, long-term survival is similar with bioprosthetic and mechanical valves. Survival after aortic valve replacement is probably better with mechanical valves. Another alternative is to use the patient's own pulmonic valve to replace the diseased aortic valve and then to implant a prosthetic pulmonic valve (the Ross procedure). In a randomized trial, this procedure was superior to homograft valve and root replacement, with a 10-year survival rate of 97% compared with 83%.[A12]

In general, a tissue valve is recommended in patients who have a life expectancy of less than 15 years or who are unable or unwilling to maintain warfarin anticoagulation. A mechanical valve is preferred in patients who already have another indication for anticoagulation or who have a longer life expectancy and want to minimize the risk of reoperation. Because many patients prefer the risk of reoperation to that of anticoagulation, the age at which bioprostheses are implanted has steadily declined, and many 60-year-old patients now request and receive a bioprosthetic valve.

TABLE 75-2 ADVANTAGES AND DISADVANTAGES OF SUBSTITUTE CARDIAC VALVES

TYPE OF VALVE	ADVANTAGES	DISADVANTAGES
Bioprosthesis (Carpentier-Edwards, Hancock)	Avoids anticoagulation in patients with sinus rhythm	Durability limited to 10-15 yr Relatively stenotic
Mechanical valves (St. Jude, Medtronic-Hall, Starr-Edwards)	Good flow characteristics in small sizes Durable	Require anticoagulation
Homografts and autografts	Anticoagulation not required Durability increased over that of bioprostheses	Surgical implantation technically demanding

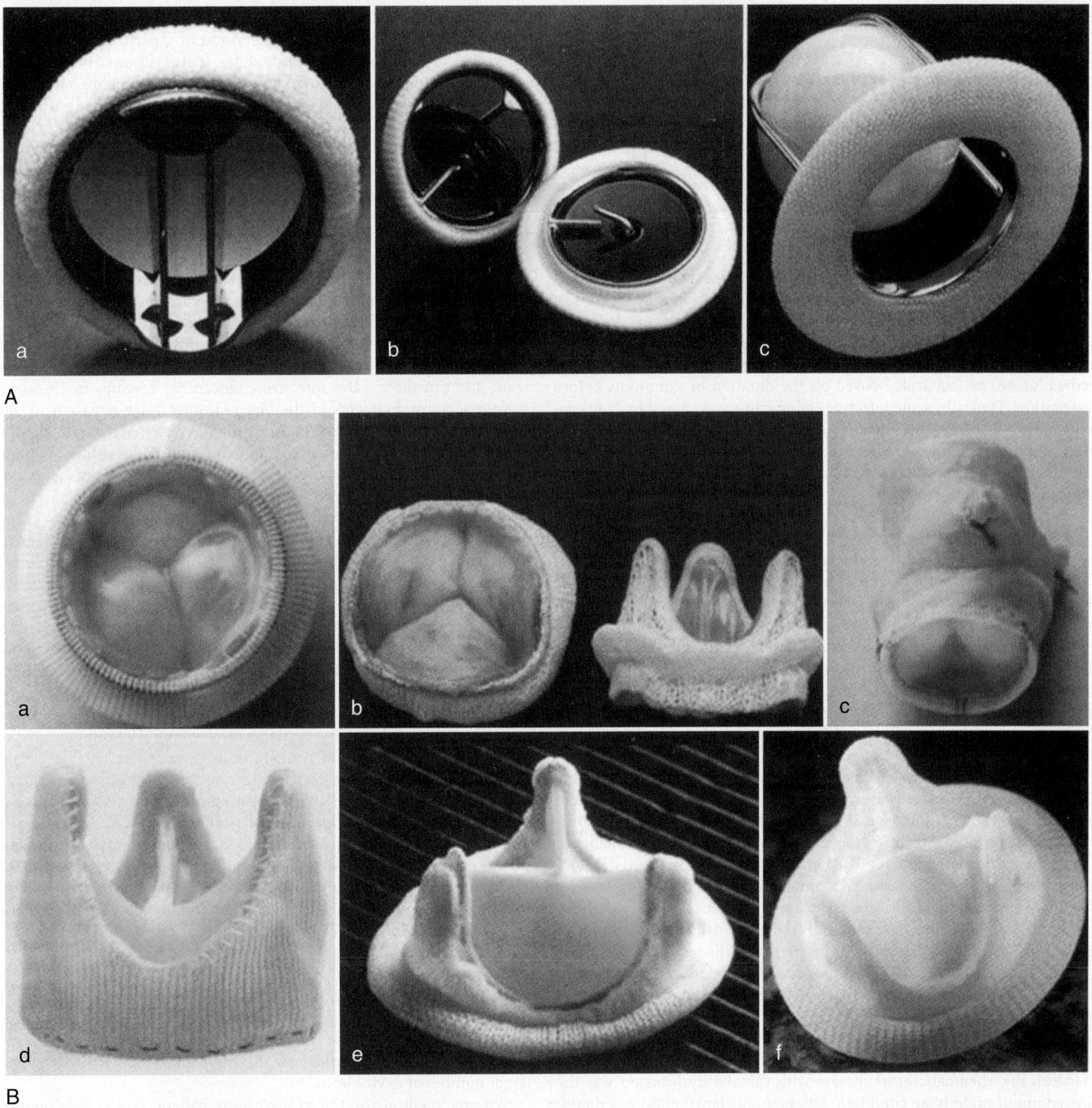

FIGURE 75-9. A, Common mechanical valves: ***a***, a bileaflet St. Jude Medical valve; ***b***, a Medtronic-Hall tilting disc valve; ***c***, a Starr-Edwards ball cage valve (no longer manufactured but still in use). (From Antunes MJ, Burke AP, Carabello B. Valvular heart disease. In: Braunwald E, Rahimtoola SH, eds. *Essential Atlas of Heart Diseases*. 3rd ed. Philadelphia: Current Medicine Group; 2005:296-297.) B, Common bioprostheses: ***a***, Hancock modified orifice stented valve; ***b***, Carpentier-Edwards stented porcine valve; ***c***, Medtronic free style stentless valve; ***d***, St. Jude Medical Toronto SPV stentless valve; ***e***, Carpentier-Edwards pericardial valve; ***f***, Autologous pericardial valve. (From Grunkemeier GL, Rahimtoola SH, Starr A. Prosthetic heart valves. In: Rahimtoola SH, ed. *Valvular Heart Disease*. Philadelphia: Current Medicine Group; 1997:13.9-13.11.)

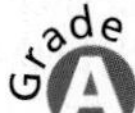

Grade A References

A1. Rossebø AB, Pedersen TR, Boman K, et al. Intensive lipid lowering with simvastatin and ezetimibe in aortic stenosis. *N Engl J Med.* 2008;359:1343-1356.

A2. Leon MB, Smith CR, Mack M, et al. Transcatheter aortic-valve implantation for aortic stenosis in patients who cannot undergo surgery. *N Engl J Med.* 2010;363:1597-1607.

A3. Makkar RR, Fontana GP, Jilaihawi H, et al. Transcatheter aortic-valve replacement for inoperable severe aortic stenosis. *N Engl J Med.* 2012;366:1696-1704.

A4. Kodali SK, Williams MR, Smith CR, et al. Two-year outcomes after transcatheter or surgical aortic-valve replacement. *N Engl J Med.* 2012;366:1686-1695.

A5. Adams DH, Popma JJ, Reardon MJ, et al. Transcatheter aortic-valve replacement with a self-expanding prosthesis. *N Engl J Med.* 2014;370:1790-1798.

A6. Acker MA, Parides MK, Perrault LP, et al. Mitral-valve repair versus replacement for severe ischemic mitral regurgitation. *N Engl J Med.* 2014;370:23-32.

A7. Smith PK, Puskas JD, Ascheim DD, et al. Surgical treatment of moderate ischemic mitral regurgitation. *N Engl J Med.* 2014;371:2178-2188.

A8. Mauri L, Foster E, Glower DD, et al. 4-year results of a randomized controlled trial of percutaneous repair versus surgery for mitral regurgitation. *J Am Coll Cardiol.* 2013;62:317-328.

A9. Eikelboom JW, Connolly SJ, Brueckmann M, et al. Dabigatran versus warfarin in patients with mechanical heart valves. *N Engl J Med.* 2013;369:1206-1214.

A10. Hammermeister K, Sethi GK, Henderson WG, et al. Outcomes 15 years after valve replacement with a mechanical versus a bioprosthetic valve: final report of the Veterans Affairs randomized trial. *J Am Coll Cardiol.* 2000;36:1152-1158.

A11. Stassano P, Di Tommaso L, Monaco M, et al. Aortic valve replacement: a prospective randomized evaluation of mechanical versus biological valves in patients ages 55 to 70 years. *J Am Coll Cardiol.* 2009;54:1862-1868.

A12. El-Hamamsy I, Eryigit Z, Stevens LM, et al. Long-term outcomes after autograft versus homograft aortic root replacement in adults with aortic valve disease: a randomised controlled trial. *Lancet.* 2010;376:524-531.

GENERAL REFERENCES

For the General References and other additional features, please visit Expert Consult at https://expertconsult.inkling.com.

76 INFECTIVE ENDOCARDITIS

VANCE G. FOWLER, JR., ARNOLD S. BAYER, AND
LARRY M. BADDOUR

DEFINITION

Infective endocarditis is defined as an infection, usually bacterial, of the endocardial surface of the heart. Infective endocarditis affects primarily the cardiac valves, although in some cases, the septa between the chambers, the mural endocardium, or cardiovascular implantable electronic devices (e.g., pacemakers) may be involved. Traditionally, infective endocarditis was categorized as "acute" or "subacute," based on the duration of symptoms before presentation. Typically, acute infective endocarditis was caused by *Staphylococcus aureus*, and subacute infective endocarditis was caused by viridans group streptococci. However, these categories have proven to be unreliable. A classification that considers the causative organism and the involved valve is much more clinically relevant.

EPIDEMIOLOGY

The true incidence of infective endocarditis is difficult to determine because of the different criteria for diagnosis and methods of reporting. An analysis based on strict case definitions reveals that only a relatively small proportion (≈20%) of clinically diagnosed cases are categorized as "definite." In 10 large surveys, infective endocarditis accounted for approximately one case per 1000 U.S. hospital admissions, with a range of 0.16 to 5.4 cases per 1000 admissions. Estimates from the American Heart Association (AHA) place the incidence of infective endocarditis in the United States at 10,000 to 20,000 new cases per year. Recent data also suggest that rates of *S. aureus* infective endocarditis have increased significantly.

Men are more commonly affected than women (mean male : female ratio, 1.7 : 1 in 18 large series). However, in patients younger than 35 years, more cases occur in women. More than 50% of patients with infective endocarditis in the U.S. are now older than 50 years of age, due in part to the low incidence of acute rheumatic heart disease (Chapter 290), the low subsequent development of rheumatic heart disease, and a simultaneous rise in the prevalence of degenerative valvular heart disease in the aging population.

Although some patients have no clearly definable risk factor for endocarditis, cardiac conditions that cause turbulent flow at the endocardial surface or across a valve (Chapter 75) predispose patients to infective endocarditis (Table 76-1). The most commonly affected valves in descending order of prevalence are the mitral valve only, the aortic valve, the mitral and aortic valves together, the tricuspid valve, mixed right- and left-sided infection, and the pulmonic valve.

Historically, rheumatic heart disease with valvular dysfunction was the most common underlying condition, although its contribution has diminished in the antibiotic era, especially in developed countries. Degenerative valvular disease is also associated with infective endocarditis, particularly in elderly patients; the increasing relevance of senile calcification as a risk factor is reflected in the increasing proportion of aortic valve involvement in infective endocarditis. Most significant congenital heart defects (Chapter 69) confer an increased risk of infective endocarditis, particularly complex cyanotic disease such as single-ventricle states, transposition of the great vessels, and tetralogy of Fallot. Similarly, surgically constructed pulmonary–systemic shunts and ventricular septal defects are risk factors associated with infective endocarditis.

TABLE 76-1 PREDISPOSING CONDITIONS ASSOCIATED WITH INCREASED RISK OF ENDOCARDITIS

MORE COMMON	LESS COMMON
Mitral valve prolapse	Rheumatic heart disease†
Degenerative valvular disease	Idiopathic hypertrophic subaortic stenosis
Intravenous drug use*	Pulmonary–systemic shunts*
Prosthetic valve*	Coarctation of the aorta
Congenital (valvular heart disease or ventricular septal defect)	Previous endocarditis*
	Complex cyanotic congenital heart disease*

*Indicates conditions with highest risk for endocarditis.
†Still common in developing countries.

Mitral valve prolapse is currently the most common underlying cardiac condition in patients with infective endocarditis, a statistic that reflects its prevalence in the general population (4%). Notably, mitral valve prolapse is a risk only in patients with thickened mitral leaflets or significant regurgitation, in which case the risk of endocarditis increases by about 10-fold over that of the general population. In addition, patients with hypertrophic cardiomyopathy are at increased risk of infective endocarditis, particularly in the presence of outflow obstruction. Finally, previous endocarditis is among the highest risk factors for subsequent infective endocarditis cases.

Prosthetic cardiac valves represent an important risk factor for infective endocarditis. More than 150,000 heart valves are implanted annually worldwide, and prosthetic valve infective endocarditis develops in 1% to 4% of prosthetic valve recipients in the first year after valve replacement and in approximately 0.8% of recipients annually thereafter. Mechanical prosthetic valves may initially be more susceptible to infective endocarditis, but bioprosthetic valves are more likely to develop infective endocarditis after 1 year; overall, the rate is similar with either type of valve.

The incidence of infective endocarditis in injection drug users (Chapter 34) may be 30 times higher than in the general population and four times higher than in adults with rheumatic heart disease. In some areas of the United States, injection drug use is the most common predisposing cause of infective endocarditis in patients younger than 40 years. *S. aureus* is the predominant organism, and tricuspid valve involvement is noted in 78% of cases, mitral involvement in 24%, and aortic involvement in 8%. More than one valve is infected in approximately 20% of cases, and some of these infections are polymicrobial.

Health care–associated infective endocarditis arises primarily as a consequence of invasive therapies, including intravenous (IV) catheters, hyperalimentation lines, pacemakers, other cardiovascular implantable electronic devices, and hemodialysis devices.[1] In a recent prospective, multinational cohort study of more than 1600 non–drug-using patients with native valve endocarditis, more than one third of patients had health care–associated endocarditis, many of which originated in the community (e.g., in patients on outpatient hemodialysis). The emerging importance of health care–associated infective endocarditis in industrialized nations has also influenced the microbiology of the disease, with an increasing prevalence of *S. aureus* and a decreasing prevalence of viridans group streptococci in much of the industrialized world.

Cardiovascular electronic devices can become infected at the time they are implanted, particularly if patients develop complications, such as a hematoma, at the incision site or need the device to be revised or replaced. Other factors that increase the risk of device infection include older age, comorbid conditions (particularly dialysis-dependent renal failure), and a larger number of device leads.[1,2]

Systemic medical conditions predispose patients to the development of infective endocarditis. For example, HIV infection is an independent risk factor for the development of infective endocarditis in injection drug users, with the risk increasing as the CD4 count decreases. Vascular catheter–related bacteremia is an important risk factor for nosocomial infective endocarditis. Patients with end-stage renal disease, particularly those receiving long-term hemodialysis, and patients with diabetes mellitus are also at increased risk, presumably because of the recurrent vascular access infections associated with the former and the low-level immunosuppression associated with both conditions.

PATHOBIOLOGY

Experimental models of infective endocarditis have demonstrated that the disease follows a predictable sequence: endocardial damage, aggregation of platelets and fibrin to create a sterile vegetation, transient bacteremia resulting in seeding of the vegetation, microbial proliferation on and invasion of the endocardial surface, and metastatic infection to visceral organs (e.g., kidneys, spleen) and brain.

Most cases of infective endocarditis begin with a damaged endocardial surface. Damage to the endocardium may be caused by a number of factors, ranging from inflammatory (e.g., rheumatic fever) to congenital (e.g., mitral valve prolapse) to senile degeneration and calcification; indeed, any excessive turbulence or high-pressure gradient can cause injury to the nearby endocardium. Next, fibrin-platelet aggregates develop at the site of damage to form sterile vegetations, also termed *nonbacterial thrombotic endocarditis*. Nonbacterial thrombotic endocarditis may occur spontaneously in patients with systemic illnesses (e.g., the marantic endocarditis of malignancy [Chapter 60] or other wasting diseases or Libman-Sacks endocarditis in systemic lupus erythematosus [Chapter 266]). When transient bacteremia occurs—for example, as a result of distant infection or gingival manipulations—the previously sterile vegetation may be seeded. Some bacterial species, such as staphylococci and streptococci, are more avidly adherent to vegetations and better able to evade innate endovascular host defenses, so they more frequently cause endocarditis. The bacteria then proliferate within the vegetation and may ultimately achieve an organism load of 10^9 to 10^{11} colony-forming units per gram of tissue. Last, the surfaces of cardiac valves and vegetations are avascular, thereby making antibiotic therapy and healing difficult. Implantable cardiac devices disrupt the endothelial surface and predispose to infection and the formation of biofilms, particularly early after their placement and before endothelialization and fibrosis occur.

CLINICAL MANIFESTATIONS

History

The initial presentation of infective endocarditis varies enormously from patient to patient. Some cases develop acutely, with symptoms progressing rapidly over several days. Other cases develop insidiously and present with progressive but nonspecific symptoms for weeks or months. In patients suspected of having infective endocarditis, the initial history should include a complete review of systems, a travel history, and a thorough discussion of health-related behaviors such as illicit drug use and sexual activity. Most patients complain of fever and nonspecific constitutional symptoms such as fatigue, malaise, or weight loss. Nearly 50% of patients complain of musculoskeletal symptoms ranging from frank arthritis to diffuse myalgias. In about 5% to 10% of patients, low back pain is the chief complaint, even in the absence of osteomyelitis or epidural abscess. In IV drug users with tricuspid valve infective endocarditis and patients with venous or right heart implantable devices, endocarditis can present as pleuritic chest pain and multilobar pneumonia. Health care–associated infective endocarditis is more likely to be clinically occult and requires a high index of suspicion.

Physical Examination

A thorough physical examination should include a search for the peripheral stigmata (Table 76-2), which are very helpful when present but are less frequent now than in the past. Although fever is present in up to 90% of patients, it is less common in elderly patients and in patients with renal or heart failure. A widened pulse pressure should alert the clinician to the possibility of acute aortic insufficiency (Chapter 75). The skin and nails should be carefully examined for suggestive but nonspecific embolic phenomena such as petechiae (Fig. 76-1), Osler nodes, Janeway lesions, and splinter hemorrhages. Petechiae are most often found on the conjunctiva, palate, and extremities. Osler nodes are small, painful nodules found most often on the palmar surfaces of the fingers and toes; they frequently wax and wane (Fig. 76-2). Classically considered to be an immunologic phenomenon, Osler nodes may have an immune complex–mediated component but are most likely initiated by microemboli. Janeway lesions (Fig. 51-11 in Chapter 51) are hemorrhagic, nonpainful macules also found primarily on the palms and soles; they are embolic in origin and are less frequently noted than the other cutaneous stigmata. Splinter hemorrhages (see Fig. 51-11 in Chapter 51) are nonblanching, linear, brownish red lesions in the nail beds parallel to the direction of nail growth; they are nonspecific and may also be found in a significant percentage of hospitalized patients without infective endocarditis.

Funduscopic examination should be performed to look for Roth spots (see Fig. 423-28 in Chapter 423), chorioretinitis, or endophthalmitis; the latter two are present in a substantial proportion of cases of fungal endocarditis. A careful cardiac examination should be performed to detect any systolic or diastolic murmurs, especially new murmurs, or evidence of heart failure, which is an ominous sign. Of note, patients with health care–associated infective endocarditis are less likely than others to have a pathologic murmur on initial presentation. The abdomen should be examined for evidence of splenomegaly (Chapter 168), which is more common in patients with subacute endocarditis. Finally, a thorough neurologic examination should be performed, both to assess for any focal neurologic deficits and to serve as a baseline during the patient's hospital stay. The neurologic examination may demonstrate evidence of major vessel embolism, cranial nerve palsies, visual field defects, or generalized toxic-metabolic encephalopathy with altered mental status. Up to 15% to 20% of patients with endocarditis have a stroke before presentation or during the course of their disease. Patients with device-related infective endocarditis often have local signs and symptoms of infection at the site of implantation.

TABLE 76-2 PHYSICAL EXAMINATION AND LABORATORY FINDINGS IN INFECTIVE ENDOCARDITIS

FINDING	% OF CASES
Fever	96
Worsening of previous murmur	20
New murmur	48
Vascular embolic event	17
Splenomegaly	11
Splinter hemorrhages	8
Osler nodes	3
Janeway lesions	5
Roth spots	2
Elevated ESR	61
Hematuria	26
Positive rheumatoid factor	5
Abnormal chest radiography findings (effusion, infiltrate, septic emboli)	67-85 (right-sided infective endocarditis)

ESR = erythrocyte sedimentation rate.
Adapted from Murdoch DR, Corey GR, Hoen B, et al. Clinical presentation, etiology, and outcome of infective endocarditis in the 21st century: International Collaboration on Endocarditis—Prospective Cohort Study. *Arch Intern Med.* 2009;169:463-473.

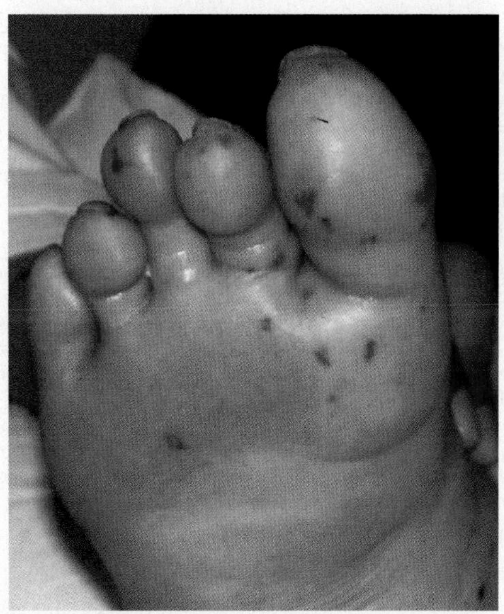

FIGURE 76-1. Petechiae in infective endocarditis.

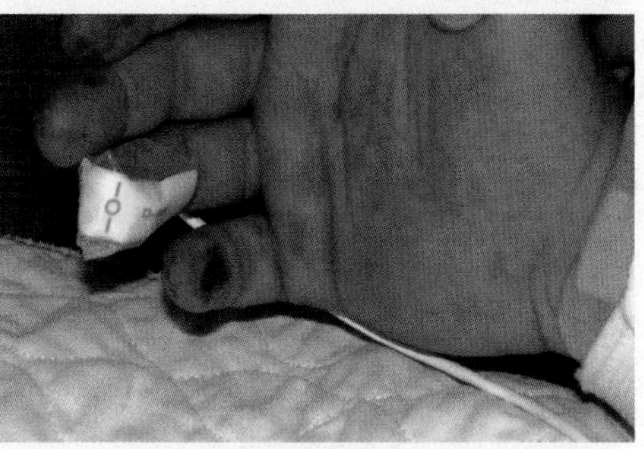

FIGURE 76-2. Osler node in infective endocarditis.

DIAGNOSIS

The "gold standard" for the diagnosis of infective endocarditis is culture of a pathologic organism from a valve or other endocardial surface. However, unless the patient undergoes valve replacement or postmortem examination, the diagnosis is made clinically. The most widely accepted clinical criteria are the modified Duke criteria (Table 76-3), which rely heavily on blood culture results and echocardiographic data and which have an estimated 76% to 100% sensitivity and 88% to 100% specificity, with a negative predictive value of at least 92%.[3,4]

Microbiology

At least three sets of blood cultures, each set consisting of one aerobic and one anaerobic bottle, should be obtained from separate sites, with careful attention to aseptic technique. Ideally, these sets should be collected at least 1 hour apart to document continuous bacteremia; however, when patients are critically ill, this approach may not be feasible.

Causative Organisms

About 90% of community-acquired, native valve infective endocarditis is caused by staphylococci, streptococci, or enterococci, which are normal inhabitants of the skin, oropharynx, and urogenital tract, respectively, and which have frequent access to the blood stream. These organisms express specific receptors for attachment and adherence to damaged endothelial surfaces. Streptococcal species (Chapter 290) are the most common cause of community-acquired infective endocarditis in patients with no history of injection drug use or health care contact. In patients with either of these latter epidemiologic risk factors, *S. aureus* (Chapter 288) is the predominant cause of infective endocarditis. Because of the emergence of health care contact as the predominant risk factor for blood stream infections, *S. aureus* is now the most common cause of infective endocarditis in most industrialized regions of the world.

Viridans group streptococci (Chapter 290) are the most common streptococci implicated in native valve endocarditis. This group of organisms, which normally inhabit the oropharynx, includes species such as *Streptococcus sanguis, Streptococcus mutans,* and *Streptococcus mitis.* Group B streptococci, β-hemolytic organisms that are also normal oropharyngeal and urogenital flora most frequently cause infective endocarditis in patients with cirrhosis or diabetes mellitus, as well as in injection drug users. In contrast, group A streptococci, although also β-hemolytic, rarely cause infective endocarditis. *Streptococcus gallolyticus,* a group D streptococcus (previously known as *Streptococcus bovis*), is now a leading cause of infective endocarditis in some parts of the world; for example, its incidence in France has increased significantly in recent years. Its presence in blood cultures should prompt endoscopic evaluation for adenocarcinoma of the colon or other malignant lesions of the gastrointestinal tract.

Pneumococcal endocarditis is decreasing in incidence but is quite fulminant when it occurs. It is associated with high morbidity and mortality rates, especially when it occurs as part of Austrian (or Osler) pneumococcal endocarditis triad of bacteremia, pneumonia, and meningitis.

S. aureus (Chapter 288) is the pathogen of primary concern among injection drug users and patients with health care contact. The clinical course of *S. aureus* endocarditis is typically acute, with a rapid progression over the course of days. Because about 10% to 15% of patients with *S. aureus* bacteremia have echocardiographic evidence of endocarditis even in the absence of classic stigmata, possible cardiac involvement should always be considered in any patient with *S. aureus* bacteremia but especially in patients with relapsing or persistent bacteremia or fever, community-acquired infection, or an implantable cardiac device. Coagulase-negative staphylococci are a relatively uncommon cause of native valve endocarditis but are important pathogens in prosthetic valve endocarditis.

Enterococcal bacteremia is far more common, particularly in hospitalized patients, than enterococcal endocarditis. However, enterococci are responsible for a significant number of cases of both community-acquired and nosocomial endocarditis. In most cases, the source of the bacteremia is thought to be the genitourinary tract, and the presentation is usually subacute. Enterococcal endocarditis, as opposed to enterococcal bacteremia, is suggested by community acquisition of infection, the absence of a clear source of infection, preexistent valvular heart disease, and the absence of polymicrobial bacteremia. As in most enterococcal infections, the overwhelming majority of cases (>90%) are caused by *Enterococcus faecalis.*

The HACEK group of gram-negative organisms (*Haemophilus* spp., *Aggregatibacter* spp. [formerly *Actinobacillus actinomycetemcomitans*], *Cardiobacterium hominis, Eikenella corrodens,* and *Kingella* spp.) accounts for about 5% of endocarditis cases. Because these fastidious organisms usually grow in blood cultures within 7 days using current methods, prolonged incubation is no longer required to isolate HACEK strains. Many other gram-negative bacilli have been reported to cause infective endocarditis but are even more unusual. Traditionally, injection drug use has been regarded as the primary risk factor for enteric gram-negative bacterial endocarditis. However, recent experience from large multinational studies shows that health care contact, not injection drug use, is the most common risk factor for enteric gram-negative endocarditis.

Fungal endocarditis is often difficult to diagnose and treat; it is most commonly found in patients with a history of injection drug use, recent cardiac valve surgery, or prolonged use of indwelling vascular catheters, especially those used for total parenteral nutrition. The most common fungi found in infective endocarditis are *Aspergillus* and *Candida* spp. *Aspergillus* (Chapter 339) rarely grows in blood cultures and must usually be cultured from a pathologic specimen (either an embolic site or vegetation); by contrast, *Candida* spp. (Chapter 338) frequently grows in blood cultures. Mortality is very high, and valve replacement surgery is usually necessary for fungal endocarditis.

TABLE 76-3 MODIFIED DUKE CRITERIA FOR THE DIAGNOSIS OF INFECTIVE ENDOCARDITIS

MAJOR CRITERIA

1. Blood culture positive
   a. Typical organism (α-hemolytic streptococcus, *Streptococcus bovis,* HACEK organisms, or community-acquired *Staphylococcus aureus* or enterococcus without a primary focus) from 2 separate blood cultures
   Or
   b. Persistent bacteremia with any organism (two positive cultures >12 hr apart or three positive cultures or a majority of ≥4 cultures positive >1 hr apart)
   Or
   c. Bacteremia with *S. aureus,* regardless of whether the bacteremia was nosocomially acquired or whether a removable focus of infection is found
2. Evidence of endocardial involvement
   a. Echocardiographic findings: mobile mass attached to valve or valve apparatus, abscess, or new partial dehiscence of prosthetic valve
   b. New valvular regurgitation
3. Serology: single positive blood culture for *Coxiella burnetii* or antiphase 1 IgG antibody titer >1 : 800

MINOR CRITERIA

1. Predisposing condition: IV drug use or predisposing cardiac condition
2. Fever ≥38° C
3. Vascular phenomena: arterial embolism, septic pulmonary emboli, mycotic aneurysm, intracranial hemorrhage, conjunctival hemorrhages, Janeway lesions
4. Immunologic phenomena: glomerulonephritis, Osler nodes, Roth spots, rheumatoid factor
5. Echocardiogram findings consistent with endocarditis but not meeting major criteria
6. Microbiologic evidence: positive blood cultures not meeting major criteria or serologic evidence of active infection consistent with endocarditis

DEFINITIVE INFECTIVE ENDOCARDITIS

1. Pathologically proven infective endocarditis
   Or
2. Clinical criteria meeting
   a. Two major criteria *or*
   b. One major and one minor criteria *or*
   c. Three minor criteria

POSSIBLE INFECTIVE ENDOCARDITIS

Findings that fall short of definitive infective endocarditis but do not reject it

REJECTED INFECTIVE ENDOCARDITIS

1. Firm alternative diagnosis *or*
2. Resolution of infective endocarditis syndrome with antibiotic therapy for ≤4 days *or*
3. No pathologic evidence of infective endocarditis at surgery or autopsy with antibiotic therapy for ≤4 days

HACEK = *Haemophilus* spp., *Aggregatibacter* spp. (formerly *Actinobacillus actinomycetemcomitans*), *Cardiobacterium hominis, Eikenella corrodens,* and *Kingella* spp.; IgG = immunoglobulin G; IV = intravenous.

Adapted from Li JS, Sexton DJ, Mick N, et al. Proposed modifications to the Duke criteria for the diagnosis of infective endocarditis. *Clin Infect Dis.* 2000;30:633-638.

Prosthetic valve endocarditis can be classified into one of two groups based on the time between valve surgery and disease onset: *early* (<2 months after surgery) and *late* (>2 months) (Table 76-4). Staphylococci, particularly *S. aureus*, predominate during the early period, when most episodes of infective endocarditis are thought to be related to perioperative infection. In the late period, the spectrum of organisms becomes more akin to that of community-acquired native valve disease, in which *S. aureus* and viridans group streptococci predominate. Of note, among the coagulase-negative staphylococci, oxacillin resistance can be seen in these late cases.

Staphylococcal species account for the large majority (≥70%) of implantable cardiac device infections. The prevalence of oxacillin resistance among *S. aureus* strains varies from study to study but is generally in the 30% to 50% range.

Endocarditis with Negative Blood Cultures

In most patients with infective endocarditis who have not received previous antibiotic therapy, every blood culture is positive because the bacteremia of endocarditis is continuous. Blood cultures are truly negative in fewer than 5% of cases of endocarditis; however, prior antibiotic administration may decrease the yield of blood cultures by up to 35%. Accordingly, most "culture-negative" cases of endocarditis occur in patients who have recently received antimicrobial agents. These cases are probably caused by the same organisms responsible for most native valve endocarditis; viridans group streptococci and the HACEK organisms are the most likely suspects because they are much more fastidious than staphylococci and enterococci and are therefore more likely to be affected by previous antibiotic administration. Ultimately, however, when blood cultures are negative and endocarditis is suspected, especially when a history of recent antimicrobial treatment is lacking, consideration should be given to fastidious organisms, fungi, and noncultivatable organisms (Table 76-5), particularly when the patient's history suggests exposure to farm animals or unpasteurized milk (*Coxiella burnetii, Brucella* spp.), cats (*Bartonella henselae*), body lice (*Bartonella quintana*), or birds (*Chlamydia psittaci*). It is important to notify the microbiology laboratory that endocarditis is suspected because special culture techniques can increase the yield for the HACEK species, nutritionally variant streptococci (*Abiotrophia* and *Granulicatella* spp.), *Brucella* spp., *Legionella* spp., and some fungi. The traditional practice of holding blood cultures for 2 to 4 weeks is no longer required routinely. Specific serologic tests can diagnose endocarditis related to *C. burnetii* (the agent of Q fever), *Brucella* spp., *Bartonella* spp., and *C. psittaci*. *Tropheryma whippelii*, the etiologic agent in Whipple disease, and multiple other organisms may be diagnosed by polymerase chain reaction. Histopathologic features of resected tissue also can provide clues in the etiologic diagnosis of culture-negative endocarditis. If the search for a causative organism is fruitless, noninfectious causes such as marantic or Libman-Sacks endocarditis and atrial myxoma (Chapter 60) should be considered.

TABLE 76-4 CAUSES OF PROSTHETIC VALVE ENDOCARDITIS*

EARLY (<2 mo POSTOPERATIVELY)	LATE (>2 mo POSTOPERATIVELY)
Staphylococcus aureus	Coagulase-negative staphylococci
Coagulase-negative staphylococci	*Staphylococcus aureus*
Gram-negative bacilli	Viridans group streptococci
Enterococci	Enterococci
Fungi	
Diphtheroids	

*Listed in order of relative frequency.
Adapted from Wang A, Athan E, Pappas PA, et al. Contemporary clinical profile and outcome of prosthetic valve endocarditis. *JAMA*. 2007; 297:1354-1361.

Laboratory Findings

Initial laboratory tests should include a complete blood count with differential, serum electrolytes, measurement of renal function, and urinalysis. Most patients with subacute infective endocarditis have the serum iron profile of anemia of chronic disease (Chapter 159). The white blood cell count is frequently elevated in acute infective endocarditis, particularly if *S. aureus* is the causative organism, but may not be elevated in more subacute forms. Microscopic hematuria is common, as is proteinuria.

The chest radiograph is abnormal—demonstrating consolidation, atelectasis, pleural effusion, or clear septic emboli—in the overwhelming majority of patients with right-sided endocarditis. In others, it may show evidence of heart failure. The electrocardiogram (ECG) should be carefully examined for evidence of atrioventricular conduction blocks, especially a prolonged PR interval (see Figs. 64-5 through 64-9 in Chapter 64), suggestive of an aortic ring abscess or frank myocardial infarction (see Figs. 73-1 and 73-2 in Chapter 73).

Rheumatoid factor, which is an ancillary test that has been included in the modified Duke criteria as a "minor criterion" in the category of "immunologic phenomenon," may be positive in subacute or chronic endocarditis. Other ancillary tests, such as the erythrocyte sedimentation rate, the C-reactive

TABLE 76-5 ORGANISMS CAUSING "CULTURE-NEGATIVE" ENDOCARDITIS*

ORGANISM	EPIDEMIOLOGY	DIAGNOSTIC TESTS
HACEK spp.	Mostly oral flora, so often history of periodontal disease	May require up to 7 days to grow
Nutritionally variant streptococci	Slow and indolent course	Supplemented culture media or growth as satellite colonies around *Staphylococcus aureus* streak
Coxiella burnetii (Q fever)	Worldwide; exposure to raw milk, farm environment, or rural areas	Serologic tests (high titers of antibody to both phase 1 and phase 2 antigens); also PCR on blood or valve tissue
Brucella spp.	Ingestion of contaminated milk or milk products; close contact with infected livestock	Bulky vegetations usually seen on echocardiography; blood cultures positive in 80% of cases with incubation time of 4-6 wk; lysis-centrifugation technique may expedite growth; serologic tests are available
Bartonella spp.	*Bartonella henselae:* transmitted by cat scratch or bite or by cat fleas *Bartonella quintana:* transmitted by human body louse; predisposing factors include homelessness and alcohol abuse	Serologic testing (may cross-react with *Chlamydia* spp.); PCR of valve or emboli is best test; lysis-centrifugation technique may be useful
Chlamydia psittaci	Exposure to birds	Serologic tests available, but must exclude *Bartonella* spp. because of cross-reactivity; monoclonal antibody direct stains on tissue may be useful; PCR now available
Tropheryma whippelii (Whipple disease)	Systemic symptoms include arthralgias, diarrhea, abdominal pain, lymphadenopathy, weight loss, CNS involvement; however, endocarditis may be present without systemic symptoms	Histologic examination of valve with PAS stain; valve cultures may be done using fibroblast cell lines; PCR on vegetation material
Legionella spp.	Contaminated water distribution systems; often nosocomial outbreaks; usually prosthetic valves	Lysis-centrifugation technique; also periodic subcultures onto buffered charcoal yeast extract medium; serologic tests and PCR available
Aspergillus and other noncandidal fungi	Prosthetic valve	Lysis-centrifugation technique; also culture and direct examination of any emboli

*Listed in approximate order of relative frequency.
CNS = central nervous system; HACEK = *Haemophilus* spp., *Aggregatibacter* spp., *Cardiobacterium hominis*, *Eikenella corrodens*, and *Kingella* spp.; PAS = periodic acid–Schiff; PCR = polymerase chain reaction.

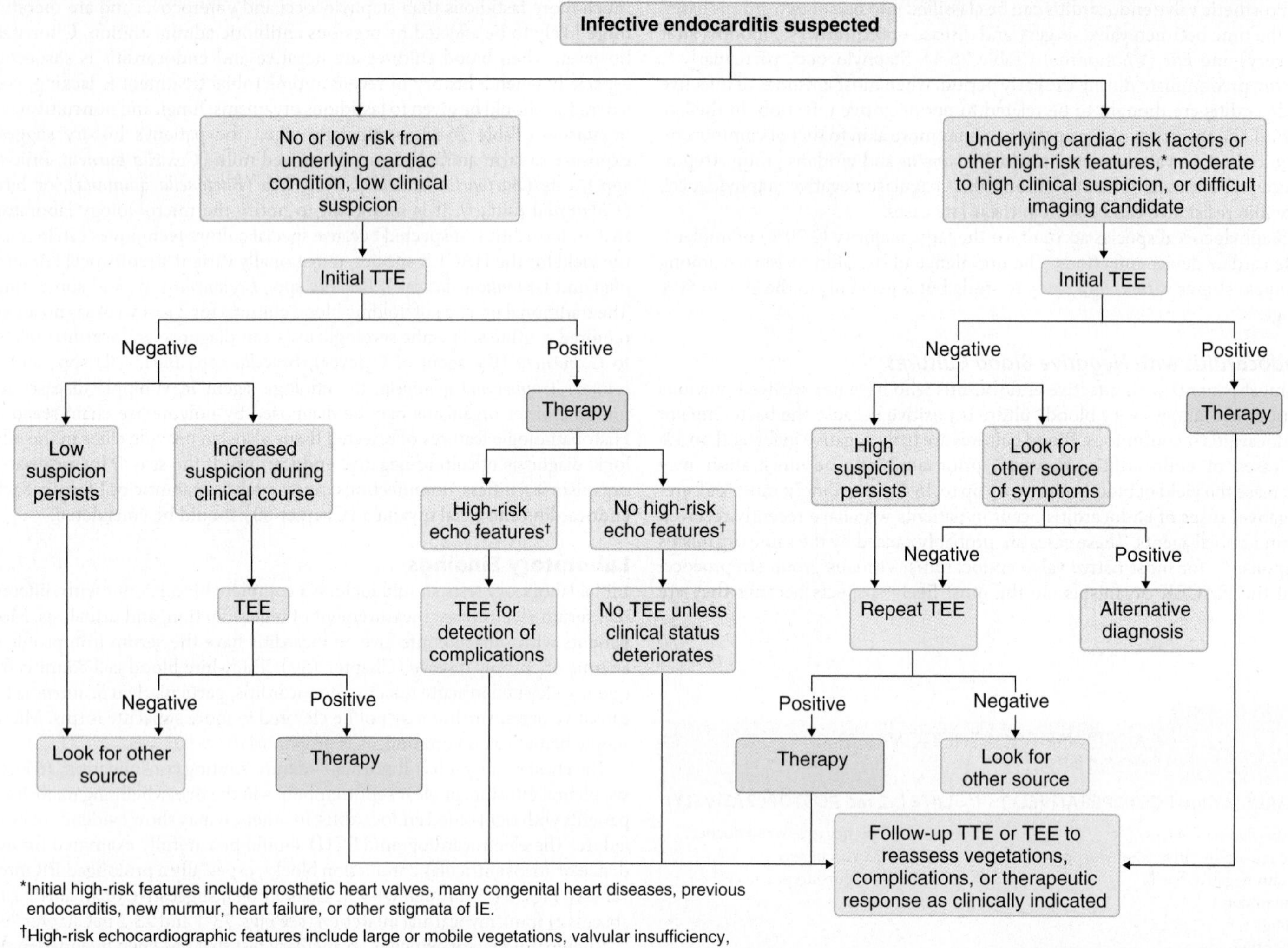

FIGURE 76-3. Algorithm for the diagnostic use of echocardiography (echo) in suspected cases of infective endocarditis (IE). TEE = transesophageal echocardiography; TTE = transthoracic echocardiography. (Adapted from Bayer AS, Bolger AF, Taubert KA, et al. Diagnosis and management of infective endocarditis and its complications. *Circulation.* 1998; 98:2936-2948.)

protein level, and the procalcitonin level, are generally not helpful in establishing an endocarditis diagnosis.

Echocardiography

Both transthoracic echocardiography (TTE) and transesophageal echocardiography (TEE) (Chapter 55) are highly specific tests (≈98%) when used as part of the diagnostic evaluation of suspected endocarditis. By contrast, TEE has a much higher sensitivity (90%-95%) in this setting than TTE (48%-63%). In most cases in which endocarditis is a serious diagnostic consideration, the evaluation should begin with TEE because negative TTE findings are not sensitive enough to exclude endocarditis (Fig. 76-3). Because TEE is the only relatively noninvasive means of detecting perivalvular extension of infection, any patient with a new conduction system abnormality or persistent fever—clinical predictors of perivalvular extension—should be evaluated with TEE. Likewise, TEE is strongly preferred in the evaluation of suspected prosthetic valve– or device-related endocarditis, although bland clots can occur on the leads of 5% to 10% of patients with intracardiac devices, and the finding of a "vegetation" on a lead is not specific for infection. The high sensitivity of TEE in detecting valvular vegetations on native valves also may be used in combination with clinical parameters (e.g., prompt resolution of bacteremia and defervescence) to support the clinical decision to abbreviate therapy in patients with vascular catheter–associated *S. aureus* bacteremia.

A negative TEE result has a negative predictive value of about 95%. Nevertheless, when clinical suspicion of endocarditis is high and the initial TEE is negative, repeat TEE in 7 to 10 days may reveal the diagnosis. If TEE is unavailable, technically impossible, or considered too invasive by the patient, it is reasonable to begin with TTE.

TREATMENT Rx

Definitive antibiotic treatment of infective endocarditis (Table 76-6) is guided by antimicrobial susceptibility testing of the responsible pathogen isolated from clinical cultures. Although it is often advisable to begin empirical treatment before definitive culture results are available, not all patients who are admitted because of possible endocarditis necessarily need to be treated empirically. Patients who are clinically stable, with a subacute presentation syndrome, and without evidence of heart failure or other end-organ complications, can be closely observed without antibiotics so that serial blood cultures can be obtained. Likewise, such stable patients who were started on empiric antibiotics before hospitalization and before blood was drawn for cultures can discontinue antibiotics so that blood cultures can be obtained, preferably as long as possible after stopping the antibiotics. By contrast, acutely ill patients, patients with evidence of complications of endocarditis, and patients who are at high risk for endocarditis (e.g., prosthetic valve recipients) should be treated empirically with antibiotics pending culture results. In most cases of infective endocarditis, an infectious diseases specialist can assist in guiding the diagnostic evaluation and designing an appropriate antibiotic regimen.

Either of two regimens provides appropriate empirical coverage for patients with suspected native valve endocarditis: nafcillin (or oxacillin)–penicillin–gentamicin or vancomycin–gentamicin (Table 76-7). Nafcillin–penicillin–gentamicin is suitable in most cases of suspected native valve endocarditis because it provides optimal coverage for viridans group streptococci, methicillin-sensitive staphylococci, enterococci, and HACEK organisms. Some experts recommend a regimen of nafcillin–ceftriaxone–penicillin–gentamicin to cover for HACEK isolates that produce β-lactamase. If methicillin-resistant *S. aureus* (MRSA) is an important consideration, as in injection drug users and patients with health care contact, empirical therapy should consist of vancomycin–ceftriaxone–gentamicin. This regimen is also acceptable for

TABLE 76-6 DEFINITIVE THERAPY OF BACTERIAL ENDOCARDITIS

ORGANISM AND REGIMEN*	COMMENTS
PCN-SUSCEPTIBLE VIRIDANS STREPTOCOCCI (MIC ≤0.1 μg/mL) AND *STREPTOCOCCUS GALLOLYTICUS* (*formerly S. bovis*)	
1. PCN 2-3 million units IV q4h × 4 wk	1. Also effective for other PCN-susceptible nonviridans streptococci
2. Ceftriaxone 2 g IV qd × 4 wk	2. Uncomplicated infection with viridans streptococci in a candidate for outpatient therapy; also for those with PCN allergy
3. PCN 2-3 million units IV q4h × 2 wk plus gentamicin 1 mg/kg IV q8h × 2 wk	3. Uncomplicated infection with none of the following features: renal insufficiency, eighth cranial nerve deficit, prosthetic valve infection, CNS complications, severe heart failure, age >65 yr; also not acceptable for nutritionally variant streptococci
4. PCN 2-4 million units IV q4h × 4 wk plus gentamicin 1 mg/kg IV q8h for at least 2 wk with ID input	4. Nutritionally variant strain; for prosthetic valve, give 6 wk of PCN
5. Vancomycin 15-20 mg/kg IV q8-12h × 4 wk	5. For PCN allergy; goal trough level of 15-20 mg/L
RELATIVELY PCN-RESISTANT VIRIDANS STREPTOCOCCI (MIC 0.12-<0.5 μg/mL)	
1. PCN 4 million units IV q4h × 4 wk plus gentamicin 1 mg/kg IV q8h × 2 wk	—
2. Vancomycin 15-20 mg/kg IV q8-12h × 4 wk	2. For PCN allergy or to avoid gentamicin; goal trough level of 15-20 mg/L
ENTEROCOCCI[†] AND PCN-RESISTANT VIRIDANS STREPTOCOCCI (PCN MIC >0.5 μg/mL)	
1. PCN[‡] 18-30 million units IV per day in divided doses × 4-6 wk or ampicillin 12 g/24 hr IV in 6 equally divided doses plus gentamicin 1 mg/kg IV q8h × 4-6 wk	1. Increase duration of both drugs to 6 wk for prosthetic valve infection or symptoms >3 mo in enterococcal infection
2. Vancomycin 15-20 mg/kg IV q8-12h × 6 wk plus gentamicin 1 mg/kg q8h × 6 wk[§]	2. For PCN allergy; PCN desensitization is also an option; high risk of nephrotoxicity with this regimen
3. Ampicillin 12 g/24 h IV in 6 equally divided doses plus ceftriaxone 2 g IV q12h	3. PCN-susceptible, aminoglycoside-resistant enterococci or patients who have significant underlying renal disease
STAPHYLOCOCCUS AUREUS	
1. Nafcillin 2 g IV q4h × 4-6 wk	1. Methicillin-susceptible strain; omit gentamicin if significant renal insufficiency
2. Vancomycin 15-20 mg/kg IV q8-12h × 6 wk	2. PCN allergy (immediate hypersensitivity or anaphylaxis) or MRSA
3. Nafcillin 2 g IV q4h × 2 wk plus gentamicin 1 mg/kg IV q8h × 2 wk	3. Methicillin-susceptible strain; 2-wk regimen only for use in IV drug abusers with only tricuspid valve infection, no renal insufficiency, and no extrapulmonary infection
4. Nafcillin 2 g IV q4h × >6 wk plus gentamicin 1 mg/kg IV q8h × 2 wk plus rifampin 300 mg PO/IV q8h × ≥6 wk	4. Prosthetic valve infection with methicillin-susceptible strain; use vancomycin instead of nafcillin for MRSA
5. Cefazolin 2 g IV q8h × 4-6 wk	5. PCN allergy other than immediate hypersensitivity
6. Daptomycin 6 mg/kg IV qd × 14-42 days	Daptomycin is FDA-approved for treatment of right-sided *S. aureus* infective endocarditis; for adults, some experts recommend 8-10 mg/kg IV
COAGULASE-NEGATIVE STAPHYLOCOCCI, PROSTHETIC VALVE INFECTION	
Vancomycin 15-20 mg/kg IV q8-12h × >6 wk plus gentamicin 1 mg/kg IV q8h × 2 wk plus rifampin 300 mg PO/IV q8h × >6 wk	Can substitute nafcillin in above doses for vancomycin if isolate is methicillin sensitive
HACEK STRAINS	
1. Ceftriaxone 2 g IV qd × 4 wk; 6 wk for prosthetic valves	—
2. Ampicillin–sulbactam 3 g IV q6h × 4 wk; 6 wk for prosthetic valves	2. HACEK strains increasingly may produce β-lactamase
NON-HACEK GRAM-NEGATIVE BACILLI	
Enterobacteriaceae	
Extended-spectrum PCN or cephalosporin plus aminoglycosides for susceptible strains	Treat for a minimum of 6-8 wk; some species exhibit inducible resistance to third-generation cephalosporins; valve surgery is required for most patients with left-sided endocarditis caused by gram-negative bacilli; consultation with a specialist in infectious diseases is recommended
Pseudomonas aeruginosa	
High-dose tobramycin (8 mg/kg/day IV or IM in once-daily doses) with maintenance of peak and trough concentrations of 15 to 20 μg/mL and ≤2 μg/mL, respectively, in combination with an extended-spectrum PCN (e.g., ticarcillin, piperacillin, azlocillin); ceftazidime, cefepime, or imipenem in full doses; or imipenem	Treat for a minimum of 6-8 wk; early valve surgery usually required for left-sided *Pseudomonas* endocarditis; consultation with a specialist in infectious diseases is recommended
Fungi	
Treatment with a parenteral antifungal agent (usually a lipid-containing amphotericin B product, 3-5 mg/kg/day IV for at least 6 weeks) and valve replacement; Fluconazole, 400 mg daily PO is an alternative for susceptible yeasts; other azoles, such as voriconazole, may be required for resistant yeasts or molds.	Long-term or lifelong suppressive therapy with PO antifungal agents often required; consultation with a specialist in infectious diseases is recommended

*Dosages are for patients with normal renal function; for those with renal insufficiency, adjustments must be made for all drugs except nafcillin, rifampin, and ceftriaxone. Gentamicin doses should be adjusted to achieve a peak serum concentration of approximately 3 μg/mL 30 min after dosing and a trough gentamicin level of <1 μg/mL.

[†]Enterococci must be tested for antimicrobial susceptibility. These recommendations are for enterococci sensitive to PCN, gentamicin, and vancomycin.

[‡]Ampicillin 12 g/day can be used instead of PCN.

[§]The need to add an aminoglycoside has not been demonstrated for PCN-resistant streptococci.

HACEK = *Haemophilus* spp., *Aggregatibacter* spp. (formerly *Actinobacillus actinomycetemcomitans*), *Cardiobacterium hominis, Eikenella corrodens*, and *Kingella* spp.; IM = intramuscular; IV = intravenous; MIC = minimum inhibitory concentration; MRSA = methicillin-resistant *Staphylococcus aureus*; PCN = penicillin; PO = oral; q = every; qd = every day.

Adapted from Baddour LM, Wilson WR, Bayer AS, et al. Infective endocarditis: diagnosis, antimicrobial therapy, and management of complications. *Circulation.* 2005;111:e394-e433.

TABLE 76-7 EMPIRICAL TREATMENT OF ENDOCARDITIS

CHARACTERISTICS OF PATIENTS	TREATMENT REGIMEN*
Native valve, community-acquired infection, MRSA unlikely	Nafcillin 2 g IV q4h plus penicillin 4 million units IV q4h plus gentamicin 1 mg/kg IV q8h
Any of the following: health care–associated infection or other reason to suspect MRSA; severe penicillin allergy	Vancomycin 15-20 mg/kg IV q8-12h† plus gentamicin 1 mg/kg IV q8h
Prosthetic valve	Vancomycin 15-20 mg/kg IV q8-12h[†] plus gentamicin 1 mg/kg IV q8h plus rifampin 300 mg PO/IV q8h

IV = intravenous; MRSA = methicillin-resistant *Staphylococcus aureus*; PO = oral; q = every.
*Dosages are for patients with normal renal function; for those with renal insufficiency, adjustments must be made for all drugs except nafcillin.
†Goal is trough level of 15-20 mg/L.

patients with a serious penicillin allergy. Patients with prosthetic valves should be empirically treated with vancomycin-gentamicin–rifampin for adequate coverage of the most important pathogens in this setting (MRSA, methicillin-sensitive staphylococci, and coagulase-negative staphylococci). Nearly 40% of patients with infective endocarditis related to implantable cardiovascular devices have concomitant valve involvement, predominantly tricuspid valve infection, with in-hospital and 1-year mortality rates of 15% and 23%, respectively. Device removal appears to reduce the mortality rate by about 50% (from about 40% to about 20%).

Treatment of Specific Organisms

When the organism is definitively identified, antibiotic treatment must be narrowed accordingly, and validated regimens should be followed[5] (see Table 76-6). More controversy exists over the treatment of unusual organisms, and consultation with infectious disease specialists is advisable in such circumstances.

Many regimens recommend consideration of low-dose gentamicin to provide antibacterial synergy with a low risk of toxicity. However, aminoglycoside toxicity is a significant risk in elderly patients and in patients with preexisting renal disease or hearing impairment; even low-dose gentamicin increases the likelihood of a decrease in creatinine clearance by about threefold.[A1] Among the organisms listed in Table 76-6, gentamicin is critical for cure only in enterococcal endocarditis. As a result of these risks and the minimal data supporting its benefit, initial low-dose gentamicin should not be routinely used.

In uncomplicated viridans group streptococcal endocarditis, outpatient therapy with once-daily ceftriaxone[A2] is as effective as more complex regimens, provided the patient has been observed in the hospital for the development of complications. The decision to administer antimicrobial therapy in the outpatient setting must, of course, take into account the patient's social situation, likelihood of compliance, and other risks involved with either an indwelling IV line or recurrent peripheral IV line placements.

Standard therapy for infective endocarditis caused by fully susceptible enterococci includes penicillin or ampicillin plus gentamicin. Although gentamicin is preferred over streptomycin, the choice of a specific aminoglycoside should be based on in vitro susceptibility testing. Nonrandomized data suggest that the duration of aminoglycoside therapy can be limited to 2 to 3 weeks in combination with either penicillin, ampicillin, or vancomycin or that aminoglycoside therapy can be avoided in favor of combination therapy with ampicillin plus high-dose (2 g IV every 12 hours) ceftriaxone. Optimal therapy for enterococci that are resistant to aminoglycosides or vancomycin is not well defined. Endocarditis caused by vancomycin-resistant enterococci may be treated with daptomycin, quinupristin–dalfopristin (7.5 mg/kg IV every 8 hours), or linezolid (600 mg orally or IV twice daily); however, clinical experience with these agents is limited. In this situation, relapse or failure rates are likely to be high, and many cases require surgical intervention (discussed later).

Semisynthetic penicillins, such as nafcillin, are advocated for endocarditis caused by methicillin-susceptible *S. aureus*. Cefazolin represents an alternative to semisynthetic penicillins in cases in which the latter are not tolerated or feasible to administer. Although vancomycin is recommended in patients who are allergic to β-lactams, the microbiologic and clinical cure rates are less than that of β-lactam therapy. In a recent randomized trial,[A3] daptomycin (6 mg/kg/day for 10 to 42 days, depending on the severity of infection) was as effective as either a semisynthetic antistaphylococcal penicillin or vancomycin for the treatment of *S. aureus* bacteremia and right-sided infective endocarditis caused by methicillin-susceptible *S. aureus* and MRSA, and this agent is now approved by the Food and Drug Administration for these indications. More recently, ceftaroline, a fifth-generation cephalosporin, has been successful in case series of patients with MRSA bacteremia and endocarditis.[6]

Rifampin or gentamicin can be added to either nafcillin or vancomycin for the treatment of prosthetic valve infection caused by methicillin-susceptible *S. aureus* or to MRSA, respectively. Gentamicin is administered for 2 weeks, and rifampin is given for the duration of either nafcillin or vancomycin therapy. Rifampin is never used as monotherapy because of the rapid development of resistance.

Fungal endocarditis is usually a consequence of extensive health care contact. Traditionally, fungal endocarditis was regarded as a primary indication for valvular surgery, and amphotericin B (Chapter 331) was considered the adjunctive treatment of choice. However, many patients with *Candida* endocarditis can be treated medically with azole-containing antimicrobial agents, with or without amphotericin. The management of fungal endocarditis should always involve the collaboration of an experienced infectious diseases specialist.

Zoonotic endocarditis is usually culture negative and most commonly caused by *Bartonella* spp. (Chapter 315), *C. burnetii* (Chapter 327), or *Brucella* species (Chapter 310). The treatments of choice for these fastidious pathogens are based on limited data, but documented *Bartonella* endocarditis is treated with doxycycline for 6 weeks plus gentamicin for the first 2 weeks.

In cases of presumed culture-negative endocarditis in which unusual organisms (see Table 76-5) and other infections have been reasonably excluded, an empirical course of treatment may be undertaken. In this situation, most authorities recommend a 4- to 6-week regimen of ceftriaxone alone, vancomycin–ceftriaxone–gentamicin, or vancomycin–gentamicin (if the clinical setting suggests a risk for enterococcal endocarditis). The vancomycin–ceftriaxone–gentamicin regimen provides optimal coverage for HACEK and *Abiotrophia* and *Granulicatella* spp. (formerly known as "nutritionally variant streptococci"), which are the two most common causes of nonzoonotic, culture-negative infective endocarditis.

Continuing Care of the Patient with Endocarditis

In addition to antibiotics, appropriate inpatient care includes surveillance for the development of complications. Widening of the pulse pressure should alert the clinician to the possible development of acute aortic insufficiency (Chapter 75). A careful cardiac examination should be performed on a daily basis to assess for new regurgitant murmurs.

Repeat echocardiography is recommended during therapy for patients with persistent fever, recurrent embolic events, a new murmur, widening of the pulse pressure, or signs or symptoms of heart failure. It is also recommended to screen for periannular complications, especially in prosthetic valve endocarditis. By comparison, repeat echocardiography is not routinely recommended if patients respond adequately to antimicrobial therapy, although serial echocardiography is usually suggested over the ensuing years to screen for long-term valvular dysfunction.

Routine serial ECGs are not recommended. ECG-documented conduction abnormalities are a late sign of perivalvular infections in patients with endocarditis; TEE is the screening method of choice if this complication is suspected.

Any new neurologic findings should prompt a search for evidence of central nervous system (CNS) complications such as embolic events, cerebral hemorrhage, mycotic aneurysm, or brain abscess. Renal function should be closely monitored so that antibiotic doses can be adjusted if necessary. If gentamicin is used for more than a few days, the patient should be alerted to watch for the signs and symptoms of vestibular or otic toxicity. Audiometric testing at baseline and periodically thereafter should be considered in patients at high risk for aminoglycoside-induced ototoxicity, including elderly patients, patients with preexisting renal dysfunction or hearing damage, patients receiving prolonged courses of gentamicin, and patients who also receive other potentially nephrotoxic agents. Serum gentamicin trough concentrations should also be assayed at regular intervals (e.g., twice weekly and more often if renal function is changing) and should be targeted for 1 to 3 μg/mL or less; higher concentrations should prompt either lower or less frequent dosing or both.

Follow-up blood cultures may be indicated toward the end of the first week of therapy in patients whose infective endocarditis is caused by organisms that commonly fail first-line treatment, such as *S. aureus* or aerobic gram-negative bacilli. Positive cultures in this setting might suggest the need to change therapy, search for metastatic abscesses, or repeat echocardiography, but negative cultures are reassuring.

Patients with infective endocarditis may continue to be febrile for some time after the institution of appropriate antibiotic treatment. About 50% of patients defervesce within 3 days of starting antibiotics, 75% by 1 week, and 90% by 2 weeks. Patients whose endocarditis is caused by *S. aureus*, aerobic gram-negative organisms, or fungi tend to defervesce more slowly than patients infected with other organisms. Prolonged fever (>1 week after the institution of appropriate antibiotics) should prompt repeat blood cultures. If such cultures are negative, several possibilities should be considered: myocardial abscess, extracardiac infection (e.g., mycotic aneurysm, psoas or splenic abscess, vertebral osteomyelitis, septic arthritis), immune complex–mediated tissue damage, or a complication of hospitalization and therapy (e.g., drug fever, nosocomial superinfection, pulmonary embolism). Appropriate studies might include TEE, computed tomography (CT) scan of the abdomen, bone scan, and urinalysis with microscopy (to elicit evidence of interstitial nephritis). IV line sites should be carefully examined for evidence of infection, and indwelling central lines should be changed according to published guidelines.

Anticoagulation in individuals with infective endocarditis is controversial. Although new anticoagulation in the setting of native valve endocarditis does not appear to provide a benefit, continuing ongoing anticoagulation may be advisable. Some authorities recommend continuing anticoagulation in patients with mechanical prosthetic valve endocarditis. However, discontinuation of all anticoagulation for at least the first 2 weeks of antibiotic therapy is generally advised in patients with *S. aureus* prosthetic valve endocarditis who have experienced a recent CNS embolic event; this approach allows the thrombus to organize and potentially prevents the acute hemorrhagic transformation of embolic lesions. Reintroduction of anticoagulation in these patients must be cautious, and the international normalized ratio must be monitored carefully. The best option for patients with other indications for anticoagulation, such as deep vein thrombosis, major vessel embolization, or atrial fibrillation, is less clear and should be decided in a multidisciplinary fashion that balances the risks and benefits for each individual patient.

High-dose (325 mg/day) aspirin does not prevent embolic events and tends to increase the incidence of bleeding in patients with infective endocarditis.[A4] Whether a patient should remain on chronic, low-dose (81 mg) aspirin if they develop subsequent infective endocarditis is uncertain.

Complications

The complications of infective endocarditis can be divided into four groups for ease of classification: direct valvular damage and consequences of local invasion, embolic complications, metastatic infections from bacteremia, and immunologic phenomena. Local damage to the endocardium or myocardium may directly erode through the involved cardiac valve or adjacent myocardial wall, resulting in hemodynamically significant valvular perforations or intra- or extracardiac fistulae. Such local complications typically present clinically with the acute onset of heart failure and carry a poor prognosis, even with prompt cardiac surgery. Valve ring abscesses also require surgical intervention and are more frequent in patients with prosthetic valves. Although a conduction defect on ECG may suggest the diagnosis, TEE is the diagnostic technique of choice for detecting paravalvular abscess, valve perforation, or intracardiac fistulae. Frank myocardial abscesses are found in up to 20% of cases on autopsy, and *Aspergillus* endocarditis invades the myocardium in more than 50% of cases. Pericarditis is rare and is usually associated with myocardial abscess. Myocardial infarction (MI), thought to be caused by embolism of vegetative material into the coronary arteries, is seen in 40% to 60% of cases on autopsy, although most cases are clinically silent and lack characteristic ECG changes. However, up to 15% of elderly patients may present with clinical evidence of acute MI, with potentially disastrous complications if the MI is thought to be the primary event and the patient is given thrombolytic therapy. Heart failure is the leading cause of death in infective endocarditis, usually related to direct valvular damage.

Embolic events are less common now than in the preantibiotic era, but about 35% of patients have at least one clinically evident embolic event. In fungal endocarditis, the majority of patients have at least one embolic event, frequently with a large embolus. The presence of large (>10 mm), mobile vegetations on the echocardiogram, particularly when the anterior mitral valve leaflet is involved, predicts a high risk of embolic complications. In addition, patients may have frank infarction of cutaneous tissue from emboli. In addition to the skin, systemic emboli most commonly lodge in the kidneys, spleen, large blood vessels, or CNS. Vegetations of right-sided endocarditis usually embolize to the lungs and cause abnormalities on the chest radiograph, although occasionally such emboli reach the left-sided circulation via a patent foramen ovale.

Renal abscesses are rare in infective endocarditis; however, bland renal infarction is a frequent asymptomatic finding on abdominal CT scanning, seen in more than 50% of cases at autopsy. Similarly, splenic infarction occurs in up to 44% of autopsy-confirmed cases. Such emboli may be asymptomatic but also can cause left upper quadrant pain radiating to the left shoulder, sometimes as the presenting symptom of infective endocarditis. A splenic infarction that progresses to form an abscess can cause persistent fever or bacteremia, so such patients should undergo abdominal CT to search for this complication. Mycotic vascular aneurysms, which frequently occur at bifurcation points, may be clinically silent until they rupture (which may be months to years after apparently successful antibiotic treatment of infective endocarditis) and have been found in 10% to 15% of cases at autopsy. Whereas peripheral mycotic aneurysms require surgical resection, intracerebral aneurysms should be resected or managed with intravascular techniques (e.g., coils) if they bleed or if they are causing a mass effect.

Many patients may have evidence of cerebrovascular emboli, which have a predilection for the middle cerebral artery distribution and may be devastating. Most emboli to the CNS occur early in the course of the disease and are evident at the time of presentation or shortly thereafter. Embolic strokes may undergo hemorrhagic transformation, with a sudden worsening of the patient's neurologic status. Many patients with fungal endocarditis present with an embolic stroke or large emboli that occlude major vessels.

Some complications of infective endocarditis result when bacteremic seeding causes metastatic infection at a distant site. Patients may present with or develop osteomyelitis, septic arthritis, or epidural abscess. Purulent meningitis (Chapter 412) is a rare complication except in pneumococcal endocarditis, although many patients with *S. aureus* infective endocarditis who undergo lumbar puncture have a pleocytosis. Intracranial abscesses are uncommon in bacterial endocarditis but frequent in *Aspergillus* endocarditis; such a finding in the setting of culture-negative endocarditis should prompt the consideration of *Aspergillus* as an etiologic agent. Importantly, the finding of one metastatic complication of infective endocarditis does not exclude the possibility of additional sites of hematogenous infection, particularly in *S. aureus* endocarditis. Thus, the need for additional diagnostic evaluations should be guided by the patient's clinical course.

The immunologic phenomena of infective endocarditis are often directly related to high levels of circulating immune complexes. Renal biopsy results nearly always are abnormal in the setting of active infective endocarditis, which classically causes a hypocomplementemic glomerulonephritis (Chapter 121). Histopathologically, the glomerular changes may be focal, diffuse, or membranoproliferative, or they may be akin to the immune complex disease found in systemic lupus erythematosus. In addition, many of the musculoskeletal conditions associated with infective endocarditis, including monoarticular and oligoarticular arthritides, are probably immune mediated. These immunologic phenomena usually abate with successful antimicrobial therapy.

Surgery

Some patients with infective endocarditis require surgical treatment, either to cure the infection or to avoid its complications[7,8] (Table 76-8). Most patients with evidence of direct extension of infection to myocardial structures,

TABLE 76-8 INDICATIONS FOR SURGERY IN ENDOCARDITIS

INDICATION	CLASS*
NATIVE VALVE ENDOCARDITIS	
Acute aortic insufficiency or mitral regurgitation with heart failure	I
Acute aortic insufficiency with tachycardia and early closure of the mitral valve on echocardiogram	I
Fungal endocarditis	I
Evidence of annular or aortic abscess, sinus or aortic true or false aneurysm, valvular dehiscence, rupture, perforation, or fistula	I
Evidence of valve dysfunction and persistent infection after a prolonged period (7-10 days) of appropriate therapy, provided there are no noncardiac causes of infection	I
Recurrent emboli after appropriate antibiotic therapy	I
Infection with enteric gram-negative organisms or organisms with a poor response to antibiotics in patients with evidence of valve dysfunction	I
Anterior mitral leaflet vegetation (especially with size >10 mm) or persistent vegetation after systemic embolization	IIa
Increase in vegetation size despite appropriate antimicrobial therapy	IIb
Early infections of the mitral valve that can probably be repaired, especially in the presence of large vegetations and/or recurrent emboli	III
Persistent fever and leukocytosis with negative blood cultures	III
PROSTHETIC VALVE ENDOCARDITIS	
Early prosthetic valve endocarditis (<2 mo after surgery)	I
Heart failure with prosthetic valve dysfunction	I
Nonstreptococcal endocarditis	I
Evidence of perivalvular leak, annular or aortic abscess, sinus or aortic true or false aneurysm, fistula formation, or new-onset conduction disturbances	I
Persistent bacteremia after 7-10 days of appropriate antibiotic therapy, with noncardiac causes for bacteremia excluded	IIa
Recurrent peripheral embolus despite therapy	IIa
Vegetation of any size seen on or near the prosthesis	IIb

*Class I = conditions for which there is evidence or general agreement that a given procedure or treatment is useful and effective; class II = conditions for which there is conflicting evidence or a divergence of opinion about the usefulness or efficacy of a procedure or treatment; class IIa = weight of evidence or opinion is in favor of usefulness or efficacy; class IIb = usefulness or efficacy is less well established by evidence or opinion; class III = conditions for which there is evidence or general agreement that the procedure or treatment is not useful and in some cases may be harmful.
Adapted with permission from Bonow RO, Carabello B, de Leon AC, et al. Guidelines for the management of patients with valvular heart disease. *Circulation.* 1998;98:1949-1984.

prosthetic valve dysfunction, or heart failure from endocarditis-induced valvular damage should undergo surgery. In addition, many cases of endocarditis caused by fungi, by aerobic gram-negative bacilli or multidrug-resistant organisms (e.g., vancomycin- or gentamicin-resistant enterococci) require surgical management. Progression of disease or persistence of fever and bacteremia for more than 7 to 10 days in the presence of appropriate antibiotic therapy may indicate the need for surgery; however, a thorough search must first be conducted to exclude other metastatic foci of infection. In a randomized trial of patients with left-sided infective endocarditis, severe valve disease, and large vegetations (>10 mm), early surgery did not significantly reduce all-cause mortality at 6 months but markedly decreased the risk of systemic embolism, including stroke and MI.[A5] Surgical management should also be considered for patients with recurrent (two or more) embolic events or those with large vegetations (>10 mm) on echocardiography and one embolic event, although the data in these situations are less convincing. The presence of *S. aureus* endocarditis involving the anterior mitral valve leaflet and large vegetations (>10 mm) may be a special circumstance calling for early surgical intervention to reduce the high risk of CNS emboli, especially when mitral valve repair, rather than valve replacement, can be accomplished. Unfortunately, only about 15% to 20% of these latter patients end up being good candidates for valve repair.

Delaying surgery in patients with deteriorating cardiac function in an attempt to sterilize the affected valve is ill advised because the risk of progressive heart failure or further complications usually outweighs the relatively small risk of recurrent infective endocarditis after prosthetic valve implantation. Relative contraindications to valve replacement include recent large CNS emboli (>2 cm) or bleed (because of the risk of bleeding in the perioperative period, when systemic anticoagulation is required), multiple prior valve replacements (because of the difficulty of sewing a new valve into tissue already weakened from previous surgeries), and ongoing injection drug use. On occasion, patients have both a compelling indication for valve replacement (e.g., acute heart failure) and a recent CNS embolic event. The risk of hemorrhagic transformation of such lesions during cardiac bypass–associated anticoagulation is controversial. However, it appears that the greatest risk of such transformation events is in larger (>2 cm) emboli, especially those that have exhibited a hemorrhagic component. In these latter scenarios, it is prudent to try to delay surgery for at least 2 to 4 weeks to allow organization and resolution of such emboli. However, there appears to be no survival benefit in delaying indicated valve replacement surgery (>7 days) after an ischemic stroke.

After definitive surgical treatment, most patients should receive further antibiotic therapy unless a full course of antibiotics was administered before surgery and there is no evidence of ongoing infection. If the patient received antibiotics for less than 1 week before surgery or the culture from the operative site is positive, the patient should receive the equivalent of a full initial course of antibiotics appropriate for the organism. If the patient received antibiotics for 2 weeks or more and the culture result from the operative site is negative (regardless of whether valve histopathology shows inflammation or a positive Gram stain result), the patient should receive whatever remains of the originally planned course of appropriate antibiotic therapy.

In patients with infective endocarditis related to implanted cardiovascular devices, complete device removal is mandatory, regardless of the pathogen, if the goal is to cure the infection. If a replacement device needs to be implanted, the optimal timing for such a procedure is unclear. However, blood culture results should be negative, and any concomitant local or pocket site infection should be completely resolved.

The duration of antimicrobial therapy after device extraction depends on the device and the infection.[9] For lead-related infective endocarditis, which is usually associated with bloodstream infection, 2 weeks of therapy is recommended if there are no infection complications. For infection caused by *S. aureus*, therapy should be extended for up to 4 weeks. In patients with valve infection, 4 to 6 weeks of therapy is recommended.

PREVENTION

Despite a lack of definitive data for dental procedures,[10] prophylactic antibiotics are recommended to prevent infective endocarditis (Table 76-9) when patients with the highest risk of adverse outcomes from endocarditis undergo dental procedures that involve manipulation of gingival tissue or the periapical region of teeth or perforation of the oral mucosa; an invasive procedure of the respiratory tract, with incision or biopsy of the respiratory mucosa, such as tonsillectomy and adenoidectomy; or invasive procedures involving infected skin, skin structures, or musculoskeletal tissue (Table 76-10).[11] Other consensus guidelines have also narrowed the indications for antimicrobial prophylaxis. In the United Kingdom, for example, no prophylaxis is advised for any dental patient, regardless of underlying cardiac valvular conditions. In contrast, French and other European guidelines are largely consistent with current AHA guidelines. Since the recent publications of these more limited recommendations from the AHA, France, and the United Kingdom, follow-up surveys in these countries have shown no appreciable increase in the incidence of viridans group streptococcal infective endocarditis.[12,13]

TABLE 76-9 HIGH-RISK CARDIAC CONDITIONS FOR WHICH ENDOCARDITIS PROPHYLAXIS WITH DENTAL PROCEDURES IS REASONABLE

Prosthetic cardiac valve or prosthetic material used for cardiac valve repair
Previous endocarditis
Complex congenital heart disease involving unrepaired cyanotic congenital heart disease (including palliative shunts and conduits), completely repaired congenital heart disease with prosthetic material within 6 mo of the procedure, or repaired congenital heart disease with residual defects at the site or adjacent to the site of prosthetic material
Cardiac transplantation recipients who develop cardiac valvuloplasty

Adapted from Wilson W, Taubert KA, Gewitz M, et al. Prevention of infective endocarditis guidelines from the American Heart Association: a guideline from the American Heart Association Rheumatic Fever, Endocarditis, and Kawasaki Disease Committee, Council on Cardiovascular Disease in the Young, and the Council on Clinical Cardiology, Council on Cardiovascular Surgery and Anesthesia, and the Quality of Care and Outcomes Research Interdisciplinary Working Group. *Circulation*. 2007;116:1736-1754.

TABLE 76-10 RECOMMENDATIONS FOR ENDOCARDITIS PROPHYLAXIS

PROPHYLAXIS IS RECOMMENDED*

Dental: all dental procedures involving manipulation of gingival tissue or the periapical region of teeth or perforation of the oral mucosa
Respiratory: procedures involving incision or biopsy of the respiratory mucosa, such as tonsillectomy and adenoidectomy
Other: procedures involving infected skin, skin structures, or musculoskeletal tissue prior to incision and drainage

PROPHYLAXIS IS NOT RECOMMENDED

Dental: routine anesthetic injections through noninfected tissue, dental radiographs, placement of removable prosthodontic or orthodontic appliances, adjustment of orthodontic appliances, placement of orthodontic brackets, shedding of deciduous teeth, bleeding from trauma to the lips or oral mucosa
Respiratory: procedures not involving incision or biopsy of the respiratory mucosa, including bronchoscopy (unless the procedure involves incision of the respiratory tract mucosa)
Genitourinary: antibiotic prophylaxis solely to prevent infective endocarditis is not recommended
Gastrointestinal: antibiotic prophylaxis solely to prevent infective endocarditis is not recommended

*Only in patients with underlying cardiac conditions associated with the highest risk for adverse outcome from endocarditis (listed in Table 76-9).
Adapted from Wilson W, Taubert KA, Gewitz M, et al. Prevention of infective endocarditis guidelines from the American Heart Association: a guideline from the American Heart Association Rheumatic Fever, Endocarditis, and Kawasaki Disease Committee, Council on Cardiovascular Disease in the Young, and the Council on Clinical Cardiology, Council on Cardiovascular Surgery and Anesthesia, and the Quality of Care and Outcomes Research Interdisciplinary Working Group. *Circulation*. 2007;116:1736-1754.

The antibiotics chosen for preprocedure prophylaxis should be active against the organisms most likely to be released into the blood stream by the procedure of interest (Table 76-11). Thus, antibiotics that cover primarily oral flora are recommended for dental and upper respiratory procedures. For patients with the conditions listed in Table 76-9 who undergo a procedure for infected skin, skin structure, or musculoskeletal tissue, the therapeutic regimen should contain an agent active against staphylococci and β-hemolytic streptococci.

Patients with implanted cardiac devices do not require antibiotic prophylaxis for dental or other invasive procedures. However, such patients require surgical site prophylaxis at the time of device placement.[2] The recommended regimens generally include a β-lactam (commonly cefazolin, 1 g IV 1 hour before device placement), regardless of whether a new device is being placed or a device is being revised.

PROGNOSIS

Untreated infective endocarditis is uniformly fatal. Aggressive medical and surgical management dramatically improves the outcome. The overall mortality rate from both native and prosthetic valve endocarditis remains fairly high, ranging from 17% to 36%. Whereas certain subgroups, such as patients with viridans group streptococcal endocarditis, have a lower risk of death,

TABLE 76-11 SUGGESTED ANTIBIOTICS FOR ENDOCARDITIS PROPHYLAXIS FOR DENTAL OR RESPIRATORY TRACT PROCEDURES* IN PATIENTS WITH HIGH-RISK CARDIAC CONDITIONS†

PATIENT CHARACTERISTICS	REGIMEN‡
Able to take oral medications	Amoxicillin 2 g PO
Unable to take oral medications	Ampicillin 2 g IV or IM; or cefazolin or ceftriaxone 1 g IM or IV
Allergic to penicillin or ampicillin and able to take oral medications	Cephalexin 2 g PO (or other first- or second-generation oral cephalosporin in equivalent adult doses); clindamycin 600 mg PO; azithromycin 500 mg PO; or clarithromycin 500 mg PO Cephalosporins should not be used in an individual with a history of anaphylaxis, angioedema, or urticaria with penicillin or ampicillin
Allergic to penicillin or ampicillin and unable to take oral medications	Cefazolin or ceftriaxone 1 g IM or IV; or clindamycin 600 mg IM or IV

*For the applicable procedures, see Table 76-10.
†For the applicable conditions, see Table 76-9.
‡All regimens consist of a single dose 30-60 min before the procedure.
IM = intramuscular; IV = intravenous; PO = oral.
Adapted from Wilson W, Taubert KA, Gewitz M, et al. Prevention of infective endocarditis guidelines from the American Heart Association: a guideline from the American Heart Association Rheumatic Fever, Endocarditis, and Kawasaki Disease Committee, Council on Cardiovascular Disease in the Young, and the Council on Clinical Cardiology, Council on Cardiovascular Surgery and Anesthesia, and the Quality of Care and Outcomes Research Interdisciplinary Working Group. *Circulation.* 2007;116:1736-1754.

patients with *S. aureus*, fungal, and zoonotic endocarditis have higher mortality rates. Heart failure and CNS events are the most frequent causes of death.

Endocarditis recurs in about 12% to 16% of patients and is more common in injection drug users, elderly people, and patients with prosthetic valves. The rate of relapse also varies depending on the causative organism. Easily treated infections, such as those with viridans group streptococci, have a low rate of relapse (5%), but more difficult-to-eradicate organisms may have significantly higher rates.

FUTURE DIRECTIONS

As cardiac imaging technology continues to improve, the duration of treatment of endocarditis may be dictated in part by the characteristics of visualized vegetations. In addition, now that large vegetations have been demonstrated to cause more embolic events, earlier interventions to remove vegetations from functionally competent valves or to introduce agents that prevent the formation or promote the dissolution of vegetations may be feasible. Moreover, advances in imaging may allow routine screening of patients for subclinical infections. Novel therapeutic and prophylactic approaches, such as antibacterial antibodies, targeted bacterial vaccines, and cell wall–specific enzymes that can act as adjuncts to antibiotics in facilitating bacteriologic clearance, are currently in development.

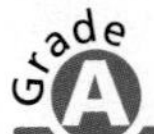

Grade A References

A1. Cosgrove SE, Vigliani GA, Fowler VG Jr, et al. Initial low-dose gentamicin for *Staphylococcus aureus* bacteremia and endocarditis is nephrotoxic. *Clin Infect Dis.* 2009;48:713-721.
A2. Sexton DJ, Tenenbaum MJ, Wilson WR, et al. Ceftriaxone once daily for four weeks compared with ceftriaxone plus gentamicin once daily for two weeks for treatment of endocarditis due to penicillin-susceptible streptococci. Endocarditis Treatment Consortium Group. *Clin Infect Dis.* 1998;27:1470-1474.
A3. Fowler VG Jr, Boucher HW, Corey GR, et al. Daptomycin versus standard therapy for bacteremia and endocarditis caused by *Staphylococcus aureus*. *N Engl J Med.* 2006;355:653-665.
A4. Chan KL, Dumesnil JG, Cujec B, et al. A randomized trial of aspirin on the risk of embolic events in patients with infective endocarditis. *J Am Coll Cardiol.* 2003;42:775-780.
A5. Kang DH, Kim YJ, Kim SH, et al. Early surgery versus conventional treatment for infective endocarditis. *N Engl J Med.* 2012;366:2466-2473.

GENERAL REFERENCES

For the General References and other additional features, please visit Expert Consult at https://expertconsult.inkling.com.

77

PERICARDIAL DISEASES

WILLIAM C. LITTLE AND JAE K. OH

The pericardium, which is a relatively avascular fibrous sac that surrounds the heart, has two layers, the visceral and parietal pericardia. The potential space between the two layers normally contains only 10 to 50 mL of fluid, which is an ultrafiltrate of plasma. The pericardium is well innervated, so pericardial inflammation may produce severe pain and trigger vagally mediated reflexes.

As a result of its relatively inelastic physical properties, the pericardium limits acute cardiac dilation and enhances mechanical interactions of the cardiac chambers. In response to long-standing stress, the pericardium dilates to allow a slowly accumulating pericardial effusion to become quite large without compressing the cardiac chambers and to allow left ventricular remodeling to occur without pericardial constriction. Conversely, a scarred or thickened pericardium can limit the filling of the heart, resulting in pericardial constriction. Despite the important functions of the normal pericardium, congenital absence or surgical resection of the pericardium does not appear to have any major untoward effects.

ACUTE PERICARDITIS

EPIDEMIOLOGY AND PATHOBIOLOGY

Acute inflammation of the pericardium, with or without an associated pericardial effusion, can occur as an isolated clinical problem or as a manifestation of systemic disease. Although about 85% of isolated cases of acute pericarditis are idiopathic or viral, the list of other potential causes is quite extensive (Table 77-1). Patients with fever greater than 38° C or a subacute course or who fail to respond promptly to therapy are most likely to have pericarditis caused by a systemic autoimmune disease, malignancy, or viral or bacterial infection.

Pericarditis can occur after an acute myocardial infarction (MI). It occurs 1 to 3 days after a transmural MI, presumably owing to the interaction between the healing necrotic epicardium and the overlying pericardium. Dressler syndrome, which is another form of pericarditis associated with MI, typically occurs weeks to months after MI. It is similar to the pericarditis that can occur days to months after traumatic pericardial injury, surgical manipulation of the pericardium, or pulmonary infarction. This syndrome is presumed to be mediated by an autoimmune mechanism and is associated with signs of systemic inflammation, including fever and polyserositis.

CLINICAL MANIFESTATIONS

Most patients with acute pericarditis experience sharp retrosternal chest pain (see Table 51-2 in Chapter 51), which can be quite severe and debilitating. In some cases, however, pericarditis is asymptomatic, such as when it accompanies rheumatoid arthritis. Pericardial pain is usually worse with inspiration and when supine, and it is generally relieved by sitting and leaning forward. Typically, pericardial pain is referred to the scapular ridge, presumably owing to irritation of the phrenic nerves, which pass adjacent to the pericardium. The chest pain of acute pericarditis must be differentiated from pulmonary embolism and myocardial ischemia or infarction (Table 77-2).

The pericardial friction rub is the classic finding in patients with acute pericarditis. A friction rub is a high-pitched, scratchy sound that can have one, two, or three components occurring when the cardiac volumes are most rapidly changing: during ventricular ejection, during rapid ventricular filling in early diastole, and during atrial systole. A pericardial rub, which is differentiated from a murmur by its scratchy quality, is sometimes localized to a small area on the chest wall and may come and go spontaneously or with changes in position. To hear a rub, it may be necessary to auscultate the heart with the patient in multiple positions, especially using the diaphragm with the patient learning forward and not breathing after full expiration. The pericardial friction rub must be differentiated from a pleural rub, which is absent during suspended respiration, but the pericardial rub is unaffected.

DIAGNOSIS

Early in the course of acute pericarditis, the electrocardiogram (ECG) typically displays diffuse ST elevation in association with PR depression (Fig. 77-1). The ST elevation is usually present in all leads except for aVR,

TABLE 77-1 CAUSES OF PERICARDITIS: INFECTIOUS AND NONINFECTIOUS

INFECTIOUS PERICARDITIS (⅔ OF CASES)

Viral (most common): echovirus and coxsackievirus (usual), influenza, EBV, CMV, adenovirus, varicella, rubella, mumps, HBV, HCV, HIV, parvovirus B19, human herpesvirus 6 (increasing reports)

Bacterial: tuberculosis (4%-5%)* and *Coxiella burnetii* (most common); other bacterial causes (rare) include pneumococcosis, meningococcosis, gonococcosis, *Haemophilus*, staphylococci, Chlamydia, *Mycoplasma, Legionella, Leptospira, Listeria*

Fungal (rare): histoplasmosis more likely in immunocompetent patients; aspergillosis, blastomycosis, candidiasis more likely in immunosuppressed patients

Parasitic (very rare): *Echinococcus, Toxoplasma*

NONINFECTIOUS PERICARDITIS (⅓ OF CASES)

Autoimmune Pericarditis (<10%)*

Pericardial injury syndromes: post–myocardial infarction syndrome; postpericardiotomy syndrome; posttraumatic pericarditis, including iatrogenic pericarditis (e.g., after percutaneous coronary interventions, pacemaker insertion, ablation)

Pericarditis in systemic autoimmune and autoinflammatory diseases: more common in systemic lupus erythematosus, Sjögren syndrome, rheumatoid arthritis, systemic sclerosis, systemic vasculitides, Behçet syndrome, sarcoidosis, familial Mediterranean fever

Autoreactive pericarditis*†

Neoplastic Pericarditis (5%-7%)*

Primary tumors (rare): pericardial mesothelioma

Secondary metastatic tumors (common): lung and breast cancer, lymphoma

Metabolic pericarditis: uremia, myxedema (common); others rare

Traumatic Pericarditis (rare)

Direct injury: penetrating thoracic injury, esophageal perforation, iatrogenic

Indirect injury: nonpenetrating thoracic injury, radiation injury

Drug-related pericarditis (rare): procainamide, hydralazine, isoniazid, and phenytoin (lupus-like syndrome), penicillins (hypersensitivity pericarditis with eosinophilia), doxorubicin, and daunorubicin (often associated with cardiomyopathy; may cause pericardiopathy)

*Percentages refer to unselected cases.

†The diagnosis of autoreactive pericarditis is established using the following criteria: (1) increased number of lymphocytes and mononuclear cells >5000/mm^3 (autoreactive lymphocytic) or the presence of antibodies against heart muscle tissue (antisarcolemmal) in the pericardial fluid (autoreactive antibody mediated); (2) signs of myocarditis on epicardial or endomyocardial biopsies by ≥14 cells/mm^2; and (3) exclusion of infections, neoplasia, and systemic and metabolic disorders.

CMV = cytomegalovirus; EBV = Epstein-Barr virus; HBV = hepatitis B virus; HCV = hepatitis C virus; HIV = human immunodeficiency virus.

From Imazio M, Spodick DH, Brucato A, et al. Controversial issues in the management of pericardial diseases. *Circulation.* 2010;121:916-928.

TABLE 77-2 DIFFERENTIATION OF PERICARDITIS FROM MYOCARDIAL ISCHEMIA OR INFARCTION AND PULMONARY EMBOLISM

FINDINGS	MYOCARDIAL ISCHEMIA OR INFARCTION	PERICARDITIS	PULMONARY EMBOLISM
CHEST PAIN			
Character	Pressure-like heavy, squeezing	Sharp, stabbing, occasionally dull	Sharp, stabbing
Change with respiration	No	Worsened with inspiration	In phase with respiration (absent when the patient is apneic)
Change with position	No	Worse when supine; improved when sitting up or leaning forward	No
Duration	Minutes (ischemia); hours (infarction)	Hours to days	Hours to days
Response to nitroglycerin	Improved	No change	No change
PHYSICAL EXAMINATION			
Friction rub	Absent (unless pericarditis is present)	Present in most patients	Pleural friction rub may occur
ELECTROCARDIOGRAM			
ST segment elevation	Localized convex	Widespread concave	Limited to leads III, aVF, and V_1
PR segment depression	Rare	Frequent	None

Modified from Little WC, Freeman GL. Pericardial disease. *Circulation.* 2006;113:1622-1632.

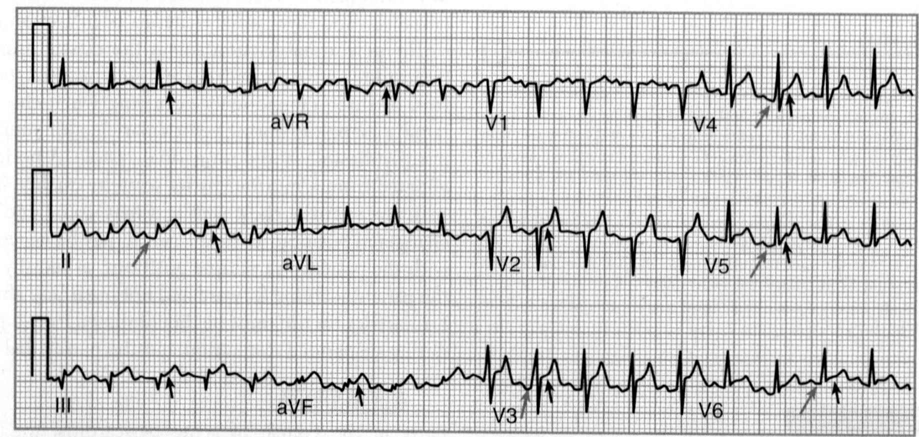

FIGURE 77-1. Electrocardiogram demonstrating typical features of acute pericarditis on presentation. There are diffuse ST elevation and PR depression except in aVR, where there is ST depression and PR elevation.

but the changes may be more localized in post-MI pericarditis. Classically, the ECG changes of acute pericarditis evolve over several days; resolution of the ST elevation is followed by widespread T-wave inversion that subsequently normalizes. Uremic pericarditis usually occurs without the typical ECG abnormalities.

Patients with acute pericarditis usually have evidence of systemic inflammation, including leukocytosis, an elevated erythrocyte sedimentation rate (ESR), and increased C-reactive protein (CRP) level. A low-grade fever is common, but a temperature greater than 38° C is unusual and suggests the possibility of bacterial pericarditis.

About 85% of cases of acute pericarditis are idiopathic or viral. Viral causes include echoviruses and group B coxsackieviruses, but obtaining specific viral titers does not alter patient management. About 6% of cases are neoplastic in origin, about 4% are caused by tuberculosis, about 3% are caused by other bacterial or fungal infections, and about 2% are caused by collagen vascular disease. A targeted evaluation (Table 77-3) can help identify the various causes (Table 77-4).

Troponin levels typically are minimally elevated in acute pericarditis owing to some involvement of the epicardium by the inflammatory process. An elevated troponin level in acute pericarditis usually returns to normal within 1 to 2 weeks and is not associated with a worse prognosis. Although the elevated troponin level may lead to the misdiagnosis of an ST elevation MI (Chapter 73), most patients with elevated troponin levels and acute pericarditis have normal coronary angiograms. An echocardiogram (Chapter 55) can help avoid a misdiagnosis of MI. Interestingly, patients with myopericarditis and elevated troponin levels tend to have a lower recurrence rate than do patients with pure pericarditis and normal troponin levels.[1]

Echocardiography may demonstrate a small pericardial effusion in the presence of acute pericarditis, but normal echocardiogram results do not exclude the diagnosis of acute pericarditis. An echocardiogram is critical, however, in excluding the diagnosis of cardiac tamponade (see later). When the diagnosis of acute pericarditis is unclear, cardiac magnetic resonance imaging (MRI) can demonstrate pericardial inflammation as delayed enhancement of the pericardium (Fig. 77-2). Diagnostic pericardiocentesis is indicated in suspected purulent tuberculosis or malignant pericarditis or if the patient has cardiac tamponade.

TABLE 77-3 SELECTED DIAGNOSTIC TESTS IN ACUTE PERICARDITIS

IN ALL PATIENTS

Tuberculin skin test (plus control skin test to exclude anergy)
BUN and creatinine to exclude uremia
Erythrocyte sedimentation rate
Electrocardiogram
Chest radiograph
Echocardiogram

IN SELECTED PATIENTS

Cardiac magnetic resonance imaging
ANA and rheumatoid factor to exclude SLE or rheumatoid arthritis in patients with acute arthritis or pleural effusion
TSH and T_4 to exclude hypothyroidism in patients with clinical findings suggestive of hypothyroidism and in asymptomatic patients with unexplained pericardial effusion
HIV test to exclude AIDS in patients with risk factors for HIV disease or a compatible clinical syndrome
Blood cultures in febrile patients to exclude infective endocarditis and bacteremia
Fungal serologic tests in patients from endemic areas or in immunocompromised patients
ASO titer in children or teenagers with suspected rheumatic fever
Heterophil antibody test to exclude mononucleosis in young or middle-aged patients with a compatible clinical syndrome or acute fever, weakness, and lymphadenopathy

AIDS = acquired immunodeficiency virus; ANA = antinuclear antibody; ASO = antistreptolysin O; BUN = blood urea nitrogen; HIV = human immunodeficiency virus; SLE = systemic lupus erythematosus; T_4 = thyroxine; TSH = thyroid-stimulating hormone.
Modified from Nishimura RA, Kidd KR. Recognition and management of patients with pericardial disease. In: Braunwald E, Goldman L, eds. *Primary Cardiology*. 2nd ed. Philadelphia: WB Saunders; 2003:625.

TABLE 77-4 PRESENTATION AND TREATMENT OF THE MOST COMMON CAUSES OF PERICARDITIS

TYPE	PATHOGENESIS OR ETIOLOGY	DIAGNOSIS	TREATMENT	COMPLICATIONS	COMMENTS
Viral	Coxsackievirus B Echovirus type 8 Epstein-Barr virus	Leukocytosis Elevated ESR Mild cardiac biomarker elevation	Symptomatic relief, NSAIDs, colchicine	Tamponade Relapsing pericarditis	Peaks in spring and fall
Tuberculous	*Mycobacterium tuberculosis*	Isolation of organism from biopsy fluid Granulomas not specific	Triple-drug antituberculosis regimen Pericardial drainage followed by early (4-6 wk) pericardiectomy if signs of tamponade or constriction develop	Tamponade Constrictive pericarditis	1%-8% of patients with tuberculosis pneumonia; rule out HIV infection
Bacterial	Group A streptococcus *Staphylococcus aureus* *Streptococcus pneumoniae*	Leukocytosis with marked left shift Purulent pericardial fluid	Pericardial drainage by catheter or surgery Systemic antibiotics Pericardiectomy if constrictive physiology develops	Tamponade in one third of patients	Very high mortality rate if not recognized early
Post–myocardial infarction	12 hr–10 days after infarction	Fever Pericardial friction rub Echo: effusion	Aspirin Prednisone	Tamponade rare	More frequent in large Q wave infarctions Anterior > inferior
Uremic	Untreated renal failure: 50% Chronic dialysis: 20%	Pericardial rub: 90%	Intensive dialysis Indomethacin: probably ineffective Catheter drainage Surgical drainage	Tamponade Hemodynamic instability on dialysis	Avoid NSAIDs ≈50% respond to intensive dialysis
Neoplastic	In order of frequency: lung cancer, breast cancer, leukemia and lymphoma, others	Chest pain, dyspnea Echo: effusion CT, MRI: tumor metastases to pericardium Cytologic examination of fluid positive in 85%	Catheter drainage Subxiphoid pericardiectomy Chemotherapy directed at underlying malignant neoplasm	Tamponade Constriction	

CT = computed tomography; ESR = erythrocyte sedimentation rate; HIV = human immunodeficiency virus; MRI = magnetic resonance imaging; NSAIDs = nonsteroidal anti-inflammatory drugs.
Modified from Malik F, Foster E. Pericardial disease. In: Wachter RM, Goldman L, Hollander H, eds. *Hospital Medicine*. 2nd ed. Philadelphia: Lippincott Williams & Wilkins; 2005:449.

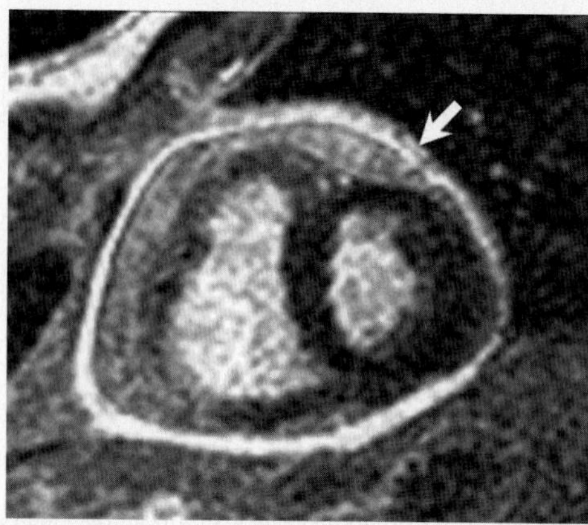

FIGURE 77-2. Cardiac magnetic resonance image of a patient with acute pericarditis shows late gadolinium hyperenhancement of the pericardium and epicardium.

TREATMENT

Rx

Acutely ill patients with fever should be hospitalized, as should patients with suspected acute MI (Chapter 73), large effusions, evidence of impending hemodynamic compromise, or a cause other than viral or idiopathic pericarditis because of the risk of a rapidly accumulating effusion with potential tamponade. Patients without effusions can usually be followed as outpatients (Fig. 77-3).

If acute pericarditis is a manifestation of an underlying disease, it often responds to treatment of the primary condition. Most cases of acute idiopathic or viral pericarditis are self-limited and respond to treatment with aspirin (650 mg every 6 hours) or another nonsteroidal antiinflammatory drug (NSAID) such as ibuprofen (300 to 800 mg every 6 to 8 hours). The dose of NSAID should be tapered after symptoms and any pericardial effusion have resolved, but the medication should be taken for at least 3 to 4 weeks to minimize the risk of recurrent pericarditis.

In addition, colchicine (0.6 to 1.2 mg/day for 3 months) should be started in all patients with acute pericarditis to reduce the rate of persistent symptoms at 72 hours, reduce the likelihood of recurrent pericarditis from 55% to 24% at 18 months, and reduce the rate of subsequent hospitalization.[A1] [A2] The major side effect of colchicine is diarrhea. The lower dose of colchicine should be used in patients who weigh less than 70 kg or who have side effects with the higher dose. Colchicine should be avoided in patients with abnormal renal or hepatic function and in patients being treated with macrolide antibiotics, which alter its metabolism.

A proton pump inhibitor, such as omeprazole (20 mg/day), should be considered to improve the gastric tolerability of NSAIDs. Warfarin and heparin should be avoided to minimize the risk of hemopericardium, but anticoagulation may be required if the patient is in atrial fibrillation or has a prosthetic heart valve. It is prudent to avoid exercise until after the chest pain completely resolves. If pericarditis recurs, the patient can be reloaded with colchicine and intravenous ketorolac (20 mg) and then continued on an oral NSAID and colchicine for at least 3 months.

Although acute pericarditis usually responds dramatically to systemic corticosteroids, observational studies strongly suggest that the use of steroids increases the probability of relapse in patients treated with colchicine. Except when needed to treat an underlying inflammatory disease, every effort should be made to avoid the use of steroids, reserving low-dose steroids for patients who cannot tolerate aspirin and other NSAIDs or whose recurrence is not responsive to colchicine and intravenous NSAIDs. If steroids are used, low-dose prednisone (0.2 to 0.5 mg/kg) appears to be as effective as higher doses and is less likely to be associated with recurrence. Steroids should be continued for at least 1 month before slow tapering, which can be guided by return of the CRP level to the normal range. Pericardiocentesis is not recommended unless purulent or tuberculous pericarditis is clinically suspected or the patient fails to respond to 2 to 3 weeks of NSAID therapy.

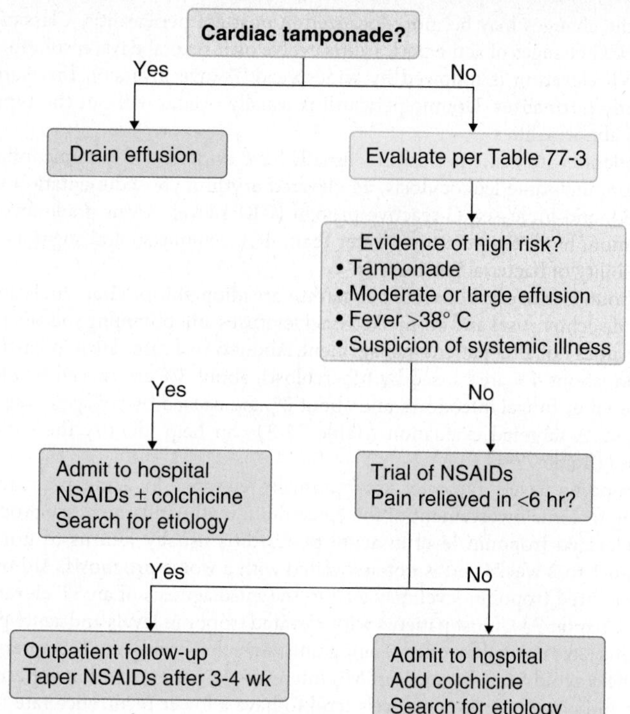

FIGURE 77-3. Initial management of patients with pericarditis. NSAID = nonsteroidal antiinflammatory drug.

TABLE 77-5 CAUSES OF MODERATE TO LARGE ASYMPTOMATIC PERICARDIAL EFFUSIONS

CAUSE	CASES (%)
Idiopathic or viral	37
Neoplastic	19
Iatrogenic or trauma	13
Tuberculous or purulent	6
Acute myocardial infarction	6
Collagen vascular disease	4
Heart failure	4
Uremia	4
Radiation induced	2
Aortic dissection	2
Hypothyroidism	1
Other	2

Modified from Nishimura RA, Kidd KR. Recognition and management of patients with pericardial disease. In: Braunwald E, Goldman L, eds. *Primary Cardiology.* 2nd ed. Philadelphia: WB Saunders; 2003:625.

PROGNOSIS

The course of viral and idiopathic pericarditis is usually self-limited, and most patients recover completely.[2] About 25% of patients, however, have recurrent pericarditis weeks to months later, probably caused by an immune response, and some patients may have multiple debilitating episodes. In patients whose acute pericarditis is accompanied by myocarditis, as evidenced by elevation of serum troponin levels, the recurrence rate is closer to 10%.[1] Recurrent pericarditis is more common in patients treated with steroids for the acute episode, especially during a rapid steroid taper. In these patients, prolonged high-dose NSAID treatment (e.g., ibuprofen 300 to 600 mg three times a day) plus colchicine (0.5 to 0.6 mg twice daily, declining to once daily after 3 to 6 months) is effective.[A3] In patients who cannot tolerate colchicine or who have recurrent episodes despite colchicine and high-dose NSAID treatment (e.g., indomethacin 50 mg three times a day or ibuprofen 800 mg four times a day), oral steroids (e.g., prednisone 0.2 to 0.5 mg/kg/day for 2 to 4 weeks; then slowly tapered over several months) are generally recommended. In patients with refractory, recurrent pericarditis, surgical pericardiectomy can be considered.[3] Patients who have tuberculous or purulent pericarditis or have recurrent episodes of pericarditis have the highest risk for progression to constrictive pericarditis (see later).

CARDIAC EFFUSION AND TAMPONADE

EPIDEMIOLOGY

A pericardial effusion can be caused by any disease that causes acute pericarditis (see Table 77-1), but a majority of cases are caused by conditions other than viral or idiopathic pericarditis (Table 77-5). For example, tamponade

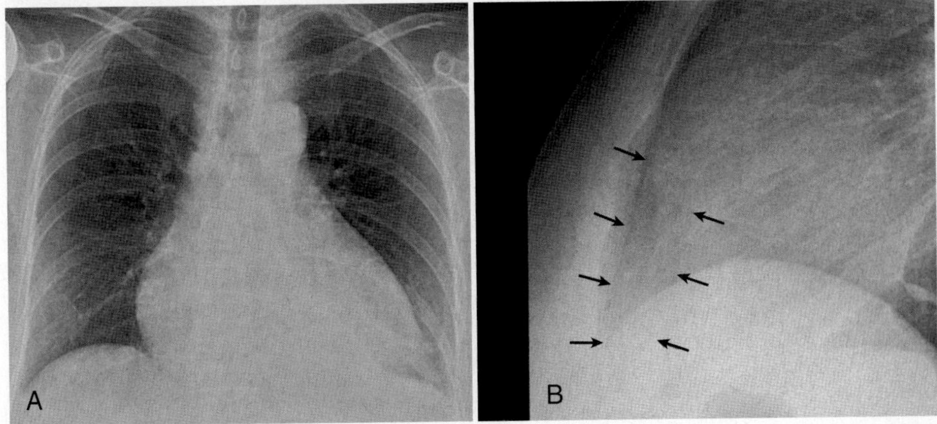

FIGURE 77-4. Chest radiographs in a patient with a large pericardial effusion. The cardiac silhouette on the posteroanterior view (**A**) is enlarged with a "water bag" configuration. The lateral view (**B**) shows a separation between the pericardial and epicardial fat stripes *(arrows)*.

occurs in about 10% to 15% of patients with idiopathic pericarditis, but it develops in more than 50% of patients with malignant, tuberculous, or purulent pericarditis. Tuberculosis and neoplastic disease are typically associated with serosanguineous effusions, but such effusions can also be seen with typical viral or idiopathic pericarditis, with uremia, and after mediastinal irradiation. Hemopericardium is seen most commonly with trauma, myocardial rupture after MI, catheter-induced myocardial or epicardial coronary artery rupture, aortic dissection with rupture into the pericardial space, or primary hemorrhage in patients receiving anticoagulant therapy, often after cardiac valve surgery. Chylopericardium is rare and results from leakage or injury to the thoracic duct.

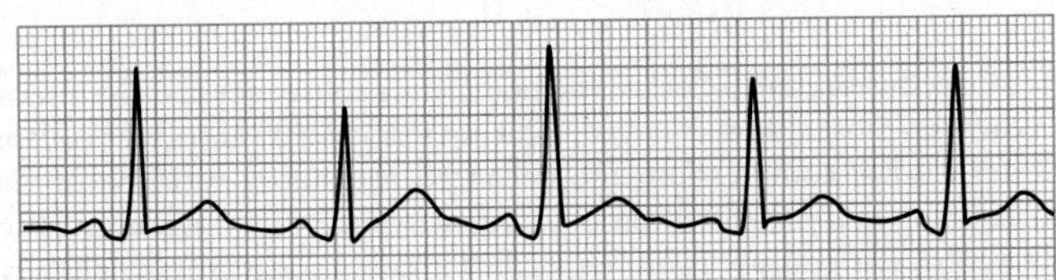

FIGURE 77-5. Electrical alternans. Lead V_5 rhythm strip from a patient with a large pericardial effusion and tamponade physiology. Note the relatively low voltage and electrical alternans.

PATHOBIOLOGY

Under normal conditions, the space between the parietal and visceral pericardium can accommodate only a small amount of fluid before the development of tamponade physiology. The clinical consequences of a pericardial effusion depend on the rate of increase. A rapidly accumulating effusion, as in hemopericardium caused by trauma or aortic dissection, may result in tamponade physiology with just 100 to 200 mL of fluid. It is not surprising, therefore, that cardiac perforation quickly results in tamponade. By comparison, a more slowly developing effusion, as is typical with uremia and hypothyroidism, may allow the gradual stretching of the pericardium, with asymptomatic or minimally symptomatic effusions of 1500 mL or more.

Tamponade physiology occurs when fluid accumulation in the intrapericardial space is sufficient to compress the heart, resulting in impaired cardiac filling. The increased pericardial pressure in cardiac tamponade accentuates the interdependence among the cardiac chambers as the total cardiac volume is limited by the pericardial effusion. With normal inspiration, right ventricular filling is enhanced, the intraventricular septum is displaced toward the left ventricle, and left ventricular filling and the resulting stroke volume are reduced. Because of its lower pressures, the right ventricle is most vulnerable to compression by a pericardial effusion, and abnormal right heart filling is the earliest sign of a hemodynamically significant pericardial effusion. In tamponade, left heart filling occurs preferentially during expiration, when there is less filling of the right heart. The small normal respiratory increase in right ventricular volume, with a concomitant decrease in left ventricular stroke volume and systolic arterial pressure is markedly accentuated in cardiac tamponade and results in the clinical finding of "paradoxical pulse." A small (<10 mm Hg) pulsus paradoxus, which is a decline in systemic blood pressure during inspiration, is normal and is related to the ventricles being confined within the pericardium and sharing a common septum. In cardiac tamponade, this phenomenon is exaggerated, and systemic blood pressure falls by more than 10 mm Hg during inspiration. A pulsus paradoxus also may be present with hypovolemic shock, chronic obstructive pulmonary disease, and bronchospasm.

CLINICAL MANIFESTATIONS

A slowly accumulating, isolated pericardial effusion is often completely asymptomatic. The physical examination results may be normal, but the heart sounds may be muffled. The diagnosis is usually suggested by a chest radiograph that shows cardiomegaly with a globular heart (Fig. 77-4; see also Fig. 56-5) or by an echocardiogram, computed tomography (CT) scan, or MRI performed for another indication. Patients with hypothyroidism, uremia, or collagen vascular disease may have asymptomatic effusions discovered during comprehensive evaluations.

Patients with impending or early tamponade are usually anxious and tachycardic, and they may complain of dyspnea, orthopnea, and chest pain. The increased venous pressure is usually apparent as jugular venous distention. The x descent (during ventricular systole) is typically the dominant jugular venous wave, with little or no y descent (during early diastole) (Chapter 51). The heart sounds are classically soft or muffled, especially if there is a large pericardial effusion. In rapidly developing cardiac tamponade, especially hemorrhagic cardiac tamponade, the jugular veins may not be distended because the time course has been insufficient for a compensatory increase in venous pressure. Such "low-pressure" tamponade may also occur with uremic pericarditis in volume-depleted patients. The patient may have signs of right heart failure, with peripheral edema, right upper quadrant pain caused by hepatic congestion, or abnormal liver enzymes and serum bilirubin level.

The hallmark of cardiac tamponade is a paradoxical pulse, which is defined as more than a 10–mm Hg drop in systolic arterial pressure during inspiration. When severe, the paradoxical pulse may be apparent as the absence of a palpable brachial or radial pulse during inspiration. A paradoxical pulse can also occur when there are wide swings in intrathoracic pressure, pulmonary embolism (Chapter 98), or hypovolemic shock (Chapter 106). A paradoxical pulse may be difficult to recognize in the presence of severe shock.

DIAGNOSIS

Cardiac tamponade, which is a treatable cause of shock (Chapter 107), can be rapidly fatal if unrecognized. As such, cardiac tamponade should be considered in the differential diagnosis of any patient with shock or pulseless electrical activity.

Cardiac tamponade is usually suspected based on jugular venous distention, sinus tachycardia with hypotension, narrow pulse pressure, elevated (>10 mm Hg) pulsus paradoxus, and distant heart sounds. Pulsus paradoxus may be obvious by palpation; it is more accurately measured with a sphygmomanometer during slow inspiration.

The ECG often shows low voltage and sometimes electrical alternans (Fig. 77-5) when the heart swings within a large pericardial effusion. The chest radiograph shows a globular, enlarged cardiac shadow (see Fig. 56-5 and Fig. 77-4) without pulmonary venous congestion.

Echocardiography, which is the key diagnostic test for cardiac tamponade, must be performed without delay in any patient suspected of having this condition. Echocardiography visualizes pericardial effusions as an echo-free space around the heart (Fig. 77-6), demonstrates the presence and size of the

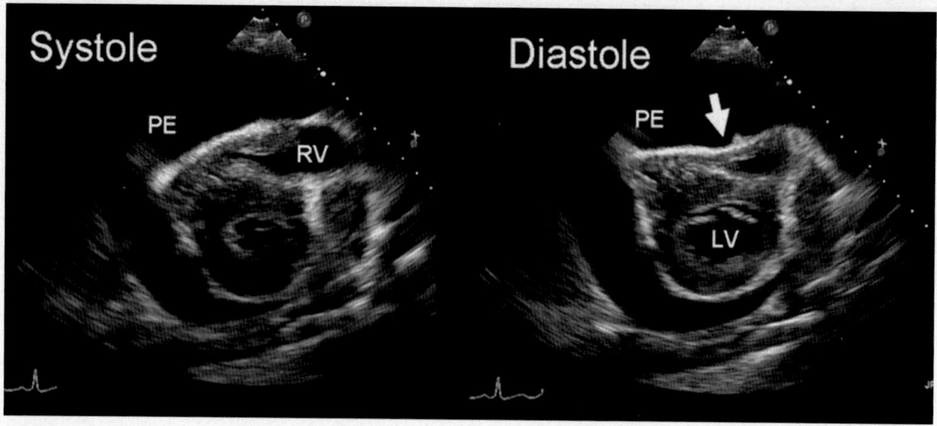

FIGURE 77-6. **Two-dimensional echocardiogram from a patient with cardiac tamponade. A large pericardial effusion (PE) is apparent as an echo-free space surrounding the left ventricle (LV) and right ventricle (RV). In diastole, there is collapse of the right ventricle *(arrow)*.**

pericardial effusion, and reflects its hemodynamic consequences. The inferior vena cava is almost always enlarged, right atrial and right ventricular collapse indicates cardiac compression, and enhanced respiratory variation of ventricular filling is a manifestation of increased ventricular interdependence. Right ventricular collapse is more specific for tamponade than is right atrial collapse, but the right-sided chambers may not collapse when tamponade occurs in patients with pulmonary hypertension. Cardiac tamponade can result from a loculated pericardial effusion after cardiac surgery or trauma. A loculated effusion may not be apparent on transthoracic echocardiography, but transesophageal echocardiography and thoracic CT or MRI can delineate loculated pericardial effusions.

On Doppler study, mitral inflow velocity (especially early diastolic velocity, designated as E velocity) normally increases with expiration and decreases with inspiration; the opposite respiratory variation is seen in tricuspid inflow velocity. Doppler findings for tamponade, which are more sensitive than two-dimensional echocardiography, include augmented respiratory variation of mitral and tricuspid inflow E velocities as a function of ventricular interdependence. These changes may be seen even before frank hemodynamic compromise caused by pericardial effusion. Although Doppler echocardiography provides important information, it must be emphasized that cardiac tamponade is ultimately a clinical diagnosis.

The routine evaluation should include an assessment of renal function, a thyroid-stimulating hormone level, a complete blood count with differential, a platelet count, coagulation parameters, and a tuberculin skin test. Common medications that can cause a pericardial effusion include cromolyn, isoniazid, and phenytoin; hydralazine, procainamide, and reserpine are others. Blood cultures are indicated if an infectious cause is suspected. Complement levels, antinuclear antibodies, and the ESR can suggest systemic lupus erythematosus (Chapter 266), which rarely presents initially as an isolated pericardial effusion.

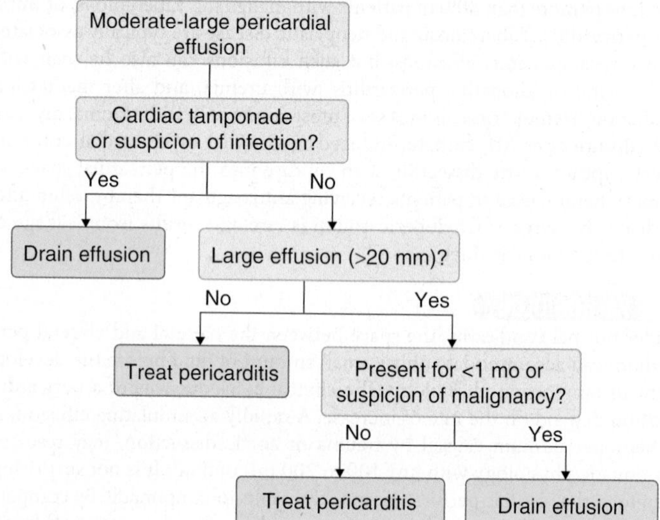

FIGURE 77-7. **Algorithm for managing patients with moderate to large pericardial effusions. (Modified from Little WC, Freeman GL. Pericardial disease. *Circulation.* 2006;113:1622-1632.)**

TREATMENT

Rx

Pericardial Effusion without Tamponade

Acute pericarditis is often accompanied by a small pericardial effusion that does not produce tamponade. If there is no hemodynamic compromise and the diagnosis can be established by other means, pericardiocentesis is not necessary (Fig. 77-7). Even small pericardial effusions may be related to underlying systemic illnesses such as systemic lupus erythematosus (Chapter 266), cardiac amyloid (Chapter 188), scleroderma (Chapter 267), hypothyroidism (Chapter 226), or AIDS, so it is important to consider and treat associated illnesses. Chylous pericardial effusion, which is usually related to obstruction of the thoracic duct, may require a surgical procedure for relief.

For suspected pericardial effusion, transthoracic echocardiography is the initial test of choice, although loculated effusions may be identified better by CT or MRI. If a small (0.5 to 1 cm) echolucent or "organized" pericardial effusion is observed, a follow-up echocardiogram in 1 to 2 weeks, or sooner if the patient deteriorates, is recommended. If the effusion is getting smaller, subsequent echocardiograms are not necessary unless the patient's clinical condition changes.

For moderate (1 to 2 cm) or large (>2 cm) effusions in patients who are hemodynamically stable and in whom tamponade is not suspected, a follow-up echocardiogram should be performed in 7 days and then every month until the effusion is minimal.[4] If bacterial or malignant pericarditis is suspected, diagnostic pericardiocentesis should be performed immediately even in the absence of clinical instability or suggestion of tamponade; tuberculous pericarditis is diagnosed best by pericardial biopsy. Anticoagulation with heparin or warfarin should be discontinued unless the patient has a mechanical heart valve or atrial fibrillation.

In hypothyroidism (Chapter 226), the effusion and the coexistent cardiomyopathy respond to hormone replacement, sometimes over several months. Uremic pericardial effusions often respond to initiation of dialysis or more intensive dialysis (Chapter 131).

Cardiac Tamponade

The treatment of cardiac tamponade is urgent drainage of the pericardial effusion, especially when there is hemodynamic compromise. Fluid resuscitation may be of transient benefit if the patient is volume depleted (hypovolemic cardiac tamponade), but inotropic agents are usually ineffective because there is already intense endogenous adrenergic stimulation. The initiation of mechanical ventilation in a patient with tamponade may produce a sudden drop in blood pressure because the positive intrathoracic pressure further impairs cardiac filling.

Echocardiographic-guided percutaneous pericardiocentesis, which can be performed at the bedside by experienced operators (Fig. 77-8), is indicated if a patient is in dire circumstances and at least 1 cm of fluid is seen anterior to the mid-right ventricular free wall throughout diastole. The ideal entry site (usually the apex) is defined using echocardiography as the minimal distance from the skin to pericardial fluid without intervening structures. The pericardial space is entered with a needle and then drained through a catheter. As much fluid as possible should be removed. The pericardial fluid should be sent for pH, glucose, lactate dehydrogenase, protein, cell count, and cytology as well as staining and culture for bacteria, fungi, and tuberculosis. Continued drainage of the pericardial fluid through an indwelling catheter minimizes the risk of recurrent effusion. For hemodynamically significant effusions of

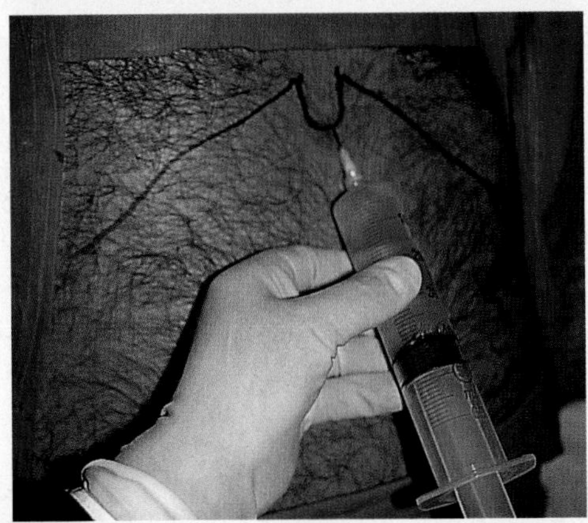

FIGURE 77-8. Aspiration of pericardial fluid is indicated in cardiac tamponade or to obtain fluid for diagnostic purposes. A wide-bore needle is inserted in the epigastrium below the xiphoid process and advanced in the direction of the medial third of the right clavicle. An alternative site is over the left ventricular apex. The procedure should be performed under echocardiographic guidance, but it may need to be performed emergently for life-saving purposes in other settings. Complications of the procedure include puncture of the heart, arrhythmias, vasovagal attack, and pneumothorax. (From Forbes CD, Jackson WF. *Color Atlas and Text of Clinical Medicine.* 3rd ed. London: Mosby; 2003.)

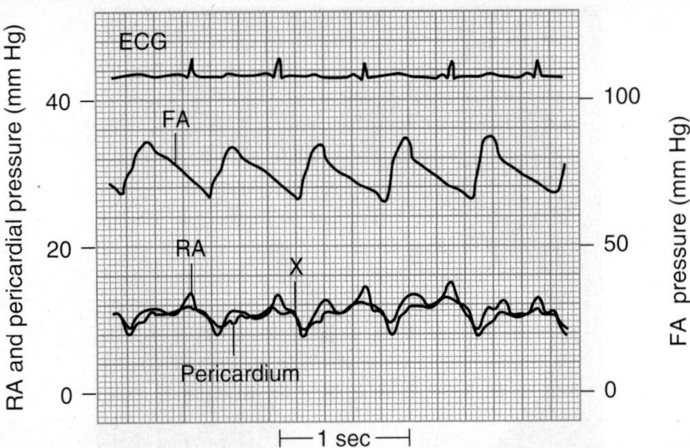

FIGURE 77-9. Right atrial (RA) pressure recording from a patient with constrictive pericarditis. Note the elevation in pressure and the prominent y descent, corresponding to rapid, early diastolic right atrial emptying. ECG = electrocardiogram; FA = femoral artery. (From Lorell BH. Profiles in constriction, restriction and tamponade. In: Baim DS, Grossman W, eds. *Cardiac Catheterization, Angiography, and Intervention.* 6th ed. Philadelphia: Williams Wilkins; 2000: 832.)

less than 1 cm, organized or multiloculated effusions, and focal effusions, a limited thoracotomy-mediastinoscopy and creation of a pericardial window are advised.

Surgical drainage may be the preferred treatment if pericardial tissue is required for diagnosis or in the case of recurrent effusions or bacterial pericarditis. Malignant pericardial effusions frequently reoccur and, similar to other recurrent pericardial effusions, may necessitate the surgical creation of a pericardial window that allows the effusion to drain into the pleural space, preventing reoccurrence of cardiac tamponade. An attractive alternative in these patients, especially if their overall prognosis is poor from the malignancy, is the percutaneous creation of a pericardial window by balloon dilation. Hemorrhagic effusions related to cardiac trauma or aortic dissection are best managed by emergency surgery.

PROGNOSIS

A pericardial effusion may recur or persist. Symptoms are usually weight loss, fatigue, dyspnea on exertion, and whatever symptoms are associated with the specific cause. Treatment of chronic or recurrent idiopathic effusions is similar to the treatment of recurrent pericarditis. If medical therapy is unsuccessful, creation of a pericardial window is indicated.

A large idiopathic, asymptomatic effusion that persists for 6 months or longer can unpredictably result in tamponade in as many as 30% of patients over long-term follow-up; diagnostic pericardiocentesis occasionally detects a neoplastic or tuberculous cause. Pericardiocentesis with prolonged drainage resolves many chronic large pericardial effusions, but pericardiectomy is often required. The long-term prognosis depends on the cause of the effusion. With pericardial tamponade, the in-hospital mortality rate is less than 10%, but the subsequent mortality rate is about 75% with a malignant effusion compared with only a 3% to 5% subsequent annual mortality rate for other causes.

PERICARDIAL CONSTRICTION

EPIDEMIOLOGY AND PATHOBIOLOGY

Pericardial constriction, which is usually the result of long-standing pericardial inflammation, occurs when a scarred, thickened, or calcified pericardium impairs cardiac filling, thereby limiting the total cardiac volume. The most frequent causes in the developed world are previous cardiac surgery, chronic idiopathic or viral pericarditis, and mediastinal radiation. Constriction may follow cardiac surgery by several weeks to months and may occur decades after chest wall irradiation. In developing countries, tuberculous pericarditis is a more common cause of constrictive pericarditis. Other less common causes include malignant disease, especially lung cancer, breast cancer, or lymphoma; histoplasmosis; rheumatoid arthritis; and uremia. However, a specific cause may not be identified in many patients.

With chronic constriction, the pericardium may thicken from its normal 2 mm or less, calcify, and adhere to the epicardium. In a subset of the patients with constriction, the pericardium may be only minimally thickened and less calcified. Fibrous scarring and adhesions of both pericardial layers obliterate the pericardial cavity. The ventricles are unable to fill because of physical constraints imposed by a thickened, rigid, and sometimes calcified pericardium. The pathophysiologic hallmark of pericardial constriction is the exaggerated interventricular dependence and differential ventricular filling with respiration.

Although both cardiac tamponade and pericardial constriction impair diastolic ventricular filling and elevate venous pressure, the impairment in ventricular filling with constriction is minimal in early diastole until cardiac volume reaches the anatomic limit set by the noncompliant pericardium, at which time diastolic pressure rises abruptly and remains elevated until the onset of systole. This prominent y descent with an elevated plateau of ventricular pressure, which has been termed the "square root" sign (Fig. 77-9), differentiates constriction from tamponade, in which the y descent is absent. Stroke volume and cardiac output are reduced because of impaired filling, but the intrinsic systolic function of the ventricles can be normal.

CLINICAL MANIFESTATIONS

Patients with pericardial constriction typically present with manifestations of elevated systemic venous pressures and low cardiac output. Because there is equalization of all cardiac pressures (including right and left atrial pressures), systemic congestion is much more marked than pulmonary congestion. Typically, patients develop marked jugular venous distention, hepatic congestion, ascites, and peripheral edema, but their lungs remain clear. The limited cardiac output typically presents as exercise intolerance and may progress to cardiac cachexia with muscle wasting. In long-standing pericardial constriction, pleural effusions, ascites, and hepatic dysfunction may be prominent clinical features. Patients with pericardial constriction are much more likely to have left-sided or bilateral pleural effusions than right-sided effusions. Because of the prominent clinical symptoms of ascites and liver enzyme abnormalities, patients may be evaluated for hepatic disease before constrictive pericarditis is recognized.

The jugular veins are distended with prominent x and y descents. The normal inspiratory drop in jugular venous distention may be replaced by a rise in venous pressure (Kussmaul sign). The classic auscultatory finding of pericardial constriction is a pericardial knock (Chapter 51), which is a high-pitched sound early in diastole when there is the sudden cessation of rapid ventricular diastolic filling, coinciding with the nadir of the y descent.

DIAGNOSIS

Pericardial constriction should be considered in any patient with unexplained systemic venous congestion. Pericardial calcification, seen best on the lateral plain chest radiograph, is a classic finding but is present in only 25% of patients with constrictive pericarditis, mostly in those with long-standing constriction. Similarly, most patients with pericardial constriction have a thickened pericardium (>2 mm) that can be imaged by echocardiography, CT, and MRI (Fig. 77-10). It is important to recognize, however, that pericardial constriction can be present without pericardial calcification and, in about 20% of patients, without any obvious pericardial thickening.

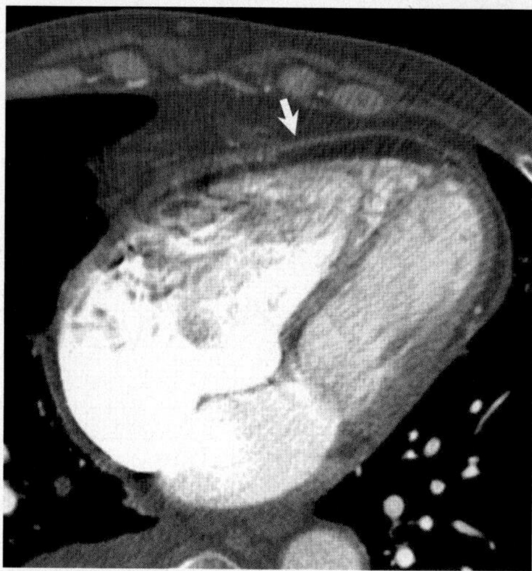

FIGURE 77-10. Computed tomography in a patient with constrictive pericarditis shows a thickened pericardium *(arrow)*.

Transesophageal Doppler echocardiography may demonstrate pericardial thickening and calcification, but increased pericardial thickness can be missed on a transthoracic echocardiogram. Echocardiography also differentiates pericardial constriction from right heart failure caused by tricuspid valve disease or associated pulmonary hypertension.

Differential Diagnosis

The most difficult differentiation is between pericardial constriction and restrictive cardiomyopathy (Chapter 60), the clinical manifestations of which may be very similar to those of pericardial constriction (Table 77-6). Doppler echocardiography is the most useful method to distinguish constriction from restriction.[5] Whereas patients with pericardial constriction usually have pronounced respiratory variation (>25%) of mitral inflow E velocity, patients with restrictive cardiomyopathies do not. In some patients with pericardial constriction and markedly elevated venous pressures, the respiratory variation may be present only after head-up tilt. The tissue Doppler measurement of early diastolic septal mitral annular velocity (e′) is almost always reduced in patients with myocardial restriction, but it remains normal or increased in patients with pericardial constriction. In addition, lateral e′, which is higher than septal or medial e′ velocity in normal and restrictive cardiomyopathy, is lower than septal e′ in most patients with constrictive pericarditis. Whereas a prominent diastolic reversal of hepatic vein flow velocity during expiration is characteristic of constriction, the reversal flow velocity occurs during inspiration in patients with right heart failure from other causes. Patients with pericardial constriction usually have only minimally elevated (<200 pg/mL) brain natriuretic peptide (BNP), but BNP levels are typically markedly increased (<600 pg/mL) in patients with restrictive cardiomyopathy.

Confirmation of the diagnosis of constriction may require cardiac catheterization in patients whose noninvasive evaluation is not clear cut. Traditional invasive hemodynamic findings of equalized end-diastolic pressures in the right and left ventricles and the "dip and plateau" pattern of left ventricular diastolic pressure do not reliably differentiate constriction from restrictive cardiomyopathy. More specific invasive hemodynamic features of constriction and restriction are based on the respiratory variation in ventricular filling; the simultaneous measurement of left and right ventricular pressures demonstrates discordant changes in their systolic pressures with respiration in constrictive pericarditis. By comparison, the direction of these pressures is concordant (both left and right sides increase with expiration and decrease with inspiration) in restrictive cardiomyopathy.

All patients with documented but otherwise unexplained pericardial constriction should be evaluated for potential tuberculosis.

TREATMENT AND PROGNOSIS Rx

In some patients with pericardial constriction of less than 3 months' duration, the symptoms and constriction may resolve over several weeks with medical therapy consisting of NSAIDs (e.g., ibuprofen 300-800 mg every 6-8 hours), colchicine (0.6 mg once or twice daily), and the cautious use of diuretics. If the patient is severely compromised hemodynamically, steroid therapy (e.g., 0.5-1.0 mg/kg up to a maximum dose of 60 mg tapered slowly over 3 months as guided by the clinical response and normalization of the CRP) can be very effective.[6] The patients with constriction who respond to medical therapy usually have high inflammatory biomarkers (ESR and CRP) and intense inflammation of the pericardium on cardiac MRI.[7] For more chronic pericardial constriction or cases that do not respond to medical therapy, the definitive treatment is surgical pericardial decortication, with a wide resection of both the visceral and parietal pericardium. This operation is a major undertaking with substantial risk (≈10% mortality rate even in the most experienced centers).[8] In many patients, surgery does not immediately restore normal cardiac function; it may take weeks after removal of the constricting pericardium to return to normal. Empirical treatment of tuberculosis (Chapter 324) may be required in patients with constriction and a high suspicion of tuberculosis, even without a definitive diagnosis.

TABLE 77-6 DIFFERENTIATION OF PERICARDIAL CONSTRICTION FROM RESTRICTIVE CARDIOMYOPATHY

FINDINGS	PERICARDIAL CONSTRICTION	RESTRICTIVE CARDIOMYOPATHY
PHYSICAL EXAMINATION		
Pulmonary congestion	Usually absent	Usually present
Early diastolic sound	Pericardial knock	S_3 (low pitched)
ECHO/DOPPLER		
Respiratory variation in E wave (%)	>25	<20
Mitral septal annular early diastolic velocity (cm/sec)	>7	<7
CT/MRI		
Pericardial thickness	>2 mm (but <2 mm in 20%)	<2 mm
BIOMARKER		
B-type natriuretic peptide (pg/mL)	<200	>600
HEMODYNAMICS		
PA systolic pressure (mm Hg)	<60	>60
PCW-LV diastolic pressure	Respiratory variation with reduction in inspiration	No variation
Respiratory variation in RV/LV peak systolic pressure	Discordant	Concordant

CT = computed tomography; LV = left ventricular; MRI = magnetic resonance imaging; PA = pulmonary artery; PCW = pulmonary capillary wedge; RV = right ventricular.
Modified from Little WC, Freeman GL. Pericardial disease. *Circulation.* 2006;113:1622-1632.

Effusive-Constrictive Pericarditis

In some patients (<10%) who present with cardiac tamponade, the elevated right atrial pressure and jugular venous distention do not resolve after removal of the pericardial fluid. In these patients, pericardiocentesis converts the hemodynamics from those typical of tamponade to those of constriction. Thus, the restriction of cardiac filling is not only attributable to pericardial effusion but also to pericardial constriction, predominantly involving the visceral pericardium. Effusive-constrictive pericarditis[9] most likely represents an intermediate transition from acute pericarditis with pericardial effusion to pericardial constriction. Frequently, the symptoms resolve after several weeks of treatment with an NSAID (e.g., ibuprofen 300-800 mg every 6-8 hours).

SPECIFIC FORMS OF PERICARDIAL DISEASE

Postcardiotomy Syndrome

Postcardiotomy syndrome is acute pericarditis occurring weeks to months after open heart surgery. Patients have typical symptoms of acute pericarditis, which is associated with antimyocardial antibodies. A similar clinical picture is seen with the postperfusion syndrome caused by cytomegalovirus (CMV) infection (Chapter 376) in patients who were previously uninfected but were exposed to CMV-positive blood during cardiopulmonary bypass or transfusions. Atypical lymphocytes and elevated liver enzymes are often seen. Treatment of postcardiotomy syndrome is similar to the treatment of acute pericarditis. One month of colchicine therapy (0.5 mg twice daily for patients weighing 70 kg or more; half that dose for smaller patients or patients with side effects) started 48 to 72 hours prior to cardiac surgery appears to reduce the rate of the postcardiotomy syndrome from about 30% to less than 20% but did not reduce the occurrence of atrial fibrillation.[A4]

Some patients who have undergone cardiac surgery develop late pericardial constriction without preceding acute pericarditis owing to bleeding in and around the open pericardium followed by inflammation, scarring, and fibrosis. If active inflammation is present, a trial of antiinflammatory agents may be instituted; however, surgical removal of the blood clot, usually accompanied by more extensive pericardiectomy, is typically required.

Post–Myocardial Infarction Pericarditis

Acute pericarditis can develop several days after an acute MI (Chapter 73), usually because of transmural extension of the infarction to the pericardial surface. This syndrome is uncommon in the reperfusion era. Anticoagulation should be temporarily withheld to avoid a bloody effusion that might progress to cardiac tamponade.

A late autoimmune pericarditis, termed *Dressler syndrome*, can develop weeks to months after a Q-wave MI, but this syndrome is very uncommon since the advent of reperfusion therapy. Diagnosis and treatment are as for acute pericarditis.

Uremic Pericarditis

Pericardial effusions develop in patients with severe renal failure, especially those on dialysis (Chapter 131). Aggressive dialysis may decrease the pericardial effusion, but sometimes the effusion persists and requires drainage or even pericardiectomy.

Infectious Pericarditis

BACTERIAL PERICARDITIS

Purulent bacterial pericarditis may result from direct extension of bacterial pneumonia; direct extension of pleural empyema; or, rarely, peritonitis or a subphrenic abscess. Most patients are acutely ill with systemic sepsis and develop acute tamponade. The most common organisms are streptococci, pneumococci, and staphylococci. Urgent pericardiocentesis, which is required for both diagnosis and therapy, shows leukocytosis and frank pus, and the fluid glucose level is markedly depressed. Persistent or recurrent drainage with an indwelling catheter or repeated taps combined with antimicrobial therapy lead to a high survival rate,[10] but late constrictive pericarditis requiring pericardiectomy develops in 30% to 40% of patients.

TUBERCULOUS PERICARDITIS

Tuberculous pericarditis is common in developing countries but accounts for less than 5% of cases of acute pericarditis in developed countries, usually in patients who are immunosuppressed, including patients infected with the human immunodeficiency virus.[11] Symptoms are often nonspecific, and acute painful pericarditis is rare. Most patients have an effusive-constrictive physiology or pericardial constriction. The chest radiograph suggests active pulmonary tuberculosis is about 30% of cases, and a pleural effusion is present in 40% to 60% of cases. The echocardiogram typically shows fibrinous strands in the pericardial effusion, with multiple echo densities adherent to the pericardial surface. Pericardiocentesis is mandatory if tuberculous pericarditis is suspected. About 75% of patients have a positive culture, and a pericardial fluid adenosine deaminase level of 40 U/L or greater is seen in 75% of patients. Polymerase chain reaction testing and pericardial biopsy are recommended when tuberculous pericarditis is strongly suspected but not otherwise confirmed.

Aggressive antituberculosis therapy (Chapter 324) yields a cure rate of about 85% to 90%. Neither corticosteroids nor adjunctive immunotherapy improves outcome.[A5] Empirical treatment may be required in patients with a consistent clinical picture but without a confirmed diagnosis.

Even with prompt treatment, 30% to 60% of patients develop constrictive pericarditis, for which surgical pericardiectomy is the treatment of choice. In cases of suspected tuberculous constriction, antituberculosis therapy (Chapter 324) should be administered before and after pericardial surgery.

FUNGAL PERICARDITIS

The most common fungal pericarditis is histoplasmosis, which usually resolves in several weeks and can be treated successfully with NSAIDs. Specific antifungal therapy (Chapter 331) is recommended only in patients with disseminated histoplasmosis (Chapter 332).

Malignant Pericarditis

About 6% of cases of acute pericarditis that initially have no obvious cause, and about 20% of cases of moderate to large pericardial effusions are related to malignant diseases; in patients with cardiac tamponade, the percentage is even higher. About 80% of malignant pericarditis is linked to breast cancer (Chapter 198), lymphoma (Chapters 185 and 186), and leukemia (Chapters 183 and 184). Melanoma (Chapter 203) is an uncommon cause of malignant pericarditis, but a large proportion of patients with melanoma have pericardial involvement.

Most patients have direct tumor extension from an adjacent malignant lesion or a tumor from hematogenous or lymphatic spread. Pericardial effusions also may be caused by pericardial irritation or compromised lymphatic drainage in patients with mediastinal lymphoma.

Pericardiocentesis is key to diagnosis and management. Fluid cytology results are positive in about 85% of patients. Complete drainage with an indwelling catheter for 2 or 3 days is the treatment of choice; if the effusion does not resolve, pericardiectomy is recommended.[12] The prognosis depends on the treatment of the underlying malignancy, but the 1-year mortality rate is 80% or higher.

Postradiation Pericarditis

Postradiation pericarditis develops in about 2% of patients after mantle radiation for Hodgkin disease (Chapter 186) and in 0.4% to 5% of patients after irradiation for breast cancer. Pericardial injury occasionally manifests during treatment, but it more commonly appears months or even a decade later. The initial pericarditis and effusion may resolve spontaneously, but constrictive pericarditis, adjacent myocarditis, and even coronary artery damage can develop. Pericardiocentesis is critical to distinguish postradiation pericarditis from malignant pericardial disease. Pericardiectomy is recommended for recurrent pericarditis and for large recurrent pericardial effusions.

Autoimmune Pericarditis

Up to 50% of patients with systemic lupus erythematosus (Chapter 266) have pericarditis, usually during an acute flare. Patients usually present with acute pericarditis or an asymptomatic effusion; cardiac tamponade is uncommon, and constrictive pericarditis is rare. If purulent pericarditis is not suspected, pericardiocentesis is not usually required. The underlying disease should be treated aggressively.

Acute pericarditis or asymptomatic pericardial effusions can develop in patients with advanced rheumatoid arthritis (Chapter 264), scleroderma (Chapter 267), or mixed connective tissue disease (Chapter 267). The process is usually self-limited or responds to aggressive treatment of the underlying disease, although cardiac tamponade can develop.

Myopericarditis

Concomitant myopericarditis (Chapter 60) may develop in patients with pericarditis, probably owing to direct extension of the inflammatory process. It is often manifested by ECG conduction delays, ventricular arrhythmias, and elevated troponin levels. No specific treatment is available.

Acute ventricular dilation and sudden or progressive heart failure develop in some patients after pericardiectomy for constrictive pericarditis or even after drainage of a large pericardial effusion. The syndrome may be underlying myocarditis.

Congenital Abnormalities

Congenital total absence of the pericardium is asymptomatic and clinically unimportant. However, partial or localized absence of the pericardium around the left atrium can cause focal herniation and lead to strangulation. CT or MRI can establish the diagnosis. Patients may present with atypical chest pain or sudden death. Surgical repair is often recommended for a partial pericardial defect.

Benign Cysts

Benign pericardial cysts are rare and are usually asymptomatic, but they can be associated with chest pain. They are typically seen as rounded or lobulated structures adjacent to the heart on the chest radiograph or adjacent to the right atrium on transthoracic echocardiography (Chapter 55). Thoracic CT and MRI are useful for the diagnosis. Cysts rarely rupture and do not require treatment unless they become symptomatic with chest pain. In this situation, the cyst can be removed surgically or drained percutaneously or with a thoracoscope.

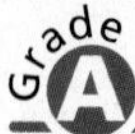

Grade A References

A1. Imazio M, Brucato A, Cemin R, et al. Colchicine for recurrent pericarditis (CORP): a randomized trial. *Ann Intern Med.* 2011;155:409-414.

A2. Imazio M, Brucato A, Cemin R, et al. A randomized trial of colchicine for acute pericarditis. *N Engl J Med.* 2013;369:1522-1528.

A3. Imazio M, Belli R, Brucato A, et al. Efficacy and safety of colchicine for treatment of multiple recurrences of pericarditis (CORP-2): a multicentre, double-blind, placebo-controlled, randomised trial. *Lancet.* 2014;383:2232-2237.

A4. Imazio M, Brucato A, Ferrazzi P, et al. Colchicine for prevention of postpericardiotomy syndrome and postoperative atrial fibrillation: the COPPS-2 randomized clinical trial. *JAMA.* 2014;312:1016-1023.

A5. Mayosi BM, Ntsekhe M, Bosch J, et al. Prednisolone and *Mycobacterium indicus pranii* in tuberculous pericarditis. *N Engl J Med.* 2014;371:1121-1130.

GENERAL REFERENCES

For the General References and other additional features, please visit Expert Consult at https://expertconsult.inkling.com.

78

DISEASES OF THE AORTA

FRANK A. LEDERLE

The ascending aorta, which is located in the anterior mediastinum, is about 3 cm in diameter and 5 cm long. The aortic root, which is just above the aortic valve, is composed of the three sinuses of Valsalva. The ascending aorta meets the aortic arch in the superior mediastinum, where the brachiocephalic arteries branch off it. The descending thoracic aorta, which is about 2.5 cm in diameter and 20 cm long, courses posteriorly, crosses the diaphragm, and becomes the abdominal aorta, which is normally 2 cm in diameter and extends for 15 cm until it bifurcates into two common iliac arteries.

The aorta itself is composed of three layers. The thin inner layer, the *intima*, is lined with endothelial cells. In the thick middle layer, the *media*, sheets of elastic tissue provide the tensile strength to withstand needed systolic pressures. The outer *adventitia*, which is composed mostly of collagen, provides arterial and venous blood supply to the aorta itself.

AORTIC ANEURYSMS

DEFINITION

An aneurysm is a pathologic dilation of the artery, often defined as a 50% increase over the expected diameter. An aneurysm can be defined based on its cause, location, shape, and size. In terms of shape, whereas a fusiform aneurysm is a symmetrical dilation of the aorta, a saccular aneurysm involves dilation mainly of one wall. A false aneurysm or pseudoaneurysm occurs when the aorta is enlarged because of dilation of only the outer layers of the vessel wall, as may occur with a contained rupture of the aortic wall.

EPIDEMIOLOGY

Although an aneurysm can develop in any part of the aorta, abdominal aortic aneurysms are much more common than thoracic aneurysms. Thoracic aortic aneurysms are most common in the ascending aorta followed in frequency by the descending aorta and the aortic arch. When an aneurysm in the descending thoracic aorta extends into the abdominal aorta, it is termed a *thoracoabdominal aortic aneurysm.*

For abdominal aortic aneurysms, risk factors include increased age, male gender, smoking, a family history of the disease, and occlusive atherosclerotic disease. Diabetes and black race are associated with a reduced risk.

Ascending thoracic aortic aneurysms are often associated with genetic mutations as in Marfan or Ehlers-Danlos syndromes (Chapter 260). Risk factors for descending thoracic and thoracoabdominal aortic aneurysms include age, smoking, and chronic obstructive pulmonary disease. Compared with abdominal aortic aneurysms, thoracic aneurysms have a stronger familial component and no gender predilection.

Deaths from abdominal aortic aneurysm increased markedly from 1950 to 1970 but have been declining in the United States since the 1990s (Fig. 78-1). The prevalence of an asymptomatic abdominal aortic aneurysm, defined as diameter larger than 3 cm, detected by screening, has also declined sharply, from more than 5% in older men in 1990 to less than 2% by 2010.[1] The most likely explanation for these changes is the increase and then decrease in U.S. rates of smoking, which accounts for about three fourths of all abdominal aortic aneurysms. By comparison, global death rates for abdominal aortic aneurysm have not declined because smoking rates and levels of other cardiovascular risk factors have not declined.[2] In the United States, deaths from rupture of thoracic aortic aneurysms also decreased by 50% from 1997 to 2010.

PATHOBIOLOGY

Atherosclerosis was once considered the most common underlying cause of abdominal aortic aneurysms, but this relationship has been called into question by a variety of observations. For example, abdominal aortic aneurysm is less common in patients with diabetes and is much more strongly associated with smoking and male gender than is atherosclerosis.[1,2] Although aortic atherosclerosis may contribute to the process, the pathogenesis of abdominal aortic aneurysms appears to include genetic, environmental, hemodynamic, and immunologic factors. The strength of the aortic wall depends on elastin and collagen within the extracellular matrix of its media. The degradation of these structural proteins by matrix metalloproteinases and inflammatory infiltrates, especially macrophages and T lymphocytes, weakens the aortic wall and allows aneurysms to develop. However, attempts to retard the

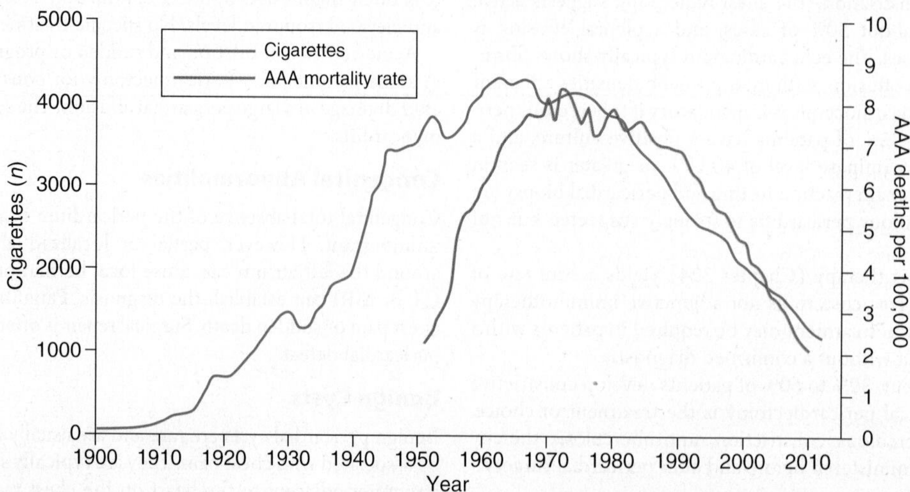

FIGURE 78-1. U.S. annual adult per capita cigarette consumption and U.S. age-adjusted abdominal aortic aneurysm (AAA) mortality rate per 100,000 white men by year. Rates include abdominal, thoracoabdominal, and unspecified aortic aneurysm and exclude thoracic aneurysm and dissection. (Adapted from Lederle FA. The rise and fall of abdominal aortic aneurysm. *Circulation.* 2011;124:1097-1099.)

process using doxycycline, which suppresses matrix metalloproteinase, have not been successful.

In the ascending thoracic aorta, the most important cause of aneurysms is cystic medial degeneration, with necrosis of smooth muscle cells and degeneration of elastic layers within the media, often related to a genetic mutation such as Marfan or Ehlers-Danlos syndrome. Almost all patients with Marfan syndrome, who are at very high risk for developing thoracic aortic aneurysms, have underlying cystic medial degeneration. In patients who develop ascending aortic aneurysms without overt evidence of connective tissue disease, a bicuspid aortic valve and familial thoracic aortic aneurysm syndrome are important congenital causes. Syphilis (Chapter 319) was formerly a common cause of thoracic aortic aneurysms in the United States but is rarely implicated now. Other uncommon causes of ascending thoracic aortic aneurysms include infectious aortitis, great vessel arteritis, aortic trauma, and aortic dissection. Descending thoracic and thoracoabdominal aortic aneurysms can also result from previous dissection, but they are usually idiopathic and degenerative.

CLINICAL MANIFESTATIONS

The majority of aortic aneurysms are asymptomatic and are discovered incidentally on an imaging study or on routine abdominal palpation. Symptoms resulting from progressive enlargement of unruptured aneurysms, such as vertebral erosion or nerve compression, are very rare.

Abdominal aortic aneurysm rupture can cause sudden death from cardiovascular collapse. Other patients present with pain in the hypogastrium, flank, lower back, or hips. The pain is often severe and frightening to the patient and may be accompanied by abdominal tenderness. Symptoms of bloating, constipation, or urinary retention may be caused by a hematoma that compresses the bowel or the urinary tract or by impaired blood supply to these organs. These symptoms typically persist for hours to a few days before death ensues or the aneurysm is repaired, although a few cases of chronic contained rupture persisting for weeks or even months have been reported.

Thoracic aortic aneurysm can expand and compress adjacent mediastinal structures. Symptoms include coughing, wheezing, dyspnea, hoarseness, recurrent pneumonia, and dysphagia. A ruptured thoracic aneurysm may present with chest or back pain. Vascular complications include aortic insufficiency, sometimes with secondary heart failure, hemoptysis, and arterial thromboembolism.

DIAGNOSIS

Abdominal aortic aneurysms may be detectable on deep abdominal palpation as a pulsatile mass, although obesity can obscure even large aneurysms. The examiner first feels deeply for the aortic pulsation, usually found a few centimeters cephalad of the umbilicus (the umbilicus marks the level of the aortic bifurcation) and slightly to the left of midline. The examiner then positions both hands on the abdomen with the palms down and an index finger on either side of the pulsation, both to confirm that it is the aorta (each systole should move the two fingers apart) and to measure the aortic width. Sufficient abdominal skin should be included between the two index fingers, and time should be taken to allow the abdominal muscles to relax. On examination, the width, not the intensity, of the pulsation guides the diagnosis. A pulsatile abdominal mass should be confirmed by ultrasonography, which provides an accurate measure of diameter; a width of 3 cm or larger establishes the diagnosis and warrants ongoing surveillance.

Clinical diagnosis of a rupturing abdominal aortic aneurysm can be challenging. The classic triad of abdominal pain, hypotension, and a pulsatile abdominal mass is insensitive because the blood pressure may be normal or near normal at presentation, and palpation may be difficult owing to guarding or bloating. Furthermore, accompanying bowel and bladder symptoms can lead to misdiagnoses. In patients with ruptured aneurysms, the white blood cell count is usually elevated, but the hematocrit can initially be normal because hemodilution does not occur acutely. The physician should have a low threshold for obtaining appropriate imaging, particularly in older men with a history of smoking.

Abdominal aortic aneurysms can be detected and measured by either abdominal ultrasonography or computed tomography (CT) (Fig. 78-2). However, CT should be obtained when rupture is considered because rupture is not reliably diagnosed by ultrasonography.

Thoracic aortic aneurysms usually cannot be palpated even when they are very large. As a result, thoracic aortic aneurysms are frequently recognized on chest radiographs, where they often are diagnosed by a widened mediastinal silhouette, enlarged aortic knob, or a trachea that is displaced from the midline. CT is accurate for detecting and measuring thoracic aneurysms and monitoring their diameter over time. Transthoracic echocardiography, which generally visualizes the aortic root and ascending aorta, is useful for screening patients with Marfan syndrome (Chapter 260), who are at particular risk for aneurysms involving this portion of the aorta.

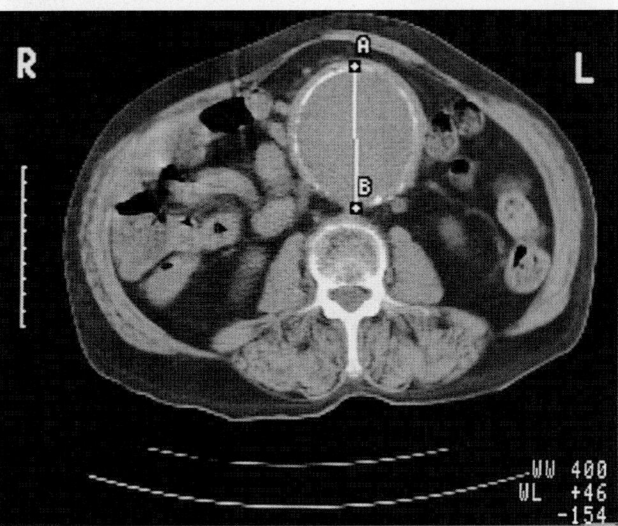

FIGURE 78-2. Abdominal aortic aneurysm on computed tomography. This sensitive imaging method allows precise measurement of size (*point A* to *point B*) and demonstrates the thickened wall of the aneurysm. (From Forbes CD, Jackson WF. *Color Atlas and Text of Clinical Medicine*. 3rd ed. London: Mosby; 2003.)

TREATMENT

The morbidity and mortality of aortic aneurysms result from both rupture and elective repair. A judicious strategy for intervention is therefore essential. Open surgical repair consists of insertion of a synthetic prosthetic tube graft. When aneurysms involve branch vessels, such as the renal or mesenteric arteries, the vessels must be reimplanted into the graft. Similarly, when a dilated aortic root must be replaced in the repair of an ascending thoracic aortic aneurysm, the coronary arteries must be reimplanted. An alternative approach to repair abdominal aortic aneurysms and some descending thoracic aneurysms is the percutaneous placement of an expandable endovascular stent graft inside the aneurysm.

In a patient with a ruptured aortic aneurysm, emergent repair by either the open or endovascular method[A1] is required. Randomized trials in patients with stab wounds and upper gastrointestinal bleeding and observational studies of ruptured abdominal aortic aneurysms have raised concerns that excessive volume expansion and transfusion before control of bleeding may increase the mortality rate.

For patients with asymptomatic abdominal aortic aneurysms smaller than 5.5 cm in diameter, elective repair, by either the open[A2,A3] or endovascular[A4,A5] method, does not reduce the overall mortality rate. The benefit of elective repair of larger abdominal aortic aneurysms has been demonstrated indirectly through randomized trials of ultrasound screening, which reduces both aneurysm-related and total mortality.[A6,A7] Elective endovascular repair has a lower postoperative mortality rate than open repair (1.5% vs. 4%), but excess late deaths after endovascular repair result in similar survival rates after 3 to 5 years.[A8,A9] Patients who have large aneurysms and who are medically unfit for open repair have a high rupture rate[3] but may not benefit from endovascular repair because of their burdens of comorbid conditions.[A10] Randomized trial data are insufficient for women, who have both a higher rate of rupture and a higher operative mortality rate.

Small aortic aneurysms should be monitored periodically to detect progressive enlargement, which may indicate the need for surgical repair. Whereas ultrasonography is the preferred modality for monitoring abdominal aneurysms, CT is used for thoracic aneurysms. Surveillance intervals are based on the probability of exceeding the operative threshold.

For abdominal aortic aneurysms, proposed screening intervals are every 3 years for aneurysms of 3.0 to 3.9 cm in diameter, 2 years for 4.0 to 4.4 cm in diameter, and yearly for 4.5 to 5.4 cm in diameter. Elective repair should be considered when the diameter exceeds 5.5 cm.[4] High-volume surgeons and hospitals have better outcomes from elective repair.

For asymptomatic thoracic aneurysms, management is less certain. No randomized trials have addressed when thoracic aortic aneurysms should be repaired or which method is preferable, and data on natural history are limited.

Endovascular repair of unruptured descending thoracic aortic aneurysms is associated with lower perioperative mortality rate than open repair (5%-6% vs. 7%-12%), but it does not improve the adjusted 5-year survival rate.[5] Normal aortic diameter is 1.5 to 2 times greater, and the operative mortality rate is two to four times higher in the thoracic aorta compared with the abdominal aorta, and the risk of rupture is low for thoracic aneurysms less than 6.0 cm in diameter. These comparisons suggest that diameter thresholds for elective repair should probably be higher than the 5.5 cm established for abdominal aortic aneurysms. An exception may be patients with Marfan syndrome, in whom the risk of dissection or rupture is higher and operative mortality rate is lower, perhaps because of their younger age. Patients with Marfan syndrome with aortic diameters less than 5 cm are at low risk, but natural history data are inadequate for larger diameters.[6] Randomized trials in patients with Marfan syndrome, which mostly involve small numbers of patients with normal aortic diameters, have suggested that several drugs (e.g., losartan) can reduce subsequent aortic root enlargement, but no differences have yet been demonstrated in the progression to aneurysm or in clinical outcomes.

PREVENTION

Ultrasonography is the safest and most practical screening method for abdominal aortic aneurysms. The U.S. Preventive Services Task Force recommends one-time ultrasound screening for men age 65 to 75 years who have ever smoked.[7] No medical therapy has been shown to reduce abdominal aortic aneurysm enlargement, but smoking cessation is important both for prevention and to slow progression.

PROGNOSIS

Most aneurysms expand over time, and the risk of rupture increases with diameter. Abdominal aortic aneurysms with diameters less than 5.5 cm have an annual rupture risk of 1% or less. Rupture rates are unknown for good operative candidates with larger aneurysms but are 10% or more per year in poor surgical candidates with large abdominal aortic aneurysms. For thoracic aortic aneurysms, a population-based study reported a 5-year rupture risk of 0% for aneurysms less than 4.0 cm in diameter, 16% for aneurysms 4.0 to 6.0 cm in diameter, and 31% for aneurysms larger than 6.0 cm in diameter.

The overall mortality rate in patients with a ruptured aortic aneurysm remains about 75%, including about a 40% mortality rate even among those who are able to undergo emergent intervention.[8] Lifelong imaging surveillance is recommended after endovascular aneurysm repair. Otherwise, the prognosis after aneurysm repair is determined largely by risk factors and comorbidities rather than the aneurysm itself. Observational data suggest that survival after repair may be improved by treatment with statins,[9] probably because it reduces the risk of death from concurrent coronary artery disease.

INTRAMURAL AORTIC HEMATOMA AND AORTIC DISSECTION

DEFINITION

An intramural aortic hematoma develops when blood accumulates within the aortic media because of either bleeding from the vasa vasorum or a tear in the intima. An aortic dissection occurs when the media of the artery becomes longitudinally cleaved, thereby forming a false lumen that communicates with the true lumen.

About two thirds of aortic dissections are classified as type A (involving the ascending aorta), and the other third are classified as type B (not involving the ascending aorta) (Fig. 78-3). Hematomas and dissections are classified as acute if they developed within the prior 2 weeks and chronic thereafter. Hematomas and dissections that are acute and involve the ascending aorta are more likely to rupture and cause severe disability or death.[10]

Aortic dissection causes about 3000 deaths per year in the United States. In patients without Marfan syndrome, the peak incidence of aortic dissection is in individuals between 60 and 80 years of age, with men affected 1.5 times more frequently than women. Hypertension and especially uncontrolled hypertension is the dominant risk factor, although patients with a bicuspid aortic valve are also at increased risk. Some patients are known to have preexisting thoracic aortic aneurysms. Aortic dissections are a rare complication in young women during the peripartum period (Chapter 239). Intraaortic catheterization procedures and cardiac surgery are iatrogenic causes of aortic dissection.

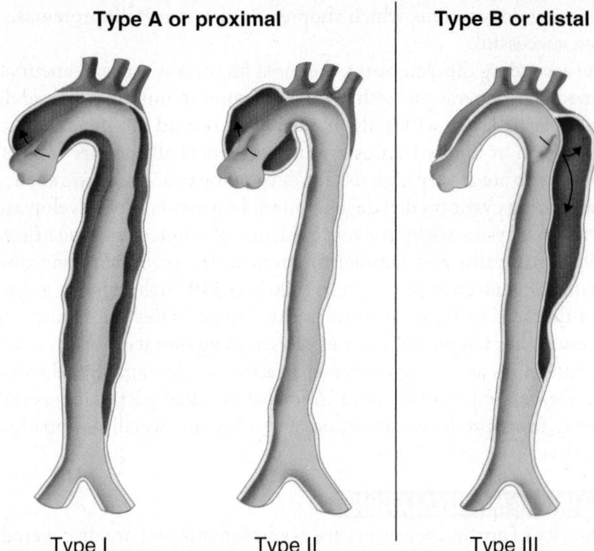

FIGURE 78-3. Classification systems for aortic dissection. (From Isselbacher EM. Diseases of the aorta. In: Braunwald E, Zipes DP, Libby P, Bonow RO, eds. *Braunwald's Heart Disease: A Textbook of Cardiovascular Medicine.* 7th ed. Philadelphia: Saunders; 2004:1416.)

PATHOBIOLOGY

The most common predisposing factor for aortic dissection is degeneration of the collagen and elastin in the aortic media. Classic cystic medial degeneration in patients with Marfan syndrome explains the particularly high risk for aortic dissection at a relatively young age.

Aortic dissection typically begins either when a tear in the aortic intima exposes the diseased medial layer to the systemic pressure of intraluminal blood or when a leaking vasa vasorum creates an intramural hematoma. This hematoma may remain relatively localized, or, alternatively may propagate longitudinally along a variable length of the aorta and rupture through the intima and into the aortic lumen. If such communication occurs, the result of an initially intramural hematoma becomes no different than a dissection that began with an intimal tear. With dissection, the media cleaves longitudinally into two layers, thereby producing a blood-filled false lumen that propagates, usually distally but sometimes retrograde, within the aortic wall for a variable distance from the site of the intimal tear. The abdominal aorta rarely dissects except as an extension of a dissecting thoracic aorta.

CLINICAL MANIFESTATIONS

Pain, which is the most common initial symptom, occurs in 96% of cases of both aortic intramural hematoma and dissection. The pain is typically severe and is usually felt in the chest or back, although it may involve the abdomen. Pain commonly begins suddenly and is worst at the start. It is often described as sharp or ripping. An isolated hematoma rarely causes symptoms other than pain. A dissection, however, can cause signs and symptoms related to its propagation, such as acute aortic insufficiency, right coronary artery occlusion, hemopericardium, cerebrovascular accident, mesenteric ischemia, or ischemic peripheral neuropathy. Syncope (Chapter 62) is associated with proximal dissection and worse outcomes.

True hypotension, which is present in more than 25% of patients, augurs a poor prognosis. Pseudohypotension occurs when measured upper extremity blood pressure is falsely low because the subclavian artery is involved in the dissection. Pulse delays or deficits, which help identify which blood vessels are compromised by the dissection, are evident on physical examination in patients whose dissections involve the subclavian, carotid, or femoral arteries.

More than one third of patients with a proximal aortic dissection develop acute aortic valve insufficiency. In some patients with acute aortic insufficiency, the murmur may be undetectable or unimpressive until the finding of a widened pulse pressure leads to more careful examinations. When aortic dissection compromises a coronary artery, especially the right coronary artery, myocardial ischemia or infarction (Chapter 73) develops. Retrograde dissection can also cause acute and even fatal hemopericardium and tamponade (Chapter 71). Whereas compromise of flow through the brachiocephalic arteries may produce stroke (Chapter 407) or coma, involvement of the

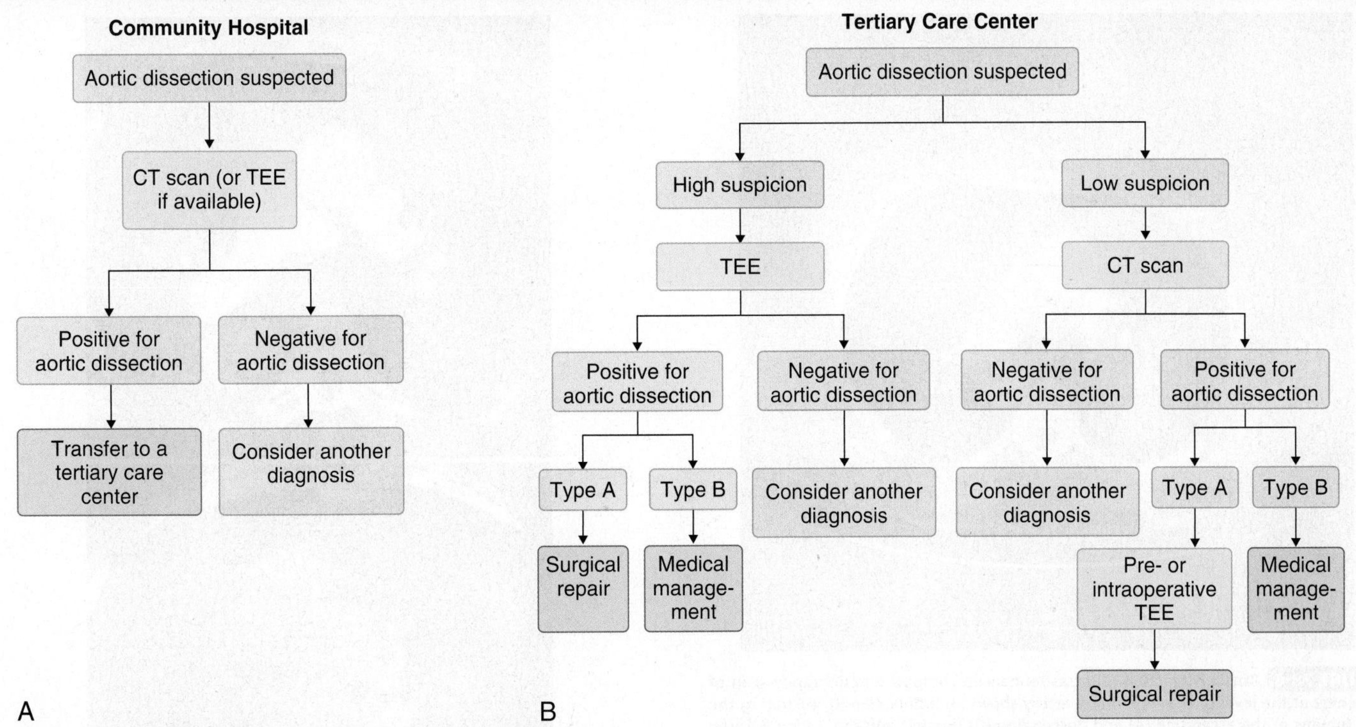

FIGURE 78-4. Algorithms for the evaluation of suspected acute aortic dissection. **A,** This approach is used in many community hospitals where cardiac surgery is not performed. **B,** This approach is used in many tertiary care centers where transesophageal echocardiography (TEE) and cardiac surgery are available. CT = computed tomography. (Courtesy of Eric M. Isselbacher, MD.)

spinal arteries may produce paraplegia. When a dissection extends into the abdominal aorta, compromised flow to one or both renal arteries may result in acute renal failure (Chapter 120). Mesenteric ischemia or infarction (Chapter 143) may manifest as abdominal pain and bloody diarrhea. Dissection distal to the aortic bifurcation can compromise or occlude one or both common iliac arteries, with a resulting femoral pulse deficit and lower extremity ischemia (Chapter 79).

DIAGNOSIS

Aortic dissection may be suspected based on a typical history or when pulse deficits are noted on physical examination. Often, however, an enlarged mediastinal silhouette on the chest radiograph of a patient who is being evaluated for chest pain (Chapter 51) and possible myocardial ischemia raises concerns even though mediastinal widening may be seen in only two thirds of patients in whom dissection is ultimately diagnosed. If the descending thoracic aorta is involved, a left pleural effusion is commonly seen, sometimes because of frank blood but often because of a small exudate from the inflamed aortic wall. Electrocardiographic findings in aortic dissection are nonspecific. Blood tests are not very helpful, but an acute aortic dissection is unlikely if the plasma D-dimer level is below 500 ng/mL.

When the clinical suspicion of aortic dissection is high, the diagnosis must be confirmed or excluded emergently with an imaging study (Fig. 78-4). Transesophageal echocardiography (Fig. 78-5) is the most rapid means of providing sufficient detail to proceed directly to the operating room. CT (Fig. 78-6) provides complementary information. Magnetic resonance (MR) imaging provides even better anatomical detail, but it is not as easy to obtain emergently, and it can be difficult to provide needed acute care in an MR suite. On cross-sectional imaging, an isolated intramural hematoma appears as a crescentic thickening around the aortic wall rather than true and false lumens separated by an intimal flap.

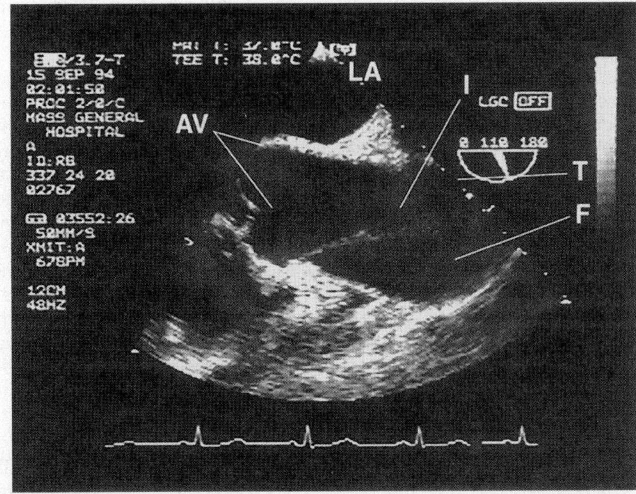

FIGURE 78-5. Transesophageal echocardiogram of the ascending aorta in the long axis in a patient with type A aortic dissection. The aortic valve (AV) is on the *left,* and the ascending aorta extends to the *right.* Within the aorta is an intimal flap (I) that originates at the level of the sinotubular junction. The true (T) and the false (F) lumens are separated by the intimal flap. LA = left atrium. (From Isselbacher EM. Diseases of the aorta. In: Braunwald E, Zipes DP, Libby P, Bonow RO, eds. *Braunwald's Heart Disease: A Textbook of Cardiovascular Medicine.* 7th ed. Philadelphia: Saunders; 2004:1423.)

TREATMENT Rx

Whenever aortic intramural hematoma or dissection is suspected, therapy should be instituted immediately even while imaging studies are ordered rather than waiting until the diagnosis is confirmed. The goal of initial medical therapy, which is to halt further progression and reduce the risk for rupture, should be the same for an isolated hematoma as for true dissection because of the risk that the hematoma will propagate.[11]

Despite the absence of randomized trials, current guidelines recommend emergent medical therapy directed at lowering the blood pressure, usually to below 120 mm Hg, and heart rate, usually to below 60 beats/min, while maintaining perfusion to the brain, heart, kidneys, and any other organs whose arterial supply may be jeopardized by dissection.[12] The most common option is intravenous (IV) labetalol (a combined α- and β-blocker, initially at 20 mg administered over a 2-minute period followed by additional doses of 20 to 80 mg every 10 to 15 minutes, up to a maximum total dose of 300 mg, and then a continuous infusion at 2 to 8 mg/min). An alternative is a pure β-blocker (e.g., IV propranolol at 1-mg boluses every 3 to 5 minutes to start followed by a continuous infusion at rates up to 20 mg/hr) combined with IV nitroprusside

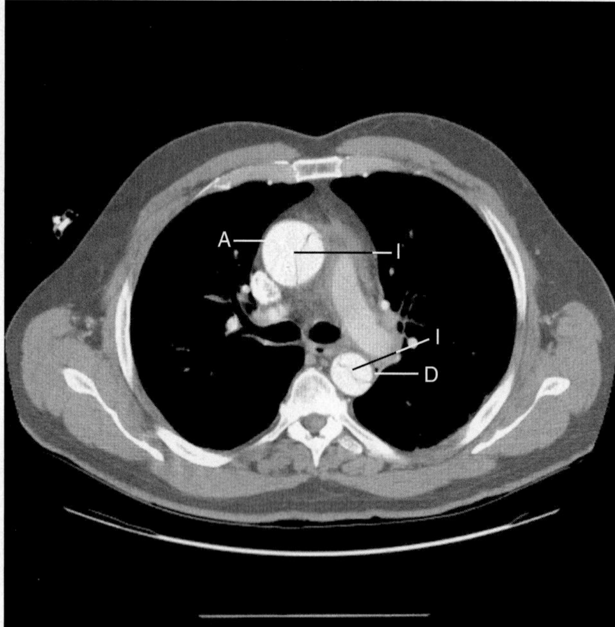

FIGURE 78-6. Aortic dissection. Contrast-enhanced computed tomography scan of the chest at the level of the pulmonary artery shows an intimal flap (I) separating the two lumens of the ascending (A) and descending (D) thoracic aorta in a type A aortic dissection. (Courtesy of Eric M. Isselbacher, MD.)

(0.5 to 8 µg/kg/min) to titrate blood pressure minute by minute as needed. If β-blockers are contraindicated, calcium channel blockers (e.g., IV diltiazem with an initial bolus of 20 mg over a 2-minute period followed by a continuous infusion of 5 to 15 mg/hr) may be useful.

For acute type A dissection, urgent surgical repair is recommended to reduce the risk of life-threatening complications such as rupture, cardiac tamponade, severe aortic insufficiency, or stroke. When patients have significant hypotension, pseudohypotension should be excluded. True hypotension may be caused by acute myocardial infarction (Chapter 73) owing to a compromise of the right coronary artery or by hemopericardium and cardiac tamponade (Chapter 77) as a result of rupture of the dissection into the pericardium. Patients with tamponade should be treated with volume expansion and taken to surgery as quickly as possible because early death is extremely high; pericardiocentesis should be performed only as a last resort because it may precipitate hemodynamic collapse and death. By comparison, patients with chronic type A dissections can often be managed medically because they have already survived the early period of high mortality associated with acute proximal dissections.

Patients with acute type B dissection are at much lower risk for life-threatening complications and are usually managed with medical therapy[13] because the addition of routine endovascular repair to medical treatment has not improved survival in small randomized trials of acute[A11] or chronic[A12] type B dissection. If, however, a type B dissection is associated with a serious complication, such as end-organ ischemia, intervention is indicated with either endovascular techniques or open surgery.

For an isolated intramural hematoma, the likelihood of progressive dissection or other complications is lower than in patients who initially have dissection, especially if the hematoma is small and aortic dimensions are normal.[14] In one series of East Asian patients, most intramural hematomas regressed, and surgery usually was not necessary. In a Western series, an estimated 10% of hematomas regressed spontaneously, and 25% to 50% progressed during the follow-up period. Hematomas in the ascending aorta have the highest risk, and surgery is often recommended for them. For distal intramural hematomas, management is generally the same as for distal dissection, with surgery reserved for patients with progressive disease (Fig. 78-7).

Before discharge, medically managed patients should be started on a regimen that will control hypertension and reduce ventricular contractility. Recommendations emphasize β-blockers (e.g., metoprolol 25 to 200 mg twice daily or atenolol 25 to 200 mg/day) as the drugs of choice in this setting, but a second (e.g., lisinopril 5 to 40 mg/day) or third (amlodipine 2.5 to 10 mg/day or hydrochlorothiazide 12.5 to 50 mg/day) agent usually is required to achieve the goal of systolic blood pressure less than 120 mm Hg (Chapter 67), although little evidence supports treatment goals different from those used for the general population.

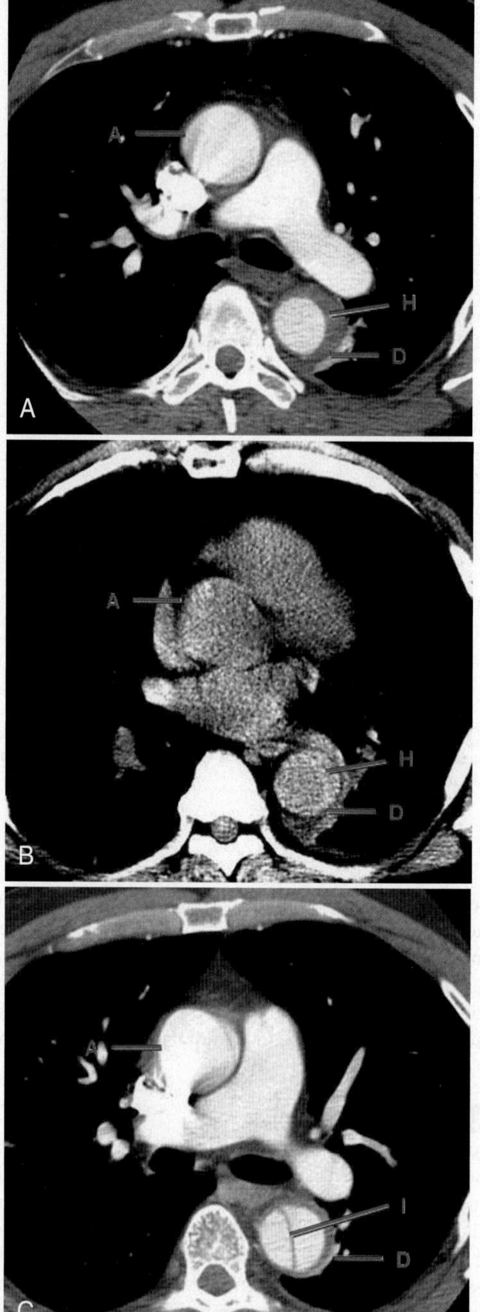

FIGURE 78-7. Intramural aortic hematoma. A, Contrast-enhanced computed tomography (CT) scan of the chest at the level of the pulmonary artery demonstrates an intramural hematoma (H) of the descending thoracic aorta (D). The hematoma appears as a crescentic thickening of the aortic wall that does not enhance from the contrast within the aortic lumen. The ascending thoracic aorta (A) is unaffected. **B,** Corresponding image from a non–contrast-enhanced CT scan in which the intramural hematoma appears as a bright crescentic thickening of the aortic wall because the density of the hematoma is greater than that of the blood within the aortic lumen. **C,** Corresponding image from a contrast-enhanced CT scan performed 1 week later for surveillance in which the intramural hematoma has evolved into a classic aortic dissection with an intimal flap (I) and contrast evident within a patent false lumen. (Courtesy of Eric M. Isselbacher, MD.)

PROGNOSIS

The acute mortality rate from untreated type A dissection is about 1% per hour, and most deaths with either type occur within 7 days of the onset of symptoms.[15] Patients are at highest risk for complications during the first 2 years, but patients who survive the initial hospitalization generally do well thereafter, regardless of whether they were treated medically or surgically. However, continued blood pressure control is critical to reduce the long-term risk of complications such as aortic insufficiency, recurrent dissection, aneurysm formation, and aneurysm rupture. Some progressive aortic expansion typically occurs without symptoms, so medically treated patients must be observed closely with serial aortic imaging at 6-month intervals for the first 2 years and annually thereafter, provided that their anatomy is stable.

TAKAYASU ARTERITIS

Takayasu arteritis is a chronic inflammatory disease of unknown cause. The median age at onset is 29 years, and it is eight times more frequent in women than in men. It occurs more often in Asia and Africa than in Europe or North America. The early stage is characterized by active inflammation involving the aorta and its branches. The disease often progresses at a variable rate to a sclerotic stage with intimal hyperplasia, medial degeneration, and obliterative changes. Most of the resulting arterial lesions are stenotic, but aneurysms may also occur.

Takayasu arteritis involves the aorta and its branches, and it occasionally involves the pulmonary artery as well. The disease tends to be most pronounced at branch points in the aorta, especially the aortic arch, brachiocephalic vessels, and abdominal aorta. Takayasu arteritis can be diffuse or patchy, and affected areas may be separated by variable lengths of normal aorta.

CLINICAL MANIFESTATIONS AND DIAGNOSIS

Most patients initially develop symptoms of a systemic inflammatory process, including fatigue, headache, fever, night sweats, arthralgia, and weight loss.[16] By the time of diagnosis, however, 90% of patients have symptoms of vascular insufficiency, typically with claudication in the upper extremities and sometimes in the lower extremities.

Physical examination commonly reveals absent pulses and diminished blood pressure in the upper extremities, consistent with why Takayasu arteritis has sometimes been called *pulseless disease*. Bruits may be heard in over the affected arteries. More than 50% of patients have significant hypertension because of renal artery involvement, but hypertension may be difficult to diagnose on routine examination because of the diminished pulses. Proximal aortic involvement can cause aortic valve insufficiency. Involvement of the ostia of the coronary arteries may cause angina or myocardial infarction, and patients may develop heart failure owing to myocardial infarction, hypertension, or aortic insufficiency. Carotid artery involvement may cause cerebral ischemia or stroke. Abdominal angina may result from compromise of the mesenteric circulation.

Laboratory abnormalities during the acute phase include elevated C-reactive protein (CRP) level, an elevated erythrocyte sedimentation rate (ESR), anemia, mild leukocytosis, and elevated immunoglobulin levels. The diagnosis is best made by aortography, CT angiography, or MR angiography, which reveal stenosis of the aorta and stenosis or occlusion of its branch vessels, often with poststenotic dilation or associated aneurysms.

TREATMENT AND PROGNOSIS

Corticosteroids (e.g., prednisone 60 to 100 mg/day, often continued for months and tapered only when symptoms or evidence of inflammation subside) are the primary therapy for the acute inflammatory stage and may be effective in improving constitutional symptoms, lowering the ESR, and slowing the progression of the disease. Additional immunosuppressive medications that are used when corticosteroid therapy alone is ineffective include methotrexate (15 to 25 mg/wk). It is unknown whether medical therapy reduces the risk for major complications or prolongs life.

Percutaneous balloon angioplasty can effectively dilate short stenotic lesions of the aorta and its branch arteries, although restenosis is common. Surgery may be necessary to bypass or reconstruct key segments, such as the coronary, carotid, or renal arteries, or to treat aortic insufficiency. Ideally, surgery should not be performed during the inflammatory phase.

The overall 15-year survival rate in patients diagnosed with Takayasu arteritis is about 85%, about 65% in patients with major complications, and about 95% in patients without major complications. Most deaths result from stroke, myocardial infarction, or heart failure.

GIANT CELL ARTERITIS

Giant cell arteritis (Chapter 271) typically affects medium-sized arteries, but in 15% of cases, it involves the aorta and branches of the aortic arch.[17] Narrowing of the aorta is rare, but weakening of the wall of the ascending aorta may lead to localized thoracic aortic aneurysms and secondary aortic valve insufficiency. If branches of the aortic arch are narrowed, symptoms will be similar to those seen in Takayasu arteritis. The arteriographic lesions of the aorta and its primary branches are generally similar to Takayasu arteritis, thereby suggesting that Takayasu arteritis and giant cell arteritis may be part of a spectrum of the same disease. Giant cell arteritis is associated with increased risks for atherosclerotic events, such as myocardial infarction and stroke.

The mean age of onset is about 67 years. Symptoms include headaches, visual disturbances, polymyalgia rheumatic, jaw claudication, and fever (Chapter 271). An elevated ESR is a universal finding; the serum CRP level is typically elevated, and anemia is common. Because the temporal artery is commonly involved, the diagnosis is usually made by temporal artery biopsy, including contralateral biopsy if the first biopsy is negative. In patients with visual symptoms, scheduling of temporal artery biopsy should not delay treatment because of the risk of sudden blindness and because biopsy specimens remain diagnostic for weeks after the onset of therapy. Management is high-dose corticosteroid therapy (e.g., prednisone 60 to 100 mg/day, often for months and tapered only after symptoms or evidence of inflammation subside), to which the disease is usually responsive. Initial use of an IV corticosteroid pulse dose or of methotrexate does not add benefit.

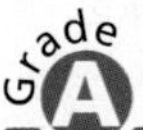

Grade A References

A1. Powell JT, Sweeting MJ, Thompson MM, et al. Endovascular or open repair strategy for ruptured abdominal aortic aneurysm: 30 day outcomes from IMPROVE randomised trial. *BMJ*. 2014;348:f7661.

A2. Powell JT, Brown LC, Forbes JF, et al. Final 12-year follow-up of surgery versus surveillance in the UK Small Aneurysm Trial. *Br J Surg*. 2007;94:702-708.

A3. Lederle FA, Wilson SE, Johnson GR, et al. Immediate repair compared with surveillance of small abdominal aortic aneurysms. *N Engl J Med*. 2002;346:1437-1444.

A4. Cao P, De Rango P, Verzini F, et al. Comparison of surveillance versus aortic endografting for small aneurysm repair (CAESAR): results from a randomised trial. *Eur J Vasc Endovasc Surg*. 2011;41:13-25.

A5. Ouriel K, Clair DG, Kent KC, et al. Endovascular repair compared with surveillance for patients with small abdominal aortic aneurysms. *J Vasc Surg*. 2010;51:1081-1087.

A6. Thompson SG, Ashton HA, Gao L, et al. Final follow-up of the Multicentre Aneurysm Screening Study (MASS) randomized trial of abdominal aortic aneurysm screening. *Br J Surg*. 2012;99:1649-1656.

A7. Takagi H, Niwa M, Mizuno Y, et al. The Last Judgment upon abdominal aortic aneurysm screening. *Int J Cardiol*. 2013;167:2331-2332.

A8. Greenhalgh RM, Brown LC, Powell JT, et al. Endovascular versus open repair of abdominal aortic aneurysm. *N Engl J Med*. 2010;362:1863-1871.

A9. Lederle FA, Freischlag JA, Kyriakides TC, et al. Long-term comparison of endovascular and open repair of abdominal aortic aneurysm. *N Engl J Med*. 2012;367:1988-1997.

A10. Greenhalgh RM, Brown LC, Powell JT, et al. Endovascular repair of aortic aneurysm in patients physically ineligible for open repair. *N Engl J Med*. 2010;362:1872-1880.

A11. Brunkwall J, Kasprzak P, Verhoeven E, et al. Endovascular repair of acute uncomplicated aortic type B dissection promotes aortic remodelling: 1 year results of the ADSORB trial. *Eur J Vasc Endovasc Surg*. 2014;48:285-291.

A12. Nienaber CA, Rousseau H, Eggebrecht H, et al. Randomized comparison of strategies for type B aortic dissection: the INvestigation of STEnt Grafts in Aortic Dissection (INSTEAD) trial. *Circulation*. 2009;120:2519-2528.

GENERAL REFERENCES

For the General References and other additional features, please visit Expert Consult at https://expertconsult.inkling.com.

79 ATHEROSCLEROTIC PERIPHERAL ARTERIAL DISEASE

CHRISTOPHER J. WHITE

DEFINITION

Lower extremity atherosclerotic peripheral arterial disease is one subset of a larger group of peripheral vascular diseases that includes all noncoronary vascular disorders that may affect the arterial, venous (Chapters 80 and 81), or lymphatic circulation. Atherosclerotic arterial diseases are characterized by arterial narrowing or occlusion caused by the accumulation of atherosclerotic plaque elements in the vessel wall (Chapter 70). Atherosclerotic vascular disease can also lead to aneurysm formation, which is the pathologic enlargement of arterial segments, and may result in rupture, dissection, or thromboembolism (Chapter 78).

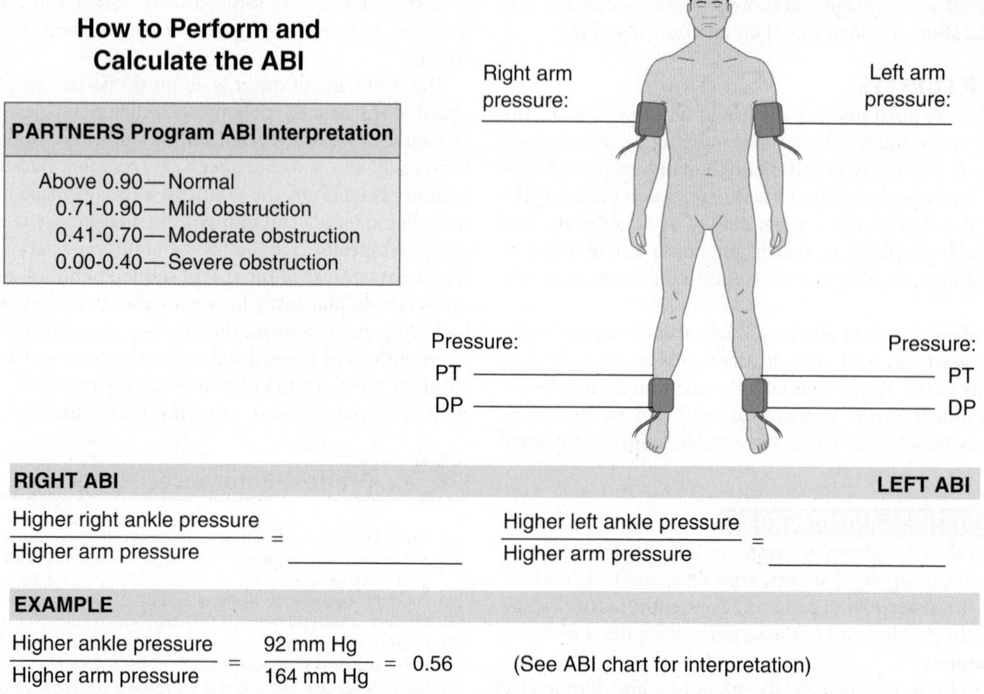

How to Perform and Calculate the ABI

PARTNERS Program ABI Interpretation
Above 0.90—Normal
0.71-0.90—Mild obstruction
0.41-0.70—Moderate obstruction
0.00-0.40—Severe obstruction

Right arm pressure: ______ Left arm pressure: ______

Pressure: PT ______ DP ______ Pressure: PT ______ DP ______

RIGHT ABI

Higher right ankle pressure / Higher arm pressure = ______

LEFT ABI

Higher left ankle pressure / Higher arm pressure = ______

EXAMPLE

Higher ankle pressure / Higher arm pressure = 92 mm Hg / 164 mm Hg = 0.56 (See ABI chart for interpretation)

FIGURE 79-1. Performing pressure measurements and calculating the ankle-brachial index (ABI). To calculate the ABI, systolic pressures are determined in both arms and both ankles with the use of a handheld Doppler instrument. The higher reading in either the dorsalis pedis (DP) or the posterior tibial (PT) arteries of the right foot and the left foot is divided by the higher systolic blood pressure reading in either the right or left arm to calculate the index. PAD = peripheral arterial disease; PARTNERS = PAD Awareness, Risk, and Treatment: New Resources for Survival.

EPIDEMIOLOGY

The prevalence of lower extremity peripheral arterial disease in the United States, Europe, and Asia continues to increase as the population ages and is exposed to atherosclerotic risk factors (Chapter 52). The presence of peripheral arterial disease is defined as an ankle-brachial index (ABI)—the ratio of the highest systolic blood pressure in the ankle divided by the highest systolic blood pressure in the arm (Fig. 79-1)—less than 0.90. Among individuals age 40 years and older, the prevalence is 4.3% (95% confidence interval [CI], 3.1%-5.5%), but the prevalence in individuals with diabetes ranges from 20% to 30%.[1]

Risk factors for atherosclerosis (Chapter 52) increase the likelihood of developing lower extremity peripheral arterial disease. More than 95% of individuals with peripheral arterial disease have at least one traditional cardiovascular risk factor, and most have multiple risk factors. More than one third of patients with peripheral arterial disease have significant coronary disease, and up to one quarter have carotid artery disease. As a result, the risk of heart attack, stroke, and death are increased severalfold in patients with peripheral arterial disease.

Among conventional atherosclerotic risk factors, cigarette smoking is two to three times more likely to cause lower extremity peripheral arterial disease than to cause coronary artery disease.

Hypertension is also associated with lower extremity peripheral arterial disease. The development of peripheral arterial disease is more likely in patients with lipid abnormalities (elevated total and low-density lipoprotein [LDL] cholesterol, decreased high-density lipoprotein [HDL] cholesterol, and hypertriglyceridemia), and the risk increases by 5% to 10% for each 10-mg/dL increase in total cholesterol. Increased homocysteine levels are associated with a two- to threefold increased risk for developing atherosclerotic peripheral arterial disease. Diabetes mellitus increases the risk of lower extremity peripheral arterial disease by two- to fourfold, and the risk of developing lower extremity peripheral arterial disease is proportional to the severity and duration of diabetes. Tight control of diabetes is important because the risk of developing peripheral arterial disease increases by 28% for every 1% increase in glycosylated hemoglobin (Chapter 229). Patients with diabetes who have lower extremity peripheral arterial disease are seven- to 15-fold more likely to undergo a major amputation than nondiabetics with lower extremity peripheral arterial disease.

Peripheral arterial disease disproportionately affects older individuals (Fig. 79-2), non-Hispanic blacks, current smokers, individuals with diabetes,

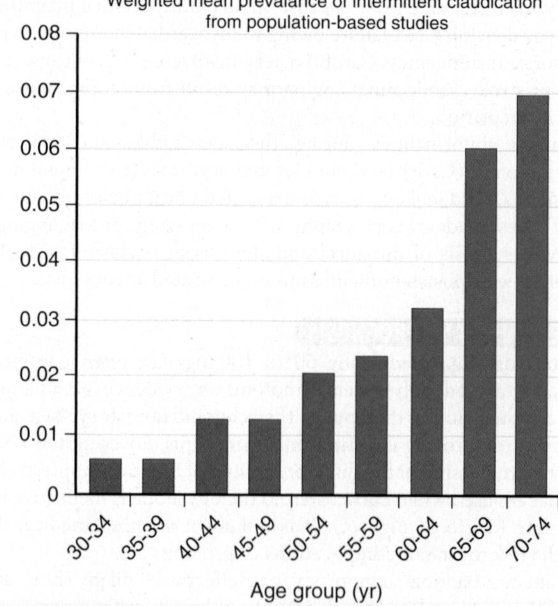

FIGURE 79-2. Weighted mean prevalence of intermittent claudication. (Modified from Dormandy JA, Rutherford RB. Management of peripheral arterial disease. TransAtlantic Inter-Society Consensus (TASC) Working Group. *J Vasc Surg*. 2000;31(suppl):S1-S296.)

and those with abnormal renal function. The overall prevalence of peripheral arterial disease in the United States among persons age 70 years and older is 14.5% (95% CI, 10.8%-18.2%), which corresponds to approximately 4 million individuals.

PATHOBIOLOGY

Acute Limb Ischemia

Acute limb ischemia occurs when blood flow to an extremity is abruptly halted or markedly diminished, resulting in hypoperfusion that threatens the viability of the limb. Acute limb ischemia is most commonly caused by either thrombosis or embolism. Most emboli originate from the heart as a mural

TABLE 79-1 CLINICAL CATEGORIES OF ACUTE LIMB ISCHEMIA

CATEGORY	DESCRIPTION	SENSORY LOSS	MUSCLE WEAKNESS	ARTERIAL DOPPLER	VENOUS DOPPLER
I. Viable	Not immediately threatened	None	None	Audible	Audible
IIa. Threatened marginally	Salvageable if promptly treated	Minimal or none	None	Inaudible	Audible
IIb. Threatened immediately	Salvageable if immediately treated	More than toes, associated with rest pain	Mild to moderate	Inaudible	Audible
III. Irreversible	Major tissue loss inevitable	Profound, anesthetic	Profound, paralysis, rigor	Inaudible	Inaudible

Adapted from Rutherford RB, Baker JD, Ernst C, et al. Recommended standards for reports dealing with lower extremity ischemia: revised version. *J Vasc Surg.* 1997;26:517-538.

thrombus from a recent myocardial infarction (MI) (Chapter 73) or from the atrial appendage in a patient with atrial fibrillation (Chapter 64). A less common cause of lower extremity emboli is an abdominal aortic aneurysm (Chapter 78) that serves as the source of cholesterol emboli (Chapter 80).

Arterial in situ thrombosis as a result of plaque rupture usually represents the final stage of a chronically diseased artery, most commonly the femoral or popliteal artery. If native artery thrombosis occurs in the absence of a preexisting stenosis, a thorough search for a hypercoagulable state should be undertaken. Thrombosis of a popliteal aneurysm may present as acute limb ischemia.

Chronic Limb Ischemia

Lower extremity peripheral artery disease may be manifest as either chronic stable disease or as critical limb ischemia. Peripheral arterial disease is most commonly caused by atherosclerosis, but it also may be caused by thromboembolism, inflammatory disease, trauma, aneurysmal disease, adventitial cysts, entrapment syndromes, or congenital abnormalities. Aneurysms may be associated with atherosclerosis, or they may be caused by underlying hereditary (familial) or acquired (e.g., smoking or trauma) causes.

Patients with critical limb ischemia have inadequate blood flow to sustain viability in the distal tissue bed. Critical limb ischemia is most often caused by atherosclerosis, but it can also be caused by atheroembolic or thromboembolic disease, vasculitis, in situ thrombosis related to hypercoagulable states, thromboangiitis obliterans, cystic adventitial disease, popliteal entrapment, or trauma. Patients presenting with critical limb ischemia typically have multisegment disease along the length of the limb.

Inflammation plays a fundamental role in the development and progression of atherosclerosis (Chapter 70). Elevated levels of C-reactive protein (CRP) are strongly associated with the development of peripheral arterial disease. Markers of inflammation such as interleukin-6, tumor necrosis factor-α, CRP, and platelet activation are increased compared with normal subjects.

No specific genetic markers have been confirmed for peripheral arterial disease, although one study identified a linkage on chromosome 1p. The proportion of low ABIs attributable to heritability is estimated at 20%. Concordance rates among twins are about 33% for monozygotic pairs and about 31% for dizygotic pairs, suggesting a limited role for heritability. Taken together, these data suggest a modest but significant heritability factor for peripheral arterial disease.

CLINICAL MANIFESTATIONS

Acute Limb Ischemia

A patient with acute limb ischemia presents with a cool, painful extremity (Table 79-1).[2] Typically, the major muscle groups below the level of obstruction are symptomatic. The absence of a pulse may help localize the site of occlusion, but pulses may be normal in cases of microemboli or cholesterol emboli (Chapter 80). Venous and capillary filling is an indicator of the severity of acute limb ischemia. The leg should be carefully examined for color and temperature abnormalities. Pallor is seen early on, but with time, cyanosis is common. Poikilothermia, or coolness, is an important finding, particularly if the opposite limb is warm. A transition level for color and temperature changes, which is often clinically obvious, should be correlated with the pulses and denoted as a baseline reference at the initial examination for comparison with subsequent examinations.

Sensory changes include numbness and paresthesias. Paralysis indicates that ischemia had advanced to jeopardize the survival of the limb unless the patient undergoes urgent revascularization. Any motor deficit indicates tissue anoxia and implies a very poor prognosis. Motor deficits progress from distal to more proximal muscle groups, so early motor weakness is seen in the intrinsic foot muscles. Complete motor paralysis is a late symptom that suggests irreversible injury. With irreversible ischemia, paralysis progresses to rigor.

TABLE 79-2 FONTAINE'S AND RUTHERFORD'S CLINICAL CLASSIFICATIONS OF CHRONIC LOWER LIMB ISCHEMIA

FONTAINE		RUTHERFORD		
STAGE	CLINICAL	GRADE	CATEGORY	CLINICAL
I	Asymptomatic	0	0	Asymptomatic
IIa	Mild claudication	I	1	Mild claudication
IIb	Moderate to severe claudication	I	2	Moderate claudication
		I	3	Severe claudication
III	Rest pain	II	4	Rest pain
IV	Ulceration or gangrene	III	5	Minor tissue loss
		IV	6	Ulceration or gangrene

Adapted from Norgren L, Hiatt WR, Dormandy JA, et al. Inter-society consensus for the management of peripheral arterial disease (TASC II). *Eur J Vasc Endovasc Surg.* 2007;33(suppl):S1-S75.

Chronic Stable Lower Limb Ischemia

Among patients with chronic stable lower extremity peripheral arterial disease, 50% of patients are asymptomatic despite abnormal pulse examinations, the presence of a vascular bruit, or an abnormal ABI (see Fig. 79-1). About 40% of patients have atypical symptoms (e.g., leg tiredness or fatigue), and only about 10% of patients have classic symptoms of intermittent claudication.

Claudication is defined as exertional discomfort, relieved with rest, in specific muscle groups at risk for ischemia during exercise (Table 79-2). Symptoms usually begin one segment below the level of the arterial narrowing. For example, whereas vascular obstructions (occlusions or stenoses) of the iliac vessels typically cause hip, thigh, and calf pain, femoral and popliteal artery obstructions typically cause symptoms in the calf and foot muscles. Claudication, which is a specific vascular syndrome, must be distinguished from other conditions that cause exertional leg pain, which have been termed *pseudoclaudication* (Table 79-3).

Symptoms in individual patients are remarkably variable despite similar degrees of vascular stenosis, in part owing to collateral vessel formation. A patient with superficial femoral artery occlusion but robust collateral formation via the deep femoral artery and geniculate collaterals, which supply blood to the infrapopliteal vessels, may have minimal or no symptoms. Another patient with similar anatomy but poor collaterals may have severe functional limitation.

Chronic Critical Lower Limb Ischemia

Critical limb ischemia, which develops in about 10% of all patients with peripheral arterial disease, presents as resting limb pain, nonhealing lower extremity ulcers, or gangrene (see Table 79-2). These patients' limbs are in jeopardy, and even the most minor trauma from a poorly fitting shoe or a carelessly clipped toenail may cause a nonhealing wound or infection that leads to amputation. Critical limb ischemia can be exacerbated by conditions that reduce blood flow to the microvascular bed, such as diabetes; severe low cardiac output states; and, rarely, vasospastic diseases.

TABLE 79-3 DIFFERENTIATION OF TRUE CLAUDICATION FROM PSEUDOCLAUDICATION

	INTERMITTENT CLAUDICATION	SPINAL STENOSIS	ARTHRITIS	VENOUS CONGESTION	COMPARTMENT SYNDROME
Character of discomfort	Cramping, tightness, or tiredness	Same as claudication or tingling, weakness, clumsiness	Aching	Tightness, bursting pain	Tightness, bursting pain
Location of discomfort	Buttock, hip, thigh, calf, foot	Buttock, hip, thigh	Hip, knee	Groin, thigh	Calf
Exercise-induced discomfort	Yes	Variable	Variable	After walking	Excessive exercise
Walking distance to discomfort	Reproducible	Variable	Variable	Variable	Excessive exercise
Occurs with standing	No	Yes	Yes, but positional	Yes, but positional	Yes, but positional
Relief of discomfort	Rapid relief with rest	Relief with sitting or changing position	Slow relief with avoidance of weight bearing	Slow relief with leg elevation	Slow relief with leg elevation
Other	Associated with atherosclerosis and decreased pulses	History of lower back problems	Discomfort at joint	History of deep vein thrombosis, signs of venous congestion	Typical in athletes

From White C. Intermittent claudication. *N Engl J Med.* 2007;356:1241-1250.

DIAGNOSIS

Acute Limb Ischemia

In patients with acute limb ischemia, the history and physical examination are the most important steps, not only for assessing the cause and severity of ischemia but also for determining the diagnostic and therapeutic path. Upon completion of the history and physical examination, the physician should be able to answer the following questions about the severity of acute limb ischemia: Is the limb viable? Is the limb's viability immediately threatened? Are there already irreversible changes that may preclude salvage of the limb? Three findings that help differentiate "threatened" from "viable" extremities are the presence of persistent pain, sensory loss, and muscle weakness.

Chronic Limb Ischemia

The clinical severity of chronic stable and chronic critical limb ischemia can be semiquantitatively assessed using either the Fontaine or the Rutherford classification (see Table 79-2). The clinician must distinguish intermittent claudication from nonvascular causes that may mimic claudication (i.e., pseudoclaudication), such as neurogenic pain from spinal stenosis or nerve root compression (Chapter 400), musculoskeletal or arthritic pain, or discomfort from venous congestion or a compartment syndrome (see Table 79-3). A typical history of claudication has a low sensitivity but a high specificity for peripheral arterial disease.

Patients presenting with peripheral arterial disease should be assessed for atherosclerotic risk factors (Table 79-4) and undergo a complete vascular physical examination with their shoes and socks removed, including measurement of the ABI (see Fig. 79-1).[3] ABI results should be uniformly reported with noncompressible values defined as greater than 1.40, normal values defined as 1.00 to 1.40, borderline values as 0.91 to 0.99, and abnormal values as 0.90 or less.

Imaging

Duplex imaging combines ultrasound imaging and Doppler blood velocity measurements to localize vascular obstructions and estimate lesion severity. The sensitivity and specificity of duplex ultrasonography for the diagnosis of a 50% or greater stenosis in the lower extremity is 90% or higher.[4]

Computed tomography angiography (CTA) and magnetic resonance angiography (MRA) offer cross-sectional images that can be reconstructed into a three-dimensional angiogram (Fig. 79-3). Whereas CTA requires iodinated intravenous contrast material and ionizing radiation, MRA uses gadolinium contrast and does not expose the patient to ionizing radiation but cannot be used in patients with ferromagnetic metallic implants such as pacemakers or defibrillators. The major toxicity of gadolinium is an uncommon but potentially lethal systemic disorder called nephrogenic systemic fibrosis or nephrogenic sclerosing dermopathy (Chapter 267); a glomerular filtration rate of 60 mL/minute or less is the major risk factor.

An advantage of CTA over MRA is its ability to visualize metallic stents and stent grafts (Fig. 79-4). CTA requires only about one fourth the radiation required for invasive digital angiography, and it can be performed more quickly and with less pretreatment planning than MRA. Vascular calcification may be a source of artifact with CTA but is inconsequential with MRA. MRA tends to overestimate lesions at the ostia of arteries owing to turbulent flow.

TABLE 79-4 INITIAL LABORATORY EVALUATION OF A PATIENT WITH PERIPHERAL ARTERIAL DISEASE

Serum electrolytes, including fasting serum glucose
Renal function (serum creatinine, blood urea nitrogen, estimated glomerular filtration rate)
Complete blood count
Fasting lipid profile
High-sensitivity C-reactive protein
Ankle-brachial index

Adapted from Rutherford RB, Baker JD, Ernst C, et al. Recommended standards for reports dealing with lower extremity ischemia: revised version. *J Vasc Surg.* 1997;26:517-538.

In a randomized trial comparing MRA with CTA for initial imaging in peripheral arterial disease, there was no difference between the two techniques in terms of ease, clinical utility, or patient outcome, but CTA reduced total diagnostic costs.[A1]

Invasive digital angiography remains the "gold standard" for the diagnosis and evaluation of peripheral arterial disease (see Fig. 79-3) despite the need for iodinated contrast material and the exposure to ionizing radiation. Invasive angiographic procedures (Chapter 57) are associated with a relatively small but nontrivial rate of complications, including severe contrast allergy in 0.1%, access-related bleeding complications, and contrast-induced nephropathy (Chapter 57).

TREATMENT Rx

The treatment of patients with atherosclerotic lower extremity peripheral arterial disease is directed at reducing the patient's risk for life-threatening cardiovascular complications of atherosclerosis, improving walking distance, and salvaging the limb. Revascularization strategies have shifted from open surgical approaches to percutaneous, catheter-based endovascular treatments because of the relative safety, success, and durability of stenting. As a result, amputation rates for peripheral arterial disease have fallen by more than 25% in the past decade or so.

Acute Limb Ischemia

Patients with irreversible limb ischemia (nonviable limb) should not undergo angiography and should be scheduled for amputation (Fig. 79-5). All other patients with acute limb ischemia should undergo emergent angiography to define the culprit lesion and to treat it endovascularly if possible. Before angiography, anticoagulation to prevent thrombus propagation or embolization (e.g., unfractionated heparin 5000 IU bolus; then 1000-IU/hr infusion) and analgesia (e.g., morphine 2 mg intravenously, as needed) should be initiated, and any underlying medical comorbidities (e.g., heart failure) should be managed aggressively to stabilize the patient.

The options for prompt revascularization include (1) endovascular therapies, with intraarterial thrombolysis (e.g., recombinant tissue plasminogen activator 0.5 mg/hr intraarterially) and/or catheter-based thrombectomy and stenting or (2) open surgical thrombectomy with or without arterial bypass. In general, endovascular therapy is recommended for patients with an onset of acute symptoms less than 14 days earlier, and surgical revascularization is

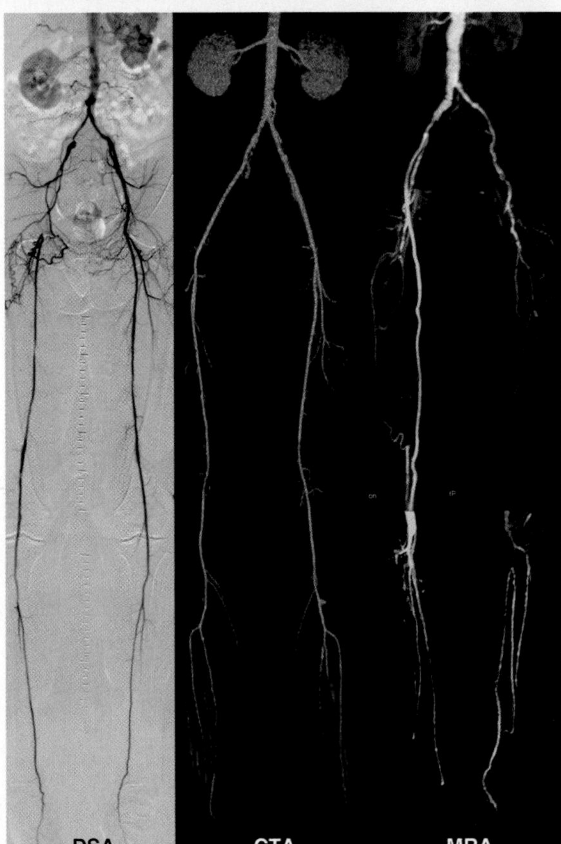

FIGURE 79-3. Aortography with distal run-off in three different patients by three different methods: digital subtraction angiography (DSA), computed tomography angiography (CTA), and magnetic resonance angiography (MRA). (From White C. Intermittent claudication. *N Engl J Med.* 2007;356:1241-1250.)

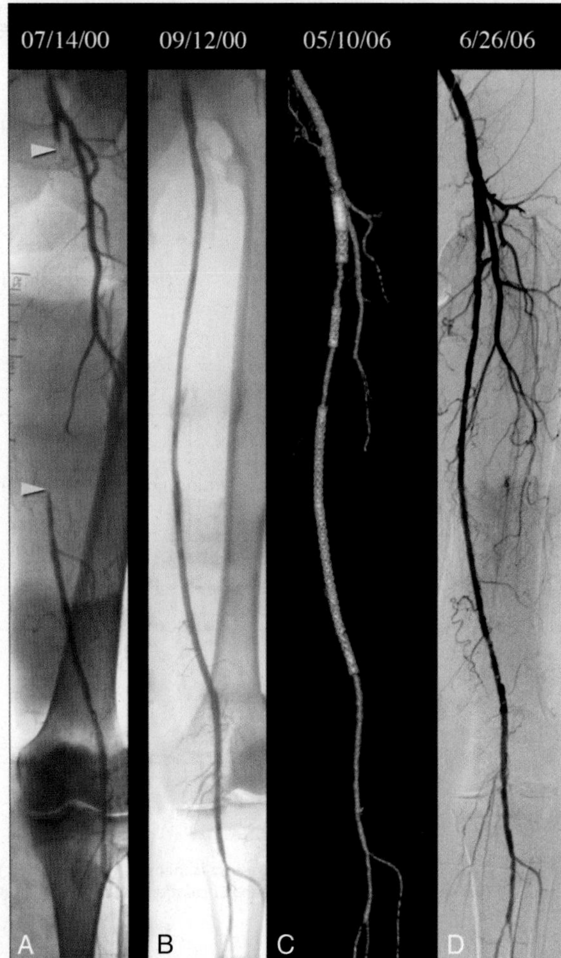

FIGURE 79-4. A, Baseline angiogram of left leg showing occlusion *(arrowheads)* of the femoral-popliteal segment. B, Post-treatment angiogram after balloon angioplasty and stent placement. C, More than 5 years later, the patient returns with claudication and a reduced ankle-brachial index. Follow-up computed tomography angiogram shows narrowing of the superficial femoral artery between the two stents. D, Final angiogram following balloon angioplasty and stent placement.

recommended for patients with a duration of symptoms longer than 14 days. These treatments are often complementary, each with its own advantages and limitations. The less invasive endovascular therapy allows simultaneous angiography to guide reperfusion therapy. Surgery offers definitive restoration of blood flow with thrombectomy or bypass surgery, but it carries higher short-term risks.

Chronic Lower Limb Ischemia

The treatment of patients with claudication is directed at both improving the walking distance and, perhaps more important, reducing the patient's risk for life-threatening cardiovascular complications of atherosclerosis. Risk factor modification (Chapter 52), an exercise prescription, antiplatelet agents (Chapter 38), and medical therapy to reduce claudication are the basic elements of treating chronic stable peripheral arterial disease.

Risk Factor Modification

Patients with known peripheral arterial disease should be encouraged to modify or eliminate atherosclerotic risk factors such as diabetes (Chapter 229), tobacco use (Chapter 32), hyperlipidemia (Chapter 206), and hypertension (Chapter 67) and to exercise regularly (Chapter 16). Specific goals include: blood pressure below 140/90 mmHg and below 130/80 mmHg for those with diabetes, LDL cholesterol below 100 mg/dL and below 70 mg/dL for those at high risk of ischemic events, HDL cholesterol above 40 mg/dL, and hemoglobin A_{1C} level below 7%.

Patients who are smokers or former smokers should be asked about their status of tobacco use at every visit. Smokers should receive counseling, usually be offered pharmacotherapy (e.g., nicotine replacement therapy, sometimes with varenicline or bupropion), and be considered for referral to a smoking cessation program (Chapter 32).[5] For patients with severe peripheral arterial disease and elevated CRP levels, statin therapy substantially improves overall survival.[A2] This finding in patients with peripheral arterial disease is consistent with findings in other studies of patients with a history of vascular disease, with or without peripheral arterial disease, and with either elevated LDL cholesterol levels or elevated CRP levels. Blood pressure control is very important, especially in patients with coexisting diabetes. β-Blockers are effective antihypertensive therapy and are not contraindicated in peripheral arterial disease. Angiotensin-converting enzyme inhibitors (e.g., ramipril 10 mg/day) improve pain-free and maximum walking distance[A3] and reduce the risk of cardiovascular death in patients with peripheral arterial disease.[A4]

Exercise Therapy

Patients should be reassured that exercising, even though it may precipitate their claudication symptoms, is not harmful and is the preferred initial treatment. A meta-analysis comparing supervised with unsupervised exercise therapy demonstrated superior improvement for claudication with supervised exercise.[A5] Improvement in walking distance can often be achieved with pharmacologic management; discontinuation of tobacco use; and a regular, supervised exercise program.[A6] For example, a randomized trial of patients with aortoiliac peripheral arterial disease who underwent a supervised exercise program showed greater improvement in walking performance compared with those who underwent primary stent therapy or home walking with cilostazol.[A7]

Supervised exercise commonly involves walking on a treadmill, with the initial workload set to elicit symptoms within 3 to 5 minutes of walking. The patient is permitted to rest until the symptoms resolve but then resumes exercising. Maximal benefits are associated with programs that require the patient to continue walking until the pain is near maximal and with sessions that last more than 30 minutes, occur three or more times per week, and continue for more than 6 months. It typically takes 1 to 2 months for the patient to begin to notice benefits, which gradually increase over several months. Recent evidence supports the benefit of home-based walking programs with group-mediated cognitive behavior intervention to improve functional performance when compared with a control arm of health education alone. These findings have implications for a large number of patients who are unable or unwilling to participate in supervised exercise programs.[A8]

Antiplatelet and Antithrombotic Therapy

Antiplatelet therapy with aspirin (usually 75 to 325 mg/day) has an established role in the secondary prevention of cardiovascular events in all patients with peripheral arterial disease because they are at high risk of MI, stroke, and

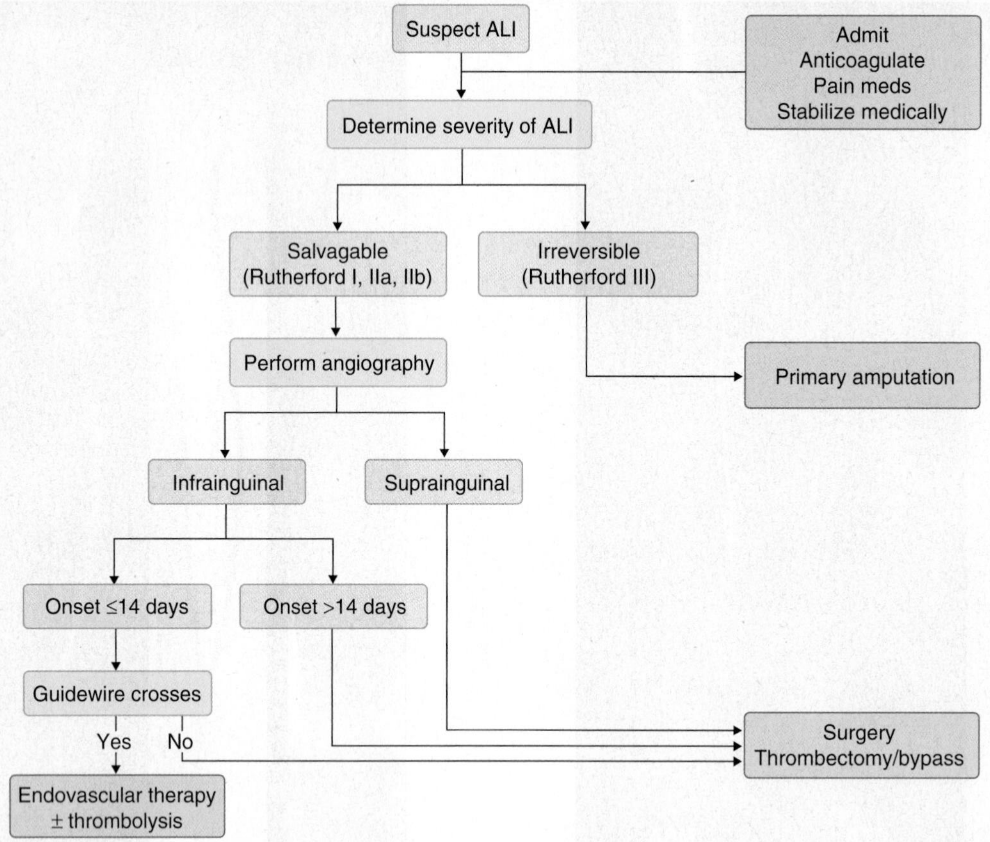

FIGURE 79-5. **Treatment algorithm for acute limb ischemia (ALI). (Modified from Gray BH, Conte MS, Dake MD, et al. Atherosclerotic Peripheral Vascular Disease Symposium II: lower-extremity revascularization: state of the art. *Circulation.* 2008;118:2864-2872.)**

vascular death, whether they are being managed medically, have had prior endovascular or surgical revascularization, or have had prior amputation. The thienopyridines, such as clopidogrel (usually 75 mg/day), are indicated only if aspirin is not tolerated, based on clopidogrel's efficacy compared with aspirin among patients with peripheral arterial disease. Another future possibility may be the novel protease-activated receptor-1 antagonist voraxapar, which can significantly reduce the incidence acute limb ischemia and the need for revascularization in patients with peripheral arterial disease.

Pharmacology

Currently, two medications are approved in the United States for the symptomatic treatment of intermittent claudication: pentoxifylline and cilostazol. Cilostazol, a phosphodiesterase inhibitor, at 50 to 100 mg twice daily improves maximal walking distance by 40% to 50% compared with placebo[A9] and has been shown in a randomized trial to reduce femoral artery stent restenosis.[A10] Cilostazol is contraindicated in patients with heart failure. By comparison, pentoxifylline has not consistently improved treadmill walking distance in randomized trials, so it cannot be recommended. Oral vasodilating prostaglandins, vitamin E, and chelation therapy with EDTA (ethylenediaminetetraacetic acid) have not been effective in improving either symptoms or walking distance.

Revascularization

The decision to perform a percutaneous or surgical revascularization procedure for the relief of claudication in a patient with chronic stable lower limb ischemia is based upon a risk-to-benefit assessment that weighs the patient's disability and discomfort against the estimated short- and long- term benefits and risks of the procedure. Because very few patients with claudication are in danger of losing their limbs, the primary goal of revascularization is long-lasting relief of symptoms, not limb salvage. Patients selected for revascularization to relieve symptoms of intermittent claudication should have significant lifestyle limitations or be unable to work and should have failed to respond to pharmacologic and exercise therapy.[6]

Superficial femoral and popliteal artery stenosis or occlusion (Fig. 79-6) are commonly associated with calf claudication. Revascularization with surgery or percutaneous transluminal angioplasty, with or without stenting, is indicated for the relief of vocational or lifestyle-limiting claudication in patients who have failed exercise and pharmacologic therapy. Angioplasty is preferred when possible in patients younger than 50 years because they have a higher risk of surgical graft failure than do older patients.

In patients with claudication, supervised exercise therapy plus balloon angioplasty improves the ABI at 1 year compared with supervised exercise therapy alone but does not improve quality-of-life measures.[A11] Randomized trials comparing surgery with angioplasty show similar rates of mortality, amputation, and patency at 4 years in patients with lower extremity ischemia. Percutaneous transluminal angioplasty with or without stenting is preferred in amenable lesions because of its lower periprocedural mortality and morbidity. Angioplasty is more cost effective than surgery if the expected 5-year patency rate of the treated vessel is 30% or greater.

To obtain a durable benefit after angioplasty, primary stenting with nitinol self-expanding stents or paclitaxel coated self-expanding stents is recommended for longer femoral lesions (7-10 cm) to reduce restenosis and to improve ABI and walking distance.[A12,A13] In more discrete femoral lesions (mean, 4.5 cm), a strategy of balloon angioplasty first, with stenting only for bailout if the primary angioplasty is unsuccessful, is as good as routine stenting.

Adjunctive angioplasty devices such as atherectomy, cryotherapy, and the cutting balloon have not been meaningfully tested in any population, and there are few data to support their use versus less expensive, more conventional therapies. In randomized trials, laser angioplasty is not superior to conventional percutaneous transluminal angioplasty or stent placement in the superficial femoral artery. Given the substantial additional expense associated with these devices, more evidence of their efficacy is needed before widespread adoption can be justified. Small randomized trials have shown superior patency when femoral angioplasty is performed using drug-coated balloons compared with standard balloon angioplasty alone, but it is too soon to know whether this approach will substitute for femoropopliteal stenting in the future.[A14]

For chronic critical lower limb ischemia, endovascular therapy has reduced the rate of amputation. For patients with critical limb ischemia and salvageable limbs, the optimal treatment is urgent revascularization. The therapeutic goal is to reestablish pulsatile, straight-line flow to the distal extremity. Establishment of uninterrupted flow to at least one infrapopliteal vessel (i.e., the anterior or posterior tibial or peroneal arteries) is a prerequisite for wound healing.

In patients with critical limb ischemia caused by infrainguinal disease, percutaneous transluminal angioplasty and surgery are comparable as first-line therapies, but endovascular therapy is less costly and is associated with lower morbidity. It is reasonable to attempt a percutaneous therapy first if a patient is a candidate for either surgery or angioplasty, particularly if the patient's life expectancy is less than 2 years.[5] The use of coronary drug-eluting stents in tibial arteries appears to be more effective than conventional therapy.[A15]

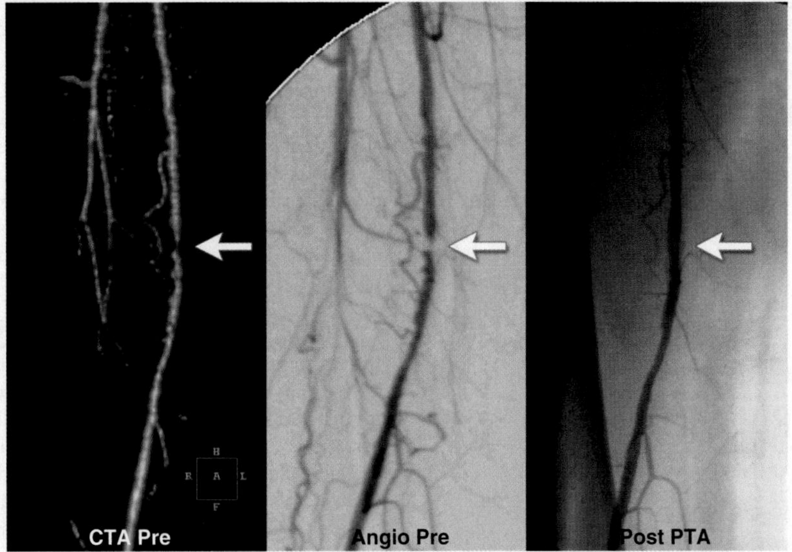

FIGURE 79-6. **Discrete stenosis *(arrows)* of the left superficial femoral artery seen on computed tomography angiography (CTA; *left*), digital subtraction angiography *(middle)*, and digital angiography after percutaneous transluminal angioplasty (PTA; *right*). (From White C. Intermittent claudication. *N Engl J Med.* 2007;356:1241-1250.)**

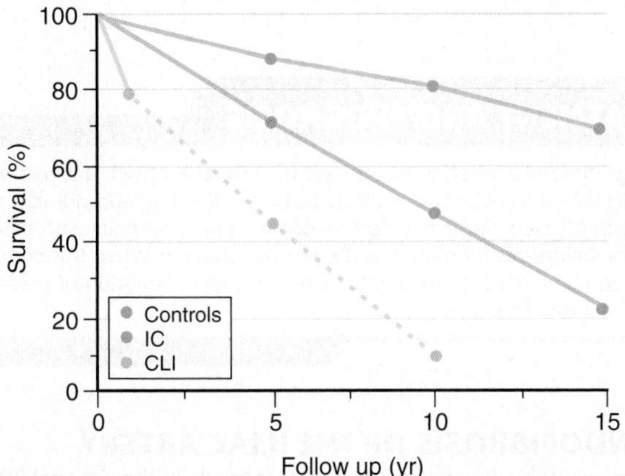

FIGURE 79-7. **Survival curve of patients with intermittent claudication (IC) versus critical limb ischemia (CLI). (Modified from Norgren L, Hiatt WR, Dormandy JA, et al. Inter-society consensus for the management of peripheral arterial disease (TASC II). *Eur J Vasc Endovasc Surg.* 2007;33(suppl):S1-S75.)**

Nevertheless, primary amputation is indicated in patients who have extensive necrosis or infectious gangrene with rest pain, are not ambulatory, and are not candidates for revascularization. Cellular therapies and growth factor therapy are being investigated for limb salvage, but none have yet proven clinically effective.

PROGNOSIS

Peripheral arterial disease is a major cause of acute and chronic illness associated with impaired functional capacity, reduced quality of life, limb loss, and increased risk of death (Fig. 79-7). Approximately two thirds of patients with peripheral arterial disease have at least one severely diseased coronary artery, and up to one quarter of patients have significant carotid artery stenosis. Consequently, patients with peripheral arterial disease face an increased risk of cardiovascular ischemic events such as MI, ischemic stroke, and death. It is estimated that coronary and cerebrovascular adverse events occur two- to fourfold more commonly than do limb adverse events in patients with peripheral arterial disease. Outcomes are improved when guideline-recommended therapy is followed.[7]

The annual mortality rate for patients with peripheral arterial disease is about 5%, but it is higher for patients with severe disease. For example, the estimated 1-year mortality rate for patients with critical limb ischemia is 25%, but this can climb to 45% for patients requiring amputation; in contrast, annual mortality rate for patients with intermittent claudication is only 1% to 2%. For patients presenting with acute limb ischemia, the 30-day amputation rate is as high as 40%, and mortality rates up to 30% have been reported.

Patients with lower extremity claudication should be reassured that the risk of limb loss is low. Moreover, a history of claudication by itself only slightly increases the risk of amputation after 10 years. However, a reduced ABI and diabetes mellitus are associated with the development of ischemic rest pain and ischemic ulceration, which may lead to limb loss. Among patients with peripheral arterial disease, those who have diabetes are 15 times more likely to have an amputation than are patients without diabetes, whose annual amputation rate is less than 1%.

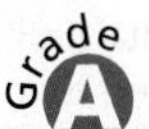

Grade A References

A1. Ouwendijk R, de Vries M, Pattynama PM, et al. Imaging peripheral arterial disease: a randomized controlled trial comparing contrast-enhanced MR angiography and multi-detector row CT angiography. *Radiology.* 2005;236:1094-1103.

A2. Schillinger M, Exner M, Mlekusch W, et al. Statin therapy improves cardiovascular outcome of patients with peripheral artery disease. *Eur Heart J.* 2004;25:742-748.

A3. Ahimastos AA, Walker PJ, Askew C, et al. Effect of ramipril on walking times and quality of life among patients with peripheral artery disease and intermittent claudication: a randomized controlled trial. *JAMA.* 2013;309:453-460.

A4. Yusuf S, Sleight P, Pogue J, et al. Effects of an angiotensin-converting-enzyme inhibitor, ramipril, on cardiovascular events in high-risk patients. The Heart Outcomes Prevention Evaluation Study Investigators. *N Engl J Med.* 2000;342:145-153.

A5. Fokkenrood HJ, Bendermacher BL, Lauret GJ, et al. Supervised exercise therapy versus non-supervised exercise therapy for intermittent claudication. *Cochrane Database Syst Rev.* 2013;8: CD005263.

A6. Lane R, Ellis B, Watson L, et al. Exercise for intermittent claudication. *Cochrane Database Syst Rev.* 2014;7:CD000990.

A7. Murphy TP, Cutlip DE, Regensteiner JG, et al. Supervised exercise versus primary stenting for claudication resulting from aortoiliac peripheral artery disease: six-month outcomes from the Claudication: Exercise Versus Endoluminal Revascularization (CLEVER) study. *Circulation.* 2012;125:130-139.

A8. McDermott MM, Liu K, Guralnik JM, et al. Home-based walking exercise intervention in peripheral artery disease: A randomized clinical trial. *JAMA.* 2013;310:57-65.

A9. Bedenis R, Stewart M, Cleanthis M, et al. Cilostazol for intermittent claudication. *Cochrane Database Syst Rev.* 2014;10:CD003748.

A10. Iida O, Yokoi H, Soga Y, et al. Cilostazol reduces angiographic restenosis after endovascular therapy for femoropopliteal lesions in the Sufficient Treatment of Peripheral Intervention by Cilostazol study. *Circulation.* 2013;127:2307-2315.

A11. Ahimastos AA, Pappas EP, Buttner PG, et al. A meta-analysis of the outcome of endovascular and noninvasive therapies in the treatment of intermittent claudication. *J Vasc Surg.* 2011;54: 1511-1521.

A12. Schillinger M, Sabeti S, Loewe C, et al. Balloon angioplasty versus implantation of nitinol stents in the superficial femoral artery. *N Engl J Med.* 2006;354:1879-1888.

A13. Dake MD, Ansel GM, Jaff MR, et al. Sustained safety and effectiveness of paclitaxel-eluting stents for femoropopliteal lesions: 2-year follow-up from the Zilver PTX randomized and single-arm clinical studies. *J Am Coll Cardiol.* 2013;61:2417-2427.

A14. Werk M, Albrecht T, Meyer DR, et al. Paclitaxel-coated balloons reduce restenosis after femoropopliteal angioplasty: evidence from the randomized PACIFIER trial. *Circ Cardiovasc Interv.* 2012;5:831-840.

A15. Feiring AJ, Krahn M, Nelson L, et al. Preventing leg amputations in critical limb ischemia with below-the-knee drug-eluting stents: the PaRADISE (PReventing Amputations using Drug eluting StEnts) trial. *J Am Coll Cardiol*. 2010;55:1580-1589.

GENERAL REFERENCES

For the General References and other additional features, please visit Expert Consult at https://expertconsult.inkling.com.

80 OTHER PERIPHERAL ARTERIAL DISEASES

MICHAEL R. JAFF AND JOHN R. BARTHOLOMEW

POPLITEAL ARTERY ENTRAPMENT SYNDROME

Popliteal artery entrapment syndrome, which is a cause of intermittent claudication in young and often athletic patients, results from extrinsic compression on the popliteal artery by muscles or ligaments within or surrounding the popliteal fossa. The artery may be entrapped by various muscle components within the popliteal fossa. The popliteal vein also can be involved, rarely, and sometimes the symptoms are functional owing to hypertrophy of the medial head of the gastrocnemius muscle.

Anatomic evidence of entrapment can be found on physical examination or imaging performed for unrelated reasons in up to 4% of apparently normal individuals and imaging evidence for popliteal artery compression with provocative maneuvers in as many of 80% of asymptomatic individuals. Clinically evident popliteal artery entrapment syndrome is rare, with one study showing a prevalence of approximately 0.16% among military recruits.

CLINICAL MANIFESTATIONS AND DIAGNOSIS

Symptoms of popliteal artery entrapment syndrome include exertional limb pain, paresthesias and cold feet after exercise, ischemic rest pain, and even tissue necrosis if undiagnosed cases progress to arterial degeneration with thromboembolization. Entrapment of the popliteal vein results in leg swelling, heaviness, varicosities, nocturnal calf cramping, and even deep vein thrombosis (Chapter 81).

The diagnosis of popliteal artery entrapment syndrome is suggested by demonstration of popliteal artery compression on active pedal plantar flexion against resistance. This compression is manifested by a decrease in the intensity of the pedal arterial pulse on physical examination and loss of the continuous wave Doppler signal over the pedal arteries. Pulse volume recordings and segmental limb pressures should be measured at rest with the knee extended and the ankle in the neutral, dorsiflexed, and plantarflexed positions. Exercise treadmill studies also may demonstrate diminished limb arterial pressure after exercise in the symptomatic limb. Arterial duplex ultrasonography, dynamic computerized tomographic (CT) arteriography, or magnetic resonance (MR) arteriography may confirm the diagnosis, and CT or MR arteriography also define the structures that cause the entrapment.

TREATMENT AND PROGNOSIS Rx

Treatment of structural popliteal artery entrapment is largely surgical with relief of the entrapment by resection or translocation of the compressing elements.[1] If popliteal artery entrapment syndrome is not identified until after the artery has been injured, arterial reconstruction or surgical bypass, ideally with a venous autologous graft, may be required. In functional popliteal artery entrapment, resection or translocation of the medial head of the gastrocnemius muscle is performed. If therapy is offered early in the course of the syndrome, patients may expect full recovery with complete resolution of symptoms.

CYSTIC ADVENTITIAL DISEASE OF THE LOWER EXTREMITY ARTERIES

In cystic adventitial disease, a mucinous cyst develops within the adventitial layers of the arterial wall and encroaches on the arterial lumen.[2,3] Cystic adventitial disease most commonly affects the popliteal artery, where it results in intermittent claudication, classically in middle-aged men. It also has been described in the external iliac, femoral, radial, and ulnar arteries.

The exact cause of cystic adventitial disease is unknown. Theories include a systemic disorder, repetitive trauma, and a persistent embryonic synovial track.

CLINICAL MANIFESTATIONS AND DIAGNOSIS

Intermittent claudication is the most common manifesting symptom of cystic adventitial disease. However, limb discomfort may persist for up to 20 minutes after the cessation of activity, unlike the classic relief of limb pain on cessation of activity in atherosclerotic peripheral artery disease (Chapter 79). The limb symptoms of cystic adventitial disease also tend to be inconsistent, often reappearing without obvious precipitants and resolving without an obvious explanation. Acute limb ischemia (Chapter 79) secondary to arterial compression and thrombosis also can occur.

The diagnosis is suspected when pedal pulses disappear with passive knee flexion and occasionally with exercise. However, cystic adventitial disease is most often confirmed with MR angiography. By comparison, arteriography may demonstrate only compression of the arterial lumen without identifying the cyst.

TREATMENT AND PROGNOSIS Rx

Image-guided aspiration of the cyst may be attempted, but recurrence is likely. Balloon angioplasty is unlikely to be an effective and durable therapy and is not advised. Surgical resection of the cyst, potentially with placement of a venous interposition graft, is the primary therapy. When this condition is identified early, patients may anticipate complete resolution of claudication after resection of the cyst.

ENDOFIBROSIS OF THE ILIAC ARTERY

Endofibrosis of the iliac artery represents stenosis of the external iliac artery, thought to be due to repetitive trauma in highly functioning and competitive athletes.[3] This condition commonly occurs in cyclists or runners 30 to 50 years of age.

Endofibrosis results from intimal hyperplasia and fibrosis of the arterial wall. Smooth muscle cell proliferation and medial and intimal proliferation also may occur.

CLINICAL MANIFESTATIONS AND DIAGNOSIS

Symptoms include exercise-interfering intermittent claudication along with a sensation of swelling or paresthesia in the proximal lower limb at the time of maximal exercise. Physical examination may be normal at rest, although a bruit may be heard over the ipsilateral pelvic fossa or inguinal region.

Diagnostic imaging includes preexercise and postexercise Doppler ankle pressure measurements at the time of maximal, symptom-limiting treadmill exercise. Ultrasound imaging and contrast angiography, preferably when the leg is flexed at the hip in the cycling position, will reveal concentric stenosis, often with lengthening of the affected iliac artery. Intravascular ultrasound and intra-arterial translesional pressure gradients may be helpful.

TREATMENT AND PROGNOSIS Rx

Surgical revascularization with patch angioplasty or interposition grafts has been the mainstay of treatment. However, percutaneous transluminal angioplasty and stent deployment may represent the optimal initial strategy, particularly among patients who agree to change their exercise routines. In patients who continue with high-intensity exercise, however, the long-term durability of a metallic stent within an artery prone to repetitive trauma is an ongoing concern.

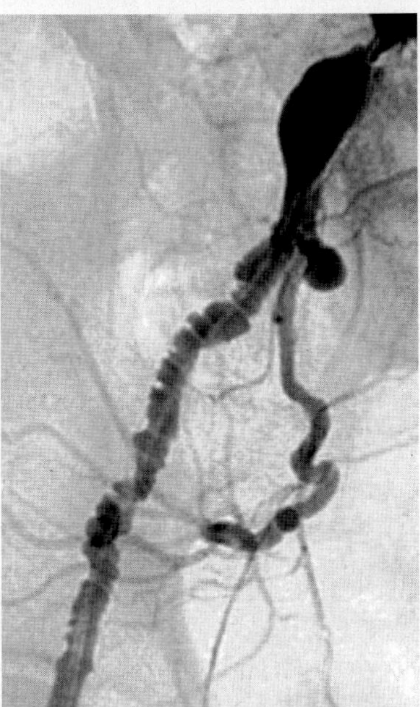

FIGURE 80-1. **Angiogram showing a typical "string of beads" pattern, typical of the medial type in fibromuscular dysplasia, in the external iliac artery. Also note the aneurysm proximal to the area of dysplasia. Courtesy Dr. Jeffrey W. Olin.**

After early detection, surgical or endovascular revascularization usually ameliorates the symptoms. With continued trauma to the arterial segment, however, careful surveillance for recurrence warranted.

FIBROMUSCULAR DYSPLASIA

Fibromuscular dysplasia[4] (Chapter 125) is a noninflammatory, nonatherosclerotic arterial disease that most commonly involves the medial layer of the artery wall and can affect any artery in the body. It is most commonly seen in women 20 to 60 years of age, with a mean age at onset of 52 years, but a range of 5 to 83 years.[5] Its true prevalence is unknown, but a series of potential renal donors showed a prevalence as high as almost 4%.

Medial fibroplasia, which is the most common type of fibromuscular dysplasia, results in the classic "string of beads" appearance on contrast arteriography (Fig. 80-1). Pathology shows alternating segments of thinning and thickening of the arterial media, but the adventitia or intima may be predominantly affected, thereby resulting in an angiographic appearance different from that for medial fibroplasia. Other types of fibromuscular dysplasia include an intimal variant that causes a single, focal, weblike stenosis within the affected artery.

CLINICAL MANIFESTATIONS AND DIAGNOSIS

The clinical presentation of patients with fibromuscular dysplasia depends on the arteries involved, and sometimes it may be incidentally discovered without any symptoms when imaging is performed for other reasons. The renal arteries are affected in almost 80% of cases (Chapter 125), and the extracranial carotid arteries are involved in almost 75% of cases. The third most commonly affected artery is the vertebral artery, which is involved in nearly 40% of patients. Not surprisingly, hypertension (Chapter 67) and headache (Chapter 398) represent the two most common manifesting signs and symptoms. Less common symptoms include dizziness, cervical bruits, and pulsatile tinnitus. Fibromuscular dysplasia may occasionally affect the iliac, femoral, or popliteal arteries.

The diagnosis of fibromuscular dysplasia relies on a combination of clinical and imaging findings. Doppler ultrasound, MR angiography, and CT angiography can identify fibromuscular dysplasia and assess possible aneurysms, but contrast angiography and intravascular ultrasound are the best diagnostic tests. Because fibromuscular dysplasia may involve several vascular beds, patients should initially undergo comprehensive MR or CT imaging of their intracranial arteries, the extracranial carotid arteries, the thoracic and abdominal aorta and its branches, and the renal arteries. If arterial aneurysms or dissections are identified without clear evidence of fibromuscular dysplasia, a genetic collagen disorder should be considered.

TREATMENT AND PROGNOSIS (Rx)

Treatment of fibromuscular dysplasia depends on the clinical presentation and extent of arterial involvement. Asymptomatic patients are empirically prescribed aspirin. In young patients with sudden onset of hypertension and renal artery fibromuscular dysplasia, percutaneous transluminal angioplasty can cure the hypertension that is often found (Chapter 125).[6] Renal and intracranial artery aneurysms should be followed closely for expansion and may require surgical repair. The decision about repair is often based on the size of the aneurysm, its rate of expansion, and the presence of associated symptoms. Carotid artery fibromuscular dysplasia is generally treated with antiplatelet therapy (e.g., aspirin 81 to 325 mg/day) or 3 to 6 months of warfarin anticoagulation in the case of carotid artery dissection; percutaneous transluminal angioplasty is reserved for patients with hemispheric cerebral ischemic symptoms and progressive dissection. Peripheral artery percutaneous transluminal angioplasty is recommended only for patients with symptoms of intermittent claudication.

In general, patients with fibromuscular dysplasia have an excellent outcome. After percutaneous transluminal angioplasty of the renal arteries, approximately one third of patients with hypertension will have normal blood pressures and most others will have substantial improvement. Optimal antiplatelet therapy (e.g., aspirin 81 to 325 mg/day) is recommended for the majority of patients with fibromuscular dysplasia. The most feared complications, which occur in less than 5% of patients, are stroke owing to progressive carotid dissection, rupture of an intracranial arterial aneurysm, or rupture of a visceral artery aneurysm.

THROMBOANGIITIS OBLITERANS (BUERGER DISEASE)

Thromboangiitis obliterans is a nonatherosclerotic, segmental inflammatory disorder that affects small and medium-sized arteries, veins, and nerves. Thromboangiitis obliterans is typically found in patients who are under the age of 50 years and who smoke or chew tobacco.[7]

Although rarely performed, biopsy of affected digits demonstrates highly cellular inflammatory thrombi with sparing of the artery wall. Thromboangiitis obliterans is one of the few vascular disorders that affects both arteries and veins, so superficial thrombophlebitis can also develop.

CLINICAL MANIFESTATIONS AND DIAGNOSIS

Patients classically present with digital or extremity pain with digital ischemia, distal limb claudication (such as in the arch of the foot or arm), and digital ulcerations (Fig. 80-2). More than 40% of patients have Raynaud phenomenon.

Clinicians must maintain a high degree of clinical suspicion in young smokers with distal extremity ischemia and pain without evidence of atherosclerosis. Many patients will demonstrate an abnormal Allen test, in which one of two of the major arteries to the hand (radial or ulnar) does not fill after the examiner compresses the other artery, as well as absent peripheral arterial pulses. The ankle brachial-index (Chapter 79) is classically abnormal, even though plethysmographic studies demonstrate essentially normal proximal artery circulation. Serologic results show no evidence for inflammatory vasculitis (Chapter 270), and proximal sources of arterial emboli are not found. Contrast arteriography is often needed to demonstrate distal arterial involvement with the absence of atherosclerosis. Segmental arterial occlusions with corkscrew collaterals are commonly found but are not pathognomonic.

TREATMENT AND PROGNOSIS (Rx)

The cornerstone of treatment is complete abstinence from tobacco use (Chapter 32). Although less effective, antiplatelet therapy (e.g., aspirin 81 to 325/day) is commonly prescribed. A 28-day course of the prostacyclin analogue iloprost (1 ng/kg/minute for 6 hours daily) can substantially improve pain and accelerate wound healing[A1][A2] compared with aspirin or lumbar sympathectomy. There are no data demonstrating benefit with vasodilators such as calcium channel antagonists, peripheral α-blockers, or sildenafil. Digital sympathectomy, bosentan, spinal cord stimulators, and intermittent pneumatic compression have all been tried with variable success.

Patients with thromboangiitis obliterans must discontinue all exposure to tobacco. However, unsuccessful patients commonly have unremitting pain, recurrent tissue necrosis, and the need for progressive limb amputation.

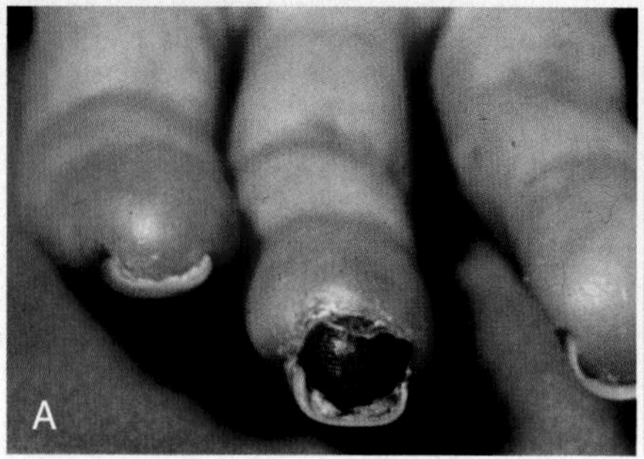

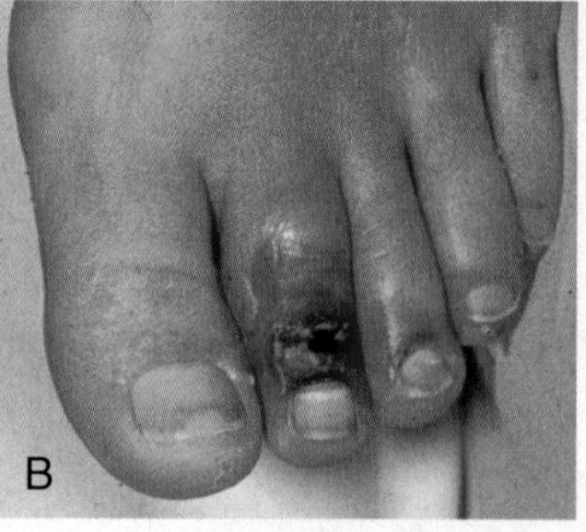

FIGURE 80-2. Buerger disease. Ischemic finger of a young male patient (A) and ischemic toe of a 28-year-old woman (B) with Buerger disease. Courtesy Dr. Jeffrey W. Olin.

LIVEDO RETICULARIS

Livedo reticularis is a vasospastic disorder that appears as a violaceous or bluish netlike discoloration surrounding a pale central area of skin. It normally involves the lower extremities.

Livedo reticularis is commonly found in healthy women during their second to fifth decade of life and strongly associated with antiphospholipid antibodies (Chapter 176). It is rare in males.

Livedo reticularis is an ischemic dermopathy caused by an increased prominence of venous beds owing to obstruction of arterial inflow, venous dilatation, or blockage of venous outflow.[8] Primary livedo reticularis is a benign condition exacerbated by cold, tobacco, or emotional upset, whereas the secondary form, referred to as livedo racemosa, is a pathologic variant seen in association with a number of disorders (Table 80-1).

CLINICAL MANIFESTATIONS AND DIAGNOSIS

The legs and to a lesser extent arms are most commonly involved in primary livedo reticularis, whereas the face, trunk, buttocks, and extremities may be involved with livedo racemosa. The discoloration of livedo reticularis is worsened by dependency and improves with elevation. It is important to differentiate the usually painless, symmetrical, unbroken vessel network of primary livedo reticularis from the frequently painful, irregular, asymmetrical, and broken pattern observed in livedo racemosa.

A thorough history should focus on exacerbating conditions. Laboratory investigation is usually not necessary for the primary form, but specific testing for diagnosing the secondary forms includes antiphospholipid antibody levels (including circulating lupus anticoagulant; anticardiolipin antibodies; P and C antineutrophil cytoplasmic antibodies) should be performed. A skin biopsy may be necessary when serologic findings are indeterminate and the diagnosis remains unclear. The differential diagnosis includes erythema ab igne, livedoid vasculopathy (a rare subtype of livedo racemosa), and acrocyanosis.

TREATMENT AND PROGNOSIS Rx

Cold temperatures, tobacco, and stressful conditions should be avoided. Primary livedo reticularis does not require treatment, although calcium channel blockers (e.g., nifedipine 10 to 20 mg PO every 6 hours or amlodipine 2.5 to 10 mg/day PO) may be beneficial for patients who are uncomfortable with their appearance. Treatment for livedo racemosa should focus on the underlying disorder. Anticoagulants, including warfarin to provide an international normalized ratio of 2.0 to 3.0, antiplatelet therapy (e.g., aspirin 81 to 325/day), or both are recommended for livedo racemosa associated with the antiphospholipid syndrome, cerebrovascular disease (Sneddon syndrome), or both. The prognosis is excellent for primary livedo reticularis, but depends on the underlying disorder for patients with livedo racemosa.

TABLE 80-1 DISORDERS ASSOCIATED WITH LIVEDO RACEMOSA

Polyarteritis nodosa, systemic lupus erythematosus, rheumatoid arthritis, Sjögren syndrome, scleroderma
Atheromatous embolization, atrial myxoma
Antiphospholipid syndrome, Sneddon syndrome
Infections
Polycythemia vera, essential thrombocythemia, cryoglobulinemia, cryofibrinogenemia, cold agglutinin disease
Calciphylaxis, hyperoxaluria
Medications: Amantadine, amphetamines, ergotamines, vasopressors (epinephrine, norepinephrine, dopamine), heparin, minocycline

ATHEROMATOUS EMBOLIZATION

Atheromatous embolization, also known as cholesterol crystal embolization, atheroembolic renal disease, or the blue or purple toe syndrome, refers to the showering of multiple small cholesterol crystals or fibrin-platelet aggregates to the extremities or any organ. The exact incidence of atheromatous embolization is unknown, in part because it is often poorly recognized. In unselected autopsy series, the prevalence ranges from 0.18% to 2%, although it is reported to be much higher in individuals who have undergone aortic manipulation, arteriography, or cardiac or vascular procedures.[9] As many as 5% to 10% of all cases of acute renal failure may result from atheroembolism (Chapter 125). Atheromatous embolization is more common in elderly individuals with advanced atherosclerosis but is less commonly diagnosed in blacks, largely owing to a failure to recognize the classic dermatologic feature because of their skin pigmentation.

Atheromatous embolization usually originates from ulcerated or stenotic atherosclerotic plaques or aneurysms of both large and small arteries. Precipitating factors include arteriography, endovascular procedures (cerebral, coronary, or peripheral), surgery, trauma, or anticoagulation. Atheroembolism also may occur spontaneously. Light microscopy demonstrates multiple biconvex, needle-shaped cholesterol crystals that lodge in arterioles and result in a foreign body reaction in which polymorphonuclear leukocytes, macrophages, and multinucleated giant cells are observed days to weeks after the initiating event. This process eventually leads to end-organ damage owing to intraluminal obliteration, ischemia, and even often infarction.

CLINICAL MANIFESTATIONS AND DIAGNOSIS

Dermatologic findings involving the lower extremities are the most common clinical presentation (Fig. 80-3), but clinical manifestations may be seen in multiple organs (Table 80-2).[10] Atheromatous embolization is frequently overlooked or misdiagnosed because the signs and symptoms are nonspecific and diverse. Once suspected, the diagnosis usually can be made on clinical grounds alone in a patient who has had a precipitating event, acute or subacute renal failure, difficult-to-control hypertension, or evidence of peripheral embolization.[11] In some cases, the definitive diagnosis may require biopsy of the skin, kidney, or gastrointestinal tract. Patients may have elevated markers of inflammation (erythrocyte sedimentation rate, C-reactive protein) or transient eosinophilia. Elevations in amylase, hepatic aminotransferase, blood urea nitrogen, serum creatinine, or serum creatinine kinase levels may be seen with involvement of the pancreas, liver, kidney, or muscle, respectively. The urine is generally nonspecific, but eosinophiluria can be seen.

Invasive diagnostic angiographic procedures should be avoided. Noninvasive procedures including multidetector CT angiography, MR angiography, or transesophageal echocardiography may be helpful if they reveal a markedly irregular and shaggy aorta.

The differential diagnosis, which depends on the end organ involved, includes contrast-induced nephropathy (Chapters 57 and 120), polyarteritis nodosa (Chapter 270), leukocytoclastic vasculitis (Chapters 270 and 439), cryoglobulinemia (Chapter 187), the antiphospholipid syndrome

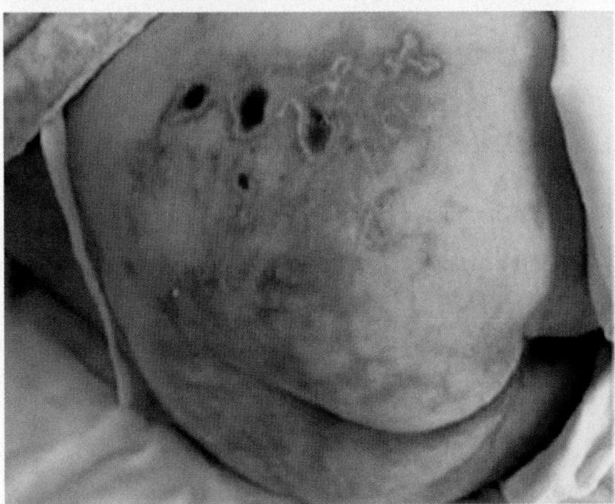

FIGURE 80-3. Livedo racemosa with ischemic ulcerations and violaceous, netlike, and broken patterns in a patient who developed atheromatous embolization after cardiac catheterization.

TABLE 80-2 CLINICAL MANIFESTATIONS OF ATHEROMATOUS EMBOLIZATION

Skin	Purple or blue toes Gangrenous digits Livedo reticularis or livedo racemosa Petechiae Ulcers, nodules Splinter hemorrhages
Kidney	Uncontrolled hypertension Advanced renal disease End-stage renal disease
Neurologic	Amaurosis fugax Hollenhorst plaque Transient ischemic attack or stroke Confusion, organic brain syndrome Spinal cord infarction
Gastrointestinal	Abdominal pain Diarrhea Gastrointestinal bleeding Ischemic bowel Acute pancreatitis Acute gangrenous cholecystitis
Cardiac	Angina pectoris Myocardial infarction
Constitutional symptoms	Fever Weight loss Malaise, myalgias Anorexia, nausea, vomiting

(Chapter 176), and thrombotic thrombocytopenia purpura (Chapter 172). An underlying malignancy is part of the differential diagnosis in patients who present with constitutional symptoms such as anorexia and weight loss. Cardiac sources such as nonbacterial thrombotic endocarditis (Chapter 76), infective endocarditis (Chapter 76), or atrial myxoma (Chapter 60) should be excluded.

TREATMENT AND PROGNOSIS Rx

The most important aspect of treatment is prevention. The prevention of recurrent atheroembolism is essential. Smoking cessation (Chapter 32) and aggressive control of hypertension (Chapter 67), diabetes (Chapter 229), and hyperlipidemia (Chapter 206) should be instituted to prevent progression of the disease. In the absence of data from randomized trials, therapy is directed toward avoiding recurrent embolization, removing the source of the athero-emboli, and providing symptomatic care of the end organ(s) involved.

Patients with ischemic ulcers require pain control and local wound care. Statins (e.g., atorvastatin 10 to 80 mg/day or rosuvastatin 10 to 40 mg/day to obtain optimal low-density lipoprotein cholesterol levels [Chapter 206]) have been reported to be beneficial, likely a result of their plaque-stabilizing activity. Other pharmacologic approaches—including antiplatelet agents (aspirin or clopidogrel), calcium channel blockers (e.g., nifedipine 10 to 20 mg PO every 6 hours or amlodipine 2.5 to 10 mg/day PO), cilostazol (100 mg PO every 12 hours), pentoxifylline (400 mg PO every 8 hours), and intravenous prostaglandins—have been tried with varying degrees of success. The use of anticoagulants is controversial because of concerns that they may lead to plaque instability, and data do not support the use of corticosteroids.

Nonpharmacologic approaches including chemical or surgical sympathectomy, a spinal cord stimulator, and arterial flow pumps may help for pain control. Endovascular therapies (angioplasty, stent placement, atherectomy, or covered-stent grafts, and the use of embolic protective devices) may help prevent future embolic events, but studies are limited and further clinical evaluation is needed. Surgical therapies including thromboendarterectomy, aortobiiliac or aortobifemoral bypass grafting, or extra-anatomic reconstruction may be necessary to eliminate the embolic source and reduce further embolization.

Patients with advanced atherosclerosis and atheromatous embolization have a poor prognosis. The estimated 1-year mortality rate is approximately 15% even with optimal medical care.

THERMAL DISORDERS

A variety of clinical syndromes can be caused by heat or cold (Fig. 80-4).

Erythromelalgia

The term *erythromelalgia* is derived from the Greek words *erythros* ("red"), *melos* ("extremities"), and *algos* ("pain"). It is characterized by episodic periods of erythema, increased warmth, and intense burning pain of the extremities.

Erythromelalgia is an uncommon disorder that affects younger to middle-aged women, adolescents, and children. The exact incidence is not known but has been reported at 1.3 per 100,000 living in Olmsted County, Minnesota. Erythromelalgia also occurs in nearly 30% of patients with polycythemia vera (Chapter 166).

Both primary (familial and sporadic/idiopathic) and secondary forms occur. The primary trigger is heat exposure or increased ambient temperature. The familial form is autosomal dominant, with symptoms most often beginning in childhood. The pathophysiology is believed to be due to a small fiber neuropathy and vasculopathy. Although the exact cause for primary erythromelalgia is unknown, it is a neuropathic disorder with neuronal hyperexcitability owing to sodium channel abnormalities because of a mutation of the gene *(SCN9A)* that encodes the Nav1.7v sodium channel (located on 2q).[12] The causes of secondary erythromelalgia (Table 80-3) are not as well understood but are thought to be due to neuropathologic and microvascular functional changes caused by the underlying condition.

CLINICAL MANIFESTATIONS AND DIAGNOSIS

A triad of clinical findings including erythema, increased warmth, and intense burning pain of the extremities is usually observed (Fig. 80-5). The lower limbs (soles of the feet) are more often affected than the hands. Involvement of the knees, elbows, ears, and face has been reported. Symptoms are generally bilateral and paroxysmal. An attack, which may last for several minutes or hours to days, is generally aggravated by dependency, alcohol, warm rooms, summer heat, exercise, or simply wearing shoes and socks or gloves. Erythromelalgia is often a disabling condition, and ulceration or even gangrene can occur in secondary forms.

The history and physical examination are keys to the diagnosis. The physical examination is usually normal unless the patient is examined during an attack. A thorough vascular and neurologic examination should include demonstration of color changes and measurement of elevated skin temperatures during an attack. A complete blood count is essential to exclude an underlying myeloproliferative disorder. Other tests including electromyography and nerve conduction studies, autonomic and small fiber nerve testing, and vascular studies may help exclude other disorders. The quantitative sudomotor axon reflex test is useful to assess for small fiber neuropathy. Genetic testing is helpful for diagnosing primary erythromelalgia.

The differential diagnosis includes complex regional pain syndrome (Chapter 30), cellulitis (Chapter 441), peripheral neuropathy (Chapter 420), osteomyelitis (Chapter 272), Raynaud syndrome, acrocyanosis, peripheral arterial disease (Chapter 79), and gout (Chapter 273).

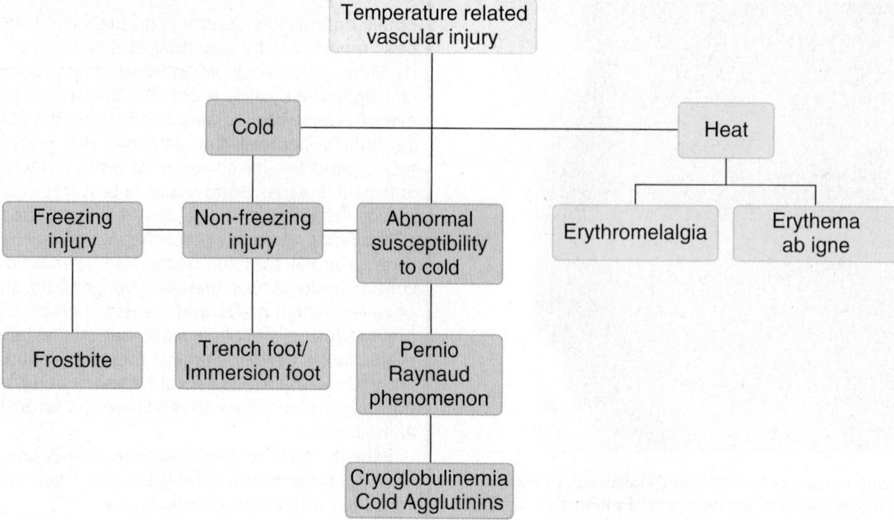

FIGURE 80-4. Clinical syndromes caused by heat or cold.

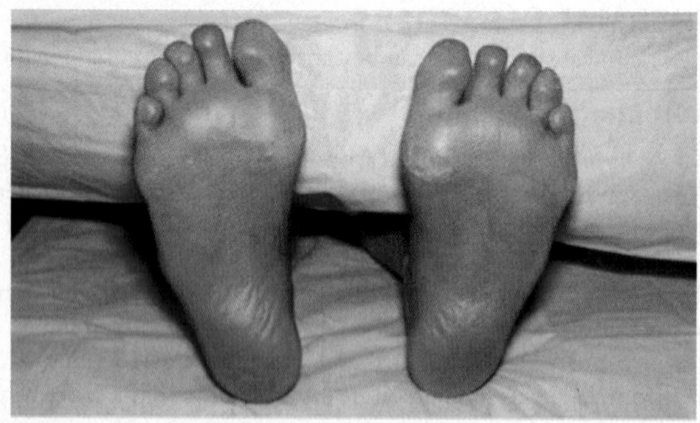

FIGURE 80-5. Erythromelalgia. Note the erythema of the feet. The patient also had pain and increased warmth on physical examination.

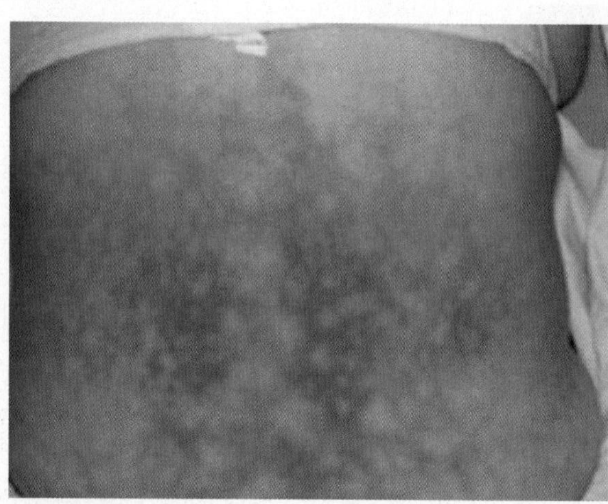

FIGURE 80-6. Erythema ab igne. Note the hyperpigmentation and livedo reticularis pattern in a patient who used a heating pad for back pain.

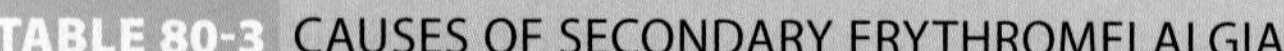

TABLE 80-3 CAUSES OF SECONDARY ERYTHROMELALGIA

Myeloproliferative neoplasms: Essential thrombocythemia, polycythemia vera, chronic myelogenous leukemia, myelodysplastic syndrome
Drugs: Calcium channel blockers, cyclosporine, bromocriptine, pergolide
Infectious diseases: Human immunodeficiency virus, hepatitis B vaccine, influenza vaccine, infectious mononucleosis, varicella virus
Connective tissue diseases: Systemic lupus erythematosus, rheumatoid arthritis
Neuropathic: Diabetic neuropathy, peripheral neuropathies, neurofibromatosis, Riley-Day syndrome, multiple sclerosis, spinal cord disease
Neoplastic: Paraneoplastic syndrome, astrocytoma, malignant thymoma, colorectal cancer, lung cancer, and thyroid cancer
Others: Mushroom ingestion, mercury poisoning

TREATMENT AND PROGNOSIS Rx

Patients must avoid aggravating conditions, such as exercise, tight shoes, and alcohol intake, as well as learn to cool their involved areas without causing tissue damage. Patients seek relief by cooling the affected area with a fan, cold towels, cooling blankets, or immersion in ice water. Elevation of the feet may help. Medications aimed at treatment of both the neuropathy and vasculopathy are often tried. In one small randomized trial, intravenous iloprost (at varying doses for up to 6 hours per day on 3 consecutive days) significantly reduced symptoms and sympathetic dysfunction.[A3] In the genetic form, a small trial showed benefit from orally administered XEN402 (an inhibitor of $Na_V1.7$ that is designated as an orphan drug by the U.S. Food and Drug Administration).[A4] Aspirin can help patients with an underlying myeloproliferative disorder. Tricyclic antidepressants (e.g., nortriptyline 25 to 100 mg/day PO), anticonvulsants (e.g., pregabalin 50 to 100 mg PO three times daily), mexiletine (10 mg/kg/day PO), topical lidocaine patches, and opioids (e.g., hydromorphone 2 to 8 mg PO every 4 to 6 hours as needed) have been used with benefit in some patients. A topical gel of 1% amitriptyline and 0.5% ketamine has demonstrated promise without systemic side effects. Other methods, including a pain rehabilitation program, biofeedback, sympathectomy, and epidural blocks, have been tried with varying degrees of success. Patients have a reduced quality of life, and life expectancy is also reduced, primarily owing to suicide.

Erythema Ab Igne

Erythema ab igne is a hyperpigmented skin condition that results from repeated or chronic exposure to a heating source or infrared radiation that is not warm enough to burn the skin. The incidence is unknown, but women are more frequently affected than men.

Skin manifestations result from damage to the dermis and venous plexus system. Dysplastic changes can predispose the patient to actinic keratosis and squamous cell carcinomas (Chapter 203). Erythema ab igne is an occupational hazard for persons whose arms are repeatedly exposed to fire in bakeries, foundries, or kitchens. It can also result from repeated application of a hot water bottle, heating pads, or electric blankets or may be seen in persons who sit too close to space heaters, wood burning stoves, or even car heaters. It also has been reported involving the anterior thighs of persons using laptop computers.[13]

CLINICAL MANIFESTATIONS AND DIAGNOSIS

Patients generally have no symptoms, although some individuals report a slight burning or itching sensation. The skin discoloration is described as reticular, erythematous, and brownish hyperpigmentation (Fig. 80-6). Ulceration and bullous lesions have been reported in chronic cases.

The diagnosis is made clinically based solely on dermatologic findings. A history of exposure to a heating source or infrared radiation should be pursued because no laboratory tests are helpful. A biopsy must be obtained if there are signs of a malignant transformation. The differential diagnosis includes livedo reticularis and livedo racemosa.

TREATMENT AND PROGNOSIS Rx

Removing the offending heat source is essential for treatment, and patients should be advised to avoid prolonged exposure to any form of infrared heat. Topical therapies including topical tretinoin or hydroquinone have been used to reduce the hyperpigmentation.

The prognosis is favorable once the source is removed, but the condition can be chronic and progressive if prolonged and repeated exposure continues. Follow-up examinations are recommended because of the potential for malignant conversion.

Raynaud Phenomenon

Raynaud phenomenon is defined as episodic attacks of discoloration of the digits brought on by cold or emotional stimuli and resulting in a characteristic triphasic color change from white to blue to red. Raynaud phenomenon affects 3 to 5% of the U.S. population. It is seen more often in young women in whom it is reported to have a prevalence as high as 5 to 15%. The prevalence is higher in cooler northern climates and in smokers. Family history, estrogen exposure, and emotional stress are commonly associated with Raynaud phenomenon in women.[14] The hand-arm vibration syndrome is more common in men, especially men who use pneumatic hammers, chain saws, sanders, and grinders. It also has been reported in typists, pianists, meat cutters, and sewing machine operators.

The pathophysiology of the vasoconstriction in Raynaud phenomenon is not well understood. It includes abnormalities of the blood vessel wall, neural control mechanisms, and intravascular factors, including platelet activation and oxidative stress. As the arterial vasoconstriction subsides, postcapillary venular constriction leads to deoxygenation of the blood and the cyanotic appearance. On rewarming, blood flow increases as a result of vasodilation, which leads to the red or hyperemic appearance of the digits.

Primary Raynaud phenomenon is a benign vasospastic disorder, whereas a number of conditions are associated with the secondary form (Table 80-4). Several clinical features can help distinguish between these two forms (Table 80-5).

CLINICAL MANIFESTATIONS AND DIAGNOSIS

Raynaud phenomenon is characterized by triphasic color change of the digits, and pallor, cyanosis, and rubor after exposure to cold or stressful stimuli (Fig. 80-7).[15] All three color changes are not seen in most individuals, and pallor may be the only finding. The middle and ring fingers are most commonly involved, whereas the thumb may be entirely spared. Raynaud phenomenon also can affect the toes, nose, ears, tongue, knees, or nipples. Patients may experience paresthesias and clumsiness of the hand during an attack. Some patients develop numbness, intense ischemic pain, and even necrosis.

TABLE 80-4 UNDERLYING CONDITIONS ASSOCIATED WITH SECONDARY RAYNAUD PHENOMENON

Rheumatologic: Scleroderma, systemic lupus erythematosus, rheumatoid arthritis, Sjögren syndrome, mixed connective tissue disorders
Obstructive arterial disease: Atherosclerosis, thromboangiitis obliterans, arterial embolism
Occupational/environmental disorders: Hypothenar hammer syndrome, hand-arm vibration syndrome, frostbite)
Endocrine: Hypothyroidism
Hematologic: Polycythemia vera, multiple myeloma, cryoglobulinemia, cryofibrinogenemia, cold agglutinins
Drugs: Amphetamines, cocaine, β-blockers, clonidine, ergot preparations, oral contraceptives, cyclosporine, certain anti-neoplastic agents
Infections: Hepatitis B and C antigenemia
Thoracic outlet syndrome, subclavian artery aneurysm
Complex regional pain syndrome
Arteriovenous fistula
Lead and arsenic poisoning

The evaluation should start with a thorough history. The physical examination is normal in primary Raynaud unless there is an ongoing attack. Findings in secondary Raynaud may include ulceration of the fingertips or an abnormal Allen test. Routine laboratory testing including a complete blood count, erythrocyte sedimentation rate and C-reactive protein, urinalysis, thyroid function tests, antinuclear antibody, serum protein electrophoresis, and chest radiograph should be performed to evaluate for secondary Raynaud phenomenon. If the antinuclear antibody is positive or if the patient's history and physical examination indicate an underlying rheumatologic disorder, specific autoantibodies should be ordered (Chapter 257). Other tests including cryoglobulin levels, cryofibrinogen, and cold agglutinins may be helpful, depending on the clinical presentation (Chapter 256).

A number of noninvasive tests may help differentiate primary and secondary Raynaud phenomenon and evaluate the extent of vasospasm, including photoplethysmography, pulse volume recordings, laser Doppler flux, duplex ultrasonography, and nail-fold capillary microscopy, often performed after a cold stress challenge, such as immersion of the hands in a bath of ice water. MR angiography or contrast angiography may be necessary, and the latter can help determine the cause of ischemia.

TREATMENT AND PROGNOSIS Rx

Lifestyle modifications, including avoidance of cold exposure and known stressful stimuli, with an emphasis on keeping the body core temperature and extremities warm, are essential for preventing attacks. Raynaud phenomenon can be treated with both pharmacologic and nonpharmacologic approaches (Table 80-6).[15]

Calcium channel blockers can reduce attacks and the severity of symptoms in primary Raynaud.[A5] Aggressive treatment of the underlying condition is essential for patients with secondary Raynaud phenomenon. Calcium channel blockers (e.g., nifedipine 10 to 20 mg PO every 6 hours or amlodipine 2.5 to 10 mg/day PO) and iloprost (1 ng/kg/minute for 6 hours daily) are clearly beneficial for secondary Raynaud[A6] as is dual endothelin receptor blockade (e.g., bosentan 62.5 to 125 mg twice daily).[A7] Phosphodiesterase-5 inhibitors also have moderate benefits.[A8] Pain control with opioids, chemical or surgical sympathectomy, and spinal cord stimulation may be necessary in the most severe cases, particularly in situations of nonhealing digital ulceration and tissue loss.

The prognosis for primary Raynaud phenomenon is excellent, whereas the prognosis for secondary Raynaud phenomenon depends on the underlying condition.

TABLE 80-5 FEATURES SUGGESTIVE OF PRIMARY OR SECONDARY RAYNAUD PHENOMENON

CLINICAL FEATURE	PRIMARY	SECONDARY
Sex	Female	Female or male
Age	<40 yr	≥ 40 yr
Involvement	Bilateral	Unilateral or bilateral
Ischemic digits or ulcerations	Absent	±
Underlying cause	Absent	Present
Systemic complaints	Absent	±

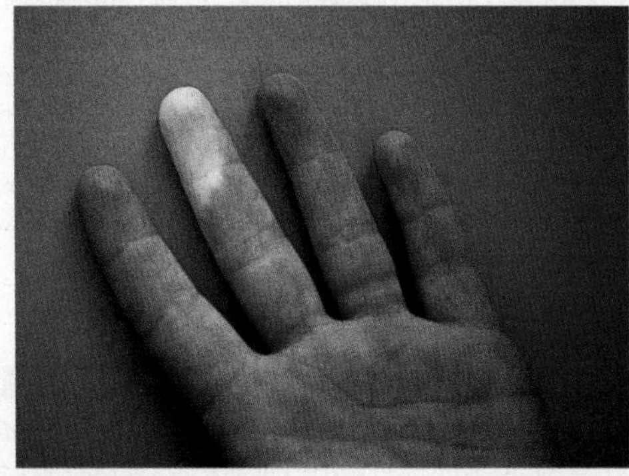

FIGURE 80-7. Unilateral Raynaud phenomenon. From Forbes CD, Jackson WF. Color Atlas and Text of Clinical Medicine, 3rd ed. London: Mosby; 2003.

TABLE 80-6 PHARMACOLOGIC AND NONPHARMACOLOGIC THERAPIES FOR RAYNAUD PHENOMENON

NONPHARMACOLOGIC THERAPIES

Educate and reassure patients about their condition
Avoid cold exposure or other triggering factors
Use warm clothing to maintain core body temperature (cover the entire body and wear a hat and scarf)
Teach how to terminate attacks: Exit from cold, warming techniques
Avoid nicotine
Biofeedback

PHARMACOLOGIC THERAPIES

Calcium channel blockers (nifedipine 10-20 mg q6h and amlodipine 2.5-10 mg q25 hr
Phosphodiesterase-5 inhibitors (sildenafil 25-50 mg TID, tadalafil 5-20 mg TID) and phosphodiesterase-3 inhibitors (cilostazol 100 mg BID)
Nitroglycerin topical 1 inch q6 hr
Angiotensin-converting enzyme inhibitors/angiotensin-receptor blockers (especially for scleroderma-associated Raynaud)
Others: Hydralazine 10-50 mg QID; reserpine 01.-0.25 mg/day PO; bosentan 125 mg PO BID
Prostaglandins: Iloprost, epoprostenol, alprostadil, beraprost
Antithrombotics/anticoagulants: (aspirin 81-325 mg/day, dipyridamole 75 mg TID, heparin [via weight-based nomogram; see Table 81-4 in Chapter 81], low-molecular-weight heparin [i.e., enoxaparin 1 mg/kg q12h; see Table 38-2 in Chapter 38])
Botulinum toxin A

Pernio

Pernio, also known as chilblains, is a cold-induced vasospastic disorder that affects the skin after exposure to nonfreezing temperatures or damp climates.[16] Pernio is seen more commonly in the northern United States and northwestern Europe. Although it can occur in children and older individuals, it is most common in young women between the ages of 15 to 30 years and in individuals with a low body mass.

The cause is unknown but is likely a result of cold-induced vasoconstriction that induces inflammation and ischemia of vessels and surrounding tissue. The histopathologic findings include dermal edema, keratinocyte necrosis, and a deep dermal lymphocytic infiltrate.

Pernio can be classified as acute or chronic. Acute pernio develops a few hours after exposure, whereas chronic pernio develops after repeated exposures to nonfreezing cold or damp conditions.

CLINICAL MANIFESTATIONS AND DIAGNOSIS

Pernio occurs most frequently in late fall to early spring in wet or nonfreezing cold environments. Acute pernio is characterized by intense itching, numbness, or a burning sensation that develops shortly after exposure to cold or damp conditions and disappears within a few weeks. Pernio is generally symmetrical. It usually involves the toes and fingers and less commonly the nose, ears, cheeks, or thighs. Pernio is associated with single or multiple erythematous, brownish or purple-blue skin lesions (macules, papules, or plaques) that may progress to blisters or ulcers (Fig. 80-8).

Chronic pernio develops after repeated cold exposure and results in cyanotic papules, macules, or nodules. Patients often report a history of similar episodes that develop each year during the cold months and typically resolve with warmer temperatures.

The diagnosis is based on the history and physical examination. Patients generally have a normal arterial examination. Pulse volume recordings may reveal vasoconstriction, but capillaroscopy is usually normal. A skin biopsy may be necessary to differentiate pernio from other disorders, such as Raynaud phenomenon, frostbite, acrocyanosis, atheromatous embolization, erythema nodosum (Chapter 440), erythema induratum (Chapter 440), lupus erythematosus (Chapter 266), sarcoidosis (Chapter 95), or atherosclerosis (Chapter 79). Laboratory testing may be necessary to exclude an underlying collagen vascular disease (Chapter 256).

TREATMENT AND PROGNOSIS (Rx)

Treatment may include the use of calcium channel blockers (nifedipine 20 to 60 mg/day or amlodipine 2.5 to 10 mg/day PO) to alleviate symptoms. Nifedipine may also be given in a topical gel form. Pentoxifylline (400 mg three times daily)[A9] and capsaicin have also been reported to be helpful.

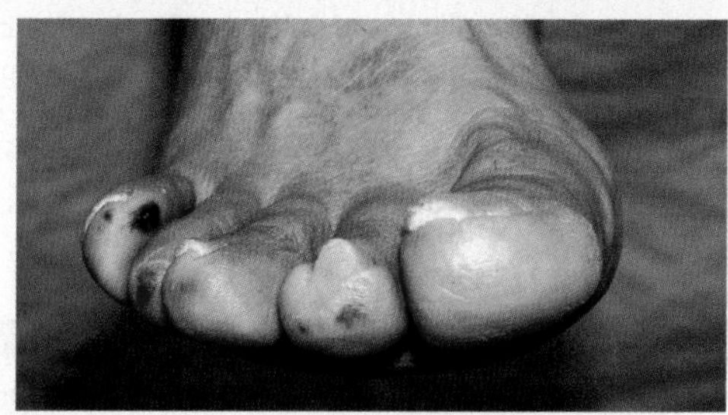

FIGURE 80-8. Pernio on the toes of the right foot. The lesions on the second, third, and fourth toes are the typical red, brown, and yellow scaling lesions. The lesion on the fifth toe can be confused with atheromatous embolization. Courtesy Dr. Jeffrey W. Olin.

PREVENTION (Rx)

Patients susceptible to pernio should be advised to avoid cold exposure. If they must go outside in cold or damp weather, they should dress appropriately with layered outdoor clothing, insulated footgear, gloves, scarf, and hat.

Pernio is usually self-limiting in the acute state. Chronic pernio can lead to scarring, atrophy, and chronic occlusive vascular disease.

Frostbite

Frostbite is a local cold-induced injury (Chapter 109) that occurs when persons are exposed to temperatures below the freezing point of intact skin, or in above-freezing temperatures in association with wet environments, high altitudes, and strong winds.

Frostbite, once considered primarily a military problem, is now seen in individuals 30 to 49 years of age who participate in winter outdoor sports, are homeless, have psychiatric illness (Chapter 397), consume excess alcohol (Chapter 33), use illegal drugs (Chapter 34), or survive outdoor trauma (Chapter 111). Patients with peripheral arterial disease (Chapter 79), a smoking history (Chapter 32), younger or older age, or diabetes (Chapter 229) are also at increased risk.[17] Frostbite injury involves three pathophysiologic components: tissue injury from extracellular and intracellular ice crystal formation, intracellular dehydration, and ischemia.

CLINICAL MANIFESTATIONS AND DIAGNOSIS

The severity of frostbite relates to the absolute temperature and to the duration of exposure. The digits of the hands and feet account for most injuries, although the ears, nose, and cheeks may be affected. Patients complain of numbness or paresthesias and report clumsiness and lack of fine coordination if the hands are involved. The numbness may persist even after rewarming. The skin may be pale, waxy, and cool to touch, and the patient may have mild to extensive swelling depending on the severity of the frostbite. Large, clear, blisters often appear (Fig. 80-9), followed by black scabs. Damage to the muscles, tendons, cartilage, joints, and bones occur in severe frostbite. Pain is often severe during the rewarming process.

The diagnosis of frostbite is made by the exposure history and physical examination. The differential diagnosis includes peripheral arterial disease, pernio, trench foot, or thermal burns.

TREATMENT AND PROGNOSIS (Rx)

Proper recognition of frostbite and removal from cold exposure is essential. Local rewarming should begin only if refreezing will not occur while the patient is being transferred to a hospital. Uninterrupted rapid rewarming in a water bath of between 40 and 42 degrees centigrade for 15 to 30 minutes is critical to help minimize tissue loss. Removal of wet or damp clothing is important, but rubbing or massage should be avoided. Splinting and elevation of the affected limb can help minimize swelling and improve perfusion. Patients should receive tetanus toxoid, analgesics (e.g., hydromorphone 2 to 8 mg either PO or parenterally every 3 to 4 hours as needed for pain), and broad-spectrum antibiotics if secondary tissue infection is present. Daily cleansing in a warm whirlpool bath and physical therapy are important. Clear blisters should be left alone, but ruptured blisters should be covered with a topical antibiotic, such as neomycin/bacitracin/polymyxin B ointment. A combination

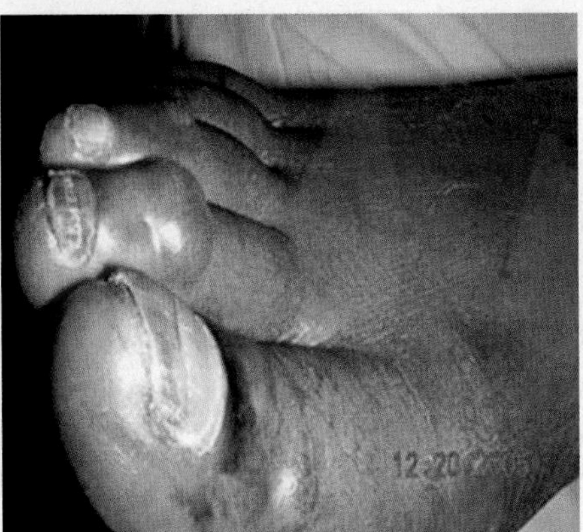

FIGURE 80-9. Blisters in a patient with frostbite.

of aspirin (250 mg), prostacyclin (0.5 to 2 ng/kg IV for 6 hours on 8 consecutive days), and tissue plasminogen activator (100 mg on day 1) has shown promise in markedly reducing the amputation rate in patients with severe frostbite, compared with aspirin plus buflomedil.[A10] If possible, surgical debridement and amputation should be avoided until complete demarcation occurs.

Patients subjected to frostbite are more susceptible to future cold injuries. They are susceptible to chronic pain, complex regional pain syndrome (Chapter 30), cold hypersensitivity, and a reduced sensitivity to touch.

Acrocyanosis

DEFINITION

Acrocyanosis is a poorly defined and often misunderstood clinical condition that manifests as painless, symmetrical, bluish or cyanotic discoloration affecting the hands, the feet, or both. Acrocyanosis occurs in primary and secondary forms. Primary acrocyanosis is generally a benign condition seen most often in young women during their second to fourth decades of life. It may be more common in cooler temperatures, and a familial predisposition has been reported. The overall incidence is not known, but its prevalence has been reported to be approximately 20 to 40% in persons with anorexia nervosa (Chapter 219) and up to 25% of all patients with cancer.

Acrocyanosis was originally thought to be a vasospastic disorder that develops when small cutaneous arteries and arterioles constrict and reduce blood flow, dilation, and oxygen desaturation in the venules. More recent data suggest that low pressures and sluggish flow result in capillary constriction.[18]

The underlying cause of primary acrocyanosis is unknown. Secondary acrocyanosis can be associated with a number of conditions, including Ehlers-Danlos syndrome (Chapter 260), hypoxemia (Chapter 104), cryoglobulins (Chapter 187), cryofibrinogens, cold agglutinins, antiphospholipid antibodies (Chapter 174), malignancy, spinal cord injury (Chapter 399), arsenic poisoning (Chapter 22), starvation, and some medications. It is also seen with the "puffy hand syndrome," a finding unique to intravenous drug abusers (Chapter 34) who inject their hands or fingers.

CLINICAL MANIFESTATIONS AND DIAGNOSIS

Persistent, painless, symmetrical bluish discoloration commonly involves the hands and feet but also can affect the forearms, nose, ears, and even nipples. Acrocyanosis may be exacerbated by cold exposure, emotional stress, or dependency of the limbs. It improves with elevation. Patients also report clamminess and hyperhidrosis of their hands and feet. Secondary acrocyanosis may be asymmetrical and associated with pain, ulceration, or tissue loss or gangrene.

The diagnosis of acrocyanosis is based on the history and physical examination. Laboratory evaluation should include a complete blood count, metabolic profile, and levels of antiphospholipid antibodies, cold agglutinins, cryofibrinogens, and cryoglobulins, as well as testing for connective tissue disorders (Chapter 256).

The differential diagnosis includes Raynaud phenomenon, pernio, erythromelalgia, and peripheral cyanosis. Acrocyanosis can be differentiated from peripheral cyanosis by the presence of cyanosis on the mucous membranes and hypoxia on an arterial blood sample.

TREATMENT AND PROGNOSIS

No treatment is necessary for primary acrocyanosis other than reassurance and avoidance of cold and damp exposures. A trial of α-adrenergic blocking agents such as prazosin may be considered. Calcium channel blockers, including amlodipine or nifedipine, are generally not helpful. Bioflavonoids and nicotinic acid derivatives have been reported beneficial in some cases, and sympathetic nerve block and sympathectomy may be tried for more severe cases. Treatment for secondary acrocyanosis depends on the underlying cause.

The prognosis of primary acrocyanosis is excellent. The prognosis of secondary acrocyanosis prognosis depends on the underlying cause.

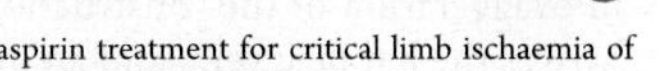

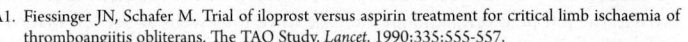

Grade A References

A1. Fiessinger JN, Schafer M. Trial of iloprost versus aspirin treatment for critical limb ischaemia of thromboangiitis obliterans. The TAO Study. *Lancet*. 1990;335:555-557.

A2. Bozkurt AK, Koksal C, Demirbas MY, et al. A randomized trial of intravenous iloprost (a stable prostacyclin analogue) versus lumbar sympathectomy in the management of Buerger's disease. *Int Angiol*. 2006;25:162-168.

A3. Kalgaard OM, Mork C, Kvernebo K. Prostacyclin reduces symptoms and sympathetic dysfunction in erythromelalgia in a double-blind randomized pilot study. *Acta Derm Venereol*. 2003;83:442-444.

A4. Goldberg YP, Price N, Namdari R, et al. Treatment of Na(v)1.7-mediated pain in inherited erythromelalgia using a novel sodium channel blocker. *Pain*. 2012;153:80-85.

A5. Ennis H, Anderson ME, Wilkinson J, et al. Calcium channel blockers for primary Raynaud's phenomenon. *Cochrane Database Syst Rev*. 2014;1:CD002069.

A6. Huisstede BM, Hoogvliet P, Paulis WD, et al. Effectiveness of interventions for secondary Raynaud's phenomenon: a systematic review. *Arch Phys Med Rehabil*. 2011;92:1166-1180.

A7. Nguyen VA, Eisendle K, Gruber I, et al. Effect of the dual endothelin receptor antagonist bosentan on Raynaud's phenomenon secondary to systemic sclerosis: a double-blind prospective, randomized, placebo-controlled pilot study. *Rheumatology (Oxford)*. 2010;49:583-587.

A8. Roustit M, Blaise S, Allanore Y, et al. Phosphodiesterase-5 inhibitors for the treatment of secondary Raynaud's phenomenon: systematic review and meta-analysis of randomised trials. *Ann Rheum Dis*. 2013;72:1696-1699.

A9. Noaimi AA, Fadheel BM. Treatment of perniosis with oral pentoxyfylline in comparison with oral prednisolone plus topical clobetasol ointment in Iraqi patients. *Saudi Med J*. 2008;29:1762-1764.

A10. Cauchy E, Cheguillaume B, Chetaille E. A controlled trial of a prostacyclin and rt-PA in the treatment of severe frostbite. *N Engl J Med*. 2011;364:189-190.

GENERAL REFERENCES

For the General References and other additional features, please visit Expert Consult at https://expertconsult.inkling.com.

81

PERIPHERAL VENOUS DISEASE

JEFFREY S. GINSBERG

DEEP VEIN THROMBOSIS

DEFINITION

Deep vein thrombosis (DVT), which is the most important disease affecting the peripheral veins, has an estimated annual incidence of 0.1% in whites. Most pulmonary emboli (Chapter 98) arise from DVT of the legs. In fact, DVT and pulmonary embolism are usually considered different clinical manifestations of one disease, venous thromboembolism (VTE), because up to 50% of patients who present with symptomatic proximal (popliteal vein or more proximal) DVT have imaging evidence of clinically silent pulmonary emboli, whereas up to 90% of patients with proved pulmonary emboli have DVT, even though only 15% of them have leg symptoms. For the most part, the cornerstones of management of DVT and pulmonary embolism are the same—long-term (>3 months of) anticoagulation.

Superficial thrombophlebitis consists of thrombosis and inflammation of one or more superficial veins. Provided the associated thrombus has not extended into the deep veins, affected patients have a negligible risk for development of pulmonary emboli and often can be effectively managed conservatively with ice, elevation, and anti-inflammatory medication.

EPIDEMIOLOGY

In nonpregnant individuals, DVT usually originates in one of the distal veins or calf veins, where it has little or no potential to cause clinically important pulmonary emboli. The true incidence of calf vein thrombosis is not known because many affected patients remain asymptomatic while the thrombus forms and spontaneously resolves. On the basis of results of studies of *symptomatic* patients with suspected DVT, approximately 10 to 25% actually have a diagnosable DVT, of whom approximately 15% have isolated calf DVT. Approximately one fourth of these thrombi that are initially isolated to a calf vein subsequently extend into the proximal veins, usually within 1 week of manifestation, where they *then* have the potential to cause pulmonary emboli.

In pregnancy, most (~90%) thrombi occur in the deep veins of the left leg and frequently involve the ileofemoral veins but not the calf or popliteal veins. These findings suggest an anatomic predisposition to left leg ileofemoral DVT, which may be a result of compression of the left iliac vein by the fetus, an exaggeration of the "obstruction" that occurs where the right iliac artery crosses the left iliac vein, and an increase in venous webs at the left iliac vein (May-Thurner syndrome). These observations strongly suggest that most, if not all, of the increase in VTE during pregnancy is attributable to the increase in left iliac DVT.

Significant triggers of hospitalization for VTE include major surgeries, fractures, immobility, and cancer, with or without chemotherapy. From a clinical perspective, risk factors can be subdivided by duration, that is, transient and finite duration (e.g., fractured fibula treated with plaster immobilization) compared with permanent or long-term duration (e.g., congenital antithrombin deficiency, metastatic cancer), and according to the magnitude of the risk, that is, major (hip or knee replacement surgery) or minor (long-distance air travel, use of oral contraceptives). Classification of patients according to the presence or absence and type of risk factor is predictive of the risk for recurrence after a prolonged (≥3 months) course of anticoagulant therapy and provides key information that helps determine the optimal duration of anticoagulant therapy. Patients in whom DVT develops in association with a major risk factor that has resolved have a much lower risk for recurrence after a 3-month course of anticoagulants than do patients whose DVT was apparently idiopathic or associated with an ongoing risk factor. Patients whose DVT was associated with a transient minor risk factor that has resolved have an intermediate risk for recurrence.

PATHOBIOLOGY

Virchow triad of hypercoagulability, venous stasis, and injury to the vessel wall provides a model for understanding many of the risk factors that lead to the formation of thrombosis. For example, in patients who have total hip or knee replacement surgery, venous endothelial injury is caused by surgery, venous stasis resulting from perioperative immobilization, and hypercoagulability as a result of postoperative fibrinolytic shutdown. In other patients, an identifiable "thrombophilia" or "tendency to clot," such as congenital antithrombin (formerly antithrombin III) deficiency or the presence of factor V Leiden (Chapter 176),[1] combined with use of oral contraceptives results in DVT in women of childbearing age. However, a relatively high proportion of patients have unexplained DVT without "clinical" risk factors that cause endothelial damage or venous stasis or identifiable thrombophilias that cause hypercoagulability. Undoubtedly, some of these patients have yet to be determined to have thrombophilias, but the DVT currently is labeled idiopathic or unprovoked.

CLINICAL MANIFESTATIONS

The clinical features of lower extremity DVT include leg pain, tenderness, swelling (Fig. 81-1), palpable cord, discoloration (red for inflammation and purplish for venous stasis), as well as dilation and prominence of the superficial veins. These signs and symptoms are nonspecific, so accurate diagnostic imaging is required for a definitive diagnosis. In patients who present with symptoms suspicious for DVT, DVT is confirmed in only 10 to 30% of cases. Moreover, patients with relatively minor symptoms and signs of DVT may have extensive DVT with or without pulmonary embolism. Conversely, approximately one third of patients with findings highly suspicious for DVT will not have it (e.g., patients with a ruptured Baker cyst).

DIAGNOSIS

By itself, clinical diagnosis of DVT is inaccurate because no individual symptom or sign is sufficiently predictive for the diagnosis to be made or excluded. Clinical assessment can categorize patients according to their pretest probability of DVT with reasonable accuracy, but should almost never be the only test used to exclude or make a diagnosis of DVT. By combining a validated prediction rule (Table 81-1) to assess pretest probability with the results of noninvasive tests, diagnostic accuracy can be improved, thereby often limiting or eliminating the need for further investigation (Fig. 81-2).

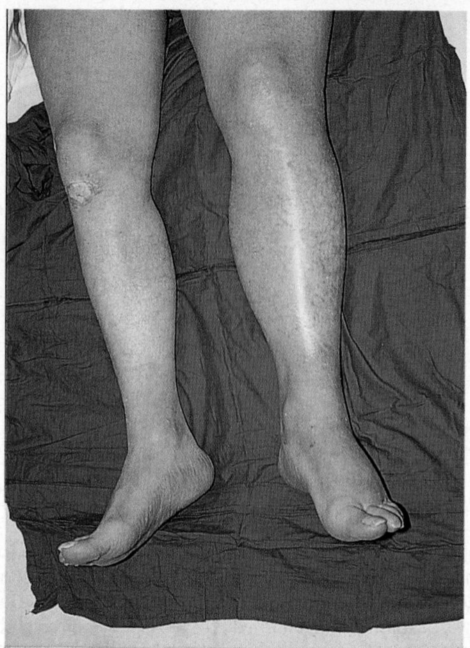

FIGURE 81-1. Deep vein thrombosis (DVT) manifesting as an acutely swollen left leg. Note the dilation of the superficial veins. The leg was hot to the touch, and palpation along the line of the left popliteal and femoral veins caused pain. Less than 50% of DVTs manifest in this way, and other conditions may mimic DVT, so further investigation is always indicated. Note the coincidental psoriatic lesion below the patient's right knee. (From Forbes CD, Jackson WF. Color Atlas and Text of Clinical Medicine, 3rd ed. London: Mosby; 2003.)

TABLE 81-1 PREDICTION RULE FOR DEEP VEIN THROMBOSIS

CLINICAL CHARACTERISTIC	SCORE*
Active cancer (treatment ongoing within previous 6 mo or palliative)	1
Paralysis, paresis, or recent plaster immobilization of the lower extremities	1
Recent bedrest of >3 days or major surgery within 3 mo requiring anesthesia	1
Localized tenderness of the deep veins of the leg	1
Entire leg swollen	1
Calf swelling of >3 cm larger than asymptomatic side measured 10 cm below tibial tuberosity	1
Pitting edema confined to the symptomatic leg	1
Collateral superficial veins (not varicosed)	1
Previously documented deep vein thrombosis	1
Alternative diagnosis as likely as or more likely than deep vein thrombosis	−2

*A score of 0 or less indicates low probability, 1 or 2 indicates moderate probability, and 3 or more indicates high probability.
Modified from Wells PS, Anderson DR, Bormanis J, et al. Value of assessment of pretest probability of deep-vein thrombosis in clinical management. *Lancet.* 1997;350:1795-1798.

Imaging

Compression Ultrasonography

Compression venous ultrasonography with or without Doppler imaging is the most widely used noninvasive test for suspected DVT because of its accuracy in detection of thrombus involving the popliteal or more proximal veins.[2] Noncompressibility (Fig. 81-3) of the proximal leg veins on

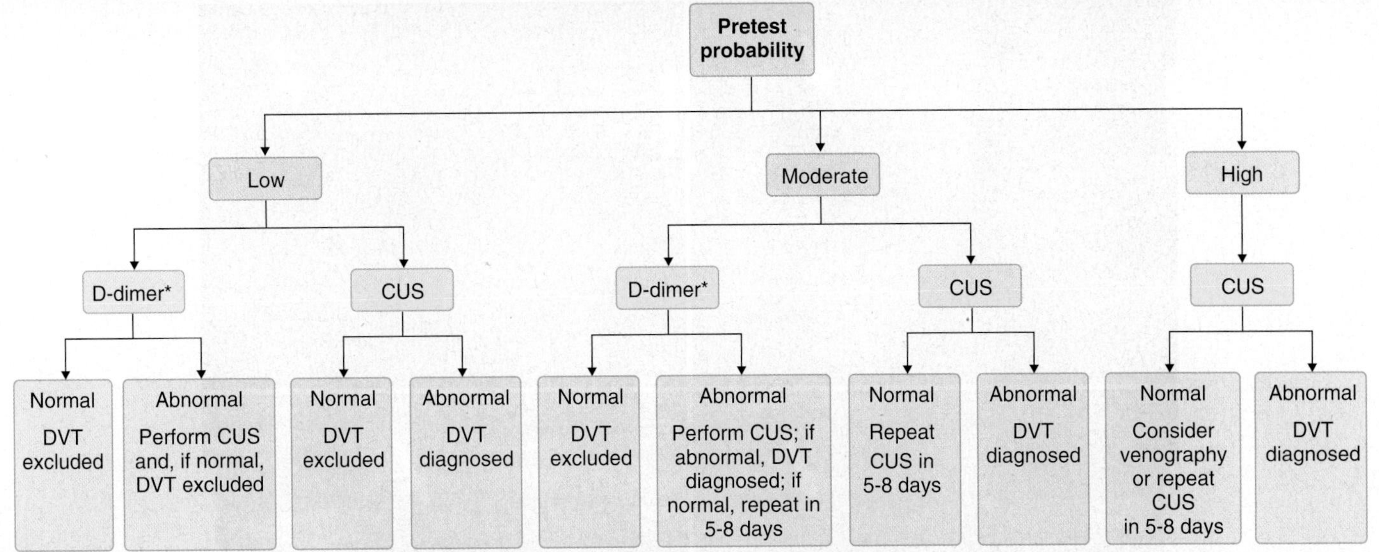

FIGURE 81-2. **Diagnostic algorithm for suspected deep vein thrombosis. This algorithm uses evaluation of pretest probability based on a clinical prediction rule (see Table 81-1) and D-dimer testing to complement compression ultrasonography (CUS). The *asterisk* indicates use of a highly sensitive (>95%) D-dimer.**

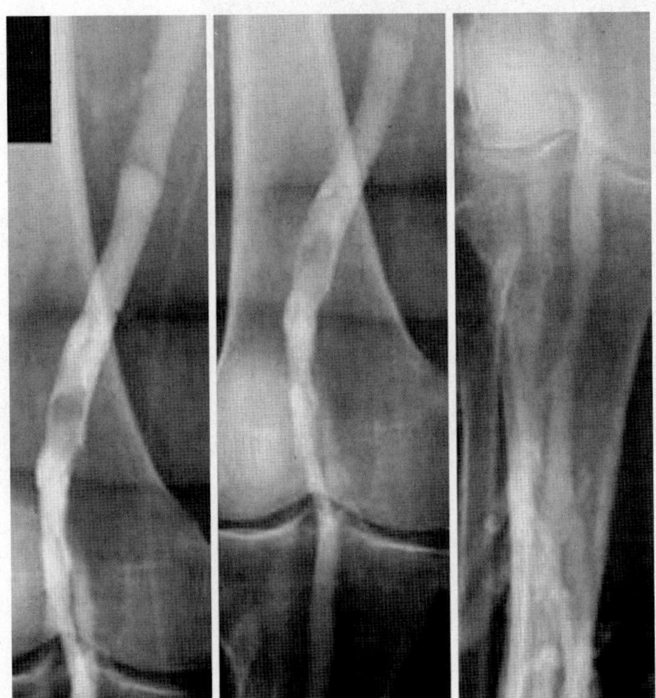

FIGURE 81-3. **Abnormal venogram demonstrates a persistent (two or more different views) intraluminal filling defect in the popliteal vein.**

ultrasonography is diagnostic of DVT in symptomatic patients and is an indication for treatment. Of patients with symptoms suggestive of DVT but with normal findings on initial ultrasound examination of the proximal veins, approximately 15% will have undetected isolated calf DVT; progression into the proximal veins occurs in a minority of patients, usually within a week of presentation. Isolated calf DVT that does not extend into the proximal veins is rarely if ever associated with clinically important pulmonary embolus. The sensitivity of ultrasonography for calf DVT is well below 90%, with a wide range of accuracies reported for different populations of patients.

Imaging of the calf veins is time-consuming and potentially inaccurate. Rather, two-point (common femoral and popliteal) or three-point (two-point plus the calf "trifurcation") compression ultrasonography should be performed. If two-point compression is normal, the test should be repeated about 1 week after the initial examination. This approach will identify the 20 to 25% of patients who have had proximal extension of distal clot in the calf veins. If the repeated ultrasound examination 1 week later also is normal, further investigation and therapy can be safely withheld. In centers with highly skilled operators, one normal ultrasound of the proximal veins and the calf veins near the popliteal vein at presentation is sufficiently accurate to exclude clinically important DVT and eliminate the need for follow-up testing. In patients with either a normal D-dimer test result or a low clinical pretest probability, normal two-point compression ultrasonography excludes DVT.

Magnetic Resonance Venography

Magnetic resonance venography (MRV), which uses the difference in magnetic resonance signals between flowing blood and stationary clot, has a high sensitivity and specificity for proximal DVT. Recent interest has focused on magnetic resonance for direct imaging of the thrombus because a thrombus produces a positive image without the use of contrast material, owing to its methemoglobin content. Although MRV is accurate in diagnosing and excluding DVT, it is expensive and not readily available in most centers outside of the United States.

Contrast Venography

Ascending contrast venography remains the gold standard for diagnosis, but because of its expense, discomfort to the patient, and potential for adverse experiences, venography is currently indicated in symptomatic patients only when diagnostic uncertainty persists after noninvasive testing or if noninvasive testing is unavailable. A constant intraluminal filling defect is diagnostic of acute thrombosis (Fig. 81-4), and DVT can be excluded in patients who have a normal, adequately performed venogram. Minor side effects of local pain, nausea, and vomiting are not uncommon, whereas more serious adverse reactions, such as anaphylaxis or other allergic manifestations, are rare. Venography also can induce DVT.

Laboratory Findings

D-Dimer

D-Dimer is a plasma protein specifically produced after lysis of cross-linked fibrin by plasmin. Levels are almost invariably elevated in the presence of acute VTE, so measurement of D-dimer levels is a sensitive test for recent DVT and pulmonary embolism. Unfortunately, numerous nonthrombotic conditions, including sepsis, pregnancy, surgery, and cardiac or renal failure, also can cause elevated levels. As a result of this nonspecificity, the role of D-dimer assays is limited to helping exclude VTE when levels are not raised.

Laboratory tests for D-dimer use enzyme-linked immunosorbent assay or agglutination techniques, both involving specific monoclonal antibodies. Sensitivity and cut points vary among assays, so results cannot be generalized. Highly sensitive tests, consisting of new rapid ELISA or immunoturbidimetric assays, have sensitivities of 95 to 100% for acute VTE but in general have low specificities (20 to 50%). Highly sensitive D-dimer assays can be

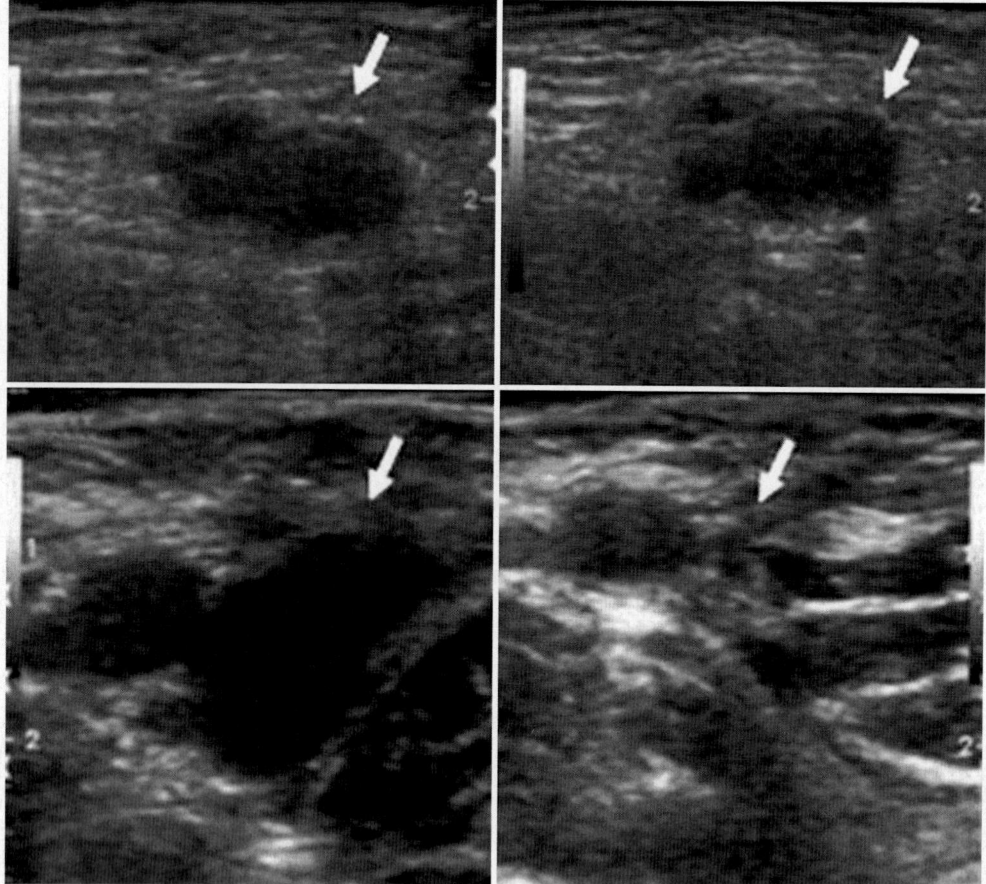

FIGURE 81-4. **Compression venous ultrasonography demonstrates thrombosis of the popliteal vein.** The sonograms in the *top row* demonstrate examination without *(left side)* and with *(right side)* gentle probe compression of the skin overlying the popliteal vein. The lack of compressibility is diagnostic of deep vein thrombosis. The *bottom row* shows analogous views of the femoral vein, which shows partial compressibility.

employed as stand-alone tests for exclusion of DVT, but clinicians must be aware of the accuracy of the assay in their institution before using the D-dimer assay to make management decisions. D-Dimer measured after a 3-month (or longer) initial treatment with warfarin also appears to be predictive of recurrent DVT. In addition, an elevated D-dimer level 1 month after stopping warfarin predicts a clinically and statistically significant higher recurrence rate than is seen in patients in whom the D-dimer levels were normal or low.

Algorithms for Diagnosis of Deep Venous Thrombosis and Their Risk for Recurrence

A number of diagnostic algorithms have been tested in prospective management trials (see Fig. 81-2).

Clinical Assessment and Venous Ultrasonography

It is safe to perform only a single ultrasound examination in patients with a low pretest probability by a validated clinical prediction rule (Table 81-2). Other patients require serial ultrasonographic testing if only clinical assessment and ultrasonography are used. Venography should be considered in patients with a high pretest probability and normal compression ultrasonography because the probability of DVT is still approximately 20% in such patients.

Clinical Assessment, D-Dimer Testing, and Venous Ultrasonography

Diagnostic imaging and treatment can be safely withheld in patients who have (1) a low pretest probability based on a validated clinical prediction rule and a negative value on a moderately sensitive D-dimer assay or (2) a low or intermediate pretest probability and a negative value on a highly sensitive D-dimer assay. Patients with a high pretest probability require ultrasonography regardless of the D-dimer result. A normal D-dimer result with use of either a moderately or highly sensitive assay can safely obviate the need for repeated imaging in patients with normal findings on the initial ultrasound examination. Algorithms for predicting the recurrence of an initially unprovoked DVT after the cessation of anticoagulant therapy are undergoing validation in prospective trials.

TABLE 81-2 ALTERNATIVE DIAGNOSES IN 87 CONSECUTIVE PATIENTS WITH CLINICALLY SUSPECTED VENOUS THROMBOSIS AND NORMAL VENOGRAMS*

DIAGNOSIS	PATIENTS (%)
Muscle strain	24
Direct twisting injury to the leg	10
Leg swelling in paralyzed limb	9
Lymphangitis, lymphatic obstruction	7
Venous reflux	7
Muscle tear	6
Baker cyst	5
Cellulitis	3
Internal abnormality of the knee	2
Unknown	26

*The diagnosis was made once venous thrombosis was excluded by venography.

Differential Diagnosis

A number of conditions can mimic DVT (see Table 81-2), but DVT often can be excluded only by accurate diagnostic testing. In some patients, however, the cause of pain, tenderness, and swelling remains uncertain.

Suspected Recurrent Deep Venous Thrombosis

Approximately 10% of patients with unprovoked VTE will experience recurrent thromboembolism in the first year after ceasing anticoagulant therapy. In addition, many patients will have positional leg swelling and pain early during treatment as a result of venous outflow obstruction or later (≥6 months after diagnosis) because of the post-thrombotic syndrome after endogenous thombolysis has maximized removal of the thrombus and venous valvular incompetence manifests. These and other nonthrombotic disorders can produce symptoms that are similar to those of acute recurrent DVT, so accurate diagnostic testing to confirm recurrence is mandatory. However, residual venous abnormalities are common after an initial event; persistent abnormalities are seen on compression ultrasonography in approximately 80% of patients at 3 months and 50% of patients at 1 year after a documented proximal DVT. Therefore comparison with previous ultrasound images is required in patients with suspected recurrence. Although an increase in diameter of 4 mm or more in the compressed vein strongly suggests recurrent DVT, a new noncompressible proximal venous segment is the most reliable criterion for the diagnosis of recurrence. When compression ultrasonography is inconclusive, venography should be considered; a new intraluminal filling defect is diagnostic of acute DVT, and the absence of a filling defect excludes the diagnosis. Nonfilling of venous segments may mask recurrent DVT and is considered a nondiagnostic finding. A normal D-dimer test result is useful in excluding recurrent DVT.

Pregnancy

Symptoms of leg pain or swelling, shortness of breath, and atypical chest pain are common during pregnancy, so objective testing is needed to diagnose VTE. As in nonpregnant patients, compression ultrasonography is the initial test of choice. A normal D-dimer test is also reassuring in excluding DVT. Because isolated iliac and iliofemoral DVT is more common in pregnancy and has the potential to be missed by ultrasonography, efforts should be made to image the iliac veins to detect such thrombi. MRV, which is sensitive for pelvic DVT, may be useful when the clinical suspicion is high or if Doppler imaging of the iliac vein is inconclusive.

TREATMENT Rx

The large majority of patients with acute DVT can now be treated on an outpatient basis, regardless of their treatment regimen (Fig. 81-5).[3] The principal indications for admission are clinical instability, the inability to adhere to outpatient therapy, or the need to use intravenous heparin for extensive iliofemoral thrombosis.

Initial Treatment

Low-molecular-weight heparin (LMWH) preparations (Chapter 38) are administered subcutaneously using weight-based dosing to provide reliable outpatient management of DVT without the need for routine laboratory monitoring. Dosage regimens differ for the various LMWH formulations (Table 81-3), but once-daily administration of LMWH is thought to be as safe and effective as twice-daily administration.[4]

Anti–factor Xa monitoring should be considered for three populations of patients: (1) patients with renal insufficiency (calculated creatinine clearance of less than 30 mL/minute); (2) obese patients, in whom the volume of distribution of LMWH might be different, so weight-adjusted dosing might not be appropriate; and (3) pregnant women, in whom it is unclear whether the dose should be adjusted according to the woman's weight change. Levels are usually determined on blood samples drawn 4 hours after subcutaneous injection; therapeutic ranges of 0.6 to 1.0 U/mL for twice-daily administration and 1.0 to 2.0 U/mL for once-daily treatment have been proposed.

Fixed-dose subcutaneous injection of LMWH is at least as effective and safe as adjusted-dose intravenous administration of unfractionated heparin for the treatment of acute DVT, with a trend toward a significant difference in mortality benefit favoring LMWH, probably because of improved survival in patients with malignant disease.[A1]

However, patients with extensive iliofemoral DVT have often been excluded from trials of LMWH, and extended-duration (i.e., >5 days) intravenous unfractionated heparin therapy is often administered to such patients. Unfractionated heparin is usually administered by continuous intravenous infusion (Table 81-4), with either fixed initial dosing or dosing according to a patient's weight, results in more rapid achievement of therapeutic activated partial thromboplastin time (aPTT) levels. The initial aPTT level should be measured 6 hours after therapy is commenced. Up to 25% of patients with acute VTE have resistance to heparin, defined as a requirement for greater than expected doses of unfractionated heparin to achieve a "therapeutic" aPTT. If it is available, anti–factor Xa monitoring is recommended in patients with heparin resistance.

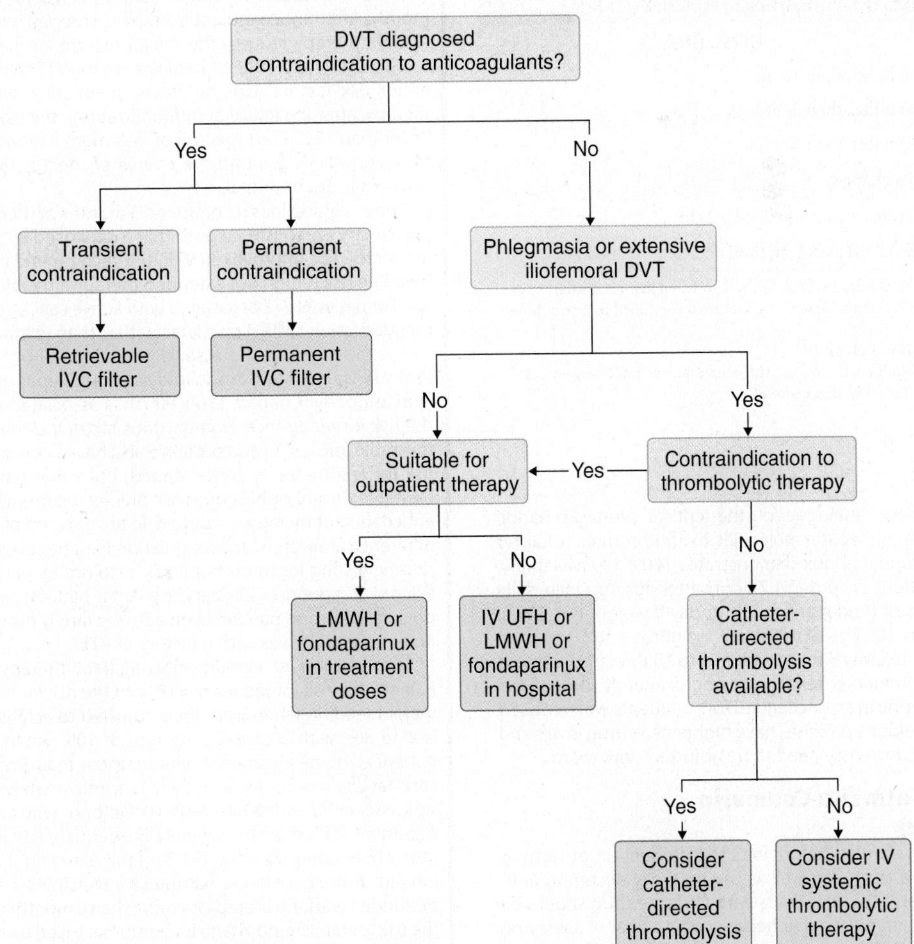

FIGURE 81-5. Guidelines for treatment of deep vein thrombosis (DVT). IVC = inferior vena cava; IV = intravenous; LMWH = low-molecular-weight heparin; UFH = unfractionated heparin.

TABLE 81-3 GUIDELINES FOR ANTICOAGULATION WITH LOW-MOLECULAR-WEIGHT HEPARIN AND FONDAPARINUX

INDICATIONS	GUIDELINES
VTE suspected	Obtain baseline aPTT, PT, CBC Check for contraindication to heparin therapy Order imaging study; consider giving IV unfractionated heparin (5000 IU) or LMWH
VTE confirmed	Give LMWH (dalteparin,* enoxaparin,† nadroparin,‡ tinzaparin,§ fondaparinux¶) Start warfarin therapy on day 1 at 5 mg and adjust the subsequent daily dose according to INR Check platelet count between days 3 and 5 Stop LMWH therapy after at least 4 or 5 days of combined therapy when the INR is > 2 Anticoagulate with warfarin for at least 3 months at an INR of 2.5, range of 2-3 (See text for alternatives to warfarin: "Oral Direct Thrombin and Factor Xa Inhibitors")

Modified from Hyers TM, Agnelli G, Hull RD, et al. Antithrombotic therapy for venous thromboembolic disease. *Chest.* 2001;119:176S-193S.
*Dalteparin sodium, 200 anti-Xa IU/kg/day SC. A single dose should not exceed 18,000 IU (approved in Canada).
†Enoxaparin sodium, 1 mg/kg q12h SC, or enoxaparin sodium, 1.5 mg/kg/day SC. A single daily dose should not exceed 180 mg (approved in both the United States and Canada).
‡Nadroparin calcium, 86 anti-Xa IU/kg two times daily SC for 10 days (approved in Canada), or nadroparin calcium, 171 anti-Xa IU/kg SC daily. A single dose should not exceed 17,100 anti-Xa IU.
§Tinzaparin sodium, 175 anti-Xa IU kg/day SC daily (approved in Canada and the United States).
¶Fondaparinux according to weight: <50 kg, 5 mg /day SC; 50-100 kg, 7.5 mg SC; and > 100 kg, 10 mg SC.
aPTT = activated partial thromboplastin time; CBC = complete blood count; INR = international normalized ratio; LMWH = low-molecular-weight heparin; PT = prothrombin time; VTE = venous thromboembolism.

TABLE 81-4 WEIGHT-BASED NOMOGRAM FOR INITIAL INTRAVENOUS HEPARIN THERAPY

aPTT	DOSE (IU/kg)
Initial dose	80 bolus, then 18/hr
<35 sec (<1.2×)*	80 bolus, then 4/hr
35-45 sec (1.2-1.5×)	40 bolus, then 2/hr
46-70 sec (1.5-2.3×)	No change
71-90 sec (2.3-3×)	Decrease infusion rate by 2/hr
>90 sec (>3×)	Hold infusion 1 hr, then decrease infusion rate by 3/hr

Modified from Raschke RA, Reilly BM, Guidry JR, et al. The weight-based heparin dosing nomogram compared with a "standard care" nomogram: a randomized controlled trial. Ann Intern Med. 1993;119:874-881.
*Figures in parentheses show comparison with control.
aPTT = activated partial thromboplastin time. In general, with contemporary aPTT reagents, the target therapeutic range is more than 1.2 to 2.3 times control.

Fondaparinux

Fondaparinux is a synthetic analogue of the critical pentasaccharide sequence required for binding of heparin molecules to antithrombin (Chapter 38). Given subcutaneously, fondaparinux demonstrates 100% bioavailability, with peak plasma concentrations occurring 1.7 hours after dosing. Once-daily subcutaneous administration of fondaparinux (5 mg/day if weight is < 50 kg; 7.5 mg/day if weight is 50 to 100 kg; 10 mg/day if weight is > 100 kg) is an effective and safe alternative to LMWH for the initial 5 to 10 days of treatment of DVT.[A2] Clearance is predominantly renal, with approximately 70% of the initial dose recovered in the urine in an unchanged form. Patients with reduced creatinine clearance, such as elderly patients, have higher peak drug levels and longer drug half-life, so their dose may need to be adjusted downward.

Transition to Oral Treatment: Coumarin Derivatives (Warfarin)

Warfarin is a vitamin K antagonist that inhibits the production of clotting factors II (prothrombin), VII, IX, and X, as well as the naturally occurring anticoagulants protein C and protein S. In patients with DVT, the drug should be started within 24 to 48 hours of initiation of heparin with a goal of achieving international normalized ratio (INR) results between 2.0 and 3.0 (Chapter 38). A higher target INR of 3.0 to 4.0 is associated with more bleeding but no better efficacy, even in patients with the antiphospholipid antibody syndrome (Chapter 176), and lower intensity warfarin therapy (target INR, 1.5 to 1.9) is significantly less effective at preventing recurrent VTE, despite similar rates of major bleeding.[A3]

The dose is empirical, but a starting dose of 5 to 10 mg is suitable for most patients. Warfarin doses are adjusted according to the prothrombin time, expressed as the INR, performed daily or every other day until the results are in the therapeutic range for at least 24 hours. After initial dosing, warfarin can be monitored two or three times per week for 1 to 2 weeks and then less frequently, depending on the stability of INR results, up to intervals as long as 4 to 6 weeks. If dose adjustment is needed, such as when medications that can interact with warfarin are introduced, the cycle of more frequent monitoring is repeated until a stable dose response is again achieved.

It is now clear that pharmacogenetics have a large impact on the relatively wide range of warfarin dose requirements among different populations and the variability of warfarin requirements over time in any individual patient.[5] Polymorphisms in the gene encoding cytochrome P-450 2C9 enzyme, the enzyme that primarily clears the S-enantiomer of warfarin, contribute to variable responses to warfarin. Vitamin K epoxide reductase (VKORC1) recycles vitamin K epoxide to the reduced form of vitamin K and is the target of warfarin. Genotyping for *CYP2C9*2, CYP2C9*3, VKORC1* can help guide warfarin dosing and increase the amount of time patients are in the the therapeutic INR range.[A4] Polymorphisms are associated with a need for lower doses of warfarin during long-term therapy. Routine pharmacogenetic testing may ultimately be recommended in candidates for long-term (>3 months) warfarin therapy to identify individuals who are likely to require higher or lower warfarin doses.

Long-Term Treatment

The preferred long-term treatment of DVT for most patients is warfarin or another coumarin derivative (e.g., acenocoumarol), continued until the benefits of treatment for reducing recurrent VTE no longer outweigh its risks for major bleeding. The decision to prolong or to stop anticoagulation should be individualized, and a patient's preferences should be considered.[6]

Patients with symptomatic proximal DVT or pulmonary emboli should be treated for at least 3 months, even if the VTE was associated with a transient risk factor,[A5] but the optimal duration of treatment for patients whose VTE is not associated with a transient risk factor is controversial. Three months of treatment is associated with a 10 to 27% risk for a recurrence during the 12 months after anticoagulant therapy is stopped, whereas 6 months of anticoagulant therapy reduces the risk for recurrence in the first year after stopping to approximately 10%. In patients whose VTE developed in association with minor risk factors (e.g., air travel, pregnancy, within 6 weeks of estrogen therapy, after leg injury or immobilization), the risk for recurrence is probably lower than 10%. Continuation of treatment beyond 6 months reduces the risk for recurrent VTE during the course of therapy, but the benefit is lost after warfarin is discontinued.

Current guidelines recommend 3 months of therapy for a first proximal DVT, pulmonary embolism, or both that is provoked by surgery or by a nonsurgical risk factor. For unprovoked VTE, the recommendation is also 3 months if the bleeding risk is high but extended therapy if the bleeding risk is low or moderate. For patients VTE associated with active cancer, extended therapy is recommended using LMWH (see later) rather than warfarin.[A6]

The most convincing association of thrombophilia with the risk for recurrent VTE is the antiphospholipid antibody (lupus anticoagulant or anticardiolipin antibody [Chapter 176]), which is associated with a two-fold increase in the risk for recurrence. Homozygous factor V Leiden, and deficiencies of antithrombin, protein C, and protein S also have been associated with an increased risk for recurrence in some reports, but other data suggest that testing for heritable thrombophilia does not predict recurrent VTE in the first 2 years after anticoagulant therapy is stopped. In the absence of randomized trials to assess different durations of anticoagulation in patients with VTE and thrombophilia, routine testing for thrombophilias need not be performed but should be considered in young (<50 years) patients, patients with venous thrombosis in unusual sites, and patients with a strong family history of VTE (i.e., one or more first-degree relatives with a history of VTE).

The decision to extend anticoagulant therapy beyond 3 months must balance the risk for recurrent VTE with the risk for bleeding. The annual risk for major bleeding when warfarin is adjusted to achieve a target INR of 2.0 to 3.0 is 1 to 3%, with a case-fatality rate of 10% when major bleeding occurs in patients who received treatment for more than 3 months. By comparison, the case-fatality rate for recurrent VTE is approximately 5%. In patients whose VTE was associated with a transient risk factor or who are at high risk for bleeding, treatment for 3 months is generally adequate because the risk for fatal recurrent VTE is lower than the risk for fatal bleeding if warfarin treatment is prolonged. Among patients without a reversible or transient cause, however, prolonged warfarin therapy for more than 6 months can be considered because the risk for fatal hemorrhage is counterbalanced by the risk for fatal recurrence. The argument to prolong therapy is stronger in patients with high-risk thrombophilia (e.g., homozygous factor V Leiden; antiphospholipid antibody; deficiency of antithrombin, protein C, or protein S; or combined heterozygous state for factor V Leiden and the prothrombin gene mutation). Indefinite therapy (preferably with LMWH) should be considered in patients with cancer-related VTE (Chapter 179) if the risk for bleeding is not high because the risk for recurrent VTE is more than 10% in the first year after anticoagulation is stopped. In motivated and capable patients, self-management of warfarin therapy is better than management by a physician or nurse.[A7]

Alternatives to Coumarin Derivatives

For patients in whom warfarin is impractical or contraindicated and for those who have recurrent VTE while being treated with appropriate doses of oral anticoagulants, therapeutic doses of LMWH are as effective as warfarin. For patients with cancer-related VTE (DVT, pulmonary embolus, or both), weight-based LMWH that is decreased to 75% of the initial dose after 1 month of treatment reduces the risk for recurrent VTE compared with warfarin, with similar bleeding rates.[A8] For patients who have had unprovoked VTE and who have discontinued anticoagulant treatment, aspirin reduces the risk for recurrent VTE with no apparent increase in the risk for major bleeding.[A9]

Oral Direct Thrombin and Factor Xa Inhibitors

Two stiochiometric or direct oral factor Xa inhibitors (rivaroxaban and apixaban) and one direct oral thrombin inhibitor (dabigatran) have been extensively evaluated (and approved by the U.S. Food and Drug Administration [FDA] and various regulatory agencies) for the prevention of stroke and systemic embolism in patients with nonvalvular atrial fibrillation (Chapter 64), and these agents also have been evaluated for the treatment of acute VTE and its secondary prevention. Currently, however, only rivaroxaban had been approved by the FDA for VTE treatment. Rivaroxaban, 15 mg twice daily for 3 weeks followed by 20 mg/day, is not inferior to enoxaparin followed by warfarin for the first 6 months of therapy and is more efficacious (recurrent VTE rates of 1.3% vs. 7.1%)[A10] than placebo when used for extended therapy for 6 to 12 months after an idiopathic DVT.

Apixaban 10 mg twice daily for 7 days followed by 5 mg twice daily for 6 months is as efficacious but safer than standard therapy with enoxaparin followed by warfarin for the treatment of acute DVT.[A11] It also is more efficacious than placebo without a significantly increased bleeding risk when used at 2.5 mg or 5 mg twice daily or placebo for another 12 months in patients who have completed 6 to 12 months of antigoagulant therapy.[A12]

In patients who have completed initial therapy with LMWH or unfractionated heparin, extended dabigatran (150 mg twice daily) is not inferior to warfarin for both efficacy and safety.[A13] Continued dabigatran at 150 mg twice daily after at least 3 months of anticoagulant therapy is as effective and safer than warfarin but causes more bleeding than placebo.[A14]

These agents are a reasonable alternative to LMWH followed by warfarin for the treatment of VTE, but their precise role has yet to be determined. They offer the advantage of fixed dosing, without a need for monitoring. Whether any are truly more effective or safer than warfarin in clinical practice and whether the lack of monitoring overrides the increase in cost remain to be determined. Another challenge is the absence of an easy antidote when patients have major bleeding (Chapter 38).[7]

Thrombolytic Therapy

Although thrombolytic therapy results in increased rates of early patency of leg veins after DVT, it has not been conclusively shown to decrease the subsequent rate of post-thrombotic syndrome or pulmonary emboli. Except for patients who have life-threatening limb ischemia as a result of massive thrombosis, thrombolysis is not recommended in patients with DVT. Ongoing trials of catheter-directed thrombolysis versus "standard therapy" should provide the definitive evidence about the relative efficacy of catheter-directed thrombolysis for the prevention of post-thrombotic syndrome.

Side Effects of Anticoagulants

Bleeding is the most common side effect of anticoagulant therapy. Major bleeding (e.g., intracranial [Chapter 408], gastrointestinal [Chapter 135], or retroperitoneal) leading to hospitalization, transfusion, or death occurs in approximately 2% of patients treated with intravenous unfractionated heparin for acute VTE. Factors such as recent surgery, trauma, and concurrent aspirin or thrombolytic therapy increase the risk for bleeding.

The risk for major bleeding with warfarin in doses adjusted to achieve a target INR of 2.0 to 3.0 ranges from 1 to 3% per year and appears to be highest soon after treatment is started or if anticoagulation is difficult to control. Risks are somewhat lower for direct thrombin and factor Xa inhibitors, but their actions cannot yet be reversed pharmaceutically (Chapter 38). The risk for major bleeding increases according to individual characteristics, such as older age, the presence of comorbid conditions (e.g., diabetes, hypertension, renal insufficiency, previous gastrointestinal bleeding, or cancer) and the use of concomitant drugs, in particular antiplatelet therapy.

Heparin-induced thrombocytopenia, which is a relatively common nonhemorrhagic complication of therapy with unfractionated heparin and a very uncommon complication of LMWH, is manifested typically with thrombocytopenia and new thrombosis (Chapter 38). Monitoring of the platelet count is recommended every other day until day 14 in patients receiving therapeutic unfractionated heparin but is not routinely recommended with LMWH or fondaparinux because of the extremely low risk with these newer medications.

When Medications Fail or Are Contraindicated

Therapeutic strategies to manage patients in whom symptomatic VTE recurs while they are receiving conventional-intensity warfarin or direct thrombin or factor Xa inhibitors include LMWH, higher-intensity warfarin (e.g., INR range of 3.0 to 4.0), and insertion of a vena caval filter. However, the optimal management of such patients is unknown because no randomized studies have been performed.

Inferior vena caval filters should be used in patients who have contraindications to anticoagulant therapy or develop major bleeding while receiving it, as well as in patients who develop recurrent VTE while receiving appropriate anticoagulation. Retrievable or removable inferior vena caval filters can be retrieved and removed within 14 days to several weeks after insertion or can be left in permanently. These filters are ideal for a patient who has a reversible cause of, or the potential for, major bleeding (e.g., DVT after craniotomy, DVT late in pregnancy).

Deep Vein Thrombosis in Pregnancy

The management of pregnant women with DVT (Chapter 239) is problematic because all coumarin derivatives cross the placenta and have the potential to cause warfarin embryopathy, consisting of nasal hypoplasia and epiphyseal stippling, if the newborn is exposed to warfarin between 6 and 12 weeks of gestation. Consequently, parenteral unfractionated heparin and LMWH, which do not cross the placenta and are safe for the fetus, are the agents of choice. The easiest approach is to initiate therapy with weight-adjusted "treatment" doses of LMWH (see Table 81-3), continued for the duration of the pregnancy. Although not proved, it is likely that the dose of LMWH can be safely decreased to approximately 80% of the therapeutic dose after 3 months of therapy. As pregnancy progresses, women normally gain weight and generally require higher doses of LMWH to achieve an anti–factor Xa level similar to that achieved at the time of diagnosis. The adequacy of the dose can be assessed by measuring a 4-hour postinjection anti–factor Xa level and targeting the dose to achieve a level of 0.5 to 1.0 U/mL for twice-daily LMWH and 0.8 to 1.5 U/mL for once-daily LMWH. Alternatively, the dose of LMWH can simply be adjusted periodically on the basis of the woman's weight.

Unfractionated heparin is less attractive than LMWH because it is associated with a greater reduction of bone density and a higher risk for heparin-induced thrombocytopenia. Unfractionated heparin can be initiated either by continuous intravenous infusion in doses adjusted to maintain an aPTT in the therapeutic range, followed by 12-hourly subcutaneous injections, or simply with 12-hourly subcutaneous injections throughout the course of pregnancy. The dose should be adjusted to target a mid-interval (6-hours after) aPTT in the therapeutic range.

Pregnant women with a DVT should probably be treated for the duration of pregnancy and for at least 6 weeks postpartum. If the DVT occurred early in pregnancy, elective induction of delivery at approximately 37 weeks with discontinuation of the heparin 24 hours earlier is recommended. If the DVT occurs in the latter part of the third trimester, intravenous heparin should be administered by continuous infusion until approximately 6 hours before the expected time of delivery. Intravenous unfractionated heparin or subcutaneous LMWH should be started postpartum as soon as hemostasis has been achieved. Maternal warfarin therapy is safe for the breast-fed infant because warfarin and its metabolites are not secreted into breast milk in doses sufficient to cause an anticoagulant effect. Consequently, warfarin (with bridging LMWH or unfractionated heparin until the INR is 2.0 or higher) can be used after delivery.

PREVENTION

Despite the plethora of large randomized trials demonstrating the efficacy and safety of mechanical and pharmacologic measures in reducing the risk for VTE in a wide range of hospitalized populations of patients, prophylaxis remains grossly underused. Factors that increase the risk for DVT include surgery (particularly major hip and knee surgery, as well as neurosurgery [Chapters 431 and 433]), major trauma (Chapter 111), prolonged bedrest or immobilization, previous episodes of VTE, presence of malignant disease, paralysis, morbid obesity, and increasing age.

Comprehensive consensus guidelines have been developed for the prevention of VTE in different populations of patients (Chapter 38). In general, mechanical prophylaxis (antiembolic stockings and intermittent pneumatic compression) should be used as an adjunct to pharmacologic prophylaxis or in patients with a high risk for bleeding. For general medical patients admitted to the hospital with a major illness and in whom mobility is likely to be reduced for 72 hours or longer, low-dose unfractionated heparin or LMWH (see Table 38-2 in Chapter 38) should be considered. In patients who undergo major hip or knee surgery, warfarin (to an INR of 2.0 to 3.0), subcutaneous LMWH, subcutaneous fondaparinux (2.5 mg/day), or oral rivaroxaban (10 mg/day) should be used for at least 7 to 14 days postoperatively. In patients with continued immobility, prophylaxis should be considered until the patient regains preoperative mobility.A6 In one randomized trial, the ultra-low-molecular-weight heparin semuloparin (20 mg/day SC) reduced the risk for VTE from 3.4% to 1.2% over 3.5 months without increasing major bleeding.

VENOUS THROMBOSIS OF THE UPPER EXTREMITIES

DVT of the upper extremities (including the arm and the axillary, subclavian, and internal jugular veins, as well as the superior vena cava) is much less common than DVT of the legs, but it is not rare,[8] especially among critically ill adults in intensive care units.[9] Factors associated with upper extremity DVT include central venous catheters, acquired or hereditary thrombophilias, and anatomic (cervical rib) and physiologic (muscular individuals) impingement of the vein. The incidence of clinically important post-thrombotic syndrome is not high if patients are treated with anticoagulants alone.

Contrast venography is the gold standard for the diagnosis of upper extremity DVT, but venous ultrasonography is accurate and less invasive. Because it is not feasible to test for compression of the subclavian vein, a diagnosis of subclavian DVT by ultrasonography is based on flow abnormalities or direct visualization of thrombus by B-mode ultrasonography. Upper extremity DVT can cause pulmonary emboli, although the exact frequency is not known.

Considerable controversy exists about the management of patients in whom DVT develops in association with a central venous catheter. If the line is not necessary or is nonfunctional, some recommend simply removing the line without subsequent anticoagulant therapy, whereas others treat with full-dose anticoagulants (a heparin-related compound, followed by 1 to 3 months of warfarin). If the line is functional and must stay in place (e.g., no alternative venous access), full-dose anticoagulants should be given. Otherwise, anticoagulant therapy should be given in all patients with upper extremity DVT, with medications, doses, regimens, and durations identical to those for treatment of DVT of the leg.

SUPERFICIAL THROMBOPHLEBITIS

Superficial thrombophlebitis usually manifests with pain, swelling, redness, and tenderness of superficial veins. Varicose veins[10] (Fig. 81-6) can be red, warm, and clustered in a circumscribed area. When superficial thrombophlebitis occurs in the short or long saphenous veins, usually redness, tenderness, and often linear induration follow the course of the involved vein (medial calf or thigh). Superficial thrombophlebitis also can occur at the insertion site of an intravenous catheter. Invariably, superficial thrombophlebitis is associated with thrombosis of the corresponding vein; particularly when the long saphenous vein is involved, venous ultrasonography should be performed to exclude extension into the deep veins, which occurs in up to 19% of patients. Approximately 25% of patients who have superficial venous thrombosis have concurrent DVT at the time of presentation, and approximately 3% of the others will subsequently develop DVT or pulmonary embolism in the next 3 months.[11]

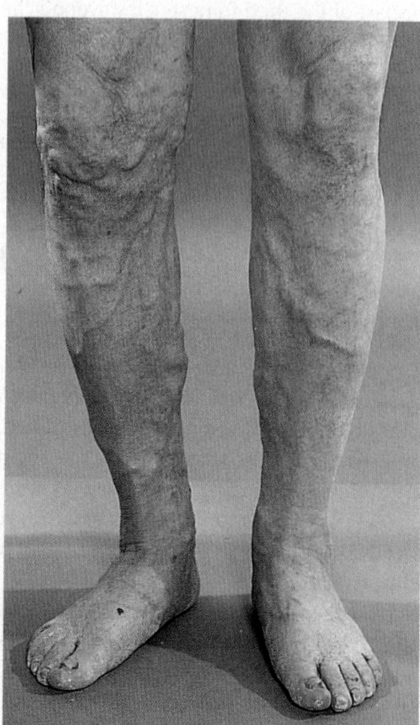

FIGURE 81-6. **Varicose veins are a risk factor for deep vein thrombosis and may result from it.** (From Forbes CD, Jackson WF. Color Atlas and Text of Clinical Medicine, 3rd ed. London: Mosby; 2003.)

Nonsteroidal anti-inflammatory drugs (NSAIDs) and either moderate or full doses of LMWH are each approximately 70% better than placebo for treating superficial thrombophlebitis.[12] LMWH relieves symptoms more quickly and prevents growth of thrombus more effectively than do NSAIDs. Fondaparinux, 2.5 mg/day for 45 days, reduces the risk for DVT or pulmonary embolism from approximately 1.3% to 0.2% without adverse effects.A15 Thus, it is reasonable to use moderate doses of LMWH or fondaparinux for the initial treatment of acute, symptomatic superficial thrombophlebitis, particularly for patients with severe symptoms, proximal saphenous vein thrombosis, recurrent disease, or evidence of thrombophilia. Alternatively, and particularly for intravenous catheter–induced superficial thrombophlebitis, an NSAID can be tried. For varicose veins, laser and surgical treatments appear to be superior to foam sclerotherapy.[13]

POST-THROMBOTIC SYNDROME

The initial pain and swelling in many patients with DVT are due to the venous obstruction or the inflammatory process mediated by the acute thrombus. Once anticoagulant therapy is initiated, the acute obstruction usually resolves during a period of several months as recanalization occurs and collateral venous channels develop, thereby leading to initial improvement in pain and swelling. However, in the long term, probably because of venous valvular incompetence produced when the thrombosed venous segments recanalize and because of residual chronic obstruction, venous hypertension and sometimes pain and swelling can recur.

This post-thrombotic syndrome develops in up to 50% of patients with proximal DVT, usually within the first 1 to 2 years after DVT.[14] The syndrome is often a chronic, progressive disease with pain, swelling, and occasionally ulceration of the leg in patients with previous DVT. In a randomized trial of patients with acute iliofemoral DVT, the addition of catheter-directed thrombolysis using alteplase reduced the development of post-thrombotic syndrome from 56% to 41% at 24 months, but at the expense of an 8% risk for clinically relevant or major bleeding.A16

PREVENTION AND TREATMENT Rx

Despite earlier enthusiasm, a large, randomized trial showed compression stockings were not beneficial in preventing post-thrombotic syndrome.A17 Consequently, it would seem reasonable to wait until the acute inflammatory process and acute outflow obstruction have subsided (usually up to 6 months) and then prescribe stockings if the patient's symptoms persist at that time.

Simple lifestyle alteration (such as frequent leg elevation, avoidance of prolonged standing or sitting, and occasional use of analgesics) relieve symptoms in many patients. If symptoms are severe, it is usually because extensive thrombus is causing massive edema. In such patients, a lightweight stocking (such as support hose) can be helpful until the edema improves. If symptoms persist or worsen despite these measures, or if ulceration seems imminent (as evidenced by severe skin changes), a full-strength stocking (30 to 40 mm Hg of pressure at the ankle) can be prescribed. However, if symptoms subside and the patient remains asymptomatic or has only trivial persistent signs or symptoms with little or no effect on quality of life, stockings can be avoided and the patient can be observed for clinically important signs and symptoms of post-thrombotic syndrome.

VENOUS ULCERS

Venous ulcers, which are the most severe complication of post-thrombotic syndrome, typically occur in the perimalleolar area of the leg. The best management is prevention by application of graduated compression stockings either at the time of diagnosis of DVT or, at the latest, when skin changes develop in association with leg swelling. When an ulcer occurs, treatment with an emollient and regular wrapping should be commenced.[A18] Once the ulcer heals, the patient should be prescribed graduated compression stockings and watched for recurrent ulceration.[15] Surgical closure or removal of the incompetent saphenous veins plus dressing management in patients with chronic venous ulceration does not reduce healing time of the acute ulcer compared with dressing management alone but significantly reduces the rate of recurrent ulceration for at least the next 4 years.

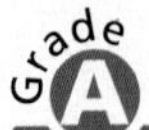

Grade A References

A1. Hull RD, Pineo GF, Brant RF, et al. Long-term low-molecular-weight heparin versus usual care in proximal-vein thrombosis patients with cancer. *Am J Med.* 2006;119:1062-1072.
A2. Buller HR, Davidson BL, Decousus H, et al. Fondaparinux or enoxaparin for the initial treatment of symptomatic deep venous thrombosis: a randomized trial. *Ann Intern Med.* 2004;140:867-873.
A3. Kearon C, Ginsberg JS, Kovacs MJ, et al. Comparison of low-intensity warfarin therapy with conventional-intensity warfarin therapy for long-term prevention of recurrent venous thromboembolism. *N Engl J Med.* 2003;349:631-639.
A4. Pirmohamed M, Burnside G, Eriksson N, et al. A randomized trial of genotype-guided dosing of warfarin. *N Engl J Med.* 2013;369:2294-2303.
A5. Kearon C, Ginsberg JS, Anderson DR, et al. Comparison of 1 month of anticoagulation with 3 months of anticoagulation for a first episode of venous thromboembolism provoked by a transient risk factor. *J Thromb Haemost.* 2003;2:743-749.
A6. Kearon C, Akl EA, Comerota AJ, et al. Antithrombotic therapy for VTE disease: antithrombotic therapy and prevention of thrombosis, 9th ed: American College of Chest Physicians evidence-based clinical practice guidelines. *Chest.* 2012;141:e419S-e494S.
A7. Bloomfield HE, Krause A, Greer N, et al. Meta-analysis: effect of patient self-testing and self-management of long-term anticoagulation on major clinical outcomes. *Ann Intern Med.* 2011;154:472-482.
A8. Lee AY, Levine MN, Baker RI, et al. Randomized comparison of low-molecular-weight heparin versus oral anticoagulant therapy for the prevention of recurrent venous thromboembolism in patients with cancer. *N Engl J Med.* 2003;349:109-111.
A9. Becattini C, Agnelli G, Schenone A, et al. Aspirin for preventing the recurrence of venous thromboembolism. *N Engl J Med.* 2012;366:1959-1967.
A10. EINSTEIN Investigators. Oral rivaroxaban for symptomatic venous thromboembolism. *N Engl J Med.* 2010;363:2499-2510.
A11. AMPLIFY Investigators. Oral apixaban for the treatment of acute venous thromboembolism. *N Engl J Med.* 2013;369:799-808.
A12. AMPLIFY-EXT Investigators. Apixaban for extended treatment of venous thromboembolism. *N Engl J Med.* 2013;368:699-708.
A13. RE-COVER Study Group. Dabigatran versus warfarin in the treatment of acute venous thromboembolism. *N Engl J Med.* 2009;361:2342-2352.
A14. RE-SONATE and RE-MEDY Study Groups. Extended use of dabigatran, warfarin, or placebo in venous thromboembolism. *N Engl J Med.* 2013;368:709-718.
A15. Decousus H, Prandoni P, Mismetti P, et al, for the CALISTO Study Group. Fondaparinux in the treatment of lower-limb superficial-vein thrombosis. *N Engl J Med.* 2010;363:1222-1232.
A16. Enden T, Haig Y, Kløw NE, et al. Long-term outcome after additional catheter-directed thrombolysis versus standard treatment for acute iliofemoral deep vein thrombosis (the CaVenT study): a randomised controlled trial. *Lancet.* 2012;379:31-38.
A17. Kahn SR, Shapiro S, Wells PS, et al. Compression stockings to prevent post-thrombotic syndrome: a randomised placebo-controlled trial. *Lancet.* 2014;383:880-888.
A18. O'Meara S, Richardson R, Lipsky BA. Topical and systemic antimicrobial therapy for venous leg ulcers. *JAMA.* 2014;311:2534-2535.

GENERAL REFERENCES

For the General References and other additional features, please visit Expert Consult at https://expertconsult.inkling.com.

82

CARDIAC TRANSPLANTATION

DONNA MANCINI AND YOSHIFUMI NAKA

Heart failure is a progressive disease that now affects over 5 million patients in the United States (Chapter 58). Recent estimates suggest that 5 to 10% of all patients with heart failure have advanced, or stage D, disease, which is associated with a very high mortality rate and very poor quality of life (Chapter 59). Heart transplantation and mechanical assist devices are the only therapies that improve quality of life and survival in patients with stage D disease. With the improving results of cardiac transplantation—that is, 1- and 5-year survival rates approaching 90 and 72%, respectively—more patients are referred for transplant evaluation. Moreover, increasing experience and excellent outcomes have resulted in an expansion of eligibility criteria (Table 82-1) to patients whose comorbid conditions would have made them ineligible in prior decades.

TABLE 82-1 INDICATIONS FOR HEART TRANSPLANTATION

1. Refractory cardiogenic shock requiring continuous intravenous inotropic support or mechanical circulatory support with an intra-aortic balloon pump, venoarterial extracorporeal membrane oxygenation, or left ventricular assist device
2. Persistent class IV New York Heart Association congestive heart failure symptoms refractory to maximal medical therapy (peak oxygen consumption < 10-12 mL/kg/min)
3. Intractable or severe symptoms of ischemia in patients with coronary artery disease not amenable to percutaneous or surgical revascularization
4. Recurrent life-threatening arrhythmias refractory to medical therapy, catheter ablation, implantation of intracardiac defibrillator, or a combination of these
5. Congenital heart disease with severe ventricular dysfunction or that cannot be corrected or palliated by either surgical or medical treatment

Based on data that the 127 active heart transplant centers in the United States report to the United Network of Organ Sharing and the Scientific Registry for Transplant Recipients, approximately 2200 to 2400 heart transplant procedures are performed annually in the United States (Fig. 82-1). The major limitation to the growth of cardiac transplantation continues to be the scarcity of donor organs. With the increasing number of potential heart transplant recipients but a relatively constant number of donors, the wait list for transplantation and time to transplantation have continued to increase.[1-3]

SELECTION CRITERIA FOR CARDIAC TRANSPLANTATION

When a patient with advanced heart failure is referred to a transplantation center, the initial evaluation requires an assessment of the severity of heart failure, the identification of any potentially reversible factors, and an assessment of the adequacy of current medical therapy. If no reversible causes are identified and therapy is optimal, the evaluation process begins by determining whether the patient meets criteria for transplantation (see Table 82-1).[4,5]

The current United Network of Organ Sharing allocation policy takes into account the intensity of therapy used to support the patient (parenteral inotropic or mechanical support), time accrued on the wait list, blood type compatibility, and geographic distance.[6] Unfortunately, these policies result in substantial regional differences in wait times.[7] In patients who depend on parenteral inotropic support because of refractory cardiogenic shock or are deteriorating on parenteral inotropic agents, cardiac replacement therapy is the only option for long-term survival. The transplant evaluation must proceed expeditiously because these patients often require several days to weeks of circulatory support with percutaneous or implantable devices before the decision can be made as to whether to transition to long-term device support, proceed directly to cardiac transplantation, or withdraw care. The proportion of patients who require mechanical support before cardiac transplantation grew from 6% in 1998 to 24% in 2011 and now exceeds 30% in some regions of the United States.

Ambulatory patients with New York Heart Association (NYHA) class IIIB/IV symptoms comprise the largest number of referrals for cardiac transplant evaluation. Patients with a preserved exercise capacity, defined as a peak oxygen consumption (VO_2) greater than 14 mL/kg/minute, have a 1-year survival that is comparable to the expected survival in newly transplanted patients. By comparison, a peak VO_2 less than 10 mL/kg/minute is an absolute indication for transplantation. For patients with a peak VO_2 of 11 to 14 mL/kg/minute, decisions regarding transplantation must be individualized. Multivariable risk models can help predict whether survival would likely be better with or without the procedure based on factors such as the resting heart rate, mean arterial blood pressure, left ventricular ejection fraction, presence or absence of an intraventricular conduction defect, and serum sodium level.

Contraindications to Cardiac Transplantation

Absolute and relative exclusion criteria for heart transplantation (Table 82-2), which have evolved over time, consist of factors that increase perioperative risk, impair patients' ability to care for themselves, or affect long-term survival. Although no absolute age cutoff for heart transplantation exists and some centers will perform transplants in patients up to age 72 years, long-term survival is clearly decreased in older patients.

The major hemodynamic factor excluding cardiac transplantation is a nonreversible pulmonary vascular resistance (PVR) greater than 6 Wood units,

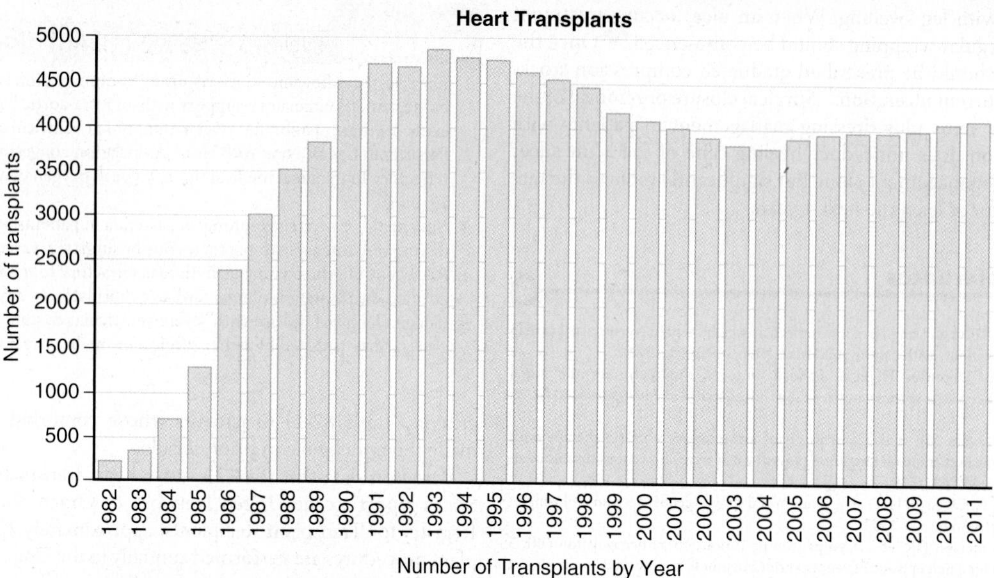

FIGURE 82-1. Heart transplant volume by year. (From Lund LH, Edwards LB, Kucheryavaya AY, et al. The Registry of the International Society for Heart and Lung Transplantation: thirtieth official adult heart transplant report—2013; focus theme: age. *J Heart Lung Transplant.* 2013;32:951-964.)

TABLE 82-2 CARDIAC TRANSPLANTATION CONTRAINDICATION CRITERIA

I. Absolute Contraindications
1. Systemic illness with a limited life expectancy despite heart transplant including:
   a. Active or recent solid organ or blood malignancy
   b. Irreversible renal or hepatic dysfunction in patients considered for heart-only transplantation
   c. Severe obstructive pulmonary disease (FEV_1 < 1 L/min)
   d. Active multisystem diseases
2. Fixed pulmonary hypertension with a mean transpulmonary gradient > 5 mm Hg or pulmonary vascular resistance > 6 Wood units not reduced with vasodilators, parenteral inotropic agents, phosphodiesterase type V inhibitors, endothelin receptor antagonists, or a mechanical assist device.

II. Relative contraindications
1. Age > 72 yr
2. Any active infection (with exception of device-related infection in ventricular assist device recipients)
3. Active peptic ulcer disease
4. Diabetes mellitus with moderate end-organ involvement (neuropathy, nephropathy, or retinopathy)
5. Severe peripheral vascular or cerebrovascular disease
6. Morbid obesity (BMI > 35) or cachexia (BMI < 18)
7. Significant chronic renal impairment with creatinine > 2.5 mg/dL or creatinine clearance < 25 mL/min*
8. Significant hepatic impairment with bilirubin > 2.5 mg/dL, serum transaminase levels > 3 times normal, INR > 1.5 off warfarin
9. Severe pulmonary dysfunction with FEV_1 < 40% normal
10. Recent pulmonary infarction within 6-8 wk
11. Irreversible neurologic or neuromuscular disorder
12. Active mental illness or psychosocial instability
13. Drug, tobacco, or alcohol abuse within 6 mo
14. Significant coagulopathies

*May be suitable for cardiac transplantation if inotropic support and hemodynamic management produce a creatinine < 2 mg/dL and creatinine clearance > 50 mL/min. Transplantation may also be advisable as combined heart-kidney transplant.
BMI = body mass index; FEV_1 = forced expiratory volume in one second; INR = international normalized ratio.

which increases the risk for immediate postoperative right ventricular failure and the 30-day mortality rate. In most patients with advanced heart failure, however, pulmonary hypertension is reversible with vasodilators (Chapter 68) or after implantation of a left ventricular assist device.

Although diabetes mellitus with evidence of significant end-organ damage (e.g., neuropathy or nephropathy) is a relative contraindication to heart transplantation, carefully selected patients with diabetes can undergo successful transplantation with morbidity and mortality similar to that in patients without diabetes. In patients with diabetes who have renal dysfunction (Chapter 124), combined heart and kidney transplantation (Chapter 131) can be considered, with a survival rate comparable to that of heart transplantation alone.

Patients with an active or recent malignancy may be offered mechanical support either before or after cancer treatment as a way to bridge them to transplant. However, any patient with a history of malignancy has an increased risk for developing a second malignancy owing to immunosuppression after the transplantation (Chapter 49).

Combined heart and stem cell transplantation (Chapter 178) is an option in patients with primary amyloid light-chain amyloidosis (Chapter 188), but survival rates are lower than in other transplant patients because of the frequent recurrence of amyloidosis in the transplanted heart. In contrast, survival of patients with familial amyloidosis caused by a mutant form of the protein transthyretin is comparable to that in other transplant recipients.

Repeat transplantation now accounts for 3% of U.S. heart transplants, usually in patients who have developed chronic allograft dysfunction because of severe transplant coronary artery disease, often with a left ventricular ejection fraction less than 45% or with restrictive cardiomyopathy, but without any other significant comorbid conditions. However, repeat transplantation is associated with greater risk for infection and malignancies, owing to the heightened immunosuppression, and a poorer long-term survival.

Currently, 3% of adults undergoing cardiac transplantation have complex congenital heart disease (Chapter 69) as the cause of their heart failure. As more patients with complex congenital heart disease survive into adulthood, however, an estimated 10 to 20% of such patients will become candidates for heart or combined heart-lung transplantation at some time during their lives. In such patients, the short-term post-transplant survival is significantly lower compared with patients who have ischemic or dilated cardiomyopathies owing to their higher rate of intraoperative and post-operative bleeding. If a patient with congenital heart disease survives the surgery, however, 10-year survival post-transplant is excellent.

Active bacterial infection is a temporary absolute contraindication to heart transplantation, except in the setting of mechanical device infection, in which transplant is felt to be curative. Patients who are positive for human immunodeficiency virus (HIV) and have end-stage cardiomyopathy can be considered for transplant, with good short-term outcome in carefully screened patients who have low or undetectable viral loads and no recent significant bacterial infections. Patients with chronic hepatitis B or C (Chapter 149) have an increased incidence of postoperative liver disease, but their post-transplant survival is not reduced.

Organ allocation

Donor Criteria

Donors and recipients are matched for ABO blood compatibility and size. Weight matching is generally within 25% of recipient body weight, though donors of equal size or larger are preferred for recipients with high PVR. Height mismatches greater than 6 inches are currently not recommended. Males under age 40 and females under age 45 are suitable donors, provided echocardiography shows no evidence of preexisting heart disease or impaired myocardial function. Older individuals also may be suitable donors if coronary atherosclerotic lesions can be excluded, optimally by cardiac catheterization. Donors with serologic findings positive for HIV, hepatitis B and C, and nonprimary brain malignancies are generally not accepted. Organs procured with ischemic times in excess of 4 hours are associated with a higher rate of primary graft failure.

Matching Donors and Recipients

Approximately 10% of transplant candidates have human leukocyte antigen (HLA) antibodies that could lead to a positive crossmatch. The sensitized candidate is typically a multiparous woman, a patient who has received multiple prior transfusions, or patients supported with a mechanical assist device. Patients with high antibody levels require a donor-specific T-cell crossmatch before transplantation to exclude the presence of lymphocytotoxic immunoglobulin G antibodies against donor HLA class I antigens, a situation that can cause hyperacute rejection. Sensitized patients are also at risk for acute humoral rejection and an earlier onset of accelerated coronary artery disease.

A donor-specific T-cell crossmatch is a contraindication to transplantation; thus, sensitized candidates have longer wait times before receiving a cardiac allograft. With technologies using solid-phase assays and flow cytometric techniques that can rapidly identify class I and II antibodies, long-distance donors can be screened for unacceptable antigens—a "virtual crossmatch" that enlarges the potential donor pool for sensitized patients.

Surgical Technique

Orthotopic cardiac transplantation can be performed by using a *biatrial* anastomosis and reconnecting the pulmonary artery and aorta above the semilunar valves. Increasingly, however, atrial function is preserved by performing a bi*caval* anastomosis, which results in improved atrial geometry, better right ventricular function, less frequent atrioventricular valve regurgitation, and less sinus node dysfunction.

Immunosuppression

Most transplant centers use a triple drug therapy regimen including a calcineurin inhibitor (cyclosporine or tacrolimus), an antiproliferative agent (usually mycophenolate mofetil), and steroids (Chapter 49). Some centers, however, use only a single agent such as tacrolimus.[A1] By the third month after surgery, most patients receive only prednisone 5 mg/day and approximately 25 to 60% of patients can tolerate total withdrawal of steroids by the end of the first year.

Acute rejection occurs most frequently in the first 3 months after transplant. Some centers use selective induction agents, such as basiliximab, that target the activated interleukin-2 (IL-2) receptor on T cells, or potent nonselective immunosuppressive agents, such as thymoglobulin, in the perioperative period to decrease early allograft rejection. However, this intensification of immunosuppression can predispose patients to more frequent opportunistic infections. Currently, approximately 50% of transplant centers use induction therapy.

For calcineurin inhibitors, prospective randomized trials have demonstrated a decreased incidence of allograft rejection, less hypertension, lower lipid levels, less hirsuitism, and less gingival hyperplasia using tacrolimus compared with cyclosporine, although most studies demonstrating no difference in survival.[A2-A5] Mycophenolate mofetil, a selective de novo purine inhibitor, is the preferred antiproliferative agent to reduce rejection and the development of transplant vasculopathy.[A6] Although everolimus may be better than mycophenolate mofetil in preventing early transplant vasculopathy, it also is associated with more side effects,[A7] so mycophenolate mofetil remains the current agent of choice.

Rejection

Allograft rejection, which can be antibody-mediated or cell-mediated, occurs most frequently in the first 6 months after the transplant. Antibody-mediated, or humoral, rejection generally occurs very early after the transplant, particularly in a previously sensitized recipient. It is characterized histologically by immunoglobulin and complement deposition in the absence of cellular rejection, and often it is associated with hemodynamic compromise. T-cell mediated rejection, triggered by the recognition of foreign antigens on the surface of engrafted cells, accounts for more than 90% of rejection episodes, usually within the first 6 months.

TABLE 82-3 HISTOLOGIC GRADING OF CELLULAR REJECTION*

Grade 0R	No rejection
Grade 1R (mild)	Interstitial, perivasicular, or both infiltrate with up to 1 focus of myocyte damage
Grade 2R (moderate)	≥2 foci of infiltrate with myocyte damage
Grade 3R (severe)	Diffuse infiltrate with multifocal myocyte damage, edema, hemorrhage, vasculitis

*Modified from Stewart S, Winters GL, Fishbein MC, et al. Revision of the 1990 working formulation for the standardization of nomenclature in the diagnosis of heart rejection. *J Heart Lung Transplant.* 2005;24:1710-1720.

TABLE 82-4 2013 INTERNATIONAL SOCIETY FOR HEART & LUNG TRANSPLANTATION CLASSIFICATION FOR DIAGNOSIS OF CARDIAC ANTIBODY-MEDIATED REJECTION (AMR)*

GRADE	DEFINITION
pAMR 0	No rejection
pAMR 1 (H+)	Histopathologic changes are present without immunopathologic findings.
pAMR 1 (I+)	Immunopathologic findings are positive without histologic findings.
pAMR 2	Both immunologic and histologic findings are present.
pAMR 3	Severe pathologic antibody-mediated rejection with interstitial hemorrhage, capillary fragmentation, mixed inflammatory infiltrates, endothelial cell pyknosis, karyorrhexis, or a combination of these, and marked edema *and* immunopathologic findings are present. These cases may be associated with profound hemodynamic dysfunction and poor clinical outcomes.

*Modified from Berry GJ, Burke MM, Andersen C, et al. The 2013 International Society for Heart and Lung Transplantation Working Formulation for the standardization of nomenclature in the pathologic diagnosis of antibody-mediated rejection in heart transplantation. *J Heart Lung Transplant.* 2013;32:1147-1162.

To diagnose allograft rejection, endomyocardial biopsies are usually performed by the transjugular approach weekly for the first month, then every other week for 2 months, then every 1 to 2 months for the first year. Biopsy grading of cellular rejection is based on the severity of lymphocyte infiltration and myocyte necrosis on hematoxylin and eosin staining (Table 82-3), whereas antibody-mediated rejection also includes immunologic staining (Table 82-4). Although the presence of donor-specific antibodies is not a requirement for the diagnosis of antibody-mediated rejection, patients suspected of having antibody-mediated rejection are frequently tested and serially monitored for donor-specific antibody. In asymptomatic patients on low doses of steroids, gene expression profiling of peripheral blood samples can reduce the number of biopsies while providing equivalent clinical outcomes.[A8]

Treatment of Rejection

The treatment of allograft rejection is determined by the presence of symptoms, the degree of left ventricular dysfunction, the time since transplant, and the pathologic grade of the biopsy. Most episodes of cellular rejection are easily treated with high-dose oral or intravenous steroids. Patients with hemodynamically significant rejection will require rescue therapy with thymoglobulin. Humoral rejection therapy includes modalities that both clear and reduce the production of the antibody, such as plasmapheresis, intravenous immunoglobulin, thymoglobulin, high-dose steroids, and B cell–specific monoclonal antibodies such as rituximab[8] (Chapter 49).

Transplant Vasculopathy

Transplant vasculopathy, which is primarily a form of chronic rejection, occurs at an annual incidence rate of 5 to 10% and remains one of the main causes of late death after cardiac transplantation. Risk factors for transplant vasculopathy include an increased number of HLA mismatches, increased number of acute rejection episodes, older donor age, prior cytomegalovirus (CMV) infection, ischemia-reperfusion injury, and the classic risk factors for atherosclerotic disease—age, smoking, obesity, diabetes, dyslipidemia, and hypertension. Histologic examination shows subendothelial accumulation of primarily T cells, myointimal proliferation of smooth muscle cells, lipid-laden foam cells, and perivascular fibrosis.

Patients rarely experience exertional angina and are more likely to present with severe fatigue, heart failure, myocardial infarction, ventricular arrhythmia, or sudden death. Patients should be screened annually either by angiography, with or without intravascular ultrasound, or by dobutamine stress echocardiography. An increase in intimal thickness of at least 0.5 mm, as detected by intravascular ultrasound, is a reliable indicator of both cardiac allograft vasculopathy and 5-year mortality.

In contrast to routine coronary artery disease, cardiac allograft vasculopathy is usually manifested by concentric narrowing, owing to neointimal proliferation of vascular smooth muscle cells throughout the length of the vessel and angiographic evidence of rapid tapering, pruning, and obliteration of vessels. Some patients may have focal coronary lesions that are amenable to stent placement, but generally the disease is diffuse and not amenable to percutaneous coronary interventions or bypass grafting.

Treatment has been predominantly aimed at prevention. Use of high-dose or low-dose statins (see Table 206-6 in Chapter 206) can reduce the development of cardiac vasculopathy.[A9] Sirolimus and everolimus also can reduce the incidence of cardiac vasculopathy and slow its progression. However, the only definitive treatment of transplant vasculopathy is repeat transplantation, and the survival of patients undergoing repeat transplantation for severe vasculopathy is comparable to that of de novo heart transplant recipients.

Malignancy

With the improved survival of heart transplant recipients and longer exposure to immunosuppressive drugs, malignancies, especially lymphomas (Chapter 185), are now almost equal to transplant vasculopathy as the leading cause of long-term mortality. Post-transplant lymphoproliferative disease (Chapters 49 and 185) includes a spectrum of predominantly B-cell lymphomas (~90%) frequently associated with Epstein-Barr virus (Chapter 377). T-cell lymphomas are much less frequent (10%) and often more difficult to treat (Chapter 185). Skin cancers (Chapter 203) are also more frequent in post-transplant patients, but the incidence of solid organ malignancies is not much different from that in the general population.

Infection

Infections (Chapter 281) account for approximately 20% of deaths within the first year after transplant surgery and continue to be a common cause of morbidity and mortality throughout the recipient's life. In the waiting period, careful attention should be given to updating immunizations against pneumococcal pneumonia, hepatitis B, and herpes zoster (Chapter 18). Young women should receive vaccination against the human papilloma virus. Patients with positive tuberculosis skin tests should be treated with isoniazid and pyridoxine (Chapter 324), and patients with latent syphilis should be treated with penicillin (Chapter 319).

Infections early after transplant are predominantly bacterial from hospital-acquired organisms (Chapter 282), catheters, the surgical site, a prior left ventricular assist device, or occasionally from donor-transmitted disease. Any infection early after transplantation increases the risk for a subsequent fatal CMV infection (Chapter 376). Any CMV-positive patient or CMV-negative patient receiving a CMV-positive organ should receive prophylactic ganciclovir followed by valganciclovir.

Fungal and viral infections are usually more frequent starting a month or so after transplant. Antibiotic prophylaxis includes perioperative antibacterial agents, such as cefazolin, and initiation of prophylaxis against CMV infection, *Pneumocystis jiroveci* pneumonia, herpes simplex virus infection, and oral candidiasis (Chapter 338). The prophylactic use of one single-strength trimethoprim-sulfamethoxazole tablet daily, typically for the first year after transplantation, has virtually eliminated *P. jiroveci* (Chapter 341) and also prevents nocardial infections (Chapter 330) and toxoplasmosis (Chapter 349). Aspergillosis (Chapter 339) and candidiasis (Chapter 338) are the most common fungal infections after heart transplantation; oral nystatin solution or clotrimazole troches are routinely used in the first 3 to 6 months (Chapter 331).

Comorbid Conditions

Within 5 years, hypertension (Chapter 67) occurs in over 92% of transplant recipients, primarily owing to the side effects of calcineurin inhibitors. Diabetes (Chapter 229) is observed in approximately 40% of patients owing to treatment with corticosteroids or tacrolimus. Hyperlipidemia is found in approximately 90% of patients and is treated with statins, with the same approach as for patients with known coronary disease (Chapter 206). Osteoporosis (Chapter 243) is also common because of chronic steroid treatment as well as the use of calcineurin inhibitors. Significant renal insufficiency (serum creatinine > 2.5 mg/dL) occurs in 20% of patients by 10 years post-transplant.

PROGNOSIS

During the first year after transplantation, early causes of death are graft failure, infection, multiorgan failure, and allograft rejection. Overall survival, which is approximately 85% at 1 year and 75% at 5 years, has been improving over time (Fig. 82-2). After 5 years, cardiac allograft vasculopathy (14%), late graft failure (18%), malignant disease (25%), and non-CMV infection (10%) are the most prominent causes of death. Of the patients, 50% will survive for more than 11 years and many survive for 20 to 30 years, often with good ventricular function.[9]

Functional capacity is usually excellent, with more than 90% of 1-year survivors reporting no functional limitations. Exercise capacity improves but remains reduced compared with that of age- and gender-matched controls, owing to denervation of the heart, side effects of immunosuppressive drugs,

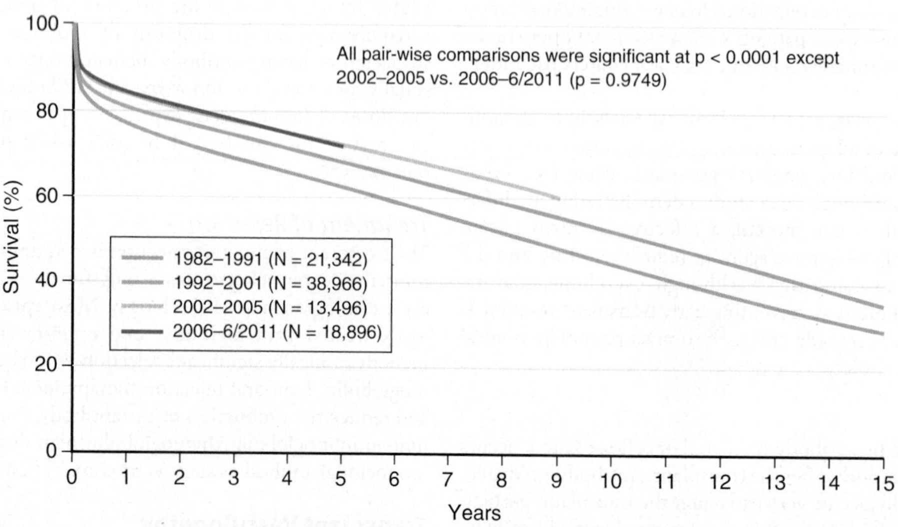

FIGURE 82-2. **Survival by transplant era. Adult heart transplants: Kaplan-Meier survival by era, January 1982-June 2011. (From Lund LH, Edwards LB, Kucheryavaya AY, et al. The Registry of the International Society for Heart and Lung Transplantation: thirtieth official adult heart transplant report—2013; focus theme: age. *J Heart Lung Transplant.* 2013;32:951-964.**

and donor-recipient size mismatch. Many patients return to full-time employment, travel extensively, and participate in vigorous sports such as skiing, running, and hiking. Some young patients may bear children of their own, though genetic counseling is recommended in patients with familial cardiomyopathies (Chapter 60). In female recipients, pregnancy, which requires modification of immunosuppression and close monitoring for allograft rejection, is recommended only in 1-year survivors with normal graft function.

FUTURE DIRECTIONS

With the continuing scarcity of donor organs, physicians must use this scarce resource wisely by selecting candidates who would benefit the greatest over time. In the future, warm preservation techniques may extend harvest time as well and enable the resuscitation of donor organs whose function may initially appear marginal. The field of mechanical circulatory support continues to evolve rapidly, and devices (Chapter 59) rather than transplantation will probably offer a greater chance for long-term survival for most patients with advanced heart failure.

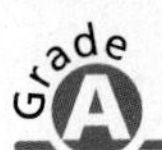

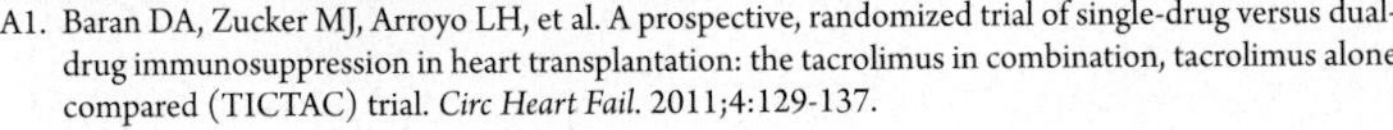

Grade A References

A1. Baran DA, Zucker MJ, Arroyo LH, et al. A prospective, randomized trial of single-drug versus dual-drug immunosuppression in heart transplantation: the tacrolimus in combination, tacrolimus alone compared (TICTAC) trial. *Circ Heart Fail.* 2011;4:129-137.
A2. Ye F, Ying-Bin X, Yu-Guo W, et al. Tacrolimus versus cyclosporine microemulsion for heart transplant recipients: a meta-analysis. *J Heart Lung Transplant.* 2009;28:58-66.
A3. Penninga L, Moller CH, Gustafsson F, et al. Tacrolimus versus cyclosporine as primary immunosuppression after heart transplantation: systematic review with meta-analyses and trial sequential analyses of randomised trials. *Eur J Clin Pharmacol.* 2010;66:1177-1187.
A4. Sanchez-Lazaro IJ, Almenar L, Martinez-Dolz L, et al. A prospective randomized study comparing cyclosporine versus tacrolimus combined with daclizumab, mycophenolate mofetil, and steroids in heart transplantation. *Clin Transplant.* 2011;25:606-613.
A5. Guethoff S, Meiser BM, Groetzner J, et al. Ten-year results of a randomized trial comparing tacrolimus versus cyclosporine a in combination with mycophenolate mofetil after heart transplantation. *Transplantation.* 2013;95:629-634.
A6. Eisen HJ, Kobashigawa J, Keogh A, et al. Three-year results of a randomized, double-blind, controlled trial of mycophenolate mofetil versus azathioprine in cardiac transplant recipients. *J Heart Lung Transplant.* 2005;24:517-525.
A7. Eisen HJ, Kobashigawa J, Starling RC, et al. Everolimus versus mycophenolate mofetil in heart transplantation: a randomized, multicenter trial. *Am J Transplant.* 2013;13:1203-1216.
A8. Pham MX, Teuteberg JJ, Kfoury AG, et al. Gene-expression profiling for rejection surveillance after cardiac transplantation. *N Engl J Med.* 2010;362:1890-1900.
A9. Som R, Morris PJ, Knight SR. Graft vessel disease following heart transplantation: a systemic review of the role of statin therapy. *World J Surg.* 2014;38:2324-2334.

GENERAL REFERENCES

For the General References and other additional features, please visit Expert Consult at https://expertconsult.inkling.com.

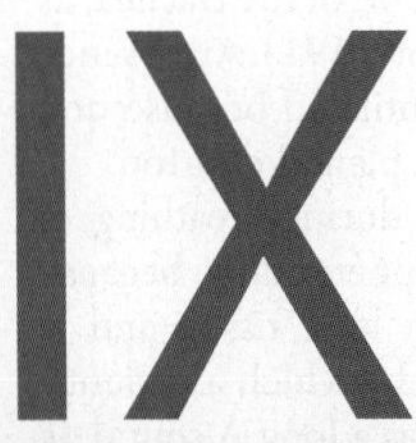

RESPIRATORY DISEASES

83

APPROACH TO THE PATIENT WITH RESPIRATORY DISEASE

MONICA KRAFT

Respiratory symptoms, which are among the most common reasons why patients seek medical care, are responsible for approximately 20% of office visits to a primary care physician. In addition to a careful history, a systematic physical examination is critical for accurate diagnosis.

A careful pulmonary examination complements the cardiac physical examination (Chapter 51). Inspection may reveal an elevated jugular pressure, indicative of right heart failure owing to cor pulmonale (Chapter 68). Cervical or supraclavicular adenopathy (Chapter 168) may be the first clue to suggest a thoracic malignancy (Chapter 191) or mycobacterial infection (Chapter 324). Unilateral arm swelling can be caused by venous thrombosis (Chapter 81), whereas venous engorgement of the head and neck can be caused by a tumor that results in superior vena cava syndrome (see Fig. 99-8 in Chapter 99). On the cardiac examination, a loud pulmonic second heart sound is suggestive of pulmonary hypertension, which also can result in a murmur of tricuspid (see Table 51-7 in Chapter 51) or pulmonic valve insufficiency.

Inspection of the chest may show hyperinflation and reduced diaphragmatic excursion, typical of chronic obstructive pulmonary disease (COPD; Chapter 88), chest wall abnormalities such as kyphoscoliosis (Chapter 99), or diaphragmatic muscle wall weakness as in many hypoventilation syndromes (Chapter 86). Percussion may reveal dullness in patients with pleural effusions or with lung that has been consolidated by pneumonia.

Auscultation of the lungs[1] includes listening at both apices and over both upper and lower lobes, anteriorly and posteriorly, and during inspiration and respiration. Normal lung sounds are heard during inspiration and early expiration as soft and non-musical sounds (Table 83-1). *Bronchial breath sounds,* which sound similar to but often somewhat harsher than normal lung sounds, are heard throughout expiration as well as inspiration, similar to what would be heard by placing a stethoscope over the trachea.

The term *rales* is no longer used and has been replaced by the term *crackles.* Fine crackles are non-musical and heard typically in late inspiration; they are most commonly a sign of heart failure (Chapter 58) or interstitial lung disease (Chapter 92). By comparison, coarse crackles, which unlike fine crackles tend to be transmitted through the mouth and cleared by coughing, are typical of bronchitis (Chapter 96) and COPD (Chapter 88). *Wheezes* are high-pitched, musical sounds heard during expiration and sometimes inspiration, most commonly in asthma (Chapter 87) and sometimes in COPD (Chapter 88). When these diseases are severe, however, the degree of airflow may be insufficient to produce wheezes. A *rhonchus* is a musical, low-pitched sound typically heard in expiration and sometimes during inspiration; it often resolves with coughing. Like coarse crackles, rhonchi are common in bronchitis (Chapter 96) and COPD (Chapter 88). A *pleural friction rub,* which classically occurs during inspiration but sometimes also during expiration, is heard in patients with inflammatory diseases or malignancies involving the pleura (Chapters 99 and 191). *Stridor* is a musical, high-pitched sound that may be audible without a stethoscope and that indicates upper airway obstruction, such as found with acute inflammatory or chronic degenerative diseases of the larynx (Chapter 429) or obstruction of the trachea, as may be caused by intrathoracic malignant diseases (Chapter 191). An absence of breath sounds would be noted if the lung is not ventilated because of a complete bronchial obstruction or if it is displaced by a pleural effusion.

Tactile fremitus, which is a vibratory sensation noted during breathing, is increased in patients who have consolidated lung from pneumonia, because the vibratory sensation conducts better through such lung tissue and is diminished in patients with pleural effusion. *Egophony,* by which a patient's recitation of the long E sound is heard on auscultation as a long A sound, is another indication of consolidation typical of pneumonia.

Evaluation of the abdomen may show a readily palpable liver, sometimes mistaken for hepatomegaly, in patients with COPD and low diaphragm. Examination of the extremities may reveal cyanosis in patients who are hypoxemic, usually with a partial pressure of oxygen less than 55 mm Hg, although it also may be observed in patients with methemoglobinemia (Chapter 158). Clubbing (Chapter 51) is indicative of chronic hypoxemia, as seen in patients with chronic right-to-left-shunting from congenital heart disease (Chapter 69) or other causes of long-standing hypoxemia (Chapters 88 and 92), but it also may be indicative of pleural-based diseases (Chapter 99) as part of the syndrome of hypertrophic pulmonary osteoarthropathy (Chapters 179 and 275).

In patients with suspected hypoxemia, careful analyses of arterial blood gases can help determine its severity and guide therapy (Chapter 103). In patients in whom it is difficult to distinguish heart failure from a pulmonary cause of hypoxemia, an elevated brain natriuretic peptide level may point to a cardiac cause (Chapter 58). Chest imaging (Chapter 84) is a crucial part of the evaluation of many potential pulmonary complaints, and pulmonary function testing (Chapter 85) can be extremely helpful in distinguishing among causes of acute and chronic lung disease.

Among the most common respiratory complaints are cough, wheezing, dyspnea, and hemoptysis. Each can and should be approached in a systematic way.

APPROACH TO THE PATIENT WITH COUGH

Cough is the single most common respiratory complaint for which patients seek care. Referrals of patients with persistently troublesome chronic cough of unknown cause account for 10 to 38% of outpatient visits to respiratory specialists.

For acute cough, defined as coughing that has been present for less than 8 weeks, a careful medical history and physical examination will usually reveal the diagnosis (Table 83-2). Although most acute coughs are of minor

TABLE 83-1 DIAGNOSTIC UTILITY OF LUNG AUSCULTATION

AUSCULTATORY FINDING	CLINICAL CORRELATION
Bronchial breathing	Pneumonia or interstitial lung disease
Fine crackle	Heart failure, interstitial lung disease, alveolar filling disorders
Coarse crackle	Bronchitis
Wheeze	Asthma, COPD
Rhonchus	Bronchitis, COPD
Stridor	Upper-airway obstruction from laryngeal or tracheal inflammation, mass lesions, or external compression
Pleural friction rub	Pleural inflammation or tumors

COPD = chronic obstructive pulmonary disease.

TABLE 83-2 SPECTRUM OF CAUSES AND FREQUENCIES OF COUGH IN IMMUNOCOMPETENT ADULTS

COMMON	LESS COMMON
ACUTE COUGH	
Common cold	Asthma
Acute bacterial sinusitis	Pneumonia
Pertussis	Heart failure
Exacerbations of COPD	Aspiration syndromes
Allergic rhinitis	Pulmonary embolism
Environmental irritant rhinitis	Exacerbation of bronchiectasis
CHRONIC COUGH	
Rhinosinus conditions/UACS	Bronchogenic carcinoma
Asthma	Chronic interstitial pneumonia
Gastroesophageal reflux	Sarcoidosis
Chronic bronchitis	Left heart failure
Eosinophilic bronchitis	Obstructive sleep apnea
Bronchiectasis	Chronic tonsillar enlargement
ACE inhibitors	
Postinfection	

ACE = angiotensin-converting enzyme; COPD = chronic obstructive pulmonary disease; UACS = upper airway cough syndrome.

consequence, cough can occasionally be a sign of a potentially life-threatening illness, such as pulmonary embolism (Chapter 98), pneumonia (Chapter 97), or heart failure (Chapter 58).

Up to 98% of all cases of chronic cough, defined as a cough that persists for more than 8 weeks, in immunocompetent adults are caused by eight common conditions: postnasal drip syndrome from a variety of rhinosinus conditions (Chapter 251), asthma (Chapter 87), gastroesophageal reflux disease (GERD) (Chapter 138), chronic bronchitis (Chapter 88), eosinophilic bronchitis, bronchiectasis (Chapter 90), use of angiotensin-converting enzyme (ACE) inhibitors, and postinfectious cough. Postinfectious cough is usually nonproductive and lasts for 3 to 8 weeks after an upper respiratory tract infection; patients have a normal chest radiograph. Uncommon causes of chronic cough include bronchogenic carcinoma (Chapter 191), chronic interstitial pneumonia (Chapter 92), sarcoidosis (Chapter 95), left ventricular failure (Chapter 58), and aspiration (Chapter 94).

DIAGNOSIS

In chronic cough (Fig. 83-1), the character and timing are not of diagnostic help. A chest radiograph should be obtained in all patients, but other tests should not be ordered in current smokers or patients taking ACE inhibitors until the response to smoking cessation or discontinuation of the drug for at least 4 weeks can be assessed. Sinus radiographs, barium esophagography, methacholine challenge, esophageal pH, and bronchoscopy can be ordered as part of the initial evaluation, depending on the history and physical examination (Table 83-3; see Fig. 83-1). If a test points toward a possible diagnosis, a trial of treatment for that condition is needed to confirm the diagnosis.[2]

TREATMENT

The specific cause of cough can be diagnosed and treated successfully 84 to 98% of the time, so nonspecific therapy[3] aimed to suppress the cough per se is rarely indicated. There is no strong evidence that nonspecific therapies such as antitussives, mucolytics, decongestants, or antihistamine-decongestant

TABLE 83-3 TESTING CHARACTERISTICS OF DIAGNOSTIC PROTOCOL FOR EVALUATION OF CHRONIC COUGH

TESTS	DIAGNOSIS	POSITIVE PREDICTIVE VALUE, %	NEGATIVE PREDICTIVE VALUE, %
Sinus radiograph	Sinusitis	57-81	95-100
Methacholine inhalation challenge	Asthma	60-82	100
Modified barium esophagography	GERD, esophageal stricture	38-63	63-93
Esophageal pH*	GERD	89-100	
Bronchoscopy	Endobronchial mass/lesion	50-89	100

*24-Hour esophageal pH monitoring.
GERD = gastroesophageal reflux disease.

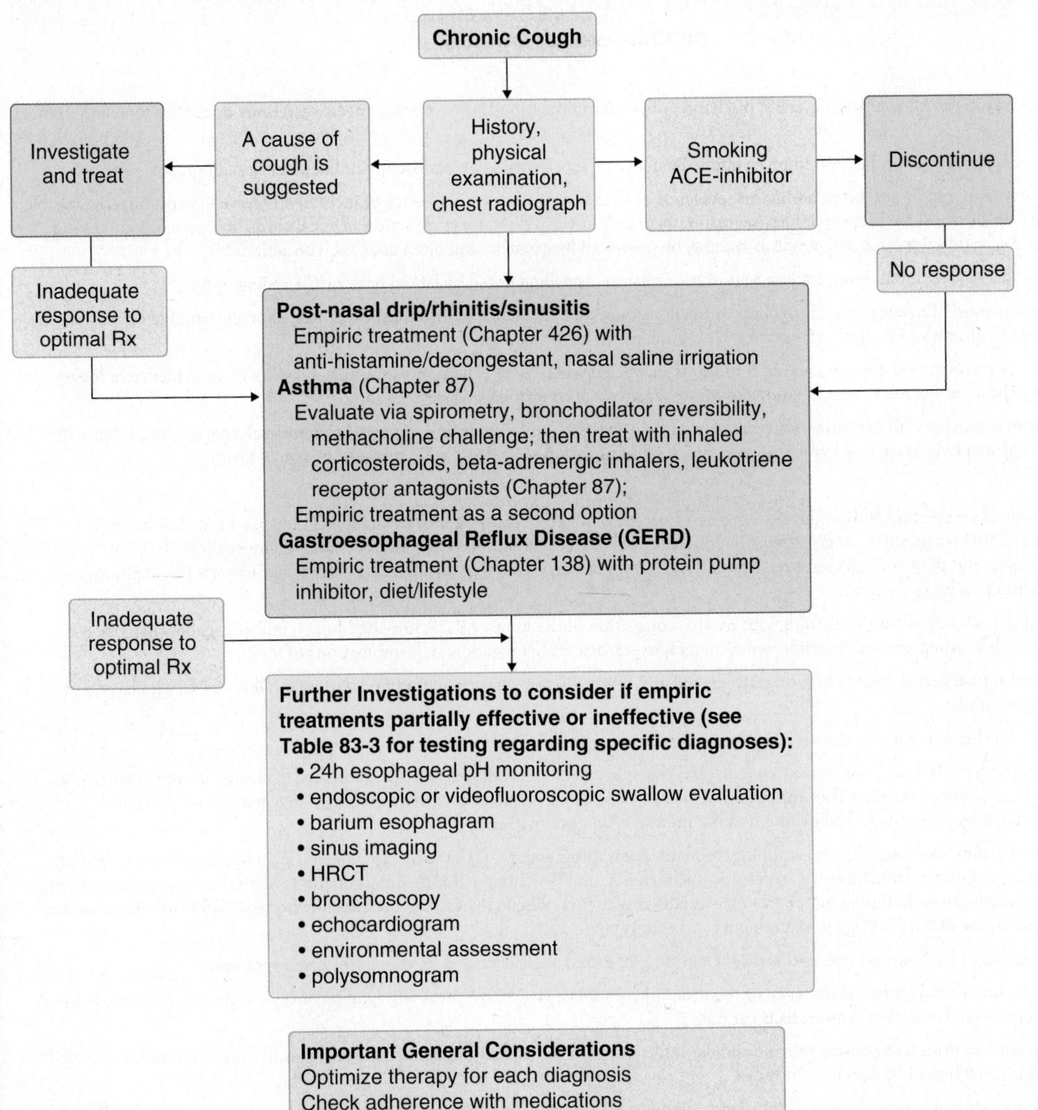

FIGURE 83-1. Algorithm for the management of chronic cough lasting longer than 8 weeks. ACE = angiotensin-converting enzyme; HRCT = high-resolution computed tomography; Rx = prescription.

combinations are efficacious for acute cough in the setting of an upper respiratory tract infection.[A1] For nonspecific persistent cough, effective treatment of chronic gastroesophageal reflux disease with a proton pump inhibitor (Chapter 138) provides no more than modest benefit, with approximately one in five patients improving.[A2] Inhaled corticosteroids can reduce cough but should be used only after evaluation by chest radiography and often spirometry.[A3] Dextromethorphan and codeine-containing cough suppressants can reduce chronic cough by approximately 40%. In adults with refractory chronic cough without active respiratory disease or infection, gabapentin (up to a maximum daily dose of 1800 mg) significantly improves cough-specific quality of life compared with placebo.[A4] For chronic refractory cough despite comprehensive evaluation and opioid therapy, a combination of education, breathing exercises, cough suppression techniques, and counseling can significantly reduce cough and its negative impact on quality of life.[A5] Coughing can also be reduced by training patients to focus externally rather than internally.[A6]

APPROACH TO THE PATIENT WITH WHEEZING

Wheeze is a continuous musical sound that lasts longer than 80 to 100 msec, likely generated by flow through critically narrowed collapsible bronchi. Although expiratory wheezing is a common physical finding in asthma (Chapter 87), the many causes of wheezing (Table 83-4) (e.g., COPD [Chapter 88], pulmonary edema [Chapter 58], bronchiolitis [Chapter 92], bronchiectasis [Chapter 90], and less common entities such as carcinoid [Chapter 232] and parasitic infections) often can be distinguished based on the history, physical examination, and pulmonary function testing (Chapter 85).[4]

DIAGNOSIS

On pulmonary function testing, the shape of inspiratory and expiratory flow-volume loops provide key information about the presence of airway obstruction and whether the obstruction is extrathoracic or intrathoracic (Fig. 83-2). An important cause of extrathoracic obstruction is vocal cord lesions (Chapter 190). Variable intrathoracic obstruction can be caused by tracheomalacia, whereas fixed upper airway obstruction can be caused by a proximal tracheal tumor.

TREATMENT Rx

Treatment of the specific cause will usually lead to complete or at least partial resolution of wheezing. However, treatment of associated asymptomatic or minimally symptomatic gastroesophageal reflux disease is not beneficial.[A7]

APPROACH TO THE PATIENT WITH DYSPNEA

Dyspnea is the sensation of difficult, labored, or unpleasant breathing. The word *unpleasant* is very important to this definition because the labored or difficult breathing encountered by healthy individuals while exercising does

TABLE 83-4 DIAGNOSIS OF SELECTED WHEEZING ILLNESSES OTHER THAN ASTHMA

DISEASES	DISTINGUISHING FEATURES
UPPER AIRWAY DISEASES	
Postnasal drip syndrome	History of postnasal drip, throat clearing, nasal discharge; physical examination shows oropharyngeal secretions or cobblestone appearance to mucosa.
Epiglottis	History of sore throat out of proportion to pharyngitis. Evidence of supraglottitis on endoscopy or lateral neck radiographs.
Vocal cord dysfunction syndrome	Lack of symptomatic response to bronchodilators, presence of stridor plus wheeze in absence of increased $P(A\text{-}a)O_2$; extrathoracic variable obstruction on flow-volume loops; paradoxical inspiratory, and/or early expiratory adduction of vocal cords on laryngoscopy during wheezing. This syndrome can masquerade as asthma, be provoked by exercise, and often coexists with asthma.
Retropharyngeal abscess	History of stiff neck, sore throat, fever, trauma to posterior pharynx; swelling noted by lateral neck or CT radiographs.
Laryngotracheal injury due to tracheal cannulation	History of cannulation of trachea by endotracheal or tracheostomy tube; evidence of intrathoracic or extrathoracic variable obstruction on flow-volume loops, neck and chest radiographs, laryngoscopy, or bronchoscopy.
Neoplasms	Bronchogenic carcinoma, adenoma, or carcinoid tumor is suspected when there is hemoptysis, unilateral wheeze, or evidence of lobar collapse on chest radiograph or combinations of these; diagnosis is confirmed by bronchoscopy.
Anaphylaxis	Abrupt onset of wheezing with urticaria, angioedema, nausea, diarrhea, and hypotension, especially after insect bite, in association with other signs of anaphylaxis such as hypotension or hives, or administration of drug or IV contrast, or family history.
LOWER AIRWAY DISEASES	
COPD	History of dyspnea on exertion and productive cough in cigarette smoker. Because productive cough is nonspecific, it should only be ascribed to COPD when other cough-phlegm syndromes have been excluded, forced expiratory time to empty more than 80% of vital capacity >4 sec, and there is decreased breath sound intensity, unforced wheezing during auscultation, and irreversible, expiratory airflow obstruction on spirometry.
Pulmonary edema	History and physical examination consistent with passive congestion of the lungs, ARDS, impaired lung lymphatics; abnormal chest radiograph, echocardiogram, radionuclide ventriculography, cardiac catheterization, or combinations of these.
Aspiration	History of risk for pharyngeal dysfunction or gastroesophageal reflux disease; abnormal modified barium swallow, 24-hr esophageal pH monitoring, or both.
Pulmonary embolism	History of risk for thromboembolic disease, positive confirmatory tests.
Bronchiolitis	History of respiratory infection, connective tissue disease, transplantation, ulcerative colitis, development of chronic airway obstruction over months to a few years rather than over many years in a nonsmoker; mixed obstructive and restrictive pattern on PFTs and hyperinflation; may be accompanied by fine nodular infiltrates on chest radiograph.
Cystic fibrosis	Combination of productive cough, digital clubbing, bronchiectasis, progressive COPD with *Pseudomonas* sp colonization and infection, obstructive azoospermia, family history, pancreatic insufficiency, and two sweat chloride determinations of > 60 mEq/L; some patients are not diagnosed until adulthood, in one instance as late as age 69 yr; when sweat test is occasionally normal, definitive diagnosis may require nasal transepithelial voltage measurements and genotyping.
Carcinoid syndrome	History of episodes of flushing and watery diarrhea; elevated 5-hydroxyindoleactic acid level in 24-hr urine specimen.
Bronchiectasis	History of episodes of productive cough, fever, or recurrent pneumonias; suggestive chest radiographs or typical chest CT findings; ABPA should be considered when bronchiectasis is central.
Lymphangitic carcinomatosis	History of dyspnea or prior malignancy; reticulonodular infiltrates with or without pleural effusions; suggestive high-resolution chest CT scan; confirmed by bronchoscopy with biopsies.
Parasitic infections	Consider in a nonasthmatic patient who has traveled to an endemic area and complains of fatigue, weight loss, fever; peripheral blood eosinophilia; infiltrates on chest radiograph; stools for ova and parasites for nonfilarial causes; blood serologic studies for filarial causes.

ABPA = allergic bronchopulmonary aspergillosis; ARDS = acute respiratory distress syndrome; COPD = chronic obstructive pulmonary disease; CT = computed tomography; IV = intravenous; $P(A\text{-}a)O_2$ = alveolar-arterial oxygen tension gradient; PFTs = pulmonary function tests.

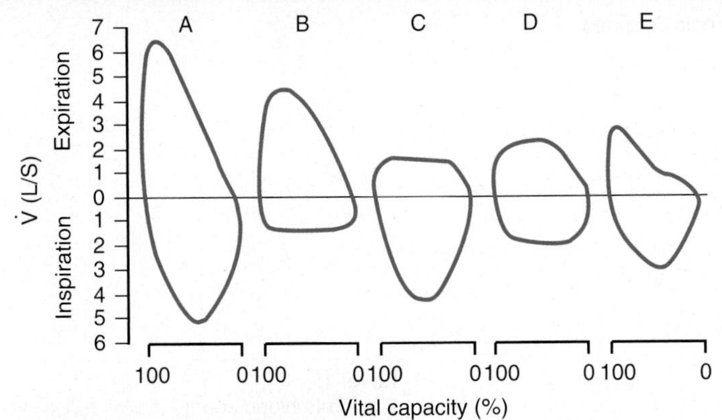

FIGURE 83-2. Schematic flow-volume loop configurations in a spectrum of airway lesions. *A* is normal; *B* is variable extrathoracic upper airway obstruction; *C* is variable intrathoracic upper airway lesion; *D* is fixed upper airway obstruction; and *E* is small airway obstruction. L/S = liters per second; = ventilation.

not qualify as dyspnea because it is at the level expected for the degree of exertion. The sensation of dyspnea is often poorly or vaguely described by the patient. The physiology of dyspnea remains unclear, but multiple neural pathways can be involved in processes that lead to dyspnea.

In acute dyspnea, or shortness of breath of sudden onset, the history, physical examination, and laboratory testing must first focus on potential life-threatening conditions, including pulmonary embolism (Chapter 98), pulmonary edema (Chapters 58 and 59), acute airway obstruction from anaphylaxis or foreign bodies, pneumothorax (Chapter 99), or pneumonia (Chapter 97). For chronic dyspnea, specific conditions to consider include COPD (Chapter 88), asthma (Chapter 87), interstitial lung disease (Chapter 92), heart failure (Chapter 58), cardiomyopathy (Chapter 60), GERD (Chapter 138), other respiratory diseases, or hyperventilation syndrome (Table 83-5).

DIAGNOSIS

A chest radiograph, electrocardiogram (ECG), pulmonary function testing, and an exercise test with electrocardiographic monitoring and pulse oximetry at rest and during exercise are key tests to assess patients with unexplained dyspnea (Fig. 83-3).[5] For acute dyspnea, B-type natriuretic peptide testing can be extremely helpful in distinguishing heart failure from other causes.[A8] The utility of more detailed pulmonary testing with maximal inspiratory and expiratory pressures, flow-volume loops, with or without methacholine challenge, computed tomographic screening of the chest, and echocardiography depends on history and physical examination and the results of these tests. When GERD is a suspected cause of dyspnea, a modified barium esophagogram or 24-hour esophageal pH monitoring, or both, should be considered (Chapter 138). Other more invasive tests such as cardiac catheterization or lung biopsy may be indicated when the results of less invasive tests have not been conclusive.

TREATMENT Rx

Whenever possible, the final determination of the cause of dyspnea is made by observing which specific therapy eliminates it. Because dyspnea may be simultaneously the result of more than one condition, it may be necessary to treat more than one condition.

TABLE 83-5 DISEASES THAT CAUSE DYSPNEA GROUPED BY PHYSIOLOGIC MECHANISMS OF ACTION*

INCREASED RESPIRATORY DRIVE
Stimulation of Chemoreceptors
Conditions leading to acute hypoxemia
Impaired gas exchanger (e.g., asthma, pulmonary embolism, pneumonia, congestive heart failure[†])
Environmental hypoxia (e.g., altitude, contained space with fire)
Conditions leading to increased dead space, acute hypercapnia
Impaired gas exchanger (e.g., acute, severe asthma; exacerbation of COPD; severe pulmonary edema)
Impaired ventilator pump (e.g., muscle weakness, airflow obstruction)
Metabolic acidosis
Renal disease (e.g., renal failure, renal tubular acidosis)
Decreased oxygen carrying capacity (e.g., anemia)
Decreased release of oxygen to tissues (e.g., hemoglobinopathy)
Decreased cardiac output
Stimulation of Pulmonary Receptors (irritant, mechanical, vascular)[‡]
Interstitial lung disease
Pleural effusion (compression atelectasis)
Pulmonary vascular disease (e.g., thromboembolism, idiopathic pulmonary hypertension)
Heart failure
Mild asthma
Behavioral Factors
Hyperventilation syndrome, anxiety disorders, panic attacks
VENTILATORY PUMP: INCREASED EFFORT OR WORK OF BREATHING
Muscle Weakness
Myasthenia gravis, Guillain-Barré syndrome, spinal cord injury, myopathy, postpoliomyelitis syndrome
Decreased compliance of the chest wall
Severe kyphoscoliosis, obesity, pleural effusion
Airflow Obstruction (including increased resistive load from narrowing of the airways and increased elastic load from hyperinflation)
Asthma, COPD, laryngospasm, aspiration of foreign body, bronchitis

*Some diseases appear in more than one category, because they act via several physiologic mechanisms.
†Heart failure includes both systolic and diastolic dysfunction. Systolic dysfunction may produce dyspnea at rest and with activity. Diastolic dysfunction typically leads to symptoms primarily with exercise. In addition to the mechanisms noted above, systolic heart failure may also produce dyspnea via metaboreceptors, which are postulated to exist in muscles and be stimulated by changes in the metabolic milieu when oxygen delivery does not meet oxygen demand.
‡These conditions probably produce dyspnea by a combination of increased ventilator drive and primary sensory input from the receptors.
COPD = chronic obstructive pulmonary disease.

APPROACH TO THE PATIENT WITH HEMOPTYSIS

Hemoptysis is the expectoration of blood from the lung parenchyma or airways.[6] Hemoptysis may be scant, with just the appearance of streaks of bright red blood in the sputum, or massive, with the expectoration of a large volume of blood. Massive hemoptysis, which is defined as the expectoration of at least 600 mL of blood in 24 to 48 hours, may occur in 3 to 10% of patients with hemoptysis. Dark red clots also may be expectorated when the blood has been present in the lungs for days.

Pseudohemoptysis, which is the expectoration of blood from a source other than the lower respiratory tract, may cause diagnostic confusion when patients cannot clearly describe the source of the bleeding. Pseudohemoptysis can occur when blood from the oral cavity, nares, pharynx, or tongue clings to the back of the throat and initiates the cough reflex, or when patients who have hematemesis aspirate into the lower respiratory tract. When the oropharynx is colonized with *Serratia marcescens*, a red-pigment–producing aerobic gram-negative rod, the sputum can also be red and be confused with hemoptysis.

Hemoptysis can be caused by a wide variety of disorders. Virtually all causes of hemoptysis (Table 83-6) may result in massive hemoptysis, but massive hemoptysis is most frequently caused by infection (e.g., tuberculosis [Chapter 324], bronchiectasis and lung abscess [Chapter 90], and cancer [Chapter 191]). Infections with aspergilloma (Chapter 339) and in patients with cystic fibrosis (Chapter 89) also are associated with massive hemoptysis. Iatrogenic causes of massive hemoptysis include rupture of a pulmonary artery after less than 0.2% of cases of balloon-guided flotation catheterization and tracheal artery fistula as a complication of tracheostomy.

In nonmassive hemoptysis, the cause is bronchitis in more than one third of cases (Chapter 96), bronchogenic carcinoma (Chapter 191) in one fifth of cases, tuberculosis (Chapter 324) in 7%, pneumonia (Chapter 97) in 5%, and bronchiectasis in 1% (Chapter 90). Using a systematic diagnostic approach (see later), the cause of hemoptysis can be found in 68 to 98% of cases. The remaining 2 to 32% have idiopathic or central hemoptysis, which occurs most commonly in men between 30 and 50 years of age. Prolonged follow-up of idiopathic hemoptysis almost always fails to reveal the source of bleeding, even though 10% continue to have occasional episodes of hemoptysis.

DIAGNOSIS

The diagnostic evaluation for hemoptysis begins with a detailed medical history and a complete physical examination. Information on the amount of

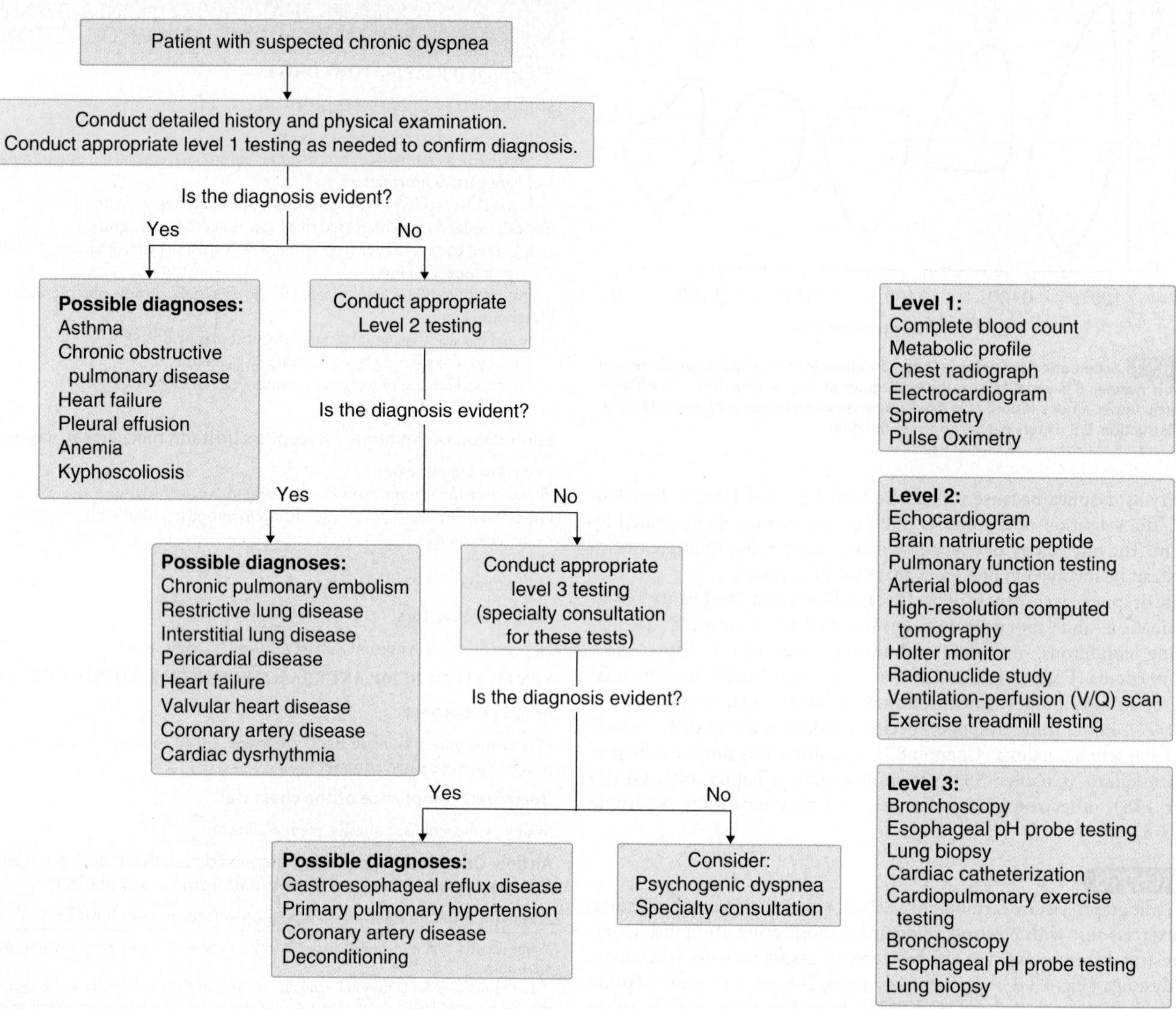

FIGURE 83-3. **Algorithm outlining the approach to chronic dyspnea.** (Modified from Karnani NG, Reisfield GM, Wilson GR. Evaluation of chronic dyspnea. *Am Fam Phys.* 2005;71:1529-1537.)

TABLE 83-6 COMMON CAUSES OF MASSIVE HEMOPTYSIS

Cardiovascular
- Arterial bronchial fistula
- Heart failure, especially from mitral stenosis
- Pulmonary arteriovenous fistula

Diffuse intrapulmonary hemorrhage

Diffuse parenchymal disease

Iatrogenic
- Malposition of chest tube
- Pulmonary artery rupture following pulmonary arterial catheterization
- Tracheoarterial fistula

Infections
- Aspergilloma
- Bronchiectasis
- Bronchitis
- Cystic fibrosis
- Lung abscess
- Sporotrichosis
- Tuberculosis

Malignancies
- Bronchogenic carcinoma
- Leukemia
- Metastatic cancer

Trauma

Drugs and toxins
- Penicillamine
- Solvents
- Crack cocaine
- Trimelletic anhydride
- Bevacizumab

bleeding should be obtained, as well as details about the frequency, timing, and duration of hemoptysis. For example, repeated episodes of hemoptysis occurring over a period of months to years suggest a bronchial adenoma or bronchiectasis as the cause, whereas small amounts of hemoptysis occurring every day for weeks are more likely to be caused by bronchogenic carcinoma. A travel history can suggest coccidioidomycosis (Chapter 333) and histoplasmosis (Chapter 332) in the United States, paragonimiasis and ascariasis (Chapter 358) in the Far East, and schistosomiasis (Chapter 355) in South America. Orthopnea and paroxysmal nocturnal dyspnea suggest heart failure (Chapter 58), especially from mitral stenosis (Chapter 75). In patients who have occupational exposure to trimellitic anhydride, which occurs when heated metal surfaces are sprayed with a corrosion-resistant epoxy resin, hemoptysis can be part of the postexposure syndrome. In a patient with the triad of upper airway disease, lower airway disease, and renal disease, granulomatosis with polyangiitis (Chapter 270) should be suspected. Pulmonary hemorrhage also may be a presenting manifestation of systemic lupus erythematosus (Chapter 266). Goodpasture syndrome, which typically occurs in young men, is also associated with renal disease (Chapter 121). Diffuse alveolar hemorrhage occurs in 20% of cases during autologous bone marrow transplantation (Chapter 178) and should be suspected in patients who have undergone recent bone marrow transplantation when they present with cough, dyspnea, hypoxemia, and diffuse pulmonary infiltrates.

On physical examination, inspection of the skin and mucous membranes may show telangiectasias suggesting hereditary hemorrhagic telangiectasia (Chapter 173) or ecchymoses and petechiae, suggesting a hematologic abnormality (Chapter 172). Pulsations transmitted to a tracheostomy cannula should heighten suspicion of a tracheal artery fistula. Inspection of the thorax should show evidence of recent or old chest trauma, and unilateral wheeze or crackles may herald localized disease such as a bronchial adenoma or carcinoma. Although pulmonary embolism (Chapter 98) cannot be definitively diagnosed on physical examination, tachypnea, phlebitis, and pleural friction rub suggest this disorder. If crackles are heard on the chest examination, heart failure as well as other diseases causing diffuse pulmonary hemorrhage (see earlier) or idiopathic pulmonary hemosiderosis (Chapter 92) should be considered. Careful cardiovascular examination may help diagnose mitral stenosis (Chapter 75), pulmonary artery fistulas, or pulmonary hypertension (Chapter 68).

Routine laboratory studies should include a complete blood count, urinalysis, and coagulation studies. The complete blood count may suggest an infection, hematologic disorder, or chronic blood loss. Urinalysis may reveal hematuria and suggest the presence of a systemic disease (e.g., Wegener granulomatosis, Goodpasture syndrome, systemic lupus erythematosus) associated with renal disease. Coagulation studies may uncover a hematologic disorder that is primarily responsible for hemoptysis or that contributes to excessive bleeding from another disease. The ECG may help suggest the presence of a cardiovascular disorder. Although as many as 30% of patients with hemoptysis have a normal chest radiograph, routine chest radiographs may be diagnostically valuable.

Bronchoscopy can localize the bleeding site in up to 93% of patients by fiberoptic bronchoscopy and in up to 86% with rigid bronchoscopy.[7] It may establish sites of bleeding different from those suggested by the chest radiograph. The best results are obtained when bronchoscopy is performed during or within 24 hours of active bleeding, and rates of diagnosis fall to approximately 50% by 48 hours after bleeding. When there is no active bleeding, bronchoscopy with bronchoalveolar lavage can be helpful in patients thought to have diffuse intrapulmonary hemorrhage. Typical findings include bright red or blood-tinged lavage fluid from multiple lobes in both lungs or a substantial number of hemosiderin-laden macrophages (i.e., at least 20% of the total number of alveolar macrophages).

Depending on the results of the initial evaluation and the likely categories of hemoptysis, additional diagnostic tests can be helpful (Table 83-7). Bronchoscopy may not be needed in patients who have stable chronic bronchitis (Chapter 88) with one episode of blood streaking or who have acute tracheobronchitis (Chapter 88). Bronchoscopy also may not be needed with obvious cardiovascular causes of hemoptysis, such as heart failure and pulmonary embolism.

TABLE 83-7 EXAMPLES OF SPECIAL EVALUATIONS FOR HEMOPTYSIS ACCORDING TO CATEGORY OF DISEASE*

TRACHEOBRONCHIAL DISORDERS
Expectorated sputum for TB, parasites, fungi, and cytology
Bronchoscopy (if not done)
High-resolution chest CT scan
LOCALIZED PARENCHYMAL DISEASES
Expectorated sputum for TB, parasites, fungi, and cytology
Chest CT scan
Lung biopsy with special stains
DIFFUSE PARENCHYMAL DISEASES
Expectorated sputum for cytology
Blood for BUN, creatinine, ANA, RF, complement, cryoglobulins, ANCA, anti-GBM antibody
Lung or kidney biopsy with special stains
CARDIOVASCULAR DISORDERS
Echocardiogram
Arterial blood gas on 21% and 100% oxygen
Ventilation-perfusion scans
Pulmonary arteriogram
Aortogram, contrast-enhanced CT scan
HEMATOLOGIC DISORDERS
Coagulation studies
Bone marrow

*This table is not meant to be all inclusive.
ANA = antinuclear antibody; ANCA = antineutrophil cytoplasmic antibody; BUN = blood urea nitrogen; CT = computed tomography; GBM = glomerular basement membrane; RF = rheumatoid factor; TB = tuberculosis.

TREATMENT

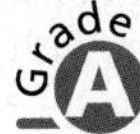

Treatment is targeted toward the cause of hemoptysis. Bronchoscopic approaches (Chapter 101) are increasingly used for endobronchial lesions.

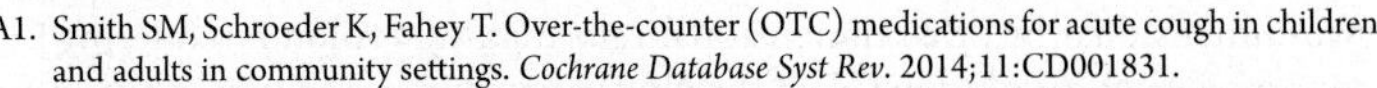

Grade A References

A1. Smith SM, Schroeder K, Fahey T. Over-the-counter (OTC) medications for acute cough in children and adults in community settings. *Cochrane Database Syst Rev.* 2014;11:CD001831.
A2. Shaheen NJ, Crockett SD, Bright SD, et al. Randomised clinical trial: high-dose acid suppression for chronic cough—a double-blind, placebo-controlled study. *Aliment Pharmacol Ther.* 2011;33:225-234.
A3. Johnstone KJ, Chang AB, Fong KM, et al. Inhaled corticosteroids for subacute and chronic cough in adults. *Cochrane Database Syst Rev.* 2013;3:CD009305.
A4. Ryan NM, Birring SS, Gibson PG. Gabapentin for refractory chronic cough: a randomised, double-blind, placebo-controlled trial. *Lancet.* 2012;380:1583-1589.
A5. Chamberlain S, Birring SS, Garrod R. Nonpharmacological interventions for refractory chronic cough patients: systematic review. *Lung.* 2014;192:75-85.
A6. Janssens T, Silva M, Davenport PW, et al. Attentional modulation of reflex cough. *Chest.* 2014;146:135-141.
A7. Mastronarde JG, Anthonisen NR, Castro M, et al. Efficacy of esomeprazole for treatment of poorly controlled asthma. *N Engl J Med.* 2009;360:1487-1499.
A8. Lam LL, Cameron PA, Schneider HG, et al. Meta-analysis: effect of B-type natriuretic peptide testing on clinical outcomes in patients with acute dyspnea in the emergency setting. *Ann Intern Med.* 2010;153:728-735.

GENERAL REFERENCES

For the General References and other additional features, please visit Expert Consult at https://expertconsult.inkling.com.

84 IMAGING IN PULMONARY DISEASE

PAUL STARK

IMAGING OF THE LUNGS, MEDIASTINUM, AND CHEST WALL

EPIDEMIOLOGY

Worldwide, chest radiography is the most commonly performed imaging procedure; more than 75 million chest radiographs are performed every year in the United States alone. Chest radiographs provide useful information about the patient's anatomy and disease at a minimal monetary cost and with radiation exposure that most experts agree is negligible (0.05 to 0.1 mSv) (Chapter 20). Although many novel imaging techniques are available, the conventional chest radiograph remains invaluable in the initial assessment of disorders of the lung, pleura, mediastinum, and chest wall.

Imaging Techniques

The standard chest radiograph is performed at 2 m from the x-ray tube focal spot to the image detector, in frontal and lateral projections. If possible, the radiographs should be obtained with the patient inhaling to total lung capacity. These images, which provide views of the lungs, mediastinum, and chest wall simultaneously, are typically acquired, stored, and distributed digitally.

Bedside Radiography

Although bedside radiography accounts for a large number of chest radiographs, especially in the intensive care unit (ICU), the images obtained are generally of lower technical quality, cost more, and are more difficult to interpret. Lung volumes are low, thereby leading to crowding of vascular structures, and the low kilovoltage technique required for the mobile equipment yields radiographs with overexposed lungs and an underpenetrated mediastinum. The anteroposterior projection and the slightly lordotic angulation of the x-ray beam combine to distort the basal lung structures and magnify the cardiac silhouette. Recumbent studies also make recognition of pleural effusions or pneumothoraces more difficult. In the ICU, chest radiography can be ordered selectively rather than as a daily routine, without compromising care.[1]

Computed Tomography

Computed tomography (CT) has multiple advantages over conventional radiography. It displays cross-sectional anatomy free of superimposition, with a 10-fold higher contrast resolution. Multislice CT scanners acquire a continuous, volumetric, near-isotropic data set with possibilities for high-quality two-dimensional or three-dimensional reformatting (volume rendering) in any plane. High-resolution CT of the lung parenchyma is an important application; narrow collimation of the beam combined with an edge-enhancing high spatial frequency algorithm results in exquisite detail of normal and abnormal lungs, and correlation with pathologic anatomy is high.

Magnetic Resonance Imaging

Magnetic resonance imaging (MRI) depends on the magnetic properties of hydrogen atoms. Magnetic coils and radio frequency coils lead to induction, excitation, and eventual readout of magnetized protons. The molecular environment of hydrogen atoms will affect the rate at which they release energy; this energy yields a spatial distribution of signals that is converted into an image by computer algorithms, similar to CT. Because of its soft tissue specificity, MRI has applications in the assessment of chest wall invasion, mediastinal infiltration, and diaphragmatic involvement by lung cancer or malignant mesothelioma.

Positron Emission Tomography

Fluorodeoxyglucose positron emission tomography (FDG-PET) uses labeled fluorodeoxyglucose to image the glycolytic pathway of tumor cells or other metabolically active tissues with affinity for glucose. This technique has proved helpful in studying intrathoracic tumors and has facilitated the work-up of solitary pulmonary nodules. Integrated PET-CT scans have improved the diagnosis and staging of intrathoracic tumors.[2]

Ultrasonography

Outside the heart, ultrasonography plays only a limited role in thoracic imaging. Its primary use is to localize pleural effusions and guide their drainage (Chapter 99). In the intensive care setting, ultrasound also may help with the diagnosis of pneumothorax and diffuse alveolar damage.

Evaluation of Chest Images

Images of the chest are best evaluated by examining regions of the lung for specific findings and relating these findings to known diagnostic groups. A number of critical radiographic features should be considered, with an appreciation for the known causes of these changes.

Diffuse Lung Disease

Diffuse lung disease is an overall term for a number of related abnormal parenchymal radiographic patterns. Although radiologists have attempted to separate alveolar from interstitial lung disease radiographically, this distinction is no longer recommended because the correlation between the radiographic localization to a compartment and the actual histopathologic findings is relatively poor.[3] For example, nodular patterns can be produced by either interstitial or alveolar disease. Conversely, so-called alveolar disease processes can induce an interstitial reaction. Ground-glass opacities can be induced by either alveolar or interstitial disease. Air bronchograms, the presumed paradigm of air space disease, can be identified in a small percentage of patients with predominantly interstitial lung disease, such as sarcoidosis, pulmonary lymphoma, and pulmonary calcinosis.

Because of such limitations, a graphically descriptive approach that combines analysis of predominant opacities, assessment of lung expansion, and distribution and profusion of disease yields a differential diagnosis. The term *infiltrate* should be avoided; instead, the term *pulmonary opacities* should be used, with opacities further classified as large (i.e., >1 cm in largest dimension) or small (i.e., <1 cm in diameter).

Large Opacities

Large opacities (Table 84-1) are characterized according to their distribution. Diffuse homogeneous opacities are typical for diffuse alveolar damage (Fig. 84-1), increased permeability (noncardiogenic) pulmonary edema, diffuse viral pneumonia (see Fig. 84-1B), or *Pneumocystis jirovecii* pneumonia. Multifocal patchy opacities (see Fig. 84-1C) are found in multifocal bronchopneumonia, recurrent aspiration, or vasculitis (Fig. 84-E1). Lobar opacities without atelectasis are typically seen in lobar pneumonia (Figs. 84-2, 84-E2, and 84-E3). Lobar opacities with atelectasis often result from obstruction of a lobar bronchus by foreign bodies, tumors, or mucous plugs. Perihilar opacities are seen in hydrostatic pulmonary edema as a result of left-sided heart failure (Figs. 84-3A and B; 84-E4), renal failure, volume overload, or pulmonary hemorrhage.

TABLE 84-1 CLASSIFICATION OF LARGE PULMONARY OPACITIES

Diffuse homogeneous
Multifocal patchy
Lobar without atelectasis
Lobar with atelectasis
Perihilar
Peripheral

TABLE 84-2 PATTERNS OF SMALL PULMONARY OPACITIES

Micronodular
Acinar
Linear
Reticular
Bronchial
Arterial
Destructive

Small Opacities

In contrast to the large pulmonary opacities, a number of radiographic patterns characterize small pulmonary opacities in diffuse lung disease. It is helpful to differentiate small nodular, linear, reticular, or combined patterns (Table 84-2).[4]

Nodular Patterns

Micronodular opacities, which include nodules 1 mm and smaller in diameter, can result from talc granulomatosis in intravenous drug abusers (Chapter 34), alveolar microlithiasis, rare cases of silicosis, talcosis, coal workers' pneumoconiosis (Chapter 93), and beryllium-induced lung diseases (Chapter 93), as well as from occasional cases of sarcoidosis (Chapter 95) or hemosiderosis. The nodular pattern includes nodules up to 1 cm in diameter. Frequent causes include infections or inflammatory granulomata such as miliary tuberculosis (Chapter 324), sarcoidosis (Chapter 95), fungal diseases, hypersensitivity pneumonia, and Langerhans cell histiocytosis (Chapter 92).

Linear Patterns

Linear patterns, also called Kerley lines, are mostly a reflection of thickened interlobular septa. Kerley A lines, which radiate 2 to 4 cm from the hilum toward the pulmonary periphery and particularly toward the upper lobes (Fig. 84-4), reflect thickening of the axial interstitial compartment and can be a feature of left ventricular failure or allergic reactions. Kerley B lines, which reflect thickening of the subpleural interstitial compartment, typically are approximately 1 cm in length and 1 mm in thickness and usually found in the periphery of the lower lobes, abutting the pleura. The B lines are characteristic of subacute and chronic left ventricular failure (Chapter 58), mitral valve disease (Chapter 75), lymphangitic carcinomatosis, viral pneumonia, and pulmonary fibrosis (Chapter 92). Kerley C lines, which are rarely diagnosed by radiologists, result from thickening of the lung parenchymal interstitium and form a reticular pattern on chest radiographs.

Reticular Patterns

Reticular patterns are small polygonal, irregular, or curvilinear opacities on chest radiographs (Fig. 84-5). The differential diagnosis varies according to the timeline of the pathologic change. Acute onset of a reticular pattern can occur in interstitial pulmonary edema (e.g., due to left-sided heart failure), atypical pneumonias (e.g., viral or mycoplasmal pneumonia), early exudative changes in a connective tissue disorder (e.g., systemic lupus

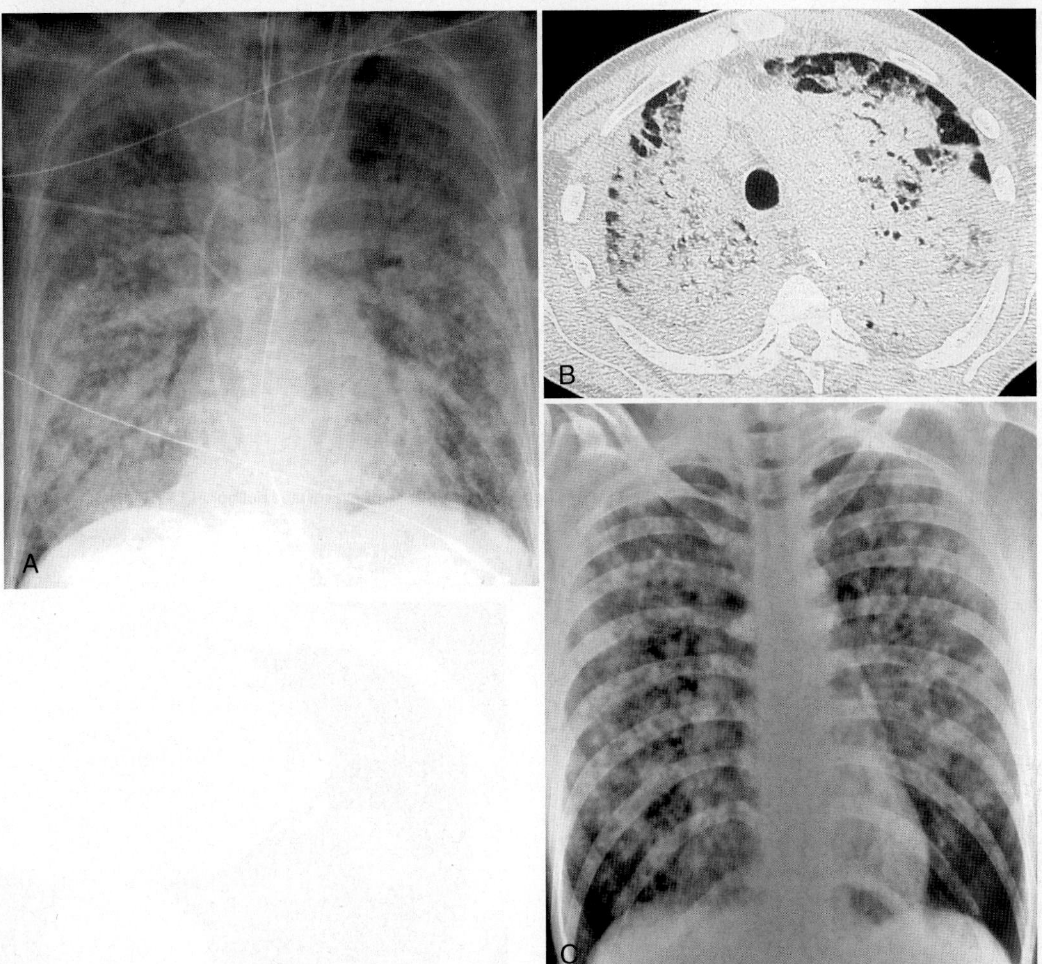

FIGURE 84-1. **Diffuse alveolar damage. A,** Chest radiograph shows diffuse homogeneous opacification of both lungs with clearly visible air bronchograms. **B,** Computed tomographic scan demonstrates diffuse consolidation with air-bronchograms extending to the periphery of both lungs in a patient with community-acquired pneumonia. **C,** Patient with acute varicella pneumonia. Chest radiograph demonstrates multiple acinar nodules with tendency for confluence, yielding multifocal patchy parenchymal opacification.

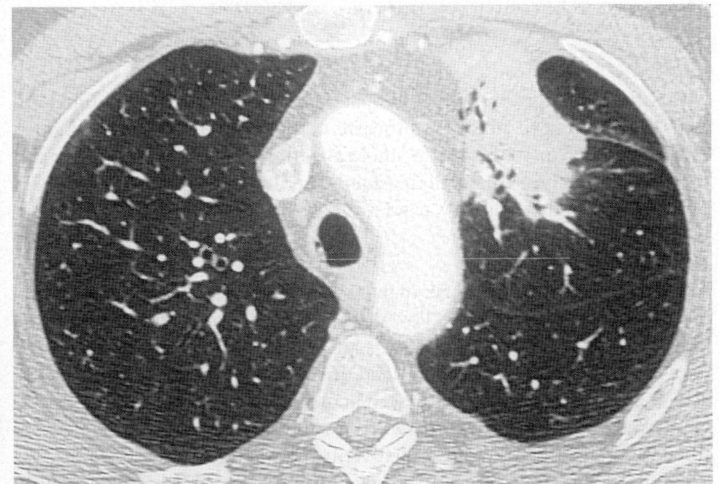

FIGURE 84-2. **Bacterial pneumonia in the left upper lobe.** Computed tomographic scan demonstrates segmental consolidation of the anterior segment of the left upper lobe with air-bronchograms.

erythematosus; Chapter 266), and acute allergic reactions (e.g., transfusion reactions [Chapter 177] or reactions to *Hymenoptera* stings). The common chronic processes resulting in a reticular pattern are idiopathic interstitial pneumonias (Chapter 92), connective tissue diseases (particularly scleroderma and rheumatoid lung), asbestosis (Chapter 93), radiation fibrosis (Chapter 92), end-stage hypersensitivity pneumonia (Chapters 92 and 93), drug reactions, lymphangitic spread of cancer, end-stage granulomatous infection, lymphoma in its bronchovascular form, Kaposi sarcoma in its bronchovascular manifestation, and sarcoidosis.

Honeycombing

Honeycombing, which is an indication of end-stage interstitial lung disease (Chapter 92), reflects a restructuring of pulmonary anatomy accompanied by bronchiolectasis. Honeycombs (Fig. 84-6) form a multilayer of small subpleural spaces between 3 and 10 mm in diameter. They can be distinguished from paraseptal emphysema by their thicker wall and multiple layers.

Alveolar Pattern

An alveolar (Chapter 91) or air space pattern is characterized by acinar nodules, 0.6 to 1 cm in diameter. These nodules encompass more than the acinus, in the strict anatomic sense, with surrounding peribronchiolar lung tissue. Other patterns include ground-glass opacities (a reflection of incomplete alveolar filling), coalescent large opacities, consolidation involving whole lobes or segments, opacification in a bronchocentric distribution, air bronchograms, and air alveolograms. These radiographic features are helpful in placing a disease into a particular radiologic category, but the radiographic pattern called *alveolar* does not simply correspond to exclusive histologic alveolar filling because the interstitial compartment is involved as well in most cases. A more accurate description is parenchymal rather than alveolar opacification or consolidation.

Bronchial Patterns

Bronchial patterns, as best depicted by diffuse bronchiectasis (Chapter 90), are seen on conventional radiographs as linear, tubular, or cystic lucencies and opacities that follow the expected path of bronchi, so-called tramlines because they resemble tram tracks. Mucoid impaction, as seen in patients

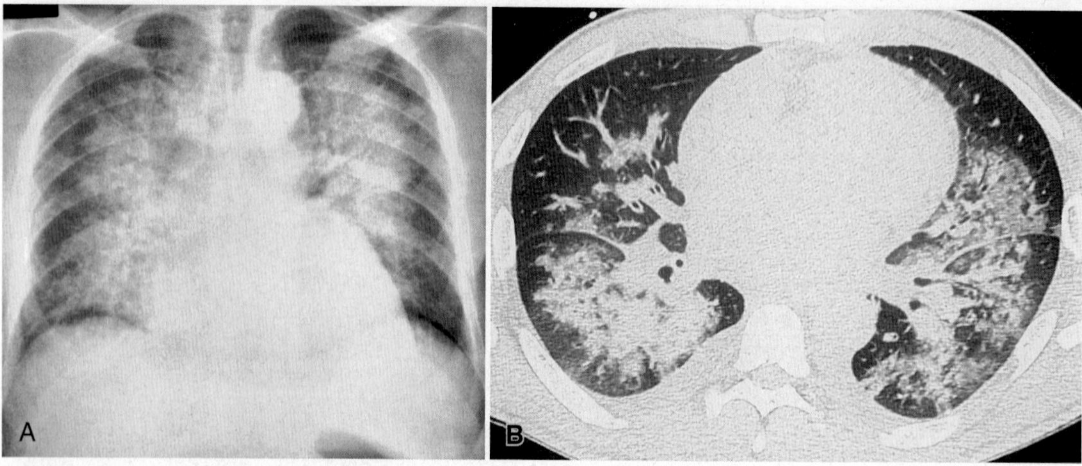

FIGURE 84-3. **A, Pulmonary edema.** Chest frontal radiograph demonstrates classic "batwing" distribution of hydrostatic pulmonary edema. **B,** Computed tomographic scan shows bilateral perihilar consolidations and a small right pleural effusion in a patient with pulmonary edema.

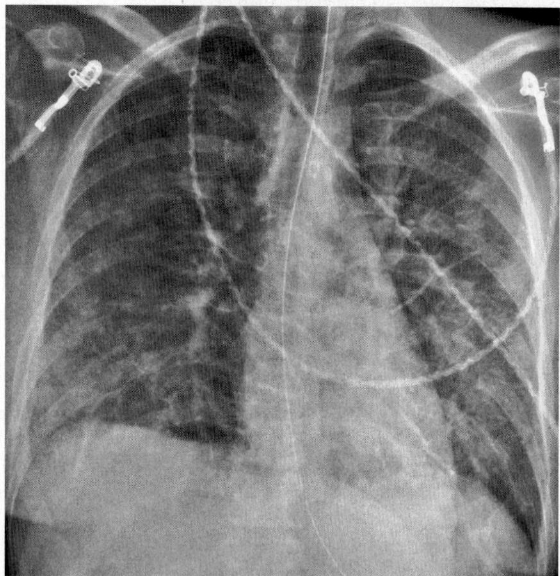

FIGURE 84-4. **Patient with known transfusion reaction.** Chest radiograph displays ground-glass opacification of both lungs and bilateral Kerley A lines, presenting as long linear structures extending from the hilar regions into the pulmonary periphery.

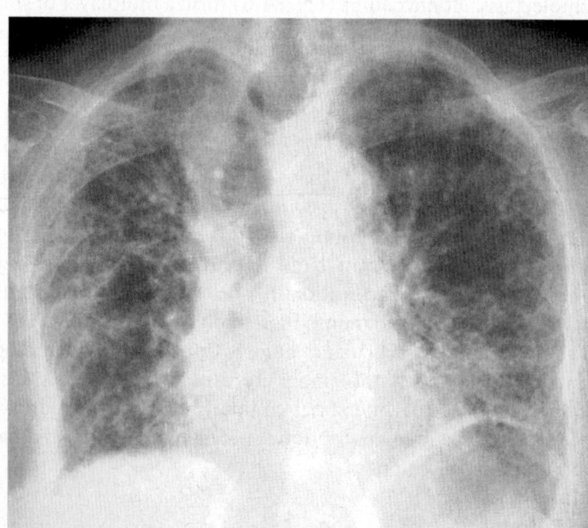

FIGURE 84-5. **Diffuse reticular lung disease.** Chest radiograph in a 94-year-old patient with diffuse reticular opacities due to idiopathic pulmonary fibrosis with honeycombing and traction bronchiectases. The lung volumes are typically reduced by a decreased pulmonary compliance.

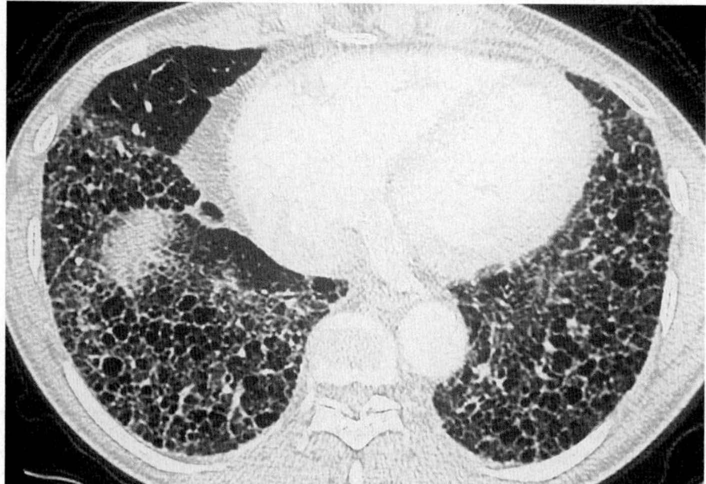

FIGURE 84-6. Honeycombing in a patient with idiopathic pulmonary fibrosis and usual interstitial pneumonia. Computed tomographic scan shows multiple bibasal reticular opacities with honeycombing and traction bronchiectases.

with asthma, allergic bronchopulmonary aspergillosis, or plastic bronchitis, leads to opacities described as toothpaste, cluster of grapes, or finger-in-glove. The "dirty lung" pattern seen in smokers with chronic bronchitis (Chapter 88) results from bronchial wall thickening, peribronchial fibrosis, respiratory bronchiolitis, and pulmonary arterial hypertension.

Vascular Patterns

Arterial patterns reflect changes in pulmonary perfusion. The term *caudalization* reflects the normal blood flow distribution pattern in an upright person in which the basal pulmonary vessels are two to three times wider than the upper lobe vasculature. *Cephalization,* in which the ratios of diameters of vessels are reversed, is frequently seen in recumbent persons, in whom it may be considered normal; however, when it is present in individuals imaged in the upright position, it indicates left ventricular failure, mitral valve disease, or basal emphysema (Fig. 84-7). Equalization, or balanced flow with well-demonstrated vessels to upper and lower lung zones, is found in hyperkinetic circulation due to anemia, obesity, pregnancy, hyperthyroidism, or left-to-right shunts. Equalization or balanced flow with oligemia can be seen in hypovolemia, diffuse emphysema, or right-to-left shunts. Centralization reflects dilation of central pulmonary vessels, with accompanying normal or diminished peripheral circulation. Typically, it is seen in pulmonary arterial hypertension (Fig. 84-8). Lateralization of flow, favoring one lung over the other, also called *asymmetrical perfusion,* is visible with unilateral emphysema, unilateral bronchiolitis obliterans (Swyer-James-McLeod syndrome), or unilateral obstruction of the pulmonary artery. Locally dilated pulmonary vessels occur adjacent to affected oligemic lung regions in patchy emphysema, multiple pulmonary emboli, arteriovenous malformations, and

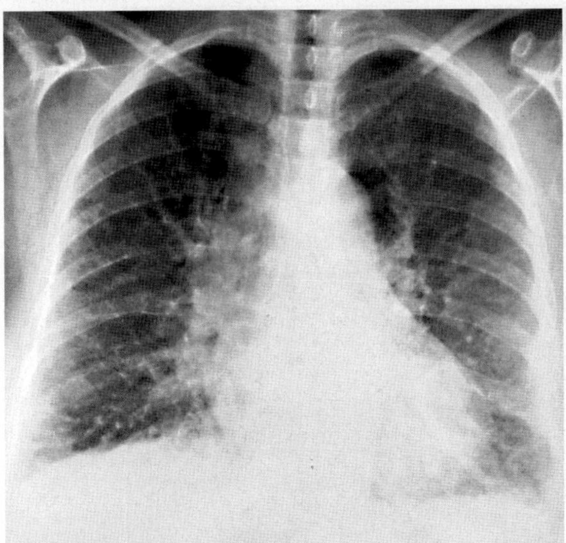

FIGURE 84-7. Patient with left ventricular failure. Chest frontal radiograph shows cephalization of pulmonary blood flow.

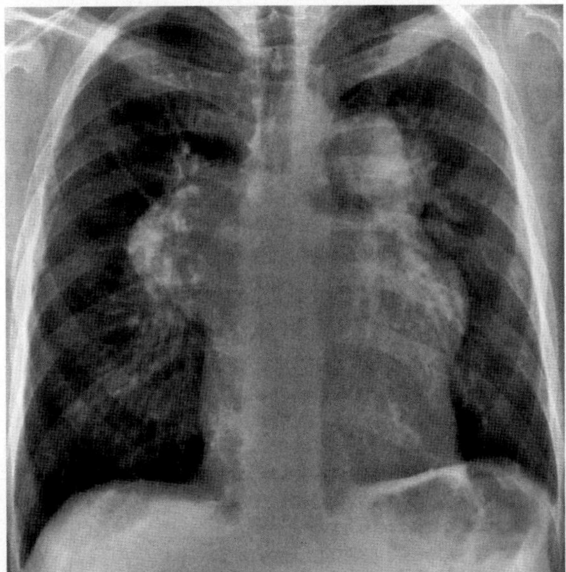

FIGURE 84-8. Patient with primary pulmonary arterial hypertension. Chest frontal radiograph shows centralization of flow with pulmonary artery aneurysms and peripheral pulmonary oligemia.

nonuniform bronchiolitis obliterans. This pattern produces mosaic attenuation on high-resolution CT scanning. Focal oligemia with vascular deficiency is characteristically seen in emphysema. Centrilobular emphysema, paraseptal emphysema, and bullous lung disease have a predilection for the upper lung regions, whereas panlobular emphysema induces basal oligemia with vascular deficiency.

Lung Volume

Conventional radiographs and CT scans are performed during a breath hold at full inspiration and total lung capacity. Low lung volumes are inferred by the high position of the diaphragm and the crowding of basal vascular structures (Table 84-3). Lung volumes larger than expected are commonly found in patients with diffuse emphysema (Fig. 84-9) (Chapter 88), chronic asthma (Chapter 87), or diffuse bronchiolitis obliterans and in highly trained athletes. With a few rare exceptions, chronic diffuse infiltrative lung diseases (Chapter 92) lead to loss of volume.

Anatomic Distribution

The anatomic distribution of disease can significantly facilitate the approach to diagnosis (Table 84-4 and Fig. 84-10). Upper zone lung disease

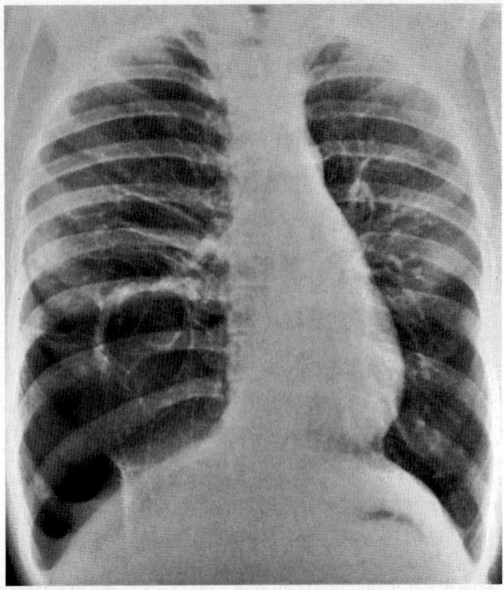

FIGURE 84-9. Patient with severe emphysema. Chest radiograph shows hyperexpansion of both lungs with bullous changes at the right lung base and leftward mediastinal shift.

TABLE 84-3 CONDITIONS ASSOCIATED WITH VARIOUS LUNG VOLUMES IN PATIENTS WITH AN UNDERLYING DIFFUSE LUNG DISEASE PATTERN

LARGE LUNG VOLUMES
Emphysema
Chronic asthma
Diffuse bronchiolitis obliterans
Highly trained athletes
Lymphangioleiomyomatosis
SMALL LUNG VOLUMES
End-stage lung fibrosis
Bilateral diaphragmatic paralysis
Massive ascites
NORMAL LUNG VOLUMES
Sarcoidosis
Langerhans cell histiocytosis
Neurofibromatosis
Combined pulmonary fibrosis and emphysema

TABLE 84-4 CONDITIONS ASSOCIATED WITH DISEASE DISTRIBUTION PATTERNS

UPPER ZONE LUNG DISEASE
Bullous lung disease
Centrilobular and paraseptal emphysema
Tuberculosis
Fungal disease
Sarcoidosis
Pneumoconioses
Langerhans cell histiocytosis
Cystic fibrosis
End-stage hypersensitivity pneumonia
Ankylosing spondylitis
Radiation pneumonia
BASAL LUNG DISEASE
Panlobular emphysema
Bronchiectasis
Aspiration
Drug reactions
Interstitial pulmonary fibrosis, nonspecific interstitial pneumonia, desquamative interstitial pneumonia, cryptogenic organizing pneumonia also called bronchiolitis obliterans with organizing pneumonia
Asbestosis
Scleroderma

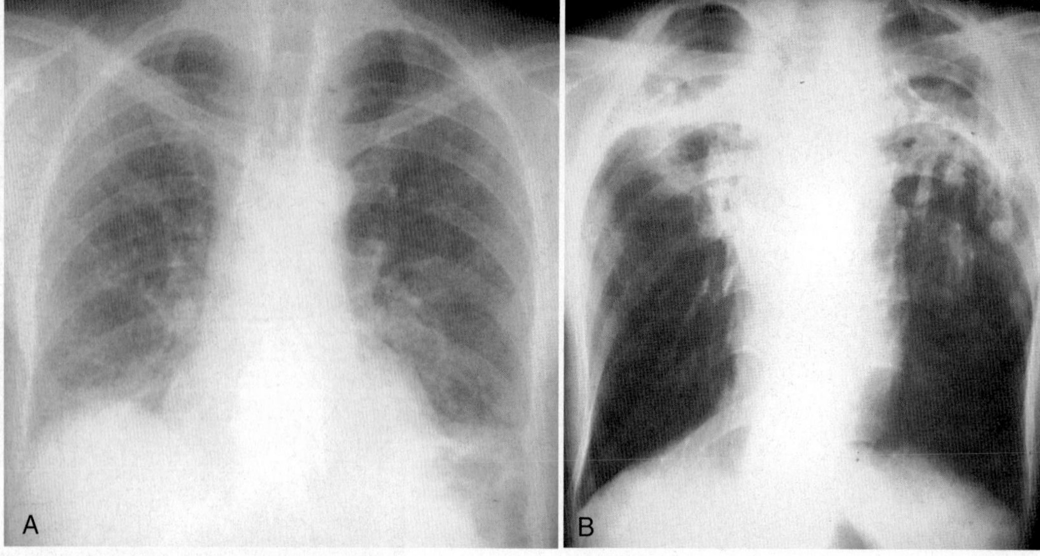

FIGURE 84-10. **A, Basal pulmonary disease.** Chest radiograph in a 48-year-old patient with known scleroderma. Bibasal fine reticular opacities and parenchymal bands are visible in both lower lobes. **B, Apical lung disease.** Chest radiograph in a 42-year-old patient with ankylosing spondylitis. Severe architectural distortion with cicatrizing atelectasis of both upper lobes, retraction of both pulmonary arteries cephalad, and bilateral bulla formation containing fungus balls are evident.

predominates in tuberculosis, fungal disease, sarcoidosis, pneumoconiosis (except asbestosis), Langerhans cell histiocytosis, ankylosing spondylitis, cystic fibrosis, cystic *P. jirovecii* pneumonia, radiation pneumonia, and end-stage hypersensitivity pneumonia. Basal lung disease is preferentially found in bronchiectases, aspiration, desquamative interstitial pneumonia, nonspecific interstitial pneumonia, usual interstitial pneumonia, drug reactions, asbestosis, scleroderma, and rheumatoid arthritis. Peripheral lung disease can be seen in eosinophilic pneumonia, cryptogenic organizing pneumonia, usual interstitial pneumonia, bronchioloalveolar cell carcinoma, adenocarcinoma in situ or minimally invasive adenocarcinoma (Chapter 191), and in occasional patients with so-called alveolar sarcoidosis (Table 84-5). However, any diffuse lung process will eventually progress to involve both lungs irrespective of zonal boundaries.

Lymph Nodes

Enlarged lymph nodes that are visible on chest CT scans and, when larger, on chest radiographs can provide diagnostic information (Table 84-6). The following entities can be associated with diffuse lung disease and concurrent enlarged lymph nodes: sarcoidosis (Chapter 95); lymphoma; fungal disease; tuberculosis (Chapter 324); pneumoconioses (Chapter 93), particularly silicosis and beryllium-associated lung disease; lung cancer; and metastatic malignant disease other than lung cancer.

Pulmonary Nodules

Solitary pulmonary nodules are covered in Chapter 191. Most patients with multiple pulmonary nodules larger than 1 cm in diameter have metastatic disease from primary cancers either within or outside the lung (Fig. 84-11). These lesions have a predilection for subpleural lung regions, including the lung subtending the interlobar fissures. In patients with human immunodeficiency virus infection, Kaposi sarcoma and lymphoma can induce the formation of such nodules. Infectious processes that present with multiple nodules include multiple abscesses from recurrent aspiration (Chapter 94) or septic emboli (Chapter 76); tuberculous and nontuberculous mycobacterial granulomata (Chapters 324 and 325); fungal processes, including histoplasmosis (Chapter 332), coccidioidomycosis (Chapter 333), and cryptococcosis (Chapter 336); and infection with flukes, such as *Paragonimus westermani* (Chapter 356). Noninfectious inflammatory conditions that can present with multiple pulmonary nodules include granulomatosis with angiitis (previously called Wegener granulomatosis, Chapter 270), rheumatoid nodules (Chapter 264), sarcoidosis (Chapter 95), and amyloidosis (Chapter 188).

Pleural Disease

Abnormalities of the pleural space (Chapter 99) can be displayed effectively by conventional radiographic methods supplemented by CT scanning. The volume of a pleural effusion (see Figs. 99-3 and 99-4 in Chapter 99) can be

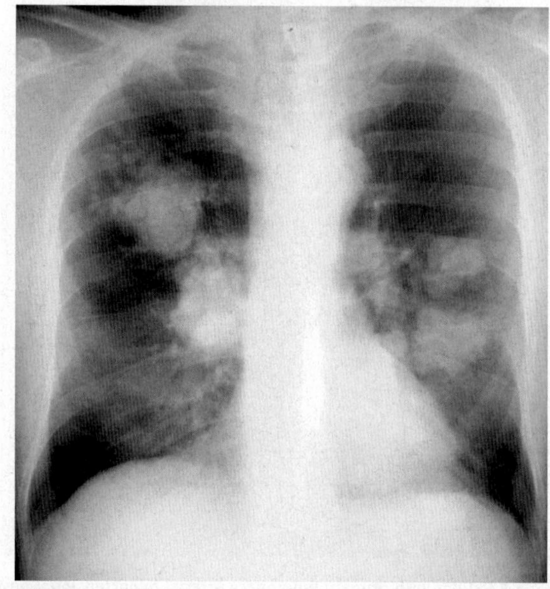

FIGURE 84-11. **Multifocal pulmonary opacities.** Chest radiograph in a 70-year-old patient with known carcinoma of the thyroid gland widening the superior mediastinum and displacing the cervical trachea to the right. Bilateral large and small pulmonary nodules and masses due to metastatic tumor are present.

TABLE 84-5 DISEASES AFFECTING THE LUNG PERIPHERY
Chronic eosinophilic pneumonia
Cryptogenic organizing pneumonia
Idiopathic interstitial fibrosis (usual interstitial pneumonia)
Bronchioloalveolar cell carcinoma (rare)
Pseudo-alveolar sarcoidosis (rare)

TABLE 84-6 CONDITIONS ASSOCIATED WITH HILAR AND MEDIASTINAL LYMPH NODE ENLARGEMENT
Sarcoidosis
Lymphoma
Fungal disease
Tuberculosis
Metastatic cancer
Silicosis, coal worker's pneumoconiosis, beryllium lung

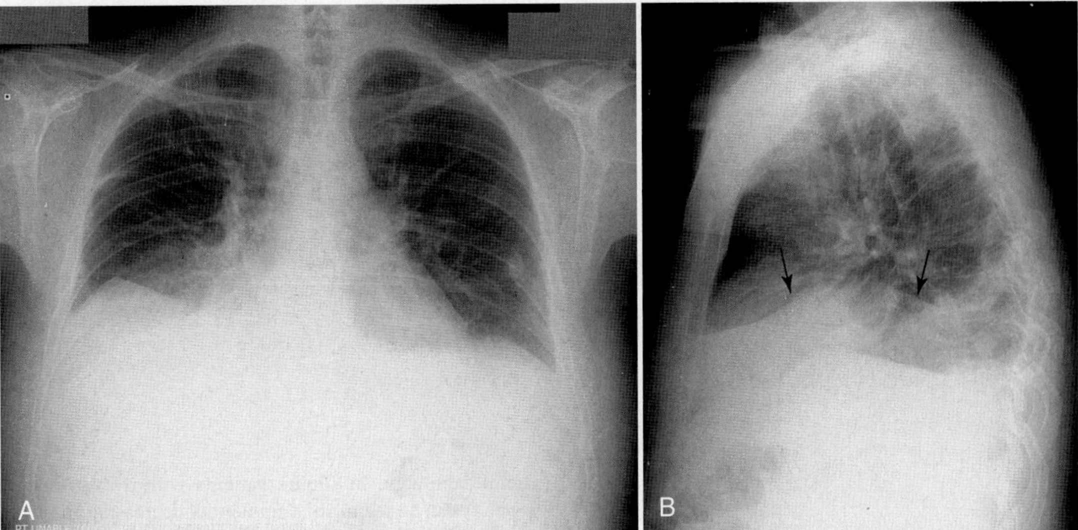

FIGURE 84-12. **Bilateral subpulmonic pleural effusions.** Chest frontal (A) and lateral (B) views. Both lung bases are elevated, with lateralization of the lung base curvature that mimics an elevated diaphragm. In the lateral projection, the configuration of the interface between the effusion and the aerated lung mimics the shape of the rock of Gibraltar (arrows).

reliably estimated on standard frontal upright chest radiograph: 75 mL obscures the posterior costophrenic sulcus; 150 mL obscures the lateral costophrenic sulcus; 200 mL produces a rind of 1 cm in thickness on decubitus films; 500 mL obscures the diaphragm and is visible on supine radiographs; and 1000-mL effusions reach the level of the fourth anterior rib on upright chest radiographs. An effusion of 200 mL or more can be sampled by thoracentesis. The smallest amount visible on decubitus radiographs is 10 mL. With care, as little as 175 mL of effusion can be detected on supine images. Free layering pleural effusions produce a veil of opacity or filter effect superimposed on the aerated lung; pulmonary vessels are clearly visible through the added opacity generated by the effusion, and air bronchograms are absent.

Subpulmonic and Loculated Pleural Effusions

Subpulmonic pleural effusions elevate the lung base, mimicking a high-riding hemidiaphragm. The highest curvature point of the pseudodiaphragm is shifted laterally with an abrupt lateral descent, the so-called Rock of Gibraltar sign; it also can be seen in the lateral projection (Fig. 84-12). Large pleural effusions can lead to diaphragmatic inversion. Separation of the lung base from the gas-containing stomach is indicative of a subpulmonic effusion, particularly when the stomach gas bubble is displaced inferomedially.

Loculated pleural effusions suggest the presence of pleural adhesions or indicate an underlying parenchymal lung abnormality with a focal decrease in adjacent pleural pressure. Such encapsulated collections have obtuse angles of interface with the chest wall, tapered borders that are incomplete towards the chest wall, and a sharply defined contour with the adjacent lung (Fig. 84-13).

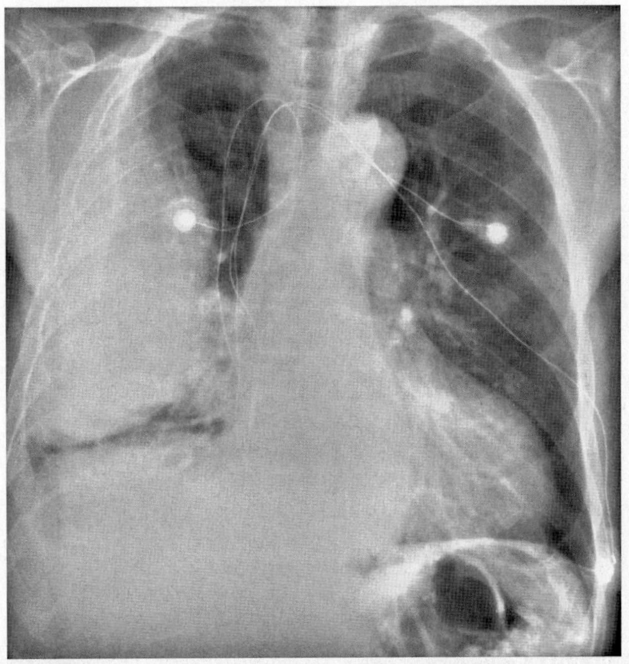

FIGURE 84-13. **Loculated right-sided pleural effusion.** Chest frontal view. A right-sided peripheral pleural mass is seen with characteristic obtuse angles of interface toward the chest wall, with tapered borders and sharp contour towards the lung. These findings localize the mass to the pleural or extrapleural compartment and not to the lung parenchyma. This loculated effusion proved to be an empyema.

Pleural Plaques

Pleural plaques result from parietal pleural accumulation of hyalinized collagen fibers (Fig. 84-14); their presence suggests asbestos exposure (Chapter 93). Plaques preferentially involve the parietal pleura adjacent to ribs six through nine and the diaphragm. They are less pronounced in the intercostal spaces and spare the costophrenic sulci as well as the apices. Calcifications are visible on chest radiographs in 20% and on CT scans in 50% of individuals with pleural plaques. Imaged in profile, pleural plaques produce focal areas of apparent pleural thickening. Over the diaphragm, they appear as curvilinear calcifications or scalloping. Pleural plaques viewed en face can simulate lung disease. Their appearance has been likened to holly leaves, sunburst patterns, or geographic patterns, and, when calcified, to a dripping candle, rolled margins, or stippled or irregular structures. Rare visceral pleural plaques that occur in interlobar fissures can mimic pulmonary nodules.

Diffuse Pleural Thickening

Diffuse pleural thickening is a response observed after exposure to any of a number of stimuli, including infection, inflammation, trauma, tumor, thromboembolism, radiation, and asbestos. Severe involvement results in formation of a generalized pleural peel with smooth margins, usually less than 2 cm in thickness. Radiologically diffuse pleural thickening is characterized by a smooth, noninterrupted pleural opacity involving at least one fourth of the chest wall circumference, obliterating the costophrenic sulci and encompassing also the apices. The CT criteria for diffuse pleural thickening include a thickness of at least 3 mm.

Malignant Disease

Malignant tumors of the pleura are more common than benign ones, and metastatic disease is more frequent than primary pleural mesothelioma. Primary tumors originate from pleural membranes. Pleural invasion by lung cancer, subpleural plaques in lymphoma, hematogenous dissemination to the pleura, and direct pleural seeding are other mechanisms of pleural involvement by tumor. Benign pleural tumors include lipomas, fibrous tumors, and neurogenic tumors. Lipomas are most common; their diagnosis is facilitated by CT scanning. Fibrous tumors of the pleura originate from pluripotent mesenchymal cells found in the visceral pleura or, less commonly, in the

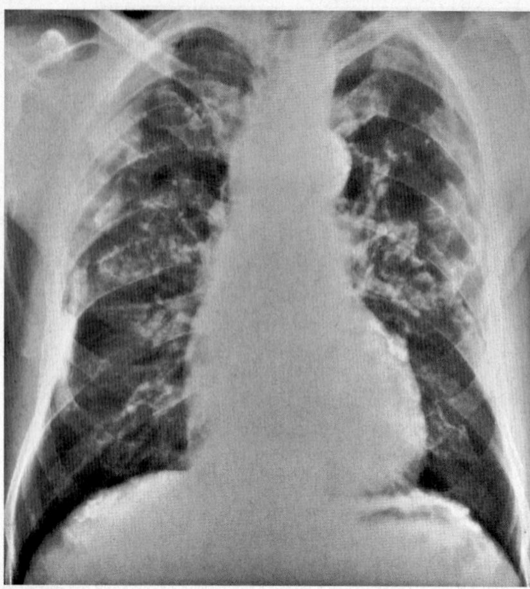

FIGURE 84-14. Patient with known prior occupational asbestos exposure. Chest radiograph shows extensive bilateral calcified plaques seen en face, in profile, and along the diaphragmatic contour.

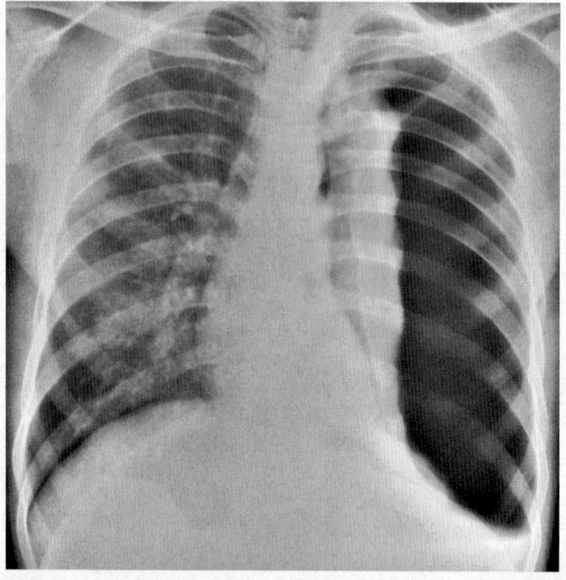

FIGURE 84-15. Patient with spontaneous tension hydropneumothorax. Chest radiograph shows complete atelectasis of the left lung with a large pneumothorax and a left basal gas-liquid level. The patient had primary tuberculosis.

parietal pleura. They can induce paraneoplastic syndromes such as hypertrophic osteoarthropathy (Chapter 179) or hypoglycemia and only rarely invade or metastasize. In nearly half of these patients, the tumor can be on a pedicle and be mobile as a patient changes position.

Pneumothorax

Pneumothorax means gas in the pleural space (Chapter 99). The most important radiologic feature of a pneumothorax is a visceral pleural line or edge that is convex or straight toward the chest wall and produces a lucent separation of the visceral and parietal pleura (Fig. 84-15). In most cases, no pulmonary vascular structures are visible beyond the visceral pleura. On upright chest radiographs, gas is primarily found in the apicolateral pleural space. Expiratory chest radiographs are not necessary for the detection of small pneumothoraces because all pneumothoraces are visible on inspiratory studies. On supine chest radiographs, pleural gas accumulates in a subpulmonic location; it outlines the costophrenic sulcus, forming the deep sulcus sign. A tension pneumothorax leads to a marked shift of the mediastinum to the contralateral side and to flattening or inversion of the ipsilateral hemidiaphragm. In supine patients with a hydropneumothorax, a veil of opacity can be seen with a gradient of decreasing attenuation toward the apex of the affected hemithorax.

TABLE 84-7 CLASSIFICATION OF MEDIASTINAL COMPARTMENTS

ANTERIOR MEDIASTINUM
Retrosternal
MIDDLE MEDIASTINUM: VISCERAL COMPARTMENT
Subcarinal space
Paratracheal region
Retrotracheal space
Aortopulmonic window
Retrocardiac space
POSTERIOR MEDIASTINUM
Paraspinal region

IMAGING OF THE MEDIASTINUM

The mediastinum encompasses midline thoracic structures that are delineated by mediastinal pleura, the diaphragm, the sternum, the spine, and the thoracic inlet. The mediastinum is commonly divided into an anterior compartment, a visceral middle compartment, and a paraspinal, posterior mediastinal compartment (Table 84-7). Each compartment contains specific pathologic entities.

Imaging Techniques

On well-penetrated chest radiographs, the anterior junction line, the posterior-superior junction line, the azygoesophageal stripe, the pleuroesophageal stripe, the paratracheal stripe, and the para-aortic and the paraspinal stripes or lines should be assessed (Fig. 84-E5). Mediastinal masses need to be detected and localized first. Their obtuse angles of interface with the mediastinal pleura, incomplete border towards the mediastinum, sharp contour towards the lung, and extension into both hemithoraces indicate the mediastinal origin of such lesions.

CT facilitates localization of a mass to a specific mediastinal compartment. When it is known whether the mass is predominantly fatty or cystic, contains soft tissue, or is calcified, the differential diagnosis can be limited. MRI of the mediastinum has a role in diagnosis of vertebral disease or neurogenic tumors with extension into the spinal canal. It is equivalent to CT in diagnosis of aortic aneurysms and dissections (Chapter 78).

Mediastinal Compartments

The anterior mediastinum is actually a potential space that may contain the fatty replaced thymus and small normal lymph nodes. Space-occupying lesions in this compartment typically include thymomas, lymphomas, teratomas and other germ cell tumors, substernal thyroid goiters, lipomas, and other connective tissue tumors, as well as hemangiomas or lymphangiomas (Fig. 84-16A).

The middle mediastinum is subdivided into the subcarinal space, paratracheal region, retrotracheal region, aortopulmonic window region, and retrocardiac space. Characteristic lesions are enlarged lymph nodes and bronchopulmonary foregut malformations (see Fig. 84-16B).

In the retrotracheal region, aberrant right subclavian arteries, posterior descending goiters, esophageal tumors, diverticula, or thoracic duct cysts can be found. In the aortopulmonic window, enlarged lymph nodes, ductus diverticula, bronchopulmonary foregut malformations, and aortic or pulmonic artery aneurysms can form compartment-specific space-occupying lesions.

The paraspinal region is considered radiologically to belong to the posterior mediastinum. Important masses in that space include neurogenic tumors that originate from the sympathetic chain or from segmental nerve roots (see Fig. 84-16C). Extramedullary hematopoiesis in patients with severe anemia can result in paravertebral masses formed by hypertrophied bone marrow that extrudes from ribs or vertebral bodies. Enlarged lymph nodes due to lymphoma or metastatic disease are occasionally seen in a paraspinal location. Vertebral disease, including bacterial or tuberculous spondylitis, tumors, and post-traumatic hematomas, can widen the paraspinal region and produce contour abnormalities.

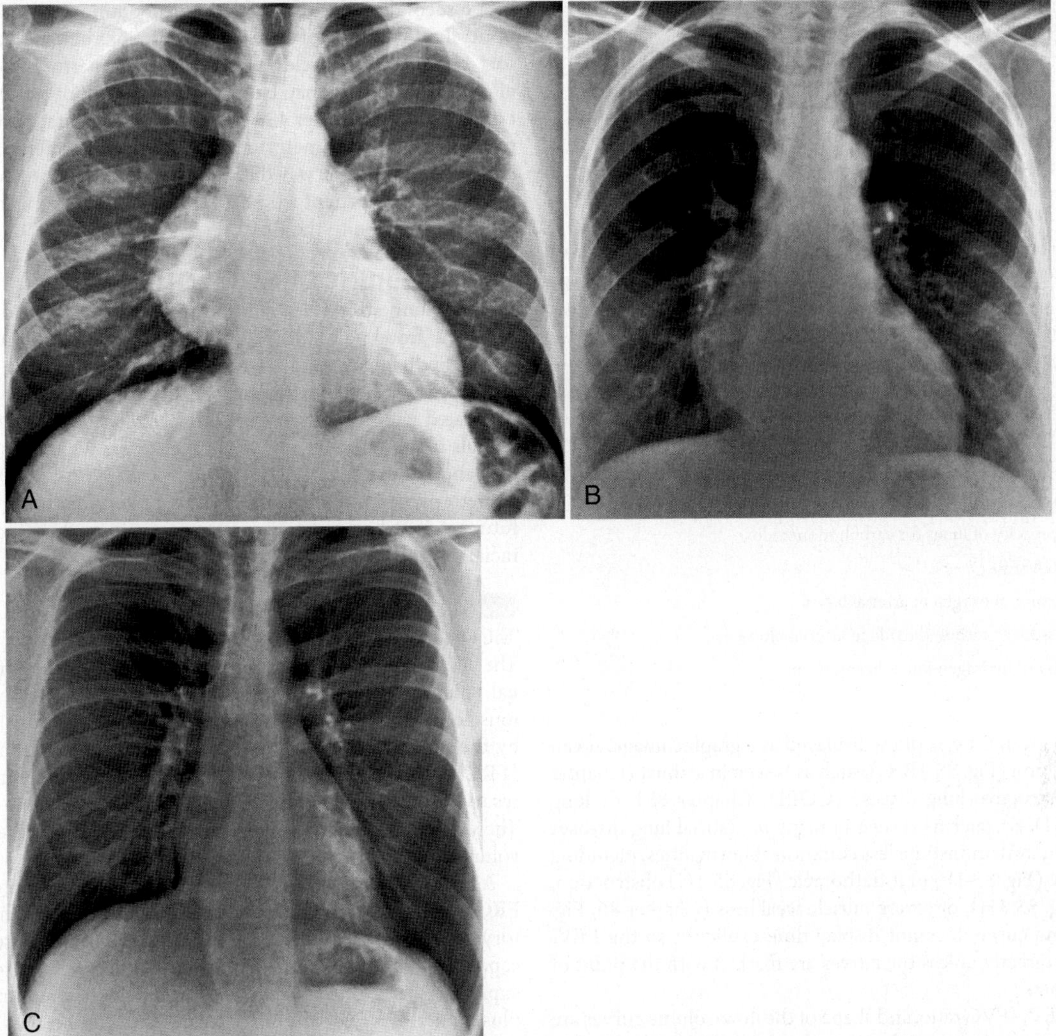

FIGURE 84-16. **A, Patient with anterior mediastinal teratoma. Chest radiograph shows a mediastinal contour abnormality due to projection of the mass into the right hemithorax. Note the obtuse angle of interface formed by the pleura covering the mass with the mediastinum. B, Patient with Castleman giant lymph node hyperplasia. Chest frontal radiograph shows large subcarinal middle mediastinal mass that projects lateral to the right atrium. C, Patient with paraspinal ganglioneuroma. Chest radiograph shows right lower paraspinal contour abnormality widening the right paraspinal region and encompassing the height of three thoracic vertebrae.**

GENERAL REFERENCES

For the General References and other additional features, please visit Expert Consult at https://expertconsult.inkling.com.

85 RESPIRATORY FUNCTION: MECHANISMS AND TESTING

PAUL D. SCANLON

Pulmonary function testing has been used in the medical evaluation of patients with respiratory issues since Hutchinson 1846 demonstration that vital capacity, the largest volume of air that can be exhaled, is an important measure of health. Data from epidemiologic studies show that lung function is one of the most important predictors of all-cause mortality.[1]

Measures of lung function include assessments of respiratory mechanics, for example, the volume of gas that is contained by the lung in various circumstances, the inspiratory and expiratory flow rates across the vital capacity, the pressures that can be generated by inspiratory and expiratory efforts, and the resistance to airflow, as well as calculations of gas exchange. Some lung function tests can be self-performed by a patient, but most are performed in pulmonary function laboratories. The analysis of bronchoalveolar lavage fluid, obtained by bronchoscopy, can also provide important insights into pulmonary disease.

SPIROMETRY

The simplest, most commonly performed, and most clinically useful pulmonary function test is spirometry (Table 85-1).[2] This test measures the forced vital capacity (FVC), which is the amount of air that can be forcefully expelled from the lungs as a function of time, beginning at maximal inhalation (termed total lung capacity) and ending when the lungs are emptied to their minimal volume (residual volume). Many secondary measures are derived from the FVC maneuver, including volume exhaled in a given time, termed the forced expiratory volume (FEV), with a subscript indicating the number of seconds during which this measurement is made (e.g., FEV_1, FEV_3). The ratio of the FEV_1/FVC is the proportion of the total vital capacity that can be expelled in the first second of a maximal expiratory effort; a low FEV_1/FVC ratio is a commonly used indicator of obstructive lung disease. In addition, expiratory flow can be measured at specific portions of exhaled vital capacity, termed forced expiratory flow (FEF), followed by a number to represent the percentage of the FVC at which the flow was measured (e.g., FEF_{75}, FEF_{50}, FEF_{25}). Expiratory flow can also be measured over a given volume range (e.g., FEF_{25-75}). Spirometry requires relatively simple equipment, modest technician training, and modest patient effort. Results are highly reproducible within a test session and over time between test sessions, thereby allowing meaningful comparisons over time for clinical evaluation and as an important outcome in research studies.

The data from a maximal exhalation can be displayed in a flow-volume curve (Fig. 85-1A), which depicts exhaled flow at any given volume as a function of exhaled volume. The flow-volume curve, which has a unique shape for

TABLE 85-1 PULMONARY FUNCTION TESTS

LUNG VOLUME	
TLC	Total lung capacity (volume of gas in lungs at the end of maximal inspiration)
FRC	Functional residual capacity (volume of gas in the lungs at relaxation point, when elastic inward pull of lungs is balanced by outward pull of the chest wall and diaphragm)
ERV	Expiratory reserve volume (volume of gas expired from FRC to maximal expiration)
RV	Residual volume (FRC − ERV, volume of gas left in lungs after maximal exhalation)
EXPIRATORY FLOW	
FEV_1	Forced expiratory volume (in 1 second)
FVC	Forced vital capacity
$FEV_{1\%}$	FEV_1/FVC ratio (expressed as percentage)
DIFFUSING CAPACITY	
DLCO	Diffusing capacity of lungs for carbon monoxide
ARTERIAL BLOOD GASES	
$Pa{O_2}$	Partial pressure of oxygen in arterial blood
$Pa{CO_2}$	Partial pressure of carbon dioxide in arterial blood
pH	Negative log of hydrogen ion concentration

any individual at any given time, is often displayed as a graphic image. It can reflect airway obstruction (Fig. 85-1B, C), such as is seen in asthma (Chapter 87) and chronic obstructive lung disease (COPD; Chapter 88), or lung restriction (Fig. 85-1D, E), such as is seen in many interstitial lung diseases (Chapter 92). It also may demonstrate less common abnormalities, including variable extrathoracic (Fig. 85-1F) or intrathoracic (Fig. 85-1G) obstruction, tracheal stenosis (Fig. 85-1H), or severe muscle weakness (Chapter 86; Fig. 85-1I). A flow-volume curve does not display time explicitly, so the FEV_1 cannot be measured directly unless the curves are marked with the point of 1 second of exhalation.

The FVC, FEV_1, FEV_1/FVC ratio, and shape of the flow-volume curves are highly reproducible measures of lung function if the tested individual makes an expiratory effort above a certain, easy-to-obtain level in a pulmonary function laboratory with modern spirometry equipment and trained staff. In the absence of quality assurance, however, measurements of lung function are neither accurate nor reproducible; poor-quality pulmonary function testing results are biased to lower values, thereby giving an incorrect impression of disease where none may exist. One way to assess a patient's performance is to compare multiple efforts and to document that the two best measures of both FVC and FEV_1 are within 150 mL of each other, a standard that most people can meet without difficulty. Poor performance should be noted by the interpreter to avoid erroneous diagnoses.

Spirometry is recommended for diagnosis of airflow obstruction in symptomatic patients. It is not recommended as a screening test for asymptomatic persons thought to be at risk for development of lung disease, such as current or former smokers,[3] but it may be part of comprehensive workplace respiratory health programs in certain occupational settings.[4] An abnormal spirometric result has not been shown to improve the likelihood that such at-risk individuals will quit smoking, and a normal screening spirometry test result might be misinterpreted as an indicator that smokers can continue smoking without risk.

Spirometry is often performed before and after administration of an inhaled bronchodilator, either a β-agonist (e.g., albuterol) or a muscarinic antagonist (e.g., ipratropium) or both, especially if it shows changes consistent with airway obstruction. Dosing may use two or four puffs from a metered dose inhaler or nebulized aerosols. The degree of improvement after bronchodilator administration indicates the degree of airway reactivity, which is generally more in asthma (Chapter 87) and less in COPD (Chapter 88). Response to bronchodilators varies with dosage, is poorly repeatable from test to test, and is not a good predictor of the clinical response to bronchodilator therapy in an individual patient.

OTHER TESTS OF VENTILATION

Maximal voluntary ventilation (MVV), which is an indication of the maximal ventilation a patient can perform, is measured during 12 seconds, using the best 6 seconds and expressed in liters per minute. MVV estimates a person's upper limit of ventilatory capacity. Reductions in MVV may be due to inspiratory obstruction, muscle weakness, or poor performance. Because MVV is effort dependent, it may be a better predictor of postoperative respiratory complications (Chapter 433) than is FEV_1. Inspiratory flows, which are not part of routine spirometry, may be useful for patients in whom there is a suspicion of upper airway disease, such as a patient referred by an otorhinolaryngologist, a patient who has stridor, or a patient whose MVV is reduced out of proportion to the FEV_1.

REFERENCE EQUATIONS

Because lung size varies substantially from person to person, the values obtained from pulmonary function testing are compared with those of normal individuals. Because test results vary as a function of sex, height, age, and ethnicity, they are usually expressed as a percentage of a reference value calculated with those four factors. Normal values in African American individuals are about 12% lower than values from white persons of the same sex, age, and height. Normal values are also about 6 to 15% smaller in Asians. Genetic markers of ethnic ancestry are predictive of lung function and, in the future, might be used to improve on traditional methods of adjusting for racial or ethnic factors.

LUNG VOLUMES

The volume of air in the lung at any given time can be partitioned (Fig. 85-2). The air that remains in the lung after a maximal expiratory effort is the residual volume. The amount of air in the lungs at the relaxation point, when muscle effort is minimized and the inward recoil of the lung is balanced by the outward recoil of the chest wall, is the functional residual capacity (FRC). The difference between FRC and residual volume is the expiratory reserve volume. The volume exhaled in a normal breath is the tidal volume. The volume that can be inhaled above tidal volume is the inspiratory reserve volume.

A series of *capacities* consist of the sum of two or more different volumes. FRC is the sum of expiratory reserve volume plus residual volume. Inspiratory capacity is the sum of tidal volume plus inspiratory reserve volume. Vital capacity is the sum of tidal volume plus inspiratory reserve volume plus expiratory reserve volume. Total lung capacity is the sum of residual volume plus expiratory reserve volume plus tidal volume plus inspiratory reserve volume.

Three of the volumes (tidal volume, inspiratory reserve volume, expiratory reserve volume) are simply volumes of exhaled gas and can be measured with a spirometer. Measurement of residual volume or any of the capacities that include it, so-called absolute lung volumes, requires more sophisticated methods, such as body plethysmography, the inert gas dilution technique, or the nitrogen washout technique.

Body Plethysmography

Body plethysmography, which is the preferred method for measuring lung volumes, is based on Boyle's law: at a given temperature, the product of the pressure and volume of a quantity of gas at one time will be equal to the product of the pressure and volume of the gas at another time ($P1 \times V1 = P2 \times V2$). The process of measuring lung volume by plethysmography consists of panting against a closed shutter to compress and to rarify gas in the chest. The body plethysmograph, a sealed box in which the patient sits, measures the changes in lung volume during panting; pressure measured at the mouth represents the pressure changes within the lung during these volume changes. A similar panting maneuver with the shutter open is used to calculate airway resistance. The clinical utility of this measurement is largely limited to instances in which airway obstruction is suspected but the FEV_1/FVC ratio is normal. Although body plethysmography is generally the most accurate method for measurement of lung volumes, particularly in patients with airway obstruction, it can overestimate lung volumes if panting is too rapid. A plethysmographic total lung capacity more than 150% of the reference value should be viewed with suspicion.

Inert Gas Dilution Technique

Lung volumes also can be measured by having the patient rebreathe from a device containing a known volume and concentration of inert gas (e.g., helium or less commonly neon or argon, which do not react with elements in the blood or tissues) until equilibrium is achieved. The final concentration of helium equals the initial helium concentration times the initial volume of the device divided by the final volume of the lungs plus the device, correcting

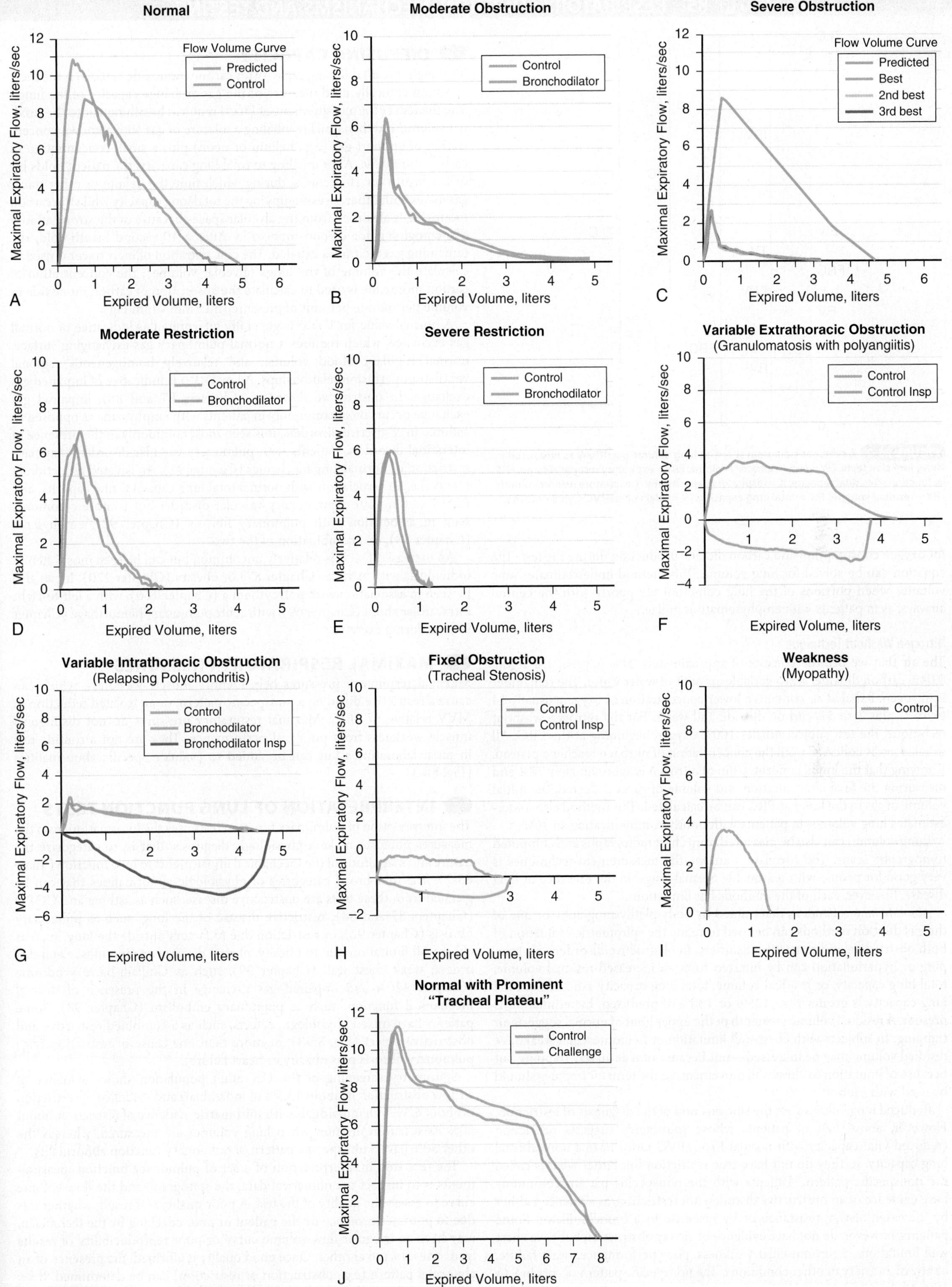

FIGURE 85-1. **Common patterns of flow-volume curve. A, Normal. B, Moderate obstruction. C, Severe obstruction. D, Moderate restriction. E, Severe restriction. F, Variable extrathoracic obstruction (granulomatosis with polyangiitis). G, Variable intrathoracic obstruction (relapsing polychondritis). H, Fixed obstruction (tracheal stenosis). I, Weak effort (myopathy). J, Normal but with a prominent tracheal plateau. FET = forced expiratory time.**

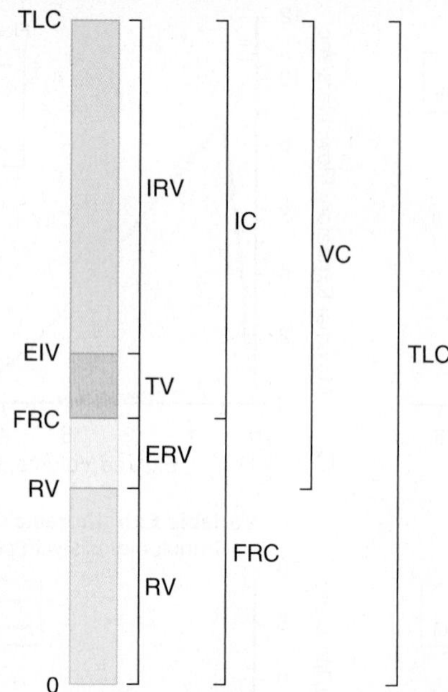

FIGURE 85-2. **A schematic diagram showing lung volume partitions as measured in lung function tests. EIV = end-inspiratory volume; ERV = expiratory reserve volume; FRC = functional residual capacity; IC = inspiratory capacity; IRV = inspiratory reserve volume; RV = residual volume; TLC = total lung capacity; TV = tidal volume; VC = vital capacity.**

for oxygen consumption and carbon dioxide production during the test. The equation can be solved for lung volume. This method underestimates lung volumes when portions of the lung communicate poorly with the central airways, as in patients with emphysematous bullae.

Nitrogen Washout Technique

The air that we breathe consists of approximately 21% oxygen, 1% argon, 0.04% carbon dioxide, and a variable amount of water vapor. The remainder is nitrogen. Exhaled air contains a lower concentration of oxygen, usually 14 to 16%, plus 3 to 5% carbon dioxide and water. For the nitrogen washout technique, the test subject inhales 100% oxygen beginning at the FRC. All exhaled gas is collected until the concentration of nitrogen reaches a plateau. Knowing that the initial concentration of nitrogen is approximately 78% and measuring the final concentration and volume of gases collected, the initial volume of gas in the lungs at FRC can be calculated. This method also underestimates lung volumes in patients with poorly communicating air spaces.

Lung volumes can also be measured from chest radiographs and computed tomography scans. The correlation among the measurement techniques is very good for people with reasonably normal lungs. In the presence of lung disease, however, each of the methods has limitations.

Absolute lung volumes as determined by body plethysmography or one of the gas dilution methods can be used to refine the spirometric evaluation of both obstructive and restrictive disorders. In obstructive disorders, air trapping or hyperinflation can be inferred from an increased residual volume, total lung capacity, or residual volume/total lung capacity ratio. If the total lung capacity is greater than 125% or 130% of predicted, hyperinflation is present. A residual volume greater than the upper limit of normal suggests air trapping. In subjects with chest wall limitation or neuromuscular weakness, residual volume may be increased—not because of true airway trapping but because of limitation to chest wall movement, so the term *air trapping* should be used with caution.

Reduced lung volumes are the sine qua non of the diagnosis of restriction. However, about half of patients whose spirometry suggests restriction (reduced vital capacity with normal FEV_1/FVC ratio) have a normal total lung capacity, so they do not have true restriction but rather what is called the nonspecific pattern.[5] Patients with the nonspecific pattern commonly have evidence of an obstructive disorder, not restriction, as evidenced either by increased airway resistance or by response to a bronchodilator. Some patients, however, do not have evidence of airway obstruction but have chest wall limitations, neuromuscular weakness, poor performance, heart failure, or any of a variety of other conditions. The nonspecific pattern occurs in 9 to 10% of all complete pulmonary function tests and is approximately as frequent as true restriction.

DIFFUSING CAPACITY

The single-breath diffusing capacity for carbon monoxide (DLCO) is the most common clinically used measure of the gas exchange capacity of the lungs. The maneuver for measurement of DLCO requires breathing out to the residual volume and then quickly inhaling a mixture of gas with a known concentration of an inert gas (e.g., helium or neon) plus a small concentration of carbon monoxide. After inhaling to total lung capacity, the patient holds his or her breath for 10 seconds, during which time the helium or other tracer gas mixes with other gases occupying the total lung capacity while the carbon monoxide is absorbed from the alveolar spaces because of the strong affinity of hemoglobin for carbon monoxide. After a 10-second breath-hold, the remaining gas mixture is exhaled. The concentration of inert tracer is used to calculate the volume of the lungs (alveolar volume); the concentration of carbon monoxide is used to calculate the absorption of carbon monoxide in volume per minute per unit of pressure (mL/min • mm Hg).

A normal value for DLCO is generally interpreted as indicative of normal gas exchange, which requires a normal pulmonary gas-exchanging surface, normal capillary blood volume, and relatively homogeneous regional ventilation-perfusion relationships. A low DLCO is indicative of impaired gas exchange. In obstructive disorders (Chapters 87 and 88), impaired gas exchange occurs most commonly in patients with emphysema as opposed to asthma. In restrictive disorders, it is seen most commonly in the presence of interstitial disorders. Patients with pulmonary vascular disorders may have restriction or normal lung mechanics (Chapter 92). An isolated reduction in DLCO (i.e., in association with normal total lung capacity, vital capacity, and FEV_1) can indicate a pulmonary vascular disorder but is more commonly seen in association with pulmonary fibrosis (Chapter 92), emphysema (Chapter 88), or a combination of the two.

An increased DLCO is relatively uncommon but can be seen most often in individuals with asthma (Chapter 87) or obesity (Chapter 220). It can also be seen in association with polycythemia (Chapter 166), with a left-to-right intracardiac shunt (Chapter 69), with acute pulmonary hemorrhage (Chapter 91), or during exercise.

MAXIMAL RESPIRATORY PRESSURES

Maximal respiratory pressures help identify muscle weakness, which can cause a restrictive disorder, a nonspecific pattern, or an isolated reduction in MVV relative to FEV_1. Maximal respiratory pressures do not distinguish muscle weakness from poor test performance. They are not a routine test in most laboratories but can be added to evaluate specific abnormalities (Fig. 85-3).

INTERPRETATION OF LUNG FUNCTION TESTS

The interpretation of pulmonary function tests uses the information from the measures noted to make a physiologic diagnosis, that is, to categorize the nature and magnitude of the mechanical impairments to lung function (Table 85-2). The four broad categories of physiologic abnormalities that can be gleaned from these tests are obstructive disease, such as asthma and COPD (Chapters 87 and 88); restrictive disease of the lung, such as pulmonary fibrosis (Chapter 92), or restriction due to factors outside the lung, such as chest wall limitation due to obesity, pleural disease, or musculoskeletal disorders; weak chest wall (Chapter 99), such as Guillain-Barré syndrome (Chapter 420); and impaired gas exchange in the presence of normal mechanical function, such as pulmonary embolism (Chapter 98). Some patients have mixed physiologic defects, such as a combined restrictive and obstructive defect (Fig. 85-3), or more than one cause of restriction (e.g., pulmonary fibrosis plus obesity or heart failure).

Spirometry screening of the U.S. adult population shows evidence of airflow obstruction in about 13.5% of individuals and evidence of restriction in about 6.5%.[6] Of individuals with spirometric evidence of restriction, about 50% have true restriction when lung volumes are measured, whereas the other 50% have a nonspecific pattern of pulmonary function abnormality.

The first step in interpretation of a set of pulmonary function measurements is to inspect the numerical data, the spirogram, and the flow-volume curve to assess the quality of the test. A poor-quality test result, whether it is due to poor performance by the patient or poor coaching by the technician, may have an irregular flow-volume curve or poor reproducibility of results from one effort to another. Once good quality is affirmed, the presence of an abnormal pattern (e.g., obstruction or restriction) can be determined. If so, attention then turns to assessing gradations of severity, subtleties of the flow-volume curve, and other physiologic data (e.g., total lung capacity, residual

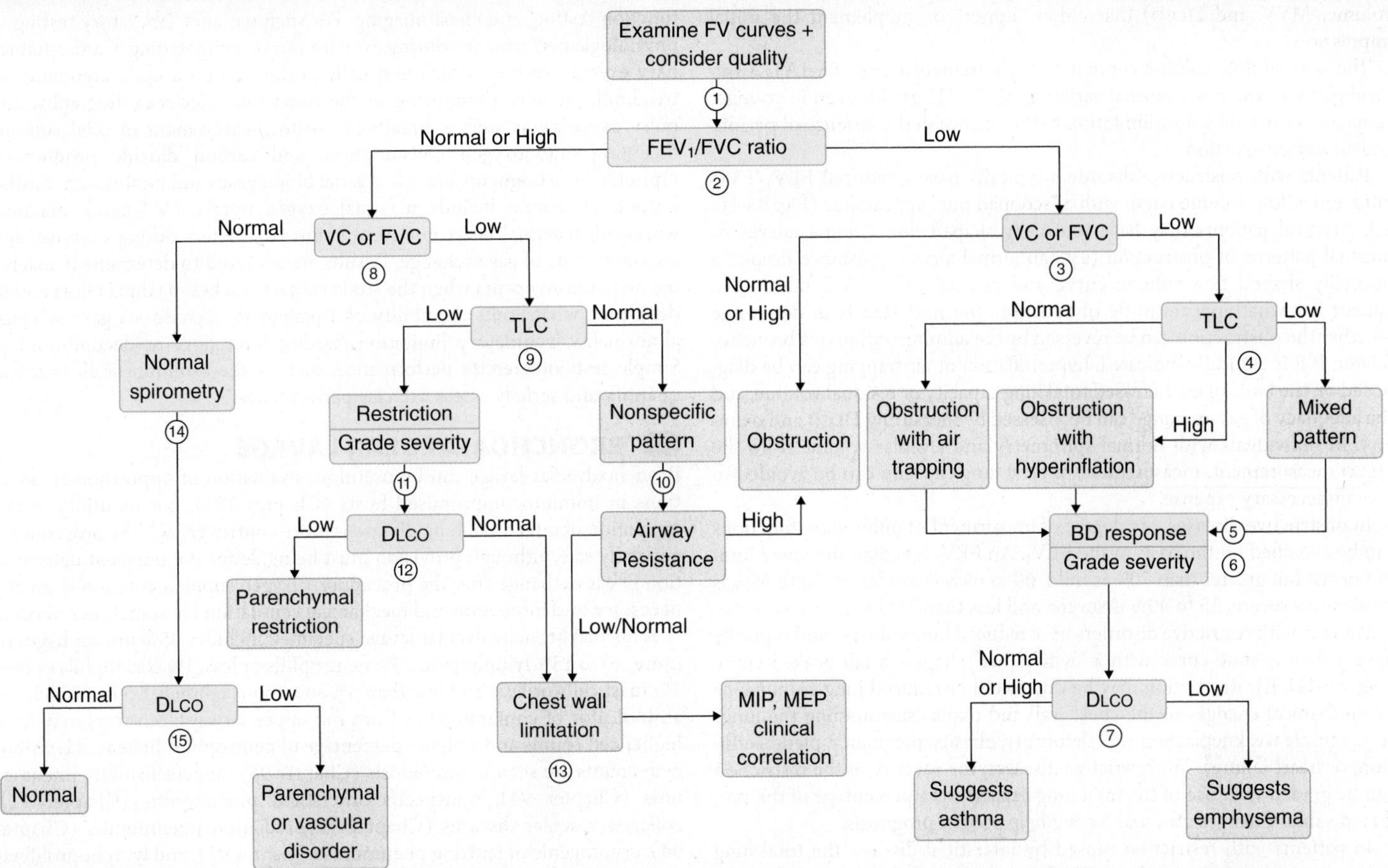

FIGURE 85-3. An algorithm for interpreting pulmonary function tests in which spirometry, lung volumes, and DLCO are measured. If only spirometry is available, interpretation is more limited. The legend keys refer to numbered branch points in the algorithm. BD = bronchodilator; DLCO = diffusing capacity of the lung for carbon monoxide; FEV_1 = forced expiratory volume in one second; FVC = forced vital capacity; MEP = maximal expiratory pressure; MIP = maximal inspiratory pressure; Nl = normal; TLC = total lung capacity; VC = vital capacity.

1. The algorithm begins at the top. Inspect the data and flow-volume (FV) curve to assess test quality and then consider the basic type of abnormality (e.g., obstruction vs. restriction).
2. A reduced FEV_1/FVC ratio suggests obstruction, and the obstruction algorithm on the right side should be followed. If the FEV_1/FVC ratio is normal or high, the restriction side (left side) of the algorithm should be followed.
3. If FEV_1/FVC is low and the VC or FVC is normal or high, simple obstruction is present. If VC or FVC is low, TLC should be checked.
4. If TLC is normal, simple obstruction is present. If TLC is high, obstruction with hyperinflation is present. If TLC is low, a mixed obstructive/restrictive pattern is present. (Note that the inert gas dilution and nitrogen washout methods commonly underestimate TLC in the presence of obstruction and can give a false impression of a mixed disorder.)
5. The response to a bronchodilator (BD) should be assessed to determine whether FEV_1 or FVC meets criteria for a positive response (i.e., a ≥12% improvement and at least a 200 mL absolute increase) and to determine the degree of positivity.
6. The severity of obstruction should be graded. Some algorithms grade severity based on post-bronchodilator values.
7. In current or former smokers with obstruction, a low DLCO suggests emphysema or other pulmonary parenchymal or vascular disorders. A normal DLCO may suggest asthma or bronchitis.
8. If FEV_1/FVC is normal or high, the restriction (left) side of the algorithm is followed. If VC or FVC is normal, spirometry is generally normal (occasional patients have an isolated abnormality of FEV_1 of uncertain significance). If VC or FVC is low, TLC should be checked.
9. If TLC is low, a restrictive disorder is present. If TLC is normal, the "nonspecific pattern" is present.
10. If the nonspecific pattern is identified, airway resistance (Raw) can be measured. An increased Raw suggests obstruction. A normal Raw suggests an alternative cause (See #13).
11. If true restriction is present, grade severity on the basis of the reduction in TLC percentage predicted.
12. If restriction is demonstrated, DLCO should be measured next. If abnormal, it indicates a pulmonary parenchymal restrictive process. If normal, it suggests an extraparenchymal or nonpulmonary cause of restriction.
13. Restriction with a normal DLCO or a nonspecific pattern with normal Raw suggests an alternative cause (chest wall limitation, weakness, heart failure, poor performance). Consider measurement of maximal respiratory pressures and review the study for test performance.
14. If spirometry is normal, lung volumes are rarely useful, but DLCO is sometimes helpful.
15. If DLCO is normal, pulmonary function is normal. An isolated reduction in DLCO is seen most often in patients with emphysema or pulmonary fibrosis or both. It less commonly indicates a pulmonary vascular disorder, such as primary pulmonary hypertension, or an obliterative vasculopathy, as sometimes seen in Sjögren syndrome.

TABLE 85-2 COMMON CHANGES ASSOCIATED WITH PATTERNS OF LUNG FUNCTION ABNORMALITY

	FORCED EXPIRATORY VOLUME IN 1 SECOND (FEV_1)	FORCED VITAL CAPACITY (FVC)	FEV_1/FVC RATIO	RESIDUAL VOLUME	TOTAL LUNG CAPACITY	MAXIMAL INSPIRATORY AND EXPIRATORY PRESSURE RATIOS
Normal	Normal*	Normal	Normal	Normal	Normal	Normal
Obstructive	↓	Normal to ↓	↓	↑ to ↑↑	Normal to ↑↑	Normal
Restrictive	↓	↓ to ↓↓	Normal or ↑	Normal or ↓	↓ to ↓↓	Normal
Weak chest wall	↓	↓ to ↓↓	Normal or ↑	↑	Normal or ↓	↓

*Normal or abnormal values are determined by comparing the measured values with those predicted from regression equations based on the patient's sex, age, height, and race. The normal range for FEV_1/FVC also varies, mainly with age, ranging from 0.70 to 0.80 among 25-year-olds to 0.63 to 0.68 among 65-year-olds.

volume, MVV, and DLCO) that either support or supplement the initial impression.

The normal flow-volume curve is roughly triangular (Fig. 85-1A). A *tracheal plateau*, which is a normal variant (Fig. 85-1J) usually seen in younger subjects, is caused by flow limitation in the trachea in the absence of peripheral airway obstruction.

Patients with obstructive disorders typically have a reduced FEV_1/FVC ratio and a flow-volume curve with a "scooped out" appearance (Fig. 85-1B, C). Atypical patients may have unusually shaped flow-volume curves or unusual patterns of obstruction (e.g., abnormal airway resistance despite a normally shaped flow-volume curve and normal FEV_1/FVC ratio). If a patient has what appears to be obstruction, the next step is to determine whether the obstruction can be reversed by the administration of a bronchodilator. If it is clinically indicated, hyperinflation or air trapping can be diagnosed on the basis of an increased total lung capacity or residual volume, and the adequacy of gas exchange can be assessed by measuring DLCO and oximetry. In individuals with normal spirometry and alveolar volume from the DLCO measurement, measurement of total lung capacity can be avoided to save unnecessary expense.

In obstructive diseases, the degree of impairment of pulmonary functions can be classified on the basis of the FEV_1. An FEV_1 less than the lower limit of normal but greater than 70% is mild, 60 to 69% is moderate, 50 to 59% is moderately severe, 35 to 49% is severe, and less than 35% is very severe.

Patients with restrictive disorders have reduced lung volumes and typically have a flow-volume curve with a "witch's hat" shape—a tall peaked curve (Fig. 85-1D, E). Restriction may be due to either reduced lung compliance or mechanical changes to the chest wall and tissues surrounding the lungs (e.g., muscle weakness, chest wall deformity, obesity, pregnancy, pleural effusion, or heart failure). For restrictive diseases, the severity of the restriction can be graded with use of the total lung capacity as a percentage of the predicted value. Changes on serial testing help predict prognosis.[7]

In patients with restriction caused by interstitial disease, the total lung capacity and the vital capacity or FVC are usually reduced by a similar proportion. In some patients with restriction, the total lung capacity as a percentage of predicted and the vital capacity percentage of predicted are quite different (>10% difference). The usual cause is the presence of more than one restrictive process, such as a parenchymal restrictive disorder plus obesity, respiratory muscle weakness, or heart failure.

Some patients have a mixed disorder with evidence of both obstruction and restriction. Common causes include cystic fibrosis (Chapter 89), sarcoidosis (Chapter 95), and heart failure (Chapters 58 and 59) as well as cases in which the cause of the obstructive disorder and the restrictive disorder are unrelated.

Disorders of the central airways can cause characteristic patterns of abnormality. In a "fixed airway obstruction" such as tracheal stenosis (Fig. 85-1H), flow is typically reduced on both inspiration and expiration. In contrast, in a variable extrathoracic upper airway obstruction (Fig. 85-1F), inspiration is disproportionately reduced; however, expiration is often abnormal, merely less so. Likewise, in variable intrathoracic obstruction (e.g., relapsing polychondritis, tracheomalacia, or a dynamic intrathoracic tracheal tumor), the expiratory flow-volume curve is reduced but in a pattern unlike that seen in asthma or COPD (Fig. 85-1G). These central airway obstructive patterns may signify a locally treatable cause of obstruction.

PROVOCATIVE TESTING

Assessing Airway Responsiveness

Hyperresponsiveness of airways to the smooth muscle–contracting effect of pharmacologic agents such as methacholine, as well as to cold air, dry air, and other physical stimuli, is characteristic of asthma (Chapter 87). It is also observed in COPD and other obstructive airway diseases. Bronchoprovocation studies, in which graded doses of a stimulus are used to elicit airway constriction, are performed to measure airway responsiveness. A responsive airway, that is, one in which a small stimulus leads to a fall in FEV_1, may be used to confirm the diagnosis of asthma (Chapter 87).

Exhaled nitric oxide is a marker of eosinophilic airway inflammation and can be used to predict the likelihood that airway obstruction will improve with corticosteroid treatment. However, the utility of exhaled nitric oxide levels for asthma management is controversial.

CARDIOPULMONARY EXERCISE TESTS

Some patients have dyspnea (Chapter 83) or exercise limitation that is not adequately explained by the clinical examination, standard pulmonary function testing, and chest imaging. For such patients, laboratory testing of physiologic performance during exercise can be enlightening. Cardiopulmonary exercise testing, which is usually performed on a cycle ergometer or treadmill, includes monitoring of the heart rate, electrocardiography, and pulse oximetry as well as breath-by-breath measurement of tidal volume, breathing rate, oxygen consumption, and carbon dioxide production. Optional measurements include arterial blood gases and noninvasive cardiac output. Outcomes include maximal oxygen uptake ($\dot{V}O_2$max), maximal workload, maximal heart rate, ventilation parameters during exercise, and measurements of gas exchange. Results are analyzed to determine if anaerobic metabolism occurs when the study subject reaches maximal effort and to determine what limits the ability of a patient to exercise—a gas exchange abnormality, ventilatory limitation, cardiac limitation, or deconditioning. Simple tests of exercise performance, such as the 6-minute walk test, can quantify and serially assess exercise performance.[8]

BRONCHOALVEOLAR LAVAGE

Bronchoalveolar lavage can be useful for evaluation of opportunistic infections in immunocompromised hosts (Chapter 281), but its utility in the evaluation of interstitial lung disease is more controversial.[9] The procedure is generally safe, although provision must be made for the transient deterioration in gas exchange after the procedure. Oxygen supplementation is usually necessary, and intubation and mechanical ventilation are sometimes needed.

A normal bronchoalveolar lavage specimen includes 85% macrophages or more, 10 to 15% lymphocytes, 3% neutrophils or less, 1% eosinophils or less, 1% mast cells or less, and less than 5% squamous epithelial cells (which are an indicator of contamination from the upper airway). Smokers may have higher cell counts and a higher percentage of neutrophils. Increased lymphocyte counts are seen in sarcoidosis (Chapter 95), hypersensitivity pneumonitis (Chapter 94), nonspecific interstitial pneumonitis (Chapter 92), collagen vascular diseases (Chapter 92), radiation pneumonitis (Chapter 94), cryptogenic organizing pneumonia (Chapter 92), and lymphoproliferative disorders. Increased neutrophil counts are seen in idiopathic pulmonary fibrosis (Chapter 92), collagen vascular diseases (Chapter 92), infectious pneumonia (Chapter 97), aspiration pneumonia (Chapter 97), acute respiratory distress syndrome (Chapter 104), diffuse alveolar damage (Chapter 91), acute interstitial pneumonia (Chapter 92), and asbestosis (Chapter 93). Increased eosinophils can be seen in asthma (Chapter 87), bronchitis (Chapter 96), allergic bronchopulmonary aspergillosis (Chapter 339), Churg-Strauss vasculitis (Chapter 270), Hodgkin lymphoma (Chapter 186), and drug-induced lung disease (Chapter 94). If eosinophils are more than 25%, eosinophilic pneumonia is likely (Chapter 170). If lymphocytes are increased and the clinical differential diagnosis includes sarcoidosis or hypersensitivity pneumonitis, analysis of T-cell populations may be helpful; the CD4:CD8 ratio is typically increased in sarcoidosis but reduced in hypersensitivity pneumonitis. If more than 20% of macrophages stain positive for hemosiderin, diffuse alveolar hemorrhage is considered likely (Chapter 91), particularly if lavage fluid is progressively bloody in successive aliquots of lavage fluid.

Cellular constituents of bronchoalveolar lavage are usually stained for cytologic analysis for malignant cells and viral inclusions. If Langerhans cell histiocytosis (Chapter 92) is considered possible, 5% or more CD1a–positive cells supports the diagnosis. If chronic beryllium disease or beryllium sensitization is possible, a lymphocyte proliferation test in response to exposure to beryllium salts can be helpful (Chapter 93). Staining of solid material from the bronchoalveolar lavage with periodic acid–Schiff (PAS) stain for the presence of PAS-positive material is essential to the diagnosis of pulmonary alveolar proteinosis (Chapter 91). A diagnosis of lipoid pneumonia (Chapter 94), caused by the aspiration of oil, can be confirmed by an excess of lipid-laden macrophages from bronchoalveolar lavage. The presence of asbestos bodies or silica is not diagnostic of lung disease related to these substances (Chapter 93) but does indicate significant exposure.

PULMONARY FUNCTION IN OBESITY

The epidemic of obesity is manifested in many organ systems. Dyspnea, exercise limitation, and respiratory failure are more common in obese persons than in the nonobese. Asthma is more common and more severe in obese patients.[10] The effects of obesity on lung function are usually relatively modest among ambulatory patients with a body mass index (BMI) of less than 40. The most commonly observed effect of obesity on lung function is a reduction in expiratory reserve volume (the amount of air exhaled between FRC and residual volume), which is substantially reduced even in persons who are overweight (BMI 25-30) or mildly obese (BMI 30-35). Vital capacity is reduced in obesity, but the effect is modest and highly variable. In large studies, on average, for each unit increase in BMI above 25, vital capacity or FVC is reduced by 0.5 to 0.8%. Effects of obesity on total lung capacity and FEV_1 are somewhat smaller. The FEV_1/FVC ratio and DLCO actually increase slightly with increase in BMI.

In exercise studies, the effects of obesity among ambulatory outpatients are likewise modest. Such patients have an increased work of breathing, but maximal oxygen uptake is often normal.

FUTURE DIRECTIONS

New test methods are likely to evolve, such as using "electronic nose" devices to identify volatile compounds in exhaled gases. Such efforts are encouraged by reports of dogs that can be trained to identify persons with malignant neoplasms and other conditions. For example, cancer-specific volatile carbonyl aldehydes and ketones can be identified in the exhaled breath condensate of patients with lung cancer, and these concentrations may return to normal after surgery.

GENERAL REFERENCES

For the General References and other additional features, please visit Expert Consult at https://expertconsult.inkling.com.

86 DISORDERS OF VENTILATORY CONTROL

ATUL MALHOTRA AND FRANK POWELL

DEFINITIONS AND PATHOGENESIS

Ventilatory Control

Ventilation is controlled by complex interactions between central chemoreceptors, which predominantly are responsive to carbon dioxide tensions in arterial blood, and peripheral chemoreceptors, which primarily respond to carbon dioxide and oxygen tensions (Table 86-1). Disorders of ventilatory control are caused by derangements in these control systems.

HYPOVENTILATION SYNDROMES

Hypoventilation syndromes are defined by a lack of adequate alveolar ventilation to maintain a normal arterial carbon dioxide tension of 40 mm Hg. The two most common clinical settings that result in chronic hypoventilation are severe chronic obstructive pulmonary disease (COPD; Chapter 88) and morbid obesity (Chapters 100 and 220); less common causes are chronic opiate therapy, neuromuscular weakness (Chapters 421 and 422), and severe kyphoscoliosis (Chapter 99). The epidemiology of these hypoventilation syndromes is poorly studied, but about 15% of patients with severe COPD or morbid obesity have an elevated $Paco_2$. Regardless of the cause, patients with hypoventilation frequently have further worsening of their ventilation at the onset of sleep due to loss of the wakefulness stimulus, which is the normal drive to breathe while awake, and some degree of upper airway collapse after the onset of sleep (Chapter 100).

Patients with central sleep apnea (Chapter 100), which is a group of conditions in which cessation of airflow occurs because of a lack of respiratory effort, are classified into those with inadequate ventilatory drive and those with excessive drive.[1] The apparent paradox of how excessive drive leads to central apnea is explained by the concept of loop gain. A negative feedback control system with a high loop gain is prone to instability that leads to periods of excessive breathing followed by periods of apnea (Table 86-2). The prototype of a condition with high loop gain is periodic breathing or Cheyne-Stokes breathing (Fig. 86-1).

Cheyne-Stokes Breathing

Cheyne-Stokes breathing is a waxing and waning pattern of breathing, which is classically described as crescendo-decrescendo and often includes periods of central apnea. Cheyne-Stokes is seen most commonly during sleep in patients with heart failure.

EPIDEMIOLOGY

Cheyne-Stokes breathing is a form of ventilatory instability that occurs in 30 to 40% of patients with left ventricular systolic dysfunction.[2] Male sex, advanced age, low baseline $Paco_2$, and atrial fibrillation are risk factors for Cheyne-Stokes breathing among patients with heart failure. Controversy remains regarding whether this breathing pattern itself is deleterious or whether it is simply a marker of the underlying severity of cardiac disease. Cheyne-Stokes breathing represents about 5 to 10% of all cases of sleep apnea (Chapter 100) and is uncommon among patients who do not have heart failure.

PATHOBIOLOGY

Individuals with Cheyne-Stokes breathing have robust chemosensitivity as evidenced by marked increases in ventilation with small increases in $Paco_2$. The drive to breathe may be further increased by neural reflexes that are triggered by extravascular lung fluid and an elevated left atrial pressure. Intermittent hypoxemia and catecholamine surges, which are frequent in these patients, contribute to oxidative stress and neuroendocrine activation, both of which are thought to contribute to worsening of the underlying heart failure.

CLINICAL MANIFESTATIONS AND DIAGNOSIS

Patients with Cheyne-Stokes breathing can sometimes be diagnosed at the bedside by careful observation of their breathing pattern. During sleep or exercise, breathing becomes dependent primarily on metabolic stimuli. Patients may complain of fatigue or sleepiness because arousals from sleep tend to occur during the hyperpneic phase. Paroxysmal nocturnal dyspnea, a classic symptom of heart failure (Chapter 58), most commonly reflects

TABLE 86-1 CLASSIFICATION OF CENTRAL SLEEP APNEA

CENTRAL SLEEP APNEA SYNDROME	MECHANISM	THERAPY
Sleep transition apneas	Carbon dioxide fluctuations during transitions from sleep to wake to sleep	Reassurance, occasionally hypnotics or oxygen
Chronic narcotic therapy	Lack of central drive	Reduce narcotic dose Consider positive-pressure device
Cheyne-Stokes breathing	High loop gain from robust chemosensitivity and ventilatory drive	Optimize medical therapy for heart failure, consider PAP devices
Idiopathic central apnea	Unknown	Supportive, bilevel PAP; consider ventilatory stimulants
Treatment of emergent central apnea or "complex apnea"	Lowering upper airway resistance at CPAP initiation improves efficiency of carbon dioxide excretion	Reassurance, generally resolves spontaneously
Sleep hypoventilation syndromes	Fall in drive with loss of wakefulness stimulus, loss of accessory muscle activity during REM sleep	Noninvasive ventilation

CPAP = continuous positive airway pressure; PAP = positive airway pressure; REM = rapid eye movement.

TABLE 86-2 CLASSIFICATION OF HYPERCAPNIC DISEASES

HYPERCAPNIC DISEASE	MECHANISM	DIAGNOSIS	TREATMENT
Narcotic overdose	Reduced central drive	History, narcotized pupils, toxicology	Supportive care, naloxone
Acute severe asthma	Severe airflow obstruction, high dead space	Typical history, wheezing on examination, low FEV_1/FVC	Bronchodilators, anti-inflammatories, mechanical ventilation (usually invasive)
Acute exacerbation of COPD	Airflow obstruction, high dead space	History, cigarette smoking, low FEV_1/FVC, infectious etiology	Bronchodilators, anti-inflammatories, noninvasive ventilation
Obesity-hypoventilation syndrome	Low respiratory system compliance, high upper airway resistance, low central drive	High BMI, lack of other diagnoses; blunted carbon dioxide response	Weight loss, nocturnal bilevel positive airway pressure
Central congenital hypoventilation syndrome	*PHOX2B* mutation, lack of central drive	Genetic testing	Supportive care, mechanical ventilation (usually noninvasive)
Neuromuscular disease (e.g., myasthenia gravis, ALS, polymyositis, GBS/AIDP)	Lack of respiratory muscle force	Immediate orthopnea, low VC, low MIPs/MEPs	Underlying cause; nocturnal noninvasive ventilation; supportive care
Severe parenchymal lung disease, e.g., COPD	Lack of alveolar surface area; high pulmonary dead space and work of breathing	Typical history, smoking, low FEV_1 and FEV_1/FVC	Bronchodilator, anti-inflammatory therapy, possible nocturnal noninvasive ventilation, smoking cessation
Kyphoscoliosis	Low respiratory system compliance	Physical examination	Supportive care, noninvasive ventilation

AIDP = acute inflammatory demyelinating polyneuropathy; ALS = amyotrophic lateral sclerosis; BMI = body mass index; COPD = chronic obstructive pulmonary disease; FEV_1 = forced expiratory volume in 1 second; FVC = forced vital capacity; GBS = Guillain-Barré syndrome; MEPs = maximal expiratory pressures; MIPs = maximal inspiratory pressures; VC = vital capacity.

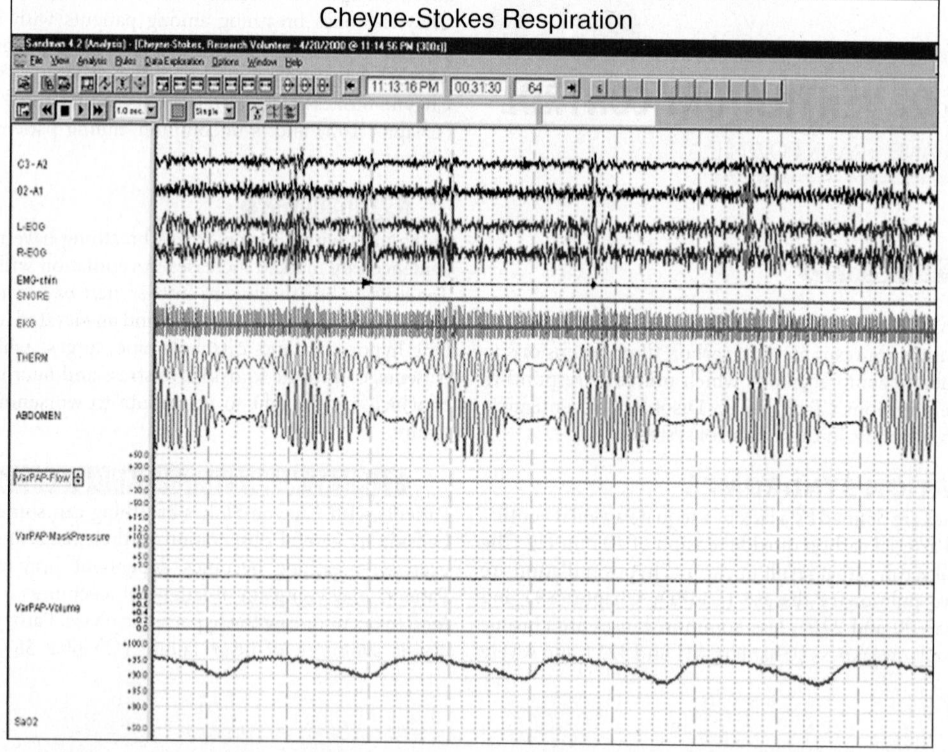

FIGURE 86-1. Cheyne-Stokes breathing with crescendo-decrescendo pattern of breathing. The thermistor detects air temperature changes at the mouth and nose. Note absences in airflow without respiratory effort seen in the abdominal belts. This breathing pattern leads to intermittent desaturations, arousals from sleep, and bursts of tachycardia. The loop gain concept can be understood by considering the thermostat analogy in which a control system is working to regulate a stable room temperature (e.g., 20°C). By analogy, the respiratory control system is working primarily to maintain a stable $Paco_2$ of 40 mm Hg and stable pH. Situations in which marked fluctuations in room temperature might occur would include one in which the thermostat is excessively sensitive (i.e., furnace turns on if room temperature falls to 19.999°C); if the furnace is too powerful, a marked overshoot in room temperature will be followed by a prolonged period when the furnace does not run. In the analogy to Cheyne-Stokes breathing, carbon dioxide is equated to room temperature and would be predicted to be unstable if chemosensitivity (i.e., the thermostat) were excessively robust (i.e., a marked increase in ventilation for a small change in carbon dioxide) or if the efficiency of carbon dioxide excretion were high (i.e., marked fall in $Paco_2$ with increased ventilation). Situations that increase the propensity for carbon dioxide fluctuations lead to elevated loop gain and thus increase the risk for Cheyne-Stokes breathing.

underlying Cheyne-Stokes breathing. Patients often are diagnosed in the sleep laboratory while undergoing investigation for possible obstructive sleep apnea.

The diagnosis of Cheyne-Stokes breathing, if it is not readily apparent, can be made during overnight polysomnography, when the typical oscillatory pattern of tidal volume is seen in the absence of ventilatory efforts during the apneic periods. In evaluating such recordings, and in contrast to obstructive apnea, it is important to note that Cheyne-Stokes breathing usually resolves during rapid eye movement (REM) sleep, that arousals on the electroencephalogram typically occur during the hyperpneic phase, and that Cheyne-Stokes breathing generally does not resolve immediately when nasal continuous positive airway pressure (CPAP) is applied.

TREATMENT

Medical management of Cheyne-Stokes breathing most often is treatment of the underlying heart failure (Chapter 59). After optimization of medical management, the Cheyne-Stokes breathing pattern frequently resolves. CPAP can improve breathing indices but is no better than standard medical therapy from the standpoint of mortality.[A1] Newer approaches to non-invasive ventilation show promise but require further evaluation.[3]

Central Congenital Hypoventilation Syndrome

DEFINITION AND EPIDEMIOLOGY

Central congenital hypoventilation syndrome is a rare congenital condition, previously referred to as Ondine curse, characterized by a diminished ventilatory response to carbon dioxide.[4] The central congenital hypoventilation syndrome was traditionally diagnosed in neonates, but more subtle forms of disease are increasingly noted in older children and adults.

PATHOBIOLOGY

The syndrome is now defined by a mutation in the *PHOX2B* gene, located on chromosome 4p12.[5] The *PHOX2B* gene is a highly conserved homeobox gene that is expressed mainly in the afferent and efferent pathways of respiratory, cardiovascular, and digestive reflexes. Deletion of the gene in mice causes irregular breathing, a reduced hypercapnic ventilatory response, and death from central apnea. These mice have neuronal loss in the retrotrapezoid nucleus and parafacial region of the brain stem, thereby suggesting the importance of this medullary region in normal breathing. Abnormalities in *PHOX2B* genes have also been associated with Hirschsprung disease (Chapter 136), neural crest tumors, cardiac asystole (Chapter 63), and other abnormalities of the autonomic nervous system (Chapter 418).

Because most parents of affected children with the central congenital hypoventilation syndrome do not carry a *PHOX2B* mutation, the mutations are de novo. About 90% of patients are heterozygous for a polyalanine repeat expansion mutation, in which the affected allele has 24 to 33 alanines rather than the normal 20 alanines. The remaining 10% of central congenital hypoventilation syndrome patients have missense, nonsense, or frameshift mutations in the *PHOX2B* gene.

CLINICAL MANIFESTATIONS AND DIAGNOSIS

Neonates can present with cyanosis at birth, recurrent central apneas, or both. Adults can present with idiopathic central sleep apnea, unexplained hypercapnia, or autonomic abnormalities (Chapter 418). Confirmation of the diagnosis requires the demonstration of an abnormality in the *PHOX2B* gene.

TREATMENT

There are currently no specific therapies for central congenital hypoventilation syndrome beyond supportive care. Genetic counseling is required for afflicted individuals and their families, given the autosomal dominant pattern of inheritance. Patients must be cautioned against the use of sedatives, which could precipitate respiratory failure. Mechanical ventilation during sleep either invasively (through tracheostomy) or noninvasively (through bilevel positive airway pressure support [Chapter 100]) is required in most patients. Some patients remain fully ventilator dependent. Alternative treatments, such as ventilatory stimulants and diaphragmatic pacing, are generally ineffective.

Acquired Hypoventilation Syndromes

DEFINITION AND EPIDEMIOLOGY

Patients with hypoventilation syndromes cannot maintain adequate minute ventilation to keep their Pa_{CO_2} at 40 mm Hg. Patients can be classified into those who lack central ventilatory drive and those who have a pulmonary mechanical or neuromuscular abnormality that prevents adequate gas exchange. The case frequency is unknown, but hypercapnic respiratory failure is one of the more common admission diagnoses in intensive care units.

PATHOBIOLOGY

Patients with conditions characterized by the lack of central drive have reasonably normal lungs and respiratory muscle function but lack adequate response to carbon dioxide and hypoxia. In contrast, most patients with mechanical or neuromuscular abnormalities have a larger work of breathing compared with normal individuals; the most common underlying conditions are severe COPD (Chapter 88) and morbid obesity (Chapter 220) with the obesity-hypoventilation syndrome. Such individuals have diminished but not absent chemoresponsiveness. Another cause of inadequate gas exchange is neuromuscular disease; common causes include disorders of neuromuscular transmission (Chapter 422), severe muscle weakness (Chapter 421), the residua from poliovirus infection (Chapter 379), Guillain-Barré syndrome (Chapter 420), and acute poisoning (Chapter 110).

CLINICAL MANIFESTATIONS AND DIAGNOSIS

Patients with hypoventilation have myriad presentations ranging from asymptomatic abnormalities in laboratory testing (e.g., elevated Pa_{CO_2}, unexplained low Sa_{O_2}, or elevated serum bicarbonate level) to respiratory failure in the intensive care unit (e.g., respiratory infection with laboratory evidence of chronic abnormalities, such as acute-on-chronic respiratory acidosis). Patients who acutely overdose on sedative-hypnotic or narcotic agents may present with acute respiratory acidosis and loss of consciousness. Patients who take chronic narcotics may present with central sleep apnea-hypopnea or otherwise unexplained oxygen desaturation at night.

Once it is suspected, the diagnosis of hypoventilation is confirmed by the finding of Pa_{CO_2} higher than 42 mm Hg on analysis of an arterial blood sample. If the increase in Pa_{CO_2} is of short duration so that renal compensation has not yet occurred (Chapter 118), the serum bicarbonate level is increased by 1 mEq/L for every rise of 10 mm Hg in Pa_{CO_2}. By comparison, if the respiratory acidosis is of sufficient duration for renal compensation to occur, the serum bicarbonate level will be increased by 4 mEq for every rise of 10 mm Hg in Pa_{CO_2} (Fig. 86-2).

Once an elevated Pa_{CO_2} is established, it is appropriate to distinguish patients who "can't breathe" from those who "won't breathe." "Can't breathe" implies that a respiratory mechanical problem or neuromuscular weakness is causing the elevation in Pa_{CO_2}. Abnormalities in pulmonary function testing (e.g., a very low vital capacity) suggest a parenchymal or chest wall disorder. Ultrasound can identify phrenic neuropathy causing diaphragmatic dysfunction.[6] Patients who "won't breathe" have central nervous system abnormalities that affect central drive, chemosensitivity, or both.

TREATMENT AND PROGNOSIS

Rx

The treatment of hypoventilation should focus on the underlying cause. Acute poisonings can be managed supportively or, in some cases, with specific antidotes (Chapter 110). Chronic conditions can be treated by addressing the underlying cause, such as weight loss in obesity-hypoventilation syndrome or cholinesterase inhibitors in myasthenia gravis (Chapter 422). For parenchymal lung disease, treatment is directed at the underlying cause, if possible (Chapters 88 and 92).

Sedative medications should be used cautiously because they can occasionally precipitate acute respiratory failure. Although profound hypoxemia can clearly be deleterious, oxygen occasionally can precipitate severe acute respiratory acidosis, particularly in patients with acute exacerbations of COPD (Chapter 88). As a result, hypoventilating patients with COPD require cautious management including the careful administration of supplemental oxygen, which should be titrated to an arterial oxygen saturation of 90% or an arterial oxygen tension of 60 mm Hg.

Severe hypoventilation requires mechanical ventilation (Chapter 105), such as noninvasive ventilation for an acute exacerbation of COPD. For other presentations in which the Pa_{CO_2} is believed to be acutely elevated, endotracheal intubation and mechanical ventilation are frequently used, especially in patients with impaired consciousness. For chronic hypoventilation in hypercapnic COPD, noninvasive bilevel positive airway pressure through a face mask during sleep can maintain alveolar ventilation, but there is no definitive evidence that noninvasive positive-pressure ventilation can prolong life or reduce hospitalizations in patients with COPD and chronic respiratory failure.[A2] In addition, the considerable difficulty of adhering to nocturnal bilevel therapy in COPD emphasizes the need for discussions with patients and families regarding its risks and benefits.

Other chronic hypoventilation syndromes are also commonly treated with bilevel positive airway pressure, although data are not compelling. In some chronic conditions, such as motor neuron disease (Chapter 419), tracheostomy should be discussed, although the impact of such interventions on quality of life should be carefully considered. Regardless of the underlying cause, an elevation in the Pa_{CO_2} level is considered a poor prognostic sign. End-of-life discussions are also important in such cases because the prognosis of patients with chronic respiratory failure is generally poor.

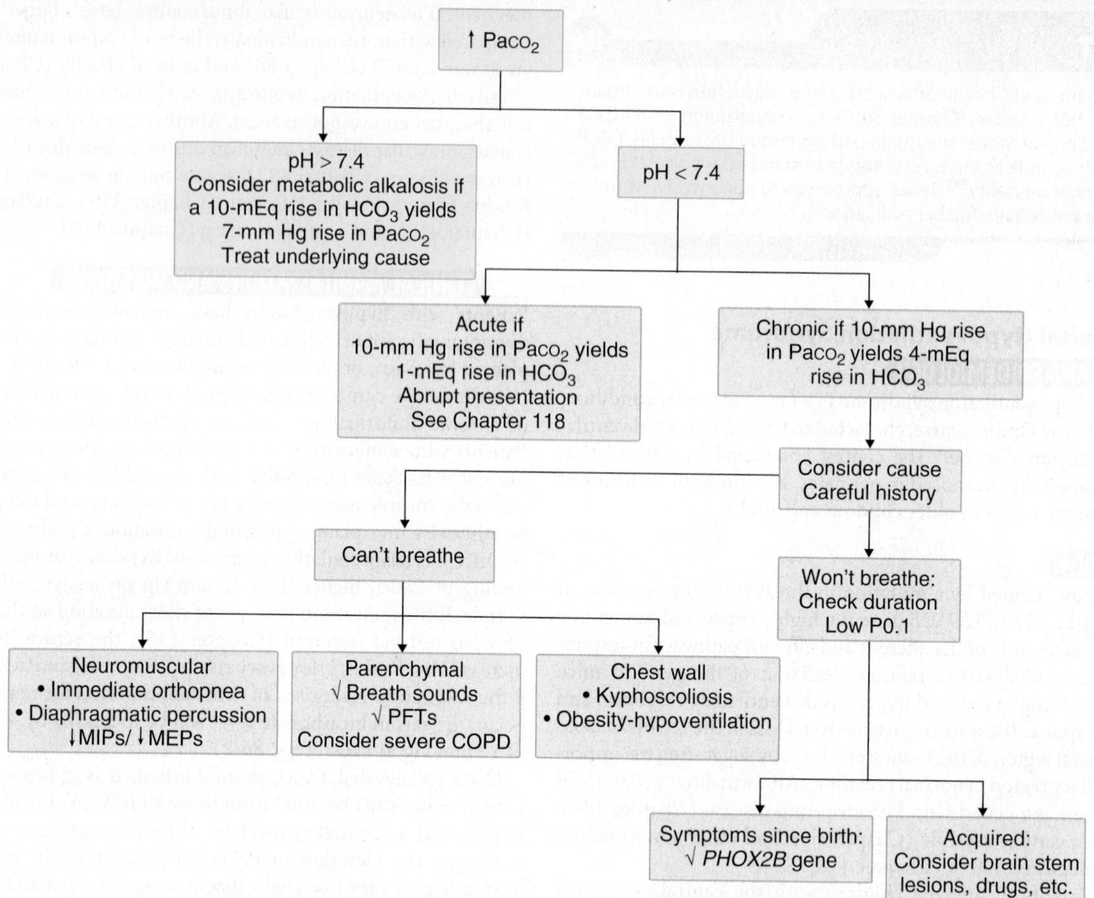

FIGURE 86-2. A flow chart of a systematic approach to hypercapnia and various causes of hypoventilation. The change in pH can help determine the cause and chronicity. A careful history and physical examination, coupled with pulmonary function testing, can help classify patients into those who "can't breathe" because of neuromuscular or mechanical abnormalities of the respiratory system compared with those who "won't breathe" because of central nervous system disease. COPD = chronic obstructive pulmonary disease; MEPs = maximal expiratory pressures; MIPs = maximal inspiratory pressures; P0.1 = the negative mouth pressure generated during the first 100 msec of an occluded inspiration; PFTs = pulmonary function tests.

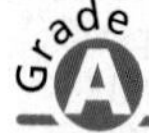

Grade A References

A1. Bradley TD, Logan AG, Kimoff RJ, et al. Continuous positive airway pressure for central sleep apnea and heart failure. *N Engl J Med.* 2005;353:2025-2033.

A2. Kohnlein T, Windisch W, Kohler D, et al. Non-invasive positive pressure ventilation for the treatment of severe stable chronic obstructive pulmonary disease: a prospective, multicentre, randomised, controlled clinical trial. *Lancet Respir Med.* 2014;2:698-705.

GENERAL REFERENCES

For the General References and other additional features, please visit Expert Consult at https://expertconsult.inkling.com.

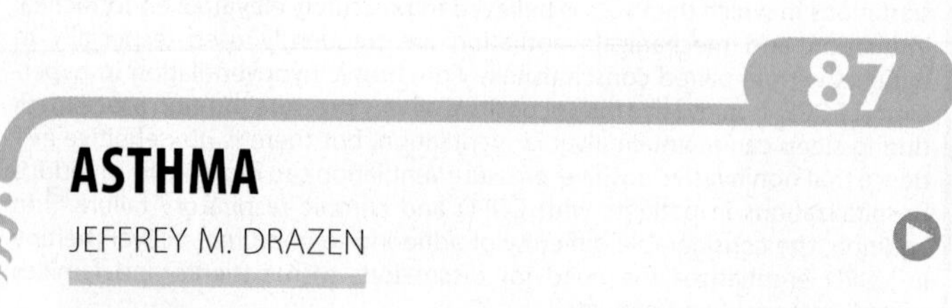

87 ASTHMA

JEFFREY M. DRAZEN

DEFINITION

Asthma is a clinical syndrome of unknown etiology characterized by three distinct components: (1) recurrent episodes of airway obstruction that resolve spontaneously or as a result of treatment; (2) exaggerated bronchoconstrictor responses to stimuli that have little or no effect in nonasthmatic subjects, a phenomenon known as airway hyperresponsiveness; and (3) inflammation of the airways as defined by a variety of criteria. Although airway obstruction is largely reversible, it is currently thought that changes in the asthmatic airway may be irreversible in some settings.

EPIDEMIOLOGY

Asthma is an extremely common disorder affecting boys more commonly than girls and, after puberty, women slightly more commonly than men; approximately 8% of the adult population of the United States has signs and symptoms consistent with a diagnosis of asthma. Although most cases begin before the age of 25 years, new-onset asthma may develop at any time throughout life.

The worldwide prevalence of asthma has increased more than 45% since the late 1970s. In the last decade alone, the prevalence of wheezing in children has increased by about 0.1% per year.

During the past four decades, the greatest increases in the prevalence of asthma have occurred in countries that adopted an "industrialized" lifestyle. For example, epidemiologic data suggest that being raised in a farming environment is associated with a much lower risk of asthma, independent of genetic factors, and this difference may be attributable to exposure to a greater diversity of environmental microbes early in life.[1]

Asthma is among the most common reasons to seek medical treatment. In the United States, it is responsible for about 15 million annual outpatient visits to physicians and for nearly 2 million annual inpatient hospital days of treatment. The estimated yearly direct and indirect costs of asthma care in the United States are more than $55 billion.

PATHOBIOLOGY

Genetics

In twin studies, asthma has about 60% heritability, indicating that both genetic and environmental factors are important in its etiology. A region on chromosome 17q21, at or near the locus for *ORMDL3*, a member of a gene family that encodes endoplasmic reticulum transmembrane proteins, has been repeatedly associated with childhood-onset asthma. Although the exact functional variant in this region has not been identified, the isolation of a locus for childhood-onset asthma supports the clinical observation that adult- and childhood-onset asthma appear to be distinct disorders. Genetic variants that influence the response to treatment also have been identified and widely replicated.

Pathology

The pathology of mild asthma, as delineated by bronchoscopic and biopsy studies, is characterized by edema and hyperemia of the mucosa and by infiltration of the mucosa with mast cells, eosinophils, and lymphocytes bearing the T_H2 phenotype. Controlled trials using antibodies against interleukin-5 or the interleukin-4 receptor α chain in patients with persistent asthma symptoms and eosinophilia, despite treatment with corticosteroids, provide solid evidence for the pathobiologic role of these inflammatory cytokines in asthma. As a result of these inflammatory stimuli coupled with the mechanical deformation of the epithelium from airway, smooth muscle constriction,[2] the airway wall is thickened by the deposition of type III and type V collagen below the true basement membrane. In addition, in severe chronic asthma, there is hypertrophy and hyperplasia of airway glands and of both surface and glandular secretory cells as well as hyperplasia of airway smooth muscle. Morphometric studies of airways from asthmatic subjects have demonstrated airway wall thickening of sufficient magnitude to increase airflow resistance and to enhance airway responsiveness. During a severe asthmatic event, the airway wall is thickened markedly; in addition, patchy airway occlusion occurs by a mixture of hyperviscous mucus and clusters of shed airway epithelial cells.

The episodic airway obstruction that constitutes an asthma attack results from narrowing of the airway lumen to airflow. Although it is now well established that asthma is associated with infiltration of the airway by inflammatory cells, the links between the presence of these cells and the pathobiologic processes that account for asthmatic airway obstruction are just beginning to be delineated. Three possible but not mutually exclusive links have been postulated: the constriction of airway smooth muscle, the thickening of airway epithelium, and the presence of liquids within the confines of the airway lumen. Among these mechanisms, the constriction of airway smooth muscle due to the local release of bioactive mediators or neurotransmitters is the most widely accepted explanation for the acute reversible airway obstruction in asthma attacks. Several bronchoactive mediators are thought to be the agents that initiate the airway obstruction characteristic of asthma. Moreover, the chronic airway narrowing, termed airway wall remodeling, that occurs in many patients with asthma likely results from the actions of inflammatory cells in the asthmatic airway.

Mediators of the Acute Asthmatic Response

Acetylcholine

Acetylcholine released from intrapulmonary motor nerves causes constriction of airway smooth muscle through direct stimulation of muscarinic receptors of the M_3 subtype. The potential role for acetylcholine in the bronchoconstriction of asthma primarily derives from the observation that tiotropium bromide, a muscarinic antagonist, can reduce bronchoconstriction.

Histamine

Histamine, or β-imidazolylethylamine, was identified as a potent endogenous bronchoactive agent more than 100 years ago. Mast cells, which are prominent in airway tissues obtained from patients with asthma, constitute the major pulmonary source of histamine. Clinical trials with novel potent antihistamines indicate only a minor role for histamine as a mediator of airway obstruction in asthma.

Leukotrienes and Lipoxins

The cysteinyl leukotrienes, namely, LTC_4, LTD_4, and LTE_4, as well as the dihydroxy leukotriene LTB_4 are derived by the lipoxygenation of arachidonic acid released from target cell membrane phospholipids during cellular activation. 5-Lipoxygenase, the 5-lipoxygenase–activating protein, and LTC_4 synthase make up the cellular protein and enzyme content needed to produce the cysteinyl leukotrienes. The production of LTB_4 requires 5-lipoxygenase, the 5-lipoxygenase–activating protein, and LTA_4 epoxide hydrolase. Mast cells, eosinophils, and alveolar macrophages have the enzymatic capability to produce cysteinyl leukotrienes from their membrane phospholipids, whereas polymorphonuclear leukocytes produce exclusively LTB_4, which is predominantly a chemoattractant molecule; LTC_4 and LTD_4 are among the most potent contractile agonists ever identified for human airway smooth muscle. The efficacy of a leukotriene receptor antagonist (i.e., pranlukast, zafirlukast, and montelukast) or a synthesis inhibitor (i.e., zileuton) in the treatment of chronic persistent asthma has led to the conclusion that the leukotrienes are important but not exclusive mediators of the asthmatic response. Lipoxins, which are double lipoxygenase products of arachidonic acid metabolism, have been shown to be endogenous downregulators of the inflammatory response. The amounts of lipoxins are decreased in the airways of patients with severe asthma.

Nitric Oxide

Nitric oxide (NO•) is produced enzymatically by airway epithelial cells and by inflammatory cells found in the asthmatic lung. Free NO• has a half-life on the order of seconds in the airway and is stabilized by conjugation to thiols to form RS-NO, where *R* designates any one of a number of molecular entities that can support this chemical linkage. Both NO• and RS-NO have bronchodilator actions and may play a homeostatic role in the airway. Paradoxically, high levels of NO•, when it is coavailable with superoxide anion, may form toxic oxidation products, such as peroxynitrite ($OONO^-$), which could damage the airway. Patients with asthma have higher than normal levels of NO• in their expired air, and these levels decrease consistently after treatment with corticosteroids.

Physiological Changes in Asthma

An increased resistance to airflow is the consequence of the airway obstruction induced by smooth muscle constriction, thickening of the airway epithelium, or free liquid within the airway lumen. Obstruction to airflow is manifested by increased airway resistance and decreased flow rates throughout the vital capacity. At the onset of an asthma attack, obstruction occurs at all airway levels; as the attack resolves, these changes are reversed—first in the large airways (i.e., mainstem, lobar, segmental, and subsegmental bronchi) and then in the more peripheral airways. This anatomic sequence of onset and reversal is reflected in the physiological changes observed during resolution of an asthmatic episode. Specifically, as an asthma attack resolves, flow rates first normalize at volumes high in the vital capacity and only later at volumes low in the vital capacity. Because asthma is an airway disease, not an air space disease, no primary changes occur in the static pressure-volume curve of the lungs. However, during an acute attack of asthma, airway narrowing may be so severe as to result in airway closure, with individual lung units closing at a volume that is near their maximal volume. This closure results in a change of the pressure-volume curve such that for a given

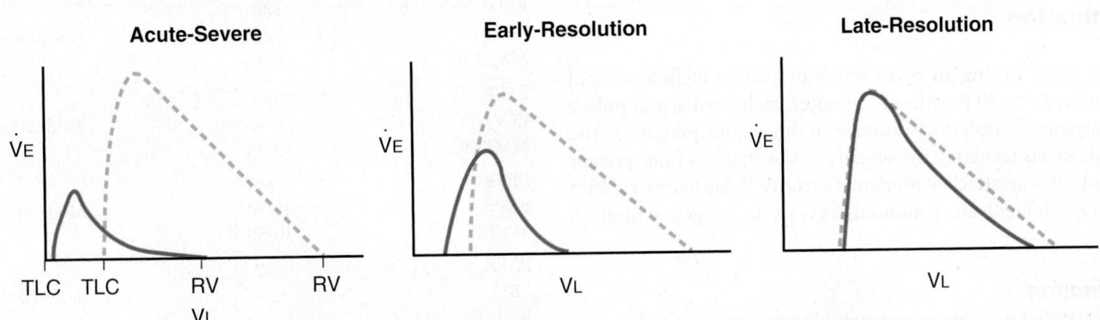

FIGURE 87-1. **Schematic flow-volume curves in various stages of asthma.** In each figure, the *dashed line* depicts the normal flow-volume curve. Predicted and observed total lung capacity (TLC) and residual volume (RV) are shown at the extremes of each curve. V̇E = expiratory flow rate; VL = lung volume.

contained gas volume within the thorax, elastic recoil is decreased, which in turn further depresses expiratory flow rates.

Additional factors influence the mechanical behavior of the lungs during an acute attack of asthma. During inspiration in an asthma attack, the maximal inspiratory pleural pressure becomes more negative than the subatmospheric pressure of 4 to 6 cm H_2O usually required for tidal airflow. The expiratory phase of respiration also becomes active as the patient tries to force air from the lungs. As a consequence, peak pleural pressures during expiration, which normally are, at most, only a few centimeters of water above atmospheric pressure, may be as high as 20 to 30 cm H_2O above atmospheric pressure. The low pleural pressures during inspiration tend to dilate airways, whereas the high pleural pressures during expiration tend to narrow airways. During an asthma attack, the wide pressure swings, coupled with alterations in the mechanical properties of the airway wall, lead to a much higher resistance to expiratory airflow than to inspiratory airflow.

The respiratory rate is usually rapid during an acute asthmatic attack. This tachypnea is driven not by abnormalities in arterial blood gas composition but rather by stimulation of intrapulmonary receptors with subsequent effects on central respiratory centers. One consequence of the combination of airway narrowing and rapid airflow rates is a heightened mechanical load on the ventilatory pump. During a severe attack, the load can increase the work of breathing by a factor of 10 or more and can predispose to fatigue of the ventilatory muscles. With respect to gas exchange, the patchy nature of asthmatic airway narrowing results in a maldistribution of ventilation (V) relative to pulmonary perfusion (Q). A shift occurs from the normal preponderance of V/Q units, with a ratio of near unity, to a distribution with a large number of alveolar-capillary units, with a V/Q ratio of less than unity. The net effect is to induce arterial hypoxemia. In addition, the hyperpnea of asthma is reflected as hyperventilation with a low arterial Pco_2.

CLINICAL MANIFESTATIONS

History

During an acute asthma attack, patients seek medical attention for shortness of breath accompanied by cough, wheezing, and anxiety. The degree of breathlessness experienced by the patient is not closely related to the degree of airflow obstruction but is often influenced by the acuteness of the attack. Dyspnea may occur only with exercise (exercise-induced asthma),[3] after aspirin ingestion (aspirin-exacerbated respiratory disease),[4] after exposure to a specific known allergen (extrinsic asthma), or for no identifiable reason (intrinsic asthma). Variants of asthma exist in which cough, hoarseness, or inability to sleep through the night is the only symptom. Identification of a provoking stimulus through careful questioning helps establish the diagnosis of asthma and may be therapeutically useful if the stimulus can be avoided. Most patients with asthma complain of shortness of breath when they are exposed to rapid changes in the temperature and humidity of inspired air. For example, during the winter months in less temperate climates, patients commonly become short of breath on leaving a heated house; in warm humid climates, patients may complain of shortness of breath on entering a cold dry room, such as an air-conditioned theater.

An important factor to consider in taking a history from a patient with asthma is the potential for occupational exposures in asthma (Chapter 93). Asthma that is brought on by occupational exposures is termed occupational asthma; preexisting asthma that is exacerbated by workplace exposures is termed workplace-exacerbated asthma. In reactive airway dysfunction syndrome, a single large exposure leads to a persistent asthma-like phenotype in a previously normal individual.[5]

Physical Examination

Vital Signs

Common features noted during an acute attack of asthma include a rapid respiratory rate (often 25 to 40 breaths per minute), tachycardia, and pulsus paradoxus (an exaggerated inspiratory decrease in the systolic pressure). The magnitude of the pulsus is related to the severity of the attack; a value greater than 15 mm Hg indicates an attack of moderate severity. Pulse oximetry, with the patient respiring ambient air, commonly reveals an oxygen saturation near 90%.

Thoracic Examination

Inspection may reveal that patients experiencing acute attacks of asthma are using their accessory muscles of ventilation; if so, the skin over the thorax may be retracted into the intercostal spaces during inspiration. The chest is usually hyperinflated, and the expiratory phase is prolonged relative to the inspiratory phase. Percussion of the thorax demonstrates hyperresonance, with loss of the normal variation in dullness due to diaphragmatic movement; tactile fremitus is diminished. Auscultation reveals wheezing, which is the cardinal physical finding in asthma but does not establish the diagnosis (Chapter 83). Wheezing, commonly louder during expiration but heard during inspiration as well, is characterized as polyphonic in that more than one pitch may be heard simultaneously (Video 87-1). Accompanying adventitious sounds may include rhonchi, which are suggestive of free secretions in the airway lumen, or rales, which should raise the suspicion of an alternative diagnosis and are indicative of localized infection or heart failure. The loss of intensity or the absence of breath sounds in a patient with asthma is an indication of severe airflow obstruction.

DIAGNOSIS

Laboratory Findings

Pulmonary Function Findings

A decrease in airflow rates throughout the vital capacity is the cardinal pulmonary function abnormality during an asthmatic episode.[6,7] The peak expiratory flow rate (PEFR), the forced expiratory volume in the first second (FEV_1), and the maximal mid-expiratory flow rate (MMEFR) are all decreased in asthma (Chapter 85). In severe asthma, dyspnea may be so severe as to prevent the patient from performing a complete spirogram. In this case, if 2 seconds of forced expiration can be recorded, useful values for PEFR and FEV_1 can be obtained. Gradation of attack severity (Table 87-1) *must* be assessed by objective measures of airflow; no other methods yield accurate and reproducible results. As the attack resolves, the PEFR and the FEV_1 increase toward normal together while the MMEFR remains substantially depressed; as the attack resolves further, the FEV_1 and the PEFR may normalize while the MMEFR remains depressed (see Fig. 87-1). Even when the attack has fully resolved clinically, residual depression of the MMEFR is not uncommon; this depression may resolve during a prolonged course of treatment. If the patient is able to cooperate such that more complete measurements of lung function can be made, lung volume measurements made during an attack demonstrate an increase in both total lung capacity and residual volume; the changes in total lung capacity and residual volume resolve with treatment. Because of the extra cooperation needed for this testing, it is not advised during an acute asthmatic event but is indicated before discharge in a patient hospitalized for the treatment of asthma or between episodes of asthma.

Pulmonary function testing obtained when the patient is relatively stable usually demonstrates airway obstruction, as indicated by low FEV_1 (as a percentage of the patient's predicted value), low forced vital capacity, and slightly elevated total lung capacity and residual volume values. These results may fully normalize after administration of a bronchodilator, but a "bronchodilator response" is canonically defined as a 12% increase in the FEV_1, provided it is at least 200 mL (E-Fig. 87-1).

TABLE 87-1 RELATIVE SEVERITY OF AN ASTHMATIC ATTACK AS INDICATED BY PEFR, FEV_1, AND MMEFR

TEST	PREDICTED VALUE (%)	SEVERITY OF ASTHMA
PEFR FEV_1 MMEFR	>80 >80 >80	No spirometric abnormalities
PEFR FEV_1 MMEFR	>80 >70 55-75	Mild asthma
PEFR FEV_1 MMEFR	>60 45-70 30-50	Moderate asthma
PEFR FEV_1 MMEFR	<50 <50 10-30	Severe asthma

FEV_1 = forced expiratory volume in the first second; MMEFR = maximal mid-expiratory flow rate; PEFR = peak expiratory flow rate.

Exhaled NO•

The fraction of NO• in the exhaled air (Fe_{NO}) is elevated in patients with asthma. Although the exact concentration considered "elevated" will vary with the details of the technique used to obtain the gas sample, a concentration of 15 parts per billion is a convenient and reliable level that can be used to distinguish people without asthma from patients with untreated asthma. However, the measurement of exhaled nitric oxide has not been shown to be of value in the day-to-day management of asthma.[A1]

Arterial Blood Gases

Blood gas analysis need not be undertaken in individuals with mild asthma. If the asthma is of sufficient severity to merit prolonged observation, however, blood gas analysis is indicated; in such cases, hypoxemia and hypocapnia are the rule. With the subject breathing ambient air, the Pao_2 is usually between 55 and 70 mm Hg and the $Paco_2$ between 25 and 35 mm Hg. At the onset of the attack, an appropriate pure respiratory alkalemia is usually evident; with attacks of prolonged duration, the pH returns toward normal as a result of a compensatory metabolic acidemia. A normal $Paco_2$ in a patient with moderate to severe airflow obstruction is reason for concern because it may indicate that the mechanical load on the respiratory system is greater than can be sustained by the ventilatory muscles and that respiratory failure is imminent. When the $Paco_2$ increases in such settings, the pH decreases quickly because the bicarbonate stores have become depleted as a result of renal compensation for the prolonged preceding respiratory alkalemia. Because this chain of events can take place rapidly, close observation is indicated for asthmatic patients with "normal" $Paco_2$ levels and moderate to severe airflow obstruction.

Other Blood Findings

Asthmatic subjects are frequently atopic; thus, blood eosinophilia is common but not universal. In addition, elevated serum levels of immunoglobulin E (IgE) are often documented; epidemiologic studies indicate that asthma is unusual in subjects with low IgE levels. If indicated by the patient's history, specific immunosorbent tests, which measure IgE directed against specific offending antigens, can be conducted. In rare instances during severe asthma attacks, serum concentrations of aminotransferases, lactate dehydrogenase, muscle creatine kinase, ornithine transcarbamylase, and antidiuretic hormone may be elevated.

Radiographic Findings

The chest radiograph of a subject with asthma is often normal. Severe asthma is associated with hyperinflation, as indicated by depression of the diaphragm and abnormally lucent lung fields. Complications of severe asthma, including subcutaneous emphysema, pneumomediastinum (E-Fig. 87-2), and pneumothorax, may be detected radiographically. In mild to moderate asthma without adventitious sounds other than wheezing, a chest radiograph need not be obtained; if the asthma is of sufficient severity to merit hospital admission, a chest radiograph is advised.

Electrocardiographic Findings

The electrocardiogram, except for sinus tachycardia, is usually normal in acute asthma. However, right axis deviation, right bundle branch block, "P pulmonale," or even ST-T wave abnormalities may arise during severe asthma and resolve as the attack resolves.

Sputum Findings

The sputum of the asthmatic patient may be either clear or opaque with a green or yellow tinge. The presence of color does not invariably indicate infection, and examination of a Gram-stained and Wright-stained sputum smear is indicated. The sputum often contains eosinophils, Charcot-Leyden crystals (crystallized eosinophil lysophospholipase), Curschmann spirals (bronchiolar casts composed of mucus and cells), or Creola bodies (clusters of airway epithelial cells with identifiable cilia that, in fresh samples, can often be seen to beat), which can affect color without the presence of infection.

DIAGNOSIS

Differential Diagnosis

Asthma is easy to recognize in a young patient without comorbid medical conditions who has exacerbating and remitting airway obstruction accompanied by blood eosinophilia. A rapid response to bronchodilator treatment is usually all that is needed to establish the diagnosis. However, in the patient with cryptic episodic shortness of breath, an elevated Fe_{NO} can help establish a diagnosis of asthma. However, in the absence of an elevated Fe_{NO}, other causes of wheezing (see Table 83-3) should be investigated.

PREVENTION AND TREATMENT Rx

There is currently no way to prevent a patient from developing an asthmatic diathesis. For example, trials of allergen avoidance in childhood have not been successful. If a patient has such a diathesis with an allergic component, avoidance of allergens can reduce the frequency of asthma attacks. For example, removal of indoor mold can improve symptoms by 25% and reduce medication use by 50%.

The treatment of asthma is directed at two distinct facets of the disease: the control of symptoms and the prevention of exacerbations. Symptomatic control is measured by the severity and frequency of asthma symptoms during the day, including limitations of activities of daily life, the need to use "rescue" β-agonist inhalers, and asthma symptoms that wake the patient from sleep. The prevention of exacerbations is less linked to symptoms than to levels of lung function, so management must include objective measures of lung function. The best measure is FEV_1, but measures of PEFR can be substituted. Inexpensive and easy-to-use peak flowmeters make the measurement feasible in virtually all cases.

Treatment of asthma has two components. The first is the use of acute reliever (rescue) agents (i.e., bronchodilators) for acute asthmatic airway obstruction. The second is the use of controller treatments, which modify the asthmatic airway environment so that acute airway narrowing, requiring rescue treatments, occurs much less frequently.

In a given individual, the intensity of asthma treatment is adjusted, for the most part, to achieve five goals:

1. to allow the patient to pursue the activities of his or her daily life without excessive interference from asthma;
2. to allow the patient to sleep without awakening because of asthmatic symptoms;
3. to minimize the use of rescue bronchodilator treatment;
4. to prevent the need for unscheduled medical care; and
5. to maintain lung function reasonably near normal.

A patient who meets these standards on the basis of a careful history, chest examination, and measurement of lung function is said to be "in control," whereas a patient whose disease activities prevent these goals from being met is said to be "out of control." Patients who are not in control should have their treatment stepped up, whereas patients whose asthma is in good control for 3 months should attempt to have their treatment stepped down (Fig. 87-2).[8]

Rescue Treatments

All patients with asthma should be prescribed a rapid-acting β-agonist rescue inhaler to use if acute asthmatic airway obstruction develops. Patients should be shown how to use the inhaler (Video 87-2) and tested for their ability to use it correctly. All albuterol inhalers now contain hydrofluoroalkane propellants. Aerosol "spacers" can help patients who have difficulty in coordinating their inspiratory effort and inhaler actuation.

β-Adrenergic Agents

Short-acting β-adrenergic agents given by inhalation are the mainstay of bronchodilator treatment of asthma.[9] Constricted airway smooth muscle relaxes in response to stimulation of β_2-adrenergic receptors. β-Adrenergic agonists with varying degrees of β_2-selectivity are available for use in inhaled (by nebulizer or metered-dose inhaler; Fig. 87-3), oral, or parenteral preparations. Most patients with mild intermittent asthma should be treated with a short-acting β_2-selective inhaler (such as albuterol) on an as-needed basis. Regardless of the specific type of medication used, rescue treatment should consist of two "puffs" from the inhaler, with the first and second puffs separated by a 3- to 5-minute interval, which is thought to allow enough time for the first puff to dilate narrowed airways, thus giving the agent better access to affected areas of the lung. Patients should be instructed to exhale to a comfortable volume, to breathe in very slowly (such as they would when sipping hot soup), and to actuate the inhaler as they inspire. Inspiration to near total lung capacity is followed by holding the breath for 5 seconds to allow the deposition of smaller aerosol particles in more peripheral airways. This treatment can be repeated every 4 to 6 hours; patients should be instructed to "advance" their asthma treatment as noted in Figure 87-2 if they need to use more than 12 puffs of a β-agonist in a 72-hour period.

Randomized trials document that the regular use (i.e., two puffs four times a day) of inhaled albuterol is not associated with adverse events. Asthma patients may notice a difference in the inhaled "feel" of albuterol inhalers compared with inhaled glucocorticoid inhalers because all albuterol inhalers are powered by hydrofluoroalkanes and the puff has a lower velocity. Randomized trials show therapeutic equivalence with chlorofluorocarbon-powered inhalers.

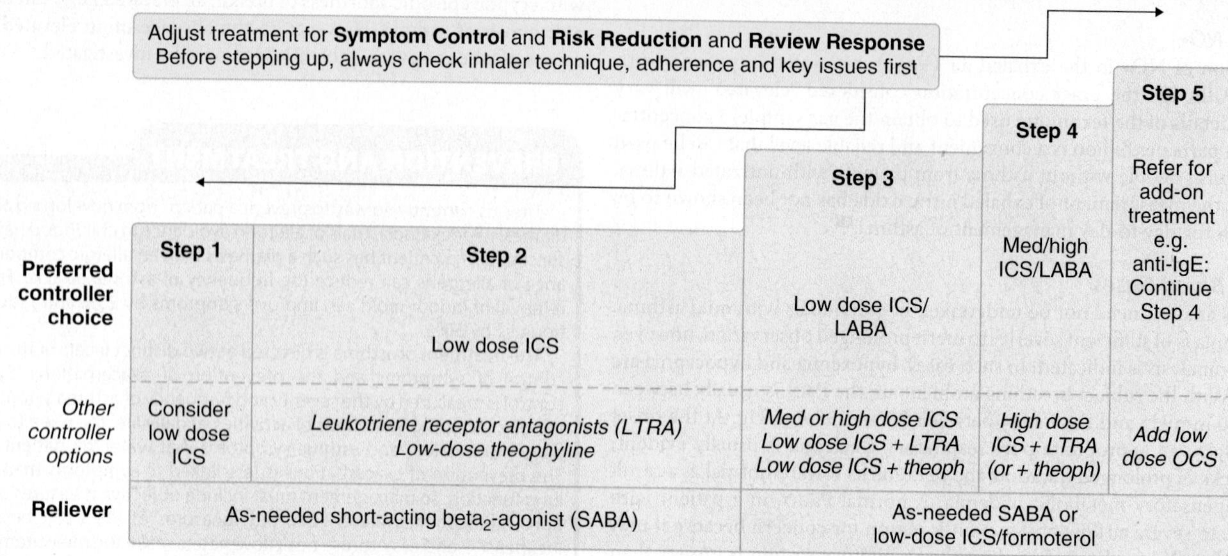

Adjust treatment for Symptom Control and Risk Reduction and Review Response
Before stepping up, always check inhaler technique, adherence and key issues first
Step 1
Step 2
Step 3
Step 4
Step 5
Preferred controller choice
Low dose ICS
Low dose ICS/LABA
Med/high ICS/LABA
Refer for add-on treatment e.g. anti-IgE: Continue Step 4
Other controller options
Consider low dose ICS
Leukotriene receptor antagonists (LTRA)
Low-dose theophyline
Med or high dose ICS
Low dose ICS + LTRA
Low dose ICS + theoph
High dose ICS + LTRA (or + theoph)
Add low dose OCS
Reliever
As-needed short-acting beta2-agonist (SABA)
As-needed SABA or low-dose ICS/formoterol
Key issues for all patients
• Assess symptom control and risk factors
• Provide ongoing self-management education (= self-monitoring + written action plan + regular review)
• Check inhaler skills and adherence, discuss barriers to regular controller use
Adjusting treatment
Always review response
• Treat modifiable risk factors and comorbidities, e.g. smoking, obesity, anxiety
• Consider stepping up if...
• Uncontrolled symptoms, exacerbations or risks (but check inhaler technique and adherence first)
• Consider stepping down if...
• Symptoms controlled for 3 months + low risk for exacerbations. Ceasing ICS is not advised.
• Provide non-pharmacological therapies and strategies
• e.g. physical activity, weight loss, avoidance of sensitizers where appropriate

FIGURE 87-2. Asthma treatment algorithm modified from the Global Initiative for Asthma (GINA 2014). There are five steps to the algorithm. First determine your patient's asthma treatment regimen and locate it on the algorithm, that is, step 1 to step 5. Next determine the level of control of your asthma patient. Your patient is in "symptom control" if he or she is able to participate in the activities of daily life without interference from asthma, if there are no nocturnal awakenings from asthma, if there have been no unscheduled visits for asthma care, and if the rescue inhaler is used minimally (twice daily at most). If the patient is in symptom control, the physician must determine whether the asthma is in functional control, that is, if lung function is normal or nearly normal. If the asthma is in symptomatic and functional control, leave the patient at the current step or step down as advised in the figure. If the asthma is not in control, step up from the current level of control. ICS = inhaled glucocorticosteroids; LABA = long-acting β-agonists; OCS = oral corticosteroids; theoph = theophylline.

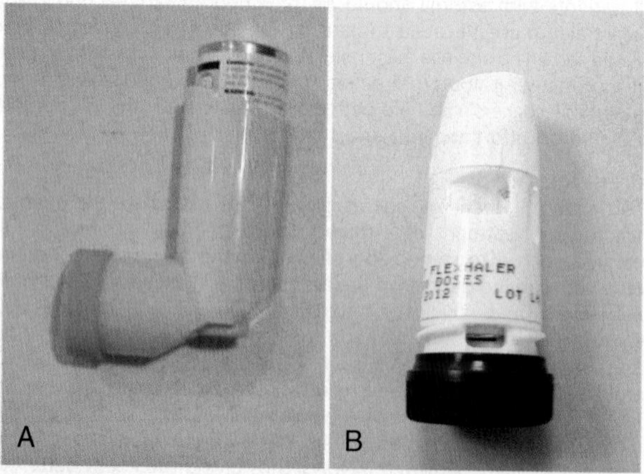

FIGURE 87-3. Commonly used inhalers. A, A pressurized metered-dose inhaler for a branded form of albuterol. Such inhalers propel the medication by means of a pressurized gas; many inhalers use propellants that do not harm the ozone layer. B, One of many types of dry powder inhalers; the one shown is a Flexhaler and dispenses budesonide. When this type of inhaler is activated, the active agent is released as a dry powder into a chamber. The patient creates the energy for airflow by means of an inspiratory effort that is directed through the device and that entrains medication into the inhaled airway.

Anticholinergics

Atropinic agents inhibit the effects of acetylcholine released from the intrapulmonary motor nerves that run in the vagus nerve and innervate airway smooth muscle. Ipratropium bromide, the atropinic agent used therapeutically in asthma, is available in a metered-dose inhaler; the recommended dose is two puffs from a metered-dose inhaler every 4 to 6 hours. Although anticholinergic inhalers are useful asthma treatments,[10] none of the inhalers marketed in the United States have a specific label indication for the treatment of asthma. In adults with uncontrolled asthma, inhaled tiotropium (18 µg every morning) added to an inhaled glucocorticoid is more effective than a double dose of glucocorticoids and similar in effect to salmeterol.[A2]

Controller Treatments

Inhaled Corticosteroids

Inhaled corticosteroids (see Fig. 87-3), which have less systemic impact than systemic steroids for a given level of therapeutic effect, are effective controller treatments for improving lung function and preventing asthmatic exacerbations in patients with persistent asthma.[A3] A *GLCCI1* polymorphism is associated with a reduced response to inhaled glucocorticoids in patients with asthma, but routine screening for this polymorphism is not currently recommended. Patients whose disease can be categorized as "mild persistent asthma" can be treated with an inhaled corticosteroid only when they have increased asthma symptoms rather than requiring an inhaled corticosteroid on a regularly scheduled basis.[A4] However, inhaled corticosteroids do not change the natural history of asthma. A wide variety of inhaled corticosteroid products are on the market (Table 87-2). All available products are effective treatments of persistent asthma but differ in terms of cost, the magnitude of adrenal suppression, and the potential for systemic effects, including growth retardation in children, loss of bone mineralization, cataracts, and glaucoma. Overall, no convincing data are available to suggest that there is reason to prefer one corticosteroid to the others. Adverse effects common to all inhaled corticosteroids are oral thrush and hoarseness (attributed to myopathy of the laryngeal muscles); the risk and severity can be reduced by aerosol spacers and good oropharyngeal hygiene (i.e., rinsing out the mouth by gargling after dosing).

Antileukotrienes

Agents with the capacity to inhibit the synthesis of the leukotrienes (zileuton, 600 mg four times a day, or controlled-release [Zyflo CR], 1200 mg twice

TABLE 87-2 ESTIMATED EQUIPOTENT DAILY DOSE FOR INHALED CORTICOSTEROIDS FOR ADULTS

DRUG	LOW DAILY DOSE (μg)*	MEDIAN DAILY DOSE (μg)	HIGH DAILY DOSE (μg)
Beclomethasone dipropionate (QVAR)†	200-500	500-1000	>1000-2000
Budesonide (Pulmicort)†	200-400	400-800	>800-1600
Ciclesonide (Alvesco)†	80-160	160-320	>320-1280
Flunisolide (AeroBid/AeroBid-M)†	500-1000	1000-2000	>2000
Fluticasone (Flovent)†	100-250	250-500	>500-1000
Mometasone furoate (Asmanex)†	200-400	400-800	>800-1200
Triamcinolone acetonide (Azmacort)†	400-1000	1000-2000	>2000

*Once-a-day dosing is acceptable for low daily dose.
†Trade name in the United States.
Note: Some doses may be outside package labeling. Metered-dose inhaler doses are expressed as the amount of drug leaving the valve, not all of which is available to the patient. Dry powder inhaler doses are expressed as the amount of drug in the inhaler after activation.
Modified from 2012 Global Initiative for Asthma guidelines. www.ginasthma.com.

daily) or the action of leukotrienes at the CysLT$_1$ receptor (montelukast [Singulair], 10 mg once a day; pranlukast [Onon, Ultair], 225 mg twice a day, not available in the United States; and zafirlukast [Accolate], 20 mg twice a day) are effective oral controller medications for patients with mild or moderate persistent asthma.[11] In patients treated with zileuton, alanine aminotransferase levels should be monitored for the first 3 to 6 months of treatment; if levels rise to more than three times the upper limit of normal, the drug should be stopped. Theophylline metabolism is slowed by zileuton, so monitoring of levels is indicated if both are prescribed. These treatments can be used on their own for mild persistent asthma or in combination with inhaled steroids for more severe asthma.

Long-Acting β-Agonists

In contrast to short- to medium-acting β-agonists, long-acting β-agonists currently available in the United States (salmeterol [Serevent, 42 μg per puff; the same dose is labeled 50 μg per puff outside of the United States; one or two puffs should be delivered every 12 hours], formoterol [Foradil, 12 μg through a proprietary dry powder inhaler every 12 hours], and bambuterol [Bambec and Oxeol, 10 to 20 mg orally each evening]) have a duration of action of nearly 12 hours and are considered controller agents rather than acute bronchodilator agents. Indacaterol (trade names: Arcapta in the United States and Onbrez in Europe), which is an ultralong-lasting β-agonist delivered by a dry powder inhaler, is used only once a day; its label indications are for chronic obstructive lung disease, not asthma, but it may be used in patients whose asthma is also being treated concomitantly with an inhaled corticosteroid.

Randomized controlled trials demonstrate that long-acting β-agonists should not be used as a sole controller agent. Other trials have shown that there are excess asthma deaths (about one for every 650 patient-years of treatment) when long-acting β-agonists are used. Therefore, long-acting β-agonists should be used in patients with asthma only when they are given in concert with inhaled corticosteroids.

A number of combination products contain both inhaled steroids and long-acting β-agonists in the same aerosol device. These products prevent patients with asthma from using inhaled long-acting β-agonists without inhaled corticosteroids. When prescribing a combination inhaler, the physician should determine the inhaled dose of corticosteroids (fluticasone, budesonide, beclomethasone, mometasone) that the patient requires and then choose a combination product that will deliver a dose of long-acting β-agonist with the inhaled corticosteroid when it is given as two puffs twice per day. The dose of long-acting β-agonist varies with brand and type of inhaler used.

Theophylline

Theophylline and its more water-soluble congener aminophylline are moderately potent bronchodilators that are useful in both inpatient and outpatient management of asthma. Treatment with theophylline is recommended only for patients who have moderate or severe persistent asthma and who are receiving controller medications, such as inhaled steroids or antileukotrienes, but whose asthma is not adequately controlled despite these treatments.

The mechanism by which theophylline exerts its effects has not been established with certainty but is probably related to the inhibition of certain forms of phosphodiesterase. Theophylline is not widely used because of its toxicity and the wide variations in the rate of its metabolism, both in a single individual over time and among individuals in a population. Because blood levels need to be monitored for optimal dosing, most physicians have reserved theophylline for third- or fourth-line therapy. For most preparations, the starting dose should be about 300 mg/day; the frequency will depend on the preparation used.

Acceptable plasma levels for therapeutic effects are between 10 and 20 μg/mL; higher levels are associated with gastrointestinal, cardiac, and central nervous system toxicity, including anxiety, headache, nausea, vomiting, diarrhea, cardiac arrhythmias, and seizures. These last catastrophic complications may occur without antecedent mild side effects when plasma levels exceed 20 μg/mL. Because of these potentially life-threatening complications of treatment, plasma levels need to be measured with great frequency in hospitalized patients receiving intravenous aminophylline and less frequently in stable outpatients receiving one of the long-acting theophylline preparations. Most asthma care providers use dosing amounts and intervals to achieve steady-state theophylline levels of 10 to 14 μg/mL, thereby avoiding the toxicity associated with decrements in metabolism.

Systemic Corticosteroids

Systemic corticosteroids are effective for the treatment of moderate to severe persistent asthma as well as for occasional severe exacerbations of asthma in a patient with otherwise mild asthma, but the mechanism of their therapeutic effect has not been established. No consensus has been reached on the specific type, dose, or duration of corticosteroid to be used in the treatment of asthma. In nonhospitalized patients with asthma refractory to standard therapy, a steroid "pulse" with initial doses of prednisone on the order of 40 to 60 mg/day, tapered to zero during 7 to 14 days, is recommended. For patients who cannot stop taking steroids without having recurrent uncontrolled bronchospasm despite the addition of multiple other controller treatments, alternate-day administration of oral steroids is preferable to daily treatment. For patients whose asthma requires in-hospital treatment but is not considered life-threatening, an initial intravenous bolus of 2 mg/kg of hydrocortisone, followed by continuous infusion of 0.5 mg/kg/hour, has been shown to be beneficial within 12 hours. In attacks of asthma that are considered life-threatening, the use of intravenous methylprednisolone (125 mg every 6 hours) has been advocated. In each case, as the patient improves, oral steroids are substituted for intravenous steroids, and the oral dose is tapered during 1 to 3 weeks; addition of inhaled steroids to the regimen is strongly recommended when oral steroids are started.

Monoclonal Antibody Treatment

Omalizumab

Subcutaneous administration of omalizumab, a humanized murine monoclonal antibody that binds circulating IgE, is associated with decreased serum free (not total) IgE levels. In patients who have moderate to severe allergic asthma with elevated levels of serum IgE and who are receiving inhaled corticosteroids, omalizumab treatment improves asthma control even as doses of inhaled steroids are decreased. Dosing is guided by weight and by pretreatment IgE levels: a monthly subcutaneous dose of 0.016 mg × body weight (kg) × IgE level (IU/mL). For example, in a patient weighing 70 kg with a pretreatment total IgE level of 300 IU/mL, 336 mg of omalizumab would be administered monthly by subcutaneous injection. Dosing calculators can be found online (e.g., http://www.xolairhcp.com/hcp/determining-the-dose.html). Anti-IgE antibodies can reduce exacerbations and improve quality of life in patients with severe allergic asthma, but their place in treatment schema has not been established. Because of the potential for anaphylaxis, all patients need to be monitored after injection; the duration of the monitoring period is not specified by the U.S. Food and Drug Administration (FDA), but most physicians monitor for 30 to 60 minutes.

Other Monoclonal Antibodies

In a randomized trial, lebrikizumab (a monoclonal antibody against interleukin-13 at 250 mg subcutaneously once per month for 6 months) enhanced lung function in adults with asthma, especially in patients with low pretreatment serum periostin levels.[A5] Mepolizumab is a monoclonal antibody directed against interleukin-5. In randomized trials using 75 to 100 mg daily, it reduced asthma exacerbations by about 50% among relatively rare patients with moderately severe asthma who still had sputum eosinophilia despite treatment with oral and inhaled corticosteroids.[A6,A7] Among patients with more conventional asthma, however, mepolizumab treatment did not have a salutary effect. A trial of a monoclonal antibody against the α subunit of the shared interleukin-4 and interleukin-13 receptor, dupilumab, in patients whose asthma and eosinophilia was not controlled with conventional doses of inhaled corticosteroids and long-acting β-agonists showed that both the inhaled long-acting β-agonists and inhaled corticosteroids could be withdrawn without losing asthma control when the monoclonal antibody was administered.[A8] None of these drugs is currently approved by the U.S. FDA.

Other Controller Drugs

Cromolyn sodium (two to four times a day by nebulizer using 20-mg nebules) is a nonsteroid inhaled treatment used in the management of mild to moderate persistent asthma. It appears to be most useful in pediatric populations or when an identifiable stimulus (such as exercise or allergen exposure) elicits an asthmatic response.

The use of systemic gold (as in rheumatoid arthritis), methotrexate, or cyclosporine has been suggested as adjunctive treatment of patients with severe chronic asthma who cannot otherwise discontinue high-dose corticosteroid treatment. However, these agents are experimental, and their routine use is not advocated. Despite initial encouraging trials, agents that inhibit the action of tumor necrosis factor-α do not benefit patients with asthma and should not be used.

Based on the concern that asthma could be caused by silent gastroesophageal reflux disease, treatment with a proton pump inhibitor has been advocated in patients with mild to moderate asthma even in the absence of gastrointestinal symptoms. Adequately powered clinical studies suggest that this approach provides no benefit for asthma control.

Vaccination for Seasonal Influenza and Pneumococcal Disease

Vaccination of patients for seasonal influenza is safe and not associated with enhanced asthma exacerbations. Vaccination against seasonal influenza and pneumococcal disease is recommended in patients with asthma.

Radio Frequency Ablation of Airway Smooth Muscle

A proprietary system to ablate airway smooth muscle by delivery of radio frequency energy through a bronchoscopically placed probe has reduced asthma exacerbations in sham-controlled trials among patients whose asthma remained out of control despite the use of multiple controller medications. Although a device for such treatment has been approved by the FDA, the long-term impacts of this treatment on airway or lung function are not known.

Control-Driven Asthma Therapy

Because all current asthma treatment is symptomatic (i.e., no current treatment changes the disease history), the approach to the management of asthma is to titrate treatment to achieve an adequate level of control. If a patient's asthma is well controlled, treatment can be continued or stepped down (see Fig. 87-2). A9 If a patient's asthma is poorly controlled, treatment intensity should be stepped up. At the mild end of the spectrum, a patient who has rare limitations in activities of daily life, has nearly normal lung function, and sleeps without interruption from asthma can be prescribed nothing more than inhaled rescue treatment on an as-needed basis. In general, if a patient can control his or her asthma with the use of a single metered-dose inhaler of rescue treatment dispensed every 7 to 8 weeks or less frequently, there is no need for background controller treatment. If a patient has a requirement for more rescue treatment, has symptoms that interfere with sleeping through the night, or has moderately deranged lung function, controller therapy should be added.

Single-agent controller therapy should consist of an inhaled corticosteroid or an antileukotriene. If control is not achieved with one of these agents, the patient can be switched to the other or have a second agent added. The best studied two-agent combination is inhaled corticosteroids and a long-acting inhaled β_2-adrenergic agonist, available in a single inhaler under the trade names of Symbicort, Advair, and Dulera in the United States; trade names vary in other parts of the world. These combinations provide excellent disease control and often allow a reduction in the dose of inhaled corticosteroids. Data indicate that another combination, an antileukotriene and inhaled steroid, is more effective than either treatment alone, but this regimen does not have as substantial an evidence base as the combination of inhaled corticosteroids and a long-acting β-agonist.

Specific Treatment Scenarios

Concurrent Pulmonary Infection

In some patients, acute exacerbations of asthma may be due to concurrent infection, which requires targeted therapy (Chapters 88, 90, and 97).

Aspirin-Exacerbated Respiratory Disease (Previously Termed Aspirin-Induced Asthma)

Approximately 5% of patients with moderate to severe persistent asthma develop asthma when they ingest agents that inhibit cyclooxygenase, such as aspirin and other nonsteroidal anti-inflammatory drugs (Chapter 37). Inhibitors of cyclooxygenase 2 are less likely to cause these reactions, but aspirin-type reactions have been reported in sensitive patients treated with selective cyclooxygenase 2 inhibitors. Although the physiologic manifestations of laboratory-based aspirin challenge can be blocked by leukotriene pathway inhibitors, these agents do not prevent clinical aspirin-exacerbated respiratory disease. Thus, patients with this form of asthma must avoid aspirin and other nonsteroidal anti-inflammatory drugs.

Asthma in the Emergency Department

When a patient with asthma presents for acute emergency care, objective measures of the severity of the attack, including quantification of pulsus paradoxus and measurement of airflow rates (PEFR or FEV_1), should be evaluated in addition to the usual vital signs. If the attack has been prolonged and failed to respond to treatment with bronchodilators (e.g., albuterol by metered-dose inhaler, two puffs every 2 to 3 hours) and high-dose inhaled steroids (e.g., more than 2000 μg/day of beclomethasone or half that amount of fluticasone) before arrival at the emergency department, intravenous steroids (40 to 60 mg of methylprednisolone or its equivalent) should be administered. If the patient has not been receiving treatment with a leukotriene receptor antagonist, such agents should be administered (10 mg of montelukast or 20 mg of zafirlukast) as soon as possible. Treatment with inhaled β-agonists (either nebulized albuterol, 0.5 mL of a 0.5% solution repeated at 20- to 30-minute intervals, or albuterol by metered-dose inhaler, two puffs every 30 minutes) should be used until the PEFR or FEV_1 increases to greater than 40% of the predicted values. If this point is not reached within 2 hours, admission to the hospital for further treatment is strongly advocated.

When patients have PEFR and FEV_1 values that are greater than 60% of their predicted value on arrival in the emergency department, treatment with inhaled β_2-agonists alone, albuterol (0.5 mL of an albuterol 0.083% solution) or equivalent, is likely to result in an objective improvement in airflow rates. If significant improvement takes place in the emergency department, such patients can usually be treated as outpatients with inhaled β_2-agonists and a controller agent (see Fig. 87-2). A good strategy is to add inhaled corticosteroids if the patient has not been receiving this treatment or has been using a single controller therapy.

For patients whose PEFR and FEV_1 values are between 40% and 60% of the values predicted at the time of initial evaluation in the emergency care setting, a plan of treatment varying in intensity between these two plans is indicated. Failure to respond to treatment by objective criteria (PEFR or FEV_1) within 2 hours of arrival at the emergency department is an indication for the use of systemic corticosteroids.

Status Asthmaticus

The asthmatic subject whose PEFR or FEV_1 does not increase to greater than 40% of the predicted value with treatment, whose $Paco_2$ increases without improvement of indices of airflow obstruction, or who develops major complications such as pneumothorax or pneumomediastinum should be admitted to the hospital for close monitoring. Frequent treatments with inhaled β-agonists (0.5 mL of an albuterol 0.083% solution every 2 hours), intravenous aminophylline (at doses to yield maximal acceptable plasma levels, that is, 15 to 20 μg/mL; 500- to 1000-mg loading dose given during an hour followed by an infusion of 30 to 60 mg/hour), and high-dose intravenous steroids (methylprednisolone, 40 to 60 mg every 4 to 6 hours) are indicated. Oxygen should be administered by face mask or nasal cannula in amounts sufficient to achieve Sao_2 values between 92% and 94%; a higher Fio_2 promotes absorption atelectasis and provides no therapeutic benefit. If objective evidence of an infection is present, appropriate treatment should be given for that infection. If no improvement is seen with treatment and if respiratory failure appears imminent, bronchodilator treatment should be intensified to the maximum tolerated by the patient as indicated by the maximum tolerated heart rate, usually 130 to 140 beats per minute. If indicated, intubation of the trachea and mechanical ventilation can be instituted; in this case, the goal should be to provide a level of ventilation just adequate to sustain life but *not sufficient to normalize arterial blood gases.* For example, a $Paco_2$ of 60 to 70 mm Hg, or even higher, is acceptable for a patient in status asthmaticus.

Asthma in Pregnancy

Asthma may be exacerbated, remain unchanged, or remit during pregnancy (Chapter 239). There need not be substantial departures from the ordinary management of asthma during pregnancy, although one randomized trial suggests that unlike in other settings, measurement of the fraction of exhaled nitric oxide can improve the management of asthma during pregnancy. However, no unnecessary medications should be administered; systemic steroids should be used sparingly to avert fetal complications, and certain drugs should be avoided, including tetracycline (as a treatment of intercurrent infection), ipratropium bromide (which may cause fetal tachycardia), terbutaline (which is contraindicated during active labor because of its tocolytic effects), and iodine-containing mucolytics (such as saturated solution of potassium iodide). Moreover, use of prostaglandin $F_{2\alpha}$ as an abortifacient should be avoided in asthmatic patients.

PROGNOSIS

Asthma is a chronic relapsing disorder. Most patients have recurrent attacks without a major loss in lung function for many years. A minority of patients experience a significant irreversible loss in lung function over and above the normal pulmonary senescence. Methods to distinguish these various clinical phenotypes have not been developed.

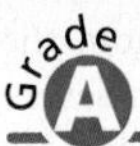

Grade A References

A1. Petsky HL, Cates CJ, Lasserson TJ, et al. A systematic review and meta-analysis: tailoring asthma treatment on eosinophilic markers (exhaled nitric oxide or sputum eosinophils). *Thorax*. 2012;67:199-208.

A2. Peters SP, Kunselman SJ, Icitovic N, et al. Tiotropium bromide step-up therapy for adults with uncontrolled asthma. *N Engl J Med*. 2010;363:1715-1726.

A3. Busse WW, Pedersen S, Pauwels RA, et al. START Investigators Group. The Inhaled Steroid Treatment As Regular Therapy in Early Asthma (START) study 5-year follow-up: effectiveness of early intervention with budesonide in mild persistent asthma. *J Allergy Clin Immunol*. 2008;121:1167-1174.

A4. Calhoun WJ, Ameredes BT, King TS, et al. Asthma Clinical Research Network of the National Heart, Lung, and Blood Institute. Comparison of physician-, biomarker- and symptom-based strategies for adjustment of inhaled corticosteroid therapy in adults with asthma: the BASALT randomized controlled trial. *JAMA*. 2012;308:987-997.

A5. Corren J, Lemanske RF, Hanania NA, et al. Lebrikizumab treatment in adults with asthma. *N Engl J Med*. 2011;365:1088-1098.

A6. Bel EH, Wenzel SE, Thompson PJ, et al. Oral glucocorticoid-sparing effect of mepolizumab in eosinophilic asthma. *N Engl J Med*. 2014;371:1189-1197.

A7. Ortega HG, Liu MC, Pavord ID, et al. Mepolizumab treatment in patients with severe eosinophilic asthma. *N Engl J Med*. 2014;371:1198-1207.

A8. Wenzel S, Ford L, Pearlman D, et al. Dupilumab in persistent asthma with elevated eosinophil levels. *N Engl J Med*. 2013;368:2455-2466.

A9. Peters SP, Anthonisen N, Castro M, et al. American Lung Association Asthma Clinical Research Centers. Randomized comparison of strategies for reducing treatment in mild persistent asthma. *N Engl J Med*. 2007;356:2027-2039.

GENERAL REFERENCES

For the General References and other additional features, please visit Expert Consult at https://expertconsult.inkling.com.

88 CHRONIC OBSTRUCTIVE PULMONARY DISEASE

DENNIS E. NIEWOEHNER

DEFINITIONS

Chronic obstructive pulmonary disease (COPD) is now the preferred term for a condition that is characterized by progressive, largely irreversible airflow obstruction, usually with clinical onset in middle-aged or elderly persons with a history of cigarette smoking, and that cannot be attributed to another specific disease, such as bronchiectasis (Chapter 90) or asthma (Chapter 87). Commonly used terms for this condition in the past included chronic bronchitis and emphysema. That terminology is outdated because nearly all patients with a clinical diagnosis of COPD have both air space destruction (i.e., emphysema) and pathologic changes of the conducting airways consistent with chronic bronchitis.

Emphysema is defined pathologically by abnormal enlargement of the air spaces due to destruction and deformation of alveolar walls. The severity of emphysema may vary widely in COPD patients with similar degrees of airflow obstruction. Chronic bronchitis is defined clinically as persistent cough and sputum production and pathologically as abnormal enlargement of the mucous glands within the central cartilaginous airways. Chronic bronchitis was once thought to be a key element in the pathogenesis of chronic airflow obstruction, but it is now known that increased airflow resistance in COPD can be attributed principally to a variety of pathologic changes within the distal airways of the lung ("small airways disease").

EPIDEMIOLOGY

COPD represents a growing global public health problem, although prevalence estimates vary widely according to the definition used. Cigarette smoking (Chapter 32) is the principal risk factor for COPD, so prevalence tends to reflect societal smoking habits with a lag phase of 20 to 30 years. Cigarette consumption has leveled off or decreased in large segments of North America and Europe, but the prevalence of COPD may continue to increase as exposed populations age. A greater future burden of COPD may be anticipated in Asia and other regions of the world because of rapidly increasing cigarette consumption.

More than 10% of the population older than 45 years in the United States has airflow obstruction of at least moderate severity as judged by spirometric criteria. COPD is the third leading cause of death in the United States, and mortality from COPD has increased during the past 30 years in both men and women.[1] Worldwide, COPD also is the third leading cause of death globally and the fifth leading cause of years lived with disability.[2,3] Medical costs and lost productivity attributable to COPD exceed $40 billion annually in the United States. Direct medical costs rise precipitously as COPD becomes more severe, with hospitalization for exacerbations accounting for more than half of the total.

Cigarette Smoking

Cigarette smoking is the principal cause of COPD, but the relationship is complex and COPD may develop without a smoking history.[4] Airflow obstruction is the sentinel physiologic disturbance in COPD, and the forced expiratory volume in the first second (FEV_1) is the single best indicator of severity. Cigarette smoking causes declines in lung function that exceed those expected from aging alone, and the magnitude of loss is dependent on both the intensity and duration of exposure to cigarette smoke. Thus, the cumulative effects of smoking largely account for the increasing prevalence of COPD with advancing age.

Individual losses of lung function vary widely, even after adjustment for smoking intensity. After the age of 30 years, everyone loses lung function on a yearly basis, but smoking further affects the rate of lung function loss. The mean annual reduction in the FEV_1 (Chapter 85) in normal nonsmoking white men is about 25 mL per year, but the loss increases to an average of about 40 mL per year among smokers (Fig. 88-1). A small minority of smokers, "susceptible smokers," suffer annual FEV_1 losses of 100 mL or more and may develop clinically significant airflow obstruction in the fourth and fifth decades of life. Factors that distinguish the susceptible smoker from the average smoker remain largely unknown.

Adverse effects of cigarette smoke on lung function may extend as far back as fetal development. Maternal smoking during pregnancy, secondhand cigarette smoke exposure during early childhood, and active smoking during adolescence impair lung growth. As a consequence, the lower lung function in early adulthood constitutes a significant risk factor for COPD later in life.

Other Environmental Exposures

Workers exposed to dust in certain workplace environments, such as mines, cotton mills, and grain-handling facilities, commonly develop symptoms of cough and sputum and may suffer permanent loss of lung function (Chapter 93). In some regions of the world, repeated exposure to biomass combustion in confined living quarters causes airflow obstruction. Current urban air

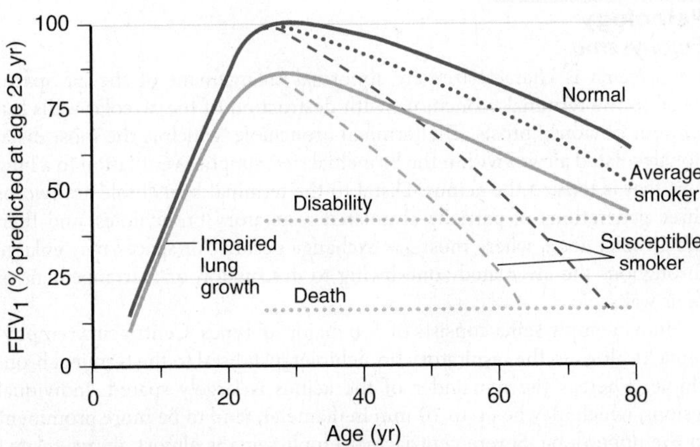

FIGURE 88-1. Lung growth occurs during childhood and adolescence, with the forced expiratory volume in 1 second (FEV_1) reaching a maximum at about 25 years of age. Thereafter, the FEV_1 steadily declines owing to normal aging effects. Lung function declines more rapidly in smokers, but the average effect is so small that clinically significant airflow obstruction would never develop. However, a proportion of "susceptible smokers" lose lung function much faster than the average, so they develop disabling chronic obstructive pulmonary disorder (COPD). If lung growth is impaired, lung function reserve is less as a young adult, and a susceptible smoker will develop disabling COPD at an earlier age.

pollution in economically advanced countries appears to have little effect on the prevalence of airflow obstruction, but this factor may be more important in heavily polluted urban centers in industrializing countries.

Respiratory Infections

Recurrent respiratory infections were once thought to be a major factor in the development of airflow obstruction, but longitudinal cohort studies have yielded inconclusive findings. An effect, if present, appears weak relative to cigarette smoking. Whether childhood respiratory infections leave residual effects on adult lung function is similarly unclear.

Airway Responsiveness

Acute bronchoconstriction after inhalation of dilute concentrations of methacholine or histamine, termed bronchial hyperresponsiveness (Chapter 87), is a defining feature of asthma but is also present in many COPD patients. Bronchial hyperresponsiveness independently predicts accelerated loss of lung function in persons with mild to moderate COPD, especially among persons who continue to smoke.

Genetic Factors

A severe deficiency of α_1-antitrypsin is the only genetic risk factor proven to have a major impact on the development of COPD.[5] This deficiency is found in about 1 to 2% of patients with an established diagnosis of COPD. α_1-Antitrypsin, which is a serine protease inhibitor that is secreted into the circulation from the liver, is thought to protect lung tissue against digestion by neutrophil elastase and related serine proteinases that have been implicated in the pathogenesis of human emphysema. The most common allele at the α_1-antitrypsin genetic locus is M, and MM homozygotes have what are considered normal levels of α_1-antitrypsin (100 to 300 mg/dL). Numerous variant alleles have been identified, but severe deficiency is most commonly found in persons who are homozygous for the Z allele, in whom serum levels are generally less than 20 to 30% of the lower range of normal. Affected persons are very susceptible to cigarette smoke–induced damage and may develop severe COPD at a relatively early age. The risk for clinically important emphysema appears to be much less if patients with the risk alleles do not smoke. Emphysema associated with severe α_1-antitrypsin deficiency is characteristically of the panacinar type with a predominant basal distribution.

About 2 to 3% of northern European populations possess the MZ heterozygote serum and have α_1-antitrypsin levels about half of normal. These individuals may be at greater risk for development of chronic airflow obstruction, but the magnitude of the effect, if present, appears to be quite small. Studies of family aggregations and of molecular genetics suggest some heritable risks beyond those associated with α_1-antitrypsin deficiency. Women with severe COPD appear to have relatively more airway disease and less emphysema compared with men with similar airflow obstruction.

PATHOBIOLOGY

Pathology

Emphysema

Emphysema is characterized by abnormal enlargement of the air spaces distal to the terminal bronchiole, with destruction of the alveolar walls but without obvious fibrosis. The terminal bronchiole, which is the most distal nonalveolated airway within the bronchial tree, supplies ventilation to a lung unit that is termed the acinus. Distal to the terminal bronchiole are two or three generations of partially alveolated respiratory bronchioles, and then the alveolar zone, where most gas exchange occurs. Air spaces may enlarge throughout the alveolated zone owing to destruction or rearrangement of their walls.

Human emphysema consists of two major subtypes. Centriacinar emphysema localizes to the respiratory bronchioles just distal to the terminal bronchiole, whereas the remainder of the acinus is largely spared. Individual lesions, which may be up to 10 mm in diameter, tend to be more prominent in the upper lobe. Severe centriacinar emphysema is almost always related to cigarette smoking, but mild centriacinar emphysema can occur from other environmental exposures. Focal areas of inflammation, fibrosis, and carbonaceous pigment are commonly present in adjacent alveolar and bronchiolar walls.

In panacinar emphysema, alveolar ducts are diffusely enlarged; adjacent alveoli may become effaced to the extent that individual units can no longer be identified. With progression of the disease, individual lesions can coalesce to form large bullae. Panacinar emphysema, which is typical of severe α_1-antitrypsin deficiency, also commonly occurs in patients in whom the major risk factor for COPD is cigarette smoking. Most patients with severe COPD appear to have mixed elements of centriacinar and panacinar emphysema, and individual subtypes cannot be reliably distinguished in advanced disease.

Chronic Bronchitis and Bronchiolitis

Mucous glands, located between the epithelial basement membrane and the cartilage plates within the central bronchial tree, and goblet cells in the airway epithelium secrete mucus into the bronchial lumen to aid in host defenses. Enlargement of the bronchial mucous glands and expansion of the epithelial goblet cell population, which occur commonly in COPD, are correlated with clinical symptoms of cough and excess sputum production but not with airflow obstruction. A low-grade inflammatory response, consisting of neutrophils, macrophages, and CD8$^+$ T lymphocytes, may also be seen in the cartilaginous airways of COPD patients.

The principal sites of increased airflow resistance in COPD are the small distal airways that have an internal diameter near the lung's functional residual capacity of less than 2 mm. The earliest pathologic changes identified in young cigarette smokers consist of focal collections of brown-pigmented macrophages in the respiratory bronchiole and a sparse infiltrate of neutrophils and lymphocytes in the walls of the terminal bronchiole. In older patients with established COPD, the inflammatory response is more intense, but still with a similar mix of neutrophils, macrophages, and lymphocytes. Other pathologic changes in the distal airways include fibrosis, goblet cell and squamous cell metaplasia of the lining epithelium, smooth muscle enlargement within the airway walls, and scattered regions of mucous plugging. Compared with normal subjects, distal airways in patients with COPD have thicker airway walls and smaller lumens.

Pulmonary Vasculature

Hypoxemia causes vasoconstriction in small pulmonary arteries and a consequent increase in pulmonary vascular resistance. Vascular remodeling in response to chronic hypoxemia results in irreversible pulmonary hypertension (Chapter 68). Medial smooth muscle enlargement and intimal fibrosis in small pulmonary arteries are the most important vascular changes. In addition, a substantial portion of the capillary bed may be destroyed by severe emphysema.

Pathogenesis

Emphysema appears to be caused by an elastase-antielastase imbalance in the lung due to either elastase excess or antielastase deficiency. Human lungs contain a rich network of elastin-containing fibers and other matrix proteins that confer structural integrity and elasticity to alveolar walls. Intratracheal instillation of proteinases, particularly those capable of hydrolyzing native elastin, induces lesions with morphologic and functional features of human emphysema in experimental animals. Chronic inflammation induced from cigarette smoke increases the burden of inflammatory cell–derived proteinases within lung parenchyma. Severe deficiency of α_1-antitrypsin, a potent inhibitor of neutrophil elastase and other serine proteinases, is associated with development of severe panacinar emphysema in humans. In addition to neutrophil elastase, other neutrophil-derived serine proteinases, such as proteinase 3 and cathepsin G, and matrix metalloproteinases degrade elastin and other matrix components, including collagen, proteoglycans, and fibronectin. A macrophage-derived metalloproteinase, MMP-12, is essential to the development of cigarette smoke–induced emphysema in an animal model, and genetic studies show that a single-nucleotide polymorphism in the promoter region of the MMP-12 gene is associated with reduced risk of COPD in adult smokers.

Relatively less is understood about the pathogenesis of distal airways disease. Particulate matter and toxic gases from inhaled cigarette smoke initiate an inflammatory response composed primarily of macrophages and neutrophils. This early inflammatory response may be mediated by the innate defense system as a response to cell injury. In more advanced disease, inflammation persists even after the patient has stopped smoking. At this stage, humoral and cellular components of the adaptive immune system may predominate, possibly in response to infection or specific antigens from other sources. Infiltration of airway walls with CD4$^+$, CD8$^+$, and B lymphocytes is a prominent feature of more advanced COPD. Repair from either type of immune response might cause airway remodeling by stimulating connective tissue matrix synthesis and smooth muscle formation and by increasing the proportion of mucus-secreting goblet cells within the epithelial layer.

Lung and Heart Mechanics

Elastic recoil refers to the lung's intrinsic tendency to deflate after inflation. A dense labyrinth of elastic fibers and other matrix elements within the lung parenchyma, along with surface tension at the alveolar air-liquid interface, confers this important mechanical property. Elastic recoil maintains the patency of small airways through radial alveolar attachments, similar to the way a tent is held up by its guy ropes, and provides a portion of the driving pressure during expiration. Age-related loss of lung elasticity largely explains the normal decline in FEV_1 with advancing age. In emphysema, loss of lung elastic recoil results from damage to elastic fibers and loss of alveolar surface area, with consequent airflow obstruction.

An increase in bronchial airflow resistance is another sentinel feature of lung mechanics in COPD. The increased resistance in COPD is due primarily to narrowing and loss in airways of less than 2 mm in diameter, known as small airways, even before emphysematous destruction occurs. As a result, peripheral airflow resistance of COPD is higher than in normal lungs by an order of magnitude or more. In contrast, airflow resistance in the central airways of lungs from COPD patients differs little from that of normal lungs. One of the key physiologic aspects of COPD is limitation of expiratory airflow (Fig. 88-2) due to loss of lung elastic recoil and increased viscous resistance to airflow in the small airways (Chapter 85). The severity of emphysema and airflow obstruction is directly related to impaired left ventricular filling, reduced stroke volume, and lower cardiac output without reducing the ejection fraction.

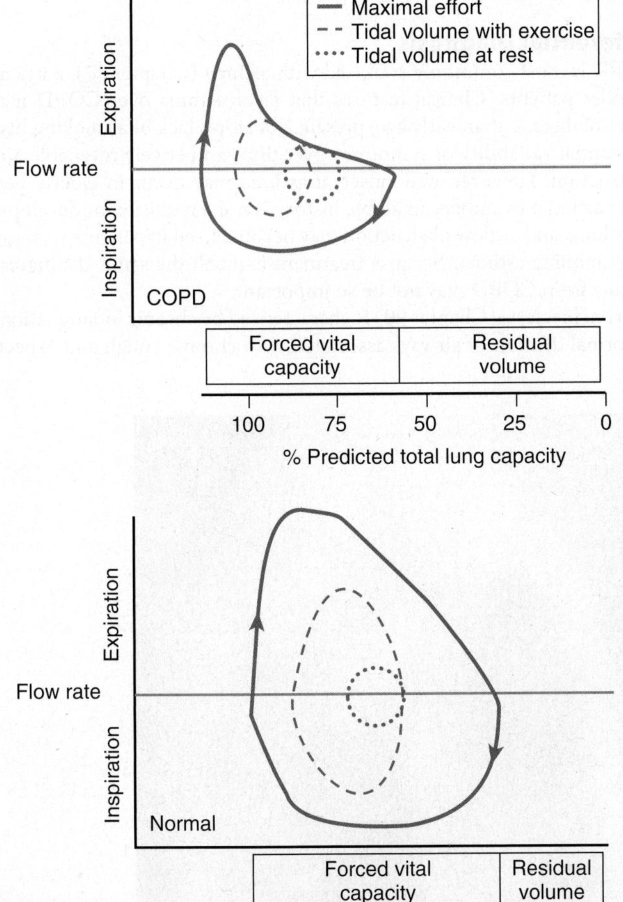

FIGURE 88-2. Inspiratory and expiratory flow-volume loops at rest, with exercise, and with maximal effort in a normal subject are compared with those in a patient with chronic obstructive pulmonary disorder (COPD). The normal subject can easily increase both tidal volume and breathing frequency to match the metabolic requirements of vigorous exercise. In contrast, the COPD patient exhibits maximal expiratory flow limitation even at rest and must breathe at larger lung volumes to optimize expiratory airflow. Lung hyperinflation requires greater respiratory work because the lung and chest wall become stiffer at larger volumes. This effect is accentuated during exercise, which causes end-expiratory lung volume to increase further. This phenomenon is described as *dynamic hyperinflation* and is an important mechanism in limiting exercise and causing dyspnea.

Gas Exchange

Mild hypoxemia may be detected in the early stages of COPD, and hypoxemia often becomes more prominent as airflow obstruction worsens. Hypercapnia usually appears only with severe COPD but is sometimes absent even in late-stage disease. Ventilation-perfusion mismatching, due to changes in both the airways and pulmonary vessels, is largely responsible for hypoxemia, with uneven ventilation being the primary event. Gas exchange is most efficient when the ratio of ventilation to perfusion is uniform in all lung regions. In COPD, there is "wasted ventilation" because some lung regions have inadequate pulmonary blood flow for the ventilation. The calculated A-a gradient for oxygen is larger than anticipated for the patient's age (Chapters 85 and 103). Thus, in most cases of COPD, modest increases in the fraction of inspired oxygen result in a resolution of clinical hypoxemia.

CLINICAL MANIFESTATIONS

History and Physical Examination

COPD should be suspected in all adults who complain of chronic respiratory symptoms, particularly dyspnea (Chapter 83) that limits activities of daily living.[6,7] Clinical features that increase the likelihood of COPD include older age, current or past cigarette use, insidious onset of dyspnea with slow progression, history of acute bronchitis for which medical care is sought, and symptoms of chronic cough, sputum production, or wheezing. Symptoms of cough and sputum may antedate dyspnea by many years. Some patients date the onset of dyspnea to a respiratory infection, but careful questioning usually elicits some history of impaired exercise tolerance before that event. Absence of cigarette smoking does not preclude a diagnosis of COPD because a few persons develop severe irreversible airflow obstruction without smoking history and even without known genetic predispositions. Some nonsmokers may relate a history of occupational dust or noxious gas exposure (Chapters 93 and 94), but in others no putative cause can be discerned.

The physical examination findings are usually normal in patients with mild to moderate disease, and characteristic physical signs may be absent even in severe disease. Physical examination findings commonly present in severe COPD include the appearance of a barrel-shaped chest, low diaphragm detected by percussion, prolonged expiratory phase, and use of accessory muscles of respiration. Heart sounds are usually distant, and auscultation of the chest may reveal diminished breath sounds or a variety of rhonchi, wheezes, and rattles. Auscultatory wheezes may be prominent, particularly during exacerbations, but this physical sign does not reliably differentiate COPD from asthma. With severe hypoxemia, cyanosis may be clinically evident. Clubbing is not associated with COPD, and its presence should suggest another diagnosis. Pedal edema, distended jugular veins, and hepatic congestion are signs of pulmonary hypertension and cor pulmonale (Chapter 68). Patients with advanced COPD may be cachectic, with loss of muscle mass and subcutaneous fat.

Clinical Phenotypes

One of the more enduring efforts to categorize COPD into subtypes is the description of the patients as either "pink puffers" or "blue bloaters."[8] The pink puffer is described as a cachectic individual with unrelenting dyspnea, clinical and radiographic signs of severe lung hyperinflation, and normal or near-normal arterial blood gases at rest. Salient features of the blue bloater are a stout body habitus, chronic cough and sputum, less troubling dyspnea, and severe hypoxemia and hypercapnia resulting in polycythemia and signs of cor pulmonale. In the original description of these phenotypes, the pink puffer phenotype was equated with severe emphysema, whereas the blue bloater was thought to have predominant chronic bronchitis.

Selected COPD patients do fit one or the other of these clinical subtypes, but most cannot be simply categorized. Limited information from clinical and pathologic correlative studies fails to show a consistent association of either clinical subtype with distinguishing pathologic features in lung parenchyma or airways. The blue bloater phenotype may now be less common, possibly because hypoxemia is recognized and treated earlier or because some COPD patients once described as blue bloaters may have had coexisting obstructive sleep apnea (Chapter 100).

COPD patients with similar degrees of airflow obstruction vary greatly with respect to severity of dyspnea, impairment of exercise tolerance, frequency of exacerbations, body habitus, and severity of arterial blood gas disturbances. There is limited understanding about the mechanisms underlying these clinical characteristics.

DIAGNOSIS

Pulmonary Function Tests

Airflow obstruction can be determined best by spirometry. If the ratio of FEV_1 to forced vital capacity (FEV_1/FVC) is less than 0.70 (Chapter 85) after administration of an inhaled bronchodilator, an obstructive defect is present (Table 88-1). A large improvement of perhaps 30 to 40% in FEV_1 after treatment with an inhaled bronchodilator may help identify a patient with predominant asthma, but the test otherwise has little clinical utility and cannot reliably identify patients who will benefit from any particular form of therapy.

Lung volume measurements may help distinguish obstructive and restrictive lung diseases in selected patients, but they are unnecessary in most COPD patients. The diffusing capacity for carbon monoxide (DLCO; Chapter 85) measures the uptake of carbon monoxide between inspired air and the blood stream. Decreases in the DLCO reflect the loss of alveolar surface area that is available for gas transfer and roughly correspond to the severity of emphysema. However, the test provides information of no practical value in the customary management of COPD.

After the diagnosis is established, follow-up spirometry may help determine whether worsening breathlessness is due to COPD, as indicated by a decrease in FEV_1, or to another cause, such as heart failure (Chapter 58). However, repeated spirometry should not be used as a guide to drug therapy because the background variability of the measurement is large relative to treatment effects.

TABLE 88-1 SEVERITY OF AIRFLOW OBSTRUCTION IN COPD ACCORDING TO POSTBRONCHODILATOR SPIROMETRY

STAGE AND SEVERITY	DEFINITION
I: Mild	$FEV_1/FVC < 0.70$, $FEV_1 \geq 80\%$ of predicted
II: Moderate	$FEV_1/FVC < 0.70$, $50\% \leq FEV_1 < 80\%$ of predicted
III: Severe	$FEV_1/FVC < 0.70$, $30\% \leq FEV_1 < 50\%$ of predicted
IV: Very severe	$FEV_1/FVC < 0.70$, $FEV_1 < 30\%$ of predicted or $FEV_1 < 50\%$ of predicted plus chronic respiratory failure

COPD = chronic obstructive pulmonary disease; FEV_1 = forced expiratory volume in the first second; FVC = forced vital capacity.
Data from *Global Initiative for Chronic Obstructive Lung Disease.* http://www.goldcopd.com.

Oximetry

Hypoxemia and hypercapnia become increasingly common as COPD worsens. Because treatment with supplemental oxygen improves mortality, patients with severe COPD should be tested for hypoxemia at regular intervals. Hypoxemia can be detected and quantified by oximetry or arterial blood gases. Oximetry is generally preferred because it is simpler, cheaper, and causes no discomfort. The added information from a set of arterial blood gases (Chapter 103) is most helpful in COPD patients with severe exacerbations.

Radiographic Studies

Common signs of severe COPD on a chest radiograph include hyperinflated lungs, flattened diaphragms, and increased retrosternal clear space (Fig. 88-3). The walls of large emphysematous bullae may be visualized as thin curvilinear lines, and severe emphysema may appear as regions of relative hyperlucency. Chest radiographs are usually normal in mild to moderate COPD and sometimes in severe COPD. Hence, a chest radiograph is not an adequate diagnostic test for COPD, and it is used mostly to exclude other pulmonary diseases. Chest computed tomography (CT), which is a superior imaging modality to assess the magnitude and distribution of emphysema (Fig. 88-4), is not helpful in the usual management of COPD.

Other Studies

Measurement of the serum level of α_1-antitrypsin deficiency may be considered, particularly if the patient has a strong family history of COPD or if the onset of airflow obstruction occurs at an early age. If the α_1-antitrypsin level is less than 20 to 30% of normal, further testing with specialized phenotyping and genotyping studies is required to confirm the diagnosis.

Differential Diagnosis

COPD is most commonly confused with asthma (Chapter 87), particularly in older patients. Clinical features that favor asthma over COPD include onset of disease at an early age, presence of atopy, lack of a smoking history, substantial variability of symptoms over time, and largely reversible airflow obstruction. However, new onset of asthma may occur in elderly people, some asthmatics smoke, an atopic history is not a requisite for development of asthma, and airflow obstruction may become fixed in patients with severe, long-standing asthma. Because treatment is much the same, distinguishing asthma from COPD may not be so important.

Bronchiectasis (Chapter 90) is characterized by chronic inflammation and abnormal dilation of airways associated with chronic cough and expectora-

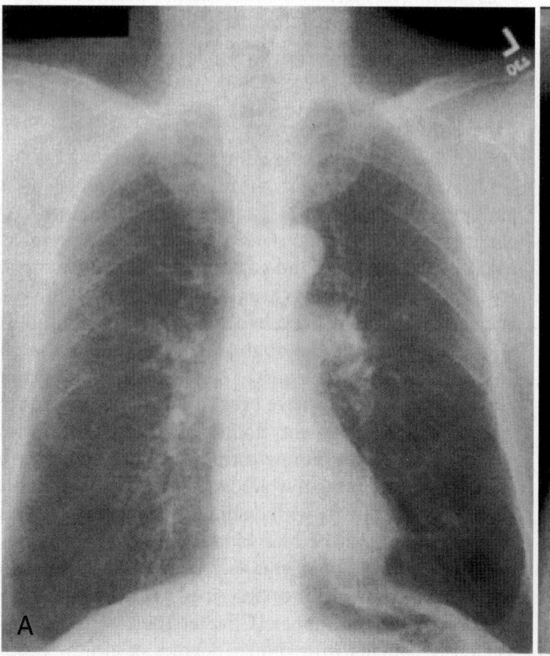

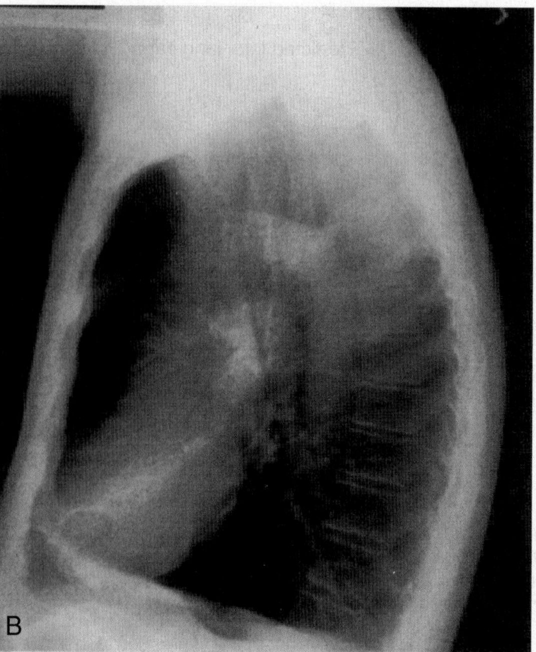

FIGURE 88-3. Posteroanterior (A) and lateral (B) radiographs of the thorax in a patient with emphysema. The most obvious abnormalities are those associated with increased lung volume. The lungs appear dark because of their increased air relative to tissue. The diaphragms are caudal to their normal position and appear flatter than normal. The heart is oriented more vertically than normal because of caudal displacement of the diaphragm, and the transverse diameter of the rib cage is increased; as a result, the width of the heart relative to the rib cage on the posteroanterior view is decreased. The space between the sternum and heart and great vessels is increased on the lateral view.

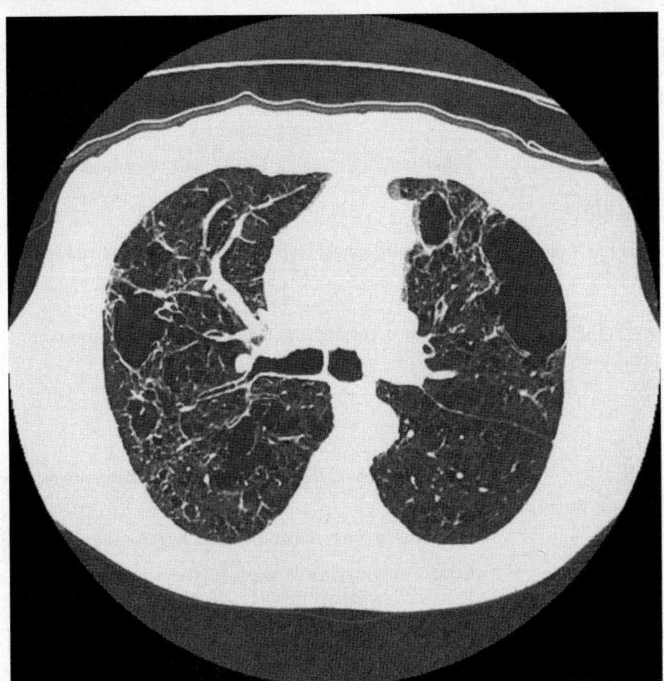

FIGURE 88-4. High-resolution axial computed tomography scan of a 1-mm section of the thorax of a patient with emphysema at the level of the tracheal carina. The right lung is on the left. Multiple large bullae—black holes—are evident. Many smaller areas of similar tissue destruction are also present in both lungs. The right upper lobe bronchus is seen entering the lung; its walls are thickened, suggesting chronic inflammation. (Courtesy Dr. Bruce Maycher.)

tion of purulent sputum. It can be distinguished from COPD with a predominant bronchitis component by chest CT imaging.

Bronchiolitis obliterans is characterized by cicatricial narrowing of the distal airways with severe irreversible airflow obstruction. The condition may occur in association with collagen vascular diseases (Chapters 264 and 266) and is commonly seen after lung transplantation (Chapter 101). A similar disorder has been described with certain industrial inhalants, such as diacetyl, a butter-like flavoring manufactured for use with microwavable popcorn (Chapter 93). In nonsmokers, the diagnosis of bronchiolitis obliterans can be reliably inferred from the history, the presence of irreversible airflow obstruction, and the absence of emphysema or other explanatory conditions on chest CT images. Attribution of cause in smokers is more difficult because the airway disease with diacetyl exposure is similar to that found with cigarette smoke.

TREATMENT Rx

Stable Disease

Smoking Cessation

Smoking cessation (Chapter 32) reduces symptoms of cough and sputum production in many patients with COPD, but it improves lung function to only a small extent. Most important, about a decade after smoking cessation, the rate of decline of FEV_1 in patients with mild to moderate disease reverts to that seen in lifelong nonsmokers, thereby making it unlikely that these former smokers will ever develop severe COPD. Smoking cessation in patients with mild to moderate COPD also improves long-term mortality by reducing both respiratory and cardiovascular deaths. Smoking cessation probably also slows the decline of lung function in patients with more severe COPD.

Limited information indicates that counseling and pharmacotherapy achieve the same low success rates for smoking cessation in COPD patients as in the general population (Chapter 32). COPD patients tend to quit smoking as the disease progresses, possibly because they have greater awareness of their disease or because cigarette smoke makes their respiratory symptoms worse. Sharing information about abnormal spirometry has not been shown to motivate patients to quit smoking.

Bronchodilators

Both β_2-adrenergic agonists and anticholinergics are widely used to treat COPD (Table 88-2). Short-acting β_2-adrenergic agonists, such as albuterol and the short-acting anticholinergic ipratropium bromide, can be administered either by oral inhaler devices or by nebulization, with little objective superiority of one delivery device over the other if a spacer is used with oral inhaler devices. Longer-acting bronchodilators have largely replaced shorter-acting drugs, but a short-acting bronchodilator, such as albuterol, is still recommended for "rescue" or "as-needed" use in patients who experience bothersome dyspnea (Table 88-3).

Inhaled long-acting β_2-adrenergic agonist bronchodilators widely used for COPD include salmeterol and formoterol, administered by one inhalation twice daily, and indacaterol, administered by one inhalation once daily (Table 88-2). Inhaled anticholinergics include tiotropium (administered by one inhalation once daily) and aclidinium (administered by one inhalation twice daily). Tiotropium (18 μg once daily) appears to be superior to salmeterol (50 μg twice daily) for reducing exacerbations,[A1] and combining a long-acting β_2-adrenergic agonist inhaler with a separate long-acting anticholinergic inhaler appears to be more effective than either agent alone.[A2] Once-daily combination inhalers likely will soon be commercially available.

Compared with placebo, each class of long-acting bronchodilators reduces exacerbation rates by about 15 to 20% in relative terms. Because the average patient with severe COPD has about one serious exacerbation per year, the number of patients that need to be treated to prevent one exacerbation is about six. Adverse symptomatic events of both classes of long-acting bronchodilators in COPD patients are generally minor.

Theophylline is a poor bronchodilator that largely has been replaced with inhaled drugs, but its effect is additive when it is given along with inhaled bronchodilators. Theophylline may also reduce exacerbations. To be used effectively and safely, it should be started with an oral daily dose of between 150 and 300 mg and titrated to achieve serum levels of 8 to 12 μg/mL. Higher levels are poorly tolerated, especially in older patients. Theophylline interacts with numerous other drugs (e.g., allopurinol, diazepam, cimetidine, ciprofloxacin), and conditions such as heart failure and liver disease may reduce its elimination rates. Patients' drug levels must be monitored on a regular basis, and toxic levels can develop even in a patient receiving a stable dose. Oral roflumilast, a phosphodiesterase 4 inhibitor at 500 μg once daily, can increase FEV_1 by 50 mL and reduce moderate to severe exacerbations in patients with COPD and chronic bronchitis, even in patients already treated with tiotropium.

Corticosteroids

Inhaled corticosteroids produce marginal improvements in lung function and respiratory health status in COPD patients, and they reduce COPD exacerbation rates by about 15 to 20% in relative terms.[A3] Inhaled corticosteroids combined with an inhaled long-acting β_2-agonist provide added benefit over that seen with either monotherapy, but added benefit appears quite small when added to both a long-acting β_2-agonist and a long-acting anticholinergic.[A4] (Table 88-3). Multiple large trials have found little effect of inhaled corticosteroids in reducing FEV_1 loss during periods of several years.

The most common adverse effects of inhaled corticosteroids are dysphonia and upper airway thrush. Less commonly, they may predispose patients to pneumonia. Observational studies suggest that long-term inhaled corticosteroids may cause osteoporosis (Chapter 243) and cataracts (Chapter 423).

A few COPD patients are prescribed systemic corticosteroids on a regular basis, usually in doses of 10 to 15 mg/day of prednisone or its equivalent. These patients are sometimes considered "prednisone dependent" because it is frequently difficult to wean them completely off drug. There are no proven benefits of chronic, low-dose prednisone in COPD, and adverse effects involving bone, eyes, and other organs are well documented (Chapter 35). Consequently, efforts should be made to reduce or to discontinue chronic systemic corticosteroids while optimizing other treatment.

Oxygen

Chronic hypoxemia in patients with COPD can induce irreversible pulmonary hypertension and cor pulmonale (Chapter 68). Long-term oxygen therapy extends life in patients who are persistently hypoxemic. The principal qualifying criteria are an arterial PaO_2 of less than 56 mm Hg and an arterial oxygen saturation of less than 89%, both while breathing ambient air at rest in a stable clinical state. Patients should also be considered for home oxygen if their PaO_2 is less than 60 mm Hg in the presence of right-sided heart failure or polycythemia. Treatment should consist of home oxygen to be used for at least 18 hours daily, to include sleep time. To determine an appropriate prescription, the oxygen flow rate should be adjusted in 1-L/minute increments at 15-minute intervals until the resting oxygen saturation remains above 90%. In qualifying patients, long-term oxygen may also decrease polycythemia and pulmonary hypertension and improve neuropsychiatric function. Oxygen does not improve mortality in patients with similarly severe airflow obstruction but milder hypoxemia.

Many patients with severe COPD may be normoxemic at rest while breathing ambient air but exhibit oxygen desaturation with exercise. Physicians commonly prescribe ambulatory oxygen in this setting, with the expectation that it will improve exercise tolerance and increase daily activity. Ambulatory oxygen modestly improves exercise endurance for such patients in a laboratory setting, but efforts to show benefit during activities of daily living have

TABLE 88-2 COMMONLY USED MEDICATIONS FOR STABLE CHRONIC OBSTRUCTIVE PULMONARY DISEASE (COPD)

	MODE OF DELIVERY	DOSE AND FREQUENCY	POSSIBLE ADVERSE REACTIONS
SHORT-ACTING INHALED BRONCHODILATORS			
Albuterol (β_2-adrenergic agonist)	Inhaler	100 µg per inhalation; 1-2 inhalations every 4-6 hours, as needed	Palpitations, tachycardia, tremor, hypersensitivity reaction
	Nebulizer	2.5 mg; every 4-6 hours, as needed	
Ipratropium (anticholinergic)	Inhaler	17 µg per inhalation; 2 inhalations 4 times daily, up to 12 inhalations a day	Dry mouth, cough, blurred vision, hypersensitivity reaction
	Nebulizer	0.5 mg; every 6-8 hours	
Albuterol/ipratropium	Inhaler device	90 µg/18 µg per inhalation; 2 inhalations 4 times daily, up to 12 inhalations per day	All those occurring with either albuterol or ipratropium
	Nebulizer	2.5 mg/0.5 mg; 4 times daily, up to 2 additional doses daily	
LONG-ACTING INHALED BRONCHODILATORS			
Formoterol (β_2-adrenergic agonist)	Inhaler Nebulizer	12 µg; 1 inhalation twice daily 20 µg; twice daily	Dizziness, tremor, throat irritation, hypersensitivity reaction
Salmeterol (β_2-adrenergic agonist)	Inhaler	50 µg; 1 inhalation twice daily	Headache, tremor, throat irritation, hypersensitivity reaction
Indacaterol (β_2-adrenergic agonist)	Inhaler	75 µg; 1 inhalation daily	Cough, oropharyngeal pain, nasopharyngitis, headache, nausea, hypersensitivity reaction
Tiotropium (anticholinergic)	Inhaler	18 µg; 1 inhalation each morning	Dry mouth, urinary retention, symptoms of narrow-angle glaucoma, hypersensitivity reaction
Aclidinium (anticholinergic)	Inhaler	400 µg; 1 inhalation twice daily	Same as for tiotropium
INHALED CORTICOSTEROIDS			
Fluticasone powder	Inhaler	250 µg; 1-2 inhalations twice daily	Sore throat, dysphonia, headache, hypersensitivity reaction
Budesonide	Inhaler	160 µg; 1-2 inhalations twice daily	Nasopharyngitis, thrush, hypersensitivity reactions
COMBINATION INHALERS			
Fluticasone/salmeterol	Inhaler	250 µg/50 µg; 1 inhalation twice daily	All those occurring with either fluticasone or salmeterol
Budesonide/formoterol	Inhaler	160 µg/4.5 µg; 2 inhalations twice daily	All those occurring with either budesonide or formoterol
ORAL DRUGS			
Theophylline (24-hour sustained release)	Pill	200-800 mg, once daily; start with daily dose of 150-300 mg and titrate to blood level of 8-12 µg/mL	Nausea and vomiting, seizures, tremor, insomnia, multifocal atrial tachyarrhythmia, hypersensitivity reaction
Roflumilast	Pill	500 µg, once daily	Depression, suicidal thought, insomnia, loss of appetite, weight loss, diarrhea

TABLE 88-3 GUIDELINE RECOMMENDATIONS FOR DIAGNOSIS AND MANAGEMENT OF STABLE COPD

Spirometry should be obtained to diagnose airflow obstruction in patients with respiratory symptoms. Spirometry should not be used to screen for airflow obstruction in individuals without respiratory symptoms.

For stable COPD patients with respiratory symptoms and FEV_1 between 60% and 80% of predicted, treatment with inhaled bronchodilators may be used.

Stable COPD patients with respiratory symptoms and $FEV_1 < 60\%$ should be treated with inhaled bronchodilators.

Clinicians should prescribe monotherapy with either long-acting inhaled anticholinergics or long-acting inhaled β-agonists for symptomatic patients with COPD and $FEV_1 < 60\%$ predicted. Clinicians should base the choice of specific monotherapy on the patient's preference, the cost, and the adverse effect profile.

Clinicians may administer combination inhaled therapies (long-acting inhaled anticholinergics, long-acting inhaled β-agonists, or inhaled corticosteroids) for symptomatic patients with stable COPD and $FEV_1 < 60\%$ predicted.

Clinicians should prescribe pulmonary rehabilitation for symptomatic patients with an $FEV_1 < 50\%$ predicted. Clinicians may consider pulmonary rehabilitation for symptomatic or exercise-limited patients with an $FEV_1 > 50\%$ predicted.

Clinicians should prescribe continuous oxygen therapy in patients with COPD who have severe resting hypoxemia (arterial oxygen partial pressure ≤ 55 mm Hg or arterial oxygen saturation ≤ 88%)

COPD = chronic obstructive pulmonary disease; FEV_1 = forced expiratory volume in 1 second.

Modified from Qaseem A, Wilt TJ, Weinberger SE, et al. Diagnosis and management of stable chronic obstructive pulmonary disease: a clinical practice guideline update from the American College of Physicians, American College of Chest Physicians, American Thoracic Society, and European Respiratory Society. *Ann Intern Med.* 2011;155:179-191.

been mostly unsuccessful.[A5] Even normoxemic COPD patients with isolated nocturnal hypoxemia have not been shown to benefit from oxygen therapy.

Immunizations and Prophylactic Antibiotics

An annual influenza vaccination (Chapter 18) is recommended for all patients with COPD, although few trials have targeted this population of patients. Observational studies suggest that influenza vaccination substantially reduces hospitalization and mortality rates in COPD patients. Polysaccharide pneumococcal vaccination (Chapter 18) is also recommended, although supporting evidence is weak. Chronic prophylactic macrolide use (e.g., azithromycin 250 mg daily) in addition to regular treatment can decrease exacerbations and improve quality of life in patients with COPD,[A6] but such treatment may cause hearing loss and may not be safe if patients have a prolonged QTc interval or if they are taking other drugs known to prolong the QTc interval.

Pulmonary Rehabilitation

COPD patients become increasingly sedentary as their disease progresses. Lack of physical activity causes muscle and cardiovascular deconditioning, which further complicates the ability to perform routine tasks. The principal goal of pulmonary rehabilitation is to reverse this process with a program of exercise endurance training. Educational and behavior modification elements are usually included in an effort to improve coping skills and psychological functioning. Most programs are hospital based and consist of 3- to 4-hour sessions, three times a week, during a 6- to 12-week period. Patients who become breathless with minimal activity or who have exercise-limiting comorbidities are not suitable candidates.

Numerous randomized, controlled trials have shown that pulmonary rehabilitation confers substantial improvements in respiratory health status and in walking distance and possibly in reduction of health care use.[A7] Unfortunately, the benefits of pulmonary rehabilitation erode rapidly in the absence of a continuation plan after completion of the initial program. Pulmonary rehabilitation is also not accessible to most patients for a variety of reasons.

Surgical Options

In lung volume reduction surgery (Chapter 101), severely emphysematous tissue is resected from the upper lobes of both lungs to permit less diseased portions of unresected lung to expand and to function more normally. Patients who are severely disabled from COPD and who have no other major comorbid conditions may be candidates for this procedure if CT imaging shows that severe emphysema is mostly localized to the upper lobes. Compared with controls receiving no surgical treatment, lung volume reduction surgery improves lung function, exercise capacity, and respiratory health status in COPD patients with severe emphysema, but there is no mortality benefit from this procedure, with a possible exception in the subset of patients with both predominant upper lobe emphysema and low exercise capacity.[A8] Procedures that deflate severely emphysematous regions of the lung by endoscopic placement of one-way bronchial valves or of transbronchial stents or that completely ablate bronchi that subtend regions of severe emphysema, with either thermal injury or biologic sealants, have not yielded clear clinical benefits and are not recommended (Chapter 101).

Lung transplantation is an option for patients who are severely incapacitated from COPD and have no major comorbid conditions (Chapter 101). Median survival after lung transplantation is only about 5 years, primarily because of the development of bronchiolitis obliterans, a form of chronic graft rejection causing severe airflow obstruction in the peripheral airways. It is unclear whether lung transplantation extends survival in patients with COPD, but patients who are fortunate enough to avoid complications are able to resume normal daily activities.

Exacerbations

Exacerbations represent an important element in the natural history of COPD.[9] An exacerbation is defined as some combination of dyspnea, cough, and productive sputum, each of which has worsened from the stable state or has newly appeared. Exacerbations may also be associated with symptoms of rhinorrhea, sore throat, fever, and chest congestion. A symptom-based clinical event, as described previously, coupled with administration of an antibiotic or a systemic corticosteroid or admission to a hospital, is a definition that has been widely used in clinical trials.

Patients with severe COPD experience an average of about one such exacerbation per year along with additional milder exacerbations that meet the symptomatic definition but do not require a medical intervention. Exacerbations are acute in onset, but recovery may require several weeks. Severe exacerbations have a major adverse impact on health status and may cause permanent loss of lung function. Hospitalization for exacerbations consumes more than half of total medical costs for COPD. For poorly understood reasons, some patients suffer frequent exacerbations, whereas others have very few, despite similar degrees of airflow obstruction. Independent risk factors include low lung function, older age, history of frequent exacerbations, elevated blood levels of inflammatory biomarkers,[10] and prior hospitalizations as well as the presence of a productive cough, gastroesophageal reflux, and cardiovascular comorbidities.

Respiratory infections are thought to cause most exacerbations, although many of these implicated microorganisms may be recovered from sputum during periods of stable disease. Bacteria commonly implicated include *Haemophilus influenzae* (Chapter 300), *Streptococcus pneumoniae* (Chapter 289), and *Moraxella catarrhalis* (Chapter 300). *Pseudomonas aeruginosa* (Chapter 306) and enteric gram-negative bacilli (Chapters 304 and 305) are less common but are seen in patients with very severe COPD who were recently hospitalized or intubated. Putative viral pathogens include rhinoviruses (Chapter 361), influenza (Chapter 364), parainfluenza (Chapter 363), and respiratory syncytial virus (Chapter 362). Periods of increased airborne pollution with diesel particulates, sulfur dioxide, ozone, and nitrogen dioxide are associated with more COPD hospitalizations, but no cause can be assigned to many exacerbations.

Evaluation and management of a patient with a suspected exacerbation vary according to severity. Mild exacerbations encountered in an office setting can be diagnosed and treated on the basis of a brief history and physical examination. Patients seen in emergency department or hospital settings generally are sicker and require a more extensive evaluation (Table 88-4). A chest radiograph should be obtained to look for signs of pneumonia (Chapter 97), pneumothorax (Chapter 99), and heart failure (Chapter 58). If pulmonary embolism (Chapter 98) is suspected, spiral CT of the chest is the test of choice. Arterial blood gases should be measured if there is any suspicion of hypercapnia because this information influences subsequent therapy. Sputum cultures need not be done routinely because they are unproven guides to antibiotic therapy. During seasonal outbreaks of influenza (Chapter 364), type A and B viruses can be identified with rapid commercially available polymerase chain reaction assays having a sensitivity of greater than 90%. These tests should not be relied on to withhold antiviral therapy if the patient is severely ill or if there is a strong clinical suspicion of influenza.

Cardiac disease is a common comorbidity in COPD patients, and distinguishing a COPD exacerbation from left ventricular failure (Chapter 58) by history and physical examination alone is often problematic. Dyspnea (Chapter 83) is common to both conditions. Peripheral edema (Chapter 51) and elevated jugular venous pressure may occur with either left ventricular failure or cor pulmonale secondary to COPD. Echocardiography (Chapter 55) and serum brain natriuretic peptide (BNP) levels (Chapter 58) are useful in this clinical setting, although echocardiography is more difficult to perform in patients

TABLE 88-4 GUIDELINE RECOMMENDATIONS FOR HOSPITAL MANAGEMENT OF COPD EXACERBATIONS

	GLOBAL INITIATIVE FOR CHRONIC OBSTRUCTIVE LUNG DISEASE*	NATIONAL INSTITUTE FOR CLINICAL EXCELLENCE†
Date of statement	2013	2010
Diagnostic testing	Chest radiograph, oximetry, ABGs, and ECG Other testing as warranted by clinical indication	Chest radiograph, ABGs, ECG, complete blood count, sputum smear and culture, blood cultures if febrile
Bronchodilator therapy	Inhaled short-acting β_2-agonist is recommended Consider ipratropium if inadequate clinical response Consider theophylline or aminophylline as second-line intravenous therapy	Administer inhaled drugs by nebulizer or hand-held inhaler with spacer device Specific agents and dosing regimens not specified Consider theophylline if inadequate response to inhaled bronchodilators
Antibiotics (see text for dosing)	Recommended if (1) increases in dyspnea, sputum volume, and sputum purulence all are present; (2) increase in sputum purulence along with increase in either dyspnea or sputum volume; or (3) need for assisted ventilation Initial empirical therapy with aminopenicillin with or without clavulanic acid, macrolide, or tetracycline, based on local bacterial resistance patterns Subsequent therapy based on sputum and blood cultures	Administer only if the patient has a history of purulent sputum Initiate with an aminopenicillin, a macrolide, or a tetracycline, taking into account local bacterial resistance patterns Adjust therapy according to sputum and blood cultures
Systemic corticosteroids	Daily prednisolone 30-40 mg (or its equivalent) for 10-14 days	Daily prednisolone 30 mg (or its equivalent) orally for 7-14 days
Supplemental oxygen	Maintain oxygen saturation 88-92% Monitor ABGs for hypercapnia and acidosis	Maintain oxygen saturation within the individualized target range Monitor ABGs
Assisted ventilation	Indications for NPPV include respiratory acidemia (arterial pH $\leq$ 7.35) or severe dyspnea with clinical signs of respiratory muscle fatigue or increased work of breathing	NPPV is the treatment of choice for persistent hypercapnic respiratory failure Consider functional status, body mass index, home oxygen, comorbidities, prior ICU admissions, age, and FEV_1 when assessing suitability for intubation and ventilation

*Data from http://www.goldcopd.com.
†Data from http://www.nice.org.uk.
ABGs = arterial blood gases; COPD = chronic obstructive pulmonary disease; ECG = electrocardiogram; ICU = intensive care unit; NPPV = noninvasive positive-pressure ventilation.

with severe COPD. BNP levels may be modestly elevated in both stable and exacerbated COPD in the absence of left ventricular dysfunction. A normal BNP level excludes a diagnosis of left-sided heart failure with a high level of confidence, but an elevated level does not confirm its presence unless it is markedly elevated.

Decisions about the need for hospitalization rely mostly on clinical judgment because there are no well-validated guidelines. Clinical assessment should consider intensity of dyspnea, use of accessory muscles of respiration, arterial blood gas disturbances, hemodynamic stability, and mental alertness.

Guideline recommendations (see Table 88-4) for treatment of patients hospitalized for COPD exacerbations emphasize that antibiotics hasten recovery.[A9] Antibiotics are most effective when cough and purulent sputum are present, but there are no well-validated methods for determining which patients should be treated. If patients are sufficiently ill to seek medical attention for an exacerbation, most should probably receive an antibiotic.

Most randomized placebo-controlled trials evaluated first-generation antibiotics, such as amoxicillin, trimethoprim-sulfamethoxazole, and tetracyclines, and it is unclear whether newer classes of antibiotics, such as macrolides and fluoroquinolones, are more effective. Choice of an antibiotic should be made with considerations to cost, safety, and local patterns of antibiotic resistance among the bacterial species commonly isolated from sputa during exacerbations. Doxycycline, 100 mg twice daily for 7 to 10 days, or trimethoprim-sulfamethoxazole, 160/800 mg twice daily for 7 to 10 days, would be reasonable choices for initial therapy in many locales.

Systemic corticosteroids improve lung function, shorten the recovery period, and prevent relapse when given to patients who are hospitalized or present to an emergency department with a COPD exacerbation. Severely symptomatic patients seen in other clinical settings are also likely to benefit. Prednisone, 40 mg once daily for 5 days, is appropriate for most patients.[A10] Longer courses of systemic corticosteroid therapy are strongly discouraged because they are no more effective and they increase the likelihood of adverse effects. Parenteral corticosteroids should be given only if gastrointestinal absorption is thought to be impaired. The major adverse effect of systemic corticosteroids is transient hyperglycemia, which may require treatment, particularly in patients with known diabetes mellitus (Chapter 229).

Patients should be encouraged to increase their use of short-acting bronchodilators during outpatient treatment of an exacerbation. For hospitalized patients, a short-acting bronchodilator should be administered on a regular schedule, every 4 to 6 hours and more frequently as needed. Anticholinergic and β_2-agonist agents are similarly effective, and a few small trials found no significant additive effect during exacerbations. Some patients express a preference for a nebulizer delivery system, although equivalent objective results can be achieved when inhalers are used with a spacer.

Sufficient oxygen should be provided to maintain arterial oxygen saturations just above 90%, usually with oxygen flow rates of 2 to 3 L/minute delivered through a nasal cannula. Even at low flow rates, oxygen therapy can be expected to increase $PaCO_2$ by an average of about 5 to 10 mm Hg in patients with chronic hypercapnia. It is prudent to use the lowest flow of oxygen that achieves the desired result. If oxygen is prescribed for hypoxemia during an exacerbation, it is important to retest the patient several weeks later after recovery to determine when long-term oxygen is needed.

The introduction of noninvasive positive-pressure ventilation (NIPPV) has significantly improved the care of patients with severe COPD exacerbations who have respiratory failure.[A11] With NIPPV, the patient wears a tightly fitting nasal or full facial mask that is attached to a positive-pressure ventilator, avoiding the need for an endotracheal tube or a tracheostomy (Chapter 105). Compared with usual care, treatment with NIPPV is associated with fewer intubations, a shorter hospital stay, and improved all-cause mortality.

PROGNOSIS

About two-thirds of patients have progressive disease.[11] Severe COPD is associated with excess mortality, and lung function, usually expressed as the percentage of predicted FEV_1, is the single strongest predictor of death. Patients with COPD have variable rates of decline in FEV_1, with more rapid average rates in smokers than in former smokers, but spirometry repeated at intervals of 1 year or more provides only limited information about prognosis. Only about half of patients with an FEV_1 that is about 40% of predicted will survive 5 years.

The severity of emphysema by CT or carbon monoxide diffusion is independently associated with a rapid annual decline in FEV_1. Additional risk factors include the severity of dyspnea, weight loss, limited walking distance, hospitalization for exacerbation, hypoxemia, hypercapnia, and impaired quality of life. The development of bronchiectasis is independently associated with an increased risk of all-cause mortality in patients with moderate to severe COPD.[12] The only interventions shown to reduce mortality are smoking cessation in patients with mild to moderate COPD, long-term oxygen therapy for the subset of patients with chronic hypoxemia, and NIPPV in selected patients who are hospitalized for respiratory failure.

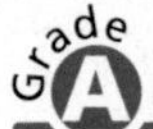

Grade A References

A1. Vogelmeier C, Hederer B, Glaab T, et al. Tiotropium versus salmeterol for the prevention of exacerbations of COPD. *N Engl J Med.* 2011;364:1093-1103.

A2. Wedzicha JA, Decramer M, Ficker JH, et al. Analysis of chronic obstructive pulmonary disease exacerbations with the dual bronchodilator QVA149 compared with glycopyrronium and tiotropium (SPARK): a randomised, double-blind, parallel-group study. *Lancet Respir Med.* 2013;1:199-209.

A3. Yang IA, Clarke MS, Sim EHA, et al. Inhaled corticosteroids for stable chronic obstructive pulmonary disease. *Cochrane Database Syst Rev.* 2012;7:CD002991.

A4. Magnussen H, Disse B, Rodriguez-Roisin R, et al. Withdrawal of inhaled glucocorticoids and exacerbations of COPD. *N Engl J Med.* 2014;371:1285-1294.

A5. Abernethy AP, McDonald CF, Frith PA, et al. Effect of palliative oxygen versus room air in relief of breathlessness in patients with refractory dyspnoea: a double-blind, randomised controlled trial. *Lancet.* 2010;376:784-793.

A6. Herath SC, Poole P. Prophylactic antibiotic therapy in chronic obstructive pulmonary disease. *JAMA.* 2014;311:2225-2226.

A7. COPD Working Group. Pulmonary rehabilitation for patients with chronic pulmonary disease (COPD): an evidence based analysis. *Ont Health Technol Assess Ser.* 2012;12:1-75.

A8. Shah PL, Slebos DJ, Cardoso PF, et al. Bronchoscopic lung-volume reduction with Exhale airway stents for emphysema (EASE trial): randomised, sham-controlled, multicentre trial. *Lancet.* 2011;378:997-1005.

A9. Vollenweider DJ, Jarrett H, Steurer-Stey CA, et al. Antibiotics for exacerbations of chronic obstructive pulmonary disease. *Cochrane Database Syst Rev.* 2012;12:CD010257.

A10. Leuppi JD, Schuetz P, Bingisser R, et al. Short-term vs conventional glucocorticoid therapy in acute exacerbations of chronic obstructive pulmonary disease. The REDUCE randomized clinical trial. *JAMA.* 2013;309:2223-2231.

A11. McCurdy BR. Noninvasive positive pressure ventilation for acute respiratory failure patients with chronic obstructive pulmonary disease (COPD): an evidence-based analysis. *Ont Health Technol Assess Ser.* 2012;12:1-102.

GENERAL REFERENCES

For the General References and other additional features, please visit Expert Consult at https://expertconsult.inkling.com.

89

CYSTIC FIBROSIS

FRANK J. ACCURSO

DEFINITION

Cystic fibrosis is an autosomal recessive disease caused by mutations in the gene that encodes the cystic fibrosis transmembrane conductance regulator (CFTR) protein, which is a membrane protein that regulates ion flux at epithelial surfaces. Cystic fibrosis affects the lungs, pancreas, intestines, liver, sweat glands, sinuses, and vas deferens, thereby resulting in substantial morbidity and premature mortality. Progressive lung disease is the cause of death in 80% of patients.

EPIDEMIOLOGY

The incidence of cystic fibrosis in the United States, Europe, and Australia is one in 3000 to 5000 births. Cystic fibrosis is most common in the non-Hispanic white population but also occurs in significant numbers in Hispanics (one in 7000), African Americans (one in 12,000), and some Native American populations. It also occurs rarely in individuals of Asian origin.

Approximately 30,000 persons in the United States have cystic fibrosis, for an estimated prevalence of approximately one in 10,000. Worldwide, an estimated 100,000 individuals are affected. Intensive daily care and exacerbations, particularly those that require hospitalization, are associated with enormous social and monetary costs.

PATHOBIOLOGY

Lung and Sinus

The pathobiology of cystic fibrosis is based on the ion transport activities of the CFTR, which is a membrane glycoprotein that functions as a chloride channel but is also involved in the regulation of transepithelial sodium and bicarbonate transport. In the airway, CFTR dysfunction reduces chloride secretion from the epithelial lining cell into the airway lumen. In addition, sodium absorption from the lumen into the cell is markedly increased. The net effect is a thinning of the airway surface's liquid lining layer, thereby crucially impairing mucociliary clearance. The subsequent chronic infection leads to an intense neutrophil-dominated inflammatory response. Neutrophil products, including proteolytic enzymes and oxidants, are thought to mediate the pathologic changes in the airway, including bronchiectasis, bronchiolectasis, bronchial stenosis, and fibrosis. Mucus plugging of airways, likely owing to chronic infection and inflammation as well as to CFTR dysfunction in mucus glands, is another prominent feature of airway disease (Fig. 89-1).

The origin of sinus disease is believed to be similar to that in the lung. Impaired mucociliary clearance leads to chronic infection and inflammation. Nasal and sinus polyps are common, but their cause is poorly understood.

Pancreas

Pathologic studies of the pancreas in infants demonstrate ductal obstruction and dilation as well as acinar dilation. The CFTR is expressed in ductal tissue, suggesting that impairment of chloride and bicarbonate secretion into the lumen of the ducts leads to the viscous secretions that obstruct the ducts and cause acinar dilation. The exposure of pancreatic tissue to proteolytic enzymes of acinar origin leads to a cystic and fibrotic pancreas in the first few years of life. Unlike the lung, injury to the exocrine pancreas does not involve infection. Almost complete exocrine pancreatic insufficiency is seen in 85% of patients and is related to genotype.

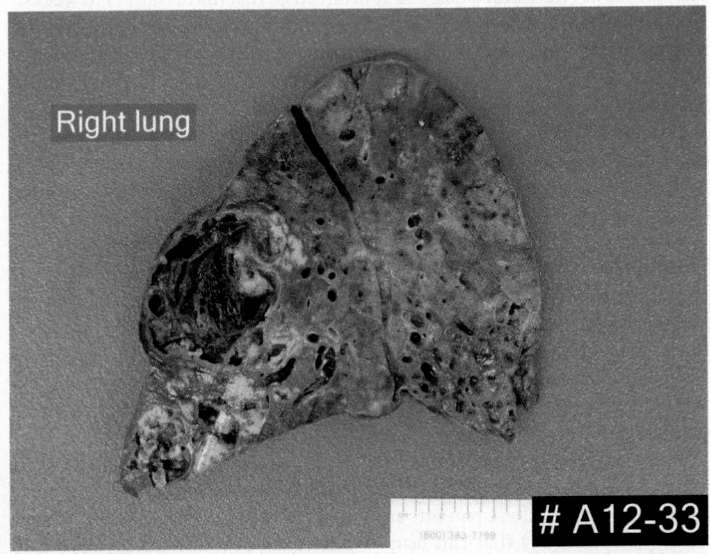

FIGURE 89-1. Section through the right lung from a 13-year-old young woman with cystic fibrosis demonstrating the gross appearance of cavity formation, bronchiectasis, and purulent mucus plugging.

Intestine and Liver

CFTR is expressed throughout the intestine. In approximately 15% of cases, cystic fibrosis is accompanied by meconium ileus as a manifestation of severe intestinal obstruction at birth. The incidence of jejunal and ileal stenoses and atresias is greatly increased compared with normal individuals. It is unclear how these severe abnormalities arise, but mucus obstruction, which is frequently seen in intestinal crypts at birth, suggests that abnormalities in CFTR lead to viscous meconium that interferes with normal intestinal development.

In the liver, bile duct obstruction is the first pathologic change noted. Focal areas of sclerosis ensue, probably owing to obstructed bile ducts. Infection is not involved in hepatic injury.

Sweat Gland

In the sweat gland, CFTR dysfunction leads to a failure of chloride absorption from the lumen into the sweat ductal lining cell. In contrast, the abnormality in the lung involves chloride secretion. The failure to absorb chloride and, by electroneutrality, sodium, results in marked elevations in the chloride and sodium content of sweat. This abnormality is not accompanied by tissue destruction.

Male Reproductive Tract

The vas deferens appears to be the organ that is most sensitive to CFTR dysfunction. It often becomes obstructed in fetuses or infants. Resorption of the vas deferens occurs very early in life, and the vas is ultimately not identifiable in most males.

Other Organ Involvement

The primary abnormalities in cystic fibrosis result in secondary involvement of a number of other systems. Diabetes (Chapter 229), which is increasingly common in adolescents and adults, has historically been attributed to the extension of scarring from the exocrine pancreas into the islets of Langerhans. Recent evidence, however, suggests that functional β-cell abnormalities related to an abnormal CFTR. Osteopenia and osteoporosis (Chapter 243), which are common in adults, result from a combination of malnutrition and chronic infection.[1] Delayed puberty (Chapters 234 and 235) is also common. Patients can experience recurrent vasculitis or arthralgias that are believed to be caused by the host response to chronic infection. Exocrine pancreatic insufficiency leads to impaired growth and to a multitude of potential nutritional complications, including deficiencies in fat-soluble vitamins and trace elements (Chapter 218).[2]

Genetics

The gene that encodes the CFTR spans more than 250,000 base pairs on the long arm of chromosome 7. The CFTR (ABCC7), which is a protein of 1480 amino acids, belongs to the adenosine triphosphate–binding cassette transporter family. More than 1500 mutations of five different classes have been described (Table 89-1).[3] In the United States, only five mutations are present in more than 1% of cases. The F508δ mutation is by far the most

TABLE 89-1 CLASSES OF CFTR MUTATIONS

CLASS	MECHANISM	GENETIC AND MOLECULAR ABNORMALITIES	REPRESENTATIVE GENOTYPE
I	Defective protein production	Unstable mRNA Truncated protein Premature stop mutations Frameshift Splicing variants	W1282X Del394TT 1717-1G to A
II	Defective protein processing	Trafficking abnormality Protein degraded in proteasome Deletion	F508del
III	Defective channel regulation	Protein at membrane Failure of gating Amino acid substitution	G551D
IV	Defective channel conductance	Protein at membrane Decreased gating Amino acid substitution	R117H
V	Decreased active CFTR	CFTR has normal activity at membrane but is decreased in amount Splice variant Substitution	3849+10kb C to T A455E

CFTR = cystic fibrosis transmembrane conductance regulator.

common and is present in approximately 90% of patients in the United States. The next most common mutation, G542X, is present in only 5% of patients.

Class 1 mutations are nonsense mutations that result in essentially no expression of the CFTR protein. Class II mutations lead to defective protein processing; in the case of 508δF, protein trafficking to the cell membrane is disrupted because the protein is recognized as defective by cellular quality control mechanisms, which direct it to the proteasome for degradation. In class III mutations, a protein is produced and processed correctly, but the channel remains closed in response to physiologic stimuli. In class IV mutations, the channel is present in the membrane but opens only partially in response to stimuli. In class V mutations, normal CFTR is produced but in reduced amounts because of defective splicing.

Different mutations lead to differing levels of CFTR dysfunction.[4] Whereas severe mutations (classes 1-3) may reduce CFTR activity to 1% to 3% of normal, mild mutations (classes 4 and 5) may be associated with CFTR activity that is 10% to 20% of normal. An important clinical correlation of CFTR activity is in the exocrine pancreas: patients with severe mutations almost always have pancreatic insufficiency, but some patients with milder mutations may retain pancreatic sufficiency. Patients with mild mutations tend, on average, to have less severe lung disease as well.

The clinical course of cystic fibrosis is variable even after controlling for the type of mutation in CFTR, suggesting additional heritable and environmental influences. Genes that code for transforming growth factor-β, mannose-binding lectin, and interferon-related developmental regulator 1 are among the identified modifiers of the severity and course of cystic fibrosis. Most modifiers have to do with the host response to infection or the development of fibrosis rather than the ion transport function of CFTR.

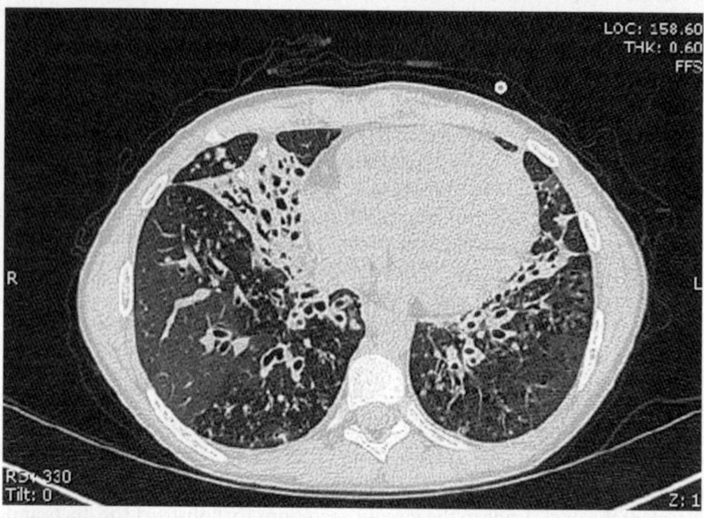

FIGURE 89-2. A computed tomography image of a 13-year-old young woman with cystic fibrosis demonstrating bronchiectasis in several different regions of the lung, right middle lobe collapse, partial lingular collapse, patchy tree-in-bud opacities, and mild hypoattenuation.

CLINICAL MANIFESTATIONS

Without specific supportive care, most patients succumb in infancy or early childhood because of malnutrition or lung disease. With the use of pancreatic enzyme replacement therapy, better pulmonary care, and the establishment of specialized centers of expertise, most patients live into their fourth or fifth decade.

Lung Disease

Cough, often persistent after viral infections, is the most prominent early feature of the disease. Viral infection may require more frequent hospitalizations in children with cystic fibrosis than in normal children.

Although lung disease begins in infancy, pulmonary function is often preserved until adolescence, when a steep decline frequently begins; at this time, pulmonary exacerbations become common. Most patients with cystic fibrosis have a daily productive cough by late adolescence or young adulthood.

Cystic fibrosis causes obstructive lung disease, initially with decreased flows at low lung volumes. Forced expiratory volume in 1 second (FEV_1) (Chapter 85) is the best correlate of outcome and starts to differ markedly from normal during late adolescence. The rate of decline in FEV_1 often predicts the clinical course.

Early in the disease, the chest radiograph demonstrates hyperinflation and peribronchial thickening. Computed tomography (Fig. 89-2) can demonstrate bronchiectasis (Chapter 90) early in the course of the disease, even before pulmonary function abnormalities are notable.

Airway infection, which is the key clinical manifestation, can be detected by culture of sputum or bronchoalveolar lavage fluid. *Pseudomonas aeruginosa* (Chapter 306) is the primary pathogen, although its prevalence is decreasing in the United States, likely owing to improved treatment. *Staphylococcus aureus* (Chapter 288), which is another prominent pathogen, can be methicillin resistant and exist in a small-colony variant form that makes antibiotic treatment difficult.

Most infections remain endobronchial and rarely cause invasive disease. An exception is *Burkholderia* infection, which can result in sepsis that leads to death. *Burkholderia* infection can also lead to an accelerated decline in lung function and result in death over months to years. Nontuberculous mycobacterial infection can cause granulomatous disease in the airway. *Aspergillus* (Chapter 339) and other fungal species, which are often identified in sputum samples, can cause allergic bronchopulmonary mycoses, but whether they contribute to endobronchitis apart from allergy is unknown.

The polymicrobial nature of airway disease is increasingly appreciated. *Stenotrophomonas maltophilia, Achromobacter xylosoxidans,* and *Inquilinus limosus* are frequently identified serially in airway cultures. Anaerobic infection may also be important.

Individuals with cystic fibrosis are subject to acute exacerbations characterized by cough, dyspnea, decreased exercise tolerance, fatigue, increased sputum production, and change in sputum color that may last days to weeks.[5] Frequently, crackles are increased on physical examination, and both the resting oxygen saturation and lung function may decline. Increasing evidence suggests that the permanent loss of lung function is accelerated during periods of exacerbation.

Pulmonary complications can also include pneumothorax (Chapter 99), hemoptysis (Chapter 83), and pulmonary hypertension (Chapter 68).[6] Some patients with more advanced disease can develop acute ventilatory failure (Chapter 104) with their exacerbations.

Gastrointestinal Disease

Exocrine pancreatic insufficiency, which is apparent in the first year of life in most patients, results in impaired growth and lifelong difficulty in maintaining a normal weight. Patients at all ages may exhibit signs of malabsorption, including bulky, foul-smelling stools and flatulence. Fat-soluble vitamin and trace element deficiencies are common and are difficult to diagnose without regular laboratory monitoring.

About 15% of patients retain exocrine pancreatic sufficiency, most of whom have mild mutations associated with 10% to 20% of CFTR function. About one sixth of these patients are subject to recurrent episodes of pancreatitis (Chapter 144) that can lead to pancreatic pseudocysts or ultimately result in exocrine pancreatic insufficiency.

Intestinal obstruction can occur at any age. Frequently, the blockage is at the ileocecal valve, but generalized chronic constipation (Chapter 136) is even more common. Intussusception of the appendix can also occur. Inflammatory bowel disease (Chapter 141) and gastrointestinal malignancies (Chapters 192 and 193) appear to be more common than in the general population. Chronic abdominal pain can occur at any time of life and is often difficult to treat.

Most patients who develop liver disease do so in childhood or adolescence. Liver abnormalities are often first appreciated when physical examination reveals splenomegaly or a palpable, firm liver. Occasionally, hematemesis leads to the identification of esophageal or gastric varices that are indicative of portal hypertension. Splenic sequestration can lead to neutropenia or thrombocytopenia. Decreased hepatic production of clotting factors can also contribute to bleeding. Occasionally, jaundice is a presenting sign of hepatobiliary disease. Except for γ-glutamyl transpeptidase (GGT) levels, liver enzymes are frequently normal, even in patients with advanced disease. Gallstones (Chapter 155) are common and may or may not lead to symptoms. The hepatopulmonary syndrome (Chapter 153) can occur.

Other Organ Involvement

Although most patients have radiographic evidence of sinus changes, acute or chronic sinusitis occurs in only a minority of individuals. Sinusitis can be accompanied by debilitating headache and anosmia. Nasal or sinus polyposis can lead to obstructed breathing during sleep.

Hypoelectrolytemia from sweat losses can occur at any age. Symptoms range from nausea, vomiting, and decreased appetite to seizures and circulatory collapse with fatal consequences. Almost all men are sterile because of the changes in the vas deferens. Spermatogenesis is normal, however.

Cystic fibrosis–related diabetes (Chapter 229) increases in frequency with age.[7] By 30 years of age, approximately one third of patients have diabetes. Although patients rarely develop ketoacidosis, the microvascular and macrovascular complications of diabetes can occur. In addition, patients with diabetes appear to have an accelerated decline in lung function. Osteoporosis (Chapter 243), osteopenia, and increased fractures also increase in frequency with age. Vasculitis accompanied by rash or arthralgia can occur at any time of life. Chronic pain and depression are other important complications that increase with age.

DIAGNOSIS

Newborn Screening and Diagnosis

In the United States, all 50 states require newborn screening for cystic fibrosis to allow early diagnosis and immediate treatment. All newborn screening programs currently measure immunoreactive trypsinogen, a marker of pancreatic injury, from a dried blood spot taken during the first few days of life as the first step in the screening process. This biochemical screen identifies a large number of infants with abnormalities, only a fraction of whom have cystic fibrosis. Most programs perform genetic mutation analysis as the next step. Sweat testing is required to establish the diagnosis if suspected patients carry only one identifiable mutation, but most programs perform confirmatory sweat testing even if two mutations are present.

Sweat testing measures the chloride concentration in sweat that is stimulated by pilocarpine iontophoresis. The result is considered abnormal in adults and children when the concentration of chloride in the sweat is greater than 60 mmol/L; in infants, a concentration greater than 40 mmol/L is considered diagnostic. Patients with milder mutations may have normal sweat chloride values. A family history of cystic fibrosis also provides supportive evidence.

Diagnosis in Adulthood

Five percent of patients are diagnosed after 18 years of age, mostly on the basis of recurrent pancreatitis, nasal polyposis, chronic sinusitis, bronchiectasis, male infertility, allergic bronchopulmonary mycoses, and nontuberculous mycobacterial infection (Table 89-2). If the predominant symptoms are respiratory, the differential diagnosis includes primary ciliary dyskinesia, immune deficiency, or postinfectious bronchiectasis (Chapter 90). If the predominant symptom is recurrent pancreatitis (Chapter 144), the differential diagnosis includes hereditary pancreatitis with abnormalities in the *SPINK* gene. Transepithelial potential differences are altered in cystic fibrosis because of abnormal transport of sodium and chloride. The measurement of nasal potential difference, therefore, can sometimes be used as a diagnostic tool, particularly in adults.

It is increasingly recognized that some patients appear to have cystic fibrosis on clinical grounds but do not meet the criteria for diagnosis, usually because their sweat test results are in the normal range or two genetic mutations cannot be identified. These patients are sometimes diagnosed as having atypical cystic fibrosis, nonclassical cystic fibrosis, or variant cystic fibrosis.

TABLE 89-2 APPROACH TO DIAGNOSIS OF CYSTIC FIBROSIS IN ADULT PATIENTS

CONDITIONS SUGGESTING THE DIAGNOSIS OF CYSTIC FIBROSIS IN ADULTS
Recurrent pancreatitis
Male infertility
Chronic sinusitis
Nasal polyposis
Nontuberculous mycobacterial infection
Allergic bronchopulmonary mycosis
Bronchiectasis
RECOMMENDED DIAGNOSTIC STUDIES
Sweat electrolyte determination
Extended CFTR mutation analysis
Nasal potential difference
High-resolution CT scan to identify bronchiectasis
CT scan of sinuses for polyposis
Sputum induction or bronchoalveolar lavage to identify bacterial and fungal pathogens

CFTR = cystic fibrosis transmembrane conductance regulator; CT = computed tomography.

Full analysis of the CFTR coding and flanking regions may be helpful in making the diagnosis. Such patients should be followed at a cystic fibrosis center so that their lung disease can be treated and they can be monitored for other complications of cystic fibrosis.

TREATMENT Rx

The general consensus is that treatment is best conducted at specialized centers that use a team approach. Much of their success is based on the education of patients and families regarding symptoms, complications, the need for daily treatment, the importance of close monitoring of pulmonary function, and the potential benefits of rapid intervention for any detected abnormalities.[8]

Much research has addressed the possibility of treating this genetic disease with gene therapy, but such approaches have not yet yielded positive results.[A1] As a result, interest has shifted to improving CFTR function by using druglike molecules.[9,10] In a randomized trial, ivacaftor, a CFTR modulator (150 mg twice daily for 48 weeks), significantly improved lung function, weight, and sweat chloride in cystic fibrosis patients with the G551D mutation.[A2] This drug was rapidly approved for clinical use by the U.S. Food and Drug Administration.

Pulmonary Infections

Pulmonary infections can be treated with oral, inhaled, or intravenous antibiotics. An increase in cough or other respiratory symptoms should be addressed with the introduction of antibiotics or a change in antibiotics within a few days. Nebulized antibiotics (4 weeks of either aztreonam 75 mg two or three times a day or tobramycin 300 mg twice daily), alone or in combination with oral antibiotics, improve lung function and decrease exacerbations in patients with chronic *Pseudomonas* infection.[A3][A4] These same antibiotic strategies have also been increasingly successful for eradicating *Pseudomonas* infection. Chronic oral macrolide treatment (e.g., azithromycin 5-15 mg/kg/day, 500 mg three times per week) can reduce exacerbations for up to 6 months.[A5] It is not yet clear whether the chronic use of antibiotics in this setting leads to the development of more resistant organisms.

More severe changes in symptoms or an acute fall in lung function requires intravenous antibiotics aimed at the cultured pathogen (Chapter 97). Nontuberculous mycobacterial infections are treated for 6 months or longer using multiple antibiotic agents (Chapter 325). Allergic bronchopulmonary mycoses are treated with corticosteroids and antifungal agents (Chapter 331).

Several agents known to decrease the viscosity of mucus have proven to be of clinical benefit in cystic fibrosis. Daily use of inhaled rhDNase (2.5 mg) is associated with improvement in lung function and fewer exacerbations. Inhaled hypertonic (7%) saline can increase pulmonary function and reduce exacerbations,[A6] and adding inhaled mannitol (400 mg twice daily) to standard therapy can produce a sustained improvement in pulmonary function for 26 to 52 weeks.[A7]

Many patients have hyperreactive airways and may benefit from inhaled bronchodilators (Chapter 87). Inhaled corticosteroids are controversial and do not have proven benefit. Oral corticosteroid "bursts" (e.g., 5 days of prednisone, 1 mg/kg twice a day in children and 60 mg a day in adults) are often useful, but chronic administration of oral corticosteroids can result in severe complications, including diabetes and stunted growth. Most patients perform physical means of airway secretion clearance one or more times a day.

Even passive smoke exposure is deleterious. Oxygen therapy is often required to maintain saturation and prevent the development of pulmonary hypertension. Noninvasive ventilation is used mainly in patients with more advanced disease. Pneumothorax almost always requires pleurodesis. Persistent or recurrent hemoptysis is treated with bronchial artery embolization. Occasionally, lobectomy is required. Patients in acute ventilatory failure should receive mechanical ventilation unless they have decided against such treatment. In patients who have advanced disease, the possible need for ventilation should be addressed before the need actually arises.

Lung transplantation (Chapter 101) is an option for many patients. Individuals with cystic fibrosis have survival rates after transplantation comparable to or better than those of other patients.

Gastrointestinal Diseases

Pancreatic enzyme replacement (Chapter 144) is the mainstay of treatment for exocrine pancreatic insufficiency. Because gastric acid decreases enzyme activity, H_2-blockers (e.g., ranitidine 150 mg twice daily in children weighing >30 kg and in adults) or proton pump inhibitors (e.g., lansoprazole 30 mg orally once daily in children weighing >30 kg and in adults) are often used. Children and adolescents frequently use multiple nutritional supplements every day to maintain weight. Fat-soluble vitamin replacement therapy is necessary in most patients. Between 10% and 20% of patients may require gastrostomy feeding to aid growth or maintain weight.

To prevent intestinal obstruction, dietary fiber should be increased, and polyethylene glycol at varying doses (e.g., 17 g orally with 8 oz of water one to three times per day) is frequently used on a daily basis. Acute obstructions can be treated with more intensive use of polyethylene glycol or Gastrografin enema. Occasionally, refractory constipation (Chapter 136) requires surgical approaches that can result in loss of intestine.

Other Organ Systems

A combination of nasal rinses and topically applied corticosteroids and antibiotics is used to treat sinus disease (Chapter 426). Surgery is often required, however, especially for polyps.

Many pediatric patients receive daily salt supplementation. Adults should be counseled on the symptoms of salt depletion and encouraged to increase the amount of salt in their diets if there are no medical contraindications to doing so.

Regular screening for the onset of impaired glucose homeostasis or frank diabetes is required in all patients older than 10 years. Diabetes is treated with insulin (Chapter 229) because the safety and efficacy of oral antihyperglycemic agents have not been demonstrated in those with cystic fibrosis. Bone health is addressed through vitamin D supplementation, calcium supplementation, and oral bisphosphonate therapy (Chapter 243). Delayed puberty and short stature require consultation with endocrinologists and sometimes hormonal administration. Most clinicians believe that both aerobic exercise and strength training can have beneficial effects, although the implementation of exercise programs has been difficult in clinical practice. Men with cystic fibrosis can father children through the use of epididymal aspiration to retrieve sperm followed by in vitro fertilization.

General Care

Given all the pulmonary, nutritional, and other therapies prescribed for individuals with cystic fibrosis, their care amounts to several hours a day. The transition from pediatric care to adult care can be challenging and requires diligent planning and execution.[11] This burden has a major influence on the quality of life in patients and their families and may contribute to the increasing incidence of depression observed in this population.

End-of-life care encompasses many complex issues. Patients are often depressed and experience chronic pain. They are asked to perform increasingly intense therapeutic regimens. They may have changed locations to await transplantation. Family, medical, and professional relationships are disrupted. Excellent communication with caregivers about advance directives and other planning is necessary.

PREVENTION

Prenatal carrier screening, which is offered in many countries, can decrease the incidence of cystic fibrosis by approximately 25%. Newborn screening programs may also decrease the incidence by influencing the future reproductive decisions of parents of an affected child.

PROGNOSIS

The median expected survival time for cystic fibrosis patients at birth in the United States is 37 years. However, the peak age at death is 26 years, demonstrating that some patients are particularly vulnerable to devastating lung disease. Late adolescence and early adulthood are high-risk times for pulmonary insufficiency. Patients who survive to their 30s and beyond are often more stable, have milder CFTR mutations, and have a very slow decline in lung function. The success of ivacaftor in treating patients with the G551D mutation has spurred research for small molecules aimed at improving CFTR function for other mutations.

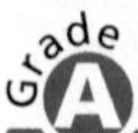

Grade A References

A1. Lee TW, Southern KW. Topical cystic fibrosis transmembrane conductance regulator gene replacement for cystic fibrosis-related lung disease. *Cochrane Database Syst Rev*. 2013;11:CD005599.

A2. Ramsey BW, Davies J, McElvaney NG, et al. A CFTR potentiator in patients with cystic fibrosis and the G551D mutation. *N Engl J Med*. 2011;365:1663-1672.

A3. Ramsey BW, Pepe MS, Quan JM, et al. Intermittent administration of inhaled tobramycin in patients with cystic fibrosis. *N Engl J Med*. 1999;340:23-30.

A4. McCoy KS, Quittner Al, Oermann CM, et al. Inhaled aztreonam lysine for chronic airway *Pseudomonas aeruginosa* in cystic fibrosis. *Am J Respir Crit Care Med*. 2008;178:921-928.

A5. Saiman L, Marshall BC, Mayer-Hamblett N, et al. Azithromycin in patients with cystic fibrosis chronically infected with Pseudomonas aeruginosa: a randomized controlled trial. *JAMA*. 2003;290:1749-1756.

A6. Elkins MR, Robinson M, Rose BR, et al. A controlled trial of long-term inhaled hypertonic saline in patients with cystic fibrosis. *N Engl J Med*. 2006;354:229-240.

A7. Aitken ML, Bellon G, De Boeck K, et al. Long-term inhaled dry powder mannitol in cystic fibrosis: an international randomized study. *Am J Respir Crit Care Med*. 2012;185:645-652.

GENERAL REFERENCES

For the General References and other additional features, please visit Expert Consult at https://expertconsult.inkling.com.

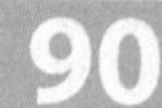

90 BRONCHIECTASIS, ATELECTASIS, CYSTS, AND LOCALIZED LUNG DISORDERS

ANNE E. O'DONNELL

BRONCHIECTASIS

DEFINITION

Bronchiectasis is an abnormal permanent dilation of the bronchi and bronchioles caused by repeated cycles of airway infection and inflammation. The distal airways become thickened; the mucosal surfaces develop edema, inflammation, and suppuration; an ultimately, there is neovascularization of the adjacent bronchial arterioles. Bronchiectasis, which can be focal or diffuse, is triggered by a variety of genetic, anatomic, and systemic processes. Abnormalities of cilia, mucus clearance, mucus rheology, airway drainage, and host defenses can result in bronchiectasis. Regardless of the cause, patients with bronchiectasis develop chronic infections, which may lead to progressive lung destruction.

EPIDEMIOLOGY

Based on insurance claims reviews, an estimated 110,000 or more patients in the United States are receiving treatment for bronchiectasis that is not related to cystic fibrosis (Chapter 89),[1] and these numbers appear to be increasing.[2] The prevalence in the United States has been reported as 4.2 per 100,000 persons age 18 to 34 years and 272 per 100,000 among those older than 75 years. In the older age category, women are disproportionally represented. Other epidemiologic surveys suggest that there is increased risk for the development of bronchiectasis in individuals with reduced access to health care and higher rates of pulmonary infection in childhood.

PATHOBIOLOGY

In up to one third of cases, the cause of bronchiectasis is not identified. Other cases are related to pulmonary infections, genetic causes, anatomic abnormalities, and immune and autoimmune diseases.[3]

Pulmonary Infections

Approximately one third of patients with bronchiectasis have an infectious trigger, usually years before the onset of the disease. Childhood viral infections, such as pertussis (Chapter 313) and bacterial infection, can cause permanent damage to the airways, leading to bronchiectasis years after the initial infection. Mycobacterial tuberculosis with its resultant granulomatous inflammation of the airway, lung parenchyma, and lymph nodes can cause subsequent bronchiectasis (Chapter 324), and nontuberculous mycobacterial infections have been recognized as an increasing cause and complication of bronchiectasis, particularly in white women older than 55 years (Chapter 325). Nontuberculous mycobacterial-related bronchiectasis typically involves the right middle lobe and lingula and can be associated with the "tree-in-bud" pattern of bronchiolar infection as well.

Genetics

Cystic fibrosis (Chapter 89) is characterized by bilateral diffuse bronchiectasis. Although many cystic fibrosis patients are diagnosed in childhood with multisystem disease, older patients may present with only pulmonary or pulmonary and sinus manifestations. Some patients with bronchiectasis may have subtle defects in the cystic fibrosis transmembrane conductance regulator channel without a clear-cut diagnosis of cystic fibrosis.[4]

In primary ciliary dyskinesia, abnormalities in the dynein arms prevent normal ciliary beating. Patients with primary ciliary dyskinesia generally have significant sinopulmonary disease and infertility, and approximately half of these patients have Kartagener syndrome with situs inversus (Chapter 69). Patients with α_1-antitrypsin deficiency also may develop bronchiectasis.

Anatomic Causes

Patients with chronic abnormalities of their swallowing mechanism or with esophageal dysfunction may develop focal or diffuse bronchiectasis with lower lobe predominance (Chapter 138). Direct lung injury caused by acid

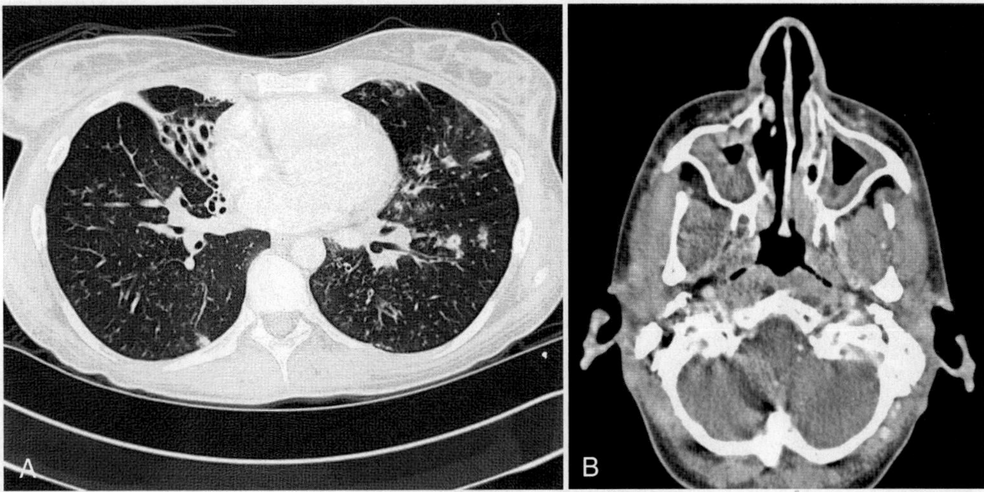

FIGURE 90-1. A and B, High-resolution computed tomographic images of bilateral bronchiectasis in a patient with primary ciliary dyskinesia.

or particulate matter aspiration or recurrent pneumonia may lead to bronchiectasis.

Chronic obstructive pulmonary disease (COPD) is sometimes complicated by bronchiectasis (Chapter 88). Patients with chronic lower airway bacterial colonization and increased airway inflammation may develop areas of bronchiectasis. Rarely, patients with asthma (Chapter 87) have been found to have bronchiectasis. Allergic bronchopulmonary aspergillosis (Chapter 339) can cause a distinct "finger-in-glove" central bronchiectasis owing to chronic inflammation and mucous plugging. Airway abnormalities such as endobronchial tumors (Chapter 191), extrinsic compression by lymph nodes (right middle lobe syndrome), and foreign bodies are also rare causes of focal bronchiectasis. Tracheobronchomegaly (Mounier-Kuhn syndrome) is associated with distal bronchiectasis.

Immune and Autoimmune Diseases

Primary hypogammaglobulinemia (Chapter 250) leads to recurrent pulmonary infections that may result in bronchiectasis. Patients with immunoglobulin G subclass deficiencies may develop bronchiectasis if the deficiency leads to reduction in antibody production. Defects of neutrophil adhesion and chemotaxis (Chapter 169) have been found to cause bronchiectasis. Patients with human immunodeficiency virus infection (Chapter 391) have a higher prevalence of bronchiectasis than individuals with a normally functioning immune system.

Bronchiectasis is an increasingly recognized complication of collagen vascular diseases, particularly rheumatoid arthritis (Chapter 264) and Sjögren syndrome (Chapter 268). The airway injury is likely attributable to chronic inflammation or esophageal dysfunction. Inflammatory bowel disease (Chapter 141) also causes bronchiectasis by undetermined mechanisms.

CLINICAL MANIFESTATIONS

Patients present with chronic cough and usually have mucopurulent or purulent sputum production. Occasionally, a dry nonproductive cough is the primary manifestation. Other symptoms include dyspnea, intermittent hemoptysis, and pleuritic chest pain. Weight loss, malaise, and fatigue sometimes develop. When patients have infectious exacerbations, they may develop fever as well as an increase in their baseline symptoms. Physical findings in patients with bronchiectasis are nonspecific and include an abnormal chest examination with wheezing, crackles, or both. Clubbing of the digits is rare.

The clinical course of patients with bronchiectasis is variable. Some patients have few to no symptoms, others have daily cough with sputum production, and some patients have occasional to frequent exacerbations. A slow decline in pulmonary function is seen with bronchiectasis; the decline is more rapid in patients infected with *Pseudomonas aeruginosa* (Chapter 306) and in patients who have more frequent exacerbations.

DIAGNOSIS

Imaging Studies

Although the diagnosis may be suspected by plain chest radiography, high-resolution computed tomography (HRCT) is the current "gold standard" for confirming bronchiectasis. The characteristic computed tomography (CT) findings are lack of bronchial tapering, bronchi visible in the peripheral 1 cm of the lungs, and an internal bronchial diameter greater than the diameter of the accompanying bronchial artery. Other associated HRCT findings are cysts off the end of a bronchus, tree-in-bud irregular branching lines (E-Fig. 90-E1) indicating mucus impaction (E-Figs. 90-E2 and 90-E3), volume loss (E-Fig. 90-E4), and occasionally associated consolidation (Fig. 90-1). The location of the bronchiectatic airways may suggest the cause: upper lobe predominance is seen in cystic fibrosis and lower lobe predominance in aspiration syndromes (E-Fig. 90-E5). Whereas right middle lobe and lingula involvement suggests the presence of nontuberculous mycobacterial infection (Fig. 90-2 and E-Figs. 90-E6A and 90-E6B), central bronchiectasis is seen with allergic bronchopulmonary aspergillosis (Fig. 90-3).

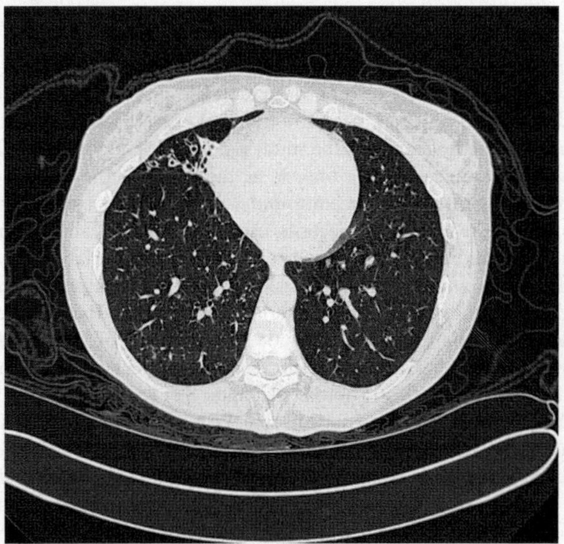

FIGURE 90-2. High-resolution computed tomography image of nodular bronchiectasis caused by a nontuberculous mycobacterium infection.

Pulmonary function testing, which should be performed on all patients with suspected bronchiectasis, usually shows airflow obstruction as measured by the ratio between the forced expiratory volume in 1 second (FEV_1) and forced vital capacity (FVC) (Chapter 85). The severity of the airflow obstruction and the rate of decline correlate with radiographic extent of disease and frequency of exacerbation. Bronchoscopy will detect airway abnormalities, including tumors, structural deformities, and foreign bodies, and hence should be considered in the evaluation of localized bronchiectasis.

Cultures of sputum and of bronchoalveolar lavage when expectorated sputum is not available have an important role in assessing the infectious complications of bronchiectasis. Molecular techniques have recently demonstrated diverse polymicrobial communities in the lungs of patients with bronchiectasis, both when they are clinically stable and also during exacerbations.[5]

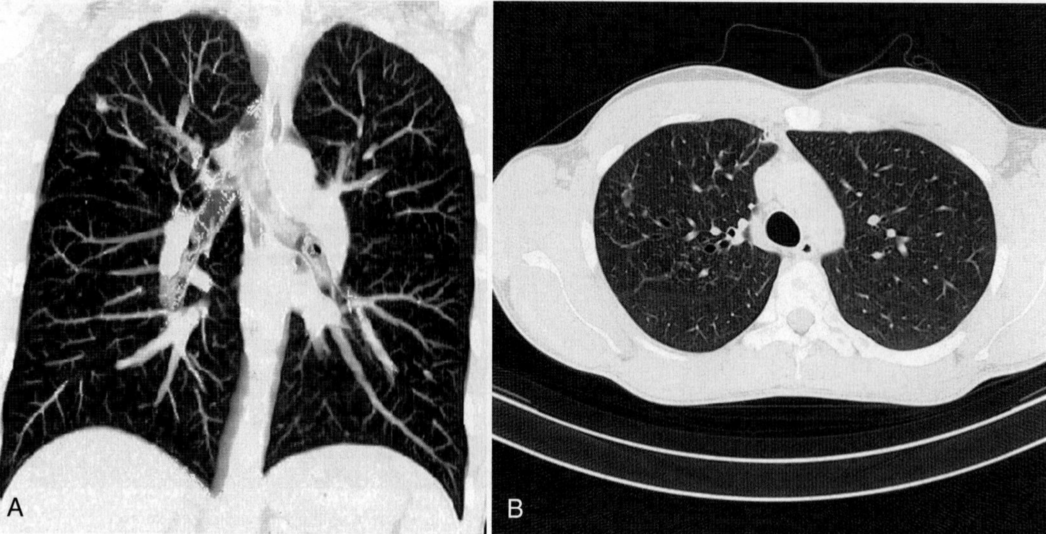

FIGURE 90-3. A and B, High-resolution computed tomography images of finger-in-glove central bronchiectasis caused by allergic bronchopulmonary aspergillosis.

The dominant organisms are *P. aeruginosa* and *Haemophilus influenzae*, but anaerobic organisms may also be detected. The presence of *P. aeruginosa* portends a worse prognosis and more frequent exacerbations. Patients with no identifiable pathogens have the mildest disease. *Staphylococcus aureus* in the airway may suggest cystic fibrosis as the cause of the bronchiectasis. Nontuberculous mycobacteria are found with increasing frequency in the airways of patients with bronchiectasis, usually as a complication of preexisting bronchiectasis but occasionally as its primary cause. The laboratory evaluation of patients with bronchiectasis should be individualized. All patients should have sputum cultures for bacterial and mycobacterial testing. Other tests that should be considered include measurement of serum immunoglobulin levels and screening for genetic diseases, particularly in patients with diffuse bronchiectasis. Cystic fibrosis (Chapter 89) is diagnosed by elevated sweat chloride levels and by genetic testing. Primary ciliary dyskinesia can be evaluated by measurement of nasal nitric oxide levels, ciliary beat frequency and pattern testing, and electron microscopy studies.[6] α_1-Antitrypsin deficiency is diagnosed by measuring levels and performing phenotyping (Chapter 88). Screening for rheumatoid arthritis (Chapter 264) or Sjögren syndrome (Chapter 268) also may be reasonable in patients with diffuse bronchiectasis.

TREATMENT

The goals of treatment are to reduce the frequency of exacerbations and potentially to improve quality of life, reduce symptoms, and alter the natural history of the disease (Table 90-1). Multimodality maintenance treatment[7] for patients with more advanced disease or three or more exacerbations may include airway clearance and anti-inflammatory therapies, as well as short and long-term antibiotic therapy, which reduces markers of airways and systemic inflammation. Exacerbations are treated based on clinical acuity. Because patients are heterogeneous and therapeutic trials are few, therapy is commonly individualized, especially because no therapies are currently approved by the U.S. Food and Drug Administration for non–cystic fibrosis bronchiectasis and because the proven treatments for cystic fibrosis are often not effective.

Preventing Exacerbations

The 23-valent pneumococcal vaccination (Chapter 18) is recommended for patients with bronchiectasis. Routine seasonal influenza vaccination is also standard. At present, no vaccines are available for prevention of the other infectious complications of bronchiectasis.

Treatment of the Underlying Etiology

For treatable conditions, such as immunoglobulin deficiency, replacement therapy (Chapter 250) should be considered even though there are few data on whether that alters the natural history of the lung disease. Patients with allergic bronchopulmonary aspergillosis (Chapter 339) should be treated with steroids to mitigate the inflammatory process that leads to the bronchiectasis.

TABLE 90-1 POTENTIAL THERAPIES FOR BRONCHIECTASIS

Treat underlying condition, if possible
Mobilization of secretions
Pharmacologic
Mechanical
Anti-inflammatory therapy
Inhaled steroids
Macrolides
Antimicrobial therapy
Pathogen specific
Surgery
Localized or refractory disease
Transplantation
End-stage disease

Adapted from O'Donnell A. Bronchiectasis. *Chest.* 2008;134:815-823.

Airway Clearance

Chest physiotherapy and the use of devices to aid mucociliary clearance appear to be beneficial in non–cystic fibrosis bronchiectasis. In a randomized trial, for example, twice-daily use of an oscillatory positive expiratory pressure device (Acapella) improved sputum volume and quality of life end points compared with no routine physiotherapy.[A1] Other techniques that may also have a role for airway clearance include traditional chest physical therapy with postural drainage and the use of chest wall oscillator vests.[8] Formal pulmonary rehabilitation and exercise also likely provide benefit to patients with bronchiectasis.

Inhaled therapy with nebulized hypertonic saline (7%) may enhance airway clearance, decrease exacerbations, and improve lung function as well as quality of life.[A2] Chronic inhalation of dry powder mannitol improves sputum clearance but does not reduce the frequency of exacerbations. Although recombinant human DNase is efficacious in cystic fibrosis bronchiectasis, a large clinical trial showed it had deleterious effects when given a maintenance therapy in patients with non–cystic fibrosis bronchiectasis, so it should not be used. Other mucolytic agents are of unproven benefit.[A3]

No randomized trials support the use of routine short-acting β-agonist or anticholinergic bronchodilators in bronchiectasis. However, a subset of patients with airway reactivity likely benefits from use of these agents (Chapter 87).

Reduction of Airway Inflammation

One clinical trial demonstrated that inhaled medium-dose budesonide, when combined with formoterol, is safe and more effective than high-dose budesonide in treating patients with non–cystic fibrosis bronchiectasis.[A4] Oral steroids, although occasionally used in patients with bronchiectasis, have never been evaluated in a clinical trial.

Antimicrobial Therapy

At present, there is no firm evidence to support the use of routine maintenance antibiotics, although such therapy may be considered in patients with frequent exacerbations and progressive lung destruction. When mycobacterial species are cultured from patients with bronchiectasis, decisions regarding whether to treat and which antimicrobial agents to use are based on published guidelines (Chapters 324 and 325).

Chronic low-dose oral macrolide therapy (e.g., azithromycin 500 mg three times per week or 250 mg/day or erythromycin ethylsuccinate 400 mg twice daily) can reduce exacerbations in patients with non–cystic fibrosis bronchiectasis.A5 A6 Whether patients will develop resistant organisms is of concern, and macrolide therapy alone should not be used in patients co-infected with nontuberculous mycobacteria.

Targeted inhaled antimicrobial therapies are also an option, particularly in patients infected with *Pseudomonas* spp.A7 For example, nebulized gentamicin (80 mg twice daily) for 12 months can provide sustained bacteriologic and clinical benefit. Clinical trials have demonstrated microbiologic benefits with inhaled tobramycin, 300 mg twice per day as a 4-week trial for one cycle and a 2-week-on, 2-week-off trial for three cycles, but clinical benefit was not firmly established, and some patients experienced unacceptable respiratory side effects. Antimicrobial resistance is also a concern. Inhaled colistin, 1 million IU twice daily delivered by nebulizer, also was recently shown to be safe and possibly effective in adherent patients with bronchiectasis and pseudomonas aeruginosa infection.A8 Additional inhaled antibiotics currently being evaluated in clinical trials include dry powder ciprofloxacin, nebulized liposomal ciprofloxacin, and dry powder tobramycin. Other off-label antibiotic strategies include prolonged intravenous antibiotics targeted at the cultured pathogens.

Surgery and Transplantation

Resectional surgery may have a role for patients who have focal disease or for patients who have hemoptysis that cannot be controlled by embolization of the bleeding vessels (Chapter 101). Surgical resection can also benefit some patients who have diffuse bronchiectasis unresponsive to conventional therapy and some patients infected with nontuberculous mycobacteria. Double-lung transplantation (Chapter 101) has been successfully performed in patients with end-stage lung disease caused by non–cystic fibrosis bronchiectasis, and the clinical outcomes parallel those seen with transplantation for other end-stage lung diseases.

Treatment of Acute Exacerbations of Bronchiectasis

When a patient with bronchiectasis experiences an acute exacerbation, antimicrobial treatments should be aimed at the known infecting organisms. Mild to moderate exacerbations can be treated with oral antibiotics, targeted to the results of the sputum culture, for 2 to 3 weeks. More severe exacerbations or exacerbations caused by resistant organisms generally require intravenous antibiotics administered in hospital or at home. No benefit has yet been demonstrated by adding an inhaled antibiotic to systemic therapy for an acute exacerbation. Patients experiencing an acute exacerbation likely benefit from airway clearance modalities and the other nonantibiotic therapies discussed previously.

PROGNOSIS

Non–cystic fibrosis bronchiectasis is a heterogeneous disease with a widely variable prognosis. Patients with more severe obstructive and restrictive findings on pulmonary function tests, poor gas transfer, and chronic pseudomonal infection have the worst prognosis.[9] Independent predictors of future hospitalization include prior hospital admissions, advanced dyspnea, FEV_1 less than 30% predicted, *P. aeruginosa* colonization, colonization with other pathogenic organisms, and three or more lobes involved on HRCT.[10] Bronchiectasis in patients with moderate to severe COPD is an independent risk factor for all-cause mortality. Radiographic extent of disease, hypoxemia, hypercapnia, and evidence of right heart failure are also predictors of outcome. Bronchiectasis patients who are admitted to an intensive care unit for respiratory failure have been reported to have a 60% 4-year survival rate.

ATELECTASIS

DEFINITION

Atelectasis, or collapse, is caused by hypoventilation of lung units. Atelectasis may involve an entire lung or a lobe, segment, or subsegment. Atelectasis can be caused by intrinsic obstruction of an airway or external compression from lymph nodes, parenchymal masses, or other entities. When lung units are atelectatic, ventilation-perfusion mismatch leads to hypoxemia. Infection may result from sustained atelectasis.

EPIDEMIOLOGY AND PATHOBIOLOGY

The lung bases and posterior segments are vulnerable to dependent atelectasis, which is caused by inadequate ventilation, particularly in an immobilized or postoperative patient. Patchy atelectasis is caused by alveolar filling processes, such as hemorrhage and edema (Chapter 91). Passive, relaxation, or compression atelectasis occurs when the lung recoils to a smaller volume because of fluid or air in the adjacent pleural space.

Obstructive or resorptive atelectasis is caused by bronchial block to the entry of air, with resultant retractile consolidation. Intrinsic airway obstruction may be caused by mucous plugs, foreign bodies, or tumors in the airway. Extrinsic airway obstruction results from compression of the airway owing to peribronchial lymph node enlargement or other masses impinging on the airway.

Rounded atelectasis is caused by pleural thickening that invaginates and traps adjacent lung. Any chronic pleural disease can cause rounded atelectasis, particularly asbestos-related pleural disease.

CLINICAL MANIFESTATIONS AND DIAGNOSIS

Atelectasis is typically asymptomatic and diagnosed on chest imaging, but it may cause dyspnea and tachypnea and result in hypoxemia. In postoperative patients, atelectasis may be a cause of low-grade fever. Plain chest radiography shows loss of lung volume and the displacement of the lobar fissure, mediastinum, or diaphragm toward the involved lung unit (Figs. 90-4 and 90-5). Platelike or discoid atelectasis manifests as horizontal or curvilinear lines on plain chest radiography. Rounded atelectasis is an ovoid masslike density abutting the pleura. The type and cause of atelectasis can sometimes be

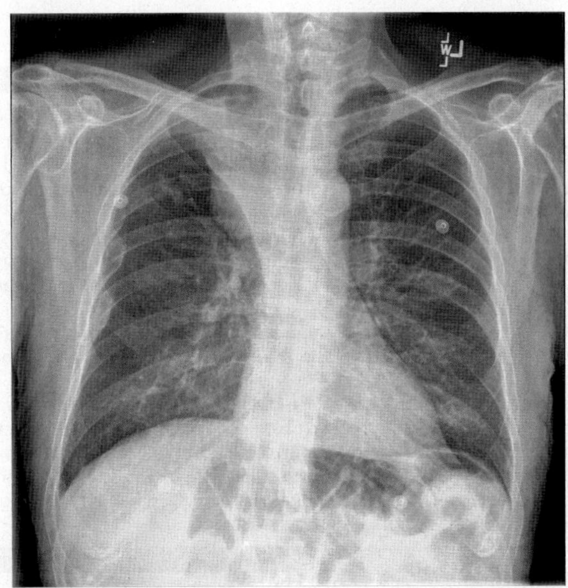

FIGURE 90-4. Plain chest radiograph demonstrating right upper lobe atelectasis (caused by an endobronchial tumor).

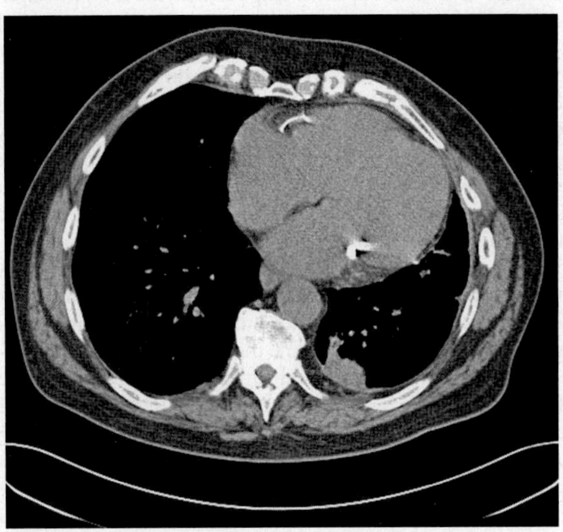

FIGURE 90-5. Computed tomography image of rounded atelectasis.

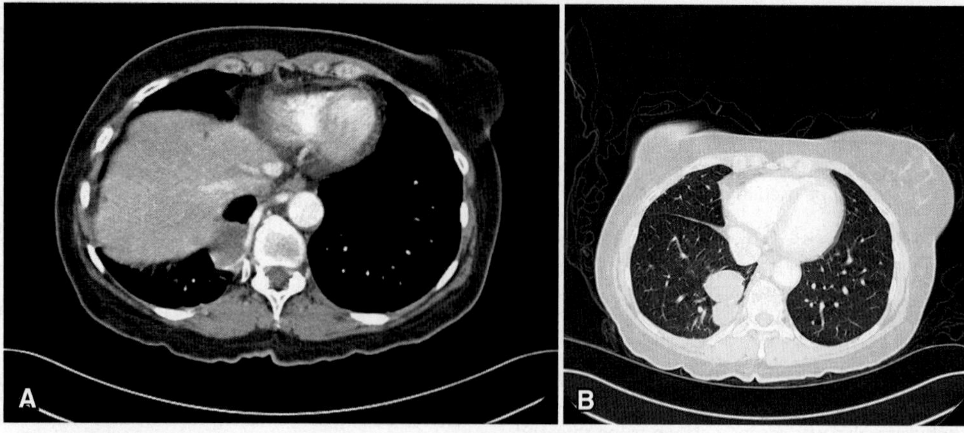

FIGURE 90-6. Pulmonary sequestration. A, Computed tomography image of pulmonary sequestration in right lower lobe. B, Feeding vessel visible arising from the aorta.

elucidated by CT or ultrasonography. Bronchoscopy is required to confirm intrinsic versus extrinsic compression in obstructive-resorptive atelectasis and to determine the exact pathology of the obstruction. An oxygen saturation concentration can help assess the severity of the atelectasis and overall lung dysfunction.

PREVENTION AND TREATMENT

Rx

Incentive spirometry is commonly prescribed to prevent or treat atelectasis in patients with limited mobility because of recent surgery, neuromuscular weakness, or any prolonged immobilization, no randomized controlled trials have proven its effectiveness. Preoperative inspiratory muscle training may reduce atelectasis in patients undergoing upper abdominal surgery,[11] and prophylactic use of noninvasive ventilation may reduce pulmonary dysfunction after lung resection surgery. Other modalities such as positive expiratory pressure devices and high-frequency chest wall oscillation airway clearance are of uncertain benefit.

Patchy atelectasis is treated by addressing the underlying disease process in the lung parenchyma. Compression atelectasis is treated by alleviating the pleural space process.

Obstructive or resorptive atelectasis often requires bronchoscopy for diagnosis and treatment. In patients with obstruction owing to retained secretions, multiple bronchoscopies are sometimes required, but the mucus often rapidly reaccumulates and will resolve only when the patient's overall status improves.

Rounded atelectasis does not require treatment. CT is helpful in distinguishing rounded atelectasis from parenchymal tumor.

CONGENITAL CYSTIC DISEASES OF THE THORAX

Thoracic cysts, which are exceedingly rare, develop because of abnormal development or branching of the foregut. Cysts may develop in the mediastinum at an early stage of gestation or in the lung parenchyma at a later stage. Abnormalities include bronchogenic cysts (mediastinal and parenchymal), congenital pulmonary airway malformation, and pulmonary sequestrations. The cysts are lined with airway and alveolar epithelium but do not communicate in a normal fashion with the airways or lung tissue.

Most patients with thoracic cysts present in childhood, but the cysts can remain asymptomatic and unnoticed until adulthood. In the absence of symptoms, these cystic lesions sometimes present as an incidental finding on chest imaging performed for another indication. Congenital cystic diseases can cause recurrent pneumonia, hemoptysis, or compression of normal structures.

Computed tomography scanning with CT angiography can usually detect congenital cystic lesions of the thorax, but pulmonary or bronchial angiography is sometimes necessary to define the blood flow to the lesion.

Bronchogenic cysts are usually found in the right paratracheal or subcarinal areas of the mediastinum but are occasionally seen in the lung parenchyma.[12] These cysts are often asymptomatic, but they can cause wheezing, dyspnea, and cough when they compress adjacent structures. Secondary infection may develop in the cysts, and there are a few case reports of malignant transformation. Complete surgical resection is generally recommended, but partial excision with de-epithelization of the cysts has also been performed. Observation is also an option when the cysts are asymptomatic.

Congenital pulmonary airway malformation, previously called *congenital cystic adenomatoid malformation of the lung*, is an exceedingly rare abnormality with reported incidence of one in every 25,000 to 35,000 pregnancies. The abnormality is caused by arrested development of the bronchial tree. Most patients are diagnosed prenatally by ultrasonography, but a few adults have first presented with complications, including pneumothorax and air embolism. Treatment is anatomic surgical resection.

Pulmonary sequestrations are areas of nonfunctioning pulmonary parenchyma with no communication to the tracheobronchial tree and abnormal arterial supply and venous drainage (Fig. 90-6). Intralobar sequestration, which accounts for about 75% of cases, does not have visceral pleura and is generally found in a lower lobe, the left more frequently than the right. Extralobar sequestrations have their own visceral pleura, are separate from the normal lobes, and may even be found below the diaphragms. Sequestrations usually have a feeding vessel that arises from the aorta. Patients with sequestrations may be asymptomatic but sometimes develop recurrent infections and or hemoptysis. Surgical excision with special care for the management of the feeding vessel is curative. Embolization of the feeding vessel is sometimes a successful treatment option.

Hyperlucent lungs are diagnosed by a paucity of vascular and interstitial markings noted on chest imaging. Lung parenchymal air collections can be caused by congenital parenchymal cysts, congenital lobar emphysema (almost exclusively diagnosed in infancy), giant bullous emphysema (vanishing lung syndrome), or Swyer-James syndrome. Lung parenchymal cysts may be a bullous alveolar type or may contain bronchial wall elements such as cartilage, smooth muscle, and glands. They may become infected and may rupture to cause pneumothorax. Surgical resection is generally recommended unless the lesions are small. Congenital lobar emphysema, otherwise known as *congenital large hyperlucent lobe*, may cause severe respiratory distress in infants owing to compression of surrounding lung tissue. Giant bullous emphysema is a rare condition that usually affects the upper lobes of young male smokers. Compression of normal lung parenchyma from these overdistended lobes may require surgical resection.

Swyer-James-Macleod syndrome, which is characterized by unilateral lucency of an entire lung, is caused by childhood bronchiolitis obliterans owing to viral or bacterial infection or toxic inhalation. CT shows air trapping and hyperlucency of the affected lung, with a normal contralateral lung. No therapy is required.

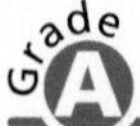

Grade A References

A1. Patterson JE, Hewitt O, Kent L, et al. Acapella versus "usual airway clearance" during acute exacerbation in bronchiectasis: a randomized crossover trial. *Chron Respir Dis.* 2007;4:67-74.

A2. Kellett F, Robert NM. Nebulised 7% hypertonic saline improves lung function and quality of life in bronchiectasis. *Respir Med.* 2011;105:1831-1835.

A3. Wilkinson M, Sugumar K, Milan SJ, et al. Mucolytics for bronchiectasis. *Cochrane Database Syst Rev.* 2014;CD001289.

A4. Martinez-Garcia MA, Soler-Cataluna JJ, Catalan-Serra P, et al. Clinical efficacy and safety of budesonide-formoterol in non-cystic fibrosis bronchiectasis. *Chest.* 2012;141:461-468.

A5. Altenburg J, de Graaff CS, Stienstra Y, et al. Effect of azithromycin maintenance treatment on infectious exacerbations among patients with non-cystic fibrosis bronchiectasis: the BAT randomized controlled trial. *JAMA.* 2013;309:1251-1259.

A6. Serisier DJ, Martin ML, McGuckin MA, et al. Effect of long-term, low-dose erythromycin on pulmonary exacerbations among patients with non-cystic fibrosis bronchiectasis: the BLESS randomized controlled trial. *JAMA*. 2013;309:1260-1267.
A7. Brodt AM, Stovold E, Zhang L. Inhaled antibiotics for stable non-cystic fibrosis bronchiectasis: a systematic review. *Eur Respir J*. 2014;44:382-393.
A8. Haworth CS, Foweraker JE, Wilkinson P, et al. Inhaled colistin in patients with bronchiectasis and chronic Pseudomonas aeruginosa infection. *Am J Respir Crit Care Med*. 2014;189:975-982.

GENERAL REFERENCES

For the General References and other additional features, please visit Expert Consult at https://expertconsult.inkling.com.

91

ALVEOLAR FILLING DISORDERS

STEPHANIE M. LEVINE

DEFINITION

Alveolar filling disorders (Table 91-1) are characterized by chest radiographic findings of alveolar involvement ranging from a ground-glass appearance to consolidation; the pathologic process shows primary involvement of the alveolar air spaces distal to the terminal bronchioles. For example, in pulmonary alveolar proteinosis, the alveoli are filled by proteinaceous fluid. By comparison, the alveolar walls are lined by adenocarcinoma cells in invasive mucinous adenocarcinoma and lepidic predominant nonmucinous adenocarcinoma, formerly called bronchioloalveolar cell cancer. In acute interstitial pneumonia, exudative organizing fibroproliferative infiltrates fill the alveolar space; in the alveolar hemorrhage disorders, blood fills the alveolar space. Alveolar spaces filled with acute inflammatory cells, as in bacterial pneumonia (Chapter 97); water, as in cardiogenic or hydrostatic pulmonary edema (Chapter 58); or high-protein fluid, as in noncardiogenic or increased permeability pulmonary edema (Chapter 104), are also part of the radiographic differential diagnosis of alveolar filling disorders and must be excluded.

A general approach to these suspected alveolar filling diseases (Fig. 91-1) can be stratified by the time elapsed since the onset of symptoms. The typical patient may present with the onset of cough (usually dry) and dyspnea of variable duration, depending on the disease process. Hemoptysis is a frequent presenting symptom in the alveolar hemorrhagic disorders. With the exception of acute interstitial pneumonia, symptoms suggesting an acute infectious process such as fever, leukocytosis, and productive cough are usually absent. If the initial chest radiograph or chest computed tomography (CT) is consistent with a possible alveolar filling process (Chapter 84) and acute pneumonia and pulmonary edema are excluded, bronchoscopy with bronchoalveolar lavage (BAL) (Chapter 85) and transbronchial biopsy should be performed, particularly if pulmonary alveolar proteinosis, invasive mucinous adenocarcinoma, lepidic predominant nonmucinous adenocarcinoma (Chapter 191), or alveolar hemorrhage is suspected. When these tests are nondiagnostic, and in many cases of suspected acute interstitial pneumonia, a surgical lung biopsy obtained by thoracoscopy or an open surgical procedure may be indicated.

PULMONARY ALVEOLAR PROTEINOSIS

EPIDEMIOLOGY

Pulmonary alveolar proteinosis is a rare alveolar filling disease caused by the accumulation of phospholipoproteinaceous surfactant material in the alveoli. The incidence is estimated to be 3.7 cases per million people. Pulmonary

TABLE 91-1 ALVEOLAR FILLING DISORDERS

DISEASES	PATHOPHYSIOLOGY	RADIOGRAPHIC FINDINGS
Pulmonary alveolar proteinosis	Impaired processing of surfactant by alveolar macrophages caused by defects in GM-CSF signaling	Bilateral alveolar opacities with "crazy paving" and diffuse areas of ground-glass attenuation on CT scan
Acute interstitial pneumonia	Diffuse alveolar damage with temporal uniformity	Diffuse alveolar filling process similar to the acute respiratory distress syndrome
Diffuse alveolar hemorrhage	Bleeding from the pulmonary microcirculation, usually from the capillaries	Acute development of bilateral alveolar opacities
Invasive mucinous adenocarcinoma and lepidic predominant nonmucinous adenocarcinoma (formerly called bronchioloalveolar cell carcinoma)	Cancer cells growing along the alveolar septa	Pneumonic opacities, consolidation with air bronchograms, ground-glass opacities (either solitary or multiple)

CT = computed tomography; GM-CSF = granulocyte-macrophage colony-stimulating factor.

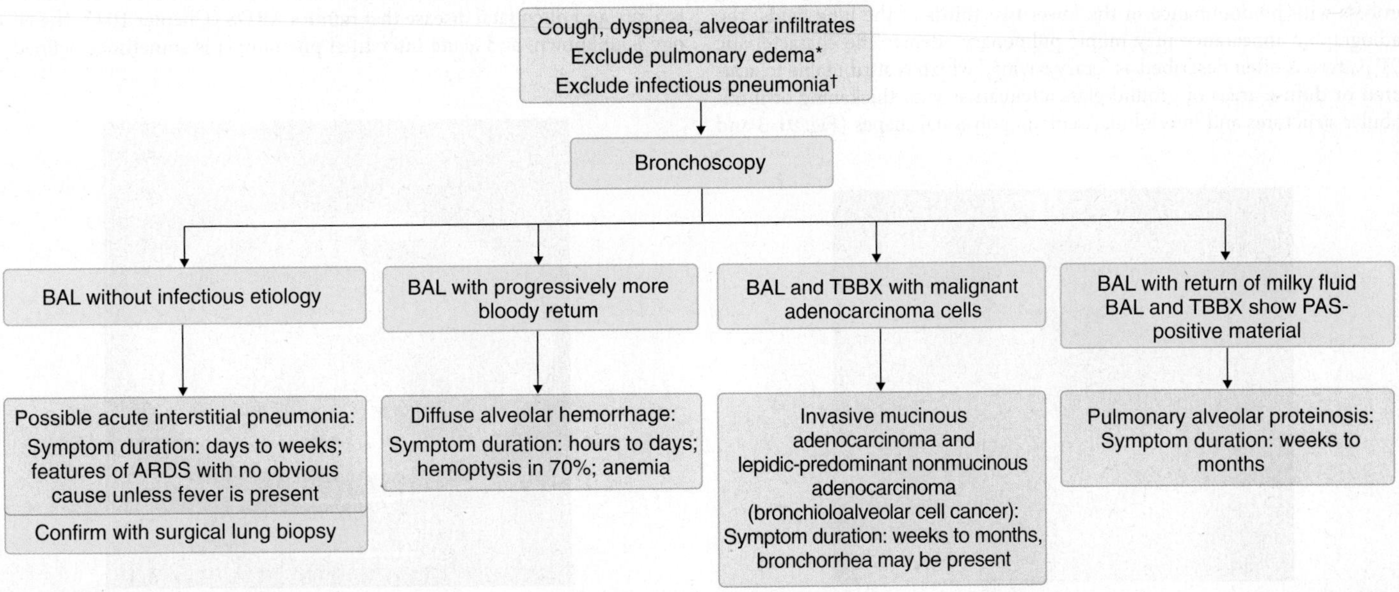

Cough, dyspnea, alveoar infiltrates
Exclude pulmonary edema*
Exclude infectious pneumonia†
↓
Bronchoscopy
↓
- BAL without infectious etiology → Possible acute interstitial pneumonia: Symptom duration: days to weeks; features of ARDS with no obvious cause unless fever is present → Confirm with surgical lung biopsy
- BAL with progressively more bloody return → Diffuse alveolar hemorrhage: Symptom duration: hours to days; hemoptysis in 70%; anemia
- BAL and TBBX with malignant adenocarcinoma cells → Invasive mucinous adenocarcinoma and lepidic-predominant nonmucinous adenocarcinoma (bronchioloalveolar cell cancer): Symptom duration: weeks to months, bronchorrhea may be present
- BAL with return of milky fluid; BAL and TBBX show PAS-positive material → Pulmonary alveolar proteinosis: Symptom duration: weeks to months

FIGURE 91-1. A general approach to the alveolar filling disorders. *See Chapter 58. †See Chapter 97. ARDS = acute respiratory distress syndrome; BAL = bronchoalveolar lavage; PAS = periodic acid–Schiff; TBBX = transbronchial biopsy.

alveolar proteinosis is a primary acquired, autoimmune disorder in more than 90% of cases, but similar histopathologic features may be found with identifiable secondary causes, such as acute silicosis (silicoproteinosis; Chapter 93), aluminum dust exposure (Chapter 93), indium dust exposure, immunodeficiency disorders (e.g., immunoglobulin G monoclonal gammopathy and severe combined immunodeficiency syndrome), hematologic malignant neoplasms (particularly myeloid leukemias; Chapters 183 and 184), and certain infections (e.g., *Pneumocystis jiroveci* pneumonia). Pulmonary alveolar proteinosis has also been described after bone marrow transplantation (Chapter 178). A congenital form also usually presents in infancy.

PATHOBIOLOGY

The pathogenesis of pulmonary alveolar proteinosis is related to impaired processing of surfactant by alveolar macrophages caused by defects in granulocyte-macrophage colony-stimulating factor (GM-CSF) signaling. This impairment may be caused by autoantibodies against GM-CSF or GM-CSF receptor gene mutations, which are found in 90% of cases. The secondary forms are caused by a relative GM-CSF deficiency, leading to macrophage dysfunction and reduced surfactant clearance. The autosomal recessive congenital form of pulmonary alveolar proteinosis, caused by a mutation in the genes encoding surfactant protein B or C, or the GM-CSF receptor results in abnormal surfactant function and severe respiratory distress in homozygous infants. The result of this impairment is accumulation of surfactant-rich material and progressive dysfunction in phagocytosis caused by excessive production or diminished clearance of surfactant by alveolar macrophages.

Histologic examination in pulmonary alveolar proteinosis reveals alveoli filled with lipoproteinaceous material that stains pink (positive reaction) with periodic acid–Schiff stain. Classically, there is no destruction of alveolar architecture. Electron microscopy reveals lamellar (phospholipid-containing) myelin bodies.

CLINICAL MANIFESTATIONS

Pulmonary alveolar proteinosis presents in patients in the third to fourth decade of life with a 2 : 1 male predominance. Most patients (72%) are smokers. Patients present with the insidious onset of dyspnea and cough, which may be dry or occasionally productive of grayish material. The duration of symptoms before diagnosis is typically 6 weeks to 6 to 8 months. Low-grade fevers, malaise, and weight loss may also be present. Hemoptysis is unusual. On physical examination, rales are present in 50% of cases. Clubbing is an unusual finding until later stages of disease.

DIAGNOSIS

Mildly elevated leukocyte counts and mildly to moderately elevated lactate dehydrogenase (LDH) levels may be found in more than 80% of patients; LDH levels may correlate with the severity of disease. Polycythemia and hypergammaglobulinemia may also be present. The chest radiograph (Fig. 91-2) and chest CT scans demonstrate a diffuse symmetrical alveolar filling process with predominance in the lower two thirds of the lung fields; the radiographic appearance may mimic pulmonary edema. The characteristic CT pattern is often described as "crazy paving," which is attributable to scattered or diffuse areas of ground-glass attenuation with thickening of intralobular structures and interlobular septa in polygonal shapes (Fig. 91-3 and E-Fig. 91-E1).[1] This radiographic pattern is not specific for this disorder and can be seen with acute respiratory distress syndrome (ARDS; Chapter 104), *P. jiroveci* pneumonia (Chapter 341), adenocarcinomas formerly described as bronchioloalveolar carcinoma (Chapter 191), lipoid pneumonia (Chapter 94), sarcoidosis (Chapter 95), organizing pneumonia, drug reactions, and pulmonary hemorrhage as well as with cardiogenic pulmonary edema (Chapter 59) and acute interstitial pneumonias. Pulmonary function tests often, but not always, show a restrictive pattern with a reduced diffusing capacity. Arterial blood gas analyses reveal hypoxemia.

Bronchoscopy should be the initial procedure when pulmonary alveolar proteinosis is suspected. The diagnosis of pulmonary alveolar proteinosis can be established in most cases by the recovery of milky white to sandy-colored or light brown fluid on BAL. When it is subjected to cytologic analysis, the BAL fluid has a positive reaction on periodic acid–Schiff staining and reveals alveolar macrophages filled with positive staining material. Transbronchial biopsy or thoracoscopic biopsy can confirm the diagnosis by providing tissue that has similar staining characteristics. Serologic analysis for GM-CSF antibodies is now often performed to support the diagnosis.

TREATMENT Rx

About 8% to 30% of cases of pulmonary alveolar proteinosis resolve spontaneously, and smoking cessation may contribute to spontaneous resolution. A second group of patients will progress to respiratory failure. The remainder will have stable disease. Superinfection with *Nocardia* spp., atypical mycobacteria, fungi, and other opportunistic organisms can occur in more than 15% of patients as a result of macrocyte phagocytic dysfunction.[2]

Therapy depends on the severity of symptoms.[3] Treatment of severely symptomatic patients with dyspnea and hypoxemia begins with multistage or sequential whole-lung lavage performed under general anesthesia with a double-lumen endotracheal tube. The recovered fluid initially has an opaque, sandy-colored appearance (E-Fig. 91-E2). This procedure may have to be repeated at variable intervals. Asymptomatic patients should be observed and followed closely. Mildly symptomatic patients should receive supportive therapy with supplemental oxygen as needed. Subcutaneous or inhaled GM-CSF can improve quality of life, oxygenation, pulmonary function, and exercise capacity in about half of treated patients.[4,5] Treatment with GM-CSF is usually reserved for patients who cannot undergo whole-lung lavage or who have failed standard treatment with whole-lung lavage. Isolated case series have reported variable responses to CD-20 monoclonal antibody, rituximab, or plasmapheresis. Corticosteroids are not routinely used. Lung transplantation can be performed, but recurrent pulmonary alveolar proteinosis has been reported.

Survival rates at 5 years approach 75%.

ACUTE INTERSTITIAL PNEUMONIA

DEFINITION

Acute interstitial pneumonia, also referred to as the *Hamman-Rich syndrome*, is a rare and often fatal disease that mimics ARDS (Chapter 104). The etiology is unknown, and acute interstitial pneumonia is sometimes defined as

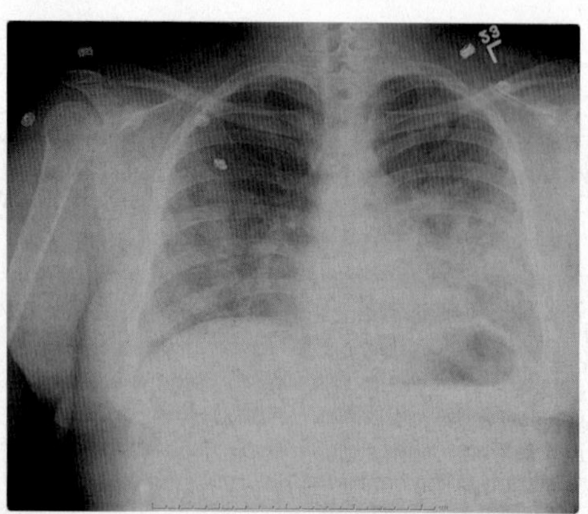

FIGURE 91-2. A chest radiograph showing bilateral alveolar opacities in a patient with pulmonary alveolar proteinosis.

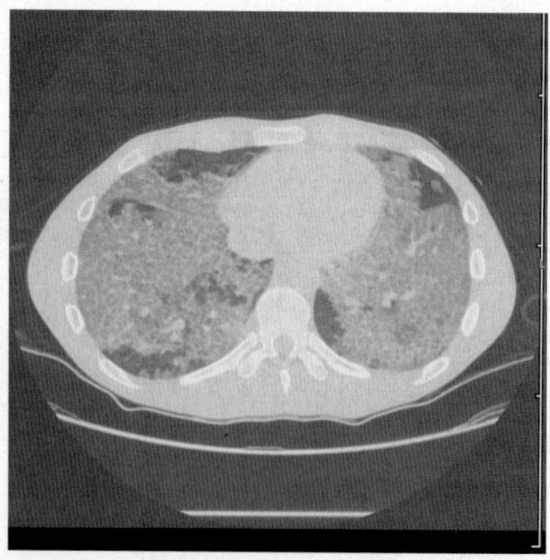

FIGURE 91-3. A chest computed tomography scan showing the "crazy paving" pattern characteristic of pulmonary alveolar proteinosis.

the development of ARDS in the absence of known triggers.[6] A similar acute presentation may be seen in patients with an acute exacerbation of idiopathic pulmonary fibrosis (Chapter 92), but most investigators believe that acute interstitial pneumonia is a separate disease process with no histologic evidence of underlying usual interstitial pneumonia.

PATHOBIOLOGY

The pathogenesis of acute interstitial pneumonia is damage to the epithelium of the alveolar membranes by a neutrophil-mediated mechanism; the result is pouring of exudate into the air space in the initial exudative phase of disease. Histologic examination reveals diffuse alveolar damage with intraalveolar hyaline membrane formation, interstitial and intraalveolar edema, acute inflammation, and epithelial cell necrosis with a nonspecific distribution and temporal uniformity. This process progresses to the organizing phase, characterized by alveolar septal thickening, type II pneumocyte hyperplasia, and fibroblast proliferation along the interstitium and alveolar spaces. In situ thrombi of small pulmonary arteries may be present. Finally, a fibrotic phase occurs with alveolar septal thickening from organizing fibrosis. One of the key pathologic findings in acute interstitial pneumonia is the temporal uniformity of the diffuse alveolar damage and of organizing and proliferating connective tissue. This uniformity supports a single acute injury at a particular point in time. Long-standing fibrosis is not a typical pathologic finding in acute interstitial pneumonia.

CLINICAL MANIFESTATIONS

Acute interstitial pneumonia manifests with equal frequency in men and women, typically in previously healthy individuals in the 50- to 55-year age range. It develops acutely to subacutely during a few days to a few weeks. The mean duration of symptoms is 15 days. Dry cough, shortness of breath, malaise, and fever (in 50% of patients) are typical clinical findings. A virus-like prodrome period has been described. Pulmonary rales are heard on physical examination, and hypoxemia is characteristic. Clubbing is rare. Acute interstitial pneumonia often progresses to hypoxemic ventilatory failure, and intensive care unit admission with mechanical ventilation is usually required. Early mortality rates are high. Radiographic features of acute interstitial pneumonia are diffuse alveolar opacities and air space consolidation similar to the appearance of ARDS (Fig. 91-4); CT scans reveal bilateral air space consolidation with areas of ground-glass opacities with little honeycombing. Septal thickening and a subpleural distribution of the opacities may also be present.

DIAGNOSIS

The diagnosis of acute interstitial pneumonia is made in the appropriate clinical setting in a patient who has a clinical presentation compatible with ARDS but without a clear etiology. The differential diagnosis histologically and clinically includes other causes of ARDS (Chapter 104), such as severe infection, trauma, and sepsis, as well as other causes of acute lung injury (Chapter 94), such as drug toxicity, inhalation injury, and collagen vascular diseases. The presentation is clinically and radiographically similar to that of diffuse alveolar hemorrhage, acute hypersensitivity pneumonitis, acute exacerbation of pulmonary fibrosis, acute eosinophilic pneumonia, and cryptogenic organizing pneumonia. Bronchoscopy with BAL is often performed to exclude alveolar hemorrhage, eosinophilic pneumonias, and infectious causes of lung injury. In a small number of cases, transbronchial biopsy may yield the diagnosis, but definitive diagnosis in most cases of acute interstitial pneumonia requires a surgical lung biopsy revealing diffuse alveolar damage.

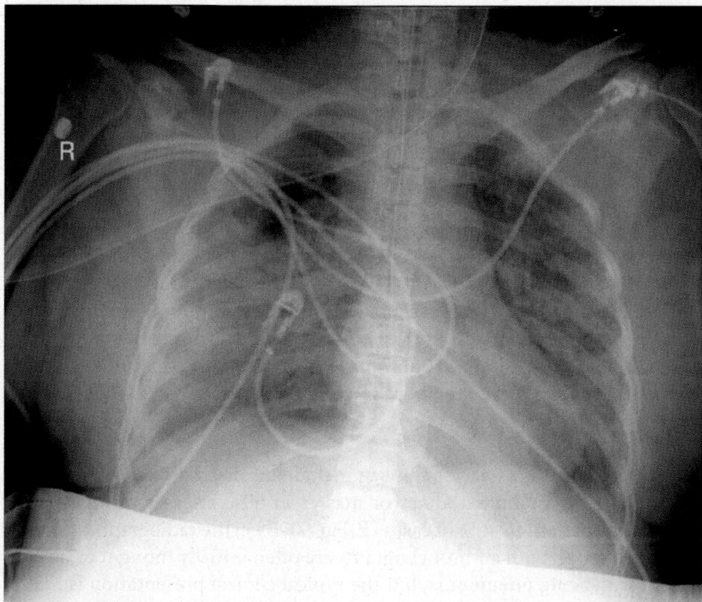

FIGURE 91-4. A chest radiograph showing bilateral alveolar opacities in a patient with acute interstitial pneumonia.

TREATMENT Rx

Treatment includes supportive intensive care unit management. In small case series, corticosteroids at doses of 1 to 2 g of methylprednisolone in divided doses intravenously per day for 3 consecutive days followed by prednisone or equivalent at 1 mg/kg/day with a taper during several weeks to months, with or without cyclophosphamide, may be of benefit, but the mortality rate remains higher than 70%. Patients also can have recurrences in months to years. Some cases of acute interstitial pneumonia may resolve without sequelae, but in some series, more than 50% of survivors may be left with residual fibrosis.

DIFFUSE ALVEOLAR HEMORRHAGE

DEFINITION

The alveolar hemorrhage syndromes cause alveolar filling disease, usually with an acute onset and often with life-threatening severity. They can be associated with ANCA- (antineutrophil cytoplasmic antibody–) associated vasculitides,[7] such as microscopic polyangiitis (Chapter 270) and granulomatosis with polyangiitis (Chapter 270); immunologic diseases, such as Goodpasture syndrome (anti–glomerular basement membrane antibody disease; Chapter 121); collagen vascular diseases, such as systemic lupus erythematosus (Chapter 266); cocaine inhalation (Chapter 34); drugs (including penicillamine, mitomycin C, trimellitic anhydride, all-*trans* retinoic acid, propylthiouracil, and isocyanates); bone marrow transplantation (Chapter 178); coagulopathy (Chapter 174); and mitral stenosis (Chapter 75). A small percentage of idiopathic and recurrent cases are termed *idiopathic pulmonary hemosiderosis.* In Goodpasture syndrome, there is a strong association with tobacco use and a male predominance, with young men most frequently affected. A viral syndrome and exposure to hydrocarbons may simulate Goodpasture disease. Idiopathic pulmonary hemosiderosis most often occurs in children and young adults.

PATHOBIOLOGY

Alveolar hemorrhage is caused by bleeding from the pulmonary microcirculation, including the capillaries, arterioles, and venules. It may be associated with injury or neutrophilic inflammation of the alveolar walls and adjacent interstitial capillaries or with a capillaritis, usually when it is associated with collagen vascular or vasculitic processes. In Goodpasture syndrome, for example, the circulating anti–glomerular basement membrane antibodies are directed against the α_3 chain of type IV collagen in the glomerular basement membrane, where they cause glomerulonephritis; these core antibodies can cross-react with the alveolar capillary basement membranes, resulting in alveolar hemorrhage. Alternatively, alveolar hemorrhage may be associated with relatively bland pathologic changes with red blood cells in the alveolar spaces. Idiopathic pulmonary hemosiderosis is an example of bland hemorrhage.

CLINICAL MANIFESTATIONS

Patients present acutely (usually in hours to a week) with dyspnea, shortness of breath, hemoptysis (which may not be present in all patients), and cough. Some patients also have low-grade fever. Lung examination reveals rales.

Laboratory examination may reveal anemia, and arterial blood gases reveal hypoxemia. In Goodpasture syndrome and the ANCA-associated vasculitides, hematuria and renal insufficiency caused by glomerulonephritis are typically present.

Radiographic features include the acute development of bilateral alveolar filling disease similar to pulmonary edema but without cardiomegaly or

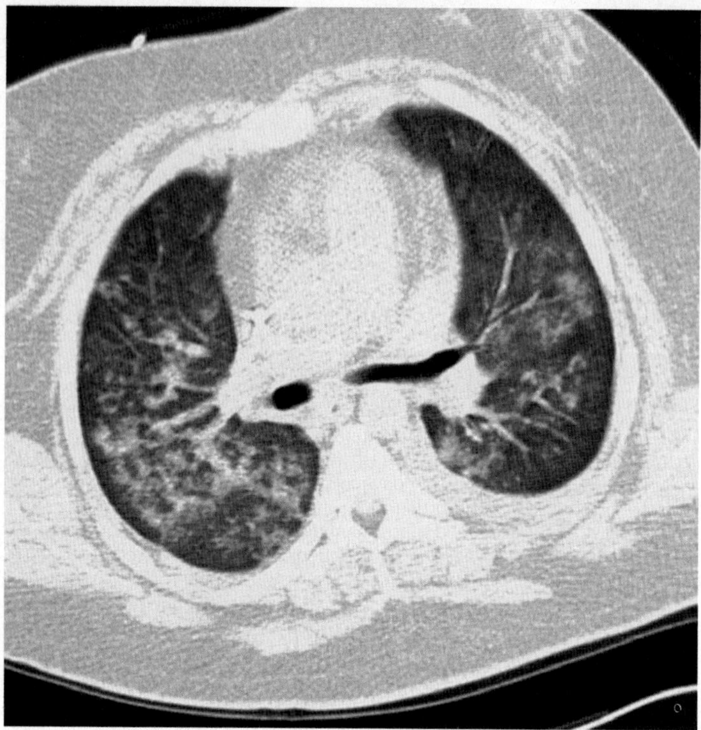

FIGURE 91-5. A chest computed tomography scan showing alveolar opacities in a patient with diffuse alveolar hemorrhage.

pleural effusions (E-Fig. 91-E3). Rapid remission and recurrences are seen with repeated episodes of bleeding, which also may result in chronic interstitial changes on the chest radiograph. Pulmonary function testing may reveal an increase in the diffusion capacity for carbon monoxide because of the presence of hemoglobin in the alveolar spaces.

DIAGNOSIS

The diagnosis of alveolar hemorrhage is usually made in the appropriate clinical setting by the triad of diffuse alveolar opacities (Fig. 91-5),[8] hemoptysis (in two thirds of patients), and anemia. BAL typically demonstrates the return of progressively more bloody aliquots of fluid (E-Fig. 91-E4), and cytologic analysis reveals that more than 20% of the macrophages are hemosiderin laden. Goodpasture syndrome is diagnosed by circulating anti–glomerular basement membrane antibodies, which are present in more than 90% of patients, or by the demonstration of linear deposition of immunoglobulin G antibodies along the alveolar or renal capillary basement membrane tissue when it is viewed by direct immunofluorescence. c-ANCA-(cytoplasmic antineutrophil cytoplasmic antibody–) associated vasculitis causes a focal, segmental, necrotizing glomerulonephritis and is associated with the presence of proteinase 3 antineutrophilic cytoplasmic antibodies in 90% of active cases of granulomatosis with polyangiitis (Chapter 270). Necrotizing granulomatous inflammation is often found in the upper airway in addition to the lungs and kidneys. A perinuclear myeloperoxidase antineutrophilic antibody is often present in association with microscopic polyarteritis (Chapter 270). Patients with systemic lupus erythematosus usually have antinuclear antibodies (Chapter 266). Patients using illicit drugs such as cocaine may have a positive drug screen. Idiopathic pulmonary hemosiderosis is a diagnosis of exclusion after other causes of diffuse alveolar hemorrhage have been eliminated.

TREATMENT Rx

Treatment of alveolar hemorrhage varies according to its underlying cause. Massive hemoptysis (Chapter 83) from any cause of alveolar hemorrhage should be managed as needed. In the case of anticoagulation-, drug-, or toxin-related alveolar hemorrhage, the offending agent should be withdrawn, and supportive care is indicated. In Goodpasture syndrome, the ANCA-associated vasculitides, and other vasculitides (Chapter 270), treatment typically includes immunosuppressant agents such as corticosteroids (methylprednisolone, 500-2000 mg/day in divided doses for 3-5 days followed by a prednisone taper beginning at 1 mg/kg/day during the next 6 to 9 months) and cyclophosphamide (2 mg/kg/day orally or 0.5 g/m^2-0.75 g/m^2 intravenously for one dose) and then if needed, every 2 weeks or change to oral therapy. Plasmapheresis (3-14 exchanges) to remove the offending circulating antibody is a mainstay therapy for Goodpasture syndrome and may also be used in some cases of alveolar hemorrhage from ANCA-associated vasculitis and systemic lupus erythematosus. In patients with ANCA-associated vasculitis, rituximab (375 mg/m^2 once a week for 4 weeks) is at least as good as cyclophosphamide followed by azathioprine for 12 to 15 months for inducing and maintaining remission (≈50% at 12 months and about 40% at 18 months),[A1] and rituximab (at 500 mg on days 0 and 14 and at 6, 12, and 18 months) is better than azathioprine for maintaining remission at 28 months.[A2]

PROGNOSIS

Alveolar hemorrhage can result in acute respiratory failure and death. Recurrent alveolar hemorrhage from any cause, such as idiopathic pulmonary hemosiderosis, can be associated with the development of pulmonary fibrosis. Alveolar hemorrhage related to collagen vascular disease, vasculitides, and idiopathic pulmonary hemosiderosis can have mortality rates ranging from 25% to 50%. With Goodpasture syndrome, renal failure is common, and the degree of renal impairment may correlate with outcome.

INVASIVE MUCINOUS ADENOCARCINOMA AND LEPIDIC PREDOMINANT NONMUCINOUS ADENOCARCINOMA (FORMERLY CALLED BRONCHIOLOALVEOLAR CELL CARCINOMA)

DEFINITION

In 2011, a multidisciplinary committee eliminated the term *bronchioloalveolar cell carcinoma* and divided pulmonary adenocarcinomas into five types: adenocarcinoma in situ, minimally invasive adenocarcinoma, lepidic predominant nonmucinous adenocarcinoma, invasive mucinous adenocarcinoma, and invasive adenocarcinoma and its subtypes.[9] The types that would most likely be correlated with an alveolar filling appearance pathologically and on chest imaging are invasive mucinous adenocarcinoma, in which consolidation and air-bronchograms may be present, and lepidic-predominant nonmucinous adenocarcinoma, in which a ground-glass appearance is characteristic. Both of these types of adenocarcinoma are among those formally characterized as bronchioloalveolar cell carcinoma. In general, these tumors are characterized by malignant cells lining the alveolar cell wall (Chapter 191). Among bronchogenic carcinomas, these subtypes are the least associated with tobacco use, and patients with these cancers are more likely to be nonsmokers. Unlike other non–small cell lung cancers, the sex ratio approaches 1 : 1 or may be slightly female predominant, and younger patients may be affected.

PATHOBIOLOGY

These types of adenocarcinoma usually arise in the periphery of the lung and may be characterized by lepidic growth, which means contiguous growth along the intact alveolar septa, with varying degrees of stromal, pleural, vascular, or lymphatic invasion and without a known primary adenocarcinoma elsewhere. The mucinous type is thought to derive from respiratory goblet cells and columnar cells, and the nonmucinous type from type II pneumocytes or Clara cells.

CLINICAL MANIFESTATIONS

Patients present with a gradual onset of shortness of breath and cough. The duration of symptoms is usually several months. Constitutional symptoms such as malaise and weight loss may be present. Hemoptysis may occur. An unusual but unique clinical finding is bronchorrhea, with patients reporting the production of copious amounts of clear sputum daily. This finding is more common in the invasive mucinous form of the disease.

DIAGNOSIS

Radiographic patterns vary[10] and can include localized disease with peripheral solitary or multiple nodules or masses in 60% of cases or a persistent pneumonic pattern in 40% of cases (E-Fig. 91-E5). The radiographic findings of consolidation with air bronchograms are often initially thought to be consistent with acute pneumonia, but the typical clinical presentation is that of a nonresolving peripheral density on chest radiograph.[11] In addition, CT may show areas of ground-glass attenuation. Positron emission tomography may be normal because of the low glucose uptake of these tumors. The diagnosis of invasive mucinous adenocarcinoma and lepidic predominant nonmucinous adenocarcinoma is most often made by bronchoscopy with transbronchial biopsy.

TREATMENT 

For staging and treatment, these types of adenocarcinoma are approached like other types of non–small cell lung cancers (Chapter 191). Testing for epidermal growth factor receptor (EGFR) mutations should be performed, and chemotherapy planned accordingly. In general, the invasive mucinous adenocarcinomas are KRAS positive, and EGFR negative. The lepidic predominant nonmucinous type tends to be EGFR positive. Bilateral lung transplantation has been performed, but recurrence in the transplanted lungs has been reported.

PROGNOSIS

Prognosis correlates with disease stage and with the histologic and radiographic patterns. Patients who undergo surgical resection for adenocarcinoma in situ or minimally invasive adenocarcinoma with a single focus of disease have a better prognosis than patients with other adenocarcinomas of like stage, with the 5-year survival rate approaching 100%. More advanced forms likely have a prognosis similar to that of other adenocarcinomas.

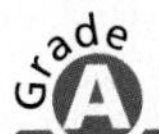

Grade A References

A1. Specks U, Merkel PA, Seo P, et al. Efficacy of remission-induction regimens for ANCA-associated vasculitis. *N Engl J Med*. 2013;369:417-427.

A2. Guillevin L, Pagnoux C, Karras A, et al. Rituximab versus azathioprine for maintenance in ANCA-associated vasculitis. *N Engl J Med*. 2014;371:1771-1780.

GENERAL REFERENCES

For the General References and other additional features, please visit Expert Consult at https://expertconsult.inkling.com.

92 INTERSTITIAL LUNG DISEASE

GANESH RAGHU

DEFINITION

In an apparently immunocompetent host, *interstitial lung disease* (ILD) is a clinical term for a heterogenous group of acute and chronic lower respiratory tract disorders with many potential causes. However, clinical and physiological features common to all ILDs include exertional dyspnea, a restrictive pattern on pulmonary function testing (Chapter 85), coexistent airflow obstruction, decreased diffusing capacity (DLCO), increased alveolar-arterial oxygen difference (PAO_2-PaO_2) (Chapter 103) at rest or during exertion, and absence of pulmonary infection or neoplasm. ILDs comprise several acute and chronic lung disorders with variable degrees of pulmonary fibrosis (Table 92-1). The term *interstitial* is a misnomer because the pathologic processes are not restricted to the interstitium, which is the microscopic space bounded by the basement membranes of epithelial and endothelial cells. Rather, all of the several cellular and soluble constituents that make up the gas exchange units (alveolar wall, capillaries, alveolar space, and acini) and the bronchiolar lumen, terminal bronchioles, and pulmonary parenchyma beyond the gas exchange units (as well as the pleura and lymphatics and sometimes the lymph nodes) are involved in the pathogenesis and manifestations of ILD.

EPIDEMIOLOGY

Among persons 18 years or older, the prevalence of all ILDs in the United States is about 81 per 100,000 men and 67 per 100,000 women. The overall incidence is also higher in men (31.5 per 100,000 per year) than in women (26.1 per 100,000 per year). Moreover, the prevalence of undiagnosed or early ILD is estimated to be 10 times that of clinically recognized disease; as

TABLE 92-1 CLINICAL CLASSIFICATION OF INTERSTITIAL LUNG DISEASE

IDIOPATHIC INTERSTITIAL PNEUMONIAS
Chronic Fibrosing Interstitial Pneumonias
Idiopathic pulmonary fibrosis
Nonspecific interstitial pneumonia
Smoking-Related Interstitial Pneumonias
Respiratory bronchiolitis–interstitial lung disease
Desquamative interstitial pneumonia
Acute or Subacute Idiopathic Interstitial Pneumonias
Cryptogenic organizing pneumonia
Acute interstitial pneumonia
Lymphoid and lymphocytic interstitial pneumonia
Rare interstitial Pneumonias
Histologic pattern of acute fibrinous and organizing pneumonia
Histological pattern of interstitial pneumonias with a bronchiolocentric distribution
Pleuroparenchymal fibroelastosis
INTERSTITIAL LUNG DISEASE ASSOCIATED WITH CONNECTIVE TISSUE DISEASE
Progressive systemic sclerosis
Rheumatoid arthritis
Systemic lupus erythematosus
Dermatomyositis and polymyositis
Sjögren syndrome
Mixed connective tissue disease
Ankylosing spondylitis
HYPERSENSITIVITY PNEUMONITIS
Occupational and environmental factors (e.g., farmer's lung; bird fancier's lung)
Iatrogenic
DRUG-INDUCED AND IATROGENIC INTERSTITIAL LUNG DISEASE
See Table 92-2
ALVEOLAR FILLING DISORDERS (Chapter 91)
Goodpasture syndrome
Pulmonary alveolar proteinosis
Pulmonary hemosiderosis
Alveolar hemorrhage syndromes
Chronic eosinophilic pneumonia
INTERSTITIAL LUNG DISEASE ASSOCIATED WITH PULMONARY VASCULITIS
Pulmonary capillaritis
Granulomatosis with polyangiitis (formerly known as Wegener granulomatosis)
Churg-Strauss syndrome
OTHER SPECIFIC FORMS OF INTERSTITIAL LUNG DISEASE
Sarcoidosis
Langerhans cell histiocytosis (histiocytosis X)
Lymphangioleiomyomatosis
INHERITED FORMS OF INTERSTITIAL LUNG DISEASE
Familial idiopathic pulmonary fibrosis
Familial pulmonary fibrosis or interstitial pneumonia
Tuberous sclerosis
Neurofibromatosis
Gaucher disease
Niemann-Pick disease
Hermansky-Pudlak syndrome

physicians' awareness of these entities increases, it is expected that the frequency of the diagnosis of ILD will rise. Among the ILDs, the most common is idiopathic pulmonary fibrosis, which represents at least 30% of incident cases. In the United States, the annual incidence of idiopathic pulmonary fibrosis is 94 per 100,000 in the Medicare population, with a mean age of onset of 79 years.[1] Recent data suggest that more than 5000 new cases are diagnosed each year in the United Kingdom.

PATHOBIOLOGY

Interstitial lung diseases are thought to result from an unknown tissue injury and attempted repair in the lung of a genetically predisposed person. Genetic variants within the *hTERT* or *hTR* components of the telomerase gene and surfactant protein gene have been associated in a subset of familial pulmonary fibrosis and in some sporadic cases.[2] An *MUC5B* promotor polymorphism is associated with familial interstitial pneumonia and idiopathic pulmonary fibrosis.[3]

In *idiopathic pulmonary fibrosis,* varying degrees of acute, subacute, and chronic fibroproliferation are present in the lungs at the time of diagnosis. Ultimately, progressive fibrosis results in honeycombing, an end-stage finding that is often associated with increased pulmonary vascular resistance and secondary pulmonary hypertension. As a reflection of these dynamic processes, histopathologic examination of lung tissue often reveals highly heterogeneous findings; for example, a single biopsy specimen may show normal alveoli adjacent to abnormal areas of inflammation and fibrosis, with or without granulomas, vasculitis, or secondary vascular changes within the pulmonary parenchyma.

CLINICAL MANIFESTATIONS

Interstitial lung diseases are typically characterized by progressive dyspnea. Nonproductive cough and fatigue are also common complaints. Pleuritic chest pain may occur with certain connective tissue or drug-induced ILDs, and acute pleuritic chest pain with dyspnea may represent a spontaneous pneumothorax (Chapter 99) in association with lymphangioleiomyomatosis, tuberous sclerosis (Chapter 417), neurofibromatosis, or Langerhans cell histiocytosis. Hemoptysis suggests a diffuse alveolar hemorrhagic syndrome, systemic lupus erythematosus (SLE) (Chapter 266), lymphangioleiomyomatosis, granulomatosis with polyangiitis (Chapter 270), or Goodpasture syndrome (Chapter 121); it is rare in other ILDs. In patients with existing ILD, new hemoptysis should prompt consideration of a superimposed malignancy, pulmonary embolus, or infection such as aspergillosis.

In some patients, the first and the only clue to the presence of an ILD may be the finding of coarse rales (crackles) on auscultation of the lungs. These coarse crackles must be distinguished from the finer rales typical of heart failure (Chapter 58) or noncardiogenic pulmonary edema (Chapter 104). Unlike patients with obstructive lung disease, wheezes are not common. A history of wheezing suggests the coexistence of occult hyperactive airways and airflow obstruction and raises the possibility of allergic bronchopulmonary aspergillosis (Chapter 339), Churg-Strauss syndrome (Chapter 270), chronic eosinophilic pneumonia (see later), or parasitic infection (Chapter 344). In some patients, the initial presentation may be with peripheral cyanosis, clubbing, or the signs and symptoms of an underlying systemic disease (see later).

DIAGNOSIS

The first key in patients with an ILD is to establish the syndromic diagnosis and then pursue the differential diagnosis of its specific cause (Fig. 92-1). However, a conclusive cause often may not be identified despite an exhaustive medical history and invasive diagnostic interventions, including bronchoalveolar lavage (BAL)[4] and sufficiently large and multiple lung biopsy specimens. Thus, the cause of several of the ILDs, even when diagnosed as specific entities, remains unknown.

History

The patient's age, sex, and cigarette smoking history may provide useful clues to the diagnosis. Idiopathic pulmonary fibrosis is an adult disorder that usually occurs in patients older than 50 years. Pulmonary sarcoidosis (Chapter 95), in contrast, is more common in young adults and middle-aged persons. Whereas pulmonary Langerhans cell histiocytosis (previously known as pulmonary histiocytosis X or eosinophilic granuloma) characteristically occurs in young cigarette-smoking men, lymphangioleiomyomatosis occurs exclusively in women of childbearing age. Respiratory bronchiolitis–associated ILD is seen almost exclusively in cigarette smokers but occurs in both men and women of all ages.

The medical history also should focus on environmental factors, especially changes in environmental exposures (including domestic, recreational, hot tub, whirlpool baths, indoor swimming pool, ventilation system at home, automobiles, and workplaces), occupational exposure, medications, and drug use (Chapters 93 and 94). A family medical history should address possible familial ILD. Environmental risk factors that may suggest the diagnosis of hypersensitivity pneumonitis include farming or exposure to overt or occult avian antigens at or in the close vicinity of home, bird droppings, feather duvets ("bird fancier's lung" or "pigeon breeder's lung"), visible molds, unkempt dusty homes, unchanged filters in furnaces, unkempt ventilatory systems, water leaks, or humidifiers in the domestic environment (hypersensitivity to thermophilic actinomycetes, *Aureobasidium pullulans*). At-risk occupations include mining (pneumoconioses), machine tool

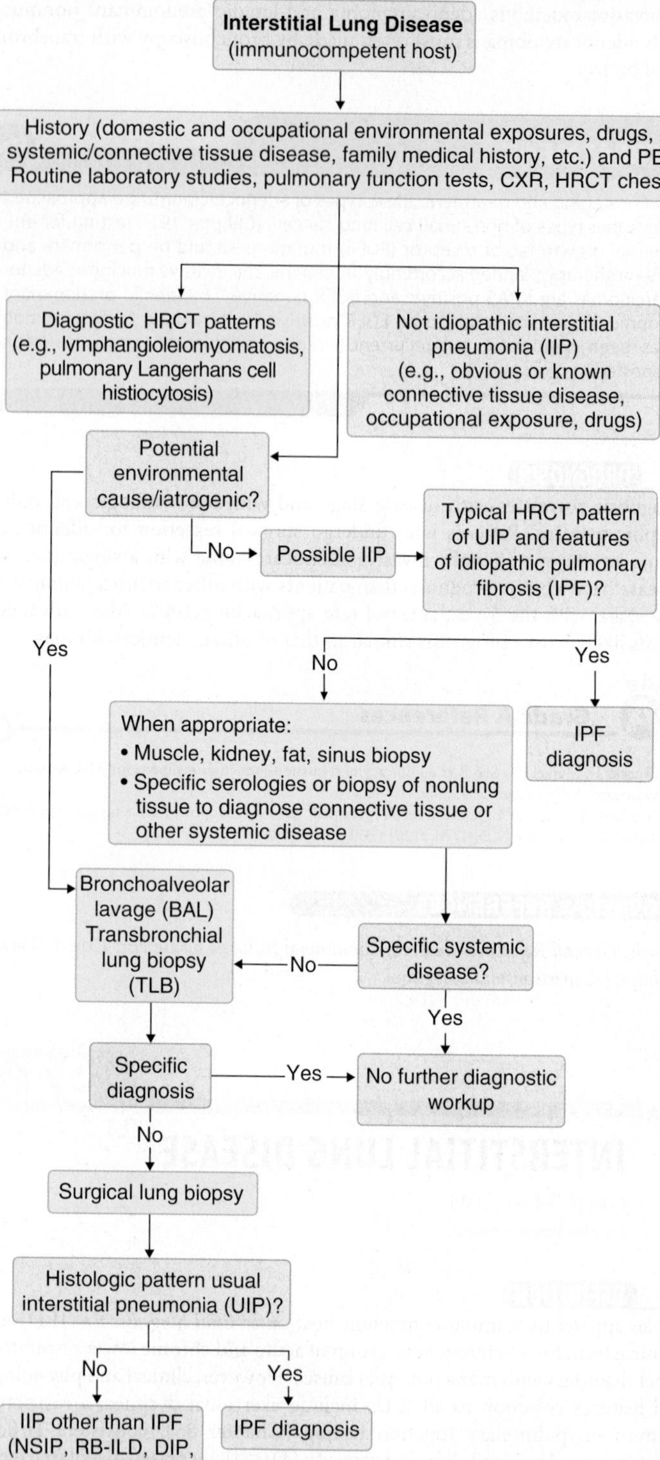

FIGURE 92-1. An approach to interstitial lung disease. DAD = diffuse alveolar damage; DIP = desquamative interstitial pneumonia; HRCT = high-resolution computed tomography; IIP = idiopathic interstitial pneumonia; IPF = idiopathic pulmonary fibrosis; LIP = lymphoid interstitial pneumonia; NSIP = nonspecific interstitial pneumonia; OP = organizing pneumonia; PE = physical examination; PFT = pulmonary function test; RB-ILD = respiratory bronchiolitis–associated interstitial lung disease; TLB = transbronchial lung biopsy; UIP = usual interstitial pneumonia. (Adapted from American Thoracic Society/European Respiratory Society: International multidisciplinary consensus classification of idiopathic interstitial pneumonias. *Am J Respir Crit Care Med.* 2002;165:277-304 and Raghu G, Collard HR, Egan JJ, et al. An official ATS/ERS/JRS/ALAT statement: idiopathic pulmonary fibrosis: evidence-based guidelines for diagnosis and management. *Am J Respir Crit Care Med.* 2011;183:788-824.)

grinding, sandblasting and working with granite (silicosis), welding and working in a shipyard (asbestosis), and working in the aerospace or electronic industries (berylliosis) (Chapters 93 and 94). Because of the long interval between the exposure and the onset of symptoms in many occupations associated with ILD, it is important to take a lifelong occupational history

TABLE 92-2 DRUG-INDUCED AND IATROGENIC INTERSTITIAL LUNG DISEASE*

ANTIMICROBIAL AGENTS
Cephalosporins
Isoniazid
Nitrofurantoin
Penicillins
Sulfonamides
ANTI-INFLAMMATORY AGENTS
Aspirin
Gold
Methotrexate
Nonsteroidal anti-inflammatory agents
Penicillamine
Phenylbutazone
Zafirlukast
CARDIOVASCULAR DRUGS
Amiodarone
Angiotensin-converting enzyme inhibitors
β-Blockers
Hydralazine
Hydrochlorothiazide
Procainamide
Protamine sulfate
Tocainide
ANTINEOPLASTIC AND CHEMOTHERAPEUTIC AGENTS
Bleomycin
Busulfan
Chlorambucil
Cyclophosphamide
Erlotinib
Gefitinib
Gemcitabine
Imatinib
Melphalan
Mercaptopurine
Methotrexate
Mitomycin
Nitrosoureas
Procarbazine
CENTRAL NERVOUS SYSTEM DRUGS
Carbamazepine
Chlorpromazine
Imipramine
Phenytoin
ORAL HYPOGLYCEMIC AGENTS
Chlorpropamide
Tolazamide
Tolbutamide
ILLICIT DRUGS
Cocaine
Heroin
Methadone
Propoxyphene
OTHER AGENTS
Antithymocyte globulin
All-*trans*-retinoic acid
Colony-stimulating factors
Interferon-α and -β
Irradiation
Mycophenolate mofetil
Tumor necrosis factor-α modulating agents
High fraction of inspired oxygen (FIO_2) with mechanical ventilation

*This list contains examples only and is not meant to be exhaustive.

(Chapter 19) as well as to establish the interval between exposure and the onset of symptoms. Because the list of medications known to cause ILD is long and continues to grow (Table 92-2), a careful history regarding recent use of prescription and over-the-counter products is essential. Risk factors for immunosuppression, including infection with human immunodeficiency virus, raise the possibility of opportunistic lung infections (Chapter 391), neoplasm (Chapter 191), and transplant-related pulmonary complications.

Particular attention should be paid to the onset and duration of symptoms; the rate of disease progression; and association with hemoptysis, fever, or extrathoracic symptoms. Symptoms that persist 4 weeks or less and the presence of fever suggest cryptogenic organizing pneumonia, drug-induced pulmonary injury, or acute hypersensitivity pneumonitis, BUT idiopathic pulmonary fibrosis, ILD associated with connective tissue diseases, and Langerhans cell histiocytosis tend to have a more subacute onset. Extrapulmonary symptoms suggest that the ILD may be associated with systemic disorders (e.g., sarcoidosis; Chapter 95), and symptoms such as dysphagia, dry eyes or mouth, skin rashes, or arthritis may suggest a connective tissue disorder (Chapters 266 to 270). Proximal muscle aches or weakness suggests the possibility of polymyositis or dermatomyositis (Chapter 269), and recurrent sinusitis suggests granulomatosis with polyangiitis (Chapter 270). Extrathoracic manifestations present in tuberous sclerosis (Chapter 417) include hematuria, epilepsy, and mental retardation.

Physical Examination

Physical examination of the respiratory system is rarely helpful in the diagnostic evaluation of ILD because findings such rhonchi and rales on auscultation and digital clubbing are nonspecific. Findings on cardiac examination, such as an accentuated P_2, a right ventricular heave, or tricuspid insufficiency, are suggestive of pulmonary hypertension (Chapter 68) and cor pulmonale in patients with advanced lung disease. However, extrathoracic findings such as skin abnormalities, peripheral lymphadenopathy, and hepatosplenomegaly may be more specifically associated with underlying sarcoidosis (Chapter 95); muscle tenderness and proximal muscle weakness may point to coexisting polymyositis (Chapter 269); and signs of arthritis may indicate connective tissue disease (Chapters 264, 266, and 270) or sarcoidosis (Chapter 95). Characteristic rashes occur in several connective tissue diseases, disseminated Langerhans cell histiocytosis, tuberous sclerosis, and neurofibromatosis. Ophthalmologic findings (Chapter 423) such as iridocyclitis, uveitis, or conjunctivitis, may be a clue to the diagnosis of sarcoidosis or a connective tissue disease, AND central nervous system abnormalities may be present in sarcoidosis, SLE, Langerhans cell histiocytosis, or tuberous sclerosis.

Laboratory Testing

Routine laboratory testing should include a complete blood count, leukocyte differential, erythrocyte sedimentation rate, chemistry panel (calcium, liver enzymes, electrolytes, creatinine), and urinalysis. Although these data rarely yield a specific diagnosis, they may provide helpful clues. Routine serology for occult connective tissue diseases (Chapter 257) may reveal typical findings of SLE (e.g., antinuclear antibodies), rheumatoid arthritis (rheumatoid factor, anticitrullinated peptide antibody), scleroderma (ScL 70), dermatomyositis or polymyositis (creatine kinase, aldolase, and anti–Jo-1 antibody), granulomatosis with polyangiitis (antineutrophil cytoplasmic antibodies), and Goodpasture syndrome (anti–basement membrane antibodies).

Mild hypoxemia is typically present on arterial blood gas analysis because of abnormal ventilation-perfusion ratios, especially in moderate to severe cases of ILD. However, carbon dioxide retention is rare and suggests possible coexisting emphysema (Chapter 88) or a hypoventilatory disorder (Chapter 86).

Noninvasive Evaluation

Chest Radiograph

The distribution and appearance of radiographic abnormalities (Chapter 84) may prove useful in differentiating the clinicopathologic syndromes in patients with ILD (Table 92-3). Comparison of previous chest radiographs with the current one is important in establishing the rate of progression of the patient's disease. A diffuse ground-glass pattern is often observed early in the course of ILD followed by progression to reticular (linear) infiltrates with nodules (reticulonodular infiltrates) or, in the case of alveolar filling disorders, ill-defined nodules (acinar rosettes) with air bronchograms. Most ILDs cause infiltrates in the lower lung zones, but upper lobe predominance is typically present in sarcoidosis, berylliosis, Langerhans cell histiocytosis, silicosis, chronic hypersensitivity pneumonitis, cystic fibrosis, and ankylosing spondylitis. The middle and lower lung zones show the most prominent abnormalities in lymphangitic carcinomatosis, idiopathic pulmonary fibrosis, subacute eosinophilic pneumonia, asbestosis, and pulmonary fibrosis caused by rheumatoid arthritis or progressive systemic sclerosis. Hilar adenopathy and mediastinal adenopathy are not common in ILDs; their presence should suggest sarcoidosis, berylliosis, silicosis, lymphocytic interstitial pneumonia (LIP), amyloidosis, or Gaucher disease. A pattern of peripherally located

TABLE 92-3 CHARACTERISTIC CHEST RADIOGRAPHIC PATTERNS IN PATIENTS WITH INTERSTITIAL LUNG DISEASE

PATTERN	SUGGESTED DIAGNOSES*
Decreased lung volumes	Idiopathic pulmonary fibrosis, nonspecific interstitial pneumonia, desquamative interstitial pneumonia, connective tissue disease, chronic eosinophilic pneumonia, asbestosis, chronic hypersensitivity pneumonitis, or drug-induced interstitial lung disease (ILD)
Increased or preserved lung volumes	Idiopathic pulmonary fibrosis with emphysema, respiratory bronchiolitis–associated ILD, cryptogenic organizing pneumonia, hypersensitivity pneumonitis, lymphangioleiomyomatosis, Langerhans cell histiocytosis, sarcoidosis, neurofibromatosis, tuberous sclerosis
Micronodules	Infection, hypersensitivity pneumonitis, sarcoidosis, respiratory bronchiolitis–associated ILD
Septal thickening	Malignancy, infection, chronic congestive heart failure, pulmonary veno-occlusive disease
Honeycombing	Idiopathic pulmonary fibrosis, fibrotic nonspecific interstitial pneumonia, connective tissue disease, asbestosis, chronic hypersensitivity pneumonitis, sarcoidosis
Recurrent infiltrates	Cryptogenic organizing pneumonia, chronic eosinophilic pneumonia, drug- or radiation-induced ILD
Migratory or fleeting infiltrates	Cryptogenic organizing pneumonia, hypersensitivity pneumonitis, Churg-Strauss syndrome, Löffler syndrome, allergic bronchopulmonary aspergillosis
Pleural disease	Connective tissue disease, asbestosis, malignancy, radiation-induced ILD, amyloidosis, sarcoidosis, lymphangioleiomyomatosis, nitrofurantoin-induced ILD
Pneumothorax	Langerhans cell histiocytosis, lymphangioleiomyomatosis, tuberous sclerosis, neurofibromatosis
Mediastinal or hilar adenopathy	Lymphocytic interstitial pneumonia, connective tissue disease, silicosis, chronic berylliosis, malignancy, infection, sarcoidosis, amyloidosis, Gaucher disease
Normal (rare)	Cellular nonspecific interstitial pneumonia, respiratory bronchiolitis–associated interstitial lung disease, connective tissue disease, hypersensitivity pneumonitis, sarcoidosis
LOCATION OF RADIOGRAPHIC ABNORMALITY	**SUGGESTED DIAGNOSES***
Mid to upper lung zone	Hypersensitivity pneumonitis, chronic berylliosis, ankylosing spondylitis, silicosis, Langerhans cell histiocytosis, sarcoidosis, pleuroparenchymal fibroelastosis, cystic fibrosis
Lower lung zone	Idiopathic pulmonary fibrosis, nonspecific interstitial pneumonia (fibrotic), connective tissue disease, asbestosis, chronic hypersensitivity pneumonitis
Peripheral	Idiopathic pulmonary fibrosis, nonspecific interstitial pneumonia (fibrotic), cryptogenic organizing pneumonia, chronic eosinophilic pneumonia

*This list is not intended to be comprehensive.
Adapted from Raghu G, Brown K. Clinical issues: patient evaluation. In: Baughman RP, du Bois RM, eds. *Diffuse Lung Disease: A Practical Approach.* New York: Oxford University Press; 2004.

pulmonary infiltrates in the upper and middle lung zones with relatively clear perihilar and central zones is a clue to chronic eosinophilic pneumonia. Recurrent infiltrates raise the possibility of cryptogenic organizing pneumonia, chronic eosinophilic pneumonia, or drug- or radiation-induced pneumonitis, and fleeting or migratory infiltrates may occur in Churg-Strauss syndrome (allergic angiitis), allergic bronchopulmonary aspergillosis, tropical eosinophilic pneumonia, or Löffler syndrome. Whereas localized pleural plaques may indicate asbestosis, diffuse pleural thickening can result from asbestosis, rheumatoid arthritis, progressive systemic sclerosis, radiation pneumonitis, nitrofurantoin, or malignancy. In the absence of left ventricular

TABLE 92-4 RADIOGRAPHIC FEATURES OF IDIOPATHIC INTERSTITIAL PNEUMONIAS

CLINICAL DIAGNOSIS	USUAL RADIOGRAPHIC FEATURES	TYPICAL FINDINGS ON HRCT
Idiopathic pulmonary fibrosis	Basal-predominant reticulation abnormality with volume loss	Pattern of usual interstitial pneumonia; peripheral, basal, subpleural reticulation; honeycombing, traction bronchiectasis
Nonspecific interstitial pneumonia	Ground-glass and reticular opacification	Peripheral, basal, subpleural, symmetrical ground-glass attenuation with irregular lines and consolidation; subpleural sparing
Cryptogenic organizing pneumonia	Patchy bilateral consolidation	Subpleural or peribronchial patchy consolidation or nodules
Acute interstitial pneumonia	Diffuse ground-glass density or consolidation	Diffuse consolidation and ground-glass opacification, often with lobular sparing and late traction bronchiectasis
Desquamative interstitial pneumonia	Ground-glass opacity	Peripheral, lower lung zone ground-glass attenuation with reticulation and/or small cysts
Respiratory bronchiolitis–associated interstitial lung disease	Bronchial wall thickening, ground-glass opacification	Diffuse bronchial wall thickening with poorly defined centrilobular nodules and patchy ground-glass opacification
Lymphocytic interstitial pneumonia	Reticular opacities and nodules	Diffuse centrilobular nodules, ground-glass attenuation, septal and bronchovascular wall thickening, and thin-walled cysts

HRCT = high-resolution computed tomography.
Adapted from American Thoracic Society/European Respiratory Society. International multidisciplinary revised classification of the idiopathic interstitial pneumonias. *Am J Respir Crit Care Med.* 2002;165:277-304; Travis WD, Costabel U, Hansell DM, et al. An official American Thoracic Society/European Respiratory Society statement: update of the international multidisciplinary classification of the idiopathic interstitial pneumonias. *Am J Respir Crit Care Med.* 2013;188:733-748; and Raghu G, Collard HR, Egan JJ, et al. An official ATS/ERS/JRS/ALAT statement: idiopathic pulmonary fibrosis: evidence-based guidelines for diagnosis and management. *Am J Respir Crit Care Med.* 2011;183:788-824.

failure, the presence of a pleural effusion (Chapter 99) raises the possibility of rheumatoid arthritis, SLE, acute hypersensitivity pneumonitis, sarcoidosis, asbestosis, amyloidosis, lymphangioleiomyomatosis, or lymphangitic carcinomatosis. A reduction of lung volumes is typical in most ILDs; the presence of preserved lung volumes or hyperinflation should raise suspicion for chronic hypersensitivity pneumonitis, Langerhans cell histiocytosis, lymphangioleiomyomatosis, neurofibromatosis, sarcoidosis, or tuberous sclerosis. However, plain chest radiographs may be normal in about 10% of patients with ILD.

High-Resolution Computed Tomography

Because of its increased sensitivity and ability to distinguish ground-glass changes, which are generally considered to be reversible areas of lung disease, from irreversible fibrotic and honeycomb changes, high-resolution computed tomography (HRCT) is essential in both the diagnosis and staging of ILD. Although microscopic ILD cannot be excluded by a normal HRCT result, HRCT allows recognition of abnormalities not apparent in plain chest radiographs and may lead to an earlier diagnosis, help narrow the differential diagnosis patterns (Table 92-4), aid in selecting the site or sites for BAL and lung biopsy, and assist in choosing among therapeutic options and in estimating the response to treatment. Whereas normal HRCT excludes the diagnosis of pulmonary fibrosis, the presence of patchy subpleural reticular and basilar septal fibrosis, traction bronchiectasis, and honeycombing increases the level of diagnostic confidence for the pattern of usual interstitial pattern, which is characteristic of idiopathic pulmonary fibrosis. The finding of bilateral cysts, including their size, configuration, distribution, and appearance, helps differentiate among lymphangioleiomyomatosis, tuberous sclerosis, and pulmonary Langerhans cell histiocytosis. HRCT can detect ILD despite normal chest radiographs in patients with asbestosis, silicosis, sarcoidosis, and scleroderma. Patients with respiratory bronchiolitis–associated ILD typically have patchy ground-glass attenuation on HRCT in concert with bilateral interstitial prominence, fine nodular radiographic infiltrates, and normal lung volumes. Images obtained in the supine and prone positions and on deep inspiration and exhalation sometimes help to differentiate fibrosis from atelectasis.

Pulmonary Function Tests

The most characteristic physiologic abnormalities in patients with ILD, regardless of etiology, are a restrictive lung defect and decreased DLCO (see Table 85-2 in Chapter 85). Forced expiratory volume in 1 second (FEV_1) and forced vital capacity (FVC) are decreased proportionally such that the ratio of the two remains normal or may even be increased. Both total lung capacity (TLC) and lung volumes measured by body plethysmography are reduced. Pulmonary function tests (PFTs) may be useful in monitoring the progression of disease and prognosis; significant changes in FVC, DLCO (corrected to hemoglobin), and physiological measurements (FVC, DLCO) at 1 year portend a worse survival in patients with idiopathic pulmonary fibrosis.

Certain PFT findings may also aid in the differential diagnosis. A mixed obstructive–restrictive pattern occurs in patients with Churg-Strauss syndrome, allergic bronchopulmonary aspergillosis, endobronchial sarcoidosis, hypersensitivity pneumonitis, cryptogenic organizing pneumonia, tropical pulmonary interstitial eosinophilia, coexisting chronic obstructive pulmonary disease or asthma, or secondary bronchiectasis. Diseases associated with respiratory muscle weakness, such as polymyositis, progressive systemic sclerosis, and SLE, may exhibit a decrease in maximal voluntary ventilation and increased residual volume out of proportion to the decrease in FEV_1.

Exercise Testing

The magnitude of the increase in PAO_2-PaO_2 on exercise correlates well with the severity of disease and the degree of pulmonary fibrosis in patients with idiopathic pulmonary fibrosis. Other exercise-induced physiologic abnormalities in ILD include a decrease in work rate and maximal oxygen consumption, abnormally high minute ventilation at submaximal work rates, decreased peak minute ventilation, and failure of tidal volumes to increase at submaximal levels of work while the respiratory rate increases disproportionately. The 6-minute walk test, performed on a flat surface, can provide quantitative data on exercise capacity and on oxygen desaturation with exercise and can justify use of supplemental oxygen based on clinical and physiological needs.

Invasive Evaluation

A collegial interaction and multidisciplinary discussions among the pulmonary clinician, chest radiologist, thoracic surgeon, and pathologist can help determine the best diagnostic approach for an individual patient (see Fig. 92-1).

Findings on BAL can be diagnostic in some patients with ILD and can narrow the differential diagnosis in others (Chapter 85). For example, a lymphocyte-predominant cellular pattern raises the possibility of sarcoidosis or hypersensitivity pneumonitis in the appropriate clinical setting. Eosinophils are seen in pulmonary Langerhans cell granulomatosis, an asbestos body count greater than 1 fiber per milliliter of BAL fluid is seen in asbestosis, and specially staining surfactant material is seen in pulmonary alveolar proteinosis. A transbronchial lung biopsy may reveal noncaseating granulomas in sarcoidosis, "loose" noncaseating granulomas in hypersensitivity pneumonitis, giant cell granulomas in hard metal pneumoconiosis, or smooth muscle proliferation in lymphangioleiomyomatosis. However, failure to establish a diagnosis on BAL and transbronchial lung biopsy does not exclude these entities.

Video-assisted thoracoscopic biopsy (Chapter 101) or open lung biopsy may be required to obtain an adequate sample for histologic evaluation of a patient with unexplained signs and symptoms when other studies have failed to establish a diagnosis, but most patients with idiopathic pulmonary fibrosis do not need to have a biopsy to confirm the diagnosis. The mortality rate for the procedure is generally less than 1%, and the morbidity rate is less than 3%.

TABLE 92-5 INTERSTITIAL LUNG DISEASE: CLINICAL RESPONSE TO SYSTEMIC CORTICOSTEROIDS ALONE*

GENERALLY RESPONSIVE	UNRESPONSIVE†
Sarcoidosis	Idiopathic interstitial pneumonia
Acute hypersensitivity pneumonitis	Idiopathic pulmonary fibrosis (usual interstitial pneumonia)
Drug induced	Desquamative interstitial pneumonia (subset)
Environmental causes (some)	Chronic secondary and advanced pulmonary fibrosis
Idiopathic interstitial pneumonia	Chronic hypersensitivity pneumonitis (subset)
Cryptogenic organizing pneumonia	Chronic radiation fibrosis
Nonspecific interstitial pneumonia (cellular)	Cryptogenic organizing pneumonia (subset)
Respiratory bronchiolitis–associated ILD	Acute interstitial pneumonia (?)
Lymphocytic interstitial pneumonia	Chronic pulmonary hemorrhage syndromes
Desquamative interstitial pneumonia (subset)	Pulmonary veno-occlusive disease
Acute interstitial pneumonia (?)	Environmental (e.g., asbestosis, pneumoconiosis)
Acute pulmonary capillaritis	End-stage ILDs, pulmonary fibrosis coexisting or associated with pulmonary hypertension
Eosinophilic pneumonia (acute and chronic)	Pulmonary Langerhans cell granulomatosis
Acute radiation pneumonitis‡	Lymphangioleiomyomatosis
Organizing pneumonia associated with connective tissue diseases	ILD in inherited disorders (?)

*The dosage plus duration of corticosteroids used is variable and based on anecdotal experience, individual expert opinion, clinical judgment, and response as judged by objective measurements (clinical, radiologic, or physiologic). Oral prednisone or prednisolone is the most common corticosteroid used. Most patients who respond during the first few weeks of 20 to 60 mg of prednisone per day require maintenance low-dose oral prednisone at 5 to 10 mg/day beyond 6 months. Some patients who require maintenance of oral prednisone doses higher than 20 mg/day beyond 4 to 6 months may tolerate lower doses of prednisone if other immune-modulating agents (e.g., azathioprine, mycophenolate) are used in combination. There is no evidence to recommend a specific regimen. Patients should be monitored carefully and regularly for known side effects of corticosteroid use (e.g., osteoporosis, glucose intolerance), and preventive and therapeutic measures must be undertaken appropriately.

†Some patients unresponsive to oral corticosteroids alone may respond to combined treatment with corticosteroids and other immune-modulating drugs (e.g., azathioprine, mycophenolate).

‡Although most patients respond to modest doses of oral prednisone (initially, 40-60 mg/day), it is important to taper the prednisone very slowly to reach a maintenance dose of 5 to 10 mg/day beyond 6 months; rapid taper of oral prednisone has been associated with "rebound," which is an exaggerated lung injury beyond the irradiated segment of the lung and in the contralateral lung.

ILD = interstitial lung disease.

TREATMENT Rx

When the cause of the ILD is clearly known (e.g., acute or subacute hypersensitivity pneumonitis, occupational ILD, iatrogenic), further avoidance of the inciting agent or agents is essential (Chapter 93). Although systemic corticosteroids are generally indicated and are associated with a favorable response in some ILDs, the dosage and duration are unclear and essentially based on anecdotal experience (Table 92-5).

Supportive oxygen supplementation is dictated by clinical needs. For selected patients with end-stage ILDs, such as those associated with significant pulmonary fibrosis and pulmonary hypertension, lung transplantation (Chapter 101) may be a feasible and viable option. Treatments for pulmonary hypertension associated with ILDs (Chapter 68) are indicated in patients with connective tissue diseases, but their clinical benefit for patients with other ILDs have been disappointing. A1

SPECIFIC TYPES OF INTERSTITIAL LUNG DISEASE

Idiopathic Interstitial Pneumonias

Idiopathic interstitial pneumonias, which are a subset of acute or chronic ILDs of unknown etiology, are characterized by the presence of varying degrees of interstitial and alveolar inflammation and fibrosis. Distinct clinicopathologic forms of idiopathic interstitial pneumonia include chronic

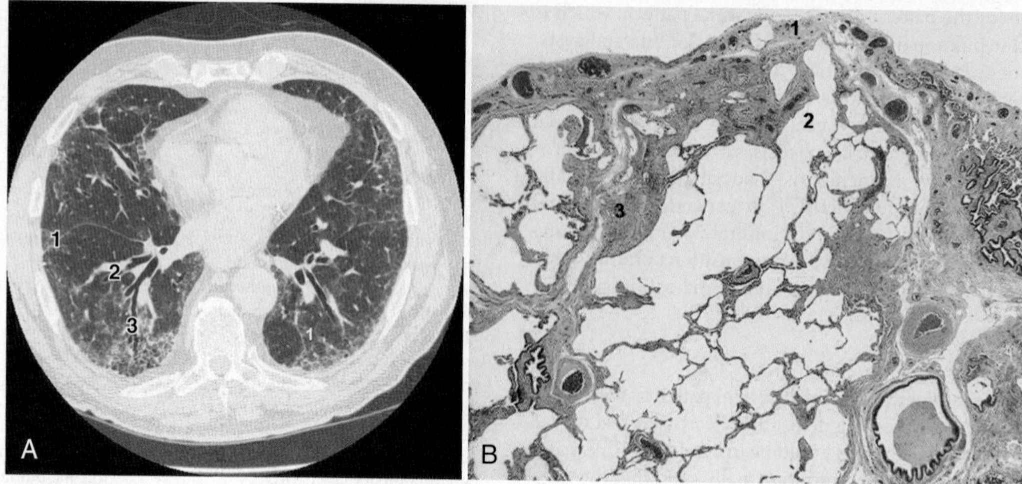

FIGURE 92-2. **Diagnosis of idiopathic pulmonary fibrosis. A, The usual interstitial pneumonia pattern of idiopathic pulmonary fibrosis in the lower lobes on high-resolution computed tomography consists of (1) subpleural fibrotic changes with (2) traction bronchiectasis and (3) honeycomb cysts in the lower lobes. B, Usual interstitial pneumonia pattern of idiopathic pulmonary fibrosis. Note the presence of (1) subpleural fibrosis with (2) traction emphysema, (3) fibroblastic foci, and temporal heterogeneity of microscopic abnormalities at low magnification. (Courtesy of Dr. Kevin Leslie.)**

fibrosing interstitial pneumonias (idiopathic pulmonary fibrosis and nonspecific interstitial pneumonia), smoking-related interstitial pneumonias (respiratory bronchiolitis–ILD and desquamative interstitial pneumonia), and acute or subacute idiopathic interstitial pneumonias (cryptogenic organizing pneumonia and acute interstitial pneumonia). Rare histologic patterns of acute fibrinous and organizing pneumonia and interstitial pneumonias with a bronchiolocentric distribution and pleuroparenchymal fibroelastosis have been recently recognized.[5] In some patients, mixed histopathologic features are evident in different segments of the same lung. When the distinct pathological forms are not evident, the diagnosis of unclassifiable interstitial pneumonia has been recently recognized. The accuracy of the diagnosis of idiopathic interstitial pneumonias is increased by multidisciplinary discussions among expert pulmonologists, radiologists, and pathologists familiar with interstitial lung diseases and idiopathic interstitial pneumonias.

Although the clinical severity may vary, the idiopathic interstitial pneumonias tend to manifest as an insidious onset of exertional dyspnea and a nonproductive cough. Chest pain and systemic symptoms such as weight loss and fatigue may be present. Bibasilar end-inspiratory crackles are often heard on auscultation. Clubbing, although not specific, is found in 25% to 50% of patients with idiopathic pulmonary fibrosis. Findings on the chest radiograph are most often nonspecific, and the presence of normal lung markings on the chest radiograph does not exclude ILD. On HRCT, many pathologic entities have characteristic image patterns that have greatly aided diagnosis (see Table 92-4). The clinical course of idiopathic pulmonary fibrosis is heterogeneous.

CHRONIC FIBROSING INTERSTITIAL PNEUMONIA

Idiopathic Pulmonary Fibrosis

Idiopathic pulmonary fibrosis accounts for 50% to 60% of all idiopathic interstitial pneumonias. Idiopathic pulmonary fibrosis occurs in adult men and women with a mean age at onset of 62 years. Some patients have familial disease, likely as an autosomal dominant with variable penetrance. The best validated genetic risk factor is a polymorphism in the promoter of the gene encoding mucin-5B (*MUC5B*), which is associated with both familial and sporadic forms.[6] Variants in the gene encoding surfactant protein C have been strongly associated with familial idiopathic pulmonary fibrosis, and mutations in the gene encoding surfactant protein A2 have been associated with familial pulmonary fibrosis and lung cancer. Telomere shortening caused by genetic variants within the human telomerase RNA or human telomerase reverse transcriptase has been associated with both familial and sporadic idiopathic pulmonary fibrosis.

Idiopathic pulmonary fibrosis is limited to the lungs in adults, usually older than 60 years, and it generally occurs in men with a history of cigarette smoking. Most often patients have otherwise been in good health and have no known connective tissue disease or exposure to drugs or environmental factors known to cause pulmonary fibrosis, although patients with significant cigarette smoking history may have coexisting emphysema. Typical clinical manifestations include a gradual onset and progression of exertional dyspnea, restrictive abnormalities on PFTs (Chapter 85), and a distinct pattern of bilateral pulmonary fibrosis on HRCT.

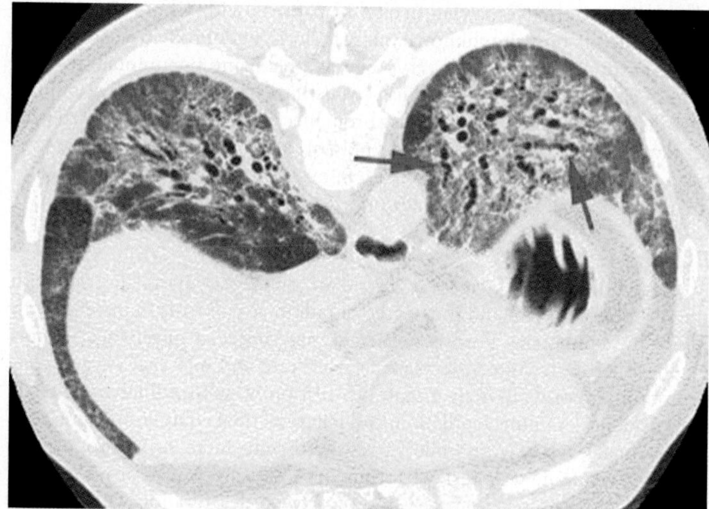

FIGURE 92-3. **Computed tomography scan showing traction bronchiectasis *(arrows)*.**

DIAGNOSIS

Chest radiographs typically show basal-predominant reticular abnormalities with low lung volumes.[7] The diagnostic features on HRCT are peripheral, predominantly basilar patchy intralobular reticulation, often with subpleural honeycomb cysts, traction bronchiectasis, and traction bronchiolectasis as the disease becomes more advanced (Fig. 92-2, *A*). Reticulation may progress to honeycombing, although neither alveolar consolidation nor parenchymal nodules are present. Compared with the other idiopathic interstitial pneumonias, the HRCT appearance of idiopathic pulmonary fibrosis is distinguished by the presence of fibrotic abnormalities, predominantly in the bases of the lower lobes (E-Fig. 92-E1), by subpleural reticulations (E-Fig. 92-E2), and by its hallmark honeycombing (E-Fig. 92-E3) and traction bronchiectasis (Fig. 92-3). There is a notable absence of extensive ground-glass opacification, micronodules, cysts, consolidation, significant air trapping in multiple lobes, pleural plaques, pleural effusion, and extensive mediastinal adenopathy, all of which are inconsistent with the radiographic pattern of usual interstitial pneumonia.

Pulmonary function tests usually show a progressive restrictive pattern. However, patients with milder disease may have normal lung volumes and a small decrease in DLCO; rarely, PFT results may be normal.

TABLE 92-6 DIAGNOSIS CRITERIA FOR IDIOPATHIC PULMONARY FIBROSIS

The diagnosis of idiopathic pulmonary fibrosis requires the presence of usual interstitial pneumonia (UIP) in the absence of other causes of interstitial lung disease (e.g., domestic, occupational, and environmental exposures, connective tissue disease, and drug toxicity) AND

a. The presence of a UIP pattern on chest HRCT in the absence of a lung biopsy or
b. Specific combinations* of chest HRCT patterns (UIP, possible UIP, inconsistent with UIP) and histopathologic features (UIP, probable UIP, possible UIP, not UIP) on surgical lung biopsy

HRCT FEATURES OF UIP	HISTOPATHOLOGIC FEATURES OF UIP
• Subpleural, basal predominance • Reticular abnormality • Honeycombing with or without traction bronchiectasis • Absence of peribronchovascular predominance, extensive ground-glass abnormality, diffuse micronodules, discrete cysts, diffuse mosaic attenuation, or consolidation	• Marked fibrosis/architectural distortion, +/− honeycombing in a predominantly subpleural/paraseptal distribution • Patchy parenchymal lung fibrosis • Fibroblast foci • No features suggesting an alternate diagnosis*

*Based on data from Raghu G, Collard HR, Egan JJ, et al. An official ATS/ERS/JRS/ALAT statement: idiopathic pulmonary fibrosis: evidence-based guidelines for diagnosis and management. *Am J Respir Crit Care Med.* 2011;183:788-824.
HRCT = high-resolution computed tomography.

The cellular pattern in BAL fluid, which is nonspecific, is marked by an excess of neutrophils in proportion to the extent of reticular change on HRCT; the percentage of eosinophils may be mildly increased. The histopathologic pattern of usual interstitial pneumonia consists of patchy interstitial changes alternating with zones of honeycombing, fibrosis, minimal inflammatory cells, collagen deposition, and normal lung (Fig. 92-2, *B*). Subepithelial fibroblastic foci, small aggregates of myofibroblasts, and fibroblasts within myxoid matrix are invariably present and represent areas of active fibrosis. The presence of temporal heterogeneity, or areas at different stages of fibrosis transitioning with normal areas and honeycomb cysts, along with fibrotic foci within the lung, is an essential feature of usual interstitial pneumonia that distinguishes it from other processes such as nonspecific interstitial pneumonia. Interstitial cellular inflammation is minimal in usual interstitial pneumonia. Although usual interstitial pneumonia characterizes the microscopic abnormality in idiopathic pulmonary fibrosis, the same histologic and radiologic pattern can also be seen in patients with rheumatologic lung diseases, chronic hypersensitivity pneumonitis, and asbestosis (Chapter 93). In the appropriate clinical setting (and after definitive exclusion of other known clinical conditions associated with ILD) (see later), a definitive diagnosis of idiopathic pulmonary fibrosis is based on the presence of a pattern of usual interstitial pneumonia on HRCT or surgical lung biopsy (Table 92-6).

TREATMENT

Rx

Pirfenidone (1800 mg/day for 1 year) decreases the rate of decline in forced vital capacity in clinical trials of patients who have idiopathic pulmonary fibrosis and mild to moderate impairment in pulmonary function,A2-A4 and pooled data suggest an improvement in survival.A5 Pirfenidone is approved for the treatment of idiopathic pulmonary fibrosis in the U.S., Japan, and Europe.[8] Treatment with nintedanib (a tyrosine kinase inhibitor at 150 mg orally twice daily) also decreases the rate of disease progression as measured by FVC over 52 weeks in patients with idiopathic pulmonary fibrosis and mild to moderate impairment in pulmonary function;A6 it is now approved in the U.S. and Europe. Sildenafil (a phosphodiesterase inhibitor at 20 mg orally three times a day) has shown small benefits in terms of dyspnea, oxygenation, and quality of life but not exercise capacity in patients with idiopathic pulmonary fibrosis and severe impairment in pulmonary function.A7 Abnormal acid gastroesophageal reflux (Chapter 138) is very common in patients with idiopathic pulmonary fibrosis, and treatment with standard doses of proton pump inhibitors, H2 receptor antagonists, or both as used for gastroesophageal reflux disease (Chapter 138) can slow the rate of progression of idiopathic pulmonary fibrosis.A8

By comparison, *N*-acetylcysteine aloneA9 or as part of triple-therapy combined with prednisone plus azathioprineA10 is not beneficial. Warfarin increases respiratory hospitalizations and death in patients with idiopathic pulmonary fibrosis.A11 Interferon-γ1b, cyclophosphamide, colchicine, D-penicillamine, dual and selective endothelin receptor antagonists, and oral corticosteroids as monotherapy or in combination with immunosuppressive agents are not beneficial.

Despite the absence of data, patients who require hospitalization and intensive care for an acute exacerbation with loss of respiratory function in the absence of infection or other complications are usually treated with empirical intravenous corticosteroids (e.g., methylprednisolone 1.0 g intravenously as a pulse dose once a day for 3 days and followed by hydrocortisone, 125 mg every 6 hours for another 3 to 5 days), with further dosing dependent on the clinical response. Ancillary treatment measures, including supplemental oxygen (based on clinical and physiologic needs); prompt detection and treatment of respiratory tract infections and pulmonary embolism (Chapter 98); pulmonary rehabilitation; and immunization for influenza, herpes zoster, and pneumococcus, are all appropriate. Pulmonary hypertension, if present, may be treated (Chapter 68), but there is no evidence that such treatment will be beneficial.A12 Lung transplantation (Chapter 101) is indicated in selected patients, but about two thirds of patients with idiopathic pulmonary fibrosis are older than 60 to 65 years, which is a relative contraindication to lung transplantation. It is important to initiate discussion of palliative care measures before patients reach the terminal stages of the disease.

PROGNOSIS

The natural course of idiopathic pulmonary fibrosis is heterogeneous. Most patients exhibit a slow and steady decline, with a mortality rate of about 7% at 1 year and 14% at 2 years after diagnosis.[9] A small subset of patients declines at a rapid rate over several months, but another subset of patients remains stable over several years before declining. Progressive impairment of lung function and gas exchange ultimately is fatal unless the patient undergoes lung transplantation. Patients who survive longer generally have less fibrosis on HRCT, less functional impairment, no evidence of pulmonary hypertension, and no significant oxygen desaturation during a modified version of the 6-minute walk test. Patients with coexisting emphysema, pulmonary hypertension, or episodes of acute exacerbation have even shorter survival times. By comparison, patients who have a polymorphism in the gene encoding *MUC5B* may have better survival times.

Nonspecific Interstitial Pneumonia

Nonspecific interstitial pneumonia is often associated with connective tissue diseases, but idiopathic nonspecific interstitial pneumonia is also recognized as a distinct clinical entity. It typically occurs in middle-aged, nonsmoking women with an average age at diagnosis of about 50 years. The prevalence of nonspecific interstitial pneumonia has been estimated at one to nine per 100,000.

Two subgroups have been described, cellular and fibrotic. Because the average age at onset is about 10 years earlier in nonspecific interstitial pneumonia than in idiopathic pulmonary fibrosis and because the clinical features of idiopathic fibrotic nonspecific interstitial pneumonia are very similar to early cases of idiopathic pulmonary fibrosis, questions persist as to whether idiopathic fibrotic nonspecific interstitial pneumonia is a separate clinical entity or represents an early form of idiopathic pulmonary fibrosis.

DIAGNOSIS

Chest radiographs show bilateral patchy pulmonary infiltrates with a lower lung zone predominance in all forms of nonspecific interstitial pneumonia. HRCT reveals a predominant ground-glass pattern of attenuation, usually bilateral and often associated with subpleural reticulation (Fig. 92-4), and loss of volume in the lower lobe. In cellular nonspecific interstitial pneumonia, HRCT shows ground-glass opacification, consolidation, or both, but the biopsy shows mild to moderate lymphoplasmacytic interstitial chronic inflammation. The major differential diagnosis to consider as an alternative to cellular nonspecific interstitial pneumonia is acute or subacute hypersensitivity pneumonitis, so a thorough history regarding environmental exposures is crucial. In contrast, fibrotic nonspecific interstitial pneumonia has a bilateral lower lobe distribution with architectural derangement on HRCT; histopathologically, it has uniformly dense interstitial fibrosis and may sometimes be difficult to distinguish from idiopathic pulmonary fibrosis and usual interstitial pneumonia in the early clinical stages. In these circumstances, the diagnosis of fibrotic nonspecific interstitial pneumonia can be ascertained only by the histologic features in a surgical lung biopsy specimen.

TREATMENT AND PROGNOSIS

Rx

Patients with cellular nonspecific interstitial pneumonia usually respond to treatment with corticosteroids (see Table 92-5), and their prognosis is generally better than that of patients with idiopathic pulmonary fibrosis. Nonetheless, some patients progress over several years, and some manifest acute exacerbations similar to patients with idiopathic pulmonary fibrosis. Immune-modulating drugs, including prednisone, azathioprine, and mycophenolate, have been used empirically, with their doses based on clinical response as assessed by clinicians and not on evidence with randomized clinical trials.

SMOKING-RELATED INTERSTITIAL PNEUMONIAS

Respiratory Bronchiolitis–Associated Interstitial Lung Disease

This ILD is almost invariably associated with chronic and current cigarette smoking, and it usually manifests clinically during the fourth or fifth decade of life. However, it may also be detected incidentally on radiographs

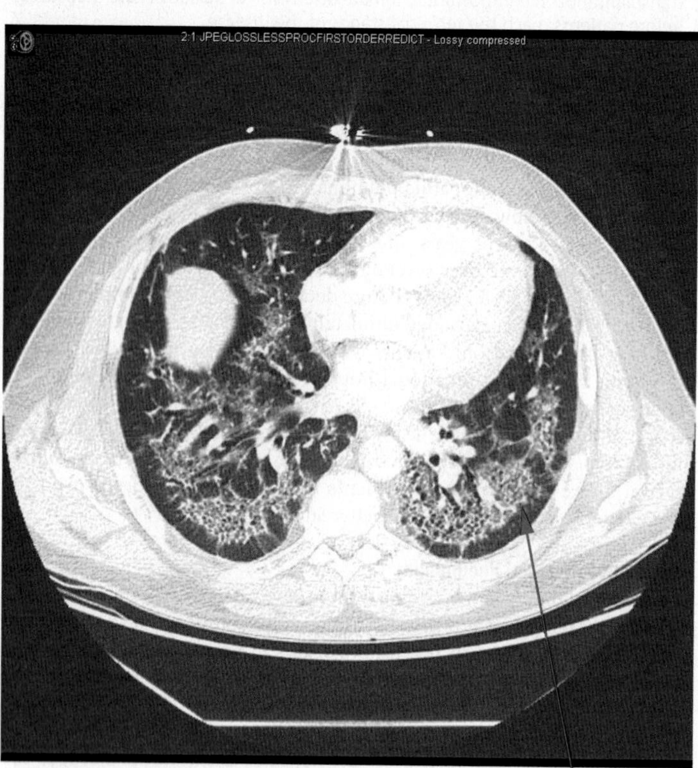

FIGURE 92-4. Nonspecific interstitial pneumonia. Computed tomography scan showing characteristic subpleural sparing.

in relatively younger and asymptomatic persons with a previous history of cigarette smoking or in people passively exposed to chronic cigarette smoke Respiratory bronchiolitis–associated ILD is always associated with chronic exposure to cigarette smoke.

DIAGNOSIS

Pulmonary function tests show varying degrees of airway obstruction, mildly decreased or preserved TLC, and decreased DLCO. The chest radiograph typically reveals bronchial wall thickening and areas of ground-glass attenuation. HRCT reveals centrilobular nodules with an upper lobe predominance, patchy ground-glass attenuation, and peribronchial alveolar septal thickening (Fig. 92-5, *A*). Areas of hypoattenuation (mosaic attenuation) represent air trapping as a result of small airways disease. The characteristic finding on BAL is numerous brown-pigmented alveolar macrophages, often with a modest increase in neutrophils. Lung biopsy is rarely needed, but its hallmark histopathologic feature is the accumulation of pigmented alveolar macrophages with glassy eosinophilic cytoplasm and granular pigmentation within respiratory bronchioles, typically with a chronic inflammatory cell infiltrate in the bronchioles and surrounding alveolar walls (Fig. 92-5, *B*). Fibroblastic foci and honeycomb change are not present, but centrilobular emphysema is frequent.

TREATMENT AND PROGNOSIS

Progression to honeycomb lung and end-stage fibrosis seldom occurs, and the prognosis is good with cessation of smoking. Discontinuation of cigarette smoking is essential, and patients may benefit from low-dose corticosteroids (e.g., prednisone, 10 to 20 mg/day) for a few months.

Desquamative Interstitial Pneumonia

Desquamative interstitial pneumonia is a rare entity (<3% of all ILDs) that may represent a form of respiratory bronchiolitis–associated ILD extending into the alveolar spaces and alveolar walls. Although most affected individuals are cigarette smokers, the histologic pattern of desquamative interstitial pneumonia may also occur in pneumoconiosis, rheumatologic disease, and drug-associated ILD. Patients are often initially seen with advanced disease and striking hypoxemia. The histopathology features of desquamative interstitial pneumonia are characterized by accumulation of pigmented alveolar macrophages within the alveoli. Histologic changes within the respiratory bronchioles and within the alveolar spaces can coexist and represent a histopathologic spectrum of alveolar macrophage accumulation.

DIAGNOSIS

Pulmonary function tests reveal a restrictive lung defect and decreased DLCO with or without coexisting airway obstruction. The chest radiograph shows patchy basal consolidation with a lower lobe and peripheral predominance (Fig. 92-6). HRCT shows bilateral symmetrical ground-glass opacities with a predominantly basal and peripheral distribution as well as diffuse alveolar septal thickening (Fig. 92-7, *A*). Irregular linear opacities, typically associated

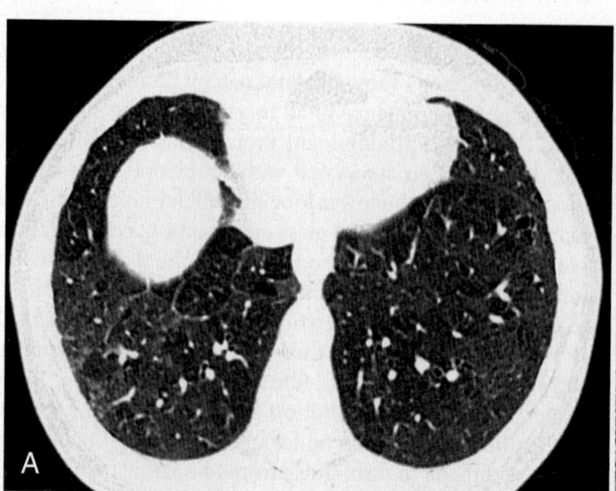

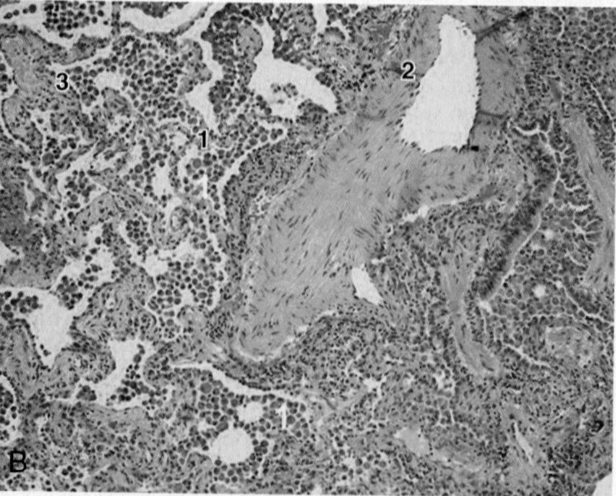

FIGURE 92-5. Respiratory bronchiolitis–associated interstitial lung disease. **A,** Ground-glass attenuation with a mosaic pattern on high-resolution computed tomography. **B,** Note the dense aggregates of (1) pigmented macrophages present in the air spaces around the terminal airways with (2) variable bronchiolar metaplasia and (3) interstitial fibrosis.

with traction bronchiectasis, may be noted. The finding of small discrete cysts, believed to represent trapped air in dilated bronchioles, within areas of ground-glass changes (E-Fig. 92-E4) and intervening normal lung parenchyma is highly suggestive of desquamative interstitial pneumonia. Fluid recovered from BAL quite often shows increased numbers of pigmented alveolar macrophages, frequently with increased neutrophils. Histopathologic findings on biopsy include diffuse alveolar septal thickening, hyperplasia of type II pneumocytes, and intense accumulation of intra-alveolar granular pigmented macrophages in a uniform manner (Fig. 92-7, *B*); fibrosis is minimal.

TREATMENT AND PROGNOSIS Rx

With cessation of smoking and administration of oral corticosteroid therapy (see Table 92-5), outcomes are generally good, with an estimated overall survival rate of 70% at 10 years. However, a subset of patients may progress despite cessation of cigarette smoking, and a trial of corticosteroid therapy and lung transplantation is an appropriate consideration for selected patients.

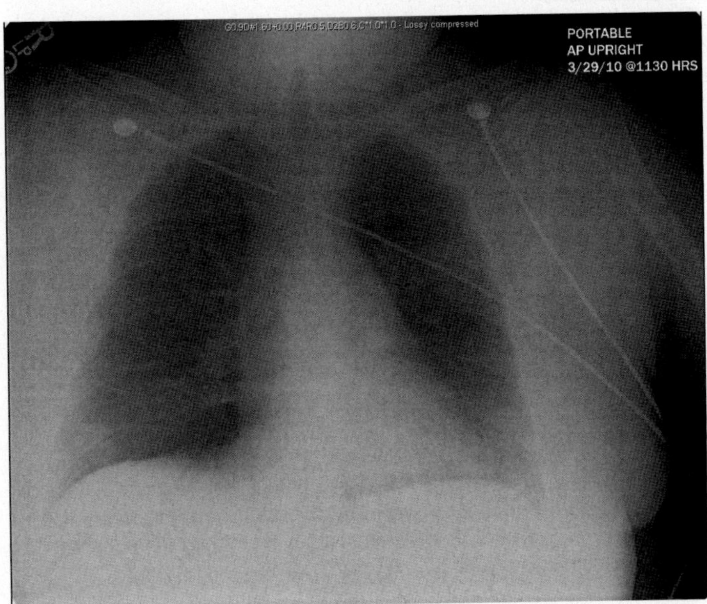

FIGURE 92-6. Anteroposterior chest radiograph showing patchy ground-glass infiltrates typical of desquamative interstitial pneumonia.

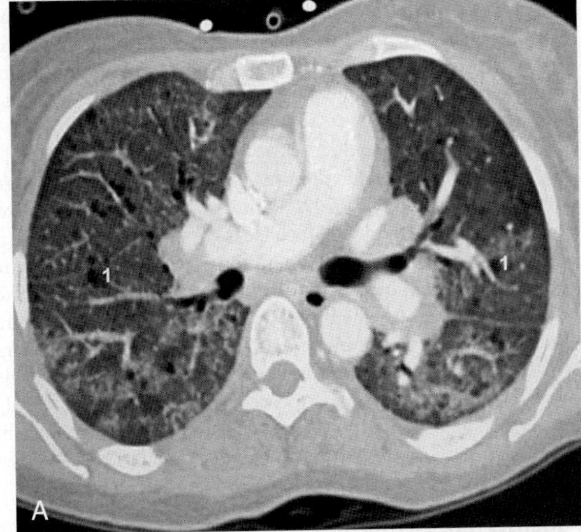

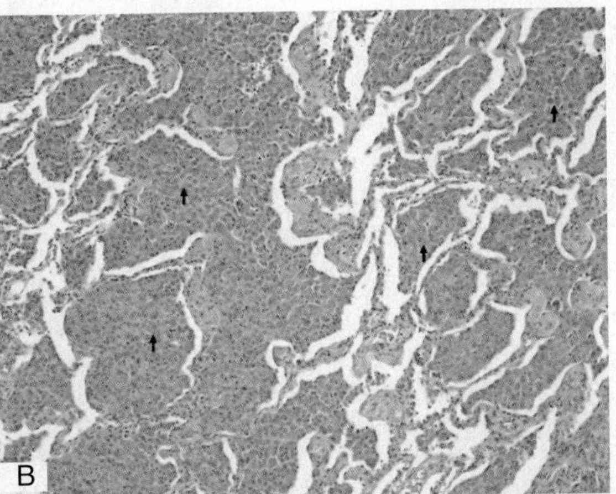

FIGURE 92-7. Desquamative interstitial pneumonia. **A,** Ground-glass attenuation with cystic spaces on high-resolution computed tomography. **B,** Note that the alveolar spaces are densely filled with macrophages *(arrowheads)*.

ACUTE OR SUBACUTE IDIOPATHIC INTERSTITIAL PNEUMONIA

Acute Interstitial Pneumonia

Acute interstitial pneumonia is seen in otherwise healthy persons usually after an apparent acute viral upper respiratory infection (Fig. 92-8). The syndrome, historically known as Hamman-Rich syndrome (Chapter 91), mimics acute respiratory distress syndrome (Chapter 104). Acute interstitial pneumonia is a rare and fulminant idiopathic interstitial pneumonia that presents with acute symptoms and leads to respiratory distress or failure.

Cryptogenic Organizing Pneumonia

Cryptogenic organizing pneumonia, previously referred to as bronchiolitis obliterans organizing pneumonia of unknown cause (BOOP), is an idiopathic form of organizing pneumonia. Organizing pneumonia affects the small airways, including the distal bronchioles, respiratory bronchioles, alveolar ducts, and alveolar walls. Although the incidence and prevalence of cryptogenic organizing pneumonia are unknown, the estimated annual incidence in the United States is six to seven cases per 100,000. The mean age at presentation is about 60 years, and there is no sex predominance.

DIAGNOSIS

Cryptogenic organizing pneumonia most commonly manifests as a flulike illness with a nonproductive cough followed by exertional dyspnea. PFTs

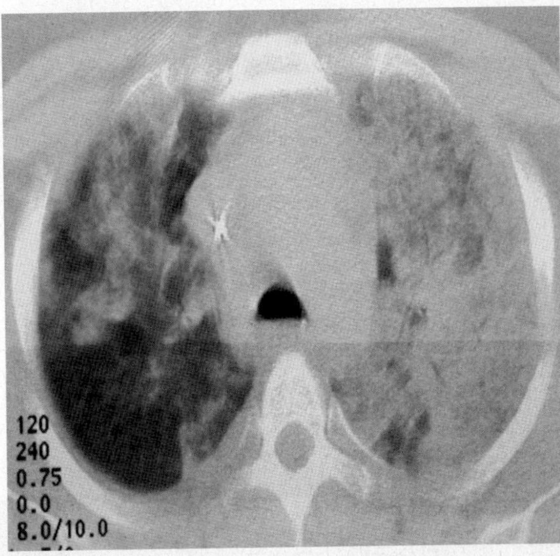

FIGURE 92-8. Acute interstitial pneumonia with diffuse alveolar damage histologically. Note the dense air space consolidation.

show a restrictive defect, but 20% of patients, most of whom are current or past smokers, also have an obstructive defect. Chest radiography reveals patchy unilateral or bilateral alveolar opacities that may be peripheral or migratory; small nodular opacities are seen in 10% to 50% of cases (Fig. 92-9). In about 90% of patients, HRCT shows areas of air space consolidation with lower lung zone predominance, frequently in a subpleural or peribronchial distribution (Fig. 92-10); other features include small nodules along bronchovascular bundles and ground-glass attenuation. BAL is nonspecific; increased lymphocytes, neutrophils, and eosinophils may be seen. On biopsy, key histologic features are excessive proliferation of granulation tissue within the small airways and alveolar ducts as well as chronic inflammation in the surrounding alveoli.

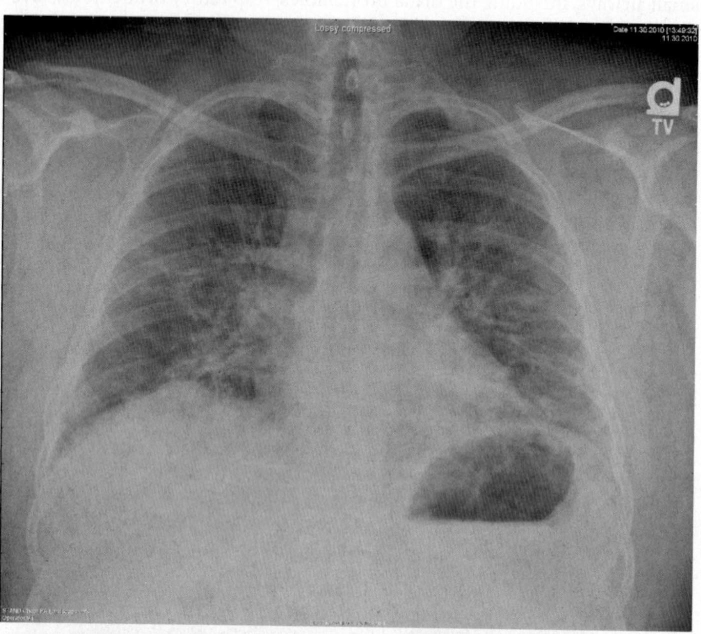

FIGURE 92-9. Chest radiograph showing cryptogenic organizing pneumonia. Note the bilateral patchy air space opacities.

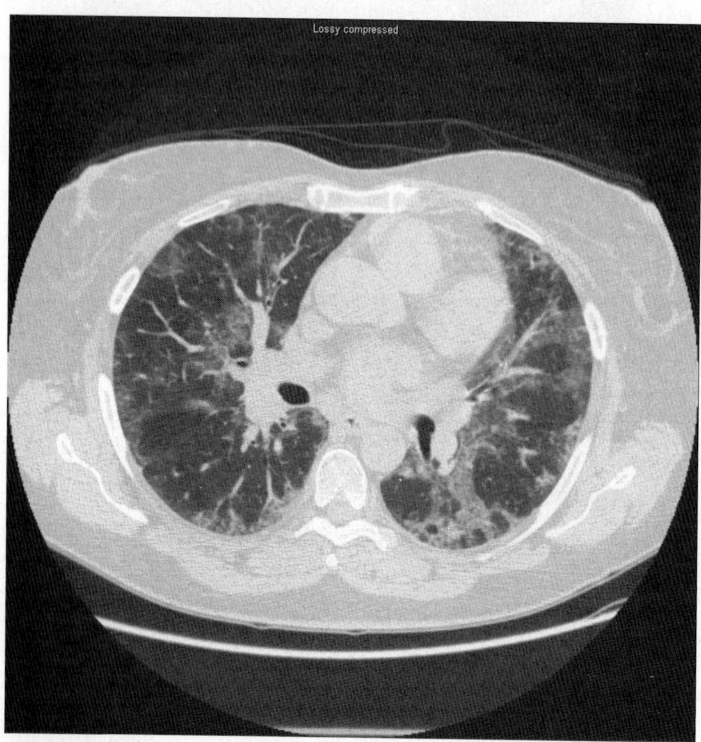

FIGURE 92-10. Peripheral ground-glass opacities in a patient with cryptogenic organizing pneumonia.

TREATMENT AND PROGNOSIS Rx

Most patients recover rapidly and completely when treated with oral corticosteroids (see Table 92-5) for 6 months but may relapse after discontinuation and require oral corticosteroids for longer periods and sometimes indefinitely, often with adjunct immunosuppressive agents such as azathioprine. A small subset of patients in whom pulmonary fibrosis develops despite corticosteroids and azathioprine behave similarly to patients with idiopathic pulmonary fibrosis. Spontaneous remissions are known to occur.

Lymphoid and Lymphocytic Interstitial Pneumonia

This condition is more common in women, especially in the fifth decade of life, but it may occur at any age. Patients should be evaluated for concurrent connective tissue disease, an autoimmune disorder (especially Sjögren syndrome; Chapter 268), or common variable immunoglobulin deficiency (Chapter 250) because idiopathic LIP is very rare. Symptoms are nonspecific and include a gradual onset of cough and exertional dyspnea. Lymphoid and LIP is within the spectrum of benign lymphoproliferative disorders, and some patients manifest pseudolymphoma or lymphoma as a complication.

DIAGNOSIS

Chest radiographs show a reticular or reticulonodular pattern predominantly involving the lower lung zones. HRCT reveals bilateral ground-glass attenuation, small or large nodules, and scattered cysts; perivascular honeycombing and reticular abnormalities may also be seen (E-Fig. 92-E5). Increased numbers of lymphocytes are found on BAL, and biopsy reveals a dense interstitial lymphocytic infiltrate.

TREATMENT AND PROGNOSIS Rx

Some patients respond to or stabilize with oral corticosteroids (see Table 92-5). The prognosis is variable, with more than one third of patients progressing to diffuse pulmonary fibrosis.

Interstitial Lung Disease Associated with Connective Tissue Disease

Many of the connective tissue diseases, including progressive systemic sclerosis (Chapter 267), rheumatoid arthritis (Chapter 264), SLE (Chapter 266), dermatomyositis and polymyositis (Chapter 269), Sjögren syndrome (Chapter 268), and mixed connective tissue disorder (Chapter 267), may have ILD as one of their manifestations. In fact, up to 20% of patients with connective tissue diseases may initially be thought to have an ILD alone. Therefore, these diagnoses must be considered in patients with ILD, even in the absence of extrathoracic findings. Conversely, because pulmonary involvement is a major cause of death in patients with connective tissue diseases, the presence of ILD should be carefully sought in affected patients. All forms of idiopathic interstitial pneumonia can occur in patients with connective tissue diseases. The natural history of ILD complicating connective tissue diseases is variable, especially because coexisting pulmonary vascular disease or nonparenchymal pulmonary involvement may be present.

PROGRESSIVE SYSTEMIC SCLEROSIS

Of the connective tissue diseases, progressive systemic sclerosis is most frequently associated with ILD. Pulmonary symptoms may antedate cutaneous or digital manifestations of the disease by several years. Most patients affected have nonspecific interstitial pneumonia, with a minority having a usual interstitial pneumonia pattern, and DLCO levels correlate with mortality. Pulmonary hypertension, which can occur in the absence of pulmonary fibrosis, may result in cor pulmonale. Patients with chronic pulmonary fibrosis also have an increased risk for bronchogenic carcinoma, usually either bronchoalveolar cell carcinoma or adenocarcinoma. In a controlled trial, treatment with cyclophosphamide (50-100 mg/day orally) for 1 year stabilized the PFT findings and improved health-related quality of life in patients with scleroderma-related ILD.[A13]

RHEUMATOID ARTHRITIS

Although rheumatoid arthritis is more common in women (2:1 to 4:1 ratio), ILD associated with rheumatoid arthritis is more common in men

(3 : 1 ratio). Most cases occur at 50 to 60 years of age, and pulmonary symptoms follow the onset of arthritis in about 75% of cases. Lung involvement in rheumatoid arthritis may take many forms, but bronchiectasis, bronchiolitis, idiopathic interstitial pneumonias, and pleural effusions or pleural thickening are some of the most common. Early in the course, the histologic changes are similar to those of idiopathic interstitial pneumonias, including pulmonary fibrosis, but are distinguished by a prominent lymphocytic infiltrate that may contain germinal follicles adjacent to vessels and airways. As the disease progresses, the infiltration becomes less pronounced and is replaced by fibrous tissue, honeycomb changes, or both. Other pulmonary manifestations include pulmonary nodules, vasculitis, pulmonary hypertension, and Caplan syndrome (progressive upper lobe nodular pulmonary fibrosis in a coal miner with rheumatoid arthritis) but are relatively rare. Treatment is directed at the underlying rheumatoid arthritis (Chapter 264).

SYSTEMIC LUPUS ERYTHEMATOSUS

Pulmonary abnormalities complicating SLE (Chapter 266) may vary greatly. Pleural disease or pleural effusions (or both) are commonly present in lung disease that complicates SLE. Acute lupus pneumonitis may mimic acute interstitial pneumonia, with widespread ground-glass attenuation admixed with consolidation, or it may manifest as diffuse alveolar hemorrhage. Chronic ILD may also occur. Infection must always be considered in acutely ill patients who have received steroids or other immunosuppressive therapy. Rarely, the restrictive lung defect, which may be predominantly a result of diaphragmatic weakness, leads to a chest radiographic pattern of small-appearing lungs that may look progressively smaller over time. This so-called "shrinking lung" is generally resistant to corticosteroids or other immunosuppressive agents used to treat SLE. Otherwise, treatment of the ILD is similar to treatment of the underlying SLE.

DERMATOMYOSITIS AND POLYMYOSITIS

In contrast to progressive systemic sclerosis, the pattern of lung involvement in dermatomyositis and polymyositis is more heterogeneous. Usual interstitial pneumonia, nonspecific interstitial pneumonia, and organizing pneumonia have all been reported. Most patients have anti–Jo-1 antibody, and the disease is typically progressive over time. An acute interstitial pneumonia–like syndrome occurs in a subset of patients and is associated with high mortality rate despite aggressive immunosuppressive agents and high-dose corticosteroids. ILD may precede the muscular manifestations by months to years or be superimposed on established muscle disease. The severity of the muscular disease does not correlate with that of the ILD. Treatment is directed at the underlying disease (Chapter 269).

SJÖGREN SYNDROME

Interstitial lung disease is seen in patients with Sjögren syndrome, particularly those with the primary form of the disease. LIP is the most frequent subtype, but cryptogenic organizing pneumonia may also be present. Respiratory infections and bronchiectasis are common in advanced stages, perhaps because of inspissated mucus. Response to corticosteroid or immunosuppressive therapy is usually good (Chapter 268).

MIXED CONNECTIVE TISSUE DISEASE

This overlap syndrome (Chapter 267) combines features of progressive systemic sclerosis, SLE, rheumatoid arthritis, and polymyositis or dermatomyositis. Pulmonary disease is common, but it is most often subclinical and identified only radiographically. Treatment includes corticosteroids and other immune-modulating agents for the underlying disease.

ANKYLOSING SPONDYLITIS

The most common pulmonary manifestation of ankylosing spondylitis (Chapter 265) is upper lobe, bilateral reticulonodular infiltrates with cyst formation as a result of parenchymal destruction. There is no known effective therapy for this apical fibrobullous disease.

HYPERSENSITIVITY PNEUMONITIS

PATHOBIOLOGY

Hypersensitivity pneumonitis, also known as extrinsic allergic alveolitis, is a syndrome caused by repeated inhalation of specific antigens from occupational or environmental exposure (Chapters 93 and 94) in sensitized individuals. Within a short period after inhalation of an inciting agent, patients develop a nonspecific diffuse pneumonitis with inflammatory cell infiltration of the bronchioles, alveoli, and interstitium, sometimes associated with a pleural effusion. In the subacute and chronic stages, loosely formed, noncaseating, epithelioid cell granulomas and a mononuclear infiltrate may be dispersed in the interstitium. Hypersensitivity pneumonitis can occur with exposure to a wide range of inhaled antigens (Chapters 93 and 94). Some of the more common exposures are farmer's lung, bird fancier's lung, parakeet keeper's lung, and pigeon breeder's lung. The exposure to an avian antigen may be occult and related to bird droppings or bird nests. Hobbies (woodworker's lung) and recreational activities (sauna taker's lung; hot tub) may be implicated as well as occupations.

CLINICAL MANIFESTATIONS

The clinical features and severity of symptoms vary according to the frequency and intensity of exposure. A history of exposure to potential agents or changes in the domestic and other environments (or both) is essential to diagnosis and treatment (Chapters 19 and 93). The interval between exposure to the antigen and the clinical manifestations of lung disease is unknown, although symptoms can occur as soon as 4 to 12 hours after exposure. In such cases, fever and chills are common symptoms, are often temporally related to the workplace or to hobbies, and may actually disappear on vacations or during absence from the site of exposure, only to recur when exposure is resumed. In more chronic and low-level exposures, however, the onset is insidious. Some patients with chronic hypersensitivity pneumonitis owing to many years of exposure may manifest clinical features similar to those of patients with idiopathic pulmonary fibrosis.

DIAGNOSIS

Findings on chest radiography are diverse, with focal patchy consolidation or a diffuse ground-glass appearance in acute hypersensitivity pneumonitis (E-Fig. 92-E6); micronodular and reticular shadowing in subacute forms; and diffuse, predominantly upper lung zone reticulation with honeycombing in the chronic form. Chest radiograph results may be normal in up to 30% of patients with significant physiologic abnormalities.

On HRCT, small centrilobular ill-defined nodules of ground-glass densities are seen, along with evidence of mosaic attenuation (trapped air) as a result of concomitant bronchiolitis and upper lobe predominance of the parenchymal abnormalities (E-Fig. 92-E7). Chronically, findings of lung fibrosis may be indistinguishable from the patterns seen in usual interstitial pneumonia and idiopathic pulmonary fibrosis (E-Fig. 92-E8).

Precipitating serum antibodies for potential causes of hypersensitivity pneumonitis confirm exposure but not cause and effect, and the absence of antibodies does not exclude hypersensitivity pneumonitis. In some cases, a thorough investigation of the patient's home and workplace by an industrial hygienist may reveal occult molds, spores, *Thermoactinomycetes* spp., *Aureobasidium pullulans*, and other precipitating causes. When such exposures are evident and suspected to be the cause of the manifested ILD, further diagnostic interventions such as BAL may be quite helpful by showing the most marked increase in T lymphocytes and an increased number of plasma cells. The characteristic histologic triad in hypersensitivity pneumonitis is cellular nonspecific interstitial pneumonia, cellular bronchiolitis, and granulomatous inflammation; however, this triad is seen in no more than 75% of affected patients. Differentiation from cellular nonspecific interstitial pneumonia may be challenging. Prompted by an elicited history of environmental exposure for an attributable antigen, bronchochallenge testing with the suspected antigen in experienced laboratories may provide further clues for the diagnosis of hypersensitivity pneumonitis in a patient otherwise suspected to have idiopathic pulmonary fibrosis. A subset of patients who meet the diagnostic criteria for idiopathic pulmonary fibrosis may be subsequently diagnosed as having chronic hypersensitivity pneumonitis after careful evaluation by experts who are familiar with hypersensitivity pneumonitis.[10]

TREATMENT AND PROGNOSIS Rx

A thorough investigation must be undertaken to identify the antigen in the patient's environment. Sometimes an industrial hygienist is needed to obtain samples for culture from potential sources in the patient's domestic or workplace environment. The identified antigen must be eradicated from the patient's environment. Avoidance of exposure to the identified antigen or antigens and treatment with corticosteroids (see Table 92-5) are important if improvement is to be obtained. However, despite thorough searches, the antigen may remain undetected in a substantial number of patients who have hypersensitivity pneumonitis confirmed by lung biopsy. Continued exposure to the unidentifiable antigens, prolonged exposure to antigens, or both can lead to chronic hypersensitivity pneumonitis and irreversible fibrosis that may not respond to any treatment regimen. In the fibrotic stages, the prognosis and clinical course may be similar to those of idiopathic pulmonary fibrosis.

OCCUPATIONAL INTERSTITIAL LUNG DISEASES

Interstitial lung diseases associated with specific occupations generally involve the inhalation and deposition of dust in the lungs followed by a tissue reaction that ultimately results in fibrosis. Examples include silicosis (inhalation of silica in crystalline form or silicon dioxide as quartz, cristobalite, or tridymite; at-risk occupations include sandblasting and working with granite), coal workers' pneumoconiosis (inhalation of coal dust), asbestosis (deposition of fibers during mining, milling, or other handling of asbestos; welding and working in a shipyard are two at-risk occupations), berylliosis (seen in aerospace workers and in electronic industries), and hard metal disease (Chapter 93). Radiographic features vary depending on the inciting inhalant. Cessation of the exposure is important, but the fibrosis is generally irreversible.

DRUG-INDUCED INTERSTITIAL LUNG DISEASE

More than 300 drugs, biomolecules, or homeopathic remedies (see Table 92-2) can cause acute, subacute, or chronic ILD, and the list continues to increase as new medications are introduced. The clinical and radiographic manifestations are quite varied. Examples of known syndromes include chronic nitrofurantoin-induced ILD that mimics idiopathic pulmonary fibrosis (and is fatal in ≈8% of cases), granulomatous pneumonitis secondary to methotrexate (<5%), sarcoid-like granulomatous ILD induced by interferon-α and tumor necrosis factor modulating agents, nonspecific bilateral alveolar and interstitial inflammatory and fibrotic abnormalities caused by bleomycin and other chemotherapeutic agents, and alveolar and interstitial abnormalities and nodular densities in acute and chronic amiodarone pulmonary toxicity. Most drug-induced ILD is reversible if recognized early and if use of the responsible drug is discontinued. In addition to discontinuing the implicated drug, treatment with corticosteroids (see Table 92-5) is indicated in patients with moderate to severe functional impairment.

Alveolar Filling Disorders

In alveolar filling disorders (Chapter 91), air spaces distal to the terminal bronchioles are filled with blood, lipid, protein, water, or inflammatory cells. The radiographic appearance is that of an alveolar infiltrate with small nodular densities and ill-defined margins; hence, the radiographic picture is similar to an ILD, and virtually all the alveolar filling disorders may result in ILD, including Goodpasture syndrome, pulmonary alveolar proteinosis (primary and secondary), alveolar hemorrhage syndromes (Chapter 91), acute interstitial pneumonia, and bronchoalveolar cell carcinoma (Chapter 191).

IDIOPATHIC PULMONARY HEMOSIDEROSIS

This rare disorder of children and young adults is characterized by intermittent, diffuse alveolar hemorrhage without evidence of vasculitis, inflammation, granulomas, or necrosis. The etiology is poorly understood. Anemia and hepatosplenomegaly may be present. Hemosiderin-laden macrophages in BAL fluid and lung tissue are part of the diagnostic picture. The chest radiograph reveals diffuse, bilateral alveolar infiltrates. A chronic interstitial infiltrate may develop after repeated episodes, infrequently with hilar and mediastinal adenopathy. Systemic corticosteroids (see Table 92-5) may be beneficial in treating acute disease.

CHRONIC EOSINOPHILIC PNEUMONIA

The clinical manifestation of chronic eosinophilic pneumonia varies over a wide spectrum, from asymptomatic to respiratory failure. The disease often occurs in women in the second to fourth decades of life; such women often manifest constitutional symptoms of fevers, sweats, weight loss, fatigue, dyspnea, and cough. Peripheral blood eosinophilia (Chapter 170), usually at levels of 10% to 40%, is common but may be absent in up to one third of affected patients at initial evaluation. On chest radiography and HRCT, the cardinal feature is peripheral multifocal consolidation, predominantly in the upper and mid lung zones. These dense peripheral infiltrates, which have sometimes been called the "photographic negative of pulmonary edema," often resolve dramatically after treatment with corticosteroids. Ground-glass attenuation commonly accompanies the consolidation. BAL fluid may show greater than 40% eosinophils during exacerbations. Treatment with corticosteroids (see Table 92-5) results in a rapid response, frequently within hours; in fact, such a dramatic resolution of symptoms with radiographic clearance of infiltrates shortly after initiation of corticosteroid therapy is considered "diagnostic." However, the rate of relapse is high, so most patients require prolonged treatment with low-dose corticosteroids (prednisone, 5-10 mg/day) to stay in remission.

Interstitial Lung Disease Associated with Pulmonary Vasculitides

GRANULOMATOSIS WITH POLYANGIITIS (FORMERLY KNOWN AS WEGENER GRANULOMATOSIS)

Granulomatosis with polyangiitis (Chapter 270) is the most common form of vasculitis that involves the lung. The systemic necrotizing granulomatous inflammation and small-vessel vasculitis are often manifested first in the upper respiratory tract as chronic rhinitis or sinusitis (or both), epistaxis, oropharyngeal ulcerations, gingival hyperplasia with clefting, or serous otitis media. Destruction of the nasal cartilage may lead to septal perforation or a saddle nose deformity. Ulcerative lesions of the tracheobronchial tree, cavitating nodules within the lung parenchyma, and diffuse alveolar hemorrhage caused by pulmonary capillaritis are lower respiratory tract manifestations. Focal segmental necrotizing glomerulonephritis is the most common extrathoracic manifestation, although pulmonary involvement may occur without renal disease. Chest radiography usually reveals multiple nodular or cavitating infiltrates, but single nodules may be found as well. The diagnosis is most commonly made serologically, with demonstration of antineutrophil cytoplasmic antibodies, although a negative test result does not exclude the disease. Treatment is usually with cyclophosphamide (50-100 mg/day or 2 mg/kg of ideal body weight per day but not more than 150 mg/day) in conjunction with oral corticosteroids (prednisone, 10-40 mg/day). Initial remission occurs in more than 90% of patients, but most patients require treatment for several years. Relapses may occur in up to 30% of patients, especially when treatment is tapered; such patients may need treatment indefinitely. Rituximab is an alternative if cyclophosphamide is unsuccessful or not tolerated (Chapter 270). Prophylaxis for *Pneumocystis jiroveci* infection is indicated in patients receiving chronic treatment.

CHURG-STRAUSS SYNDROME (ALLERGIC ANGIITIS)

This systemic necrotizing vasculitis (Chapter 270) affects both the upper and lower respiratory tracts and is almost invariably preceded by allergic disorders such as asthma, allergic rhinitis, sinusitis, or a drug reaction. Peripheral and lung eosinophilia, bronchospasm, increased immunoglobulin E levels, and rashes are common manifestations. The pulmonary radiographic findings are bilateral patchy, fleeting infiltrates; diffuse nodular infiltrates; or diffuse reticulonodular disease. Histopathologic examination of lung tissue is generally diagnostic with features of granulomatous angiitis or vasculitis. Although treatment with corticosteroids is indicated, the dosage and duration are unclear (see Table 92-5).

IDIOPATHIC PULMONARY CAPILLARITIS

Idiopathic pulmonary capillaritis may involve the pulmonary vasculature within the alveolar walls and be manifested as ILD. Patients may also have subclinical alveolar hemorrhage, often associated with the presence of perinuclear antineutrophilic cytoplasmic antibodies. Corticosteroids are the mainstay of treatment, but the doses and duration of treatment are unclear. Frequently, patients need adjunctive treatment with cyclophosphamide or rituximab, similar to patients with vasculitis and granulomatosis with polyangiitis (Chapter 270).

Other Forms of Interstitial Lung Disease

SARCOIDOSIS

See Chapter 95.

PULMONARY LANGERHANS CELL HISTIOCYTOSIS

This condition, previously known as pulmonary histiocytosis X or eosinophilic granuloma of the lung, is an idiopathic, granulomatous ILD that typically occurs in the second or third decade of life; there is a male preponderance. The currently accepted term is *Langerhans cell histiocytosis*. Pulmonary Langerhans cell histiocytosis is rare, with an estimated incidence of two to five cases per million population. The large majority (~90%) of affected individuals are male smokers, and current evidence suggests that the disorder results from an abnormal immune response to a component or derivative of cigarette smoke.

CLINICAL MANIFESTATIONS

The clinical findings are variable and range from an abnormal chest radiograph in an asymptomatic patient to progressive dyspnea with a nonproductive cough. Systemic symptoms of malaise, fever, and weight loss may be present. Hemoptysis is rare. Spontaneous pneumothorax, which occurs in approximately 25% of patients and is caused by rupture of subpleural cysts, may be an initial finding. Langerhans cell histiocytosis may be confined to the lung or may be a component of a multisystem disease that includes painful cystic bone lesions and diabetes insipidus (Chapter 225).

DIAGNOSIS

The chest radiograph shows diffuse symmetrical reticulonodular opacities superimposed on multiple small cysts in the upper and mid lung zones. HRCT reveals subpleural nodules; scattered ground-glass densities; and irregular cysts of varying number, size, and configuration in both lungs, with sparing of the lung bases (E-Fig. 92-E9). In the appropriate clinical setting, this pattern may be pathognomonic. As the disease progresses, the increase in fibrosis and cysts may lead to honeycombing of the lung. PFTs are characterized by a mixed restrictive and obstructive pattern, including a reduction in diffusing capacity. Vital capacity is disproportionately reduced compared with TLC because of air trapping within the cysts; the result is an increased residual volume. BAL reveals Langerhans cells (atypical histiocytes) that have the characteristic "x body" (i.e., Birbeck granule) on electron microscopy; immunostaining shows CD1 antigen on the cell surface and S-100 protein in the cytoplasm. However, the absence of these findings does not exclude the diagnosis. The diagnosis is usually made by transbronchial biopsy or open lung biopsy, which reveals interstitial and peribronchiolar collections of histiocytes, eosinophils, and lymphocytes; peribronchiolar nodules; and cysts with areas of central stellate fibrosis.

TREATMENT AND PROGNOSIS

Although definitive regression after discontinuation of smoking has not been proved, small series report improvement, so patients should be encouraged to discontinue smoking. The prognosis in pulmonary Langerhans cell histiocytosis is usually favorable, with approximately 75% of patients improving or stabilizing, especially with cessation of smoking; some patients, however, may progress to end-stage lung disease. In patients with progressive disease, corticosteroids (see Table 92-5) with or without vincristine, arabinoside, cyclosporine, cyclophosphamide, and azathioprine have been used with some anecdotal reports of success. Lung transplantation has been performed, but recurrent disease has been reported in the allograft.

LYMPHANGIOLEIOMYOMATOSIS

This rare ILD is limited to women, primarily of childbearing age. Proliferation of abnormal smooth muscle around bronchioles leads to bilateral small cysts, which give an appearance of ILD on chest radiographs, and progressive impairment of lung function. Hemoptysis, pneumothorax (from rupture of subpleural cysts), and chylothorax (from lymphatic obstruction) may be initial symptoms that distinguish this disorder from other diffuse lung diseases. Although lymphangioleiomyomatosis is usually limited to the lungs, an association with angiomyolipomas of the mediastinal and retroperitoneal lymph nodes and kidney has been described, so the disease may mimic the manifestations of tuberous sclerosis (Chapter 417). Coarse reticulonodular infiltrates, often with cysts or bullae, are typically seen on chest radiographs. In contrast to most other ILDs, increased lung volumes may be present and should prompt consideration of this diagnosis in a nonsmoking woman of reproductive age. HRCT shows characteristic diffuse thin-walled cysts, generally less than 2 cm in diameter. BAL may show occult alveolar hemorrhage (E-Fig. 92-E10). Lung biopsy reveals abnormal smooth muscle cells lining the airways, lymphatics, and blood vessels, with concurrent airflow obstruction and replacement of the lung parenchyma with cysts.

TREATMENT AND PROGNOSIS

In a randomized trial, sirolimus, an inhibitor of rapamycin signaling, initially at 2 mg/day and titrated to maintain trough levels between 5 and 15 ng/mL, was safe and stabilized lung function.[A14] Treatment with progesterone or tamoxifen has been tried, but no randomized trials support the use of interventions to alter the estrogen–progesterone balance. Although lung transplantation is indicated as the patient reaches severe functional impairment, the disease may recur in the transplanted lung. Most patients currently die of respiratory failure about 10 years after the onset of symptoms.

Inherited Disorders

Several rare genetic disorders are associated with ILD and pulmonary fibrosis. Inheritance is autosomal dominant with variable penetrance for most cases of familial idiopathic pulmonary fibrosis and familial idiopathic interstitial pneumonia and for tuberous sclerosis (Chapter 417), neurofibromatosis (Chapter 417), and familial hypocalciuric hypercalcemia (Chapter 245). Inheritance is autosomal recessive for Gaucher disease (Chapter 208), Niemann-Pick disease (Chapter 208), and Hermansky-Pudlak syndrome (Chapter 208). The congenital form of the alveolar filling disorder pulmonary alveolar proteinosis also is inherited in an autosomal recessive manner.

Tuberous sclerosis (Chapter 417), an autosomal dominant disease of variable penetrance, is characterized pathologically by the presence of hamartomas in multiple organs. The most well-known clinical manifestations include epilepsy, mental retardation, adenoma sebaceum, and renal angiomyolipomas. ILD occurs in only 1% of patients with tuberous sclerosis, usually in women older than 30 years with little or no mental retardation. The pulmonary involvement, which is indistinguishable from lymphangioleiomyomatosis both radiographically and histopathologically, may be manifested as exertional dyspnea, recurrent pneumothorax, and hemoptysis. HRCT reveals thin-walled cysts and a diffuse reticulonodular infiltrate. Recurrent parenchymal hemorrhage may lead to hemosiderin deposition and interstitial pulmonary fibrosis. There is no cure, and treatment is supportive.

Neurofibromatosis (Chapter 417) may affect all age groups and both sexes. Type 1 (von Recklinghausen disease) is characterized by cafe au lait spots, neurofibromas, optic glioma, and bony lesions; the more rare type 2 is associated with bilateral acoustic neuromas. Diffuse ILD is manifested as bilateral lower lobe fibrosis as well as bullae or cystic changes. Interstitial fibrosis and alveolitis with thickening of the alveolar septa, accompanied by a cellular infiltrate, are seen on lung biopsy. Management is as for idiopathic pulmonary fibrosis.

Gaucher disease (Chapter 208), a lysosomal glycolipid storage disorder, has a predilection for the Ashkenazi Jewish population. Pulmonary manifestations, which occur most frequently in type 2 disease, may be a result of interstitial infiltration by Gaucher cells with fibrosis, alveolar consolidation, and filling of alveolar spaces; capillary plugging by Gaucher cells may cause secondary pulmonary hypertension. Treatment is as for the systemic disease, and the general approaches for idiopathic interstitial pneumonias and pulmonary arterial hypertension may be followed for these patients.

Niemann-Pick disease (Chapter 208) is a rare lipid storage disease that may cause infiltration of the characteristic "foam cell" throughout the pulmonary lymphatics, the pulmonary arteries, and the pulmonary alveoli. Patients with type B may survive into adulthood. Treatment is as for the systemic disease.

Hermansky-Pudlak syndrome (Chapter 208) is characterized by oculocutaneous albinism, a bleeding diathesis, and ceroid inclusions in macrophages. Most patients are of Puerto Rican ancestry, and women are affected more frequently than men. Pulmonary fibrosis, with onset in the third or fourth decade, is slowly progressive. Treatment principles and interventions are largely supportive and extrapolated from other related conditions, especially idiopathic pulmonary fibrosis.

Grade A References

A1. Corte TJ, Keir GJ, Dimopoulos K, et al. Bosentan in pulmonary hypertension associated with fibrotic idiopathic interstitial pneumonia. *Am J Respir Crit Care Med.* 2014;190:208-217.

A2. Taniguichi H, Ebina M, Kondoh Y, et al. Pirfenidone in idiopathic pulmonary fibrosis. *Eur Respir J.* 2010;35:821-829.

A3. Noble PW, Albera C, Bradford WZ, et al. Pirfenidone in patients with idiopathic pulmonary fibrosis (CAPACITY): two randomised trials. *Lancet.* 2011;377:1760-1769.

A4. King TE Jr, Bradford WZ, Castro-Bernardini S, et al. A phase 3 trial of pirfenidone in patients with idiopathic pulmonary fibrosis. *N Engl J Med.* 2014;370:2083-2092.

A5. Xaubet A, Serrano-Mollar A, Ancochea J. Pirfenidone for the treatment of idiopathic pulmonary fibrosis. *Expert Opin Pharmacother.* 2014;15:275-281.

A6. Richeldi L, du Bois RM, Raghu G, et al. Efficacy and safety of nintedanib in idiopathic pulmonary fibrosis. *N Engl J Med.* 2014;370:2071-2082.

A7. Zisman DA, Schwarz M, Anstrom KJ, et al. A controlled trial of sildenafil in advanced idiopathic pulmonary fibrosis. *N Engl J Med.* 2010;363:620-628.

A8. Lee JS, Collard HR, Anstrom KJ, et al. Anti-acid treatment and disease progression in idiopathic pulmonary fibrosis: an analysis of data from three randomised controlled trials. *Lancet Respir Med.* 2013;1:369-376.

A9. Martinez FJ, de Andrade JA, Anstrom KJ, et al. Randomized trial of acetylcysteine in idiopathic pulmonary fibrosis. *N Engl J Med.* 2014;370:2093-2101.
A10. Raghu G, Anstrom KJ, King TE Jr, et al. Prednisone, azathioprine, and N-acetylcysteine for pulmonary fibrosis. *N Engl J Med.* 2012;366:1968-1977.
A11. Noth I, Anstrom KJ, Calvert SB, et al. A placebo-controlled randomized trial of warfarin in idiopathic pulmonary fibrosis. *Am J Respir Crit Care Med.* 2012;186:88-95.
A12. Raghu G, Behr J, Brown KK, et al. Treatment of idiopathic pulmonary fibrosis with ambrisentan: a parallel, randomized trial. *Ann Intern Med.* 2013;158:641-649.
A13. Tashkin DP, Elashoff R, Clements PJ, et al. Cyclophosphamide versus placebo in scleroderma lung disease. *N Engl J Med.* 2006;354:2655-2666.
A14. McCormack FX, Inoue Y, Moss J, et al. Efficacy and safety of sirolimus in lymphangioleiomyomatosis. *N Engl J Med.* 2011;364:1595-1606.

GENERAL REFERENCES

For the General References and other additional features, please visit Expert Consult at https://expertconsult.inkling.com.

93

OCCUPATIONAL LUNG DISEASE

SUSAN M. TARLO

Occupational lung diseases include a wide spectrum of respiratory disorders with symptoms, signs, and diagnostic test results that often present with features similar to nonoccupational diseases (Table 93-1). For example, adult-onset asthma (Chapter 87) may be occupational asthma, presumed sarcoidosis (Chapter 95) may actually be chronic beryllium disease, apparent idiopathic pulmonary fibrosis may be asbestosis, or a suspected viral pneumonia (Chapter 97) may be hypersensitivity pneumonitis from an occupational cause such as contaminated metal-working fluid.

When evaluating any respiratory disease, the clinician should consider the possibility of an occupational cause or contribution (see E-Fig. 19-1; see Table 93-1). The onset of disease after an occupational exposure may occur with a short latency period, as for an acute toxic inhalation injury, or over a period of months to years, as for occupational asthma or hypersensitivity pneumonitis. Latency can be 20 years or more in chronic beryllium disease or lung cancer from chromium, asbestos, or other carcinogens. The most relevant job and occupational exposure history will therefore depend in part on the type of lung disease: for acute syndromes, the recent job exposure is most relevant; for asthma or hypersensitivity pneumonitis, the exposures at the onset of symptoms and ongoing exposures are most relevant; but for chronic diseases or diseases that may result from a long latency exposure, a full working history is essential. Consideration also should be given to potentially relevant exposures that may be related to a patient's hobbies or avocations (e.g., woodworking, model building, or insect collecting).

The clinical relevance of a correct occupational attribution is most apparent for diseases with a close temporal relationship between exposure and the onset of symptoms because intervention to reduce or remove exposure may reverse the disease or prevent progression. In addition, interventions in the workplace may reduce or prevent disease in other workers. However, even for diseases with a potential long latency, such as chronic beryllium disease, identification of disease in one worker should be regarded as a sentinel event that can lead to investigation of the workplace exposures and introduction of preventive measures. With the assistance of their physicians, workers with occupational lung diseases also often can qualify for workers' compensation.

EPIDEMIOLOGY

No reliable figures exist for the total incidence or prevalence of occupational lung diseases, and regional variation in occupations and exposures is substantial. Work-related asthma has become the most common chronic occupational lung disease in developed countries, where occupational asthma (asthma caused by work) accounts for about 15% of all adult-onset asthma, and work-exacerbated asthma occurs in 25 to 52% of asthmatic workers. The occupational contribution of workplace dusts, fumes, and gases to chronic obstructive pulmonary disease (COPD) is estimated at 15%.

In contrast, pneumoconiosis from silica or coal dust, although still important in developing countries, has declined in incidence in developed countries (E-Fig. 93-1A and B)[1] as a result of occupational hygiene measures. For example, approximately 100,000 Americans received benefits from the Federal Black Lung Program in 2005, compared with about 500,000 in 1980, and the percentage of coal miners with pneumoconiosis has fallen from 11% in the mid-1970s down to 3%. In some states, however, mortality rates have started to rise again, especially in smaller mines. Newer exposures that can cause silicosis include the textile industry's use of jet silica blasting of denim jeans, the use of artificial stone for kitchen counters, and hydraulic fracturing (fracking). Newly recognized asbestos-related diseases continue to occur, owing to the long latency period between exposure and clinical disease, despite the declining exposure to asbestos in developed countries. Although annual deaths from asbestosis have now reached a plateau in North America (E-Fig. 93-1C) and will likely decline, new cases of mesothelioma, which has a latency of up to 35 years or more, are not estimated to plateau until 2020.

Chronic beryllium disease declined in frequency and severity after the elimination of beryllium from fluorescent light bulbs in the 1950s, but then increased because of the increasing use of beryllium in nuclear facilities, aerospace, electronics, dental ceramics, metal alloys, recycling of metals, and products such as golf clubs and bicycles. The beryllium lymphocyte proliferation test can identify beryllium sensitization, which can be found in up to 10% of exposed workers and facilitates earlier diagnosis of chronic beryllium disease.

SPECIFIC OCCUPATIONAL LUNG DISORDERS

Occupational lung diseases are often misdiagnosed as other common nonoccupational diseases, but a careful history and appropriate investigations can lead to a correct diagnosis. For many occupational lung diseases, the diagnosis can significantly improve prognosis and lead to measures to prevent illness in other workers.

Work-Related Asthma

Work-related asthma includes both occupational asthma that is caused by work[2] and asthma that is not caused by work but is exacerbated by work exposures.

SENSITIZER-INDUCED OCCUPATIONAL ASTHMA

EPIDEMIOLOGY

Occupational asthma is most commonly associated with a specific immune response to a high- or low-molecular-weight sensitizer (Table 93-2). Sensitizer-induced occupational asthma usually affects no more than 5 to 10% of workers exposed to the sensitizing agent, but exposure to complex platinum salts or detergent enzymes may result in symptoms in about 50% of highly exposed workers. In most studies, higher levels of exposure are associated with higher rates of sensitization in the exposed populations, but there is no clear threshold exposure below which all workers are protected from the risk for sensitization.

PATHOBIOLOGY

Genetic factors increase the risk for sensitization, but the risks appear to be polygenic and may differ for different allergens and sensitizers. Underlying atopy, as exemplified by a history of allergy or positive skin tests to common environmental allergens (Chapter 249), carries an increased risk for sensitization to the high-molecular-weight allergens, and smoking (Chapter 32) has been reported as a risk factor for sensitization to complex platinum salts. Currently, no host factors are sufficiently specific to justify exclusion of workers from settings with exposure to potential sensitizers.

Occupational asthma from a high-molecular-weight allergen is associated with specific immunoglobulin E (IgE) antibody production. Low-molecular-weight sensitizers may act as haptens or may induce neoantigens by reacting with proteins in vivo, but specific IgE antibodies have been demonstrated with only a few low-molecular-weight sensitizers, such as complex platinum salts and acid anhydrides used in epoxy compounds.

CLINICAL MANIFESTATIONS

Sensitizer-induced occupational asthma has a latency period ranging from weeks to several years before it develops, but most patients develop symptoms within the first few years of exposure. After a patient has become sensitized and has developed asthma, even very small subsequent exposures can trigger asthma, sometimes including exposures that may be below the limit of measurable detection. Pulmonary function and histologic changes are similar to those in nonoccupational asthma (Chapter 87). Sensitizer-induced occupational asthma from a high-molecular-weight agent sensitizer typically causes a prompt asthmatic response within minutes after exposure with or

TABLE 93-1 EXAMPLES OF OCCUPATIONAL RESPIRATORY DISEASES THAT COULD BE MISDIAGNOSED AS COMMON NONOCCUPATIONAL RESPIRATORY DISEASE

DISEASE THAT IS MIMICKED	POSSIBLE OCCUPATIONAL DISEASE	EXAMPLES OF SUGGESTIVE FEATURES LEADING TO A CORRECT DIAGNOSIS
Asthma	Occupational asthma from a work sensitizer	Asthma symptoms begin and are worse during a working period, with some improvement on days or weeks off work. Exposure to a high- or low-molecular-weight workplace sensitizer
	Occupational asthma—irritant induced, including reactive airways dysfunction syndrome	Asthma begins within days after a high-level (accidental) workplace exposure
	Work-exacerbated asthma	Asthma usually began before starting the job or exposure, but severity is worse on days of work, or work exposures to expected asthma triggers or common allergens at work.
COPD	Occupational COPD	Prolonged exposure at work to dusts, fumes, or gases
Pneumonia	Acute hypersensitivity pneumonitis	Symptoms typically resolve within days and recur on re-exposure to the same work trigger (e.g., metal-working fluid, moldy hay, humidifiers)
Acute viral respiratory illness or pneumonia	Humidifier fever, organic dust toxic syndrome, metal fume fever, polymer fume fever, cotton dust fever	Exposure triggers the episodes
Sarcoidosis	Chronic beryllium disease	History of exposure to beryllium dust or fumes up to 30 years or more before onset of disease
	Silicosis	History of exposure; typical radiographic findings of rounded opacities with upper lobe predominance and progressive massive fibrosis, biopsy
Idiopathic pulmonary fibrosis	Asbestosis	History of moderate or high previous asbestos exposure and appropriate latency period, often with other markers of asbestos exposure, such as radiographic evidence of pleural plaques
	Chronic hypersensitivity pneumonitis	± Work exposure to a known trigger, ± improvement during periods away from exposure
	Flock-worker's lung	Lymphocytic bronchiolitis and interstitial lung disease from nylon/synthetic textile microfibers
Idiopathic pulmonary fibrosis or alveolar proteinosis	Indium lung	Exposure to indium-tin oxide in making of flat screens
Idiopathic pulmonary fibrosis or hypersensitivity pneumonitis	Hard metal disease	History of exposure to hard metal (tungsten, cobalt), and histologic findings of giant cell pneumonitis on lung biopsy
Chest infections	Occupational causes of chest infections, e.g., SARS or TB in health care workers, histoplasmosis in construction workers, anthrax in wool workers or farmers	History of occupation and exposures
Pleural effusion	Asbestos-related benign pleural effusion	Previous asbestos exposure with appropriate latency; pleural plaques commonly present
Incidental pulmonary nodule	Rounded atelectasis from asbestos	Previous asbestos exposure with appropriate latency; pleural plaques commonly present
Multiple nodules	Silicosis or pneumoconiosis	History of exposure, distribution of nodules, presence of progressive massive fibrosis
Lung cancer	Occupational lung cancer	History of exposure to carcinogens at work, with an appropriate latency period (e.g., asbestos, radon, chromium)
Bronchiolitis obliterans	Popcorn lung	History of working with microwave popcorn or flavorings
	Bronchiolitis in military personnel	History of deployment in South-East Asia with exposure to burn-pits and other irritants

COPD = chronic obstructive pulmonary disease; SARS = severe acute respiratory syndrome; TB = tuberculosis.

without a late asthmatic response starting 4 to 6 hours after exposure. By comparison, responses to low-molecular-weight sensitizers typically start 4 to 6 hours after exposure.

DIAGNOSIS

The diagnosis of sensitizer-induced occupation asthma is clinically suspected by history and should be considered in all cases of new-onset asthma in patients who work. Supportive features include symptomatic improvement when away from work, such as weekends off work or holidays, but not necessarily in the evenings after a work shift, when symptoms from a late asthmatic response may occur. In patients who are exposed to high-molecular-weight sensitizers, allergic rhinitis or conjunctivitis associated with work frequently appears before the development of asthma. A detailed occupational history (Chapter 19) or review of material safety data sheets or occupational hygiene reports may reveal a known occupational sensitizer. However, more than 300 occupational respiratory sensitizers are currently known, and new agents or exposures are reported each year; as a result, the absence of a recognized sensitizer does not exclude occupational asthma.

Although the history can be very helpful, the evaluation should always include objective pulmonary function testing (Chapter 85) to confirm asthma, either when the patient has symptoms or within 24 hours of the typical suspected work exposure (Fig. 93-1). Allergy skin-prick tests, blood samples, or both should be obtained to test for specific IgE antibodies to any relevant sensitizer if feasible. Serial monitoring of peak expiratory flow rates, symptom diaries, or use of rescue inhalers can provide supportive information. The results of a methacholine challenge test (Chapter 87) toward the end of a typical work week can help when compared with results after 10 days or more without exposure. A comparison of eosinophil counts in induced sputum at work and after a period away from exposure, showing higher levels when exposed, provides supportive diagnostic information. If the diagnosis is still in doubt, a carefully controlled specific inhalation challenge with the suspected workplace sensitizer can be performed. Each investigation can be falsely positive or negative, so a combination of investigations is advised while the patient continues to work until the diagnosis is confirmed. Given the specialized nature of many of these studies, consultation with a specialist is recommended. The main differential diagnosis for patients with confirmed asthma is the coincidental onset of asthma with subsequent work-exacerbated asthma. Other conditions, such as vocal cord dysfunction, may explain symptoms or may coexist with asthma and confound the diagnosis.

TABLE 93-2 COMMON CAUSES OF SENSITIZER-INDUCED OCCUPATIONAL ASTHMA

OCCUPATION	ALLERGEN BY SETTING
Bakers	Wheat, rye, fungal amylase in flour
Laboratory workers	Animal allergens, e.g., proteins in rat urine, mouse or rabbit dander
Detergent-making, medical instrument cleaning, pharmaceuticals or laboratory workers	Enzymes: e.g., *Bacillus subtilis*, pancreatic enzymes
Farmers	Grains, plant, and animal allergens; mites
Greenhouse workers and florists	Pollen, fungi, mites
Food workers	Airborne food allergens, e.g., powdered milk or eggs and vegetables
Some office workers	Fungal allergens in moldy or "sick" buildings
Health care workers	Latex allergens from gloves, glutaraldehyde, orthophthaldehyde, aerosolized medications
Factory or other industrial workers	Chemicals in spray paints, glues, polyurethane, coatings and spray insulation, adhesives
Electronic workers	Soldering flux with colophony

TREATMENT AND PREVENTION (Rx)

The optimal management of patients with sensitizer-induced occupational asthma includes complete removal from further exposure to the sensitizer and cross-reacting agents combined with the usual pharmacologic approach to the treatment of asthma (Chapter 87) and advocacy for appropriate workers' compensation.[3] Consideration of the other exposed workers typically includes communication with the workplace or public health officials, in the hope that measures may be instituted to protect other workers from similar exposures and symptoms. Recommendations for primary prevention have been to reduce exposures to occupational sensitizers as far as possible, removing unnecessary sensitizing agents (e.g., removing high-powdered and high-protein latex gloves) and limiting exposures to sensitizers with occupational hygiene measures. Ongoing medical surveillance measures in the workplace may also be of value.

PROGNOSIS

Outcome is best if an early diagnosis results in removal from further exposure while asthma is relatively mild. Improvement may continue to occur up to 10 years after removal from exposure, but asthma does not completely resolve in most patients. For patients with occupational asthma from natural rubber latex, use of powder-free, low-protein latex gloves by coworkers and direct avoidance of natural rubber products by the sensitized worker result in improvement that is similar to the improvement in patients who are completely removed from work.

WORK-EXACERBATED ASTHMA

EPIDEMIOLOGY AND CLINICAL MANIFESTATIONS

Work-exacerbated asthma is defined as asthma that is not caused by work but is aggravated or exacerbated by work conditions.[4] Asthma may have been present before starting employment or may begin coincidentally during employment, but it is not caused by work. Work exposures that commonly exacerbate asthma include extreme temperature or humidity, exertion, dusts, fumes, and gases. Patients may be exposed at work to common environmental allergens (e.g., fungal allergens in an office setting or dust mites or animals in domestic settings) that exacerbate asthma in patients who are sensitized to these allergens. Symptoms of work-exacerbated asthma may occur transiently with an unusual work exposure (e.g., during renovation in a work building) or may occur on a daily basis (e.g., daily exposure to fumes while performing physical exertion in an industrial setting).

DIAGNOSIS AND TREATMENT (Rx)

Transient work-exacerbated asthma is commonly diagnosed on the basis of the history of work exposures and the associated increase in asthmatic symptoms, medication requirements, or unscheduled physician visits. The recommended evaluation of patients with daily or frequent work exacerbations of asthma is similar to that for patients with suspected occupational asthma. Work-related changes in serial peak flow recordings mimic those seen in occupational asthma, but sputum eosinophil counts typically show less of a work-related increase than is observed with occupational asthma. If the workplace exposure includes a potential work sensitizer, immunologic testing or a controlled challenge exposure may confirm whether respiratory sensitization has occurred.

Management includes the same pharmacologic measures as for non-work-related exacerbations, including the optimization of pharmacologic asthma management (Chapter 87) and, when needed, adjusting the work exposures to avoid ongoing exacerbations. Occupational hygiene measures can reduce exposures, but some patients require a change in job description or work area. Workers' compensation may be available for some patients who miss work owing to work-exacerbation of asthma.

Irritant Exposure and Reactive Airways Dysfunction Syndrome

A high level of usually accidental exposure to an irritant agent can cause asthma. Although the clinical manifestations can be dramatic, irritant-induced occupational asthma represents a relatively small proportion of all occupational asthma. The most definitive criteria for this condition are those applied to the term *reactive airways dysfunction syndrome*: the onset of asthma symptoms within 24 hours of the exposure, generally severe enough to lead to an unscheduled physician visit; exposure to a single high-level irritant; asthma symptoms that persist for at least 3 months; pulmonary function testing that confirms asthma with a significant beneficial response to bronchodilators or a bronchoconstrictor response to a methacholine challenge; and the lack of preexisting lung disease or other conditions to explain the symptoms. When these criteria are not completely met (e.g., symptoms start later than 24 hours after exposure or resolve within weeks after exposure), the term *irritant-induced asthma* is commonly applied, recognizing that this diagnosis is less certain than reactive airways dysfunction syndrome. Chronic low-level exposures to cleaning products and other irritants also may precipitate asthma.

Irritant-induced asthma and reactive airways dysfunction syndrome may clear after weeks or months. Management is the same as for other causes of asthma (Chapter 87), although these patients are often less responsive to the usual pharmacologic treatment.

Occupational hygiene measures at the workplace should be improved to prevent similar future exposures. Affected patients may need a modified work environment to prevent subsequent exacerbations of asthma.

OCCUPATIONAL CHRONIC OBSTRUCTIVE PULMONARY DISEASE

Chronic exposure to dusts, fumes, and gases can cause occupationally induced COPD, with pathophysiologic changes essentially identical to those seen in COPD that is related to smoking[5] (Chapter 88). Symptoms of chronic bronchitis, including chronic cough and sputum production, may occur with or without changes on pulmonary function testing. Causes include mineral dusts such as silica and organic dust exposures such as those of farmers and woodworkers; particulate matter in diesel exhaust fumes; and nitrogen oxides, ozone, and ultrafine particles in welding fumes.[6] Occupational exposures such as diacetyl in artificial flavorings and styrene can cause constrictive bronchiolitis.[7]

No specific diagnostic tests distinguish an occupational from a nonoccupational cause of COPD. The history of exposure, with objective documentation, is helpful. Confirmation of the absence of a smoking history can assist in determining probability of an occupational cause. However, a positive smoking history does not exclude an occupational contribution because the two can be synergistic.

Management is the same as for patients with nonoccupational COPD (Chapter 88). In addition, however, further exposure to dusts, fumes, and gases that are likely to worsen disease should be minimized.

HYPERSENSITIVITY PNEUMONITIS

Many exposures that lead to hypersensitivity pneumonitis (Chapters 92 and 94) occur in the workplace, and several bear the name of the occupation or

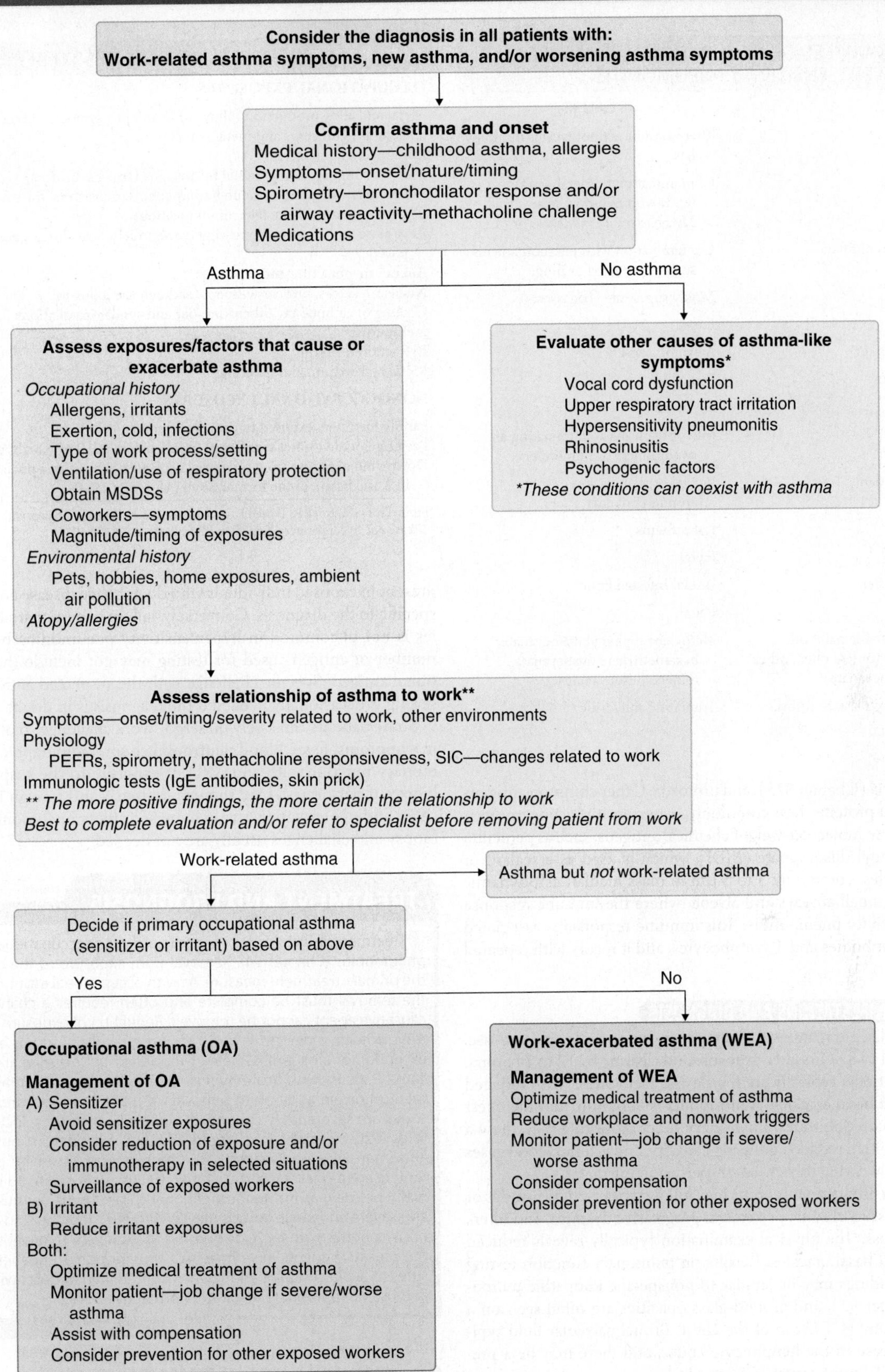

Consider the diagnosis in all patients with:
Work-related asthma symptoms, new asthma, and/or worsening asthma symptoms
Confirm asthma and onset
Medical history—childhood asthma, allergies
Symptoms—onset/nature/timing
Spirometry—bronchodilator response and/or airway reactivity–methacholine challenge
Medications
Asthma
No asthma
Assess exposures/factors that cause or exacerbate asthma
Occupational history
Allergens, irritants
Exertion, cold, infections
Type of work process/setting
Ventilation/use of respiratory protection
Obtain MSDSs
Coworkers—symptoms
Magnitude/timing of exposures
Environmental history
Pets, hobbies, home exposures, ambient air pollution
Atopy/allergies
Evaluate other causes of asthma-like symptoms*
Vocal cord dysfunction
Upper respiratory tract irritation
Hypersensitivity pneumonitis
Rhinosinusitis
Psychogenic factors
*These conditions can coexist with asthma
Assess relationship of asthma to work**
Symptoms—onset/timing/severity related to work, other environments
Physiology
PEFRs, spirometry, methacholine responsiveness, SIC—changes related to work
Immunologic tests (IgE antibodies, skin prick)
** The more positive findings, the more certain the relationship to work
Best to complete evaluation and/or refer to specialist before removing patient from work
Work-related asthma
Asthma but not work-related asthma
Decide if primary occupational asthma (sensitizer or irritant) based on above
Yes
No
Occupational asthma (OA)
Management of OA
A) Sensitizer
Avoid sensitizer exposures
Consider reduction of exposure and/or immunotherapy in selected situations
Surveillance of exposed workers
B) Irritant
Reduce irritant exposures
Both:
Optimize medical treatment of asthma
Monitor patient—job change if severe/worse asthma
Assist with compensation
Consider prevention for other exposed workers
Work-exacerbated asthma (WEA)
Management of WEA
Optimize medical treatment of asthma
Reduce workplace and nonwork triggers
Monitor patient—job change if severe/worse asthma
Consider compensation
Consider prevention for other exposed workers

FIGURE 93-1. **Clinical evaluation and management of work-related asthma. IgE = immunoglobulin E; MSDS = Material Safety Data Sheet; PEFR = peak expiratory flow rates; SIC = specific inhalation challenge. (From American College of Chest Physicians. Consensus statement: diagnosis and management of work-related asthma. *Chest.* 2008;134:1S-41S.)**

job associated with them: farmer's lung; maple bark stripper's lung; cheese washer's lung; thatcher's lung; mushroom worker's lung, and metal-working fluid hypersensitivity pneumonitis (Table 93-3).[8] Occupational causes also include exposure to contaminated humidifiers (with protozoa or fungi) in factories or office buildings (humidifier lung), as well as lifeguards exposed to sprays of water from pool fountains contaminated with microorganisms. Metal workers or machinists can develop hypersensitivity pneumonitis from recirculated coolants that can become contaminated with gram-negative bacteria or atypical mycobacteria, which then are aerosolized in the coolant mist and inhaled.

PATHOBIOLOGY

Most antigenic exposures that lead to hypersensitivity pneumonitis are organic, especially thermophilic actinomycetes (Chapter 329), fungi,

TABLE 93-3 EXAMPLES OF OCCUPATIONAL CAUSES OF HYPERSENSITIVITY PNEUMONITIS

OCCUPATION	CAUSE
Farmer	Thermophilic actinomycetes in moldy hay
Metal worker	Contamination of metal-working fluids with microorganisms such as *Mycobacteria immunogens* or fungi
Worker exposed to humidifiers	Contamination with microorganisms such as protozoa or fungi
Sugarcane worker	Moldy sugarcane (bagassosis)
Maple bark stripper	Fungi
Chicken or turkey worker	Avian proteins
Pharmaceutical worker	Penicillin
Food handler	Soybeans
Office worker	Microorganisms contaminating air conditioners or humidifiers
Swimming pool attendant	Fungal contamination in sprays around pool area
Animal worker	Rat proteins
Mushroom worker	Fungi
Wheat farmer or handler	Weevil-infested flour
Greenhouse worker	Fungi
Workers spraying urethane paint or adhesives/sealants (or less often, other workers using diisocyanate)	Methylene diphenyl diisocyanate, hexamethylene diisocyanate, toluene diisocyanates
Chemical worker using plastics, resins, paints	Trimellitic anhydride

atypical mycobacteria (Chapter 325), and protozoa. Other common antigens include avian and rat proteins. Less commonly, hypersensitivity pneumonitis can be induced by low-molecular-weight chemical antigens, such as penicillin or methylene diphenyl diisocyanate (MDI), which is used as a sealant or binder. Small particles, commonly 3 to 5 μm in mass median aerodynamic diameter, reach the small airways and alveoli, where the immune response leads to hypersensitivity pneumonitis. This immune response is associated with specific IgG antibodies and T lymphocytes, and it recurs with repeated exposures.

CLINICAL MANIFESTATIONS AND DIAGNOSIS

The acute form of disease manifests as cough, dyspnea, chills, and malaise, typically occurring 4 to 8 hours after exposure and clearing by 12 to 24 hours. On examination, patients typically are febrile and tachypneic, with reduced chest expansion and basal crackles. Neutrophilia is common, and the chest radiograph shows acute infiltrates. Pulmonary function testing may show a restrictive pattern, with a reduced diffusing capacity, and arterial blood gases may show hypoxemia owing to ventilation-perfusion mismatch.

Chronic hypersensitivity pneumonitis may follow repeat acute episodes or start de novo. It causes a chronic dry cough, progressive dyspnea, and often, significant weight loss. The physical examination typically reveals reduced chest expansion and basal crackles. Results on pulmonary function testing and radiographic findings may be similar to nonspecific idiopathic pulmonary fibrosis (Chapter 92), and ground-glass opacities are often seen on a computed tomography (CT) scan of the chest. Bronchoalveolar fluid typically shows an increase in the lymphocyte count, and there may be a predominance of CD8 T lymphocytes (Chapter 85).

The specific occupational cause for hypersensitivity pneumonitis may be suspected from a temporal relationship to work exposures. The differential diagnosis in the chronic form includes idiopathic pulmonary fibrosis, although clubbing is less common in hypersensitivity pneumonitis. Radiographic and pulmonary function test findings may also mimic idiopathic pulmonary fibrosis, but a distinguishing finding is often a bronchoalveolar lavage that shows lymphocytes as high as 60 to 80% of the cells, usually with a predominance of $CD8^+$ T lymphocytes but sometimes with $CD4^+$ cells in chronic forms of disease.

Laboratory investigations include determining the presence of serum IgG antibodies to the suspected antigen. However, IgG antibodies may also be

TABLE 93-4 POTENTIAL EXPOSURES TO BERYLLIUM

OCCUPATIONAL EXPOSURES
Metal and alloy production (alloys of aluminum, copper, and nickel; recently includes golf clubs and metal pen clips)
Ceramic manufacturing
Metal casting, including dental technicians (crowns, bridges)
Electronics, including computer components, transistors, microwave and x-ray windows, heat sinks, telecommunications
Aerospace and atomic engineering (rocket fuels, heat shields, nose cones, and metal parts)
Aircraft manufacture and repair
Nuclear reactors, nuclear weapons, and defense industry
Coating of cathode ray tubes for radar and similar installations
Laboratories
Extraction from ore
Metal reclamation and recycling
NONOCCUPATIONAL EXPOSURES
Family members exposed to dust from workers' clothing
Breakage of old fluorescent lamps (made before 1950 in North America)
Downwind exposure from industrial accidents (e.g., from a nuclear processing plant in Kazakhstan, in the former Soviet Union in 1990)

From Tarlo SM, Rhee K, Powell E, et al. Marked tachypnoea in siblings with chronic beryllium disease due to copper-beryllium alloy. *Chest.* 2001;119:647-650.

present in exposed individuals who do not have disease and are therefore not specific to the diagnosis. Conversely, failure to demonstrate specific antibodies is not uncommon in hypersensitivity pneumonitis because the limited number of antigens used for testing may not include the relevant occupational antigen. Specific challenge with the suspected antigen in a laboratory setting is occasionally needed if the diagnosis is in doubt.

Some patients can safely undergo "work challenge" that monitors changes in symptoms, fever, blood neutrophil count, radiographic findings, and pulmonary function with and without exposure to the suspected agent. Lung biopsy, if performed, may show granulomas and foreign body giant cells. If other findings are supportive of hypersensitivity pneumonitis, however, open biopsy and challenges usually are not needed.

TREATMENT AND PROGNOSIS — Rx

Treatment principles are the same as for nonoccupational hypersensitivity pneumonitis (Chapter 94). Removal from exposure to the causative agent is the primary treatment measure. As with occupational asthma from a sensitizer, the removal must be complete and often requires a change in work if the causative agent cannot be removed. Reduction of exposure by use of respiratory protective devices is generally not practical and not effective, with the exception of air-supplied helmet respirators for occasional short-term exposures. Patients with acute hypersensitivity pneumonitis may not require any medications in addition to removal from antigen exposure, but if acute episodes are severe, they may need supportive measures, including corticosteroids (e.g., 20 to 60 mg of prednisone orally per day), supplemental oxygen, and intensive care (Chapter 94). Chronic hypersensitivity pneumonitis may require additional oral corticosteroid treatment (e.g., 5 to 10 mg of prednisone orally per day) as for nonoccupational chronic hypersensitivity pneumonitis, and severe end-stage fibrosis may lead to need for lung transplantation. Prognosis is better with early diagnosis and complete removal from exposure to the causative agent. Preventive measures include occupational hygiene measures to avoid contamination of aerosolized fluid or dusts with bio-organisms and use of appropriate respiratory protective devices.

CHRONIC BERYLLIUM DISEASE

EPIDEMIOLOGY AND PATHOBIOLOGY

Acute toxic pneumonitis was described in workers who had high exposure to beryllium in the manufacture of fluorescent light bulbs in the 1940s, and a hypersensitivity response causing chronic beryllium disease was described in the 1950s. Acute toxic effects are now rare, but chronic beryllium disease remains a problem because of the expanded use of beryllium (Table 93-4) and better recognition of sensitization by development of an immunologic blood test.

Chronic beryllium disease is a hypersensitivity disease with a strong genetic association with HLA-DPB1 gene variants that code for Glu69 and that have been identified in 83 to 97% of patients with disease. However, this gene variant occurs in 30 to 48% of the general population and, as a result, is not useful as a screening test.

CLINICAL MANIFESTATIONS

The pulmonary clinical features of chronic beryllium disease are similar to those of sarcoidosis (Chapter 95), ranging from asymptomatic histologic or radiographic findings, to potential progression, to severe granulomatous restrictive lung disease. Onset can occur up to 20 years or more after exposure to beryllium, even if the patient no longer is exposed. The clinical history in all patients with apparent sarcoidosis must include inquiry about possible beryllium exposure, even many years ago.

DIAGNOSIS AND TREATMENT Rx

The chest radiograph shows changes that appear identical to sarcoidosis with enlarged hilar or mediastinal lymph nodes or multiple lung nodules, or both (Fig. 93-2). Sensitization to beryllium can be detected by a beryllium lymphocyte proliferation test that demonstrates the presence of sensitized lymphocytes in blood or bronchoalveolar lavage fluid. This test also can detect sensitization to beryllium among asymptomatic exposed workers, who can then be evaluated to assess possible chronic beryllium disease and provided with advice for reducing or eliminating further work exposures.

After disease develops, removal from exposure is advised, but the disease may still worsen. Progressive deterioration in lung function is treated similarly to sarcoidosis (Chapter 95), with oral corticosteroids and supportive measures.

ASBESTOS-RELATED DISEASES

Although the use of asbestos has declined, and better protective equipment has been mandated, asbestos-related disease has continued to occur owing to the long latency between exposure and disease. Chrysotile asbestos has less effect on the lungs than other forms of asbestos, that is, amphiboles. Effects of exposure include benign and malignant disease.

Benign asbestos disease is often asymptomatic and identified on chest imaging. Pleural thickening and pleural plaques, commonly with calcification, can occur 20 to 30 years after first exposure and may initially appear on the chest radiograph as calcified linear opacities over the hemidiaphragms and cardiac border (see Fig. 84-14). If extensive, it may be difficult to exclude intrapulmonary opacities except by CT scan. Pleural plaques are a marker of asbestos exposure but do not occur in all workers with significant asbestos exposure. They generally do not cause significant changes in lung function, except that diffuse pleural thickening may result in exertional dyspnea and extrapulmonary restrictive lung disease. Pleural thickening may cause rounded atelectasis (Chapter 90) when encasement of a portion of the peripheral lung tissue by thickened pleura causes an apparent lung nodule, typically with a "comet sign" showing the thickened pleura. Benign pleural effusion can develop, typically about 10 to 15 years after asbestos exposure. It requires further investigation because the differential diagnosis includes malignant pleural effusion (Chapter 99).

Asbestosis is the term for interstitial lung disease caused by asbestos. The clinical presentation is usually with dry cough and dyspnea on exertion. Physical examination usually reveals digital clubbing and basal crackles on lung auscultation. Chest imaging shows basal interstitial lung disease, with or without additional pleural changes as described earlier. Pulmonary function testing shows restrictive lung disease (Chapter 85), and histologic findings are the same as in usual interstitial pneumonia (Chapter 92). Findings supporting the diagnosis of asbestosis rather than usual interstitial pneumonia include a significant duration and level of exposure to asbestos, an appropriate latency of usually 20 to 40 years after first exposure, and the finding of ferruginous asbestos bodies in sputum or lung tissue (Fig. 93-3). Unfortunately, pharmacologic treatment is not effective, and the lung disease may progress to end-stage fibrosis. Management is supportive, including supplemental oxygen and consideration for lung transplantation (Chapter 101). As with the other diseases of long latency, preventing exposure is paramount.

Mesothelioma (Chapter 191), a malignant tumor of the pleura, peritoneum, or both, is the one complication of asbestos exposure that can occur after even relatively minor exposure, such as second-hand exposure from dust on clothing in the families of those working with exposure. It typically occurs 30 to 40 years after exposure to asbestos and may present incidentally on chest imaging or with chest pain or weight loss. Radiographs show pleural thickening, and a pleural effusion may be present. Mesothelioma often is difficult to distinguish from benign pleural thickening without a biopsy. No treatment has proved effective (Chapter 191), so routine screening to detect mesothelioma in exposed persons is not currently recommended. The risk for lung cancer (Chapter 191) increases after significant exposure to asbestos, with a usual latency period of 20 to 30 years. Smoking and asbestos exposure have additive effects, whereas smoking and asbestosis have even greater effects on the risk for lung cancer.

SILICOSIS AND OTHER PNEUMOCONIOSES

The incidences of silicosis and other inorganic dust diseases of the lungs (Table 93-5) have declined substantially in recent decades owing to better worksite protection in mines, sandblasting, and other settings. There is an association between silicosis and the development of collagen vascular disease, especially rheumatoid arthritis. Patients with pneumoconiosis and rheumatoid arthritis may be at higher risk for developing rheumatoid nodules in the lung, so-called Caplan syndrome, and mycobacterial infections.

Patients may initially be identified incidentally during a medical surveillance program or by a chest radiograph that shows multiple small lung nodules, often with enlarged mediastinal lymph nodes that can mimic sarcoidosis (Fig. 93-4).[9] Nodules can coalesce and lead to progressive massive fibrosis, especially in the upper lungs, sometimes mimicking malignancy, and can be positive on PET scanning due to their metabolic activity. There can be compensatory emphysema in the lower lung fields. On chest imaging,

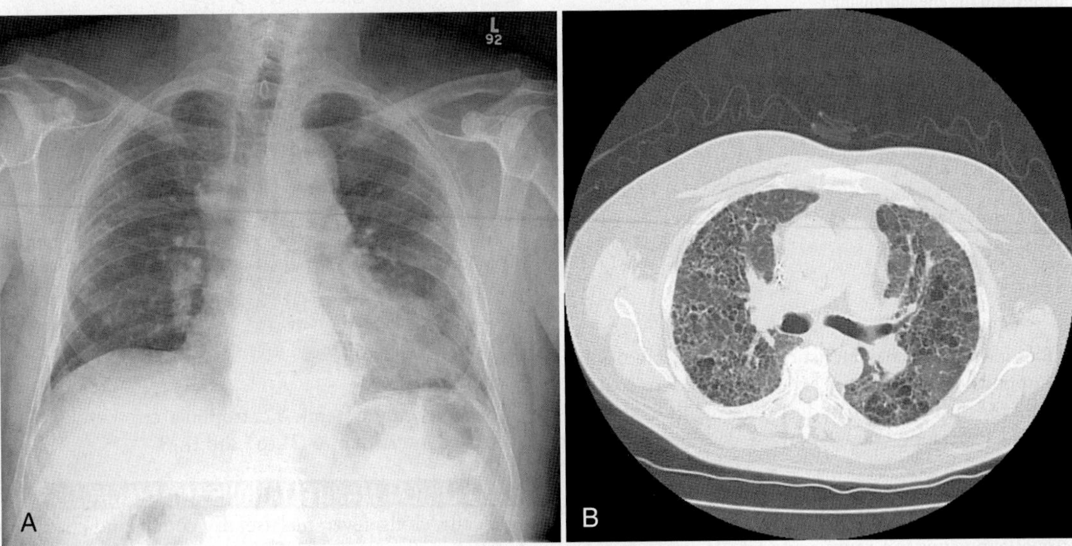

FIGURE 93-2. Posteroanterior chest radiograph (A) and high-resolution computed tomography scan (B) from patients with chronic beryllium disease. The chest radiograph demonstrates hilar adenopathy and infiltrates, and the scan shows air space destruction and infiltrates.

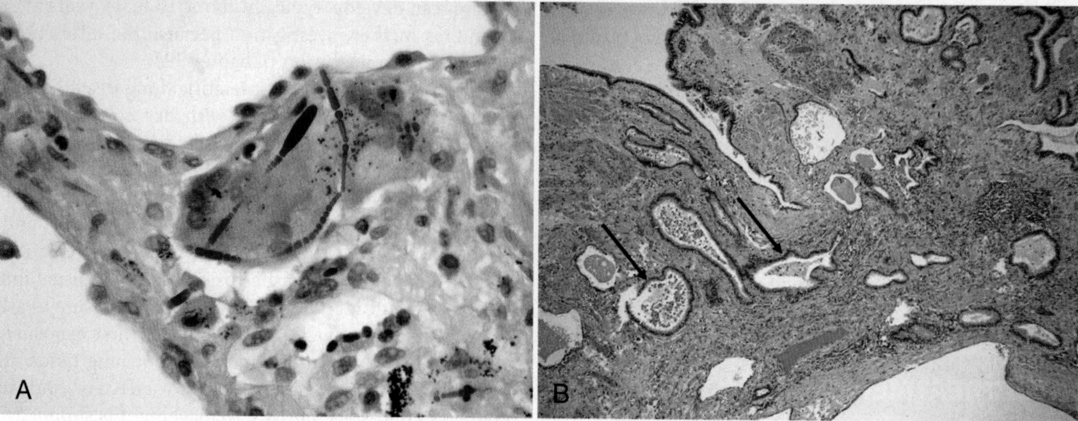

FIGURE 93-3. Histology from a lung biopsy showing asbestos bodies. Ferruginous bodies consisting of asbestos fibers coated by iron-protein-mucopolysaccharide material with typical golden-brown, beaded appearance. The two longest asbestos bodies at the center of the figure are present within a multinucleated giant cell. (Hematoxylin and eosin stain, × 400). (Courtesy of Dr. David Hwang, Toronto General Hospital.)

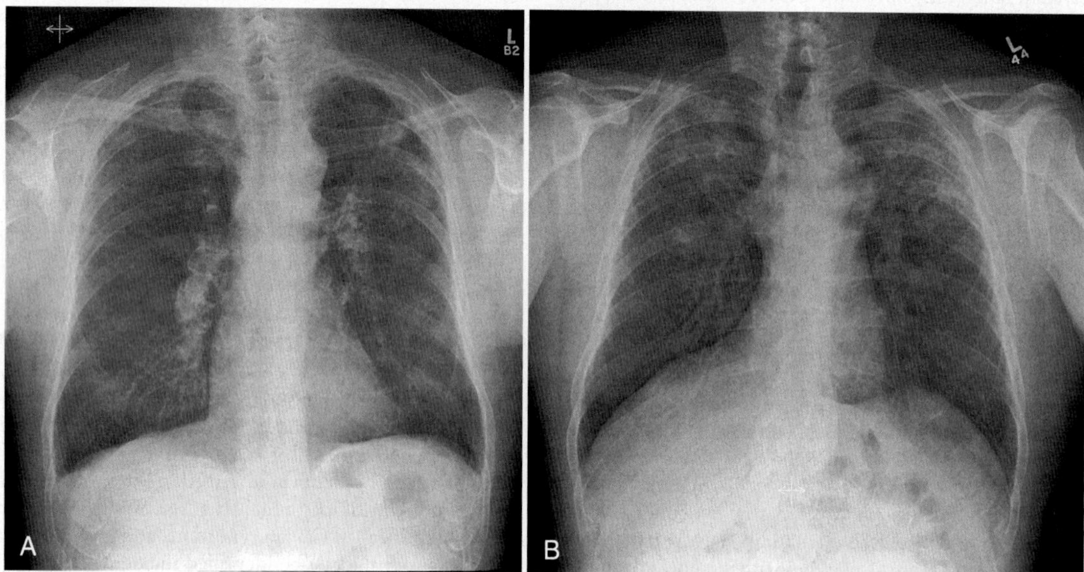

FIGURE 93-4. Posteroanterior chest radiographs from two patients with silicosis. A, Small nodules and eggshell calcification of hilar lymph nodes. B, Progressive massive fibrosis of the upper lung zones with compensatory emphysema.

TABLE 93-5 JOBS THAT CAN LEAD TO SILICOSIS

Mining: surface or underground mining (tunneling)
Milling: ground silica for abrasives and filler
Quarrying
Sandblasting: e.g., of buildings, preparing steel for painting
Pottery; ceramic or clay work
Grinding, polishing using silica wheels
Stone work
Foundry work: grinding, molding, chipping
Refractory brick work
Glass making: to polish and as an abrasive
Boiler work: cleaning boilers
Manufacture of abrasives

mediastinal lymph nodes may have a characteristic "eggshell" calcification in silicosis. Treatment is supportive. Patients with exposure to silica or coal dust may develop COPD from the dust exposure or dust-related diffuse fibrosis.[10] Patients who develop end-stage lung disease may be considered for lung transplantation.

ACUTE FEBRILE SYNDROMES

A variety of occupational exposures can cause acute febrile respiratory syndromes that may mimic acute viral respiratory illnesses (Table 93-6). The mechanism of these syndromes is incompletely understood, but they are associated with systemic neutrophilia and cytokine activation, often with increased interleukin-6 (IL-6) and IL-8.

TABLE 93-6 OCCUPATIONAL CAUSES OF AN ACUTE FEBRILE SYNDROME

SYNDROME	CAUSE
Polymer fume fever or Teflon fever	Polytetrafluoroethylene and other fluorocarbon polymer fumes
Metal fume fever	Zinc fumes from welding of galvanized steel, less commonly other metal fumes
Cotton mill fever	Dust and endotoxins from bacterial contamination of unprocessed cotton, flax, and hemp
Humidifier fever	Microorganisms found in reservoirs, e.g., humidifiers, air conditioners, aquariums
Organic dust toxic syndrome	Grain dust, moldy wood chips

CLINICAL MANIFESTATIONS AND DIAGNOSIS

Typically, chills, fever, malaise, dry cough, and chest tightness start about 6 to 8 hours after onset of an exposure at work and generally resolve by the next day. Occasionally, shortness of breath and other respiratory symptoms are severe enough for patients to seek emergency medical attention. Infiltrates on the chest radiograph can occur with neutrophilia and hypoxemia that can mimic acute pneumonia or acute hypersensitivity pneumonitis. Symptoms and signs generally resolve in 24 to 48 hours without antibiotics and recur with further exposures, although the clinical manifestations generally become milder with repeated daily exposures (e.g., Monday morning fever in cotton mill workers). Workers are often familiar with the syndrome because it commonly affects up to 30% of exposed workers. If the diagnosis is not provided by the patient, however, careful elicitation of potential work exposures is needed.

TREATMENT Rx

Treatment is supportive. If the causative exposure can be removed (e.g., cleaning a contaminated humidifier), symptoms can be prevented. If the cause cannot be removed and symptoms are severe, the patient may need reduction or change of the work exposure.

OCCUPATIONAL LUNG CANCER

A significant duration and level of exposure to a recognized carcinogen such as asbestos, hexavalent chromium (as in chromate production and the pigment industry), soluble radon compounds or radon gas, polycyclic aromatic hydrocarbons, chloromethyl ethers, arsenic, or silica can increase the risk for lung cancer (Chapter 191). Such a history should be elicited in all patients, and exposure to these agents represents a risk factor when considering whether to recommend patients for CT screening for lung cancer. The International Agency for Research on Cancer provides a listing of occupational lung carcinogens and the likelihood of their association with cancer.[11]

GENERAL REFERENCES

For the General References and other additional features, please visit Expert Consult at https://expertconsult.inkling.com.

94

PHYSICAL AND CHEMICAL INJURIES OF THE LUNG

DAVID C. CHRISTIANI

SUBMERSION INCIDENTS: DROWNING

DEFINITION

Drowning is defined as the process of experiencing respiratory impairment from submersion/immersion in liquid. The term *near-drowning* was previously used to describe individuals who survived a submersion incident, at least temporarily, but it has been abandoned on the basis of recommendations of the First World Congress of Drowning in Amsterdam in 2002.

EPIDEMIOLOGY

The estimated annual number of deaths worldwide due to drowning is 500,000. About 4200 persons are treated per year for nonfatal drowning in U.S. emergency departments, and about another 3400 suffer fatal drowning. Alcohol use, age younger than 4 years, and male gender are associated with increased rates of both nonfatal and fatal drowning.

PATHOBIOLOGY

The initial response to submersion/immersion is apnea, followed almost invariably by aspiration.[1] Laryngospasm may result in aspiration of a variable quantity of liquid medium into the lungs. Hypoxemia, hypercapnia, and acidemia develop acutely. Aspiration of either fresh or salt water results in occlusion of the airway, reduced surfactant activity, direct alveolar injury, and bronchospasm. Acute lung injury or the acute respiratory distress syndrome (ARDS)—associated with noncardiogenic pulmonary edema, respiratory failure, and severe hypoxemia—may develop hours or days after the incident. Acute renal failure may also occur. Alcohol consumption also increases the risk for hypothermia. Changes to serum electrolytes with drowning in either fresh water or salt water are not clinically significant.

The most serious secondary consequence of hypoxemia is anoxic brain injury. Fortunately, a reduction of brain temperature by 10° C during drowning decreases adenosine triphosphate (ATP) consumption by approximately 50%, thereby doubling the duration of time that the brain can survive. Mortality is primarily due to the cardiovascular sequelae of severe early or late hypoxemia.

CLINICAL MANIFESTATIONS

The initial presentation of a drowning victim varies widely. Hypothermia, which is common in drowning victims, may be associated with bradycardia or cardiac arrest due to asystole or ventricular fibrillation. Tachypnea, tachycardia, and low-grade fever are typical in nonhypothermic patients. Cyanosis may be present, and a coughing patient may produce pink frothy sputum. Neurologic evaluation may reveal agitation with or without intoxication or coma. The patient should be examined carefully for signs of associated trauma.

Expected laboratory findings include mild electrolyte abnormalities independent of whether submersion occurs in salt water or fresh water, moderate leukocytosis, and slight decrease in hematocrit in the first 24 hours or slight increase in free hemoglobin with a stable hematocrit in fresh water submersion due to hemolysis, severe hypoxemia, and metabolic acidosis. Evidence of disseminated intravascular coagulation (DIC) may occur. Initial electrocardiographic changes include sinus tachycardia and nonspecific ST segment and T wave changes, which revert to normal within hours. Life-threatening ventricular arrhythmias, complete heart block, or evidence of myocardial infarction can occur early or late in the course. Chest radiographs may initially be normal, despite severe respiratory impairment. Bilateral patchy alveolar infiltrates, which indicate progression to ARDS, may develop.

DIAGNOSIS

The diagnosis of drowning is made on clinical history of submersion in liquid medium with resulting respiratory impairment. Patients with unusual presenting circumstances should be carefully examined for evidence of trauma or assault.

PREVENTION

Drowning incidents are largely preventable, particularly in children. Pool fencing is a proven, effective strategy to prevent drowning. The primary cause of drowning of infants and toddlers is lack of adult supervision, and supervision of all young children near any form of water is strongly recommended. The role of alcohol in teenage and adult drowning incidents is substantial, and all individuals participating in water-based activities should restrict alcohol intake. The use of personal flotation devices is recommended for children and adults.

TREATMENT Rx

When the victim has been recovered from submersion, treatment should focus on basic life support, including notification of emergency response personnel, establishment of an adequate airway, and cardiopulmonary resuscitation, if necessary (Chapter 63). If the victim is apneic, rescue breathing should occur immediately, even before removal from the water. Cervical spine stabilization is needed if there is a history of diving, use of a water slide, signs of injury, or signs of alcohol intoxication. Spinal cord injury (Chapter 399) is otherwise unlikely, and cervical spine stabilization techniques and equipment may impede timely and effective treatment. Attempts to remove water from the airway are unnecessary. Cardiac arrhythmias should be treated with Advanced Cardiac Life Support protocols, including the use of automated external defibrillators when appropriate (Chapter 63). A majority of drowning victims who receive cardiopulmonary resuscitation or rescue breathing will vomit; if vomiting occurs, the head should be turned to the side, and any visible vomitus remaining in the oral cavity should be removed with a finger. When vomiting occurs in patients who may have spinal cord injury, log-rolling techniques are recommended for turning the patient to the side.

All victims of a submersion incident should be transported to a hospital for further evaluation, treatment of potential respiratory failure (Chapter 104), and monitoring for up to 24 hours. Bronchoscopy may be required to evaluate localized wheezing or persistent atelectasis. Prophylactic antibiotics are not useful, but evidence of pneumonia (Chapter 97) should be treated with appropriate antibiotics. Because unusual microorganisms may be isolated from the lower airways, efforts should be made to identify specific microbial flora pertinent to the locus of the drowning incident. Randomized controlled trials of specific ventilator strategies have not been conducted, but lung-protective ventilation (i.e., a tidal volume of 4 to 6 mL/kg ideal body weight) with sufficient positive end expiratory pressure of 5 to 10 cm H_2O to avoid atelectasis is commonly recommended.

Treatment of neurologic injury is focused on supportive care while the extent of cerebral edema is minimized. To decrease cerebral edema and intracranial pressure, intravenous hypertonic saline (7.5 to 23% to target serum sodium values of 145 to 155 mmol/L) or mannitol (1g/kg bolus of 20% mannitol, with repeat dosing every 6 to 8 hours as necessary to target serum osmolality of less than 300-320 mOsm/kg) may be used, although their benefit in this setting is unproved. Hyperventilation to a $Paco_2$ of 34 to 36 mm Hg may be helpful. Intracranial pressure may increase in response to shivering or purposeless movements, which should be reduced. Induced therapeutic hypothermia to 36°C improves neurologic outcome after cardiac arrest (Chapter 109), and current recommendations for drowning victims who remain comatose after rescue are to avoid rewarming to core or tympanic temperatures above 34°C and to maintain temperature of 32° to 34°C for 24 to 48 hours. Hyperthermia should be avoided at all times.

PROGNOSIS

The mortality rate for drowning victims who present alive to an emergency department is about 25%. Long-term neurologic deficits persist in approximately 6% of nonfatal drowning victims. Prolonged duration of submersion is associated with a worse prognosis, and the risk for death or severe permanent neurologic deficits increases from 10% after less than 5 minutes of submersion, to about 55% with 6 to 10 minutes of submersion, nearly 90% with 11 to 25 minutes of submersion, and nearly 150% with more than 25 minutes of submersion.[1] However, young children who are hypothermic when they are rescued after submersion times of up to 60 minutes have recovered without neurologic damage. Other factors associated with poor prognosis include hypotension, persistent apnea, coma, more than a 10-minute delay in receiving basic life support, and duration of resuscitation of more than 25 minutes.

DISEASES OF HIGH ALTITUDE

DEFINITION

Neurologic and pulmonary disturbances, primarily due to direct tissue effects of hypoxia, occur in individuals who either ascend to or reside at altitudes of 7000 feet (2133 meters) or more (Table 94-1).[2]

EPIDEMIOLOGY

Acute mountain sickness is the most common high-altitude syndrome. It occurs in approximately 20% of individuals who ascend to altitudes of 7000 to 9000 feet, 40% at 10,000 to 14,000 feet, and more than 50% above 14,000 feet. The incidence of chronic mountain sickness, also known as Monge disease, is thought to be between 5 and 18%. More severe neurologic disturbances due to high-altitude cerebral edema are rare, occurring in approximately 1 to 2% of individuals who ascend to altitudes above 15,000 feet. High-altitude pulmonary edema occurs in approximately 2 to 6% of otherwise healthy individuals who ascend to altitudes of 8000 to 15,000 feet. However, the incidence in individuals with a prior history of high-altitude pulmonary edema may be as high as 60%, or higher during rapid ascents. The occurrence of high-altitude retinal hemorrhage is approximately 33% among individuals who ascend to very high altitudes (up to 19,000 feet) and is thought to be common at lower altitudes as well. High-altitude retinal hemorrhage is not associated with high-altitude cerebral edema or long-term visual consequences.

TABLE 94-1 HIGH-ALTITUDE SYNDROMES

SYNDROME	CLINICAL DESCRIPTION
Acute mountain sickness	Common after recent ascent to altitudes above 7,000 feet; symptoms include headache, anorexia, and malaise
Chronic mountain sickness	Occurs in 5-18% of people dwelling above 10,000 feet; symptoms include headache, fatigue, dyspnea, and digestive disturbances
High-altitude pulmonary edema	Occurs in 2-6% of people above 9500 feet; symptoms include dyspnea, cough, and tachycardia
High-altitude retinal hemorrhage	Common above 15,000 feet; asymptomatic or reversible vision changes
High-altitude cerebral edema	Occurs in 1-2% of people above 15,000 feet; symptoms include confusion, ataxia, hallucinations, coma, or death

PATHOBIOLOGY

Clinically significant hypoxemia is the underlying factor in all high-altitude diseases. The decrease in barometric pressure during an ascent to altitude causes a decrease in the alveolar pressure of oxygen (PAO_2). For example, PAO_2 drops from 105 mm Hg at sea level to 60 mm Hg at 10,000 feet and to 40 mm Hg at 18,000 feet. Below 60 mm Hg, oxygen dissociates from hemoglobin more readily (see Fig. 158-2), thereby decreasing oxygen saturation and oxygen delivery to tissues. The effect is even more noticeable in patients with impaired diffusion capacity, such as occurs in emphysema, interstitial lung diseases, or heart failure. Furthermore, increased ventilatory drive induces an acute respiratory alkalosis. In the brain, tissue hypoxia causes cerebral vasodilation, whereas hypobaria causes cerebral vasoconstriction. In severe hypoxemia, vasodilation is the likely cause of cerebral edema in susceptible individuals. The response to hypoxemia in the lungs is primarily increased pulmonary arterial pressures due to hypoxic pulmonary vasoconstriction, which results in reversible injury to pulmonary capillaries, increased capillary permeability, and eventually pulmonary edema. Reduced oxygen consumption also occurs, perhaps because of impaired mitochondrial function. Sleep disordered breathing has also been noted but has minimal if any clinical significance.

CLINICAL MANIFESTATIONS

Symptoms of acute mountain sickness begin 2 to 3 hours after ascent and include breathlessness, lightheadedness, fatigue, nausea, anorexia, headache, and insomnia. Most symptoms resolve within 2 to 3 days, although insomnia may persist. Chronic symptoms of headache, fatigue, sleep disturbances, dyspnea, and digestive complaints are seen with chronic mountain sickness in individuals residing at higher elevations. Chronic mountain sickness may be associated with polycythemia (hemoglobin concentrations above 21 g/dL). Severe neurologic symptoms with high-altitude cerebral edema include ataxia and confusion that may progress to coma or death. Symptoms of high-altitude pulmonary edema that usually begin 2 to 4 days after ascent to higher altitudes include dyspnea, cough, and tachycardia. Fundoscopic changes of flame-shaped hemorrhages are seen with high-altitude retinal hemorrhage.

DIAGNOSIS

Diagnosis of most high-altitude disease is made on the basis of clinical manifestations at high altitude. Diagnosis of chronic mountain sickness, and a milder form often termed subacute mountain sickness, is more challenging because it may mimic other cardiopulmonary, neurologic, or psychiatric disease. Individuals with chronic mountain sickness typically have higher hemoglobin concentrations, higher serum erythropoietin levels, higher nocturnal heart rates, lower nocturnal oxygen saturation, and higher systolic and diastolic arterial pressure than do normal individuals living at similar altitude.

PREVENTION

Prevention of high-altitude disease can be achieved by avoidance in high-risk individuals, such as young children and persons with a history of high-altitude disease. Gradual ascent and acclimatization are crucial to prevention of high-altitude illness, particularly at extreme altitudes. At altitudes up to 10,000 feet, 2 to 3 days or more may be needed for adjustment to the effects of hypoxemia. For mountaineers, current recommendations are to ascend no more than approximately 984 feet (300 meters) per day at altitudes higher than 9843 feet (3000 meters).

When rapid ascent is unavoidable, such as flights to high-altitude locales, the carbonic anhydrase inhibitor acetazolamide (125 mg orally twice daily) provides effective prophylaxis of acute mountain sickness, and 125 mg at night may improve sleep[A1] (Table 94-2). Other medications shown to be effective in the prevention of acute mountain sickness in randomized, controlled trials include ibuprofen (600 mg three times daily),[A2] sumatriptan

TABLE 94-2 RECOMMENDED MEDICATION FOR THE PREVENTION AND TREATMENT OF ALTITUDE SICKNESS

MEDICATION	INDICATION	ROUTE	DOSE
Acetazolamide	Prevention of AMS, HACE	Oral	125 mg twice per day Pediatrics: 2.5 mg/kg every 12 hr
	Treatment of AMS*	Oral	250 mg twice per day Pediatrics: 2.5 mg/kg every 12 hr
Dexamethasone	Prevention of AMS, HACE	Oral	2 mg every 6 hr or 4 mg every 12 hr Pediatrics: should not be used for prophylaxis
	Treatment of AMS, HACE	Oral, IV, IM	AMS: 4 mg every 6 hr HACE: 8 mg once then 4 mg every 6 hr Pediatrics: 0.15 mg/kg/dose every 6 hr
Nifedipine	Prevention of HAPE	Oral	30 mg SR version every 12 hr, *or* 20 mg of SR version every 8 hr
	Treatment of HAPE	Oral	30 mg SR version every 12 hr, *or* 20 mg of SR version every 8 hr
Tadalafil	Prevention of HAPE	Oral	10 mg twice per day
Salmeterol	Prevention of HAPE	Inhaled	125 μg twice per day†

*Acetazolamide can also be used at this dose as an *adjunct* to dexamethasone in HACE treatment, but dexamethasone remains the primary treatment for that disorder.
†Should not be used as monotherapy and should only be used in conjunction with oral medications.
AMS = acute mountain sickness; HACE = high altitude cerebral edema; HAPE = high altitude pulmonary edema; SR = sustained release; IV = intravenous; IM, intramuscular.

(50 mg orally once after ascent),[A3] dexamethasone (2 mg every 6 hours or 4 mg every 12 hours),[A4] and prednisolone (20 mg daily). For the prevention of high-altitude pulmonary edema in susceptible individuals, options include the long-acting β-adrenergic agonist salmeterol (125 μg inhaled twice daily), the phosphodiesterase inhibitor tadalafil (10 mg twice daily), the calcium-channel blocker nifedipine (20 mg of slow-release formulation every 8 hours, or 30 mg of slow-release formulation every 12 hours), and dexamethasone (8 mg twice daily).

TREATMENT Rx

For acute, life-threatening symptoms such as high-altitude pulmonary edema and high-altitude cerebral edema, the best treatment is immediate descent, if possible, combined with supplemental oxygen therapy and, if needed, use of a portable hyperbaric chamber. For individuals who develop less severe symptoms, sildenafil (50 mg, one time dose) can increase exercise capacity at altitude by 10 to 35%.[A5] Increasing inspired oxygen concentrations in high-altitude working facilities also improves productivity and quality of sleep. Sustained-release theophylline (300 mg daily) significantly reduces the symptoms of acute mountain sickness compared with placebo, and acetazolamide (250 mg twice daily) is useful in treating symptoms of acute as well as chronic mountain sickness.[A6] Milder forms of acute mountain sickness, such as headache, can be treated with typical doses of nonsteroidal anti-inflammatory medications, including aspirin or acetaminophen.

PROGNOSIS

Symptoms of high-altitude disease respond rapidly to immediate descent. However, high-altitude cerebral edema and high-altitude pulmonary edema can be fatal, particularly at extreme altitudes and weather when descent may be impossible.

DECOMPRESSION ILLNESS: DECOMPRESSION SICKNESS, BAROTRAUMA, AND ARTERIAL GAS EMBOLISM

DEFINITION

Exposures to changes in ambient pressure cause a spectrum of illness, either by increasing or decreasing the volume of gas in air-filled body cavities or by causing the release of inert gas bubbles from solution in tissues or blood vessels. Symptoms associated with decreasing ambient pressure, which occur most commonly with ascent from depth during recreational or occupational diving, are known as decompression illness. The most common form of decompression illness is decompression sickness, which is classified as either type I (mild symptoms, such as general fatigue or joint pain) or type II (more severe neurologic or cardiopulmonary disturbances). Life-threatening forms of decompression illness include pulmonary barotrauma and arterial gas embolism syndromes. During the descent of a dive, increasing ambient pressure may cause mild symptoms of facial or sinus pain, often called "the squeezes."

EPIDEMIOLOGY

In addition to the approximately 9 million recreational divers in the United States, aviators, astronauts, and compressed air workers are also exposed to changes in ambient pressure that may cause decompression illness. Among recreational divers, the annual incidence rate for either type I or type II decompression sickness is estimated at 1 case per 5000 to 10,000 dives. Approximately 1000 episodes of decompression illness severe enough to warrant recompression therapy occur each year, up to 10% of which are fatal. Well-recognized risk factors for decompression illness include long duration of dives, deep dives, repetitive dives, heavy exertion at depth, cold water, and rapid ascent. Additional risk occurs in individuals who experience further decreases in ambient pressure after the dive, such as on commercial or private aircraft or driving over mountainous areas.[3]

PATHOBIOLOGY

The principles of Boyle's law and Henry's law describe the properties of gases during changes in ambient pressure. Boyle's law states that the volume of a gas varies inversely to changes in pressure, $P_1V_1 = P_2V_2$. During the descent of a dive, pain due to the "squeezes" is caused by increasing ambient pressures that are not equalized by a compensatory increase in gas volume. The resulting negative pressure causes a vacuum effect in the mask associated with engorgement of the blood vessels in adjacent tissues, such as periorbital and ocular vessels, and may result in swelling, pain, and subconjunctival hemorrhages. Facial sinuses, the middle ear, and the external auditory canals may also be affected.

Barotrauma in sinus, otic, or pulmonary tissues may be due to changes in ambient pressures and the resulting increase or decrease in the volume of gas. During descent, the decreasing volume of gas causes vascular engorgement in the sinuses and otic compartments and may result in rupture of the tympanic or inner ear membranes. During ascent, breath holding, particularly with compressed air devices (SCUBA diving), and the presence of obstructive lung disease with delayed exhalation times and air trapping impair equilibration and increase the risk for pulmonary barotrauma (E-Figure 94-1). If the expanding volume of gas causes a pressure gradient between the alveoli and pulmonary interstitium that exceeds the compliance of the lung, alveolar rupture will lead to pulmonary interstitial emphysema. Further extension of gas along pulmonary tissues may cause additional barotrauma, leading to pneumothorax, mediastinal emphysema, pneumopericardium, and soft tissue emphysema.

Arterial gas embolism, which is a serious consequence of pulmonary barotrauma, results in the development of free gas in the pulmonary arterial circulation. The resulting bubbles may then enter the systemic circulation by overwhelming the filtering mechanism of the pulmonary capillaries or through a right-to-left intracardiac shunt (Chapter 69), such as a patent foramen ovale. Bubbles may then migrate to the brain, spinal cord, heart, lung, or kidney and lead to tissue ischemia or infarct.

Henry's law states that the solubility of a gas in liquid is proportional to the partial pressure of that gas above the liquid. An increase in partial pressure of gases during descent will therefore cause the amount of gas dissolved in the pulmonary capillaries to increase. Dissolved oxygen is used during normal body metabolism; however, inert nitrogen, which is abundant in inspired air, becomes dissolved in the blood and tissues, particularly in fat, where it is five-fold more soluble than in water. During ascent, decreasing ambient pressure causes tissues to become supersaturated with nitrogen, and nitrogen is subsequently released into blood vessels and tissues as gas bubbles. Decompression-induced gas bubbles cause decompression illness by either mechanical compression of tissues or embolization through blood vessels to end organs. Bubbles that obstruct capillaries or venules damage the endothelium and cause tissue ischemia, which leads to activation of inflammatory mediators or tissue reperfusion injury. Although not well understood, toxic effects due to increased partial pressure of gases also are likely to contribute to symptoms of decompression illness, possibly by denaturing of proteins and release of fatty acids from cell membranes.

CLINICAL MANIFESTATIONS AND DIAGNOSIS

Symptoms of decompression illness can occur within minutes and up to 24 hours or more after exposure to changes in ambient pressure associated with dives of 20 feet in depth or more. The severity of symptoms depends on the rate and the magnitude of the change of ambient pressure and can vary among individuals. Diagnosis is based on clinical manifestations, which can be classified according to whether they are caused by formation of inert nitrogen gas bubbles or the localized toxic effects of gas (associated with decompression sickness), barotrauma associated with descent (sinus or otic barotrauma), barotrauma associated with ascent (pulmonary barotrauma), or more severe arterial gas embolism syndromes.

Symptoms vary according to location of bubble formation. For example, type I decompression sickness, also known as the bends or caisson disease, is typically associated with pain in the joints, from mild to severe, and numbness of the extremities. Rashes and lymphedema may also occur. Symptoms of type II decompression sickness may be systemic (fatigue, hypovolemic shock), cardiopulmonary (cough, substernal chest pain, tachypnea, asphyxia), otic (vertigo, hearing loss), or neurologic (ataxia, aphasia, speech disturbances, incontinence, confusion, personality changes, depression, paralysis, and loss of consciousness).

Otic barotrauma, which typically occurs during descent, can affect the external, middle, or inner ear (Chapter 426). External ear symptoms, such as a sensation of ear fullness or otalgia, are caused by a blockage of the canal, for example, with the use of ear plugs or presence of cerumen. Middle ear symptoms of otalgia, vertigo, tinnitus, transient conductive hearing loss, and facial nerve palsy occur when inadequate equalization of pressures results from blocked eustachian tubes, typically in association with allergic rhinitis or upper respiratory infections. Inner ear barotrauma, which is a more serious form of otic barotrauma, is associated with elevated intracranial pressure and rupture of the inner ear membrane. Inner ear barotrauma causes symptoms of sensorineural deafness, tinnitus, vertigo, nausea, and vomiting. Sinus barotrauma typically occurs during descent, is associated with facial pain and epistaxis, and occurs more frequently in individuals with mucosal inflammation from allergies or infection.

Pulmonary barotrauma, which is the second leading cause of death among divers, should be suspected in postdive individuals, particularly at-risk individuals, with symptoms of sudden pleuritic pain, dyspnea, or coughing. Physical examination findings include tachypnea, subcutaneous emphysema, and dullness to percussion or decreased breath sounds over a pneumothorax. Development of tension pneumothorax (Chapter 99) or severe pneumomediastinum may lead to decreased venous return of systemic blood and reduced cardiac preload, a situation that is characterized by hypotension and may lead to refractory shock or cardiac arrest. Chest and neck radiographs are recommended for diagnosis, particularly because pneumothoraces must be treated with chest tube thoracostomy before recompression therapy.

Because arterial gas embolism syndromes are caused by pulmonary barotrauma, careful neurologic assessment is critical. The neurologic findings are similar to those of an acute stroke (Chapter 407), with manifestations of focal or unilateral motor deficits, visual disturbances, sensory deficits, speech difficulties, and cognitive disturbances, including loss of consciousness. Symptoms typically occur within 10 minutes after ascent. Delayed neurologic symptoms are more likely to be due to type II decompression sickness.

PREVENTION

Education is the most effective method of preventing decompression illness.[4] Before participation in diving-related activities, all individuals should undergo a thorough and intensive training program. Instruction of proper pressure equalization techniques is critical in the prevention of decompression illness. Persons with asthma who wish to dive should be assessed by a physician (preferably knowledgeable in the field of diving medicine), have no wheezing on physical examination, and have normal spirometry before and after exercise. The presence of structural lung disease (e.g., lung cysts or bullae) is associated with a significant increase in the risk for pneumothorax and is a contraindication to diving. Presence of a known right-to-left intracardiac shunt, such as a patent foramen ovale, is not an absolute contraindication to diving, although conservative diving is recommended, and patients should be cautioned that they are at increased risk for decompression illness.

TREATMENT Rx

Symptoms of decompression illness at altitude should be treated with supplemental oxygen and return to the lowest attainable altitude. Serious decompression illness associated with diving requires immediate medical evaluation by emergency personnel, including basic and advanced life support (Chapter 63) when hemodynamic instability is present. Pneumothorax (Chapter 99) should be treated immediately with needle decompression or chest tube thoracostomy. Symptoms that persist for more than 2 hours or increase in intensity require recompression therapy, preferably with 100% oxygen or transfer to a facility with a hyperbaric chamber, where standard protocols should be followed. The only two randomized controlled trials to evaluate recompression therapy found that the addition of tenoxicam (20 mg daily, not available in the United States) or a helium-oxygen mixture (rather than pure oxygen) decreases the number of recompression treatments needed in divers with decompression illness, but neither improved the overall effectiveness of recompression treatment.[A7]

PROGNOSIS

Survival of patients with decompression illness depends on prompt medical evaluation and treatment. Immediate hyperbaric oxygen therapy per standard protocols is associated with resolution of symptoms in 95% of cases. However, symptoms of decompression illness, even neurologic deficits, may respond to recompression therapy after delays of 24 hours or more.

INHALATION INJURIES

Smoke Inhalation and Thermal Injury

DEFINITION

Pulmonary complications, largely caused by smoke inhalation, occur in a large proportion of burn victims (Chapter 111) and account for a substantial number of deaths in these patients. Even patients who do not sustain surface burns in a fire can inhale sufficient smoke to result in injury to the lungs or airways.

EPIDEMIOLOGY

Modern building codes and the widespread presence of firefighting personnel in communities have decreased the importance of fire as a cause of death in the United States. However, fire continues to cause several thousand deaths annually. Also, larger scale fires with mass casualties and wildfires that affect large geographic areas still occur occasionally.

PATHOGENESIS

Smoke loses heat rapidly as it traverses the upper airway, so direct thermal injury is often limited to the mucosa of the supraglottic airway. A notable exception is steam inhalation, which can produce thermal injury throughout the airways. Smoke inhalation injury affects the entire respiratory tract. The pathogenesis of smoke inhalation is complicated by the wide variety of pulmonary irritants in smoke, many of which are directly toxic to respiratory epithelial or alveolar cells: aldehydes such as acrolein, acetaldehyde, and formaldehyde; acids such as hydrochloric, hydrofluoric, and hydrocyanic acid; and ammonia, nitrogen oxides, and phosgene.

Irritants can rapidly induce intense neutrophilic inflammation, which evolves during 12 to 24 hours after injury and is characterized by mucosal edema and ulceration, abnormally increased permeability of pulmonary capillaries with resultant capillary leak, and epithelial, alveolar, and immune cellular dysfunction. Bronchospasm or bronchorrhea may occur, and the processes may result in ARDS. In addition, because oxygen is consumed in fires, breathing of hypoxic air for prolonged periods may potentiate other injuries or cause clinically significant hypoxemia in its own right.

CLINICAL MANIFESTATIONS

Thermal injury to upper airway mucosa can cause airway compromise, particularly due to laryngeal edema, sometimes rapidly and sometimes over the first 12 to 24 hours. Burns to the face, mouth, and neck can externally damage and distort structures of the upper airway and cause airway compromise, both subacutely and late in the course. Inhalation injury manifests primarily with bronchospasm and bronchorrhea, which cause cough, dyspnea, or wheezing and may progress rapidly to respiratory failure. Accumulation of secretions, failure of mucociliary clearance and immune mechanisms, and epithelial necrosis predispose to pulmonary infection, particularly 3 to 5 days after injury. Late pulmonary complications can also be caused indirectly by eschar formation and restriction of thoracic motion.

DIAGNOSIS

Patients with apparent or suspected burn injuries (Chapter 111) should be assessed emergently for airway patency. Head or neck burns, respiratory distress, stridor, or visibly erythematous or edematous oral mucosa should prompt immediate laryngoscopic evaluation of the oropharynx and supraglottic airway. Hypoxemia may develop and may be severe enough to meet criteria for ARDS. Chest radiography should be performed serially to detect the evolution of lung injury or superinfection.

TREATMENT Rx

If airway patency is threatened, endotracheal intubation should be performed immediately. Delay can result in increased edema and greater technical difficulty of intubation. Patients who cannot be intubated should have emergent tracheostomy performed surgically. Because of the risk for ARDS, mechanical ventilation with a goal tidal volume of 4 to 6 mL/kg of ideal body weight should be considered. All patients should receive supplemental oxygen with the goal of providing a high fractional concentration of inspired oxygen (FIO_2) to reverse the effects of hypoxemia and carbon monoxide inhalation (see later). Preliminary data suggest a role for inhaled anticoagulants to mitigate the development of acute lung injury, although well-designed prospective trials are currently lacking.[5] Pulmonary toilet is essential to clear secretions in the face of bronchorrhea and epithelial sloughing. Because of the risk for superinfection, surveillance for infection should be vigilant, including diagnostic bronchoscopy if ventilator-associated pneumonia is suspected.

PROGNOSIS

Patients who survive burns and recover generally do not have long-term pulmonary sequelae. Tracheostomies placed at the time of injury can usually be removed later, unless airway structures are damaged or distorted. Impaired pulmonary function is uncommon but may be manifested as airway hyperresponsiveness that has been termed reactive airway dysfunction syndrome.

Carbon Monoxide Poisoning

DEFINITION AND EPIDEMIOLOGY

Carbon monoxide is a colorless, odorless gas produced by the combustion of carbon-based fuels. Because of the ubiquity of these substances, carbon monoxide inhalation is often coincident with smoke inhalation in fires or may occur accidentally in association with malfunctioning equipment or improper venting of emissions from heaters, stoves, combustion motors, or other similar devices. In addition, intentional inhalation of carbon monoxide is a method commonly used in suicide attempts. Carbon monoxide inhalation is the leading cause of death from poisoning (Chapter 110) worldwide.

PATHOBIOLOGY

Carbon monoxide readily diffuses across the alveolar-capillary interface and binds to hemoglobin with extremely high affinity. When the resulting carboxyhemoglobin molecule undergoes an allosteric change at oxygen-binding sites, the ability of bound oxygen to dissociate and to be delivered to peripheral tissues is greatly reduced. This tissue hypoxia can cause severe functional impairment and ischemic injury of oxygen-sensitive tissues, particularly in the brain and heart.

CLINICAL MANIFESTATIONS

Mild carbon monoxide intoxication may go unrecognized because the symptoms are nonspecific and may include headache, nausea, malaise, fatigue, and dizziness. With more severe intoxications, neuropsychiatric symptoms may range from minor disturbances in attention and cognition to agitation, confusion, hallucination, or, in the worst intoxications, seizures or frank coma. Physical findings, which are generally nonspecific, can include tachycardia or hyperthermia. The classic "cherry-red" skin thought to be associated with carbon monoxide intoxication is rarely seen. Other manifestations of severe intoxications may include lactic acidosis, cardiac dysfunction with arrhythmia or ischemia, pulmonary edema, and rhabdomyolysis.

DIAGNOSIS

A high index of suspicion is required for diagnosis because clinical findings are nonspecific. All patients known to have been involved in fires, suicide attempts, or other scenarios compatible with exposures should have arterial carboxyhemoglobin levels checked by co-oximetry. Although levels do not correlate well with clinical findings or risk for complications, symptoms generally occur at carboxyhemoglobin concentrations of 10% or higher.

TREATMENT Rx

All patients should be treated with 100% supplemental oxygen, which competes with carbon monoxide for hemoglobin-binding sites and gradually eliminates it from the blood. If patients require mechanical ventilation because of a depressed neurologic status or respiratory problems, 100% oxygen should be administered by endotracheal tube. Rigorously conducted randomized controlled trials are lacking, but most expert guidelines endorse treatment with hyperbaric oxygen at a pressure of 2.5 to 3.0 atm, which can increase the dissolved oxygen content of blood by more than 10-fold.[6] At least one treatment of approximately 2 hours should be considered in severe cases to reverse the effects of acute intoxication; three hyperbaric oxygen treatments within 24 hours of diagnosis reduce neurocognitive sequelae. A8

PROGNOSIS

The mortality rate is highly variable according to the severity of intoxication but can approach 30% in severe cases. Approximately two thirds of patients who survive acute intoxication will recover without sequelae. Many of the remainder will suffer from long-term neuropsychiatric symptoms, including cognitive dysfunction, abnormal mood or affect, memory disturbances, and other motor or sensory abnormalities, which can often occur within the first month but may be delayed for up to 6 to 9 months.

Cyanide and Other Gases

PATHOBIOLOGY

In addition to carbon monoxide and pulmonary irritants, cyanide gas may be formed when a number of commonly found substances, particularly plastics and textiles, are combusted. This gas is highly toxic and can rapidly cause morbidity and death by binding to cytochrome enzymes and inhibiting cellular respiration.

Other inhaled gases that can injure the lungs in occupational settings include ammonia, chlorine, nitrogen dioxide, organic dust, paraquat, phosgene (which has also been used as a chemical weapon), sulfur dioxide, and toxic metal fumes such as cadmium and mercury.

CLINICAL MANIFESTATIONS AND DIAGNOSIS

Cyanide intoxication typically includes shock, lactic acidosis, and coma; it can rapidly lead to death before results of laboratory studies are available. In the setting of possible exposure, an elevated venous oxygen saturation indicates that cyanide is preventing cells from extracting oxygen from arterial blood.

Other inhaled gases that can produce potent irritant responses include ammonia, chlorine, and nitrogen dioxide ("silo-filler's lung"). Phosgene is notable for its propensity to cause delayed symptoms, up to 24 hours after exposure. Other inhalants may produce an acute chemical pneumonitis with respiratory distress (Chapter 93). A diverse group of inhaled toxins can cause syndromes of inhalational fever, including heavy metal fumes, polymer fumes, and organic dust aerosols that contain thermophilic bacteria, gram-negative bacteria and their associated endotoxins, and fungal elements. These inhalations are characterized by fever and malaise with mild respiratory symptoms and are also notable for tachyphylaxis with repeated exposure (and thus referred to as Monday morning fever in some occupational settings).

TREATMENT Rx

Cyanide intoxication is treated by use of a Taylor Cyanide Antidote Package (Taylor Pharmaceuticals) that contains amyl nitrate gas ampules (one 0.3-mL ampule each minute until sodium nitrate infusion begins) for inhalation. This treatment is followed by intravenous administration of sodium nitrite (300 mg one-time dose; can give an additional 150 mg if symptoms return), which converts hemoglobin to methemoglobin by attracting bound and unbound cyanide. Finally, patients are treated with intravenous sodium thiosulfate (12.5 g one-time dose; can repeat half the original dose if symptoms return), which converts cyanide to less harmful thiocyanate ions. If carboxyhemoglobinemia is present or the patient has heart disease or lung disease, sodium thiosulfate should be used alone because of the additive toxicity of methemoglobinemia.

Hydroxocobalamin (5 mg given intravenously once, can be repeated for a total of 10 mg), which directly binds cyanide, can be used in conjunction with sodium thiosulfate. It is thought to be safer than the amyl nitrate gas ampules because it does not cause methemoglobinemia and is better suited to prehospital care.

The mainstay for treatment of other irritating inhalations is to remove the patient immediately from the toxic environment and to provide supportive care for respiratory injury. Depending on the intensity and duration of exposure, most patients will recover completely without sequelae.

OXYGEN TOXICITY

DEFINITION

Hypoxemic respiratory failure often requires treatment with supplemental oxygen to maintain tissue oxygenation. In some settings, such as ARDS, patients may require high FIO_2 for prolonged periods to combat severe hypoxia. However, it has long been recognized that oxygen may be toxic to the lungs when it is present in concentrations higher than those found in ambient air.[7]

PATHOBIOLOGY

When the concentration of oxygen in the airways is high, formation of reactive oxygen species and free radicals is increased. Under normal circumstances, innate antioxidant mechanisms in airway epithelia and alveoli are sufficient to abrogate the effect of these molecules. However, under conditions of critical illness, prolonged exposure to increased concentrations of these toxins may overwhelm these defenses. Superoxide, hydrogen peroxide, and hydroxyl radicals may directly oxidize cellular components. Cellular damage potentiates inflammation and may be synergistic with inflammatory processes already underway in the diseased lung; the result can be alveolar edema, formation of hyaline membranes, hypoxemia, and progression to fibrosis and obliteration of alveolar and capillary structures. In addition, washout of nitrogen from air spaces can result in absorptive atelectasis if oxygen is removed by the circulation faster than it can be replenished by ventilation (especially in the setting of ventilation-perfusion mismatch). Hyperoxia can also worsen hypercapnia through multiple mechanisms, as occurs in patients with chronic obstructive pulmonary disease who suffer from carbon dioxide retention.

CLINICAL MANIFESTATIONS AND DIAGNOSIS

Although the exact levels of hyperoxia that cause lung injury are unclear, it appears to occur with exposure to FIO_2 of 50 to 60% after exposures as short as 6 hours in duration. Because of the high flow of supplemental oxygen required to deliver this FIO_2, oxygen toxicity is observed primarily in mechanically ventilated patients being treated for hypoxemic respiratory failure. This level of exposure can cause a clinically detectable tracheobronchitis, demonstrable by symptoms of cough and dyspnea, as well as airway erythema that is visible macroscopically on bronchoscopy. This syndrome may impair mucociliary clearance and result in impaction of secretions, especially in conjunction with absorptive atelectasis.

Patients who may be susceptible to oxygen toxicity generally already have a significant degree of parenchymal injury from other processes. Thus, although some patients may appear to display a syndrome of worsening air space disease, atelectasis, consolidation, hypoxia, and diffuse alveolar damage, it is not clear when these changes are related to oxygen therapy or merely occur as part of the acute lung injury from other causes.

TREATMENT

Rx

Because the threshold level for oxygen toxicity is unknown, a general guideline for treatment of hypoxemic respiratory failure (Chapter 104) is that patients be ventilated with the lowest possible FIO_2 that is required to restore an acceptable oxygen saturation. A SaO_2 of 90%, corresponding to PaO_2 of 55 to 60 mm Hg, is generally considered the minimum acceptable level. Unfortunately, under conditions of severe hypoxia, such as ARDS, patients often require an FIO_2 approaching 100% to achieve this oxygen level. Maneuvers to improve oxygenation without increasing FIO_2 include paralysis with continuous infusions of neuromuscular blocking agents; inhaled pulmonary vasodilators; red blood cell transfusions to improve the delivery of oxygen; alternative ventilatory strategies, such as high-frequency oscillatory ventilation, airway pressure-release ventilation, inverse-ratio ventilation, and prone positioning; and alveolar recruitment maneuvers using positive end-expiratory pressure or transiently increased inflation pressures (Chapter 105).

PROGNOSIS

Patients who sustain oxygen toxicity in the setting of prior bleomycin exposure may be left with residual pulmonary fibrosis. In other patients, the incremental impact of oxygen toxicity on prognosis is unknown.

LUNG INJURY

Radiation Lung Injury

DEFINITION

Accidental or occupational radiation exposures (Chapter 20) are generally characterized by systemic toxicity that outweighs any injury to the lungs. As such, radiation lung injury refers to a pneumonitis that can progress to pulmonary fibrosis and that results from therapeutic use of ionizing radiation, usually in the treatment of malignant neoplasms.[8]

EPIDEMIOLOGY

As many as 50% of patients receiving thoracic radiation will display radiographic abnormalities after treatment; duration and dose of therapy affect the odds for development of lung injury. However, most of these patients will never have clinically significant radiation lung injury. For unclear reasons, the incidence of lung injury appears to vary by the type of underlying malignant disease and modality of treatment. The highest frequency is in lung cancer (10 to 20%).

PATHOBIOLOGY AND CLINICAL MANIFESTATIONS

The pathogenesis of radiation lung injury is often divided into three or four phases on the basis of time course. Typically, the early phase occurs immediately after exposure and is characterized by injury to alveolar cells, resulting in mild alveolitis, recruitment of inflammatory cells, capillary leak, and pulmonary edema. These changes are usually asymptomatic; patients do not usually come to clinical attention, although the chest radiograph will be abnormal if it is performed. In most patients, these changes resolve without progression within 1 to 3 months.

A minority of patients will progress to the next phase, in which alveolar cells desquamate and the air spaces fill with protein-rich fluid. In this phase, referred to as radiation pneumonitis, patients will complain of cough, dyspnea, and occasionally fever or pleuritic chest pain. Severe cases may present with hypoxemic respiratory failure. This phase generally resolves within 3 to 6 months after exposure and is followed by an organizing phase, in which alveolar edema resolves and the damaged alveoli heal. Clinically, patients generally show improvement in symptoms during this period. However, this phase is also characterized by fibroblast proliferation and deposition of collagen in the lung. In a minority of patients, this process will proceed unchecked and result in clinically significant fibrosis, with progressive loss of alveolar-capillary surface and development of restrictive lung disease.

DIAGNOSIS

Clinical history and radiographic evaluation are often sufficient for diagnosis of radiation lung injury as patients typically present with respiratory symptoms and opacities on chest radiography after undergoing radiation therapy. Radiography may show air space disease with alveolar filling or consolidation during the pneumonitis phase, which may progress to an interstitial pattern and eventual honeycombing with parenchymal distortion in the chronic phase. Because radiation characteristically causes injury only within directly affected lung tissue, radiography may show opacities that are well delineated and form straight lines that cross anatomically distinct regions of lung. This finding is rarely if ever seen in other conditions.

The differential diagnosis may include pneumonia, recurrence, and metastatic malignant disease. On occasion, invasive evaluation with bronchoalveolar lavage or even biopsy is required to exclude these possibilities if the clinical history and imaging do not provide a diagnosis.

TREATMENT AND PREVENTION Rx

Corticosteroids, such as prednisone 1 mg/kg body weight per day for 2 to 3 weeks followed by a slow taper over several weeks or months, are the mainstay of therapy. Patients often show a dramatic response to treatment, and symptoms may recur after treatment is discontinued. Other immunosuppressive agents have been used successfully in case reports of patients who failed to respond to corticosteroids. Prophylactic amifostine, a cytoprotective agent, significantly reduces the risk for radiation pneumonitis but does not improve survival in patients who receive radiation treatment for lung cancer.[A9] Ambroxol, a free-radical scavenger given at 90 mg three times daily for 3 months, decreases the production of harmful cytokines and lessens the decrement in the diffusion capacity for carbon monoxide (DLCO), a marker of interstitial lung damage, in patients with locally advanced lung cancer.[A10] Dixiong decoction, a Chinese herbal preparation, has also been reported to decrease the incidence and severity of radiation pneumonitis in patients with non–small cell lung cancer.

PROGNOSIS

Within 2 years after initial exposure, progression will usually slow, and symptoms and lung function will stabilize or improve. After this time, further improvement or worsening is uncommon. In severe cases that become chronic, patients may develop features of advanced interstitial lung disease, including pulmonary hypertension and hypoxic respiratory failure.

Aspiration Injury

DEFINITION

Aspiration, which is defined as the inhalation of any nongaseous foreign substance into the lungs, generally refers specifically to the inhalation of gastric contents or secretions from the oropharynx. Aspiration is a common occurrence, and in most cases it resolves spontaneously without clinical manifestations. Clinically significant aspiration can range from acute pneumonitis and respiratory failure caused by a single massive aspiration to chronic symptoms of respiratory disease caused by recurrent small-scale aspiration. These syndromes may overlap with pneumonia that occurs when the lungs are exposed to bacteria from the gastrointestinal tract (Chapter 97).

PATHOBIOLOGY

The common element of clinically significant aspiration is impairment of normal airway protective mechanisms. Under normal circumstances, the airway is protected by the normal swallowing mechanism, the cough reflex, and the anatomy of the supraglottic airway. However, even healthy individuals experience microaspiration despite having functional protective mechanisms. These secretions are handled by normal pulmonary clearance mechanisms.

Any disturbance of these protective mechanisms can result in aspiration injury to the lungs. An altered level of consciousness can impair normal swallowing and suppress the cough reflex. Even in patients who are alert, neurologic injury can result in dysphagia and concomitant aspiration, as in patients who have bulbar neurologic deficits in association with ischemic stroke. Patients with altered airway or oropharyngeal anatomy, such as patients who have received surgical or radiation therapy for head and neck malignant neoplasms, may also be highly susceptible to aspiration of oral secretions.

The nature of the aspirated material is also important in determining whether an injury occurs. Materials with a pH lower than 2.5, such as acidic gastric contents, are much more likely to cause a significant chemical pneumonitis. Particulate matter also increases the likelihood for development of clinically significant inflammation. A large-volume aspiration with distribution throughout the lungs is more likely to produce an acute, severe pneumonitis.

When material has been aspirated into the lungs, the injury that occurs is similar to a chemical burn. Acid rapidly injures airway epithelial and alveolar cells; within hours, cells become dysfunctional and capillary leak occurs, resulting in profound noncardiogenic pulmonary edema. In severe cases, diffuse alveolar damage may result.

CLINICAL MANIFESTATIONS

The classic eponym applied to aspiration pneumonia is Mendelsohn syndrome, which refers to a single, large-volume aspiration of gastric contents followed by rapidly progressive hypoxemic respiratory failure that develops within hours. Patients may suffer from cough, dyspnea, fever, and respiratory distress. Physical examination may reveal diffuse crackles, wheezing, cyanosis, and hypotension. Chest radiography may show a pattern of alveolar filling with diffuse bilateral involvement or involvement of dependent regions, particularly the right lower lobe if the patient is upright at the time of aspiration. In many patients, this period of acute deterioration is followed by stabilization and resolution within 2 or 3 days. In other patients, deterioration may continue, and patients may meet clinical criteria for ARDS. If the volume of aspirated material is large enough, the initial aspiration may be sufficient to cause tracheal obstruction and asphyxiation.

In patients who initially improve, a small percentage will show further deterioration after 2 or 3 days. This deterioration should prompt an investigation for bacterial superinfection.

DIAGNOSIS

The clinical history and presentation are generally sufficient for diagnosis of aspiration pneumonitis. Bacterial pneumonia and other causes of ARDS also should be considered, as should cardiogenic pulmonary edema. Airway erythema and edema on bronchoscopy can be suggestive of aspiration. Bronchoalveolar lavage may help evaluate for the presence of bacterial infection.

PREVENTION

Prevention should focus on identification of patients who are at risk for aspiration and then use of strategies to minimize the risk. Patients with swallowing dysfunction or airway abnormalities can work with speech pathologists to learn effective strategies for swallowing. Patients who are unsuccessful or not suitable for this approach may benefit from tracheostomy or enteral tube feedings, which do not prevent microaspiration but can prevent large-volume aspiration. However, the risk for aspiration pneumonia is no different among patients with nasogastric tubes compared with patients who have percutaneous endoscopy gastrostomy tubes.[A11] In hospitalized patients, particularly patients with an altered mental status due to illness or sedation, simple strategies such as avoidance of oral feeding and semirecumbent positioning can effectively reduce the risk for aspiration. Use of histamine-2 blockers or proton pump inhibitors (Chapter 139) can alter gastric pH to reduce the risk for injury from acidic secretions.

TREATMENT Rx

Because of the acuity and severity of aspiration pneumonitis, immediate attention should be paid to maintaining a patent airway. The oropharynx and trachea should be suctioned to clear any potentially obstructing material, and endotracheal intubation should be performed if necessary (Chapter 105). Bronchoscopy is often performed to clear residual particulate or solid matter, but it cannot remove acidic secretions, which damage airways and parenchyma quickly and then are rendered neutral. Oxygen supplementation should be provided as needed for hypoxia. Corticosteroids have not been shown to be beneficial. Antibiotics should be reserved for patients who appear to have developed bacterial superinfection (Chapter 97).

PROGNOSIS

For patients with severe respiratory failure or ARDS, mortality can be high. In others, improvement should be expected within days. If the underlying factor that led to aspiration is irreversible, patients have an increased likelihood of recurrent episodes.

Lipoid Pneumonia

DEFINITION

Lipoid pneumonia is a chronic inflammatory reaction of the lungs to the presence of lipid substances. Exogenous lipoid pneumonia results from the aspiration of vegetable, animal, or (most commonly) mineral oils.

PATHOBIOLOGY

The most frequently implicated agent is mineral oil used as a laxative and to reduce dysphagia, either in clear liquid form or as petroleum jelly. Mineral oil is bland and, when introduced into the pharynx, can enter the bronchial tree without eliciting the cough reflex. It also mechanically impedes the ciliary action of the airway epithelium. The risk for mineral oil aspiration is increased in debilitated or senile patients, in those with neurologic disease that interferes with deglutition, and in patients with esophageal disease. Mineral oil taken as nose drops to relieve nasal dryness can also cause lipoid pneumonia. Inhalation of mineral oil mist by airplane and automobile mechanics has also been implicated as a cause.

Mineral oils, which cannot be hydrolyzed in the body, provoke a chronic inflammatory reaction that may not become clinically overt until years later. In the alveolar spaces, macrophages accumulate and phagocytose the emulsified oil. Some macrophages disintegrate, releasing their lysosomal enzymes and oil. The alveolar septa become thickened and edematous, containing lymphocytes and lipid-laden macrophages. Oil droplets are seen in the pulmonary lymphatics and hilar nodes. Later, fibrosis develops, and the normal lung architecture is effaced. A single pathologic specimen may include both the early inflammatory and the later fibrotic picture, in keeping with repetitive aspirations during many months or years. Nodular lesions may grossly resemble tumor and be called paraffinomas.

CLINICAL MANIFESTATIONS

Most patients are asymptomatic and come to the physician's attention because of an abnormal chest radiograph. When patients are symptomatic, cough and exertional dyspnea are the most frequent complaints. Chest pain (sometimes pleuritic), hemoptysis, fever (usually low grade), chills, night sweats, and weight loss may occur. Findings on physical examination may be completely normal, but fever, tachypnea, dullness on percussion of the chest, bronchial or bronchovesicular breath sounds, rales, and rhonchi may be found. Clubbing and cor pulmonale are rare.

DIAGNOSIS

In mild lipoid pneumonia, arterial blood gas values may be normal with the patient at rest but may show hypoxemia after exercise. In more severe disease, resting hypoxemia, hypocapnia, and mild respiratory alkalosis develop. Pulmonary function testing reveals a restrictive ventilatory defect; lung compliance is decreased. The only specific laboratory finding is the presence in sputum of macrophages with clusters of vacuoles that are 5 to 50 µm in diameter and that stain deep orange with Sudan IV; extracellular droplets may stain similarly.

On radiographic examination, the earliest abnormalities are air space infiltrates, most often in the dependent portions of the lung. The infiltrates may be unilateral or bilateral, localized or diffuse. Air bronchograms may be seen. Hilar adenopathy and pleural reaction are rare. As fibrosis develops, volume loss occurs, and linear and nodular infiltrates appear. A solid lesion that closely resembles bronchogenic carcinoma may develop. High-resolution computed tomography usually shows consolidated areas of low attenuation and "crazy paving" (Fig. 94-1).

The differential diagnosis is extensive, particularly in the late phase, when multiple other causes of pulmonary fibrosis must be considered. The key to the correct diagnosis before biopsy is the history of chronic oral or intranasal use of an oil- or a lipid-based product or an occupational exposure to oil mists. The presence of lipid-laden macrophages in sputum or bronchoalveolar lavage fluid also can be used to confirm the diagnosis, particularly in conjunction with typical findings on high-resolution computed tomography.

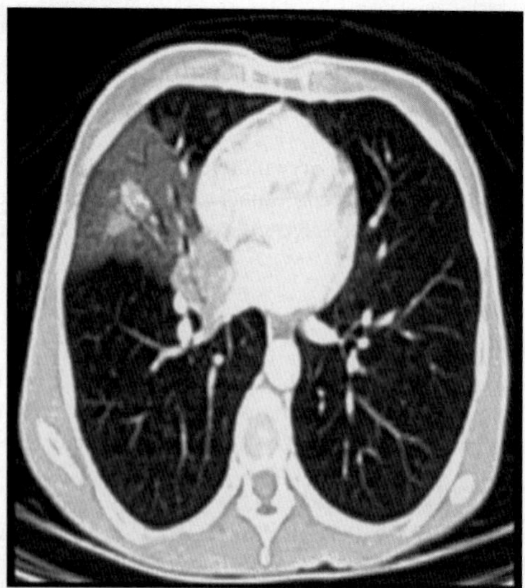

FIGURE 94-1. Lipoid pneumonia on a computed tomographic scan.

TREATMENT AND PREVENTION Rx

When the diagnosis has been made and the aspiration stopped, the subsequent course is variable. Because the only way the lung can dispose of mineral oil is by expectoration, the patient should be instructed in coughing exercises to be performed many times each day for months. Expectorants have not been shown to help. In some uncontrolled case reports, systemic corticosteroids have been used successfully at varying doses and length, but the literature suggests that they cannot be routinely recommended for treatment.

Transfusion-Related Acute Lung Injury

DEFINITION

The syndrome of transfusion-related acute lung injury (TRALI; Chapter 177) involves the rapid onset of respiratory distress within minutes to hours after the transfusion of blood products (fresh-frozen plasma, platelets, and red blood cells).[9] The initial clinical picture is indistinguishable from acute lung injury or ARDS due to other causes, such as sepsis, multiple trauma, and lung injury. TRALI may similarly be confused with pulmonary edema due to volume overload (Chapter 58).

EPIDEMIOLOGY

The true incidence of TRALI is unknown; incidence rates are underestimated because of the difficulty in distinguishing TRALI from other causes of acute respiratory failure and the labor-intensive and costly diagnostic evaluation required. Reported incidences range from 1 in 1000 to 1 in 100,000 units of blood products transfused. The risk for TRALI varies according to the type of blood product transfused, with pooled products associated with a higher incidence. Only 8 to 21 TRALI-related deaths are reported to the U.S. Food and Drug Administration annually, and even liberal estimates accounting for underreporting suggest the number may be only as high as 300 per year of an estimated 25 million transfusions in the United States.

PATHOBIOLOGY

The physiologic manifestations of TRALI are caused by alveolar filling with fluid and protein. This alveolar process is the result of increased microvascular permeability due to pulmonary endothelial damage mediated by either leukocyte antibodies or the priming and activation of neutrophils in the pulmonary circulation by bioactive substances.

TRALI most commonly occurs when human leukocyte antigen (HLA) type I or II or neutrophil-specific antigen antibodies from the donor attach to the recipient's leukocytes, leading to the release of injurious oxidative and nonoxidative products. Development of HLA antibodies occurs commonly in women during pregnancy, and increasing parity in female blood donors is associated with an increased risk for TRALI.

Episodes of TRALI occurring in patients without HLA or neutrophil-specific antigen antibodies in either the donor or recipient are thought to be caused by a two-hit process of neutrophil priming and activation. Neutrophils are primed and sequestered in the lung by conditions that often occur in patients requiring blood products, such as multiple trauma, surgery, or sepsis. Primed neutrophils are then activated by bioactive lipids and cytokines stored in the blood products, thereby leading to lung injury and alveolar damage. Levels of these bioactive lipids or cytokines may increase after prolonged storage of blood products.

CLINICAL MANIFESTATIONS

Although most cases of TRALI present within 1 to 2 hours after the transfusion of blood products, tachypnea, hypoxemia, cyanosis, dyspnea, and fever can develop during the transfusion or up to 6 hours later. Hypertension or hypotension commonly occurs, depending on the severity of the reaction. Copious amounts of pink, frothy edema fluid may be present. Lung auscultation generally reveals bilateral crackles and decreased breath sounds in dependent lung zones.

DIAGNOSIS

Bilateral patchy infiltrates consistent with alveolar edema are found on plain chest radiographs, typically without effusions. Arterial blood gas analysis demonstrates reduced Po_2, and further laboratory testing may reveal thrombocytopenia or a transient leukopenia. Diagnosis of TRALI requires the presence of the following: acute onset of hypoxemia with Pao_2/Fio_2 of less than 300 mm Hg or room air oxygen saturation of less than 90% during or within 6 hours after a transfusion; bilateral infiltrates on the chest radiograph; no evidence of left atrial hypertension; no preexisting acute lung injury before transfusion; and no temporal relationship to an alternative risk factor for acute lung injury.

The diagnosis of "possible TRALI" is made in patients who have a concurrent diagnosis of another risk factor for acute lung injury, including direct lung injury due to aspiration, pneumonia, toxic inhalation, lung contusion, or nonfatal drowning, and indirect lung injury due to severe sepsis, shock, multiple trauma, burn injury, acute pancreatitis, cardiopulmonary bypass, or drug overdose. Absolute confirmation of the diagnosis requires testing for HLA and neutrophil-specific antigen antibodies, usually performed first in female donors, then in male donors, and finally in the recipient.

TREATMENT

Most cases are self-limited and resolve within hours to days with supplemental oxygen and supportive care. Volume resuscitation, with or without vasopressors, is required for hypotension. Mechanical ventilation should be managed as for any other case of acute lung injury, with the implementation of a low tidal volume ventilation strategy to prevent further ventilator-induced lung injury. Diuresis should be attempted cautiously and may even be detrimental because intravascular filling pressures are often low.

PROGNOSIS

The mortality rate of TRALI is approximately 5%. If an implicated donor can be identified, the recipient should not receive any further transfusions from that donor, but patients are not at increased risk for further episodes of TRALI from nonimplicated donor transfusions.

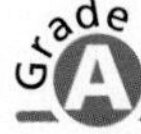

Grade A References

A1. Low EV, Avery AJ, Gupta V, et al. Identifying the lowest effective dose of acetazolamide for the prophylaxis of acute mountain sickness: systematic review and meta-analysis. *BMJ*. 2012;345:e6779.

A2. Lipman GS, Kanaan NC, Holck PS, et al. Ibuprofen prevents altitude illness: a randomized controlled trial for prevention of altitude illness with nonsteroidal anti-inflammatories. *Ann Emerg Med*. 2012;59:484-490.

A3. Jafarian S, Gorouhi F, Salimi S, et al. Sumatriptan for prevention of acute mountain sickness: randomized clinical trial. *Ann Neurol*. 2007;62:273-277.

A4. Tang E, Chen Y, Luo Y. Dexamethasone for the prevention of acute mountain sickness: systematic review and meta-analysis. *Int J Cardiol*. 2014;173:133-138.

A5. Xu Y, Liu Y, Liu J, et al. Meta-analysis of clinical efficacy of sildenafil, a phosphodiesterase type-5 inhibitor on high altitude hypoxia and its complications. *High Alt Med Biol*. 2014;15:46-51.

A6. Richalet JP, Rivera-Ch M, Maignan M, et al. Acetazolamide for Monge's disease: efficiency and tolerance of 6-month treatment. *Am J Respir Crit Care Med*. 2008;177:1370-1376.

A7. Bennett MH, Lehm JP, Mitchell SJ, et al. Recompression and adjunctive therapy for decompression illness. *Cochrane Database Syst Rev*. 2012;5:CD005277.

A8. Buckley NA, Juurlink DN, Isbister G, et al. Hyperbaric oxygen for carbon monoxide poisoning. *Cochrane Database Syst Rev*. 2011;4:CD002041.

A9. Bourhis J, Blanchard P, Maillard E, et al. Effect of amifostine on survival among patients treated with radiotherapy: a meta-analysis of individual patient data. *J Clin Oncol*. 2011;29:2590-2597.

A10. Xia DH, Xi L, Xv C, et al. The protective effects of ambroxol on radiation lung injury and influence on production of transforming growth factor beta1 and tumor necrosis factor alpha. *Med Oncol*. 2010;27:697-701.

A11. Gomes CA Jr, Lustosa SA, Matos D, et al. Percutaneous endoscopic gastrostomy versus nasogastric tube feeding for adults with swallowing disturbances. *Cochrane Database Syst Rev*. 2012;3:CD008096.

GENERAL REFERENCES

For the General References and other additional features, please visit Expert Consult at https://expertconsult.inkling.com.

95

SARCOIDOSIS

MICHAEL C. IANNUZZI

DEFINITION

Sarcoidosis, a systemic granulomatous disease of unknown cause, is characterized by a variable clinical presentation and course. More than 90% of patients exhibit thoracic involvement with mediastinal and hilar lymph node enlargement or parenchymal lung disease, but any organ may be involved. The presentation and course vary from asymptomatic disease with spontaneous resolution to organ system failure and even death.

EPIDEMIOLOGY

Sarcoidosis occurs worldwide, affects people of all racial and ethnic groups, and may present at any age. Sarcoidosis usually develops before the age of 50 years, with the incidence peaking at 20 to 39 years. The incidence of sarcoidosis fluctuates throughout the world, most likely because of differences in the presentation of the disease and the surveillance methods used. The annual incidence of sarcoidosis is highest in northern European countries, where it is 5 to 40 cases per 100,000 people. The incidence in Japan is about 1 to 2 cases per 100,000 people. In the United States, the adjusted annual incidence among black Americans is about 3.5 times higher than among white Americans (35.5 cases per 100,000 compared with 10.9 per 100,000). Regardless of ethnic or racial group, sarcoidosis affects women more often. The reportedly low incidence in certain regions such as Africa, China, India, and Russia may be due to decreased access to health care, minimal surveillance, and misdiagnosis of sarcoidosis as tuberculosis or leprosy.

Black women in the United States have the highest lifetime risk for developing sarcoidosis (2.7%). In both black men and women, sarcoidosis occurs later in life, peaks in the fourth decade, and is more likely to be chronic and fatal. Socioeconomic status does not affect the incidence of sarcoidosis, but low income and other financial barriers to care are associated with more severe sarcoidosis, even after adjustment for age, sex, and race or ethnic group.

Sarcoidosis clusters in families, and monozygotic twins are more often concordant for disease than are dizygotic twins. Familial sarcoidosis occurs in 10% of cases from the Netherlands, 7.5% from Germany, 6% from the United Kingdom, 4.7% from Finland, and 0.8% from Spain. In the United States, sarcoidosis patients are five times as likely to have siblings or parents with sarcoidosis as control subjects. However, less than 1% of the first-degree relatives of patients with sarcoidosis are affected, so screening for disease in asymptomatic relatives is ineffective.

PATHOBIOLOGY

The development and accumulation of granulomas represent the basic pathologic abnormality in sarcoidosis (E-Fig. 95-1). Sarcoidal granulomas are tightly organized collections of macrophages and macrophage-derived epithelioid cells encircled by lymphocytes. Fused epithelioid cells, which become multinucleated giant cells, are often found scattered throughout the granuloma. This appearance suggests that the granuloma is meant to contain an inciting agent, but no such agent has been identified.

Granuloma formation begins with HLA-mediated processing of antigens by macrophages. T-cell activation follows, with oligoclonal expansion of $CD4^+$ (helper-inducer) lymphocytes. These $CD4^+$ cells, primarily of the T_H1 phenotype, produce interleukin-2 (IL-2) and interferon-γ (IFN-γ). A complex interplay of cytokines, along with macrophage-derived tumor necrosis factor-α, organizes the inflammatory cells into granulomas. In some cases, fibroblasts and collagen encase the granulomas with subsequent fibrosis. Fibrosis has been associated with a shift in the involved lymphocytes from the T_H1 (IL-2 and IFN-γ) to the T_H2 phenotype (IL-4, -10, and -13). This fibrotic process irreversibly alters organ architecture and function. Increased 1-α hydroxylase activity in macrophages within granulomas and the alveoli converts 25-hydroxyvitamin D to the biologically active form 1,25-dihydroxyvitamin D (calcitriol), thereby resulting in increased intestinal absorption of calcium.

In sarcoidosis, an immune paradox exists: patients often develop anergy as indicated by a suppressed response to tuberculin, despite active granulomatous inflammation. This anergy results in part from an expansion of CD25^{bright} regulatory T cells, which are a subgroup of CD4^{+} T lymphocytes and which can abolish production of IL-2 and inhibit T-cell proliferation. Although sarcoidosis is predominantly a T-cell-driven disease, the presence of polyclonal hyperglobulinemia indicates that B lymphocytes may also play a role.

Multiple inciting agents rather than a single pathogen are likely to cause sarcoidosis. Airborne antigens are suspected because the lungs, followed by the eyes and skin, are the most commonly involved organs. A microbial origin of the antigens is favored because sarcoidosis occurs sporadically in clusters and is worldwide. Furthermore, sarcoidosis may recur in transplanted organs and can develop in recipients of tissues from donors with sarcoidosis.

Several environmental exposures are modestly associated with the risk for sarcoidosis, each with odds ratios of about 1.5: mold or mildew, musty odors at work, agricultural employment, and pesticide-using industries. Highly sensitive methods for detecting microbial DNA and proteins, such as polymerase chain reaction and mass spectrometry, have yielded potential etiologic agents. One promising candidate of microbial origin is the mycobacterial KatG protein.

Major histocompatibility complex (MHC) genes and non-MHC genes located on the short arm of chromosome 6p have been implicated as genetic risk factors for sarcoidosis.[1] HLA-DQB1*0201 and HLA-DRB1*0301 alleles are strongly associated with acute disease and good prognosis. The HLA-DRB1*1501/DQB1*0602 haplotype predicts a chronic course and severe pulmonary sarcoidosis. Genome-wide scans have identified the gene candidates *BTNL2* (butyrophilin-like 2 gene) and *ANXA11* (annexin A11).[2]

CLINICAL MANIFESTATIONS

Patients may present with any organ involved, with or without concomitant intrathoracic involvement.[3,4] The severity of symptoms and organ dysfunction also varies, and as many as 30 to 50% of patients have no symptoms at the time of diagnosis. Clinical manifestations also vary by ethnicity, race, and sex as well as by the particular organ system predominantly affected.[5]

Sarcoidosis often first comes to attention during routine screening when enlarged mediastinal and hilar lymph nodes are detected on a chest radiograph (Figs. 95-1 and 95-2). Symptomatic individuals commonly experience fatigue, night sweats, and weight loss. Fatigue often remains a prominent problem and can lead to impaired quality of life.

Symptomatic sarcoidosis may present insidiously or as an acute illness. Löfgren syndrome, an acute form of the disease, consists of erythema nodosum (see Fig. 440-24), arthritis, and bilateral hilar adenopathy. Fever and uveitis may also accompany Löfgren syndrome. Erythema nodosum occurs predominantly in women, whereas arthritis predominates in men.

Respiratory System Disease

More than 90% of patients have respiratory tract involvement, sometimes with symptoms and sometimes with asymptomatic radiographic abnormalities. The most common respiratory symptoms are dry cough and dyspnea. Chest pain, when present, is vague and nonspecific.

Upper respiratory tract involvement occurs in 2 to 6% of patients, with most having nasal mucosal involvement. Severe upper respiratory tract disease may lead to anosmia, erosion of septal cartilage, and nasal deformity. Supraglottic and glottic involvement can lead to stridor, dysphonia, cough, and dysphagia.

Examination of the chest often reveals few or no findings. Localized wheezing suggests endobronchial granulomatous disease, whereas diffuse wheezing suggests hyperreactive airways disease. Crackles may be heard when bronchiectasis and fibrosis are present. Hemoptysis may occur with bronchiectasis or cavitary disease.

The most common radiographic finding is intrathoracic lymph node enlargement with or without parenchymal lung involvement. Mediastinal lymphadenopathy without hilar adenopathy is extremely rare. Hilar lymph node enlargement is usually symmetrical, and less than 3% of patients have unilateral enlargement. Concurrent enlargement of right paratracheal and aortic-pulmonary window lymph nodes is common.

The chest radiograph is traditionally categorized into five stages (Table 95-1), but these stages do not necessarily denote the severity or chronologic progression of disease, particularly when extrathoracic involvement is present. Furthermore, 50 to 94% of patients will have hilar or mediastinal lymphadenopathy on computed tomography (CT) scans irrespective of their stage on a plain chest radiograph.

Chest CT may demonstrate nodules, ground-glass opacities, bronchiectasis, cysts, and thickening of the pleural surface (Fig. 95-3). In more advanced cases, patients develop fibrotic changes (Fig. 95-4) and evidence of pulmonary hypertension (Fig. 95-5). CT, however, generally adds little to diagnosis and management, particularly for those with a stage I chest radiograph. CT can be justified when atypical clinical and chest radiographic findings are present, a normal chest radiograph is found during the evaluation of suspected extrathoracic disease, or complications are suspected.

TABLE 95-1 CHEST RADIOGRAPHIC STAGING

Stage 0: Normal
Stage 1: Bilateral hilar adenopathy, often with right paratracheal adenopathy
Stage 2: Bilateral hilar adenopathy and parenchymal infiltration
Stage 3: Parenchymal infiltration without lymphadenopathy
Stage 4: Advanced parenchymal disease demonstrating fibrosis and possibly including honeycombing, cysts, bullae, and traction bronchiectasis

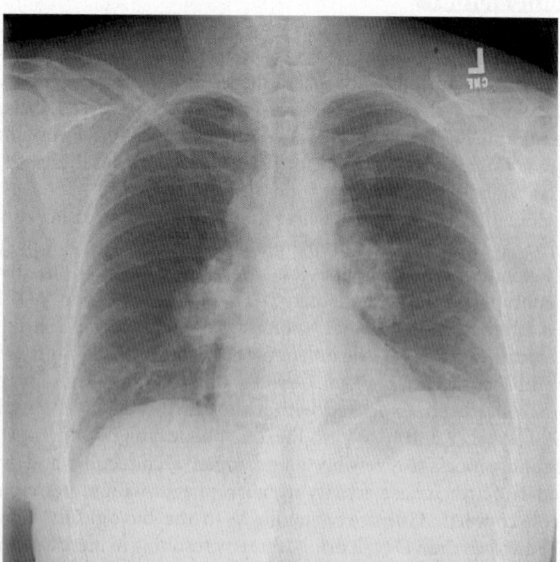

FIGURE 95-1. Chest radiograph demonstrating a stage I disease with enlarged mediastinal and hilar lymph nodes.

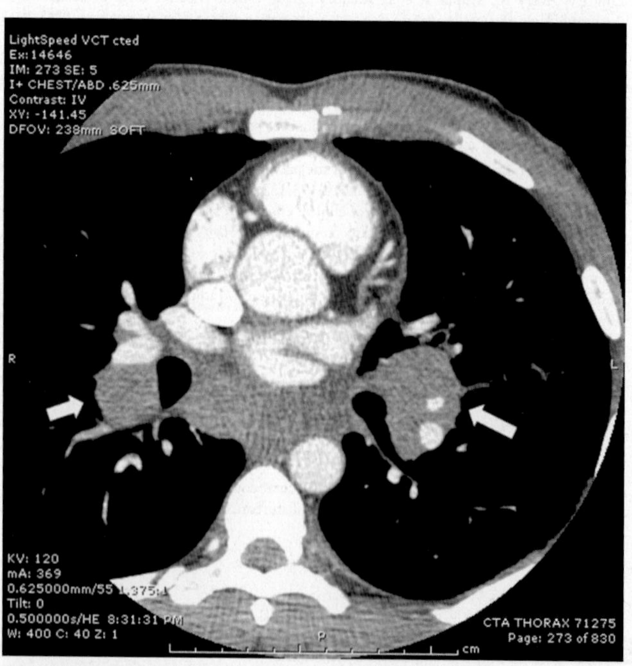

FIGURE 95-2. Chest computed tomographic scan showing typical hilar adenopathy, which correlates with stage I.

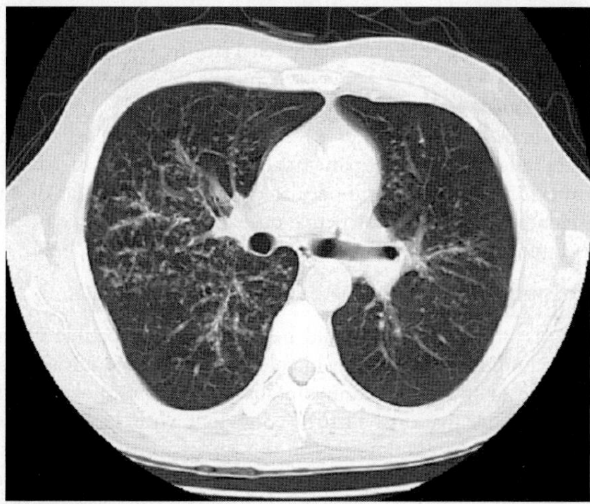

FIGURE 95-3. High-resolution chest computed tomographic scan demonstrating numerous small nodules in a predominantly bronchovascular distribution.

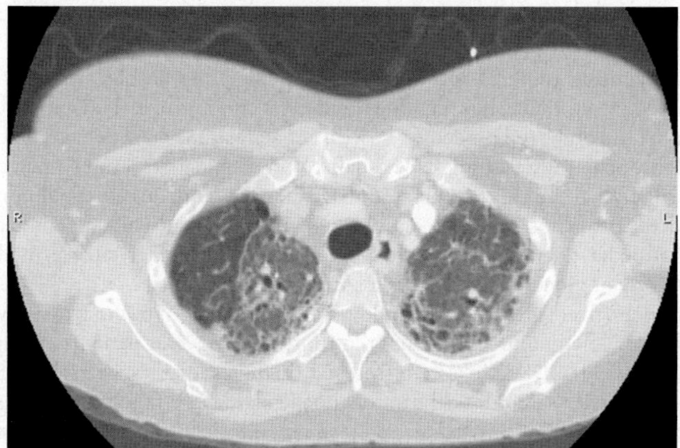

FIGURE 95-4. Chest computed tomographic scan showing fibrotic changes in the upper lobes with bronchiectasis.

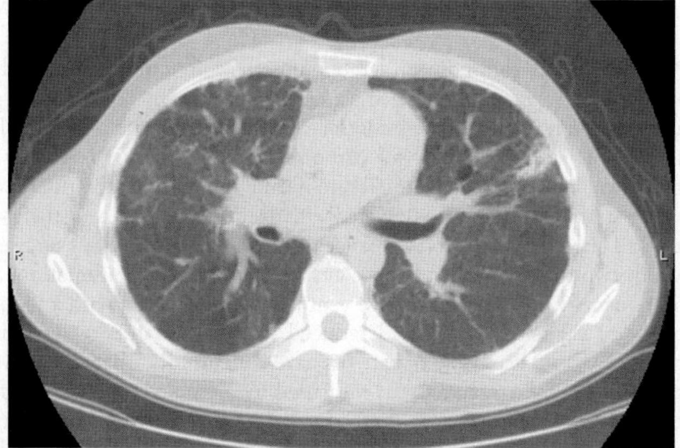

FIGURE 95-5. Chest computed tomographic scan showing diffuse bilateral fibrosis along with severe pulmonary artery enlargement consistent with pulmonary hypertension.

Endobronchial sarcoidosis may lead to bronchial stenosis and recurrent obstructive pneumonias. Pleural effusions on plain radiography are uncommon (1 to 3% of patients). Pulmonary hypertension (Chapter 68) may complicate sarcoidosis, particularly when pulmonary fibrosis is present.

Skin Disease

Skin involvement occurs in 25 to 35% of patients, but lesions are commonly misdiagnosed because they can present as macules, papules, plaques, subcutaneous lesions, areas of increased or decreased pigmentation, and ulcerations. Lesions are commonly found on the upper back, the nape of the neck, and extremities (Fig. 95-6) and have a predilection for scars and tattoos. The most common skin manifestation is a maculopapular eruption, consisting of firm, flesh-colored to violaceous lesions that have a predilection for the eyelids and perioral area. Scalp involvement with alopecia may occur. Skin lesions in black American patients frequently leave hyperpigmented scars and pale or depigmented areas.

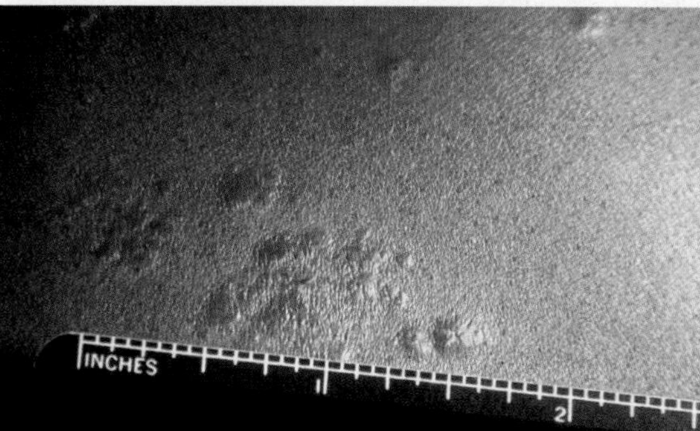

FIGURE 95-6. Skin lesions of sarcoidosis. Sarcoidal lesions may occur at any site. This patient's papules have a waxy appearance and are located on the upper part of the back.

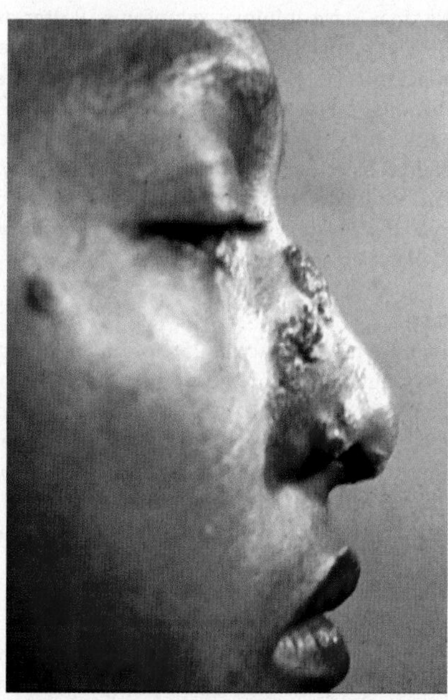

FIGURE 95-7. *Lupus pernio* is the term used to describe infiltrative skin lesions affecting the nose, cheeks, and ears in chronic sarcoidosis.

Erythema nodosum occurs in about 10% of patients and commonly occurs as part of Löfgren syndrome. It presents as raised, red, hot, tender subcutaneous nodular lesions, most commonly on the shins, but sometimes also on the arms and buttocks (see Fig. 440-24). Lesions persist for 1 to 3 weeks and may recur. The lesions of erythema nodosum typically show nonspecific septal panniculitis without sarcoidal granulomas, so biopsy is not usually helpful. Erythema nodosum portends a good prognosis, with up to 85% of patients resolving their sarcoidosis within 2 years.

Lupus pernio (Fig. 95-7) consists of chronic, lumpy, violaceous, indurated plaques and nodules distributed around the nose, cheeks, lips, and ears; it is specific to sarcoidosis. Patients with lupus pernio more commonly have a chronic course, fibrotic lung disease, and upper respiratory tract involvement.

Eye Disease

More than 25% of patients have ocular involvement (Chapter 423), and any part of the eye and adnexa may be involved. Lacrimal gland enlargement and conjunctival involvement are common. Conjunctival involvement consists of pale yellow nodules, which demonstrate granulomas on biopsy. Corneal involvement is rare. Acute anterior uveitis presents with pain, photophobia,

TABLE 95-2 NEUROSARCOIDOSIS

Cranial neuropathies
- VII—Facial nerve palsy (unilateral, bilateral)
- II—Optic nerve (unilateral and bilateral)
- VIII—Hearing loss
- Other cranial neuropathies

Myelopathy (sensory and motor)
Seizure
Basilar meningitis
Central diabetes insipidus
Panhypopituitarism
Intraparenchymal mass
Hydrocephalus
Peripheral neuropathy

lacrimation, and redness. Chronic anterior uveitis, which is more common than acute uveitis, may have minimal symptoms. Posterior uveitis, which occurs in about 30% of patients with ocular sarcoidosis, is frequently accompanied by central nervous system involvement. Choroidal lesions may occur anywhere in the fundus and may be multifocal. In 10 to 15% of patients with uveitis, both the anterior and posterior segments are affected.

Uveitis can herald the nonocular signs of sarcoidosis and may precede the diagnosis of sarcoidosis by decades. Chronic anterior uveitis may lead to cataracts and glaucoma. Heerfordt syndrome consists of anterior uveitis accompanied by parotid gland enlargement and fever.

Cardiac Disease

Cardiac granulomas are found in about 25% of sarcoidosis patients who are examined at autopsy, but cardiac sarcoidosis is suspected in only about 5% of patients. In cardiac sarcoidosis (Chapter 60), granulomas most often infiltrate the left ventricular free wall. Next most frequently, sarcoidal granulomas infiltrate the intraventricular septum, where they often involve the conduction system. Cardiac manifestations include atrioventricular block, ventricular arrhythmias, left ventricular dysfunction, and sudden death.[6]

Neurologic Disease

Nervous system granulomas are found in up to 25% of sarcoidosis patients who undergo autopsy, but only 10% of patients present with neurologic symptoms (Table 95-2). In patients with neurologic involvement, the neurologic signs or symptoms precede the diagnosis of sarcoidosis in up to 75% of patients and may be the only manifestation of sarcoidosis.

Neurosarcoidosis has a predilection for the base of the brain, hypothalamus, and pituitary gland.[7] Myelopathy may occur anywhere in the spinal cord and carries a poor prognosis. Peripheral neuropathy (Chapter 420) may manifest as mononeuropathy or polyneuropathy.

Liver and Spleen

Liver involvement is twice as common in black Americans as in white Americans. Symptoms due to liver disease are infrequent, but abdominal pain and pruritus are the most common symptoms. Fever, weight loss, and jaundice are present in less than 5% of those with liver involvement. About 20% of patients will have hepatomegaly on physical examination, and 35% will have an elevated serum aminotransferase or alkaline phosphatase level. Sarcoidosis can rarely (<1%) cause progressive liver disease that leads to portal hypertension with variceal bleeding; the hepatopulmonary syndrome, with refractory hypoxemia, cirrhosis, and liver failure, may also occur.

Splenomegaly is found on physical examination in 5 to 15% of patients with sarcoidosis. Massive splenomegaly is rare.

Bone and Joint

Most patients complain of arthralgias, but only about 35% develop arthritis. Acute sarcoid arthritis (Chapter 275) consists of large joint periarthritis, particularly involving the ankles and knees, and commonly occurs with Löfgren syndrome. These patients often report difficulty walking related to joint pain. Acute sarcoid arthritis usually persists for up to 3 months but is self-limited. Chronic sarcoid arthritis with direct granulomatous synovial infiltration is rare. Osseous sarcoidosis usually does not produce symptoms.

Calcium Metabolism

Aberrant calcium and vitamin D metabolism occurs in up to 50% of patients and may result in renal stones (Chapter 126), nephrocalcinosis with renal insufficiency, and hypercalciuria (urine calcium > 300 mg/24 hours) with or without hypercalcemia (Chapter 245). In chronic sarcoidosis, 10 to 14% of patients have at least one symptomatic renal stone.

Renal Involvement

Renal involvement, other than as a result of dysregulated calcium metabolism, occurs in less than 1% of patients. Renal disease may include granulomatous interstitial nephritis, glomerular disease, renal tubular dysfunction, renal vascular disease, and obstructive uropathy. Granulomatous interstitial nephritis is more common in white men.

DIAGNOSIS

The diagnosis of sarcoidosis should be based on compatible clinical and radiographic findings supported by histologic evidence of noncaseating granulomas in one or more organs in the absence of any foreign particles or organisms.[8] An occupational history consistent with beryllium exposure (Chapter 93), such as employment in the aerospace, automotive, ceramic, or computer industries, requires further investigation because chronic beryllium disease cannot be clinically or histologically distinguished from sarcoidosis.

A diagnosis of sarcoidosis is reasonably certain even without histologic confirmation in patients who present with Löfgren syndrome. In all other cases, a biopsy specimen from an involved organ should be obtained. The organ for which biopsy is safest, such as the skin, peripheral lymph nodes, lacrimal glands, or conjunctiva, should be sampled.

If diagnosis requires intrathoracic sampling, fine-needle aspiration of enlarged intrathoracic lymph nodes guided by endobronchial ultrasound has become the preferred procedure,[A1] with a diagnostic yield of 80% or higher.[9] Endobronchial ultrasound also visualizes mediastinal structures, including the subcarinal region, the paraesophageal space, and the aortopulmonary window. Bronchoscopy and endobronchial ultrasound-guided fine-needle aspiration have generally replaced more invasive approaches, such as mediastinoscopy or video-assisted thoracoscopic surgical biopsies.

Bronchoalveolar lavage sampling demonstrates lymphocytosis with normal or low granulocyte counts in more than 85% of patients (Chapter 85). The CD4/CD8 ratio is increased in bronchoalveolar lavage in about 50% of patients with sarcoidosis, but bronchoalveolar lavage findings are nonspecific and should not be used to diagnose sarcoidosis. Bronchoalveolar lavage findings also cannot predict prognosis or responsiveness to corticosteroid therapy.

Sarcoidal granulomas produce angiotensin-converting enzyme (ACE). Although serum ACE levels are elevated in 60% of patients with sarcoidosis, the value of a serum ACE level in diagnosing sarcoidosis remains limited because positive and negative predictive values are only about 84% and 74%, respectively.

Patients should routinely undergo pulmonary function testing, which often does not correlate with the chest radiographic stage. For example, pulmonary function tests may be abnormal even in patients with a normal chest radiograph. Diffusion capacity for carbon monoxide (DLCO) is usually the first abnormality detected and the last to normalize on remission. A DLCO of less than 50% of predicted is associated with exercise-induced oxygen desaturation and should prompt formal oxygen saturation testing with exercise.

About two thirds of patients have airflow limitation at presentation. Spirometry usually indicates restrictive ventilatory dysfunction with a reduced forced vital capacity (FVC) and reduced forced expiratory volume in 1 second (FEV_1). At least 50% of patients have concurrent obstructive airways disease. Airway hyperreactivity, as measured by increased responsiveness to methacholine, occurs in up to 83% of patients. In patients with abnormal spirometric findings at diagnosis, spirometry returns to normal in 80%. Alterations in cardiopulmonary exercise testing have been reported in nearly 50% of patients with sarcoidosis. Abnormalities, including a ventilatory limitation with exercise and a widened alveolar-arterial O_2 gradient, may be present. FVC is the single best test for following respiratory involvement and correlates well with FEV_1, total lung capacity, and DLCO.

Because ocular involvement is common and vision loss may occur, complete ocular evaluation with slit lamp and funduscopic examinations should be routinely performed during the initial evaluation and then annually in patients with active systemic disease.

An electrocardiogram (ECG) should be performed at the initial encounter. Screening for cardiac symptoms (palpitations, dizziness, and syncope) should be performed during the initial evaluation and routinely during follow-up visits if the disease is active. Any cardiac symptoms or abnormalities on the ECG should prompt further cardiac event monitoring (Chapter 62) and testing by echocardiography (Chapter 55). Endomyocardial biopsy has less than 20% diagnostic yield because cardiac involvement is patchy and is usually most dense in the left ventricle and basal ventricular septum where endomyocardial biopsies are avoided. If cardiac involvement is suspected, positron emission tomography (PET) or cardiac magnetic resonance imaging (MRI) with contrast should be performed.[10] In patients who have arrhythmias, decreased ventricular function, or septal involvement detected on MRI or PET, electrophysiologic studies should be considered, and the need for an automatic implantable cardioverter-defibrillator (AICD) should be evaluated (Chapters 65 and 66).

The criteria for the diagnosis of neurosarcoidosis in the absence of histologic confirmation are not established. Compatible MRI findings, a characteristic presentation, and exclusion of other neurologic diseases are required. Histologic confirmation of disease elsewhere supports the diagnosis of neurosarcoidosis. Cerebrospinal fluid (CSF) analysis typically demonstrates nonspecific lymphocytic inflammation (Chapter 412). The CSF glucose can be as low as 14 mg/dL, with a white blood cell count as high as 350 cells/μL and a protein concentration as high as 670 mg/dL. CSF ACE levels are neither sensitive nor specific. CSF oligoclonal immunoglobulin bands are elevated in one third of patients, thereby making it difficult to differentiate sarcoidosis from multiple sclerosis (Chapter 411).

Up to 65% of patients will have granulomas on liver biopsy, but hepatic granulomas (Chapter 151) occur commonly with other disorders such as infection and drug-induced hepatitis. As a result, the diagnosis of sarcoidosis should not be based solely on detection of hepatic granulomas.

On plain radiographic images, most skeletal lesions of sarcoidosis are seen in the small bones of the hands and feet. MRI and PET scanning show much greater involvement of the axial skeleton and long bones, and osseous sarcoidosis may appear similar to metastatic disease on a PET scan.

Sarcoidosis Complicating Type 1 Interferon Therapy

Type 1 interferons, IFN-α and IFN-β, used to treat viral hepatitis (Chapter 149), multiple sclerosis (Chapter 411), and autoimmune and malignant disease may increase the T_H1 cytokines, IFN-γ, and IL-2 and rarely (<1 to 5%) result in sarcoidosis. Most reported cases of interferon-induced sarcoidosis occur within 6 months of therapy and manifest primarily with lung and skin involvement.

TREATMENT Rx

Because the inciting agent has not yet been identified nor genetic risk factors firmly established, no means exist to prevent sarcoidosis. Most patients with sarcoidosis are not disabled by their illness, so the decision to recommend treatment should weigh the risks of using corticosteroids (Chapter 35), which are the most common treatment, against potential benefits (Table 95-3). Hypercalcemia, cardiac disease, and neurologic disease are indications for treatment, and immediate treatment is appropriate whenever organ function is threatened or when symptoms are severe. Detection of granulomatous inflammation on physical examination, biopsy, or imaging or the presence of an elevated serum ACE level is not a mandate to provide treatment.

Treatment is, however, recommended for patients who have a progressive decline in their pulmonary function, which sometimes is accompanied by progressive changes on chest imaging.[11] Oral prednisone at a dose of 20 to 40 mg per day for 3 months is usually the initial recommended therapy.[3] Response to treatment is indicated by improvement in symptoms or objective measures, such as decreased size and number of skin lesions, increased FVC, or a reduction of detectable cardiac or brain lesions. For pulmonary involvement, steroids improve symptoms, pulmonary function test results, and chest radiographic findings.[A2] If a response is noted at 3 months, the prednisone dose should be tapered to 10 to 15 mg per day for an additional 6 to 9 months and then tapered off. Because recurrence is possible, patients should be followed closely for 1 to 2 years after discontinuing treatment. The indications for restarting treatment are the same as those used to begin treatment. Lack of response after a 3-month trial suggests nonadherence to therapy, an inadequate dose of prednisone, or irreversible fibrotic disease. Inhaled corticosteroids should be used only in patients with bronchial hyperreactivity or persistent cough.

Despite the absence of definitive randomized trials, cytotoxic and immunosuppressive drugs have been used to treat patients who do not respond to corticosteroid therapy or who cannot tolerate it (see Table 95-3) and both methotrexate and azathioprine appear to have significant steroid-sparing effects.[12,13] Generally, 3 to 6 months of cytotoxic and immunosuppressive treatment is required to determine whether a response has occurred. For patients who respond, the duration of treatment should be 9 to 12 months. In patients who are steroid dependent but have ongoing extrapulmonary disease, the addition of infliximab, 3 to 5 mg/kg for 24 weeks, can be efficacious.[A3]

TABLE 95-3 TREATMENT

ORGAN	CLINICAL FINDINGS	TREATMENT
Respiratory	Dyspnea, persistent cough, FVC < 70%	Prednisone, 20-40 mg/day
	Mild cough, wheezing	Inhaled corticosteroid
Skin	Lupus pernio	Prednisone, 20-40 mg/day Hydroxychloroquine, 400 mg/day Methotrexate, 10-15 mg/wk Infliximab, 3-5 mg/kg every 2-4 wk
	Maculopapular eruptions	Topical corticosteroid Hydroxychloroquine, 400 mg/day Prednisone, 20-40 mg/day
	Erythema nodosum	NSAID*
Eyes	Anterior uveitis	Topical corticosteroid
	Posterior uveitis	Prednisone, 20-40 mg/day
Cardiac	Complete heart block, ventricular arrhythmias	AICD, prednisone, 20-40 mg/day
	Decreased LVEF (<35%)	AICD, prednisone, 20-40 mg/day
Central nervous system	Cranial nerve palsies	Prednisone, 20-40 mg/day
	Myelopathy	Prednisone, 40-60 mg/day, and azathioprine, 150 mg/day (or mycophenolate mofetil, or cyclophosphamide)
	Intracerebral involvement	Prednisone, 40-60 mg/day, and azathioprine, 150 mg/day (or mycophenolate mofetil, 1000-2000 mg/day, or cyclophosphamide, 1-5 mg/kg/day)
Liver	Cholestatic hepatitis	Prednisone, 20-40 mg/day
Bone and joint	Arthralgias	NSAID
	Granulomatous arthritis	Prednisone, 20-40 mg/day Methotrexate, 10-15 mg/wk
	Bone destruction/pain	Prednisone, 20-40 mg/day Methotrexate, 10-15 mg/wk
Hypercalciuria and hypercalcemia	Kidney stones	Prednisone, 20-40 mg/day Hydroxychloroquine, 400 mg/day

*For example, ibuprofen, 200-800 mg three times a day.
AICD = automatic implantable cardioverter-defibrillator; FVC = forced vital capacity; LVEF = left ventricular ejection fraction; NSAID = nonsteroidal anti-inflammatory drug.

Bosentan (up to 125 mg daily) can significantly reduce pulmonary hypertension but has not been shown to improve exercise tolerance in patients with sarcoidosis.[A4] Adalimumab may be effective for treating skin lesions.

Moderate doses of corticosteroids (15 to 20 mg prednisone) reduce the elevated serum and urinary calcium within a few days of starting treatment. Failure of serum calcium to normalize within 2 weeks should alert the clinician to an alternative diagnosis such as hyperparathyroidism or malignancy (Chapter 245). With treatment, most patients with granulomatous interstitial nephritis regain renal function but are often left with chronic kidney disease of varying severity.

Less than 1% of heart and liver and about 3% of lung transplantations are performed in patients with sarcoidosis. The 1- and 5-year graft survival rates for lung, liver, and heart transplantations in patients with sarcoidosis compare favorably with the results obtained for patients with other disorders.

PROGNOSIS

Patients with Löfgren syndrome have a good prognosis characterized by spontaneous resolution with few consequences. Overall, spontaneous remission with few or no consequences occurs in more than 50% of patients within 3 years of diagnosis and in two thirds of patients within a decade. After one or more years of remission without treatment, recurrence occurs in fewer than 5% of patients. Up to one third of patients have unrelenting disease that leads to significant organ impairment, but less than 5% of patients die from sarcoidosis. Black Americans tend to have a worse prognosis with more chronic disease and more extrathoracic involvement of the eyes, liver, bone marrow, extrathoracic lymph nodes, and skin. In the absence of extrathoracic disease, patients with stage I radiographs generally have the best prognosis. Pulmonary function testing is more reliable in determining prognosis than is radiograph staging. Patients with neurologic and cardiac involvement have a poorer prognosis.

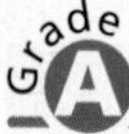

Grade A References

A1. von Bartheld MB, Dekkers OM, Szlubowski A, et al. Endosonography vs conventional bronchoscopy for the diagnosis of sarcoidosis: the GRANULOMA randomized clinical trial. *JAMA.* 2013;309:2457-2464.
A2. Paramothayan S, Jones PW. Corticosteroid therapy in pulmonary sarcoidosis: a systematic review. *JAMA.* 2002;287:1301-1307.
A3. Judson MA, Baughman RP, Costabel U, et al. Efficacy of infliximab in extrapulmonary sarcoidosis: results from a randomized trial. *Eur Respir J.* 2008;31:1189-1196.
A4. Baughman RP, Culver DA, Cordova FC, et al. Bosentan for sarcoidosis-associated pulmonary hypertension: a double-blind placebo controlled randomized trial. *Chest.* 2014;145:810-817.

GENERAL REFERENCES

For the General References and other additional features, please visit Expert Consult at https://expertconsult.inkling.com.

96 ACUTE BRONCHITIS AND TRACHEITIS

RICHARD P. WENZEL

DEFINITION

The term *acute bronchitis and tracheitis* defines a self-limited (1 to 3 weeks) inflammation of the large airways of the lung that extends to the tertiary bronchi (Fig. 96-1).[1] In patients with a primary symptom of cough (Chapter 83), the diagnosis is made if there is no clinical or radiologic evidence of pneumonia. At the bedside, the absence of criteria for systemic inflammatory response syndrome (SIRS) (Chapter 108) suggests bronchitis and tracheitis and makes a diagnosis of pneumonia (Chapter 97) unlikely. The SIRS criteria are met if the patient has more than two of the following: temperature lower than 36° C or higher than 38° C, pulse greater than 90 beats per minute, respiratory rate higher than 20 breaths per minute, or white blood cell count less than 4000 cells/mm^3 or higher than 12,000 cells/mm^3 or with greater than 10% bands.

The definition of acute bronchitis and tracheitis also seeks to differentiate the illness from acute inflammation of the small airways (bronchiolitis), even though the accompanying symptoms with the former may include sputum production, wheezing, and shortness of breath.[1,2] Among patients with primarily small airways disease, some might be expected to have prominently decreased breath sounds in the areas involved. Acute bronchitis and tracheitis is also different from bronchiectasis (Chapter 90), which is associated with permanent dilation of bronchi and a chronic cough. Furthermore, a diagnosis of chronic bronchitis (Chapter 88) is reserved for patients who have prolonged cough and sputum production: at least 3 months of the year for 2 consecutive years.

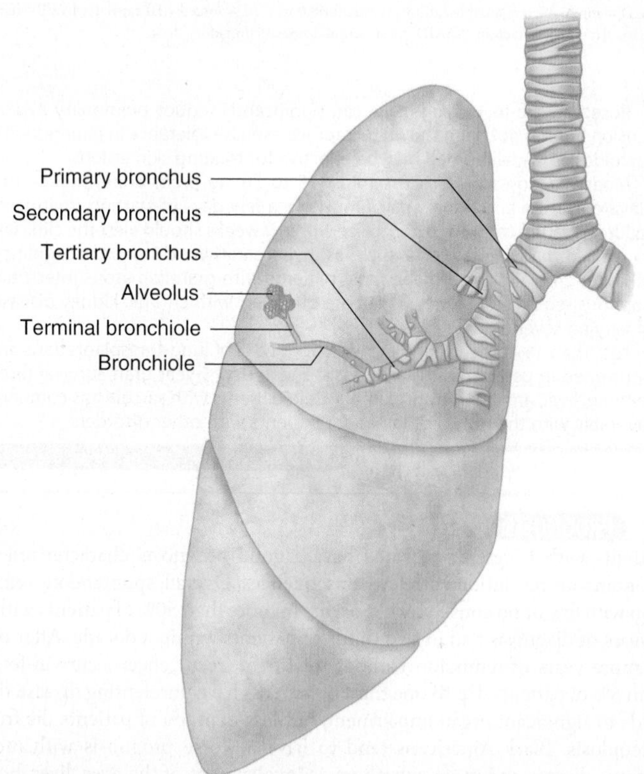

FIGURE 96-1. Many infecting agents that cause bronchitis and tracheitis can infect both large and small airways of the lung and occasionally the alveoli. Not surprisingly, a wide spectrum of signs and symptoms are associated with bronchitis, including cough, wheezing, and shortness of breath.

EPIDEMIOLOGY

Occurring at a rate of 44 per 1000 adults per year, acute bronchitis and tracheitis affects approximately 5% of adults annually. A higher incidence is observed in the winter and fall than in the summer and spring. In the United States, acute bronchitis and tracheitis is the ninth most common illness in outpatients as reported by physicians.

The disorder is thought to be viral in origin almost all the time. However, viruses have been isolated in only 8 to 37% of patients. Thus, the true causes of the illness are unknown in most cases. Nevertheless, at least 70% of patients with acute bronchitis and tracheitis in the United States receive antibacterial antibiotics after visiting a physician. Importantly, although the same bacteria that are commonly implicated in community-acquired pneumonia are also isolated from the sputum in half the patients, their role in the pathobiology of acute bronchitis and tracheitis or its attendant symptoms is unclear, and bronchial biopsies have not shown bacterial invasion.

PATHOBIOLOGY

Infections of the epithelium of the bronchi and trachea are thought to incite an inflammatory response. Pathologically, there is an accompanying microscopic thickening of bronchial and tracheal mucosa corresponding to the inflamed areas. Such pathologic findings are also consistent with the occasional case report of upper airway inflammation confined to the bronchi and trachea detected by ^{18}F-labeled fluorodeoxyglucose positron emission tomography (FDG-PET).

In various studies, specific pathogens have been found in more than half of patients with acute bronchitis.[1] These pathogens include common respiratory viruses, typical respiratory bacteria, and atypical bacteria. At least three variables can influence the yield of specific pathogens: the presence of epidemics, the season of the year, and the population's influenza vaccination status. Furthermore, there are probably wide variations in the anatomic distribution of all pathogens causing acute bronchitis and tracheitis, extending from the nasal mucosa to the bronchiolar epithelium.

The viruses implicated in acute bronchitis and tracheitis include influenza A and B (Chapter 364), parainfluenza (Chapter 363), respiratory syncytial virus (Chapter 362), coronavirus (Chapter 366), adenovirus (Chapter 365), and rhinoviruses (Chapter 361), usually in this order from the most to the least common. Human metapneumovirus (Chapter 361) also has been identified as an etiologic agent. In children, bronchiolitis has been associated with respiratory syncytial virus, influenza virus, parainfluenza virus, and metapneumovirus.

Typical bacteria implicated in acute bronchitis include *Haemophilus influenzae* (Chapter 300) and *Moraxella catarrhalis* (Chapter 300). Severe bronchiolitis has also been reported with *Mycoplasma pneumoniae* (Chapter 317), even though this pathogen is usually associated with either pneumonia or acute bronchitis and tracheitis in adults. Up to 25% of cases of acute bronchitis and tracheitis may be due to "atypical" bacteria: *Bordetella pertussis* (Chapter 313), *Chlamydophila (Chlamydia) pneumoniae* (Chapter 318), and *Mycoplasma pneumoniae* (Chapter 317).

CLINICAL MANIFESTATIONS

The cardinal clinical symptom is cough (Chapter 83) of recent onset. Because most upper respiratory infections resolve within 1 week, a more extended period of cough is useful for considering the diagnosis of acute bronchitis. Patients usually seek care from their physician after 4 to 7 days of coughing that is not resolving. With acute bronchitis, there is often a continued cough and sometimes a worsened cough that lasts an initial 1 to 3 weeks. Associated symptoms vary and include sputum production, fever, malaise, wheezing, and dyspnea. Adults with pertussis may exhibit paroxysms of coughing, whooping, or vomiting, although less commonly than seen in children with this infection.

DIAGNOSIS

Acutely ill patients may not be able to distinguish their early symptoms from those accompanying very mild upper respiratory infections. However, with acute bronchitis and tracheitis, a protracted phase of coughing persists beyond 1 to 5 days, during which time pulmonary function tests may become abnormal. A substantial proportion of patients will have significant declines in forced expiratory volume in 1 second (FEV_1) (Chapter 85).

When "atypical" bacteria are identified by culture or serology, patients tend to be seen later in the course of their illness than patients with viral causes and more often have wheezing. In some studies, 12 to 32% of patients with coughing that persists for longer than 1 week have pertussis. In other studies, however, pertussis has been confirmed in only 1% of such patients.

Because a major issue is whether symptoms are caused by an organism that could be responsive to antibiotics, the differentiation between bacterial infection compared with viral infection is often more important than determining the precise organism responsible for the infection. Measurement of serum levels of procalcitonin, which is the prohormone of calcitonin, can help detect the presence of bacterial infection and thereby guide the initiation or discontinuation of antibacterial antibiotics.[3] A level lower than 0.1 ng/L makes bacterial infection highly unlikely, and limiting treatment to patients with levels higher than 0.25 ng/L can markedly reduce the use of antibiotics without adverse clinical outcomes.[A1][A2] If the test is available, the finding of very low levels may help the clinician decide against prescribing antibiotics.

In the occasional instance in which it is important to diagnose specific viral cause, rapid diagnostic tests exist for most viruses linked to acute bronchitis and tracheitis. However, their value lies in identifying a virus for which there is therapy or avoiding antibacterial antibiotics if any virus is identified. Not all rapid tests are widely available, and they are expensive and rarely cost-effective in an outpatient setting.

For diagnosing specific bacterial causes, polymerase chain reaction (PCR) testing of nasopharyngeal swabs or aspirates is the easiest and most sensitive way to diagnose infections by *B. pertussis, M. pneumoniae,* and *C. pneumoniae;* most experts recommend calcium alginate swabs for pertussis because cotton inhibits growth. Dacron swabs with aluminum handles are preferred for specimens used to diagnose *Chlamydophila* because cotton, calcium alginate, and the wooden shaft can all inhibit growth of the organism. Cultures for *M. pneumoniae* are slow and insensitive. In general, testing for atypical organisms should not be done because of the cost of PCR and both the insensitivity and slowness of cultures. However, if the clinician suspects an outbreak in the community or the likelihood of pertussis, rapid testing with PCR may be quite beneficial.

TREATMENT

Rx

Although fewer than 50% of cases of acute bronchitis are probably caused by bacterial pathogens, antibiotics are used in 50 to 85% of cases worldwide. In a meta-analysis of randomized trials of antibacterial antibiotics for acute bronchitis, patients receiving antibiotics were significantly less likely to have a cough, but their 0.58 fewer days with cough, 0.46 fewer days of productive cough, and 0.64 fewer days of feeling ill were not statistically significant and were generally offset by the adverse effects of the antibiotics themselves.[A3] When antibiotics are prescribed, azithromycin (500 mg daily for three days) is probably better than other alternatives.[A4] Another option is to delay the initiation of antibiotics and to use them only in patients with persistent symptoms. This strategy slightly reduces patient satisfaction but has had no detectable adverse clinical implications.[A5] Of note is that discolored sputum per se does not appear to predict responsiveness to antibiotics.[A6]

Antibiotics may be used in patients with known atypical pathogens, but even then their effect on outcomes is not clear except to limit the spread of pertussis, especially during a defined outbreak. In adults suspected of having pertussis, erythromycin, 500 mg four times a day for 14 days, is thought to be most effective. However, many patients cannot tolerate erythromycin, and either doxycycline, 100 mg every 12 hours, or a newer macrolide such as azithromycin, 500 mg on day 1 and 250 mg/day thereafter, is effective. The latter two drugs are also active against *C. pneumoniae* and *M. pneumoniae,* although the optimal duration of therapy for acute bronchitis is unknown. A useful range is 5 to 14 days.

During influenza season, anti-influenza agents may be useful in decreasing symptoms by approximately 1 day and may lead to a 0.5-day earlier return to normal activity in patients with influenza.[A7] The first-generation drugs amantadine and rimantadine are ineffective against H3N2 influenza A viruses and are not recommended. Second-generation drugs such as zanamivir (two inhalations of 5 mg each, twice a day) or oseltamivir (75 mg twice a day) can be given for 5 days. Up to 20% of patients given oseltamivir will have nausea or vomiting.

Antihistamines and over-the-counter antitussives and expectorants have no apparent value. Although some subsets of patients with bronchial hyperresponsiveness may benefit from β-agonists, overall they appear to confer no benefit.[A8] No data support the routine use of inhaled steroids. Mucolytic agents may be of small benefit.[A9]

In experimental rhinovirus colds, nonsteroidal drugs, alone or in combination with antihistamines, reduce the severity of symptoms, including cough. However, the widespread use of either type of drug alone or as a combination in naturally occurring, community-acquired bronchitis and tracheitis has not been evaluated. In patients with acute bronchitis, various alternative medicines include *Pelargonium sidoides* (a herbaceous perennial widely used in Europe), extracts of thyme herb and primrose root, and a phytomedicine from essential oils; these medicines have shown some benefit compared with placebo in acute bronchitis, but corroborating studies are needed before they can be routinely recommended.

Because antibiotics are overused and probably lead to community-wide alterations in antibiotic resistance, interventions to reduce overuse could have substantial long-term benefits while also reducing health care costs. Unfortunately, such interventions have had only very modest success.[4,5]

PROGNOSIS

Coughing usually lasts 10 to 14 days, during which time the illness causes significant transient decrements in vitality and social functioning. Limited data on short- and long-term outcomes show that up to 20% of patients have persistent or recurrent symptoms for a month. Antibiotics may reduce symptoms by a fraction of a day, but side effects, the emergence of antibiotic resistance, and cost must be weighed against their modest benefits. The mean duration of an office visit for adults in the United States with upper respiratory tract infections is 14.2 minutes when patients are prescribed antibiotics versus 15.2 minutes without prescription of antibiotics, but antibiotic use is not an independent predictor of visit length. Future widespread use of rapid diagnostic tests for specific bacterial and viral pathogens will be useful in targeting effective therapies.

Grade A References

A1. Albrich WC, Dusemund F, Bucher B, et al. Effectiveness and safety of procalcitonin-guided antibiotic therapy in lower respiratory tract infections in "real life": an international, multicenter poststudy survey (ProREAL). *Arch Intern Med.* 2012;172:715-722.

A2. Schuetz P, Muller B, Christ-Crain M, et al. Procalcitonin to initiate or discontinue antibiotics in acute respiratory tract infections. *Cochrane Database Syst Rev.* 2012;9:CD007498.

A3. Smith SM, Fahey T, Smucny J, et al. Antibiotics for acute bronchitis. *Cochrane Database Syst Rev.* 2014;3:CD000245.

A4. Panpanich R, Lerttrakarnnon P, Laopaiboon M. Azithromycin for acute lower respiratory tract infections. *Cochrane Database Syst Rev.* 2008;1:CD001954.

A5. Spurling GK, Del Mar CB, Dooley L, et al. Delayed antibiotics for respiratory infections. *Cochrane Database Syst Rev.* 2013;4:CD004417.

A6. Llor C, Moragas A, Bayona C, et al. Efficacy of anti-inflammatory or antibiotic treatment in patients with non-complicated acute bronchitis and discoloured sputum: randomised placebo controlled trial. *BMJ.* 2013;347:f5762.

A7. Jefferson T, Jones M, Doshi P, et al. Neuraminidase inhibitors for preventing and treating influenza in healthy adults: systematic review and meta-analysis. *BMJ.* 2009;339:b5106.

A8. Becker LA, Hom J, Villasis-Keever M, et al. Beta2-agonists for acute bronchitis. *Cochrane Database Syst Rev.* 2011;7:CD001726.

A9. Poole P, Black PN, Cates CJ. Mucolytic agents for chronic bronchitis or chronic obstructive pulmonary disease. *Cochrane Database Syst Rev.* 2012;8:CD001287.

GENERAL REFERENCES

For the General References and other additional features, please visit Expert Consult at https://expertconsult.inkling.com.

97

OVERVIEW OF PNEUMONIA

DANIEL M. MUSHER

Pneumonia, which has been a major cause of death throughout recorded history, affects people of all ages without regard to social class or economic status. It remains a major cause of morbidity and mortality in both the developed and the developing world.

DEFINITION

Pneumonia occurs when an infection of the lung parenchyma causes lower respiratory symptoms, and a pulmonary infiltrate is detected on a chest radiograph. Pneumonias are commonly classified as community acquired,[1] health care associated, and health care acquired. Health care–associated pneumonia occurs in patients who live in a skilled nursing facility, have been hospitalized for more than 2 days in the preceding 90 days, have repeated exposure to a medical facility (e.g., for hemodialysis, wound care, or intravenous antibiotics or chemotherapy) or are immunosuppressed. Hospital-acquired pneumonia either appears 48 hours or more after admission in a patient who did not already have or was incubating pneumonia at the time of admission or develops soon after discharge from a hospital. All other pneumonias are considered to be community acquired.

EPIDEMIOLOGY

Pneumonia is the most common potentially lethal acute infection in the United States, each year affecting 1% of the population and causing more than 1.25 million hospitalizations. The incidence of pneumonia is high among infants and toddlers, declines greatly in childhood, remains relatively uncommon among young adults, but begins to increase after 50 years of age and especially after 65 years of age (E-Fig. 97-1). Not only is bacterial pneumonia more prevalent in elderly patients, it is also more severe, with the risk for death rising steadily with increasing age. Factors predisposing older adults to pneumonia include diminished gag and cough reflexes, poor glottal function, diminished toll-like receptor responses, and less robust antibody responses. These factors are far more prominent in persons who are bedridden—whether at home, in a nursing facility, or in a hospital—than they are in healthy aging persons.

Most adults of any age who develop bacterial pneumonia are likely to have one or more underlying predisposing conditions (Table 97-1). Most common is an antecedent viral respiratory infection, which increases adherence of bacteria to respiratory epithelial cells and damages clearance mechanisms by interfering with ciliary action. Influenza virus (Chapter 364) greatly increases the susceptibility to pneumonia caused by *Streptococcus pneumoniae* (Chapter 289), *Haemophilus influenzae* (Chapter 300), or *Staphylococcus aureus* (Chapter 288), and recent studies have confirmed that most of the deaths attributed to influenza virus during the great pandemic of 1918-1919 were due to bacterial superinfection. Bacterial pneumonia generally does not affect perfectly healthy young adults. Even when outbreaks of pneumococcal pneumonia occur among seemingly healthy adults, such as in military recruits, concurrent viral infection, physical exhaustion, and stress are all thought to play a contributory role. *Haemophilus* and *Moraxella* pneumonia almost always occur in persons with chronic obstructive pulmonary disease (COPD; Chapter 88), and *Pseudomonas* pneumonia (Chapter 306) occurs in patients with COPD, cystic fibrosis (Chapter 89), bronchiectasis (Chapter 90), or other structural abnormalities of the lung, especially if they are also taking corticosteroids.

Other predisposing factors include malnutrition (Chapter 215), which weakens the immune system; excessive alcohol intake (Chapter 33), which suppresses the cough reflex and affects migration of white blood cells (WBCs); cigarette smoking, which increases pulmonary secretions and damages ciliary action; hepatic or renal disease, which decrease antibody formation and WBC function; diabetes mellitus, which decreases WBC function; and immunoglobulin deficiencies of any cause. The nearly 100-fold increase in bacterial pneumonia in young adults who have AIDS (Chapter 391) is thought to be related largely to defective antibody production.

In contrast to bacterial pneumonia, viral or mycoplasmal pneumonia occurs when organisms are transmitted to immunologically naïve hosts. The presence or absence of preexisting immunity and the competence of the immune system itself appear to be principal determinants of whether infection occurs. Immune compromise contributes greatly to the severity of pneumonia due to respiratory syncytial virus (Chapter 362), influenza virus (Chapter 364), and parainfluenza virus (Chapter 363), and pregnancy predisposes to severe pneumonia due to influenza virus or measles virus.

TABLE 97-1 CONDITIONS SUGGESTING VARIOUS CAUSES OF PNEUMONIA

UNDERLYING CONDITION	ASSOCIATED MICROORGANISM
Active smoking/chronic obstructive lung disease	*Streptococcus pneumoniae, Haemophilus influenzae, Moraxella catarrhalis, Pseudomonas aeruginosa*
Nursing home resident	*S. pneumoniae*, gram-negative bacilli, *H. influenzae, Staphylococcus aureus*, microaerophilic and anaerobic mouth flora
Alcoholism	*S. pneumoniae*, gram-negative bacilli, microaerophilic and anaerobic mouth flora, *Mycobacterium tuberculosis,*
Gross aspiration/poor dentition	Microaerophilic and anaerobic mouth flora
Travel to southwestern United States	*Coccidioides immitis*
Residence in Mississippi River basins, exposure to bats	*Histoplasma capsulatum*
Exposure to birds	*Cryptococcus neoformans, Chlamydia psittaci, H. capsulatum*
Exposure to sick psittacine birds	*Chlamydia psittaci*
Exposure to rabbits	*Francisella tularensis*
Exposure to farm animals	*Coxiella burnetii* (Q fever)
Influenza active in community	Influenza virus, *S. aureus, S. pneumoniae, H. influenzae, Streptococcus pyogenes*
Bronchiectasis, cystic fibrosis	*Pseudomonas aeruginosa, Burkholderia cepacia, S. aureus, Aspergillus* species, nontuberculous mycobacteria
Cavitary lung lesion	Microaerophilic and anaerobic mouth flora, *S. aureus*, tuberculous and nontuberculous mycobacteria, endemic fungi
Intravenous drug use	*S. aureus, M. tuberculosis, S. pneumoniae*
Endobronchial obstruction	Microaerophilic and anaerobic mouth flora, gram-negative bacilli, *S. aureus,*
Recent antibiotic therapy	Drug-resistant *S. pneumoniae*
HIV (early)	*S. pneumoniae, H. influenzae, M. tuberculosis*
HIV (late)	The pathogens listed for early HIV infection, plus *Pneumocystis jirovecii, Cryptococcus, Histoplasma, Aspergillus, Mycobacterium kansasii, Mycobacterium avium* complex, *P. aeruginosa,*
Travel to Middle East	Middle East respiratory syndrome (MERS) coronavirus
In the context of bioterrorism	*Bacillus anthracis* (anthrax), *Yersinia pestis* (plague), *Francisella tularensis* (tularemia)

CA-MRSA = community-acquired methicillin-resistant *Staphylococcus aureus*; HIV = human immunodeficiency virus.
Data from Infectious Diseases Society of America/American Thoracic Society. Consensus guidelines on the management of community acquired pneumonia in adults. *Clin Infect Dis.* 2007;44:S27-S72.

PATHOBIOLOGY

Infecting microorganisms may reach alveoli and trigger pneumonia because of aspiration of small amounts of nasopharyngeal secretions or mouth contents, especially during sleep. Some degree of aspiration is a normal occurrence. More substantial aspiration, however, is prominent in older persons, especially those who are frail or bedridden, in whom it can be documented by applying radiopaque material to the posterior pharynx at bedtime and then documenting its presence in the bronchi and lungs by a plain chest radiograph the following morning. Aspiration is the usual cause of *S. pneumoniae* (Chapter 289) or *H. influenzae* (Chapter 300) bacterial pneumonia, in which the upper airways are colonized with potentially infective bacteria. Aspiration probably is also responsible for the large number of cases in which no causative organism is found but which may be due to mixed microaerophilic and anaerobic organisms of the mouth and upper respiratory tract.

This aspiration of small amounts of secretions should be distinguished from gross aspiration (Chapter 94). Gross aspiration occurs, for example, in persons who have seizures, in persons who choke while vomiting, or in people whose gag reflex is markedly suppressed by alcohol, drugs, or neurologic diseases. In such patients, the clinical syndrome of aspiration pneumonia includes the effects of the aspirated microorganisms and material as well as the accompanying gastric acid.

Another cause of pneumonia is the direct inhalation of aerosolized material into the lungs. This process is uncommon for most bacterial pneumonias but is characteristic of pneumonia due to *Mycobacterium tuberculosis* (Chapter 324) and *Bacillus anthracis* (Chapter 294). This mechanism also explains infection by some viruses, such as influenza virus or respiratory syncytial virus. Some viruses that infect the lung—such as influenza virus (Chapter 364), respiratory syncytial virus (Chapter 362), and human metapneumovirus (Chapter 361)—replicate and spread along cells that line the lower respiratory tract, usually but not always after first gaining entry by inhalation.

Bacteria also may reach the lungs through the blood stream, be filtered by normal host clearance mechanisms, but then escape and cause pneumonia. *S. aureus* pneumonia (Chapter 288) is commonly caused by hematogenous spread, especially if an endovascular infection such as endocarditis is present. *Escherichia coli* (Chapter 304) and other gram-negative rods also may precipitate pneumonia through hematogenous spread.

An array of host defense factors protects the lower respiratory tract against the entry of infectious organisms. The configuration of the upper airways ensures that a thin, laminar flow of air passes over hairs and sticky surfaces that can trap potentially infectious particles. Secretory immunoglobulin A (IgA), which constitutes 10% of the protein in nasal secretions, neutralizes viruses. Immunoglobulins also inhibit bacterial colonization. Closure of the epiglottis prevents food particles from passing into the trachea during swallowing. The larynx prevents the passage of secretions into the trachea and allows the generation of intrapulmonic pressure needed for an effective cough. When microorganisms bypass these mechanisms, ciliary action of the epithelial cells moves them steadily upward toward the larynx, and the cough reflex propels them more rapidly in the same direction. Tracheobronchial secretions maintain moist surfaces, and pulmonary surfactant probably helps to prevent atelectasis, which might interfere with distal clearance.

When potentially infective organisms reach the alveoli, innate and specific defenses come into play. Cells that line the respiratory tract produce substances that inhibit or kill microorganisms, including lysozyme, lactoferrin, β-defensins, and surfactant. Bacterial cell wall components, such as lipopolysaccharide in gram-negative bacteria and peptidoglycan in gram-positive bacteria, activate the alternative complement cascade, leading to opsonization or killing of bacteria. They also upregulate toll-like receptors, with subsequent enhancement of humoral and cellular immune mechanisms. Antibodies to surface-expressed bacterial components greatly enhance the host defense response, and serotype-specific antibodies against bacterial capsular polysaccharide are especially important in protecting against pneumococcal infection.

If these defense mechanisms fail, bacteria may replicate in the alveoli, where they stimulate the local production of cytokines and cause capillary leakage and the accumulation of plasma and inflammatory cells. This sequence initiates a vicious cycle, in which additional inflammatory cells are attracted, and further cytokine release is stimulated. In bacterial pneumonia, the host inflammatory response is responsible for most of the manifestations of disease.

Pathology

Pathologically, pneumonia results from the replication and spread of microorganisms through the pulmonary interstitium and alveoli. The presence of microorganisms and the resulting inflammatory response, characterized by the accumulation of plasma and WBCs in alveoli, explains most of the clinical manifestations of pneumonia. This progressive inflammatory exudate, which is detected radiographically as pneumonia, causes a ventilation-perfusion mismatch and hypoxemia.

Unlike bacterial pneumonia, influenza virus directly invades columnar epithelium cells, thereby resulting in pathologic changes that range from vacuolization of some respiratory epithelial cells to desquamation of the entire epithelial layer. These widespread changes, which lead to a diffuse interstitial pattern on the chest radiograph, also predispose to secondary bacterial invasion. *Chlamydophila pneumoniae* (Chapter 318) adheres to specific receptors and replicates within cells, thereby producing microcolonies that stimulate an inflammatory response and result in focal pneumonia. Mycoplasma also damages respiratory epithelial cells (Chapter 317) but, rather than invading cells, adheres to the cell surface, where it impairs ciliary activity and generates toxic substances. Secondary bacterial pneumonia is uncommon in *Mycoplasma* pneumonia, perhaps because these organisms, unlike the influenza virus, do not adversely affect phagocytic cells.

CLINICAL MANIFESTATIONS

Pneumonia is generally characterized by an acute onset of fever, a cough often with sputum production, and a newly recognized pulmonary infiltrate detected on a chest radiograph. However, patients with pneumonia may not cough, do not always produce sputum, can be afebrile when first evaluated, and may not have obvious radiographic infiltrates, especially if they are high-risk adults with chronic lung disease, are obese, or are evaluated with only a portable chest radiograph. In young adults who have bacterial pneumonia, acute severe malaise and subjective fever are common, often with chills, cough, and sputum production, or at least a sensation of needing to produce sputum. Some patients also have pleuritic chest pain. When sputum is produced, it may be tinged with blood. With advancing age, patients are increasingly likely to have only some or even few of these specific manifestations of pneumonia, in part because they produce lower levels of cytokines and may exhibit a less vigorous response to them. As a result, elderly patients with pneumonia may present with disorientation, confusion, fatigue, or more subtle changes in mental status. Diarrhea, which can be a prominent manifestation of *Legionella* pneumonia (Chapter 314), is also frequent in pneumococcal and probably in other bacterial pneumonias, likely because of a nonspecific gastrointestinal response to circulating cytokines.

Viral pneumonia is more likely to present with upper respiratory symptoms such as rhinorrhea or a sore throat and a dry cough. Patients often recall being exposed to someone with a respiratory infection.

DIAGNOSIS

Physical Examination

Younger patients with bacterial or influenza pneumonia appear acutely ill, in contrast to elderly and frail persons, who may simply appear listless. Younger adults with noninfluenzal viral, *Mycoplasma*, or *Chlamydophila* pneumonia (Chapters 317 and 318) often do not look as acutely ill. Patients with tuberculosis or other more chronic forms of pneumonia may appear chronically ill or may look relatively well.

A respiratory rate more than 20 breaths per minute is distinctly abnormal, and a rate of more than 25 breaths per minute should cause serious concern. An oxygen saturation (Sa_{O_2}) of less than 92% is likely to indicate a very low partial pressure of oxygen, and a low saturation together with a rapid respiratory rate suggests serious respiratory compromise. In a patient with pneumonia and tachypnea, an Sa_{O_2} of less than 90% should raise concern about impending respiratory distress (Chapter 104).

In bacterial pneumonia, crackles or rales are generally present over the affected area. Bronchial breath sounds and egophony strongly suggest pneumonia when present but are not sensitive for diagnosis. Dullness to percussion over the affected area may be detected in about one half of cases. Increased tactile fremitus is often present and is especially useful in distinguishing a pulmonary infiltrate from a pleural effusion, in which fremitus is diminished or absent. The failure to detect excursion of the diaphragm by percussion suggests an effusion. Unfortunately, the overall sensitivity and specificity of the physical examination for pneumonia is fairly low. As a result, the diagnosis of pneumonia requires radiographic validation.

Radiographic Findings

Pneumonia is usually diagnosed by the presence of an infiltrate on a chest radiograph or excluded by the absence of an infiltrate. A dense consolidation that involves a segment or a lobe of the lung is very likely to reflect an acute bacterial infection. Many patients with bacterial pneumonia, however, have radiographic infiltrates that are not clearly segmental. Small areas of alveolar consolidation may be missed by a chest radiograph, especially an anterior-posterior portable radiograph, but be detected by the far more sensitive computed tomography (CT) scan.[2] However, small areas of consolidation (ground-glass appearance) are often described on the CT scan of patients who do not have pneumonia.

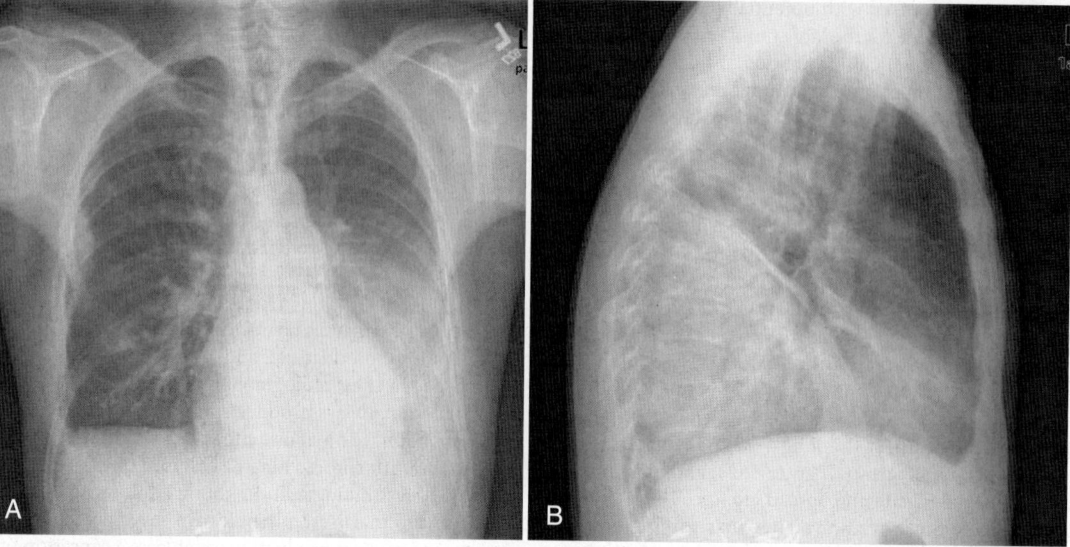

FIGURE 97-1. Pneumococcal left lower lobe pneumonia as seen in posterior-anterior (A) and lateral (B) views.

Although the presence of an infiltrate is the key to making a diagnosis of pneumonia, its radiographic appearance provides very little insight into the etiology. Dense consolidation of a segment or lobe is usually bacterial (Fig. 97-1), especially pneumococcal, but other bacteria, including *Legionella* (Fig. 97-2), may cause a similar picture, but many bacterial pneumonias do not cause segmental or lobar infiltrates.

Aerogenous *S. aureus* pneumonia (Chapter 288) presents as a segmental or lobar pneumonia, whereas hematogenous *S. aureus* pneumonia and gram-negative bacilli often cause necrotizing pneumonia, which is defined as a cavitary lesion in a pneumonic infiltrate. However, pneumococcal pneumonia also causes lung necrosis that is visible on a chest radiograph in 2% of cases and on a CT scan in 11% of cases (see Fig. 97-2).

Hematogenous *S. aureus* pneumonia (Chapter 288), especially when seen with endocarditis or an infected intravascular source (Chapter 76), can present with a distinctive radiographic appearance of several 1- to 3-cm round lesions, which are likely to cavitate (Fig. 97-3A and B). Subsegmental or "patchy" pneumonia (Fig. 97-4) may be due to bacteria, viruses, *Mycoplasma*, or *Chlamydophila* (Chapters 317 and 318). *Pneumocystis jiroveci* (Chapter 341) causes a diffuse interstitial infiltrate that may, in its earlier clinical stages, be mistaken for prominent pulmonary markings. Aspiration of mixed anaerobic, microaerophilic, and facultative bacteria from the mouth may cause pneumonia but may also lead to a lung abscess (Chapter 90) with a thick wall, a fluid level, and surrounding consolidation, especially in the superior segments of the lower lobes or posterior segments of the upper lobes. A cavitary lesion of an upper lobe without a fluid level, especially if confined to the posterior segment, suggests tuberculosis (Chapter 324). Occasionally, more acute presentations of tuberculosis may mimic acute bacterial pneumonia. *Aspergillus* (Chapter 339) can grow as a mass within a cavity, causing the distinctive appearance of an intracavitary mycetoma (fungus ball) surrounded by an arc or halo of air (E-Fig. 97-2).

Rapidly progressive pneumonia of any cause may result in diffuse pulmonary infiltrates consistent with the acute respiratory distress syndrome (Chapter 104). Although the appearance or enlargement of infiltrates after hospitalization is often attributed to fluid repletion, such progression more likely reflects the ongoing inflammatory response. A chest CT scan may help clarify the nature of an infiltrate and determine whether an effusion or mass is present, but it is usually not necessary at hospital admission for patients in whom a good-quality chest radiograph can be obtained.

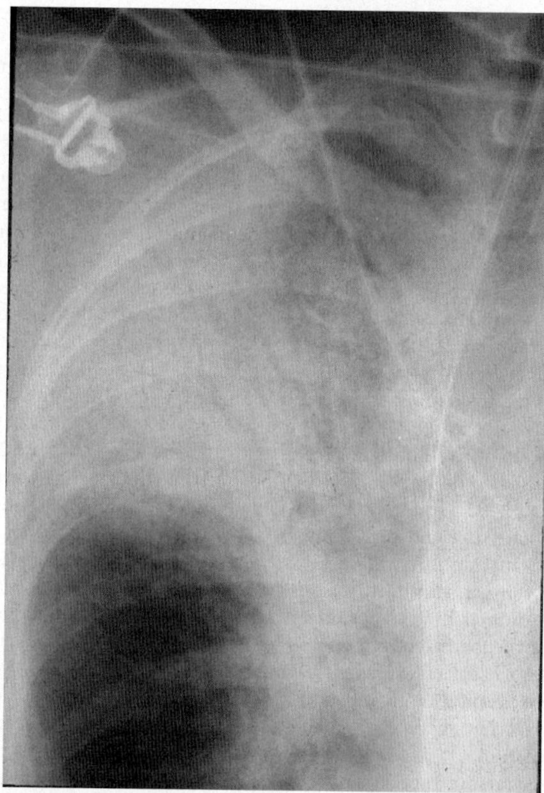

FIGURE 97-2. Dense lobar consolidation with air bronchograms in a patient with proven *Legionella* pneumonia.

Laboratory Findings

Most patients with bacterial pneumonia have a WBC count higher than 11,500/μL at the time of admission to hospital, and about one third have a WBC count higher than 15,000 WBC/μL. A low WBC count should not be interpreted as reassuring because WBC counts of 6000/μL or less may be seen in overwhelming bacterial infection. When overwhelming bacterial infection suppresses the WBC count, immature (band) cells are almost always elevated. About 40% of uninfected patients who present to the hospital with a syndrome consistent with community-acquired pneumonia, such as patients with pulmonary edema or lung cancer, also have WBC counts higher than 11,500/μL, so an elevated WBC count is by no means specific for pneumonia. Nevertheless, WBC counts higher than 20,000/μL are unusual in acute pulmonary conditions other than bacterial pneumonia. Mild nonspecific elevations in the serum bilirubin level, aminotransferase levels, and lactate dehydrogenase (LDH) level are often noted. Marked elevations of the LDH level can be seen in *Pneumocystis* and *Histoplasma* pneumonia (Chapters 332 and 341) in AIDS patients.

An elevated serum procalcitonin level increases the likelihood of a bacterial infection, whereas a low level opposes such a diagnosis. In randomized trials of patients who present with lower respiratory tract symptoms, even rather severe symptoms, treatment guided by a procalcitonin level

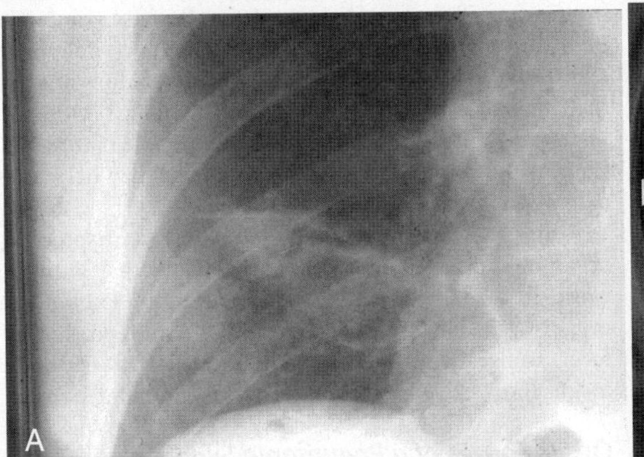

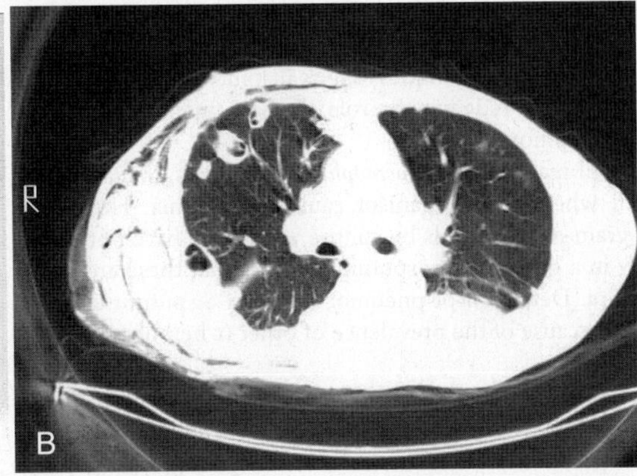

FIGURE 97-3. Hematogenous *Staphylococcus aureus* pneumonia. **A,** The chest radiograph shows the characteristic round lesions with cavitation. **B,** The same lesions confirmed by computed tomographic scan.

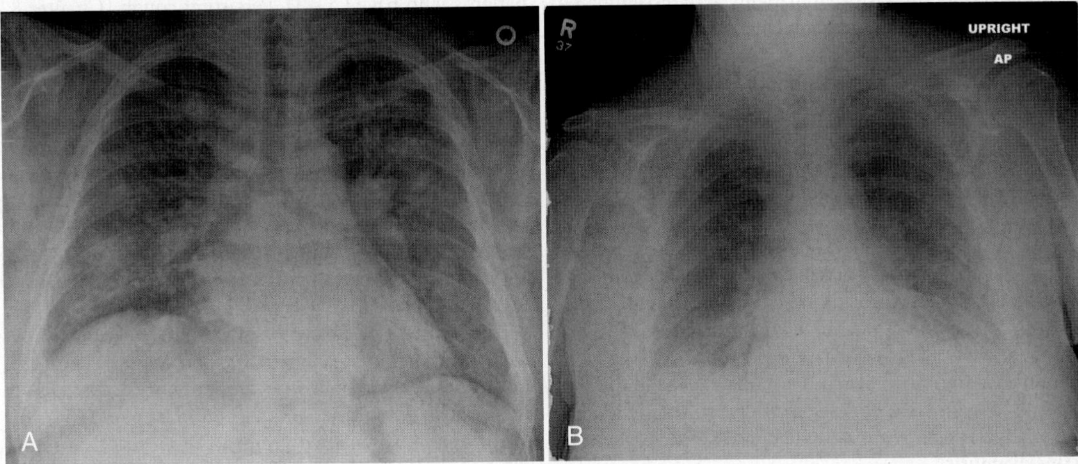

FIGURE 97-4. **A,** Bilateral "patchy" infiltrates in a patient with coronavirus pneumonia. **B,** Chest radiograph of community-acquired pneumonia ultimately proved to be caused by human metapneumovirus infection.

(antibiotics discouraged if the level is ≤0.25 µg/L and strongly discouraged if <0.1 µg/L) has resulted in less use of antibiotics without any adverse overall effects.[A1][A2] However, up to 25% of patients with bacterial pneumonia have a normal procalcitonin level, and about 25% of patients with a pneumonia syndrome but no evidence for bacterial infection have an elevated procalcitonin level, so this test cannot be used alone to determine therapeutic decisions.

Microbiologic Diagnosis

The respiratory tract clears inflammatory exudate by the ciliary action of cells that line the bronchi and trachea as well as by the cough reflex. Sputum is composed of this exudate—plasma, white blood cells, and bacteria—with a greater or lesser admixture of saliva. The presence of large numbers of a single type of bacterium in an inflammatory specimen that is relatively free of contaminating epithelial cells strongly suggests this organism as the etiologic agent of the pneumonia (Fig. 97-5). *Haemophilus* (Chapter 300), *Moraxella* (Chapter 300), and gram-negative rods (Chapters 305 and 306) are even more distinctive in their microscopic appearance. If antibiotics have not already been administered, the absence of visible organisms in an inflammatory specimen suggests that the cause of pneumonia is either a bacterium that does not readily accept Gram stain (e.g., *Legionella* or *Mycobacteria*), or another kind of organism such as *Mycoplasma, Chlamydophila,* or a virus that lacks typical bacterial cell walls and does not take up Gram stain. Reports of the poor sensitivity of sputum to detect bacteria largely reflect the inclusion of specimens that are inadequate or have been obtained after antibiotic therapy has been begun. In patients with bacteremic pneumococcal pneumonia who cough up a valid specimen and have not received antibiotics, the sensitivity of Gram stain or culture is each about 90% for detecting pneumococci. Because the sensitivity of these standard microbiologic tests falls dramatically after 18 hours of antibiotic treatment, specimens are useful diagnostically only if they are collected in a timely fashion.

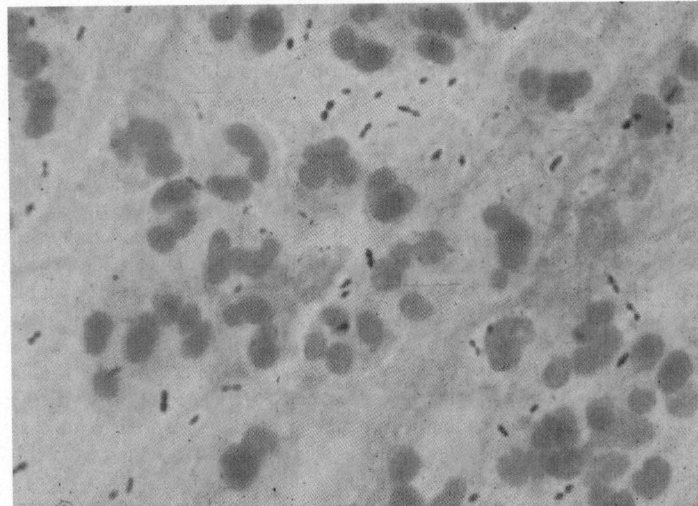

FIGURE 97-5. Gram stain of sputum from a patient with pneumococcal pneumonia shows large numbers of polymorphonuclear leukocytes and many lancet-shaped gram-positive cocci with no epithelial cells, indicating that this specimen originated in the lower airways. Such a specimen is diagnostic of pneumococcal pneumonia, although it cannot exclude coexisting infection by an organism such as a virus that is not seen by Gram stain.

Examination of a Gram-stained sputum specimen is also useful if it does not show bacteria. If antibiotics have not already been administered, the absence of visible organisms in an inflammatory specimen suggests that the cause of pneumonia is either a bacterium that does not readily accept Gram stain (e.g., *Legionella* or *Mycobacteria*), an organism such as *Mycoplasma* or

Chlamydophila that lacks typical bacterial cell walls, or a virus that does not take up Gram stain. In the past, diagnosis of infection due to these organisms relied upon unreliable serologic techniques. The availability of modern diagnostic techniques is likely to redefine the role of these agents in causing community-acquired pneumonia.

Bacterial cultures will readily yield *Haemophilus, Moraxella, S. aureus,* or gram-negative bacilli when these organism cause pneumonia. However, finding *S. aureus* or gram-negative rods by culture when they have not been seen microscopically in a good-quality sputum suggests that these are contaminating mouth flora. Detection of pneumococcus on a sputum culture may be more difficult because of the prevalence of other α-hemolytic streptococci in saliva.

Enzyme-linked immunosorbent assay (ELISA) can detect pneumococcal cell wall or capsular polysaccharide in the urine of 60 to 80% of patients with bacteremic pneumococcal pneumonia and a smaller proportion of those with nonbacteremic disease. An ELISA for urinary *Legionella* antigen detects only the most common *Legionella* serotype but is positive in about 70% of cases of *Legionella* pneumonia (Chapter 314), with higher sensitivity in more severe disease. *Histoplasma* (Chapter 332) urine and *Cryptococcus* (Chapter 336) serum antigen tests are positive in patients with disseminated disease but are less likely to be positive in patients with discrete pulmonary infiltrates.

Polymerase chain reaction (PCR) testing of sputum is a highly sensitive technique that may be nonspecific because it can detect colonization rather than infection. When used in African patients with AIDS and suspected pneumonia, quantitative PCR testing on a nasopharyngeal swab reliably identified pneumococcal pneumonia.[3] The generalizability of this method to patients in developed countries remains to be determined. For organisms that do not normally colonize the upper airways, PCR is specific as well as sensitive. PCR on a throat swab can reliably detect *Chlamydophila* and *Mycoplasma* as well as 15 respiratory viruses (including influenza, parainfluenza, respiratory syncytial virus, human metapneumovirus, coronavirus, and adenovirus) with very high sensitivity and specificity. As a result, PCR has generally replaced viral culture as the gold standard for diagnosing influenza virus infection (Chapter 364). Sputum PCR also can detect *M. tuberculosis* (Chapter 324) and is now part of the recommended evaluation in patients suspected of having this diagnosis.

Bacteremia is documented in about 10% of patients who are hospitalized for community-acquired pneumonia, including in about 25% of patients with pneumococcal pneumonia, 10 to 15% of patients who are hospitalized for aerogenous pneumonia due to *S. aureus* or gram-negative rods, and a lower proportion of patients with nontypable *H. influenzae* pneumonia, and only rarely in pneumonia caused by *Moraxella catarrhalis*. By comparison, patients with hematogenous *S. aureus* pneumonia virtually always have positive blood cultures.

Differential Diagnosis

Streptococcus pneumoniae (Chapter 289), which is the most commonly identified infectious cause of community-acquired pneumonia, causes up to 20% of cases in hospitalized patients in the United States[4] but a greater proportion of cases in Europe, perhaps because of higher rates of smoking in Europe and higher rate of pneumococcal vaccination in the U.S. *H. influenzae* (Chapter 300), *S. aureus* (Chapter 288), *P. aeruginosa* (Chapter 306), and other gram-negative bacilli (Chapters 304 and 305) are the next most common bacterial causes of community-acquired pneumonia. *Haemophilus* generally causes pneumonia only in persons who have preexisting bronchopulmonary disease. *Pseudomonas* and other gram-negative rods generally cause pneumonia in patients who have structural lung disease and who are receiving corticosteroids or are otherwise immunocompromised.

When influenza is active in the community, this virus is identified in a substantial proportion of patients admitted to an intensive care unit because of community-acquired pneumonia.[5] Identification of influenza virus in a patient with pneumonia should lead to appropriate antiviral treatment (Chapter 360), even if more than 48 hours have passed since the onset of symptoms. Evidence for viral infection is found in 20 to 30% of all adults hospitalized for community-acquired pneumonia. Rhinovirus (Chapter 361) is most commonly recognized, but its role as a cause of pneumonia is not well established. Respiratory syncytial virus (Chapter 362), coronavirus (Chapter 366), and human metapneumovirus (Chapter 361) are clearly implicated as causes of pneumonia and are the next most commonly found viruses in adults hospitalized for pneumonia. Outbreaks of adenovirus (Chapter 365) pneumonia may occur in military recruits. Because coinfecting bacteria are also detected in about half of cases of documented viral pneumonia,[6] identifying a virus by PCR in a patient with pneumonia does not prove that the virus is the cause or especially the sole cause of illness. Other features, such as the history, severity of illness, sputum production, nature of the pulmonary infiltrate, WBC count, and procalcitonin level may help to establish or refute a diagnosis of viral pneumonia.

Although *Mycoplasma* and *C. pneumoniae* (Chapters 317 and 318) may be common causes of pneumonia in the ambulatory setting, they less frequently cause disease that requires hospitalization. Pneumonia caused by these organisms is characterized by prolonged nonproductive cough, low-grade fever, and scattered pulmonary infiltrates. PCR is preferred over serologies for diagnosing *Chlamydophila* or *Mycoplasma* infections.

Other Causes of a Pneumonia Syndrome

Fever, cough, and sputum production without an infiltrate is called acute bronchitis (Chapter 96). In persons who do not have chronic lung disease, acute bronchitis is generally a self-limited viral illness, but bacterial infection, for example with *H. influenzae* (Chapter 300), may cause bronchitis in patients who have COPD. Persistent cough (Chapter 83) of several weeks' duration without fever or sputum suggests pertussis (Chapter 313) or a post-viral infection syndrome due, for example, to adenovirus.

Epidemiologic clues may suggest specific infectious causes of pneumonia (Table 97-2). *Coccidioides immitis* (Chapter 333), found in arid regions of the Americas, or *Histoplasma capsulatum* (Chapter 332), found worldwide but especially in river basins of North America, cause a variable proportion of community-acquired pneumonia in endemic regions. Exposure to livestock or late summer residence in a hot and dry ranching area suggests *Coxiella burnetii* (Q fever) (Chapter 327), especially if patients have a severe headache and abnormal liver enzymes. Exposure to sick psittacine birds raises concern for *Chlamydia psittaci* (Chapter 318).

Tuberculosis (Chapter 324) should be suspected in persons who have lived in endemic areas, patients who have served time in prison or been homeless, and patients who are immunocompromised, especially patients with AIDS. *Mycobacterium kansasii* (Chapter 325) may cause an identical syndrome in patients with none of those risk factors. *Mycobacterium avium*, often called *Mycobacterium avium-intracellulare* (MAI) or *Mycobacterium avium* complex (MAC), causes diffuse bilateral pneumonia in immunocompromised patients (Chapter 325). *Mycobacterium intracellulare* also is a well-known cause of pneumonia in adults, usually in men with bronchiectasis (Chapter 90) or extensive lung scarring owing to emphysema (Chapter 88) or previously treated tuberculosis. This organism also causes disease in

TABLE 97-2 COMMON CAUSES OF PNEUMONIA SYNDROME

REQUIRING HOSPITAL ADMISSION	
Common	**Uncommon**
Streptococcus pneumoniae	*Nocardia*
Haemophilus influenzae	*Legionella*[‡§]
Staphylococcus aureus	*Chlamydophila*[§]
Influenza virus,[†] other respiratory viruses	*Mycoplasma*[§]
Lung cancer	Anaerobic bacteria
Pulmonary edema	Cryptogenic organizing, eosinophilic, and other noninfectious pneumonias
Mycobacterium tuberculosis	Sarcoidosis
Pneumocystis jiroveci	Kaposi sarcoma
Less Common	Q fever[‡]
Moraxella catarrhalis	*Coccidioides immitis*[‡]
Pseudomonas	**OUTPATIENT TREATMENT MAY BE ADEQUATE**
Klebsiella	
Nontuberculous mycobacteria	*Streptococcus pneumoniae*
Histoplasma[‡]	*Mycoplasma pneumoniae*
Cryptococcus	*Haemophilus influenzae*
Pulmonary infarction	*Chlamydophila pneumoniae*
	Respiratory viruses*

*Routine use of polymerase chain reaction (PCR) technology substantially increases the recognition of these agents.
†Likely to be associated with secondary bacterial infection.
‡Strong dependence on geographic exposure.
§True incidence of pneumonia caused by these organisms will be clarified by routine use of PCR technology.

middle-aged women who lack these risk factors; in such patients, subtle infiltrates may be missed by routine chest radiography.

Patients with HIV infection are susceptible to a variety of pulmonary infections depending on how immunocompromised they are (see Table 97-2 and Chapter 391). These opportunistic infections include typical and atypical tuberculous and nontuberculous mycobacteria, *Pneumocystis* (Chapter 341), *Histoplasma* (Chapter 332), and *Cryptococcus* (Chapter 336). AIDS patients also have a 50- to 100-fold increased risk for developing pneumococcal disease.

Even after an exhaustive evaluation, no causative organism is identified in about half of patients who are hospitalized for symptoms, physical examination findings, laboratory abnormalities, and radiographic changes consistent with community-acquired pneumonia. The presumption is that bacterial infection is responsible for most of these pneumonias because they generally respond to antibiotic therapy.

Noninfectious Considerations

Many noninfectious conditions cause patients to present with a syndrome consistent with acute or subacute pneumonia (see Table 97-1). Cryptogenic organizing pneumonia (Chapter 91), acute interstitial pneumonia, eosinophilic pneumonia, and other interstitial pneumonias (Chapter 92) are uncommon conditions that almost always are initially misdiagnosed as community-acquired pneumonia. Pulmonary hemorrhage and vasculitis may also cause pulmonary infiltrates and fever. In ANCA-associated granulomatous vasculitis, these infiltrates may also be associated with cavitary lesions. Attention to the patient's history may reveal a longer history of symptoms, and careful review of earlier chest radiographs may reveal prior radiographic abnormalities, consistent with a chronic, noninfectious process. Pulmonary embolus with infarction can cause pleuritic chest pain and pulmonary infiltrates, with sputum that contains neutrophils but few or no bacteria. Patients with septic pulmonary emboli should be assessed for other foci of infection, such as an infected heart valve or intravascular device.

Pulmonary edema (Chapter 58) is the most common noninfectious cause of a community-acquired pneumonia-like syndrome in middle-aged and older patients. The diagnosis should be made based on history, physical examination, and radiographic findings, supported by elevated B-natriuretic peptide levels. Patients with lung cancer (Chapter 191) commonly present with fever and a pulmonary infiltrate, which sometimes is attributed to a postobstructive pneumonia. Acute respiratory distress syndrome (Chapter 104) in response to a serious nonpulmonary infection is often indistinguishable from pneumonia because it commonly presents with fever, lung crackles, an elevated WBC count, and pulmonary infiltrates. In light of all these possibilities, at least brief consideration should be given to other infectious and noninfectious causes before treating presumptive community-acquired pneumonia with guideline-recommended empirical therapy.

TREATMENT Rx

Hospital Admission

Scoring systems can help determine whether a patient with community-acquired pneumonia requires hospitalization (Tables 97-3 and 97-4). A corollary decision, whether a patient should be admitted to an intensive care unit (ICU), can be guided by the respiratory rate, heart rate, systolic blood pressure, oxygenation, mental status, extent of pulmonary involvement, serum albumin level, and arterial pH (Table 97-5).[7] This decision aid is 92% sensitive in detecting patients who will require ICU transfer for intensive respiratory or vasopressor support. Other indicators of overwhelming infection that indicate a need for ICU admission include a WBC count of 6000/μL or lower in bacterial pneumonia (especially if increased band forms are present), thrombocytopenia, and hypothermia.

Supportive therapy should include fluid replacement to maintain blood pressure (e.g., an average of 4.5 liters of fluids with electrolytes will be needed in a patient with pneumonia and septic shock [Chapter 108]), oxygen for hypoxemia, and mechanical ventilation (Chapter 105).

Antibiotic Therapy

Based on good evidence that outcomes are worse with prolonged delays, initial antibiotics should be given as soon as the diagnosis of pneumonia is considered likely, regardless of whether that be in a physician's office or an emergency department. Guidelines for the empirical antibiotic therapy of community-acquired pneumonia (Table 97-6)[8,9] focus on common infectious causes of pneumonia and are generally successful because a specific etiologic agent is infrequently determined in outpatients who have pneumonia. However, this approach should not discourage the careful consideration of possible noninfectious causes of fever and pulmonary infiltrates or discourage

TABLE 97-3 PNEUMONIA OUTCOMES RESEARCH TRIAL (PORT) SEVERITY INDEX

	POINTS ASSIGNED FOR EACH CRITERION
VITAL SIGNS	
Pulse >125/min	10
Systolic BP <90 mm Hg	20
Temp <35 or >40°C	15
Respiratory rate >30/min	20
HISTORY OF CO-MORBID CONDITIONS	
Neoplasm (active, not skin)	30
Cirrhosis or chronic hepatitis	20
Heart failure, stroke, chronic renal insufficiency	10
Altered mental status	20
DEMOGRAPHY	
Age	age (subtract 10 for women)
Nursing home resident	10
LABORATORY DATA	
Arterial pH <7.35	30
BUN >30 mg/dL	20
Serum sodium <130 mEq/L	20
Glucose >250 mg/dL	10
Hematocrit <30%	10
pO2 <60 mm Hg or O2 saturation <90%	10
Pleural effusion on chest radiograph	10

For mortality associated with various PORT scores, see Table 97-4.
Data from Fine MJ, Auble TE, Yealy DM, et al. A prediction rule to identify low-risk patients with community-acquired pneumonia. *N Engl J Med.* 1997;336:243-250.

TABLE 97-4 PORT SEVERITY INDEX (PSI) AND MORTALITY AT 30 DAYS

		MORTALITY		
POINT SCORE	**CLASS**	***Community-Acquired Pneumonia*** *	***Community-Acquired Pneumonia*** †	***S. pneumoniae*** ‡
≤70	II	<1%	3%	—
71-90	III	3%	4%	3%
91-130	IV	8%	8%	21%
>130	V	29%	22%	35%

*Original calculation in patients with community-acquired pneumonia report of PORT score (Fine MJ, Auble TE, Yealy DM, et al. A prediction rule to identify low-risk patients with community-acquired pneumonia. *N Engl J Med.* 1997;336:243-250.)
†Mortality in patients admitted for pneumonia during a 1-year period, Veterans Affairs Medical Center, Houston (patients with noninfectious causes were excluded) (Musher DM, Roig IL, Cazares G, et al. Can an etiologic agent be identified in adults who are hospitalized for community-acquired pneumonia: results of a one-year study. *J Infect.* 2013;67:11-18.)
‡Results in patients with proven pneumococcal pneumonia (Musher DM, Alexandraki I, Graviss EA, et al. Bacteremic and nonbacteremic pneumococcal pneumonia. A prospective study. *Medicine [Baltimore].* 2000;79:210-221.)

reasonable attempts to establish a specific infectious diagnosis, especially in patients who do not respond promptly.

Outpatient Antibiotic Regimens

For empirical outpatient therapy, guidelines from the Infectious Diseases Society of America and the American Thoracic Society[8] recommend a macrolide, doxycycline, a "respiratory" quinolone (levofloxacin or moxifloxacin, but not ciprofloxacin, which is thought to be slightly less effective against pneumococci), or a β-lactam together with a macrolide. These recommendations are based on a desire to provide therapy effective for common bacterial causes of pneumonia such as *S. pneumoniae* (Chapter 289), *H. influenzae* (Chapter 364), *M. catarrhalis* (Chapter 300), and *Legionella* (Chapter 314), as well as infections due to *Mycoplasma* (Chapter 317) or *Chlamydophila* (Chapter 318).

In contrast, the Swedish Society of Infectious Diseases[9] recommends outpatient treatment for acute pneumonia with oral penicillin or amoxicillin. The rationale for this approach is that pneumococcus, which is the most likely potentially dangerous cause of community-acquired pneumonia, is much better treated by penicillin or amoxicillin than by doxycycline[A3] or macrolides, whereas a patient who fails to respond to penicillin or amoxicillin within a few days can be switched to a macrolide or doxycycline to treat potential *Mycoplasma* and *Chlamydophila*. *Legionella* pneumonia presents with an acute syndrome that is indistinguishable from pneumococcal pneumonia but, in the absence of a specific history of exposure, only rarely causes pneumonia in an outpatient setting. In the United States, one third of *Haemophilus* and the majority of *Moraxella* produce β-lactamase, which would make amoxicillin plus clavulanic acid a better choice in patients who have underlying lung disease. Patients with pneumonia and a history of low-grade fever and cough for more than 5 to 6 days should be treated with a macrolide or doxycycline.

In-Hospital Antibiotic Regimens

In a patient who is sick enough to be hospitalized, the physician should make a conscientious effort to determine an etiologic agent; initial therapy may be empirical, but antibiotics should be tailored to an identified causative organism. Recommended initial empirical antibiotic treatment of pneumonia that does not require ICU care (see Table 97-6) includes a respiratory fluoroquinolone (levofloxacin or moxifloxacin, but not ciprofloxacin) or a β-lactam (cefotaxime, ceftriaxone, ampicillin, or ampicillin-sulbactam), together with a macrolide. Either of these regimens will treat pneumonia due to *S. pneumoniae*, and they will also be effective against *Haemophilus, Moraxella, Legionella, Mycoplasma*, and *Chlamydophila*, as well as some less common organisms. However, this approach risks both overtreatment and undertreatment.

To avoid overtreatment,[10] every effort should be made to identify the responsible organism and narrow treatment accordingly. However, the

TABLE 97-5 SMART-COP SCORING SYSTEM*

	POINTS
Low **S**ystolic blood pressure (<90 mm Hg)	2
Multilobar involvement (on chest radiograph)	1
Low **A**lbumin (<3.5 g/dL)	1
High **R**espiratory rate (≥25 if <50 years old, ≥30 if >50 years old)	1
Tachycardia (heart rate >125 beats/min)	1
New-onset **C**onfusion	1
Poor **O**xygenation (Pa_{O_2} <70 mm Hg if <50 years old, <60 mm Hg if >50 years old)	2
Low arterial **p**H (<7.35)	2

*The risk for needing intensive respiratory or ventilatory support is low if ≤2 points, about 10-15% if 3-4 points, about 35% if 5-6 points, and about 65% if ≥7 points.

Data from Chalmers JD, Singanayagam A, Hill AT. Predicting the need for mechanical ventilation and/or inotropic support for young adults admitted to the hospital with community-acquired pneumonia. *Clin Infect Dis.* 2008;47:1571-1574; and Charles PG, Wolfe R, Whitby M, et al. SMART-COP: a tool for predicting the need for intensive respiratory or vasopressor support in community-acquired pneumonia. *Clin Infect Dis.* 2008;47:375-384.

TABLE 97-6 EMPIRICAL TREATMENT FOR COMMUNITY-ACQUIRED PNEUMONIA

OUTPATIENTS*

For syndromes suggesting "typical" bacterial pneumonia (acute onset of cough, sputum, high fever, high white cell count, elevated procalcitonin level):
- Amoxicillin-clavulanic acid (500-125 mg every 6 hr for 5-7 days); add azithromycin (500 mg orally on day 1, followed by 250 mg orally each day on days 2-5) if *Legionella* is a consideration, *or*
- Levofloxacin (750 mg daily), moxifloxacin (400 mg daily), or gatifloxacin (320 mg daily) for 5 days

For syndromes suggesting influenza pneumonia:
- Oseltamivir (75 mg twice daily for 5 days); observe for secondary bacterial infection

For syndromes suggesting viral pneumonia other than influenza (exposure to someone with viral infection, upper respiratory tract symptoms, patient doesn't look very ill, WBC <10,500, procalcitonin level not elevated):
- Symptomatic therapy

For subacute syndromes suggesting *Mycoplasma* or *Chlamydophila* pneumonia:
- Azithromycin (500 mg on day 1, followed by 250 mg daily for 5 days) or doxycycline (100 mg twice daily for 7 days)

INPATIENTS

Patients hospitalized for pneumonia are sufficiently likely to have a bacterial infection that antibacterial agents are nearly always prescribed unless an alternate diagnosis is strongly suspected. In every hospitalized patient, all reasonable efforts should be made to determine an etiologic diagnosis. For initial empiric therapy:
- A beta-lactam (ceftriaxone 1gm daily, cefotaxime 1 gm every 6 hr, or ceftaroline 600 mg every 12 hr) AND a macrolide (azithromycin 500 mg)
- *or*
- A quinolone (levofloxacin 750 mg, moxifloxacin 400 mg or gatifloxacin 320 mg daily)
- Initial therapy is IV until patient is clinically stable; thereafter switch to oral therapy, tailoring therapy based on culture results or selecting agent(s) that provide similar coverage. Total duration of antibiotic therapy generally 5-8 days (see text).

If influenza is likely:
- Oseltamivir (75 mg twice daily for 5 days) with vigilant observation for possible secondary bacterial infection

If influenza is complicated by secondary bacterial pneumonia, add to oseltamivir:
- Ceftaroline, ceftriaxone or cefotaxime plus either vancomycin or linezolid (ceftaroline alone may suffice if it is licensed to treat *S. aureus* pneumonia)

If *S. aureus* is likely, add to the usual empiric antibacterial regimen:
- Vancomycin (15-20 mg/kg every 8-12 hr, monitoring to maintain trough serum levels at 15-20 mcg/ml or linezolid (600 mg every 12 hr); see above comment regarding ceftaroline. Duration of treatment for proven *S. aureus pneumonia* is 10-14 days.

If *Pseudomonas* or other Gram negative organism is likely:
- Antipseudomonal beta-lactam: piperacillin-tazobactam (4.5 gm every 6 hr), cefepime 1-2 gm every 6-8 hr
- *or*
- A carbapenem (meropenem 500mg IV every 6 hr or 1 gm every 8 hr or imipenem-cilastatin 500mg IV every 6 hr or 1 gm every 8 hr; extended infusions of carbapenems may be preferable), plus azithromycin as above†

Adapted from Musher DM, Thorner AT. Community-acquired pneumonia. *N Engl J Med.* 2014;371:1619-1628; and from Infectious Diseases Society of America/American Thoracic Society. Consensus guidelines on the management of community acquired pneumonia in adults. *Clin Infect Dis.* 2007;44:S27-S72.

*A decision to treat pneumonia as an outpatient should be made after assessing need for hospitalization and only if follow-up contact is planned.

†Add an aminoglycoside in patients with severe community-acquired pneumonia in whom *P. aeruginosa* or an antibiotic-resistant Gram-negative organism is likely because susceptibility is difficult to predict. Narrow therapy to one agent with activity against gram-negative bacilli once susceptibility results are available.

IM = intramuscularly; IV = intravenously.

addition of a macrolide to a β-lactam may improve outcomes in pneumococcal pneumonia.

To avoid undertreatment, possible *S. aureus* infection is an important consideration, especially in patients who may have influenza or a history of injection drug use, chronic renal failure, prior corticosteroid therapy, or progression despite outpatient antibiotics.[11] In such patients, the prevalence of methicillin-resistant *S. aureus* (MRSA) in the community mandates further consideration of vancomycin or linezolid; ceftaroline (not yet approved for this purpose) also may prove to be useful in the future. The absence of nasal carriage of MRSA on PCR testing reduces the likelihood that this organism is causing pneumonia.

ICU Antibiotic Regimens

For patients who require ICU admission, a β-lactam (cefotaxime, ceftriaxone, or ampicillin-sulbactam) should be given in combination with either azithromycin or a respiratory fluoroquinolone. When *Pseudomonas* is a consideration (e.g., in patients who have predominantly gram-negative rods on sputum examination; patients with COPD, bronchiectasis, or other structural lung disease; or patients who have been treated with glucocorticoids or other immunosuppressive drugs), an antipseudomonal β-lactam or carbapenem (piperacillin-tazobactam, cefepime, imipenem, or meropenem) should be selected. Whether adding a second antipseudomonal drug, such as a quinolone or aminoglycoside, is helpful is less clear. A more important principle is that treatment of gram-negative pneumonia should focus on using the optimal dose of an appropriate antibiotic based on susceptibility testing. Whether low-dose corticosteroid treatment is beneficial in patients with community-acquired pneumonia, especially with more severe disease, is uncertain.[12]

Hospital Course

The value of aggressive attempts to determine the cause of pneumonia becomes obvious during a patient's hospital course. The expected response to therapy includes defervescence, return of the WBC count to normal, and disappearance of the systemic signs of acute infection within a few days after antibiotics have been begun. Cough may persist for weeks, and fatigue may persist for months, especially in elderly persons.

Patients may not respond or may even deteriorate during the first day or two despite correct antibiotic therapy, and physicians need diagnostic information to avoid the temptation to simply add antibiotics that may provide no further benefit and may have deleterious side effects. For patients who do respond, identification of the causative organism allows broad-spectrum antibiotics to be replaced by a simpler regimen, thereby potentially shortening the hospitalization, reducing the risk for complications such as *Clostridium difficile* colitis (Chapter 296), and avoiding uncertainty about the culprit medication should an adverse drug reaction occur.

Failure to Respond to Antibiotic Therapy

The failure to respond to antibiotic therapy raises a number of concerns (Table 97-7).[13] The initial diagnosis of community-acquired pneumonia may be incorrect, and one of the many other causes of a pulmonary infiltrate, cough, and fever (e.g., a *Mycobacterium* or a fungus) may be responsible. Alternatively, an entirely different class of disease such as lung cancer or an inflammatory lung condition may be present. If the patient simply does not improve, the antibiotic therapy may not be appropriate for the infecting organism. The first step should be to review culture results and antibiotic susceptibilities to ensure that the patient has received an adequate dose of an appropriate antibiotic. The antimicrobial therapy may have been correct, and the causative organism may be susceptible, but there may be a loculated infection such as empyema (Chapter 99), especially in patients who initially improve but then have persistent low-grade fever and leukocytosis.

When antibiotics have been given empirically and cultures have not been obtained, the failure to respond promptly creates a difficult therapeutic dilemma. In patients with a partial or inadequate response to initial therapy, additional diagnostic measures—such as additional cultures, a chest CT scan, a thoracentesis if an effusion is present, bronchoscopy with bronchoalveolar lavage, and possibly transbronchial biopsy—should be aggressively considered rather than simply adding antibiotics.

TABLE 97-7 REASONS FOR FAILURE OF ANTIMICROBIAL THERAPY IN TREATING PNEUMONIA

Correct organism, inappropriate antibiotic choice or dose
- Organism not susceptible
- Wrong dosage (e.g., morbidly obese or fluid-overloaded patient)
- Antibiotic not given

Correct organism and antibiotic, but infection is loculated
- Empyema (the most common)
- Obstruction (e.g., lung cancer, foreign body)

Unidentified causative organism responsible

Noninfectious cause
- Malignancy
- Inflammatory infiltrate

Duration of Treatment

The optimal duration of therapy is uncertain. In general, outpatients with community-acquired pneumonia should be treated for 5 to 7 days. Patients who are hospitalized should receive parenteral therapy until they are hemodynamically stable and able to ingest and absorb oral antibiotics, after which oral antibiotics can be given. Three to 5 days of parenteral therapy and a final few days of oral treatment after the patient has become afebrile (temperature <99°F) may be the best approach for pneumococcal pneumonia. Treatment for community-acquired pneumonia of undetermined etiology should generally not exceed a total of 7 to 8 days,[A4] and 3 days of treatment is as effective as 8 days for mild to moderately severe pneumonia.[A5] In contrast, pneumonia due to *S. aureus* (Chapter 288) or gram-negative bacilli (Chapters 304, 305, and 306) probably requires 10 to 14 days of treatment, whereas bacteremic *S. aureus* pneumonia requires 4 weeks of treatment because of concerns regarding endocarditis, either as a cause or as a result of the pneumonia. For documented *Legionella* pneumonia (Chapter 314), the recommendation is 5 to 10 days of treatment with azithromycin, 14 days with a fluoroquinolone, or 3 weeks with either regimen if the patient is immunocompromised.

Patients may be discharged when they are clinically stable, have no other medical problems requiring continued hospitalization, and have a suitable discharge environment. Reported markers of clinical stability include temperature of 37.8°C or lower, heart rate of 100 beats per minute or lower, respiratory rate of 24 breaths per minute or lower, systolic blood pressure of 90 mm Hg or greater, oxygen saturation of 90% or higher, or Po_2 of 60 mm Hg or higher on room air (for patients not previously dependent on supplemental oxygen), and mental status at baseline. More rigorous criteria are for temperature to be less than 99°F, respiratory rate to be normal or nearly normal, and oxygen saturation and blood pressure to be back to baseline. Patients are commonly observed in an inpatient setting for up to 24 hours after switching from intravenous to oral therapy, but there is no evidence to support this practice, and it is not necessary for patients who are otherwise stable.

Infectious Complications

Empyema (Chapter 99), which is the most common infectious complication of pneumonia, should be considered in patients who have persisting fever and leukocytosis after 4 to 5 days of appropriate antibiotic therapy for pneumonia. A repeat chest radiograph and a CT scan are important diagnostic tools. Other extrapulmonary infections occur when bacteria are carried by the blood stream to bones or joints (especially intervertebral spaces), peritoneal cavity (if peritoneal fluid was present when bacteremia occurred), meninges, heart valves, or even large muscle groups. Such infections will usually declare themselves by causing symptoms, to which the physician must remain attuned in patients whose recovery is not a rapid as was expected.

Noninfectious Complications

Myocardial infarction (Chapter 73) and new arrhythmias, especially atrial fibrillation (Chapter 64), are seen in 7 to 10% of patients admitted for community-acquired pneumonia, and worsening of heart failure is even more frequent. These cardiac events are associated with substantial increases in morbidity and mortality.

PREVENTION

Maintaining good general health, smoking cessation, avoidance of excessive alcohol ingestion, and control of blood sugar in diabetic patients are good general measures to reduce the risk for bacterial pneumonia. Vaccination against influenza (Chapters 18 and 364) reduces the risk not only of influenza but also of all causes of pneumonia because influenza infection predisposes to secondary bacterial pulmonary infection. Two currently available pneumococcal vaccines[14] specifically reduce the risk for pneumococcal pneumonia (Chapter 18): a polysaccharide vaccine that contains capsular polysaccharide from 23 different pneumococcal serotypes (marketed in the United States as Pneumovax 23 or Pnu-Imune), and a pneumococcal conjugate vaccine, in which capsular polysaccharides are conjugated to an immunogenic protein (originally marketed in the United States as Prevnar7 and now as Prevnar13. Unlike polysaccharide vaccine, conjugate vaccine also eliminates detectable nasopharyngeal carriage of pneumococci and, as a result, the spread of pneumococci to unvaccinated individuals. Pneumococcal infection caused by strains contained in the 7-valent vaccine has fallen in children by 95% and in adults by 85% since widespread vaccination of children has taken place. This same decline has already begun to be observed for strains contained in the 13-valent vaccine.

Pneumococcal polysaccharide vaccine is recommended for all persons 65 years of age or older and for all persons 19 to 64 years of age who are immunocompromised (e.g., congenital or acquired immunodeficiency, HIV infection, chronic renal failure, nephrotic syndrome, hematologic malignancies, iatrogenic immunosuppression, generalized malignancy, and organ transplantation) or have conditions that predispose to pneumococcal infection or that put an individual at particularly high risk for complications (e.g., asplenia, cigarette smoking, asthma, chronic lung disease, heart failure, diabetes, alcoholism, chronic liver disease, cerebrospinal fluid leak, and cochlear implant).

Patients who received pneumococcal polysaccharide vaccine before age 65 years should receive another dose at or after age 65 years, provided at least 5 years have passed since the last dose. Multiple revaccinations after age 65 years are not recommended.

Pneumococcal conjugate vaccine is recommended for all immunocompromised adults 19 years of age and older (see earlier), and individuals who have had a splenectomy or who have cerebrospinal fluid leak or cochlear implant should receive a single lifetime dose of conjugate vaccine. If they have not previously received any pneumococcal vaccine, they should receive conjugate vaccine, followed at least 8 weeks later by the 23-valent polysaccharide vaccine. There is no recommendation to administer more than one dose of conjugate vaccine to an adult.

PROGNOSIS

In developed countries, the mortality among outpatients with pneumonia is less than 2%, but it exceeds 10% in patients who are hospitalized and approaches 40% in patients who require admission to an ICU. In patients with pneumococcal pneumonia, a WBC count of less than 6000/μL is associated with greater than 65% mortality. In community-acquired pneumonia, a serum sodium level of less than 130 mEq/L, a newly elevated serum creatinine level, or a serum glucose level of greater than 250 mg/dL in a nondiabetic patient is also associated with a poor prognosis.

Patients often recuperate only slowly, with residual fatigue and weakness persisting for months. After recovery from bacterial pneumonia requiring hospitalization, mortality is substantially increased at 1 year and, at least in the case of pneumococcal pneumonia, is still significantly increased 3 to 5 years later,[15] presumably because the pneumonia has served as a marker for comorbid conditions that limit lifespan. There is a good correlation between the severity of the pneumonia and the later risk for death.

ASPIRATION PNEUMONIA

EPIDEMIOLOGY AND PATHOBIOLOGY

Although microaspiration underlies most cases of pneumonia, some patients experience repeated gross aspiration of oropharyngeal contents. In such patients, predisposing social factors include alcoholism, cigarette smoking, poor dental hygiene, and homelessness. Predisposing medical conditions include acute or chronic mental status changes, neuromuscular disease, esophageal obstruction, and severe esophageal reflux (Chapter 138). Aspiration pneumonia may not be infectious if it results from damage produced by gastric acid or as a response to gastric contents other than bacteria. However, in practice, a distinction between infectious and noninfectious aspiration pneumonia cannot be made, and aspiration initially should be treated as if it is due to infection.

CLINICAL MANIFESTATIONS

Patients with aspiration pneumonia can present acutely because of the aspiration of food or the acute irritant effects of gastric acid. In most cases, however, clinical deterioration, decreased oxygenation, fever, dyspnea, purulent sputum, and leukocytosis evolve over a number of days.[16] In cases of lung abscess, patients state that their sputum has a foul taste and odor. Physical examination generally reveals malnutrition, findings of chronic comorbid conditions, poor dentition, signs of chronic lung disease, and coarse rhonchi in the lower lobes or dependent lung regions.

DIAGNOSIS

On chest radiography, aspiration pneumonia is most commonly seen as a parenchymal bronchopneumonia process in the superior segments of the right lower lobe and the posterior segments of the upper lobes,[17] but aspiration can involve any part of the lung depending on the patient's position during aspiration. The finding of a thick-walled abscess (Chapter 90) with a fluid level provides strong confirmatory evidence.

Microbiology

Because oropharyngeal secretions contain massive numbers of aerobic and anaerobic organisms, aspiration pneumonia is usually a polymicrobial infection. The diagnosis of aspiration pneumonia can be made by examination of gram-stained sputum that shows many WBCs, few or no epithelial cells, and profuse numbers of mixed bacteria. Because the usual pathogens are mixed normal flora, cultures of sputum are not often helpful, although they might demonstrate other pathogenic bacteria such as *S. aureus* or a multidrug-resistant gram-negative rod that requires therapy. Cultures of resected lung abscess or of transtracheal aspirates in patients with lung abscess typically yield expected mouth organisms, including microaerophilic streptococci and staphylococci, *Bacteroides* species, *Fusobacteria,* and *Prevotella* species. *S. pneumoniae, S. aureus,* and *H. influenzae* may also be present. Because the oropharynx of hospitalized patients and residents of long-term care facilities is regularly colonized by facultative gram-negative bacteria, *P. aeruginosa,* and *S. aureus,* these organisms are also likely to be implicated in aspiration pneumonia.

TREATMENT Rx

Patients who are admitted from the community with aspiration pneumonia or lung abscess should be treated initially with parenteral ampicillin-sulbactam (1.5 to 3 g intravenously every 6 hours) or clindamycin (600 mg intravenously every 8 hours) for at least 5 days. Results of cultures might suggest that other antibiotics be used as well, but the prominence of microaerophilic and anaerobic organisms that will not be identified by routine cultures mandates that one of these drugs be continued. When the patient is stable, treatment can be switched to oral therapy (e.g., clindamycin 600 mg three times daily or ampicillin-sulbactam 750 mg three times daily). Aspiration pneumonia is treated for 7 to 10 days unless cavitation is present, in which case treatment is continued for several weeks or even until the cavity is no longer detectable. In elderly, bedridden patients, especially patients in nursing units or hospitals, intravenous piperacillin-tazobactam (3.375 g intravenously every 6 hours), meropenem (1 g intravenously every 8 hours), or imipenem (1 g intravenously every 6 to 8 hours) for at least 5 days is probably more appropriate initial therapy because of the likelihood of gram-negative bacteria, especially multidrug-resistant organisms that may produce extended-spectrum β-lactamases or a carbapenemase. If MRSA is suspected or is documented by culture, appropriate therapy needs to be added for it as well (Chapter 288).

The most common, serious complication of anaerobic pneumonia or a lung abscess is the development of an empyema. Insertion of one or more chest tubes may control the disease, but thoracotomy with pleural stripping may be the only way to remove the infected material.[18] Unfortunately, patients who develop this complication are often unable to undergo such an aggressive procedure, thereby creating a major therapeutic dilemma. In patients with underlying neurologic disease or malignancy, a gastrostomy or jejunostomy feeding tube can be inserted to provide palliative nutrition, fluids, and medications.

PROGNOSIS

Unless an empyema has developed, the prognosis for aspiration pneumonia or lung abscess is largely determined by the comorbid conditions that led to its occurrence rather than a failure of the pneumonia or abscess to respond.

HOSPITAL-ACQUIRED PNEUMONIA, VENTILATOR-ASSOCIATED PNEUMONIA, AND HEALTH CARE–ASSOCIATED PNEUMONIA

EPIDEMIOLOGY

Hospital-acquired pneumonia, ventilator-associated pneumonia, and health care–associated pneumonia represent the second most common nosocomial infections (Chapter 282) in the United States. Hospital-acquired pneumonia, which increases costs and the length of hospital stay, is responsible for up to 25% of all ICU infections. Hospital-acquired pneumonia and ventilator-associated pneumonia occurring within the first 4 hospital days tend to be caused by antibiotic-susceptible bacteria, whereas late-onset infections are more frequently caused by multidrug-resistant organisms (Table 97-8).

TABLE 97-8 EMPIRICAL ANTIBIOTIC TREATMENT OF HOSPITAL-ACQUIRED PNEUMONIA, VENTILATOR-ASSOCIATED PNEUMONIA, AND HEALTH CARE–ASSOCIATED PNEUMONIA

GROUP A: PATIENTS WITH EITHER HOSPITAL-ACQUIRED PNEUMONIA OR VENTILATOR-ASSOCIATED PNEUMONIA, WITHOUT RISK FACTORS FOR MULTIDRUG-RESISTANT PATHOGENS, AND WITH EARLY-ONSET PNEUMONIA

POTENTIAL PATHOGENS	RECOMMENDED THERAPY
Streptococcus pneumoniae *Haemophilus influenzae* Methicillin-sensitive *Staphylococcus aureus* Antibiotic-sensitive enteric gram-negative bacilli *Escherichia coli* *Klebsiella pneumoniae* *Enterobacter* species *Proteus* species *Serratia marcescens*	Ceftriaxone, 1-2 g IV/IM every 12-24 hr, maximum of 4 g/day, with duration dependent on clinical response and individualized, as discussed in text *or* Levofloxacin, 500-750 mg IV every day, with duration dependent on clinical response and individualized; or ciprofloxacin, 400 mg IV every 8 hr, with duration dependent on clinical response and individualized; or moxifloxacin, 400 mg IV or orally every 24 hr, with duration dependent on clinical response and individualized *or* Ampicillin-sulbactam, 1.5-3 g (1-2 g ampicillin and 0.5-1 g sulbactam) IV/IM every 6 hr, maximum of 4 g sulbactam/day, depending on type and severity of infection, with duration dependent on clinical response and individualized *or* Ertapenem, 1 g IV/IM once a day, with duration dependent on clinical response and individualized

GROUP B: PATIENTS WITH HOSPITAL-ACQUIRED PNEUMONIA, VENTILATOR-ASSOCIATED PNEUMONIA, OR HEALTH CARE–ASSOCIATED PNEUMONIA AND WITH LATE-ONSET PNEUMONIA OR WITH RISK FACTORS FOR MULTIDRUG-RESISTANT PATHOGENS

ORGANISMS	THERAPY
S. pneumoniae *H. influenzae* Methicillin-sensitive *S. aureus* Antibiotic-sensitive enteric gram-negative bacilli *E. coli* *K. pneumoniae* *Enterobacter* species *Proteus* species *S. marcescens* Multidrug-resistant pathogens *Pseudomonas aeruginosa* *K. pneumoniae* (extended spectrum β-lactamase producing) *Acinetobacter* species Methicillin-resistant *S. aureus* Legionella pneumophila	Antipseudomonal cephalosporin (ceftazidime, 2 g IV every 8 hr, or cefepime, 1-2 g every 8-12 hr, with duration dependent on clinical response and individualized) *or* Antipseudomonal carbapenems (meropenem, 1 g every 8 hr, or imipenem, 500 mg every 6 hr or 1 g every 8 hr, with duration dependent on clinical response and individualized) *or* β-Lactam/β-lactamase inhibitor (piperacillin-tazobactam, 4.5 g IV every 6 hr, with duration dependent on clinical response and individualized) *plus* Antipseudomonal fluoroquinolone (levofloxacin, 750 mg IV every day, or ciprofloxacin, 400 mg IV every 8 hr, with duration dependent on clinical response and individualized) *or* Aminoglycoside (amikacin, 15-20 mg/kg/day, divided every 8-12 hr, with monitoring to maintain trough lower than 4-5 μg/mL; or gentamicin, 7 mg/kg/day as a single daily dose, with monitoring to maintain trough levels lower than 1 μg/mL; or tobramycin, 4-7 mg/kg/day as a single daily dose, with monitoring to maintain trough levels lower than 1 μg/mL and duration dependent on clinical response and individualized) *plus* Vancomycin (15 mg/kg IV every 12 hr, with monitoring to maintain trough at 10-15 μg/mL and duration dependent on clinical response and individualized) or linezolid (600 mg IV every 12 hr, with duration dependent on clinical response and individualized)

Data from American Thoracic Society. Guidelines for management of adults with hospital-acquired ventilator associated, and healthcare-associated pneumonia. *Am J Respir Crit Care Med*. 2005:171:388-416.

PATHOBIOLOGY

When pneumonia occurs in the first few days after hospitalization, including the 3 to 4 days after an elective surgical procedure, the most likely organisms include microaerophilic and anaerobic bacteria of the mouth and bacteria that normally cause community-acquired pneumonia, such as *S. pneumoniae* and *H. influenzae*. Thereafter, *S. aureus* and facultative gram-negative bacilli, (e.g., *P. aeruginosa, E. coli, Klebsiella pneumoniae,* and *Acinetobacter* species) become increasingly more common. Many cases are polymicrobial and include gram-positive agents such as *S. aureus*, particularly MRSA strains, especially in patients with severe underlying chronic disease. *P. aeruginosa, Acinetobacter* species, *Stenotrophomonas maltophilia,* and *Burkholderia cepacia* complex rapidly become resistant to multiple classes of antibiotics, so routine local surveillance and monitoring are critical to help predict drug susceptibilities.

CLINICAL MANIFESTATIONS AND DIAGNOSIS

Hospital-acquired pneumonia, ventilator-associated pneumonia,[19] and health care–associated pneumonia can present with typical signs, such as fever, leukocytosis, and purulent sputum or as increased tracheal secretions in an intubated patient. Chest radiographs are often difficult to interpret, but they may show new or worsening pulmonary infiltrates. Oxygen levels fall, and acute respiratory distress (Chapter 104) may result.

If microscopic examination of a gram-stained sputum or tracheal secretions does not show many inflammatory cells with a single organism, cultures of specimens obtained by bronchoscopy, using a protected brush with quantitative analysis, may be needed to determine the causative organism. Sterile culture of lower respiratory tract secretions in the absence of a new antibiotic in the past 72 hours essentially excludes most bacterial pneumonias, although *Legionella* and viral infection are still possible in this situation.

TREATMENT Rx

If the patient is unstable, or if there is a high suspicion for hospital-acquired pneumonia, ventilator-associated pneumonia, or health care–associated pneumonia, prompt empirical antibiotic therapy (see Table 97-8) is required because delays in antimicrobial therapy increase mortality. For early-onset disease in the first 4 days of hospitalization, options include either ceftriaxone, an intravenous fluoroquinolone (levofloxacin, moxifloxacin, or ciprofloxacin), ampicillin-sulbactam, or ertapenem. These options will cover *S. pneumoniae, H. influenzae,* MSSA, and most antibiotic-sensitive gram-negative bacilli, including *E. coli, K. pneumoniae, Proteus* species, *Enterobacter* species, and *Serratia marcescens.*

With late-onset hospital-acquired pneumonia, ventilator-associated pneumonia, or health care–associated pneumonia, or when risk factors for multidrug-resistant infection have been identified, the initial choice of antibiotics should be guided by knowledge of the antibiotic susceptibility of commonly isolated organisms in the facility in question. Because such prediction can be very difficult, multiagent regimens are recommended, but this recommendation emphasizes the importance of obtaining good culture specimens so that therapy can later be narrowed. Options include an antipseudomonal cephalosporin such as ceftazidime or cefepime, an antipseudomonal carbapenem (meropenem or imipenem), or a β-lactam/β-lactamase inhibitor agent such as piperacillin-tazobactam; in addition, either an antipseudomonal fluoroquinolone (ciprofloxacin) or an aminoglycoside such as amikacin, gentamicin, or tobramycin should be considered. If *Legionella* is strongly suspected, the fluoroquinolone should suffice; otherwise a macrolide such as azithromycin should be added. Finally, either vancomycin or linezolid should be added for coverage of MRSA unless the presence of this organism can be excluded.

If the patient improves over the first 48 to 72 hours, strong consideration should be given to de-escalating antibiotic therapy based on culture results. If lower respiratory cultures remain negative but the patient has not improved, an extrapulmonary site of infection should be considered, and additional radiographic studies or cultures may be helpful. In general, aminoglycosides should be limited to 5 to 7 days; overall antibiotic therapy can be as short as 7 days if the patient has improved, but some patients require 14 to 21 days of therapy.

PREVENTION

Prevention centers first on staff education and compliance with alcohol-based hand disinfection. Patients with documented multidrug-resistant organisms should be isolated or, if isolation is not possible, cohorted, in order to reduce the risk for patient cross-contamination. Ventilator-associated pneumonia can be reduced by elevation of the head of the patient's bed, regular aspiration of subglottic secretions, daily "sedation vacations," and daily assessment of the patient's readiness for extubation.

PROGNOSIS

The overall mortality attributed to hospital-acquired pneumonia may be as high as 30 to 50%. Mortality is due, in part, to the severity of the pneumonia and the difficulty of providing adequate antibiotic coverage for some gram-negative bacilli but also to the underlying health of the patient.

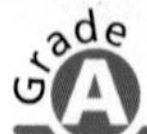

Grade A References

A1. Schuetz P, Christ-Crain M, Thomann R, et al. Effect of procalcitonin-based guidelines vs standard guidelines on antibiotic use in lower respiratory tract infections: the ProHOSP randomized controlled trial. *JAMA*. 2009;302:1059-1066.

A2. Schuetz P, Muller B, Christ-Crain M, et al. Procalcitonin to initiate or discontinue antibiotics in acute respiratory tract infections. *Cochrane Database Syst Rev*. 2012;9:CD007498.

A3. Zhanel GG, Wolter KD, Calciu C, et al. Clinical cure rates in subjects treated with azithromycin for community-acquired respiratory tract infections caused by azithromycin-susceptible or azithromycin-resistant *Streptococcus pneumoniae*: analysis of Phase 3 clinical trial data. *J Antimicrob Chemother*. 2014;69:2835-2840.

A4. Li JZ, Winston LG, Moore DH, et al. Efficacy of short-course antibiotic regimens for community-acquired pneumonia: a meta-analysis. *Am J Med*. 2007;120:783-790.

A5. el Moussaoui R, de Borgie CA, van den Broek P, et al. Effectiveness of discontinuing antibiotic treatment after three days versus eight days in mild to moderate-severe community acquired pneumonia: randomised, double blind study. *BMJ*. 2006;332:1355.

GENERAL REFERENCES

For the General References and other additional features, please visit Expert Consult at https://expertconsult.inkling.com.

98 PULMONARY EMBOLISM

JEFFREY I. WEITZ

DEFINITIONS

Pulmonary embolism (PE) refers to an obstruction of a pulmonary artery by material that has traveled to the lungs from elsewhere in the body through the blood stream.[1] Thrombus from the deep veins of the legs or arms represents the most common type of material to embolize to the lungs—a process known as venous thromboembolism (VTE).[2] In addition to thrombotic pulmonary emboli, nonthrombotic material also can embolize to the lungs. Such material includes fat, air, amniotic fluid, tumor cells, talc in intravenous drug users, and various medical devices. Regardless of the type of embolic material, blockage of blood flow through the lungs and the resultant increased pressure in the right ventricle are responsible for the symptoms and signs of PE.

THROMBOTIC PULMONARY EMBOLISM

EPIDEMIOLOGY

VTE, which includes deep vein thrombosis (DVT; Chapter 81) and PE, represents the third most common cause of cardiovascular death after myocardial infarction and stroke. A first episode of VTE occurs in about 1 to 2 persons per 1000 each year in the United States. The incidence rises exponentially with age, with 5 cases per 1000 persons per year by the age of 80 years. Although men and women are affected equally, the incidence is higher in whites and African Americans than in Hispanic persons and Asian Pacific Islanders.

Approximately one third of patients with symptomatic VTE present with PE; the remainder present with DVT alone but have clinically silent PE in 10 to 15% of cases.[3] Up to half of the patients with a first episode of VTE have no identifiable risk factors and are described as having unprovoked or idiopathic VTE. The remainder develop VTE secondary to well-recognized, transient risk factors, such as surgery or immobilization. PE accounts for an estimated 15% of deaths in hospitalized patients, with at least 100,000 deaths from PE each year in the United States.

PATHOBIOLOGY

PE and DVT are part of the spectrum of VTE and share the same genetic and acquired risk factors, which determine the intrinsic risk for VTE for each individual (E-Fig. 98-1). Genetic risk factors include abnormalities associated with hypercoagulability of the blood (Chapter 176), the most common of which are factor V Leiden and the prothrombin 20210 gene mutation. Acquired risk factors include advanced age, history of previous VTE, obesity, and active cancer, all of which limit mobility and may be associated with hypercoagulability. Superimposed on this background risk, VTE often occurs in the presence of triggering factors, which increase the risk above the critical threshold. The triggering factors, including surgery and pregnancy or estrogen therapy, lead to endothelial cell activation, stasis, and hypercoagulability, which are the components of Virchow triad.

In at least 90% of patients, PE originates from DVT in the lower limbs, and up to 70% of patients with proven PE still have demonstrable DVT on presentation. Thrombi usually start in the calf veins. About 20% of these calf vein thrombi then extend into the popliteal and more proximal veins of the leg, from which they are more likely to embolize. Although often asymptomatic, PE can be detected in about 50% of patients with proximal DVT (Chapter 81). Upper extremity DVT involving the axillary or subclavian veins also can give rise to PE, but only 10 to 15% of such patients develop PE. Upper extremity DVT most often occurs in patients with cancer (Chapter 179), particularly those with indwelling central venous catheters. Unprovoked upper extremity DVT, usually involving the dominant arm, can occur with strenuous effort—the so-called Paget-Schroetter syndrome.

PE often involves both lungs, with the lower lobes affected more frequently than the upper. Larger emboli tend to lodge in the main pulmonary artery or its branches, whereas smaller emboli occlude more peripheral arteries. Peripheral PE can lead to pulmonary infarction, which is characterized by intra-alveolar hemorrhage and necrosis that may be pleura based. Because the circulation to the lungs arises from bronchial as well as pulmonary arteries, pulmonary infarction occurs in only about 10% of patients without underlying cardiopulmonary disease. In contrast, pulmonary infarction occurs in up to 30% of patients who have compromised oxygenation of the affected areas of lung because of preexisting disorders, such as airways disease or increased pulmonary venous pressure because of left ventricular dysfunction.

The clinical impact of PE depends on the extent of reduction in pulmonary blood flow, the time frame over which vascular obstruction occurs, and the absence or presence of underlying cardiopulmonary disease. With acute PE, most patients develop tachypnea and some degree of hypoxemia. Stimulation of irritant receptors in the lungs likely accounts for the increase in respiratory rate. Obstruction of pulmonary arteries contributes to the hypoxemia and the increase in alveolar-arterial oxygen tension gradient, which reflects inefficient oxygen transfer across the lungs. These abnormalities result mainly from the increase in alveolar dead space that occurs because ventilation to alveoli exceeds blood flow in parts of the lung affected by PE. Other contributing factors to the hypoxemia include ventilation-perfusion mismatch because of relative overperfusion of normal areas of the lung, and shunting of blood through nonventilated atelectatic or collapsed areas of lung that retain at least some perfusion.

Pulmonary vascular resistance increases with PE because of vascular occlusion by thrombi. In addition, humoral mediators, such as serotonin and thromboxane, are released from activated platelets and may trigger vasoconstriction in unaffected areas of lung. Consequently, the increase in pulmonary vascular resistance may be disproportionate to the extent of pulmonary vascular occlusion. With obstruction of less than 50% of the pulmonary vascular bed, the mean pulmonary artery pressure rarely exceeds 25 mm Hg. Under these circumstances, the right ventricle maintains its output, so cardiac output and systemic blood pressure remain normal.

With acute occlusion of more than 50% of the pulmonary circulation, the pulmonary artery systolic pressure increases, thereby increasing right ventricular afterload. The pulmonary artery systolic pressure rarely exceeds 55 mm Hg with sudden occlusion because of insufficient time for right ventricular hypertrophy to occur. If the thin-walled right ventricle fails to maintain output in the face of the increased pulmonary artery pressure, it dilates, and right heart failure ensues. Right ventricular end-diastolic and right atrial pressures increase as the right ventricle fails. Dilation of the right ventricle may result in tricuspid regurgitation, which can compromise left ventricular filling and lead to reduced cardiac output and subsequent hypotension. Rightward bulging of the interventricular septum may also contribute to left ventricular diastolic dysfunction. The decrease in aortic pressure, together with the increase in right ventricular pressure, can produce right ventricular ischemia because of decreased perfusion of the right coronary artery despite increased demand by the dilated right ventricle. If this process occurs over a rapid time frame (i.e., minutes to hours), syncope or sudden death, often associated with electromechanical dissociation, may be the first manifestation of severe PE.

With multiple pulmonary emboli over an extended period of time, the right ventricle has an opportunity to adapt to the increased pulmonary vascular resistance. The subsequent increase in right ventricular systolic pressure results in less right heart failure than occurs with acute large PE. Patients with multiple smaller PEs over an extended period of time often have increasing dyspnea with progressively decreasing exercise tolerance. With maintained cardiac output, hypotension does not develop. Additional emboli, however, may convert the clinical picture to one of severe acute PE.

Patients who have underlying cardiopulmonary disease or who are elderly, frail, and debilitated will be more sensitive to the effects of PE than patients who were previously healthy. Consequently, even a small PE may be fatal in patients with limited reserve.

CLINICAL MANIFESTATIONS

Patients with PE most often present with a history of dyspnea, which may be sudden in onset and tends to progress in severity over time. Dyspnea may be associated with pleuritic chest pain, cough, and hemoptysis, particularly in patients with pulmonary infarction. Although the symptoms and signs of PE can be nonspecific, the diagnosis should be suspected in patients with risk factors for VTE, such as prolonged immobility, recent surgery, or active malignancy. Patients with associated DVT (Chapter 81) may present with recent onset of leg pain or with swelling and tenderness along the course of the deep veins. The superficial veins of the leg may be dilated, and the affected leg may be warm to touch with skin that is red or dusky blue in color.

Most patients with PE have tachypnea and tachycardia associated with hypoxemia, but these findings also can occur with disorders such as heart failure, pneumonia, or chronic obstructive pulmonary disease. Other nonspecific symptoms include palpitations, anxiety, and lightheadedness.

Patients with acute severe PE often complain of dyspnea at rest or with minimal exertion, and they may present with syncope (Chapters 51 and 62) because of hypoxemia and low cardiac output. The combination of hypotension, hypoxemia, and increased cardiac workload may trigger angina (Chapter 71) or overt myocardial infarction (Chapter 73).

Central and peripheral cyanosis can occur, and a gallop rhythm may develop as a consequence of heart failure. The jugular veins may be distended if right heart failure develops. The second heart sound can be widely split and the pulmonic component may be loud because of delayed emptying of the right ventricle. A right ventricular heave may be present with massive PE and acute pulmonary hypertension.

DIAGNOSIS

Most patients with PE will have one or more of the following clinical features: dyspnea, often of sudden onset; tachypnea, with a respiratory rate of more than 20 breaths per minute; and chest discomfort, which is usually substernal and often pleuritic in nature. When patients present with these features, the differential diagnosis includes pulmonary disorders, such as pneumonia (Chapter 97), an exacerbation of chronic obstructive lung disease (Chapter 88), or asthma (Chapter 87); pleurisy secondary to connective tissue disease (Chapter 99); cardiac disorders, such as heart failure (Chapter 58), acute coronary syndrome (Chapter 72), or pericarditis (Chapter 77); and musculoskeletal disorders, such as rib fracture.

TABLE 98-1 WELLS' CLINICAL PREDICTION RULE FOR LIKELIHOOD OF PULMONARY EMBOLISM

VARIABLE	POINTS
PREDISPOSING FACTORS	
Previous VTE	1.5
Recent surgery or immobilization	1.5
Cancer	1
SYMPTOMS	
Hemoptysis	1
SIGNS	
Heart rate > 100 beats/min	1.5
Clinical signs of DVT	3
CLINICAL JUDGMENT	
Alternative diagnosis less likely than PE	3
CLINICAL PROBABILITY	**TOTAL POINTS**
Low	<2
Moderate	2-6
High	>6

DVT = deep vein thrombosis; PE = pulmonary embolism; VTE = venous thromboembolism.
Adapted from Wells PS, Ginsberg JS, Anderson DR, et al. Use of a clinical model for safe management of patients with suspected pulmonary embolism. *Ann Intern Med.* 1998;129:997-1005.

Because the clinical features are nonspecific, the diagnosis of PE requires objective testing. Patients who require such testing can be identified by their pretest likelihood of PE using validated clinical prediction rules (Table 98-1) that include components of the clinical assessment, presence of risk factors for VTE, and absence of an alternative diagnosis to explain the symptoms and signs. Some clinical prediction rules also include the results of simple tests, such as the electrocardiogram (ECG) and the chest radiograph.

Based on the results of such an assessment, the pretest likelihood of PE can be designated as low, moderate, or high, and this likelihood then guides the subsequent selection of blood tests, such as the D-dimer assay, and noninvasive or invasive tests for diagnosis of PE or DVT (Fig. 98-1) (Chapter 81). Tests for diagnosis of DVT are relevant because a diagnosis of DVT in a patient with suspected PE provides sufficient grounds for initiation of treatment, and the treatment of DVT and PE is usually the same. Noninvasive tests include computed tomography (CT) pulmonary angiography or ventilation-perfusion lung scanning for diagnosis of PE and venous compression ultrasound for diagnosis of DVT. These tests have largely replaced pulmonary angiography to diagnose PE and venography to diagnose DVT.

Diagnostic Tests

D-Dimer

A plasmin-derived degradation product of cross-linked fibrin, D-dimer can be measured in whole blood or plasma to provide an indirect index of ongoing activation of the coagulation system. An elevated D-dimer level has an 85% to 98% sensitivity for the diagnosis of PE, but all available D-dimer assays have low specificities.[4] False-positive D-dimer elevations can occur with advanced age, chronic inflammatory conditions, and malignancy. In addition, hospitalized patients are more likely to have an elevated D-dimer level than outpatients. Because of this lack of specificity, the value of the D-dimer assay resides with its high negative predictive value and the ability of a normal D-dimer to reduce the probability of PE sufficiently to avoid further diagnostic testing in patients with a low or moderate pretest likelihood, who represent up to 30% of patients with suspected VTE.

Computed Tomography Pulmonary Angiography

Multidetector CT pulmonary angiography has largely replaced ventilation-perfusion lung scanning for PE diagnosis because of its wide availability and the rapidity of its results. In contrast to lung scanning, CT pulmonary angiography not only permits direct visualization of thrombi in the pulmonary arteries of patients with PE (Fig. 98-2) but also provides an alternative

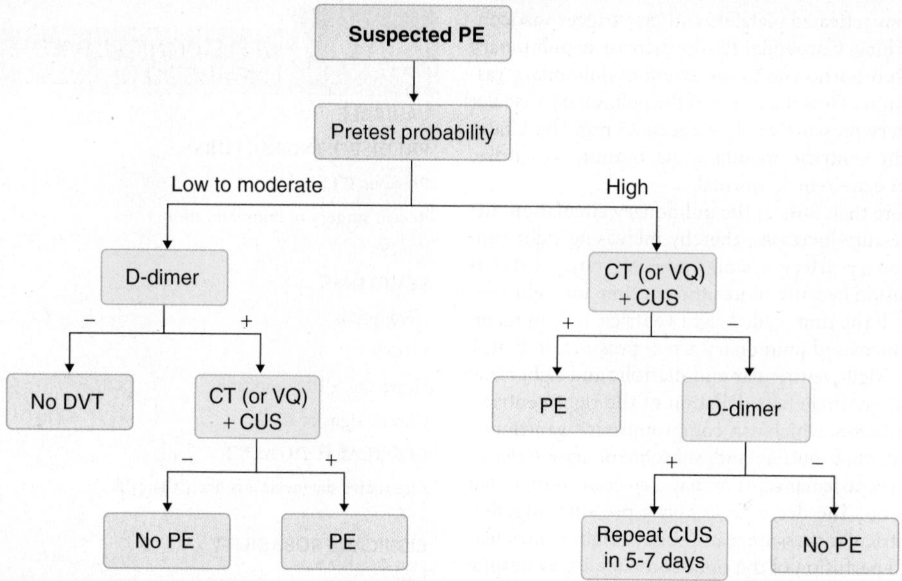

FIGURE 98-1. Clinical approach to patients with suspected pulmonary embolism (PE). CT = computed tomography; CUS = venous compression ultrasound; DVT = deep vein thrombosis; VQ = ventilation-perfusion lung scan.

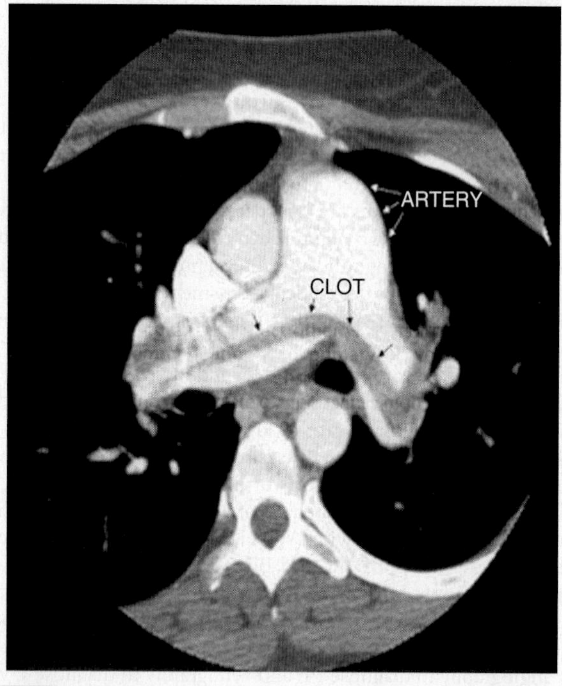

FIGURE 98-2. Computed tomographic pulmonary arteriogram demonstrating a pulmonary embolus.

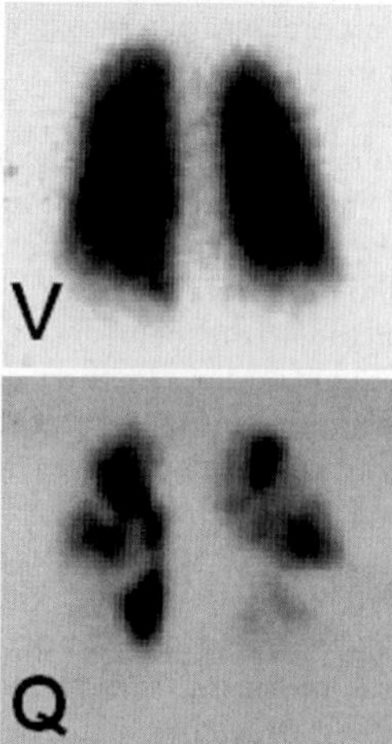

FIGURE 98-3. Ventilation-perfusion lung scan demonstrating pulmonary emboli. The ventilation scan (V) is normal, whereas the perfusion scan (Q) shows multiple defects.

diagnosis in many of those who prove not to have PE. With the evolution from single-detector to multidetector CT scanners, the sensitivity and specificity of CT pulmonary angiography are sufficient for its use as a stand-alone test: a CT pulmonary angiogram showing thrombus in pulmonary arteries up to the segmental level provides evidence of PE, whereas a negative CT pulmonary angiogram excludes PE and is associated with subsequent clinical outcomes that are at least as good as in patients with negative lung scanning.[A1] Compared with lung scanning, CT pulmonary angiography detects more isolated subsegmental thrombi in about 1 to 5% of patients, but the importance of such thrombi is unclear because patients with isolated subsegmental defects appear to have uneventful outcomes without treatment. A negative D-dimer and/or a normal venous compression ultrasound examination may help to exclude the possibility of VTE in this setting.

CT pulmonary angiography can be combined with CT venography so that the diagnosis of PE and DVT can be established with a single test and only one injection of contrast dye. Compared with CT pulmonary angiography alone, the combination of CT pulmonary angiography and CT venography increases the sensitivity for diagnosing PE from 83% to 90%, but the specificity remains unchanged, thereby resulting in only a modest increase in negative predictive value. CT venography adds significant radiation exposure and only marginally increases the overall detection rate, so venous compression ultrasound is preferred for the diagnosis of DVT because it provides the same information without exposing patients to ionizing radiation. Standard venography is not recommended in patients with suspected PE.

Ventilation-Perfusion Lung Scanning

This two-part test consists of a ventilation phase and a perfusion phase. The ventilation phase involves inhalation of an aerosol form of radioactive isotopes of xenon or technetium to assess air delivery to the various parts of the lung. In contrast, the perfusion phase involves the intravenous injection of technetium-labeled macroaggregates of albumin, which enables assessment of blood flow within the lungs after the aggregates lodge in the pulmonary microcirculation. Images for both parts of the test are acquired using a gamma counter. Areas of lung affected by PE do not light up on the perfusion scan because the macroaggregates of albumin fail to reach sites where the pulmonary arteries are occluded (Fig. 98-3). By comparison, areas with abnormal perfusion because of PE will ventilate normally, yielding a ventilation-perfusion mismatch.

A normal ventilation-perfusion lung scan effectively excludes the diagnosis of PE, but only 25% of patients with suspected PE have a normal scan. One or more segmental or larger perfusion defects that ventilate normally characterize a high probability lung scan, which establishes the diagnosis of PE. However, even with single-photon emission CT technology, only about 10% of patients with suspected PE have a high-probability lung scan. The remaining 65% of lung scans exhibit smaller areas of mismatch or matched defects and fall within the non-high-probability category. Because up to 40% of patients with non-high-probability scans have PE, such patients require additional investigations to exclude the diagnosis.

Although CT pulmonary angiography has largely replaced lung scanning, the lung scan is the diagnostic test of choice for patients with renal impairment or a history of allergy to angiographic contrast media and for women younger than 40 years to reduce radiation exposure to the breasts. For diagnosis of PE in pregnancy, lung scanning produces less maternal and fetal radiation exposure and is preferred over CT pulmonary angiography.

Magnetic Resonance Imaging

In contrast to CT pulmonary angiography, gadolinium-enhanced magnetic resonance imaging (MRI) does not subject patients to ionizing radiation, and gadolinium can safely be given to patients with a history of allergy to contrast dye. Although originally promoted as the test of choice to diagnose PE in patients with renal impairment, the emergence of nephrogenic systemic fibrosis (Chapter 267) as a complication of gadolinium administration in patients with renal impairment has tempered enthusiasm for the test. The accuracy of MRI for the detection of PE appears to be similar to that of CT pulmonary angiography, but magnetic resonance (MR) pulmonary angiography is more technically demanding. The combination of MR pulmonary angiography with MR venography has a higher sensitivity than MR pulmonary angiography alone for the diagnosis of PE. With these limitations, MRI should be used to diagnose PE only in centers with experience with the test and in patients for whom standard tests are contraindicated.

Pulmonary Angiography

Pulmonary angiography requires direct contrast injection into the pulmonary arteries, followed by imaging using digital subtraction technology to provide high-quality images. Presence of a thrombus, which appears as a filling defect or as a sudden cutoff of blood flow in a pulmonary arterial branch, establishes the diagnosis of PE. Although direct angiography allows visualization of small thrombi in subsegmental pulmonary arteries, high interobserver variability in the interpretation of isolated filling defects at this level limits the specificity of this finding. As an invasive test, the mortality rate associated with pulmonary angiography is 0.2%, with deaths usually occurring in patients with hemodynamic compromise or respiratory failure. Because of its associated risks and because CT pulmonary angiography offers similar or better information, direct pulmonary angiography is now rarely performed, except in patients who may undergo pulmonary embolectomy.

Other Tests

Routine blood tests in PE patients should include a complete blood count, including a platelet count, and a baseline international normalized ratio (INR), and activated partial thromboplastin time (aPTT). A serum creatinine and blood urea nitrogen level are needed to help guide the choice of anticoagulant therapy, and serum electrolytes and liver enzymes provide useful baseline information.

Blood markers of right ventricular dysfunction, which occurs with extensive PE, include brain natriuretic peptide (BNP) or its precursor, N-terminal proBNP, which are released in response to myocardial stretching (Chapter 58). Elevated levels of troponin I or T provide evidence of myocardial injury (Chapter 72). Although these markers are associated with a worse prognosis in patients with PE, their positive predictive value for making the diagnosis is low.

The ECG may show new changes suggestive of right ventricular strain, such as T wave inversion in leads V_1 to V_4; the classic S1, Q3, T3 pattern (Fig. 98-4); and complete or incomplete right bundle branch block. However, these ECG changes have limited sensitivity and are seen predominantly in patients with more severe pulmonary emboli.

Echocardiographic findings suggestive of right ventricular dysfunction include right ventricular dilation or hypokinesis, increased right ventricular diameter relative to that of the left ventricle, and increased velocity of the jet of tricuspid regurgitation. Echocardiography can also detect a right-to-left shunt through a patent foramen ovale and may provide evidence of right ventricular thrombus, both of which are associated with increased mortality in patients with PE. With no universal criteria for the diagnosis of right ventricular dysfunction, however, the utility of routine echocardiography remains uncertain. In general, routine echocardiography is recommended only in patients with severe hypoxemia or other evidence to suggest hemodynamic compromise.

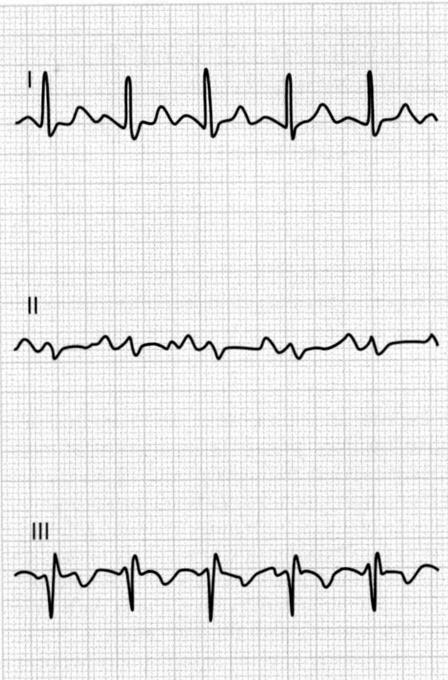

FIGURE 98-4. Classic electrocardiogram of pulmonary embolus. Note the "S1, Q3, T3" pattern.

Diagnostic Strategies

Patients with a low to moderate pretest likelihood of PE should undergo D-dimer testing (see Fig. 98-2). A negative D-dimer test excludes the diagnosis of PE in these patients, whereas a positive test should prompt multidetector CT pulmonary angiography. Patients with a high pretest likelihood of PE should be sent directly for multidetector CT pulmonary angiography. A positive CT pulmonary angiogram establishes the diagnosis of PE, whereas a negative test excludes it.

The role of venous compression ultrasound, which is used to establish the diagnosis of DVT (Chapter 81), remains controversial. Because of the suboptimal sensitivity of single-detector CT pulmonary angiography for the diagnosis of PE, bilateral venous compression ultrasound should also be performed if multidetector technology is not available. Although a negative multidetector CT pulmonary angiogram safely excludes PE, at least in patients with low to moderate pretest likelihood, bilateral venous compression ultrasound can still be helpful. For example, the finding of proximal DVT in the lower or upper extremities, which obviates the need for further testing, can be particularly helpful in patients who are poor candidates for CT pulmonary angiography, such as those with renal impairment or a history of allergy to contrast dye. Patients with a non-high-probability lung scan or with equivocal CT pulmonary angiographic findings should undergo serial venous compression ultrasound examination of the lower extremities to exclude the possibility of calf DVT, which then extends into the proximal veins.

TREATMENT

Rx

Although anticoagulant therapy remains the mainstay of treatment of PE, patients with severe hemodynamic compromise may require reperfusion therapy or surgical thrombectomy to restore blood flow rapidly to the pulmonary arteries and to reduce pulmonary artery pressure. By comparison, outpatient treatment is as safe as routine inpatient treatment in low-risk patients with acute PE.[A2][A3] In PE patients at intermediate risk (Table 98-2), outpatient management can be considered, but brief admission to hospital may be a safer approach. Therefore, rapid risk stratification is crucial to help guide treatment. PE patients who have contraindications to anticoagulant therapy may require insertion of an inferior vena cava filter.

Severe Pulmonary Embolism

High-risk patients can be identified at the bedside (see Table 98-2) based on the presence or absence of hemodynamic compromise. Such patients also have right ventricular dysfunction and have elevated levels of biomarkers. The most common cause of death in patients with severe PE is acute right ventricular failure, which causes low systemic output. To prevent this complication, patients with severe PE require hemodynamic and respiratory support and may benefit from reperfusion therapy. Patients with right ventricular failure often require modest fluid expansion and may need inotropic agents,

TABLE 98-2 RISK STRATIFICATION OF PATIENTS WITH PULMONARY EMBOLISM AND TREATMENTS IN ADDITION TO ANTICOAGULATION

CLASSIFICATION	HEMODYNAMIC COMPROMISE	RIGHT VENTRICULAR DYSFUNCTION	INCREASED TROPONIN AND/OR BNP LEVELS*	TREATMENT
Severe	Yes	Yes	Yes	Fibrinolytic therapy
Moderate	No	Yes	Yes	May consider fibrinolytic therapy if very symptomatic
Mild	No	No	No	Consider outpatient treatment

*Blood markers include troponin, brain natriuretic peptide (BNP), and N-terminal proBNP.

such as dobutamine (starting at a dose of 0.5 to 1.0 µg/kg/minute and then titrated according to the blood pressure), dopamine (starting at a dose of 5 µg/kg/minute and then increased gradually in 5- to 10-µg/kg/minute increments, according to the blood pressure, up to 20 to 50 µg/kg/minute) or norepinephrine (starting at a dose of 2 to 4 µg/minute and then titrated according to the blood pressure) for severe hypotension or shock. Emerging data raise the possibility that endothelin antagonists and phosphodiesterase-5 inhibitors may attenuate the pulmonary hypertension in patients with severe PE, but these drugs are not currently approved for this indication.

Patients with PE frequently have hypoxemia and hypocapnia. Hypoxemia can usually be reversed with nasal oxygen. Measures to reduce fever and agitation with acetaminophen and mild sedation may help minimize oxygen consumption. In patients who have severe PE and who require mechanical ventilation, low tidal volumes should be used, and positive end-expiratory pressure should be applied with caution because it can reduce venous return and worsen right ventricular failure (Chapter 105).

Reperfusion Therapy

Patients with severe PE associated with hypotension or shock may benefit from pharmacologic[5], mechanical, or surgical reperfusion[6] therapy. Pharmacologic reperfusion therapy involves the systemic administration of a fibrinolytic agent (Table 98-3), preferably within 48 hours of the onset of symptoms, but later treatment may still be of benefit. Up to 13% of patients who receive fibrinolytic therapy experience a major bleed, and the rate of intracranial or fatal bleeding can reach 1.8%. Consequently, fibrinolytic therapy currently is justified only in patients who have severe PE and no contraindications (Table 98-4). In patients at intermediate risk, fibrolytic therapy prevents hemodynamic deterioration but increases bleeding and stroke.

Mechanical reperfusion includes percutaneous catheter embolectomy with thrombus fragmentation, an approach that avoids the need for fibrinolytic drugs altogether, or catheter-directed fibrinolytic therapy, which requires lower doses of fibrinolytic agents than are used for systemic administration. In some centers, surgical pulmonary embolectomy may be an option for patients who have severe PE, such as a saddle embolus occluding the main pulmonary artery (Fig. 98-5), and who are at high risk for bleeding with systemic fibrinolytic therapy or who have failed such treatment. Mechanical techniques require skilled operators and should only be performed in high-volume centers.

Anticoagulation Therapy

Anticoagulation therapy is the cornerstone of PE treatment and should be initiated immediately, even while patients with suspected PE are awaiting the results of confirmatory tests. Treatment starts with a rapidly acting parenteral anticoagulant (e.g., heparin, low-molecular-weight heparin (LMWH), fondaparinux, or with a direct orally active factor Xa inhibitor (e.g., rivaroxaban 15 mg twice daily). Patients with severe PE should be treated with heparin because the other agents have not been extensively evaluated in this setting. In addition, the short half-life of heparin is beneficial should reperfusion therapy be necessary. Heparin should also be used in patients with severe renal impairment (creatinine clearance <30 mL/minute) because LMWH, fondaparinux, and rivaroxaban are cleared by the kidneys. If LMWH or fondaparinux is used in patients with moderate renal impairment (creatinine clearance of 30 to 50 mL/minute), lower doses should be considered and anti–factor Xa levels should be measured at trough to ensure there is no accumulation.

Heparin should be administered by continuous intravenous infusion and dosed using weight-based nomograms (see Table 81-4). Typically, an 80 U/kg bolus is followed by an infusion at the rate of 18 U/kg per hour, and subsequent doses are adjusted based on the results of the aPTT. Rapid achievement and maintenance of a therapeutic aPTT are important to reduce the risk for recurrent PE. In addition to monitoring the aPTT, the platelet count should be measured at least two to three times per week because of the risk for heparin-induced thrombocytopenia (Chapter 172).

Subcutaneous LMWH or fondaparinux or oral rivaroxaban can be used for intermediate- or low-risk PE patients (see Table 98-2) using the regimens illustrated in Table 98-5. Unlike heparin, these agents do not require coagulation monitoring. The risk for heparin-induced thrombocytopenia is lower with LMWH than with heparin, is minimal with fondaparinux, and is nonexistent with rivaroxaban.

TABLE 98-3 APPROVED REGIMENS FOR FIBRINOLYTIC THERAPY FOR TREATMENT OF SEVERE PULMONARY EMBOLISM

AGENTS	RECOMMENDED REGIMENS
Streptokinase	250,000 IU as a loading dose over 30 min, followed by 100,000 IU/hr over 12 to 24 hr
Tissue plasminogen activator	100 mg over 2 hr, or 0.6 mg/kg over 10 to 15 min (maximal dose of 50 mg)

TABLE 98-4 CONTRAINDICATIONS TO FIBRINOLYTIC THERAPY

ABSOLUTE CONTRAINDICATIONS

Any hemorrhagic stroke or stroke of unknown origin
Central nervous system damage or neoplasm
Major trauma, surgery, or head injury in past 3 weeks
Gastrointestinal bleeding in past month
Significant ongoing bleeding

RELATIVE CONTRAINDICATIONS

Ischemic stroke or transient ischemic attack in past 6 months
Treatment with a vitamin K antagonist
Pregnancy or within 1 week of delivery
Noncompressible puncture site
Traumatic resuscitation
Advanced liver disease
Infective endocarditis
Active peptic ulcer disease

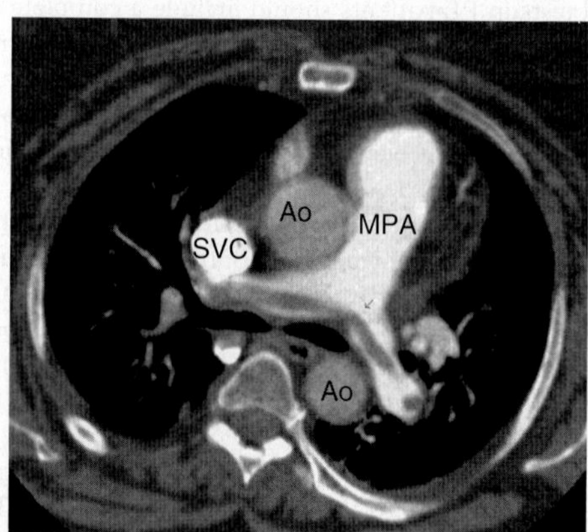

FIGURE 98-5 Thrombotic pulmonary embolism. Computed tomographic pulmonary angiogram revealing a saddle embolism in the main pulmonary artery (MPA). Ao = aorta; SVC = superior vena cava.

After initial treatment with a parenteral anticoagulant, patients with PE require long-term therapy with a vitamin K antagonist, such as warfarin (Chapter 81), or with an oral factor Xa inhibitor to prevent recurrent VTE. In PE patients at low or intermediate risk (see Table 98-2), warfarin can be started on the same day that parenteral anticoagulant therapy is initiated. Parenteral anticoagulant therapy should be continued for at least 5 days and should only be stopped when the INR has been within the therapeutic range of 2 to 3, which is the target range for long-term therapy, for at least 24 hours. Initiation of warfarin therapy should be delayed in patients with severe PE; such patients should receive heparin until they have stabilized.

TABLE 98-5 LOW-MOLECULAR-WEIGHT HEPARIN, FONDAPARINUX, RIVAROXABAN, AND APIXABAN REGIMENS FOR TREATMENT OF PULMONARY EMBOLISM

AGENT	DOSE	INTERVAL
Enoxaparin	1 mg/kg 1.5 mg/kg	Twice daily Once daily
Dalteparin	100 U/kg 200 U/kg	Twice daily Once daily
Tinzaparin	175 U/kg	Once daily
Fondaparinux	5 mg (weight < 50 kg) 7.5 mg (weight 50-100 kg) 10 mg (weight > 100 kg)	Once daily Once daily Once daily
Rivaroxaban	15 mg 20 mg	Twice daily × 3 weeks Once daily thereafter
Apixaban	10 mg 5 mg	Twice daily × 7 days Twice daily thereafter

Oral rivaroxaban (15 mg twice daily for 3 weeks, followed by 20 mg once daily thereafter) is as efficacious as enoxaparin followed by warfarin for the initial treatment of acute PE and causes less major bleeding. Alternatives include oral apixaban (10 mg twice daily for 7 days followed by 5 mg twice daily), or enoxaparin for at least 5 days followed by dabigatran (150 mg twice daily), and edoxaban (60 mg once daily or 30 mg once daily for a creatinine clearance 30 to 50 mL/minute or weight below 60 kg). A5 A6 A7 Edoxaban is not yet licensed for this indication.

Duration of Anticoagulant Therapy

Patients who develop PE as a complication of a reversible risk factor, such as surgery, trauma, or medical illness, have a low risk for recurrence when anticoagulant therapy is stopped. Consequently, a 3-month course of warfarin therapy represents adequate treatment in such patients provided that their risk factors have resolved.[7] Women who develop PE with estrogen therapy also can be treated for 3 months, provided that hormonal treatment is withdrawn. In contrast, patients with unprovoked PE have a higher rate of recurrent VTE when anticoagulant therapy stops and require longer treatment, perhaps indefinitely provided that the risk for bleeding remains low. An elevated D-dimer level 1 month after stopping anticoagulant therapy may help to identify such patients. A8 After a minimum 3-month course of usual-intensity warfarin (target INR between 2 and 3), a lower-intensity regimen (target INR between 1.5 and 2.0) may simplify management by decreasing the frequency of INR monitoring and reducing the risk for bleeding, but the risk for recurrent VTE is slightly higher with this lower intensity warfarin regimen. Rivaroxaban (20 mg once daily), apixaban (2.5 mg twice daily), or dabigatran (150 mg twice daily) are long-term alternatives. These agents produce less bleeding than extended warfarin and no difference in the risk for recurrent VTE. There may be a higher risk for myocardial infarction with dabigatran than with warfarin. A9

Inferior Vena Cava Filters

Inferior vena cava filters, which are inserted percutaneously, are usually placed below the level of the renal veins but can be placed higher if thrombus extends into the inferior vena cava. Both permanent and retrievable filters reduce the risk for recurrent PE but have not been shown to prolong survival, in part because permanent filters can be associated with long-term complications, including inferior vena cava occlusion because of thrombus, recurrent DVT, and post-thrombotic syndrome. Retrievable filters, designed to be removed within 2 to 4 weeks of implantation, can circumvent these long-term complications, but device migration or thrombosis occurs in up to 10% of patients with temporary filters because most are not removed.[8] Because of these potential problems, vena cava filters should be restricted to patients who have high risk for recurrent PE and an absolute contraindication for anticoagulation, such as patients who develop a PE after major surgery, patients who experience major bleeding with anticoagulant therapy, and pregnant women who suffer a PE shortly before delivery. Retrievable filters should be used in these cases, and the devices should be removed as soon as anticoagulant therapy can safely be administered. Permanent filters are suitable for patients who have ongoing contraindications to anticoagulation.

Specific Patient Subgroups

Patients with PE in the setting of active cancer, women who suffer a PE during pregnancy, and patients with chronic thromboembolic pulmonary hypertension (Chapter 68) require special treatment.

Cancer

Active cancer and its treatment with chemotherapy, radiation therapy, and growth factors or other biologic agents increase the risk for VTE (Chapter 179). Patients with advanced cancer often have limited mobility, which adds to their risk for VTE.[9] In addition, indwelling percutaneously inserted or central venous access catheters can trigger upper extremity DVT, which can lead to PE. Therefore, the index of suspicion should be high in cancer patients who present with symptoms and signs suggestive of PE or DVT, or both. With advances in diagnostic imaging, incidental PE may be discovered on CT scans performed for staging purposes or for monitoring response to treatment. Although 20% of patients with VTE have an underlying malignancy, patients with PE should not undergo routine extensive screening for cancer.

Like patients without cancer, initial treatment of PE in cancer patients involves administration of a rapidly acting parenteral anticoagulant. For extended treatment, however, LMWH reduces the risk for recurrent VTE to a greater extent than warfarin. In addition, in the face of poor nutritional intake, severe nausea and vomiting, transient thrombocytopenia, or invasive procedures, LMWH is easier to manage than warfarin. The role of the new oral anticoagulants in cancer patients with PE is uncertain.

Cancer patients who develop PE after curative surgery or with adjuvant chemotherapy for limited-stage disease should be treated for at least 3 months or until they have completed their chemotherapy. Those with PE on the background of advanced cancer have a risk for recurrence of at least 20% in the first year after stopping anticoagulant therapy, so they often require extended treatment.[10]

Pregnancy

Treatment of PE in pregnancy (Chapter 239) centers mainly on heparin or LMWH because, unlike warfarin or the new oral anticoagulants, these agents do not cross the placenta.[11] Although both heparin and LMWH can be given subcutaneously, weight-adjusted LMWH is preferred over heparin because it can be given once daily without routine monitoring and because the risks of heparin-induced thrombocytopenia and osteoporosis are lower with LMWH than with heparin. Anti–factor Xa monitoring of LMWH should be considered in women at extremes of body weight and in those with renal impairment. Fondaparinux should only be considered for pregnant women who have a history of heparin-induced thrombocytopenia or who develop injection-site reactions to heparin or LMWH.

LMWH should be continued throughout pregnancy. Warfarin should be avoided because it crosses the placenta and can cause bone and central nervous system abnormalities, fetal hemorrhage, or placental abruption. During labor and delivery, epidural analgesia should be avoided unless prophylactic LMWH has been stopped at least 12 hours before insertion of the epidural catheter and therapeutic LMWH has been stopped at least 24 hours before. Treatment can be resumed within 6 hours of epidural catheter withdrawal.[12] After delivery, anticoagulation therapy should be continued for at least 3 months; warfarin can be used in place of LMWH because it does not appear in breast milk.

Fibrinolytic agents have been used successfully for treatment of severe PE in pregnancy but can cause bleeding, usually from the urogenital tract. If PE develops late in pregnancy, a retrievable filter may prevent recurrence during delivery when anticoagulant therapy must be withheld.

Chronic Thromboembolic Pulmonary Hypertension

A rare complication of PE, chronic thromboembolic pulmonary hypertension develops in 0.5 to 5% of patients over the course of months or years when emboli in major pulmonary arteries are replaced by fibrous tissue that becomes incorporated into the vessel wall, thereby narrowing or obstructing it.[13] Chronic obstruction of the pulmonary vascular bed increases pulmonary arterial resistance and can lead to right heart failure. Although patients initially may be asymptomatic, they experience increasing dyspnea on exertion and hypoxemia as the disease progresses. Chronic thromboembolic pulmonary hypertension should be suspected in patients with pulmonary hypertension (Chapter 68), and the diagnosis can be established with a combination of echocardiography and lung scanning or CT pulmonary angiography.

Medical therapy focuses on treatment of right heart failure and the use of prostacyclin, endothelin receptor antagonists, or phosphodiesterase-5 inhibitors, or a combination of these, to lower pulmonary artery pressure (see Table 68-2 and Fig. 68-6). Riociguat, a soluble guanylate cyclase stimulator, is a new option. A10 These agents may be of limited utility, however, because of the fibrotic nature of the obstructing material. Definitive treatment involves surgical thromboendarterectomy to remove the occluding material from the pulmonary arteries. This procedure is associated with a perioperative mortality rate that can be as high as 4%, depending on the severity of the disease, and a 3-year survival rate of about 80%.

PREVENTION

At least half of the outpatients with newly diagnosed VTE have a history of recent hospitalization, and most failed to receive thromboprophylaxis during their hospital stay; as a result, PE is the most common preventable cause of death in hospitalized patients in the United States. Guidelines for primary prophylaxis are available and should be followed (see Tables 38-2 and 38-3).

PROGNOSIS

With the diagnosis established and adequate anticoagulant therapy initiated, most patients with PE survive. Case-fatality rates 1 month after diagnosis of DVT or PE are 6% and 12%, respectively. Patients with severe PE who present with shock have the highest mortality rate, and many die within an hour of presentation. Although the case-fatality rate in patients with PE is twice that in those with DVT, many of the deaths are the result of comorbid conditions rather than the PE itself. Factors associated with early mortality after VTE include presentation as PE, advanced age, cancer, and underlying cardiovascular disease. The most serious long-term complication of PE is chronic thromboembolic pulmonary hypertension (Chapter 68).

Despite anticoagulant therapy, recurrent VTE occurs in up to 6% of patients during the first 6 months. While on anticoagulation treatment, patients with provoked and unprovoked VTE have similar risks for recurrence. In contrast, when anticoagulant therapy is stopped, patients with unprovoked VTE have a risk for recurrence of 10% at 1 year and 30% at 5 years, whereas those with provoked VTE have recurrence rates of 3% at 1 year and 10% at 5 years. Recurrent events often mirror the index events; after an initial PE, about 60% of recurrences are PE. Because of the high risk for recurrence in patients with unprovoked VTE, many experts recommend indefinite anticoagulant therapy for such patients. In contrast, because of the lower risk for recurrence in patients with provoked VTE, anticoagulation therapy can be stopped after 3 months provided that transient risk factors for VTE have resolved.

In patients with unprovoked VTE, anticoagulants reduce the risk for recurrence by 80 to 90%, whereas aspirin reduces the risk by only about 35%. Therefore, anticoagulation treatment is preferred over aspirin. Extended warfarin therapy can be cumbersome, and emerging data indicate that the new oral anticoagulants, such as dabigatran, rivaroxaban and apixaban, are effective for long-term secondary VTE prevention.

NONTHROMBOTIC PULMONARY EMBOLISM

DEFINITION

Nonthrombotic material that can embolize to the lungs includes fat, air, amniotic fluid, tumor cells, talc in intravenous drug abusers, and medical devices.

Fat Embolism Syndrome

EPIDEMIOLOGY

Fat embolism syndrome usually occurs in the setting of trauma, particularly after fracture of long bones or the pelvis. The risk increases with the number of fractured bones, and the syndrome occurs more often with closed fractures than with open ones. Fat embolism also can complicate orthopedic surgery or trauma to tissues rich in fat, such as may occur with liposuction.

PATHOBIOLOGY

Characterized by a combination of respiratory, neurologic, hematologic, and cutaneous manifestations, fat embolism syndrome reflects a combination of vascular obstruction by fat globules (E-Fig. 98-2) as well as the deleterious effects of free fatty acids released from these fat globules by the action of lipoprotein lipases. These free fatty acids increase vascular permeability, induce a capillary leak syndrome, and can trigger platelet aggregation.

CLINICAL MANIFESTATIONS

Symptoms typically develop 24 to 72 hours after trauma or surgery. Patients often complain of vague chest pain and shortness of breath. Tachypnea and fever associated with disproportionate tachycardia are common. The syndrome can rapidly progress to severe hypoxemia that requires mechanical ventilation. Neurologic manifestations, which often start after the respiratory distress, include drowsiness, confusion, decreased level of consciousness, and seizures. Patients may have petechiae, particularly involving the conjunctiva, oral mucosa, and upper half of the body.

DIAGNOSIS

Fat embolism syndrome should be suspected when respiratory distress occurs a day or more after major trauma or orthopedic surgery, particularly when there are associated neurologic defects and petechiae. The chest radiograph may reveal diffuse alveolar infiltrates. Although fat droplets may be found in bronchoalveolar lavage fluid, this finding lacks specificity for the fat embolism syndrome.

PREVENTION, TREATMENT, AND PROGNOSIS (Rx)

Early stabilization of long bone fractures reduces the risk for fat embolization. Supportive treatment should be provided, including oxygen and mechanical ventilation. The utility of corticosteroids remains controversial.

Although mortality rates as high as 10% have been reported, the prognosis is generally good.

Venous Air Embolism

EPIDEMIOLOGY

Venous air embolism, which involves entrapment of environmental air or exogenous gas in the venous system, requires direct communication between the air and a vein, as well as a pressure gradient that favors entry of the air into the vein. Air can be introduced through indwelling central venous catheters as a consequence of invasive surgical or medical procedures or after barotrauma.

PATHOBIOLOGY

Large venous air emboli obstruct the right ventricular pulmonary outflow tract, whereas mixtures of air bubbles and fibrin thrombi can obstruct pulmonary arterioles. In either case, right ventricular failure can result. With a patent foramen ovale (Chapter 69), venous air emboli can enter the coronary, cerebral, or systemic circulation.

CLINICAL MANIFESTATIONS

Symptoms and signs depend on the volume of air and the rapidity of its entry into the circulation. Large, rapid boluses of air are tolerated less well than slow entry of smaller amounts. Small air emboli may be asymptomatic. With larger emboli, patients often complain of dyspnea and retrosternal chest discomfort, and they may feel lightheaded. Physical findings include tachypnea, tachycardia, and evidence of respiratory distress. Patients may have signs of right heart failure. A continuous, drum-like, mill-wheel murmur, which reflects air in the right ventricle, may be heard.

DIAGNOSIS

Patients may present with ECG evidence of right ventricular dysfunction associated with elevated levels of troponin, indicative of myocardial injury. Echocardiography or chest CT may reveal air in the right ventricle. Patients may have hypoxemia and hypercapnia, and the platelet count may be low.

PREVENTION AND TREATMENT (Rx)

All catheters should be removed using techniques that minimize air embolism, air should be removed from syringes before injection, and care should be taken during surgery to ensure that air bubbles do not form in blood vessels. To avoid air embolism associated with barotrauma, divers require training in how to dive and surface safely (Chapter 94).

The source of any air embolism should be identified so that further embolism can be prevented. Left lateral decubitus positioning may benefit patients who have a large air bubble trapped in the right ventricular outflow tract; such positioning places the outflow tract below the right ventricular cavity, thereby allowing the air bubble to migrate into a nonobstructing position. Aspiration of the right ventricle through a central venous catheter may also be of benefit. Patients should receive high-flow supplemental oxygen, and hyperbaric oxygenation should be considered for patients with cardiac or neurologic dysfunction.

PROGNOSIS

The outcome depends on the extent of air embolism. With good supportive care, the mortality rate can be less than 10%, even in patients with major air emboli. However, residual neurologic defects often persist.

Amniotic Fluid Embolism

EPIDEMIOLOGY AND PATHOBIOLOGY

Amniotic fluid embolism is a rare but catastrophic complication of pregnancy, occurring in about 1 in 8000 to 1 in 80,000 pregnancies. The syndrome develops when amniotic fluid and fetal cells enter the maternal blood stream through small tears in the uterine veins during labor. Emboli to the heart and lungs (E-Fig. 98-E3) cause cardiac dysfunction and respiratory distress. In addition, amniotic fluid and other debris activate the coagulation system, and the resultant thrombin then triggers fibrin formation and platelet activation to induce disseminated intravascular coagulation (Chapter 175).

CLINICAL MANIFESTATIONS AND DIAGNOSIS

The syndrome often starts with the abrupt onset of dyspnea, cyanosis, and hypotension that can rapidly progress to cardiovascular collapse and death. Patients who survive this stage often develop manifestations of disseminated intravascular coagulation (Chapter 175) characterized by diffuse bleeding, petechiae, and ecchymoses.

The diagnosis should be suspected in women late in pregnancy, often in labor, who present with sudden onset of respiratory distress followed by cyanosis, hypotension, and shock. These findings are often associated with confusion or reduced level of consciousness, seizures, and evidence of a consumptive coagulopathy.

TREATMENT

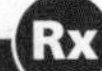

Supportive measures include oxygen, mechanical ventilation, and hemodynamic support. Fresh-frozen plasma, cryoprecipitate, and platelets transfusion can be given to replace consumed clotting factors and platelets. Heparin, often in low therapeutic doses, may be useful in some cases. If amniotic fluid embolism occurs before or during delivery, the fetus often has a poor outcome. As soon as the mother stabilizes, therefore, every attempt should be made to deliver the fetus.

PROGNOSIS

Although rare, amniotic fluid embolism remains the leading cause of maternal death during labor and the first few hours after delivery. Despite advances in critical care management, maternal and fetal mortality rates continue to be about 60% and 20%, respectively, with up to half of the survivors, both mother and baby, suffering from permanent hypoxia-induced neurologic dysfunction.

Other Embolic Material

Many substances, such as talc, starch, and cellulose are used as fillers in the manufacture of illicit drugs. Some of these drugs are ground up by drug users (Chapter 34), mixed in liquids, and then injected intravenously. The filler particles can then be trapped in the pulmonary vasculature, where they can induce granuloma formation.

Tumor emboli in the lung can mimic pneumonia, tuberculosis, or interstitial lung disease on the chest radiograph. Cancers of the prostate and breast are the most common sources of such emboli, followed by hepatocellular cancer and cancers of the stomach and pancreas. Although found in up to 26% of autopsies in patients with advanced cancer, tumor emboli are infrequently identified before death.

Various types of intravascular devices can embolize to the lungs, including vena cava filters, broken catheter tips, guidewires, stent fragments, and coils used for embolization. Many of these devices lodge in the right atrium, right ventricle, or pulmonary arteries. Intravascular retrieval can recover most of these devices; open surgery may be required for the remainder.

Grade A References

A1. Anderson DR, Kahn SR, Rodger MA, et al. Computed tomographic pulmonary angiography vs ventilation-perfusion lung scanning in patients with suspected pulmonary embolism: a randomized controlled trial. *JAMA*. 2007;298:2743-2753.

A2. Aujesky D, Roy PM, Verschuren F, et al. Outpatient versus inpatient treatment for patients with acute pulmonary embolism: an international, open-label, randomised, non-inferiority trial. *Lancet*. 2011;378:41-48.

A3. Zondag W, Kooiman J, Klok FA, et al. Outpatient versus inpatient treatment in patients with pulmonary embolism: a meta-analysis. *Eur Respir J*. 2013;42:134-144.

A4. Meyer G, Vicaut E, Danays T, et al. Fibrinolysis for patients with intermediate-risk pulmonary embolism. *N Engl J Med*. 2014;370:1402-1411.

A5. Schulman S, Kearon C, Kakkar AK, et al. Dabigatran versus warfarin in the treatment of acute venous thromboembolism. *N Engl J Med*. 2009;361:2342-2352.

A6. Agnelli G, Buller HR, Cohen A, et al. Oral apixaban for the treatment of acute venous thromboembolism. *N Engl J Med*. 2013;369:799-808.

A7. Büller HR, Décousus H, Grosso MA, et al. Edoxaban versus warfarin for the treatment of symptomatic venous thromboembolism. *N Engl J Med*. 2013;369:1406-1415.

A8. Prandoni P, Prins MH, Lensing AW, et al. for the AESOPUS Investigators. Residual thrombosis on ultrasonography to guide the duration of anticoagulation in patients with deep venous thrombosis: a randomized trial. *Ann Intern Med*. 2009;150:577-585.

A9. Schulman S, Kearon C, Kakkar AK, et al. Extended use of dabigatran, warfarin, or placebo in venous thromboembolism. *N Engl J Med*. 2013;368:709-718.

A10. Ghofrani HA, D'Armini AM, Grimminger F, et al. Riociguat for the treatment of chronic thromboembolic pulmonary hypertension. *N Engl J Med*. 2013;369:319-329.

GENERAL REFERENCES

For the General References and other additional features, please visit Expert Consult at https://expertconsult.inkling.com.

99 DISEASES OF THE DIAPHRAGM, CHEST WALL, PLEURA, AND MEDIASTINUM

F. DENNIS MCCOOL

DIAPHRAGM

The diaphragm is a dome-shaped structure that separates the thorax from the abdomen. It consists of a central tendon and a peripheral muscular component that inserts into the rib cage laterally along the inner surface of the lower six ribs, the costal cartilages anteromedially, and the upper three lumbar vertebral bodies posteriorly. The diaphragm is innervated by the phrenic nerve, which originates from cervical nerve roots 3 through 5.

Diaphragmatic Weakness and Paralysis

EPIDEMIOLOGY AND PATHOBIOLOGY

When the diaphragm is activated, it contracts and descends caudally. The downward descent of the diaphragm increases abdominal pressure, expands the lower rib cage, and lowers pleural pressure, thereby resulting in lung inflation. It is the major muscle of inspiration, and its action accounts for approximately 70% of the inspired tidal volume in the normal individual. Diaphragm function can be impaired by disorders that affect the brain (Chapter 404), spinal cord (Chapter 400), phrenic nerve (Chapter 420), neuromuscular junction (Chapter 422), and muscle itself (Chapter 421). The incidence and prevalence of diaphragm paralysis and weakness are unknown.

CLINICAL MANIFESTATIONS

Diaphragmatic weakness or paralysis can involve either one or both hemidiaphragms.[1] With unilateral diaphragmatic paralysis, patients are generally asymptomatic at rest but may have dyspnea with exertion or when supine, especially with comorbid conditions such as obesity. If they are asymptomatic, the abnormality may be discovered as an incidental finding of an elevated hemidiaphragm on chest radiography.

Bilateral diaphragmatic paralysis is not as common as unilateral paralysis. Generally, the disability with bilateral paralysis is more dramatic than with unilateral paralysis. Orthopnea is an especially prominent symptom, and patients are often unable to sleep in the supine position. These individuals, who also experience significant dyspnea with exertion when they are lifting objects or bending, are at an increased risk to hypoventilate during sleep, especially during rapid eye movement (REM) sleep. Consequently, initial symptoms of individuals with bilateral or unilateral diaphragm weakness or paralysis may be related to nocturnal hypoventilation and include frequent nocturnal awakenings, nocturia, vivid nightmares, night sweats, daytime hypersomnolence, depression, and morning headaches.

With bilateral diaphragmatic paralysis, the physical examination is remarkable for use of accessory muscles of inspiration and paradoxical inward motion of the abdominal wall during inspiration, which is especially noticeable when these individuals are asked to lie flat. Percussion during inspiration and expiration can detect the absence of diaphragmatic movement.

DIAGNOSIS

Disorders that can cause unilateral diaphragmatic weakness or paralysis (Table 99-1) include traumatic phrenic nerve injury, herpes zoster (Chapter 375), cervical spinal disease (Chapter 400), compressive tumors, and phrenic nerve injury related to cardiac or thoracic surgery, or mechanical ventilation. Diagnosis is often suggested by elevation of a hemidiaphragm on a chest radiograph (Fig. 99-1). The diagnosis can be confirmed by performing a "sniff test" using fluoroscopy or ultrasound, in which paradoxical (cephalad) movement of the hemidiaphragm dome occurs during a sniff maneuver.

TABLE 99-1 CAUSES OF DIAPHRAGMATIC WEAKNESS AND PARALYSIS

TRAUMA
Cardiac surgery with cold cardioplegia
Blunt trauma
Spinal cord injury
Cervical manipulation
Scalene and brachial nerve block
TUMOR COMPRESSION
Lung cancer
Metastatic mediastinal tumor
METABOLIC
Diabetes
Vitamin deficiency (B_6, B_{12}, folate)
Hypothyroidism
Acid maltase deficiency
INFLAMMATORY NEURITIS
Neuralgic amyotrophy (Parsonage-Turner)
Mononeuritis multiplex
Vasculitis
Paraneoplastic
MUSCULAR DYSTROPHIES
Limb-girdle
Duchenne and Becker
MISCELLANEOUS
Amyloidosis
Malnutrition
Radiation injury
Cervical spondylosis
Poliomyelitis
Amyotrophic lateral sclerosis
IDIOPATHIC

The presence of bilateral diaphragmatic paralysis can be much more difficult to ascertain than unilateral paralysis. Chest radiography, which typically shows elevation of both hemidiaphragms, may be interpreted as a "poor inspiratory effort" or "low lung volumes." Tests that can support or refute the diagnosis include pulmonary function testing (Chapter 85), which typically shows a moderate to severe reduction of vital capacity (VC) and total lung capacity (TLC) (30 to 60% predicted). The restriction becomes more severe (10 to 30% further decrease for unilateral and 30 to 50% further decrease for bilateral paralysis) when the individual assumes the supine position. Maximal static inspiratory pressure measured at the airway opening (PImax) is reduced to 20 to 30% of predicted in individuals with bilateral diaphragmatic paralysis. The diagnosis of bilateral diaphragmatic paralysis can be confirmed if measurements of transdiaphragmatic pressure (the pressure difference between the thoracic and abdominal cavity) do not change with inspiration. Diaphragm electromyography and phrenic nerve conduction studies may be useful to distinguish neuropathy or myopathy. Unlike unilateral diaphragmatic paralysis, a sniff test is not helpful in individuals with bilateral diaphragmatic paralysis because it can yield both false-negative and false-positive results. Using two-dimensional ultrasound, the normal thickening of the diaphragm during inspiration will not be observed. If the diagnosis of bilateral diaphragmatic paralysis is confirmed, an evaluation for nocturnal hypoventilation (Chapter 86) should be undertaken. Computed tomography (CT) of the chest may be needed to exclude a mediastinal mass, and magnetic resonance imaging (MRI) of the neck may be necessary to evaluate the spinal cord and nerve roots (E-Fig. 99-1).

TREATMENT AND PROGNOSIS Rx

Bilateral diaphragmatic paralysis may not be reversible unless the underlying cause is treatable. For example, myopathies (Chapter 421) related to metabolic disturbances may be improved by correcting electrolyte imbalances or replacing thyroid hormone. Toxic or metabolic disturbances related to diabetes, alcohol, or viral infections may resolve with treatment of the underlying disease. Idiopathic diaphragmatic paralysis or paralysis due to neuralgic amyotrophy (brachial plexus neuritis) may spontaneously improve or resolve completely in approximately 60% of individuals, but recovery can take 18 months to 3 years. The phrenic nerve courses through the pericardium and can be injured during

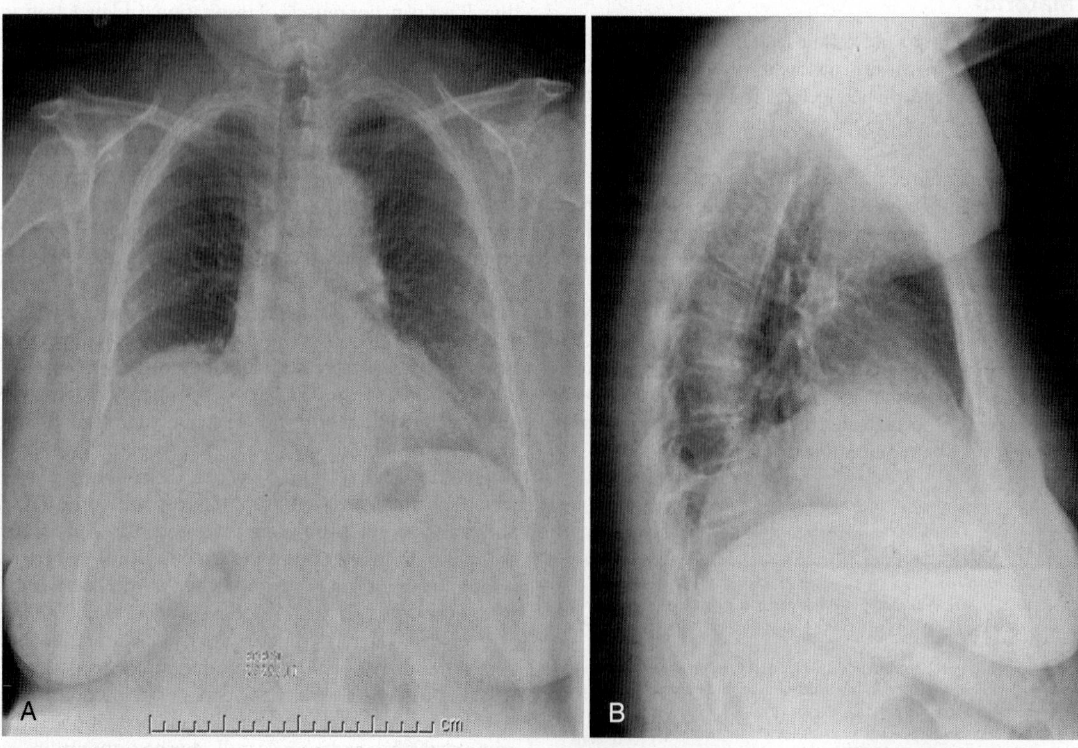

FIGURE 99-1. Patient with paralysis of the right hemidiaphragm as seen on the posteroanterior radiograph of the chest (A) and lateral radiograph of the chest (B).

TABLE 99-2 THERAPEUTIC BENEFITS OF NONINVASIVE MECHANICAL VENTILATION IN PATIENTS WITH CHEST WALL AND NEUROMUSCULAR DISORDERS*

GAS EXCHANGE INDICES	
Pa_{O_2}	Increase
Pa_{CO_2}	Decrease
Bicarbonate	Decrease
RESPIRATORY MECHANICS	
MIP, MEP	No change or slight increase
HEMODYNAMIC PARAMETERS	
PAP	Decrease
VENTILATORY CONTROL	
Hypercapnic ventilatory response	Increase
SLEEP	
Epworth sleepiness score	Decrease
OTHER PARAMETERS	
Quality of life	Improvement
Survival	Increase

*Efficacy data derived from mostly nonrandomized, noncontrolled studies.
MEP = maximal expiratory pressure; MIP = maximal inspiratory pressure; PAP = pulmonary artery pressure.

thoracic surgery. Phrenic nerve damage related to cardiac surgery usually resolves spontaneously but may persist if the phrenic nerve is transected. For a high spinal cord injury, in which the phrenic nerve roots remain intact (injury above C3), phrenic nerve pacing can provide ventilation.

As in sleep-disordered breathing (Chapter 100), noninvasive positive-pressure ventilation (NPPV) is the preferred method of treatment for patients with diaphragmatic paralysis because it can improve both symptoms and physiologic derangements.

Nocturnal positive-pressure ventilation is associated with a number of benefits in patients with neuromuscular disease (Table 99-2). The improvement in ventilation may be related to resting the diaphragm during periods of mechanical ventilation; this reduced work appears to reverse chronic respiratory muscle fatigue and improve daytime function. Other benefits may be related to changes in the control of breathing by reversing the brain's adaptation to high levels of CO_2 by "resetting" the central controller toward normal. When patients with unilateral paralysis have severe symptoms, surgical plication of the paralyzed hemidiaphragm may improve vital capacity, but this intervention has no role in bilateral diaphragm paralysis.

Miscellaneous Diaphragmatic Disorders

Diaphragmatic eventration results from localized atrophy of the diaphragm muscle or from part of the diaphragm being replaced with fibroelastic tissue. Eventration most often results in an elevation of the right anteromedial portion of the diaphragm. Metastatic tumors to the diaphragm usually are related to direct extension of lung cancer. Primary tumors of the diaphragm are very rare. Lipomas are the most common benign tumor, and fibrosarcomas are the most common malignant neoplasm.

CHEST WALL

The chest wall is a key component of the "inspiratory pump" and allows for maintenance of normal alveolar ventilation. It consists of the bony structures of the rib cage, the articulations between the ribs and the vertebrae, the diaphragm, intercostal muscles, and the abdomen. Disorders that affect any of the components of the chest wall can result in impaired breathing.

Kyphoscoliosis

EPIDEMIOLOGY AND PATHOBIOLOGY

Kyphoscoliosis, which is a common spinal disorder, affects approximately 1 in 1000 individuals, and about 1 in 10,000 affected individuals has a severe spinal deformity.[2] Deformities include excessive spinal curvature in the coronal (scoliosis) and sagittal (kyphosis) planes as well as rotation of the spinal axis. Kyphoscoliosis can be idiopathic or can be secondary (paralytic) and associated with neuromuscular diseases, such as muscular dystrophy and polio (Chapters 421 and 379). Kyphoscoliosis also may be associated with congenital vertebral malformations.

Idiopathic kyphoscoliosis, in which there may be a familial predominance, usually manifests in late childhood or early adolescence and involves females more than males with a ratio of 4 : 1. Although a defect in the chromatin-remodeling gene family (*CHD7*) has been associated with idiopathic kyphoscoliosis, other genes have also been identified.

Kyphoscoliosis produces one of the most severe restrictive impairments of all the chest wall diseases. TLC and VC may be reduced to as low as 30% of predicted values, which are based on arm span rather than height. This restrictive pathology becomes most severe as the degree of spinal angulation increases. The patient's age, degree of spinal rotation, presence of respiratory muscle weakness, and involvement of the thoracic vertebrae are all factors that promote the restrictive process. Respiratory failure is a common cause of morbidity and mortality in patients with kyphoscoliosis.

CLINICAL MANIFESTATIONS

Individuals with mild to moderate kyphoscoliosis may have complaints of back pain and have psychosocial problems as a result of their deformity. Kyphoscoliosis may be classified as mild, moderate, or severe based on the angle of spinal deformity. Adolescents with mild idiopathic kyphoscoliosis usually have normal exercise capacity, whereas those with moderate idiopathic kyphoscoliosis have reduced exercise capacity with additional exercise limitation due to deconditioning. With severe deformities, patients may experience dyspnea with minimal exertion or at rest.

Severe kyphoscoliosis can be readily diagnosed on physical examination. Typical findings are the dorsal hump, which is due to the angulated ribs and shoulder asymmetry, as well as the hip tilt that is related to the spinal rotation. In younger individuals with milder spinal deformities, the initial changes may be subtle. The Adams forward bend test, in which the examiner observes for thoracic or lumbar region asymmetry while the patient bends forward at the waist until the spine becomes parallel to the floor, can help detect minor deformities. With severe kyphoscoliosis, signs of right heart failure (Chapter 58) may be present, such as cyanosis, distended neck veins, peripheral edema, and hepatomegaly.

Individuals with kyphoscoliosis are particularly prone to hypoventilation during sleep, especially REM sleep. Because sleep-related abnormalities and their effects on cardiorespiratory function are potentially treatable, individuals with kyphoscoliosis should be evaluated for nocturnal hypoventilation well in advance of the development of daytime hypercapnia.

DIAGNOSIS

Although spinal deformity is often readily apparent on physical examination, the degree of spinal deformity should be assessed by calculation of the angle of spinal curvature (the Cobb angle) from radiographs. This angle is formed by the intersection of lines parallel to the top and bottom vertebrae of the scoliotic or kyphotic curves (Fig. 99-2). Angles more than 100 degrees are severe and usually associated with respiratory symptoms such as dyspnea. Angles more than 120 degrees can be associated with respiratory failure. Factors associated with progression of the spinal deformity include inspiratory muscle weakness, a large spinal curvature at the time of presentation, skeletal immaturity, and a thoracic location of the curve apex. Individuals with inspiratory muscle weakness and kyphoscoliosis are more prone to develop respiratory failure than those with normal inspiratory muscle strength.

TREATMENT Rx

Patients should be encouraged to remain physically active to minimize peripheral muscle deconditioning.[A1] In addition, general supportive measures including immunizations against influenza and pneumococci (Chapter 18), smoking cessation (Chapter 32), maintenance of a normal body weight (Chapter 220), and treatment of respiratory infections in a timely fashion should be instituted. Patients with severe kyphoscoliosis and Cobb angles of more than 100 degrees should be monitored closely for respiratory complications and nocturnal hypoventilation. Respiratory failure may be precipitated by respiratory infections or by medications that produce central nervous system depression.

Nocturnal hypoventilation, which typically precedes findings of daytime hypercapnia and hypoxemia, should be treated with NPPV. This is typically delivered through a nasal or full face mask. Indications for instituting NPPV include symptoms of nocturnal hypoventilation or signs of cor pulmonale (Chapter 68) with either an elevated daytime Pa_{CO_2} or nocturnal oxygen saturation of less than 89% for 5 consecutive minutes. Supplemental oxygen will be needed if hypoxemia persists despite correction of hypoventilation. NPPV

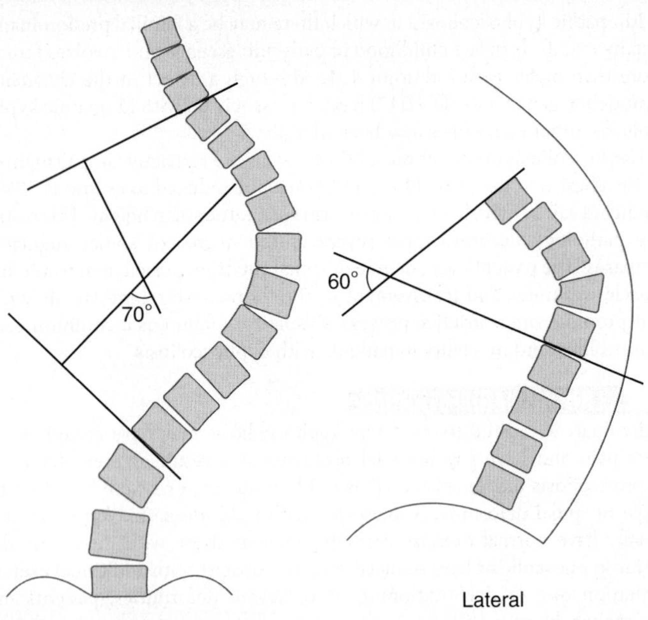

FIGURE 99-2. Schematic drawings of the spine illustrating the lines constructed to measure the Cobb angle of scoliosis and kyphosis. The angle can be calculated either from the intersection of the lines parallel to the vertebrae (as shown for kyphosis, on the *right*) or from the intersection of lines perpendicular to these lines (as shown for scoliosis, on the *left*).

can reduce the number and duration of hospitalizations and improve gas exchange, daytime blood gases, quality of life, and survival (see Table 99-2).

Surgical and nonsurgical (back-brace) treatments have been used in skeletally immature patients with idiopathic kyphoscoliosis in an effort to correct or prevent progression of the spinal deformity. Braces have been used for growing children with Cobb angles between 25 and 40 degrees, whereas surgery has been used for adolescents with a Cobb angle of more than 45 degrees.[A2] Surgical techniques have improved since the introduction of Harrington rods in the 1960s, but the overall role of surgical management in restoring pulmonary function to that of scoliotic individuals and minimizing the possibility of respiratory failure is not clear.[3]

PROGNOSIS

Idiopathic kyphoscoliosis has a better prognosis than kyphoscoliosis secondary to neuromuscular diseases. In general, individuals with mild idiopathic kyphoscoliosis have an overall benign course. Patients with moderate or severe deformities are at higher risk for developing respiratory complications.

In secondary kyphoscoliosis, early age of onset, rapid curve progression during growth, progression of scoliosis after skeletal maturity, large curves at the time of presentation, and a thoracic rather than a thoracolumbar or lumbar location of the curve apex are risk factors for respiratory complications. Respiratory failure may occur in individuals with mild or moderate kyphoscoliosis owing to concurrent respiratory muscle dysfunction. Muscle strength should be evaluated in individuals with respiratory failure and Cobb angles of less than 100 degrees. When cor pulmonale develops (Chapter 68), the prognosis is poor, and death may occur within 1 year without therapy.

Pectus Excavatum

EPIDEMIOLOGY AND PATHOBIOLOGY

Pectus excavatum, a common congenital chest wall deformity that occurs in approximately 0.5 to 2% of the population, is characterized by excessive depression of the sternum and its adjacent costal cartilages. The ratio of affected males to females is 4 : 1, and a family history is common. Pectus excavatum produces minimal functional impairment of the respiratory system. Occasionally, a restrictive defect will be present with mild reductions in VC and TLC. Individuals with the most severe pectus deformities may exhibit a mild reduction in maximal exercise capacity.

CLINICAL MANIFESTATIONS

Cosmetic concerns are the usual reason for seeking medical attention. Dyspnea with activity or exercise may be present but is usually out of proportion to any measurable abnormality in cardiopulmonary function. On physical examination, sternal depression is readily apparent, and there is normal excursion of the rib cage during inspiration. A mild degree of scoliosis may be present in 40 to 60% of individuals.

DIAGNOSIS

Pectus excavatum, which is diagnosed by inspecting the rib cage, usually becomes noticeable before or at puberty. Chest CT is the best means of assessing the sternal deformity. The anteroposterior diameter of the rib cage and the transverse diameter of the rib cage are measured at the level of the deepest sternal depression. Normally, the transverse-to-anteroposterior diameter ratio is 2.5. A ratio of greater than 3.5 signifies a significant pectus deformity.

TREATMENT AND PROGNOSIS Rx

Surgical correction of the deformity is considered for patients with a CT ratio of more than 3.5 in conjunction with symptoms of dyspnea or laboratory evidence of cardiac or pulmonary restriction. However, there is no convincing evidence that correction of the deformity improves either cardiopulmonary function or exercise capacity. Invasive surgical approaches include resecting costal cartilage and repositioning the sternum. Sternal necrosis and infection may complicate invasive surgical procedures, and sternal osteotomy should be avoided in early childhood because it may be complicated by arrested growth of the rib cage. Minimally invasive approaches insert curved metal rods into the sternum through small incisions on each side of the rib cage; over time, the rod is rotated to force the sternum outward. After approximately 2 years, the rods are removed. Complications do not differ between these surgical approaches. The prognosis is excellent in individuals who have only mild deformity and patients who have undergone minimally invasive surgical correction of more severe deformities.

Flail Chest

EPIDEMIOLOGY AND PATHOBIOLOGY

Flail chest occurs following trauma in which there have been either double fractures of three or more contiguous ribs or combined sternal and rib fractures. The result is an unstable segment of the chest wall, which moves paradoxically inward with inspiration and outward with expiration. When multiple single rib fractures produce an unstable segment of the chest wall, this condition is referred to as *nonintegrated chest wall* rather than *flail chest*. In adults, flail chest is most commonly a consequence of blunt chest wall trauma owing to automobile accidents or falls (Chapter 111). In children, the chest wall is more compliant, and flail chest is infrequent.

With a flail chest, inspiratory capacity is limited, and VC may be reduced by 50% or more. Reductions in lung compliance, owing to concomitant pulmonary contusion or microatelectasis, will worsen the restrictive dysfunction and impair gas exchange. The most common location for a flail segment is the lateral chest wall, and this location is generally associated with more clinical derangement. By contrast, a posterior flail segment has less impact on the respiratory system because of splinting provided by the paraspinal muscles. Patients with flail chest may have concomitant lung contusion, pneumothorax, or hemothorax; appropriate diagnostic studies should be undertaken (Chapter 111).

Hypoventilation and flail-induced changes in respiratory muscle function are key factors in the development of respiratory failure in individuals with flail chest (E-Fig. 99-2). Excessive shortening of the inspiratory muscles related to the flail segment and excessive pressure requirements related to lung stiffness increase the work of breathing. The increased work, in concert with reduced oxygen supplies due to pulmonary contusion or hypoventilation, predisposes these individuals to developing respiratory muscle fatigue. Pain associated with the rib fractures and the disordered motion of the flail segment during expiration impair cough. Flail chest and its associated pain promote atelectasis, impair cough, and may lead to respiratory failure.

DIAGNOSIS

Bedside inspection and gentle palpation of the rib cage and abdomen can reveal the characteristic paradoxical movement of the flail segment during spontaneous breathing. Chest radiographs will confirm the presence of multiple rib fractures, but a three-dimensional reconstruction of a thoracic CT can provide better visualization of thoracic injuries, including lung contusion.

The diagnosis may be less apparent in a sedated mechanically ventilated patient, in whom paradoxical motion of a segment of the rib cage may not occur because the positive alveolar and pleural pressures act as a "pneumatic splint" and allow for uniform inflation of the chest wall. However, after withdrawal of sedation, spontaneous breathing should reveal the flail segment.

TREATMENT

Rx

Nonsurgical management of flail chest consists of adequate analgesia, clearance of bronchial secretions, and mechanical ventilatory assistance if needed. Pain relief (Chapter 30) can be accomplished by oral medications, patient-controlled analgesic pumps, intercostal nerve blocks, or epidural anesthesia. Pain control is crucial in averting atelectasis and achieving an effective cough. These interventions often produce a successful outcome with avoidance of respiratory failure and mechanical ventilation, and as the rib cage heals, function is restored. If respiratory failure ensues, not only will mechanical ventilation enhance gas exchange, but also the positive pleural pressure provided by the ventilator during inspiration provides a pneumatic splint, which will stabilize the flail segment. Ventilation delivered by a nasal or face mask to patients who are spontaneously breathing improves gas exchange and may allow for early mobilization and access to physical therapy.

Surgical techniques, none of which is supported by large randomized clinical trial evidence, include open thoracotomy with stabilization of the fractured ribs.[4] The indications for operative fixation are not fully defined, but patients who are unable to wean from mechanical ventilation owing to chest wall instability or patients who are undergoing thoracotomy for concomitant injuries may be candidates for surgical fixation.[A3]

PROGNOSIS

A flail chest is a marker of increased mortality, both in patients with isolated chest wall trauma and in patients with multiple sites of trauma. The overall mortality from chest wall trauma is high, ranging from 7 to 16%.[5] If concomitant lung contusion and flail are present, the mortality rate increases further and may be as high as 70%. The associated high mortality rate is also partly due to the coexistence of other injuries, such as fractures of the long bones, head trauma, or rupture of major vascular structures (Chapter 111). Older age is another poor prognostic factor.

In patients with flail chest without lung contusion, the restrictive impairment can resolve, and the VC can return to baseline values within 6 months after the acute injury. By contrast, individuals with flail chest and concomitant lung contusion often have impairment of pulmonary function that may persist for up to 4 years after injury. Operative fixation of the chest wall may reduce long-term respiratory dysfunction in these individuals.

Ankylosing Spondylitis

EPIDEMIOLOGY AND PATHOBIOLOGY

Ankylosing spondylitis (Chapter 265) is a chronic progressive inflammatory disease that involves the ligamentous structures of the spine, sacroiliac, and large peripheral joints. It affects men more than women, with the most common age of onset between 15 and 25 years. There is a genetic predisposition, with the HLA-B27 antigen present in 95% of whites with ankylosing spondylitis. Chronic inflammation of the spine and peripheral joints may cause fibrosis and ossification of structures adjacent to the spine. Fusion of the costovertebral and sternoclavicular joints produces relative fixation of the rib cage in an inspiratory position, with limited motion of the rib cage during inspiration and a mild restrictive respiratory impairment. The degree of restriction is proportional to disease activity and duration as well as to the degree of spinal and rib cage immobility. Concomitant kyphosis, which may occur in advanced disease or be secondary to osteoporosis, will further impair respiratory function. Because the rib cage is less distensible, the diaphragm shortens to a greater degree for a given tidal volume, thereby increasing the work performed by the diaphragm. Intercostal muscle atrophy secondary to decreased rib cage mobility may cause inspiratory muscle weakness.

About 1 to 4% of patients with ankylosing spondylitis develop fibrobullous upper lobe disease. The cause of this apical disease is unknown, but its presence may impair gas exchange. Occasionally, individuals with ankylosing spondylitis develop nonapical interstitial lung disease (Chapter 92). When these complications occur, lung compliance, which otherwise is usually normal despite a pronounced reduction in rib cage mobility, may be reduced.

CLINICAL MANIFESTATIONS AND DIAGNOSIS

Ankylosing spondylitis is diagnosed when there is a history of low back pain and stiffness for more than 3 months, limited chest wall expansion, limited lumbar spine motion in the sagittal and frontal planes, and radiographic evidence of sacroiliitis. Radiographic findings include calcifications and ossifications of the vertebrae and paravertebral tissues.

Low back pain and spinal stiffness are the most common presenting symptoms. Dyspnea may be present as the disease progresses and chest wall expansion becomes more restricted. Physical examination may reveal loss of lateral flexion of the lumbar spine, tenderness over the sacroiliac joints, and kyphosis. Respiratory function may be further impaired and kyphosis worsened by fractures involving the rigid spine. Endotracheal intubation should be performed with caution because hyperextension of a rigid cervical spine may lead to fracture because of frequent involvement of the cricoarytenoid joint.

TREATMENT AND PROGNOSIS

Rx

Exercise and physiotherapy programs can enhance cardiorespiratory fitness and spinal mobility.[A4] When ankylosing spondylitis is treated with nonsteroidal anti-inflammatory agents and biologic agents, such as tumor necrosis factor antagonists (Chapter 265), rib cage expansion can also improve. A high index of suspicion for possible reactivation of latent tuberculosis is required for patients treated with anti–tumor necrosis factor-α (anti-TNF-α) agents. Corticosteroids do not prevent the progression of fibrobullous disease, which can be complicated by major hemoptysis. Thoracic surgery may be indicated for hemoptysis, but surgical intervention carries major risk, with 50 to 60% of patients developing bronchopleural fistulas. Ankylosing spondylitis rarely leads to pulmonary disability unless individuals develop fibrobullous disease.

Obesity

PATHOBIOLOGY

The degree of obesity (Chapter 220) can be assessed by measuring the body mass index (BMI), which is the ratio of body weight (BW) in kilograms to the square of the height (Ht) in meters (BW/Ht^2). Individuals with a BMI between 18.5 and 24.9 kg/m^2 are normal, whereas those with a BMI greater than 40 kg/m^2 are considered morbidly obese.

Obesity can be accompanied by changes in pulmonary function or alterations in respiratory control. Obesity characteristically reduces end-expiratory lung volume or functional reserve capacity (FRC) and expiratory reserve volume (ERV). TLC and VC may be normal or only mildly reduced, except in the most severe cases. Obesity can be accompanied by alterations in respiratory control, resulting in elevated levels of $Paco_2$ (Chapter 86), because chronic hypoxemia or hypercapnia resets the central chemoreceptors.

Dyspnea and exercise intolerance, which are the most frequent respiratory complaints of obese individuals, may be related to disordered chest wall mechanics, altered respiratory control, or the presence of inflammatory mediators, such as those linking obesity to airway hyper-responsiveness. The increase in intra-abdominal pressure when supine will further reduce FRC, may result in expiratory flow limitation during tidal breathing, and can cause orthopnea. The worsening of respiratory mechanics in the supine position must be considered when evaluating the risk for general anesthesia in obese patients (Chapter 431). Weight loss (Chapter 220) is the optimal therapy, and it improves lung volumes, respiratory muscle performance, gas exchange, dyspnea, and sleep apnea. In individuals with obesity-hypoventilation syndrome (Chapter 100), nocturnal positive-pressure ventilation can reverse gas exchange abnormalities.

PLEURA

The pleura, which is a thin membrane that covers the inner surfaces of the thoracic cavity, consists of a layer of mesothelial cells supported by a network of connective and fibroelastic tissue. The visceral pleura lines the lung, whereas the parietal pleura lines the rib cage, diaphragm, and mediastinal structures. The closed space between the visceral and parietal pleura is referred to as the pleural space. The vascular supply of the parietal pleural surface is from the systemic circulation, and it contains sensory nerves and lymphatics. By contrast, the visceral pleura is supplied with blood vessels from the pulmonary circulation and has no sensory nerves.

Pleural Effusion

EPIDEMIOLOGY AND PATHOBIOLOGY

The overall frequency of pleural effusion on a chest radiograph ranges from 0.3 to 1% but varies widely depending on the underlying disease. Pleural effusions occur most frequently in patients with pneumonia (Chapter 97) or heart failure (Chapter 58).

Normally, a small amount of fluid in the pleural space forms a thin layer between the visceral and parietal pleural surfaces and acts as a lubricant to minimize friction between the chest wall and lung as they move against each other during inspiration and expiration. There is continual movement of fluid into and out of the pleural space. This flux of fluid depends on the oncotic and hydrostatic pressures within the parietal and visceral pleura as well as the pressure within the pleural space itself. Hydrostatic pressure in the parietal pleura is similar to systemic circulation (30 cm H_2O), whereas that of the visceral pleura is similar to the pulmonary circulation (10 cm H_2O). Accordingly, most fluid in the pleural space is filtered from the higher pressure vascular structures in the parietal pleura. Because the pressure within the pleural space itself is more subatmospheric at the apex than at the base, most of the fluid filters in from the less dependent upper lung zones. Fluid is drained out primarily through lymphatics in the parietal pleura. The fluid enters through lymphatic stomas on the surface of the parietal pleura, which are located beneath the mesothelial monolayer. The normal turnover of fluid within the pleural space is 10 to 20 mL/day, with only 0.2 to 1 mL remaining in the pleural space.[6] Excess fluid can accumulate in the pleural space because of decreased removal (owing to obstruction of pleural lymphatics) or increased production (owing to an increase in hydrostatic pressure, a decrease in oncotic pressure, decreased pressure in the pleural space, or increased pleural membrane permeability; Table 99-3).

An increase in hydrostatic pressure or decrease in oncotic pressure will result in a low-protein collection of pleural fluid characterized as *transudates* (Table 99-4). For example, heart failure (Chapter 58) can produce transudates by increasing hydrostatic pressure in the pulmonary venous system, atelectasis (Chapter 90) can promote transudates by making pleural pressure more subatmospheric, and occasionally, oncotic pressure may be sufficiently reduced to cause transudates (e.g., with hypoalbuminemia). Changes in pleural membrane permeability can produce high-protein effusions, which are characterized as *exudates* and can be seen in malignancy or inflammatory states such as pneumonia, tuberculosis, or rheumatoid arthritis. Tumors can disrupt the integrity of the mesothelial layer or the integrity of the capillary epithelium, thereby resulting in exudative effusions, or they may block lymphatic drainage either through interference with stomal openings into the pleural space or obstruction of lymphatic channels.

CLINICAL MANIFESTATIONS

Patients with pleural effusions may be asymptomatic or may experience dyspnea. When the parietal pleura is actively inflamed, pain can be present, and it is generally unilateral, is sharp, and worsens with inspiration. At times, effusions may be sufficiently large to contribute to respiratory failure. Physical findings include dullness to percussion in the area of the effusion, along with diminished breath sounds and absent tactile fremitus.[7]

DIAGNOSIS

Chest radiography (Chapter 84) is often the first imaging method used to detect an effusion (Fig. 99-3). The volume of fluid in the pleural space needs to exceed 250 mL to be visualized on the chest radiograph. When an effusion is present, there is blunting of the costophrenic angle on the posteroanterior chest radiograph (see Fig. 99-3), and a meniscus can be seen posteriorly on the lateral chest radiograph (see Fig. 99-3B). Fluid may also collect in either the minor or major fissures. Occasionally, pleural fluid collections in the major or minor fissures may appear as a pulmonary mass and are referred to as *pseudotumors*. Apparent elevation or changes in the contour of the diaphragm on a posteroanterior chest radiograph may signify a subpulmonic effusion, named because it does not distort the general shape of the diaphragm but will be evident on the lateral film. A lateral decubitus chest radiograph can be obtained to determine whether fluid is free flowing or loculated. Chest CT provides much better characterization of pleural and parenchymal abnormalities by better defining loculated effusions, distinguishing between atelectasis and effusion, and distinguishing loculated effusion from lung abscess or other parenchymal processes (Fig. 99-4). The edge of a parenchymal process usually touches the chest wall and forms an acute angle, whereas the edge of an empyema is usually an obtuse angle.

To determine the etiology of the effusion, a sample of fluid can be removed from the pleural space by thoracentesis, preferably using ultrasound or CT guidance to minimize procedural complications (Fig 99-5). The tests needed to make a diagnosis require a relatively small amount of fluid (30 to 50 mL). Larger volumes of fluid can be removed (1 to 1.5 L) in an attempt to alleviate symptoms. Removing volumes greater than 1.5 L may result in re-expansion

TABLE 99-3 MECHANISMS PROMOTING PLEURAL FLUID ACCUMULATION

MICROVASCULAR CIRCULATION
Increased hydrostatic pressure (heart failure)
Decreased oncotic pressure (severe hypoalbuminemia)
Increased permeability (pneumonia)

PLEURAL SPACE
Decreased pressure (lung collapse)

LYMPHATICS
Impaired lymphatic drainage (malignant effusion)

DIAPHRAGM
Movement of fluid from the peritoneal space (hepatic hydrothorax)

TABLE 99-4 CONDITIONS THAT CAUSE PLEURAL EFFUSION

TRANSUDATES
Heart failure
Nephrotic syndrome
Hepatic hydrothorax
Superior vena cava syndrome
Peritoneal dialysis
Atelectasis
Urinothorax

EXUDATES
Parapneumonic effusions
- Simple
- Complicated
- Empyema

Other infections
- Tuberculosis
- Fungal
- Parasites
- Nocardia

Esophageal rupture
Malignancy
- Carcinoma
- Lymphoma
- Mesothelioma
- Metastatic disease

INFLAMMATORY DISORDERS
Connective tissue disease
- Rheumatoid arthritis
- Systemic lupus erythematosus
- Churg-Strauss syndrome
- Wegener granulomatosis
- Familial Mediterranean fever

Abdominal disease
- Subdiaphragmatic abscess (hepatic, splenic)
- Pancreatitis, pancreatic pseudocyst
- Postoperative

Iatrogenic
- Drug induced
- Misplacement of enteral feeding tube
- Esophageal endoscopic interventions

Miscellaneous
- Asbestos exposure
- Atelectasis
- Cholesterol effusion
- Chylothorax
- Dressler syndrome
- Meigs syndrome
- Pulmonary embolus
- Radiation
- Sarcoidosis
- Trapped lung
- Uremia
- Yellow nail syndrome

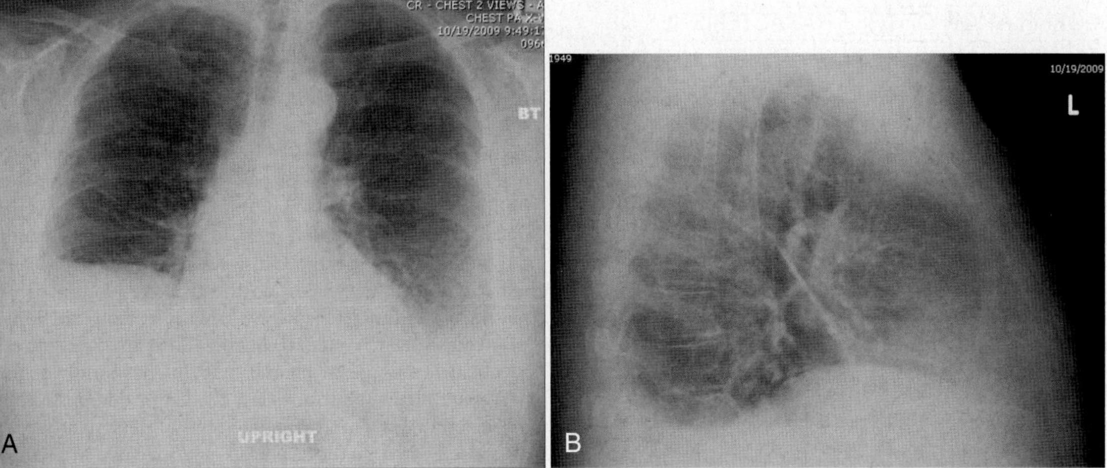

FIGURE 99-3. Patient with bilateral pleural effusions as seen on the posteroanterior radiograph of the chest (A) and lateral radiograph of the chest (B).

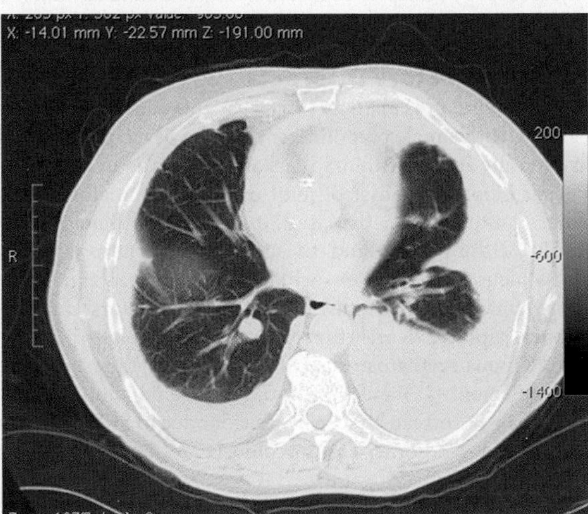

FIGURE 99-4. Chest computed tomography showing pleural effusion in the same patient as in Figure 99-3.

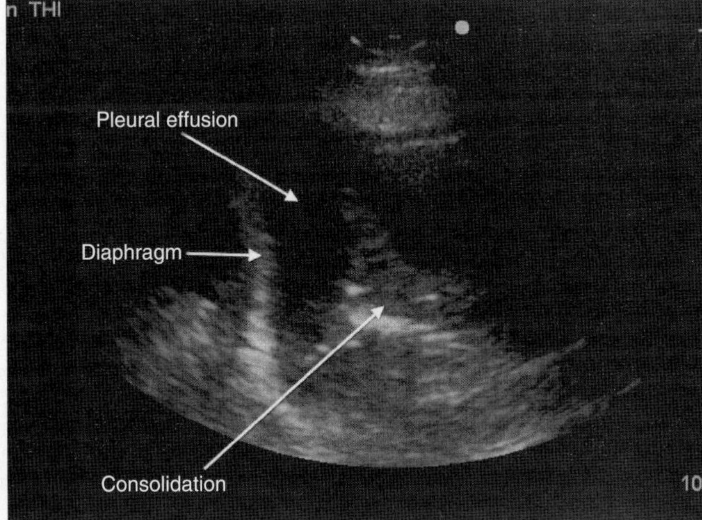

FIGURE 99-5. A right-sided pleural effusion as seen on ultrasound. The ultrasound can be performed at the bedside to aid in needle placement for thoracentesis.

pulmonary edema. Most thoracenteses can be performed at the bedside, using ultrasound guidance to enhance the procedure's safety. Relative contraindications to a diagnostic thoracentesis include a bleeding diathesis, a very small volume of pleural fluid, and a low benefit-to-risk ratio.

After fluid is obtained, a definitive diagnosis may be achieved, and the fluid can be classified as either a transudate or exudate (Table 99-5). To differentiate an exudate from a transudate, the pleural fluid needs to be analyzed for protein and lactate dehydrogenase (LDH). Simultaneous serum values of protein and LDH also need to be obtained. A pleural fluid exudate is characterized by a pleural fluid–to–serum protein ratio greater than 0.5, a pleural fluid–to–serum LDH ratio greater than 0.6, and a pleural fluid LDH greater than two thirds the normal serum value for LDH. An exudate can also be defined if the pleural fluid cholesterol is higher than 45 mg/dL.

TABLE 99-5 PLEURAL FLUID CHARACTERISTICS OF EXUDATES

LIGHT'S CRITERIA	
Protein	>0.5 pleural fluid/serum value
LDH	>0.6 pleural fluid/serum value
LDH	>⅔ upper limit of normal serum value

LDH = lactate dehydrogenase.

Transudates

Effusions that accumulate owing to changes in osmotic and hydrostatic forces usually form transudates. Transudative effusions are most commonly due to heart failure, in which the effusions are often bilateral or, if unilateral, preferentially involve the right hemithorax. Effusions caused by heart failure are usually related to elevated left and right heart pressures (Chapter 58), although right heart failure alone (such as seen in advanced pulmonary arterial hypertension) may rarely cause an effusion. Transudates may also be seen in cirrhosis (Chapter 153), nephrotic syndrome (Chapter 121), myxedema (Chapter 226), pulmonary embolism (Chapter 98), superior vena caval obstruction, and peritoneal dialysis (Chapter 131). With cirrhosis, ascites may cross from the peritoneum into the pleural space through small defects in the diaphragm (hepatic hydrothorax) (see Table 99-4). Unusual causes of transudates include peritoneal dialysis and atelectasis. Although malignancy typically causes an exudate, it can occasionally produce a transudate. Urinothorax, which is a rare cause of transudate, results from obstruction of the urinary system.

Exudates

Exudative effusions, which occur because of an alteration in vascular permeability and/or pleural fluid resorption, can be seen in inflammatory states, infection, or neoplasm. An effusion is characterized as an exudate if it meets one of the following criteria: pleural fluid–to–serum protein ratio higher than 0.5, pleural fluid–to–serum LDH ratio higher than 0.6, or pleural fluid LDH concentration higher than two thirds the normal serum value. When all three criteria are met, the sensitivity, specificity, and positive predictive value exceed 98% for defining an exudative effusion. Cholesterol levels also may be increased in exudates (>45 mg/dL). The pleural fluid analysis helps distinguish among the causes of pleural exudates (Table 99-6).

Parapneumonic Effusions

Parapneumonic effusions, which are the most common type of exudative pleural effusion, occur in up to 40% of patients with pneumonia. They

TABLE 99-6 CORRELATION OF THE CHARACTERISTICS OF PLEURAL EXUDATES WITH SPECIFIC DISEASE

TEST	DISEASE
pH < 7.2	Empyema, malignancy, esophageal rupture; rheumatoid, lupus, and tuberculous pleuritis
Glucose (<60 mg/dL)	Infection, rheumatoid pleurisy, tuberculous and lupus effusions, esophageal rupture
Amylase (>200 μg/dL)	Pancreatic disease, esophageal rupture, malignancy, ruptured ectopic pregnancy
RF, ANA, LE cells	Collagen vascular disease
↓ Complement	SLE, RA
RBCs (>5000/μL)	Trauma, malignancy, pulmonary embolus
Chylous effusion (triglycerides > 110 mg/dL)	Tuberculosis, disruption of thoracic duct (trauma, malignancy)
Cytology or biopsy (+)	Malignancy
ADA (>50 μg/L)	Tuberculosis

ADA = adenosine deaminase; ANA = antinuclear antibody; RA = rheumatoid arthritis; RBC = red blood cell; RF, rheumatoid factor; SLE = systemic lupus erythematosus.

typically occur in patients with bacterial pneumonia (Chapter 97) and can be classified as uncomplicated or complicated. With uncomplicated parapneumonic effusion, the pH is generally greater than 7.3, the glucose content more than 60 mg/dL, and the pleural fluid LDH less than 1000 IU/L. Elevated pleural fluid levels of proinflammatory markers, such as interleukin-1β (IL-1β) and IL-1 receptor antagonist, show promise in distinguishing complicated from uncomplicated effusions. Uncomplicated parapneumonic effusions are usually free flowing, do not require drainage, and will respond to the same antibiotic therapy as the pneumonia itself. Uncomplicated parapneumonic effusions can, however, rapidly transition to complicated effusions, sometimes within 24 hours. Complicated effusions, which are characterized by a pH of less than 7.2 and which often have a glucose content of less than 60 mg/dL, generally will not respond to antibiotic therapy alone but require drainage to prevent formation of an empyema, cutaneous fistulas, bronchopleural fistulas, or a thick pleural peal (fibrothorax).

Empyema

An empyema is present when frank pus is aspirated from the pleural space or when the Gram stain of the fluid is positive for bacteria or bacteria are cultured from the fluid. Pneumonia due to *Streptococcus pneumoniae* (Chapter 289) or *Staphylococcus aureus* (Chapter 288) infection can cause empyema. Individuals who aspirate are at high risk for empyema caused by anaerobic organisms, and patients with tuberculosis (Chapter 324) can develop a tuberculous empyema. Methicillin-resistant staphylococci, *Klebsiella* species pneumonia, and *Pseudomonas* species infections may cause an empyema that is difficult to treat. Uncommon infectious causes of effusions include *Actinomyces* species (Chapter 329), *Nocardia* species (Chapter 330), amebiasis (Chapter 352), *Echinococcus* species (Chapter 354), and paragonimiasis (Chapter 356).

Individuals with empyema often complain of pleuritic chest pain and have refractory fevers several days or more into the course of their pneumonia, but immunocompromised patients may develop empyema sooner and more rapidly.

Tuberculous Effusions

Tuberculosis (Chapter 324) can cause pleural effusion in up to 30% of patients who reside in locations endemic for tuberculosis. The pleural effusion typically is not due to direct mycobacterial infection but rather to increased vascular permeability of the pleural membrane because of a hypersensitivity reaction to mycobacterial proteins. The pleural fluid is generally lymphocyte predominant and culture negative for acid-fast bacilli. Adenosine deaminase levels higher than 50 U/L may be helpful in identifying tuberculous pleural effusions. A tuberculous empyema, which is distinct from a tuberculous effusion, is characterized by direct extension of the infection from thoracic lymph nodes or hematogenous spread of tuberculosis into the pleural space.

Malignancy

Malignant effusions are the second most common cause of exudative pleural effusions and may be due to seeding of the parietal or visceral pleura with malignant cells that change vascular permeability and/or impede resorption. Tumor cells also may amplify the production of mediators that promote leakage of fluid into the pleural space.[8] Rarely, a malignant effusion may be transudative. Lung cancer (Chapter 191) is the most frequent cause of malignant pleural effusion, and other malignancies that can involve the pleural space include breast cancer (Chapter 198), ovarian cancer (Chapter 199), gastric cancer (Chapter 192), and lymphoma (Chapters 185 and 186). When malignancy involves the pleural space, the prognosis is poor. However, the finding of a pleural effusion in an individual with underlying malignancy does not necessarily imply that there is a metastatic malignant process involving the pleural space. Benign effusions in patients with underlying malignancy may be due to atelectasis, postobstructive pneumonia, hypoalbuminemia, pulmonary emboli (Chapter 98), lymphatic obstruction, and complications from radiation (Chapter 20) or chemotherapy. For this reason, it is important to obtain a sample of pleural fluid in these individuals. The diagnosis of malignant pleural effusion is established by demonstrating malignant cells in the pleural fluid. Approximately 60% of malignant pleural effusions can be diagnosed with one thoracentesis, and the yield increases to 80% with repeat thoracenteses. If needed, a biopsy of the pleura may be useful in identifying the malignancy. Pleural biopsies are optimally obtained either by medical or surgical thoracoscopy (Chapter 101) rather than in a blind fashion (e.g., using a Cope or Abrams needle).

Systemic Inflammatory Disorders

Effusions may be seen in as many as 15% of patients with rheumatoid arthritis (Chapter 264), with a male preponderance to the development of effusions. Effusions typically appear within 5 years after the onset of disease but occasionally occur before the onset of joint disease. Rheumatoid factor in the pleural fluid is often greater than 1 : 320, and pleural fluid glucose is low (<60 mg/dL, or the pleural fluid–to–serum glucose ratio is <0.5). Other causes of low pleural fluid glucose include complicated parapneumonic effusions or empyema, malignant effusions, tuberculous pleurisy, lupus pleuritis, and esophageal rupture. Pleural effusions can be seen in 15 to 50% of patients with systemic lupus erythematosus (SLE). Lupus erythematosus cells, low levels of complement (C3 and C4), and pleural fluid antinuclear antibody titer of more than 1 : 160 can be seen in effusions due to SLE. Wegener granulomatosis, Sjögren syndrome, and sarcoidosis are less common causes of pleural effusions.

Pancreatitis

Patients with pancreatitis or pancreatic pseudocysts (Chapter 144) may develop exudative pleural effusions that often involve the left hemithorax. A pleural fluid amylase concentration that is greater than the upper limit of normal for serum amylase is consistent with acute or chronic pancreatitis as a cause of the effusion. Extremely high amylase levels have been reported in effusions due to pancreaticopleural fistulas. Amylase also may be seen in the pleural fluid with an esophageal rupture or malignancy. Pancreatic disease is associated with pancreatic isoenzyme amylase, whereas malignancy and esophageal rupture are characterized by a predominance of salivary amylase isoenzymes.

Chylothorax

A chylothorax has a milky-white appearance and is characterized by high levels of triglycerides (>110 mg/dL) and chylomicrons. A chylothorax is caused by leakage of lymph from the thoracic duct into the pleural space, most commonly related to mediastinal malignancy but also occurring after trauma to the thoracic duct. Major complications from a chylothorax are malnutrition and immunologic compromise when fat, protein, and lymphocytes are depleted by repeated thoracentesis or chest tube drainage. Chylous effusions must be distinguished from pseudochylous effusions, which have a white appearance but are devoid of chylomicrons, and are indicative of a chronic long-standing effusion.

Hemothorax

Blood in the thorax is easily recognized during a thoracentesis. A hemothorax has a pleural fluid hematocrit that is at least half that of the circulating hematocrit. By contrast, a bloody pleural effusion will appear red but have a lower hematocrit. A bloody effusion often suggests a malignant process. Other causes include trauma, pulmonary infarction (Chapter 98), tuberculosis (Chapter 324), collagen vascular disease (Chapters 264 and 266), and hematologic disorders. Generally, blood removed from the pleural space does not clot, whereas blood due to the trauma of the thoracentesis itself will clot when collected. Because blood in the pleural space does not clot, it can be removed by lymphatics if the volume is small. Larger hemothoraces may require chest tube drainage.

Asbestos Exposure

Pleural effusion may occur after exposure to asbestos. The effusion is often small, unilateral, and serosanguineous, with fewer than 6000 cells/mL. The effusion tends to resolve within a year, resulting in pleural plaques that may calcify over time. Malignant mesothelioma should be excluded in these individuals.

Other Causes of Pleural Exudates

Meigs syndrome is the triad of ovarian tumor (Chapter 199), ascites, and pleural effusion. The effusion, which is usually large and on the right side, is formed when fluid moves from the abdomen to the pleural space through diaphragmatic defects. Meigs syndrome usually occurs in postmenopausal women and resolves following removal of the tumor.

Dressler syndrome may occur from 3 to 30 days after open heart surgery or myocardial infarction. The patient usually experiences pleuritic pain and has a small to moderate left-sided effusion. Treatment is as for the accompanying pericardial effusion (Chapter 77).

Uremia (Chapter 130), which can cause a polyserositis with effusion, must be distinguished from the transudate that commonly is seen in the nephrotic syndrome (Chapter 121). Subdiaphragmatic processes, such as hepatic or splenic abscesses (Chapter 151), may cause effusions. Trapped lung occurs when a lobe or segment is unable to re-expand owing to a restrictive visceral pleural peel or an endobronchial mass. Increased negative intrapleural pressures associated with trapped lung promote the formation of an effusion. A number of drugs, including amiodarone, bleomycin, dantrolene, hydralazine, isoniazid, methotrexate, methysergide, mitomycin, procainamide, and procarbazine, can cause pleural effusions. Treatment consists of discontinuing the offending agent, although treatment with oral corticosteroids may be needed (Chapter 254).

TREATMENT AND PROGNOSIS Rx

Empyemas and complicated parapneumonic effusions require drainage by tube thoracostomy in concert with appropriate antibiotic therapy. When an empyema is present, it must be drained immediately using an indwelling chest tube. The combination of intrapleural t-PA (10 mg) and DNase (5 mg) therapy can improve chest tube drainage in patients with pleural infections.[A5][A6] If chest tube drainage is unsuccessful in resolving the empyema, video-assisted thoracic surgery (Chapter 101) is preferred, with intrapleural streptokinase reserved for patients who are poor candidates for video-assisted thoracic surgery or are in situations in which it is not available. Occasionally, empyema requires thoracotomy and decortication.

Treatment options for malignant pleural effusion include observation, chemical pleurodesis with talc or tetracycline derivatives, and treatment of the underlying malignancy. For patients with recurrent malignant effusions, the tunneled placement of an indwelling pleural catheter can permit intermittent drainage to relieve symptoms.[9,10] In a randomized trial of patients with malignant pleural effusion and no previous pleurodesis, indwelling pleural catheters and talc pleurodesis were equivalent for relieving patient-reported dyspnea; catheter-based treatment shortened hospital length of stay but also produced more adverse effects.[A7] A complete response occurs in perhaps 50% of patients. A low pleural fluid pH (<7.2) tends to impart a poor response to chemical pleurodesis. Malignant effusions with a tendency to respond to generalized chemotherapy include those related to breast cancer (Chapter 198) and small cell carcinoma of the lung (Chapter 191). Malignant effusions related to lymphomas and obstruction of lymphatic drainage of the pleural space may also respond to treatment of the underlying disease.

Treatment of inflammatory effusions centers on the use of anti-inflammatory agents and corticosteroids (Chapters 264 and 266). Treatment of chylous effusions may involve chest tube drainage, although fat malnutrition may ensue. Attempts to decrease chyle formation can be accomplished by intravenous hyperalimentation, decreased oral fat intake, and the intake of medium- and light-chain fatty acids, which are absorbed directly into the portal circulation. Ligation of the thoracic duct should be considered for traumatic chylous effusions. Thoracic duct embolization has been performed successfully for nontraumatic chylous effusion.[11]

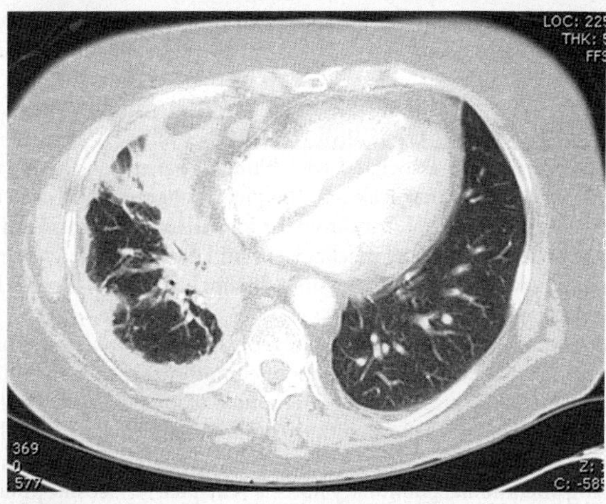

FIGURE 99-6. Computed tomographic angiogram of the chest in a patient with mesothelioma. There is diffuse thickening of the pleura and pericardium on the right with a rind-like appearance.

Mesothelioma

EPIDEMIOLOGY AND PATHOBIOLOGY

Malignant mesotheliomas (Chapter 191) are neoplasms arising from the serosal membrane of body cavities. Eighty percent of mesotheliomas originate in the pleural space, and most others arise from the peritoneum. Individuals are usually older than 55 years and often have a history of asbestos exposure in the distant past (frequently, 30 to 40 years ago). Smoking is not a risk factor for developing mesothelioma, but smoking in concert with asbestos exposure increases the risk for lung cancer. Approximately 3000 cases of mesothelioma occur in the United States each year. The annual incidence is decreasing in the United States owing to better control of occupational exposure, but it may still be increasing in other countries where there are fewer regulations.

CLINICAL MANIFESTATIONS AND DIAGNOSIS

Patients with mesothelioma often complain of dyspnea, weight loss, and pain. Malignant mesothelioma may present as an extremely large mass or pleural effusion occupying the entire hemithorax at times. Chest CT may demonstrate either localized or circumferential pleural thickening associated with various amounts of calcified pleural plaque (Fig. 99-6). Elevated levels of hyaluronic acid in the pleural fluid may be seen with mesotheliomas, but pleural fluid cytology frequently is insufficient for diagnosis. The most efficient way of obtaining a diagnosis is by CT-guided core biopsy or thoracoscopy. Special stains and electron microscopy of biopsy tissue may help to make the difficult distinction between metastatic adenocarcinoma and mesothelioma. The use of biomarkers such as fibulin-3 in plasma and pleural effusions may aid in detecting mesothelioma at an earlier stage and in distinguishing it from other malignancies involving the pleura.

A fraction of mesotheliomas are benign. Benign mesotheliomas are usually large and often pedunculated at the time of diagnosis.

TREATMENT AND PROGNOSIS Rx

Unfortunately, no particular therapy, surgical or chemotherapy, has met with great success in malignant mesothelioma, and median survival is only 8 to 12 months after diagnosis.[A8] Pleurodesis with talc or pleurectomy is usually performed for palliation and control of symptoms related to any pleural effusion. In highly selected patients with localized disease and no comorbid illnesses, surgical resection or radical extrapleural pneumonectomy may be attempted. Radiation therapy can provide symptom palliation and has been used following attempts at curative surgery. Treatment of benign mesothelioma involves surgical resection.

Pneumothorax

Pneumothorax refers to the accumulation of air in the pleural space (see Fig. 84-15). Normally, the pressure within the pleural space is slightly subatmospheric. However, when more than a very small amount of air accumulates within the pleural space, pressure within it becomes positive, and there is compression of underlying lung. Typically, the visceral pleura separates from the parietal pleura, and air can be seen between the visceral pleural lining and the rib cage.

EPIDEMIOLOGY AND PATHOBIOLOGY

Pneumothorax is often associated with blunt or penetrating trauma. With penetrating trauma, air may leak into the pleural space through the injured chest wall or into the pleural space from the injured lung. Patients with underlying lung disease undergoing mechanical ventilation may acutely develop a pneumothorax when high local pressures disrupt lung tissue, thereby leading to a leak (Chapter 105).

Pneumothorax also may occur spontaneously or be secondary to underlying lung disease. Typically, spontaneous pneumothorax occurs in tall, young, thin men, presumably as a result of rupture of preexisting apical blebs. Diseases that are associated with pneumothorax include emphysema (Chapter 88), cystic fibrosis (Chapter 89), granulomatous inflammation, necrotizing pneumonia, pulmonary fibrosis (Chapter 92), eosinophilic granulomatous disease, sarcoidosis (Chapter 95), and endometriosis (Chapter 236). Catamenial pneumothorax occurs in patients who have subpleural and diaphragmatic endometriosis (Chapter 236); rupture of the endometrial nodules at the time of menstruation causes pneumothorax.

CLINICAL MANIFESTATIONS AND DIAGNOSIS

Symptoms typically include acute shortness of breath and sharp chest pain. Physical examination is characterized by tachycardia, decreased breath sounds, decreased tactile fremitus, a pleural friction rub, subcutaneous emphysema, hyper-resonance to percussion, and a tracheal shift toward the uninvolved hemithorax.

Diagnosis can be made by obtaining an upright chest radiograph, and rapid assessment with point-of-care ultrasound is increasingly being used as well. Air within the pleural space appears as an area of lucency on the chest radiograph (Fig. 99-7). With a small pneumothorax, the lucency is best appreciated at the lung apex when the patient is upright. An end-expiratory radiograph is particularly helpful in diagnosing a small pneumothorax. During expiration, the density of the lung will increase because of a reduction in volume, thereby highlighting the difference between lung parenchymal and pleural gas. When a portable chest radiograph is obtained with the patient in the supine position, such as a patient in an intensive care unit, the lucent area may be most noticeable over the lower rib cage (superior sulcus sign).

A *tension pneumothorax* is defined as a pneumothorax associated with a mediastinal shift and hemodynamic compromise, usually because high intrathoracic pressures compress the vena cava and atrium. This physiology implies an ongoing leak of air into the pleural space without opportunity for the air to escape.

TREATMENT AND PROGNOSIS Rx

If the pneumothorax is small and the patient is not in distress, tube thoracostomy is not needed, and observation alone may be sufficient.[12] However, if a patient is symptomatic, the pneumothorax occupies more than 50% of the hemithorax, or a tension pneumothorax develops, management requires insertion of a thoracostomy tube, suction, and water-seal drainage. If there is a continuing leak despite tube thoracostomy, a bronchopleural fistula may be suspected. In this instance, chemical pleurodesis or surgical correction, usually by video-assisted thoracoscopic surgery, may be necessary (Chapter 101). In a randomized trial of patients with primary spontaneous pneumothorax, simple aspiration and drainage followed by 300 mg of minocycline pleurodesis was a safe and effective treatment, with a 30% 1-year recurrence rate, compared with a 50% 1-year recurrence rate for simple aspiration and drainage only.[A9]

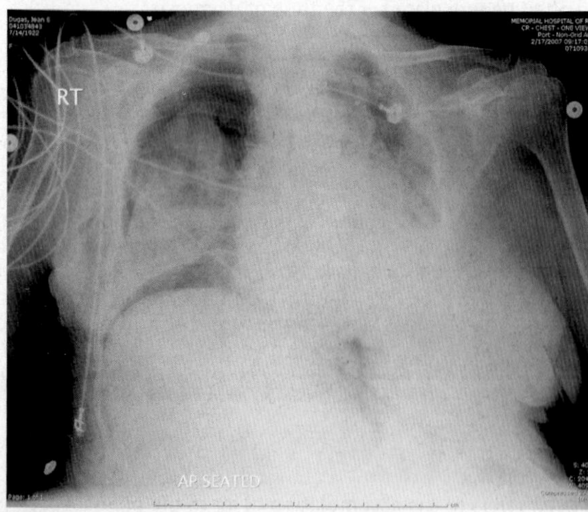

FIGURE 99-7. A portable anteroposterior chest radiograph demonstrating a right-sided pneumothorax. Note that the right lung has collapsed to less than half the size of the right hemithorax. In addition, there is a pneumoperitoneum best seen as a collection of air under the right hemidiaphragm.

MEDIASTINUM

The mediastinum, which is the central part of the thoracic cavity, lies between the right and left lungs. It contains the heart and aorta, esophagus, trachea, lymph nodes, thymus, and great vessels. It is bordered by the two pleural cavities laterally, the diaphragm inferiorly, and the thoracic inlet superiorly.

Mediastinal Masses

PATHOBIOLOGY

For clinical purposes, the mediastinum has been divided into three compartments: anterior, middle, and posterior (E-Fig. 99-E3). The anterior compartment contains the thymus, substernal extensions of the thyroid, blood vessels, pericardium, and lymph nodes. The middle compartment contains the heart, great vessels, trachea, main bronchi, lymph nodes, and the phrenic and vagal nerves. The posterior compartment contains the vertebrae, descending aorta, esophagus, thoracic duct, azygous and hemizygous veins, lower portion of the vagus, sympathetic chain, and lymph nodes.

CLINICAL MANIFESTATIONS

Mediastinal masses usually are not accompanied by symptoms, and most masses are incidentally found on either a chest radiograph or a chest CT scan. If present, however, symptoms include chest pain, cough, hoarseness, stridor, dysphasia, and dyspnea. One third of patients with a mediastinal thymoma have symptoms or weakness owing to myasthenia gravis (Chapter 422), and individuals with mediastinal lymphoma (Chapters 185 and 186) may have systemic symptoms such as fever, night sweats, and weight loss. Occasionally, a mass may compress the superior vena cava, causing partial obstruction and resulting in facial edema and dilated neck and chest veins (Fig. 99-8).

DIAGNOSIS

When a mass is identified by chest radiography or chest CT, further evaluation is mandatory. If a benign process is suspected, follow-up CT may be indicated. If a malignant process is suspected, radiologic evaluation may include angiography, positron emission tomography, or MRI. Biopsies can be obtained either with mediastinoscopy or mediastinotomy. Less invasive approaches include ultrasound-guided transbronchial needle aspiration biopsy, and direct sampling by transthoracic CT-guided needle aspiration may be useful in evaluating anterior or posterior mediastinal masses. The evaluation and differential diagnosis of mediastinal masses are guided by the compartment in which they arise (Table 99-7). The *anterior mediastinal compartment* includes lesions such as thymomas, germ cell tumors (teratomas), lymphomas, and intrathoracic thyroid tissue.[13] Thymomas make up about

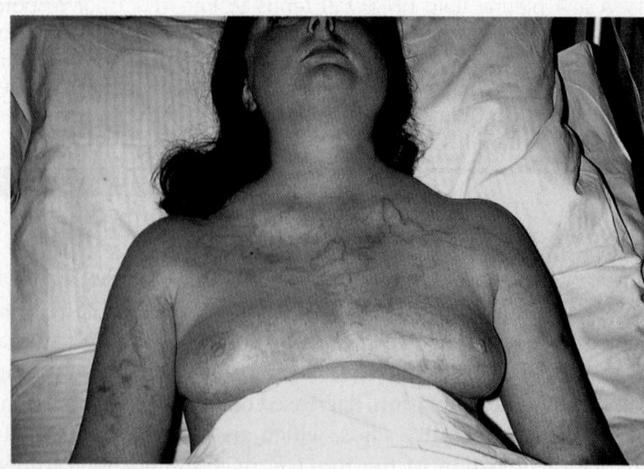

FIGURE 99-8. Superior vena cava obstruction in bronchial carcinoma. Note the swelling of the face and neck and the development of collateral circulation in the veins of the chest wall.

TABLE 99-7 CAUSES OF MEDIASTINAL MASSES

ANTERIOR	MIDDLE	POSTERIOR
Teratoma	Pericardial cyst	Neurogenic tumor
Thymoma	Lymph node hyperplasia	Esophageal tumor
Thyroid tumor	Bronchogenic tumor	Bronchogenic tumor
Goiter	Bronchogenic cyst	Bronchogenic cyst
Aneurysm	Aneurysm	Aneurysm
Lymphoma	Lymphoma	Lymphoma
Parathyroid tumor		Meningocele
Lipoma		Enteric cyst
Morgagni diaphragm hernia		Esophageal diverticula
		Bochdalek diaphragm hernia

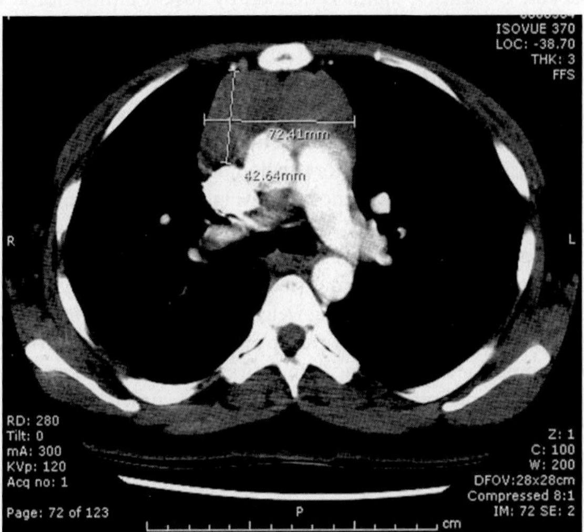

FIGURE 99-9. Chest computed tomography of a patient with an anterior mediastinal mass that proved to be a substernal goiter.

20% of mediastinal neoplasms in adults, in whom they are the most common anterior mediastinal primary neoplasm. Patients with systemic lymphoma often have involvement of the mediastinum, but only 5 to 10% of patients with lymphoma present with primary mediastinal lesions. When lung cancer (Chapter 191) presents with mediastinal adenopathy, it is at an advanced stage. Teratomas, which account for 10% of mediastinal tumors, may contain squamous cells, hair follicles, sweat glands, cartilage, and linear calcifications; about one third are malignant. Intrathoracic goiters (Chapter 226) (Fig. 99-9) may compress the trachea and cause stridor, cough, dyspnea, and, occasionally, superior vena cava obstruction. Anterior masses in the right cardiophrenic angle, which are rare and may be associated with pericardial defects or obesity, may be due to herniation of liver or intestinal contents through the foramina of Morgagni.

In the posterior mediastinum, neurogenic tumors are the most common lesions. Many of these tumors are benign and originate in the nerve sheath or sympathetic ganglion cells (ganglioneuroma). Posterior mediastinal masses also include cysts, meningocele, lymphoma (Chapter 185 and 186), aortic aneurysm (Chapter 78), and esophageal disorders (Chapter 138) such as diverticula and neoplasm. Herniation of abdominal contents into the thorax can result in posterior mediastinal masses. Herniation of abdominal contents through the foramina of Bochdalek results in a mass in the posterolateral area of the diaphragm, usually on the left side; it is the most common congenital hernia and may contain spleen or kidney. Herniation of the stomach through the esophageal hiatus (Chapter 138), which is the most common type of diaphragmatic herniation, produces a mass posterior to the heart, often with an air-fluid level.

Benign cysts can occur in the anterior, middle, or posterior compartments. They can arise in the pericardium, bronchi, thymus, thoracic duct, esophagus, and stomach and can produce compressive symptoms. Pericardial cysts, which are often located in the cardiophrenic angle, contain clear liquid. Bronchogenic cysts occur in the middle or posterior compartments and are filled with liquid and lined with respiratory epithelium; they often develop around the paratracheal area or carina and do not communicate with the tracheal bronchial tree.

TREATMENT Rx

The treatment of a mediastinal mass depends on the underlying pathology. Some lesions, such as thymomas, teratomas, cysts, neurogenic tumors, and hernias, require surgical resection. Others, such as lymphoma, are treated with radiation or chemotherapy. Some can be carefully monitored over time.

Mediastinitis

Acute mediastinitis is most commonly caused by bacterial infection. Mediastinal infections are most commonly seen as complications after cardiothoracic surgical procedures, such as sternotomy, or procedures involving the esophagus or tracheobronchial tree. Rupture of the esophagus or trachea from trauma or tissue necrosis can cause mediastinitis. Treatment of acute mediastinitis requires antibiotics, pleural drainage, and evacuation of necrotic tissue. Chronic mediastinitis (fibrosing mediastinitis) is a progressive illness that may be idiopathic or can be caused by granulomatous infection, fungus, neoplasm, radiotherapy, or drugs (such as methysergide). Patients with chronic mediastinitis remain asymptomatic until vascular or neurologic structures are affected. When respiratory structures are involved, tracheobronchial narrowing is the most common presentation. The diagnosis and treatment often require surgical exploration, and further treatment is often not necessary unless it is due to tuberculosis (Chapter 324) or a fungal infection (Chapter 331).

Pneumomediastinum

Pneumomediastinum occurs when air infiltrates the mediastinal structures after a rupture of the esophagus, trachea, or lung dissects into the mediastinum. Loss of esophageal or tracheal integrity often results from trauma, whereas leaks from alveoli may result from trauma, occur spontaneously, or can be a complication of mechanical ventilation (Chapter 105). Pneumomediastinum rarely is seen as a complication of an asthma exacerbation (Chapter 87), violent coughing, or emesis. The diagnosis can be made by seeing thin columns of hyperlucency between mediastinal structures on chest radiography or CT scan. Pneumomediastinum may present as a sore throat, neck pain, or shortness of breath. Often, the mediastinal air dissects into the subcutaneous tissues of the neck and chest wall, where it results in subcutaneous emphysema. A characteristic crepitus is palpable when subcutaneous emphysema is present. A rare tension pneumomediastinum may compress the right ventricle. Spontaneous pneumomediastinum generally resolves without treatment. When more severe collections of subcutaneous air occur, surgical decompression is often warranted.

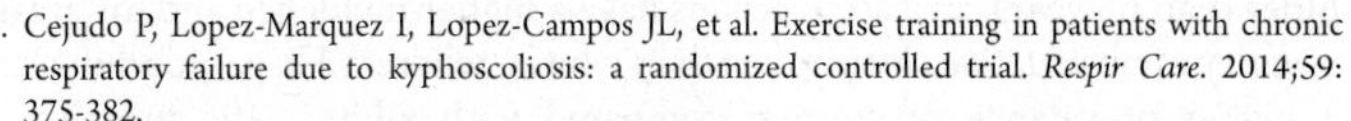

Grade A References

A1. Cejudo P, Lopez-Marquez I, Lopez-Campos JL, et al. Exercise training in patients with chronic respiratory failure due to kyphoscoliosis: a randomized controlled trial. *Respir Care.* 2014;59:375-382.

A2. Weinstein SL, Dolan LA, Wright JG, et al. Effects of bracing in adolescents with idiopathic scoliosis. *N Engl J Med.* 2013;369:1512-1521.

A3. Slobogean GP, MacPherson CA, Sun T, et al. Surgical fixation vs nonoperative management of flail chest: a meta-analysis. *J Am Coll Surg.* 2013;216:302-311.

A4. Kjeken I, Bo I, Ronningen A, et al. A three-week multidisciplinary in-patient rehabilitation programme had positive long-term effects in patients with ankylosing spondylitis: randomized controlled trial. *J Rehabil Med.* 2013;45:260-267.

A5. Rahman NM, Maskell NA, West A, et al. Intrapleural use of tissue plasminogen activator and DNase in pleural infection. *N Engl J Med.* 2011;365:518-526.

A6. Nie W, Liu Y, Ye J, et al. Efficacy of intrapleural instillation of fibrinolytics for treating pleural empyema and parapneumonic effusion: a meta-analysis of randomized control trials. *Clin Respir J.* 2014;8:281-291.

A7. Davies HE, Mishra EK, Kahan BC, et al. Effect of an indwelling pleural catheter vs chest tube and talc pleurodesis for relieving dyspnea in patients with malignant pleural effusion: the TIME2 randomized controlled trial. *JAMA.* 2012;307:2383-2389.

A8. Muers MF, Stephens RJ, Fisher P, et al. Active symptom control with or without chemotherapy in the treatment of patients with malignant pleural mesothelioma (MS01): a multicentre randomised trial. *Lancet.* 2008;371:1685-1694.

A9. Chen JS, Chan WK, Tsai KT, et al. Simple aspiration and drainage and intrapleural minocycline pleurodesis versus simple aspiration and drainage for the initial treatment of primary spontaneous pneumothorax: an open-label, parallel-group, prospective, randomised, controlled trial. *Lancet.* 2013;381:1277-1282.

GENERAL REFERENCES

For the General References and other additional features, please visit Expert Consult at https://expertconsult.inkling.com.

100

OBSTRUCTIVE SLEEP APNEA

ROBERT C. BASNER

DEFINITION

Obstructive sleep apnea is a chronic condition of cyclic obstruction of the upper airway during sleep, characteristically combined with associated symptoms or signs of disturbed sleep (Chapter 405), the most common being excessive daytime sleepiness and loud snoring. A frequency of at least five obstructive events (apneas, hypopneas, and/or respiratory effort–related arousals; see Pathogenesis) per hour of sleep is a minimal criterion for diagnosing obstructive sleep apnea in adults, although a higher frequency of obstructive events is more consistently correlated with an increased risk for cardiovascular and neurocognitive disorders. For continuous positive airway pressure (CPAP) treatment to be covered by Medicare in the United States, patients must be documented to have at least 15 such events per hour, or to have between 5 and 14 events per hour and also have at least one of the following: documented symptoms of excessive daytime sleepiness, impaired cognition, mood disorders, or insomnia; or documented hypertension, ischemic heart disease, or history of stroke.

EPIDEMIOLOGY

Obstructive sleep apnea is underrecognized by clinicians and underreported by patients, and most adults with moderate to severe disease remain undiagnosed. In adults, obstructive sleep apnea is characteristically found in overweight persons, although other anatomic (primarily upper airway and craniofacial) and ventilatory abnormalities may also predispose to the disorder. The presence of at least five obstructive events per hour of sleep has been found in 9 to 28% of adults without specific risk factors for, or symptoms of, obstructive sleep apnea, whereas the prevalence of such obstructive events and associated excessive daytime sleepiness is closer to 3 to 7% for adult men and 2 to 5% for adult women. Although overall prevalence appears to be much greater in men than in women, postmenopausal and obese women are at increased risk. Populations with a particularly high prevalence of obstructive sleep apnea include people older than 60 years of age and patients with systemic hypertension, particularly poorly controlled hypertension (Chapter 67); prior strokes (Chapter 407); heart failure (Chapter 58); atrial fibrillation (AF; Chapter 64), particularly recurrent AF following electrical cardioversion; prior acute myocardial infarction (Chapter 73); obesity-hypoventilation syndrome (Chapters 86 and 220); metabolic syndrome (Chapter 229); idiopathic pulmonary fibrosis (Chapter 92); and medically refractory epilepsy (Chapter 403). African Americans, particularly those younger than 25 and older than 65 years, and adult Asians have a higher incidence and/or greater severity of obstructive sleep apnea than whites, whereas Hispanic adults have a higher prevalence of snoring compared with whites. The presence of obstructive sleep apnea in a given patient more than doubles the chance of family members having the disorder compared with controls. Mean annual medical costs for patients with untreated obstructive sleep apnea are almost double those of otherwise normal people, and the costs increase in proportion to its severity.

PATHOBIOLOGY

Genetics

Despite the familial aggregation of obstructive sleep apnea, no specific genes or genetic loci have been identified to date. Most identified candidate genes share linkages to pathobiologic correlates, including obesity, craniofacial dysmorphisms, leptin, serotonin, ventilatory responsiveness, and carbonic anhydrase isoenzymes.

Pathogenesis

Obstructive sleep apnea involves complete or partial closure of the collapsible segments of the pharynx, including the velopharynx, oropharynx, and hypopharynx. *Obstructive apnea* is defined by absent airflow for at least 10 seconds associated with continued ventilatory effort (Fig. 100-1). *Obstructive hypopnea*, which is partial airway obstruction, is recognized functionally by a discrete decrease in, rather than cessation of, airflow for at least 10 seconds, associated with either a pathologic decrease in the oxygen saturation of hemoglobin (Sao_2) or an abrupt arousal from sleep. Typically the patient will display progressive ventilatory effort, flattening of the transduced nasal pressure tracing, and/or crescendo snoring (E-Fig. 100-1). A respiratory effort–related arousal occurs when such limitations of airflow are not severe enough to define hypopnea, but the progressive ventilatory effort is nevertheless associated with abrupt arousal from sleep.

Both excess weight and increasing weight are closely linked to the development and worsening of obstructive sleep apnea in adults. Conversely, weight loss, both surgical and nonsurgical, improves it (see Treatment). Anatomic and physiologic explanations of how excess weight contributes to obstructive sleep apnea include restriction of chest wall movement, with resultant mechanical and reflex upper airway narrowing; increased compliance and narrowing of the upper airway; ventilatory instability; and impaired ability to compensate for increased upper airway resistance in sleep.

The final common pathway in each obstructive event is attainment of a critical pharyngeal closing pressure. When narrowed or collapsed, the pharynx is more difficult to expand during the next inspiratory effort, thereby resulting in the characteristic generation of progressively more forceful inspiratory efforts against the obstructed upper airway and increasingly negative intrathoracic pressure excursions. Subsequent reopening of the airway is usually associated with arousal. After several hyperpneic breaths, re-transition into sleep generally occurs. The cycling of blood gases and the recurrent awake-to-asleep transitions interfere with the respiratory controllers' need to find a set point during sleep. Hypopnea or outright apnea followed by hyperpnea is the hallmark of obstructive sleep apnea.

The pathogenic importance of respiratory periodicity in obstructive sleep apnea varies by sleep stage (Chapter 405). The transition into "light" stages of sleep, termed *stages N1* and *N2 non–rapid eye movement* (NREM) *sleep*, is characterized by a tendency for arousal and sleep-wake cycling. These stages are most likely to demonstrate the periodicity of obstructive events characteristic of obstructive sleep apnea. In contrast, "deep" NREM sleep, termed *stage N3* or *slow-wave sleep*, is characteristically a time of relatively regular central nervous system output, with a decreased tendency for arousal, a

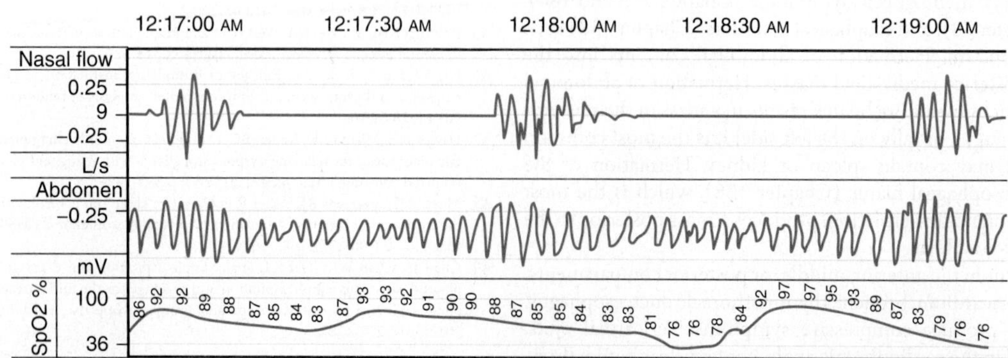

FIGURE 100-1. Polysomnographic tracing of a patient with obstructive sleep apnea during 2 minutes of non–rapid eye movement sleep. Displayed are airflow in the upper airway ("nasal flow"), recorded with a nasal pressure transducer; respiratory effort ("abdomen"), recorded by inductance plethysmography; and oxygen saturation of hemoglobin (Spo_2), recorded with pulse oximetry.

regularization of breathing, and a relative paucity of obstructive events, even with generally increased upper airway resistance when compared with N1 and N2 sleep. During rapid eye movement (REM) sleep, erratic neural drive and descending neural inhibition of accessory ventilatory and upper airway muscles may lead to severe alveolar hypoventilation and apnea. Severe hypoxemia, caused by a combination of obstructive events and ventilation-perfusion mismatch, is characteristic of REM sleep in patients with obstructive sleep apnea.

Pathophysiology

With each obstructive event, the combination of progressive asphyxia, increasingly negative intrathoracic pressure, and sudden autonomic and behavioral arousal leads to acute cardiac and cerebrovascular perturbations, including increased afterload of both the left and right ventricles, decreased left ventricular compliance, increased pulmonary artery pressure, decreased coronary artery blood flow, and increased myocardial oxygen demand (Chapter 53). The abrupt arousal at the termination of the majority of obstructive events is associated with sympathetic discharge, leading to peripheral vasoconstriction and an abrupt increase in the heart rate and in systolic and diastolic blood pressure, even as cardiac output continues to fall when ventilation resumes with the airway reopened. Accordingly, systemic blood pressure characteristically fluctuates; it is relatively low during apnea and acutely elevated at termination of the obstructive event (Chapter 67). Electrocardiographic abnormalities include sinus bradycardia during obstructive events and acceleration at arousal; in REM sleep, which is a time of increased vagal tone, sinoatrial and atrioventricular block may be seen. Ventricular and supraventricular ectopy and dysrhythmia can occur with obstructive sleep apnea. At the termination of obstructive apnea, cerebral blood flow and oxygenation are decreased. The recurrent abrupt, transient arousal from sleep at the termination of each obstructive event is associated with fragmented sleep and a decreased ability to consolidate restorative sleep.

CLINICAL MANIFESTATIONS

Symptoms and Signs

The cardinal manifestations of obstructive sleep apnea include loud, chronic snoring; excessive daytime somnolence; and apneas witnessed by third parties. The snoring reflects vibratory noise from partially occluded pharyngeal soft tissue, usually with the mouth open, and it typically occurs in a crescendo pattern, with a burst of louder noise at resolution of the event. Loud snoring without obstructive sleep apnea may progress to obstructive sleep apnea, particularly if the patient gains weight.

The most useful observation for identifying patients with obstructive sleep apnea is nocturnal choking or gasping (a three-fold increase in risk). Snoring is very common in patients with obstructive sleep apnea but is not nearly as predictive, and normal-weight people with mild snoring are unlikely to have moderate or severe obstructive sleep apnea.[1]

In the hospital setting, obstructive sleep apnea may be detected because of apnea or refractory decreases in Sa_{O_2} during surgical or endoscopic procedures that require sedation or anesthesia. In other cases, the diagnosis may be suspected when hospital staff note nocturnal heart block or dysrhythmias during sleep.

Excessive Daytime Somnolence

Patients with excessive daytime somnolence (Chapter 405) fall asleep unexpectedly; this is typically microsleep rather than sustained sleep episodes. Excessive daytime somnolence may be quantified by laboratory tests that monitor the propensity to fall asleep during the day or by questionnaires or subjective scales that assess sleepiness or decrements in quality of life. Resolution of obstructive sleep apnea does not necessarily resolve excessive daytime somnolence, thereby suggesting the possibility of sustained neurologic perturbation from chronic intermittent hypoxemia and highlighting the association of obstructive sleep apnea with metabolic, neurocognitive, respiratory, and cardiovascular perturbations. Further, many patients with otherwise clinically significant obstructive sleep apnea do not complain of excessive daytime somnolence, nor are patients typically aware of their degree of sleep fragmentation. Mood disorders, including depression and irritability, as well as perturbations in visual memory and working memory appear to be related to the severity of sleep fragmentation and hypoxemia.

Obstructed Breathing

The bed partners of obstructive sleep apnea patients often describe breathing cessation rather than obstructed breathing; close questioning usually elicits the obstructive nature of the breathing. Patients may be aware of their own snoring or complain of choking or dyspnea, particularly in relation to an inability to sleep supine. Morning dry mouth is a common symptom, as is morning headache.

Insomnia and Parasomnia

Insomnia, which is the subjective complaint of difficulty falling asleep or staying asleep (Chapter 405), is associated with the consistent sleep interruption characteristic of obstructive sleep apnea. Transient arousals during N3 sleep may result in confusional parasomnias, such as sleep walking and sleep talking. Arousals and increased work of breathing may result in restless sleep and night sweats. Nocturia, possibly mediated by atrial natriuretic receptors, may resolve with treatment.

Upper Airway Abnormalities

Nasal congestion, rhinitis, chronic sinusitis, and nasopharyngeal anatomic abnormalities are often associated with obstructive sleep apnea, as are craniofacial abnormalities such as micrognathia and retrognathia. Large tonsils, redundant soft palate tissue, and a large tongue may all be associated with a "crowded" oropharynx, but the precise role of these upper airway abnormalities in the pathogenesis of the disorder is unclear.

DIAGNOSIS

The spectrum of sleep-related breathing disorders other than obstructive sleep apnea includes hypoventilation and gas exchange disorders that may worsen with sleep, including nocturnal asthma (Chapter 87), chronic obstructive pulmonary disease (Chapter 88), neuromuscular and chest wall disorders (Chapter 99), and obesity-hypoventilation syndrome (Chapter 220), as well as other disorders in which central apnea (Chapter 405) is prominent, such as idiopathic central apnea, Cheyne-Stokes breathing, and central alveolar hypoventilation (Chapter 86). Patients with obstructive sleep apnea alone characteristically do not hypoventilate while awake, unlike patients with other disorders of hypoventilation. In patients with suspected obstructive sleep apnea, clinicians must also consider other disorders that are associated with hypersomnia, such as narcolepsy, insufficient sleep, poor sleep hygiene, and periodic limb movement disorder, as well as circadian rhythm disorders, such as shift work sleep disorder (Chapter 405). The use of standardized questionnaires such as the STOP-Bang questionnaire (Table 405-5) and the Epworth Sleepiness Scale (Table 405-3) can select patients for definitive testing.

Polysomnography

The definitive diagnostic study is polysomnography (see Fig. 100-1),[2] which generally involves all-night monitoring in a sleep laboratory by electroencephalography, electro-oculography (primarily to determine rapid eye movements characteristic of REM sleep), electrocardiography, leg and chin electromyography, and measures of respiratory effort, airflow, Sa_{O_2}, and alveolar or arterial carbon dioxide (usually end-tidal or transcutaneous CO_2). Audiovisual recordings can identify crescendo snoring and thoracoabdominal paradoxical breathing efforts to help differentiate obstructive from nonobstructive hypopnea.

The severity of obstructive sleep apnea is usually described by the apnea-hypopnea index, which is the number of obstructive apneas plus hypopneas per hour of sleep (Fig. 100-2). The term *respiratory disturbance index* includes obstructive apneas, hypopneas, and respiratory effort–related arousals. Oxygen desaturation more directly reflects the chronic intermittent hypoxia that has been increasingly linked to adverse health effects and outcomes.

It is possible to diagnose obstructive sleep apnea by means of unattended home studies that include cardiorespiratory monitoring and/or use of an autotitrating positive airway pressure (PAP) machine, which continuously self-adjusts the level of positive pressure delivered to the airway on a breath-to-breath basis in response to upper airway impedance changes. Such autotitration allows the immediate diagnosis and treatment of a patient suspected of having severe obstructive sleep apnea, with equivalent outcomes at lower cost compared with studies performed at sleep centers.[A1]

TREATMENT Rx

The goal of treatment is to decrease sleep fragmentation and repetitive asphyxia, the resultant cardiovascular, metabolic, and cerebrovascular stress, and the increased work of breathing associated with obstructive sleep apnea.

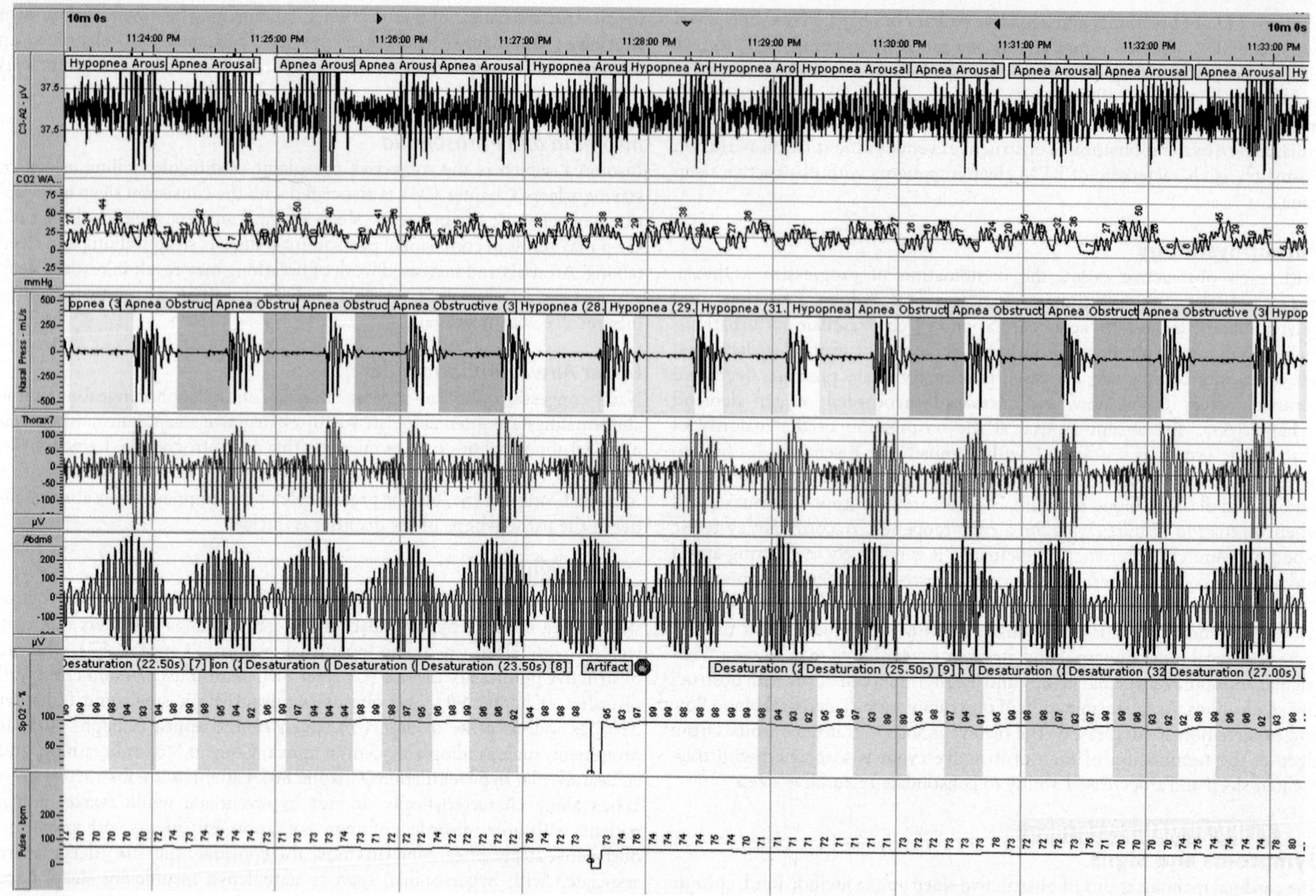

FIGURE 100-2. Continuous 10-minute polysomnographic tracing in a patient with severe obstructive sleep apnea. The 14 repetitive obstructive apneas constitute an apnea-hypopnea index of 84/hour. Each obstructive event is associated with a cyclic waxing-waning respiratory effort (seen in the thoracic and abdominal effort tracings), absent airflow (in the nasal pressure transducer), electroencephalographic arousal (C3-A2, top tracing), oxygen desaturation, and increased end-tidal P_{CO_2}.

Mechanical Therapy

Positive Airway Pressure

CPAP, which is the current first-line therapy for obstructive sleep apnea,[3,4] consistently lowers the apnea-hypopnea index while also decreasing daytime sleepiness, oxygen desaturation, diurnal and nocturnal blood pressure[A2], and pulmonary artery pressures. CPAP also improves sleep efficiency, quality of life, and executive mental function. CPAP is superior to oral appliances or no treatment at an acceptable cost, especially in patients with an apnea-hypopnea index greater than 30/hour. For patients with lower apnea-hypopnea index levels, CPAP is generally recommended for patients with prominent oxygen desaturation, daytime sleepiness, or concurrent respiratory, cardiovascular, or cerebrovascular disease. In that setting, CPAP improves cognitive function, improves left ventricular function in patients with heart failure, and decreases the risk for motor vehicle accidents.[5]

The major equipment required to administer PAP includes an interface with appropriate headgear, anchoring straps, and hosing and a compact airflow generator (Fig. 100-3). With CPAP, the fixed level of positive pressure delivered to the upper airway acts as a physiologic splint throughout the respiratory cycle, allowing the patient to achieve normal ventilation as well as more continuous and deeper sleep. CPAP does not supply ventilation above this splinting; the positive end-expiratory pressure may, however, result in improved oxygenation.

Prescribing PAP

PAP is typically prescribed after therapeutic titration in the sleep laboratory, beginning with CPAP of 2 to 4 cm H_2O and increasing by 1- to 2-cm H_2O increments to the minimum level that eliminates obstructive events in all sleep stages. Such a level should reduce other evidence of increased upper airway resistance and increased work of breathing (e.g., snoring, use of accessory inspiratory muscles, thoracoabdominal paradoxical respiration), while improving sleep continuity. Although CPAP is typically prescribed in the 8- to 12-cm H_2O range, it is not uncommon for patients with severe obstructive sleep apnea to need pressures up to 20 cm H_2O. However, as pressures increase above 12 to 14 cm H_2O, the likelihood of air leak and discomfort rises. When laboratory titration is not available, starting CPAP at a level of 10 cm H_2O is reasonable. Adding a feature that decreases expiratory pressure ("pressure relief") does not improve outcomes or adherence, or reduce side effects.

The first night of CPAP is often associated with a "rebound" of slow-wave NREM sleep and REM sleep, along with amelioration of acute fluctuations in heart rate and blood pressure. Daytime sleepiness and vigilance consistently improve with chronic use of CPAP; diurnal and nocturnal blood pressure and catecholamine levels decrease, and left ventricular ejection fraction and diastolic function improve. However, obstructive sleep apnea returns when CPAP is removed, so CPAP must be used nightly throughout sleep. The term *complex sleep apnea* refers to the commonly noted emergence of central apneas during initial CPAP titration; such an effect is generally not long-term, and the significance of this phenomenon remains to be elucidated.

Bilevel PAP

In some cases, a specific ventilatory mode of pressure delivery—generally bilevel PAP, wherein inspiratory pressure is set higher than expiratory pressure—may be helpful after the level of expiratory positive pressure necessary to prevent closure of the airway during expiration is established. Bilevel PAP may be delivered with a backup rate, similar to assist/control mode ventilation. Bilevel PAP should be considered in those with hypoventilation syndromes that overlap obstructive sleep apnea, such as obese patients who continue to have significant hypoventilation or ventilation-perfusion mismatch–related hypoxemia despite CPAP. For most obstructive sleep apnea patients beginning treatment, however, no high-quality data show improved outcomes or cost-effectiveness of bilevel PAP compared with CPAP, even when bilevel PAP is used as secondary therapy when CPAP is unsuccessful.

Autotitrating PAP

CPAP and bilevel PAP can be delivered so that the pressure automatically adjusts to the patient's breathing, based on either breath-to-breath detection of changes in airway resistance or the pattern of breathing. Short-term outcomes, including apnea-hypopnea index, symptomatic sleepiness, and quality of life, are similar, regardless of whether CPAP is guided by titration at a sleep

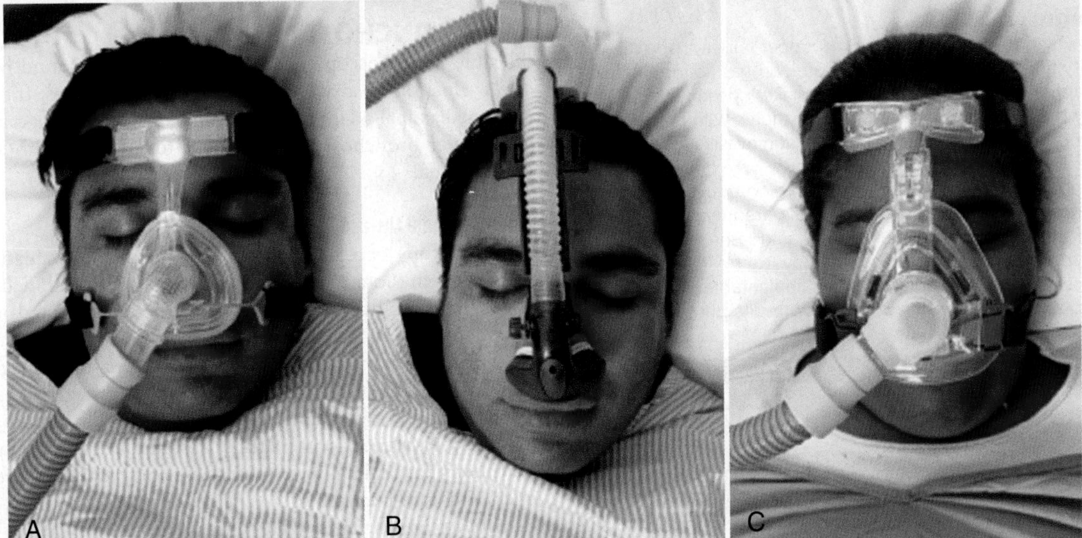

FIGURE 100-3. Positive airway pressure–patient interfaces. A, Subject wearing a nasal mask and headgear with positive airway pressure being delivered. Positive pressure is delivered only to the nasal airway; opening of the mouth may cause air to leak and decrease the efficacy of the positive-pressure regimen. B, Subject wearing nasal pillows. Positive pressure is delivered directly into the nares rather than covering the nose or mouth; only minimal headgear is necessary to anchor the interface in place. C, Subject wearing a full face mask. Positive pressure is delivered to both the nose and the mouth based on the subject's own breath-to-breath partitioning of nasal and oral airflow.

center or use of an autotitrating machine at home to determine a fixed pressure.[A3] However, autotitrating PAP does not improve adherence or outcomes compared with fixed-pressure CPAP.

PAP-Patient Interface

The choice of interface is important for achieving optimal efficacy and adherence. Aside from many different shapes, sizes, and consistencies of nasal masks (see Fig. 100-3A), flexible nasal "pillows" or "prongs" (see Fig. 100-3B) can fit directly into the nares, avoiding the discomfort of a mask over the nose and pain and pressure at the bridge of the nose and over the upper teeth. Although nasal PAP is commonly used, nasal delivery may be ineffective because of nasal congestion, nasopharyngeal anatomic abnormalities, or inability to keep the mouth closed, allowing air to leak from the mouth so that ineffective pressure is delivered to the collapsible airway. Soft "hybrid" interfaces, which have a mouthpiece and nasal prongs to permit both mouth and nose breathing, may be tried in such settings. Full face masks (see Fig. 100-3C) may also improve CPAP efficacy in such situations, but gastrointestinal bloating secondary to air swallowing is a common side effect, and the risks for vomiting and aspiration are a concern. Regardless of the interface used, the patient must be vigilant to maintain the interface throughout sleep, particularly after changes in position. Cold or heated humidification may be added directly to the circuit to improve comfort and adherence, but contamination of the humidifier with pathogenic organisms must be avoided.

Adherence and Outcome

PAP adherence is generally similar to that for treatments of other chronic medical disorders, although most studies suggest that CPAP is not used optimally for maximizing restorative sleep. Adherence may be improved by systematic cognitive behavioral and educational strategies, as well as strategies that address patient-specific issues.[A4] Treatment with PAP can be accurately monitored by systems that track the amount of time that physiologically successful PAP levels are delivered.

Oxygen

Although supplemental oxygen alone during sleep may ameliorate hypoxemia and improve sleep quality in obstructive sleep apnea, such treatment alone may lengthen apneas, cause paradoxical worsening of SaO_2, and fail to improve sleep fragmentation. Therefore, oxygen alone should not be used as first-line treatment for suspected or proven obstructive sleep apnea without nocturnal monitoring.

When sleep SaO_2 remains low despite otherwise optimal levels of CPAP or bilevel PAP, oxygen can be added directly to the mask, to an adapter near the mask, or beneath the mask by nasal cannulae.[6,A5] Higher flow rates of oxygen may be necessary as PAP levels increase, particularly if bilevel PAP is used.

Other Ways to Relieve or Bypass Obstruction

Oral appliances, specifically in the form of mandibular advancement devices fitted by an expert, improve symptoms in patients with obstructive sleep apnea, particularly with predominantly supine sleep apnea.[A6] However, such devices are generally less effective than CPAP in improving apnea-hypopnea index and oxygen desaturation during sleep. They are currently recommended specifically for patients with mild or moderate obstructive sleep apnea who do not benefit from CPAP or who prefer such an appliance rather than CPAP. Other recently developed alternatives include expiratory positive airway pressure, hypoglossal nerve stimulation, and oral pressure therapy, but few data are available on their efficacy.

General Measures

Sleep Positioning and Nasal Treatments

Sleep positioning may benefit many patients who have obstructive sleep apnea predominantly in the supine position, although such positioning does not appear to be as effective as CPAP in decreasing the apnea-hypopnea index. Treatment of chronic nasal congestion and inflammation with nasal steroids, saline washes, and systemic antihistamine-decongestant regimens sometimes may ameliorate obstructive sleep apnea. Otolaryngologic consultation can be useful to identify treatable nasopharyngeal disorders, including the rare nasopharyngeal neoplasm.

Weight Loss

Weight loss is a primary goal in an overweight patient with obstructive sleep apnea. It not only affects the severity of the breathing disorder during sleep but also may contribute to regression of the associated metabolic and cardiovascular perturbations.[A7] Non–morbidly obese patients who achieve nonsurgical weight loss also have significantly greater improvements in obstructive sleep apnea than do controls without such weight loss. In severely obese patients with marked obstructive sleep apnea, bariatric surgery significantly reduces weight compared with conventional medical therapy, but the incremental weight loss does not necessarily result in incremental improvement in obstructive sleep apnea itself.[7]

Treatment of Underlying Conditions

It is important to diagnose and treat underlying conditions such as diabetes (Chapter 229) and heart failure (Chapter 59) in patients with obstructive sleep apnea, but such treatment does not necessarily optimally treat the obstructive sleep apnea. For example, in patients with obstructive sleep apnea and heart failure, cardiac atrial overdrive pacing provides small improvements in the apnea-hypopnea index and sleep-related oxygen desaturation, but it is not as effective as CPAP.

Medical Therapy

There is no acceptably efficacious pharmacologic therapy for obstructive sleep apnea.[A8] Respiratory stimulants, including medroxyprogesterone and acetazolamide, have not proved effective in patients with normal $PaCO_2$ levels. Selective serotonin reuptake inhibitors, including fluoxetine and paroxetine, have been associated with a decreased apnea index during NREM but not REM sleep in a small number of patients. Tricyclic antidepressants have shown some utility in predominantly REM sleep–associated obstructive sleep apnea by decreasing REM volume, although side effects have hindered the use of such agents. Hormone replacement therapy may ameliorate the breathing disorder in postmenopausal women.

Surgical Procedures

Tracheostomy, which bypasses the site of upper airway obstruction, decreases morbidity and mortality and improves blood gas abnormalities in obstructive sleep apnea. However, tracheostomy makes speech difficult and is reserved for only the most severe cases and for patients with concomitant hypoventilation syndromes that do not respond to noninvasive forms of PAP.

Procedures to reduce uvular or palatal tissue, which were once widely recommended, have not shown a consistent benefit in high-quality studies.[8] As a result, surgical uvulopalatopharyngoplasty, radio frequency volumetric tissue reduction of the palate or tongue (or both), and laser-assisted uvuloplasty are not recommended as first-line therapy to treat symptomatic patients. A newer experimental approach is an implantable upper airway stimulator, which has shown promising preliminary results but has not been tested in randomized trials.[9]

PROGNOSIS

Population studies show an increased risk for all-cause and cerebrovascular and coronary mortality in patients with untreated severe obstructive sleep apnea and in patients with apnea-hypopnea indices of 30 or more per hour, independent of other major risk factors.[10] When patients with severe obstructive sleep apnea are prescribed CPAP, 5-year survival rates are significantly higher in those with good CPAP adherence (>6 hours/day) than in those with poor adherence. Like other patients with sleep disorders (Chapter 405), patients with obstructive sleep apnea and moderate to severe sleepiness are at greater risk for morbidity and mortality from motor vehicle accidents compared with drivers without obstructive sleep apnea.

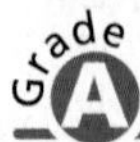

Grade A References

A1. Rosen CL, Auckley D, Benca R, et al. A multisite randomized trial of portable sleep studies and positive airway pressure autotitration versus laboratory-based polysomnography for the diagnosis and treatment of obstructive sleep apnea: the HomePAP study. *Sleep*. 2012;35:757-767.

A2. Iftikhar IH, Valentine CW, Bittencourt LR, et al. Effects of continuous positive airway pressure on blood pressure in patients with resistant hypertension and obstructive sleep apnea: a meta-analysis. *J Hypertens*. 2014;32:2341-2350.

A3. Berry RB, Hill G, Thompson L, et al. Portable monitoring and autotitration versus polysomnography for the diagnosis and treatment of sleep apnea. *Sleep*. 2008;31:1423-1431.

A4. Wozniak DR, Lasserson TJ, Smith I. Educational, supportive and behavioural interventions to improve usage of continuous positive airway pressure machines in adults with obstructive sleep apnoea. *Cochrane Database Syst Rev*. 2014;1:CD007736.

A5. Gottlieb DJ, Punjabi NM, Mehra R, et al. CPAP versus oxygen in obstructive sleep apnea. *N Engl J Med*. 2014;370:2276-2285.

A6. Phillips CL, Grunstein RR, Darendeliler MA, et al. Health outcomes of continuous positive airway pressure versus oral appliance treatment for obstructive sleep apnea: a randomized controlled trial. *Am J Respir Crit Care Med*. 2013;187:879-887.

A7. Chirinos JA, Gurubhagavatula I, Teff K, et al. CPAP, weight loss, or both for obstructive sleep apnea. *N Engl J Med*. 2014;370:2265-2275.

A8. Mason M, Welsh EJ, Smith I. Drug therapy for obstructive sleep apnoea in adults. *Cochrane Database Syst Rev*. 2013;5:CD003002.

GENERAL REFERENCES

For the General References and other additional features, please visit Expert Consult at https://expertconsult.inkling.com.

101

INTERVENTIONAL AND SURGICAL APPROACHES TO LUNG DISEASE

DAVID J. FELLER-KOPMAN AND MALCOLM M. DECAMP

Interventional pulmonology and minimally invasive thoracic surgery have drastically changed the approach to the diagnosis and staging of lung cancer, the management of central airway obstruction, and the treatment of patients with pleural disease.

BRONCHOSCOPY

Flexible bronchoscopy and endobronchial ultrasound have revolutionized the evaluation of airway and parenchymal diseases, the approach to hilar and mediastinal adenopathy, and the staging of lung cancer. New technologies offer bronchoscopic treatment for patients with severe asthma and emphysema.

Endobronchial Ultrasound

Bronchoscopy is a standard component of the evaluation and staging of patients with thoracic tumors. Convex-probe endobronchial ultrasound uses a curvilinear ultrasound probe, which is incorporated into the tip of the bronchoscope, to visualize structures outside of the airway and sample hilar and mediastinal lymph nodes under direct, real-time imaging. This approach has largely replaced mediastinoscopy in the staging of patient with lung cancer[1,2] and in the diagnosis of sarcoidosis (Chapter 95) and certain lymphomas. Adding endobronchial ultrasound to surgical staging improves the sensitivity for finding nodal metastases and can reduce the unnecessary thoracotomy rate from 18 to 7%.[A1] It is important to note, however, that the sensitivity of endobronchial ultrasound is not 100%, so nondiagnostic samples must be confirmed as true negatives with either surgical staging or clinical and radiologic follow-up.

In radial-probe endobronchial ultrasound, an ultrasound probe is passed through the working channel of the bronchoscope to visualize parenchymal lesions as well as to discriminate tumor invasion compared with compression of the central airways. When used with smaller bronchoscopes and advanced navigational technologies, such as electromagnetic navigation or virtual bronchoscopic navigation, this technique can improve the diagnostic yield when sampling pulmonary nodules.

Bronchial Thermoplasty

Bronchial thermoplasty uses radio frequency energy to ablate airway smooth muscle in patients whose severe asthma (Chapter 87) remains symptomatic despite medical therapy. The patient must undergo three bronchoscopic procedures to treat all of the visible airways. The right lower lobe is treated during the first procedure, the left lower lobe in the second, and both upper lobes in the third (the right middle lobe is not treated). Although asthma may be exacerbated in the immediate peritreatment period, this approach can significantly improve asthma-related quality of life, days lost from work or school, and emergency department visits in carefully selected patients for at least five years.[A2]

Bronchoscopy for Central Airway Obstruction

A variety of malignant and nonmalignant diseases can obstruct the central airways (Table 101-1). Malignant causes include bronchogenic carcinoma (Chapter 191) or metastatic malignancy to the airways, as well as extrinsic compression from adenopathy. Nonmalignant causes include granulation tissue arising after an intubation or tracheostomy, adenopathy from sarcoidosis (Chapter 95), inflammatory conditions such as relapsing polychondritis (Chapter 275), amyloidosis (Chapter 188), and infectious causes such as tuberculosis (Chapter 324) and respiratory papillomatosis.

CLINICAL MANIFESTATIONS AND DIAGNOSIS

A high index of suspicion is essential because significant airway obstruction can be present before the development of symptoms or the characteristic abnormalities on the inspiratory and expiratory flow-volume curves (Chapter 85). Patients with central airway obstruction often develop exertional dyspnea when the tracheal lumen is less than 8 mm in diameter (normal is about 18 to 20 mm) but do not develop stridor, which usually is a sign of impending respiratory failure and the need for urgent intervention, until the tracheal diameter is less than 5 mm.

Hemoptysis (Chapter 83) may be present in patients with malignancies but is also seen in infectious and inflammatory conditions. Some patients may present with a postobstructive pneumonia that responds poorly to antibiotic treatment. Most patients, however, present with nonspecific symptoms including dyspnea and cough.

Patients who have risk factors for chronic airway obstruction and present with symptoms consistent with obstruction unresponsive to conventional therapy should undergo airway imaging by computed tomography (CT) (Fig. 101-1) and flexible bronchoscopy (Fig. 101-2). Because loss of airway patency can be lethal, evaluation of these patients should be performed by individuals experienced in the management of critical airway disorders.

TABLE 101-1 CAUSES OF CENTRAL AIRWAY OBSTRUCTION

NONMALIGNANT	MALIGNANT
Congenital vascular sling	Primary airway tumors (e.g., bronchogenic, mucoepidermoid, adenoid cystic carcinoid)
Cartilage	Tumors metastatic to the airway (e.g., bronchogenic, renal cell, breast, melanoma, thyroid, colon, esophageal)
Relapsing polychondritis	External compression
Tracheobronchomalacia	Lymphadenopathy from any malignancy
Lymphadenopathy	Mediastinal tumors (e.g., thyroid, thymus, germ cell, lymphoma)
Infectious (e.g., histoplasmosis, tuberculosis)	
Sarcoidosis	
Granulation tissue associated with artificial airways, airway stenosis, aspirated foreign bodies, surgical anastomosis	
Inflammatory lesions (e.g., granulomatosis with polyangiitis, amyloidosis, papillomatosis)	
External compression (e.g., goiter)	
Internal	
Secretions	
Blood clot	

Adapted from Feller-Kopman D, Mehta AC, Wahidi MM. Therapeutic bronchoscopy. In: Broaddus VC, Mason RJ, Ernst JD, et al, eds. *Murray & Nadel's Textbook of Respiratory Medicine.* 6th ed. Philadelphia, PA: Saunders; in press (2016).

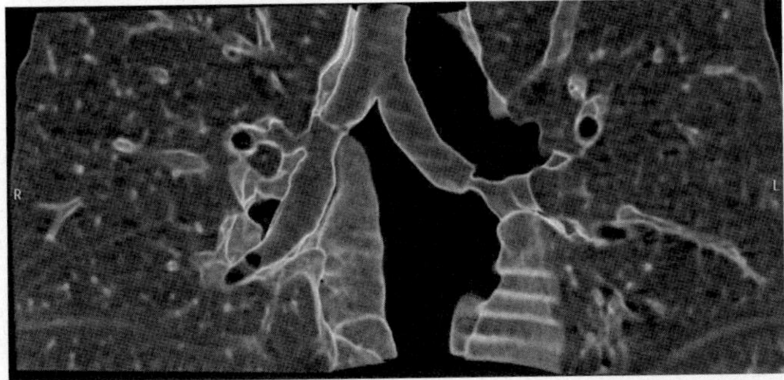

FIGURE 101-1. Three-dimensional reconstruction of a computed tomographic scan in a 20-year-old woman after bilateral lung transplantation. The image clearly shows the high-grade stenosis at the level of the left mainstem anastomosis. The right-sided airways are normal.

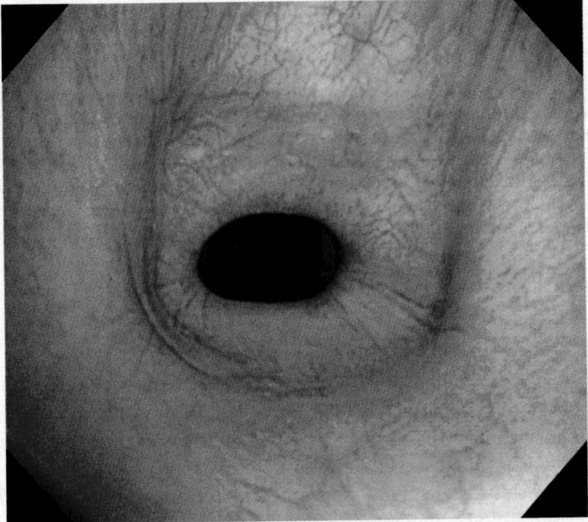

FIGURE 101-2. Bronchoscopic view of the proximal trachea in a 54-year-old man with shortness of breath and stridor. Significant circumferential narrowing is noted in the subglottic space, consistent with gastric reflux–induced subglottic stenosis.

TREATMENT

Rx

Relief of airway obstruction requires a multidisciplinary approach by expert physicians. Techniques for achieving a patent airway include coring out the tissue with the barrel of the rigid bronchoscope; laser treatment to vaporize the tissue; electrocautery or argon plasma coagulation to carbonize the tissue, so it will later slough; cryotherapy; and mechanical débridement with forceps or a microdebrider.[3] In the absence of definitive randomized trials, the choice of modality is often left to the expertise and resources of the bronchoscopist.

In contrast to endobronchial disease, airway stenting is the primary treatment for airway obstruction caused by extrinsic compression. Because airway stents can be associated with long-term complications, including stent fractures, the formation of granulation tissue, infection, and migration, they are primarily a palliative approach for malignant diseases and should be used sparingly in patients with nonmalignant airway obstruction.

PROGNOSIS

Successful endoscopic treatment can significantly improve the quality of life of patients with malignant airway obstruction and improve their survival rates to be the equivalent of similar stage patients without airway obstruction. Patients with nonmalignant disease similarly experience significant improvements in physiology (pulmonary function), exercise capacity, and quality of life.

Surgical Approaches

Open Approaches

Thoracotomy has been the standard approach to evaluate the contents of the pleural space, lung parenchyma, pulmonary hilum, and ipsilateral mediastinum and diaphragm. Selective lung ventilation, achieved by use of a double-lumen endotracheal tube or mainstem bronchial blocker, allows one lung to be collapsed and visualized. Given the precision and accuracy of contemporary preprocedure CT and magnetic resonance imaging (MRI), many procedures can be performed using smaller targeted incisions, with a muscle-sparing technique that allows specific access to regional pathology. Many lung processes can also be approached through a median sternotomy, which affords access to both lungs, although access to the left lower lobe through this approach can be challenging.

Video-Assisted Thoracoscopic Surgery

Thoracoscopy, or video-assisted thoracoscopic surgery (VATS), requires two or three incisions, termed *ports*, to place instruments in any intercostal space. A common configuration is to place one port for the video thoracoscope and two ports for endoscopic instrumentation. With the VATS approach, recovery is shorter than after an open thoracotomy because little if any muscle is divided and no mechanical rib spreading retractors are used.

The size of the surgical incisions depends on the goals of the procedure and the anatomic findings at the time of exploration. Unexpected pleural symphysis or incomplete lobar fissures may require extension of the incision to facilitate visualization. In patients undergoing anatomic resection, such as segmentectomy or lobectomy, at least one of the port incisions is extended to 4 to 8 cm in length to permit extraction of the resected lung from the hemithorax.

SURGERY FOR BENIGN LUNG DISEASE

A variety of benign lung diseases present as focal parenchymal lesions or diffuse processes that require a tissue biopsy for diagnosis. Thoracoscopy has essentially replaced a limited thoracotomy and wedge resection for this purpose. VATS provides a more complete view of the ipsilateral hemithorax, including the visceral, parietal, and mediastinal pleura, as well as access to all lung lobes. In addition, subpleural nodules that are too small to be visualized by preoperative radiography can be identified so that representative biopsy samples can be obtained.

Spontaneous Pneumothorax

Although most spontaneous pneumothoraces (Chapter 99) are uncomplicated, up to 20% of patients with pneumothoraces experience complications such as tension pneumothorax, persistent air leak despite tube drainage, or recurrent pneumothoraces either ipsilaterally or contralaterally. Patients in whom a second pneumothorax develops have a 70 to 80% chance of a third recurrence within 2 years. The current surgical approach to the treatment of recurrent pneumothoraces is VATS resection of the subpleural blebs responsible for the pneumothorax, usually combined with mechanical abrasion of the parietal pleura or chemical pleurodesis (e.g., with 300 mg of minocycline[A3] or with insufflated talc) to induce an inflammatory reaction that will cause the visceral and parietal pleural surfaces to fuse, thereby preventing subsequent recurrence.

Giant Bullae

Most patients with chronic obstructive pulmonary disease (COPD) have diffuse parenchymal disease, but a small number of patients with COPD have dominant or giant bullae that may occupy 50% or more of the volume of the hemithorax and that compress relatively preserved lung parenchyma. The indications for bullectomy include progressive symptoms with demonstrated disability, obstructive spirometry (Chapter 85), and a single or dominant bullous lesion with radiographic demonstration of compression of the surrounding preserved lung parenchyma. Either excision or plication can remove the bullous lesion.

Malignant Lung Disease

Solitary Pulmonary Nodules

Most small pulmonary nodules (see Fig. 191-2) present in the periphery of the lung beyond the reach of diagnostic bronchoscopy. For such lesions, VATS excisional biopsy (see Video 101-1) of a small pulmonary nodule leads to a definitive diagnosis in almost all cases and is generally preferred over transthoracic needle biopsy.[4] Furthermore, thoracoscopy can allow concurrent nodal staging should a primary malignancy (Chapter 191) be confirmed. In the absence of regional adenopathy, patients with primary malignant lesions can undergo definitive resection at the same time.

Primary Lung Cancer

In patients with node-negative primary lung cancer and adequate pulmonary reserve, lobectomy or pneumonectomy is indicated to obtain optimal survival and to decrease the risk for local recurrence. Similar oncologic outcomes can be achieved by performing an open thoracotomy or by lobectomy through VATS or robotic assistance, and VATS lobectomy generally is associated with fewer complications, less pain, a shorter hospitalization, and a speedier recovery.[5] Achieving a complete lobectomy is important because sublobar resection (segmentectomy or wedge) for stage I lung cancers is associated with a two- to three-fold higher incidence of locoregional recurrence.

Metastatic Cancer

The lung is a frequent site of metastatic recurrence. Common histologies include colorectal cancer (Chapter 193), renal cell carcinoma (Chapter 197), sarcoma (Chapter 202), melanoma (Chapter 203), breast cancer (Chapter 198), and head and neck cancer (Chapter 190). VATS is often the diagnostic procedure of choice to locate and excise nodules that are too small for reliable percutaneous biopsy.

The role of pulmonary metastectomy as therapy for advanced disease remains controversial. Five-year survival rates of 20 to 30% have been reported for selected patients, especially if the disease-free interval from original diagnosis to lung metastasis is greater than 3 years. These cases often require resection of bilateral lung nodules, which in turn mandate either a median sternotomy, clamshell incision, staged thoracotomies, or bilateral VATS.

SURGERY FOR ADVANCED LUNG DISEASES: LUNG VOLUME REDUCTION SURGERY

Emphysema (Chapter 88) is the most common chronic progressive disabling lung disease treated by pulmonologists and thoracic surgeons. In eligible patients (Table 101-2), lung volume reduction surgery confers durable symptomatic, physiologic, and survival benefits compared with medical therapy (Fig. 101-3) for patients who have severe emphysema but who do not have a forced expiratory volume in 1 second (FEV_1) measure of less than 20% of predicted with either a homogeneous distribution of emphysema on CT or a diffusing capacity of less than 20% of predicted.[6,7] However, subgroup analyses suggest that the benefit is mainly in patients with upper lobe predominant disease.

For eligible patients, most programs require a 6- to 10-week preoperative pulmonary rehabilitation followed by a cardiopulmonary exercise test to assess the risks and benefits of surgery. Patients with upper lobe predominant emphysema and a low preoperative exercise capacity have a nearly 50% lower risk for death after lung volume reduction surgery compared with continued medical therapy.[A4] High-risk patients with severe airflow obstruction (FEV_1 < 20%) should be assessed for lung transplantation evaluation unless their disease is localized to the upper lobes and their gas exchange as defined by diffusing capacity is preserved (Table 101-3).

In experienced centers, bilateral stapled resection approaches yield nearly twice the physiologic benefit of unilateral lung volume reduction surgery without adversely affecting operative morbidity or mortality. Bilateral lung volume reduction surgery using the VATS approach also may reduce intensive care unit and hospital length of stay and increase the likelihood of living independently 60 days after surgery compared with median sternotomy.

TABLE 101-2 INCLUSION AND EXCLUSION CRITERIA FOR LUNG VOLUME REDUCTION SURGERY

INCLUSION CRITERIA
Radiographic evidence of emphysema, especially involving upper lobes
Hyperinflation evidenced by TLC > 100% predicted and RV > 150% predicted
FEV_1 > 20 and < 45% predicted (after bronchodilator)
DLCO > 20% predicted
Severe dyspnea
Restricted activities of daily living
Decreased quality of life
Abstinence from tobacco
EXCLUSION CRITERIA
Active smoking
Bronchiectasis
Pulmonary nodule requiring evaluation
Excessive daily sputum production
Previous thoracotomy
Obvious pleural disease
Active or inducible coronary ischemia
Pulmonary hypertension
Depressed LVEF (<45%)
Obesity (BMI > 32)
Unable or unwilling to participate in pulmonary rehabilitation
Systemic steroids, ≥20 mg prednisone/day

BMI = body mass index; DLCO = diffusion capacity for carbon monoxide; FEV_1 = first second forced expiratory volume; LVEF = left ventricular ejection fraction; RV = residual capacity; TLC = total lung capacity.

Adapted from DeCamp MM Jr, McKenna RJ Jr, Deschamps CC, et al. Lung volume reduction surgery: technique, operative mortality and morbidity. *Proc Am Thorac Soc.* 2008;5:442-446; and DeCamp MM Jr, Lipson D, Krasna M, et al. The evaluation and preparation of the patient for lung volume reduction surgery. *Proc Am Thorac Soc.* 2008;5:427-431.

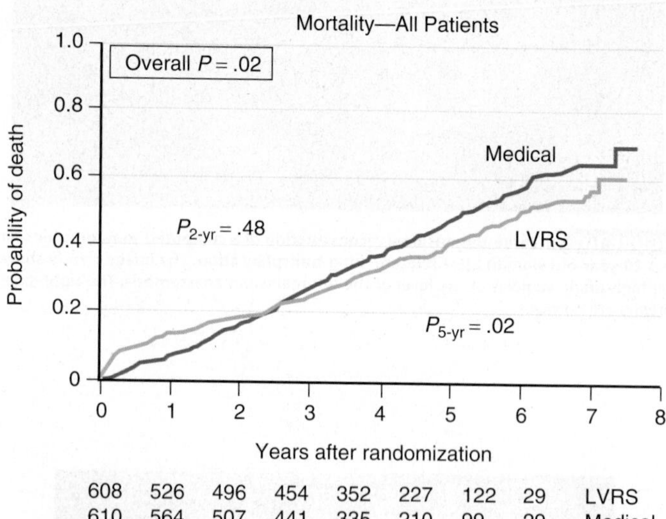

FIGURE 101-3. Long-term mortality of all patients treated with lung volume reduction surgery (LVRS) versus maximal medical therapy in the National Emphysema Treatment Trial. Note the statistically significant (P = .02) reduction in relative risk for death (RR = 0.85) in the surgical cohort. (Adapted from Naunheim KS, Wood DE, Mohsenifar Z, et al, for the National Emphysema Treatment Trial Research Group. Long-term follow-up of patients receiving lung-volume-reduction surgery versus medical therapy for severe emphysema in the National Emphysema Treatment Trial. *Ann Thorac Surg.* 2006;82:431-443.)

TABLE 101-3 DECISION GUIDE FOR SELECTION OF LUNG VOLUME REDUCTION SURGERY VERSUS TRANSPLANTATION FOR SEVERE CHRONIC OBSTRUCTIVE PULMONARY DISEASE

FACTORS FAVORING LVRS	FACTORS FAVORING TRANSPLANTATION
Age > 65 yr	$FEV_1 \le 20\%$ predicted
Upper lobe predominant disease	DLCO ≤ 20% predicted
Chronic medical conditions	Homogeneous or lower lobe distribution of disease
Hepatitis B and/or C	TLC < 100% predicted
HIV infection	RV < 150% predicted
Renal insufficiency	$PaCO_2$ > 60 mm Hg
Cirrhosis	PaO_2 < 45 mm Hg
Neuropathy	6 MWD < 140 m or
Poorly controlled diabetes	<3 min unloaded pedaling cycle ergometer
Osteoporosis	Pulmonary hypertension
Severe GERD	Bronchiectasis
Poor esophageal motility	Recurrent pulmonary infections
Malignancy	
Unable to maintain long-term follow-up	
Psychiatric issues limiting compliance	
Insufficient social support	

6 MWD = 6-minute walk distance; DLCO = diffusion capacity of carbon monoxide; FEV_1 = first second forced expired volume; GERD = gastroesophageal reflux disease; HIV = human immunodeficiency virus; LVRS = lung volume reduction surgery; RV = residual volume; TLC = total lung capacity.
Adapted from Patel N, DeCamp M, Criner GJ. Lung transplantation and lung volume reduction surgery versus transplantation in chronic obstructive pulmonary disease. *Proc Am Thorac Soc.* 2008;5:447-453.

ENDOSCOPIC MANAGEMENT OF EMPHYSEMA

The only therapies that have a proven survival advantage in the management of patients with severe emphysema are the use of oxygen and surgical lung volume reduction. A5 Endoscopic approaches to lung volume reduction may offer a less invasive way to achieve some of the benefits of surgical lung volume reduction.[8] As with surgical lung volume reduction, the goals of these technologies are to reduce the magnitude of overdistended and poorly perfused lung tissue, thereby increasing elastic recoil, diminishing dynamic hyperinflation, and redistributing airflow to better perfused areas of the lung. Bronchoscopic options include one-way valves, coils, foam, and steam. Although some of these devices are approved in Europe, none is currently approved in the United States because randomized trials have not shown significant benefits. A6 A7

LUNG TRANSPLANTATION

About 180 worldwide lung transplant centers perform more than 3700 transplantations per year.[9] Lung transplantation is now an accepted therapy for all forms of advanced lung disease. The use of ex vivo perfusion to resuscitate lungs considered unsuitable for transplant by traditional procurement criteria appears to be expanding the availability of donor organs.[10]

The most common indications for transplantation (Table 101-4) are diseases or conditions that share the following features: they produce extreme disability in affected patients, they are unresponsive to medical therapy, and they are responsible for limited life expectancy in affected patients. With the exception of a small number of cases of sarcoidosis and lymphangioleiomyomatosis, the original lung disease does not usually recur after lung transplantation.

Types of Procedures

Currently, four types of lung transplantation procedures are performed. *Single-lung transplantation,* which is typically performed through a posterolateral thoracotomy incision, requires three anastomoses: the mainstem bronchus, pulmonary artery, and pulmonary veins and left atrium. The contralateral lung is not removed, so single-lung transplantation is not performed in patients with bilaterally infected lungs (e.g., patients with cystic fibrosis or bronchiectasis) (see Table 101-3).

Bilateral lung transplantation is performed in a sequential fashion that is functionally equivalent to two single-lung transplantations completed during a single operation, most commonly through a transverse sternotomy ("clamshell") incision. It requires six anastomoses: both mainstem bronchi, both pulmonary arteries, and both sets of pulmonary veins. It is the procedure of choice for patients with bilaterally infected lungs and is also performed in certain patients with emphysema, primary pulmonary hypertension, and other diseases (see Table 101-3). Bilateral transplantation is preferred for nearly all indications because a double-lung recipient can expect a half-life of 6.9 years compared with 4.6 years for a single-lung recipient. As a result, about 75% of the world's reported lung transplants are now bilateral.

Heart-lung transplantation is now performed in only about 75 cases per year. It is an en bloc procedure with right atrial, aortic, and distal tracheal anastomoses. It is performed in patients with advanced lung disease and coexistent irreparable cardiac disease, usually associated with fixed pulmonary hypertension, and in those with Eisenmenger syndrome (Chapter 69).

Living donor lobar transplantation involves the removal of a lower lobe from each of two living donors. One is implanted into each hemithorax of the recipient in a manner similar to bilateral lung transplantation.[11]

TABLE 101-4 INDICATIONS AND CONTRAINDICATIONS FOR LUNG TRANSPLANTATION

SINGLE-LUNG TRANSPLANT	PATIENTS (%)	DOUBLE-LUNG TRANSPLANT	PATIENTS (%)
INDICATIONS			
COPD	44	CF, bronchiectasis	30
Pulmonary fibrosis, sarcoid	40	Emphysema	27
α_1-Antitrypsin deficiency	65	α_1-Antitrypsin deficiency	6
PPH, Eisenmenger	1.4	PPH, Eisenmenger	6.2
CF, bronchiectasis	2.4	Pulmonary fibrosis, sarcoid	17
Retransplantation	3	Retransplantation	2
Other*	4	Other*	6

ABSOLUTE CONTRAINDICATIONS

Untreatable advanced extrapulmonary organ dysfunction (e.g., heart, liver, kidney)
- CAD not amenable to PCI or bypass
- Poor LV function (could consider heart-lung transplantation)

Malignancy within 2 years (excludes cutaneous squamous or basal cell carcinoma)
- 5-year disease-free interval preferred

Noncurable extrapulmonary infection
- Infection with human immunodeficiency virus
- Hepatitis B antigen positivity
- Hepatitis C with histologic evidence of active liver disease

Active substance abuse (including cigarettes)
Severe musculoskeletal disease affecting the thorax
Documented noncompliance
Untreatable psychiatric condition that impairs compliance
Absence of consistent and reliable social support

RELATIVE CONTRAINDICATIONS

Physiologic age > 65 yr
Poor nutritional status (<70% ideal body weight)
Severe obesity (BMI > 30 kg/m)
Symptomatic osteoporosis
Colonization with highly virulent and/or highly resistant fungi, mycobacteria, or bacteria
Requirement for invasive ventilation and/or circulatory support
Uncontrolled chronic medical conditions (e.g., diabetes, hypertension, GERD)
Severely limited functional status with poor rehabilitation potential
Psychosocial problems likely to affect the outcome adversely
High-dose (>20 mg of prednisone daily) corticosteroid use

*Other includes lymphangioleiomatosis, non-retransplantation-related obliterative bronchiolitis, and miscellaneous indications.
BMI = body mass index; CAD = coronary artery disease; CF = cystic fibrosis; COPD = chronic obstructive pulmonary disease; GERD = gastroesophageal reflux disease; LV = left ventricle; PCI = percutaneous coronary intervention; PPH = primary pulmonary hypertension.
Adapted from Yusen RD, Christie JH, Edwards LB, et al. Twenty-sixth official adult lung and heart-lung transplant report—2013. *J Heart Lung Transplant.* 2013;32:965-978; and Orens JB, Estenne M, Arcasoy S, et al. International guidelines for the selection of lung transplant candidates: 2006 update—a consensus report from the Pulmonary Scientific Council of the International Society for Heart and Lung Transplantation. *J Heart Lung Transplant.* 2006;25:745-755.

Evaluation of Potential Transplant Recipients

The ideal candidate for lung transplantation has lung disease unresponsive to medical therapy but is in otherwise good health. Patients who experience critical illness as a result of lung disease often have poor nutritional status, coexistent major organ dysfunction, refractory infection, or other contraindications to transplantation. The specific evidence-based recommendations for referral for transplant evaluation vary with the underlying disease.

In the United States, the lung allocation system is based on expected disease-specific and patient-specific survival during the waiting period and after engraftment, thereby reflecting net transplant benefit. Early evaluations of the system, which was introduced in 2005, indicate shorter waiting times, an increase in the total number of transplantations performed, a decreased waitlist mortality, and an unchanged overall survival after transplantation.

Post-transplantation Issues

Most of the medical issues that patients and physicians face after lung transplantation are the consequence of the transplantation and post-transplantation medication rather than the underlying disease for which the transplantation was performed. Examples include immunosuppression, infections and their prophylaxis, acute allograft rejection, chronic allograft rejection, and nonpulmonary complications of transplantation.

Immunosuppression

The standard chemotherapeutic regimen for immunosuppression after lung transplantation consists of a calcineurin inhibitor such as cyclosporine or tacrolimus, azathioprine or mycophenolate mofetil, and corticosteroids. More than 50% of centers add an antilymphocyte antibody preparation in the first days after transplantation, and this practice has led to a small but statistically significant improvement in long-term survival.

Infections and Prophylaxis after Lung Transplantation

Lung transplant recipients are at high risk for bacterial, viral, fungal, and protozoal infections; infections are the leading causes of death during the early post-transplantation period. In the first 3 months after transplantation, bacterial infections are responsible for most deaths. In approximately one third of patients, pneumonia is diagnosed in the first weeks after transplantation, with gram-negative organisms as the cause in 75% of cases. Colonization and recurrent infections, usually with *Pseudomonas* species, often develop in patients with chronic rejection.

Among potential viral pathogens, *cytomegalovirus* (CMV; Chapter 376) is the most important in lung transplant recipients. Seronegative patients who receive an allograft from a seropositive donor are at particularly high risk for the development of a clinically significant CMV infection. Seronegative patients who have a seronegative donor are at low risk for infection if they are treated with seronegative blood products. Epstein-Barr virus (EBV) has been associated with the development of post-transplantation lymphoproliferative disorder.

Aspergillus species are the most common cause of invasive fungal infection (Chapter 339). Colonized patients and those deemed at risk may receive prophylactic inhaled amphotericin B.

Because of the nature of the immunosuppressive chemotherapeutic regimen used, patients are at high risk for infection by the protozoan *Pneumocystis jirovecii* (Chapter 341). The use of trimethoprim-sulfamethoxazole prophylaxis (typically 1 double-strength tablet three times weekly indefinitely) has virtually eliminated *Pneumocystis* pneumonia.

Acute Rejection

Histologically, the initial manifestation of acute rejection is a lymphocyte-predominant inflammatory response, usually centered on blood vessels, airways, or both. By convention, acute rejection is graded histologically from 0 (normal) to 4 (severe), with subclasses defined by the presence or absence of airway inflammation.

The risk for acute allograft rejection is highest in the early months after transplantation and declines with time. Multiple episodes of acute rejection are the major risk factor for the subsequent development of chronic rejection.

Clinically, patients may have fever, cough, and exertional dyspnea. Evaluation may demonstrate rales or rhonchi on chest examination, a decline in pulmonary function by spirometry, leukocytosis, opacities on chest radiography, and exertional desaturation. The clinical manifestation is often indistinguishable from infectious pneumonia, and the clinical impression is accurate in only 50% of cases.

Treatment of acute rejection most often consists of high-dose corticosteroids (typically, 1 g/day of methylprednisolone administered intravenously for 3 days).

Chronic Rejection

PATHOBIOLOGY

The bronchiolitis obliterans syndrome is thought to be a manifestation of chronic rejection. Risk factors for development of the syndrome include the number of acute rejection episodes and, in some series, previous symptomatic CMV infection. Pathologically, "early" lesions demonstrate inflammation and disruption of the epithelium of small airways, followed by growth of granulation tissue into the airway lumen and subsequent complete or partial obstruction. The granulation tissue then organizes in a stereotypical pattern with resultant fibrosis that obliterates the lumen of the airway.

CLINICAL MANIFESTATIONS

Clinically, bronchiolitis obliterans is accompanied by nonspecific symptoms.[12] Progressive exertional breathlessness typically develops, and pulmonary function testing usually demonstrates evidence of progressive airflow obstruction (Chapter 85). Bronchiolitis obliterans is classified according to the FEV_1: 0 (no significant abnormality) if FEV_1 is greater than 80% of baseline; 1 (mild) if FEV_1 is 65 to 80% of baseline; 2 (moderate) if FEV_1 is 50 to 65% of baseline; and 3 (severe) if FEV_1 is 50% or less of baseline. In early stages, chest radiography is notable only for hyperinflation, but it may show bronchiectasis as the syndrome progresses. Later stages of bronchiolitis obliterans may include a syndrome of bronchiectasis with chronic productive cough and airway colonization with *Pseudomonas* species.

DIAGNOSIS

The diagnosis of bronchiolitis obliterans is made on both clinical and pathologic grounds. Transbronchial biopsy has a low yield for demonstrating histologic evidence of bronchiolitis obliterans, but when such evidence is seen, it is diagnostic. In patients with a compatible clinical syndrome, exclusion of anastomotic stenosis and occult pulmonary infection is sufficient to establish the diagnosis.

TREATMENT Rx

A variety of therapies have been tried for chronic rejection, including pulse corticosteroids, antilymphocyte antibodies, total lymphoid irradiation, photopheresis, and nebulized cyclosporine, but none has been clearly established as effective. Most patients with bronchiolitis obliterans experience a progressive decline in pulmonary function despite immunosuppression.

PROGNOSIS

Bronchiolitis obliterans is the leading cause of late mortality after lung transplantation. Half of lung transplant recipients surviving to 5 years will have either biopsy-proven bronchiolitis obliterans or the clinical diagnosis of bronchiolitis obliterans syndrome.

Nonpulmonary Medical Complications of Lung Transplantation

Most of the nonpulmonary medical complications that arise in patients after lung transplantation are the result of immunosuppressive therapy. One or more of these complications develop in virtually all lung transplant recipients.

Osteoporosis (Chapter 243) is common because of the long-term use of corticosteroids and cyclosporine. Bone density should be monitored periodically, and pharmacologic therapy should be instituted if excessive bone loss is identified.

Chronic renal insufficiency (Chapter 130) is common and is the result of therapy with the calcineurin inhibitors cyclosporine or tacrolimus, both of which affect afferent vascular tone in the kidneys and result in an average 50% drop in the glomerular filtration rate in the first 12 months after lung transplantation. Systemic arterial hypertension is also common and is caused by corticosteroids and cyclosporine. Calcium-channel blockers, which are often used to treat hypertension, raise serum cyclosporine levels; appropriate monitoring and dose adjustment are needed when starting such therapy. Both corticosteroids and tacrolimus contribute to the development of diabetes mellitus and hyperlipidemia.

Solid organ transplantation is associated with an increased incidence of malignancy, thought to be due to pharmacologic immunosuppression and

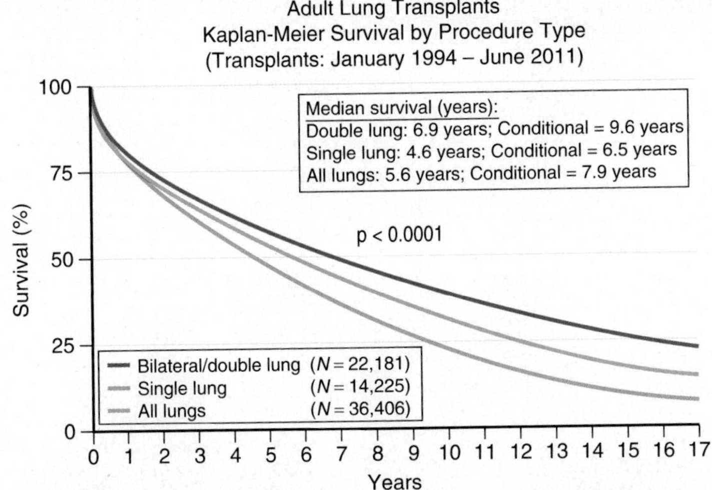

FIGURE 101-4. **Kaplan-Meier survival estimates for all adult lung transplantations reported to the International Registry for Heart and Lung Transplantation from 1994 to 2011. Note the highly statistically significant survival advantage conferred by double lung grafts. Because the decline in survival is greatest during the first year after transplantation, the conditional survival (i.e., when 50% of the recipients who survive to at least 1 year have died) provides a more realistic expectation of survival time for recipients who survive the early post-transplant period. (Adapted from Yusen RD, Christie JH, Edwards LB, et al. Twenty-sixth official adult lung and heart-lung transplant report—2013. *J Heart Lung Transplant.* 2013;32:965-978.)**

alteration in immune surveillance. Patients are at increased risk for lymphoproliferative malignancies and other types of cancers. Post-transplantation lymphoproliferative disorders occur in about 4% of patients after organ transplantation; most are associated with EBV. These syndromes can be polyclonal or monoclonal. Reduction in immunosuppression is sometimes therapeutic in those with polyclonal disease. The prognosis in patients with monoclonal disease is poor, with little response to modification of immunosuppression or antineoplastic chemotherapy. Patients are also at increased risk for skin, bladder, lung, cervical, and hepatobiliary malignancy after solid organ transplantation.

Outcomes after Lung Transplantation

Currently, the annual mortality rate following lung transplantation is 8 to 10% per year, largely owing to bronchiolitis obliterans syndrome. The median survival after lung transplantation is about 5.5 years (Fig. 101-4).

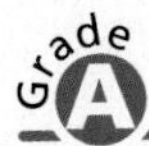

Grade A References

A1. Annema JT, van Meerbeeck JP, Rintoul RC, et al. Mediastinoscopy vs endosonography for mediastinal nodal staging of lung cancer: a randomized trial. *JAMA.* 2010;304:2245-2252.
A2. Wechsler ME, Laviolette M, Rubin AS, et al. Bronchial thermoplasty: Long-term safety and effectiveness in patients with severe persistent asthma. *J Allergy Clin Immunol.* 2013;132:1295-1302.
A3. Chen JS, Chan WK, Tsai KT, et al. Simple aspiration and drainage and intrapleural minocycline pleurodesis versus simple aspiration and drainage for the initial treatment of primary spontaneous pneumothorax: an open-label, parallel-group, prospective, randomised, controlled trial. *Lancet.* 2013;381:1277-1282.
A4. Naunheim KS, Wood DE, Mohsenifar Z, et al. Long-term follow-up of patients receiving lung-volume-reduction surgery versus medical therapy for severe emphysema by the National Emphysema Treatment Trial Research Group. *Ann Thorac Surg.* 2006;82:431-443.
A5. Fishman A, Martinez F, Naunheim K, et al. A randomized trial comparing lung-volume-reduction surgery with medical therapy for severe emphysema. *N Engl J Med.* 2003;348:2059-2073.
A6. Sciurba FC, Ernst A, Herth FJF, et al. A randomized study of endobronchial valves for advanced emphysema. *N Engl J Med.* 2010;363:1233-1244.
A7. Shah PL, Slebos DJ, Cardoso PF, et al. Bronchoscopic lung-volume reduction with Exhale airway stents for emphysema (EASE trial): randomised, sham-controlled, multicentre trial. *Lancet.* 2011;378:997-1005.

GENERAL REFERENCES

For the General References and other additional features, please visit Expert Consult at https://expertconsult.inkling.com.

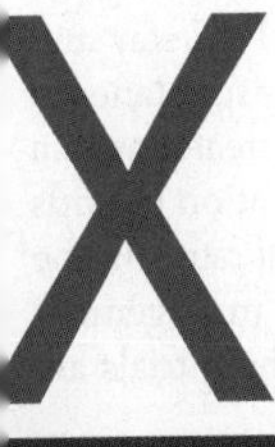

CRITICAL CARE MEDICINE

102

APPROACH TO THE PATIENT IN A CRITICAL CARE SETTING

DEBORAH J. COOK

THE INTENSIVIST-LED MULTIDISCIPLINARY TEAM

Patients with critical illness in the intensive care unit (ICU) usually require advanced life support, such as mechanical ventilation, vasopressors, inotropic agents, or renal replacement therapy. Morbidity associated with critical illness includes complications of both acute and chronic diseases, nosocomial and iatrogenic consequences, and impaired quality of life among survivors. Critically ill patients are at a higher risk of death than any other hospital population. Accordingly, the goals of critical care are to reduce morbidity and mortality, to maintain organ function, and to restore health. Unlike many other specialties, critical care medicine is not limited to a particular population, disease, diagnosis, or organ system.

Staffing of ICUs with critical care physicians, often referred to as *intensivists*, who provide mandatory consultations or principal ongoing care is associated with a significantly reduced ICU and hospital mortality and reduced ICU and hospital lengths of stay. The addition of nighttime intensivist staffing appears to reduce mortality by 38% in ICUs with low-intensity daytime staffing but not in centers with high-intensity daytime staffing, such as academic ICUs.[A1] These findings emphasize the value of the on-site availability of trained physicians who are dedicated to appropriate triaging, diagnosis, monitoring, treatment, and palliation of critically ill patients.

Daily rounds by an ICU physician who leads the coordinated work of nurses, pharmacists, respiratory therapists, physiotherapists, dietitians, chaplains, and other physicians appear to improve outcomes. Observational studies suggest that a standardized, goal-oriented approach to care delivered by multidisciplinary clinicians, with explicitly defined roles and best practices checklists, can help improve the quality of ICU rounds.[1] The critical care process can be optimized by interprofessional leadership, communication, and a positive organizational culture.

FLUID RESUSCITATION

Intravenous fluids to maintain or to restore intravascular volume are an important component of ICU therapy. Both crystalloid and colloid solutions are in widespread use. Crystalloids are readily available and inexpensive, whereas colloids generally require less volume to achieve a specific physiologic goal.

Fluid replacement with either normal saline or 4% albumin results in similar rates of death, organ failure, and other clinical outcomes,[A2] but crystalloids may lower mortality for patients with traumatic brain injury (Chapter 399). Fluid management with hydroxyethyl starch increases the need for renal replacement therapy and increases mortality compared with crystalloid infusions.[A3] On the basis of these data, either crystalloid- or albumin-based colloid fluid resuscitation is recommended for most critically ill patients, crystalloids are recommended for head-injured patients, and starches are not recommended.

SEDATION, ANALGESIA, AND SPONTANEOUS BREATHING TRIALS

Endotracheal intubation, central venous catheterization, postoperative pain management, and other ICU procedures require that most patients receive sedation, analgesia, or both. Sedatives and analgesics are used to ensure ongoing tolerance to mechanical ventilation, particularly in patients with shock or severe acute respiratory distress syndrome (ARDS). As long as pain and anxiety are well treated, bolus injections are preferred to continuous infusions because of emerging concerns about drug-induced delirium and delayed weaning from the ventilator. If patients are receiving drug infusions, daily interruption of sedatives and analgesics, by protocols that provide an opportunity for the patient to be observed safely in a less sedated state, are associated with a shorter duration of mechanical ventilation and ICU length of stay than continuous infusions. A second key component of managing sedation and analgesia is to use a drug titration protocol and nurse-led sedation scale; in these situations, daily interruption of sedation infusions may confer no additional benefit.[A4]

Discontinuation of ventilation is affected by sedation and analgesic infusions, and vice versa. A daily sedation vacation followed by a spontaneous breathing test increases the days of breathing without assistance and shortens ICU stay and hospital stay compared with usual sedation management plus a daily spontaneous breathing test.[A5] In the year after enrollment, patients who were treated with a "wake up and breathe" protocol, which linked daily sedation vacation periods with daily spontaneous breathing trials, had a 32% better survival rate. On the basis of these data, a nurse-implemented sedation and analgesic management scale with daily drug interruption and daily spontaneous breathing trials are recommended for mechanically ventilated critically ill patients.

LONG-TERM OUTCOMES FOR SURVIVORS

Biomarkers of inflammation, residual organ dysfunction, and functional disabilities persist in most ICU survivors even after transfer out of the ICU. Treatments administered in the ICU also have serious sequelae. For example, neuromuscular blockers and corticosteroids may contribute to critical illness polyneuropathy. These problems have particularly serious adverse consequences for elderly critically ill patients who are deconditioned before hospitalization.

In addition, anxiety, post-traumatic stress, and major mood disorders are common among patients and their caregivers during recovery. Therefore, although ICU discharge and hospital discharge are milestones in a patient's trajectory, sequelae of critical illness have rarely resolved completely when patients are on the regular hospital unit. For example, residual muscle weakness is common,[2] even 5 years after ICU discharge.

The legacy of critical care and the resulting residual functional impairment increase postdischarge morbidity and costs, thereby encouraging rehabilitation interventions to improve long-term outcomes. In a randomized trial of patients who received mechanical ventilation for 72 hours or less, the addition of graduated, individualized, early physical therapy and occupational therapy during daily sedation vacation periods improved functional capacity at hospital discharge, reduced the duration of delirium, and reduced the number of ventilator days during the 28-day follow-up.[A6] Discontinuation of physiotherapy as a result of patient instability, usually patient-ventilator asynchrony, occurred in only 4% of all sessions. This trial highlights how the recovery of critically ill patients potentially can be improved by coordinated multidisciplinary care.

APPLYING EVIDENCE TO PREVENT COMPLICATIONS OF CRITICAL ILLNESS

Considerable evidence of effective preventive and therapeutic ICU interventions has emerged in randomized trials during the past decade. For example, evidence-based initial management of a patient with urosepsis and ARDS includes low tidal volume ventilation,[A7] avoidance of early high-frequency oscillation,[A8] high positive end-expiratory pressure,[A9] inotrope or vasopressor infusion, low-dose corticosteroids, early enteral small bowel nutrition, avoidance of antioxidants,[A10] head of bed elevation, oral antisepsis with chlorhexidine, stress ulcer prophylaxis,[3] thromboprophylaxis with low-molecular-weight heparin,[A11] and insulin therapy aimed at avoiding marked hyperglycemia but not achieving normoglycemia[A12] (Chapters 104 and 105). In mechanically ventilated adults, chest radiographs on demand provide clinical outcomes equivalent to those of routine radiographs, despite about one-third fewer radiographs.[A13] Later during the stabilization and recovery phase of critical illness, evidence-based management includes targeted protocol-driven sedation, daily interruption of sedation infusions, daily spontaneous breathing trials, and early mobilization.

Potential barriers to applying evidence in fast-paced ICUs include a perceived lack of responsibility, unclear decisional authority, and errors of omission. Passive dissemination of information, whether written or verbal, is generally ineffective in modifying physicians' behavior. More effective strategies to encourage the implementation of evidence-based recommendations are interactive education, audit and feedback, reminders (written or computerized), involvement of local opinion leaders, and multifaceted approaches. In the high-acuity ICU setting, preprinted physician orders may help guide (but not dictate) management (Table 102-1). For example, a statewide intervention coached local safety teams to lead multidisciplinary education about central venous catheter management strategies known to decrease infection risk, including a procedural checklist that incorporated handwashing, full barrier precautions for catheter insertion, chlorhexidine skin cleansing, avoidance of the femoral site, and removal of unnecessary catheters. This multimethod approach, which included periodic site-specific feedback,

TABLE 102-1 ICU ADMISSION ORDERS: EXAMPLE FOR A PATIENT WITH UROSEPSIS AND ARDS

MANAGEMENT STRATEGY	ORDERS	REEVALUATE
ACUTE PHASE		
Mechanical ventilation	Target TV 5-7 mL/kg of ideal body weight, PC 16 cm, rate 12, FIO_2 0.7, PEEP 16 cm, plateau pressure <35 cm	PRN
Maintenance fluid	Lactated Ringer 75 mL/hr IV	PRN
Norepinephrine	Titrate to mean arterial pressure >65 mm Hg	PRN
Corticosteroids	Hydrocortisone 50 mg IV q6h while vasopressor dependent	Daily
Sedation	Midazolam 2-8 mg/hr IV, bolus 2-4 mg PRN	PRN
Analgesia	Morphine 1-4 mg IV PRN	PRN
Antibiotics	Ampicillin 2 g IV q6h	Daily
Head of bed	45-degree elevation from horizontal	PRN
Oral antisepsis	Chlorhexidine 15 mL q6h	Daily
Small bowel enteral nutrition	10 mL/hr of a commercial balanced feed containing about 1 kcal/mL; increase by 20 mL q4h to 70 mL/hr	Daily
Stress ulcer prophylaxis	Pantoprazole 40 mg IV daily	Daily
Thromboprophylaxis	Dalteparin 5000 U SC daily	Daily
Intensive insulin therapy if glucose >180 mg/dL	50 U insulin in 50 mL NS; start at 0.5 U/hr, repeat glucose q1h for 4 hr, and reassess; target 110-150 mg/dL	Daily
Glucometer calibration	Calibrate glucose from glucometer and central laboratory every morning	Daily
Tests	Glucose q4h when stable, ABG with each ventilator change, other tests as per ICU team	PRN
Monitoring	Arterial catheter for systolic blood pressure, central venous catheter for central venous pressure and mixed venous oxygen saturation, ECG, oximetry, ABGs, sedation scale, Foley catheter, others as per ICU monitoring protocols	PRN
STABILIZATION AND RECOVERY PHASES		
Sedation vacation	Daily interruption of sedation from 0700 h until 0900 h; restart at half prior infusion rate at 0900 h if necessary; aim to discontinue infusion as soon as possible	Daily
Spontaneous breathing trials	Spontaneous breathing trial when weaning readiness criteria met	Daily
Early mobility	Titrated physiotherapy and occupational therapy when able	Daily

ABG = arterial blood gas; ARDS = acute respiratory distress syndrome; ECG = electrocardiogram; FIO_2 = fraction of inspired oxygen; ICU = intensive care unit; IV = intravenous; NS = normal saline; PC = pressure control; PEEP = positive end-expiratory pressure; PRN = as needed; SC = subcutaneous; TV = tidal volume.

decreased catheter-related blood stream infections from 7.7 per 1000 catheter-days at baseline to 1.4 at 18 months' follow-up.[4] In a provincial cluster randomized trial addressing six evidence-based critical care practices in community ICUs, a multimethod approach including video conferencing, education, provision of algorithms, audit, and feedback resulted in a threefold increased adoption of the six management strategies.[A14]

PREDICTIONS, PREFERENCES, AND PALLIATIVE CARE

The prognosis of many critically ill patients improves once they are in the ICU. For others, treatment responsiveness is delayed or not realized, organ dysfunction evolves but does not resolve, and complications arise. Despite best efforts of the multidisciplinary ICU team, critical illness proves fatal to between 5 and 40% of adults. Approximately 2% of ICU patients discharged to the ward are readmitted within 48 hours and about 4% within 120 hours.[5] When a therapeutic trial of critical care is started, and particularly when it is failing, it is crucial to discuss prognosis openly with families (Chapter 3). Among medical ICU patients older than 80 years at one tertiary care university hospital, ICU mortality was 46%, hospital mortality was 55%, and mortality among hospital survivors was 53% at 2 years.[6] About 15% of patients who are admitted to an ICU have clinical courses that probably should generate discussion about palliative care.[7] Families bring key information about the patient's prior function and preferences.

In the shared decision-making model dominant in many settings today, these exchanges often result in plans to withhold or to withdraw basic or advanced life support.[8] Mechanical ventilation is the most frequent life support administered to and withdrawn from critically ill patients. Ventilator withdrawal very often precedes death in the ICU. Patients undergoing ventilator withdrawal or who die while mechanically ventilated have a shorter ICU stay than patients successfully weaned from the ventilator. When life support modalities are withdrawn because their further use would be futile,[9] each can be discontinued or weaned, with attendant considerations and cautions (Table 102-2). Withdrawal may be guided by the severity of the illness and other physiologic characteristics, but it is more heavily influenced by the contemporary life support model that is attentive to a patient's values and the physician's predictions about future quality of life. This complexity underscores the need for ICU teams to be expert communicators, sensitive in eliciting patients' preferences, timely in relieving suffering, and compassionate in

TABLE 102-2 CONSIDERATIONS AND CAUTIONS IN THE WITHDRAWAL OF LIFE SUPPORT

ISSUE	RISKS	OTHER CONSIDERATIONS
Weaning from inotropes or vasopressors	No risk of physical distress	May prolong the dying process, particularly if patient requires low doses and this is the only life support withdrawn
Discontinuation of inotropes or vasopressors	No risk of physical distress	Death may not occur quickly if the patient requires low doses, particularly if mechanical ventilation is ongoing Death may occur quickly if the patient requires high doses, with or without withdrawal of mechanical ventilation
Weaning from mechanical ventilation	Low risk of dyspnea	May prolong the dying process, particularly if the patient requires low pressure settings or low oxygen levels and this is the only life support withdrawn
Discontinuation of mechanical ventilation	Risk of dyspnea	Death may not occur quickly if the patient requires low pressure settings or low oxygen levels Death may occur quickly if the patient requires high pressure settings or high oxygen levels Preemptive sedation is typically needed to blunt air hunger due to rapid changes in mechanical ventilation
Extubation	Risk of dyspnea Risk of stridor (steroids) Risk of airway obstruction (jaw thrust) Risk of noisy breathing (glycopyrrolate)	Avoids discomfort and suctioning of endotracheal tube Can facilitate oral communication Informing families about possible physical signs after extubation can prepare and reassure them Allows for the most natural appearance Not advised if the patient has hemoptysis
Discontinuation of renal replacement therapy	Low risk of physical distress	Death may take several days if this is the only advanced life support withdrawn

Reprinted with permission from Cook D, Rocker G. Dying with dignity in the intensive care unit. *N Engl J Med*. 2014;370:2506-2514. Copyright © 2014 Massachusetts Medical Society.

providing dignity to the dying while administering culturally competent, family-centered end-of-life care. A death with dignity in the ICU infers that whereas some treatments may be foregone, care can be enhanced as death ensues. Fundamental to maintaining dignity is the need to understand a patient's unique perspectives on what gives life meaning in a setting replete with depersonalizing devices. The goal is caring for patients in a manner consistent with their values at a time of incomparable vulnerability, when they cannot speak for themselves.[10]

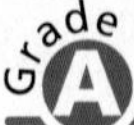

Grade A References

A1. Kerlin MP, Small DS, Cooney E, et al. A randomized trial of nighttime physician staffing in an intensive care unit. *N Engl J Med.* 2013;368:2201-2209.

A2. Finfer S, Bellomo R, Boyce N, et al. A comparison of albumin and saline for fluid resuscitation in the intensive care unit. *N Engl J Med.* 2004;350:2247-2256.

A3. Rochwerg B, Alhazzani W, Sindi A, et al. Fluid resuscitation in sepsis: a systematic review and network meta-analysis. *Ann Intern Med.* 2014;161:347-355.

A4. Mehta S, Burry L, Cook D, et al. Daily sedation interruption in mechanically ventilated critically ill patients cared for with a sedation protocol: a randomized controlled trial. *JAMA.* 2012;308:1985-1992.

A5. Girard T, Kress JP, Fuchs BD, et al. Efficacy and safety of a paired sedation and ventilator weaning protocol for mechanically ventilated patients in intensive care (Awakening and Breathing Controlled trial): a randomised controlled trial. *Lancet.* 2008;371:126-134.

A6. Schweickert WD, Pohlman MC, Pohlman AS, et al. Early physical and occupational therapy in mechanically ventilated, critically ill patients: a randomised controlled trial. *Lancet.* 2009;373:1874-1882.

A7. Burns KE, Adhikari NK, Slutsky AS, et al. Pressure and volume limited ventilation for the ventilatory management of patients with acute lung injury: a systematic review and meta-analysis. *PLoS ONE.* 2011;6:e14623.

A8. Ferguson ND, Cook DJ, Guyatt GH, et al. High-frequency oscillation in early acute respiratory distress syndrome. *N Engl J Med.* 2013;368:795-805.

A9. Briel M, Meade M, Zhou Q, et al. Higher versus lower positive end-expiratory pressure in patients with acute lung injury and acute respiratory distress syndrome: systematic review and individual patient data meta-analysis. *JAMA.* 2010;303:865-873.

A10. Heyland D, Muscedere J, Wischmeyer PE, et al. A randomized trial of glutamine and antioxidants in critically ill patients. *N Engl J Med.* 2013;368:1489-1497.

A11. Cook D, Meade M, Guyatt G, et al. Dalteparin versus unfractionated heparin in critically ill patients. *N Engl J Med.* 2011;364:1305-1314.

A12. Finfer S, Chittock DR, Su SY, et al. Intensive versus conventional glucose control in critically ill patients. *N Engl J Med.* 2009;360:1283-1297.

A13. Hejblum G, Chalumeau-Lemoine L, Ioos V, et al. Comparison of routine and on-demand prescription of chest radiographs in mechanically ventilated adults: a multicentre, cluster-randomized, two-period crossover study. *Lancet.* 2009;374:1687-1693.

A14. Scales DC, Dainty K, Hales B, et al. A multifaceted intervention for quality improvement in a network of intensive care units. *JAMA.* 2011;305:363-372.

GENERAL REFERENCES

For the General References and other additional features, please visit Expert Consult at https://expertconsult.inkling.com.

103 RESPIRATORY MONITORING IN CRITICAL CARE

JAMES K. STOLLER AND NICHOLAS S. HILL

Monitoring of the respiratory system involves a broad array of assessment techniques ranging from low-technology approaches like a careful physical examination to sophisticated technologies to monitor oxygenation and ventilation.

PHYSICAL EXAMINATION

The physical examination can provide important information about the patient's ventilation and oxygenation. Ventilation can be assessed by recording the respiratory rate (normally 12 to 20 breaths/minute in adults) as well as by closely inspecting the pattern of chest wall movement during inspiration and by noting the use of accessory inspiratory muscles (e.g., the scalene, trapezius, and sternocleidomastoid muscles). Hypopnea (shallow or slow breathing) or a slowed respiratory rate (bradypnea) can indicate decreased ventilation. Shallow breathing may relate to muscle weakness (Chapter 421) or increased lung stiffness, which is commonly accompanied by a compensatory increase in the ratio of the respiratory rate to maintain ventilation. Bradypnea may relate to a suppressed respiratory drive (e.g., excessive use of narcotics, slowing the respiratory rate). Conversely, sustained tachypnea (e.g., >35 breaths/minute in an adult) can indicate ongoing increased work of breathing, impending respiratory failure, and the need for mechanical assistance, such as noninvasive ventilation or intubation and mechanical ventilation, depending on the etiology of the respiratory failure.

Contraction of the sternocleidomastoid muscles or scalene muscles, often with a seated, bent posture, is called the tripod sign (E-Fig. 103-1). This response indicates inadequate diaphragmatic function, most commonly in the setting of emphysema with associated diaphragmatic flattening, which causes a mechanical disadvantage of diaphragmatic contraction. In this circumstance, patients may demonstrate Hoover sign, which is inspiratory retraction of the rib cage at the level of the zone of apposition, where the diaphragm inserts on the chest wall.

The physical examination of the nail beds and lips may also reveal cyanosis, which suggests hypoxemia. Cyanosis occurs when saturation falls, but it requires the presence of 5 g of desaturated hemoglobin. As such, polycythemic patients may show cyanosis with relatively high oxyhemoglobin saturation values, whereas patients with profound anemia may not demonstrate cyanosis even in the face of low values of oxyhemoglobin saturation.

SYSTEMIC ARTERIAL BLOOD GAS ANALYSIS

Sampling of arterial blood, either through a percutaneous arterial puncture or by withdrawal of blood from an indwelling arterial catheter, provides important information about the patient's oxygenation and ventilation status as well as the acuity of and compensation for derangements. The partial pressure of carbon dioxide ($PaCO_2$) reflects ventilation, the elimination of carbon dioxide. In many but not all cases, $PaCO_2$ is close to the mixed alveolar $PaCO_2$. The $PaCO_2$ in the arterial blood is closely related to the ratio of metabolic carbon dioxide production to alveolar ventilation:

$$PaCO_2 = (K)(CO_2 \text{ production rate})/(\text{alveolar ventilation } [VA]) \quad (1)$$

The partial pressure of oxygen (PaO_2) reflects the level of oxygenation. Normal levels of oxygenation are defined by the alveolar-arterial oxygen gradient, $P(A\text{-}a)O_2$, which is calculated as

$$P(A\text{-}a)O_2 = FIO_2(PB - PH_2O \text{ at standard pressure and body temperature}) - (PaO_2 + PaCO_2/\text{respiratory quotient}) \quad (2)$$

where the respiratory quotient equals the number of moles of carbon dioxide produced for each mole of oxygen consumed (generally ~0.8 under normal metabolic conditions at rest but variable with dietary intake and metabolic rate). The normal value of the alveolar-arterial oxygen gradient varies with age and position and can be approximated by the simple equation

$$P(A\text{-}a)O_2 = (\text{age}/4) + 4 \quad (3)$$

Normal age-related values of PaO_2 in the sitting position can be determined by the equation

$$PaO_2 \text{ sitting} = 104.2 - (0.27 \times \text{age in years}) \quad (4)$$

Normal values of PaO_2 are generally in the range of 70 to 95 mm Hg, depending on the patient's age.

The $PaCO_2$ helps assess the adequacy of the patient's ventilation. At sea level, normal values of $PaCO_2$ range from 35 to 45 mm Hg. Values of $PaCO_2$ below 35 mm Hg indicate hyperventilation, either as a primary respiratory event (e.g., with anxiety) or in response to another insult (e.g., hypoxemia, sepsis, liver disease). Similarly, values of $PaCO_2$ exceeding 45 mm Hg indicate hypoventilation, hypercapnia, and respiratory acidosis, which may result either from suppression of the ventilatory drive (Chapter 86) (e.g., excess narcotics; Chapter 34) or from respiratory insufficiency (e.g., respiratory muscle weakness; Chapter 421).

Assessment of the patient's bicarbonate level (HCO_3^-) helps define the chronicity of changes in the patient's $PaCO_2$, where the value of bicarbonate is defined by the Henderson-Hasselbalch equation:

$$pH = 6.1 + \log_{10}[HCO_3^-]/0.003\ PaCO_2 \quad (5)$$

Acute increases in $PaCO_2$ drive the normal kidney to retain bicarbonate (Chapter 118), whereas acute decreases in $PaCO_2$, as in hyperventilation from anxiety or liver disease, would be expected to cause the normal kidney to waste bicarbonate to preserve the body's pH (normally 7.35 to 7.45).

The clinician can also assess whether the patient's ventilatory response to metabolic acidosis is appropriate or inadequate by the Winter equation, which predicts the expected $PaCO_2$ in the face of a decreased bicarbonate from a metabolic acidosis (Equation 6). Specifically, a measured $Pa{CO_2}$ above the expected value indicates an inadequate ventilatory response, whereas a value of $Pa{CO_2}$ that falls within the expected range indicates an expected, appropriate ventilatory response to the metabolic derangement (i.e., the acidosis).

$$Pa{CO_2} = (1.5[HCO_3^-] + 8) \pm 2 \quad (6)$$

When the patient is hypercapnic and hypoxemic, a useful step is to calculate the ambient air $P(A\text{-}a)O_2$ and to determine whether it is normal or increased for the patient's age. Of the six mechanisms of hypoxemia, only two (hypoventilation and breathing decreased ambient oxygen, as at altitude or from a hypoxic gas mixture) are associated with a preserved $P(A\text{-}a)O_2$ (Table 103-1). Under clinical circumstances at sea level, hypoxemia in the face of a normal $P(A\text{-}a)O_2$ indicates that the patient's hypoxemia is caused by hypoventilation and should prompt the clinician to consider the various causes of suppressed respiratory drive (Chapter 86) or respiratory insufficiency that interferes with a normal ventilatory response (e.g., respiratory muscle weakness; Chapter 421).

PULSE OXIMETRY

Pulse oximetry is a noninvasive method to assess arterial blood oxygenation.[1] The percentage of hemoglobin that is oxygenated is measured by passing light of two different wavelengths (660 nm [for deoxyhemoglobin] and 940 nm [for oxyhemoglobin]) through a blood-carrying tissue (e.g., finger, earlobe, forehead), identifying the pulsatile component (which contains arterial blood and background tissue elements), and subtracting the nonpulsatile component to isolate the arterial component. The device can estimate the percentage of oxygenated hemoglobin over the range of 100% to about 75%. Most clinicians regard the output of pulse oximeters to be inaccurate for percentage saturation values of less than 70%, although the probability of a low saturation should not be discounted (Fig. 103-1). Pulse oximetry measurements may help identify significant drops in $Pa{O_2}$ below 60 to 65 mm Hg but are relatively insensitive to changes in $Pa{O_2}$ from 90 to 65 mm Hg. The true value of pulse oximetry for decision-making in the emergency department setting remains uncertain. A1

TABLE 103-1 PHYSIOLOGIC MECHANISMS OF HYPOXEMIA AND ACCOMPANYING VALUES OF THE ALVEOLAR-ARTERIAL OXYGEN GRADIENT ON BREATHING OF ROOM AIR

MECHANISM/ PHYSIOLOGIC PROCESS	EXAMPLE	ALVEOLAR-ARTERIAL OXYGEN GRADIENT ON ROOM AIR
Ventilation-perfusion mismatch	Pneumonia	Increased
Diffusion impairment	Interstitial lung disease	Increased
Anatomic right-to-left shunt	Pulmonary arteriovenous malformation	Increased
Hypoventilation	Neuromuscular weakness	Normal
Breathing decreased ambient oxygen (from either hypobaric conditions [e.g., altitude] or breathing a gas mixture with decreased inspired oxygen fraction)	Altitude exposure	Normal
Diffusion-perfusion impairment	Hepatopulmonary syndrome	Increased

CARBON DIOXIDE MONITORING: CAPNOMETRY AND TRANSCUTANEOUS CARBON DIOXIDE MEASUREMENT

The fraction of carbon dioxide in exhaled air can be measured in real time by infrared capnometry.[2] Partial pressures can then be calculated on the basis of knowledge of atmospheric pressure. The expiratory capnogram (Fig. 103-1) represents a continuous plot of exhaled $P{CO_2}$ versus time or exhaled volume and reflects the sequential appearance of gas from various compartments (e.g., the endotracheal tube, central airways, and finally the alveoli, where the $P{CO_2}$ is in equilibrium with end-capillary blood). The shape of the capnogram provides clues to the presence of chronic obstructive pulmonary disease, in that emptying of areas of lung with increased dead space (see later) can cause the capnogram to have a rising contour (Fig. 103-1A), whereas the attainment of a so-called alveolar plateau on the normal capnogram (Fig. 103-1B) indicates that alveolar gas is composed of a mix with a relatively small contribution from areas of increased dead space. The value of $PE{CO_2}$ measured at the end of expiration on the capnometer (i.e., the highest value recorded) represents the end-tidal $PET{CO_2}$. Notably, the value of $PET{CO_2}$ is always below the $Pa{CO_2}$ because there is a normal component of dead space ventilation (VD/VT) related to the anatomic dead space of the conducting airways (i.e., the trachea and airways to the level of gas-exchanging alveolar ducts and alveoli). The numerical difference between the $Pa{CO_2}$ and the mixed exhaled carbon dioxide tension ($PE{CO_2}$, defined as the partial pressure of carbon dioxide that would be measured in a balloon in which the entire exhaled volume is gathered) is related to the magnitude of dead space ventilation (i.e., areas of the lung that are ventilated without accompanying blood flow, normally ~0.3 to 0.4) as defined by the Bohr equation:

$$V_D/V_T = (Pa{CO_2} - PE{CO_2})/Pa{CO_2} \quad (7)$$

The difference between $Pa{CO_2}$ and $PE{CO_2}$ may be as low as several millimeters of mercury, but changing conditions of ventilation-perfusion matching (e.g., with pulmonary embolism [Chapter 98], atelectasis [Chapter 90]) may change the gradient over time. Measurement of the $PET{CO_2}$ can be clinically useful to assess trends, to help detect esophageal intubation, to detect disconnection from the ventilator, and to detect perfusion during cardiopulmonary resuscitation, but it is not a reliable surrogate for $Pa{CO_2}$. Furthermore, measurement of the dead space fraction has prognostic value in patients with early acute respiratory distress syndrome (Chapter 104), in whom rising dead space is linearly related to increased mortality risk.

Measurement of transcutaneous $P{CO_2}$ by heated probes applied to the skin represents an alternative noninvasive method for estimating $P{CO_2}$. This

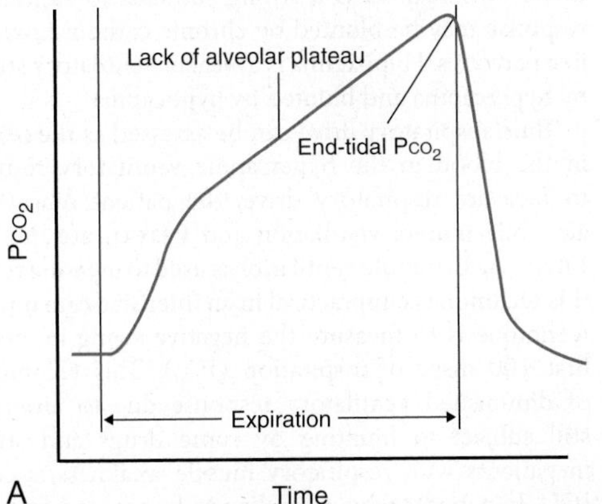

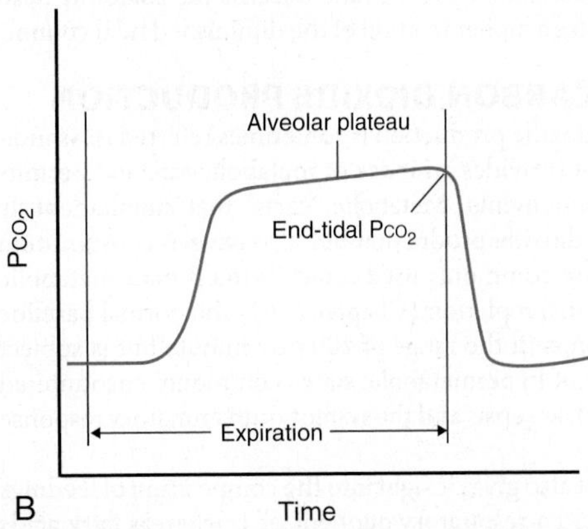

FIGURE 103-1. Abnormal and normal end-tidal capnograms. A, Illustration of a capnogram from a patient with chronic obstructive pulmonary disease in which the end-tidal $P{CO_2}$ rises throughout expiration as carbon dioxide excretion varies from different parts of the lung. B, Illustration of a normal capnogram in which the end-tidal $P{CO_2}$ reaches a plateau with more uniform carbon dioxide excretion. The end-tidal $P{CO_2}$ is the highest point of the alveolar plateau.

approach is less widely used clinically, at least in adults, because of technical requirements, such as site rotation for the probes and repetitive calibration, and its generally lower accuracy in estimating PCO_2.

ARTERIAL OXYGEN CONTENT AND SYSTEMIC OXYGEN DELIVERY

Arterial (CaO_2) and venous oxygen content (CvO_2) are used to calculate cardiac output by the Fick equation (Equation 8), which is an alternative to determining cardiac output by the thermodilution method with a flow-directed pulmonary artery (Swan-Ganz) catheter (Chapter 57). The Fick equation is

$$\text{Oxygen consumption}\,(\text{mL } O_2/\text{min}) = \text{cardiac output} \times (CaO_2 - CvO_2) \quad (8)$$

where oxygen content has the units of milliliters of oxygen per 100 mL of blood and is calculated as

$$\text{Oxygen content} = 1.34\,(\text{hemoglobin})\,(\%\ \text{saturation}) + 0.0031(PaO_2) \quad (9)$$

Under normal conditions (with, for example, an arterial percentage saturation of 95% and a hemoglobin level of 15 g/100 mL and an oxygen consumption of 250 mL/minute), arterial oxygen content is about 20 mL/100 mL, and because mixed venous oxygen saturation is about 75%, central venous oxygen content is about 15 mL/100 mL, making the normal arteriovenous oxygen content difference with a normal cardiac output about 5 mL/100 mL.

Systemic oxygen transport defines the amount of oxygen delivered to the tissues and multiplies the arterial oxygen content by the cardiac output:

$$\text{Systemic oxygen transport}\,(\text{mL/min}) = \text{cardiac output} \times CaO_2 \quad (10)$$

where the normal value is about 1000 mL/minute.

MEASURING VENTILATION: MINUTE VENTILATION AND ALVEOLAR VENTILATION

Minute ventilation (V_E), which is the amount of gas exhaled from the airway per minute, is the product of the respiratory rate times the exhaled tidal volume, measured at body temperature and standardized to barometric pressure at sea level, saturated with water vapor (BTPS). The BTPS is a standard condition under which many measurements for most pulmonary function equipment and mechanical ventilators are made. These devices use an airflow meter to measure exhaled airflow and integrate the signal to derive tidal volume. An alternative way to measure tidal volume in an intensive care setting is respiratory impedance plethysmography, which uses calibrated magnetic coils in belts strapped around the chest and abdomen to monitor respiratory frequency and changes in thoracic volume.

Alveolar ventilation is the rate of gas delivery in liters per minute to gas-exchanging areas of the lung (i.e., the alveoli and alveolar ducts). The portion of minute ventilation that fails to undergo gas exchange is dead space ventilation (V_D) and is determined by Equation 7. Minute, alveolar (V_A), and dead space ventilation are related as follows:

$$V_E = V_A + V_D \quad (11)$$

It follows that conditions such as acute lung injury and acute respiratory distress syndrome (ARDS; Chapter 104) that are associated with very high dead space ratios require high V_E to achieve a sufficient V_A. Conversely, conditions that cause neuromuscular weakness (Chapter 421) are associated with small tidal volumes and have a high V_D/V_T ratio because the anatomic dead space is fixed and constitutes a higher fraction of the diminished tidal volume.

MEASURING CARBON DIOXIDE PRODUCTION

Measurement of carbon dioxide production is sometimes referred to as indirect calorimetry because it provides an index of metabolic rate and permits estimation of calorie requirements. Metabolic "carts" that simultaneously measure not only carbon dioxide production but also oxygen consumption and respiratory quotient are commonly used clinically to estimate metabolic needs to prescribe nutritional repletion (Chapter 216). The normal baseline carbon dioxide production is in the range of 200 mL/minute but is subject to wide variation because of hypermetabolic states commonly encountered in critically ill patients, such as sepsis and the systemic inflammatory response syndrome.

The respiratory quotient also gives insight into the composition of feedings because carbohydrates yield a respiratory quotient of 1, whereas fatty acids yield a ratio of 0.8 and amino acids a ratio of 0.7. Thus, balanced nutrition should yield a respiratory quotient of approximately 0.85. A respiratory quotient of 1 in combination with a high carbon dioxide production suggests that the dietary proportion of carbohydrates is excessive.

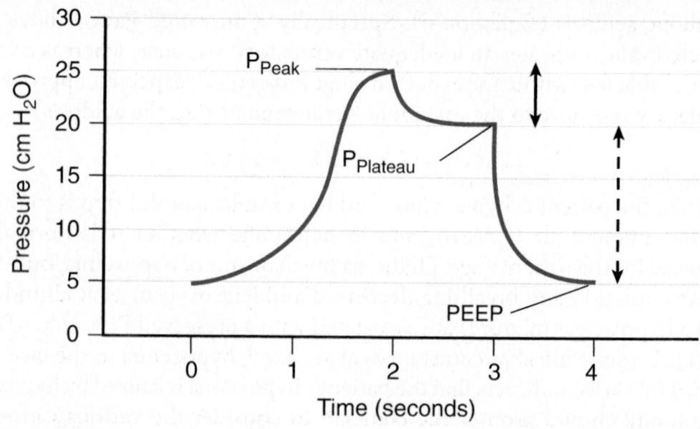

FIGURE 103-2. Illustration of inspiratory hold maneuver to determine plateau pressure ($P_{plateau}$). Airway pressure during volume-targeted mechanical ventilation rises as the tidal volume is delivered and reaches a peak. An inspiratory hold is initiated at peak pressure that prevents exhalation, so pressure falls to a "plateau" of about 20 cm H_2O. The drop in pressure reflects the pressure needed to overcome airway resistance. After slightly more than 1 second, the inspiratory hold is released, and airway pressure falls to positive end-expiratory pressure (PEEP). The difference between $P_{plateau}$ and PEEP is used to calculate static compliance by dividing the difference into the tidal volume.

MEASURING RESPIRATORY COMPLIANCE

Respiratory compliance is the change in respiratory system volume induced by a change in applied pressure (i.e., inspiratory pressure) and is the mathematical inverse of elastance. Compliance diminishes in conditions like lung injury and ARDS (Chapter 104) or pulmonary fibrosis (Chapter 92), in which diffuse inflammation and scarring alter lung structure and contribute to increased lung "stiffness." Static respiratory compliance is measured in patients receiving volume-limited mechanical ventilation by imposing a brief inspiratory hold at end inspiration. Assuming the patient has no spontaneous breathing effort, the airway pressure measured when airflow ceases is referred to as the plateau pressure ($P_{plateau}$). The difference between this pressure and the positive end-expiratory pressure (PEEP) is taken as the driving pressure required to deliver the tidal volume (Fig. 103-2). Static respiratory system compliance (C_{RS}) is then calculated as

$$C_{RS} = \Delta V(\text{exhaled tidal volume})/\Delta P\,(P_{plateau} - \text{PEEP}) \quad (12)$$

This compliance not only reflects the status of the lung but also includes contributions of the chest wall and abdomen. Thus, patients with chest wall deformities or morbid obesity have lower values of respiratory compliance even in the absence of lung abnormalities (Chapter 99). The normal respiratory compliance is in the range of 50 to 70 mL/cm H_2O, and patients with ARDS usually have values of C_{RS} of less than 30 cm H_2O. If respiratory compliance is below 20 to 25 cm H_2O, weaning from mechanical ventilation (Chapter 105) is difficult or impossible because of the high work of breathing requirements (see later).

MEASURING RESPIRATORY DRIVE

The respiratory center, located in the pons and medulla, regulates respiratory drive. Hypercapnia is a strong stimulus to ventilation (Chapter 86). This response may be blunted by chronic carbon dioxide retention or by drugs like narcotics. Hypoxemia is a weaker ventilatory stimulus that is potentiated by hypercapnia and blunted by hypocapnia.

Thus, respiratory drive can be assessed as the response to carbon dioxide in the blood in the hypercapnic ventilatory response. In one technique to measure respiratory drive, the patient rebreathes his or her exhaled air while minute ventilation and $PETCO_2$ are monitored; a graph relating $PETCO_2$ with minute ventilation is used to measure respiratory drive. However, this technique is impractical in an intensive care unit (ICU) setting. Another technique is to measure the negative swing in airway pressure during the first 100 msec of inspiration (P_{100}). This technique avoids the problem of diminished ventilatory response due to airway obstruction, but it is still subject to blunting by some drugs and still underestimates drive in patients with respiratory muscle weakness, a common problem in the ICU. In patients who are failing to be weaned from mechanical ventilation, a practical way to assess the integrity of respiratory drive is to determine whether the respiratory rate increases, usually into the range of 30 to 40 breaths/minute, as $PaCO_2$ rises after the patient is removed from ventilatory support.

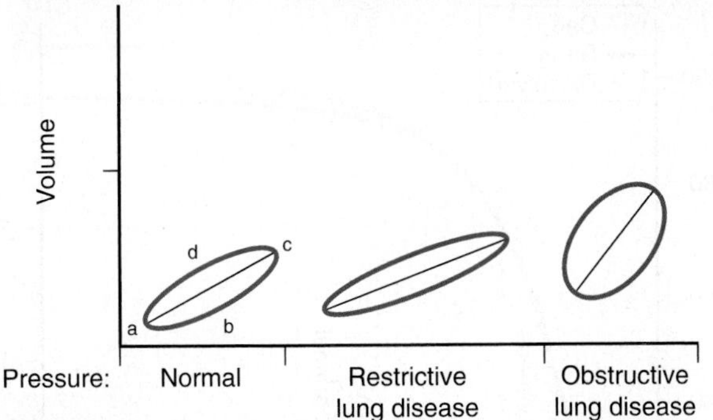

FIGURE 103-3. Pressure-volume curves illustrating components of work in a normal subject and in patients with restrictive or obstructive disease. The line between *a* and *c* represents elastic work as the lung expands, but this work is a net zero because static forces return the lung to its neutral position. The restrictive curve is flatter than normal because the lung is stiffer and volume changes less for a given unit change in pressure. The obstructive curve has a greater slope because (e.g., in emphysema) the lung is more compliant and starts inhalation from a higher volume. The *abc* curve represents resistive work during inspiration, and *cda* represents resistive work during exhalation. Resistive work during exhalation is greater in patients with obstructive lung disease.

MEASURING RESPIRATORY MUSCLE STRENGTH

Respiratory muscle weakness has long been recognized as a contributor to respiratory failure and failure to be weaned from mechanical ventilation in the ICU (Chapter 105). This recognition has intensified in recent years with the increased awareness of ICU-acquired weakness after critical illness. However, measurement of respiratory muscle strength remains challenging because of the need to differentiate between actual weakness and reduced muscle performance due to inability to cooperate or to exert a full inspiratory effort.

The most commonly used measures of respiratory muscle strength are the maximal inspiratory and expiratory pressures (PImax or MIP and PEmax or MEP). These values are obtained by measuring the pressure change with a manometer when the patient inhales with maximal force from residual volume and exhales with maximal force from total lung capacity. Normal MIP is usually more negative than −75 cm H_2O, and normal MEP is usually more positive than 125 cm H_2O. When the value for MIP is less negative than −20 or −30 cm H_2O, weaning from mechanical ventilation may be difficult, and values less positive than 60 cm H_2O suggest cough insufficiency.[3] However, these values have poor predictive value in mechanically ventilated patients because many of these patients are unable to cooperate. This problem may be addressed by attaching a one-way valve to the end of an endotracheal tube that permits exhalation but not inhalation and then measuring the inspiratory pressure efforts for 20 to 25 seconds.

MEASURING WORK OF BREATHING

Work of breathing is the product of pressure and volume for each breath (Fig. 103-3). The components include work needed to overcome elastic recoil of the lung and to displace the chest wall and abdomen as well as work needed to overcome airway resistance and lung viscosity and work needed to overcome inertia. With restrictive lung diseases, the inspiratory work of breathing is increased because of the decreased lung elasticity. With obstructive diseases, the work of breathing is increased because of increased airway resistance.

In clinical settings, a more practical way to assess the inspiratory work of breathing is to calculate the pressure-time product (in cm H_2O-seconds). The pressure-time product can be calculated by the decrease in airway pressure during inspiration, esophageal pressure (measured with an esophageal balloon manometer), or transdiaphragmatic pressure (measured with esophageal and gastric balloon manometers) as an index of diaphragmatic work. The work can be calculated as work of breathing per breath or as work of breathing per minute by multiplying the work per breath by the respiratory frequency. Commercially available devices using esophageal manometry automatically calculate the inspiratory work of breathing, which may be of some value in assessing the likelihood of weaning from mechanical ventilation. If the drop in inspiratory pressure necessary to achieve an adequate tidal volume is too large, the calculated work of breathing will be high, and the likelihood of successful weaning will be reduced.

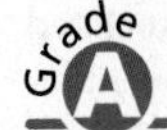

Grade A Reference

A1. Schuh S, Freedman S, Coates A, et al. Effect of oximetry on hospitalization in bronchiolitis: a randomized clinical trial. *JAMA*. 2014;312:712-718.

GENERAL REFERENCES

For the General References and other additional features, please visit Expert Consult at https://expertconsult.inkling.com.

104

ACUTE RESPIRATORY FAILURE

MICHAEL A. MATTHAY AND ARTHUR S. SLUTSKY

DEFINITION

Acute respiratory failure occurs when dysfunction of the respiratory system results in abnormal gas exchange that is potentially life-threatening. Each element of this definition is important to understand. The term *acute* implies a relatively sudden onset (from hours to days) and a substantial change from the patient's baseline condition. *Dysfunction* indicates that the abnormal gas exchange may be caused by abnormalities in any element of the respiratory system (e.g., a central nervous system abnormality affecting the regulation of breathing or a musculoskeletal thoracic abnormality affecting ventilation [Chapter 83]) in addition to abnormalities of the lung itself. The term *respiration* refers, in a broad sense, to the delivery of oxygen (O_2) to metabolically active tissues for energy use and the removal of carbon dioxide (CO_2) from these tissues (Table 104-1). Respiratory failure is a failure of the process of delivery of O_2 to the tissues or removal of CO_2 from the tissues. Abnormalities in the periphery (e.g., cyanide poisoning, circulatory shock, pathologic distribution of organ blood flow in sepsis) can lead to tissue hypoxia; although these conditions represent forms of respiratory failure in the broadest terms, this chapter focuses on respiratory failure resulting from dysfunction of the lungs, chest wall, and control of respiration.

PATHOBIOLOGY

Abnormal gas exchange is the physiologic hallmark of acute respiratory failure, which can be classified in several ways (Table 104-2). Although gas exchange can be abnormal for either oxygenation or CO_2 removal, significant hypoxemia is nearly always present when patients with acute respiratory failure breathe ambient air. If CO_2 is retained at a potentially life-threatening level under these conditions, it must be accompanied by significant hypoxemia (see later). The *life-threatening* aspect of the condition places the degree of abnormal gas exchange in a clinical context and calls for urgent treatment.

The diagnosis of acute respiratory failure requires a significant change in arterial blood gases from baseline. Many patients with chronic respiratory problems can function with blood gas tensions that would be alarming in a physiologically normal individual. Over time, patients with so-called chronic respiratory failure or chronic respiratory insufficiency develop mechanisms to compensate for inadequate gas exchange. Conversely, this chronic condition makes patients vulnerable to insults that could be easily tolerated by a previously healthy individual.

In acute respiratory failure, the O_2 content in the blood (available for tissue use) is reduced to a level at which the possibility of end-organ dysfunction increases markedly. The value of the partial pressure of O_2 in the arterial blood (PaO_2) that demarcates this vulnerable zone is often considered to be the point of the oxyhemoglobin dissociation relationship at which any further decrease in the PaO_2 results in sharp decreases in the amount of hemoglobin saturated with O_2 (SaO_2) and in the arterial blood O_2 content (CaO_2). Thus, acute respiratory failure is often defined in practice as occurring when the PaO_2 is less than about 55 mm Hg (Fig. 104-1). The oxyhemoglobin dissociation curve of venous blood, which is the partial pressure at which O_2 is being unloaded to the tissues, is a critical determinant of how much O_2 is available for the cells and their mitochondria. Other than under conditions of an extremely hypoxic environment (e.g., in utero or on the summit of Mt. Everest), the enhanced ability to unload O_2 at the tissue level more than compensates for small decreases in the amount of O_2 picked up in the lungs when the oxyhemoglobin dissociation curve is shifted rightward. With a leftward shift in the curve, O_2 is bound more tightly to hemoglobin, so less O_2 is available for tissue delivery.

These clinical considerations imply that any definition of acute respiratory failure based on an absolute level of PaO_2 is arbitrary. A healthy, young, conditioned individual climbing at high altitude may have a PaO_2 of less than

TABLE 104-1 ABBREVIATIONS COMMONLY USED IN ACUTE RESPIRATORY FUNCTION

ABG	Arterial blood gas or arterial blood gas analysis
ALI	Acute lung injury
ARDS	Acute respiratory distress syndrome
ARF	Acute respiratory failure
cm H_2O	Centimeters of water
Cao_2	Content of oxygen in arterial blood
Cco_2	Content of oxygen in end-capillary blood
CO_2	Carbon dioxide
COPD	Chronic obstructive pulmonary disease
CPAP	Continuous positive airway pressure (used when positive pressure during exhalation is applied with spontaneous ventilation)
Cvo_2	Content of oxygen in mixed venous blood
F_{IO_2}	Fraction of inspired oxygen
g/dL	Grams per deciliter
HbO_2	Saturation of hemoglobin by oxygen
L/min	Liters per minute
mL/kg	Milliliters per kilogram
mL/min	Milliliters per minute
mm Hg	Millimeters of mercury
NIPPV	Noninvasive positive-pressure ventilation
O_2	Oxygen
$P(A\text{-}a)o_2$	Difference of partial pressure of oxygen between mean alveolar gas and arterial blood (alveolar-to-arterial oxygen difference)
P_{ACO_2}	Partial pressure of carbon dioxide in alveolar gas
$Paco_2$	Partial pressure of carbon dioxide in arterial blood
P_{AO_2}	Partial pressure of oxygen in alveolar gas
Pao_2	Partial pressure of oxygen in arterial blood
Pao_2/F_{IO_2}	Ratio of partial pressure of oxygen in arterial blood to fraction of inspired oxygen
PBW	Predicted body weight
P_{cCO_2}	Partial pressure of carbon dioxide in end-capillary blood
P_{CO_2}	Partial pressure of carbon dioxide
P_{cO_2}	Partial pressure of oxygen in end-capillary blood
PEEP	Positive end-expiratory pressure (used when positive pressure during exhalation is applied with mechanical ventilation)
P/F	Pao_2/F_{IO_2} ratio
P_{IO_2}	Partial pressure of oxygen in inspired gas
Po_2	Partial pressure of oxygen
$P\bar{v}co_2$	Partial pressure of carbon dioxide in mixed venous blood
$P\bar{v}o_2$	Partial pressure of oxygen in mixed venous blood
$\dot{Q}$	Blood flow or perfusion
RR	Respiratory rate
Sao_2	Percentage of saturation of hemoglobin by oxygen in arterial blood
$\dot{V}$	Ventilation
$\dot{V}/\dot{Q}$	Ventilation-perfusion ratio
V_T	Tidal volume

50 mm Hg because of the reduction in inspired O_2 pressure.[1] This individual is not in acute respiratory failure, even though the Pao_2 may be in the low 40s. A patient who has chronic obstructive pulmonary disease (COPD) and whose usual range of Pao_2 is 50 to 55 mm Hg would not be considered to be in acute respiratory failure if the Pao_2 was 50 mm Hg. However, if a patient's usual Pao_2 is 80 mm Hg, a sudden drop to a Pao_2 of 50 mm Hg could be associated with a substantial risk for a further life-threatening reduction in oxygenation; this patient should be considered to have acute respiratory failure.

Traditionally, the level of arterial CO_2 partial pressure ($Paco_2$) that defines acute respiratory failure has been 50 mm Hg or greater, if it is accompanied by arterial acidosis with a pH of less than about 7.30. The $Paco_2$ is linked to pH in this definition because of the general belief that acidosis is what leads to tissue dysfunction and symptoms. Patients with severe COPD may have chronic CO_2 retention, but renal compensation for the respiratory acidosis protects them against abnormalities related to the elevation in CO_2. A further acute rise in $Paco_2$ can precipitate symptoms and other organ dysfunction; however, even severe respiratory acidosis (pH 7.1) seems to be better tolerated than metabolic acidosis of the same pH in most previously healthy individuals if arterial and tissue oxygenation is adequate.

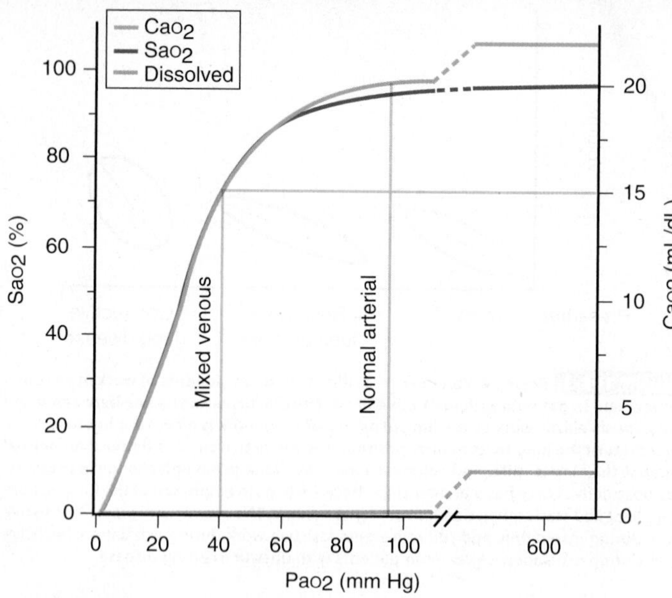

FIGURE 104-1. Oxyhemoglobin association-dissociation curve. The axis for oxygen saturation in the arterial blood (Sao_2) is on the left, and the axis for arterial content of oxygen (Cao_2) is on the right. Cao_2 is the sum of the oxygen dissolved in plasma (denoted as "Dissolved" in the figure) plus the oxygen bound to hemoglobin. With a normal hemoglobin, most of the oxygen is carried in combination with hemoglobin, with only a relatively small amount of oxygen dissolved in plasma. When the value of the arterial partial pressure of oxygen (Pao_2) is on the "flat" portion of the curve ($Pao_2 \geq 60$ to 65 mm Hg, normal partial pressure of arterial carbon dioxide [$Paco_2$], and normal pH), raising the Pao_2 further has relatively little effect on total oxygen content. Increases in temperature, P_{CO_2}, hydrogen ion concentration, or 2,3-diphosphoglycerate cause a rightward shift in the oxyhemoglobin association-dissociation curve.

Pathophysiology

Five mechanisms can lead to a reduction in Pao_2: (1) decreased inspired partial pressure of O_2 (P_{IO_2}) (e.g., at high altitude or when breathing a reduced percentage O_2 mixture); (2) hypoventilation; (3) ventilation-perfusion ($\dot{V}/\dot{Q}$) mismatch; (4) shunting of blood from the pulmonary to systemic circulation, bypassing the alveoli anatomically or functionally; and (5) any barrier for diffusion of O_2 from the alveoli into the capillary blood. In essence, a shunt is an extreme $\dot{V}/\dot{Q}$ mismatch in which blood perfuses alveoli with *no* ventilation; it is differentiated clinically from other $\dot{V}/\dot{Q}$ mismatching by the response to breathing of supplemental O_2 (see later).

For clinical purposes, diffusion abnormalities are not usually important causes of hypoxemia at sea level because there is sufficient time for adequate diffusion of O_2 during the transit of a red blood cell through the pulmonary capillary bed, even in the presence of severe lung disease. When diffusion abnormalities are present and contribute to hypoxemia, $\dot{V}/\dot{Q}$ mismatch nearly always coexists with the shunting, and this mismatch is an important cause of hypoxemia. Except at high altitude or when a subject is breathing a gas mixture low in O_2, hypoventilation, $\dot{V}/\dot{Q}$ mismatch, and shunting are the dominant causes of hypoxemia.

If only hypoventilation is present, the resulting hypoxemia is associated with a normal difference between the calculated alveolar and the measured arterial oxygenation levels [$P(A\text{-}a)o_2$]. In this setting, an elevated $Paco_2$ suggests disease processes that affect nonpulmonary respiratory function (e.g., central respiratory depression resulting from drug overdose, neuromuscular diseases such as Guillain-Barré syndrome, or chest wall disease such as flail chest; Chapter 86). In contrast, $\dot{V}/\dot{Q}$ mismatch and shunting are associated with an elevated $P(A\text{-}a)o_2$, which may or may not coexist with hypoventilation. The normal value for $P(A\text{-}a)o_2$ varies as a function of the fraction of inspired O_2 (F_{IO_2}), increasing as F_{IO_2} increases.

TABLE 104-2 SYSTEMS TO CLASSIFY ACUTE RESPIRATORY FAILURE

HYPOXIC VERSUS HYPERCAPNIC-HYPOXEMIC	ACUTE RESPIRATORY FAILURE WITH AND WITHOUT CHRONIC LUNG DISEASE
Causes of Hypoxemic Acute Respiratory Failure	**With Chronic Lung Disease**
Acute lung injury/ARDS	COPD
Pneumonia	Asthma
Pulmonary thromboembolism	Parenchymal lung diseases
Acute lobar atelectasis	Restrictive lung/chest wall diseases
Cardiogenic pulmonary edema	**Without Chronic Lung Disease**[‡]
Lung contusion	Acute lung injury/ARDS
Acute collagen vascular disease (Goodpasture syndrome, systemic lupus erythematosus)	Pneumonia
Causes of Hypercapnic-Hypoxemic Acute Respiratory Failure	Pulmonary thromboembolism
Pulmonary disease	**ACUTE RESPIRATORY FAILURE BY ORGAN SYSTEM INVOLVED**
COPD	**Respiratory (Lungs and Thorax)**
Asthma: advanced, acute, severe asthma	Airway/airflow obstruction
Drugs causing respiratory depression	COPD
Neuromuscular	Asthma
Guillain-Barré syndrome	Pulmonary parenchyma
Acute myasthenia gravis	Pneumonia
Spinal cord tumors	ARDS
Metabolic derangements causing weakness (including hypophosphatemia, hypomagnesemia)	Acute flare of chronic collagen vascular disease (e.g., Goodpasture syndrome, systemic lupus erythematosus)
Musculoskeletal	**Central Nervous System**
Kyphoscoliosis	Respiratory depression
Ankylosing spondylitis	Increased sedatives, tranquilizers with respiratory effect; opiates; alcohol
Obesity hypoventilation syndrome (often with additional acute, superimposed abnormality as cause of acute respiratory failure)	Brain stem and spinal cord involvement
ETIOLOGIC MECHANISMS OF HYPOXEMIA	Tumors, trauma, vascular accidents
Normal $P(A\text{-}a)O_2$*	**Neuromuscular**
$\downarrow P_{IO_2}$	Guillain-Barré syndrome
High altitude; inadvertent administration of low F_{IO_2} gas mixture	Myasthenia gravis
Hypoventilation	**Cardiovascular**
See causes of hypercapnic-hypoxic acute respiratory failure above	Cardiogenic pulmonary edema
Increased $P(A\text{-}a)O_2$*	Pulmonary thromboembolism
Ventilation-perfusion ($\dot{V}/\dot{Q}$) mismatch	**Renal/Endocrine**
Airway disease	Volume overload
Vascular disease, including pulmonary thromboembolism	Metabolic abnormalities
Shunt	
Acute lung injury/ARDS	
Pneumonia	
Parenchymal lung disease	
Cardiogenic pulmonary edema	
Pulmonary infarction	
Diffusion limitation[†]	

*Calculated by the alveolar-air equation; see text for description.
[†]See text for discussion.
[‡]These can also be superimposed on chronic disease.
ARDS = acute respiratory distress syndrome; COPD = chronic obstructive pulmonary disease; F_{IO_2} = fraction of inspired oxygen; $P(A\text{-}a)O_2$ = alveolar-to-arterial oxygen difference; P_{IO_2} = partial pressure of inspired oxygen; $\dot{V}/\dot{Q}$ = ventilation-perfusion ratio.

When $\dot{V}/\dot{Q}$ mismatch or shunting is the cause of hypoxemia, some alveolar regions have increased levels of P_{CO_2} and associated reduced levels of P_{O_2}; the blood in the vessels perfusing these alveoli reflects these abnormal gas tensions. The resulting increased arterial P_{CO_2} (Pa_{CO_2}) usually can be reversed by increasing overall ventilation, but this increased ventilation usually does not correct the decreased arterial P_{O_2} (Pa_{O_2}).

$\dot{V}/\dot{Q}$ mismatch is distinguished from shunting by assessing the Pa_{O_2} response to enhanced O_2 administration. Hypoxemia caused by $\dot{V}/\dot{Q}$ mismatch can be corrected to a nearly complete O_2 saturation of the hemoglobin in most patients by a relatively small increase in F_{IO_2}, such as from 0.24 to 0.28 by face mask or 1 to 2 L/minute O_2 by nasal prongs, in patients with acute exacerbations of COPD. If the airways to poorly ventilated alveoli remain open and the enriched O_2 mixture is administered for an adequate length of time (ranging from a few minutes to about 20 minutes, depending on the degree of $\dot{V}/\dot{Q}$ inequality), the increased P_{IO_2} is reflected by an increased P_{AO_2} and an increased Pa_{O_2}. When a shunt is present (no ventilation but continued perfusion), a relatively small increase in the F_{IO_2} has little or no effect on the Pa_{O_2}, and even large increases in F_{IO_2} up to 1.0 result in only modest increases in Pa_{O_2} (Fig. 104-2).

CLINICAL MANIFESTATIONS

The hallmark of acute respiratory failure is the inability to maintain adequate oxygenation or the inability to maintain an appropriate Pa_{CO_2}. Patients are typically dyspneic and tachypneic, unless progressive respiratory failure causes fatigue—sometimes leading to respiratory arrest—or a drug overdose or neuromuscular condition prevents an appropriate respiratory response to hypoxemia or hypercapnic acidosis. Neurologic function may deteriorate, and myocardial ischemia or even infarction may be precipitated by hypoxemia. In addition, each cause has its own specific manifestations (see later).

DIAGNOSIS

As part of the diagnosis of acute respiratory failure, the physician has three objectives: (1) to confirm the clinical suspicion that acute respiratory failure is present, (2) to classify the type of acute respiratory failure (e.g., hypoxemia caused by hypoventilation vs. hypoxemia caused by $\dot{V}/\dot{Q}$ mismatch or shunting), and (3) to determine the specific cause (e.g., the acute respiratory distress syndrome [ARDS]) secondary to pulmonary or nonpulmonary sepsis or decompensated COPD because of acute bronchitis. Defining the type of acute respiratory failure and determining the specific cause are prerequisites to optimal management.

The initial approach to diagnosis consists of considering information from four sources: (1) clinical history and physical examination; (2) physiologic abnormalities, particularly arterial blood gas derangements, which help establish the mechanisms of hypoxemia; (3) chest radiographic findings; and (4) other tests aimed at elucidating specific causes. In many cases, the clinical picture from the history is so clear that the presumptive type of acute respiratory failure (and sometimes the cause) is obvious, so treatment can be started

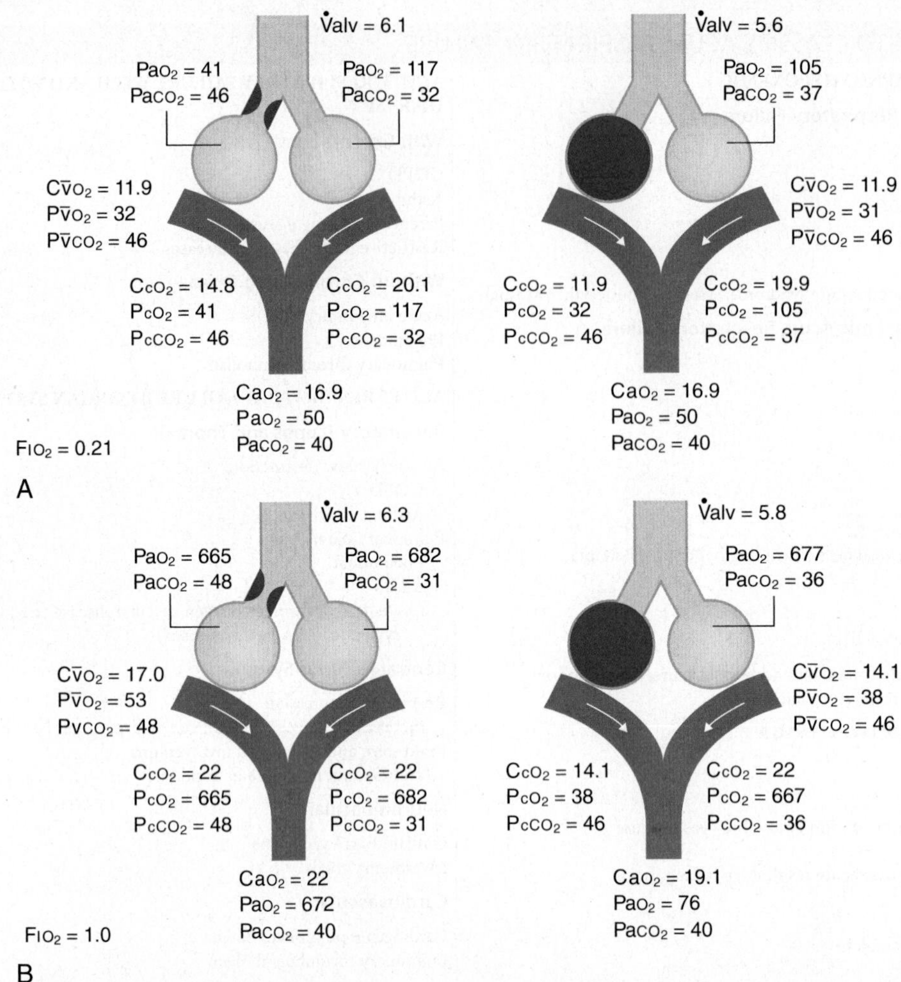

FIGURE 104-2. Arterial oxygenation. Comparison of the effect on arterial oxygenation of increasing the fraction of inspired oxygen (FIO_2) from breathing of ambient air (FIO_2 = 0.21) (A) and breathing of 100% oxygen (FIO_2 = 1.0) (B) with a low ventilation-perfusion ratio ($\dot{V}/\dot{Q}$) (*left*) and a shunt (*right*), using a two-compartment lung model. Shunting and decreased $\dot{V}/\dot{Q}$ can lead to identical arterial blood gases (partial pressure of oxygen in arterial blood [PaO_2] = 50 mm Hg; partial pressure of carbon dioxide in arterial blood [$PaCO_2$] = 40 mm Hg). The response to supplemental oxygen administration is markedly different. Hypoxemia is only partially corrected by breathing of 100% oxygen when a shunt is present because arterial oxygenation represents an average of the end-capillary oxygen content (CcO_2) from various parts of the lung, not an average of the partial pressures of oxygen (partial pressure of carbon dioxide in the end-capillary blood [$PcCO_2$]). When the CcO_2 values are mixed, the PaO_2 is determined from the resultant content of oxygen in the arterial blood (CaO_2) by the oxyhemoglobin association-dissociation relationship (see Fig. 104-1). With low $\dot{V}/\dot{Q}$ (as is often the case in patients with chronic obstructive pulmonary disease), an increase in FIO_2 increases the alveolar partial pressure of oxygen (PO_2) of the low $\dot{V}/\dot{Q}$ unit and leads to a marked increase in arterial PO_2. The values in this figure were generated from modeling to result in the same $PaCO_2$ (40 mm Hg) for all four situations shown; this is the reason for slight changes in alveolar ventilation ($\dot{V}alv$) for some of the conditions. Several assumptions are made: no diffusion limitation is present; oxygen consumption = 300 mL/minute, and CO_2 production = 240 mL/minute; cardiac output = 6.0 L/minute; the low $\dot{V}/\dot{Q}$ regions in the left panels represent 60% of the cardiac output perfusing alveoli with a $\dot{V}/\dot{Q}$ 25% of normal; and the shunts in the right panels represent a 37% shunt (i.e., 37% of the cardiac output is perfusing alveoli with no ventilation).

while confirmatory laboratory studies are ordered. In other cases, a clinician may be asked to see a patient because of an abnormal chest radiograph or abnormal arterial blood gases ordered by someone else and may elicit the pertinent history based on these clues. When the degree of hypoxemia is life-threatening, therapeutic decisions must be made quickly, even if data are limited. The clinician must obtain updated information continually and should view most therapeutic decisions as therapeutic trials, with careful monitoring to assess desired benefits and possible detrimental effects.

Clinical Evaluation

The presentation often reflects one of three clinical scenarios: (1) the effects of hypoxemia or respiratory acidosis, (2) the effects of primary (e.g., pneumonia) or secondary (e.g., heart failure) diseases affecting the lungs, and (3) the nonpulmonary effects of the underlying disease process. The clinical effects of hypoxemia and respiratory acidosis are manifested mainly in the central nervous system (e.g., irritability, agitation, changes in personality, depressed level of consciousness, coma) and the cardiovascular system (e.g., arrhythmias, hypotension, hypertension) (Table 104-3). In patients with underlying COPD (Chapter 88) with a gradual onset of acute respiratory failure, central nervous system abnormalities may be the major presenting findings. Cyanosis, which requires at least 5 g/dL of unsaturated hemoglobin to be detectable, may not be seen before serious tissue hypoxia develops, especially in patients with underlying anemia.

TABLE 104-3 CLINICAL MANIFESTATIONS OF HYPOXEMIA AND HYPERCAPNIA

HYPOXEMIA	HYPERCAPNIA
Tachycardia	Somnolence
Tachypnea	Lethargy
Anxiety	Restlessness
Diaphoresis	Tremor
Altered mental status	Slurred speech
Confusion	Headache
Cyanosis	Asterixis
Hypertension	Papilledema
Hypotension	Coma
Bradycardia	Diaphoresis
Seizures	
Coma	
Lactic acidosis*	

*Usually requires additional reduction in oxygen delivery because of inadequate cardiac output, severe anemia, or redistribution of blood flow.

Pulmonary symptoms and signs often reflect the respiratory disease causing the acute respiratory failure. Examples include cough and sputum with pneumonia (Chapter 97) or chest pain from pulmonary thromboembolism with infarction (Chapter 98). Dyspnea and respiratory distress are nonspecific reflections of the respiratory system's difficulty in meeting the increased demands from pulmonary and nonpulmonary diseases.

Physical findings may be associated with a particular pathologic lung process, such as pneumonia (Chapter 97), which often results in bronchial breathing and crackles on auscultation, or the crackles (rales) of cardiogenic pulmonary edema (Chapter 58). Abnormal findings may be minimal or absent in patients with ARDS or pulmonary thromboembolism (Chapter 98).

In some patients, the clinical picture is dominated by the underlying disease process, particularly with diseases that cause ARDS, such as sepsis (Chapter 108), severe pneumonia (Chapter 97), aspiration of gastric contents (Chapter 94), and trauma. In these conditions, the physical examination findings are often nonspecific, with no obvious clues except, for example, fever with sepsis or pneumonia and hypotension with septic shock.

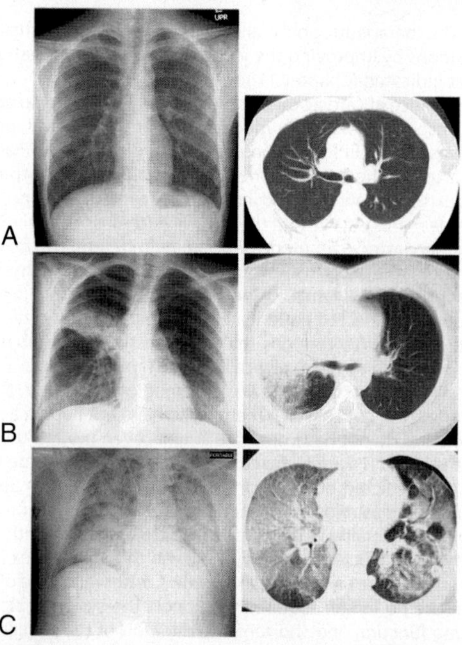

FIGURE 104-3. **Chest radiographs (*left*) and computed tomography scans (*right*) of the three most common findings in diseases causing acute respiratory failure. A, Relatively clear chest, consistent with an acute exacerbation of airway disease (e.g., asthma, chronic obstructive pulmonary disease) or a central nervous system or neuromuscular disease as the cause of acute respiratory failure. B, Localized alveolar filling opacity, most commonly seen with acute pneumonia. C, Diffuse bilateral alveolar filling opacities consistent with acute lung injury and acute respiratory distress syndrome. The computed tomography scan in C shows a small left pneumothorax and cavities or cysts that are not apparent on the anteroposterior chest radiograph.**

Assessment of Physiologic Abnormalities

The clinical suspicion of acute respiratory failure must be addressed by arterial blood gas analysis to answer several questions.

Is hypoxemia present? The answer is based largely on the value of the Pao_2 or Sao_2. The degree of the hypoxemia not only confirms the diagnosis of acute respiratory failure but also helps define its severity.

Is hypoventilation present? If the $Paco_2$ is elevated, alveolar hypoventilation is present.

Does the degree of hypoventilation fully explain the hypoxemia? If the $P(A\text{-}a)o_2$ is normal, hypoventilation fully explains the presence and degree of hypoxemia. When this is the case, the most likely causes of acute respiratory failure are central nervous system abnormalities or a chest wall abnormality. If the $P(A\text{-}a)o_2$ is increased but hypoventilation does not fully explain the hypoxemia, another condition must be present; common diagnoses include COPD (Chapter 88), severe asthma (Chapter 87), pneumonia (Chapter 97), and early stages of ARDS.

If hypoxemia exists without hypoventilation, an elevated $P(A\text{-}a)o_2$ should be confirmed, and the response to breathing of an enhanced O_2 mixture would answer this question: *Is the increase in $P(A\text{-}a)O_2$ the result of a $\dot{V}/\dot{Q}$ abnormality or of shunting?* If hypoxemia is primarily the result of a $\dot{V}/\dot{Q}$ abnormality, the likely cause is an airway disease, either COPD or acute severe asthma, or a vascular disease, such as pulmonary thromboembolism. If shunting is the major explanation for the hypoxemia, processes that fill the air spaces (e.g., cardiogenic pulmonary edema, noncardiogenic pulmonary edema or ARDS, or purulent pulmonary secretions in acute pneumonia) or, less commonly, an intracardiac or anatomic intrapulmonary shunt is the likely cause. Conditions that fill air spaces should be confirmed by abnormal findings on a chest radiograph; if the radiograph is normal, the possibility of intracardiac shunt (Chapter 69) or thromboembolism (Chapter 98) should be evaluated.

Chest Radiography

The chest radiograph in acute respiratory failure is likely to show one of three patterns (Fig. 104-3): (1) normal (or relatively normal), (2) localized alveolar filling opacities, or (3) diffuse alveolar filling opacities. Diffuse interstitial opacities are also possible, but diseases that cause this pattern usually have a more gradual onset and are associated with chronic respiratory failure. If the chest radiograph is normal (i.e., it is clear or relatively clear), airway diseases, such as COPD and asthma, or pulmonary vascular diseases, such as thromboembolism, are more likely. If a localized alveolar filling abnormality is present, pneumonia is the major consideration, but pulmonary embolism and infarction should also be considered. When diffuse (bilateral) alveolar filling abnormalities are present, cardiogenic pulmonary edema and ARDS (e.g., as seen after sepsis, trauma, pneumonia, or aspiration of gastric contents) are the major considerations. The combination of the chest radiograph and the arterial blood gas interpretation can be helpful. The finding of a significant shunt may suggest ARDS in a patient in whom this diagnosis was not clinically obvious; the chest radiograph should help confirm that possibility.

Other Evaluations

All patients with acute respiratory failure should have a complete blood count including a platelet count, routine blood chemistry tests, prothrombin time, and urinalysis to screen for possible underlying causes and comorbid conditions. Other blood tests should be guided by the clinical picture. Examples include a serum amylase level if pancreatitis is a possible cause of ARDS and thyroid indices if severe hypothyroidism is a possible cause of hypoventilation. Blood cultures are recommended when an infectious cause such as sepsis is suspected.

Any abnormal fluid collections, especially pleural effusion (Chapter 99), should be aspirated for diagnostic purposes. Sputum Gram stain and culture are indicated when pneumonia is suspected.

Other specific tests should be directed by the history, physical examinations, arterial blood gas levels, and chest radiograph. An abdominal computed tomography (CT) scan may be indicated to search for the source of infection in a patient with sepsis and ARDS. A chest CT scan may help define pulmonary disease if the chest radiograph is not definitive. CT arteriography of the pulmonary circulation may diagnose pulmonary thromboembolism (Chapter 98). A head CT scan may be indicated if a stroke involving the respiratory center is suspected. Routine blood chemistry studies can detect diabetic ketoacidosis or renal failure as contributing causes.

TREATMENT Rx

General Measures

The management of acute respiratory failure depends on its cause, its clinical manifestations, and the patient's underlying status. Certain goals apply to all patients: improvement of the hypoxemia to eliminate or markedly reduce the acute threat to life; improvement of the acidosis if it is considered life-threatening; maintenance of cardiac output or improvement if cardiac output is compromised; treatment of the underlying disease process; and avoidance of predictable complications.

The precise methods for improving hypoxemia depend on the cause of the acute respiratory failure. However, an increase in the inspired O_2 concentration is a cornerstone of treatment for nearly all patients, even though it may not produce a marked increase in Pao_2 in patients whose underlying pathophysiologic process involves a significant amount of lung with low ventilation-perfusion ratios or true shunting.

The level of acidosis that requires treatment other than for the underlying disease process is a matter of debate. Although normalization of the arterial pH was suggested in the past, respiratory acidosis is apparently well tolerated in many patients with severe ARDS, so a patient with a pH of 7.15 or higher may not require bicarbonate therapy. If the acidemia coexists with clinical complications, such as cardiac arrhythmias or a decreased level of consciousness, that have no other obvious cause, treatments to increase pH should be considered. The therapeutic goal is alleviation or reduction of the accompanying complications by improving the level of acidosis; normalization of the pH usually is not indicated (Chapter 118).

The maintenance of cardiac output is crucial for O_2 delivery in acute respiratory failure, especially because mechanical ventilation and positive end-expiratory pressure (PEEP) may compromise cardiac output. Placement of a pulmonary artery catheter allows measurement of cardiac output and filling pressures, but most patients who have these catheters do no better than similar patients managed without them.[A1] Nevertheless, selective use of diagnostic pulmonary artery catheterization can help determine the cause of the pulmonary edema (cardiogenic vs. noncardiogenic) and the physiologic basis for shock (sepsis, hypovolemia, or decreased cardiac output from impaired cardiac function) in selected patients in whom either is not clear.[2]

Many therapeutic interventions that improve short-term physiologic variables may worsen long-term, clinically important outcomes. For example, transfusing all patients to maintain a hemoglobin greater than 10 g/dL *increases* mortality in critically ill patients who have not had an acute myocardial infarction and do not have unstable angina, even though the O_2-carrying capacity of the blood is acutely increased. Use of a relatively large tidal volume (e.g., 12 mL/kg predicted body weight, which is equivalent to approximately 10 to 10.5 mL/kg measured body weight in patients who are somewhat overweight) *increases* mortality in patients with ARDS compared with a lower tidal volume (6 mg/kg predicted body weight), even though it raises PaO_2 more in the short term than does a lower tidal volume. Conservative use of fluids when vasopressors are no longer required to support the systemic blood pressure improves lung function and shortens the duration of mechanical ventilation and intensive care.[A2]

Improvements in oxygenation, acid-base status, and cardiac output are of no more than temporary benefit unless the underlying disease processes are diagnosed and treated properly. In patients with ARDS, sepsis may worsen injury to the lung and other organs despite optimal supportive care. Similarly, if the precipitating cause of acute respiratory failure in a patient with COPD is not identified and treated, supportive care is likely to be futile. Complications may arise from the physiologic effects of the gas exchange abnormality, from the disease processes causing the acute respiratory failure, from being critically ill and its associated incursions on homeostasis (e.g., sleep deprivation), or from iatrogenic complications of therapy.

Mechanical Therapy to Improve Oxygenation

A PaO_2 greater than 60 mm Hg is usually adequate to produce an SaO_2 in the low to middle 90s. The PaO_2 can be increased by the administration of supplemental O_2, by pharmacologic manipulations, by continuous positive airway pressure (CPAP), by mechanical ventilation with or without maneuvers such as PEEP, and by the prone position. PEEP, pharmacologic manipulations, and positioning are used primarily in patients with ARDS (see later).

The initial choice of the concentration and amount of supplemental O_2 is based on the severity of the hypoxemia, the clinical diagnosis, the likely mechanism causing the hypoxemia, and the O_2 delivery systems available. For the tracheal FIO_2 to be the same as the delivered FIO_2, the O_2 delivery system must deliver a flow that matches the patient's peak inspiratory flow rate with gas of a known FIO_2. High-flow O_2 blenders can achieve this goal by delivering gas at 80 L/minute or more to a nonintubated patient. These systems require a large flow of O_2 (from a wall unit or tank), however, and are not universally available. Other systems for nonintubated patients (including nasal prongs, simple face masks, and non-rebreather and partial rebreather masks) use a simple regulator that mixes room air with O_2 from a wall unit or tank, with resulting flows that are frequently unable to match the patient's peak inspiratory flow rate. The patient entrains more air from the environment, and the resulting tracheal FIO_2 or partial pressure of oxygen in inspired gas (PaO_2) is unknown. The amount of air entrained depends on the patient's inspiratory pattern and minute ventilation. Although the resulting FIO_2 is unknown, these systems are satisfactory if the delivery is constant and if they result in adequate arterial O_2 saturation, as monitored by arterial blood gases or oximetry. Nasal prongs can deliver a tracheal FIO_2 of approximately 0.50, and non-rebreather masks can deliver 50 to 100% O_2; in both cases, this depends on the inspiratory pattern and flow rate. If only hypoventilation or $\dot{V}/\dot{Q}$ mismatch is present, only a small increment in FIO_2 (e.g., an FIO_2 of 0.24 or 0.28 delivered by a Venturi principle face mask or by mechanical ventilation; or 1 to 2 L/minute O_2 delivered by nasal prongs) is likely to be required. By comparison, if marked shunting or many lung units with low but not zero $\dot{V}/\dot{Q}$ are the cause of hypoxemia, a considerably higher FIO_2 (e.g., >0.7) may be required, and even this high FIO_2 may not reverse the hypoxemia. A common practice when a significant shunt is suspected is to give an FIO_2 of 1.0, then adjust the FIO_2 downward as guided by the resulting PaO_2 or SaO_2.

The O_2 concentration that is toxic to the lungs in critically ill patients is not known, but prior injury may provide tolerance to O_2 toxicity, whereas other conditioning agents, such as bleomycin, may enhance oxidative injury. An FIO_2 of 0.7 or higher is generally considered injurious to the normal human lung. Because it is unknown what lower concentration is safe, however, patients should be given the lowest FIO_2 that provides an adequate SaO_2 (≥90%). If an FIO_2 equal to or greater than 0.5 to 0.7 is required for adequate oxygenation, other measures, especially PEEP or CPAP, should be considered. Even a lower FIO_2 of about 0.5 may be associated with impaired ciliary action in the airways and impaired bacterial killing by alveolar macrophages, but the clinical importance of these effects is not known.

A low concentration of supplemental O_2 can be administered by nasal prongs or nasal cannula, which most patients find comfortable and allows them to cough, speak, eat, and drink while receiving O_2. When the nasal passages are open, the PIO_2 does not depend too much on whether the patient breathes through the nose or the mouth because O_2 is entrained from the posterior nasal pharynx during a breath taken through the mouth. The level of O_2 can be adjusted by the flow rate to the nasal prongs. In patients with COPD, flows as low as 0.5 to 2 L/minute are usually adequate unless an intrapulmonary shunt is contributing to the hypoxemia, as usually occurs in acute pneumonia. At flows greater than approximately 6 L/minute, only a small further augmentation in the PIO_2 can be achieved. Because gas flow through the nose has a drying and irritating effect, a face mask should be considered at high flow rates. O_2 face masks using the Venturi principle allow the regulation of FIO_2 and can be particularly useful when COPD is suspected, and it is important to avoid the CO_2 retention that can be associated with the unregulated administration of O_2. A higher FIO_2 of 0.5 to nearly 1.0 can be administered through a non-rebreathing face mask with an O_2 reservoir. If an FIO_2 equal to or greater than 0.70 is required for more than several hours, particularly in an unstable patient, endotracheal intubation should be considered so O_2 can be administered by a closed system with reliable maintenance of the patient's SaO_2. Indications for placement of an artificial airway in a patient with acute respiratory failure are to protect the airway against aspiration of gastric contents, to deliver an increased FIO_2, to facilitate prolonged mechanical ventilation, and possibly to aid in the control of respiratory secretions (Chapter 105).

Ventilatory maneuvers that may increase arterial oxygenation include mechanical ventilation itself and the administration of PEEP or CPAP, all of which allow ventilation of areas of the lung that were previously poorly ventilated or unventilated. Although large tidal volumes with mechanical ventilation may open areas of atelectasis and may improve oxygenation initially, these higher tidal volumes can cause lung injury, particularly if the lung is already injured (Chapter 105).[2]

CPAP refers to the maintenance of positive pressure during the respiratory cycle while breathing spontaneously. PEEP refers to the maintenance of positive pressure throughout the expiratory cycle when it is applied together with mechanical ventilation (Chapter 105). CPAP and PEEP can result in recruitment of microatelectatic regions of the lung that are perfused but were not previously ventilated, thus contributing substantially to hypoxemia. CPAP and PEEP have the theoretical advantage of keeping some of these regions open during exhalation, thus preventing cyclic closure and reopening of lung units, which may result in alveolar wall stress and injury.

Supportive Measures

Every patient with acute respiratory failure is at risk for deep venous thrombosis, pulmonary thromboembolism, and gastric stress ulceration. Prophylactic anticoagulation is recommended in patients who are not at high risk for bleeding complications; sequential leg compression therapy may be preferred for high-risk patients (Chapter 81). Nutrition is important to maintain strength needed for weaning. In patients with ARDS, limited enteral feeding for up to 6 days is as good as full enteral feeding in terms of ventilator-free days, 60-day mortality, and infectious complications, and limited feedings induce less gastrointestinal intolerance.[A3]

The best means of preventing gastric stress ulceration is not known, but current evidence indicates that the use of an H_2-receptor blocker is superior to the gastric administration of sucralfate on the basis of a large randomized, controlled trial that found a higher incidence of significant bleeding in patients receiving sucralfate than in those receiving ranitidine. Evidence also indicates that proton pump inhibitors may be useful in the acute care setting (Chapter 217).

Current evidence supports maintaining the head of the bed at a 45-degree angle to reduce aspiration in critically ill patients. Attempts should be made to ensure a normal day-night sleep pattern, including minimizing activity and reducing direct lighting at night. The patient should change position frequently, including sitting in a chair and walking short distances if possible, even while receiving mechanical ventilatory support. Mobilization can enhance the removal of secretions, help maintain musculoskeletal function, reduce the risk of deep venous thrombosis, and provide psychological benefits.

SPECIFIC ACUTE RESPIRATORY FAILURE SYNDROMES

Chronic Obstructive Pulmonary Disease

EPIDEMIOLOGY AND PATHOBIOLOGY

The epidemiology and pathobiology of COPD are discussed in Chapter 88.

CLINICAL MANIFESTATIONS

When patients with COPD develop acute respiratory failure, they commonly have a history of increasing dyspnea and sputum production. Acute respiratory failure may be manifested in more cryptic ways, however, such as changes in mental status, arrhythmias, or other cardiovascular abnormalities. Acute respiratory failure must be considered whenever patients with COPD have significant nonspecific clinical changes.

DIAGNOSIS

The diagnosis can be confirmed or excluded by arterial blood gas analysis. The pH is helpful in assessing whether the hypoventilation is partly or exclusively acute. The pH declines by approximately 0.08 for each rise of 10 mm Hg in the $PaCO_2$ in acute respiratory acidosis without renal compensation. By comparison, in chronic respiratory acidosis with normal renal compensation, the pH drops only about 0.03 for each rise of 10 mm Hg in the $PaCO_2$.

TREATMENT Rx

General Care

As soon as acute respiratory failure is confirmed in a patient with COPD, attention must focus on detecting potential precipitating events (Table 104-4), including decreased ventilatory drive, commonly because of oversedation; decreased muscle strength or function, often related to electrolyte abnormalities, including hypophosphatemia and hypomagnesemia; decreased chest wall elasticity, possibly related to rib fracture, pleural effusion, ileus, or ascites; atelectasis, pneumonia, or pulmonary edema; increased airway resistance, caused by bronchospasm or increased secretions; or increased metabolic O_2 requirements, such as may occur with systemic infection. Many of these abnormalities can impair the cough mechanism, diminish the clearance of airway secretions, and precipitate acute respiratory failure.

Infection

The most common specific precipitating event is airway infection, especially acute bronchitis. The role played by viral agents, *Mycoplasma pneumoniae*, chronic contaminants of the lower airway such as *Haemophilus influenzae* and *Streptococcus pneumoniae*, and other acute pathogens is difficult to determine on a clinical or even microbiologic basis. Acute exacerbations of COPD commonly result from new infections rather than from reemergence of an infection by preexisting colonization. Antibiotics modestly shorten the duration of the exacerbation, with no significant increase in toxicity, compared with placebo; the impact of antibiotics on the subsequent emergence of resistant organisms is not known. It is standard practice to use antibiotics to treat a patient with COPD who has an exacerbation severe enough to cause acute respiratory failure and who has evidence consistent with acute tracheobronchitis (Chapters 88 and 96). Pneumonia may account for 20% of cases of acute respiratory failure in patients with COPD. Compared with the physiologically normal population, patients with COPD who have community-acquired pneumonia are more likely to have gram-negative enteric bacteria or *Legionella* infections and are more likely to have antibiotic-resistant organisms.

Other Precipitating Causes

Other common precipitating causes of acute respiratory failure include heart failure and worsening of the underlying COPD, often related to noncompliance with medications. Less common and often difficult to diagnose in this setting is pulmonary thromboembolism.

Site of Care

Many patients with COPD and acute respiratory failure can be managed on a general medical hospital unit rather than in an intensive care unit if the precipitating cause of acute respiratory failure has been diagnosed and is potentially responsive to appropriate therapy, provided blood gas abnormalities respond to O_2 therapy, the patient can cooperate with the treatment, and appropriate nursing and respiratory care is available (Chapter 88). An unstable patient who requires closer observation and monitoring should be admitted to an intensive care unit.

Mechanical Therapy

The decision to institute mechanical ventilation in patients with COPD and acute respiratory failure must be made on clinical grounds and is not dictated by any particular arterial blood gas values. In general, if the patient is alert and is able to cooperate with treatment, mechanical ventilation often is not necessary. If ventilatory support is required (Chapter 105), the decision is whether to use noninvasive positive-pressure ventilation therapy (without endotracheal intubation) or endotracheal intubation with positive-pressure ventilation. A number of studies have demonstrated that noninvasive positive-pressure ventilation is preferred for patients with COPD and can decrease mortality if it is applied in appropriate patients with no factors that are likely to lead to complications.[A4]

TABLE 104-4 KEY PRINCIPLES IN THE MANAGEMENT OF CHRONIC OBSTRUCTIVE PULMONARY DISEASE PATIENTS WITH ACUTE RESPIRATORY FAILURE

1. Monitor and treat life-threatening hypoxemia (these measures should be performed virtually simultaneously).
   a. Assess the patient clinically, and measure oxygenation by arterial blood gases and/or oximetry.
      (1) If the patient is hypoxemic, initiate supplemental oxygen therapy with nasal prongs (low flows [0.5-2. L/min] are usually sufficient) or by Venturi face mask (24 or 28% oxygen delivered).
      (2) If the patient needs ventilatory support, consider noninvasive ventilation.
      (3) Determine whether the patient needs to be intubated; this is almost always a clinical decision. Immediate action is required if the patient is comatose or severely obtunded.
   b. A reasonable goal in most patients is PaO_2 of 55-60 mm Hg or SaO_2 of 88-90%.
   c. After changes in FIO_2, check blood gases and check regularly for signs of carbon dioxide retention.
2. Start to correct life-threatening acidosis.
   a. The most effective approach is to correct the underlying cause of acute respiratory failure (e.g., bronchospasm, infection, heart failure).
   b. Consider ventilatory support, based largely on clinical considerations.
   c. With severe acidosis, the use of bicarbonate can be considered, but it is often ineffective, and there is little evidence of a clinical benefit.
3. If ventilatory support is required, consider noninvasive mechanical ventilation.
   a. The patient must have intact upper airway reflexes and be alert, cooperative, and hemodynamically stable.
   b. Careful monitoring is required; if the patient does not tolerate the mask, becomes hemodynamically unstable, or has a deteriorating mental status, consider intubation.
4. Treat airway obstruction and the underlying disease process that triggered the episode of acute respiratory failure.
   a. Treat airway obstruction with pharmacologic agents: systemic corticosteroids and bronchodilators (ipratropium and/or β-adrenergic agents).
   b. Improve secretion clearance: encourage the patient to cough, administer chest physical therapy if cough is impaired and a trial appears effective.
   c. Treat the underlying disease process (e.g., antibiotics, diuretics).
5. Prevent complications of the disease process and minimize iatrogenic complications.
   a. Pulmonary thromboembolism prophylaxis: use subcutaneous heparin if no contraindications exist.
   b. Gastrointestinal complications: administer prophylaxis for gastrointestinal bleeding.
   c. Hemodynamics: if the patient is ventilated, monitor and minimize auto-PEEP.
      (1) Treat the underlying obstruction.
      (2) Minimize minute ventilation; use controlled hypoventilation.
      (3) Use small tidal volumes; increase the inspiratory flow rate to decrease the inspiratory time and lengthen the expiratory time.
   d. Cardiac arrhythmias: maintain oxygenation and normalize electrolytes.

FIO_2 = fraction of inspired oxygen; PaO_2 = partial pressure of oxygen in arterial blood; PEEP = positive end-expiratory pressure; SaO_2 = oxygen saturation.

PROGNOSIS

Acute respiratory failure in patients with severe COPD is associated with an in-hospital mortality of 6 to 20%. The severity of the underlying disease and the severity of the acute precipitating illness are important determinants of hospital survival. Hospital mortality is higher if the respiratory failure is associated with a pH lower than 7.25 and if the patient requires invasive mechanical ventilation. However, the pH, the $PaCO_2$, and other clinical characteristics are not reliable in predicting a particular patient's chances of survival.

Acute Lung Injury/Acute Respiratory Distress Syndrome

DEFINITION

ARDS is the abrupt onset of diffuse lung injury characterized by severe hypoxemia (shunting) and generalized pulmonary infiltrates on the chest radiograph in the absence of left-sided cardiac failure.[3,4] The term *acute lung injury* has been used to include "traditional" ARDS as well as less severe forms of lung injury. Acute lung injury and its more severe manifestation, ARDS, are diagnosed by bilateral pulmonary infiltrates compatible with pulmonary edema in the absence of clinical heart failure (usually determined by the lack of elevated left atrial pressures). A recent Berlin consensus conference recommended that the term *acute lung injury* should no longer be used, with ARDS diagnosed on the basis of a PaO_2/FIO_2 of less than 300 mm Hg. With this new definition, the severity of ARDS is defined on the basis of the PaO_2 divided by the FIO_2 (PaO_2/FIO_2, also called the P/F ratio) as mild ARDS ($200 < P/F \leq 300$ mm Hg), moderate ARDS ($100 < P/F \leq 200$ mm Hg), or severe ARDS ($P/F \leq 100$ mm Hg).[5]

EPIDEMIOLOGY

ARDS is a clinical syndrome triggered by some other cause (Table 104-5), with an annual incidence of about 80 cases per 100,000 adult population. This underlying precipitating factor may affect and injure the lungs directly, such as in diffuse pneumonia or aspiration of gastric contents, or it may affect the lungs indirectly, as in severe sepsis from a nonpulmonary or a pulmonary source (Chapter 108) or severe nonthoracic trauma associated with shock (Chapter 111).[6] Severe sepsis is the most common precipitating cause of ARDS worldwide. The organisms vary widely, ranging from gram-negative and gram-positive bacteria and viruses (e.g., H1N1 influenza in 2009) to leptospiral infections or malaria. It can be difficult to determine whether pneumonia is diffuse, with endobronchial spread involving most of the lungs, or whether localized pneumonia has precipitated a sepsis syndrome, with secondary injury to other parts of the lung.

PATHOBIOLOGY

Pathology

Despite the variety of underlying disease processes leading to ARDS, the response to these insults in the lung is monotonously characteristic, with similar clinical findings, physiologic changes, and morphologic abnormalities. The pathologic abnormalities in ARDS are nonspecific and are described as *diffuse alveolar damage* by pathologists. The initial process is inflammatory, with neutrophils usually predominating in the alveolar fluid. Hyaline membranes are present in some but not all patients,[7] similar to those seen in premature infants with infant respiratory distress syndrome, presumably related to the presence of large-molecular-weight proteins that have leaked into the alveolar space. Alveolar flooding leads to impairment of surfactant, which is abnormal in quantity and quality. The result is microatelectasis, which may be associated with impaired immune function. Cytokines and other inflammatory mediators are usually markedly elevated, although with different patterns over time in the bronchoalveolar lavage fluid and the systemic blood. The resolution of ARDS depends in part on restoration of a functional alveolar epithelial barrier, capable of removing alveolar edema fluid by sodium-dependent vectorial fluid transport.[8] Lung repair is also disturbed; early evidence of profibrotic processes includes the appearance of breakdown products of procollagen in the bronchoalveolar lavage fluid, followed by fibrosis in some patients. Lung function improves over time in survivors of ARDS; however, the fibrosis is often reversible.

Pathophysiology

The physiologic abnormalities are dominated by severe hypoxemia with shunting, decreased lung compliance, decreased functional residual capacity, increased pulmonary dead space, and increased work of breathing. Initially, the $PaCO_2$ is low or normal, usually associated with increased minute ventilation. The initial abnormalities in oxygenation are thought to be related to alveolar flooding and collapse. As the disease progresses, especially in patients who require ventilatory support, fibroproliferation may develop; the lungs (including alveoli, blood vessels, and small airways) remodel and scar, with a loss of microvasculature. In some patients, these changes may lead to pulmonary hypertension and increased pulmonary dead space; marked elevations in minute ventilation are required to achieve a normal $PaCO_2$, even as oxygenation abnormalities are improving.

TABLE 104-5 DISORDERS ASSOCIATED WITH THE ACUTE RESPIRATORY DISTRESS SYNDROME

COMMON
Sepsis (gram-positive or gram-negative bacterial, viral, fungal, or parasitic infection)
Diffuse pneumonia (bacterial, viral, or fungal)
Aspiration of gastric contents
Trauma (usually severe)
LESS COMMON
Near-drowning (fresh or salt water)
Drug overdose
Acetylsalicylic acid
Heroin and other narcotic drugs
Massive blood transfusion (likely a marker of severe trauma, but also seen with severe gastrointestinal bleeding, especially in patients with severe liver disease)
Leukoagglutination reactions
Inhalation of smoke or corrosive gases (usually requires high concentrations)
Pancreatitis
Fat embolism
UNCOMMON
Miliary tuberculosis
Paraquat poisoning
Central nervous system injury or anoxia (neurogenic pulmonary edema)
Cardiopulmonary bypass

CLINICAL MANIFESTATIONS

In most cases of ARDS, the onset either coincides with or occurs within 72 hours of the onset of the underlying disease process; the mean time from onset of the underlying cause to onset of acute lung injury is 12 to 24 hours. The presenting picture is dominated by respiratory distress and the accompanying laboratory findings of severe hypoxemia and generalized infiltrates or opacities on the chest radiograph. Alternatively, it may be dominated by manifestations of the underlying disease process, such as severe sepsis with hypotension and other manifestations of systemic infection.

DIAGNOSIS

The key to diagnosis is to distinguish ARDS from cardiogenic pulmonary edema (Table 104-6). No specific biochemical test exists to define ARDS. Certain blood or bronchoalveolar lavage (Chapter 85) abnormalities are frequent but are not sufficiently specific to be useful clinically.

TREATMENT Rx

Treatment of ARDS consists predominantly of respiratory support and treatment of the underlying disease (Fig. 104-4). Sepsis, which is a common predisposing condition for the development of ARDS, must be treated aggressively (Chapter 108).

Current recommendations for lung-protective mechanical ventilation by endotracheal intubation (Table 104-7) emphasize lower tidal volumes based on the patient's predicted body weight (Chapter 105).[A5,A6] This approach also includes achieving a plateau airway pressure less than 30 cm H_2O. PEEP is a mainstay in the ventilatory strategy for ARDS; although the method for determining the optimal level of PEEP has not been established, higher PEEP levels may have some benefit for patients with moderate to severe ARDS.[A6-A8] PEEP may allow a lower FIO_2 to provide adequate oxygenation, thereby reducing the risk of O_2 toxicity. It also may prevent the cyclic collapse and reopening of lung units, a process that is thought to be a major cause of ventilator-induced lung injury, even when adequate oxygenation can be obtained at relatively low levels of FIO_2.[9] On the basis of one clinical trial, the early use of cisatracurium besylate (15 mg rapid infusion followed by 37.5 mg/hour for 48 hours), a neuromuscular blocker, can reduce ARDS mortality rates by about 25% in patients with moderately severe ARDS with a P/F below 150 mm Hg.[A9] In patients with severe ARDS who do not respond to standard therapy but otherwise have a reasonable life expectancy and do not have multiorgan failure, extracorporeal membrane oxygenation is an acceptable albeit not fully proven rescue therapy.[10,A10] Data also indicate that prone positioning reduces mortality in patients with moderate to severe ARDS (initial P/F < 150 mm Hg).[A11]

PROGNOSIS

Case-fatality rates are 30 to 50% and are highly dependent on disease severity and the underlying predisposing condition. Based on the degree of hypoxemia (mild, 200 mm Hg $< PaO_2/FIO_2 <$ 300 mm Hg; moderate, 100 mm Hg $< PaO_2/FIO_2 <$ 200 mm Hg; and severe, $PaO_2/FIO_2 <$ 100 mm Hg), inpatient mortality rates are about 27%, 32%, and 45%, respectively, not including patients with severe underlying conditions, such as end-stage cancer.[5] Memory, verbal fluency, and executive function are impaired in about 13%, 16%, and 49% of long-term survivors after ARDS.[11,12] Lower PaO_2 during hospitalization is associated with cognitive and psychiatric impairment.

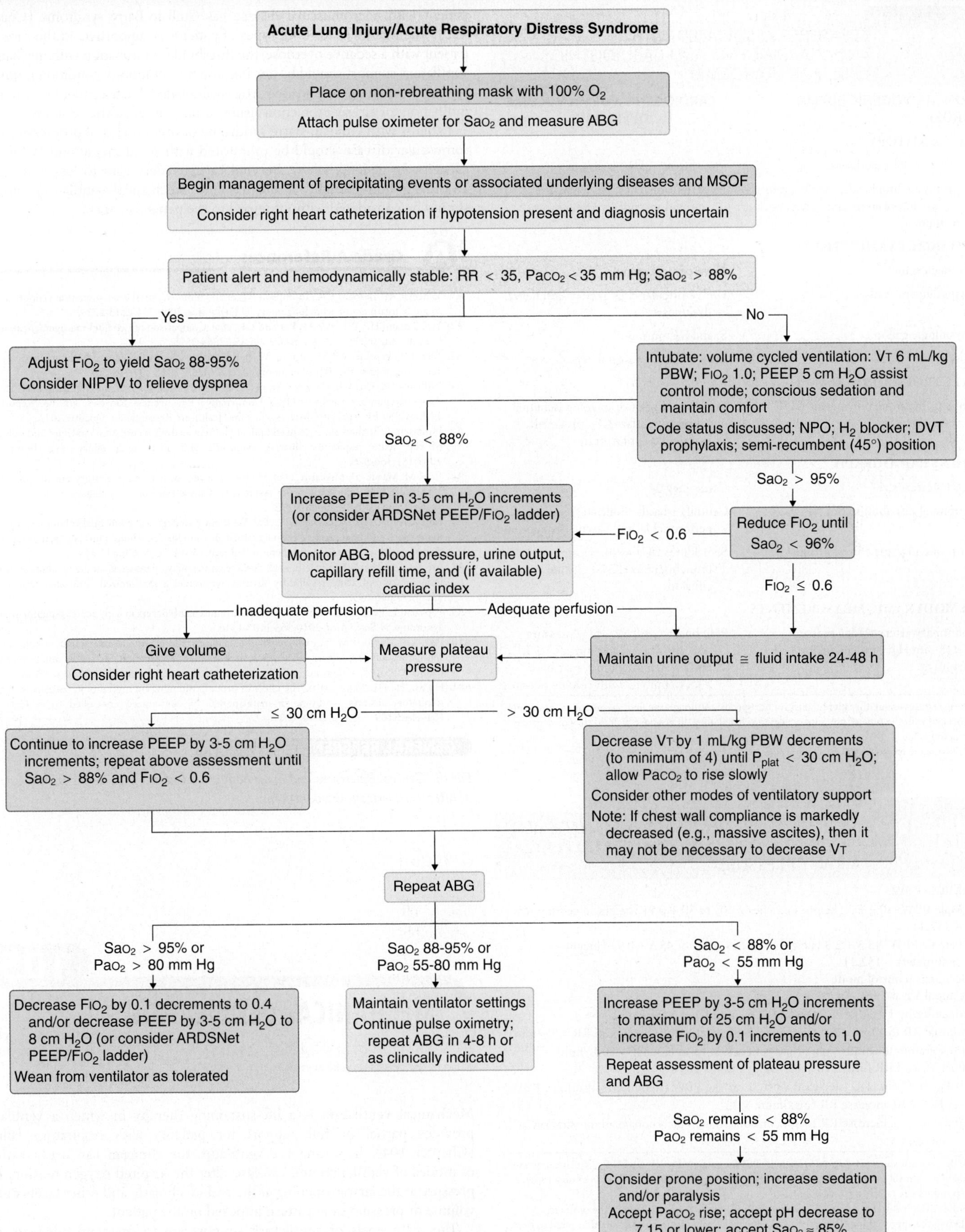

FIGURE 104-4. **Algorithm for the initial management of acute respiratory distress syndrome.** ABG = arterial blood gas analysis; CO_2 = carbon dioxide; DVT = deep venous thrombosis; FIO_2 = inspired oxygen concentration; MSOF = multisystem organ failure; NIPPV = noninvasive intermittent positive-pressure ventilation; O_2 = oxygen; $PaCO_2$ = arterial partial pressure of carbon dioxide; PaO_2 = arterial partial pressure of oxygen; PBW = predicted body weight; PEEP = positive end-expiratory pressure; P_{plat} = plateau pressure; RR = respiratory rate; SaO_2 = arterial oxygen saturation; VT = tidal volume.

TABLE 104-6 FEATURES ASSOCIATED WITH NONCARDIOGENIC AND CARDIOGENIC PULMONARY EDEMA*

NONCARDIOGENIC EDEMA (ARDS)	CARDIOGENIC EDEMA/VOLUME OVERLOAD
PRIOR HISTORY	
No history of heart disease	Prior history of heart disease
Appropriate fluid balance (difficult to assess after resuscitation from shock or trauma)	Hypertension, chest pain, new-onset palpitations; positive fluid balance
PHYSICAL EXAMINATION	
Flat neck veins	Elevated neck veins
Hyperdynamic pulses	Left ventricular enlargement, lift, heave, dyskinesis
Physiologic gallop	S_3 and S_4; murmurs
Absence of edema	Edema: flank, presacral, legs
ELECTROCARDIOGRAM	
Sinus tachycardia, nonspecific ST-T wave changes	Evidence of prior or ongoing ischemia, supraventricular tachycardia, left ventricular hypertrophy
CHEST RADIOGRAPH	
Normal heart size	Cardiomegaly
Peripheral distribution of infiltrates	Central or basilar infiltrates; peribronchial and vascular congestion
Air bronchograms common (80%)	Septal lines (Kerley lines), air bronchograms (25%), pleural effusion
HEMODYNAMIC MEASUREMENTS	
Pulmonary artery wedge pressure <15 mm Hg, cardiac index >3.5 L/min/m^2	Pulmonary capillary wedge pressure >18 mm Hg, cardiac index <3.5 L/min/m^2 with ischemia, may be >3.5 L/min/m^2 with volume overload

*These features are neither highly sensitive nor specific. Although the findings are more commonly associated with the type of pulmonary edema as listed, they do not have high positive or negative predictive value.
ARDS = acute respiratory distress syndrome.

TABLE 104-7 ARDS NETWORK VENTILATORY MANAGEMENT PROTOCOL FOR TIDAL VOLUME AND PLATEAU AIRWAY PRESSURE

Calculate PBW:
- Male PBW: 50 + 2.3 (height in inches – 60) or 50 + 0.91 (height in centimeters – 152.4)
- Female PBW: 45.5 + 2.3 (height in inches – 60) or 45.5 + 0.91 (height in centimeters – 152.4)

Select assist control mode
Set initial VT at 8 mL/kg PBW
Reduce VT by 1 mL/kg at intervals < 2 hr until VT = 6 mL/kg PBW
Set initial RR to approximate baseline minute ventilation (maximum RR = 35/min)
Set inspiratory flow rate higher than patient's demand (usually > 80 L/min)
Adjust VT and RR further to achieve P_{plat} and pH goals
- If P_{plat} > 30 cm H_2O: decrease VT by 1 mL/kg PBW (minimum = 4 mL/kg PBW)
- If pH ≤ 7.30, increase RR (maximum = 35)
- If pH < 7.15, increase RR to 35; consider sodium bicarbonate administration or increase VT

ARDS = acute respiratory distress syndrome; PBW = predicted body weight; P_{plat} = plateau pressure (airway pressure at the end of delivery of a tidal volume breath during a condition of no airflow); RR = respiratory rate; VT = tidal volume.
See the ARDSNet website (http://www.ardsnet.org) for further details about the protocol, including the approach for setting positive end-expiratory pressure and fraction of inspired oxygen.

Acute Respiratory Failure without Lung Disease

Acute respiratory failure without pulmonary abnormalities (see Table 104-2) develops in patients with depressed ventilatory drive secondary to central nervous system dysfunction and in patients with severe neuromuscular disease. The prototypical patient with suppressed ventilatory drive has taken an overdose of a sedative or tranquilizing medication (Chapter 110). The prototypical patient with neuromuscular disease has Guillain-Barré syndrome (Chapter 420). The treatment for both types of patients is supportive. In the case of a patient with a sedative overdose, the threshold for intubation with mechanical ventilatory support should be low because this temporary condition is quickly reversible when the responsible drug is eliminated. Such a patient may require intubation for airway protection against aspiration of gastric contents.

Patients with Guillain-Barré syndrome or other forms of progressive neuromuscular disease should be monitored with serial measurements of vital capacity. In general, when the vital capacity decreases to less than 10 to 15 mL/kg body weight, intubation and mechanical ventilatory support should be considered without regard to the patient's $Paco_2$.

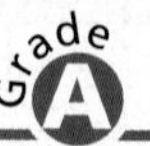

Grade A References

A1. Wheeler AP, Bernard GR, Thompson BT, et al. Pulmonary-artery versus central venous catheter to guide treatment of acute lung injury. *N Engl J Med*. 2006;354:2213-2224.
A2. Wiedemann HP, Wheeler AP, Bernard GR, et al. Comparison of two fluid-management strategies in acute lung injury. *N Engl J Med*. 2006;354:2564-2575.
A3. Rice TW, Wheeler AP, Thompson BT, et al. Initial trophic vs full enteral feeding in patients with acute lung injury: the EDEN randomized trial. *JAMA*. 2012;307:795-803.
A4. Williams JW, Cox CE, Hargett CW, et al. Noninvasive Positive-Pressure Ventilation (NPPV) for Acute Respiratory Failure. AHRQ Comparative Effectiveness Reviews, No. 68. Report No. 12-EHC089-EF. Rockville, MD: Agency for Healthcare Research and Quality; 2012.
A5. Putensen C, Theuerkauf N, Zinserling J, et al. Meta-analysis: ventilation strategies and outcomes of the acute respiratory distress syndrome and acute lung injury. *Ann Intern Med*. 2009;151:566-576.
A6. Briel M, Meade M, Mercat A, et al. Higher vs lower positive end-expiratory pressure in patients with acute lung injury and acute respiratory distress syndrome: systematic review and meta-analysis. *JAMA*. 2010;303:865-873.
A7. Meade MO, Cook DJ, Guyatt GH, et al. Ventilation strategy using low tidal volumes, recruitment maneuvers, and high positive end-expiratory pressure for acute lung injury and acute respiratory distress syndrome: a randomized controlled trial. *JAMA*. 2008;299:637-645.
A8. Mercat A, Richard JC, Vielle B, et al. Positive end-expiratory pressure setting in adults with acute lung injury and acute respiratory distress syndrome: a randomized controlled trial. *JAMA*. 2008;299:646-655.
A9. Papazian L, Forel JM, Gacouin A, et al. Neuromuscular blockers in early acute respiratory distress syndrome. *N Engl J Med*. 2010;363:1107-1116.
A10. Peek GJ, Mugford M, Tiruvoipati R, et al. Efficacy and economic assessment of conventional ventilatory support versus extracorporeal membrane oxygenation for severe adult respiratory failure (CESAR): a multicentre randomised controlled trial. *Lancet*. 2009;374:1351-1363.
A11. Hu SL, He HL, Pan C, et al. The effect of prone positioning on mortality in patients with acute respiratory distress syndrome: a meta-analysis of randomized controlled trials. *Crit Care*. 2014;18:R109.

GENERAL REFERENCES

For the General References and other additional features, please visit Expert Consult at https://expertconsult.inkling.com.

105

MECHANICAL VENTILATION

ARTHUR S. SLUTSKY

Mechanical ventilation is a life-sustaining therapy in which a ventilator provides partial or full support for patients with respiratory failure (Chapter 104). In setting the ventilator, the clinician can use a variety of modes of ventilation and can also alter the inspired oxygen tension, the pressure at the airway opening at the end of a breath, and other facets of the volume or pressure time pattern imposed on the patient.

The main goals of ventilatory support are to maintain adequate gas exchange, to rest the respiratory muscles, and to decrease the oxygen cost of breathing. Modern ventilation strategies focus on minimizing its iatrogenic consequences, such as iatrogenic hyperinflation (from endogenously derived positive pressure at the end of a breath, i.e., auto-PEEP) and ventilator-induced lung injury. In some patients, the physician should be willing to accept arterial blood gases that are not in the normal range to avoid these complications by using lower levels of minute ventilation or relatively smaller tidal volumes.

TYPES OF MECHANICAL VENTILATORS

Negative-Pressure Ventilators

Delivery of gas to the lungs requires a hydrostatic pressure gradient between the airway opening and the alveoli. During spontaneous breathing, this pressure gradient is generated by developing negative pleural pressure due to respiratory muscle contraction. Some ventilators operate by generating negative pressure around the chest wall (e.g., cuirass) or around the entire body below the neck (e.g., iron lung). The cuirass has the major advantage of minimizing detrimental hemodynamic consequences, but it is difficult to apply because the device must have an adequate seal to the body so that the negative pressure is not dissipated to the room—a task that is not always easy to accomplish in a way that is comfortable for the patient. The iron lung makes nursing care difficult because it encircles the patient's entire body. Although iron lungs were widely used during the polio epidemic of the mid-1950s, they are rarely used today.

Positive-Pressure Ventilators

The most widely used approach to mechanical ventilation is to deliver gas to the lung with positive-pressure ventilation (PPV) applied through an endotracheal tube, a tracheostomy, or a tight-fitting mask. The approach with a mask is considered noninvasive ventilation (NIV) and is considered separately.

The most basic mode of PPV is controlled ventilation, in which a preset tidal volume at a predetermined rate is delivered, regardless of the patient's requirements or efforts. This form of ventilation is usually used in patients who cannot initiate spontaneous breaths (e.g., heavily sedated or paralyzed patients) or in those who need full ventilatory support because of extremely severe pulmonary or cardiovascular disease (e.g., severe shock). This ventilator mode may be beneficial when it is used for relatively short periods (~48 hours) in patients with the acute respiratory distress syndrome (ARDS) early in their clinical course, when they may be treated with neuromuscular blocking agents (see later).[A1] However, a paralyzed patient without any ability to make breathing efforts is at risk of asphyxia in the event of an inadvertent disconnection from the ventilator. If the patient is not making any respiratory efforts, controlled ventilation can rapidly lead to respiratory muscle atrophy. For these reasons, clinicians usually try to limit the time that a patient is paralyzed and receiving controlled ventilation. Assisted ventilation is the term used when the patient's spontaneous ventilatory efforts trigger the ventilator to deliver breaths, rather than having the breaths delivered by the ventilator at a fixed rate without regard to the patient's efforts.

Mechanical ventilation can be applied by either volume-controlled or pressure-controlled modes. In volume-controlled ventilation, the desired tidal volume and respiratory rate are set by the user, and the airway pressure is the dependent variable. The airway pressure profile depends on the mechanical properties of the patient's respiratory system and on the ventilator's flow settings. In pressure-controlled ventilation, the pressure imposed at the airway opening along with the respiratory rate is set by the user, and the tidal volume becomes the dependent variable.

Positive End-Expiratory Pressure

A key characteristic that can be combined with most ventilatory modes is the level of the end-expiratory pressure. Positive end-expiratory pressure (PEEP) is used in patients with diffuse pulmonary diseases (e.g., pulmonary edema or ARDS) to recruit collapsed alveolar regions and to maintain them in a recruited state, to reopen collapsed airways, to redistribute fluid in the lung, to increase functional residual capacity, and to redistribute ventilation to dependent regions. All these changes can improve the matching of ventilation to perfusion, thereby leading to improved oxygenation and allowing the fractional inspiratory concentration of oxygen (FIO_2) to be reduced. PEEP does not usually improve alveolar ventilation and, in fact, may increase dead space by overdistending alveoli, with a concomitant decrease in alveolar capillary blood flow in certain regions of the lung. PEEP can also be administered to spontaneously breathing subjects by a technique termed continuous positive airway pressure (CPAP). In patients with exacerbations of chronic obstructive pulmonary disease (COPD), PEEP and CPAP can overcome some of the mechanical consequences of auto-PEEP (see later) to minimize the work of breathing, provided the magnitude of the PEEP is low enough that it does not cause additional hyperinflation.

Volume-Controlled Ventilation

Volume-controlled ventilation (or volume-limited ventilation) refers to mechanical ventilation in which the tidal volume is preset. The major advantage is that the delivered tidal volume is maintained even if lung mechanics change, thereby ensuring a more constant partial pressure of arterial carbon dioxide ($PaCO_2$). The potential disadvantage is that if lung mechanics deteriorate, higher pressures may be required to achieve the tidal volume goal, and regions of overinflation may result in regional lung injury. Although controlled ventilation as described earlier can be either volume limited (preset tidal volume) or pressure limited (preset peak airway pressure), clinicians usually use the term *controlled mechanical ventilation* to refer to volume-limited ventilation with a set ventilatory rate. In volume-controlled ventilation, an upper limit to applied airway pressure is commonly used for safety reasons.

The most common form of volume-controlled ventilation is one in which the patient assists the ventilator, thus triggering at least some of the breaths. The term *assisted mechanical ventilation* can refer to either volume-limited ventilation or pressure-limited ventilation when the patient triggers some or all of the breaths, but in either case the ventilator should be set to deliver breaths if apnea occurs. This mode is also referred to as assist/control (A/C).

Intermittent Mandatory Ventilation

Intermittent mandatory ventilation (IMV) refers to a mode in which the patient is allowed to breathe spontaneously through an endotracheal tube or tracheostomy but also receives some preset (and thus mandatory) volume-limited breaths from the ventilator. In current ventilators, the mandatory breaths are triggered by the patient and are synchronized (synchronized IMV); however, if the patient ceases spontaneous ventilatory efforts, breaths at the rate set on the ventilator will still be delivered. Synchronized IMV is a form of partial ventilatory support because some breaths are spontaneous, in contrast to full ventilatory support, in which all breaths are delivered by the ventilator. This mode allows the patient to do a variable amount of the respiratory work but with the security of a set minimal backup rate should spontaneous ventilatory efforts stop.

Pressure-Controlled Ventilation

Pressure-controlled ventilation is a type of ventilation in which the ventilator delivers pressure-limited breaths to the patient; delivered volume becomes a dependent variable. The initiation of each breath may be triggered by the patient (assisted breaths) or may be initiated by the ventilator (controlled breaths). In the assist mode, a backup control rate protects any patients who cease to make inspiratory efforts on their own. The delivered tidal volume depends on the preset pressure, the ventilatory rate, the inspiratory-to-expiratory ratio, and the patient's respiratory mechanics (resistance, compliance, and auto-PEEP). At a fixed preset pressure and inspiratory-to-expiratory ratio, tidal volume decreases as respiratory frequency increases. In patients with COPD, the tidal volume at low frequencies is relatively high but decreases substantially as the respiratory rate is increased; whereas in patients with stiff respiratory systems (e.g., ARDS), the tidal volume does not change much with respiratory frequency because the lung fills with gas quickly.

Pressure-Support Ventilation

Pressure-support ventilation is a pressure-limited, patient-triggered ventilatory mode. Once the patient triggers the ventilator by creating either a small negative pressure or a low inspiratory flow at the airway opening, the ventilator switches to inspiratory mode and provides the airflow needed to maintain a preset level of pressure. In contrast to pressure-controlled ventilation, inspiration terminates when the inspiratory airflow decreases to a threshold level (the specific algorithm varies from ventilator to ventilator). This mode provides flexibility for the patient with respect to tidal volume, inspiratory flow, and ratio of time allowed for inspiration compared with expiration. Tidal volume depends on patient-related factors (effort), respiratory system mechanics, and level of pressure set for support. During pressure-support ventilation, the size of each breath is determined partially by the patient's muscle effort and partially by the ventilator. This mode can compensate for the added work of breathing imposed by the resistance of the endotracheal tube. Pressure-support ventilation has been used to wean patients from ventilatory support because it provides a simple way to reduce the magnitude of mechanical support while the patient assumes a larger fraction of the ventilatory work.

High-Frequency Ventilation

High-frequency ventilation refers to modes that have the common feature of providing ventilation at frequencies that are substantially greater than those used during normal breathing. During high-frequency ventilation, tidal volumes may be less than the dead space, so adequate gas transport takes place by various convective and diffusive mechanisms. Interest in these modes of ventilation has waned because it appears to be no better or even worse than conventional ventilation for adults with ARDS.[A2,A3]

Proportional Assist Ventilation and Neurally Adjusted Ventilatory Assist

One of the difficulties in providing assisted ventilation is ensuring that there is adequate synchrony between the patient's respiratory drive and the delivery of the ventilator's breaths. This issue is a particular problem for patients with severe obstructive airways disease, especially if they have significant auto-PEEP. Two newer modes of ventilation, proportional assist ventilation (PAV) and neurally adjusted ventilatory assist (NAVA), have been developed and implemented on some ventilators in part to address this concern. Both these modes deliver ventilation in proportion to the instantaneous effort of the patient, but the underlying principles are different. Although both of these modes improve patient-ventilator synchrony, data are insufficient to know whether either will improve clinically important outcomes.

PAV is based on the mathematical relationships between airway pressure and airflow; these state that the pressure applied by the respiratory muscles is used to overcome the elastic losses (i.e., compliance) and the resistive losses of the respiratory system. With PAV, the pressure that is applied during inspiration varies on the basis of the patient's inspiratory effort and respiratory system mechanics. This form of ventilation is not in widespread use, in part because of its complexity and the need to estimate the patient's compliance and resistance on a regular basis. This latter issue has been addressed in new versions of the technique in which measurements of compliance and resistance are automatically measured repeatedly.

NAVA makes use of the electrical activity of the diaphragm (E_{di}) as measured by an array of electrodes attached to a nasogastric tube inserted into the esophagus. Pressure is then delivered by the ventilator in direct proportion to the (virtually) instantaneous E_{di}. Because the initiation and delivery of the breath by the ventilator are not dependent on measurement of pressures in the lung, patient-ventilator synchrony is improved in patients with auto-PEEP. Once the array of electrodes has been inserted, the mode is relatively easy to use; the only parameter to set is the proportionality factor linking the E_{di} and the pressure delivered by the ventilator.

Noninvasive Positive-Pressure Ventilation

PPV can be provided through a mask rather than through an endotracheal tube. This method, which has been termed noninvasive because the patient is not intubated, is conceptually simple but requires appropriate implementation and monitoring for its successful application.[1] Of particular importance are patient selection and appropriate training of hospital personnel. Patients must be alert, cooperative, and hemodynamically stable. Patients must also have intact upper airway reflexes to prevent aspiration of material from the upper airway into the lung, and they must not have any facial trauma that would preclude the use of a mask. Once patients are started on NIV, they should be carefully monitored, and NIV should be discontinued if the patient's clinical condition deteriorates, if the patient develops cardiovascular instability, or if it appears that the patient is likely to aspirate. NIV can also be delivered through a "helmet" that avoids some of the problems associated with the use of face masks.

NIV has potential advantages compared with invasive ventilation. It is relatively easy to apply and can be used for short intervals because it can be started and stopped easily. The major advantages are that it avoids the complications associated with intubation, it is usually more comfortable for the patient, and it reduces the need for sedation. Patients receiving NIV are able to communicate verbally with medical staff and family members, are probably able to sleep better, and are able to eat if they are sufficiently stable to remove the mask for short periods.

However, NIV has several disadvantages. Implementation of NIV takes more time from caregivers at the bedside initially, and the time course of correction of blood gases is slower than usually occurs in patients who are intubated and ventilated. Gastric distention is an unusual occurrence; medical staff should be aware of this complication and should watch for signs of abdominal distention. Data strongly support the use of NIV for patients with COPD (see later),[A4] and it is preferred in cardiogenic pulmonary edema,[A5] but whether it provides better outcomes in other forms of respiratory failure is uncertain.

COMPLICATIONS OF MECHANICAL VENTILATION

Intubation

Endotracheal intubation can be used to secure a patient's airway, to act as a conduit to deliver gas from the ventilator to the patient, to prevent aspiration, and to help with pulmonary toilet when secretions are increased. However, intubation can be associated with complications including the risk of aspiration during insertion of the endotracheal tube, difficulty in swallowing and communicating, disruption of normal host defense mechanisms, and upper airway trauma. Pressure from the cuff of the tube that provides a pneumatic seal between the tube and trachea can lead to regions of tracheal ischemia and may eventually cause tracheal stenosis.

The endotracheal tube increases airway resistance because its diameter is smaller than the airway into which it is inserted. The magnitude of the increase depends on the length, diameter, and shape of the tube as well as on the buildup of secretions and mucus that narrow the tube's diameter. Furthermore, the upper airway is normally an effective means of heating and humidifying inspiratory gases. This natural system is bypassed by an endotracheal tube; inadequately humidified inspiratory gases can reduce mucociliary clearance and can lead to inspissation of tracheal secretions.

Intubation affects a number of factors that increase the likelihood of nosocomial pneumonia (Chapters 97 and 282). Normally, cough involves an increase in airway pressure as respiratory muscles are contracted against a closed glottis. When the glottis opens, expiratory flow sharply increases, resulting in dynamic compression of major airways. The presence of an endotracheal tube limits the buildup of airway pressure and alters the dynamics of expiratory flow, thereby greatly impairing the efficacy of the patient's cough. A cuffed endotracheal tube helps prevent gross aspiration, but pharyngeal secretions that pool at the top of the cuff often seep into the lungs. Endotracheal tubes also can often become colonized with the microorganisms that cause ventilator-associated pneumonia (Chapter 97). Silver-coated tubes can reduce this risk but are considerably more expensive than conventional endotracheal tubes and are unlikely to be used routinely for initial intubation. Endotracheal tubes with a port that allows suctioning of secretions above the cuff may also reduce the incidence of ventilator-associated pneumonia, although results of studies have been mixed.

In addition, endotracheal intubation is often not well tolerated in awake patients, and there is always the danger that the tube will inadvertently be dislodged—a complication that can have tragic consequences. For these reasons and to improve oral care and feeding, a tracheostomy can be performed. However, tracheostomy is associated with its own set of complications, and performing a tracheostomy in the first week is no better than waiting until the patient has been ventilated for about 10 days,[A6,A7] in part because clinicians are not accurate in predicting which patients will require prolonged ventilatory support. Early tracheostomy should be avoided in patients in whom uncertainty exists as to how long invasive ventilation will be needed.

Hemodynamic Compromise

The major mechanical determinants of cardiovascular hemodynamics during mechanical ventilation are intrathoracic pressure, changes in lung volume, and the patient's circulatory volume status. An increase in lung volume can cause a beneficial decrease in pulmonary vascular resistance, if lung units that had been closed are opened as a result of mechanical ventilation, or it can lead to a detrimental increase in pulmonary vascular resistance related to overdistention of the lung with concomitant compression and lengthening of alveolar vessels.

PPV can affect cardiovascular hemodynamics through its effect on pleural pressure, an effect that is directly related to changes in lung volume and not necessarily directly reflected in measurements of airway pressure; the relation between alveolar pressure and lung volume depends on respiratory system mechanics. For example, in a patient with stiff lungs (e.g., ARDS), a given increase in airway pressure will lead to much less of an increase in lung volume than in a patient with COPD, so the increase in pleural pressure will be much less in the patient with ARDS. As a result, patients with ARDS tolerate relatively high PEEP levels, whereas similarly high levels in patients with normal lungs (e.g., in a drug overdose) or in patients with COPD would markedly reduce cardiac output. At very high lung volumes, a direct effect of the pressure of the lung on the heart can increase pericardial pressure and can thereby decrease cardiac filling.

Auto-PEEP and Dynamic Hyperinflation

A key factor that affects cardiovascular hemodynamics and other physiologic variables during mechanical ventilation is the development of auto-PEEP, which is defined as the difference between alveolar pressure and airway pressure at end expiration. Auto-PEEP is associated with dynamic hyperinflation, which is an increase in the end-expiratory lung volume above the value that would be obtained if there was complete exhalation to the static functional residual capacity. This phenomenon occurs whenever there is insufficient time for a complete exhalation to occur; the respiratory system is thus prevented from reaching its static end-expiratory volume. The major determinants of auto-PEEP and hence dynamic hyperinflation are increased expiratory airway resistance, high minute ventilation, increased respiratory system compliance, and decreased expiratory time.

Auto-PEEP may not be detected by routine measurements of pressure at the airway opening because most of the pressure drop occurs across the airways. Moreover, measurements of auto-PEEP are difficult to make in spontaneously breathing patients. When patients are not making spontaneous breathing efforts, auto-PEEP can be assessed as the difference in pressure between the set PEEP and the pressure obtained when the airway opening is occluded at the end of expiration (Fig. 105-1). It can also be assessed by the change in plateau pressure after a prolonged pause during volume cycle ventilation. If it is considered safe for the patient, a rapid estimate of the effect of auto-PEEP on cardiovascular hemodynamics can be obtained by transiently disconnecting the ventilator and allowing the auto-PEEP to approach zero during a long expiration. If the auto-PEEP is less than 5 cm H_2O, it is unlikely to cause clinically important changes in the measured intravascular pressures.

If auto-PEEP is not considered in the interpretation of respiratory mechanics, measurements of respiratory system compliance will be falsely low. Dynamic hyperinflation can be measured as the volume of gas that is released when the expiratory time of a given breath is lengthened by 20 to 30 seconds. The techniques for measuring auto-PEEP are based on the assumptions that no respiratory efforts are made and that the alveoli communicate with the airway opening, thereby allowing equilibration of pressures or exhalation of trapped gas. However, this assumption is not necessarily correct in patients with severe airways obstruction (e.g., status asthmaticus) because some airways may be completely closed.

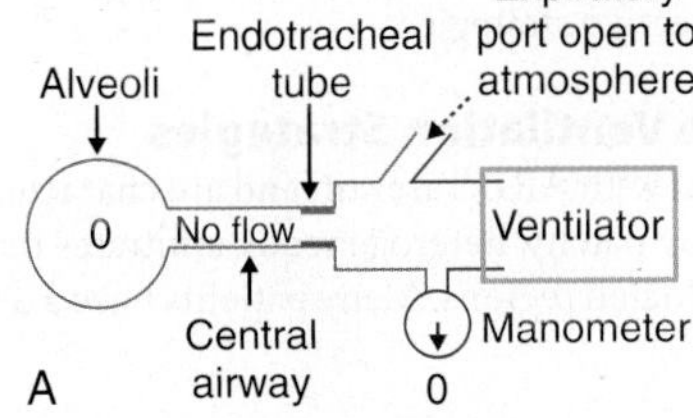

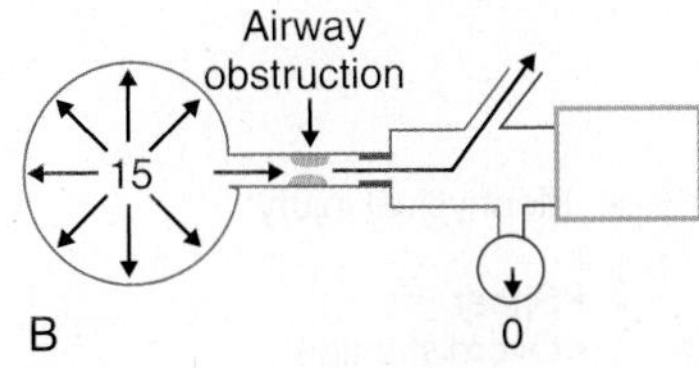

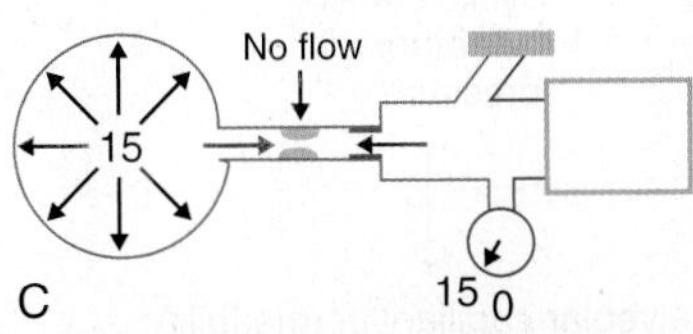

FIGURE 105-1. The relationships among alveolar, central airway, and ventilator circuit pressure at the end of exhalation under the following conditions: A, Normal conditions (no auto–positive end-expiratory pressure [auto-PEEP]). B, Severe dynamic airway obstruction with the expiratory port open. C, Severe dynamic airway obstruction with the expiratory port occluded at the end of exhalation. The auto-PEEP level is identified by creating an end-expiratory hold, thereby allowing the alveolar, central airway, and ventilator circuit pressures to equilibrate because there is no flow in the circuit. During equilibration, the level of auto-PEEP can be read on the manometer in the ventilator circuit. (Modified from Pepe PE, Marini JJ. Occult positive end-expiratory pressure in mechanically ventilated patients with airflow obstruction: the auto-PEEP effect. *Am Rev Respir Dis.* 1982;126:166-170.)

Auto-PEEP should be suspected whenever flow at end expiration is detectable or when a patient fails to trigger the ventilator consistently with inspiratory efforts. This failure to trigger the ventilator occurs because the patient must generate sufficient pressure to overcome the level of auto-PEEP before a negative deflection of pressure or generation of inspiratory flow (either of which may be used by the ventilator to detect the onset of inspiration) is sensed at the airway opening.

Auto-PEEP and the attendant dynamic hyperinflation have numerous detrimental consequences. In a patient who is not breathing spontaneously, dynamic hyperinflation increases pleural pressure and right atrial pressure, thereby leading to a decrease in the driving pressure for venous return, with a concomitant decrease in cardiac output. This effect can be magnified in patients with airway obstruction immediately after intubation and initiation of mechanical ventilation because compensatory mechanisms to enhance venous return are impaired by pharmacologic agents that are often used to prepare the patient for endotracheal tube insertion and that also reduce venous and arterial tone. In such patients, auto-PEEP can also lead to gross misinterpretation of vascular pressures. For example, the absolute value of capillary wedge pressure will be directly affected by the increase in intrathoracic pressure during auto-PEEP. The clinician may interpret this high (absolute) capillary wedge pressure as indicating adequate ventricular filling when, in fact, transmural capillary wedge pressure is low because intrathoracic pressure is also high. This misinterpretation, coupled with the decreased cardiac output related to the high intrathoracic pressure, may suggest the diagnosis of cardiogenic shock rather than the correct diagnosis of auto-PEEP.

In a spontaneously breathing patient, dynamic hyperinflation can markedly increase the oxygen cost of breathing for two reasons. First, because the respiratory system is stiffer at higher lung volumes, more energy is required to complete each ventilatory cycle. Second, to initiate flow into the lung, the patient must generate a pressure in the alveolar zone that is lower than atmospheric pressure. However, if dynamic hyperinflation is present, the patient first has to generate an inspiratory effort sufficient to overcome the (positive) end-expiratory alveolar pressure before he or she begins to lower alveolar pressure to less than atmospheric pressure to initiate airflow. The increase in lung volume associated with dynamic hyperinflation also has an impact on the effectiveness of the ventilatory muscles; at high lung volumes, the diaphragm is relatively flat, so it is at a mechanical disadvantage in producing changes in pleural pressure.

Auto-PEEP is more likely to occur in patients with airway obstruction. Avoidance of high levels of auto-PEEP by approaches such as controlled hypoventilation—during which minute ventilation is minimized, with the attendant hypercapnia—is a fundamental approach to consider in ventilating patients who have severe airway obstruction. Treatment of the detrimental hemodynamic consequences of auto-PEEP include infusion of fluids and, most important, decreasing the level of auto-PEEP, which can usually be accomplished by increasing expiratory time, decreasing airway resistance (e.g., bronchodilators, when appropriate), or decreasing minute ventilation. The last approach is usually the most effective ventilatory maneuver, but it results in an increase in the $Paco_2$.

Ventilator-Induced Lung Injury

Mechanical ventilation itself can lead to numerous types of lung injury[2,3] (Fig. 105-2) in addition to oxygen toxicity[4] when high levels of inspired oxygen concentrations are administered. Barotrauma refers to pulmonary air leaks, such as pneumothorax and pneumomediastinum. However, a much more subtle injury—diffuse alveolar damage presenting as pulmonary edema—can also occur. For both types of injury, the critical factor is the degree of overdistention of the lung, best assessed by the transpulmonary pressure (P_{tp}), the airway opening minus pleural pressure (P_{pl}). The esophageal pressure, measured with an esophageal balloon, estimates P_{pl}, although this measurement is not routinely performed in clinical practice.

The usual pressures measured during mechanical ventilation are airway pressures referenced to atmospheric pressure. The peak inspiratory pressure (PIP) is easy to measure, but its interpretation is not always simple. PIP represents the sum of the pressure needed to overcome the resistance to flow plus the pressure required to inflate the lungs. Thus, a high PIP does not necessarily indicate an increased propensity to overdistending the lung with subsequent ventilator-induced lung injury. For example, for a given inspiratory flow, use of a smaller endotracheal tube will increase PIP, but the danger of pulmonary overdistention is no greater than would be present if the patient was ventilated with a larger-bore tube and a lower PIP. The plateau pressure (P_{plat}) is the airway pressure at the end of an end-inspiratory pause (usually

>0.5 second) and is relatively easy to measure at the bedside if the patient is passive (e.g., receiving a paralytic agent). Depending on P_{pl}, it has some relationship with the development of overdistention. Although P_{pl} can vary greatly and no single value of P_{plat} can be defined as "dangerous" from a lung injury perspective, a reasonable maximal value of P_{plat} in patients with ARDS is 30 cm H_2O.

Certain caveats should be noted in interpreting P_{plat} and PIP, related to associated changes in P_{pl}. If the patient is breathing spontaneously, P_{pl} will be negative, and overdistention may occur even with a P_{plat} much lower than 30 cm H_2O. Conversely, in a patient who is either paralyzed or not making ventilatory efforts and who has a stiff chest wall (e.g., due to ascites, obesity, pregnancy), as airway pressure increases, most of the pressure drop will be dissipated across the chest wall, thus leading to values of P_{pl} that are positive. In this setting, a high P_{plat} may not be indicative of a high P_{tp} and hence may not indicate increased lung distention. Thus, the physician caring for a patient receiving mechanical ventilatory support must interpret the measured airway pressures within the clinical context. Measurement of P_{pl}, as noted earlier, may help resolve these difficulties.

During mechanical ventilation, some areas of the lung may undergo cyclic recruitment and de-recruitment. This process, which is of particular importance in patients who have ARDS, has been termed atelectrauma and can cause significant lung injury. The precise mechanisms of injury are not entirely clear but are thought to result from shear stress due to opening and closing of lung units, regional hypoxia in atelectatic lung units, and effects on surfactant. Prevention of this type of injury provides part of the rationale for the use of PEEP to maintain recruitment of lung units during tidal ventilation (Video 105-1).

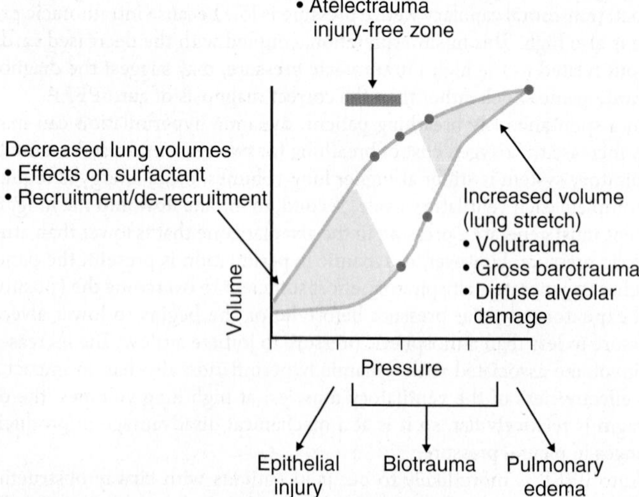

FIGURE 105-2. Schematic representation of the pressure-volume curve of a lung with diffuse alveolar edema. Mechanical ventilation can induce or worsen lung injury by numerous mechanisms when ventilation occurs at high lung volumes or when ventilation occurs at low lung volumes. Lung-protective strategies during ventilation of patients with acute respiratory distress syndrome should try to keep the ventilatory pattern in the *injury-free zone*. Data in patients confirm the benefit of ensuring that overdistention does not occur.

Finally, evidence suggests that mechanical ventilation strategies that promote overdistention and atelectrauma can lead to an inflammatory response in the lung, a mechanism of injury termed biotrauma, with the release of proinflammatory cytokines and chemokines. To the extent that these mediators can translocate from the lung into the systemic circulation, they could potentially lead to dysfunction of other organs (Fig. 105-3). This concept suggests that optimal ventilatory strategies are important not only to maintain lung function but also to prevent the development of multiple-organ dysfunction (Chapter 104), a condition that is reasonably frequent in very sick, ventilated patients. This hypothesis may explain the decreased mortality recently observed with a strategy designed to avoid overdistention in a large randomized trial of mechanical ventilation in patients with ARDS.

SPECIFIC COMMON TREATMENT SCENARIOS

Initiation of Mechanical Ventilation

The initiation of mechanical ventilation involves several steps in clinical decision making (Table 105-1). Despite the utility of such guidelines, each patient must be evaluated for specific factors that could modify the recommendation or mandate an alternative.

Acute Respiratory Distress Syndrome

Patients with ARDS (Chapter 104) have noncardiogenic pulmonary edema, with a reduced functional residual capacity and a mortality rate that commonly exceeds 25%. Although therapy may be available for the underlying disease process that led to the development of ARDS (e.g., antibiotics for a predisposing pneumonia), no effective therapy directly reverses diffuse alveolar damage. These patients require mechanical ventilation as supportive therapy to improve oxygenation and to decrease the oxygen cost of breathing until their lungs recover from the primary insult that led to the alveolar damage. The major goal in treating these patients is to provide adequate gas exchange while ensuring that damaged lungs are not further injured by whatever ventilatory strategy is required to provide sufficient oxygenation. The balanced approaches to minimize lung injury are termed lung-protective ventilation or lung-protective strategies.

Lung-Protective Ventilation Strategies

The lungs of a patient with ARDS are stiff and are characterized on computed tomographic scans by patchy, heterogeneous infiltrates that consist of airless atelectatic or consolidated regions. Many patients have a dependent zone that

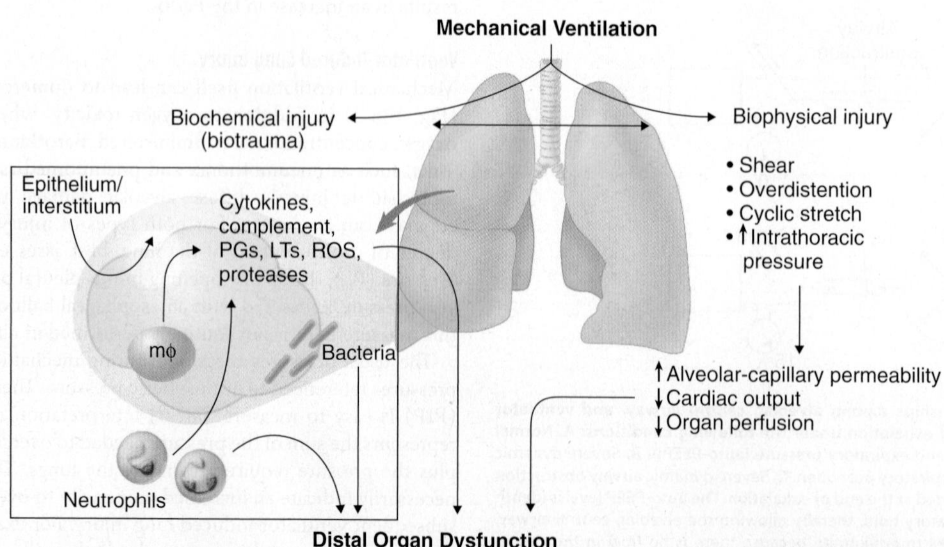

FIGURE 105-3. Mechanisms by which mechanical ventilation may lead to distal organ dysfunction. LTs = leukotrienes; mϕ = macrophages; PGs = prostaglandins; ROS = reactive oxygen species. (Modified from Slutsky AS, Tremblay LN. Multiple system organ failure: is mechanical ventilation a contributing factor? *Am J Respir Crit Care Med.* 1998;157:1721-1725.)

TABLE 105-1 STEPS AND GUIDELINES FOR INITIATION OF MECHANICAL VENTILATION*

1. Ventilatory mode
   Unintubated patients
   - NIV for patients with COPD and acute hypercapnic respiratory failure if alert, cooperative, and hemodynamically stable
   - NIV not routinely recommended for acute hypoxemic respiratory failure

   Intubated patients
   - Assist/control with volume-limited ventilation as initial mode
   - Consider specific indications for PCV or HFOV (see text) in acute lung injury
   - SIMV: consider if some respiratory effort, dyssynchrony
   - PSV: consider if patient's effort good, ventilatory needs moderate to low, and patient more comfortable during PSV trial
2. Oxygenation
   - If infiltrates on chest radiograph, then
     F_{IO_2}: begin with 0.8-1.0, reduce according to Sp_{O_2}
     PEEP: begin with 5 cm H_2O, increase according to Pa_{O_2} or Sp_{O_2}, F_{IO_2} requirements, and hemodynamic effects; consider PEEP/F_{IO_2} "ladder" (see Fig. 105-4); goal of Sp_{O_2} >90%, $F_{IO_2} \le 0.6$
   - No infiltrates on chest radiograph (COPD, asthma, PTE)
     F_{IO_2}: start at 0.4 and adjust according to Sp_{O_2} (consider starting higher if pulmonary embolism is strongly suspected)
3. Ventilation
   - Tidal volume: begin with 8 mL/kg PBW (see Fig. 105-4 for formulas); decrease to 6 mL/kg PBW over a few hours if acute lung injury present (see Fig. 105-4)
   - Rate: begin with 10-20 breaths/min (10-15 if not acidotic; 15-20 if acidotic); adjust for pH; goal pH > 7.3 with maximal rate of 35; may accept lower goal if minute ventilation high
4. Secondary modifications
   - Triggering: in spontaneous modes, adjustment of sensitivity levels to minimize effort
   - Inspiratory flow rate of 40-80 L/min; higher if tachypneic with respiratory distress or if auto-PEEP present, lower if high pressure in ventilator circuit leads to a high-pressure alarm
   - Assessment of auto-PEEP, especially in patients with increased airways obstruction (e.g., asthma, COPD)
   - I/E ratio: 1 : 2, either set or as function of flow rate; higher (1 : 3 or more) if auto-PEEP present
   - Flow pattern: decelerating ramp reduces peak pressure
5. Monitoring
   - Clinical: blood pressure, ECG, observation of ventilatory pattern including assessment of dyssynchrony, effort or work by the patient; assessment of airflow throughout expiratory cycle
   - Ventilator: tidal volume, minute ventilation, airway pressures (including auto-PEEP), total compliance
   - Arterial blood gases, pulse oximetry

*Decisions within this algorithm will be influenced by the specific conditions of the individual patient.
COPD = chronic obstructive pulmonary disease; ECG = electrocardiogram; F_{IO_2} = fraction of inspired oxygen; HFOV = high-frequency oscillatory ventilation; I/E ratio = inspiratory-to-expiratory ratio; NIV = noninvasive ventilation; Pa_{O_2} = partial pressure of oxygen in arterial blood; PBW = predicted body weight; PCV = pressure-controlled ventilation; PEEP = positive end-expiratory pressure; PSV = pressure-support ventilation; PTE = pulmonary thromboembolism; SIMV = synchronized intermittent mandatory ventilation; Sp_{O_2} = arterial oxygen saturation by pulse oximetry.

is consolidated, atelectatic, or fluid filled; a nondependent zone that looks relatively normal; and a middle zone that has some collapsed regions that can be recruited to resemble the nondependent regions if sufficiently increased levels of airway pressure are transiently used (these approaches are called recruitment maneuvers). Arterial oxygen saturation can often be increased by high tidal volumes but at the expense of regional overdistention of those lung units that were not affected by the disease process itself—a treatment strategy that can lead, over time, to worse lung injury and poorer clinical outcomes.

The injury caused by mechanical ventilation can be reduced by ventilatory strategies that avoid or minimize regional lung overdistention: limiting inspiratory pressure to some "safe" level or using smaller tidal volumes to limit end-inspiratory stretch, or both. However, in some patients, this lower "dose" of ventilation results in higher levels of Pa_{CO_2} (so-called permissive hypercapnia) and a lower pH. Higher tidal volumes (12 mL/kg predicted body weight) yielded more normal blood gases, but lower tidal volumes (6 mL/kg predicted body weight) decreased mortality by 22% (from an absolute value of 40 to 31%) in a large clinical trial (Fig. 105-4).[A8]

Data also suggest that limiting tidal volumes in ventilated patients who are intubated for reasons other than ARDS prevents injury later in the course of their intensive care unit stay.[5] A lung-protective strategy with limitation of tidal volume should be considered in ventilated patients who are at high risk for development of acute lung injury or ARDS.

Positive End-Expiratory Pressure

PEEP traditionally has been used to improve oxygenation while at the same time allowing reduction in F_{IO_2} to relatively nontoxic levels. Within the context of the current paradigm of trying to minimize iatrogenic complications of mechanical ventilation, PEEP is a therapy that can potentially minimize the injury caused by ventilation at low lung volumes by recruiting lung units and keeping them open. The critical issues are how to assess the level of PEEP in an individual patient and how to determine whether the procedures to recruit the lung units and keep them open are less harmful than allowing the lung units to remain de-recruited. One experimental option is chest computed tomography to assess whether areas of the lung are recruited, but this technique is not practical for routine assessment.

Data are inconclusive regarding the benefits of higher (≈13 cm H_2O) compared with lower (≈8 cm H_2O) PEEP levels, and PEEP levels often are individualized on the basis of a PEEP/F_{IO_2} table (Fig. 105-4). Higher PEEP levels appear to be associated with decreased mortality in ARDS patients with Pa_{O_2}/F_{IO_2} of less than 200 mm Hg but not in patients with higher Pa_{O_2}/F_{IO_2} ratios.[A9] PEEP guided by esophageal pressure measured by an intraesophageal balloon[6] can significantly increase P_{O_2} levels and respiratory compliance compared with treatment guided by a standard protocol.[A10]

Adjunctive Approaches for Ventilating ARDS Patients

The neuromuscular blocking agent cisatracurium (15 mg intravenous bolus followed by 37.5 mg/hour infusion) can decrease mortality in ARDS patients with Pa_{O_2}/F_{IO_2} ratios below 150 mm Hg when it is given for 48 hours in patients with early ARDS.[A11] The putative mechanism is a decrease in ventilator-induced lung injury.

The use of prone position in patients with ARDS can improve oxygenation compared with the supine position by permitting a more even distribution of pleural pressure, thereby reducing ventilator-induced lung injury and decreasing F_{IO_2}. Use of the prone position has decreased mortality by an absolute 9% in patients who have Pa_{O_2}/F_{IO_2} below 100 mm Hg[A12] and by an absolute 16% in patients with PaO_2/FIO_2 below 150 mm Hg.[A13] A critical factor in the use of the prone position is proper training of medical personnel in how to place patients safely in the prone position.

Obstructive Airways Diseases

The major physiologic abnormality in patients with obstructive airways diseases (e.g., COPD, asthma) is an increase in airway resistance leading to expiratory airflow limitation; patients may also have a concomitant increase in minute ventilation. These factors may lead to dynamic hyperinflation, which is associated with numerous complications (described earlier), including respiratory muscle compromise, increased oxygen cost of breathing, and hemodynamic compromise. Thus, the main goals in the ventilatory support of patients with obstructive airway diseases are to minimize auto-PEEP, to rest the respiratory muscles, to maintain adequate gas exchange, and to decrease the oxygen cost of breathing while simultaneously minimizing the iatrogenic complications of mechanical ventilation. These strategies allow time for the diagnosis and treatment of the primary cause of the exacerbation (Chapters 87 and 88).

Noninvasive Ventilation

For patients who have acute respiratory failure resulting from an exacerbation of COPD and who require ventilatory support, the preferred approach is NIV if the patient is hemodynamically stable, alert, and cooperative and does not need to be intubated to protect the airway.[7] It is important to choose a comfortable mask and to reassure the patient because some patients find the mask difficult to tolerate. This strategy may be applied with several ventilation modes, including pressure support and bilevel positive airway pressure. The ventilation settings are adjusted to improve gas exchange and to ensure the patient's comfort. Despite this approach, some patients with COPD require intubation and ventilation because of cardiac or respiratory arrest, agitation, increased sputum, worsening respiratory failure, or other concomitant severe disorders.

Intubation and Ventilation

The key goal after intubation is to minimize the detrimental effects of dynamic hyperinflation. The most effective way to do this is to decrease the minute

Ventilatory Strategy for Patients with ARDS*

Goal 1: Low Vt /P_{plat}

Initiation:

Calculate PBW
—Male:
50 + 2. 3 (height [inches] – 60)
—Female:
45.5 + 2.3 (height [inches] – 60)
Initiate volume assist control
—start with 8 mL/kg, and ↓ to
6 mL/kg over a few hours

↓

Keep P_{plat} (based on 0.5-sec pause) < 35 cm H_2O
If P_{plat} > 30 cm H_2O, ↓ Vt by 1 mL/kg to 5 or 4 mL/kg
If P_{plat} < 25 AND Vt < 6 mL/kg, ↑Vt by 1 mL/kg until P_{plat} > 25 cm H_2O OR Vt = 6 mL/kg
If patient severely distressed and/or breath stacking, consider ↑Vt to 7 or 8 mL/kg, as long as P_{plat} ≤ 30 cm H_2O†

Goal 2: Adequate Oxygenation

Specific goal:

Pa_{O_2} 55-80 mm Hg
or
Sp_{O_2} 88-95%

Use only F_{IO_2} /PEEP combinations shown below to achieve this target
- if oxygenation is low, choose F_{IO_2} /PEEP combination (from F_{IO_2} /PEEP table) to the right
- if oxygenation is high, choose F_{IO_2} /PEEP combination to the left

Goal 3: Arterial pH

Goal:

pH: 7.30–7.45
Acidosis algorithm
If pH 7.15–7.30
- ↑set rate until pH > 7.30 or Pa_{CO_2} < 25 mm Hg (max RR = 35)
- if RR = 35 & pH < 7.30 $NaHCO_3$ may be given

If pH < 7.15
- ↑set RR to 35
- if set RR = 35 & pH < 7.15, Vt may be ↑in 1 mL/kg steps until pH > 7.15

(P_{plat} target may be exceeded)

Alkalosis algorithm
If pH > 7.45
- ↓set RR until patient RR > set RR

(minimum set RR = 6/min)

F_{IO_2}/PEEP Table

F_{IO_2}	0.3	0.4	0.4	0.5	0.5	0.6	0.7	0.7	0.7	0.8	0.9	0.9	0.9	1.0
PEEP	5	5	8	8	10	10	10	12	14	14	14	16	18	18–24

*Based on ARDS Network Algorithm
†If compliance of the chest wall is markedly decreased (e.g., massive ascites), it may be reasonable or necessary (if the patient is very hypoxemic) to allow a P_{plat} >30 cm H_2O.

FIGURE 105-4. Ventilatory strategy for patients with the acute respiratory distress syndrome (ARDS). Several caveats should be considered in using the low tidal volume strategy. (1) Tidal volume (Vt) is based on predicted body weight (PBW), not actual body weight; PBW tends to be about 20% lower than actual body weight. (2) The protocol mandates decreases in the Vt lower than 6 mL/kg of PBW if the plateau pressure (P_{plat}) is greater than 30 cm H_2O and allows small increases in Vt if the patient is severely distressed or if there is breath stacking, as long as P_{plat} remains at 30 cm H_2O or lower. (3) Because arterial carbon dioxide (CO_2) levels will rise, pH will fall; acidosis is treated with increasingly aggressive strategies dependent on the arterial pH. (4) The protocol has no specific provisions for the patient with a stiff chest wall, which in this context refers to the rib cage and abdomen; in such patients, it seems reasonable to allow P_{plat} to increase to more than 30 cm H_2O, even though it is not mandated by the protocol; in such cases, the limit on P_{plat} may be modified on the basis of analysis of abdominal pressure, which can be estimated by measuring bladder pressure. RR = respiratory rate; Sp_{O_2} = oxygen saturation based on pulse oximeter.

ventilation, even if this means an increase in Pa_{CO_2}—a strategy known as permissive hypercapnia or controlled hypoventilation. Judicious use of sedation may decrease carbon dioxide production and improve patient-ventilator synchrony, although the avoidance of sedation can reduce the duration of ventilation and hospitalization.[A14] In a randomized study, no difference was found between dexmedetomidine and midazolam in time at targeted sedation level, but dexmedetomidine resulted in less time on mechanical ventilation, less delirium, and less hypertension and with less tachycardia but more bradycardia.[A15] Care must be taken in the use of paralytic agents, especially when patients with asthma are also receiving corticosteroids, because they may lead to prolonged muscle weakness and resulting difficulty in extubation and post–intensive care unit recovery.

Increasing expiratory time by use of a higher peak inspiratory flow may be somewhat helpful, but it is not nearly as effective as decreasing minute ventilation. What level of Pa_{CO_2} (and pH) should be tolerated is not known with certainty, but maintaining pH higher than approximately 7.20 is a reasonable target if the patient is not having side effects (e.g., arrhythmias, increasing right-sided heart failure), although much lower values have been reported in clinical studies.

In patients with COPD who are spontaneously breathing, the addition of external (set) PEEP at a level that is just less than what is necessary to overcome the auto-PEEP fully may not increase P_{plat} and may decrease the inspiratory effort that the patient needs to generate to initiate inspiratory airflow. This strategy does not appear to be as effective in patients with status asthmaticus, in whom it may cause an increase in P_{plat}. Measurements of auto-PEEP by airway occlusion may be inaccurate in some patients with status asthmaticus, probably because of gas trapping at the end of expiration with closed-off lung regions that do not communicate with the central airways.

DISCONTINUATION OF MECHANICAL VENTILATION

To minimize the iatrogenic consequences of intubation and mechanical ventilation, discontinuation of ventilatory support and extubation should occur as expeditiously as possible. However, if discontinuation is attempted too early, patients may deteriorate and require urgent reintubation.

From the moment that mechanical ventilation is instituted, it is important that the clinician start planning for eventual discontinuation of ventilatory support. A key aspect of this approach is serial evaluation, with aggressive treatment of the factors contributing to the patient's ventilatory dependence, including respiratory systems factors (e.g., respiratory muscles), cardiovascular factors (e.g., myocardial ischemia), neurologic factors (e.g., respiratory muscle weakness), and metabolic factors (e.g., increased oxygen consumption).

Two major types of weaning strategies have been used historically: a ventilatory mode thought to hasten the weaning process; and daily monitoring of the patient for criteria suggesting the likelihood of successful weaning, with a trial of spontaneous breathing for patients deemed likely to succeed. Studies of ventilatory modes of weaning have included trials in which patients are allowed to breathe spontaneously from a fresh gas supply delivered to the endotracheal tube (a so-called T-tube), trials of IMV, and trials of pressure-support ventilation. With all approaches, the level of support is gradually decreased until extubation is tolerated by the patient. These methods have been compared in randomized controlled trials, with mixed results, although weaning with IMV appeared less favorable in most trials. Likewise, use of ventilatory criteria to predict weaning success has been disappointing, mainly because some patients who fail to meet the criteria will be successfully weaned if they are given the opportunity to breathe spontaneously. An easily measured variable is the so-called rapid shallow breathing index, in which the respiratory rate is divided by tidal volume (in liters), with a value of less than 105 suggesting the ability to be weaned; however, false-negative and false-positive test results commonly occur.

More recently, the approach to weaning has been based on the concept that a patient is ready to be removed from ventilatory support when the underlying disease process that led to the intubation has resolved or improved substantially. Rather than applying rigorous ventilatory criteria, the only requirements are that the patient be clinically stable (i.e., has shown improvement in the underlying process), be hemodynamically stable, and have oxygen requirements that can be met by face mask once the patient is extubated.[8] If the patient meets these general criteria, a spontaneous breathing trial is recommended (Fig. 105-5); if the patient passes the trial, the patient

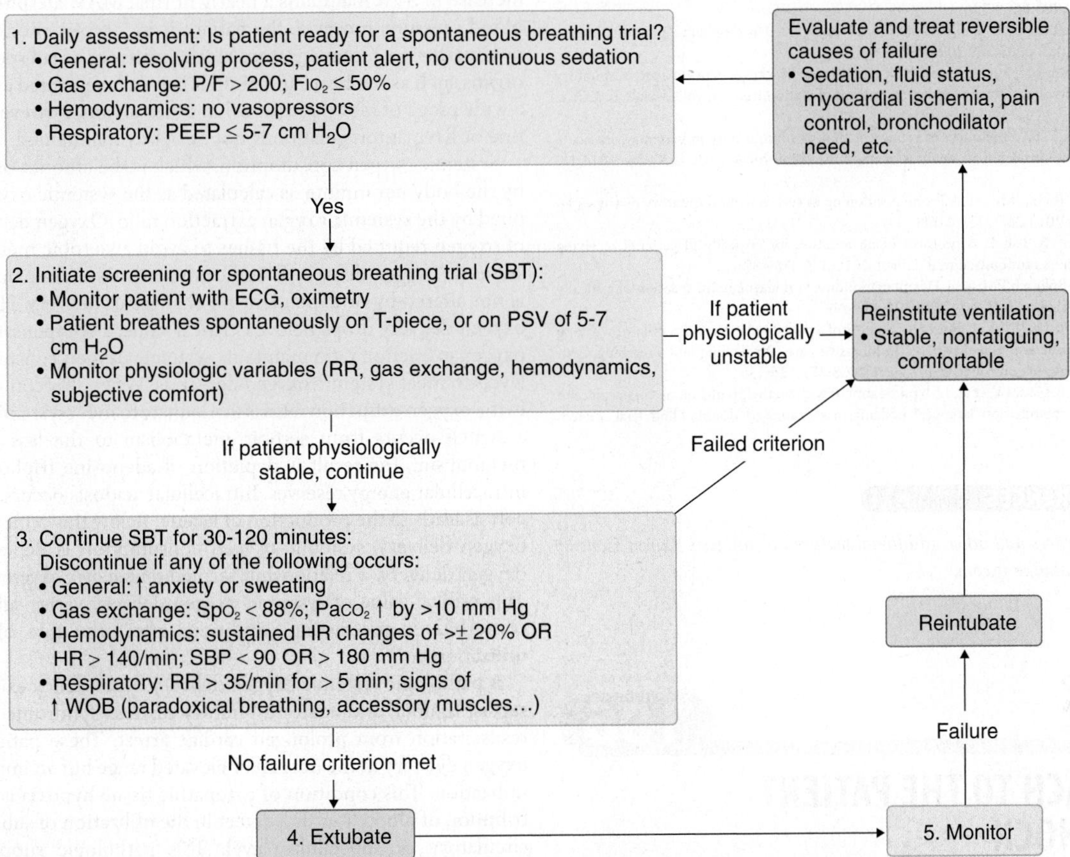

FIGURE 105-5. **Algorithm for assessing whether a patient is ready to be liberated from mechanical ventilation and extubated.** ECG = electrocardiogram; HR = heart rate; P/F = PaO_2/FIO_2 ratio; PSV = pressure support ventilation; RR = respiratory rate; SBP = systolic blood pressure; SpO_2 = oxygen saturation based on pulse oximeter; WOB = work of breathing.

can be extubated. A corollary is that gradual weaning is not necessary; instead, patients should be assessed on a daily basis regarding their suitability for removal from ventilatory support, and if they are not ready, a comfortable, nonfatiguing form of mechanical ventilation should be used between the assessments. Assisted modes of ventilation are preferred between the spontaneous breathing trials. After extubation, evidence suggests that noninvasive ventilation may be beneficial in hypercapnic or high-risk patients.[9]

An important recommendation in relation to weaning or discontinuation of mechanical ventilation relates to evidence that intensive care units should develop weaning or discontinuation protocols that can be implemented by health care professionals other than physicians. Three large randomized trials demonstrated that protocols implemented by health care professionals other than physicians improved care and were associated with substantial savings in costs compared with standard management approaches, even though the specifics of the protocols were different. A strategy that paired spontaneous awakening, based on the interruption of sedatives, with spontaneous breathing trials improved extubation rates, reduced intensive care length of stay, and decreased mortality by 32%.[A16]

A major issue to assess before extubation is the patency of the patient's airway and whether the patient will be able to clear secretions after extubation. Assessment of the likely patency of the upper airway can be achieved by use of the *cuff-leak volume*, which is the difference between the inspiratory and expiratory tidal volume when the cuff of the endotracheal tube is deflated. If this volume is more than 110 mL, it is usually an indication that major upper airway obstruction will not occur after extubation. Although this test is not required before extubation, a low cuff-leak volume warrants added precautions, such as the availability of equipment and personnel for managing a difficult intubation, when the patient is extubated. In patients who have been ventilated for more than 36 hours, methylprednisolone (20 mg intravenously) started 12 hours before a planned extubation and repeated every 4 hours until tube removal substantially reduces postextubation laryngeal edema and reduces the need for reintubation by 50%.[A17]

Despite the use of all these techniques, approximately 5 to 25% of patients will have to be reintubated and have mechanical ventilation reinstituted. Once a patient is reintubated, it is again necessary to reevaluate the respiratory and nonrespiratory reasons for the failure.

The choice of the specific weaning protocol should be left to the individual institution and should be individualized to the specific group of patients considered. In instituting such protocols, several key issues should be recognized. First, protocols are guides that should not replace clinical judgment. If a clinician does not follow some aspect of the protocol, there should be a mechanism in place for keeping track of what recommendations were not accepted, with an explanation of the rationale; these data should be collated and used to reassess the protocol. Second, protocols should be viewed as dynamic structures that are open to change and should be reevaluated on a regular basis. Third, implementation of a protocol requires adequate resources, and an institution must make a commitment not only to develop protocols but also to implement and regularly assess them.

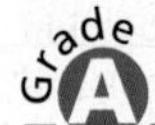

Grade A References

A1. Papazian L, Forel JM, Gacouin A, et al. Neuromuscular blockers in early acute respiratory distress syndrome. *N Engl J Med*. 2010;363:1107-1116.

A2. Ferguson ND, Cook DJ, Guyatt GH, et al. High-frequency oscillation in early acute respiratory distress syndrome. *N Engl J Med*. 2013;368:795-805.

A3. Young D, Lamb S, Shah S, et al. High-frequency oscillation for acute respiratory distress syndrome. *N Engl J Med*. 2013;368:806-813.

A4. Williams JW, Cox CE, Hargett CW, et al. Noninvasive Positive-Pressure Ventilation (NPPV) for Acute Respiratory Failure. AHRQ Comparative Effectiveness Reviews, No. 68. Report No. 12-EHC089-EF. Rockville, MD: Agency for Healthcare Research and Quality; 2012.

A5. Gray A, Goodacre S, Newby DE, et al. Noninvasive ventilation in acute cardiogenic pulmonary edema. *N Engl J Med*. 2008;359:142-151.

A6. Terragni PP, Antonelli M, Fumagalli R, et al. Early vs late tracheotomy for prevention of pneumonia in mechanically ventilated adult ICU patients: a randomized controlled trial. *JAMA*. 2010;303:1483-1489.

A7. Young D, Harrison DA, Cuthbertson BH, et al. Effect of early vs late tracheostomy placement on survival in patients receiving mechanical ventilation: the TracMan randomized trial. *JAMA*. 2013;309:2121-2129.

A8. The Acute Respiratory Distress Syndrome Network. Ventilation with lower tidal volumes as compared with traditional tidal volumes for acute lung injury and the acute respiratory distress syndrome. *N Engl J Med*. 2000;342:1301-1308.

A9. Briel M, Meade M, Mercat A, et al. Higher vs lower positive end-expiratory pressure in patients with acute lung injury and acute respiratory distress syndrome: systematic review and meta-analysis. *JAMA*. 2010;303:865-873.
A10. Talmor D, Sarge T, Malhotra A, et al. Mechanical ventilation guided by esophageal pressure in acute lung injury. *N Engl J Med*. 2008;359:2095-2104.
A11. Alhazzani W, Alshahrani M, Jaeschke R, et al. Neuromuscular blocking agents in acute respiratory distress syndrome: a systematic review and meta-analysis of randomized controlled trials. *Crit Care*. 2013;17:R43.
A12. Hu SL, He HL, Pan C, et al. The effect of prone positioning on mortality in patients with acute respiratory distress syndrome: a meta-analysis of randomized controlled trials. *Crit Care*. 2014;18:R109.
A13. Guerin C, Reignier J, Richard JC, et al. Prone positioning in severe acute respiratory distress syndrome. *N Engl J Med*. 2013;368:2159-2168.
A14. Strom T, Martinussen T, Toft P. A protocol of no sedation for critically ill patients receiving mechanical ventilation: a randomised trial. *Lancet*. 2010;375:475-480.
A15. Riker RR, Shehabi Y, Bokesch PM, et al. Dexmedetomidine vs midazolam for sedation of critically ill patients: a randomized trial. *JAMA*. 2009;301:489-499.
A16. Girard TD, Kress JP, Fuchs BD, et al. Efficacy and safety of a paired sedation and ventilator weaning protocol for mechanically ventilated patients in intensive care (Awakening and Breathing Controlled trial): a randomised controlled trial. *Lancet*. 2008;371:126-134.
A17. Francois B, Bellissant E, Gissot V, et al. 12-h pretreatment with methylprednisolone versus placebo for prevention of postextubation laryngeal oedema: a randomised double-blind trial. *Lancet*. 2007;369:1083-1089.

GENERAL REFERENCES

For the General References and other additional features, please visit Expert Consult at https://expertconsult.inkling.com.

106

APPROACH TO THE PATIENT WITH SHOCK

EMANUEL P. RIVERS

DEFINITION

The key feature of shock is tissue hypoperfusion, not a specific level of systemic arterial blood pressure. The clinical picture may be cryptic or obvious.

EPIDEMIOLOGY

More than 1.2 million patients present in shock or develop shock in U.S. hospitals each year, at an annual cost of more than $100 billion. Shock can be categorized as hypovolemic, cardiogenic (Chapter 107), extracardiac/obstructive, distributive, or dissociative.[1]

PATHOBIOLOGY

The delivery and utilization of oxygen are essential for cellular viability, and the failure to deliver or to use oxygen is central to the concept of shock and its pathogenesis (Fig. 106-1). Systemic oxygen delivery (i.e., the amount of oxygen delivered to tissues by the arterial blood) depends on the concentration of hemoglobin in the blood, the fractional saturation of the hemoglobin with oxygen (Sa_{O_2}), the amount of oxygen dissolved in the blood (Pa_{O_2}), and cardiac output. Cardiac output is a product of stroke volume and heart rate. Stroke volume is determined by ventricular preload and afterload as well as by contractility of the right or left side of the heart. Systemic vascular resistance (SVR), the force resisting cardiac contraction, can be calculated by Equation 1:

$$SVR = (MAP - CVP) * 80 / CO \quad (1)$$

$$MAP = \text{diastolic blood pressure} + (\text{systolic} - \text{diastolic blood pressure})/3 \quad (2)$$

MAP denotes the mean systemic arterial blood pressure, CVP denotes central venous pressure, and CO denotes cardiac output. SVR is determined primarily by the degree of vasomotor tone in the precapillary smooth muscle sphincters.

The systemic circulation is normally autoregulated, so that when systemic arterial pressure increases, vessel diameter decreases to maintain flow at a steady level. The clinical significance of these relationships is apparent when a patient presents with a decrease in cardiac output, but a compensatory increase in SVR maintains a nearly normal MAP. Despite the nearly normal blood pressure, however, the patient is in "cryptic shock" because of tissue hypoperfusion. Compensatory mechanisms are organ specific. Blood flow to organs such as the heart and brain is carefully regulated and maintained over a wide range of blood pressures. In other organs, however, such as the intestine or liver, autoregulation is not as tightly maintained.

Systemic oxygen consumption, which is the amount of oxygen consumed by the body per minute, is calculated as the systemic oxygen delivery multiplied by the systemic oxygen extraction ratio. Oxygen demand is the amount of oxygen required by the tissues to avoid anaerobic metabolism. Normally, systemic oxygen delivery is sufficient so that systemic oxygen consumption is not altered by or dependent on changes in delivery. However, if systemic oxygen delivery drops below a critical value, a compensatory increase in the oxygen extraction ratio maintains systemic oxygen consumption at adequate levels to meet systemic oxygen demands. When this compensatory response in the oxygen extraction ratio is inadequate to meet systemic oxygen demands, a switch occurs from aerobic metabolism to the less efficient anaerobic metabolism. The result is depletion of adenosine triphosphate (ATP) and intracellular energy reserves. Intracellular acidosis occurs, and anaerobic glycolysis leads to the production of lactate. Below this critical value of systemic oxygen delivery, systemic oxygen consumption is dependent on systemic oxygen delivery, a relationship termed *physiologic oxygen supply dependency*. This critical value of systemic oxygen delivery varies substantially because comorbid or preexisting conditions affect the rate of systemic oxygen utilization.

A pathologic systemic oxygen delivery dependency exists in patients with sepsis, trauma, and acute respiratory distress syndrome (ARDS) and after resuscitation from prolonged cardiac arrest. These patients have systemic oxygen delivery in the normal or elevated range but an impairment of oxygen utilization. This condition of cytopathic tissue hypoxia is a result of maldistribution of blood flow or a defect in the utilization of substrate at the microcirculatory or subcellular level. This pathologic supply dependency is accompanied by very high mixed venous oxygen saturation levels or venous hyperoxia as well as by elevated lactate levels. This process is believed to be an important mechanism of cellular damage in various forms of shock.

Compensatory Responses

Minor decreases in arterial blood pressure and systemic oxygen delivery activate the baroreceptor reflex through stretch receptors or sensing mechanisms located in the carotid sinus, splanchnic vasculature, aortic arch, right atrium, and juxtaglomerular apparatus of the kidney as well as through chemoreceptors sensitive to concentrations of carbon dioxide or oxygen located in the central nervous system, mostly in the medulla. These compensatory responses mediated by activation of the sympathetic nervous system include the following: release of cortisol, aldosterone, and epinephrine; activation of the renin-angiotensin system; release of arginine vasopressin from the posterior pituitary; augmentation of myocardial contractility and heart rate; constriction of arterial and venous capacitance vessels, particularly in the splanchnic bed, thereby augmenting venous return; redistribution of blood flow away from skeletal muscle beds and the splanchnic viscera; and creation of a local tissue environment to enhance the unloading of oxygen to tissues and to improve its extraction because of acidosis, pyrexia, and increased red blood cell 2,3-diphosphoglycerate.

Noncompensatory Responses

Noncompensatory responses develop when physiologic adjustments are exaggerated or lead to pathologic results. Vasodilatory shock results from many sources, including unregulated nitric oxide synthesis, inadequate ATP synthesis in vascular smooth muscle cells, activation of the enzyme poly(ADP-ribose) polymerase 1, lipid mediators, and opening of ATP-sensitive potassium channels in vascular smooth muscle cells. This multifaceted insult leads to interstitial fluid and cellular edema, which impairs oxygen diffusion from capillary to cell, causing a failure of energy-dependent ion transport, the production of lactate, and the inability to maintain normal transmembrane gradients of potassium, chloride, and calcium. Cells lose their ability to use available oxygen as a result of mitochondrial dysfunction, abnormal carbohydrate metabolism, and failure of many energy-dependent enzyme reactions.

Acidosis commonly accompanies shock. When a molecule of ATP is hydrolyzed to adenosine diphosphate (ADP) and inorganic phosphate, the reaction also generates a proton. The net yield of protons is positive when ATP is hydrolyzed in the cell and then regenerated only by the anaerobic

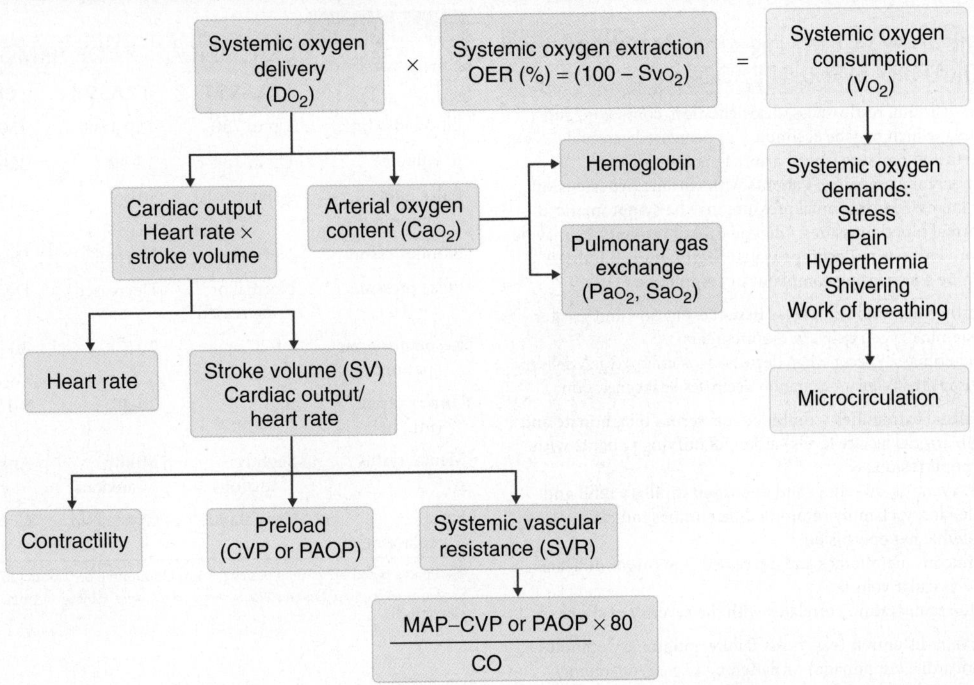

FIGURE 106-1. The hemodynamic, oxygen transport, and oxygen utilization components of shock management. Systemic oxygen delivery (Do_2) is affected by cardiac output (CO) and arterial oxygen content. The cardiac, pulmonary, and blood determinants of Do_2 are shown. CVP = central venous pressure; MAP = mean arterial pressure; OER = oxygen extraction ratio; PAOP = pulmonary artery occlusion pressure.

breakdown of glucose. Thus, during anaerobic glycolysis, the use of ATP to power cellular processes, coupled with the anaerobic production of ATP by substrate-level phosphorylation reactions, results in the development of acidosis.

Cells in organs such as the kidneys, liver, and brain can convert lactate into glucose through gluconeogenesis or oxidize lactate to pyruvate and then, ultimately, to carbon dioxide and water. Lactate levels are a reflection of tissue hypoxia, clearance, and alternative sources of production. When the splanchnic circulation is compromised in shock, hepatic lactate clearance is impaired, contributing to the buildup of lactate levels in the circulation. In sepsis, however, the rate of glycolysis increases even in the absence of tissue hypoxia. This phenomenon, which has been termed accelerated aerobic glycolysis, may reflect a change in the ratio of the active to the inactive form of pyruvate dehydrogenase, which is the rate-limiting step for the entry of substrate into the mitochondrial tricarboxylic acid cycle.

When systemic oxygen delivery continues to fail to meet systemic oxygen demands, the oxygen debt accumulates. Three stages of shock can ensue. The first stage, which is called early, reversible, or compensated shock, is characterized by compensatory responses to minimize tissue injury. This stage of shock can be self-limited, with full recovery and minimal residual morbidity, if the cause is recognized and treated early. If substantial oxygen debt persists without timely repayment or resolution, inflammation and cellular and microvascular injury define the second stage of shock, which is associated with a prolonged recovery and is typically complicated by organ failure, such as acute lung injury and acute kidney injury. The third stage is late, irreversible, or decompensated shock. In this situation, the oxygen debt is large, and repayment is slow or nonexistent. When shock reaches this point, cellular and tissue injury is extensive and largely irreversible. Progression to multisystem organ failure or death is inevitable, regardless of therapy.

CLINICAL MANIFESTATIONS

The five general types of shock are cardiogenic, distributive, hypovolemic, obstructive, and dissociative. The distinction among these five shock syndromes can be made by combining the history, clinical picture, and hemodynamic measurements. Cardiogenic shock (Chapter 107) and shock syndromes related to sepsis (Chapter 108) are covered in detail elsewhere.

The clinical manifestation of shock is variable and depends on the initiating cause and the response of multiple organs. Shock typically is manifested as absolute or relative systemic arterial hypotension and evidence of end-organ dysfunction (Table 106-1). Even a one-time hypotensive episode on hospital admission is associated with increased in-hospital mortality. The extremities are cool and pale if shock is associated with peripheral vasoconstriction, which is typical of hypovolemic, cardiogenic, and obstructive shock, but they are typically warm and pink with the peripheral vasodilation of distributive shock and dissociative shock (cyanide poisoning). Skin mottling is a physical finding that correlates with hemodynamic compromise, organ failure, and mortality.[2]

The most frequent neurologic finding in shock is alteration in the level of consciousness, ranging from confusion to coma. Many of the clinically apparent manifestations of cardiac involvement in shock result from sympathoadrenal stimulation, with tachycardia being the most sensitive indicator that shock is present. Acute lung injury, which can be immediate or delayed, results in impaired gas exchange; the work of breathing is increased, and respiratory muscle fatigue and ventilatory failure require mechanical ventilation. Hypovolemia with or without acute tubular necrosis results in oliguria, although polyuria may be seen in early shock.

Typical clinical manifestations of gut involvement during shock include abdominal pain, ileus, erosive gastritis, pancreatitis, acalculous cholecystitis, and submucosal hemorrhage. If the integrity of the gut barrier is compromised, bacteria and their toxins are translocated into the blood stream. The most common manifestation of liver involvement in shock is a mild increase in serum levels of aminotransferases and lactate dehydrogenase. With severe hypoperfusion, shock liver may be manifested with massive aminotransferase elevations and extensive hepatocellular damage.

Thrombocytopenia may result from dilution during volume repletion or from immunologic platelet destruction, which is especially common during septic shock. Activation of the coagulation cascade can lead to disseminated intravascular coagulation (Chapter 175), which results in thrombocytopenia, decreased fibrinogen, elevated fibrin split products, and microangiopathic hemolytic anemia. The finding of nucleated red blood cells on a peripheral blood smear is associated with increased in-hospital mortality.[3]

Hypovolemic Shock

Hemorrhagic shock, whether from internal or external bleeding, is the most common cause of hypovolemic shock (Table 106-2). Nonhemorrhagic hypovolemic shock can be caused by severe dehydration due to massive urinary or gastrointestinal fluid losses. Such losses are common in conditions such as diabetic ketoacidosis (Chapter 229) and diarrhea from some infectious diseases, such as cholera (Chapter 302). Massive insensible losses of water or perspiration can precipitate shock in patients with major burn injuries (Chapter 111) or heatstroke (Chapter 109). Sequestration of fluid in the extravascular compartment, commonly referred to as third spacing, can cause shock in patients as a result of surgery, bowel obstruction, hepatic failure (Chapter 154), systemic inflammation, acute pancreatitis (Chapter 144), or

TABLE 106-1 PHYSICAL EXAMINATION AND SELECTED LABORATORY SIGNS IN SHOCK

Central nervous system	Acute delirium, restlessness, disorientation, confusion, and coma, which may be secondary to decreased cerebral perfusion pressure (mean arterial pressure minus intracranial pressure). Patients with chronic hypertension or increased intracranial pressure may be symptomatic at normal blood pressures. Cheyne-Stokes respirations may be seen with severe decompensated heart failure. Blindness can be a presenting complaint or complication.
Temperature	Hyperthermia results in excess tissue respiration and greater systemic oxygen delivery requirements. Hypothermia can occur when decreased systemic oxygen delivery or impaired cellular respiration decreases heat generation.
Skin	Cool distal extremities (combined low serum bicarbonate and high arterial lactate levels) aid in identifying patients with hypoperfusion. Pallor, cyanosis, sweating, and decreased capillary refill and pale, dusky, clammy or mottled extremities indicate systemic hypoperfusion. Dry mucous membranes and decreased skin turgor indicate low vascular volume. Low toe temperature correlates with the severity of shock.
General cardiovascular	Neck vein distention (e.g., heart failure, pulmonary embolus, pericardial tamponade) or flattening (e.g., hypovolemia), tachycardia, and arrhythmias Decreased coronary perfusion pressures can lead to ischemia, decreased ventricular compliance, and increased left ventricular diastolic pressure. A "mill wheel" heart murmur may be heard with an air embolus.
Heart rate	Usually elevated. However, paradoxical bradycardia can be seen in patients with preexisting cardiac disease and severe hemorrhage. Heart rate variability is associated with poor outcomes.
Systolic blood pressure	May actually increase slightly when cardiac contractility increases in early shock and then fall as shock advances A single episode of undifferentiated hypotension with a systolic blood pressure <80 mm Hg carries an in-hospital mortality of 18%.
Diastolic blood pressure	Correlates with arteriolar vasoconstriction and may rise early in shock and then fall when cardiovascular compensation fails
Pulse pressure	Defined as systolic minus diastolic pressure and related to stroke volume and the rigidity of the aorta Increases early in shock and decreases before systolic pressure decreases
Pulsus paradoxus	An exaggerated change in systolic blood pressure with respiration (systolic blood pressure declines >10 mm Hg with inspiration) seen in asthma, cardiac tamponade, and air embolus
Mean arterial blood pressure	Diastolic blood pressure + [pulse pressure/3]
Shock index	Heart rate/systolic blood pressure. Normal = 0.5 to 0.7. A persistent elevation of the shock index (>1.0) indicates impaired left ventricular function (as a result of blood loss or cardiac depression) and is associated with increased mortality.
Respiratory	Tachypnea, increased minute ventilation, increased dead space, bronchospasm, hypocapnia with progression to respiratory failure, acute lung injury, and adult respiratory distress syndrome
Abdomen	Low-flow states may result in abdominal pain, ileus, gastrointestinal bleeding, pancreatitis, acalculous cholecystitis, mesenteric ischemia, and shock liver.
Renal	Because the kidney receives 20% of cardiac output, low cardiac output reduces the glomerular filtration rate and redistributes renal blood flow from the renal cortex toward the renal medulla, thereby leading to oliguria. Paradoxical polyuria in early sepsis may be confused with adequate hydration.
Metabolic	Respiratory alkalosis is the first acid-base abnormality, but metabolic acidosis occurs as shock progresses. Hyperglycemia, hypoglycemia, and hyperkalemia may develop.

TABLE 106-2 CLASSIFICATION OF HEMORRHAGIC SHOCK*

	CLASS I	CLASS II	CLASS III	CLASS IV
Blood loss (mL)	Up to 750	750-1500	1500-2000	>2000
% Volume	Up to 15	15-30	30-40	>40
Pulse rate (per minute)	<100	>100	>120	>140
Blood pressure	Normal	Normal	Decreased	Decreased
Pulse pressure	Normal or increased	Decreased	Decreased	Decreased
Respiratory rate (per minute)	14-20	20-30	30-40	>35
Urine output (mL/hr)	>30	20-30	5-15	Negligible
Mental status	Slightly anxious	Mildly anxious	Anxious, confused	Confused, lethargic
Fluid replacement	Crystalloid	Crystalloid	Crystalloid and blood	Crystalloid and blood

*Estimates based on a 70-kg patient. From Committee on Trauma of the American College of Surgeons. *Advanced Trauma Life Support for Doctors.* Chicago: American College of Surgeons; 1997:108.

thermal injuries (Chapter 111).[4] Regardless of whether hypovolemic shock is due to hemorrhage or fluid losses, the rate of loss is a critical component of the presentation. If volume is lost at a slow rate, compensatory mechanisms are usually effective, and any given amount of volume depletion is often better tolerated than if the same volume were lost acutely. In addition, underlying diseases, especially those that limit cardiac reserve, can substantially influence the clinical severity of a hypovolemic insult. As the importance of the microcirculation continues to be elucidated, it may become a target of future management strategies.

Distributive Shock

The most important and prevalent cause of distributive shock is septic shock (Chapter 108), but anaphylaxis (Chapter 253), drug overdose (Chapter 34), neurogenic insults, and addisonian crisis (Chapter 227) can also produce vasodilatory shock. Sepsis can be a combination of hypovolemia, vasodilation, myocardial suppression, and impaired tissue oxygen use (dissociative shock). In approximately 10 to 15% of septic shock patients, myocardial dysfunction results in a low cardiac output form of shock. Early interventions (Chapter 108) can improve outcomes substantially.

Cardiogenic Shock

Cardiogenic shock (Chapter 107) is defined by a decrease in systemic oxygen delivery caused by an acute or chronic deterioration of cardiac function due to myocardial, valvular, structural, toxic, or infectious causes. The clinical picture of cardiogenic shock is variable, depending on which structural component of the ventricle is impaired.

Extracardiac Obstructive Shock

This form of shock results from acute obstruction to flow in the circulation. Examples include impaired diastolic filling of the right ventricle (e.g., superior vena cava syndrome; Chapter 179), obstruction of right ventricular output (e.g., massive pulmonary embolism; Chapter 98), and an air embolus from cardiopulmonary bypass or central line placement (Chapter 98). Systemic arterial hypertension (Chapter 67) severe enough to impair left ventricular function or acute pericardial tamponade or constrictive pericarditis (Chapter 77) can also produce an obstructive shock pattern.

Dissociative Shock

Dissociative shock results from microvascular abnormalities, with maldistribution or shunting of blood flow, or cytopathic tissue hypoxia. Dissociative shock includes disorders that inhibit oxygen utilization, such as cyanide poisoning (Chapter 110), sodium nitroprusside use, and sepsis.

Mixed Shock States

Shock may arise from multiple causes. For example, a patient with pneumonia and a history of ischemic cardiomyopathy may present in a hypodynamic rather than in a hyperdynamic state when combined with sepsis. Thus, a mixture of hypovolemic, distributive, cardiogenic, obstructive, and dissociative shock can potentially be seen in the same patient.

DIAGNOSIS

A key element in the approach to shock is a problem-directed history and physical examination. Some patients present with few symptoms other than generalized weakness, lethargy, or altered mental status. A discussion with the patient and family members should specifically address symptoms that suggest volume depletion, including bleeding, vomiting, diarrhea, excessive urination, insensible losses due to fever, and orthostatic lightheadedness. The history should also inquire about prior or current evidence of cardiovascular disease, especially episodes of chest pain (Chapter 51) or symptoms of heart failure (Chapter 58). Prior neurologic diseases can render patients more susceptible to complications from hypovolemia. Medication use, both prescribed and nonprescribed, must be ascertained. Some medications cause volume depletion (e.g., diuretics), whereas others depress myocardial contractility (e.g., β-blockers, calcium-channel blockers). The possibility of an anaphylactic reaction to a new medication or cardiovascular depression due to drug toxicity should be considered. A recent or remote history of steroid use may suggest adrenal insufficiency (Chapters 35 and 227).

The physical examination can provide critical information to aid in the diagnosis (see Table 106-1). Traditionally, shock is defined by a systolic blood pressure less than 90 mm Hg or 40 mm Hg less than the baseline systolic blood pressure if the patient has a history of hypertension. Ultrasound can be incorporated into a formal protocol to evaluate cardiac function, cardiac chamber filling, and certain aspects of the peripheral vasculature (Table 106-3).[5]

Acidosis

A common theme in shock is that tissue hypoxia leads to acidosis (Chapter 118), which develops as a consequence of anaerobic metabolism and generally parallels the severity of shock. Laboratory manifestations may include a base deficit, low arterial and venous pH levels, and an elevated serum lactate level. Base deficit is the absolute decrease in the serum concentration of bicarbonate (normal minus the patient's bicarbonate). A mild base deficit is −2 to −5, moderate is −6 to −14, and severe is −15 mmol/L or greater. When patients are resuscitated with large volumes of normal saline, the large fluid load can cause a dilutional acidosis, and the large chloride load can induce metabolic acidosis even in the absence of tissue hypoxia and anaerobic metabolism. Base deficit can also be caused by cocaine, alcohol (Chapter 33), and diabetic ketoacidosis (Chapter 229). Despite its limitations, base deficit provides the clinician with a quick indicator to assess the severity of tissue hypoperfusion and the adequacy of resuscitation in relieving anaerobic metabolism and oxygen debt.

The low blood pH of metabolic acidosis can result from different acids. Acidosis caused by lactate and unidentified anions produces an anion gap. The blood lactate concentration rises with increased anaerobic metabolism, as is seen in shock but also in diabetic ketoacidosis (Chapter 229), total parenteral nutrition (Chapter 217), seizures (Chapter 403), thiamine deficiency (Chapter 218), treatment of HIV infection with protease inhibitors (Chapter 388), and administration of metformin, salicylate, isoniazid, propofol, and cyanide (Chapter 110). A lactate concentration greater than 4 mmol/L is unusual in normal and non–critically ill hospitalized patients and warrants concern. A lactate concentration greater than 4 mmol/L is associated with an in-hospital mortality exceeding 25%, regardless of the cause, and failure to decrease lactate levels during the first 6 hours of shock is associated with an increased inflammatory response, the development of organ failure, and mortality. The arterial-venous difference in carbon dioxide content is inversely related to cardiac output. Whether the samples are taken from the pulmonary artery or the central venous circulation, the relationship and clinical interpretation are the same.

Urine Output

The kidneys normally receive 20% of the systemic oxygen delivery, and because of this large amount of blood flow per gram of tissue, they are highly sensitive to changes in renal blood flow. Urine output is a valuable indicator of renal perfusion and vital organ blood flow. Although a significant drop in urine output indicates reduced renal blood flow, an adequate urine output does not always indicate successful resuscitation. In fact, paradoxical polyuria may be present. Other factors that may affect urine output include the use of mannitol or diuretics. Preexisting conditions, such as renal failure, may also limit the ability of this measure to reflect the adequacy of resuscitation.

TREATMENT

Rx

The goal of initial management is to restore global and microvascular perfusion to levels that sustain aerobic cellular respiration. Multiple randomized trials have shown significant and consistent reductions in mortality when shock is reversed aggressively before organ failure develops. Once this initial management is accomplished, the definitive diagnosis leads to more specific therapy based on the cause of shock.

Markers of shock serve not only as diagnostic tools for risk stratification but also as targets or end points for the early restoration of adequate tissue perfusion. Clinical monitoring of tissue oxygenation and organ function commonly involves measuring traditional end points of resuscitation, such as heart rate, blood pressure, mentation, urine output, and skin perfusion. Many clinicians continue to use these parameters as indicators that systemic oxygenation imbalances have been corrected. However, there is increasing evidence that clinical parameters may be poor indicators of the ongoing tissue hypoxia and microcirculatory dysfunction that are associated with increased mortality.

Initial Management

The initial management of shock requires immediate diagnostic and therapeutic interventions, including attention to airway, breathing, and circulation and definitive diagnosis and treatment (Chapter 63). The first step to optimize systemic oxygen delivery is to provide supplemental oxygen to increase arterial oxygen content. If any doubt exists about the patency of the airway or the adequacy of ventilation, endotracheal intubation should be performed and mechanical ventilation initiated (Chapter 105). Mechanical ventilation helps provide adequate oxygenation and carbon dioxide elimination and decreases oxygen utilization by the respiratory muscles, which may be responsible for up to 40% of systemic oxygen consumption and lactate production.

Although endotracheal intubation and mechanical ventilation may be critical for patients in shock, the sudden increase in airway pressure can lead to a series of deleterious hemodynamic complications, especially in patients who are hypovolemic or vasodilated or have compromised cardiac function. In such patients, the resulting decreased venous return, increased pulmonary

TABLE 106-3 RAPID ULTRASOUND IN SHOCK (RUSH) PROTOCOL*

RUSH EVALUATION	HYPOVOLEMIC SHOCK	CARDIOGENIC SHOCK	OBSTRUCTIVE SHOCK	DISTRIBUTIVE SHOCK
Heart	Hypercontractile LV Small LV chamber size	Hypocontractile or dilated LV	Hypercontractile LV Pericardial effusion Cardiac tamponade RV strain Cardiac thrombus	Hypercontractile LV in early sepsis, hypocontractile LV in late sepsis
Fluid status	Flat IVC Flat jugular veins Peritoneal fluid (fluid loss) Pleural fluid (fluid loss)	Distended IVC Distended jugular veins Pulmonary edema Pleural or peritoneal fluid	Distended IVC Distended jugular veins Pneumothorax	Normal or small IVC in early sepsis Peritoneal or pleural fluid
Extracardiac circulatory system	Abdominal aneurysm Aortic dissection	Normal	DVT	Normal

*Modified from Perera P, Mailhot T, Riley D, et al. The RUSH exam: Rapid Ultrasound in SHock in the evaluation of the critically ill. *Emerg Med Clin North Am.* 2010;28:29-56.
DVT = deep venous thrombosis; IVC = inferior vena cava; LV = left ventricle; RV = right ventricle.

TABLE 106-4 VASOPRESSOR AGENTS

		PERIPHERAL VASCULATURE		CARDIAC EFFECTS			
AGENT	**DOSE RANGE**	***Vasoconstriction***	***Vasodilation***	***Heart Rate***	***Contractility***	***Dysrhythmias***	**TYPICAL USE**
Dopamine	1-4 μg/kg/min	0	1+	1+	1+	1+	"Renal dose" does not improve renal function; may be used with bradycardia and hypotension
	5-10 μg/kg/min	1-2+	1+	2+	2+	2+	
	11-20 μg/kg/min	2-3+	1+	2+	2+	3+	Vasopressor range
Vasopressin	0.04-0.1 units/min	3-4+	0	0	0	1+	Septic shock, post–cardiopulmonary bypass shock state, no outcome benefit in sepsis
Phenylephrine	20-200 μg/min	4+	0	0	0	1+	Vasodilatory shock; best for supraventricular tachycardia
Norepinephrine	1-20 μg/min	4+	0	2+	2+	2+	First-line vasopressor for septic shock, vasodilatory shock
Epinephrine	1-20 μg/min	4+	0	4+	4+	4+	Refractory shock, shock with bradycardia, anaphylactic shock
Dobutamine	1-20 μg/kg/min	1+	2+	1-2+	3+	3+	Cardiogenic shock, septic shock
Milrinone	37.5-75 μg/kg bolus followed by 0.375-0.75 μg/min	0	2+	1+	3+	2+	Cardiogenic shock, right-sided heart failure, dilates pulmonary artery; caution in renal failure

vascular resistance, and decreased ventricular compliance may lead to hypotension and cardiovascular collapse.[6,7] Early sedation and muscle relaxation with mechanical ventilation have been shown to have outcome benefit, especially with acute lung injury.[A1] However, early use of sedatives, anxiolytics, or induction agents during and after intubation can decrease catecholamine levels, peripheral vascular resistance, and cortisol levels and may result in hypotension. If possible, preparations should be made to monitor physiologic variables, to ensure adequate fluid administration, and to provide rapid access to vasopressors should systemic arterial pressure fall to dangerously low levels.

On initial presentation, it is good practice to place one or two large-bore (≥16 gauge) peripheral intravenous catheters and to administer a crystalloid solution (normal saline or lactated Ringer solution). If MAP is less than 60 to 65 mm Hg, systolic blood pressure is less than 90 mm Hg, or evidence of tissue hypoperfusion is present, an intravenous fluid challenge (20 to 40 mL/kg crystalloid or colloid) should be given rapidly. A bolus of 500 mL every 30 minutes titrated to MAP or measurement of preload is recommended. In an 80-kg person, the average intravascular volume is 5 L. In shock states, such as septic shock, in which intravascular hypovolemia is a predominant feature, 5 to 6 L of fluid during the first 6 hours is considered an average volume resuscitation. If hemorrhage is the likely cause of shock, blood should be used to replace volume. Fluids should not be withheld, even in patients with end-stage renal disease.

Central venous access and arterial blood pressure monitoring should be established to administer vasopressors and to monitor hemodynamics and venous and arterial blood gases, respectively. Electrocardiographic monitoring and continuous measurement of oxygen saturation by pulse oximetry are useful adjuncts. Because the Trendelenburg position may impair gas exchange and promote aspiration, an alternative is to raise the patient's legs above the level of the heart with the patient in the supine position.

If the patient remains hypotensive, vasopressors such as norepinephrine, dopamine, or phenylephrine (Table 106-4) should be administered to restore adequate systemic arterial pressure while the diagnostic evaluation is ongoing. Treatment with vasopressors should not be postponed while trying to achieve euvolemia by using fluid boluses because patients with cerebrovascular and coronary artery disease may be intolerant of the hypotensive interval. However, vasopressors may also mask hypovolemia when they increase blood pressure. If the volume status remains undefined or the hemodynamic condition requires repeated fluid challenges or vasopressor treatment, a central venous catheter should be placed to determine central venous oxygen saturation, ventricular filling pressures, and intravascular volume status while echocardiography is performed. On the basis of these data, patients can usually be classified and managed according to their hemodynamic and oxygen transport patterns (Figs. 106-2 and 106-3).

Fluid Replacement

Rapid and appropriate restoration of vascular volume decreases the need for vasopressor therapy, adrenal replacement therapy, and invasive monitoring; in addition, it modulates the inflammation that arises when a patient progresses to severe shock. The goal of fluid resuscitation is not merely to achieve a predetermined volume or pressure but rather to titrate fluid to optimize systemic oxygen delivery and to meet tissue oxygen demands.[8]

To assess the adequacy of cardiac preload during the resuscitation of a patient with shock, decisions based on monitoring of CVP lead to the same outcomes as those based on measuring equivalence to wedged pulmonary artery occlusion pressure.[A2] However, the CVP does not correlate well with left ventricular end-diastolic volume; although a low CVP indicates hypovolemia, a "normal" CVP does not exclude inadequate preload as a cause of shock. A fluid challenge in a volume-responsive patient increases cardiac output by about 20% for each change of 2 cm H_2O in CVP; by comparison, cardiac output does not change if the CVP is raised in a patient with adequate left ventricular volume.

When intrathoracic pressure increases during the application of positive airway pressure in a mechanically ventilated patient, venous return decreases, and as a consequence, left ventricular stroke volume also decreases. The variation in pulse pressure or stroke volume during a positive-pressure breath can also predict the responsiveness of cardiac output to changes in preload. Pulse pressure variation is defined by Equation 3:

$$100 \times (PPmax - PPmin)/[(PPmax + PPmin)/2] \quad (3)$$

PPmax and PPmin are the maximal and minimal pulse pressures, respectively, in a respiratory cycle; these measurements must be made when the patient is not making any respiratory efforts on his or her own. Pulse pressure variation values of 13 to 15% suggest that hypovolemia is present and that the cardiac index will increase by at least 15% after the rapid infusion of 500 mL of crystalloid. Pulse pressure variation is a reasonable predictor of volume status and response to fluids, although atrial arrhythmias can interfere with the usefulness of this technique.

Types of Fluids

The two most commonly used crystalloid solutions are 0.9% sodium chloride solution (normal saline) and lactated Ringer solution (Table 106-5). Although these two solutions have been regarded as essentially interchangeable, accumulating data suggest that large volumes of normal saline, but not of lactated Ringer solution, promote the development of hyperchloremic metabolic acidosis and coagulopathy. Hypertonic saline is not recommended for routine use in trauma patients.[A3]

Colloids are higher-molecular-weight solutions that increase plasma oncotic pressure; they are classified as natural (albumin) or artificial (starches, hetastarch, pentastarch, dextrans, and gelatins). Colloids are dissolved in either normal saline or a balanced salt solution. Colloids stay in the intravascular space significantly longer than crystalloids do, with an intravascular half-life of 16 hours for albumin versus 30 to 60 minutes for normal saline and lactated Ringer solution. When they are titrated to the same volume status, colloids and crystalloids restore tissue perfusion to the same magnitude, but a two to four times greater volume of crystalloids is required to achieve the same end point. The outcomes of patients with hypovolemic shock are equivalent for crystalloids and albumin (see Table 106-5).[A4,A5] By comparison, hetastarch increases renal failure and mortality in intensive care unit (ICU) patients with shock.[A6]

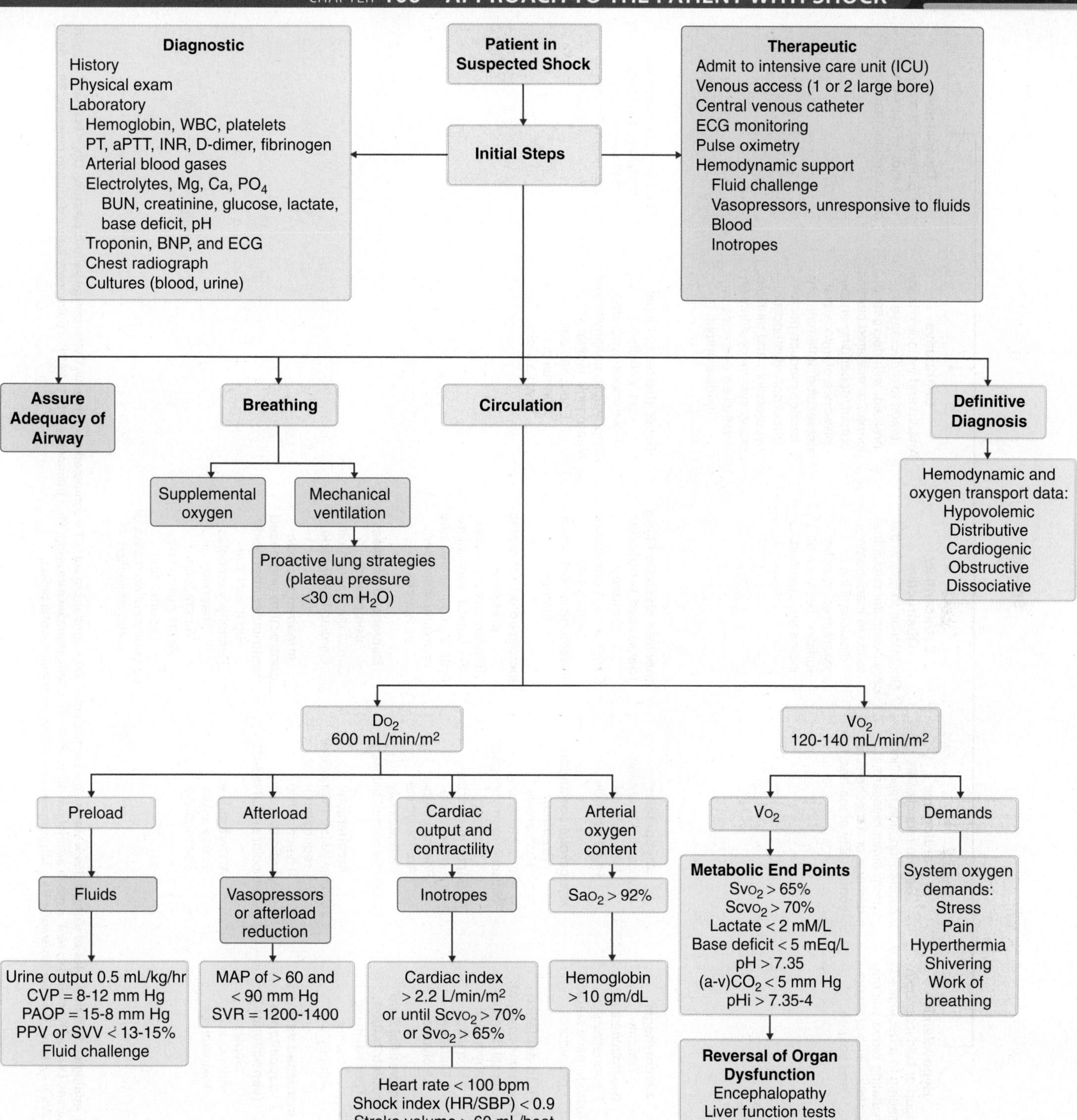

FIGURE 106-2. General hemodynamic management. aPTT = activated partial thromboplastin time; BNP = brain natriuretic peptide; bpm = beats per minute; BUN, blood urea nitrogen; CVP = central venous pressure; Do_2 = (systemic) oxygen delivery; ECG = electrocardiogram; HR = heart rate; INR = international normalized ratio; MAP = mean arterial pressure; PAOP = pulmonary artery occlusion pressure; pHi = intestinal mucosal pH; PPV = pulse pressure variation; PT = prothrombin time; SBP = systolic blood pressure; SVR = systemic vascular resistance; SVV = stroke volume variation; Vo_2 = (systemic) oxygen consumption; WBC = white blood cell.

Fluid Management Strategies

After initial aggressive fluid resuscitation within 6 hours of presentation, controversy exists regarding fluid management strategies in the next 2 days or so, especially in patients with ARDS. Beginning an average of about 48 hours after admission to the ICU and 24 hours after the establishment of ARDS, conservative fluid therapy to maintain euvolemia provides significantly better lung and central nervous system function as well as a decreased need for sedation, mechanical ventilation, and ICU care compared with more aggressive fluid therapy.[A7] However, patients who receive conservative volume replacement transiently may need more vasopressor support. One of the negative attributes of an open-ended and oftentimes aggressive fluid resuscitation strategy is that patients may develop an intra-abdominal compartment syndrome in which elevated abdominal pressures impair gas exchange, decrease renal perfusion, decrease visceral organ perfusion, impair venous return, and thereby decrease cardiac output and systemic oxygen delivery.[9]

Hemoglobin

In hemorrhagic shock, the rapid administration of packed red blood cells and, if indicated, platelets and thawed fresh-frozen plasma can be life-saving. Whenever possible, fully crossmatched packed red blood cells are preferable, but type-specific blood can often be given safely when immediate therapy is warranted (Chapter 177). In dire emergencies, type O Rh-negative blood can be administered to women of childbearing potential, and type O Rh-negative or Rh-positive blood can be given to men or postmenopausal women.

Shock

	Hypovolemic	Cardiogenic	Extracardiac/Obstructive	Distributive	Dissociative
Definition	Blood or fluid loss, both leading to a decreased circulating blood volume, diastolic filling pressure, and volume.	Severe reduction in cardiac function resulting from direct myocardial damage or a mechanical abnormality of the heart.	Obstruction to flow in the cardiovascular circuit that leads to inadequate diastolic filling or decreased systolic function because of increased afterload.	Arterial and venous dilation leads to a decrease in preload, with decreased, normal, or elevated cardiac output, depending on the presence of myocardial depression. Inflammatory causes produce micro-circulatory dysfunction, hypotension, and multiple organ system dysfunction without a decrease in cardiac output.	Impairment of oxygen utilization or impairment of the cellular machinery.
Etiologies	**Hemorrhagic:** Trauma Gastrointestinal Retroperitoneal Postoperative surgical procedures **Fluid depletion (nonhemorrhagic):** External fluid loss Dehydration Vomiting Diarrhea Polyuria **Interstitial fluid redistribution:** Thermal injury Trauma Anaphylaxis **Increased vascular capacitance (venodilation):** Sepsis Anaphylaxis Toxins/drugs	**Myopathic:** Myocardial infarction Left ventricle Right ventricle **Myocardial contusion (trauma):** Myocarditis Cardiomyopathy Postischemic myocardial stunning Septic myocardial depression Pharmacologic Anthracycline cardiotoxicity Calcium-channel blockers **Mechanical:** Valvular failure (stenotic or regurgitant) Hypertrophic cardiomyopathy Ventricular septal defect **Arrhythmias:** Bradycardia Tachycardia	**Impaired diastolic filling (decreased ventricular preload):** Direct venous obstruction (vena cava) Intrathoracic obstructive tumors **Increased intrathoracic pressure:** Tension pneumothorax Mechanical ventilation (with excessive pressure or volume depletion) Asthma **Decreased cardiac compliance:** Constrictive pericarditis Cardiac tamponade **Impaired systolic contraction (increased ventricular afterload):** Right ventricle Pulmonary embolus (massive) Air embolus Acute pulmonary hypertension Left ventricle occlusion or aortic dissection	Septic (bacterial, fungal, viral, rickettsial) Toxic shock syndrome Anaphylactic anaphylactoid Neurogenic (spinal shock) Endocrinologic Adrenal crisis Thyroid storm	Toxic (e.g., nitroprusside, bretylium, cyanide) End-stage sepsis Catecholamine toxicity

A

FIGURE 106-3. Definitions, etiologies, and therapies of various shock states. CI = cardiac index; CO = cardiac output; CT = computed tomography; CVP = central venous pressure; Do_2 = systemic oxygen delivery; ECG = electrocardiogram; LV = left ventricular; MAP = mean arterial pressure; MRI = magnetic resonance imaging; PA = pulmonary artery; PAOP = pulmonary artery occlusion pressure; RA = right atrial; RV = right ventricular; SVR = systemic vascular resistance; US = ultrasonography; VSD = ventricular septal defect.

Hemodynamic Characterization					
CVP/RA	↓	↑	↑↑	↓ early, normal later	↓ early, normal to ↑ later
PAOP	↓	↓ early, ↑ later	↓	↓ early, normal later	↓ early, normal to ↑ later
CO/CI/Do_2	↓	↓↓	↕	↓ early, ↑ later	↓ early, ↑ later
SVR	↑	↑	↑	↑ early, ↓ later	↑ early, ↓ later
Svo_2/$Scvo_2$	↓	↓	↓	↓ early, ↑ later	↑ early, ↑↑ later
Comments	Preexisting heart disease may alter the filling pressures	If there is a VSD, there may be $Scvo_2$/Svo_2 or a step up from the right atrium to right ventricle to the pulmonary artery. Large V wave is seen on PA catheter with mitral regurgitation.	Equalization of intracardiac diastolic pressure is consistent with pericardial tamponade. A rapid x and blunted y descent on CVP wave form indicates the inability of the heart to fill.	In the early stage, filling pressures are low, leading to low to normal cardiac output and variable $Scvo_2$/Svo_2. If myocardial depression accompanies, then a similar profile of cardiogenic shock is seen. After resuscitation a hyperdynamic circulation is seen.	Filling pressures can be variable, depending on stage of the disease. Cardiac output is generally increased. SVR is decreased and $Scvo_2$/Svo_2 and lactate are increased.
Therapy	Rapid replacement of blood, colloid or crystalloid Identify source of blood/fluid loss Replace deficient coagulation factors Consider factor VIIa Endoscopy/colonoscopy Angiography CT/MRI/US or other	LV infarction: intra-aortic balloon pump (IABP) coronary angiography Recanalization: thrombolytic therapy, angioplasty, coronary bypass surgery RV infarction: fluids and inotropes with PA catheter Mechanical abnormality: echocardiography, cardiac catheterization Corrective surgery: mechanical assist devices, transplantation	Pericardial tamponade: pericardiocentesis, surgical drainage (if needed) Pneumothorax: chest tube Pulmonary embolism: heparin, ventilation-perfusion lung scan, pulmonary angiography, consider thrombolytic therapy, embolectomy Severe hypertension: afterload reduction	Identify site of infection Antimicrobial agents Early goal-directed therapy: fluids, vasopressors, inotropic agents Goals: Sco_2 > 70%; CVP > 8 mm Hg; MAP > 65 mm Hg; Improving organ function; Decreasing lactate levels Consider activated protein C Requiring vasopressors, consider corticosteroids	Toxin antidote or remove agent, hyperbaric oxygen therapy Recombinant activated protein C Nitroglycerin (speculative) Prostacyclin (speculative)

B

FIGURE 106-3, cont'd.

TABLE 106-5 FLUID THERAPY

Normal saline	Normal saline is a slightly hyperosmolar solution containing 154 mEq/L of both sodium and chloride. Because of the relatively high chloride concentration and low pH, normal saline carries a risk of inducing hyperchloremic metabolic acidosis when it is given in large amounts.
Lactated Ringer solution (LR)	Lactate is metabolized to carbon dioxide (CO_2) and water by the liver, leading to the release of CO_2 in the lungs and excretion of water by the kidneys. LR is preferred to normal saline and buffers acidemia. Because LR contains a very small amount of potassium, there is a small risk of inducing hyperkalemia in patients with renal insufficiency or renal failure. LR may be incompletely metabolized in severe hepatic failure.
Albumin	Albumin is a protein derived from human plasma and is available in varying concentrations from 4 to 25%. A study comparing fluid resuscitation with albumin versus saline found similar 28-day mortalities and secondary outcomes in each arm. However, a post hoc subset analysis of patients with sepsis and acute lung injury resuscitated with albumin showed a trend toward a decrease in mortality. There was a significant increase in mortality in trauma patients, particularly those with head injury.
Hydroxyethyl starch (HES)	HES, which is a synthetic colloid derived from hydrolyzed amylopectin, causes renal impairment at recommended doses and impaired long-term survival at high doses. HES can also cause coagulopathy and bleeding complications from reduced factor VIII and von Willebrand factor levels as well as impaired platelet function. HES increases the risk of acute renal failure and reduces the probability of survival in patients with sepsis.
Dextrans	Dextrans are artificial colloids synthesized by *Leuconostoc mesenteroides* bacteria grown in sucrose media. Dextrans are used more frequently to lower blood viscosity than for rapid plasma expansion. They can cause renal dysfunction as well as anaphylactoid reactions.
Gelatins	Gelatins are produced from bovine collagen. Because they have a small molecular weight, they are not very effective at expanding plasma volume, but they cost less than other options. They have been reported to cause renal impairment as well as allergic reactions ranging from pruritus to anaphylaxis. Gelatins are not currently available in North America.

The appropriate hemoglobin level in shock remains controversial, but a transfusion threshold value of ≥7 g/dL is as good as a transfusion threshold of 9 g/dL in septic shock.[A8] A hemoglobin value of 7 to 10 g/dL is appropriate when the patient is in the acute but stable phase of upper gastrointestinal bleeding.[A9]

Vasopressor Therapy

To optimize end-organ perfusion, the second phase of intervention after adequate fluid therapy is to maintain perfusion pressure. A specific MAP goal has not been established for all shock states, but a MAP of at least 60 to 65 mm Hg is a reasonable target.

The most common vasopressors are agonists at various adrenergic receptors. Receptors include peripheral α-adrenergic receptors that lead to vasoconstriction; cardiac β_1 receptors with both chronotropic and inotropic effects; β_2 receptors located in the circulation and airways that mediate vasodilation and bronchodilation; and dopaminergic receptors located throughout the cardiovascular, mesenteric, and renal circulations. On the basis of these mechanisms, therapy can be tailored to a specific circumstance. For example, a patient with severe tachycardia would be best served by an agent with more α-selective activity and less β activity to avoid tachycardia and increased myocardial oxygen consumption (see Table 106-4).

Norepinephrine, which is a vasoconstrictor and an inotrope, provides better splanchnic oxygen utilization compared with dopamine. It is generally considered the first-line vasopressor for treating persistent hypotension in septic patients despite adequate resuscitation, and it may be superior to dopamine in treating cardiogenic shock. For example, a randomized trial comparing dopamine with norepinephrine in patients with shock showed no significant difference in mortality for hypovolemic and septic shock but a significant benefit of norepinephrine in cardiogenic shock.[A10] In addition, there was a significant two-fold increase in arrhythmic events with dopamine compared with norepinephrine (24.1 vs. 12.4%).

Dopamine's effects result from transduction at dopaminergic receptors in the renal, mesenteric, coronary, and systemic circulations. The positive chronotropic and inotropic effects of dopamine can lead to tachycardia and tachyarrhythmias; this effect frequently limits its dosing because the increased myocardial oxygen requirements promote the development of myocardial ischemia, especially in the presence of coronary artery disease.

Phenylephrine is a synthetic catecholamine that is a selective α-adrenergic agonist and is ideal in patients with tachycardia. However, the resulting increase in myocardial oxygen consumption, decrease in splanchnic blood flow, and decrease in cardiac output can be detrimental for patients with septic shock.

Epinephrine, which is a potent α-, β_1-, and β_2-adrenergic agonist, increases peripheral arteriolar tone as well as cardiac contractility. It is the first-line agent for the treatment of anaphylactic shock and is used to support myocardial contractility after cardiac surgery. Epinephrine increases the white blood cell count and the blood lactate concentration because of accelerated aerobic glycogenolysis or maldistribution of blood flow.

Vasopressin deficiency accompanies vasodilatory shock, and administration of low doses of vasopressin (0.03–0.04 units/minute) increases arterial blood pressure in septic patients with intractable hypotension. In patients with septic shock, the addition of low-dose vasopressin to norepinephrine does not have any overall benefit,[A11] but it may benefit patients who have less severe forms of shock and who also receive glucocorticoids.[10]

Adrenal Dysfunction

Beyond their metabolic functions, glucocorticoids are required to maintain responsiveness to vasopressors, intravascular volume, vascular permeability, and myocardial contractility. If the hypothalamic-pituitary-adrenocortical axis is depressed in shock, clinical findings can include unexplained fever, hypoglycemia, hyponatremia, hyperkalemia, metabolic acidosis, hypotension refractory to fluid resuscitation, and eosinophilia. Cortisol levels and the results of cosyntropin stimulation testing may not be clinically helpful.[11] If adrenal insufficiency is strongly suspected, or if patients have refractory hypotension despite vasopressors and hemodynamic optimization, stress doses of intravenous hydrocortisone (e.g., 50 mg every 6 hours) are recommended.[A12]

Mechanical Support

Mechanical hemodynamic support with an intra-aortic balloon may be indicated in cardiogenic shock, but it does not improve survival in patients with acute myocardial infarction.[A13] Extracorporeal membrane oxygenation is another temporary option for cardiopulmonary support in patients with ARDS until more definitive long-term interventions can be performed.[12]

PROGNOSIS

Clinical characteristics associated with a poor outcome include the severity of shock; its temporal duration, underlying cause, and reversibility; and preexisting vital organ dysfunction. Decreased systemic oxygen consumption, persistently elevated lactate levels, size of the base deficit, and severity of the anion gap are associated with increased organ failure and are prognostic in trauma, in septic shock, and after cardiac arrest. Regional measurements of pH are highly predictive of outcome; for example, if the gastric mucosal pH remains below 7.3 for 24 hours, the hospital mortality rate is about 50%. Although many of these poor prognostic signs are suggestive of microcirculatory failure, no targeted therapies yet exist to reverse this disorder. The mortality for an undiagnosed patient who is sent to a general medical ward and develops shock is three times higher than for a patient who is admitted directly to the ICU.

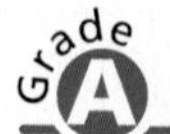

Grade A References

A1. Papazian L, Forel JM, Gacouin A, et al. Neuromuscular blockers in early acute respiratory distress syndrome. *N Engl J Med*. 2010;363:1107-1116.

A2. Wheeler AP, Bernard GR, Thompson BT, et al. Pulmonary-artery versus central venous catheter to guide treatment of acute lung injury. *N Engl J Med*. 2006;354:2213-2224.

A3. Wang JW, Li JP, Song YL, et al. Hypertonic saline in the traumatic hypovolemic shock: meta-analysis. *J Surg Res*. 2014;191:448-454.

A4. Rochwerg B, Alhazzani W, Sindi A, et al. Fluid resuscitation in sepsis: a systematic review and network meta-analysis. *Ann Intern Med*. 2014;161:347-355.

A5. Annane D, Siami S, Jaber S, et al. Effects of fluid resuscitation with colloids vs crystalloids on mortality in critically ill patients presenting with hypovolemic shock: the CRISTAL randomized trial. *JAMA*. 2013;310:1809-1817.

A6. Zarychanski R, Abou-Setta AM, Turgeon AF, et al. Association of hydroxyethyl starch administration with mortality and acute kidney injury in critically ill patients requiring volume resuscitation: a systematic review and meta-analysis. *JAMA*. 2013;309:678-688.
A7. Wiedemann HP, Wheeler AP, Bernard GR, et al. Comparison of two fluid-management strategies in acute lung injury. *N Engl J Med*. 2006;354:2564-2575.
A8. Holst LB, Haase N, Wetterslev J, et al. Lower versus higher hemoglobin threshold for transfusion in septic shock. *N Engl J Med*. 2014;371:1381-1391.
A9. Villanueva C, Colomo A, Bosch A, et al. Transfusion strategies for acute upper gastrointestinal bleeding. *N Engl J Med*. 2013;368:11-21.
A10. De Backer D, Biston P, Devriendt J, et al. Comparison of dopamine and norepinephrine in the treatment of shock. *N Engl J Med*. 2010;362:779-789.
A11. Russell JA, Walley KR, Singer J, et al. Vasopressin versus norepinephrine infusion in patients with septic shock. *N Engl J Med*. 2008;358:877-887.
A12. Sprung CL, Annane D, Keh D, et al. Hydrocortisone therapy for patients with septic shock. *N Engl J Med*. 2008;358:111-124.
A13. Thiele H, Zeymer U, Neumann FJ, et al. Intra-aortic balloon counterpulsation in acute myocardial infarction complicated by cardiogenic shock (IABP-SHOCK II): final 12 month results of a randomised, open-label trial. *Lancet*. 2013;382:1638-1645.

GENERAL REFERENCES

For the General References and other additional features, please visit Expert Consult at https://expertconsult.inkling.com.

107 CARDIOGENIC SHOCK

STEVEN M. HOLLENBERG

DEFINITION

Cardiogenic shock is the syndrome that ensues when the heart is unable to deliver enough blood to maintain adequate tissue perfusion.[1] The hemodynamic picture includes sustained systemic hypotension, pulmonary capillary wedge pressure (PCWP) greater than 18 mm Hg, and cardiac index less than 2.2 L/minute/m^2 (Table 107-1). Although systolic blood pressure less than 90 mm Hg is a commonly accepted threshold for shock, a decrease of 30 mm Hg from baseline is also used. The diagnosis of cardiogenic shock is often made on clinical grounds—hypotension combined with signs of poor tissue perfusion, including oliguria, clouded sensorium, and cool extremities, all in the setting of myocardial dysfunction. To make the diagnosis, it is important to document myocardial dysfunction and to exclude or to correct factors such as hypovolemia, hypoxemia, and acidosis.

EPIDEMIOLOGY

The predominant cause of cardiogenic shock (Fig. 107-1) is left ventricular failure secondary to acute myocardial infarction (MI)—an extensive first acute MI, the cumulative loss of myocardial function in a patient with previous MI or cardiomyopathy, or a mechanical complication of MI (Chapter 73). However, any cause of severe left ventricular (LV) or right ventricular (RV) dysfunction can lead to cardiogenic shock, including end-stage cardiomyopathy (Chapter 60), prolonged cardiopulmonary bypass, valvular disease (Chapter 75), myocardial contusion (Chapter 111), sepsis with unusually profound myocardial depression (Chapter 108), and fulminant myocarditis (Chapter 60) (Table 107-2). Stress-induced (takotsubo) cardiomyopathy (Chapter 60), a syndrome of acute apical LV dysfunction that occurs after emotional distress, may also be manifested with cardiogenic shock. Acute valvular regurgitation, most often caused by endocarditis (Chapter 76) or chordal rupture (Chapter 75), can lead to shock, as can physiologic stress in the setting of severe valvular stenosis. Cardiac tamponade (Chapter 77) and massive pulmonary embolism (Chapter 98) with acute RV failure can cause shock without pulmonary edema.

The incidence and mortality associated with cardiogenic shock appear to be declining.[2] In the past 30 years, the incidence has fallen from about 8% to 6% of MIs, largely because of the benefit of early perfusion strategies (Chapter 73). In parallel, mortality from cardiogenic shock has decreased from 70 to 80% to 50% or less, suggesting that increasingly effective early treatment and more widespread adoption of early revascularization have improved the outcomes of patients in whom shock has already developed.

TABLE 107-1 DIAGNOSIS OF CARDIOGENIC SHOCK

CLINICAL SIGNS
Hypotension
Oliguria
Clouded sensorium
Cool and mottled extremities
HEMODYNAMIC CRITERIA
Systolic blood pressure < 90 mm Hg or > 30 mm Hg decrease from baseline for > 30 minutes
Cardiac index < 2.2 L/min/m^2
Pulmonary capillary wedge pressure > 18 mm Hg
OTHER
Documented myocardial dysfunction
Exclusion of hypovolemia, hypoxia, and acidosis

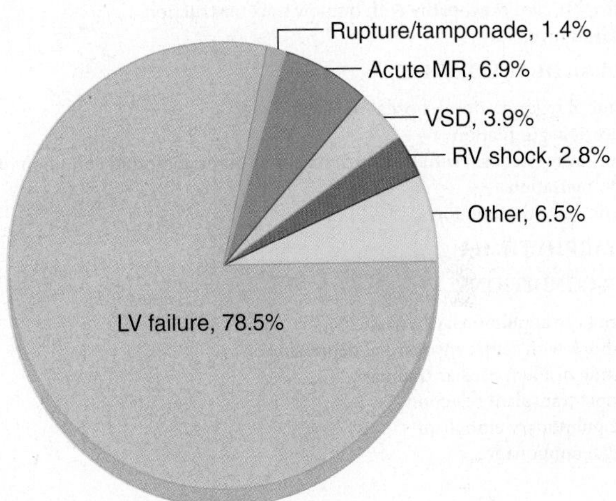

FIGURE 107-1. Causes of cardiogenic shock in patients with myocardial infarction in the SHOCK trial registry. LV = left ventricular; MR = mitral regurgitation; RV = right ventricular; VSD = ventricular septal defect. (Modified from Hochman JS, Boland J, Sleeper LA, et al. Current spectrum of cardiogenic shock and effect of early revascularization on mortality. Results of an International Registry. SHOCK Registry Investigators. *Circulation*. 1995;91:873-881).

Risk factors for the development of cardiogenic shock in MI parallel those for LV dysfunction and the severity of coronary artery disease (CAD). Characteristics of patients include older age, anterior MI, diabetes, hypertension, multivessel CAD, previous MI, and peripheral vascular and cerebrovascular disease. Clinical risk factors include decreased ejection fractions, larger infarctions, and lack of compensatory hyperkinesis in myocardial territories remote from the infarction. Clinical harbingers of impending shock include the degree of hypotension and tachycardia at hospital presentation. The factors that predict mortality reflect the severity of the acute insult as well as comorbid conditions.

Coronary angiography most often demonstrates multivessel CAD. About 30% of patients have a left main coronary artery occlusion, about 60% have three-vessel coronary disease, and only about 20% have single-vessel disease. Multivessel CAD helps explain the failure to develop compensatory hyperkinesis in remote myocardial segments because of either previous infarction or high-grade coronary stenoses.

Only one fourth of patients who develop cardiogenic shock are in shock when they initially present to the hospital; in the others, shock usually evolves during several hours, suggesting that early treatment may prevent shock. Comparison of the clinical characteristics of patients with early and late shock shows similar demographic, historical, clinical, and hemodynamic characteristics, but shock tends to develop earlier in patients with single-vessel CAD than in those with triple-vessel disease. This finding suggests that early shock in the setting of acute MI may be more amenable to revascularization of the culprit vessel by thrombolysis or angioplasty (Chapter 73), whereas shock developing later may require more complete revascularization with multivessel percutaneous coronary intervention (PCI) or coronary artery bypass graft (CABG) surgery (Chapter 74).

TABLE 107-2 CAUSES OF CARDIOGENIC SHOCK

ACUTE MYOCARDIAL INFARCTION
Pump failure
Large infarction
Smaller infarction with preexisting left ventricular dysfunction
Infarct extension
Reinfarction
Infarct expansion
Mechanical complications
Acute mitral regurgitation due to papillary muscle rupture
Ventricular septal defect
Free wall rupture
Pericardial tamponade
Right ventricular infarction
CARDIOMYOPATHY
Myocarditis
Peripartum cardiomyopathy
End-stage low-output heart failure
Hypertrophic cardiomyopathy with outflow tract obstruction
Stress cardiomyopathy
VALVULAR HEART DISEASE
Acute mitral regurgitation (chordal rupture)
Acute aortic regurgitation
Aortic or mitral stenosis with tachyarrhythmia or other comorbid condition causing decompensation
Prosthetic valve dysfunction
TACHYARRHYTHMIA
OTHER CONDITIONS
Prolonged cardiopulmonary bypass
Septic shock with severe myocardial depression
Penetrating or blunt cardiac trauma
Orthotopic transplant rejection
Massive pulmonary embolism
Pericardial tamponade

PATHOBIOLOGY

Cardiogenic shock is characterized by a downward cascade in which myocardial dysfunction reduces stroke volume, cardiac output, and blood pressure; these changes compromise myocardial perfusion, exacerbate ischemia, and further depress myocardial function, cardiac output, and systemic perfusion. Concomitant diastolic dysfunction increases left atrial pressure, which leads to pulmonary congestion and hypoxemia that can exacerbate myocardial ischemia and impair ventricular performance.

Compensatory mechanisms include sympathetic stimulation, which increases heart rate and contractility, and renal fluid retention, which increases preload. Increases in heart rate and contractility raise output but also increase myocardial oxygen demand. Another compensatory mechanism, vasoconstriction to maintain blood pressure, increases myocardial afterload, further impairing cardiac performance and increasing myocardial oxygen demand. In the face of inadequate perfusion, this increased demand can worsen ischemia and perpetuate a vicious circle that, if unbroken, may culminate in death. Interruption of this circle of myocardial dysfunction and ischemia is the basis for therapeutic regimens for cardiogenic shock.

In cardiogenic shock, LV dysfunction is not always severe. In one large study, the mean LV ejection fraction was 30%, indicating that mechanisms other than primary pump failure were operative. Furthermore, systemic vascular resistance is not always elevated, suggesting that compensatory vasoconstriction is not universal. Inflammatory responses may contribute to the vasodilation and myocardial dysfunction in cardiogenic shock.

Patients in cardiogenic shock may have areas of nonfunctional but viable myocardium due to stunning or hibernation. Myocardial stunning represents postischemic dysfunction that persists despite restoration of normal blood flow. Hibernating myocardial segments have persistently impaired function at rest because of severely reduced coronary blood flow. Although hibernation is conceptually different from stunning, the two conditions may not differ much clinically. Repetitive episodes of myocardial stunning can occur in areas of viable myocardium subtended by a critical coronary stenosis. Such episodes can recapitulate the hibernation phenotype, blurring the distinction between myocardial stunning and hibernation. Regardless of the degree of overlap, their therapeutic implications differ in cardiogenic shock. The contractile function of hibernating myocardium improves with revascularization, whereas stunned myocardium retains inotropic reserve and can respond to inotropic stimulation. In addition, the severity of the antecedent ischemic insult determines the intensity of stunning, providing a rationale for reestablishing the patency of occluded coronary arteries in patients with cardiogenic shock. Finally, the notion that some myocardial tissue may recover function emphasizes the importance of measures to support the patient hemodynamically and to minimize myocardial necrosis in patients with shock.

TABLE 107-3 CLINICAL SIGNS OF VOLUME STATUS AND PERFUSION

SIGNS AND SYMPTOMS OF CONGESTION
Orthopnea, paroxysmal nocturnal dyspnea
Jugular venous distention
Abdominojugular reflux
Rales
Hepatomegaly
Edema
Right upper quadrant tenderness
POSSIBLE EVIDENCE OF LOW PERFUSION
Narrow pulse pressure
Obtundation
Cool extremities
Cachexia, muscle loss
Decreased exercise tolerance
Renal/hepatic dysfunction
Hypotension with angiotensin-converting enzyme inhibition

CLINICAL MANIFESTATIONS

The physical examination should be geared toward evaluating congestion and systemic perfusion to characterize the patient's hemodynamic profile (Table 107-3). An assessment of whether the patient is "wet" or "dry" and "cold" or "warm" is integral to management. Signs of congestion (Chapter 58) include jugular venous distention (see Fig. 51-3) and pulmonary rales and may include peripheral edema and ascites. Whether the patient is cold or warm is an indication of systemic perfusion.

The majority of the cardiogenic shock patients present wet and cold. Patients with shock are usually ashen or cyanotic, and they have cool skin and mottled extremities. Cerebral hypoperfusion may cloud the sensorium. Pulses, which are rapid and faint, may be irregular in the presence of arrhythmias. Jugular venous distention and pulmonary rales are usually present, although their absence does not exclude the diagnosis. A precordial heave resulting from LV dyskinesis may be palpable. The heart sounds may be distant, and third and fourth heart sounds are usually present. A systolic murmur of mitral regurgitation or a ventricular septal defect may be heard, but either complication can occur without an audible murmur (Chapter 73).

DIAGNOSIS

After recognizing the clinical manifestations of apparent cardiogenic shock, the clinician must confirm its presence and assess its cause while simultaneously initiating supportive therapy before irreversible damage to vital organs ensues. The clinician must balance overzealous pursuit of an etiologic diagnosis before achieving stabilization with overzealous empirical treatment without establishing the underlying pathophysiologic process.

An electrocardiogram (ECG) should be performed immediately. In cardiogenic shock caused by acute MI, the ECG most commonly shows ST elevation, but ST depression or nonspecific changes are found in 25% of cases. If RV infarction is suspected, ST elevation in modified right-sided leads may be diagnostic (Chapter 73). The ECG may also provide information on previous MIs and rhythm abnormalities. A relatively normal ECG or one showing only diffuse, nonspecific changes in a patient with clinical cardiogenic shock should suggest myocarditis (Chapter 60), especially if the patient has arrhythmias. In end-stage heart failure, the ECG may show Q waves or bundle branch block, indicative of extensive disease.

Other initial diagnostic tests include a chest radiograph, complete blood count, and measurement of arterial blood gases, electrolytes, and cardiac biomarkers. A high-quality chest film can assess signs of pulmonary edema and is helpful when signs suggest an alternative diagnosis, such as a widened mediastinum indicative of aortic dissection (Chapter 78).

Echocardiography

Echocardiography should be performed as early as possible, preferably with color flow Doppler, to provide an expeditious assessment of cardiac chamber size, LV and RV function, valvular structure and motion, atrial size, and the pericardium (Chapter 55). Echocardiography can also assess or diagnose overall and regional systolic function, diastolic function, papillary muscle rupture, acute ventricular septal defect, free wall rupture, degree of mitral regurgitation, presence of RV infarction, cardiac tamponade, and valvular stenosis.

Right-Sided Heart Catheterization

If the history, physical examination, chest radiograph, and echocardiogram demonstrate systemic hypoperfusion, low cardiac output, and elevation of venous pressures, right-sided heart catheterization may not be necessary for diagnosis. However, therapy with vasopressors and inotropic agents is best optimized with hemodynamic measurements. Right-sided heart catheterization can exclude other causes of shock, such as volume depletion and sepsis. A step-up in oxygen saturation between the right atrium and pulmonary artery can indicate a ventricular septal defect (Chapter 69), and large *v* waves in the PCWP waveform can reflect acute severe mitral regurgitation. RV infarction should be suspected when the PCWP is normal but right-sided filling pressures are notably elevated.

Right-sided heart catheterization is most useful, however, to optimize therapy in unstable patients. In such patients, clinical estimates of filling pressures can be unreliable, and changes in myocardial performance or therapeutic interventions can change cardiac output and filling pressures precipitously. Although patients with a low cardiac index (<2.2 L/minute/m^2) and a PCWP greater than 18 mm Hg meet the definition of cardiogenic shock, optimal filling pressures may be even higher in individual patients with LV diastolic dysfunction.

TREATMENT Rx

Initial Management

Initial stabilization of the patient with suspected cardiogenic shock consists of venous access, supplemental oxygen, and continuous ECG monitoring (Fig. 107-2). Many patients require endotracheal intubation and mechanical ventilation (Chapter 105), if only to reduce the work of breathing and to facilitate sedation and stabilization before cardiac catheterization. Electrolyte abnormalities should be corrected. Morphine (1 to 2 mg every 5 minutes) relieves pain and anxiety, reduces excessive sympathetic activity, and decreases oxygen demand, preload, and afterload. Atrial bradyarrhythmias or tachyarrhythmias (Chapter 64) or ventricular tachyarrhythmias can reduce cardiac output and should be corrected promptly with antiarrhythmic drugs (see Table 64-6), cardioversion, or pacing (Chapter 66).

If the cause is likely to be an acute MI, aspirin and heparin should be given immediately (Chapter 73). Some therapies routinely used in acute MI (e.g., nitrates, β-blockers, angiotensin-converting enzyme inhibitors) have the potential to exacerbate hypotension in cardiogenic shock and have recently been associated with poorer outcomes in hypotensive patients.[3] As a result, they should be avoided in patients with a tenuous hemodynamic status until they stabilize.

An initial assessment of fluid status and systemic perfusion should be performed. Patients are commonly diaphoretic, and relative hypovolemia may be present. Ischemia produces diastolic dysfunction, so high filling pressures may be necessary to maintain stroke volume in some patients. Some patients may benefit from judicious fluid replacement with predetermined rapid bolus infusions of 100 to 200 mL of normal saline titrated to clinical end points. Patients who do not respond rapidly to initial treatment should be considered for invasive hemodynamic monitoring to identify the filling pressure at which cardiac output is maximized. Maintenance of adequate preload is particularly important in patients with RV infarction.

After initial stabilization and restoration of adequate blood pressure, tissue perfusion should be assessed. If tissue perfusion is adequate but significant pulmonary congestion remains, low-dose diuretics may be used, with care taken not to remove too much fluid. If tissue perfusion remains inadequate, inotropic support or mechanical support should be initiated.

Vasopressors and Inotropes

Maintenance of adequate blood pressure is essential to break the vicious circle of progressive hypotension and further myocardial ischemia. When arterial pressure remains inadequate, therapy with vasopressor agents, titrated not only to blood pressure but also to clinical indices of perfusion and mixed venous oxygen saturation, may be required.[3] Norepinephrine and dopamine are considered first-line drugs for hypotension in this situation. Dopamine acts as both an inotrope (particularly at 3 to 10 μg/kg/minute) and a vasopressor (10 to 20 μg/kg/minute). Norepinephrine (0.02 to 1.0 μg/kg/minute) acts primarily as a vasoconstrictor, has a mild inotropic effect, and increases coronary flow. In a randomized trial of patients with shock, there was no significant difference overall in 28-day mortality between those receiving dopamine and those receiving norepinephrine, but norepinephrine reduced mortality in a prespecified subgroup of patients with cardiogenic shock.[A1] Vasopressor infusions need to be titrated carefully in patients with cardiogenic shock to maximize coronary perfusion pressure with the least possible increase in myocardial oxygen demand. Invasive hemodynamic monitoring with an arterial line and temporary right-sided heart catheterization are advisable during the initial titration of vasoactive agents.[4]

If tissue perfusion remains inadequate despite norepinephrine, inotropic therapy should be initiated. Dobutamine (2.5 to 20 μg/kg/minute), a selective β_1-adrenergic receptor agonist, can improve myocardial contractility and increase cardiac output, and it is the initial agent of choice in patients with a low-output syndrome and systolic blood pressures greater than 90 mm Hg. Dobutamine may exacerbate hypotension in some patients because of its vasodilatory effects, and it can precipitate tachyarrhythmias. Milrinone (0.125 to 0.75 μg/kg/minute), a phosphodiesterase inhibitor, has fewer chronotropic and arrhythmogenic effects than catecholamines, but it has a long half-life and can cause hypotension; in patients whose clinical status is tenuous, it is usually reserved for situations in which other agents have proved ineffective. Levosimendan (0.05 to 0.2 μg/kg/minute) is a calcium sensitizer that has both inotropic and vasodilatory properties and does not increase myocardial oxygen consumption. Levosimendan may be more effective than dobutamine in treating low-output heart failure,[A2] but it also may cause hypotension, and it must be used with caution in patients with cardiogenic shock. A randomized trial of nitric oxide inhibition did not show benefit.[A3]

Intra-aortic Balloon Counterpulsation

An intra-aortic balloon pump (IABP) reduces systolic afterload and augments diastolic perfusion pressure without increasing oxygen demand. Despite a convincing hemodynamic rationale for its use, however, a recent randomized trial failed to show improvement in 30-day[A4] or 1-year mortality[A5] with IABP insertion in patients who have cardiogenic shock and who undergo early revascularization, perhaps because IABPs do not produce a significant improvement in blood flow distal to a critical coronary stenosis. Although this finding has dampened enthusiasm for their routine use, these trial results may not be applicable to all patients. Use of an IABP still may be a reasonable stabilizing measure in appropriately selected patients, such as supporting patients through a critical period of shock until definitive therapy is undertaken.

Reperfusion

Supportive therapy may improve blood pressure and cardiac output in cardiogenic shock, but it does not interrupt the vicious circle of myocardial dysfunction and ischemia. Rapid restoration of myocardial blood flow is the cornerstone of therapy for patients with cardiogenic shock due to MI (Chapter 73). Reperfusion therapy (see Fig. 73-3) restores patency of the infarcted artery and decreases the likelihood of progression to cardiogenic shock. After cardiogenic shock has already developed, however, fibrinolytic therapy is less effective at achieving and maintaining reperfusion, probably because of a combination of hemodynamic, mechanical, and metabolic factors that prevent the achievement and maintenance of patency in the infarct-related artery.

Prompt revascularization is the only intervention that consistently reduces mortality rates in patients with cardiogenic shock. In a randomized trial of patients with LV failure complicating ST elevation MI, cardiac catheterization with PCI or CABG within 48 hours of presentation reduced all-cause mortality marginally at 30 days (47% in the revascularization group vs. 56% in the medical therapy group; $P = 0.11$) and significantly at 6 months, 1 year,[A6] and 6 years[A7] compared with optimal medical management, including IABP, in 86% of patients. Subgroup analyses also revealed benefits in patients younger than 75 years, those with prior MI, and those randomized less than 6 hours from the onset of infarction. Another similarly designed trial, which was terminated early because of difficulties in patient recruitment, also showed a trend toward reduced 30-day and 1-year mortality. Together, these

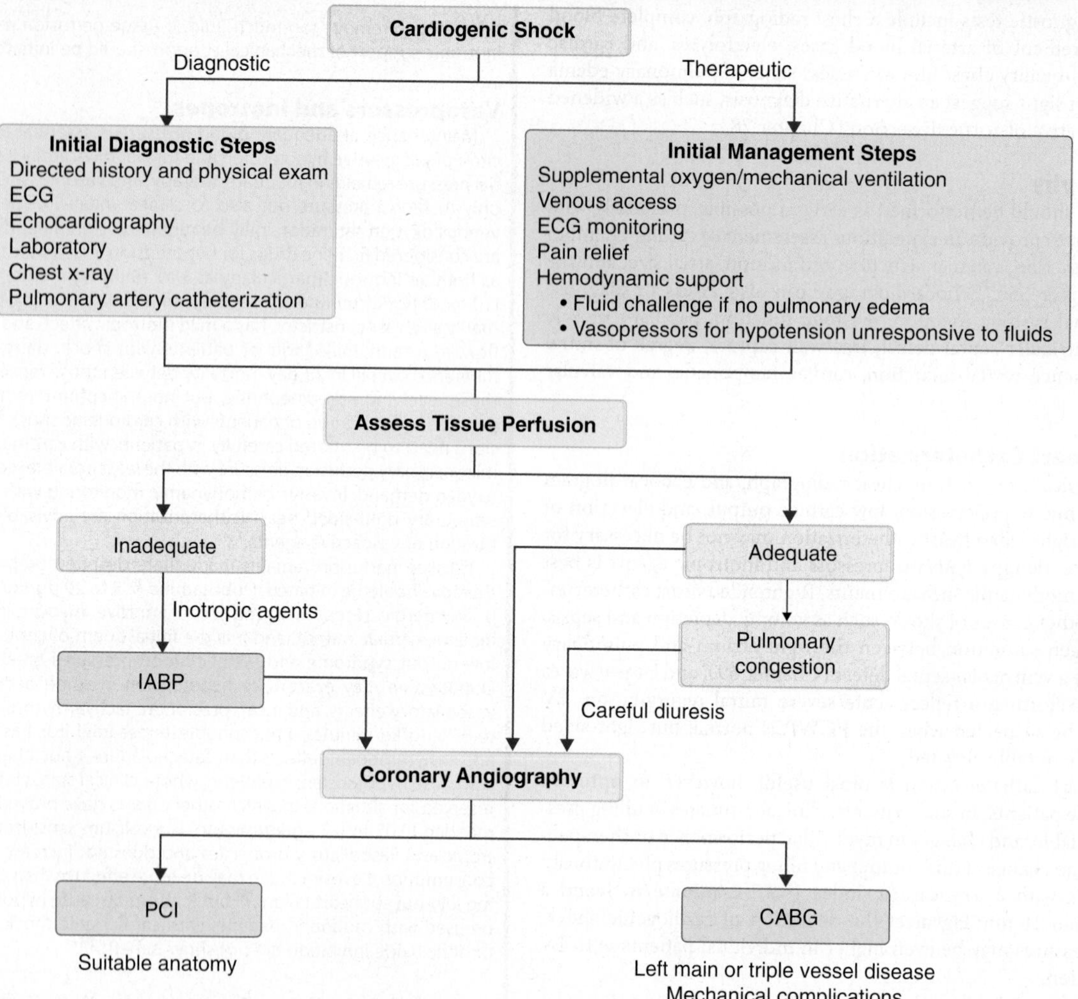

FIGURE 107-2. **Approach to the diagnosis and treatment of cardiogenic shock caused by myocardial infarction. Right ventricular infarction and mechanical complications are discussed in the text. CABG = coronary artery bypass graft; ECG = electrocardiogram; IABP = intra-aortic balloon pump; PCI = percutaneous coronary intervention. (Modified from Hochman JS, Boland J, Sleeper LA, et al. Current spectrum of cardiogenic shock and effect of early revascularization on mortality. Results of an International Registry. SHOCK Registry Investigators. *Circulation*. 1995;91:873-881.)**

trials suggest that about 13 patients will be saved at 1 year for each 100 patients treated.[A8]

On the basis of these results, emergent coronary revascularization, most often with PCI and stents, is the standard of care for cardiogenic shock due to pump failure in acute MI. Outcomes are best when PCI is performed within 6 hours after the onset of symptoms, but survival benefits are still demonstrable up to 48 hours after the onset of MI and 18 hours after the onset of shock. Elderly patients who are suitable for aggressive therapy also appear to benefit.

CABG surgery is more likely to provide complete revascularization and achieves long-term survival rates comparable to those of PCI, often despite worse coronary anatomy and a higher prevalence of diabetes. In practice, however, emergency CABG is performed less than 10% of the time.

When cardiogenic shock results from mechanical complications of MI (Chapter 73), surgery is recommended when feasible. For acute mitral regurgitation due to papillary muscle rupture, supportive therapy with an IABP and vasoactive agents is a temporizing measure; definitive therapy requires expeditious surgical valve repair or replacement (Chapter 75). Although mortality is 20 to 40%, survival and ventricular function are improved compared with medical therapy.

Timely surgery is also critical in patients whose cardiogenic shock is caused by ventricular septal or free wall rupture. Because perforations are exposed to shear forces, the rupture site can expand abruptly. Repair can be technically difficult because of the need to suture in areas of necrosis. Surgical mortality is 20 to 50% and is especially high for serpiginous inferoposterior ruptures, which are typically less well circumscribed than anteroapical ruptures. RV function is an important determinant of outcome in this setting. Timing of surgery has been controversial, but guidelines now recommend that operative repair be undertaken early, within 48 hours of the rupture. Placement of a septal occluding device may be helpful in selected patients.

Circulatory Support

Mechanical support with a left ventricular assist device (LVAD; Chapter 73) can interrupt the downward spiral of myocardial dysfunction, hypoperfusion, and ischemia in cardiogenic shock, allowing time for stunned or hibernating myocardium to recover. In cardiogenic shock after acute MI, percutaneous LVADs can be placed in the catheterization laboratory. These devices provide short-term support and are usually intended as a bridge to recovery or, occasionally, as a bridge to transplantation. Percutaneous LVADs provide better hemodynamics compared with IABPs, with higher cardiac indices and mean arterial pressures as well as lower filling pressures, but they have not been shown to improve mortality at 30 days.[A9] Extracorporeal support has been used in selected patients.[5]

Management of Special Conditions

At the end stage of a dilated or restrictive cardiomyopathy (Chapter 60), low cardiac output can result in cardiogenic shock. A search for reversible precipitating causes should be undertaken. Some patients will respond to inotropic therapy and will have a brief period of relative improvement. Appropriate candidates should be referred for evaluation for possible cardiac transplantation (Chapter 82). In selected patients, a surgically placed LVAD, such as a continuous-flow device, can provide 45% 2-year survival free of device surgery or disabling stroke.[6] LVADs can be used either as a bridge to transplantation or as destination therapy. A discussion about end-of-life care is also warranted.

Acute myocarditis (Chapter 60) can have a fulminant course leading to shock in 10 to 15% of cases. Patients with acute myocarditis are typically younger than those with cardiogenic shock due to MI, and they present more commonly with dyspnea rather than chest pain. Echocardiography usually shows global LV dysfunction. Supportive therapy is indicated; some patients may require circulatory support and even consideration of cardiac transplantation. Immunosuppressive therapy does not improve outcome in this setting.

Patients with hypertrophic cardiomyopathy (Chapter 60) may present with severe outflow tract obstruction and shock. Recognition of this condition is important because diuretic and inotropic therapy may worsen the obstruction. Careful volume resuscitation and use of a pure α-agonist, such as phenylephrine (0.1 to 0.3 mg/kg/minute), can increase afterload and cavity size. β-Blockers (esmolol, 0.05 to 0.2 mg/kg/minute; metoprolol, 2.5 to 5 mg IV every 2 to 5 minutes, up to 15 mg) or calcium blockers with negative inotropic properties (e.g., diltiazem, 5 mg IV every 2 minutes, up to 20 mg) can also be helpful.

Some patients with stress (takotsubo) cardiomyopathy (Chapter 60) may have LV dysfunction severe enough to produce shock. Because the presentation is similar to that of acute MI, with chest pain and ECG changes, the diagnosis is usually made in the catheterization laboratory, when significant coronary obstruction is excluded and the characteristic apical hypokinesis or dyskinesis is documented. Treatment is supportive and may include an IABP. Most patients have recovery of LV function within days to weeks, and the long-term prognosis is excellent.

Acute valvular regurgitation (Chapter 75) is manifested with pulmonary edema and decreased forward cardiac output. The regurgitant murmur may be soft or inaudible, and the diagnosis is best made by echocardiography. Acute ischemic mitral regurgitation is usually associated with rupture of the posterior papillary muscle, which has a single blood supply. Other causes include spontaneous chordal rupture, infective endocarditis (Chapter 76), rheumatic fever (Chapter 290), and trauma (Chapter 111). Immediate management includes afterload reduction (Chapter 59) and an IABP as temporizing measures. Inotropic or vasopressor therapy may also be needed to support cardiac output and blood pressure. Definitive therapy, however, consists of surgical valve repair or replacement (Chapter 75).

Acute aortic regurgitation most commonly results from infective endocarditis (Chapter 76) with leaflet destruction, but it may also be due to traumatic injury (Chapter 111) or acute aortic dissection (Chapter 78). The pulse pressure is usually narrow, indicating decreased forward stroke volume, and the bounding pulsations seen with chronic aortic regurgitation are usually absent. Temporizing measures include afterload reduction, with vasopressor and inotropic support as needed. IABP is contraindicated, and excessive slowing of the heart rate may worsen hemodynamics by prolonging diastole. Definitive therapy is surgical.

PROGNOSIS

Cardiogenic shock is still the most common cause of death in acute MI. Survival rates are improving, however, coincident with the increasing use of reperfusion therapy in appropriately selected patients. Hemodynamics predict short-term but not long-term mortality. Among patients undergoing revascularization, age, time to revascularization, and restoration of coronary blood flow independently predict survival, but the benefits of revascularization are seen at every level of risk, with an average 1-year survival of 50 to 55%. Encouragingly, the survival benefit of early revascularization is maintained at 6-year follow-up, with 5-year survival approaching 45%. The quality of life in survivors is usually excellent, with 83% either asymptomatic or having only mildly symptomatic heart failure.[A7] For patients with end-stage nonischemic myocardial disease, the prognosis is very poor in the absence of heart transplantation.

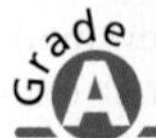

Grade A References

A1. De Backer D, Biston P, Devriendt J, et al. Comparison of dopamine and norepinephrine in the treatment of shock. *N Engl J Med*. 2010;362:779-789.

A2. Unverzagt S, Wachsmuth L, Hirsch K, et al. Inotropic agents and vasodilator strategies for acute myocardial infarction complicated by cardiogenic shock or low cardiac output syndrome. *Cochrane Database Syst Rev*. 2014;1:CD009669.

A3. Alexander JH, Reynolds HR, Stebbins AL, et al. Effect of tilarginine acetate in patients with acute myocardial infarction and cardiogenic shock: the TRIUMPH randomized controlled trial. *JAMA*. 2007;297:1657-1666.

A4. Thiele H, Zeymer U, Neumann FJ, et al. Intraaortic balloon support for myocardial infarction with cardiogenic shock. *N Engl J Med*. 2012;367:1287-1296.

A5. Thiele H, Zeymer U, Neumann FJ, et al. Intra-aortic balloon counterpulsation in acute myocardial infarction complicated by cardiogenic shock (IABP-SHOCK II): final 12 month results of a randomised, open-label trial. *Lancet*. 2013;382:1638-1645.

A6. Hochman JS, Sleeper LA, White HD, et al. One-year survival following early revascularization for cardiogenic shock. *JAMA*. 2001;285:190-192.

A7. Hochman JS, Sleeper LA, Webb JG, et al. Early revascularization and long-term survival in cardiogenic shock complicating acute myocardial infarction. *JAMA*. 2006;295:2511-2515.

A8. Jeger RV, Urban P, Harkness SM, et al. Early revascularization is beneficial across all ages and a wide spectrum of cardiogenic shock severity: a pooled analysis of trials. *Acute Card Care*. 2011;13:14-20.

A9. Cheng JM, den Uil CA, Hoeks SE, et al. Percutaneous left ventricular assist devices vs. intra-aortic balloon pump counterpulsation for treatment of cardiogenic shock: a meta-analysis of controlled trials. *Eur Heart J*. 2009;30:2102-2108.

GENERAL REFERENCES

For the General References and other additional features, please visit Expert Consult at https://expertconsult.inkling.com.

108 SHOCK SYNDROMES RELATED TO SEPSIS

JAMES A. RUSSELL

DEFINITION

Sepsis is defined by presence of at least two of the four signs of the systemic inflammatory response syndrome (SIRS): (1) fever (>38° C) or hypothermia (<36° C); (2) tachycardia (>90 beats/minute); (3) tachypnea (>20 breaths/minute), hypocapnia (partial pressure of carbon dioxide <32 mm Hg), or the need for mechanical ventilatory assistance; and (4) leukocytosis (>12,000 cells/μL), leukopenia (<4000 cells/μL), or a left shift (>0% immature band cells) in the circulating white blood cell differential and suspected or proven infection. *Bacteremia* is defined as the growth of bacteria in blood cultures, but infection does not have to be proved to diagnose sepsis at the onset. *Severe sepsis* is sepsis in addition to dysfunction of one or more organ systems (e.g., hypoxemia, oliguria, lactic acidosis, thrombocytopenia, decreased Glasgow Coma Scale score). *Septic shock* is defined as severe sepsis in addition to hypotension (systolic blood pressure <90 mm Hg or a >40 mm Hg decrease from baseline) despite adequate fluid resuscitation.[1]

EPIDEMIOLOGY

Approximately 750,000 cases of severe sepsis or septic shock occur every year in the United States. Sepsis causes as many deaths as acute myocardial infarction, and septic shock and its complications are the most common causes of death in noncoronary intensive care units (ICUs). The medical care costs associated with sepsis are approximately $16.7 billion a year in the United States alone. The frequency of septic shock is increasing as physicians perform more aggressive surgery, as more resistant organisms are present in the environment, and as the prevalence of immune compromise resulting from disease and immunosuppressive drugs increases. Studies suggest that African Americans have a higher incidence of severe sepsis than whites do (6.0 vs. 3.6 per 1000 population) and a higher mortality in ICUs (32.1 vs. 29.3%; $P < .0001$), even after adjustment for poverty levels. The mechanisms of this apparent difference in risk for and mortality from sepsis are not known.

Gram-positive or gram-negative bacteria, fungi, and, very rarely, protozoa or rickettsiae can cause septic shock. Increasingly common causes of septic shock are gram-positive bacteria, especially methicillin-resistant *Staphylococcus aureus*, vancomycin-resistant enterococci, penicillin-resistant *Streptococcus pneumoniae*, and resistant gram-negative bacilli.

The common infections causing septic shock are pneumonia, peritonitis, pyelonephritis, abscess (especially intra-abdominal), primary bacteremia, cholangitis, cellulitis, necrotizing fasciitis, and meningitis. Nosocomial pneumonia is the most common cause of death from nosocomial infection.

PATHOBIOLOGY

At onset, septic shock activates inflammation, leading to enhanced coagulation, activated platelets, increased neutrophils and mononuclear cells, and diminished fibrinolysis. After several days, a compensatory anti-inflammatory response with immunosuppression may contribute to death. Several pathways amplify one another: inflammation triggers coagulation, and coagulation triggers inflammation, resulting in a positive feedback loop that is proinflammatory and procoagulant. Tissue hypoxia in septic shock also amplifies inflammation and coagulation. Many mediators that are critical for the homeostatic control of infection may be injurious to the host (e.g., tumor necrosis factor-α [TNF-α]), so therapies that fully neutralize such mediators are largely ineffective.

Widespread endothelial injury is an important feature of septic shock; an injured endothelium is more permeable, so the flux of protein-rich edema fluid into tissues such as the lung increases. Injured endothelial cells release nitric oxide, a potent vasodilator that is a key mediator of septic shock. Septic shock also injures epithelial cells of the lung and intestine. Intestinal epithelial injury increases intestinal permeability; this leads to epithelial translocation of intestinal bacteria and endotoxin, which further augments the inflammatory phenotype of septic shock.

Early Infection, the Innate Immune Response, Inflammation, and the Endothelium

Host defense is organized into innate and adaptive immune responses. The innate immune system responds by using pattern recognition receptors (e.g., toll-like receptors [TLRs]) to pathogen-associated molecular patterns, which are extremely well conserved molecules of microorganisms. Surface molecules of gram-positive and gram-negative bacteria (peptidoglycan and lipopolysaccharide, respectively) bind to TLR-2 and TLR-4, respectively (E-Fig. 108-1). TLR-2 and TLR-4 binding initiates an intracellular signaling cascade that culminates in nuclear transport of the transcription factor nuclear factor κB (NF-κB), which triggers transcription of cytokines such as TNF-α and interleukin (IL)–6. Cytokines upregulate adhesion molecules of neutrophils and endothelial cells, and neutrophil activation leads to bacterial killing. However, cytokines also directly injure host endothelial cells, as do activated neutrophils, monocytes, and platelets. Inhibition of early cytokine mediators of sepsis, such as TNF-α and IL-1β, has not proved successful, probably because TNF-α and IL-1β peak and then decline quickly, before these antagonist therapies can be applied clinically.

After the early cytokine inflammatory response, immune cells, including macrophages and neutrophils, release later mediators, such as high-mobility group box 1 (HMGB-1). HMGB-1 activates neutrophils, monocytes, and endothelium. Unlike TNF-α antagonists, inhibitors of HMGB-1 decrease mortality even when they are given 24 hours after the induction of experimental peritonitis.

Another adverse effect of sepsis is widespread endothelial injury that leads to increased endothelial permeability with loss of protein and fluids to the interstitial space. This endothelial permeability is a final common pathway for widespread tissue injury. Cytokines and other inflammatory mediators induce intercellular endothelial cell gaps by disrupting intercellular junctions, by changing cytoskeletal structure, or by direct damage to endothelial cells. Several pathways of altered endothelial permeability have been implicated in sepsis, including protease-activated receptor 1 (PAR-1) and disruption of the intercellular VE-cadherin, β-catenin, and p120-catenin complex. PAR-1 binding by activated protein C and low-dose thrombin is cytoprotective, whereas PAR-1 stimulation by high-dose thrombin increases endothelial permeability. Binding of Slit to Robo4 maintains the integrity of the intercellular VE-cadherin, β-catenin, and p120-catenin complexes and thus maintains healthy endothelial permeability.

Adaptive Immunity Adds Specificity and Amplifies the Immune Response

Microorganisms stimulate specific humoral and cell-mediated adaptive immune responses that amplify innate immunity. B cells release immunoglobulins that bind to microorganisms and thereby facilitate delivery of microorganisms to natural killer cells and neutrophils. In sepsis, type 1 helper T (T_H1) cells generally secrete proinflammatory cytokines (TNF-α, IL-1β), and type 2 helper T (T_H2) cells secrete anti-inflammatory cytokines (IL-4, IL-10).

Coagulation Response to Infection

Septic shock activates the coagulation system (E-Fig. 108-2) and ultimately converts fibrinogen to fibrin, which is bound to platelets to form microvascular thrombi. Microvascular thrombi further amplify endothelial injury by the release of mediators and by tissue hypoxia because of obstruction to blood flow.

Normally, natural anticoagulants (protein C, protein S, antithrombin, and tissue factor pathway inhibitor) dampen coagulation, enhance fibrinolysis, and remove microthrombi. Thrombin-α binds to thrombomodulin, which activates protein C when protein C is bound to the endothelial protein C receptor (EPCR). Activated protein C dampens the procoagulant phenotype because it inactivates factors Va and VIIIa and inhibits the synthesis of plasminogen activator inhibitor 1 (PAI-1). Activated protein C also decreases apoptosis, leukocyte activation and adhesion, and production of cytokines.

Septic shock decreases the levels of the natural anticoagulants protein C, protein S, antithrombin, and tissue factor pathway inhibitor. Furthermore, lipopolysaccharide and TNF-α decrease thrombomodulin and EPCR, thereby limiting the activation of protein C. Lipopolysaccharide and TNF-α also increase levels of PAI-1, inhibiting fibrinolysis.

Tissue Hypoxia in Septic Shock

Tissue hypoxia independently activates inflammation (by activation of NF-κB and cytokines, synthesis of nitric oxide, and activation of HMGB-1), induces coagulation (through tissue factor and PAI-1), and activates neutrophils, monocytes, and platelets. Hypoxia induces hypoxia-inducible factor-1α (HIF-1α), which upregulates erythropoietin, and vascular endothelial growth factor (VEGF). Erythropoietin is protective to brain and other tissues. VEGF inhibits fibrinolysis and increases inducible nitric oxide synthase, which augments nitric oxide–induced vasodilation. Nitric oxide has a further injurious effect: excessive nitric oxide inhibits the beneficial actions of HIF-1α (e.g., upregulating synthesis of erythropoietin) during hypoxia.

Late Septic Shock, Immunosuppression, and Apoptosis of Immune and Epithelial Cells

After about 1 week of septic shock, death can result from immunosuppression, which is suggested by anergy, lymphopenia, hypothermia, and nosocomial infection (E-Fig. 108-3). Multiple organ dysfunction may be an anti-inflammatory phenotype because of the apoptosis of immune, epithelial, and endothelial cells. Activated $CD4^+$ T cells evolve into either a T_H1 proinflammatory (TNF-α, IL-1β) or a T_H2 anti-inflammatory (IL-4, IL-10) phenotype. Sepsis leads to migration from a T_H1 to a T_H2 phenotype; for example, persistent elevation of IL-10 is associated with an increased risk of death. Immunosuppression also develops because of apoptosis of lymphocytes. Proinflammatory cytokines, activated B and T cells, and glucocorticoids induce lymphocyte apoptosis, whereas TNF-α and endotoxin induce apoptosis of lung and intestinal epithelial cells. The fact that glucocorticoids also stimulate apoptosis could be the biologic explanation for the observation that patients with septic shock who are treated with hydrocortisone have more superinfections than do patients treated with placebo.

Death from infectious disease appears to be highly heritable. Sepsis is a prime example of a polygenic disease related to the interaction of multiple genes and an environmental insult (infection). Single-nucleotide polymorphisms of cytokines (TNF-α, IL-6, IL-10), coagulation factors (protein C, fibrinogen-β), the catecholamine pathway (β-adrenergic receptor), and innate immunity genes (CD14, TLR-1, TLR-2) have been variably associated with an increased risk of death from sepsis.

Cardiovascular Dysfunction

Inadequate tissue perfusion and tissue hypoxia are the cardinal features of all types of shock. Early in septic shock, most patients have sinus tachycardia and, by definition, decreased blood pressure (<90 mm Hg systolic, a decrease of ≥40 mm Hg from baseline systolic pressure, or mean arterial pressure <65 mm Hg; Table 108-1). Septic shock is the classic form of distributive shock (Chapter 106), characterized by increased pulse pressure (bounding pulses), decreased systemic vascular resistance (warm, flushed skin), and functional hypovolemia (low jugular venous pressure). Distributive shock means that the distribution of systemic blood flow is abnormal, such that areas of both low flow (and low venous oxygen saturation) and high flow (and increased venous oxygen saturation) are present. Nevertheless, about one third of patients with septic shock initially present with findings more typical of hypovolemic shock (low central venous pressure and low central venous oxygen saturation) because the clinical features depend on the stage and severity of septic shock as well as on the degree of fluid resuscitation that has occurred. After fluid resuscitation, patients typically develop the characteristic clinical and hemodynamic features of classic distributive shock.

Ventricular preload is commonly decreased in early septic shock, for several reasons.[2] First, patients may be volume depleted because of decreased fluid intake and because of increased fluid losses as a result of fever, vomiting, and

TABLE 108-1 HEMODYNAMIC VARIABLES, ABBREVIATIONS, AND NORMAL VALUES

Arterial pressure: systolic pressure (SAP) (>100 mm Hg), diastolic pressure, pulse pressure, mean arterial pressure (MAP) (>65 mm Hg)
Central venous pressure (CVP): normal, 6-12 mm Hg
Pulmonary artery pressure (PAP): normal, 25/15 mm Hg
Pulmonary vascular resistance (PVR): normal, 150-250 dynes/sec/cm

$$\left(\equiv \frac{PAP - PAOP}{CO} \times 80\right)$$

Pulmonary artery occlusion pressure (PAOP) or pulmonary artery wedge pressure (PAWP): normal, 8-15 mm Hg
Systemic vascular resistance (SVR): normal, 900-1400 dynes/sec/cm

$$\left(\equiv \frac{MAP - CVP}{CO} \times 80\right)$$

Cardiac output (CO): normal, 5 L/min
Left ventricular stroke work index (LVSWI): normal, (60-100 grams × meters/beats) = (SV × [MAP − PAWP] × 0.0136)
Oxygen delivery (Do_2): normal, 1 L/min (= CO × [Hg × 1.38 × Sao_2] + [0.003 × Po_2])
Oxygen consumption (Vo_2): normal, 250 mL/min (= CO × Hg × 1.38 × [Sao_2 − Svo_2] + [0.003 × (Pao_2 − Pvo_2)])
Oxygen extraction ratio: normal, 0.23-0.32 (= Vo_2/Do_2)
Hemodynamic variables are often normalized to account for different body mass by dividing by body surface area (BSA)
- Pulmonary vascular resistance index (PVRI): normal (= PVR/BSA)
- Systemic vascular resistance index (SVRI): normal (= SVR/BSA)
- Cardiac index (CI): normal, 2.5-4.2 L/min/m^2 (= CO/BSA)
- Left ventricular stroke work index (LVSWI): normal (= LVSW/BSA)
- Oxygen delivery index (Do_2I): normal, 460-650 mL/min/m^2 (= Do_2/BSA)
- Oxygen consumption index (Vo_2I): normal, 95-170 mL/min/m^2 (= Vo_2/BSA)

diarrhea if gastrointestinal disease is present. Second, fluid loss from the intravascular to the interstitial space (capillary leak) is caused by mediators that induce widespread endothelial injury, which increases capillary permeability. Increased capillary permeability leads to loss of protein-rich edema fluid into the interstitial space. In the lung, increased permeability is a key component of acute lung injury. A third reason that ventricular preload is decreased in septic shock is venodilation induced by mediators such as nitric oxide. Venodilation increases venous capacitance, leading to relative volume depletion, which compounds the absolute volume depletion. Ventricular afterload is decreased because of excessive release of potent vasodilators such as nitric oxide, prostaglandin I_2, adenosine diphosphate, and other vasodilators.

In addition to abnormal vasodilation, patients have concurrent microvascular vasoconstriction. Microvascular vasoconstriction may not be apparent clinically or hemodynamically, but it can lead to tissue hypoxia, detected by increased arterial lactate concentrations. Microvascular vasoconstriction is caused by increased norepinephrine, thromboxanes, and other local vasoconstrictors. Microvascular vasoconstriction causes focal hypoxia, which is exacerbated by microvascular obstruction by platelets and leukocytes.

The abnormal mismatch of oxygen delivery to oxygen demand can disturb the global relationship of oxygen delivery to oxygen consumption. Normally, oxygen consumption is independent of oxygen delivery over a wide range. When oxygen delivery decreases to less than the critical oxygen delivery level, oxygen consumption decreases and leads to a state in which oxygen consumption depends on oxygen delivery. At levels lower than the critical oxygen delivery level, arterial lactate increases as a result of tissue hypoxia. The clinical implication is that oxygen delivery should be increased (e.g., by increasing cardiac output by volume resuscitation, infusion of dobutamine, or transfusion of erythrocytes) to more than the critical level.

Cardiovascular function is further compromised in septic shock because of decreased ventricular contractility.[3] Decreased ventricular contractility may be difficult to detect clinically and may be diagnosed only by hemodynamic or echocardiographic assessment. Numerous circulating mediators of sepsis, including endotoxin, cytokines (e.g., IL-6, TNF-α), and nitric oxide (locally released into the coronary circulation), decrease contractility. Endotoxin signals through TLRs to upregulate the expression of proteins such as S110A8 and S100A9 to cause a receptor for advanced glycation end products (RAGE)–dependent decrease in calcium flux, which decreases the ejection fraction. Coronary ischemia resulting from microvascular obstruction by leukocytes and oxygen free radicals, which are released by neutrophils adherent to the coronary capillary endothelium, is another mechanism of decreased contractility.

Early in septic shock, patients who survive have increased left ventricular end-diastolic volume, which likely allows them to maintain cardiac output despite decreased contractility. In contrast, nonsurvivors do not have increased left ventricular end-diastolic volume, so their cardiac output is compromised. In some patients with septic shock, concurrent acute lung injury and secondary pulmonary hypertension increase right ventricular afterload, with a secondary shift of the interventricular septum from right to left. This septal shift decreases left ventricular end-diastolic volume and can also limit cardiac output.

CLINICAL MANIFESTATIONS

Cardiovascular dysfunction in septic shock is characterized by decreased preload (because of decreased intake, fluid losses, third spacing resulting from increased permeability, and venodilation), decreased afterload, and often decreased ventricular contractility. Decreased ventricular volume is detected clinically by low jugular venous pressure and hemodynamically by decreased central venous pressure. Left ventricular resistance, or afterload, is also commonly decreased and is detected clinically by warm, flushed skin and hemodynamically by decreased systemic vascular resistance.

DIAGNOSIS

Even as the diagnostic evaluation is beginning, the initial assessment of a critically ill patient must focus immediately on the airway (need for intubation), breathing (respiratory rate, respiratory distress, pulse oximetry), circulation (heart rate, blood pressure, jugular venous pressure, skin perfusion), and rapid initiation of resuscitation (Fig. 108-1). Vital signs and the leukocyte count quickly establish whether the patient has SIRS (two of the four criteria). Arterial blood gases and lactate levels are useful complementary tests. A secondary survey is designed to determine the likely source of infection and the status of organ function. Pneumonia (Chapter 97) is suggested by cough, sputum, and respiratory distress; empyema (Chapter 99) is suggested by pleuritic chest pain. Signs of peritonitis, an abdominal mass, and right upper quadrant tenderness suggest abdominal sepsis. Pyelonephritis (Chapter 284) is likely in patients with dysuria and costovertebral angle tenderness. Integumentary assessment for erythema (cellulitis), line site erythema (line sepsis), tenderness (necrotizing fasciitis), crepitus (anaerobic myonecrosis), and petechiae and purpura (meningococcemia) can be illuminating. Headache, stiff neck, and signs of meningismus raise the suspicion of meningitis (Chapter 412). Focal neurologic signs suggest brain abscess (Chapter 413).

Laboratory investigations that are helpful to identify the source of infection include appropriate cultures and Gram stains (blood, sputum, urine, fluids, and cerebrospinal fluid). Blood cultures are positive in 40 to 60% of patients who have septic shock. The chest radiograph aids in the diagnosis of pneumonia, empyema, and acute lung injury. Abdominal ultrasound and computed tomography are indicated if abdominal sepsis is suspected.

Hemodynamic assessment of the patient includes diagnostic central venous or pulmonary artery catheterization. In early septic shock, central venous pressure is usually low and increases in response to volume resuscitation. Central venous oxygen saturation, cardiac output, and ventricular filling pressures may be determined continuously. Pulmonary artery pressure is usually normal but may be increased because septic shock can cause pulmonary hypertension. Pulmonary artery occlusion (or wedge) pressure is usually low before resuscitation, but it may be normal or increased if the patient has underlying preexisting heart disease (e.g., heart failure or coronary artery disease with prior myocardial infarction) or if left ventricular contractility is decreased by sepsis. Cardiac output may be low or normal before fluid resuscitation and typically increases to higher than normal after fluid resuscitation. If fluid resuscitation increases central venous pressure and pulmonary artery occlusion pressure but cardiac output does not increase, left ventricular dysfunction is presumably present.

Echocardiographic features of decreased ventricular contractility include decreased right and left ventricular ejection fractions and increased end-diastolic and end-systolic volumes. Early in septic shock, the left ventricular ejection fraction is decreased, and it remains low in nonsurvivors. In survivors, the left ventricular ejection fraction usually returns to normal during 5 to 10 days. Bedside echocardiography can also be used to assess intravascular volume status, which can be diagnosed on the basis of collapse of the inferior vena cava, and valvular dysfunction.

Renal, hepatic, and coagulation function tests are helpful to evaluate organ function. After determination of the source of sepsis, it is crucial to address

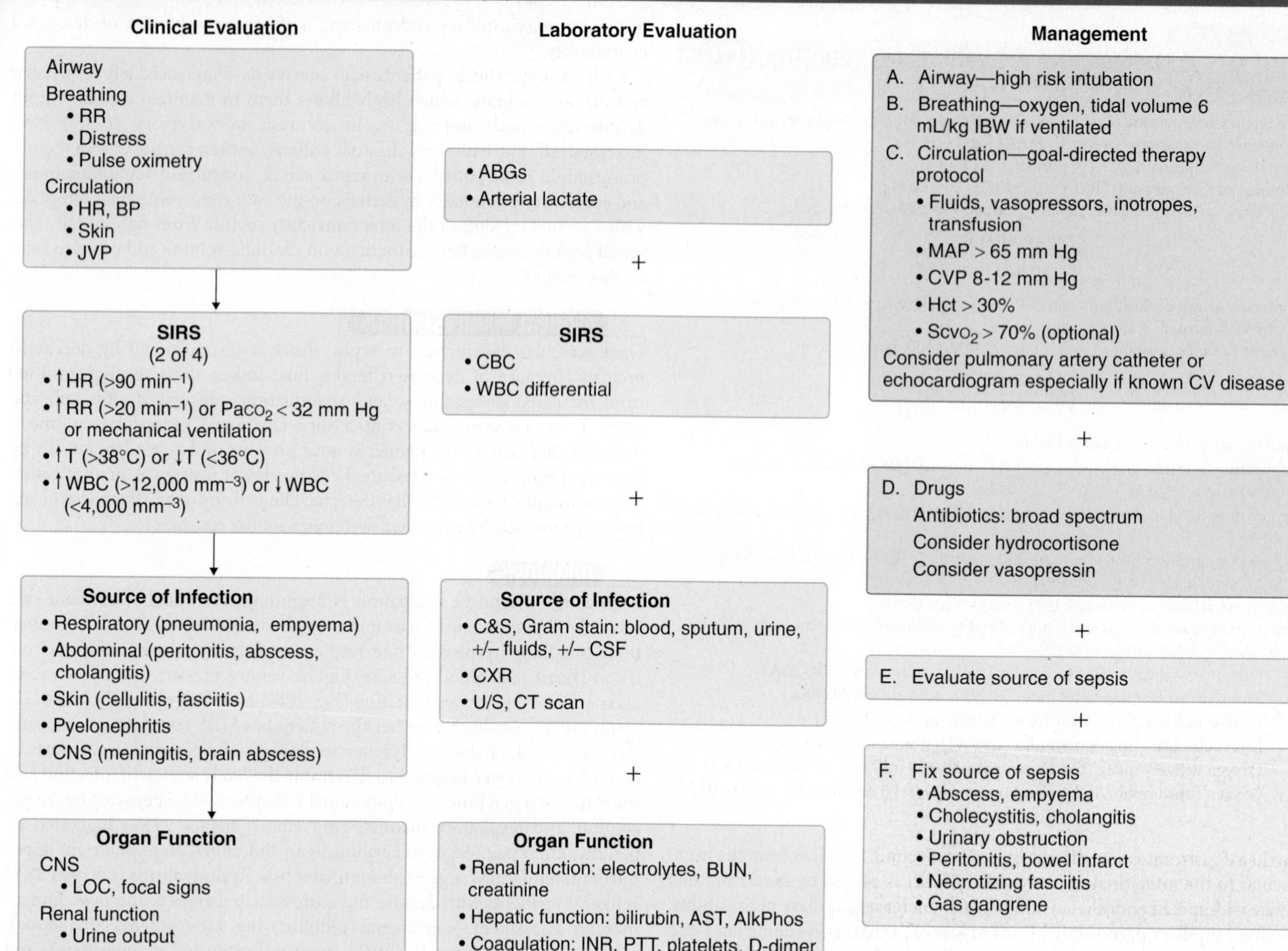

FIGURE 108-1. Algorithm for the clinical and laboratory evaluation and management of septic shock. ABGs = arterial blood gases; AlkPhos = alkaline phosphatase; AST = aspartate aminotransferase; BP = blood pressure; BUN = blood urea nitrogen; C&S = culture and sensitivity; CBC = complete blood count; CNS = central nervous system; CSF = cerebrospinal fluid; CT = computed tomography; CV = cardiovascular; CVP = central venous pressure; CXR = chest radiograph; Hct = hematocrit; HR = heart rate; IBW = ideal body weight; INR = international normalized ratio; JVP = jugular venous pressure; LOC = level of consciousness; MAP = mean arterial pressure; $Paco_2$ = partial pressure of carbon dioxide; PTT = partial thromboplastin time; RR = respiratory rate; $Scvo_2$ = central venous oxygen saturation; SIRS = systemic inflammatory response syndrome; T = temperature; U/S = ultrasound; WBC = white blood cell count.

that source by draining abscesses and empyemas; radiologically or surgically correcting urinary tract obstruction; and surgically managing peritonitis, bowel infarction, cholecystitis, cholangitis, necrotizing fasciitis, and gas gangrene.

Differential Diagnosis

The major differential diagnoses of classic septic shock are other nonseptic causes of SIRS, such as acute pancreatitis (Chapter 144), acute respiratory distress syndrome (Chapter 104), aspiration pneumonitis (Chapter 94), multiple trauma (Chapter 111), and recent major surgery without infection (Chapter 433). Other causes of distributive shock are anaphylactic shock (suggested by angioedema and hives; Chapter 440), spinal shock (recent trauma and paraplegia; Chapter 399), acute adrenal insufficiency ("tanned skin," hyperkalemia, metabolic alkalosis; Chapter 227), and acute or acute-on-chronic hepatic failure (jaundice, ascites, encephalopathy; Chapter 153).

The differential diagnosis of septic shock must include the other causes of shock: hypovolemic, cardiogenic, and obstructive shock (Chapters 106 and 107). Patients with hypovolemic shock (from internal or external fluid losses, hemorrhage) present with a suggestive history and signs of hypovolemia (low jugular venous pressure) and skin hypoperfusion (cool, clammy, cyanotic extremities). Cardiogenic shock (resulting from myocardial infarction or acute-on-chronic congestive heart failure or occurring after cardiovascular surgery) is suggested by the history, signs of increased filling pressure (increased jugular venous pressure, crackles, S_3, pulmonary edema, cardiomegaly), and skin hypoperfusion (Chapter 107). Some patients who have acute myocardial infarction and cardiogenic shock have features of SIRS without infection. Obstructive shock (from pulmonary thromboembolism, cardiac tamponade, pneumothorax) is manifested similarly to cardiogenic shock.

PREVENTION

Measures to prevent sepsis include handwashing, elevation of the head of the bed, scrupulous sterile techniques for the insertion of catheters, and possibly the use of antibiotic-impregnated catheters. New catheter insertion sites for catheter changes, isolation of patients who have resistant organisms, and isolation of significantly immunocompromised patients may also prevent infection.

Preventing the progression from sepsis to septic shock requires early diagnosis and aggressive resuscitation.[4] Early fluid resuscitation, lung-protective ventilation, and antibiotics are critical therapies in early septic shock (Table 108-2).

TREATMENT Rx

Respiratory Therapy

All patients in septic shock require oxygen initially, and many require mechanical ventilation. Mechanical ventilation is required in most patients who have septic shock because acute lung injury is the most common complication. Lung-protective ventilation (mechanical ventilation that minimizes lung injury by using a relatively low tidal volume, such as >6 mL/kg of

TABLE 108-2 POTENTIAL ANTIBIOTIC REGIMENS FOR PATIENTS WITH SEPTIC SHOCK*

SOURCE OF SEPSIS	INITIAL ANTIBIOTIC REGIMEN	ALTERNATIVE ANTIBIOTIC REGIMEN
Community-acquired pneumonia	Third-generation cephalosporin (cefotaxime 2 g IV q6h; ceftriaxone 2 g IV q12h; ceftizoxime 2 g IV q8h) *plus* Fluoroquinolone (e.g., ciprofloxacin 400 mg IV q12h, levofloxacin 750 mg IV q24h, moxifloxacin 400 mg IV q24h) *or* Macrolide (azithromycin 500 mg IV q24h)	Piperacillin-tazobactam 3.375 g IV q6h *plus* Fluoroquinolone *or* Macrolide
Hospital-acquired pneumonia	Imipenem 0.5 g IV q6h *or* Meropenem 1 g IV q8h	Fluoroquinolone (ciprofloxacin 400 mg IV q12h) *plus* Vancomycin 1.5 g IV q12h *or* Piperacillin-tazobactam 3.375 g IV q6h *plus* Tobramycin 1.5 mg/kg q8h *plus* Vancomycin
Abdominal (mixed aerobic/anaerobic)	Piperacillin-tazobactam 3.375 g IV q6h *or* Imipenem 0.5 g IV q6h (or meropenem 1 g IV q8h)	Ampicillin 2 g IV q4h *plus* Metronidazole 500 mg IV q8h *plus* Fluoroquinolone (ciprofloxacin 400 mg IV q12h)
Urinary tract	Fluoroquinolone (ciprofloxacin 400 mg IV q12h)	Ampicillin 2 g IV q4h *plus* Gentamicin 1.5 mg/kg IV q8h *or* Third-generation cephalosporin (cefotaxime 2 g IV q6h, ceftriaxone 2 g IV q12h, or ceftizoxime 2 g IV q8h)
Necrotizing fasciitis	Imipenem 0.5 g IV q6h	Penicillin G (if confirmed group A streptococci)
Primary bacteremia (normal host)	Piperacillin-tazobactam 3.375 g IV q6h *plus* Vancomycin 1.5 g IV q12h	Imipenem 0.5 g IV q6h *plus* Vancomycin 1.5 g IV q12h
Primary bacteremia (intravenous drug user)	Vancomycin 1.5 g IV q12h *plus* Fluoroquinolone (ciprofloxacin 400 mg IV q12h)	Piperacillin-tazobactam 3.375 g IV q6h *plus* Vancomycin 1.5 g IV q12h
Febrile neutropenia	Cefepime 2 g IV q8h *plus* Vancomycin 1.5 g IV q12h	Piperacillin-tazobactam 3.375 g IV q6h *plus* Gentamicin 1.5 mg/kg q8h *or* Imipenem 0.5 g IV q6h *plus* Gentamicin 1.5 mg/kg q8h
Bacterial meningitis	Ceftriaxone 2 g IV q12h *plus* Ampicillin 3 g IV q6h *plus* Vancomycin 1.5 g IV q12h *plus* Dexamethasone 0.15 mg/kg IV q6h for 2-4 days	Gram-positive cocci: vancomycin *plus* ceftriaxone 2 g IV q12h Gram-negative diplococci: cefotaxime 2 g IV q4-6h Gram-positive bacilli: ampicillin 3 g IV q6h *plus* gentamicin Gram-negative bacilli: ceftazidime 2 g IV q8h *plus* gentamicin 1.5 mg/kg IV q8h All above *plus* dexamethasone
Cellulitis	Ciprofloxacin 400 mg IV q12h *plus* Clindamycin 900 mg IV q8h	Imipenem 0.5 g IV q6h

*Most antibiotic doses must be adjusted if there is hepatic or renal dysfunction. Some antibiotics require adjustment based on levels (e.g., gentamicin). In selecting a drug, carefully consider the patient's history of antibiotic (especially penicillin) allergy.

predicted body weight) decreases mortality from acute lung injury and acute respiratory distress syndrome (Chapter 105).[A1]

Patients who require ventilation need adequate but not excessive sedation, which can worsen hemodynamic instability, prolong ventilation, and increase the risk for development of nosocomial pneumonia. Sedation should be titrated by objective assessment. Daily interruption of sedation decreases the duration of mechanical ventilation and intensive care. Weaning from mechanical ventilation is often associated with fluid overload from prior fluid resuscitation and from the reduction in intrathoracic pressure. Patients whose weaning is guided by brain natriuretic peptide levels are weaned more quickly and have more ventilator-free days because they generally receive more aggressive diuretic therapy, without a concomitant increased need for vasopressors, an increased risk of renal dysfunction, or more electrolyte abnormalities.[A2]

Circulatory Therapy

Early therapy is the cornerstone of emergency management, but such therapy need not achieve specific central hemodynamic targets or require the placement of a central venous catheter or the administration of inotropic agents or blood transfusions.[A3][A4] Standard therapies should have the goal of increasing tissue oxygen delivery by increasing profoundly low blood pressure, increasing inadequate blood flow, increasing low arterial oxygen saturation, and increasing mixed venous oxygen saturation. Although oxygen delivery is higher in survivors than in nonsurvivors, it is not clear that a specific oxygen delivery target is more beneficial than clinical end points. Several trials have shown that supernormal global oxygen delivery does not decrease mortality rates in sepsis and septic shock.

A mean arterial blood pressure goal of 65 to 70 mm Hg is as good as a goal of 80 to 85 mm Hg.[A5] However, a higher mean arterial pressure target (80 to 85 mm Hg) may decrease the risk of renal injury and the need for renal replacement therapy in patients with preexisting hypertension. In patients who have acute lung injury, no difference in outcomes is seen with management using a pulmonary artery catheter versus a central venous catheter. Patients whose acute lung injury is managed after 24 to 48 hours with a conservative fluid strategy (compared with a liberal fluid strategy) have significantly improved lung function and shorter duration of ventilation and ICU stay.

Fluids should be used to maintain central venous pressure at 8 to 12 mm Hg; at present, no convincing data indicate that albumin is better than normal saline solution.[5][A6] In patients with severe sepsis, large randomized trials confirm that modified lactated Ringer solution or albumin is preferred to 10% hetastarch (a colloid) because of lower rates of acute kidney injury, less need for renal replacement therapy, and fewer deaths.[A7] As a result, hetastarch should not be used in septic shock. If central venous oxygen saturation is less than 70%, packed red cell transfusions should be used to maintain a hematocrit greater than 30%.

Vasopressors (e.g., norepinephrine, 1 to 50 μg/minute; epinephrine, 1 to 30 μg/minute) should be added if the mean arterial pressure is less than 65 mm Hg. Dobutamine (2.5 to 20 μg/kg/minute) is required if central venous pressure, mean arterial pressure, and hematocrit are optimized but the central venous oxygen saturation remains less than 70%. In a randomized trial of patients with septic shock, the combination of norepinephrine plus dobutamine resulted in a mortality similar to that with epinephrine alone, with no differences in organ dysfunction, time to resolution of shock, or adverse events.[A8] In another randomized trial, norepinephrine was slightly but not significantly better than dopamine for reducing mortality when used as the first-line vasopressor for patients with septic shock[A9]; however, norepinephrine was associated with a lower rate of arrhythmias, especially atrial fibrillation. These accumulated data suggest that norepinephrine may be preferable to dopamine as the first vasopressor in septic shock.

Clinicians can use epinephrine alone, norepinephrine alone, or norepinephrine plus dobutamine in patients with low cardiac output. As a strategic approach to persistent hypotension despite adequate fluid resuscitation, a vasopressor such as norepinephrine (1 to 50 µg/minute) can be added first. If the cardiac index is low or if the mixed venous oxygen saturation is low (>70%) despite an adequate central venous pressure, an inotropic agent such as dobutamine should be added, initially at approximately 2 to 5 µg/kg/minute and increasing until the mixed venous oxygen saturation is adequate. In some patients in septic shock, the cardiac index is inadequate, as reflected by a low mixed venous oxygen saturation despite a high central venous pressure (>12 mm Hg) or pulmonary artery wedge pressure (>18 mm Hg) because of underlying cardiovascular dysfunction or because of acute left ventricular dysfunction resulting from sepsis. In such patients, earlier use of an inotropic agent such as dobutamine should be considered to increase left ventricular contractility. The overall goal is to achieve an adequate mean arterial pressure (>65 mm Hg), central venous pressure, and mixed venous oxygen saturation while other indices of adequate perfusion are monitored, such as hourly urine output (>0.5 mL/kg/hour), arterial lactate levels (<2 mmol/L), mental status, and skin perfusion. To assess the adequacy of early resuscitation of severe sepsis and septic shock and to guide ongoing therapy, a central venous oxygen saturation goal greater than 70% or a lactate clearance of at least 10% is an equally good measure.A10

Fever, which is common in septic shock, may have some beneficial effects for resisting infection but also increases oxygen demand. Reducing fever can decrease the need for vasopressors and possibly the risk of septic encephalopathy. In one large trial, external cooling for 48 hours to maintain core body temperature between 36.5° C and 37° C was safe and decreased the need for vasopressors as well as 14-day mortality rates (from 34% to 19%).A11 Cooling to reduce fever to normothermia is especially promising for febrile septic shock patients who are receiving high doses of vasopressors, require inotropic agents, or have marked tachycardia.

Transfusion of Erythrocytes and Erythropoietin

Anemia is common in septic shock, but the optimal hemoglobin level for resuscitation has been controversial. Recently, however, a randomized trial of transfusion in critically ill patients with septic shock found that a transfusion threshold of a hemoglobin level of 7 g/dL was equivalent to a threshold of 9 g/dL in terms of ischemic events, the need for life support, or death, while reducing transfusions from a median of 4 units to a median of 1 unit.A12

Drugs

Antibiotics

The infected site and infecting organisms of septic shock are often not known initially, and clinicians usually need to decide on an empirical antibiotic regimen before knowing culture results in patients with septic shock. After appropriate culture specimens are obtained, intravenous broad-spectrum antibiotics should be administered on an emergency basis (within 1 hour) while considering host factors such as immune and allergic status (Chapters 280 and 281; see Fig. 108-1). Emergency, empirical antibiotic therapy (Table 108-2) should be guided by the greater frequency of gram-positive bacteria, the possibility of resistant organisms, and the local bacteriologic features. In one large trial, meropenem alone was equivalent to the combination of meropenem and moxifloxacin in terms of mortality rates and organ dysfunction.A13 Adding empirical fluconazole treatment does not result in better outcomes in critically ill, non-neutropenic patients.

Because outcomes in patients with septic shock are worse if the organisms causing the sepsis are not sensitive to the initial antibiotic regimen, a central question is the relative value of using a single antibiotic compared with multiple antibiotics. Broad-spectrum antibiotics should be used for as short a time as possible. If a causative organism is identified (<20% of septic patients have negative cultures), the antibiotic regimen should be quickly narrowed with 3 to 5 days to decrease the emergence of resistant organisms. The duration of antibiotics should be guided by the cause of septic shock, but patients generally require 10 to 14 days of therapy.

Corticosteroids

High-dose corticosteroids do not improve outcomes in the full spectrum of patients with sepsis or acute respiratory distress syndrome, but the evidence supporting the use of low-dose corticosteroids in septic shock is controversial. In one trial, corticosteroids (hydrocortisone, 50 mg intravenously every 6 hours, plus fludrocortisone, 50-µg tablet/day per nasogastric tube or orally for 7 days) increased survival in septic patients whose serum cortisol response after stimulation with an intravenous infusion of 250 µg of corticotropin was 9 µg/dL or less. In a subsequent randomized trial of hydrocortisone (50 mg every 6 hours intravenously for 5 days) versus placebo, however, mortality was not improved, regardless of the patient's response to corticotropin stimulation.A14 Adding fludrocortisone to hydrocortisone does not appear to be better than hydrocortisone alone, and aggressive insulin therapy to address the hyperglycemia that often accompanies corticosteroid treatment is no better than usual glucose control.A15 Hydrocortisone treatment is often associated with a shorter duration of septic shock but can increase the risk of superinfections. Current sepsis guidelines suggest that corticosteroids should be considered only in patients who are poorly responsive to vasopressors.

Corticosteroids administered before antibiotics also decrease the neurologic sequelae of bacterial, especially pneumococcal, meningitis (Chapter 412). Enthusiasm for corticosteroid therapy must be tempered by the risk of complications such as superinfection, neuromyopathy, hyperglycemia, immune suppression, and impaired wound healing.

Recombinant Human Activated Protein C

In septic shock, a deficiency of activated protein C is nearly universal, and low levels of activated protein C are associated with increased mortality. However, recombinant human activated protein C infusion does not reduce mortality in patients who receive guideline-driven therapy for septic shock,A16 and the drug has been removed from the worldwide market.

Vasopressin

Although vasopressin deficiency and downregulation of vasopressin receptors are common findings in septic shock, a low-dose vasopressin infusion added to norepinephrine is not significantly better than a norepinephrine infusion alone in septic shock.A17 Whether vasopressin infusion may be beneficial in patients with less severe shock is uncertain.

Hyperglycemia and Intensive Insulin Therapy

Hyperglycemia and insulin resistance are common in septic shock, but intensive insulin therapy to control hyperglycemia is not beneficial in patients in medical ICUs because of significantly higher rates of hypoglycemia and perhaps increased mortality.A18 Therefore, intensive insulin therapy cannot be recommended for patients with septic shock.

Renal Dysfunction and Dialysis

Acute renal failure is an important complication of septic shock because of its associated morbidity, mortality, and resource use (Fig. 108-2). In critically ill patients who have acute kidney injury, hemodialysis six times per week is no better than conventional hemodialysis, and intensive renal replacement therapy is no better than standard therapy overall or in patients who have sepsis.A19

Low-dose dopamine (2 to 4 µg/kg/minute) does not decrease the need for renal support, does not improve outcomes, and is not recommended. Lactic acidosis is a common complication of septic shock, but administration of sodium bicarbonate in the setting of lactic acidosis does not improve hemodynamics or the response to vasopressors.

A small randomized controlled trial evaluated the use of polymyxin B hemoperfusion in patients with abdominal sepsis to reduce blood endotoxin levels. Polymyxin B hemoperfusion increased blood pressure, decreased vasopressor requirements, improved organ dysfunction, and reduced mortality by one third. However, this intervention requires further evaluation before it can be recommended.

Other Therapies

Deep venous thrombosis prophylaxis with low-dose heparin is recommended for patients who do not have active bleeding, coagulopathy, or a contraindication to heparin (see Fig. 108-2). Low-molecular-weight heparin does not decrease risk of deep venous thrombosis compared with unfractionated heparin, but it may decrease the risk of pulmonary emboli in the critically ill.A20 Stress ulcer prophylaxis with H_2-receptor antagonists decreases the risk of gastrointestinal hemorrhage. Proton pump inhibitors may also be effective, but they have not been fully evaluated in septic shock.

Enteral nutrition is generally safer and more effective than total parenteral nutritionA21, but total parenteral nutrition is sometimes required in patients with abdominal sepsis, surgery, or trauma.[6] Initial trophic feeding, which provides about 25% of normal calorie requirements, appears to be as good as full enteral feeding and is therefore recommended after stabilization of patients in septic shock.A22 The use of sedation, neuromuscular blocking agents, and corticosteroids should be minimized because they can exacerbate septic encephalopathy and the polyneuropathy or myopathy of sepsis. Neutropenic patients may benefit from granulocyte colony-stimulating factor (Chapter 167). The risk of nosocomial infection is decreased by narrow-spectrum antibiotics, early weaning from ventilation, and periodic removal and replacement of catheters (Chapter 282).

B. Breathing—Oxygen, with a tidal volume 6 mL/kg IBW if ventilated. Wean according to ARDSNet protocol (Chapters 105 and 106)

C. Circulation

- Fluids, vasopressors, inotropes, transfusion; goals include:
  - MAP > 65 mm Hg
  - CVP 8-12 mm Hg
  - Hg 70-90 g/L
  - $Scvo_2$ > 70% (optional)

Consider pulmonary artery catheter or echocardiogram especially if known cardiovascular disease; goals include:

- Wedge pressure 8-15 mm Hg
- Cardiac index: normal or increased

D. Drugs:

- Antibiotics: Narrow spectrum to cause of infection
- Hydrocortisone (if evidence of relative adrenal insufficiency [see text]): hydrocortisone 50 mg intravenously every 6 hours and fludrocortisone 50-μg tab orally or per NG tube daily for 7 days

Other Organ Support

- Renal function: Continuous renal replacement
- DVT prophylaxis: Low-dose heparin 5000 IU subcutaneously every 12 hours
- Stress ulcer prophylaxis: H_2-receptor antagonist (e.g., ranitidine 50 mg intravenously every 8 hours)
- Nutrition: Enteral preferred
- Sedation: Intermittent with daily awakening

FIGURE 108-2. Ongoing critical care support and management in septic shock. CVP = central venous pressure; DVT = deep venous thrombosis; Hg = hemoglobin; IBW = ideal body weight; MAP = mean arterial pressure; NG = nasogastric; $Scvo_2$ = central venous oxygen saturation.

PROGNOSIS

The 28-day mortality of septic shock has decreased during the past 20 years from about 50% to about 25 to 35%,[7] especially in academic centers,[8] probably because of the earlier initiation of appropriate therapies at appropriate doses for limited periods. Early deaths (in the first 72 hours) are usually the result of refractory, progressive shock despite escalating life support. Later deaths from septic shock (after day 3) are usually secondary to multiple organ dysfunction. The number of dysfunctional organs and the progression or lack of improvement of organ dysfunction are indicators of increased risk of death. Other factors that portend a poor prognosis are increased age, underlying medical conditions, more severe illness, increased arterial lactate concentrations, and the need for high-dose vasopressors. Furthermore, a delay in achieving adequate resuscitation is associated with increased mortality.

As the number of survivors of septic shock has increased, so have the numbers with significant long-term sequelae, including cognitive dysfunction,[9] depression, and post-traumatic stress disorder. Survivors of septic shock who also had acute lung injury (Chapter 104) can have weakness, fatigue, and dyspnea on exertion after hospital discharge due to pulmonary dysfunction, neuromuscular dysfunction, or other persistent organ dysfunction. Patients who have an episode of acute kidney injury during septic shock have a significantly decreased long-term survival than patients without it.[10] Overall, the survival and quality of life after hospital discharge after septic shock remain poorer than expected for at least the next 10 years.[11,12]

Grade A References

A1. Acute Respiratory Distress Syndrome Network. Ventilation with lower tidal volumes as compared with traditional tidal volumes for acute lung injury and the acute respiratory distress syndrome. *N Engl J Med.* 2000;342:1301-1308.

A2. Mekontso Dessap A, Roche-Campo F, Kouatchet A, et al. Natriuretic peptide–driven fluid management during ventilator weaning: a randomized controlled trial. *Am J Respir Crit Care Med.* 2012;186:1256-1263.

A3. Yealy DM, Kellum JA, Huang DT, et al. A randomized trial of protocol-based care for early septic shock. *N Engl J Med.* 2014;370:1683-1693.

A4. Peake SL, Delaney A, Bailey M, et al. Goal-directed resuscitation for patients with early septic shock. *N Engl J Med.* 2014;371:1496-1506.

A5. Asfar P, Meziani F, Hamel JF, et al. High versus low blood-pressure target in patients with septic shock. *N Engl J Med.* 2014;370:1583-1593.

A6. Caironi P, Tognoni G, Masson S, et al. Albumin replacement in patients with severe sepsis or septic shock. *N Engl J Med.* 2014;370:1412-1421.

A7. Rochwerg B, Alhazzani W, Sindi A, et al. Fluid resuscitation in sepsis: a systematic review and network meta-analysis. *Ann Intern Med.* 2014;161:347-355.

A8. Annane D, Vignon P, Renault A, et al. Norepinephrine plus dobutamine versus epinephrine alone for management of septic shock: a randomized trial. *Lancet.* 2007;370:676-684.

A9. De Backer D, Biston P, Devriendt J, et al. Comparison of dopamine and norepinephrine in the treatment of septic shock. *N Engl J Med.* 2010;362:779-789.

A10. Jones AE, Shapiro NI, Trzeziak S, et al. Lactate clearance vs. central venous oxygen saturation as goals of early sepsis therapy: a randomized clinical trial. *JAMA.* 2010;303:739-746.

A11. Schortgen F, Clabault K, Katsahian S, et al. Fever control using external cooling in septic shock: a randomized controlled trial. *Am J Respir Crit Care Med.* 2012;185:1088-1095.

A12. Holst LB, Haase N, Wetterslev J, et al. Lower versus higher hemoglobin threshold for transfusion in septic shock. *N Engl J Med.* 2014;371:1381-1391.

A13. Brunkhorst FM, Oppert M, Marx G, et al. Effect of empirical treatment with moxifloxacin and meropenem vs meropenem on sepsis-related organ dysfunction in patients with severe sepsis: a randomized trial. *JAMA.* 2012;307:2390-2399.

A14. Sprung CL, Annane D, Keh D, et al. Hydrocortisone therapy for patients with septic shock. *N Engl J Med.* 2008;358:111-124.

A15. Annane D, Cariou A, Maxime V, et al. Corticosteroid treatment and intensive insulin therapy for septic shock in adults: a randomized controlled trial. *JAMA.* 2010;303:341-348.

A16. Ranieri VM, Thompson BT, Barie PS, et al. Drotrecogin alfa (activated) in adults with septic shock. *N Engl J Med.* 2012;366:2055-2064.

A17. Russell JA, Walley KR, Singer J, et al. Vasopressin versus norepinephrine infusion in patients with septic shock. *N Engl J Med.* 2008;358:877-887.

A18. Finfer S, Chittock DR, Su SY, et al. Intensive versus conventional glucose control in critically ill patients. *N Engl J Med.* 2009;360:1283-1297.

A19. Palevsky PM, Zhang JH, O'Connor TZ, et al. Intensity of renal support in critically ill patients with acute kidney injury. *N Engl J Med.* 2008;359:7-20.

A20. Cook D, Meade M, Guyatt G, et al. Dalteparin versus unfractionated heparin in critically ill patients. *N Engl J Med.* 2011;364:1305-1314.

A21. Harvey SE, Parrott F, Harrison DA, et al. Trial of the route of early nutritional support in critically ill adults. *N Engl J Med.* 2014;371:1673-1684.

A22. Rice TW, Wheeler AP, Thompson BT, et al. Initial trophic vs full enteral feeding in patients with acute lung injury: the EDEN randomized trial. *JAMA.* 2012;307:795-803.

GENERAL REFERENCES

For the General References and other additional features, please visit Expert Consult at https://expertconsult.inkling.com.

109 DISORDERS DUE TO HEAT AND COLD

MICHAEL N. SAWKA AND FRANCIS G. O'CONNOR

TEMPERATURE REGULATION

Body temperature is regulated through two parallel processes that modify body heat balance: behavioral (clothing, shelter, physical activity) and physiologic (skin blood flow, sweating, shivering). Both peripheral (skin) and central (core) thermal receptors provide afferent input to a central nervous system integrator (hypothalamic thermoregulatory center), and any deviation between the controlled variable (body temperature) and a theoretical reference variable ("set point" temperature) results in a heat loss or conservation response (E-Fig. 109-1).

Humans normally regulate body (core) temperature at about 37° C (98.6° F), and fluctuations within the narrow range of 35° C to 41° C (95° F to 105.8° F) can be tolerated by healthy acclimatized persons; core temperatures outside this range can induce morbidity and mortality. There is no single core temperature because it varies at different deep body sites and during rest and physical exercise. Arterial blood temperature, which provides the best invasive measurement of core temperature, is slightly lower than brain temperature. The most accurate noninvasive index of core temperature is esophageal temperature, followed in order of preference by rectal, gastrointestinal tract (telemetry pill), and oral temperature. Ear (tympanic and auditory meatus) or scanned temporal artery temperature should not be relied on for clinical judgment. Rectal temperatures are most commonly recommended because they are easy to measure and are not biased by environmental conditions.

HEAT ILLNESS

DEFINITION

Minor heat-related illnesses include miliaria rubra, heat syncope, and heat cramps. Serious heat illness represents a continuum from heat exhaustion to heat injury and heatstroke.

EPIDEMIOLOGY

Heat illness accounts for considerable morbidity and mortality in the world today. Serious heat illness is associated with a variety of individual factors, health conditions, drugs, and environmental factors (Table 109-1). Exertional heat illness is among the leading causes of death in young athletes,[1] and its incidence appears to be increasing in the United States. Classic heat illness caused by high environmental temperatures remains a problem especially in homebound elderly persons without air conditioners.[2] Anticholinergic and sympathomimetic poisoning (Chapter 110) can induce hyperthermia. Malignant hyperthermia (Chapter 432) is a rare disorder occurring in genetically predisposed individuals; rapid and massive skeletal muscle contraction from exposure to certain anesthetic agents, most commonly halothane and succinylcholine, can trigger core temperature elevations well above 43° C (110° F). Neuroleptic malignant syndrome (Chapter 434) is an idiosyncratic hyperthermic reaction caused by skeletal muscle rigidity from treatment with neuroleptic medications (e.g., antipsychotics, antidepressants, antiemetics). Both malignant hyperthermia and neuroleptic malignant syndrome are potentially fatal without prompt recognition and early intervention.

TABLE 109-1 FACTORS PREDISPOSING TO SERIOUS HEAT ILLNESS

INDIVIDUAL FACTORS
Lack of acclimatization
Low physical fitness
Excessive body weight
Dehydration
Advanced age
Young age
HEALTH CONDITIONS
Inflammation and fever
Viral infection
Cardiovascular disease
Diabetes mellitus
Gastroenteritis
Rash, sunburn, and previous burns to large areas of skin
Seizures
Thyroid storm
Neuroleptic malignant syndrome
Malignant hyperthermia
Sickle cell trait
Cystic fibrosis
Spinal cord injury
DRUGS
Anticholinergic properties (atropine)
Antiepileptic (topiramate)
Antihistamines
Glutethimide (Doriden)
Phenothiazines
Tricyclic antidepressants
Amphetamines, cocaine, Ecstasy
Ergogenic stimulants (e.g., ephedrine, ephedra)
Lithium
Diuretics
β-Blockers
Ethanol
ENVIRONMENTAL FACTORS
High temperature
High humidity
Little air motion
Lack of shade
Heat wave
Physical exercise
Heavy clothing
Air pollution (nitrogen dioxide)

Heat illness can also occur in low-risk individuals who have taken appropriate precautions relative to situations to which they have been exposed in the past. Historically, such unexpected cases were attributed to dehydration (which impairs thermoregulation and increases hyperthermia and cardiovascular strain), but it is now suspected that a previous heat exposure or a concurrent event (e.g., sickness or injury) might make these individuals more susceptible to serious heat illness. One theory is that previous heat injury or illness primes the acute phase response and augments the hyperthermia of exercise, inducing unexpected serious heat illness. Another theory is that previous infection produces proinflammatory cytokines that deactivate the cells' ability to protect against heat shock.

PATHOBIOLOGY

Body temperature can increase from a number of mechanisms: exposure to environmental heat (impeded heat dissipation); physical exercise (increased heat production); fever from systemic illness (elevated set point with subsequent activation of shivering); and medications (neuroleptic malignant syndrome and malignant hyperthermia). In addition, febrile persons have accentuated elevations in core temperature when they are exposed to high ambient temperature, physical exercise, or both. Environmental temperature and humidity, medications, and exercise heat stress in turn challenge the cardiovascular system to provide high blood flow to the skin, where blood pools in warm, compliant vessels such as those found in the extremities. When blood flow is diverted to the skin, reduced perfusion of the intestines and other viscera can result in ischemia, endotoxemia, and oxidative stress (E-Fig. 109-2). In addition, excessively high tissue temperatures (heat shock: >41° C [105.8° F]) can produce direct tissue injury; the magnitude and duration of the heat shock influence whether cells respond by adaptation (acquired thermal tolerance), injury, or death (apoptotic or necrotic). Heat shock, ischemia, and systemic inflammatory responses can result in cellular dysfunction, disseminated intravascular coagulation, and multiorgan dysfunction syndrome. In addition, reduced cerebral blood flow, combined with abnormal local metabolism and coagulopathy, can lead to dysfunction of the central nervous system.

CLINICAL MANIFESTATIONS AND DIAGNOSIS

Minor heat illness is common and can be recognized by its clinical features. Miliaria rubra (heat rash) results from the occlusion of eccrine sweat gland ducts and can be complicated by secondary staphylococcal infection. Heat syncope (fainting) is caused by temporary circulatory insufficiency as a result of blood pooling in the peripheral veins, especially the cutaneous and lower extremity veins. Skeletal muscle cramps most commonly occur during and after intense exercise and are probably related to dehydration, loss of sodium or potassium, and neurogenic fatigue rather than to overheating itself.

Serious heat illness includes heat exhaustion, which can progress to heat injury, which then can progress to heatstroke. In many patients, the degree of severity of heat illness often is not initially clear. Patients who exhibit symptoms (e.g., dizziness, unsteady gait, ataxia, headache, confusion, weakness, fatigue, nausea, vomiting, diarrhea) should have an immediate assessment of their mental status, core (rectal) temperature, and other vital signs. Until it is proved otherwise, heatstroke should be the initial working diagnosis in anyone who is a heat casualty and has an altered mental status.

Heat exhaustion is defined as a syndrome of hyperthermia (temperature at time of event usually ≤40° C or 104° F) and debilitation that occur during or immediately after exertion in the heat, accompanied by no more than minor central nervous system dysfunction (headache, dizziness), which resolves rapidly with intervention. It is primarily a cardiovascular event (insufficient cardiac output) frequently accompanied by sweaty hot skin, dehydration, and collapse.

Heat injury is a moderate to severe illness characterized by evidence of damage to organs (e.g., liver, renal, gut) and tissues (e.g., rhabdomyolysis) without sufficient neurologic symptoms to be diagnosed as heat stroke. It is usually associated with body temperatures above 40° C (104° F).

Heatstroke is a severe illness characterized by profound mental status changes with high body temperatures, usually but not always higher than 40° C (104° F). However, patients with a core temperature higher than 40° C do not universally have a heat injury or heatstroke, and core temperatures this high can be seen transiently after stressful exercise in the heat. To establish the diagnosis of heatstroke, the entire clinical picture, including mental status and laboratory results, must be considered. Heatstroke is often categorized as classic or exertional; classic heatstroke is observed primarily in otherwise sick and compromised individuals, and exertional heatstroke is observed

TABLE 109-2 COMPARISON OF CLASSIC AND EXERTIONAL HEATSTROKE

PATIENT CHARACTERISTICS	CLASSIC	EXERTIONAL
Age	Young children or elderly	15-55 years
Health	Chronic illness	Usually healthy
Fever	Unusual	Common
Prevailing weather	Frequent in heat waves	Variable
Activity	Sedentary	Strenuous exercise
Drug use	Diuretics, antidepressants, anticholinergics, phenothiazines	Ergogenic stimulants or cocaine
Sweating	Often absent	Common
Acid-base disturbances	Respiratory alkalosis	Lactic acidosis
Acute renal failure	Uncommon	Common (≈15%)
Rhabdomyolysis	Uncommon	Common (≈25%)
CK	Mildly elevated	Markedly elevated (500-1000 U/L)
ALT, AST	Mildly elevated	Markedly elevated
Hyperkalemia	Uncommon	Common
Hypocalcemia	Uncommon	Common
DIC	Mild	Marked
Hypoglycemia	Uncommon	Common

ALT = alanine aminotransferase; AST = aspartate aminotransferase; CK = creatine kinase; DIC = disseminated intravascular coagulation.

TABLE 109-3 MANAGEMENT OF HEAT ILLNESS

HEAT EXHAUSTION

Rest and shade
Loosen and remove clothing
Supine position and elevate legs
Actively cool skin
Fluids by mouth
Monitor core temperature
Monitor mental status

HYPERTHERMIA

Protect the airway
Insert at least two large-bore intravenous lines
Monitor core temperature; options include rectal, pulmonary artery, esophageal probe
Actively cool the skin until core temperature reaches <39° C (<102.2° F)
Ice baths or cool water (≈22° C [71.6° F]) immersion
Wetting with water (avoid alcohol rubs)
Continuous fanning
Exposure to cool environment
Axillary or perineal ice packs and ice sheets
Infusion of room-temperature saline
Gastric or colonic iced saline lavage
Peritoneal lavage with cool saline
Monitor electrocardiogram for arrhythmia
Obtain serial diagnostic studies*

*Electrocardiogram, chest radiograph, complete blood count with differential, platelet count, urinalysis, aminotransferases, alkaline phosphatase, bilirubin, creatine kinase, blood urea nitrogen, creatinine, phosphate, calcium, glucose, electrolytes, uric acid, prothrombin time and partial thromboplastin time, fibrin split products, fibrinogen, arterial blood gases, toxicology screen.

primarily in apparently healthy and physically fit individuals during or after vigorous exercise (Table 109-2). In heatstroke, neuropsychiatric impairments (e.g., marked confusion, disorientation, combativeness, and seizures) develop early and universally[3] but are readily reversible with early cooling. In addition, heatstroke can be complicated by liver damage, rhabdomyolysis, disseminated intravascular coagulation, water and electrolyte imbalance, and renal failure. In fulminant heat stroke, patients have the full spectrum of abnormalities associated with the systemic inflammatory response syndrome (Chapter 108).

PREVENTION AND TREATMENT Rx

Heat illness can be prevented by heat acclimatization and acquired thermal tolerance, maintenance of adequate hydration, and avoidance of overwhelming heat exposure. Adequate fluid intake is critical, and oral rehydration solutions may be preferable to other forms of hydration for patients with heat exhaustion.[A1]

Management of serious heat illness, which should begin in the field setting, includes cooling,[4] rehydration, and monitoring (Table 109-3). The first priority should be immediately to initiate whole body cooling and to continue cooling until the core temperature falls below 38.8° C (102° F). Body cooling lowers tissue temperatures, thereby facilitating conduction and convection from the core to the shell, and reduces cardiovascular stress by causing arterial and venous constriction that redirects blood back to the heart. Immersion or soaking of the skin in cool or ice water with skin massage is the most effective method, but other effective methods include soaking of the skin followed by accelerated evaporation with fans or the use of ice sheets and ice packs. These noninvasive treatments can be supplemented with the infusion of chilled (≈5° C) normal saline. Cooling can induce shivering, which is usually not sufficient to increase body temperature, so shivering need not be treated.

In the hospital, the priority for patient care remains urgent cooling. Patients who are unconscious are at risk of poor airway control and may require endotracheal intubation to prevent aspiration. Fluid and electrolyte deficits should be corrected; restoration of plasma volume with isotonic fluids (e.g., normal saline) sufficient to sustain adequate perfusion, as judged by carefully monitored urine output, is also a priority. Rapid overcorrection of serum electrolytes (e.g., sodium) should be avoided. If rhabdomyolysis (Chapter 113) and myoglobinuria are present, maintaining urine flow helps minimize renal injury.

For exercise-induced and environmental heat illness, no pharmacologic interventions have been proved to augment cooling. For patients with malignant hyperthermia, however, dantrolene should be administered as a loading bolus of 2.5 mg/kg intravenously, with subsequent bolus doses of 1 mg/kg intravenously until the signs have abated.[5]

Patients should be carefully monitored to detect possible metabolic abnormalities (e.g., hyperkalemia), renal or hepatic failure, disseminated intravascular coagulation, cardiac arrhythmias, and acute respiratory failure. Medications to be avoided include antipyretics and sedatives with hepatic toxicities. Lorazepam (1 to 2 mg administered intravenously during a 2- to 5-minute period, repeated if necessary) is a safe sedative because of its low hepatotoxicity and rapid metabolism and may be indicated in patients who are combative or exhibit seizure activity.

PROGNOSIS

A single episode of heat exhaustion does not imply a predisposition to heat illness, and most patients recover within several hours after cooling and rehydration. For patients who present to a hospital with heatstroke, however, mortality rates can range from 21 to 63%. Mortality in both classic and exertional heat stroke correlates directly with the magnitude and duration of temperature elevation, the delay in time to initiation of cooling, and the number of organ systems affected.

Patients who have suffered heat injury or heatstroke should not be reexposed to heat until recovery is complete, which can be many weeks or months, and about 10% of heatstroke patients remain intolerant of heat. The long-term consequences of heatstroke likely include sustained organ damage, which presumably explains why such patients have a higher long-term mortality from cardiovascular, liver, and digestive diseases.

COLD INJURY

DEFINITION

Cold injuries are classified as hypothermia and peripheral cold injuries. Hypothermia is whole body cooling, whereas peripheral cold injuries are localized to the extremities and exposed skin. Hypothermia is further divided into three categories: mild (≈33° C to ≈35° C), moderate (≈27° C to ≈32° C), and profound (<27° C). Peripheral cold injuries can be divided into nonfreezing (chilblain, trench foot) and freezing (frostbite). Both hypothermia and peripheral cold injuries often occur simultaneously, and treatment priority should be given to rewarming in moderate and profound hypothermia.

EPIDEMIOLOGY

A variety of individual factors, health conditions, medications, and environmental factors are associated with a predisposition to cold injury

TABLE 109-4 FACTORS PREDISPOSING TO COLD INJURY

INDIVIDUAL FACTORS
Inadequate clothing and shelter
Lean and low body fat
Low physical fitness
Advanced age
Young age
Black race (men and women)
HEALTH CONDITIONS
Burns
Diabetes mellitus
Hypoglycemia
Neurologic lesions
Dementia
Hypoadrenalism, hypopituitarism, hypothyroidism
Prior frostbite or trench foot
Raynaud phenomenon
Sickle cell trait
Trauma
Spinal cord injury
DRUGS
Alcohol
Anesthetics
Antidepressants
Antithyroid agents
Sedatives and narcotics
ENVIRONMENTAL FACTORS
Cold temperatures
High air motion
Rain and immersion
Skin contact with metal and fuels
Repeated cold exposure
Physical fatigue
Immobility
High-altitude and low-oxygen-tension environments

(Table 109-4). In trauma patients (Chapter 111), hypothermia is associated with increased morbidity and mortality.

PATHOBIOLOGY

Cold exposure elicits peripheral vasoconstriction to reduce heat transfer between the body's core and shell (skin, subcutaneous fat). If sufficiently cold, the underlying tissues (e.g., muscle) constrict to thicken the isolative shell while reducing the body's core area. This vasoconstrictor response defends core temperature but at the expense of declining peripheral tissue temperatures, which contribute to peripheral cold injuries. Hypothermia depresses enzymatic activity, interferes with physiologic functions (e.g., clotting, respiration, cardiac conduction and rhythm), impairs the expression of cytokines, and can induce cellular injury and death.

The pathophysiologic mechanism of frostbite includes four overlapping pathologic phases: prefreeze, freeze-thaw, vascular stasis, and late ischemic.[6] The prefreeze phase consists of tissue cooling with accompanying vasoconstriction and ischemia but does not involve actual ice crystal formation. In the freeze-thaw phase, intracellular ice crystals form, thereby causing protein and lipid derangement, cellular electrolyte shifts, cellular dehydration, cell membrane lysis, and subsequent cell death. In the vascular stasis phase, vessels may fluctuate between constriction and dilation; blood may leak from vessels or coagulate within them. The late ischemic phase results from progressive tissue ischemia and infarction due to a cascade of inflammatory cytokines and prostaglandins, intermittent vasoconstriction with continued thrombus formation, and secondary reperfusion injury.

CLINICAL MANIFESTATIONS AND DIAGNOSIS

Hypothermia is a core temperature below 35° C (95° F), and clinical manifestations are related to the core temperature achieved (Table 109-5). The classic J wave on the electrocardiogram (Fig. 109-1) appears at a core temperature below about 33.8° C (93° F).

Chilblain (Chapter 80) appears as localized inflammatory lesions of the skin, most often involving the dorsal surface of fingers but also involving the ears, face, and exposed shins. Trench foot is caused by prolonged cold, wet exposure (e.g., wet socks or gloves), which can cause skin breakdown and

TABLE 109-5 HYPOTHERMIA: STAGES AND ASSOCIATED CLINICAL MANIFESTATIONS

STAGE	CORE TEMPERATURE °F	CORE TEMPERATURE °C	CLINICAL MANIFESTATIONS
Normothermia	98.6	37.0	
Mild hypothermia	95.0	35.0	Cold diuresis, maximal shivering
	93.0	33.8	Ataxia, poor judgment, J wave
	91.0	32.7	Amnesia, blood pressure difficult to measure
Moderate hypothermia	89.0	31.6	Stupor, pupils dilated
	87.0	30.5	Shivering ceases
	85.0	30.0	Cardiac arrhythmias, insulin inactive
	82.0	27.8	Unconsciousness, ventricular fibrillation likely
	80.0	26.6	No muscle reflexes
Profound hypothermia	78.0	25.5	Acid-base disturbances, no response to pain
	75.0	23.8	Pulmonary edema, hypotension
	73.0	22.7	No corneal reflexes
	66.0	18.8	Heart standstill
	62.0	16.6	Isoelectric electrocardiogram
	57.6	14.2	Lowest infant survival from accidental hypothermia
	48.2	9.0	Lowest adult survival from accidental hypothermia

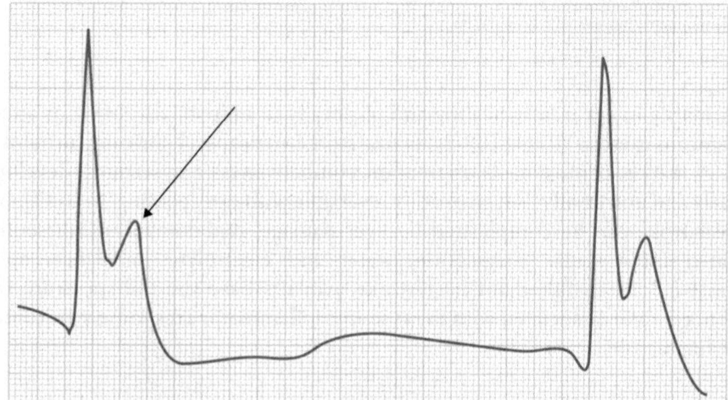

FIGURE 109-1. J (Osborne) wave.

nerve damage. Trench foot is often accompanied by infection and increased sensitivity to pain.

Frostbite, which is actual freezing of tissues, has traditionally been categorized as first degree (superficial, "frostnip"), second degree (full skin), third degree (subcutaneous tissue), and fourth degree (extensive tissue and bone). For patients with frostbite, early surgical consultation is advised.

PREVENTION AND TREATMENT Rx

Humans demonstrate minimal cold acclimatization, so prevention depends primarily on avoiding cold exposure and having adequate protection and calorie intake to support metabolism. Management of hypothermia depends on the core temperature (Table 109-6). Patients' wet clothing should be removed, and they should be provided with dry insulation. Shivering is an effective physiologic rewarming mechanism and should not be pharmacologically suppressed.

Moderately and profoundly hypothermic patients require active rewarming. Rewarming of the hypothermic patient includes both passive (insulation of the patient to prevent further heat loss) and active core (e.g., warmed saline and humidified oxygen) and external (e.g., warmed water bottles, electric blankets) techniques. Rewarming at a rate of 0.5° C to 1.0° C (0.9° F to 1.8° F) per hour is acceptable in most cases, except that aggressive rewarming is warranted in patients with significant trauma (because coagulation is hindered by hypothermia) or cardiac arrest.

Complications commonly associated with rewarming of the hypothermic individual include both afterdrop (reduction of core temperature by cold blood returning to the circulation from the periphery) and aftershock (hypotension caused by peripheral vasodilation). Another potential complication of

TABLE 109-6 TREATMENT OF HYPOTHERMIA

STAGE	MANAGEMENT	BODY REWARMING
Mild hypothermia	Monitor vital signs Warm intravenous saline Oxygen Monitor electrocardiogram for arrhythmia	Insulate Shivering Warm bath Active warming blanket
Moderate hypothermia	Diagnostic studies* Intensive care Anticipate infection and multiorgan dysfunction	Prevent extra heat loss by supplementing with airway rewarming Colonic irrigation Peritoneal dialysis
Profound hypothermia	Diagnostic studies*	Central rewarming

*See Table 109-3. Also lactate dehydrogenase, serum lactate, cortisol, thyroid-stimulating hormone, T_3, and T_4.

rewarming is ventricular fibrillation, which is more difficult to treat in the presence of moderate or profound hypothermia. If ventricular tachycardia or ventricular fibrillation develops, defibrillation should be attempted (Chapter 63). If ventricular tachycardia or ventricular fibrillation persists after a single shock, additional defibrillation attempts should be made, concurrent with rewarming but without waiting for the patient to warm to a particular target body temperature. Standard resuscitation approaches generally should be followed (Chapter 63).

Body cooling induces cold diuresis, so plasma volume must be reestablished to support adequate perfusion. Patients should receive an intravenous infusion of 250 to 1000 mL of heated (40° C to 42° C [104° F to 108° F]) 5% dextrose in normal saline. Lactated Ringer solution should be avoided because the liver cannot metabolize lactate efficiently during hypothermia. Patients should be monitored for disturbances in potassium and glucose. If hypoglycemia, alcohol, or opiate intoxication is contributing to hypothermia, intravenous glucose (50 to 100 mL of 50% dextrose), thiamine[7] (100 mg), or naloxone (1 to 2 mg), respectively, may be indicated.

Frostbitten tissues should be protected from friction or trauma but should not be thawed until there is confidence in the ability to maintain warmth because refreezing causes more injury. Gentle rewarming in a water bath (38° C to 43° C [100° F to 108° F]) is recommended. Ibuprofen should be started in the field at a dose of 12 mg/kg per day (divided twice daily) to inhibit harmful prostaglandins and increased up to a maximum dose of 2400 mg/day (divided four times daily) if the patient is experiencing pain. Common practice for blister care is selective draining of clear blisters while leaving hemorrhagic blisters intact. Case reports suggest that intravenous or intra-arterial thrombolysis within 24 hours of injury at experienced centers may mitigate the morbidity of frostbite injury.[8]

PROGNOSIS

Although noninvasive imaging with technetium pyrophosphate or magnetic resonance imaging can often predict the likelihood of tissue viability, it may take weeks to determine the precise demarcation of tissue that will require amputation. As morbidity may result from premature or unnecessary surgical intervention, consultation with a surgeon with experience evaluating and treating frostbite should be obtained to assess the need for and the timing of any amputations.

Hypothermic Syndromes

Exercise-induced bronchospasm (Chapter 87) can be triggered by exercise in cold air, particularly in patients with asthma. Livedo reticularis is patchy mottling of the limbs with cold exposure. Cryoglobulinemia (Chapter 187) occurs when immunoglobulins (IgM, IgG) reversibly precipitate after being cooled and contribute to impaired capillary blood flow in hypothermic tissues. Cold urticaria (Chapters 252 and 440) is the development of localized and general erythema and wheals in skin exposed to cold. Paroxysmal hypothermia is periodic lowering of the thermoregulatory set point and is often associated with hypothalamic abnormalities. Raynaud phenomenon (see Fig. 80-7) is intense vasoconstriction with sensitivity to pain in limbs exposed to cold.

Trauma Hypothermia

In trauma patients (Chapter 111), unintended hypothermia (<34° C [93° F]) is associated with increased morbidity and mortality due to impaired coagulation, peripheral vasoconstriction, respiratory depression, and increased risk for cardiac arrhythmias. Shivering aggravates perfusion problems by requiring blood flow to support increased metabolism in contracting muscles. Trauma patients become hypothermic because of heat loss from exposed cavities, environmental exposure, infusion of cool fluids, and ischemia, which depletes cell energy stores. Body temperature should be measured, and appropriate actions should be taken to restore normothermia during the early treatment of trauma patients.

THERAPEUTIC HYPOTHERMIA AND HYPERTHERMIA

Therapeutic Hypothermia

Therapeutic hypothermia theoretically can provide benefits by suppressing metabolism, free radical production, lipid peroxidation, inflammatory products, excitatory amino acid release, and calcium release. Among children with neonatal encephalopathy, whole body hypothermia reduces death and the combined end point of death or an IQ score of less than 70 at 6 to 7 years of age by 15%.[A2] It is being tested for spinal cord injury but has not consistently shown a benefit in children with traumatic brain injury.

For post–cardiac arrest adults, therapeutic hypothermia improves survival and neurologic outcomes.[A3] It should be initiated as soon as possible by skin cooling (e.g., cooling packs to the axilla, groin, head, and neck while simultaneously treating the patient with a cooling blanket, water mattress, or fan), endovascular cooling, or both. Endovascular cooling can be achieved either by the infusion of cool fluids (e.g., 30 mL/kg crystalloids at 4° C [40° F]) or by indwelling heat transfer devices. Cooling by peritoneal and pleural lavage is not generally used. Endovascular cooling provides a more rapid and better-controlled cooling than skin cooling. Thermoregulatory responses (shivering and peripheral vasoconstriction) will resist induced hypothermia and elevate blood pressure and should therefore be pharmacologically blunted. Low-dose meperidine (e.g., 12.5 mg intravenously) can blunt shivering without excessive toxicity. By comparison, mild pre-hospital hypothermia to a temperature of 34° C does not improve survival or neurologic outcomes,[A4] and a target temperature of 33° C is no better than a target temperature of 36° C among unconscious adults after out-of-hospital cardiac arrest.[A5]

Therapeutic Hyperthermia

Hyperthermia treatment (whole body or regional) is an experimental technique used as an adjunct to chemotherapy or radiation therapy in patients with advanced cancer. Hyperthermia (40° C to 43° C [104° F to 109° F]) alone can damage or kill cancer cells, but more important, hyperthermia might potentiate the effectiveness of chemotherapy and radiation by softening the tumor tissue, thus reducing its interstitial pressure.

Externally applied radiant heat, microwaves, or extracorporeal circulation usually induces whole body hyperthermia. Target temperatures are usually achieved during 1 to 2 hours and then maintained for approximately 1 hour, followed by a 1-hour cooling phase. Patients are usually sedated while core and skin temperatures are monitored. In regional hyperthermia, the part of the body where the tumor is located is heated while being perfused or bathed by a warmed solution containing anticancer drugs. The potential benefit of regional hyperthermia as an adjunct treatment of advanced prostate cancers is currently under investigation.[9]

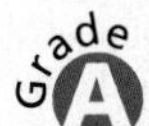

Grade A References

A1. Ishikawa T, Tamura H, Ishiguro H, et al. Effect of oral rehydration solution on fatigue during outdoor work in a hot environment: a randomized crossover study. *J Occup Health.* 2010;52:209-215.

A2. Shankaran S, Pappas A, McDonald SA, et al. Childhood outcomes after hypothermia for neonatal encephalopathy. *N Engl J Med.* 2012;366:2085-2092.

A3. Arrich J, Holzer M, Havel C, et al. Hypothermia for neuroprotection in adults after cardiopulmonary resuscitation. *Cochrane Database Syst Rev.* 2012;9:CD004128.

A4. Kim F, Nichol G, Maynard C, et al. Effect of prehospital induction of mild hypothermia on survival and neurological status among adults with cardiac arrest: a randomized clinical trial. *JAMA.* 2014;311:45-52.

A5. Nielsen N, Wetterslev J, Cronberg T, et al. Targeted temperature management at 33°C versus 36°C after cardiac arrest. *N Engl J Med.* 2013;369:2197-2206.

GENERAL REFERENCES

For the General References and other additional features, please visit Expert Consult at https://expertconsult.inkling.com.

110 ACUTE POISONING

LEWIS S. NELSON AND MARSHA D. FORD

EPIDEMIOLOGY

Each year, more than 4 million poisoning cases, suspected or verified, and 300,000 related hospital admissions occur in the United States. Poisoning-related deaths total more than 30,000 per year and are increasing. Poisonings are now the leading cause of injury-related death in the United States, where approximately 90% of these deaths involve drugs, predominantly prescription opioid analgesics.[1] Worldwide, however, pesticides and insecticides[2] are also common causes, as are intentional ingestions of toxic plants. The incidence of recurrent, purposeful self-poisoning is 12 to 18%, with most events occurring within 3 months of the original attempt. Poison centers provide support and collect data on more than 2 million exposures annually.[3] These facts emphasize the need for regulatory measures to improve the safety of prescription drugs, especially opioid analgesics, including appropriate prescribing, and aggressive treatment of poisoned patients, including early psychiatric intervention for suicidal behavior, to reduce fatalities and repeated attempts (Chapter 397).

DIAGNOSIS

Despite the vast array of toxins to which a patient may be exposed, the clinical manifestations of poisoning are fairly limited. In most cases, it is less important to predict exactly which toxin is responsible for the acute poisoning than it is to create a differential diagnosis based on a careful history and physical examination as well as basic laboratory assays. The recognition of the specific toxic syndrome, or *toxidrome*, guides the clinician toward the likely diagnosis based on reasonably solid evidence. On this basis, treatment, including initial stabilization, critical care, decontamination, and even the empirical administration of antidotes, can be guided by an understanding of the pharmacology and physiology of the patient's toxidrome. More advanced care, such as methods to enhance the elimination of specific toxicants, commonly requires serial examinations, additional history, and subsequent laboratory testing. Even then, however, the clinical picture may be clouded by exposures to multiple toxicants and an ill-defined time course since the initial exposure.

History

Details elicited about toxic exposures should include the involved drugs and other toxicants, their estimated or known amounts, the time and routes of exposure, the patient's symptoms and signs, and any treatment already administered. Intoxication may result from acute, chronic, or acute-on-chronic exposure. A *toxicant* is defined as a chemical capable of harming a biologic organism; this definition encompasses toxins, which are derived from living organisms, as well as medications, drugs of abuse, dietary supplements, and industrial and other chemicals. Determination of chronicity is important because signs and symptoms of chronic intoxication (Chapter 22) can differ from those of acute and acute-on-chronic intoxication. For example, a history of acute multisystem organ failure narrows the toxicant possibilities to a few gases, chemicals, and drugs. A listing of available medications (e.g., medications of the patient, spouse, relatives, or friends), use of nonprescription medications and herbal or dietary supplements or ethnic remedies, and occupational and avocational activities should be obtained. Occupational and avocational histories should include present and all past jobs and hobbies, with a focus on chemicals, metals, and gases. Known medical conditions may suggest classes of medications available to the patient. The patient's history, which may be incomplete if the patient is confused or suicidal, should be correlated with the clinical manifestations and course. Further history from relatives and friends and findings from the scene as reported by the transporting emergency medical services personnel may be relevant.

Physical Examination

The physical examination should focus on vital signs; the eye, ear, nose, and throat examination; and the neurologic, cardiopulmonary, gastrointestinal, and dermatologic systems. Findings can suggest certain toxidromes, which are clusters of signs and symptoms typical of poisoning. Among the dozens of toxidromes that assist in patient assessment and guide management, those due to adrenergic, anticholinergic, cholinomimetic, opioid, and sedative-hypnotic agents are most relevant to the emergency management of poisoned patients (Table 110-1). Patients may have some or all of these signs and symptoms; an incomplete clinical picture does not exclude a particular toxidrome, but it can still assist the clinician in identifying the correct category of toxicant involved.

Vital Signs

Tachycardia, which can occur with numerous toxicants, is most prominent in patients with anticholinergic and sympathomimetic toxidromes. However, because tachycardia also may occur with anxiety and other nontoxicologic conditions, it is not generally a helpful finding. The differential diagnosis for toxicant-induced *bradycardia* is more limited and includes β-adrenergic receptor antagonists, L-type calcium-channel antagonists (diltiazem or verapamil), cardioactive steroids, α-adrenergic receptor agonists (e.g., phenylephrine, whose

TABLE 110-1 TOXIDROMES AND ASSOCIATED DRUGS AND TOXICANTS

TOXIDROME	SYNDROME FEATURES: *Vital Signs*	SYNDROME FEATURES: *End Organ*	COMMON DRUGS AND TOXICANTS
Adrenergic	Hypertension, hyperthermia, tachycardia, tachypnea	Agitation, arrhythmias, diaphoresis, mydriasis, seizures	Amphetamines, caffeine, cathinone derivatives, cocaine, ephedrine, pseudoephedrine, *Ephedra* sp, phenylephrine,* theophylline
Anticholinergic	Hyperthermia, tachycardia, blood pressure generally normal	Agitation, delirium, decreased or absent bowel sounds, dry flushed skin and mucous membranes, mydriasis or blurred vision, seizures, urinary retention	First-generation H_1-receptor antagonists (e.g., diphenhydramine), belladonna alkaloids (e.g., scopolamine, atropine) from plants (e.g., *Datura* sp—deadly nightshade, henbane), benztropine, cyclic antidepressants, dicyclomine, muscle relaxants (e.g., orphenadrine, cyclobenzaprine), trihexyphenidyl
Cholinomimetic	Tachycardia or bradycardia[†]	Agitation, delirium, coma; bronchorrhea, bronchospasm; diaphoresis; fasciculations; lacrimation; miosis; urination; diarrhea, vomiting; seizures	Carbamate cholinesterase inhibitors (e.g., physostigmine, neostigmine, edrophonium), organophosphorus compounds including pesticides and nerve agents (e.g., somin, sarin) *Inocybe* or *Clitocybe* mushroom sp
Opioid, opiate	Bradycardia, bradypnea or apnea, hypotension (rare), hypothermia	CNS depression; hypotonia; miosis	Codeine, fentanyl, ultrapotent fentanyls, heroin, opioids (e.g., hydrocodone, oxycodone, meperidine, morphine), central α_2-agonists (e.g., clonidine, imidazolines)
Sedative-hypnotic	Generally near normal with benzodiazepines, but bradypnea or apnea, mild hypotension, and mild hypothermia can occur	Ataxia, CNS depression, hyporeflexia, slurred speech, stupor, or coma	Barbiturates, benzodiazepines, bromides, chloral hydrate, ethanol, ethchlorvynol, etomidate, glutethimide, meprobamate, methaqualone, methyprylon, propofol, zolpidem

*Reflex bradycardia can occur as a result of a pure α-adrenergic agonist effect.
[†]Tachycardia can occur early as a result of a preganglionic nicotinic effect; as toxicity progresses, postganglionic muscarinic effects predominate, and bradycardia develops.
CNS = central nervous system.

effects are mediated by baroreceptor reflexes), γ-hydroxybutyric acid, opioids, sedative-hypnotics, baclofen, central α_2-agonists like clonidine, organophosphorus and carbamate pesticides, muscarine-containing mushrooms (*Clitocybe, Inocybe* sp), plant- and animal-derived toxins (e.g., aconitine, andromedotoxin, ciguatoxin, and veratridine, all of which open sodium channels in the myocardium), therapeutic cholinesterase inhibitors (e.g., physostigmine), and some antiarrhythmic drugs (e.g., procainamide, flecainide, and other class IA, IC, and III drugs, such as amiodarone and sotalol). Bradycardia also is a preterminal sign for many consequential toxicants, such as cyclic antidepressants and cyanide.

Many toxicants cause *hypotension* (Chapter 8). The primary mechanisms are decreased peripheral vascular resistance, decreased myocardial contractility, hypovolemia secondary to gastrointestinal or dermal loss of intravascular volume, and, occasionally, arrhythmias. Common causes of *hypertension* (Chapter 67), generally due to vasoconstriction with or without enhanced inotropy, include amphetamines, cocaine, ephedrine and similar agents, ergots, phencyclidine, nicotine, phenylephrine, thyroid hormones, yohimbine, and chronic lead toxicity. Blood pressure can rise early in poisoning with central α_2-adrenergic agonists and monoamine oxidase inhibitors, but subsequent hypotension should be expected and is more concerning.

Hyperthermia (Chapter 109) occurs with toxicants that cause agitation or excessive psychomotor activity (e.g., cocaine, phencyclidine, monoamine oxidase inhibitors, strychnine), uncouple oxidative phosphorylation (e.g., salicylates, 2,4-dinitrophenol), increase the metabolic rate (thyroid hormones), impair sweating (e.g., first-generation antihistamines, anticholinergics, cocaine, phenothiazines, zonisamide), cause vasoconstriction (e.g., amphetamines, ephedrine), or impair vasodilation and alter perception of heat (cocaine). Other toxicant-induced states associated with hyperthermia include malignant hyperthermia, neuroleptic malignant syndrome, serotonin syndrome, metal fume fever, and aspiration. Toxicant-induced *hypothermia* is typically due to sedative-hypnotics, opioids, barbiturates, ethanol, phenothiazines, or hypoglycemic agents (such as insulin, sulfonylureas, and meglitinides) or rarely to unripe ackee fruit. Oxygen saturation (see Fig. 158-2) as measured by *pulse oximetry* decreases with true hypoxemia (see Fig. 104-1) or methemoglobinemia (Chapter 158) but remains normal or may be increased in patients with carbon monoxide poisoning (Chapter 94).

Eyes, Ears, Nose, and Throat

Toxicant-induced bilateral miosis (Fig. 110-1) has a limited differential diagnosis that includes central α_2-agonists such as clonidine, guanfacine, and the imidazolines; olanzapine; opioids; organophosphorus compounds or carbamates; therapeutic cholinesterase inhibitors (e.g., physostigmine); topical miotic ophthalmic drugs (e.g., pilocarpine, carbachol); and, variably, phencyclidine, phenothiazines, ethanol, and some sedative-hypnotics (Chapter 424). Pontine hemorrhage is a major nontoxicologic diagnosis to consider in a comatose patient with miotic pupils (Chapter 408). Mydriasis is a nonspecific finding. A unilateral dilated pupil may be due to topical ocular application of sympathomimetics (e.g., phenylephrine), antihistamines, or anticholinergic agents (e.g., inhaled anticholinergics such as ipratropium or tiotropium, dust or sap from *Datura* sp) and can be caused by a postauricular scopolamine patch. Failure of topical 4% pilocarpine ophthalmic drops to constrict the pupil supports the diagnosis of pupillary dilation from a topical mydriatic agent. Visual disturbances, including partial or total blindness as a result of systemic toxicity, have been reported with anticholinergic agents, carbon monoxide, digitalis, ethambutol, methanol, methyl bromide, quinine, and agents that are associated with pseudotumor cerebri, including antimicrobials (e.g., ampicillin, metronidazole, nalidixic acid, nitrofurantoin, sulfa drugs, tetracycline), glucocorticosteroids, lead, lithium, oral contraceptives, phenothiazines, phenytoin, and vitamin A. Nonarteritic anterior ischemic optic neuropathy has developed after the use of sildenafil and other related drugs (Chapter 234); the causal relationship is unknown.

Acute hearing loss (Chapter 428) can occur as a toxic effect of aminoglycosides, bromates, chloroquine, cisplatin, carboplatin, high-dose loop diuretics, nitrogen mustard, quinine, opioids, salicylates, vinblastine, and vincristine. Nasal septal erosions and perforations may be due to chronic exposure to intranasal cocaine (Chapter 34) or inhalation of fumes from chromium and nickel (Chapters 93 and 94).

Neurologic Signs

Many toxicants affect the central nervous system (CNS) and can produce agitated delirium, depression, or seizures (Table 110-2). Distinguishing features of various toxicants may assist in making the correct diagnosis. Patients who are withdrawing from opioids because of abstinence (as opposed to use of naloxone) are alert and oriented, whereas patients withdrawing from alcohol, barbiturates, benzodiazepines, and other sedative-hypnotics can be disoriented. Initial CNS depression can also develop with large ingestions of acetaminophen or ibuprofen. Isoniazid and theophylline are noted for producing seizures refractory to the usual doses of benzodiazepines and barbiturates. Pyridoxine treats isoniazid-induced seizures by increasing CNS γ-aminobutyric acid, which is depleted by isoniazid. Phenytoin is relatively ineffective for the majority of toxicant-induced seizures, perhaps because of the absence of a discrete seizure focus in most patients. Plant or mushroom ingestion can also produce CNS depression (e.g., *Rhododendron* sp, *Solanum* [bittersweet], *Taxus* [yew], *Sophora* [mescal bean]), CNS stimulation (e.g., *Catha edulis* [khat], *Strychnos nux-vomica* [contains strychnine], *Cicuta* sp [water hemlock], *Ephedra* [Mormon tea]), atropine-like effects (e.g., *Atropa belladonna* [deadly nightshade], *Datura* sp [jimsonweed]), and cholinomimetic effects (e.g., *Nicotiana* genus [tobacco], *Conium maculatum* [poison

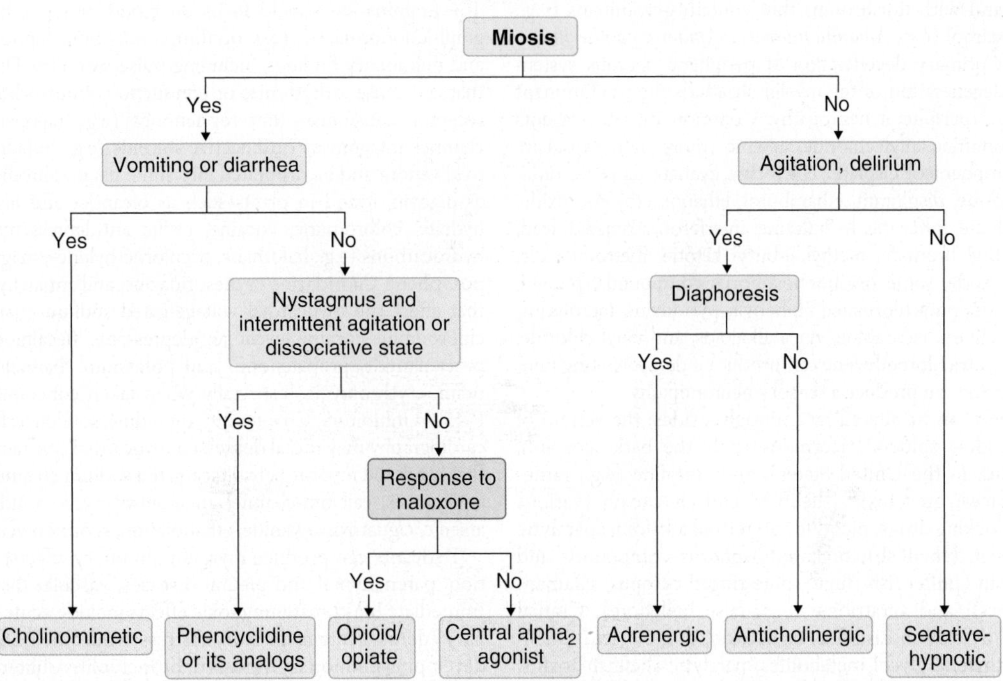

FIGURE 110-1. Diagnostic algorithm using the size of the pupils.

TABLE 110-2 CENTRAL NERVOUS SYSTEM EFFECTS OF TOXICANTS

	CNS EFFECTS		
TOXICANT CATEGORIES AND AGENTS	***Agitated Delirium***	***Decreased Level of Consciousness***	***Seizures***
CATEGORIES			
Adrenergic agonists	•		•
Anticholinergic agents	•	•	•
Anticonvulsants		•	• (paradoxical with some agents)
Antipsychotic drugs	•	•	•
β-Adrenergic receptor antagonists		•	•
Hallucinogenic agents	•		•
Monoamine oxidase inhibitors	•	•	•
Opioids	• (meperidine, tramadol)	•	• (meperidine, tramadol)
Sedative-hypnotics		•	• (rare)
Serotonin agonists	•	•	•
AGENTS			
Amphetamines, cocaine	•	•	•
Antidepressants	•	•	• (can be delayed with bupropion)
Antihistamines (first generation, e.g., diphenhydramine)	•	•	•
Barbiturates		•	
Benzodiazepines		•	
Cytochrome oxidase inhibitors (e.g., carbon monoxide, cyanide, hydrogen sulfide, azides)		•	•
Ephedra alkaloids and similar agents	•		•
Ethylene glycol, methanol	•	•	•
γ-Hydroxybutyrate and precursors	•	•	• (rare)
Lithium	•	•	•
Organophosphorus compounds (e.g., diazinon, malathion) and carbamates (e.g., carbaryl)		•	•
Salicylates	•	•	•
SSRIs/SRIs	•	•	• (uncommon)
Withdrawal from alcohol, barbiturates, benzodiazepines, other sedative-hypnotics	•	•	•
Withdrawal from opioids			• (reported only in neonates)

CNS = central nervous system; SRIs = serotonin re-uptake inhibitors; SSRIs = selective serotonin re-uptake inhibitors.

hemlock], *Inocybe* and *Clitocybe* mushrooms). Seizures can also occur with many of these plants and with mushrooms that contain gyromitrins (e.g., *Gyromitra* sp) and muscimol (e.g., *Amanita muscaria, Amanita pantherina*).

Distal axonopathy, a primary degeneration of peripheral nervous system axons with secondary degeneration of the myelin sheath, is the predominant type of toxicant-induced peripheral neuropathy. Common causative agents include acrylamide monomer, allyl chloride, arsenic (inorganic), capsaicin, carbon disulfide, chloramphenicol, cisplatin, colchicine, cyanate, dapsone, dideoxycytidine, dideoxyinosine, disulfiram, ethambutol, ethanol, ethylene oxide, gold salts, hexachlorophene, *n*-hexane, hydralazine, interferon, isoniazid, lead, linezolid, mercury, methyl bromide, methyl *n*-butyl ketone, metronidazole, nitrofurantoin, nitrous oxide, some organophosphorus compounds, phenol, platinum, podophyllotoxin, polychlorinated biphenyls, pyridoxine, tacrolimus, taxoids, thalidomide, thallium, vidarabine, vinca alkaloids, and vinyl chloride. Amiodarone, arsenic, and trichloroethylene can produce a demyelinating neuropathy, whereas pyridoxine can produce a sensory neuronopathy.

Neuronal transmission can be altered by aminoglycosides; the venom of *Latrodectus* species (widow spiders), scorpions (only the bark scorpion, *Centruroides sculpturatus*, in the United States), and crotaline (e.g., rattlesnakes) and elapid snakes; brevetoxin (shellfish) and ciguatoxin (various fish); neuromuscular blocking drugs; nicotine and related alkaloids; paralytic shellfish toxins; saxitoxin (shellfish); organophosphorus compounds and carbamates; tetrodotoxin (puffer fish [fugu], blue-ringed octopus, salamanders, newts, and others); and veratridine (e.g., false hellebore). Cranial nerves can be affected by carbon disulfide, ciguatoxin, domoic acid (shellfish), elapid venom, ethylene glycol metabolites, paralytic shellfish toxins, bark scorpion, saxitoxin, tetrodotoxin, thallium, and trichloroethylene. Mononeuropathies and vasculitic neuropathies are unlikely to be induced by toxicants (Chapter 112).

Cardiopulmonary Effects

The examination should focus on blood pressure, heart rate, electrocardiographic abnormalities (e.g., rhythm, conduction, depolarization, repolarization), and pulmonary findings, including pulse oximetry. Drugs and other toxicants that can cause arrhythmias or conduction abnormalities include β-adrenergic receptor antagonists, butyrophenones (e.g., haloperidol), L-type calcium-channel antagonists, cardioactive steroids (e.g., bufadienolides, found in toxic toad venom and incorporated into some illicit aphrodisiacs; cardenolides, such as digoxin, found in plants such as oleander and lily of the valley), chloral hydrate, chloroquine, cocaine, cyclic antidepressants, ethanol, halogenated hydrocarbons (e.g., halothane, trichloroethylene), magnesium, potassium, propoxyphene, thioridazine or mesoridazine, and antiarrhythmics and other agents that affect the myocardial voltage-gated sodium channels (e.g., bupivacaine, chloroquine, cocaine, cyclic antidepressants, flecainide, mexiletine, quinidine, procainamide, propafenone) and potassium channels (e.g., cisapride, citalopram, erythromycin [especially when taken concomitantly with cytochrome P-450 A inhibitors; Chapter 29], quinidine, sotalol, terfenadine). Bedside echocardiography may reveal depressed myocardial contractility as a result of agents that block the myocardial voltage-gated sodium channel, β-adrenergic receptor antagonists, calcium-channel antagonists, cyclic antidepressants, magnesium, arsenic, ciguatoxin, cyanide, ethanol, iron, scorpion venom, and tetrodotoxin.

Toxicants can produce myriad pulmonary effects, including airway irritation, parenchymal and pleural diseases, vascular diseases, and barotrauma. Immediate life-threatening toxic effects include acute lung injury and pulmonary edema, acute respiratory distress syndrome (Chapter 104), and rapidly developing pulmonary fibrosis or bronchiolitis obliterans. Typical syndromes and etiologic agents include pulmonary edema (β-adrenergic receptor antagonists, calcium-channel antagonists, antiarrhythmics, daunorubicin, doxorubicin), acute lung injury or acute respiratory distress syndrome (amphetamines, cadmium, chlorine, cocaine, ethchlorvynol, methotrexate, opioids, heroin, paraquat, salicylates; inhalation of smoke, zinc chloride, methyl bromide, methyl chloride), and rapidly developing pulmonary fibrosis or bronchiolitis obliterans (nitrogen dioxide, paraquat).

Gastrointestinal Effects

Symptoms of nausea, vomiting, diarrhea, and abdominal pain are nonspecific and must be interpreted in the context of other findings. Agents that produce severe or life-threatening toxicity with early gastrointestinal findings include acid or large alkali ingestions; cardiac glycosides, colchicines, and other microtubular toxicants (e.g., podophyllin); iron; metals such as arsenic, mercury salts, and thallium; mushrooms containing amanitin (*Amanita phalloides, Amanita virosa, Amanita verna, Lepiota chlorophyllum*), gyromitrins (*Gyromitra esculenta*), orellanines (*Cortinarius orellanus*), or allenic norleucine (*Amanita smithiana*); nicotine; organophosphorus compounds; and theophylline. Severe abdominal pain and rigidity can occur with envenomation by *Latrodectus* species (widow spiders). Hepatotoxicity can occur as an adverse effect of the therapeutic use of many drugs; in the United States, acetaminophen and ethanol are the most common causes of toxicant-induced hepatotoxicity (Chapter 150). Other notable hepatotoxicants include aflatoxins (in food contaminated with *Aspergillus flavus*), arsenicals, carbon tetrachloride, copper sulfate, cyclopeptide mushrooms (e.g., *Amanita phalloides*), *Ephedra* species (e.g., ma huang), iron, methamphetamine, pennyroyal oil, pyrrolizidine alkaloids (various plant species used in herbal teas), and vitamin A in chronic excessive doses.

Dermatologic Signs

The skin, hair, nails, and mucous membranes should be examined for evidence of intravenous drug use; the presence or absence of skin and mucous membrane moisture; abnormal skin coloration, including erythema and cyanosis; alopecia; and nail abnormalities. Bullous skin lesions have been reported with chronic barbiturate use, glutethimide, carbon monoxide, meprobamate, methadone, and valproic acid. Cyanosis may reflect hypoxemia or methemoglobinemia. Commonly used agents that can cause methemoglobinemia include aniline dyes, benzocaine and other amide anesthetics, dapsone, naphthalene, nitrates, nitrites, phenazopyridine, rifampin, and sulfonamides. Skin erythema or flushing occurs with anticholinergic agents, boric acid ingestion, monosodium glutamate, niacin, scombroid toxicity as a result of the ingestion of inadequately refrigerated fish with a high histidine content (e.g., tuna, mahi-mahi, amberjack), vancomycin, and interactions between ethanol and numerous agents that produce disulfiram or disulfiram-like reactions (e.g., carbon disulfide, some cephalosporins, *Coprinus atramentarius* mushroom, disulfiram, griseofulvin, metronidazole, thiuram herbicides, trichloroethylene).

Specific Toxicants

Some common toxicants can be suspected from their characteristic manifestations (Table 110-3). These suspicions should guide specific diagnostic and therapeutic strategies that complement general decontamination and supportive treatments.

Diagnostic Tests

Drug testing should be guided by the history and physical examination, with emphasis on tests that can influence management. Rapid qualitative urine drug screening tests are readily available in most hospitals, but their clinical value is limited by the number of drugs that can be tested and the reliability of the tests themselves. Although such testing may be valuable for subsequent psychiatric evaluation, it is less reliable for urgent diagnosis and therapy. For example, a positive test result may be unrelated to the patient's condition because drug analytes may be detectable for days after drug use, depending on the drug, dose, and frequency of use. In addition, both false-positive and false-negative results occur (Table 110-4), so the screening result must be verified with a second method, such as gas chromatography–mass spectrometry. The type of drug use in a population should be considered in determining the drugs to be screened to decrease the incidence of false-positive results. A test with 99% specificity for a drug with a prevalence of 0.1% in a population would produce 10 false-positive results for

TABLE 110-3 PATHOPHYSIOLOGY, CLINICAL EFFECTS, AND MANAGEMENT OF SPECIFIC DRUGS AND TOXICANTS

DRUG OR TOXICANT	PATHOPHYSIOLOGY	CLINICAL EFFECTS	LABORATORY	SPECIFIC THERAPY
Acetaminophen[7]	NAPQI (toxic metabolite) binds hepatic and renal tubular cells; acetaminophen itself induces transient decrease in functional factor VII	Initial: nausea, vomiting, coma, lactic acidosis in severe cases Days 1-3: elevated INR, aminotransferase levels; RUQ tenderness; increased creatinine level in severe cases Days 4-14: gradual recovery or continued increase in INR and creatinine, lactic acidosis, coma, cerebral edema, death	Potentially toxic level ≥150 μg/mL 4 hours after ingestion* INR may be transiently elevated in first 24 hours because of decrease in functional factor VII; further increases indicate hepatic necrosis; elevated aminotransferase and bilirubin levels not predictive of hepatic failure Creatinine elevated in severe cases	NAC (see dosing guidelines in Table 110-6); NAC can increase INR but not aPTT[†]
Amphetamines	Increased release of presynaptic norepinephrine and dopamine Increased serotonin release (especially MDMA, PMA, DOB, other synthetic amphetamines)	Mild: euphoria, decreased appetite, repetitive behavior Moderate: vomiting, agitation, hypertension, tachycardia, mydriasis, bruxism, diaphoresis Severe: hypertension or hypotension, arrhythmias, hyperthermia, seizures, coma, multisystem organ failure, hyponatremia (SIADH), cerebral infarction or hemorrhage	Not helpful; many false-positives and false-negatives on screening tests (see Table 110-4)	IV crystalloids External cooling Benzodiazepines to control agitation or seizures Benzodiazepines or phentolamine for hypertension See SSRIs/SRIs for features and treatment of serotonin syndrome
β-Adrenergic receptor antagonists	Blocks catecholamines from β-adrenergic receptors α- and β-adrenergic receptor antagonism: carvedilol, labetalol Delayed rectifier potassium-channel blockade: sotalol	Bradyarrhythmias (with high doses), decreased myocardial contractility, hypotension, respiratory depression, decreased consciousness with seizures or coma (lipophilic agents, e.g., propranolol), prolonged QT interval (sotalol)	ECG No specific tests	IV glucagon, 3-5 mg over 2-minute period; if no increase in BP or HR, can repeat up to 10 mg; if effective, immediately start continuous infusion at 2-10 mg/hr; if still unstable, options include (1) regular insulin, 1 U/kg by IV bolus, followed by 1 U/kg/hr, plus dextrose to maintain euglycemia; (2) norepinephrine or dobutamine infusion titrated to desirable BP and HR Electrical pacing, IABP, or intravenous lipid emulsion therapy in refractory cases

TABLE 110-3 PATHOPHYSIOLOGY, CLINICAL EFFECTS, AND MANAGEMENT OF SPECIFIC DRUGS AND TOXICANTS—cont'd

DRUG OR TOXICANT	PATHOPHYSIOLOGY	CLINICAL EFFECTS	LABORATORY	SPECIFIC THERAPY
L-type calcium-channel antagonists	Blocks L-type voltage-sensitive calcium channels, thereby decreasing calcium entry into myocardial and vascular smooth muscle cells Decreases pancreatic insulin release and increases insulin resistance	Bradyarrhythmias (verapamil, diltiazem), hypotension, hyperglycemia Tachycardia and hypotension (dihydropyridines such as amlodipine, nifedipine)	ECG No specific tests	IV 10% calcium chloride, 10-20 mg/kg (0.1-0.2 mL/kg); can repeat once; if BP improves, continuous infusion at 0.2-0.5 mL/kg/hr (20-50 mg/kg/hr) Ionized Ca^{2+} levels should not exceed 2× normal (severe cases will be refractory to calcium therapy) Glucagon, high-dose insulin and dextrose, catecholamines, and milrinone (as for β-adrenergic antagonists) Intravenous lipid emulsion therapy for verapamil and diltiazem, unclear for dihydropyridines
Cardiac glycosides, including digoxin, bufadienolides (toxic toad venom), and cardenolides (e.g., oleander, lily of the valley, dogbane)	Inhibits Na^+,K^+-ATPase Decreased CNS sympathetic output Decreased baroreceptor sensitivity Increased vagal acetylcholine discharge	Bradyarrhythmias, including second- and third-degree AV block and asystole Ventricular ectopy, tachycardia, fibrillation Junctional tachycardia, paroxysmal atrial tachycardia with block Weakness, visual disturbances, nausea, vomiting	Serum digoxin level Serum potassium (hyperkalemia occurs in acute poisoning and is prognostic for poor outcome without Fab; hypokalemia may be present in chronic poisoning due to concomitant medications), magnesium, and creatinine levels	Correct hypokalemia and hypomagnesemia; do not give calcium Digoxin-specific antibody fragments (Fab) indicated if patient has hemodynamically significant arrhythmias, serum potassium ≥5 mEq/L if acute overdose, Mobitz II or third-degree AV block, ingestion of bufadienolide- or cardenolide-containing agents, or renal insufficiency Empirical dose Chronic: 2-5 vials Acute: 10-20 vials Calculated dose Chronic: number of vials = 2 × serum digoxin level (ng/mL) × 5.6 × weight (kg)/1000 Acute: number of vials = 2 × oral digoxin dose (mg) × 0.8 If hypokalemic (generally chronic overdose), replete serum potassium
Cyclic antidepressants	Myocardial sodium- and potassium-channel blockade Blockade of α-adrenergic and cholinergic muscarinic receptors Inhibition of norepinephrine re-uptake	Decreased level of consciousness (can develop rapidly), myoclonus, seizures, coma Anticholinergic toxidrome (see Table 110-1) Sinus tachycardia, ventricular conduction delays, ventricular arrhythmias, asystole Hypotension	Serum levels not helpful in management	Intermittent IV boluses of $NaHCO_3$ (1 mEq/kg) to narrow QRS to <100 msec; infusion of $NaHCO_3$ is less effective; maintain arterial pH at 7.5 because alkalemia and sodium ions can improve cardiovascular performance Contraindicated drugs: types IA and IC antiarrhythmic agents, physostigmine, flumazenil
Ethylene glycol, methanol (e.g., antifreeze, window cleaners, camping stove fuels)	Ethylene glycol: toxic metabolites produce cytotoxicity in CNS, kidneys, lungs, heart, liver, muscles; metabolic acidosis is due to glycolate accumulation; oxalate complexes with calcium, so hypocalcemia can develop Methanol: metabolized to formic acid, which is responsible for metabolic acidosis and inhibition of cytochrome aa_3; target organs include retina, optic nerve, CNS	Ethylene glycol: CNS depression, cerebral edema, seizures, anion gap metabolic acidosis, renal failure with acute tubular necrosis, pulmonary edema, myositis Methanol: nausea, vomiting; cerebral edema, hemorrhage, infarcts; necrosis of thalamus and putamen; anion gap metabolic acidosis; visual disturbances, papilledema, hyperemic optic disc, nonreactive pupils	Serum ethylene glycol and methanol levels; levels may be low or undetectable if significant metabolism has occurred Ethylene glycol: serum calcium, creatinine, BUN levels; examine urine for calcium oxalate crystals; false hyperlactatemia occurs with certain analyzers using L-lactate oxidase, which cross-reacts with glycolic and glyoxylic acid metabolites	For both: fomepizole[8] (inhibits alcohol dehydrogenase and blocks formation of toxic metabolites), 15 mg/kg IV loading dose, then 10 mg/kg IV for 4 doses during the next 48 hours, then 15 mg/kg for subsequent doses; interval dosing is q12h (q4h during hemodialysis, with dosing interval adjustments at start and finish); continue until ethylene glycol or methanol is no longer detectable Use of ethanol is no longer recommended Hemodialysis: initiate if level is ≥50 mg/dL or metabolic acidosis with end-organ toxicity; continue until acidosis resolves and serum level of ethylene glycol or methanol is undetectable (if available) Monitor for cerebral edema with possible herniation Ethylene glycol: IV calcium for symptomatic hypocalcemia Methanol: folinic acid, 50 mg IV q4h until methanol not detectable and acidosis cleared

TABLE 110-3 PATHOPHYSIOLOGY, CLINICAL EFFECTS, AND MANAGEMENT OF SPECIFIC DRUGS AND TOXICANTS—cont'd

DRUG OR TOXICANT	PATHOPHYSIOLOGY	CLINICAL EFFECTS	LABORATORY	SPECIFIC THERAPY
γ-Hydroxybutyrate (GHB) and its precursors (γ-butyrolactone and 1,4-butanediol)	Agonist effect on CNS GHB receptors; indirect action with opioid receptors (may increase proenkephalins); metabolized to GABA, interacts with $GABA_B$ receptors; decreases dopamine release	CNS: rapid loss of consciousness, with recovery typical within 2-4 hours; myoclonus (possible seizures) Respiratory depression; bradycardia; nausea, vomiting	No specific tests	Supportive care, including respiratory support as needed Withdrawal resembles sedative-hypnotic withdrawal and can be treated with benzodiazepines or pentobarbital
Lithium	Decreases brain inositol; alters CNS serotonin, dopamine, and norepinephrine; inhibits adenylate cyclases, including those that mediate vasopressin-induced renal concentration and thyroid function	Chronic toxicity usually more severe than acute toxicity: tremor, hyperreflexia, drowsiness, incoordination, clonus, confusion, ataxia; in severe cases, seizures, coma, death; recovery may take weeks, and CNS deficits may persist Sinus node dysfunction, QT prolongation, T wave abnormalities, U waves Nephrogenic diabetes insipidus, hypothyroidism, hyperthyroidism, hypercalcemia, pseudotumor cerebri Acute toxicity: nausea, vomiting, diarrhea, and milder neurologic findings	Peak serum levels: Normal dose, 2-3 hours; up to 5 hours for sustained-release lithium Acute overdose: peak may be delayed ≥4-12 hours	Replenish intravascular volume, maintain urinary output at 1-2 mL/kg/hr Consider gastrointestinal decontamination with oral polyethylene glycol electrolyte solution within 1-2 hours after acute overdose of sustained-release drug Hemodialysis[†] in patients with altered mental status, ataxia, seizures, or coma or in patients with mild symptoms in the setting of acute overdose or renal insufficiency Ineffective or contraindicated therapies include oral activated charcoal, diuretics, and aminophylline
Opioids (e.g., opiate [natural]: morphine, codeine; semisynthetic: heroin, oxycodone, hydrocodone; synthetic: methadone, fentanyl)	Agonist effect at CNS μ, κ, and δ opioid receptors; result is cell hyperpolarization and decreased neurotransmitter release	CNS depression, respiratory depression, miosis (see Table 110-1) Dextromethorphan increases CNS serotonin and inhibits NMDA receptors, which causes hallucinations Seizure risk with tramadol, meperidine QTc prolongation and torsades de pointes with methadone	Rapid urine drug screens detect morphine, poorly detect semisynthetic opioids, and do not detect synthetic opioids; some interferents/irrelevants (see Table 110-4)	Ventilate and oxygenate IV naloxone, 0.04 mg initial dose and titrate every 2-3 minutes in patients with likely opioid dependence; in patients known to be naïve, start 0.4 mg; repeat up to 10 mg if no response Continuous infusion for recurrent symptoms or sustained-release opioid ingestion; give 50% of dose that produces desired effect 15 minutes after initial effect is obtained, then infuse two thirds of this dose every hour; infusion rate can be increased or decreased to maintain normal respiration and to avoid withdrawal symptoms Contraindicated therapies: naltrexone should not be used for acute opioid reversal[9]
Organophosphorus compounds and carbamates (e.g., diazinon, mevinphos, fenthion, aldicarb)	Inhibits acetylcholinesterase, resulting in excessive acetylcholine stimulation of nicotinic and muscarinic receptors in autonomic and somatic motor nervous systems and CNS	Nicotinic-mediated effects: tachycardia, mydriasis, hypertension, delirium, coma, seizures, muscle weakness, fasciculations Muscarinic-mediated effects: salivation, lacrimation, urination, vomiting, defecation, miosis, bronchorrhea, bronchospasm, bradycardia	Serum (butyrylcholinesterase) or RBC (acetylcholinesterase) activity <50% of normal (see Table 110-6) Clinical recovery occurs before serum cholinesterase levels normalize	Atropine, 1-2 mg by initial IV bolus; double the dose every 5 minutes (2 mg, 4 mg, 8 mg, 16 mg, and so on) until drying of bronchial secretions, adequate oxygenation, pulse >80 beats/min, systolic blood pressure >80 mm Hg achieved; continuous infusion at 10-20% of total stabilizing dose per hour; stop infusion when patient develops concerning signs or symptoms of anticholinergic toxidrome (see Table 110-1); restart infusion at lower rate when signs or symptoms abate Pralidoxime chloride 30 mg/kg (maximum 2 g) IV bolus during 30 minutes, then 8-10 mg/kg/hr (maximum 650 mg/hr) continuous infusion; administer as soon as possible after poisoning; continue 12-24 hours after atropine no longer required and symptoms resolve[§]

TABLE 110-3 PATHOPHYSIOLOGY, CLINICAL EFFECTS, AND MANAGEMENT OF SPECIFIC DRUGS AND TOXICANTS—cont'd

DRUG OR TOXICANT	PATHOPHYSIOLOGY	CLINICAL EFFECTS	LABORATORY	SPECIFIC THERAPY
Salicylates	Inhibit cyclooxygenase; decrease formation of prostaglandins and thromboxane A_2; stimulate CNS medullary respiratory center and chemoreceptor trigger zone; impair platelet function; disrupt carbohydrate metabolism; uncouple oxidative phosphorylation; increase vascular permeability	Acute toxicity Mild: nausea, vomiting, diaphoresis, tinnitus, decreased hearing, hyperpnea, tachypnea Moderate-severe: confusion, delirium, coma, seizures, hyperthermia, ARDS; death can occur within hours of overdose Chronic toxicity: same as acute, but may not have diaphoresis or vomiting Consider diagnosis in patients with new-onset confusion, anion gap metabolic acidosis, or acute lung injury	Serum salicylate level: toxic ≥30 mg/dL; level ≥100 mg/dL indicates life-threatening toxicity with possible sudden, rapid clinical deterioration; in chronic toxicity, levels may be minimally elevated (>30 mg/dL), and clinical evaluation is more reliable for gauging degree of toxicity Arterial blood gases: respiratory alkalosis with metabolic acidosis Anion gap metabolic acidosis Prolonged PT and PTT, ketonuria, ketonemia	Multidose activated charcoal q2-3h in acute overdose Hemodialysis with progressive symptoms, particularly neurologic, hyperthermia, renal failure, ARDS, or salicylate level >100 even with minor clinical findings
SSRIs/SRIs	Inhibit re-uptake of serotonin SRIs have additional effects (e.g., duloxetine inhibits norepinephrine re-uptake, nefazodone inhibits serotonergic 5-HT_2 receptors, trazodone inhibits peripheral α-adrenergic receptors, venlafaxine inhibits norepinephrine and dopamine re-uptake)	Vomiting, blurred vision, CNS depression, tachycardia Seizures and coma rare Torsades de pointes reported with citalopram Serotonin toxicity: clonus, agitation, tremor, diaphoresis, hyperreflexia; hyperthermia and hypertonicity in severe cases	No specific tests If serotonin toxicity suspected: electrolytes, BUN, glucose, liver enzymes, coagulation panel, blood gases, chest radiograph	Respiratory support as needed Benzodiazepines for agitation or seizures Serotonin toxicity: consider cyproheptadine, 12 mg PO initial dose, then 2 mg PO q2h (to a maximum of 32 mg/day) until symptoms resolve Critical therapies for hyperthermia, rhabdomyolysis, DIC, ARDS, renal and hepatic dysfunction, torsades de pointes

*A nomogram to evaluate the potential toxicity of levels drawn more than 4 hours after ingestion is provided in Rumack BH, Matthew H. Acetaminophen poisoning and toxicity. *Pediatrics.* 1975;55:871-876. The nomogram is valid only for levels drawn after a single acute ingestion.
†Intravenous *N*-acetylcysteine (NAC) has generally replaced oral NAC for the majority of cases, largely because of convenience, not efficacy. The full 21-hour course of intravenous NAC should be administered in most situations in which it is used. Oral NAC, which remains an acceptable alternative, can be discontinued in patients with uncomplicated disease after a loading dose plus six maintenance doses if hepatic aminotransferase levels are normal and acetaminophen is not detected; otherwise, the full regimen should be administered.
‡Continue hemodialysis until the serum lithium level is less than 1 mEq/L. Recheck the level 4 to 8 hours after dialysis, and restart hemodialysis if the level is higher than 1 mEq/L. Repeat this cycle until the serum lithium level remains lower than 1 mEq/L.
§Randomized, placebo-controlled trials of pralidoxime in acute organophosphorus poisoning have not found a significant difference in mortality rates or need for intubation. A3
aPTT = activated partial thromboplastin time; ARDS = acute respiratory distress syndrome; AV = atrioventricular; BP = blood pressure; BUN = blood urea nitrogen; CNS = central nervous system; DIC = disseminated intravascular coagulation; DOB = 4-bromo-2,5-dimethoxyamphetamine; ECG = electrocardiogram; GABA = γ-aminobutyric acid; HR = heart rate; IABP = intra-aortic balloon counterpulsation; INR = international normalized ratio; MDMA = 3,4-methylenedioxymethamphetamine; Na^+,K^+-ATPase = sodium, potassium adenosine triphosphatase; NAC = *N*-acetylcysteine; NAPQI = *N*-acetyl-*p*-benzoquinone imine; NMDA = *N*-methyl-D-aspartate; PMA = paramethoxyamphetamine; PT = prothrombin time; PTT = partial thromboplastin time; RBC = red blood cell; RUQ = right upper quadrant (abdomen); SIADH = syndrome of inappropriate antidiuretic secretion; SRIs = serotonin re-uptake inhibitors; SSRIs = selective serotonin re-uptake inhibitor.

TABLE 110-4 QUALITATIVE URINE DRUG SCREENS: CAUSES OF ERRONEOUS RESULTS*

DRUG/TOXICANT	INTERFERENTS/IRRELEVANTS†	COMMENTS
Amphetamines	Amantadine, bupropion, chlorpromazine, ephedrine, pseudoephedrine, desoxyephedrine, ephedra alkaloids (from *Ephedra* sp), mexiletine, phenylephrine, phenylpropanolamine, selegiline, trazodone	Many false positives; Vicks nasal inhaler (desoxyephedrine) and selegiline also cause positive GC-MS findings; chiral confirmation is required; newer immunoassays have eliminated false-positive results from desoxyephedrine
Benzodiazepines	Oxaprozin, sertraline	Most assays directed against oxazepam; poor detection of benzodiazepines without the oxazepam metabolite (e.g., alprazolam, lorazepam, triazolam)
Cocaine	Coca leaf teas (clinical false positive)	Few analytical false positives; urine is reliable for detecting true positives
Opiates, opioids	Poppy seeds (contain morphine), quinine, quinolones, rifampin	Assay directed against morphine; poorly detects semisynthetic opiates and does not detect synthetic opiates (e.g., fentanyls, meperidine, methadone, propoxyphene)
Phencyclidine	Dextromethorphan, diphenhydramine, doxylamine, ibuprofen, ketamine, tramadol, venlafaxine	Can be used, although not reliably, to identify dextromethorphan or ketamine misuse and abuse
Tetrahydrocannabinol	Dronabinol, efavirenz, proton pump inhibitors	Positive result is seldom clinically relevant; synthetic cannabinomimetics (e.g., spice, K2) are not reliably detected
Tricyclic antidepressants	Carbamazepine, cyclobenzaprine, cyproheptadine, diphenhydramine, phenothiazines, quetiapine	

*Advances in drug screening and variability in immunoassay results should be considered by the clinician when interpreting qualitative drug screening results. Consultation with the testing laboratory is advised. Positive screening results are considered presumptive and should be verified by GC-MS.
†Irrelevants are agents causing true-positive but clinically irrelevant results on laboratory screening tests; they vary, depending on the screening method.
GC-MS = gas chromatography–mass spectrometry.

every true-positive result. Clinically irrelevant true-positive findings also occur, such as when poppy seeds produce a positive opiate test result. Failure to consider these limitations of drug screens can result in misdiagnosis.

For a limited number of drugs and toxicants, levels in blood or urine are useful for diagnosis, therapy, or monitoring (Table 110-5). Threshold levels of certain toxicants indicate the need for specific therapies: acetaminophen (*N*-acetylcysteine), ethylene glycol (fomepizole and hemodialysis), iron (deferoxamine), methanol (fomepizole and hemodialysis), methemoglobin (methylene blue), and salicylates (urine alkalinization and hemodialysis). In chronic poisoning with some drugs, such as salicylates or theophylline, these therapies may be indicated at lower drug levels. In general, any end-organ toxicity that is evident or anticipated (on the basis of the toxicant, amount

TABLE 110-5 CLINICALLY IMPORTANT QUANTITATIVE DRUG LEVELS

DRUG OR TOXICANT	LEVELS	
	Therapeutic	***Toxic****
SOURCE: BLOOD OR SERUM		
Acetaminophen[†]	10-30 μg/mL	≥150 μg/mL 4 hours after ingestion[‡]
Carbamazepine	4-12 μg/mL	>15 μg/mL
Carboxyhemoglobin	Nonsmoker: 0.5-1.5% Smoker: 4-9%	>20%[§]
Cholinesterase[‖]		
Serum (butyrylcholinesterase)	3100-6500 U/L	<50% of normal value
Red blood cell (acetylcholinesterase)	26.7-49.2 U/g of hemoglobin	<50% of normal value
Digoxin (≥6 hours after oral dose for long-term therapy)	0.8-2.0 ng/mL[¶]	>2.0 ng/mL
Ethanol	None measured	>80 mg/dL**
Ethylene glycol	None measured	>25 mg/dL
Iron	50-175 μg/dL	>350 g/dL
Lead	<10 μg/dL	>25 g/dL
Lithium	0.6-1.2 mEq/L	>1.2 mEq/L[††]
Methanol	None measured	>25 mg/dL
Methemoglobin	1-2%	>15%
Phenobarbital	15-40 μg/mL	>40 g/mL
Phenytoin	10-20 μg/mL	>20 g/mL
Salicylates	≤30 mg/dL	>30 mg/dL
Theophylline	8-20 μg/mL	>20 g/mL
Valproic acid	50-100 μg/mL	>100 g/mL
SOURCE: URINE	***Normal***	***Toxic****
Arsenic	< 50 μg/day	>100 g/24-hr urine[††]
Mercury	< 20 μg/L	>20 g/L[††]
Thallium	< 5.0 μg/L	>200 g/L[††]

*The "toxic" level is provided for perspective. For many toxicants, simply being above this value does not imply a specific need for therapy or a necessarily poor prognosis. It does, however, suggest a need for additional evaluation, observation, or monitoring.
[†]False-positive levels of 16 to 28 μg/mL have been reported in patients with bilirubin levels greater than 17 mg/dL.
[‡]Levels drawn more than 4 hours after ingestion should be plotted on the nomogram provided by Rumack and Matthew (Rumack BH, Matthew H. Acetaminophen poisoning and toxicity. *Pediatrics.* 1975;55:871-876) to assess the potential for toxicity.
[§]Lower levels may be toxic in pregnant patients and in those with prolonged exposure to carbon monoxide.
[‖]Consult a reference laboratory for normal values; results are assay dependent.
[¶]Some patients may require levels above the therapeutic range to control symptoms.
**The value of 80 mg/dL for ethanol is the statutory limit for operating a motor vehicle. Toxic clinical effects are uncommon with concentrations below 200 mg/dL.
[††]Lower values may indicate toxicity if appropriate clinical findings are present.

ingested, and time required to produce toxic effects) is more important than a specific level in determining the need for treatment.

Occult acetaminophen ingestion with toxic serum levels occurs in 0.3 to 1.9% of intentional ingestions. Given that these patients may be asymptomatic until hepatotoxicity develops and that administration of an antidote can prevent this hepatotoxicity, the current recommendation is to test the serum for acetaminophen in all patients with intentional self-harm ingestions.

Other Blood Tests

Anion gap metabolic acidosis resulting from primary lactic acidosis can be caused by cyanide, hydrogen sulfide, iron, isoniazid, metformin, nucleoside reverse transcriptase inhibitors, phenformin, sodium azide, and, rarely, acetaminophen with high serum levels. Anion gap metabolic acidosis not related to lactic acidosis occurs with diethylene glycol, ethylene glycol, nonsteroidal anti-inflammatory drugs, methanol, salicylates, and toluene. In poisonings resulting from ibuprofen, methanol, propylene glycol, and salicylates, lactic acid can also be produced, but the level is insufficient to account for the anion gap. Anion gap metabolic acidosis can also develop in patients with ongoing agitation, hyperthermia, and muscle rigidity, such as in neuroleptic malignant syndrome (Chapter 434), or in some cases of rhabdomyolysis (Chapter 113) secondary to toxicants such as doxylamine, phencyclidine, strychnine, cocaine, and amphetamines. Elevated serum creatinine and blood urea nitrogen levels indicative of declining renal function may be seen with numerous toxicants. Direct toxicity occurs with acetaminophen, aminoglycosides, cadmium, Chinese weight-loss botanicals (containing *Stephania tetrandra* or *Magnolia officinalis*), chromium, *Crotalus durissus* venom, diethylene glycol, diquat, ethylene glycol, fluorinated anesthetics, gold, heroin, lithium (diabetes insipidus), mercury salts, mushrooms (*Amanita smithiana* and *Cortinarius* sp), paraquat, radiocontrast agents, solvents (e.g., carbon tetrachloride, trichloroethylene, tetrachloroethylene, toluene), and sulfonamides. Agents that decrease glomerular perfusion by reducing renal blood flow include amphotericin, angiotensin-converting enzyme inhibitors, angiotensin receptor blockers, cocaine, cyclosporine, mannitol (excessive chronic doses), methotrexate, and nonsteroidal anti-inflammatory drugs.

Imaging

A computed tomographic scan of the head can detect life-threatening cerebral edema secondary to toxicant-induced hepatic failure, ethylene glycol, and methanol. It also detects intracranial bleeding caused by anticoagulants, scorpion venom, and sympathomimetics (e.g., amphetamines, cocaine, phenylpropanolamine). An abdominal radiograph can reveal radiopaque ferrous sulfate tablets or metals such as arsenic, lead, mercury, and thallium.

Diagnostic Syndromes

Given the myriad combinations of signs, symptoms, and laboratory findings, making the correct diagnosis in a noncommunicative patient can be daunting. A thorough history from bystanders, friends, and prehospital medical personnel may yield crucial information. In addition, the diagnostic possibilities can be narrowed by findings that can narrow the differential diagnosis with modest certainty. For example, consider a patient with sudden loss of consciousness, anion gap metabolic acidosis, and bradycardia without hypoxemia. Among the possible causes of anion gap metabolic acidosis (see earlier) and sudden loss of consciousness are hydrogen sulfide, cyanide, and severe poisoning with sodium azide; however, sinus bradycardia in the absence of acute ischemic cardiac injury is typical only of cyanide poisoning.

TREATMENT

Rx

Initial Stabilization

Intubation and Respiratory Support

Appropriate airway management should be instituted to correct hypoxemia and respiratory acidosis and to protect against pulmonary aspiration (Fig. 110-2); intubation should be considered if the patient has depressed consciousness and a decreased gag reflex. Rapid-sequence intubation facilitates airway management. Anatomic difficulties should be anticipated in patients with caustic ingestions (e.g., hypopharyngeal burns that may perforate); angioedema caused by angiotensin-converting enzyme inhibitor therapy or envenomation by some rattlesnakes, such as the canebrake (*Crotalus horridus atricaudatus*) and eastern diamondback (*Crotalus adamanteus*; Chapter 112); and swelling secondary to direct tissue injury (e.g., huffing compressed hydrocarbons, smoking crack) or secondary to anaphylactoid and anaphylactic reactions. Endotracheal intubation by flexible fiberoptic nasopharyngoscopy may be indicated in these cases. Hypoxemia can occur with toxicants that produce CNS depression, such as antidepressants, barbiturates, sedative-hypnotics, and central α_2-adrenergic receptor agonists (clonidine), or agents causing peripheral neuromuscular impairment, such as nicotine, organophosphorus compounds, strychnine, tetrodotoxin (puffer fish, blue-ringed octopus), botulinum, or envenomation from elapids (coral snake), Mojave rattlesnakes, or certain coelenterates (box jellyfish; Chapter 112).

Respiratory acidosis can rapidly worsen the toxicities of cyclic antidepressants and salicylates; sedation of these patients should be accompanied by immediate airway support. Intoxicated patients may have an increased risk for pulmonary aspiration because of concomitant CNS depression, attenuated airway reflexes, full stomachs, and delayed gastric emptying.

Succinylcholine can cause prolonged paralysis in patients with organophosphorus poisoning and can exacerbate hyperkalemia from cardioactive steroids (e.g., digoxin), hydrofluoric acid, or rhabdomyolysis (Chapter 113).

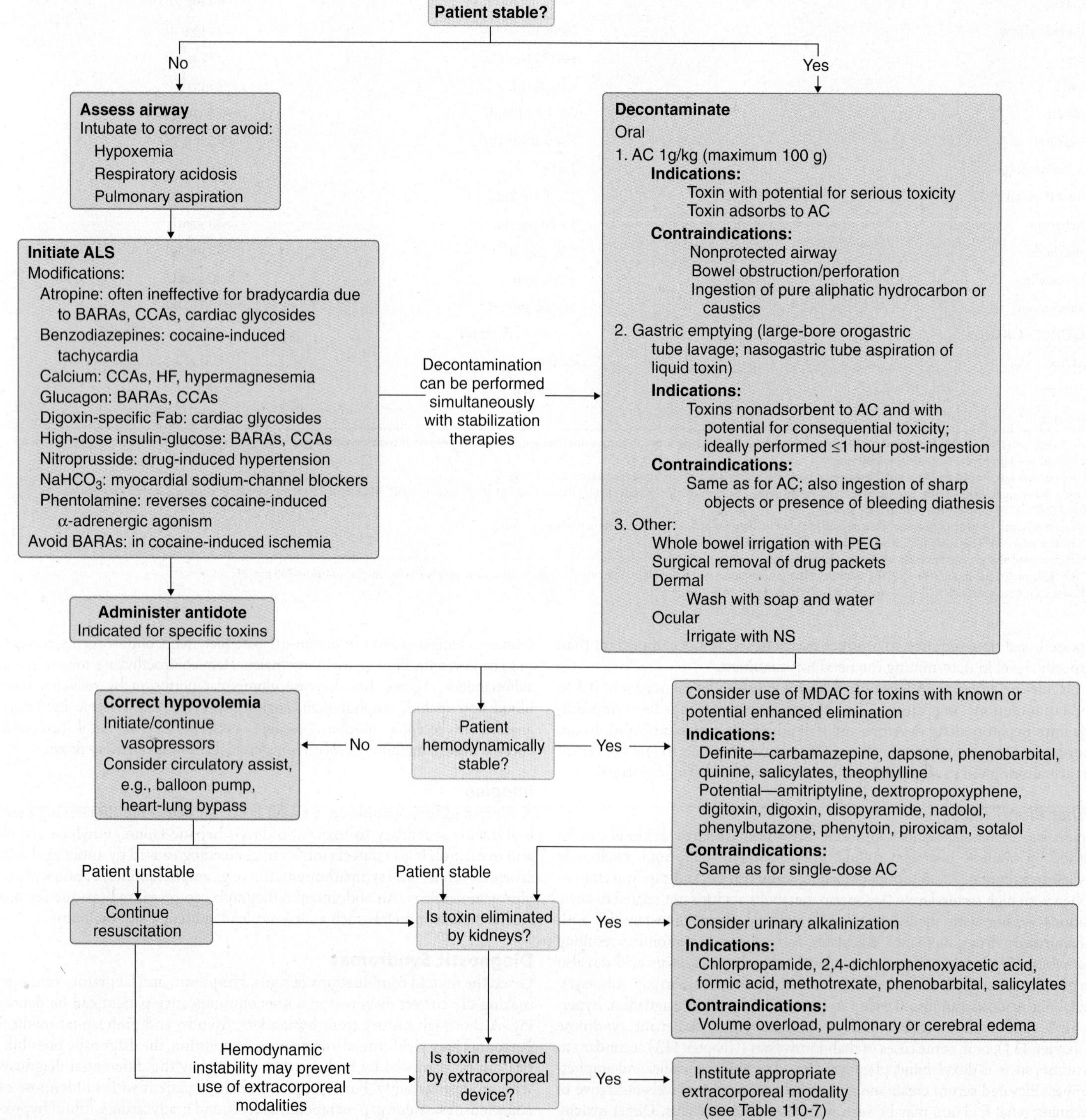

FIGURE 110-2. Algorithm for the management of acute poisoning. AC = activated charcoal; ALS = advanced life support; BARAs = β-adrenergic receptor antagonists; CCAs = L-type calcium-channel antagonists; HF = hydrofluoric acid; MDAC = multidose activated charcoal; NS = 0.9% saline solution; PEG = nonabsorbable polyethylene glycol solution.

Rhabdomyolysis has been reported with adrenergic agents, doxylamine, phencyclidine, heroin, *Tricholoma equestre* mushrooms, and envenomation by crotaline snakes, scorpions, or widow spiders (*Latrodectus* sp); short-acting nondepolarizing agents, such as vecuronium and rocuronium, are preferable in these cases.

Advanced Life Support

Standard emergency cardiovascular care algorithms (Chapter 63) must be modified for effects caused by specific poisons. Atropine often does not reverse bradycardia secondary to β-adrenergic receptor antagonists, L-type calcium-channel antagonists, or cardiac glycosides, and it may actually impair the ability to do adequate gastrointestinal decontamination. In these cases, more specific therapy with intravenous calcium (calcium-channel antagonists), high doses of glucagon (β-adrenergic receptor antagonists, calcium-channel antagonists), or digoxin-specific Fab antibody (cardiac glycosides) is indicated. High-dose insulin-glucose therapy can successfully reverse myocardial depression and conduction abnormalities in humans poisoned with β-adrenergic receptor antagonists and calcium-channel antagonists. Intravenous sodium bicarbonate may reverse cardiac conduction delays caused by antiarrhythmic drugs with sodium-channel blockade recovery rates of greater than 1 second (Vaughn-Williams classification IA and IC), cocaine, cyclic antidepressants, diphenhydramine, and quinine. β-Adrenergic receptor antagonists are contraindicated in patients with cocaine-induced myocardial syndromes because they can result in unopposed α-adrenergic–mediated vasoconstriction, but phentolamine can reverse the agonistic effects of cocaine on α-adrenergic receptors. Benzodiazepines can reverse significant sinus tachycardia from sympathomimetic agents. Calcium may also be life-saving in systemic hydrofluoric acid poisoning and severe hypermagnesemia, and it is indicated for symptomatic hypocalcemia caused by ethylene glycol toxicity. Drug-induced hypertension may be transitory; nitroprusside should be used if treatment is clinically indicated. In patients with toxicant-induced circulatory collapse refractory to maximal therapy, including vasopressors, circulatory assist devices may support the patient until sufficient toxicant is eliminated (Chapter 107).

Decontamination

Activated Charcoal

Single-dose activated charcoal without prior gastric emptying has been the preferred method of treatment for the ingestion of substances that have the potential to cause moderate to life-threatening toxicity and are known to adsorb to activated charcoal. The absence of clinical signs and symptoms does not preclude administration of activated charcoal because drug absorption and toxicity can be delayed. Activated charcoal can also be administered when the ingested toxicant cannot be identified but significant toxicity is a concern. Activated charcoal consists of pyrolysis products that have been specially cleaned to produce an internal pore structure to which substances can adsorb, thereby limiting their systemic absorption. Activated charcoal can be administered with antiemetic drugs or given through a nasogastric tube, when necessary. The oral dose is approximately 1 g/kg body weight, with a maximum single dose of 100 g. Efficacy in preventing toxicant absorption declines with time, so activated charcoal should be given as soon as possible after ingestion. However, the documented efficacy of activated charcoal for reducing toxicant blood levels has not translated into reduced mortality in reports[4] or in randomized trials.[A1][A2] The decision to administer activated charcoal should be based on a risk/benefit assessment that includes nature of the exposure, clinical effects displayed during evaluation, and abilities of the medical facility and staff. For patients likely to have a good outcome, the risk and effort associated with activated charcoal administration are not worthwhile. Its use is justified in patients who present early (1 to 2 hours) after exposures to a large amount of a concerning toxin that is likely to be adsorbed to charcoal. Activated charcoal should not be used in patients at risk for aspiration until the airway is secure to minimize aspiration; the patient's head should also be elevated unless it is contraindicated. Activated charcoal is contraindicated in patients with a perforated bowel, functional or mechanical bowel obstruction, ingestion of a pure aliphatic hydrocarbon such as gasoline or kerosene (no benefit and increased risk for aspiration), and ingestion of caustic acid and alkali (no benefit and obscures endoscopy). Certain agents, such as lithium, iron, metals, and ethanol, do not adsorb significantly to activated charcoal, but its use is not precluded if the patient has ingested other toxicants that do adsorb to activated charcoal. Pulmonary aspiration and bowel obstruction from inspissated activated charcoal are the most common complications; both occur more frequently when multidose activated charcoal is administered, but they can be avoided by withholding treatment in patients who have suboptimal bowel function or decreased fecal elimination.

Gastric Emptying

Two methods of gastric emptying, syrup of ipecac[5] and orogastric lavage through a large-bore tube, are no longer routinely used. Both are relatively ineffective therapies that potentially increase the risk for aspiration. No well-designed study has documented any benefit of gastric emptying, either by lavage or by syrup of ipecac, compared with the use of activated charcoal alone. Gastric emptying by lavage or, rarely, by syrup of ipecac may be of benefit and should be performed in patients who have ingested toxicants that do not adsorb to activated charcoal and are known to produce significant morbidity or for which aggressive decontamination may offer the best chance for survival (e.g., colchicine, sodium azide, sodium fluoroacetate). Removal of a liquid toxicant, such as ethylene glycol, may be accomplished by aspiration of gastric contents through a nasogastric tube. Contraindications to gastric emptying include those for activated charcoal, a bleeding diathesis, and the ingestion of sharp objects. Placement of an endotracheal tube before gastric lavage may be necessary to protect the airway in patients who have a decreased level of consciousness and impaired gag reflex but is not required in all cases. Major complications of gastric emptying include pulmonary aspiration, esophageal tears and perforations, and laryngospasm (with lavage).

Whole Bowel Irrigation

Whole bowel irrigation with a nonabsorbable polyethylene glycol solution has been recommended for iron and sustained-release medications, for agents not adsorbed to activated charcoal, and for body packers (smugglers who swallow packets of illicit drugs). The most common complication is vomiting, and whole bowel irrigation is contraindicated in patients with bowel perforation, obstruction, hemorrhage, or hemodynamic or respiratory instability. The initial recommended dose is 500 mL/hour given orally or by nasogastric tube, with titration to 2000 mL/hour as tolerated; treatment continues until the rectal effluent clears. Rarely, surgery may be necessary to remove packets in smugglers who have symptoms of cocaine toxicity or are obstructed; endoscopic removal of these packets should never be attempted because of the risk of packet rupture.

Antidotes

Few toxicants have specific therapies (Table 110-6). Although antidotes may be essential in treating patients exposed to certain toxicants, their use does not preclude the need for ongoing supportive care and, in some cases, extracorporeal elimination.

Enhanced Elimination

Methods to accelerate the elimination of toxicants or drugs from the body include multiple doses of activated charcoal, urinary alkalinization, and extracorporeal removal. Another method, using the oral ion exchange resins sodium polystyrene sulfonate and cholestyramine, has experimentally enhanced the elimination of lithium, digoxin, digitoxin, and organochlorines but has limited clinical usefulness.

Multiple Doses of Oral Activated Charcoal

The rationale for administering multiple doses of oral activated charcoal includes the adsorption of any toxic agent remaining in the gastrointestinal tract (e.g., sustained-release drugs or drugs that retard their absorption, such as anticholinergics); interference with the enterohepatic and enteroenteric recirculation of toxicants; and enhancement of the elimination of drugs with a long half-life, a volume of distribution less than 1 L/kg body weight, and low protein binding (termed gastrointestinal dialysis). The existing evidence shows enhanced elimination of carbamazepine, dapsone, phenobarbital, quinine, salicylates, and theophylline, but multiple doses of activated charcoal may also be effective for amitriptyline, dextropropoxyphene, digitoxin, digoxin, disopyramide, nadolol, phenylbutazone, phenytoin, piroxicam, and sotalol. Whether enhanced elimination provided by repeated doses of activated charcoal translates into decreased morbidity and mortality has not been adequately examined in large controlled clinical trials, except for yellow oleander and organophosphate ingestion, for which it has shown no benefit.[A1] The usual recommendations are an average dose of 12.5 g of activated charcoal (after the initial dose of 1 g/kg body weight, with a maximum single dose of 100 g) administered every 4 to 6 hours after the previous dose. The contraindications to single-dose activated charcoal also apply to multidose activated charcoal. Reported complications include pulmonary aspiration, bowel obstruction from inspissated charcoal, and fluid and electrolyte imbalance from multiple doses of a simultaneously administered cathartic.

Urinary Alkalinization

Alkalinization of the urine, which increases the renal elimination of weak acids, is used primarily to enhance the elimination of salicylates, but the elimination of chlorpropamide, 2,4-dichlorophenoxyacetic acid, formic acid, methotrexate, and phenobarbital may be increased with this method. Urinary alkalinization is accomplished by an intravenous bolus of 1 to 2 mEq of sodium bicarbonate per kilogram body weight, followed by three ampules (150 mL) of sodium bicarbonate (44 mEq/50 mL) in 850 mL of 5% dextrose in water infused at two to three times the normal maintenance fluid rate. Urinary pH should be checked hourly, and the infusion should be adjusted to maintain a urine pH of 7.5 to 8.0. Potassium should be administered simultaneously to avoid hypokalemia, which prevents urinary alkalinization because the distal tubule excretes hydrogen ion in exchange for potassium (Chapters 116 and 117). Serum pH should be monitored and kept at 7.55 or lower to avoid excessive alkalemia. Contraindications to this therapy include volume overload and cerebral or pulmonary edema. Urinary acidification is not recommended to enhance the elimination of weak bases, such as amphetamines, because of the danger of precipitating tubular myoglobin in patients with rhabdomyolysis.

Extracorporeal Removal

Extracorporeal techniques enhance the elimination of a few drugs and toxicants, especially those that exist in the blood and are otherwise poorly eliminated. Such drugs generally have single-compartment kinetics, a volume of distribution less than 1 L/kg, and endogenous clearance of less than 4 mL/minute/kg (Table 110-7). For hemodialysis, the toxicant must be water soluble, have a molecular weight less than 500, and exhibit low protein binding. For continuous renal replacement therapy, the toxicant must have a molecular weight less than the permeability limit of the filter membrane. As a group, these latter forms of elimination are slow and likely to be of limited benefit to most patients with acute poisoning.[6] Rarely, extracorporeal removal has been used for aminoglycosides, atenolol, bromide, carbamazepine, diethylene glycol, isopropanol, magnesium, metformin, methotrexate, *N*-acetylprocainamide, phenobarbital, procainamide, sotalol, and trichloroethanol (chloral hydrate).

TABLE 110-6 ANTIDOTES AND INDICATIONS FOR USE

ANTIDOTE	INDICATION FOR USE	DOSE*	TREATMENT END POINT	COMMENTS
Antivenom, *Crotalidae* (Fab)†	Crotaline snake (e.g., rattlesnakes, copperhead)	4-6 vials; repeat for persistent or worsening clinical condition; repeated doses of 2 vials at 6, 12, and 18 hours after initial antivenom dose are recommended	Halt in progression of circumferential and proximal swelling Resolving systemic effects	Better safety profile than historical equine-derived antivenom Repetitive dosing indicated for recurrent soft tissue swelling Less effective at correcting hematologic (i.e., coagulation and platelet) disorders
Antivenom, *Latrodectus* (equine)†	Black widow spider (*Latrodectus* sp)	1 vial diluted in 50-100 mL NS, infused during 1 hour; can repeat	Resolution of symptoms, vital signs normal	Dilution and slow infusion rate are **critical** to avoid anaphylactoid reaction Indications include severe pain unresponsive to opioids and severe hypertension Serum sickness can occur IV calcium is ineffective
Atropine	Carbamates Nerve agents Organophosphorus compounds	2 mg IV; double the dose every 5 minutes to achieve atropinization and hemodynamic stability; then start continuous infusion of 10-20% of total stabilizing dose per hour	Cessation of excessive oral and pulmonary secretions, >80 beats/min, systolic blood pressure >80 mm Hg	Doubling of the dose every 5 minutes (e.g., 2 mg, 4 mg, 8 mg, 16 mg) estimated to achieve atropinization within 30 minutes Stop infusion when patient develops concerning signs or symptoms of anticholinergic toxidrome (see Table 110-1); restart infusion at lower rate when signs or symptoms abate
Calcium salt†	Calcium-channel antagonists	Calcium chloride 10%, 10 mL (1 g) during 10 minutes; can be given in 1 minute if critically ill Calcium gluconate 10%, 30 mL (3 g) during 10 minutes; can be given in 1 minute if critically ill	Reversal of hypotension; may not reverse bradycardia	*All indications:* Monitor ionized calcium levels IV extravasation causes tissue necrosis, especially with calcium chloride Can administer at faster than stated rates for immediate life-threatening conditions (i.e., in 1 minute) Calcium chloride contains three times more elemental calcium than calcium gluconate does
	Hydrofluoric acid	Systemic toxicity: calcium gluconate 10%, 1-3 g (10-30 mL) per dose IV during 10-minute period; repeat as needed every 5-10 minutes	Reversal of life-threatening manifestations of hypocalcemia and hyperkalemia	Can dilute and give intra-arterially or IV with a Bier block for extremity exposures and burns
	Hyperkalemia (except cardiac glycosides)	Calcium gluconate 10%, 1 g (10 mL) per dose IV during 10-minute period; repeat as needed every 5-10 minutes	Reversal of myocardial depression and conduction delays	May precipitate ventricular arrhythmias
	Hypermagnesemia	Calcium gluconate 10%, 1-2 g (10-20 mL) per dose IV during 10-minute period; repeat as needed every 5-10 minutes	Reversal of respiratory depression, hypotension, and cardiac conduction blocks	Simultaneous therapies to increase magnesium elimination should be instituted
	Hypocalcemia (e.g., ethylene glycol)	Calcium gluconate 10%, 0.5-1.0 g (5-10 mL) per dose during 10-minute period; repeat as needed every 10 minutes	Reversal of tetany	Correct symptomatic hypocalcemia; avoid excessive administration that may increase production of calcium oxalate crystals in ethylene glycol poisoning
L-Carnitine	Valproate-induced hyperammonemia or hepatotoxicity	100 mg/kg (maximum 6 g) IV during 30 minutes, then 15 mg/kg IV during 30-minute period q4h (maximum 6 g/day)	Treat until clinical improvement occurs	Levocarnitine is active form Adjust dose for end-stage renal disease
Cyanide antidote kit Amyl nitrite Sodium nitrite Sodium thiosulfate [Hydroxocobalamin is preferred if available, see below]	Cyanide	Amyl nitrite: 0.3-mL pearls, crush and inhale during 30-second period Sodium nitrite 3%: 10 mL IV during 10-minute period Sodium thiosulfate 25%: 50 mL (12.5 g) IV during 10-minute period	Resolution of lactic acidosis and moderate to severe clinical signs and symptoms: seizures, coma, dyspnea, apnea, hypotension, bradycardia	Coordinate amyl nitrite with continued oxygenation and give only until sodium nitrite infusion is begun; nitrites may produce hypotension and excess methemoglobinemia Sodium nitrite dose must be adjusted if patient has hemoglobin <12 g/dL Sodium thiosulfate dosing can be repeated

TABLE 110-6 ANTIDOTES AND INDICATIONS FOR USE—cont'd

ANTIDOTE	INDICATION FOR USE	DOSE*	TREATMENT END POINT	COMMENTS
Deferoxamine	Iron	Initiate at 5 mg/kg/hr, titrate to 15 mg/kg/hr IV (maximum 8 g/day) Mild to moderate: administer for 6-12 hours Severe toxicity: administer 24 hours	Resolution of clinical signs and symptoms Do not use urine color, which is an unreliable marker for iron clearance Laboratory testing is unreliable while antidote is being received	Indications: symptomatic patients with lethargy, severe abdominal pain, hypovolemia, acidosis, shock; any symptomatic patient with peak serum iron level >350 g/dL Prolonged therapy can cause pulmonary toxicity
Digoxin-specific antibody fragments (Fab)	Digoxin Digitalis and related plants (e.g., oleander, lily of the valley) Other cardiac glycosides (e.g., bufadienolides [Bufo toads])	Unknown digoxin dose or serum level, or for plant or toad source: acute toxicity—10-20 vials; chronic toxicity—3-6 vials Digoxin dose known: number of vials = (mg ingested × 0.8) ÷ 0.5 Digoxin serum level known: number of vials = [serum level (ng/mL) × weight (kg)] ÷ 100 Infuse dose during 30 minutes	Resolution of hyperkalemia, symptomatic bradydysrhythmias, ventricular arrhythmias, Mobitz II or third-degree heart block	Each vial binds 0.5 mg of digoxin or digitoxin Monitor ECG and potassium levels Digoxin serum levels unreliable after antidote administered unless test is specific for free serum digoxin
Dimercaprol (BAL)	Arsenic Lead Mercury, elemental and inorganic salts	Arsenic: 3-5 mg/kg IM q4h Lead: 75 mg/m^2 (4 mg/kg) IM q4h for 5 days Inorganic mercury: 5 mg/kg IM, then 2.5 mg/kg IM q12h for 10 days or until patient is clinically improved	Arsenic: 24-hour urinary arsenic <50 µg/L Lead: encephalopathy resolved, blood lead level <100 µg/dL, and succimer therapy can be started Mercury, elemental and inorganic: 24-hour urinary mercury <20 µg/L	Formulated in peanut oil; painful IM injection and caution with allergy Maximum adult dose is 3 g/day BAL started 4 hours before initiation of concomitant $CaNa_2EDTA$ for lead encephalopathy Dosing not well established for arsenic and elemental or inorganic mercury toxicity; not used for organic mercury poisoning Adverse effects: painful injections, fever, diaphoresis, agitation, headache, salivation, nausea and vomiting, hemolysis in G6PD-deficient patients, chelation of essential metals Check essential metal levels if chelation is prolonged Succimer is replacing BAL for many indications except lead encephalopathy Treatment end points for arsenic and mercury include improving clinical condition
Edetate calcium disodium ($CaNa_2EDTA$)	Lead	1500 mg/m^2/24 hr (maximum 3 g) by continuous infusion	Treat for 5 days, followed by 2-day hiatus; repeat until encephalopathy resolved, lead level <100 µg/dL, and succimer therapy can be started	Use in patients with lead encephalopathy or lead level >100 g/dL Administer BAL 4 hours before initiating $CaNa_2EDTA$ Hydrate patient and establish good urinary output before starting therapy Avoid thrombophlebitis by diluting in NS or D_5W to a concentration ≤0.5% Substitution of Na_2EDTA can cause fatal hypocalcemia
Flumazenil	Benzodiazepines	0.1 mg/min IV to a total dose of 1 mg	Reversal of coma	Limit use to reversal of inadequate ventilation in benzodiazepine-toxic patients Acute benzodiazepine withdrawal may occur in patients dependent on benzodiazepines Increases intracranial pressure and risk for seizures in presence of underlying seizure disorder or ingestion of seizure-producing toxicants Monitor for resedation up to 2 hours after last dose
Folinic acid (tetrahydrofolic acid [leucovorin])	Methanol Methotrexate	Methanol: 50 mg IV q4h Methotrexate: 100 mg/m^2 IV during 15-30 minutes q3-6h; dosing lower when used as "rescue" in chemotherapy	Methanol: methanol undetectable, metabolic acidosis cleared Methotrexate: serum level <1 × 10^{-8} mol/L	Essential therapy for both toxicants Little concern with excessive dosing when used for methotrexate overdose Methotrexate: large overdoses may require increased dose Glucarpidase administered 2-4 hours before or after folinic acid

TABLE 110-6 ANTIDOTES AND INDICATIONS FOR USE—cont'd

ANTIDOTE	INDICATION FOR USE	DOSE*	TREATMENT END POINT	COMMENTS
Fomepizole[8]	Ethylene glycol Methanol	Dose 1: 15 mg/kg IV Doses during next 48 hours: 10 mg/kg IV All subsequent doses: 15 mg/kg IV Administer q12h, except when HD performed: HD initiation: ½ next dose if >6 hours since last dose HD ongoing: q4h End of HD (based on time of last dose): <1 hour, no dose; 1-3 hours, ½ next dose; >3 hours, next dose	For both: serum level <25 mg/dL and metabolic acidosis resolved	Start immediately if toxic alcohol suspected, without waiting for confirmatory levels Dose amount is not affected by interval timing of doses
Glucagon	β-Adrenergic receptor antagonists Calcium-channel antagonists	Bolus of 3-5 mg IV; can repeat to achieve clinical effect, then infusion of 2-10 mg/hr	Reversal of hypotension and bradycardia; taper infusion	Can precipitate vomiting; be prepared to protect airway Mild hyperglycemia occurs Maximum dosing amounts unknown; bolus doses up to 30 mg reported Duration of effect is 15 minutes; thus infusion must be started immediately
Hydroxocobalamin	Cyanide	Initial: 5 g IV during 15-minute period Second dose: 5 g IV during 15 minutes to 2 hours; maximum total dose is 10 g Follow each hydroxocobalamin dose with sodium thiosulfate 25%: 50 mL (12.5 g) IV during 10-minute period	Resolution of lactic acidosis and moderate to severe clinical signs and symptoms: seizures, coma, dyspnea, apnea, hypotension, bradycardia	Can be administered IV push if patient is in cardiac arrest Do not give hydroxocobalamin and sodium thiosulfate through the same IV line Adverse effects: red discoloration of plasma, urine, mucous membranes, skin; transient hypertension Interference with laboratory colorimetric assays: Levels increased: bilirubin; creatinine; glucose; hemoglobin; magnesium; co-oximetry total Hb, COHb%, MetHb% Levels decreased: AST, ALT, creatinine, co-oximetry O_2Hb%
Hyperbaric oxygen (HBO)	Carbon monoxide Experimental: carbon tetrachloride, cyanide, hydrogen sulfide	3.0 atm pressure for 60 minutes (25 minutes O_2, 5 minutes air, 25 minutes O_2, 5 minutes air), then 2.0 atm for 65 minutes (30 minutes O_2, 5 minutes air, 30 minutes O_2), then "surface" to 1.0 atm	One treatment Repeated treatment controversial	Carbon monoxide: treatment protocols may vary HBO indicated for loss of consciousness; seizures; cerebellar dysfunction; impaired cognition; headache, nausea/vomiting persisting after 4 hours of O_2 therapy regardless of carboxyhemoglobin level
Insulin-glucose	Calcium-channel antagonists β-Adrenergic receptor antagonists	Regular insulin, 1 U/kg bolus, followed by 0.5-1 U/kg/hr Titrate 50% dextrose IV to avoid hypoglycemia	Reversal of myocardial depression	Initiate early to reverse myocardial depression Monitor glucose and potassium; hypoglycemia can occur during and after therapy Hyperglycemia results from calcium-channel antagonist–induced insulin resistance, and initial dextrose requirements may be less than anticipated Recovery may be heralded by normalization of glucose levels, with increased dextrose required to avoid hypoglycemia
Lipid emulsion	Cardiac toxicity from local anesthetics (e.g., bupivacaine, ropivacaine) Experimental: verapamil, diltiazem, tricyclic antidepressants, bupropion, propranolol and other lipophilic toxicants	Use 20% formulation Initial bolus: 1.5 mL/kg IV during 1 minute, followed immediately by infusion of 0.25 mL/kg/min for 30-60 minutes Can repeat bolus for asystole	Return of hemodynamic stability	Use for other than bupivacaine based on animal experiments and human case reports; numerous dosing regimens have been used Use if advanced life support measures fail; continue CPR as needed during drug administration
Methylene blue	Methemoglobin-producing agents	1-2 mg/kg body weight (0.1-0.2 mL/kg of 1%) methylene blue during 5-minute period; repeat dose for persistent or recurrent symptoms or signs	Resolution of dyspnea and altered mental status	Use if patient is symptomatic (i.e., dyspneic, altered mental status) Maximum dose should not exceed 7 mg/kg (0.7 mL/kg) Contraindicated in G6PD-deficient patients; may cause hemolysis Some toxicants (e.g., dapsone) may require prolonged therapy

TABLE 110-6 ANTIDOTES AND INDICATIONS FOR USE—cont'd

ANTIDOTE	INDICATION FOR USE	DOSE*	TREATMENT END POINT	COMMENTS
N-Acetylcysteine (NAC)[7]	Acetaminophen Experimental: carbon tetrachloride, chloroform, pennyroyal oil	Oral (total 72 hours) Load: 140 mg/kg Maintenance (starting 4 hours after load): 70 mg/kg q4h × 17 doses IV (total 21 hours) Load: 150 mg/kg during 1-hour period Maintenance infusion: 12.5 mg/kg/hr during 4-hour period, then 6.25 mg/kg/hr over 16 hours as continuous infusion	At the end of therapy, repeat AST and APAP levels: if AST normal and APAP not detected, treatment complete; if AST normal and APAP detected, continue NAC; if AST elevated, continue NAC After patient has received full course of NAC therapy, if INR ≥2.0 or severe hepatotoxicity present (AST > 1000 U/L), continue NAC until INR <2.0 and aminotransferases normalize	Most effective if initiated within 8 hours after ingestion; may be started any time after ingestion and is beneficial in severe hepatotoxic states Longer duration of treatment may be required in patients with hepatotoxicity Treatment end points simplified for ease of use INR result not valid indicator if FFP recently administered
Naloxone[9]	Opioids	Opioid dependence possible: 40-50 μg (0.04-0.05 mg) IV titrated upward to reversal, while avoiding withdrawal if concerns for opioid dependence Opioid dependence not likely: 0.4 mg by any route and titrate up to 10 mg Continuous infusion: establish bolus dose required to reverse respiratory depression; begin infusing two thirds of reversal dose every hour and titrate to maintain adequate respirations; repeated bolus with half of reversal dose 15 minutes after reversal of respiratory depression	Initial: reversal of respiratory depression with resolution of hypoxia and hypercapnia Final: resolution of CNS and respiratory depression	Pre-ventilate patients with respiratory depression by bag-valve-mask or intubation before administration Use smaller doses in opioid-dependent patients Some opioids (e.g., buprenorphine) may require larger doses of naloxone Use continuous infusion for recurrent symptoms and prolonged action of some formulations (e.g., sustained-release morphine, methadone) Re-sedation can occur Do not use naltrexone to reverse acute toxicity
Octreotide	Sulfonylurea-induced hypoglycemia	50 mg SC q6h	Resolution of hypoglycemia and dextrose not required	Maintain dextrose infusion as needed Not for insulin-induced hypoglycemia
Physostigmine	Anticholinergic agents (e.g., diphenhydramine, jimsonweed [*Datura* sp], scopolamine)	1-2 mg IV during 5-minute period; can repeat in 5 minutes if no effect and cholinergic effects do not occur	Reversal of anticholinergic effects	Duration of effect is 60-90 minutes Benzodiazepine used for subsequent treatment of agitation and seizures; additional physostigmine used rarely (e.g., refractory seizures or agitation) Adverse effects include seizures, excessive oral secretions, bradyarrhythmias; contraindicated in cyclic antidepressant toxicity
Pralidoxime chloride	Organophosphorus compounds Nerve agents: sarin, VX	30 mg/kg IV bolus (maximum 2 g) during 30 minutes, followed by continuous infusion of 8-10 mg/kg/hr (maximum 650 mg/hr)	Resolution of signs and symptoms, atropine no longer required	Can give initial dose during 2-minute period for life-threatening clinical effects Administer early when diagnosis known or strongly suspected Efficacy variable, depending on the organophosphate Fat-soluble organophosphates may require prolonged treatment
Pyridoxine	Ethylene glycol Isoniazid Monomethylhydrazine (*Gyromitra esculenta* mushrooms)	100 mg IV 5 g IV, repeat for refractory seizures	One dose Resolution of seizures	Efficacy theoretical for ethylene glycol to enhance elimination of toxic metabolites Pyridoxine may be required even with benzodiazepines to stop seizures, but patient can remain comatose (isoniazid, *Gyromitra* mushrooms) Excessive dosing can cause neuropathy
Sodium bicarbonate ($NaHCO_3$)	Reversal of myocardial sodium-channel blockers (e.g., cyclic antidepressants, cocaine, sodium-channel–blocking antiarrhythmics with $\tau_{recovery}$ >1 second, piperidine phenothiazines (thioridazine, mesoridazine)	1-2 mEq $NaHCO_3$/kg by intermittent bolus; repeat as needed	Narrowing of prolonged QRS, resolution of ventricular arrhythmias, reversal of hypotension	Monitor blood pH (optimal pH approximately 7.50); avoid pH > 7.55

TABLE 110-6 ANTIDOTES AND INDICATIONS FOR USE—cont'd

ANTIDOTE	INDICATION FOR USE	DOSE*	TREATMENT END POINT	COMMENTS
Sodium bicarbonate ($NaHCO_3$) (cont'd)	Altered tissue distribution or enhanced elimination of salicylates; may be used for chlorophenoxy herbicides, formic acid, methotrexate, phenobarbital	1-2 mEq $NaHCO_3$/kg, followed by 3 ampules (150 mL) $NaHCO_3$ (44 mEq per 50 mL) in 850 mL of D_5W, infused at 2-3 times normal maintenance fluid rate	Serum salicylate <30 mg/dL and patient clinically stable	Target blood pH: 7.50-7.55 Monitor urinary pH hourly; adjust infusion to maintain urine pH of 7.5-8.0 (avoid blood pH >7.55) Monitor ABGs Maintain normokalemia
Succimer (DMSA)	Arsenic Lead Mercury, all forms	10 mg/kg/dose q8h for 5 days, followed by q12h for 14 days Drug holiday for 2 weeks; repeat if treatment end point not reached	Arsenic: 24-hour urinary arsenic <50 μg/L Lead: resolution of encephalopathy, gastrointestinal symptoms, neuropathy, nephropathy, arthralgias, myalgias, and blood lead level <70 μg/dL Mercury, elemental and inorganic: 24-hour urinary mercury <20 μg/L Mercury, organic: end point not well established	Oral chelator; adverse effects include rash, transient AST and alkaline phosphatase elevations, and gastrointestinal distress; minimal chelation of essential metals occurs Dosing for arsenic and mercury not well established Therapeutic end point for organic mercury not established; neurotoxicity not responsive to chelation therapy; suggest chelation until blood mercury level within normal value range for reference laboratory
Vitamin K	Vitamin K antagonist anticoagulants (e.g., warfarin, long-acting anticoagulant rodenticides [LAARs]) [note this is not for normalizing a supratherapeutic INR in patients prescribed Warfarin]	Subcutaneous: AquaMEPHYTON (K_1), 10-25 mg, repeat every 6-12 hours until oral vitamin K_1 started Oral: 25-50 mg q6h; larger doses may be required	INR is normal 48-72 hours after stopping vitamin K_1 therapy Can also monitor factor VII activity	Anaphylactoid reaction can occur with rapid IV administration Severe bleeding may also require FFP, prothrombin protein concentrate (off label), or factor concentrates Base decision to treat on finding of elevated INR; do not administer prophylactic vitamin K_1 Oral therapy may be required for months with LAAR poisoning because of lipophilicity of toxicant, with slow body clearance

*Dose concentrations and infusion times are not given. Drug dosages may require adjustment in patients with renal or hepatic failure.
†Administer antivenom in a monitored setting; antivenom must be reconstituted and then diluted; initially infuse at a rate of 2 to 5 mL/hr, and double the infusion rate every 5 minutes as tolerated to administer antivenom during a 1-hour period.
‡Ten percent calcium chloride solution = 100 mg/mL (27.2 mg/mL elemental calcium); 10% calcium gluconate solution = 100 mg/mL (9 mg/mL elemental calcium).
ABGs = arterial blood gases; ALT = alanine aminotransferase; APAP = acetyl-*p*-aminophenol (acetaminophen); AST = aspartate aminotransferase; BAL = British antilewisite; CNS = central nervous system; COHb% = percentage carboxyhemoglobin; CPR, cardiopulmonary resuscitation; D_5W = 5% dextrose in water; DMSA = 2,3-dimercaptosuccinic acid; ECG = electrocardiogram; FFP = fresh-frozen plasma; G6PD = glucose-6-phosphate dehydrogenase; Hb = hemoglobin; HD = hemodialysis; INR = international normalized ratio; MetHb% = percentage methemoglobinemia; NS = normal saline; O_2Hb% = percentage oxyhemoglobin; $\tau_{recovery}$ = drug blockade recovery rate.

TABLE 110-7 COMMON TOXICANTS REMOVED BY HEMODIALYSIS

TOXICANT	INDICATIONS	COMMENTS
Ethylene glycol	Serum level ≥50 mg/dL, or lower levels with concomitant metabolic acidosis and evidence of end-organ toxicity	Not routinely required in a patient with normal creatinine clearance and acid-base status who is receiving fomepizole
Lithium*	Clinical indications	Clinical indication is CNS toxicity (e.g., decreased mental status, ataxia, coma, seizures) Use dialysate containing bicarbonate to decrease Na^+/K^+ antiporter intracellular sequestration of lithium
Methanol	Serum level ≥50 mg/dL, or lower levels with concomitant metabolic acidosis and evidence of end-organ toxicity	Usually required because of slow elimination half-life in presence of fomepizole (mean, 52 hours; range, 22-87 hours), even in patients with no metabolic acidosis or evidence of end-organ toxicity
Phenobarbital	Clinical indications	Rarely necessary except when a patient is hemodynamically unstable despite aggressive support
Salicylates	Acute toxicity: serum level ≥100 mg/dL without clinical abnormality or <100 mg/dL in the presence of a clinical indication Chronic toxicity: any clinical indication	Serum protein binding decreases with increasing toxic levels, increasing the amount of free salicylate available for HD removal; clinical indications are one or more of the following: altered mental status, seizures, pulmonary edema, intractable acidosis, renal failure
Valproic acid	Severe intoxication with serum concentration >850 mg/L	Clinical indications include hepatic dysfunction; coma, especially with hyperammonemia; deteriorating clinical status despite aggressive support

*Hemodiafiltration removes lithium; the clinical benefit of this technique is unknown.
CNS = central nervous system; HD = hemodialysis.

PROGNOSIS

Almost all patients who reach the hospital alive survive with appropriate care. Inpatient mortality rates are 0.2 to 0.5%.

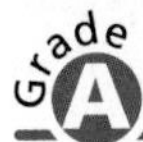

Grade A References

A1. Eddleston M, Juszczak E, Buckley NA, et al. Multiple-dose activated charcoal in acute self-poisoning: a randomised controlled trial. *Lancet*. 2008;371:579-587.

A2. Cooper GM, Le Couteur DG, Richardson D, et al. A randomized clinical trial of activated charcoal for the routine management of oral drug overdose. *QJM*. 2005;98:655-660.

A3. Buckley NA, Eddleston M, Li Y, et al. Oximes for acute organophosphate pesticide poisoning. *Cochrane Database Syst Rev*. 2011;2:CD005085.

GENERAL REFERENCES

For the General References and other additional features, please visit Expert Consult at https://expertconsult.inkling.com.

111 MEDICAL ASPECTS OF INJURIES AND BURNS

ROBERT L. SHERIDAN

Injured or burned patients are complex to manage not only because of the vast number of potential anatomic derangements but also because of the complex physiologic cascades triggered by injury. Although burns are associated with the most profound physiologic derangements, most medical issues are fairly similar across a wide range of injuries. As a result, needed interventions are often predictable regardless of the mechanism of injury.

EPIDEMIOLOGY

Trauma is an enormous public health issue. In the United States alone each year, about 2.5 million people are injured and 40,000 killed in automobile crashes, and about 78,000 are injured and 32,000 killed by gunshots. Burns and falls follow in frequency. Worldwide, injury by trauma and burns is the leading cause of death in children and young adults. In the middle-aged and elderly, injury follows only cancer and heart disease as a cause of death. Many long-term survivors of trauma and burns have high degrees of disability, which creates a particularly difficult problem given the young age of many victims.

Death after injury has a trimodal distribution.[1] At least 50% of fatalities occur within minutes of the injury as a result of massive hemorrhage or nonsurvivable brain injury. Because no medical interventions are possible in such cases, the importance of prevention is paramount. Approximately one third of deaths occur within a few hours after the injury and are usually caused by hemorrhage, anoxia, or progressive brain trauma. This interval provides an opportunity for emergent intervention. Later fatalities are usually the result of multisystem organ dysfunction or overwhelming infection in the days and weeks after the injury.

PATHOBIOLOGY

Early Local Response to Injury

The local response to blunt, penetrating, electrical, crush, thermal, blast, or other injury varies with the energy transferred. All are associated with some degree of secondary injury by progressive microvascular thrombosis, progressive edema, and secondary compromise of perfusion. The most common preventable mechanisms are related to progressive edema beneath an inelastic eschar or fascial compartments or direct injury to vascular inflow or outflow.

Early Systemic Response to Injury

The early systemic response to burns and local trauma is driven by fluid loss and release of vasoactive mediators from injured tissue. In more severe injuries, including surface burns greater than about 20% of the body surface, interstitial edema develops in unburned skin as well as in distant organs and soft tissues. These distant microvascular effects, which can compromise the function of organs that were not directly injured, explain the frequent occurrence of pulmonary and other organ dysfunctions in patients with large burns.

The capillary leak syndrome, in which the leak is typically proportional to the scope of the injury, is caused by the release of vasoactive substances from the injured and reperfused tissue. As a result, during the first 18 to 24 hours after a serious burn, both electrolytes and large colloid molecules freely diffuse into the interstitial space.

Late Local Response to Injury

At about 72 hours after the initial trauma, local wound issues are particularly important in patients who have extensive soft tissue damage, especially after burns or crush injury with extensive volumes of devitalized tissue. Even wounds that initially are generally clean can be rapidly colonized by endogenous bacteria. As these bacteria multiply in the avascular tissue during the succeeding days, proteases liquefy the eschar and necrotic tissue, which then separates and leaves a bed of granulation tissue. In healthy patients with smaller wounds and burns (<20% of the body surface), this septic process is usually tolerated. When injuries are larger, however, systemic infection results and explains the rare survival of patients who have burns in excess of 40% of body surface area or who have massive soft tissue injuries that were managed without early wound excision.

Late Hypermetabolic Systemic Response to Injury

Successfully resuscitated patients with large burns and, to a lesser extent, those with serious non-burn trauma demonstrate an initial decrease in cardiac output and metabolic rate. After successful resuscitation, a hypermetabolic response occurs, with a near doubling of cardiac output and resting energy expenditure during the next 24 to 72 hours. The magnitude of the response, which becomes greater with larger burns and more severe injuries, peaks at up to twice the normal metabolic rate in otherwise healthy patients with burn involving 60% or more of the body surface area. This hypermetabolic response is characterized by enhanced gluconeogenesis, insulin resistance, and increased protein catabolism. Although the causes of these physiologic changes are not well understood, they seem to involve the systemic release of bacterial products, the breakdown of gastrointestinal barrier dysfunction with translocation of bacteria and their byproducts into the circulation, and increases in the secretion of glucagon, cortisol, and catecholamines.

CLINICAL MANIFESTATIONS

All injuries involve the transmission of energy to viable tissue. Classic injury mechanisms include blunt, penetrating, electrical, thermal, blast, and crush (Table 111-1), but combined mechanisms are common. For example, patients crushed in building collapses frequently suffer a concomitant penetrating component, and patients who suffer high-voltage injury frequently fall from a height, such as a utility pole. In all mechanisms, edema or vascular injury can compromise perfusion and lead to secondary injury.

Blunt injury is commonly seen in motor vehicle accidents and falls. Injuries are often multisystem. Penetrating soft tissue injuries vary widely (Fig. 111-1), but the overarching concern is the possibility of occult injury to vascular, bone, or visceral structures. The degree of trauma is directly related to the energy of the injury. For example, high-velocity gunshots cause greater injury than lower velocity rounds because they create a local blast effect, called cavitation, along their trajectory.

Thermal injury (Fig. 111-2) by whatever mechanism (flame, scald, contact) is associated with a graded soft tissue injury described in degrees.[2] As thermal injuries increase beyond about 15% of the body surface, a clinically important systemic phenomenon occurs. A major manifestation of severe burns is a diffuse capillary leak that continues for 18 to 24 hours after injury and involves both burned and unburned tissue. This phenomenon can result in cardiovascular collapse and is the key physiologic derangement underlying the shock state accompanying burns.

The severity of electrical injuries (Fig. 111-3) varies with voltage, current flow, and contact quality. Low-voltage injuries are rarely associated with distant sequelae, whereas high-voltage injuries are commonly associated with compartment syndromes, cardiac complications, pigmenturia, and other trauma.

Crush injuries (Fig. 111-4) include direct soft tissue injuries as well as secondary ischemic damage due to a compartment syndrome or

TABLE 111-1 INJURY CLASSES

INJURY CLASS	CLINICAL IMPLICATIONS	COMMON ERRORS
Blunt	Graded soft tissue and bone injury, edema Occult vascular or visceral injury	Delayed consequences of edema Missed visceral injury and secondary consequences
Penetrating	Soft tissue and bone injuries vary with energy of injuring object (e.g., knife vs. fragment vs. bullet) Occult vascular or visceral injury	Missed vascular or visceral injury Secondary consequences of missed vascular injury
Thermal	Graded soft tissue injury (first- to fourth-degree burns) Capillary leak phenomenon	Inadequate appreciation of capillary leak phenomenon and consequent under-resuscitation Inaccurate wound evaluation and over-resuscitation Unanticipated local injury progression
Electrical	Range of soft tissue injury with increasing voltage and contact duration and quality	Occult cardiac and muscle injury Secondary compartment syndrome complications
Crush	Graded soft tissue, bone, and visceral injury with secondary consequences of edema and of reperfusion	Underappreciation of injury severity Missed muscle ischemia due to primary ischemia and to reperfusion edema
Blast	Graded injury severity (primary to quaternary injury patterns) Occult visceral injury	Underappreciation of secondary, tertiary, and quaternary components of injury Missed associated visceral injury
Fragmentation injury	Multiple unpredictable penetrations with associated visceral and vascular injury	Missed visceral and vascular injury Associated blast trauma

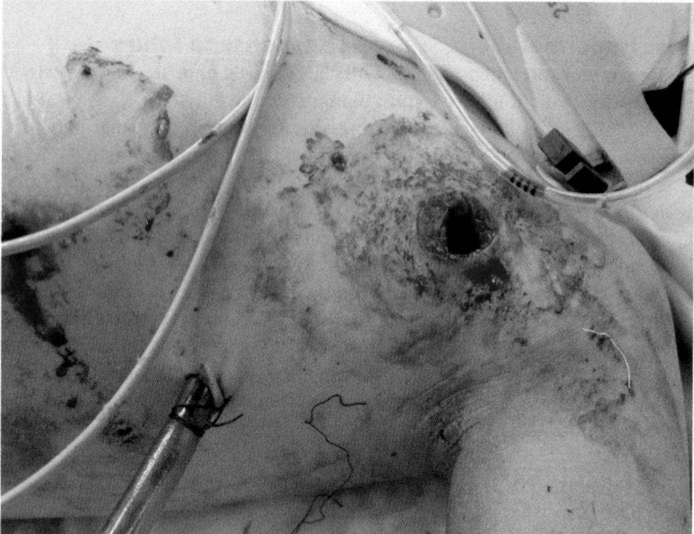

FIGURE 111-1. **Penetrating injury is associated with often occult visceral and bone trauma.**

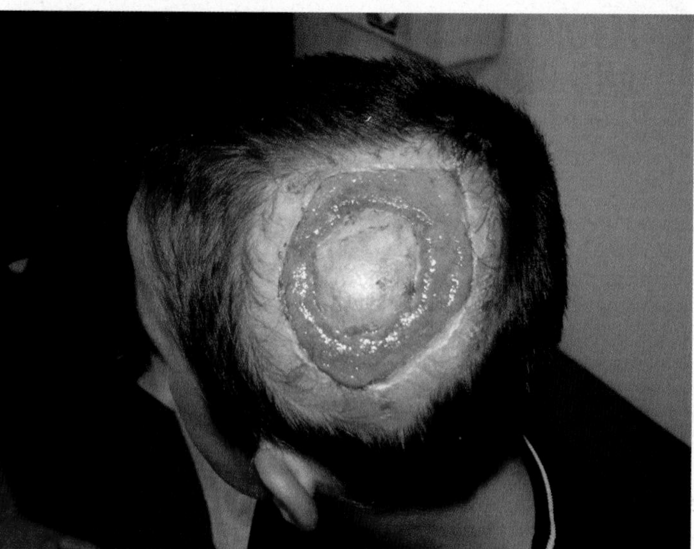

FIGURE 111-3. **Electrical injury can be associated with a number of systemic sequelae, depending on current strength and pattern of flow.**

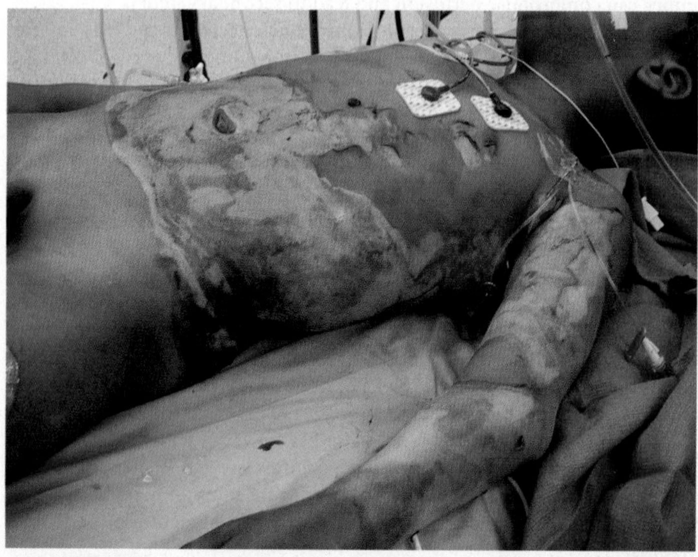

FIGURE 111-2. **Thermal injury is of variable depth.** Initial evaluation usually underestimates this depth.

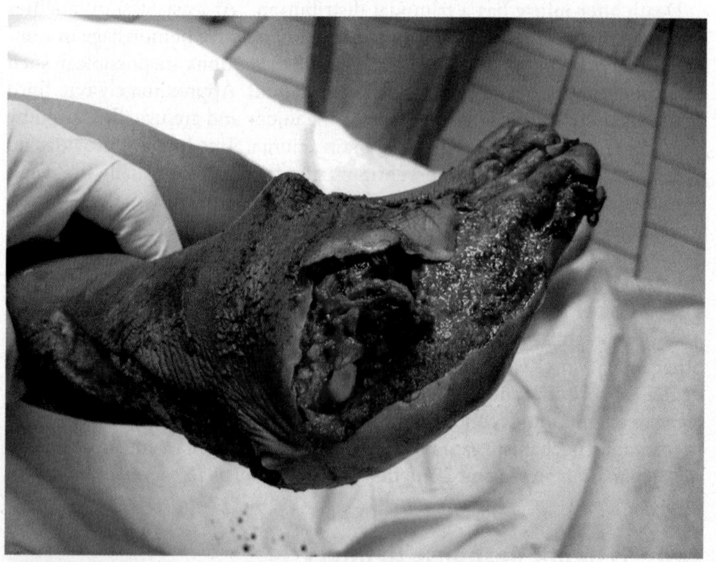

FIGURE 111-4. **Crush injury is often associated with underappreciated deep muscle injury.**

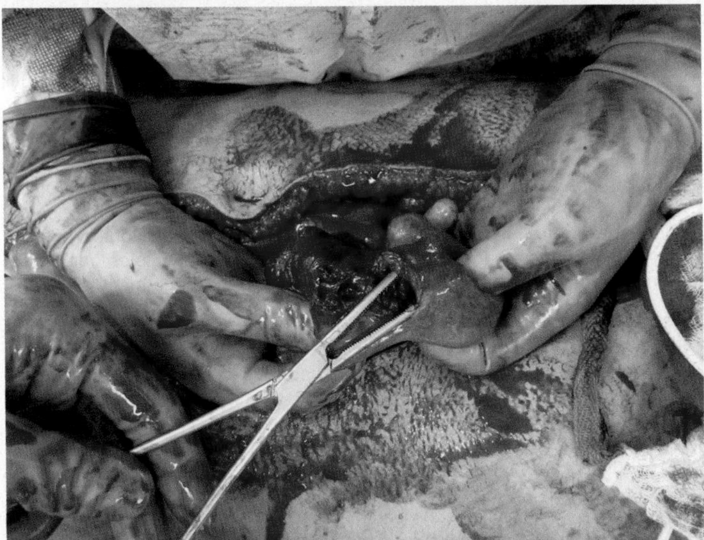

FIGURE 111-5. Blast injury is a complex of four injury subtypes. Missed injuries are common.

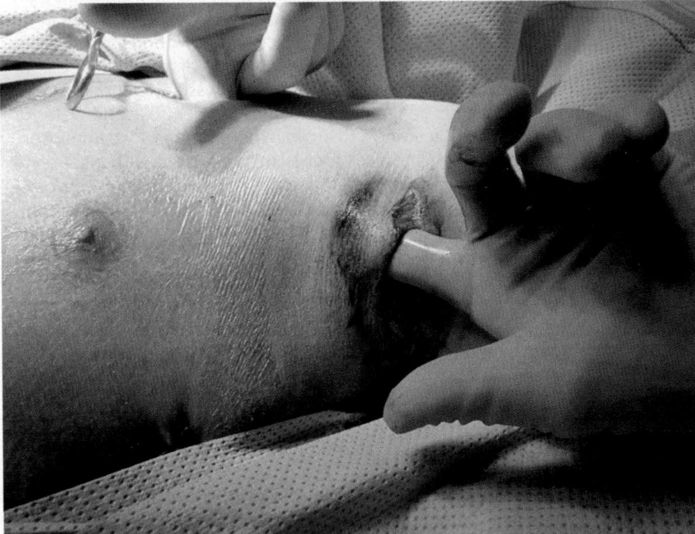

FIGURE 111-6. Fragmentation injury is a particular form of penetrating injury frequently associated with missed injuries.

ischemia-reperfusion. Associated bone, visceral, and vascular injuries are common. Major septic complications are common when necrotic soft tissues are left unexcised.

Blast injuries (Fig. 111-5) are graded complex injuries with four characteristics: primary injury to air-filled structures and the central nervous system, secondary injury from flying debris, tertiary injury from collisions with stationary objects, and quaternary injury from associated crush or other trauma. Blast injuries of all types can be subtle or have a delayed clinical presentation, and visceral injuries often are not diagnosed promptly.

Fragmentation injuries (Fig. 111-6) are penetrating injuries characterized by multiple foreign bodies of variable size and energy as well as unpredictable trajectories. As with blast injuries, the full extent of injury is often underestimated initially.

DIAGNOSIS AND TREATMENT

Rx

Complex burns and trauma are most successfully and cost-effectively managed in high-volume programs.[3] Trauma and burn center programs emphasize the comprehensive nature of injury care, including community involvement with injury prevention programs, thorough prehospital care, early resuscitation and surgery, and long-term rehabilitation and reconstruction. Most programs include imbedded specialty intensive care units and operating rooms. Multidisciplinary staff include physicians, physician assistants, nurse practitioners, nurses, physical and occupational therapists, respiratory therapists, psychiatrists, social workers, and nurse administrators. Coordination and scheduled communication are essential.

Care of individual patients with serious multisystem injury is complex and requires a longitudinal four-phase approach. Phase One, which describes the initial evaluation and resuscitation, generally is completed in the first 24 hours. Phase Two includes initial wound excision for burn patients and initial resuscitative surgery and fracture stabilization for non-burn trauma patients. This phase frequently overlaps with Phase One but is usually completed within 72 hours. Phase Three involves definitive wound closure for burns and the completion of surgery for trauma patients. The duration of this phase varies greatly with injury but is usually complete at the time of discharge. Phase Four describes the sometimes long process of reconstruction, rehabilitation, and reintegration. This phase of care commonly spans the later part of the acute hospitalization, inpatient rehabilitation, and variable amounts of time in the home-based setting.

Prehospital Care and Interhospital Transport

When prehospital and interhospital transfers are being arranged, key issues include control of the airway, secure venous access, placement of bladder and nasogastric catheters, maintenance of body temperature, fluid administration if transport time will be more than 1 hour, documentation of the events of the injury from personnel who will not be available to the receiving facility, efforts to notify family members, and clear documentation of all interventions. Hypothermia (Chapter 109) is a particular problem in burn patients because of their evaporative heat losses. Transporting vehicles and emergency department receiving areas should be heated before the patient's arrival. Initial burn dressings should be dry, clean sheets rather than wetted dressings. Cooling of a wound involving less than 15% of the body surface within minutes may help limit burn depth without causing systemic hypothermia, whereas cooling after a few minutes is generally unhelpful.

Phase One: Initial Evaluation and Resuscitation

Primary Survey

The organized approach to the initial evaluation of injured patients requires primary and subsequent patient surveys. The primary survey is an initial look for major aberrations in airway, circulatory, or neurologic status that justify emergent intervention. The airway is controlled with intubation if needed. Clinically obvious pneumothoraces (Chapter 99) should be decompressed, and hemothoraces must be diagnosed and drained. In suspicious cases, pericardial tamponade (Chapter 77) can usually be documented or excluded by handheld bedside ultrasonography. Vascular access is obtained and fluid resuscitation started. A very brief neurologic assessment (Chapter 396), including use of the Glasgow Coma Scale, is critical.

Secondary Survey

The secondary survey includes a much more detailed head-to-toe physical examination after the patient has a reliable airway and has been hemodynamically stabilized. The physical examination should assess for evidence of closed head injury, skull and facial fractures, and eye and ear injuries, with a low threshold for a head computed tomography (CT) scan. The neck must be stabilized and assessed for possible injury. Burns should be categorized as first-degree burns, involving only the epidermis; second-degree burns, involving variable amounts of dermis; third-degree burns, involving the entire dermis; and fourth-degree burns, involving fat, muscle, and bone.

A constant concern is the potentially missed injury. In the chaos of initial care, major issues can be missed if they do not have a dramatic initial presentation. Unfortunately, many injuries, such as epidural hematoma and small bowel perforations, are initially subtle and become catastrophic hours or days later. The best way to deal with this difficult reality is to have a highly organized approach to initial evaluation so that all potential injuries are considered and reasonably excluded.

Projectiles often follow an unpredictable course through tissue and bone, thereby increasing the likelihood of missed injury. Missed visceral injury is also common with fragmentation injuries, especially because surgical exploration of all potential sites of injury is often impossible. Selected exploration is guided by initial and serial examination and by imaging when it is available.

Appropriate laboratory and imaging studies should be obtained. The fundamental goal is to consider carefully the injury mechanism and to exclude all potential occult injuries to a reasonable level of confidence. High-energy injuries, such as electrical burns, motor vehicle crashes, and blasts, are notorious for generating significant injuries that are missed during the initial evaluation. Bedside ultrasonography has emerged as a routine, rapid, and repeatable method to assess for abdominal fluid, usually blood. CT scanning of the head, chest, abdomen, and pelvis is justified if the mechanism of injury is consistent with head or abdominal trauma. Rapid imaging has largely supplanted operative exploration for diagnostic purposes, except in unstable patients, in whom immediate operative exploration is performed for ongoing hemorrhage.

Chest Injuries

Life-threatening tension pneumothorax (Chapter 99), massive hemothorax, cardiac tamponade (Chapter 77), flail chest, open pneumothorax, and disruption of the thoracic aorta (Chapter 78) may be missed in the primary survey but must be diagnosed in the secondary survey. All trauma patients should have a supine chest radiograph to examine the lung fields, the mediastinal contour, and the chest wall. Thoracic aortic injury is usually an immediately fatal complication of severe acceleration-deceleration injury, but some patients may have a contained mediastinal hematoma that requires urgent evaluation and repair.

Myocardial contusion should be suspected in patients with blunt trauma, especially if they have a sternal fracture or anterior rib fractures. Life-threatening myocardial contusion can be manifested with electrocardiographic abnormalities, ventricular arrhythmias, and even cardiogenic shock. Coronary artery injuries are uncommon, although lacerations and dissections can occur and require emergent percutaneous coronary intervention similar to a typical ST elevation myocardial infarction (Chapter 73).

Commotio cordis is sudden cardiac arrest (Chapter 63) after acute blunt chest trauma from softballs, baseballs, hockey pucks, or collisions. The trauma presumably occurs during an electrically vulnerable period between 30 and 15 msec before the T wave peak and produces ventricular fibrillation. Death is essentially universal unless the victim receives immediate resuscitation.

Abdominal Injuries

The spleen is the most frequently injured intra-abdominal organ, and splenic injury is suggested by left-sided rib fractures, left upper quadrant pain or tenderness, and pain referred to the left shoulder secondary to diaphragmatic irritation. CT scanning is the test of choice. High-grade injuries require splenectomy or, infrequently, splenorrhaphy for salvage of the damaged spleen with preservation of splenic function. Right-sided rib fractures and right upper quadrant tenderness suggest liver injury, which can also be assessed by CT. Most isolated blunt liver injuries can be managed nonoperatively. Focused abdominal sonography has a sensitivity of 95% for detection of free blood in the abdomen (Fig. 111-7) but is not usually able to identify the source. An alternative is diagnostic peritoneal aspiration or lavage. If blood is found by either approach, laparotomy is necessary to identify and to correct the source. Abdominal CT is a reliable determinant of both intraperitoneal and retroperitoneal injury in a stable patient (Fig. 111-8). CT evaluation also can identify sources of blood loss and help decide whether the problem requires operative exploration.

Head and Spine Injuries

Neurologic issues often dominate the quality of long-term outcome. The initial evaluation of the neurotrauma patient focuses on detection of reversible causes of elevated intracranial pressure or reduced perfusion (Chapter 399),[4] but routine measurement of intracranial pressures does not improve outcome.[A1] Although many outcomes are fixed from the time of injury, opportunities for early intervention should not be missed. It is particularly important to avoid secondary neurologic injury, most commonly due to reduced perfusion from hypotension and cerebral edema.

Prevention of spinal cord injury (Chapter 399) and evaluation of the spine for bone and ligamentous disruption are also important components of the early evaluation. Multidetector CT images can be obtained quickly to detect occult spinal injuries.

A multidisciplinary approach to the evaluation and management of pain and anxiety in injured patients has important short- and long-term benefits.[5] An organized approach facilitates dealing with the inevitable pain and anxiety in an organized and consistent manner and allows the unit to determine the effectiveness of new interventions.

Tertiary Survey

The tertiary survey is a planned and careful repeated physical examination, usually 1 or 2 days after admission, often accompanied by focused imaging tests. The goal again is to exclude subtle injuries that might otherwise cause significant long-term morbidity. Examples include minor fractures of the wrist or foot, small deep lacerations of the scalp, subtle eye injuries, and some abdominal injuries, particularly retroperitoneal duodenal or colonic perforations. Such injuries can become the patient's dominant source of long-term morbidity if they are missed during initial evaluation and treatment.

Key Management Issues

Fluid Resuscitation and Transfusion

The clinical goal is to administer adequate but not excessive fluid while ensuring that soft tissues are not rendered ischemic by increasing pressure beneath inelastic eschar or tense muscle compartments. The severity of hemorrhagic shock should be assessed and treated appropriately (Table 111-2).

For burn patients, several formulas based on weight, surface area, and burn size have been developed over the years. These are general guides, and physiologic monitoring is needed with individual titration of infusions to meet set resuscitation end points, such as urine output, base deficit, and vital signs (E-Table 111-1).

In resuscitation of burn patients, capillary integrity generally returns if resuscitation has been successful at 18 to 24 hours, and fluid needs markedly decrease toward approximately 1.5-fold maintenance in most patients. Overadministration of fluid should be avoided at this phase of resuscitation. With the reduction in the infusion rate of isotonic crystalloid, topical care of large wounds will have a major impact on serum electrolytes. Wounds treated with nonaqueous topical antimicrobials, such as silver sulfadiazine cream or mafenide acetate cream, promote transeschar water loss and generate a free water requirement, which is generally provided as 5% dextrose and water or free water added to enteral feedings, to avoid hypernatremia. By comparison, wounds treated with aqueous topical agents are associated with electrolyte leeching and secondary hyponatremia (Chapter 116). Serum levels of potassium, calcium, and magnesium (Chapters 117-119 and 245) should be monitored frequently and replaced as needed. In most patients, enteral feedings (Chapter 216) can be started.

Modern fluid resuscitation in trauma patients emphasizes initial "permissive hypotension" to reduce early bleeding (Chapters 104 and 106). Patients with systemic arterial pressures in the range of 60 to 80 mm Hg are resuscitated initially to modest hypotension (i.e., the range of 80 to 90 mm Hg) if they are otherwise alert and well perfused. They are then taken expeditiously to the operating room for surgical control before targeting a normotensive state. Early use of blood products such as fresh-frozen plasma and red cells rather than crystalloid can minimize the coagulopathy and improve outcomes in rapidly hemorrhaging patients.[6] Liberal use of tourniquets and compressive dressings before surgery further improves outcome by reducing blood loss. Among the various crystalloids, none seems to have any obvious advantages or disadvantages for treatment of hemorrhage.[A2] Tranexamic acid (e.g., loading dose of 1 g during 10 minutes, then infusion of 1 g during 8 hours), which inhibits thrombolysis, beginning within 8 hours of injury may reduce bleeding in selected patients who require massive transfusion.[A3]

Pigmented urine is commonly seen in the setting of high-voltage, crush, blast, or very deep thermal injury. Myoglobin and hemoglobin that are liberated from lysed muscle (Chapter 113) and red cells cause the pigmentation.

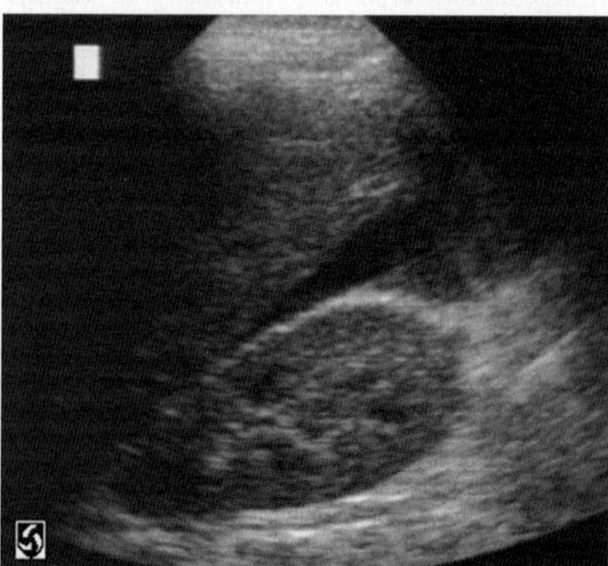

FIGURE 111-7. Positive focal abdominal sonography in trauma (FAST) study. There is a collection of fluid that shows up as a black strip between the liver and kidney. The white appearance is fat around the kidney. These findings are consistent with a fluid collection in Morison pouch. (Courtesy Robert H. Demling, MD.)

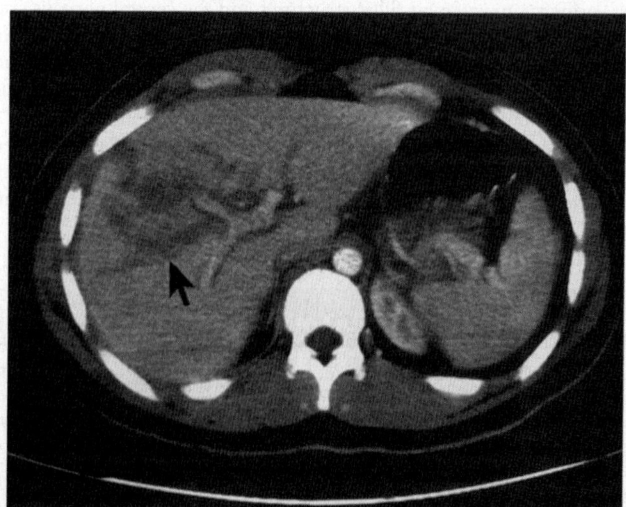

FIGURE 111-8. Abdominal injury. **An abdominal computed tomography scan shows an injury to the right lobe of the liver (*arrow*). (Courtesy Robert H. Demling, MD.)**

TABLE 111-2 CATEGORIZATION AND INITIAL TREATMENT OF HEMORRHAGIC SHOCK*

	CLASS I	CLASS II	CLASS III	CLASS IV
Blood loss (mL)	≤750	750-1500	1500-2000	≥2000
Blood loss (% of blood volume)	≤15	15-30	30-40	≥40
Pulse rate	<100	>100	>120	≥140
Blood pressure	Normal	Normal	Decreased	Decreased
Capillary refill test	Normal	Positive	Positive	Positive
Respiratory rate	14-20	20-30	30-40	>35
Urine output (mL/hr)	≥30	20-30	5-15	Negligible
Mental status	Slightly anxious	Mildly anxious	Anxious and confused	Confused and lethargic
Fluid replacement (3 : 1 rule)	Crystalloid	Crystalloid	Crystalloid + blood	Crystalloid + blood

*Based on a 70-kg adult. From Demling RH, Gates JD. Medical aspects of trauma and burn care. In: Goldman L, Schafer AI, eds. *Goldman's Cecil Medicine*. 24th ed. Philadelphia: Saunders-Elsevier; 2012.

To avoid renal tubular injury (Chapter 120), crystalloids should be administered to achieve a urine output of 2 mL/kg/hour (Chapter 113).

Decompression Procedures

An important component of the initial evaluation of the trauma and burn patient is to find and to rectify compartment syndromes before irreversible tissue ischemia occurs. Perfusion of the extremities can be compromised by inelastic near-circumferential burns, and the normal fascial envelopes of major muscle groups can cause high soft tissue pressure if muscles are injured by crush, thermal, or electrical injury or in association with major fractures. Even if pressures are normal in large vessels, edematous soft tissues can cause ischemia and necrosis because capillary perfusion is compromised. Extremities at risk should be dressed simply to facilitate frequent assessment for temperature, pliability, voluntary motion, pain with passive motion, detectable pulsations, and low-pressure flow by capillary refill and Doppler signals in the digital vessels and digital pulp. In assessing capillary refill, it is important to elevate the extremity, as even a mottled nonperfused extremity will demonstrate venous refill when it is dependent. Serial measurements of compartment pressures may be valuable in selected patients, with decompression recommended when measured pressures are above 30 cm H_2O. In most situations, serial clinical examination is sufficient to determine the need for escharotomy or fasciotomy, thereby avoiding the risk of bacterial seeding posed by passing pressure-monitoring catheters through contaminated wounds. Compromised extremities should be promptly decompressed by escharotomy or fasciotomy before the development of irreversible tissue necrosis (Fig. 111-9).

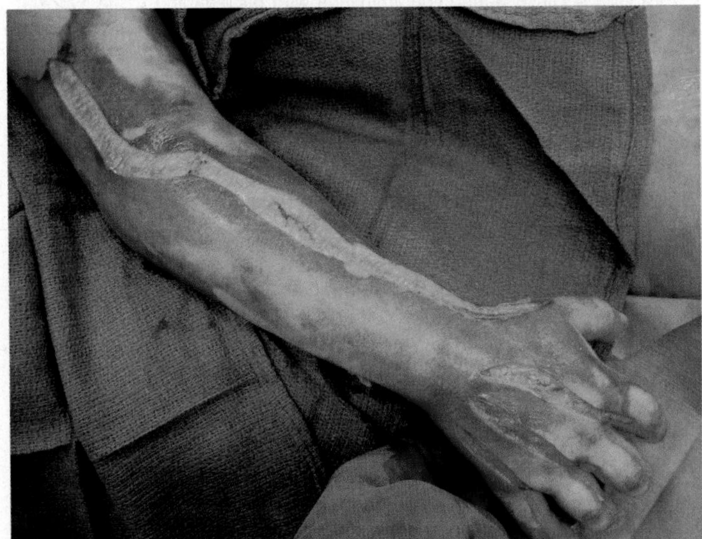

FIGURE 111-9. Tight extremities should be promptly decompressed by escharotomy or fasciotomy before the development of irreversible tissue necrosis.

Abdominal Compartment Syndrome

If abdominal viscera become extremely edematous, abdominal compartment syndrome may result.[7] This syndrome, which is usually caused by edema of the bowel wall, occurs after abdominal trauma or after the gut is reperfused by resuscitative therapies. When intra-abdominal pressures exceed 25 mm Hg (34 cm H_2O), renal blood flow, inferior vena cava blood return, and diaphragmatic excursion are impaired. This syndrome typically is manifested with oliguria, hypotension, and difficult ventilation. Diagnosis is by physical examination and measurement of bladder pressure. Treatment is by laparotomy with temporary abdominal closure.

Phase Two: Initial Surgical Care

Phase Two includes initial wound excision for burn patients and initial resuscitative surgery and fracture stabilization for non-burn trauma patients. This phase frequently overlaps with Phase One but is usually completed within 72 hours. Multiple subspecialty surgical teams may need to be coordinated by a trauma surgeon who directs overall care and reconciles conflicting priorities.

Early Wound Excision

Early wound excision within the first 72 hours of injury, before heavy microbial colonization occurs, is important for patients with significant burns, crush, or other soft tissue trauma. Early identification, excision, and closure of full-thickness wounds can avoid otherwise inevitable sepsis, systemic infection, and systemic inflammatory response. Excisional débridement of nonviable soft tissues or deep burns is critically important.

Damage Control Surgery

Damage control surgery identifies the most important surgical tasks that must be done to save the patient's life and only these are performed initially, thereby allowing a more stable patient to return to the operating room later for a subsequent definitive and often time-consuming operation.[8] The prototypical example is for abdominal trauma, when bleeding and gastrointestinal contamination are addressed initially but the abdomen is left open so a warmed and more stable patient can return to the operating room in 12 to 36 hours for a definitive bowel anastomosis and abdominal closure. This concept can also be applied to the trauma care system. If multiple patients need to share limited operating room resources, truncating individual operations allows more patients to be treated urgently.

Early Fracture Fixation

Early surgical fixation of long bone fractures benefits injured patients by reducing the complications of immobilization, enhancing rehabilitation, and likely reducing the systemic inflammatory state and proclivity to thromboembolic complications.[9]

Prophylaxis for Thromboembolic Complications and Gastrointestinal Hemorrhage

Trauma incites a hypercoagulable state, and seriously injured patients are prone to deep venous thrombosis and pulmonary embolism.[10] Pharmacologic prophylaxis, such as low-molecular-weight heparin, is recommended. Mechanical prophylaxis with automatic compression stockings is also routine in most trauma programs.

During the early hypodynamic phase with reduced splanchnic blood flow, gastrointestinal hemorrhage may occur in the seriously injured and burned patient. This complication can be sharply reduced with routine pharmacologic prophylaxis, including proton pump inhibitors or histamine-2 receptor blockers, such as with immediate-release omeprazole oral suspension (40 mg twice daily on the first day and 20 mg daily thereafter).[A4] [11]

Critical Care of the Injured or Burned

Many injured patients require transient intubation and mechanical ventilation (Chapter 105) to facilitate resuscitation, evaluation, and initial care. Some will go on to develop respiratory failure (Chapter 104) requiring protracted ventilator support.

Multiple mechanical and injury factors contribute to respiratory insufficiency in trauma patients, including chest wall trauma and pulmonary contusion. In patients with more severe injuries including flail chest, rib fixation is a useful intervention.[12]

In burn patients, inhalation injury (Chapter 94) is an important cause of respiratory failure. The diagnosis of inhalation injury is best made by history and clinical examination revealing singed nasal vibrissae and carbonaceous debris in the mouth and pharynx (E-Fig. 111-1). Chest radiographs are usually normal initially. Carbon monoxide poisoning (Chapter 94) can be seen in conjunction with inhalation injury; the standard of care is 100% oxygen at the prevailing atmospheric pressure for 6 hours, with hyperbaric oxygen reserved for patients with a carboxyhemoglobin level above 30% or neurologic changes.

Pneumonia (Chapter 97) or tracheobronchitis (Chapter 96) occurs in about 30% of burn patients with inhalation injury. The acute respiratory distress syndrome (Chapter 104) also is common in trauma patients, particularly those who go on to develop sepsis, pneumonia, and multiple organ failure. Antibiotic therapy is directed by sputum Gram stain and cultures and should not be prolonged beyond a 7- to 10-day therapeutic course. Vigorous pulmonary toilet, with directed bronchoscopy to clear secretions in selected patients, is an important component of therapy.

Post-Resuscitation Metabolic Issues

In the days that follow successful resuscitation, a hyperdynamic state predictably occurs, characterized by a high cardiac output and low peripheral resistance. Because wound contamination with bacteria and tissue hypoxia drive much of the hypermetabolic response, early excision of burned tissue and closure of burn wounds with autografting shorten hospital stays and enhance functional outcomes in patients with deep dermal and full-thickness burns. Prevention of tissue ischemia by repair of vascular injuries and decompression of edematous limbs by escharotomy or fasciotomy minimize the burden of necrotic tissue (E-Fig. 111-2). Early excision of necrotic or ischemic tissue will minimize the incidence of wound contamination and systemic sepsis and inflammation.

Several formulas have been devised to predict non-protein calorie needs (E-Table 111-2). A very rough estimate of calorie needs is a range of 25 to 35 kcal/kg/day, with the lower number applying to more stable and older patients and the upper number applying to more seriously injured and younger patients. Protein administration of 2 to 3 g per kilogram per day will adequately support the needs of most injured patients.

The route of nutritional support is ideally enteral (Chapter 216), with tube feeding beginning during resuscitation. However, some patients, particularly those with very severe and abdominal injuries or those with intervening sepsis, will not tolerate enteral feedings at goal rates and will require supplemental parenteral nutrition to ensure delivery of all needed nutrients (Chapter 217).

Safe and reliable modification of adverse components of the hypermetabolic response, particularly protein catabolism, has proved an elusive goal. Anabolic agents such as recombinant human growth hormone and anabolic steroids may help restore positive nitrogen balance, but they are not widely used because of their complications, expense, and conflicting data regarding the efficacy in most injured patients. Other attempted interventions, such as antipyretics, β-adrenergic blockade, β-adrenergic supplementation, nonsteroidal anti-inflammatory agents, recombinant growth hormone, insulin-like growth factor-I, and anabolic steroids, have been tried, but available data are inadequate to support any of these therapies as standard care.

Septic Complications and Multiple Organ Failure

Injured patients are at elevated risk for all types of infectious complications (Chapter 282). Multiple organ dysfunction and septic shock (Chapter 108) are manifestations of uncontrolled systemic inflammation for severe infection.

Phase Three: Definitive Surgical Care

Phase Three involves definitive wound closure for burns and completion surgery for trauma patients. In non-burn trauma patients, this phase may involve removal of vacuum wound dressings and definitive closure, closure of fasciotomy sites, and fixation of facial fractures. The duration of this phase varies greatly with injury, but it is usually complete at the time of acute hospital discharge. For example, in burn patients, this phase of care is defined by replacement of temporary membranes with permanent grafts and the important but time-consuming grafting of hands and face.

Phase Four: Rehabilitation and Reintegration

Phase Four describes the sometimes long process of reconstruction, rehabilitation, and reintegration.[13] This phase of care may begin in an inpatient rehabilitation setting and progress into the home environment. Depending on the specifics of the injury, the process may be a few weeks to months or years. Daily passive range of motion movements, splinting, anti-deformity positioning, and strengthening can reduce the frequency of these complications.

The environment of recovery is an important therapeutic consideration. Data suggest that specific qualities of the family have a major impact on multiple aspects of recovery, some that can potentially be modified. Community resources can be used to enhance recovery and are an important part of discharge planning.

REHABILITATION OF THE INJURED PATIENT

Rehabilitation in the Critically Ill Patient

Passive range of motion movement, splinting, and anti-deformity positioning will minimize the capsular contraction and shortening of tendon and muscle groups that otherwise occur with protracted immobilization.

Emotional recovery after severe trauma can be limited by neurologic injury and post-traumatic stress. These issues can be anticipated and their adverse effects blunted by early and continuous involvement of emotional supports for the family and patient. Ideally, psychiatric, social service, and psychological resources are available.

SPECIAL CONSIDERATIONS

Electrical Injury

Cardiopulmonary arrest can be caused by low-voltage electrical injury[14] but is more common with high-voltage electrical injury. Extensive tissue necrosis may also liberate enough potassium to cause cardiac dysfunction. Because cardiac arrhythmias may recur after resuscitation or develop 24 to 48 hours after injury, all patients who have sustained high-voltage electrical injury should undergo continuous electrocardiographic monitoring for at least 48 hours after the last documented arrhythmia.

A detailed neurologic examination must be performed on all patients with high-voltage electrical injury because dysfunction may be apparent immediately or may appear later. Recovery of function after direct electrical nerve damage is rare. Conversely, the nerves that are not injured directly commonly recover. A polyneuritic syndrome of relatively late onset can cause deficits in the function of peripheral nerves far removed from the points of contact. Delayed-onset spinal cord deficits can be manifested as quadriplegia, hemiplegia, localized nerve deficits with signs of ascending paralysis, transverse myelitis, and even an amyotrophic lateral sclerosis–like syndrome.

Among patients hospitalized with serious high-voltage electrical injuries, about 8% die and another 22% have permanent neurologic deficits despite optimal care. Most patients with low-voltage injuries, such as can be caused by electrical flash burns, also develop long-term sequelae, including neurologic (memory loss, numbness, headache, chronic pain, weakness) and musculoskeletal (pain, reduced range of motion, contracture) symptoms.

Lightning Injury

Cardiopulmonary arrest is common in patients struck by lightning.[15] Coma is also common acutely but typically resolves in a few hours. Keraunoparalysis, which is lightning-induced paralysis, is characterized by usually transient paresthesias and paralysis that develop during several days and typically involve the lower limbs. Ruptured tympanic membranes and hearing loss may also occur. With immediate cardiopulmonary resuscitation, about two thirds of lightning victims survive, and persistent neurologic deficits are relatively uncommon.

Considerations at the Extremes of Age

Injured patients at the extremes of age bring with them a number of important physiologic and psychosocial issues that directly affect their care (E-Table 111-3). Older adults do not have the depth of physiologic reserve of the young (Chapter 25). Cardiopulmonary function may be compromised, and peripheral vascular disease is common. Muscle mass and respiratory muscle strength are often reduced. Reduced renal reserve increases sensitivity to nephrotoxic drugs. The skin is relatively atrophic and consequently tolerates burning and donor harvest poorly. Nutritional needs are not well predicted by standard equations.

As a result, a major injury is often the event that changes the subsequent living condition of an elderly person.[16] Injuries are often the result of cognitive or functional changes (Chapter 27) and may be associated with syncopal episodes (Chapter 62) that need to be concurrently evaluated. Resuscitation should be carefully considered if burns are very large or trauma is severe. Data suggest that mortality is nearly 90% in patients who are older than 60 years, have burns of more than 40% of their body surface, and have concomitant inhalation injury. Patients may have advanced directives, interested families, or health care proxies who should be consulted as early as possible in the care of such patients (Chapter 3).

Older adults bring unique psychosocial issues to the trauma and burn center. They may live alone or have a spouse who cannot meet their discharge care needs for wound care, transportation, or general support. Children may live far away and be unable to support them. Discharge planning can be very involved, requiring orchestration of many community resources, and must be started early.

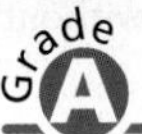

Grade A References

A1. Chesnut RM, Temkin N, Carney N, et al. A trial of intracranial-pressure monitoring in traumatic brain injury. *N Engl J Med*. 2012;367:2471-2481.

A2. Gruen RL, Brohi K, Schreiber M, et al. Haemorrhage control in severely injured patients. *Lancet*. 2012;380:1099-1108.

A3. Shakur H, Roberts I, Bautista R, et al. Effects of tranexamic acid on death, vascular occlusive events, and blood transfusion in trauma patients with significant haemorrhage (CRASH-2): a randomised, placebo-controlled trial. *Lancet*. 2010;376:23-32.

A4. Conrad SA, Gabrielli A, Margolis B, et al. Randomized, double-blind comparison of immediate-release omeprazole oral suspension versus intravenous cimetidine for the prevention of upper gastrointestinal bleeding in critically ill patients. *Crit Care Med*. 2005;33:760-765.

GENERAL REFERENCES

For the General References and other additional features, please visit Expert Consult at https://expertconsult.inkling.com.

112

ENVENOMATION

GEOFFREY K. ISBISTER AND STEVEN A. SEIFERT

GENERAL CONCEPTS OF ENVENOMATION

EPIDEMIOLOGY

Terrestrial and marine envenomations result in a wide range of clinical syndromes and remain an important and unrecognized cause of morbidity and mortality, especially in the developing world. An estimated 5.5 million people are bitten by snakes each year, and snake envenomation is the most important envenomation syndrome worldwide, especially in tropical and subtropical countries. Snake bites cause an estimated 440,000 envenomation cases and 20,000 deaths each year.[1] Scorpions and spiders,[2] which also cause envenomation, are discussed in Chapter 359.

Marine envenomation is less common, except in coastal regions where hundreds of thousands and potentially millions of minor jellyfish stings occur each year. Venomous fish stings and injuries from other creatures such as sponges and sea urchins also occur, but the annual incidence is unknown. Worldwide, ciguatera is also a major clinical syndrome because of the large number of cases and morbidity in the Pacific region, where people rely on fish as a major food source. Fortunately few deaths occur. Other marine poisonings, including puffer fish poisoning and shellfish poisoning, often result in severe and potentially life-threatening effects but are rare.[3]

Venoms, Toxins, and Poisons

Envenomation includes any injury caused by a venomous creature that produces venom in a specialized gland and can deliver it to other organisms by means of fangs (e.g., snakes and spiders), stings (e.g., scorpions and jellyfish), or spines (e.g., fish). Venoms can be any combination of procoagulant, neurotoxic, myotoxic, and cytotoxic substances, not all of which affect humans because humans are not the intended victim of envenomation. Envenomation differs from poisoning, which occurs when mainly marine animals containing toxic substances (e.g., ciguatera) are ingested.

TREATMENT OF ENVENOMATION (Rx)

Very few first-aid techniques have been shown to be clinically effective for envenomations, so rapid transport to the hospital for definitive medical care is of utmost importance. Because envenomations such as snake bites and box jellyfish stings can result in early hypotensive collapse and cardiac arrest, the most important first aid is basic life support (Chapter 63).

Many snake venoms contain local tissue cytotoxins and techniques that concentrate venom at the bite site for prolonged periods and may result in greater local injury. Nonetheless, immobilization of the bitten extremity is recommended to minimize the venom's spread or systemic uptake, provided immobilization does not delay access to definitive therapy. With envenomations from Australasian elapids, kraits, and coral snakes, where there is likely to be only minor local tissue injury, a pressure bandage should be applied.[4] Pharmacologic agents that slow lymphatic flow (e.g., topical nifedipine or lidocaine) also may be useful as adjuncts in slowing venom uptake.[5] Other popular first-aid treatments that are often found in snake bite kits actually cause harm, including arterial or venous tourniquets, incision, suction, heat, cold, and electric shock.

Antivenom

Antivenom, which is the major treatment for envenomation, consists of a mixture of polyclonal whole or fractionated antibodies against the toxins in a specific venom. Because these antivenoms are produced in animals that are exposed to one or more venoms, they are generally specific to the venoms and their local species. Most antivenoms have never been tested in randomized controlled trials, so their true effectiveness is rarely known despite proven efficacy in preclinical studies. Antivenoms also cause a number of side effects, the most important being hypersensitivity reactions that can range from skin reactions to anaphylaxis (Chapter 253) that is not immunoglobulin E mediated and is characterized mainly by hypotension. Microbial contamination of antivenoms also can cause pyogenic reactions, which are characterized by fevers, rigors, and chills and may be associated with headache, gastrointestinal symptoms, and rarely hypotension. Anywhere from 6% to more than 30% of patients develop delayed antivenom serum sickness (Chapter 47), with influenza-like fever, arthralgia, myalgia, rash, urticaria, lymphadenopathy, headache, and gastrointestinal symptoms about 4 to 14 days after antivenom administration.[6]

The high frequency of reactions to some snake antivenoms has prompted the use of premedication, and one large randomized trial supports premedication with epinephrine (0.25 mL of 1 : 1000 solution subcutaneously) for antivenoms with a high reaction rate.[A1] By comparison, no evidence supports corticosteroids or antihistamines for premedication.

Other treatments for envenomation and poisoning focus on the specific but wide-ranging clinical effects caused by the various toxins and are not aimed at neutralizing the toxins or eliminating them. Examples include intubation and ventilation (Chapters 104 and 105) for neurotoxicity that leads to ventilatory muscle failure, hydration and renal replacement therapy in severe myotoxicity and acute kidney injury (Chapter 120), blood product replacement for severe coagulopathy with or without hemorrhage (Chapters 174 and 175), cardiac support for cardiac toxicities (Chapter 63), and pain relief (Chapter 30) in toxin-mediated pain syndromes such as scorpion stings and latrodectism and jellyfish stings.

SNAKE ENVENOMATION

Venomous snakes belong to one of five families: Viperidae, with its two subfamilies, Viperinae, or Old World vipers (e.g., saw-scaled vipers, puff adders), and Crotalinae, or pit vipers, named for the heat-sensitive organ between the eye and nostril used for hunting warm-blooded prey (e.g., rattlesnakes, copperheads); Elapidae (e.g., cobras, kraits, coral snakes); Hydrophiidae (e.g., sea snakes); Atractaspididae (e.g., asps); and Colubridae (e.g., garter snakes, corn snakes, boomslangs). Although all five families contain venomous species, the two responsible for more than 90% of venomous bites are Viperidae and Elapidae.

CLINICAL SYNDROMES

Local swelling and bruising after a bite are caused by increased vascular permeability as a result of endothelial cell damage and are mediated by hydrolases, proteases, phospholipase A_2, polypeptide toxins, metalloproteinases, and the release of endogenous autacoids such as bradykinin and histamine. Some venoms (e.g., some cobras) may cause necrotic skin lesions or extensive swelling and bruising. Other venoms (e.g., European adders and North American rattlesnakes) increase vascular permeability and result in significant regional swelling and edema. In rare cases, the loss of fluid into the tissues can cause hypovolemic shock.

One type of toxin will usually predominate in a particular snake, and the combination of toxins will result in a somewhat unique clinical syndrome for each snake. For example, bites from *Bungarus* spp (kraits) usually result in neurotoxicity, whereas *Echis* spp (saw-scaled or carpet vipers) primarily cause a coagulopathy with spontaneous bleeding.

Abnormal Coagulation

Coagulopathy (Chapters 175 and 176) is the most important snake envenomation syndrome, and venom-induced consumption coagulopathy is the most common form.[7] The syndrome results from the activation of the clotting pathway at a number of specific points due to procoagulant toxins in snake venoms. (See also http://wikitoxin.toxicology.wikispaces.net/Venom+induced+consumption+coagulopathy+-+VICC.) Important procoagulant toxins include fibrinogenolytic toxins or thrombin-like enzymes (e.g., Malaysian pit viper, American vipers), prothrombin activators (e.g., Australian elapids), and factor X activators (e.g., Russell's viper venom), all of which result in low or undetectable fibrinogen levels.

Venom-induced consumption coagulopathy is an acquired acute clotting factor deficiency that persists until clotting factors can be resynthesized. Venom-induced consumption coagulopathy results in an abnormal international normalized ratio (INR), activated partial thromboplastin time (aPTT), and thrombin clotting time as well as elevated D-dimer levels and fibrinogen degradation products. The coagulopathy may not result in hemorrhage unless it is accompanied by associated injury or trauma. Unlike disseminated intravascular coagulation (Chapter 175), the syndrome has a rapid onset and resolution and is not associated with systemic microthrombi, end-organ failure, or poor clinical outcomes.

Some venoms can cause a thrombotic microangiopathy, with clinical manifestations (e.g., thrombocytopenia, microangiopathic hemolytic anemia, and acute renal failure) similar to what is seen in other microangiopathies, such as thrombotic thrombocytopenic purpura and the hemolytic-uremic syndrome (Chapter 172). This syndrome has been reported for Australian elapids, Russell's viper, saw-scaled viper, and desert horned viper.

Conversely, venom-induced anticoagulant coagulopathy is characterized by an elevated aPTT and a mildly abnormal INR. It has been reported in Australian black snake envenomation but does not appear to cause a clinically important coagulopathy. Thrombocytopenia occurs in many snakes and is prominent in North American Crotalinae spp because of decreased production, aggregation, and sequestration of platelets.

Neuromuscular Toxicity

Snake neurotoxins, which occur mainly with elapid and some viperid venoms, are usually classified as presynaptic neurotoxins (e.g., β-bungarotoxins, taipoxin), which injure the presynaptic neuromuscular terminal and prevent acetylcholine release, or postsynaptic toxins (e.g., α-bungarotoxins), which bind to acetylcholine receptors on the motor end plate. Presynaptic neurotoxins generally result in irreversible neurotoxicity that may take days to weeks to resolve if it is not treated early with antivenom. The clinical presentation is initially with ptosis and extraocular ophthalmoplegia, which progress to bulbar palsy, and finally respiratory and peripheral muscle paralysis.

Myotoxic envenomation syndromes are divided into two clinical types, local myotoxicity and systemic myotoxicity or rhabdomyolysis (Chapter 421). Local myotoxicity is most commonly seen when viper envenomation affects muscles near the bite site. Symptoms range from local myalgia with swelling and pain to myonecrosis. Moderate (10-fold) transient creatine kinase (CK) concentration elevations are seen for up to 48 hours. In systemic myotoxicity, widespread muscle injury results in generalized myalgia, a raised CK concentration to as high as 100,000 U/L for several days, and myoglobinuria (Chapter 113). Systemic myotoxicity is seen with sea snakes, Australian elapids, and the South American rattlesnake *Crotalus durissus*. However, acute renal failure is uncommon.

Other Effects

Some snakes (primarily vipers and Australian elapids) produce an acute hypotensive syndrome within minutes of the bite, apparently due to the release of vasodilating autacoids. *Bothrops* species inhibit the breakdown of bradykinin and angiotensinogen, which are naturally occurring, rapid-acting angiotensin-converting enzyme inhibitors. Other cardiovascular effects include vasodilation, diffuse vascular permeability, myocardial depression (Chapter 58), and atrioventricular block (Chapter 64), which may contribute to the hypotension caused by crotalines and elapids. Acute kidney injury (Chapter 120) is uncommon but can be caused by a direct renal toxin, hypotension with resulting acute tubular necrosis, or rhabdomyolysis or as part of a thrombotic microangiopathy.

Many envenomations cause nonspecific systemic symptoms, including nausea, vomiting, headache, abdominal pain, diarrhea, and diaphoresis. Although these effects are not life-threatening, they may be useful early markers of envenomation and may require symptomatic treatment.

DIAGNOSIS

Most patients present with an obvious history of a snakebite, but they may not have envenomation. The initial assessment and investigation needs to determine

- whether the patient has snake envenomation or a bite without envenomation;
- what snake or snake group is likely to have caused the bite; and
- whether antivenom is indicated and, if so, what antivenom is available and should be used.

In some patients, signs or symptoms of envenomation may be obvious. Other patients, however, initially may not have any evidence of envenomation and should be observed with serial clinical and laboratory assessment, depending on the region and type of snake potentially involved (e.g., vipers may inject large amounts of venom with delayed absorption) as well as the severity of the patient's clinical syndrome.

Laboratory Investigations

If they are available, the most important laboratory studies are coagulation studies: INR, aPTT, and platelet count. Point-of-care testing devices for measuring the INR are insensitive to the changes caused by venom-induced consumption coagulopathy and should not be relied on. If they are available, measures of fibrinogen and D-dimer can assist in the diagnosis of venom-induced consumption coagulopathy.

A complete blood count can identify thrombocytopenia and thrombotic microangiopathy; nonspecific leukocytosis and lymphopenia can occur in snake envenomation and may provide support for the diagnosis. An elevated CK level indicates systemic myotoxicity but lags behind the muscle injury by 12 to 24 hours. A serum creatinine level is important to assess possible acute kidney injury. Measurements of venom and antivenom in serum are available only in the research setting.

TREATMENT Rx

The most important first-aid measures in snake bite are to move a safe distance from the snake, to immobilize the patient as well as the bitten body part, and to organize transport to medical care. Unproven and potentially dangerous first-aid techniques that should not be used include suction, cutting the bite site, electrocution, and the application of heat, cold, or tourniquets. Pressure bandaging with immobilization (at lymphatic obstruction pressures of 55 to 70 mm Hg) is recommended for Australian snake bites and some other elapids but should not be used for the majority of other snakes, including all viperid snakes.

Patients whose envenomation is manifested as coagulopathy, myotoxicity, or neurotoxicity should be administered antivenom and admitted until the clinical effects have resolved. The specific antivenom, the indications for its use, and the dosing regimens depend on the type of snake and the geographic region. Regional and national guidelines should be consulted.

Local Tissue Injury and Local Myotoxicity

Most local injuries can be treated with supportive care, including analgesia (e.g., an anti-inflammatory such as ibuprofen, 400 to 800 mg, and opioids such as morphine, 2.5 to 10 mg intravenously, titrated to the pain), elevation, and standard wound care. Some viperid bites will cause significant local and regional swelling with increased tissue pressures, but early surgical treatment is not indicated and may be associated with worse outcomes. Late surgical débridement of necrotic tissue may be required. There does not appear to be a role for prophylactic antibiotics, which should be reserved for documented infection.

Abnormal Coagulation

The treatment of venom-induced consumption coagulopathy includes antivenom to neutralize the procoagulant toxins, supportive or interventional care for any spontaneous or traumatic hemorrhage, and blood or factor replacement. The clinical effectiveness of antivenom is supported by a number of observational studies but depends on the type of procoagulant toxin and the timing of antivenom administration. In one of the most striking observational studies, *Echis* antivenom corrected coagulopathy within 24 to 48 hours, whereas untreated patients had deranged hemostasis for 8 to 10 days.[8] Similar benefits have been reported for other antivenoms.[A2] In one randomized trial of Australian elapid bites, fresh-frozen plasma restored clotting function more rapidly but did not decrease major hemorrhage or death, and it may even worsen the coagulopathy if it is given within 6 hours of the bite.[A3]

Thrombotic microangiopathy (Chapter 172) requires close monitoring and supportive care. Antivenom may prevent thrombotic microangiopathy, but repeated doses are of no benefit. Major hemorrhage such as intracranial (Chapter 408) and gastrointestinal bleeding (Chapter 135) should be managed per standard protocols, including blood transfusion as required (Chapter 177). There is no evidence to support the use of plasmapheresis in snakebite-induced thrombotic microangiopathy.

Neuromuscular Toxicity

Antivenom is the only specific treatment for neurotoxicity, and numerous studies have demonstrated that early antivenom can prevent neurotoxicity. However, because most neurotoxicity is presynaptic, antivenom will not reverse neurotoxicity once it appears, and delayed administration may be of no benefit. For snakes that cause neurotoxicity (Chapters 420 and 422), repeated examinations should look for ptosis, extraocular muscle weakness, bulbar palsy, and respiratory abnormalities. Intubation and mechanical ventilation may be required for respiratory muscle weakness.

Systemic myotoxicity with rhabdomyolysis (Chapter 113) is irreversible but can be prevented with early antivenom administration. Serial measurement of the CK level is essential to monitor systemic myotoxicity.

Specific Snake Syndromes

The worldwide distribution of the most common snakes of medical importance is available at either www.toxinology.com or http://apps.who.int/bloodproducts/snakeantivenoms/database/snakeframeset.html.

NORTH AMERICAN SNAKES

In the United States, an estimated 8000 bites by native venomous snake species occur annually, mostly by pit vipers—rattlesnakes (*Crotalus* and *Sistrurus* spp), copperheads, and cottonmouths (*Agkistrodon* spp); fewer than 100 bites occur by coral snakes, which are the only native elapid (*Micrurus* spp and *Micruroides euyxanthus*). Fortunately, the number of fatalities, primarily caused by rattlesnakes, is fewer than 10 per year. Because the crotaline antivenom in the United States (CroFab) is effective against all North American crotaline species, because envenomations are readily clinically diagnosable, and because coral snakes are easily recognized, there is no need to capture or kill the offending snake for identification. In the prehospital setting, management priorities include avoidance of further interaction with the snake, removal of jewelry, loosening of tight-fitting clothing, loose splinting of the bitten body part, and rapid transportation to a health care facility capable of treating snakebite.

Envenomation by North American viperids invariably produces local tissue injury, with progressive swelling and pain. However, frank necrosis occurs in only about 5% of cases, and rates of hematologic (prothrombin time/INR and aPTT prolongation, thrombocytopenia, or hypofibrinogenemia), neurologic, hemodynamic, and nonspecific symptoms and signs vary. Definitive management is antivenom plus elevation of the bitten body part. Surgical intervention is not beneficial in the acute phase. Infection is uncommon, and prophylactic antibiotics are not recommended. Antibiotics may also be added if there is tissue necrosis or signs of infection. Unless there are signs of an immediate hypersensitivity reaction to the venom, there is no role for antihistamines or steroids. Local venom effects may recur within the first 24 hours. Hematologic effects may recur after several days and persist for days or weeks, and about 1% of patients may develop late bleeding complications.[9] Monitoring and management strategies are complex, and expert assistance is suggested.[10]

Clinical effects of coral snakes, primarily the Eastern coral snake (*Micrurus fulvius*), include neurotoxicity and minimal local effects. With severe envenomation, perioral paresthesias, nausea, vomiting, hypersalivation, and euphoria progress to cranial nerve paralysis (e.g., ptosis, diplopia, and dysphagia) and respiratory failure. Respiratory failure may develop within minutes of the onset of neurologic signs. Because of a shortage of antivenom, some clinicians have elected to wait for signs of envenomation before administering antivenom. If this approach is taken, patients should be given antivenom at the first signs of neurotoxicity and observed for at least 24 hours before it is concluded that no envenomation has occurred.

There are approximately 50 venomous snake bites a year in the United States by non-native (exotic) species. Antivenoms for these snakes as well as expert assistance in the management of envenomations can be obtained by contacting the appropriate poison center (1-800-222-1222).

CENTRAL AND SOUTH AMERICA

Snake envenomation in Central and South America is associated with more morbidity and mortality than in North America, despite the availability of antivenom for most venomous species. One reason is the larger variety of snakes, most importantly viperid snake species (*Crotalus*, *Bothrops*, and *Lachesis*) and the coral snakes (elapids) (see http://wikitoxin.toxicology.wikispaces.net/Latin+American+Snakebite). Various South and Central American vipers induce bite site necrosis, consumption coagulopathy, and bleeding. As in North America, coral snake envenomation causes a descending paralysis but few local effects. Polyvalent antivenoms are available in Central and South America to cover the particular vipers in different geographic regions. (See http://apps.who.int/bloodproducts/snakeantivenoms/database/snakeframeset.html.)

ASIAN SNAKES

The incidence of snake envenomation in Asia, particularly in south Asia, is potentially the highest in the world, with significant mortality and morbidity. (See http://wikitoxin.toxicology.wikispaces.net/Asian+Snakebite.) As a general rule, vipers cause coagulopathy and elapids cause neurotoxicity. Russell's vipers, saw-scaled vipers, and pit vipers (e.g., Malayan pit vipers) cause venom-induced consumption coagulopathy, except the mechanism of action of the procoagulant toxin differs (see http://wikitoxin.toxicology.wikispaces.net/Venom+induced+consumption+coagulopathy+-+VICC). Viper bites are also associated with local tissue injury and nonspecific systemic effects. Neurotoxicity, which is a major problem with krait envenomation and some cobras, results in an irreversible descending paralysis that develops during hours. Many krait bites occur at night when the snakes are active and patients are often not aware of the bite, so patients often present late with established neurotoxicity.

Treatment protocols for snake bite differ throughout Asia and depend on local resources, the availability of antivenom, and the presumed venomous snakes. Antivenom is the main treatment and is manufactured in a number of countries (http://apps.who.int/bloodproducts/snakeantivenoms/database/snakeframeset.html). Venom-induced consumption coagulopathy resulting from Asian snakes appears to respond to antivenom treatment, which may be effective days after the bite. The irreversibility of neurotoxicity means that intubation and mechanical ventilation are often required, particularly for patients presenting late when antivenom is unlikely to be effective. In krait envenomation, patients may require ventilation for days to weeks.

AFRICAN SNAKES

Snake envenomation is a major problem in Africa (see http://wikitoxin.toxicology.wikispaces.net/African+Snakebite), especially in locations with limited health care and availability of antivenom. In addition, the offending species of snakes are not as well known or categorized.

The puff adder is widely distributed and likely to cause many bites, but most of the bites cause only local swelling, blistering, and uncommonly necrosis. Systemic envenomation causes early hypotension, bradycardia, thrombocytopenia, and uncommonly coagulopathy.

Carpet vipers (*Echis*), which are the most important snakes in western and northern Africa and across to the Middle East, cause a significant coagulopathy that may persist for 7 to 14 days without antivenom. The desert vipers (*Cerastes*) of northern Africa and across into the Middle East cause local effects and rarely a mild coagulopathy.

Cobras are widely distributed elapids divided into the cytotoxic/spitting cobras (*Naja nigricolis*, *Naja mossambica*) and the neurotoxic cobras. The cytotoxic/spitting cobras can spit venom into the eye and cause venom ophthalmia. Bites by cytotoxic cobras cause nonspecific systemic symptoms and necrosis. In contrast, the neurotoxic cobras (e.g., Egyptian cobras, or *Naja haje*) cause progressive descending paralysis. Mambas are large elapids that cause neurotoxicity characterized by paresthesia, muscle fasciculations, and weakness, associated with nonspecific and autonomic effects (sweating, hypertension, tachycardia, vomiting). The boomslang (*Dispholidus typhus*) is a Colubrid that causes a severe venom-induced consumption coagulopathy that results in spontaneous and major bleeding and uncommonly thrombotic microangiopathy. The burrowing asps are reported to cause local effects and nonspecific symptoms.

Although a number of snake antivenoms are available for African snakes, they often are not readily available, and many patients do not present to a hospital. Polyvalent antivenom from South Africa covers many of the important snakes. Other antivenoms are available and details are at http://apps.who.int/bloodproducts/snakeantivenoms/database/snakeframeset.html.

EUROPEAN SNAKES

Snake envenomation is uncommon in Europe, and the only medically important species are *Vipera* spp (true vipers) that occur across most of Europe including England, almost all of continental Europe down to the Mediterranean, and also across into north Asia and northern Africa (Morocco, Algeria, and Tunisia). The most important species are *Vipera berus*, *Vipera aspis*, and

Vipera ammodytes, although the epidemiology of snake envenomation is not well defined for many countries.

The major effects of *Vipera* bites are local swelling and regional swelling, tissue injury, hematomas, nonspecific systemic symptoms (vomiting, diarrhea, abdominal pain), and hypotension. Coagulopathy and neurotoxicity are uncommon. The severity of envenomation can be graded (see table at http://wikitoxin.toxicology.wikispaces.net/European+Snakebite). Antivenoms for *Vipera* bites are available in a number of countries and are regarded as the main treatment.[11] Supportive care, including intravenous fluids for hypotension and elevation of the bitten limb, is also important.

AUSTRALASIAN SNAKES

In Australasia, the medically important venomous snakes include brown snakes (*Pseudonaja* spp), tiger snakes (*Notechis* spp), black snakes (*Pseudechis* spp), taipans (*Oxyuranus* spp), and death adders (*Acanthophis* spp). All are elapids and all look similar, except the death adder. As a result, the choice of antivenom is usually based on geography and clinical effects and only rarely on the identification of the snake.

Each snake group causes a characteristic clinical syndrome. Venom-induced consumption coagulopathy is the most common with all except black snakes and death adders. Myotoxicity occurs with black snakes and tiger snakes, and it also occurs less commonly with taipans. Neurotoxicity is the only clinical effect of death adder envenomation, is the major clinical effect in taipan envenomation, and can occur with tiger snakes. (See http://wikitoxin.toxicology.wikispaces.net/Australian+Snakebite.) Local effects are uncommon, so pressure bandaging is the current standard first-aid method.

About 90% of suspected snake bites in Australia are nonenvenomed cases or dry bites, so treatment focuses on excluding envenomation. Five monovalent antivenoms are available, depending on the clinical features and geography. A snake venom detection kit can detect venom on a wound swab from the five major snake groups and may assist in determining the type of snake. If the type of snake remains unclear on the basis of clinical effects and geography, polyvalent antivenom should be administered. The dose is one vial for all antivenoms, and redosing is not required. (See http://wikitoxin.toxicology.wikispaces.net/Australian+Snakebite.)

SNAKE HANDLERS AND EXOTIC SNAKE BITE

A considerable number of snake bites occur in snake handlers, including zoo keepers, private collectors, wild-life rescuers, and venom researchers. In the United States, for example, bites were reported from more than 90 different non-native species during a 10-year period. The case-fatality rate of exotic envenomation can be an order of magnitude higher than for native species, in part because of an immunoglobulin E–mediated anaphylactic reaction (Chapter 253) to the venom in individuals who handle snakes or who have been bitten previously. Early expert advice and contact with a poison center are essential to access information and antivenom.

MARINE ENVENOMATION

A wide variety of venomous marine creatures exist worldwide, including invertebrates and vertebrates. Fortunately, the limited number of types of marine envenomation result in only a few major envenomation syndromes, with more similarities than differences.[12] Perhaps the most important venomous marine creatures are the jellyfish, including the major box jellyfish (*Chironex fleckeri*), which is regarded as the most toxic venomous creature. Other important venomous marine creatures are the venomous fish, echinoderms (including sea urchins), sea snakes, and sponges.

Jellyfish Envenomation

EPIDEMIOLOGY

More than 100 jellyfish (Cnidaria) of medical importance exist worldwide, with a range of envenomation from very minor to potentially life-threatening. The epidemiology remains unclear, with millions of minor unreported injuries occurring in some coastal parts of the developed world and an unknown number of cases in other parts of the world. Deaths from major box jellyfish stings are rare and occur mainly in northern Australia, but such events may be underestimated in resource-poor countries.

PATHOBIOLOGY

Jellyfish are covered by millions of nematocysts (stinging cells), mainly on their tentacles. When these nematocysts are triggered by chemical or physical stimuli, such as contact with human skin, venom released from these stinging cells results in dermal injection and clinical envenomation. The severity of the envenomation depends on the amount of tentacle contact and the potency of the venom. Envenomation with the major box jellyfish, which have multiple long tentacles and highly potent venom, can be life-threatening, whereas stings with *Physalia* species tend to be minor.

CLINICAL MANIFESTATIONS

Envenomation by jellyfish can be broadly divided into two major clinical syndromes. With linear/tentacle stings, contact with one or more jellyfish tentacles results in local pain of varying severity and a raised linear erythematous or urticarial lesion that persists for a few hours to a day. Rarely these stings are associated with nonspecific systemic symptoms such as dizziness, nausea, vomiting, and malaise. With Irukandji-like stings, there is minimal local pain and evidence of the sting, but the envenomation syndrome results in systemic effects, including severe generalized back, chest, abdominal, and large muscle pain associated with nausea, vomiting, and headache within about 20 to 30 minutes after contact with the jellyfish. Sympathomimetic-like effects, including tachycardia, hypertension, anxiety, and agitation, also occur. With severe envenomation, cardiac effects, likely secondary to this catecholaminergic excess, can include electrocardiogram changes (T wave changes and ST segment depression), elevated troponin levels, myocardial depression, and even cardiogenic pulmonary edema.

Common and Important Jellyfish Groups and Syndromes

Numerous jellyfish result in specific syndromes. (See http://wikitoxin.toxicology.wikispaces.net/Jellyfish.) *Physalia* species are widespread and have different common names throughout the world, including Portuguese man-of-war, Pacific man-of-war, and blue bottle. They are the most common jellyfish stings and are responsible for hundreds of thousands of stings in America, Australia, and Europe each year, although most victims do not seek medical attention. *Physalia* stings cause typical linear erythematous reactions with moderate to severe local pain persisting for a few hours. The linear markings, which may have a characteristic ladder-like or beaded appearance, persist for several days. Localized bullous reactions and scarring can occur, but systemic effects are rare and deaths are extremely rare. *C. fleckeri*, which is a box jellyfish (Cubozoa), is reported to be the most venomous creature in the world. *C. fleckeri* has resulted in more than 70 deaths in northern Australia, the majority in young children in remote areas. Like all box jellyfish, they are cube shaped with long tentacles attached to each corner. Contact with them can result in several meters of skin involvement and severe envenomation. Fortunately, however, most stings are minor linear tentacle stings. Linear erythematous eruptions are similar to other linear tentacle stings but usually more severe, with severe pain persisting for hours and requiring opioid analgesia (Chapter 30). Local necrosis can occur along the sting line, but permanent scarring is rare. Severe envenomation is characterized by profound hypotension and early cardiovascular collapse, which can result in death in 20 to 30 minutes. Delayed hypersensitivity reactions occur in more than 50% of patients, with papular urticarial lesions developing along the stings. Numerous other jellyfish include the sea nettle (*Chrysaora quinquecirrha*), which is important in the Chesapeake Bay area of America but also occurs in Japan and the Philippines. It has effects similar to those of *Physalia*. Hair jellyfish cause stings to the eyes and cornea because the tentacles break off. *Pelagia* spp (moon jellyfish) are also common in parts of the world and cause effects similar to those of *Physalia*.

TREATMENT Rx

The treatment of the majority of jellyfish stings occurs out of the hospital. The jellyfish is rarely identified, so treatment is based on the clinical effects and the known local jellyfish. Most victims do not seek formal medical care unless they have severe, persistent pain or systemic effects that require medical intervention. First aid can be given by bystanders, surf life-savers, first-aid personnel, or ambulance services.

First aid includes washing off tentacles or any jellyfish material with sea water or carefully removing them by hand.[13] The use of fresh water may cause additional nematocyst discharge and potentially worsen the effects. For some major box jellyfish (including *C. fleckeri*) that can cause severe systemic envenomation, vinegar, which is often available on beaches where these jellyfish stings occur, should be applied immediately. Despite limited evidence, the aim of the vinegar is to prevent further nematocyst discharge and severe systemic envenomation from major jellyfish stings. Vinegar may increase the pain and is not recommended for these less severe jellyfish stings.

Box jellyfish stings have the potential to cause severe systemic envenomation within the first 30 minutes. Cardiovascular collapse or arrest should be treated with standard advanced life support (Chapter 63). Antivenom is unlikely to be effective for *C. fleckeri*, but guidelines still recommend its use in severe envenomation if it is available to be given by the intravenous route. Patients who arrive at the hospital without cardiovascular effects are highly unlikely to develop severe envenomation after arrival.

Physalia stings should be treated with hot-water immersion (45°C for 20 minutes) to treat local pain.[A4] An alternative is a hot shower or a constant flow of hot water. Analgesia or local dressings are rarely required for skin reactions.

For more severe stings, such as *C. fleckeri* stings, oral or parenteral opioids (Chapter 30) may be required. Numerous topical treatments, such as bicarbonate slurry, urine, or sand, are not supported by any evidence and are not recommended. Most stings do not require any local treatment, but necrosis can occur in severe cases and should be treated similar to burns (Chapter 111) with appropriate dressings.

Irukandji syndrome or Irukandji-like stings often require in-hospital treatment for severe pain and systemic symptoms. Titrated intravenous opiates (Chapter 30) should be given in combination with an antiemetic (e.g., metoclopramide, 10 mg; see Table 132-5). Benzodiazepines may be useful for agitation and anxiety. All patients with Irukandji syndrome should have an electrocardiogram and measurement of the serum troponin level because of the risk of cardiac toxicity. Patients can be discharged if they have a normal electrocardiogram and troponin level and are pain free. However, patients with evidence of cardiac involvement should be admitted for monitoring and an echocardiogram. Acute pulmonary edema should be treated per standard protocols (Chapter 59).

Evidence for the treatment of other jellyfish stings is limited, but first aid should include washing off the tentacles with sea water. Hot water may be effective, but it has not been rigorously tested.

Venomous Fish and Stingray Injuries

EPIDEMIOLOGY

Venomous fish occur in tropical and sometimes in temperate oceans. The important venomous fish, which differ throughout the world, include catfish (Siluriformes), stonefish (Synanceiidae), bullrout, weever fish (Trachinidae), scorpion fish, and lionfish (Scorpaenidae). Venomous fish are also kept in private aquariums, and many injuries in North America are due to lionfish in captivity. Stingrays, which vary in size from smaller than a hand to more than a meter, can live in tropical and temperate oceans as well as in fresh water.

PATHOBIOLOGY

Venomous fish and stingrays have a venomous sheath-covered spine that is formed on the dorsal or ventral spine of the fish and the tail of a stingray. The venom, which is between the spine and the sheath, is injected as the spine penetrates the skin. However, the majority of the injury is simply due to penetrating trauma, particularly in the case of stingrays with their much larger spines. Although the venoms differ among types of venomous fish and stingrays, they appear to be responsible for the severe pain out of proportion to the trauma and possibly contribute to the slow recovery and risk of infection with some wounds.

The site of injury varies for different fish and depends on how they encounter humans. Stingrays most commonly cause injuries to the ankle when they are stepped on, stonefish and bullrout cause injuries to the foot when they are stepped on, and catfish cause injuries to the hands when they are being caught.

CLINICAL MANIFESTATIONS

Symptoms vary among different fish and stingrays (see http://wikitoxin.toxicology.wikispaces.net/Penetrating+Marine+Envenoming). The main effects are a puncture wound or laceration associated with pain that varies on the basis of the size of the injury and the venom injected.[14] Severe and prolonged site pain may occur with stonefish, bullrout, some marine catfish, and weever fish. In addition, local bleeding, particularly with stingrays, and surrounding swelling and edema can occur. The spines rarely remain in the wound, but small amounts of foreign material often do and represent a considerable risk of secondary marine infection. Systemic effects are rarely reported but may include nonspecific symptoms such as nausea, vomiting, and malaise.

Catfish injuries most commonly occur when fishermen remove them from fishing lines. The pain of the puncture wound varies from mild with nonvenomous spines to severe with venomous spines such as the striped catfish (*Plotosus lineatus*). Bleeding and secondary infection are rare.

Stonefish typically cause injuries to the sole of the foot. The pain is usually very severe and out of proportion to the local trauma. Significant swelling and edema of the foot may extend up the lower leg. Systemic effects have been reported but are uncommon.

Most lionfish injuries, which are the most common venomous fish injury in the United States, usually occur in private aquariums when they are being cleaned. Stings cause severe local pain that may be associated with swelling and edema. Systemic effects are rare and minor.

Stingray injuries, which cause more trauma than venom-mediated effects, generally occur when people tread on them in shallow water, although they are occasionally picked up and rarely cause thoracoabdominal trauma to divers who are swimming too close to them. Laceration, local pain, and bleeding are the major effects. The wound may become necrotic and there is a risk of secondary infection, worse with larger wounds and those with foreign debris.

TREATMENT

Rx

The first aid for penetrating venomous marine injuries is washing the site and immersing it in hot water (45°C) for up to 90 minutes if this improves the pain. Unlike for jellyfish, there is limited evidence to support hot water for penetrating injuries, and the pain often recurs as soon as the hot water is removed. It is essential to test the temperature and not to immerse for more than 90 minutes so that superficial burns do not occur.

If the pain does not respond to hot water, a combination of ibuprofen (200 to 400 mg every 8 hours), acetaminophen (1 g every 4 to 6 hours), and oxycodone (5 to 10 mg every 4 hours) can be used. The pain rarely persists for more than 12 to 24 hours. Titrated intravenous opiates (Chapter 30) may be required, but local or regional local anesthetic infiltration is often more effective and can also assist with cleaning of the wound.

Careful wound management, which is key in all cases of penetrating marine injuries, includes cleaning and irrigating the wound. In some cases, radiographic images or ultrasound may be useful to evaluate or to exclude any retained foreign bodies. Most wounds do not require closure, and larger wounds will heal by secondary intention, although they may require surgical exploration and débridement. The use of prophylactic antibiotics remains unclear, with limited evidence supporting their use. Wounds that enter sterile body cavities (e.g., joints) require surgical exploration. Stingray injuries to the abdomen or chest should be managed as major thoracoabdominal trauma (Chapter 111).

Secondary infections that may uncommonly complicate penetrating marine injuries are usually *Vibrio* spp (Chapter 302) in the marine environment or *Aeromonas* spp (Chapter 359) in fresh water. Both are associated with significant morbidity and mortality if they are not treated early and aggressively. It is essential that all cases be observed closely in the first week. If there is any evidence of infection, wound swabs or aspirates for marine organisms should be sent and antibiotics (e.g., ciprofloxacin, 400 mg twice daily) should be commenced while awaiting culture and sensitivity test results. Surgical drainage may sometimes be required.

An antivenom is available for stonefish stings if the pain does not resolve with analgesia. Antivenom is given diluted by the intravenous route.

Sea Snake Envenomation

Sea snakes are found in the tropical parts of the Indian and Pacific oceans. They differ from eels because they have scales and do not have fins or gills. Sea snakes have small fangs similar to elapids, and their venom contains myotoxins and neurotoxins. Among the number of different species, the beaked sea snake (*Enhydrina schistosa*) is the most medically important.

Sea snake bites cause minimal pain, and the patient may not be aware of the bite. Systemic effects, which develop during hours, include nausea, vomiting, and headache as well as myotoxicity with myalgia of the face, neck, limbs, and trunk, sometimes with trismus. The CK level rapidly rises and usually is diagnostic. Rhabdomyolysis (Chapter 113) occurs in severe cases and may precipitate acute kidney injury. A rare sea snake bite may cause predominant neurotoxicity.

First aid is with a pressure bandage and immobilization. Polyvalent sea snake antivenom is manufactured in Australia (CSL Ltd, Melbourne). If it is available, one vial should be administered early. Intravenous fluids should be given, and renal function should be monitored.

Echinoderms

The two major echinoderms that cause human injury are sea urchins and the crown-of-thorns sea star. Sea urchins, which are worldwide in distribution, cause injuries when they are picked up or more commonly when they are stepped on. The spines, which range from chalky material to much stronger thorns, are usually nonvenomous. Crown-of-thorns sea stars are found in the Indo-Pacific region and cause injuries similar to those of sea urchins.

Local pain is rarely severe, and the major issue is the presence of retained spines, which are often multiple, are difficult to find, and may cause ongoing pain. The treatment of sea urchin injuries is similar to that of venomous fish stings, with hot-water immersion and local wound cleaning. However, removal of the spines can be a major problem because of the potential for multiple difficult-to-remove foreign bodies. Radiography and ultrasound may assist in locating spines. Any spines close to the surface should be removed, and the patient should be observed carefully until the symptoms resolve. If patients have ongoing pain from retained spines, surgical consultation is required.

Sponges

Tedania spp (fire sponges) and *Neofibularia* spp are among a number of medically important sponges that produce toxic secretions. Stinging sponge dermatitis, which is uncommon, results from contact with the sponge.[15]

The majority of sponge stings are minor with local pain, paresthesia, itchiness, and numbness. The symptoms develop during hours and may persist for several days. Symptoms are associated with local erythema and sometimes with vesicular reactions and stiffness. An unusual manifestation of fire sponge contact is delayed pain, swelling, and erythema at the contact site 2 to 3 weeks later, followed by desquamation.

The sting site should be washed as soon as possible. Most cases can be treated with analgesia (e.g., ibuprofen, 400 mg three times daily; see Table 30-3).

MARINE POISONING

Marine poisoning is uncommon except for ciguatera, which remains a major problem in many parts of the Pacific where fish are the main source of protein in the diet. Although marine poisoning is rare, the transport of fish by air has meant that marine poisoning can occur anywhere the fish are served. Most marine poisonings, including ciguatera, shellfish poisoning, and tetrodotoxin poisoning, result in neurotoxic effects.

Ciguatera

Ciguatera is endemic to parts of the Caribbean and Indo-Pacific, but it can occur anywhere fish are transported. Ciguatera poisoning affects about 60 individuals annually in the United States.[16] It results from toxins that are accumulated in tropical reef fish. A large number of fish have been implicated, including Spanish mackerel, bass, moray eels, some cod species, coral trout, and emperors (see online table at http://wikitoxin.toxicology.wikispaces.net/Ciguatera). A major issue is that it is not possible to determine if a particular serving of fish can cause ciguatera.

The clinical manifestations of ciguatera are mainly gastrointestinal in the Caribbean and a combination of gastrointestinal and neurologic in the Indo-Pacific region. The gastrointestinal effects, which include vomiting, diarrhea, and abdominal cramping, start within hours and may persist for up to 24 hours. The major neurologic effect is a sensory polyneuropathy (Chapter 420), which is delayed and develops within 24 hours. The almost pathognomonic feature of ciguatera is cold allodynia, which is often referred to as heat reversal but is in fact an unpleasant discomfort or sensation when touching cold objects. Other neurologic features are perioral and distal paresthesia and numbness. Patients may also develop myalgia, arthralgia, and pruritus (see online table at http://wikitoxin.toxicology.wikispaces.net/Ciguatera). The clinical diagnosis is based on the history of eating fish combined with the gastrointestinal or neurologic effects.

No antidote exists for ciguatera, and treatment is symptomatic relief and supportive care. Intravenous fluids should be given for dehydration, but there is no evidence for the use of mannitol.[A5] Nonsteroidal anti-inflammatory agents (ibuprofen, 200 to 800 mg three times daily) should be given for acute symptoms. Tricyclic antidepressants, gabapentin, and calcium antagonists have been suggested for chronic symptoms, but data on their efficacy are lacking.

Tetrodotoxin (Puffer Fish) Poisoning

Tetrodotoxin poisoning results from the ingestion of a number of types of bony fish, including puffer fish and toad fish; it is also known as fugu poisoning in Japan. Tetrodotoxin is a sodium-channel blocker that interrupts nerve conduction and results in paralysis (Chapter 420).

Tetrodotoxin poisoning causes a sensorimotor neuropathy and mild gastrointestinal symptoms with mainly nausea and occasional vomiting. The rate of onset of toxicity is more rapid with more severe poisoning, which usually develops within an hour. The major clinical effects are perioral numbness and paresthesia, ataxia due to weakness, distal to proximal muscle weakness, and respiratory muscle paralysis that can be fatal. A clinical grading system is available at http://wikitoxin.toxicology.wikispaces.net/Tetrodotoxin+Poisoning.

The treatment for tetrodotoxin poisoning is supportive care because no antidote exists. Prehospital management of the airway and breathing is required in severe cases. Patients may require mechanical ventilation for 2 to 5 days.

Shellfish Poisoning

Shellfish poisoning is rare and occurs sporadically when there are algal blooms in areas where shellfish are collected. Shellfish poisoning is divided into four types, three that are neurologic and one that is gastrointestinal. Paralytic shellfish poisoning, which is the most common shellfish poisoning, is clinically indistinguishable from tetrodotoxin poisoning because it is due to other sodium-channel blockers, including saxitoxin and gonyautoxins. It has a high fatality rate because of the respiratory paralysis. Treatment is the same as for tetrodotoxin poisoning. Neurotoxic shellfish poisoning is much rarer and is a neuroexcitatory syndrome that is similar to ciguatera. Treatment is supportive.

Encephalopathic shellfish poisoning has been reported only once in North America. It results from domoic acid, and there is no specific treatment. Diarrhea from shellfish poisoning causes a severe gastroenteritis, which is rapid in onset and can be severe with fluid loss and hypovolemic shock. Treatment is supportive with aggressive fluid therapy.

Scombroid

Scombroid, which is similar to an acute hypersensitivity reaction (Chapter 47), results from ingestion of fish that contain high concentrations of histamine.[17] The high histamine concentrations are due to spoilage when the fish are stored or transported after they are caught. The most commonly implicated fish are from the Scombridae family, including kingfish, mackerel, wahoo, and tuna.

The clinical manifestations, which are due to the histamine in the fish, may resemble an acute hypersensitivity reaction. Signs and symptoms develop within a few hours and continue for about 6 hours. They include diffuse erythema, flushing, itchiness, and urticaria with nausea, vomiting, abdominal pain, and diarrhea. More severe cases can be manifested with hypotension, wheezing, and bronchospasm. The clinical diagnosis is confirmed by measurement of histamine in the ingested fish.

Treatment is supportive with intravenous fluids for dehydration and hypotension. Both H_1- and H_2-receptor antagonists (e.g., diphenhydramine, 25 to 50 mg orally or intravenously; ranitidine, 150 mg orally or 50 mg intravenously) should be given as required. Epinephrine is rarely required.

Other Marine Invertebrates

The blue-ringed octopus in Australia has saliva that contains tetrodotoxin. Bites cause effects similar to tetrodotoxin poisoning. Cone snails are a rare cause of envenomation, and their stings cause minor pain, numbness, and sometimes partial or complete paralysis. In both cases, treatment is supportive but may require mechanical ventilation.

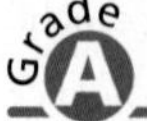

Grade A References

A1. de Silva HA, Pathmeswaran A, Ranasinha CD, et al. Low-dose adrenaline, promethazine, and hydrocortisone in the prevention of acute adverse reactions to antivenom following snakebite: a randomised, double-blind, placebo-controlled trial. *PLoS Med.* 2011;8:e1000435.

A2. Maduwage K, Isbister GK. Current treatment for venom-induced consumption coagulopathy resulting from snakebite. *PLoS Negl Trop Dis.* 2014;8:e3220.

A3. Isbister GK, Buckley NA, Page CB, et al. A randomized controlled trial of fresh frozen plasma for treating venom-induced consumption coagulopathy in cases of Australian snakebite (ASP-18). *J Thromb Haemost.* 2013;11:1310-1318.

A4. Loten C, Stokes B, Worsley D, et al. A randomised controlled trial of hot water (45°C) immersion versus ice packs for pain relief in bluebottle stings. *Med J Aust.* 2006;184:329-333.

A5. Schnorf H, Taurarii M, Cundy T. Ciguatera fish poisoning: a double-blind randomized trial of mannitol therapy. *Neurology.* 2002;58:873-880.

GENERAL REFERENCES

For the General References and other additional features, please visit Expert Consult at https://expertconsult.inkling.com.

113

RHABDOMYOLYSIS

FRANCIS G. O'CONNOR AND PATRICIA A. DEUSTER

DEFINITION

Rhabdomyolysis, an acute, potentially fatal clinical syndrome, reflects the dissolution and disintegration of striated muscle, with the release of muscle cell contents into the systemic circulation.[1] Myoglobinemia and myoglobinuria are common sequelae. Skeletal muscle destruction can cause systemic effects mediated by substances released from affected muscle cells (e.g., myoglobin, calcium, potassium). Prerenal azotemia, complicated by the toxicity of free myoglobin on the renal tubules, may lead to acute kidney injury (Chapter 120), which exacerbates other metabolic abnormalities. At the extreme, arrhythmias, caused by the release of intracellular potassium and organic acids, coupled with hypocalcemia may be fatal.

EPIDEMIOLOGY

In the absence of a widely accepted laboratory definition or of clinical diagnostic criteria, the true incidence of rhabdomyolysis is unclear, but about 26,000 hospitalized cases are seen each year in the United States. The U.S. military also reports about 400 annual cases of exertional rhabdomyolysis.[2] Among patients with rhabdomyolysis, anywhere from 13 to 67% may develop acute kidney injury, accounting for 5 to 10% of all cases of acute kidney failure in the United States.

ETIOLOGY

Rhabdomyolysis is a complex and multifactorial clinical disorder, with multiple potential inherited and acquired causes (Table 113-1). In urban adults, abuse of alcohol and other drugs, muscle compression, and status epilepticus are common causes of rhabdomyolysis. In pediatric patients, the most common cause is trauma, followed by nonketotic hyperosmolar coma, viral myositis, dystonia, and malignant hyperthermia. However, exertional rhabdomyolysis from repetitive exercise is also a concern in young athletes. Importantly, children and adolescents with recurrent rhabdomyolysis are increasingly being recognized as possibly having inherited metabolic disorders.

Drugs and Intoxications

Among intoxications, which are a common cause of rhabdomyolysis, the most frequent illegal drug-associated causes are cocaine and heroin (Chapter 34), with nearly 20% of cocaine overdoses complicated by rhabdomyolysis. Other recreational drugs, such as "bath salts" (of which methylenedioxypyrovalerone is the primary ingredient) and synthetic cannabinoids (or "spice"), have been associated with rhabdomyolysis.[3] Other substances that can induce rhabdomyolysis include ethanol (Chapter 33), amphetamines, phenylalkylamine derivatives, caffeine, and statins. Statins (Chapter 206) may result in myalgias in up to 10% of patients receiving treatment, but reported rates of statin-induced rhabdomyolysis range from 0 to 2.2 cases per 1000 person-years, with cerivastatin being associated with the highest rates.[4] Dietary supplements, in particular those with combinations of stimulants, have also been associated with rhabdomyolysis and other complications.

Exertional Rhabdomyolysis

Rhabdomyolysis can also be a consequence of excessive exertion,[5] prolonged heat exposure (Chapter 109), coexisting sickle cell trait (Chapter 163), and the use of dietary supplements (e.g., ephedra). In one series, 35 of 225,000 emergency department visits to an urban tertiary care center were for exertional rhabdomyolysis. The average creatine kinase (CK) level was 40,000 U/L, but no patient developed acute kidney injury. In another series, 57% of participants in an ultramarathon had evidence of myoglobinemia, but none progressed to acute kidney injury. Exertional rhabdomyolysis has also been diagnosed in other sports settings (e.g., baseball, football, track, wrestling), but none with a higher frequency than seen with endurance events.

In the military, acute exertional rhabdomyolysis occurs in 2 to 40% of individuals undergoing basic training, usually within the first 6 days. Resolution of myoglobinuria typically occurs after 2 or 3 days, with clinical improvement within 1 week. Consistent risk factors for exertional rhabdomyolysis are low levels of physical fitness and early introduction of repetitive exercises (e.g., squats, push-ups, sit-ups). Although most cases are self-limited, with no long-term evidence of kidney or muscle injury, patients who demonstrate systemic signs, generalized clinical findings, or acute kidney injury often have an underlying metabolic myopathy. Importantly, 25% of all heatstroke cases in the military between 1980 and 2000 were associated with rhabdomyolysis; acute kidney injury developed in 33%. A retrospective review of deaths in a military basic trainee population found an increased risk for nontraumatic, exertional sudden death in African Americans with sickle cell trait; several deaths were associated with fulminant exertional rhabdomyolysis.

The extreme exertion characteristics of military service carry over to the population of correctional inmates and civil servant first responders. Unsupervised repetitive exercise in prison populations can lead to exertional rhabdomyolysis. Among New York City firefighters, 32 of 16,506 candidates (0.2%) were hospitalized for exertional rhabdomyolysis after a physical fitness test, with four requiring hemodialysis. In a group of 50 prospective police officers from Massachusetts, 13 trainees were hospitalized with exertional rhabdomyolysis and had CK levels higher than 32,000 U/L; six required dialysis, and one died 44 days later as a result of complications of heatstroke, exertional rhabdomyolysis, and kidney and hepatic failure.

PATHOBIOLOGY

Pathophysiology

The final common pathway for all cases of rhabdomyolysis is from direct or indirect injury or destruction of muscle cells, with displacement of their intracellular contents into extracellular fluid, the circulation, or both (E-Fig. 113-1). Cell function is critically dependent on the relationship

TABLE 113-1 INHERITED AND ACQUIRED CAUSES OF RHABDOMYOLYSIS

INHERITED	ACQUIRED
Glycolytic/glycogenolytic, e.g., McArdle disease (myophosphorylase deficiency)	Exertion, e.g., exercise, status epilepticus, delirium, electrical shock, status asthmaticus, cardiopulmonary resuscitation (see also Table 113-2)
Fatty acid oxidation, e.g., carnitine palmitoyltransferase II deficiency	Crush, e.g., external weight, prolonged immobility, bariatric surgery
Krebs cycle, e.g., aconitase deficiency	Ischemia, e.g., arterial occlusion, compartment syndrome, sickle cell disease, disseminated intravascular coagulation
Pentose phosphate pathway, e.g., glucose-6-phosphate dehydrogenase deficiency	Extremes of body temperature, e.g., fever, exertional heatstroke, burns, malignant hyperthermia, hypothermia, lightning
Purine nucleotide cycle, e.g., myoadenylate deaminase deficiency	Metabolic, e.g., hypokalemia, hypernatremia or hyponatremia, hypophosphatemia, pancreatitis, diabetic ketoacidosis, renal tubular acidosis, hyperthyroidism or hypothyroidism, nonketotic hyperosmolar states
Mitochondrial respiratory chain, e.g., succinate dehydrogenase deficiency	Drugs or toxins, e.g., anticholinergics, amphetamines, antihistamines, arsenic, ethanol, opiates, statins, cocaine, succinylcholine, halothane, corticosteroids, cyclosporine, itraconazole, phenothiazines, bath salts, synthetic cannabinoids
Malignant hyperthermia susceptibility, e.g., familial malignant hyperthermia (*RYR1*) mutations, myotonic dystrophy, Duchenne and Becker dystrophies	Infections, e.g., Epstein-Barr virus, human immunodeficiency virus, herpes simplex, influenza A and B, *Borrelia burgdorferi*, tetanus
Other, e.g., familial recurrent myoglobinuria	Inflammatory and autoimmune disorders, e.g., polymyositis, dermatomyositis

Modified and reproduced with permission from Warren JD, Blumbergs PC, Thompson PD. Rhabdomyolysis: a review. *Muscle Nerve.* 2002;25:332-347.

between intracellular calcium (Ca^{2+}) and sodium (Na^+) concentrations. Sarcolemmal Na^+,K^+-ATPase regulates extracellular Ca^{2+} concentrations by exchanging Na^+ for Ca^{2+} across the sarcolemma. A low intracellular Na^+ concentration creates a gradient that actively results in efflux of Ca^{2+} as it is exchanged for Na^+ ions. This process maintains intracellular Ca^{2+} levels at several orders of magnitude lower than extracellular Ca^{2+}.

When the cell is subjected to mechanical stress, stretch-activated channels in the sarcolemma can open and cause an influx of Na^+ and Ca^{2+}. With excessive intracellular Ca^{2+}, several pathologic processes begin: persistent contraction of myofibers, depletion of adenosine triphosphate (ATP), production of free radicals, activation of vasoactive molecules, release of proteases, and, ultimately, cell death. Cell death is followed by an invasion of neutrophils, which amplify the damage by further release of proteases and increased production of free radicals. Rather than simple necrosis, a self-sustaining, inflammatory myolytic reaction develops.

Rhabdomyolysis can be further complicated by reperfusion injury and compartment syndrome. In reperfusion injury, restoration of vascular flow after a prolonged period of ischemia results in the delivery of activated neutrophils in combination with an abundance of oxygen, which contributes to the development of highly reactive free radicals. Because most muscle groups are contained within rigid fascial compartments, rhabdomyolysis can quickly precipitate a secondary acute compartment syndrome. The swelling associated with traumatized tissue can also increase intracompartmental pressure, which can provoke additional damage by compromising both venous and arterial blood flow. Thus, compartment syndrome can also result in rhabdomyolysis.

Inherited and Acquired Rhabdomyolysis

Rhabdomyolysis can be classified as inherited or acquired (see Table 113-1). Patients who have recurrent episodes of high levels of CK in the blood triggered by low levels of stress or exertion should be evaluated for a metabolic myopathy. A number of pathways leading to the formation of ATP can be disrupted by genetic defects (e.g., inherited disorders of glycogenolysis, glycolysis, and lipid and purine metabolism). In one series of 77 patients who underwent biopsy for idiopathic myoglobinuria, 47% were found to have enzymatic defects; the most common disorders were deficiencies of carnitine palmitoyltransferase II and myophosphorylase. Recent work suggests that carnitine palmitoyltransferase, acid maltase, and lipin deficiencies are common causes of rhabdomyolysis.

Inherited Rhabdomyolysis

Malignant hyperthermia (Chapters 432 and 434) is a potentially fatal, heterogeneous, pharmacogenetic disorder triggered by volatile anesthetics in predisposed individuals. The disorder is most commonly inherited in an autosomal dominant pattern. Evidence from molecular studies indicates that 25% of patients who are susceptible to malignant hyperthermia have mutations in the ryanodine receptor (*RYR1*) gene, which encodes the protein for one of the primary Ca^{2+} release channels involved in triggering muscle contraction. When a susceptible patient is exposed to a triggering anesthetic agent, excessive release of Ca^{2+} into the myoplasm leads to a hypermetabolic state manifested by hypercapnia, tachycardia, and metabolic acidosis. Although a genetic predisposition to malignant hyperthermia may be linked to a predisposition to exertional rhabdomyolysis and exercise-induced heat injury, this association has not been proved.

Acquired Rhabdomyolysis

Drugs and Toxins

Drugs and toxins, also common causes of rhabdomyolysis, operate through a number of mechanisms, including direct membrane toxicity (e.g., herbicides), indirect metabolic derangements (e.g., anticholinergics), ischemia (e.g., cocaine), and agitation (e.g., hemlock).[6] The most commonly cited drugs precipitating rhabdomyolysis are alcohol, statins, cocaine, amphetamines, and phenothiazines, although new designer drugs (spice, bath salts) are also implicated. Alcohol can induce rhabdomyolysis through a combination of mechanisms, including immobilization, direct myotoxicity, and electrolyte abnormalities. Statins, which inhibit 3-hydroxy-3-methylglutaryl-coenzyme A (HMG-CoA) reductase, can be directly myotoxic and appear to trigger sustained increases in intracellular Ca^{2+}. Although the precise mechanisms underlying statin-induced myopathy are currently incompletely understood, it can be aggravated by the concomitant administration of cytochrome P-450 3A4 inhibitors (e.g., itraconazole, erythromycin, cyclosporine, danazol) and fibrates as well as by physical exercise, excessive alcohol intake, and pre-existing comorbid medical conditions. Amphetamines and phenothiazines may lead to a clinical picture of rhabdomyolysis through the serotonin syndrome (Chapter 434) and the neuroleptic malignant syndrome (Chapter 418), respectively. The mechanism whereby bath salts lead to rhabdomyolysis may be direct muscle toxicity, severe hyperthermia, or electrolyte disorders.

Infections

Both viral and bacterial infections can trigger rhabdomyolysis. Either cellular invasion or generation of various toxins may precipitate infection-induced rhabdomyolysis. Influenza A and B (Chapter 364) are the most common viral causes, followed by human immunodeficiency virus (Chapter 386), coxsackievirus (Chapter 379), and Epstein-Barr virus (Chapter 377). The most common bacterial organisms that induce rhabdomyolysis are *Legionella* species (Chapter 314), followed by *Francisella tularensis* (Chapter 311) and *Streptococcus pneumoniae* (Chapter 289). Acute kidney injury develops in approximately 57% (33 to 100%) and 34% (0 to 100%) of bacterial and viral cases of rhabdomyolysis, respectively.

Trauma

Trauma is the most common cause of rhabdomyolysis. Wars, natural disasters, and traffic and occupational accidents are frequent causes of trauma-induced "crush injury syndrome" (Chapter 111). Other less frequent causes of trauma- or compression-induced rhabdomyolysis include struggling against restraints, direct blows, child abuse, torture, prolonged immobilization (e.g., anesthesia, coma, drug- or alcohol-induced stupor), and bariatric and other forms of surgery. The primary mechanism of crush syndrome and compression-induced rhabdomyolysis is reperfusion of damaged tissue after a period of ischemia.

Exertional rhabdomyolysis can result from excessive exercise in fit and unfit individuals, particularly eccentrically based activities (lengthening contractions, such as lowering a weight), but it can also be triggered by exertion in combination with thermal stress, sickle cell trait, or altitude or by the use of medications (e.g., anticholinergics) or dietary supplements (e.g., caffeine, ephedra). The spectrum of exertional rhabdomyolysis is broad and can range from a subclinical event to catastrophic collapse and death; underlying mechanisms may be either mechanical or metabolic in nature, but all are associated with elevated myoplasmic Ca^{2+} concentrations.

A number of underlying genetic polymorphisms and inherited disorders are associated with exertional rhabdomyolysis (Table 113-2).[7] Multiple mutations in the carnitine palmitoyltransferase II and myophosphorylase genes have been found, and although each mutation has been associated with exercise-induced myoglobinuria, the mutations alone may not explain the clinical episodes. Mutations and variants in the ryanodine receptor 1 (*RYR1*) gene, which are common in malignant hyperthermia (Chapter 432), have also been found in persons with exertional rhabdomyolysis. Other single-nucleotide polymorphisms associated with severe exertional rhabdomyolysis are found in the genes encoding CK muscle isoform (*CKMM* NcoI), α-actinin-3 (*ACTN3* R577X), or myosin light chain kinase (*MYLK* C37885A). However, data are insufficient to use these or other variants to predict an individual's clinical susceptibility to infection-, toxin-, exertion-, or drug-induced rhabdomyolysis.

TABLE 113-2 GENETIC MUTATIONS/VARIANTS ASSOCIATED WITH EXERTIONAL RHABDOMYOLYSIS

GENE	
Ryanodine receptor 1	*RyR1*
Myoadenylate deaminase	*AMPDA1*
Carnitine palmitoyltransferase II	*CPT2*
Myophosphorylase	*PYGM*
Phosphofructokinase	*PFKM*
Phosphorylase *b* kinase	*PHKA1*
Very long chain acyl–coenzyme A dehydrogenase	*ACAD9*
Phosphoglycerate mutase	*PGAMM*
Phosphoglycerate kinase	*PGK1*
Lactate dehydrogenase	*LDHA*
Cytochrome *c* oxidase	*COX I, II,* and *III*
Cytochrome *b* (complex III)	*CYTB*
Mitochondrial tRNA	*Mt-tRNA*
β-Sarcoglycan	*SGCB*
Mitochondrial DNA	*MT-CO2*

CLINICAL MANIFESTATIONS

The classic manifestations of rhabdomyolysis include acute myalgia and pigmenturia as a result of myoglobinuria in association with elevated serum muscle enzymes (CK in particular). Many clinical features are nonspecific, however, and the course and initial signs, symptoms, and laboratory abnormalities are clearly dependent on the underlying cause and severity of the event.

Rhabdomyolysis can be accompanied by both local and systemic features. Local features, generally noted in the area of the traumatized muscle groups, can occur within hours of the trauma and include muscle pain, tenderness, and swelling. Systemic features include tea-colored urine, chills, fever, and malaise. In extreme cases, patients complain of nausea and vomiting and demonstrate confusion, agitation, or delirium. Whenever systemic features such as chills, fever, malaise, or generalized muscle involvement are observed, an underlying metabolic myopathy should be considered.

Clinical findings may also include compartment syndrome, which can occur in muscle groups encased by fascia, especially the lower leg, forearm, and thigh muscle groups. Sensory abnormalities caused by nerve compression are an early manifestation of compartment syndrome; the loss of a pulse as a result of vascular compromise is a later finding. If compartment syndrome is not addressed within 6 to 8 hours, irreversible ischemic muscle and nerve damage may occur.

Laboratory findings are related to the degree of muscle involvement. Early findings include elevated blood levels of CK, myoglobin, potassium, urea, and phosphorus. CK levels typically peak 2 to 5 days after the initial insult; levels higher than 15,000 U/L are more likely to be associated with acute kidney injury than are lower levels.[8] Hypocalcemia, caused by the influx and deposition of Ca^{2+} in damaged muscle tissue, may accompany rhabdomyolysis. Moreover, an anion gap metabolic acidosis may develop because of the release of organic acids from damaged muscle. With resolution of rhabdomyolysis, sequestered Ca^{2+} may be released back into the circulation and cause hypercalcemia.

DIAGNOSIS

Creatine Kinase Levels

A diagnosis of rhabdomyolysis is made when there is clinical evidence of myonecrosis and release into the systemic circulation of muscle cell contents, including myoglobin, creatinine, CK, organic acids, potassium, aldolase, lactate dehydrogenase, and hydroxybutyrate dehydrogenase. The skeletal muscle subtype CK-MM is abundantly present in skeletal muscle and released as a result of muscle destruction. Serum levels exceeding 100,000 U/L are not uncommon with rhabdomyolysis. Because CK remains in the circulation longer than myoglobin and can be detected easily and efficiently, it is the most frequently used marker to diagnose rhabdomyolysis. No universally accepted clinical or laboratory definition of rhabdomyolysis currently exists, but CK elevations ranging from more than five times to more than 50 times the upper limits of normal, as well as varying requirements for serum creatinine elevation, have been proposed. Importantly, sex, ethnicity, and baseline physical activity levels all affect individual baseline CK levels. For example, African American males and young athletic men have the highest baseline CK levels, whereas non–African American women have the lowest. Thus, modifying factors such as sex, ethnicity, and physical fitness must be considered when CK is used for the diagnosis of rhabdomyolysis. In general, CK levels in excess of at least five times normal, in combination with the appropriate clinical presentation, are accepted as evidence of muscle breakdown, which may be consistent with a diagnosis of rhabdomyolysis.

Myoglobin Testing

Because myoglobinuria does not occur in the absence of rhabdomyolysis, myoglobin should be the most specific marker of rhabdomyolysis. However, testing for serum or urine myoglobin is problematic and not always consistent. Because myoglobin is normally bound to plasma globulins, only a small fraction of the myoglobin that is released into the circulation reaches the glomeruli. In the presence of severe muscle damage, blood levels of myoglobin overwhelm the binding capacity of the circulating proteins, so free myoglobin reaches the glomeruli and eventually the renal tubules. Elevations in serum myoglobin occur before the rise in serum CK, but the elimination kinetics of serum myoglobin is more rapid than that of CK, which makes the often evanescent rise in serum myoglobin a less reliable marker of muscle injury. Furthermore, the liver can quickly metabolize myoglobin.

Because most laboratories will perform urine myoglobin testing no more often than once per day, urine myoglobin is neither a timely nor accurate predictor of acute kidney injury.[9] Nevertheless, urine screening for rhabdomyolysis may be performed by dipstick. The orthotoluidine portion of urine dipsticks turns blue in the presence of hemoglobin or myoglobin, so if the urine sediment does not contain erythrocytes, one can assume, in the appropriate clinical setting, that a positive dipstick reading reflects the presence of myoglobin.

Other Laboratory Tests

Other associated laboratory findings in acute rhabdomyolysis can include hypocalcemia or hypercalcemia, hyperphosphatemia, metabolic (lactic) acidosis, thrombocytopenia, and disseminated intravascular coagulation. Muscle biopsy is not required to make a diagnosis of rhabdomyolysis, but it can be confirmatory, especially in cases of recurrent rhabdomyolysis or when the diagnosis is not clear. Histopathologic evaluation usually demonstrates muscle necrosis, loss of the cell nucleus, and muscle stria with the absence of inflammatory cells.

Differential Diagnosis

The clinical findings of acutely swollen muscles or muscle weakness (or both) with reddish brown urine are not always the result of rhabdomyolysis, and the examining clinician must be careful to scrutinize all information. The differential diagnosis includes disorders that may indirectly affect myocytes, such as Guillain-Barré syndrome and periodic paralysis. Guillain-Barré syndrome (Chapter 420) differs from rhabdomyolysis in that it is characterized as a fulminant polyneuropathy, usually after an antecedent viral infection. Periodic paralysis (Chapter 421) is frequently associated with transient electrolyte disturbances and is distinguished from rhabdomyolysis in that most cases follow periods of rest or sleep.

Myoglobinuria causes the urine to be reddish brown, but tea-colored (or cola-colored) urine does not necessarily indicate the presence of myoglobin. Other conditions associated with discoloration of urine include hemoglobinuria from hemolysis, intrinsic renal disease, porphyria, acute glomerulonephritis, "athletic pseudonephritis," and external factors such as ingestion of beets and various drugs (e.g., phenytoin, rifampin, riboflavin, or vitamin B_2).

The diagnosis of rhabdomyolysis is complete when the clinician determines the cause. This step, although it is frequently established during the history and physical examination, may require further diagnostic assessment after initiation of clinical treatment during the acute phase. Individuals with recurrent rhabdomyolysis, a positive family history of rhabdomyolysis or malignant hyperthermia, low exercise tolerance, no apparent cause, or a fulminant or explosive form of rhabdomyolysis appear to warrant further testing.

Testing may include a nonischemic forearm test, which involves isometric exercise at 70% of maximal voluntary contraction for 30 seconds under nonischemic conditions; electromyography; more in-depth blood tests for muscle enzymes (e.g., mitochondrial myopathies [Chapter 421], fatty acid transport defects [Chapter 421], glycogen storage diseases [Chapter 207], diseases associated with myoglobinuria); muscle biopsy to investigate specific metabolic myopathies and other enzyme or genetic defects; or any combination of such testing. The forearm exercise test may help identify metabolic and genetic causes of rhabdomyolysis. Patients who have had an episode of malignant hyperthermia or exertional heat illness may be candidates for a caffeine halothane contracture test, which evaluates the force produced by biopsied muscle samples after separate exposures to caffeine, halothane, and caffeine/halothane in the laboratory. Isolated, perfused muscle fibers must show an increase in tension of at least 0.2 g when exposed to 2 mM of caffeine or at least 0.7 g of tension after exposure to 3% halothane. In addition, genetic investigation for mutations of the *RYR1* receptor gene may be warranted.

PREVENTION

Approaches for preventing rhabdomyolysis induced by infections, medications, toxins, heat stress, or exercise may emerge in the future, but no definitive guidelines currently can be presented. To prevent further muscle injury, blood flow to ischemic areas must be promptly restored to minimize ischemia-reperfusion damage.

TREATMENT Rx

Treatment of rhabdomyolysis begins with a careful history and physical examination to identify and to manage any underlying illness. Vital signs, urine output, and serial electrolyte and CK levels should be obtained as soon as possible. Patients require aggressive early management to preserve renal function (Table 113-3). Careful observation and treatment of potential early and late complications are critical, and intensive care monitoring may be required.

TABLE 113-3 STEPS IN THE PREVENTION AND TREATMENT OF RHABDOMYOLYSIS-INDUCED ACUTE KIDNEY INJURY

Check for extracellular volume status, central venous pressure, and urine output.*
Measure serum creatine kinase levels. Measurement of other muscle enzymes (myoglobin, aldolase, lactate dehydrogenase, alanine aminotransferase, aspartate aminotransferase) adds little information relevant to diagnosis or management.
Measure levels of plasma and urine creatinine, potassium, and sodium; blood urea nitrogen; total and ionized calcium, magnesium, and phosphorus; and uric acid and albumin. Evaluate acid-base status, blood cell count, and coagulation.
Perform a urine dipstick test and examine the urine sediment.
Initiate volume repletion with normal saline promptly at a rate of approximately 400 mL/hr (200-1000 mL/hr, depending on the patient size, setting, and severity) and monitor the clinical course or central venous pressure.
Target urine output of approximately 3 mL/kg body weight/hr (200-300 mL/hr).
Check serum potassium levels frequently.
Correct hypocalcemia only if symptomatic (e.g., tetany, seizures) or severe hyperkalemia occurs.
Investigate the cause of rhabdomyolysis.
Consider treatment with bicarbonate. Check urine pH: if it is <6.5, alternate each liter of normal saline with 1 L 5% dextrose or 0.45% saline plus 100 mmol bicarbonate. Avoid potassium- and lactate-containing solutions.
Consider treatment with mannitol (up to 200 g/day; cumulative dose up to 800 g). Check for plasma osmolality and calculate the plasma osmolal gap (Chapter 120). Discontinue if diuresis (>20 mL/hr) is not established.
Maintain volume repletion until myoglobinuria is cleared (as evidenced by clear urine or urine dipstick test that is negative for blood).
Consider kidney replacement therapy with resistant hyperkalemia (>6.5 mmol/L) that is symptomatic (as assessed by electrocardiography), rapidly rising serum potassium levels, oliguria (<0.5 mL of urine/kg/hr for 12 hours), anuria, volume overload, or resistant metabolic acidosis (pH < 7.1).

*In the case of crush syndrome (e.g., earthquake, building collapse, bariatric surgery), institute aggressive volume repletion promptly before evacuating the patient if creatine kinase level is >15,000 U/L.
Modified from Bosch X, Poch E, Grau JM. Rhabdomyolysis and acute kidney injury. *N Engl J Med.* 2009;361:62-72.

Hydration

Hydration is the cornerstone of preserving kidney function in patients with rhabdomyolysis, and delay of fluid administration for more than 6 hours increases the risk for acute kidney injury. Inpatient hydration is indicated for victims of collapse, trauma, or exertional heat injury as well as for patients who have moderate early symptoms, more than mild elevations in CK, or abnormal serum levels of creatinine, potassium, calcium, phosphate, or bicarbonate. In adults, the target urine output is 300 mL/hr for at least 24 hours to prevent acute kidney injury. Hydration is accomplished by the aggressive administration of isotonic intravenous fluids at a rate that results in a urine output of 200 to 300 mL/hour until CK levels begin to decline. If fluid resuscitation fails to correct intractable hyperkalemia and acidosis, renal replacement therapy should be considered (Chapter 120). By comparison, adults with mild symptoms and serum CK levels less than 3000 U/L are considered to be at low risk and may be treated as outpatients with vigorous oral hydration, limited physical activity, and careful follow-up.

Specific Therapeutic Measures

Alkalinization of the urine decreases cast formation, minimizes the toxic effects of myoglobin on the renal tubules, inhibits lipid peroxidation, and decreases the risk for hyperkalemia. However, bicarbonate therapy can cause calcium to precipitate in the soft tissues and contribute to a hyperosmolar state. Mannitol is an osmotic diuretic, volume expander, and free radical scavenger, but it should be used only after adequate kidney function is established and must be used with great caution in patients with marginal cardiac function. To date, no convincing evidence demonstrates that adding sodium bicarbonate or mannitol is superior to fluid therapy alone.[8] Sodium bicarbonate should be used only in patients with evidence of systemic acidosis, and mannitol should be used only when it is needed to maintain a urine output of 300 mL/hour.

Deposition of calcium, which occurs early in rhabdomyolysis, is directly related to the degree of muscle destruction and to the administration of calcium. Furthermore, reversal of hypocalcemia early in the patient's course may worsen ectopic calcification and exacerbate hypercalcemia during the resolution phase.[10] Accordingly, hypocalcemia should be treated only when patients develop clinical symptoms, signs of tetany, or severe hyperkalemia.

Management of Compartment Syndrome

Compartment syndrome (Chapter 111) is a well-described late complication as well as a potential cause of rhabdomyolysis. Compartment syndrome can occur as a direct consequence of muscle injury associated with increased vascular permeability, aggressive fluid resuscitation, or restoration of reperfusion. Compartment syndrome should be suspected when the muscles are tense and swollen, previously declining CK levels start to rise, or neurovascular compromise occurs. In these cases, compartment pressures should be measured; if pressures exceed 30 mm Hg, prompt fasciotomy should be considered. However, because late fasciotomy (>12 hours after the onset of symptoms) can convert a closed injury into an open wound and thereby increase the risk of uncontrollable infection, late fasciotomy is relatively contraindicated.

Management of Crush Injury

For victims of crush injury (Chapter 111), aggressive on-site hydration with intravenous normal saline is recommended. For massive damage, amputation of the extremity may be required to protect the patient's overall health. The Mangled Extremity Severity Score can identify nonsalvageable extremities on the basis of the degree of skeletal and soft tissue injury, the patient's blood pressure, the presence of a detectable pulse, and age (see http://www.mdcalc.com/mangled-extremity-severity-score-mess-score/).

Malignant Hyperthermia

Rhabdomyolysis caused by malignant hyperthermia (Chapter 432) requires rapid diagnosis and aggressive management. Anesthetics should be discontinued, and the patient should be treated with dantrolene sodium, 2.5 to 4 mg/kg intravenously, followed by about 1 mg/kg every 4 hours for up to 48 hours to avoid recrudescence.

PROGNOSIS

The most serious consequence of rhabdomyolysis is acute kidney injury, which occurs in up to 67% of all cases, regardless of cause. Predictors of the risk of needing renal replacement therapy or death in patients with rhabdomyolysis include age older than 50 years; initial serum creatinine level of 1.4 mg/dL or higher; initial serum calcium level below 7.5 mg/dL; initial serum phosphate level above 4.0 mg/dL; initial serum bicarbonate level below 19 mEq/L; and a cause other than syncope, seizures, exercise, statins, or myositis.[11] Event rates range from 0% in patients with none of these criteria to 20% or more in patients with four or more criteria. For compartment syndrome, a poor prognosis is associated with an ischemic period lasting longer than 6 hours.

The prognosis of patients with rhabdomyolysis improves markedly when treatment is started soon after the diagnosis is made. With mild episodes, the prognosis is customarily excellent, and the patient can typically resume usual activities within several weeks after CK levels have normalized. However, some patients do not return to normal and continue to experience extreme fatigue and muscle pain on exertion. These patients require additional testing (nonischemic forearm test, electromyography, muscle disease enzyme panel, muscle biopsy; Chapter 421) to determine whether an underlying metabolic myopathy exists. The results of these tests will help determine future recommendations, but the patient's tolerance and response to light and more strenuous exercise are important factors. Most authorities agree that statin-induced rhabdomyolysis is an indication for discontinuation of their use.

GENERAL REFERENCES

For the General References and other additional features, please visit Expert Consult at https://expertconsult.inkling.com.

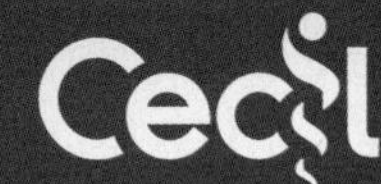

XI RENAL AND GENITOURINARY DISEASES

114

APPROACH TO THE PATIENT WITH RENAL DISEASE

DONALD W. LANDRY AND HASAN BAZARI

The prominent functions of the kidney include the excretion of nitrogenous waste; the regulated excretion of water, sodium, potassium, and acid; and the synthesis of a variety of hormones, including 1,25-dihydroxyvitamin D, erythropoietin, and renin. The kidney's elaboration of a protein-free and cell-free ultrafiltrate is uniquely responsible for the excretion of nitrogenous wastes. The approach to the patient with renal disease is largely focused on disordered ultrafiltration and not on defects in the isolated renal tubular processing of individual ions, water, or acids. A patient may, for example, present with an isolated defect in renal acid excretion (Chapter 118), but in this case the "approach to the patient" is framed for the evaluation of metabolic acidosis, an abnormality for which the kidney is only one among the many causes in a broad differential diagnosis. In contrast, acute kidney injury (Chapter 120) and chronic kidney disease (Chapter 130) refer specifically and exclusively to defects in the filtration function of the kidney. In the context of a diminished magnitude of filtration, many of the other individual functions of the kidney (e.g., hormone synthesis, electrolyte homeostasis) may fail as well.

Primary diseases of the tubules, such as acute tubular necrosis (Chapter 120) and tubulointerstitial disease (Chapter 122), also impair the rate of glomerular filtration and cause acute kidney injury and chronic kidney disease. In contrast, an impairment in ultrafiltration may, in early chronic kidney disease, be reflected solely in a decreased *quality* of glomerular filtration (e.g., the presence of albuminuria) rather than in a decreased *quantity* of filtrate with increased concentrations of nitrogenous waste. Similarly, the glomerular filtration rate (GFR) may be normal in nephrotic syndrome despite ultrafiltration defects that result in massive proteinuria. Defects in the filter can also allow passage of cells, such as red blood cells (RBCs), as is seen in the acute nephritic syndrome (Chapter 121), with or without heavy proteinuria. The paradox of glomerular hematuria without albuminuria is also possible. For example, in mild forms of immunoglobulin A (IgA) nephropathy (Chapter 121), relatively few defects in the glomerular filter will permit a detectable number of RBCs per high-power field in the urine despite a urine albumin level that still remains within normal limits (Fig. 114-1).

In this context, this chapter considers the approach to the patient with acute kidney injury, glomerular syndromes (nephrotic vs. nephritic), tubulointerstitial disease, vasculitis and vascular diseases of the kidney, papillary necrosis, and chronic kidney disease.

PATHOBIOLOGY

The approximately 2 million renal glomeruli normally filter about 180 L/day. The renal glomerulus is not simply a filter but rather a size- and charge-dependent ultrafilter that excludes not only cells but also proteins larger than 60 kD from the ultrafiltrate. Smaller proteins are variably filtered at the glomerulus and endocytosed in the proximal tubule so that the protein concentration of the urine is normally low. Kidney disease reflects a failure in the quantity or quality of the glomerular ultrafiltrate.

The normal GFR may decline in hours to days in acute kidney injury or during months to years in chronic kidney disease. An acute decline in glomerular filtration is the necessary and sufficient condition for the diagnosis of acute kidney injury, but abnormal urinary findings can assist with elucidating the etiology of the injury. Proteinuria, ranging from microscopic to nephrotic range (Chapter 121), and urinary findings, from a few cells per microscopic high-power field to gross hematuria or pyuria, may be the only evidence of the earliest stages of chronic kidney disease. As chronic kidney disease advances, the decline in the GFR progresses until dialysis or transplantation (Chapter 131) is required to forestall or to treat the syndrome of uremia.

DIAGNOSIS

Measuring Kidney Function

Although the most accurate method of evaluating kidney function is a formal measurement of GFR with iothalamate, iohexol, or similar markers, these tests are too expensive and time-consuming to be recommended for routine clinical practice. Currently, the most common methods used to estimate GFR are the serum creatinine concentration, the calculated creatinine clearance, and estimation equations based on serum creatinine.[1]

Serum creatinine is, to a first approximation, neither secreted nor reabsorbed, so the amount appearing in the urine per unit time is a measure of the amount that was filtered at the glomerulus during that period. As a result, the rate of creatinine clearance is a reasonably close estimate of the GFR. A decrement in the GFR diminishes creatinine clearance but has no immediate effect on creatinine production by muscle; as a result, the serum creatinine concentration rises. The change in serum creatinine over time indicates the tempo of the renal disease and can distinguish acute injury from chronic kidney disease. Problems with the routine use of serum creatinine alone to infer GFR stem from the differing rates of creatinine production among individuals, mainly because of variations in muscle mass. Women and the elderly can have deceptively low serum creatinine levels despite significant declines in GFR.[2] In addition, the shape of the curve relating the GFR to serum creatinine (Fig. 114-2) has an important and potentially easily overlooked clinical implication, namely, that an initial small absolute rise in creatinine usually reflects a marked fall in GFR.

Creatinine clearance can be calculated with a 24-hour urine collection to measure the creatinine concentration. The patient must be instructed to discard the first morning urine before initiating the collection and to conclude the collection by including the next morning void. The formula for calculating creatinine clearance is as follows:

$$CCr = (\text{urine Cr} \times V)/(\text{plasma Cr})$$

where *CCr* is creatinine clearance, *urine Cr* is urine creatinine concentration, *V* is urine flow rate, and *plasma Cr* is plasma creatinine. The creatinine clearance overestimates GFR by about 10% owing to tubular secretion of creatinine. Calculation of creatinine clearance from a 24-hour urine collection can be cumbersome for patients and is prone to error because of inaccurate urine collection.

Because of the logistical and practical limitations of a 24-hour urine collection, several equations have been developed to estimate GFR on the basis of easily obtainable clinical data and laboratory results. To date, the most widely used equations are the Cockcroft-Gault, the Modification of Diet in Renal Disease (MDRD) Study, and the Chronic Kidney Disease Epidemiology Collaboration (CKD-EPI) equations (Table 114-1). Weight estimations or ideal weight estimations can make calculation and reporting of Cockcroft-Gault results problematic. The MDRD equations (both the full and abbreviated forms) use data that are readily available to laboratories, but the equations systematically underestimate GFR at higher serum creatinine values, thereby raising concern for false diagnoses of chronic kidney disease. The CKD-EPI equation appears to be more precise and accurate than the MDRD equation, especially at higher GFRs.[3] Cystatin C may provide a more accurate and prognostic measurement of GFR in patients whose creatinine levels are in the upper end of the normal range, but it does not replace estimated GFR measurements for most clinical purposes.[4,5]

Urinalysis

The normal color of the urine is derived from urochromes, which are pigments excreted in the urine. Abnormal color or appearance of the urine may be explained by many conditions (Table 114-2). The basic analysis of the urine sample involves measurements with commercially available dipsticks or microscopic analyses.

Urine Dipstick

The *specific gravity* of the urine generally is related linearly with osmolality. However, it can be raised by the presence of molecules with relatively high molecular weight, such as glucose or contrast dye. A fixed specific gravity of 1.010, so-called isosthenuria, is characteristic of chronic kidney disease (Chapter 130).

Urine pH typically is 5 as a result of daily net acid excretion. An alkaline pH often is noted after meals, when an "alkaline tide" to balance gastric acid excretion increases urine pH. A high urine pH also is seen in patients who are on a vegetarian diet. An exceptionally high urine pH is indicative of an infection with a urea-splitting organism, such as *Proteus* species (Chapter 284). An inappropriately high urine pH in the setting of systemic non–anion gap metabolic acidosis may be seen in certain forms of renal tubular acidosis (Chapter 118). In a proximal renal tubular acidosis, the urine pH is high until the tubular reabsorption threshold for bicarbonate, which is abnormally low,

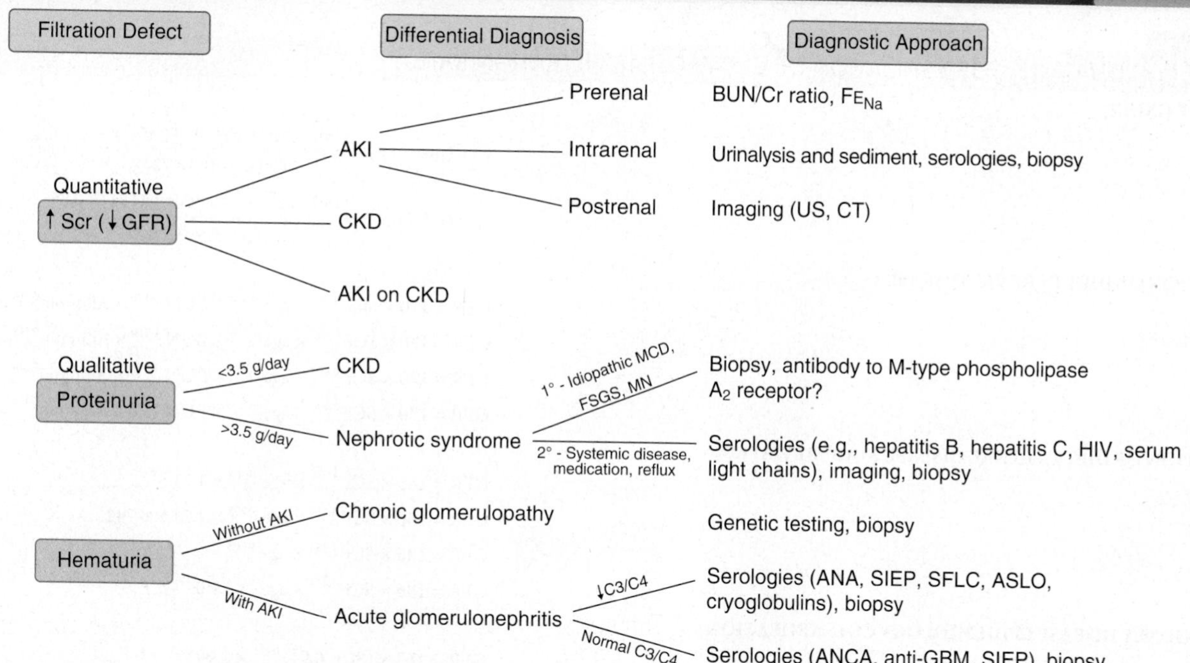

FIGURE 114-1. **Overview of approach to kidney disease. Quantitative defects in filtration, manifested by elevated serum creatinine (Scr) and reduced glomerular filtration rate (GFR), should lead to a query into acute kidney injury (AKI) versus chronic kidney disease (CKD). AKI, in turn, is generally divided into prerenal, postrenal, and intrinsic causes. Qualitative defects in filtration, manifested by proteinuria or hematuria, can occur in the absence of changes in GFR and often require biopsy for diagnosis. Proteinuria of more than 3.5 g/day signals nephrotic syndrome, which may be idiopathic or secondary to systemic diseases, such as hepatitis B or C, human immunodeficiency virus (HIV) infection, or diabetes. Glomerular hematuria without AKI is consistent with a chronic glomerulopathy, such as IgA nephropathy, or familial diseases, such as thin basement membranes disease. When hematuria accompanies AKI, acute glomerulonephritis should be suspected and can diagnostically be divided into low-complement glomerulonephritides (immune complex–mediated lesions such as lupus nephritis, postinfectious glomerulonephritis, and cryoglobulinemic glomerulonephritis) and normocomplementemic glomerulonephritides (classically seen in the rapidly progressive glomerulonephropathies due to antineutrophil cytoplasmic antibody [ANCA] and anti–glomerular basement membrane [anti-GBM] antibody). ANA = antinuclear antibody; ASLO = antistreptolysin O; BUN = blood urea nitrogen; Cr = creatinine; CT = computed tomography; MCD = minimal change disease; FE_{Na} = fractional excretion of sodium; FSGS = focal segmental glomerulosclerosis; MN = membranous nephropathy; SFLC = serum free light chain; SIEP = serum immunoelectrophoresis; US, ultrasonography.**

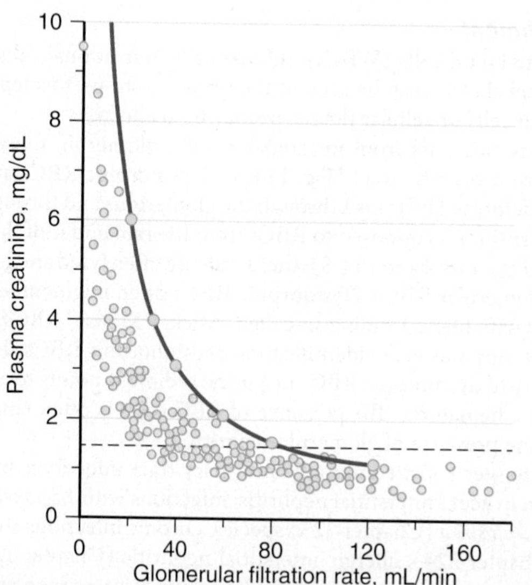

FIGURE 114-2. **Relationship between plasma creatinine and glomerular filtration rate measured by inulin clearance in 171 patients (*circles*). The *continuous line* reflects the idealized relationship between these parameters if creatinine were excreted solely by glomerular filtration; the *dashed line* represents an upper limit of "normal" for the creatinine concentration of 1.4 mg/dL. (Redrawn from Shemesh O, Golbetz H, Kriss JP, et al. Limitations of creatinine as a filtration marker in glomerulopathic patients. *Kidney Int.* 1985;28:830-838.)**

is reached. At this point, the urine pH decreases to 5. In distal renal tubular acidosis, the inability to create a sufficient gradient for hydrogen ions results in a urine pH that is always higher than 5.5. In type 4 renal tubular acidosis, the urine pH is often 5, and the urine net charge is often positive, thereby confirming the absence of significant amounts of ammonium in the urine; this defect is exacerbated by the accompanying hyperkalemia.

Glucose in the urine is detected by an assay using dipsticks impregnated with the enzyme glucose oxidase. Glycosuria is seen in diabetes mellitus (Chapter 229), when pregnancy causes the tubular threshold for glucose reabsorption to change, and in tubular diseases that affect the proximal convoluted tubule and cause tubular glycosuria. Evidence for pan–proximal tubular dysfunction (e.g., glycosuria, aminoaciduria, phosphaturia) indicates that Fanconi syndrome is present.

The dipstick for *protein* is a sensitive assay based on color change induced by the presence of proteins at a given pH. It is most sensitive to the presence of albumin and is much less sensitive to other proteins, such as the light chains of Bence Jones protein (Chapter 187). The presence of 1+ protein correlates with about 30 mg/dL of albuminuria, and 3+ protein correlates with more than 500 mg/dL of proteinuria. Because the dipstick is not a quantitative measurement, small amounts of proteinuria in an oliguric patient may give the false appearance of high-grade proteinuria. The excretion of abnormal quantities of albumin below the level detectable by the urine dipstick is called *microalbuminuria*. Normal albumin excretion, which is less than 30 mg/day, is best detected by radioimmunoassay or enzyme immunoassay. Microalbuminuria is the earliest clinically detectable stage of diabetic nephropathy (Chapter 124). Proteinuria of increasing severity is associated with a more rapid decline in the GFR, regardless of the GFR,[6] except in minimal change disease (Chapter 121).

The dipstick for *heme* uses the peroxidase-like activity of hemoglobin and myoglobin molecules to detect the presence of heme pigment. The reaction occurs on exposure to hemoglobin, myoglobin, or intact RBCs. The presence of myoglobin, which is found in patients with rhabdomyolysis (Chapter 113), or free hemoglobin, which is seen in patients with intravascular hemolytic anemias (Chapter 160), is suspected if the heme reaction is intensely positive and there is a paucity of cellular elements in the sediment. Persistent, isolated, asymptomatic, microscopic hematuria in adolescents and young adults is associated with a nearly 20-fold increased risk of subsequent end-stage renal disease.[7]

The dipstick detection of *leukocytes* depends on the presence of leukocyte esterase. Leukocyte esterase is usually present in infections (Chapter 284) and in inflammatory conditions.

TABLE 114-1 EQUATIONS FOR ESTIMATION OF GLOMERULAR FILTRATION RATE

COCKCROFT-GAULT	
Male	$CCr\,(mL/min) = \frac{(140 - age) \times lean\ body\ wt\,(kg)}{SCr\,(mg/dL) \times 72}$
Female	$CCr\,(mL/min) = \frac{(140 - age) \times lean\ body\ wt\,(kg) \times 0.85}{SCr\,(mg/dL) \times 72}$
MODIFICATION OF DIET IN RENAL DISEASE 1	
Black male	$GFR = 170 \times SCr^{-0.999} \times age^{-0.176} \times BUN^{-0.170} \times Albumin^{0.318} \times 1.18$
Black female	$GFR = 170 \times SCr^{-0.999} \times age^{-0.176} \times BUN^{-0.170} \times Albumin^{0.318} \times 1.18 \times 0.762$
White male	$GFR = 170 \times SCr^{-0.999} \times age^{-0.176} \times BUN^{-0.170} \times Albumin^{0.318}$
White female	$GFR = 170 \times SCr^{-0.999} \times age^{-0.176} \times BUN^{-0.170} \times Albumin^{0.318} \times 0.762$
MODIFICATION OF DIET IN RENAL DISEASE 2 (ABBREVIATED)	
Black male	$GFR = 186 \times SCr^{-1.154} \times age^{-0.203} \times 1.21$
Black female	$GFR = 186 \times SCr^{-1.154} \times age^{-0.203} \times 1.21 \times 0.742$
White male	$GFR = 186 \times SCr^{-1.154} \times age^{-0.203}$
White female	$GFR = 186 \times SCr^{-1.154} \times age^{-0.203} \times 0.742$
CHRONIC KIDNEY DISEASE EPIDEMIOLOGY COLLABORATION	
Black male, SCr ≤0.9 mg/dL	$GFR = 163 \times (SCr/0.9)^{-0.411} \times 0.993^{age}$
Black male, SCr >0.9 mg/dL	$GFR = 163 \times (SCr/0.9)^{-1.209} \times 0.993^{age}$
Black female, SCr ≤0.7 mg/dL	$GFR = 166 \times (SCr/0.7)^{-0.329} \times 0.993^{age}$
Black female, SCr >0.7 mg/dL	$GFR = 166 \times (SCr/0.7)^{-1.209} \times 0.993^{age}$
White male, SCr ≤0.9 mg/dL	$GFR = 141 \times (SCr/0.9)^{-0.411} \times 0.993^{age}$
White male, SCr >0.9 mg/dL	$GFR = 141 \times (SCr/0.9)^{-1.209} \times 0.993^{age}$
White female, SCr ≤0.7 mg/dL	$GFR = 144 \times (SCr/0.7)^{-0.329} \times 0.993^{age}$
White female, SCr >0.7 mg/dL	$GFR = 144 \times (SCr/0.7)^{-1.209} \times 0.993^{age}$

BUN = blood urea nitrogen; GFR = glomerular filtration rate; SCr = serum creatinine.

TABLE 114-2 MACROSCOPIC APPEARANCE OF URINE

APPEARANCE	CAUSE
Milky	Acid urine: urate crystals Alkaline urine: insoluble phosphates Infection: pus Spermatozoa Chyluria
Smoky pink	Hematuria (>0.54 mL blood/L urine)
Foamy	Proteinuria
Blue or green	*Pseudomonas* urinary tract infection Bilirubin Methylene blue
Pink or red	Aniline dyes in sweets Porphyrins (on standing) Blood, hemoglobin, myoglobin Drugs: phenindione, phenolphthalein Anthocyaninuria (beetroot, "beeturia")
Orange	Drugs: anthraquinones (laxatives), rifampicin Urobilinogenuria
Yellow	Mepacrine Conjugated bilirubin Phenacetin Riboflavin
Brown or black	Melanin (on standing) Myoglobin (on standing) Alkaptonuria
Green or black	Phenol Lysol
Brown	Drugs: phenazopyridine, furazolidone, L-dopa, niridazole Hemoglobin and myoglobin (on standing) Bilirubin

From Forbes CD, Jackson WF. *Color Atlas and Text of Clinical Medicine*. 3rd ed. London: Mosby; 2003.

Urine Sediment

RBCs, white blood cells (WBCs), tubular cells, transitional cells, and squamous epithelial cells may be seen in the urine. Casts are formed in tubules, may contain cells or cellular debris, or may be acellular.

RBCs may originate from intrarenal vessels, glomeruli, tubules, or anywhere in the urogenital tract (Fig. 114-3). Dysmorphic RBCs are cells that have been deformed by transit through the glomerulus and through the medullary interstitium, as opposed to RBCs from the remainder of the genitourinary tract (Figs. 114-4 and 114-5); these cells are often lysed and less refractile than nonglomerular RBCs. Dysmorphic RBCs often fragment with poikilocytosis and with blebs, forming so-called "Mickey Mouse" RBCs. Phase contrast microscopy aids in the identification of dysmorphic RBCs. The presence of a majority of dysmorphic RBCs in a urine sediment points to a glomerular origin of the hematuria. The presence of RBC casts is often conclusive evidence for the presence of glomerulonephritis.

WBCs are seen most commonly in urinary tract infections, but they also can be seen in acute interstitial nephritis, infections with *Legionella* (Chapter 314) and *Leptospira* (Chapter 323) species, chronic infections such as tuberculosis (Chapter 324), allergic interstitial nephritis (Chapter 122), atheroembolic diseases (Chapter 125), granulomatous diseases such as sarcoidosis (Chapter 95), IgG4-related interstitial nephritis, and tubulointerstitial nephritis and uveitis syndrome. Mononuclear cells often appear with transplant rejection. Tubular cells, which are seen in many conditions involving tubulointerstitial diseases, also are seen in ischemic and nephrotoxic injury, such as with myeloma kidney (Chapter 187) or cast nephropathy. Eosinophils require special stains, with the Giemsa stain being much less sensitive than the Hansel stain (Chapter 122). Urine eosinophils classically are seen in allergic interstitial nephritis (Chapter 122), but they also are seen in atheroembolic disease (Chapter 125), prostatitis (Chapter 129), and vasculitis.

Casts, which are formed in tubules, are characterized by the arrangement of the cells in a clearly formed matrix composed of Tamm-Horsfall protein. Because casts are formed in the renal parenchyma, they may give a clue to the origin of accompanying cellular elements.

Hyaline casts are composed of Tamm-Horsfall proteins that are formed normally and are seen in increased numbers after exercise (Fig. 114-6).

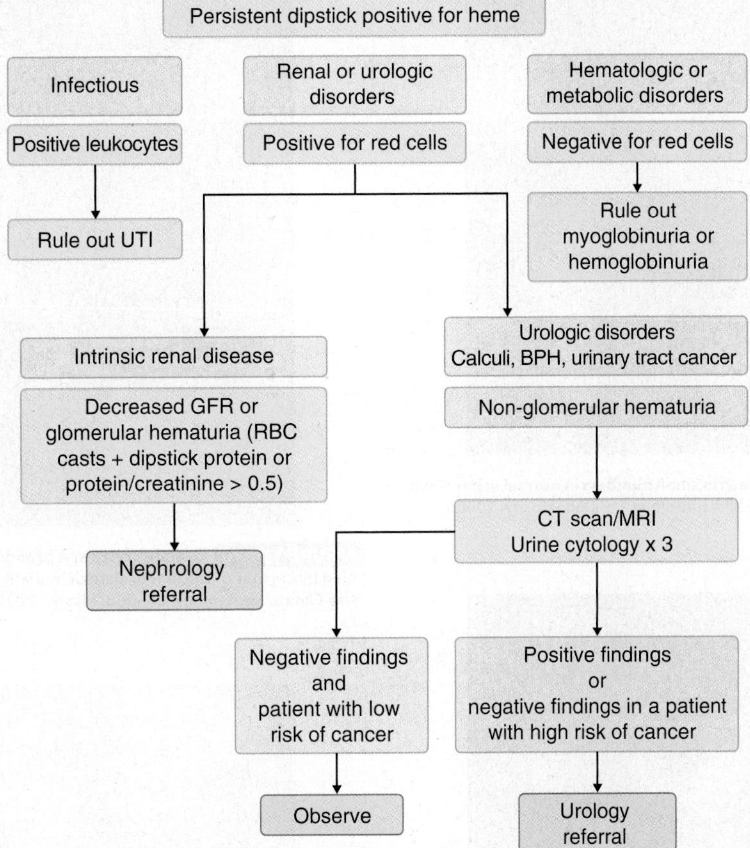

FIGURE 114-3. **Algorithm for the evaluation of asymptomatic hematuria.** BPH = benign prostatic hyperplasia; CT = computed tomography; GFR = glomerular filtration rate; MRI = magnetic resonance imaging; RBC = red blood cell; UTI = urinary tract infection. (Courtesy Ali Gharavi, MD. Modified from Cohen RA, Brown RS. Microscopic hematuria. *N Engl J Med.* 2003;348:2330-2338).

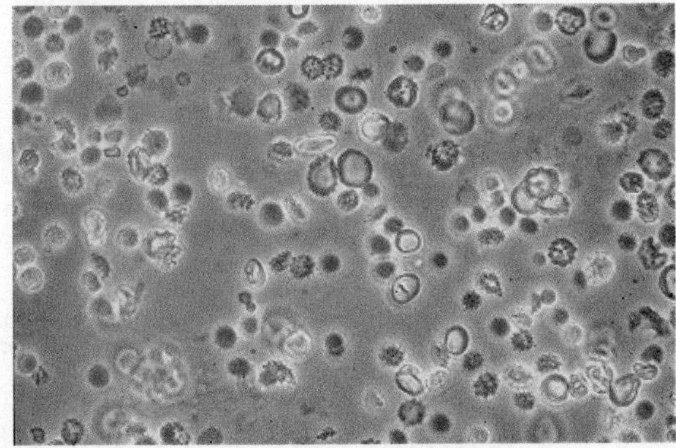

FIGURE 114-4. **Dysmorphic erythrocytes.** These dysmorphic erythrocytes vary in size, shape, and hemoglobin content and reflect glomerular bleeding. (From Johnson RJ, Feehally J. *Comprehensive Clinical Nephrology*. London: Mosby; 2000.)

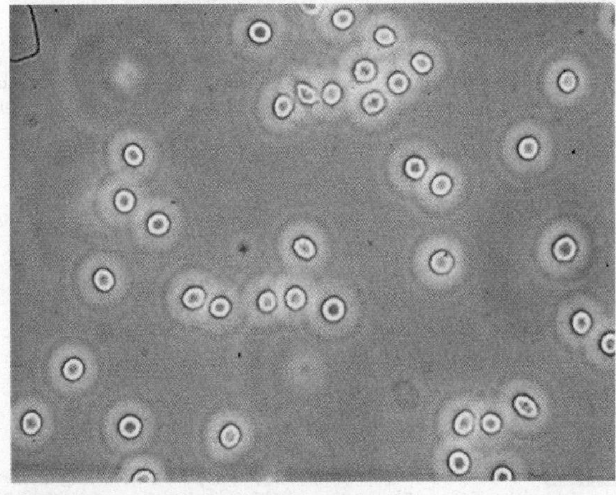

FIGURE 114-5. **Isomorphic erythrocytes.** These erythrocytes are similar in size, shape, and hemoglobin content. Isomorphic cells reflect nonglomerular bleeding from lesions such as calculi and papillomas or hemorrhage from cysts in polycystic renal disease. (From Johnson RJ, Feehally J. *Comprehensive Clinical Nephrology*. London: Mosby; 2000.)

Granular casts are degenerated tubular cell casts that are seen in the setting of tubular injury (Fig. 114-7). *Pigmented granular casts* are seen in rhabdomyolysis (Chapter 113) with myoglobinuria or, rarely, hemoglobinuria. *RBC casts* (Fig. 114-8) are rarely seen in allergic interstitial nephritis and diabetic nephropathy, but they are frequently seen in acute glomerulonephritis (Chapter 121). The presence of RBC casts in a patient with microscopic hematuria can narrow the focus of the evaluation to a glomerular lesion. *WBC casts* are seen commonly in pyelonephritis (Chapter 284) and in acute and chronic nonbacterial infections. They also are seen in other conditions in which WBCs are associated with parenchymal renal processes, such as allergic interstitial nephritis (Chapter 122), atheroembolic diseases (Chapter 125), and granulomatous diseases such as sarcoidosis (Chapter 95). Rarely, WBC casts can be a dominant feature of many diseases that traditionally are thought of as glomerular diseases, such as lupus nephritis (Chapter 266) and antineutrophil cytoplasmic antibody (ANCA)–associated glomerulonephritis (Chapter 270). *Tubular cell casts* are seen with any acute tubular injury and are the dominant cellular casts in ischemic acute tubular necrosis (Chapter 120). They also can be seen with nephrotoxic injury, such as with aminoglycosides and cisplatin. Some casts may contain both leukocytes and tubular cells.

Crystals can be a normal finding in the urine or serve as clues to pathophysiologic processes. Certain crystals, such as the hexagonal crystals seen with cystinuria (Chapter 128), are always abnormal (Fig. 114-9). Others, such as the octahedral calcium oxalate crystals (Fig. 114-10), may be a normal finding or may be evidence for ethylene glycol intoxication (Chapter 110). Triple phosphate crystals, which are composed of ammonium magnesium phosphate and are coffin shaped (Fig. 114-11), are seen in urinary tract infections with urea-splitting organisms (Chapter 284). Uric acid crystals,

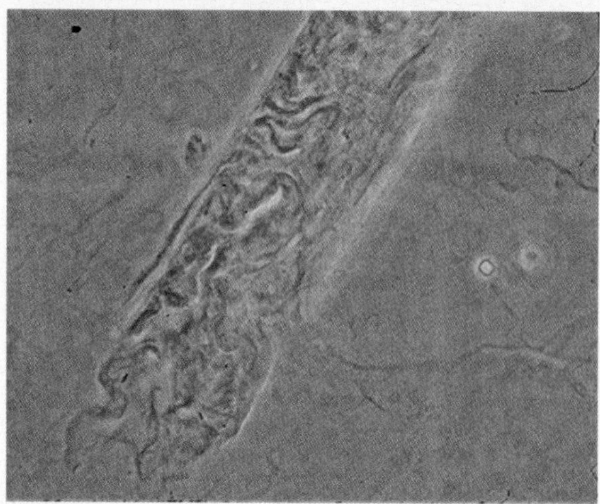

FIGURE 114-6. Hyaline cast of the type seen in small numbers in normal urine. (From Johnson RJ, Feehally J. *Comprehensive Clinical Nephrology*. London: Mosby; 2000.)

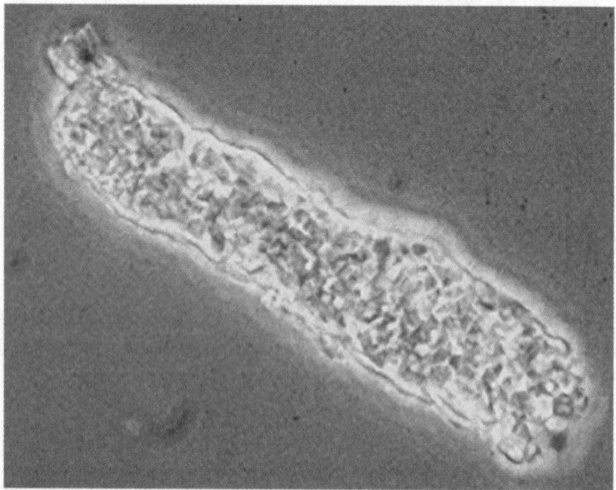

FIGURE 114-7. Number and type of granules and their density in the cast vary in different casts. The presence of erythrocytes in this cast may mean that the granules are derived partly from disrupted erythrocytes. (From Johnson RJ, Feehally J. *Comprehensive Clinical Nephrology*. London: Mosby; 2000.)

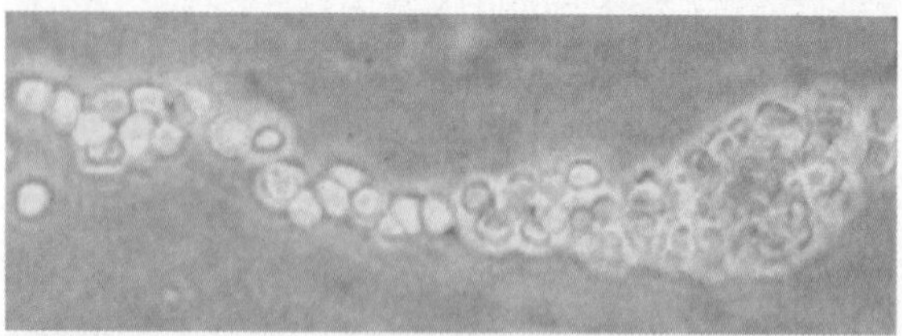

FIGURE 114-8. A cast composed entirely of erythrocytes reflects heavy hematuria and active glomerular disease. Crescentic nephritis is likely to be present if erythrocyte cast density is greater than 100/mL. (From Johnson RJ, Feehally J. *Comprehensive Clinical Nephrology*. London: Mosby; 2000.)

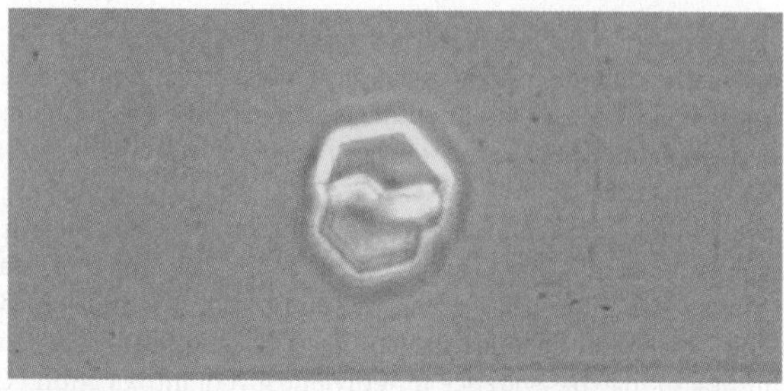

FIGURE 114-9. Typical hexagonal cystine crystal. A single crystal provides a definitive diagnosis of cystinuria. (From Johnson RJ, Feehally J. *Comprehensive Clinical Nephrology*. London: Mosby; 2000.)

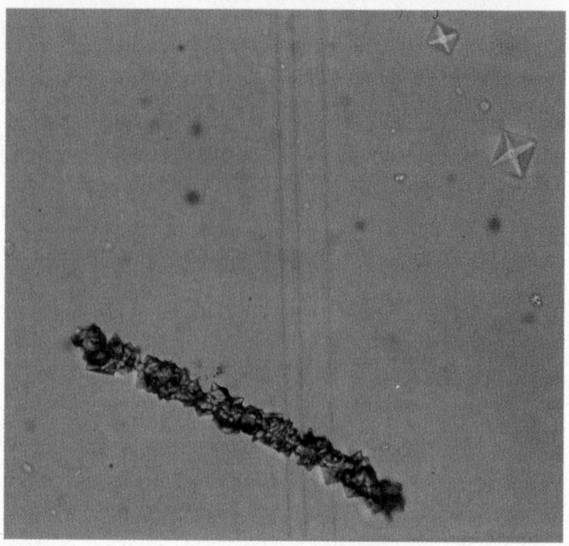

FIGURE 114-10. Oxalate crystals. A pseudocast of calcium oxalate crystals accompanied by crystals of calcium oxalate dehydrate. (From Johnson RJ, Feehally J. *Comprehensive Clinical Nephrology*. London: Mosby; 2000.)

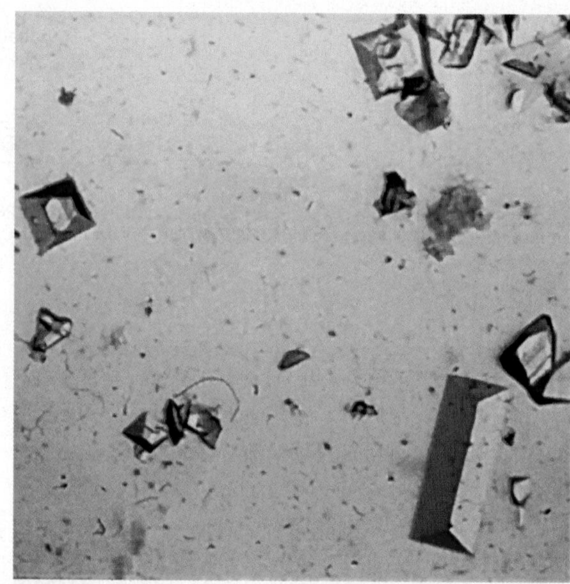

FIGURE 114-11. Coffin-lid crystals of magnesium ammonium phosphate (struvite). (From Johnson RJ, Feehally J. *Comprehensive Clinical Nephrology*. London: Mosby; 2000.)

sodium urate crystals (Fig. 114-12), and calcium phosphate amorphous crystals are common and do not usually have pathologic significance.

Other Elements

Bacteria may be seen in the urine sediment. A spun urine sediment may show rods or cocci in chains, but bacteria are identified best by Gram staining of the urine sediment. Budding yeast forms (which are highly refractile), trichomonads, and spermatozoa also may be seen in the urinary sediment.

SPECIFIC RENAL SYNDROMES

This chapter considers the approach to the patient with acute kidney injury (Chapter 120), glomerular syndromes (nephrotic vs. nephritic; Chapter 121), tubulointerstitial disease (Chapter 122), vasculitis and vascular diseases of the kidney (Chapter 125), papillary necrosis, and chronic kidney disease (Chapter 130).

Acute Kidney Injury

Acute kidney injury (Chapter 120) is a syndrome in which glomerular filtration declines during a period of hours to days. The serum creatinine level is elevated in both acute and chronic kidney disease, but an actively rising serum creatinine level confirms an acute or acute-on-chronic insult to kidney

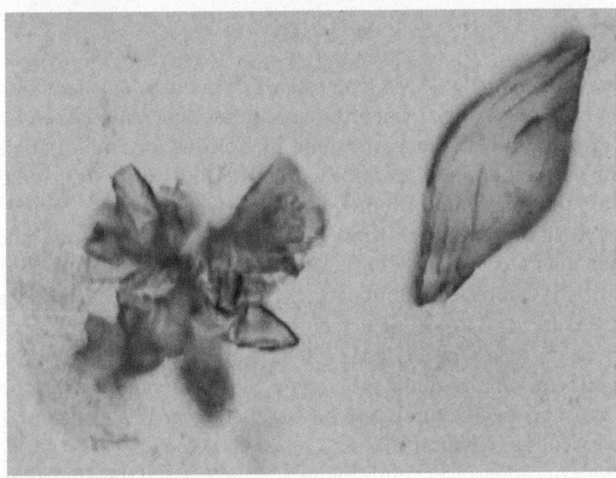

FIGURE 114-12. Urate crystals. Complex crystals suggestive of acute urate nephropathy or urate nephrolithiasis. (From Johnson RJ, Feehally J. *Comprehensive Clinical Nephrology*. London: Mosby; 2000.)

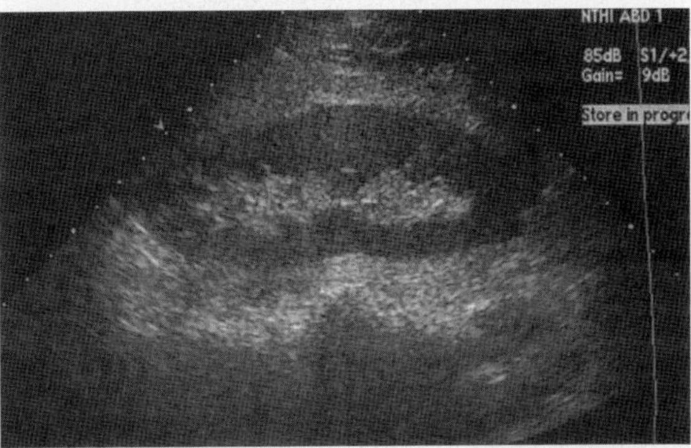

FIGURE 114-13. Normal findings on sagittal renal ultrasound. The cortex is hypoechoic compared with the echogenic fat containing the renal sinus. (From Johnson RJ, Feehally J. *Comprehensive Clinical Nephrology*. London: Mosby; 2000.)

function. As a blood filtration organ, the kidney is susceptible to an acute compromise of renal arterial perfusion (Chapter 125), such as prerenal kidney injury, or blockage in urine outflow, such as urinary obstruction due to benign prostatic hypertrophy (Chapter 129). Thus, the patient with acute renal failure is best approached by evaluation for prerenal, renal, and postrenal causes. The intrarenal causes of acute kidney injury include acute tubular necrosis (Chapter 120), acute interstitial nephritis (Chapter 122), acute glomerulonephritis (Chapter 121), and acute vasculitis and vascular disease (Chapters 121 and 125). The careful and systematic evaluation of the patient should start with a thorough history and physical examination, which should be followed by selected laboratory tests and often an imaging test, such as renal ultrasonography. Most cases of acute renal failure in the hospital have hemodynamic or toxic causes, so prerenal azotemia and acute tubular necrosis must be considered carefully and distinguished from one another.

ETIOLOGY

Prerenal Kidney Injury

Prerenal kidney injury can be caused by shock or renal hypoperfusion from a variety of conditions, including arterial underfilling secondary to edematous states (e.g., severe heart failure, decompensated cirrhosis) or, more variably, cases of nephrotic syndrome. History relevant to renal hypoperfusion states, such as a history of acute gastroenteritis, should be sought. Patients should also be asked about use of nonsteroidal anti-inflammatory drugs or blockers of the renin-angiotensin-aldosterone system (e.g., angiotensin-converting enzyme inhibitors, angiotensin receptor blockers) that can exacerbate prerenal injury. Relative hypotension compared with a patient's baseline blood pressure and orthostatic changes in blood pressure and pulse indicate arterial underfilling. Relatively minor orthostatic hypotension may explain the acute decompensation of kidney function in a patient with chronic kidney disease (Chapter 130) or renal artery stenosis (Chapter 125). Lower extremity edema is common in cirrhosis (Chapter 153), heart failure (Chapter 58), and nephrotic syndrome (Chapter 121).

Acute Tubular Necrosis

Acute tubular necrosis can arise from ischemic or toxic injury to the kidneys. Prerenal azotemia can progress to acute tubular necrosis, particularly if frank hypotension occurs in the setting of infection and persists. The transition of prerenal renal failure to acute tubular necrosis may be revealed by a rise in the fractional excretion of sodium to a value greater than 1%. Alternatively, acute tubular necrosis may arise from a toxic effect, so a medication and ingestion history is critical to the evaluation of the patient.

DIAGNOSIS

Laboratory Testing

The normal concentration of blood urea nitrogen (BUN), which is a product of protein catabolism, is about 10-fold higher than the creatinine concentration. Because the BUN-to-creatinine ratio commonly rises with arterial underfilling, BUN typically is used as a marker of effective volume status. Classically, the BUN-to-creatinine ratio will be higher than 15 to 20 in prerenal azotemia but 10 or close to it in acute tubular necrosis. However, the BUN concentration (and hence its ratio to creatinine concentration) may be inappropriately high in other circumstances, such as with high protein intake, gastrointestinal bleeding, or the use of steroids or tetracyclines. The BUN concentration and its ratio to creatinine concentration may be low in patients who have a poor dietary intake of protein, malnutrition, or liver disease.

The excretion of sodium in the setting of oliguria and acute kidney injury (Chapter 120) often gives insight into the appropriateness of tubular function. The fractional excretion of sodium (FE_{Na}) is calculated as follows:

$$FE_{Na} = (\text{urine Na/plasma Na})/(\text{urine Cr/plasma Cr}) \times 100$$

where *Na* is the sodium concentration (in mmol/L) and *Cr* is the creatinine concentration (in mmol/L or mg/dL). In the setting of oliguria, FE_{Na} below 1% often denotes prerenal azotemia, whereas FE_{Na} above 1% suggests intrinsic renal damage. Although this measurement is generally useful, FE_{Na} below 1% may be seen without evidence of a prerenal component, including contrast nephropathy (Chapter 120), hepatorenal syndrome (Chapter 154), obstructive uropathy (Chapter 123), interstitial nephritis (Chapter 122), glomerulonephritis (Chapter 121), and rhabdomyolysis (Chapter 113). Conversely, a high FE_{Na} can be seen in cases in which there is a prerenal component, including diuretic use, adrenal insufficiency (Chapter 227), cerebral salt wasting, and salt-wasting nephropathy (Chapter 116). The FE_{Na} must be evaluated in the context of the clinical situation because it can be low or high in a normal patient or in a patient with chronic kidney disease. Ultimately, a patient's volume status is best at the bedside and should not be deduced solely from a measurement of electrolytes.

Imaging

Ultrasonography, which is the most commonly used renal imaging study (Fig. 114-13), provides reliable information about obstruction, kidney size, presence of masses, and renal echotexture. Ultrasonography has only a 90% sensitivity for the detection of hydronephrosis and hence is not sufficient to exclude obstruction (Chapter 123) with certainty. In addition, its inability to detect stones in the ureters and bladder limits its utility in the evaluation for kidney stones (Chapter 126). Ultrasonography can detect vascular disease, and Doppler imaging permits evaluation of the renal vessels with resistive indices. Resistive indices are crucial in ascribing renal dysfunction to the detected vascular disease (Chapter 125). A high resistive index reflects parenchymal disease with scarring and indicates that intervention on the vascular disease itself is unlikely to improve renal function.

A computed tomography (CT) scan stone protocol to assess the kidneys, ureters, and bladder is the study of choice for detecting kidney stones (Chapter 126) because of its ability to detect stones of all kinds, including uric acid stones and nonobstructing stones, as well as stones in the ureters (Fig. 114-14). Masses in the kidney can be evaluated with either contrast CT or a renal ultrasound examination. CT angiography with iodinated contrast material can assess possible renal artery stenosis (Chapter 125) with an accuracy comparable to that of magnetic resonance (MR) angiography.

Glomerular Syndromes: Nephrotic versus Nephritic

The nephrotic syndrome (Chapter 121) is characterized by the presence of proteinuria of more than 3.5 g/day/1.73 m^2, with accompanying edema, hypertension, and hyperlipidemia. Other consequences include a predisposition to infection and hypercoagulability. In general, the diseases associated

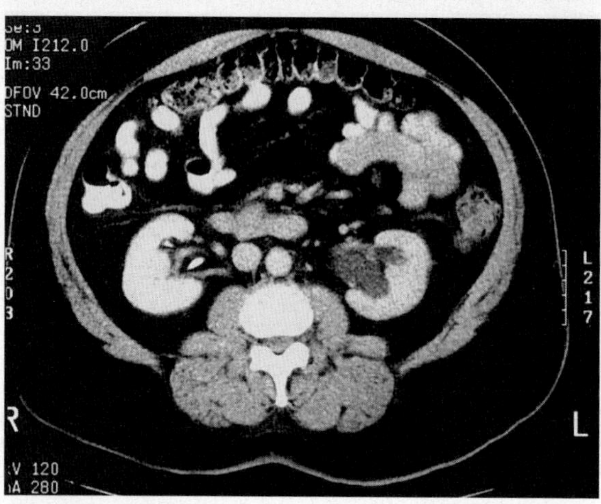

FIGURE 114-14. Delayed excretion in the left kidney secondary to a distal calculus. Contrast-enhanced computed tomography scan shows dilated left renal pelvis. (From Johnson RJ, Feehally J. *Comprehensive Clinical Nephrology*. London: Mosby; 2000.)

with nephrotic syndrome do not cause acute kidney injury, although acute kidney injury may be seen with minimal change disease, human immunodeficiency virus (HIV)–associated nephropathy, and bilateral renal vein thrombosis (Chapter 125). The causes of primary idiopathic nephrotic syndrome, in decreasing order of prevalence, are focal and segmental glomerulosclerosis, membranous nephropathy, minimal change disease, and membranoproliferative glomerulonephritis. Membranous nephropathy has been associated with antibodies to the M-type phospholipase A_2 receptor. Secondary causes of the nephrotic syndrome include diabetic nephropathy (Chapter 124), amyloidosis (Chapter 188), and membranous lupus nephritis (Chapters 121 and 266).

The acute nephritic syndrome is an uncommon but dramatic presentation of an acute glomerulonephritis (Chapter 121). The hallmark of the acute nephritic syndrome is the presence of dysmorphic RBCs and RBC casts, but their absence does not exclude the syndrome. The acute nephritic syndrome can be caused by any of the rapidly progressive glomerulonephropathies with ANCA-associated vasculitis (granulomatosis with polyangiitis, microscopic polyangiitis, and eosinophilic granulomatosis with polyangiitis), anti–glomerular basement membrane (anti-GBM) glomerulonephritis, and immune complex–mediated glomerulonephritis (including systemic lupus erythematosus, cryoglobulinemia, postinfectious glomerulonephritis, endocarditis, IgA nephropathy, and Henoch-Schönlein purpura). The rapid decline in renal function often warrants urgent and usually inpatient evaluation.

DIAGNOSIS

Laboratory Testing

Proteinuria (as albuminuria) of more than 3.5 g in 24 hours generally indicates glomerular disease (Chapter 121). Lesser quantities do not preclude glomerular disease, and electrophoresis gives valuable insight into the composition of the proteinuria (Chapter 187). On occasion, overflow proteinuria of a low-molecular-weight protein, such as light chains in Bence Jones proteinuria, can be higher than 3.5 g/day without any of the manifestations or implications of the nephrotic syndrome; a urine protein electrophoresis study is important in making the distinction. A comparison of the microalbumin-to-creatinine ratio with the protein-to-creatinine ratio will give an insight into the presence of Bence Jones protein because of the absence of albuminuria despite significant proteinuria. Collection must be done by discarding the first morning void and collecting all urine output for the next 24 hours, including the first morning void the next day.

The 24-hour urine collection for protein excretion is cumbersome and subject to inaccuracies. Instead, a spot urine sample for protein and creatinine can be used to estimate the amount of protein excreted. A protein-to-creatinine ratio of 3 translates to a 24-hour protein excretion of about 3 g. The ratio is most accurate when the first morning urine collection is used and may be inaccurate in patients with orthostatic proteinuria.

The evaluation of proteinuric renal dysfunction, particularly when glomerular diseases are suspected, should follow a stepwise progression from noninvasive serologic evaluation to a definitive or confirmatory diagnostic evaluation, such as a renal biopsy.[8] Sometimes an expeditious diagnosis is needed, and a biopsy may be done relatively early in the evaluation.

Serologies

An *antinuclear antibody* (ANA) titer can be useful to evaluate glomerular disease in either nephrotic or nephritic presentations. A high ANA titer (e.g., 1:320), especially if it is accompanied by a more specific finding such as anti–double-stranded DNA antibody or anti-Smith antibody, can be highly specific for the diagnosis of lupus nephritis (Chapter 266), which usually requires a renal biopsy. Lower titers (e.g., 1:80 or 1:40) are nonspecific.

A *rheumatoid factor* titer will usually be elevated in patients with rheumatoid arthritis (Chapter 264), but vasculitis is a relatively late and rare event. Rheumatoid factor can be detected in some forms of cryoglobulinemia (Chapter 187); for example, IgM, which is present in type II and type III cryoglobulinemia, has rheumatoid factor activity. Rheumatoid factor also can be seen as a nonspecific finding in bacterial endocarditis (Chapter 76) and systemic vasculitis (Chapter 270).

The levels of *complement* components C3 and C4 and the 50% hemolyzing dose of complement (CH_{50}) usually are measured to evaluate suspected rapidly progressive glomerulonephritis (Chapter 121). Complement levels are usually low in active systemic lupus erythematosus (Chapter 266), poststreptococcal glomerulonephritis (Chapter 121), endocarditis (Chapter 76), membranoproliferative glomerulonephritis, cryoglobulinemia (Chapter 187), shunt nephritis with infection of a ventriculoatrial shunt, and glomerulonephritis associated with visceral abscesses. A particularly depressed C4 compared with C3 should raise the suspicion of cryoglobulinemia.

Serum immunoelectrophoresis will detect elevated polyclonal IgA levels in about 50% of cases of IgA nephropathy (Chapter 121) and Henoch-Schönlein purpura (Chapter 121). Polyclonal elevation of IgG may occur in a variety of systemic diseases and is a nonspecific finding. The presence of a monoclonal protein in the serum should raise the suspicion for a monoclonal gammopathy–associated disease (Chapter 187). The differential diagnosis includes monoclonal gammopathy of uncertain significance, myeloma kidney, lymphomas (Chapter 185), amyloidosis (Chapter 188), light chain deposition disease, heavy chain deposition disease, immunotactoid glomerulonephritis, and cryoglobulinemia. The concentration of the monoclonal protein is higher when the diagnosis of multiple myeloma is made, but even small quantities of Bence Jones proteins in the serum can have clinical significance.

A *urine immunoelectrophoresis* always should be obtained concomitantly if myeloma is suspected. Because a substantial fraction of multiple myelomas can have no heavy chain excretion and small quantities of light chains may be difficult to detect by serum immunoelectrophoresis, a urine immune electrophoresis test for Bence Jones protein complements the serum immunoelectrophoresis. In light chain myeloma, patients may have Bence Jones proteinuria even in the absence of an M component in the serum immunoelectrophoresis. Bence Jones proteinuria may be present in myeloma kidney, amyloidosis, light chain deposition disease, lymphoma, or, occasionally, monoclonal gammopathy of uncertain significance. However, some patients with systemic AL (light chain) amyloidosis have a normal serum immunoelectrophoresis and no Bence Jones proteinuria (Chapter 187). More sensitive assays for serum free light chains and an assessment of the ratio of κ to λ lights chains increase the sensitivity for detection of monoclonal gammopathies.

The *antineutrophil cytoplasmic antibody* (ANCA) assay has allowed earlier and more definitive recognition of vasculitic causes of rapidly progressive glomerulonephritis (Chapter 270), especially granulomatosis with polyangiitis, microscopic polyangiitis, and eosinophilic granulomatosis with polyangiitis, when it is confirmed by enzyme-linked immunosorbent assay. The antibodies cause two different patterns of staining: perinuclear staining (p-ANCA) and cytoplasmic staining (c-ANCA). Both antigens actually have a cytoplasmic distribution, and the perinuclear staining pattern is an artifact of the fixation method. In most cases, the antigen for p-ANCA is myeloperoxidase (MPO), whereas the antigen for c-ANCA is proteinase 3 (PR3). Anti-MPO antibodies are associated with microscopic polyangiitis, idiopathic crescentic glomerulonephritis, or Churg-Strauss syndrome (eosinophilic granulomatosis with polyangiitis; Chapter 270). Anti-PR3 antibodies often correlate with the classic disease of granulomatosis with polyangiitis (formerly known as Wegener granulomatosis) (Chapter 270).

Anti–glomerular basement membrane (anti-GBM) antibodies are autoantibodies to the Goodpasture antigen (Chapter 121), which resides in a domain of the α chain of type 4 collagen. An early and accurate diagnosis of Goodpasture syndrome can be made by immunofluorescence and confirmed by Western blot analysis. Anti-GBM antibody staining also may occur in the presence of a positive ANCA. In these cases, the theory is that exposure of the Goodpasture antigen, as a result of the glomerular injury, leads to anti-GBM antibody formation as a secondary process.

Cryoglobulins (Chapter 187) are thermolabile immunoglobulins. They are a single monoclonal type in type I cryoglobulinemia. In type II and type III cryoglobulinemia, however, the mixture of immunoglobulins includes one with rheumatoid factor activity against IgG. Type I and type II cryoglobulins are more likely to be associated with clinical disease, especially at higher titers. Type III cryoglobulinemia is often of less clinical significance. Type I cryoglobulinemia is seen with Waldenström macroglobulinemia and multiple myeloma (Chapter 187); type II, with hepatitis C infection (Chapters 148 and 149), Sjögren syndrome (Chapter 268), lymphomas (Chapters 185 and 186), and systemic lupus erythematosus (Chapter 266); and type III, with hepatitis C (Chapters 148 and 149), chronic infections, and inflammatory conditions. When cryoglobulinemia is associated with hepatitis C, the hepatitis C virus (HCV) RNA is concentrated in the cryoprecipitate; the diagnosis can be made by an RNA assay of the cryoprecipitate at 37° C.

Membranous nephropathy is associated with chronic hepatitis B infection with hepatitis B surface antigenemia (Chapter 149). Classic polyarteritis nodosa (Chapter 270) occasionally is seen with chronic hepatitis B infection, often with surface antigenemia and hepatitis B e antigenemia. M-type phospholipase A_2 receptor antibodies also have been detected as autoantibodies in idiopathic membranous nephropathy.

Hepatitis C serology is associated with a variety of renal diseases, including cryoglobulinemia, membranoproliferative glomerulonephritis, and membranous nephropathy. The evaluation may include the antibody test and an assay for HCV RNA. On occasion, the HCV RNA analysis may have to be conducted on the cryoprecipitate at 37° C.

HIV-associated nephropathy (Chapter 121) is associated with nephrotic syndrome and acute kidney injury. In the appropriate clinical setting, HIV serology and viral titers are warranted tests for both clinical syndromes.

Streptococcal infection can be confirmed as the cause of postinfectious glomerulonephritis (Chapter 121) with an anti-DNase or antistreptolysin assay. Acute and convalescent serology assays are used to confirm recent infection.

The erythrocyte sedimentation rate (ESR) is a relatively nonspecific test in the evaluation of renal disease. However, a high ESR often points to systemic vasculitis (Chapter 270), multiple myeloma (Chapter 187), or malignant disease as the underlying cause. However, the ESR often is elevated in the nephrotic syndrome (Chapter 121), including diabetic nephropathy (Chapter 124).

Renal Biopsy

No formal guidelines exist for the indications to perform a renal biopsy. Most nephrologists will perform a biopsy for adults with idiopathic nephrotic syndrome and for children with steroid-dependent or steroid-resistant nephrotic syndrome. In addition, acute kidney injury without an identifiable inciting cause is a clear indication for biopsy. Notably, patients with hospital-acquired kidney failure rarely meet this indication. Other abnormal clinical findings, such as gross or microscopic hematuria or subnephrotic proteinuria, often but not always lead to a kidney biopsy. Renal biopsy usually is performed percutaneously with real-time ultrasound or CT guidance. About 1 to 2% of patients without an underlying coagulopathy will develop bleeding that requires a transfusion. The transjugular approach can be used in patients in whom the risks for bleeding are high.

The decision to pursue a kidney biopsy should be individualized for each patient, but a renal biopsy generally is justified for most patients with two or more of the following four findings: hematuria, proteinuria above 1 g/day, renal insufficiency, or positive serologies for systemic diseases with known potential for kidney involvement (e.g., hepatitis B or C virus infection, systemic lupus erythematosus, ANCA seropositivity). The decision about whether to perform a renal biopsy in diabetic patients with suspected diabetic nephropathy should be individualized and is usually driven by the presence of atypical features or an active urine sediment.[9] In addition, in patients with renal transplants (Chapter 131) and acute or chronic renal failure, biopsy of the allograft kidney provides crucial information in guiding diagnosis and treatment.

Tubulointerstitial Diseases

Tubulointerstitial diseases (Chapter 122) vary in presentation from acute kidney injury to chronic kidney dysfunction that initially is manifested as asymptotic mild renal insufficiency (Table 114-3). The urine sediment often contains small to moderate amounts of proteinuria, usually less than 1 g/day, as well as WBCs, RBCs, tubular cells, and WBC casts. RBC casts are rare in acute interstitial nephritis and are more characteristic of glomerular disease.

TABLE 114-3 MAJOR CAUSES OF TUBULOINTERSTITIAL DISEASE

Ischemic and toxic acute tubular necrosis
Allergic interstitial nephritis
Interstitial nephritis secondary to immune complex–related collagen vascular disease, such as Sjögren disease or systemic lupus erythematosus
Granulomatous diseases: sarcoidosis, tubulointerstitial nephritis with uveitis
IgG4-related interstitial nephritis
Pigment-related tubular injury: myoglobulinuria, hemoglobinuria
Hypercalcemia with nephrocalcinosis
Tubular obstruction: drugs such as indinavir, uric acid in tumor lysis syndrome
Myeloma kidney or cast nephropathy
Infection-related interstitial nephritis: *Legionella, Leptospira* species
Infiltrative diseases, such as lymphoma

Vasculitis and Vascular Diseases of the Kidney

Vascular diseases of the kidney can be divided into large-vessel obstruction and medium- to small-vessel diseases (Chapter 125). Renovascular disease is a common cause of hypertension, heart failure, and renal insufficiency. About 90% of renal artery stenosis is atherosclerotic in origin, with most of the remaining caused by fibromuscular dysplasia, which is more common in women 20 to 50 years of age. Medium-sized arterial vessel diseases include polyarteritis nodosa, which is seen in patients with hepatitis B (Chapters 148 and 149), HIV infection (Chapter 121), or, rarely, hepatitis C (Chapters 148 and 149). Symptoms include abdominal pain, hypertension, and mild renal insufficiency, often with a benign sediment; diagnostic findings include microaneurysms at the bifurcation of medium-sized arteries. Other diseases involving small vessels include atheroembolic disease (Chapter 125), which is seen either spontaneously or after arteriography or surgery. This syndrome typically affects the kidneys, gastrointestinal tract, and lower extremities, but it can also involve the central nervous system when the aortic arch is affected.

The thrombotic microangiopathies include hemolytic-uremic syndrome (HUS) and thrombotic thrombocytopenic purpura (Chapter 172). Thrombocytopenic purpura is associated with an acquired inhibitor to or the congenital inherited absence of a protease that cleaves large-molecular-weight von Willebrand multimers. HUS is caused by endothelial injury. In diarrhea-positive (or typical) HUS, the endothelial injury is induced by Shiga toxin from *Escherichia coli* O157:H7 infection. In diarrhea-negative (atypical) HUS, dysregulation of the alternative complement pathway is the underlying cause of endothelial injury. The antiphospholipid antibody syndrome (Chapter 176) can cause large-vessel thrombosis and stenosis as well as a thrombotic microangiopathy with proteinuria, hypertension, and renal insufficiency. Scleroderma renal crisis, which is a manifestation of systemic sclerosis (Chapter 267), often leads to an inexorable progression to end-stage renal insufficiency if untreated.

A systemic vasculitis may be manifested in a variety of ways, including skin manifestations such as petechial rash, purpura, digital gangrene, and splinter hemorrhages. Otitis, sinusitis, epistaxis, hemoptysis, and nasal septal ulcers are common manifestations of granulomatosis with polyangiitis (Chapter 270). Pulmonary hemorrhage can be a catastrophic manifestation of Goodpasture syndrome (Chapter 121) or anti-GBM disease as well as the ANCA-associated vasculitis (Chapter 270). Abdominal pain and tenderness and gastrointestinal hemorrhage may be observed in Henoch-Schönlein purpura and classic polyarteritis nodosa (Chapter 270). Neurologic symptoms may be a manifestation of vasculitis, such as microscopic polyangiitis (Chapter 270) and cryoglobulinemia (Chapter 187).

DIAGNOSIS

Radiologic Evaluation

Magnetic resonance imaging (MRI) with MR angiography (Fig. 114-15) is highly sensitive for detecting atherosclerotic renovascular disease (Chapter 125), but it tends to overestimate the degree of stenosis. Its accuracy in detecting fibromuscular dysplasia, however, is less well validated. MRI also can be used to evaluate renal masses. MRI does not require iodinated contrast material, but gadolinium-based contrast agents for vascular studies are

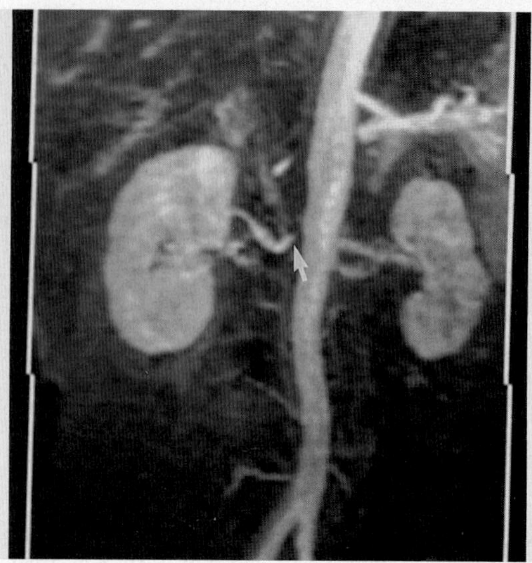

FIGURE 114-15. **Magnetic resonance angiography.** Coronal three-dimensional image shows right renal artery stenosis *(arrow)*. (From Johnson RJ, Feehally J. *Comprehensive Clinical Nephrology*. London: Mosby; 2000.)

associated with the syndrome of nephrogenic systemic fibrosis in patients with advanced renal failure (Chapter 267).

Renal arteriography, which is the "gold standard" in the evaluation of renal artery stenosis (Chapter 125), also is used for the evaluation of arteriovenous malformations, polyarteritis nodosa, and other vascular lesions of the kidneys. This invasive study uses iodinated contrast material and incurs a small risk for atheroembolic disease (Chapter 125). Therapeutic angioplasty and stenting can be done at the time of angiography.

Papillary Necrosis

Acute necrosis of the renal papilla is associated with sickle cell anemia (Chapter 163), analgesic nephropathy (Chapter 122), diabetic nephropathy (Chapter 124), and obstructive pyelonephritis (Chapter 284). In sickle cell disease (Chapter 163)[10], the hypoxic and hypertonic milieu of the inner medulla promotes sickling, and chronic sickling at the vasa recta results in medullary ischemia. Massive and prolonged consumption of analgesics, particularly the combination of aspirin, caffeine, and acetaminophen, is associated with chronic interstitial nephritis and a predisposition to papillary necrosis (Chapter 122); medullary ischemia is thought to be caused by inhibition of synthesis of vasodilatory prostaglandins by aspirin, and direct toxicity is attributed to metabolites of phenacetin. Similarly, medullary perfusion is thought to be compromised in diabetic nephropathy (Chapter 124) and obstructive pyelonephritis (Chapter 123).

The clinical manifestations of papillary necrosis can include flank pain and hematuria. If the papilla is sloughed, obstruction may occur at the renal pelvis or ureter of the affected kidney, with referred pain migrating from the flank to the groin. A sloughed papilla may precipitate frank renal failure if the function of the contralateral kidney is impaired or if obstruction occurs at the level of the bladder or urethra (Chapter 123).

Classically, papillary necrosis is diagnosed on an excretory pyelogram as a calyceal defect after sloughing of a papilla, but CT with contrast enhancement is as good for advanced lesions. If the necrotic papilla is retained, however, the defect will be more subtle. Transitional cell carcinoma (Chapter 197) can occur in the setting of papillary necrosis or can mimic its appearance. Obstruction, if present, must be relieved, but treatment otherwise is limited to pain control and hydration.

Chronic Kidney Disease

Chronic kidney disease, which is defined as either kidney damage or a GFR of less than 60 mL/min/1.73 m^2 for longer than 3 months, includes five stages (Table 114-4). Kidney damage is defined as pathologic abnormalities or markers of kidney damage, including abnormalities in the composition of blood or urine or abnormalities on imaging tests. The excretion of 30 to 300 mg of albumin in a 24-hour period defines microalbuminuria. An estimated 12% of the adult U.S. population has abnormal albumin excretion in the urine, and the frequency increases with age. Kidney failure is defined as either a GFR of less than 15 mL/min/1.73 m^2 that is accompanied by signs and symptoms of uremia or a need for initiation of kidney replacement therapy for treatment of complications of decreased GFR (Fig. 114-16). End-stage renal disease includes all cases requiring treatment by dialysis or transplantation regardless of the level of GFR.

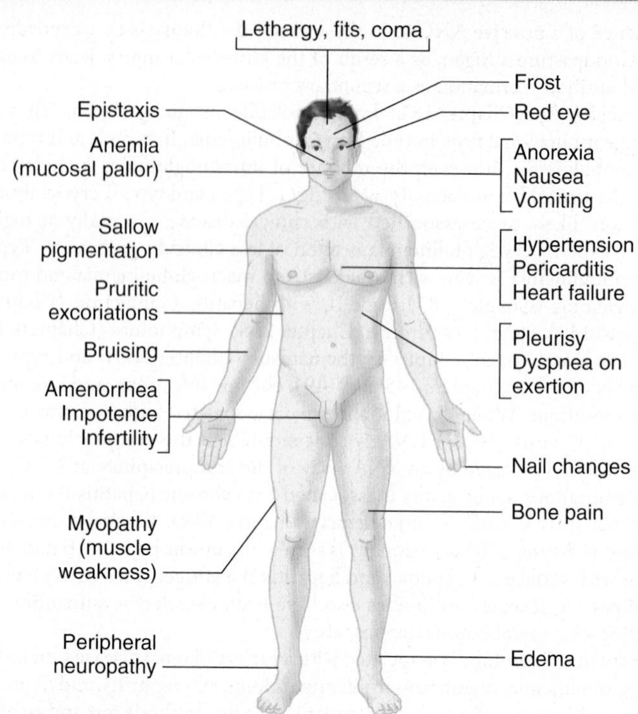

FIGURE 114-16. Common symptoms and signs of chronic renal failure. (Redrawn from Forbes CD, Jackson WF. *Color Atlas and Text of Clinical Medicine*. 3rd ed. London: Mosby; 2003.)

TABLE 114-4 STAGES OF CHRONIC KIDNEY DISEASE*

STAGE	DESCRIPTION	GFR (mL/min/1.73 m^2)
1	Kidney damage with normal or ↑GFR	≥90
2	Kidney damage with mild or ↓GFR	60-89
3	Moderate ↓GFR	30-59
4	Severe ↓GFR	15-29
5	Kidney failure	<15 (or dialysis)

*Chronic kidney disease is defined as either kidney damage or GFR <60 mL/min/1.73 m^2 for ≥3 months. Kidney damage is defined as pathologic abnormalities or presence of markers of damage, including abnormalities in blood or urine test results or imaging studies.
GFR = glomerular filtration rate.

Patients with chronic kidney disease warrant referral to a nephrologist. Care of these patients should focus on efforts to slow disease progression, to optimize medical management, and to make a seamless transition to renal replacement therapy (Chapter 130).[11] The care should include optimal blood pressure control, use of angiotensin-converting enzyme inhibitors and angiotensin receptor blockers if indicated, dietary counseling, careful management of calcium and phosphorus levels, control of the parathyroid hormone level, and management of anemia with the use of erythropoietin and iron supplements. Early referral for placement of access for dialysis and initiation of transplant evaluation (Chapter 131) are important components of the care of patients with chronic kidney disease.

GENERAL REFERENCES

For the General References and other additional features, please visit Expert Consult at https://expertconsult.inkling.com.

115

STRUCTURE AND FUNCTION OF THE KIDNEYS

QAIS AL-AWQATI AND JONATHAN BARASCH

The kidney regulates the ionic composition and volume of body fluids, the excretion of nitrogenous waste, the elimination of exogenous molecules (e.g., many drugs), the synthesis of a variety of hormones (e.g., erythropoietin), and the metabolism of low-molecular-weight proteins (e.g., insulin). Befitting such an array of responsibilities, the kidney receives 25% of the cardiac output. The gross anatomy of the kidney is notable for a weight of approximately 150 g and a characteristic bean shape with approximate dimensions of 11 × 6 × 2.5 cm. On bisection, a simple gross structure is evident with an outer cortex and a more central medulla that narrows to multiple papillae at the apices of so-called pyramids (Fig. 115-1).

Understanding of the kidney, however, requires an appreciation of the intricate microstructure that underlies its complex functions. Although the kidney is an organ, the *nephron* is actually the organ's definable and independent unit. The human kidney is composed of approximately 1 million essentially identical nephrons. All the functions of the kidney are performed by each individual nephron, and to a first approximation, all nephrons are independent of each other because they have their own innervation and blood supply. The nephron is made up of two functional subunits, the glomerulus and the tubules and ducts (Fig. 115-2). The glomerulus begins with the branching of the afferent arteriole, an end artery of the corresponding renal artery, to a tuft of capillaries. The glomerular capillaries invaginate an epithelium with the visceral epithelial cells adjacent to the capillary and the parietal epithelial cells outside this tuft. The space between the epithelial layers is the urinary space. The fenestrated glomerular capillary endothelium, the intervening basement membrane, and the foot processes of the visceral epithelium, so-called podocytes, make up the glomerular filtration barrier. The balance of hydrostatic and oncotic pressures drives the extrusion of a protein-free filtrate through this barrier into the urinary space. The urinary space then leads to a series of tubules and ducts: the proximal tubule, the thin limb of the loop of Henle, the thick limb of the loop of Henle, the distal convoluted tubule, the cortical collecting duct, and the medullary collecting duct. The papillary collecting duct empties through the renal papilla into the renal pelvis and then to the ureter. The glomerular capillary bed coalesces to form the efferent arteriole, a vessel that is exquisitely sensitive to angiotensin II, and then the peritubular (proximal) capillaries. This system allows efferent arteriole constriction to regulate proximal tubule reabsorption, as described later.

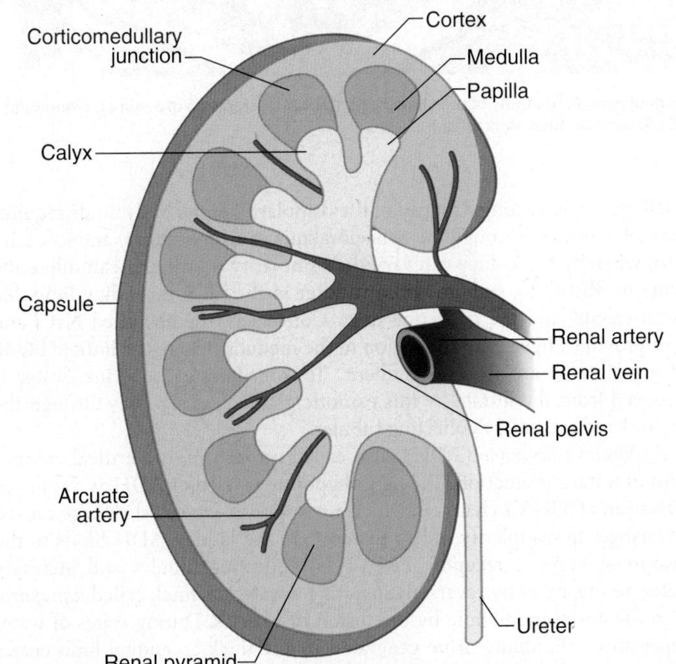

FIGURE 115-1. Sagittal section of the human kidney depicting gross anatomy and organization.

The nephron regulates homeostasis by three actions. First, in the glomerulus, nephrons produce as much as 120 mL/minute of an ultrafiltrate of blood. Second, different segments of the nephron change the composition of the filtrate by the transfer of nearly 99% of its components (e.g., glucose, NaCl, water) from the lumen to the blood. Third, additional electrolytes (e.g., NH_4^+, K^+, HCO_3^-) are secreted from the blood into the lumen.

To perform these functions, each nephron segment, with the exception of the collecting ducts, is composed of a single epithelial cell type whose luminal or apical surface (facing the urine) and basolateral surface (facing the blood) differentially express various proteins and lipids. For example, the apical membrane often has microvilli or cilia, whereas the basolateral membrane does not. Apical polarized endocytosis and exocytosis are often important in the regulation of the number of transport proteins on the apical surface. In addition, epithelia are connected to one another by tight junctions, which confer a characteristic ionic permeability on the epithelial sheet. Transepithelial transport occurs largely through the cell, but transport through the tight junction (the *paracellular pathway*) can also be important in different segments of the tubule. For instance, sodium transport begins with entry at the luminal surface down an electrochemical gradient, whereas its exit at the basolateral surface is uphill and requires adenosine triphosphate (ATP) hydrolysis. The Na^+, K^+-ATPase is located at the basolateral surface of all epithelia, and all "active" energy-consuming transport is coupled directly or indirectly to it with the exception of H^+ transport. Each segment has a distinct composition of channels, carriers, and ATPases, and each segment is regulated by different chemical and physical sensors, so the "final urine" contains the components that must be discarded to maintain constancy of body composition.

THE KIDNEY REGULATES EXTRACELLULAR FLUID VOLUME BY REGULATING ITS SODIUM CONTENT

Filtration of 180 L/day containing 24,000 mEq of sodium is followed by the reabsorption of more than 99% of the filtered sodium. Sodium reabsorption accounts for more than 90% of the oxygen consumed by the kidney. It is regulated by volume receptors that are located in the carotid artery and increase β-sympathetic output, which in turn releases renin, an aspartate protease from the granular cells of the juxtaglomerular apparatus. The renin-releasing cells are close to the afferent arterioles, where renin cleaves angiotensinogen to angiotensin I, which is then converted locally to angiotensin II. Angiotensin II binds to angiotensin receptors and constricts the efferent arteriole, thereby affecting glomerular hemodynamics. The increased hydrostatic pressure within the glomerular capillaries drives the formation of an ultrafiltrate of plasma. As filtration progresses, a protein-rich, oncotically active solution in the capillary opposes the glomerular capillary hydrostatic pressure until a pressure equilibrium is achieved before the efferent arteriole is reached. Consequently, angiotensin II may not change glomerular filtration rate (GFR) markedly, but it can increase proximal reabsorption by reducing the hydrostatic pressure and increasing the oncotic pressure in the peritubular capillaries that surround the proximal tubule in a plexus, thereby favoring reabsorption of water and solutes such as urea.

The glomerular filtrate next enters the tubular portion of the nephron, where Na^+ traverses the cell by entering the apical membrane either through a cotransporter or countertransporter or through a sodium channel, depending on the specific mechanisms of different segments. In the apical membrane of the proximal tubule, an Na^+/H^+ (NHE3) exchanger, an Na^+-coupled glucose carrier, and an Na^+-coupled amino acid and phosphate cotransporter are present. Subsequently, Na^+ is actively transported by the basolateral Na^+, K^+-ATPase into the paracellular space, thereby resulting in local hypertonicity, which causes osmosis through low-resistance tight junctions of the initial segments of the proximal tubule (Fig. 115-3).

In the thick ascending limb of Henle, Na^+ is absorbed by an Na-K-2Cl cotransporter. The driving force for this neutral carrier allows Na^+ and Cl^- to enter the cell, but K^+ is then recycled across the apical membrane, thereby resulting in depolarization of the transepithelial membrane potential. In the distal convoluted tubule, Na^+ is absorbed by a thiazide-sensitive cotransporter, which conducts Na^+ and Cl^- in a strict 1 : 1 stoichiometry. Na^+ exits as usual by the Na^+, K^+-ATPase, but there is also a basolateral Na/Ca exchanger. In this short segment, the macula densa helps control the GFR by regulating renin release through secretion of adenosine and prostaglandins.

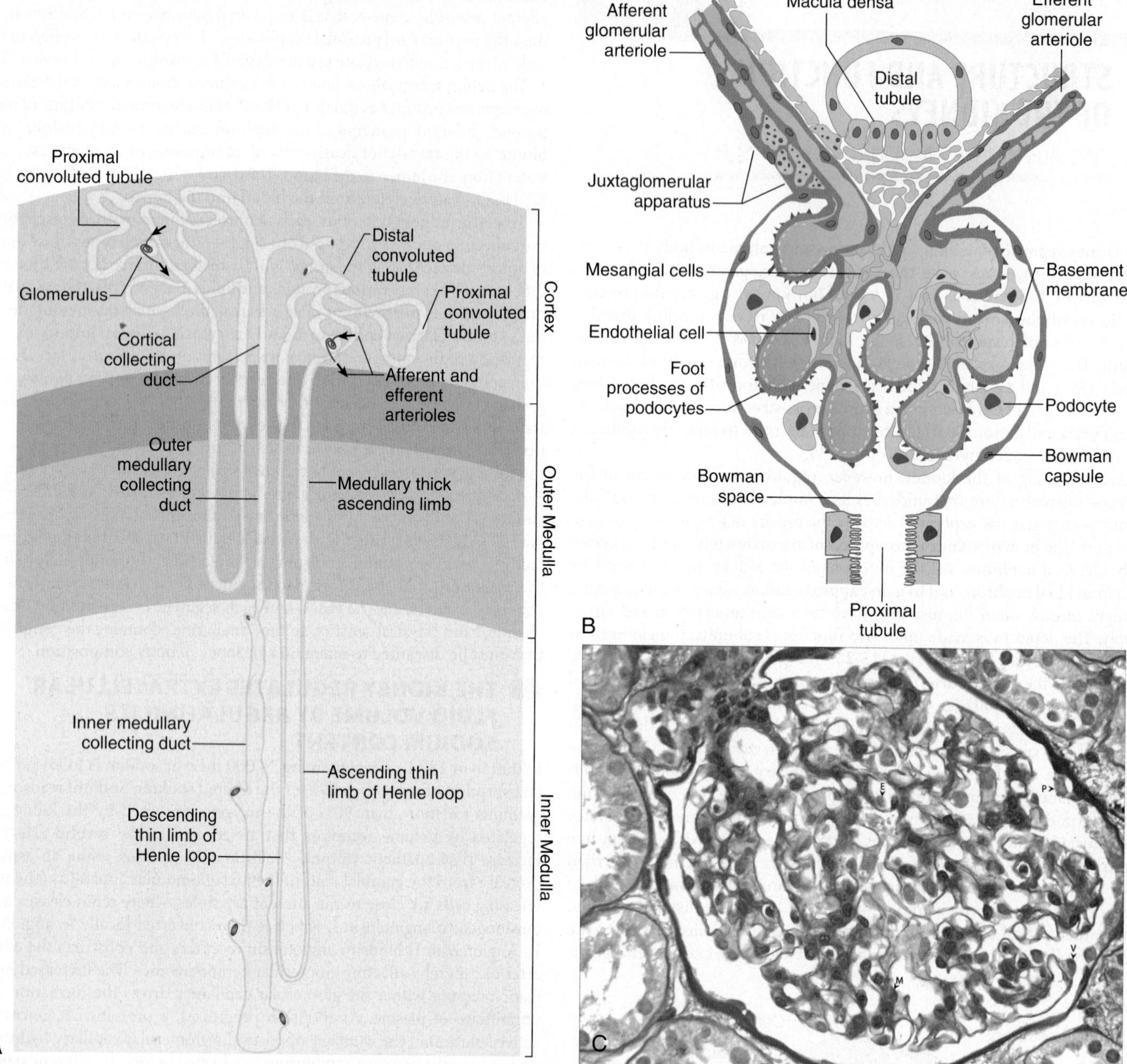

FIGURE 115-2. Structure of the nephron. A, Components of the cortical and juxtaglomerular nephrons. B, Anatomy of the glomerulus. C, Light micrograph of a human glomerulus. E = endothelial cell; M = mesangial cell; P = parietal epithelial cell; V = visceral epithelial cell. (C courtesy Dr. Glen Markowitz.)

In the principal cells of the collecting duct, aldosterone, derived from the zona glomerulosa of the adrenal cortex, increases reabsorption of the final 50 to 100 mEq/day of sodium remaining in the lumen by increasing the number of open sodium channels (ENac), by activating expression of α-subunits, and by increasing the activity of the basolateral Na^+, K^+-ATPase.[1] Aldosterone is the final critical regulator of sodium balance.

A number of the steps that regulate sodium reabsorption can be counteracted by atrial natriuretic peptide (ANP), which is released from the atria in response to volume overload. ANP increases filtration in the glomerulus by dilating the afferent arteriole, thereby increasing glomerular capillary pressure and lowering the oncotic pressure. In addition, ANP increases sodium excretion by inhibiting the release of renin, the production of aldosterone, and the tubular reabsorption of sodium in the terminal collecting duct.

THE KIDNEY REGULATES BODY FLUID OSMOLARITY BY REGULATING ITS WATER CONTENT

Water moves freely among all cells and compartments of the body owing to the presence of water-conducting channels called aquaporins.[2] The concentration of water (its osmolarity) is strictly regulated to prevent cells from swelling or contracting. Control of the osmolarity of the body fluids requires control of intake (through the behavioral mechanism of thirst) and its excretion, whereby the kidney can vary the osmolarity of urine. It can dilute the urine by absorbing sodium without water in the thick ascending limb, the distal tubule, and the collecting duct. Conversely, the absorbed NaCl and urea provide a hyperosmotic region in the medulla, where the limited blood flow maintains an osmotic gradient. To concentrate the urine, water is removed from the filtrate by this osmotic gradient as it passes through the cortical and medullary collecting tubules.

Antidiuretic hormone (ADH), also called *vasopressin*, is a critical component of water reclamation. The neurohypophysis releases ADH as a result of activation of TRPV1 channels, which are responsive to cell shrinkage caused by changes in osmolarity of less than 1%. In the kidney, ADH binds to the vasopressin type 2 receptor TRPV1 on collecting tubules and increases water permeability by reversibly inserting a water channel, called *aquaporin* 2, in the apical membrane by the fusion of vesicles. During states of water deprivation, the dilute urine generated by the thick ascending limb enters vasopressin-sensitive segments in the cortical collecting tubule, where the bulk of the water is absorbed into the cortex to increase the osmolarity of the urinary filtrate to 300 mOsm, which is the osmolarity of plasma. Subsequently, the urine becomes concentrated when it equilibrates with the

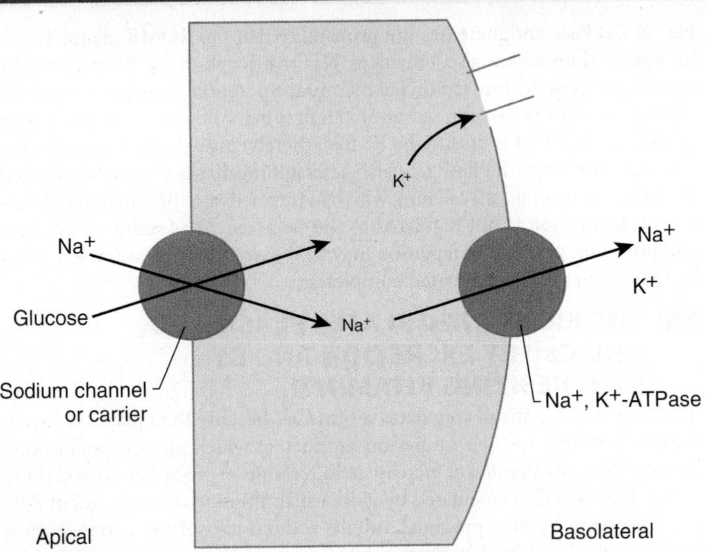

FIGURE 115-3. Sodium reabsorption in the proximal tubular cell.

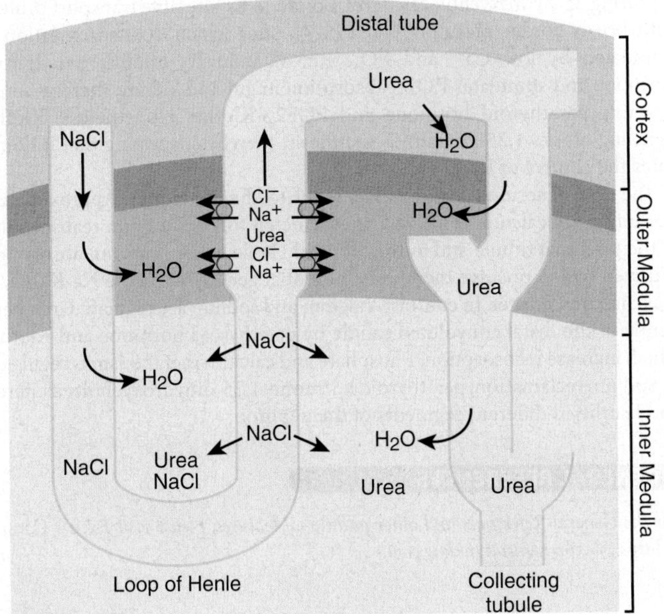

FIGURE 115-4. Regulation of water content.

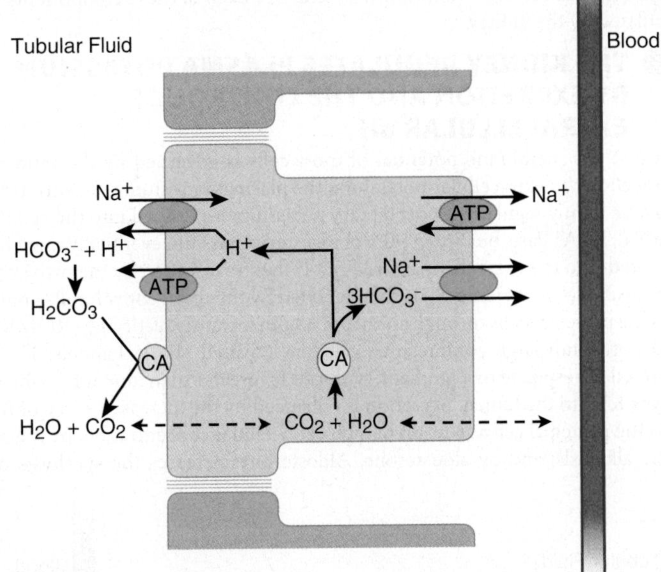

FIGURE 115-5. Ion transport in the proximal tubule. ATP = adenosine triphosphate; CA = carbonic anhydrase.

osmolarity of the medulla as the urine courses down the medullary collecting duct (Fig. 115-4).

THE KIDNEY REGULATES PLASMA pH BY REGULATING HCO_3 CONTENT

The concentration of free H^+ in the intracellular and extracellular fluids is maintained at about 40 nM (pH 7.4) by the daily excretion of acid or base in amounts equal to what is generated by dietary intake and by cellular activity. The complete oxidation of carbohydrates and fats generates approximately 15 to 20 mol/day of the volatile acid CO_2, and nonvolatile acids generated by the metabolism of protein-rich diets account for 60 to 80 mEq/day. HCO_3^- is the most important buffer not only because it is consumed by metabolic acid, thereby producing CO_2 that can be exhaled, but also because it can be regenerated by the kidney. The overall relationship of this buffer system is described by the Henderson-Hasselbalch equation:

$$pH = pK_a + \log[HCO_3^-]/\alpha P_{CO_2}$$

where pK_a is 6.1 and α represents the solubility coefficient of P_{CO_2} (which is 0.03). Because all the body buffers (e.g., bone, intracellular proteins) are in equilibrium, changes in the concentration of HCO_3^- regulate the pH of body fluids.

Although one task of the kidney is to replace the HCO_3^- that is lost as a consequence of the production of acid by oxidative metabolism, it must first reabsorb the 5000 mEq/day HCO_3^- that is filtered every day. The proximal tubule reabsorbs luminal HCO_3^- by secreting H^+ through an apical Na^+/H^+ exchanger, which is directly stimulated by angiotensin II to secrete H^+ in strict 1:1 exchange for Na^+, thereby mediating both sodium absorption and H^+ secretion. An H^+-ATPase is also present in the microvilli and apical endocytic vesicles that fuse with the apical membrane in response to elevated blood P_{CO_2}. H^+ secretion titrates filtered HCO_3 and, catalyzed by carbonic anhydrase, converts it to CO_2 and water, thereby allowing CO_2 reabsorption. H^+ secretion leads to an excess of OH^- in the cell, where it combines with this CO_2 to produce cellular HCO_3^-, which then exits across the basolateral membrane through an Na-HCO_3^- cotransporter (Fig. 115-5).

Given that the proximal tubule regulates bicarbonate reabsorption, the collecting duct must produce "new" HCO_3 to replace what is lost during titration by nonvolatile acids. The cortical collecting tubules contain intercalated cells that mediate H^+ secretion (α-intercalated cell) or β-cell types that mediate HCO_3 secretion, whereas only α cells are present in the medulla. H^+ secretion is mediated in the α-intercalated cell by the H^+-ATPase that is delivered to the apical membrane by fusion of apical vesicles as stimulated by ambient P_{CO_2} (Fig. 115-6).

In a reaction catalyzed by carbonic anhydrase II, the excess OH^- is carboxylated by CO_2 to form HCO_3^-. HCO_3^- is subsequently transported across the basolateral surface in exchange for Cl^- by an alternately spliced form of the red cell anion exchanger (band 3). In contrast, β cells secrete HCO_3^- by an apical Cl/HCO_3 exchanger (pendrin) and a basolateral H^+-ATPase. An H^+, K^+-ATPase in the collecting tubule may also play a role in potassium absorption and perhaps in H^+ secretion.

The collecting tubule is a "tight epithelium" that can maintain electrical and concentration gradients. Secretion of H^+ reduces the pH of the filtrate; the maximal gradient is 3 pH units or 180 mV, but both the size of the pH gradient and its transepithelial membrane potential can be modified to regulate H^+ secretion. For example, Na^+ absorption by the principal cell hyperpolarizes the epithelium and can thus drive H^+ secretion. Aldosterone can stimulate not only Na^+ absorption but also independently H^+ secretion; hence, it is the major hormone that stimulates acid secretion in the collecting tubule. Finally, chronic metabolic acidosis converts the β-intercalated cells into α-intercalated cells, thereby increasing the number of acid-secreting cells and reducing the amount of HCO_3^- secretion in this segment.[3]

The secreted H^+ titrates urinary NH_3 and HPO_4^{2-}. NH_3, which is synthesized by the conversion of glutamine to α-ketoglutarate, is secreted into the proximal lumen. In the loop of Henle and distal segments, the protonated ammonium ion is transferred into the interstitium, from where it reenters the nephron as ammonia gas. Once in the lumen, ammonia gas becomes reprotonated to ammonium, thus trapping a proton. The amount of NH_3 generated from glutamine increases up to four- to five-fold in the setting of metabolic acidosis. Net acid secretion is consequently urinary NH_4^+ plus titratable weak acids (such as HPO_4^{2-}) minus urinary HCO_3^-. Each of these components is regulated by the kidney.

THE KIDNEY REGULATES PLASMA POTASSIUM BY EXCRETION AND THE CONTROL OF EXTRACELLULAR pH

Because the membrane potential of most cells is governed by the ratio of intracellular to extracellular potassium, the plasma potassium concentration must be tightly regulated. Most dietary potassium is pumped into the cell by the Na^+, K^+-ATPase, but about 90% of ingested potassium eventually must be excreted into the urine. K^+ is filtered but is then reabsorbed by the proximal tubule and loop of Henle. K^+ is then secreted by the distal convoluted tubule and the principal cells through apical potassium inwardly rectifying (ROMK) and potassium large conductance calcium-activated (BK) channels. K^+ is secreted in response to a gradient, with cell K^+ greater than lumen K^+, which drives K^+ into the lumen. Secretion is enhanced by the increased entry of K^+ into the principal cell as a result of high extracellular concentration, by metabolic alkalosis, and by aldosterone. Aldosterone increases the synthesis of Na^+, K^+-ATPase and increases the probability that the ROMK channels will be open. Aldosterone also enhances Na^+ reabsorption by ENaC, thereby hyperpolarizing the transepithelial membrane potential, which increases the driving force for potassium secretion. High urinary flow rates deliver a large volume of fluid that is essentially K^+ free, thereby providing a concentration gradient. However, the flow rate also activates mechanosensory flagella that lead to an increase in cell calcium, which in turn activates BK channels. Potassium reabsorption is not regulated to the same extent as sodium retention, and profound potassium depletion may be required for potassium excretion by the kidneys to be eliminated completely.

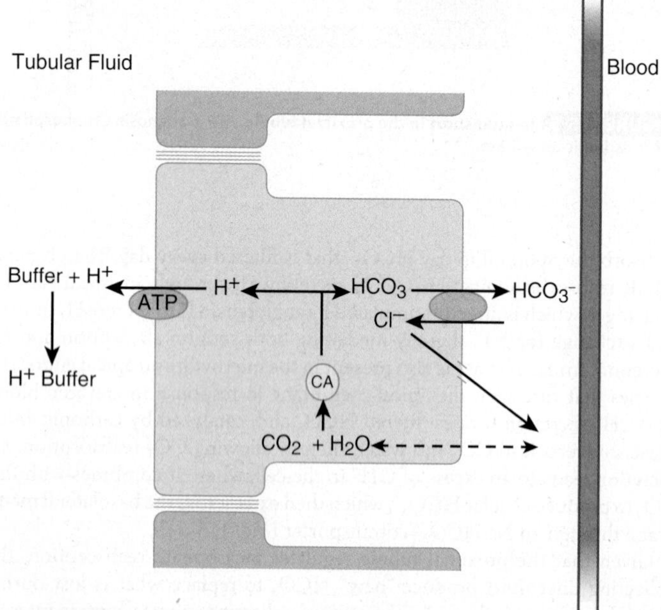

FIGURE 115-6. **Mechanism of acid secretion in the collecting duct. ATP = adenosine triphosphate; CA = carbonic anhydrase.**

THE KIDNEY REGULATES PLASMA PO_4 AND Ca^{2+} BY EXCRETION AND BY SYNTHESIZING VITAMIN D_3

The level of PO_4 critically regulates serum Ca^{2+} because their plasma concentrations are close to their saturation product, at which point crystallization occurs. Thus, any significant increase in PO_4 results in precipitation of $CaPO_4$.

The level of PO_4 is regulated by glomerular filtration. Initially, about 85% is reabsorbed by the proximal tubule sodium-phosphate cotransporters NaPi-2a and NaPi-2c. Parathyroid hormone and the heteromeric receptor FGFR/Klotho, which binds fibroblast growth factor 23 (FGF23), inhibit the expression of NaPi and hence increase excretion of PO_4. Conversely, the proximal tubule generates vitamin D_3 (1,25-dihydroxycholecalciferol) by capturing 25-hydroxycholecalciferol, bound to its filterable transport protein with brush border megalin (Fig. 115-7), after which 1α-hydroxylation is stimulated by low Ca^{2+} and PO_4. 1,25-Vitamin D_3 inhibits parathyroid hormone and stimulates PO_4 reabsorption in gut and kidney, thereby counteracting parathyroid hormone and FGF23-Klotho. Nonetheless, Klotho signaling blocks 1,25-vitamin D_3 synthesis, thereby suggesting that it dominates the control of PO_4.[4]

The level of serum calcium is also regulated by the kidney. Approximately 60% of serum calcium is filtered, after which it follows sodium reabsorption in the proximal tubule and in the loops of Henle, where calcium absorption is driven by the positive membrane potential generated by the Na-K-2Cl/K recycling transporter. In contrast, calcium and sodium are regulated independently in the distal convoluted tubule by parathyroid hormone and Klotho, which increase reabsorption. Phosphate and calcium metabolism is regulated by sodium reclamation, parathyroid hormone, 1,25-dihydroxycholecalciferol, and Klotho in different segments of the nephron.

GENERAL REFERENCES

For the General References and other additional features, please visit Expert Consult at https://expertconsult.inkling.com.

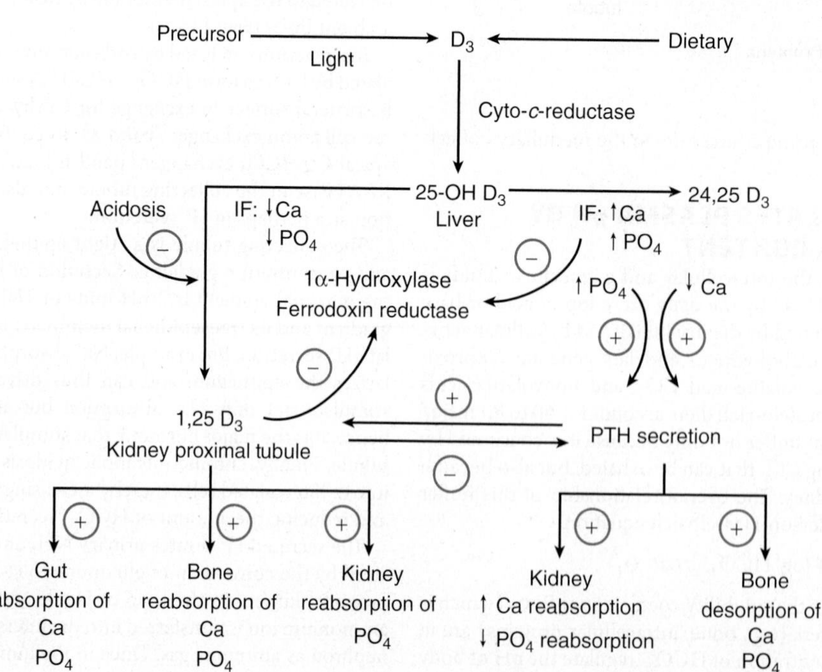

FIGURE 115-7. **Calcium and phosphate metabolism. PTH = parathyroid hormone.**

116

DISORDERS OF SODIUM AND WATER HOMEOSTASIS

ITZCHAK SLOTKI AND KARL SKORECKI

SODIUM AND WATER HOMEOSTASIS

EPIDEMIOLOGY

Disturbances in sodium and water balance or distribution, with attendant perturbations in the volume or solute composition of body fluid compartments, are among the most frequently encountered abnormalities in clinical medicine. The principal manifestations of these disturbances are *hypovolemia, hypervolemia, dysnatremia* (*hyponatremia* or *hypernatremia*), and *polyuria*. Disturbances in body tonicity, reflected by hyponatremia or hypernatremia, are estimated to affect up to 15 to 20% of hospitalized patients, with severe disturbances (>10% deviation from normal values) affecting 1 to 2% of patients. Prevalence rates for these abnormalities in ambulatory populations are lower, and elderly individuals and patients treated with multiple medications are the most susceptible.

PATHOBIOLOGY

Approximately 60% of body mass is composed of solute-containing fluid solutions that are divided into extracellular fluid (ECF) and intracellular fluid (ICF) compartments. Water flows freely across cell membranes through specific water channels (aquaporin family of transmembrane proteins) according to the dictates of osmotic forces, thereby maintaining near equality of the solute-to-water ratio (osmolality) in the ICF and ECF. However, the composition of the major solutes differs between the ECF and ICF (Fig. 116-1A). Sodium and potassium are the major cations in the ECF and ICF, respectively. Chloride and bicarbonate are the major accompanying anions in the ECF, and negative charges on organic molecules maintain electroneutrality with potassium in the ICF. The difference in cationic solute composition between these two compartments is maintained by a pump-leak mechanism involving the activity of Na^+, K^+-adenosine triphosphatase (ATPase) operating in concert with cell membrane sodium and potassium conductance pathways. The free movement of water ensures that the sodium concentration in ECF is nearly equivalent to the potassium concentration in ICF. The magnitude of free water movement is determined by the *tonicity*, which refers to the concentration of solutes that are "effective" in eliciting a water shift between body fluid compartments. Tonicity should be distinguished from *osmolality*, which refers to the concentration of all solutes, some of which permeate freely and equilibrate across most cell membranes. Molecules in this category include urea and glucose. However, urea and glucose do contribute to the laboratory measurement of fluid osmolality. Addition or removal of effective solutes causes a sustained shift of water to restore the near equality of concentrations. The restriction of sodium to the ECF compartment by virtue of the pump-leak mechanism, together with maintenance of osmotic equilibrium between the ECF and ICF, ensures that ECF volume is determined principally by the total body fluid sodium content, which governs the partitioning of fluid between the ECF and ICF compartments. The addition or removal of water without solutes results in a proportionate reduction or increase, respectively, in both osmolality and tonicity of all body fluid compartments.

The mechanisms that govern body fluid homeostasis preserve near constancy of the volumes of the ECF and ICF compartments despite variations in dietary intake and extrarenal losses of sodium and water and adjust this balance in response to variations in the capacity of these compartments. Thus, the overriding principle of body fluid and solute homeostasis is mass balance of total body intake and output of water as well as balance of osmotically active particles. Even the slightest perturbations in these parameters activate neural and hormonal mediators for restoration of balance. This restoration of balance is achieved through adjustments in the urinary excretion of sodium and water in response to perceived changes in ECF or ICF volume. Constancy of ECF volume together with control of vascular capacitance ensures a high degree of circulatory stability.

Intracellular Water (2/3)		Extracellular Water (1/3): Interstitial (2/3) / Blood (1/3)
25	Na	140
150	K	4.5
15	Mg	1.2
0.01	Ca	2.4
2	Cl	100
6	HCO_3	25
50	Phos	1.2

A

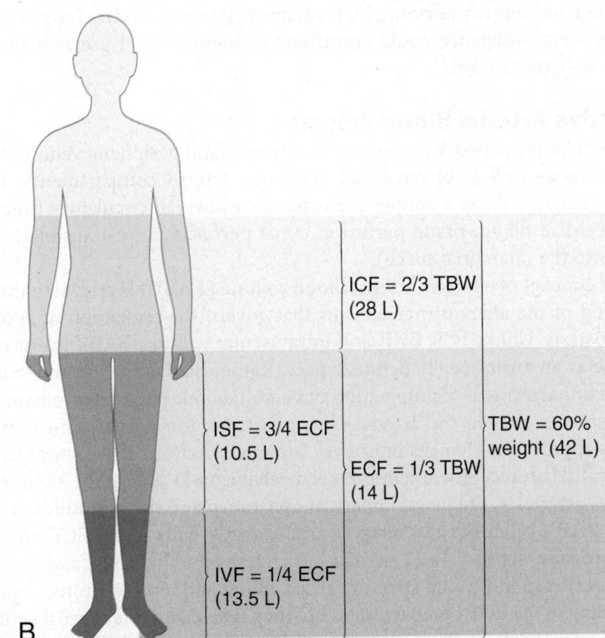

FIGURE 116-1. Composition of body fluid compartments. Schematic representation of (A) electrolyte composition of compartments in humans and (B) body fluid compartments. In A, electrolyte concentrations are in millimoles per liter; intracellular concentrations are typical values obtained from muscle. In B, shaded areas depict the approximate size of each compartment as a function of body weight. In a normally built individual, the total body water content is roughly 60% of body weight. Because adipose tissue has a low concentration of water, the relative water–to–total body weight ratio is lower in obese individuals. Relative volumes of each compartment are shown as fractions; in parentheses are shown approximate absolute volumes of the compartments (in liters) in a 70-kg adult. ECF = extracellular fluid; ICF = intracellular fluid; ISF = interstitial fluid; IVF = intravascular fluid; TBW = total body water. (B from Verbalis JG. Body water osmolality. In: Wilkinson B, Jamison R, eds. *Textbook of Nephrology*. London: Chapman & Hall; 1997:89-94. Reproduced with permission of Hodder Arnold.)

Sodium Balance

Sodium balance refers to the difference between intake and excretion. In the nonclinical setting, sodium intake is controlled by dietary habits. In the clinical setting, prescribed adjustments in sodium intake and the administration of sodium-containing medications or solutions cause variation to overall sodium intake. Although nonrenal loss is under some regulatory influence (e.g., aldosterone-mediated regulation of sodium concentration in stool and sweat), the fine adjustment of sodium balance in response to changes in intake is mediated by regulation of urinary sodium excretion. In the steady state, urinary excretion of sodium is closely matched to dietary salt intake. This balance depends on a series of afferent mechanisms that sense the volume of the ECF compartment relative to its capacitance and trigger effector mechanisms that modify the rate of renal sodium excretion to maintain ECF volume homeostasis. Normal functioning of these mechanisms in turn is affected by the partitioning of the ECF into two subcompartments: intravascular and extravascular (interstitial) (Fig. 116-1B). The composition and concentration of small, noncolloid electrolyte solutes in these two ECF subcompartments are nearly equivalent, but there is a higher concentration of colloid osmotic particles, mostly molecules of albumin and globulin proteins, in the intravascular compartment. Opposing transcapillary hydraulic and colloid osmotic (oncotic) pressure gradients (Starling forces) favor the net transudation of fluid from the intravascular to the interstitial compartment. At the same time, lymphatic fluid movement from interstitial sites back to the circulation through the thoracic duct ensures that the intravascular subcompartment is replenished and maintains a nearly constant proportion of approximately 25% of the overall ECF, which corresponds to 3.5 L of plasma. The remaining approximately 75% of ECF volume (equivalent to 10.5 L in a normal 70-kg man) is contained in the interstitial space. Because intravascular volume is one of the key determinants of circulatory integrity, preservation of the constancy of ECF volume and appropriate partitioning of the ECF volume between the intravascular and interstitial subcompartments are critical for hemodynamic stability.

A hypertonic interstitial fluid compartment also exists in the skin, where it is associated with a macrophage-mediated increased vasoreactivity in precapillary arterioles, the major resistance vessel of the skin (Chapter 435). Although not directly affecting ECF volume responses, the resulting increase in peripheral resistance could contribute to higher blood pressure in salt-sensitive hypertension.[1]

Effective Arterial Blood Volume

The circulatory network is composed of central and peripheral venous compartments as well as of renal and extrarenal arterial compartments. Each compartment reflects a unique characteristic of overall circulatory function (e.g., cardiac filling, tissue perfusion, renal perfusion, and transudation of fluid into the interstitial space).

The concept of effective arterial blood volume (EABV) is crucial to understanding of the afferent mechanisms that govern the regulation of sodium homeostasis. Unlike ICF, ECF, and intravascular volume, EABV is not measurable as an anatomically defined space. Rather, EABV is best understood in functional terms as an integration of hemodynamic parameters emanating from specific sites in the arterial circuit that monitor tissue perfusion and trigger appropriate changes in urinary sodium excretion. These sites include the carotid baroreceptor and intrarenal mechanisms located at the glomerular afferent arterioles, the juxtaglomerular apparatus, and the peritubular capillaries. EABV often but not always varies directly with actual ECF volume. Low-pressure sensors (e.g., cardiac atrial transmural stretch and tension receptors) respond to the state of cardiac filling and tend to protect against overfilling of the ECF compartment, but they also have a role in renal sodium retention in states of perceived underfilling (Table 116-1). Taken together, the integrated ECF volume–sensing signals elicit an appropriate renal response for modulating sodium excretion in an effort to maintain a constant ECF volume.

The filtered load of sodium vastly exceeds net intake, so tubular reabsorption usually serves as the principal modulator of urinary sodium excretion, the preservation of sodium balance, and the maintenance of a constant ECF volume. Specific luminal membrane sodium transporters or channels at each tubular segment mediate movement of sodium from the luminal fluid into the cell in a carefully regulated manner, followed by extrusion of sodium across the basolateral surface through Na^+, K^+-ATPase and other sodium transporters. Among many others, these regulated luminal transporters include the Na/H exchanger (proximal tubule), the Na-K-2Cl cotransport pathway (loop of Henle), the NaCl cotransporter along the distal convoluted tubule, and the epithelial sodium channel along the connecting and cortical collecting tubule. At some nephron sites, sodium reabsorption is isotonic (e.g., proximal tubule), whereas at other sites, sodium reabsorption exceeds water reabsorption, so tubular fluid has a sodium concentration less than that of plasma (e.g., thick ascending limb of the loop of Henle). Sodium reabsorptive transport pathways are subject to a series of regulatory influences that sense EABV, including the renin-angiotensin-aldosterone pathway, natriuretic peptides, endothelium-derived endothelins and nitric oxide, the eicosanoid-prostaglandin system, guanylin peptides of gut origin, and urotensins. This redundancy of multiple hormonal mediators, which act together with the sympathetic nervous system, renal neural stimulation, and intrarenal physical factors (e.g., peritubular capillary Starling forces, tubule lumen sodium chloride delivery, and tubuloglomerular feedback), underscores the evolutionary importance of regulating urinary sodium excretion to maintain volume homeostasis.

TABLE 116-1 MECHANISMS FOR SENSING REGIONAL CHANGES IN BODY FLUID VOLUME

Cardiopulmonary volume sensors
Atria (neural and humoral pathways)
Ventricular and pulmonary sensing sites
Arterial volume sensors
Carotid and aortic arch baroreceptors
Renal volume sensors
Central nervous system sensors
Hepatic and gastrointestinal tract sensors

Water Balance

Water balance refers to the difference between intake (oral, enteral, or parenteral) and excretion (insensible, gastrointestinal, perspiratory, and renal). Maintaining equivalency of intake and excretion of water ensures constancy of body fluid tonicity (osmoregulation). Osmoregulation ensures that the content of effective solutes in each body fluid compartment determines the volume of that compartment. Positive water balance or negative water balance and the corresponding changes in tonicity and cell volume are sensed by osmoreceptor and thirst center cells in the hypothalamus. The osmoreceptors are situated in the supraoptic and paraventricular nuclei of the hypothalamus; the thirst center is situated in the organum vasculosum of the anterior hypothalamus. Just a 2% change in effective osmolality or tonicity elicits a change in release of the hormone arginine vasopressin (AVP) from the posterior pituitary gland and the perception of thirst (Fig. 116-2A). Endothelin-1 also is released from the posterior pituitary in response to water deprivation and increases plasma AVP levels. Stimulation of thirst depends on centrally produced angiotensin II. A reduction of more than approximately 8% of ECF volume serves as an overriding afferent signal (carried by the ninth and tenth cranial nerves) for the nonosmotically driven release of AVP and also stimulates thirst by means of angiotensin II, even when body tonicity is not elevated (Fig. 116-2B).

The urinary excretion of water depends on the delivery of isotonic sodium-containing filtrate to the thick ascending limb of the loop of Henle, reabsorption of sodium and accompanying electrolytes in the thick ascending limb of the loop of Henle and the distal tubule, and the AVP-regulated reabsorption of the appropriate volumes of solute-free water through aquaporin 2 water channels in the cells of the collecting tubule. The hydro-osmotic movement of water from the collecting tubule lumen to the hyperosmotic milieu of the renal medulla minimizes urinary excretion of the hypotonic fluid generated in the thick ascending limb of the loop of Henle and the distal tubule, thereby promoting positive water balance. In the absence of AVP, this hypotonic fluid is excreted, and negative water balance ensues. Typical levels of urine osmolality that can be achieved in the human kidney by fluctuations in AVP action range between 50 and 1200 mOsm/kg, but this range narrows at the extremes of age or in the presence of intrinsic renal disease.

PATHOPHYSIOLOGY

Disturbances in sodium balance primarily affect ECF volume, and disturbances in water balance primarily affect body fluid tonicity. A cumulative negative balance of sodium (sodium deficit) in the absence of a change in tonicity results in ECF volume contraction (hypovolemia), whereas a cumulative positive balance of sodium (sodium surfeit) results in ECF volume expansion (hypervolemia). In contrast, a cumulative positive body water balance (water surfeit) results in volume expansion of all the body fluid compartments, whereas negative water balance (water deficit) results in volume contraction of all the body fluid compartments. However, because ICF volume is double that of ECF at baseline, the more prominent expansion or contraction in absolute volume terms involves the ICF compartment. Furthermore, maintenance of a surfeit or deficit of water relative to solutes results in a uniform decrease or increase in body fluid tonicity in all fluid compartments. Because the solute composition of the plasma component of the ECF compartment is sampled, a disturbance in tonicity is most commonly detected as an abnormality in plasma sodium concentration (hyponatremia for water surfeit and hypernatremia for water deficit). Disturbances in water and sodium balance frequently occur together, and all combinations of surfeit or deficit can occur (Table 116-2). The clinical approach to a patient with a sodium or water balance disturbance (or both) can be facilitated by careful consideration of which states apply.

SODIUM BALANCE DISORDERS

Hypovolemia

DEFINITION

Hypovolemia is a reduction in the volume of the ECF compartment in relation to its capacitance. In states of absolute hypovolemia, a deficit in sodium

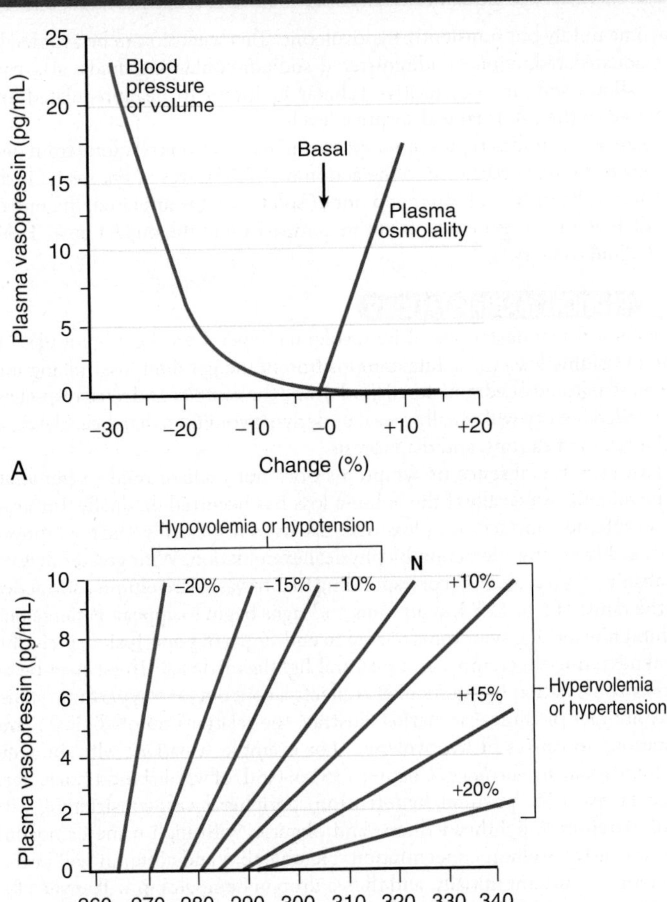

FIGURE 116-2. Relationship between arginine vasopressin (AVP) and osmolality. A, Comparative sensitivity of AVP secretion in response to increases in plasma osmolality versus decreases in blood volume or blood pressure in human subjects. The *arrow* indicates the low plasma AVP concentrations found at basal plasma osmolality. Note that AVP secretion is much more sensitive to small changes in blood osmolality than to changes in volume or pressure. B, The relationship between the osmolality of plasma and the concentration of AVP in plasma is modulated by blood volume and pressure. The line labeled N shows plasma AVP concentrations across a range of plasma osmolality in an adult with normal intravascular volume (euvolemic) and normal blood pressure (normotensive). The lines to the left of N show the relationship between plasma AVP concentration and plasma osmolality in adults whose low intravascular volume (hypovolemia) or blood pressure (hypotension) is 10%, 15%, and 20% below normal. Lines to the right of N are for volumes and blood pressure 10%, 15%, and 20% above normal. Note that hemodynamic influences do not disrupt the osmoregulation of AVP but rather raise or lower the set point and possibly also the sensitivity of AVP secretion in proportion to the magnitude of the change in blood volume or pressure.

TABLE 116-2 PATHOGENIC PROCESSES LEADING TO DISORDERS OF BODY SODIUM AND FLUID HOMEOSTASIS

CLINICAL STATE	EXTRACELLULAR FLUID VOLUME	BODY FLUID TONICITY	PATHOGENIC PROCESS
Normal	↔	↔	
Hypovolemic hypernatremia	↓	↑	Net loss of water in excess of sodium
Hypovolemic normonatremia	↓	↔	Isotonic net loss of sodium and water
Hypovolemic hyponatremia	↓	↓	Net loss of sodium in excess of water
Normovolemic hyponatremia	↔	↓	Net water gain ± sodium loss
Normovolemic hypernatremia	↔	↑	Net water loss ± sodium gain
Hypervolemic normonatremia	↑	↔	Isotonic net gain of sodium and water
Hypervolemic hyponatremia	↑	↓	Hypotonic net gain of sodium and water
Hypervolemic hypernatremia	↑	↑	Hypertonic net gain of sodium and water

↔ = unchanged.

TABLE 116-3 CAUSES OF ABSOLUTE AND RELATIVE HYPOVOLEMIA

EXTRARENAL

Absolute
- Bleeding
- Gastrointestinal fluid loss (diarrhea, vomiting, ileostomy or colostomy secretions)
- Fluid loss from skin (burns, sweat)
- Respiratory fluid loss

Relative
- Third space loss
- Sepsis

RENAL

Absolute
- Diuretics
- Inherited sodium-wasting tubulopathies
- Tubulointerstitial diseases
- Partial obstruction or postobstruction etiology
- Endocrine disorders (e.g., hypoaldosteronism, adrenal insufficiencies)

Relative
- Nephrotic syndrome

reflects past or ongoing negative sodium balance. The volume of the ECF intravascular and extravascular (interstitial) subcompartments may vary in the same or opposite directions. ICF volume is reflected by the measurement of plasma osmolality and sodium concentration and may be concomitantly disturbed (see Table 116-2).

EPIDEMIOLOGY

Causes of absolute and relative hypovolemia can be categorized into extrarenal and renal causes (Table 116-3). Gastrointestinal fluid loss and massive bleeding are the most frequent and direct causes of a reduction in the absolute volume of the intravascular subcompartment of the ECF (Chapters 106 and 135). Infectious diarrhea remains a leading cause of death from hypovolemia in many areas of the world. Another extrarenal cause of absolute hypovolemia is fluid loss from the integumentary and respiratory systems. Burns (Chapter 111), which allow the loss of large volumes of plasma and interstitial fluid, can rapidly lead to profound hypovolemia similar to what is seen with bleeding (Chapter 135). Enhanced evaporative water loss from the respiratory tract can occur with exercise, in response to heat stress (Chapter 109), in febrile states, and in patients undergoing mechanical ventilation with inadequate humidification.

In *relative hypovolemia*, ECF volume is not reduced in absolute terms but the capacitance of the ECF or intravascular compartment is expanded, thereby leading to clinical manifestations that mimic those of absolute hypovolemia. Relative hypovolemia can be classified into two categories: states of vasodilation and states of generalized edema. Vasodilation occurs in response to endogenous endothelial substances (e.g., nitric oxide) or exogenous agents (such as vasodilator drugs). Peripheral vasodilation occurs in sepsis (Chapter 108) and normal pregnancy (Chapter 239). "Third space" loss refers to states in which ECF is sequestered into compartments within the body without an evident history of fluid loss. Included in this category are gastrointestinal obstruction, sequestration of fluids in subcutaneous tissue after trauma or burns (Chapter 111), and sequestration in the retroperitoneal or peritoneal space in patients with pancreatitis (Chapter 144) or peritonitis (Chapter 142), respectively.

Renal causes of absolute hypovolemia include any situation in which tubular reabsorption of the filtered sodium load does not match the sum of this filtered load plus dietary intake, thereby leading to a renal sodium-wasting state. Most of the widely used diuretic (or, more appropriately, natriuretic) medications inhibit specific pathways for sodium reabsorption at various sites along the nephron. Loop diuretics (furosemide, bumetanide, torsemide, and ethacrynic acid) are the most potent, and their potential to induce renal sodium loss is augmented when they are combined with other classes of diuretic agents (thiazides, carbonic anhydrase inhibitors, aldosterone antagonists, and distal epithelial sodium-channel blockers). Tubular sodium reabsorption also may be disrupted by inherited or acquired renal tubulopathies, such as various forms of proximal tubulopathy and different forms of Bartter and Gitelman syndromes (Chapter 128).

Impairment of renal tubule sodium reabsorption may also occur with nonoliguric acute kidney injury and the recovery phase after oliguric acute kidney injury or after release of urinary obstruction (Chapters 120 and 123). Interstitial renal disease (Chapter 122) may result in fluid and electrolyte abnormalities, which can include renal sodium wasting. Nonelectrolyte urinary solutes such as glucose (in severe hyperglycemia) and mannitol cause polyuria and hypovolemia. Mineralocorticoid deficiency and resistance, including adrenal insufficiency (Chapter 227), should always be considered in a patient with evidence of urinary sodium loss in the face of hypovolemia. In cerebral salt wasting (also referred to as renal salt wasting), tubular sodium reabsorption is impaired in the setting of acute head injury (Chapter 399) or intracranial hemorrhage.

PATHOBIOLOGY

Extrarenal Causes of Absolute Hypovolemia

The immediate effect of bleeding is a proportionate net loss in plasma and erythrocytes and hence an isotonic reduction in ECF volume. Compensatory hemodynamic responses include tachycardia and vasoconstriction, followed by a shift of fluid from the interstitial to the intravascular compartment because of altered transcapillary Starling hydraulic forces. Additional neural and hormonal responses result in renal sodium and water retention, with the aim of restoring intravascular volume and stabilizing the circulation.

Besides dietary intake, approximately 7 L of isotonic fluid enters the gastrointestinal tract on a daily basis, the bulk of which is reabsorbed to minimize fecal fluid loss. Because this fluid contains varying concentrations of sodium and accompanying anions, enhanced secretion or impaired reabsorption causes absolute ECF volume depletion. The composition of the fluid and electrolyte loss differs according to the cause and source of gastrointestinal fluid loss (Chapters 132 and 140).

Given its large surface area, it is not surprising that fluid losses from the integumentary system can be an important cause of hypovolemia. In the absence of medical intervention, hemoconcentration and hypoalbuminemia ensue; however, because of the isotonic composition of the lost fluid, no changes in plasma osmolality or sodium concentration are expected. Exertion in hot environments increases thermoregulatory fluid losses from the skin in the form of sweat. Fluid loss through perspiration can reach 1 L/hour or more, depending on exertion and environment. The sodium concentration in sweat varies among individuals (range, approximately 20 to 50 mmol/L). Thus, although the fluid loss is hypotonic, a significant sodium deficit and ECF volume contraction can ensue. The extent of hypovolemia and the resulting body fluid composition (plasma osmolality and sodium concentration) will depend on fluid replacement, which is determined primarily by thirst and availability.

All extrarenal causes of hypovolemia are expected to invoke a renal response, whose hallmark is sodium and fluid conservation. Obviously, this expected response is absent when the kidney itself is responsible for sodium loss, whether it is due to the effect of pharmacologic or hormonal influences or to intrinsic renal disease.

Renal Causes of Absolute Hypovolemia

When the glomerular filtration rate (GFR) and plasma sodium concentration are normal, approximately 24,000 mmol of sodium is filtered per day. Even when the GFR is markedly impaired, the quantities of sodium filtered far exceed normal dietary intake. Thus, the small quantities of sodium excreted in urine relative to the filtered load depend on the integrity of tubular sodium reabsorptive mechanisms to match urinary sodium excretion to dietary intake through volume sensing and effector mechanisms. Impairment in the integrity of one or more of these sodium reabsorptive mechanisms can result in a profound sodium deficit and absolute volume depletion.

An underappreciated but frequent clinical setting for renal sodium loss occurs after the administration of high volumes of volume-expanding, salt-containing solutions to hospitalized patients. Such patients are usually in the postoperative or post-trauma setting and may be administered many liters of saline or other sodium-containing maintenance intravenous fluids for several consecutive days, during which tubular reabsorption of sodium is downregulated. There may be a lag in the restoration of full tubular reabsorptive capacity when intravenous fluids are discontinued, and high volumes of urine rich in sodium continue to be excreted. During this lag phase, the patient may become mildly but transiently hypovolemic. This scenario can be avoided by a graduated reduction in administered sodium-containing fluids, at a pace that allows sodium reabsorptive tubular pathways to be upregulated and restored to their normal reabsorptive levels.

Diabetes insipidus represents a spectrum of conditions resulting from deficiency or tubular resistance to the action of AVP. However, because it is the tubular reabsorption of water and not of solutes that is impaired, the impact on ECF volume is generally minor in comparison to the impact on ICF and body fluid tonicity.

CLINICAL MANIFESTATIONS

The clinical manifestations of hypovolemia depend on the magnitude and rate of volume loss, the solute composition of the net fluid loss (taking into account ingested or administered fluids), and the vascular and renal responses. A detailed history will usually reveal underlying vomiting, diarrhea, bleeding, polyuria, medications, and diaphoresis.

However, the absence of symptoms does not exclude mild to moderate hypovolemia, especially if the volume loss has occurred gradually. Intravascular volume contraction of less than 5% does not usually elicit symptoms and readily escapes detection by physical examination. With greater degrees of absolute hypovolemia (corresponding to intravascular volume contraction in the range of 5 to 15%), symptoms and signs begin to appear. Patients may exhibit nonspecific symptoms related to end-organ hypoperfusion, including weakness, muscle cramps, and postural lightheadedness. Thirst may be an early manifestation but more likely reflects a concomitant hypertonic state.

A number of clinical scenarios illustrate the relationship of clinical manifestations to causes of hypovolemia. For example, a patient with an acute *gastrointestinal hemorrhage* (Chapter 135) of 0.5 L of whole blood can experience tachycardia, postural hypotension, peripheral vasoconstriction with cool extremities, lightheadedness, and oliguria, with high urine osmolality and low urine sodium concentration. Hemoglobin and albumin will probably remain constant initially, and then a drop in hemoglobin will ensue after movement of ECF from the interstitial to the intravascular compartment. The plasma solute composition (sodium and potassium concentrations, acid-base parameters) is not likely to change initially. The plasma concentration of urea may rise somewhat as a result of increased proximal tubular reabsorption of urea and the increased nitrogen load from the destruction of erythrocytes in the gastrointestinal tract. Jugular venous pressure is expected to fall, and central venous pressure (CVP) will generally be less than 5 cm H_2O in the absence of confounding factors. Urine output is expected to be low, with a high specific gravity and osmolality and a low urine sodium concentration.

In another scenario, a patient inappropriately receiving potent *loop diuretics* during a period of many days for localized peripheral edema may suffer a cumulative net ECF loss of 3 L, or about 20%; approximately one third of this lost volume will have originated from the intravascular compartment, with the remainder coming from the interstitial compartment. This degree of intravascular loss usually induces weakness, tachycardia, low jugular venous pressure, and hypotension. However, because the deficit may have accumulated over time, a degree of adaptation would attenuate the severity of these clinical manifestations and lead the clinician to underestimate the extent of hypovolemia. The plasma sodium concentration may remain unaltered because disruption of the urine-concentrating mechanism by loop diuretics attenuates the tendency to water retention, and an intact thirst mechanism prevents hypertonicity. Because loop diuretics enhance urinary potassium and ammonium excretion, hypokalemic metabolic alkalosis is expected. The ongoing effect of the loop diuretic would mitigate oliguria and lead to inappropriately high concentrations of solutes including sodium and potassium in urine. After cessation of the loop diuretic, the appropriate renal response of oliguria, high urine osmolality, and sodium concentration would be expected.

A third scenario is a patient with relative hypovolemia due to the vasodilation that typically accompanies *sepsis* (Chapter 108). No source of fluid loss would be identified in the history, but the patient would usually manifest symptoms of weakness and even prostration, accompanied by tachycardia and hypotension. The extremities might be warm, but reduced tissue perfusion could reduce the level of consciousness and cause oliguria, elevated plasma urea and creatinine levels, and lactic acidosis.

DIAGNOSIS

The most readily appreciated physical findings related to contraction of the intravascular compartment include tachycardia, orthostatic hypotension, and reduced jugular venous pressure. Although low CVP often reliably reflects intravascular volume contraction, an elevated CVP does not necessarily exclude hypovolemia because of the possible confounding influence of cardiac or lung disease. Severe degrees of hypovolemia (corresponding to intravascular volume contraction exceeding 10 to 20%) cause hypotension (even in the supine position), peripheral cyanosis, cold extremities, and reduced levels of consciousness (extending even to coma) as a result of end-organ and cerebral hypoperfusion. Hemodynamic collapse (hypovolemic shock; Chapter 106) also can occur with more rapid volume loss, comorbid conditions, and greater degrees of hypovolemia. When the source of volume loss is purely extrarenal, oliguria is expected. Physical findings, such as reduced skin or eyeball turgor and dry mucous membranes, are not reliable indicators of hypovolemia.

Laboratory Findings

Laboratory measurements are an adjunct to clinical assessment but do not replace symptoms and physical examination findings as a primary diagnostic tool. Decreases in *hemoglobin* may indicate past or ongoing bleeding, but a normal or stable hemoglobin level does not exclude acute bleeding. Hemoconcentration is often observed when hypovolemia is not the consequence of bleeding, but comorbid disease processes that produce anemia may mitigate this rise.

The *albumin* concentration may rise with gastrointestinal, urinary, or skin losses of albumin-free fluids. Conversely, fluid losses that are accompanied by albumin loss (e.g., proteinuria, protein-losing enteropathy) may mitigate this rise or even result in hypoalbuminemia. Similarly, burns and hepatic disease are often accompanied by hypoalbuminemia as a result of the loss or third spacing of protein-rich fluid.

Serum levels of *sodium* and *other electrolytes* also can vary widely. Even subtle and subclinical degrees of hypovolemia trigger urinary water retention and result in a hypotonic, hyponatremic plasma if the patient is exposed to solutions that are more hypotonic than the fluid lost. In contrast, loss of hypotonic fluids with inadequate water ingestion or replacement results in a hypertonic plasma composition and hypernatremia.

Acid-base (Chapter 118) and *potassium* (Chapter 117) changes point to specific causes of hypovolemia. For example, hypokalemia with metabolic alkalosis frequently accompanies vomiting and some causes of diarrhea (e.g., a villous adenoma). More often, diarrheal fluid loss is associated with a non–anion gap metabolic acidosis. Loop and thiazide diuretic-induced hypovolemia is often associated with hypokalemic metabolic alkalosis, as are the inherited tubulopathies (Bartter and Gitelman syndromes) (Chapter 128), which disrupt sodium reabsorptive mechanisms at the loop of Henle and distal convoluted tubule, respectively. Severe hypovolemia with circulatory compromise and tissue hypoperfusion is often accompanied by lactic acidosis.

Increases in *plasma urea* and *creatinine* concentrations are frequently observed in hypovolemic states and reflect reduced renal plasma flow. If acute tubular injury does not supervene, the rise in plasma urea concentration is often disproportionate to the rise in plasma creatinine concentration (see Prerenal Azotemia in Chapter 120). The rise in plasma urea and creatinine concentrations is particularly common when hypovolemia is a consequence of urinary fluid losses. In such conditions, the patient is not oliguric, even though renal plasma flow and GFR are compromised. Other causes of urinary sodium loss, such as occur with adrenal insufficiency or aldosterone unresponsiveness, are accompanied by a tendency toward hyperkalemia and mild metabolic acidosis.

Urinary biochemical parameters may also help in the clinical assessment of hypovolemic states.[2] When fluid loss is extrarenal, the expected renal response of water and sodium conservation occurs, thereby resulting in oliguria with an elevated urine specific gravity (>1.020), an elevated osmolality (>400 mOsm/kg), and a sodium concentration of less than 20 mmol/L because of enhanced renal tubule reabsorptive activity. More complex indices of the appropriate renal response to hypovolemia include fractional excretion of sodium of less than 1% and fractional excretion of urea of less than 30 to 35%. Intrinsic renal injury confounds the diagnostic value of these urinary indices.

Differential Diagnosis

Relative hypovolemia secondary to arterial vasodilation mimics some of the clinical manifestations of absolute hypovolemia. With vasodilation, as seen, for example, in sepsis (Chapter 108), tachycardia and hypotension are common, but the extremities may be warm. However, tissues are actually underperfused, as reflected by reduced renal and cerebral function and lactic acidosis.

TREATMENT Rx

Absolute Hypovolemia

The major goal in treatment of hypovolemia is to restore hemodynamic integrity and tissue perfusion. The management approach includes treatment of the underlying disease state when possible, replacement of the volume deficit, and fluid administration to maintain ECF volume in the event of continuing losses. Irrespective of specific treatments, the mainstay of therapy involves fluid administration. The important issues are the volume, rate of administration, and composition of the replacement and maintenance fluids. These factors may vary during different stages of treatment and should be adjusted according to the patient's response as determined by closely monitored clinical parameters.

The choice of oral or intravenous replacement fluids (or both) for hypovolemic states is dictated by the integrity of gastrointestinal absorptive function, by the magnitude of the volume deficit, and by the disturbances in other electrolyte and acid-base parameters. The rate of replacement is a function of the urgency of the threat to circulatory integrity and consideration of complications related to overzealous or too rapid correction.

Fluid therapy for hypovolemic states sometimes begins with a diagnostic fluid challenge. In situations in which clinical parameters do not permit a firm diagnosis of hypovolemia, the response to a fluid challenge can be informative and serve as the initial treatment step. For example, a patient with known long-standing compensated heart failure who is being maintained on a therapeutic regimen that includes diuretics may have tachycardia, reduction in blood pressure from baseline values, poor cognition, and renal dysfunction. Such a clinical scenario could have a number of different explanations, including superimposed volume depletion with inadequate left ventricular filling volume. CVP, whether measured directly or assessed by jugular venous pressure, may be misleading in the face of right ventricular dysfunction, but direct measurement of pulmonary capillary wedge pressure does not significantly improve clinical outcomes.[3] Conversely, interventional hemodynamic monitoring to guide fluid resuscitation has been shown, in randomized controlled trials, to lead to lower mortality and a reduced incidence of acute kidney injury in certain postsurgical settings.[A1]

Another example is a patient with hyponatremia in the setting of suspected volume depletion. The degree of volume depletion is often too subtle to be detected by clinical examination, and a therapeutic challenge with fluid of the appropriate composition may be the only option.

The initial volume and rate of therapeutic replacement fluid should be determined by ongoing monitoring of clinical parameters rather than by a priori estimates of volume deficit.[3] In some settings, the clinical state will dictate rapid fluid replacement, as in a patient with unambiguous hypovolemic shock and life-threatening circulatory collapse. In such cases, fluids can be administered at the most rapid rate possible, limited only by intravenous access, until blood pressure and tissue perfusion are restored. However, in most cases, much slower rates are indicated, especially in elderly patients, patients whose medical background is unclear, or those with known comorbid conditions. Replacement fluids of different compositions have disparate volumes of distribution in the body fluid compartments and therefore differ in their efficiency of restoring ECF volume. *Crystalloid solutions* with sodium as the principal cation are the mainstay in fluid replacement therapy for hypovolemic states and are indicated primarily for hypovolemic states that are caused by renal, gastrointestinal, or sweat-based sodium losses. These solutions also are useful initial agents and adjuncts to therapy for the hypovolemia of hemorrhage and burns. *Isotonic saline* is confined to the ECF compartment (except in cases of severe dysnatremia). Thus, retention of 1 L of infused isotonic saline increases plasma volume by about 300 mL, with the remaining portion distributed in the interstitial subcompartment of the ECF. In contrast, a solution of *5% dextrose in water* (D_5W) is equivalent to administering solute-free water and distributes uniformly throughout all body fluid compartments (one third of the retained volume of infusate remains in the ECF compartment and only approximately 10 to 15% in the intravascular compartment). Infusing a given volume of *half-isotonic saline (0.45% sodium chloride plus 5% glucose)* can be considered equivalent to infusing half that volume as solute-free water (distributed throughout body fluid compartments) and the other half as isotonic saline (confined to the ECF compartment). The retained solute-free volume reduces body tonicity and the plasma sodium concentration, potentially beneficial in the follow-up treatment of patients whose hypovolemia is accompanied by hypertonicity and hypernatremia but detrimental for patients with normotonic or hypotonic hypovolemia.[4]

When hypovolemia is accompanied by hypobicarbonatemia (metabolic acidosis), it may be appropriate to design a solution in which a portion of the sodium is accompanied by bicarbonate (Chapter 118). For example, it is possible to add a given quantity of hypertonic sodium bicarbonate to a solution of half-isotonic saline (in which chloride is the anion accompanying sodium) to obtain an isotonic replacement fluid appropriate for the given acid-base status of the patient. Similarly, in patients with concomitant potassium depletion (Chapter 117), especially when it is accompanied by metabolic alkalosis, addition of potassium chloride to the replacement solution may be indicated. A number of crystalloid solutions with predetermined concentrations of potassium, lactate (converted to bicarbonate by the liver), and other electrolytes are commercially available, but it is more appropriate to begin with a sodium chloride–containing solution at a concentration appropriate to body tonicity, then to add other solutes as indicated or at a separate intravenous administration site. This approach provides maximal flexibility in tailoring individualized fluid replacement therapy to the patient's needs. Administration of chloride-restricted intravenous fluids rather than of chloride-liberal intravenous fluids may decrease the incidence of acute kidney injury in critically ill patients.[5]

Colloid-containing solutions include albumin or high-molecular-weight carbohydrate molecules (e.g., hydroxyethyl starch or dextran) at concentrations that exert a colloid osmotic pressure equal to or greater than that of plasma. Banked human plasma is also considered a colloid solution. Because large molecules such as albumin and high-molecular-weight carbohydrates do not readily cross the transcapillary barrier, they are thought to expand the intravascular compartment more rapidly and efficiently than crystalloid solutions. However, randomized trials have not shown any benefit of colloids compared with crystalloids for fluid resuscitation.[A2] Moreover, some large-molecular-weight carbohydrates, such as hydroxyethyl starch, appear to be nephrotoxic and probably should not be used.[A3] In patients with multiorgan system failure and capillary leakage, albumin is both rapidly catabolized and redistributed into the interstitial compartment, so it can aggravate interstitial edema without providing the benefit of intravascular volume repletion. Nevertheless, albumin-containing solutions may be useful in hypovolemia associated with burns (Chapter 111), when cutaneous protein losses are appreciable. Furthermore, because of the capacity for rapid intravascular volume expansion with just a small volume of replacement fluid, colloid-containing solutions are frequently used when rapid intravascular expansion is desired, such as at trauma sites outside of the hospital setting. Overall, crystalloid-containing solutions should be the mainstay of volume replacement therapy.

In theory, blood products can be used for volume replacement in hypovolemic states, and a unit of packed red blood cells remains entirely in the vascular compartment. However, erythrocytes are actually considered part of the intracellular compartment and do not contribute to organ plasma flow. The role of packed red cells in the treatment of hemorrhage is to restore the principal function of the erythrocyte in oxygen carriage and delivery, not as a means of ECF volume replacement.

In addition to replacement fluids, maintenance fluids must be provided to counteract ongoing losses. Such ongoing losses may be a continuation of the underlying disease state (e.g., continued vomiting, diarrhea, polyuric states, or severe burns). The volume, rate of administration, and composition of these replacement fluids are best determined by actual measurements of the corresponding ongoing fluid losses, with appropriate adjustments for the patient's clinical assessment parameters.

Relative Hypovolemia

The treatment approach to relative hypovolemia is more complex than for absolute hypovolemia. When relative hypovolemia is the result of peripheral vasodilation, therapy should be directed toward reversal of the underlying cause and restoration of normal vascular reactivity. Bridging to maintain circulatory integrity until the underlying cause is successfully reversed can be achieved by infusion of an *isotonic crystalloid solution* such as normal saline. In such situations, selection of volumes and rates must be done with extreme caution because there is no absolute deficit and the administered volume will have to be excreted or removed once systemic vascular resistance and vascular capacitance are restored to normal. Furthermore, it is more difficult to estimate an increase in vascular capacitance than it is to estimate an absolute volume deficit. On occasion, it is appropriate to consider the use of vasoconstrictor agents.

Hypervolemia

DEFINITION

Hypervolemia refers to expansion of ECF volume, which varies, even in normal individuals, with dietary sodium intake. Thus, an individual in steady state with low daily dietary sodium intake (e.g., 20 mmol/day, corresponding to approximately 1.2 g of table salt per day) will have correspondingly low urinary sodium excretion, equivalent to dietary intake minus extrarenal losses. A shift to much higher sodium intake (e.g., 200 mmol/day, corresponding to approximately 12 g of table salt per day) will bring the individual to a new steady state characterized by a correspondingly higher urinary sodium excretion rate. This shift is accompanied by an increase in ECF volume, which triggers the sensor and effector mechanisms for increased urinary sodium excretion (described earlier). In most individuals, this increase in ECF volume is not clinically detectable and does not have pathologic consequences. In some individuals, however, this upward shift in ECF volume increases systemic arterial blood pressure. When the sodium surfeit expands the ECF volume beyond the range necessary for the adjustment needed to restore sodium balance, a state of pathologic hypervolemia ensues.

TABLE 116-4 PRIMARY AND SECONDARY RENAL SODIUM-RETAINING STATES

PRIMARY
Oliguric renal failure
Chronic kidney disease
Glomerular disease, including nephrotic syndrome
Severe bilateral renovascular obstruction
Mineralocorticoid excess
Inherited sodium-retaining tubulopathies
SECONDARY
Cardiac failure
Cirrhosis
Idiopathic edema

EPIDEMIOLOGY

Primary and secondary renal sodium retention (Table 116-4) can lead to hypervolemia. Patients with oliguric renal failure of any cause (Chapters 120 and 130) have a limited ability to excrete both sodium and water. Urinary sodium retention can be one of the cardinal manifestations of primary glomerular diseases (Chapter 121), even when the GFR is well preserved. States of *mineralocorticoid excess* (Chapter 227) or enhanced activity are associated with a phase of sodium retention; however, because of the phenomenon of "mineralocorticoid escape," the clinical manifestation is generally that of hypertension rather than hypervolemia. Both heart failure (Chapter 58) and cirrhosis (Chapter 153) are associated with renal sodium retention.

PATHOBIOLOGY

Two pathophysiologic mechanisms can lead to sodium retention with ECF volume expansion. The first involves renal sodium retention that is primary and unrelated to the activation of afferent sensor mechanisms. This category includes primary renal diseases and endocrine disorders characterized by excess mineralocorticoid action. In the second category, EABV is reduced, and afferent sensory mechanisms activate effector responses that drive renal sodium retention. In these conditions, total ECF volume is expanded, but intravascular volume is contracted. Therefore, the volume homeostatic mechanisms of the body mimic those of hypovolemia because of the perception of reduced EABV. The degree of solute-free water retention that accompanies the sodium surfeit has a relatively small influence on the extent of hypervolemia but influences the accompanying tonicity state and determines whether the hypervolemia is hypotonic or isotonic.

When the ECF volume is expanded, the relative distribution between the intravascular and extravascular (interstitial) compartments depends on a number of factors. When cardiac and hepatic functions are normal and peripheral transcapillary Starling forces are intact, the excess ECF volume is evenly distributed between the intravascular and interstitial fluid compartments. In such cases, edema does not occur until there is a substantial surfeit of sodium, and hypertension is expected. In contrast, concomitant disruption of transcapillary Starling forces in a given microcirculatory bed would favor the accumulation of retained fluid at one or more such interstitial locations (e.g., dependent edema progressing to anasarca, ascites, pleural effusion, pulmonary congestion).

Primary Renal Sodium Retention

Patients who retain ingested or administered sodium and water loads expand their ECF volume. In patients with chronic kidney disease, the filtered load of sodium remains well above dietary intake until very late stages of severely reduced GFR; even when the GFR is decreased by as much as 90%, the daily filtered load of approximately 2400 mmol still greatly exceeds dietary intake. Nevertheless, the relationship between tubular reabsorption and filtered load may be disrupted in kidney disease.

Monogenic disorders that cause or mimic enhanced mineralocorticoid activity or are associated with enhanced activity of the distal nephron sodium reabsorptive pathways include Liddle syndrome and pseudohypoaldosteronism type 2 (Chapters 67, 117, and 128). In these conditions and in other causes of mineralocorticoid excess, the only clue to mild hypervolemia may be hypertension, which can be severe. Mineralocorticoid excess, glucocorticoid-remediable hypertension, apparent mineralocorticoid excess, and Liddle syndrome are associated with hypokalemia, whereas pseudohypoaldosteronism type 2 (Gordon syndrome) is often accompanied by hyperkalemia.

Secondary Renal Sodium Retention

With both low-output and high-output heart failure and both systolic and diastolic dysfunction, sodium retention is typical (Chapter 58). Low cardiac output, diversion of cardiac output away from arterial intravascular volume–sensing sites, or a high cardiac output that still is not sufficient to meet tissue demands appears to be a necessary and sufficient condition for initiating renal sodium retention. In the case of cirrhosis with ascites (Chapter 153), hepatic intrasinusoidal hypertension is a sufficient and necessary condition for initiating renal sodium retention. These pathophysiologic disturbances in cardiac or hepatic function disrupt afferent signals that govern normal sodium homeostasis and trigger effector mechanisms that lead to enhanced tubular reabsorption of sodium at multiple nephron sites. At the very earliest stages of disease, sodium retention occurs independently of any measurable or detectable reduction in the volume of the intravascular compartments or any of its measurable subcompartments. At more advanced stages of disease, reduced intravascular volume serves as the overriding stimulus for renal sodium retention and thereby leads to a decompensated state of intractable ECF volume accumulation. The more advanced stages, which often are accompanied by a disproportionate degree of positive water balance and consequent hyponatremia, herald imminent compromise of the GFR. Among the many neuronal and humoral abnormalities that characterize the sodium retention associated with heart failure and cirrhosis are endothelial dysfunction, enhanced sympathetic nerve activity, activation of the renin-angiotensin-aldosterone axis, and resistance to natriuretic peptides. In cirrhosis with ascites (Chapter 153), portosystemic shunting together with translocation of intravascular volume to the splanchnic and venous circulation further compromises EABV. In addition, synthetic dysfunction with resulting hypoalbuminemia favors transudation of fluid into the interstitial compartment. At the level of intrahepatic hemodynamics, intrasinusoidal hypertension results in enhanced hepatic lymph formation. When the rate of enhanced hepatic lymph formation exceeds the capacity for return to the intravascular compartment through the thoracic duct, hepatic lymph accumulates in the form of ascites, and the intravascular compartment is further compromised.

CLINICAL MANIFESTATIONS

In addition to the clinical manifestations of the underlying disease, the clinical manifestations of *hypervolemia* depend on the amount and relative distribution of accumulated fluid in the various ECF subcompartments, including the venous and arterial components of the intravascular compartment (jugular venous distention and hypertension), the interstitial spaces of the extremities, the subcutaneous tissues of the lower back and the periorbital region (peripheral pitting edema, the predominant location of which depends on the patient's position), the peritoneal and pleural spaces (ascites and pleural effusion, respectively), and the alveolar space (pulmonary edema). When cardiac and hepatic function are normal and the transcapillary Starling forces are not disrupted, the excess volume is distributed proportionately throughout the ECF compartment. *Hypertension* may be an early manifestation, depending on cardiac function and the state of systemic vascular resistance. Jugular venous distention (see Fig. 51-3) and peripheral edema (see Fig. 51-7) may be present. Clinically detectable pitting peripheral edema usually signifies the accumulation of at least 3 L of excess interstitial volume. Because intravascular plasma volume is itself only 3 L, any state of generalized peripheral edema must signify ECF volume expansion and therefore past or ongoing renal sodium retention or both.

When cardiac function is impaired because of myocardial disease, valvular disease, or pericardial disease, pulmonary and systemic venous hypertension predominates and systemic arterial pressure may be low as a result of disproportionate accumulation of intravascular volume in the venous as opposed to the arterial circulation (Chapter 58). The presence of transudative ascites (see Fig. 146-4) signifies the substantial accumulation of excess ECF volume in the peritoneal cavity, most commonly secondary to disruption of intrahepatic hemodynamics in the setting of liver disease. Pleural effusions can also be a manifestation of hypervolemia, particularly in the setting of heart failure or advanced cirrhosis with ascites.

DIAGNOSIS

Hypervolemia usually is easily detected by findings of generalized edema, ascites, elevated jugular venous pressure, inspiratory pulmonary crackles, or evidence of the presence of pleural effusion. The prevailing systemic arterial blood pressure often provides a clue about whether the hypervolemic state is secondary to reduced EABV or instead due to primary renal sodium retention. The history and physical examination are often sufficient to yield the diagnosis of an underlying secondary cause of sodium retention, such as heart failure or cirrhosis. Adjunctive laboratory tests providing evidence of cardiac dysfunction or liver disease may be helpful. The presence of glomerular-range proteinuria with hypoalbuminemia indicates a glomerular cause of the sodium retention and hypervolemia. Elevated creatinine points to renal failure, which can be intrinsic or may occur in association with advanced stages of some of the aforementioned conditions, such as heart failure (cardiorenal syndrome) or hepatic cirrhosis (hepatorenal failure). Hypoalbuminemia is characteristic of both cirrhosis and nephrotic syndrome.

A low urine sodium concentration and low fractional excretion of sodium confirm renal sodium retention secondary to a perceived decrease in EABV in the edema states, even in the face of overall hypervolemia. More recently, elevated concentrations of brain natriuretic peptide have been used to support the diagnosis of hypervolemia, particularly in the setting of cardiac failure and renal disease.

TREATMENT Rx

The most important step in ameliorating renal sodium retention is recognition and treatment of the underlying disease. Optimization of hemodynamic parameters in heart failure (Chapter 59), improvement of liver function (Chapter 154), or remission of nephrotic syndrome (Chapter 121) improves or reverses sodium retention. Therapeutic intervention to reduce ECF volume without addressing the underlying disease is often met by complications, especially when ECF volume expansion is associated with decreased intravascular volume or EABV. Nevertheless, three treatment modalities are available to reduce ECF volume directly by inducing negative sodium balance: dietary sodium restriction, diuretics, and extracorporeal fluid removal by ultrafiltration. The modality and the desired rate of sodium removal vary with the clinical setting and depend on the relative distribution of the sodium surfeit and excess volume in the body fluid compartments. Therefore, before initiating any treatment, the clinician should identify the specific disturbances in clinical parameters that are harmful to the patient and monitor the improvement in these parameters during the course of treatment. Harmful manifestations of hypervolemia include hypertension, pulmonary congestion and edema or pleural effusions with compromised respiratory function, hepatic congestion and ascites, and degrees of peripheral edema that compromise skin integrity and predispose the patient to cellulitis. Once ECF volume reduction has removed these threats to the patient's well-being, rates of sodium removal should be slowed significantly. Thus, a patient with mild peripheral edema, small pleural effusions, minimal ascites, jugular venous distention, and normal blood pressure might be managed with sodium restriction and limited use of natriuretic medications to induce a gradual negative sodium balance during a period of many days to weeks. In contrast, a patient with limb- or life-threatening anasarca, pulmonary congestion, or hypervolemia-induced hypertension might require the continuous intravenous infusion of natriuretics or in some cases extracorporeal ultrafiltration therapy.

Sodium Restriction

In the management of chronic hypervolemia, other modalities are futile if they are not accompanied by restriction of sodium intake because renal sodium avidity results in the reaccumulation of ECF fluid as soon as the influence of diuretics has ceased. Dietary sodium restriction in the range of 50 to 100 mmol/day is often recommended and requires abstention from added salt as well as from foods rich in sodium. In acute decompensated heart failure, however, sodium restriction does not augment negative fluid balance over what can be achieved by furosemide alone.[A4] Sodium substitutes can be useful, although caution needs to be exercised in patients with a tendency to hyperkalemia because some salt substitutes contain potassium. Calorie intake and nutritional parameters should be monitored to ensure that an overly draconian diet does not induce protein-energy malnutrition. In hospitalized patients, it is particularly important to ensure that the sodium content of administered intravenous fluids and sodium-containing medications is monitored and reduced to the minimum possible. The practice of infusing sodium-containing solutions on the one hand and simultaneously treating with diuretics has no sound physiologic or therapeutic basis. In one randomized trial, however, the combination of high-dose furosemide and small doses of hypertonic saline was better than furosemide alone for treatment of patients with refractory heart failure[A5] or with ascites.[A6] Water restriction is not appropriate in hypervolemic edema states unless the plasma sodium concentration is less than 135 mmol/L or symptomatic hyponatremia supervenes.

Diuretics

Diuretics and natriuretics (Table 116-5) enhance the urinary excretion of sodium-containing fluid by inhibiting tubular reabsorption at specific nephron sites (Fig. 116-3).

Proximal Tubule Natriuretics

The cardinal example of a proximal tubule natriuretic is acetazolamide, a carbonic anhydrase inhibitor that blocks proximal reabsorption of sodium bicarbonate. Consequently, prolonged use of acetazolamide may lead to hyperchloremic acidosis, in contrast to all other natriuretics, which act at loci before the late distal nephron. Metolazone, a congener of the thiazide class of natriuretics, blocks sodium chloride absorption in the proximal tubule as well as in the early distal tubule. Because the major locus for phosphate absorption is in the proximal nephron, the phosphaturia accompanying metolazone administration considerably exceeds that observed with other thiazide-class diuretics. Proximal tubule natriuretics rarely are used as primary therapy but are used as supplements to loop natriuretics when loop natriuretics alone are insufficiently effective.

Loop Natriuretics

Loop natriuretics, such as furosemide, bumetanide, torsemide, and ethacrynic acid, induce natriuresis by inhibiting the coupled entry of Na^+, Cl^-, and K^+ across apical plasma membranes in the thick ascending limb of the loop of Henle, which is responsible for the reabsorption of approximately 25% of filtered sodium. Loop diuretics, which are the most potent diuretics, continue to be effective even in patients with relatively compromised kidney function.

Distal Tubule Natriuretics

Distal tubule natriuretics, such as hydrochlorothiazide, chlorthalidone, and metolazone, interfere primarily with sodium chloride absorption in the earliest segments of the distal convoluted tubule, where they block the sodium chloride cotransport mechanism across apical plasma membranes. Distal tubule natriuretics generally are used in the same conditions as loop natriuretics are, but not in chronic kidney disease and in disorders of calcium metabolism. Whereas loop natriuretics are calciuretic and are valuable for managing acute

TABLE 116-5 DIURETICS AND OTHER NATRIURETIC MEDICATIONS

DIURETICS IN COMMON USE	DAILY DOSE RANGE	ADVERSE REACTIONS	COMMENTS
Thiazides (oral)		Rash, neutropenia, thrombocytopenia, hyperglycemia, hyperuricemia	Usually not effective below GFR of 30-40 mL/mm (metolazone, 20-30 mL/mm)
Hydrochlorothiazide	25-100 mg		
Metolazone	2.5-5 mg		
Chlorthalidone	20-50 mg		
Loop diuretics (oral or intravenous)			Rapid onset, short duration Split doses in normal renal function; give intravenously in acute situations or if reduced gastrointestinal absorption Can use up to 500 mg furosemide (or equivalent) in severe renal insufficiency
Furosemide	20-320 mg	Ototoxicity at high doses	
Bumetanide	1-8 mg		
Torsemide	20-200 mg		
Potassium sparing		Hyperkalemia	Not very potent
Spironolactone	25-400 mg		
Triamterene	25-100 mg		
Amiloride	5-20 mg		
Eplerenone	25-50 mg		

GFR = glomerular filtration rate.

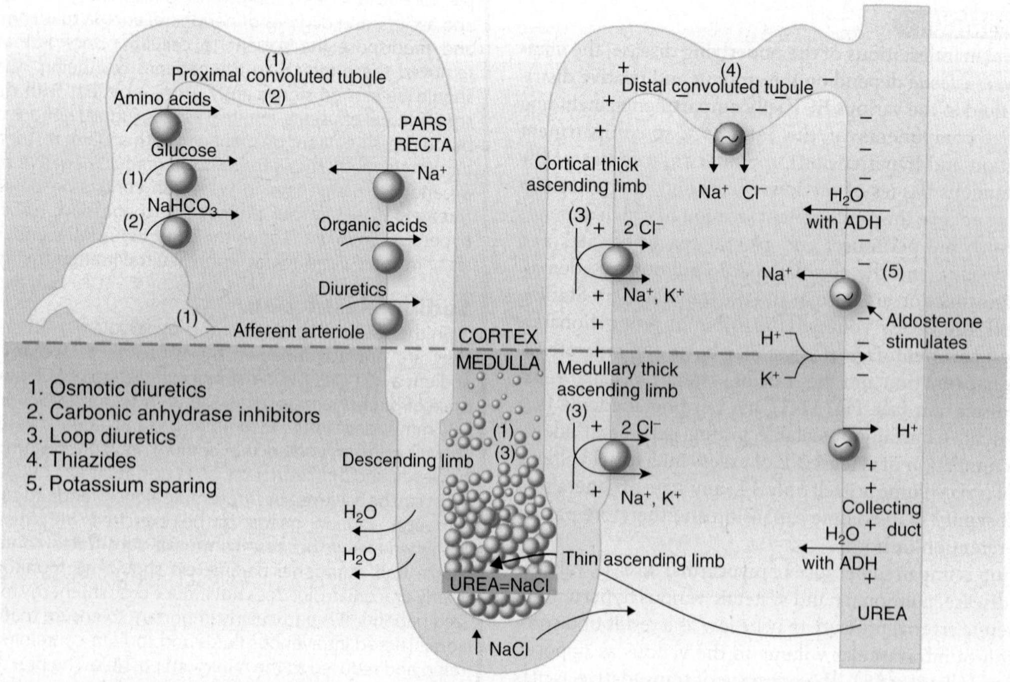

FIGURE 116-3. **Major transport processes along the nephron segments and primary sites of action of diuretics. The site of action of diuretics is shown by numbers in parentheses in each nephron segment; numbers correspond to those next to the diuretics listed in the lower left section of the figure. ADH = antidiuretic hormone. (From Kokko JP. Diuretics. In: Alexander RW, Schlant RC, Fuster V, eds. *The Heart*. 9th ed. New York: McGraw-Hill; 1998.)**

hypercalcemia (Chapter 245), thiazide natriuretics promote hypocalciuria and calcium retention and are useful in managing hypercalciuric states. With the exception of acetazolamide, which impairs bicarbonate absorption, the natriuretics discussed so far can cause hypokalemia and metabolic alkalosis.

Collecting Duct Natriuretics

Spironolactone and eplerenone compete with aldosterone and inhibit sodium absorption in the collecting duct while concomitantly suppressing potassium and proton secretion. Triamterene and amiloride directly block sodium uptake by collecting duct cells and concomitantly suppress potassium and proton secretion. These agents are used in combination with thiazide and loop natriuretics to offset hypokalemia. However, hyperkalemia and hyperchloremic metabolic acidosis may complicate the injudicious use of any of these agents. Spironolactone and eplerenone are useful in managing disorders characterized by secondary hyperaldosteronism (such as cirrhosis with ascites), in promoting natriuresis in hypokalemic patients, and in competitively blocking nonepithelial mineralocorticoid receptors in patients with left ventricular dysfunction (Chapter 59).

Nesiritide is the recombinant version of a naturally occurring brain natriuretic peptide with unique vasodilator and natriuretic actions. Nesiritide given alone may compromise renal function, especially when high levels are achieved after an initial bolus, so its usefulness appears to be limited; frequent monitoring of urine output and of plasma urea and creatinine concentrations is required. However, a recent randomized trial showed therapeutic benefit with the combination of an angiotensin-converting enzyme inhibitor (enalapril) and the endopeptidase inhibitor AHU-377 (a neprilysin inhibitor prodrug, which blocks the breakdown and, hence, augments the levels and activity of endogenous natriuretic peptides) for patients with heart failure.[A7]

Patients with severe degrees of renal sodium avidity can be resistant to conventionally recommended doses of individual classes of diuretic agents. In such patients, combinations of diuretic agents acting at different sites along the nephron may overcome this resistance and induce a natriuretic response.[6] The continuous intravenous infusion of furosemide, sometimes in conjunction with intermittent bolus infusions of albumin, also can overcome natriuretic resistance in some hospitalized patients. Monitoring of plasma sodium, potassium, magnesium, calcium, and phosphate concentrations is mandatory in patients treated with high or frequent doses or continuous infusions of natriuretic agents. Besides body tonicity and electrolyte disturbances, other potential adverse consequences include a reduction in GFR. Drug-specific idiosyncratic adverse responses, such as allergic cutaneous reactions, interstitial nephritis, pancreatitis, and blood dyscrasias, are much less common.

Extracorporeal Ultrafiltration

In a small subset of patients, either superimposed renal impairment or extreme resistance to natriuretic action may require the direct removal of excess ECF volume by ultrafiltration, hemodialysis, or peritoneal dialysis (Chapter 131). Chronic ambulatory peritoneal dialysis has been used for the symptomatic relief of pulmonary congestion and anasarca in some patients with chronic heart failure who are unresponsive to other therapeutic modalities and are not candidates for cardiac transplantation.

WATER BALANCE DISORDERS

Water balance disorders generally come to medical attention because of one or more of three clinical manifestations: hyponatremia,[7] hypernatremia,[8] or polyuria.

Hyponatremia

DEFINITION

Hyponatremia, which is defined as a plasma sodium concentration of less than 136 mmol/L, is the most frequently encountered electrolyte abnormality in hospitalized patients. Hyponatremia, irrespective of the underlying cause, is independently associated with higher mortality.[9]

EPIDEMIOLOGY AND PATHOBIOLOGY

Hyponatremia may be hypertonic, isotonic, or hypotonic. *Hypertonic hyponatremia* occurs when there is an accumulation in the ECF compartment of non–sodium-containing effective solutes, such as very high concentrations of glucose in diabetic patients or exogenously administered mannitol or glycerol. These non-sodium solutes lead to a shift of water from the ICF to the ECF compartments and consequent ICF shrinkage. The accumulation of a solute such as urea, which contributes to the measured plasma osmolality but is not an osmotically effective solute in terms of transcellular water shift, should not be included in the category of hypertonic hyponatremic states. *Isotonic hyponatremia* signifies the laboratory finding of hyponatremia in patients with no disturbances in body fluid tonicity and almost always reflects the interference of marked hyperlipidemia or marked hyperglobulinemia with certain laboratory techniques for the measurement of the plasma sodium concentration; these situations are termed *pseudohyponatremia* and should always be excluded before embarking on diagnostic or therapeutic measures to alter water balance or body tonicity.

True *hypotonic hyponatremia* always reflects an important underlying disorder that leads to abnormal body water retention and either past or ongoing expansion of ICF volume. Even in chronic hypotonic hyponatremic states in which cell volume has been restored to normal by osmotic adaptive mechanisms, the compensation occurs at the price of loss of intracellular solutes and compromised cell function.

Hypotonic hyponatremia can be further classified according to volume status. Heart failure (Chapter 59) and cirrhosis with ascites (Chapter 153) are examples of hypervolemic hyponatremia. In these conditions, reduced EABV stimulates the release of AVP and also may limit the delivery of glomerular ultrafiltrate to the diluting segments of the nephron, thereby leading to impaired water excretion. The hyponatremia that is seen in advanced renal failure (Chapter 130) because of impaired excretion of water may also be associated with hypervolemia.

Hypovolemic hyponatremia occurs when relatively more sodium than water is lost through the gastrointestinal tract (e.g., diarrhea) or in urine (e.g., thiazide diuretics). Decreased body tonicity can also develop even when fluid loss is isotonic or hypotonic (e.g., sweat) if the ingested or administered replacement fluid is more hypotonic than the lost fluid (e.g., ingestion of water or intravenous administration of D_5W).

Another important consideration is the potassium concentration in the lost fluid. For example, diarrheal fluid and natriuretic medication–induced polyuric urine are often rich in potassium as well as in sodium. Because water moves freely across most cell membranes, the ECF and ICF are in osmotic equilibrium. As a result, plasma tonicity is equal to the sum of the effective osmolalities of the ICF and total body water. Given that sodium is the principal determinant of ECF tonicity and potassium is the main contributor to ICF tonicity, plasma sodium is directly proportional to the sum of sodium and potassium concentrations in total body water. Therefore, even if the concentration of lost sodium alone is less than that in the ECF, combined loss of sodium plus potassium can cause hypotonicity.

CLINICAL MANIFESTATIONS

The finding of hyponatremia is often incidental on routine laboratory testing, on laboratory testing of patients with nonspecific complaints, or as part of the investigation of other clinical syndromes. The symptoms of hypotonic hyponatremia depend on its duration, severity, and rate of development. When hyponatremia develops rapidly (hours to days), acute brain swelling or cerebral edema occurs and is manifested as headache, lethargy, seizures, and a progressively decreased level of consciousness that can lead to coma and death. In addition, women between menarche and menopause are particularly susceptible to the life-threatening neurologic manifestations of acute hyponatremia, even of relatively mild degree. In contrast, when the rate of decline in plasma sodium concentration is more gradual, osmotic adaptation ensues, and even severe hyponatremia (plasma sodium concentration <120 mmol/L) may induce few or only subtle clinical manifestations.

DIAGNOSIS

After immediate assessment of the clinical urgency of the situation, the first step in the diagnostic approach to a patient with hyponatremia is to establish the presence of true hypotonic hyponatremia. Plasma electrolytes, urea, glucose, and osmolality should be checked to allow comparison of the measured with the calculated plasma osmolality according to the following equation:

$$\text{Plasma osmolality (mOsm/kg)} = 2\text{Na}^+ \text{(mmol/L)} + (\text{blood urea nitrogen [mg/dL]}/2.8) + (\text{glucose [mg/dL]}/18)$$

A careful history, including a search of the medical record for previous plasma sodium values, will help to indicate the rate of decline. The history and physical examination usually provide important clues to underlying disorders, disease states, or medication exposures that can inform the diagnosis. A history of weight gain or loss also can be helpful in the assessment of recent fluid mass balance. The physical examination should focus on attempts to establish the state of ECF volume. The presence of generalized edema with jugular venous distention and ascites, especially in the setting of heart or liver disease, points clearly to hypervolemic hyponatremia. Conversely, orthostatic hypotension and tachycardia, particularly in the setting of a history of

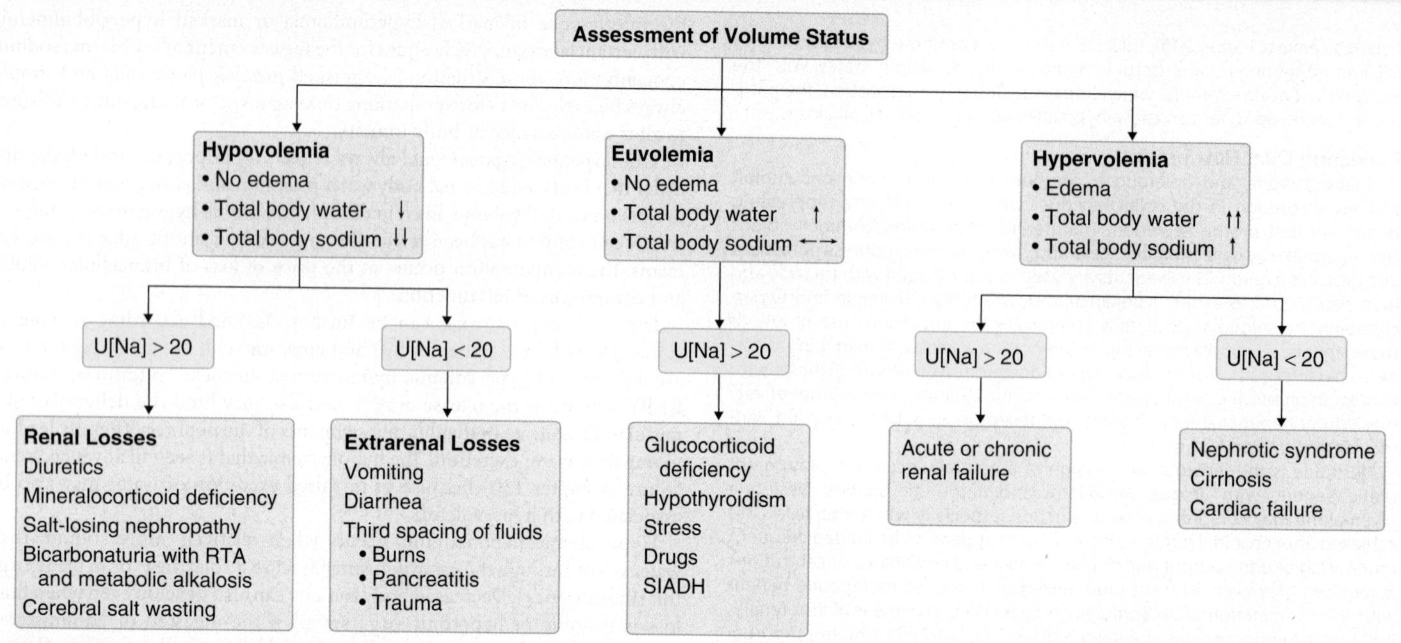

FIGURE 116-4. Diagnostic approach to hyponatremia. RTA = renal tubular acidosis; SIADH = syndrome of inappropriate antidiuretic hormone secretion. (Modified from Halterman R, Berl T. Therapy of dysnatremic disorders. In: Brady H, Wilcox C, eds. *Therapy in Nephrology and Hypertension*. Philadelphia: Saunders; 1999:256.)

natriuretic medication use or gastrointestinal fluid losses, suggest hypovolemia, but the absence of these findings does not exclude hypovolemia.

Further laboratory tests should include a repeated set of plasma electrolyte concentrations, including potassium and chloride levels, which together with determination of acid-base parameters (pH, P_{CO_2}, and bicarbonate) can point to processes not always detectable in the history, such as vomiting, diarrhea, or natriuretic medication exposure. Other laboratory tests should include liver function tests and measurement of plasma urea, creatinine, uric acid, thyroid-stimulating hormone, and cortisol concentrations and, if indicated, an adrenocorticotropic hormone stimulation test. High levels of both urea and creatinine point to intrinsic renal disease, whereas a disproportionate elevation of urea over creatinine might support hypovolemia with a tendency to prerenal azotemia (Chapter 120). In contrast, very low levels of urea and uric acid are typical of both the syndrome of inappropriate antidiuretic hormone secretion (SIADH) and the cerebral salt-wasting syndrome.

Marked elevation in the plasma glucose concentration increases both measured and calculated plasma osmolality and indicates a state of hypertonic hyponatremia that should be approached as a state of body fluid hypertonicity with cell shrinkage (see later) rather than hypotonicity. The plasma sodium concentration declines by approximately 1.6 mmol/L for each increase of 100 mg/dL (5.5 mmol/L) in plasma glucose concentration. However, this decline in plasma sodium is variable and is greater in states of progressively severe hyperglycemia. In contrast to hyperglycemia, an elevated urea concentration should not be considered as contributing to plasma or ECF tonicity, even though urea does contribute to the laboratory measurement of plasma osmolality. Thus, a hyponatremic patient with a normal or elevated laboratory measurement of plasma osmolality that can be fully attributed to an increased urea concentration should be considered as having hypotonic hyponatremia. A discrepancy in which measured plasma osmolality exceeds calculated plasma osmolality and that cannot be attributed to either glucose or urea indicates the presence of an unidentified small solute (osmolar gap), including alcohols (e.g., ethanol, methanol, ethylene glycol, and isopropyl alcohol) and the organic anions of weak acids, which raise the plasma anion gap. Because these small molecules are not effective solutes in terms of water movement, the water balance and tonicity status of the patient is determined by the plasma sodium concentration. Just as for urea, a patient with hyponatremia and normal or elevated measured plasma osmolality as a result of one of these small solutes should be approached as having a true hypotonic hyponatremia, notwithstanding the normal or elevated plasma osmolality measurement. However, the finding of such an osmolar gap should prompt a thorough investigation for poisoning, intoxication, or an organic acidosis (Chapter 118).

Once a state of true hypotonic hyponatremia has been established, determination of the cause and further diagnostic approach follow a classification into one of three categories based on assessment of the volume status of the patient (Fig. 116-4). Abnormal liver function test results can provide adjunctive support for hepatic disease and a hypervolemic hyponatremic state. The diagnosis of heart failure should be made clinically, but it can be assisted by a brain natriuretic peptide level, chest radiograph, or echocardiograph (Chapter 58). A radiograph or chest computed tomography scan may help identify intrathoracic lesions that are associated with SIADH.

Approximately 85% of hyponatremic inpatients have true hypotonic hyponatremia. Among these patients, about 25% are hypovolemic, about 25% have an edema state, about one third are normovolemic, and most of the remainder have renal failure.

In the absence of a clinically obvious edema state, a low urine sodium concentration (<20 mmol/L) or a low fractional excretion of sodium (<1%) supports the diagnosis of hypovolemic hyponatremia secondary to extrarenal losses or past renal losses that have since abated. If hypovolemia is due to ongoing renal losses, the urine sodium concentration may remain high in the face of hypovolemia, but a low fractional excretion of urea (<35%) may still be evident. High urinary concentrations of potassium point to persistent renal loss, such as from the ongoing effect of potassium-depleting natriuretic drugs. Conversely, potassium loss due to diarrhea or vomiting would lead to renal potassium retention and low urinary concentrations of potassium (<20 mmol/L). In SIADH, the urine sodium concentration often reflects sodium intake as well as mild volume expansion and is therefore most often higher than 40 mmol/L and frequently higher than 100 mmol/L. Hypotonic hyponatremia in a patient without evidence of either hypovolemia or hypervolemia, together with low plasma urea and uric acid concentrations without hypothyroidism or adrenal insufficiency, strongly suggests SIADH. If there is any doubt about the presence of hypovolemia, a carefully monitored volume challenge can be of diagnostic as well as therapeutic benefit (see later). Lack of sustained improvement after an adequate salt-containing volume challenge lends further support to the diagnosis of SIADH. Once the diagnosis of SIADH has been established in this manner, the cause should be sought, including a thorough review of medication exposure, review of the history for symptoms and signs of malignant disease, and magnetic resonance imaging or computed tomography of the brain and chest (Table 116-6).

Hypervolemic Hyponatremia

A patient with hypervolemic hyponatremia suffers from a surfeit of both sodium and water, but the surfeit of water is disproportionate to that of sodium. Once the hypervolemic state has been established, the cause of the sodium surfeit should be determined. The most frequent causes are heart failure, decompensated cirrhosis with ascites, and renal failure. The occurrence of hyponatremia in any of these conditions often signifies advanced disease, although it may be due to overzealous sodium deprivation while the patient is taking natriuretic medications. Patients who have heart failure or cirrhosis with ascites experience avid renal sodium retention with urine sodium concentrations of less than 20 mmol/L and fractional sodium excretion of less than 1% in the face of clear-cut clinical evidence of ECF volume

TABLE 116-6 CAUSES OF THE SYNDROME OF INAPPROPRIATE ANTIDIURETIC HORMONE SECRETION

MALIGNANT NEOPLASIA
Carcinoma: bronchogenic, pancreatic, duodenal, ureteral, prostatic, bladder
Lymphoma and leukemia
Thymoma and mesothelioma
CENTRAL NERVOUS SYSTEM DISORDERS
Trauma
Infection
Tumors
Porphyria
PULMONARY DISORDERS
Tuberculosis
Pneumonia
Fungal infections
Lung abscesses
Mechanical positive-pressure ventilation
DRUG INDUCED
Carbamazepine
Desmopressin
Oxytocin
Vinca alkaloids
Alkylating agents/antimetabolites
Interferons
Anticonvulsants
Antipsychotic agents
Nicotine
Cyclophosphamide
Morphine
Amitriptyline
Selective serotonin reuptake inhibitors
3-4-Methylenedioxymethamphetamine (Ecstasy)

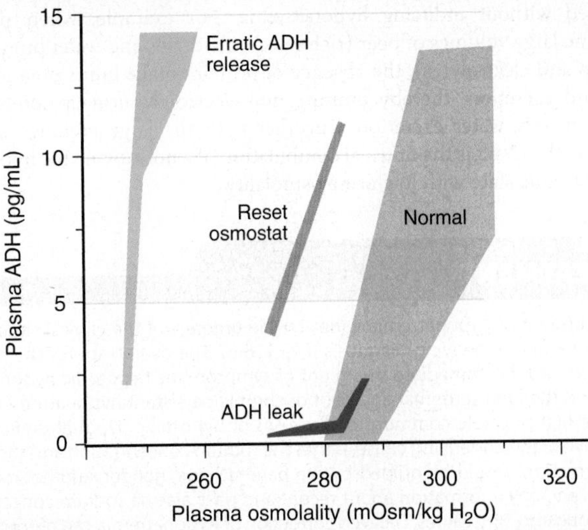

FIGURE 116-5. Patterns of serum antidiuretic hormone (ADH) abnormalities in the syndrome of inappropriate ADH secretion (SIADH). The shaded area to the right indicates the normal relationship between increases in effective extracellular osmolality and ADH levels; the normal osmotic threshold is lower than the normal serum osmolality. The three other shaded areas indicate ADH patterns in SIADH from various causes. (Modified from Zerbe R, Strope L, Robertson G. Vasopressin function in the syndrome of inappropriate diuresis. *Annu Rev Med.* 1980;31:315-327.)

expansion, usually with generalized edema. However, these urine parameters can be masked by the ongoing influence of natriuretic agents. The edema state of the nephrotic syndrome is less commonly associated with hyponatremia unless the patient has been exposed to severe salt restriction and natriuretic therapy. Water retention with hyponatremia is a feature of renal failure only in its more advanced stages (stage 4 and stage 5 chronic kidney disease; Chapter 130).

Normovolemic and Hypovolemic Hyponatremia

It is often difficult to distinguish normovolemic from hypovolemic hyponatremia because mild hypovolemia can easily escape clinical detection. The initial history and physical examination should try to establish or to exclude a cause of hypovolemia. In extrarenal hypovolemia, a low urine sodium concentration and low fractional excretion of sodium are characteristic. When the hypovolemia is due to urinary loss, the urine sodium concentration is usually elevated rather than decreased.

Hypovolemic hyponatremia always signifies past or ongoing sodium loss (often with potassium), accompanied by a degree of net water loss that does not match the electrolyte loss and hence leaves the patient hypotonic. The high levels of AVP that are associated with hypovolemic hyponatremia are usually an appropriate response to the physiologic stimulus of hypovolemia. The most common extrarenal causes of hypovolemia leading to hyponatremia are gastrointestinal fluid losses and excessive sweating. In gastrointestinal fluid losses, any concomitant nausea and vomiting may be independent triggers for the central release of AVP. In unaccompanied patients with impaired consciousness or cognitive dysfunction, clues to vomiting include the characteristic plasma and urine biochemical parameters of metabolic alkalosis (Chapter 118), often with higher than expected urinary concentrations of sodium and bicarbonate. Hyponatremia is a more common complication of diarrhea when the diarrheal fluid is secretory and rich in electrolytes. Sweating-induced hyponatremia occurs when individuals ingest high volumes of hypotonic fluid, often pure water, while losing sodium in sweat.

The renal causes of hypovolemic hyponatremia (see Fig. 116-4) include thiazide-induced hyponatremia and the cerebral salt-wasting syndrome. Thiazide-induced hyponatremia occurs when patients with impaired urinary diluting capacity excrete concentrated urine because thiazides do not affect the ability of the renal medulla to concentrate urine. Thiazide-treated patients are particularly susceptible to hyponatremia when they ingest or receive hypotonic solutions that exceed their maximal capacity to excrete electrolyte-free water in their urine. In cerebral salt wasting (also known as renal salt wasting), patients who have suffered a head injury or intracranial hemorrhage experience a state of negative sodium balance due to inappropriate renal sodium wasting. The consequent ECF volume depletion stimulates the release of AVP, and these patients are prone to the development of hyponatremia if hypotonic fluid is then ingested or administered. The combination of a high urine sodium concentration and hyponatremia makes the syndrome difficult to distinguish from hyponatremia caused by the syndrome of inappropriate secretion of AVP (see later). However, persistently low plasma uric acid levels and high fractional excretion of uric acid, even after correction of the hyponatremia, may be observed in cerebral salt wasting but not in SIADH.

In normovolemic hypotonic hyponatremia, there is neither an osmolar nor a volume stimulus to the release of AVP. Thus, concentrated urine, usually containing concentrations of sodium higher than 40 mmol/L as a result of dietary intake plus the effects of mild ECF volume expansion, indicates either inappropriate secretion or an augmented renal response to AVP. Conditions that can result in inappropriate AVP secretion or responsiveness include tumors, central nervous system lesions or disorders, intrathoracic or chest wall disease, and numerous drugs and medications (see Table 116-6). All syndromes in which the AVP level or the kidney's responsiveness is inappropriately high and not attributable to osmolar or volume stimuli are known collectively as SIADH (Chapter 225). Patterns of abnormal AVP secretion (Fig. 116-5) include an erratic release of AVP from the neurohypophysis without any apparent coordination with incoming volume or osmotic stimuli (type A pattern), a constant low-level leak of AVP from the neurohypophysis (type B pattern), a reduced threshold for osmotic release of AVP at a lower than normal plasma osmolality (type C pattern), and an abnormal renal response to circulating AVP in patients whose neurohypophysial regulation is intact (type D pattern). However, no consistent correlation between these various patterns and an underlying cause has emerged. A specific monogenic disorder involves a mutation in which the AVP V_2 receptor is constitutively active in the absence of ligand. Hypothyroidism (Chapter 226) and adrenal glucocorticoid insufficiency (Chapter 227) can be associated with hypotonic hyponatremia without clinically evident hypovolemia and with a clinical and biochemical profile that mimics SIADH; abnormal regulation of the aquaporin 2 water channel and reduced distal tubular delivery may be involved. Pregnancy, which also is associated with a reduction in both the osmotic threshold for AVP release and thirst, results in mild hyponatremia (Chapter 239). Another unusual setting for normovolemic hyponatremia is the "beer potomania" syndrome. Because the minimal urine osmolarity, even in the absence of AVP, is 30 to 50 mOsm/L, the upper limit of solute-free water excretion depends on total obligate solute excretion. A paucity of available urinary solutes sets an upper limit on the total water intake that can be tolerated without inducing hyponatremia. For example, when patients consume large volumes of beer (rich in carbohydrates and water but poor in sodium and electrolytes), the absence of protein intake limits urea production and excretion, thereby limiting non-electrolyte urinary solutes and hence urinary water excretion. Together with the large volumes of beer ingested, the result is the unusual combination of a normovolemic hypotonic hyponatremic state with low urine osmolality.

TREATMENT

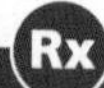

Treatment of hyponatremia varies by the urgency of the clinical situation, its cause, and underlying diagnosis (Fig. 116-6). The overall approach can be divided into the immediate treatment of symptomatic hypotonic hyponatremia and the long-term management of chronic persistent hyponatremia.

The first principle common to all causes of hypotonic hyponatremia, irrespective of the underlying cause, is that the sodium concentration and the rate of correction should be guided by the patient's age, gender, and neurologic status and any information about recent and past plasma sodium concentrations or osmolality values. Delayed correction of hyponatremia can perpetuate cerebral edema and result in irreversible neurologic damage and death, especially in women of reproductive age and in patients whose hyponatremia developed at a rapid pace that outstripped the rate of osmotic adaptation by brain cells. In contrast, overly rapid correction or correction to a sodium concentration that is above the level needed to safeguard the patient from the neurologic sequelae of cerebral edema can result in the *osmotic demyelination syndrome*.[10] This devastating and often irreversible syndrome is characterized by fluctuating levels of consciousness, pseudobulbar palsy, ataxia, dysarthria, difficulty in swallowing, and characteristic abnormalities in the region of the brain stem on magnetic resonance imaging. Osmotic demyelination syndrome can be fatal, and recovery in nonfatal cases is either slow or incomplete, often with irreversible residual neurologic sequelae.

The second principle is the importance of identifying and treating any underlying disorder. Thus, in a patient with hypervolemic hyponatremia associated with heart failure, measures to optimize cardiac function are the most appropriate and effective means of restoring a normal sodium concentration. Indeed, restoration of normal sodium concentration provides one of the most reassuring indices for successful management of this underlying disorder. Conversely, in hypovolemic hyponatremia, appropriate correction of ECF volume will lead to the resolution of hyponatremia.

Acute Hyponatremia

Current guidelines suggest that if the hyponatremia is known to be acute (<24 to 48 hours) and is accompanied by severe neurologic symptoms such as seizures or decreased level of consciousness, correction should be rapid; 4 to 6 mmol/L in 4 to 6 hours should be sufficient to reverse the most severe neurologic symptoms. The total increase in sodium concentration should not exceed 9 to 12 mmol/L (some experts recommend no more than 6 to 8 mmol/L) in the first 24 hours or surpass 18 mmol/L within 48 hours.

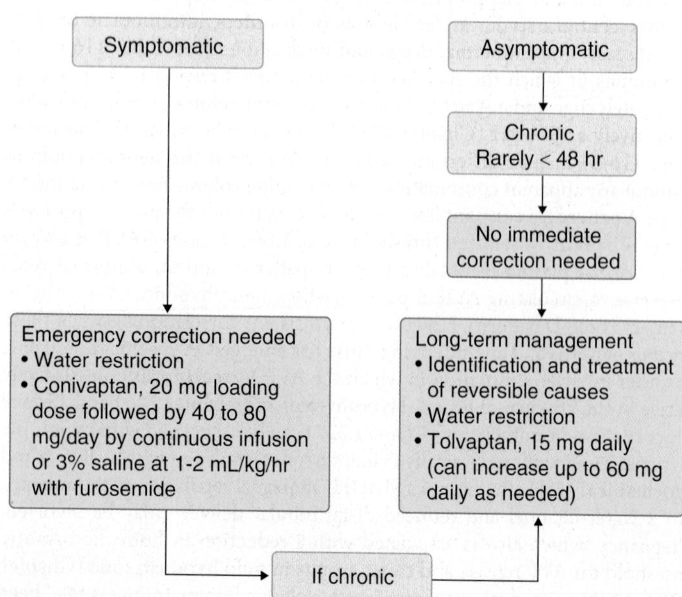

FIGURE 116-6. Treatment of severe normovolemic hyponatremia. (From Thurman J, Halterman R, Berl T. Therapy of dysnatremic disorders. In: Brady H, Wilcox C, eds. *Therapy in Nephrology and Hypertension*. 2nd ed. Philadelphia: Saunders; 2003.)

Chronic Hyponatremia

Mild degrees of hyponatremia can be tolerated for long periods but have been associated with increased risk of hip fractures.[11] Current recommendations are that only symptomatic hyponatremia or sodium concentrations below 125 to 130 mmol/L require specific additional treatment.

If the rate of decline in plasma sodium concentration has been slow, brain cells have the opportunity to undergo osmotic adaptation by extruding or eliminating intracellular solutes. It is this subgroup of patients who are most susceptible to osmotic demyelination after too rapid or overzealous correction of hyponatremia. Patients in whom there is no previous record of sodium concentration or osmolality should be considered in the same category and treated accordingly. In such cases, the targeted rate of increase in sodium concentration should not exceed 0.5 mmol/L/hour, and the total rise in sodium concentration should not exceed 8 mmol/L in any 24-hour period, even (and especially) if the initial sodium concentration is extremely low (<110 mmol/L), provided the hyponatremia is not accompanied by severe neurologic symptoms. Patients with severe degrees of chronic hyponatremia in the setting of malnutrition, alcoholism, or chronic illness are particularly susceptible to osmotic demyelination. Frequent monitoring of the plasma sodium concentration and osmolality is crucial. If the safe target rate of correction is exceeded, osmotic demyelination can be prevented by slowing the correction rate, returning to a lower plasma sodium concentration by the judicious readministration of hypotonic solutions, or administering vasopressin analogues (see later).

A target goal and rate of correction having been established, the approach varies with the underlying diagnosis. In hypervolemic hyponatremia, there is a surfeit of both sodium and water, but in tonicity terms, the excess water is disproportionate to the excess sodium. Thus, the goal of treatment is to remove both sodium and water but to replace proportionately less water than sodium. Water restriction is helpful but is often inadequate or impractical because patients are thirsty, and their adequate nutrition requires calorie intake that is accompanied by obligate water ingestion and metabolic water production. The AVP V_2-receptor antagonists tolvaptan (starting at 15 mg once daily, with a maximal dose of 60 mg once daily) ameliorates hyponatremia and improves symptoms and outcomes in patients with hypervolemic hyponatremic syndromes, including decompensated heart failure and hepatic cirrhosis.[12] Moreover, in a randomized trial in patients with acute decompensated heart failure, tolvaptan alone was found to have a diuretic effect superior to that of furosemide alone; the combination of the two drugs produced a diuresis similar to that of tolvaptan alone.[A8] In another randomized placebo-controlled trial, a newer member of the vaptan group, lixivaptan, also was effective as an add-on diuretic to standard therapy in the management of acute decompensated heart failure.[A9] Vaptans are also useful in normovolemic hyponatremic states, such as SIADH (see later), but should be assiduously avoided in hypovolemic hyponatremic states.

Hypovolemic Hypotonic Hyponatremia

A frequent diagnostic dilemma is the distinction between hypovolemic and normovolemic hypotonic hyponatremia. When hypovolemia is clearly evident (appropriate clinical history, orthostatic hypotension, low urine sodium concentration in the setting of extrarenal fluid losses, elevated plasma urea disproportionate to the rise in the serum creatinine level, and elevated uric acid concentrations), administration of volume repletion in the form of isotonic saline is the treatment of choice. The salutary effect of saline derives mostly from the effect of volume repletion to remove the hypovolemic stimulus to release of AVP, thereby inducing a water diuresis, with a minor contribution of the osmolar effect of the infused solute. However, great caution should be exercised in the administration of isotonic saline to these patients because the administration of small volumes of isotonic saline can sometimes induce a brisk and rapid decrease in urine osmolality and an accompanying water diuresis, with an overly rapid correction of hyponatremia. Accordingly, whenever isotonic saline or other forms of volume repletion therapy are administered to patients with known or suspected hypovolemic hyponatremia, careful hour-by-hour monitoring of urine output, urine osmolality, plasma sodium concentration, and plasma osmolality is required. A rapid drop in urine osmolality accompanied by water diuresis should prompt cessation of volume repletion and, in some cases, administration of hypotonic solutions or even analogues of AVP itself (see later) to halt or to reverse the rapid rise in sodium concentration to within the recommended guidelines so as to prevent osmotic demyelination. When hypovolemia is not clearly evident but cannot be excluded, a brisk drop in urine osmolality in response to a saline challenge confirms the suspicion of hypovolemia and simultaneously initiates therapy. In contrast, failure to induce such a response lends support to the diagnosis of normovolemic hyponatremia.

Normovolemic Hyponatremia

In patients with normovolemic hyponatremia, the appropriate therapeutic approach is to address the underlying disease. Hypothyroidism (Chapter 226) and adrenal insufficiency (Chapter 227) should be corrected with appropriate hormonal replacement therapy. Medication-induced SIADH mandates identification and cessation of the offending medication when possible. If the underlying disease cannot be identified or reversed, treatment is aimed at removal of the water surfeit. The therapeutic outcome depends on the minimal urine osmolality that can be achieved, which in turn depends on the severity of SIADH. In many cases, when urine osmolality cannot be suppressed below certain high levels, the severity of water restriction required would not be consistent with the need for calorie intake or compatible with reasonable expectations for the patient's adherence. Therefore, maneuvers to generate a gradual net negative water balance are required. In such cases, titrated dose oral tolvaptan (beginning at 15 mg once daily and increasing to a maximum of 60 mg once daily) and reliance on an intact thirst mechanism are crucial to avoid polyuria or hypernatremia. In rare cases with an urgent need to correct the hyponatremia because of a neurologic emergency or definitive documentation that the sodium concentration has decreased acutely during a 24- to 72-hour period, intravenous conivaptan (20 mg loading dose followed by 40 to 80 mg/day by continuous infusion) can be used cautiously to avoid overly rapid correction of hyponatremia.[13] When volume status is in doubt, however, these agents are better avoided until the possibility of hypovolemic hyponatremia has been addressed. Hemodialysis, which can rapidly raise the plasma sodium concentration, should be reserved for the most extreme cases of acute life-threatening hyponatremia for which no other solution is available (Chapter 131).

Hypernatremia

DEFINITION

Hypernatremia, defined as a plasma sodium concentration higher than 144 mmol/L, always reflects a state of hypertonicity, with an increase in the ratio of the concentration of osmotically active solutes to water throughout all body fluid compartments.

EPIDEMIOLOGY AND PATHOBIOLOGY

Because sodium is an osmotically effective ECF solute, hypernatremic patients have undergone a process whereby water has moved from the ICF to the ECF compartment, accompanied by a reduction in ICF volume and cell shrinkage. Cell shrinkage in the brain is associated with intracerebral hemorrhage, which is often punctate but sometimes due to ruptured blood vessels, particularly at the brain surface and arachnoid interface. In an effort to restore their cell volume, brain cells undergo osmotic adaptation by accumulating sodium and other electrolytes and then subsequently producing non-electrolyte small solutes (osmolytes) such as inositol, taurine, glutamine, and glutamate, among others. This process partially reverses cell shrinkage, but at the price of an altered intracellular solute composition with consequent perturbations in neuronal function.

Hypernatremia is the most frequent but not the only hypertonicity state in clinical medicine. Glucose, mannitol, and glycerol can produce hypertonicity states that may not be accompanied by hypernatremia and in fact are frequently accompanied by hyponatremia (see earlier). In hypertonicity states, the measured plasma osmolality is always high, but elevated plasma osmolality is not necessarily associated with hypertonicity because a number of solutes that contribute to the measured plasma osmolality are not osmotically effective in terms of movement of water from the ICF to the ECF compartment. Thus, patients with high concentrations of urea or small alcohols (e.g., methanol, ethylene glycol, ethanol) often have elevated plasma osmolality but should not be considered to have a hypertonicity state.

Although hypernatremia can be diagnosed as an incidental laboratory abnormality, it most commonly occurs in the setting of a severe underlying disease with other accompanying disturbances in body fluid homeostasis (Table 116-7).

In *hypervolemic hypernatremia,* a disproportionate excess of sodium over water expands ECF volume, but owing to water egress from cells in an attempt to restore normal plasma tonicity, ICF volume is decreased. Hypervolemic hypernatremia usually occurs in the hospital setting because of inadvertent or overzealous administration of hypertonic saline, the administration of hypertonic sodium bicarbonate solutions during cardiopulmonary resuscitation, or dialysis against a hypertonic dialysate.

In *normovolemic hypernatremia,* a pure water deficit with no disturbance in total body sodium content or clinically perceptible decrease in ECF volume occurs owing to proportionally greater water loss from the ICF (approximately two thirds) than from the ECF compartment. Thus, for example, a 3-L pure net water deficit will consist of 2 L lost from the ICF but a clinically undetectable loss of only 1 L from the ECF compartment. Nevertheless, a 3-L or greater deficit certainly increases body fluid tonicity and the measured plasma sodium concentration. Clinical conditions in this category require a

TABLE 116-7 CAUSES OF HYPERNATREMIA CLASSIFIED BY TOTAL BODY SODIUM CONTENT

Hypervolemia	Hypertonic saline excess Hypertonic sodium bicarbonate solutions
Hypertonicity with near normovolemia	Diabetes insipidus Febrile fluid loss
Hypovolemia	Gastrointestinal loss (diarrhea, vomiting) Skin fluid loss (burn, sweat) Loop diuretics Osmotic diuresis Impaired thirst perception

source of fluid loss that has a relatively low content of osmotically effective solutes (principally sodium and potassium and their accompanying anions), such as the various forms of diabetes insipidus or the use of AVP V_2-receptor antagonists (vaptans) without adequate monitoring. In these conditions, profuse volumes of low-osmolality urine are excreted. Even so, hypernatremia is actually uncommon as long as thirst perception and availability of water remain intact. The principal clinical manifestation is polyuria and polydipsia (see later). Insensible evaporative losses from the skin and respiratory tract also are a source of hypotonic fluid loss. Increased fluid loss can occur in febrile patients (skin and respiratory tract), patients on mechanical ventilation (respiratory tract), and patients with profuse sweating. The sweat sodium concentration decreases with increasing volumes of perspiration. These conditions also will lead to hypernatremia with body fluid hypertonicity only if the thirst mechanism or access to water is impaired.

Hypovolemic hypernatremia is by far the most common hypertonicity state. Patients with hypovolemic hypernatremia have lost both sodium and water, but the net loss of water is disproportionately greater than the net loss of sodium. The actual plasma sodium concentration resulting from loss of hypotonic fluid depends not only on the sodium concentration of the fluid lost but also on the concentration of other osmotically active solutes, such as potassium, and on the solute composition of concomitantly ingested or administered fluids. The extrarenal and renal causes of such fluid losses are similar to those of isotonic hypovolemia. Among gastrointestinal causes of hypovolemic hypernatremia, diarrhea is more common than vomiting, and osmotic diarrheas result in disproportionately greater loss of water than electrolytes, with a greater propensity to hypernatremia than is seen with secretory diarrheas. Among the renal sources of sodium and water loss, the two most common causes are loop natriuretic medications and osmotic diuresis. Loop natriuretic agents interfere with the countercurrent mechanism and generate large volumes of urine with an iso-osmolar composition. Because some of the solutes are non-electrolyte (urea), the impact on body tonicity may be to increase tonicity, unless there is concomitant intake or administration of hypotonic fluids. In contrast, thiazides do not interfere with the countercurrent mechanism and therefore rarely promote hypernatremia. The presence of non-electrolyte solutes in urine causes an osmotic diuresis. Such solutes can be either endogenous (e.g., urea or glucose) or exogenous (e.g., mannitol or glycerol). The presence of these solutes in tubular fluid impairs both sodium and water reabsorption, but the excretion of urine that is relatively rich in non-electrolyte solutes tends to promote body fluid hypertonicity, unless sufficient hypotonic fluids are ingested or administered concomitantly.

Failure to replace hypotonic fluid losses generally reflects impairment in thirst, disability or infirmity that prevents the patient from responding to thirst, or failure of the clinician to recognize the need for hypotonic fluid replacement. Rarely, impaired thirst in patients who are awake and alert can be caused by damage to the hypothalamic osmoreceptors that control thirst perception and response, a condition known as *primary hypodipsia.* This condition usually tends to be associated with an abnormality in the osmotic regulation of AVP secretion. However, cases have been described in which the osmotic regulation of AVP secretion has been dissociated from the osmotic regulation of thirst. Such patients suffer hypernatremia only when extrarenal fluid losses exceed their habitual water intake, as might occur in settings of thermal stress or exercise.

CLINICAL MANIFESTATIONS

The clinical features of patients with hypernatremia can be divided into those associated with the underlying disease state, those associated with a concomitant disturbance in ECF volume, and those associated with an increase in body fluid tonicity. The main clinically relevant consequence of increased body fluid tonicity is decreased brain cell volume, with the attendant risk for intracerebral hemorrhage. Thus, the major symptoms are neurologic and include confusion, seizures, focal neurologic deficits, and a progressively decreasing level of consciousness that can progress to coma. In the absence of an underlying neurologic problem or disturbance in the thirst mechanism, the patient would be expected to complain of thirst unless the neurologic injury has disturbed consciousness.

In patients with hypernatremia of sufficient duration to enable brain cells to undergo osmotic adaptation, the risk for intracerebral hemorrhage from cell shrinkage is decreased, but a hypertonic intracellular environment with the accumulation of new intracellular solutes can perturb normal cellular function. However, few if any clinical manifestations would be observed in this situation.

DIAGNOSIS

The diagnosis of hypernatremia is made by laboratory testing of the sodium concentration, which always should be repeated to confirm its accuracy, corroborated by measurement of plasma osmolality, which is expected to be elevated in all cases. The underlying cause of the hypernatremia is usually evident from the history and physical examination. The history should include a review of recent and current medication use and questions about exercise, heat exposure, sweating, vomiting, diarrhea, urine output, recent fluid intake, and presence of thirst. Physical examination should include an assessment of ECF volume and a complete neurologic evaluation. Urine volume should be monitored, urine osmolality should be measured in several spot urine samples, and 24-hour urine osmolar excretion should be measured if polyuria is present. In the less common situation of hypervolemic hypernatremia, there is often an antecedent history of the administration of sodium-containing solutions, and the findings on physical examination are consistent with ECF volume expansion. In the absence of underlying intrinsic renal disease or diuretic action, urine osmolality should be high because of the hypertonic stimulus to AVP release, which overrides the attenuating effect of hypervolemia. In such patients, the urine sodium concentration should be elevated in response to hypervolemia.

In the more common condition of hypovolemic hypernatremia with extrarenal fluid loss, urine output should be reduced to less than 500 mL/day, and urine osmolality should be the maximum expected for age (>1000 mOsm/kg in young adulthood decreasing to >600 mOsm/kg by the seventh decade of life and beyond). Polyuria with a submaximal urine osmolality in the presence of hypernatremia suggests impaired urine-concentrating ability, such as occurs with preexisting or underlying intrinsic renal disease or exposure to diuretic agents. A spot urine osmolality measurement of less than 100 to 200 mOsm/kg or polyuria (>3 L/day) together with 24-hour urine solute excretion of less than 600 mOsm/day in the face of hypernatremia suggests diabetes insipidus. In contrast, daily solute excretion exceeding 800 to 1000 mOsm/day suggests an osmotic diuresis, which can be confirmed by measurement of glucose and urea in urine.

TREATMENT Rx

The main components of treatment are to correct the underlying disorder and the abnormality in ECF volume, to replace the water deficit, and to provide maintenance fluids to match continuing ongoing fluid losses if they persist.

The management of serious symptomatic hypovolemic hypernatremia is challenging and often controversial. It is best to divide the therapeutic approach into two separate phases: rapid correction of the depleted ECF volume, followed by gradual replacement of the water deficit, including provision for ongoing fluid losses. When ECF volume contraction is severe, as evidenced by tissue hypoperfusion and shock, administered fluid should have a sodium concentration as close as possible to that of the patient and should distribute to the ECF, especially the intravascular compartment. Isotonic saline is generally the fluid of choice, and the volume and rate of administration should be guided by clinical parameters related to reversal of hypovolemia. After the patient's tissue perfusion has been restored, further fluid replacement should be aimed at correction of the estimated water deficit. This estimate begins with a simple calculation of the percentage deficit based on the measured sodium concentration:

$$\text{Total body water deficit} = 0.4 \times \text{premorbid weight} \times ([\text{Na}/140] - 1)$$

Total body water is used because the sodium concentration reflects tonicity in all body fluid compartments, including the ICF. Unlike the isotonic fluid replacement for ECF volume, the water replacement should be administered gradually during a period of hours to days, unless there is clear documentation that the hypernatremia has itself evolved during minutes to hours. The necessity for gradual replacement is dictated by the process of osmotic adaptation described previously, and, ideally, the rate of water replacement should match the rate at which brain intracellular solutes can be adaptively extruded or removed. More rapid rates of administration could result in brain cell swelling with attendant dangerous neurologic consequences. It is recommended that the estimated volume of the water deficit be replaced at a rate that will lead to a reduction of approximately 0.5 to 1.0 mmol/L in measured plasma sodium concentration per hour and no more than 10 to 12 mmol/L but no less than 6 mmol/L in 24 hours. In addition to the estimated water deficit, the estimated ongoing water loss during replacement should include at least 1 L per 24 hours of insensible fluid losses (greater volumes in patients who are febrile or mechanically ventilated), supplemented with any ongoing water losses (renal or gastrointestinal) resulting from continuation of the underlying disease process. Because of the need to distribute replacement of the initial water deficit, which can amount to several liters in a number of days during which ongoing water losses continue, it is not unusual for patients to require large volumes of water, sometimes reaching 5 to 10 L, for the duration of the correction period. This water deficit, together with ongoing losses, can be replaced by the dietary ingestion of tap water, if the patient's condition is suitable, or by an enteral feeding tube. If a gastrointestinal or other disease process precludes these preferred routes, a hypotonic intravenous solution such as D_5W or half-isotonic saline can be used. When D_5W is used, the glucose is either stored as glycogen or fat or metabolized into carbon dioxide and water, thus effectively providing the patient with solute-free water replacement. In the case of half-isotonic saline, for any given liter administered, only half can be considered as replacement of the water deficit, and the sodium content will either replace any remaining sodium deficit that has not been fully corrected in the first phase of treatment or be excreted if there is no impairment in urinary sodium excretion. In elderly patients with known or possible underlying cardiac, hepatic, or renal disease, caution should be exercised in the provision of excessive volumes of salt-containing solutions. In any case, the sodium concentration should be monitored at regular intervals of no less than every 4 hours to avoid too slow or too rapid correction, and ECF volume parameters should be monitored to avoid hypervolemic complications.

Special considerations apply for hypertonic states in the setting of uncontrolled diabetes with hyperglycemia (Chapter 229). The unusual cases of patients with hypervolemic hypernatremia in the hospital setting also need special attention and sometimes require continuous infusions of loop diuretics together with the administration of hypotonic solutions or, in some cases, extracorporeal means to remove both the sodium and water excess in a controlled and safe manner under careful monitoring, preferably in the intensive care unit.

The route of administration should change in accordance with the patient's response. Although an initial parenteral or nasogastric enteral route might be appropriate when the patient's neurologic status is compromised, subsequent therapy can consist of simple dietary intake of water. Once a patient is awake and alert, and if thirst mechanisms are intact, the patient will generally correct the hypertonic state by spontaneous oral fluid intake.

Polyuria

Polyuria (Table 116-8), which is defined as a urine output of more than 3 L/day, should be distinguished from urinary frequency, which can occur with frequent voiding of small volumes totaling less than this amount per day. Polyuria occurs when urine-concentrating mechanisms are not being used at any time of the day (water diuresis) or urine solute excretion is excessive (solute diuresis).

SOLUTE DIURESIS

Polyuria in association with a urine osmolality of 300 mOsm/kg or more generally indicates solute (or osmotic) diuresis. On a typical Western diet, solute excretion (mainly sodium, potassium, and urea) is 600 to 900 mOsm/day. Therefore, normal maximum urine output cannot be greater than 3 L (= 900 mOsm/300 mOsm/kg). Hence, if urine volume exceeds 3 L/day in the presence of a urine osmolality greater than 300 mOsm/kg, extra solute must be present in the urine. The composition of these excess solutes can be electrolyte or non-electrolyte. Electrolyte solute diuresis usually occurs in response to the iatrogenic administration of high volumes of electrolyte-containing solutions, which are eliminated by the kidney through normal physiologic mechanisms. Non-electrolyte solute diuresis (glucose or urea, resulting from hyperglycemia or high-protein feeding, respectively) is equivalent to osmotic diuresis in which the presence of a non-reabsorbable non-electrolyte solute in the tubular fluid prevents reabsorption of sodium and other electrolytes as well as water.

TABLE 116-8 REASONS FOR POLYURIA

WATER DIURESIS
Diabetes insipidus
- Central (neurogenic)
  - Inherited
  - Acquired (e.g., tumors, trauma, hypoxia)
- Nephrogenic
  - Hypercalcemia
  - Amyloidosis
  - Drugs (e.g., lithium, foscarnet, cidofovir, vaptans)
  - Sjögren syndrome
  - Sickle cell disease
  - Inherited

Polydipsia
- Primary (e.g., hypothalamic)
- Psychogenic

SOLUTE DIURESIS
Sodium
- Excess sodium intake (oral, enteral, parenteral)
- Renal sodium wasting (e.g., inherited tubulopathies, interstitial nephritis, natriuretic drugs)

Anion based (sodium is usually the associated cation)
- Chloride excretion (e.g., Bartter syndrome, loop diuretic)
- Bicarbonate excretion (e.g., exogenous bicarbonate, carbonic anhydrase inhibition)

Glucose/keto acids
- Diabetic ketoacidosis
- Hyperglycemic-hyperosmolar syndrome
- Renal glycosuria

Sugar alcohols
- External loading (e.g., mannitol, glycerol)

Urea
- Exogenous loading (e.g., urea, protein, amino acids)
- Diuretic phase of acute kidney injury
- Post-obstructive diuresis
- Hypercatabolic states
- Hemoglobin/myoglobin driven (post-rhabdomyolysis or reabsorption of a hematoma)

Other
- Radiocontrast agents

WATER DIURESIS

When polyuria is associated with a urine osmolality of less than 250 mOsm/kg, a defect in urine-concentrating ability is generally suggested. In some cases, this defect occurs in association with a more general state of intrinsic renal injury and can be part of the spectrum of interstitial injury in chronic renal disease. More specific defects in urine-concentrating ability fall into the category of diabetes insipidus (Chapter 225).

TREATMENT Rx

Once a patient with polyuria has been classified as having a solute or water diuresis (see Table 116-8), the clinical manifestations and treatment will be those of the underlying disease, and the consequences of changes in ECF volume and tonicity are the same as discussed earlier. Depending on the nature of fluid intake and medication used at the onset of polyuria, a significant percentage of polyuric patients will have alterations in plasma sodium and ECF volume and will need attention to the underlying disease as well as correction of fluid and electrolyte abnormalities. Thus, for example, although antihyperglycemic treatment effectively corrects the solute diuresis and polyuric state of uncontrolled diabetes mellitus, initial correction of the concomitant electrolyte and ECF volume disorders takes precedence (Chapter 229).

Grade A References

A1. Prowle JR, Chua HR, Bagshaw SM, et al. Clinical review: volume of fluid resuscitation and the incidence of acute kidney injury—a systematic review. *Crit Care*. 2012;16:230.

A2. Roberts I, Blackhall K, Alderson P, et al. Human albumin solution for resuscitation and volume expansion in critically ill patients. *Cochrane Database Syst Rev*. 2011;11:CD001208.

A3. Myburgh JA, Finfer S, Bellomo R, et al. Hydroxyethyl starch or saline for fluid resuscitation in intensive care. *N Engl J Med*. 2012;367:1901-1911.

A4. Aliti GB, Rabelo ER, Clausell N, et al. Aggressive fluid and sodium restriction in acute decompensated heart failure: a randomized clinical trial. *JAMA Intern Med*. 2013;173:1058-1064.

A5. Paterna S, Fasullo S, Parrinello G, et al. Short-term effects of hypertonic saline solution in acute heart failure and long-term effects of a moderate sodium restriction in patients with compensated heart failure with New York Heart Association class III (Class C) (SMAC-HF Study). *Am J Med Sci*. 2011;342:27-37.

A6. Licata G, Tuttolomondo A, Licata A, et al. Clinical Trial: High-dose furosemide plus small-volume hypertonic saline solutions vs. repeated paracentesis as treatment of refractory ascites. *Aliment Pharmacol Ther*. 2009;30:227-235.

A7. McMurray JJ, Packer M, Desai AS, et al. Angiotensin-neprilysin inhibition versus enalapril in heart failure. *N Engl J Med*. 2014;371:993-1004.

A8. Udelson JE, Bilsker M, Hauptman PJ, et al. A multicenter, randomized, double-blind, placebo-controlled study of tolvaptan monotherapy compared to furosemide and the combination of tolvaptan and furosemide in patients with heart failure and systolic dysfunction. *J Card Fail*. 2011;17:973-981.

A9. Ghali JK, Orlandi C, Abraham WT. The efficacy and safety of lixivaptan in outpatients with heart failure and volume overload: results of a multicentre, randomized, double-blind, placebo-controlled, parallel-group study. *Eur J Heart Fail*. 2012;14:642-651.

GENERAL REFERENCES

For the General References and other additional features, please visit Expert Consult at https://expertconsult.inkling.com.

117 POTASSIUM DISORDERS

JULIAN L. SEIFTER

DEFINITION

Maintenance of a normal and narrow range of blood plasma potassium concentration, usually on the order of 3.5 to 5.0 mmol/L, is vital for health. *Hyperkalemia* refers to an increased plasma potassium concentration and *hypokalemia* to a decreased concentration. Within the human body, potassium is not equally distributed in the total body water. Approximately two thirds of body water is intracellular, and potassium is the major cation within that compartment, reaching concentrations as high as 140 mEq/L. Consequently, more than 98% of potassium resides within cells. An *excess* of total body potassium stores is less common than potassium *depletion* unless renal function is compromised.

Discordance between total body stores and the plasma concentration can cause hyperkalemia despite potassium depletion, and it can cause hypokalemia even with potassium excess. Potassium *adaptation* defines changes in regulatory mechanisms resulting from potassium excesses or deficits.

EPIDEMIOLOGY

Potassium is ubiquitous in both plant and animal dietary sources, so avoiding potassium is difficult. Nevertheless, disorders of potassium balance are common in both inpatient and outpatient settings. Diets high in potassium and low in sodium are associated with lower blood pressure and decrease the risk of cardiovascular disease, including stroke. By comparison, hypokalemia is associated with increased mortality, especially in patients with heart disease,[1] whereas renal dialysis patients with hyperkalemia have a higher cardiovascular mortality.[2] Mild decreases in plasma potassium are seen in healthy well-trained athletes and during normal pregnancy. Patients with chronic kidney disease (Chapter 130) and insulin-deficient diabetes (Chapter 229) have a tendency to development of hyperkalemia in association with high-potassium diets or treatment with medications that interfere with potassium balance. Starvation, gastrointestinal disease, commonly used diuretics, and other medications may cause hypokalemia. Some renal disorders, such as urinary tract obstruction (Chapter 123), may be associated with hyperkalemia, whereas others, such as aminoglycoside nephrotoxic injury, result in hypokalemia. Endocrine diseases, including adrenal insufficiency (Chapter 227), characteristically cause hyperkalemia, whereas hypokalemia is a common finding in patients who have adrenal aldosterone-secreting adenomas or tumors with ectopic secretion of adrenocorticotropic hormone (ACTH).

PATHOBIOLOGY

Potassium Balance

Most cells express sodium-potassium adenosine triphosphatase (Na^+, K^+-ATPase) on the cell plasma membranes and thereby use metabolic energy in the form of ATP to develop gradients of potassium and sodium. As a result, cellular potassium may exceed extracellular concentrations 35-fold. Established electrochemical gradients enable normal muscle and neural function as well as facilitate cellular nutrient uptake and transcellular solute transport in the intestine and kidney. Potassium entry into cells is balanced by extrusion by potassium channels and transporters in a regulated and coordinated fashion.

The total amount of potassium is usually on the order of 50 mmol/kg of body weight, so a 70-kg individual has a store of about 3500 mmol of potassium, mostly in skeletal muscle. By comparison, the entire extracellular fluid, which is approximately 20% of body weight, or 14 L in a 70-kg person, may have a potassium content of only 50 to 60 mmol. As a result, total body potassium is poorly reflected by the extracellular or plasma potassium concentration. Changes in the distribution between the cells and extracellular fluid can occur rapidly, within minutes, in contrast to the matching of dietary potassium intake to potassium elimination from the body, which occurs within hours. Potassium ingestion at the time of a meal may be equal to a large fraction of the total extracellular potassium. An average daily consumption on the order of 50 to 100 mmol would cause a rapid rise in extracellular potassium concentration after meals if it were not for the ability of potassium to distribute rapidly from the extracellular space to the intracellular space. The intracellular space, given its large volume and potassium content, can accommodate, or buffer, an extra load of potassium without significant changes in plasma or cellular concentration.

The Importance of Potassium

Potassium is essential for a number of critical body functions, including enzymatic reactions that regulate protein and glycogen synthesis, as well as for cell growth and division. The ability of cells to take up or to extrude potassium contributes to the regulation of cell volume during periods of osmotic stress. In excitable cells, such as cardiac myocytes, the relationship of intracellular to extracellular potassium concentration is critical in establishing the resting membrane potential. Because of the relative magnitude of cellular and extracellular concentrations, larger percentage changes tend to occur in the extracellular potassium concentration, which consequently has the greatest impact on the electrical properties across cell membranes.

Potassium has critical effects on excitable tissues, especially cardiac and skeletal muscle. A low serum potassium concentration not only hyperpolarizes most cells, thereby leading to an increase in the resting potential, but also alters potassium channels required for repolarization (Chapter 61). Thus, hypokalemia decreases or slows potassium conductance in some potassium channels.

Because of an increased potassium conductance, hyperkalemia antagonizes the normal slow depolarization of pacemaker tissue that is usually associated with a decrease in potassium conductance. Certain muscle-depolarizing anesthetic agents, such as succinylcholine, may potentiate the effects of hyperkalemia, as may gentamicin, particularly in patients with renal failure.

Potassium is as important a body fluid osmole as sodium, and losses of potassium obligate sodium to replace it in the intracellular space, thereby resulting in hyponatremia (Chapter 116). Hypokalemia contributes to the hyponatremia associated with thiazide diuretics. Iso-osmotic losses of combined potassium and sodium salts in watery diarrhea (Chapter 140) may result in isotonic extracellular volume depletion. Similarly, if potassium chloride is added to isotonic saline, a hypertonic solution results, and potassium may enter cells as sodium exits, thereby contributing to hypernatremia.

Potassium is also an important local mediator of vascular tone in muscle beds. During exercise, local interstitial fluid potassium concentrations may rise 10-fold, thereby causing local vasodilation to allow more blood supply to the exercising muscle but also resulting in sarcolemmal depolarization that creates muscle fatigue. Very little of that potassium enters the total extracellular fluid, so severe hyperkalemia does not usually occur with exercise. The trained athlete develops an adaptive increase in Na^+, K^+-ATPase to allow efficient re-uptake of potassium into muscle cells. For example, experienced marathoners know that their diet must provide adequate potassium stores needed for muscle endurance because overexertion during a state of potassium depletion can lead to rhabdomyolysis (Chapter 113).

Potassium excretion[3] follows a circadian rhythm. This rhythm appears to be a feed-forward mechanism that anticipates the highest level of urinary potassium excretion to coincide with dietary intake of potassium. The relationship likely involves potassium sensing within the gastrointestinal tract or splanchnic or hepatic circulation.[4] In healthy humans, potassium excretion is greatest during the daytime hours, and it can increase several-fold, without requiring a change in the blood potassium level. Independent of aldosterone, a relationship between increased potassium and sodium excretion may account for the beneficial association of high-potassium diets with lower blood pressures. The distribution of potassium between the extracellular and intracellular spaces also shows a circadian variation that may contribute to the diurnal variance in cardiac arrhythmias and sudden death in patients at risk.

Renal Potassium Handling

In the kidney, potassium excretion begins with filtration. Because the extracellular concentration of potassium is approximately 4 mmol/L and that of sodium is 140 mmol/L, far less potassium is filtered than sodium (about 3%). The renal proximal tubule reabsorbs potassium, primarily by the paracellular pathway, in the process of reabsorbing sodium and water. In the thick ascending limb of the loop of Henle, potassium is reabsorbed both by the apical sodium–potassium–2 chloride cotransporter (NKCC) and, like calcium and magnesium, by paracellular reabsorption of the cation. The latter mechanism is a consequence of the electropositive lumen created by the recycling of potassium from the cell to the lumen through renal outer medullary potassium channels (ROMK). Potassium that is reabsorbed in the thick ascending limb re-enters the tubular fluid when it is secreted into the thin descending limb in a process known as medullary potassium recycling. The resulting high interstitial potassium concentrations may enable potassium excretion from the medullary collecting duct by limiting potassium backleak. Luminal ammonium (NH_4^+) can substitute for potassium on the thick limb NKCC; the resulting increase in medullary interstitial fluid NH_4^+ concentrations enhances medullary collecting duct net acid excretion. In hyperkalemic states, less NH_4^+ appears in the urine because the high concentration of luminal potassium competes with NH_4^+ for reabsorption in the thick limb. As a consequence, metabolic acidosis may develop in hyperkalemic states, and lowering of elevated plasma potassium levels helps treat acidosis.

In hypokalemia, whether through proximal tubule intracellular acidosis or other mechanisms, glutaminase enzymes are increased, and more ammonia is produced. This ammonia leads to greater medullary interstitial fluid concentrations and therefore to enhanced net acid elimination. Ammonium production in hypokalemia could be considered an adaptation to allow potassium to be reabsorbed as NH_4^+ accompanies excreted anions into the urine. The increase in ammonia production may have a deleterious effect in that it may contribute to the chronic tubulointerstitial nephritis of chronic hypokalemia.

By the time the tubular fluid reaches the distal tubule and collecting duct, more than 90% of potassium has been reabsorbed. In potassium depletion, an increase in the apical membrane hydrogen-potassium ATPase (H^+, K^+-ATPase) of the collecting duct intercalated cell allows near-complete removal of potassium from the urine. However, potassium reabsorption is seldom as complete as that of sodium. It is unusual to see potassium concentrations in the urine lower than 5 to 10 mmol/L. When dietary potassium is abundant, the reabsorption of 90% of filtered potassium by the proximal and distal nephron is followed by net potassium secretion.

The secretion of potassium in the cortical collecting duct (E-Fig. 117-1), which may vary according to need by as much as 400%, is controlled by three major mechanisms: (1) development of a lumen-negative transepithelial potential difference that provides the driving force for potassium secretion into the lumen, (2) regulated apical membrane secretory potassium channels, and (3) tubular fluid flow dependency. The urinary potassium most closely reflects potassium secreted by the distal nephron.

The Aldosterone Paradox

The traditional view of regulating potassium secretion and therefore excretion has focused on the central role of aldosterone, the steroid hormone synthesized and secreted by the zona glomerulosa of the adrenal cortex.[5] Aldosterone is stimulated by angiotensin II, predominantly in the hyperreninemic states of extracellular volume depletion, and independently by potassium loading, usually from an excess of potassium in the diet. The renal effects of aldosterone show overlap of functions to conserve sodium and to eliminate potassium. In what has been called the *aldosterone paradox,* the kidney can prevent undesired losses of potassium from occurring when sodium retention is required to maintain extracellular volume (the angiotensin II stimulus), and it also can prevent undesired retention of sodium from occurring while maintaining normal potassium balance when the stimulus to aldosterone is potassium loading. The feedback mechanism coupling aldosterone with serum potassium is important in regulating the degree of potassium losses in the urine. For example, hyperaldosteronism results in potassium loss, and then the resulting hypokalemia reduces aldosterone production and subsequent potassium losses. Hyperkalemia has the opposite effect: it is an important stimulus of aldosterone synthesis and release. Thus, with volume expansion and low angiotensin II, the rise in potassium stimulates aldosterone release from the zona glomerulosa of the adrenal cortex, thereby allowing potassium to be secreted into the urine.

Mechanism of Sodium Reabsorption and Electrochemical Forces

The major regulatory site for potassium secretion resides in the aldosterone-sensitive distal nephron, which is composed of the late distal convoluted tubule as well as the principal cells of the connecting tubule and the cortical collecting duct. Aldosterone regulates sodium reabsorption in these segments: by the NaCl cotransporter in the late distal convoluted tubule and connecting tubule, and by the apical epithelial sodium channel (ENaC) in the principal cells of the connecting tubule and cortical collecting duct. Thiazide-sensitive NaCl cotransport is independent of aldosterone in the early distal convoluted tubule.

To optimize potassium secretion, sodium must be delivered in ample amounts (depending on the flow rate and sodium concentration of the tubular fluid) to result in sodium reabsorption through the apical ENaC in the principal cells. In severe prerenal states of avid sodium reabsorption, including hypovolemic states, the hepatorenal syndrome, and severe heart failure, sodium delivery from more proximal sites may become rate limiting for potassium secretion. Assuming that sodium delivery is not limiting, reabsorption of the sodium cation creates a lumen-negative transepithelial potential difference. Aldosterone affects the transepithelial potential difference in several ways. The intracellular mineralocorticoid receptor functions to increase the activity and density of ENaC and of basolateral Na^+, K^+-ATPase enzymes. Cortisol, which is normally present in higher concentrations than aldosterone, has equal affinity for the aldosterone receptor and therefore could lead to increased ENaC activity. However, the enzyme 11β-hydroxysteroid dehydrogenase type 2 is present in the principal cells and converts cortisol to inactive cortisone.

The reabsorption of sodium is dependent on the low intracellular sodium concentrations that result from the energy-requiring Na^+, K^+-ATPase on the basolateral membrane. Both increased intracellular Na^+ and extracellular K^+ also stimulate the Na^+, K^+-ATPase. Increased Na^+ entry through an apical mechanism will increase Na^+, K^+-ATPase, thereby bringing more potassium into the cells for transepithelial secretion, independent of aldosterone. However, oral potassium loads in the intestine may increase potassium secretion without prior increments in plasma potassium.

Most of the potassium that enters the principal cell from the extracellular fluid through the Na^+, K^+-ATPase is secreted into the lumen because of the lumen-negative transepithelial voltage. Some is then either recycled back to the extracellular fluid by basolateral potassium transport mechanisms or, after secretion into the cortical collecting duct lumen, reabsorbed back to the blood by neighboring intercalated cell H^+, K^+-ATPase.

Role of Potassium Secretory Channels and Tubular Flow Rate

Optimal potassium secretion requires adequate function of several types of potassium secretory channels on the luminal membranes of distal nephron cells. Two predominant potassium channels are present in the apical membranes of the collecting duct cells.

The renal outer medullary potassium channel (ROMK), which is located on the apical membrane of the principal cell in the connecting tubule and cortical collecting duct, is aldosterone sensitive, is increased by dietary potassium loads, and likely subserves constitutive K^+ secretion under basal conditions. ROMK undergoes new synthesis and increased cycling to the apical membrane under the control of aldosterone. The principal cell also mediates vasopressin-responsive water reabsorption. Factors regulating ROMK channels include antidiuretic hormone (ADH) and intracellular pH. The increase in ROMK channel activity in response to ADH, combined with an ADH effect to increase ENaC and osmotic water flow, allows the highest possible potassium concentration in the urine with the low tubular flow that accompanies antidiuresis. When ADH is suppressed, luminal potassium concentrations are lower, thereby favoring gradients for potassium secretion, but ROMK activity is reduced because of the low ADH. Cellular acidification inhibits potassium secretion through an effect on ROMK, thereby providing a renal mechanism for decreased electrogenic potassium secretion when proton secretion is necessary during metabolic and respiratory acidoses. In alkalosis, ROMK activity is increased, thereby favoring increased potassium secretion, but the result may be significant potassium loss.

Additional potassium channels, known as maxi-K or big-K channels, are prominent in the principal cells and intercalated cells of the cortical collecting duct, thereby implying that the intercalated cell also has a role in potassium secretion. The big-K channels are highly regulated by tubular fluid flow rate. One mechanism by which flow rate influences this potassium secretory channel is by the deformation by flow of the primary cilium of the principal cell, which leads to a secondary increase in cellular calcium that has both direct and indirect effects to enhance BK potassium secretion.

Excretion Mechanisms and Normal Function

Because the major regulatory site for potassium secretion resides in the aldosterone-sensitive distal nephron, the mechanisms for Na^+ and K^+ transport in each of these cell types are central to the proposed role of a network of protein kinases, including the "with no lysine" or WNK kinases in the aldosterone paradox. Note that aldosterone regulates sodium reabsorption in all segments: NaCl cotransport in the late distal convoluted tubule and connecting tubule, and ENaC in the connecting tubule and principal cells of the cortical collecting duct. ROMK is increased by aldosterone in the cortical collecting duct.

In hypovolemia, sodium reabsorption is increased by angiotensin II in the proximal tubule, the early and late distal convoluted tubule, and the connecting tubule so that very little sodium is delivered to the principal cells of the cortical collecting duct. Potassium losses are diminished because of decreased delivery of sodium, and an angiotensin II–induced switch involving WNK kinase decreases ROMK activity. Although aldosterone will still activate principal cell ENaC, the decrease in sodium delivery and decreased potassium secretion (favoring chloride reabsorption instead), will allow greater NaCl reabsorption while limiting potassium loss.

When aldosterone is present in the absence of angiotensin II, as in potassium loading, there is no earlier stimulation of sodium reabsorption, so sodium delivery to late aldosterone-sensitive distal nephron segments that contain ROMK, the NaCl cotransporter, and ENaC is increased. In the absence of angiotensin II, the WNK network of protein kinases favors increased ROMK, whereas aldosterone increases ENaC activity. The result favors potassium secretion, but overall sodium reabsorption is not increased because increased NaCl delivery from proximal sites offsets the increase in sodium reabsorption through ENaC.

Internal Potassium Balance and Associated Disorders

Because of the delay in hours before renal excretion matches dietary intake and because potassium first enters the extracellular fluid from the gastrointestinal tract, it is critical that the process of cellular buffering be effective (Table 117-1). Essentially, increases in postprandial blood potassium are minimized before potassium is eliminated from the body. A major factor in this regulation after meals is the feedback loop involving insulin and potassium. An increase in serum potassium stimulates insulin release from the β cells of the pancreatic islets. Insulin increases potassium uptake into cells, primarily muscle, independent of its effect on glucose uptake. Acutely, potassium uptake is chiefly the result of increased Na^+, K^+-ATPase activity, whereas chronically there is increased abundance in the plasma membranes in these cells.

Another important mechanism of regulating the distribution of potassium between extracellular and cellular spaces involves the sympathoadrenal

TABLE 117-1 FACTORS REGULATING INTERNAL POTASSIUM BALANCE

Circadian rhythm
Insulin
β-Adrenergic activity
Acid-base balance
Magnesium
Aldosterone
Osmolality
Thyroid hormone
Extracellular potassium
Intracellular sodium

system. β-Adrenergic activation, particularly through the β_2-receptor, increases potassium uptake into muscle and fat cells. As with insulin, potassium uptake is the consequence of increased Na^+, K^+-ATPase activity associated with increased intracellular cyclic adenosine monophosphate. The adrenergic effect is important in regulating the serum potassium concentration during exercise and is independent of the additional effect that catecholamines may have on blood glucose with the expected increases in insulin. In the trained athlete, a chronic increase in Na^+, K^+-ATPase on cell membranes may cause a transient lowering of the serum potassium concentration after exertion. Conversely, a severe stress may contribute to hypokalemia, through both direct β_2 effects and insulin action secondary to the blood glucose rise.

Phenylephrine, an α-adrenergic agonist, increases serum potassium. Importantly, epinephrine, which also has α-adrenergic effects, is associated with a transient increase in potassium release from the liver before a more prolonged period of decreased serum potassium mediated by the β_2-receptor.

Metabolic acidosis raises the potassium level more than does respiratory acidosis; both metabolic alkalosis and respiratory alkalosis lower the potassium level. Anion gap acidosis does not raise the potassium level, probably because of the movement of the organic anion (e.g., lactate) from cells into the extracellular space with an accompanying proton, whereas the ingestion of chloride salts has the most profound effect on the potassium level because chloride is restricted to the extracellular space and protons enter cells in exchange for the exit of the potassium cation. The ingestion of excessive chloride salts of arginine and lysine is associated with hyperkalemic acidosis. ε-Aminocaproic acid has also been associated with hyperkalemia and is hypothesized to exchange for cellular potassium, much like the other cationic amino acids.

Just as multiple simultaneous acid-base disturbances lead to a single blood pH level, many processes that affect the net potassium concentration can be simultaneously present. Metabolic acidosis may be associated with diarrheal or urinary losses of potassium, so that the potassium concentration is low, not high. Metabolic acidosis in diabetes can also be associated with insulin deficiency and renal failure, in which case the plasma potassium level might be elevated despite osmotically driven urinary losses of potassium and total body potassium depletion.

Other hormonal effects on potassium include thyroid and growth hormone, but patients with disorders of these hormones do not usually have significant changes in their blood potassium levels. Some patients with hyperthyroidism may have mild hypokalemia, perhaps related to increased sympathetic activity. Growth states are associated with a greater need for potassium; for example, in normal pregnancy, the maternal potassium concentration may fall as the developing fetus grows.

Hypomagnesemia frequently accompanies hypokalemia. Both magnesium and potassium are found predominantly in cells, but Na^+, K^+-ATPase requires magnesium for function. If magnesium is deficient, potassium distributes more to the extracellular fluid, thereby masking the degree of potassium deficiency. Moreover, magnesium deficiency leads to renal potassium wasting, so potassium depletion is difficult to correct until magnesium is repleted.

External Potassium Balance and Associated Disorders

Normally, no more than 10 to 20% of total potassium excretion is accomplished by the gastrointestinal tract, but colonic excretion is increased in renal failure, primarily through potassium-induced increases in epithelial Na^+, K^+-ATPase activity and aldosterone. In renal failure, the normal mechanisms to distribute potassium acquire increased importance.

Some conditions that cause the greatest losses of gastrointestinal potassium include secretory diarrheas of the colon, the result of infection or laxative abuse. Disorders of the small intestine, which may lead to large quantities of liquid stool with a low potassium concentration, engender favorable gradients for marked potassium secretion by the colon. A syndrome of watery diarrhea and hypokalemia is associated with neuroendocrine tumors (Chapter 195) that secrete vasoactive intestinal peptide. Rectosigmoid secretion of potassium may result in particularly high potassium losses, and potassium deficiency is seen in patients who have ureterosigmoidostomies. Potassium can be lost from a variety of other sources, including excess sweat or salivation, vomiting, and diarrhea.

Potassium can be depleted by vomiting or diarrhea. Urinary losses may exceed intake in renal tubular disorders, when excessive quantities of osmotic or anionic products are excreted in the urine, or in patients who take diuretics.

It is unusual for hyperkalemia to be caused by excessive potassium intake unless the patient has renal dysfunction. However, in patients who have brisk hemolysis, internal hemorrhage, or rhabdomyolysis, particularly if the hemoglobinuria or myoglobinuria also results in acute kidney injury, life-threatening hyperkalemia can quickly develop by the rapid release of cellular potassium stores.

CLINICAL MANIFESTATIONS

Hypokalemia

Clinical manifestations of potassium depletion include hypertension, decreased growth, and muscle symptoms such as weakness, cramps, fasciculations, and even paralysis. In severe cases, the diaphragm may be paralyzed, leading to respiratory failure. Cardiac arrhythmias are a critical component of low potassium states and are usually seen when the serum potassium falls below 3 mmol/L or when ischemia, hypercalcemia, or drugs such as digoxin are simultaneously present. A patient who has a chronically low potassium level (e.g., from diuretic use) may be particularly vulnerable to supraventricular and ventricular tachyarrhythmias during periods of stress, such as head trauma, or during the acute coronary syndrome, to which cardiac ischemia also contributes. The prolonged cardiac repolarization phase of hypokalemia accounts for the characteristic electrocardiographic findings of broad, flattened T waves. U waves are also indicative of this delay in repolarization (Fig. 117-1). In the intestine, hypokalemia may result in paralytic ileus, which may interfere with oral replacement. Hypokalemia may result in acute skeletal muscle weakness and even paralysis.

In addition to these systemic effects of potassium imbalance, the kidney is particularly sensitive to depletion of potassium. Structural changes in the glomeruli and tubules lead to a decreased glomerular filtration rate, increased proximal tubule ammoniagenesis, increased sodium bicarbonate reabsorption, and net acid excretion, thereby causing metabolic alkalosis. A condition of nephrogenic diabetes insipidus results when potassium depletion decreases expression of vasopressin-dependent water channels (aquaporin 2) in the collecting duct luminal plasma membranes. Hypokalemia diminishes insulin secretion and may be associated with glucose intolerance.

Hyperkalemia

In hyperkalemia, the depolarizing effect on the resting membrane potential and increased potassium channel conductance lead to the classic

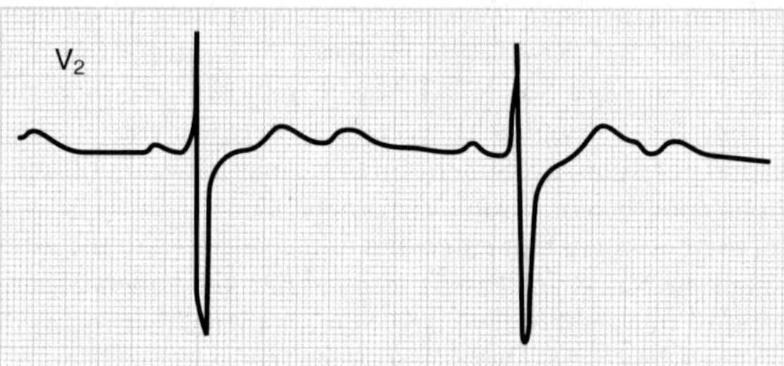

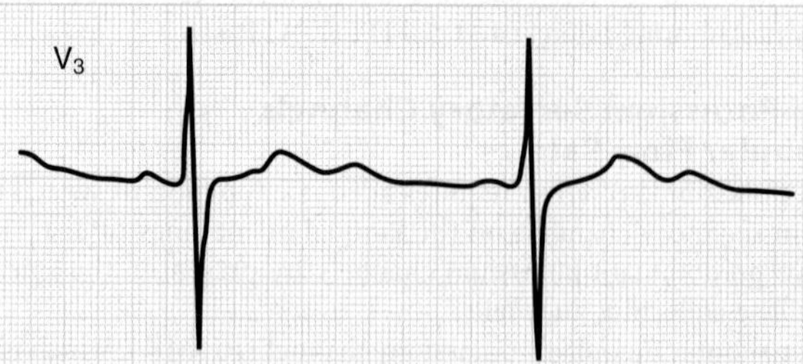

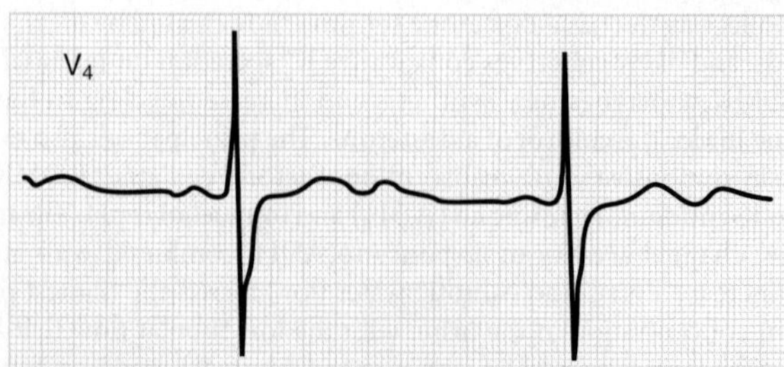

FIGURE 117-1. The electrocardiographic manifestations of hypokalemia. The serum potassium concentration was 2.2 mEq/L. The ST segment is prolonged, primarily because of a U wave following the T wave, and the T wave is flattened.

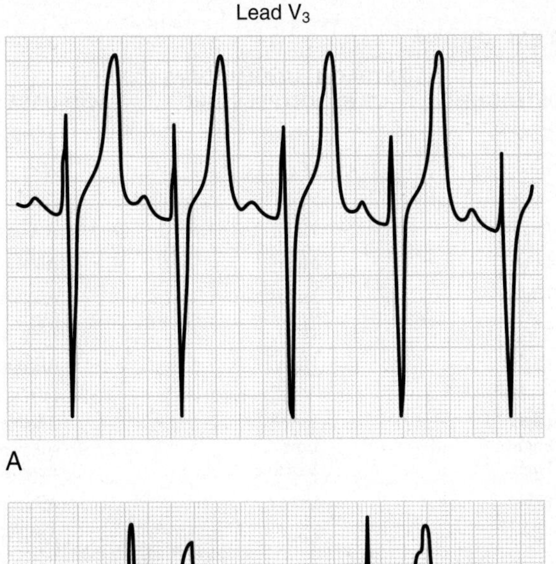

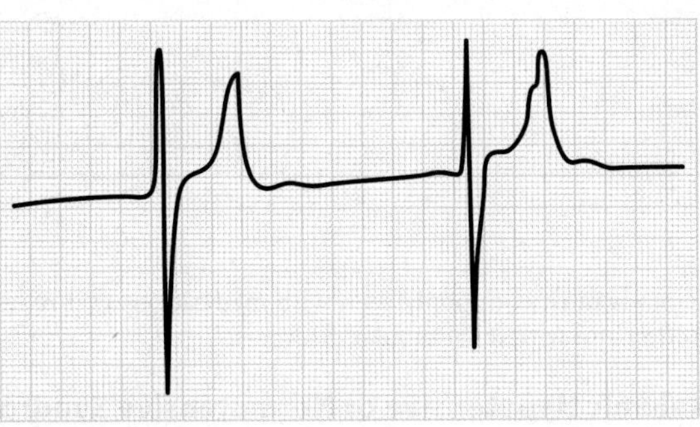

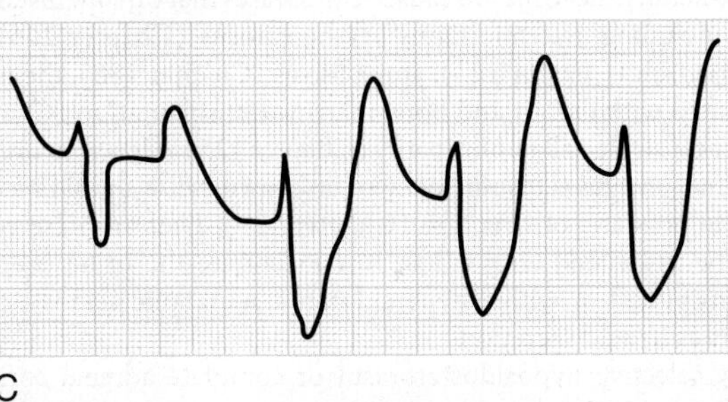

FIGURE 117-2. **The effects of progressive hyperkalemia on the electrocardiogram. All of the illustrations are from lead V_3. A, Serum potassium concentration ([K^+]) = 6.8 mEq/L; note the peaked T waves together with normal sinus rhythm. B, Serum [K^+] = 8.9 mEq/L; note the peaked T waves and absent P waves. C, Serum [K^+] > 8.9 mEq/L; note the classic sine wave with absent P waves, marked prolongation of the QRS complex, and peaked T waves.**

electrocardiographic changes of hyperacute peaked T waves associated with rapid repolarization (Fig. 117-2). Hyperkalemia commonly results in sinus bradycardia. Heart block, loss of P waves on the electrocardiogram, and prolonged QRS intervals are all seen in cases of severe hyperkalemia, usually in excess of 6 mmol/L. The electrocardiogram, however, is not a sensitive indicator of severe hyperkalemia, and cardiac arrest may occur without warning. Like hypokalemia, severe hyperkalemia can cause skeletal muscle paralysis; unlike hypokalemic paralysis, it is often ascending in nature.

DIAGNOSIS

The first clue to a disorder in potassium balance usually is an abnormal serum potassium concentration obtained as part of a laboratory evaluation, not because an abnormal potassium level itself is suspected.[6] When the potassium concentration is elevated above normal, it is imperative to exclude common artifacts, known as pseudohyperkalemia. Hemolysis in the test tube is a common artifact; in cases of cold-induced hemolysis (Chapter 161), it is important to collect the blood and to allow it to clot in a warm environment. Some patients have pseudohyperkalemia resulting from high platelet counts, usually in excess of 1 million/μL, or myelogenous leukemia (Chapters 183 and 184); in such cases, potassium is released during clot formation in the test tube. Plasma potassium levels should be within the normal range. The serum potassium level may sometimes be elevated because of local ischemia related to application of the tourniquet and clenching of the fist.

A detailed medical history should focus on medications, family history, and sources of potassium excess or loss. The physical examination should pay particular attention to blood pressure, extracellular volume status, heart rate and rhythm, and muscle strength and reflexes.

Laboratory testing should include a complete blood count as well as serum levels of sodium, chloride, bicarbonate, creatinine, and blood urea nitrogen. In more serious cases, arterial blood gases and levels of creatine kinase and magnesium should be obtained. A 12-lead electrocardiogram also should be obtained.

A low urinary potassium level is expected in hypokalemia. In a hypokalemic patient, a urinary potassium concentration higher than 30 mEq/L suggests renal potassium wasting, whereas extrarenal losses are usually reflected by concentrations lower than 20 mEq/L. In a state of potassium excess, urinary potassium excretion should exceed about 35 mEq/L, unless urinary underexcretion was the cause of the hyperkalemia. A high aldosterone level causes a high urinary potassium-to-sodium ratio, whereas hypoaldosteronism may cause the opposite.

Hypokalemic Disorders

The most common cause of hypokalemia (Table 117-2) in medical practice is the use of thiazide or loop diuretics.[7] Patients may have low, normal, or high blood pressures, depending on their volume status and whether the diuretics were prescribed for hypertension or heart failure. The most common acute causes of hypokalemia are diarrhea and vomiting.

Hypokalemic Hypertensive Syndromes

If the renal principal cells develop a transepithelial electrical gradient that is more lumen negative than is needed to maintain potassium balance, urinary potassium wasting, inappropriate to the blood potassium level, occurs. Because a parallel increase in H^+ secretion will occur, it is common to see an accompanying metabolic alkalosis. If the abnormality is related to a primary increase in sodium reabsorption, hypertension or extracellular volume expansion also will develop.[8]

Evaluation of plasma renin and aldosterone levels can help distinguish among specific diagnoses (see Table 117-2).[9] Primary hyperaldosteronism is associated with low renin levels due to volume expansion. If it is corrected for plasma potassium, an aldosterone-to-renin ratio of 30 : 1 suggests a primary adrenal cortical tumor (aldosteronoma) or hyperplasia (Chapter 227). However, such ratios must be used with caution, and the absolute value of aldosterone is important, especially when the renin and aldosterone levels are both low. The tubular delivery of large amounts of sodium chloride in a setting of volume expansion and nonsuppressible aldosterone results in hypokalemia, which improves after sodium restriction and worsens with the administration of intravenous saline. In congenital adrenal hyperplasia (Chapter 227), such as 11β-hydroxylase deficiency, hypokalemic alkalosis is associated with excessive androgen production. In patients with renin-secreting tumors or unilateral renal artery stenosis, high renin levels stimulate angiotensin II and then aldosterone secretion, with a resulting increase in sodium reabsorption, hypertension, and hypokalemic metabolic alkalosis.

In some patients with overproduction of ACTH, as in ectopic production from lung and other malignant neoplasms (Chapter 179), cortisol may overwhelm the aldosterone receptor and result in hypertensive, hypokalemic alkalosis. The patient may not show signs of Cushing syndrome unless the syndrome is prolonged. In glucocorticoid-remediable aldosteronism, which is a familial disorder in which episodes of hypokalemia and hypertension develop, a chimeric gene duplication couples the ACTH-responsive 11β-hydroxylase promoter to the coding region of aldosterone synthase.

Glycyrrhizic acid, which is found in licorice and anisette, inhibits the renal enzyme 11β-hydroxysteroid dehydrogenase and thereby causes hypokalemia, metabolic alkalosis, and hypertension. A rare genetic disorder known as apparent mineralocorticoid excess syndrome produces the same effect due to deficiency of 11β-hydroxysteroid dehydrogenase. The syndrome produces a high ratio of cortisol to cortisone; as a result, renin and aldosterone are suppressed by the volume expansion. Hypokalemia may be precipitated by ACTH stimulation of cortisol.

Activating mutations of ENaC cause increased sodium reabsorption (Liddle syndrome; Chapter 128). The syndrome can be distinguished from primary or secondary hyperaldosteronism by a decrease in renin and aldosterone levels.

Hypokalemic Hypotensive Syndromes

In contrast to the hypokalemic hypertensive syndromes, in which an increased sodium reabsorption is a primary event, many hypokalemic alkaloses are

TABLE 117-2 CAUSES OF HYPOKALEMIA AND INCREASED POTASSIUM EXCRETION

CAUSES OF INCREASED K⁺ EXCRETION AND HYPOKALEMIA	RENIN	ALDOSTERONE	EXTRACELLULAR VOLUME OR BLOOD PRESSURE	ACID-BASE STATUS
Increased ENaC: Liddle syndrome	Low	Low	High	Alkalosis
Decreased β-hydroxysteroid dehydrogenase: apparent mineralocorticoid excess, licorice	Low	Low	High	Alkalosis
Adrenal tumor or hyperplasia	Low	High	High	Alkalosis
Ectopic ACTH: Cushing syndrome	Low	Low	High	Alkalosis
Congenital adrenal hyperplasia	Low	High	High	Alkalosis
Unilateral renal artery stenosis	High	High	High	Alkalosis
Renin-secreting tumor	High	High	High	Alkalosis
Diuretics				
Thiazides	High	High	Low	Alkalosis
Furosemide	High	High	Low	Alkalosis
Acetazolamide	High	High	Variable	Acidosis
Bartter syndrome	High	High	Low	Alkalosis
Gitelman syndrome	High	High	Low	Alkalosis
Fanconi syndrome	High	High	Low	Acidosis
Distal RTA	High	High	Low	Acidosis

ACTH = adrenocorticotropic hormone; ENaC = epithelial Na^+ channel; RTA = renal tubular acidosis.

associated with extracellular volume depletion. With a physiologic response to volume depletion, the potassium losses may be a result of appropriate sodium reabsorption; signs of hypotension or extracellular volume depletion will be observed. Secretory diarrheas, whether associated with hypochloremic alkalosis or hyperchloremic acidosis, lead to extracellular volume depletion and secondary increases in renin and aldosterone; the result is both gastrointestinal and urinary potassium losses. However, because alkalosis increases potassium secretion, urinary potassium losses are most severe in gastric alkalosis or other chloride-wasting syndromes associated with alkalemia.

Diuretic use, Bartter syndrome (Chapter 128), and Gitelman syndrome (Chapter 128) are renal tubular causes of extracellular volume depletion, hypotension, and hypokalemic, hypochloremic alkalosis; sodium and chloride are lost in the urine, and secondary rises in renin and aldosterone occur. Increased urinary flow rates are important contributors to the increased potassium losses in each of these examples. Bartter syndrome affects the function of the thick ascending limb through mutations in NKCC or in potassium or chloride channels, whereas Gitelman syndrome is characterized by inactivating mutations or dysregulation of the Na^+-Cl^- cotransporter in the distal tubule. The hypokalemia in Gitelman syndrome may be caused by secondary hyperaldosteronism, bicarbonaturia, and hypomagnesemia.

Classic type 1 distal renal tubular acidosis (Chapters 118 and 128) is often associated with hypokalemia, which may improve with correction of the acidemia. In contrast, proximal renal tubular acidosis, when it is corrected with bicarbonate, often results in worsening of the hypokalemia because of greater bicarbonate wasting associated with increases in the filtered bicarbonate load.

Acetazolamide, when it is given to an alkalotic patient, is a particularly potent kaliuretic agent. Volume depletion and hyperaldosteronism contribute to the potassium losses, as does the bicarbonate wasting, which appears to have a direct effect on potassium secretion. Whenever the urine is alkaline, potassium will usually be present in significant amounts.

Tubular toxins that may be associated with severe potassium losses include aminoglycosides, cisplatinum, and ifosfamide. Amphotericin B results in significant potassium wasting accompanied by renal tubular acidosis. In many of these conditions, simultaneous use of amiloride may diminish potassium losses by as much as 50%.

Patients who present with unexplained hypokalemia and alkalosis with volume depletion should have urinary electrolytes measured to determine whether the urine chloride is low, as with vomiting or laxative abuse. If the urine contains chloride, a diuretic screen should be considered; Gitelman syndrome and Bartter syndrome are other possibilities.

Hyperkalemic Disorders

In clinical practice, acute hyperkalemia is seen most commonly with renal failure (Chapter 131), with acidosis (Chapter 118), and with acute muscle damage from rhabdomyolysis (Chapter 113) (Table 117-3). Chronic hyperkalemia is most commonly seen with medications that reduce potassium secretion and with renal tubular disorders.

Hyperkalemic Hypotensive or Normotensive Syndromes

Type 4 renal tubular acidoses (Chapter 118) that are associated with an inability to acidify the urine are caused by diseases that disrupt distal nephron function, including systemic lupus erythematosus (Chapter 266), urinary tract obstruction (Chapter 123), amyloidosis (Chapter 188), the nephropathy associated with kidney and bone marrow transplantation (Chapters 131 and 178), and sickle cell nephropathy (Chapter 125). Men who present with hyperkalemia and renal insufficiency of unknown cause should be evaluated for possible prostatic obstruction (Chapter 129). Each of these conditions may also be associated with failure to concentrate the urine (nephrogenic diabetes insipidus) or with a hyperchloremic metabolic acidosis caused by abnormalities in acid secretion.

Primary selective hypoaldosteronism or complete adrenal cortical deficiency (Chapter 227) is associated with elevated renin and low aldosterone. Secondary hypoaldosteronism may be seen in hyporenin states caused by β-blockers, renin antagonists, or nonsteroidal anti-inflammatory drugs (NSAIDs). Angiotensin-converting enzyme inhibitors and angiotensin receptor blockers increase renin and decrease aldosterone. Heparin, including low-molecular-weight and fractionated forms (Chapter 38), can lead to hyperkalemia even in small subcutaneous doses.

Disorders that affect the transepithelial potential difference and can result in hyperkalemia, acidosis, and extracellular volume depletion include inactivating mutations of ENaC (autosomal recessive pseudohypoaldosteronism type 1), which may be accompanied by high renin and aldosterone levels. The ENaC may also be inhibited by the potassium-sparing diuretics (i.e., amiloride and triamterene) and certain medications secreted by the proximal tubule organic cation transporters, such as trimethoprim and pentamidine, as well as by lithium. Inhibition of the aldosterone receptor may be the result of antagonists such as spironolactone and eplerenone.

Hyperkalemic Hypertensive Syndromes

NSAIDs can cause hyperkalemia, particularly in patients with renal disease, by decreasing sodium delivery, increasing water reabsorption, and decreasing renin and aldosterone. Hypertension with the NSAIDs is most likely caused by renal salt and water retention.

Cyclosporine or tacrolimus may produce a hyperkalemic acidosis. The mechanism may involve inhibition of cyclooxygenase 2 and therefore hyporenin-hypoaldosteronism. There may also be a decrease in apical potassium secretion in the collecting duct. Gordon syndrome is a genetic disorder (pseudohypoaldosteronism type 2) associated with hyperkalemia, volume expansion, and metabolic acidosis. It is caused by activation of the thiazide-sensitive distal convoluted tubule NaCl cotransporter related to a dysfunction of the WNK kinase regulatory role.

TABLE 117-3 CAUSES OF HYPERKALEMIA AND DECREASED POTASSIUM EXCRETION

CAUSE OF DECREASED K^+ EXCRETION AND HYPERKALEMIA	RENIN	ALDOSTERONE	EXTRACELLULAR VOLUME OR BLOOD PRESSURE	ACID-BASE STATUS
Decreased ENaC Drugs: amiloride, triamterene, trimethoprim, lithium Pseudohypoaldosteronism type 1 autosomal recessive ENaC mutation	High	High	Low or normal	Normal or acidosis
Pseudohypoaldosteronism type 1 autosomal dominant MR mutation	High	High	Low	Acidosis
MR blockade: spironolactone, eplerenone, progesterone	High	High	Low	Acidosis
Hypoaldosteronism: adrenal insufficiency	High	Low	Low	Acidosis
Hyporenin-hypoaldosteronism: NSAIDs, β-blockers, autonomic neuropathy	Low	Low	Low	Acidosis
Pseudohypoaldosteronism type 2	Low	Low	High	Acidosis

ENaC = epithelial Na^+ channel; MR = mineralocorticoid receptor; NSAIDs = nonsteroidal anti-inflammatory drugs.

TREATMENT Rx

It may be difficult to determine the exact state of total body potassium stores from the serum potassium level because as much as 100 to 300 mmol of potassium may be lost from the body with a fall in serum potassium of only 1 mmol/L.

Hypokalemia

The goal of acute therapy for hypokalemia is to prevent or to manage potentially life-threatening arrhythmias or paralysis. Patients at greatest risk are elderly patients, patients with known liver disease or cardiac disturbances, and patients who have had an abrupt fall in serum potassium concentration to less than 2.5 mEq/L. Potassium must traverse the extracellular space before repleting intracellular stores, so it is dangerously easy to replete potassium too quickly. Oral potassium should be given, if possible. If the potassium level is greater than 3 mEq/L, an increase in dietary potassium can be considered, along with removal of the underlying cause of hypokalemia. Usual oral replacement is with potassium chloride at a dose of 40 to 100 mmol/day. The chloride salt has the advantage of treating concomitant metabolic alkalosis, but other available forms include potassium citrate (in the acidotic patient) and potassium phosphate (in patients with a phosphate deficit). Giving potassium with a non-reabsorbable anion, such as gluconate, may not replace the potassium deficit adequately. Intravenous potassium is reserved for patients who are unable to take enteral potassium and patients with symptomatic hypokalemia, paralysis, or cardiac arrhythmias. It is usually given as a solution of 20 to 40 mmol of potassium in 1 L of solution at a rate that does not exceed 10 to 20 mmol/hour. In some cases of severe hypokalemia (<2.5 mEq/L) and in symptomatic patients, higher concentrations (up to 40 mmol in 100 mL) have been used. If the potassium level is less than 3 mmol/L or if more than 10 mmol/hour is to be delivered, it may be best to treat the patient in a monitored setting to observe for cardiac complications. A central venous catheter may be required for these higher concentrations. In these unusual circumstances, it is best to consult with a renal specialist and the pharmacy.

In patients who have prerenal azotemia associated with hyperglycemia or severe metabolic alkalosis, volume expansion with sodium chloride solutions alone can result in life-threatening potassium losses, despite improvement in the extracellular volume. Potassium must be given in anticipation of such events.

In a hypokalemic patient, care must be exercised when glucose-containing solutions are given because the resulting increase in insulin may further decrease the blood potassium level. Attention to the urine output and ongoing losses is crucial. If ongoing losses of potassium are severe, it may be necessary to provide a potassium-sparing diuretic (e.g., amiloride, 5 to 10 mg orally) and to treat the cause of the ongoing losses (e.g., diarrhea). Magnesium should be measured and replaced, if necessary, in any hypokalemic patient.

In the inpatient setting, hypokalemia is a common complication of intravenous fluid administration. In patients with normal renal function, a maintenance dose of intravenous potassium can avoid hypokalemia.[10] In the outpatient setting, hypokalemia is a common side effect of diuretic therapy. The serum potassium level should be maintained within the normal range (>3.5 mEq/L), especially in high-risk patients. Addition of 40 to 100 mmol of potassium per day as the chloride salt is the usual treatment, depending on the patient's response.

Hyperkalemia

If hyperkalemia is severe, the goal is to achieve a rapid reduction in potassium concentration.[11] If hyperkalemia is associated with cardiac arrhythmias, however, the cardiac effects of the hyperkalemia require interim treatment in a monitored setting, before the serum potassium level can be expected to decline, even with aggressive therapy. Calcium gluconate, 10 mL of a 10% solution (8.9 mg calcium) during 10 to 20 minutes, is often indicated to stabilize electrical effects on cardiac excitation. Calcium chloride (3 to 4 mL of a 10% solution) is used as another alternative, but it should be administered through a central access line because extravasation of the chloride salt may result in tissue necrosis.

However, calcium does not lower the potassium concentration. Nebulized or inhaled β-agonists and intravenous insulin and glucose, either alone or the two in combination, are the best treatments.[A1] To lower the potassium level acutely, alternatives include 100 mL of 50% glucose alone or in combination with 10 units of regular insulin; the combination will, on average, provide a significantly greater reduction in the serum potassium level (0.8 mmol/L vs. 0.5 mmol/L) at 60 minutes, but about 20% of insulin-treated patients will develop hypoglycemia.[A2] Alternatively, 10 mg of regular insulin can be given with 10% glucose solution during 1 hour for a total of 30 to 50 g in the normoglycemic patient. The blood glucose level should be monitored because an abrupt increase in plasma osmolality with glucose may worsen hyperkalemia if it causes potassium to leak from cells with osmotic water flow. Albuterol by nebulizer (10 to 20 mg in 4 mL of saline during 10 minutes) can redistribute potassium acutely but should not be the sole treatment because some patients are not responsive. In some cases, intravenous β-adrenergic agonists (e.g., albuterol, 0.5 mg in 100 mL of 5% dextrose during 15 minutes) have been used to lower the serum potassium level by about 1 mmol/L within minutes to hours. Sodium bicarbonate, as an isotonic mixture calculated to correct acid-base status, should be reserved for acidemic patients who otherwise require alkalinization, while being careful to avoid hypocalcemia; complications of sodium bicarbonate infusions include hypernatremia, volume expansion, and decreased ionized calcium, potentially resulting in tetany. Diabetic patients may be potassium depleted even though they present with hyperkalemia; as they are volume repleted, they typically require potassium replacement (Chapter 229). The hyperkalemia of Gordon syndrome is highly responsive to thiazide diuretics.

During the longer term, potassium loss may be sustained by use of cation exchange resins such as sodium polystyrene sulfonate, given orally or as an enema (Chapter 131).[12] A dose of 30 to 50 g can reduce potassium levels during several hours. This resin will also provide a sodium load and bind calcium, thereby resulting in volume expansion and hypocalcemia. These resins may interfere with the absorption of lithium and thyroxine. A serious complication of sodium polystyrene sulfonate resins when they are used in combination with sorbitol is colonic ulceration and necrosis. These resins also should not be given in combination with aluminum-based antacids because the resulting concretions can obstruct the gastrointestinal tract. If the patient is volume expanded, furosemide (40 to 100 mg), chlorothiazide (500 mg), or, if the patient is also alkalotic, acetazolamide (250 to 500 mg) may enhance renal potassium clearance. If the patient is volume depleted, isotonic saline expansion may improve urine output and, with it, potassium excretion.

New medications that reduce potassium levels in high-risk patients include patiromer (a non-absorbed calcium-potassium exchange resin that works in the colon at 4.2 to 8.4 g twice daily[A3]) in patients with chronic kidney disease who are taking renin-angiotensin-aldosterone system inhibitors, or zirconium cyclosilicate (an oral crystalline agent with high binding affinity for potassium within the gastrointestinal tract at 1.25 to 10 g three times daily[A4,A5]). However, the long-term utility and safety of these agents remains to be determined, and they are not currently FDA-approved.

Specific Clinical Syndromes

Hypokalemia

Patients with pernicious anemia who receive vitamin B_{12} to stimulate erythropoiesis may deplete extracellular potassium and suffer from hypokalemia as a cost of producing new red blood cells. Leukemias with rapid growth rates (Chapter 183) also may cause a drop in the serum potassium level, and some forms of myelogenous leukemia are associated with a high level of lysozyme, which leads to urinary potassium loss as well (Chapter 184).

Familial hypokalemic periodic paralysis is an autosomal dominant disorder usually caused by mutations in certain voltage-gated skeletal muscle sodium channels or L-type calcium channels.[13] Characteristically, periodic attacks of severe hypokalemia are precipitated by stimuli, such as the insulin response to carbohydrate ingestion or rest after exercise, that usually induce mild hypokalemia by distributing potassium into cells. In individuals with these channel mutations, the same stimuli cause progressive and severe hypokalemia, enough to result in muscle paralysis due to hyperpolarization of the sarcolemma. The cause of the syndrome is an imbalance between outwardly directed K^+ current and inwardly directed cation leaks of Na^+ and Ca^{2+}. In the familial mutations, the cation depolarizing influx, normally very small under hyperpolarizing conditions, is instead increased and, when balanced with the outward K^+ current, results in a paradoxical depolarization. In turn, the depolarization inactivates the sodium channel needed for the rapid action potential, so the muscle cell is inexcitable. In nonfamilial hypokalemic periodic paralysis, a loss in function of outwardly directed potassium channels (Kir) accounts for paradoxical depolarization, inactivation of sodium channels, and decreased excitability.

The clinical presentation of hypokalemic periodic paralysis is usually in the teenage years or early adulthood. In some familial cases, a progressive proximal myopathy (Chapter 421) may develop. Asian patients, usually males with hyperthyroidism (Chapter 226), have a decrease-in-function mutation of an outwardly directed potassium channel that causes them to develop episodic paralysis, which is precipitated by high-carbohydrate meals (insulin secretion) or by rest after exercise (when plasma potassium falls because of reuptake of potassium by the ATPase pumps). In Anderson syndrome, which is another form of hypokalemic periodic paralysis, cardiac potassium channels are also affected, and serious cardiac arrhythmias may result.

The condition is treated by a high-potassium diet as well as with β_2-blockers (e.g., propranolol, 20 to 40 mg twice daily) and carbonic anhydrase inhibitors (e.g., acetazolamide, 125 to 500 mg), which in part work by creating a hyperchloremic acidosis that offsets the urinary potassium wasting they cause.

Hyperkalemia

The abnormal distribution of potassium between cells and the extracellular space results in the hyperkalemia that is associated with acidosis, insulin-deficient states, and β_2-adrenergic blockade. Although it is not always possible, it is best to know the levels of serum glucose and potassium in an unconscious diabetic patient before infusing concentrated glucose solutions because of the risk for aggravating an already elevated potassium concentration.

Familial hyperkalemic periodic paralysis is a myopathy caused by a genetic defect in voltage-gated sodium channels in skeletal muscle. Exercise or dietary increases in plasma potassium result in mild depolarization of skeletal muscle that then unmasks the sodium channel defect, rendering the cells unexcitable. Treatment is frequent meals and acetazolamide (125 to 500 mg).

Potassium competes with digoxin-binding sites on the Na^+, K^+-ATPase, so that if hypokalemia coexists, digoxin will have an intensified effect and may lead to drug toxicity. In extreme cases of digitalis overdose, severe hyperkalemia develops as a result of generalized blockade of Na^+, K^+-ATPase.

PROGNOSIS

The prognosis of patients with hypokalemia and hyperkalemia depends on the severity and underlying illness. Most hypokalemic cases are mild (potassium concentration, 3 to 3.5 mEq/L). However, mortality of hospitalized patients with hypokalemia is increased 10-fold. Hyperkalemia is reported in 1 to 10% of hospitalized patients, of whom 10% have severe hyperkalemia (potassium concentration, >6.0 mEq/L). Hyperkalemia is associated with increased mortality (14 to 41%), and it accounts for 2 to 5% of deaths in patients with end-stage renal disease.

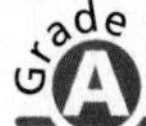

Grade A References

A1. Mahoney BA, Smith WA, Lo DS, et al. Emergency interventions for hyperkalaemia. *Cochrane Database Syst Rev.* 2005;2:CD003235.
A2. Chothia MY, Halperin ML, Rensburg MA, et al. Bolus administration of intravenous glucose in the treatment of hyperkalemia: a randomized controlled trial. *Nephron Physiol.* 2014;126:1-8.
A3. Weir MR, Bakris GL, Bushinsky DA, et al. Patiromer in patients with kidney disease and hyperkalemia receiving RAAS inhibitors. *N Engl J Med.* 2015;372:211-221.
A4. Packham DK, Rasmussen HS, Lavin PT, et al. Sodium zirconium cyclosilicate in hyperkalemia. *N Engl J Med.* 2015;372:222-231.
A5. Kosiborod M, Rasmussen HS, Lavin P, et al. Effect of sodium zirconium cyclosilicate on potassium lowering for 28 days among outpatients with hyperkalemia: the HARMONIZE randomized clinical trial. *JAMA.* 2014;312:2223-2233.

GENERAL REFERENCES

For the General References and other additional features, please visit Expert Consult at https://expertconsult.inkling.com.

118 ACID-BASE DISORDERS

JULIAN L. SEIFTER

DEFINITION

If arterial pH is below 7.35, acidemia is said to exist. If pH is above 7.45, alkalemia exists. However, several processes may simultaneously drive the pH upward or downward; these individual processes are known as *acidoses* or *alkaloses.* Because multiple processes may coexist, an abnormal pH is not always noted in acid-base disturbances. Because pH is related to the ratio of HCO_3^- to PCO_2, the finding of an abnormal bicarbonate level alone cannot define acidosis or alkalosis.

EPIDEMIOLOGY

An acid-base disturbance should alert the clinician to the possible presence of an important underlying condition. Anion gap acidoses represent serious underlying metabolic disorders, ranging from sepsis (Chapter 108) to uremia (Chapter 130) to diabetic ketoacidosis (Chapter 229) to serious poisonings (Chapter 110). Specific renal abnormalities as well as diarrhea (Chapter 140) can cause hyperchloremic acidosis (Table 118-1). Metabolic alkaloses are commonly caused by diuretics or renal tubular abnormalities or the loss of acid from the stomach due to vomiting or nasogastric suction (Table 118-2). Respiratory acidosis and alkalosis are related to ventilation, which is increased by conditions such as sepsis (Chapter 108) and anxiety and decreased in many pulmonary conditions (Chapters 86 and 104).

PATHOBIOLOGY

One of the major requirements for cell survival, along with maintaining electrical gradients and cell volume, is the regulation of the H^+ ion concentration, or pH (defined as the negative logarithm of the hydrogen ion concentration).

TABLE 118-1 CAUSES OF HYPERCHLOREMIC ACIDOSIS

TYPE	CAUSE
Renal with hypokalemia	Proximal RTA, type 2 Distal RTA, type 1 Some anion gap acidoses with high anion clearance
Renal with hyperkalemia	Type 4 RTA; hyporenin-hypoaldosteronism
Nonrenal with hypokalemia	Diarrhea Urinary diversions: ureteroileostomy, ureterosigmoidostomy
Nonrenal with hyperkalemia	NaCl, KCl, NH_4Cl, $CaCl_2$, Arg-HCl, Lys-HCl

RTA = renal tubular acidosis.

TABLE 118-2 CAUSES OF METABOLIC ALKALOSIS

TYPE	CAUSES
Renal, hypochloremic alkalosis: chloride responsive with urine chloride concentration >20 mEq/L	Loop and distal tubule diuretics Bartter syndrome Gitelman syndrome Post-hypercapnic status
Nonrenal, hypochloremic alkalosis: chloride responsive with urine chloride concentration <20 mEq/L	Vomiting, nasogastric suction Chloridorrhea Villous adenoma
Renal, alkalosis with extracellular expansion: chloride unresponsive with urine chloride concentration >20 mEq/L	Hyperaldosteronism, primary and secondary to unilateral renal artery stenosis Liddle syndrome
Nonrenal alkalosis, chloride unresponsive	$NaHCO_3$, acetate, citrate, lactate
Other causes of metabolic alkalosis	Excessive non-reabsorbable anion excretion Hypoproteinemia

Growth, cell division, fertilization, and protein and glucose metabolism are examples of pH-sensitive processes. Acids are generated within cells during metabolism, and each cell must maintain a pH appropriate for its function. For example, cardiac contractility (Chapter 53) is reduced when cardiac myocytes are too acid. Bone and muscle develop and grow poorly in an acidic environment. Intracellular pH may be lower than extracellular pH because cells are electronegative with respect to extracellular fluid, but they are not as acidic as they would be if H^+ reached electrochemical equilibrium with the extracellular fluid, which means that all cells require energy to lose acid actively. Cells are capable of buffering an acid load, and intracellular vacuoles may use hydrogen adenosine triphosphatases (H^+-ATPases) to sequester excess acid before transport from the cell. The transport processes located on the plasma membranes can protect cells from both acid and alkaline loads. The specific mechanisms may differ from one cell type to another, but they are similar to those used by the excretory organs that finally eliminate the net acid produced by the body into the external world.[1]

At a normal arterial blood pH of 7.36 to 7.45, the hydrogen ion concentration is in the range of 40 nanoequivalents (nEq) per liter, a very small concentration in comparison to a normal plasma sodium concentration of 140 mEq/L. In severe disease states, arterial pH may fall as low as 6.8 and rise as high as 7.7. Strenuous exercise with the metabolic production of lactate may transiently but severely lower pH, even in normal healthy individuals.

The hydrogen ion concentration of body fluids is in equilibrium with each of multiple weak acids or buffers, such as proteins and phosphate, but acid-base equilibria in the body are often described and analyzed by use of the CO_2/HCO_3^- system and the relationship of the proton concentration (thus pH) to the ratio of HCO_3^- to CO_2.[2] The Henderson-Hasselbalch equation is a logarithmic expression of the relationship.

$$CO_2 + H_2O \leftrightarrow H_2CO_3 \leftrightarrow H^+ + HCO_3^-$$

$$pH = pK + \log[HCO_3]/0.03\,(P\text{CO}_2)$$

In this equation, p*K*, or the log of the equilibrium constant for the reaction, is 6.1; 0.03 (mM/mm Hg) is the solubility factor for CO_2 in solution. The product of 0.03 × $P\text{CO}_2$ represents dissolved CO_2; the "total CO_2" in plasma is the sum of HCO_3^-, normally about 25 mM, and 0.03 × $P\text{CO}_2$, normally about 1.2 mM. It is important to note that pH is a function of the *ratio* of HCO_3^- to $P\text{CO}_2$. The HCO_3^- concentration in the numerator is regulated by the kidney, and $P\text{CO}_2$ is regulated by the lung.

Production of Carbonic Acid and the Elimination of Carbon Dioxide by the Lung

Volatile acid is the term used for the approximately 20,000 mmol/day of CO_2 produced, with an equimolar amount of water, by tissue respiration. This CO_2 is carried from tissues to the lung, where it is eliminated by alveolar ventilation. Steady-state arterial $P\text{CO}_2$ is normally 38 to 42 mm Hg.

Oxidation of carbohydrates, fat, and the carbon skeleton of amino acids results in the production of water and CO_2. To maintain a steady state, any acid (or base) produced per day must be equivalent to what is eliminated. If tissue CO_2 production exceeds CO_2 elimination by the lungs, respiratory acidosis characterized by a high $P\text{CO}_2$ will develop. If the rate of CO_2 eliminated exceeds production, respiratory alkalosis develops. The inverse relationship between alveolar ventilation (the clearance of CO_2) and $P\text{CO}_2$ is demonstrated as

$$\text{alveolar ventilation} \sim CO_2\ \text{elimination} \div P\text{CO}_2$$

The circulation plays a critical role in transporting tissue CO_2 to the lungs. The process depends not only on cellular respiration but also on tissue capillary flow as well as diffusion of CO_2 into the blood and across red blood cell membranes, where it may react with hemoglobin and proteins to form carbamino compounds or combine with water for conversion to H^+ and HCO_3^- in a reaction catalyzed by carbonic anhydrase. The intracellular H^+ can combine with hemoglobin (the Bohr effect) and the HCO_3^- exchanged with plasma Cl^- through red cell anion exchangers. Most tissue CO_2 is brought to the lung as venous plasma HCO_3^-. Compared with arterial blood, venous blood has the characteristics of a respiratory acidosis. Venous pH is normally approximately 0.05 pH unit more acid than arterial pH, its $P\text{CO}_2$ is 5 to 6 mm Hg higher than that of arterial blood, and its bicarbonate concentrations are normally greater than arterial concentrations.

In disease, changes in $P\text{CO}_2$ are most often caused by changes in alveolar ventilation rather than by production of CO_2. Thus, respiratory acidosis is a consequence of decreased pulmonary ventilation because of lung, skeletal muscle, or central nervous system (CNS) disease. However, if alveolar ventilation is compromised, increased production of CO_2 will worsen CO_2 retention. Similarly, respiratory alkalosis develops because of hyperventilation rather than decreased CO_2 production. In either case, when the elimination rate of CO_2 (alveolar ventilation × $P\text{CO}_2$) again equals CO_2 production, a new steady-state $P\text{CO}_2$ will prevail, with no net retention or loss of carbonic acid.

Production of Acids and Excretion by the Kidney

Nonvolatile or fixed acid describes non-carbonic acids that are formed primarily from protein metabolism. The usual rate of formation is approximately 1 to 2 mEq of H^+ per kilogram of body weight per day. Most diets that contain animal protein have a net positive quantity of nonvolatile acids, primarily sulfates from the sulfur-containing amino acids cysteine and methionine. Other acids are produced in the form of phosphates (from phosphoproteins, phospholipids, and phosphonucleotides) and nonmetabolizable organic acids (e.g., uric acid) and chloride from salts of lysine, arginine, and histidine.

From the Henderson-Hasselbalch equation, consider the addition of metabolic acid HA (where the anion A^- could be Cl^-, lactate$^-$, HSO_4^-, or $H_2PO_4^-$) to blood that contains Na^+ and HCO_3^-.

$$HA + NaHCO_3 \rightarrow Na^+ + A^- + H^+ + HCO_3^-$$

and

$$H^+ + HCO_3^- \leftrightarrow H_2CO_3 \leftrightarrow CO_2 + H_2O$$

The CO_2 produced by this process will not raise the blood $P\text{CO}_2$ if the system is well ventilated because the contribution of metabolic acid is a small part of the daily production of CO_2. Note that the addition of protons to body fluids by these acid end products consumes bicarbonate ("lost bicarbonate"), which then must be replenished by the kidney as it eliminates the proton and A^- in the urine. The process of excreting net H^+ and A^- is equivalent to producing a "new" HCO_3^- to restore the HCO_3^- that is lost by the addition of HA, the metabolic acid. The kidney must excrete any nonvolatile acid (or alkali) load to maintain a steady-state serum HCO_3^- concentration in the 22- to 28-mEq/L range.

When the diet requires the excretion of acids, the urine pH will fall to a value as low as 5.0, and the urine will become nominally free of bicarbonate. With an alkaline load, by comparison, the kidney will reject the excess filtered HCO_3^-, and the urine pH may approach a maximal value of 8.0 to 8.5. In most humans, particularly those who eat animal protein or an "acid-ash" diet, the requirement for net acid *excretion* predominates. However, some vegetarians may have an overall "alkaline-ash" diet, for which net alkali must be excreted to match intake.

Bicarbonate and the Kidney in Acid-Base Balance

The first role of the kidney in achieving acid excretion is to reabsorb all filtered HCO_3^- (E-Fig. 118-1). At a normal glomerular filtration rate (e.g., ~180 L/day in an adult) and plasma HCO_3^- concentration of 25 mEq/L, about 4500 mEq of HCO_3^- is filtered in 1 day. Loss of even a small fraction of that amount would result in metabolic acidosis if not replaced by HCO_3^- intake. Just as reabsorption of all filtered glucose does not add glucose to the body, reabsorption of all filtered HCO_3^- will maintain the status quo but will not fulfill the need to generate new HCO_3^-. Therefore, the kidney must perform two functions: reabsorb all filtered HCO_3^- and eliminate enough additional H^+ (producing HCO_3^- in the process) to maintain balance. Without urinary buffers, the urinary pH cannot be lowered enough to excrete the amount of acid needed for this purpose.

The Proximal Tubule

About 80 to 90% of HCO_3^- reabsorption is accomplished in the proximal tubule by a proton secretory process that renders the proximal tubular fluid more acid (pH ~6.5). The brush border membranes facing the lumen of the proximal tubule cell contain transporters known as Na/H exchangers (NHE3), which carry out the greatest proportion of acidification, and vacuolar H^+-ATPases, which provide a smaller contribution. Through the normal function of basolateral membrane Na^+, K^+-ATPase, cell Na^+ is kept at low concentration so that filtered Na^+ in the lumen will be favored to enter the cell in exchange for H^+ secreted into the lumen. This H^+ rapidly combines with filtered HCO_3^- to form H_2CO_3, which then dehydrates in the lumen to form CO_2 and H_2O. This last process is greatly facilitated by the large surface area of microvillous membranes and by luminal carbonic anhydrase (CA_{IV}). The CO_2 enters the proximal cell by diffusion through apical water channels (aquaporin 1). CO_2 within the cell re-forms HCO_3^-, a reaction catalyzed by intracellular carbonic anhydrase (CA_{II}). The cell, more alkaline by apical H^+ secretion, favors the reaction $OH^- + CO_2$ to form HCO_3^- catalyzed by carbonic anhydrase at the higher cell pH. The HCO_3^- is then transported back toward the blood by a sodium bicarbonate cotransporter (NBC), which couples 1Na and $3HCO_3^-$, thereby completing net Na^+ and HCO_3^- reabsorption. The 1 : 3 stoichiometry of NBC is necessary to provide sufficient energy to couple Na^+ and HCO_3^- in this electrogenic process, which protects the cell from an alkaline load, accomplishes HCO_3^- reabsorption, and drives uphill Na^+ reabsorption without further direct requirement for adenosine triphosphate (ATP). The entire process requires a mitochondrial source of ATP for the Na^+/K^+ pump, intact NHE3 and NBC, and two isoforms of carbonic anhydrase. In addition, there must be favorable ion gradients for luminal Na^+ entry, H^+ secretion, and basolateral HCO_3^- transport. A disturbance in any of these factors may disrupt proximal HCO_3^- reabsorption enough to cause loss of HCO_3^- in urine. It is also clear that the acidifying process in the proximal tubule provides a significant mechanism for Na^+ reabsorption, consistent with the finding that HCO_3^- reabsorption is increased by angiotensin II and the sympathetic nervous system in the defense of extracellular volume. Another 10 to 15% of filtered HCO_3^- is reabsorbed in the thick ascending limb of Henle through a mechanism similar to the mechanism in the proximal tubule, so that only small amounts of the filtered HCO_3^- are normally delivered to more distal nephron segments.

The Cortical Collecting Duct

The cortical connecting tubules and collecting ducts reabsorb less than 10% of the filtered HCO_3^-. In principal cells, Na^+ is reabsorbed from lumen to cell by the epithelial sodium channel (ENaC), driven by the inwardly directed Na^+ gradient and favorable electrical potential. With the reabsorption of Na^+, the lumen becomes electronegative, thus favoring the secretion of both K^+, through potassium channels, and H^+, through vacuolar H^+-ATPases on the luminal surface of neighboring α-intercalated cells, which are acid-secreting cells. The secreted H^+ will combine with the remaining HCO_3^- in the lumen to generate CO_2, with subsequent reabsorption of CO_2, re-formation of cellular HCO_3^- with the help of cellular carbonic anhydrase (CA_{II}), and then exchange of HCO_3^- from cell to blood for entry of Cl^- through Cl^-/HCO_3^- exchangers, similar to the erythrocytic anion exchangers (AE1) that participate in blood CO_2 transport. The distal nephron, which has a smaller requirement for bicarbonate reabsorption than the proximal tubule, lacks both brush border and luminal carbonic anhydrase. It is at this distal site that tubular fluid pH starts to fall to levels below pH 6.0.

Some collecting duct cells have reverse polarity and secrete HCO_3^- into the lumen in exchange for Cl^- entry into the cell. In these cells, the H^+-ATPase faces the blood side of the cell (β-intercalated cells). An elevated extracellular HCO_3^- concentration, as seen with an alkaline-ash diet or metabolic alkalosis, will increase HCO_3^- secretion by these cells through pendrin, which is the apical Cl^-/HCO_3^- exchanger.

The Medullary Collecting Duct

The medullary collecting duct continues to secrete protons into the luminal fluid, where the pH reaches its lowest values of close to 5.0. The mechanism is based on continued function of H^+-ATPases with an additional role of an ATP-dependent K^+/H^+ exchanger, a member of the family of K^+, H^+-ATPases found in the stomach and colon.

Once the filtered HCO_3^- is fully reabsorbed, the kidney is still required to eliminate an additional net amount of acid equivalent to that produced in metabolism. Most of this net acid excretion is in the form of ammonium (NH_4^+), which is derived from the renal synthesis of ammonia from glutamine in the proximal tubule and the titration of filtered phosphate to acid phosphate (titratable acidity).

$$NH_3 + H^+ \leftrightarrow NH_4^+ \quad pK\ 9.1$$

and

$$HPO_4^{2-} + H^+ \leftrightarrow H_2PO_4^- \quad pK\ 6.8$$

Urinary Buffers

As the collecting duct cells continue to secrete H^+ into urine with a diminishing luminal HCO_3^- concentration and decreasing pH, H^+ is captured by the urinary buffers. The resulting alkalinization of the cells after H^+ leaves results in the formation of cellular HCO_3^- ready for transport into blood. This process generates new HCO_3^- that is not a result of the reabsorption of filtered HCO_3^-. The amount of new HCO_3^- matches the amount of net acid eliminated and is also equal to each of the following: the amount of acid produced; the amount of body buffer consumed by that acid; and the amount of fixed acid anions, such as sulfate, phosphate, and Cl^-, that accompanied the H^+. The result is maintenance of normal acid-base equilibrium.

The ability of the kidney to lower urinary pH to values as low as 5.0 enables the buffers to capture a proton. Net acid excretion in urine is accomplished not simply by a decrease in urine pH but mostly by titration of these important urinary buffers. For example, a typical daily urine volume of 1 L at pH 5.0 contains only 10^{-5} molar hydrogen ion, or 0.01 mmol, a trivial amount compared with the amount of produced acid (~1 mmol/kg/day). In chronic kidney disease, it is the failure to produce enough ammonium that leads to a poorly buffered, although acid, urine and an inability to excrete enough net acid to stay in normal balance.

Regulation of Urinary Acid Secretion

Renal mechanisms of urinary acidification are adaptable. Transport processes such as H^+-ATPases, Na^+/H^+ exchange, and Cl^-/HCO_3^- exchange can increase or decrease their capacity to handle acid-base equivalents, depending on the challenge presented. Renal ammoniagenic mechanisms are also critically regulated to serve the acid-base needs of the individual. Metabolic acidosis and respiratory acidosis increase the capacity to reabsorb HCO_3^-, including increased expression of the transporters involved in acidifying the urine. At the same time, increased glutamine uptake into proximal cells and ammonia production enable increased acid excretion and the generation of new HCO_3^- in the distal nephron. Metabolic alkalosis and respiratory alkalosis have the opposite effects.

Ammoniagenesis, which is a key element in urinary acid excretion, provides the major acceptor for protons. Ammonia is produced predominantly in the proximal tubule cell by mitochondrial glutaminase enzymes. Production is increased by increasing the metabolic acid load in the body, respiratory acidosis, and hypokalemia. NH_4^+ can preserve potassium in the hypokalemic state by serving as a cation needed for anion excretion. Similarly, in response to metabolic acidosis, the kidney would ideally excrete chloride with ammonium and preserve the ability to retain Na^+ and K^+.

Ammonia can be secreted by nonionic diffusion into the proximal fluid, where it will pick up a proton and form ammonium (NH_4^+), or it could form ammonium within the proximal tubule cell and be secreted by Na^+/NH_4^+ exchange, a mode of operation of the Na^+/H^+ exchanger. Ammonium may be reabsorbed by the thick ascending limb of Henle on the Na-K-2Cl transporter, where it can substitute for K^+. By countercurrent multiplication, NH_3/NH_4^+ concentrates in the medullary interstitial fluid rather than remaining in the ascending limb fluid as it reaches the highly perfused renal cortex, where it would otherwise dissipate into renal venous blood. The countercurrent mechanism also allows ammonia to diffuse into the lumen of the medullary collecting duct, where it will be trapped as ammonium in the acid tubular fluid. Collecting duct cells also secrete NH_3 by way of glycoproteins that are in the family of the Rh factor, red blood cell ammonia transporters.

Regulation is accomplished at a number of levels. Hormones such as angiotensin II and catecholamines stimulate Na^+ reabsorption in the proximal tubule by increasing sodium-hydrogen exchange and $NaHCO_3$ cotransport. Aldosterone increases H^+-ATPase in the collecting duct cell and stimulates Na^+ reabsorption, thereby increasing proton secretion. Low extracellular fluid volume increases proximal HCO_3^- reabsorption, as does hypokalemia and high P_{CO_2}. Hyperkalemia (Chapter 117) may limit urinary acidification by decreasing the NH_3 entering the countercurrent multiplier in the loop of Henle and decreasing H^+ secretion by ATPases in the collecting duct as the need to secrete K^+ predominates.

The liver also contributes to urinary net acid excretion. Acidosis decreases activity of the urea cycle, which otherwise consumes NH_3 and HCO_3^- to form carbamoyl phosphate. In acidosis, NH_3 produces hepatic glutamine, which is delivered to the proximal tubule cell, where mitochondrial enzymes produce $2NH_3$ to assist in urinary net acid excretion; the associated increased α-ketoglutarate provides a substrate for renal gluconeogenesis.

CLINICAL MANIFESTATIONS AND DIAGNOSIS

Assessment of clinical acid-base disturbances usually begins with measurement of arterial blood gases (Fig. 118-1 and Table 118-3). In some situations, venous blood can be used as an alternative.

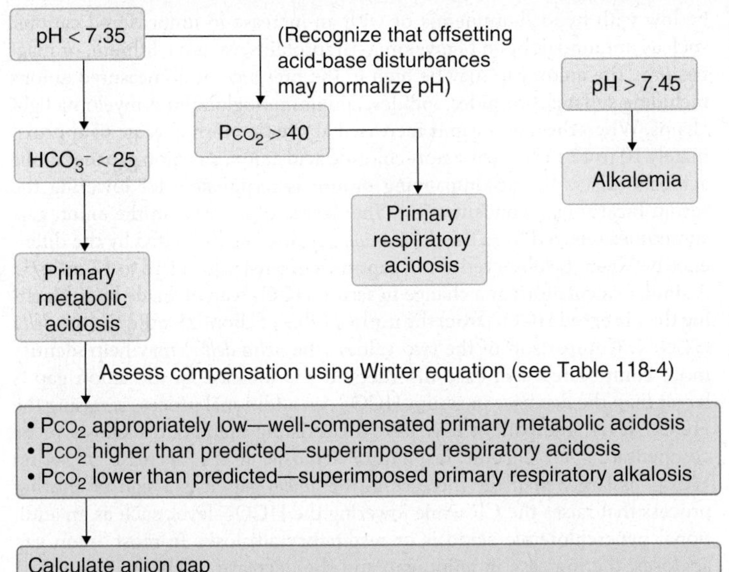

FIGURE 118-1. Evaluation of acidemia.

TABLE 118-3 LABORATORY STEPS IN IDENTIFYING ACID-BASE DISORDERS

EVALUATE pH	ACIDEMIC	ALKALEMIC
Elevated Pco_2	Respiratory acidosis	Metabolic alkalosis
Elevated HCO_3	Respiratory acidosis	Metabolic alkalosis
Decreased Pco_2	Metabolic acidosis	Respiratory alkalosis
Decreased HCO_3	Metabolic acidosis	Respiratory alkalosis
EVALUATE FOR EXPECTED COMPENSATION		
Meets expectation: simple disorder with compensation or could be offsetting metabolic alkalosis and acidosis		
Does not meet expectation: complex disorder, but pH indicates whether acidosis or alkalosis is dominant		
If a metabolic disorder is dominant, a Pco_2 greater than predicted indicates an additional respiratory acidosis. A Pco_2 less than predicted indicates an additional respiratory alkalosis.		
If a respiratory disorder is dominant, an HCO_3 concentration greater than predicted indicates additional metabolic alkalosis. An HCO_3 concentration less than predicted indicates an additional metabolic acidosis.		
ASSESS ANION GAP		
Elevated: metabolic acidosis is present whether acidemic or alkalemic. If alkalemic, an additional metabolic or respiratory alkalosis is present.		
If the gap is greater than the fall in HCO_3, consider an additional metabolic alkalosis or respiratory acidosis.		
If the gap is less than the fall in HCO_3, consider an additional nongap acidosis or respiratory alkalosis.		

It is useful to conceptualize acid-base disorders by a mass action shift of the variables to the right or left in the following relationship:

$$H^+ + HCO_3^- \leftrightarrow H_2CO_3 \leftrightarrow CO_2 + H_2O$$

The addition of CO_2, as in respiratory acidosis, will increase the hydrogen and bicarbonate concentrations (left shift). Removal of CO_2, as in respiratory alkalosis, will decrease CO_2, protons, and bicarbonate (shift right). The addition of protons with an anion other than HCO_3^-, as in metabolic acidosis, will lead to increased concentrations of protons and a decreased bicarbonate concentration. Removal of HCO_3^- with a cation such as Na^+, also a cause of metabolic acidosis, will increase the proton concentration and lower the HCO_3^- concentration. Metabolic alkalosis might be caused by the addition of $NaHCO_3$ with a resulting decrease in the proton concentration or by removal of H^+ with chloride, thereby leading to a decreased proton concentration and increased HCO_3^-. Because of the relationship of metabolic acidosis and alkalosis to the gain or loss of fluids and electrolytes, one could consider acid-base disorders a consequence of electrolyte imbalance.[3]

TABLE 118-4 EXPECTED DEGREES OF COMPENSATION IN ACID-BASE DISORDERS

DISORDER	EXPECTED COMPENSATION
Metabolic acidosis	Steady state in 12-36 hours Expected Pco_2 = 1.5 (measured HCO_3) + 8 ± 2 (Winter equation)
Metabolic alkalosis	Less predictable Expected Pco_2 increases 0.5 mm Hg per 1-mEq/L increase in HCO_3
Respiratory acidosis	
Acute	Expected 1-mEq/L increase in HCO_3 per 10-mm Hg rise in Pco_2
Chronic, 24-36 hours	Expected 3- to 5-mEq/L increase in HCO_3 per 10-mm Hg rise in Pco_2
Respiratory alkalosis	
Acute	Expected 1- to 2-mEq/L fall in HCO_3 per 10-mm Hg fall in Pco_2
Chronic, after 24-36 hours	Expected 5-mEq/L fall in HCO_3 per 10-mm Hg fall in Pco_2

Compensatory Changes

Few patients have an isolated acid-base disturbance. In nearly all cases, a respiratory or renal compensation (or both) occurs in response to counteract a primary acid-base process.

When they are functioning normally, the lungs may maintain a normal pH and Pco_2 during changes in volatile acid production. The kidneys will also maintain normal acid-base balance during changes in fixed acid production. Only excesses beyond the capacity to eliminate an acid or alkali load will lead to clinical disturbances. It follows that patients with renal or lung disease may do less well in response to metabolic and respiratory disorders.

When an acid-base disturbance develops, the initial response to modulate its severity depends on the titration of various body buffer pairs. For example, phosphate, hemoglobin, and albumin change their protonated and unprotonated concentrations. The body will then further attempt to correct the extracellular pH toward normal but usually not to normal. For metabolic disturbances caused by increased or decreased nonvolatile acid, the response is respiratory; for primary respiratory acidosis and alkalosis, the compensation is renal (Table 118-4). The direction of change in HCO_3^- and Pco_2 is the same when the primary disturbance is compensated; the ratio of HCO_3^- to Pco_2 and thus pH become more normal. These compensations tend to take time, so acid-base disturbances, particularly the respiratory conditions, are classified as acute (lasting less than 24 to 48 hours) or chronic.

Peripheral blood does not demonstrate complete compensation for most acid-base disturbances, with the occasional exception of chronic respiratory alkalosis. Full compensation for metabolic acidosis would expend large amounts of respiratory muscle energy, which could limit a prolonged response. Full compensation for metabolic alkalosis would result in excessive hypoventilation and adverse effects on oxygenation. In contrast, the CNS closely regulates its pH, with nearly full correction within 1 to 2 days. Before this compensation occurs, acute alkalemia may be associated with cerebral vasoconstriction and ischemia, whereas acidemia may result in vasodilation and cerebral edema. Rapid changes in blood Pco_2 affect the CNS chemosensors more quickly than do changes in HCO_3^- because of the more rapid movement of nonionic CO_2 across the blood-brain barrier. Increases in CNS CO_2 lead to acidification of the medullary center interstitial fluid and an increased ventilatory drive. Decreases in CNS CO_2 (alkalinization of the respiratory center) lead to hypoventilation. Acid-base changes are reflected in the composition of the cerebrospinal fluid (CSF).

In metabolic acidosis, peripheral chemosensors in the carotid body stimulate the CNS to increase ventilation to reduce Pco_2. The fall in peripheral Pco_2 will lead to dissolved CO_2 leaving the CNS ahead of HCO_3^-; the alkalinization of the medullary center interstitial fluid will then slow the hyperventilatory response until a new steady state of hypocapnia is achieved. Patients may sense dyspnea or air hunger acutely with rapid and shallow respirations. In severe cases of metabolic acidemia, the respirations are deep and gasping, typical of Kussmaul breathing.

When the bicarbonate concentration increases as a result of metabolic alkalosis, a hypoventilatory response, signaled from the peripheral chemosensors, raises Pco_2. As Pco_2 rises, the dissolved CO_2 will enter the CSF and will acidify the medullary respiratory center. The stimulus to breathe will, in part, antagonize the peripheral signal until a steady state of hypoventilation is reached.

The acute stimulus of hypercapnia to increase net renal acid excretion disappears in chronic respiratory acidosis when, at the elevated Pco_2, carbonic acid production and elimination are again equal. However, the hypochloremia, brought about by the compensatory early excretion of NH_4Cl, and elevated serum HCO_3^-, maintained by the high Pco_2, persist.

In respiratory alkalosis, the primary event is a fall in Pco_2 because of increased alveolar ventilation. On transition from acute to chronic respiratory alkalosis, the compensatory mechanisms that initially helped maintain a more normal systemic pH are no longer required as CO_2 production and elimination become equal. Thus, the initial compensatory decrease in renal acid excretion brought about by increased loss of filtered $NaHCO_3$ ceases, but low serum HCO_3^- and high serum Cl^- concentrations are maintained.

In identifying whether an acid-base disturbance is simple (a single disturbance with its compensation) or complex (multiple primary processes simultaneously present), it is useful to compare the expected compensation for a simple process with the observed parameters of the blood gases (see Table 118-3). For example, if Pco_2 is lower than would be predicted in a patient with a simple, compensated metabolic acidosis, an additional respiratory alkalosis must be driving the Pco_2 down. If Pco_2 is higher than would be predicted for a low bicarbonate level in a patient with metabolic acidosis, a coexistent respiratory acidosis is present.

METABOLIC ACIDOSIS

EPIDEMIOLOGY AND PATHOBIOLOGY

In metabolic acidosis, the primary change is a fall in serum bicarbonate. The compensatory response is to increase ventilation to reduce Pco_2. Worsening acidosis elicits increasing alveolar ventilation.

Primary metabolic acidosis results from an imbalance between net acid production and net acid excretion (NAE) in the form of urinary ammonium excretion and acid phosphate excretion. Consider the following relationship, where U_x represents the urinary concentration and the urinary flow rate $\dot{V}$:

$$NAE = (U_{NH_4} \times \dot{V}) + (U_{phos} \times \dot{V}) - (U_{HCO_3^-} \times \dot{V})$$

In a normal steady-state condition, the rate of excretion of net acid must be equal to the rate of production. The normal production rate depends on diet. If net acid production is normal, metabolic acidosis could occur because of a failure to reabsorb bicarbonate or a failure to elaborate enough urinary buffers, as is the case in renal failure and renal tubular acidosis. An inequality also could develop if net acid production were excessive or if large extrarenal bicarbonate losses were unable to be matched by maximal adaptive increases in net acid excretion. Endogenous sources of acid include ketoacidosis and lactic acidosis, whereas exogenous sources might be acid metabolic products of ingested ethylene glycol or methanol. On occasion, strong inorganic acids may be ingested. When net acid is retained in body fluids, the serum bicarbonate concentration falls. However, maintenance of a constant low serum HCO_3^- concentration does not guarantee that there is a new steady state in which net acid production is equal to net acid excretion because body buffers such as carbonate salts of bone may become depleted by relentless acid retention, as in chronic kidney disease and distal renal tubular acidosis.

The causes of metabolic acidosis are usually categorized according to the presence of either hyperchloremia or an elevated serum anion gap. The serum anion gap is the net charge difference when the sum of chloride and bicarbonate is subtracted from the serum sodium concentration.[4]

$$\text{Anion gap} = Na^+ - (Cl^- + HCO_3^-)$$

The normal anion gap is due to the net unmeasured anionic charge associated predominantly with albumin. When acidemia is present, albumin is in a more protonated form, which lowers the normal gap. In alkalemia, the effect of pH is to increase the gap attributed to albumin. Each 1 g/dL of albumin contributes approximately 2.5 mEq/L to the normal anion gap. The anion gap may be low with hypoalbuminemia or with an increase in unmeasured cations, such as immunoglobulin G myeloma paraproteins, calcium, lithium, or magnesium. The anion gap may be high in the presence of unmeasured anions including sulfates, bromides, iodides, and immunoglobulin A myeloma light chains. When the anion gap is increased above the normal value of approximately 10 to 12 mEq/L by a non-chloride acid anion, an anion gap metabolic acidosis exists. The accompanying proton is responsible for lowering the serum bicarbonate concentration. The degree of increase in the anion gap, sometimes referred to as the *delta anion gap*, may be estimated by the difference between the observed anion gap and a normal value of 10 to 12 mEq/L. A similar calculation for a change in serum HCO_3^- can be made by subtracting the observed HCO_3^- from the normal value of about 25 mEq/L (the *delta* HCO_3^-). Comparison of the two values (the *delta-delta*) may help identify more complicated acid-base disorders. If the increase in the anion gap is larger than the decrease in serum HCO_3^-, an additional process is raising the HCO_3^- level. The patient may have a coexisting metabolic alkalosis or be compensating for chronic respiratory acidosis. If the decrease in serum HCO_3^- is larger than the increase in the anion gap, it is a sign of another process that raises the Cl^- while lowering the HCO_3^- level, such as an additional hyperchloremic acidosis or respiratory alkalosis. In most anion gap acidoses, the increase in anion gap and the decrease in HCO_3^- is not 1:1 because the excretion of urinary anions with Na^+ results in a hyperchloremic component to the acidosis. Conversely, any buffering of H^+ with non-HCO_3^- buffers will decrease the drop in HCO_3^- compared with the increase in anion gap. In severe cases of anion gap acidosis, Cl^- may be displaced into cells, thereby resulting in a higher anion gap compared with the decrease in HCO_3^-—a hypochloremic anion gap acidosis.

CLINICAL MANIFESTATIONS

The effects of metabolic acidosis depend on its rapidity of onset and severity.[5] Patients often complain of fatigue and dyspnea, particularly on exertion. Nausea and vomiting are common. On examination, deep respirations, often labored with the use of accessory muscles, may be detected acutely, but hyperventilation may be less notable with long-standing metabolic acidemia. Metabolic acidemia also may be associated with vasodilation, tachycardia, and hypotension (Chapter 106). The negative inotropic effect of acidemia on the heart can exacerbate septic shock (Chapter 108). The stress of either an underlying illness or an increase in adrenergic and corticosteroid activity associated with acidemia may elevate the peripheral white blood cell count and cause hyperglycemia. Other laboratory findings include variable degrees of hyperkalemia, hyperphosphatemia, and hyperuricemia as well as hypocalcemia as a result of decreased renal synthesis of 1,25-dihydroxyvitamin D.

Anion Gap Metabolic Acidoses

A variety of abnormalities can cause anion gap acidoses. One mnemonic for the common ones is *gold mark*, for glycols (ethylene and propylene), oxoproline, *l*-lactate, *d*-lactate, methanol, aspirin, renal failure, and ketoacidosis.[6] Because some causes are life-threatening, a rapid diagnosis is required. The osmolar gap should be calculated in all cases of anion gap acidosis (Table 118-5) because unmeasured toxic, nonionic alcohols that contribute to body osmolality but not to acidity oxidize to dangerous unmeasured organic acid anions that contribute only to the anion gap. The osmolar gap is defined as the difference between the measured and the calculated serum osmolality.

TABLE 118-5 CAUSES OF INCREASED ANION AND OSMOLAR GAPS

ANION GAP METABOLIC ACIDOSIS	OSMOLAR GAP
Uremia	No
Lactic acidosis	Variable/no
D-Lactic acidosis	No
Diabetic ketoacidosis	No
Starvation ketoacidosis	No
Alcoholic ketoacidosis	If ethanol is present
Ethylene glycol	Yes
Methanol	Yes
Salicylates	No
5-Oxoprolinuria (acetaminophen)	No

The serum osmolality should be measured by a freezing point depression technique and compared with the calculated osmolality.

$$\text{Calculated osmolality} = 2\,(\text{Na}^+) + (\text{Glucose}\,[\text{mg/dL}] \div 18) + (\text{Blood urea nitrogen}\,[\text{mg/dL}] \div 2.8)$$

UREMIC ACIDOSIS

The metabolic acidosis of advanced chronic kidney disease (Chapter 130) may be due to tubular leakage of HCO_3^-, but it is often present when inadequate ammonia production is unable to facilitate excretion of the normal metabolic acid load. Many patients with renal failure can acidify their urine, but the lack of buffering capacity diminishes net acid excretion. Many organic and inorganic anions, such as phosphate and sulfates, are retained at glomerular filtration rates of less than 25 mL/minute and constitute an increased anion gap in association with the metabolic acidosis. The magnitude of the gap is usually less than 20 mEq/L consisting of poorly filtered sulfates and phosphates. The renal patient who is maximally producing NH_3 to stay in balance with daily acid production may be unable to accommodate any further acid production, such as a metabolic or respiratory acidosis, that would require increased ammoniagenesis. The patient with a poor glomerular filtration will retain HCO_3^-, thereby worsening both metabolic and respiratory alkalosis. The systemic acid-base disturbance in renal diseases with prominent tubular dysfunction is attributable to the kidney's inability to secrete hydrogen and to reabsorb and generate HCO_3^-. It is particularly pronounced in oliguric acute kidney injury and is exacerbated by hypercatabolic states such as infection. A significant metabolic acidosis in a patient with chronic kidney disease of unknown cause should raise the possibility of urinary tract obstruction (Chapter 123) or chronic tubulointerstitial diseases (Chapter 122), including amyloidosis (Chapter 188), myeloma (Chapter 187), autoimmune disorders, and analgesic nephropathy (Chapter 122).

It is important to treat the metabolic acidosis of chronic kidney disease.[7,8] Maintaining the serum HCO_3^- concentration above 20 to 22 mEq/L, by administering $NaHCO_3$ at a rate of 1 mEq HCO_3^-/kg/day, will slow the progression of chronic kidney disease, delay end-stage renal failure,[A1] and improve nutritional status.[A2]

PROGNOSIS

In population studies, a low serum bicarbonate level is associated with higher all-cause mortality. The relative risk of death is about 2.6-fold higher in patients with chronic kidney disease and about 1.7-fold higher even without it.

OVERPRODUCTION OF ENDOGENOUS ACIDS

Lactic Acidosis

EPIDEMIOLOGY AND PATHOBIOLOGY

Overproduction of lactate may occur with severe exertion, but true lactic acidosis is frequently associated with critical illness, multiorgan failure, and increased mortality. Lactate, which is the final product in the anaerobic pathway of glucose metabolism, is produced from pyruvate in a reaction catalyzed by lactate dehydrogenase:

$$\text{NADH} + \text{pyruvate} + \text{H}^+ \rightarrow \text{lactate} + \text{NAD}$$

A high reduced nicotinamide adenine dinucleotide (NADH)/NAD ratio will favor the formation of lactate. Conversion of ethanol to acetaldehyde and conversion of β-hydroxybutyrate to acetoacetate use NAD and produce NADH. Alcohol metabolism may be associated with excessive β-hydroxybutyrate and lactic acidosis.

Lactic acidosis is caused by an imbalance in the rates of lactate production and its clearance, primarily in the liver. Lactic acidosis, which increases the anion gap, is most often due to circulatory failure, hypoxia, and mitochondrial dysfunction that each increase anaerobic glycolysis and the rate of conversion of pyruvate to lactate. Sepsis (Chapter 108) is associated with an elevated lactate level because of poor clearance and impaired gluconeogenesis. Lactic acidosis can also result from seizure activity (Chapter 403) when lactate is released from muscle cells that have sustained a period of anaerobic metabolism. Other causes include thiamine deficiency (Chapter 214), hypophosphatemia (Chapter 119), isoniazid toxicity (Chapter 110), and hypoglycemic states (Chapter 230).[9] Metformin may cause lactic acidosis, particularly in elderly patients with cardiac, hepatic, or renal dysfunction.

Nucleoside antivirals (Chapter 388), including zidovudine, may cause lactic acidosis and abnormal liver function as a result of toxic mitochondrial effects. Abnormal mitochondrial function is also a feature of aspirin overdose (Chapter 37) or toxicity with hypoglycin from ingestion of the unripe ackee fruit (Jamaican vomiting sickness). The antibiotic linezolid is another cause of lactic acidosis.

Lactic acidosis can also be caused by the overproduction of lactate, which may occur with severe exertion and malignant neoplasms, particularly with a large tumor burden from lymphoma or widely metastatic cancer. Malignant cells can upregulate glycolytic activity, which may increase their uptake of glucose and decrease their dependence on mitochondrion-derived energy. These tumors can use large amounts of available glucose and inorganic phosphate, thereby leading to a syndrome of hypoglycemia, hypophosphatemia, and lactic acidosis.

CLINICAL MANIFESTATIONS AND DIAGNOSIS

In any patient with an anion gap acidosis, the serum lactate level should be directly measured. Glucose, creatinine, and blood urea nitrogen levels also should be obtained. In cases in which a toxic ingestion is suspected (see Table 118-5), a screen for such toxins in the serum should be performed.

TREATMENT Rx

Treatment of lactic acidosis is aimed at correction of the underlying cause. Central venous oxygen saturation should be increased, with a goal of at least 70%, by restoring tissue perfusion and ventilation, but specific therapy to increase the clearance of lactate is not of significant incremental value.[A3] In a randomized trial of patients with lactic acidosis (pH of 6.9 to 7.2 and an average lactate level of 7.8 mM) in an intensive care unit, for example, sodium bicarbonate infused at a rate of 2 mEq/kg per 15 minutes did not improve hemodynamics, despite improvement in pH, but adversely lowered ionized serum calcium compared with saline.[A4] Sodium bicarbonate can be considered when the arterial pH is below 7.0 or when acidemia has resulted in decreased cardiac inotropy or systemic vasodilation and shock. It is preferable to give $NaHCO_3$ as an isotonic mixture in 5% dextrose and water, rather than as a hypertonic bolus, because a hypertonic bolus carries the risk of pulmonary edema and hypernatremia. The quantity of administered sodium bicarbonate to raise arterial pH to 7.2 should be estimated by multiplying the desired minus observed bicarbonate concentration by 50% of body weight. Full correction should be avoided.

In patients with a metabolic acidosis after seizures (Chapter 403), the lactate is quickly metabolized to HCO_3^- by the liver and kidneys, and the acidosis often resolves within 60 minutes. The administration of HCO_3^- is usually unnecessary and may precipitate an overshoot metabolic alkalosis as the lactate is metabolized, which lowers the seizure threshold.

In patients with intestinal bacterial overgrowth (Chapter 140), a syndrome of disorientation, ataxia, and anion gap metabolic acidosis may develop after a carbohydrate meal because of bacterial production of D-lactate. This isomer of the mammalian L-lactate can be measured only by a specific D-lactate assay. The condition is treated with oral antibiotics and appropriate diet.

PROGNOSIS

Lactic acidosis, when severe, is associated with a high early mortality. When the pH is less than 7.2, only 17% of patients who are admitted to an intensive care unit are ultimately discharged from the hospital.

Diabetic Ketoacidosis

EPIDEMIOLOGY AND PATHOBIOLOGY

Diabetic ketoacidosis is defined as hyperglycemia with metabolic acidosis resulting from generation of the acid anions β-hydroxybutyrate (a hydroxy acid) and acetoacetate (a keto acid) in response to insulin deficiency and elevated counter-regulatory hormones such as glucagon. It is most commonly seen in cases of type 1 diabetes mellitus but can occasionally be seen in type 2 diabetes mellitus (Chapter 229). In an urban population, African Americans of low socioeconomic status were found to have more frequent episodes of diabetic ketoacidosis.[10]

The lack of insulin increases lipolysis in adipose tissue; free fatty acids are transported to the liver, where hepatic mitochondria produce ketone bodies, including acetoacetate, from acetyl coenzyme A. In the presence of high NADH/NAD ratio, the more reduced form of β-hydroxybutyrate is produced.

CLINICAL MANIFESTATIONS

Symptoms include nausea, vomiting, anorexia, polydipsia, and polyuria. Patients often exhibit Kussmaul respirations and volume depletion.

Neurologic symptoms include fatigue and lethargy with depression of the sensorium. CSF exhibits a change in acid-base status with treatment of diabetic ketoacidosis. Even without bicarbonate administration, CSF pH falls as a result of the ventilatory response to the correction of acidosis and the sudden rise in P_{CO_2}. However, no correlation between decreased CSF pH and depression of sensorium has been established. Ketoacidosis is also seen in cases of starvation, in which it is generally mild and not associated with hyperglycemia.

Keto acids in the urine may be accompanied by cations, including sodium and potassium, thereby contributing to volume depletion, potassium depletion, relative chloride retention, and a mixed anion gap and hyperchloremic acidosis. The delta HCO_3^- will exceed the delta anion gap, especially if the glomerular filtration rate and the filtered load of keto acids are high. The serum anion gap in general will be greatest when renal failure is present because the additional anions cannot be cleared from extracellular fluid.

DIAGNOSIS

The urinary dipstick nitroprusside test for ketones may underestimate the degree of ketosis because it does not detect β-hydroxybutyrate; in fact, the ketone test result may become more positive as treatment helps metabolize β-hydroxybutyrate to acetoacetate. This problem should be addressed by direct measurement of serum β-hydroxybutyrate. Diabetic patients also are more prone to lactic acidosis because an increase in NADH favors the formation of lactate from pyruvate, and pyruvate dehydrogenase is inhibited in the absence of insulin.

TREATMENT Rx

Treatment of diabetic ketoacidosis (Chapter 229) consists of volume repletion, insulin administration with dextrose if necessary to avoid hypoglycemia, and potassium replacement (Chapter 117). Bicarbonate administration should be considered only if ketoacidosis is accompanied by shock or if arterial pH is less than 7.0 or 7.1, and bolus infusion should be avoided. The administration of bicarbonate occasionally results in cerebral edema significant enough to lead to loss of consciousness and even death.

PROGNOSIS

Most patients with diabetic ketoacidosis recover. In the less than 0.5% of patients who present with coma from cerebral edema, the mortality rate ranges from 20% to as high as 90%. The cerebral edema may be exacerbated by bicarbonate administration, which is discouraged in this situation.

Salicylate Intoxication

EPIDEMIOLOGY AND PATHOBIOLOGY

Salicylate intoxication can be caused by accidental overdose, therapeutic overdose, or a suicide attempt (Chapters 37 and 110). Salicylate functions as an uncoupler of oxidative phosphorylation and consequently results in increased oxygen consumption and CO_2 production. However, the increase in alveolar ventilation resulting from stimulation of central chemoreceptors overcomes this increase in CO_2.

CLINICAL MANIFESTATIONS AND DIAGNOSIS

The most common clinical manifestation is a combined anion gap metabolic acidosis and respiratory alkalosis, although the condition also can be manifested as either one or the other only. Children are often seen with metabolic acidosis, whereas adults often have predominant respiratory alkalosis. Hypoglycemia, ketoacidosis, and lactic acidosis may result. Other manifestations of intoxication include hemorrhage, fever, nausea and vomiting, hyperventilation, diaphoresis, tinnitus, and occasionally polyuria followed by oliguria. Severe cases may lead to seizures, respiratory depression, and coma. Noncardiogenic pulmonary edema is sometimes seen in adults.

Respiratory alkalosis is the result of a direct stimulatory effect of salicylate on the medullary respiratory control center. Salicylate intoxication also increases the metabolic rate. Diagnosis is suspected by the clinical presentation and confirmed by the salicylate level (Chapters 37 and 110).

Treatment of salicylate intoxication (Chapter 110) is aimed at correction of the metabolic acidosis and removal of salicylate. Bicarbonate as a sodium salt should be administered according to an estimated calculation of the deficit if metabolic acidosis predominates. Salicylates are removed by alkaline diuresis because the less reabsorbable salicylate anion will predominate when the urine pH increases. Urinary alkalinization with acetazolamide should be used cautiously because carbonic anhydrase inhibition may impair CO_2 transport from tissue to blood and potentially worsen acidosis in the respiratory center. In severe intoxication (salicylate concentrations greater than 35 mg/dL) or when renal failure is present, dialysis may be required.

PROGNOSIS

The prognosis of salicylate toxicity is better with early diagnosis and prompt management, in which case most patients do well. Patients who ingest oil of wintergreen (methylsalicylate) may have more severe deterioration because of the high lipid solubility of the drug.

Alcoholic Ketoacidosis

EPIDEMIOLOGY AND PATHOBIOLOGY

Alcoholic ketoacidosis occurs in a patient who has been drinking very heavily without eating. The pathophysiologic mechanism is based on the overproduction of β-hydroxybutyrate and, to a lesser extent, acetoacetate because of an increased production of free fatty acids from adipose tissue. Alcohol inhibits the conversion of lactate to glucose in the liver. The oxidation of ethanol increases the ratio of NADH to NAD^+ and favors the production of β-hydroxybutyrate from acetoacetate. Damage to mitochondria by alcohol can further elevate the ratio of β-hydroxybutyrate to acetoacetate by preventing reoxidation of NADH to NAD. The oxidative metabolism of ethanol favors the reaction of dehydrogenase enzymes to form β-hydroxybutyrate and lactate (opposing glucose production).

CLINICAL MANIFESTATIONS

Alcoholic ketoacidosis usually follows binge drinking and may be associated with withdrawal symptoms (Chapters 33 and 416) and the associated hyperadrenergic state. Alcoholic ketoacidosis is associated with abdominal pain, vomiting, starvation, and volume depletion. In contrast to diabetic ketoacidosis, coma is rare. Blood glucose levels are generally low or normal, and the insulin level is frequently low, with elevated glucagon (favoring ketogenesis) and cortisol levels. Some patients have hyperglycemia because of the increased catecholamine response.

DIAGNOSIS

Patients typically have a high osmolal gap initially. Blood alcohol levels may be absent or elevated on initial evaluation. A clue to the diagnosis of toxic alcohol ingestion is the simultaneous presence of an anion gap metabolic acidosis and an osmolal gap. This osmolal gap, if secondary to ethanol, should be equal to the ethanol concentration in milligrams per deciliter divided by 4.6. If this calculation does not yield the expected gap based on the ethanol concentration, ingestion of another alcohol, such as methanol, isopropanol, or ethylene glycol, should be suspected (see Table 118-2).

If possible, ethanol, ethylene glycol, propylene glycol, and methanol levels should be measured directly; each is associated with a metabolic acidosis. In contrast, isopropanol metabolizes to acetone and causes ketosis without acidosis. An osmolar gap may be present.

TREATMENT Rx

Treatment of alcoholic metabolic acidosis consists of volume repletion with normal saline in dextrose; the administration of thiamine (50 to 100 mg intravenously) and enough glucose to treat hypoglycemia; and the correction of any hypophosphatemia (Chapter 119), hypokalemia (Chapter 117), and hypomagnesemia (Chapter 119) that may be present. The acid-base disturbance usually resolves after several hours. Both hypophosphatemia and thiamine deficiency, which may not be apparent until 12 to 24 hours after the initiation of treatment in an undernourished patient, are exacerbated by glucose administration and may contribute to an associated lactic acidosis.

PROGNOSIS

The prognosis of alcoholic ketoacidosis is usually favorable. The long-term outlook is more closely tied to other complications of continued alcohol abuse.

5-Oxoprolinuria

5-Oxoprolinuria, which is an acquired form of anion gap metabolic acidosis, is increasingly recognized in patients who have glutathione depletion associated with underlying chronic illness, malnutrition, diabetes, alcoholism, or cancer, especially in the context of a high therapeutic level or overdose of acetaminophen.[11] It has been observed without concomitant hepatic failure. Glutathione, which is a tripeptide consisting of glutamate, cysteine, and glycine, has many functions, including protection from cellular toxins, combating of oxidative stress, and shuttling of amino acids into the cytosol by the γ-glutamyl transpeptidase pathway. Hereditary forms of 5-oxoprolinuria are associated with γ-glutamyl transpeptidase cycle enzyme deficiencies (5-oxoprolinase and glutathione synthase). The usual production of 5-oxoproline is by release of the transported amino acid from the γ-glutamyl–amino acid dipeptide. The enzyme 5-oxoprolinase re-forms glutamate to re-enter the cycle as glutamylcysteine. Acetaminophen causes further depletion of glutathione due to binding of an acetaminophen metabolite, *N*-acetyl-*p*-benzoquinone imine (NAPQI), to glutathione. Treatment with *N*-acetylcysteine, in doses similar to those used for acetaminophen toxicity (Chapter 110), should be considered to decrease further glutathione depletion.

Ethylene Glycol

Ethylene glycol (Chapter 110)[12] is commonly found in antifreeze and is used as an industrial solvent. It has a sweet taste, and patients occasionally ingest it as a substitute for ethanol. Although ethylene glycol itself is not particularly damaging, its highly toxic metabolites include glyoxylate, glycolate, oxalic acid, and ketoaldehydes. Glycolic acid appears to be primarily responsible for the metabolic acidosis observed in this condition.

Intoxication is characterized by profound CNS symptoms, including diplopia, seizures and coma, severe metabolic acidosis, cardiac failure, pulmonary failure, and renal failure. Patients are often dehydrated and hypernatremic because of osmotic diuresis from the renal excretion of the alcohol.

An increased anion gap is attributable to ethylene glycol metabolites. A high osmolal gap will also be present because of the uncharged alcohol. However, an osmolal gap may not be present if all of the alcohol has been converted to the toxic anionic forms. Calcium oxalate crystals in the urine may cause intratubular obstruction and acute kidney injury. Treatment is aimed at rehydration with saline and correction of acidosis with $NaHCO_3$ based on an estimate of the bicarbonate deficit. When an osmolal gap exists, competitive inhibition of alcohol dehydrogenase should be initiated with fomepizole at a loading dose of 15 to 20 mg/kg intravenously in 100 mL normal saline during 30 minutes to 1 hour, followed by a maintenance dose of 10 mg/kg every 12 hours (Chapter 110). If ethanol is used, a solution of 10% ethanol in 5% dextrose can be given as a loading dose of 0.6 g/kg intravenously followed by a maintenance dose of 150 mg/kg per hour in alcoholic patients or 65 mg/kg per hour in nonalcoholic patients. The ethanol level should be maintained at 100 to 200 mg/dL. The goal of therapy is early recognition to prevent metabolism of the uncharged glycol to acidic products. Hemodialysis is required in severe cases. If the diagnosis is made promptly and appropriate therapy is instituted, outcomes are favorable. Renal failure may be reversible.

Methanol

Methanol, wood alcohol, is a component of shellac and windshield wiper fluid and is highly toxic to the CNS after metabolism to formaldehyde and formic acid. Some automotive fluids now contain the less toxic propylene glycol. Optic papillitis may cause blindness. Detection may be made easier if fluorescein has been added to the methanol-containing fluid.

Treatment consists of competitive inhibitors for alcohol dehydrogenase, including ethanol and fomepizole, in similar amounts as for ethylene glycol poisoning, to reduce the formation of acid anions and the anion gap while maintaining a higher level of methanol in the blood (Chapter 110). Hemodialysis may be necessary to increase elimination. Early diagnosis and treatment are associated with a favorable outcome, but visual loss may be permanent. Late presentation is associated with a poor prognosis, particularly if the amount consumed exceeds 30 mL. As with ethylene glycol, the simultaneous presence of ethanol on presentation may help slow the metabolism of methanol and improve outcome.

Isopropyl Alcohol

Toxic ingestion of isopropyl alcohol (Chapter 110), as in rubbing alcohol, does not cause an increased anion gap or ketoacidosis because the metabolite is acetone, but test results for ketones are positive, and a high osmolal gap will be present.

Propylene Glycol

On occasion, patients in the intensive care unit setting are given high doses of intravenous benzodiazepines, such as lorazepam or diazepam, that contain propylene glycol as a diluent. Other intravenous medications that also contain this diluent include phenobarbital, phenytoin, nitroglycerine, and esmolol. Propylene glycol has also been used as a less toxic substitute for methanol in windshield wiper fluid. A high osmolal gap may develop because of the propylene glycol and lead to a clinical picture of sedation, failure to be weaned from the respirator, and an increased lactate level. Propylene glycol, a 3-carbon glycol, oxidizes to lactate and pyruvate. Treatment, which consists of early recognition and withdrawal of the offending agent, usually results in a favorable prognosis.

Hyperchloremic (Normal Anion Gap) Acidosis

Hyperchloremic metabolic acidoses (see Table 118-1) can be caused by renal or nonrenal mechanisms and can be associated with an elevated, normal, or low serum potassium level.

HYPERCHLOREMIC METABOLIC ACIDOSIS OF NONRENAL ORIGIN ASSOCIATED WITH NORMAL OR INCREASED POTASSIUM LEVEL

Hyperchloremic metabolic acidoses with a normal or elevated potassium concentration can develop as a result of the addition of chloride salts such as NaCl, KCl, $CaCl_2$, NH_4Cl, arginine and lysine hydrochlorides, or HCl itself. If the quantity of Cl^- introduced exceeds the ability of the kidney to eliminate Cl^- salts in urine, hyperchloremia will develop. Electroneutrality is maintained by a decrease in the serum HCO_3^- concentration, and a hyperchloremic acidosis ensues. Renal production of NH_3 increases in an attempt to improve HCl (NH_4Cl) excretion. Hyperkalemia can occur because the acidemia favors the exit of K^+ from cells. Acidemia also inhibits K^+ secretion in the renal collecting duct.

HYPERCHLOREMIC METABOLIC ACIDOSIS OF NONRENAL ORIGIN ASSOCIATED WITH HYPOKALEMIA

Hypokalemic, hyperchloremic acidosis may result from loss of a body fluid that is low in Cl^- relative to Na^+ and K^+ compared with the ratio of Cl^- to Na^+ in extracellular fluid. For example, stool losses of Na^+, K^+, and HCO_3^- in small bowel diarrhea or organic acid anions of bacterial origin, such as butyrate, in colonic diarrhea lead to hyperchloremic acidosis (Chapter 140). Pancreatic secretions (Chapter 195) or heavy losses from ileostomy sites may lead to loss of bicarbonate-containing fluids. Secretagogues such as vasoactive intestinal peptide (VIP), which is associated with neoplasms of the pancreas or sympathetic chain (Chapter 195), cause large losses of HCO_3^- in stool, with a resulting hypokalemic, hyperchloremic metabolic acidosis. Concomitant gastric achlorhydria is part of the syndrome known as *watery diarrhea, hypokalemic, hypochlorhydric acidosis.* Urinary diversions, such as ureterosigmoidostomies and ileal loops, may increase chloride absorption in exchange for bicarbonate in the intestinal segment and lead to hyperchloremic acidosis. In the presence of urea-splitting bacteria, the net absorption of NH_4Cl can result in both hyperchloremic acidosis and hyperammonemia.

RENAL TUBULAR ACIDOSIS TYPES 1 AND 2

Proximal Renal Tubular Acidosis

Renal tubular acidosis causes the cations Na^+ and K^+ to be lost in the urine with HCO_3^- rather than with Cl^-, thereby leading to hyperchloremia. Proximal renal tubular acidosis (type 2) is characterized by a decreased threshold for bicarbonate reabsorption. HCO_3^- wasting and concomitant urinary losses of potassium occur until a lower level of serum bicarbonate reduces the filtered HCO_3^- to a level that the combined function of the dysfunctional proximal tubule and distal nephron can completely reabsorb. At that point, the urine becomes acid (pH < 5.3), and net acid production equals net acid excretion, with a steady-state low plasma HCO_3^-.

Isolated proximal renal tubular acidosis may result from mutations of specific transporters of the proximal tubule, such as the $NaHCO_3$ cotransporter, or from hereditary deficiency of carbonic anhydrase. More commonly, proximal renal tubular acidosis is associated with the Fanconi syndrome or generalized proximal tubule dysfunction. Causes (Table 118-6) include genetic diseases such as glucose-6-phosphatase deficiency (Chapter 161), cystinosis (Chapter 128), hereditary fructose intolerance (Chapter 205), and Wilson disease (Chapter 211). Multiple myeloma (Chapter 187) and Sjögren

TABLE 118-6 CAUSES OF RENAL TUBULAR ACIDOSIS*

HYPOKALEMIC DISTAL (TYPE 1) RTA

Hereditary tubule disorders
- Vacuolar H^+-ATPase β-subunit gene mutations
- Carbonic anhydrase type II deficiency
- Cl^-/HCO_3^- exchanger (AE1) mutations

Genetic causes
- Sickle cell
- Fabry disease
- Wilson disease
- Elliptocytosis
- Paroxysmal nocturnal hemoglobinuria
- Medullary cystic kidneys

Autoimmune disorders
- Systemic lupus erythematosus
- Sjögren syndrome

Multiple myeloma and amyloidosis

Drugs: amphotericin, cisplatinum, aminoglycosides

Nephrocalcinosis and hypercalcemic disorders

Tubulointerstitial diseases
- Acute tubulointerstitial nephritis
- Reflux nephropathy
- Analgesic nephropathy

PROXIMAL (TYPE 2) RTA

Hereditary tubule disorders
- $NaHCO_3$ cotransport (NBC) mutations
- Carbonic anhydrase deficiency

Generalized proximal tubular dysfunction
- Hereditary Fanconi syndrome
- Genetic diseases: cystinosis, glycogen storage disease (glucose-6-phosphatase deficiency), Wilson disease
- Hormonal: hyperparathyroidism, vitamin D deficiency
- Multiple myeloma, lysozymuria
- Sjögren syndrome
- Renal transplantation
- Heavy metals: cobalt, mercury, lead
- Drugs: ifosfamide, outdated tetracycline, tenofovir, tacrolimus, aminoglycosides

HYPERKALEMIC (TYPE 4) RTA

Renal diseases—aldosterone resistance
- Diabetes mellitus
- Amyloidosis
- Systemic lupus erythematosus
- Urinary tract obstruction

Hyporeninism
- Autonomic neuropathy (diabetic)
- Sickle cell anemia

Primary hypoaldosteronism

Adrenal insufficiency: Addison disease

Tubular mutations: pseudohypoaldosteronism

Drugs: potassium-sparing diuretics, amiloride, triamterene, spironolactone, nonsteroidal anti-inflammatory drugs, lithium, trimethoprim, cyclosporine, tacrolimus, renin inhibitors, angiotensin-converting enzyme inhibitors, angiotensin II receptor antagonists

*Type 3 renal tubular acidosis (RTA) is not listed separately because it is an overlap of proximal and distal dysfunction.

syndrome (Chapter 268) should be considered in an adult patient. Primary hyperparathyroidism (Chapter 245) results in proximal renal tubular acidosis and hypophosphatemia secondary to inhibition of Na^+/H^+ exchange and sodium phosphate cotransport in the proximal tubule by parathyroid hormone through cyclic adenosine monophosphate. Hyperparathyroidism is one of the few causes of metabolic acidosis with hypercalcemia. The Cl^-/phosphate ratio in plasma may be elevated. Drug toxicity with aminoglycosides, cisplatin, and ifosfamide may cause proximal tubule dysfunction. The antiretroviral drug tenofovir, a nucleotide analogue reverse transcriptase inhibitor, is a cause of the Fanconi syndrome. The syndrome also may be seen after kidney transplantation (Chapter 131).

Distal Renal Tubular Acidosis

In distal renal tubular acidosis (type 1), failure to produce ammonia leads to an inability to excrete adequate net acid, thereby leading to continuous retention of acid in the body. The degree of acidemia is often severe, with pH reaching values as low as 7.2, whereas urine pH usually exceeds 5.3.

Kindreds have been described in which mutations in genes for the distal vacuolar H^+-ATPase cause an autosomal recessive distal renal tubular acidosis with deafness. Mutations resulting in defective Cl^-/HCO_3^- exchange protein (AE1) have been linked to an autosomal dominant form of distal renal tubular acidosis.

Distal renal tubular acidosis (see Table 118-6) is also associated with autoimmune disorders, including systemic lupus erythematosus (Chapter 266) and Sjögren syndrome (Chapter 268), and genetic diseases, including sickle cell anemia (Chapter 163), Wilson disease (Chapter 211), Fabry disease (Chapter 208), cystic kidney diseases (Chapter 127), and hereditary elliptocytosis (Chapter 161). Hypercalciuria and hyperoxaluria may cause distal renal tubular acidosis; nephrocalcinosis and nephrolithiasis may be present. Increased proximal tubular citrate reabsorption, as a consequence of the chronic acidosis, also leads to hypocitraturia, which is a risk factor for calcium nephrolithiasis (Chapter 126). A chronically alkaline urine is a risk for pure $CaHPO_4$ stones (brushite). Amyloidosis (Chapter 188) may be manifested as severe acidemia and other tubular dysfunction, including nephrogenic diabetes insipidus. Chronic tubulointerstitial diseases of the kidney (Chapter 122), including reflux nephropathy (Chapter 128) and urinary obstruction (Chapter 123), may result in renal tubular acidosis with hypokalemia or hyperkalemia. Acute tubulointerstitial nephritis also may result in renal tubular acidosis. Drugs such as amphotericin B can cause hypokalemic distal renal tubular acidosis. Topiramate, used for migraines, is a carbonic anhydrase inhibitor that may cause mixed proximal and distal renal tubular acidosis.

HYPERCHLOREMIC METABOLIC ACIDOSIS OF RENAL ORIGIN ASSOCIATED WITH HYPERKALEMIA

Hyperkalemic, hyperchloremic acidosis (type 4) suggests dysfunction of the cortical collecting duct, where acidification of urine and disorders in potassium secretion may occur. Some patients with high blood potassium and hyperchloremic acidosis can lower urinary pH below 5.3, whereas others appear to have defects in both potassium balance and urinary acidification. Hyperkalemia itself may worsen metabolic acidosis by decreasing NH_3 accumulation by countercurrent multiplication in the medullary interstitium.

Causes include hyporenin-hypoaldosteronism, as seen in diabetic renal disease (Chapter 124); other tubulointerstitial diseases (Chapter 122), usually with some renal impairment; sickle cell anemia (Chapter 163); and the use of drugs such as β-blockers and nonsteroidal anti-inflammatory drugs. Low renin and aldosterone levels can also be found in cases of volume expansion with hypertension. Cyclosporine and tacrolimus may lead to decreased electrical driving forces for K^+ and H^+ secretion. Hyperkalemic acidosis with elevated renin and low aldosterone is found in adrenal insufficiency (Chapter 227), in isolated hypoaldosteronism (Chapter 227), and with the use of angiotensin-converting enzyme inhibitors, renin inhibitors, and angiotensin II receptor blockers. High renin and aldosterone levels are anticipated when the renal collecting duct cell is insensitive to aldosterone, as in urinary tract obstruction, sickle cell anemia, amyloidosis, and systemic lupus erythematosus. Inhibition of aldosterone action with spironolactone or eplerenone may cause hyperkalemic acidosis, as does ENaC inhibition by amiloride, triamterene, trimethoprim, and lithium.

Pseudohypoaldosteronism type 1 is due to autosomal recessive, inactivating mutations of the sodium channel ENaC, whereas autosomal dominant pseudohypoaldosteronism type 1 is due to mutations of the mineralocorticoid receptor. Both cause hypovolemia, metabolic acidosis, and hyperkalemia with secondary increases in renin and aldosterone. In Gordon syndrome (pseudohypoaldosteronism type 2), increases in Na^+ and Cl^- reabsorption through increased activity of the distal thiazide-sensitive NaCl transporter lead to hypertension, hyperkalemic acidosis, volume expansion, and consequently low renin and aldosterone.

CLINICAL MANIFESTATIONS AND DIAGNOSIS

The urinary anion, or charge, gap helps distinguish renal tubular acidosis[13] from extrarenal bicarbonate loss (e.g., from diarrhea). Because the normal renal response to metabolic acidosis is an increase in ammoniagenesis, the urine should contain large amounts of NH_4Cl while the kidney retains sodium and potassium; the urinary charge gap, which is $(Na^+ + K^+) - Cl^-$, should be strongly negative because of the unmeasured NH_4^+.

In renal diseases such as distal renal tubular acidosis, however, the urinary anion gap will be zero or positive because of either the failure of ammoniagenesis or the excretion of sodium plus potassium with bicarbonate. With type 2 (proximal) renal tubular acidosis, patients often have Fanconi

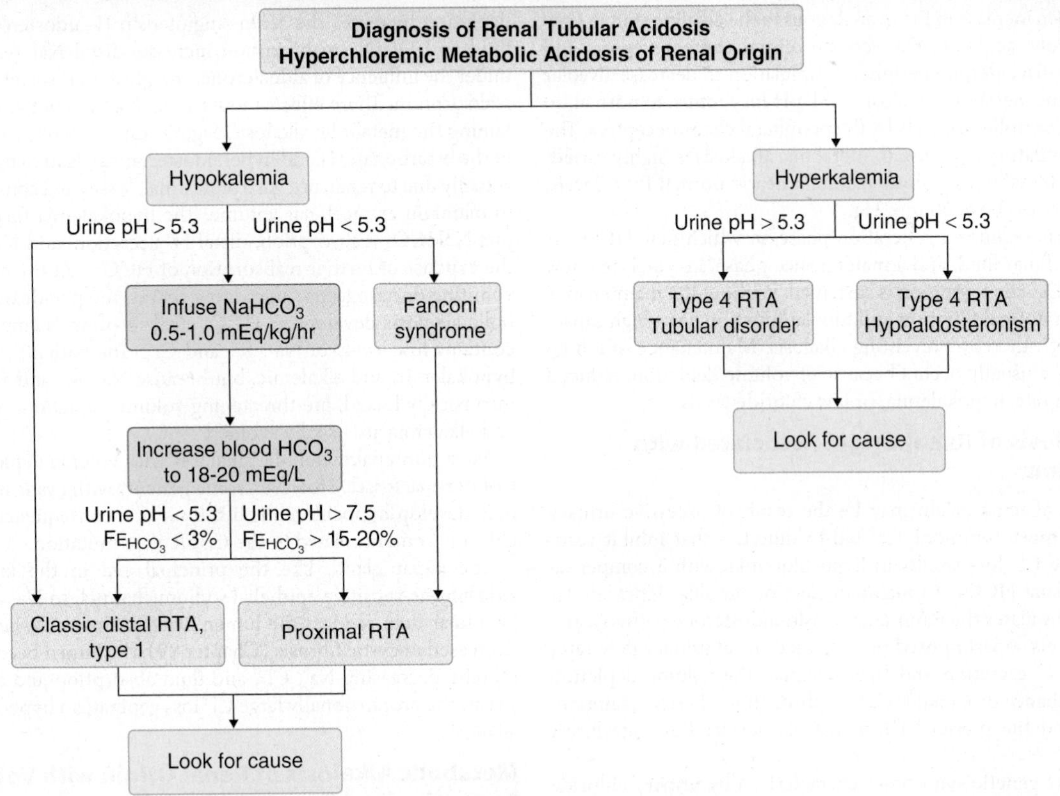

FIGURE 118-2. Diagnosis of renal tubular acidosis (RTA). FE = fractional excretion; $NaHCO_3$ = sodium bicarbonate.

syndrome with glycosuria, phosphaturia, aminoaciduria, and uricosuria. In proximal renal tubular acidosis, the steady-state urine pH is usually less than 5.3, the acidosis is not severe (i.e., HCO_3^- usually not less than 16), and acid excretion may balance acid production at this new steady state.

In contrast to proximal renal tubular acidosis, distal renal tubular acidosis (type 1) is generally a more severe metabolic disorder that may be accompanied by hypercalciuria, nephrocalcinosis, calcium phosphate kidney stones (Chapter 126), and bone disease that includes rickets in children and osteomalacia in adults. Proximal and distal renal tubular acidoses usually can be distinguished by a careful clinical evaluation (Fig. 118-2). Helpful findings include the presence of a urine pH greater than 5.3 in distal but not in proximal renal tubular acidosis during acidemia; a fractional excretion of bicarbonate as high as 10 to 15% in proximal renal tubular acidosis; and the lowering of serum potassium on correction of proximal but not of distal tubular acidosis.

In patients with an elevated serum anion gap, unmeasured anions such as keto acids and lactate, rather than NH_4^+, are present in urine, so a positive urinary anion gap does not indicate renal tubular acidosis. On occasion, however, the prompt renal excretion of organic anions with sodium and potassium may minimize the increase in the serum anion gap. In the metabolic acidosis of glue sniffers, hippurate, which is a product of toluene, is rapidly excreted, thus giving the appearance of a nongap metabolic acidosis with a positive urinary anion gap. Similarly, if keto acids are completely cleared into the urine, ketoacidosis may be manifested as a hyperchloremic acidosis rather than as an anion gap acidosis.

TREATMENT

Rx

If possible, treatment of metabolic acidosis should focus on correction of the underlying cause, such as discontinuation of an offending drug, permitting the body's homeostatic mechanisms to correct the acid-base disturbance.

Patients whose pH is less than 7.2 are typically treated with infusions of sodium bicarbonate, guided by the estimated base deficit in milliequivalents, calculated by the serum HCO_3^- concentration in milliequivalents per liter:

$$\text{Amount of } HCO_3^- = (25 - [HCO_3^-]) \times \text{wt (kg)}/2$$

In general, the correction of metabolic acidemia should be based on a calculated amount, with not more than 50% of the estimate given before recalculation. Moreover, this equation is used for deficit correction only; the ongoing losses of 1 to 2 mEq/kg per day, equivalent to the daily acid load, should be replaced in distal renal tubular acidosis with $NaHCO_3$, $KHCO_3$, or citrate salts in divided doses. Hypokalemia may accompany distal renal tubular acidosis and may improve with treatment. Citrate should be avoided as an alkalinizing salt in patients with low glomerular filtration rate.

Proximal renal tubular acidosis in children may affect growth and require large quantities of bicarbonate in excess of 1 to 2 mEq/kg per day to correct the acidosis because ingested alkali is promptly excreted in alkaline urine. In adults, treatment is often deferred because the steady-state acidosis allows a normal acid excretion rate. Hypokalemia may worsen with bicarbonate treatment of proximal tubular acidosis.

In type 4 renal tubular acidosis, treatment of hyperkalemia with a low-potassium diet, thiazide, or loop diuretics or sodium polystyrene sulfonate often improves urinary acidification without the use of bicarbonate salts.

PROGNOSIS

The prognosis of renal tubular acidosis generally depends on the presence of an underlying systemic disease, such as myeloma (Chapter 187). In children, disorders such as medullary cystic kidney disease (Chapter 127) and cystinosis (Chapter 128) usually result in renal failure by the teenage years. These patients are candidates for renal replacement therapy, including transplantation. Chronic metabolic acidosis in children, if not well treated, is associated with rickets (Chapter 244) and short stature.

METABOLIC ALKALOSIS

EPIDEMIOLOGY AND PATHOBIOLOGY

In metabolic alkalosis, the primary event is elevation of the plasma bicarbonate concentration. In response to increased systemic pH, alveolar ventilation is decreased to increase P_{CO_2} and thereby decrease pH. However, respiratory compensation is generally less effective in cases of metabolic alkalosis than in cases of metabolic acidosis. Contributing factors may include the fact that hypoventilation also decreases P_{O_2}, which is a potent stimulus for the peripheral chemoreceptors to increase alveolar ventilation when P_{O_2} falls below about 60 mm Hg. A second mechanism that may blunt respiratory compensation is intracellular acidosis in the brain in the setting of hypokalemia. In acute metabolic alkalosis, an initial paradoxical acidotic shift in CSF pH secondary to a sudden increase in P_{CO_2}, analogous to the alkaline shift in CSF pH in acute metabolic acidosis, may activate central chemoreceptors and increase ventilatory drive despite peripheral stimulation to decrease alveolar ventilation. In chronic metabolic alkalosis, CSF pH may return to normal, so respiratory drive is controlled entirely by the peripheral chemoreceptors. The result is that the ventilatory response to metabolic alkalosis is highly varied: many patients with metabolic alkalosis maintain nearly normal P_{CO_2} levels, and the level rarely rises above 60 mm Hg.

Metabolic alkalosis requires a generation phase, in which new HCO_3^- is added to the extracellular fluid, and a maintenance phase, in which the new elevated serum HCO_3^- concentration is sustained. Without the maintenance phase, a kidney with normal filtration and tubular function has a high capacity to excrete HCO_3^-, thereby preventing alkalosis. Maintenance of a high HCO_3^- concentration usually occurs because of volume depletion, reduced glomerular filtration rate, hypokalemia, or low chloride levels.

Metabolic Alkalosis of Renal Origin Associated with Volume Depletion

Metabolic alkalosis of renal origin may be the result of excessive urinary chloride excretion, most commonly related to diuretics that inhibit reabsorption of Cl^-. The Cl^- loss results in hypochloremia, with a compensatory increase in plasma HCO_3^- to maintain electroneutrality. Extracellular volume depletion stimulates the renin-angiotensin-aldosterone pathway, and high aldosterone levels superimposed on increased distal urinary flow rates result in increased K^+ excretion and hypokalemia. The volume depletion and hypokalemia enhance proximal HCO_3^- reabsorption, thereby maintaining the alkalosis, and the prerenal fall in the glomerular flow rate limits HCO_3^- filtration.

Important but rare genetic syndromes characterized by urinary chloride wasting include Bartter syndrome and Gitelman syndrome. Bartter syndrome is an autosomal recessive salt-losing state associated with extracellular volume depletion and excessive urinary chloride loss that results in hypokalemia and hypochloremic metabolic alkalosis. Secondary increases of plasma renin and aldosterone occur, as does renal juxtaglomerular cell hyperplasia. The syndrome resembles the effects of furosemide on the thick ascending limb of Henle; gene mutations in the Na-K-2Cl cotransporter, the renal outer medullary potassium channel (ROMK), and chloride channels have been described. Because calcium reabsorption occurs in the thick ascending limb of Henle, Bartter syndrome (Chapter 128), like furosemide, causes hypercalciuria and nephrocalcinosis as well as polyuria due to decreased urinary concentrating ability.

Gitelman syndrome is an autosomal recessive cause of extracellular volume depletion, urinary chloride wasting, and hypokalemic metabolic alkalosis. It is due to inactivating mutations in the *SLC12A3* gene encoding the thiazide-sensitive NaCl cotransporter of the renal distal tubule. Urinary concentrating ability is preserved, and patients are hypocalciuric because decreased NaCl reabsorption in the distal tubule is associated with a decrease in calcium excretion. Hypomagnesemia may also be severe.

Metabolic Alkalosis of Nonrenal Origin with Extracellular Volume Depletion

Metabolic alkalosis may develop as a result of gastrointestinal Cl^- loss from vomiting, nasogastric suctioning, or secretory diarrhea. In such cases, extracellular volume is usually contracted, hypochloremia develops, and the urinary chloride level is usually less than 20 mEq/L.

In Zollinger-Ellison syndrome (Chapter 195), excessive gastrin-induced gastric acid secretion may result in an acidic stool with high chloride content. Diarrhea does not cause metabolic alkalosis unless the electrolyte relationship $[(Na^+ + K^+) - Cl^-]$ in the stool is less than plasma HCO_3^-.

Infectious gastroenteritis, congenital chloridorrhea, and villous adenomas also cause chloride losses in stool. Congenital chloridorrhea is an autosomal recessive disorder of defective intestinal apical Cl^-/HCO_3^- exchange associated with the downregulated adenoma (*DRA*) gene.

With vomiting, the initiating event is loss of HCl. This secretion of HCl into the stomach lumen by the parietal cell is coupled to the absorption of HCO_3^- in exchange for chloride at the basolateral membrane. When gastric acid is normally secreted, a mild increase in serum HCO_3^- spills into urine and causes an "alkaline tide." With vomiting, however, the net loss of HCl generates the alkalosis. Initially, this increased HCO_3^- is filtered by the glomeruli and excreted in urine accompanied by Na^+ and K^+; volume depletion begins to develop. As vomiting continues, extracellular volume depletion worsens, glomerular filtration falls, HCO_3^- filtration is limited, volume depletion increases the renin–angiotensin II–aldosterone system, proximal fluid and HCO_3^- reabsorption increase, distal Na^+ reabsorption increases under the influence of aldosterone, and greater H^+ secretion enhances HCO_3^- reabsorption. These effects reduce renal Na^+ loss but at the expense of maintaining the metabolic alkalosis. Significant K^+ losses, which occur as a result of the bicarbonaturia and hyperaldosteronism, lead to hypokalemia, which is actually due to renal, not gastrointestinal, losses as a consequence of attempts to maintain extracellular volume. The hypokalemia further increases proximal $NaHCO_3$ reabsorption, distal H^+ secretion, and K^+ reabsorption, all at the expense of further reabsorption of HCO_3^-. At the new steady state after vomiting or nasogastric suctioning ceases, the paradoxical aciduria of metabolic alkalosis develops as HCO_3^- reabsorption is complete, and the urine contains low levels of Na^+, K^+, and Cl^-. The patient may be hypovolemic, hypokalemic, and alkalemic, but because Na^+, K^+, and acid-base balance are intrinsically linked, life-threatening volume depletion, potassium depletion, and alkalemia are usually avoided.

Most nonrenal metabolic alkaloses with volume depletion are due to gastrointestinal losses. However, some patients with cystic fibrosis (Chapter 89) may develop hypochloremic alkalosis as a consequence of excessive sweat chloride content related to the *CFTR* gene mutation.

The sweat gland, like the principal cell in the kidney, contains the aldosterone-sensitive epithelial sodium channel, so Na^+ absorption from the glandular duct renders the lumen electronegative. When Cl^- absorption is decreased in cystic fibrosis (Chapter 89), the lumen becomes more negative, thereby decreasing Na^+, Cl^-, and fluid absorption and also leading to salty sweat; the proportionally large Cl^- loss generates a hypochloremic metabolic alkalosis.

Metabolic Alkalosis of Renal Origin with Volume Expansion and Hypertension

The renal conditions that cause metabolic alkalosis and volume expansion are due to a proportionately greater increase in Na^+ reabsorption above what is required to maintain a steady state of Na^+ balance, rather than primary loss of the Cl^- anion. As Na^+ is reabsorbed, electroneutrality is maintained by an increase in plasma HCO_3^-. The plasma Na^+ concentration may be increased, and Cl^- balance is normal; Cl^- appears in urine, and hypochloremia is not present. In the kidney, the loss of net acid as NH_4Cl in excess of the acid produced generates a metabolic alkalosis, in which the new bicarbonate generated is due to proton secretion by the distal nephron through H^+-ATPases. The H^+ then combines with NH_3 to form NH_4^+ in urine.

Na^+ is reabsorbed independently of Cl^- in the cortical collecting duct through the aldosterone-sensitive cells containing the ENaC. When Na^+ is reabsorbed by the principal cells of the cortical collecting duct, the tubule lumen becomes electronegative and stimulates both K^+ and H^+ secretion by the electrogenic H^+-ATPases. To the extent that HCO_3^- remains in the lumen, the secreted protons complete HCO_3^- reabsorption. Additional secreted protons combine with NH_3 and phosphates and lead to net acid excretion. Any increase in the distal H^+ secretory mechanism will produce more urinary net acid; more new HCO_3^- will be generated and returned to the now expanded extracellular fluid, and metabolic alkalosis will develop. The increased plasma HCO_3^- will be filtered, but in the absence of a stimulus to increase proximal HCO_3^- reabsorption, the HCO_3^- will flow distally to be reabsorbed by the increased H^+ secretion of the collecting duct. At first, the alkalosis is mild, but increased cortical collecting duct Na^+ reabsorption will also lead to increased K^+ secretion and hypokalemia. Hypokalemia increases the capacity for proximal HCO_3^- reabsorption, thereby opposing the effect of volume expansion, so that distal delivery of HCO_3^- decreases. The higher than normal distal H^+ secretion titrates urinary buffers, so further new HCO_3^- is formed and the alkalosis worsens. Metabolic alkaloses in the hypermineralocorticoid syndromes are sustained by hypokalemia.

Metabolic Alkalosis of Nonrenal Origin Associated with Normal or Expanded Volume

If an alkalotic patient is not hypochloremic, electroneutrality must be maintained either by depletion of an alternative anion or by an excessive concentration of a cation. An example of a metabolic alkalosis associated with depletion of a non-chloride anion is hypoproteinemic alkalosis, with hypoalbuminemia and a small anion gap. Chloride balance is normal and chloride appears in urine.

Alkalosis also may result from the addition of alkali salts of organic anions. The normal response to the ingestion of $NaHCO_3$ is rapid urinary alkalinization because of an unaltered threshold for HCO_3^- reabsorption. However, a marked excess of HCO_3^-, as may be administered in an attempt to alkalinize a patient's urine, expands volume and causes an alkalemia, especially in the presence of volume depletion or low glomerular filtration. Milk-alkali syndrome, usually seen when patients in renal failure ingest milk or calcium antacids, is associated with hypercalcemia, alkalemia, and normal chloride concentration.

Other situations in which intake of alkali salts results in metabolic alkalosis include infusion of large quantities of sodium salts of metabolizable organic compounds, such as acetate, citrate, lactate, or bicarbonate; hyperalimentation with acetate salts; chronic peritoneal dialysis with acetate or lactate dialysate; and excessive transfusions or plasmapheresis, in which large quantities of citrate, used as an anticoagulant, are delivered.

CLINICAL MANIFESTATIONS

Mild metabolic alkalosis up to a pH of 7.50 is usually asymptomatic. When the pH exceeds 7.55, however, the alkalosis itself and the compensatory hypoventilation are frequently associated with metabolic encephalopathy. Symptoms include confusion, obtundation, delirium, and coma. The seizure threshold is lowered; tetany, paresthesias, muscle cramping, and other symptoms of low calcium are seen. In patients with hypocalcemia, these signs may be seen at pH values above 7.45. Other findings include cardiac tachyarrhythmias and hypotension. Lactate production increases as a result of the increased anaerobic glycolysis.

DIAGNOSIS

In diagnosis of the cause of metabolic alkalosis, it is important to distinguish whether the condition is chloride responsive or chloride unresponsive. Metabolic alkalosis is generally divided into two categories on the basis of its responsiveness to chloride (see Table 118-2). Chloride-responsive metabolic alkalosis is associated with extracellular fluid and chloride depletion and is seen in cases of gastric fluid loss and diuretic use. A diagnostic clue comes from the serum electrolytes. HCO_3^- is increased with a corresponding fall in serum chloride (hypochloremic alkalosis). Chloride-unresponsive metabolic alkalosis is seen in patients with extracellular fluid expansion in conditions such as primary aldosteronism and hypokalemia. Entry of hydrogen ions into cells can also lead to metabolic alkalosis in patients with hypokalemia.

Vomiting, nasogastric suction, and diarrhea are usually obvious sources of metabolic alkalosis. However, the Zollinger-Ellison syndrome (Chapter 195), villous adenomas (Chapter 193), and VIPomas (Chapter 195) may be more difficult to diagnose unless the index of suspicion is high.

Patients who present with hypokalemic metabolic alkalosis with normal or low blood pressure and have urinary chloride concentrations above 25 mEq/L may be taking diuretics such as furosemide or thiazides surreptitiously; a diuretic screen can document the presence of the drug. If the screen is negative, Bartter or Gitelman syndrome (Chapter 128) should be considered. Bartter syndrome is less common, is usually more severe, and presents in young patients. The presence of hypercalciuria favors Bartter syndrome, whereas hypocalciuria and hypomagnesemia suggest Gitelman syndrome.

Specific causes of renal alkalosis with volume expansion and hypertension can be classified according to levels of renin and aldosterone. Primary increases in renin with secondary increases in aldosterone can be seen in patients with unilateral renal artery stenosis (Chapter 125), renin-secreting tumors of the kidney (Chapter 67), and malignant hypertension (Chapter 67). Low renin and elevated aldosterone levels are characteristic of primary hyperaldosteronism from adrenal adenoma or hyperplasia (Chapter 227). A high cortisol level with volume expansion is seen in hypercortisolism and adrenocorticotropic hormone–secreting tumors (Chapter 227). Inhibition of the intracellular enzyme 11β-hydroxysteroid dehydrogenase Type 2, which normally inactivates cortisol to form cortisone in the principal cell, will also result in low renin levels, low aldosterone levels, and hypokalemic alkalosis. Both genetic mutations (the apparent mineralocorticoid excess syndrome) and an excess consumption of glycyrrhizic acid found in licorice and anisette are causes of this enzyme block. Another cause of hypertension with hypokalemic alkalosis but with low renin and aldosterone levels is Liddle syndrome (Chapter 128), in which an activating mutation in the cortical collecting duct sodium channel (ENaC) leads to increased Na^+ reabsorption.

Metabolic alkalosis may also develop without volume expansion when a non-reabsorbable anion is presented to the cortical collecting duct lumen. Nitrates, sulfates, and certain antibiotics such as nafcillin, carbenicillin, and ticarcillin may obligate K^+ and H^+ secretion as Na^+ is reabsorbed. Topical administration of silver nitrate to burn victims may result in alkalosis.

TREATMENT Rx

In chloride-responsive patients (see Table 118-2), treatment is directed at increasing urinary excretion of bicarbonate. In patients with mild to moderate alkalosis, liberalizing salt intake and administering potassium chloride is effective in increasing renal HCO_3^- excretion. The K^+ deficit is likely to be at least 100 mEq for every decrease of 1 mEq/L in serum potassium. Unless potassium chloride is also replenished, the improvement in filtration and proximal reabsorption will result in severe potassium wasting as bicarbonaturia develops and aldosterone's effects remain. In addition, complete resolution of alkalosis will not occur until K^+ is normalized. In a patient with renal failure and vomiting, the elevation in HCO_3^- may be more severe because of poor HCO_3^- filtration. In cases of volume expansion and alkalosis, acetazolamide may be administered carefully while monitoring its potential for losing K^+. If this agent fails to work, dilute solutions of HCl (0.1N HCl) may be cautiously administered. The amount of H^+, in milliequivalents, to be given may be calculated as the product of the desired change in serum HCO_3^- concentration (mEq/L) times 0.5 of body weight in kilograms. It is likely that this calculation will overestimate the amount of acid needed for correction, so no more than one third of the amount should be given before recalculating to avoid metabolic acidosis. Full correction of HCO_3^- should not be the goal. In the absence of renal failure, intravenous acetazolamide (250 to 500 mg every 8 hours) may be effective but may greatly increase K^+ losses.

Chloride-unresponsive patients (see Table 118-2) include those with mineralocorticoid excess. In these patients, the metabolic alkalosis can be lessened by potassium replacement or by blocking Na^+ reabsorption with aldosterone antagonists such as spironolactone, starting with 25 mg orally, or amiloride, beginning with 5 mg orally. Indomethacin effectively treats Bartter syndrome (Chapter 128) by interfering with prostaglandin E_2 to allow greater NaCl reabsorption in the thick ascending limb. Gitelman and Bartter syndromes are best treated with combinations of potassium chloride, a potassium-sparing diuretic, and magnesium if needed.

RESPIRATORY ACIDOSIS

Respiratory acidosis is characterized by a primary elevation in Pco_2 as reflected by reduced arterial pH with variable elevation in the HCO_3^- concentration. It is most frequently caused by a decrease in alveolar ventilation due to pulmonary disease (Chapter 104), respiratory muscle fatigue, musculoskeletal abnormalities of the chest wall, or abnormalities in ventilatory control (Chapter 86).

CLINICAL MANIFESTATIONS

Clinical findings in respiratory acidosis are related to the degree and duration of the respiratory acidosis and whether hypoxemia is present. A precipitous rise in Pco_2 can lead to confusion, anxiety, psychosis, asterixis, seizures, and myoclonic jerks, with progressive depression of the sensorium and coma at an arterial Pco_2 greater than 60 mm Hg (CO_2 narcosis). Hypercapnia, which increases cerebral blood flow and volume, can lead to symptoms and signs of elevated intracranial pressure, including headaches and papilledema. Other findings in acute respiratory acidosis include signs of catecholamine release, such as skin flushing, diaphoresis, and increased cardiac contractility and output. Symptoms of chronic hypercapnia include fatigue, lethargy, and confusion, in addition to the findings seen in acute hypercapnia.

The slow time course of many of these diseases allows the kidney to compensate adequately as the disease progresses by increasing its excretion of hydrogen ion as ammonium and generating and reabsorbing bicarbonate to restore systemic pH toward normal values. This compensatory process is not maximal until 3 to 5 days after the onset of respiratory acidosis. Chronic $NaHCO_3$ retention and edema often accompany chronic respiratory acidosis.

DIAGNOSIS

Disorders that cause a respiratory acidosis include central effects of drugs, stroke, and infection; airway obstruction; primary parenchymal processes, such as chronic obstructive pulmonary disease (Chapter 88) and acute respiratory distress syndrome (Chapter 104); disorders of ventilation (Chapter 86); and neuromuscular diseases, such as myasthenia gravis (Chapter 422) and muscular dystrophies (Chapter 421). Permissive hypercapnia has been used clinically in patients with acute respiratory distress syndrome to limit pulmonary damage secondary to mechanical ventilation (Chapter 105).

TREATMENT

Treatment of both chronic and acute respiratory acidosis aims primarily to correct the underlying cause and to ensure adequate ventilation. In acute respiratory acidosis, measures to relieve severe hypoxemia and acidemia should be instituted immediately, including intubation and assisted mechanical ventilation (Chapter 105) if necessary. Patients with myxedema coma require thyroid replacement (Chapter 226).

In patients with compensated chronic respiratory acidosis, rapid and complete correction of hypercapnia can result in post-hypercapnic metabolic alkalosis. Patients who are chronically hypercapnic and hypoxemic should receive necessary oxygen even though their P_{CO_2} will rise. The rise is not necessarily due to loss of a hypoxic drive to ventilation but may instead be because of release of CO_2 from hemoglobin in the presence of oxygen or because oxygen-induced pulmonary arteriolar vasodilation increases perfusion to poorly ventilated alveoli. Patients recovering from an acute-on-chronic respiratory acidosis should be monitored carefully to correct hypokalemia, hypochloremia, and hypovolemia so that adequate renal excretion of bicarbonate can occur.

Bicarbonate therapy is not indicated for respiratory acidosis unless the pH falls below 7.0 and the patient is about to be intubated. There is a role for bicarbonate therapy in patients with renal failure (Chapter 130), in whom adequate compensatory acid excretion cannot take place.

RESPIRATORY ALKALOSIS

EPIDEMIOLOGY AND PATHOBIOLOGY

In respiratory alkalosis, a primary decrease in P_{CO_2} is reflected by increases in arterial pH and variable decreases in plasma bicarbonate concentration. The most common cause is alveolar hyperventilation, not underproduction of CO_2.

Acute hypocapnia results in an initial increase in the pH of both the CSF and the brain's intracellular environment. However, this increase is quickly offset by a decrease in bicarbonate levels. In acute respiratory alkalosis, one of the primary mechanisms of this fall in bicarbonate appears to be the generation of lactate as a result of vasoconstriction, hypoxia, and increased hemoglobin affinity for oxygen. The combination of increased oxygen demand and decreased oxygen delivery may contribute to adverse clinical outcomes in hypocapnic alkalosis.

Cerebral blood flow is significantly decreased by hypocapnia, which is a potent vasoconstrictor. As in respiratory acidosis, the CNS is immediately affected by decreases in systemic P_{CO_2} because of the blood-brain barrier's permeability to CO_2. In addition, as in respiratory acidosis, CSF and intracellular pH show an initial short-lived response that parallels the systemic increase in pH.

Renal compensation for sustained hypocapnia is complete in 36 to 72 hours. The mechanism rests primarily in the kidney's net reduction of hydrogen ion excretion, which it accomplishes largely by decreasing ammonium and titratable acid excretion. The threshold for bicarbonate excretion is also lowered, and bicarbonaturia develops. As a result, systemic bicarbonate levels decrease, and arterial pH returns toward normal values.

Acute exposure to high altitude (Chapter 94) results in hypoxia-induced hyperventilation. Compensation requires at least several days and is characterized by a gradual further increase in hyperventilation, a steadily decreasing P_{CO_2}, and a recovering P_{O_2}. The effect of the hypoxic stimulus to ventilate is initially modulated by the effects of alkalosis, both peripherally and centrally. However, as HCO_3^- falls in the CSF, inhibition of the central stimulus to ventilate decreases. Once a steady state is achieved, the drive to ventilate is determined by the effects of hypoxemia and alkalemia on the peripheral chemoreceptors.

CLINICAL MANIFESTATIONS

The clinical manifestations of respiratory alkalosis depend on the degree and duration of the condition but are primarily those of the underlying disorder. Chronic hypocapnia does not appear to be associated with any significant clinical symptoms.

Symptoms of acute hypocapnia are largely attributable to the alkalemia and include dizziness, perioral or extremity paresthesias, confusion, asterixis, hypotension, seizures, and coma. Most symptoms, which are manifested only when the P_{CO_2} falls below 25 or 30 mm Hg, can be related to decreased cerebral blood flow or reduced free calcium because alkalosis increases calcium's protein-bound fraction. Shortness of breath and chest wall pain, which frequently may be seen when patients hyperventilate because of pain or anxiety, do not appear to be related to hypocapnia.

DIAGNOSIS

Alveolar hyperventilation leading to respiratory alkalosis is seen with hypoxemia from pulmonary disease (Chapter 83), heart failure (Chapter 58), high altitudes (Chapter 94), or anemia. Mechanical ventilation (Chapter 105) is also a common cause of respiratory alkalosis.

Another common cause of respiratory alkalosis is primary stimulation of the central chemoreceptor, as seen in sepsis (Chapter 108), hepatic cirrhosis (Chapter 153), salicylate intoxication (Chapters 37 and 110), correction of metabolic acidosis, hyperthermia (Chapter 109), and pregnancy, as well as cortical hyperventilation from anxiety and pain. In these situations, central signals override peripheral chemoreceptors until the primary stimulus is removed.

Primary neurologic diseases that can stimulate alveolar hyperventilation include acute stroke, infection, trauma, and tumors. Two patterns of respiration are seen: central hyperventilation and Cheyne-Stokes respiration (Chapter 86). Central hyperventilation, which is associated with lesions at the pontine-midbrain level, is regular, but with an increased rate and tidal volume. Cheyne-Stokes breathing, which is characterized by periods of hyperventilation alternating with apnea, is seen in patients with bilateral cortical and upper pontine lesions and in patients with heart failure.

TREATMENT

Treatment of respiratory alkalosis must address the underlying cause of the disturbance. Hyperventilation syndrome is a diagnosis of exclusion, but patients who exhibit symptoms, such as tetany and syncope, and who do not have more serious causes of hyperventilation can be treated with a rebreathing mask. Hypophosphatemia can be seen in these patients, but it usually improves with treatment of the alkalosis. Patients with respiratory alkalosis associated with mountain sickness can be pretreated with acetazolamide to induce a metabolic acidosis, thereby preventing extreme elevations in pH (Chapter 94).

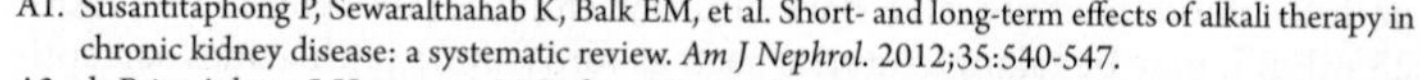

Grade A References

A1. Susantitaphong P, Sewaralthahab K, Balk EM, et al. Short- and long-term effects of alkali therapy in chronic kidney disease: a systematic review. *Am J Nephrol.* 2012;35:540-547.

A2. de Brito-Ashurst I, Varagunam M, Raftery MJ, et al. Bicarbonate supplementation slows progression of CKD and improves nutritional status. *J Am Soc Nephrol.* 2009;20:2075-2084.

A3. Jones AE, Shapiro NI, Trzeciak S, et al. Lactate clearance vs central venous oxygen saturation as goals of early sepsis therapy: a randomized clinical trial. *JAMA.* 2010;303:739-746.

A4. Cooper DJ, Walley KR, Wiggs BR, et al. Bicarbonate does not improve hemodynamics in critically ill patients who have lactic acidosis. A prospective, controlled clinical study. *Ann Intern Med.* 1990;112:492-498.

GENERAL REFERENCES

For the General References and other additional features, please visit Expert Consult at https://expertconsult.inkling.com.

119 DISORDERS OF MAGNESIUM AND PHOSPHORUS

ALAN S. L. YU

MAGNESIUM METABOLISM

Magnesium is an important mineral component of the bony skeleton, a cofactor for many metabolic enzymes, and a regulator of ion channels and transporters in excitable tissues.

Normal Magnesium Metabolism

The majority of total body magnesium is intracellular or in bone, with only 1% in extracellular fluid. The normal serum magnesium concentration is 1.8 to 2.3 mg/dL (1.5 to 1.9 mEq/L). The average daily intake of magnesium is 300 mg, the main sources of which are green vegetables, nuts, whole grain cereals, milk, and seafood. Magnesium is absorbed mainly in the jejunum and ileum. In the kidney, 70 to 80% of serum magnesium is filtered at the glomerulus, with the majority being reabsorbed along the length of the tubule, particularly in the thick ascending limb of Henle. In states of magnesium deficiency or excess, renal tubule reabsorption is tightly regulated so that magnesium excretion is adjusted accordingly.

MAGNESIUM DEFICIENCY

PATHOBIOLOGY

Magnesium deficiency is usually detected when hypomagnesemia becomes evident. However, because magnesium is stored primarily intracellularly, substantial depletion of total body magnesium can occur before serum magnesium levels drop appreciably.

Magnesium deficiency may be due to nutritional deficiency, intestinal malabsorption, redistribution into bone, or losses via cutaneous, lower gastrointestinal, or renal routes (Table 119-1). The recommended daily allowance of magnesium is 420 mg for males and 320 mg for females. Approximately 25% of alcoholics are chronically hypomagnesemic because of a combination of poor nutritional intake and increased renal loss. Magnesium deficiency can occur, rarely, in protein-calorie malnutrition and may be associated with acute hypomagnesemia during refeeding because of rapid cellular magnesium uptake. Fat malabsorption in conditions such as celiac disease, Crohn disease, and small intestinal resection causes magnesium deficiency because free fatty acids accumulate in the intestinal lumen, where they combine with magnesium to form insoluble soaps. Proton pump inhibitors also can cause hypomagnesemia, primarily in patients concurrently using diuretics.[1] This is thought to be due to inhibition of intestinal absorption. Lower gastrointestinal tract secretions are rich in magnesium, so diarrhea of colonic origin is a common cause of hypomagnesemia. Sweat contains significant amounts of magnesium, and transient hypomagnesemia can occur after prolonged, intense exercise such as marathon runs. Magnesium is also lost from burned skin surfaces, and 40% of patients with severe burns (Chapter 111) are hypomagnesemic.

In patients with severe hyperparathyroidism (Chapter 245) and high bone turnover, continued sequestration of minerals within bone may continue for several days after parathyroidectomy and cause transient hypocalcemia, hypomagnesemia, and hypophosphatemia. Renal magnesium losses can occur in any polyuric state, including the recovery phase of acute tubular necrosis or urinary tract obstruction. Hypomagnesemia is common in diabetes mellitus (Chapter 229), in which it is thought to be due to a combination of poor intestinal absorption owing to autonomic neuropathy, osmotic diuresis, and decreased renal tubule reabsorption. Failure of sodium reabsorption in the thick ascending limb of Henle as a result of the use of loop diuretics and in the distal convoluted tubule as a result of thiazide diuretics inhibits tubular magnesium reabsorption and leads to urinary magnesium wasting. Drugs that are tubular toxins are also common causes of renal magnesium wasting. Such drugs include cisplatin, carboplatin, amphotericin B, and aminoglycosides, which are commonly associated with hypokalemia and rarely with renal tubule acidosis, as well as calcineurin inhibitors such as cyclosporine and tacrolimus, which also cause hyperkalemia. Antibodies to the epidermal growth factor receptor, such as cetuximab and panitumumab, which are used to treat metastatic colorectal cancer, downregulate a distal tubule magnesium channel and are an increasingly common cause of isolated severe hypomagnesemia.[2]

Inherited hypomagnesemia is usually caused by renal magnesium loss and can be subdivided into three main types, depending on the coexistence of other electrolyte disturbances: Bartter and Gitelman syndromes, which are associated with renal salt wasting and hypokalemic metabolic alkalosis; familial hypomagnesemia with hypercalciuria and nephrocalcinosis; and isolated hypomagnesemia, which is usually associated with hypocalcemia.[3]

TABLE 119-1 CAUSES OF MAGNESIUM DEFICIENCY

Nutritional deficiency
- Alcoholism*
- Malnutrition
- Refeeding syndrome

Intestinal malabsorption*

Proton pump inhibitors

Lower gastrointestinal losses
- Colonic diarrhea*
- Intestinal fistula
- Laxative abuse

Cutaneous losses
- Burns*
- Exercise-induced sweating

Redistribution into bone
- Hungry bone syndrome

Renal losses
- Polyuria (including diabetes mellitus)*
- Volume expansion
- Hyperaldosteronism
- Bartter and Gitelman syndromes
- Hypercalcemia
- Loop and thiazide diuretics*
- Nephrotoxins (cisplatin, amphotericin, aminoglycosides, pentamidine, cyclosporine)*

Epidermal growth factor monoclonal antibodies (cetuximab, panitumumab)*

*Common causes.

CLINICAL MANIFESTATIONS

Mild-to-moderate hypomagnesemia or magnesium deficiency is frequently asymptomatic. Manifestations of increased neuronal excitability are the most common symptoms, including paresthesias, tetany, and seizures. These may be associated with Chvostek's sign (twitching of the cheek muscles in response to tapping the facial nerve in front of the ear) or Trousseau sign (carpal spasm induced by compressing the upper arm with a tourniquet or blood pressure cuff). Cardiac disturbances also may occur and range in severity from mild electrocardiographic abnormalities (nonspecific T wave changes, U waves, prolonged QT interval, and repolarization alternans) to ventricular tachycardia, torsades de pointes, and ventricular fibrillation (Chapter 65).

Coexistent hypokalemia is very common, for two reasons: many of the causes of hypomagnesemia are also causes of potassium loss, and hypomagnesemia itself causes renal potassium wasting. Severe hypomagnesemia also impairs parathyroid hormone secretion and induces tissue resistance to its actions, thereby leading to hypocalcemia.

DIAGNOSIS

The cause of the magnesium deficiency is often obvious from the history. In difficult diagnostic cases, a random urine sample should be collected and the fractional excretion of magnesium (FE_{Mg}) determined.

$$FE_{Mg} = \frac{\text{Urine magnesium} \times \text{Serum creatinine}}{0.7 \times \text{Serum magnesium} \times \text{Urine creatinine}}$$

With extrarenal magnesium loss (usually malabsorption or laxative abuse), the FE_{Mg} is appropriately suppressed (<4%). Higher FE_{Mg} levels indicate renal magnesium wasting, often secondary to surreptitious diuretic use or one of the familial magnesium-wasting disorders.

TREATMENT Rx

It is unclear whether mild, asymptomatic hypomagnesemia needs to be treated. Magnesium repletion is recommended in hypomagnesemic patients if they are symptomatic, have underlying cardiac or seizure disorders, exhibit concurrent severe hypocalcemia or hypokalemia, or have severe hypomagnesemia (<1.4 mg/dL). In mild cases or in the outpatient setting, oral magnesium salts such as magnesium oxide (250 to 500 mg four times daily) can be used for repletion, but these substances frequently cause diarrhea, particularly at high doses. In the inpatient setting, intravenous magnesium sulfate (1 to 2 g every 6 hours) can be used for repletion. Because the redistribution of magnesium from extracellular to intracellular compartments is relatively slow, the serum magnesium concentration may normalize before total body magnesium stores are replete. It is therefore prudent to continue intravenous magnesium for an additional 1 to 2 days after restoration of normomagnesemia. In patients with normal renal function, any excess magnesium is simply excreted renally. Adverse effects from intravenous magnesium administration are primarily due to transient hypermagnesemia and include flushing, hypotension, and flaccid paralysis. Amiloride (10 to 20 mg PO once daily) abrogates renal magnesium wasting in some patients with this problem, but the mechanism is unknown.

PROGNOSIS

Hospitalized patients with hypomagnesemia have a longer length-of-stay and higher mortality, presumably because it is a marker of more severe illness.[4] In patients with a self-limited cause of magnesium deficiency, repletion is easily accomplished. However, in patients with persistent magnesium wasting, such as in Gitelman syndrome (Chapter 128), it can be difficult to keep up with the ongoing losses with oral therapy. Fortunately, these individuals tend to adapt to their chronic hypomagnesemia and tolerate it fairly well

HYPERMAGNESEMIA

Transient hypermagnesemia can occur in patients given large doses of intravenous magnesium, for example, in the setting of preeclampsia. It has also been reported in individuals taking large doses of magnesium-containing antacids or cathartics, particularly in settings in which intestinal absorption is enhanced, such as inflammatory bowel disease and intestinal obstruction. However, the kidney has a very large capacity to excrete excess magnesium. Thus, persistent hypermagnesemia is seen almost exclusively in patients who have chronic renal insufficiency (Chapter 130) who are also taking excessive amounts of magnesium in the form of antacids, cathartics, or enemas.

CLINICAL MANIFESTATIONS

Magnesium toxicity is a serious and potentially fatal condition. Mild hypermagnesemia (serum magnesium level > 4 to 6 mg/dL) causes hypotension, nausea, vomiting, facial flushing, urinary retention, and ileus. Above serum levels of 8 to 12 mg/dL, flaccid skeletal muscle paralysis and hyporeflexia may ensue, along with bradyarrhythmias, respiratory depression, coma, and cardiac arrest. A low or even negative serum anion gap is sometimes seen.

TREATMENT

Mild hypermagnesemia in a patient with good renal function usually requires no treatment because renal clearance is rapid and the normal serum half-life of magnesium is approximately 1 day. In the event of serious toxicity, the effects of magnesium can be temporarily antagonized by the administration of intravenous calcium salts (5 to 10 mL of 10% calcium chloride). Renal magnesium excretion can be enhanced by administering furosemide (20 to 40 mg every 4 hours) together with a saline infusion (0.9% NaCl at 150 mL/hour, titrated to replace urinary losses). In patients with advanced renal insufficiency, the most effective method of magnesium removal is hemodialysis.

PROGNOSIS

Severe hypermagnesemia is potentially fatal. Lesser degrees of hypermagnesemia usually respond well to treatment.

PHOSPHORUS METABOLISM

Phosphorus has many critical roles. It is a major component of bone mineral, of phospholipids in cell membranes, and of nucleic acids. It forms high-energy phosphate bonds in compounds such as adenosine triphosphate (ATP), is post-translationally bound to proteins as an intracellular signal, and acts as a major pH buffer in serum and urine.

Normal Phosphorus Metabolism

Of the total body phosphorus content, 85% is in bone, 14% is in intracellular compartments, and only 1% is in extracellular fluid. The normal concentration of phosphorus in plasma is 3 to 4.5 mg/dL (1 to 1.5 mM). Daily intake of phosphorus is 800 to 1500 mg. Phosphorus is present in many foods, including dairy products, meats, and grains, and it is absorbed in the small intestine. The kidneys excrete excess phosphorus, which is the principal mechanism by which the body regulates extracellular phosphate balance. Ninety percent of serum phosphate is filtered at the glomerulus, of which 80 to 97% is reabsorbed along the nephron, primarily in the proximal tubule. Parathyroid hormone increases renal phosphate excretion by inhibiting the sodium-phosphate cotransporter in the proximal tubule, whereas vitamin D enhances intestinal phosphate absorption.

HYPOPHOSPHATEMIA

PATHOBIOLOGY

Hypophosphatemia may be caused by decreased intake, impaired intestinal absorption, redistribution into cells or bone, and renal losses (Table 119-2). Phosphate is frequently depleted in alcoholism (Chapter 33) because of the intake of a carbohydrate-rich, phosphate-poor diet, as well as renal phosphate wasting. Divalent cation-containing antacids bind phosphate in the intestinal lumen to form insoluble salts, thereby preventing their absorption. Vitamin D deficiency also leads to decreased intestinal phosphate absorption and hence to hypophosphatemia. Respiratory but not metabolic alkalosis (Chapter 118) may cause transient hypophosphatemia. In this disorder, intracellular pH is increased, thereby stimulating glycolysis, which depletes the intracellular inorganic phosphate pool and leads to a shift of phosphate into cells.

TABLE 119-2 CAUSES OF HYPOPHOSPHATEMIA

Nutritional deficiency
Alcoholism*
Impaired intestinal absorption
Antacids
Vitamin D deficiency*
Redistribution into cells
Respiratory alkalosis*
Insulin*
Refeeding syndrome
Burns*
Redistribution into bone
Hungry bone syndrome
Tyrosine kinase inhibitors (imatinib, sorafenib)
Renal losses
Hyperparathyroidism*
Renal tubulopathy
Fanconi syndrome
Drugs (pentamidine, foscarnet, acetazolamide)
Phosphatonin excess syndrome
Oncogenic osteomalacia
Familial hypophosphatemic rickets

*Common causes.

Insulin is also a strong stimulus for shifting phosphate into cells. Patients with diabetic ketoacidosis (Chapter 229) are often hyperphosphatemic because of a shift of phosphate out of cells under insulinopenic conditions, but their total body phosphate is actually depleted as a result of urinary losses. Subsequent treatment with insulin may uncover severe hypophosphatemia. Similarly, in malnourished patients (Chapter 215), whose total body phosphate stores may be depleted, overzealous intravenous refeeding with carbohydrate-rich fluids may stimulate insulin release and cause acute hypophosphatemia. The tyrosine kinase inhibitors imatinib, sorafenib, and nilotinib, which are used in the treatment of various cancers (Chapter 184), can cause profound hypophosphatemia, which appears to be due either to inhibition of bone resorption or a partial Fanconi syndrome.[5]

Renal phosphate wasting is usually due to impaired proximal tubule phosphate reabsorption. In primary hyperparathyroidism (Chapter 245), hypercalcemia is typically associated with hypophosphatemia. Fanconi syndrome is a generalized proximal tubule disorder characterized by hypophosphatemia in association with glycosuria, aminoaciduria, hypokalemia, and type II renal tubular acidosis; it can be caused by a variety of inherited metabolic disorders, multiple myeloma (Chapter 187), heavy metal intoxication (Chapter 22), and drugs such as ifosfamide, cidofovir, and tenofovir.[6] Phosphaturia also can occur with diuretics, particularly carbonic anhydrase inhibitors, and with antimicrobial agents such as pentamidine and foscarnet.

Oncogenic osteomalacia is a paraneoplastic syndrome (Chapter 179) associated primarily with mesenchymal tumors that secrete a variety of phosphaturic factors collectively known as phosphatonins. A similar phenotype is found in X-linked and autosomal dominant hypophosphatemic rickets; these inherited disorders are characterized by an increase in a circulating phosphatonin called *fibroblast growth factor*-23.[7] Phosphatonins inhibit both renal tubular phosphate reabsorption and 1α-hydroxylation of 25-hydroxycholecalciferol, thereby leading to hypophosphatemia, rickets, or osteomalacia (Chapter 244) and inappropriately low serum levels of 1,25-dihydroxycholecalciferol.

CLINICAL MANIFESTATIONS

Clinical complications, which are usually observed only with severe hypophosphatemia (<1 mg/dL), are thought to be due to the disruption of cell membrane composition, depletion of ATP (which particularly affects high energy–consuming tissues such as skeletal and cardiac muscle), and depletion of 2,3-diphosphoglycerate in erythrocytes, with impaired tissue oxygen delivery. Manifestations of severe hypophosphatemia include encephalopathy, dilated cardiomyopathy, generalized muscle weakness that can lead to respiratory failure, rhabdomyolysis, and hemolysis. Hypophosphatemia also impairs renal ammoniagenesis and reduces the availability of urinary buffer, thereby impairing renal acid excretion and causing metabolic acidosis. Chronic hypophosphatemia leads to resorption of bone and osteomalacia.

DIAGNOSIS

The cause of hypophosphatemia is often evident from the history and physical examination. If not, measurement of either 24-hour urinary phosphate excretion or fractional excretion of phosphate (FE_{PO4}) in a spot urine sample is often helpful.

$$FE_{PO4} = \frac{\text{Urine phosphate} \times \text{Serum creatinine}}{\text{Serum phosphate} \times \text{Urine creatinine}}$$

In the setting of hypophosphatemia, the normal response of the kidney is to reduce urinary phosphate excretion to less than 100 mg/day or to reduce FE_{PO4} to less than 5%. Higher values suggest one of the causes of renal phosphate wasting.

TREATMENT Rx

Patients with asymptomatic mild-to-moderate hypophosphatemia, normal total body phosphorus stores, and minimal ongoing phosphorus losses (e.g., a patient with hypophosphatemia as a result of acute respiratory alkalosis) do not require treatment. Phosphate should be repleted in patients who are symptomatic, are suspected of having severely depleted intracellular phosphorus stores (malnourished or alcoholic patients), have ongoing gastrointestinal or renal losses, or have severe hypophosphatemia (<1 mg/dL).[8] Oral repletion can be accomplished with sodium or potassium phosphate salts (1 to 2 g/day) or with skimmed milk. Intravenous phosphorus repletion at a dose of 0.16 to 0.64 mmol/kg over 4 to 8 hours is recommended for severe hypophosphatemia but is contraindicated in patients with renal insufficiency or hypercalemia. Complications of phosphate therapy include hypocalcemia, metastatic calcification, hypotension, acute renal failure, and arrhythmias, as well as concomitant hypernatremia or hyperkalemia, depending on which salt is administered.

PROGNOSIS

Most patients with hypophosphatemia respond well to treatment.

HYPERPHOSPHATEMIA

PATHOBIOLOGY

Pseudohyperphosphatemia may occur in blood specimens that are hemolyzed or hyperglobulinemic, such as in multiple myeloma (Chapter 187). True hyperphosphatemia is caused by excessive phosphate intake, increased intestinal absorption, redistribution from intracellular stores, or impaired renal excretion (Table 119-3 and Fig. 119-1).[9] Overzealous phosphate repletion can obviously cause hyperphosphatemia. The phosphorus in some laxatives and enemas may be absorbed and cause hyperphosphatemia. Intoxication with vitamin D or its analogues increases intestinal absorption of both calcium and phosphorus. Conditions associated with massive cell lysis, such as rhabdomyolysis (Chapter 113) and tumor lysis syndrome (Chapter 179), cause the release of intracellular phosphate into the extracellular fluid. Patients with diabetic ketoacidosis (Chapter 229) are often hyperphosphatemic at initial evaluation because of the redistribution of phosphate out of cells in the insulin-deficient state. Decreased phosphate excretion is most commonly due to acute or chronic renal failure (Chapter 130). With a normal diet, serum phosphate levels can be maintained within the normal range until the glomerular filtration rate falls below 25 mL/minute. However, even mild degrees of renal insufficiency may predispose to hyperphosphatemia if there is a concurrent excessive intake of phosphate-containing compounds such as laxatives. Finally, because parathyroid hormone stimulates proximal tubule phosphate excretion, primary hypoparathyroidism (Chapter 245) is often associated with mild hyperphosphatemia together with hypocalcemia.

CLINICAL MANIFESTATIONS

Acute hyperphosphatemia increases the risk for precipitation of calcium phosphate and subsequent metastatic calcification in soft tissues, including the kidney, in which it can cause acute renal failure. The resultant hypocalcemia (Chapter 245) can cause tetany, hypotension, seizures, and cardiac arrhythmias. In the chronic hyperphosphatemia of chronic renal insufficiency, patients with a serum phosphate concentration greater than 6.5 mg/dL have higher mortality. Hyperphosphatemia in this setting is a risk factor for coronary and other vascular calcification, which is associated with increased mortality.

TABLE 119-3 CAUSES OF HYPERPHOSPHATEMIA

Phosphate intake
Phosphate repletion
Phosphate-containing laxatives and enemas*
Increased intestinal absorption
Vitamin D toxicity
Redistribution from intracellular stores
Rhabdomyolysis*
Tumor lysis syndrome
Diabetic ketoacidosis
Decreased renal excretion
Renal failure*
Hypoparathyroidism
Pseudohypoparathyroidism
Familial tumoral calcinosis

*Common causes.

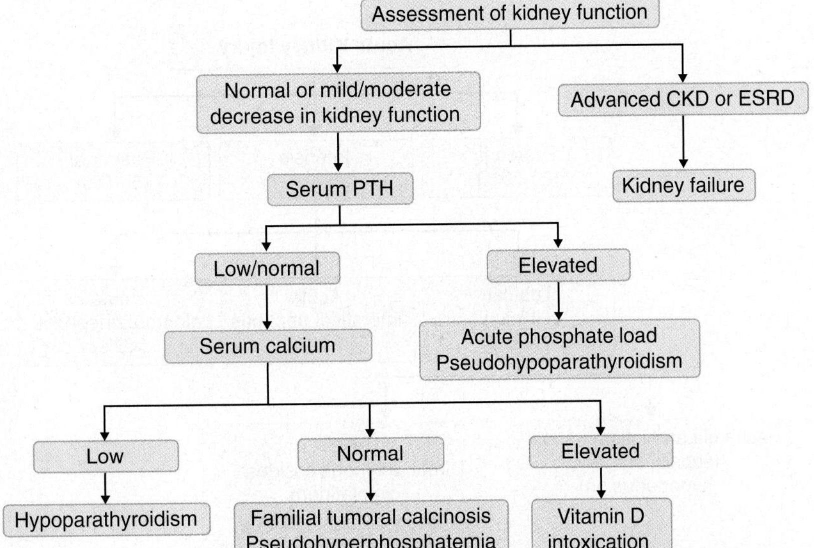

FIGURE 119-1. Diagnostic approach to chronic hyperphosphatemia, a parathyroid hormone (PTH)-based diagnostic algorithm. CKD = chronic kidney disease; ESRD = end-stage renal disease; PTH = parathyroid hormone. (Redrawn from Leaf DE, Wolf M. A physiologic-based approach to the evaluation of a patient with hyperphosphatemia. *Am J Kidney Dis.* 2013;61:330-336).

TREATMENT Rx

Acute hyperphosphatemia in an asymptomatic patient with normal renal function often resolves spontaneously as excess phosphate is excreted. In symptomatic patients and those with impaired renal function, phosphate should be removed by extracorporeal therapy. Because of the slow rate of phosphate mobilization from intracellular stores, continuous venovenous hemodiafiltration is considerably more effective than intermittent hemodialysis. Chronic hyperphosphatemia (Chapter 130) can be managed by minimizing dietary phosphorus intake and administering oral phosphate binders such as calcium salts (e.g., calcium acetate 1334 mg with each meal), lanthanum carbonate (500 mg with each meal), or sevelamer (800 to 1600 mg with each meal) (Table 119-4).[10] Aluminum hydroxide (300 to 600 mg with meals) is also a very effective phosphate binder, but prolonged use leads to aluminum accumulation and results in encephalopathy and osteomalacia. Cinacalcet (30 to 180 mg/day), a calcimimetic used in patients with chronic renal insufficiency to treat secondary hyperparathyroidism, also reduces the serum phosphate concentration and calcium-phosphate product. However, it does not significantly reduce the risk for death or major cardiovascular events in patients undergoing dialysis.[A1]

TABLE 119-4 MEDICATIONS FOR HYPERPHOSPHATEMIA

MEDICATION	USUAL DOSE WITH EACH MEAL	COMMENTS
CALCIUM SALTS		
Calcium acetate	1334 mg	Calcium level will increase approximately 0.5 mg/dL
Calcium carbonate	500-1000 mg	Calcium level will increase approximately 0.5 mg/dL
MAGNESIUM SALTS		
Magnesium hydroxide	311-622 mg	Can cause diarrhea or hypermagnesemia
Magnesium carbonate	63-126 mg	Can cause diarrhea or hypermagnesemia
ALUMINUM SALTS		
Aluminum hydroxide	300-600 mg	Encephalopathy and osteomalacia with prolonged use
OTHERS		
Sevelamer hydrochloride	800-1600 mg	Gastrointestinal side effects
Sevelamer carbonate	800-1600 mg	Gastrointestinal side effects
Lanthanum carbonate	250-500 mg	Monitor serum bicarbonate and chloride levels as well as folic acid and vitamin D, E, and K levels

PROGNOSIS

Severe acute hyperphosphatemia can be life-threatening owing to metastatic calcification and multiorgan failure, but it generally responds well to prompt therapy. Chronic hyperphosphatemia in patients with chronic kidney failure (Chapter 130) is often fairly resistant to treatment, particularly in poorly compliant individuals, and is associated with increased long-term mortality.

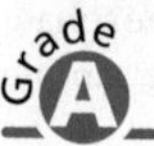

Grade A Reference

A1. Chertow GM, Block GA, Correa-Rotter R, et al. Effect of cinacalcet on cardiovascular disease in patients undergoing dialysis. *N Engl J Med*. 2012;367:2482-2494.

GENERAL REFERENCES

For the General References and other additional features, please visit Expert Consult at https://expertconsult.inkling.com.

120

ACUTE KIDNEY INJURY

BRUCE A. MOLITORIS

DEFINITION

Acute kidney injury (AKI) is a clinical syndrome defined as a functional or structural kidney abnormality that manifests with an increase in serum creatinine (Cr) of 0.3 mg/dL or greater within 48 hours, an increase in serum Cr of 1.5 or greater times baseline within 7 days or a urine volume less than 0.5 mL/kg/hour for 6 hours (Table 120-1).[1] Diagnostically, the reduction in kidney function in AKI is staged according to the maximal rise in serum Cr or reduction in urine output with oliguria. The use of a 50% change in serum Cr over baseline should not be used in patients with a very low baseline volume.[2]

EPIDEMIOLOGY

Most episodes of AKI occur in the hospital, with an incidence of 20% among all hospitalized patients[3] and up to 50% among patients in intensive care units. AKI is the number one reason for hospital nephrology consult. By contrast, the incidence of community-acquired AKI is no more than 1%.

The various causes of AKI are divided broadly into three anatomic categories: prerenal, intrarenal or intrinsic, and postrenal (Fig. 120-1). Each of the categories represents a unique pathophysiologic process with distinctive diagnostic parameters and prognosis.

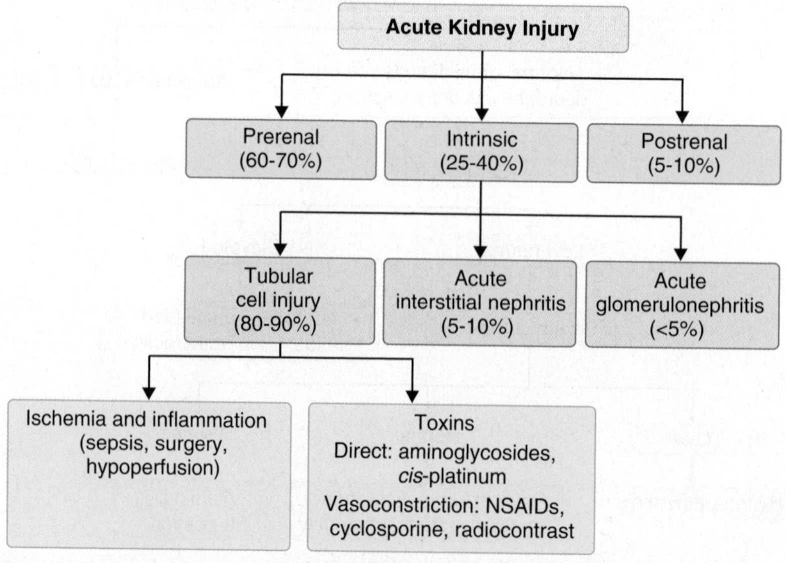

FIGURE 120-1. Main categories of acute kidney injury. NSAIDs = nonsteroidal anti-inflammatory drugs.

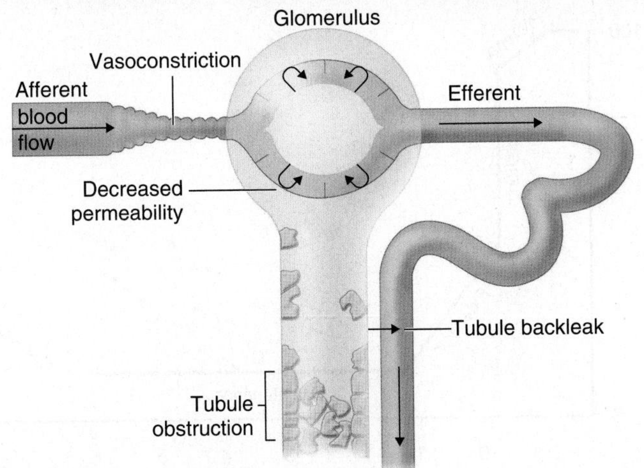

FIGURE 120-2. Mechanisms of prerenal and intrinsic acute renal injury. See text for descriptions.

TABLE 120-1 KDIGO ACUTE KIDNEY INJURY CLASSIFICATION

STAGE	SERUM CREATININE	URINE OUTPUT
1	1.5-1.9 times baseline OR ≥0.3 mg/dL (≥26.5 μmol/L) increase	<0.5 mL/kg/hr for 6-12 hr
2	2.0-2.9 times baseline	<0.5 mL/kg/hr for ≥12 hr
3	3.0 times baseline OR Increase in serum creatinine to ≥4.0 mg/dL (≥353.6 μmol/L) OR Initiation of renal replacement therapy OR In patients <18 yr, decrease in eGFR to <35 mL/min per 1.73 m^2	<0.3 mL/kg/hr for ≥24 hr OR Anuria for ≥12 hr

eGFR = estimated glomerular filtration rate; KDIGO = Kidney Disease Improving Global Outcomes

TABLE 120-2 COMMON RENAL TUBULAR TOXINS

Aminoglycosides
Radiocontrast agents
Acyclovir
Cisplatin
Sulfonamides
Methotrexate
Cyclosporine
Tacrolimus
Amphotericin B
Foscarnet
Pentamidine
Ethylene glycol
Toluene
Cocaine
HMG-CoA reductase inhibitors

HMG-CoA = 3-hydroxy-3-methylglutaryl coenzyme A.

TABLE 120-3 MEDICATIONS ASSOCIATED WITH ACUTE INTERSTITIAL NEPHRITIS

β-LACTAM ANTIBIOTICS
Penicillin
Cephalosporins
Ampicillin
Methicillin
Nafcillin

DIURETICS
Furosemide
Hydrochlorothiazide
Triamterene

OTHER ANTIBIOTICS
Sulfonamides
Vancomycin
Rifampin
Acyclovir
Indinavir

NSAIDS
Ibuprofen
Naproxen
Indomethacin

NSAIDs = nonsteroidal anti-inflammatory drugs.

Prerenal Azotemia

Prerenal azotemia, which is the most common cause of AKI, is a result of renal hypoperfusion. It accounts for approximately 60 to 70% of community-acquired and 40% of hospital-acquired cases. Hypoperfusion occurs in disease states that reduce effective intravascular volume, such as volume depletion from bleeding over-diuresis, sepsis (Chapter 108), heart failure (Chapter 58), or liver failure (Chapter 154). Additionally, medications that act directly to reduce glomerular capillary perfusion, such as angiotensin-converting enzyme (ACE) inhibitors, angiotensin-receptor blockers (ARBs), and nonsteroidal anti-inflammatory drugs (NSAIDs), also can cause prerenal AKI. The use of these agents in a patient with underlying renal hypoperfusion is to be avoided.

Intrinsic Acute Kidney Injury

Intrarenal AKI often results when untreated or untreatable severe hypoperfusion leads to cellular injury and ischemic AKI. The diverse causes of intrinsic AKI can involve any portion of the renal vasculature, nephron, or interstitium (Fig. 120-2). Ischemic and septic injury are major causes. Renal toxins, such as radiocontrast agents and aminoglycosides, also can damage tubules both directly and indirectly (Table 120-2). Fortunately, AKI does not develop in every patient exposed to these agents, but elderly patients with diabetes mellitus, hemodynamically unstable patients, and patients with a reduced effective arterial volume (heart failure, burns, cirrhosis, hypoalbuminemia) are the most susceptible to toxic renal injury. In fact, the incidence of aminoglycoside antibiotic nephrotoxicity increases from 3 to 5% to 30 to 50% in these high-risk patients.

AKI secondary to injury to the renal interstitium is termed *acute interstitial nephritis*. Commonly implicated medications for interstitial nephritis include penicillins, cephalosporins, sulfonamides, and NSAIDs (Table 120-3) (Chapter 122). Bacterial and viral infections also can be the causative agents. Interstitial nephritis is also associated with a kidney-confined or systemic autoimmune process, such as systemic lupus erythematosus (Chapter 266), Sjögren syndrome (Chapter 268), cryoglobulinemia (Chapter 187), and primary biliary cirrhosis (Chapter 153).

Postrenal Acute Kidney Injury

Postrenal AKI can occur in the setting of bilateral urinary outflow obstruction or in a patient with a solitary kidney when a single urinary outflow tract is obstructed (Chapter 123). Most commonly, this type of outflow obstruction is observed in patients with prostatic hypertrophy (Chapter 129), prostatic or cervical cancer (Chapter 199), or retroperitoneal disorders, including lymphadenopathy. A functional obstruction also can be observed in patients with a neurogenic bladder. In addition, intraluminal obstruction can be seen in patients with bilateral renal calculi (Chapter 126), papillary necrosis, blood clots, and bladder carcinoma, whereas extraluminal obstruction can develop in connection with retroperitoneal fibrosis, colon cancer, and lymphomas. Finally, intratubular crystallization of compounds such as uric acid, calcium oxalate, acyclovir, sulfonamide, and methotrexate, as well as myeloma light chains, can result in tubular obstruction.

PATHOBIOLOGY

The causes of AKI are diverse, and it can arise from a number of physiologic insults that injure the kidney and reduce the glomerular filtration rate (GFR). Decreased kidney perfusion and a reduced GFR can occur with or without cellular injury; toxic, ischemic, or obstructive injury to the nephron; inflammation and edema of the tubulointerstitium; and a primary glomerular disease process.

TABLE 120-4 CONDITIONS THAT LEAD TO ISCHEMIC ACUTE RENAL FAILURE

MECHANISM	CONDITION
Intravascular volume depletion and hypotension	Hemorrhage; gastrointestinal, renal, and dermal losses
Decreased effective intravascular volume	Heart failure, cirrhosis, hepatorenal syndrome, peritonitis
Systemic vasodilation, renal vasoconstriction	Sepsis, hepatorenal syndrome
Large-vessel renal vascular disease	Renal artery thrombosis or embolism, intraoperative arterial cross-clamping, renal artery stenosis, cholesterol emboli
Small-vessel renal vascular disease	Sepsis, vasculitis, atheroembolism, hemolytic-uremic syndrome, malignant hypertension, scleroderma, preeclampsia, sickle cell anemia, hypercalcemia, transplant rejection
Impaired renal blood flow	Cyclosporine, tacrolimus, ACEIs, ARBs, NSAIDs, radiocontrast agents

ACEIs = angiotensin-converting enzyme inhibitors; ARBs = angiotensin-receptor blockers; NSAIDs = nonsteroidal anti-inflammatory drugs.

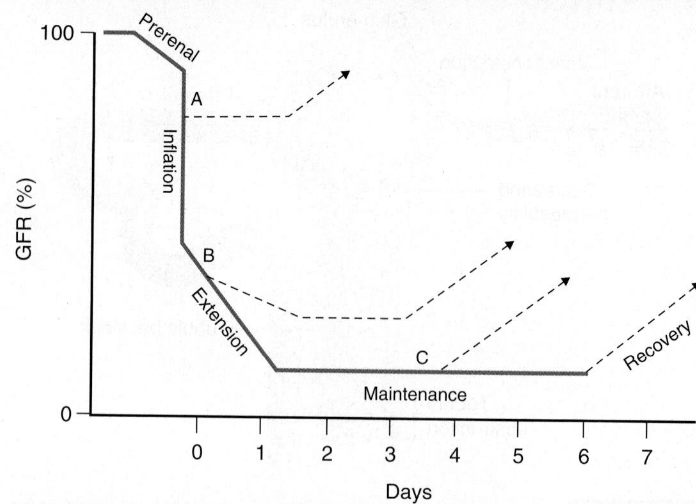

FIGURE 120-3. **Phases of acute kidney injury.** GFR = glomerular filtration rate. (From Sutton TA, Fisher CJ, Molitoris BA. Microvascular endothelial injury and dysfunction during ischemic acute renal failure. *Kidney Int.* 2002;62:1539-1549.)

Prerenal Acute Kidney Injury

The precipitating event for prerenal AKI is hypoperfusion of the kidney (see Fig. 120-2), which can be caused by a reduction in the total or intravascular fluid volume or disease states associated with normal or even increased total or intravascular fluid volumes but decrements in effective arterial volume, such as in sepsis, heart failure, and advanced cirrhosis. Prerenal azotemia is also divided functionally into volume responsive and nonresponsive azotemia, based on the response to hydration. For example, in severe heart failure (Chapter 58), additional intravascular volume may not improve kidney perfusion, whereas afterload reduction may improve perfusion by increasing cardiac output. Early in the course of prerenal AKI, the renal parenchyma remains intact and functional. During this initial phase, the GFR remains largely intact because kidney hypoperfusion initiates a neurohormonal cascade that results in afferent arteriolar dilation and efferent arteriolar constriction, thereby maintaining glomerular perfusion pressure. Because prerenal azotemia is often easily reversible, and mortality rates are low, early diagnosis and correction of the underlying pathophysiology are of critical importance. However, without early medical corrective intervention, prerenal azotemia progresses, ischemia worsens, and the resulting injury to tubular epithelial cells further decreases the GFR. This progression from prerenal azotemia to ischemic AKI is a continuum that depends on the severity and duration of the pathophysiologic insult.

Intrarenal Acute Kidney Injury

Intrinsic AKI is classified according to the primary histologic site of injury: tubules, interstitium, vasculature, or glomerulus. Renal tubular epithelial cell injury, commonly termed *acute tubular necrosis* (ATN), occurs more commonly in the setting of ischemia, although the renal tubules also can be damaged by specific kidney toxins. Ischemia can arise from a number of different clinical scenarios, but the common underlying pathogenesis is reduced renal blood flow (Table 120-4) with progression from prerenal azotemia to ischemic AKI in four distinct clinical and cellular phases: initiation, extension, maintenance, and recovery. Each of these phases encompasses distinct cellular events and declines in GFR as the kidneys respond to the insult and attempt to maintain and reestablish function (Fig. 120-3).[4] The initiation phase, which marks the transition from prerenal to tubular cell injury and dysfunction, is characterized by severe cellular depletion of adenosine triphosphate. Renal tubular epithelial cell injury, especially of proximal tubular cells, is a prominent feature during this phase, but injury to endothelial and vascular smooth muscle cells also has been documented. During this phase, extensive signaling between the proximal tubular cells and adjacent endothelial cells results in endothelial dysfunction and an inflammatory endothelial response.[5] Leukocytes of all types play a role in ongoing inflammation and cell injury. Dendritic cells, macrophages, neutrophils, and lymphocytes have been shown to play either a detrimental or protective role. The time course of involvement varies according to the cell type, and changes in macrophage phenotype from M1 to M2 mediate conversion from a proinflammatory form to a repair-mediating form.

During the extension phase, microvascular congestion with continued hypoxia and inflammation are most pronounced in the corticomedullary junction of the kidney, where reperfusion is limited owing to endothelial dysfunction at the capillary and postcapillary venule levels, with white blood cell adhesion and rouleaux formation.[6] The GFR is at its ebb during the maintenance phase as cells undergo repair, migration, and proliferation and as the kidney attempts to reestablish cellular and tubular integrity. Finally, during the recovery phase, the GFR begins to improve as cellular differentiation continues and normal cellular and organ function returns. Proximal tubular cells undergo cellular repair, and terminally differentiated epithelial cells re-express stem cell markers and divide to repopulate the nephron.[7] This last phase is often heralded by increasing urine output.

The S3 segment of the proximal tubule is located in the outer stripe of the medullary region of the nephron. This region is particularly susceptible to continued reduced perfusion after injury, and ongoing or worsening hypoxia results in continued cellular injury. Proximal tubular cell injury during the initiation phase of renal ischemia is first manifested as bleb formation in the apical membranes, with loss of the brush border. Proximal tubule cells also lose the polarity of the surface membrane and the integrity of their tight junctions. As the injury progresses, both live and necrotic proximal cells detach and enter the tubular lumen, where they ultimately form casts in the distal tubule. Casts contribute to a reduction in GFR by obstructing tubular urine flow, thereby preventing further filtration into that nephron. In addition, loss of the epithelial cell barrier and cell tight junctions allows back-leak of the glomerular filtrate into the interstitium, thus further compromising GFR (see Fig. 120-2).

Common agents that can cause direct tubular cell toxicity (see Table 120-2) include the aminoglycoside antibiotics, intravenous radiocontrast agents, and cisplatin. Other agents such as radiocontrast dyes, NSAIDs, and cyclosporine induce vasoconstriction and reduce kidney perfusion. Cocaine and the 3-hydroxy-3-methylglutaryl coenzyme A (HMG-CoA) reductase inhibitors can damage skeletal muscle and cause rhabdomyolysis (Chapter 113), thereby resulting in the release of myoglobin that is toxic to the tubular epithelium. Finally, the precipitation of some compounds or their metabolites can cause intratubular obstruction; agents in this category include acyclovir, sulfonamides, ethylene glycol (calcium oxalate metabolite; Chapter 110), methotrexate, and the light chains of multiple myeloma (Chapter 187).

Sepsis is a very common cause of intrinsic AKI. Although the causes of septic AKI are often multifactorial, ischemia owing to poor microvascular perfusion is a major factor. Interestingly, proximal tubular cells act as part of the innate immune system to detect danger-associated molecular patterns and establish pathogen-associated recognition patterns via toll-like receptors (TLRs).[8] Lipopolysaccharide is a prime example of proximal tubule TLR4-mediated uptake that results in subsequent signaling via cytokines and oxidative stress. The resulting histology in humans is patchy involvement of cells with apoptosis and minimal cellular necrosis that cannot fully explain the severity of sepsis-induced kidney dysfunction. Coagulation abnormalities of the microvasculature also play an important role in kidney dysfunction and ongoing ischemia.

In AKI caused by the interstitial injury, a mixed inflammatory infiltrate composed of T lymphocytes, monocytes, and macrophages, is seen. These inflammatory lesions can be diffuse or patchy in distribution. Occasionally, granulomas also can be observed, especially in drug hypersensitivity reactions. Acute interstitial nephritis that persists and becomes chronic is characterized by interstitial fibrosis and tubular atrophy, although foci of inflammatory cells can persist. This process can lead to chronic and even end-stage kidney disease requiring chronic dialysis.

Vascular causes of intrinsic AKI can include microvascular and macrovascular processes. Classic microvascular disorders, which include thrombotic thrombocytopenic purpura (Chapter 172), sepsis (Chapter 108), hemolytic-uremic syndrome (Chapter 172), and the HELLP syndrome (*h*emolysis, *e*levated *l*iver enzymes, and *l*ow *p*latelet count; Chapters 146 and 239), cause AKI as a result of glomerular capillary thrombosis and microvascular occlusion. Macrovascular disease such as atherosclerosis can cause AKI secondary to atheroembolization (Chapter 125), especially during or after an invasive or interventional vascular procedure in a patient with preexisting atherosclerotic disease.

A less common cause of AKI is glomerulonephritis (Chapter 121), which can be seen in systemic lupus nephritis (Chapter 266), granulomatosis with polyangiitis (Chapter 270), polyarteritis nodosa (Chapter 270), Goodpasture syndrome (Chapter 121), Henoch-Schönlein purpura (Chapter 270), and hemolytic-uremic syndrome (Chapter 172). AKI in this setting is termed *rapidly progressive glomerulonephritis* and results from direct inflammatory glomerular or vascular injury.

Postrenal Acute Kidney Injury

Postrenal AKI is caused by obstruction to luminal flow of the glomerular filtrate. This obstruction results in a relatively complex pathophysiology that begins with transmission of backpressure to Bowman space of the glomerulus. Intuitively, this backpressure would be expected to reduce the GFR. However, by dilation of the glomerular afferent arteriole, the GFR remains largely preserved. Unfortunately, such compensation is only transient, and the GFR will begin to attenuate if the obstruction is not rapidly relieved. With continued obstruction for more than 12 to 24 hours, renal blood flow and intratubular pressure decline and large unperfused and underperfused areas of the kidney cortex result in a reduction in GFR.

CLINICAL MANIFESTATIONS

AKI, even when advanced, frequently is first diagnosed by abnormalities observed in a patient's laboratory studies and not by any specific symptom or sign. The clinical manifestations associated with AKI are frequently protean, occur late in the course, and are often not apparent until kidney dysfunction has become severe. The clinical findings of AKI also depend on the stage at which it is diagnosed. Patients with AKI may report symptoms such as anorexia, fatigue, nausea and vomiting, and pruritus, as well as a decline in urine output or dark-colored urine. Furthermore, if the patient has become volume overloaded, shortness of breath and dyspnea on exertion may be noted.

A thorough physical examination with special emphasis on determination of volume status and effective arterial volume is essential. If volume overload is present, jugular venous distention, pulmonary crackles, and peripheral edema may be found (Chapter 58). Findings such as asterixis, myoclonus, or a pericardial rub may be seen in severe AKI.

DIAGNOSIS

A systematic approach that considers each of the three major categories in the pathogenesis of AKI will ensure that an accurate diagnosis and an appropriate therapeutic plan will be achieved. An appropriate diagnostic strategy is to exclude prerenal and postrenal causes first and then, if needed, begin an evaluation for possible intrinsic causes.

Laboratory analysis of blood and urine samples of patients with AKI reveals the level of dysfunction, will frequently suggest a cause, and may also direct the rapidity with which a specific therapy needs to be instituted. All patients with clinical findings of AKI should be evaluated with serum measurements of electrolytes, Cr, calcium, and phosphorus; a blood urea nitrogen level; and complete blood count with differential. In addition, urine studies, including sodium, potassium, chloride, and Cr determinations for calculation of the fractional excretion of sodium (FE_{Na}), are important. The formula for calculating FE_{Na} is as follows:

$$FE_{Na} = \frac{\text{Urine Na} \times \text{Plasma Cr}}{\text{Plasma Na} \times \text{Urine Cr}} \times 100$$

TABLE 120-5 FE_{NA} VALUES FOR THE VARIOUS CAUSES OF ACUTE KIDNEY INJURY

CAUSE OF ACUTE KIDNEY INJURY	FE_{Na}	BUN-TO-SERUM CREATININE RATIO
Prerenal	<1%	>20
Intrarenal		<10-15
Tubular necrosis	≥1%	
Interstitial nephritis	≥1%	
Glomerulonephritis (early)	<1%	
Vascular disorders (early)	<1%	
Postrenal	≥1%	>20

TABLE 120-6 COMMON URINALYSIS FINDINGS IN ACUTE KIDNEY INJURY

CAUSE OF ACUTE KIDNEY INJURY	URINALYSIS
Prerenal	Normal or hyaline casts
Intrarenal	
Tubular cell injury	Muddy-brown, granular, epithelial casts
Interstitial nephritis	Pyuria, hematuria, mild proteinuria, granular and epithelial casts, eosinophils
Glomerulonephritis	Hematuria, marked proteinuria, red blood cell casts, granular casts
Vascular disorders	Normal or hematuria, mild proteinuria
Postrenal	Normal or hematuria, granular casts, pyuria

The numerical value of FE_{Na} can be helpful in determining the potential cause of the AKI (Table 120-5). In some cases, it is better to use FE_{Cl} because urinary sodium can be elevated during systemic alkalosis when a high urinary bicarbonate level obligates the loss of sodium. Urine dipstick and microscopy (Table 120-6) should be performed on a fresh urine sample because important cellular elements that could indicate potential causes degrade rapidly with time. Finally, renal ultrasound to determine the presence or absence of outlet obstruction also should be included in the initial evaluation. Measurement of urine and serum levels of structural biomarkers, such as kidney injury molecule 1 (KIM-1) and inflammatory markers, such as neutrophil gelatinase–associated lipocalin (NGAL) and interleukin 18, may aid in the diagnosis of AKI, although the data are not yet conclusive.[9]

Prerenal Azotemia

Prerenal azotemia, which is the most common cause of renal dysfunction, often can be determined by the patient's history. Common historical features in patients with prerenal azotemia include vomiting, diarrhea, and poor oral intake. Heart failure can suggest a possible prerenal cause of reduced renal perfusion from over-diuresis or as exacerbation of the heart failure itself. Other medications that can attenuate renal perfusion, such as NSAIDs, ACE inhibitors, and ARBs, can cause prerenal azotemia. Common physical examination findings include tachycardia, systemic or orthostatic hypotension (or both), and dry mucous membranes.

Laboratory studies in patients with prerenal azotemia demonstrate elevated serum Cr and blood urea nitrogen (BUN) levels. FE_{Na} is typically less than 1%. However, in a patient taking diuretics such as furosemide, FE_{Na} may be greater than 1% even though the patient has prerenal azotemia because of diuretic-induced natriuresis. For these clinical situations, the fractional excretion of urea can be used and is calculated in similar fashion:

$$FE_{urea} = \frac{\text{Urine Urea} \times \text{Plasma Cr}}{\text{Plasma Urea} \times \text{Urine Cr}} \times 100$$

FE_{urea} less than 35% suggests prerenal AKI. Other causes of an FE_{Na} greater than 1% include the presence of a non-reabsorbable solute such as bicarbonate, glucose, or mannitol. Chronic kidney disease, ATN, and late obstructive nephropathy are also associated with FE_{Na} greater than 1%. Therefore, in these disease states, FE_{Na} cannot provide reliable diagnostic information regarding AKI unless the FE_{Na} is less than 1%. Moreover, FE_{urea} has not been validated for these clinical entities.

Another laboratory parameter to assist in diagnosing prerenal AKI is the ratio of BUN to serum Cr. Commonly, a patient with prerenal azotemia will have a ratio of BUN to serum Cr of greater than 20 : 1.

Intrarenal Acute Kidney Injury

A history of hypotension or exposure to a nephrotoxin or medication is a common finding in patients with intrarenal AKI. The nephrotoxin can be a specific tubular toxin that causes ATN or a medication that causes an allergic reaction as in acute interstitial nephritis (see Tables 120-2 and 120-3). Physical examination may reveal signs and symptoms of volume depletion or fluid overload. It is important to remember that ATN often results from a persistent severe prerenal state and the prerenal state must first be corrected to prevent ongoing or worsening ATN. Rash may accompany acute interstitial nephritis. Cholesterol embolism in patients with severe atherosclerotic disease (Chapter 125) may manifest classically as cyanotic digits and AKI; this finding is frequently seen after invasive vascular surgery or an interventional study.

Laboratory studies will demonstrate elevated serum Cr and BUN levels in intrarenal AKI. ATN and acute interstitial nephritis are frequently associated with FE_{Na} greater than 1, whereas FE_{Na} is typically less than 1 in early radiocontrast-induced AKI, sepsis, glomerulonephritis, and vascular disorders. Peripheral eosinophilia and urinary eosinophils may be present in acute interstitial nephritis, although the latter are neither sensitive nor specific for this type of AKI. Urinary eosinophils are also associated with cholesterol microembolic disease (Chapter 125). Intrarenal AKI has specific urinalysis findings that can be helpful in making diagnostic and therapeutic decisions (see Table 120-6).

Postrenal Acute Kidney Injury

A history of prostatic hypertrophy (Chapter 129), prostate cancer (Chapter 201), lymphoma (Chapter 185), cervical cancer (Chapter 199), or retroperitoneal disease often can be found in patients with postrenal AKI. Postrenal AKI should always be in the differential diagnosis of patients with severe oliguria (urine output < 450 mL/day) or anuria (urine output < 100 mL/day). However, many patients with postrenal AKI are neither oliguric nor anuric. Beyond an elevation in a patient's serum Cr and BUN levels, laboratory studies generally yield benign results. Bladder catheterization can be both diagnostic and therapeutic in postrenal AKI. However, renal ultrasound is the diagnostic test of choice, although it may be falsely negative early in postrenal AKI.

TREATMENT Rx

The cornerstones of therapy for AKI are rapid recognition and correction of reversible causes such as hypoperfusion, avoidance of any further renal injury, and correction and maintenance of a normal electrolyte and fluid volume milieu. Preventive therapy or medical interventions performed during the initiation and extension phases of AKI provide the greatest chance for minimizing the extent of injury (see Fig. 120-3, *lines A* and *B*) and hastening renal recovery (see Fig. 120-3, *line B*); interventions provided during the maintenance phase of AKI have not proved beneficial (see Fig. 120-3, *line C*). If prerenal AKI is not addressed early in a patient's course or if the patient is seen late in the course, ATN may occur and markedly increase morbidity and mortality.[10]

Prerenal azotemia in its early stages often can be rapidly corrected by aggressive normalization of effective arterial volume, although more care must be taken during volume resuscitation in patients with a history of heart failure, cirrhosis, and sepsis. Key approaches include administering volume (e.g., normal saline) to achieve euvolemia, improving cardiac output by afterload reduction (Chapter 59), or normalizing systemic vascular resistance.

Postrenal AKI secondary to prostatic hypertrophy frequently can be corrected by placement of a bladder catheter. However, outlet obstruction from a neoplastic process will usually require urologic consultation for consideration of ureteral stenting or placement of a percutaneous nephrostomy tube.

Intrarenal AKI can be the most complex and difficult to treat. AKI caused by glomerulonephritis (Chapter 121) or vasculitis (Chapters 266 and 270) will frequently require immunosuppressive therapy. For suspected acute interstitial nephritis, the offending medication must be determined and discontinued; a 2-week tapering course of glucocorticoids, beginning with 1 mg/kg of prednisone (up to 60 mg) for 3 days, is commonly recommended despite the absence of data from randomized trials.

General supportive measures include avoiding any further nephrotoxins and paying careful attention to the patient's fluid balance by monitoring weight and daily input and output. In addition, serum electrolytes, Cr, and BUN should be monitored at least daily more frequently if the patient's renal function appears to be tenuous. Patients with AKI also should receive a diet low in sodium, potassium, and protein, which can be liberalized as the patient's renal function improves. A phosphate binder (e.g., calcium acetate [1334 mg], lanthanum carbonate [500 mg], sevelamer [300 to 1000 mg], or aluminum hydroxide [300 to 600 mg] with each meal; see Table 119-4) is also usually helpful in controlling the serum phosphate level by minimizing the absorption of dietary phosphate.

Early nephrology consultation will ensure that the patient receives optimal care. Some patients will warrant urgent hemodialysis because of marked metabolic acidosis unresponsive to sodium bicarbonate infusions; electrolyte abnormalities, such as hyperkalemia that is unresponsive to medical management; pulmonary edema not responding to diuretic therapy; and uremic symptoms of encephalopathy, seizures, and pericarditis. In the absence of acute indications, however, when to initiate dialysis in AKI remains unresolved.

For AKI, early initiation of dialysis (Cr level 7.5 mg/dL) is no better than standard dialysis beginning at a Cr level of approximately 10 mg/dL.[A1] Furthermore, intensive dialytic renal support therapy is no better than standard dialytic therapy, and intermittent hemodialysis and continuous renal replacement therapy lead to similar clinical outcomes in acute renal failure. However, it is important to verify that the prescribed dialysis is received and that standardized measures are achieved. Some patients—especially patients in an increased catabolic state, trauma patients, and patients receiving glucocorticoids—may require dialysis more than three times per week to achieve adequate therapy (Chapter 131). Neither furosemide nor low-dose dopamine improve outcome, even though low-dose dopamine may temporarily improve metrics of renal physiology.

PREVENTION

Given the marked increase in morbidity and mortality associated with AKI, especially for critically ill patients, potential measures to prevent AKI are essential. The first step in prevention, however, is being aware of patients who are at highest risk for AKI because of known kidney disease or comorbid medical conditions, such as chronic kidney disease, diabetes, hypertension, nephrotic syndrome, heart failure, age, and peripheral vascular disease.

Of all the risk factors for acquiring AKI, the presence of preexisting chronic kidney disease is the most predictive. Recent data document a vicious cycle involving AKI and CKD (Fig. 120-4). Appropriate hospital surveillance measures include avoiding nephrotoxic medications (e.g., NSAIDs and aminoglycosides); minimizing diagnostic procedures that require radiocontrast material, especially in the prerenal patient; and careful monitoring of urinary output with daily determination of serum electrolyte and Cr levels after any procedures known to induce AKI. Additionally, educating the patient regarding common nonprescription nephrotoxins such as NSAIDs can reduce the risk for AKI in outpatients.

Before a potentially nephrotoxic exposure, early consultation with a nephrologist is warranted for this high-risk group to advise whether a specific medication or intervention may reduce the risk for AKI or whether an alternative medication or procedure, such as magnetic resonance imaging instead of computed tomography with intravenous radiocontrast agents, may be preferred. All potential nephrotoxins, such as NSAIDs, should be discontinued before a potentially nephrotoxic procedure and avoided after it. The patient's volume and hemodynamic status must be maximized both before and after the event.

In high-risk patients, a renal protective intervention is often instituted before exposure to the agent. Interventions that may be useful for preventing AKI associated with intravenous radiocontrast agents include hydration with intravenous sodium chloride[A2][A3] and short-term rosuvastatin (40 mg on admission then 20 mg/day or 10 mg/day for 2 days before and 3 days after

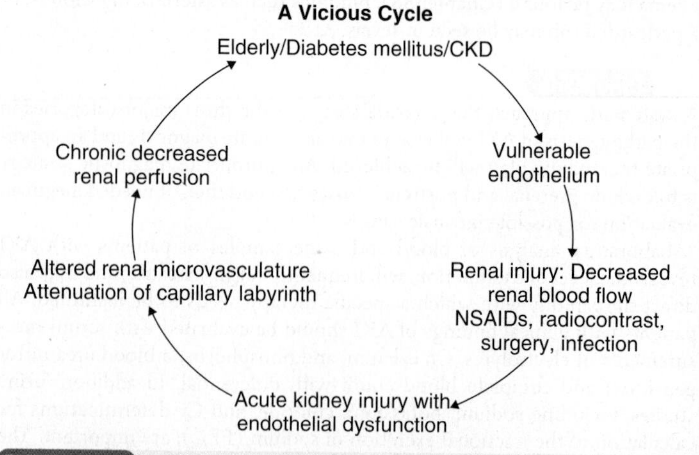

FIGURE 120-4. A vicious cycle exists between acute kidney injury (AKI) and chronic kidney disease (CKD), with CKD increasing the risk for developing AKI, and AKI accelerating progression of CKD.

the procedure).[A4,A5] *N*-Acetylcysteine is no longer recommended for this purpose.[A6]

PROGNOSIS

Typically, AKI secondary to prerenal causes, if diagnosed and treated early, has the best prognosis for renal recovery. Patients with prerenal AKI commonly return to their baseline level of renal function and have a mortality rate of less than 10%. Similarly, patients with postrenal AKI also have a good prognosis for renal recovery if the outlet obstruction is promptly diagnosed and definitively treated.

In contrast, patients with intrarenal AKI have a less predictable renal outcome, and mortality in this group varies between 30 and 80%, depending on the severity of injury. Higher mortality rates occur in older patients with hospital-acquired AKI admitted to ICUs. Furthermore, mortality in patients with AKI is incremental, and seemingly modest increases in serum Cr can result in marked increases in the mortality rate. Even a rise in serum Cr of only 0.3 mg/dL results in a significantly increased mortality risk.

The clinical course after recovery from ATN is subsequent tubular regeneration with recovery of renal function. However, this outcome is less ensured in patients with preexisting kidney disease. In addition, given the frequent systemic nature of their illness, patients with ATN, glomerulonephritis, and vasculitic causes of AKI may not fully recover to their baseline renal function.[11] Recovery is often difficult to quantify using serum creatinine because muscle wasting alone results in lower creatinine values.[12] Patients who have a severe episode of AKI requiring hemodialysis may not recover their renal function and may need hemodialysis indefinitely (Chapter 131), especially if they have a preexisting history of chronic kidney disease.[13] AKI hastens progression of chronic kidney disease to end-stage kidney disease and is often the major factor that causes such progression. It is also important that a nephrologist see most patients with hospital-acquired AKI and follow them in terms of any progression, hypertension, or other abnormalities.

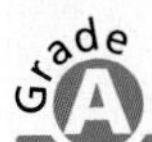

Grade A References

A1. Jamale TE, Hase NK, Kulkarni M, et al. Earlier-start versus usual-start dialysis in patients with community-acquired acute kidney injury: a randomized controlled trial. *Am J Kidney Dis.* 2013;62:1116-1121.

A2. Koc F, Ozdemir K, Altunkas F, et al. Sodium bicarbonate versus isotonic saline for the prevention of contrast-induced nephropathy in patients with diabetes mellitus undergoing coronary angiography and/or intervention: a multicenter prospective randomized study. *J Investig Med.* 2013;61:872-877.

A3. Brar SS, Aharonian V, Mansukhani P, et al. Haemodynamic-guided fluid administration for the prevention of contrast-induced acute kidney injury: the POSEIDON randomised controlled trial. *Lancet.* 2014;383:1814-1823.

A4. Han Y, Zhu G, Han L, et al. Short-term rosuvastatin therapy for prevention of contrast-induced acute kidney injury in patients with diabetes and chronic kidney disease. *J Am Coll Cardiol.* 2014;63:62-70.

A5. Leoncini M, Toso A, Maioli M, et al. Early high-dose rosuvastatin for contrast-induced nephropathy prevention in acute coronary syndrome: results from the PRATO-ACS Study (Protective Effect of Rosuvastatin and Antiplatelet Therapy On contrast-induced acute kidney injury and myocardial damage in patients with Acute Coronary Syndrome). *J Am Coll Cardiol.* 2014;63:71-79.

A6. Acetylcysteine for prevention of renal outcomes in patients undergoing coronary and peripheral vascular angiography: main results from the randomized Acetylcysteine for Contrast-Induced Nephropathy Trial (ACT). *Circulation.* 2011;124:1250-1259.

GENERAL REFERENCES

For the General References and other additional features, please visit Expert Consult at https://expertconsult.inkling.com.

121

GLOMERULAR DISORDERS AND NEPHROTIC SYNDROMES

GERALD B. APPEL AND JAI RADHAKRISHNAN

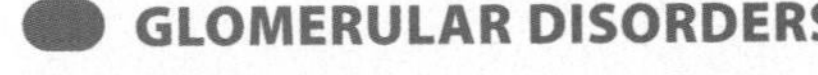

GLOMERULAR DISORDERS

DEFINITION

Each *glomerulus,* the basic filtering unit of the kidney, consists of a tuft of anastomosing capillaries formed by the branching of the afferent arteriole. Approximately 1 million glomeruli comprise approximately 5% of the kidney weight and provide almost 2 m^2 of glomerular capillary filtering surface. The glomerular basement membrane (GBM) provides both a size- and charge-selective barrier to the passage of circulating macromolecules. Renal pathologic processes involving all glomeruli are called *diffuse* or *generalized;* if only some glomeruli are involved, the process is called *focal.* When dealing with the individual glomerulus, a process is *global* if the whole glomerular tuft is involved and *segmental* if only part of the glomerulus is involved. The modifying terms *proliferative, sclerosing,* and *necrotizing* are often used (e.g., focal and segmental glomerulosclerosis; diffuse global proliferative lupus nephritis). Extracapillary proliferation or crescent formation is caused by the accumulations of macrophages, fibroblasts, proliferating epithelial cells, and fibrin within Bowman space. In general, crescent formation in any form of glomerular damage conveys a serious prognosis. Scarring of the tissue between the tubules and glomeruli, interstitial fibrosis, is also a poor prognostic sign in every glomerular disease.

EPIDEMIOLOGY

At present, more than 10% of the U.S. population may have proteinuria or renal dysfunction, often caused by glomerular diseases. More than 500,000 Americans are in end-stage renal disease (ESRD) programs, which cost approximately $33 billion per year and account for approximately 28% of all Medicare spending, largely as a result of renal involvement by glomerular diseases. Diabetic renal damage alone affects many millions of persons and is the major cause of ESRD in the United States (Chapter 124). Glomerular diseases associated with infectious agents such as malaria (Chapter 345), schistosomiasis (Chapter 355), human immunodeficiency virus (HIV) and the hepatitis B and C viruses (Chapter 149) are major worldwide health problems. Manifestations of glomerular injury range from asymptomatic microhematuria and albuminuria to rapidly progressive oliguric renal failure. Some patients develop massive fluid retention and edema at onset of their glomerular disease, whereas others present with only the slow insidious signs and symptoms of chronic renal failure (Chapter 130).

PATHOBIOLOGY

Common mechanisms, such as breaks in the glomerular capillary wall leading to hematuria and loss of the selective barrier to particles based on size and charge associated with proteinuria, are characteristic of glomerular diseases. Nevertheless, the nature of the initiating processes varies among different glomerular diseases. In some, such as diabetes and amyloidosis, structural and biochemical alterations are clearly present in the glomerular capillary wall. In others, immune-mediated renal injury is caused by deposition of circulating immune complexes, in situ formation of immune complexes, or the localized effects of anti–glomerular basement membrane (anti-GBM) antibodies. In still other diseases, genetic or acquired defects in the glomerular podocytes are associated with proteinuria and progressive renal dysfunction.

CLINICAL MANIFESTATIONS

Findings indicative of a glomerular origin of renal disease include erythrocyte casts and dysmorphic red blood cells (RBCs) in the urinary sediment, as well as large amounts of albuminuria. Persistent urinary excretion of more than 500 to 1000 erythrocytes per milliliter (or more than 5 RBCs per high-power field on microscopy) is abnormal. Dysmorphic RBCs, which are deformed as a result of their passage through the glomerular capillary wall and tubules, as well as RBC casts, which are formed when these erythrocytes become enmeshed in a proteinaceous matrix in the lumen of the tubules, are also indicative of glomerular disease.

In a normal person, the urinary excretion of albumin is less than 30 mg/day and the total urinary excretion of protein is less than 150 mg/day. Although increases in urinary protein excretion may come from the filtration of abnormal circulating proteins (e.g., light chains in multiple myeloma) or from the deficient proximal tubular reabsorption of normal, filtered low-molecular-weight proteins (e.g., β_2-microglobulin), the most common cause of proteinuria, and specifically albuminuria, is glomerular injury. Proteinuria associated with glomerular disease may range from several hundred milligrams to more than 30 g daily. In some diseases, such as minimal change nephrotic syndrome, albumin is the predominant protein in the urine. In others, such as focal sclerosing glomerulonephritis and diabetes, the proteinuria, although still largely composed of albumin, is nonselective and contains many higher-molecular-weight proteins.

DIAGNOSIS

Some patients have asymptomatic microhematuria or proteinuria discovered by routine evaluations. Microscopic hematuria associated with deformed RBCs or RBC casts is likely to be glomerular in origin. Subnephrotic levels of proteinuria may arise from orthostatic proteinuria, exercise, hypertension, tubular disease, or glomerular damage.

In patients with asymptomatic urinary abnormalities of glomerular origin, the underlying renal lesion may represent the early phase of a progressive glomerular disease or may be due to a benign, nonprogressive glomerular lesion. In general, if patients have less than 1 g of proteinuria daily or only glomerular microhematuria but a normal glomerular filtration rate (GFR) and no evidence of systemic disease, it is not necessary to proceed to a diagnostic renal biopsy. Most of these patients need no immunosuppressive therapy. The patient can be followed closely, and biopsy need be performed only in patients with progressively increasing proteinuria or evidence of a decreasing GFR.

THE NEPHROTIC SYNDROME

DEFINITION

The nephrotic syndrome (Table 121-1) is defined by albuminuria of more than 3 to 3.5 g/day accompanied by hypoalbuminemia, edema, and hyperlipidemia. In practice, many clinicians refer to "nephrotic range" proteinuria regardless of whether patients have the other manifestations of the full syndrome, because these are a consequence of the proteinuria.

EPIDEMIOLOGY

The nephrotic syndrome may be primary and idiopathic (Table 121-2), or it may be caused by a known underlying condition, such as diabetes, amyloidosis, or systemic lupus erythematosus (Table 121-3). Although minimal change disease is the most common cause of nephrotic syndrome in children, idiopathic membranous nephropathy and focal segmental glomerular sclerosis are the most common causes in adults, with the former being most common in whites and the latter in blacks.

PATHOBIOLOGY

Hypoalbuminemia, which is largely a consequence of urinary protein loss, also may be due to proximal tubular catabolism of filtered albumin, the redistribution of albumin within the body, and reduced hepatic synthesis of albumin. As a result, the relationship among urinary protein loss, the level of the serum albumin, and other secondary consequences of heavy albuminuria is inexact.

The salt and volume retention in the nephrotic syndrome may occur through at least two different major mechanisms. The classic teaching is that hypoalbuminemia reduces the oncotic pressure of plasma, the resulting intravascular volume depletion leads to activation of the renin-angiotensin-aldosterone axis, and this activation increases the retention of renal sodium and fluid. However, primary salt retention in the distal nephron also may occur independently of the renin-angiotensin-aldosterone axis.

Venous thrombosis often occurs in patients with the nephrotic syndrome. Explanations include urinary loss of antithrombin III, protein C, and protein S, which prevent thrombosis, as well as increased synthesis of acute phase reactants that promote thrombosis.

CLINICAL MANIFESTATIONS

Patients may present with weight gain, peripheral edema, and periorbital edema. Hypertension is common, and varying degrees of hematuria may be present. A 24-hour urine sample usually shows more than 3 to 3.5 g of proteinuria. Nephrotic patients often have a hypercoagulable state and are predisposed to deep vein thrombosis (Chapter 81), pulmonary emboli (Chapter 98), and renal vein thrombosis (Chapter 125). Patients with nephrotic syndrome have increased risk for atherosclerotic complications. Most nephrotic patients have elevated levels of total and low-density lipoprotein (LDL)

TABLE 121-1 TYPICAL FINDINGS OF NEPHROTIC SYNDROME VERSUS NEPHRITIS

NEPHROTIC SYNDROME	NEPHRITIS
RENAL INSUFFICIENCY	
Uncommon at presentation	Common at presentation
PROTEINURIA	
Typically high (>3 g/day)	Variable
Urine RBCs	
Few	Prominent
Urine RBC CASTS	
Unlikely	Likely

RBCs = red blood cells.

TABLE 121-2 CAUSES OF IDIOPATHIC NEPHROTIC SYNDROME IN ADULTS

CAUSE	INCIDENCE (%)
Minimal change disease	5-10
Focal segmental glomerulosclerosis	20-25
Membranous nephropathy	25-30
Membranoproliferative glomerulonephritis	5
Other proliferative and sclerosing glomerulonephritides	15-30

TABLE 121-3 NEPHROTIC SYNDROME ASSOCIATED WITH SPECIFIC CAUSES (SECONDARY NEPHROTIC SYNDROME)

SYSTEMIC DISEASES
Diabetes mellitus
Systemic lupus erythematosus and other collagen vascular diseases
Amyloidosis (amyloid AL- or AA-associated)
Vasculitic-immunologic disease (mixed cryoglobulinemia, granulomatous polyangiitis, microscopic polyangiitis, rapidly progressive glomerulonephritis, Henoch-Schönlein purpura, anti-GBM disease)
INFECTIONS
Bacterial (post-streptococcal, congenital and secondary syphilis, subacute bacterial endocarditis, cerebral ventriculoatrial shunt nephritis)
Viral (hepatitis B, hepatitis C, HIV infection, infectious mononucleosis, cytomegalovirus infection)
Parasitic (malaria, toxoplasmosis, schistosomiasis, filariasis)
MEDICATION RELATED
Gold, mercury, and the heavy metals
Penicillamine
Nonsteroidal anti-inflammatory drugs, including COX2 inhibitors
Lithium
Paramethadione, trimethadione
Captopril
"Street" heroin
Others: Probenecid, chlorpropamide, rifampin, tolbutamide, phenindione, pamidronate
ALLERGENS, VENOMS, AND IMMUNIZATIONS
NEOPLASMS
Hodgkin lymphoma and leukemias/lymphomas (with minimal change lesion)
Solid tumors (with membranous nephropathy)
HEREDITARY AND METABOLIC DISEASES
Alport syndrome
Fabry disease
Sickle cell disease
Congenital (Finnish type) nephrotic syndrome
Familial nephrotic syndrome
Nail-patella syndrome
Partial lipodystrophy
OTHER
Pregnancy related (includes preeclampsia)
Transplant rejection
Serum sickness
Accelerated hypertensive nephrosclerosis
Unilateral renal artery stenosis
Massive obesity–sleep apnea
Reflux nephropathy

COX = cyclooxygenase; GBM = glomerular basement membrane; HIV = human immunodeficiency virus.

TABLE 121-4 SERUM COMPLEMENT LEVELS IN GLOMERULAR DISEASES

DISEASES WITH A REDUCED COMPLEMENT LEVEL
Post-streptococcal glomerulonephritis
Subacute bacterial endocarditis, visceral abscess, shunt nephritis
Systemic lupus erythematosus
Cryoglobulinemia
Idiopathic membranoproliferative glomerulonephritis
DISEASES ASSOCIATED WITH A NORMAL SERUM COMPLEMENT
Minimal change nephrotic syndrome
Focal segmental glomerulosclerosis
Membranous nephropathy
Immunoglobulin A nephropathy
Henoch-Schönlein purpura
Anti–glomerular basement disease
Pauci-immune rapidly progressive glomerulonephritis (e.g., granulomatous polyangiitis and microscopic polyangiitis)

cholesterol with low or normal high-density lipoprotein (HDL) cholesterol. Lipoprotein(a) levels are elevated as well and normalize with remission of the nephrotic syndrome.

DIAGNOSIS

Initial evaluation of the nephrotic patient includes laboratory tests to define whether the patient has primary, idiopathic nephrotic syndrome (see Table 121-2) or a secondary cause related to a systemic disease, toxin, or medication (see Table 121-3).[1] Common screening tests include the fasting blood sugar and glycosylated hemoglobin tests for diabetes, an antinuclear antibody test for collagen vascular disease, and a serum complement level, which screens for many immune complex–mediated diseases (Table 121-4). In selected patients, cryoglobulins, hepatitis B and C serologies, HIV testing, antineutrophil cytoplasmic antibodies (ANCAs), anti-GMB antibodies, serum protein and immunoelectrophoresis, and other tests may be useful.

After exclusion of secondary causes, a renal biopsy is often required in the adult nephrotic patient. Biopsy results in patients with heavy proteinuria and the nephrotic syndrome are likely to provide a specific diagnosis, determine prognosis, and guide therapy.

TREATMENT Rx

Treatment varies by the specific cause.[2] Elevated lipid levels should be treated (Chapter 206). Anticoagulation is not recommended routinely but is needed if any thrombotic complications occur. It is commonly recommended in patients with additional risk factors for thrombosis (e.g., a prior idiopathic thromboembolic event, immobilization, severe heart failure, or morbid obesity), and may be considered in patients who have membranous nephropathy and are at low risk for bleeding. Edema is treated with a low-salt diet and diuretics. The combination of a loop diuretic plus albumin may be more effective than a loop diuretic alone for some patients who have refractory edema and evidence of intravascular volume depletion.[A1] In childhood-onset relapsing or steroid-dependent nephrotic syndrome, rituximab (375 mg/m² once weekly for 4 weeks) can provide a median relapse-free interval of about 9 months.[A2]

Idiopathic Nephrotic Syndrome

MINIMAL CHANGE DISEASE

Minimal change disease, which is the most common pattern of nephrotic syndrome in children, accounts for only approximately 5 to 10% of cases of idiopathic nephrotic syndrome in adults. A similar histologic pattern may be seen as an adverse reaction to certain medications (nonsteroidal anti-inflammatory drugs [NSAIDs], lithium) or in association with certain tumors (e.g., Hodgkin disease).

CLINICAL MANIFESTATIONS

Patients typically present with weight gain and periorbital and peripheral edema related to the proteinuria. Proteinuria in adult patients can average as much as 10 g/day, and subnephrotic levels are rare. Approximately 30% of adults are hypertensive and 30% have microscopic hematuria. However, an active urinary sediment with RBC casts is not typical of this disease. Many

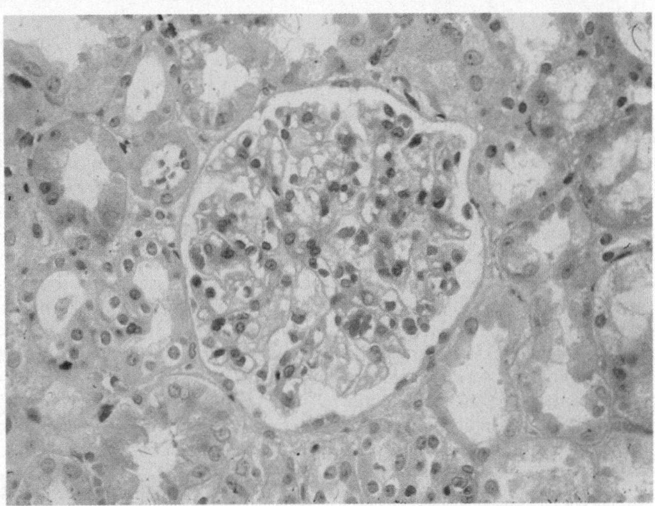

FIGURE 121-1. Unremarkable light microscopic appearance of minimal change disease glomerulopathy. Glomerular basement membranes are thin, and there is no glomerular hypercellularity.

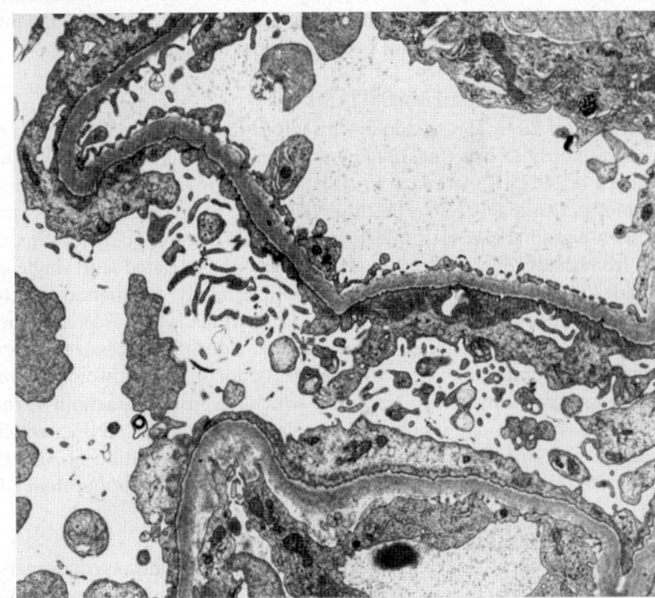

FIGURE 121-2. Minimal change disease. Electron micrograph shows widespread effacement of foot processes with microvillous transformation of the visceral epithelium. No electron-dense deposits are present (uranyl acetate, lead citrate stain; 6000×).

adult patients have mild-to-moderate azotemia, which may be related to hypoalbuminemia and intravascular volume depletion. Complement levels and serologic test results are normal.

DIAGNOSIS

In true minimal change disease, histopathology typically reveals no glomerular abnormalities on light microscopy (Fig. 121-1). The tubules may show lipid droplet accumulation from absorbed lipoproteins (hence the older term *lipoid nephrosis*). Immunofluorescence staining and electron microscopy (Fig. 121-2) show no immune-type deposits. By electron microscopy, the GBM is normal and effacement or "fusion" of the visceral epithelial foot processes is noted along virtually the entire distribution of every capillary loop.

TREATMENT Rx

The course of minimal change nephrotic syndrome is often one of remissions followed by relapses, which are typically responsive to corticosteroids.[3] When treated with corticosteroids for 8 weeks, 85 to 95% of children experience a remission of proteinuria. In adults, the response rate is somewhat lower, with 75 to 85% of patients responding to regimens of daily prednisone (1 mg/

kg, maximum 80 mg) or alternate-day therapy (2 mg/kg, maximum 120 mg), tapered after 2 months of treatment for a total of 5 to 6 months of therapy. The time to clinical response is slower in adults, and they are not considered steroid resistant until they have failed to respond to 16 weeks of treatment. Tapering of the steroid dose after remission should be gradual over 1 to 2 months. Approximately 40% of adults relapse by 1 year. Most clinicians treat the first relapse similarly to the initial episode. Patients who relapse a third time or who become corticosteroid dependent (unable to decrease the prednisone dose without proteinuria recurring) may be treated with a 2- to 3-month course of the alkylating agent cyclophosphamide at a dose of up to 2 mg/kg/day. Up to 50% of patients will have a remission of at least 5 years, but the response rate is lower in corticosteroid-dependent patients. Other alternative treatments for patients who frequently relapse or are steroid dependent include rituximab (375 mg/m^2 weekly for 4 weeks), low-dose cyclosporine (3 to 5 mg/kg/day for 4 months), tacrolimus (0.05 to 0.1 mg/kg/day), and mycophenolate mofetil (750 to 1000 mg twice daily). All provide approximately equivalent remission and relapse rates, but cyclosporine and tacrolimus are potentially nephrotoxic, so their trough blood levels must be monitored.

PROGNOSIS

The prognosis of minimal change disease is excellent, and most patients who have a decline in kidney function actually have focal segmental glomerulosclerosis on a subsequent kidney biopsy. However, more than 50% of patients have relapses and 10 to 20% may become steroid dependent.

FOCAL SEGMENTAL GLOMERULOSCLEROSIS

Approximately 20 to 25% of adults with idiopathic nephrotic syndrome are found on biopsy to have focal segmental glomerulosclerosis (FSGS).[4] The incidence of FSGS is increasing in all races, but it is especially common in African Americans. FSGS may be either idiopathic or secondary (e.g., associated with heroin abuse, HIV infection, sickle cell disease, obesity, reflux of urine from the bladder to the kidneys, and lesions associated with single or remnant kidneys). FSGS can occur in multiple family members owing to genetic defects in components of the podocyte, which is the visceral epithelial cell. The most common defects include an autosomal recessive pattern caused by mutations in the structural protein podocin; and autosomal dominant forms, caused by mutations in the structural protein α-actinin 4, the TRPC6 glomerular slit diaphragm-associated channel, or INF2, which encodes a formin (actin-regulating protein). The predisposition of African Americans to FSGS is partly related to alleles of the gene apolipoprotein L1.

CLINICAL MANIFESTATIONS

Patients with idiopathic FSGS typically present with either asymptomatic proteinuria or edema. Although two thirds are fully nephrotic at presentation, proteinuria may vary from less than 1 to more than 30 g/day. Hypertension is found in 30 to 50% of patients, and microscopic hematuria occurs in approximately half of patients. The GFR is decreased at presentation in 20 to 30% of patients. Complement levels and other serologic test results are normal.

DIAGNOSIS

By light microscopy, only some glomeruli initially have areas of segmental scarring (Fig. 121-3). As renal function declines, repeat biopsy specimens show more glomeruli with segmental sclerosing lesions and increased numbers of globally sclerotic glomeruli. By immunofluorescence staining, immunoglobulin M (IgM) and C3 commonly are trapped in the areas of glomerular sclerosis. Electron microscopy, however, shows no immune-type deposits and only visceral epithelial cell foot process effacement. The histopathologic variants of FSGS are associated with epidemiologic, clinical, and prognostic differences. For example, the "tip lesion" variant has a relatively benign course, whereas the "collapsing variant" progresses more rapidly to renal failure.

TREATMENT

Rx

For primary (idiopathic) FSGS, corticosteroids are used as initial therapy (e.g., prednisone, 1 mg/kg/day, maximum 80 mg, or 2 mg/kg every other day, maximum 120 mg, as tolerated) for a minimum of 3 to 4 months and slowly tapered over the next 3 to 6 months if remission is achieved. A complete or partial remission may be seen in up to 40 to 60% of patients, with preservation of long-term renal function. In patients who relapse after initial therapy or who are steroid resistant, cyclosporine (5 to 6 mg/kg/day) appears to be as good as the combination of pulse dexamethasone (0.9 mg/kg per dose [maximum 40 mg] daily on 2 consecutive days weekly for the first 8 weeks, every other week for weeks 8 to 26, then every 4 weeks until week 50) plus mycophenolate mofetil (25 to 36 mg/kg/day, maximum 2 g/day).[A3] Tacrolimus (0.05 to 0.1 mg/kg/day) is as good as cyclophosphamide.[A4] As a result, either cyclosporine or tacrolimus is recommended for 12 to 24 months in steroid-resistant patients who respond, with slow tapering thereafter. With these calcineurin inhibitors, careful monitoring of renal function and serum levels are necessary to avoid nephrotoxicity. Abatacept, a cytotoxic T lymphocyte–associated antigen 4-immunoglobulin fusion protein, has been used in small numbers of resistant patients.

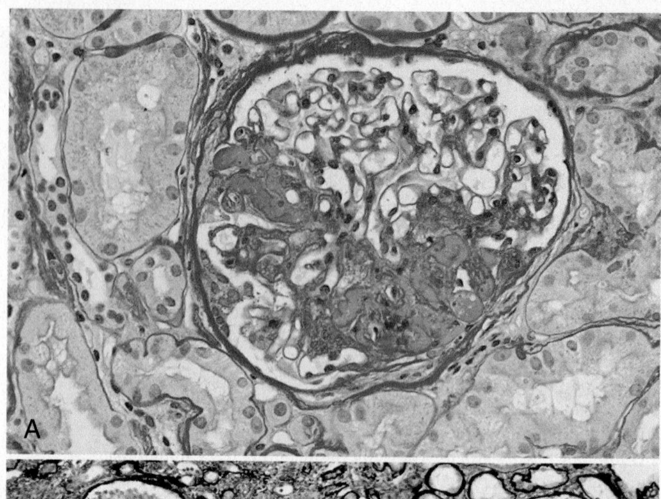

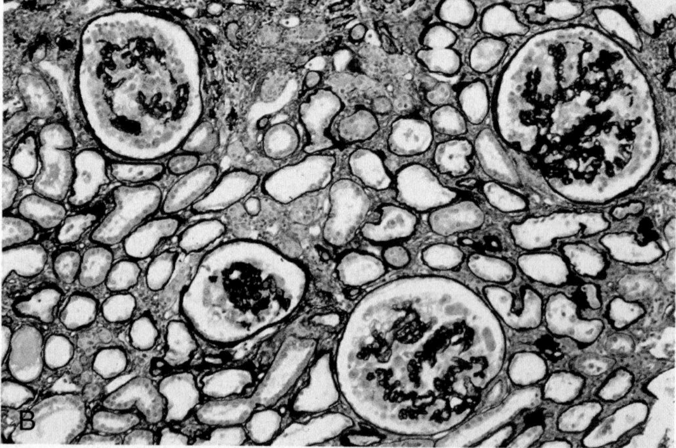

FIGURE 121-3. Focal segmental glomerulosclerosis. A, Light micrograph of classic focal segmental glomerulosclerosis. B, Silver stain of collapsing focal segmental glomerulosclerosis showing collapse of the glomerular tufts.

PROGNOSIS

The course of untreated FSGS is usually one of progressive proteinuria and declining GFR. Only a minority of patients experiences a spontaneous remission of proteinuria, and most untreated patients who do not remit eventually develop ESRD within 5 to 20 years. Patients with a sustained remission of their nephrotic syndrome are unlikely to progress to ESRD.

Most patients with genetic forms of FSGS are steroid resistant, have a progressive course, and do not experience recurrences of the FSGS if they receive a renal transplant. Overall, however, FSGS recurs in the transplanted kidney in up to 30% of cases, often in association with elevated levels of a circulating permeability factor. Younger patients, those with a rapid course to renal failure, and those with a prior recurrence are more likely to have allograft recurrence.

MEMBRANOUS NEPHROPATHY

Membranous nephropathy is the most common pattern of idiopathic nephrotic syndrome in white patients. It also may be associated with infections (syphilis [Chapter 319] and hepatitis B and C [Chapter 149]), systemic

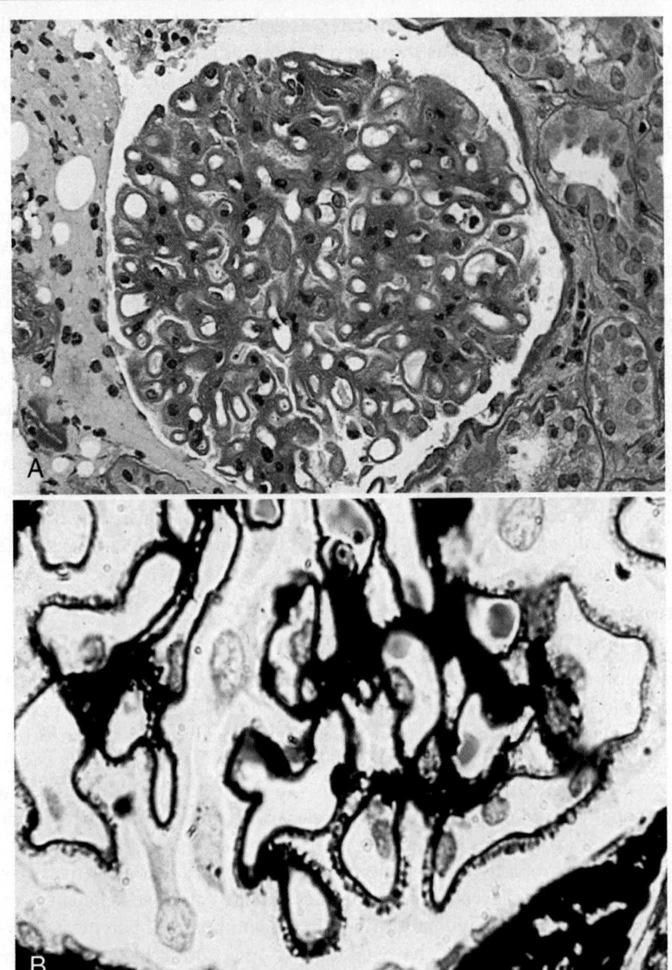

FIGURE 121-4. **Membranous nephropathy. A, Light micrograph of membranous nephropathy demonstrating thickening of the glomerular capillary wall but no hypercellularity. B, Silver stain of idiopathic membranous nephropathy showing spike formation along the outer aspect of the glomerular basement membrane corresponding to projections of the basement membrane between the epimembranous deposits.**

lupus erythematosus (SLE; Chapter 266), medications (gold salts, NSAIDs), and certain tumors (solid tumors and lymphomas). In most patients with idiopathic membranous nephropathy, the antigen in the immune deposits is the M-type phospholipase A_2 receptor, which is present in podocytes. Circulating antibodies combine with this antigen to form in-situ immune complexes on the epithelial side of the basement membrane, thereby leading to proteinuria.

CLINICAL MANIFESTATIONS

Membranous nephropathy typically manifests with proteinuria and edema. Hypertension and microhematuria are not infrequent, but renal function and GFR are usually preserved at presentation. Despite the finding of complement in the glomerular immune deposits, serum complement levels are normal. Membranous nephropathy is the most common pattern of the nephrotic syndrome to be associated with a hypercoagulable state and renal vein thrombosis (Chapter 125). The presence of sudden flank pain, deterioration of renal function, or symptoms of pulmonary disease in a patient with membranous nephropathy should prompt an investigation for renal vein thrombosis and pulmonary emboli.

DIAGNOSIS

On light microscopy, the glomerular capillary loops often appear rigid or thickened (Fig. 121-4), but there is no cellular proliferation. Immunofluorescence staining and electron microscopy show subepithelial immune dense deposits all along the glomerular capillary loops (Fig. 121-5). The presence of circulating antibodies to the M-type phospholipase A_2 receptor are highly sensitive and specific for idiopathic membranous nephropathy.

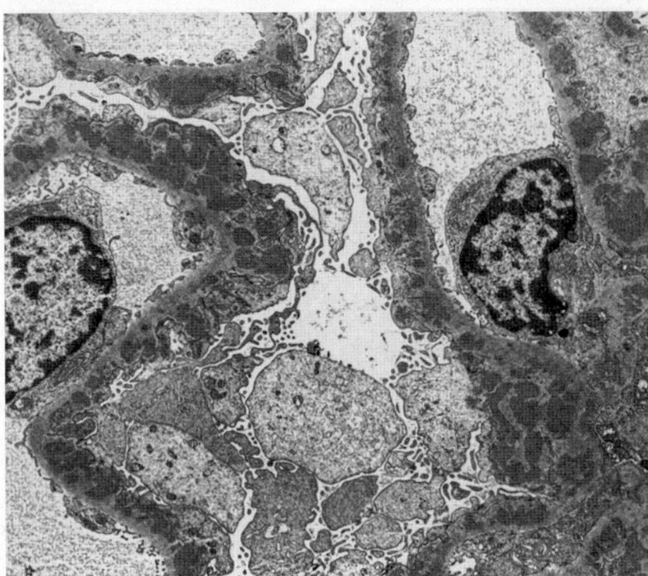

FIGURE 121-5. **Membranous glomerulopathy. On ultrastructural examination, there are numerous, closely apposed epimembranous electron-dense deposits separated by basement membrane spikes (uranyl acetate, lead citrate stain; 2500×).**

TREATMENT

Rx

Most studies using corticosteroids alone to treat membranous nephropathy have not shown significant benefit in terms of remission of the nephrotic syndrome or preservation of renal function. By comparison, the combination of corticosteroid therapy (methylprednisolone, 1 g intravenously (IV) daily for 3 days, then prednisone, 0.5 mg/kg/day orally (PO) for 27 days, in months 1, 3, and 5) plus oral cytotoxic therapy (cyclophosphamide, 2 to 2.5 mg/kg/day, for 30 days in months 2, 4, and 6) given in alternating months over 6 months results in more remissions and better preservation of renal function compared with symptomatic therapy.[A5] The combination of cyclosporine (3.5 mg/kg/day adjusted to serum levels of 125 to 225 μg/L) plus prednisone (0.15 mg/kg/day up to a maximum of 15 mg/day) for 6 months also is more likely to induce remission of nephrotic syndrome compared with placebo or prednisone alone. Success with tacrolimus has been similar to that with cyclosporine. Other agents used successfully in uncontrolled or small controlled trials in membranous nephropathy include mycophenolate mofetil, adrenocorticotropic hormone, and the monoclonal anti-CD20 antibody, rituximab. In one report, two thirds of 100 consecutive patients treated with rituximab (375 mg/m^2 weekly or subsequent doses based on CD20 count recovery > 5/μL) achieved complete or partial remission, with a median time to remission of 7.1 months. Patients with membranous nephropathy are at increased risk for developing renal vein thrombosis, especially when their serum albumin levels decline. A risk benefit approach to this problem is recommended; however, no clear guidelines exist on when to start anticoagulation.[5]

PROGNOSIS

In most large series, renal survival is more than 75% at 10 years,[6] with a spontaneous remission rate of 20 to 30%. In general, older patients, males, and those with heavy persistent proteinuria are most likely to progress to renal failure and hence to benefit from therapy.

MEMBRANOPROLIFERATIVE GLOMERULONEPHRITIS

Idiopathic membranoproliferative glomerulonephritis was formerly divided into three types (type I, II, and II) based on the location of electron dense deposits. Now, however, the classification is based on immunofluorescence findings into immunoglobulin-mediated and complement-mediated membranoproliferative glomerulonephritis. Immunoglobulin-mediated membranoproliferative glomerulonephritis is associated with immune complex diseases, including systemic lupus erythematosus (Chapter 266), infections such as hepatitis C (Chapter 149), and monoclonal gammopathy (Chapter 187).[7] Complement-mediated membranoproliferative glomerulonephritis includes dense deposit disease and C3 glomerulonephritis. All these stimuli have been proposed to incite the glomerular mesangial cells to grow out along the capillary wall and split the GBM.[8]

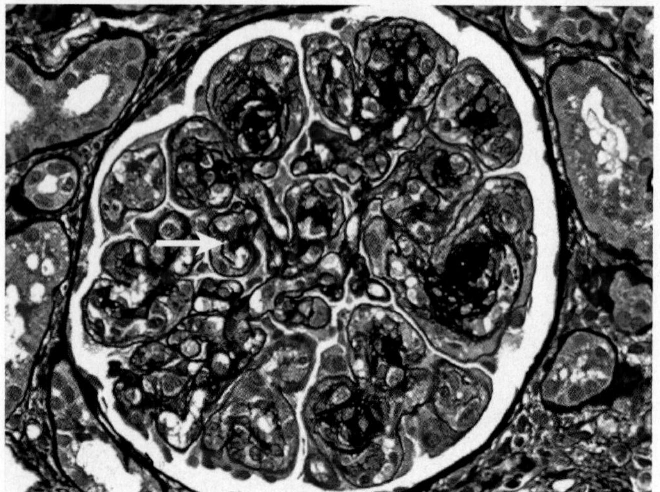

FIGURE 121-6. Membranoproliferative glomerulonephritis with lobulation of the glomerular tuft and splitting of the basement membrane as seen by silver stain.

The entity formerly called type II membranoproliferative glomerulonephritis, or dense deposit disease, and the associated C3 glomerulonephritis are rare glomerular diseases associated with uncontrolled systemic activation of the alternative complement pathway. Many patients have C3 nephritic factor, an autoantibody directed against the C3 convertase of the alternate complement pathway, whereas others have deficiencies of factor H or I or other inhibitors of the alternate complement cascade. Dense deposit disease may be associated with partial lipodystrophy. Patients with alternate complement pathway activation also may have a proliferative glomerulonephritis with electron-dense deposits dissimilar to dense deposit disease. These patients have C3 glomerulonephritis. Indeed, some of the patients originally classified as having membranoproliferative glomerulonephritis type I are found to have a pathogenesis closer to those of dense deposit disease and C3 glomerulonephritis.

CLINICAL MANIFESTATIONS AND DIAGNOSIS

Most patients with idiopathic membranoproliferative glomerulonephritis are children or young adults who present with proteinuria or the nephrotic syndrome. A low serum complement level is found intermittently in immunoglobulin-associated membranoproliferative glomerulonephritis, whereas the C3 level is usually reduced in dense deposit disease. The diagnosis of dense deposit disease requires a renal biopsy that shows complement C3 in a characteristic ribbon-like pattern around the capillary loops (Fig. 121-6).

TREATMENT AND PROGNOSIS Rx

Attempts to treat idiopathic membranoproliferative glomerulonephritis have included corticosteroids, other immunosuppressive medications, anticoagulants, and antiplatelet agents. No therapy has been proved effective in a randomized trial in adults, but corticosteroids have had some success in children. Dense deposit disease and C3 glomerulonephritis have recently been treated with eculizumab, a blocker of the complement system, with variable efficacy. Some may also respond to immunosuppressive therapies.

ACUTE GLOMERULONEPHRITIS AND THE NEPHRITIC SYNDROME

EPIDEMIOLOGY AND PATHOBIOLOGY

Known inciting causes of acute glomerulonephritis include infectious agents, such as type 12 and type 49 "nephritogenic" strains of group A streptococci and endocarditis caused by *Staphylococcus aureus* and *Streptococcus viridans*. Acute glomerulonephritis can also be caused by the deposition of immune complexes in autoimmune diseases such as SLE (Chapter 266) and the damaging effect of circulating antibodies directed against the GBM, as in Goodpasture syndrome.

Invading neutrophils and monocytes, as well as resident glomerular cells, can damage the glomerulus through a number of mediators, including oxidants, chemoattractant agents, proteases, cytokines, and growth factors. Some factors, such as transforming growth factor-β, have been related to eventual glomerulosclerosis and chronic glomerular damage.

CLINICAL MANIFESTATIONS AND DIAGNOSIS

Patients with acute glomerulonephritis often present with a nephritic picture characterized by a decreased GFR, azotemia, oliguria, hypertension, and an active urinary sediment (see Table 121-1). Hypertension is common and is caused by intravascular volume expansion, although renin levels may not be appropriately suppressed for the degree of volume expansion. Patients may note dark, smoky, or cola-colored urine in association with an active urinary sediment, which is composed of erythrocytes, leukocytes, and a variety of casts, including RBC casts. Although many patients with acute glomerulonephritis have proteinuria, sometimes even in the nephrotic range, most have lesser degrees of albuminuria, especially when the GFR is markedly reduced. Regardless of the inciting cause, acute glomerulonephritis is characterized on light microscopy by hypercellularity of the glomerulus, which may be composed of infiltrating inflammatory cells, proliferation of resident glomerular cells, or both.

Immunoglobulin A Nephropathy

EPIDEMIOLOGY AND PATHOBIOLOGY

IgA nephropathy, the most frequent form of idiopathic glomerulonephritis worldwide, represents 15 to 40% of primary glomerulonephritides in parts of Europe and Asia.[9] In geographic areas where renal biopsies are performed for milder urinary findings, a higher incidence of IgA is noted. In the United States, some centers report this diagnosis in up to 20% of all primary glomerulopathies. Males outnumber females, with peak occurrence in the second to third decades of life.

In IgA nephropathy, most patients and their direct blood relatives have elevated circulating levels of IgA molecules that are galactose deficient at the hinge region. The predominant form of IgA is composed of polymeric IgA1. Patients, but not relatives, have circulating IgG and IgA autoantibodies against this galactose-deficient IgA. It is thought that a second "hit" phenomenon (e.g., infection, oxidative stress, etc.) stimulates production of these antibodies, and then the resulting immune complexes deposit in the glomeruli, thereby leading to an inflammatory reaction and consequent glomerulosclerosis and interstitial fibrosis.

CLINICAL MANIFESTATIONS AND DIAGNOSIS

IgA nephropathy often presents either as asymptomatic microscopic hematuria with or without proteinuria (the most common presentation in adults) or as episodic gross hematuria after an upper respiratory tract infection or exercise (the most common presentation in children and young adults).[10] Approximately 20 to 50% of all patients have hypertension. Increased serum IgA levels, noted in one third to half of cases, do not correlate with the course of the disease. Serum complement levels are normal. The diagnosis of IgA nephropathy is established by finding glomerular IgA deposits as either the dominant or the codominant immunoglobulin on immunofluorescence microscopy (Fig. 121-7). Deposits of C3 and IgG also are often found. Light microscopy varies from the most common pattern of mild mesangial proliferation to severe crescentic glomerulonephritis. By electron microscopy, immune-type dense deposits are typically found in the mesangial and paramesangial areas.

TREATMENT Rx

The pathogenesis of IgA nephropathy may involve abnormal antigenic stimulation of mucosal IgA production and subsequent immune complex deposition in the glomeruli. Efforts to treat the disease by preventing antigenic stimulation, including broad-spectrum antibiotics (e.g., doxycycline), tonsillectomy, and dietary manipulations (e.g., gluten elimination), generally have been controversial or unsuccessful. Trials using fish oils to decrease proteinuria and slow progressive disease have given conflicting results. Controlled trials support the use of angiotensin-converting enzyme (ACE) inhibitors and angiotensin receptor blockers (ARBs) (see Table 67-7, in Chapter 67) to decrease proteinuria and protect renal function.[A6] Randomized trials suggest that a 6-month course of glucocorticoids (e.g., 6 months of oral prednisone, starting with 0.8 to 1 mg/kg/day for 2 months and then reduced by 0.2 mg/kg/day per month for the next 4 months) reduces both proteinuria and the risk for kidney failure.[A7] ACE inhibitors or ARBs with glucocorticoid

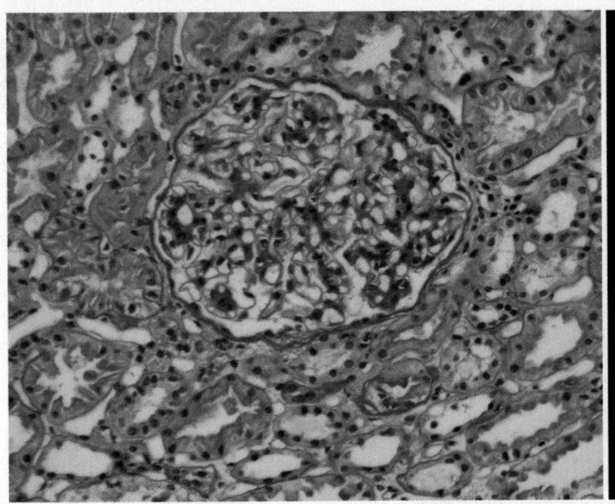

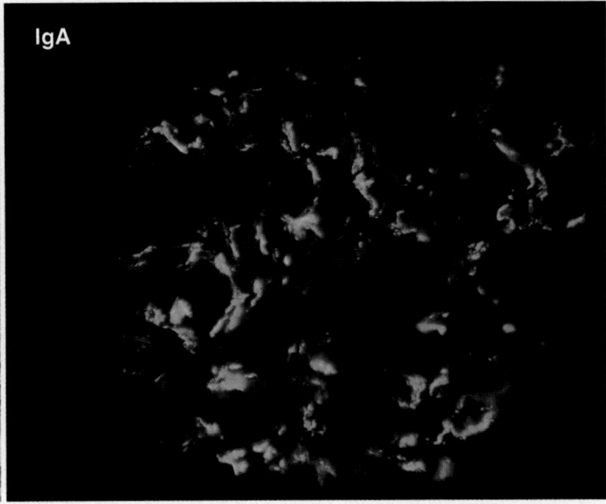

FIGURE 121-7. Immunoglobulin A (IgA) nephropathy with mesangial cell proliferation by light microscopy and IgA deposition on immunofluorescence.

therapy appear to be of incremental benefit. There are conflicting data on the benefit of immunosuppressive agents (e.g., cyclophosphamide, azathioprine, mycophenolate mofetil). For the few patients with crescentic IgA nephropathy, cytotoxic agents have been used.

PROGNOSIS

The course is variable, with some patients showing no decline in GFR over decades and others developing the nephrotic syndrome, hypertension, and renal failure. Factors predictive of a poor outcome in IgA nephropathy include hypertension, persistent proteinuria greater than 1 g/day, male gender, an elevated serum creatinine level, and the histologic features of mesangial and endothelial proliferation and sclerosis or of tubulointerstitial damage and crescent formation. Levels of galactose-deficient IgA and levels of autoantibodies against this galactose-deficient IgA correlate with renal prognosis. Renal survival rates are estimated at 80% to 85% at 10 years and 65% at 20 years. A significant percentage of transplant recipients have a morphologic recurrence in the allograft, but graft loss is uncommon.

Henoch-Schönlein Purpura

Henoch-Schönlein purpura (HSP; Chapter 270) is characterized by a small-vessel vasculitis with arthralgias, skin purpura, and abdominal symptoms, as well as a proliferative acute glomerulonephritis. HSP is predominantly a disease of childhood, although cases occur at all ages. As with IgA nephropathy, patients and their relatives have elevated levels of circulating IgA molecules that are galactose deficient. Renal biopsies are identical to those seen in IgA nephropathy. Some investigators feel IgA nephropathy and HSP are two sides of a spectrum of the same pathogenetic disease. No infectious agent or allergen has been defined as causative, and serum complement levels are normal.

CLINICAL MANIFESTATIONS AND DIAGNOSIS

The clinical manifestations of HSP (Chapter 270) include dermatologic, gastrointestinal, rheumatologic, and renal findings. Skin involvement typically starts with a macular rash that coalesces into purpuric lesions (see Fig. 270-2 in Chapter 270) on the ankles, legs, and occasionally arms and buttocks. Gastrointestinal symptoms include cramps, diarrhea, nausea, and vomiting, with melena and bloody diarrhea in the most severely involved cases. Although arthralgias of the knees, wrists, and ankles are common, true arthritis is uncommon. Symptoms of different organ system involvement may occur concurrently or separately, and recurrent episodes during the first year are not uncommon. The renal histopathology of HSP is similar to that of IgA nephropathy. Skin biopsies typically show a small-vessel leukocytoclastic angiitis with immune deposition of IgA.

TREATMENT AND PROGNOSIS Rx

Like IgA nephropathy, HSP has no proved therapy. Episodes of rash, arthralgias, and abdominal symptoms usually resolve spontaneously. Some patients with severe abdominal findings have been treated with short courses of high doses of corticosteroids. Patients with severe glomerular involvement may benefit by modalities used to treat patients with severe IgA nephropathy, that is, ACE inhibitors and ARBs, and a 6-month course of corticosteroids. Although most patients with HSP recover fully, patients with a more severe nephritic or nephrotic presentation and more severe glomerular damage on renal biopsy have an unfavorable long-term prognosis.

Post-streptococcal Glomerulonephritis

Acute post-streptococcal glomerulonephritis may occur in either an epidemic form or as sporadic cases after infection with nephritogenic strains of group A β-hemolytic streptococci (Chapter 290). Post-streptococcal glomerulonephritis is largely a disease of childhood, but severe disease in adults is well documented. The disease is most common after episodes of pharyngitis, but it can follow streptococcal infections at any site and subclinical cases greatly outnumber clinical cases. Post-streptococcal glomerulonephritis is an acute immune complex disease characterized by the formation of antibodies against streptococci with the localization of immune complexes and complement in the kidney.

CLINICAL MANIFESTATIONS AND DIAGNOSIS

Most cases manifest with hematuria, proteinuria, hypertension, and the nephritic syndrome (see Table 121-1) 10 days to several weeks after a streptococcal infection. Throat cultures and skin cultures of suspected sites of streptococcal involvement often are no longer positive for group A β-hemolytic streptococci. A variety of antibodies (e.g., antistreptolysin O [ASLO], antihyaluronidase [AHT]) and a streptozyme panel of antibodies against streptococcal antigens (which includes ASLO, AHT, antistreptokinase, and anti-DNase) often show high titers, but a change in titer over time is more indicative of a recent streptococcal infection. More than 95% of patients with post-streptococcal glomerulonephritis secondary to pharyngitis and 85% of patients with streptococcal skin infections have positive antibody titers. The serum total hemolytic complement levels and C3 levels are decreased in more than 90% of patients during the episode of acute glomerulonephritis.

In a patient with a classic acute nephritic episode after a documented streptococcal infection, with a change in streptococcal antibody titer and a depressed serum complement level, a renal biopsy adds little to the diagnosis. In other cases, a biopsy may be necessary to confirm or refute the diagnosis. On light microscopy (Fig. 121-8), glomeruli are markedly enlarged and often fill Bowman space. Glomeruli exhibit hypercellularity with infiltration of monocytes and polymorphonuclear cells and a proliferation of the glomerular cellular elements. The capillary lumens often are compressed. Some cases demonstrate extracapillary proliferation with crescents. On immunofluorescence microscopy, there is coarse granular deposition of IgG, IgM, and complement, especially C3, along the capillary wall. Electron microscopy shows large dome-shaped, electron-dense subepithelial deposits resembling the humps of a camel at isolated intervals along the GBM.

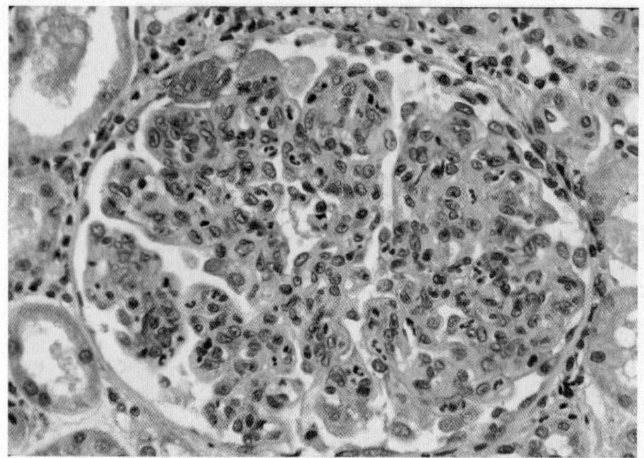

FIGURE 121-8. Post-streptococcal glomerulonephritis with hypercellular glomerulus filling Bowman space and infiltrated by polymorphonuclear and other cells.

TREATMENT AND PROGNOSIS Rx

Therapy is symptomatic and directed at controlling the hypertension and fluid retention with antihypertensive agents (see Table 67-7 in Chapter 67) and diuretics. In most patients, this is a self-limited disease, with recovery of renal function and disappearance of hypertension in several weeks. However, the presence of underlying renal disease, especially diabetic nephropathy, is associated with a worse prognosis. Proteinuria and hematuria may resolve more slowly over months.

Glomerulonephritis with Endocarditis and Visceral Abscesses

Various glomerular lesions are found in patients with acute and chronic bacterial endocarditis (Chapter 76). Although embolic phenomena can lead to glomerular ischemia and infarcts, a common finding is an immune complex glomerulonephritis. With *S. viridans* endocarditis, both focal and diffuse proliferative glomerulonephritides are common. With the increased incidence of *S. aureus* endocarditis, 40 to 80% of patients have clinical evidence of an immune complex proliferative glomerulonephritis. Glomerulonephritis is now more common with acute than subacute bacterial endocarditis.

Patients often have hematuria and urinary RBC casts, proteinuria ranging from less than 1 g/day to nephrotic levels, and progressive renal failure. Serum total complement and C3 levels are usually reduced. Renal insufficiency may be mild and reversible with appropriate antibiotic therapy, or it may be progressive and lead to dialysis and irreversible renal failure.

A proliferative immune complex glomerulonephritis also can occur in patients with deep visceral bacterial abscesses and infections, such as empyema of the lung (Chapter 99) and osteomyelitis (Chapter 272). Immune complex forms of acute glomerulonephritis also have been noted in patients with bacterial pneumonias, including *Mycoplasma* (Chapter 317), and patients with chronically infected cerebral ventriculoatrial shunts for hydrocephalus. Many of these patients have nephrotic-range proteinuria and only mild renal dysfunction. With appropriate antibiotic therapy, most patients' glomerular lesions heal, and renal function recovers.

RAPIDLY PROGRESSIVE GLOMERULONEPHRITIS

Rapidly progressive glomerulonephritis (RPGN) includes glomerular diseases that progress to renal failure in a matter of weeks to months (Table 121-5). The renal biopsy in all RPGN shows extensive extracapillary proliferation, that is, crescent formation. Patients with primary RPGN can be divided into three patterns as defined by immunologic pathogenesis: those with anti-GBM disease (e.g., Goodpasture syndrome); those with immune complex deposition (e.g., SLE, HSP, post-streptococcal); and those without immune deposits or anti-GBM antibodies (so-called pauci-immune, usually ANCA-positive RPGN).

TABLE 121-5 CLASSIFICATION OF RAPIDLY PROGRESSIVE (CRESCENTIC) GLOMERULONEPHRITIS

PRIMARY
Anti–glomerular basement membrane antibody disease, Goodpasture syndrome (with pulmonary disease)
Immune complex mediated
Pauci-immune (usually antineutrophil cytoplasmic antibody-positive)
SECONDARY
Membranoproliferative glomerulonephritis
IgA nephropathy, Henoch-Schönlein purpura
Post-streptococcal glomerulonephritis
Systemic lupus erythematosus

Anti–Glomerular Basement Membrane Disease

The disease has two peaks of occurrence: in the third decade of life predominantly in men and after 60 years of age predominantly in women. Anti-GBM disease (Table 121-6) is caused by circulating antibodies that are directed against the noncollagenous domain of the α_3 chain of type IV collagen. These antibodies damage the GBM, thereby resulting in an inflammatory response, breaks in the GBM, and the formation of a proliferative and often crescentic glomerulonephritis. If the anti-GBM antibodies cross-react with and damage the basement membrane of pulmonary capillaries, the patient develops pulmonary hemorrhage and hemoptysis, an association called *Goodpasture Syndrome.*

TABLE 121-6 COMMON RENAL DISEASES WITH ASSOCIATED PULMONARY DISEASES

DISEASE	MARKER
Goodpasture syndrome	+Anti–glomerular basement membrane antibodies
Small vessel vasculitis (granulomatous polyangiitis and microscopic polyangiitis)	+Antineutrophil cytoplasmic antibodies
Systemic lupus erythematosus	+Anti-DNA antibodies, low complement
Nephrotic syndrome, renal vein thrombosis, pulmonary embolus	+Lung scan or +CT angiography
Pneumonia with immune complex glomerulonephritis	Low complement, circulating immune complexes
Uremic lung	Elevated creatinine level

CT = computed tomography.

CLINICAL MANIFESTATIONS AND DIAGNOSIS

Patients present with a nephritic picture (see Table 121-1). Renal function may deteriorate from normal to dialysis-requiring levels in a matter of days to weeks. Patients with pulmonary involvement may have life-threatening hemoptysis with dyspnea and with diffuse alveolar infiltrates on chest radiograph. The pathology of anti-GBM disease shows a proliferative glomerulonephritis, often with severe crescentic proliferation in Bowman space. There is linear deposition of immunoglobulin (usually IgG) along the GBM by immunofluorescence (Fig. 121-9), but electron microscopy does not show electron-dense deposits.

Although the treatment of this rare disease has not been studied in large controlled trials, intensive immunosuppressive therapy with cyclophosphamide (e.g., 2 mg/kg/day as tolerated) and corticosteroids (e.g., pulse methylprednisolone, 15 to 30 mg/kg to a maximum of dose of 1000 mg IV daily for three doses, followed by prednisone, 1 mg/kg/day PO to a maximum of 60 to 80 mg/day and slowly tapered after achieving clinical remission) to reduce the production of anti-GBM antibodies, combined with daily plasmapheresis to remove circulating anti-GBM antibodies, has been successful in many patients. Rapid treatment is recommended to prevent irreversible renal damage and is necessary in patients with pulmonary hemorrhage. The optimal duration of therapy is uncertain, but daily plasmapheresis should be performed, preferably until anti-GBM antibody is undetectable, and corticosteroids and cyclophosphamide should be continued until clinical remission is achieved, typically between 3 and 6 months. Patients who already require dialysis at the time of treatment generally do not regain renal function despite aggressive therapy. Relapses of the disease are rare.

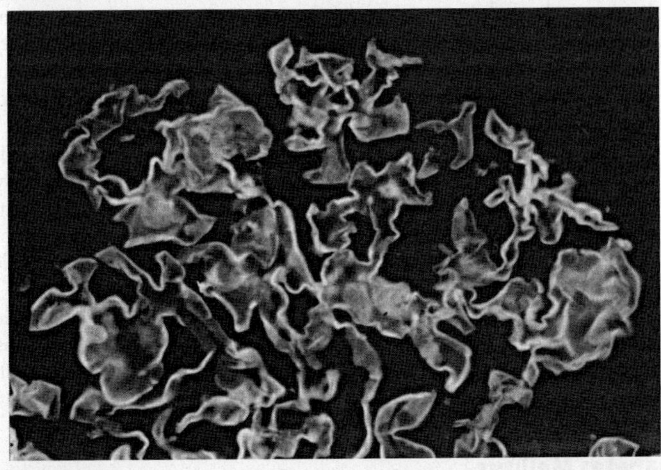

FIGURE 121-9. **Anti–glomerular basement membrane (GBM) glomerulonephritis.** An immunofluorescence micrograph of a portion of a glomerulus with anti-GBM glomerulonephritis shows linear staining of GBM for immunoglobulin G (IgG) (fluorescein isothiocyanate anti-IgG stain, 600×). (From Falk RJ, Jennette JC, Nachman PH. Primary glomerular disease. In: Brenner BM, ed. *Brenner and Rector's The Kidney.* 7th ed. Philadelphia: Elsevier; 2004.)

Immune Complex Rapidly Progressive Glomerulonephritis

RPGN-associated immune complex–mediated damage to the glomeruli can be seen with idiopathic glomerulopathies, such as IgA nephropathy and idiopathic membranoproliferative glomerulonephritis, or with systemic diseases such as postinfectious glomerulonephritis and SLE. Many cases of crescentic postinfectious glomerulonephritis resolve with successful treatment of the underlying infection. The treatment of severe lupus nephritis is described later.

Pauci-immune and Vasculitis–Associated Rapidly Progressive Glomerulonephritis

Pauci-immune RPGN includes patients with and without evidence of systemic vasculitis. Most patients have circulating ANCAs that are directed against components of neutrophil primary granules. Some patients have granulomatous polyangiitis (formerly called Wegener granulomatosis) with upper and lower respiratory tract involvement by granulomatous angiitis (Chapter 270) along with the pauci-immune glomrulonephritis. Others have microscopic polyangiitis akin to what was formerly called a subgroup of polyarteritis. Finally, others have eosinophilic polyangitis, formerly called Churg-Strauss disease (Chapter 270).

CLINICAL MANIFESTATIONS AND DIAGNOSIS

Patients often present with progressive renal failure and a nephritic picture (see Table 121-1). Patients with microscopic polyangiitis often have circulating perinuclear ANCA (antibodies directed against granulocyte myeloperoxidase) and a systemic clinical picture (Chapter 270) with arthritis, dermal leukocytoclastic angiitis, pulmonary disease, and constitutional and systemic signs. Patients with granulomatous polyangiitis often have circulating cytoplasmic ANCA (antibodies directed against a granulocyte serine proteinase, anti-PR3), upper and lower respiratory tract involvement by granulomatous angiitis, as well as pauci immune glomrulonephritis (Chapter 270). However, there is considerable overlap among these groups, and some patients have both ANCA and anti-GBM antibodies (Fig. 121-10). Patients with eosinophilic polyangiitis usually have a history of asthma, pulmonary infiltrates, and circulating eosinophila. If they are ANCA positive, they often have associated glomerular disease. Although there is no direct correlation between ANCA titers and disease activity, patients with high titers (especially high anti-PR3 titers) and patients with a major recent increase in titers are more likely to have flares of their disease.

TREATMENT AND PROGNOSIS

Rx

For induction therapy, combination therapy with corticosteroids (e.g., pulse methylprednisolone, 10 to 15 mg/kg/day up to a maximum of 500 to1000 mg IV daily, for 3 days, followed by prednisolone, 1 mg/kg/day PO) and cyclophosphamide (e.g., 15 mg/kg IV every 2 to 3 weeks or 1.5 to 2 mg/kg/day PO), with or without plasmapheresis, has markedly improved renal and patient survival rates in patients with granulomatous polyangiitis and microscopic polyangiitis (Chapter 270). Rituximab, a monoclonal antibody against CD20-positive B cells (375 mg/m^2 weekly for 4 weeks), is as effective and safe as a cyclophosphamide at 6 and 18 months.[A8] Methotrexate is as effective as cyclophosphamide in achieving remission, but it leads to a higher relapse rate, so it is not an initial alternative to cyclophosphamide or rituximab in most patients. In severe renal vasculitis, renal survival, but not patient survival, is improved with the addition of plasmapheresis.[A9] Maintenance regimens using rituximab (500 mg at months 6, 12, and 18)[A10], azathioprine (1.5 mg/kg/day), mycophenolate mofetil (1000 mg twice daily) or methotrexate (20 to 25 mg/week) should be administered for 12 to 18 months after achieving remission. Corticosteroids should be slowly tapered, as determined by the presence of clinical symptoms.

As in all forms of RPGN, renal function may deteriorate rapidly. In pauci-immune RPGN, high-risk patients include older patients, patients with severe pulmonary involvement, and patients with severe renal failure. Analyses have found no difference in prognosis in patients who have systemic vasculitis compared with isolated crescentic RPGN.

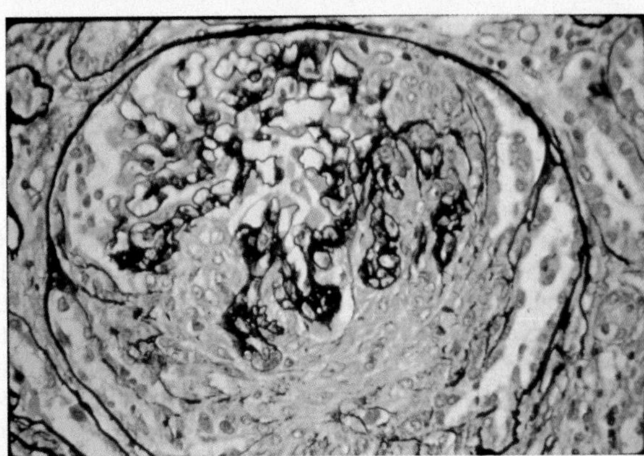

FIGURE 121-10. Crescentic glomerulonephritis typical of both anti–glomerular basement membrane disease and antineutrophil cytoplasmic antibody–positive pauci-immune glomerulonephritis.

GLOMERULAR DISEASES ASSOCIATED WITH GENETIC DEFECTS

As described earlier, some patients with FSGS have abnormalities in genes encoding for podocyte proteins or channels. Other patients, often with a history of clinical renal disease in siblings and other relatives, have other forms of hereditary nephritis.

Alport syndrome is a hereditary form of glomerulonephritis that often manifests with asymptomatic urinary findings. In approximately 85% of cases, it is an X-linked condition with hematuria and proteinuria, often in association with high-pitched hearing loss and abnormalities of the lens of the eye (lenticonus). Most of these patients have a localized mutation in the α_5 chain of type IV collagen (COL4A5). Other families have different patterns of inheritance, more often with mutations in the α_3 and α_4 chains of type IV collagen (COL4A3, COL4A4). Although the light microscopy findings vary from mild mesangial proliferative to advanced sclerosing lesions depending on the stage of biopsy, electron microscopy typically shows areas of GBM thinning and other areas of GBM splitting with lamellations. Some patients with mutations in the collagen IV gene have microhematuria and proteinuria with only areas of extreme GBM thinning on electron microscopy (so-called thin basement membrane disease). In males, Alport syndrome often leads to progressive glomerulosclerosis and ESRD. Use of ACE-inhibitors (Table 67-7) at the onset of proteinuria may slow progression of renal failure.

Fabry disease (Chapter 208), which is caused by an X-linked recessive genetic defect of α-galactosidase, leads to the deposition of ceramide trihexose in the kidneys and other organs. It may cause progressive proteinuria and renal insufficiency in males and in some female carriers. It is associated with telangiectasias of the skin, typically in the bathing suit area, acroparesthesias, cardiac abnormalities, and eye changes. Replacement with intravenous recombinant enzyme agalsidase β is associated with clinical improvement.

Nail-patella syndrome, associated with skeletal and nail deformities, is a rare cause of the nephrotic syndrome. It is due to an autosomal dominant mutation in the LMX1B transcription factor that regulates collagen, nephrin, and podocin gene expression.

OTHER GLOMERULAR DISEASES

Systemic Lupus Erythematosus

The pattern and degree of renal involvement greatly influences the course and therapy of SLE (Chapter 266). Although the incidence of clinical renal disease in SLE varies from 15 to 75%, histologic evidence of renal involvement is found in most biopsy specimens.

The International Society of Nephrology biopsy classification of lupus nephritis can provide a guide to therapy and prognosis (see Table 121-7). In general, class I and II patients have mild lesions that require no therapy directed at the kidney. All patients with class IV lesions (diffuse proliferative lupus nephritis) on biopsy deserve some form of vigorous therapy for their nephritis. Many class III (focal proliferative lupus nephritis) patients, especially those with active necrotizing lesions and large amounts of subendothelial deposits (Fig. 121-11), also benefit from vigorous therapy. For class V (membranous lupus nephritis) patients, the optimal therapy is less clear, and recommendations vary from uniform vigorous treatment to reserving such therapy for patients with serologic activity or more severe nephrotic syndrome.[11]

Induction therapy for severe proliferative lupus nephritis (either active class III or class IV) includes one of two regimens: corticosteroids (prednisone up to 1 mg/kg PO), tapering according to the clinical response over 6 to 12 months) with either daily mycophenolate mofetil (up to 1500 mg PO twice daily) or with cyclophosphamide pulses (0.5 to 1 g/m^2 IV/month for 6 months or 500 mg every 2 weeks for 6 doses) followed by maintenance therapy to prevent flares of disease or progression to renal failure.[A11] The addition of plasamapheresis has not been shown to improve outcome. Maintenance therapy with mycophenolate mofetil (1000 mg twice daily) or azathioprine (2 mg/kg/day) is more effective and less toxic than continued intravenous cyclophosphamide therapy after the 6-month induction period.[A12]

TABLE 121-7 CLASSIFICATION OF LUPUS NEPHRITIS

CLASS	CLINICAL FEATURES
I. Minimal mesangial LN	No renal findings
II. Mesangial proliferative LN	Mild clinical renal disease; minimally active urinary sediment; mild-to-moderate proteinuria (never nephrotic) but may have active serology
III. Focal proliferative LN < 50% glomeruli involved A. Active A/C. Active and chronic C. Chronic	More active sediment changes; often active serology; increased proteinuria (~25% nephrotic); hypertension may be present; some evolve into class IV pattern; active lesions require treatment, chronic do not
IV. Diffuse proliferative LN (>50% glomeruli involved); all may be with segmental or global involvement (S or G) A. Active A/C. Active and chronic C. Chronic	Most severe renal involvement with active sediment, hypertension, heavy proteinuria (frequent nephrotic syndrome), often reduced glomerular filtration rate; serology very active. Active lesions require treatment
V. Membranous LN glomerulonephritis	Significant proteinuria (often nephrotic) with less active lupus serology
VI. Advanced sclerosing LN	More than 90% glomerulosclerosis; no treatment prevents renal failure

LN = lupus nephritis.

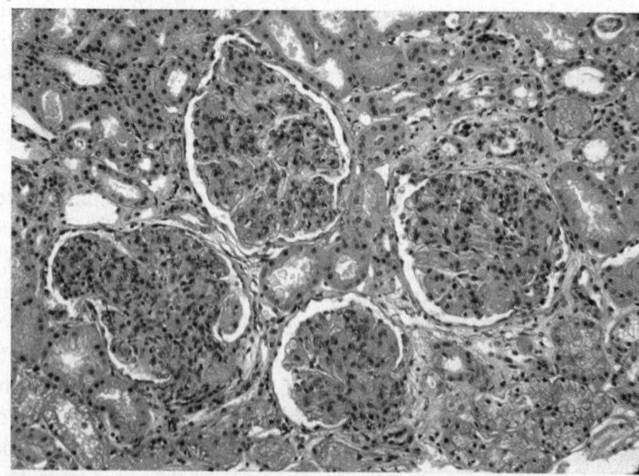

FIGURE 121-11. Diffuse proliferative lupus nephritis with involvement of all glomeruli.

Rituximab, an anti-CD20 monoclonal antibody, has not proved beneficial in inducing remissions when added to full doses of other immunosuppressive agents in controlled trials of patients with lupus nephritis. It may have a role in refractory or relapsing disease or as a steroid-sparing agent. Other agents under investigation include blockers of T- and B-cell costimulatory molecules, and anti-B LyS therapy.

Many patients with lupus nephritis (40 to 50%) produce autoantibodies against certain phospholipids, including anticardiolipin antibodies. Those patients who experience clotting in the glomeruli and arterioles, require anticoagulation or antiplatelet agents, or both, as well as immunosuppressive medications.

Diabetes Mellitus

Diabetic nephropathy, which is the most common form of glomerular damage seen in developed countries, is discussed in detail in Chapter 124.

Amyloidosis

Renal amyloid deposits, whether due to AL, AA, or hereditary-genetic forms of amyloid, are predominantly found within the glomeruli, where they often appear as amorphous eosinophilic extracellular nodules (Chapter 188). All amyloid is due to fibril formation of proteins that have a tendency to conform into β-pleated sheets. All stain positively with Congo red and display apple-green birefringence under polarized light. By electron microscopy, amyloid appears as nonbranching rigid fibrils 8 to 10 nm in diameter. In AL amyloid, overproduction of an abnormal light chain (λ 80%, κ 20%) can be detected by immunofluorescence staining for only λ or only κ light chains. Most patients have a clonal proliferation of plasma cells that typically does not reach levels seen with symptomatic multiple myeloma. In AA amyloid, antisera to the AA protein stain the glomeruli. Some patients with renal amyloidosis have genetically abnormal forms of proteins such as transthyretin, LECT2, and lipoproteins that lead to fibrillogenesis and deposition of amyloid fibrils in the kidney.

Almost 80% of patients with AL amyloid have renal disease. Renal manifestations include albuminuria and renal insufficiency. Approximately 25% of these patients present with nephrotic syndrome, which eventually is diagnosed in up to half of patients. Extrarenal amyloid involvement may cause cardiac disease (Chapter 60) or neuropathy (Chapter 420). Diagnosis may be made from organ biopsy other than the kidney (e.g., myocardial, gingival, rectal, or fat pad biopsy). Treatment strategies for renal AL amyloidosis are similar to those for multiple myeloma and other plasma cell dyscrasias (Chapter 187).

AA amyloid is usually associated with chronic inflammatory conditions such as rheumatoid arthritis (Chapter 264), familial Mediterranean fever (Chapter 261), inflammatory bowel disease (Chapter 141), osteomyelitis (Chapter 272), and other chronic infections. Treatment is directed at the underlying inflammatory process. Specific therapy against the primary inflammatory disease (e.g., anti–tumor necrosis factor therapy in rheumatoid arthritis and colchicine in familial Mediterranean fever) can prevent fibrillogenesis in AA amyloid patients. Eprodisate, a compound that inhibits polymerization and deposition of amyloid fibrils, can slow the progression of renal disease in patients with AA amyloidosis.[A13]

Light-Chain Deposition Disease

Light-chain deposition disease, like AL amyloidosis, is a systemic disease caused by the overproduction and extracellular deposition of a monoclonal immunoglobulin light chain (Chapter 187). However, the deposits do not form β-pleated sheets, do not stain with Congo red, and are granular rather than fibrillar. Most patients with light chain deposition disease have a lymphoplasmacytic B-cell disease similar to multiple myeloma (Chapter 187).

Albuminuria is common, and the nephrotic syndrome is found in half of patients at presentation, often accompanied by hypertension and renal insufficiency. On light microscopy, most glomeruli contain eosinophilic mesangial glomerular nodules. Some biopsy samples show associated light-chain cast nephropathy with eosinophilic laminated and fracturing casts obstructing the tubules, as seen in myeloma. By immunofluorescence, a single class of immunoglobulin light-chain (κ in 80% of cases) stains in a diffuse linear pattern along the GBM, in the nodules and along the tubular basement membranes.

The treatment for most patients with light-chain deposition disease is chemotherapy similar to that for myeloma (Chapter 187).

Fibrillary Glomerulopathy–Immunotactoid Glomerulopathy

Some patients with renal disease have glomerular lesions with deposits of nonamyloid fibrillar proteins ranging in size from 12 to more than 50 nm. Patients with these lesions have been divided into two groups: those with fibrillary glomerulonephritis with fibrils of 20 nm in diameter and those with immunotactoid glomerulonephritis, a much rarer disease often associated with lymphoproliferative disorders, in which the fibrils are much larger (30 to 50 nm). Proteinuria is found in almost all patients, and hematuria, the nephrotic syndrome, and renal insufficiency eventually develop in most. There is no proved therapy for fibrillary glomerulopathy. In patients with immunotactoid glomerulopathy, a search for a treatable underlying B cell disorder is important.

Human Immunodeficiency Virus–Associated Nephropathy

Infection with human immunodeficiency virus (HIV) (Chapter 386) is associated with a number of patterns of renal disease, including acute kidney injury and a unique form of glomerulopathy now called HIV-associated nephropathy.[12] HIV-associated nephropathy is characterized by heavy proteinuria and rapid progression to renal failure. On light microscopy, biopsies show global collapse of the glomerular tufts, severe tubulointerstitial changes with interstitial inflammation, edema, microcystic dilation of tubules, and severe tubular degenerative changes. On electron microscopy, tubuloreticular inclusions can be seen in the glomerular endothelium. The use of ACE inhibitors or ARBs (see Table 67-7 in Chapter 67) and antiretroviral therapy may slow the progression to renal failure and decrease proteinuria. Corticosteroids (e.g., prednisone, 1 mg/kg for 1 month followed by a taper over several months) may be beneficial in selected patients with HIV-associated nephropathy.

Mixed Cryoglobulinemia

Cryoglobulinemia (Chapter 187) is caused by the production of circulating immunoglobulins that precipitate on cooling and resolubilize on warming. Cryoglobulinemia may be found in association with infections, collagen vascular disease, and lymphoproliferative diseases such as multiple myeloma and Waldenström macroglobulinemia. Many patients with what was originally described as glomerulonephritis resulting from essential mixed cryoglobulinemia have been found to have hepatitis C–associated renal disease. Some patients develop an acute nephritic picture with acute renal insufficiency. Most patients have proteinuria, and approximately 20% present with the nephrotic syndrome. Most patients with renal disease have a slow, indolent course characterized by proteinuria, hypertension, hematuria, and renal insufficiency. Hypocomplementemia, especially of the early components C1q to C4, is a characteristic finding in cryoglobulinemic glomerulonephritis, whether hepatitis C–related or idiopathic. Treatment of hepatitis C–associated cryoglobulinemia includes antiviral therapy (Chapter 149). When significant renal disease is present, various combinations of corticosteroids with or without rituximab or cyclophosphamide or plasmapheresis have been used.

Thrombotic Microangiopathies

A number of systemic diseases, including hemolytic-uremic syndrome (Chapters 125 and 172), thrombotic thrombocytopenic purpura (TTP; Chapter 172), and the antiphospholipid syndrome (Chapter 176), as well as microangiopathy associated with drugs such as mitomycin and cyclosporine, are characterized by microthromboses of the glomerular capillaries and small arterioles. The renal findings may be dominant or only part of a more generalized picture of microangiopathy.

Renal manifestations of the thrombotic microangiopathies may include gross or microscopic hematuria, proteinuria that is typically less than 2 g/day but may reach nephrotic levels, and renal insufficiency. Patients may have oliguric or nonoliguric acute kidney injury. The histologic findings in all of the microangiopathies resemble each other and include glomerular capillary thromboses, areas of ischemic damage, and intimal proliferation with luminal narrowing by thrombi of arterioles and small arteries. In all thrombotic microangiopathies, treatment includes correcting hypovolemia, controlling hypertension, and the use of dialytic support for those with severe renal failure. In TTP associated with an acquired or hereditary deficiency of the von Willebrand convertase ADAMTS-13 and in some other cases, plasmapheresis with fresh-frozen plasma is beneficial (Chapter 172). In some patients whose hemolytic-uremic syndrome is not associated with Shiga toxin, defects in the alternate complement system are found. These patients with atypical hemolytic-uremic syndrome may benefit from a monoclonal blocker of the fifth component of complement, eculizumab (Chapter 172). In the antiphospholipid syndrome, anticoagulation with heparin and then warfarin is useful (Chapter 176).

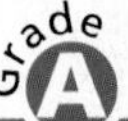

Grade A References

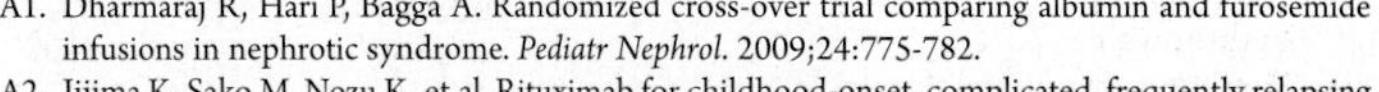

A1. Dharmaraj R, Hari P, Bagga A. Randomized cross-over trial comparing albumin and furosemide infusions in nephrotic syndrome. *Pediatr Nephrol.* 2009;24:775-782.

A2. Iijima K, Sako M, Nozu K, et al. Rituximab for childhood-onset, complicated, frequently relapsing nephrotic syndrome or steroid-dependent nephrotic syndrome: a multicentre, double-blind, randomised, placebo-controlled trial. *Lancet.* 2014;384:1273-1281.

A3. Gipson DS, Trachtman H, Kaskel FJ, et al. Clinical trial of focal segmental glomerulosclerosis in children and young adults. *Kidney Int.* 2011;80:868-878.

A4. Ren H, Shen P, Li X, et al. Tacrolimus versus cyclophosphamide in steroid-dependent or steroid-resistant focal segmental glomerulosclerosis: a randomized controlled trial. *Am J Nephrol.* 2013;37:84-90.

A5. Chen Y, Schieppati A, Cai G, et al. Immunosuppression for membranous nephropathy: a systematic review and meta-analysis of 36 clinical trials. *Clin J Am Soc Nephrol.* 2013;8:787-796.

A6. Cheng J, Zhang W, Zhang XH, et al. ACEI/ARB therapy for IgA nephropathy: a meta analysis of randomised controlled trials. *Int J Clin Pract.* 2009;63:880-888.

A7. Lv J, Xu D, Perkovic V, et al. Corticosteroid therapy in IgA nephropathy. *J Am Soc Nephrol.* 2012;23:1108-1116.

A8. Specks U, Merkel PA, Seo P, et al. Efficacy of remission-induction regimens for ANCA-associated vasculitis. *N Engl J Med.* 2013;369:417-427.

A9. Jayne DR, Gaskin G, Rasmussen N, et al. Randomized trial of plasma exchange or high-dosage methylprednisolone as adjunctive therapy for severe renal vasculitis. *J Am Soc Nephrol.* 2007;18:2180-2188.

A10. Guillevin L, Pagnoux C, Karras A, et al. Rituximab versus azathioprine for maintenance in ANCA-associated vasculitis. *N Engl J Med.* 2014;371:1771-1780.

A11. Henderson LK, Masson P, Craig JC, et al. Induction and maintenance treatment of proliferative lupus nephritis: a meta-analysis of randomized controlled trials. *Am J Kidney Dis.* 2013;61:74-87.

A12. Dooley MA, Jayne D, Ginzler EM, et al. Mycophenolate versus azathioprine as maintenance therapy for lupus nephritis. *N Engl J Med.* 2011;365:1886-1895.

A13. Dember LM, Hawkins PN, Hazenberg BP, et al. Eprodisate for the treatment of renal disease in AA amyloidosis. *N Engl J Med.* 2007;356:2349-2360.

GENERAL REFERENCES

For the General References and other additional features, please visit Expert Consult at https://expertconsult.inkling.com.

122 TUBULOINTERSTITIAL NEPHRITIS

ERIC G. NEILSON

DEFINITION

Interstitial nephritis can be primary and begin in the tubulointerstitium or appear as a secondary event and spread from blood vessels, including the glomerular capillaries. Injury to the tubulointerstitial compartment can be the result of autoimmunity, toxic insult, infection, or exposure to drugs. In all cases, however, the inflammatory process has an immunologic component that leads to the release of tissue cytokines, which attract T lymphocytes and other monocytes, which eventually convert tubular epithelia into fibroblasts to produce fibrosis.

Tubulointerstitial nephritis can be arbitrarily divided into acute and chronic types. The acute form of interstitial nephritis often begins abruptly. When inciting events subside, so does the nephritis, and the glomerular filtration rate tends to normalize, with little residual damage except in patients with preexisting disease. Chronic interstitial nephritis is persistent and over time reduces the number of functioning nephrons by encasing and dismantling them with irreversible fibrosis. So-called toxic nephropathy is similar to this form of nephritis. Sometimes acute and chronic injury is difficult to distinguish because global destruction of the tubulointerstitium can occur within a matter of weeks.

EPIDEMIOLOGY

Acute interstitial nephritis appears unexpectedly in otherwise healthy individuals from a variety of causes. Approximately 1% of patients with hematuria and proteinuria have acute interstitial nephritis, and it is seen in 1 to 15% of

TABLE 122-1 CAUSES OF ACUTE INTERSTITIAL NEPHRITIS

DRUGS
Antibiotics
Penicillins
Rifampin, ethambutol
Sulfa
Vancomycin
Ciprofloxacin
Cephalosporins
Erythromycin
Trimethoprim-sulfamethoxazole
Acyclovir
Nonsteroidal Anti-Inflammatory Drugs
Selective and Nonselective
Cyclooxygenase-2 Inhibitors
Diuretics
Thiazides
Furosemide
Triamterene
Miscellaneous
Captopril
Ranitidine
Omeprazole
Phenobarbital
Phenytoin
Sodium valproate
Carbamazepine
Allopurinol
Interferon
Interleukin-2
All-*trans*-retinoic acid
INFECTIONS
Bacteria
Legionella
Brucella
Diphtheria
Streptococcus
Staphylococcus
Yersinia
Salmonella
Escherichia coli
Campylobacter
Viruses
Epstein-Barr virus
Cytomegalovirus
Hantavirus
Herpes simplex virus
Hepatitis B virus
Other
Mycoplasma
Rickettsia
Leptospira
Mycobacterium tuberculosis
Schistosoma mekongi
Toxoplasma
Chlamydia
AUTOIMMUNE DISEASES
Anti–tubular basement membrane disease
Tubulointerstitial nephritis and uveitis (TINU) syndrome
Kawasaki disease

TABLE 122-2 CAUSES OF CHRONIC INTERSTITIAL NEPHRITIS

HEREDITARY DISEASES
Mitochondrial mutations
METABOLIC DISTURBANCES
Hypercalcemia, nephrocalcinosis
Hyperoxaluria
Hypokalemia
Hyperuricemia
Cystinosis
Methylmalonic acidemia
DRUGS AND TOXINS
Analgesics
Cadmium
Lead
Health food botanicals, herbs
Lithium
Cyclosporine, tacrolimus
Cisplatin, methotrexate
Nitrosoureas
AUTOIMMUNE DISEASES
Renal allograft rejection
Granulomatosis with polyangiitis
Immunoglobulin G4–related tubulointerstitial nephropathy
Sjögren syndrome
Systemic lupus erythematosus, vasculitis
Tubulointerstitial nephritis and uveitis (TINU) syndrome
Sarcoidosis
HEMATOLOGIC DISTURBANCES
Multiple myeloma, light chains
Lymphoma
Sickle cell disease
INFECTIONS
Complicated pyelonephritis
Human immunodeficiency virus (HIV)
Epstein-Barr virus
Malakoplakia
Xanthogranulomatous pyelonephritis
OBSTRUCTIVE NEPHROPATHY
Tumors
Stones
Outlet obstruction
Vesicoureteral reflux
MISCELLANEOUS
Age-related vascular disease
Hypertension
Ischemia
Balkan (endemic) nephropathy
Radiation nephritis

autopsy series. In recent decades its prevalence has increased in individuals over 65 years of age, perhaps owing to their more frequent exposure to prescription drugs.[1]

Although acute interstitial nephritis is largely due to the use of pharmaceuticals,[2] other important causes include infection and idiopathic autoimmune diseases (Table 122-1). Penicillin moieties (less so nafcillin and piperacillin), cephalosporins, sulfa-like drugs, and nonsteroidal anti-inflammatory drugs (NSAIDs) top the list. NSAIDs cause both acute interstitial nephritis and chronic analgesic nephropathy. Diphtheria in children (Chapter 292), legionellosis (Chapter 314), leptospirosis (Chapter 323), histoplasmosis (Chapter 332), tuberculosis (Chapter 324), and DNA viruses such as cytomegalovirus (Chapter 376) and Epstein-Barr virus (Chapter 377) are well-recognized agents of acute interstitial nephritis. Anti–tubular basement membrane disease is a rare cause of autoimmune interstitial nephritis. Although sarcoidosis or the tubulointerstitial nephritis and uveitis (TINU) syndrome can manifest as acute interstitial nephritis on biopsy, they often quickly evolve into chronic disease.

All forms of injury to the kidney, regardless of origin, progress to end-stage renal disease through a terminal phase of chronic interstitial nephritis. In addition to glomerulonephritides (Chapter 121), cystic diseases (Chapter 127), and diabetes (Chapter 229), a wide variety of renal conditions start slowly in the tubulointerstitium and often go unrecognized until late in the course, when biopsy shows chronic interstitial nephritis.

Primary chronic interstitial nephritis can be caused by a variety of toxic, metabolic, hematologic, obstructive, and infectious processes. Ingestion of six or more tablets per day of acetaminophen, aspirin, or NSAIDs, alone or together, for at least 3 years puts patients at risk for analgesic nephropathy. A careful history of drug or toxin exposure, previous renal images, and a family history often point to a probable diagnosis (Table 122-2).

PATHOBIOLOGY

Pathophysiology

Regardless of the origin of renal inflammation, the kidneys do not fail until interstitial nephritis, fibrosis, and tubular atrophy develop. Interstitial nephritis is the pathologic equivalent of clinical progression because it is the final common pathway to permanent tissue damage.[3] The degree of reduction in the glomerular filtration rate correlates with the degree of interstitial injury. Urinary flow is impeded by tubular obstruction. Increased vascular resistance causes progressive tubular injury and fibrosis. A net reduction in the cross-sectional area of peritubular vessels increases postglomerular resistance to the extent that the compensatory increase in glomerular hydrostatic pressure cannot fully restore filtration to normal levels. Tubuloglomerular feedback assumes increasing importance in the transition from acute to chronic glomerulonephritis when autoregulation of renal blood flow is disrupted by tubulointerstitial fibrosis. Loss of autoregulation by tubuloglomerular feedback results from the absence or insensitivity of the afferent arteriole. Perhaps more significant is the effect of interstitial pressure on the sensitivity of the feedback mechanism. Tubular atrophy may disrupt the normal renal osmotic gradient by decreasing sodium chloride transport along the proximal tubule or thick ascending loop of Henle. The result is poor abstraction of water from the filtrate, with hyposthenuria and polyuria. Such an increase in solute and water within the tubular fluid results in adaptive downregulation of the glomerular filtration process.

The antigen targets engaging the inflammasome and the immune system in interstitial nephritis are slowly unfolding. Drugs act as haptens, mimic endogenous structures in the interstitium, alter regulation of the immune system, or function in some combination of the foregoing. Bacteria, fungi, and viruses can infect the kidney and cause mononuclear cell infiltration or activate toll-like receptors on tubular epithelia, which subsequently educate the adaptive immune response to events in the interstitium. Autoimmune diseases such as anti–tubular basement membrane disease or spontaneous interstitial nephritis remain confined to the kidney, whereas systemic diseases spread to the kidney, where they cause persistent, chronic interstitial nephritis.

Although the adaptive immune response is similar to that of other tissues, T-cell activation figures prominently in interstitial nephritis. Antibodies (anti–tubular basement membrane disease) and immune complex deposition along the tubular basement membrane (systemic lupus erythematosus) are rarely seen. Antigens presented by class II major histocompatibility complex molecules on macrophages, dendritic cells, and adjacent tubular epithelia, in conjunction with associative recognition molecules, engage the CD4/CD8 T-cell repertoires. The resultant cytokine and protease activity injures tubular nephrons and basement membranes and causes fibroblasts to form locally by epithelial-mesenchymal transition and to proliferate. Transforming growth factor-β (TGF-β), fibroblast growth factor 2, and platelet-derived growth factor are particularly active in this transition. If the nephritis persists, fibrogenesis dismantles nephrons and causes tubular atrophy; in late stages, the inflammatory reaction outgrows its survival factors and lymphocytes and fibroblasts disappear by apoptosis and leave an acellular fibrotic scar.[4]

Viruses, including Epstein-Barr virus, have long been suspected of contributing to idiopathic, chronic interstitial nephritis. Malakoplakia and xanthogranulomatous pyelonephritis are probably not defects in nephrogenesis but rather are destructive responses to bacterial inflammation in the interstitium. Focal abnormalities in kidney structure can be a nidus for infections associated with perinephric, psoas, or peritoneal abscesses. Children with vesicoureteral reflux can have chronic or repeating episodes of pyelonephritis, but whether the reflux or the infection is more important to progression to renal failure is unclear. There is also no agreement on whether recurrent pyelonephritis by itself produces chronic interstitial nephritis in adults.

Pathology

Both kidneys are typically involved, except in cases of unilateral infection, obstruction, or trauma. The inflammatory reaction in acute interstitial nephritis consists mainly of T lymphocytes and monocytes, but neutrophils, plasma cells, and eosinophils can be present. The T cells are of a mixed phenotype with a distinct preference for CD4+ lymphocytes. The infiltrative process is associated with interstitial edema, which displaces tubules away from one another and causes the kidneys to swell. The tubular basement membrane may be disrupted in more severe cases, but immune deposits are rarely found by immunofluorescence.

In chronic interstitial nephritis, the kidney assumes an irregular or contracted appearance. The tubular epithelia sit on thickened or disrupted tubular basement membranes and are often effaced against dilated lumens; the tubules eventually dismantle and atrophy. *Chronic* is a relative term, because fibrotic changes can be seen within 7 to 10 days of continuing inflammation. Normal glomeruli in primary interstitial nephritis are eventually surrounded by periglomerular fibrosis and subsequently undergo segmental or global sclerosis. Chronic vascular thickening and glomerular changes are present in advanced stages of disease, so pathologic determination of the primary cause may be difficult in some biopsy samples. Progressive glomerular sclerosis also occurs with aging and must be factored in when interpreting the biopsy findings.

A third pathologic category, granuloma formation, can be seen in either acute or chronic interstitial nephritis. In acute granulomatous interstitial nephritis, granulomas are sparse and non-necrotic and giant cells are rare. The granulomas in chronic interstitial nephritis contain an abundance of giant cells, and those caused by tuberculosis may become necrotic. Drugs are a common cause of this lesion in the acute setting, and most of the drugs associated with acute interstitial nephritis have been reported to cause granuloma formation. In the absence of drug exposure, sarcoidosis (Chapter 95), Wegener granulomatosis with polyangiitis (Chapter 270), histoplasmosis (Chapter 332), or tuberculosis (Chapter 324) should be considered, depending on the context, when numerous granulomas are present. The renal granulomas seen in granulomatosis with polyangiitis are almost always accompanied by glomerular and vascular pathology.

ACUTE INTERSTITIAL NEPHRITIS

CLINICAL MANIFESTATIONS

Most patients present with an asymptomatic rise in the serum creatinine level or an abnormal urinalysis, and it is important to consider acute interstitial nephritis in any patient with an unexplained precipitous diminution in renal function.[5] Because injury is often asymptomatic, patients already may have substantial renal failure on initial presentation. Patients also may present with nonspecific symptoms such as lethargy or weakness, and many patients have fever and oliguria owing to severe acute kidney injury (Chapter 120).

Several features can distinguish acute interstitial nephritis from acute tubular necrosis (Chapter 120) or glomerulonephritis (Chapter 121) (Table 122-3). Fever and occasional flank pain over the kidneys occur in infection or with drug-induced acute interstitial nephritis. Lumbar pain, sometimes unilateral, is due to distention of the renal capsule. Allergic reactions are associated with maculopapular rash, fever, and eosinophilia, but the entire triad is seen in less than 33% of patients, and such signs are uncommon when NSAIDs cause acute interstitial nephritis. These signs and symptoms of drug reaction have been codified and referred to as the DRESS syndrome (*d*rug *r*ash, *e*osinophilia, and *s*ystemic *s*ymptoms; Chapter 440), which is associated with interstitial nephritis in up to 40% of patients with persistent exposure to selected drugs.[6]

The course of renal failure in acute interstitial nephritis takes several days to weeks and follows the kinetics of the primary immune response. However, renal failure can be precipitous, especially in patients re-exposed to a previous agent. Rarely, the course can be protracted, with the glomerular filtration rate declining over a period of months if the diagnosis is not recognized. This protracted course is more common with diuretic-induced interstitial nephritis. The onset of drug-induced nephritis ranges from days to weeks after the initiation of therapy, and a previous allergic history is rare. The classic setting for a drug reaction is a febrile patient with an infectious process and who defervesces while taking antibiotics but then develops recurrent fever several days later.

DIAGNOSIS

Urinalysis is particularly helpful. Mild-to-moderate proteinuria and hematuria are seen in most cases, and gross hematuria is observed rarely. The sediment typically shows red and white blood cells, and white blood cell casts are commonly seen. Conversely, red blood cell casts suggest a glomerular

TABLE 122-3 TYPICAL CLINICAL MANIFESTATIONS OF ACUTE INTERSTITIAL NEPHRITIS

History of drug hypersensitivity or recent infection and taking antibiotics
Sudden onset of fever lasting several days to weeks
Variable degrees of hypertension
Rise in creatinine with $FE_{Na} > 1.0$; no expected acute tubular necrosis or glomerulonephritis
Kidney size normal or increased
Hematuria with mild proteinuria (<1.0 g)
Presence of WBC casts and WBCs on urinalysis; rarely eosinophils

FE_{Na} = fractional excretion of sodium; WBC = white blood cell.

TABLE 122-4 WHEN TO CONSIDER A RENAL BIOPSY TO DIAGNOSE NEPHRITIS

The setting, history, or clinical findings do not support a diagnosis of acute tubular necrosis or volume depletion
The clinical setting warrants a tissue diagnosis to determine the type of lesion, the extent of involvement, or the degree of fibrosis
The patient is stable enough to undergo biopsy and receive immunosuppressive drugs
The physician believes that the choice of therapy or the length of treatment is partially determined by the type of tissue injury

diagnosis. The finding of eosinophils in the urine supports the diagnosis of allergic interstitial nephritis, but the positive predictive value is low, even with more than 5% eosinophils in the urine, and the absence of eosinophiluria does not exclude the diagnosis of acute interstitial nephritis.[7]

An elevated serum creatinine level is usually the first abnormal laboratory result in renal injury. The normal serum creatinine of 0.6 to 1.3 mg/dL varies with muscle mass, age, and gender. Early recognition of acute interstitial nephritis requires a high degree of clinical suspicion because the serum creatinine level may be only mildly elevated even after the kidneys lose half their function.

The magnitude of proteinuria in acute interstitial nephritis is nearly always less than 3 g/24 hours and is typically less than 1 g/24 hours. Nephrotic-range proteinuria is not seen unless there is a coexisting glomerular lesion, such as a concurrent minimal-change lesion, or after exposure to NSAIDs. Many patients with acute interstitial nephritis also have a fractional excretion of sodium (FE_{Na}) greater than 1, but occasionally they are oliguric.

Imaging is of little diagnostic value. The kidney in acute interstitial nephritis is usually normal or slightly increased in size on echographic or tomographic images. Increased cortical echogenicity may correlate with diffuse interstitial infiltrates on renal biopsy. Gallium scanning is not particularly useful because a variety of other renal processes can cause gallium uptake, including minimal change glomerulonephritis, cortical necrosis, and acute tubular necrosis; in addition, acute interstitial nephritis can be found on biopsy in those with a normal scan.

DIFFERENTIAL DIAGNOSIS

It is sometimes difficult to distinguish among nonoliguric acute tubular necrosis, acute interstitial nephritis, and glomerulonephritis without a biopsy. Exposure to pharmaceuticals, particularly antibiotics and NSAIDs, is responsible for most cases of acute interstitial nephritis, followed by infections and autoimmune disease. Selective tubular defects and tubular syndromes, such as proximal acquired Fanconi syndrome or distal renal tubular acidosis, can be seen in subacute or chronic interstitial nephritis but argue against acute interstitial nephritis.

Biopsy

Ultimately, the diagnosis can be established with certainty only by renal biopsy, which confirms and assesses the extent of acute interstitial inflammation. A biopsy should be performed in patients with acute renal failure who have suggestive signs or symptoms of an interstitial process and in whom prerenal azotemia and obvious acute tubular necrosis cannot be excluded on clinical grounds (Table 122-4). In primary acute interstitial nephritis, the biopsy demonstrates inflammatory cells that typically spare the glomeruli until late in the course (Fig. 122-1A). Lesions that reduce renal function are usually diffuse, but drug-induced interstitial injury is often patchy, beginning deep in the cortex before spreading.

TREATMENT Rx

Biopsy is important to confirm acute interstitial nephritis, because chronic interstitial fibrosis rarely responds to aggressive treatment. The principal intervention for acute interstitial nephritis is to remove the inciting drug or treat the infection. Switching to different derivatives of a suspected drug is unwise. Concomitantly, or if the serum creatinine concentration does not fall after a few days, steroids (prednisone 0.75 to 1.0 mg/kg PO) can be given daily for approximately 1 week. If no further improvement occurs, cyclophosphamide (1 to 2 mg/kg/day PO) can be added for several more weeks. In patients who respond, cyclophosphamide can be steroid sparing, particularly in those with persistent sarcoidosis. It is important not to continue high-dose immunosuppression without some evidence of benefit because immunosuppressive drugs in patients with azotemia can lead to serious infection and even death. It is better to reserve these drugs for use with kidney transplantation if the primary disease does not respond.

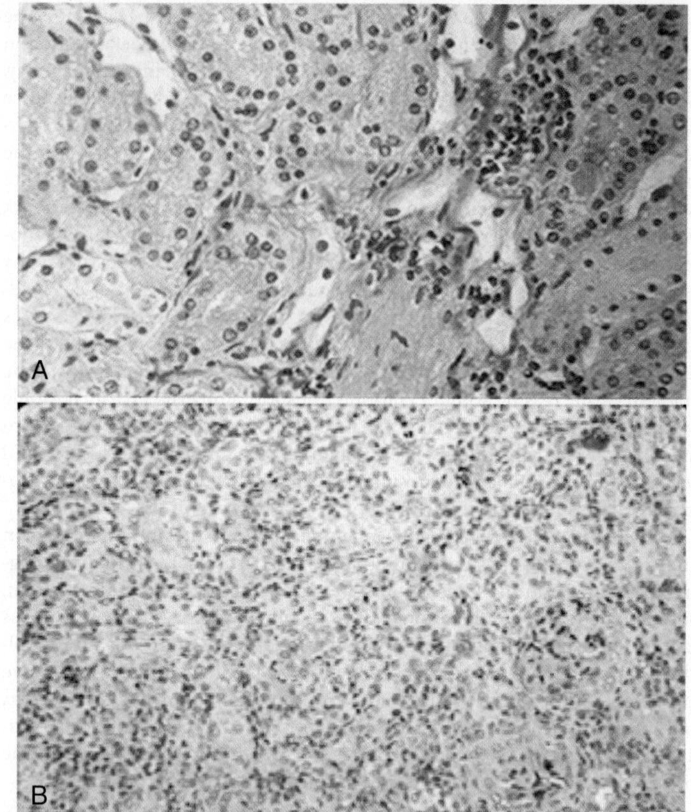

FIGURE 122-1. **Tubulointerstitial nephritis on biopsy. A,** Acute interstitial nephritis can be most aggressive when the interstitium is crowded with mononuclear cells and giant cells that destroy nearly all tubular nephrons (hematoxylin-eosin). **B,** Chronic interstitial nephritis is a slower process, with substantial collagen deposition (*blue color;* trichrome), tubular dropout, and fibroblasts in the interstitial spaces widened by fibrosis.

PROGNOSIS

The prognosis for acute interstitial nephritis is good if it is recognized early in the setting of minimal fibrosis. In nonrandomized, observational series, patients treated with steroids tend to do somewhat better.[8] Early removal of offending agents or prompt treatment with antibiotics or immunosuppressive drugs can be renoprotective.

CHRONIC INTERSTITIAL NEPHRITIS

CLINICAL MANIFESTATIONS

Patients with primary chronic interstitial nephritis typically have elevated levels of serum creatinine and signs and symptoms of renal failure, including hematuria, hyposthenuria, nocturia, fatigue, and nausea. Urinalysis shows a fixed specific gravity of about 1.010, occasional glycosuria, and non-nephrotic-range proteinuria (often <1 g/L), with red and white blood cells and granular casts. Pyuria and positive urine cultures for bacteria are seen occasionally, and varying degrees of metabolic acidosis and hyperphosphatemia may be present. Before the glomerular filtration rate falls below 25 to 30 mL/minute, tubular acidosis is common. Anemia is often out of proportion to the degree of renal failure, and many patients have hypertension but only minimal edema until advanced stages of renal failure. Acquired Fanconi syndrome can be seen in patients with a serum creatinine level less than 2.5 mg/dL in the setting of drug exposure, myeloma, human immunodeficiency virus (HIV) infection, lead exposure, and herbal nephropathy.

DIAGNOSIS

A careful dietary history is critical. As for any patient with evidence of renal failure, the evaluation includes laboratory tests to determine possible causes and severity. These tests include measures of renal function (serum creatinine level and blood urea nitrogen level), as well as levels of serum electrolytes, calcium, phosphate, uric acid, and albumin. Urinalysis shows a fixed specific gravity of approximately 1.010, occasional glycosuria, proteinuria (often < 1 g/L), and red cells, white cells, and granular casts. Depending on the clinical situation, the search for specific causes may include serum and urine protein electrophoresis, blood cultures, serologic tests for autoimmune diseases (e.g., cryoglobulin level, antinuclear antibodies, anti–neutrophil cytoplasmic antibody, and anti–glomerular basement membrane antibody levels [see Table 257-2]), or viral infection, particularly after renal transplantation (Chapter 131).

Selective tubular defects and tubular syndromes, such as proximal acquired Fanconi syndrome (bicarbonaturia with a plasma carbon dioxide [CO_2] content < 20 mEq/L, aminoaciduria, phosphate wasting, uricosuria, and glycosuria) or distal renal tubular acidosis type 1 (urine pH > 5.6, plasma CO_2 content < 20 mEq/L, with low or high potassium) can be seen occasionally in subacute or chronic interstitial nephritis. Patients with Fanconi syndrome, in particular, exhibit proximal tubular epithelium alterations that variably impair transporter function in the area of injury. These tubular defects are classically and occasionally seen in light-chain myeloma, cystinosis, Lowe syndrome, TINU syndrome, biliary cirrhosis, or after exposure to selected drugs, such as tenofovir or ifosfamide. Patients with Fanconi syndrome quickly develop an alkaline urine (pH > 7.5) and increased fractional excretion of urine bicarbonate when serum bicarbonate is elevated above 20 mEq/L by intravenous infusion.

Classic images of analgesic nephropathy on tomography are quite specific (Fig. 122-2) and show a decrease in overall kidney size, with atrophic scars and an irregular cortical contour, sometimes accompanied by papillary necrosis.

On biopsy (see Table 122-4), chronic interstitial nephritis is manifest by a cellular infiltrate that is eventually replaced by tubulointerstitial fibrosis (see Fig. 122-1B). Infiltrates of lymphocytes and rare neutrophils are scattered and less abundant than in acute interstitial nephritis.

Specific Causes

Analgesics

Aspirin, acetaminophen, and NSAIDs alone or together are a source of toxic metabolites and can induce medullary ischemia and papillary necrosis, sometimes with papillary calcification. The likelihood of analgesic nephropathy from taking acetaminophen alone is much less than with the others. Uroepithelial malignancies also occur with increased frequency in this group of patients.

Aristolochic Acid Nephropathy

Aristolochic acid has been implicated as a cause of Balkan nephropathy and so-called Chinese herbal nephropathy. A growing number of people are taking vitamins and herbal preparations purchased from health food stores (Chapter 39), and some of these remedies contain botanicals that produce chronic interstitial nephritis.[9] Patients who are dieting often use these remedies and are first seen when they already have late-stage disease, which increases the risk for uroepithelial malignancies (Chapter 197).

Human Immunodeficiency Virus Tubulointerstitial Nephropathy

Predominate tubulointerstitial nephropathy accounts for about 25% of the renal lesions seen on biopsy in HIV-infected patients. Biopsies show two general forms: a tubulopathy or an interstitial nephritis. In the tubulopathy, damage is to the proximal tubule; 80% of cases are associated with drug exposure, particularly tenofovir (Chapter 360), and approximately 30% improve with time. Patients in the tubulointerstitial nephritis group have a mononuclear infiltration and more persistent viral loads, but 50 to 60% recover.[10]

Tubulointerstitial Nephritis with Uveitis Syndrome

Seen at any age but more commonly in young women and children, the TINU syndrome may be idiopathic, genetic, or in response to pharmaceutical exposure.[11] Unilateral or bilateral anterior panuveitis (Chapter 423) may precede or follow evidence of interstitial nephritis that starts acutely but may persist as chronic renal injury. If the renal function is not greatly impaired, concomitant Fanconi syndrome may suggest proximal tubular involvement. In the absence of controlled trials, treatment with varying doses of methylprednisolone followed by oral prednisone may be beneficial in some patients. Varying durations of supplemental or steroid-sparing immunosuppression with mycophenolate mofetil or cyclophosphamide also have been used.

Vascular Disease

Chronic renal ischemia from vascular injury can lead to interstitial nephritis, nephrosclerosis, and fibrosis, which are the classic renal lesions of untreated

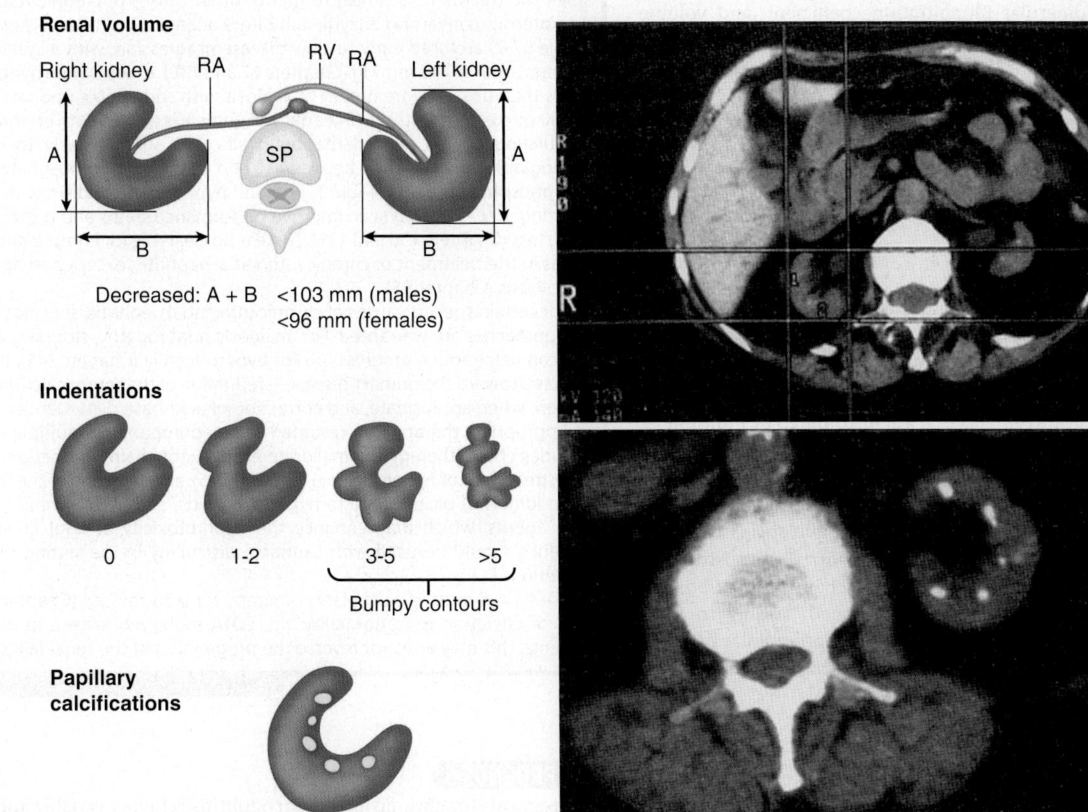

FIGURE 122-2. Renal changes in analgesic nephropathy seen by tomographic imaging. Structural changes, including reduced volume, nodularity, and calcifications, are seen on computed tomography. RA = right artery; RV = right vein; SP = spinal vertebra. (From Elseviers MM, De Schepper A, Corthouts R, et al. High diagnostic performance of CT scan for analgesic nephropathy in patients with incipient to severe renal failure. *Kidney Int.* 1995;48:1316.)

essential hypertension (Chapter 67). Similar injury is seen with aging, diabetes (Chapter 124), sickle cell disease (Chapter 163), and radiation nephritis (Chapter 20). This tubulointerstitial injury from the vascular diseases is quite different from the aggressive necrosis seen with acute vasculitis. In patients taking calcineurin inhibitors such as cyclosporine or tacrolimus, renal ischemia from vasoconstriction can cause interstitial fibrosis that is sometimes difficult to distinguish from chronic allograft rejection (Chapter 131).

Immunoglobulin G4–Related Tubulointerstitial Nephritis

Immunoglobulin G4 (IgG4)-related tubulointerstitial nephritis is a relatively new systemic syndrome that expresses in the kidney as inflammatory masses associated with plasma cells and interstitial mononuclear cell infiltrates. Patients may have lesions in other organs, such as the liver, pancreas, thyroid, and myocardium. Eosinophilia and low complement levels can be seen. Serum IgG4 levels and tissue plasma cells are increased, but it is not clear whether the IgG4 antibodies are a biomarker or causative. The renal lesions in many patients respond briskly to corticosteroid treatment.[12] IgG4 is also separately associated with membranous nephropathy (Chapter 121) and nephrotic-range proteinuria.

Obstruction

Significant urinary obstruction (Chapter 123) owing to occlusion of both ureters by bladder tumors, cervical carcinoma, ureteral valve disease, or bladder outlet obstruction is an important cause of chronic interstitial nephritis. Complete or partial urinary tract obstruction is accompanied by a decline in glomerular filtration and classic tubular abnormalities, including diminished reabsorption of solutes, impaired excretion of H^+ and K^+, and a vasopressin-resistant concentrating defect in the medulla. Obstruction is associated with a fall in the glomerular filtration rate because of reduced plasma flow and hydraulic pressure associated with the release of angiotensin II, leukotrienes, and nitric oxide, a process leading to mononuclear cell infiltration. Growth factors such as TGF-β, released by infiltrating cells, may contribute to the interstitial and glomerular fibrosis. Obstruction is more common in men than in women and is part of the routine assessment of renal failure by renal ultrasound (Chapters 120 and 123). Almost all obstructed kidneys eventually become infected if the obstruction is not relieved.

Hypercalcemia

Hypercalcemia can decrease glomerular filtration through renal vasoconstriction, a decrease in the glomerular ultrafiltration coefficient, and volume depletion as a result of a vasopressin-resistant concentrating defect associated with nephrocalcinosis and calcium deposition around the basement membranes of the distal tubules and collecting ducts. Such deposition secondarily leads to mononuclear cell infiltration and tubular death. Nephrocalcinosis also occurs in normocalcemic disorders of augmented calcium absorption through the gut (sarcoidosis [Chapter 95], vitamin D intoxication [Chapter 245]), skeletal breakdown (neoplasms or multiple myeloma [Chapter 187]), or classic distal renal tubular acidosis.

Myeloma

The chronic renal failure of multiple myeloma (Chapter 187) is caused by several mechanisms, including cast nephropathy ("myeloma kidney"), coexistent volume depletion, hypercalcemia (Chapter 245), nephrocalcinosis (Chapter 245), and uric acid nephropathy.[13] Proteinaceous casts form in dilated, atrophic distal nephron segments that are surrounded by multinucleated giant cells in interstitial infiltrates. The casts typically contain both Tamm-Horsfall protein and a pathologic light chain. Interstitial plasma cells and mononuclear infiltrates, calcifications in the interstitium, and amyloid deposits in the vessels and glomeruli are often present. Light chains are nephrotoxic by direct injury to tubular cells or through intrarenal obstruction from cast formation. In the setting of excess light chain production, the proximal tubule reabsorptive capacity is overwhelmed, leading to their urinary excretion as Bence Jones proteins. An elevated intratubular pressure partly accounts for the decline in glomerular filtration in experimental cast nephropathy.

Lead Toxicity

Epidemiologic analyses support the association between excess lead burden (Chapter 22) and chronic renal failure.[14] Blood lead levels reflect only recent, not chronic, exposure and can be normal in patients with a significant lead burden. Lead preferentially deposits in the proximal tubule, and nuclear inclusions within proximal tubular cells are characteristic of lead nephropathy.

Ingestion of moonshine liquor, with its high lead content, can be an important historical clue to the diagnosis. In adults, lead nephropathy produces chronic interstitial nephritis, fibrosis, and nephrosclerosis. Proximal tubular dysfunction may produce isolated tubule defects or a full Fanconi syndrome. Patients often have recurrent gout, and hyperuricemia and hypertension may be present. Some laboratories can measure δ-aminolevulinic acid dehydratase, which is inhibited by lead. Although chelation studies may document lead burden, this test is difficult to perform in patients with renal failure. X-ray fluorescent measurements of in vivo skeletal lead stores correlate well with ethylenediaminetetraacetic acid (EDTA) chelation tests and have the advantage of being rapid and noninvasive.

Cadmium Toxicity

Cadmium nephropathy (Chapter 22) is seen in regions with contamination from smelters that result in prolonged low-level exposure. Cadmium is bound to metallothionein, and proximal tubular cells take up these complexes. The liver and kidney are the two major organs in which cadmium accumulates. Its half-life in the body is longer than 10 years. Like blood levels of lead, blood levels of cadmium fall after acute exposure because of extensive tissue deposition. Once a threshold of renal deposition is exceeded, excess cadmium is excreted in urine. Cadmium intoxication produces irreversible proximal tubular dysfunction, hypercalciuria, nephrolithiasis, and metabolic bone disease with pain (called "ouch-ouch" disease in Japan).

Hyperuricemia

Hyperuricemia, especially in acutely treated myeloproliferative disease, can cause acute renal failure. Many patients with chronic renal failure have serum uric acid levels higher than 10 mg/dL, attributable to diminished glomerular filtration and the effects of diuretics. However, most studies have not demonstrated an independent association of hyperuricemia with chronic interstitial disease that could not otherwise be attributed to hypertension, vascular disease, calculi, or aging.

TREATMENT

Chronic interstitial nephritis tends to progress slowly. Inciting factors such as obstruction, infection, drugs, or toxins should be removed whenever possible. The treatment is similar to that of other causes of chronic renal failure. Angiotensin-converting enzyme inhibitors or angiotensin II receptor blockers (Table 67-7) are used early to slow disease progression, with a systolic blood pressure goal of 140 mm Hg (Chapters 67 and 130), except when hyperkalemia limits their use. Early treatment of acidosis with sodium bicarbonate, starting at 600 mg orally (PO) three times daily.[A1] Anemia is treated with erythropoiesis-stimulating agents (e.g., darbepoetin alfa 0.45 µg/kg weekly to keep the hemoglobin concentration between 10 and 12 g/L), hyperphosphatemia with oral phosphate binders (Table 119-4) and hyperparathyroidism with calcitriol (starting at 0.25 µg/day) can improve performance status and protect against bone loss (Chapters 130 and 131). There is no clear role for immunosuppressive drugs in the treatment of chronic interstitial nephritis, except perhaps in early sarcoidosis (Chapter 95).

For certain specific causes of chronic interstitial nephritis, specific therapeutic approaches are warranted. For analgesic nephropathy, stopping analgesic use can help reduce progression. For hypercalcemia (Chapter 245), therapy is directed toward the primary disease—reduction of the serum calcium concentration, when appropriate, and correction of acid-base disturbances.

Appropriate therapy for presumed cast nephropathy in multiple myeloma includes chemotherapy to ameliorate excess light chain production (Chapter 187); treatment of hypercalcemia (Chapter 245); alkalinization of the urine with the addition of bicarbonate to hypotonic fluids; and avoidance of radiocontrast agents, which may enhance the nephrotoxicity of light chains. Loop diuretics should be used with caution, particularly in the setting of volume depletion.

EDTA is advocated as chelation therapy for lead toxicity (Chapter 22). The goal of chelation is to normalize the EDTA mobilization test. In occasional patients, this may arrest or reverse the progression of the renal failure.

PROGNOSIS

The prognosis for chronic interstitial nephritis is highly variable and depends on the underlying condition and on comorbid conditions, including cardiovascular disease and diabetes mellitus, which become increasingly common in these patients over time.

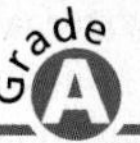

Grade A Reference

A1. de Brito-Ashurst I, Varagunam M, Raftery MJ, et al. Bicarbonate supplementation slows progression of CKD and improves nutritional status. *J Am Soc Nephrol.* 2009;20:2075-2084.

GENERAL REFERENCES

For the General References and other additional features, please visit Expert Consult at https://expertconsult.inkling.com.

123 OBSTRUCTIVE UROPATHY

MARK L. ZEIDEL

DEFINITION

Each day an average adult produces 1.5 to 2 L of urine, which must flow from the kidneys to the end of the urethra, a process that requires proper functioning of each renal pelvis, the ureters, bladder, and urethra. *Obstructive uropathy* occurs when a structural or functional defect in the urinary tract blocks or reduces urine flow. *Obstructive nephropathy* ensues when obstructive uropathy impairs renal function. Increased hydrostatic pressure from downstream obstruction may dilate upstream elements of the urinary tract, thereby causing *hydronephrosis.* Because recovery of renal function relates inversely to the duration and severity of the obstruction, prompt recognition and treatment of obstructive uropathy is essential for preserving renal function in this condition.

EPIDEMIOLOGY

Although there are few studies of unselected populations, in autopsy series hydronephrosis occurs at a rate of 3.1% in all subjects (2.9% in females, 3.3% in males). Autopsy in children younger than 16 years reveal hydronephrosis in 2.2% of boys and 1.5% of girls; 80% of hydronephrosis occurs in children younger than 12 months. In adults, hydronephrosis occurs with equal frequency in both sexes in those younger than 20 years, but owing to pregnancy and uterine cancer, it is more common in women than in men between the ages of 20 and 60 years. In individuals older than age 60 years of age, obstructive uropathy occurs more commonly in men because of prostate disease. The annual frequency of hospitalization for obstructive uropathy in the United States is 166 per 100,000. Each year, the 2000 or so patients who begin treatment for end-stage renal disease (ESRD) because of a presumed diagnosis of obstructive nephropathy represent approximately 2% of patients with ESRD. Among these patients, 4% are younger than 20 years of age, 44% are 20 to 64 years, and the others are older than 64 years.

PATHOBIOLOGY

Rhythmic, coordinated contractions of the renal pelvis "milk" urine from the renal papilla into the proximal end of the ureter. Peristaltic contractions of the ureter coordinate with periodic openings of the ureterovesical junction to propel the urine to the bladder. As the bladder fills, stretch is detected in its muscular wall and possibly its lining epithelium, the urothelium, thereby activating relaxation reflexes that suppress contraction of the bladder wall musculature and tighten the urethral sphincter to allow the bladder to expand without large increases in intravesicular pressure (E-Fig. 123-1; Chapter 26). When filling reaches a critical level, the relaxation reflex is suppressed and the voiding reflex is initiated. Suppression of detrusor muscle contraction ends and stimulation begins while the urethral sphincter is relaxed, leading to the buildup of pressure needed for voiding.

Obstructive uropathy results from functional or mechanical defects of the entire urinary tract. Functional failures include an inability to open the ureteropelvic or ureterovesical junction, failure to open the urethrovesical junction, or failure of bladder reflexes. Partial or complete mechanical blockade of the urinary tract at any level can lead to obstruction.

Functional or mechanical obstruction can occur at any point along the urinary tract from the renal pelvis and proximal urethra to the end of the urethra (phimosis). Because diagnosis and treatment depend heavily on the location of the obstruction, disorders are classified by anatomic location and whether the obstruction is due to factors within the urinary tract (intrinsic obstruction) or factors outside the tract (extrinsic obstruction) (Table 123-1). Intrinsic obstruction may be due to intraluminal or intramural causes. Intraluminal causes include stones or sludging of material, such as sloughed papillae or clots in papillary necrosis. Intramural causes may be anatomic (e.g., tumors or strictures) or functional (e.g., uncoordinated ureteral peristalsis or failure to open the ureteropelvic or ureterovesical junction). Extrinsic

TABLE 123-1 CAUSES OF URINARY TRACT OBSTRUCTION

INTRARENAL

Uric acid nephropathy
Sulfonamide precipitates
Acyclovir, indinavir precipitates
Multiple myeloma

URETERAL

Intrinsic

Intraluminal
- Nephrolithiasis
- Papillary necrosis
- Blood clots
- Fungus balls

Intramural
- Ureteropelvic junction dysfunction
- Ureterovesical junction dysfunction
- Ureteral valve, polyp, or tumor
- Ureteral stricture
  - Schistosomiasis
  - Tuberculosis
  - Scarring from instrumentation
  - Drugs (e.g., nonsteroidal anti-inflammatory agents)

Extrinsic

Vascular system
- Aneurysm: Abdominal aorta or iliac vessels
- Aberrant vessels: Ureteropelvic junction
- Venous: Retrocaval ureter

Gastrointestinal tract
- Crohn disease
- Diverticulitis
- Appendiceal abscess
- Colon cancer
- Pancreatic tumor, abscess, or cyst

Reproductive system
- Uterus: Pregnancy, prolapse, tumor, endometriosis
- Ovary: Abscess, tumor, ovarian remnants
- Gartner duct cyst, tubo-ovarian abscess

Retroperitoneal disease
- Retroperitoneal fibrosis: Radiation, drugs, idiopathic
- Inflammatory: Tuberculosis, sarcoidosis
- Hematoma
- Primary tumor (e.g., lymphoma, sarcoma)
- Metastatic tumor (e.g., cervix, ovarian, bladder, colon)
- Lymphocele
- Pelvic lipomatosis

BLADDER

Neurogenic bladder
- Diabetes mellitus
- Spinal cord defect
- Trauma
- Multiple sclerosis
- Stroke
- Parkinson disease
- Spinal anesthesia
- Anticholinergics

Bladder neck dysfunction
Bladder calculus
Bladder cancer

URETHRA

Urethral stricture
Prostate hypertrophy or cancer
Obstruction from instrumentation

causes of obstruction are grouped according to the organ system causing the obstruction.

Pathology and Pathophysiology

Acute obstruction of urine flow out of the nephron reversibly alters renal blood flow, glomerular filtration, and tubular function. Acute unilateral obstruction may cause minimal systemic clinical disturbance because, absent other disease, the contralateral kidney compensates for the loss of function in the affected kidney. Obstructive uropathy is most often partial and of prolonged duration; this chronic obstruction leads to fibrosis and permanent damage.

Because of ease of study in animal models, the pathophysiology of acute complete obstruction is better understood than is partial obstruction. In acute complete obstruction, glomerular filtration ceases and tubular transport is markedly reduced. Immediately after the onset of complete ureteral obstruction, blockage of urine flow markedly increases tubular intraluminal pressure, which is transmitted back to the glomerulus. Initial dilation of the afferent arteriole maintains glomerular filtration. However, local production of the potent vasoconstrictors angiotensin II and thromboxane A_2 soon decreases the renal blood flow, glomerular filtration pressure, and glomerular filtration rate (GFR). Angiotensin and thromboxane also contract glomerular mesangial cells, reducing the glomerular capillary bed surface area available for filtration. At the same time, prostaglandin E_2 and I_2 levels rise and attenuate the level of vasoconstriction.

Obstruction also shuts down the ability of renal tubules (including the proximal tubule, the medullary thick ascending limb of Henle, and the cortical and medullary collecting ducts) to absorb sodium, secrete potassium and acid, and concentrate and dilute the urine. Reduced tubular transport results from the local release of mediators, such as prostaglandin E_2, that inhibit transport, the local accumulation of macrophages, and the release of inflammatory mediators, as well as mechanisms intrinsic to tubular epithelial cells. When urine flow is halted or markedly slowed, reduced delivery of solutes to tubular cells slows the rate of apical sodium entry, resulting in reduced synthesis and deployment to the plasma membrane of crucial transporter proteins, such as Na^+, K^+-ATPase, and apical sodium entry pathways, such as the epithelial sodium channel and Na/K/Cl cotransporter. As obstruction becomes more prolonged, renal fibrosis and permanent damage ensue. In addition to attenuation of salt reabsorption, reduced solute reabsorption in the thick ascending limb leads to loss of high solute concentrations in the medullary interstitium. Obstruction also markedly reduces the synthesis and membrane trafficking of aquaporins, especially aquaporin 2. The combined impact of the absence of medullary solute accumulation and reduced aquaporin activity leads to an inability to concentrate and dilute the urine.

With bilateral complete obstruction, the loss of function of both kidneys leads to the accumulation of salt, water, and uremic toxins; acidosis; and hyperkalemia. Accumulation of salt and water leads to elevated levels of salt-wasting hormones, such as atrial natriuretic peptide, kinins, and prostaglandins, and reduced levels of salt-retaining hormones, such as angiotensin II, catecholamines, and aldosterone. If the kidneys have not been severely damaged by the obstruction, these hormonal changes act synergistically with the postobstructive state of the kidneys to enhance glomerular filtration and reduce tubular salt reabsorption after the obstruction is released.

Obstructive nephropathy markedly attenuates the ability of distal nephron segments to secrete potassium and acid, so it can lead to hyperkalemia (Chapter 117) and a non–anion gap metabolic acidosis (Chapter 118) in patients with chronic partial obstruction. With acidemia, failure to acidify the urine may be revealed by a high urine pH (>5.5) and a positive urine anion gap (urine sodium and potassium higher than urine chloride), which indicates distal nephron failure to excrete ammonium in urine. In elderly patients, especially those with azotemia, chronic partial obstruction is associated with hyporeninemic hypoaldosteronism. In this condition, hyperkalemia and non–anion gap metabolic acidosis result from a combination of inadequate aldosterone production for the level of potassium and blood pH and an inadequate tubular response to aldosterone secondary to tubular dysfunction.

Chronic partial urethral obstruction, such as that caused by prostatic hypertrophy in men, can lead to dilation and remodeling of the bladder. Under normal circumstances, as the bladder fills, stretch receptors in the bladder wall and possibly in the epithelium sense the filling. Signaling via afferents to brain stem centers transmits efferent impulses to inhibit bladder wall contraction, permitting the bladder to fill with a modest increase in hydrostatic pressure (see E-Fig. 123-1). These bladder-filling reflexes also tighten the internal urethral sphincter and allow the maintenance of continence without the need for voluntary contraction of the external sphincter. However, bladder filling to volumes of 200 to 300 mL in women and 300 to 400 mL in men activates additional stretch receptors, stimulating brain stem micturition centers (see E-Fig. 123-1). Efferents from these centers augment reflex contraction of the bladder detrusor musculature, relax the internal sphincter, and alert the cortex of the need to void. As the bladder fills further, the micturition reflex becomes stronger, the urge to void becomes uncomfortable and urgent, and the bladder begins to contract against the voluntary, external sphincter, rendering it difficult to maintain continence.

With chronic urethral obstruction, micturition requires higher contractile pressure, resulting in detrusor muscle hypertrophy. The bladder empties less completely, and residual volumes increase. Initially, retained urine owing to incomplete emptying diminishes the volume capacity of the bladder between micturitions, thereby resulting in frequency and nocturia. Over time, with bladder remodeling and changes in autonomic reflexes, the transition from bladder accommodation to the micturition reflex may be delayed and occur at increasingly higher bladder-filling volumes. When the micturition reflex is suddenly activated in patients whose bladders are dilated, urgency, dribbling, and frank incontinence ensue. Some of these same features occur in women with pelvic floor disturbances that impede normal bladder function. Bladder wall remodeling and elevated pressures on voiding may increase back pressure up the ureters and result in the physiologic changes of chronic obstruction, including diminished ability to acidify and concentrate the urine, as well as reduced glomerular filtration.

The renal response to the release of obstruction depends on several factors, including whether the obstruction is unilateral or bilateral and the extent and duration of the obstruction. Release of acute unilateral obstruction leads to gradual reversal of renal vasoconstriction and rapid recovery of the glomerular filtration rate. Because tubular transport mechanisms may still be inhibited, postobstructive salt wasting, inability to secrete potassium and acid, and inability to concentrate and dilute the urine persist and lead to the production of a high quantity of isosthenuric urine (urine with a tonicity similar to that of plasma) from the affected kidney. However, the normal contralateral kidney compensates for these abnormalities in tubular transport. Release of an acute bilateral obstruction can lead to high volumes of urine output and striking salt wasting.

CLINICAL MANIFESTATIONS

The clinical appearance of obstructive uropathy depends on the extent (partial or complete), duration (acute or chronic), and location of the obstruction, as well as on whether one or both kidneys are affected (Table 123-2). Patients may be asymptomatic even with severe obstruction, especially when the obstruction has developed gradually.

TABLE 123-2 CLINICAL MANIFESTATIONS AND LABORATORY FINDINGS IN URINARY TRACT OBSTRUCTION

No symptoms (chronic hydronephrosis)
Intermittent pain (chronic hydronephrosis)
Elevated levels of blood urea nitrogen and serum creatinine with no other symptoms (chronic hydronephrosis)
Renal colic (usually caused by ureteral stones or papillary necrosis)
Changes in urinary output
- Anuria or oliguria (acute renal failure)
- Polyuria (incomplete or partial obstruction)
- Fluctuating urinary output

Hematuria
Palpable masses
- Flank (hydronephrotic kidney, usually in infants)
- Suprapubic (distended bladder)

Hypertension
- Volume dependent (usually caused by chronic bilateral obstruction)
- Renin dependent (usually caused by acute unilateral obstruction)

Repeated urinary tract infections or infection refractory to treatment
Hyperkalemic, hyperchloremic acidosis (usually caused by defective tubular secretion of hydrogen and potassium)
Hypernatremia (seen in infants with partial obstruction and polyuria)
Polycythemia (increased renal production of erythropoietin)
Lower urinary tract symptoms: Hesitancy, urgency, incontinence, postvoid dribbling, decreased force and caliber of the urinary stream, nocturia

Symptoms

In patients with acute obstruction, bladder distention caused by the inability to relax the urethral sphincter (e.g., postoperatively) gives rise to sharp pain. By contrast, in the setting of gradual urethral obstruction, as can occur from prostatic enlargement (Chapter 129), the bladder may be able to fill to enormous volumes without causing significant pain.

Renal colic from the abrupt distention of the ureter is a common manifestation of the passage of a renal calculus (Chapter 126), with or without acute ureteral obstruction. Renal colic is a severe, stabbing pain localized to the flank (when the stone is in the upper third of the ureter) or radiating to the groin or pelvic structures (when the stone is located in the lower two thirds of the ureter).

Patients with chronic partial obstruction may have no symptoms or may have intermittent pain. Chronic partial ureteral obstruction may cause intermittent flank pain. Abdominal pain that radiates to the flank during voiding may indicate vesicoureteral reflux. Increasing the urine volume with the administration of fluid loads or diuretics may elicit pain in patients with partial obstruction by stretching the ureteral wall.

In patients with complete bilateral ureteral obstruction, complete obstruction of a solitary functioning kidney, or complete obstruction to urine flow beyond the bladder, anuric acute renal failure occurs. Patients with partial obstruction may have normal urine volumes or polyuria. In some cases, partial obstruction prevents urinary concentration, leading to polyuria, increased thirst, and sometimes hypernatremia. Although unusual, a history of oligoanuria alternating with polyuria or the sudden onset of anuria strongly suggests obstructive uropathy.

Bilateral complete obstruction or complete obstruction of a single functioning kidney may cause signs, symptoms, and laboratory evidence of acute renal failure (Chapter 120), with volume overload, hypertension, and metabolic disturbances. By contrast, unilateral obstruction with a functioning contralateral kidney usually does not lead to manifestations of renal failure because the functioning kidney may compensate in large part for the failure of filtration and tubular transport in the obstructed kidney. If the obstruction affects both kidneys, patients may have symptoms of impaired renal function, including nocturia and polyuria from failure to concentrate the urine and increased levels of potassium, phosphate, creatinine, and blood urea nitrogen (Chapter 120).

Given the complexity of bladder filling and emptying, a variety of disorders of these processes can lead to distressing lower urinary tract symptoms, such as incontinence (Chapter 26), urgency, frequency, and dysuria. These disorders, which include interstitial cystitis and urethral symptoms, are present in varying severity in 20 to 40% of adults over age 50 years.

Symptoms such as reduced force and caliber of the urine stream, urinary frequency, hesitancy, incontinence, nocturia, postvoid dribbling, and urgency often arise with urethral obstruction. Neurogenic bladder may alter micturition and result in frequency, urgency, and incontinence. Incontinence (Chapter 26) may occur because an inadequate sensation of bladder fullness or an inability to void properly leads to overfilling of the bladder and reflex emptying (overflow incontinence).

Physical Examination

In patients with acute ureteral obstruction, the physical examination may be normal or it may reveal flank tenderness. Flank tenderness can denote obstruction or pyelonephritis (Chapter 284). Renal colic may cause abdominal distention and evidence of reduced peristalsis with diminished bowel sounds. Kidneys enlarged by chronic hydronephrosis may be palpable on the abdominal examination or may cause costovertebral angle tenderness and flank rigidity. In patients with acute obstruction below the bladder, acute bladder distention may be detectable as a suprapubic mass, and the bladder may be tender. In the setting of bladder distention, the rectal examination in men may reveal prostatic enlargement, whereas the pelvic examination in women may reveal pelvic masses. Obstructive uropathy may cause hypertension owing to salt and water retention. Examination of the sensory and reflex pathways of the sacral nerves may reveal neurologic causes of urinary retention.

Laboratory Findings

Patients with obstruction may exhibit gross hematuria, especially in the setting of ureteral stones, which may abrade the urothelium and cause bleeding as they pass. Microscopic examination of the urine reveals round, regular red blood cells, which can be distinguished from the dysmorphic red blood cells that are typically seen in the hematuria of glomerular disease, in which red cells cross the glomerulus and remain in the tubules for a prolonged period. Gross hematuria from any cause may lead to clots, which themselves can cause obstruction.

A urinary tract infection in a younger man or repeated urinary tract infections in women without apparent cause suggest a structural lesion in the urinary tract (Chapter 128) and may be associated with partial or complete obstruction. Infection occurs more commonly in patients with obstruction involving the bladder or urethra, likely as a result of disruption of normal defenses against bacterial access and adherence to the bladder urothelium. The finding of unusual organisms (e.g., *Pseudomonas* or *Proteus* sp) in noninstrumented patients suggests the disruption of normal defense mechanisms and possible obstruction.

Depending on the extent and duration of obstruction, obstructive uropathy impairs renal function. Hyperkalemia and a nonanion acidosis, owing to distal renal tubular acidosis (Chapter 118), commonly develop. Chronic and more complete obstruction causes permanent renal damage and can lead to ESRD. Any patient with no previous history of kidney disease who has significant renal impairment should be evaluated for obstructive uropathy, especially if the urinary sediment is bland (Chapter 120). In addition, obstruction should be considered as a potential cause of accelerating deterioration of renal function in patients with underlying disease. In some obstructed kidneys, vasoconstriction may reduce cortical blood flow and oxygen tension, leading to increased erythropoietin production and polycythemia, which reverses with relief of the obstruction.

DIAGNOSIS

Because obstructive uropathy may be asymptomatic or may manifest in many different ways, the diagnosis may not be apparent. However, early diagnosis (Table 123-3) and prompt treatment reduce the extent of long-term renal damage.

Age, gender, and concomitant conditions often help identify the cause of obstruction. In children, congenital sources of obstruction at the ureteropelvic or ureterovesical junction are a major cause of ESRD. In adult women, complications of pregnancy or reproductive malignancies such as cervical or uterine cancer may cause obstruction resulting from compression of the ureters or ureterovesical junction. Infravesical obstruction explains less than 50% of lower urinary tract symptoms in men. In older men, prostatic hypertrophy (Chapter 129) or cancer (Chapter 201) often causes urethral obstruction.[1]

In outpatients, a history of renal colic, flank pain, or hematuria may suggest stone disease leading to ureteral obstruction. Changes in the volume or frequency of urination, including anuria, polyuria, or swings from oligoanuria to polyuria, may suggest obstruction. Bladder dysfunction is suggested by symptoms of frequency, urgency, and nocturia. In addition, a history of conditions that predispose to obstructive uropathy, such as sickle cell disease (Chapter 163), chronic ingestion of high levels of pain relievers (papillary necrosis; Chapter 125), previous stone disease (Chapter 126), or abdominal cancer (which may lead to ureteral obstruction), should raise the suspicion

TABLE 123-3 DIAGNOSTIC TESTS FOR OBSTRUCTIVE UROPATHY

UPPER URINARY TRACT OBSTRUCTION
Sonography (ultrasound)
Plain films of the abdomen (KUB)
Excretory or intravenous pyelography
Retrograde pyelography
Isotopic renography
Computed tomography
Magnetic resonance imaging
Pressure flow studies (Whitaker test)
LOWER URINARY TRACT OBSTRUCTION
Computed tomography
Magnetic resonance imaging
Cystoscopy
Voiding cystourethrography
Retrograde urethrography
Urodynamic tests
Cystometrography
Electromyography
Urethral pressure profile

From Klahr S. Obstructive uropathy. In: Jacobson HR, Striker GE, Klahr S, eds. *The Principles and Practice of Nephrology*. Toronto: BC Decker; 1991:432-441.
KUB = kidneys, ureter, bladder.

of obstruction. Finally, the presence of a single functioning kidney should raise the possibility that unilateral obstruction may be causing azotemia. In the inpatient setting, monitoring the pattern of urine output may reveal oligoanuria or polyuria.

Laboratory Studies

Initial laboratory evaluation includes a careful urinalysis and standard chemistry panel. The urine may reveal hematuria in the case of stones, bacteriuria and numerous granulocytes in the setting of obstruction or infection, or a urine pH greater than 7.5 in the case of chronic infection with urea-splitting organisms. Serum chemistries may reveal hyperkalemia, non–anion gap acidosis, and, more rarely, hypernatremia. Corresponding urine chemistry evaluation may reveal a pH higher than 5.5, lack of a negative anion gap (see earlier), and isosthenuria. The urine sediment also may reveal evidence of crystals (uric acid or calcium oxalate) that suggest stone disease. In addition, laboratory measurements should include blood urea nitrogen and creatinine levels to assess the adequacy of glomerular filtration.

DIAGNOSTIC TESTING

When obstructive uropathy is suspected, ultrasonography is the best screening modality because it is highly sensitive, safe, and inexpensive and does not expose the patient to contrast material or ionizing radiation. Because of its safety and low cost, ultrasonography is often used in patients with acute renal failure to exclude obstruction, although ultrasound performed in the absence of clinical suspicion of obstruction rarely finds a clinically significant obstructive nephropathy.[2] Ultrasound may reveal dilation of the calyces, renal pelvis, and, on occasion, proximal ureter (Fig. 123-1). It is also the preferred test to diagnose a renal calculus (see Fig. 126-2, Chapter 126). In patients with stones, measurement of the renal resistive index by bilateral color Doppler ultrasound can help predict which patients will progress to ureteral dilatation and obstruction.[3] False-positive findings (dilation in the absence of obstruction) occur in patients with congenital anomalies, during diuresis, and in many patients with ileal conduits. False-negative findings may occur because the pelvis and calyces fail to dilate despite obstruction, as may occur with retroperitoneal fibrosis or volume depletion. In such situations, the addition of color Doppler ultrasound can sometimes detect obstruction and its causes.[4] Because of the possibility of false-negative ultrasound results, computed tomography (CT) is warranted when the clinical setting strongly suggests obstruction and the ultrasound findings are negative. CT scanning may define the anatomic location of obstruction in patients found to have hydronephrosis on ultrasound, or it may identify obstruction in patients with negative ultrasound studies. In the setting of cancer or other structural lesions obstructing the ureters or invading the bladder, CT may help identify the cause of obstruction. CT, or in some centers magnetic resonance imaging (MRI), is the optimal method for diagnosing retroperitoneal fibrosis (Fig. 123-2), a rare condition that can cause partial or total bilateral ureteral obstruction.

Diffusion-weighted MRI can noninvasively detect changes in renal perfusion and in tissue density that occur during acute ureteral obstruction, and MRI is highly sensitive for detecting suspected obstructive uropathy.[5] However, the use of MRI is limited by the risk for nephrogenic systemic fibrosis in patients who are azotemic, especially if the glomerular filtration rate is below 30 mL/minute. Definitive diagnosis of the location of obstruction can be obtained by retrograde pyelography, in which contrast material is injected directly into the ureters via catheters inserted into the urethra and bladder, or by antegrade pyelography, in which the contrast material is injected into the renal pelvis via a percutaneous catheter. Retrograde pyelography is performed when obstruction has been diagnosed or is strongly suggested. This procedure precisely localizes the site of obstruction and guides the urologist in the placement of stents to clear the obstruction.

When bladder dysfunction or lesions in the bladder have been identified, retrograde cystograms may define bladder anatomy. In addition, cystometrography with urodynamic testing can define the force of detrusor function, determine whether the detrusor and sphincter act in a coordinated fashion (lack of coordination is referred to as *dyssynergy*), and define the extent to which pressure within the bladder is elevated and is causing obstruction to urine flow (Chapter 26).

DIFFERENTIAL DIAGNOSIS

Because obstructive uropathy may have subtle manifestations that mimic many other conditions, the differential diagnosis depends on the initial clinical symptoms and signs. Though suggestive of obstructive uropathy, anuria and acute renal failure (Chapter 120) may result from intrarenal diseases such

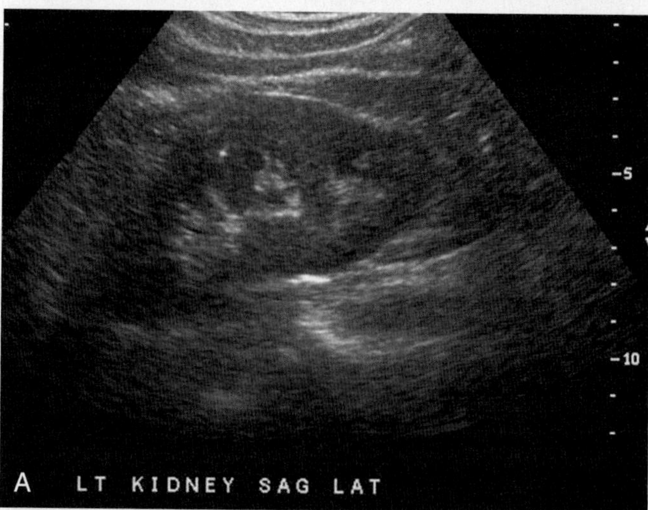

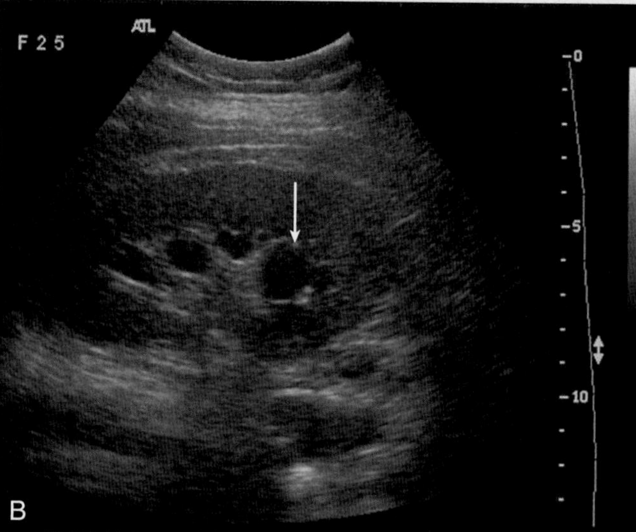

FIGURE 123-1. **A, Renal ultrasound of a normal kidney. The outline of the kidney is clearly seen, and the calyces (*darker areas*) are small and somewhat indistinct. B, Renal ultrasound of an obstructed kidney. The *arrow* points directly at a dilated renal calyx. Other dilated calyces are seen as large, round, dark areas adjacent to the calyx indicated by the *arrow*. For orientation, the tail end of the *arrow* overlies the margin of the renal cortex. (Courtesy Jonathan Kruskal, MD, PhD.)**

as glomerulonephritis or acute tubular necrosis. Patients with polyuria, hypernatremia, and dilute urine may have nephrogenic or central diabetes insipidus (Chapter 225). Obstructive uropathy is a rare cause of nephrogenic diabetes insipidus. Patients with hyperkalemic hyperchloremic metabolic acidosis may have hyporeninemic hypoaldosteronism, which is associated with chronic mild obstruction or other tubular disorders (Chapter 122). Renal colic may resemble abdominal pain secondary to diseases of the gastrointestinal or reproductive tract, such as appendicitis (Chapter 142) or an ovarian cyst, especially when the colic is associated with nausea, vomiting, and diaphoresis.

In some patients, the cause of disturbing lower urinary tract symptoms may be elusive. Men should be evaluated for prostatic disease (Chapter 129), and both men and women should be evaluated in terms of their bladder function (Chapter 26).[6]

TREATMENT Rx

Once obstructive nephropathy has been identified, therapy focuses on the rapid restoration of normal urine flow, treatment of any accompanying infection, and management of postobstructive complications. The degree to which renal function recovers depends on several factors, including the extent and duration of the obstruction and the extent of previous renal dysfunction.

Acute Obstruction

Complete obstruction causes acute renal failure. Because the extent and rate of recovery of renal function depend on the speed of relief, prompt

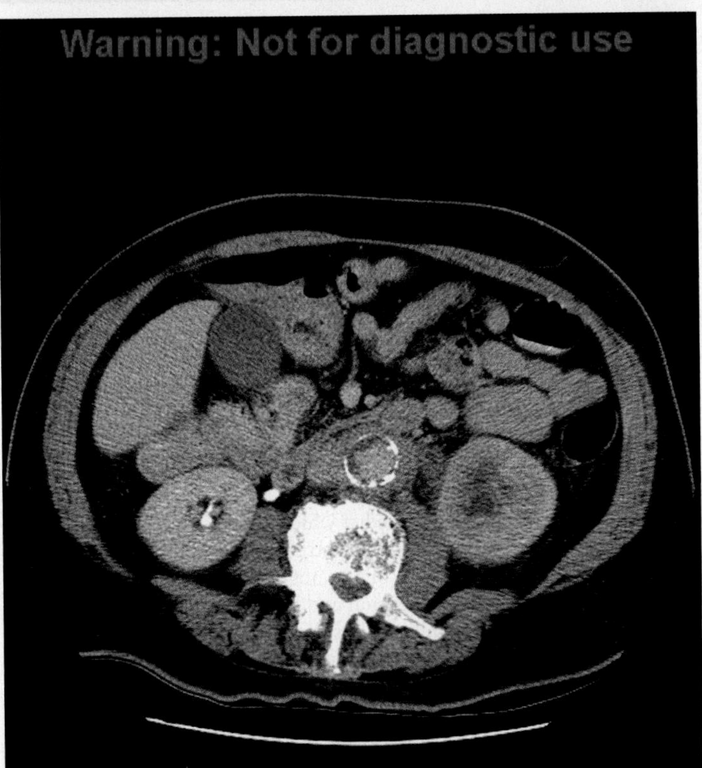

FIGURE 123-2. Contrast-enhanced axial computed tomography scan through the mid-abdomen, showing retroperitoneal fibrosis encircling the aorta and causing left-sided hydronephrosis owing to ureteral obstruction. (Courtesy of Jonathan Kruskal, MD, PhD.)

resolution of obstruction obviates the complications of uremia and the need for acute dialysis in patients with bilateral obstruction or obstruction of a single functioning kidney. In the setting of antecedent renal disease, partial obstruction may lead to permanent renal damage, so prompt relief can salvage significant renal function. In all cases of obstruction, the urine should be examined and cultured to identify and treat infections (Chapter 284). In patients with urinary sepsis and obstruction, the sepsis cannot be treated successfully until the obstruction is relieved; in such patients, it is also crucial to look for perinephric abscesses and drain them if present.

The site of the obstruction and its cause determine the therapeutic approach. Obstruction in the urethra or owing to bladder dysfunction may be relieved by placement of a urethral catheter. If catheters cannot be passed through the urethra, urgent suprapubic cystotomy is needed, followed by a more permanent approach, such as surgical diversion or ileal conduits, to prevent recurrent obstruction. If the obstruction is in the upper urinary tract, retrograde ureteral catheters with stents or nephrostomy tubes may be needed to relieve the obstruction. Retrograde catheters have the advantage that internal stents can be left in place to restore normal voiding, avoiding the need to maintain percutaneous drainage tubes.

Acute Obstruction Caused by Calculi

Calculi (Chapter 126) are the most common cause of ureteral obstruction. The cornerstones of therapy include analgesia, relief of the obstruction, and treatment of concomitant infections (Chapter 284). Stones 5 mm or less often pass without procedural intervention, but larger (7 to 15 mm) stones are more likely to cause complete obstruction and are progressively less likely to pass without intervention. If the stone is above the pelvic brim and is less than 15 mm, extracorporeal shock wave or ultrasonic lithotripsy is 90% effective, with passage of the fragments within 3 months. It is important to increase the volume of urine flow after these approaches to help the patient pass the fragments. For stones located below the pelvic brim or for larger stones, endoureteroscopy with direct removal may be performed via catheters passed through the urethra. In all patients with stone disease, it is crucial to identify the cause and initiate appropriate measures to prevent further stones (Chapter 126). The common practice of routinely placing a ureteral stent after ureteroscopy increases irritative lower urinary symptoms without any demonstrable clinical benefit.

Chronic Partial Obstruction

Although patients with chronic partial obstruction may do well for prolonged periods, the obstructive process should be relieved because it poses a long-term threat to renal function. Prompt relief is mandatory when partial obstruction progresses to frank urinary retention, the obstruction is accompanied by urinary sepsis or repeated urinary tract infections, the obstruction is causing renal damage, or the patient has symptoms such as voiding dysfunction, flank pain, or dysuria. Most often, chronic partial obstruction results from lesions in the lower urinary tract, including urethral blockage from prostate enlargement (Chapter 129). In men, benign prostatic hypertrophy, which may remain stable for long periods, usually responds to medications, but therapeutic decisions, including surgery, depend on symptoms, the presence of infection, and the risk for permanent bladder or renal dysfunction. The possibility of prostate cancer also must be considered (Chapter 201).

Idiopathic retroperitoneal fibrosis, which is an unusual cause of chronic ureteral obstruction, can progress to complete acute obstruction.[7] Treatment has not been definitively established, but prednisone (1 mg/kg/day tapered over 6 months), A1 has been shown to be effective in up to 90% of patients for avoiding or delaying interventional treatments.

Chronic obstruction at the bladder neck or urethra can lead to bladder dilation and remodeling, with attendant persistence of dysfunction and symptoms even after relief of the obstruction. On this basis, it may be appropriate to relieve the obstruction before infection, major symptoms, or renal dysfunction occurs. Urethral strictures can be treated by dilation or urethrotomy.[8]

Postobstructive Diuresis

Though usually self-limited, postobstructive diuresis can last several days to a week and may result in clinically important depletion of sodium, potassium, and chloride. Because postobstructive diuresis is prolonged and promoted by excessive fluid replacement, administration of volume is justified only when excessive losses result in clear volume depletion. Proper replacement is guided by measurement of urine chemistries and osmolality. Because the urine is generally isosthenuric, with relatively high sodium levels as a result of residual tubular dysfunction, appropriate replacement fluid is often 0.45% saline given at a rate somewhat slower than that of urine output. By careful monitoring of vital signs, volume status, urine output, and serum and urine chemistry and osmolality, coupled with judicious fluid replacement, the diuresis can be limited and will not cause serious volume or electrolyte abnormalities. As basic research continues to unravel the signaling mechanisms that induce fibrosis rather than repair in obstructed kidneys, new therapeutic approaches may be possible after obstruction.[9]

Lower Urinary Tract Symptoms

Because lower urinary tract symptoms in the absence of demonstrable obstruction, infection (Chapter 284), or prostatic disease (Chapter 129) are so poorly understood, therapy is empirical and often ineffective.[10] Options in men usually focus on treatments for prostatic hyperplasia.[11] For women, treatments tend to focus on bladder function (Chapter 26) and menopause-related changes in the urogenital tract (Chapter 240).[12]

PROGNOSIS

The recovery of renal function depends on the duration and completeness of the obstruction. If the obstruction involves only one kidney and the other kidney has relatively normal function, the preserved kidney will compensate for the loss of function in the obstructed kidney. If obstruction is of relatively short duration and is partial, renal function will likely improve, leaving the patient with no symptoms of renal failure. However, if obstruction is bilateral, complete, or near-complete and persists for a week or more, significant permanent renal damage ensues, particularly if renal function was impaired before the onset of obstruction. Vigorous postobstructive diuresis is associated with renal recovery, but it may take weeks for renal function to recover. Approximately 20% of patients may have persistent chronic renal failure, and 5 to 10%[13] may need chronic renal replacement therapy (Chapter 131). Patients with lower urinary tract symptoms of unknown cause often have persisting symptoms despite therapies aimed at prostatic or bladder disease.[14]

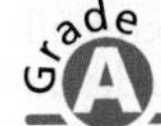

Grade A Reference

A1. Vaglio A, Palmisano A, Alberici F, et al. Prednisone versus tamoxifen in patients with idiopathic retroperitoneal fibrosis: an open-label randomised controlled trial. *Lancet.* 2011;378:338-346.

GENERAL REFERENCES

For the General References and other additional features, please visit Expert Consult at https://expertconsult.inkling.com.

124

DIABETES AND THE KIDNEY

RAYMOND C. HARRIS

EPIDEMIOLOGY

In the industrialized world, diabetes mellitus is the single leading cause of end-stage renal disease (ESRD). Despite the improved care of patients with diabetes, both the incidence and prevalence of ESRD secondary to diabetes continue to rise. In the United States, more than 30% of patients undergoing either dialytic therapy or renal transplantation have ESRD as a result of diabetic nephropathy, and 40% of the new (incident) cases of ESRD are attributable to diabetes. Currently, more than 200,000 patients receive ESRD care as a result of diabetic nephropathy.

In the United States, Europe, and Japan, more than 90% of patients with diabetes have type 2 rather than insulinopenic type 1 diabetes (Chapter 229). The incidence of renal disease is equivalent, and more than 80% of the ESRD secondary to diabetes is also seen in patients with type 2 diabetes. Although it was previously supposed that ESRD secondary to type 2 diabetes was less common than with type 1 diabetes, when cohorts of patients with type 1 and type 2 diabetes are monitored for an extended period, the degree of renal involvement is similar. The demographics of ESRD secondary to type 2 diabetes mirror the prevalence of type 2 diabetes in the U.S. population, with a higher incidence in women and in African Americans, Hispanic Americans, Native Americans, and Asian Americans and a peak incidence in the fifth to seventh decade. Much of the increased mortality in type 2 diabetes is associated with the prevalence of nephropathy.[1] Given the global epidemic of obesity in developed countries, an increasing incidence of diabetic nephropathy is being widely appreciated. Smoking and elevated blood cholesterol may be predisposing factors for the development of diabetic nephropathy in type 2 patients with diabetes.

PATHOBIOLOGY

Hyperglycemia

The metabolic sequelae of hyperglycemia appears to be the most important causative factor in the development of diabetic nephropathy. Hyperglycemia leads to increased generation of reactive oxygen species; depletion of the reduced form of nicotinamide dinucleotide (phosphate); activation of the polyol pathway, which can lead to de novo synthesis of diacylglycerol and increased protein kinase C activity; alterations in the hexosamine pathway; and nonenzymatic protein glycation (advanced glycosylation end products), all of which have been implicated in the development of diabetic nephropathy, as well as other diabetic microvasculopathies. Although this can be marked by individual variations, better glucose control generally reduces the risk of nephropathy and other microvascular complications. For example, in a cohort of patients who had glucokinase mutations, which are associated with milder hyperglycemia (average hemoglobin A_{1c} [HbA_{1c}] levels, 6.9%), they had far less proteinuria, microalbuminuria, or nephropathy than patients with long-standing type 2 diabetes with HbA_{1c} levels averaging 7.8%.[2] Furthermore, randomized interventional studies clearly demonstrate that relatively better control of blood sugar decreases the development of nephropathy in type 1 diabetes, and observational studies with repeat renal biopsies show that the renal lesions of diabetic nephropathy may reverse after long-term functioning pancreas transplantation.

Hemodynamics

Patients with type 1 and, to a lesser extent, type 2 diabetes exhibit an increased glomerular filtration rate (GFR), so-called hyperfiltration, that is mediated by proportionately greater relaxation of the afferent arteriole than the efferent arteriole. This hyperfiltration leads to increased glomerular blood flow and elevated glomerular capillary pressure. With poorly controlled diabetes, patients also develop glomerular hypertrophy, with an increased glomerular capillary surface area. These intraglomerular hemodynamic and structural alterations may contribute to the development or progression (or both) of diabetic renal injury. Because angiotensin-converting enzyme (ACE) inhibitors and decreased dietary protein reduce this elevated intraglomerular capillary pressure in experimental animals, the hyperfiltration hypothesis provides one rationale for the success of these interventions in resisting the progression of diabetic nephropathy (see later discussion).

Hormones and Cytokines

Studies in experimental animals have implicated a number of cytokines, hormones, and intracellular signaling pathways in either development or progression of diabetic nephropathy, notably transforming growth factor ß, connective tissue growth factor, angiotensin II, vascular endothelial growth factor, endothelin, prostaglandins, and nitric oxide. Because these factors have also been implicated in a variety of nondiabetic kidney diseases, it is likely that they will not prove to be specific for diabetic nephropathy. However, agents that interrupt angiotensin II production and signaling have proven to be very effective in slowing the progression of diabetic nephropathy. Furthermore, agents that interrupt intracellular pathways activated by these factors or by other consequences of hyperglycemia may provide future therapeutic opportunities.

Genetics

At present, it is not possible to predict which patients will develop diabetic nephropathy. Although poor glycemic and blood pressure control undoubtedly contribute, nephropathy may or may not develop in an individual patient even after many years of hypertension and hyperglycemia. Both type 1 and type 2 diabetes cluster in families. Those with type 1 diabetes with siblings who have diabetic nephropathy have a greater than 70% lifetime risk of diabetic nephropathy developing in themselves. Patients with type 2 diabetes also appear to have a hereditary predisposition for or against the development of diabetic nephropathy.

However, diabetic nephropathy is likely to be a polygenic disease, and its development and progression are likely related to the inheritance of multiple polymorphisms with variable effect sizes.[3] For example, African Americans with the apolipoprotein-1 gene do not have an increased predisposition to develop diabetic nephropathy, but nephropathy will have an accelerated progression in such patients.[4] In addition, the lack of nephropathy in patients with glucokinase mutations may be more pronounced than can be explained just by their relatively lower HgA_{1c} levels. Studies also suggest a long-term programming or memory effect in the development of diabetic kidney disease, such that patients whose type 1 diabetes was poorly controlled in the past will develop nephropathy at an increased rate despite subsequent excellent glycemic control. These findings suggest the possible role for epigenetic programming in the development of diabetic nephropathy.[5]

CLINICAL MANIFESTATIONS

Natural History

Although a minority of patients with diabetic nephropathy have type 1 diabetes, the natural history of the disease is best exemplified in this population because the onset of diabetes is more clearly definable and typically occurs at an early enough age to permit long-term follow-up. Furthermore, patients with type 1 diabetes usually do not initially have comorbid essential hypertension, atherosclerotic cardiovascular disease, obesity, and other conditions that are often associated with type 2 diabetes and that may independently produce chronic renal injury. However, the similarity of the nephropathic progressions in type 1 and 2 diabetes is exemplified by the Pima Indians, who exhibit a strong genetic predisposition for the development of type 2 diabetes by the fourth decade of life and in whom the diabetic nephropathy progresses in a similar pattern as seen in type 1 diabetic patients.

Diabetic nephropathy progresses through four relatively distinct stages (Fig. 124-1).

Stage I

In stage I, which commences soon after the overt manifestations of diabetes, renal blood flow and GFR increase by up to 50%, and the kidneys' glomeruli and tubules hypertrophy compared with age- and weight-matched normal control subjects. Although patients with type 2 diabetes also tend to have an elevated GFR during the early course of their disease, the GFR increases are not usually as pronounced as seen with insulin-dependent diabetes mellitus. At this stage, no macroalbuminuria is detectable, but transient microalbuminuria can occasionally be measured by radioimmunoassay, enzyme-linked immunosorbent assay, or special dipsticks, especially when induced by stress, physical exertion, concurrent illness, or poor glycemic control. Hypertension is usually absent in the early stages in patients with type 1 diabetes but is present in 10% to 25% of type 2 patients with diabetes at their initial evaluations.

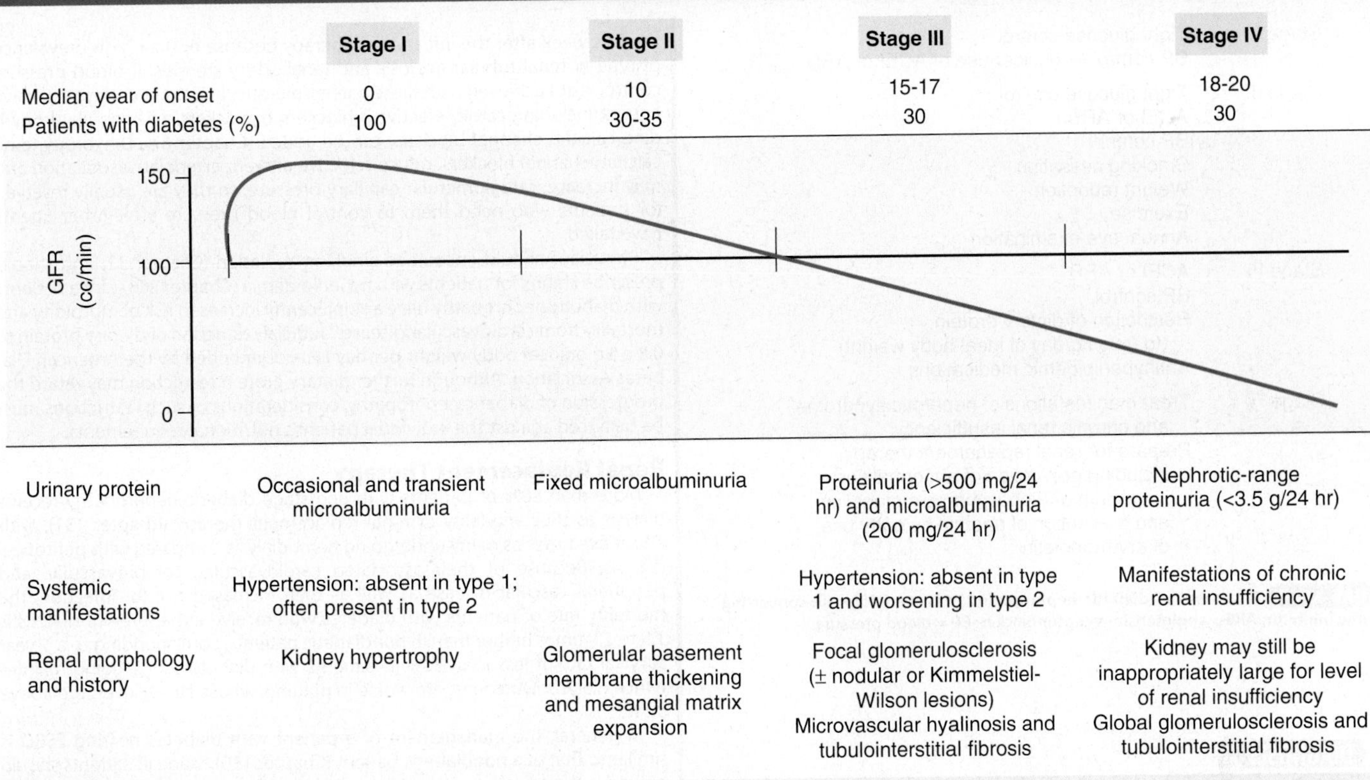

Stage I
Stage II
Stage III
Stage IV
Median year of onset
0
10
15-17
18-20
Patients with diabetes (%)
100
30-35
30
30
GFR (cc/min)
150
100
0
Urinary protein
Occasional and transient microalbuminuria
Fixed microalbuminuria
Proteinuria (>500 mg/24 hr) and microalbuminuria (200 mg/24 hr)
Nephrotic-range proteinuria (<3.5 g/24 hr)
Systemic manifestations
Hypertension: absent in type 1; often present in type 2
Hypertension: absent in type 1 and worsening in type 2
Manifestations of chronic renal insufficiency
Renal morphology and history
Kidney hypertrophy
Glomerular basement membrane thickening and mesangial matrix expansion
Focal glomerulosclerosis (± nodular or Kimmelstiel-Wilson lesions)
Microvascular hyalinosis and tubulointerstitial fibrosis
Kidney may still be inappropriately large for level of renal insufficiency
Global glomerulosclerosis and tubulointerstitial fibrosis

FIGURE 124-1. Stages of diabetic nephropathy. GFR = glomerular filtration rate.

Stage II

Approximately 30% of patients with type 1 diabetes progress to stage 2, which is characterized by fixed microalbuminuria of at least 30 mg/24 hr, after a median of about 10 years of diabetes. Although the GFR either remains elevated or is within the normal range at this stage, renal histology becomes abnormal and is manifested as glomerular and tubular basement membrane thickening and the inception of mesangial matrix expansion. Microalbuminuria is more likely in patients who have evidence of other microvascular insults, especially proliferative retinopathy. Microalbuminuria is a more specific sign of diabetic nephropathy in type 1 diabetes than in type 2 diabetes because of the high incidence of hypertension, which itself may lead to microalbuminuria, in the latter.

Stage III

The great majority of patients who are initially seen with fixed microalbuminuria progress to overt nephropathy (stage III) within 5 to 7 years. In this stage, patients have overt proteinuria (>500 mg of total protein per 24 hours) and macroalbuminuria (>200 mg/24 hr), which are detectable with a routine urinary protein dipstick. With the onset of stage III, estimated GFR (eGFR) is usually below normal levels for age and continues to decrease as the disease progresses. Blood pressure begins to rise in patients with type 1 diabetes with stage III nephropathy. In patients with type 2 diabetes, who frequently have preexistent hypertension, blood pressure commonly becomes more difficult to control.

Renal biopsy reveals diffuse or nodular (Kimmelstiel-Wilson) glomerulosclerosis. Although the Kimmelstiel-Wilson lesion is considered pathognomonic of advanced diabetic nephropathy, only approximately 25% of patients manifest this lesion. A nodular pattern of glomerulopathy mimicking Kimmelstiel-Wilson lesions may also be seen in light-chain nephropathy (Chapter 187), and historic descriptions of "diabetic nephropathy without overt hyperglycemia" based solely on light microscopic analysis actually may have represented light-chain disease. Nodular glomerular lesions can also be observed in amyloidosis (Chapter 188) and membranoproliferative glomerulonephritis type II (Chapter 121).

An additional pathognomonic feature of diabetic nephropathy is the finding of both afferent and efferent arteriolar hyalinosis, which can be distinguished from the isolated afferent arteriolar lesion of essential hypertension. In overt diabetic nephropathy, progressive tubulointerstitial fibrosis correlates most closely with the decline in renal function. The GFR begins to decline from the normal range, but the serum creatinine level may remain in the normal range.

Stage IV

Stage IV, or advanced diabetic nephropathy, is characterized by a relentless decline in renal function and progression to ESRD. Patients typically have heavy or nephrotic-range proteinuria (>3.5 g/24 hr) and systemic hypertension but have no evidence of inflammatory glomerular (red blood cell casts) or tubulointerstitial (white blood cells, white blood cell casts) lesions. The kidneys may be inappropriately large for the observed degree of renal insufficiency. However, a subset of patients with type 2 diabetes develops chronic kidney disease without nephrotic-range proteinuria. Whether this difference represents a fundamental difference in the pathophysiology of the two conditions or represents the synergistic effects of other kidney injuries, such as hypertensive renal disease, is unclear.

Other Renal Complications

Patients with diabetes also have an increased rate of other kidney and genitourinary abnormalities. Type IV (hyporeninemic, hypoaldosteronemic) metabolic acidosis (Chapter 118) with hyperkalemia is commonly encountered in patients with diabetes and mild to moderate renal insufficiency. These patients should be carefully monitored for the development of severe hyperkalemia (Chapter 117) in response to volume depletion or after the initiation of drugs that interfere with the renin-angiotensin system, such as ACE inhibitors, AT1 receptor blockers (ARBs), β-adrenergic blockers, both nonselective and selective cyclooxygenase-2 (COX-2) nonsteroidal anti-inflammatory agents, and heparin, as well as potassium-sparing diuretics.

Patients with diabetes have an increased incidence of bacterial and fungal infections of the genitourinary tract (Chapter 284). In addition to lower urinary tract infections, they have an increased risk for pyelonephritis and intrarenal and perinephric abscess formation (Chapter 284).

Unilateral or bilateral renal artery stenosis (Chapter 125) is more frequent in the type 2 diabetic population than in age-matched nondiabetic individuals and should be considered if a patient with diabetes has intractable hypertension or a rapidly rising serum creatinine level immediately after initiation of therapy with an ACE inhibitor or AT1 receptor blocker. Other causes of acute deterioration in renal function include papillary necrosis with ureteral obstruction owing to sloughing of a papilla, obstructive uropathy (Chapter 123) caused by bladder dysfunction as a result of autonomic neuropathy, and contrast media–induced acute tubular necrosis (Chapter 120). In addition, prerenal azotemia or acute tubular necrosis may develop in patients with diabetes as a result of heart failure or volume depletion owing to vomiting induced by gastroparesis (Chapter 229) or diarrhea from autonomic neuropathy.

Stage I	Tight glucose control BP control—consider use of ACEI or ARB
Stage II	Tight glucose control ACEI or ARB BP control Smoking cessation Weight reduction Exercise Annual eye examination
Stage III	ACEI or ARB BP control Restriction of dietary protein (to 0.8g/kg/day of ideal body weight) Antihyperlipidemic medications
Stage IV	Treat manifestations of nephrotic syndrome and chronic renal insufficiency Prepare for renal replacement therapy, including prevention of abnormalities in calcium and phosphorus metabolism and prevention of anemia by early use of erythropoietin

FIGURE 124-2. Treatment of diabetic nephropathy. ACEI = angiotensin-converting enzyme inhibitor; ARB = angiotensin-receptor blocker; BP = blood pressure.

DIAGNOSIS

The diagnosis of overt diabetic nephropathy is made by three main criteria: the presence of proteinuria within an appropriate time frame, the presence of retinopathy (found in 90%-95% of patients with type 1 diabetes and in 60%-65% of patients with type 2 diabetes), and the absence of other causes of nephrotic syndrome or renal insufficiency. For patients with type 1 diabetes who develop diabetic nephropathy, significant proteinuria is seen within 17 ± 6 years of the onset of diabetes. Although microalbuminuria does not always progress to overt proteinuria in these patients, it always precedes overt proteinuria in patients who do progress. The American Diabetes Association recommends screening all patients with type 1 diabetes for microalbuminuria 5 years after the diagnosis and yearly thereafter. For patients with type 2 diabetes, the recommendation is screening for microalbuminuria at the time of diagnosis and yearly thereafter.

PREVENTION AND TREATMENT

Rx

Glycemic control significantly lessens the incidence of nephropathy in patients with type 1 diabetes for at least 20 or more years[A1] but does not completely eliminate the risk (Fig. 124-2). However, tight glycemic control to reduce to a $HgBA_{1c}$ target level of 6.5% or less in patients with type 2 diabetes does not reduce the risk of nephropathy compared with standard therapy to a goal of 7% to 7.9%.[A2][A3]

Elevated blood pressure is an important risk factor in the progression of diabetic nephropathy, and it was previously believed that blood pressure goals should be lower than for the general population. However, recent studies have shown detrimental effects of low blood pressures in patients with diabetic nephropathy, and more moderate blood pressure control with systolic blood pressures of 130 to 140 mm Hg is advocated.[A4]

In latent (stage II) and overt (stage III) diabetic nephropathy, renal function declines. With declining renal function, oral hypoglycemic agents become contraindicated. Because of the increased risk of prolonged hypoglycemia, sulfonylureas are contraindicated in patients with eGFRs less than 45 mL/min. Because of the potentially increased risk of lactic acidosis with metformin therapy in patients with renal insufficiency, treatment guidelines currently recommend it be avoided in patients with a serum creatinine level greater than 1.7 mg/dl, although this strict guideline is currently debated and may be changed in the future. As GFR declines, insulin requirements may decrease owing to reduced insulin degradation and clearance by the failing kidney.

Medications that interfere with the renin–angiotensin system, either ACE inhibitors or ARBs, are the preferred agents and appear to have additional benefits beyond lowering systemic blood pressure.[A5][A6] However, combination therapy using both an ACE inhibitor and an ARB is contraindicated because of increased side effects.[A7]

Patients whose diabetic nephropathy is treated with ACE inhibitors or ARBs should have their serum potassium and creatinine levels monitored closely in the first week after the initiation of therapy because of their high prevalence of type IV renal tubular acidosis and renal artery stenosis. If blood pressure control is not achieved with these agents, diuretics and other antihypertensive agents, including cardioselective β-blockers, α-blockers, and nondihydropyridine calcium channel blockers, can be added (Chapter 67). Dihydropyridine calcium channel blockers induce selective afferent arteriolar vasodilation and may increase intraglomerular capillary pressure, so they are usually reserved for patients who need them to control blood pressure after other agents have failed.

Physicians should encourage smoking cessation (Chapter 32) and should prescribe statins for patients with hyperlipidemia (Chapter 206), since patients with diabetic nephropathy have a significantly increased risk of morbidity and mortality from cardiovascular disease.[6] Judicial restriction of dietary protein to 0.8 g/kg of ideal body weight per day is recommended by the American Diabetes Association. Although further dietary protein restriction may retard the progression of diabetic nephropathy, considerations of such restrictions must be balanced against the individual patient's nutritional requirements.

Renal Replacement Therapy

More than 80% of patients with end-stage diabetic nephropathy receive dialysis as their modality of renal replacement therapy (Chapter 131), with about five times as many undergoing hemodialysis compared with peritoneal dialysis. Because of their associated cardiovascular, cerebrovascular, and peripheral vascular disease as well as their increased risk for infection, the mortality rate of patients with diabetes who receive either type of dialysis is 1.5 to 2.0 times higher than in nondiabetic patients, corresponding to a 5-year survival rate of less than 20% in patients with diabetes undergoing maintenance dialysis. Outcomes are worse in patients whose HbA_{1c} levels are above 8.5%.[7]

In general, the management of a patient with diabetes nearing ESRD is similar to that of a nondiabetic patient (Chapter 130). Stage III patients should be under the care of a nephrologist, and planning should be initiated for the modality of dialysis. Although dialysis is generally initiated when the GFR declines to less than 10 mL/min, earlier initiation of dialysis is sometimes necessary in patient with diabetes because their volume-dependent hypertension or hyperkalemia is not otherwise manageable or when their uremia and gastroparesis lead to malnutrition or uncontrollable recurrent emesis.

Approximately 25% of renal transplants performed in the United States are in patient with diabetes, and more than 90% of these are in patient with type 1 diabetes because of their younger age and lesser degrees of macrovascular comorbidity. Long-term survival and quality of life are generally superior after transplantation compared with chronic dialysis. However, the other microvascular complications (retinopathy, neuropathy) are not improved by renal transplantation alone. Pancreas and combined kidney and pancreas transplantation can significantly improve the quality of life of patients with diabetic nephropathy by improving autonomic neuropathy, retarding or possibly correcting retinopathy, and avoiding the potential complications of insulin administration. However, all transplantation options remain limited by organ availability.

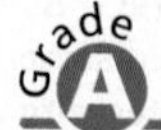

Grade A References

A1. de Boer IH, Sun W, Cleary PA, et al. Intensive diabetes therapy and glomerular filtration rate in type 1 diabetes. *N Engl J Med.* 2011;365:2366-2376.

A2. Gerstein HC, Miller ME, Byington RP, et al. Effects of intensive glucose lowering in type 2 diabetes. *N Engl J Med.* 2008;358:2545-2559.

A3. Patel A, MacMahon S, Chalmers J, et al. Intensive blood glucose control and vascular outcomes in patients with type 2 diabetes. *N Engl J Med.* 2008;358:2560-2572.

A4. Cushman WC, Evans GW, Byington RP, et al. Effects of intensive blood-pressure control in type 2 diabetes mellitus. *N Engl J Med.* 2010;362:1575-1585.

A5. Lv J, Perkovic V, Foote CV, et al. Antihypertensive agents for preventing diabetic kidney disease. *Cochrane Database Syst Rev.* 2012;12:CD004136.

A6. Wu HY, Huang JW, Lin HJ, et al. Comparative effectiveness of renin-angiotensin system blockers and other antihypertensive drugs in patients with diabetes: systematic review and bayesian network meta-analysis. *BMJ.* 2013;347:f6008.

A7. Fried LF, Emanuele N, Zhang JH, et al. Combined angiotensin inhibition for the treatment of diabetic nephropathy. *N Engl J Med.* 2013;369:1892-1903.

GENERAL REFERENCES

For the General References and other additional features, please visit Expert Consult at https://expertconsult.inkling.com.

125

VASCULAR DISORDERS OF THE KIDNEY

THOMAS D. DUBOSE, JR., AND RENATO M. SANTOS

Vascular disorders that significantly alter renal perfusion can impact the glomerular filtration rate (GFR); tubular function; and, ultimately, kidney function. Stenosis, thrombosis, emboli, atherosclerosis, inflammation, and hypertension may involve the renal arteries, arterioles, microvasculature, and renal veins.

RENAL ARTERY STENOSIS

DEFINITION

Renal artery stenosis is the prototype for secondary hypertension. It is defined as narrowing of the renal arteries, resulting in hypoperfusion of one or both kidneys. The two most common forms are atherosclerotic disease and fibromuscular dysplasia, but other causes include vasculitis (Chapter 270), neurofibromatosis (Chapter 417), congenital bands, extrinsic compression, and radiation injury (Chapter 20).

EPIDEMIOLOGY

The prevalence of renal artery stenosis is estimated to be about 2% in the fifth decade of life rising to 20% to 25% in the ninth decade. The prevalence may be somewhat higher in African Americans and Latinos compared with whites.

An estimated 2% of all patients with systemic hypertension (Chapter 67) have renal artery stenosis,[1] although the prevalence is much higher in patients whose hypertension is resistant to multiple medications.[2] Atherosclerotic disease, which is the most common form of renal artery stenosis, accounts for approximately 90% of all lesions. As with other forms of atherosclerosis, it is more common in elderly adults and in patients with cardiovascular risk factors such as hypertension, hyperlipidemia, smoking, and diabetes (Chapter 229). It is also more common in patients with heart failure (Chapter 58), multivessel coronary disease (Chapter 71), and peripheral vascular disease (Chapters 79 and 80).

In contrast, fibromuscular dysplasia is more common in young patients, with 90% of cases occurring in women at a mean age of 52 years at diagnosis.[3] Its true prevalence is unknown, but in one study of more than 2500 individuals evaluated as possible kidney donors by renal computed tomography angiography (CTA), the prevalence was 26%, 31% of whom had previously diagnosed hypertension.[4] It is an important cause of treatable hypertension in young patients without cardiovascular risk factors and is pathologically and angiographically distinct from atherosclerotic disease. The cause remains unknown, but genetic, hormonal, and mechanical factors may predispose to this disorder.

PATHOBIOLOGY

The pathobioloy of atherosclerotic renal artery stenosis is identical to that of atherosclerotic disease in other arterial beds (Chapter 70). Fibromuscular dysplasia, by contrast, includes four distinct histopathologic types: medial fibroplasia, which is the most common type and accounts for 75% to 80% of cases; perimedial fibroplasia, with irregular thickening of the media; medial hyperplasia, with smooth muscle hyperplasia without fibrosis; and intimal fibroplasia. Unlike atherosclerotic disease, which localizes at ostial and proximal segments of the renal arteries, fibromuscular dysplasia more commonly involves the middle and distal arterial segments.

The renal hypoperfusion caused by renal artery stenosis activates the renin–angiotensin–aldosterone system (RAAS) and results in an increase in systemic blood pressure. This mechanism explains the ability of angiotensin-converting enzyme (ACE) inhibitors and angiotensin receptor blockers (ARBs) to control the resulting hypertension in animal models and in patients with fibromuscular dysplasia. Although hypoperfusion-stimulated activation of the RAAS is essential for initiating the pressor response, this effect is transient. Over time, the pathophysiology of atherosclerotic disease transitions to pressor mechanisms independent of the RAAS, including vasoconstriction from oxidative stress, endothelial dysfunction, endothelin release, and sympathetic activation. Confounding risks—including smoking, advanced age, dyslipidemia, diabetes, and hypertension—can also contribute to vascular injury. This activation of inflammatory pathways combined with typical atherosclerotic risk factors contribute to chronic pressor mechanisms that may not respond to revascularization.

Ischemic nephropathy, which is defined as impairment of renal function beyond the decrease in perfusion typical of hemodynamically significant renal artery stenosis, is difficult to assess. Unlike cardiac or cerebral tissue, perfusion to the kidneys is primarily determined by glomerular ultrafiltration and exceeds its own metabolic needs by more than 10-fold. Therefore, a severe reduction in perfusion to the entire renal parenchyma is necessary to cause kidney injury. This relationship is supported by the observation that hemodynamically significant lesions of the fibromuscular dysplasia are rarely associated with renal dysfunction. Conversely, a decline in kidney function that is common in atherosclerotic renal artery stenosis may be caused in part by atherogenic stimuli, which can magnify oxidative stress and activate pro-inflammatory and profibrogenic pathways. Repetitive bouts of hypoperfusion in atherosclerotic disease may lead to renal tubular injury and, over time, can lead to tubulointerstitial fibrosis. Thus, a combination of repetitive perfusion insults superimposed on atherogenic risk factors, not hypoperfusion alone, likely explains renal dysfunction.

CLINICAL MANIFESTATIONS AND DIAGNOSIS

The clinical features of renal artery stenosis are related primarily to renovascular hypertension and ischemic nephropathy. Patients typically present with resistant hypertension unresponsive to high doses of multiple antihypertensive agents.

Patients with fibromuscular dysplasia often complain of headache and pulsatile tinnitus. Fibromuscular dysplasia should be suspected in young patients, especially young women, who have a recent onset of hypertension without other cardiac risk factors or a family history of hypertension. Because patients with fibromuscular dysplasia often benefit from renal artery revascularization, renal Doppler ultrasonography, which is the preferred screening test in these patients, is recommended. If the renal artery ultrasonography suggests significant renal artery stenosis, then renal angiography (Fig. 125-1) should be considered.

In patients at risk for atherosclerotic renal artery stenosis, any enthusiasm for making the diagnosis must be tempered by the lack of efficacy of renal artery revascularization for reducing blood pressure or improving outcomes

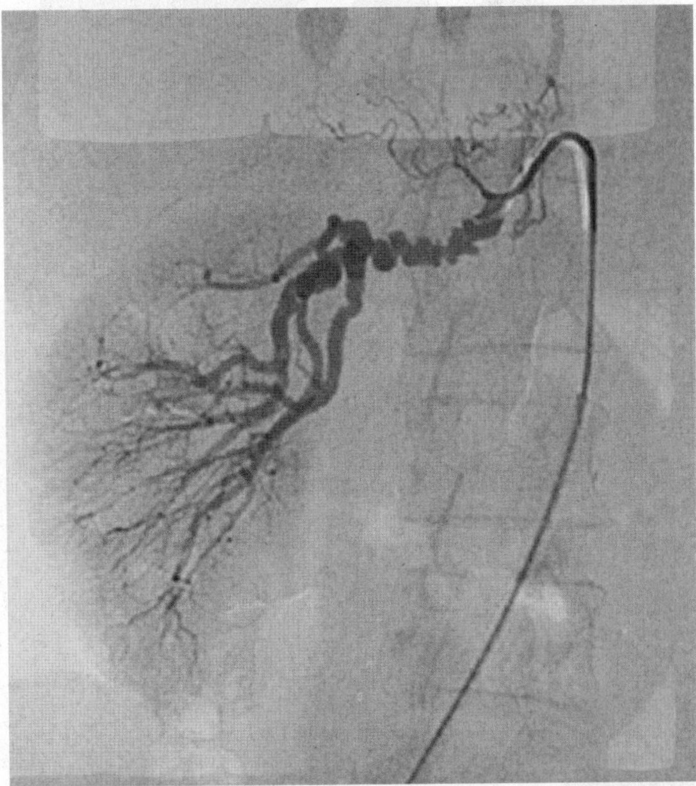

FIGURE 125-1. Selective right renal arteriogram demonstrating fibromuscular dysplasia. Typical features of medial form of fibromuscular dysplasia are illustrated by the "beads on a string" appearance.

(Chapter 67). For the small subgroup of patients whose atherosclerotic vascular artery stenosis may benefit from revascularization (see later), screening by renal Doppler or magnetic resonance angiography (MRA) is reasonable (Fig. 125-2). MRA requires gadolinium enhancement, which may precipitate a rare but severe condition called nephrogenic systemic fibrosis (Chapter 267), particularly when the linear gadolinium chelate gadodiamide is used in patients with advanced chronic kidney disease or acute kidney injury. Gadolinium is contraindicated if the estimated GFR is less than 30 mL/min. The risk of nephrogenic systemic fibrosis limits the applicability of gadolinium-enhanced MRA for patients with advanced renal dysfunction, but these patients are also less likely to benefit from renal revascularization. CTA of the renal artery may be required in some cases, but it has the disadvantages of requiring iodinated contrast as well as exposure to ionizing radiation. Digital subtraction angiography is used when revascularization is planned (Fig. 125-3). Although the complication rates are low, the usual risks of catheterization should be considered, including access site trauma, contrast reactions, contrast nephropathy (Chapter 57), and atheroembolic renal disease (Chapter 29).

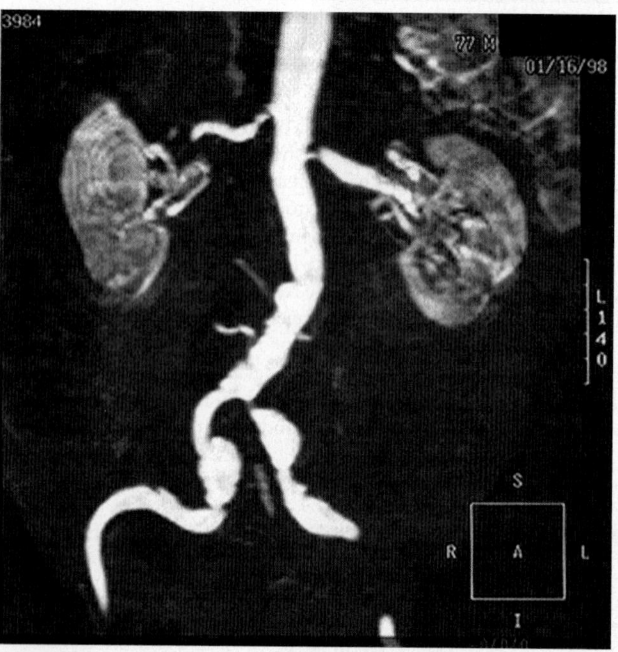

FIGURE 125-2. Magnetic resonance angiogram of the abdominal aorta showing bilateral renal artery stenosis. Significant iliac stenosis is also demonstrated.

TREATMENT

Rx

In patients with fibromuscular dysplasia, balloon angioplasty is the treatment of choice[5] because the stenosis can progress to renal artery occlusion despite adequate blood pressure control (Video 125-1). Stenting is rarely needed, and restenosis rates are generally low. Close follow-up with serial blood pressure measurements and evaluation of renal function should be performed every 3 to 4 months.

By comparison, routine renal artery revascularization is no longer recommended even for patients with severe atherosclerotic renal artery stenosis[A1-A3] because medical therapy, especially with an ACE inhibitor or ARB, is superior to revascularization. Atherosclerotic renal artery stenosis should be viewed as a biologic marker of cardiovascular disease and cardiac morbidity. The goals of therapy are to control blood pressure, stabilize renal function, and reduce cardiovascular complications. Efforts to optimize medical therapy for secondary prevention include aspirin (81 mg/day), statins to treat dyslipidemia (Chapter 206), management of diabetes (Chapter 229), and control of blood pressure (Chapter 67). Medical therapy for blood pressure control should include ACE inhibitors or ARBs because of their proven benefit in renal protection. Although both ACE inhibitors and ARB therapy are usually well tolerated, the serum creatinine and estimated GFR must be monitored carefully during the first weeks after their initiation, particularly in elderly patients. An increase of 1.0 mg/dL or more in the serum creatinine level suggests significant bilateral renal artery stenosis, renal artery stenosis in a unilateral functional kidney, or renal artery stenosis in the kidney transplant allograft. This complication, which arises as a result of inhibition of autoregulation, is an absolute indication to discontinue ACE inhibitor or ARB therapy. Smoking cessation, weight control, and increased exercise should be universally recommended.

In selected circumstances, renal artery intervention may be considered for patients whose atherosclerotic renal artery stenosis is associated with recurrent episodes of pulmonary edema that cannot be explained by cardiac lesions, particularly if left ventricular function is preserved.[6] Revascularization may also be considered for acute reversible renal dysfunction associated with an ACE inhibitor or ARB therapy. Finally, critical bilateral renal artery stenosis or stenosis in a single functioning kidney may be an indication for intervention. Procedures should be performed at high-volume centers with capability for digital subtraction angiography and experienced operators to minimize the risk of contrast-induced nephropathy.

PROGNOSIS

When adjusted for baseline variables, atherosclerotic renal artery stenosis remains an independent predictor of cardiovascular mortality, with a 4-year adjusted mortality rate of 25% to 40%. Factors associated with higher mortality rates include an elevated baseline serum creatinine level, more severe renal artery stenosis, worsening renal function, age, advanced diabetes, other cardiovascular disease, and heart failure. Improvement of blood pressure control or renal function after revascularization is associated with improved survival even though revascularization does not affect overall survival.

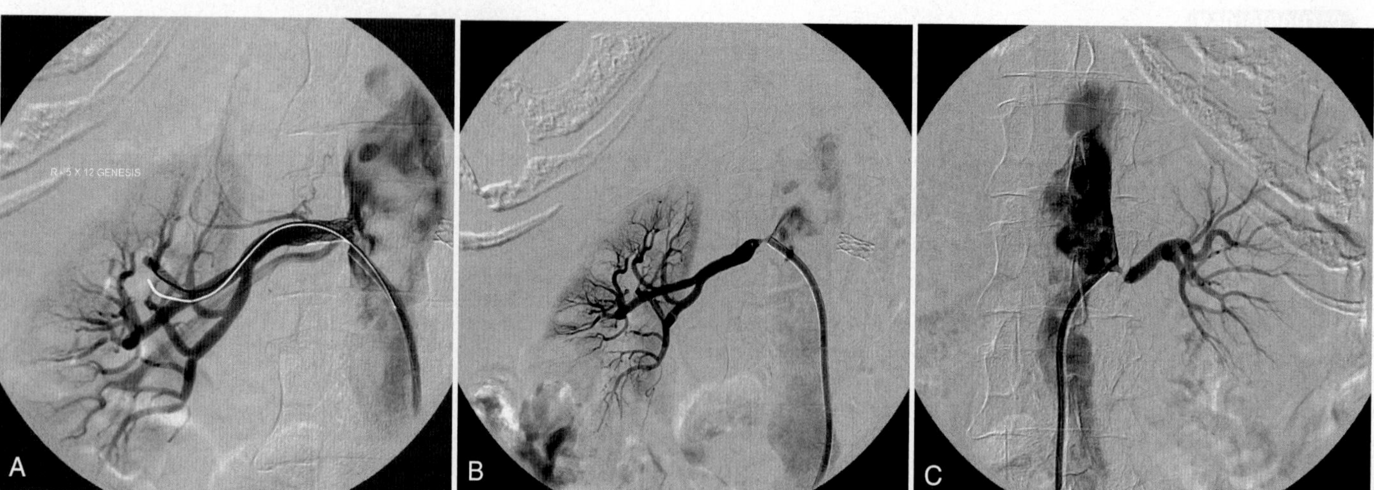

FIGURE 125-3. **Renal angiograms from an elderly patient with heart failure.** Cardiac catheterization revealed normal coronary arteries, but after initiation of therapy with an angiotensin-converting enzyme inhibitor and spironolactone, progressive kidney disease with hyperkalemia and poor blood pressure control ensued. Renal Doppler ultrasonography suggested bilateral renal artery stenosis, as confirmed by angiography (**A** and **B**). The patient underwent successful percutaneous revascularization in stages, leading to a return to normal left ventricular function and improved blood pressure control (**C**).

For fibromuscular dysplasia, angioplasty corrects the hypertension in approximately 45% of patients.[7] Younger age, milder hypertension, and shorter duration of hypertension are associated with successful outcomes. An atrophic kidney (<8 cm), however, is unlikely to recover with revascularization.

THROMBOEMBOLIC OCCLUSION OF THE RENAL ARTERIES

EPIDEMIOLOGY AND PATHOBIOLOGY

Acute occlusion of the renal arteries and segmental branches may arise as a result of intrinsic pathology of the renal arteries, abdominal trauma, or embolization of thrombi arising in the heart or proximal aorta. Thrombosis can occur as a complication of progressive atherosclerosis, in which case it may be an important cause of progressive renal insufficiency. In other patients, thrombosis may be associated with thrombophilic states (Chapter 176), such as the antiphospholipid antibody syndrome. Thrombosis also may occur as a consequence of inflammatory disorders, including Takayasu arteritis (Chapter 78); syphilis (Chapter 319); thromboangiitis obliterans (Chapter 80); and systemic vasculitides, especially granulomatosis with polyangiitis (Chapter 270). It has also been reported after infliximab infusions. In situ thrombosis has been observed in structural lesions of the renal arteries, such as fibromuscular dysplasia or renal artery aneurysms. In patients younger than 60 years, traumatic thrombosis is the most common cause. Blunt trauma and deceleration injuries can cause acute thrombosis as a result of intimal tears, contusion against the vertebral column, or compression from a retroperitoneal hematoma. Iatrogenic causes include diagnostic angiography or arterial intervention in the renal arteries or vessels proximal to the kidneys.

Embolization, which is a more common cause of renal artery occlusion than in situ thrombosis, is generally unilateral but is bilateral in 15% to 30% of cases. Total infarction of the kidney is much less common than segmental infarction or ischemia. Approximately 90% of thromboemboli to the renal arteries originate in the heart. Atrial fibrillation with embolization of atrial thrombus is the most common cause (Chapter 64), but left ventricular thrombus (Chapter 73), valvular heart disease (Chapter 75), bacterial endocarditis (Chapter 76), nonbacterial (aseptic) endocarditis (Chapter 76), and atrial myxoma (Chapter 60) are other instigators. Noncardiac sources include aortic atheroma (Chapter 78) and mural thrombus, as well as paradoxical emboli through an atrial septal defect or patent foramen ovale (Chapter 69).

CLINICAL MANIFESTATIONS

The clinical presentation of a renal infarction can be variable, and the diagnosis is often confused with more common disorders such as renal colic or pyelonephritis. Occlusion of a primary or secondary branch of the renal artery in a patient with preexisting disease and established collateral circulation, such as in long-standing renal artery stenosis, may produce little or no infarction and minimal symptoms. Acute thrombosis and infarction may cause a sudden onset of flank pain, fever, nausea, vomiting, and, on occasion, hematuria. Pain may be localized to the abdomen, back, or even the chest, but pain is absent in more than 50% of cases. Hypertension, which occurs with infarction, is a result of the release of renin from the ischemic renal parenchyma and may be severe.

Anuria suggests bilateral involvement or occlusion of the artery to a solitary kidney. Urinalysis usually, but not always, reveals microscopic hematuria, and mild proteinuria may be present.

If infarction occurs, leukocytosis usually develops, and serum enzyme levels of aspartate aminotransferase, lactate dehydrogenase (LDH), and alkaline phosphatase may be elevated. These laboratory findings are nonspecific, but elevation of the urinary LDH level is more specific because its concentration should be normal in extrarenal disorders. Blood urea nitrogen and creatinine levels typically increase transiently with unilateral infarction, but more severe and protracted renal dysfunction may follow bilateral renal infarction or infarction of a solitary kidney.

DIAGNOSIS

The diagnosis of renal artery occlusion is most reliably established by computed tomography (CT), with and without contrast. CT is accurate, can be performed rapidly, and can identify associated traumatic injury. Findings may include filling defects in the main or segmental renal arteries, as well as the absence of enhancement of renal tissue, indicating a lack of perfusion (Fig. 125-4). The complication of contrast nephropathy is a major concern in patients with a creatinine level of 2.0 mg/dL or greater or an estimated GFR less than 60 mL/m. Alternatives to contrast administration should always be considered in patients with chronic kidney disease, acute renal failure, or diabetes mellitus and in elderly patients. MRA has a high diagnostic accuracy and may be preferable to contrast CT in elderly patients and in patients with diabetes mellitus, although it is contraindicated in patients with renal insufficiency. Radioisotope renograms, excretion urograms, and duplex ultrasound scanning are not recommended for the diagnosis of acute occlusions. Invasive angiography carries inherent risks but is occasionally required if the diagnosis remains uncertain or if percutaneous reperfusion is considered.

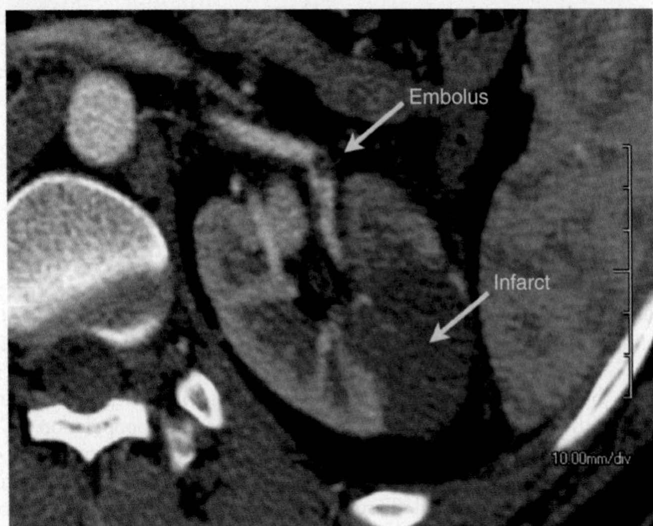

FIGURE 125-4. Computed tomography demonstrating a clot in the main renal artery and segmental renal infarction.

In patients with suspected embolic renal artery occlusion, echocardiography is indicated to search for a possible intracardiac thrombus. In nontraumatic thrombotic occlusion, evaluation for thrombophilia (Chapter 176), vasculitides (Chapter 270), or progressive atherosclerosis (Chapter 79) should be considered.

TREATMENT Rx

The human kidney can tolerate 60 to 90 minutes of warm ischemia, although the presence of collateral circulation may permit longer ischemic times. As a result, acute renal artery thrombosis requires urgent treatment in an attempt to reopen the artery. Options for nontraumatic renal artery thrombosis include systemic anticoagulation with unfractionated heparin (see Table 81-4 in Chapter 81) or low-molecular-weight heparin (LMWH) (see Table 81-3 in Chapter 81) for about 7 to 10 days, with oral warfarin begun at about day 3 and continued for 1 year to maintain an international normalized ratio of 2.0 to 3.0. Alternatively, intraarterial thrombolytic therapy may be considered. Surgical revascularization is associated with a higher mortality rate than medical therapy without improved renal salvage rates, so it is not recommended as primary therapy; it can be considered, however, for patients with bilateral renal artery occlusion or occlusion of the renal artery of a solitary kidney. Percutaneous endovascular therapies (e.g., local thrombolysis, thrombectomy, stent placement) have also been successful in acute renal artery occlusion, but there have been no comparative studies of endovascular intervention compared with medical therapy for renal artery occlusion.

For traumatic renal artery thrombosis, surgery is the treatment of choice but usually can salvage renal function only if accomplished immediately. For iatrogenic occlusion of the renal artery as a result of angiographic manipulations or angioplasty, intraarterial stent placement may be considered.

Patients with renal artery thrombosis also require rigorous medical care with assiduous attention to control of their blood pressure. To achieve a target blood pressure between 140/90 and 110/70 mm Hg may require multiple parenteral agents, as is recommended for malignant hypertension, before switching to oral agents, preferably a combination of ACE inhibitors, ARBs, or nondihydropyridine calcium channel blockers (Chapter 67). Adequate hydration is also imperative.

PROGNOSIS

The mortality rate is high, especially in patients who require hemodialysis, and it correlates with the severity of the underlying conditions. For patients undergoing surgical revascularization for complete acute renal artery occlusion, the mortality rate is 11% to 25%. The risk of end-stage renal disease (ESRD) is variable, and rates of 0% to greater than 50% have been reported. Hypertension, which may develop as a late sequela of treated renal artery occlusion, is preferably treated with ACE inhibitors, ARBs, or nondihydropyridine calcium channel blockers (see Table 67-7 in Chapter 67).

ARTERIOLES AND MICROVASCULATURE

Atheroembolic Disease of the Renal Arteries

EPIDEMIOLOGY AND PATHOBIOLOGY

Cholesterol crystal embolization is a potential complication of widespread atherosclerosis. The risk factors are similar to those for all atherosclerotic disease (Chapter 52), including smoking, hypertension, hyperlipidemia, diabetes, and older age. Atheroembolic disease appears to be more common in whites, but the condition may be underdiagnosed in African Americans owing to the difficulty of assessing livedo reticularis in this population.

The most common triggering events are manipulation of a thrombus or of the abdominal aorta or renal arteries during angiography or transluminal angioplasty. It is not unusual, therefore, for cholesterol crystal embolization to be mistaken for contrast-induced nephropathy. Atheroemboli can also be associated with anticoagulant or thrombolytic therapy and may be accompanied by the finding of a cyanotic toe on physical examination. Spontaneous atheroembolism after detachment of a mural plaque is uncommon. Cholesterol crystals typically do not occlude arterial flow but induce an inflammatory response and subsequent endothelial proliferation, so the clinical manifestations may occur some time after the initial insult.

CLINICAL MANIFESTATIONS

Although all organ systems can be affected (Chapter 80), the kidneys are most commonly involved followed by the spleen and gastrointestinal tract.[8] Acute renal failure, hypertension, or both typically occur, and many patients progress to chronic kidney disease or even ESRD.[9] Nonspecific complaints may include fever, myalgias, headaches, and weight loss. Evidence of cholesterol embolization may be present in the retina, muscles, or skin, where livedo reticularis (see Fig. 80-3 in Chapter 80) or cyanotic digits may be observed. Embolization can also result in cerebrovascular events, acute pancreatitis, ischemic bowel, and gangrene of the extremities (Chapter 80).

DIAGNOSIS

Although most atheroembolic events are diagnosed because of an acute clinical change, clinically silent, chronic, low-grade embolization may be overlooked because patients at risk for this complication often have other chronic illnesses associated with renal failure, hypertension, and atherosclerosis. Urinalysis may not be helpful because cholesterol crystals often are not present, but mild proteinuria, eosinophiluria, and increased cellularity are frequently observed. Transient eosinophilia is common, and an elevated erythrocyte sedimentation rate (ESR), hypocomplementemia, anemia, and leukocytosis may also be present. Up to 80% of patients may have a serum creatinine level exceeding 2 mg/dL.

Although the demonstration of cholesterol crystals in the renal microvasculature with subsequent vessel occlusion is considered a diagnostic feature, a kidney biopsy generally is not necessary for patients with typical clinical features, including livedo reticularis and violaceous mottling of the toes, eosinophilia, and an elevated ESR. When uncertainty exists, noninvasive biopsy of the skin of the lower extremity, muscle of the calf or thigh, or gastric mucosa can be diagnostic in up to 80% of patients.

TREATMENT Rx

There is no curative therapy for atheroembolic disease, so supportive care is often all that can be offered. Aggressive control of dyslipidemia with statins (Chapter 206) is recommended and may have the added benefit of stabilizing the endothelial surface. Anticoagulants are of no value and may delay the healing of ulcerating atherosclerotic lesions; if possible, anticoagulant therapy should be discontinued. Adequate hydration is important to sustain renal perfusion. Hypertension should be treated with angiotensin II antagonists and vasodilators (see Table 67-7 in Chapter 67), and volume should be controlled with diuretics, with care to avoid hypotension. Intravascular radiologic procedures and vascular surgery should be avoided if possible.

PROGNOSIS

Recent series suggest up to an 80% survival rate at 1 year. Most patients die of cardiovascular complications. With adequate blood pressure control for several months or years, renal function may recover sufficiently to avoid dialysis. Patients who develop ESRD have a significantly higher mortality rate.

RENAL VEINS

Renal Vein Thrombosis

EPIDEMIOLOGY

Unilateral or bilateral thrombosis of the major renal veins or their segments is often a subtle disorder that can develop in a variety of conditions but is especially prominent with nephrotic syndrome[10] (Chapter 121) or renal cell carcinoma (Chapter 197). Cases have also been associated with trauma, oral contraceptive use, hypovolemia, renal transplantation (Chapter 131), and thrombophilic states (Chapter 176). The reported incidence of renal vein thrombosis ranges from 5% to 62% in patients with nephrotic syndrome and is typically associated with membranous nephropathy, but it may also occur with membranoproliferative glomerulonephritis, focal glomerular sclerosis, sickle cell nephropathy, amyloidosis, diabetic nephropathy, renal vasculitis, and lupus nephritis. Spontaneous renal vein thrombosis is unusual in patients without underlying risk factors.

PATHOBIOLOGY

The precipitating factors are apparently abnormalities in coagulation or fibrinolysis. Antithrombin III and plasminogen levels may be depressed as a result of urinary excretion of antithrombin III in patients with nephrotic syndrome. Thrombocytosis, increased platelet activation, hyperfibrinogenemia, inhibition of plasminogen activation, and altered circulating levels of proteins S and C in nephrotic syndrome contribute to thromboembolic complications.

Extrinsic compression of the renal veins from retroperitoneal sources such as lymph nodes, fibrosis, abscess, aortic aneurysm, or tumor may cause renal vein thrombosis as a result of sluggish renal venous flow. Acute pancreatitis, trauma, and retroperitoneal surgery also may predispose to renal vein thrombosis. Renal cell carcinoma characteristically invades the renal vein and compromises venous flow, resulting in renal vein thrombosis. Renal vein thrombosis in the setting of severe volume depletion and impaired renal blood flow has been described in young adults.

CLINICAL MANIFESTATIONS

The manifestations of renal vein thrombosis depend on the extent and rapidity of the development of the occlusion. Patients with acute renal vein thrombosis may have nausea, vomiting, flank pain, leukocytosis, hematuria, compromised renal function and an increase in kidney size. These features may be confused with renal colic or pyelonephritis. Adult patients with nephrotic syndrome and chronic renal vein thrombosis may have more subtle findings, such as a dramatic increase in proteinuria or evidence of tubular dysfunction, including glycosuria, aminoaciduria, phosphaturia, and impaired urinary acidification. Chronic renal vein thrombosis may first present in association with a pulmonary embolus.

DIAGNOSIS

For acute renal vein thrombosis, which is typically associated with thrombophilia, contrast-enhanced CT shows an enlarged kidney, stretching of the calyces, and notching of the ureters. A venogram is rarely required but can be considered in cases of acute renal failure in which thrombectomy or thrombolysis is considered. In chronic renal vein thrombosis, an incidentally noted renal vein thrombus may be seen on imaging studies ordered for other reasons. The tumor thrombus associated with renal cell carcinoma often extends into the inferior vena cava and occasionally to the level of the right heart. Routine screening for thrombus is not recommended for patients with nephrotic syndrome, but contrast-enhanced CT is recommended in patients with suggestive clinical manifestations.

TREATMENT Rx

The most widely accepted form of therapy for both acute and chronic renal vein thrombosis is anticoagulation with LMWH (see Table 81-3 in Chapter 81) or unfractionated heparin (see Table 81-4 in Chapter 81) for about 7 to 10 days, with oral warfarin begun on about day 3 and continued for at least 1 year to hieve an international normalized ratio of 2.0 to 3.0. In patients with ongoing k factors, such as persistent nephrotic syndrome, or recurrent thrombosis, ticoagulation should be continued indefinitely. In patients who have an nderlying renal cell carcinoma, long-term LMWH is preferred over warfarin ecause it is better for preventing cancer-related thrombosis (Chapter 176). brinolytic therapy may be considered in patients with acute renal vein rombosis associated with acute renal failure.

PROGNOSIS

e prognosis of patients with renal vein thrombosis depends entirely on the lerlying condition causing or associated with it. Renal vein thrombosis ociated with membranous glomerulonephritis and nephrotic syndrome hapter 121) usually resolves if the underlying condition responds to rapy or spontaneously resolves. In contrast, renal vein thrombosis associ- d with renal cell carcinoma (Chapter 197) has a very poor prognosis. nal vein thrombosis associated with trauma or hypovolemia may resolve r appropriate therapy.

de

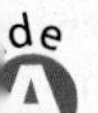

Grade A References

Wheatley K, Ives N, Gray R, et al. Revascularization versus medical therapy for renal-artery stenosis. *N Engl J Med*. 2009;361:1953-1962.

Bax L, Woittiez AJ, Kouwenberg HJ, et al. Stent placement in patients with atherosclerotic renal artery stenosis and impaired renal function: a randomized trial. *Ann Intern Med*. 2009;150: 840-848.

Cooper CJ, Murphy TP, Cutlip DE, et al. Stenting and medical therapy for atherosclerotic renal-artery stenosis. *N Engl J Med*. 2014;370:13-22.

GENERAL REFERENCES

· the General References and other additional features, please visit Expert Consult https://expertconsult.inkling.com.

126

NEPHROLITHIASIS

DAVID A. BUSHINSKY

Kidney stones are composed of crystals in a protein matrix. Most crystals contain calcium, which is generally complexed with oxalate, phosphate, or both; other stones are composed of uric acid, magnesium ammonium phosphate (struvite), or cystine, alone or in combination. Kidney stones form when the urinary saturation of their components exceeds the solubility of the solid phase.

EPIDEMIOLOGY

The annual incidence of kidney stones in industrialized nations exceeds one per 1000 persons, with a lifetime risk of about 7% in women and about 11% in men.[1] The incidence of stone formation peaks in the third and fourth decades of life, and the prevalence increases with age until approximately 70 years in men and 60 years in women. In the United States, the increase in lifetime risk of nephrolithiasis from 3% in the late 1970s to almost 9% in 2010 is far faster than can be accounted for by alterations in our genome. The increasing prevalence suggests that changes to our diets and lifestyle may account for this increased stone formation. The estimated yearly economic cost of kidney stones exceeds $5 billion in the United States.

In the United States, whites are more likely to develop renal stones than are other ethnic groups. Stones are more common in hot, dry climates, perhaps because greater fluid loss through the skin and respiration leads to more concentrated urine. Many occupations make it inconvenient to use a restroom, and these individuals often avoid fluids in an effort to avoid urination, thereby leading to excretion of a concentrated urine. Insufficient rehydration among people who engage in physical activity and have large insensible losses also leads to concentrated urine.

Obesity is correlated with the risk for kidney stone formation. Individuals weighing more than 220 lb or having a body mass index (BMI) greater than 30 are significantly more likely to form stones than are individuals who weigh less than 150 lb or have a BMI between 21 and 22.9.[2]

The types of stones vary around the world. In the United States, the majority of stones are calcium oxalate or calcium phosphate (>80%), and fewer than 10% are pure uric acid stones. By comparison, about 70% of stones in the Mediterranean and Middle East are composed of uric acid. Magnesium ammonium phosphate (struvite) stones account for 10% to 25% of stones, and cystine stones comprise 2% of stones.

PATHOBIOLOGY

Human bone is composed of calcium and phosphate, principally in the form of apatite. When humans reach their adult height and their skeletons are fully mineralized, the net amount of calcium that is absorbed by nonpregnant individuals must be excreted in the urine. Similarly, absorbed phosphate that is not needed for bone mineralization or cell growth must be excreted. Oxalate is an end product of metabolism, and it too must be excreted in the urine. The need for water conservation by terrestrial man often leads to excretion of these ions in relatively scant amounts of urine, thereby leading to increasing saturation with respect to the solid phases of calcium oxalate and calcium phosphate. Increasing saturation drives the formation of the solid crystal phase and is expressed as the ratio of calcium oxalate (or phosphate) ion activity to its solubility. At ratios of greater than 1, termed *supersaturation*, a solid phase can form, but the substances remain in solution at ratios less than 1. When urine is supersaturated, ions can bond to form the more stable, solid phase, which is termed *nucleation*. Homogeneous nucleation refers to the bonding of similar ions into crystals. The more common and thermodynamically favored heterogeneous nucleation occurs when crystals grow on dissimilar crystals or substances as cellular debris in the urine. Although humans produce inhibitors of stone formation, such as osteopontin and Tamm-Horsefall protein, supersaturation can overwhelm this inhibition, and a solid phase will form.

Calcium Stones

About 70% to 80% of kidney stones contain calcium, which is often complexed with oxalate or phosphate.[3] Calcium-containing kidney stones are most often caused by excessive excretion of calcium (hypercalciuria), oxalate (hyperoxaluria), or urate (hyperuricosuria), or an insufficient excretion of citrate (hypocitraturia)

Calcium-containing stones have a strong genetic component. Idiopathic hypercalciuria is thought to be a polygenic disorder in which a generalized dysregulation of calcium transport in the kidney, intestine, and bone leads to excessive urine calcium excretion.[4]

An initial genome-wide association study has identified sequence variants in genes encoding claudin 14, which regulates calcium reabsorption in the thick ascending limb of Henle loop.

Urinary oxalate is derived from endogenous metabolism of glyoxylate and ascorbic acid or from dietary sources, such as cocoa, nuts, tea, and certain leafy green vegetables (e.g., spinach). The three main causes of hyperoxaluria are excessive oxalate ingestion (dietary oxaluria), the excessive intestinal absorption of oxalate (enteric oxaluria) that is paradoxically observed in malabsorptive gastrointestinal (GI) disorders, and the excessive endogenous oxalate production seen in certain hepatic enzyme deficiencies (primary hyperoxaluria; Chapter 205). Additionally, ethylene glycol, a common automobile antifreeze, is metabolized to oxalate and can cause excessive urinary oxalate excretion in conjunction with severe metabolic acidosis and renal failure (Chapter 110).

Enteric oxaluria results in elevated urinary oxalate levels (60-100 mg/day). In GI malabsorptive conditions such as Crohn disease (Chapter 141), celiac sprue (Chapter 140), jejunoileal bypass (Chapter 220), and chronic pancreatitis (Chapter 144), malabsorbed fatty acids bind dietary calcium, thereby allowing oxalate to be readily absorbed in the colon. The colonic mucosa becomes more permeable to oxalate owing to exposure to bile acids.

Primary hyperoxaluria (Chapter 205) results from hepatic enzyme deficiencies that lead to substantial endogenous oxalate production and a marked elevation of urinary oxalate (80-300 mg/day).[5] Oxalate deposits in numerous organs, including the heart, bone marrow, muscle, and renal parenchyma, where they lead to renal failure, cardiomyopathy, and bone marrow suppression at an early age. In type 1 primary hyperoxaluria, the hepatic enzyme alanine glyoxylate aminotransferase is deficient because of one of several mutations in the *AGXT* gene. In the less common type 2 primary hyperoxaluria, patients lack D-glycerate reductase and glyoxylate reductase owing to mutations in the *GRHPR* gene. Type 3 is a pediatric disease that is due to mutations in the *HOGA1* gene and does not lead to kidney failure.

Nephrolithiasis and nephrocalcinosis can also result from a variety of monogenic disorders, such as Dent disease (X-linked recessive nephrolithiasis), McCune-Albright syndrome (Chapters 231 and 248), osteogenesis imperfecta type 1 (Chapter 260), and congenital lactase deficiency (Chapter 140).

Citrate combines with calcium to form a soluble complex that reduces the availability of calcium to bind with oxalate or phosphate. The principal risk factor for hypocitraturia is a high protein intake. Men often have lower urinary citrate concentrations than women. Distal renal tubular acidosis (Chapter 118) leads to calcium phosphate stones owing to bone demineralization and an alkaline tubular pH.

Calcium oxalate kidney stones form on calcium phosphate deposits, termed Randall plaques, which are located in the renal papillae. Randall plaque formation is positively correlated with urine calcium excretion and negatively correlated with urine volume and pH. These calcium phosphate crystals, in the form of apatite, originate around the thin loop of Henle and then extend into the interstitium without eroding into the tubular lumen or damaging the tubular cells. The crystals move toward the urinary space, where they form Randall plaques, which are visible on cystoscopy but not generally visible on a routine CT scan. In the presence of urine that is supersaturated with respect to calcium oxalate, calcium oxalate crystals bind to these plaques and increase in size. If the calcium oxalate crystals then break off from the Randall plaques, the free stone can enter, migrate, irritate, and possibly obstruct the ureter, where it can cause severe pain.

Uric Acid Stones

The incidence of uric acid stones in the United States appears to be rising in parallel with the increase in obesity, which leads to renal insulin resistance and a very low urine pH.[6] Most patients with uric acid stones have a reduced urinary pH, and some have low urine volumes or elevated urinary uric acid levels. More than five times as much uric acid is soluble in a urine with a pH of 6.5 compared with a pH of 5.3. Diarrhea and diets high in animal protein can contribute to an acidic urinary pH. Uric acid stone formers have greater body weight and a higher incidence of insulin resistance and type 2 diabetes mellitus. Insulin resistance leads to impaired urinary ammonium excretion, thereby resulting in the excretion of more hydrogen ions as titratable acids than as ammonium and, therefore, a lower urinary pH.

Hyperuricosuria may be seen in patients who ingest large quantities of dietary purine, such as found in organ meats, shellfish, certain fish (e.g., anchovies, sardines, herring, and mackerel), and meat extracts such as bouillon and consommé, and protein. Hyperuricemic disorders, including gout (Chapter 273), myeloproliferative disorders, tumor lysis syndrome, and certain inborn errors of metabolism, can also contribute to an increased urinary uric acid. Medications such as salicylates and probenecid can be hyperuricosuric.

Struvite Stones

Struvite stones, sometimes called *triple phosphate stones, magnesium ammonium phosphate stones,* and *infection stones,* comprise only about 10% to 25% of all stones but constitute the majority of staghorn calculi, which are large stones that extend beyond a single renal calyx.[7] Struvite stones are far more common in women than in men, in large part owing to women's increased susceptibility to urinary tract infections (UTIs) (Chapter 284). Similarly, any patient with urinary stasis, such as patients with neurogenic bladders, indwelling urinary catheters, or spinal cord lesions, is susceptible to struvite stones.

Struvite stones form only in the presence of both ammonium ions and an alkaline urinary pH of 7 or greater, which only occur with urease-producing bacteria. *Proteus* spp. (Chapter 305) are common urease-producing bacteria, but other gram-negative and gram-positive bacteria (e.g., *Klebsiella* spp. and *Staphylococcus epidermidis*) as well as *Mycoplasma* spp. (Chapter 317) and yeast species have been implicated in urease production. By comparison, *Escherichia coli* does not produce urease.

Cystine Stones

Cystinuria (Chapter 128), which is an autosomal recessive disorder caused by mutations of the *SLC3A1* gene or the *SCLC7A9* gene, results in decreased renal tubular reabsorption and excessive urinary excretion of the dibasic amino acids cystine, ornithine, lysine, and arginine.[8] The resulting urinary excretion of cystine in the typical volume of urine exceeds its solubility of about 300 mg/L, so stones form. Although normal people excrete about 30 to 50 mg/day of cystine, heterozygotes for cystinuria excrete about 400 mg/day, and homozygotes often excrete about 600 mg/day. Thus, homozygotes must continually excrete 2 L or more of urine each day to avoid stone formation. Cystinuria is unrelated to the much more severe disorder *cystinosis* (Chapter 128), which results in extensive intracellular cystine accumulation.

CLINICAL MANIFESTATIONS

Patients with kidney stones often present with pain or hematuria (or both) and less often with UTIs (Chapter 284) or acute kidney injury (Chapter 120), either owing to bilateral obstruction or unilateral obstruction of a single functioning kidney (Chapter 123). Patients often complain of severe ureteral colic. The pain is of abrupt onset and can intensify into severe, excruciating flank pain. The pain may migrate anteriorly along the abdomen and inferiorly to the groin, testicles, or labia majora as the stone moves down the ureter toward the ureterovesical junction. The pain resolves only after the stone passes or is removed. Hematuria, even gross hematuria, is common, and patients occasionally present with painless hematuria (see Fig. 114-1 in Chapter 114), and the finding of a stone on radiographic examination does not preclude another cause. Conversely, even large calculi may be asymptomatic and be discovered during the investigation of unrelated symptoms. Obstruction caused by calculi may also be painless, and nephrolithiasis should always be considered in the differential diagnosis of unexplained acute or chronic kidney disease (Chapters 120, 123, and 130).

DIAGNOSIS

The physical examination can provide clues to the diagnosis of kidney stones but is not diagnostic. Some patients have demonstrable flank tenderness, and a rare patient with hyperuricemia will have tophi (Chapter 273). However, the physical examination is most helpful for not showing other potential causes of pain (Fig. 126-1). The suspicion of a kidney stone generally obligates radiographic evaluation. Radiographic studies can be deferred, however, in patients in whom the clinical diagnosis is clear, who have no evidence of infection, who are able to eat and drink, and who can be managed on oral analgesics.[A1]

Ultrasonography is an easy and rapid way to detect possible urinary obstruction. Ultrasonography can detect clinically significant renal calculi, although it has only a 19% sensitivity in detecting the ureteral stones that cause acute symptoms in many patients. The main advantage of ultrasonography is that it does not use radiation and is clearly the modality of choice when radiation exposure must be minimized.

A helical computed tomographic (CT) scan without radiographic contrast can detect kidney stones with both a sensitivity and a specificity exceeding 95% (Fig. 126-2). Based on the density of the stone, it also can often differentiate a calcium-containing stone from a cysteine or uric acid stone. An added benefit is that helical CT is often helpful in determining the cause of non–stone-induced abdominal pain.

However, a helical CT scan, especially when performed both with and without contrast, exposes the patient to ionizing radiation, which increases the risk of cancer. In a recent trial, initial ultrasonography was associated with lower cumulative radiation exposure than an initial helical CT, without significant differences in high-risk diagnoses with complications.[A2]

In certain situations, however, such as in patients with HIV thought to have stones induced by protease inhibitor, a helical CT scan with contrast is often required because the stones are not radiopaque and do not obstruct the ureter.

Approximately 90% of kidney stones are radiopaque and may be detected on a simple abdominal radiograph. Unfortunately, however, the stone is often obscured by stool, vertebrae, or abdominal gas, so the sensitivity of a plain abdominal radiograph is about 50%, and its specificity is only about 75%. Uric acid stones are radiolucent and cannot be detected radiographically without contrast.

Intravenous pyelography (IVP) has a sensitivity of about 75% and a specificity of more than 90% for detecting renal calculi. IVP is also useful for identifying structural abnormalities of the urinary tract such a medullary sponge kidney (Chapter 127) that predisposes to stone formation. However, an IVP often does not detect nonobstructing radiolucent stones because they do not create a filling defect. An IVP exposes the patient to more radiation than a plain radiograph but less than a CT scan. It also carries the risk of radiographic contrast material, which is greater in individuals with underlying renal compromise. With the widespread availability of ultrasonography and helical CT scans, an IVP is rarely indicated.

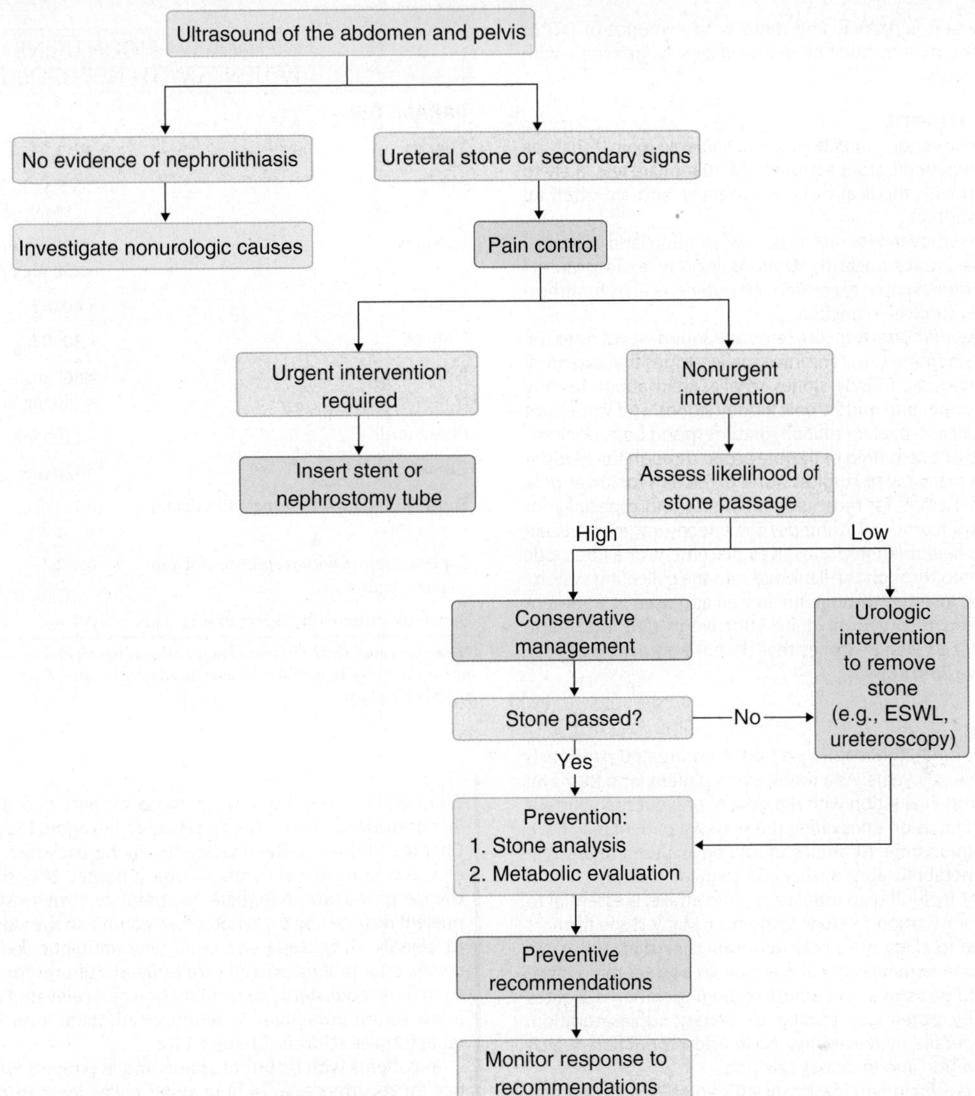

FIGURE 126-1. Algorithm for evaluation of suspected renal colic. CT = computed tomography; ESWL = extracorporeal shock-wave lithotripsy.

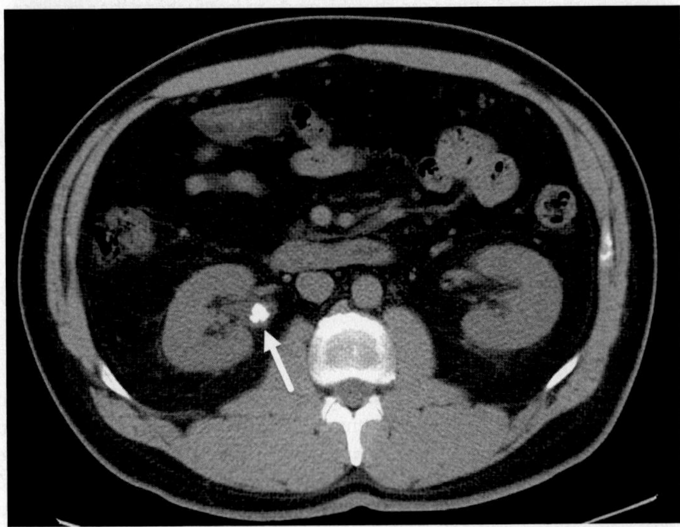

FIGURE 126-2. High-resolution helical computed tomography scan of the upper part of the abdomen demonstrating a stone in the right renal pelvis and a smaller stone in the left kidney *(arrows)*. There is no hydronephrosis. (Courtesy of Marc Brown, MD, and Lawrence H. Schwartz, MD, Department of Radiology, Columbia University Medical Center.)

TREATMENT Rx

Medical Therapy

Because the pain of renal colic can be excruciating, pain control is critical after the definitive diagnosis has been made (see Fig. 126-1). If nausea and vomiting prevent the use of oral medication, parenteral medication is typically required. Nonsteroidal anti-inflammatory drugs (NSAIDs) are as effective as opiates for renal colic and are preferred because they have fewer side effects.[A3] An intravenous (IV) option is ketorolac (30 mg), and ibuprofen (200-400 mg/dose every 4-6 hours with a maximum daily dose of 1.2 g) is a common oral option in patients who can tolerate oral medication. Morphine (5-10 mg IV) and hydromorphone (1-2 mg IV) are options if ketorolac is insufficient to control pain. Oral oxycodone (5-15 mg every 4 to 6 hours as needed) may be added to ibuprofen for outpatient pain control. Ondansetron (2-4 mg IV) is helpful if antiemetics are required. Because NSAIDs can cause acute kidney injury, especially in patients who are dehydrated or who have chronic underlying kidney disease, adequate hydration (e.g., normal saline with dextrose at 75-150 mL/hr) is essential, but neither high-volume fluid therapy nor diuretics promote the passage of the stone.[A4]

Medical Expulsive Therapy

Kidney stones 5 mm or smaller in size have about a 70% probability of passing spontaneously; stones between 5 and 10 mm have less than a 50% chance of passing spontaneously. Medical expulsive therapy using α-adrenergic receptor blockers, such as tamsulosin (0.4 mg/day orally [PO]), terazosin, and doxazosin,[A5] or the calcium-channel blocker nifedipine (nifedipine XL 30 mg/day or twice daily) reduces spasm of the ureteral smooth muscle, allows peristalsis to move the stone more effectively, and increases spontaneous passage rates by about 50%. Medical expulsive therapy may be cautiously attempted with ureteral stones smaller than 10 mm in diameter for 4 to 6 weeks if pain is controlled, kidney function is normal, and there is no evidence of UTI or significant obstruction. The patient must be followed closely, generally with repeat ultrasound examinations.

Initial Surgical Treatment

Stones that cause obstruction, infection, or intractable pain must be removed expeditiously. In general, stones larger than 10 mm are less likely to pass spontaneously, even with medical expulsive therapy, and are often an indicator for earlier intervention.

The approach to stone removal depends on its size, location, and composition, as well as on urinary tract anatomy. Options include extracorporeal shock-wave lithotripsy, ureteroscopic extraction, percutaneous nephrolithotomy, and only rarely open surgical extraction.

Extracorporeal shock-wave lithotripsy focuses external sound waves onto the kidney stone, thereby fragmenting the stone into smaller stones that can more easily be passed spontaneously. Kidney stones smaller than about 15 mm, proximal ureteral stones, upper and middle pole kidney stones, and stones not composed of cystine or calcium oxalate monohydrate respond best. *Ureteroscopy* involves the passage of a semirigid or flexible scope through the bladder and into the ureter. It is a mainstay of surgical stone extraction for lower pole renal calculi smaller than 1 cm,[A6] for most ureteral stones and especially for distal ureteral stones.[A7] Endocorporeal lithotripsy can directly fragment visualized stones. *Percutaneous nephrolithotomy* involves placement of a fiberoptic catheter with an open lumen through the flank and into the collecting system. Instruments and lasers are inserted through the lumen and used to fragment and remove the stone. This technique is quite effective in removing large (>2 cm) or staghorn calculi, as well as stones that do not fragment well with extracorporeal shock-wave lithotripsy.

Medical Evaluation

After an initial stone episode, the recurrence rate in nontreated patients is estimated to be about 50% at 5 years. As a result, every patient who forms an initial stone should undergo evaluation with the goal of preventing recurrent stones. The history should focus on uncovering the reason a patient may have formed a stone at this point in time. All stones should be analyzed to assist in defining the underlying metabolic abnormality and to guide therapy.

A careful dietary history, including an estimate of fluid intake, is essential to determine its potential contribution to stone formation. Many stone formers are erroneously instructed to eliminate all calcium from their diet, a practice that not only increases stone formation but also enhances bone demineralization. Sodium intake should be estimated because sodium excretion obligates calcium excretion, thereby potentially leading to urinary supersaturation. Excessive animal protein intake increases metabolic acid production, which induces bone demineralization and increases calciuria.

Hypercalcemic disorders—including malignancy (Chapter 245), hyperparathyroidism (Chapter 245), and sarcoidosis (Chapter 95)—often result in hypercalciuria, increased urinary supersaturation, and calcium stone formation. Malabsorptive GI disorders, such as Crohn disease (Chapter 141) and celiac disease (Chapter 140), or weight reduction surgery (Chapter 220), such as ileal resection or jejunoileal bypass, will often result in calcium oxalate stone formation owing to increased oxalate absorption and excretion and volume depletion.

Medications that can cause calcium stone formation include loop diuretics, which increase urinary calcium excretion, as well as salicylates and probenecid, which increase urinary uric acid excretion. Other medications that can themselves precipitate into stones include IV acyclovir, high-dose sulfadiazine, triamterene, and the antiretroviral agents indinavir and nelfinavir. Still other medications, such as acetazolamide and topiramate, inhibit tubular carbonic anhydrase activity, thereby leading to metabolic acidosis, bone resorption, hypercalciuria, lower urinary citrate excretion, and higher urinary pH, all of which can result in the formation of calcium phosphate stones.

The number and frequency of stones formed, the patient's age at the time of the first stone, the size of the stone, and an analysis of the composition of the stone are also important clues. Stones that develop at a young age suggest a genetic disorder, such as primary hyperoxaluria or cystinuria. Large staghorn calculi in elderly patients are consistent with struvite stones. A stone's response to intervention is also helpful: cystine stones do not fragment well with lithotripsy, and stones that recur frequently in a single kidney suggest a unilateral anatomic abnormality.

The basic evaluation of a stone patient includes measurement of serum electrolytes (sodium, potassium, chloride, and bicarbonate), creatinine, calcium, phosphorus, and uric acid, as well as a 25 hydroxyvitamin D level and the level of thyroid stimulating hormone. If the serum calcium is above the midrange of normal and the serum phosphorus is below the midrange of normal, a serum parathyroid hormone level should be obtained.

An elevated urine specific gravity suggests inadequate fluid intake. Patients with struvite stones generally have an elevated urine pH (>7.4) owing to the splitting of urea into ammonia and bicarbonate, but a low urinary pH (<5.5) raises the suspicion of uric acid stones. Hematuria may indicate irritation to the urothelial lining by a stone. Characteristic crystals (see Fig. 114-10 in Chapter 114) may be seen in stone formers and are more common than in nonstone formers. The presence of hexagonal crystals (see Fig. 114-9 in Chapter 114) mandates that cystinuria be excluded. The combination of an elevated urine pH with bacteriuria (Chapter 284) suggests struvite stones. Urease production adequate to stimulate struvite stone formation may be present despite low bacterial colony counts, so the laboratory should be asked to identify all bacteria and determine antibiotic sensitivities even with low colony counts. If no bacteria are isolated, cultures for *Ureaplasma urealyticum* should be requested. The combination of an elevated urinary pH (6.5-7.2) with a low serum potassium or serum bicarbonate level strongly suggests distal renal tubular acidosis (Chapter 118).

In patients with recurrent stones and in patients with high-risk characteristics for recurrence, a 24-hour urine collection can determine the levels of calcium, oxalate, citrate, sodium, urate, phosphorus, and creatinine, as well as supersaturation with respect to calcium oxalate, calcium phosphate, and uric acid (Table 126-1). The presence of supersaturation should lead the clinician to determine the individual urinary components that are causing the increased supersaturation, and efforts can then be made to rectify these abnormalities. Cystine should also be measured at least once in every stone former to exclude cystinuria and regularly in patients who form cysteine stones. Multivitamins should be discontinued about 5 days before the collection to prevent any antioxidant effect on the urine sample.

TABLE 126-1 OPTIMAL 24-HOUR URINE VALUES IN PATIENTS WITH NEPHROLITHIASIS*

PARAMETER	VALUE
Volume	>2-2.5 L
pH	>5.5 and <7.0 (24-hr specimen not required)
Calcium	<300 mg or <3.5-4.0 mg/kg in men; <250 mg or <3.5-4.0 mg/kg in women
Oxalate	<40 mg
Sodium	<3000 mg
Uric acid	<800 mg in men <750 mg in women
Phosphorus	<1100 mg
Citrate	>320 mg
Supersaturation with respect to calcium oxalate	<5
Supersaturation with respect to calcium phosphate	0.5-2
Supersaturation with respect to uric acid	0-1

*Urine creatinine should be measured to ensure adequacy of collection and should be >15 mg/kg in men and >10 mg/kg in women. Supersaturation is the ratio of the ion activity product and its solubility product.

PREVENTING RECURRENT STONES

General treatment to prevent recurrent stone formation (Fig. 126-3) consists of advising the patient to increase oral fluid intake to result in a urine volume greater than 2 L/day,[9] which will decrease recurrent stone formation by about 50%.[A8]

Calcium Stones

Because urine sodium excretion is directly correlated with urine calcium excretion, decreasing dietary sodium intake will decrease urine calcium excretion and reduce supersaturation. Patients with calcium stones should be instructed to limit their daily sodium intake to no more than 2 g/day. As the metabolism of animal protein leads to hypercalciuria, patients should also reduce animal protein intake to 0.8 to 1.0 g/kg/day.[A9]

The recommended calcium intake for a 19- to 50-year-old man or woman is 1000 mg of elemental calcium per day, and a number of studies demonstrate decreased formation of calcium stones when people consume diets adequate in calcium, presumably because appropriate calcium intake is needed for intestinal binding of dietary oxalate by dietary calcium. Dairy products are preferred over calcium supplements because data suggest that women taking supplemental vitamin D and calcium have a significant increase in stone formation.

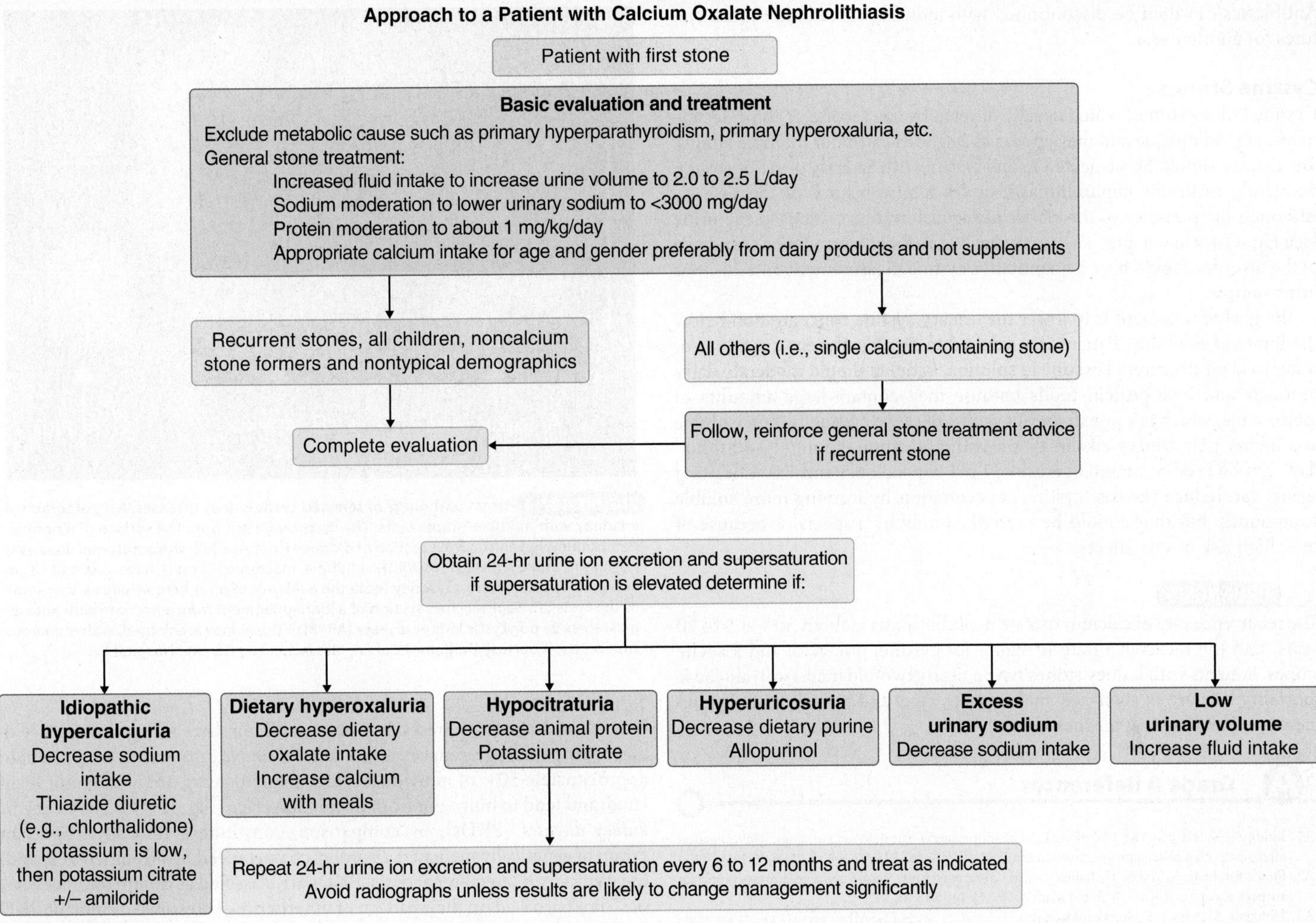

FIGURE 126-3. Approach to a patient with calcium oxalate nephrolithiasis.

Patients with persistent hypercalciuria often benefit from thiazide diuretics (e.g., chlorthalidone [12.5-25 mg/day]), which directly lower urinary calcium and reduce recurrent stone formation by about 50%.[A8] Thiazides are effective only if patients restrict dietary sodium. In patients with hypercholesterolemia or hyperglycemia, indapamide (1.25-5 mg/day) can be used because it has less effect on these parameters. If patients develop hypokalemia, dietary potassium intake should be increased or a potassium supplement can be administered. Potassium citrate (10-40 meq/day) will increase urinary citrate excretion, bind urinary calcium, and further decrease recurrent stone formation. Potassium citrate is available as a wax-matrix tablet. A 24-hour urine collection can be repeated in a month or two to assess the response to therapy.

Patients with dietary hyperoxaluria should be instructed to limit or avoid foods, such as cocoa, nuts, tea, and leafy green vegetables such as spinach, that have a high oxalate content. Because dietary calcium binds dietary oxalate, patients should consume these foods with calcium-containing foods. For enteric hyperoxaluria, treatment is first directed at the underlying disorder and then at instituting therapy for cause of the steatorrhea (Chapter 140). Dietary oxalate should be restricted, and dietary calcium and oxalate should be ingested at the same meal. A diet that is low in fat; high in fruits, vegetables, and low-fat dairy products; that is rich in grains, fish, poultry, beans, seeds, and nuts; and that contains less sweets, added sugar, and red meat appears to be a reasonable alternative to a low-oxalate diet.[A10] Additional fluid intake and potassium citrate are often beneficial.

In some patients with type 1 primary hyperoxaluria, pyridoxine (vitamin B_6) can increase enzyme activity and reduce oxalate production. All patients with primary hyperoxaluria should be treated with measures that reduce calcium oxalate precipitation, such as ample fluid supplementation and potassium citrate (10-40 meq/day). These patients should be seen by specialists because prompt and effective treatment can forestall kidney failure. Liver transplantation (Chapter 154) can be curative.

Calcium stones may be found in patients with hyperuricosuria.[10] These patients often excrete excess amounts of urinary uric acid but normal amounts of urinary calcium and oxalate. Compared with patients with pure uric acid stones, they generally have a higher urinary pH (≈5.5). The mechanism by which uric acid promotes calcium stone formation is unclear. Therapy generally consists of dietary purine restriction, increased fluid intake, and the addition of allopurinol (300 mg/day) if necessary.

If moderation of dietary protein is not successful in patients with hypocitraturia, oral potassium citrate is given in a wax-matrix formulation (10 to 40 mEq/day). Serum levels of potassium and bicarbonate must be closely monitored, especially in patients with chronic kidney disease.

Uric Acid Stones

Uric acid stones are radiolucent and are thus most often visualized with ultrasonography or CT. Therapy for patients with uric acid stones begins with nonspecific measures such as increasing fluid intake, a low purine diet, and lowering animal protein intake to increase urinary pH. Ideally, the urinary pH should be elevated to approximately 6.5 to 7.0, a level that not only prevents new stone formation but also can dissolve existing uric acid stones without promoting calcium phosphate deposition. Potassium citrate, again in a wax-matrix formulation (10-40 mEq/day), may be required to raise the urinary pH sufficiently. If all else fails, the carbonic anhydrase inhibitor acetazolamide (250-500 mg/day) may be initiated to raise urine pH. Because hyperuricemia usually persists, allopurinol (100-300 mg/day) is commonly indicated to lower the serum uric acid level.

Struvite Stones

Struvite stones rapidly grow to a large size and may promptly recur if they are not completely removed. As a result, struvite stone therapy requires complete surgical stone removal coupled with appropriate long-term antibiotic therapy (Chapter 284) selected on the basis of cultures of stone fragments retrieved from surgery. Antibiotics should be continued at full doses until the urine is sterile and then continued at a lower dose. Monthly surveillance cultures should be continued until the urine remains sterile for 3 consecutive months.

Antibiotics can then be discontinued with monthly surveillance urine cultures for another year.

Cystine Stones

Cystine kidney stones, which usually develop by the second or third decade of life, are radiopaque and may appear as staghorn calculi or multiple stones. The disease should be suspected in any patient with an early onset of stones, frequently recurrent nephrolithiasis, and a family history of the disease. Although the presence of the classic hexagonal cystine crystals in the urine (see Fig. 114-9 in Chapter 114) may suggest the diagnosis, anyone suspected of the disorder should have a quantitative cystine measurement on a 24-hour urine sample.

The goal of treatment is to lower the urinary cystine concentration below the limits of solubility. Patients are advised to drink sufficient quantities of water to keep all excreted cystine in solution. Patients should moderate dairy products and high-protein foods because they contain large amounts of methionine, which is a precursor of cystine. Because cystine is more soluble at a higher pH, urinary alkalinization with potassium citrate (10-40 mEq/day) can be used to maintain a urinary pH between 6.5 and 7.0. Chelating agents can reduce the free cystine concentration by forming more soluble compounds, but they should be prescribed only by a specialist because of their high risk of side effects.

PROGNOSIS

The recurrence rate of calcium oxalate nephrolithiasis is about 50% at 5 to 10 years, and the recurrence rate is higher for cystine, uric acid, and struvite stones. Patients with kidney stones have a nearly twofold increase in all-cause mortality because of their age, male gender, race, and poverty level but no increase after adjusting for these factors.[11]

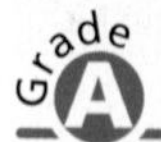

Grade A References

A1. Lindqvist K, Hellstrom M, Holmberg G, et al. Immediate versus deferred radiological investigation after acute renal colic: a prospective randomized study. *Scand J Urol Nephrol.* 2006;40:119-124.
A2. Smith-Bindman R, Aubin C, Bailitz J, et al. Ultrasonography versus computed tomography for suspected nephrolithiasis. *N Engl J Med.* 2014;371:1100-1110.
A3. Holdgate A, Pollock T. Nonsteroidal anti-inflammatory drugs (NSAIDs) versus opioids for acute renal colic. *Cochrane Database Syst Rev.* 2005:CD004137.
A4. Worster AS, Bhanich Supapol W. Fluids and diuretics for acute ureteric colic. *Cochrane Database Syst Rev.* 2012;2:CD004926.
A5. Campschroer T, Zhu Y, Duijvesz D, et al. Alpha-blockers as medical expulsive therapy for ureteral stones. *Cochrane Database Syst Rev.* 2014;4:CD008509.
A6. Srisubat A, Potisat S, Lojanapiwat B, et al. Extracorporeal shock wave lithotripsy (ESWL) versus percutaneous nephrolithotomy (PCNL) or retrograde intrarenal surgery (RIRS) for kidney stones. *Cochrane Database Syst Rev.* 2014;11:CD007044.
A7. Aboumarzouk OM, Kata SG, Keeley FX, et al. Extracorporeal shock wave lithotripsy (ESWL) versus ureteroscopic management for ureteric calculi. *Cochrane Database Syst Rev.* 2012;5:CD006029.
A8. Fink HA, Wilt TJ, Eidman KE, et al. Medical management to prevent recurrent nephrolithiasis in adults: a systematic review for an American College of Physicians Clinical Guideline. *Ann Intern Med.* 2013;158:535-543.
A9. Escribano J, Balaguer A, Roque IFM, et al. Dietary interventions for preventing complications in idiopathic hypercalciuria. *Cochrane Database Syst Rev.* 2014;2:CD006022.
A10. Noori N, Honarkar E, Goldfarb DS, et al. Urinary lithogenic risk profile in recurrent stone formers with hyperoxaluria: a randomized controlled trial comparing DASH (Dietary Approaches to Stop Hypertension)-style and low-oxalate diets. *Am J Kidney Dis.* 2014;63:456-463.

GENERAL REFERENCES

For the General References and other additional features, please visit Expert Consult at https://expertconsult.inkling.com.

127 CYSTIC KIDNEY DISEASES

M. AMIN ARNAOUT

DEFINITION AND EPIDEMIOLOGY

The term *cystic kidney diseases* refers to a heterogeneous group of hereditary and acquired disorders characterized by the presence of unilateral or bilateral renal cysts. When acquired singly or in small numbers and in the absence of any other pathology, renal cysts are termed *simple cysts,* which are present in approximately 50% of individuals older than 40 years, are usually not loculated, and tend to bulge out from the renal surface (Fig. 127-1). The *polycystic kidney diseases* (PKDs), by comparison, constitute a clinically important group of genetically mediated disorders characterized by prominent, expanding, typically bilateral renal cysts. PKDs are classified as dominant, recessive, or X-linked, based on their pattern of inheritance. Autosomal dominant PKD (ADPKD), with a prevalence rate between one in 400 and one in 1000, is the most common monogenic disease in humans and accounts for about 8% to 10% of all end-stage renal disease (ESRD) in the United States. ADPKD develops in an age-dependent manner and affects mainly adults. Autosomal recessive PKD (ARPKD), by contrast, is a relatively rare childhood disorder that appears in one in every 6000 to 50,000 live births. Renal cysts are also seen in several other rare hereditary kidney diseases and in several syndromic PKDs (Table 127-1). Collectively, the hereditary PKDs generally affect both genders and all races equally and cost more than $1 billion annually to manage in the United States alone. *Acquired cystic kidney disease* refers to the multiple bilateral renal cysts that occur in 90% of patients who have been receiving renal replacement therapy for 8 years or longer and are associated with increased rates of renal cell carcinoma.

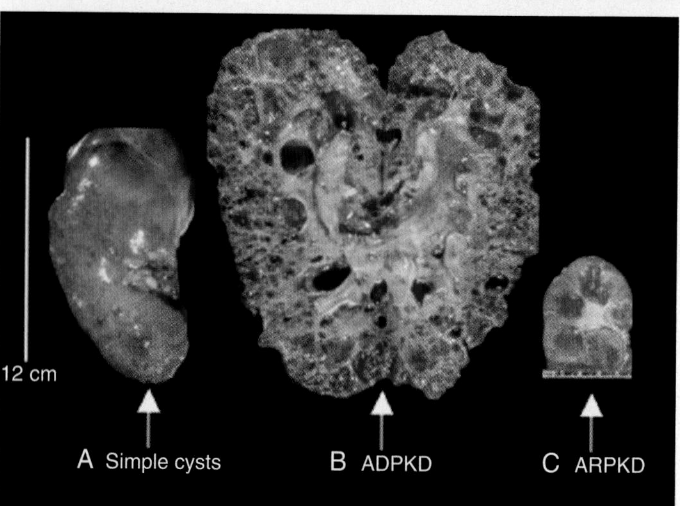

FIGURE 127-1. Gross pathology of selected cystic kidney diseases. A, Photograph of a kidney with multiple simple cysts. The cysts bulge out from the surface of a normal-sized kidney. B, Sagittal cross section of a kidney from an adult with autosomal dominant polycystic kidney disease (ADPKD). Multiple macroscopic cysts have resulted in an enlarged but still reniform kidney (note the evidence of prior hemorrhage within some of the cysts). C, Sagittal cross section of a kidney segment from a neonate with autosomal recessive polycystic kidney disease (ARPKD). The kidney is enlarged, with numerous small cysts. (Courtesy Dr. Robert Colvin, Massachusetts General Hospital.)

AUTOSOMAL DOMINANT POLYCYSTIC KIDNEY DISEASE

PATHOBIOLOGY

ADPKD is a systemic disorder characterized by cyst formation in multiple organs, including the kidneys, other ductal organs, and the cardiovascular system. Renal cysts originate as outpouchings of tubules and may arise from any portion of the nephron, with up to 1% of nephrons involved. The outpouchings expand and eventually separate from the parent tubules, yielding cysts (Fig. 127-2). Cyst growth is caused by proliferation of the cyst lining cells and by abnormal fluid accumulation that results when chloride-driven fluid secretion outpaces absorption.[1] Cyst expansion and fibrosis (induced by cystic epithelium-derived chemokines, cytokines, and growth factors that attract macrophages and fibroblasts) cause compression and obstruction of noncystic normal tubules, thereby resulting in upstream tubular dilation. The kidneys become massively enlarged, and kidney function progressively declines.

Genetics

Heterogeneous mutations in two genes, *PKD1* and *PKD2,* cause ADPKD. Heterogeneous mutations in *PKD1* and PKD2 account for approximately

TABLE 127-1 COMPARISON OF CLINICAL FEATURES OF CYSTIC KIDNEY DISEASES

DISEASE	INHERITANCE	FREQUENCY	GENE PRODUCT	AGE OF ONSET	CYST ORIGIN	RENOMEGALY	CAUSE OF ESRD	OTHER MANIFESTATIONS
ADPKD	AD	1:400-1000	Polycystin-1 Polycystin-2	20s and 30s	Anywhere (including Bowman capsule)	Yes	Yes	Liver cysts Cerebral aneurysms Hypertension Mitral valve prolapse Kidney stones, UTIs
ARPKD	AR	1:6000-10,000	Fibrocystin/ polyductin	First year of life	Distal nephron, CD	Yes	Yes	Hepatic fibrosis Pulmonary hypoplasia Hypertension
ACKD	No	90% of ESRD patients at 8 yr	None*	Years after onset of ESRD	Proximal and distal tubules	Rarely	No	None
Simple cysts	No	50% in those older than 40 yr	None*	Adulthood	Anywhere (usually cortical)	No	No	None
NPHP	AR	1:80,000	Nephrocystins (NPHP1–11)	Childhood or adolescence	Medullary DCT	No	Yes	Retinal degeneration; neurologic, skeletal, hepatic, cardiac malformations
MCKD	AD	Rare	MUC1 and Uromodulin	Adulthood	Medullary DCT	No	Yes	Hyperuricemia, gout
MSK	No	1:5000-20,000	None*	30s	Medullary CD	No	No	Kidney stones
Tuberous sclerosis	AD	1:10,000	Hamartin (TSC1), tuberin (TSC2)	Childhood	Loop of Henle, DCT	Rarely	Rarely	Renal cell carcinoma Tubers, seizures, angiomyolipoma, hypertension
VHL syndrome	AD	1:40,000	VHL protein	20s	Cortical nephrons	Rarely	Rarely	Retinal angioma, CNS hemangioblastoma, renal cell carcinoma, pheochromocytoma
Oral-facial-digital syndrome-1	XD	1:250,000	OFD1 protein	Childhood or adulthood	Renal glomeruli	Rarely	Yes	Malformation of the face, oral cavity, and digits; liver cysts; mental retardation
BBS	AR	1:65,000-160,000	BBS 1-14	Adulthood	Renal calyces	Rarely	Yes	Syndactyly and polydactyly, obesity, retinal dystrophy, male hypogenitalism, hypertension, mental retardation

*No known genetic susceptibility.
ACKD = acquired cystic kidney disease; AD = autosomal dominant; ADPKD = autosomal dominant polycystic kidney disease; AR = autosomal recessive; ARPKD = autosomal recessive polycystic kidney disease; BBS = Bardet-Biedl syndrome; CD = collecting duct; CNS = central nervous system; DCT = distal convoluted tubule; ESRD = end-stage renal disease; MCKD = medullary cystic kidney disease; MSK = medullary sponge kidney; NPHP = nephronophthisis; UTI = urinary tract infection; VHL = von Hippel-Lindau; XD = X-linked dominant.

85% and 15% of cases of ADPKD, respectively. In a minority of ADPKD cases, no demonstrable *PKD1* or *PKD2* mutations are found, suggesting that a third gene may be involved.

PKD1 is 54 kb long and is located on chromosome 16p13.3, adjacent to the tuberous sclerosis 2 (*TSC2*) gene. *PKD1* has 46 exons, generates a 14-kb transcript, and encodes a 4302- residue protein called polycystin-1 (PC1), the first described member of an expanding polycystin protein family. The 5′ region of human *PKD1* (to exon 33) is replicated on the same chromosome, resulting in approximately six copies of *PKD1*-like pseudogenes, which must be distinguished from the *PKD1* gene in direct mutational analysis. To date, 1923 truncating mutations have been identified throughout the gene (http://pkdb.mayo.edu/) but especially in the 3′ half. Mutations in the 5′ half of the gene are associated with more severe disease, with only 19% of patients retaining adequate renal function at 60 years of age (vs. 40% of those with 3′ mutations), and they are more likely to have intracerebral aneurysms and aneurysm rupture.

The 68-kb *PKD2* gene is located on chromosome 4q13-23, transcribes 15 exons, and generates a 5-kb transcript, which encodes a protein of 968 residues called polycystin-2 (PC2). To date, 241 heterogeneous mutations in *PKD2* have been identified. The greater number of cysts that occur at an early age in PKD1 compared with PKD2 disease is likely a result of a higher frequency of mutations in the longer *PKD1* coding region and the presence of six *PKD1*-like pseudogenes that may be involved in recombination-based gene conversion and rearrangements.

Because renal cysts develop from approximately 1% of nephrons, somatic inactivation of the normal *PKD1* or *PKD2* allele (somatic second hit model) has been proposed as the main mechanism of cyst initiation. The *PKD1* or *PKD2* haploinsufficiency state may produce wide stochastic fluctuations in level of the normal gene product and may reduce it to below a critical disease-causing threshold in the absence of a somatic second hit (haploinsufficiency model). Increasing evidence seems to support the latter model. It remains plausible that the genomic instability associated with the *PKD1* or *PKD2* haploid state may increase the likelihood of somatic second hits, which contribute to disease progression by providing cysts with a growth or survival advantage.

There are wide variations in the onset and severity of ADPKD even among affected members of the same family. This variability could arise from variable frequency and timing of the somatic inactivation of the respective normal allele. Variability in disease onset and severity can also result from bilineal inheritance of *PKD1* and *PKD2* mutant alleles or by inheritance of hypomorphic or incompletely penetrant variants of either gene. Mosaicism in a parent in whom a mutation has arisen de novo could result in one sibling having the disease while another is disease free despite sharing the identical inherited haplotype at the *PKD* locus. Digeneic inheritance of mutant *PKD1*, *PKHD1*, *TSC2*, or *HNF1B* alleles can result in ADPKD in infancy. Paradoxically, combining conditional inactivation of the polycystins with ablation of cilia (by inactivating, for example, the ciliopathy genes encoding heterotrimeric kinesin component Kif3a or the intraflagellar transport [protein ift20]) suppress cyst growth in developing and adult kidney and liver. Other modifier loci beyond known disease genes as well as nongenetic risk factors (e.g., smoking, caffeine and male hormones) also likely influence disease variability.

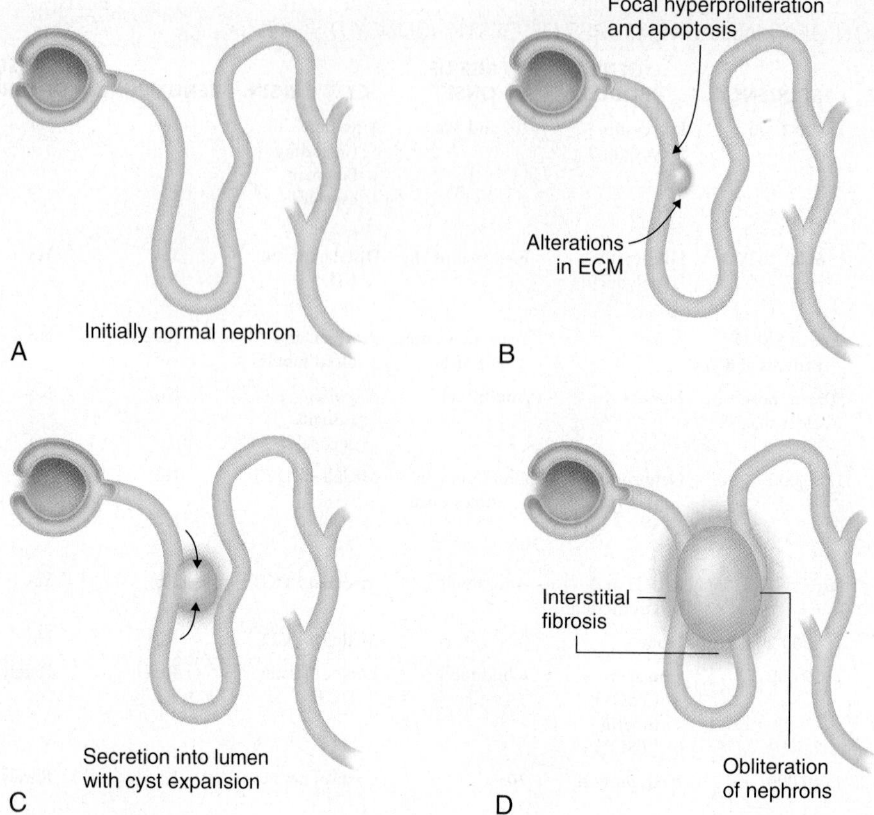

FIGURE 127-2. A to D, Steps involved in cyst formation in autosomal dominant polycystic kidney disease. Note that this process occurs hundreds or thousands of times during the natural history of the disease. ECM = extracellular matrix.

Gene Products

PKD1 encodes PC1, which consists of a large extracellular modular ectodomain followed by an 11-pass transmembrane segment and a short cytoplasmic carboxyl terminus (E-Fig. 127-1). The PC1 ectodomain contains multiple functional motifs, which are also present in cell adhesion receptors, thereby suggesting a role in cell–cell or cell–matrix interactions (or both). Cleavage of PC1 at a membrane proximal G protein–coupled receptor proteolytic site found within the G-protein–coupled receptor autoproteolysis inducing domain is necessary for normal function and results in N-terminal and C-terminal fragments that remain tethered. PC2, the protein encoded by *PKD2*, is a six-membrane spanner that acts as a nonselective voltage-dependent, calcium-permeable ion channel with cytoplasmic amino- and carboxy termini. Its six-transmembrane segment bears topologic and sequence similarity to the carboxyl terminal six-transmembrane segment of PC1. The coiled–coil domains within the carboxyl termini of PC1 and PC2 interact, thereby facilitating PC1 translocation to the plasma membrane and stabilizing the channel activity of PC2. The latter function is regulated by casein kinase 2 (CK2β), which binds the intracellular PLAT domain of PC1.

PC1 and PC2 are widely expressed in tissues, with some overlap consistent with their direct interaction. PC1 expression is highest in fetal tissue and progressively declines thereafter, becoming mainly limited to the collecting duct in the normal adult kidney. PC1 expression is induced in injured adult kidney. By comparison, renal expression of PC2 is maintained throughout development and predominates in the medullary thick ascending limb and distal cortical tubules in the normal adult kidney. PC1 is found at multiple cell membrane sites, including primary cilia, adherens junctions, desmosomes, and focal adhesions, as well as in intracellular vesicles. PC2 is found in primary cilia as well as the basolateral membrane, endoplasmic reticulum, centrosome, and mitotic spindles in dividing cells. Both PC1 and PC2 are also found in urinary exosome-like vesicles.

Experimental studies have suggested that developing renal tubules with high proliferative indices are more sensitive to the reduction in PC1 or PC2 levels, with disease severity radically altered depending on the time of gene inactivation. Whereas *Pkd1* or *Pkd2* inactivation in mice during proliferation of immature tubular epithelium leads to massive cysts and embryonic or neonatal death, inactivation when the renal epithelium has already differentiated into recognizable nephron segments causes mild disease. Maintenance of higher proliferative indices in distal nephron epithelium relative to that in the proximal nephron may explain the predominance of cysts in the distal nephron in adult human ADPKD.

CLINICAL MANIFESTATIONS

ADPKD has a highly variable presentation, even within families. The clinical features of *PKD2*-associated ADPKD are indistinguishable from those of *PKD1*-associated disease. However, *PKD2* disease is milder, with an older average age of onset—74 years versus about 54 years for *PKD1*-associated disease—owing to the development of fewer cysts at an early age rather than to a slower cyst growth rate.[2]

Despite an estimated 100% penetrance by age 90 years, only half the individuals with heterozygous mutations in *PKD1* or *PKD2* are ever diagnosed clinically with ADPKD. Of these patients, the majority present in the third or fourth decade of life with symptoms referable to renal cystic disease. However, ADPKD can develop at any age, including infancy, and it can have a nonrenal presentation. Renomegaly may predominate the clinical picture, with abdominal distention, discomfort, or pain; however, renomegaly can also be discovered incidentally on physical examination or after radiographic studies of the abdomen.

Nocturia, one of the earliest signs of abnormal renal function in ADPKD, reflects the early impairment in urinary concentration owing to disruption of renal architecture by the cysts. Hematuria is typical, but proteinuria is less prominent than in many other renal diseases. Cyst hemorrhage and sometimes rupture, which can occur spontaneously or after trauma, present as sharp pain and hematuria. Anemia features less prominently than in other renal diseases, probably because of the relatively well-preserved erythropoietin secretion. Kidney stones (Chapter 126) occur in 20% to 36% of patients, with uric acid stones slightly more common than calcium oxalate stones; predisposing factors include urinary stasis, defective trapping of urea in the medulla, low urine pH, hypocitraturia, hyperoxaluria, hypercalciuria, and hypomagnesuria. Recurrent cyst infection (Chapter 284), usually by common urinary tract–infecting organisms, is characterized by flank or abdominal pain, fever, rigors, leukocytosis, and occasionally sepsis.

Cardiovascular disease, which is common in ADPKD, manifests as biventricular diastolic dysfunction even in young patients with normal blood pressure and renal function, thoracic and abdominal aortic aneurysms, and cervicocephalic and coronary aneurysms.[3] Arterial hypertension is present in approximately 70% of cases before renal dysfunction is detected. Development of hypertension at a young age is associated with a fourfold increased risk of ESRD and increased cardiovascular morbidity. The risk for preeclampsia is also higher than in the general population.

An estimated 4% to 17% of individuals with ADPKD develop saccular cerebral aneurysms (Chapter 408),[4] a prevalence rate that is four to 10 times greater than in the general population. These aneurysms tend to segregate in families, making ADPKD one of a group of diseases characterized by autosomal dominant inheritance of cerebral aneurysms. ADPKD-associated aneurysms tend to rupture at a smaller size and in younger individuals—on average, 10 years younger than among the general population. Although usually clinically silent, intact cerebral aneurysms can present with focal neurologic symptoms and headaches. By contrast, aneurysms that rupture lead to subarachnoid hemorrhage (Chapter 408) and have dramatic presentations that include severe headaches, seizures, altered sensorium, and death. Aortic and coronary artery aneurysms are also more prevalent in patients with ADPKD, and the frequency of aortic insufficiency is increased.

Although almost never severe enough to cause end-stage liver disease, age-dependent hepatic cysts occur in 30% to 80% of patients with ADPKD and can lead to signs and symptoms of mass effect, infection, hemorrhage, and rupture.[5] Estrogen intake and multiparity in women are risk factors in developing larger and more symptomatic cysts. The cysts that occasionally form in other organs, such as the pancreas, spleen, brain, ovaries, epididymis, and prostate, are usually asymptomatic.[6] Sperm abnormalities and defective motility may occur but rarely cause male infertility. Bronchiectasis (Chapter 90) is threefold more common, inguinal hernias may be more prevalent, and colonic diverticulosis and diverticulitis are more common in ESRD patients with ADPKD.

DIAGNOSIS

Renomegaly, typically presenting in the third or forth decade of life with a positive family history and common extrarenal manifestations, such as hypertension, are useful findings in making a presumptive diagnosis of ADPKD. In these cases, renal ultrasonography is frequently diagnostic. Because only about 60% of individuals give a family history of ADPKD, ultrasound screening of asymptomatic parents or grandparents may be required to uncover diagnostically relevant silent ADPKD.

A diagnosis of ADPKD can be made in an asymptomatic individual by ultrasonography (Fig. 127-3A).[7] To account for the common age-dependent appearance of simple cysts, ADPKD is diagnosed if at least three renal cysts (distributed in one or both kidneys) are present in individuals 15 to 29 years old (sensitivity, 0.82; specificity, 1.0), 30 to 39 years old (sensitivity, 0.96; specificity, 1.0), if at least two renal cysts are present in each kidney in individuals age 40 to 59 years (sensitivity, 1.0; specificity, 0.99), or if at least four renal cysts are detected in each kidney in individuals 60 years of age or older (sensitivity, 1.0; specificity, 1.0). Fewer than two renal cysts in an individual from an ADPKD family with an unknown genotype age 40 years or older or the absence of renal cysts in such an individual age 30 to 39 years is sufficient to exclude the disease, with negative predictive values of 100% and 99.3%, respectively. A negative ultrasound result is less accurate in excluding disease in individuals younger than 30 years, so computed tomography (CT) or magnetic resonance imaging (MRI) is recommended. When a young relative is being considered as a potential kidney donor to a family member with end-stage ADPKD, contrast-enhanced, three-dimensional CT or magnetic resonance angiography (MRA) is required because these tests can detect 3-mm cysts compared with ultrasonography's ability to detect 10-mm cysts.

Cerebral aneurysms are increasingly being detected with MRI in ADPKD patients. Four-vessel cerebral angiography remains the gold standard and is often used for surgical planning.

DNA-based diagnosis of ADPKD by means of direct sequencing is commercially available and detects mutations in more than 90% of affected individuals. Next-generation exome sequencing may have a much higher sensitivity and specificity for the diagnosis.[8] Testing is recommended when imaging study results are equivocal, in a young transplant donor from an ADPKD family when imaging study results are negative, or to facilitate pre-implantation genetic diagnosis. The marked allelic heterogeneity of the *PKD1* and *PKD2* mutations, as well as the paucity of phenotype–genotype correlations, contributes to the complexity of DNA-based diagnostics.

Monitoring Renal Disease Progression

Despite ongoing renal cyst expansion, the glomerular filtration rate (GFR) and the serum creatinine level are generally maintained within the normal range in ADPKD patients until the fourth to sixth decade of life. These markers are therefore insensitive for monitoring disease progression, especially in young patients. Reduced renal blood flow is the most sensitive prognostic indicator of renal progression. Estimating height-adjusted total kidney volume from measurements of kidney length, width, and thickness using MRI, CT, or ultrasonography can also reliably monitor disease progression in the early stages of ADPKD when the GFR is still in the normal range. A baseline kidney volume of 600 cm^3 or greater predicts the development of renal insufficiency with a 75% accuracy within an 8-year follow-up period. Although gadolinium-enhanced MRI provides excellent detail of kidney structures, MRI without gadolinium is recommended to monitor kidney volume, especially in ADPKD patients with a reduced GFR, because of concern about nephrogenic systemic fibrosis (Chapter 267) and further impairment of renal function associated with its use. The kidney volume in ADPKD patients progressively increases in most cases but at widely differing rates, ranging from less than 1% to more than 10% annually, and renal function declines as the kidneys enlarge.[9] Kidney volumes greater than 1,500 mL are frequently associated with a decreased GFR and gross hematuria and invariably with arterial hypertension.

PREVENTION AND TREATMENT Rx

Management strategies are aimed at monitoring for complications of ADPKD and treating them, as well as providing counseling. Frequent monitoring and effective treatment of hypertension (Chapter 67; see Tables 67-7 and 67-8) are essential because hypertensive patients have a greater annual increase in kidney volume, as well as a higher prevalence of left ventricular

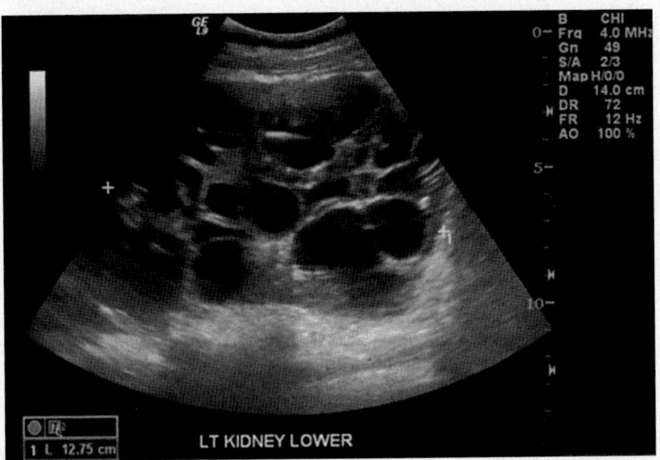

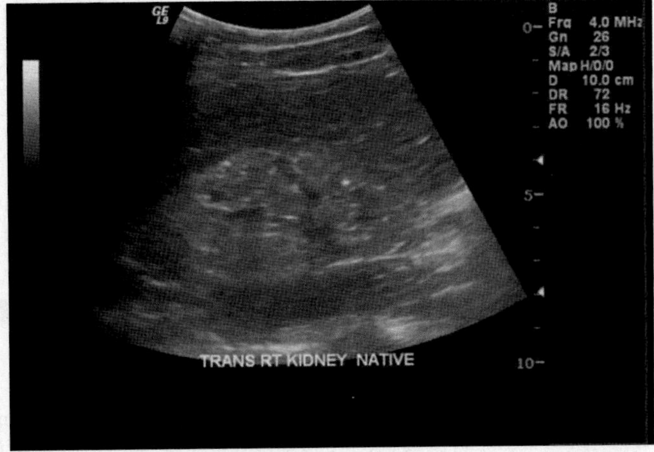

FIGURE 127-3. A, Ultrasound image of a kidney from a patient with autosomal dominant polycystic kidney disease. B, Ultrasound image of a kidney from a patient with autosomal recessive polycystic kidney disease. (Courtesy Dr. Javier M. Romero and Jennifer A. McDowell, Massachusetts General Hospital.)

hypertrophy, ischemic heart disease, and stroke, compared with normotensive patients. The goals of blood pressure control are the same as for other patients with renal disease, including the attainment of a symptom-free blood pressure of 120/80 mm Hg or less. Experimental and clinical data suggest that angiotensin-converting enzyme (ACE) inhibitors may be the preferred type of medication because they promote more reversal of left ventricular hypertrophy for the same of blood pressure reduction compared with calcium channel blockers in patients with ADPKD.

Treatment of urinary tract infection (Chapter 284) and prevention of nephrolithiasis (Chapter 126) are the same as in the general population and include standard antimicrobial therapy and increased fluid intake, respectively. Renal and hepatic cyst infections are optimally treated with lipophilic antibiotics that possess cyst-penetrating capabilities, including ciprofloxacin, trimethoprim, clindamycin, and vancomycin. Blood or urine cultures and sensitivities are used to guide the choice of antibiotic therapy.

Cyst hemorrhage and rupture, with resultant pain and hematuria, are usually managed conservatively with rest and analgesics; nonsteroidal anti-inflammatory drugs (NSAIDs) are avoided owing to their antiplatelet action and potential renal toxicity. Alternatives include acetaminophen 500 mg up to every 4 hours for mild to moderate pain, nonopiates such as tramadol 50 mg up to every 4 hours for moderate to severe pain, and the addition of an oral or transdermal opioid (see Table 30-5 in Chapter 30) as needed. Patients with enlarged kidneys should be advised to avoid playing contact sports, and those with massively enlarged kidneys should refrain from wearing belts and seatbelts. Some patients with unusually painful cysts respond to cyst fluid aspiration, cyst deroofing, or ethanol-induced sclerosis.

Nephrectomy is rarely indicated before the onset of ESRD. Renal replacement therapies, including renal transplantation (Chapter 131), are at least as effective as in other causes of ESRD.

The massive cystic enlargement of the liver commonly seen by midlife in women with ADPKD makes it prudent to avoid estrogen intake and repeated pregnancies. Partial hepatectomy has been successful in improving the quality of life in patients with massive liver enlargement.

Magnetic resonance angiography screening is not routinely recommended for asymptomatic patients without a family history of cerebral aneurysm or subarachnoid hemorrhage, but it is recommended for patients with a positive personal or family history and for patients who experience a new onset of severe headache or central nervous system symptoms or signs. It may also be considered in those with high-risk occupations, such as airline pilots, and for patients with incapacitating anxiety. The risk of a patient with a positive family history developing a new aneurysm after an initially negative MRA result is 2.6% at a mean follow-up period of 9.8 years, so rescreening every 5 to 10 years in such cases may be appropriate, especially in patients with early-onset hypertension or a history of heavy smoking. Asymptomatic patients with positive family history of cerebral aneurysms and positive MRA results should be followed closely with a neurosurgeon and monitored by annual MRA screening. The decision to perform surgical clipping or endovascular embolization should take into consideration the age of the patient, the size of the aneurysm and its location, and a previous history of cerebral bleeding (Chapter 408).

Patients should be advised that their children have a 50% probability of inheriting a disease-causing germline mutation. DNA-based diagnostics are most useful in identifying the germline mutation prenatally or preimplantation. As DNA-based diagnostics become more widely available and less expensive and as promising new treatment options are developed, counseling will become an increasingly important component of prevention.

Experimental Therapies

Current therapeutic efforts are targeting increased cell proliferation of cystic epithelium and abnormal fluid secretion into cysts (E-Fig. 127-2). So far, the only effective specific therapy is oral tolvaptan (45-90 mg in the morning and 15-30 mg in the afternoon as tolerated), which slows the increase in total kidney volume and the decline in kidney function over a 3-year period compared with placebo.[A1] However, tolvaptan also is associated with a fourfold increase in liver injury and could not be tolerated by nearly 25% of patients. As a result, tolvaptan has not been approved by the Food and Drug Administration for the treatment of ADPKD. The metabolically stable somatostatin analogue octreotide (at a dose of 40 mg every 28 days) can slow the expansion of renal cysts but does not slow the decline in renal function, and it also is associated with substantial side effects.[A2-A4] In meta-analyses, rapamycin complex 1 inhibitors, such as sirolimus and everolimus, also have not been beneficial.[A4,A5] These data suggest that cyst growth may not be the key determinant of renal function decline.

PROGNOSIS

The rate of progression of renal disease is highest in men with poorly controlled hypertension, an early age at diagnosis, and mutations in *PKD1*. Kidney cysts develop earlier in *PKD1* than in *PKD2* disease, but the rate of expansion is similar, indicating that the basic difference in phenotype is in cyst initiation not expansion. Whereas the presence of one affected family member who developed ESRD by age 60 years is highly predictive of PKD1 disease (positive predictive value, 100%; sensitivity, 75%), the development of ESRD after age 70 years in a family member is highly predictive of PKD2 disease (positive predictive value, 95%; sensitivity, 75%). Approximately 5% of all ADPKD patients with cerebral aneurysms die from aneurysmal rupture.

AUTOSOMAL RECESSIVE POLYCYSTIC KIDNEY DISEASE

DEFINITION AND EPIDEMIOLOGY

ARPKD is a multisystem childhood disorder characterized by severe and early PKD dominated by dilation of the kidney collecting ducts, systemic hypertension, biliary ductal plate dysgenesis in neonates, and portal tract fibrosis in older children.

PATHOBIOLOGY

ARPKD has been linked to heterogeneous mutations in a single gene, *PKHD1* (polycystic kidney and hepatic disease 1). Located on chromosome 6q21, *PKHD1* has 67 exons and spans a genomic region of approximately 470 kb, the longest open reading frame of which is 12,222 base pairs long. *PKHD1* encodes a unique type I membrane protein, fibrocystin/polyductin, comprising 4074 amino acids, with a large extracellular segment and a short cytoplasmic carboxyl terminus. The precise physiologic function of fibrocystin/polyductin in collecting duct and biliary duct epithelium is not clear, but its domains are known to mediate cell motility and invasion, extracellular protein and carbohydrate binding, and catalysis of polysaccharide hydrolysis. Alternatively-spliced transcripts of *PKHD1* encode a membrane protein with variable extracellular domains, as well as forms lacking the transmembrane segment. Homozygous truncating mutations in *PKHD1* are associated with perinatal renal disease, whereas patients with homozygous missense mutations present later because some functional protein is produced.

Fibrocystin/polyductin protein encoded by *PKHD1* is predominantly expressed in the cortical and medullary collecting ducts and the thick ascending limbs of Henle. It is also found to a lesser degree in the pancreas, liver, and lungs, which are also affected in ARPKD. In common with many cystogenic proteins, fibrocystin/polyductin is found in basal bodies and primary apical cilia, suggesting that it is important in maintaining the structural integrity of cilia.

Loss of the fibrocystin/polyductin protein downregulates PC2. Fibrocystin/polyductin–PC2 interactions may regulate calcium influx mediated by PC2. It has been proposed that cystogenesis in ADPKD and ARPKD share a common mechanism, with the variability in the ARPKD phenotype traced to the degree of PC2 expression among patients. However, renal cysts can originate from any part of the nephron and are detached from the nephron proper in ADPKD, but they originate from and remain attached to the distal nephron in ARPKD, suggesting that additional signaling pathways specific for each disease and gene product likely explain these anatomic differences.

CLINICAL MANIFESTATIONS

Although ARPKD can present as renal cysts discovered radiographically either antenatally or during adulthood, it usually manifests as bilateral abdominal masses and renal insufficiency in infancy. It carries a 30% mortality rate owing to severe pulmonary hypoplasia; oligohydramnios, presumably linked to in utero renal disease, likely accounts for the pulmonary hypoplasia. Hypertension is almost universal, typically develops before renal impairment is apparent, and probably accelerates the decline in renal function. Findings related to renal tubular dysfunction may be present and include polyuria, enuresis, hyponatremia, and hyperchloremic metabolic acidosis. Cystic complications related to infection and rupture also occur, although hematuria is an infrequent finding. ESRD can take up to 20 years to develop, and in rare instances, it never occurs.

Hepatic fibrosis, secondary to dilation of the intrahepatic and extrahepatic bile ducts, manifests as recurrent ascending cholangitis (Chapter 155) and portal hypertension with splenomegaly and esophageal varices. Pancreatic fibrosis is rarely a clinical concern.

DIAGNOSIS

The demonstration by abdominal ultrasonography (see Fig. 127-3, *B*) or CT of symmetrically enlarged polycystic kidneys that retain their reniform shape (owing to uniform microcystic dilation of collecting ducts) and hepatic fibrosis is sufficient to diagnose ARPKD. In contrast to ADPKD cysts, ARPKD cysts tend to retain their connections with the originating nephron. Aside from an occasional affected sibling, a family history is often not elicited. Distinguishing ARPKD from ADPKD, especially in patients presenting in childhood or adulthood, may require a liver biopsy to document otherwise undetectable hepatic fibrosis. Gene-based diagnostics in ARPKD are helpful in making a firm diagnosis, especially in patients with late-onset disease, and they are useful in preimplantation and in prenatal diagnosis.

PREVENTION AND TREATMENT Rx

In the absence of specific therapy for ARPKD, management goals focus on early detection and on treatment of the complications of hypertension, urinary tract or cyst infection, ESRD, and portal hypertension. Kidney transplantation may be necessary in late childhood in patients with ARPKD who present with renal disease perinatally. Treatment of portal hypertension may require liver transplantation or portosystemic shunting (Chapter 154). Treatment of hypertension begins with ACE inhibitors and angiotensin receptor blockers (see Tables 67-7 and 67-8 in Chapter 67), which are generally effective. As in all children with ESRD, attention to nutrition and renal osteodystrophy is paramount (Chapter 130). With improving sensitivity of gene-based diagnostics, genetic counseling will play a more active role in prevention.

PROGNOSIS

For patients with ARPKD, the highest mortality rates occur during the first year of life. Approximately 50% to 80% of patients survive to 15 years of age.

NEPHRONOPHTHISIS

DEFINITION AND EPIDEMIOLOGY

Nephronophthisis (NPHP) is the most common genetic cause of ESRD in childhood and adolescence, accounting for 5% to 15% of cases of ESRD.[10] It is an autosomal recessive disorder caused by mutations in a number of genes that encode nephrocystins, which are expressed in the centrosome and basal body of primary cilia, with some also localizing to adherens junctions or focal adhesions in epithelia. Homozygotic and compound heterozygotic mutations in at least 11 known genes (*NPHP1* through *NPHP11*) account for about 30% of cases. Infantile, juvenile, and adolescent variants have been described based on the median age of onset of ESRD. Infantile NPHP is characterized by mutations in the *NPHP2* gene. Whereas the juvenile form caused by mutations in *NPHP1* is the most common, the adolescent form is caused by mutations in *NPHP3*. As in other genetic renal diseases, the rate of progression to ESRD is determined in part by type and severity of the genetic defect.

Nephronophthisis is characterized pathologically by renal interstitial fibrosis, tubular atrophy with basement membrane thickening and disruption, and renal cysts and diverticula that are largely restricted to the loops of Henle and distal tubules at the corticomedullary junctions. Kidney size is generally normal or reduced, except in the rare infantile variant that leads to ESRD by 3 years of age. Expression of NPHP genes at extrarenal sites accounts for the associated retinal, neural, liver, and skeletal abnormalities. Each of the NPHP genes is associated with a somewhat different phenotype, although some share common phenotypes, explained by protein–protein interactions between two or more nephrocystins. Cerebello-ocular-renal syndromes associated with NPHP can sometimes include early-onset retinitis pigmentosa, when the syndrome is caused by mutations in *NPHP5* and *NPHP6*.

CLINICAL MANIFESTATIONS

Presenting symptoms include polyuria, growth failure, and anemia. Polyuria occurs early, owing to reduced urinary concentrating ability and to salt wasting. Decreased growth rate is related to chronic dehydration, and growth failure and anemia occur with the onset of ESRD. Blood pressure is normal, and edema is absent before the onset of renal failure. Hematuria and proteinuria are absent or minimal. Patients with mutations in specific NPHP genes may also present with eye defects, oculomotor apraxia, congenital amaurosis, retinitis pigmentosa, neural anomalies, cerebellar ataxia, seizures, liver fibrosis, skeletal defects, scoliosis, cleft palate, and situs inversus.

DIAGNOSIS

The diagnosis relies on clinical suspicion of the disorder in a pediatric or adolescent patient who presents with ESRD and extrarenal manifestations such as abnormal eye movements, blindness, mental retardation, and polydactyly. Differential diagnosis includes renal dysplasia, early-onset ADPKD, urinary tract obstruction, and ARPKD. Abdominal ultrasonography, MRI (without gadolinium), electroretinography, and full neurologic and ophthalmologic evaluations should assess the patient's renal, liver, retinal, and neurologic status. Renal ultrasonography showing loss of corticomedullary differentiation, increased parenchymal echogenicity, and occasionally small medullary or corticomedullary cysts in normal-sized or moderately small kidneys is highly suggestive of juvenile NPHP in a child with severe uremia. Genetic testing may be required for a conclusive diagnosis. A renal biopsy showing evidence of chronic tubulointerstitial nephritis may be necessary to confirm the diagnosis if genetic testing is not available.

PREVENTION AND TREATMENT Rx

Treatment is largely supportive, focusing on the progressive renal failure and the need for dialysis and transplantation. Prenatal genetic testing in families with a genetic diagnosis of NPHP is feasible. DNA-based diagnostics are most useful in identifying the germline mutation prenatally or preimplantation.

MEDULLARY CYSTIC KIDNEY DISEASE

Medullary cystic kidney disease is an autosomal dominant interstitial kidney disease that results in renal failure after the fourth decade of life. It is more rare than autosomal recessive NPHP, with which it shares a number of histologic features, including tubular basement membrane disintegration, tubular cyst formation, and tubulointerstitial inflammation and fibrosis.

Mutations in two genes, *MCKD1* and *MCKD2*, cause medullary cystic kidney disease. *MCKD1* encodes mucin 1 (MUC1), a transmembrane protein expressed in the kidney but with unknown function. Knockout studies in mice show that *Muc1* is not essential, suggesting a dominant-negative and/or gain-of-function mode of action for the mutant protein in humans. *MCKD2* encodes an 85-kD nonciliary protein, uromodulin, which is expressed on the luminal side of renal epithelium in the thick ascending limb of Henle loop and early distal convoluted tubules. Uromodulin has been associated with urate metabolism, inhibition of stone formation and renal immune response. Familial juvenile hyperuricemic nephropathy and glomerulocystic kidney disease, rare but distinct disorders, are allelic to *MCKD2*. The former is characterized by glomerular cysts, hyperuricemia-associated gouty arthritis, and early-onset ESRD, and the latter is characterized by impaired urine concentrating ability and reduced uric acid excretion.

Mutations in *MCKD1* and *MCKD2* result in a similar clinical picture except for an earlier onset of ESRD and precocious gout with mutations in *MCKD2*. Polyuria and anemia are usually not clinically present in the early stages of the renal disease. Hypertension is likely secondary to renal failure.

Corticomedullary cysts, which are present in most adult patients, cannot always be recognized on ultrasonography or CT because they tend to be very small. Except for the treatment of gout (Chapter 273), management is similar to that of patients with NPHP.

MEDULLARY SPONGE KIDNEY

Medullary sponge kidney, which is a rare disorder of unknown pathogenesis, is characterized by congenitally acquired inner medullary and papillary collecting duct dilations, hypercalciuria, and a mild defect in urinary concentration and acidification owing to tubular dysfunction.[11] Patients present with hematuria and recurrent kidney stones, usually by the second or third decade of life. Medullary sponge kidney may also be an incidental finding on an intravenous pyelogram that shows the characteristic pooling of contrast material within the cystic collecting ducts. ESRD is uncommon, and the long-term prognosis is excellent.

OTHER INHERITED CYSTIC SYNDROMES

Bardet-Biedl syndrome (BBS) is an autosomal recessive disorder characterized by vision loss; obesity; hypertension; dystrophy of the hands, kidneys, and male genitalia; delayed development of motor skills; and behavioral problems. Mutations in at least 14 BBS genes involved in maintenance and function of cilia have been identified. About 45% of cases result from mutations in *BBS1* or *BBS10*, but in about 25% of cases, the defective gene remains to be identified. Calyceal cysts and calyceal clubbing predominate the renal lesion and are best diagnosed by intravenous urography rather than ultrasonography. Renal impairment is frequent and is an important cause of death.

Oral-facial-digital syndrome is a rare neurodevelopmental ciliopathy characterized by malformations of the brain, face, oral cavity, and digits. It is inherited in an X-linked dominant pattern and is caused by defects in the *OFD1* gene, which encodes OFD1 protein expressed in the centrosome and basal body of primary cilia but has an undetermined function. Renal (primarily glomerular) cysts are found in as many as 50% of patients, all females; males carrying the mutation die in utero. ESRD has been reported in affected girls and women ranging in age from 11 to 72 years.

Autosomal dominant renal cyst formation is also seen in tuberous sclerosis and von Hippel-Lindau syndrome (Chapter 417). In tuberous sclerosis, cyst formation is commonly associated with hypertension; this disorder can resemble ADPKD and is associated with about a 5% incidence of renal cell carcinoma. In von Hippel-Lindau syndrome, cyst formation can also lead to features of ADPKD; more important, the syndrome is associated with a 25% incidence of renal cell carcinoma.

ACQUIRED CYSTIC KIDNEY DISEASE

Acquired cystic kidney disease is largely confined to the ESRD population on dialysis (Chapter 131). Cysts arise from proximal and distal tubule dilations in small end-stage kidneys regardless of cause, mode of dialysis, or presence of a functioning kidney transplant. Identifiable risk factors include duration of ESRD, older age, male gender, black race, and chronic hypokalemia.

CLINICAL MANIFESTATIONS AND DIAGNOSIS

Acquired cystic kidney disease is usually asymptomatic, but it occasionally leads to enlarged kidneys with associated abdominal discomfort and pain. Cyst hemorrhage, which is more common than cyst infection, presents with flank pain, anemia, or hematuria. The most significant complication of acquired cystic kidney disease is malignant conversion of cysts into renal cell carcinoma (Chapter 197). Carcinomas commonly present as hematuria and are two to 200 times more common in patients with acquired cystic kidney disease than in the general dialysis population.

Acquired cystic kidney disease is diagnosed by ultrasonography or CT demonstrating multiple and bilateral renal cysts in a patient with preexisting chronic renal failure or ESRD. In contrast to ADPKD and ARPKD, the kidneys are usually not enlarged, and there is no family history of PKD. Renal CT or MRI is preferable to detect cysts in small kidneys and to assess for malignant conversion.

PREVENTION AND TREATMENT

Rx

There are no strategies to prevent the appearance or delay the expansion of renal cysts in patients on hemodialysis, but cysts may stabilize or regress after successful renal transplantation. New or frank hematuria raises the concern of renal cell carcinoma (Chapter 197), which should be assessed using ultrasonography and contrast-enhanced CT. Any evidence of septa formation, solid material, or contrast enhancement within a cyst is suspicious for carcinoma and warrants consideration of nephrectomy.

PROGNOSIS

Asymptomatic acquired cystic kidney disease does not affect survival. The incidence of renal cell carcinoma in patients with acquired cystic kidney disease is approximately 0.18% per year. Although metastasis is less common at the time of diagnosis in patients with acquired cystic kidney disease than in other patients with renal cell carcinoma, the 5-year mortality rates are higher, likely related to the almost invariable coexistence of ESRD.

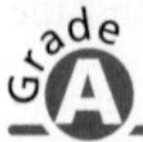

Grade A References

A1. Torres VE, Chapman AB, Devuyst O, et al. Tolvaptan in patients with autosomal dominant polycystic kidney disease. *N Engl J Med.* 2012;367:2407-2418.

A2. Hogan MC, Masyuk TV, Page LJ, et al. Randomized clinical trial of long-acting somatostatin for autosomal dominant polycystic kidney and liver disease. *J Am Soc Nephrol.* 2010;21:1052-1061.

A3. Caroli A, Perico N, Perna A, et al. Effect of longacting somatostatin analogue on kidney and cyst growth in autosomal dominant polycystic kidney disease (ALADIN): a randomised, placebo-controlled, multicentre trial. *Lancet.* 2013;382:1485-1495.

A4. Myint T, Rangan G, Webster A. Treatments to slow progression of autosomal dominant polycystic kidney disease: systematic review and meta analysis of randomized trials. *Nephrology (Carlton).* 2014;19:217-226.

A5. Liu YM, Shao YQ, He Q. Sirolimus for treatment of autosomal-dominant polycystic kidney disease: a meta-analysis of randomized controlled trials. *Transplant Proc.* 2014;46:66-74.

GENERAL REFERENCES

For the General References and other additional features, please visit Expert Consult at https://expertconsult.inkling.com.

128 HEREDITARY NEPHROPATHIES AND DEVELOPMENTAL ABNORMALITIES OF THE URINARY TRACT

LISA M. GUAY-WOODFORD

HEREDITARY NEPHROPATHIES

The proximal tubule is responsible for reclaiming most of the filtered glucose, amino acids, uric acid, phosphate, bicarbonate, and low-molecular-weight proteins. The loop of Henle and the distal nephron reabsorb approximately 30% of the filtered sodium chloride and 50% of the filtered divalent cations. The collecting duct, under the regulatory control of aldosterone, fine-tunes sodium reabsorption and secretes hydrogen and potassium ions. In the terminal collecting duct, antidiuretic hormone regulates water reabsorption and urine concentration.

Inherited renal tubular disorders are a group of conditions in which the normal renal tubular reabsorption of ions, organic solutes, and water (Chapter 116) is disrupted because of defects in single genes.[1] These defects can be categorized by the nephron segment affected (Table 128-1).

Disorders of Proximal Tubule Function

CYSTINURIA

Cystinuria is characterized by defective proximal tubular reabsorption of cystine and dibasic amino acids, resulting in increased excretion of cystine and the risk of forming cystine-containing urinary stones (Chapter 126).[2] This autosomal recessive trait has an estimated prevalence of 1 in 7000 individuals. Two cystinuria genes have been identified: *SLC7A9*, which encodes the luminal transport channel itself; and *SLC3A1*, which encodes the transporter regulatory subunit. Several large studies indicate that mutations in *SLC3A1* are more common than mutations in *SLC7A9*. Mutations in *SLC3A1* cause cystinuria type A, mutations in *SLC7A9* cause cystinuria type B, and mutations in both genes (compound heterozygotes) cause cystinuria type AB.

Although the severity of the disease is similar in all types of cystinurias, the clinical presentation can be variable, and the onset of disease may occur from infancy to the seventh decade of life. Cystine stones are radiopaque and often form the nidus for secondary calcium oxalate stones. Symptoms include renal colic, which may be associated with urinary tract obstruction or infection. Affected children can be identified by elevated urinary cystine levels, but testing must be performed after tubular transport has fully matured (at 2 years of age). Genetic testing is available, but at this point it does not offer any clinical therapeutic benefit. Conservative therapy with high urine volume and urinary alkalinization is sufficient for many patients with cystinuria. However, recurrent stone formation may cause renal damage and warrants treatment with thiol-containing agents, such as D-penicillamine (pediatric dose, 15 to 30 mg/kg/day in four divided doses; adult dose, 2 g/day in four divided doses), α-mercaptopropionylglycine (pediatric dose, 10 to 15 mg/kg/day in three divided doses; adult dose, 0.8 to 1.0 g/day in three divided doses), or captopril (pediatric dose, 12.5 mg/kg/day in two divided doses), to form soluble mixed disulfides with cystine and to maintain free urine cystine levels below 200 mg per gram of creatinine.

CYSTINOSIS

Cystinosis is the most common inherited cause of renal Fanconi syndrome; it also affects the eyes, muscles, central nervous system, lungs, and various endocrine organs. Cystinosis is an autosomal recessive disorder caused by mutations in the gene *CTNS*, which encodes cystinosin, a lysosomal cystine transporter. Defects in this transporter lead to the accumulation of intralysosomal cystine crystals and widespread cellular destruction.

TABLE 128-1 HEREDITARY NEPHROPATHIES BY NEPHRON SEGMENT

NEPHRON SEGMENT	DISORDER	INHERITANCE	OMIM	MAJOR RENAL FEATURES
PROXIMAL TUBULE				
	Renal glycosuria	AR	233100	Isolated glycosuria
	Proximal renal tubular acidosis	AR	604278	Hyperchloremic, hypokalemic, metabolic acidosis
	Carbonic anhydrase II deficiency	AR	259730	Mixed proximal and distal renal tubular acidosis
	Hartnup disease	AR	234500	Neutral aminoaciduria
	Cystinuria	AR	Type A: 220100 Type B: 604144	Urinary calculi
	Cystinosis	AR	Infantile: 219800 Late-onset: 219900 Non-nephropathic: 219750	Renal Fanconi syndrome
	Dent disease	X-linked	Dent disease 1: 300009 Dent disease 2: 300555	Nephrocalcinosis, urinary calculi; low-molecular-weight proteinuria
	Lowe syndrome	X-linked	309000	Renal Fanconi syndrome
	Hereditary fructose intolerance	AR	229600	Renal Fanconi syndrome
	Tyrosinemia, type I	AR	276700	Renal Fanconi syndrome
	Wilson disease	AR	277900	Renal Fanconi syndrome
LOOP OF HENLE				
	Bartter syndrome	AR AD	Type 1: 601678 Type 2: 241200 Type 3: 607364 Type 4: 602522 Type 5: 601199	Hypokalemic, hypochloremic metabolic alkalosis
DISTAL TUBULE				
	Gitelman syndrome	AR	263800	Hypokalemic, hypochloremic, metabolic alkalosis
	Familial hypomagnesemia with hypercalciuria	AR	248250, 248190	Severe renal magnesium and calcium wasting
	Isolated hypomagnesemia	AD	154020	Renal magnesium wasting
COLLECTING DUCT				
	Liddle syndrome	AD	177200	Low-renin hypertension
	Glucocorticoid-remediable hyperaldosteronism	AD	103900	Low-renin hypertension
	Apparent mineralocorticoid excess	AR	218030	Low-renin hypertension
	Pseudohypoaldosteronism, type 1	AR, AD	AR: 264350 AD: 177735	Hyponatremic, hypokalemic, metabolic acidosis
	Pseudohypoaldosteronism type 2 (Gordon syndrome)	AD	114300	Low-renin hypertension with hyperkalemia
	Distal renal tubular acidosis	AR, AD	AR: 602722, 605239 AD: 179800, 611590	Hyperchloremic, hypokalemic, metabolic acidosis
	Carbonic anhydrase II deficiency	AR	259730	Mixed proximal and distal renal tubular acidosis
	Nephrogenic diabetes insipidus	X-linked AR and AD	X-linked: 304800 AD and AR: 125800	Urinary concentrating defect

AD = autosomal dominant; AR = autosomal recessive; OMIM = entries in Online Mendelian Inheritance in Man, available at www.ncbi.nlm.nih.gov/omim.

Three clinical presentations have been described.[3] The most severe is infantile (classic) cystinosis, which is manifested in the first year of life with renal tubular acidosis, impaired growth, and evidence of renal Fanconi syndrome, including aminoaciduria, glucosuria, phosphaturia, and low-molecular-weight proteinuria. Progressive renal failure reaches end-stage renal disease in childhood. A less severe, late-onset (juvenile or intermediate) form causes renal dysfunction in adolescence and involves cystine deposits in the cornea. The mildest form, an ocular, non-nephropathic form, features photophobia but no renal problems.

The mainstay of cystinosis therapy is oral cysteamine (dose: 60 to 90 mg/kg/day or 1.35 to 1.90 g/m^2/day, divided every 6 hours), an aminothiol that can lower intracellular cystine content by 90%. In well-treated adolescent and young adult patients, cysteamine delays renal glomerular deterioration, enhances growth, prevents hypothyroidism, and lowers muscle cystine content. Therefore, early diagnosis and prompt, proper treatment are critical for preventing or significantly delaying the complications of cystinosis. In a randomized trial, twice-daily dosing with delayed-release cysteamine bitartrate (at approximately 70% of the patient's usual dose) was as efficacious as cysteamine for reducing white blood cell cystine levels in patients with nephropathic cystinosis,[A1] thereby suggesting that it is an equally effective therapy.

Disorders of Loop of Henle and Distal Tubule Function

THE BARTTER-GITELMAN DISORDERS

The Bartter-Gitelman syndromes are a group of disorders characterized by markedly reduced salt transport in the thick ascending limb of Henle (Bartter syndrome) or in the distal convoluted tubule (Gitelman syndrome).[4] Most patients with Gitelman syndrome have defects in *SLC12A3*, the gene encoding the sodium-chloride cotransporter NCCT. However, a minority of patients with the Gitelman phenotype have mutations in *CLCNKB*.

Bartter syndrome can be caused by mutations in one of four genes: *SLC12A2*, encoding the sodium-potassium-chloride cotransporter NKCC2; *KCNJ1*, encoding the ROMK1 potassium ion channel; *CLCNKB*, encoding the ClC-Kb basolateral chloride ion channel; and *BSND*, encoding barttin, a regulatory subunit required for basolateral chloride channel targeting to the membrane. These mutations cause autosomal recessive Bartter syndrome

TABLE 128-2 FEATURES OF THE INHERITED RENAL TUBULAR ACIDOSES

DISORDER	RENAL TRANSPORT DEFECT	MINIMAL URINE pH DURING ACIDOSIS	ALKALI SUPPLEMENTATION	UAG DURING ACIDOSIS
Proximal renal tubular acidosis	↓Proximal bicarbonate reabsorption	<5.5	Children: 10-15 mEq HCO_3^-/kg/day	0 or +
Carbonic anhydrase II deficiency	↓Proximal bicarbonate reabsorption and ↓distal acidification	Variable	Variable	0 or +
Distal renal tubular acidosis	↓Distal acidification	>5.5	Adults: 1-3 mEq HCO_3^-/kg/day Children: 3-6 mEq HCO_3^-/kg/day	+

HCO_3^- = bicarbonate; UAG = urinary anion gap = $[Na^+] + [K^+] - [Cl^-]$. In renal tubular acidosis, the UAG is usually 0 or positive. By comparison, the UAG is negative in metabolic acidosis associated with diarrheal illness.

types 1, 2, 3, and 4, respectively. Defects in any of these genes disrupt salt transport in the thick ascending limb, causing a furosemide-like effect (E-Fig. 128-1). In addition, severe gain-in-function mutations in *CASR*, the gene encoding the extracellular calcium ion–sensing receptor CaSR, can cause a Bartter-like phenotype (referred to as Bartter syndrome type 5) that is distinguished from the others by autosomal dominant transmission and associated hypocalcemic hypercalciuria.

Individuals with Bartter syndrome exhibit renal salt wasting, lowered blood pressure, polyuria, hypokalemic metabolic alkalosis, and hypercalciuria with a variable risk of nephrocalcinosis. In comparison, individuals with Gitelman syndrome exhibit milder renal salt wasting, normal blood pressure, hypokalemic metabolic alkalosis, hypomagnesemia, and hypocalciuria. This clinical disorder resembles the effects of long-term thiazide administration. Clinical differences between Bartter and Gitelman syndromes relate to the severity of salt wasting, whereas phenotypic differences among Bartter syndrome types 1 through 5 correlate with the specific physiologic roles played by the individual transporters or channels in the kidney and other organs.

The mainstay of treatment includes replacing salt and water losses and providing potassium supplementation to maintain serum levels greater than 3 mEq/dL. In patients with perinatal (type 1 or 2) Bartter syndrome, cyclooxygenase inhibitors (e.g., indomethacin, 2 to 4 mg/kg/day in two to four divided doses) may be beneficial. In patients with Gitelman syndrome and some patients with Bartter syndrome type 3, oral magnesium supplementation may be required to maintain serum levels above 1.2 mg/dL.

Disorders of Collecting Duct Function

LIDDLE SYNDROME (PSEUDOALDOSTERONISM)

Liddle syndrome is an autosomal dominant form of salt-sensitive hypertension (Chapter 67) caused by mutations in the α-, β-, or γ-subunits of the epithelial sodium channel, which is expressed at the apical surface of collecting duct cells and plays a critical role in maintaining salt balance and blood pressure. Both the β- and the γ-subunits regulate the channel activity of the α-subunit. Mutations in either of these regulatory subunits result in increased epithelial sodium channel activity and Liddle syndrome.

Severe hypertension typically is manifested in childhood, with features of hypokalemic metabolic alkalosis that resemble primary aldosteronism. However, renin and aldosterone secretion is suppressed in this disorder. The clinical abnormalities can be ameliorated by a low-salt diet plus a potassium-sparing diuretic (e.g., amiloride, 5 to 10 mg/day), which acts as an antagonist of the epithelial sodium channel.

DISTAL RENAL TUBULAR ACIDOSIS

Distal renal tubular acidosis (dRTA) results from failure of the collecting duct α-intercalated cells to excrete fixed acids (see Fig. 118-1). Both autosomal dominant and autosomal recessive forms of dRTA have been described. These heritable disorders include mutations in genes encoding carbonic anhydrase II, the chloride-bicarbonate exchanger AE1, and subunits of the hydrogen adenosine triphosphatase (H^+-ATPase) proton pump. Mutations in the *SLC4A1* gene encoding AE1 cause autosomal dominant dRTA and are rarely associated with recessive forms of the disease. Mutations in subunits of H^+-ATPase are the primary causes of autosomal recessive dRTA. Vacuolar H^+-ATPases (V-type ATPases) are ubiquitous, multisubunit protein complexes that mediate the ATP-dependent transport of protons. In the kidney, V-type ATPases are the major proton-secreting pumps in the distal nephron and are involved in net proton secretion (bicarbonate generation) or proton reabsorption (net bicarbonate secretion). Defects in two genes, *ATP6B1* and *ATP6N1B*, cause dRTA with or without associated sensorineural deafness.

Clinical consequences include hypokalemic, hyperchloremic metabolic acidosis; impaired growth; hypercalciuria; hypocitraturia; nephrocalcinosis; nephrolithiasis; rickets in children; and osteomalacia in adults. Classic dRTA can be distinguished from other metabolic acidoses by an inappropriately high urine pH (>5.5), diminished net acid excretion, positive urinary anion gap, and low urinary ammonium concentration (Table 128-2). Treatment with alkali supplementation (1 to 3 mEq/kg/day in adults and 3 to 6 mEq/kg/day in children) is usually effective in correcting the acidosis. In contrast to proximal RTA, urinary potassium wasting can be ameliorated with alkali therapy alone.

DEVELOPMENT OF THE KIDNEY AND URINARY TRACT

The human kidney and urogenital tract develop from three principal embryonic structures: the metanephric mesenchyme, the mesonephric (wolffian) duct, and the cloaca (Fig. 128-1). At 4 to 5 weeks of gestation, the ureteric bud originates as a diverticulum of the mesonephric duct. Reciprocal interactions between the branching ureteric bud and the metanephric mesenchyme induce kidney development, with the metanephros undergoing an epithelial transformation to form the glomeruli and the proximal and distal tubules. The ureteric bud branches give rise to the collecting ducts, the renal pelvis, the ureter, and the bladder trigone. Nephrogenesis is completed by 36 weeks of gestation.

Concurrent with the initial nephrogenic events, the urorectal fold divides the cloaca into the urogenital sinus and the future rectum. The mesonephric duct opening into the bladder becomes the vesicoureteric orifice of the trigone. Between 5 and 6 weeks of gestation, the second genital duct (müllerian duct) appears and runs in parallel with the wolffian duct. In males, the müllerian duct subsequently regresses; the wolffian duct proceeds to form the epididymis, the vas deferens, the seminal vesicle, and the ejaculatory duct. In females, the wolffian duct regresses, and the müllerian ducts fuse to form the ureterovaginal primordium, which merges with the urogenital sinus and eventually gives rise to the uterus, the oviducts, and the proximal vagina. The remnants of the allantois form the urachus, a fibrous cord that connects the bladder to the umbilicus.

Congenital abnormalities of the kidney and urinary tract are detected in about 1 in 500 fetal ultrasound examinations and account for approximately 20 to 30% of all anomalies identified in the prenatal period. Some urinary tract anomalies are asymptomatic and inconsequential, but many renal tract malformations are important causes of infant mortality as well as morbidity in older children and adults, including the progression to renal failure.[5]

ABNORMALITIES OF THE URINARY TRACT

Renal Parenchymal Malformations

Congenital defects in renal development may result in the absence of a kidney (agenesis) or abnormalities in kidney size, structure, or position. Irregularities in the renal contour may arise from the persistence of fetal lobulation or a depression in the midpole of the left kidney caused by the spleen (a "dromedary hump"). Neither irregularity impairs renal function.

RENAL AGENESIS

Renal agenesis reflects a complete failure of nephrogenesis. Unilateral agenesis can occur as an isolated abnormality or as a component of syndromic

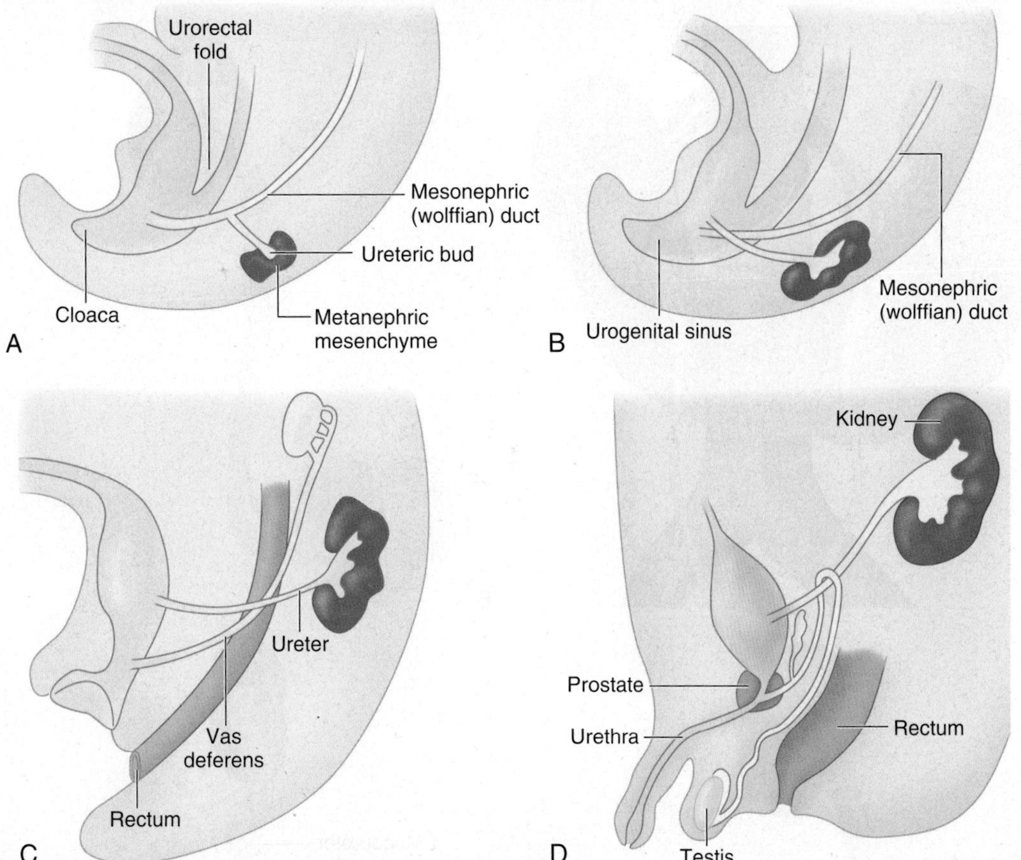

FIGURE 128-1. Key events in the development of the urinary tract. In the 4-week embryo, the ureteric bud emerges from the wolffian duct (A). Reciprocal interactions between the branching ureteric bud and the metanephric mesenchyme induce kidney development. Concurrently, the cloaca is divided by the urorectal fold into the urogenital sinus and the future rectum (B). In the 8-week male embryo, the wolffian duct begins to give rise to the epididymis, the seminal vesicles, and the caudal part of the vas deferens (C). By 9 weeks, axial growth of the fetal spine prompts the developing kidney to ascend from the pelvis to its final lumbar position. The external genitalia develop between 8 and 16 weeks, and testicular descent begins in month 7 of gestation (D).

disorders, such as Turner syndrome (Chapter 233). As an isolated entity, the complete absence of one kidney occurs in 1 in 1000 to 1500 individuals. The incidence is higher in males and occurs somewhat more frequently on the left side; in about half the patients, the ipsilateral ureter and hemitrigone are also absent. The remaining kidney is usually enlarged as a result of compensatory hypertrophy, but it may be ectopic or malrotated. Vesicoureteral reflux is observed on the contralateral side in about 30% of patients.

Renal agenesis is commonly associated with genital anomalies, suggesting that it represents a developmental field defect. In females, absence of the ipsilateral oviduct and malformation of the uterus and vagina result from maldevelopment of the müllerian duct; whereas in males, wolffian duct–derived structures, such as the vas deferens and the seminal vesicles, are often absent. Other associated anomalies can involve the cardiovascular system (30%), the musculoskeletal system (14%), and the adrenal gland (10%). Unilateral renal agenesis is found in 30% of patients with the vertebral, imperforate anus, trachea-esophageal, and renal (VATER) syndrome.

Bilateral renal agenesis has an estimated incidence of 1 in 4000 births and is associated with the Potter phenotype, which includes pulmonary hypoplasia, a characteristic facies, and deformities of the spine and limbs. At birth, these neonates have a critical degree of pulmonary hypoplasia that is incompatible with survival. The familial association of unilateral and bilateral renal agenesis, renal dysplasia, and congenital hydronephrosis occurs in hereditary renal adysplasia syndrome (Online Mendelian Inheritance in Man entry 191830), a rare autosomal dominant disorder with variable penetrance.

RENAL HYPOPLASIA

The term *renal hypoplasia* describes small kidneys with normally differentiated nephrons that are reduced in number. *Oligomeganephronia* describes a form of bilateral renal hypoplasia with a marked reduction in nephron number and associated hypertrophy of individual glomeruli and tubules. This abnormality occurs sporadically as an isolated developmental defect that must be differentiated from acquired renal atrophy and the nephronophthisis–medullary cystic disease complex. Renal function declines slowly, with progression to end-stage renal failure in the second to third decade of life.

RENAL DYSPLASIA

Renal dysplasia, which can be associated with various abnormalities of kidney size, results from abnormal metanephric differentiation that causes anomalous or incompletely differentiated renal elements. Small dysplastic kidneys are commonly referred to as *aplastic.* Large dysplastic kidneys are often cystic; the most extreme type is referred to as *multicystic dysplastic kidney.*

Unilateral dysplasia may be asymptomatic well into adult life. Small aplastic and large multicystic dysplastic kidneys are nonfunctioning and can be distinguished from renal agenesis by imaging studies. The ipsilateral ureter is typically atretic. Contralateral malformations, including obstruction and vesicoureteral reflux, are common. Unilateral multicystic kidneys involute over time and often disappear. Unilateral aplasia and multicystic dysplasia may be manifestations of the hereditary renal adysplasia syndrome. Bilateral multicystic dysplastic kidneys are incompatible with neonatal survival.

Renal and Ureteral Structural Abnormalities

RENAL MALROTATION AND ECTOPIA

Metanephric kidney development begins caudally. By 9 weeks of gestation, the kidney has ascended to its normal level (L1 to L3), and the renal pelvis has rotated 90 degrees toward the midline. Anomalies of ascent and failure of rotation are common. Mutations in the dual serine-threonine and tyrosine protein kinase gene (*DSTYK*) are found in 2.3% of patients with congenital abnormalities of the kidney or urinary tract.[6] Bilateral renal ectopia is often associated with kidney fusion. The most common fusion anomaly is the horseshoe kidney, which occurs in 1 in 500 newborns with a 2 : 1 male predominance. Renal ascent is prevented by the root of the inferior mesenteric artery (Fig. 128-2A). Crossed renal ectopia can occur with or without fusion. Supernumerary (extra) kidneys are typically ectopic and vary in location.

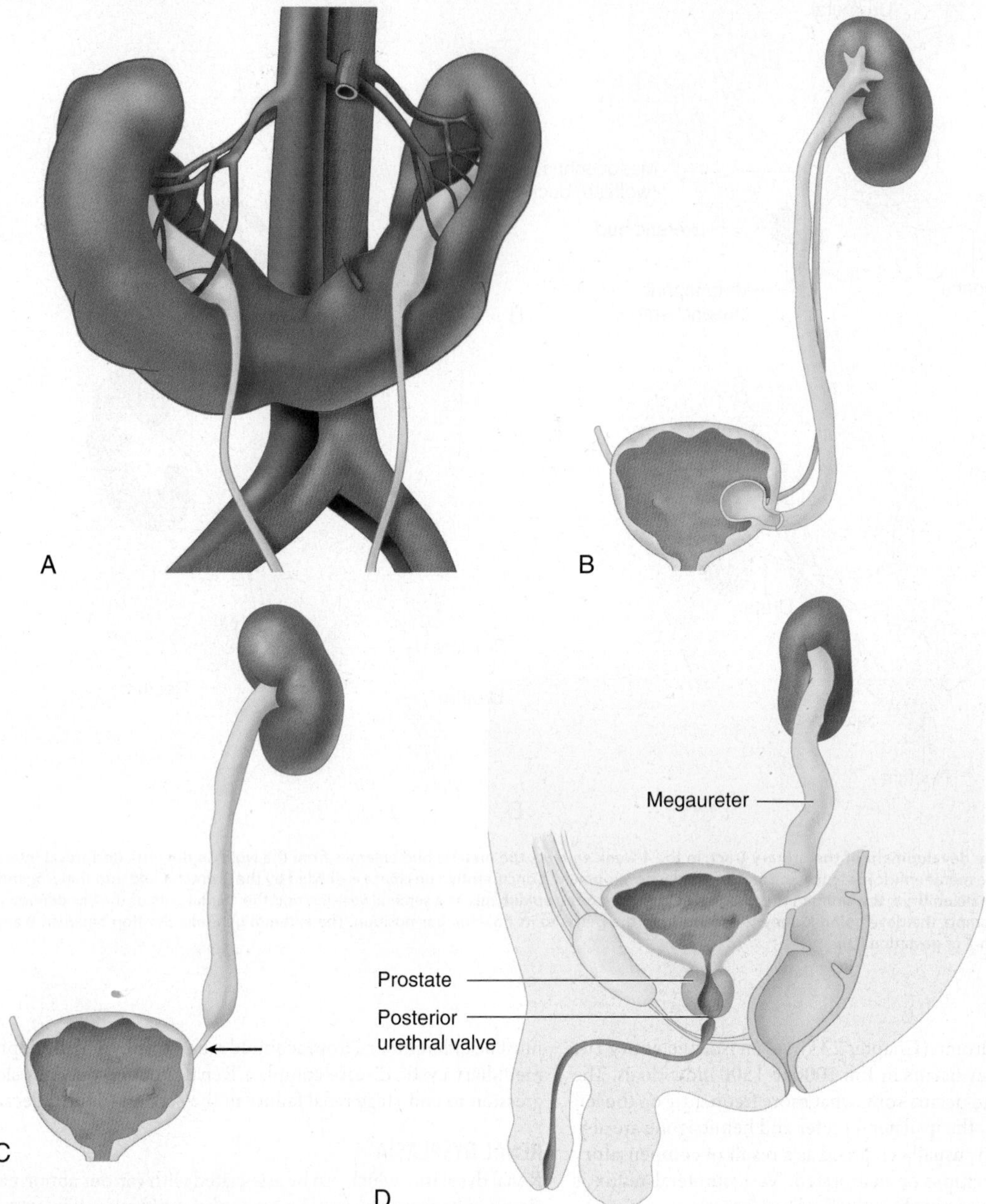

FIGURE 128-2. **Developmental abnormalities of the urinary tract. A, Horseshoe kidney. B, Ectopic ureter associated with a ureterocele. C, Megaureter with the aperistaltic segment (*arrow*). D, Bladder outlet obstruction caused by posterior urethral valves.**

Although almost one third of patients with renal ectopia remain asymptomatic, the associated malrotation of the renal pelvis increases the risk of hydronephrosis, infection, and stone formation.

PELVIURETERAL ABNORMALITIES

Obstruction of the ureteropelvic junction impedes the flow of urine from the renal pelvis into the ureter. It is one of the most frequently occurring urinary tract anomalies in infants, occurring in 1 in 500 live births. In congenital obstruction of the ureteropelvic junction, urologic anomalies in the contralateral system are common, including renal agenesis, renal dysplasia, multicystic dysplasia, ureteropelvic junction obstruction, and vesicoureteral reflux. Ureteropelvic junction obstruction may occur in adults secondary to external compression, kinking, or stenosis of the proximal ureter. Surgical intervention is indicated if there is associated renal function impairment, pyelonephritis, stones, or pain.

Hydrocalyx or *hydrocalycosis* refers to dilation of a major calyx that occurs in the context of intrinsic obstruction, as in infundibular stenosis, or in the context of extrinsic compression of the pelvis, as caused by a vessel or a parapelvic cyst. In comparison, *megacalycosis* represents a nonobstructive, dysplastic lesion seen primarily in males, in which the calyces are dilated and usually increased in number. Associated renal medullary hypoplasia causes malformation of the renal papillae.

Calyceal diverticula are cystic structures connected by a narrow channel to an adjacent minor calyx. In imaging studies, these diverticula typically fill with contrast material, which distinguishes them from renal parenchymal cysts.

Partial duplication of the renal pelvis and ureter is a common anomaly that occurs more frequently in females, is typically unilateral, and is clinically insignificant.

URETERIC ANOMALIES

Ectopic ureters usually reflect complete ureteric and renal duplication. Approximately 10% are bilateral. The ectopic ureter typically drains the dysplastic upper pole of a duplex kidney and inserts below the normal vesicoureteral junction into the lower trigone or the proximal urethra. Ectopic ureters occur much more frequently in females, and the insertion sites can include the vagina and the vulva, with resulting incontinence. An ectopic ureter is often associated with a ureterocele, a cystic dilation of the terminal ureter (Fig. 128-2B). In children, ureteroceles can be associated with urinary tract infection and obstruction of the bladder neck or even of the contralateral ureter. In adults, the clinical presentation usually involves an associated infection, ureteric stones, or both.

A megaureter, or grossly dilated ureter, has multiple potential causes, including intrinsic ureteric obstruction by a stone, bladder outflow obstruction, vesicoureteral reflux, and external compression of the distal ureter. In contrast, primary megaureter results from a functional obstruction of the distal ureter caused by an aperistaltic segment (Fig. 128-2C).

VESICOURETERAL REFLUX

In the normal urinary tract, urinary reflux from the bladder into the ureters is prevented by a functional valve-like mechanism at the vesicoureteral junction. The competence of this valve is dependent on several critical factors, such as the intramural length of the ureter, the position of the ureteric orifice in the bladder, and the integrity of the bladder wall musculature.

Primary vesicoureteral reflux results from incompetence of the vesicoureteral junction due to the shortened length of the ureter's submucosal segment and the lateral, ectopic position of its orifice. It is estimated to occur in 1 to 2% of children. Genetic factors appear to contribute to the pathogenesis of primary vesicoureteral reflux because there is a 30- to 50-fold increased risk in immediate relatives of an index case. A deleterious heterozygous mutation (T3257I) in the gene encoding tenascin XB (*TNXB* in 6p21.3), which is expressed in the human uroepithelial lining of the ureterovesical junction and may be important for generating tensile forces, is associated with familial vesicoureteral reflux.[7] As the intramural ureter lengthens with age, primary vesicoureteral reflux tends to remit or to disappear. Vesicoureteral reflux can also be secondary to obstructive maldevelopment of the lower urinary tract in children, such as in triad syndrome and posterior urethral valves, or secondary to masses that obstruct the bladder or urethra (in adults). In both primary and secondary vesicoureteral reflux, intrarenal reflux can lead to the development of reflux nephropathy, a tubulointerstitial lesion (Chapter 122) associated with gross scarring at the renal poles. In addition, the development of a glomerular lesion consistent with focal and segmental glomerulosclerosis (Chapter 121) can cause proteinuria, hypertension, and progressive loss of renal function.

Primary vesicoureteral reflux is diagnosed in about 30 to 40% of children who have imaging studies after urinary tract infections (Chapter 284). Management of these children has been controversial with respect to both antibiotic prophylaxis and surgical correction. Nevertheless, there is general agreement that frequent urinary tract infection, higher grades of vesicoureteral reflux, and the presence of bladder and bowel dysfunction are particular risk factors for renal cortical scarring and that the rates of spontaneous resolution of reflux and of endoscopic surgical success depend on bladder and bowel dysfunction.[8,9] In a randomized trial, antibiotic prophylaxis substantially reduced recurrent urinary tract infections but did not reduce renal scarring[A2] in children with vesicoureteral reflux.

Surgical correction is the current standard of care for severe grades of vesicoureteral reflux and for recurrent symptomatic infections despite medical management, particularly for patients with secondary forms associated with maldevelopment of the lower urinary tract. However, endoscopic polyacrylate polyalcohol copolymer injection can correct grade IV and grade V vesicoureteral reflux with an 83% success rate that is comparable to surgical correction, so this alternative should be considered as a minimally invasive treatment option.[10]

Lower Urinary Tract Abnormalities

TRIAD SYNDROME (PRUNE-BELLY SYNDROME, EAGLE-BARRETT SYNDROME)

Triad syndrome, also referred to as prune-belly syndrome or Eagle-Barrett syndrome, involves a constellation of anomalies including congenital absence or deficiency of the abdominal wall musculature, gross ureteral dilation, bladder wall thickening, prostatic hypoplasia, and bilateral undescended testes (cryptorchidism). The full syndrome is expressed only in males, and surviving individuals are typically infertile. Patients with an incomplete syndrome can have anomalies of the abdominal wall musculature, bladder, and upper urinary tract; 3% of these patients are females. Although the specific molecular events have yet to be defined, defects in mesenchymal development appear to cause poor prostate and bladder differentiation, ureteral smooth muscle aplasia with consequent ureteral aperistalsis, and varying degrees of renal dysplasia. Three fourths of patients with triad syndrome have associated malformations in the cardiopulmonary system, gastrointestinal tract, and skeleton. In the immediate postnatal period, prognosis depends on the severity of extragenitourinary anomalies. Long-term outcome is based on the degree of renal dysplasia and the success of urodynamic management.

BLADDER ABNORMALITIES

Bladder exstrophy results from a midline closure defect involving the lower anterior abdominal wall, the bladder, and the external genitalia. These abnormalities have been attributed to a primary defect in the differentiation of the cloacal membrane, but the precise molecular events are unclear. In severe cases, bladder exstrophy may be associated with imperforate anus and rectal atresia. However, other congenital anomalies are rarely associated. Clinical studies indicate that there is a correlation between the success of bladder reconstruction and long-term preservation of renal function.

In adults, neuropathic or neurogenic bladder (Chapter 26) has numerous etiologic contributors, including central nervous system trauma, stroke, disorders such as Parkinson disease, spinal trauma, multiple sclerosis, and peripheral nerve damage caused by trauma or surgery. In children, myelomeningocele (spina bifida) is the most common cause of neurogenic bladder dysfunction. Other forms of myelodysplasia, such as spinal dysraphism (spina bifida occulta) and sacral agenesis, are less common causes.

POSTERIOR URETHRAL VALVES

In male infants, posterior urethral valves are the most common cause of bladder outflow obstruction, with resulting bilateral hydronephrosis and megaureters. However, among all infants with hydronephrosis, only 10% have posterior urethral valves. The urethral obstruction results from defective reabsorption of mucosal folds in the posterior urethra, just distal to the verumontanum. As a result, dilation of the proximal urethra, bladder wall hypertrophy and trabeculation, associated vesicoureteral reflux, and varying degrees of renal dysplasia are present (Fig. 128-2D). Surgical management strategies are dictated by the age of the child and the degree of associated renal insufficiency. Survival and long-term renal outcome depend on the severity of the associated renal dysplasia.

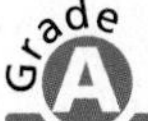

Grade A References

A1. Langman CB, Greenbaum LA, Sarwal M, et al. A randomized controlled crossover trial with delayed-release cysteamine bitartrate in nephropathic cystinosis: effectiveness on white blood cell cystine levels and comparison of safety. *Clin J Am Soc Nephrol*. 2012;7:1112-1120.

A2. Hoberman A, Greenfield SP, Mattoo TK, et al. The RIVUR Trial Investigators. Antimicrobial prophylaxis for children with vesicoureteral reflux. *N Engl J Med*. 2014;370:2367-2376.

GENERAL REFERENCES

For the General References and other additional features, please visit Expert Consult at https://expertconsult.inkling.com.

129

BENIGN PROSTATIC HYPERPLASIA AND PROSTATITIS

STEVEN A. KAPLAN

BENIGN PROSTATIC HYPERPLASIA

DEFINITION

The prostate gland is composed of four zones: peripheral, central, transitional, and stroma. It can also be divided by lobes: anterior, posterior, lateral, and median (Fig. 129-1). Benign prostatic hyperplasia (BPH) is a condition that can lead to lower urinary tract symptoms, which can have a significant negative impact on quality of life.[1] Complaints associated with BPH may relate to difficulty with voiding (e.g., urinary hesitancy, weak stream, straining, and prolonged voiding) or difficulty with controlling urinary storage (e.g., urinary urgency, nocturia). BPH is a histologic diagnosis defined by the proliferation of smooth muscle and epithelial cells within the prostatic transition zone.

EPIDEMIOLOGY

Age is the major risk factor for BPH. A histologic diagnosis of BPH will develop in approximately 50% of men older than 40 years. Of these men, approximately 50% will develop notable lower urinary tract symptoms,

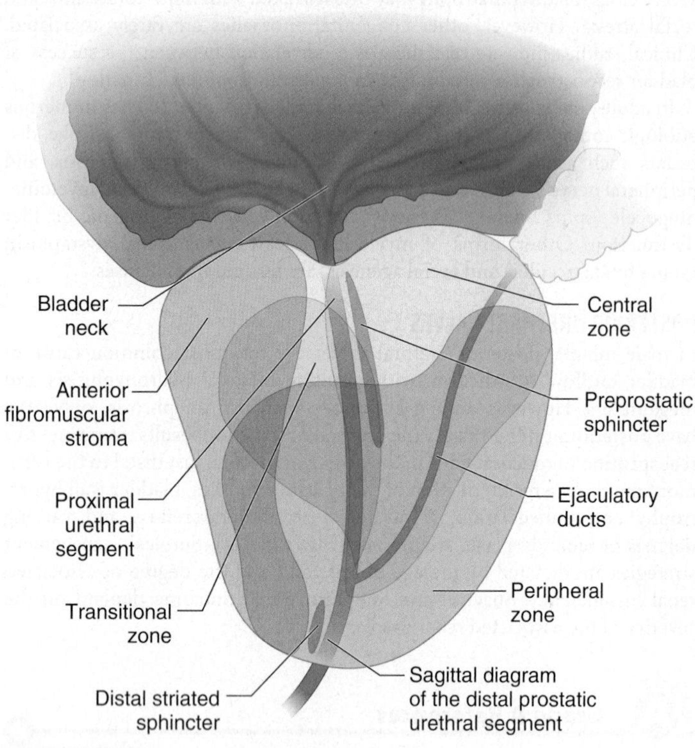

FIGURE 129-1. **Anatomy of the prostate.**

which increase in prevalence in a linear fashion between the ages of 40 and 80 years.[2]

PATHOBIOLOGY

An enlarged prostate may cause lower urinary tract symptoms by directly obstructing the flow of urine or by increasing the muscle tone of the prostate. In addition, changes in the vascularity of the prostate or the urinary bladder can contribute to the development of symptoms. The degree of prostatic enlargement, which can contribute to and affect the severity of the symptoms, is highly variable. Enlargement typically is a combination of stromal hypertrophy and glandular hyperplasia, mostly in the central zone. In BPH the calculated volume exceeds 30 mL.

CLINICAL MANIFESTATIONS

The presence of lower urinary tract symptoms is often indicative of bladder outlet obstruction secondary to BPH. Symptoms may significantly impair health-related quality of life and are classified as voiding (hesitancy, weak stream, straining, and prolonged voiding), storage (frequency, urgency, nocturia, urge incontinence, and voiding of small volumes), or postmicturition (postvoid dribble, incomplete emptying). Most patients who have lower urinary tract symptoms present with a combination of these symptoms. The symptoms of overactive bladder (Chapter 26) and lower urinary tract symptoms secondary to BPH often overlap.

DIAGNOSIS

Assessment should begin with a medical history and review of the patient's medications. The medical history should include any causes that may lead to bladder dysfunction, such as cerebrovascular disease, previous surgical procedures, and a history of prostatic disease. Diuretics and over-the-counter preparations, such as nasal decongestants and antihistamines, may exacerbate the patient's urinary symptoms. Furthermore, dietary factors such as water, caffeine, alcohol, and artificial sweeteners can be important contributors to the overall clinical manifestations of symptoms because they serve as direct bladder irritants and diuretics. Urinary symptoms should be assessed in a standardized fashion with validated instruments such as the International Prostate Symptom Score (IPSS) (Fig. 129-2) and observed over time.

	Not at all	Less than 1 time in 5	Less than half the time	About half the time	More than half the time	Almost always
1. Over the past month or so, how often have you had a sensation of not emptying your bladder completely after you finished urinating?	0 ☐	1 ☐	2 ☐	3 ☐	4 ☐	5 ☐
2. Over the past month or so, how often have you had to urinate again less than two hours after you finished urinating?	0 ☐	1 ☐	2 ☐	3 ☐	4 ☐	5 ☐
3. Over the past month or so, how often have you found you stopped and started again several times when you urinated?	0 ☐	1 ☐	2 ☐	3 ☐	4 ☐	5 ☐
4. Over the past month or so, how often have you found it difficult to postpone urination?	0 ☐	1 ☐	2 ☐	3 ☐	4 ☐	5 ☐
5. Over the past month or so, how often have you had a weak urinary stream?	0 ☐	1 ☐	2 ☐	3 ☐	4 ☐	5 ☐
6. Over the past month or so, how often have you had to push or strain to begin urination?	0 ☐	1 ☐	2 ☐	3 ☐	4 ☐	5 ☐

7. Over the past month, how many times did you most typically get up to urinate from the time you went to bed at night until the time you got up in the morning?

0 ☐ none	1 ☐ 1 time	2 ☐ 2 times	3 ☐ 3 times	4 ☐ 4 times	5 ☐ 5 or more times

Total IPSS Score = sum of questions 1–7 =

Quality of life due to urinary symptoms

If you were to spend the rest of your life with your urinary condition just the way it is now, how would you feel about that?

Delighted	Pleased	Mostly satisfied	Mixed—about equally satisfied and dissatisfied	Mostly dissatisfied	Unhappy	Terrible
0 ☐	1 ☐	2 ☐	3 ☐	4 ☐	5 ☐	6 ☐

FIGURE 129-2. **International Prostate Symptom Score (IPSS). The seven symptom questions constitute a scale initially developed by the American Urological Association. The eighth question about quality of life is scored separately. (From Barry MJ, Fowler FJ Jr, O'Leary MP, et al. The American Urological Association symptom index for benign prostatic hyperplasia: the Measurement Committee of the American Urological Association. *J Urol.* 1992;148:1549.)**

Abdominal examination should be performed to identify the presence of a palpable bladder, which could be a sign of urinary retention. The physical examination should include a prostate examination to evaluate its size and the possible presence of nodules. The digital rectal examination gives only an approximate estimate of size because only the posterior half is palpated. A focused neurologic examination is also important to assess a patient's mental status, ambulatory status, lower extremity neuromuscular function, and anal sphincter tone.

Laboratory Findings

Urinalysis should be performed to screen for hematuria and urinary tract infection (Chapter 284). A serum prostate-specific antigen (PSA) level should be measured because it can detect symptomatic prostate cancer (Chapter 201) that may require treatment even in men who would not be candidates for treatment if they were asymptomatic. However, the results must be interpreted with caution because the serum PSA level correlates with prostatic volume even in the absence of cancer.[3] Objective parameters such as maximum urinary flow by uroflowmetry and postvoid residual by ultrasound should also be measured if the diagnosis is in question.[4] Although there is not a direct correlation between lower urinary tract symptoms and objective parameters such as prostate size or flow rate, prostate volume and serum PSA levels generally predict worsening of symptoms.

Other causes of bladder dysfunction that should be considered during the assessment of men presenting with lower urinary tract symptoms include bladder cancer (Chapter 197), diabetes (Chapter 229), urethral strictures, and bladder stones. The absence of hematuria makes bladder cancer very unlikely, but patients with BPH symptoms require cystoscopy if they also have hematuria. Neurologic disorders including Parkinson disease (Chapter 409) and multiple sclerosis (Chapter 411) may also cause lower urinary tract symptoms in men.

TREATMENT Rx

The treatment of BPH aims to improve subjective symptoms and quality of life as well as to prevent progression of the disease. Over time, treatment has evolved away from surgical therapy and largely to medical therapy.

Men who are mildly symptomatic, defined as a score of 7 or less on the IPSS questionnaire, can be observed (Fig. 129-3). Lifestyle changes that may improve symptoms include fluid restriction, timed voiding, and double voiding. Patients who have moderate symptoms, defined as 8 to 19 points on

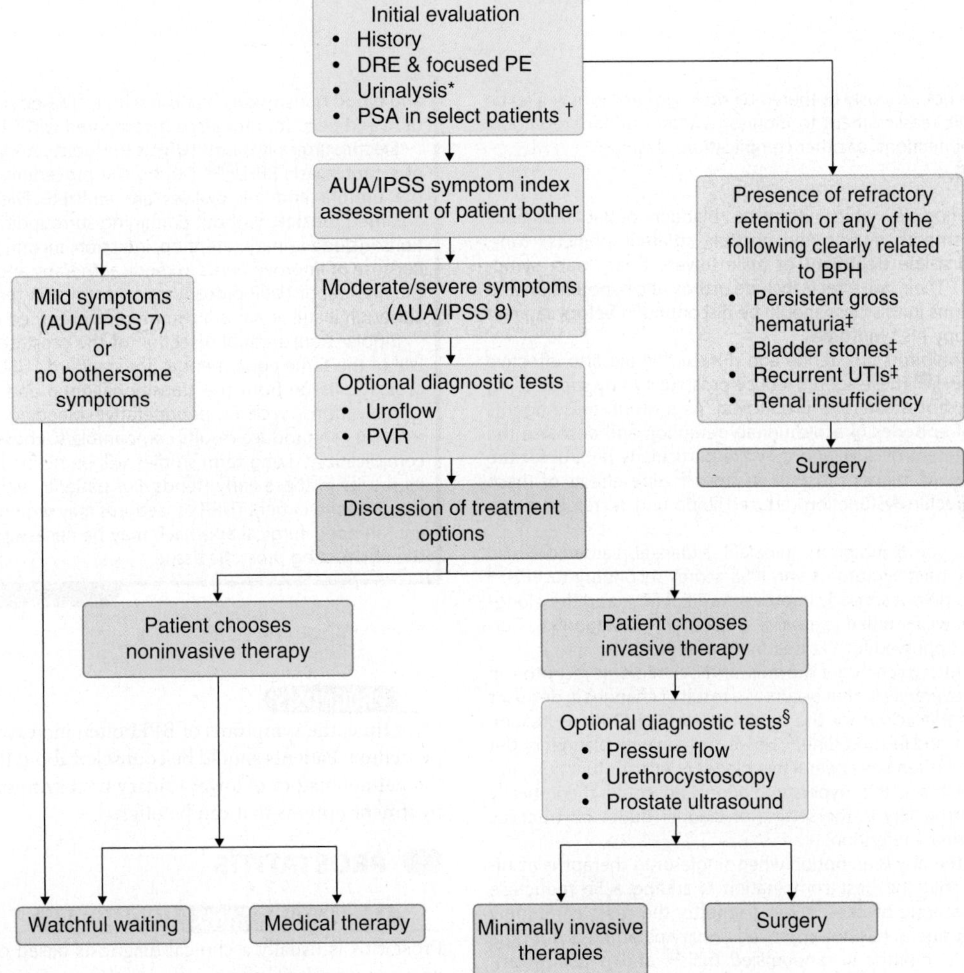

*In patients with clinically significant prostatic bleeding, a course of a 5 alpha-reductase inhibitor may be used. If bleeding persists, tissue ablative surgery is indicated.
†Patients with at least a 10-year life expectancy for whom knowledge of the presence of prostate cancer would change management or patients for whom the PSA measurement may change the management of voiding symptoms.
‡After exhausting other therapeutic options.
§Some diagnostic tests are used in predicting response to therapy. Pressure-flow studies are most useful in men prior to surgery.

AUA, American Urological Association; DRE, digital rectal exam; IPSS, International Prostate Symptom Score; PE, physical exam; PSA, prostate-specific antigen; PVR, postvoid residual urine; UTI, urinary tract infection.

FIGURE 129-3. Algorithm of management of benign prostatic hyperplasia (BPH). (©2003 American Urological Association Educations and Research, Inc.)

TABLE 129-1 MEDICATIONS AND RECOMMENDED DAILY DOSES FOR MALE LOWER URINARY TRACT SYMPTOMS

α-BLOCKERS	5α-REDUCTASE INHIBITORS	α-BLOCKER AND 5α-REDUCTASE INHIBITOR	ANTICHOLINERGICS	ANTICHOLINERGIC PATCHES	PHOSPHODIESTERASE TYPE 5 INHIBITORS
Alfuzosin 10 mg	Dutasteride 0.5 mg	Dutasteride and tamsulosin 0.5/0.4 mg	Darifenacin 7.5, 15 mg	Oxybutynin transdermal 3.9 mg	Tadalafil 2.5, 5, 10, 20 mg
Doxazosin 1-8 mg	Finasteride 5 mg		Fesoterodine 4, 8 mg		Sildenafil 20, 50, 100 mg
Tamsulosin 0.4 mg			Oxybutynin 5, 10, 15 mg		Vardenafil 10, 20 mg
Terazosin 1-10 mg			Oxybutynin XL 5, 10, 15 ER mg		
Silodosin 4, 8 mg			Tolterodine 1, 2 mg Tolterodine LA 2, 4 ER mg Trospium 20, 60 mg Solifenacin 5, 10 mg		

ER = extended-release.

the IPSS, and who are not seriously bothered by their symptoms may also be observed with periodic reassessment to monitor whether urinary retention, refractory hematuria, infections, or other complications develop.

Medications

α-Adrenergic antagonists, which decrease bladder outlet resistance by relaxing urethral smooth muscle and possibly striated sphincter tone, are considered the first-line treatment of male lower urinary tract symptoms[A1,A2] (Table 129-1). Their side effects include orthostatic hypotension and dizziness. All medications in this class should be discontinued before cataract surgery for fear of floppy-iris syndrome.

The 5α-reductase inhibitors finasteride and dutasteride are also effective for the treatment of BPH.[A3] These agents reduce prostate size by suppressing testosterone and dihydrotestosterone production. As a result, these agents reduce the number of episodes of acute urinary retention and decrease the need for surgical treatment of BPH, and they are particularly helpful for the treatment of patients with higher prostate volumes.[A4] Side effects of these medications include erectile dysfunction, reduced libido, and decreased ejaculate volume.

Phosphodiesterase type 5 inhibitors (tadalafil, sildenafil, vardenafil) also improve lower urinary tract symptoms and IPSS scores secondary to BPH,[A5] although these agents do not similarly improve maximal flow, and their long-term efficacy is not as well studied as that of α-adrenergic antagonists. Currently, only tadalafil is approved for the treatment of BPH.

Antimuscarinic agents, which target the muscarinic cholinergic receptors in the bladder to reduce overactivity that occurs as a result of changes in detrusor function, are safe and efficacious for the treatment of BPH. Options include tolterodine, solifenacin, and fesoterodine.[A6] However, men with bladder outlet obstruction due to BPH often have overactive bladder detrusor function, and antimuscarinic agents block this hyperstimulation and could theoretically decrease detrusor contractility in the setting of bladder outlet obstruction, thereby resulting in urinary retention.

Combination drug therapy is an option when single-drug therapy is insufficient. Data suggest that the best combination is adding a 5α-reductase inhibitor to an α-adrenergic blocker.[A7] Saw palmetto, the most commonly used phytotherapeutic agent, has not improved urinary parameters during a treatment period of 12 months in randomized trials[A8] and is not recommended even as add-on therapy.[A1,A2]

If oral medications are insufficient to control symptoms, another option is onabotulinumtoxinA (Botox). Injection of onabotulinumtoxinA into the prostate, through either a transrectal or transperineal route, improves IPSS scores and maximum flow rates.[A9] However, its role in the treatment of lower urinary tract symptoms secondary to BPH remains to be elucidated.

Surgical Treatments

A variety of minimally invasive treatment options are available for BPH.[5] Transurethral needle ablation uses interstitial radiofrequency needles to necrotize tissue. Various laser options can ablate, coagulate, resect, enucleate, or vaporize tissue. Data suggest that these techniques provide results that are similar to open transurethral resection of the prostate (TURP),[A10] but many of the reports of their use are from single-site trials, and their efficacy requires further study. Transurethral microwave therapy, during which the prostate is heated by a microwave antenna mounted on a urethral catheter, is associated with lower risks for retrograde ejaculation, treatment for strictures, hematuria, and blood transfusions but also with increased risks for dysuria, urinary retention, and need for retreatment compared with TURP.[A11]

Electrosurgically based TURP is the "gold standard" in endoscopic treatment of symptomatic BPH.[A1,A2] During the procedure, an antenna is inserted into the urethra and microwaves are emitted. This heat energy destroys the enlarged prostate without damaging surrounding tissue. Potential complications include urinary retention, infection, incontinence, and urethral stricture. Because of improvements in medical therapy and minimally invasive options, the number of TURP procedures performed in the United States has declined, although it still remains a commonly performed urologic procedure.

Bipolar transurethral resection of the prostate is another alternative. With use of the same equipment as for standard TURP, it resects large amounts of prostatic tissue from the transitional zone and central zone but decreases complications, such as perioperative bleeding requiring transfusion. As a result, it can produce results comparable to those of regular TURP with fewer complications. Long-term studies will be needed to confirm the durability of its results in these early trends. For patients with very large prostate glands (i.e., 80 g and larger), TURP procedures may require prolonged operative times, and an open surgical approach may be necessary for adequate debulking of the obstructing prostatic tissue.

PROGNOSIS

Over time, the symptoms of BPH often increase, requiring medications or a procedure. Patients should be counseled about the likelihood of progression, the natural history of lower urinary tract symptoms related to BPH, and the treatment options that can be offered.

PROSTATITIS

EPIDEMIOLOGY AND PATHOBIOLOGY

Prostatitis is usually a clinical diagnosis based on signs and symptoms that occur as a result of inflammation of the prostate gland. The overall prevalence of prostatitis is approximately 8%, and it affects men of a wide age range. Swelling or inflammation of the prostate gland, which may be due to various causes, can have a significant impact on quality of life. The current classification system defines the various types of prostatitis on the basis of whether it is acute or chronic, associated with infection, or associated with pelvic pain (Table 129-2).

The causative organisms of acute bacterial prostatitis are usually similar to those that cause other common genitourinary infections (Chapter 284) and include *Escherichia coli* and *Enterococcus* spp. About 60% of patients with chronic bacterial prostatitis have evidence of ongoing infection based on polymerase chain reaction (PCR) testing of their expressed prostatic secretions, with *Chlamydia trachomatis*, *Ureaplasma urealyticum*, *Mycoplasma genitalium*, and *Mycoplasma hominis* the most common organisms detected.[6] The pathogenesis of chronic prostatitis/chronic pelvic pain syndrome, however, remains unclear.

TABLE 129-2 CLASSIFICATION OF PROSTATITIS

	CATEGORIES			
	I	II	III	IV
Term	Acute bacterial prostatitis	Chronic bacterial prostatitis	Chronic prostatitis/chronic pelvic pain syndrome (CP/CPPS) IIIa. Inflammatory CPPS IIIb. Noninflammatory CPPS	Asymptomatic inflammatory prostatitis
Characteristics	Acute infection of prostate gland	Recurrent or relapsing infection caused by the same organism; not acute	90% of cases of chronic prostatitis are presumed to be nonbacterial; diagnosis of exclusion Characteristic symptoms Discomfort or pain in pelvic region for more than 3 months within the past 6 months Pelvic, perineal, penile, or ejaculatory pain; irritative or obstructive voiding symptoms, sexual dysfunction No documented recurrent urinary tract infections; repeated negative cultures Classification into IIIa or IIIb determined by presence of leukocytes in semen, post–prostate massage urine, or prostatic secretion	No symptoms of prostatitis Leukocytes or inflammatory cells present in prostate tissue, semen, or expressed prostatic secretions

CLINICAL MANIFESTATIONS

Acute bacterial prostatitis (type I) is characterized by acute infection of the prostate gland. Presenting symptoms include pelvic, perineal, penile, or ejaculatory pain as well as irritative or obstructive voiding symptoms and sexual dysfunction. Patients with severe infections can present with fever and chills and can become septic (Chapter 108). Type II prostatitis is characterized by recurrent or relapsing infection caused by the same organism. These patients tend to be less sick during each episode and usually present with voiding symptoms and pain.

Type III prostatitis is characterized by pelvic discomfort or pain for more than 3 of the 6 months before evaluation. Type III patients have repeatedly negative urine cultures. Classification into type IIIa or IIIb is contingent on the presence of leukocytes in semen, post–prostate massage urine, or prostatic secretions. Patients with type IV prostatitis do not experience any symptoms of prostatitis. Leukocytes or inflammatory cells are found in prostate tissue, semen, or expressed prostatic secretions.

DIAGNOSIS

The diagnosis of prostatitis requires a careful history, physical examination, and examination of the urine. The physician must ask pertinent questions about voiding history, sexual history, symptoms, pain, neurologic disorders, and prior pelvic surgery. The National Institutes of Health Chronic Prostatitis Symptom Index (NIH-CPSI), which is a standardized tool for the evaluation and assessment of prostatitis, consists of nine parts that outline three major areas of prostatitis: pain, urinary symptoms, and quality of life (Fig. 129-4). The NIH-CPSI is not specific for making the diagnosis of prostatitis, but it is very useful for longitudinally monitoring changes in symptoms over time after a diagnosis of prostatitis has been established.[7] The physical examination should include an abdominal, external genital, perineal, and digital rectal examination. Attention should be placed on identifying pelvic wall discomfort, structural abnormalities, or prostatic pain on digital rectal examination.

Laboratory Evaluation

Urinalysis and urine culture should be performed for every patient. Historically, the four-specimen test was recommended, with specimens obtained from the initial voided bladder urine, midstream voided bladder urine, expressed prostatic secretions obtained during prostate massage, and voided bladder urine collected after prostate massage. Leukocytes in the third specimen suggest the diagnosis of prostatitis. Leukocytes without bacteria suggest inflammation consistent with nonbacterial prostatitis. However, this four-step approach is rarely used today because it has not proved to be useful as a diagnostic tool or for directing treatment. It has been replaced by either a semen culture or a midstream urine culture and by examination of a voided urine specimen after prostate massage.

Urodynamic methods offer valuable insight for patients experiencing predominantly voiding symptoms. Other conditions, such as prostatic obstruction, primary bladder neck obstruction, dysfunctional voiding, urethral obstruction, and detrusor-sphincter dyssynergia, may be defined with the help of postvoid residual, pressure-flow urodynamics, or videourodynamics. These conditions, in comparison to prostatitis, have many effective treatment options.

Measurement of a postvoid residual urine volume by ultrasound can be used to assess incomplete emptying because urinary retention can be a risk factor for recurrent infections. Low maximum urine flow rates suggest bladder outlet obstruction, decreased detrusor contractility, or both as an alternative explanation for lower urinary tract symptoms and poor flow. However, for those who fail to respond to treatment, PCR analysis of semen to evaluate for possible fastidious organisms (e.g., *C. trachomatis*, *U. urealyticum*, *Mycoplasma* species, and *Neisseria gonorrhoeae*) may be useful for the evaluation of chronic prostatitis. Cultures of urethral swabs may be used to evaluate patients with potentially undiagnosed sexually transmitted diseases (Chapter 285). Other diagnostic tests include semen analysis and culture, which are useful for patients with complaints of abnormal-smelling semen or infertility.

Cystoscopy is an adjunct to urodynamics in the evaluation of chronic prostatitis/chronic pelvic pain syndrome, especially before any surgical intervention. Cystoscopy is also performed for evaluation of hematuria or abnormal cytology findings because prostate cancer (Chapter 201) or bladder cancer (Chapter 197) can cause symptoms similar to chronic pelvic pain syndrome.

PSA testing should be ordered on the basis of prostate cancer screening (Chapter 201) but has no specific role in evaluation of prostatitis symptoms. Acute prostatitis can increase the serum level of PSA, but it usually returns to normal levels with appropriate antibiotics within 1 to 3 months. PSA can be elevated and even can wax and wane in patients with chronic prostatitis/chronic pelvic pain syndrome. Patients with chronic prostatitis have a less well defined decrease in PSA after a course of antibiotics. Anywhere from one third to two thirds of men undergoing prostate biopsy have chronic inflammation, but the correlation with symptoms of prostatitis is unclear.

Transrectal ultrasound can identify a prostatic abscess and is generally recommended for patients who have recurrent prostatitis or who do not respond to treatment. The potential utility of pelvic computed xerographic scanning and transrectal magnetic resonance imaging is unclear.

TREATMENT Rx

Acute Bacterial Prostatitis

Oral or intravenous antibiotics are usually effective for curing acute prostatitis, and progression to chronic bacterial prostatitis is uncommon. Typical first-course antibiotics include oral fluoroquinolones (e.g., levofloxacin 500 mg once daily or ofloxacin 300 mg twice daily) and sulfonamides (e.g., trimethoprim/sulfamethoxazole 160 mg/800 mg twice daily) for 6 weeks. Patients who are unable to tolerate oral medications and patients with signs of sepsis may require broad-spectrum intravenous antibiotics (e.g., ampicillin 2 g every 6 hours plus gentamicin 1.5 mg/kg every 8 hours until afebrile) followed by 6 weeks of oral therapy as before.[8]

Chronic Bacterial Prostatitis

Antibiotic therapy is the mainstay of treatment for chronic bacterial prostatitis. Antibiotics with good lipid solubility, good enteric bacterial coverage, and a high pK_a have the best prostatic penetration. These antibiotics include quinolones, sulfa-based preparations, macrolides, tetracyclines, and aminoglycosides. The fluoroquinolones (e.g., ciprofloxacin 500 mg twice daily, levofloxacin 500 mg twice daily, or ofloxacin 300 mg twice daily) have equivalent success rates in patients with chronic bacterial prostatitis and are generally the first-line treatment.A12 In cases in which atypical bacteria, such as chlamydia, are suspected to be the cause of chronic bacterial prostatitis, better results may be achieved by macrolide antibiotics, such as azithromycin (500 mg twice daily).

NIH-Chronic Prostatitis Symptom Index (NIH-CPSI)

Pain or Discomfort

1. In the last week, have you experienced any pain or discomfort in the following areas?

	Yes	No
a. Area between rectum and testicles (perineum)	☐1	☐0
b. Testicles	☐1	☐0
c. Tip of the penis (not related to urination)	☐1	☐0
d. Below your waist, in your pubic or bladder area	☐1	☐0

2. In the last week, have you experienced:

	Yes	No
a. Pain or burning during urination?	☐1	☐0
b. Pain or discomfort during or after sexual climax (ejaculation)?	☐1	☐0

3. How often have you had pain or discomfort in any of these areas over the last week?

☐0 Never
☐1 Rarely
☐2 Sometimes
☐3 Often
☐4 Usually
☐5 Always

4. Which number best describes your AVERAGE pain or discomfort on the days that you had it, over the last week?

☐ ☐ ☐ ☐ ☐ ☐ ☐ ☐ ☐ ☐ ☐
0 1 2 3 4 5 6 7 8 9 10
NO PAIN — PAIN AS BAD AS YOU CAN IMAGINE

Urination

5. How often have you had a sensation of not emptying your bladder completely after you finished urinating, over the last week?

☐0 Not at all
☐1 Less than 1 time in 5
☐2 Less than half the time
☐3 About half the time
☐4 More than half the time
☐5 Almost always

6. How often have you had to urinate again less than two hours after you finished urinating, over the last week?

☐0 Not at all
☐1 Less than 1 time in 5
☐2 Less than half the time
☐3 About half the time
☐4 More than half the time
☐5 Almost always

Impact of Symptoms

7. How much have your symptoms kept you from doing the kinds of things you would usually do, over the last week?

☐0 None
☐1 Only a little
☐2 Some
☐3 A lot

8. How much did you think about your symptoms, over the last week?

☐0 None
☐1 Only a little
☐2 Some
☐3 A lot

Quality of Life

9. If you were to spend the rest of your life with your symptoms just the way they have been during the last week, how would you feel about that?

☐0 Delighted
☐1 Pleased
☐2 Mostly satisfied
☐3 Mixed (about equally satisfied and dissatisfied)
☐4 Mostly dissatisfied
☐5 Unhappy
☐6 Terrible

Scoring the NIH-Chronic Prostatitis Symptom Index Domains

Pain: Total of items 1a, 1b, 1c,1d, 2a, 2b, 3, and 4 = ______
Urinary Symptoms: Total of items 5 and 6 = ______
Quality of Life Impact: Total of items 7, 8, and 9 = ______

FIGURE 129-4. NIH Chronic Prostatitis Symptom Index. (Modified from Litwin MS, McNaughton-Collins M, Fowler FJ Jr, et al. The National Institutes of Health chronic prostatitis symptom index: development and validation of a new outcome measure. Chronic Prostatitis Collaborative Research Network. *J Urol.* 1999;162:369-375.)

Most studies demonstrate effective treatment with 30 days of therapy, but some clinicians prescribe 6 weeks of therapy as for acute prostatitis because the recurrence rate is as high as 40% within a year. Delivery of antibiotics by intraprostatic injection or anal submucosal injection is rarely used today.

Treatments for Chronic Prostatitis/Chronic Pelvic Pain Syndrome

The optimal regimen for the treatment of chronic prostatitis/chronic pelvic pain syndrome is not known, and the response to treatment is often disappointing.[9] Prolonged courses of antibiotics are not generally effective. A13 One option is to perform PCR testing of expressed prostatic secretions and to use antibiotics only if the test result is positive. Current empirical therapy uses a combination of α-blockers, adrenergic antagonists, and anti-inflammatory agents (e.g., ibuprofen 400 mg three times daily or naproxen 200 mg twice daily). A14 Neuroleptics, such as gabapentin, have been tried but appear to be no better than placebo and have side effects. A15 The potential value of allopurinol is unclear. Many phytotherapies have been tried, but improvements have not been dramatic or consistent in various trials.

Conservative supportive therapies include warm sitz baths and special diets that avoid spicy foods, caffeine, alcohol, and other urinary irritants. Behavioral therapies and stress reduction have also been used. Therapies that aim to improve relaxation and to reeducate pelvic floor muscle function can improve symptoms in highly stressed individuals with dysfunctional voiding. Options include biofeedback and bladder retraining. Unproven treatments include trigger point massage combined with relaxation and electromagnetic pelvic floor therapy, acupuncture, and percutaneous tibial nerve stimulation. Prostate massage can be combined with other therapies, but its efficacy has been variable.

PROGNOSIS

Most patients with type I prostatitis are effectively treated with oral or intravenous antibiotics, although some cases do not respond to treatment and progress to type II prostatitis. The natural history of type II, type III, and type IV prostatitis remains undefined.

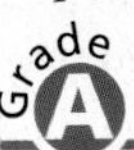

Grade A References

A1. McVary KT, Roehrborn CG, Avins AL, et al. Update on AUA guideline on the management of benign prostatic hyperplasia. *J Urol.* 2011;185:1793-1803.

A2. Oelke M, Bachmann A, Descazeaud A, et al. EAU guidelines on the treatment and follow-up of non-neurogenic male lower urinary tract symptoms including benign prostatic obstruction. *Eur Urol.* 2013;64:118-140.

A3. Park T, Choi JY. Efficacy and safety of dutasteride for the treatment of symptomatic benign prostatic hyperplasia (BPH): a systematic review and meta-analysis. *World J Urol.* 2014;32:1093-1105.

A4. Kaplan S, McConnell J. Combination therapy with doxazosin and finasteride for benign prostatic hyperplasia in patients with lower urinary tract symptoms and a baseline total prostate volume of 25 mL or greater. *J Urol.* 2006;175:217-220.

A5. Gacci M, Corona G, Salvi M, et al. A systematic review and meta-analysis on the use of phosphodiesterase 5 inhibitors alone or in combination with alpha-blockers for lower urinary tract symptoms due to benign prostatic hyperplasia. *Eur Urol.* 2012;61:994-1003.

A6. Abrams P, Kaplan S, De Koning Gans HJ, et al. Safety and tolerability of tolterodine for the treatment of overactive bladder in men with bladder outlet obstruction. *J Urol.* 2006;175:999-1004.

A7. Fullhase C, Chapple C, Cornu JN, et al. Systematic review of combination drug therapy for non-neurogenic male lower urinary tract symptoms. *Eur Urol.* 2013;64:228-243.

A8. Barry MJ, Meleth S, Lee JY, et al. Effect of increasing doses of saw palmetto extract on lower urinary tract symptoms: a randomized trial. *JAMA.* 2011;306:1344-1351.

A9. Marberger M, Chartier-Kastler E, Egerdie B, et al. A randomized double-blind placebo-controlled phase 2 dose-ranging study of onabotulinumtoxinA in men with benign prostatic hyperplasia. *Eur Urol.* 2013;63:496-503.

A10. Lee SW, Choi JB, Lee KS, et al. Transurethral procedures for lower urinary tract symptoms resulting from benign prostatic enlargement: a quality and meta-analysis. *Int Neurourol J.* 2013;17:59-66.

A11. Hoffman RM, Monga M, Elliott SP, et al. Microwave thermotherapy for benign prostatic hyperplasia. *Cochrane Database Syst Rev.* 2012;9:CD004135.

A12. Perletti G, Marras E, Wagenlehner FM, et al. Antimicrobial therapy for chronic bacterial prostatitis. *Cochrane Database Syst Rev.* 2013;8:CD009071.

A13. Zhu Y, Wang C, Pang X, et al. Antibiotics are not beneficial in the management of category III prostatitis: a meta analysis. *Urol J.* 2014;11:1377-1385.

A14. Anothaisintawee T, Attia J, Nickel JC, et al. Management of chronic prostatitis/chronic pelvic pain syndrome: a systematic review and network meta-analysis. *JAMA.* 2011;305:78-86.

A15. Aboumarzouk OM, Nelson RL. Pregabalin for chronic prostatitis. *Cochrane Database Syst Rev.* 2012;8:CD009063.

GENERAL REFERENCES

For the General References and other additional features, please visit Expert Consult at https://expertconsult.inkling.com.

130

CHRONIC KIDNEY DISEASE

WILLIAM E. MITCH

DEFINITION

Chronic kidney disease (CKD) refers to the many clinical abnormalities that progressively worsen as kidney function declines. CKD results from a large number of systemic diseases that damage the kidney or from disorders that are intrinsic to the kidney (Table 130-1). The severity of CKD is graded by the depressed level of the glomerular filtration rate (GFR); a GFR persistently below 60 mL/min/1.73 m^2 serves to identify patients who will most likely develop clinical manifestations as a result of progressive loss of kidney function. Measurement of GFR is cumbersome, so estimates of GFR (eGFR) based on a patient's serum creatinine and demographics (Chapter 114) are used to monitor the course of CKD.

TABLE 130-1 CAUSES OF CHRONIC RENAL FAILURE

Diabetic glomerulosclerosis*
Hypertensive nephrosclerosis
Glomerular disease
Glomerulonephritis
Amyloidosis, light chain disease*
Systemic lupus erythematosus, granulomatosis with polyangiitis
Tubulointerstitial disease
Reflux nephropathy (chronic pyelonephritis)
Analgesic nephropathy
Obstructive nephropathy (stones, benign prostatic hypertrophy)
Myeloma kidney*
Vascular disease
Scleroderma*
Vasculitis*
Renovascular renal failure (ischemic nephropathy)
Atheroembolic renal disease*
Cystic disease
Autosomal dominant polycystic kidney disease
Medullary cystic kidney disease

*Systemic disease involving the kidney.

Unlike acute kidney damage (Chapter 120), which can be repaired with a resulting improvement in kidney function, the kidney damage in CKD is rarely repaired, so loss of function persists. In most CKD patients, in fact, loss of kidney function generates more kidney damage, so CKD can progressively worsen even if the disorder that initially caused it becomes inactive.

CKD includes a spectrum of clinical dysfunctions that range from abnormalities detectable only by laboratory testing to a syndrome known as uremia. *Uremia*, which literally means "urine in the blood," results from the accumulation of unexcreted ions and waste products and the metabolic abnormalities they induce. When the kidney fails to perform most of its functions, the clinical state is called *end-stage renal disease* (ESRD), and dialysis or transplantation is required to sustain life (Chapter 131). Before this stage, treatment strategies are directed at slowing the loss of kidney function, postponing the onset of ESRD, and ameliorating the symptoms of uremia.

EPIDEMIOLOGY

The most widely used method for identifying degrees of CKD is the 2009 Chronic Kidney Disease Epidemiology Collaboration (CKD-EPI) equation, which has been modified to include information about creatinine or cystatin C to ascertain the risks for development of complications of CKD (see Table 114-1).[1] On the basis of these equations plus demographic and medical information from the National Health and Nutrition Examination Survey, from the National Institutes of Health United States Renal Data System,[2] and from the Kidney Disease Improving Global Outcomes work group,[3] an estimated 23.1 million Americans, representing 11.5% of noninstitutionalized adults older than 20 years, have evidence of CKD (Table 130-2). The largest group of CKD patients has an eGFR below 60 mL/min/1.73 m^2 (i.e., stages 3 to 5). These individuals are at higher risk for having their GFR decline below a threshold that will precipitate progressive CKD and its complications (e.g., hypertension, anemia, hyperphosphatemia, and acidosis). The overall prevalence of adults with stage 3 CKD is increasing, probably related to the aging of the population as well as the increasing prevalence of obesity and type 2 diabetes.[4] Fortunately, data suggest that an individual's risk for development of CKD has not been rising since 2001. Nevertheless, the number of adults with ESRD is estimated to be about 615,000, mainly because increasing numbers of CKD patients are 70 years of age and older.

Besides the elderly, CKD occurs more widely in African Americans, Asian Americans, Hispanics, and Native Americans, including Hawaiians and Pacific Islanders. Two disorders account for more than 70% of all adult CKD patients in the United States: 44% have diabetes mellitus (Chapter 229), and 28% have hypertension. The frequency of CKD is also increased in patients with albuminuria and in patients with a family member with CKD. Data on the genetic epidemiology of CKD are limited, but African Americans with two copies of high-risk variants of the *APO1* gene encoding apolipoprotein-1 have about a 2-fold higher probability of suffering rapid decline in eGFR and

TABLE 130-2 PREVALENCE OF STAGES OF CHRONIC KIDNEY DISEASE AND FREQUENCY OF COMPLICATIONS

STAGE	DESCRIPTION	GFR* (mL/min/1.73 m²)	ADULT PREVALENCE (MILLIONS)	SYMPTOMS OR SIGNS
1	Chronic kidney damage; normal or increased GFR	>90	4.6	Anemia 4% Hypertension 40% 5-year mortality 19%
2	Mild GFR loss	60-89	5.0	Anemia 4% Hypertension 40% 5-year mortality 19%
3	Moderate GFR loss	30-59	12.5	Anemia 7% Hypertension 55% 5-year mortality 24%
4	Severe GFR loss	15-29	0.8	Hyperphosphatemia 20% Anemia 29% Hypertension 77% 5-year mortality 46%
5	Kidney failure	<15 or dialysis	0.2	Hyperphosphatemia 50% Anemia 69% Hypertension >75% 3-year mortality 14%

*The formula for estimating the glomerular filtration rate (GFR) of adults with chronic kidney disease (CKD) is derived from data obtained during the National Health and Nutrition Examination Survey (NHANES 2001-2008). The 2009 Chronic Kidney Disease Epidemiology Collaboration (CKD-EPI) creatinine equation is

$$eGFR = 141 \times \min(SCr/\kappa, 1)^{\alpha} \times \max(SCr/\kappa, 1)^{-1.209} \times 0.993^{age} [\times 1.018 \text{ if female}][\times 1.159 \text{ if black}]$$

where SCr is serum creatinine (in mg/dL), κ is 0.7 for females and 0.9 for males, α is −0.329 for females and −0.411 for males, min is the minimum of SCr/κ or 1, and max is the maximum of SCr/κ or 1.

TABLE 130-3 FUNCTIONS OF THE KIDNEY AND IMPAIRMENT OF KIDNEY FUNCTION IN PATIENTS WITH CHRONIC KIDNEY DISEASE

KIDNEY FUNCTION	CONSEQUENCES OF DYSFUNCTION
Maintain concentration and body content of electrolytes and fluid volume	Hyponatremia, hyperkalemia, low total potassium content, hypocalcemia, hyperphosphatemia, decreased tolerance to electrolyte or mineral loading
Regulate blood pressure	Hypertension, cardiovascular disease
Endocrine mediator	Anemia (low erythropoietin), hypertension (renin system activation), bone disease (secondary hyperparathyroidism), low vitamin D activation, prolonged half-lives of peptide hormones (e.g., insulin)
Waste product excretion	Anorexia, nausea, soft tissue deposition of oxalates and phosphates, neurologic dysfunction, loss of muscle protein

adverse renal outcomes.[5] Other epidemiologic factors associated with an increasing risk of progressive CKD are cardiovascular disease, smoking, and hyperlipidemia.

PATHOBIOLOGY

The intact nephron hypothesis helps explain the importance of GFR as a measure of remaining kidney function. The nephron consists of the glomerulus, proximal tubule, loop of Henle, distal tubule, and collecting duct. Individuals are born with 0.75 million to 1.25 million nephrons per kidney, but if nephrons are lost, new ones are not regenerated. The intact nephron hypothesis is that each nephron functions as an independent unit, so the sum of the functions of all remaining nephrons determines the whole kidney's GFR, the most accurate estimate of remaining kidney function.

Physiologic and metabolic functions of the kidney include the regulation of blood pressure, several endocrine functions, and ion concentrations in the extracellular and intracellular fluids as well as the excretion of waste products (Table 130-3). Loss of these functions yields several direct and derivative consequences of CKD. For example, a limitation in the ability to excrete acid causes hyperventilation and a decrease in P_{CO_2}. In muscle, acidosis activates the ubiquitin-proteasome enzymatic process to degrade protein, causing loss of muscle mass. Bone buffers acid by releasing calcium and phosphates, a response that leads to demineralization and secondary hyperparathyroidism, both of which make bones more susceptible to fracture.

Balance and Steady-State Considerations

Metabolic balance is the state in which the intake or production of a substance equals its elimination. In response to CKD, the ability to excrete sodium falls as nephrons are lost, but the remaining nephrons respond at least partially by excreting a greater fraction of the sodium filtered by each glomerulus. Similar phenomena adjust the excretion of other ions and substances, thereby allowing the patient with CKD to reduce the accumulation of ions and to avoid adverse consequences such as hyperkalemia. The ability to achieve balance between intake and excretion, however, has a limit; if the sodium balance is positive because the intake of sodium exceeds its excretion by the kidney, hypertension and edema will develop.

A related concept is that of steady state. A patient is in steady state when the internal environment is constant and the intake and production of an ion or compound equal its output and metabolism. Although a constant weight indicates that sodium intake is equal to sodium output, this steady state does not necessarily indicate normal conditions. For example, a patient who is grossly edematous may be in the steady state because the intake of sodium equals its excretion but at the price of sodium accumulation in the extracellular fluid.

The Tradeoff Hypothesis

Another important principle, the tradeoff hypothesis, refers to the activation of pathophysiologic responses that produce adverse consequences. In response to CKD, the loss of nephrons will initially reduce salt excretion, thereby leading to sodium retention, expansion of extracellular fluid, and a rise in weight and blood pressure. The pathophysiologic response to sodium retention triggers adaptations that increase sodium excretion by raising blood pressure and suppressing the reabsorption of filtered sodium. The tradeoffs include the development of volume-dependent hypertension and the persistence of impaired reabsorption of filtered sodium by the remaining tubules. An abrupt decrease in salt intake will elicit only a sluggish increase in sodium reabsorption, and the result will be a loss of sodium and a reduction in extracellular and intravascular volume, which will impair kidney perfusion and decrease GFR.

The most extensively studied tradeoff is the adaptation that stimulates secondary hyperparathyroidism (Fig. 130-1). In CKD, the loss of nephrons impairs the kidney's ability to excrete phosphates, which accumulate and result in an increased formation of calcium-phosphate complexes. The resulting reduction in the level of ionized calcium stimulates calcium-sensing receptors in the parathyroid gland. These responses stimulate the production and secretion of parathyroid hormone (PTH). The increase in PTH is beneficial because it suppresses Na/Pi type II, the cotransporter of phosphates, thereby reducing phosphate reabsorption by the kidney and promoting the excretion of the accumulated phosphates. Besides stimulating PTH

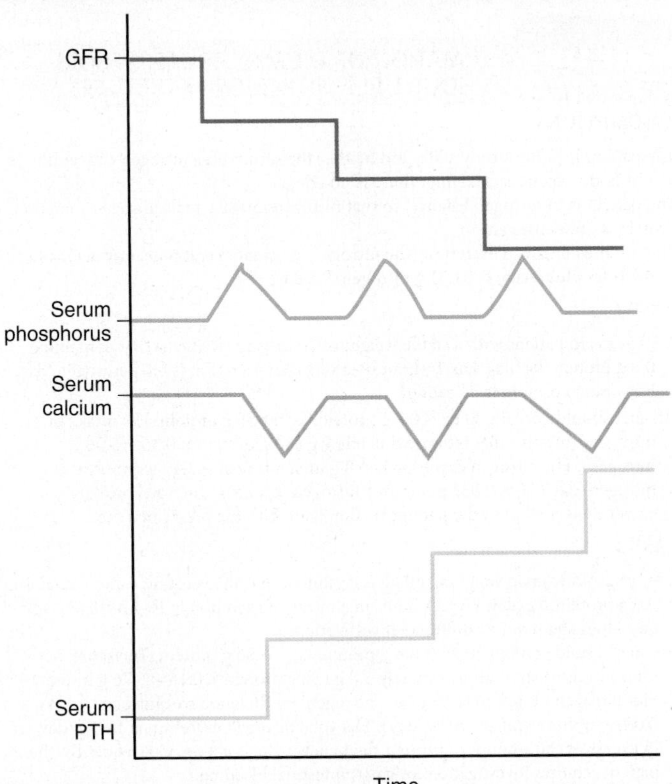

FIGURE 130-1. A decrease in glomerular filtration rate (GFR) is followed by an increase in serum phosphorus and a decrease in serum calcium. An increase in serum parathyroid hormone (PTH) returns phosphorus and calcium to normal levels, but the tradeoff is PTH-induced bone disease.

secretion, an increase in the levels of circulating phosphates will suppress the production of 1,25-dihydroxycholecalciferol (calcitriol), which is the most potent form of vitamin D. Finally, the increase in circulating phosphates stimulates bone osteoclasts to secrete fibroblast growth factor 23 (FGF23). FGF23 can interact with the cofactor Klotho in the proximal tubule, thereby suppressing the Na/Pi type II phosphate transporter. The result is that the increase in PTH and FGF23 stimulates urinary phosphate excretion. The tradeoff for eliminating phosphates is the development of renal osteodystrophy because the steady-state increase in ionized calcium and reduction in circulating phosphates can be maintained only if the circulating concentrations of PTH and FGF23 are increased to cause phosphate excretion (see Fig. 130-1). The adverse consequences of these responses include PTH-mediated stimulation of osteoclasts and an increase in mortality associated with a high FGF23 level (see later).

Hypertension

Hypertension, like anemia, is almost universal in CKD patients and is often the first clinical indication of CKD. The coincidence of CKD and high blood pressure is particularly important because hypertension contributes to the development of cardiovascular disease, which is the leading cause of morbidity and mortality in CKD patients. Hypertension in CKD patients largely reflects an expanded extracellular volume due to a salt-rich diet plus impaired capacity to excrete sodium; activation of the renin-angiotensin-aldosterone system also plays a role. In terms of a tradeoff, when sodium retention raises extracellular volume, blood pressure and sodium excretion increase, thereby contributing to a balance between sodium intake and its excretion; salt balance can be maintained only as long as blood pressure is high. Two practical implications arise from these relationships. First, treatment of hypertensive patients with vasodilating drugs alone is frequently unsuccessful because the initial reduction in blood pressure stimulates sodium retention and expansion of the extracellular volume, which raise blood pressure. Second, a salt-rich diet cancels the benefits of diuretics even in normal adults.

Another mechanism for hypertension in CKD patients is activation of the renin-angiotensin-aldosterone system and the sympathetic nervous system. When inhibitors of the renin-angiotensin-aldosterone system, such as angiotensin-converting enzyme (ACE) inhibitors or angiotensin receptor blockers (ARBs), are given to patients with CKD, they can slow the loss of GFR. Evidence for activation of the sympathetic nervous system includes higher circulating levels of norepinephrine, which can contribute to vasoconstriction, and suppressed production of nitric oxide. Inhibition of this system in CKD patients, unlike blocking of the renin-angiotensin-aldosterone system, does not, however, slow the loss of GFR.

Endocrine Disorders

CKD, even in patients with serum creatinine values as low as 2.5 mg/dL, reduces the ability of insulin to stimulate glucose uptake by muscle and other organs, an abnormality known as *insulin resistance* (Chapter 229). The resulting reduction in glucose uptake raises blood glucose levels and causes a compensatory increase in the release of insulin, which acts to maintain blood glucose levels near normal. Insulin resistance in nondiabetic CKD patients is generally associated with blood glucose values within the normal range, and blood glucose levels rarely exceed 200 mg/dL. Insulin resistance also impairs intracellular signaling and interferes with the metabolism of both glucose and protein, thereby causing loss of muscle proteins.

The metabolic acidosis (Chapter 118) of CKD contributes to the development of insulin resistance, impairs the ability of growth hormone to stimulate insulin-like growth factor-I, and depresses circulating levels of thyroxine and triiodothyronine (Chapter 226). Fortunately, most of these metabolic changes, like the acidosis-induced loss of bone density and muscle protein, are reversed simply by treating CKD patients with sodium bicarbonate or other alkalizing agents.[A1]

Another mechanism that affects endocrine status in CKD patients is the kidney's impaired ability to degrade small proteins, including several hormones. For example, diabetic patients with CKD can progressively lose the ability to degrade insulin, thereby lengthening its half-life. This response can cause hypoglycemia in patients with progressive CKD who are treated with standard doses of insulin. Second, incomplete degradation of PTH by the damaged kidney can affect the interpretation of the circulating PTH concentration. Fragments of partially degraded PTH are recognized by the PTH immunoassay, thereby leading to a misinterpretation that levels of PTH are excessively high.

In patients with advanced, stage 4 CKD, normochromic, normocytic anemia (Chapter 158) is almost universal, principally because of impaired production of erythropoietin by interstitial cells in the damaged kidney. Other factors contributing to anemia in CKD patients include a shortened half-life of erythrocytes, gastrointestinal bleeding, and deficiencies of vitamins and iron.

Renal Bone Disease

Renal bone disease, also called *renal osteodystrophy*, afflicts virtually all CKD patients to different degrees. Findings on bone biopsies of patients with renal bone disease range from features indicative of increased bone turnover (i.e., greater numbers of osteoclasts, osteoblasts, and osteocytes) to abnormalities reflecting low bone turnover (i.e., reduced numbers of osteoclasts and osteoblasts and the accumulation of demineralized matrix). PTH is a major stimulus for the development of renal osteodystrophy in CKD patients; patients with high bone turnover have increased circulating PTH levels, whereas patients with low bone turnover exhibit only a small increase in circulating PTH. A third type of disease is mixed uremic osteodystrophy, which has features of hyperparathyroidism plus defective mineralization. The pathophysiologic process of this bone disorder involves an increase in circulating phosphates, which increase circulating PTH, which in turn activates osteoclasts to reduce bone mass. Besides stimulating PTH, the increase in circulating phosphates suppresses the activation of calcitriol, and this decrease in calcitriol limits intestinal absorption of calcium and phosphates and also suppresses PTH production. The physicochemical interaction between circulating phosphates and "free" or ionized calcium lowers the level of ionized calcium. Consequently, the binding of ionized calcium to calcium receptors on parathyroid chief cells is blunted, thereby stimulating the production and secretion of PTH. Second, hyperphosphatemia can act directly on parathyroid cells to stimulate PTH production. Other factors that contribute to CKD-induced bone disease include defects in cellular signaling by the calcium receptor and changes in vitamin D metabolism. Hyperphosphatemia also can blunt the ability of ACE inhibitors or ARBs to slow the loss of GFR.

A G protein–coupled plasma membrane receptor present in chief cells of the parathyroid gland and in certain renal tubular cells responds directly to changes in calcium ions. This receptor can then interact with calcium or with cinacalcet, a small, orally available molecule that activates the calcium receptor, thereby leading to suppression of the expression and a release of PTH from parathyroid chief cells. In contrast, hyperphosphatemia and a reduced level of circulating ionized calcium increase the production and release of PTH (see Fig. 130-1). Stimulation of PTH secretion is negated by cinacalcet even when there is hyperphosphatemia and low ionized calcium levels. Because of the complexity of its action, use of cinacalcet requires careful monitoring to avoid hypoparathyroidism and hypocalcemia.

Another factor that regulates the circulating calcium level and affects the development of renal bone disease is vitamin D. Under normal conditions, activation of vitamin D proceeds by repeated hydroxylation of the parent molecule, cholecalciferol (vitamin D_3). The initial hydroxylation occurs in the liver, where 25-hydroxyvitamin D_3 is formed. This form of vitamin D stimulates the absorption of calcium and phosphates from the intestines and is believed to change the function and metabolism of muscle and possibly other organs by mechanisms that are poorly defined. Moreover, low circulating values of 25-hydroxyvitamin D_3 in CKD patients are associated with an increase in the risk of all-cause mortality.

Calcitriol, the most active form of vitamin D, is produced when 25-hydroxyvitamin D_3 is hydroxylated by 25-hydroxycholecalciferol 1α-hydroxylase in the proximal tubules of the kidney. Activity of the 1α-hydroxylase is regulated by factors that change mineral metabolism; for example, its activity is reduced by hyperphosphatemia, which decreases the production of calcitriol and hence absorption of calcium and phosphates from the intestine. Alternatively, the β-glucuronidase Klotho is a tissue-specific, locally secreted cofactor of FGF23. It increases the excretion of phosphates by the kidney. In addition, the Klotho-FGF23 combination can bind to the FGF receptor to decrease the expression of the 1α-hydroxylase, thereby suppressing the production of calcitriol. Finally, the Klotho-FGF23 combination interacts with its receptor in the parathyroid gland and down-regulates the secretion of PTH. These complex regulatory processes emphasize how loss of kidney function disrupts the normal function and turnover of bone.

Accumulation of Uremic Toxins

When diets contain protein-rich foods, the protein is metabolized to amino acids that can be used to build body protein stores (E-Fig. 130-1). Amino acids not used for this purpose are metabolized to form urea or are converted into potentially toxic products that are accumulated in patients with CKD.[6] Because urea production is directly proportional to the amount of protein eaten, it follows that excess protein in the diet increases the production of urea and uremic toxins. Another source of uremic toxins results when bacteria in the colon metabolize amino acids into uremic toxins (e.g., tryptophan or histidine can be converted into *p*-cresol and indoxyl sulfate).

The concentration of creatinine in serum is determined by the degree of renal insufficiency and the rate of creatinine production, which is proportionate to lean body mass. For example, a serum creatinine concentration of 1.4 mg/dL in an adult with a small muscle mass signifies a much greater loss of kidney function than it does in an individual with a large muscle mass. Creatinine is formed from creatine and creatine phosphate by a nonenzymatic reaction, so creatinine production in subjects with a stable weight should be constant. The production of creatinine is affected by the diet; creatine and creatine phosphate are highly concentrated in muscle, and extensive cooking of meat converts creatine to creatinine. At least 4 months are required to reach a new steady state of the conversion of creatine and creatine phosphate to creatinine when CKD patients change the protein in their diets. Consequently, if serum creatinine rises or falls in response to a treatment affecting kidney function, conclusions that the treatment has slowed the loss of GFR must be delayed until 4 months have passed.

With CKD, the accumulation of peptides (also known as *middle molecules*) has been associated with disorders that range from the induction of anorexia to neurologic abnormalities. Alternatively, high uric acid levels, which are related to excess protein intake, can cause gout (Chapter 273) and may participate in the development of hypertension and inflammatory responses in blood vessels. Another association between protein-rich diets and increased levels of uremic toxins arises because foods rich in protein invariably raise the intake of phosphates, sodium, acid, potassium, and other ions.[A2] These ions aggravate phosphate-induced renal osteodystrophy, volume-dependent hypertension, and acidosis-stimulated loss of muscle protein.

Ideally, circulating levels of uremic toxins should be monitored, but such measurements are not practical. Fortunately, the blood urea nitrogen (BUN) provides a readily available index of the level of uremic toxins because the production of urea is directly proportional to the intake of proteins and hence the accumulation of ions and other unexcreted waste products (see E-Fig. 130-1). The amount of protein in the diet can be reliably estimated from the 24-hour excretion of urea nitrogen as long as the patient is in the steady state (i.e., BUN and weight are stable; Table 130-4). When the ratio of BUN to serum creatinine is chronically below 10 : 1, the patient is eating a protein-restricted diet. When the BUN concentration exceeds 10 times the serum creatinine concentration, three possibilities should be considered. First, the patient may have gastrointestinal bleeding or may be suffering from a severely catabolic condition (e.g., trauma or high-dose glucocorticoid administration) that results in catabolism of endogenous proteins to amino acids and hence to urea. Second, the patient may be eating excessive amounts of protein, which yields more urea than the impaired kidney can excrete. Finally, extracellular volume depletion or severe liver or heart disease can stimulate active reabsorption of sodium and fluid by the proximal tubule and thereby increase the passive reabsorption of urea and raise the BUN level. The corollary is that a decrease in urea production is associated with a decrease in the load of uremic toxins. Consequently, the goal of dietary manipulation in CKD is to minimize production of urea while ensuring an adequate intake to maintain body protein stores. To accomplish this goal, the dietary content of protein should be monitored to limit the excessive production of urea (see later).

TABLE 130-4 ESTIMATION OF DIETARY PROTEIN FROM 24-HOUR UREA NITROGEN EXCRETION

ASSUMPTIONS

The patient is in the steady state, and neither the serum urea nitrogen concentration nor body weight is changing; there is no edema.
The patient is in nitrogen balance, so that nitrogen intake equals nitrogen excretion.
Protein is 16% nitrogen.
The nonurea nitrogen excretion (the nitrogen in urinary creatinine, uric acid, and peptides plus feces) is 0.031 g nitrogen/kg/day.

CASE 1

A 50-year-old patient with a stable weight of 70 kg is prescribed a diet containing 0.8 g protein/kg/day. His 24-hour urea nitrogen excretion is 6.8 g nitrogen/day. How much protein is he eating?
His diet should contain 70 kg × 0.8 g protein/kg, or 56 g protein. His intake of nitrogen from this diet is approximately 9 g (56 g protein × 0.16 = 8.96 g nitrogen). His nitrogen excretion is 6.8 g urea nitrogen + 2.17 g nonurea nitrogen/day (70 × 0.031 g nonurea nitrogen/kg/day). The total nitrogen excretion is 8.97 g, so the patient is compliant with the prescribed diet.

CASE 2

A 40-year-old woman weighing 60 kg is confident that she is eating a diet containing 0.6 g protein/kg/day. Her 24-hour urea nitrogen excretion is 10 g nitrogen/kg/day. Does she require additional investigation?
Her diet should contain 60 kg × 0.6 g protein/kg, or 36 g protein. Therefore, her intake of nitrogen is approximately 5.8 g (36 g protein × 0.16 = 5.76 g nitrogen). Her nitrogen excretion is 10 g urea nitrogen + 1.86 g nonurea nitrogen (60 kg × 0.031 g nonurea nitrogen/kg/day). Her total nitrogen excretion is 11.9 g/day, far in excess of the amount of protein she believes she is eating. Consequently, the patient requires investigation for gastrointestinal bleeding.

Progression of Chronic Kidney Disease

Persistence of diseases affecting the kidney (e.g., diabetes or inflammatory conditions such as systemic lupus erythematosus) is not the only factor that determines the rapidity of the loss of kidney function. Even when diseases that initially damage the kidney are no longer active, kidney function continues to decline, perhaps because of systemic hypertension, hemodynamic injury to the kidney, proteinuria, and the accumulation of nephrotoxins.

There is no agreement that treatment of hypertension aggressively will change the course of progressive loss of kidney function. Clinical observations suggest that hypertension adversely affects the kidney; malignant hypertension damages endothelial cells of both the afferent arteriole and the glomerulus and may even cause thrombosis in these vessels. Chronic hypertension is frequently associated with ischemic injury to glomeruli and can result in glomerulosclerosis. Furthermore, the degree of hypertension in CKD patients is directly correlated with the rate of loss of kidney function.

Experimentally, angiotensin II–related, progressive glomerular damage (Table 130-5) arises because it preferentially constricts the glomerular efferent arteriole to a greater extent than the afferent arteriole. This imbalance raises intracapillary pressure and tends to increase glomerular filtration, thereby leading to the hyperfiltration mechanism, but the tradeoff for the

TABLE 130-5 ANGIOTENSIN II RESPONSES IN CHRONIC KIDNEY DISEASE*

Hemodynamic responses
- Systemic hypertension
  - Vasoconstriction
  - Salt retention (aldosterone)
  - Intraglomerular hypertension
  - Efferent arteriolar vasoconstriction

Nonhemodynamic responses in the kidney
- Macrophage infiltration and inflammation
- Interstitial matrix accumulation
  - Increased transforming growth factor-β
  - Increased plasminogen activator inhibitor type 1
  - Increased aldosterone

*Includes the proposed actions of angiotensin II that can contribute to the development of cardiovascular disease and progressive loss of kidney function.

increase in GFR is damage to glomerular capillaries. Because angiotensin II is the mediator of preferential efferent arteriolar constriction, ACE inhibitors and ARBs are used to prevent both hyperfiltration and damage to the kidney.

ACE inhibitors and ARBs not only lower blood pressure but also block growth factor properties of angiotensin II and its ability to activate transforming growth factor-β, plasminogen activator inhibitor type 1, and other cytokines that can contribute to the development of interstitial damage to the kidney (see Table 130-5). Aldosterone may also contribute to the development of interstitial damage and collagen deposition in the kidney. ACE inhibitors or ARBs also generally reduce albuminuria, and a decrease in albuminuria is highly associated with a slowing of progressive CKD, perhaps because albumin or molecules bound to albumin can directly injure kidney cells.

CLINICAL MANIFESTATIONS

Unfortunately, progressive loss of kidney function produces no clinically distinct signs or symptoms. Findings that should raise the possibility of CKD include hypertension, urinary abnormalities such as hematuria or repeated urinary tract infections, and edema.

As the GFR declines, clinical abnormalities become more frequent, but symptoms are mostly nonspecific even with stage 4 CKD (see Table 130-2). Some patients complain only of exercise intolerance, fatigue, or anorexia. If these symptoms are present, serum creatinine and BUN levels should be measured, and the urine should be examined for albuminuria. For this assessment, a "spot" urine can suffice if the urine albumin and creatinine concentrations are measured; an albumin-to-creatinine ratio of more than 30 mg/g in urine is associated with more adverse outcomes. As CKD progresses, patients frequently develop anemia (Chapter 158), metabolic acidosis (Chapter 118), hyperkalemia (Chapter 117), hyperphosphatemia (Chapter 119), hypocalcemia (Chapter 245), and hypoalbuminemia (Chapter 215), each of which may be associated with symptoms (Table 130-6).

Specific syndromes can be associated with proteinuria and CKD. For example, severe albumin losses (>3 g/day) plus edema and hypercholesterolemia define the nephrotic syndrome (Chapter 121), which can lead to the loss of the relatively small (59 kD) vitamin D–binding protein that is attached to 25-hydroxyvitamin D_3, thereby aggravating renal osteodystrophy. Advanced proteinuria also can be associated with losses of clotting factors IX, XI, and XII, causing coagulation defects (Chapter 174). Conversely, urinary losses of antithrombin III can result in thrombosis (Chapter 171), especially when inflammation increases levels of acute phase reactant proteins, including fibrinogen.

Some patients with renal bone disease complain of vague, ill-defined pain in the lower back, hips, knees, and other locations. In advanced renal osteodystrophy, pain can be so severe that it decreases exercise tolerance, and the resulting immobilization can increase the risk of fractures even with minimal trauma.

Another clinical syndrome related to hyperphosphatemia and hence to the development of renal bone disease is vascular calcification, which causes vascular stiffness, an increase in systolic blood pressure, and the development of left ventricular hypertrophy. A more disabling manifestation is calcification in the tunica media of blood vessels (i.e., Mönckeberg sclerosis) as well as calcifications that impair the function of multiple organs, including the lungs, myocardium, and skin. Calcification of the skin and cutaneous vessels defines the syndrome of calciphylaxis.

TABLE 130-6 COMPLICATIONS OF CHRONIC KIDNEY DISEASE

AFFECTED SYSTEM	CAUSE OR MECHANISM	CLINICAL SYNDROME
Systemic symptoms	Anemia, inflammation	Fatigue, lassitude
Skin	Hyperparathyroidism, calcium-phosphate deposition	Rash, pruritus, metastatic calcification
Cardiovascular disease	Hypertension, anemia, hyperhomocysteinemia, vascular calcification	Atherosclerosis, heart failure, stroke
Serositis	Unknown	Pericardial or pleural pain and fluid, peritoneal fluid
Gastrointestinal	Unknown	Anorexia, nausea, vomiting, diarrhea, gastrointestinal tract bleeding
Immune system	Leukocyte dysfunction, depressed cellular immunity	Infections
Endocrine	Hypothalamic-pituitary axis dysfunction	Amenorrhea, menorrhagia, impotence, oligospermia, hyperprolactinemia
Neurologic	Unknown	Neuromuscular excitability, cognitive dysfunction progressing to coma, peripheral neuropathy (restless leg syndrome or sensory deficits)

DIAGNOSIS

If CKD is suspected, emphasis should be placed on eliciting a history of hypertension, urinary abnormalities, and treatment with drugs that might affect kidney function (e.g., ACE inhibitors, ARBs, and nonsteroidal anti-inflammatory drugs; see Chapter 120). The family history should focus on family members with kidney diseases, kidney stones, surgery involving the urinary tract, diabetes, and hypertension. The physical examination should include lying and standing blood pressure measurements in both arms and a search for findings associated with CKD, such as skin abnormalities, persistent itching, a palpable polycystic kidney (Chapter 127), evidence of lost lean body mass, peripheral edema, and neurologic abnormalities.

Staging

The severity of CKD is divided into five stages based on persistent reductions in estimated GFR (see Table 130-2). Two assessments of impaired kidney function are required: estimated GFR (eGFR) and the degree of albuminuria. The eGFR is calculated from the serum creatinine concentration or the serum level of the protease inhibitor cystatin C plus age, body weight, gender, and race (see Table 130-2).

Shortcomings of the creatinine-based method of assessing kidney function are that it is influenced by both kidney function and creatinine production, the latter of which is directly proportional to lean body mass and is also influenced by the amount of well-cooked meat in the diet. Another shortcoming is that the serum creatinine concentration can remain in the nominally normal range until as much as 50% of kidney function is lost. The assessment of eGFR from cystatin C is limited because the level of this protein is influenced by inflammation, cigarette smoke, and excess acid. In addition, the measurement of cystatin C concentration is not as standardized as the measurement of serum creatinine concentration. Regardless, a low eGFR estimated by the cystatin C method or by a combination of the creatinine and cystatin C methods is closely associated with the development of complications of CKD.[7]

The progression of CKD, which can be estimated by the decline in the reciprocal of the creatinine level (1/serum creatinine), is linear in most patients (Fig. 130-2), and deviations from this linearity suggest a change in the course of CKD. Other markers are not as accurate for estimating changes in kidney function; the BUN concentration, for example, is determined not only by the remaining kidney function but also by the amount of protein in the diet.

A careful microscopic examination of the urine is critical for diagnosis of CKD or changes in progression. The presence of erythrocytes and

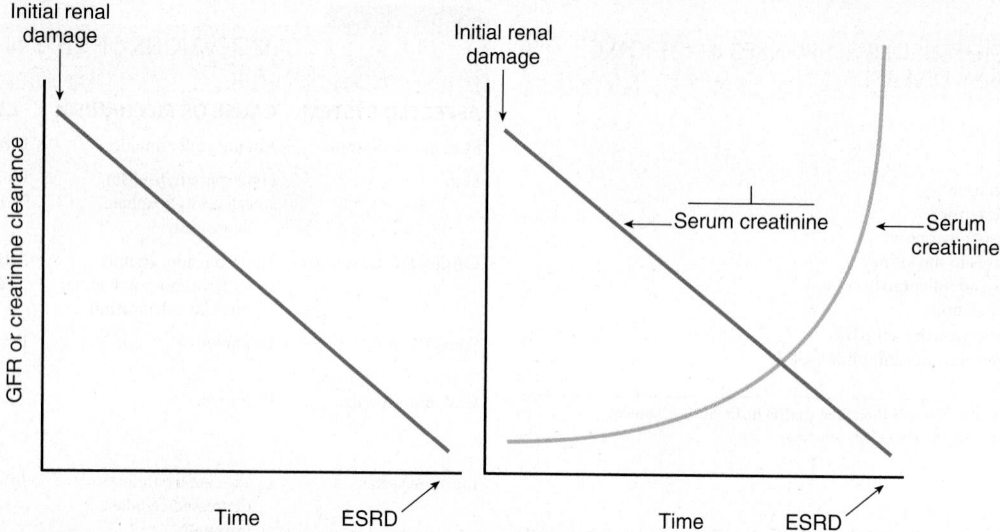

FIGURE 130-2. The loss of kidney function in chronic kidney disease is constant from initial damage to end-stage renal disease (ESRD, ***left panel***). The constant loss of glomerular filtration rate (GFR) or creatinine clearance is estimated most easily by plotting the reciprocal of serum creatinine against time. (Reprinted with permission from *Annual Review of Medicine* 35. ©1984 by Annual Reviews, www.annualreviews.org.)

erythrocyte casts in the urine sediment is consistent with glomerulonephritis (Chapter 121), the presence of fine granular casts plus protein suggests diabetic kidney disease (Chapter 124), urine samples containing leukocytes plus fine and coarse granular casts suggest interstitial nephritis (Chapter 122), and eosinophils in the urine suggest a drug reaction with interstitial damage (Chapter 122).

Microalbuminuria is defined as 30 to 300 mg albumin/24 hours in a urine specimen, and the abnormality should be present in at least two specimens. A urinary albumin-to-creatinine ratio higher than 30 mg/g in at least two specimens is also associated with high risks of morbidity and mortality in patients with CKD. However, it is uncertain whether albuminuria precedes and potentially causes the loss of eGFR or whether it is a marker of kidney damage.[8] Albuminuria (>300 mg/24 hours) is defined as a persistent excretion rate exceeding that of microalbuminuria.

The urea nitrogen content of the 24-hour urine collection can be used to calculate the amount of dietary protein, which is composed of 16% nitrogen (see E-Fig. 130-1 and Table 130-4). When the amount of urea nitrogen excreted in the steady state (i.e., stable values of weight and BUN) is added to the amount of nonurea nitrogen excreted daily (i.e., 0.031 g nitrogen per kilogram of ideal body weight per day, which includes the nitrogen present in proteinuria of 5 g), the total daily intake of nitrogen can be calculated. If the calculated total of nitrogen excreted exceeds the nitrogen contained in a prescribed diet, the physician should suspect dietary nonadherence, gastrointestinal bleeding, or a catabolic illness.

Other Laboratory Tests

Blood chemistries that evaluate the consequences of CKD include concentrations of sodium, potassium, chloride, bicarbonate, calcium, and phosphorus as well as uric acid levels. The blood glucose level and hemoglobin A_{1c} level should be monitored in diabetics. In patients with suspected glomerulonephritis (Chapter 121), testing commonly includes measurement of antinuclear antibodies, double-stranded DNA antibodies, serum complement levels, antineutrophil cytoplasmic antibody levels, and serologies for hepatitis viruses. The hematocrit or hemoglobin level should be monitored because anemia can develop even with mild renal dysfunction and tends to worsen as CKD progresses because of reduced erythropoietin production and iron deficiency. Iron deficiency can be recognized if the serum iron level is low, the serum ferritin concentration is less than 200 ng/mL, and the transferrin saturation is less than 20% (Chapter 159). Such findings should raise the possibility of gastrointestinal bleeding. To detect CKD-induced bone disease, serum levels of PTH, alkaline phosphatase, calcium, and phosphorus should be obtained.

Imaging

The initial evaluation should include an ultrasound examination of the kidney and bladder to ensure that there is no obstruction of urine flow (Chapter 123) or evidence of polycystic kidney disease (Chapter 127). Enlarged kidneys suggest that CKD may be caused by diabetes (Chapter 124), HIV-associated nephropathy (Chapter 121), infiltrative diseases (e.g., amyloidosis; Chapters 121 and 188), or polycystic kidney disease. Small kidneys, especially with a shrunken kidney cortex, suggest chronic glomerular (Chapter 121) or interstitial (Chapter 122) diseases. If the size of the two kidneys differs substantially, stenosis of the renal artery (Chapter 125) of the smaller kidney should be considered, especially in hypertensive patients.

TREATMENT

Cardiovascular disorders are common in patients with CKD, in part because hypertension is almost universal. The 2014 Eighth Joint National Committee (JNC 8) for the management of high blood pressure in adults concludes that results from randomized, controlled trials of blood pressure control support lowering of blood pressure to 140/90 mm Hg,[9] although some suggest a lower target of 130/80 mm Hg. Lowering of blood pressure to 140/90 mm Hg with ACE inhibitors or ARBs in combination with a diuretic should be included in the initial treatment plan to slow the loss of kidney function and to reduce cardiovascular events[A3] (see Table 67-7). Combining an ACE inhibitor and an ARB provides no additional benefit in terms of protecting the kidney and is associated with more frequent adverse events, so this combination is not recommended. In patients with type 2 diabetes, a systolic blood pressure goal of 135 to 140 mm Hg is preferable to a blood pressure below 120 mm Hg, and the goal for those with hypertensive renal diseases is about 140/85 mm Hg because lowering of blood pressure to 130/80 mm Hg does not further reduce the loss of GFR.[A4]

If the serum creatinine concentration increases shortly after ACE inhibitor or ARB therapy is started, it should not trigger an automatic discontinuation of the drug but rather a search for other mechanisms that cause kidney damage (e.g., an increase in blood pressure, urinary infection, use of drugs that adversely affect kidney function, or an exacerbation of the underlying renal disease) and an evaluation to be sure that the patient does not have bilateral renal artery stenosis (Chapter 125). Hyperkalemia also occurs with ACE inhibitor or ARB treatment because a reduced angiotensin II level will suppress aldosterone release. Other causes of an increase in serum potassium concentration should be sought and corrected (e.g., stop treatment with nonsteroidal anti-inflammatory drugs or potassium-sparing diuretics, the development of metabolic acidosis, or increased intake of potassium-rich foods). The abnormality will be corrected in some hyperkalemic patients by reducing dietary potassium-rich foods and adding a loop diuretic (e.g., 40 mg furosemide when the serum creatinine level is below 2 to 3 mg/dL, with higher doses for patients with more advanced CKD). If ACE inhibitor or ARB therapy produces persistent hyperkalemia or an increase in serum creatinine concentration, the dose should be reduced by 50% and amlodipine should be instituted. If the increase in serum potassium concentration persists, the potassium-binding resin Kayexalate can be added to control hyperkalemia (Chapter 117).

For blood pressure goals to be achieved, patients almost always must restrict dietary salt to 2 g sodium/day, which is the equivalent to 86 mEq sodium/day in the urine. Dietary salt restriction to 60 to 80 mEq/day alone (approximately 1.5 to 2 g of sodium) can reduce blood pressure by 10/4 mm Hg A1 [10] and is routinely recommended. This goal is achievable if patients are taught to avoid salt-rich foods. If blood pressure remains above 140/90 mm Hg, a loop diuretic such as furosemide should be added because it does not compromise renal blood flow (see Table 67-11). A critical strategy is to monitor body weight; an increase in weight and edema signifies salt retention. Conversely, a rapid loss of weight and edema would be the first clue that the diuretic dose should be reduced.

Despite the ability of calcium-channel blockers to combat hypertension, they are not as effective as ACE inhibitors or ARBs in reducing albuminuria, and they can cause peripheral edema. The loop diuretics are preferred for patients with more advanced CKD because they maintain renal blood flow, have few adverse effects, and, unlike thiazide diuretics, remain effective even at GFRs below 25 mL/minute. As renal insufficiency advances, higher daily doses of loop diuretics (e.g., 80 to 160 mg furosemide orally) may be required to reduce extracellular volume. The dose-response relationship of loop diuretics is sigmoidal, so once a dose that reduces edema and decreases body weight is identified, it should not be changed or given in divided doses because its effectiveness will be sharply reduced.

Stage 1 and Stage 2 Chronic Kidney Disease

In patients with stage 1 or stage 2 CKD, uremic symptoms are unusual because kidney function is sufficient to control the levels of potential uremic toxins. Therapy therefore emphasizes reducing blood pressure to 140/90 mm Hg plus intensive treatment of the underlying disease (e.g., treating infections, normalizing the blood glucose concentration in diabetic patients). Physicians often monitor changes in albuminuria and the rate of loss of GFR (Fig. 130-3), but there is no proven benefit of doing so.[11]

Stage 3 and Stage 4 Chronic Kidney Disease

Patients with stage 3 CKD should be referred to a nephrologist to maximize preventive measures and to search for remediable disorders. When stage 4 CKD is reached, a nephrologist should instruct patients about the advantages of therapies such as hemodialysis, peritoneal dialysis, and transplantation (Chapter 131).

In stage 3 and stage 4 CKD, the doses of many drugs that are excreted by the kidney must be reduced to prevent overdosing (Chapter 29). Treatable complications of CKD, including hypertension, secondary hyperparathyroidism, acidosis, and uremic symptoms, must be addressed. Radiologic tests with nephrotoxic contrast dye should be avoided if possible.

The development of many CKD complications (see Table 130-6) requires modification of the diet. Current levels of the estimated intake of protein in the diets of CKD patients substantially exceed recommended amounts.[12] These unrestricted high-protein diets also increase the intake of salt, acid precursors, and phosphates and can lead to the development of metabolic acidosis, hyperkalemia, hyperphosphatemia, edema, hypertension, and uremic symptoms. Recommended diets for CKD patients and especially for patients with complications of CKD should contain 0.8 g protein per kilogram of ideal body weight per day, not the patient's actual weight, which may be a function of edema or obesity. This amount will maintain body protein stores and reduce the likelihood for development of other complications. Calorie intake should be reduced to 30 kcal or fewer calories per kilogram of ideal body weight per day for largely sedentary patients; more calories are needed by those who exercise vigorously. If CKD-induced uremic symptoms persist, dietary protein can be restricted to a minimum of 0.6 g protein/kg/day, with a calorie intake of 30 kcal/kg/day. With both diets, successful implementation requires the advice, guidance, and close monitoring of a dietitian to take

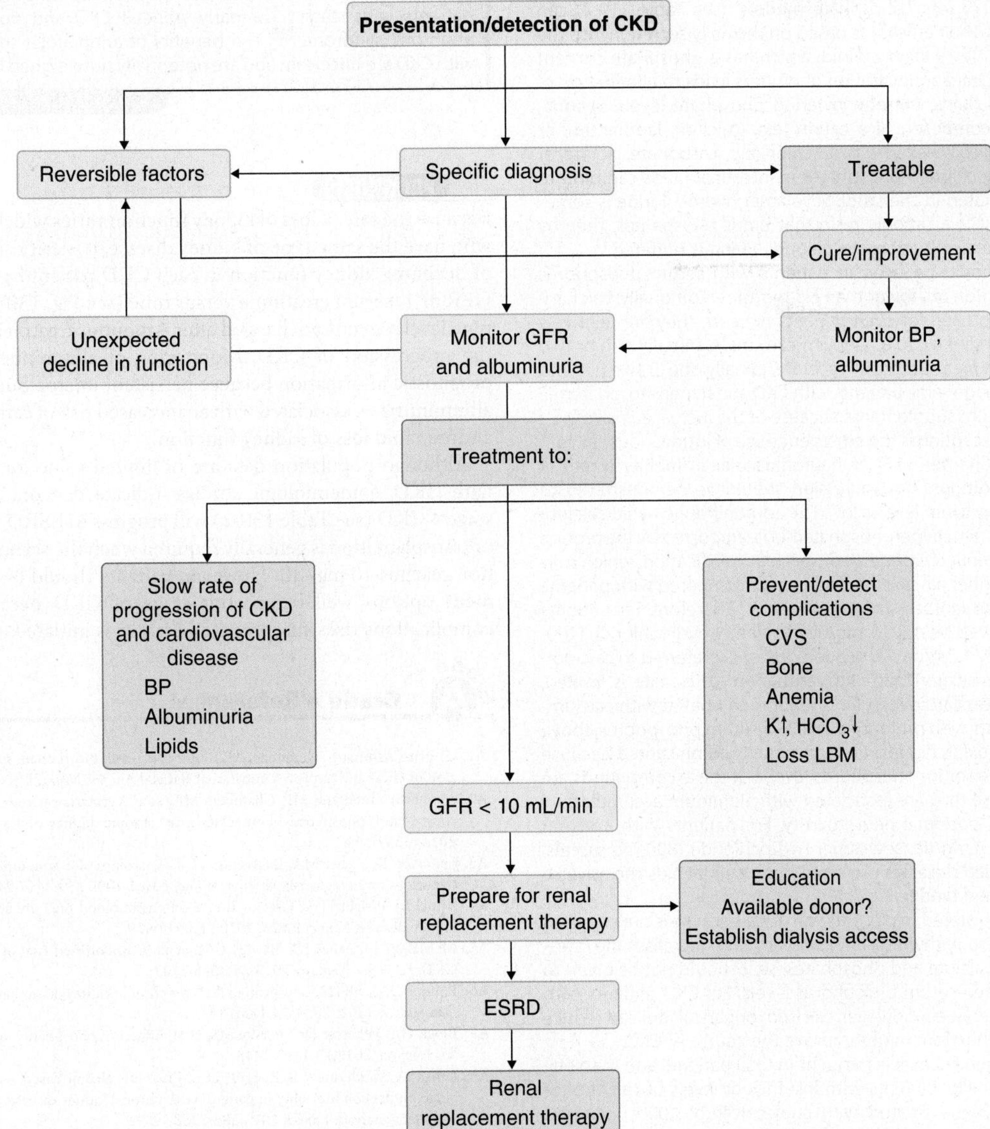

FIGURE 130-3. Management of patients in the various stages of chronic kidney disease (CKD). BP = blood pressure; CVS = cardiovascular system; ESRD = end-stage renal disease; GFR = glomerular filtration rate; LBM = lean body mass.

advantage of the patient's food preferences. Dietary compliance with protein and salt restriction can be monitored by measuring the 24-hour excretion of urea nitrogen and sodium (see Table 130-4), and the adequacy of protein stores should be assessed regularly by measuring body weight and serum protein levels. Although low-protein diets may not slow the loss of kidney function, they reduce uremic symptoms and can delay the need for dialysis without compromising the maintenance of protein stores.[A6] Most patients on a protein-restricted diet should be given a daily supplement of water-soluble vitamins (Chapter 218); fat-soluble vitamins should be prescribed for documented deficiencies.

Renal Bone Disease

Successful treatment of renal bone disease depends on correction of the principal disorder, which is the accumulation of phosphates. Even in patients with serum phosphorus levels below 5.5 mg/dL, abnormalities in calcium and phosphate metabolism can be detected by measuring the serum level of the intact PTH (i.e., the fraction that does not include PTH fragments) or by measuring the serum phosphorus level after a normal meal. A high PTH level means that kidney damage has limited the capacity to excrete phosphates despite the presence of two counterbalancing hormones, PTH and FGF23, both of which increase renal phosphate excretion. For such patients, the dietary content of phosphates must be reduced to less than 800 mg/day. Because the dietary content of phosphates is proportional to dietary protein and because phosphates are present in so many foods, CKD patients require training from a skilled dietitian or nutritionist to interpret labels on prepared foods and to change their diet successfully. The need to modify dietary phosphates and salt is emphasized because excesses of either nutrient can block the beneficial effects of ACE inhibitors or ARBs on slowing the loss of GFR. Fortunately, carefully planned diets are nutritionally sound even when the protein content is markedly restricted, provided there is adequate monitoring.

If dietary restriction proves insufficient to maintain serum phosphorus concentration of 5.5 mg/dL or less, "phosphate binders" (see Table 119-4) can lower phosphate levels.[13] Their efficacy is based on the daily secretion into the intestines of approximately 13 liters of fluid, which has a phosphate content similar to that in blood. Oral administration of binders leads to elimination of phosphates in intestinal fluids, thereby lowering phosphate levels. Second, phosphate binders are composed of a cation (e.g., calcium, lanthanum, or aluminum) that is loosely complexed with an anion (e.g., carbonate, lactate, or hydroxide), so negatively charged phosphates in intestinal fluids can bind to the cation and be eliminated in the stool. Sevelamer hydrochloride is somewhat different because it is a cationic resin that binds phosphates, thereby promoting their intestinal elimination; the chloride anion is buffered.[14]

Phosphate binders should be used in patients with serum phosphorus levels higher than 5.5 mg/dL but lower than 6.5 mg/dL. Traditionally, calcium-based binders have been used for such patients because they are relatively inexpensive and can be effective (e.g., calcium carbonate, initially one or two 500-mg tablets with each meal, or calcium acetate, initially one or two 667-mg tablets with each meal). In general, patients with CKD and hyperphosphatemia should not be given calcium supplements because of the increased risk of soft tissue calcification. The exception is the emergency use of intravenous calcium to treat hyperkalemia (Chapter 117) or neuromuscular irritability (Chapter 245). Even in these conditions, Trousseau sign should be demonstrated to confirm that the ionized calcium level is low. The admonition to avoid calcium supplements for patients with hyperphosphatemia is supported by the reports that these patients have an increased risk of vascular calcification, which may contribute to the 22% higher all-cause mortality rate compared with patients treated with sevelamer or lanthanum carbonate.[A7,A8] Therefore, for patients with serum phosphate levels below 6.5 mg/dL, sevelamer hydrochloride (400- to 800-mg tablets, initially 1.2 g/day in divided doses) is preferred to calcium-based binders. Long-term experience with lanthanum carbonate is limited, but it also may cause fewer cardiovascular problems compared with calcium-based binders. For patients with prolonged levels of serum phosphorus above 8 mg/dL, aluminum hydroxide binders are occasionally administered because they can rapidly lower the serum phosphorus level, but these compounds are generally avoided because they are associated with aluminum accumulation, deposition in bone, and potential neurotoxicity. For patients with a serum phosphorus level above 8 mg/dL, sevelamer hydrochloride (800-mg tablets, initially 1.6 g/day in divided doses) is preferred because it avoids the adverse responses to calcium-based binders.

Calcitriol is often administered to patients with CKD because it can suppress the development of hyperparathyroidism. However, it also increases the intestinal absorption of both calcium and phosphates, so it should not be given to patients who have elevated serum phosphorus levels. For CKD patients with normal serum phosphorus levels, however, calcitriol or paricalcitol can reduce proteinuria by 16% and therefore might improve the course of CKD.

A low 25-hydroxyvitamin D_3 level is frequent in CKD patients and is associated with increased mortality. Patients with insufficient levels of calcitriol or 25-hydroxyvitamin D_3 can be treated with cholecalciferol 1000 units/day. Careful monitoring is needed to avoid hypercalcemia or urinary calcium values above 250 mg/day because this level increases the risk for development of kidney stones.

Calciphylaxis, which results from deposition of calcium phosphate crystals and the secondary inflammation in blood vessels and soft tissues, is an unusual complication in patients with unrelenting hyperphosphatemia and high PTH levels. Calciphylaxis is painful, and treatment options are directed at aggressively restricting dietary phosphates and reducing serum phosphorus with phosphate binders. If the disorder persists despite correction of the serum phosphorus level, a trial of cinacalcet (initial dose of 30 mg and increasing the dose as needed to reduce circulating PTH) is warranted. However, successful treatment generally requires parathyroidectomy.

Anemia

Because of the decreased absorption of oral iron in patients with advanced CKD, ferumoxytol (two 500-mg intravenous injections separated by 3 to 8 days) provides a better response than oral iron supplements and has a low risk of side effects.[A9] In predialysis patients, treatment with erythropoietin (e.g., weekly injections of darbepoetin alfa 0.45 μg/kg) corrects anemia and improves quality of life. The hemoglobin concentration should not be raised above 12 g/dL to avoid an increased risk of stroke.[A10] Consequently, erythropoietin-stimulating agents should be used to maintain the hemoglobin concentration between 10 and 12 g/dL.

Acidosis

Treating metabolic acidosis of CKD with $NaHCO_3$ (initially with two tablets of 650 mg each two or three times daily) to raise the serum bicarbonate concentration above 22 mM can slow the loss of kidney function and improve the metabolism of muscle and bone.[A1,15]

Atherosclerosis

Cardiovascular disease is the most common cause of mortality in CKD. Contributing factors include hypertension, diabetes, increased low-density-lipoprotein cholesterol levels, and vascular calcification. Statins benefit patients with stage 2 or early stage 3 CKD and possibly those with the nephrotic syndrome.[A11] The benefits of antiplatelet therapy among persons with CKD are uncertain and are potentially outweighed by bleeding hazards.[A12]

PROGNOSIS

Because the rate of loss of kidney function varies widely, even among patients who have the same type of kidney disease, it is critical to monitor the course of declining kidney function in each CKD patient by plotting the estimated GFR or 1/serum creatinine versus time (see Fig. 130-2). If the serum creatinine level remains unchanged after 4 months, treatment has probably slowed the progression of CKD. Monitoring of albuminuria provides additional prognostic information because persistent microalbuminuria, and especially albuminuria, is associated with an increased risk of cardiovascular disease and a more rapid loss of kidney function.

Although population data are of limited value for the individual patient with CKD, epidemiologic studies indicate that one third of patients with stage 4 CKD (see Table 130-2) will progress to ESRD within 3 years. Dialysis or transplantation is generally required when the serum creatinine concentration reaches 10 mg/dL. However, patients should be informed about treatment options well before this stage of CKD because the frequency of complications rises sharply when dialysis is initiated on an emergency basis.

Grade A References

A1. de Brito-Ashurst I, Varagunam M, Raftery MJ, et al. Bicarbonate supplementation slows progression of CKD and improves nutritional status. *J Am Soc Nephrol.* 2009;20:2075-2084.

A2. Moe SM, Zidehsarai MP, Chambers MA, et al. Vegetarian compared with meat dietary protein source and phosphorus homeostasis in chronic kidney disease. *Clin J Am Soc Nephrol.* 2011;6:257-264.

A3. Jamerson K, Weber MA, Bakris GL, et al. Benazepril plus amlodipine or hydrochlorothiazide for hypertension in high-risk patients. *N Engl J Med.* 2008;359:2417-2428.

A4. Appel LJ, Wright JT Jr, Greene T, et al. Intensive blood-pressure control in hypertensive chronic kidney disease. *N Engl J Med.* 2010;363:918-929.

A5. McMahon EJ, Bauer JD, Hawley CM, et al. A randomized trial of dietary sodium restriction in CKD. *J Am Soc Nephrol.* 2013;24:2096-2103.

A6. Fouque D, Laville M. Low protein diets for chronic kidney disease in non diabetic adults. *Cochrane Database Syst Rev.* 2009;3:CD001892.

A7. Block GA, Wheeler DC, Persky MS, et al. Effects of phosphate binders in moderate CKD. *J Am Soc Nephrol.* 2012;23:1407-1415.

A8. Jamal SA, Vandermeer B, Raggi P, et al. Effect of calcium-based versus non-calcium-based phosphate binders on mortality in patients with chronic kidney disease: an updated systematic review and meta-analysis. *Lancet.* 2013;382:1268-1277.

A9. Lu M, Cohen MH, Rieves D, et al. FDA report: ferumoxytol for intravenous iron therapy in adult patients with chronic kidney disease. *Am J Hematol.* 2010;85:315-319.

A10. Pfeffer MA, Burdmann EA, Chen CY, et al. A trial of darbepoetin alfa in type 2 diabetes and chronic kidney disease. *N Engl J Med.* 2009;361:2019-2032.

A11. Tonelli M, Wanner C. Lipid management in chronic kidney disease: synopsis of the Kidney Disease: Improving Global Outcomes 2013 clinical practice guideline. *Ann Intern Med.* 2014;160:182-189.

A12. Palmer SC, Di Micco L, Razavian M, et al. Effects of antiplatelet therapy on mortality and cardiovascular and bleeding outcomes in persons with chronic kidney disease: a systematic review and meta-analysis. *Ann Intern Med.* 2012;156:445-459.

GENERAL REFERENCES

For the General References and other additional features, please visit Expert Consult at https://expertconsult.inkling.com.

131

TREATMENT OF IRREVERSIBLE RENAL FAILURE

DAVID COHEN AND ANTHONY MICHAEL VALERI

Chronic kidney disease (Chapter 130) tends to progress over time owing to progressive nephron dropout, glomerular capillary hypertension, and glomerular hyperfiltration, whether it is caused by primary glomerular injury or by tubulointerstitial or vascular injury. Irreversible and advanced end-stage renal disease (ESRD) requires renal replacement therapy, which can be broadly categorized as hemodialysis, peritoneal dialysis, and renal transplantation.[1] In the United States, about 640,000 people receive some form of renal replacement therapy each year.

Renal replacement therapy must be initiated when fluid and electrolyte derangements, particularly hyperkalemia and acidosis, can no longer be adequately controlled with dietary modifications and medications (Chapter 130) or if uremic symptoms, such as anorexia, nausea, vomiting, gastritis, pericarditis, or encephalopathy, develop (Table 131-1). Renal replacement therapy typically is required when the estimated glomerular filtration rate (eGFR) is below 10 mL/minute, although it may be needed at an eGFR of 10 to 15 mL/minute when comorbid conditions, particularly heart failure, make medical management even more challenging and difficult. However, preventive earlier initiation of renal replacement therapy at an eGFR of 10 to 14 mL/minute is no better than later initiation at an eGFR of 5 to 7 mL/minute or when uremic symptoms require it.[A1]

Hemodialysis relies on diffusion across a semipermeable artificial membrane, whereas peritoneal dialysis brings the blood and the dialysate solution in contact across a natural biologic membrane. The diffusion of solutes along their respective concentration gradients across a semipermeable membrane removes nitrogenous waste products and corrects imbalances of potassium, calcium, magnesium, phosphorus, and acid. In addition, plasma water filters across the membrane and, by convection, drags solutes across the membrane in approximately the same concentration as in the plasma water. The electrolyte concentrations in the dialysate solution are not necessarily physiologic but are intentionally varied with respect to their potassium, calcium, magnesium, and bicarbonate concentrations to favor correction of the plasma toward a more normal physiologic state. For example, a typical dialysate solution might use a potassium concentration of 2 mEq/L and a bicarbonate concentration of 35 mEq/L to produce concentration gradients that favor correction of hyperkalemia and uremic metabolic acidosis. Convection across the dialysis membrane is driven by either a hydrostatic pressure gradient applied across the membrane (hemodialysis) or an oncotic pressure gradient using high-dextrose concentrations or a large, poorly absorbed carbohydrate polymer in the dialysate solution (peritoneal dialysis) for the removal and filtration of excess salt and water from the body.[2]

TABLE 131-1 INDICATIONS FOR DIALYSIS IN CHRONIC KIDNEY DISEASE

Uremic encephalopathy or neuropathy
Pericarditis or pleuritis
Bleeding attributable to uremia
Fluid overload refractory to diuretics
Hypertension poorly responsive to medication
Persistent hyperkalemia, metabolic acidosis, hypercalcemia, hypocalcemia, or hyperphosphatemia refractory to medical therapy
Malnutrition or weight loss
Persistent nausea and vomiting

From Tolkoff-Rubin N. Treatment of irreversible renal failure. In: Goldman L, Schafer AI, eds. *Goldman's Cecil Medicine*. 24th ed. Philadelphia: Elsevier Saunders; 2012.

DIALYSIS

Hemodialysis

Conventional hemodialysis is typically provided at an outpatient dialysis unit where patients are treated three times per week for 3 or 4 hours per session. The measures used for determining the adequacy of treatment are based on urea clearance (as a surrogate marker molecule for the generation and clearance of small-molecular-weight nitrogenous waste products, <500 daltons). The simplest measure is the urea reduction ratio, which is the percentage fall in the blood urea nitrogen level with each dialysis session, with the goal being a 65% or greater fall in blood urea nitrogen with each dialysis session on a thrice-weekly dialysis schedule. More precise measurements can fine-tune the dialysis in an individual patient.[3] A more intensive protocol for increased urea clearance on a thrice-weekly schedule does not improve survival of patients,[A2] perhaps because it increases the likelihood of hypotension during dialysis.[4] More frequent hemodialysis, whether as in-center hemodialysis or nocturnal home hemodialysis six times per week, improves outcomes such as kidney-specific measures of quality of life, blood pressure, regression of left ventricular hypertrophy, and serum phosphorus levels, but it has not reduced mortality.[A3][A4]

Patients on hemodialysis are exposed to a large volume of dialysate solution (typically 36 to 48 L/hour during dialysis) and must be protected against even small quantities of impurities, such as trace minerals, bacteria, and bacterial endotoxins, in the dialysis solution. To this end, dialysate solutions are prepared from concentrates diluted with water prepared by reverse osmosis systems or deionizer tanks to remove undesired trace cations and anions and then filtered through small micron-sized pore filters to remove bacteria and their byproducts. Exposure to low levels of bacteria and bacterial byproducts may contribute to the chronic inflammation seen in some patients on hemodialysis.

In critically ill patients who are hemodynamically unstable, one alternative is continuous venovenous hemofiltration, which requires central venous access (double-lumen catheter) and blood flows between 150 and 200 mL/minute. Plasma water under pressure passes across one side of a highly permeable membrane, thereby allowing both water and solutes up to about 60 kD to be removed. In contrast to hemodialysis, urea, creatinine, and phosphate are cleared at similar rates (convective clearance) during hemofiltration. The filtrate is discarded, and the fluid lost is partially replaced with a solution containing the major crystalloid components of the plasma at physiologic levels. However, there is no evidence from randomized trials that continuous venovenous hemofiltration offers a survival advantage compared with intermittent hemodialysis in patients with acute renal failure.

New modes of hemodialysis, used predominantly outside the United States, have sought to take advantage of convection to increase the clearance of middle molecules by using high-flux dialysis membranes and ultrafiltration rates of more than 20 L of fluid per dialysis session. In a large randomized trial, this approach, termed high-efficiency postdilution online hemofiltration, reduced all-cause mortality by 30%.[A5]

The most common complications during hemodialysis are vascular access problems, hypotension, muscle cramps, nausea, vomiting, headache, and chest pain. Excessive fluid removal is the most frequent cause of hypotension, but persistent hypotension may be caused by sepsis (Chapter 108), myocardial ischemia (Chapter 72), pericardial tamponade (Chapter 77), arrhythmias (Chapters 62-65), and active bleeding. A rare complication is an air embolus (Chapter 98), which is manifested with agitation, cough, dyspnea, and chest pain. The patient should be given 100% oxygen and be positioned with the left side down in an attempt to trap air in the right ventricle.

Peritoneal Dialysis

Peritoneal dialysis, which is an alternative mode of renal replacement therapy, is usually performed at home by the patient or the patient's family. A peritoneal dialysis catheter is implanted through a surgically created tunnel in the abdominal wall and inserted into the peritoneal cavity. The catheter's tip in the pelvis is used to instill a dialysis solution into the peritoneal cavity and then to drain the solution from it. Peritoneal dialysis uses the peritoneal membrane, which consists of the visceral peritoneum, the interstitial tissues, and the mesenteric capillaries, as the filter across which the diffusion of solutes and convection of plasma water occur. Different forms include continuous ambulatory peritoneal dialysis, which is typically performed with 1.5- to 3-L exchanges of peritoneal dialysis solution instilled in the abdomen through a Tenckhoff catheter four times per day; automated peritoneal dialysis, which is performed with a cycler machine at night cycling 1.5 to 3 L of peritoneal dialysis fluid into and out of the abdomen four or five times overnight; and continuous cyclic peritoneal dialysis, a hybrid of continuous ambulatory peritoneal dialysis and automated peritoneal dialysis that uses cycler therapy at night combined with one or two manual exchanges during the day. *Kt/V* urea is the total volume clearance of urea (*Kt*) normalized to the urea space, *V*, which is approximately equal to total body water.

Clearance of small solutes is a key predictor of survival in patients undergoing peritoneal dialysis, and residual renal function also plays a critical role. Current guidelines advocate a minimal target *Kt/V* urea of at least 1.7 per week.[A6] Every effort should be made to maintain residual renal function as long as possible by avoiding nephrotoxins such as nonsteroidal anti-inflammatory drugs, iodinated contrast agents, and aminoglycosides. As residual renal function diminishes over time, the peritoneal dialysis prescription needs to be adjusted accordingly.

MEDICAL ISSUES

Renal replacement therapy is concerned not only with adequate dialytic clearance of nitrogenous waste products, the restoration of acid-base and electrolyte balance, and the control of salt and water balance but also with preserving adequate access sites for dialysis, nutrition, and the management of anemia, bone diseases, and cardiovascular risk.

Access Issues

The optimal dialysis access for hemodialysis is a native vein arteriovenous fistula, which can be created by the surgical anastomosis of the radial artery to the cephalic vein or of the brachial artery to either the brachiocephalic or the basilic vein. If a patient's veins are inadequate, a synthetic graft can be placed between the radial, brachial, or axillary artery and the brachiocephalic, basilic, or axillary vein as an alternative. Most commonly, these grafts are made from a synthetic polymer, expanded polytetrafluoroethylene. Less frequently, urgent temporary access can be obtained with a dual-lumen central venous dialysis catheter that is inserted into the internal jugular (preferable) or subclavian vein (right preferred to left). Dialysis access requires periodic Doppler monitoring to detect stenoses that develop as a result of intimal hyperplasia from high turbulent flow and that can lead to reduced or even inadequate blood flow and recirculation within the access. These stenoses can be treated by percutaneous transluminal angioplasty, although stenting is sometimes required to maintain adequate luminal patency.

Nutrition

Adequate nutrition is important for optimizing outcome with renal replacement therapy, and rates of hospitalization are reduced when patients ingest at least 1 g/kg/day of protein. Another marker of nutritional status is the serum albumin level, which generally serves as a good predictor of outcomes with renal replacement therapy.

Anemia

Anemia in ESRD is due to the reduced production of erythropoietin by the diseased kidneys, a shortened half-life of red blood cells, and the potential loss of red blood cells in the extracorporeal dialysis circuit and the gastrointestinal tract (related to intermittent anticoagulation for the hemodialysis procedure). Erythropoietic stimulating agents should aim to avoid transfusion[5] by keeping the hemoglobin level generally above 9 g/dL but not higher than 11 g/dL[A7-A9] because higher levels are associated with more cardiovascular complications. Patients who have relative or absolute iron deficiency, as evidenced by a transferrin saturation below 20% or a serum ferritin level below 200, are often relatively resistant to erythropoietic stimulating agents and may benefit from the concurrent administration of a 1-g course (during 8 to 10 dialysis sessions) of intravenous iron (iron sucrose, ferric gluconate, or ferumoxytol).[A10]

Metabolic Bone Disease

Metabolic bone disease and phosphorus balance are common in ESRD. Clinical manifestations of renal osteodystrophy (Chapter 130) can range from adynamic bone disease to osteomalacia (Chapter 244) to secondary hyperparathyroidism (Chapter 245) and osteitis fibrosa cystica. The goals of therapy are to achieve a serum phosphorus level within or close to the normal physiologic range, typically about 2.5 to 5.5 g/dL; a corrected calcium ($0.8 \times [4 -$ the serum albumin level$]$ + the serum calcium level])–phosphorus product less than 55; and an intact parathyroid hormone level within two to nine times the upper limit of normal.[6] Management includes the restriction of dietary phosphate to 750 to 1000 mg/day of elemental phosphorus; the use of phosphate binders (calcium carbonate or acetate, sevelamer carbonate, lanthanum carbonate, or potentially other cationic agents, magnesium or ferric ion) with meals to bind phosphate in the intestines and to reduce its absorption (see Table 119-4); the use of activated forms of vitamin D (e.g., calcitriol [0.25 to 5.0 μg], paricalcitol [1 to 15 μg], or doxercalciferol [1 to 7 μg] intravenously at each hemodialysis session or 50% of that dose orally daily) to stimulate the parathyroid cells to suppress parathyroid hormone secretion; and cinacalcet (30 to 180 mg daily) to significantly reduce secondary hyperparathyroidism by nearly 70%,[A11] even though it does not provide a survival benefit over activated vitamin D therapy alone.[A12]

Cardiovascular Disease

Cardiovascular disease is the leading cause of morbidity and mortality in patients on dialysis. The mainstay of blood pressure control in renal replacement therapy is to achieve the lowest tolerated postdialysis weight to facilitate blood pressure control and to enhance the body's sensitivity to antihypertensive agents. The general approach to antihypertensive medication therapy is similar to the approach for other patients, with the exception that diuretics are not helpful (see Tables 67-7 and 67-11).

Dialysis-dependent chronic kidney disease is an indicator for the same type of aspirin therapy and β-adrenergic blockade used in survivors of a myocardial infarction (Chapters 72 and 73). Statin therapy (Chapter 206) is often recommended, but statins are not of proven benefit for reducing major cardiovascular events or overall mortality in dialysis patients despite clinically relevant reductions in low-density lipoprotein cholesterol levels.[A13] The addition of spironolactone (25 mg daily) can reduce the risk of a cardiovascular or cerebrovascular event by about 50%.[A14] Control of diabetes (Chapter 229) is important, but mortality in hemodialysis patients is not increased until the hemoglobin A_{1c} level is 8.5% or higher.[7]

Amyloidosis

Dialysis-associated amyloidosis (Chapter 188), which is typically seen in patients who have been on dialysis for more than 10 to 12 years, is caused by the deposition of end-products of β_2-microglobulin catabolism as amyloid fibrils. The clinical syndrome includes carpal tunnel syndrome (Chapter 420), arthropathy, and autonomic neuropathy (Chapter 418).

Infection

Infection is the second leading cause of morbidity and mortality in dialysis patients. In hemodialysis, vascular access sites are the primary sources of bacteria and account for about 75% of all cases of bacteremia. In a patient with possible catheter-related bacteremia, blood culture specimens should be obtained both from the catheter and from a peripheral vein. Most vascular access infections are caused by staphylococcal organisms (Chapter 288) and should be treated empirically with 1 g of vancomycin, continued every 3 days for at least 2 weeks while blood levels are monitored, unless another organism is cultured. In patients with systemic sepsis (Chapter 108) with hemodynamic instability, the line should be pulled promptly and be reinserted only after blood cultures are negative for at least 48 hours and the patient has defervesced. Interim dialysis can use an alternative access site, such as a temporary nontunneled catheter. A prolonged course of antibiotic therapy (4 to 8 weeks) is recommended for bacteremia or fungemia that persists after the catheter is removed or in patients with evidence of endocarditis (Chapter 76), septic arthritis (Chapter 272), osteomyelitis (Chapter 272), epidural abscess (Chapter 413), or other metastatic infection.

With peritoneal dialysis, infection is the most frequent reason that the catheter must be removed and therapy must be discontinued. Infection is suspected by erythema, tenderness, induration, or purulent or bloody drainage. Peritonitis must be suspected in patients with abdominal pain and cloudy dialysate; the physical examination usually shows abdominal tenderness, often with rebound. The peritoneal fluid white blood cell count is typically above 100/μL with a predominance of neutrophils, although lymphocytes may predominate with fungal or mycobacterial infections. Polymicrobial infections should raise the possibility of a perforated diverticulum (Chapter

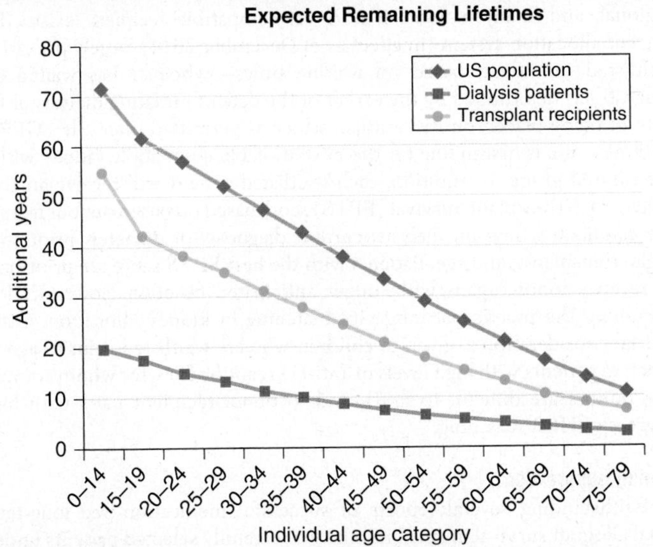

FIGURE 131-1. Life expectancy in end-stage renal disease compared with the general population. (Source: Organ Procurement and Transplantation Network. *Concepts for Kidney Allocation*. http://optn.transplant.hrsa.gov/SharedContentDocuments/KidneyConceptDocument.PDF. Accessed February 2, 2015.)

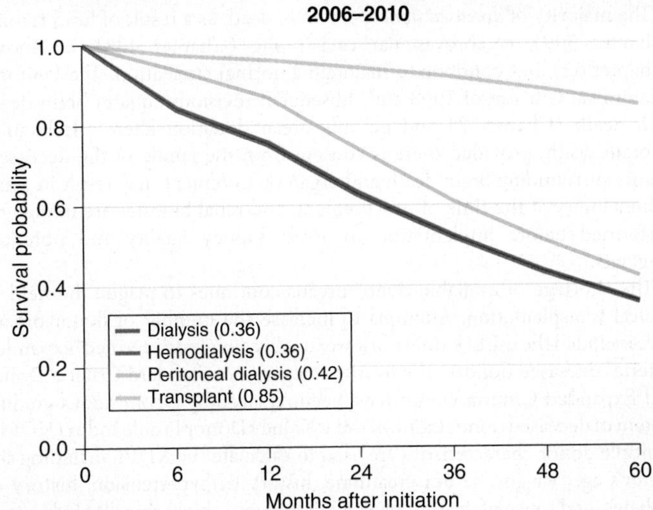

FIGURE 131-2. Adjusted 5-year survival, by modality. (Source: The U.S. Renal Data System. *USRDS 2013 Annual Data Report: Atlas of Chronic Kidney Disease and End-Stage Renal Disease in the United States*. Bethesda, MD: National Institutes of Health, National Institute of Diabetes and Digestive and Kidney Diseases; 2013.)

142), ruptured appendix (Chapter 142), ischemic bowel (Chapter 143), incarcerated hernia (Chapter 142), pancreatitis (Chapter 144), or gynecologic conditions (Chapters 199, 235, and 236) and should prompt an emergent abdominal computed tomography scan. *Staphylococcus epidermidis* (Chapter 288) is the most common cause of peritonitis, but *Pseudomonas* species (Chapter 306) account for 5 to 8% of cases. Recommended initial empirical treatment is intraperitoneal, unless there is evidence of bacteremia or hematogenous spread of the infection. Options include vancomycin (e.g., 1 g every 5 to 7 days, as guided by serum levels, for at least 2 weeks) or a cephalosporin (e.g., cefazolin, 15 mg/kg in one exchange per day) together with intravenous or intraperitoneal administration of a third-generation cephalosporin with antipseudomonal activity (e.g., ceftazidime, 1 to 1.5 g in one exchange per day) or gentamicin (0.6 mg/kg in one exchange per day or 80 mg intravenously) for at least 2 weeks.

Staphylococcus aureus (Chapter 288) is the most common organism for exit site and tunnel infections. Treatment options include empirical oral penicillinase-resistant penicillins (e.g., dicloxacillin, 250 to 500 mg twice daily for 14 days), fluoroquinolones (e.g., ciprofloxacin, 250 to 500 mg twice daily for 14 days), trimethoprim-sulfamethoxazole (e.g., 40/800 mg for 14 days), and cephalosporins (e.g., cephalexin, 500 mg twice daily for 14 days). Vancomycin should be avoided as first-line therapy except for methicillin-resistant *S. aureus*. Mupirocin nasal ointment applied to the exit site twice daily for 5 days every 4 weeks significantly reduces the incidence of *S. aureus* exit site infections.

RENAL TRANSPLANTATION

The success of renal transplantation has increased dramatically during the past several decades owing to improved surgical technique, improved medical care, and more effective and safe immunosuppressive medications. Although transplant recipients do not have a normal life expectancy (Fig. 131-1), current 5-year survival rates are nearly twice as high as for similar patients who remain on dialysis or on the transplant waiting list (Fig. 131-2). Several long-held axioms have been proved false, most notably the need for long-term steroid therapy, the impossibility of transplantation in the face of a positive crossmatch, the inability to transplant ABO-incompatible donor-recipient pairs, and the inability to create long-term tolerance. Despite this remarkable progress, the number of patients on the waiting list far exceeds the number of available kidneys, and the long-term survival rates for kidneys and patients remain disappointing.

EPIDEMIOLOGY AND DEMOGRAPHICS

Between 17,000 and 18,000 total renal transplants, including combined kidney-pancreas, kidney-liver, and kidney-heart, are performed annually in the United States. The most common disease leading to renal transplantation is diabetic nephrosclerosis (Chapter 124), followed by hypertensive nephrosclerosis (Chapter 125) and other forms of glomerulonephritis (Chapter 121). Kidney transplant recipients vary in age from infants to older than 80 years, with the majority being between 35 and 64 years of age. About 65% of the kidneys transplanted in the United States are from deceased donors (E-Fig. 131-1), with the other 35% from living donors, who include both living genetically related family members and genetically unrelated donors, most often spouses or friends. Unfortunately, the number of kidney donors, both living and deceased, has remained relatively constant, whereas the number of patients awaiting transplant continues to increase. The number of patients on the active waitlist is currently three times larger than the supply of kidneys (E-Fig. 131-2), and as a result, the median waiting time for a patient listed for kidney transplantation is currently about 4.3 years. About 10% of newly listed candidates die within 3 years of listing without having received a transplant.[1]

Renal Transplant Success Rates

For deceased donor kidney transplants, the overall 1-year success rate is approximately 91%, and the 10-year success rate is just below 50%. For recipients of live donor kidney transplants, the overall 1-year success rate is more than 96%, and the 10-year success rate is more than 60% (E-Fig. 131-3).

Kidney Donation

Potential *living kidney donors* undergo a thorough evaluation to ensure that age-adjusted renal function is normal, that the surgical risk of donor nephrectomy is acceptably low, and that there are no medical conditions that would increase the risk of future renal disease in the donor. In addition, all donors are screened for transmissible infections or malignant neoplasms. Potential donors must be capable of understanding the risks and benefits of live kidney donation, cannot be coerced into donating, and cannot condition the donation on the receipt of money or other valuable goods. Federal law prohibits the buying and selling of organs. Recent data suggest that live kidney donors have a slightly elevated relative risk[8] for development of ESRD compared with healthy nondonors during the 10 years after donation, but this risk remains less than 1%.

Potential recipients who have a willing and medically and psychosocially suitable live donor but who either have preformed antidonor HLA antibodies or are blood group incompatible with their donor can receive successful transplants by protocols that involve intravenous immune globulin and plasmapheresis to reduce the level of antidonor HLA antibodies or isoagglutinins. Despite remarkable short-term success, the high incidence of antibody-mediated rejection has made long-term success rates somewhat disappointing, at about 60 to 70% at 5 years. An increasingly popular alternative is kidney-paired donation, in which two live donor-recipient pairs are found and each donor is immunologically incompatible with his/her intended recipient but is compatible with and donates to the other recipient. These paired donations now represent nearly 10% of all live donor kidney transplants in the United States. In some situations, even more complicated chains may involve three or more donor-recipient pairs.

The majority of *deceased donors* are brain dead, as a result of head trauma (Chapter 399), cerebrovascular catastrophe (Chapter 408), or anoxia (Chapter 63), but continue to maintain a normal circulation. The Uniform Anatomical Gift Act of 1968 and subsequent revisions equates brain death with death (Chapter 2) and permits organ donation after a declaration of brain death, provided there is consent from the family of the deceased. Events surrounding brain death and organ procurement may result in acute kidney injury at the time of procurement, and renal biopsies are frequently performed before implantation to assess kidney quality and potential longevity.

The shortage of available donor organs continues to plague the field of clinical transplantation. Attempts to increase the number of donor organs have included the use of kidneys of lower quality, previously termed "expanded criteria" deceased donors. The former categories of Standard Criteria Donor and Expanded Criteria Donor have been replaced by a continuous grading system of deceased donor kidneys—the Kidney Donor Profile Index (KDPI). Multiple donor characteristics are used to calculate the KDPI, including the donor's age, weight, serum creatinine, history of hypertension, history of diabetes, and cause of death. Lower KDRI values—higher quality kidneys—are associated with a lower inherent estimated risk of kidney failure (longer anticipated function after transplantation), whereas transplantation of kidneys with higher KDRI values will result in shorter estimated allograft survival times. This prognosis allows for better informed decision-making on the part of both patients and physicians. Developing algorithms to facilitate the optimal use of sub-optimal kidneys—those with higher KDRI—will continue to be a challenge. Protocols have also been developed to allow organ recovery from deceased donors after cessation of cardiac function (Donation after Cardiac Death or DCD donors). These kidneys function as well as those recovered by traditional donation after brain death.

Who Is a Candidate for Renal Transplantation?

All patients with advanced chronic kidney disease must be informed about the option of transplantation. Candidates must undergo a comprehensive medical and psychosocial evaluation to determine their suitability. Because cardiovascular disease is common in ESRD patients, cardiovascular testing is often undertaken in patients older than 50 years and in patients with a history of diabetes (see Table 431-5).[9] Up to 30% of patients never complete their evaluation or are determined not to be suitable candidates for transplantation.

Allocation

The national system for the allocation of deceased donor organs in the U.S. is divided into 58 donor service areas, each with an organ procurement organization responsible for procuring and allocating deceased donor organs. The distribution of these organs is first local (within the donor service area), then regional, and finally national if no local compatible recipient exists. The current allocation system (in effect as of December 2014) largely prioritizes waitlisted candidates based on waiting times—whoever has waited the longest—as determined by the earlier of the date of initiating dialysis or the date of being placed on the waitlist, which is permitted once the eGFR is <20 mL/min, is first in line for the next available compatible kidney within their blood group. In addition, each waitlisted patient will receive an Estimated Post-Transplant Survival (EPTS) score based on based on four factors: the candidate's time on dialysis, current diagnosis of diabetes, prior solid organ transplants, and age. Patients with the best EPTS score are prioritized to receive donor organs with longer anticipated function (lower KDPI), beginning the practice of longevity matching in kidney allocation. Other special consideration is given to children who are waitlisted prior to age 18 years, to patients with high levels of anti-HLA antibodies (for whom compatible donors are difficult to find), and to donor-recipient pairs with high degrees of HLA matching.[10]

Immunosuppression

Notwithstanding several reports of successful medication-free long-term renal allograft survival in small numbers of carefully selected patients undergoing complicated conditioning regimens, long-term immunosuppression continues to remain obligatory in virtually all patients to achieve long-term renal allograft survival. The principal drivers of the immune response to an organ allograft and the principal obstacle to organ acceptance are the HLA antigens (Chapter 49). HLA-identical siblings enjoy the best long-term survival rates, and increasing degrees of HLA antigen *mis*match continue to be associated with inferior long-term outcomes (Chapter 49).

Immunosuppressive treatment can be divided into three phases: induction, maintenance, and antirejection (Table 131-2). Induction immunosuppression consists of antilymphocyte antibodies given within the first week immediately after transplantation. Maintenance immunosuppression refers to those medications given daily as long as the allograft is functioning. Antirejection therapy is given to treat acute rejection episodes when they occur.

For about two thirds of patients, the standard maintenance therapy for the long-term prevention of renal allograft rejection is a three-drug regimen: tacrolimus, mycophenolate, and prednisone. In one third of patients, steroids are withdrawn within the first week after transplantation, but patients are maintained with a dual-therapy regimen of mycophenolate and tacrolimus. Outcomes appear to be similar with either regimen.[A15]

Induction therapy consists of either polyclonal or monoclonal antilymphocyte antibodies administered in the first week after transplantation. Approximately 80% of kidney transplant recipients are in centers that administer induction therapy, the majority with rabbit-derived polyclonal antilymphocyte serum (usually 600 mg/kg total dose) and the others with either basiliximab (20 mg, day 0 and day 4) or alemtuzumab (30-mg single dose).

TABLE 131-2 IMMUNOSUPPRESSIVE MEDICATIONS USED IN RENAL TRANSPLANTATION

CLASS	DRUGS	HOW USED	MECHANISM OF ACTION	MAJOR ADVERSE EFFECTS
Steroids	Prednisone, methylprednisolone	Induction, maintenance, antirejection	Multiple sites, anti-inflammatory; inhibit production of multiple cytokines	Poor wound healing, weight gain, diabetes, acne, hypertension, cushingoid appearance
Calcineurin inhibitors	Tacrolimus and cyclosporine	Maintenance	Inhibit calcineurin, prevent interleukin-2 production	Nephrotoxicity, hypertension, diabetes mellitus
Purine synthesis inhibitors	Azathioprine	Maintenance	Metabolized to 6-mercaptopurine	Anemia, leukopenia, thrombocytopenia
	Mycophenolic acid	Maintenance	Inhibits purine synthesis by the inhibition of inosine monophosphate dehydrogenase, specific for the purine de novo pathway on which lymphocytes depend	Anemia, leukopenia, thrombocytopenia; teratogenic
mTOR inhibitors	Sirolimus, everolimus	Maintenance	Inhibit mTOR (mammalian target of rapamycin), block lymphocyte response to growth factors	Poor wound healing, proteinuria, hyperlipidemia
Costimulation blockade	Belatacept	Maintenance	Human recombinant fusion protein combining the extracellular portion of cytotoxic T lymphocyte–associated antigen-4 (CTLA-4) with the Fc fragment of human IgG; this binds to the CTLA-4 receptor, preventing engagement of CTLA-4 on the T cell, preventing costimulation	Central nervous system post-transplantation lymphoproliferative disease
T cell–depleting antibodies	Thymoglobulin	Induction, antirejection	Rabbit-derived polyclonal antilymphocyte serum (multiple targets)	Infusion reaction, leukopenia, thrombocytopenia
	Alemtuzumab	Induction	Anti-CD52	Infusion reaction, leukopenia, thrombocytopenia
Anti-IL2R monoclonal antibodies	Basiliximab	Induction	Block interleukin-2 receptor	Rare infusion reaction

The goals of induction therapy include a reduction in the number of acute rejection episodes in the first several weeks or months after transplantation, a long-term reduction in the overall number of acute rejection episodes, and a resulting improvement in long-term success rates.

Rejection and Its Treatment

Despite the availability of more effective and safer immunosuppressive medications, rejection remains an ever-present threat, and a significant proportion of allograft failures are ultimately caused by immune-mediated injury. Classically, there are three types of rejection: hyperacute, acute, and chronic.

Hyperacute rejection occurs when a kidney is transplanted into a recipient who is presensitized to the donor, that is, has preformed, circulating antibodies reactive against antigens expressed on the donor kidney. Antidonor antibodies causing hyperacute rejection may target donor HLA antigens, blood group (ABO) antigens, or endothelial cell antigens. The result is immediate endothelial injury and irreversible thrombosis of the transplant. Because of the prescreening of all donor-recipient pairs for the presence of such antidonor antibodies, hyperacute rejection occurs in less than 1% of all renal transplants.

Acute rejection is characterized clinically by an increase in the serum creatinine level during a period of days to weeks, most often in the absence of any symptoms. On pathologic examination, acute rejection is most frequently "cellular" and characterized by T-lymphocyte infiltration of the tubules, of the interstitium, and sometimes into the vascular structures in more severe rejection. Acute rejection now occurs in only 10 to 15% of transplant patients during the first post-transplantation year and in only about another 10% in the second year. The majority of acute rejections occur in the first 3 to 6 months after transplantation and are clinically mild, treatable, and reversible. Other causes of allograft dysfunction (e.g., hemodynamic factors such as hypotension and volume depletion, urinary tract obstruction, drug-induced nephrotoxicity, and BK polyomavirus nephropathy) must be excluded. Percutaneous biopsy of the allograft is required to establish the diagnosis with certainty, to determine the type and severity of the rejection, and thereby to guide therapeutic decisions. Acute cellular rejection should be treated immediately, either with high-dose intravenous corticosteroid therapy for milder forms or with polyclonal antilymphocyte sera for steroid-resistant or more severe acute rejection episodes. Such treatment is usually effective.

About 10 to 20% of patients have acute antibody-mediated rejection injury, usually as evidenced by the deposition of C4d, which is a metabolite of a complement component C4, in the peritubular capillaries, accompanied by inflammatory cells in the peritubular capillaries. This antibody-mediated rejection may occur[11] alone or in combination with cellular rejection. Early antibody-mediated rejection is much more common in patients with a prior history of exposure to alloantigen through transfusion, pregnancy, or prior transplantation. The development of sensitive reagents for detection of circulating antidonor antibodies has greatly facilitated the diagnosis of antibody-mediated rejection. Treatment for antibody-mediated rejection is more problematic and usually involves plasmapheresis to remove antidonor antibodies and the administration of various regimens of intravenous immune globulin. Although this treatment is often effective in reversing acute antibody-mediated rejection, the successful elimination of antidonor antibody and the prevention of alloantibody resynthesis are much more difficult, and chronic antibody-mediated rejection frequently follows an episode of acute antibody-mediated rejection. Anti–B cell and anti–plasma cell drugs have also been tried, but none are currently approved by the Food and Drug Administration for this use. High-dose corticosteroids and polyclonal antilymphocyte serum are often administered as well.

Although *chronic rejection* can occur in the absence of any documented episodes of acute rejection and after many years of stable allograft function, early acute rejection is a major risk factor for later chronic rejection and allograft failure. Chronic rejection is characterized by a slow decline in allograft function, generally during a period of months to years, and frequently accompanied by proteinuria. The development of donor-specific antibodies appears to be a strong risk factor for subsequent allograft failure, and antidonor antibodies are detectable in a high percentage of cases of chronic allograft dysfunction. Biopsy characteristically shows evidence of T cell–induced injury, antibody-induced injury with deposits of C4d, or a combination of the two. In many patients with long-term deterioration of allograft function, however, the only findings are interstitial fibrosis and tubular atrophy without clear-cut evidence as to the cause. Unfortunately, no treatment has been proved to be effective for chronic rejection.

Other Complications of Renal Transplantation

Immunosuppression in renal transplant recipients is associated with a number of adverse effects, the most important of which are infection, malignant neoplasia, and nephrotoxicity.

Infection

Infections occurring in the first few weeks after transplantation are generally nosocomial (Chapter 282), donor derived, present in the recipient at the time of transplantation, or a result of complications of the surgical procedure, such as wound, catheter-associated, or urinary tract infections (Chapter 284) (Fig. 131-3).[12] Next is a period of 5 to 6 months during which opportunistic infection or reactivation of latent infection, such as cytomegalovirus (CMV) infection (Chapter 370) or Epstein-Barr virus (EBV) infection (Chapter 370), is most likely to occur. Later in the course, when the doses of immunosuppressive medication are decreased, community-acquired infections are most common. This timeline is partly a function of infection prophylaxis, which is given to all renal transplant recipients to minimize infectious complications during periods of highest risk, including perioperative antibiotics to prevent wound infection and urinary tract infection (Chapter 284), trimethoprim-sulfamethoxazole to prevent *Pneumocystis jiroveci* pneumonia (Chapter 341), oral nystatin or clotrimazole to prevent oral candidiasis (Chapter 338), and oral valganciclovir (see Table 360-4) to prevent CMV disease (Chapter 376). Urinary tract infections (Chapter 284) are the most frequent bacterial infections that lead to hospitalizations in kidney transplant recipients, and the most common organism is *E. coli*.

Up to 30% of patients develop active infection with the BK polyomavirus,[13] which is tropic for the urinary epithelia. In 5 to 10% of patients, this infection leads to tubulitis and interstitial nephritis, which may result in significant allograft injury. BK polyoma nephritis is often difficult to distinguish from acute rejection without the use of a special SV40 stain that identifies the large T antigen of BK virus. Approximately 80 to 90% of the general population has serologic evidence of exposure to BK polyomavirus, so infection in the renal transplant recipient may be due to reactivation, superinfection, or primary infection. Interestingly, BK nephropathy is very rare in equally immunosuppressed recipients of other transplants. The most important noninvasive indicator of possible BK viral nephropathy is BK viremia, which can be documented in about 10 to 20% of renal transplant recipients. It is presently estimated that 5 to 10% of all renal transplant recipients develop BK virus–induced nephritis and allograft dysfunction, which leads to allograft failure in about half of the patients with nephritis. Monitoring for BK viremia or viruria is strongly recommended. BK viremia and BK viral nephropathy are treated initially with a reduction in immunosuppression, but effective antiviral therapy has yet to be developed.

CMV infection (Chapter 370) continues to be a major cause of morbidity in renal transplant recipients. Like BK polyomavirus, CMV is widely distributed in the general population, with seroprevalence rates ranging from 40 to 90%, depending on the population, so infections may be due to reactivation, superinfection, or primary infection. CMV disease may be limited to fever and malaise, but it frequently causes significant morbidity and even mortality after infecting the gastrointestinal tract, the lungs, or the liver. Most transplant centers use oral valganciclovir (see Table 360-4) for CMV prophylaxis for 7 months or more after transplantation for all patients at risk of CMV disease, especially seronegative recipients who receive transplants from seropositive donors. Another alternative is frequent post-transplantation monitoring, with treatment reserved only for patients who develop viremia. Regardless of the initial strategy, approximately 10% of patients have later viral activation and require additional treatment. Antiviral therapy (Chapters 360 and 370) is usually highly effective.

EBV infection (Chapter 370) also may represent a primary infection, reactivation, or superinfection. EBV may cause a mononucleosis-like syndrome, but the more serious concern in renal transplant patients is a form of lymphoma termed post-transplantation lymphoproliferative disease (Chapters 370 and 185).

Malignant Neoplasia

Renal transplant patients develop some malignant neoplasms at higher rates than in the general population. These include post-transplantation lymphoproliferative disorder related to EBV, Kaposi sarcoma (Chapter 392) caused by human herpesvirus 8 (Chapter 374), and cervical (Chapter 199) and anal (Chapter 145) carcinomas caused by human papillomavirus (Chapter 373). Post-transplantation lymphoproliferative disease most commonly involves

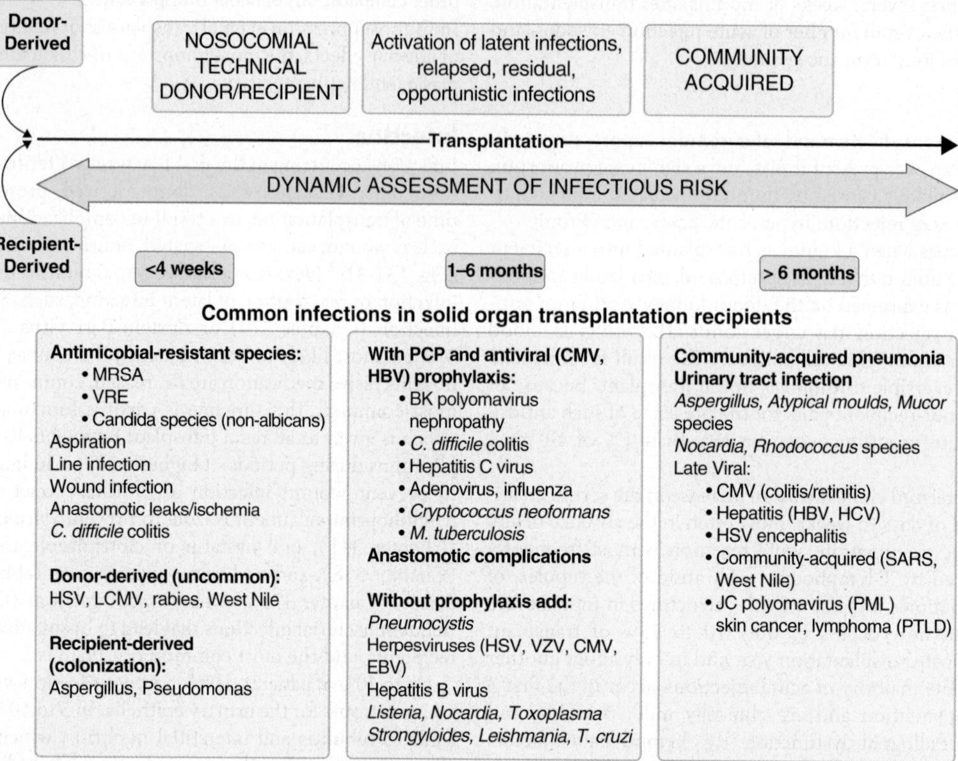

FIGURE 131-3. **Timeline of post-transplantation infections.** CMV = cytomegalovirus; EBV = Epstein-Barr virus; LCMV = lymphocytic choriomeningitis virus; MRSA = methicillin-resistant *Staphylococcus aureus*; PCP = *Pneumocystis* pneumonia; HBV = hepatitis B virus; HCV = hepatitis C virus; HSV = herpes simplex virus; PML = progressive multifocal leukoencephalopathy; PTLD = post-transplantation lymphoproliferative disease; SARS = severe acute respiratory syndrome; VRE = vancomycin-resistant enterococci; VZV = varicella-zoster virus. (From Fishman JA. Introduction: infection in solid organ transplant recipients. *Am J Transplant.* 2009;9(Suppl 4):S3-6.)

the renal allograft, but it may involve any organ, including the gastrointestinal tract, lung, and central nervous system.[14] Treatment usually involves a reduction in immunosuppression along with chemotherapy (Chapter 185). Long-term patient survival rates approach 75%.

The relative risks of many common solid carcinomas are also elevated about 2-fold, but with the exception of nonmelanoma skin cancers, the absolute risks remain low.[15] For nonmelanoma skin cancers (Chapter 203), the lifetime risk may be as high as 70%. Annual skin screening and the attentive use of ultraviolet-blocking skin creams are strongly recommended.[16] Otherwise, transplant recipients should follow the same standard guidelines as the general population for screening for breast (Chapter 198), colon (Chapter 193), prostate (Chapter 201), and lung (Chapter 191) cancer. Whether immunosuppression should be reduced in patients who develop malignant neoplasms other than post-transplantation lymphoproliferative disease is unknown.

Calcineurin Inhibitor–Induced Nephrotoxicity

Calcineurin inhibitors (cyclosporine and tacrolimus)—arguably the most effective antirejection medications used in kidney transplantation—ironically cause a chronic, usually mild and stable, impairment of GFR in virtually all patients who receive them. Superimposed, acute reversible cyclosporine or tacrolimus nephrotoxicity may occur in patients who experience sudden elevations in drug blood levels. These acute episodes usually resolve when the dose of cyclosporine or tacrolimus is reduced. Of greater concern is long-term, irreversible calcineurin inhibitor–induced nephrotoxicity, which can cause allograft failure. This diagnosis is often difficult to make because there are few if any absolutely specific histologic biopsy findings. As a result, careful monitoring of blood calcineurin inhibitor levels is essential to avoid supratherapeutic levels (risking nephrotoxicity and infection) or subtherapeutic levels (risking rejection).

New-Onset Diabetes

By 36 months after transplantation, between 30 and 40% of patients develop glucose intolerance or frank diabetes, which may be caused by corticosteroids, tacrolimus, and, to a lesser extent, cyclosporine. Treatment is as for diabetes in the general population (Chapter 229), with the understanding that doses of insulin and oral agents may need to be adjusted for renal function. Patients who develop diabetes have poorer outcomes, including higher rates of cardiovascular events, graft failure, and death.[17]

Management of the Patient after Renal Transplantation

In the initial few months after transplantation, patients are generally seen weekly. The interval then gradually expands to once monthly for the remainder of the first year and every 2 to 6 months thereafter, depending on the patient. Routine testing includes measurement of blood pressure, renal function, calcineurin inhibitor blood levels, lipid levels, glucose levels, BK polyomavirus assays, and proteinuria. Polymerase chain reaction analysis for CMV or EBV is indicated in selected patients. Monitoring for metabolic bone disease is also recommended, by parathyroid hormone and vitamin D levels as well as by bone densitometry. Influenza and pneumococcal vaccinations are strongly recommended for renal transplant recipients, but live vaccines are contraindicated (Chapter 18).

PROGNOSIS

Approximately 6% of long-term transplants fail each year. Allograft failure with return to dialysis or retransplantation accounts for about 50% of long-term allograft failures. Progressive loss of function in the long-term renal allograft is most commonly the result of chronic rejection but may also be due to nonimmunologic causes, such as calcineurin inhibitor–induced nephrotoxicity, hypertension, diabetes, or recurrent glomerular disease (Table 131-3). A standardized evaluation (Table 131-4) can help establish the cause.

The importance of immunologic (or alloantigen-dependent) factors is illustrated by the fact that living donor transplants between HLA-identical siblings have a 70 to 80% 10-year graft survival, compared with 50 to 60% for parental or other less well matched living donor kidneys and 40 to 50% overall for cadaveric kidney recipients. Deceased donor kidneys with zero and one HLA-A, B, or DR mismatchs have a higher success rate (close to 65% at 10 years) than do deceased donor kidneys with two or more antigen mismatches, which have 15 to 30% lower absolute survival rates.

TABLE 131-3 COMMON CAUSES OF RENAL ALLOGRAFT DYSFUNCTION

Volume depletion: Nausea, vomiting, diarrhea, poor fluid intake, hemorrhage
Medication induced: Diuretics, antihypertensive medications, nonsteroidal anti-inflammatory drugs, calcineurin inhibitors, angiotensin-converting enzyme inhibitors
Urinary tract obstruction: Bladder outlet obstruction, ureteral obstruction
Transplant renal artery stenosis
Infection: Bacteremia, urinary tract infection
Rejection: Cell mediated, antibody mediated

TABLE 131-4 EVALUATION OF RENAL ALLOGRAFT DYSFUNCTION

History: Fluid intake and loss, medication changes, fever
Physical examination: Blood pressure, pulse rate, temperature, weight, edema, allograft tenderness or swelling
Laboratory tests: Serum creatinine level, BK virus detection by polymerase chain reaction analysis of urine or blood, calcineurin inhibitor levels, antidonor antibody testing, urine protein analysis, urine and blood cultures
Doppler ultrasound to assess for possible urinary tract obstruction or transplant renal artery stenosis
Renal biopsy

Factors unrelated to antiallograft immunity are also associated with reduced long-term success rates. These characteristics include hypertension, a kidney from an older (>50 years) donor, hyperlipidemia, diabetes mellitus, calcineurin inhibitor nephrotoxicity, recurrent glomerular disease, and a maladaptive response to hemodynamic injury, which is caused by elevated glomerular flow and pressure. Chronic calcineurin inhibitor toxicity leads to ESRD in at least 5 to 10% of recipients of nonrenal transplants and is likely to have at least a comparable long-term impact in renal transplant patients. Virtually all primary glomerular diseases (Chapter 121), including focal segmental glomerulosclerosis, membranous nephropathy, membranoproliferative glomerulonephritis, and immunoglobulin A nephropathy, can recur after transplantation. Recurrent glomerulonephritis is a common cause of proteinuria and nephrotic syndrome after transplantation, and recurrent glomerulonephritis may be responsible for up to 10% of all graft failures.[18] Renal biopsy is required to establish the diagnosis in a long-term renal allograft with deteriorating function or proteinuria and to distinguish immune-related from non–immune-related causes. For long-term allograft survival rates to improve significantly, the discovery of biomarkers of actual or impending allograft injury is essential.[19]

In the other 50% of failures, a patient dies with a functioning allograft. The most common cause of death in these patients is cardiovascular, due to the high prevalence of diabetes, hypertension, and hyperlipidemia as well as the high burden of preexisting cardiovascular disease in transplant candidates. Although there are no specific guidelines for the prevention, monitoring, or management of cardiovascular disease after renal transplantation, standard risk factor reduction guidelines are generally considered applicable, including the use of statins (Chapter 206)[20] 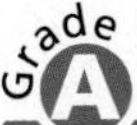 and the use of antihypertensive medications to meet blood pressure targets (Chapter 67).[21] The other leading causes of long-term death in renal transplant recipients are infection, sepsis, and malignant disease.

Grade A References

A1. Cooper BA, Branley P, Bulfone L, et al. A randomized, controlled trial of early versus late initiation of dialysis. *N Engl J Med.* 2010;363:609-619.
A2. Eknoyan G, Beck GJ, Cheung AK, et al. Effect of dialysis dose and membrane flux in maintenance hemodialysis. *N Engl J Med.* 2002;347:2010-2019.
A3. Chertow GM, Levin NW, Beck GJ, et al. In-center hemodialysis six times per week versus three times per week. *N Engl J Med.* 2010;363:2287-2300.
A4. Rocco MV, Lockridge RS Jr, Beck GJ, et al. The effects of frequent nocturnal home hemodialysis: the Frequent Hemodialysis Network Nocturnal Trial. *Kidney Int.* 2011;80:1080-1091.
A5. Maduell F, Moreso F, Pons M, et al. High-efficiency postdilution online hemodiafiltration reduces all-cause mortality in hemodialysis patients. *J Am Soc Nephrol.* 2013;24:487-497.
A6. Paniagua R, Amato D, Vonesh E, et al. Effects of increased peritoneal clearances on mortality rates in peritoneal dialysis: ADEMEX, a prospective, randomized, controlled trial. *J Am Soc Nephrol.* 2002;13:1307-1320.
A7. Drueke TB, Locatelli F, Clyne N, et al. Normalization of hemoglobin level in patients with chronic kidney disease and anemia. *N Engl J Med.* 2006;355:2071-2084.
A8. Singh AK, Szczech L, Tang KL, et al. Correction of anemia with epoetin alfa in chronic kidney disease. *N Engl J Med.* 2006;355:2085-2098.
A9. Pfeffer MA, Burdmann EA, Chen CY, et al. A trial of darbepoetin alfa in type 2 diabetes and chronic kidney disease. *N Engl J Med.* 2009;361:2019-2032.
A10. Coyne DW, Kapoian T, Suki W, et al. Ferric gluconate is highly efficacious in anemic hemodialysis patients with high serum ferritin and low transferrin saturation: results of the Dialysis Patients' Response to IV Iron with Elevated Ferritin (DRIVE) Study. *J Am Soc Nephrol.* 2007;18:975-984.
A11. Parfrey PS, Chertow GM, Block GA, et al. The clinical course of treated hyperparathyroidism among patients receiving hemodialysis and the effect of cinacalcet: the EVOLVE trial. *J Clin Endocrinol Metab.* 2013;98:4834-4844.
A12. Chertow GM, Block GA, Correa-Rotter R, et al. Effect of cinacalcet on cardiovascular disease in patients undergoing dialysis. *N Engl J Med.* 2012;367:2482-2494.
A13. Palmer SC, Navaneethan SD, Craig JC, et al. HMG CoA reductase inhibitors (statins) for dialysis patients. *Cochrane Database Syst Rev.* 2013;9:CD004289.
A14. Matsumoto Y, Mori Y, Kageyama S, et al. Spironolactone reduces cardiovascular and cerebrovascular morbidity and mortality in hemodialysis patients. *J Am Coll Cardiol.* 2014;63:528-536.
A15. Woodle ES, First MR, Pirsch J, et al. A prospective, randomized, double-blind, placebo-controlled multicenter trial comparing early (7 day) corticosteroid cessation versus long-term, low-dose corticosteroid therapy. *Ann Surg.* 2008;248:564-577.
A16. Palmer SC, Navaneethan SD, Craig JC, et al. HMG CoA reductase inhibitors (statins) for kidney transplant recipients. *Cochrane Database Syst Rev.* 2014;1:CD005019.

GENERAL REFERENCES

For the General References and other additional features, please visit Expert Consult at https://expertconsult.inkling.com.

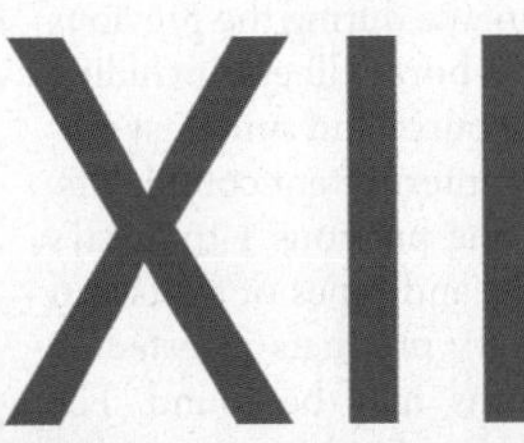

XII GASTROINTESTINAL DISEASES

132

APPROACH TO THE PATIENT WITH GASTROINTESTINAL DISEASE

KENNETH R. MCQUAID

The luminal gastrointestinal (GI) tract (esophagus, stomach, duodenum, small and large intestine, and anus) and pancreas are responsible for digestion, for the absorption of nutrients and fluids, and for the temporary storage and excretion of undigested waste. The GI tract has an epithelial lining with an enormous surface area that provides nutrient absorption and serves as a barrier to microorganisms. In addition, the GI tract has a large innate and adaptive immune system that interfaces with luminal food antigens, host proteins, commensal and pathogenic bacteria, and parasites and must decide which antigens to tolerate and which require immune activation.[1] The GI tract also contains an extensive enteric endocrine system that regulates food intake, weight control, and glucose homeostasis as well as secretions from the stomach, intestine, and pancreas. Finally, it has an enteric nervous system that is integrated with the autonomic and central nervous systems to control gastric emptying, intestinal motility, and defecation.[2]

Numerous diseases within and outside the GI tract may alter normal function by causing structural damage (erosion, ulceration, perforation, stenosis, or obstruction), bleeding, inflammation, abnormal absorption or secretion of nutrients and electrolytes, or abnormal motility. Despite its anatomic and physiologic complexity, the GI system has only a limited repertoire of symptoms and signs to express conditions that may be either serious or clinically insignificant: abdominal pain, heartburn, regurgitation, dysphagia, odynophagia, dyspepsia, nausea and vomiting, gas and bloating, weight loss, diarrhea, constipation, overt or occult GI tract bleeding, and incontinence.

GENERAL APPROACH TO PATIENTS WITH GASTROINTESTINAL SIGNS AND SYMPTOMS

An appropriate history and physical evaluation usually can narrow the differential diagnosis of GI complaints. A specific diagnosis can almost always be established thereafter by the judicious use of laboratory, endoscopic, or imaging studies (Table 132-1).

Clinical History

The clinician should elicit the nature of the complaint, including its acuity, severity, location, radiation, duration, pattern (steady vs. colicky; abrupt vs. gradual onset), and relationship to food, meals, and bowel movements. Symptoms that arise from the GI tract are almost always improved or worsened by eating or by bowel movements. For symptoms of recent onset, it is important to elicit recent dietary intake, a medication history, potential exposure to enteric infections or sexually transmitted diseases (Chapter 285), and recent travel. It is also useful to establish whether there are signs or symptoms that suggest a systemic illness, including fever, weight loss, arthralgias, fatigue, weakness, and rash.

Most nonsurgical GI diseases are manifested with mild to moderate symptoms that develop gradually and do not require immediate attention. Acute symptoms that require urgent assessment are severe abdominal pain and overt GI bleeding (Chapter 135) that is manifested by hematemesis, melena, or large-volume hematochezia. Severe or dramatic abdominal pain that develops acutely during minutes to hours requires urgent evaluation to determine whether surgical intervention is required. Severe vomiting or diarrhea with signs of dehydration also warrants urgent attention.

Mild to moderate chronic or intermittent symptoms that have been present for a long period can be evaluated in a deliberate fashion. A substantial proportion of chronic GI complaints has no obvious organic or biochemical basis and ultimately is classified as *functional* GI disorders (Chapter 137). Complaints that have been ongoing for years rarely are attributable to readily remedied structural disorders. In patients with chronic GI symptoms, it is important to elicit and to address the current reason for seeking evaluation, which may include concern for underlying serious illness (especially cancer), a change in the character or severity of symptoms, life stressors, and depression. Asking the patient what he or she thinks or fears may provide insights into the proportion of the complaint attributable to these amplifying issues, regardless of whether the problem is functional or structural in origin.

A dietary history (Chapter 214) should be obtained. For acute symptoms of nausea, vomiting, diarrhea, or abdominal pain, intake during the previous 24 to 48 hours should be reviewed for clues to a food-borne illness, including possible exposure to a contaminated food or water source and similar symptoms in other people (Chapter 283). For chronic or intermittent complaints, a recall of meals and types of foods eaten during the previous 1 to 2 days provides insight into eating habits and the amounts and types of fruits and vegetables, whole grains, fiber, protein, fat, and dairy products ingested. A relationship between specific foods and symptoms may be found. For example, dairy products (lactose intolerance), whole grains, legumes or cruciferous vegetables, or fatty meals (malabsorption) may cause pain, flatulence, or diarrhea, and a low-fiber diet may cause chronic constipation. Recent and long-term changes in body weight should be elicited. Involuntary loss of more than 5% of body weight during the prior 12 months is worrisome for serious disease and significant malnutrition (Chapter 215).

The number and consistency of bowel movements should be elicited, and any change in bowel habits must be explored. Signs of acute GI bleeding (melena or hematochezia) or inflammatory colitis (blood, mucus, or pus) should be elicited. Improvement in symptoms after passage of flatus or a bowel movement suggests a disorder of the colon or anorectum.

Past Medical History

The past medical history should be reviewed for conditions that may cause acute or chronic GI symptoms, including endocrine disorders such as diabetes (Chapter 229) and thyroid dysfunction (Chapter 226), cardiovascular diseases such as heart failure (Chapter 58) and peripheral vascular disease (Chapter 79), chronic liver disease and portal hypertension (Chapter 153), neurologic conditions such as Parkinson disease (Chapter 409) and neuromuscular disorders (Chapter 396), and rheumatologic and collagen vascular disorders (Chapter 256). In addition to their impact on GI tract function, the severity of these conditions must be considered in weighing the risks of diagnostic studies, especially endoscopy. Patients with symptomatic or advanced respiratory insufficiency (Chapter 104), sleep apnea (Chapter 100), valvular heart disease (Chapter 75), coronary artery disease (Chapter 51), heart failure (Chapter 58), cirrhosis (Chapter 153), cerebrovascular disease (Chapter 406), neuromuscular disease (Chapter 422), or dementia (Chapter 402) have an increased risk of sedation-related complications during endoscopy.

A list of prescription and nonprescription medications, vitamins, minerals, and other nutritional supplements should be obtained, paying particular attention to any that were recently initiated or changed. Herbal supplements (Chapter 39) are commonly used but are seldom reported without direct questioning. Medications are potential causes of odynophagia, dyspepsia, nausea or vomiting, abdominal pain, diarrhea, and constipation. The use of antiplatelet agents, including aspirin and anticoagulants, should be determined. The risks of stopping versus continuing these medications must be weighed in patients who have acute or chronic GI bleeding or in whom a therapeutic procedure is to be performed.[3]

Social History

The patient's personal relationships, employment history, quality of life, alcohol intake (Chapter 33), and smoking (Chapter 32) history should be determined. It can be very informative to observe both verbal and nonverbal interactions between the patient and a partner or caregiver during an interview. Alcohol may cause heartburn, dyspepsia, nausea, diarrhea, or chronic liver disease. Many patients are reluctant to disclose the full extent of their alcohol intake on direct questioning; therefore, in addition to asking how often they imbibe (days/week and drinks/day), it may be revealing to inquire about their preferred beverage and how it is purchased (location, volume, and frequency). Cigarette smoking is associated with an increased risk of heartburn, peptic ulcer disease, Crohn disease, and GI malignant neoplasms.

Clinicians should inquire about the degree to which GI symptoms are disrupting a patient's life. GI illness may affect dietary and bowel habits, sleep, and sense of vitality. Concerns about dietary intolerances, inability to eat, inability to have comfortable bowel movements, uncontrolled diarrhea or gas, fecal urgency, or fecal incontinence may affect a patient's social life, personal and sexual relationships, employment, and sense of optimism.

The social history should also be reviewed for recent stressors that may precipitate or exacerbate GI symptoms, including marital or interpersonal discord, personal or family illness, bereavement, financial pressures, job loss, and change in employment. To elicit such information, it may be helpful to tell patients that stress worsens many conditions and to inquire whether they believe stress may be contributing to their problem.

For elderly, disabled, or marginally housed patients, it is important to elicit how they obtain and prepare their meals and how they access toilet facilities. For patients undergoing GI procedures, it is important to determine whether they have mental, physical, or social barriers that would make it difficult to comply with preprocedure instructions (including bowel preparation) and whether they have an able-bodied adult who can accompany them to the procedure and observe them at home, if necessary, afterward.

Family History

The family history should be reviewed for GI disorders with a heritable component, especially celiac disease (Chapter 140), inflammatory bowel diseases (Chapter 141), and neoplasms of the GI, gynecologic, and genitourinary tracts.

Physical Examination

Nonabdominal Examination

The nonabdominal examination should assess nutritional status (Chapter 214) and any signs of systemic conditions that may cause GI symptoms or that must be considered in weighing the risks and benefits of further testing, especially endoscopy. Vital signs should be obtained in all patients. Low-grade fever (<100.5° F) is common in inflammatory conditions, including gastroenteritis, inflammatory bowel disease, appendicitis, cholecystitis, and diverticulitis. High fever (>102° F) suggests sepsis, pelvic or intra-abdominal infections (e.g., cholangitis, pelvic inflammatory disease, pyelonephritis), or peritonitis. Hemodynamic instability (hypotension or tachycardia) suggests intravascular depletion due to poor oral intake, acute GI or intra-abdominal bleeding, severe diarrhea, or peritonitis. A body mass index of less than 18 suggests malnourishment.

A general survey should be performed to assess for signs of weight loss (fat and muscle wasting), malnutrition (dry or thin skin, hair loss, edema, anasarca), and vitamin deficiencies (pellagra, scurvy). Skin lesions may provide clues to systemic conditions such as liver disease (jaundice, spider telangiectasias, palmar erythema), inflammatory bowel disease (erythema nodosum, pyoderma gangrenosum), celiac disease (dermatitis herpetiformis), vasculitis, and rare GI malignant neoplasms, polyposis syndromes, and pancreatic endocrine tumors (Chapters 192, 193, and 195). An oral examination looks for mucocutaneous candidiasis (which may reflect immunosuppression), ulcerations (which may reflect inflammatory bowel disease, vasculitis, viral infection, or vitamin deficiencies), and glossitis or angular cheilitis (which may reflect vitamin deficiencies). With the exception of supraclavicular lymph nodes, peripheral lymph nodes are uninvolved with GI diseases but should be examined when systemic infection or advanced malignant disease is suspected (Chapter 168). Examination of the lungs and cardiovascular system should focus on evidence of conditions that might increase the risk of moderate sedation in the event that endoscopy is required (respiratory insufficiency, heart failure) and of conditions that increase the risk of intestinal ischemia (atrial fibrillation, valvular heart disease, peripheral vascular disease) (Chapter 143). The extremities should be evaluated for edema and peripheral pulses. Finally, a brief neurologic assessment should be performed to screen for intracranial mass lesions or other neurologic disorders that may be manifested with GI symptoms.

Abdominal Examination

The abdominal examination begins with a visual inspection of the abdomen and inguinal region for scars (due to prior surgeries or trauma), asymmetry (suggesting a mass or organomegaly), distention (due to obesity, ascites, or intestinal ileus or obstruction), prominent periumbilical veins (suggesting portal hypertension), or hernias (umbilical, ventral, inguinal). The examination proceeds with auscultation followed by percussion, and it ends with light and deep palpation.

In patients *without* abdominal pain, auscultation of bowel sounds to assess intestinal motility has limited usefulness and may be omitted. Percussion may be performed before or in conjunction with light and deep palpation. Initial cursory light percussion across the upper, mid, and lower abdomen is useful to denote areas of dullness and tympany as well as to elicit unanticipated areas of pain or tenderness before palpation. More extensive percussion provides limited but useful information about the size of the liver and spleen, gastric or intestinal distention, bladder distention, and ascites (Chapters 146 and 153). Gentle, light palpation promotes abdominal relaxation and allows the detection of muscle resistance (guarding), abdominal tenderness, and superficial masses of the abdominal wall or abdomen. Deeper palpation of the abdominal organs (liver, spleen, kidneys, aorta) and abdominal cavity may detect enlargement or abnormal masses. Superficial or deep masses should be assessed for size, location, mobility, content (solid, liquid, or air), and the presence or absence of tenderness. The consistency of a patient's response to palpation with and without distraction is particularly useful in those with suspected chronic functional abdominal discomfort. Superficial masses include hernias, lymph nodes, subcutaneous abscesses, lipomas, and hematomas. Neoplasms (liver, gallbladder, pancreas, stomach, intestine, kidney), abscesses (appendicitis, diverticulitis, Crohn disease), or aortic aneurysms may represent deep abdominal masses.

Examination of the right upper quadrant should assess the liver size, contour, texture, and tenderness. Liver size is crudely estimated by percussion of the upper and lower borders of liver dullness in the midclavicular line. Liver contour and tenderness are best assessed during held inspiration by deep palpation along the costal margin. Examination of the left upper quadrant is useful to detect splenomegaly (Chapter 168), although a normal-sized or even an enlarged spleen often cannot be detected. Percussion in the left upper quadrant near the tenth rib (posterior to the midaxillary line) may detect splenic dullness that is distinct from gastric or colonic tympany. The tip of an enlarged spleen may be palpated during inspiration if the examiner supports the left costal margin with the left hand while palpating below the costal margin with the right hand. Ascites should be suspected in a patient with a protuberant abdomen and bulging flanks. To screen for ascites, percussion of the flanks should be performed to assess the level of dullness. If the level of flank dullness appears to be increased, the most sensitive test for ascites is to check for "shifting" dullness when the patient rolls from the supine to the lateral position.

Digital Rectal and Pelvic Examinations

The digital rectal examination is intrusive and uncomfortable and should be performed only when necessary, such as in patients with perianal or rectal symptoms, incontinence, difficult defecation, suspected inflammatory bowel disease, and acute abdominal pain. The digital examination, with or without fecal occult blood testing, is not a useful screening test for colorectal cancer (Chapter 193). However, in patients with acute or chronic GI bleeding (Chapter 135), it is a rapid means of assessing the stool for color and occult blood. The perianal area should be visually inspected for rashes, soilage (suggesting incontinence or fistula), fistulas, fissures, skin tags, external hemorrhoids, and prolapsed internal hemorrhoids (Chapter 145). After gentle digital insertion, the anal canal should be assessed for resting tone and voluntary squeeze. The distal rectal vault should be swept circumferentially to palpate for mass lesions, tenderness, or fluctuance.

Laboratory Studies

Blood Tests

Blood tests routinely obtained in the evaluation of patients with GI symptoms include a complete blood count, liver tests (Chapter 147), serum chemistries, and, in selected cases, pancreatic enzymes and markers of inflammation. GI causes of anemia include acute or chronic GI blood loss, inflammatory bowel disease, nutrient malabsorption (folate, iron, or vitamin B_{12}), and chronic liver disease. Microcytosis suggests iron deficiency due to chronic GI blood loss or malabsorption. Macrocytosis may be attributable to folate or B_{12} malabsorption, medications (e.g., immunomodulators used for inflammatory bowel disease), or chronic liver disease. An elevated platelet count suggests chronic inflammation (e.g., inflammatory bowel disease) or GI blood loss with compensatory marrow production. A low platelet count may be attributable to portal hypertension with splenic sequestration. Low serum albumin may be caused by chronic GI disorders that result in weight loss, nutrient malabsorption, chronic inflammation, loss of protein across abnormal GI mucosa (i.e., protein-losing enteropathy), or decreased hepatic synthesis (e.g., chronic liver disease). Abnormal liver test results may be due to acute or chronic liver diseases, disorders of the pancreas or biliary tract, and medications (Chapter 147). Serum amylase and lipase are obtained to screen for pancreatitis (Chapter 144) in patients with acute abdominal pain. Increased levels of inflammatory markers, such as an elevated erythrocyte sedimentation rate and C-reactive protein, are nonspecific but useful in the management of patients with inflammatory bowel disease (Chapter 141).

Serum ferritin reflects total body iron and may be decreased in patients with chronic GI blood loss or intestinal malabsorption (e.g., celiac disease). Deficiencies in the fat-soluble vitamins (A, D, E, K) (Chapter 140) may reflect disorders of malabsorption that result in steatorrhea. The serum

TABLE 132-1 APPROACH TO COMMON GASTROINTESTINAL SYMPTOMS AND SIGNS

	ABDOMINAL PAIN	GI BLEEDING	DIARRHEA	STEATORRHEA	CONSTIPATION
History (ascertain the following)	Duration: acute vs. chronic Onset: sudden vs. 1-2 hr vs. gradual Character: visceral (vague or dull, steady or cramping, diffuse) or parietal (severe, well localized, worse with movement) Location: upper, middle, or lower; radiation Associated symptoms: vomiting, hematemesis, diarrhea, hematochezia, melena, constipation, obstipation, jaundice Previous episodes Other diseases	Acute vs. chronic (duration); intermittent vs. continuous; quantity; hematemesis, melena, or hematochezia; associated pain and location; symptoms of anemia (e.g., dyspnea, chest pain, lightheadedness); medication use (especially aspirin, NSAIDs, anticoagulants); previous episodes; risk factors for chronic liver disease (alcohol, hepatitis)	Acute (<2 wk) vs. chronic (duration); fever, weight loss, or abdominal pain; stool character: number per 24 hr, watery or bloody, large vs. small volume, change in volume with eating, greasy; dietary history (especially lactose); history of IBD, pancreatic disease, intestinal surgery, DM; recent change in medications or antibiotic use; community outbreak or similar symptoms in family members; potential exposure to contaminated food; elderly immunosuppressed host; risk of HIV or sexually transmitted disease	Duration; weight loss; stool number, consistency (greasy), presence of blood; abdominal pain; flatulence; history of excessive alcohol, chronic liver disease, pancreatitis, intestinal dysmotility, surgery, DM; history of easy bruising, night blindness, bone pain, osteoporosis, dermatitis herpetiformis	Acute vs. chronic (duration); age; number of stools per week; difficulty with defecation (straining, incomplete evacuation, digital manipulation); bloating or discomfort; blood on stools, weight loss; dietary fiber and fluid intake; chronic illness (DM, neuromuscular, endocrine); abdominal surgeries; medications, impaired mobility
Physical findings (evaluate for the following)	Fever, HR, BP Appearance: calm, restless, motionless Inspect: skin, distention, hernias Bowel sounds: present, absent, roaring Percussion and palpation: organomegaly, mass (abscess), focal tenderness, guarding Peritoneal signs: sharp pain with cough, shaking, percussion, light palpation	HR, BP, orthostatic findings; abdominal pain present or absent; signs of chronic liver disease and portal hypertension (which may indicate varices); jaundice, spider angiomas, hepatosplenomegaly; ascites; examine nasogastric aspirate for blood ("coffee grounds" vs. bright red); examine stool for blood (Hemoccult) and color (melena, maroon, or bright red)	HR, BP, orthostatic findings; fever; wasting; presence of abdominal tenderness or mass; perianal disease; extraintestinal symptoms of IBD (e.g., oral ulcers, arthritis, erythema nodosum)	Wasting, presence or absence of abdominal mass or tenderness; rash (vitamin deficiencies) or excessive bruising (vitamin K deficiency); jaundice or signs of chronic liver disease	Assess mobility and chronic medical conditions; abdominal distention; palpable stool within bowel in left lower quadrant; rectal examination—impacted stool, anal fissure, rectal prolapse, pelvic floor descent with straining, rectocele
Laboratory tests	CBC, BUN, Cr, glucose, amylase, lipase, liver tests (ALT, AST, bilirubin, alkaline phosphatase), albumin, INR, U/A, urine β-HCG	CBC, BUN, Cr, liver tests, INR, type and cross	CBC, BUN, Cr, glucose, electrolytes, liver tests, albumin, C-reactive protein Selected cases: consider serum chromogranin A, VIP, calcitonin, gastrin, glucagon, urinary 5-HIAA; stool for culture, ova, parasites; consider fecal weight, fat, electrolytes, laxative screen	CBC, glucose, liver tests, albumin, electrolytes, celiac disease antibodies (anti-tTG or antiendomysial); assessment of vitamin and mineral absorption (A, D) and INR (K is fat soluble), folate, iron, calcium, phosphate, B_{12}; stool for fecal elastase and qualitative fat; stool for quantitative fecal fat; hydrogen breath test for bacterial overgrowth	CBC, Chem-7, calcium, magnesium, phosphate, TFTs; selected patients with severe constipation may undergo colonic transit studies or anal manometry with balloon expulsion
Endoscopy	EGD, colonoscopy	EGD, colonoscopy, enteroscopy, wireless capsule study	Colonoscopy (including ileal inspection) with biopsies; EGD with duodenal biopsies; wireless capsule study	EGD with duodenal biopsies	Colonoscopy if recent change in bowel habits
Imaging	CT scan or ultrasound; angiography; small bowel enterography	Tagged RBC scan, angiography	Small bowel enterography: CT, MRI, or barium (Crohn disease); somatostatin scintigraphy	CT of the abdomen (pancreatic calcifications; biliary dilation)	Usually not necessary; MRI or defecography

ALT = alanine transaminase; AST = aspartate transaminase; BP = blood pressure; BUN = blood urea nitrogen; CBC = complete blood count; CNS = central nervous system; COPD = chronic obstructive pulmonary disease; Cr = creatinine; CT = computed tomography; DM = diabetes mellitus; EGD = esophagogastroduodenoscopy; ESR = erythrocyte sedimentation rate; GERD = gastroesophageal reflux disease; GI = gastrointestinal; HbA_{1C} = hemoglobin A_{1C}; HCG = human chorionic gonadotropin; 5-HIAA = 5-hydroxyindoleacetic acid; HIV = human immunodeficiency virus; HR = heart rate; IBD = inflammatory bowel disease; INR = international normalized ratio; MRI = magnetic resonance imaging; NSAIDs = nonsteroidal anti-inflammatory drugs; RBC = red blood cell; TFTs = thyroid function tests; tTG = tissue transglutaminase; U/A = urinalysis; VIP = vasoactive intestinal polypeptide.

Modified from Proctor DD. Approach to the patient with gastrointestinal disease. In: Goldman L, Ausiello D, eds. *Cecil Textbook of Medicine.* 23rd ed. Philadelphia: Saunders-Elsevier; 2008.

NAUSEA AND VOMITING	DYSPHAGIA	ODYNOPHAGIA	HEARTBURN AND REGURGITATION	ANOREXIA	WEIGHT LOSS
Nausea with or without emesis; acute vs. chronic (duration); intermittent vs. constant; presence or absence of severe abdominal pain, comorbid illnesses, especially peptic ulcer, endocrine (DM), cardiac, psychiatric; medications; history of excessive alcohol	Oropharyngeal vs. esophageal dysphagia; solids vs. liquids; acute vs. chronic (duration); intermittent vs. progressive; GERD symptoms present or absent; weight loss; history of food impactions, allergies, atopic conditions, skin changes, cold hands (Raynaud phenomenon)	Duration of pain with swallowing; underlying immunosuppression (e.g., HIV infection, DM); caustic ingestion; use of medications that cause topical injury (especially NSAIDs, KCl, bisphosphonates, iron, antibiotics, zidovudine)	Duration of symptoms; location; relation to meals or specific foods; nocturnal symptoms; dysphagia or chest pain; extraesophageal manifestations: cough, hoarseness, asthma	Acute vs. chronic (duration); association with different foods; psychiatric disease (e.g., depression, dementia); chronic or undiagnosed medical conditions (e.g., DM, thyroid or adrenal disease, COPD, advanced heart failure, renal insufficiency, malignant disease, HIV infection); medication use	Acute vs. chronic (duration); age; total amount (>5% is significant); intentional vs. unintentional; appetite increased or decreased; rapid vs. gradual; change in physical activity; documented vs. undocumented; fever or sweats; anorexia, nausea, vomiting; diarrhea, steatorrhea, blood in stool; abdominal pain; history or symptoms of chronic medical, neurologic, or psychiatric illness; medications; alcohol and substance abuse
Acute with severe abdominal pain: evaluate for GI obstruction, pancreatitis, mesenteric ischemia, biliary colic, appendicitis, or other conditions causing peritonitis Acute without abdominal pain: evaluate for pregnancy, medications, food poisoning, infectious gastroenteritis, hepatitis, CNS disease, postoperative ileus Chronic: evaluate for medications, chronic gastric outlet obstruction (due to ulcer disease or malignant disease), impaired GI motility (gastroparesis), other chronic medical conditions, intracranial disorders, psychiatric disease (bulimia)	Usually normal; examine oropharynx and neck for lymphadenopathy and masses; evaluate the skin for sclerodermatous changes	Usually normal; evaluate oropharynx for thrush, herpetic lesions, caustic injury; general examination for signs of underlying immunosuppression	Usually normal, unless extraesophageal manifestations are present	Wasting; fever; signs of bulimia (e.g., loss of tooth enamel, knuckle ulcerations and calluses); abdominal masses; enlarged lymph nodes	Wasting; malnutrition; poor dentition or poorly fitting dentures; thyromegaly; COPD or heart failure; abdominal masses; enlarged lymph nodes; pelvic masses in women; diabetic neuropathy; signs of depression, dementia, or bulimia
β-HCG, CBC, serum electrolytes, BUN, Cr, glucose, HbA_{1c}, liver tests, albumin, TFTs, cortisol	CBC; eosinophilia or elevated IgE in some patients with eosinophilic esophagitis	CBC, HIV test, fasting glucose	Usually normal	CBC, Chem-7, liver tests, albumin, HIV test, TFTs	CBC, Chem-7, HbA_{1c}, TFTs, liver tests, C-reactive protein or ESR, calcium, phosphate, albumin, HIV test, morning cortisol
EGD to exclude gastric outlet obstruction	EGD with biopsies or dilation, esophageal motility study	EGD with biopsies	EGD (to detect erosive esophagitis or Barrett esophagus); ambulatory pH/impedance probe	Directed at detecting underlying disease, e.g., if a GI cause is suspected, EGD or colonoscopy with biopsies may be helpful	Directed at detecting underlying disease, e.g., if a GI cause is suspected, EGD or colonoscopy with biopsies may be helpful
CT of the abdomen; if chronic, also consider head CT, gastric emptying study, small bowel enterography	Esophagogram (barium swallow) will show stricture, Schatzki ring, mass	Usually not necessary	Usually not necessary	Directed at detecting underlying disease, e.g., if a GI cause is suspected, abdominal CT may be helpful	Directed at detecting underlying disease, e.g., chest or abdominal CT may be helpful

international normalized ratio may be elevated in patients with cholestasis because of malabsorption of vitamin K or in patients with chronic liver disease because of decreased hepatic synthetic function. Serum B_{12} may be decreased in patients with autoimmune gastritis (pernicious anemia), gastric bypass surgery, or malabsorption because of small bowel bacterial overgrowth or disease of the terminal ileum (e.g., Crohn disease).

Specialized laboratory tests that may be useful for the diagnosis of specific diseases include stool *Helicobacter pylori* antigen in patients with duodenal ulcer disease or dyspepsia, antibodies to tissue transglutaminase IgA in celiac disease, antibodies to microbial antigens or autoimmune markers in inflammatory bowel disease (anti–*Saccharomyces cerevisiae*, perinuclear antineutrophil cytoplasmic antibody), and CA19-9 in pancreaticobiliary malignant disease. Because of their limited sensitivity and specificity, these tests are not useful for screening but may be helpful in circumscribed situations in which the results may shift the diagnostic probability.

Stool Examination

Fecal occult blood testing is useful to evaluate iron deficiency anemia and acute or chronic GI blood loss. In patients with acute diarrhea, assessment of fecal leukocytes or culture of common pathogens is routine, and in selected patients, testing for parasites (*Giardia, Entamoeba histolytica*), *Clostridium difficile, Escherichia coli* O157:H7, or other specific organisms may be warranted. To distinguish among the causes of chronic diarrhea (Chapter 140), stool samples may be sent for assessment of electrolytes, leukocytes, and fecal fat.

Endoscopy and Radiology

Endoscopy (Chapter 134) and radiographic studies (Chapter 133) play a major role in the evaluation and management of many GI disorders. Esophageal manometry and esophageal pH and impedance monitoring can be useful for the evaluation of heartburn, reflux, and other esophageal symptoms (Chapter 138). Anorectal manometry may be useful in some patients with fecal incontinence and defecatory dysfunction (Chapter 145). Breath tests are commonly used to diagnose *H. pylori* infection (a urease breath test; Chapter 139), lactose intolerance, and small bowel bacterial overgrowth (a hydrogen breath test with lactulose or glucose; Chapter 140).

The diagnosis of a functional GI disorder is made after organic disorders have been excluded by clinical evaluation and limited, directed diagnostic testing. "Overtesting" should be avoided. Thereafter, the emphasis should switch from finding a "cause" of the symptoms to implementing successful coping and adaptive behaviors.

ABDOMINAL PAIN

Abdominal pain, which is a frequent complaint among outpatients in the office setting and emergency department, may be benign and self-limited or the presenting symptom of severe, life-threatening disease. Chronic abdominal pain that has been present for months or years in the absence of other organic illness is almost always functional in origin and does not require urgent evaluation. By contrast, most patients with severe acute abdominal pain require a thorough but emergent evaluation, which may quickly reveal an acute surgical illness (Chapter 142).

PATHOBIOLOGY

Stimulation of hollow abdominal viscera is mediated by splanchnic afferent fibers within the muscle wall, visceral peritoneum, and mesentery that are sensitive to distention and contraction. Visceral afferent nerves are loosely organized, innervate several organs, and enter the spinal cord at several levels. Thus, visceral pain is vague or dull in character and diffuse; patients attempting to localize the pain often move their entire hand over the upper, middle, or lower abdomen. Most visceral pain is steady, but cramping, intermittent pain or "colic" results from peristaltic contractions caused by partial or complete obstruction of the small intestine, ureter, or uterine tubes. In contrast to visceral innervation, a dense network of nerve fibers that follow a spinal T6 to L1 somatic distribution innervates the parietal peritoneum. Pain fibers of the parietal peritoneum are stimulated by stretch or distention of the abdominal cavity or retroperitoneum; direct irritation from infection, pus, or secretions (e.g., caused by a ruptured viscus); or inflammation caused by contact between the parietal peritoneum and an adjacent inflamed organ (e.g., appendicitis). Parietal pain is sharp, well characterized, and localized by the patient to a precise location on the abdomen, often by pointing with one finger.

The GI viscera (liver, biliary system, pancreas, and GI tract) arise during embryologic development from midline structures that have bilateral innervation. Thus, GI visceral pain is typically localized to the abdominal midline.

Acute Abdominal Pain

CLINICAL MANIFESTATIONS

History

The history should determine the time course, character, and location and radiation pattern of the pain (Table 132-2). Severe abdominal pain that begins suddenly during seconds to minutes indicates a catastrophic event, such as esophageal rupture, perforated peptic ulcer or viscus, ruptured ectopic pregnancy, ruptured aortic aneurysm, acute mesenteric ischemia, or myocardial infarction. Pain that progresses within 1 to 2 hours is consistent with a rapidly progressive inflammatory disorder (e.g., cholecystitis, appendicitis, pancreatitis), acute obstruction of a viscus (small intestinal obstruction, ureteral colic), or organ ischemia caused by a strangulated blood supply (volvulus, strangulated hernia, ovarian torsion). Pain that is less severe and develops during several hours is more commonly caused by a medical rather than a surgical condition, including upper GI disorders (dyspepsia), intestinal disorders (gastroenteritis, inflammatory bowel disease), liver disorders (hepatitis, abscess), urinary disorders (cystitis, pyelonephritis), and gynecologic infections; however, the slow evolution of surgical disorders such as cholecystitis (Chapter 155), appendicitis or diverticulitis (Chapter 142), and intra-abdominal abscesses must not be overlooked.

The character of the pain provides important information about whether the symptoms are due to visceral stimulation or parietal stimulation (peritonitis). Patients with peritonitis may report severe localized pain or irritation with activities or maneuvers that stretch or move the parietal peritoneum, such as walking, moving in bed, and coughing; as a result, they tend to lie quietly to avoid painful stimulation. By contrast, patients with visceral pain may move or walk restlessly or attempt a bowel movement in an effort to relieve their symptoms.

The location of pain in the upper, middle, or lower abdomen is a crude but important indicator of the diagnosis (Fig. 132-1). Visceral pain arising from the foregut (esophagus, stomach, proximal duodenum, bile duct, gallbladder, pancreas) most often is manifested in the epigastrium. Pain derived from the midgut (small intestine, appendix, ascending colon, proximal transverse colon) occurs in a periumbilical location. Pain derived from the hindgut (distal transverse colon, left colon, rectum) localizes to the lower midline between the umbilicus and symphysis pubis. Paired intra-abdominal organs such as the kidneys, ureters, ovaries, and fallopian tubes have unilateral innervation that localizes pain to the side of the involved organ. As some surgical conditions progress, the character and location of the pain shift from a visceral to a parietal pain pattern. Thus, early cholecystitis (Chapter 155) may be manifested with vague midline epigastric pain that progresses to sharp right upper quadrant pain as localized peritoneal irritation develops. Likewise, appendicitis (Chapter 142) commonly begins with vague, diffuse periumbilical pain that evolves to sharp, well-localized right lower quadrant pain as peritonitis ensues.

Anorexia, vomiting, diarrhea, distention, and constipation are commonly seen with abdominal pain caused by both medical and surgical disorders. Although nonspecific, the *absence* of any of these symptoms is evidence against an emergent surgical or medical disorder because severe illness usually leads to reflex stimulation or inhibition of gastric and intestinal peristalsis. Vomiting is common in medical and surgical disorders involving the upper GI tract, including acute gastroenteritis, pancreatitis, gastric and small intestinal obstruction, and biliary tract disease. Pain that precedes the onset of vomiting is typical of surgical conditions, whereas the reverse is true of medical conditions (e.g., food poisoning, gastroenteritis). Abdominal pain with prominent diarrhea is most commonly caused by a medical condition (e.g., gastroenteritis, inflammatory bowel disease). Although constipation alone is a nonspecific complaint, the absence of stool passage and flatus is consistent with complete bowel obstruction or paralytic ileus.

Jaundice accompanying acute abdominal pain virtually always indicates a hepatobiliary disorder (Chapter 147), including obstruction of the biliary duct (choledocholithiasis, pancreatic carcinoma, cholangiocarcinoma), complications of acute cholecystitis, acute hepatitis (viral, ischemic), and hepatic malignant neoplasms. The possibility of cholangitis should be considered and excluded in all patients with acute abdominal pain and jaundice, especially if the patient has fever, chills, hypotension, altered mental status, or leukocytosis. Hematemesis with upper abdominal pain suggests a Mallory-Weiss tear, alcoholic gastritis, or peptic ulcer disease. Hematochezia with abdominal pain is most commonly caused by medical conditions such as infectious

TABLE 132-2 TYPICAL MANIFESTATIONS OF KEY CAUSES OF ACUTE AND CHRONIC ABDOMINAL PAIN

CONDITION	LOCATION	QUALITY	ONSET	AGGRAVATING OR RELIEVING FACTORS	ASSOCIATED SYMPTOMS OR SIGNS	DIAGNOSTIC STUDIES
Peptic ulcer disease (Chapter 139)	Epigastric, occasionally RUQ, rarely LUQ	Dyspepsia: mild to moderate aching discomfort, pain, burning, gnawing, postprandial fullness	Days	Variable relief with antacids; may be relieved by, worsened by, or unrelated to meals	Recurrent; associated factors (e.g., *Helicobacter pylori*, aspirin, NSAIDs)	Anemia, upper endoscopy, *H. pylori* testing
Acute pancreatitis (Chapter 144)	Epigastric, radiates to midback (occasionally RUQ or LUQ)	Diffuse, steady, stabbing, penetrating	1-2 hr	Aggravated by food; better when lying still and with narcotics	Severe nausea and vomiting; reduced or absent bowel sounds; associated factors (e.g., alcohol, gallstones)	Elevated amylase and lipase, CT
Acute cholecystitis (Chapter 155)	Epigastric, then moves to RUQ; may radiate to right scapula	Gradual, steady increase, moderate to severe	Hours	May follow a fatty meal; better with narcotics and surgery	Nausea, some vomiting, fever	Elevated WBC count, US or CT
Acute appendicitis (Chapter 142)	Periumbilical, then moves to RLQ	Vague initially; gradual, steady increase to intense, localized, pain	Hours	Unprovoked; better with narcotics and surgery	Anorexia, nausea, obstipation; occasional vomiting, fever late	Elevated WBC count, US or CT
Diverticulitis (Chapter 142)	LLQ or suprapubic	Moderate to severe, steady or cramping, sharp or aching, localized	Hours to days	Unprovoked; better with narcotics and antibiotics or surgery	Anorexia, nausea, distention, constipation or loose stools; partial relief with passage of flatus or BM; fever late	Elevated WBC count, CT
Ruptured viscus and peritonitis (Chapter 142)	Diffuse	Intense	Minutes to hours	Worse with cough or movement; better when lying still or with narcotics or surgery	Fever, anorexia, nausea, vomiting; lack of bowel sounds; tenderness with percussion, light touch, rebound; guarding and rigidity (late); loath to move	Elevated WBC count, CT
Intestinal ischemia (Chapter 143)	Small intestine—periumbilical; proximal (right) colon—periumbilical or RLQ; distal colon—LLQ	Severe, stabbing pain out of proportion to physical findings	Minutes	Chronic ischemia—occurs after eating; acute ischemia—usually unprovoked; better with narcotics, thrombus dissolution, stenting, surgical resection	Nausea, bloody diarrhea; associated factors (e.g., hypotension, cardiac arrhythmias)	Elevated WBC count, CT or MR with angiography, or colonoscopy (colonic ischemia)
Strangulated hernia (Chapter 142)	Localized	Sharp, localized, intense; crampy or steady	Minutes to hours	Previous hernia history; unprovoked; better with narcotics and decompression, including surgery	Anorexia, nausea, vomiting, no stool or flatus passage if obstruction; bowel sounds variable—hyperactive early if obstruction present, but absent bowel sounds late, especially with peritonitis	Elevated WBC count, CT, US
Small or large bowel obstruction (Chapter 142)	Small intestine—periumbilical; proximal (right) colon—periumbilical or right abdomen; distal (left) colon—LLQ	Early—diffuse, colicky, crampy; late—steady and better localized	Hours to days	Aggravated by food; better with narcotics, NGT decompression, or surgery	Distention, anorexia, nausea, vomiting; no stool or flatus passage; small intestine—increased hyperperistaltic (rushes) bowel sounds (early) or quiet abdomen (late); large intestine—bowel sounds variable; associated factors (e.g., hernia, previous surgery)	CT
Abdominal abscess (Chapter 142)	Located over the abscess, usually LLQ or RLQ	Insidious, intense, constant	Days	May be aggravated by movement; better with abscess drainage	Fever, anorexia, nausea, abdominal mass	Elevated WBC count, CT
Acute hepatitis (Chapter 148)	RUQ	Dull or intense; localized	Days	Worse with deep inspiration	Jaundice, anorexia, nausea; liver enlarged and tender to palpation; associated factors (e.g., alcohol, infection)	Abnormal liver test results
GERD (Chapter 138)	Substernal or epigastric	Burning, gnawing	Days to years	Provoked by large or fatty meals or recumbency; relief with antacids	Recurrent; may have regurgitation, dysphagia, or extraesophageal manifestations (e.g., asthma, chronic cough, laryngitis)	Upper endoscopy (usually normal), ambulatory pH/impedance probe

TABLE 132-2 TYPICAL MANIFESTATIONS OF KEY CAUSES OF ACUTE AND CHRONIC ABDOMINAL PAIN—cont'd

CONDITION	LOCATION	QUALITY	ONSET	AGGRAVATING OR RELIEVING FACTORS	ASSOCIATED SYMPTOMS OR SIGNS	DIAGNOSTIC STUDIES
Nonulcer (functional) dyspepsia (Chapter 137)	Epigastric	Mild to moderate discomfort, pain, burning, gnawing, postprandial fullness	Years	May be worsened by meals; cannot be reliably distinguished from ulcer disease by history alone	Other symptoms of functional disorders (IBS, fibromyalgia, pelvic pain)	Normal EGD
IBS (Chapter 137)	Variable; usually lower abdomen	Vague, crampy, sense of urgency	Years	Pain may be precipitated by dietary factors or stress; associated with change in bowel characteristics (e.g., frequency, form, difficulty with passage); relieved with stool passage	Bloating and abdominal distention	Normal sigmoidoscopy, colonoscopy, and CT, but these are usually not necessary for diagnosis
Chronic pancreatitis (Chapter 144)	Epigastric or periumbilical, radiates to midback	Intense, localized	Days to years	Aggravated by food; better with narcotics	Anorexia, nausea, vomiting; associated factors (e.g., alcohol); DM (with advanced disease)	Amylase and lipase may be normal; CT may show calcifications, dilated pancreatic duct, pseudocyst; increased fecal fat and decreased fecal elastase if pancreatic insufficiency
Inflammatory or infectious enterocolitis (Chapters 142 and 283)	Small intestine—periumbilical; large intestine—right or left side of the abdomen over the colon; rectum—tenesmus	Crampy	Hours to days	Better with stool passage and treatment of underlying cause	Nausea, vomiting, bloody diarrhea; associated factors (e.g., infectious—food transmission; IBD—prolonged duration, family history)	Stool studies for culture, colonoscopy with biopsies
Malignant disease (Chapter 193)	Variable, depending on cancer location	Variable; intense and crampy if bowel obstruction; steady and vague if local invasion	Days	Better with narcotics and cancer therapy	Primary vs. metastatic disease	CT and biopsies, PET
Pneumonia/pleurisy (Chapters 97 and 99)	Upper abdomen: epigastric, RUQ, or LUQ	Localized; worse with deep breathing	Hours to days	Painful breathing; better with antibiotics	Cough, fever, dyspnea	CXR
Angina and myocardial infarction (Chapters 71-73)	Retrosternal or epigastric	Pressure, squeezing, heaviness, or intense	Minutes	Worse with exertion; relief with nitroglycerin	Dyspnea, diaphoresis	ECG, cardiac enzymes, stress testing
Genitourinary disorders (Chapters 126, 284, and 285)	Bladder—suprapubic; renal colic—abrupt, excruciating LLQ or RLQ pain radiating to the groin; prostate—dull, suprapubic; kidney—CVA	Constant or colicky; stone passage—restless, cannot find a comfortable position	Minutes to days	Better with antibiotics and pain medications (pyelonephritis or nephrolithiasis)	Hematuria, dysuria, prostate tenderness, fever	Urinalysis, urine culture, CT for stone disease
Ovarian cysts or torsion (Chapters 199 and 235)	LLQ or RLQ	Constant, intense	Minutes	Better with NSAIDs or surgery (torsion)	Nausea, vomiting; may be recurrent	US
Ruptured ectopic pregnancy (Chapter 239)	LLQ or RLQ	Constant, intense, stabbing	Minutes	Better with surgery	Rebound and guarding present, abnormal menses or amenorrhea	Acute anemia, elevated β-HCG, US
Musculoskeletal disorders	Specific muscle groups	Aching	Days	Better with heat or NSAIDs; aggravated by movement	History of muscle injury or exertion	Normal laboratory results
Herpes zoster (Chapter 375)	Dermatomal distribution	Burning, itching, neuropathic, constant	Days	Aggravated by touching the dermatome; better with pain or antiviral medications	Recurrent; rash may or may not be present	Skin culture or biopsy

TABLE 132-2 TYPICAL MANIFESTATIONS OF KEY CAUSES OF ACUTE AND CHRONIC ABDOMINAL PAIN—cont'd

CONDITION	LOCATION	QUALITY	ONSET	AGGRAVATING OR RELIEVING FACTORS	ASSOCIATED SYMPTOMS OR SIGNS	DIAGNOSTIC STUDIES
Metabolic disorders (e.g., DM; Chapter 229)	Epigastric or generalized	Intense, constant	Hours to days	Worse with poor metabolic control (e.g., poor glucose control)	Recurrent; nausea, vomiting, diabetic neuropathy	Specific metabolic parameters abnormal (e.g., elevated glucose in DM)
Abdominal epilepsy (Chapter 403)	Epigastric or umbilical	Constant	Hours to days	Unprovoked; better with antiseizure therapy	Recurrent; may have associated seizure disorder	EEG
Dissecting or leaking abdominal aortic aneurysm (Chapter 78)	Over the aneurysm, radiates to the back or groin	Severe, searing, constant	Minutes to hours to days	History of HTN or CAD	Shock, pulsatile mass; bruit *not* usually present	Acute anemia, CT, angiography

BM = bowel movement; CAD = coronary artery disease; CT = computed tomography; CVA = costovertebral angle; CXR = chest radiograph; DM = diabetes mellitus; ECG = electrocardiography; EEG = electroencephalography; EGD = esophagogastroduodenoscopy; GERD = gastroesophageal reflux disease; HCG = human chorionic gonadotropin; HTN = hypertension; IBD = irritable bowel disease; IBS = irritable bowel syndrome; LLQ = left lower quadrant; LUQ = left upper quadrant; MR = magnetic resonance; NGT = nasogastric tube; NSAIDs = nonsteroidal anti-inflammatory drugs; PET = positron emission tomography; RLQ = right lower quadrant; RUQ = right upper quadrant; US = ultrasonography; WBC = white blood cell.

Modified from Proctor DD. Approach to the patient with gastrointestinal disease. In: Goldman L, Ausiello D, eds. *Cecil Textbook of Medicine*. 23rd ed. Philadelphia: Saunders-Elsevier; 2008.

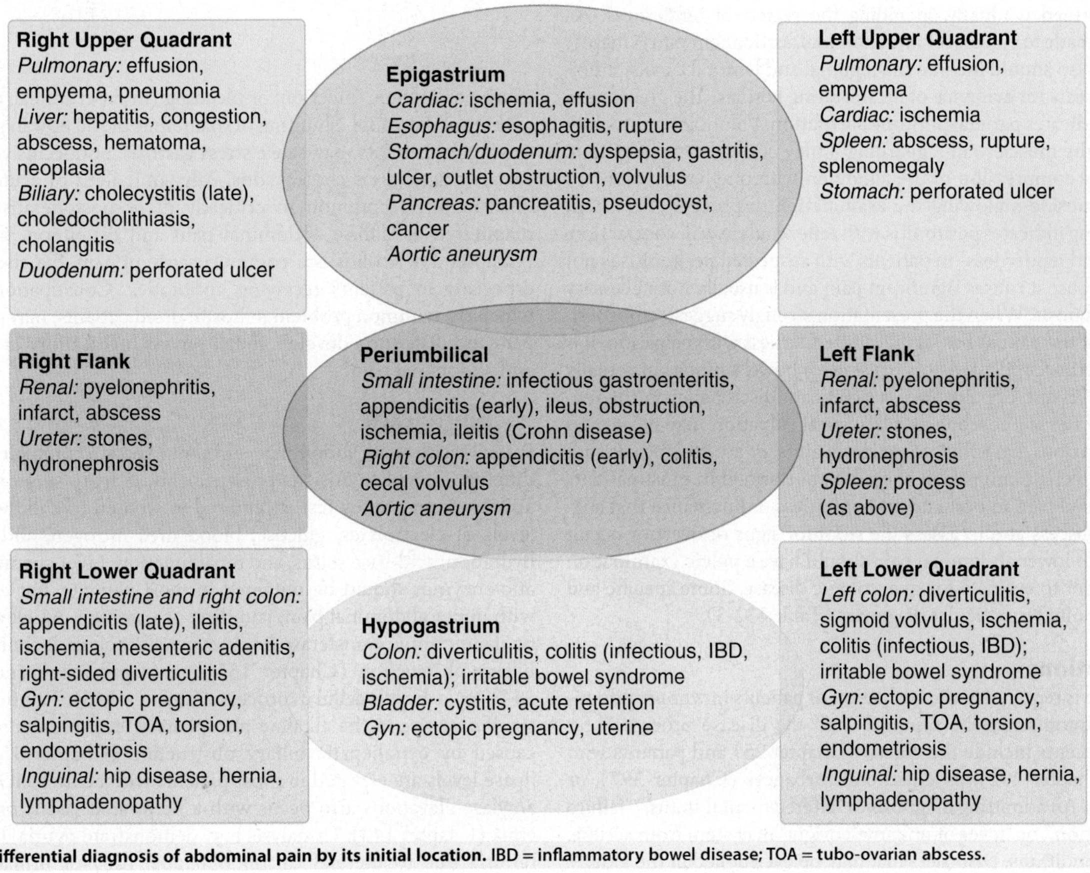

FIGURE 132-1. Differential diagnosis of abdominal pain by its initial location. IBD = inflammatory bowel disease; TOA = tubo-ovarian abscess.

gastroenteritis or inflammatory bowel disease, but it also may be caused by ischemic colitis or mesenteric ischemia. Gross hematuria may be due to cystitis (Chapter 284) or a ureteral stone (Chapter 126). Abdominal pain with weight loss may be due to inflammatory bowel disease, chronic mesenteric ischemia, or advanced GI malignant neoplasms. In women, a missed menstrual period, adnexal pain, spotting, or cramping may suggest pregnancy, ectopic pregnancy, or spontaneous abortion. Acute pain between cycles may be caused by ovarian follicles or ruptured corpus luteum cysts. Pelvic pain with fever, chills, or cervical discharge suggests pelvic inflammatory disease.

The past medical history and review of systems can provide clues about systemic and extra-abdominal conditions that may be manifested with abdominal pain. Acute coronary syndromes (Chapter 72), heart failure (Chapter 58), pneumonia (Chapter 97), or empyema may cause dyspepsia, epigastric or right or left upper quadrant pain, nausea, and vomiting. Metabolic conditions such as uremia (Chapter 130), diabetes with hyperglycemia or ketoacidosis (Chapter 229), hypercalcemia (Chapter 245), or acute adrenocortical insufficiency (Chapter 227) may cause pain, nausea, vomiting, and diarrhea. Acute intermittent porphyria (Chapter 210) and familial Mediterranean fever (Chapter 275) may cause recurrent episodes of severe pain and peritonitis that may be misdiagnosed, leading to unnecessary surgeries. Other causes of acute abdominal pain include narcotic withdrawal (Chapter 34), insect or reptile bites (Chapter 112), and lead or arsenic poisoning (Chapter 22).

Physical Examination

The physical examination must identify life-threatening illnesses that require urgent surgical evaluation. Nevertheless, the examination must be orderly, careful, and complete. If the examiner immediately palpates the site of maximal pain, the patient is unlikely to relax and to cooperate for the remainder of the examination.

First, the patient should be observed and the abdomen inspected. Most patients remain calm, cooperative, and freely capable of moving during the examination. Patients who are writhing or restless may have pain due to visceral distention (e.g., renal colic, intestinal obstruction), whereas patients who lie motionless may have peritonitis. Gentle shaking of the bed or having the patient cough may elicit sharp, well-localized pain in patients with parietal but not with visceral pain. Auscultation should be performed before percussion or palpation so that intestinal activity is undisturbed. An abdomen that is quiet except for infrequent squeaks or tinkles suggests peritonitis or ileus. Loud peristaltic rushes that occur in synchrony with abdominal pain suggest small bowel obstruction. Light percussion across the upper, middle, and lower abdomen can determine any site of focal tenderness suggestive of peritonitis. Light palpation should be performed with one or two fingers (not the whole hand), beginning away from where the patient localizes the pain and gradually moving to the site of pain. Thereafter, gentle, deeper palpation of the entire abdomen is performed gradually, including the region of tenderness. An attempt should be made to palpate for an abdominal aortic aneurysm (Chapter 78). Examination also should include the inguinal and femoral canals, umbilicus, and surgical scars for evidence of incarcerating hernias. The presence of focal tenderness indicates parietal peritoneal irritation. Voluntary or involuntary tightening of the muscle wall ("guarding") may occur during palpation. With gentle, steady compression of the abdomen with one hand, voluntary guarding usually subsides, allowing the examination to proceed. Persistent involuntary guarding indicates peritonitis with reflex muscle wall contraction. Testing for "rebound tenderness" in patients with suspected peritonitis is not recommended because it causes significant pain and is usually not necessary to establish the diagnosis. When the presentation strongly suggests a nonserious GI disorder but the patient has significant tenderness with palpation, it is useful to use the stethoscope ostensibly to listen for bowel sounds but actually to reproduce the pressure of palpation. A significant discrepancy in the tenderness elicited by the stethoscope and by digital palpation may be seen in patients who are anxious, have functional complaints, or are seeking secondary gain. A digital rectal examination should be performed in most patients with acute abdominal pain to evaluate for tenderness or fluctuance that suggests a perirectal abscess and to assess the stool for signs of overt or occult blood. Women with lower abdominal pain should have a pelvic examination by a skilled examiner to evaluate for gynecologic disease. Some specific and dramatic findings point to particular diagnoses (Table 132-3).

TABLE 132-3 PHYSICAL SIGNS IN PATIENTS WITH ACUTE ABDOMINAL PAIN

SIGN	DESCRIPTION	DIAGNOSIS
Murphy sign	Cessation of inspiration during right upper quadrant examination	Acute cholecystitis
McBurney sign	Tenderness located midway between anterior superior iliac spine and umbilicus	Acute appendicitis
Cullen sign	Periumbilical bluish discoloration	Retroperitoneal hemorrhage Pancreatic hemorrhage Ruptured abdominal aortic aneurysm
Grey Turner sign	Bluish discoloration of flanks	Retroperitoneal hemorrhage Pancreatic hemorrhage Ruptured abdominal aortic aneurysm
Kehr sign	Severe left shoulder pain	Splenic rupture Ectopic pregnancy rupture
Obturator sign	Pain with flexed right hip rotation	Appendicitis
Psoas sign	Pain with straight leg raising against resistance (right side)	Appendicitis

Special Populations

Increased diligence is required in the evaluation of patients in whom abdominal signs and symptoms may be minimal until the disease process is far advanced. Such patients include the elderly (Chapter 25) and patients who have dementia (Chapter 402), psychiatric disturbances (Chapter 397), or spinal cord injuries. An admitting diagnosis of "altered mental status," "failure to thrive," "obstipation," or "fever of unknown origin" may stem from serious intra-abdominal conditions. Disorders that may be overlooked in the elderly include bowel perforation, bowel obstruction, cholecystitis, diverticulitis, volvulus, mesenteric ischemia, and abdominal aortic aneurysm. In patients with chronic liver disease, the presence of ascites may mask the signs and symptoms of serious surgical conditions such as cholecystitis, appendicitis, and diverticulitis. Even in the presence of perforation, signs of peritonitis may be lacking because the ascites fluid separates the visceral peritoneum and parietal peritoneum. Likewise, immunocompromised populations, who are at risk for infectious, drug-related, and iatrogenic complications, may manifest few physical findings or laboratory abnormalities. Owing to the limitations of the clinical evaluation in these vulnerable populations, there should be a low threshold for the use of abdominal imaging.

Abdominal Pain Developing in the Hospital

When pain develops as a new problem in a hospitalized patient, it is usually caused by a limited number of conditions. Postprocedural complications may cause perforation, infection, or bleeding (intraperitoneal, retroperitoneal, or within solid organs). Shunting of splanchnic blood flow in severely ill medical or surgical patients may cause stress gastritis, nonocclusive mesenteric ischemia, or acalculous cholecystitis. Adynamic ileus or acute colonic pseudo-obstruction is common in critically ill or postoperative patients and is manifested as diffuse abdominal pain and distention. *Clostridium difficile* (Chapter 296) colitis is a common cause of pain, diarrhea, and distention, especially in patients receiving antibiotics. Constipation (Chapter 136), which is a common problem in hospitalized patients, may go unnoticed until pain and distention develop. Finally, many medications can cause dyspepsia and abdominal pain.

DIAGNOSIS

Patients with acute abdominal pain should have a complete blood count with differential; leukocytosis is present in most acute surgical conditions (Fig. 132-2). A pregnancy test is required in women of childbearing age. Serum levels of electrolytes, glucose, blood urea nitrogen, and creatinine assess hydration, acid-base status, and renal function. Liver chemistries and pancreatic enzymes should be obtained in most patients, but especially in those with upper abdominal pain, jaundice, or vomiting. An elevation in aspartate or alanine aminotransferase levels may reflect choledocholithiasis with acute biliary obstruction (Chapter 155), acute gallstone pancreatitis (Chapter 144), or a hepatocellular process (Chapter 148). Painful jaundice with a significant rise in the alkaline phosphatase level usually reflects cholestasis caused by extrahepatic biliary obstruction (Chapter 155). Amylase and lipase levels are elevated in most patients with acute pancreatitis, but minor amylase elevations also occur with a perforated viscus or mesenteric ischemia (Chapter 143). Urinalysis may demonstrate pyuria, hematuria, or bacteriuria due to ureteral calculi (Chapter 126) or urinary tract infection (Chapter 284).

Imaging

Ultrasound is preferred in suspected pregnancy and to evaluate for other acute gynecologic disorders, such as tubo-ovarian abscess, ruptured corpus luteum cyst, or ovarian torsion; it is also preferred for the initial evaluation of suspected acute cholecystitis (Chapter 155) and ureteral stones with hydronephrosis (Chapter 123) and for the bedside evaluation of unstable patients. In most other settings, abdominal computed tomography (CT) with oral and intravenous administration of contrast material (when possible) is preferred and can provide a definitive diagnosis in up to 90% of patients with acute severe abdominal pain[A1] (Chapter 133). Abdominal CT may be falsely negative early in the course of acute pancreatitis, mesenteric ischemia, cholecystitis, appendicitis, and diverticulitis, especially if it is performed without contrast enhancement.

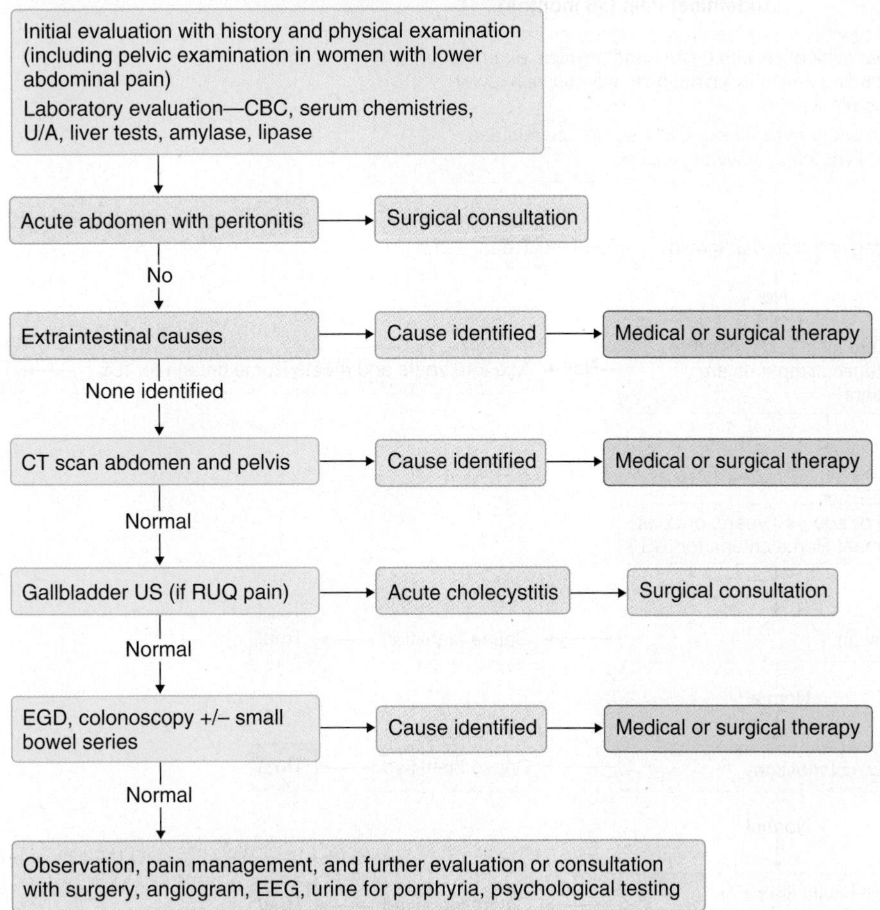

FIGURE 132-2. Approach to the patient with acute abdominal pain. CBC = complete blood count; CT = computed tomography; EEG = electroencephalography; EGD = esophagogastroduodenoscopy; RUQ = right upper quadrant; U/A = urinalysis; US = ultrasonography.

TREATMENT Rx

Once the diagnosis is clear, treatment of the underlying condition is initiated. In patients with nonspecific acute abdominal pain and no clear diagnosis, early laparoscopy is useful for diagnosis, but outcomes such as complication rates, readmission rates, and length of hospitalization are no better than with a strategy of active observation.

Chronic Abdominal Pain

Chronic or recurrent abdominal pain that has been present for months to years may be caused by structural (organic) disease, but the majority of patients have a functional disorder such as irritable bowel syndrome (Chapter 137). Common organic causes of chronic abdominal pain include medications with GI side effects, peptic ulcer disease (Chapter 139), inflammatory bowel disease (Chapter 141), chronic pancreatitis (Chapter 144), biliary tract disease (Chapter 155), GI cancers (Chapters 192 and 193), and endometriosis (Chapter 236). The clinician should attempt to distinguish patients with symptoms or signs of organic disease, in whom further diagnostic investigation is warranted, from those with probable functional disease (Fig. 132-3). Although functional disorders occur in all age groups, the symptoms usually begin before the age of 40 years. "Alarm" features that suggest a structural disorder and are inconsistent with a functional disorder are fever, severe pain, significant weight loss, jaundice, progressive dysphagia, recurrent vomiting, nocturnal pain or diarrhea, and stools that are bloody or positive for fecal occult blood. Laboratory study findings should be normal with functional disorders; therefore, an unrevealing evaluation for anemia, leukocytosis, and levels of iron, albumin, C-reactive protein, and vitamins A, D, or B_{12} argues against structural or organic disease.

In patients younger than 50 years with a suspected functional disorder and no alarm features (e.g., family history of colon cancer or inflammatory bowel disease or abnormalities on screening blood tests), further testing should be minimized, and the emphasis should be shifted to managing symptoms, coping, and making lifestyle changes (Chapter 137).[A2] In patients who may have organic disease, testing often includes a combination of upper GI endoscopy, colonoscopy, and ultrasound or CT imaging.

GAS AND BLOATING

Belching

Belching (eructation), which is the involuntary or voluntary release of gas from the esophagus or stomach, commonly occurs during or after a meal. Virtually all belching is caused by swallowed air, which may be increased by eating quickly, drinking carbonated beverages, chewing gum, and smoking. Gas also may be produced within the stomach by antacids, especially sodium bicarbonate, which rapidly neutralize gastric acid and release carbon dioxide. Belching seldom reflects serious GI dysfunction but may be increased in patients with gastroesophageal reflux (Chapter 138), functional dyspepsia (Chapter 137), or gastroparesis (Chapter 136). Chronic, excessive, repetitive belching is a functional disorder caused by transient ingestion of air into the esophagus (caused by subconscious diaphragmatic contraction and upper esophageal sphincter relaxation) and its subsequent expulsion; it is treated with behavioral modification.[4]

Flatus

Flatus or "gas" is a normal byproduct of digestion. Otherwise healthy adults pass flatus 10 to 20 times daily and excrete up to 1500 mL. Thus, it is difficult to distinguish patients with abnormal or excessive gas production from those with only a heightened awareness of or sensitivity to normal production. Increased flatulence with diarrhea may be symptomatic of

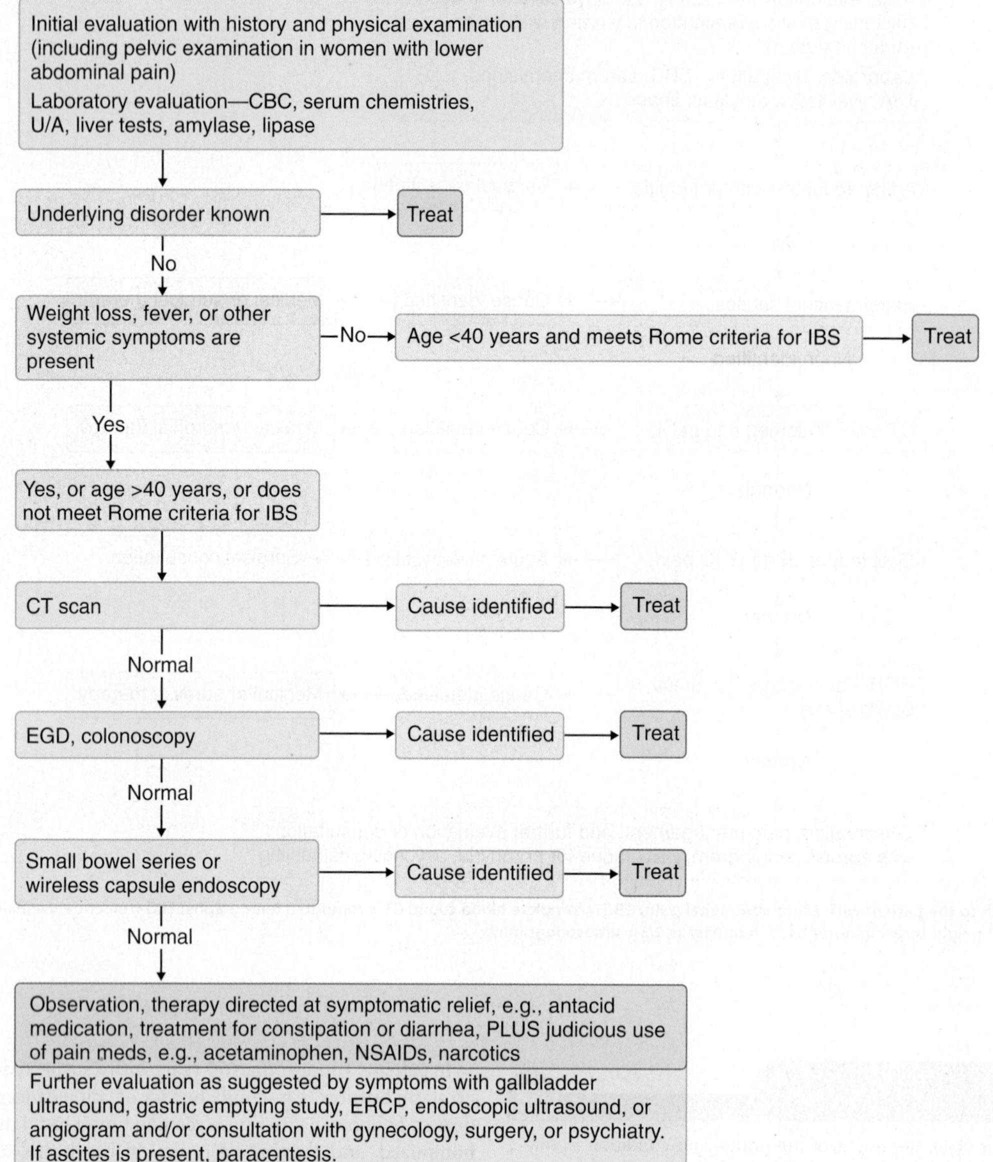

FIGURE 132-3. Approach to the patient with chronic abdominal pain. CBC = complete blood count; CT = computed tomography; EGD = esophagogastroduodenoscopy; ERCP = endoscopic retrograde cholangiopancreatography; IBS = irritable bowel syndrome; NSAIDs = nonsteroidal anti-inflammatory drugs; U/A = urinalysis.

disorders of malabsorption, including celiac disease (Chapter 140), pancreatic insufficiency (Chapter 144), and small intestinal bacterial overgrowth (Chapter 140).

In normal adults, flatus is derived from two sources: swallowed air and colonic bacterial fermentation of FODMAPs (fermentable oligosaccharides, disaccharides, and monosaccharides and polypols), which are short-chain carbohydrates that may be incompletely absorbed in the small intestine and result in the colonic production of carbon dioxide or methane. FODMAPs include lactose (dairy products), fructose, fructans, polypols, and galacto-oligosaccharides. Fructose is present in fruit, especially apples and pears, and is a major component of corn syrups that are widely used as sweeteners. Polyols include sorbitol, which is a natural sugar in stone fruit (peaches, apricots, plums, prunes) and a common added sweetener in sugar-free candies, as well as trehalose, which is present in mushrooms. Fructans and oligosaccharides are plentiful in cruciferous vegetables (cabbage, broccoli, cauliflower, Brussels sprouts, turnips, rutabagas), garlic, onions, legumes (beans, soy, lentils, peas), pasta, and whole grains.[5]

TREATMENT Rx

Patients with long-standing flatulence in the absence of other symptoms or signs of GI disease can be treated conservatively. Avoidance of carbonated beverages, chewing gum, sorbitol- and fructose-containing sweeteners, and gas-producing vegetables improves symptoms in most patients.[A3,A4] Lactase deficiency may be confirmed by a lactose breath test. Underlying GI illness is suggested by the recent onset of flatulence with other symptoms of organic disease, including weight loss, abdominal pain, diarrhea, distention, and abnormal laboratory studies (Chapter 140). A positive fecal fat analysis confirms malabsorption and merits further investigation (see Table 140-6). Suspected small bowel bacterial overgrowth may be confirmed by carbohydrate breath tests or treated empirically with antibiotics.

Bloating and Distention

Bloating and distention are common complaints among patients with functional GI disorders (Chapter 137). As chronic, isolated symptoms, they are almost never caused by serious structural disease. Functional bloating may be caused by heightened sensitivity to minor increases in intestinal gas or impaired transit of gas, even though the total volume of intestinal gas is within normal limits. The acute onset of distention in conjunction with alarm symptoms such as cramping pain, weight loss, nausea, vomiting, obstipation, or diarrhea warrants further evaluation for disorders that cause intestinal obstruction (Chapter 142) or malabsorption (Chapter 140). Rifaximin (550 mg three times daily for 2 weeks) is effective for functional bloating, pain, and loose or watery stools[6]; but dietary and behavioral changes and reassurance may also be useful.

INVOLUNTARY WEIGHT LOSS

The unintentional loss of more than 5% of baseline weight within a 12-month period is frequently due to a serious underlying medical or psychiatric illness. Weight loss is seldom the sole presenting sign of medical disorders, but it is often revealed during the clinical evaluation of other complaints. Chronic weight loss in the elderly is commonly caused by depression, dementia, difficulty with chewing or swallowing, malignant disease, medications, alcoholism, or physical and social limitations to procuring, preparing, and eating meals (Table 132-4) (Chapter 24). Gradual, mild weight loss occurs in some elderly patients because of the loss of lean body mass. In young patients, weight loss is more commonly caused by eating disorders (Chapter 219), endocrine disorders (Chapters 226 and 227), or chronic GI conditions such as inflammatory bowel disease (Chapter 141) or celiac disease (Chapter 140). In chronic medical conditions, involuntary weight loss is usually caused by a combination of decreased appetite (anorexia) and varying degrees of cachexia; examples include advanced malignant disease, chronic infections (HIV, tuberculosis), heart failure, chronic kidney or liver disease, end-stage lung disease, and adrenal insufficiency. Weight loss that occurs in the presence of normal or increased appetite suggests increased metabolism and energy expenditure caused by endocrine disorders, such as poorly controlled diabetes (Chapter 229) or hyperthyroidism (Chapter 226), or GI disorders that result in food malabsorption (Chapter 140). Chronic GI disorders that cause progressive narrowing or obstruction of the esophagus (cancer, achalasia), stomach (cancer, peptic ulcer disease with gastric outlet obstruction), small intestine (Crohn disease), or arterial circulation (chronic mesenteric ischemia) may cause weight loss as a result of dysphagia, vomiting, or postprandial pain that limits the ability to ingest sufficient calories.

DIAGNOSIS

The cause of weight loss (see Table 132-4) is usually evident from the history, physical examination, and routine laboratory studies, including complete blood count, electrolytes, liver chemistries, thyroid-stimulating hormone, urinalysis, and, when appropriate, HIV serology (Fig. 132-4). A chest radiograph should be obtained in patients who smoke, have any respiratory symptoms, or are older than 40 years. Signs of dehydration or severe malnutrition may require an assessment for nutritional deficiencies (Chapter 214) and nutritional support (Chapters 216 and 217).

Other symptoms and signs necessitate consideration of additional diagnostic testing. Weight loss with increased appetite merits an assessment of thyroid function (Chapter 226), glucose intolerance (Chapter 229), and malabsorption (Chapter 140). Suspected malabsorption may be confirmed by a positive fecal fat analysis. GI symptoms suggesting obstruction or occult GI malignant disease can be evaluated with upper GI endoscopy, upper GI radiographic series, colonoscopy, or abdominal CT. Psychiatric evaluation may be warranted in patients with signs of depression, early dementia, or eating disorders. In up to 25% of patients, no cause of weight loss is found.

NAUSEA AND VOMITING

Nausea is an unpleasant feeling of the impending need to vomit. *Vomiting* is the forceful oral expulsion of gastric contents as a result of retrograde contraction of the duodenum and antrum with compression of the thoracoabdominal musculature. Nausea and vomiting may be caused by a number of GI and non-GI disorders, but they are best categorized according to chronicity and the presence of abdominal pain. The acute onset of vomiting *with* severe abdominal pain suggests a serious illness potentially requiring surgical intervention, including GI obstruction (Chapter 142), mesenteric ischemia (Chapter 143), pancreatitis (Chapter 144), biliary colic (Chapter 155), and conditions causing peritonitis (Chapter 142), such as appendicitis or a perforated viscus. Acute vomiting *without* abdominal pain is most commonly caused by medications (including chemotherapy), motion sickness (Chapter 428), food poisoning (Chapter 283), infectious gastroenteritis (Chapter 283), hepatitis (Chapters 148 and 149), upper GI bleeding, postoperative ileus, or acute central nervous system disease. Chronic or recurrent nausea and vomiting *with* abdominal pain are commonly caused by GI disorders that result in the partial or intermittent obstruction of the stomach or small intestine. Chronic nausea and vomiting *without* abdominal pain may be due to disorders that impair gastric emptying or small intestine motility and non-GI causes, including medications, pregnancy, intracerebral disorders, cardiac disease, endocrine disease, labyrinth disorders, psychiatric disease (including bulimia), and functional disorders. Vomiting of undigested food eaten hours earlier suggests gastric obstruction or gastroparesis. Abdominal distention or feculent emesis suggests obstruction of the small intestine.

DIAGNOSIS

Most cases of acute vomiting without abdominal pain are self-limited and require no evaluation (Fig. 132-5). Medication-related symptoms and pregnancy should be excluded. With severe vomiting, serum electrolyte values should be obtained. Hyperglycemia may cause acute gastroparesis. Increased liver chemistries or pancreatic enzymes suggest hepatobiliary or pancreatic disease. In patients with acute abdominal pain and vomiting, abdominal plain radiography or CT is performed to look for evidence of GI obstruction, a perforated viscus, or pancreaticobiliary disease. In patients with chronic vomiting of uncertain cause, the goal is to distinguish structural GI disorders, GI motility disorders, and non-GI disorders. Esophagogastroduodenoscopy, enterography, abdominal cross-sectional imaging, GI motility studies, and head CT or magnetic resonance imaging may be indicated.

TREATMENT Rx

The approach to the medical treatment of nausea and vomiting depends on the cause (Table 132-5). Patients who are receiving moderately emetogenic chemotherapy are frequently managed with a 5-HT_3 receptor antagonist and dexamethasone; aprepitant is added for highly emetogenic regimens.[A5] For patients with mildly emetogenic regimens or vomiting from other causes, treatment with single or combinations of anticholinergic agents, dopamine receptor antagonists, or 5-HT_3 receptor antagonists usually provides symptomatic relief.[7]

OTHER GASTROINTESTINAL COMPLAINTS

Heartburn, esophageal regurgitation, dysphagia, odynophagia, and noncardiac chest pain suggest esophageal disease (Chapter 138). *Dyspepsia*, which refers to bothersome, intermittent, mild to moderate upper abdominal or epigastric symptoms (burning, pain, early satiation, postprandial fullness) can be caused by peptic ulcer disease (Chapter 139) or esophageal disease (Chapter 138), or it can be functional in origin (Chapter 137). An orderly diagnostic approach (Fig. 132-6) can help distinguish among the various causes, avoid unnecessary testing, and minimize symptoms.[8,A6]

Diarrhea, which is defined pathophysiologically as an increase in stool weight to more than 200 g/day, can be caused by malabsorption of osmotically active substances or by increased intestinal secretion of electrolytes and water. In clinical practice, however, stool weight is seldom quantified, and the term *diarrhea* refers to an increase in stool liquidity or frequency (more than three bowel movements per day). Acute and chronic diarrhea should be distinguished because the evaluation and treatment are different[9] (Chapter 140).

Constipation (Chapter 136), which is the most common digestive symptom, occurs in 15% of the population. Constipation may refer to fewer than three bowel movements per week; hard or lumpy stools; or difficulty during defecation, characterized by straining, a sensation of obstruction or incomplete evacuation, or the need to engage in manual manipulations to promote evacuation. Constipation may be caused by systemic conditions that slow colonic transit, including neuromuscular disease, endocrine disorders, and electrolyte abnormalities, or by lesions that obstruct the passage of stool through the distal colon or anorectum, such as neoplasms, strictures, prolapse, and aganglionosis (Hirschsprung disease). Most patients, however, do not have an apparent cause and are deemed to have functional constipation.[10]

TABLE 132-4 CAUSES OF INVOLUNTARY WEIGHT LOSS

CONDITION	QUALITY	DURATION	AGGRAVATING OR RELIEVING FACTORS	ASSOCIATED SYMPTOMS OR SIGNS	DIAGNOSTIC STUDIES
WEIGHT LOSS SECONDARY TO GASTROINTESTINAL CAUSES					
GI, pancreatic, or hepatobiliary malignant disease (Chapters 192-196)	Progressive, fast	Months	Better with cancer therapy (e.g., surgery, XRT, chemotherapy)	Dysphagia (esophageal); anorexia, nausea, vomiting (gastric, small or large bowel obstruction); visible or occult blood in stool; altered bowel habits; jaundice or hepatomegaly (biliary obstruction, hepatic tumor, metastatic disease); iron deficiency anemia	CBC, FOBT, ferritin, CEA, CA19-9, AFP, EGD, colonoscopy, abdominal CT, PET
Malabsorption (Chapter 140) (poor absorption of nutrients due to pancreatic insufficiency, small intestinal mucosal disorders, or bacterial overgrowth)	Progressive, slow	Months to years	Diarrhea or steatorrhea, excessive flatulence; worse with eating and resolves with NPO status	Usually associated with increased appetite; may have anemia (iron, B_{12}, folate), osteoporosis, or osteomalacia (vitamin D, calcium, phosphorus); easy bruising (vitamin K), night blindness (vitamin A)	72-hr stool for fecal fat; fecal elastase; vitamins A and D and INR; calcium, ferritin, B_{12}, albumin; celiac disease antibodies (e.g., anti-tTG, antiendomysial antibodies); EGD with small bowel biopsy; breath test for bacterial overgrowth
Inflammatory bowel disease (especially Crohn disease) (Chapter 141)	Progressive, slow	Months	Eating causes pain, cramps, increased diarrhea and urgency; improved by low-residue diet or NPO status	Bloody stools, abdominal cramps and pain, perianal disease, extraintestinal manifestations (e.g., oral ulcers, uveitis, erythema nodosum, arthralgias)	CBC, albumin, ESR, CRP, colonoscopy with biopsies, CT or MR enterography, wireless capsule study
GI motility disorders (Chapter 136)	Intermittent, slow	Years	Worse with eating	Nausea, vomiting, distention, diarrhea, or constipation may be present	EGD and colonoscopy, gastric emptying study, CT or MR enterography, surgical full-thickness intestinal biopsies
Cirrhosis (Chapter 153)	Muscle wasting with edema, so weight may increase	Months to years	Worse with salt or fluid intake	Ascites, peripheral edema	Liver biopsy
Chronic intestinal ischemia (Chapter 143)	Progressive	Months to years	Worse with eating	Afraid to eat; postprandial abdominal pain, nausea; associated atherosclerotic disease	CT or MR angiography
WEIGHT LOSS SECONDARY TO NONGASTROINTESTINAL CAUSES					
Poor or inadequate calorie intake due to social factors (Chapter 215)	Intermittent or progressive, acute (hospitalized) or chronic	Days to months to years	Common in elderly, teenagers; exacerbated by poor dentition or poorly fitting dentures	Will eat if food is made available	Review dietary log and how food is obtained and prepared
Medications	Intermittent or progressive	Months	Worse with medication; resolves with discontinuation of offending drug	Anorexia, nausea, vomiting	Review drug profile
Non-GI malignant disease	Progressive	Months	Better with cancer therapy (e.g., surgery, XRT, chemotherapy)	Anorexia, nausea, vomiting; pain; metastatic disease	Calcium, cortisol; CT for underlying disease, PET
Endocrine disorders: DM, hyperthyroidism, adrenal insufficiency (Chapters 226, 227, and 229)	DM—appetite increased or decreased, early satiety; hyperthyroidism—increased appetite	Months to years	Worse with disease chronicity	DM: gastroparesis, neuropathy, retinopathy, nephropathy Adrenal insufficiency: nausea, vomiting, diarrhea, abdominal pain	Serum glucose, TFT, cortisol
Chronic infections, including HIV and TB (Chapters 324 and 390)	Progressive, fast	Months	Better with directed therapy, megestrol acetate (Megace)	Nausea, anorexia, other infections	HIV test, PPD, cultures, biopsies if necessary
Systemic inflammatory disorders	Progressive, moderate	Months to years	Better with directed therapy, megestrol acetate (Megace)	Arthritis, rash, vasculitis	ANA, RF, ESR, CRP
Chronic renal failure (Chapter 130)	Progressive, slow; edema may increase weight	Months to years	Better with dialysis, megestrol acetate (Megace)	Nausea, anorexia, weight gain	BUN, Cr, 24-hr creatinine clearance
Advanced COPD or heart failure (Chapters 58 and 88)	Progressive, slow	Months to years	Better with oxygen and specific treatment	Fatigue, dyspnea, edema, wasting	Pulmonary function testing or two-dimensional echocardiography
Psychiatric illness: depression, manic-depressive illness (Chapter 397)	Progressive, slow	Months to years		Depression common in elderly; flat affect; manic phase associated with hyperactivity and decreased intake	Psychological testing

TABLE 132-4 CAUSES OF INVOLUNTARY WEIGHT LOSS—cont'd

CONDITION	QUALITY	DURATION	AGGRAVATING OR RELIEVING FACTORS	ASSOCIATED SYMPTOMS OR SIGNS	DIAGNOSTIC STUDIES
Psychogenic eating disorders—anorexia nervosa, bulimia (Chapter 219)	Intermittent or progressive	Months to years	Worse with stressors	Refusal to eat, loss of tooth enamel, calluses and healing ulcerations of hand	Psychiatric testing
Substance abuse (alcohol, opiates, CNS stimulants)	Intermittent or progressive	Months	Resolves with discontinuation	Anorexia, nausea, vomiting	Careful interview; patients may deny or minimize

AFP = α-fetoprotein; ANA = antinuclear antibody; BUN = blood urea nitrogen; CBC = complete blood count; CEA = carcinoembryonic antigen; CNS = central nervous system; COPD = chronic obstructive pulmonary disease; Cr = creatinine; CRP = C-reactive protein; CT = computed tomography; DM = diabetes mellitus; EGD = esophagogastroduodenoscopy; ESR = erythrocyte sedimentation rate; FOBT = fecal occult blood test; GI = gastrointestinal; HIV = human immunodeficiency virus; INR = international normalized ratio; MR = magnetic resonance; NPO = nothing orally; PET = positron emission tomography; PPD = purified protein derivative; RF = rheumatoid factor; TB = tuberculosis; TFT = thyroid function test; tTG = tissue transglutaminase; XRT = x-ray therapy.
Modified from Proctor DD. Approach to the patient with gastrointestinal disease. In: Goldman L, Ausiello D, eds. *Cecil Textbook of Medicine.* 23rd ed. Philadelphia: Saunders-Elsevier; 2008.

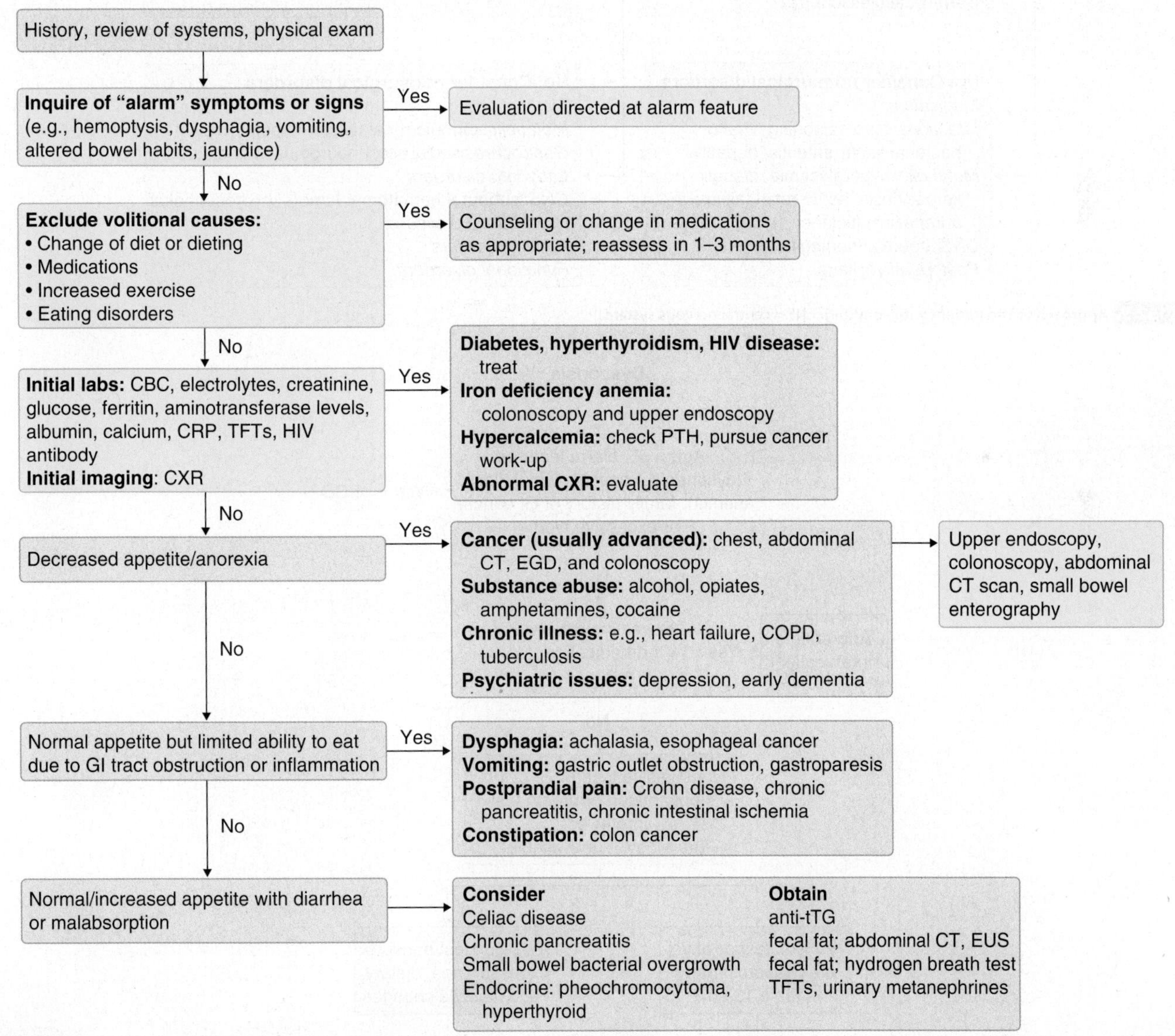

FIGURE 132-4. Approach to the patient with unintentional weight loss of more than 5%. CBC = complete blood count; COPD = chronic obstructive pulmonary disease; CRP = C-reactive protein; CT = computed tomography; CXR = chest radiograph; EGD = esophagogastroduodenoscopy; EUS = endoscopic ultrasound; GI = gastrointestinal; HIV = human immunodeficiency virus; PTH = parathyroid hormone; TFTs = thyroid function tests; tTG = tissue transglutaminase; U/A = urinalysis.

GI bleeding (Chapter 135) may be acute and clinically apparent (overt) or chronic, slow, and clinically inapparent (occult). The location of acute GI bleeding is described as either upper or lower, according to whether the source is proximal or distal to the ligament of Treitz (distal duodenum). Upper GI bleeding, which is three times more common than lower GI bleeding, is manifested by bloody emesis (hematemesis), coffee ground emesis, and, in most cases, black stools (melena). Common causes of significant bleeding are peptic ulcer disease, esophageal varices, Mallory-Weiss tears, erosive gastritis or esophagitis, and vascular ectasias.[11] Major lower GI bleeding is manifested by large-volume maroon or bright red bloody stools (hematochezia). Although 80 to 90% of patients with hematochezia have a lower source of bleeding, massive upper GI bleeding also may cause hematochezia.

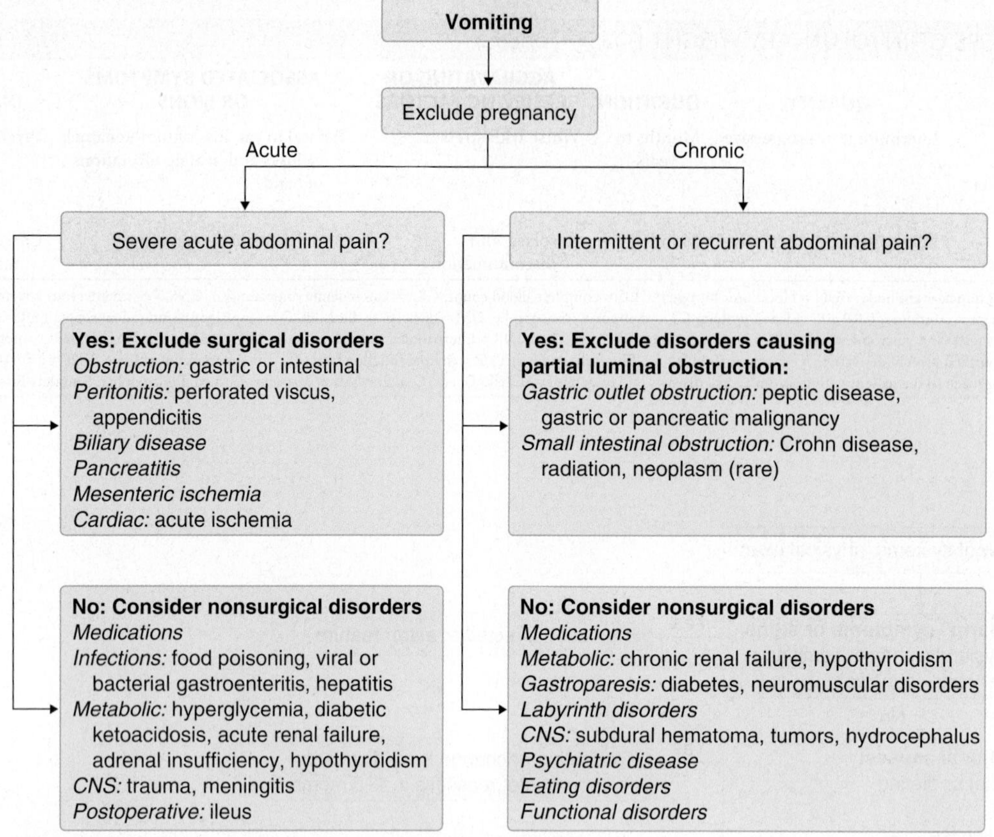

FIGURE 132-5. Approach to the patient with vomiting. CNS = central nervous system.

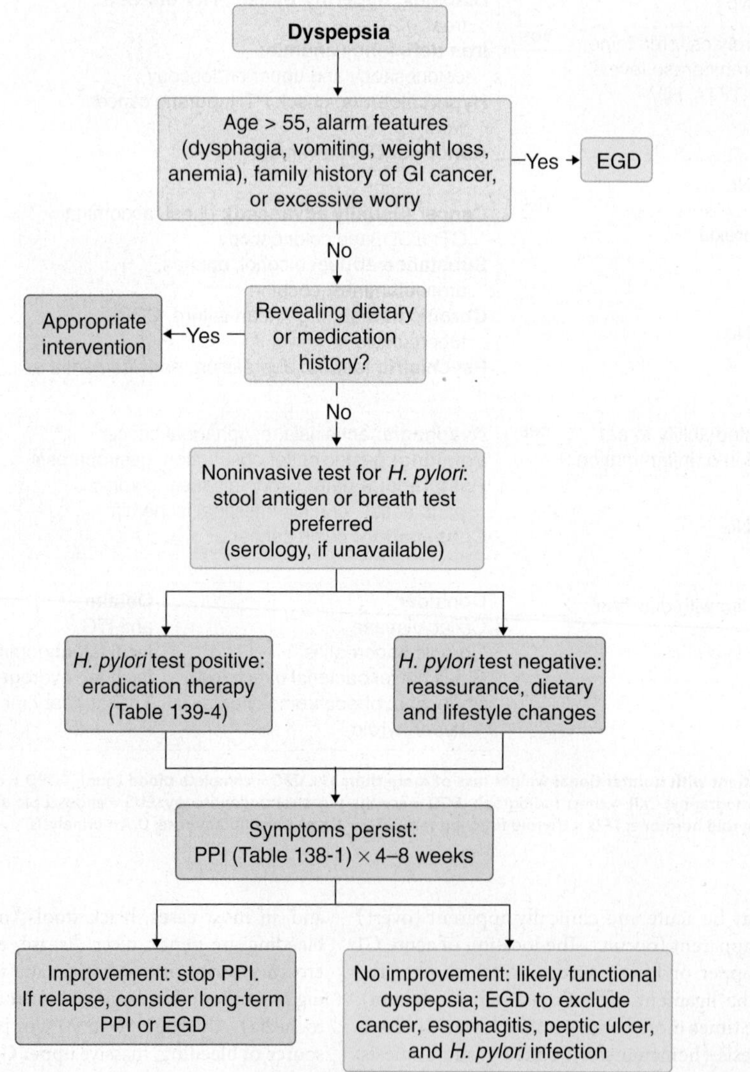

FIGURE 132-6. Approach to the patient with dyspepsia. EGD = esophagogastroduodenoscopy; GI = gastrointestinal; PPI = proton pump inhibitor.

TABLE 132-5 MEDICAL TREATMENT OF NAUSEA AND VOMITING

DRUG	USUAL INDICATIONS	USUAL DOSE (RANGE)	ROUTE	COMMENTS
ANTICHOLINERGIC-ANTIHISTAMINE AGENTS				Side effects: sedation, dizziness, delirium, blurred vision, glaucoma, bronchospasm, tachycardia, urinary retention Avoid concomitant alcohol or CNS depressants; use with caution in elderly patients
Scopolamine patch	MS	1.5 mg/72 hr	Patch	
Dimenhydrinate	MS	50 mg (50-100 mg) q4-6h	PO, IM, IV	Maximum 400 mg/24 hr
Cyclizine	MS, GIDz	50 mg q8h	PO, IM	Maximum 200 mg/24 hr
Meclizine	MS, V	25-50 mg q24h	PO	
Diphenhydramine	GIDz	25-50 mg q6h 50-100 mg q6h	PO, IV IM	
Promethazine	GIDz, PONV, MS	25 mg (12.5-25 mg) q6-12h 25 mg (12.5-50 mg) q4-6h	PO, PR IV, IM	Phenothiazine derivative, but lacks significant antidopaminergic effects Avoid perivascular extravasation or subcutaneous injection (severe tissue necrosis)
Trimethobenzamide	GIDz, PONV	200 mg q6-8h	IM	
DOPAMINE RECEPTOR ANTAGONISTS				Side effects: neuromuscular (extrapyramidal) symptoms—agitation, restlessness, involuntary movements, dystonia, torticollis, laryngospasm, Parkinson-like features
Prochlorperazine	GIDz, PONV, CTX	5-10 mg q6-8h 25 mg q12h	PO, IV, IM PR	Maximum dose 20-40 mg/24 hr; avoid subcutaneous injection (irritation)
Metoclopramide	GIDz CTX	10 mg (10-20 mg) q6-8h 1-2 mg/kg before and 2 hr after CTX	PO, IV, IM IV	Modest efficacy at these doses High doses infrequently used owing to availability of safer, more effective CTX regimens; use with diphenhydramine to reduce adverse side effects
Droperidol	PONV	2.5 mg (1.25-5 mg) preinduction and q4-6h as needed	IV, IM	May cause QTc prolongation and torsades de pointes; use is restricted to patients who fail to respond to other agents
CORTICOSTEROIDS				
Dexamethasone	PONV CTX	4-8 mg once preinduction 8-20 mg on day 1; 8 mg on days 2-4	PO, IV PO, IV	Most beneficial when used with other agents (e.g., 5-HT_3 RA, neurokinin-1 RA)
BENZODIAZEPINES				Used to reduce anxiety and anticipatory vomiting
Lorazepam	CTX	1-2 mg q4-6h	PO, IV	
CANNABINOIDS				May stimulate appetite; adverse side effects (sedation, dizziness, dysphoria, dry mouth) limit use
Dronabinol	GIDz, CTX	5-10 mg q6-8h	PO	
Nabilone	GIDz, CTX	1-2 mg q12h	PO	
5-HT_3 RECEPTOR ANTAGONISTS	PONV, CTX			PONV prevention: give IV immediately before anesthesia induction Prevention of CTX-induced vomiting: give 30 min (IV) to 1 hr (PO) before chemotherapy
Ondansetron	PONV CTX, RadTx	4 mg once 4-8 mg 8 mg once, 8 mg twice daily	IV PO PO	
Granisetron	CTX, RadTx	1 mg twice daily 1 mg once	PO IV	
Dolasetron	CTX, PONV	100 mg once daily	PO only	
Palonosetron	CTX PONV	0.25 mg once 0.5 mg 0.075 mg	IV PO, 1-3 days IV	
NEUROKININ-1 RECEPTOR ANTAGONISTS	Highly emetogenic CTX			Used exclusively in combination with a 5-HT_3 RA or dexamethasone
Aprepitant		125 mg on day 1 80 mg on days 2-3	PO	
Fosaprepitant		150 mg on day 1	IV	Aprepitant 80 mg PO on days 2-3
ANTIEMETIC REGIMENS FOR CHEMOTHERAPY				
Mildly emetogenic CTX	Option 1 Option 2	Dexamethasone 8 mg Dopamine receptor antagonist	IV or PO	One dose only One dose only
Moderately emetogenic CTX		Day 1: 5-HT_3 RA plus dexamethasone 8 mg	IV or PO	Days 2-3: continue oral 5-HT_3 RA and dexamethasone 8 mg to reduce delayed emesis
Highly emetogenic CTX		Day 1: 5-HT_3 RA plus dexamethasone 12 mg plus neurokinin-1 RA	IV or PO	Give aprepitant 80 mg PO days 2-3 and dexamethasone 8 mg PO days 2-4 to reduce delayed emesis

CNS = central nervous system; CTX = chemotherapy; GIDz = gastrointestinal disorders associated with nausea and vomiting; 5-HT_3 = serotonin or 5-hydroxytryptamine$_3$; MS = motion sickness; PONV = postoperative nausea and vomiting; PR = per rectum; RA = receptor antagonist; RadTx = radiation therapy–induced nausea and vomiting; V = vertigo.

Modified from Proctor DD. Approach to the patient with gastrointestinal disease. In: Goldman L, Ausiello D, eds. *Cecil Textbook of Medicine*. 23rd ed. Philadelphia: Saunders-Elsevier; 2008.

Approximately 95% of major lower GI bleeding arises from the colon and 5% from the small intestine. Lower GI bleeding is increased in patients older than 50 years, in whom diverticulosis accounts for 60% of cases; the remainder are due to ischemia, neoplasms, ulcers, vascular ectasias, or hemorrhoids. In patients younger than 50 years, bleeding is more commonly attributable to inflammatory bowel disease, hemorrhoids, or infectious colitis.

Occult GI bleeding refers to GI blood loss that is small in volume and not apparent to the patient but is detectable by tests for fecal occult blood. Chronic occult bleeding may result in iron deficiency anemia. Both upper endoscopy and colonoscopy should be performed to look for a source of occult bleeding, most commonly gastroesophageal or colonic neoplasia, erosive esophagitis or gastritis, ulcer disease, or vascular ectasia. In patients with recurrent iron deficiency and occult blood loss in whom no source is found on upper and lower endoscopy, video capsule endoscopy or enteroscopy is performed to look for a small bowel source (vascular ectasia, ulcer, or neoplasm).

Fecal incontinence (Chapter 145) is dependent on a number of factors, including a solid or semisolid stool, a compliant and distensible rectal reservoir, the ability to sense rectal fullness, an intact internal anal sphincter (an involuntary muscle innervated by the enteric nervous system), an intact external anal sphincter and puborectalis (voluntary muscles innervated by the pudendal nerve), and the mental and physical ability to reach a toilet facility when needed.[12] Minor incontinence, which occurs in 10% of people older than 70 years, is characterized by the inability to control flatus or by the seepage of fecal matter that results in soiling of the perianal area and undergarments. It tends to be intermittent, occurring after bowel movements; when coughing, lifting, or passing flatus; or when stools are loose. Major incontinence is characterized by the partial or complete inability to reliably control bowel movements, resulting in gross, involuntary loss of feces and the need to wear a diaper. It occurs in less than 1% of the population and is virtually always caused by a central nervous system disorder that results in diminished awareness of bowel needs, neuropathy, or damage to the anal sphincters.

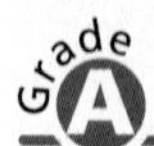

Grade A References

A1. Kim K, Kim YH, Kim SY, et al. Low-dose abdominal CT for evaluating suspected appendicitis. *N Engl J Med.* 2012;366:1596-1605.

A2. Begtrup LM, Engsbro AL, Kjeldsen J, et al. A positive diagnostic strategy is noninferior to a strategy of exclusion for patients with irritable bowel syndrome. *Clin Gastroenterol Hepatol.* 2013;11:956-962.

A3. Biesiekierski JR, Peters SL, Newnham ED, et al. No effects of gluten in patients with self-reported non-celiac gluten sensitivity after dietary reduction of fermentable, poorly absorbed, short-chain carbohydrates. *Gastroenterology.* 2013;145:320-328.

A4. Halmos EP, Power VA, Shepherd SJ, et al. A diet low in FODMAPs reduces symptoms of irritable bowel syndrome. *Gastroenterology.* 2014;146:67-75.

A5. dos Santos LV, Souza FH, Brunetto AT, et al. Neurokinin-1 receptor antagonists for chemotherapy-induced nausea and vomiting: a systematic review. *J Natl Cancer Inst.* 2012;104:1280-1292.

A6. Mazzoleni LE, Sander GB, Francesconi CF, et al. *Helicobacter pylori* eradication in functional dyspepsia: HEROES trial. *Arch Intern Med.* 2011;171:1929-1936.

GENERAL REFERENCES

For the General References and other additional features, please visit Expert Consult at https://expertconsult.inkling.com.

133

DIAGNOSTIC IMAGING PROCEDURES IN GASTROENTEROLOGY

DAVID H. KIM AND PERRY J. PICKHARDT

A wide range of diagnostic imaging modalities are available for evaluation of diseases of the gastrointestinal (GI) tract and the hepatopancreaticobiliary system. Once the workhorses of GI radiology, conventional radiography and fluoroscopy are still relevant but have largely given way to more advanced cross-sectional imaging studies, such as ultrasonography, computed tomography (CT), and magnetic resonance imaging (MRI). Many of the visceral vascular evaluations undertaken by conventional angiography have been replaced by these noninvasive modalities as well. These cross-sectional technologies have become the preferred methods of evaluation, allowing more precise and accurate diagnoses. In addition, cross-sectional techniques can be used to guide a wide variety of interventional procedures. With the emergence of molecular imaging, there has been renewed interest in nuclear medicine, most notably positron emission tomography (PET) and the combination modalities of PET/CT and PET/MR.

CONVENTIONAL RADIOGRAPHY

Conventional radiographs, often referred to as plain films, remain useful for a limited number of abdominal indications but are generally much less sensitive and specific for disease compared with techniques such as CT. Advantages of radiography include its wide availability, low cost, and portability, allowing the acquisition of images in acute clinical situations. Supine and upright frontal abdominal radiographs can assess rapidly for bowel obstruction or perforation in the setting of an acute abdomen (Fig. 133-1). Serial abdominal radiographs remain a practical approach for observing patients

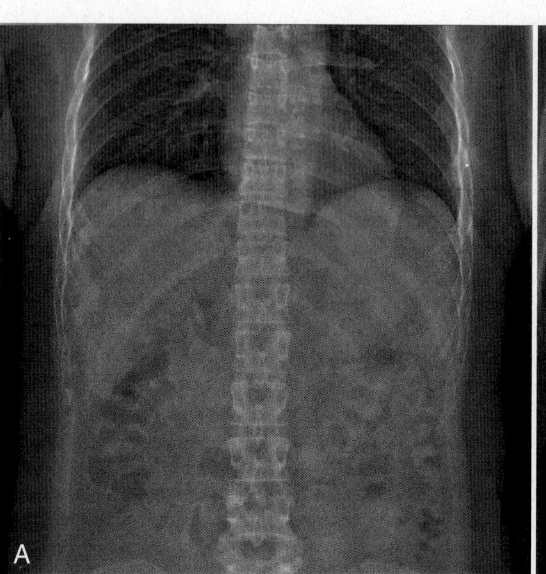

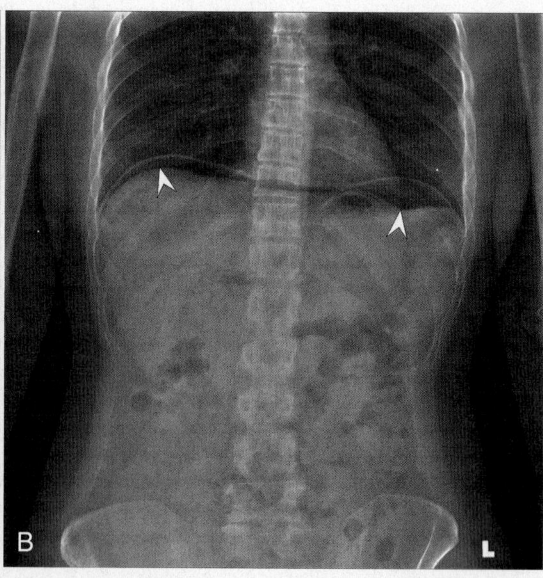

FIGURE 133-1. Pneumoperitoneum from bowel perforation on conventional radiography. A 36-year-old renal transplant patient presents with abdominal pain after colonoscopy. A, Supine abdominal radiograph is grossly normal with scattered nondistended bowel. B, Upright radiograph centered over the diaphragm reveals a lucent area below the diaphragm (*arrowheads*) consistent with free intraperitoneal air. This view is required for the detection of pneumoperitoneum because the supine examination does not show free air unless it is present in large amounts.

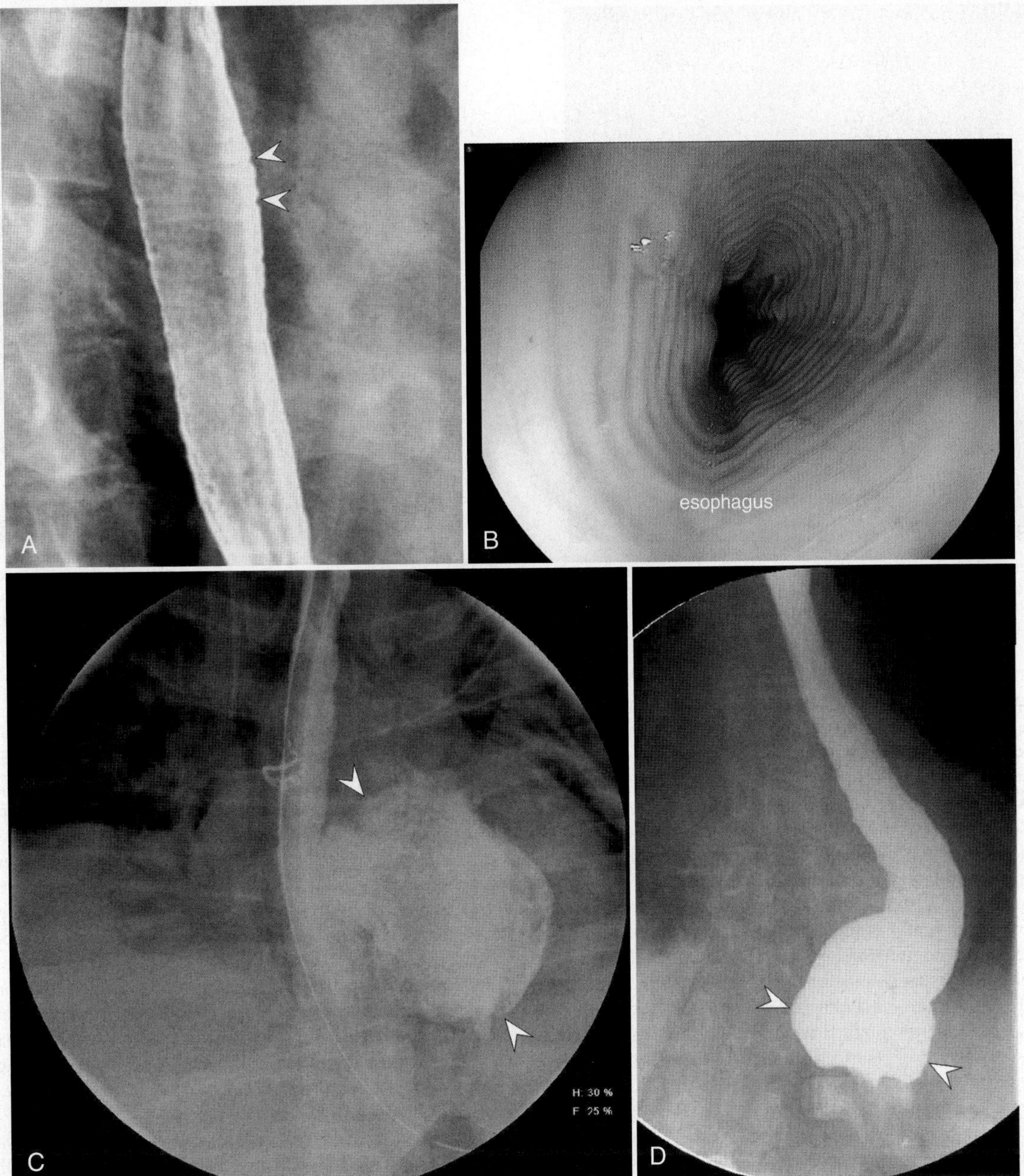

FIGURE 133-2. **Evolving nature of contrast fluoroscopy. A, Double-contrast image of the esophagus shows fine mucosal constrictions or rings (*arrowheads*) in a young adult man with dysphagia suggestive of eosinophilic esophagitis. This imaging approach is now used less commonly. B, Digital photograph from esophagogastroduodenoscopy confirms the diagnosis (numerous eosinophils at biopsy). C, Single-column esophagography is a more modern radiographic technique to confirm a leak (*arrowheads*) of water-soluble contrast material from the esophagus after trauma or to demonstrate obstruction and dilation (D, *arrowheads*) of the esophagus and proximal stomach upstream of an overly tight gastric band placed for weight control.**

with an abnormal bowel gas pattern suggestive of either evolving small bowel obstruction or adynamic ileus.[1] Conventional radiographs can demonstrate abnormal abdominal calcifications and radiopaque foreign bodies. In each of these cases, however, cross-sectional modalities, such as CT, have increased sensitivity and provide better delineation of disease processes. CT is often undertaken when the findings on initial plain film evaluation are normal or to provide better information when the findings on conventional radiography are abnormal.

FLUOROSCOPIC PROCEDURES

The role of contrast fluoroscopy has changed dramatically during the past two decades.[2] Double-contrast radiographic images (Fig. 133-2) to depict mucosal details of the esophagus, stomach, small bowel, and colon have largely been supplanted by endoscopy (Chapter 134) and advanced radiologic techniques. The diagnoses of an erosion, ulcer, polyp, or mass are now largely in the domain of endoscopy, supplemented by the newer cross-sectional modalities, such as CT or MR enterography for the small bowel (replacing the double-contrast small bowel enteroclysis) and CT colonography (replacing the double-contrast barium enema).

Single-column contrast images to depict overall anatomic structure and for problem-solving now constitute the bulk of fluoroscopic studies. In single-column examinations, the luminal structure of concern is distended by contrast material only, either thin barium or a water-soluble iodinated contrast agent, to delineate the gross structure and without trying to determine fine mucosal detail. In the esophagus and stomach, single-column luminal examinations are commonly used to assess for postoperative anastomotic breakdown after esophagectomy, gastrectomy, or bariatric surgery (see Fig 133-2). In the small bowel, single-contrast examinations (i.e., small bowel series/follow-through) can be used preoperatively as anatomic "road maps" to delineate fistulas or to guide bowel resection in Crohn disease. For the colorectum, the single-contrast barium enema remains an important diagnostic tool in such settings as suspected colonic obstruction, postoperative leak or fistula, and ileocolic intussusception in children (Chapter 142). Many institutions continue to perform fluoroscopic defecography to help delineate functional abnormalities in patients with evacuation disorders (Chapter 145), although dynamic MR cine series have replaced defecography at some institutions.

In addition to these single-column examinations, videofluoroscopy remains a mainstay for evaluation of swallowing problems. In this examination, the

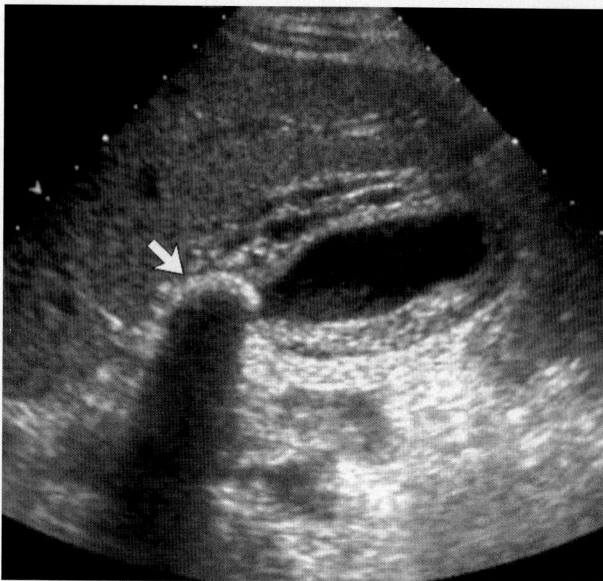

FIGURE 133-3. Acute cholecystitis on ultrasound examination. Image from right upper quadrant sonography shows diffuse gallbladder wall thickening and a shadowing impacted gallstone (*arrow*). A sonographic Murphy sign was present. These findings are diagnostic for acute calculous cholecystitis.

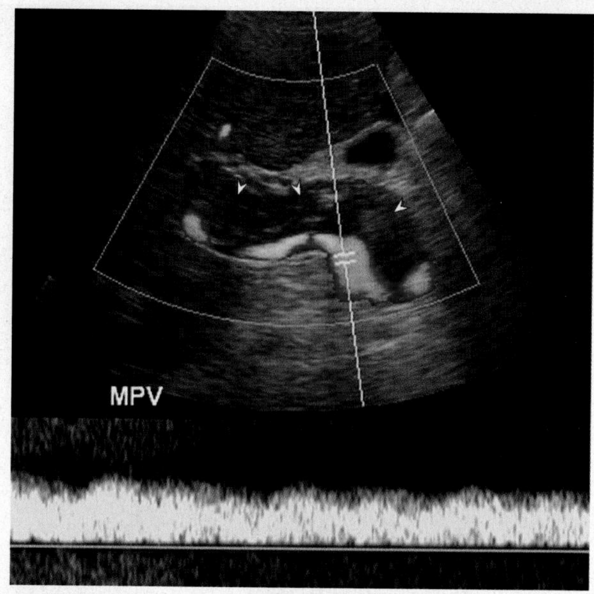

FIGURE 133-4. Portal vein thrombosis on ultrasound examination. Ultrasound gray-scale image with both power color Doppler and spectral Doppler interrogation shows a tubular hypoechoic structure (*arrowheads*) consistent with nonocclusive thrombus filling the majority of the main portal vein (MPV). Flow patency is seen in the deep peripheral aspect of the vessel.

patient swallows varying consistencies of barium, ranging from thin liquids to solids, typically in the form of a barium cookie. This test is an excellent way to assess the swallowing mechanism dynamically and to exclude aspiration.

ULTRASONOGRAPHY

The introduction of harmonic and compound imaging, advances in high-resolution transducers, and improvements in color Doppler evaluation have all combined to enhance the diagnostic capabilities of portable ultrasound. In general, ultrasound is useful for imaging solid organs and fluid-filled structures, but it is unable to penetrate gas-filled structures. For example, overlying bowel gas often precludes a complete sonographic evaluation of the pancreas. Ultrasound is a relatively versatile imaging technique in that it can be performed by many different routes, including transabdominal, endoscopic (as part of esophagogastroduodenoscopy), transrectal, intravascular, and endovaginal approaches. In addition, it is excellent for many image-guided interventions because of its real-time capabilities.

Ultrasonography is the most frequently used initial modality to evaluate the liver and biliary system. Suspected acute cholecystitis (Chapter 155) in the setting of right upper quadrant pain is a common indication for right upper quadrant sonography; classic findings include cholelithiasis, gallbladder wall thickening, and a sonographic Murphy sign (reproducible pain when the transducer is pressed over the gallbladder) (Fig. 133-3). The sensitivity for detection of gallstones with ultrasonography exceeds 95%. Acalculous cholelithiasis can be a more challenging diagnosis because the findings overlap with nonspecific gallbladder wall thickening in critically ill patients. Ultrasound is typically the first imaging test obtained in patients with new-onset jaundice or cholestatic laboratory findings because it offers a rapid, noninvasive evaluation of the biliary tree to differentiate obstruction from other causes.[3] If biliary ductal dilation is present, the level and cause of the obstruction can sometimes be demonstrated on ultrasound; common causes include choledocholithiasis and pancreatic head masses. In most cases of biliary obstruction, additional imaging tests will be necessary, consisting of CT, MR cholangiopancreatography (MRCP), endoscopic retrograde cholangiopancreatography, or percutaneous transhepatic cholangiography, depending on the specific circumstances.

Although ultrasonography is typically less sensitive and specific than CT or MRI for the detection or characterization of focal liver lesions (Chapters 151 and 196), it is useful for distinguishing cystic lesions from solid lesions. Although they are not approved for use in the United States, intravenous contrast agents for ultrasound have been studied fairly extensively in other countries and appear to offer similar advantages seen with CT and MRI contrast agents.

In diffuse liver disease, ultrasound is an alternative to CT or MR in screening of patients with viral hepatitis for possible cirrhosis and hepatocellular carcinoma (Chapters 153 and 196). Although it is less sensitive for hepatocellular carcinoma, ultrasound holds the advantages of being relatively inexpensive, convenient, and not requiring ionizing radiation. Sonographic findings in cirrhosis include a heterogeneously coarsened parenchymal echotexture, nodular surface contour, predominantly right-sided volume loss, and evidence of portal hypertension, including ascites, splenomegaly, and portosystemic collaterals. Ultrasound elastography uses either an acoustic pulse or mechanical vibration to create a shear wave that can assess the stiffness of the liver as a nonspecific measurement of the degree of liver fibrosis.[4] Studies have shown good agreement between this technique and histology, particularly at the extremes (none and severe fibrosis). Recently, the FibroScan or transient elastrography has been used for the longitudinal evaluation of liver fibrosis, but it is not yet ready for integration with routine clinical practice.

Ultrasonography can be used to detect hepatic steatosis (fatty liver; Chapter 152) when the parenchyma demonstrates increased echogenicity and decreased penetration of the sound beam. The findings of steatosis can be focal, multifocal, or diffuse; ultimately, MRI is more specific and can confirm the diagnosis.

Color and power Doppler evaluation allows the noninvasive sonographic assessment of vascular patency. Doppler evaluation of the liver is commonly performed in patients with end-stage liver disease (Chapter 154) to evaluate the portal system and to search for portosystemic collaterals. Abnormal portal vein findings include hepatofugal flow and thrombosis (Fig. 133-4). Doppler ultrasound is also used for the evaluation of transjugular intrahepatic portosystemic shunts (TIPS), both before and after stent placement. In orthotopic liver transplant recipients, Doppler evaluation is frequently performed to assess the hepatic vasculature, with particular attention to the hepatic arterial supply.

COMPUTED TOMOGRAPHY

CT has revolutionized the imaging of abdominal disease, providing a rapid, reproducible, and comprehensive evaluation. The introduction of single-detector helical or spiral CT, followed by multidetector scanners, has resulted in improved resolution and faster acquisition of true volumetric data. High-resolution scans of the entire abdomen and pelvis can now be easily acquired in a single short breath-hold. With the automated, high-rate injection of intravenous contrast materials and advanced processing, specialized CT examinations are replacing many traditional modalities.

A major challenge of CT scanning, however, is to minimize radiation doses as CT use increases, especially in patients who may undergo these because of the possibility of multiple scans for nonmalignant indications throughout their lifetime.[5] Newer image reconstruction techniques hold the promise of markedly decreasing the dose of radiation while maintaining the fidelity of the CT images.

The clinical indications for abdominal CT are broad. One common use is the diagnostic evaluation of a nontraumatic acute abdomen (Chapter 142). Common inflammatory conditions such as appendicitis[A1] and diverticulitis are diagnosed by CT. Other common indications include evaluation for intra-abdominal abscess, pancreatitis, and small bowel obstruction. In cases of relatively high-grade bowel obstruction, CT can often localize the transition point, elucidate the underlying cause, and evaluate for vascular compromise. In the setting of an acute abdomen due to blunt trauma (Chapter 111), CT has become invaluable for the prompt detection of significant abdominal injury.

In the nonacute setting, multiphase CT with intravenous administration of contrast material can characterize lesions and often results in a noninvasive diagnosis, particularly in combination with the clinical history (Fig. 133-5). Primary abdominal malignant neoplasms, such as hepatocellular carcinoma and pancreatic cancer, are often first detected on CT. CT has become the modality of choice for abdominal staging for metastatic disease, including hematogenous, lymphatic, peritoneal, and local spread, and in assessing the response to various therapies.

A rapidly growing indication of CT is to replace traditional fluoroscopy in the diagnostic evaluation of bowel complaints because of its better sensitivity and specificity. CT enterography protocols combine neutral (i.e., water density) oral contrast agents with dynamic, high-resolution imaging that provides detailed multiplanar evaluation of the small bowel. Indications include evaluation of occult GI bleeding due to small bowel masses and low-grade chronic obstruction. Dedicated CT enterography and capsule endoscopy yield a complementary and comprehensive evaluation of the small bowel. Although it is accurate and useful for the diagnosis of Crohn disease,[6] CT enterography has been largely supplanted by its MR counterpart for follow-up assessments so that radiation exposure can be limited. For the large bowel, CT colonography, also referred to as virtual colonoscopy, combines two- and three-dimensional evaluation of the prepared and distended colon for the detection of colorectal polyps and masses (Fig. 133-6; Video 133-1). CT colonography, which has replaced the double-contrast barium enema at many institutions, can be used to screen for colorectal cancer in average-risk

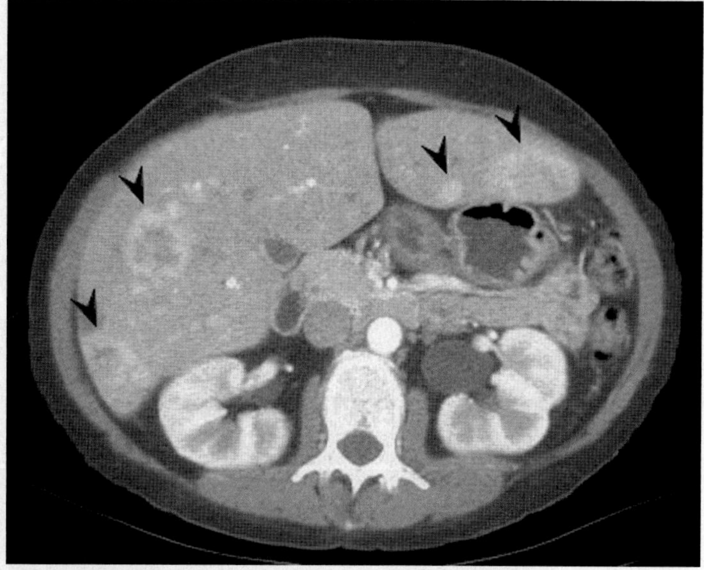

FIGURE 133-5. Multiple hypervascular liver lesions on CT. Dynamic contrast-enhanced CT image obtained during the arterial phase shows multiple hypervascular liver lesions (*arrowheads*), which proved to be hepatic adenomas in a patient with von Gierke disease.

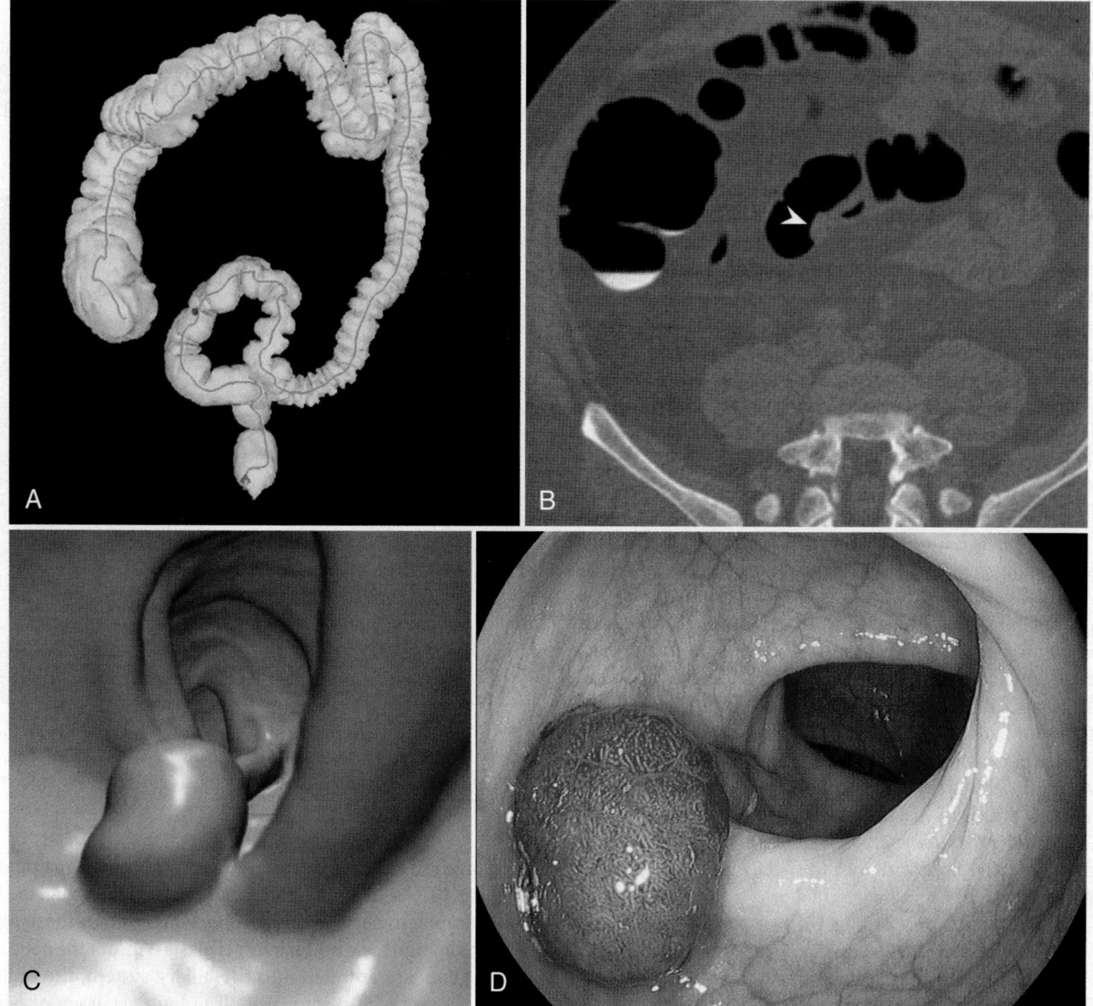

FIGURE 133-6. Pedunculated tubulovillous adenoma on screening virtual colonoscopy (CT colonography). A, Colonic color map allows precise documentation of location of this sigmoid polyp (*red dot*). **B,** Transverse two-dimensional image confirms that the lesion is composed of soft tissue (*arrowhead*). **C,** Three-dimensional endoluminal view nicely matches the pedunculated appearance at colonoscopy (**D**).

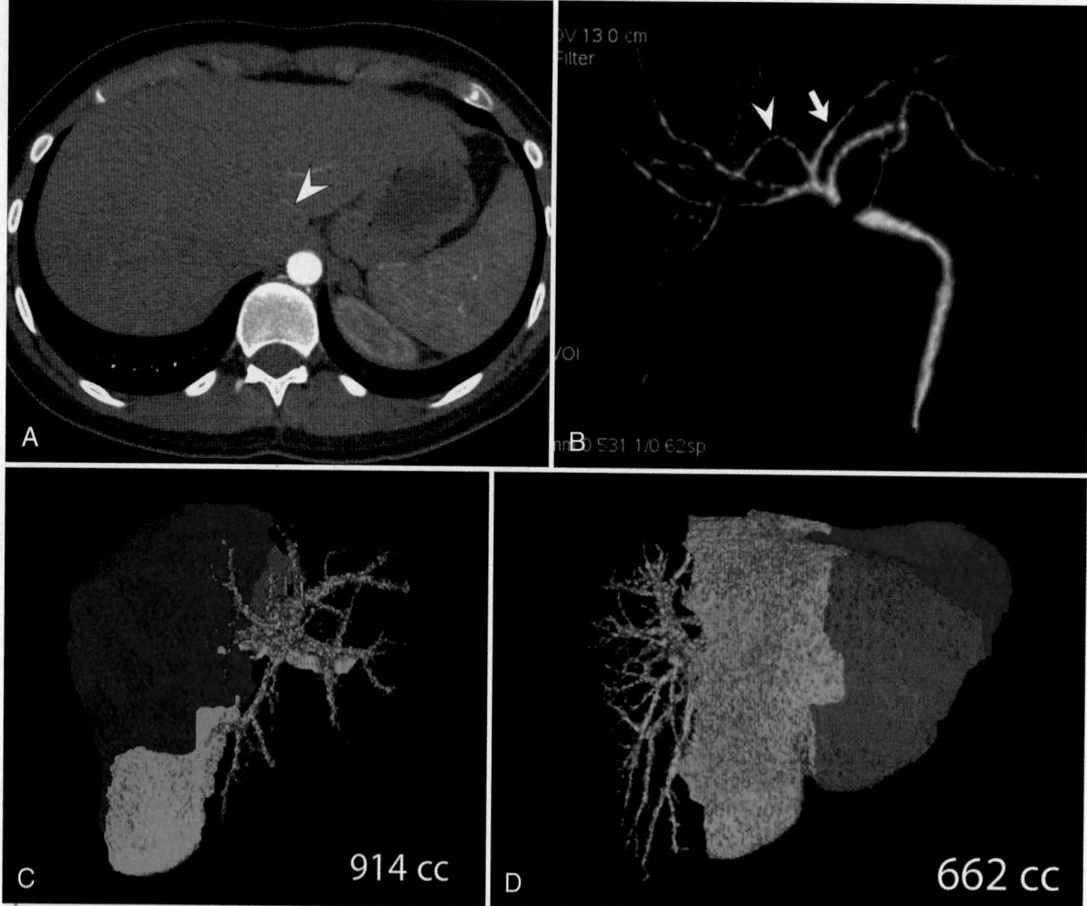

FIGURE 133-7. **Preoperative anatomic evaluation of potential living related liver donors.** Specialized CT protocols with vascular and cholangiographic contrast can allow complete evaluation. **A,** Transverse CT image shows a small-caliber accessory left hepatic artery (*arrowhead*). Other levels (not pictured) show normally branching right and left intrahepatic arteries at the porta hepatis. **B,** Three-dimensional cholangiographic reconstruction shows an anatomic variant, in which a posterior segment hepatic duct (*arrowhead*) does not join the anterior segment but rather drains anomalously into a left hepatic duct (*arrow*), thereby potentially influencing the choice of the transplant donor. **C** and **D,** Segmented liver volumes allow prediction of hepatic adequacy for both the donor and the recipient.

individuals, with reported sensitivity of 90% for detection of polyps 10 mm and larger. Optical colonoscopy is still required for polypectomy.

The technologic advances in CT drive an ever-expanding number of applications in abdominal imaging. Visceral CT angiography is largely replacing conventional diagnostic angiography. For example, in many institutions, evaluation of the vascular anatomy before hepatic transplantation (Chapter 154) is now undertaken by CT rather than by catheter angiography. Similarly, CT cholangiography can accurately map the biliary system of a living related liver transplant donor, and CT volumetric analysis can help assess whether enough liver will remain after such donation (Fig. 133-7).[7]

MAGNETIC RESONANCE IMAGING

The advantages of MRI over CT for abdominal evaluation include superior soft tissue contrast resolution and lack of ionizing radiation. Drawbacks include decreased spatial resolution, longer examination times, increased expense, decreased availability, and inability to scan some patients due to claustrophobia or implanted devices such as cardiac pacemakers. Imaging artifacts can also make MRI interpretation more difficult and less uniform across different readers. At many institutions, MRI primarily is used to assess a specific known condition. For example, MR is commonly used to characterize a liver lesion seen on another modality or to determine the local staging of a rectal cancer rather than ordered to evaluate nonspecific abdominal pain or to detect possible abdominal abscesses in a patient with fever of unknown origin.

Contrast-enhanced MRI offers a dynamic evaluation comparable to CT for the solid abdominal organs. Its sensitivity and specificity for detection of focal lesions are better than CT when image quality is good. For example, many institutions screen cirrhotic populations for hepatocellular cancer by MR rather than by CT because of its high accuracy and lack of ionizing radiation. MR also is a good examination in assessing response to local ablative therapies (Fig 133-8). Unfortunately, patient factors (e.g., the inability to hold a breath adequately or large amounts of ascites in cirrhotic patients) can often limit the quality of the MR image, thereby decreasing accuracy.

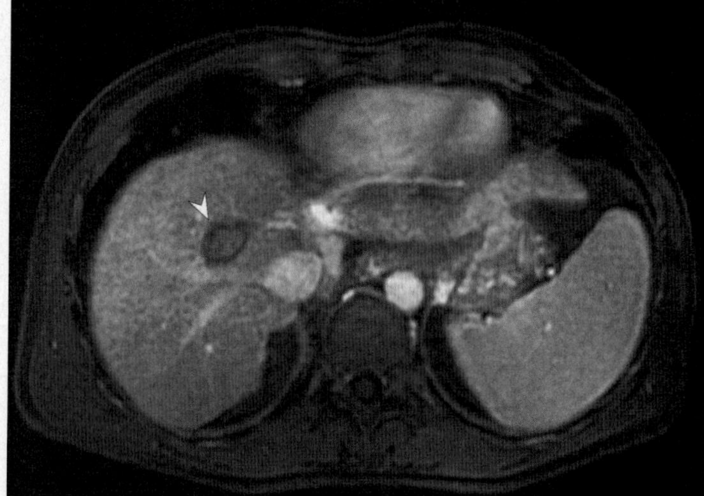

FIGURE 133-8. **Surveillance after microwave ablation of hepatocellular carcinoma.** Contrast-enhanced fat-suppressed gradient echo MRI shows a bland postablation site (*arrowhead*) with central carbonaceous "char" and no evidence of enhancing recurrence in the periphery.

Intravenous gadolinium-based agents with hepatocyte-specific uptake increase MRI's diagnostic capabilities in evaluating focal hepatic lesions. For example, hypervascular lesions, which retain these agents, can be diagnosed as benign focal nodular hyperplasia without the need for biopsy. Because these agents are excreted into the biliary system, the evaluation of possible biliary disease is also improved. The high accuracy of MRI in diagnosis of hepatic steatosis (Chapter 152) can sometimes prevent unnecessary biopsy, particularly in cases of focal fatty infiltration that simulates metastatic disease.

MRI is also sensitive for detection of iron overload within the liver and other organs related to primary hemochromatosis (Chapter 212) and secondary hemosiderosis (most often due to multiple transfusions). Similar to CT, MRI can provide quality arterial and venous angiographic imaging, such that conventional angiography is generally reserved for therapeutic interventions.

Patients with decreased renal function should not receive gadolinium because of their risk for development of the rare nephrogenic systemic fibrosis (Chapter 267), which is characterized by involvement of the skin, eyes, joints, and internal organs. Whether newer formulations of MR gadolinium-based contrast agents may decrease this risk is under investigation.

Three specialized MR examinations have significantly changed practice patterns in recent years. MRCP, a heavily T2-weighted imaging technique for the noninvasive diagnostic evaluation of the biliary and pancreatic ductal systems, relies not on the administration of contrast material but on the presence of static fluid.[8] MRCP can be a useful screening tool to select appropriate candidates for more invasive therapeutic procedures, such as endoscopic retrograde cholangiopancreatography and percutaneous transhepatic cholangiography (Fig. 133-9). MRCP is useful for diagnosis of biliary and pancreatic ductal obstruction, choledocholithiasis, primary sclerosing cholangitis, and cystic conditions such as Caroli disease. T1-weighted MR cholangiography with intravenous administration of contrast agents that undergo biliary excretion can be useful in evaluating for bile leaks, analogous to hepatobiliary scintigraphy.

MR enterography has become the preferred approach for assessment of disease activity in patients with Crohn disease (Chapter 141). Given the lack of ionizing radiation, it is particularly advantageous in young patients who require multiple examinations over a lifetime. Oral contrast agents such as polyethylene glycol and nonabsorbable low-concentration barium preparations are given to distend the small bowel; spasmolytics are typically administered to decrease bowel peristalsis. Similar to CT, fast breath-held imaging with intravenous administration of contrast material allows evaluation of mucosal and wall enhancement or thickening, suggesting active disease. Unlike CT, MRI can assess intrinsic signal characteristics on T2-weighted images to improve specificity and to distinguish active inflammation from chronic fibrostenotic disease (Fig. 133-10).

The use of neoadjuvant rather than adjuvant chemoradiation for stage II to stage IV rectal cancer has made MR staging an important preoperative test[9] before surgical resection. MR is preferred to endoscopic rectal ultrasound for determination of the relationship of the cancer to the mesorectal fascia as well as for detection of lateral pelvic lymph nodes, which cannot be seen by ultrasound because of its limited field of view (Fig. 133-11).

INTERVENTIONAL PROCEDURES

Ultrasound, CT, fluoroscopy, and even MR techniques have been used for guidance in performing a wide variety of abdominal interventional procedures. Percutaneous image-guided biopsy, whether by fine-needle aspiration or core biopsy, is a relatively safe procedure that is commonly performed for tissue diagnosis[10] and has drastically reduced the need for open surgical biopsy. Other common nonvascular procedures that use image guidance include abscess drainage, biliary interventions, gastrostomy, and tumor ablation. In the case of peridiverticular and periappendiceal abscesses, CT-guided drainage can often simplify the ultimate operative approach and turn high-risk emergent surgery into a safer elective procedure. Biliary interventions include transhepatic access of an obstructed system for stenting or external drainage and cholecystostomy tube placement. Percutaneous CT- or ultrasound-guided tumor ablation is a rapidly evolving technique that is particularly useful in poor operative candidates or in conjunction with surgical resection of other lesions.[11] A variety of ablation methods have been employed, including radio frequency, alcohol, microwave, and cryoablation.

Diagnostic conventional angiography has been replaced largely by noninvasive CT and MR techniques, but direct catheter angiography remains an important procedure for directing various therapies. Vascular interventions include angioplasty, stenting, embolization, and thrombolysis. TIPS placement (Chapter 153) is a commonly performed angiographic procedure in patients with portal hypertension complicated by variceal bleeding or

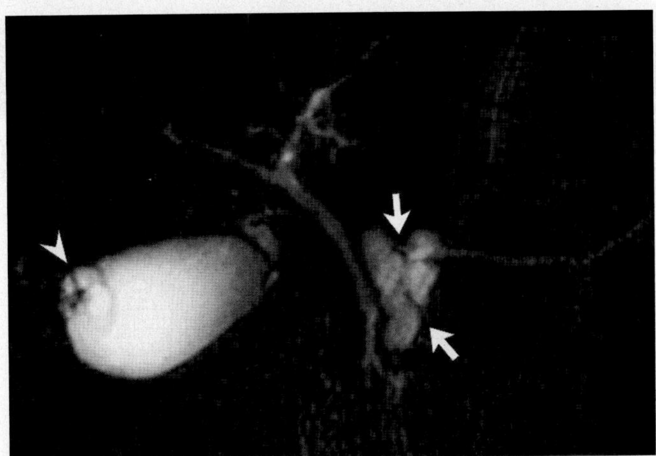

FIGURE 133-9. Pancreatic intraductal papillary mucinous neoplasm on MRCP. Heavily T2-weighted MR image shows a lobulated cystic lesion in the pancreatic head region (*arrows*) that represents a side branch intraductal papillary mucinous neoplasm. Note the mild focal irregularity of the gallbladder (*arrowhead*), consistent with the fundal form of adenomyomatosis. The intrahepatic and extrahepatic biliary ducts are normal.

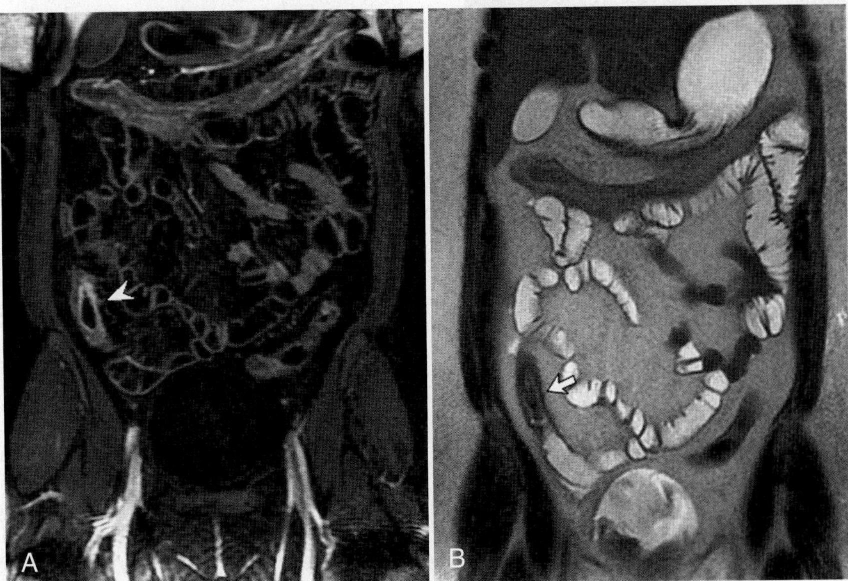

FIGURE 133-10. Active Crohn disease on MR enterography. A, Coronal three-dimensional volume-acquired breath-hold, T1-weighted, gradient-echo image with dynamic gadolinium administration and fat saturation shows wall thickening and enhancement (*arrowhead*) of an abnormal segment of terminal ileum. B, Coronal two-dimensional single-shot, fast spin-echo, T2-weighted image shows increased signal in this area (*arrow*), signifying edema and active disease.

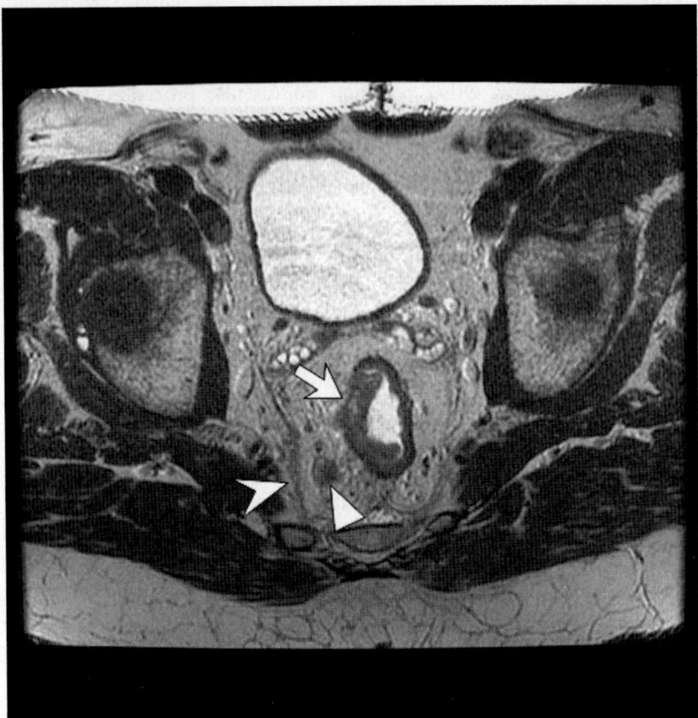

FIGURE 133-11. Preoperative rectal cancer staging by MR. Fast spin-echo T2 image shows the clear margin between the mesorectal fascia (*arrowhead*) and primary cancer (*arrow*) as well as a metastatic lymph node (*triangle*).

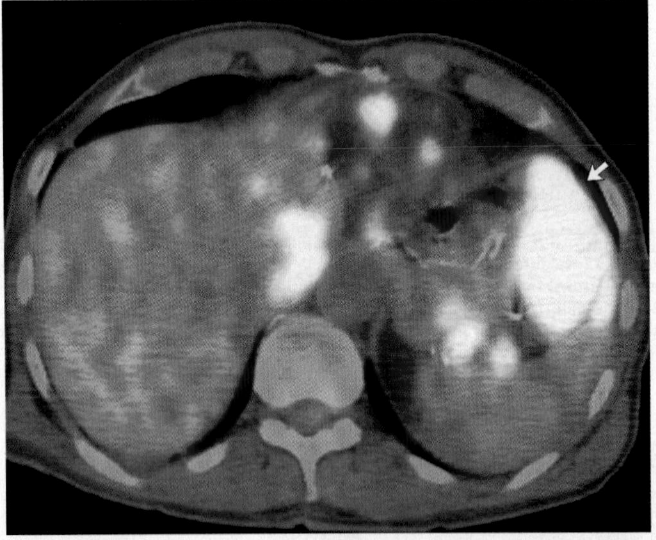

FIGURE 133-12. Metastatic gastrointestinal stromal tumor (GIST) on fused PET/CT. Transverse fused PET/CT image shows a dominant hypermetabolic mass (*arrow*) representing a gastric GIST. Multiple smaller peritoneal and hepatic hypermetabolic foci are consistent with metastatic deposits. Note the utility of combining the functional information from PET with the anatomic localization provided by CT.

intractable ascites. Placement of a TIPS stent creates a low-pressure communication between the portal and hepatic venous systems. Chemoembolization can provide palliation for those with advanced hepatic malignant disease, whether primary or metastatic.

NUCLEAR MEDICINE (RADIONUCLIDE SCINTIGRAPHY)

Owing to the emergence of PET/CT for oncologic evaluation, nuclear medicine is more relevant now than ever before in abdominal imaging. PET/CT is a powerful diagnostic tool that combines functional and anatomic imaging. PET is useful for both initial staging and evaluating the response to therapy for a wide range of primary malignant tumors, especially when it is combined with CT (Fig. 133-12). Currently, clinical PET imaging most often uses ^{18}F-fluorodeoxyglucose, but other positron-emitting agents may be used for specific purposes. PET/MR also is a newer combined modality.[12]

Several other nuclear medicine studies are used to evaluate GI and hepatobiliary diseases. Injection of red blood cells labeled with technetium Tc 99m provides a useful test for GI bleeding. Advantages of performing this as the initial diagnostic imaging study include its noninvasive nature, high sensitivity for active bleeding, and ability to rescan the patient hours later without the need for repeated injection. Disadvantages include relatively poor anatomic localization and lack of therapeutic ability. The use of tagged red blood cell scintigraphy for the diagnosis of hepatic cavernous hemangioma has decreased significantly owing to advances in CT and MRI. Hepatobiliary scintigraphy remains a useful tool in equivocal cases of cholecystitis, particularly acalculous disease, and it can confirm suspected biliary leaks. Scintigraphic imaging with ^{111}In-octreotide is valuable for the diagnosis, staging, and follow-up of GI neuroendocrine tumors, such as carcinoid and pancreatic islet cell tumors.

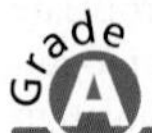

Grade A Reference

A1. Kim K, Kim YH, Kim SY, et al. Low-dose abdominal CT for evaluating suspected appendicitis. *N Engl J Med.* 2012;366:1596-1605.

GENERAL REFERENCES

For the General References and other additional features, please visit Expert Consult at https://expertconsult.inkling.com.

134 GASTROINTESTINAL ENDOSCOPY

PANKAJ JAY PASRICHA

IMPORTANCE AND USE OF ENDOSCOPY

Technologic advances in radiologic and endoscopic imaging have transformed medicine in the past few decades. With its remarkable accessibility, the gastrointestinal tract, perhaps more than any other organ system, has benefited particularly from the endoscopic approach. The major advantages of endoscopy over contrast radiography for evaluation of diseases of the alimentary tract include direct visualization, resulting in a more accurate and sensitive evaluation of mucosal lesions; the ability to obtain biopsy specimens from superficial lesions; and the ability to perform therapeutic interventions. These advantages make endoscopy the procedure of choice in most cases in which mucosal lesions or growths are suspected. Conversely, computed tomography (CT) or, occasionally, contrast radiography may be indicated when extrinsic or intrinsic distortions of anatomy are suspected, such as volvulus, intussusceptions, subtle strictures, or complicated postsurgical changes (Chapter 133).

On the therapeutic front, the endoscopic approach (transorally or transrectally) is increasingly being used to replace traditional and more invasive forms of surgery, a trend that is expected to gain strength in the years to come. In this context, the flexible endoscope is rapidly becoming an essential tool for both gastroenterologists and surgeons alike.

INSTRUMENTS AND PROCEDURES

Endoscopic procedures and their therapeutic applications are described in Table 134-1.

Luminal Endoscopy: Conventional and Wireless

The modern gastrointestinal endoscope is a "videoscope," with a charged couple device chip at its tip. The scope itself is tethered to a light source and video processer, and the image is displayed on one or more monitors. The endoscopic shaft not only carries the optical elements for imaging but also contains channels that enable various functions, such as air insufflation, water irrigation, suction, and passage of diagnostic and therapeutic devices.

Endoscopy no longer requires tethering to a light source. The capsule endoscope, a disposable plastic capsule that is approximately the size of a large vitamin pill, contains a chip camera, batteries, and a radio transmitter

TABLE 134-1 ENDOSCOPIC PROCEDURES AND GENERAL APPLICATIONS

ENDOSCOPIC PROCEDURE	THERAPEUTIC APPLICATIONS
LUMINAL ENDOSCOPY	
Common procedures Esophagogastroduodenoscopy Colonoscopy Flexible sigmoidoscopy	Hemostasis Luminal restoration (dilation, ablation, stenting) Lesion removal (e.g., polypectomy, mucosal ablation) Provision of access (percutaneous endoscopic gastrostomy and jejunostomy)
Less common procedures Enteroscopy Capsule endoscopy	Barrier strengthening (antireflux procedures)
PANCREATOBILIARY IMAGING	
Endoscopic retrograde cholangiopancreatography	Lesion (stone) removal Luminal restoration (dilation, stenting) Provision of access (sphincterotomy) Drainage (bile, pancreatic pseudocyst)
TRANSLUMINAL IMAGING	
Endoscopic ultrasonography	Analgesic block Delivery of therapeutic agents (experimental)

that wirelessly sends images to a device that the patient wears as a belt. At the end of the procedure, the information is downloaded to a computer, and the capsule itself passes out harmlessly in the stool. The capsule endoscope has allowed routine evaluation of the entire length of the small bowel, a feat that was challenging and oftentimes impossible with conventional instruments. Variations of the capsule endoscope have been developed for esophageal and colonic imaging, but the utility of these capsules in routine clinical practice has not been established.

Ancillary Organ Imaging: Endoscopic Retrograde Cholangiography and Pancreatography

Endoscopic retrograde cholangiopancreatography (ERCP) uses a side-viewing endoscope that accesses the second part of the duodenum, where a small catheter is then introduced into the bile or pancreatic duct to inject radiographic contrast medium under fluoroscopic monitoring. Successful cannulation and imaging can be achieved in up to 95% of cases. In some instances, a fine-caliber endoscope can also be introduced into the duct of interest (cholangioscopy or pancreatoscopy) for direct visualization of intraductal disease.

Mural and Transmural Imaging: Endoscopic Ultrasonography

An ultrasonic transducer in the tip of a flexible endoscope or a stand-alone ultrasound probe inserted through the channel of a regular endoscope can image lesions within the wall of the gut as well as adjacent lymph nodes, vascular structures, and neighboring organs such as the pancreas. Endoscopic ultrasonography (EUS) can guide fine-needle aspiration of suspicious lesions more accurately than abdominal ultrasonography or CT.

COMPLICATIONS AND PRE-ENDOSCOPIC PREPARATION

Diagnostic endoscopy is a remarkably safe and well-tolerated procedure.[1] It can be performed under conscious sedation with a combination of benzodiazepines and narcotics or increasingly in the United States with propofol. Although propofol provides faster and deeper sedation with rapid recovery (Chapter 432), it adds significantly to the cost of the procedure, principally because of the need for monitored anesthesia care. Recent Food and Drug Administration approval of a computer-assisted semiautomated delivery and monitoring system for propofol may address some of these concerns.

Although rare, potential complications (Table 134-2) must be carefully explained to the patient as part of the informed consent process.[2,3] In general, routine blood tests, radiographs, or electrocardiograms are not necessary before endoscopy unless a careful history and physical examination suggest possible hematologic, cardiovascular, or pulmonary and airway problems. Women of childbearing age should be questioned about the possibility of pregnancy and tested if there is any doubt.

Diagnostic endoscopies, including those with mucosal biopsies, are considered low enough risk that they do not warrant discontinuation

TABLE 134-2 COMPLICATIONS OF ENDOSCOPY

ENDOSCOPIC COMPLICATION	INCIDENCE (%)	SPECIFIC PROPHYLAXIS
GENERAL COMPLICATIONS		
Complications related primarily to sedation (cardiovascular and respiratory depression, aspiration)	0.6-0.7	Airway protection with massive upper gastrointestinal bleeding Preprocedure medical evaluation, intraprocedure and postprocedure monitoring Anesthesiology consultation for high-risk patients
Perforation	0.1-0.3 (upper endoscopy) 0.14-0.25 (colonoscopy)	None (except careful technique)
Bleeding	0.3 (upper endoscopy) 0.7-2.5 (polypectomy)	Carefully balance risk and benefits Discontinue or reduce anticoagulant use before high-risk procedures
Bacteremia and infectious complications (endocarditis, bacterial ascites)	<0.1	Antibiotics for patients at risk for endocarditis (patients with artificial valves, pulmonary-systemic shunts, previous history of endocarditis), with synthetic vascular grafts, and with bacterial ascites (cirrhotics)
Death	0.6 (upper endoscopy) 0.2 (colonoscopy)	
COMPLICATIONS ASSOCIATED WITH SPECIALIZED PROCEDURES		
Pancreatitis (ERCP)	3-20	Rectal indomethacin
Cholangitis (ERCP)	0.1-2	Preprocedure antibiotics
Wound infections (PEG)	3-4	Preprocedure antibiotics

ERCP = endoscopic retrograde cholangiopancreatography; PEG = percutaneous endoscopic gastrostomy.

of anticoagulant medication. Similarly, patients undergoing screening colonoscopy can continue aspirin or other nonsteroidal anti-inflammatory agents. In high-risk elective procedures, the decision to withhold anticoagulants and antiplatelet agents should be individualized. Depending on the underlying thromboembolic risk, patients may require "bridging" therapy with agents in the heparin family (Chapters 38 and 431). For patients with acute bleeding, reversal therapy or platelet replacement may be considered (Chapters 171 through 175).

ERCP is associated with the highest risk of serious complications, with about 5% of cases developing pancreatitis. Most experts will place a short-term pancreatic stent in high-risk cases as a reasonable preventive measure. Prophylactic rectal indomethacin (two 50-mg suppositories immediately after the completion of the procedure) reduces the incidence of post-ERCP pancreatitis by almost 50%[A1] and is becoming the standard of care.

SPECIFIC INDICATIONS

Most indications for gastrointestinal endoscopy are based on the presenting symptoms of the patient (e.g., dysphagia, bleeding, diarrhea). In other instances, endoscopy is required to evaluate specific lesions found by other diagnostic imaging, such as a gastric ulcer or colon polyp discovered by barium radiography. Finally, screening endoscopy is often performed in asymptomatic individuals on the basis of their risk for commonly occurring and preventable conditions, such as colon cancer (see later).

Implicit in the decision to perform endoscopy is the assumption that it will have a bearing on future management strategy. In evaluating gastrointestinal symptoms, several questions need to be addressed by the referring physician and the endoscopist. Which patients need endoscopy? When should the endoscopy be done? What is the endoscopist looking for? What endoscopic therapy, if any, should be planned?

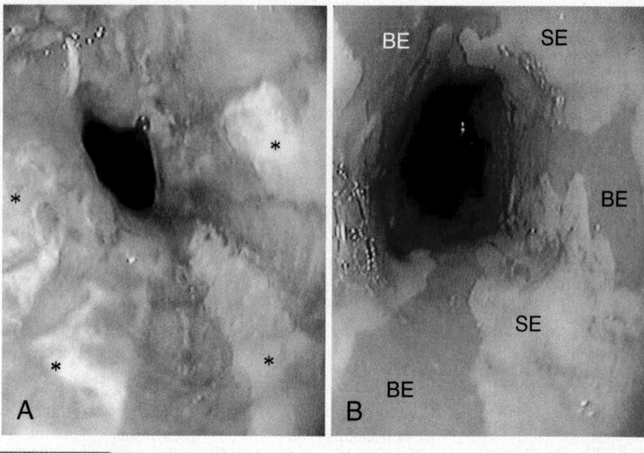

FIGURE 134-1. Severe reflux esophagitis (*left*) with mucosal erythema and linear ulcers with yellow exudates (*asterisks*). It is thought that such changes eventually lead to Barrett esophagus (*right*), in which the normal white squamous epithelium (SE) is replaced by red columnar epithelium (BE). These pictures are from different patients.

Gastroesophageal Reflux and Heartburn (Chapters 138 and 139)

Gastroesophageal reflux disease (GERD) is an extremely common condition in the general population. The fact that its cardinal symptom, heartburn, is relatively specific for this condition justifies an empirical approach to treatment by a combination of lifestyle modifications and over-the-counter or even prescription drugs. Endoscopy is not therefore necessary to make the diagnosis of GERD. Indeed, normal findings on endoscopy do not exclude the diagnosis of GERD because the overall sensitivity of endoscopy in GERD is only about 70%. If necessary, further evaluation with ambulatory esophageal manometry and pH monitoring may be indicated to establish the diagnosis. However, there are several circumstances in which endoscopy should be considered for patients with reflux, including patients with associated warning symptoms ("red flags"), such as dysphagia, odynophagia, regurgitation, weight loss, gastrointestinal bleeding, or frequent vomiting (Fig. 134-1). These symptoms imply either the development of a GERD-related complication (erosive esophagitis, stricture, or adenocarcinoma) or another disorder masquerading as GERD (esophageal cancer or a gastric-duodenal lesion such as cancer or peptic ulcer). Another group of patients who are candidates for endoscopy are those with severe, persistent, or frequently recurrent symptoms that suggest significant esophagitis and hence a risk for complications, such as stricture or Barrett esophagus, which is intestinal metaplasia of the esophageal epithelium.

If a significant length of Barrett esophagus, especially more than 3 cm, is discovered (see Fig. 134-1), most experts recommend some form of periodic surveillance endoscopy because of the increased risk for the development of adenocarcinoma. Control of reflux by either pharmacologic or surgical means does not generally lead to regression of established Barrett esophagus (Chapter 138). For patients whose high-grade dysplasia associated with Barrett esophagus poses a serious risk for future cancer, endoscopic ablation or resection may provide a potentially curative alternative to surgical esophagectomy.[A2] Ablation can be achieved by a variety of modalities, including radio frequency, cryotherapy, electrical cautery, argon plasma coagulation, and photodynamic therapy. An alternative to ablation is endoscopic mucosal resection, which is en bloc resection of the mucosa to allow a complete pathologic analysis and to minimize the risk for regrowth of the abnormal mucosal lining.

Several endoscopic techniques are potential alternatives to surgical fundoplication for patients whose reflux is not satisfactorily managed by medical therapy.[4] These include methods that provide thermal energy to the lower esophageal sphincter and others that serve to tighten the gastroesophageal "valve" area. Other procedures that are in clinical trials include electrical stimulation by implantable electrodes.

Heartburn in immunocompromised patients often indicates an esophageal infection with an opportunistic organism, such as *Candida albicans*, cytomegalovirus, or herpesvirus. Because most patients with the acquired immunodeficiency syndrome (AIDS) and esophagitis have candidiasis, an empirical course of antifungal therapy may be justified. Patients who do not respond to this approach, however, should almost always have endoscopy and biopsy so that more specific therapy can be instituted.

Dysphagia (Chapter 138)

Dysphagia can often be categorized as oropharyngeal on the basis of the clinical features of nasal regurgitation, laryngeal aspiration, or difficulty in moving the bolus out of the mouth. These symptoms are usually associated with a lesion in the central or peripheral nervous system. Although endoscopy is often performed in these patients, videofluoroesophagography (modified barium swallow or cine-esophagogram) is the procedure of choice because it allows a frame-by-frame evaluation of the rapid sequence of events involved in transfer of the bolus from the mouth to the esophagus. Common causes of dysphagia in the esophageal body include malignant as well as benign processes (peptic strictures secondary to reflux, Schatzki ring) and motility disturbances. Endoscopic examination is considered mandatory in all patients with esophageal dysphagia. However, contrast esophagography is helpful; it can provide guidance for endoscopy that is anticipated to be difficult (e.g., a patient with a complex stricture or diverticulum), suggest a disturbance in motility, and occasionally detect subtle stenoses that are not appreciated on endoscopy (the scope diameter is typically ≤10 mm, whereas some symptomatic strictures can be considerably wider).

Endoscopic treatment options are available for many causes of esophageal dysphagia. Tumors can be ablated by thermal means (cautery or laser) or stented with prosthetic devices. Metallic expandable stents have become the palliative procedure of choice for most patients with symptomatic esophageal cancer. Benign lesions of the esophagus, such as strictures or rings, can also be dilated endoscopically, usually with excellent results. Finally, some motility disturbances, such as achalasia, may be approached endoscopically with the use of large balloon dilators for the lower esophageal sphincter or, in the case of high-risk patients, local injection of botulinum toxin.

Dyspepsia (Chapter 137)

Dyspepsia, which is chronic or recurring pain or discomfort centered in the upper abdomen, is a common condition that can be caused by a variety of disorders, including peptic ulcer, reflux esophagitis, gallstones, gastric dysmotility, and, rarely, gastric or esophageal cancer. However, up to 60% of patients with chronic (>3 months) dyspepsia belong to the so-called functional category in which there is no definite structural or biochemical explanation for the symptoms. Although *Helicobacter pylori* gastritis is found frequently in these patients, there is no definite evidence to prove a cause-and-effect relationship between these two findings. If a diagnostic test is to be performed, endoscopy, sometimes with biopsies to detect *H. pylori*, is clearly the procedure of choice (see Fig. 139-2), with accuracy of about 90% compared with about 65% for double-contrast radiography. Because dyspepsia is a recurrent condition and because patients who do not respond to empirical therapy eventually almost always undergo endoscopy, many gastroenterologists opt for early endoscopy, if only for the reassurance that a normal examination provides.

Upper Gastrointestinal Bleeding (Chapter 135)

Acid peptic disease (including ulcers, erosions, and gastritis), variceal bleeding, and Mallory-Weiss tears account for most cases of upper gastrointestinal bleeding. Other less common but important lesions are angiomas, gastric vascular ectasia ("watermelon" stomach), and the uncommon Dieulafoy lesion (a superficial artery that erodes through the gut mucosa). Finally, upper gastrointestinal cancers are occasionally associated with significant bleeding. Endoscopy is mandatory in all patients with upper gastrointestinal bleeding, with the rare exception being the terminally ill patient in whom the outcome is unlikely to be affected. Endoscopy is able to detect and to localize the site of the bleeding in 95% of cases and is clearly superior to contrast radiography (with an accuracy of only 75 to 80%). The endoscopic appearance of bleeding lesions can also help predict the risk of rebleeding, thus facilitating the triage and treatment process. Bleeding can be effectively controlled during the initial endoscopic examination itself in the majority of cases. The risk of recurrent bleeding is diminished, thereby resulting in a shorter duration of hospital stay as well as a reduction in the need for surgery.

In general, endoscopy should be performed only after adequate stabilization of hemodynamic and respiratory parameters. The role of gastric lavage before endoscopy is controversial; some endoscopists prefer that it be done, occasionally even with use of a large-bore tube, whereas others avoid such preparation because of the fear of producing artifact. The timing of subsequent endoscopy depends on two factors: the severity of the hemorrhage and the risk status of the patient. Patients with active, persistent, or severe bleeding (>3 units of blood) require urgent endoscopy. In these patients,

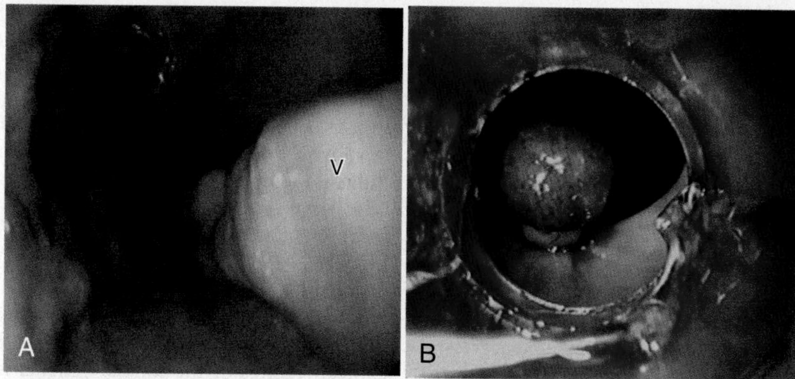

FIGURE 134-2. Endoscopic view of esophageal varices (*left*) in the wall of the esophagus (V). *Right*, Image of a varix that has been endoscopically ligated with a band.

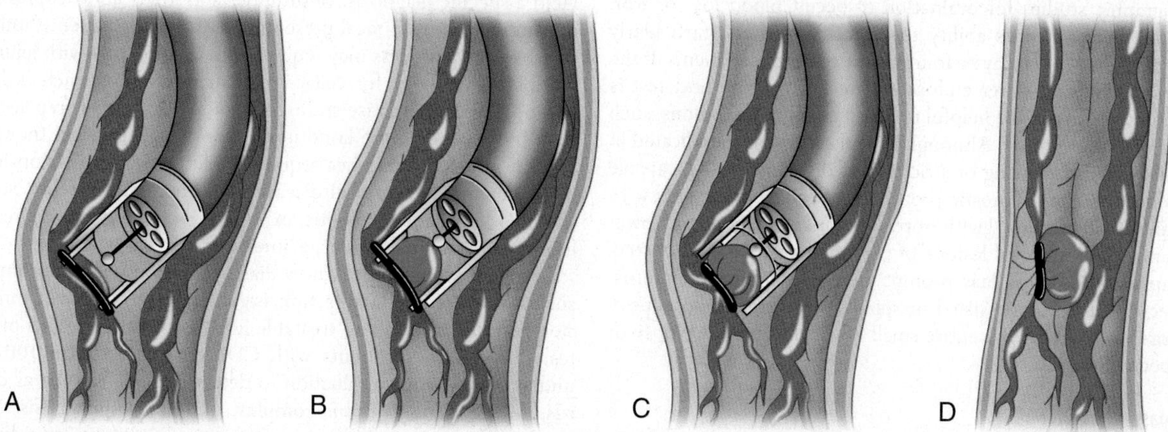

FIGURE 134-3. Endoscopic variceal ligation technique. A, The endoscope, with attached ligating device, is brought into contact with a varix just above the gastroesophageal junction. B, Suction is applied, drawing the varix-containing mucosa into the dead space created at the end of the endoscope by the ligating device. C, The tripwire is pulled, releasing the band around the aspirated tissue. D, Completed ligation.

endoscopy is best performed in the intensive care unit because of the risk for aspiration and the occasional need for emergent intubation to provide respiratory protection and ventilation. Patients with slower or inactive bleeding may be evaluated by endoscopy in a "semielective" manner (usually within 12 to 20 hours), but a case can be made to perform endoscopy early even in these stable patients (perhaps in the emergency department itself) to allow more confident triage and efficient resource management.[5]

Nonvariceal bleeding vessels can be treated by a variety of means, including injections of various substances (epinephrine, saline, sclerosants), thermal coagulation (laser or electrocautery), and mechanical means (clipping). In the United States, the most popular approach to a bleeding peptic ulcer lesion is a combination of injection with dilute epinephrine and electrocoagulation. Initial hemostasis can be achieved in more than 90% cases; rebleeding, which may occur in up to 20% of cases, responds about half of the time to a second endoscopic procedure. Patients who continue to bleed (typically patients with large ulcers in the posterior wall of the duodenal bulb) are usually managed by interventional angiography (with embolization of the bleeding vessel) or surgically.

Variceal bleeding is also effectively managed endoscopically, with a success rate similar to that with bleeding ulcers (Fig. 134-2). Hemostasis with band ligation (Fig. 134-3) has replaced the older methods of sclerotherapy because of fewer side effects. Even if initial endoscopic hemostasis is successful, long-term prevention of rebleeding requires a program of ongoing endoscopic sessions until variceal obliteration is complete. Patients who do not respond to endoscopic treatment are considered candidates for a transjugular intrahepatic portosystemic shunt. In patients whose large esophageal varices have never bled, β-blockers are considered first-line treatment, but endoscopic band ligation may be useful in selected patients.

Acute Lower Gastrointestinal Bleeding

The most common cause of acute lower gastrointestinal bleeding is angiodysplasia, followed by diverticulosis, neoplasms, and colitis. In about 10% of patients presenting with hematochezia, a small bowel lesion may be responsible. In contrast to upper gastrointestinal bleeding, there is no single best test for acute lower gastrointestinal bleeding (Fig. 134-4). In young patients (<40 years old) with minor bleeding, features that are highly suggestive of anorectal origin (e.g., blood on the surface of the stool or on the wipe) may warrant only flexible sigmoidoscopy. Conversely, patients presenting with hemodynamic compromise may need upper endoscopy first to exclude a lesion in the upper gastrointestinal tract (typically postpyloric) bleeding so briskly that it presents as hematochezia. Colonoscopy has been traditionally recommended after bleeding has slowed or stopped and the patient has been given an adequate bowel purge. However, a disadvantage of delaying endoscopy is that when a pathologic lesion such as an arteriovenous malformation (see Fig. 134-4) or diverticulum is found, it may be impossible to implicate it confidently as the site of bleeding (complementary information by radiography or scintigraphy becomes particularly important in this situation). Some

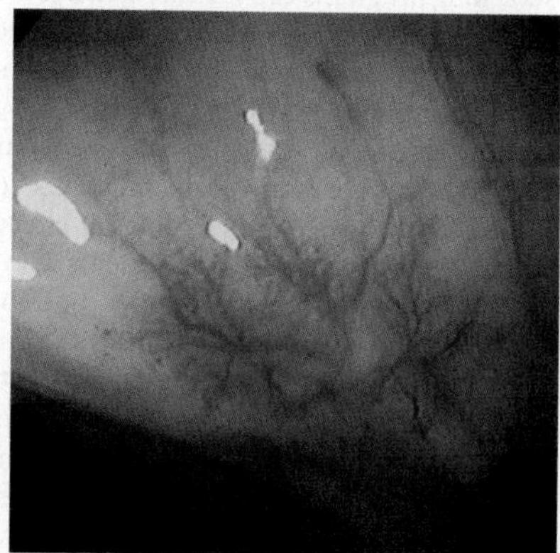

FIGURE 134-4. Mucosal telangiectasia (arteriovenous malformation) in the colon. The patient presented with hematochezia. The lesion was subsequently cauterized endoscopically.

experts therefore recommend urgent diagnostic endoscopy with little or no preparation for acute lower gastrointestinal hemorrhages and have reported significant diagnostic as well as therapeutic success rates. However, such recommendations have not been universally accepted and remain logistically difficult to implement in most hospital settings. If an acute bleeding site cannot be identified by upper and lower gastrointestinal endoscopy, capsule endoscopy is better than angiography to find the source of bleeding.[A3]

Occult Gastrointestinal Bleeding or Iron Deficiency Anemia

Normal fecal blood loss is usually less than 2 to 3 mL/day. Most standard fecal occult blood tests detect blood loss of only 10 mL/day or more. Therefore, even if this test result is negative, patients with iron deficiency anemia and no other obvious source of blood loss should always undergo aggressive gastrointestinal evaluation, which uncovers a gastrointestinal lesion in the majority of cases. Although most lesions that cause overt gastrointestinal bleeding can also cause occult blood loss, occult bleeding should almost never be ascribed to diverticulosis or hemorrhoids. Endoscopy is always preferable to radiographic studies for evaluation of occult blood loss or iron deficiency anemia because of its ability to detect flat lesions, particularly vascular malformations, which may be found in 6% or more of patients. If the findings on both upper and lower endoscopy are normal, the next test is capsule endoscopy, which may be helpful to detect small bowel lesions, such as erosions, tumors, or angiomas. Although it is relatively contraindicated in patients with suspected narrowing or strictures of the small bowel, capsule endoscopy has become the diagnostic procedure of choice in patients with obscure gastrointestinal bleeding (with normal findings on upper and lower endoscopies) and when mucosal lesions of the small bowel are suspected. Findings on capsule endoscopy may prompt the consideration of enteroscopy (with specialized balloon-assisted or spirally advancing endoscopes), which can theoretically access the entire small bowel and permit biopsy or therapy of suspected lesions.

Colorectal Neoplasms (Chapter 193)

Colonoscopy is the most accurate test for detection of mass lesions of the large bowel or colon that are suspected on clinical or radiologic grounds. However, the greatest impact of endoscopy on colorectal neoplasia may be in the area of screening and prevention. The adenoma to carcinoma sequence of progression in colorectal cancer provides a unique opportunity for prophylaxis. Thus, if screening programs can identify patients with polyps and if these polyps are removed, cancer can largely be prevented. Various techniques are available for safe and effective polypectomy, depending on the size, presence of a stalk, and location (Fig. 134-5). Colonoscopy is currently recommended for screening of patients at average risk, that is, anyone older than 50 years. Adenomatous polyps are removed, and patients are entered into a surveillance program with follow-up colonoscopies at intervals that depend on the nature and number of the initial lesions. Patients who do not have any polyps generally do not require follow-up colonoscopies more than once every 10 years. More aggressive screening strategies are required for patients considered at high risk for colorectal cancer, including patients with well-defined hereditary syndromes as well as those with a history of colorectal cancer in a first-degree relative. In addition, patients with ulcerative colitis (Chapter 141) with long-standing (>8 years) disease affecting the entire colon have an increased risk for development of colon cancer, about 0.5 to 3% after 20 years.

CT colonography (Chapter 133), which involves the digital construction of an endoluminal view of the colon on the basis of data from abdominal CT, has generally replaced barium enema as an alternative method for colon cancer screening.[A4] It has not, however, generally replaced colonoscopy, in part because it misses smaller polyps and in part because any abnormalities found on CT colonoscopy require colonoscopic follow-up.[A5] Its major utility is for screening patients who have an incomplete colonoscopy. Imaging of the colon by capsule endoscopes is currently not adequate and not recommended.

Chronic Diarrhea (Chapter 140)

Endoscopy may be a valuable aid in the evaluation of patients with persistent diarrhea. The timing of the endoscopy in these patients often depends on the clinical features of the illness. Patients with bloody diarrhea should have lower endoscopy as part of their initial evaluation to determine if inflammatory bowel disease is present (Chapter 141). In most patients with chronic diarrhea, endoscopy is often done when initial routine testing does not yield a specific diagnosis. Both upper and lower endoscopies may be used, depending on the clinical presentation. Thus, the patient thought to have a malabsorptive process may require upper endoscopy with jejunal or duodenal biopsies to look for celiac sprue or rare lesions such as lymphoma or Whipple disease because endoscopic biopsy has largely replaced blind intestinal biopsies for these conditions. Conversely, patients thought to have a secretory cause of diarrhea require a colonoscopy with biopsies to look for overt inflammatory bowel disease or more subtle variants such as microscopic or lymphocytic colitis, in which cases the diagnosis requires careful examination of the biopsy specimens.

The endoscopic approach to diarrhea in immunocompromised patients, such as those with HIV infection, is guided by the degree of immunosuppression and the need to find treatable infections. When results of routine stool tests are negative, patients with CD4 counts less than $100/mm^3$ should undergo endoscopic evaluation to detect pathogens, such as cytomegalovirus, *Mycobacterium avium* complex, and microsporidiosis. Small-volume stools with tenesmus suggest proctocolitis, for which sigmoidoscopy (rather than a full colonoscopy) with biopsies is usually adequate. In patients with upper gastrointestinal symptoms (large-volume diarrhea, bloating, and dyspepsia), upper endoscopy with small bowel biopsy may be attempted first.

Miscellaneous Indications

The upper endoscope has provided a relatively quick and noninvasive means for removal of accidentally or deliberately ingested foreign bodies. Timing is critical for removal, however, because objects are usually beyond endoscopic retrieval when they reach the small bowel. Any foreign object that is causing symptoms should be removed, as should potentially dangerous devices such as batteries and sharp objects. In general, objects larger than 2.5 cm in width or 13 cm in length are unlikely to leave the stomach and so should also be removed. On occasion, patients with food impacted in the esophagus require endoscopic removal (Fig. 134-6). This condition almost always indicates an underlying functional or structural problem (Chapter 138) and should prompt a thorough diagnostic evaluation after the acute problem has been addressed.

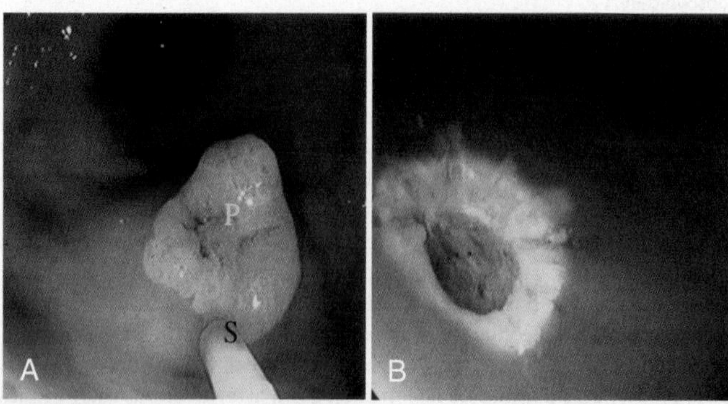

FIGURE 134-5. Endoscopic polypectomy. *Left,* A snare (S) has been passed through the endoscope and positioned around the polyp (P). *Right,* Subsequently, cautery was applied and the polyp guillotined, leaving behind a clean mucosal defect.

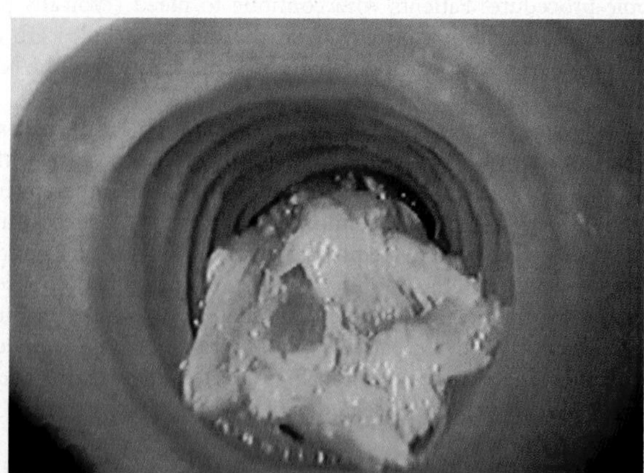

FIGURE 134-6. Impacted food bolus in a young male patient who was found to have a ringed esophagus on endoscopy. This presentation is characteristic and may be either congenital or acquired secondary to reflux-induced or eosinophilic esophagitis.

Because of the relatively poor correlation between oropharyngeal lesions and more distal visceral injury, upper endoscopy is usually recommended urgently in patients with corrosive ingestion (Chapter 110). Endoscopy allows patients to be divided into high- or low-risk groups for complications, with institution of appropriate monitoring and therapy.

Malignant obstruction of the gastrointestinal lumen including the esophagus (Fig. 134-7), pylorus or duodenum, and colon can now be safely and effectively palliated endoscopically by expandable metal stents, thereby avoiding the need for surgery. Colonoscopy is also useful in patients with pseudo-obstructive (nonobstructive) colonic dilation or Ogilvie syndrome; such patients are at risk for colonic rupture at diameters of more than 9 to 12 cm, and colonoscopic decompression is often required, sometimes on an emergent basis.

A major advance in enteral feeding has been the introduction of percutaneous endoscopic gastrostomy (PEG), a relatively quick, simple, and safe endoscopic procedure that has virtually eliminated surgical placement of gastric tubes. The most common indication for these procedures is the need for sustained nutrition in patients with neurologic impairment of swallowing or with head and neck cancers. Patients with a short life expectancy are not suitable candidates for PEG and can be managed by nasoenteral tubes. Further, despite its intuitive appeal, there is little or no evidence that PEG feeding alters clinical or nutritional outcomes or significantly improves quality of life. A variation of PEG is percutaneous endoscopic jejunostomy (PEJ), in which a long tube is passed through the gastric tube, past the pylorus, and into the jejunum. PEJ does not prevent aspiration, but it is effective in patients who have significant impairment of gastric emptying. Retrograde tube migration with PEJ is common, however, and may require frequent replacement.

Therapeutic endoscopy is increasingly an option for patients who have leaks, perforations, or even fistulas.[6] However, its precise role in these situations remains to be clarified.

PANCREATOBILIARY ENDOSCOPY (IMAGING)

Suspected Biliary Disease (Chapter 155)

The diagnostic approach to patients with cholestasis begins with an attempt to differentiate obstructive from hepatocellular causes. The most common causes of obstructive jaundice are common bile duct stones and tumors of the pancreatic and bile ducts. Less invasive conventional imaging with ultrasonography, CT, or magnetic resonance imaging demonstrates dilated bile ducts and mass lesions but is not sensitive or specific for the detection or delineation of pathologic changes in the distal common bile duct and pancreas, two regions where the majority of obstructing lesions are found. Furthermore, some biliary diseases, such as sclerosing cholangitis, do not result in dilated ducts but have a characteristic appearance on cholangiography. Finally, the ability to use devices such as cytology brushes and biopsy forceps during cholangiography provides an additional aid in the diagnosis of biliary lesions. Both percutaneous and endoscopic cholangiographic techniques are associated with a high rate of success in experienced hands, but the endoscopic approach allows visualization of the ampullary region and the performance of sphincterotomy and also avoids the small risk of a biliary leak associated with puncture of the liver capsule.

In the last few years, magnetic resonance cholangiopancreatography (MRCP), a digital reconstruction technique based on an abdominal MR imaging scan, has become popular as an imaging modality for the pancreatobiliary system, with excellent sensitivity and specificity. Because of its relative safety, this procedure should be routinely used for screening of patients with a low likelihood of disease because it avoids the risk of pancreatitis associated with ERCP. In patients with a higher probability of having a definite lesion, however, ERCP is still the procedure of choice because of its therapeutic options.

Of the approximately 600,000 patients undergoing cholecystectomy in the United States, 5 to 10% may present with bile duct stones before or after surgery. Endoscopic stone removal is successful in 90% or more of these cases and usually requires a sphincterotomy (Fig. 134-8). The sphincter of Oddi is a band of muscle that encircles the distal common bile duct and pancreatic duct in the region of the ampulla of Vater; cutting of this muscle, or sphincterotomy, is one of the mainstays of endoscopic biliary treatment and is accomplished with a special tool called a papillotome or sphincterotome. This procedure is often sufficient for the treatment of small stones in the bile ducts, but larger stones may require additional procedures, such as mechanical, electrohydraulic, or laser lithotripsy, which can be performed endoscopically. In addition to stone disease, sphincterotomy can be curative for patients with papillary stenosis. In other patients with suspected spasm of the biliary sphincter (termed sphincter of Oddi dysfunction), sphincter pressures can be measured by manometry, although the role of sphincterotomy in the treatment of these patients is much more controversial and associated with some of the highest risks for pancreatitis. Finally, by enlarging the access to the bile duct, sphincterotomy facilitates the passage of stents and other devices into the bile duct.

Endoscopic placement of indwelling metal stents for malignant biliary obstruction is superior to both radiologic and surgical techniques.

Pancreatic Neoplasms

EUS is probably the single best test for diagnosis of pancreatic tumors (Chapter 195), particularly the small endocrine varieties, with sensitivities approaching 95% (Fig. 134-9). It is also the procedure of choice for imaging of submucosal and other mural lesions of the gastrointestinal tract (overall accuracy of 65 to 70%) as well as for staging of a variety of gastrointestinal tumors (overall accuracy of 90% or more), especially esophageal and pancreatic cancer. EUS-directed celiac plexus neurolysis appears to be effective for

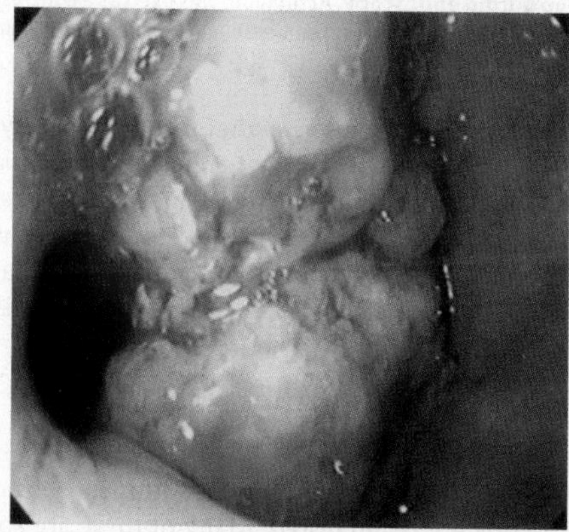

FIGURE 134-7. Large malignant mass at the gastroesophageal junction as seen endoscopically.

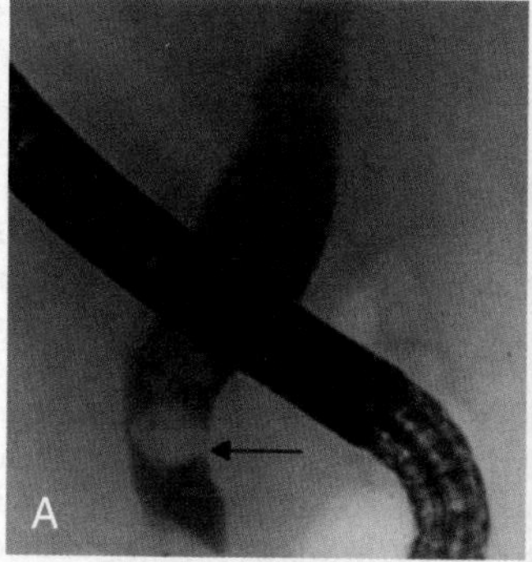

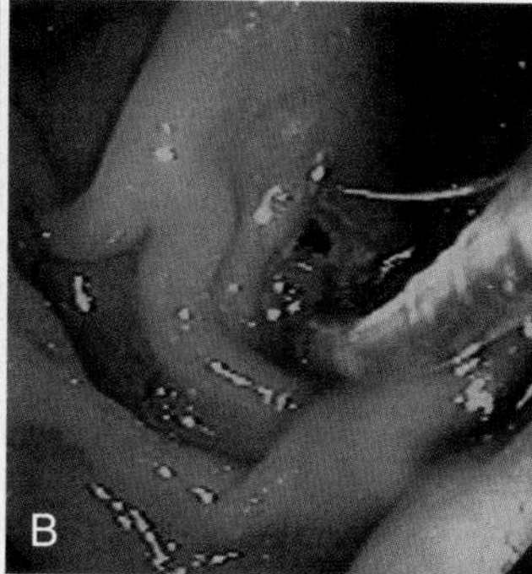

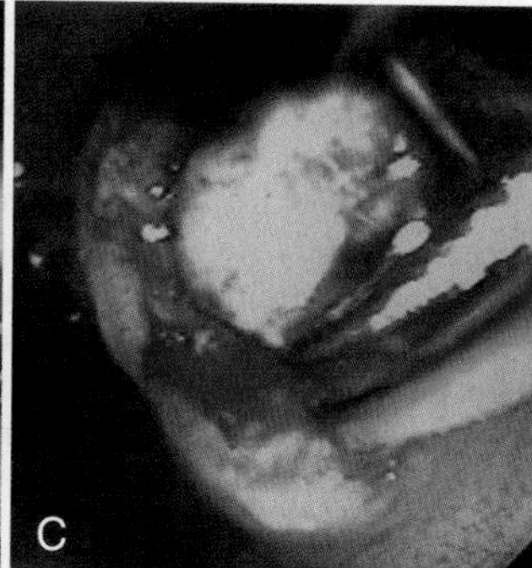

FIGURE 134-8. **Biliary sphincterotomy and stone removal from the bile duct.** *Left,* Endoscopic retrograde cholangiographic image showing stones (*arrow*) in the distal common bile duct. *Center,* Endoscopic image of a sphincterotome in the bile duct with the wire cutting the roof of the ampulla (sphincter). *Right,* A stone is being removed from the bile duct by an endoscopically passed basket.

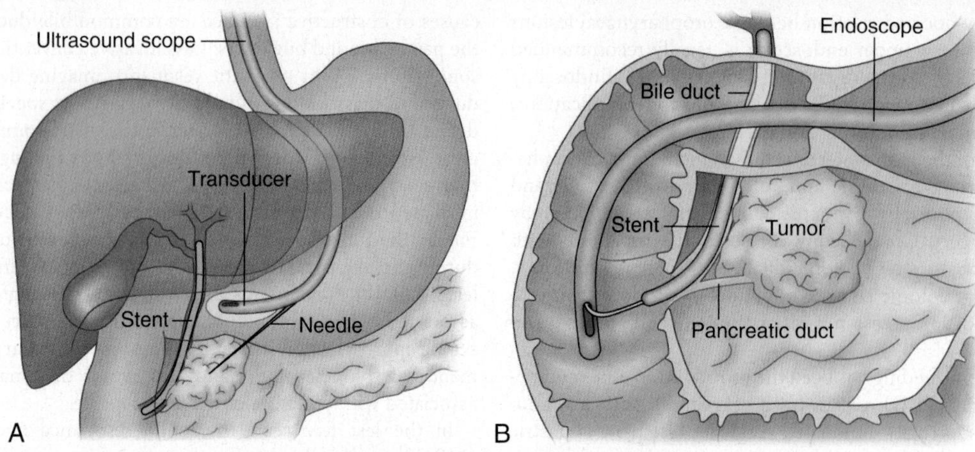

FIGURE 134-9. **Biopsy of a pancreatic mass guided by endoscopic ultrasonography (A) and the placement of a stent into a malignant bile duct stricture with endoscopic retrograde cholangiopancreatography (B).** (From Brugge WR, Van Dam J: Pancreatic and biliary endoscopy. *N Engl J Med.* 1999;341:1808-1816. Copyright ©1999 Massachusetts Medical Society. All rights reserved.)

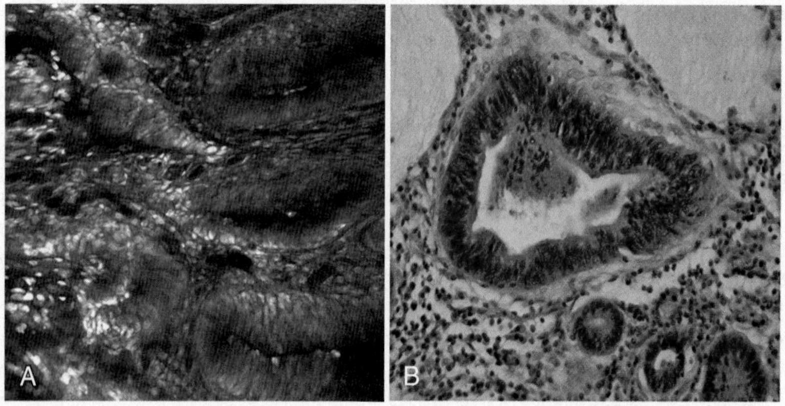

FIGURE 134-10. **Confocal microscopy (*left*) showing high-grade intraepithelial neoplasia of a colorectal polyp during endoscopy. Acriflavine was used as a contrast agent (0.02%), highlighting the cellular and nuclei architecture. The histologic picture on the right was taken from the same polyp.** (Courtesy Dr. Ralph Kiesselich, University of Mainz.)

the treatment of pain in patients with pancreatic cancer, although it does not appear to work as well in patients with chronic pancreatitis.

Nonmalignant Pancreatic Disease (Chapter 144)

ERCP has replaced MRCP as the test of choice for patients with acute or recurrent pancreatitis without any obvious risk factors on history or routine laboratory evaluation. Imaging of the pancreatic duct by either method may delineate anatomic abnormalities that may be responsible for the pancreatitis, such as congenital variants (pancreas divisum, annular pancreas) or intraductal tumors. In patients with chronic pancreatitis, which is most often due to excessive alcohol intake, pancreatography can confirm the diagnosis, provide useful information about the severity of the disease, and identify ductal lesions that may be amenable to therapy by either endoscopic or surgical means. Adjunctive diagnostic measures include the collection and analysis of bile or pancreatic juice in the duodenum. Bile duct crystals (so-called microlithiasis) can result in pancreatitis in some patients even in the absence of macroscopic stones. In more subtle cases, collection and analysis of the electrolyte content of pancreatic juice after stimulation with secretin may be useful in establishing exocrine impairment and hence in confirming chronic pancreatic injury.

ERCP also has a role in some patients with acute pancreatitis (Chapter 144) that is caused by obstructing biliary stones. Patients presenting with severe biliary pancreatitis may benefit from urgent ERCP early in their course, with the intention of detecting and removing stones from the common bile duct. Similarly, patients who have smoldering acute pancreatitis that does not appear to be improving satisfactorily with conservative treatment may require ERCP for identification and treatment of any obstructing lesions in the pancreatic or distal biliary duct.

Therapeutic endoscopy for chronic pancreatic disease is still evolving. Relief of ductal obstruction (e.g., by endoscopic removal of pancreatic stones or dilation of strictures) can provide short to intermediate pain relief in some patients with chronic pancreatitis, although it is not as effective as surgery in the long term.[A6] Endoscopic pseudocyst drainage by a variety of techniques is now technically feasible, with results that appear to be comparable to those of surgical or radiologic techniques. Patients with ductal disruptions (e.g., those with pancreatic ascites) can often be treated successfully with endoscopic stent placement. Pancreatic papillotomy may also be useful for some patients with recurrent pancreatitis, such as when pancreas divisum is thought to play a role.

EVOLVING TECHNIQUES AND FUTURE DIRECTIONS

Significant technologic and procedural innovations in both diagnostic and therapeutic endoscopy are being tested. Many of these are so-called optical biopsy techniques that include confocal microscopy (Fig. 134-10), optical coherence tomography, and a variety of different forms of spectroscopy. These techniques have the ability to provide microscopic images of cells at the surface as well as within deeper layers, thereby providing virtual real-time histology.[7] Furthermore, with use of targeted probes, it is possible to image function as well as form (E-Fig. 134-1), thereby adding another dimension to diagnosis. Innovations in endoscopic therapy include natural orifice transluminal endoscopic surgery, by which the endoscopist or surgeon introduces an endoscope through a natural orifice (mouth, vagina, or anal canal), traverses the wall of the viscus, and accesses the peritoneal cavity to perform diagnostic and therapeutic procedures. Although this approach remains controversial, it has paved the way for much more aggressive forms of intraluminal endoscopic therapy. Thus, removal and resection of large tumors is possible with endoscopic approaches, sometimes requiring the closure of real or potential leaks with adjunctive measures, such as clipping or suturing. Another example is the so-called POEM procedure (*per*oral *e*ndoscopic *m*yotomy) for achalasia,[8] in which esophageal myotomy is performed by a submucosal tunneling technique from within the esophagus. Yet another example will be the ability to obtain full-thickness biopsy specimens of the intestinal tract to allow systematic analysis of changes in nerves and muscle in motility disorders. Endoscopic methods also may become viable and less morbid alternatives to more traditional forms of bariatric surgery for obesity and diabetes.

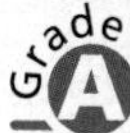

Grade A References

A1. Elmunzer BJ, Scheiman JM, Lehman GA, et al. A randomized trial of rectal indomethacin to prevent post-ERCP pancreatitis. *N Engl J Med.* 2012;366:1414-1422.

A2. Phoa KN, van Vilsteren FG, Weusten BL, et al. Radiofrequency ablation vs endoscopic surveillance for patients with Barrett esophagus and low-grade dysplasia: a randomized clinical trial. *JAMA.* 2014;311:1209-1217.

A3. Leung WK, Ho SS, Suen BY, et al. Capsule endoscopy or angiography in patients with acute overt obscure gastrointestinal bleeding: a prospective randomized study with long-term follow-up. *Am J Gastroenterol.* 2012;107:1370-1376.

A4. Atkin W, Dadswell E, Wooldrage K, et al. Computed tomographic colonography versus colonoscopy for investigation of patients with symptoms suggestive of colorectal cancer (SIGGAR): a multicentre randomised trial. *Lancet.* 2013;381:1194-1202.

A5. Halligan S, Wooldrage K, Dadswell E, et al. Computed tomographic colonography versus barium enema for diagnosis of colorectal cancer or large polyps in symptomatic patients (SIGGAR): a multicentre randomised trial. *Lancet.* 2013;381:1185-1193.

A6. Cahen DL, Gouma DJ, Nio Y, et al. Endoscopic versus surgical drainage of the pancreatic duct in chronic pancreatitis. *N Engl J Med.* 2007;356:676-684.

GENERAL REFERENCES

For the General References and other additional features, please visit Expert Consult at https://expertconsult.inkling.com.

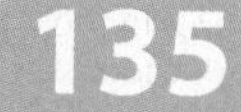

135 GASTROINTESTINAL HEMORRHAGE

THOMAS O. KOVACS AND DENNIS M. JENSEN

BACKGROUND

Gastrointestinal (GI) hemorrhage can be manifested clinically as overt bleeding from the upper GI tract (esophagus, stomach, and duodenum), lower GI tract (colon), or obscure locations (usually in the small intestine). Alternatively, it can occur as occult bleeding detected by iron deficiency anemia (Chapter 159) or by a positive result of fecal occult blood testing (Chapter 193).

GI hemorrhage is a common worldwide clinical problem and continues to be associated with significant morbidity and mortality. The annual hospitalization rate for upper GI bleeding is estimated to be 30 to 100 patients per 100,000, or about 400,000 hospitalizations per year for acute nonvariceal upper GI bleeding in the United States. A report using a national inpatient database showed that hospitalizations for upper GI hemorrhage decreased by more than 20% in the decade of 2001 to 2009. Lower GI bleeding occurs less frequently, with an incidence of 6 to 20 per 100,000, and also has decreased during the past decade. The incidence of lower GI bleeding increases substantially with age (200 per 100,000 by the age of 80 years), and lower GI hemorrhage may occur more frequently than upper GI bleeding in the elderly. Overall, for patients hospitalized for GI bleeding, 40% occurred in the upper GI tract, 25% in the lower GI tract, and 35% in an undefined location.[1] Mortality rates from upper GI hemorrhage are high, varying from 3.5 to 7% in the United States.

UPPER GASTROINTESTINAL BLEEDING

CLINICAL MANIFESTATIONS

Upper GI bleeding occurs proximal to the ligament of Treitz. Patients with upper GI bleeding usually present with hematemesis (vomiting blood or coffee-ground material) or melena (black, tarry stool). In large series, about 50% of patients have hematemesis and melena, about 30% have hematemesis alone, and about 20% have only melena. On occasion, however, hematochezia (passage per rectum of red blood or clots) may be the only manifestation of a bleeding ulcer, and about 15% of all patients who present with hematochezia have an upper GI source.[2] Peptic ulcer disease is the most common cause of acute upper GI hemorrhage, accounting for about 40% of cases.[3] Other common causes are esophageal and gastric varices (Fig. 135-1) and erosive esophagitis (see Fig. 134-1). Variceal bleeding, which occurs in the setting of portal hypertension, is discussed in Chapter 153. Other conditions, such as Mallory-Weiss tears (Fig. 135-2; Chapter 138), angiodysplasia, watermelon stomach, tumors, and Dieulafoy lesion, occur less frequently than peptic ulcer (Table 135-1). The mortality from nonulcer bleeding is comparable to that from ulcer hemorrhage in high-risk patients,[4] so all causes of upper GI hemorrhage contribute to the morbidity and cost of care associated with it.

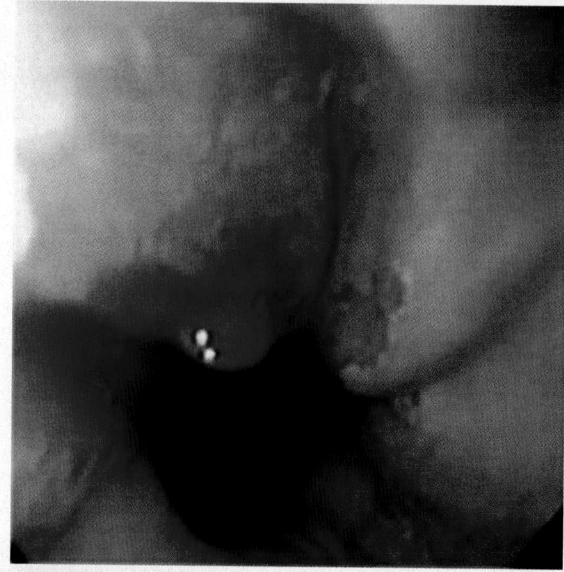

FIGURE 135-1. Bleeding esophageal varix at the gastroesophageal junction. (Courtesy Pankaj Jay Pasricha, MD.)

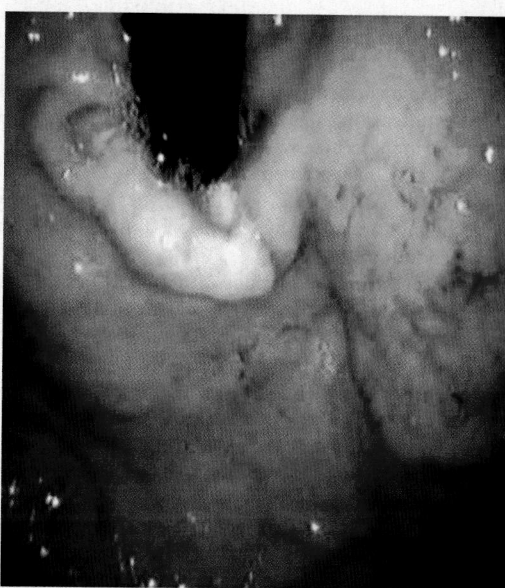

FIGURE 135-2. Retroflexed endoscopic image of a Mallory-Weiss tear at the gastroesophageal junction.

DIAGNOSIS

Initial assessment includes a medical history, vital signs, physical examination (including digital rectal examination), and nasogastric lavage in an attempt to localize the source of melena or hematochezia to the upper GI tract. Patients should be asked questions that can help determine the diagnostic possibilities for the bleeding source. For example, peptic ulcer bleeding (Chapter 139) should be suspected in patients taking daily aspirin or nonsteroidal anti-inflammatory drugs (NSAIDs). For patients with known or suspected liver disease, bleeding related to portal hypertension (such as varices or portal hypertensive gastropathy; Chapter 153) should be strongly considered. Heavy alcohol intake or vomiting should suggest a Mallory-Weiss tear (Chapter 138). A feeding tube or a chronic nasogastric tube and a history of

TABLE 135-1 CAUSES OF SEVERE UPPER GASTROINTESTINAL (GI) BLEEDING IN ONE LARGE CENTER

DIAGNOSIS	%
Peptic ulcer (gastric or duodenal)	38
Gastric or esophageal varices	16
Erosive esophagitis	13
Upper GI tumors	7
Upper GI angiomas*	6
Mallory-Weiss tear	4
Gastric or duodenal erosions	4
Dieulafoy lesion	2
Other†	2
No upper GI cause found‡	8

*Upper GI angiomas include single or multiple angiectasia, watermelon stomach, and Osler-Weber-Rendu telangiectasia.
†Other lesions were surgical anastomoses, Cameron ulcers, aortoenteric fistulas, and hemobilia.
‡No cause found in esophagus, stomach, or duodenum, but 2% had mouth, nose, or pharyngeal bleeding sites. From Kovacs TO, Jensen DM. Endoscopic therapy for severe ulcer bleeding. *Gastrointest Endosc Clin N Am.* 2011;21:681-696.

TABLE 135-2 ENDOSCOPIC STIGMATA OF RECENT ULCER HEMORRHAGE

ENDOSCOPIC APPEARANCE	FREQUENCY (%)	RISK OF REBLEEDING (%)	REBLEEDING RISK AFTER ENDOSCOPIC HEMOSTASIS (%)*
Active arterial bleeding	12	80-90	15-30
Nonbleeding visible vessel	22	40-50	15-30
Adherent clot	10	30-35	0-5
Oozing without other stigmata	14	10-20	0-5
Flat spot	10	5-10	—†
Clean ulcer base	32	3	—†

*Reduction in bleeding risk is with the administration of a proton pump inhibitor, after successful endoscopic hemostasis.
†Endoscopic hemostasis is not recommended for these stigmata.
From Kovacs TO, Jensen DM. Endoscopic therapy for severe ulcer bleeding. *Gastrointest Endosc Clin N Am.* 2011;21:681-696.

gastroesophageal reflux disease raise the suspicion for severe erosive esophagitis (Chapter 138).

The physician should check the vital signs with attention to signs of hypovolemia, such as hypotension, tachycardia, and orthostasis. The patient's skin should be examined for petechiae (see Fig. 436-5), purpura (see Fig. 436-11), spider angiomas, and palmar erythema (see Fig. 146-2), and the abdomen should be assessed for ascites (see Fig. 146-4), hepatomegaly, or splenomegaly, which may indicate portal hypertension. Tenderness or a mass may indicate an intra-abdominal tumor.

Nasogastric or orogastric tube placement to aspirate gastric contents can potentially be useful to localize bleeding to the upper GI tract and to determine the amount of red blood, coffee-ground material, or nonbloody fluid present. There is little use in testing of nasogastric tube aspirates for blood because the trauma of tube placement may cause bleeding and false-positive results. Patients who have witnessed coffee-ground emesis or fresh bloody emesis do not require a nasogastric tube for diagnostic purposes but may need one to help clear the gastric blood for better endoscopic visualization and to minimize the risk of aspiration.

Peripheral blood should be sent for standard hematology, chemistry, liver, and coagulation studies as well as for typing and crossmatching for packed red blood cells (Chapter 177). Hemoglobin concentration and hematocrit may not accurately reflect blood loss because equilibration with extravascular fluid requires 24 to 72 hours. A low platelet count suggests chronic liver disease, dilution, drug reaction, or a hematologic disorder. In upper GI bleeding, the blood urea nitrogen level typically increases to a greater extent than the creatinine level owing to increased intestinal absorption of urea after the breakdown of blood proteins. However, this phenomenon can be misleading in the setting of renal insufficiency or rapid transit of blood. An elevated international normalized ratio can be observed in chronic liver disease and in patients who are taking warfarin.

TREATMENT Rx

Acute Management

Resuscitation efforts should be initiated simultaneously with assessment in the emergency department and continue during the hospitalization. Large-bore (14- or 16-gauge) intravenous catheters are recommended, with normal saline infused as fast as necessary to maintain hemodynamic stability.[5,6] A restrictive transfusion strategy (red blood cell transfusions given only at hemoglobin level <7 g/dL, with a post-transfusion target of 7 to 9 g/dL) is better than a liberal strategy for reducing 45-day mortality and further bleeding in patients with acute upper GI hemorrhage.[A1] However, these results cannot be generalized to patients with upper GI bleeding who are hypotensive due to severe hemorrhage or have associated cardiovascular disease, in whom a hemoglobin target of 9 to 10 g/dL is recommended. General guidelines are also to use blood products as needed to maintain the platelet count above 50,000/μL and the international normalized ratio below 2. To prevent aspiration, which can cause considerable morbidity and mortality, endotracheal intubation should be considered in patients with active hematemesis or altered mental status.

Endoscopic Evaluation and Therapy

Endoscopy can identify the site of bleeding and provide therapeutic hemostasis in most patients.[7,8] Patients with evidence of active bleeding (red blood by nasogastric lavage or hypotension) should undergo emergency endoscopy as soon as possible after medical resuscitation.[A2] An intravenous prokinetic agent (either erythromycin, 250 mg, or metoclopramide, 10 mg) 30 to 60 minutes before endoscopy may help move blood out of the stomach and into the small intestine, improving endoscopic visualization.[A3]

In addition to localization of the bleeding source, endoscopic evaluation can provide prognostic information and stratify the risk of rebleeding on the basis of the presence or absence of stigmata of recent hemorrhage (Table 135-2). In addition to endoscopic stigmata, other clinical and laboratory factors that predict a poor prognosis include older age, bleeding onset in the hospital, medical comorbidities, shock, coagulopathy, fresh blood in the nasogastric lavage, and the need for multiple blood transfusions. Clinical scoring systems, such as the Rockall score (Table 135-3), use clinical information and endoscopic findings to predict clinical outcomes. Endoscopic Doppler ultrasound may also help in the risk stratification of patients with ulcer hemorrhage. Persistence of a positive Doppler signal after endoscopic treatment correlates with rebleeding.

The goal of endoscopic therapy is to stop acute bleeding and to reduce the risk of recurrent bleeding. Most endoscopic therapies were designed for peptic ulcer hemorrhage, but they can be used for other causes of nonvariceal upper GI bleeding, in which underlying arteries are the source of bleeding. Available treatments include injection (epinephrine or sclerosants), thermal coagulation (with multipolar/bipolar or heater probe), and mechanical compression (hemostatic clips). Injection therapy is effective, safe, and inexpensive, but it is sometimes inadequate for definitive hemostasis when it is used alone. When epinephrine injection is combined with either thermal coagulation or hemoclips, hemostasis is achieved in more than 95% of patients with active bleeding, and rebleeding rates are decreased by more than 50%.[A4] Endoscopic therapy is reserved for lesions that have high-risk stigmata for rebleeding (e.g., active arterial bleeding, nonbleeding visible vessel, or adherent clot) or moderate-risk stigmata, such as oozing blood without associated clot or nonbleeding visible vessel. It is not warranted for low-risk stigmata (clean-based ulcer or flat pigmented spot), which have the lowest risk of rebleeding (Fig. 135-3). Some causes of upper GI bleeding, such as gastric or duodenal erosions and neoplasms, generally are not amenable to endoscopic treatment and require appropriate medical or surgical therapy.

Medical Therapy

The most common cause of upper GI bleeding is peptic ulcer disease, and the most common cause of peptic ulcer disease is NSAID use. Aspirin and other NSAIDs should be discontinued in patients with bleeding peptic ulcers, unless there is a contraindication to do so (e.g., secondary prophylaxis for stroke). Patients with documented *Helicobacter pylori* infection should be treated with combination antibiotics and proton pump inhibitors (Chapter 139).[9] After documentation of *H. pylori* eradication, maintenance antisecretory treatment is not needed unless the patient also requires NSAIDs or anticoagulation therapy.

Proton pump inhibitors (see Table 138-1) are the mainstay of medical therapy for hemostasis and healing of peptic lesions. Acid suppression can promote platelet aggregation and clot formation as well as reduce the risk of rebleeding. High-dose intravenous proton pump inhibitors (bolus followed by

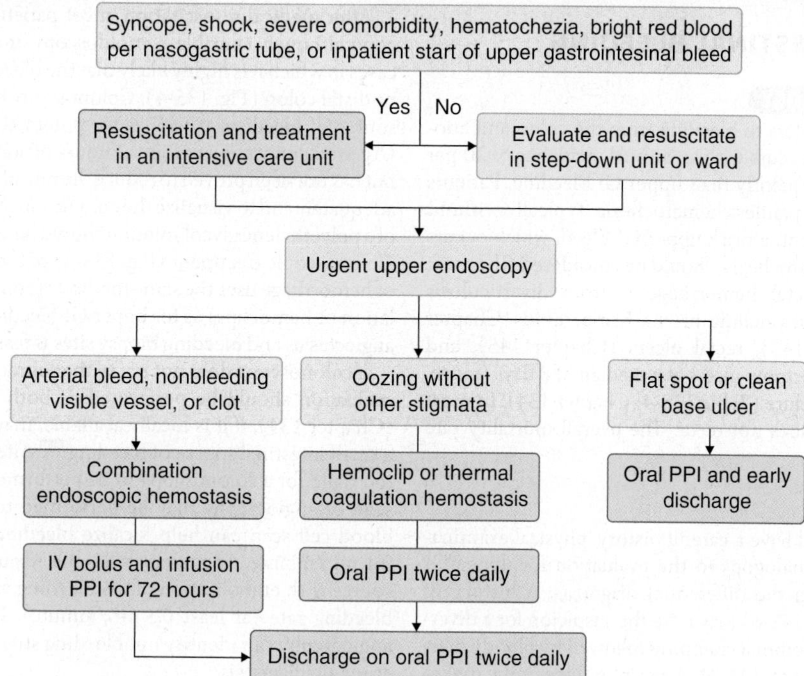

FIGURE 135-3. **Management algorithm for nonvariceal upper gastrointestinal hemorrhage.** IV = intravenous; PPI = proton pump inhibitor.

TABLE 135-3 COMPLETE ROCKALL SCORING SYSTEM FOR UPPER GASTROINTESTINAL BLEEDING

VARIABLE	0 POINTS	1 POINT	2 POINTS	3 POINTS
Age (years)	<60	60-79	>80	—
Shock				
Pulse rate (beats/min)	<100	>100	—	—
Systolic blood pressure	>100	>100	<100	—
Comorbidity	None	—	Ischemic heart disease, cardiac failure, other major illness	Renal failure, hepatic failure, metastatic cancer
Endoscopic stigmata of recent hemorrhage	No stigmata or dark spot in ulcer base	—	Blood in upper gastrointestinal tract, adherent clot, visible vessel, active bleeding	—
Diagnosis	Mallory-Weiss tear or no lesion seen	All other diagnoses	Malignant lesions	—
PRE-ENDOSCOPY SCORE	**MORTALITY (%)**	**POST-ENDOSCOPY SCORE**	**REBLEED RATE (%)**	**MORTALITY (%)**
0	0.2	0	4.9	0
1	2.4	1	3.4	0
2	5.6	2	5.3	0.2
3	11	3	11.2	2.9
4	24.6	4	14.1	5.3
5	39.6	5	24.1	10.8
6	48.9	6	32.9	17.3
7	50	7	43.8	27
—	—	8+	41.8	41.1

From Rockall TA, Logan RFA, Devlin HB, Northfield TC. Risk assessment after acute upper gastrointestinal haemorrhage. *Gut.* 1996; 38:316-321.

continuous infusion [e.g., pantoprazole, 80 mg, followed by 8 mg/hour for 72 hours]) after successful endoscopic hemostasis reduce rebleeding rates and mortality in patients with high-risk stigmata of recent hemorrhage.[A5] For patients with high-risk stigmata, either this same regimen or intermittent high-dose proton pump inhibitor therapy appears to be equally effective.[A6] Patients with low-risk or no stigmata can be treated with an oral proton pump inhibitor (e.g., esomeprazole or pantoprazole, 40 mg twice daily) and considered for early discharge. Pre-endoscopic proton pump inhibitor therapy does not alter clinical outcomes,[A7] but it may downstage the severity of the lesion and decrease the need for endoscopic intervention. Therefore, in patients with suspected ulcer bleeding, proton pump inhibitors given as an intravenous bolus may be considered while waiting for the endoscopy, but this therapy cannot substitute for endoscopy and should not delay it.

The optimal management approach for patients who develop peptic ulcer–related GI bleeding while receiving antiplatelet or anticoagulant therapy is controversial. In a randomized trial of patients who had a bleeding peptic ulcer while receiving low-dose aspirin therapy followed by successful endoscopic hemostasis and high-dose intravenous proton pump inhibitor therapy, the incidence of recurrent ulcer bleeding at 30 days was twice as high (10% vs. 5%) in patients who continued low-dose aspirin compared with those who did not. However, the patients who continued low-dose aspirin had a significantly lower mortality rate compared with the placebo group because of lower rates of cardiovascular and cerebrovascular complications.[A8] Current recommendations suggest that patients with upper GI hemorrhage who need secondary cardiovascular prophylaxis should resume low-dose aspirin treatment as soon as the cardiovascular risks outweigh the gastrointestinal risks, usually within 7 days, while continuing proton pump inhibitors (e.g., esomeprazole or pantoprazole, 40 mg daily).[10] Patients with idiopathic (non–*H. pylori*, non-NSAID) peptic ulcers should receive long-term proton pump inhibitor therapy.

LOWER GASTROINTESTINAL BLEEDING

DEFINITION AND EPIDEMIOLOGY

Lower GI hemorrhage generally refers to bleeding from the colon and anorectum. Severe lower GI bleeding occurs with an annual incidence of 20 per 100,000 population, much less frequently than upper GI bleeding. Patients are usually older and present with painless hematochezia, typically without orthostasis.[11] If orthostasis is present, a brisk upper GI bleed, which occurs in 15 to 20% of cases of severe hematochezia, should be considered. The most common cause of severe colorectal hemorrhage is from diverticulosis (Chapter 142). Other frequent causes include internal hemorrhoids (Chapter 145), ischemic colitis (Chapter 143), rectal ulcers (Chapter 145), and delayed bleeding from post-polypectomy ulcers at a median of 8 days (range, 5 hours to 17 days) after the procedure (Table 135-4; Chapter 134). In most patients, the bleeding stops and does not recur. The overall mortality rate from lower GI bleeding is 2 to 4%.

DIAGNOSIS

Patients with hematochezia should have a careful history, physical examination, and laboratory evaluation, analogous to the evaluation for upper GI bleeding. The history may help in the differential diagnosis. A history of diverticulosis (see Figs. 142-5 and 142-6) may raise the suspicion for a diverticular bleed (Chapter 142).[12] Abdominal cramping followed by bloody diarrhea suggests ischemic colitis (see Fig. 143-2). A recent polypectomy makes a post-polypectomy bleed more likely.

TABLE 135-4 MOST COMMON COLONIC SOURCES OF SEVERE HEMATOCHEZIA IN A SERIES OF 486 CASES (EXPRESSED AS PERCENTAGE OF COLONIC SOURCES)*

Diverticulosis	32%
Internal hemorrhoids	13%
Ischemic colitis	12%
Rectal ulcers	8%
Colonic angiodysplasia, angiectasia, angiomas, or radiation telangiectasias	7%
Ulcerative colitis, Crohn, other colitis	6%
Post-polypectomy ulcer	5%
Other lower gastrointestinal tract sources	6%

*Less common causes include surgical anastomotic ulcers or sutures, nonsteroidal anti-inflammatory agent colopathy, metastases, portal hypertensive colopathy, lymphoma, and endometriosis.
Modified from Jensen DM. Management of patients with severe hematochezia—with all current evidence available. *Am J Gastroenterol.* 2005;100:2403-2406.

After medical resuscitation, most patients will need to undergo colonoscopy, although a flexible sigmoidoscopy or anoscopy may be an alternative in cases in which it is highly likely that the bleeding source is from the anorectum or distal colon (Fig. 135-4). Colonoscopy is critical for identifying a luminal source of bleeding as well as for potential hemostasis of amenable lesions. Urgent colonoscopy within 12 hours of admission improves diagnostic yield but has not been proved to reduce the rate of rebleeding.[A9] To cleanse the colon adequately and to visualize the colonic mucosa, a bowel purge with 6 L or more of a polyethylene glycol solution should be administered before the procedure. Colonoscopic treatment (Fig. 135-4) of focal bleeding sources with stigmata of hemorrhage uses the same methods (epinephrine and either thermocoagulation or hemoclips) as for upper GI bleeding.[13,14] In addition, coagulation of angiectasias and bleeding biopsy sites is feasible during colonoscopy.

If colonoscopy does not reveal the source of bleeding, an upper endoscopic evaluation should be performed. If both are negative, capsule endoscopy (Chapter 134), if it is locally available, may be the preferred way to look for a small intestinal source of bleeding.[A10] Alternatively, if bleeding persists or is too rapid for a colonoscopy to be performed, a tagged red blood cell nuclear scan or angiography may be performed to localize the bleeding.[15] The red blood cell scan can help localize bleeding if it occurs at a rate of at least 0.1 mL/minute. Angiography has the advantage that it can treat the bleeding source with embolization of the bleeding vessel. However, it requires a faster bleeding rate (at least 0.5 mL/minute). Neither red blood cell scans nor angiography can identify nonbleeding stigmata, and usually neither yields an etiologic diagnosis.

Surgical management rarely is needed for hemostasis of lower GI bleeding because most bleeding is either self-limited or easily managed with medical or endoscopic therapy. The main indications for surgery are malignant lesions (Chapters 145 and 193), diffusely bleeding lesions that fail to respond to medical therapy (such as ischemia), and recurrent diverticular hemorrhage (Chapter 142). If the bleeding source can be localized preoperatively to a particular area of the colon, a segmental colonic resection can be performed rather than a subtotal colectomy.

OBSCURE AND OCCULT GASTROINTESTINAL BLEEDING

DEFINITION AND EPIDEMIOLOGY

Obscure GI bleeding is persistent or recurrent bleeding, despite negative initial GI evaluation, including upper endoscopy, colonoscopy, and radiologic evaluation of the small intestine, such as small bowel follow-through. Obscure GI bleeding can be classified as either overt (melena, maroon stool, or hematochezia) or occult bleeding (positive result of fecal occult blood testing, usually in the setting of iron deficiency anemia).

In most large series of hospitalized patients, 5% of overt GI bleeding cases are considered to be obscure, and 75% of these patients have bleeding from the small intestine that is beyond the reach of an upper endoscope or

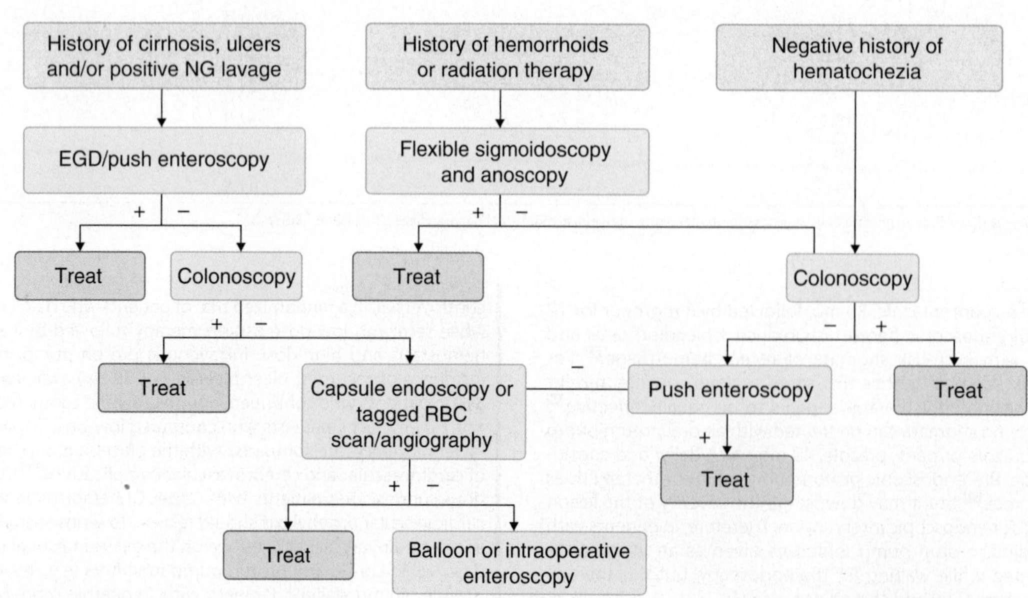

FIGURE 135-4. Management algorithm for severe hematochezia. EGD = esophagogastroduodenoscopy; NG = nasogastric; RBC = red blood cell.

colonoscope. Angiectasias (see Fig. 134-4) are the most common source of small intestinal bleeding, followed by ulcers and tumors (Table 135-5). Other causes for obscure GI bleeding include lesions that are within reach of standard endoscopes but that were not recognized as the bleeding site (e.g., a large hiatal hernia with lesions known as Cameron ulcers on endoscopy, or internal hemorrhoids on colonoscopy) and intermittently bleeding lesions such as a Dieulafoy lesion (Fig. 135-5), which is an aberrant submucosal vessel without an ulcer.

Iron deficiency (Chapter 159) has a prevalence of 2 to 5% among adult men and postmenopausal women. It can occur from overt or occult blood loss (e.g., GI tract lesions, menorrhagia), iron malabsorption (celiac disease, atrophic gastritis), and red blood cell destruction (hemolysis). It should be suspected in patients with low mean corpuscular volume, low ferritin level, or low transferrin saturation.

DIAGNOSIS

The approaches to overt and occult obscure GI bleeding are similar (Fig. 135-6). In the case of recurrent overt bleeding, upper endoscopy and colonoscopy should be repeated, with the type of bleeding dictating which endoscopic procedure to do first. Colonoscopy with anoscopy should be done first if there is hematochezia. If there is melena, a push small bowel enteroscopy

TABLE 135-5 SMALL INTESTINAL LESIONS FOUND IN 488 PATIENTS DURING DOUBLE-BALLOON ENTEROSCOPY FOR OBSCURE GASTROINTESTINAL BLEEDING

LESION	FREQUENCY (RANGE)
None	40% (0-57)
Angiectasias	31% (6-55)
Ulcerations	13% (2-35)
Malignancy	8% (3-26)
Other	6% (2-22)

From Rajir GS, Gerson L, Das A, et al. American Gastroenterological Association (AGA) Institute technical review on obscure gastrointestinal bleeding. *Gastroenterology.* 2007;133:1697-1717.

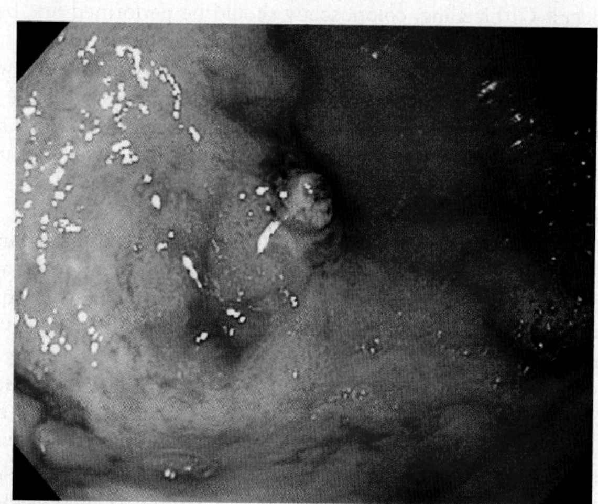

FIGURE 135-5. Dieulafoy lesion.

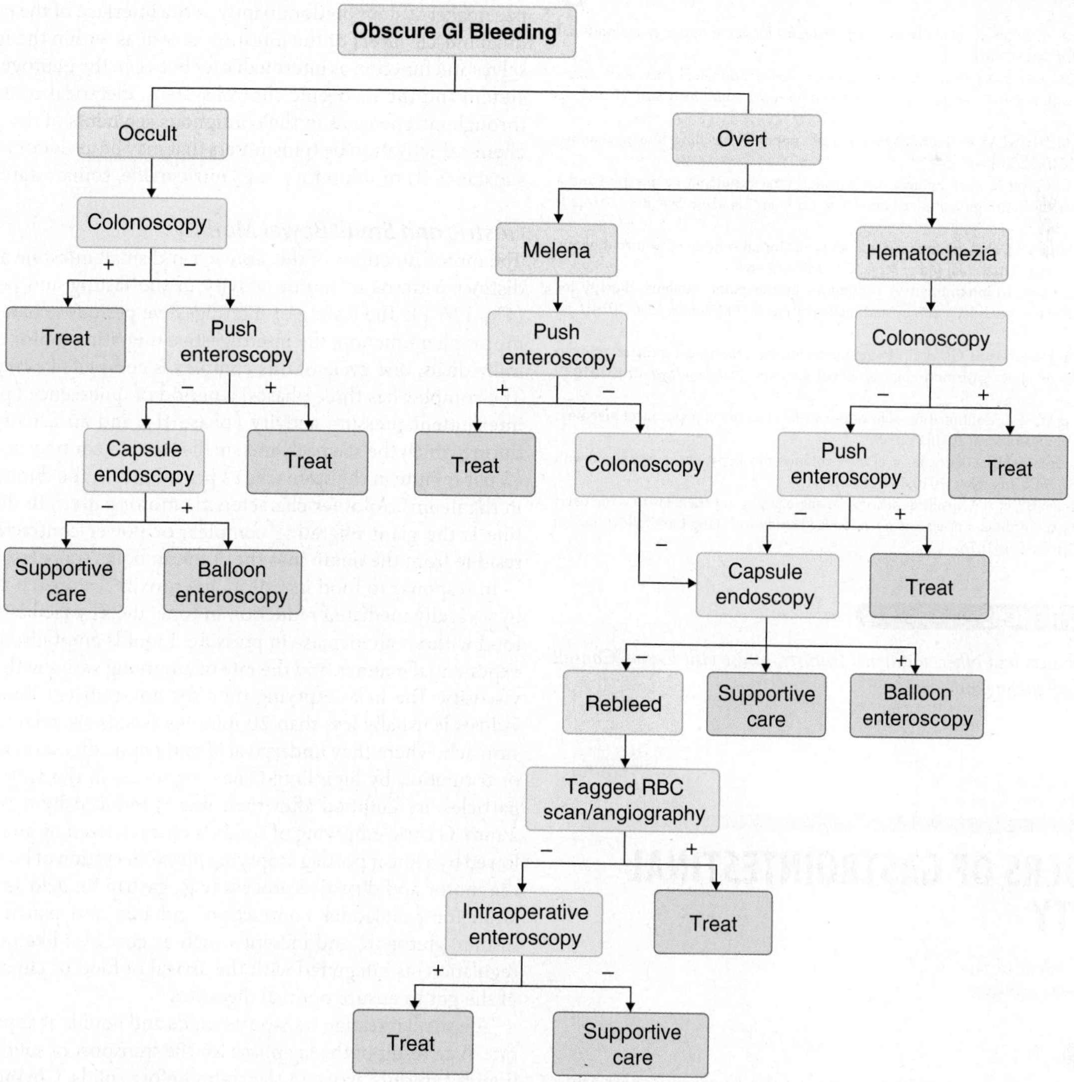

- Obscure GI Bleeding
  - Occult
    - Colonoscopy
      - + Treat
      - − Push enteroscopy
        - + Treat
        - − Capsule endoscopy
          - − Supportive care
          - + Balloon enteroscopy
  - Overt
    - Melena
      - Push enteroscopy
        - + Treat
        - − Colonoscopy
          - − Capsule endoscopy
    - Hematochezia
      - Colonoscopy
        - + Treat
        - − Push enteroscopy
          - + Treat
          - − Capsule endoscopy
            - − Rebleed
              - Tagged RBC scan/angiography
                - + Treat
                - − Intraoperative enteroscopy
                  - + Treat
                  - − Supportive care
            - − Supportive care
            - + Balloon enteroscopy

FIGURE 135-6. Management algorithm for obscure gastrointestinal bleeding. GI = gastrointestinal; RBC = red blood cell.

should be performed. If the first procedure is unremarkable, evaluation should be undertaken from the opposite end. If the second test result is negative, capsule endoscopy should be performed (Chapter 134).[16] If bleeding from the small intestine is seen on capsule endoscopy, further attempts to diagnose and to treat the bleeding should be performed with either deep enteroscopy (using a balloon overtube to slide much farther along into the small intestine) or intraoperative enteroscopy. All of these long enteroscopes facilitate diagnosis and hemostasis. If the capsule endoscopy is negative and rapid rebleeding recurs, a tagged red blood cell scan or angiography may be used to localize the bleeding site and assist with subsequent intraoperative enteroscopy.

For occult GI bleeding, colonoscopy should be performed first because fecal occult blood testing was designed to screen for colorectal cancer (Chapter 193). Upper endoscopy and push enteroscopy should follow if the colonoscopy is unremarkable. Afterward, the algorithm is the same as for overt bleeding; however, if the capsule endoscopy is negative, efforts should be focused toward providing supportive care rather than further evaluation.

Iron Deficiency Anemia

GI evaluation of iron deficiency anemia (Chapter 159) is indicated in adult men, regardless of age, and postmenopausal women. Women who have not reached menopause may warrant a GI evaluation after obvious or potential causes of iron deficiency and blood loss, such as chronic menorrhagia, have been excluded. Colonoscopy should be performed first, followed by upper endoscopy and push enteroscopy if the colonoscopy is negative. Duodenal biopsy specimens should be taken to look for evidence of celiac disease (Chapter 140). If all three of these endoscopic procedures are unrevealing, capsule endoscopy should be performed. If the capsule study is negative, investigation into non-GI causes of iron deficiency (Chapter 159) may be pursued.

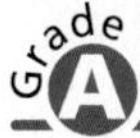

Grade A References

A1. Villanueva C, Colomo A, Bosch A, et al. Transfusion strategies for acute upper gastrointestinal bleeding. *N Engl J Med.* 2013;368:11-21.
A2. Barkun AN, Bardou M, Kuipers EJ, et al. International consensus recommendations on the management of patients with nonvariceal upper gastrointestinal bleeding. *Ann Intern Med.* 2010;152: 101-113.
A3. Barkun AN, Bardou M, Martel M, et al. Prokinetics in acute upper GI bleeding: a meta-analysis. *Gastrointest Endosc.* 2010;72:1138-1145.
A4. Vergara M, Bennett C, Calvet X, et al. Epinephrine injection versus epinephrine injection and a second endoscopic method in high-risk bleeding ulcers. *Cochrane Database Syst Rev.* 2014;10: CD005584.
A5. Sung JJ, Barkun A, Kuipers EJ, et al. Intravenous esomeprazole for prevention of recurrent peptic ulcer bleeding: a randomized trial. *Ann Intern Med.* 2009;150:455-464.
A6. Sachar H, Vaidya K, Laine L. Intermittent vs continuous proton pump inhibitor therapy for high-risk bleeding ulcers: a systematic review and meta-analysis. *JAMA Intern Med.* 2014;174: 1755-1762.
A7. Sreedharan A, Martin J, Leontiadis GI, et al. Proton pump inhibitor treatment initiated prior to endoscopic diagnosis in upper gastrointestinal bleeding. *Cochrane Database Syst Rev.* 2010;7: CD005415.
A8. Sung JJ, Lau JY, Ching JY, et al. Continuation of low-dose aspirin therapy in peptic ulcer bleeding: a randomized trial. *Ann Intern Med.* 2010;152:1-9.
A9. Laine L, Shah A. Randomized trial of urgent vs. elective colonoscopy in patients hospitalized with lower GI bleeding. *Am J Gastroenterol.* 2010;105:2636-2641.
A10. Leung WK, Ho SS, Suen BY, et al. Capsule endoscopy or angiography in patients with acute overt obscure gastrointestinal bleeding: a prospective randomized study with long-term follow-up. *Am J Gastroenterol.* 2012;107:1370-1376.

GENERAL REFERENCES

For the General References and other additional features, please visit Expert Consult at https://expertconsult.inkling.com.

136

DISORDERS OF GASTROINTESTINAL MOTILITY

MICHAEL CAMILLERI

DEFINITION

Motility disorders result from impaired control of the neuromuscular apparatus of the gastrointestinal tract. Associated symptoms include recurrent or chronic nausea, vomiting, bloating, abdominal discomfort, and constipation or diarrhea in the absence of intestinal obstruction.

PATHOBIOLOGY

Normal Physiology

Neuroenteric Control

Motor function of the gastrointestinal tract depends on the contraction of smooth muscle cells and their integration and modulation by enteric and extrinsic nerves as well as the interstitial cells of Cajal. Extrinsic neural control of gastrointestinal motor function comprises the cranial and sacral parasympathetic outflow (excitatory to nonsphincteric muscle) and the thoracolumbar sympathetic supply (excitatory to sphincters, inhibitory to nonsphincteric muscle). The cranial outflow is predominantly through the vagus nerve, which innervates the gastrointestinal tract from the stomach to the right colon. Parasympathetic innervation of the colon is provided by the vagal fibers coursing along the ileocolonic branches of the superior mesenteric artery and the S2 to S4 parasympathetic supply to the distal colon. Sympathetic fibers to the stomach and small bowel arise from T5 to T10 levels of the intermediolateral column of the spinal cord. Sympathetic innervation of the colon arises from T11 to L3 levels of the spinal cord. The prevertebral ganglia play an important role in the integration of afferent impulses between the gut and the central nervous system and in the reflex control of abdominal viscera.

The enteric nervous system is an independent nervous system comprising approximately 100 million neurons organized into ganglionated plexuses. The larger myenteric or Auerbach plexus is situated between the longitudinal and circular muscle layers of the muscularis externa; this plexus contains neurons responsible for gastrointestinal motility. The submucosal or Meissner plexus controls absorption, secretion, and mucosal blood flow. The enteric nervous system also plays an important role in visceral afferent function.

The interstitial cells of Cajal are spontaneously active pacemaker cells that coordinate muscle contraction and sense distortion. They form a non-neural pacemaker system predominantly at the interface of the circular and longitudinal muscle layers of the intestine as well as within the muscle layers themselves and function as intermediaries between the neurogenic enteric nervous system and the myogenic control system. Electrical control activity spreads through interneurons in the contiguous segments of the gut through neurochemical activation by transmitters that may be excitatory (e.g., acetylcholine, substance P) or inhibitory (e.g., nitric oxide, somatostatin).

Gastric and Small Bowel Motility

The motor functions of the stomach and small intestine are characterized by distinct patterns of motor activity in the fasting and postprandial periods (Fig. 136-1). The fasting or interdigestive period is characterized by a cyclic motor phenomenon, the interdigestive migrating motor complex. In healthy individuals, one cycle of this complex is completed every 60 to 90 minutes. The complex has three phases: a period of quiescence (phase I), a period of intermittent pressure activity (phase II), and an activity front (phase III) during which the stomach and small intestine contract at highest frequencies (3 per minute in the stomach, 12 per minute in the duodenum, 8 per minute in the ileum). Another characteristic motor pattern in the distal small intestine is the giant migrating complex, or power contraction, which empties residue from the ileum into the colon in bolus transfers.

In response to food ingestion, the proximal stomach accommodates food by a vagally mediated reduction in tone, thereby facilitating the ingestion of food without an increase in pressure. Liquids empty from the stomach in an exponential manner, and the rate of emptying varies with calorie content and viscosity. The half-emptying time for non-nutrient liquids in healthy individuals is usually less than 20 minutes. Solids are retained selectively in the stomach, where they undergo acid and peptic digestion as well as "churning" or trituration by high liquid shearing forces in the antrum. Digestible food particles are emptied after their size is reduced by trituration to less than 2 mm. Gastric emptying of solids is characterized by an initial lag period followed by a linear postlag emptying phase. Secretion of hormones that mediate the motor and digestive process (e.g., gastrin for acid secretion; cholecystokinin for gallbladder contraction and bile and pancreatic secretion; and insulin, glucagon, and incretins such as glucagon-like peptide 1 for glucose regulation) is integrated with the arrival of food or chyme at different levels of the gut to ensure optimal digestion.

The small intestine transports solids and liquids at approximately the same rate. As a result of the lag phase for the transport of solids from the stomach, liquids typically arrive in the colon before solids. Chyme moves from ileum to colon intermittently in boluses propelled by contractions.

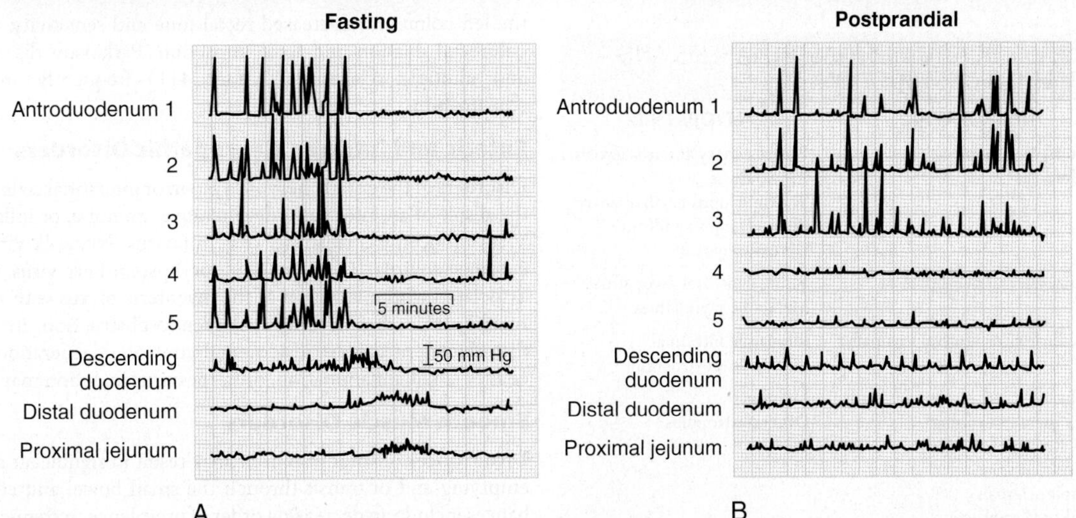

FIGURE 136-1. **Fasting and postprandial gastroduodenal manometric recordings in a healthy volunteer. A 535-kcal meal is ingested during the study. Note the cyclic interdigestive migrating motor complex (A) and the sustained, high-amplitude but irregular pressure activity after a meal (B). (From Coulie B, Camilleri M. Intestinal pseudo-obstruction. *Annu Rev Med*. 1999;50:37-55.)**

In the postprandial period, the interdigestive migrating motor complex is replaced by an irregular pattern of variable amplitude and frequency. This pattern, which enables mixing, digestion, and absorption, is observed in the gastrointestinal regions in contact with food. The maximum frequency of contractions is lower than during phase III of the interdigestive motor complex, and the duration of this postprandial contractile activity is proportional to the number of calories consumed (about 1 hour for each 200 kcal ingested). Segments of the small intestine that are not in contact with food continue with interdigestive motor patterns.

Vomiting is characterized by a stereotypic sequence of motor events, including contractions of the stomach, abdominal muscles, and diaphragm. This sequence is followed immediately in the proximal small bowel by a propagated, rhythmic contractile response similar to the migrating motor complex.

Colonic Motility

The normal colon displays short-duration (phasic) contractions and a background contractility or tone. Nonpropagated phasic contractions have a role in segmenting the colon into haustra, which compartmentalize the colon and facilitate mixing, retention of residue, and formation of solid stool. High-amplitude propagated contractions, which are characterized by an amplitude greater than 75 mm Hg, propagation over a distance of at least 15 cm, and a propagation velocity of 0.15 to 2.2 cm/second, contribute to the mass movements in the colon. In health, these contractions occur on average five or six times per day, most often postprandially and between 6 AM and 2 PM.

Colonic transit is a discontinuous process, slow most of the time and rapid at other times. Residue may be retained for prolonged periods in the right colon, and a mass movement may deliver the contents to the sigmoid colon in seconds. Feeding stimulates movement of colonic content (referred to as the gastrocolonic response). In health, the average mouth-to-cecum transit time is about 6 hours, and transit times through the right colon, left colon, and sigmoid colon are about 12 hours each. As the ingestion of dietary fiber increases, mean colonic transit time decreases, stool frequency increases, and stool consistency is softer. Decreased calorie intake slows colonic transit, whereas a meal (typically >500 kcal, especially a fat-rich meal) stimulates colonic motor function and propulsion of colonic content. Outlet obstruction in patients with pelvic floor dysfunction or voluntary suppression of defecation often is associated with slow colonic transit and decreased motor response to feeding.

Fluid reabsorption influences gastrointestinal transit.[1] Approximately 9 L of fluid enters the gut from oral intake and endogenous secretions. The small intestine delivers about 1.5 L of fluid to the colon, where most is reabsorbed, leaving a maximum of 200 mL of water excreted in normal stool. Up to 3 L of fluid can be reabsorbed by the colon in a 24-hour period, unless the rate of ileocolonic flow or colonic motility overwhelms the colon's capacity or reabsorptive ability.

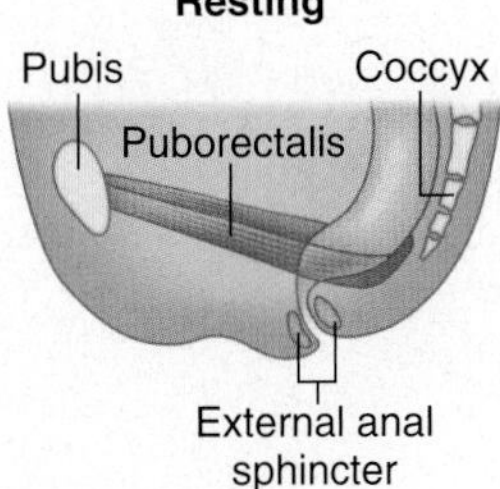

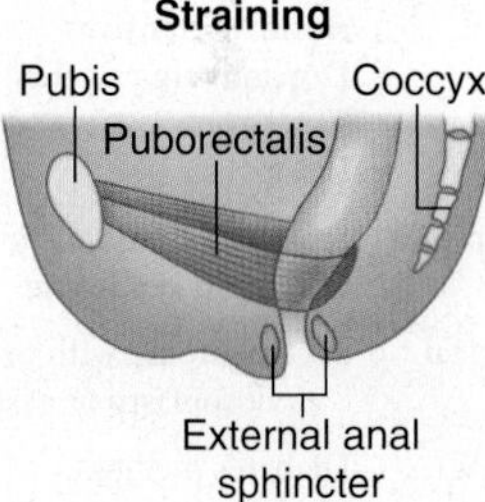

FIGURE 136-2. **Pelvic floor and anorectal functions during continence and defecation. Sagittal view through the pelvis in the resting (A) and straining (B) postures. Coordinated functions of pelvic floor (puborectalis) and anal sphincter are essential for continence and defecation.**

Defecation and Continence

Normal defecation requires a series of coordinated actions of the colon, rectum, pelvic floor, and anal sphincter muscles (Fig. 136-2). Filling of the rectum by a volume of 10 mL may be sensed, although the rectum can accommodate 300 mL before a sense of fullness and urge to defecate develop. Distention of the rectum results in the relaxation of the internal anal sphincter (rectoanal inhibitory reflex) and simultaneous contraction of the external anal sphincter to maintain continence. The anal transition zone can sense the difference between solid or liquid stool and gas.

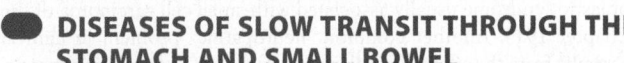

DISEASES OF SLOW TRANSIT THROUGH THE STOMACH AND SMALL BOWEL

PATHOBIOLOGY

Gastrointestinal motility disturbances (Table 136-1) result from disorders of the extrinsic nervous system, enteric nervous system, interstitial cells of Cajal (or intestinal pacemakers), or smooth muscle. Neuropathic patterns are characterized by normal amplitude but incoordinated contractions, whereas myopathies are characterized by low-amplitude contractions (average of less than 40 mm Hg in the antrum and less than 10 mm Hg in the small bowel). Combined disorders occur in systemic sclerosis (Chapter 267), amyloidosis (Chapter 188), and mitochondrial cytopathy (Chapter 421), which can be manifested initially with neuropathic patterns and later display myopathic characteristics with disease progression.

TABLE 136-1 CLASSIFICATION OF GASTROPARESIS AND PSEUDO-OBSTRUCTION

TYPE	NEUROPATHIC	MYOPATHIC
Infiltrative	Progressive systemic sclerosis Amyloidosis	Progressive systemic sclerosis Amyloidosis Systemic lupus erythematosus Ehlers-Danlos syndrome Dermatomyositis
Familial	Familial visceral neuropathies	Familial visceral myopathies Metabolic myopathies
Idiopathic	Sporadic hollow visceral myopathy	Idiopathic intestinal pseudo-obstruction
Neurologic	Porphyria Heavy metal poisoning Brain stem tumor Parkinson disease Multiple sclerosis Spinal cord transection	Myotonia Other dystrophies
Infectious	Chagas disease Cytomegalovirus Norwalk virus Epstein-Barr virus	
Drug induced	Tricyclic antidepressants Narcotic agents Anticholinergic agents Antihypertensives Dopaminergic agents Vincristine Laxatives	
Paraneoplastic	Small cell lung cancer Carcinoid syndrome	
Postsurgical	Postvagotomy with or without pyloroplasty or gastric resection	
Endocrine	Diabetes mellitus Hypothyroidism or hyperthyroidism Hypoparathyroidism	

Genetic defects that result in congenital dysmotilities include abnormalities of *RET*, the gene that encodes the tyrosine kinase receptor, and abnormalities in the endothelin B system. Neural crest cells migrate from the vagal and sacral crest to the developing gut and, over time, colonize the entire developing alimentary canal and its appendages. Endothelin B serves to retard maturation of migrating neural crest cells, thus facilitating colonization of the entire gut with nerve cells. Other abnormalities resulting in congenital dysmotility involve other transcription factors, such as Sox10, which enhances maturation of neural precursors, and Kit, a marker for the interstitial cells of Cajal. Defects of *RET*, endothelin B, and Sox10 are associated with the phenotypic picture recognized in Hirschsprung disease, whereas *KIT* defects have been associated with idiopathic hypertrophic pyloric stenosis and congenital megacolon. c-*KIT* mutations are associated with gastrointestinal stromal tumors (Chapter 192).

Extrinsic Neuropathic Disorders

Extrinsic neuropathic processes include vagotomy, trauma, Parkinson disease (Chapter 409), diabetes (Chapter 229), amyloidosis (Chapter 188), and a paraneoplastic syndrome usually associated with small cell carcinoma of the lung (Chapter 191). Another common "neuropathic" problem in clinical practice results from the effect of medications, such as α_2-adrenergic agonists, glucagon-like peptide 1 analogues, opiates, and anticholinergics, on neural control.

Damage to the autonomic nerves by trauma, infection, neuropathy, and neurodegeneration may lead to motor, secretory, and sensory disturbances, most frequently resulting in constipation. Patients with spinal cord injury (Chapter 399) above the level of the sacral segments have delayed proximal and distal colonic transit attributable to parasympathetic denervation. In these patients, fasting colonic motility and tone are normal, but the response to feeding generally is reduced or absent. Spinal cord lesions involving the sacral segments and damage to the efferent nerves from these segments disrupt the neural integration of rectosigmoid expulsion and anal sphincter control. In patients with these injuries, there is loss of contractile activity in the left colon and decreased rectal tone and sensitivity, which may lead to colorectal dilation and fecal impaction. Parkinson disease (Chapter 409) and multiple sclerosis (Chapter 411) frequently are associated with constipation.

Enteric and Intrinsic Neuropathic Disorders

Disorders of the enteric nervous system or interstitial cells of Cajal are usually the result of an infectious, degenerative, immune, or inflammatory process. Virus-induced gastroparesis (e.g., rotavirus, Norwalk virus [Chapter 380], cytomegalovirus [Chapter 376], or Epstein-Barr virus [Chapter 377]) is associated with infiltration of the myenteric plexus with inflammatory cells. In idiopathic chronic intestinal pseudo-obstruction, in which there is no disturbance of the extrinsic neural control, degeneration of the interstitial cells of Cajal, inflammation, or herpesvirus infection may contribute.

Smooth Muscle Disorders

Disturbances of smooth muscle may result in significant disorders of gastric emptying and of transit through the small bowel and colon. These disturbances include, in decreasing order of prevalence, systemic sclerosis (Chapter 267), amyloidosis (Chapter 188), dermatomyositis (Chapter 269), myotonic dystrophy (Chapter 421), and metabolic muscle disorders (Chapter 421). Motility disturbances may be the result of metabolic disorders, such as hypothyroidism (Chapter 226) and hyperparathyroidism (Chapter 245), but these patients more commonly present with constipation. Scleroderma may result in focal or general dilation, wide-mouthed diverticula, and delayed transit in the stomach, small bowel, and colon. The amplitude of contractions is reduced, and bacterial overgrowth may result in steatorrhea or pneumatosis intestinalis. Mitochondrial neurogastrointestinal encephalomyopathy, or familial visceral myopathy type II, is an autosomal recessive condition that may be manifested with hepatic failure in neonates, seizures or diarrhea in infants, and hepatic failure or chronic intestinal pseudo-obstruction in adults.

Gastroparesis and Pseudo-Obstruction

CLINICAL MANIFESTATIONS

The clinical features of gastroparesis[2] and chronic intestinal pseudo-obstruction[3] are similar and include nausea, vomiting, early satiety, abdominal discomfort, distention, bloating, and anorexia. Severe cases, which occur mostly in patients with disorders of smooth muscle, may be accompanied by considerable dilation as well as by weight loss, with depletion of mineral and vitamin stores. Diarrhea and constipation indicate that the motility disorder extends beyond the stomach. Vomiting may result in aspiration pneumonia (Chapter 94) or Mallory-Weiss esophageal tears (Chapters 135 and 138), and patients with a generalized motility disorder may have abnormal swallowing or delayed colonic transit.

A careful family and medication history is essential. Review of systems may reveal an underlying collagen vascular disease (e.g., scleroderma) or disturbances of extrinsic autonomic neural control, including orthostatic dizziness, difficulties with erection or ejaculation, recurrent urinary tract infections, dry mouth, dry eyes, dry vagina, difficulties with visual accommodation in bright lights, and absence of sweating.

On physical examination, a succussion splash indicates stasis, typically in the stomach. The hands and mouth may reveal signs of Raynaud phenomenon or scleroderma (Chapter 267). Testing of pupillary responses (to light and accommodation), external ocular movements, blood pressure in the lying and standing positions, and general features of a peripheral neuropathy can identify patients with an associated neurologic disturbance (e.g., diabetic neuropathy) or with the oculogastrointestinal dystrophy that typically is found with mitochondrial cytopathies (see under the Smooth Muscle Disorders section in this chapter).

The differential diagnosis includes mechanical obstruction, functional gastrointestinal disorders, anorexia nervosa, and the rumination syndrome. The rumination syndrome is a relatively common, underdiagnosed condition that is manifested with early (0 to 30 minutes) postprandial, effortless regurgitation of undigested food after virtually every meal.

DIAGNOSIS

A motility disorder of the stomach or small bowel should be suspected whenever large volumes are aspirated from the stomach, particularly after an overnight fast, or when undigested solid food or large volumes of liquids are observed during esophagogastroduodenoscopy. The clinician should assess the acuity of symptoms and the patient's state of hydration and nutrition. The

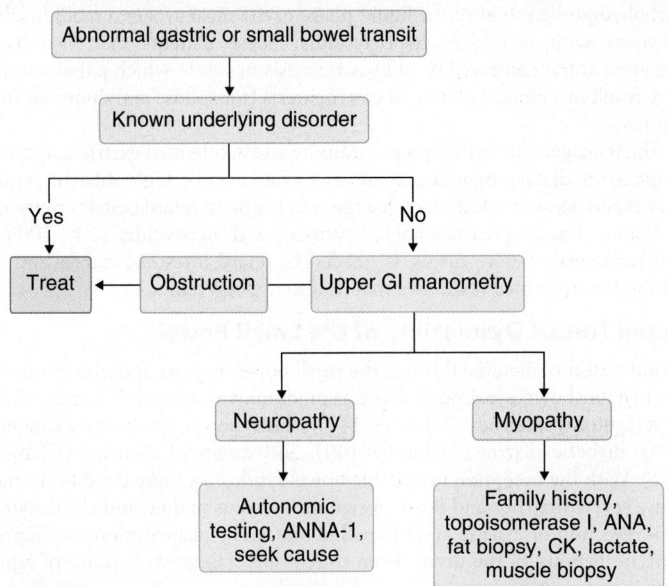

FIGURE 136-3. Flow diagram outlines steps in diagnosis of idiopathic gastroparesis and intestinal pseudo-obstruction. ANA = antinuclear antibody; ANNA-1 = type 1 antineuronal nuclear antibody; CK = creatine kinase; GI = gastrointestinal.

goals of the evaluation are to determine what regions of the digestive tract are malfunctioning and whether the symptoms are due to a neuropathy or a myopathy (Fig. 136-3). Key steps include the following:

1. *Suspect and exclude mechanical obstruction.* In symptomatic patients with pseudo-obstruction, plain radiographs of the abdomen typically show dilated loops of small bowel with associated air-fluid levels. Mechanical obstruction should be excluded by upper gastrointestinal endoscopy and small bowel imaging studies, including a small bowel follow-through, computed tomographic enterography, and magnetic resonance enteroclysis. Capsule endoscopy should be avoided because of the potential risk of retention of the capsule. Barium studies may suggest the presence of a motor disorder, particularly if there is gross dilation, dilution of barium, or retained solid food within the stomach. These studies rarely identify the cause, however, except for systemic sclerosis and mitochondrial cytopathy, which are characterized by megaduodenum, multiple small bowel diverticula, and pneumatosis intestinalis.
2. *Assess gastric and small bowel motility.*[4] After mechanical obstruction and alternative diagnoses such as Crohn disease (Chapter 141) have been excluded, a transit profile of the stomach or small bowel should be performed. The preferred test is a gastric emptying study, in which ingestion of a radiolabeled solid meal is followed by scintigraphy at 0, 1, 2, 3, 4, and 6 hours. An alternative is measurement of gastric emptying by a stable isotope breath test. If the cause of the motility disturbance is obvious, such as gastroparesis in a patient with long-standing diabetes mellitus, it is usually unnecessary to pursue further diagnostic testing. If the cause is unclear, gastroduodenal manometry by use of a multilumen tube with sensors in the distal stomach and proximal small intestine can differentiate a neuropathic process (normal-amplitude contractions but abnormal patterns of contractility) from a myopathic process (low-amplitude contractions in the affected segments). An alternative that can assess contraction amplitude is the wireless motility capsule.
3. *Identify the pathogenesis* (see Table 136-1). In patients with neuropathic causes of uncertain origin, tests should assess autonomic dysfunction (Chapter 421), measure type 1 antineuronal nuclear autoantibodies and other autoantibodies associated with paraneoplastic syndromes, and consider the possibility of a brain stem lesion. In patients with a myopathic disorder of unclear cause, the evaluation should consider amyloidosis (immunoglobulin electrophoresis, fat aspirate, or rectal biopsy; Chapter 188), systemic sclerosis (topoisomerase I; Chapter 267), and thyroid disease (Chapter 226). In appropriate settings, porphyria (Chapter 210) and Chagas disease (Chapter 347) may need to be excluded. In refractory cases, referral to a specialized center may result in genetic testing or full-thickness biopsy of the small intestine (Fig. 136-4) to identify metabolic muscle disorders and mitochondrial cytopathies.

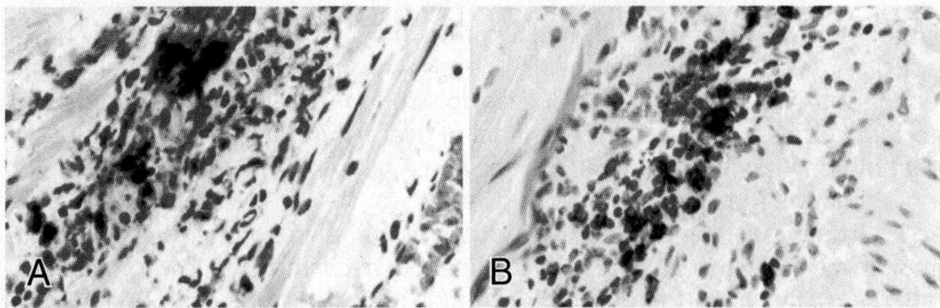

FIGURE 136-4. Micrographs showing both types of T lymphocytes, CD4 (A) and CD8 (B), detectable within the myenteric plexus of the small intestine (proximal ileum) of a 20-year-old man with chronic intestinal pseudo-obstruction. Note the intense CD4 and CD8 immunoreactivities that represent the predominant component of the immune infiltrate observed in cases of lymphocytic ganglionitis. Alkaline phosphatase anti–alkaline phosphatase immunohistochemical technique (×120) in A and B. (From De Giorgio R, Camilleri M. Human enteric neuropathies: morphology and molecular pathology. *Neurogastroenterol Motil.* 2004;16:515-531.)

Diabetes mellitus (Chapter 229) is associated with gastroparesis, pylorospasm, intestinal pseudo-obstruction, diarrhea, constipation, and fecal incontinence.[5] All of these manifestations may be caused by poor glycemic control, autonomic dysfunction, or changes in the structure and function of the interstitial cells of Cajal and enteric nervous system. Patients may become poorly nourished with vitamin deficiencies. The prevalence of constipation is 22% among diabetic patients with neuropathy but only 9.2% in diabetic patients without neuropathy, a rate that is not significantly different from that of nondiabetic controls.

4. *Identify complications of the motility disorder, including bacterial overgrowth, dehydration, and malnutrition.* In patients presenting with diarrhea, it is important to assess nutritional status and to exclude bacterial overgrowth by culture of small bowel aspirates or glucose-hydrogen breath test (Chapter 140). Bacterial overgrowth is relatively uncommon in neuropathic disorders but is found more often in myopathic conditions, such as scleroderma, that are associated more often with dilation or low-amplitude contractions. An empirical trial of antibiotics (see later) often is used instead of formal testing.

TREATMENT

Rx

Rehydration, electrolyte repletion, and nutritional supplementation are particularly important during acute exacerbations of gastroparesis and chronic intestinal pseudo-obstruction. Initial nutritional measures include low-fiber supplements with the addition of iron, folate, calcium, and vitamins D, K, and B_{12} at the usually recommended daily levels. In patients with more severe symptoms, enteral or parenteral supplementation may be required. If it is anticipated that enteral supplementation may be needed for more than 3 months, a jejunostomy feeding tube is recommended. These tubes may be placed with the aid of endoscopy. Gastrostomy tubes should be avoided in patients with gastroparesis except for venting purposes. The rumination syndrome is treated with behavioral approaches such as diaphragmatic breathing in the early postprandial period.

Medical Therapy

Medications increasingly are being used to treat neuromuscular motility disorders, but there is little evidence of effectiveness in myopathic disturbances except for the rare case of dystrophia myotonica affecting the stomach and for small bowel systemic sclerosis. Small randomized trials demonstrate symptomatic benefit of metoclopramide and domperidone over placebo in patients with gastroparesis. Metoclopramide is a dopamine antagonist with prokinetic and antiemetic properties. Antiemetic effects are due in part to its anti–5-hydroxytryptamine type 3 (HT_3) antagonist actions. The recommended duration of treatment with metoclopramide is 3 months; longer-term use may result in tremor and parkinsonian-like symptoms. It is available in tablet or elixir form or as a parenteral preparation and, typically, is taken orally 30 minutes before meals and at bedtime. Usual doses are 5 to 10 mg four times daily, but patients may experience side effects (changes in affect, anxiety) at relatively low doses (even 30 to 40 mg/day). The U.S. Food and Drug Administration recommends its use only in patients who do not respond to other treatments and for periods of less than 3 months.

Domperidone (10 to 20 mg, three times per day before meals) is another dopamine antagonist that is approved in some countries but not in the United States, where it may be available through an investigational drug application to the U.S. Food and Drug Administration and local Institutional Review Board. Its efficacy appears similar to metoclopramide, with a lower incidence of somnolence and much lower incidence of involuntary movements.

Domperidone-induced cardiac arrhythmias may occur in patients who have specific genetic polymorphisms in the cytochrome P-450 3A4 gene, which encodes the enzyme that metabolizes domperidone. Clinically, it is important to modify dose if the patient has renal or liver failure or ingests medications that inhibit cytochrome P-450 3A4 enzyme (Chapter 29). Genetic screening is not recommended in any guidelines.

Erythromycin, a macrolide antibiotic that stimulates motilin receptors at higher doses (250 to 500 mg) and cholinergic mechanisms at lower doses (40 to 80 mg), results in the dumping of solids from the stomach. It accelerates gastric emptying in gastroparesis, increases the amplitude of antral contractions, and improves antroduodenal coordination. Erythromycin is most effective when it is used intravenously (3 mg/kg every 8 hours by slow infusion) during acute exacerbations of gastroparesis. For oral erythromycin, tolerance and gastrointestinal side effects often prevent use for longer than 1 month, but sometimes liquid erythromycin can be tolerated at 40 to 80 mg three times daily before meals. Because of the limited availability of medications approved for long-term treatment, older medications such as pyridostigmine (30 to 60 mg every 6 hours) are sometimes used.

Octreotide (50 µg subcutaneously at bedtime), a cyclized analogue of somatostatin, induces small intestinal activity that mimics phase III of the interdigestive migrating motor complex. It retards gastric emptying, decreases postprandial gastric motility, and inhibits small bowel transit. Octreotide appears to be useful in the treatment of dumping syndromes associated with accelerated transit. Octreotide may be used before sleep at night to induce migrating motor complex activity, to sweep residue toward the colon, and to avoid bacterial overgrowth. If it is required during the daytime, octreotide often is combined with an oral prokinetic to "normalize" the gastric emptying rate.

Antiemetics, including diphenhydramine (25 mg orally up to two times per day for up to 3 months), promethazine (orally or by suppository, 25 mg up to two times per day), and metoclopramide (5 to 10 mg orally up to three times per day for up to 3 months), can treat nausea and vomiting in patients with gastroparesis and intestinal pseudo-obstruction. The more expensive serotonin 5-HT_3 antagonists (e.g., ondansetron) or NK_1 antagonists (e.g., aprepitant) have not proved to be of greater benefit than these less expensive alternatives in these patients. Nortriptyline is not effective in patients with idiopathic gastroparesis.[6]

Antibiotic therapy is indicated in patients with documented, symptomatic bacterial overgrowth. Although formal clinical trials have not been conducted, it is common practice to use different antibiotics for 7 to 10 days each month, in an attempt to avoid bacterial resistance. Common antibiotics include doxycycline, 100 mg twice daily; metronidazole, 500 mg three times daily; ciprofloxacin, 500 mg twice daily; double-strength trimethoprim-sulfamethoxazole, two tablets twice daily; and rifaximin, 275 mg twice daily. Use of antibiotics in patients with diarrhea and fat malabsorption secondary to bacterial overgrowth results in significant symptomatic relief.

Surgical Therapy

Surgical decompression is rarely necessary in patients with chronic pseudo-obstruction. Venting enterostomy (jejunostomy) is effective, however, in relieving abdominal distention and bloating and in reducing the frequency with which nasogastric intubations and hospitalizations are required for acute exacerbations compared with the period before vent placement. Access to the small intestine by enterostomy also provides a means to deliver nutrients and should be considered in patients with intermittent symptoms. Surgical treatment should be considered whenever the motility disorder is localized to a resectable portion of the gut: completion gastrectomy for patients with post-gastric surgical stasis syndrome, and colectomy with ileorectostomy for intractable constipation associated with chronic colonic pseudo-obstruction.

Gastric electrical stimulation, a treatment approved for humanitarian use, may improve symptoms in some patients with severe gastroparesis, but data on its efficacy are inconclusive, and its use is restricted to a few centers in the United States. Small bowel transplantation currently is limited to patients with intestinal failure who have reversible liver disease induced by total parenteral nutrition or who have life-threatening or recurrent catheter-related sepsis. Isolated transplantation of the small intestine is associated with higher graft and patient survival and fewer complications related to rejection and infection.

DISEASES OF RAPID TRANSIT THROUGH STOMACH AND SMALL BOWEL

Dumping Syndrome and Accelerated Gastric Emptying

Dumping syndrome and accelerated gastric emptying typically follow truncal vagotomy and gastric drainage procedures (Chapter 139) or fundoplication for gastric esophageal reflux disease (Chapter 138). With the widespread use of highly selective vagotomy and the advent of effective antacid secretory therapy, these problems are becoming rare. A high calorie (usually carbohydrate) content of the liquid phase of the meal evokes a rapid insulin response with secondary hypoglycemia. These patients may also have impaired antral contractility and gastric stasis of solids, which paradoxically may result in a clinical picture of gastroparesis (for solids) and dumping (for liquids).

The management of dumping syndrome and accelerated gastric emptying emphasizes dietary maneuvers, such as avoidance of high-nutrient liquid drinks and possibly addition of guar gum or pectin to retard gastric emptying of liquids. Rarely, pharmacologic treatment with octreotide, 25 to 100 µg subcutaneously before meals, is needed to retard intestinal transit and to inhibit the hormonal responses that lead to hypoglycemia.

Rapid Transit Dysmotility of the Small Bowel

Rapid transit of material through the small bowel may occur in the setting of the irritable bowel syndrome–diarrhea predominant subtype (Chapter 137), postvagotomy diarrhea (Chapter 140), short bowel syndrome (Chapter 140), diabetic diarrhea (Chapter 140), and carcinoid diarrhea (Chapter 232). With the exception of irritable bowel syndrome, these conditions may cause severe diarrhea and result in significant losses of fluid and electrolytes. Ileal resection or disease and idiopathic bile acid malabsorption may represent an inability of the distal ileum to reabsorb bile acids because of rapid transit and reduced contact time with the ileal mucosa; this condition may induce colonic secretion and secondary diarrhea. Accelerated transit may be confirmed by scintigraphic studies.

Treatment goals are to restore hydration and nutrition and to slow small bowel transit. Dietary interventions include avoiding hyperosmolar drinks and replacing them with iso-osmolar or hypo-osmolar oral rehydration solutions. The fat content in the diet should be reduced to approximately 50 g/day to avoid delivery of unabsorbed fat to the colon. All electrolyte and nutritional deficiencies of calcium, magnesium, potassium, and water-soluble and fat-soluble vitamins should be corrected. In patients with less than 1 m of residual small bowel, it may be impossible to maintain fluid and electrolyte homeostasis without parenteral support. In patients with a longer residual segment, oral nutrition, pharmacotherapy, and supplements are almost always effective.

The opioid agent loperamide (4 mg 30 minutes before meals and at bedtime for a total dose of 16 mg/day) suppresses the motor response to feeding and improves symptoms but may be ineffective or cause side effects (e.g., hypotension). Bile acid binding, such as with cholestyramine (4 g three times daily) or colesevelam (1.875 g twice daily), is indicated for patients with suspected or proven bile acid malabsorption. Verapamil (40 mg twice daily), clonidine (0.1 mg twice daily), or a 5-HT_3 antagonist (e.g., ondansetron, 4 to 8 mg three times daily) is used rarely in addition to loperamide. Octreotide (50 µg subcutaneously three times daily before meals) may be used in patients for whom the oral agents are ineffective or poorly tolerated. 5-HT_3 antagonists (e.g., alosetron, 0.5 to 1 mg orally up to two times per day) may be efficacious in the treatment of carcinoid diarrhea and diarrhea-predominant irritable bowel syndrome, but it should be reserved for patients with severe, unresponsive diarrhea, and the dose should be titrated to avoid constipation.

COLONIC MOTILITY DISORDERS

Constipation

EPIDEMIOLOGY

Constipation is a common clinical problem, reported by about 20% of the population, and 40% of Americans report needing to strain excessively to pass their bowel movements.[7]

PATHOBIOLOGY

In functional constipation, transit is normal, and there is no evacuation disorder. These patients may have pain in association with constipation, and there is overlap with constipation-predominant irritable bowel syndrome (Chapter 137). In patients with acquired slow-transit constipation, unassociated with colonic dilation, the number of interstitial cells of Cajal in the different layers of the colon is reduced compared with controls.

Idiopathic megarectum and megacolon can be either congenital or acquired; an enteric nervous system defect is suspected. In megacolon, the dilated segment shows normal phasic contractility but decreased colonic tone, with smooth muscle hypertrophy and fibrosis of the muscularis mucosa, circular muscle, and longitudinal muscle layers.

Acquired defects in the enteric nervous system may result in constipation in Chagas disease (Chapter 347), which is caused by infection with

TABLE 136-2 CLINICAL CLUES SUGGESTIVE OF AN EVACUATION DISORDER

HISTORY

Prolonged straining to expel stool
Taking up unusual postures on the toilet to facilitate stool expulsion
Support of perineum or digitation of rectum or vagina to facilitate rectal emptying
Inability to expel enema fluid
Constipation after subtotal colectomy for constipation

RECTAL EXAMINATION (WITH PATIENT IN LEFT LATERAL POSITION)

Inspection

Anus "pulled" forward during attempts to simulate strain during defecation
Anal verge descends <1 cm or >4 cm during attempts to simulate strain during defecation
Perineum balloons down during straining, and rectal mucosa prolapses through anus

Palpation

High anal sphincter tone at rest precludes easy entry of examining finger (in absence of painful perianal condition, e.g., anal fissure)
Anal sphincter pressure during voluntary squeeze is minimally higher than tone at rest
Perineum descends <1 cm or >4 cm during attempts to simulate strain during defecation
Puborectalis muscle palpable through posterior rectal wall is tender
Palpable mucosal prolapse during straining
"Defect" in anterior wall of the rectum, suggestive of rectocele

ANORECTAL MANOMETRY AND BALLOON EXPULSION (WITH PATIENT IN LEFT LATERAL POSITION)

Average anal sphincter resting tone >80 cm H_2O or squeeze pressure >240 cm H_2O
Failure of balloon expulsion despite addition of 200 g weight

Trypanosoma cruzi and results in the destruction of myenteric neurons. Acquired aganglionosis also has been reported with circulating antineuronal antibodies, with or without associated neoplasm.

DIAGNOSIS

It is essential to distinguish an evacuation disorder, also called functional outlet obstruction (Table 136-2), from constipation resulting from slow transit or other causes. In a tertiary center, about 25% of 1411 patients presenting with constipation had impaired evacuation, and the remainder had constipation associated with either normal transit (also called functional constipation) or delayed colonic transit (also called slow-transit constipation). Characterization of constipated patients (Fig. 136-5) relies on the measurement of transit with radiopaque markers or scintigraphy.

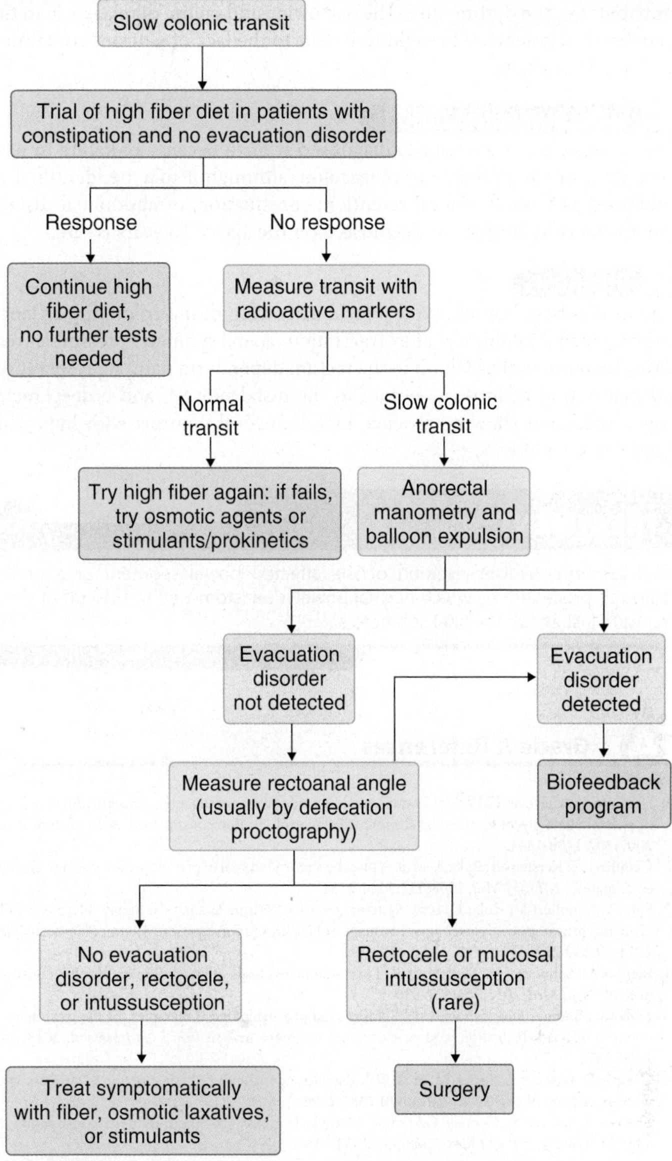

FIGURE 136-5. Algorithm in the management of constipation.

TREATMENT Rx

The average daily fiber intake is around 12 g/day. In patients with normal-transit constipation, 12 to 30 g/day is effective in relief of constipation. In patients with slow-transit constipation, drug-induced constipation, or evacuation disorders, however, supplementation of 30 g of fiber per day does not result in any improvement in constipation. A second step is to add an osmotic laxative, such as a magnesium salt or polyethylene glycol solution, to enhance the retention of fluid within the lumen by osmotic forces, to increase the fluidity, and to ease aboral transport of colonic content. Polyethylene glycol solutions (such as GoLYTELY, NuLYTELY, MiraLAX, OCL solution) are used frequently as a first-line therapy.[A1] If these measures do not suffice, a prokinetic or stimulant agent, such as bisacodyl (5 to 10 mg every 1 to 2 days) may be added.

Newer medications that accelerate colonic transit include prucalopride (2 mg daily), which is beneficial in chronic constipation[A2,A3]; lubiprostone (24 µg twice daily), a chloride channel activator; and linaclotide (145 µg or 290 µg daily), a guanylate cyclase C agonist that induces chloride and fluid secretion.[A4] These drugs[A5] as well as naloxegol (a peripheral µ-opioid antagonist at 12.5 or 25 mg daily)[A6] and methylnaltrexone (0.15 mg/kg subcutaneously every other day for 2 weeks) are effective in patients with opiate-induced constipation as a complication of advanced illness.[A7]

When these approaches do not work, the patient should be reassessed to exclude an evacuation disorder. For evacuation disorders, a biofeedback treatment program with muscle relaxation of the anal sphincters and pelvic floor results in a 70% or greater cure rate for the constipation. The response to this treatment program is influenced by comorbidity, such as the coexistence of eating disorders or a psychological or psychiatric diagnosis.

Surgical Therapy

In patients whose constipation is not associated with an evacuation disorder and does not respond to aggressive medical therapies (including combinations described earlier), subtotal colectomy with ileorectostomy is effective in relieving constipation. Laparoscopic colectomy with ileorectostomy achieves the same success rate with less morbidity compared with open colectomy with ileorectostomy.

Hirschsprung Disease

DEFINITION

Hirschsprung disease occurs in 1 in 5000 live births. It is characterized by a localized segment of narrowing of the distal colon as a result of failure of local development of intrinsic nerves in the myenteric plexus.[8]

PATHOBIOLOGY

A relative deficiency of *KIT*-positive interstitial cells of Cajal has been reported in Hirschsprung disease and chronic intestinal pseudo-obstruction. The majority of familial and sporadic Hirschsprung disease is associated with *RET* oncogene mutations, but mutations in *EDNRB*, *GDNF*, and *EDN3* have been reported as well. Hirschsprung disease is well characterized histologically by the absence of ganglion cells in the myenteric and submucosal plexus and the presence of hypertrophied nerve trunks in the space normally occupied by the ganglion cells. In the muscle layers of the colon involved with Hirschsprung disease, deficiency of nerve growth factor receptors also contributes to the dysfunction. The narrowing and failure of relaxation in the aganglionic segment are thought to be due to the lack of neurons containing nitric oxide synthase.

CLINICAL MANIFESTATIONS

Hirschsprung disease is usually diagnosed at birth because of failure to pass meconium or the presence of megacolon, although it may be identified in childhood as a result of fecal retention, constipation, or abdominal distention. Onset of symptoms or diagnosis after the age of 10 years is rare.

DIAGNOSIS

Diagnosis is based on the typical focal narrowing of the colon, the absence of the rectoanal inhibitory reflex (relaxation of anal sphincter pressure at rest during distention of a balloon in the rectum depends on natural preservation and maturation of intrinsic nerves in the distal bowel), and a deep rectal biopsy specimen showing absence of submucosal neurons with hypertrophied nerve trunks.

TREATMENT

Treatment involves excision of the affected bowel segment or a pull-through procedure by which normal bowel is anastomosed to the cuff of the rectum, just above the anal sphincters.

Grade A References

A1. Dipalma JA, Cleveland MV, McGowan J, et al. A randomized multicenter, placebo-controlled trial of polyethylene glycol laxative for chronic treatment of chronic constipation. *Am J Gastroenterol.* 2007;102:1436-1441.

A2. Camilleri M, Kerstens R, Rykx A, et al. A placebo-controlled trial of prucalopride for severe chronic constipation. *N Engl J Med.* 2008;358:2344-2354.

A3. Shin A, Camilleri M, Kolar G, et al. Systematic review with meta-analysis: highly selective 5-HT_4 agonists (prucalopride, velusetrag or naronapride) in chronic constipation. *Aliment Pharmacol Ther.* 2014;39:239-253.

A4. Lembo AJ, Schneier HA, Shiff SJ, et al. Two randomized trials of linaclotide for chronic constipation. *N Engl J Med.* 2011;365:527-536.

A5. Ford AC, Brenner DM, Schoenfeld PS. Efficacy of pharmacological therapies for the treatment of opioid-induced constipation: systematic review and meta-analysis. *Am J Gastroenterol.* 2013;108:1566-1574.

A6. Chey WD, Webster L, Sostek M, et al. Naloxegol for opioid-induced constipation in patients with noncancer pain. *N Engl J Med.* 2014;370:2387-2396.

A7. Thomas J, Karver S, Cooney GA, et al. Methylnaltrexone for opioid-induced constipation in advanced illness. *N Engl J Med.* 2008;358:2332-2343.

GENERAL REFERENCES

For the General References and other additional features, please visit Expert Consult at https://expertconsult.inkling.com.

137

FUNCTIONAL GASTROINTESTINAL DISORDERS: IRRITABLE BOWEL SYNDROME, DYSPEPSIA, CHEST PAIN OF PRESUMED ESOPHAGEAL ORIGIN, AND HEARTBURN

EMERAN A. MAYER

DEFINITIONS

Irritable bowel syndrome (IBS), functional dyspepsia, functional chest pain of presumed esophageal origin, and functional heartburn are characterized by chronic, recurrent symptoms of pain and discomfort referred to the lower abdomen, the epigastrium and upper abdomen, and the retrosternum, respectively. They belong to the family of functional gastrointestinal (GI) disorders that comprise a wide spectrum of chronic GI disorders common in both the adult and pediatric populations. In the absence of disease-specific biomarkers, each syndrome is classified by symptoms and the absence of other conditions that can account for the symptoms. Despite the benign prognoses, functional GI diseases can affect health-related quality of life at least as much as organic diseases. Because effective pharmacologic therapies are limited, disease management may include cognitive behavioral approaches and alternative medicine approaches (Chapter 39).

PATHOBIOLOGY

The pathophysiology of functional GI diseases remains incompletely understood, but these diseases are characterized by alterations in bidirectional interactions between the brain and the gut (brain-gut axis; E-Fig. 137-1), with variable contributions of peripheral (gut microbiota, mucosal immune activation, motility, bile acids) and central factors (enhanced perception of visceral signals by the central nervous system). In addition, altered signaling from the nervous system to the GI tract through the autonomic nervous system can modulate esophagogastrointestinal function. Each diagnostic category of functional GI disease is defined by symptomatic criteria that include different subsets of patients who exhibit different patterns of the brain-gut axis dysregulation and that result in varying abnormalities in GI motility, secretion, immune function, or visceral sensitivity. Despite this heterogeneity, however, functional GI diseases all share certain features, including a greater prevalence in women, enhanced sensitivity to stress, enhanced perception of visceral signals, the frequent coexistence of psychiatric and chronic pain disorders, and the response to centrally targeted pharmacologic and nonpharmacologic therapies.

Enhanced Perception of Visceral Pain

About 30 to 70% of patients with functional GI diseases have an altered perception of visceral afferent stimuli ("visceral hypersensitivity"), in which normally innocuous stimuli, such as physiologic contractions, distentions by food or gas, or chemical stimulation of the intestine (bile salts, microbial signaling molecules), stomach, or esophagus (hydrochloric acid, bile acids) lead to the sensation of pain or discomfort. The stimulus may be spontaneous peristaltic activity or result from distention by luminal contents, such as ingested food, liquids, gas, or feces. Visceral hypersensitivity may be associated with aberrant referral of visceral sensations to a particular body area, and this referral is often atypical in location and larger compared with most individuals. Many patients also have enhanced perception of somatic pain owing to alterations in sensory processing and modulation systems.

Altered Stress Responsiveness

Abnormal autonomic and neuroendocrine responses to psychosocial stressors are a key feature of functional GI disease and may play an important role in both its cause and its exacerbation. For example, stressful events are more likely to lead to abdominal pain and a change in stool pattern in patients with IBS compared with healthy controls, and stress has been correlated with bowel symptoms and physician visit. Patients with functional GI disease report more lifetime stressful events than healthy controls, including a higher frequency and severity of early adverse life events.

IRRITABLE BOWEL SYNDROME

DEFINITION

IBS is defined as chronic, recurring abdominal pain or discomfort that is associated with defecation or a change in bowel habits; the diagnosis also requires the absence of detectable organic disease that may explain the symptoms[1] (Table 137-1). Given the high prevalence of IBS in the general population, comorbid organic GI syndromes may coexist with IBS, including ulcerative colitis (Chapter 141), microscopic and collagenous colitis (Chapter 140), and celiac disease (Chapter 140). As a result of such comorbidity, some colitis patients report symptom severity disproportionate to the degree of mucosal inflammation and may continue to have GI symptoms after their inflammatory bowel disease or other types of colitis have been successfully treated. For example, a small subset of ulcerative colitis patients exhibit IBS-like symptoms and have demonstrable changes in colonic motility when they are in clinical remission.

IBS is further subdivided into IBS with diarrhea, IBS with constipation, or IBS with mixed bowel habits depending on the predominant bowel habit. Another subset is postinfectious IBS, which includes patients who develop

TABLE 137-1 ROME III DIAGNOSTIC CRITERIA FOR IRRITABLE BOWEL SYNDROME

1. Recurrent abdominal pain or discomfort at least 3 days per month in the last 3 months (but with symptom onset for at least 6 months) associated with two or more of the following:
   - Improvement with defecation
   - Onset associated with a change in frequency of stool
   - Onset associated with a change in form (appearance) of stool

   Symptoms that cumulatively support the diagnosis of irritable bowel syndrome
   - Abnormal stool frequency: ≤3 bowel movements per week or >3 bowel movements per day
   - Abnormal stool form: lumpy/hard stool or loose/watery stool
   - Defecation straining
   - Urgency
   - Feeling of incomplete bowel movement
   - Passing mucus
   - Bloating or feeling of abdominal distention
2. Absence of alarm symptoms:
   - Weight loss
   - Bloody stool
   - Anemia
   - Family history of inflammatory bowel disease
   - Colon cancer
   - Celiac disease

persistent IBS-like symptoms despite the resolution of an episode or episodes of bacterial gastroenteritis. When patients do not fulfill criteria for these subtypes, their disease is classified as unspecified IBS.

EPIDEMIOLOGY

IBS is a common disorder, with a worldwide prevalence that ranges between 5 and 15%. As is the case with many related functional pain disorders, it is more common in women, with a female-to-male ratio of 2 : 1 to 2.5 : 1. It is generally assumed that IBS most commonly presents between the ages of 30 and 50 years, but IBS is also common in the pediatric population, in which such symptoms have traditionally been referred to as recurrent abdominal pain.

The socioeconomic burden of IBS is substantial, with patients taking three times as many days of sick leave compared with individuals without IBS; about 8% of patients retire early because of their symptoms. IBS is estimated to account for about 12% of primary care visits and 19% of GI specialty visits. In the United States, IBS is estimated to account for $1.6 billion in direct costs and $19.2 billion in indirect costs annually.

PATHOBIOLOGY

Although IBS is the most common and best studied functional GI disease, there is no general agreement on its pathophysiology. Both peripheral and central alterations are implicated in the brain-gut axis that best explains the clinical manifestations of IBS.[2]

Altered Gastrointestinal Motility and Secretion

GI motility is quantitatively but not qualitatively different in 25 to 75% of IBS patients compared with healthy controls, but these measured differences are not sufficiently reliable to be used as diagnostic markers. Colonic transit is accelerated in about 45% of IBS patients with diarrhea, and high-amplitude propagating contractions occur more frequently in such patients than in controls. These high-amplitude propagating contractions correlate with crampy abdominal pain and may be the mechanism underlying urgency, diarrhea, and associated fecal incontinence in this patient subgroup. By contrast, slowed colonic transit is observed in about 25% of IBS patients with constipation. Exaggerated or prolonged colonic motility responses to food intake (gastrocolonic response) may be present in approximately 30% of patients who report an exacerbation of abdominal pain after food intake. Likely contributors to alterations in bowel habits include abnormalities in intestinal water and electrolyte secretion and absorption as well as altered synthesis and secretion of bile acids.

Acute stress-induced activation of contractions and secretions of the hindgut is mediated by sacral parasympathetic pathways, and IBS patients have increased activation of these pathways in response to severe laboratory stressors. Tonic upregulation of sympathetic and sacral parasympathetic activity may result in neuroplastic changes in peripheral target mechanisms within the gut, including the enteric nervous system.

Evidence supports increased intestinal permeability predominantly in IBS patients with diarrhea. Metabolites from gut microbiota, GI infections, and chronic psychological stress can decrease epithelial barrier function in susceptible individuals.

In response to luminal signals such as bile acids, moving intestinal contents, and microbial products, serotonin is released from enterochromaffin cells on the basolateral side of the intestinal epithelium, where it stimulates vagal afferent nerves and enteric neurons involved in secretion and motility. An increased release of serotonin from these cells following a meal may contribute to increased motility and secretion in IBS patients with diarrhea.

Data indicate decreased diversity in small bowel microbiota of patients with IBS, with an increased abundance of gram-negative organisms and a decrease of *Bifidobacterium* and *Lactobacillus*, as well as increased ratios of Firmicutes to Bacteroidetes.[3,4] Metabolites produced by microbiota, including short-chain fatty acids and neurotransmitter substances, have been implicated in mediating the effects of dysbiosis on the gut. Small bowel bacterial overgrowth may contribute to IBS symptoms in some patients, especially those with predominant bloating-type symptoms, in whom treatment with nonabsorbable antibiotics may reduce symptoms.

Altered synthesis and secretion of bile acids may result in increased fluid secretion and motility patterns. Certain foods that may trigger symptoms include milk, wheat products, and fermentable oligosaccharides, disaccharides, monosaccharides, and polyols (FODMAP).

Genetics

Familial aggregation has been demonstrated in several studies of IBS patients, and the genetic heritability of functional GI diseases has been estimated to be between 22 and 57%. Candidate gene association studies suggest possible association of IBS with polymorphisms in genes related to signaling systems within the brain-gut axis, including bile acid physiology, serotonin, noradrenaline, corticotropin-releasing factor, and voltage-gated sodium channels.[5] Epigenetic factors, including the influence of certain types of stress, have been identified as an important influence on the risk for developing IBS.

CLINICAL MANIFESTATIONS

Symptoms

The location of abdominal symptoms in IBS is highly variable, but pain is most typically referred to the lower abdomen. Pain and discomfort, which occur mainly while the patient is awake, are frequently aggravated by emotion or stress, poor sleep, and intake of food, but these aggravating factors cannot be elicited in all patients. By definition, abdominal symptoms are relieved by defecation, but this relief may be temporary. IBS symptoms vary widely, from mild to very severe. Most patients seen by primary care physicians have mild symptoms, whereas most patients seen by gastroenterologists have moderate to severe symptoms.

Psychological symptoms and psychiatric diagnoses (Chapter 397), such as anxiety disorders (e.g., generalized anxiety disorder, panic disorder, and post-traumatic stress syndrome), depression, somatization, hypochondriasis, and phobias, are more common in patients with IBS, even in mildly symptomatic patients. The prevalence of coexisting psychiatric disorders can be as high as 40% to more than 90% in patients seen in tertiary referral centers but is lower in patients seen in primary care practices. Even in the absence of demonstrable psychiatric comorbidity, psychosocial stressors play an important role in exacerbating IBS symptoms in patients seen in all settings.

Patients with IBS have a three-fold or higher prevalence of fibromyalgia (Chapter 274) and migraine headaches (Chapter 398) compared with patients without IBS. IBS also frequently coexists with chronic fatigue syndrome, and 60% or more of patients with chronic fatigue syndrome have IBS symptoms. Interstitial cystitis, chronic prostatitis (Chapter 129), chronic pelvic pain, and temporomandibular disorders are also common in IBS patients.

These associations of IBS with comorbid conditions and other symptoms are more common in female patients, but all patients with IBS on average see primary care physicians for non-GI complaints three times more frequently than do healthy subjects. IBS patients also often complain of extraintestinal symptoms such as dyspareunia, fatigue, loss of energy, impotence, urinary frequency, backache, and dysmenorrhea.

DIAGNOSIS

The Rome III criteria (see Table 137-1) can establish the diagnosis of IBS without additional extensive testing. Alternative diagnoses should be considered if symptoms awaken patients from sleep, are unrelated to defecation or

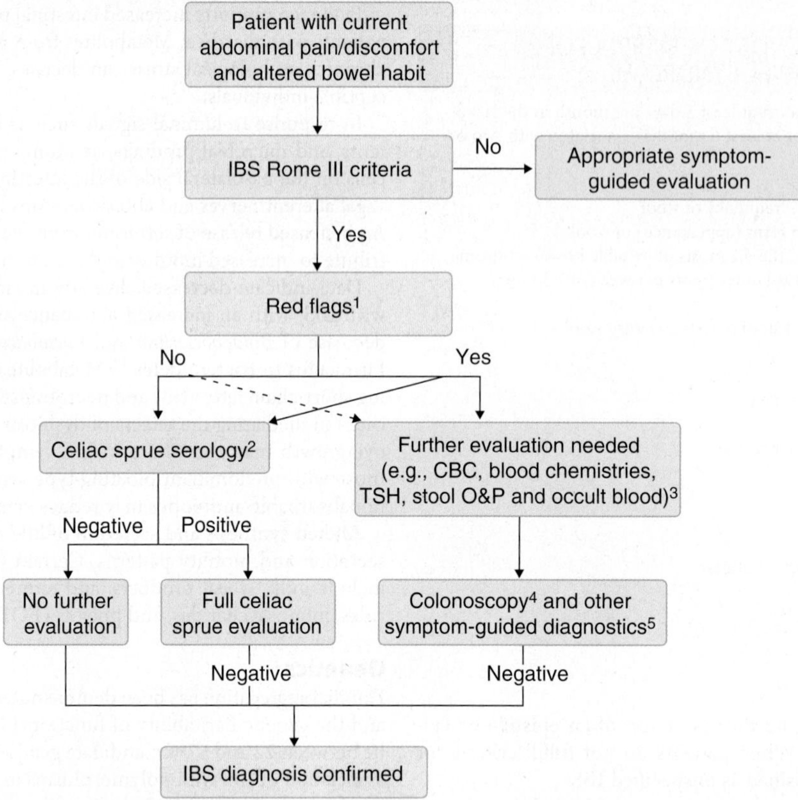

FIGURE 137-1. **Diagnostic algorithm for irritable bowel syndrome (IBS). (1) Red flags include rectal bleeding, anemia, weight loss, fever, family history of colon cancer, first symptom onset after age 50 years, or major symptom change. (2) Testing for celiac sprue may be useful in patients meeting Rome criteria, in particular in irritable bowel syndrome with diarrhea, if there are red flags, and in populations in which the background prevalence of celiac sprue is high. (3) In the absence of red flags, basic complete blood count (CBC), serum biochemistry, stool testing for occult blood and ova and parasites (O&P), and thyroid-stimulating hormone (TSH) levels are only indicated in cases of a supportive clinical history. (4) Colonoscopy is only recommended in the patient with positive red flags. However, according to colon cancer screening guidelines, routine colonoscopy should be performed in IBS patients at age 50 years or older regardless of IBS symptoms. (5) If there has been a major qualitative change in the pattern of chronic symptoms, a new comorbid condition producing these symptoms should be suspected, and a more comprehensive diagnostic approach is warranted. (From Mayer EA. Clinical perspectives: irritable bowel syndrome. *N Engl J Med*. 2008;358:1692-1699.)**

food intake, are constant, or are not relieved by any physiologic intervention. Weight loss is uncommon in IBS except in patients with depression (Chapter 397) or eating disorders (Chapter 219), and its presence mandates investigation of an underlying organic cause. Other alarm features raising concern for serious alternative diagnosis include bloody stools, anemia, and a family history of inflammatory bowel disease, colon cancer, or celiac disease.

Careful review of medications and dietary supplements may reveal an etiologic agent because many prescribed medications can cause constipation and some diet supplements can lead to the inadvertent ingestion of laxatives. Specific dietary agents rarely cause IBS symptoms, but lactose malabsorption can be assessed by history or by a short trial of a lactose-free diet (Chapter 140), and the diagnosis of celiac disease (Chapter 140) should be excluded. A brief psychosocial assessment is useful in identifying risk factors for chronic pain, such as traumatic early life events or somatization, as well as potential symptom triggers or exacerbating factors, such as anxiety, depression, and significant life stress.

The physical examination in IBS is usually normal but may reveal abdominal tenderness, especially in the left lower quadrant, or a tender, palpable sigmoid colon. In patients with constipation-predominant IBS and associated defecatory dysfunction, rectal examination may reveal paradoxical contraction of the puborectalis muscle or decreased descent of the pelvic floor when simulating a bowel movement.

Diagnostic Testing

In an otherwise healthy person who is younger than 50 years and who fulfills the Rome III criteria, further diagnostic testing should be minimal and guided by the individual presentation (Fig. 137-1). It remains controversial when to order a complete blood count, sedimentation rate, or thyroid studies, but most agree that it is not cost-effective to obtain these tests in all patients with presumed IBS. Serologic screening for celiac disease (Chapter 140) should be pursued in patients with diarrhea-predominant or mixed bowel habits, in patients with a family history of celiac disease, and in patients who have identified gluten-containing foods as a trigger of their symptoms. Colonic biopsies for collagenous or microscopic colitis (Chapter 140) should be considered in the setting of severe persistent diarrhea. The onset of symptoms after age 50 years and the presence of rectal bleeding or unexpected weight loss are indications for colonoscopy to assess for colorectal cancer (Chapter 193). Lower abdominal discomfort occurring with menses or with associated weight loss should trigger gynecologic evaluation. If the duration of diarrhea symptoms is short, it may be useful to assess for giardiasis (Chapter 351) or *Campylobacter* species infection (Chapter 303), but routine stool testing of all patients with diarrhea is not indicated.

Differential Diagnosis

Differential diagnosis for IBS with diarrhea predominance or mixed bowel habit includes inflammatory bowel diseases (e.g., Crohn disease, ulcerative colitis, collagenous or microscopic colitis) (Chapters 140 and 141), celiac disease (Chapter 140), infection, small bowel bacterial overgrowth (Chapter 140), malabsorptive syndromes (including lactose intolerance) (Chapter 140), bile salt malabsorption (Chapter 140), and pancreatic insufficiency (Chapter 144) or malignancy (including neuroendocrine tumors [Chapter 195] and colorectal adenocarcinoma [Chapter 193]). The differential diagnosis for constipation-predominant IBS includes colonic inertia, GI manifestations of Parkinson disease, pseudo-obstruction, paradoxical pelvic floor contraction, or pelvic outlet obstruction from structural causes such as rectal prolapse, rectocele, or short-segment Hirschsprung disease (Chapter 136).

TREATMENT Rx

General Principles

Symptomatic treatment attempts to normalize bowel habits and decrease abdominal pain, in part by providing the patient with a plausible biologic explanation for their symptoms as well as reassurance that the symptoms are real and the prognosis is benign. Dietary intervention can be helpful, and

TABLE 137-2 MEDICATIONS USED IN THE TREATMENT OF IRRITABLE BOWEL SYNDROME*

SYMPTOMS AND MEDICATION	INITIAL DOSE (mg/day)†	TARGET DOSE (mg/day)†	COMMON OR SERIOUS SIDE EFFECTS	DEGREE OF EVIDENCE of the Symptom	DEGREE OF EVIDENCE of IBS	FDA APPROVED for the Symptom	FDA APPROVED for IBS
CONSTIPATION							
Laxatives‡ and Secretory Stimulators							
Polyethylene glycol 3350 (MiraLAX)	17,000	70,000	Diarrhea, bloating, cramping	+++	–		
Lactulose (Kristalose)	10,000-20,000	20,000-40,000	Diarrhea, bloating, cramping	+++	–		
Lubiprostone (Amitiza)		24, twice a day	Nausea, diarrhea, headache, abdominal pain and discomfort	+++	–	Yes§	No
Linaclotide (Linzess)		145,000 (IBS-C) 290,000 (Constip)	Diarrhea, abdominal pain, flatulence	+++	+++	Yes	Yes
DIARRHEA							
Loperamide (Imodium)	2	2-8	Constipation	+++	–	Yes	No
Alosetron (Lotronex)			Constipation, ischemic colitis (rare)	–	+++	No	Yes¶
BLOATING							
Antibiotics							
Rifaximin		400, three times a day	Abdominal pain, diarrhea, bad taste	–	+	No	No
Probiotics**							
Bifidobacterium infantis 35624		1 capsule per day	None	+	+	No	No
Activia *Bifidus regularis*		1 pod, twice a day	None	+		N/A	N/A
PAIN							
Tricyclic Antidepressants††			Dry mouth, dizziness, weight gain				
Amitriptyline (Elavil)	10, at bedtime	10-75, at bedtime		++	+	No	No
Desipramine (Norpramin)	10, at bedtime	10-75, at bedtime		++	+	No	No
Selective Serotonin Reuptake Inhibitors‡‡			Sexual dysfunction, headache, nausea, sedation, insomnia, sweating, withdrawal symptoms				
Paroxetine (Paxil CR)		10-60		–	+	No	No
Citalopram (Lexapro)		5-20		+	+	No	No
Fluoxetine (Prozac)		20-40	Somnolence, dizziness, headaches, insomnia	+	–	No	No
Nonselective Reuptake Inhibitors							
Duloxetine (Cymbalta)	30	60	Nausea, dry mouth, headache, dizziness	++	-	Yes	No

*This list is not exhaustive but includes major medications for which there is evidence from well-designed clinical trials of effectiveness for global irritable bowel syndrome (IBS) symptoms or for individual symptoms (e.g., constipation, diarrhea, or abdominal pain and discomfort). In the column about evidence, + denotes some evidence from at least one controlled trial; ++, moderate evidence from several controlled trials or from meta-analysis of such trials; +++, strong evidence from well-designed, controlled clinical trials; and –, no evidence. FDA = U.S. Food and Drug Administration.
†Dosages are in milligrams per day unless otherwise noted.
‡A wide range of osmotic and irritant laxatives, including fiber products, are available over the counter.
§Lubiprostone is FDA approved for the treatment of chronic constipation.
Linaclotide is FDA approved for the treatment of chronic constipation (145 mcg/day) and IBS with constipation (290 mcg/day).
¶Lotronex use is restricted for women with severe diarrhea-predominant IBS, unresponsive to other medications, because of side effects.
**Many probiotics are available over the counter and are not listed. Align is a probiotic for which a beneficial effect for IBS symptoms has been shown in a high-quality, randomized, controlled trial.
††A wide range of tricyclic antidepressants with various side effects and side-effect profiles are available. Two commonly prescribed tricyclic antidepressants are listed.
‡‡Many selective serotonin reuptake inhibitors are available. Only those that have been evaluated in IBS trials are listed.

specific medications can be targeted to the management of individual symptoms, such as constipation, diarrhea, and abdominal pain (Table 137-2).

Physician-Patient Relationship and Patient Education

The doctor-patient relationship is of utmost importance in the treatment of IBS and other functional GI diseases. Many patients have been told previously that their symptoms are "all in their head" and have had their concerns dismissed. The physician must listen to and determine the patient's understanding of the illness and related concerns because patients frequently seek validation from the physician that their symptoms are real. Patients with functional GI disease typically visit a physician because of a flare of their usual symptoms, and it is important to identify such triggering factors, in particular various psychosocial stressors or, less commonly, a gastroenteric infection.

A thorough explanation of the symptoms and relationship to functional GI disease should be provided to the patient, including the natural history and benign prognosis of the disorder. Patients who are not properly informed tend to have more health care visits, whereas symptoms generally are reduced when diagnostic and prognostic information is explained. The physician must then set realistic short-term and long-term goals, including methods of adapting to symptoms that are not amenable to treatment. Patients often benefit from being involved in their treatment, and the maintenance of a symptom diary is one such example. Apart from providing the patient with a sense of empowerment, the symptom diary can help identify erroneous beliefs as well as lifestyle or dietary factors that may exacerbate symptoms; lifestyle modifications based on this information may provide symptomatic relief.

Dietary Modification

Some patients with functional GI disease, especially patients with IBS and functional dyspepsia, often complain that certain types of food exacerbate their symptoms. Others complain that any type of food, even a sip of water, may trigger symptoms. Perceived food sensitivity may be related to a variety of factors, including conditioned fear responses related to anticipatory anxiety, food intake in general, volume of the meal, or sensitivities to certain food items. For example, a diet low in fermentable oligosaccharides, disaccharides, monosaccharides, and polyols (FODMAP) can effectively reduce symptoms of IBS in some patients.[A1] Some IBS patients report an exacerbation of symptoms with high-fat food, milk products, gas-producing food, gluten-containing food, alcohol, and caffeine. It is important to inform the patient that there is no universal diet that is successful in every IBS patient. However, a therapeutic trial of a lactose-free diet or a gluten-free diet[6] may benefit some patients, even in the absence of obvious lactose intolerance or documentable celiac disease. If, however, such dietary changes are not effective in consistently reducing symptoms, patients should resume consumption of the eliminated foods.

Pharmacologic Therapy

Medications for Bowel Habit Abnormalities and Bloating

Few medications have been proved to benefit patients with IBS.[7] In IBS with constipation, osmotic laxatives, such as polyethylene glycol or lactulose, or secretory stimulators, such as lubiprostone, or linaclotide[A2] can be useful. Dietary fiber supplements often increase symptoms of gas, bloating, and flatulence and should not be used as first-line therapy.

In the IBS patient with diarrhea, loperamide is generally effective in reducing urgency and uncontrollable bowel movements. The 5-HT_3 receptor antagonist alosetron (0.5 to 1 mg orally twice per day) is clinically effective but should be considered only in patients who have severe diarrhea and who have failed all other therapies because of its infrequent but potentially serious side effects.

Manipulation of the intestinal flora with antibiotics (rifaximin 550 mg three times daily for 2 weeks)[A3] may be effective in some patients, particularly patients with abdominal bloating symptoms. It should not be used as a first-line drug, however, because its long-term effects on the gut microbiome are unknown. Clinical evidence supports the use of probiotics[A4] for nonpainful symptoms, but the response rate is low. Herbal laxatives such as aloe, rhubarb root products, and peppermint oil may be of use in some patients.

Antidepressants and Psychological Therapies

Low doses of tricyclic antidepressants (e.g., nortriptyline, amitriptyline, or imipramine, 10 to 50 mg at bedtime) are frequently used to treat IBS based on data that about one patient in four may benefit. Doses should be started as low as 5 mg once daily and gradually advanced to a maximum of 50 mg once daily if tolerated. The therapeutic effect should be expected within days to 2 weeks of initiating therapy; if no beneficial effect is observed at 50 mg once daily or if significant side effects are experienced, the drug should be discontinued. Amitriptyline may be most useful in patients with prominent abdominal pain and diarrhea symptoms and in patients with sleep problems, but other tricyclics should be tried if side effects are experienced.

To maximize compliance and reduce side effects, the patient should be informed about the rationale of the treatment choice (i.e., the goal is the treatment of pain and not psychiatric symptoms) and informed about the much lower risk for side effects at the low dose range compared with full psychiatric doses.

If the treatment goal is aimed at comorbid depression or anxiety disorders, a selective serotonin reuptake inhibitor (SSRI) should be tried. In such patients, either a combination of a low-dose tricyclic antidepressant with a full therapeutic dose of an SSRI (see Table 137-2) or the use of a nonselective uptake inhibitor (SNRI) such as duloxetine, milnacipran, or venlafaxine should be considered.

Cognitive-behavioral therapy, which involves relaxation, change in beliefs, and self-management, can reduce gastrointestinal symptoms in at least 50% of patients.[A5] Novel delivery forms of cognitive-behavioral therapy, such as minimal contact therapy or Internet-assisted therapy, are cost-effective approaches where available. Several controlled trials support the effectiveness of hypnotherapy.

PROGNOSIS

The natural history of IBS is periods of exacerbation followed by periods of remission, but about 50% of IBS patients become asymptomatic. Patients with coexisting psychiatric disorders are less likely to have their IBS symptoms resolve.

FUNCTIONAL DYSPEPSIA

As with other functional GI diseases, the diagnosis of functional dyspepsia is based on specific symptoms (Tables 137-3 and 137-4). Functional dyspepsia is thought to originate from the upper GI tract, but no detectable organic disease can explain the symptoms. Symptoms may include epigastric pain, epigastric burning, postprandial fullness, and early satiation. Abdominal bloating and nausea also may be experienced, but they are less specific and are not considered cardinal symptoms of functional dyspepsia. Symptoms

TABLE 137-3 ROME III DIAGNOSTIC CRITERIA FOR FUNCTIONAL DYSPEPSIA*

1. One or more of the following:
   - Bothersome postprandial fullness
   - Early satiation
   - Epigastric pain
   - Epigastric burning

and

2. No evidence of structural disease (including at upper endoscopy) that is likely to explain the symptoms

*The criteria must be fulfilled for the last 3 months with symptom onset at least 6 months before diagnosis.

TABLE 137-4 ROME III DIAGNOSTIC CRITERIA FOR SUBGROUPS OF PATIENTS WITH FUNCTIONAL DYSPEPSIA*

POSTPRANDIAL DISTRESS SYNDROME

One or both of the following:
1. Bothersome postprandial fullness, occurring after ordinary sized meals, at least several times per week
2. Early satiation that prevents finishing a regular meal, at least several times per week

Supportive criteria

1. Upper abdominal bloating or postprandial nausea or excessive belching can be present.
2. Epigastric pain syndrome may coexist.

EPIGASTRIC PAIN SYNDROME

One or more of the following:
1. Pain or burning localized to the epigastrium of at least moderate severity at least once per week
2. Intermittent pain
3. Pain not generalized or localized to other abdominal or chest regions
4. Pain not relieved by defecation or passage of flatus
5. Pain not fulfilling criteria for gallbladder and sphincter of Oddi disorders

Supportive criteria

1. The pain may be of a burning quality but without a retrosternal component.
2. The pain is commonly induced or relieved by ingestion of a meal but may occur while fasting.
3. Postprandial distress syndrome may coexist.

*The criteria must be fulfilled for the last 3 months with symptom onset at least 6 months before diagnosis.

overlap with atypical manifestations of gastroesophageal reflux disease (GERD; Chapter 138), and previous studies on functional dyspepsia may have inadvertently included patients with atypical GERD symptoms.

In the current Rome III criteria, symptoms are divided into the meal-related postprandial distress syndrome and the meal-unrelated epigastric pain syndrome (see Table 137-4). The clinical utility of these subgroups is controversial because these two entities often overlap in the same patient. Moreover, the concept of distinct pathophysiologies correlating with distinct symptom patterns has not been confirmed.[8]

EPIDEMIOLOGY

Functional dyspepsia is a common disorder, with an estimated prevalence of 3 to 10% based on Rome III criteria and of up to 40% when less restrictive criteria are used. The socioeconomic burden of functional dyspepsia is substantial; patients with functional dyspepsia take three times as much sick leave as patients with duodenal ulcers. In the United Kingdom, an estimated 2 to 5% of primary care visits and more than 10% of primary care drug expenditures are related to functional dyspepsia. Approximately one of two individuals with functional dyspepsia seeks health care for symptoms at some time in their life. In the United States, the diagnosis, treatment, and work absenteeism related to functional dyspepsia have been estimated to cost $18.4 billion per year.

Pain or discomfort in the upper abdomen may be assumed to be related to the upper GI tract, but on detailed questioning, the "dyspepsia" may be related to bowel disturbances. One third of patients with functional dyspepsia have concurrent symptoms of IBS, and approximately 40% of IBS patients also report symptoms of functional dyspepsia. Moreover, transitions between the two syndromes in the same patient over time are common. In a 1-year follow-up of patients with IBS or dyspepsia, 22% of IBS patients reported a change in their symptom profile to that of functional dyspepsia, and 16% of patients with functional dyspepsia reported a change to an IBS symptom profile. This transition of patients between different diagnostic categories puts into question the concept that these symptom-based entities are really distinct pathophysiologic syndromes. Compared with patients with non-life-threatening organic GI disease, patients with functional dyspepsia have higher anxiety but not depression or neuroticism scores.

PATHOBIOLOGY

The pathobiology of functional dyspepsia is not fully understood, but both central and peripheral mechanisms have been proposed. Although enhanced perception of gastric stimuli may be a key central mechanism, the roles of gastric acid, acute and chronic gastric mucosal infections, and gastroduodenal dysmotility remain to be determined. Attempts to classify subtypes of functional dyspepsia based on pathophysiologic abnormalities or predominant symptoms have been unsuccessful so far.

As with IBS patients, visceral hypersensitivity is common in functional dyspepsia, and 34 to 65% of patients with functional dyspepsia report pain and discomfort at lower volumes of gastric distention than healthy control subjects or patients with dyspepsia from organic causes. Chemical sensitivity to capsaicin also has been reported. Central sensory augmentation of painful and nonpainful stimuli also likely contribute to the observed gastric hypersensitivity. For example, the presence of lipids in the duodenum increases the sensitivity of patients with functional dyspepsia to gastric balloon distention compared with controls. This abnormal modulation of gastric perception thresholds to distention by lipid in a distant site supports the concept of a centrally mediated mechanism and is consistent with the clinical observation that fatty foods worsen symptoms in such patients. Furthermore, about 50% of patients with functional dyspepsia experience altered viscerosomatic referral patterns in response to gastric balloon distention. Some patients are hypersensitive to either intraduodenal or intra-antral acid or suffer from atypical manifestations of GERD.

In a small subset of patients, chronic *Helicobacter pylori* infection (Chapter 139) may be related to functional dyspepsia. About 20% of patients with functional dyspepsia develop their symptoms after an acute episode of presumed viral or bacterial gastroenteritis or *Giardia* species infection (Chapter 351).

Alterations in gastroduodenal motility, such as delayed gastric emptying, are found in some patients with functional dyspepsia, but the low concordance between symptoms and altered motility argues against a pathophysiologic link. Anxiety, depression, somatization, and stress contribute to the severity of symptoms and their impact on quality of life.

CLINICAL MANIFESTATIONS AND DIAGNOSIS

Dyspepsia can be suspected to be functional based on a clinical history consistent with the Rome III criteria (see Tables 137-3 and 137-4) and the absence of alarm features (see Table 137-1). The presence of anxiety, in particular symptom-related anxiety and comorbid IBS, increases the likelihood of functional dyspepsia. Nonsteroidal anti-inflammatory medications, alcohol, and certain foods can trigger dyspeptic symptoms. A psychosocial history may reveal underlying stressors that contribute to symptoms.

The physical examination is generally normal, although epigastric tenderness may be present. In contrast to gastroparesis, a succussion splash indicative of delayed gastric emptying is typically absent. Although confirmation of the functional dyspepsia diagnosis requires a normal upper endoscopic examination, invasive testing in the absence of alarm features should be considered only in a minority of symptomatic patients, such as patients older than 50 years with new-onset or changing symptoms or a poor response to initial therapy. Evaluation for *H. pylori* (Chapter 139) may be performed by stool antigen, urea breath test, or gastric biopsy.

Differential Diagnosis

Common organic causes of dyspepsia include gastroesophageal reflux disease (Chapter 138) and peptic ulcer disease (Chapter 139). Mild to moderately delayed gastric emptying is present in about 30% of patients with functional dyspepsia but is characteristic and more pronounced in patients with diabetic or idiopathic gastroparesis (Chapter 136). Delayed vomiting of undigested food is characteristic of these forms of gastroparesis, but not of dyspepsia. Gastric and esophageal cancers (Chapter 192) may also present with symptoms of dyspepsia but are much less common. Pancreaticobiliary disorders (Chapters 144 and 155) (including sphincter of Oddi dysfunction, chronic pancreatitis, or pancreatic cancer) also occasionally mimic dyspepsia.

TREATMENT Rx

H. pylori infection, if present, should be eradicated[9] (Chapter 139), and then symptoms should be reassessed. About 10 to 15% of patients with functional dyspepsia respond to acid suppression therapy,[A6] and options include histamine (H_2)-receptor antagonists (e.g., famotidine, 20 mg twice per day) and proton pump inhibitors (e.g., omeprazole, 20 mg per day).[10] Young patients who respond well to a trial of proton pump inhibitor (see Table 138-1) therapy or *H. pylori* eradication (see Table 139-4) do not require further investigation unless alarm features are identified. If symptoms persist, some patients respond to treatment with a low-dose tricyclic antidepressant (e.g., amitriptyline, desipramine, or imipramine 10 to 50 mg every night at bedtime). In patients with comorbid depression or anxiety, the combination of low-dose tricyclics with a full dose of an SSRI or the use of an SNRI (see Table 137-2) should be considered.

The benefits of cognitive-behavioral therapy and hypnosis for functional dyspepsia have not been studied in high-quality trials, but such therapies may be reasonable in patients who do not respond to pharmacotherapy. Prokinetic drugs such as domperidone and acotiamide are of uncertain benefit and are not approved by the U.S. Food and Drug Administration for this purpose.

PROGNOSIS

As with all functional disorders, functional dyspepsia has a benign prognosis with a high rate of spontaneous remissions, although symptoms can be persistent.

FUNCTIONAL CHEST PAIN OF PRESUMED ESOPHAGEAL ORIGIN AND FUNCTIONAL HEARTBURN

DEFINITION

Functional chest pain of presumed esophageal origin (Table 137-5) is a chronic, unexplained midline chest pain that is thought to be of esophageal origin. To make the diagnosis, cardiac causes, gastroesophageal reflux, and well-defined motility disorders (achalasia, scleroderma) must be excluded. Functional heartburn is defined as a burning retrosternal discomfort of pain that persists for at least 3 months in the absence of GERD or an esophageal motility disorder.[11]

EPIDEMIOLOGY

Functional chest pain is quite common, with prevalence rates as high as 25%, evenly divided between men and women. Its prevalence appears to decline with advancing age. Most patients who present to a physician with acute chest pain (see Table 51-2) have a noncardiac cause, and many are cases of functional chest pain. Risk factors for developing functional chest pain are not well defined but include younger age, adversity in childhood, and a history of other functional gastrointestinal conditions. Once symptoms occur, more than 50% of patients have persisting symptoms for longer than 6 months. Even after the initial diagnosis, however, many patients with chronic pain undergo repeated and unnecessary diagnostic cardiac evaluations. Patients with functional chest pain may have comorbid anxiety or panic attacks, but formal referral for psychological treatment is infrequent. When compared with patients who have known cardiac chest pain, patients with functional chest pain report

TABLE 137-5 ROME III DIAGNOSTIC CRITERIA FOR FUNCTIONAL CHEST PAIN OF PRESUMED ESOPHAGEAL ORIGIN*

Must include all of the following:

- Midline chest pain or discomfort that is not of burning quality
- Absence of evidence that gastroesophageal reflux is the cause of symptoms
- Absence of histopathology-based esophageal motility disorders

*The criteria must be fulfilled for the last 3 months with symptom onset at least 6 months before diagnosis.

greater impairment of health-related quality of life in the domains of mental health and vitality. These findings suggest a link between psychological disturbance and functional chest pain, at least in a subgroup of patients.

Functional heartburn has been reported in about 20% of patients evaluated in a tertiary referral population for heartburn that is refractory to proton pump inhibitor therapy. However, its prevalence in the general population is unknown.

PATHOBIOLOGY

The pathophysiology of both functional chest pain and functional heartburn are incompletely understood, although visceral hypersensitivity, altered esophageal motility, and psychological factors have all been implicated. A substantial proportion of patients show enhanced sensitivity to esophageal distention by a balloon. These same patients will often also have increased perceptual responses to intraesophageal acid infusion. The origin of such findings is not clear, although alterations in central processing of sensory signals from the esophagus (central sensory augmentation) have been implicated. In addition, altered esophageal motility can be observed in a subset of patients with functional chest pain, with or without visceral hypersensitivity. Increased contraction of the esophageal muscle has long been considered a source of chest pain, although reproducible studies to prove this hypothesis are lacking.

CLINICAL MANIFESTATIONS

Patients with functional chest pain may complain of pain that is typical for myocardial ischemia or of pain with a variety of characteristics that would be considered atypical for ischemia (Chapters 51 and 71). The location of pain is typically substernal, but radiation to the arm and neck can be described. The pain typically is not precipitated by exertion and may persist for hours. Nitroglycerin may sometimes be helpful acutely in patients with coexisting esophageal spasm. Patients may describe the discomfort using a variety of adjectives, and those descriptions may be indistinguishable from angina.

Patients with functional heartburn complain of typical heartburn symptoms that usually are triggered by food intake and psychosocial stress but are refractory to acid suppressive therapy with proton pump inhibitors. By definition, they also have negative endoscopic and acid monitoring evaluations of the esophagus.

DIAGNOSIS

Patients who present with chest pain suspicious for angina should undergo prompt cardiac evaluation (Chapters 51 and 71). In patients with an initial negative cardiac evaluation, causes of functional chest pain can be categorized based on historical features (Table 137-6), and repeated cardiac evaluation for recurrent pain is of low yield. Clinical features, such as association with certain foods or pain location, can help differentiate well between acid-induced and non-acid-related causes. Patients with prominent chest wall pain and tenderness on palpation or with changes in pain with movement usually have musculoskeletal rather than esophageal pain. The remaining patients may have an esophageal source of pain (Chapter 138) and should be divided into patients with and without alarm symptoms, such as weight loss, progressive dysphagia, or anemia. Upper endoscopy is useful in patients with alarm features but is of lower yield in patients without them.

Many patients with functional chest pain or heartburn will have atypical GERD and should be given a therapeutic trial of a proton pump inhibitor (e.g., omeprazole, 20 mg daily).[12] Patients who respond to a 1- to 2-week trial of daily proton pump inhibitor likely have acid-related symptoms and should be treated for GERD. In patients whose response is equivocal, a longer proton pump inhibitor trial of 4 to 8 weeks, endoscopy, or 24-hour pH testing can be considered.

For patients who do not respond to a proton pump inhibitor, a disorder of esophageal motility or visceral hypersensitivity may be present. Esophageal motility disorders such as high-amplitude contractions ("nutcracker esophagus") or diffuse esophageal spasm can be identified by esophageal manometry, but the low concordance between symptoms and manometric findings suggests that such testing should be performed only in highly selected patients based on the advice of a gastroenterologist.

TABLE 137-6 DIFFERENTIAL DIAGNOSIS OF FUNCTIONAL CHEST PAIN

ORGANIC ESOPHAGEAL CAUSES
Gastroesophageal reflux disease
Achalasia
Virus- or pill-induced esophagitis
NONGASTROINTESTINAL CAUSES
Cardiac chest pain
Chest wall pain
Pulmonary disease
Panic attack

TREATMENT

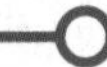

For both functional chest pain and functional heartburn, low-dose tricyclic antidepressants (e.g., amitriptyline, imipramine, or desipramine, 10 to 50 mg per day) may be useful, particularly in patients suspected to have visceral hypersensitivity.[13] Comorbid psychological symptoms should be addressed with either pharmacologic (addition of an SSRI to the tricyclic antidepression or trial with an SNRI [see Table 137-2]) or cognitive behavioral approaches. Even in the absence of a specific psychiatric diagnosis, relaxation therapy or cognitive behavioral therapy may be of benefit.

In the patient with functional chest pain, fears of cardiac disease should be addressed explicitly, and the significance of a negative cardiac evaluation must be reinforced. If the functional chest pain is responsive to a proton pump inhibitor trial, patients should be continued on such therapy or treated with alternative acid-suppressing medications. The optimal duration of treatment is unclear, but it is reasonable to attempt withdrawal of medication and observe patients who have remained asymptomatic for several months.

PROGNOSIS

The natural course of functional chest pain is not well understood, likely because most patients undergo a cardiac evaluation but then may have no further evaluation of their symptoms. However, both functional chest pain and functional heartburn have a benign prognosis, although symptoms may persist and continue to diminish quality of life.

Grade A References

A1. Halmos EP, Power VA, Shepherd SJ, et al. A diet low in FODMAPs reduces symptoms of irritable bowel syndrome. *Gastroenterology*. 2014;146:67-75.

A2. Atluri DK, Chandar AK, Bharucha AE, et al. Effect of linaclotide in irritable bowel syndrome with constipation (IBS-C): a systematic review and meta-analysis. *Neurogastroenterol Motil*. 2014;26:499-509.

A3. Menees SB, Maneerattannaporn M, Kim HM, et al. The efficacy and safety of rifaximin for the irritable bowel syndrome: a systematic review and meta-analysis. *Am J Gastroenterol*. 2012;107:28-35.

A4. Moayyedi P, Ford AC, Talley NJ, et al. The efficacy of probiotics in the treatment of irritable bowel syndrome: a systematic review. *Gut*. 2010;59:325-332.

A5. Pajak R, Lackner J, Kamboj SK. A systematic review of minimal-contact psychological treatments for symptom management in irritable bowel syndrome. *J Psychosom Res*. 2013;75:103-112.

A6. Wang WH, Huang JQ, Zheng GF, et al. Effects of proton-pump inhibitors on functional dyspepsia: a meta-analysis of randomized placebo-controlled trials. *Clin Gastroenterol Hepatol*. 2007;5:178-185.

GENERAL REFERENCES

For the General References and other additional features, please visit Expert Consult at https://expertconsult.inkling.com.

138 DISEASES OF THE ESOPHAGUS

GARY W. FALK AND DAVID A. KATZKA

NORMAL ANATOMY AND PHYSIOLOGY

The esophagus, which averages about 27 cm in length, is a hollow muscular tube consisting of the mucosa, submucosa, and muscularis layers, with the notable absence of a serosal layer. The mucosa is a stratified squamous nonkeratinized epithelium that transitions to a columnar epithelium at the gastroesophageal junction. The muscular layer of the esophagus is composed of striated muscle in the upper one third and smooth muscle in the lower two thirds. These muscular components are arranged as an inner circular and an outer longitudinal layer. Located between the circular and longitudinal muscle layers is Auerbach (myenteric) plexus, whereas Meissner plexus is located within the submucosa and innervates the muscularis mucosae. The esophagus is bound by an upper esophageal sphincter proximally and the lower esophageal sphincter distally. The upper esophageal sphincter contains functional contributions from the inferior pharyngeal constrictor proximally and the cricopharyngeus distally. By contrast, the lower esophageal sphincter is anatomically and histologically indistinguishable from the lower esophagus. Blood supply for the cervical portion is derived from branches of the inferior thyroid artery. The intrathoracic segment of the esophagus receives its blood supply from bronchial arteries and direct branches from the aorta, and the left gastric and the inferior phrenic arteries supply the abdominal portion of the esophagus. Venous drainage follows the arterial supply in the cervical and abdominal portions, whereas the thoracic esophagus drains into the azygous and hemiazygos system. Likewise, the lymphatic drainage of the esophagus is segmental, with the cervical portion draining into deep cervical lymph nodes, the thoracic portion into the superior and posterior mediastinal lymph nodes, and the abdominal portion into the gastric and celiac lymph nodes.

The motor functions of the esophagus are to transport a food bolus from the oropharynx into the stomach and then to keep food from returning to the esophagus after it has entered the stomach. The upper esophageal sphincter and the proximal third of the esophagus compose the first portion of the esophagus. The upper esophageal sphincter is approximately 2 to 4 cm in length. The recurrent laryngeal nerve inferiorly and a pharyngeal plexus superiorly supply the upper esophageal sphincter, which is approximately 2 to 4 cm in length. The muscle layers close the esophageal lumen and shorten the esophagus to facilitate forward transport through the proximal esophagus. After food traverses the proximal esophagus, it moves into the distal two thirds of the esophagus, where peristalsis is achieved by sequential muscular contraction mediated through an interplay of inhibitory and excitatory neurotransmitters. Peristalsis may be primary, that is, initiated by a swallow, or secondary, that is, stimulated by refluxed gastric contents. Although local mechanisms control most esophageal motor function, vagal input is important in the distal esophagus, where smooth muscle myopathies and autonomic neuropathies can cause dysfunction. The distal esophagus is separated from the stomach by the lower esophageal sphincter, which is 4 to 5 cm in length and is functionally distinct because it maintains a tonic high-pressure zone. This sphincter relaxes nearly completely upon swallowing to allow the passage of food and then regains its tone to provide a barrier against reflux. It also relaxes transiently during normal functions, such as belching and vomiting. The vagus nerve, acetylcholine, and nitric oxide influence tone, but the lower esophageal sphincter tone is influenced by the crural diaphragm as the esophagus traverses the diaphragmatic hiatus.

Esophageal Functional Testing

Options for esophageal functional testing include barium esophagography, high-resolution esophageal manometry, and esophageal impedance testing. Barium esophagography (Chapter 133) reveals both anatomic and physiologic information about luminal lesions, such as malignancies, ulceration, diverticula, hiatal hernia, and strictures; intramural lesions, such as leiomyomas; and extrinsic lesions, such as occur from vascular (aorta, right atrium, subclavian artery) impingement or solid lesions (pulmonary malignancy, adenopathy) that compress the esophagus. Radiography is also an excellent tool for studying motility patterns, such as peristalsis with either liquid or solid contrast material, while precisely visualizing how the esophagus handles a bolus rather than by implying function from pressure or impedance changes.

High-resolution esophageal manometry measures pressure changes generated by esophageal wall contraction and changes in tone using multiple sensors that simultaneously measure pressure from the pharynx to the lower esophageal sphincter. Esophageal impedance testing detects the movement of an intraluminal bolus by measuring conductance between catheter-based electrodes based on the substance that is in contact with each electrode. Air, which is a poor conductor of electric current, will yield high impedance, whereas swallowed or refluxed liquids, which are excellent conductors of electricity, will generate a low impedance signal. From these measurements, the direction and velocity of the transport of air and bolus can help assess peristaltic function and the reflux of acid and nonacid gastric contents.

Symptoms of Esophageal Disease

The most common symptom of esophageal disease is heartburn, which is defined as a sensation of substernal burning. Chest pain without typical heartburn may occur in a variety of esophageal disorders, including gastroesophageal reflux and motor disorders such as in achalasia. However, esophageal pain and even heartburn can be indistinguishable from cardiac angina (Chapter 51), so care must be taken when a patient at risk for coronary artery disease complains of heartburn for the first time.

Dysphagia, or difficulty swallowing, is another cardinal symptom of esophageal disease. Dysphagia with only solid food tends to occur with structural lesions, which cause esophageal constriction, whereas dysphagia with both liquids and solids occurs more often with motility disorders. Patients with oropharyngeal dysphagia will commonly complain of a feeling of food "sticking" in the throat or the inability to propel the bolus from the mouth to the pharynx; they may also complain of the need for multiple swallowing motions to clear the bolus. Since the cranial nerves that generally control the initial phases of swallowing are responsible for other functions as well, symptoms that may be associated with oropharyngeal dysphagia include drooling, dysarthria (due to tongue dysfunction), nasal regurgitation (due to failure to seal off the nasal passage), or coughing and aspiration (due to failure to elevate and cover the laryngeal vestibule). Dysphagia that results from abnormalities in the body of the esophagus may be referred to the chest or the neck, so the location of pain does not predict the location of the disease. Dysphagia may also lead to a variety of behavioral accommodations, including maneuvers such as slow eating, food aversion, avoidance of hard solid food, and drinking of large amounts of liquids with solid meals.

Regurgitation, which is another typical esophageal symptom, may be described as the feeling of food coming up into the chest or, more dramatically, into the mouth. When regurgitation occurs early in the meal, it suggests a proximal lesion. Regurgitation later in the meal suggests a motility abnormality such as achalasia.

Food impaction is an extreme esophageal symptom. When impaction occurs in the oropharynx, patients may develop a "steakhouse" syndrome, in which an impacted food bolus leads to tracheal impaction or compression. With more distal esophageal lesions, impaction may occur any time during the meal, almost always from a mechanical cause. Patients experience the sudden onset of chest pain and the sensation of food sticking, typically after solids such as meats, raw vegetables, and sticky rice. With complete impaction, patients who cannot handle secretions because of the obstructing bolus are at risk for aspiration, esophageal rupture, and perforation.

GASTROESOPHAGEAL REFLUX DISEASE

DEFINITION

Gastroesophageal reflux disease (GERD) develops when the reflux of stomach contents into the esophagus causes troublesome symptoms or complications.

EPIDEMIOLOGY

It is estimated that GERD, defined as at least weekly heartburn or acid regurgitation, has a prevalence ranging from 10 to 20% in the Western world and less than 5% in Asia. The prevalence also tends to be higher in North America than Europe and higher in northern Europe than in southern Europe. Risk factors for developing GERD include obesity, particularly central obesity, and possibly increasing age. A genetic component may also play a role because GERD is more common in patients with a positive family history and in monozygotic twins than in dizygotic twins.

PATHOBIOLOGY

The esophagus is protected from the harmful effects of refluxed gastric contents by the antireflux barrier at the gastroesophageal junction, by esophageal clearance mechanisms, and by epithelial defensive factors. The antireflux barrier consists of the lower esophageal sphincter, crural diaphragm, phrenoesophageal ligament, and angle of His, which causes an oblique entrance of the esophagus into the stomach. The attachment of the lower esophageal sphincter to the crural diaphragm results in increased pressure during inspiration and when intra-abdominal pressure increases. Disruption of normal defense mechanisms leads to pathologic amounts of reflux.[1]

Reflux of gastric contents from the stomach into the esophagus occurs in healthy individuals, but refluxed gastric contents are normally cleared in a two-step process: volume clearance by peristaltic function and neutralization of small amounts of residual acid by weakly alkaline swallowed saliva. In normal healthy individuals, physiologic reflux occurs primarily when the lower esophageal sphincter transiently relaxes in the absence of a swallow because of a vagally mediated reflex that is stimulated by gastric distention. In GERD patients, transient relaxation of the lower esophageal sphincter or a low resting lower esophageal sphincter pressure can result in regurgitation, especially when intra-abdominal pressure is increased.

A hiatal hernia, which results in axial and vertical spatial separation between the augmenting effects of the crural diaphragm and the lower esophageal sphincter, predisposes to reflux events by widening the opening of the gastroesophageal junction and decreasing the pressure of the lower esophageal sphincter. The result is an increased exposure of the esophagus to acid and gastric contents, with increased reflux events during transient physiologic relaxation of the lower esophageal sphincter and/or increased gastric pressure. Hernias also act as a reservoir for gastric contents when normal esophageal clearance mechanisms result in trapping of fluids in the hernia sac. These contents can reflux into the esophagus when the lower esophageal sphincter relaxes during subsequent swallowing.

Normal individuals also have an unbuffered acid pocket in the gastric cardia, which escapes the buffering effects of a meal in the postprandial period. This region is a source of postprandial reflux and may explain the chronic inflammation often seen in the cardia and distal esophagus. In reflux patients, the acid pocket is more common and longer in length than in normal individuals. Displacement of the acid pocket into a hiatal hernia also appears to increase acidic reflux in patients with GERD.

Increased intra-abdominal fat associated with obesity increases intragastric pressure, which increases the gastroesophageal pressure gradient and the frequency of transient lower esophageal sphincter relaxation, thereby predisposing gastric contents to migrate into the esophagus. In addition, obesity enhances the spatial separation of the crural diaphragm and the lower esophageal sphincter, thereby predisposing obese individuals to a hiatal hernia. The metabolic syndrome (Chapter 229) that is associated with obesity may also have an independent effect in promoting esophageal injury in GERD.

The normal defense mechanisms based on peristalsis and saliva can also be impaired. Peristaltic dysfunction is associated with an increasing severity of esophagitis, and ineffective peristaltic clearance may occur when the amplitude of esophageal contractions is less than 20 mm Hg. Saliva production may be impaired by a variety of mechanisms, such as smoking and Sjögren syndrome (Chapter 268).

The esophageal mucosa contains several lines of defense. A pre-epithelial barrier constitutes a small unstirred water layer combined with bicarbonate from swallowed saliva and from the secretions of submucosal glands. A second epithelial defense is composed of cell membranes and tight intercellular junctions, cellular and intercellular buffers, and cell membrane ion transporters. The postepithelial line of defense is composed of the blood supply to the esophagus. Acid and acidified pepsin in the refluxate are the key factors that damage the intercellular junctions, increase intracellular permeability, and dilate intercellular spaces. If sufficient quantities of refluxate diffuse into the intercellular spaces, cellular damage may occur. Signs and symptoms of GERD occur when defective epithelium comes into contact with refluxed acid, pepsin, or other noxious gastric contents. In addition to the direct noxious effects of refluxed acid, pepsin, and bile, refluxed gastric juice stimulates esophageal epithelial cells to secrete chemokines that attract inflammatory cells into the esophagus, thereby damaging the esophageal mucosa.

CLINICAL MANIFESTATIONS

The classic symptoms of GERD are heartburn and acid regurgitation; atypical symptoms include chest pain, dysphagia, and odynophagia. Extraesophageal manifestations of reflux disease can include cough (Chapter 83), laryngitis (Chapter 429), asthma (Chapter 87), and dental erosions, but these symptoms are more easily attributable to GERD if accompanied by classic signs and symptoms of reflux disease. Other proposed associations that are not clearly established include pharyngitis, sinusitis, otitis media, and idiopathic pulmonary fibrosis (Fig. 138-1).

When excessive gastric contents overwhelm the mucosal protective factors in the esophagus, esophagitis may be manifest as erosions or ulceration of the esophagus and may also lead to fibrosis with stricturing, columnar metaplasia (Barrett esophagus) or esophageal adenocarcinoma (Chapter 192). However, approximately two thirds of individuals with reflux symptoms have no evidence of esophageal damage by endoscopy.

DIAGNOSIS

When GERD is associated with typical signs and symptoms, such as heartburn or acid regurgitation, that are responsive to antisecretory therapy, no diagnostic evaluation is warranted.[2,3] Diagnostic endoscopy is warranted in individuals who fail to respond to 4 to 8 weeks of therapy or have alarm symptoms or signs such as dysphagia, weight loss (Fig. 132-4), anemia, gastrointestinal bleeding, or persistent heartburn (Fig. 138-2).[4] Endoscopy permits the detection of erosive esophagitis and complications such as a peptic stricture (Fig. 138-3) and Barrett esophagus (Fig. 138-4); mucosal biopsy, which is crucial in these settings, also excludes conditions that can mimic GERD, such as eosinophilic esophagitis. However, most patients have no mucosal damage seen on endoscopy, regardless of whether they are on or off antisecretory therapy.

Esophageal manometry is useful to exclude achalasia in patients with suggestive symptoms. Esophageal reflux testing may be performed using 24-hour transnasal pH monitoring, 48-hour devices attached to the esophageal lumen, or 24-hour combined impedance and pH monitoring. Testing of a patient who is not receiving antisecretory therapy can document abnormal esophageal acid exposure and establish the relationship between symptoms and reflux events. Testing of a patient who is on therapy is best accomplished by combined impedance pH monitoring, which can establish the relationship, if any, between symptoms and reflux events, thereby permitting exclusion of GERD as the cause of persistent symptoms. Barium radiography has no role in the diagnostic evaluation of patients with reflux disease.

TREATMENT Rx

Although avoidance of foods or beverages that may provoke symptoms, such as alcohol, coffee, spicy foods, and late meals, makes physiologic sense, data from clinical trials to support these maneuvers are lacking. Similarly, elevation of the head of the bed for patients with nocturnal regurgitation or

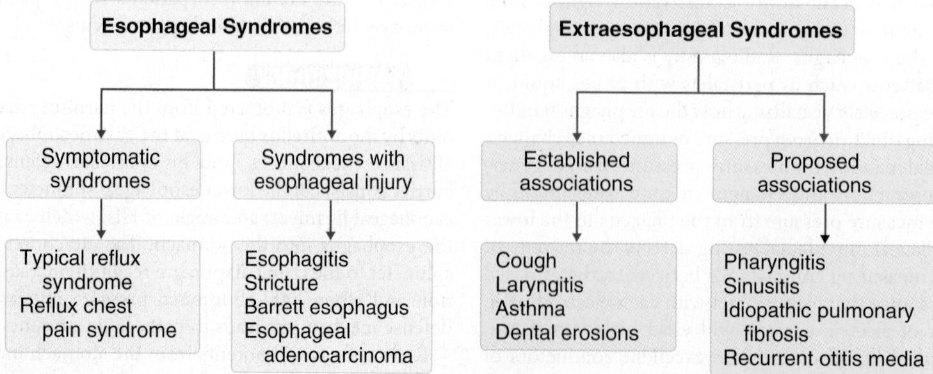

FIGURE 138-1. Montreal classification of gastroesophageal reflux disease (GERD). (From Vakil N, van Zanten S, Kahrilas P, et al. The Montreal definition and classification of gastroesophageal reflux disease: a global evidence-based consensus. *Am J Gastroenterol.* 2006;101:1900-1920.)

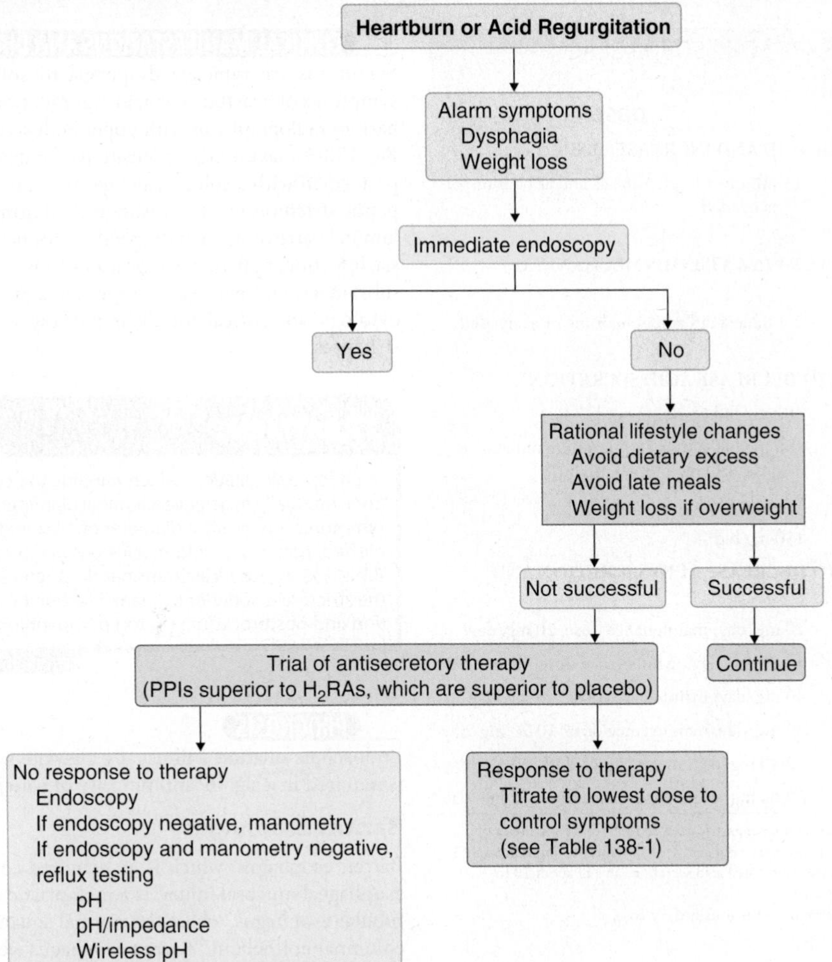

FIGURE 138-2. Algorithm for the management of heartburn or regurgitation symptoms. Surgery is indicated only for patients who are intolerant of antisecretory therapy or who have ongoing symptoms, especially regurgitation if reflux is well documented. H_2RA = histamine-2 receptor antagonist; PPI = proton pump inhibitor. (Based on Kahrilas PJ, Shaheen NJ, Vaezi MF. American Gastroenterological Association Institute technical review on the management of gastroesophageal reflux disease. *Gastroenterology.* 2008;135:1392-1413.)

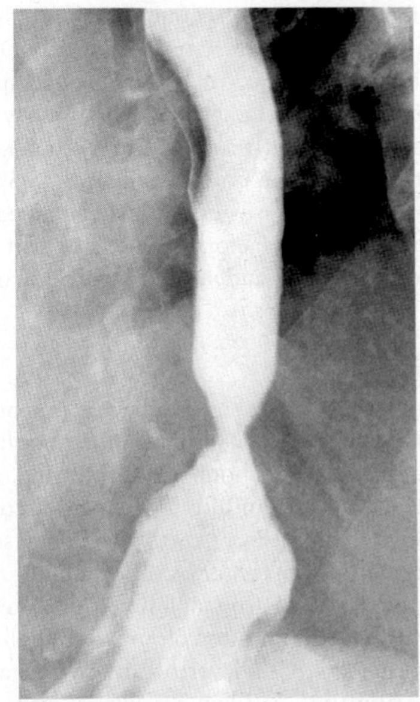

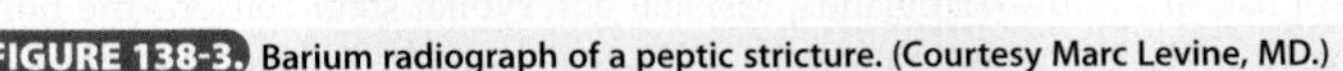
FIGURE 138-3. Barium radiograph of a peptic stricture. (Courtesy Marc Levine, MD.)

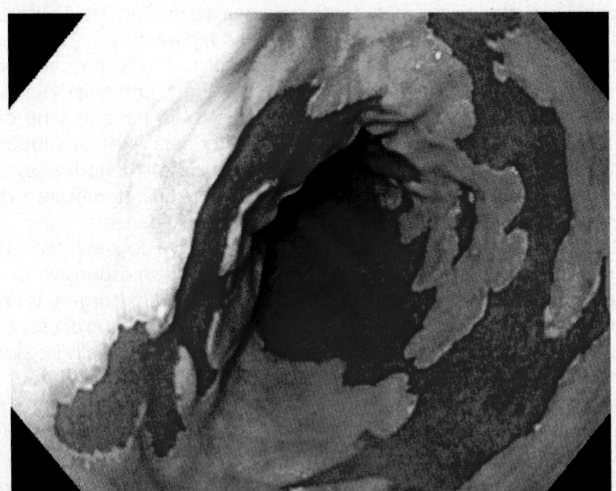

FIGURE 138-4. Endoscopic appearance of Barrett esophagus. Note the white-appearing normal squamous mucosa displaced above the true end of the esophagus. The intervening mucosa appears salmon-pink.

heartburn also is logical. Given the association of obesity and GERD symptoms, weight loss should be part of any treatment program for obese patients.

Inhibition of gastric acid secretion (Table 138-1) is the cornerstone of the acute treatment of GERD, and proton pump inhibitors are superior to histamine (H_2)-receptor antagonists for both the healing of esophagitis and the control of symptoms.[A1] However, the healing of esophagitis is more predictable than improvement in heartburn symptoms, even with proton pump inhibitors. There are no major differences in treatment efficacy among the various proton pump inhibitors, and once-daily dosing is adequate in most patients.

Given the chronicity of reflux symptoms, long-term maintenance therapy with proton pump inhibitors is typically required and is mandatory for patients with erosive esophagitis. Dosing should be titrated to the lowest dose necessary to control symptoms. Data to support the use of proton pump inhibitors in the management of extraesophageal GERD syndromes are weak, although selected patients may benefit. The safety profile of proton pump inhibitors is

TABLE 138-1 DRUG THERAPY FOR ESOPHAGEAL DISORDERS

AGENT	DOSE
ANTACIDS: LIQUID (TO BUFFER ACID AND INCREASE LESP)	
For example, Mylanta II/Maalox TC (acid-neutralizing capacity, 25 mEq/5 mL)*	15 mL qid 1 hr after meals and at bedtime or as needed
GAVISCON (TO DECREASE REFLUX VIA A VISCOUS MECHANICAL BARRIER AND BUFFER ACID)	
$Al(OH)_3$, $NaHCO_3$, Mg trisilicate, alginic acid	2-4 tablets qid and at bedtime or as needed
H_2-RECEPTOR ANTAGONISTS (TO DECREASE ACID SECRETION)	
Cimetidine	400 mg bid or 200 mg qid
Ranitidine	150 mg bid-qid or 10 mL qid; maintenance dose, 150 mg bid, 10 mL bid
Famotidine	20-40 mg bid or 2.5-5 mL bid
Nizatidine	150 mg bid
PROTON PUMP INHIBITORS (TO DECREASE ACID SECRETION AND GASTRIC VOLUME)†	
Omeprazole	20 mg/day; maintenance dose, 20 mg/day
Lansoprazole	15-30 mg/day; maintenance dose, 15 mg/day
Pantoprazole	40 mg/day; maintenance dose, 40 mg/day
Rabeprazole	20 mg/day; maintenance dose, 10-20 mg/day
Esomeprazole	20-40 mg/day; maintenance dose, 20 mg/day
Dexlansoprazole	30-60 mg/day; maintenance dose, 30 mg/day

*Patients with reflux are not generally hypersecretors of gastric acid, so the therapeutic doses of antacids are based on their capacity to buffer (normal) basal acid secretion rates of approximately 1 to 7 mEq/hr (mean, 2 mEq/hr) and peak meal-stimulated acid secretion rates of about 10 to 60 mEq/hr (mean, 30 mEq/hr).
†High-dose therapy is a twice-daily administration of the usually daily dose.
LESP = lower esophageal sphincter pressure.

excellent, but short-term adverse events such as headaches and diarrhea may occur. Long-term proton pump inhibitors use is associated with vitamin B_{12} deficiency[5] and may be associated with an increased risk for *Clostridium difficile* infection, community-acquired pneumonia, and hip fracture.

Although proton pump inhibitors are superior to H_2-receptor antagonists for long-term maintenance therapy as well as for short-term relief, H_2-receptor antagonists are superior to placebo and are useful in patients who cannot tolerate proton pump inhibitors. No high-quality data exist to support the common practice of using metoclopramide as either monotherapy or an adjunct to acid suppression therapy; furthermore, its significant adverse effects argue against the use of this drug in any GERD patients.

Antireflux surgery is an option for patients who have documented esophagitis, who are intolerant of proton pump inhibitors or unresponsive to them, or who regurgitate large volumes. Laparoscopic antireflux surgery is equivalent to continued proton pump inhibitor therapy for the healing of esophagitis and for the treatment of chronic GERD in patients who initially respond to proton pump inhibitors.[A2][A3] However, surgery has a number of serious complications that may affect quality of life, including dysphagia, vagal nerve injury, gas bloat syndrome, and diarrhea. Endoscopic approaches to GERD are being studied but are not currently part of routine care.

PROGNOSIS

Patients with GERD generally do well with conservative antireflux measures and proton pump inhibitor therapy. When surgery is required, the outcome is usually excellent.

Peptic Strictures

Esophageal strictures are a well-recognized complication of GERD, especially in older patients with long-standing reflux symptoms, but population-based studies suggest that the incidence of new and recurrent strictures is declining. Peptic strictures are thought to be a consequence of severe inflammation, which leads to fibrosis, scarring, esophageal shortening, and loss of compliance of the lumen.

CLINICAL MANIFESTATIONS AND DIAGNOSIS

Symptoms are typically dysphagia to solids with or without antecedent symptoms of heartburn or acid regurgitation. Strictures may be diagnosed by barium radiography or with upper endoscopy, but barium esophagrams (see Fig. 138-3) have a higher sensitivity for detecting subtle lesions, especially if performed with a solid challenge such a barium-impregnated pill. However, peptic strictures must be distinguished from a wide variety of other causes of luminal narrowing, including pills, prior nasogastric tube intubation, neoplasia, infection, radiation, surgical anastomosis, some systemic diseases, caustic substances, and extrinsic compression. As a result, endoscopic biopsy and cytology are critical for distinguishing benign from malignant causes of strictures.

TREATMENT Rx

Endoscopic dilation, which remains the cornerstone of therapy, should be done gradually to achieve a luminal diameter that is sufficiently large to relieve symptoms—typically a diameter of 13 mm or greater. After dilation is accomplished, patients should receive chronic proton pump inhibitor therapy (see Table 138-1). For recalcitrant peptic strictures, injection of triamcinolone into the stricture is superior to sham injection in patients who receive balloon dilation and postprocedure proton pump inhibitors.[A4]

PROGNOSIS

Endoscopic dilation will usually alleviate symptoms, but repetitive dilation is required in a significant minority of patients.

Barrett Esophagus

Barrett esophagus, which is an acquired condition that results from severe esophageal mucosal injury, is a metaplastic change in the lining of the distal tubular esophagus, where the normal squamous epithelium is replaced by a columnar epithelium.[6] Barrett esophagus would be of little importance if not for its well-recognized association with adenocarcinoma of the esophagus (Chapter 192). However, the risk for cancer in an individual patient with Barrett esophagus is low.[7]

EPIDEMIOLOGY

It is estimated that Barrett esophagus is found in approximately 5 to 15% of patients who undergo endoscopy for symptoms of GERD. Population-based studies suggest that the prevalence of Barrett esophagus is approximately 1.3 to 1.6%, but about 45% of affected patients do not have reflux symptoms. Barrett esophagus is predominantly a disease of middle-aged white men, but about 25% of patients are women or are younger than 50 years. The prevalence of Barrett esophagus increases until a plateau is reached between the seventh and ninth decades. Risk factors include frequent and long-standing reflux episodes, smoking, male gender, older age, and central male pattern obesity.

PATHOBIOLOGY

Barrett esophagus results from severe esophageal mucosal injury. Patients who develop Barrett esophagus typically have more esophageal acid and bile exposure, the former based on 24-hour pH monitoring, and almost always have a hiatal hernia, which is typically longer and associated with larger defects than in patients without Barrett. However, why some patients with GERD develop Barrett esophagus whereas others do not remains unclear, as does the cell of origin of columnar metaplasia. Candidates include dedifferentiation of squamous epithelium into columnar epithelium or stimulation of stem cells from either the basal layer of the esophageal epithelium, the esophageal submucosal glands, residual embryonal stem cells, or the bone marrow. The transcription factor CDX2, which can be induced by both acid and bile salts, appears to play a role in promoting the development of the columnar epithelium in the distal esophagus and gastroesophageal junction. A small subset of patients may have an inherited predisposition to Barrett esophagus, although the genetics of the disease are unknown.

CLINICAL MANIFESTATIONS

The development of reflux symptoms at an earlier age, an increased duration of reflux symptoms, an increased severity of nocturnal reflux symptoms, and prior complications of GERD such as esophagitis, ulceration, stricture, and bleeding may raise the likelihood of Barrett's esophagus. Nevertheless, patients with Barrett's esophagus are difficult to distinguish clinically from patients whose GERD is uncomplicated by a columnar-lined esophagus. Patients with Barrett's esophagus may paradoxically have impaired sensitivity to esophageal acid perfusion compared with patients with uncomplicated GERD.

DIAGNOSIS

Endoscopically, Barrett's esophagus is characterized by displacement of the squamocolumnar junction so that it is now proximal to the gastroesophageal junction, which is defined by the proximal margin of gastric folds (see Fig. 138-4). The diagnosis of Barrett's esophagus is established if the squamocolumnar junction is displaced proximal to the gastroesophageal junction and if intestinal metaplasia, which is characterized in part by acid mucin-containing goblet cells, is detected by biopsy.

The precise junction of the stomach and the esophagus may be difficult to determine endoscopically owing to the presence of a hiatal hernia, inflammation, and the dynamic nature of the gastroesophageal junction. If the squamocolumnar junction is above the level of the esophagogastric junction, as defined by the proximal margin of the gastric folds, biopsy specimens should be obtained for confirmation of columnar metaplasia.

Intestinal or columnar metaplasia may be seen in the cardia of normal individuals as well as in persons with chronic reflux disease, and the prevalence of intestinal metaplasia at a normal-appearing gastroesophageal junction varies from 5 to 36%. Dysplasia and an increased risk for carcinoma have been reported in patients who have intestinal metaplasia of the gastroesophageal junction or cardia, but the magnitude of that risk appears to be less than that of Barrett's esophagus.

TREATMENT Rx

Patients who are diagnosed with Barrett esophagus require surveillance endoscopy at regular intervals (Fig. 138-5). They characteristically worry about cancer risk, which they may overestimate, face higher life insurance premiums, and may receive conflicting information on how best to treat their condition.

Proton pump inhibitors (see Table 138-1), which are the cornerstone of medical therapy for Barrett esophagus, consistently relieve symptoms and heal esophagitis. However, proton pump inhibitors, even at high doses, provide no more than modest regression of Barrett histology, perhaps because alleviation of reflux symptoms is not necessarily equivalent to normalization of esophageal acid exposure. In fact, abnormal acid exposure persists in approximately 25% of Barrett esophagus patients despite twice-daily proton pump inhibitors. The importance of complete control of esophageal acid exposure in patients with Barrett esophagus remains unknown, although data suggest that effective therapy can protect against the development of cancer.[8] Antireflux surgery effectively alleviates GERD symptoms, and the indications for surgery are the same as those for patients with GERD without Barrett esophagus. Surgery should not, however, be viewed as a better cancer prevention tool.

Current practice guidelines, based on observational data, recommend endoscopic surveillance of patients with documented Barrett esophagus in an attempt to detect dysplasia and cancer at an early and potentially curable stage.[9] Before entering into a surveillance program, patients should be advised about risks and benefits, including the limitations of surveillance endoscopy as well as the importance of adhering to appropriate surveillance intervals. Other considerations include age, likelihood of survival over the next 5 years, and ability to tolerate either endoscopic or surgical interventions for early esophageal adenocarcinoma.

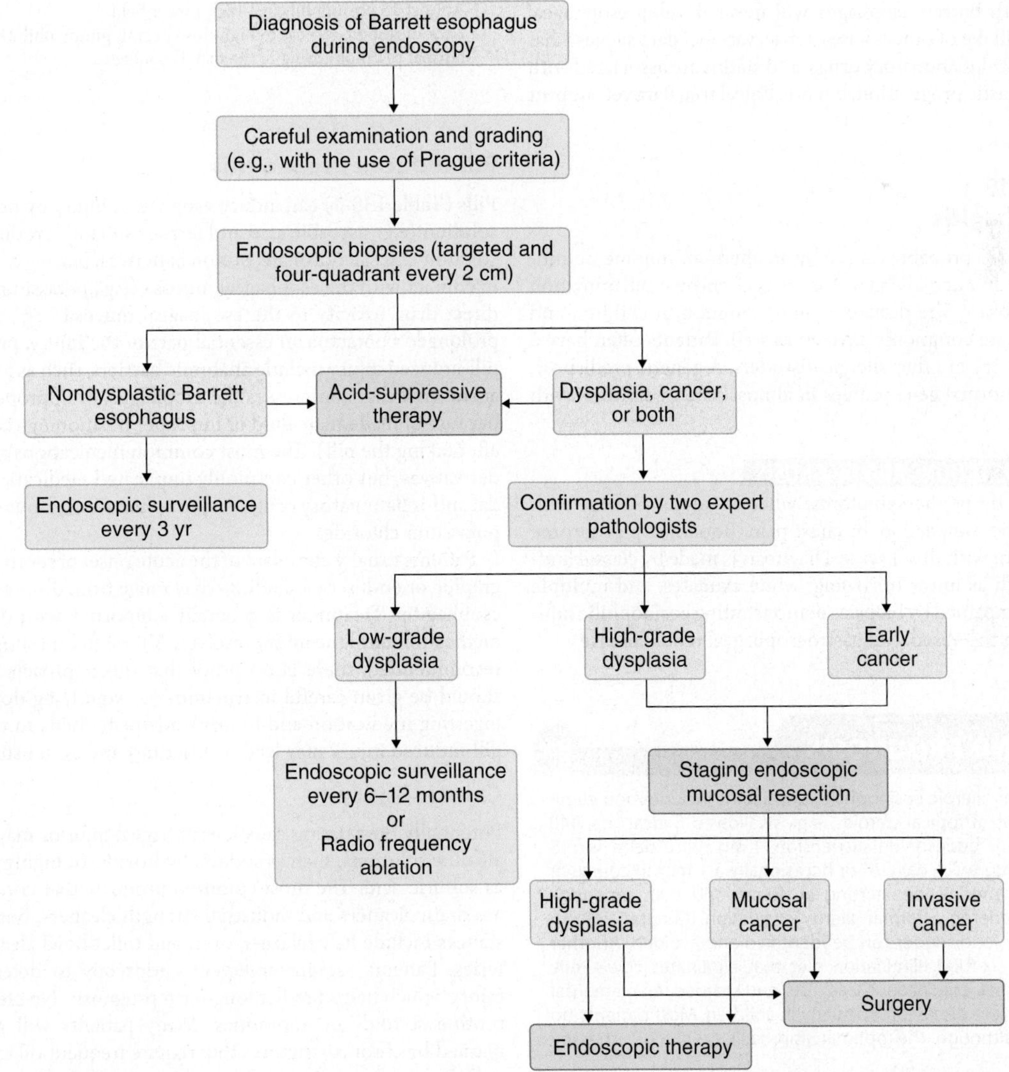

FIGURE 138-5. Proposed treatment algorithm for patients with Barrett esophagus. (From Sharma P. Barrett's esophagus. *N Engl J Med.* 2009;361:2548-2556, Fig. 3).

Systematic four-quadrant biopsies should be obtained at 2-cm intervals along the entire length of the Barrett segment after inflammation related to GERD is controlled with antisecretory therapy. Mucosal abnormalities, especially in the setting of high-grade dysplasia, should be resected endoscopically. Surveillance intervals, determined by the presence and grade of dysplasia, are based on a limited understanding of the biology of esophageal adenocarcinoma. Surveillance for patients without dysplasia should occur every 3 to 5 years after an initial negative examination. If low-grade dysplasia is found, the diagnosis should first be confirmed by an expert gastrointestinal pathologist because of the marked interobserver variability in the interpretation of these biopsies. If confirmed, aggressive proton pump inhibitor therapy (see Table 138-1) is recommended to decrease inflammation and regeneration, which may make pathologic interpretation difficult. A repeat endoscopy should then be performed within 6 months of the initial diagnosis. If low-grade dysplasia is confirmed, options include continued surveillance at 6- to 12-month intervals or radiofrequency ablation, but ablation significantly reduces the risk for progression to high-grade dysplasia or to adenocarcinoma over the next 3 years.[A5]

If high-grade dysplasia is found, an experienced independent gastrointestinal pathologist should confirm the diagnosis. For patients with confirmed high-grade dysplasia, endoscopic ablation therapy with radio frequency ablation, endoscopic mucosal resection, or a combination is now recommended instead of surgery or continued surveillance.[A6][A7] For high-grade dysplasia patients with any visible abnormality, endoscopic mucosal resection is recommended for optimal diagnosis and staging.[10] Surgery with esophagectomy is reserved only for patients who fail to respond to endoscopic ablation therapy.

PROGNOSIS

The risk that a patient with Barrett esophagus will develop esophageal adenocarcinoma is now estimated to be approximately 0.1 to 0.3% annually,[11] and thus, most patients with Barrett esophagus will never develop esophageal adenocarcinoma but will die of other causes. Observational data suggest that aspirin, nonsteroidal anti-inflammatory drugs, and statins are associated with a reduced risk for neoplastic progression, but no clinical trial data yet support their routine use.

ESOPHAGITIS

Eosinophilic Esophagitis

Eosinophilic esophagitis is probably caused by an aberrant immune or antigenic response to food and aeroallergens that trigger chronic inflammation in the esophageal mucosa.[12] The disease is most common in children and adolescents, but adults are commonly affected as well. Patients often have a personal and family history of other allergic disorders. A genetic predisposition is suggested by abnormal gene profiles in almost 50% of children with this disorder.[13]

CLINICAL MANIFESTATIONS AND DIAGNOSIS

Children present with dyspeptic symptoms, whereas adults present with solid food dysphagia, food impaction, or chest pain. Booerhaave syndrome (see later) may also occur with this disease. Diagnosis is made by classic findings on endoscopy, such as linear furrowing, white exudates, and multiple rings (Fig. 138-6), accompanied by biopsies demonstrating eosinophilic infiltration (Table 138-2) in the absence of gastroesophageal reflux disease.

TREATMENT AND PROGNOSIS Rx

Treatment options for allergic eosinophilic esophagitis include food elimination diets[A8], 2 months of topical steroids (e.g., swallowed fluticasone, 440 to 880 µg twice daily, or budesonide suspension, 1 mg twice daily, for 15 days, followed by 0.25 mg twice daily),[A9] or occasionally a 1-month course of systemic steroids (e.g., prednisone, starting at 40 mg and then tapering). Patients also should undergo a formal allergy evaluation (Chapter 249) to determine whether any food trigger can be identified and avoided. Another option is an empirical six-food elimination diet that eliminates cow's milk protein (casein), soy, wheat, egg, peanut/tree nuts, and seafood. An elemental diet may be used for severe disease, particularly in children. Most patients do well after treatment, although the optimal approach to chronic therapy remains uncertain.

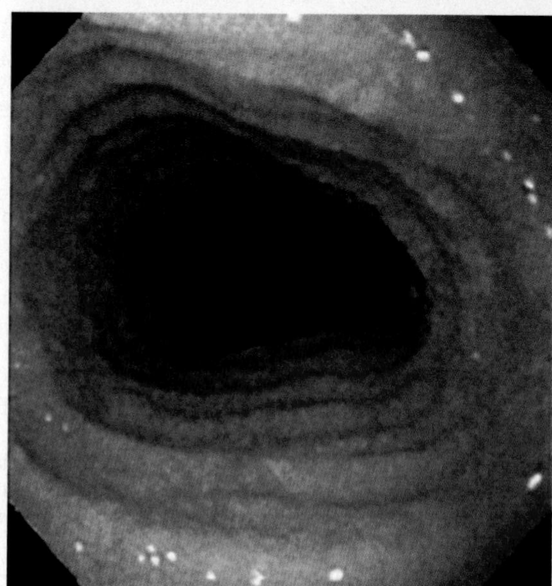

FIGURE 138-6. Endoscopic corrugated (ringed) appearance of esophagus in eosinophilic esophagitis.

TABLE 138-2 GUIDELINES FOR THE DIAGNOSIS OF EOSINOPHILIC ESOPHAGITIS

- Clinical symptoms of esophageal dysfunction
- At least 15 eosinophils in 1 high-power field
- Lack of responsiveness to high-dose proton pump inhibition (see Table 138-1) or normal pH monitoring of the distal esophagus

Pill-Induced Esophagitis

Pills (Table 138-3) can induce esophageal injury by producing a caustic acid solution (e.g., ascorbic acid and ferrous sulfate), producing a caustic alkaline solution (e.g., alendronate, button batteries), placing a hyperosmolar solution in contact with the esophageal mucosa (e.g., potassium chloride), or causing direct drug toxicity to the esophageal mucosa (e.g., tetracycline). Because prolonged contact is an essential part of the injury, predisposing factors for pill-induced injury include anatomic barriers, such as a stricture, a prominent aortic arch that compresses the esophagus, or improper ingestion of the pill because of inadequate fluid or improper positioning (i.e., lying down directly after taking the pill). The most common medications are tetracycline and its derivatives, but other commonly implicated medications include nonsteroidal anti-inflammatory drugs, bisphosphonates, ferrous sulfate, quinidine, and potassium chloride.

Patients usually complain of the acute onset of severe odynophagia. Radiographic or endoscopic findings may range from discrete ulceration to diffuse esophagitis. Treatment is generally supportive with discontinuation of the medication until the injury resolves. Although acid suppression is commonly recommended, there is no proof that this approach is beneficial. Patients should be given careful instructions to avoid lying down immediately after ingesting medication and to drink adequate fluids to prevent injury. Rarely, pill-induced injury may lead to strictures and even fistulas.

Caustic Injury

Potentially devastating caustic esophageal injuries may be caused by highly alkaline solutions, such as sodium hydroxide, or highly acidic solutions, such as sulfuric acid. The most common products that contain these substances are drain cleaners and industrial strength cleaners, but other corrosive substances include hair relaxers, oven and toilet bowl cleaners, and button batteries. Patients require emergent endoscopy to determine the degree of injury, which helps predict long-term prognosis. No clear evidence supports routine steroids or antibiotics. Many patients will have lifelong disease marked by chronic strictures that require frequent dilation and even esophageal reconstruction. In patients with a severe initial injury, the risk for esophageal cancer is significantly increased.

TABLE 138-3 MEDICATIONS COMMONLY ASSOCIATED WITH ESOPHAGITIS OR ESOPHAGEAL INJURY

ANTIBIOTICS
Tetracycline
Doxycycline
Clindamycin
Penicillin
Rifampin
ANTIVIRAL AGENTS
Zalcitabine
Zidovudine
Nelfinavir
BISPHOSPHONATES
Alendronate
Etidronate
Pamidronate
CHEMOTHERAPEUTIC AGENTS
Dactinomycin
Bleomycin
Cytarabine
Daunorubicin
5-Fluorouracil
Methotrexate
Vincristine
NONSTEROIDAL ANTI-INFLAMMATORY DRUGS
Aspirin
Naproxen
Ibuprofen
OTHER MEDICATIONS
Quinidine
Potassium chloride
Ferrous sulfate
Ascorbic acid
Multivitamins
Theophylline

ESOPHAGEAL MOTOR DISORDERS

Oropharyngeal Dysfunction

The cricopharyngeus and inferior pharyngeal constrictor are composed of striated muscle and innervated by upper motor neurons, the brain stem, and the cerebral cortex. Both primary myopathic and neuropathic disorders can result in dysfunction. The most common neurologic cause of oropharyngeal dysphagia is a cerebrovascular accident (Chapter 407). Other neuropathic disorders that may also affect function include myasthenia gravis (Chapter 422), brain stem tumors (Chapter 189), amyotrophic lateral sclerosis (Chapter 419), Parkinson disease (Chapter 409), Alzheimer disease (Chapter 402), postpolio syndrome (Chapter 379), Guillain-Barré syndrome (Chapter 420), and botulism (Chapter 296). Myogenic disorders that cause dysfunction include paraneoplastic antibody-mediated syndromes (Chapter 179), thyroid disease (Chapter 226), primary myopathies (Chapter 421) such as dermatomyositis and inclusion body myositis, and drugs that cause myopathy such as statins and amiodarone.

Patients with oropharyngeal abnormalities experience dysphagia, often accompanied by postprandial coughing, hoarseness, and aspiration pneumonia. Treatment focuses on the underlying myopathic or neurologic cause and swallowing therapy, but prognosis is often poor owing to limited treatment options.

Achalasia

Achalasia, which is the prototypic esophageal motility disorder, is characterized by insufficient relaxation of the lower esophageal sphincter accompanied by loss of esophageal peristalsis.[14]

EPIDEMIOLOGY AND PATHOBIOLOGY

Achalasia can occur in patients of almost any age, from infants to nonagenarians, but it most commonly presents between 30 and 60 years of age. The prevalence is 10 per 100,000 in the United States, with all races affected and an equal distribution in men and women. The pathophysiology of achalasia most likely reflects an antibody-mediated autoimmune myenteric plexopathy in the lower esophageal sphincter and a generalized neuropathy in the esophageal body. The triggering event is unclear, but a viral cause is suggested. Injury to the lower esophageal sphincter neurons leads to a relative selective deficiency of nitric oxide. With this loss of the main functional inhibitory neurotransmitter, the sphincter loses its ability to relax. The neurochemical process that leads to aperistalsis is unclear.

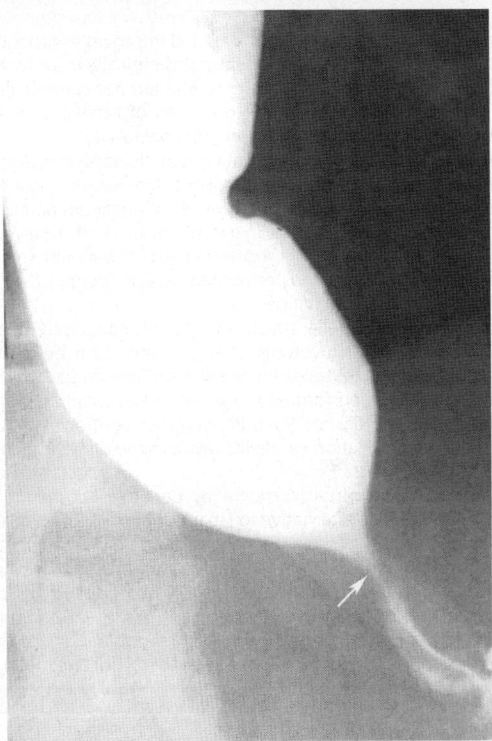

FIGURE 138-7. Esophagogram of a patient with idiopathic achalasia. Note the dilated esophagus with an air-fluid level and distal tapering providing a "bird's beak" deformity in the area of the lower esophageal sphincter. (Courtesy Marc Levine, MD.)

CLINICAL MANIFESTATIONS AND DIAGNOSIS

The cardinal symptoms of achalasia are dysphagia to both liquids and solids, regurgitation, and chest pain. Some patients may have more subtle symptoms, including heartburn, presumably caused by esophageal stasis of acidic food content, weight loss, and aspiration pneumonia; in these settings, diagnosis is often delayed.

The diagnosis of achalasia relies on esophageal manometry and barium radiography. The classic radiographic appearance is esophageal dilation, stasis of contrast material, and a "bird's beak" appearance to the lower esophageal sphincter (Fig. 138-7).[15] Manometry demonstrates high residual pressures of the lower esophageal sphincter and either simultaneous contractions or complete absence of peristaltic contractions. Whether classification systems based on manometric findings can predict response is being studied. Endoscopy is recommended to exclude secondary causes of achalasia, such as gastroesophageal junctional cancer. Occasionally, patients present with a massively dilated esophagus and marked food retention. Radiographically, these patients develop a "sigmoid" esophagus with a radiographic picture similar to a sigmoid colon.

Achalasia may represent a paraneoplastic presentation of some malignancies, particularly small cell lung cancer (Chapter 191); in these patients, the tumor produces an antineuronal antibody (anti-Hu) that mediates the autoimmune lower esophageal sphincter plexopathy and produces a syndrome identical to primary achalasia. Some tumors, such as proximal gastric cancer, may also metastasize to or directly extend into the lower esophageal sphincter and produce an achalasia-like picture, possibly owing to extrinsic compression or tumor infiltration.

TREATMENT Rx

Treatment options to decrease the functional obstruction at the level of the lower esophageal sphincter include the intrasphincteric injection of botulinum toxin, pneumatic dilation, and surgical myotomy. Injection of botulinum toxin during endoscopy reduces symptoms and improves esophageal emptying in up to 90% of patients. Because symptoms typically recur within 6 to 24 months, this treatment is best for patients who are not candidates for more definitive therapies or to confirm the diagnosis of achalasia when clinical, radiographic, and manometric criteria are not conclusive.

In pneumatic dilation, a 30- to 40-mm pneumatic balloon is placed fluoroscopically to straddle the lower esophageal sphincter; the balloon is then inflated to tear the muscle fibers of the lower esophageal sphincter. In general, one pneumatic dilation will achieve 5 years of symptomatic remission in 70% of patients, and three dilations will succeed in 90% of patients. The downside of this procedure is the risk for perforation, which occurs in up to 2% of patients, even in experienced hands.

The third approach is a Heller myotomy, which is now typically performed laparoscopically. This long myotomy starts at least 2 cm below the lower esophageal sphincter and extends for about 6 cm upward past the sphincter; a loose fundoplication is performed to prevent gastroesophageal reflux. The 5-year success rate approaches 90%. Randomized controlled trials suggest that either pneumatic dilation or Heller myotomy will provide comparable clinical results over 2 years. A10

A new endoscopic approach known as peroral endoscopic myotomy (referred to as POEM) is an alternative to laparoscopic myotomy.[16] Early results are encouraging, but this approach is not yet standard clinical practice.

In patients with massive dilation, esophageal dysfunction may warrant total esophagectomy because of life-threatening symptoms such as continued weight loss, recurrent aspiration pneumonia, or tracheal compression. In patients with underlying paraneoplastic malignancy, treatment of the tumor may be helpful, and botulinum toxin has been tried with anecdotal success.

PROGNOSIS

No treatment approach is curative, and all are palliative. Recurrent symptoms may be related to an incomplete myotomy, herniation or unwrapping of the fundoplication, esophageal strictures, Barrett esophagus, or just the natural history of the disease. Achalasia patients may also be predisposed to squamous cell carcinoma of the esophagus, although current evidence does not support cancer screening.

Diffuse Esophageal Spasm

Diffuse esophageal spasm is found in fewer than 5% of patients who undergo manometry for symptoms of chest pain, dysphagia, or both. The pathophysiology of diffuse esophageal spasm is not well understood, but a deficiency of nitric oxide in the esophageal body may lead to a loss of control of esophageal peristalsis, high pressures, and rapid velocity contractions.

CLINICAL MANIFESTATIONS AND DIAGNOSIS

Classically, patients have symptoms of intermittent chest pain (Chapter 137), dysphagia, or both. On endoscopic ultrasound, patients may demonstrate thickening of the circular and longitudinal muscle layers. Diffuse esophageal spasm is defined manometrically by premature rapid contractions in at least 20% of all swallows, accompanied by normal peristalsis. Radiographically, diffuse esophageal spasm is characterized by a "corkscrew" esophagus with multiple simultaneous contractions that obliterate the lumen (Fig. 138-8).

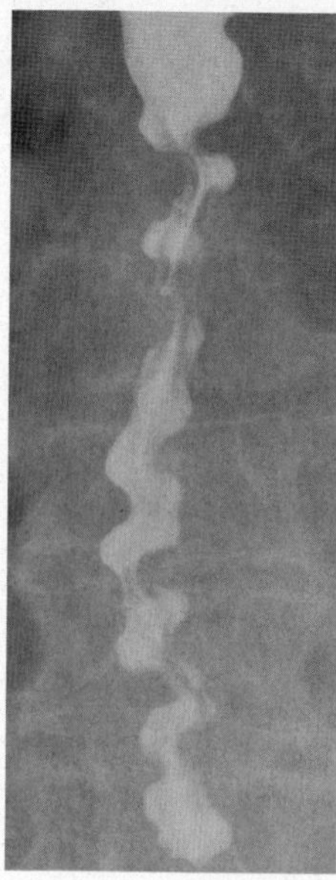

FIGURE 138-8. Barium esophagogram showing a "corkscrew" esophagus in a patient with diffuse esophageal spasm. The patient had dysphagia, chest pain, and normal endoscopic findings. (Image courtesy of Marc Levine, MD.)

TREATMENT AND PROGNOSIS Rx

Treatment of these patients is challenging, and clinical trials have not demonstrated efficacy of any therapy. Empirical therapy may be tried with agents that relax smooth muscle or augment the nitric oxide content, such as hyoscyamine (0.125 mg sublingually), calcium-channel antagonists (nifedipine, 10 mg sublingually), nitroglycerin (0.3 mg sublingually), and sildenafil (50 mg orally). Injection of botulinum toxin into the esophageal body has had equivocal results. Antidepressants, particularly low-dose tricyclics (e.g., imipramine, 10 to 50 mg before bedtime), have had some success. For patients with dysphagia, sphincter options include botulinum toxin injection and pneumatic dilation, but surgery is not indicated unless there is evidence of achalasia. In general, these disorders can be difficult to manage but are not life-threatening.

Other Motility Disorders

Jackhammer esophagus and hypertensive peristalsis are recently described manometric diagnoses that formerly were called nutcracker esophagus. Both are characterized by high-amplitude peristaltic contractions and are of uncertain clinical significance. Antisecretory therapy with proton pump inhibitors (see Table 138-1) is often warranted.

A hypertensive lower esophageal sphincter is of unknown significance, but isolated incomplete relaxation of the lower esophageal sphincter may represent an achalasia variant and should be treated as such in patients with dysphagia. Patients with manometric findings of low-amplitude contractions, failed contractions, or contractions with large breaks have weak peristalsis, which is commonly seen in patients with severe underlying GERD.

STRUCTURAL ABNORMALITIES

Cricopharyngeal Bars

A cricopharyngeal bar, which is caused by a prominent impression of the cricopharyngeus, reflects an inability to relax the upper esophageal sphincter maximally during the flow of barium, with a sustained decrease in compliance. The decrease in cross-sectional area of the upper esophageal sphincter is likely caused by fibrosis. This condition may be asymptomatic or accompanied by symptoms of oropharyngeal dysphagia to solids. Treatment of symptomatic patients is usually surgical, and the response is generally excellent.

Esophageal Diverticula

Esophageal diverticula are encountered in fewer than 1% of upper gastrointestinal radiographic studies and account for less than 5% of cases of dysphagia. Esophageal diverticula may occur in one of three locations: above the upper esophageal sphincter, in the mid-esophagus, and just above the lower esophageal sphincter.

Zenker diverticulum is a pouch that protrudes posteriorly above the upper esophageal sphincter (Fig. 138-9). This protrusion occurs through a triangular region known as Killian triangle, which is bordered above by fibers of the inferior constrictor muscle and below by the cricopharyngeal muscle. It is thought to be caused by increased hypopharyngeal pressure that results from decreased compliance and impaired opening of the upper esophageal sphincter. Small diverticula may be asymptomatic, but increasing size is associated with globus, dysphagia to solids or liquids, regurgitation of undigested food, halitosis, and aspiration. Although no treatment is needed for asymptomatic patients, open or endoscopic surgery is indicated when symptoms occur. Prognosis after surgery is excellent.

Mid-esophageal diverticula, which are focal outpouchings of the middle of the esophagus, are thought to be related to an underlying abnormality of esophageal motility. Past tuberculosis disease may result in such diverticula. Symptoms typically include dysphagia with or without regurgitation, and diagnosis is usually made with barium contrast radiography. Surgical diverticulectomy with myotomy is reserved for patients with symptoms.

Epiphrenic diverticula are herniations of mucosa and submucosa through the muscular layers of the distal 10 cm of the esophagus. They are most

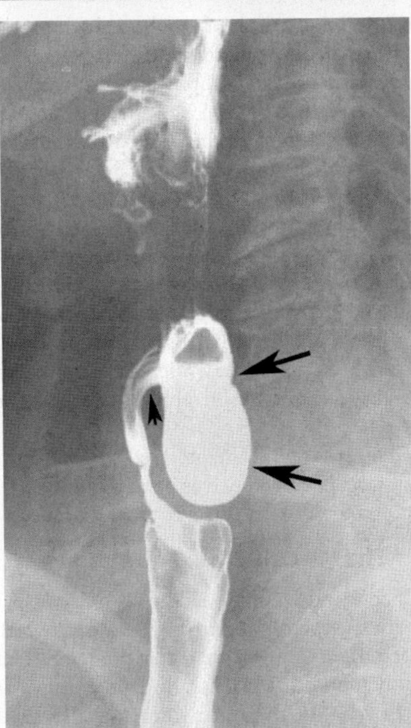

FIGURE 138-9. Barium radiograph of Zenker diverticulum *(arrow)* and cricopharyngeus *(arrowhead)*. (Courtesy Marc Levine, MD.)

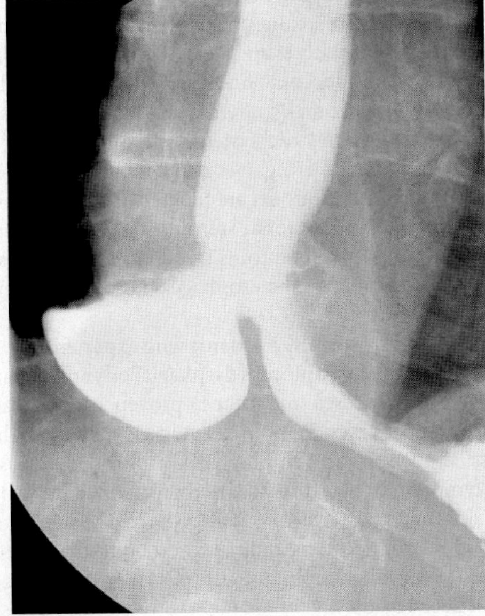

FIGURE 138-10. Barium radiograph of an esophageal epiphrenic diverticulum. (Courtesy Marc Levine, MD.)

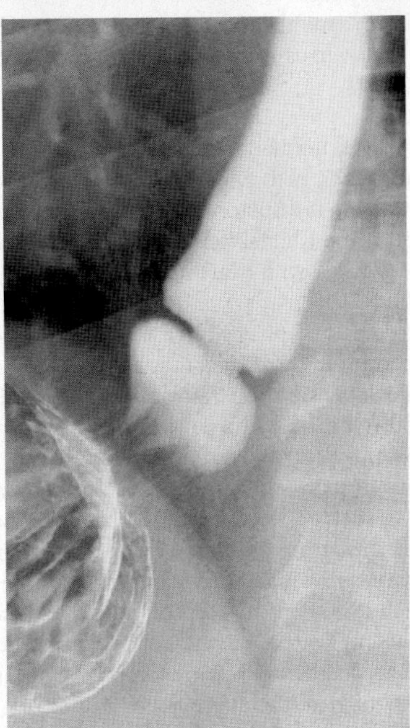

FIGURE 138-11. Barium radiograph of Schatzki ring. (Courtesy Marc Levine, MD.)

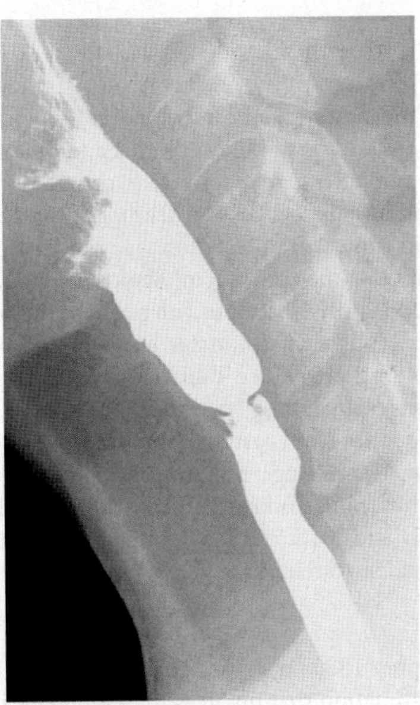

FIGURE 138-12. Barium radiograph of an esophageal web. (Courtesy of Marc Levine, MD.)

commonly caused by functional lower esophageal sphincter obstruction, owing to underlying motility abnormalities such as achalasia or diffuse esophageal spasm, but may also be associated with mechanical obstruction, owing to a leiomyoma, prior surgery, stenosis, stricture tumor, or web. Epiphrenic diverticula may be asymptomatic or cause dysphagia, regurgitation, odynophagia, chest pain, heartburn, or aspiration. Diagnosis is typically made by barium radiography (Fig. 138-10), but endoscopy is recommended to exclude a structural cause of obstruction, and esophageal manometry is recommended to evaluate for underlying motility abnormalities. No therapy is warranted in asymptomatic patients, but symptomatic patients generally do well with surgical diverticulectomy, repair of the defect in the esophageal wall, and relief of the underlying obstruction, usually with a myotomy and partial fundoplication.

Rings and Webs

Esophageal rings are concentric areas of narrowing, usually in the distal esophagus. *Schatzki ring* (Fig. 138-11) is a thin, fixed, circumferential membrane-like narrowing at the gastroesophageal junction, typically at the proximal border of a hiatal hernia. The cause may be congenital, secondary to a pleat of redundant mucosa, or related to gastroesophageal reflux. Symptoms typically occur if the ring results in a lumen that is 13 mm or less in diameter. Classic symptoms are intermittent dysphagia to solids or impaction of solid food. Diagnosis is best accomplished with barium radiography, especially for rings larger than 13 mm in diameter, which may be missed at the time of endoscopy. Treatment involves use of large-caliber dilators at least 18 mm in diameter. Long-term therapy with proton pump inhibitors (see Table 138-1) may prevent relapses. Most patients relapse after a single dilation.

Muscular rings, which are located several centimeters above the squamocolumnar junction, are composed of mucosa, submucosa, and muscle. Barium radiography and endoscopy reveal a focal constriction of variable diameter. Optimal therapy is unclear. Dilation leads to only partial or temporary relief. Other treatment modalities include injection of botulinum toxin and anticholinergic agents.

Esophageal webs are thin, eccentric, membranous areas of narrowing that may be found anywhere in the esophagus but most commonly are in the proximal region (Fig. 138-12). The pathogenesis of webs is unknown, but they are associated with a number of systemic diseases, including bullous skin disorders, chronic graft-versus-host disease, and iron deficiency anemia.

Hiatal Hernia

A hiatal hernia involves herniation of elements of the abdominal cavity through the diaphragmatic hiatus. A sliding or type I hernia, in which the gastroesophageal junction is displaced above the diaphragmatic hiatus, is the most common type. Type I hiatal hernias typically are not associated with symptoms or are associated with heartburn or acid regurgitation. Treatment is the same as for GERD.

In a type II or true paraesophageal hernia, which is uncommon, the gastroesophageal junction is in its normal location, but the fundus and parts of the greater curvature of the stomach herniate into the mediastinum alongside the esophagus. With type III or mixed paraesophageal hernia, the gastroesophageal junction and a large part of the stomach herniate into the mediastinum. Both types of paraesophageal hernias present with symptoms of postprandial distress, such as epigastric pain, chest pain, substernal fullness, shortness of breath, nausea, or vomiting. Iron deficiency anemia may be seen with large hiatal hernias in which at least one third of the stomach is in the chest; linear gastric erosions at the top of gastric folds at the level of the diaphragm have been implicated as a cause of chronic blood loss. Asymptomatic paraesophageal hernias do not require surgery. Symptomatic paraesophageal hernias warrant surgical therapy because of the risk for strangulation, bleeding, perforation, or obstruction.

THE ESOPHAGUS IN SYSTEMIC DISEASES

Scleroderma

Up to 90% of patients with scleroderma (Chapter 267) have esophageal involvement, thereby making it the most common gastrointestinal abnormality in the disease. The classic manometric and radiologic findings are aperistalsis of the distal two thirds of the esophagus and hypotensive or patulous lower esophageal sphincter on manometry or radiography, respectively. These findings result initially because of neuropathy and later because of the myopathy. The main clinical manifestation is severe gastroesophageal reflux. Delayed gastric emptying may also occur. Marked esophageal stasis may also lead to *Candida* esophagitis. A patulous (on radiography) or hypotensive (on manometry) lower esophageal sphincter strongly supports the diagnosis. Proton pump inhibitor therapy (see Table 138-1) is the cornerstone of treatment. Lifestyle changes, including small frequent meals and avoiding nighttime meals, may reduce the gastric symptoms. Antireflux surgery can exacerbate dysphagia by creating a functional high-pressure zone in the distal esophagus and is thus contraindicated. Unfortunately, many patients suffer from chronic GERD and are at risk for developing Barrett esophagus, recurrent strictures, and adenocarcinoma.

Amyloidosis

Amyloidosis (Chapter 188) may lead to smooth muscle and autonomic nervous system dysfunction that involves the esophagus in a pattern similar to scleroderma. Patients will have both dysphagia and severe reflux because of esophageal aperistalsis and a hypotensive lower esophageal sphincter. Dysphagia may result not only from the motility changes but also from diffuse esophageal rigidity and loss of compliance owing to amyloid infiltration of the esophageal wall. Rarely, an achalasia-like pattern may develop. No treatment improves the esophageal manifestations of amyloidosis, other than treatment for the underlying disease and high-dose proton pump inhibitors given twice daily.

Other Systemic Diseases

Dermatomyositis (Chapter 269) principally involves the striated muscle of the oropharynx and proximal esophagus, but sometimes the distal esophagus may lose normal peristaltic function. Symptoms can be oropharyngeal or esophageal depending on the site of greatest muscular involvement. Dysphagia may be an early presenting symptom of dermatomyositis, and the esophagus may be involved in 10 to 50% of patients. Treatment is directed at the generalized myositis because there are no specific treatments for the esophagus. Swallowing therapy may sometimes be helpful. Return of swallowing commonly lags behind recovery of other striated muscle symptoms.

Esophageal involvement in *systemic lupus erythematosus* (Chapter 266) is not as prominent as in scleroderma, dermatomyositis, or mixed connective tissue disease. Dysphagia occurs in fewer than 15% of patients and may be caused by decreased salivation from secondary Sjögren syndrome or reduced esophageal peristalsis. Other causes of esophageal symptoms in patients with systemic lupus erythematosus include GERD, esophageal ulcers, esophageal infection, and medication-induced esophagitis. *Behçet disease* (Chapter 270) causes esophageal ulcers in less than 15% of affected patients. Ulcers are typically located in the middle third of the esophagus and are often associated with ulcers in the stomach, ileum, or colon. Rare esophageal lesions include strictures, varices, and fistulas connecting with the trachea. These complications can be severely debilitating.

Esophageal involvement in *Crohn disease* (Chapter 141) is uncommon but has been described in up to 1 to 2% of patients. Occasionally, isolated esophageal disease may occur. Ulceration is the most common manifestation, but strictures, fissures, esophagobronchial fistulas, mediastinal abscesses, and aphthoid lesions have been described. Patients typically complain of dysphagia and odynophagia. Treatment and prognosis are as for the underlying Crohn disease.

In the *Ehlers-Danlos syndrome* (Chapter 260), hiatal hernias are common, and structural esophageal defects such as giant epiphrenic diverticula, megaesophagus, and spontaneous esophageal rupture may also be seen.

Skin Disorders That Involve the Esophagus

Lichen planus (Chapter 438) involves the esophagus. Patients generally present in the fourth to seventh decade of life. Histologically, the lesions in up to 25 to 50% of patients show a characteristic lymphohistiocytic inflammatory infiltrate and apoptotic basal keratinocytes known as Civatte bodies. Lesions classically occur on the buccal mucosa and the tongue, but the disease may also involve other areas of the oral cavity and the esophagus, conjunctiva, nose, larynx, stomach, bladder, and anus. Most patients are asymptomatic or have only minor symptoms, but patients with severe esophageal lichen planus often develop strictures and may present with dysphagia, odynophagia, and weight loss. Strictures are typically proximal but may be variable in length and location, sometimes involving most of the esophageal body. Patients may present with esophageal lichen planus in the absence of extraesophageal disease. Endoscopic findings, which can be subtle and nonspecific, include peeling mucosa, hyperemic focal abnormalities, and submucosal plaque or papules. High-dose systemic steroids, starting with at least 40 mg prednisone and then tapering over 1 to 2 months, are often successful, but relapse is common when steroids are tapered. Topical steroids have also been tried. Dilation and intralesional steroids can alleviate the symptoms associated with strictures, but symptoms frequently recur in less than a year and necessitate repeat dilations. The esophageal lesions of lichen planus may rarely have malignant potential.

Pemphigus vulgaris (Chapter 439) patients who experience acute flares may have upper gastrointestinal symptoms (dysphagia, odynophagia, or retrosternal burning) in 80% of cases and biopsy-proven esophageal pemphigus lesions in nearly 50% of cases. Pemphigus vulgaris may rarely be isolated to the esophagus. Paraneoplastic pemphigus (Chapter 439), most commonly reported with lymphoreticular disease, also may involve the esophagus. Like lesions on the skin, esophageal lesions may be flaccid blisters or erosions, but they may also appear as red longitudinal lines along the entire esophagus. Like cutaneous and oral pemphigus, esophageal pemphigus is generally treated with corticosteroids.

In *mucous membrane pemphigoid* (cicatricial pemphigoid, Chapter 439), the esophagus is the most common site of gastrointestinal involvement, but esophageal disease occurs in less than 15% of patients. The esophageal disease can present as many as 10 years after disease onset and may be the only presentation of the disease. Patients complain of dysphagia and odynophagia. Imaging typically shows erosions, strictures, bullae, or webs. Treatment generally is as for the skin disease.

In *dystrophic epidermolysis bullosa* (Chapter 439), approximately 70 to 95% of patients develop esophageal stenosis or strictures. Strictures are especially common in children with recessive dystrophic epidermolysis bullosa, whereas fewer than 10% of patients with dominant dystrophic epidermolysis bullosa develop strictures by age 50 years.

ESOPHAGEAL INFECTIONS

Herpes Simplex Virus

Herpes simplex virus (HSV; Chapter 374) esophagitis, which is usually caused by HSV-1, is a well-recognized disease in immunocompromised patients but may also occur in immunocompetent hosts. HSV typically presents as severe odynophagia. Endoscopy and radiology characteristically demonstrate multiple ulcers and friable mucosa, predominantly involving the

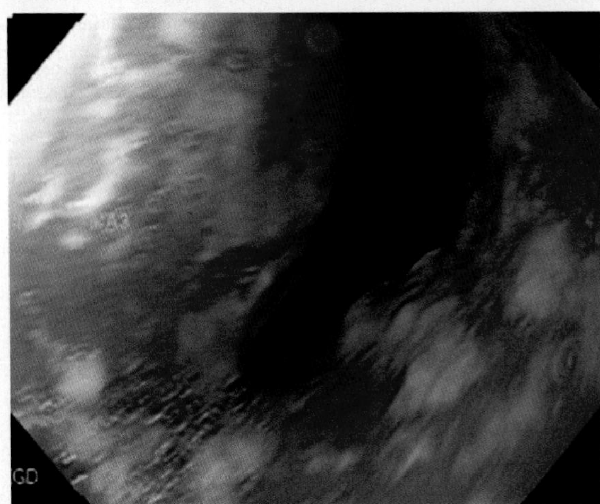

FIGURE 138-13. Candidal esophagitis.

distal esophagus. Mucosal biopsies demonstrate typical intranuclear inclusion bodies. Depending on the severity of the esophageal disease and the underlying health of the patient, treatment options may include intravenous acyclovir, 5 mg/kg every 8 hours for 7 days, or oral acyclovir, 800 mg five times daily for 7 days, combined with symptomatic treatment.

Candidiasis

Esophageal candidiasis is common in patients with HIV infection or with impaired cellular immunity owing to hematologic malignancies, immunosuppressive therapy, or diabetes mellitus. Esophageal candidiasis is also occasionally seen in immunocompetent patients with marked esophageal stasis, such as patients with advanced achalasia or scleroderma. Esophageal candidiasis characteristically presents with symptoms of odynophagia, dysphagia, and chest pain. Endoscopy demonstrates scattered or coalescent yellow-white mucosal plaques (Fig. 138-13). Given the high prevalence of esophageal candidiasis in HIV patients, some recommend treating symptomatic HIV patients empirically and reserving endoscopy for refractory symptoms. Mild oropharyngeal candidiasis may be treated with topical clotrimazole (10 mg troche five times daily for 7 to 14 days) or nystatin (600,000 units four times daily for 7 to 10 days), whereas oral fluconazole (100 mg daily for 7 to 14 days) is needed for moderate to severe oropharyngeal and esophageal candidiasis. Intravenous fluconazole or amphotericin B deoxycholate (Chapter 331) are appropriate options for severe esophageal candidiasis or for patients who cannot tolerate oral therapy.

Cytomegalovirus

Cytomegalovirus (CMV; Chapter 370) infection of the esophagus is exclusively found in immunocompromised patients. Patients infected with the HIV virus with low CD4 counts are most commonly affected, but CMV also occurs in transplant recipients on immunosuppressive therapy and in immunosuppressed patients with malignancy. Patients typically have severe odynophagia with evidence of radiographic or endoscopic esophageal ulcers. Treatment is usually with intravenous ganciclovir (5 mg/kg once or twice daily for 10 to 14 days) or foscarnet (90 mg/kg every 8 to 12 hours until healing occurs).

Bacterial Esophagitis

Bacterial infection of the esophagus is uncommon but can occur in immunosuppressed patients, typically those with neutropenia and malignancy. Patients present with chest pain or odynophagia, or both, and endoscopy reveals extensive erosions, usually in the distal esophagus. Biopsy and Gram stain reveal acute and chronic inflammation and bacteria, commonly gram-positive organisms, especially Viridans-group streptococci, *Staphylococcus aureus*, *Staphylococcus epidermidis*, and *Bacillus* species. Treatment is with the appropriate antibiotics administered parenterally.

Human Papillomavirus

Esophageal infections with human papillomavirus (HPV; Chapter 373) are typically asymptomatic. HPV lesions are most frequently found in the mid to distal esophagus as erythematous macules, white plaque, nodules, or exuberant frond-like lesions. The diagnosis is made by histologic demonstration of koilocytosis (an atypical nucleus surrounded by a ring), giant cells, or immunohistochemical stains. Treatment is usually not necessary, although large lesions may require endoscopic removal. Other treatments, such as interferon, bleomycin, and etoposide, have yielded varying results. HPV infection is a risk factor for esophageal squamous cell carcinoma (Chapter 192), but the value of endoscopic surveillance is not known.

MISCELLANEOUS ESOPHAGEAL CONDITIONS

Esophageal Emergencies

BOERHAAVE SYNDROME

Boerhaave syndrome, or spontaneous rupture of the esophagus, is a transmural full-thickness tear of the esophageal wall. A sudden rise in intraesophageal pressure during forceful vomiting is the cause in most cases. The tear is most commonly in the lower third of the esophagus, 2 to 3 cm proximal to the gastroesophageal junction.

CLINICAL MANIFESTATIONS AND DIAGNOSIS

The classic presentation is vomiting, lower thoracic pain, and subcutaneous emphysema. Other findings may include pleural effusions, especially left sided, tachypnea, abdominal rigidity, fever, and hypotension. Because the condition is rare and classic antecedent vomiting is not always reported, rupture is often recognized only after the development of mediastinitis.

The chest radiograph may demonstrate mediastinal widening, a unilateral pleural effusion, hydropneumothorax, and pneumomediastinum. The esophagram, typically with a water-soluble agent, reveals extravasation, although false-negative results may be encountered. Computed tomography (CT) scanning with an oral contrast agent, which is perhaps the best diagnostic option, typically demonstrates air in the mediastinum.

TREATMENT AND PROGNOSIS Rx

Successful therapy depends on early recognition and the underlying condition of the patient. The classic approach is operative repair in conjunction with broad-spectrum antibiotics and nutritional support, especially if the diagnosis is made within the first 24 hours. Aggressive conservative therapy with percutaneous drains, broad-spectrum parenteral antibiotics, and nutrition has also been successful. In selected individuals, endoscopic insertion of self-expanding covered metallic stents is an option. The mortality rate can be as high as 100% without treatment.

MALLORY-WEISS TEAR

A Mallory-Weiss tear (see Fig. 135-2) is a mucosal tear, often at the gastroesophageal junction, usually caused by severe vomiting or retching. The syndrome is more common in alcoholic patients. In about 85% of patients, it is associated with acute upper gastrointestinal bleeding, which requires transfusion in about 70% of patients and urgent intervention in about 10% of cases. Mortality is about 5%, similar to the mortality in severe bleeding ulcers.[17] Most tears heal spontaneously within about 48 hours.

IATROGENIC PERFORATION

Esophageal perforation may occur as a result of a variety of iatrogenic causes, including endoscopy, dilation, endosonography, or surgery as well as with foreign body ingestion. Typical symptoms include chest pain with or without abdominal pain, subcutaneous emphysema, and fever. Diagnosis may be made immediately at the time of endoscopy or radiography. Chest radiographs may show pneumomediastinum, subcutaneous emphysema, hydrothorax, or hydropneumothorax. A Gastrografin swallow may show a leak, and chest CT may show mediastinal air. Acute perforations are life-threatening emergencies that warrant immediate closure before contamination of the mediastinum. For acute perforation caused by endoscopy, endoscopic clips or stents are an option. Conservative therapy also is an option for well-contained perforations with minimal mediastinal, pleural, or peritoneal contamination and no obvious signs of sepsis. Prognosis is generally good if the perforation is recognized and treated early, preferably within 12 to 24 hours.

FOREIGN BODIES

Impaction of food or foreign bodies is a common gastrointestinal emergency. Meat impaction is most commonly seen in adults, but other foreign objects that also may be ingested accidentally or by design include batteries, coins, and bones. Many patients have an underlying esophageal abnormality, such as Schatzki ring, stricture, eosinophilic esophagitis, tumor, or achalasia. The clinical presentation includes dysphagia, odynophagia, foreign body sensation, chest pain, excessive salivation, and difficulty handling secretions. Immediate endoscopic extraction with concomitant airway protection is recommended because prolonged impaction may result in penetration into the esophageal wall followed by perforation and mediastinitis.[18]

ESOPHAGEAL VARICES

Esophageal varices are described in Chapters 135 and 153.

ESOPHAGEAL FISTULA

Tracheoesophageal fistulas may arise from a variety of different causes, including trauma, infectious esophagitis, necrosis after prolonged endotracheal intubation, esophageal cancer, and radiation therapy. Patients are often critically ill and may not tolerate surgery. Metallic stents are a treatment option.

Atrial-esophageal fistulas are a rare complication after radiofrequency ablation (Chapter 66) for atrial fibrillation. The clinical presentation is nonspecific and includes features such as dysphagia, fever, leukocytosis, bacteremia, massive intestinal bleeding, and septic shock. Diagnosis requires a high index of suspicion and is aided by a chest CT scan. Surgery is required; the prognosis is excellent with early recognition and treatment but can be dire if treatment is delayed.

Congenital Abnormalities

ESOPHAGEAL ATRESIA AND TRACHEOESOPHAGEAL FISTULA

Children with congenital esophageal anomalies commonly survive into adulthood after successful surgery. As adults, these patients typically have gastroesophageal reflux that warrants proton pump inhibitor therapy. Strictures at prior surgical anastomoses are common, and patients may require periodic endoscopic dilation.

HETEROTOPIC GASTRIC MUCOSA (INLET PATCH)

Inlet patches, which are areas of gastric columnar epithelium, are present in up to 4.5% of adults and are usually found incidentally at the time of routine endoscopy. Typically, a red columnar patch varying in size from a few millimeters to a few centimeters is seen just below the cricopharyngeus. Inlet patches can be associated with hoarseness, sore throat, and globus sensation. Strictures, ulcers, and rare malignant transformation have also been described. Treatment options include proton pump inhibitors (see Table 138-1) and endoscopic ablation.

OTHER CONGENITAL ESOPHAGEAL DISORDERS

Duplication cysts, which may be located anywhere in the esophagus, may be in continuity with or separate from the esophageal lumen. Symptoms, which may present initially in adulthood, include dysphagia owing to luminal compression, chest pain, and regurgitation. Treatment is surgical.

Dysphagia lusoria is caused by an aberrant right subclavian artery that originates from the right aortic arch and causes partial compression of the esophagus as it crosses over to the left side. Patients may complain of dysphagia. This condition is most commonly detected incidentally during barium radiography, where it is visualized as a crossing diagonal impression at the junction of the proximal and middle thirds of the esophagus. Surgery is rarely indicated because of the complexity of the operation and the difficulty in establishing a clear relationship between the radiographic findings and symptoms.

Grade A References

A1. Sigterman KE, van Pinxteren B, Bonis PA, et al. Short-term treatment with proton pump inhibitors, H2-receptor antagonists and prokinetics for gastro-oesophageal reflux disease-like symptoms and endoscopy negative reflux disease. *Cochrane Database Syst Rev.* 2013;5:CD002095.

A2. Lundell L, Miettinen P, Myrvold HE, et al., for the Nordic GEORD Study Group. Seven-year follow-up of a randomized clinical trial comparing proton-pump inhibition with surgical therapy for reflux oesophagitis. *Br J Surg.* 2007;94:198-203.

A3. Galmiche JP, Hatlebakk J, Attwood S, et al. Laparoscopic antireflux surgery vs esomeprazole treatment for chronic GERD: the LOTUS randomized clinical trial. *JAMA.* 2011;305:1969-1977.

A4. Ramage JI Jr, Rumalla A, Baron TH, et al. A prospective, randomized, double-blind, placebo-controlled trial of endoscopic steroid injection therapy for recalcitrant esophageal peptic strictures. *Am J Gastroenterol.* 2005;100:2419-2425.

A5. Phoa KN, van Vilsteren FG, Weusten BL, et al. Radiofrequency ablation vs endoscopic surveillance for patients with Barrett esophagus and low-grade dysplasia: a randomized clinical trial. *JAMA.* 2014;311:1209-1217.

A6. Shaheen NJ, Sharma P, Overholt BF, et al. Radiofrequency ablation in Barrett's esophagus with dysplasia. *N Engl J Med.* 2009;360:2353-2355.

A7. van Vilsteren FG, Pouw RE, Seewald S, et al. Stepwise radical endoscopic resection versus radio-frequency ablation for Barrett's oesophagus with high-grade dysplasia or early cancer: a multicentre randomised trial. *Gut.* 2011;60:765-773.

A8. Arias A, Gonzalez-Cervera J, Tenias JM, et al. Efficacy of dietary interventions for inducing histologic remission in patients with eosinophilic esophagitis: a systematic review and meta-analysis. *Gastroenterology.* 2014;146:1639-1648.

A9. Straumann A, Conus S, Degen L, et al. Budesonide is effective in adolescent and adult patients with active eosinophilic esophagitis. *Gastroenterology.* 2010;139:1526-1537.

A10. Boeckxstaens GE, Annese V, des Varannes SB, et al. Pneumatic dilation versus laparoscopic Heller's myotomy for idiopathic achalasia. *N Engl J Med.* 2011;364:1807-1816.

GENERAL REFERENCES

For the General References and other additional features, please visit Expert Consult at https://expertconsult.inkling.com.

139

ACID PEPTIC DISEASE

ERNST J. KUIPERS AND MARTIN J. BLASER

Acid peptic diseases can involve the esophagus (Chapter 138), the stomach, and the duodenum. Dyspeptic symptoms also can occur in patients who have no endoscopic abnormalities, in whom it is termed *nonulcer dyspepsia* (Chapter 137).

DEFINITIONS

Gastric and duodenal ulcers usually occur in an area of inflamed mucosa. This inflammation, termed *gastritis, duodenitis, or bulbitis,* can sometimes be recognized during endoscopy by signs of edema and erythema of the mucosa, but microscopic evaluation of endoscopic biopsy specimens is required for a definitive diagnosis of mucosal inflammation.

Gastritis is categorized by endoscopic and histologic criteria, with granulocytes predominating in active gastritis and mononuclear cells in chronic gastritis. Gastritis is further classified by the segment of the involved stomach: antral-predominant gastritis, corpus-predominant gastritis, or pangastritis. Finally, the absence or presence of premalignant stages of damage to the mucosa as a result of long-standing inflammation defines the categories of nonatrophic and atrophic gastritis, respectively. Endoscopic findings usually are not specific, unless the gastric mucosa has either a typical miniature cobblestone appearance, termed *nodular gastritis* (a finding particularly in children colonized by *Helicobacter pylori*), or grossly enlarged folds without evidence of cancer, termed *hypertrophic gastritis.*

A *peptic ulcer* is a mucosal defect at least 0.5 cm in diameter that penetrates the muscularis mucosae. Smaller mucosal defects are called *erosions* (Fig. 139-1). Gastric ulcers are subdivided into proximal ulcers, located in the body of the stomach, and distal ulcers, located in the antrum and angulus of the stomach. Gastric ulcers are located mainly along the lesser curvature, in particular at the transitional zone of corpus- to antral-type mucosa. This transitional zone is often in the area of the angulus but may shift proximally. Duodenal ulcers usually are located on the anterior or posterior wall of the duodenal bulb (Fig. 139-2), or occasionally at both sites ("kissing" ulcers). Lesions distal to the duodenal bulb are termed *postbulbar ulcers.* Patients who previously underwent a distal gastric resection (Billroth I or II procedure) can develop ulceration at the gastroduodenal anastomosis (anastomotic ulcer). However, ulcers occurring after Billroth II resection are located predominantly in the jejunal mucosa at the junction between the afferent and efferent loops. Anastomotic ulcers also occur after gastric bypass surgery (Chapter 220), for instance, bariatric Roux-en-Y gastric bypass. Other peptic ulcers can occur at sites of metaplastic or heterotopic gastric mucosa, for example, in Meckel diverticulum, the rectum, or Barrett esophagus. Patients with a large hiatal hernia can develop gastric ulceration, known as *Cameron ulcers,* at the level of the herniation. *Dieulafoy ulcers,* which are small mucosal defects over an intramural arteriole, can lead to severe bleeding. Although these lesions can occur throughout the gastrointestinal tract, two thirds occur in the stomach.

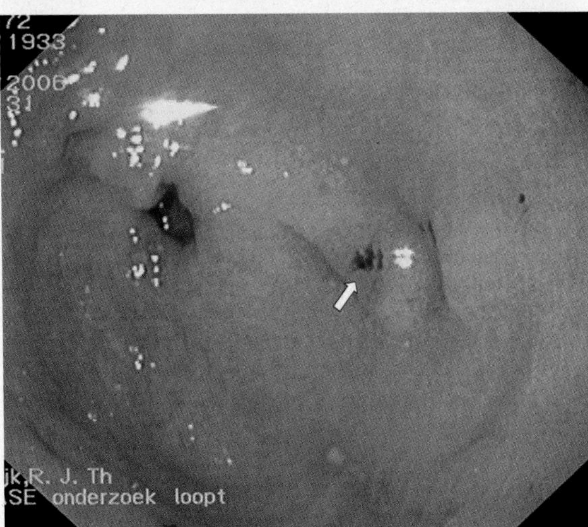

FIGURE 139-1. **Endoscopic view of uncomplicated erosive gastritis. The erosion appears as a small, superficial mucosal break with a black base** ***(arrow)*****.**

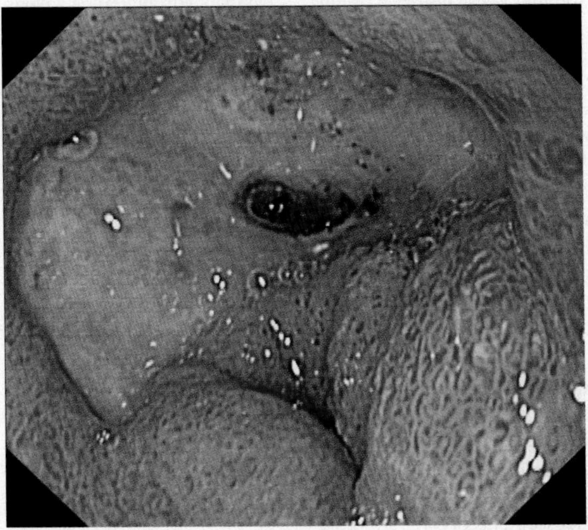

FIGURE 139-2. **Endoscopic view of an ulcer at the anterior wall of the duodenal bulb.** The ulcer has a clean base, with a visible vessel appearing as a dark red protruding spot close to the lower ulcer rim. The surrounding mucosa is inflamed and swollen.

EPIDEMIOLOGY

The worldwide prevalence of gastritis reflects the prevalence of *H. pylori.* Colonization with this bacterium is virtually always associated with chronic active gastritis, which persists as long as an individual remains colonized and only slowly disappears 6 to 24 months after the eradication of *H. pylori.* Colonization with *H. pylori* usually occurs in the first decade of life and then remains lifelong. In developing countries, high colonization rates result in a high prevalence of *H. pylori* gastritis (often ≥80%) in all age groups, including children. In Western countries, the colonization pressure in children has decreased markedly in recent decades, thereby leading to a birth-cohort phenomenon for the prevalence of *H. pylori* gastritis—currently less than 20% in young adults but 40 to 60% in elderly persons. Some recent studies suggest that this decrease in *H. pylori* prevalence in children has slowed or stopped,[1] owing to factors such as the increasing use of daycare facilities.[2] Nevertheless, the decline of *H. pylori* in developed country populations has been inexorable.

Although peptic ulcer disease is strongly related to *H. pylori* gastritis and duodenitis, the epidemiology of ulcer disease has shown secular variation even when *H. pylori* was ubiquitous. The incidence of peptic ulcer disease rose steeply in Western countries in the late 19th and early 20th centuries and has decreased over the past 40 years; nevertheless, peptic ulceration remains a common disorder. The decline in incidence, associated with a decrease in hospital admissions and surgery for ulcer disease, is believed mostly to reflect the decreasing prevalence of gastric colonization with *H. pylori.* The declining incidence of ulcer disease is also the result of the widespread application of eradication therapy, which strongly reduced recurrent ulcers in *H. pylori*–positive patients. Other factors may include the widespread use of acid suppressive medications. Nevertheless, hospital admissions for complications of ulcers and mortality from ulcer disease have shown a far less marked decline in both the United States and other countries because the reduction in *H. pylori*–associated ulcers in younger persons has been counterbalanced by an increase in ulcers related to nonsteroidal anti-inflammatory drugs (NSAIDs) in older persons.

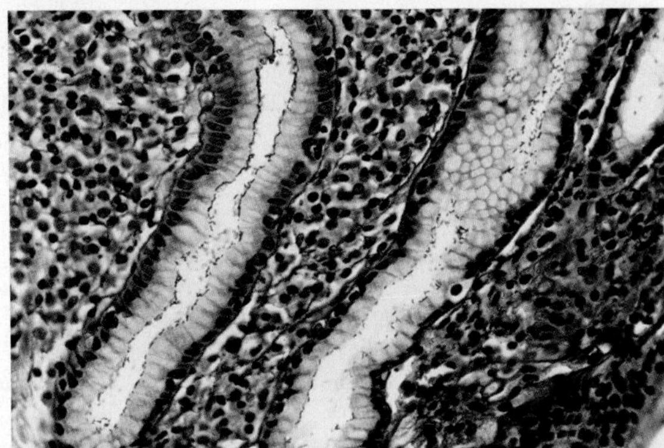

FIGURE 139-3. **Gastric mucosa colonized with** ***Helicobacter pylori*** **appearing as curved bacilli on the mucosal surface.**

In Western countries, duodenal ulcers occur more frequently than gastric ulcers. The predominant age at which duodenal ulcers occur is between 20 and 50 years, whereas gastric ulcers most commonly occur in patients older than 40 years. The incidence of gastroduodenal ulcer disease is approximately 1 to 2 per 1000 inhabitants per year. Although the prevalence of *H. pylori* colonization is nearly identical in males and females, two thirds of patients with ulcers are male. The risk for recurrent disease after initial healing is high; more than 50% of patients have a recurrent ulcer within 12 months of healing in the absence of treatment. Maintenance acid suppressive therapy reduces this recurrence rate, but only therapeutic measures that remove the underlying cause of the ulcer can prevent most ulcer recurrences.

PATHOBIOLOGY

Helicobacter pylori

Most peptic ulcers are associated with colonization with *H. pylori* (Fig. 139-3). Initial clinical studies of the association between *H. pylori* and ulcer disease reported that approximately 85% of patients with gastric ulcer disease and 95% of patients with duodenal ulcer disease were colonized by *H. pylori.* Most persons who are *H. pylori* positive do not have any specific complaints, nor do they develop ulcer disease. The estimated risk for the development of ulcer disease during persistent *H. pylori* colonization is 5 to 15%—that is, three- to eight-fold higher than the risk in patients who are *H. pylori* negative. The risk for the development of an ulcer in the presence of *H. pylori* is determined by a combination of host- and bacteria-related factors. Host factors include immune response, smoking, and stress. A recent genome-wide association study in two independent European cohorts and a subsequent meta-analysis identified a relationship between specific genetic variations in the toll-like receptor (TLR)-1 gene and the prevalence of *H. pylori.*[3] This relationship may in part explain the variation in risk for *H. pylori* colonization and thus the risk for *H. pylori*-associated disease, including peptic ulcer. Bacterial factors that increase the risk for ulcer include a high production of the *VacA* product, which reflects the presence of the s1m1 genotype; a high level of cytokine induction, owing to the presence of genes in the *cag* pathogenicity island; and enhanced adherence, resulting from bacterial *babA* expression.

Nonsteroidal Anti-inflammatory Drugs and Aspirin

The other common cause of gastroduodenal ulcer disease is the use of NSAIDs. At least 2 to 4% of the population in many countries use acetylsalicylic acid, acetic acid derivatives (diclofenac, indomethacin, sulindac), or propionic acid derivatives (ibuprofen, ketoprofen, naproxen) on a daily basis. The risk for ulcer disease is dose and duration dependent. Within 14 days after the start of such treatment, about 5% of patients develop mucosal breaks, that is, erosions and ulcers. In patients who continue therapy for 4 weeks or longer, this proportion increases to 10%, but many are clinically silent. The concomitant presence of *H. pylori* infection increases the incidence of NSAID-related ulcers.

TABLE 139-1 DIFFERENTIAL DIAGNOSIS OF PEPTIC ULCER DISEASE

ORIGIN	CONDITION	FREQUENCY*	DIAGNOSTIC TEST	FINDINGS
Microbes	*Helicobacter pylori*	Very common	*H. pylori* tests Histology	Bacteria, enzymes, antigens, antibodies Gastritis
	Helicobacter heilmannii	Rare	Histology	Spiral bacteria, gastritis
	Treponema pallidum	Very rare	Serology	Antibodies
	Mycobacterial infection	Very rare	Histology, immune response testing, chest radiograph	Acid-fast bacteria, granuloma, immune response, pulmonary infiltrate
	Cytomegalovirus, herpes simplex virus type 1; Epstein-Barr virus	Rare	Histology, serology	Virus inclusions, antibodies
Drug use	NSAIDs, aspirin	Very common	History, urine test	NSAID use
	Bisphosphonates	Rare	History	Bisphosphonate use
	Corticosteroids	Rare	History	Corticosteroid use, comorbidity
	Amphetamines, cocaine	Rare	History, drug testing	Drug use
	Anticoagulants, coagulopathy	Rare	Endoscopy	Ulcer after intramural bleed
Malignancy	Gastric cancer	Common	Histology	Malignancy
	Duodenal cancer	Rare	Histology, CT	Malignancy
	Pancreatic cancer	Common	Histology, CT	Malignancy
	Mucosa-associated lymphoid tissue lymphoma	Rare	Histology	Malignancy
	Metastatic cancer	Rare	Histology	Malignancy
Gastritis syndromes	Eosinophilic gastritis	Rare	Histology	Eosinophilic infiltration
	Lymphocytic gastritis	Rare	Histology, celiac disease screening	Lymphocytic infiltration, villous atrophy
Hyperacidicity syndromes	Zollinger-Ellison syndrome	Rare	Serum gastrin, secretin test	Extreme hypergastrinemia, positive secretin test
	Antral G-cell hyperfunction	Very rare	Serum gastrin, secretin test	Moderate hypergastrinemia, negative secretin test
	Retained gastric antrum	Very rare	Medical history, gastrin	Billroth II resection, hypergastrinemia
	Systemic mastocytosis	Very rare	Histology of affected sites	Mast cell infiltration
	Chronic myelogenous leukemia	Very rare	Leukemia evaluation	Leukemia
Ischemia	Mesenteric vascular occlusion	Common	Angiography	Vascular disease
	Polycythemia vera	Rare	Blood counts	Polycythemia
Specific ulcer types	Cameron ulcer	Common	Endoscopy	Ulcer in large hiatal hernia
	Marginal ulcer	Common	Endoscopy	Ulcer at anastomosis
	Dieulafoy ulcer	Common	Endoscopy	Singular bleeding focus with minimal mucosal disruption
Systemic inflammation	Crohn disease	Common	Histology, ileocolonoscopy	Inflammation, granulomas
	Vasculitides	Rare	Histology, systemic evaluation	Vasculitis, signs of systemic disease
	Gastric amyloidosis	Very rare	Histology	Amyloid deposition
Other conditions	Stress ulcer	Fairly common in patients in intensive care units	Endoscopy	—
	Radiation therapy, chemotherapy	Rare	Endoscopy, history	—

*Frequency as a cause of gastroduodenal ulcer disease.
CT = computed tomography; NSAID = nonsteroidal anti-inflammatory drug.

The risk for developing an ulcer during NSAID use is higher in patients who are older than 60 years; patients with a previous ulcer; patients who use corticosteroids, selective serotonin reuptake inhibitors, or aldosterone antagonists[4]; and patients with major comorbid diseases. In patients who use anticoagulants, such as warfarin and new oral anticoagulants (thrombin and factor Xa inhibitors), or who have severe comorbid disease, an NSAID-induced ulcer is more likely to lead to life-threatening gastroduodenal hemorrhage.

On the basis of their activities, NSAIDs are divided into cyclooxygenase 1 (COX1) and COX2 inhibitors (Chapter 37). The COX1 enzyme is involved in the production of prostaglandins, which play a role in normal cell regulation. The COX2 enzyme, which is also involved in the production of prostaglandins, is induced by inflammatory responses. Most NSAIDs have a nonselective COX inhibitory effect; selective COX2 inhibitors are associated with fewer gastroduodenal ulcers, but their use is limited by adverse coronary effects (Chapter 37). Because of the strong association between NSAIDs and ulcer disease and the risk for recurrence of ulcers with their continued use, patients with ulcers must be thoroughly assessed for any use of NSAIDs.

Helicobacter pylori–Negative, Non-NSAID Ulcer Disease

In most series, *H. pylori* and NSAID use account for 80 to 95% of cases of ulcer disease. The remaining cases are often referred to as *idiopathic* or *H. pylori–negative, non-NSAID* acid peptic disease. The proportion of ulcer disease that is idiopathic is increasing throughout the world as the prevalence of *H. pylori* decreases. Further, it is likely that some ulcers in *H. pylori*–positive patients were not caused by *H. pylori.* Consistent with this notion is the fact that some *H. pylori*–positive patients develop recurrent ulcers after successful bacterial eradication, so presumably their ulcer disease was idiopathic. It is not known whether the increase in idiopathic ulcer disease is simply proportional to the decrease in *H. pylori*–associated ulcers or whether it reflects a true increase in the incidence of idiopathic ulcers.

In patients with idiopathic ulcer disease, specific clues to the underlying cause are often provided by the medical history, including comorbidity and drug use; the endoscopic appearance of the ulcer; and the histologic features of the ulcer's margins and surroundings. In most cases, these initial data can be used to direct further diagnostic studies (Table 139-1).

Malignant Ulcer Disease

Gastroduodenal ulcers can result from underlying malignancies. In the stomach, such tumors are related to gastric adenocarcinoma and, rarely, to mucosa-associated lymphoid tissue (MALT) lymphomas (Chapter 192). Malignant ulcers in the duodenum may result from primary duodenal carcinomas or from penetrating pancreatic cancers. Duodenal cancers have an association with polyposis syndromes, especially familial adenomatous polyposis and, to a much lesser extent, MYH-associated polyposis and Peutz-Jeghers syndrome (Chapter 193). In both the stomach and the duodenum, ulcer disease also may be caused by metastatic tumors, including cancers of the breast, colon, thyroid, or kidney, or by melanoma, disseminated lymphoma, or Kaposi sarcoma. Malignant ulcers are characteristically irregular in shape with heaped borders, but they also may be flat or depressed lesions.

Current high-resolution and magnification endoscopes allow visualization of the altered mucosal structure surrounding an ulcer, including changes in the microvascular pattern. For a definite diagnosis of malignancy, multiple biopsy specimens are needed, usually from the ulcer margins.

Systemic Inflammatory Disorders

A few gastroduodenal ulcers are caused by systemic inflammatory diseases, in particular, Crohn disease (Chapter 141). Patients with Crohn disease affecting the proximal gastrointestinal tract often have multiple ulcers characterized by irregular longitudinal shapes. Ulcers in the duodenum occur on top of Kerckring folds. Patients with gastroduodenal ulcers from Crohn disease do not invariably have evidence of disease elsewhere in the digestive tract, nor do blood tests always suggest an active inflammatory bowel disorder. The demonstration of ulcerative inflammation elsewhere in the digestive tract, in particular in the terminal ileum and colon, strongly supports the diagnosis of Crohn disease, as do noncaseating granulomas on biopsy specimens. However, the absence of granulomas does not exclude Crohn disease, and these lesions are not specific for Crohn disease; they also are associated with *H. pylori* gastritis and other conditions, particularly sarcoidosis (Chapter 95). Sarcoidosis can also lead to gastroduodenal ulcer disease.

Other inflammatory disorders that can cause gastritis or gastroduodenal ulcers include various forms of vasculitis affecting the mesenteric system, in particular Behçet disease (Chapter 270), Henoch-Schönlein purpura (Chapter 270), Takayasu arteritis (Chapters 78 and 270), polyarteritis nodosa (Chapter 270), systemic lupus erythematosus (Chapter 266), Churg-Strauss syndrome (Chapter 270), and granulomatosis with polyangiitis (Chapter 270). Lymphocytic gastroduodenitis, which is strongly associated with celiac disease (Chapter 140), may lead to duodenal ulceration and subsequent stenotic web formation. Ulcer disease also may occur in patients with polycythemia vera (Chapter 166), possibly in relation to reduced mucosal blood flow. Vasculitis underlying ulcer disease should be considered in patients with chronic or recurrent ulceration in whom other causes have been excluded. Lymphocytic phlebitis, which is a rare vasculitic inflammatory disorder that affects the mesenteric veins, may cause gastric ulcers. Systemic amyloidosis (Chapter 188) affecting the stomach wall may lead to gastric ulcers. Rare cases of duodenal ulceration have been described in the presence of annular pancreas or congenital bands obstructing the descending duodenum.

Hypergastrinemic Syndromes

Peptic ulcers can result from chronic gastric hyperacidity related to hypergastrinemia. The most important hypergastrinemic disorder is Zollinger-Ellison syndrome (Chapter 195), a condition of marked hyperacidity leading to severe peptic ulcer disease caused by a gastrin-producing endocrine tumor. These patients usually have multiple bulbar and postbulbar duodenal ulcers that are resistant to conventional acid suppressive therapy. The diagnosis can be confirmed by the presence of a high fasting serum gastrin level (often but not always ≥10-fold increased and >1000 pg/mL). Similar gastrin levels are sometimes seen in patients treated for chronic ulcer disease with high-dose proton pump inhibitors. For clarification, secretin testing can be performed: in patients with Zollinger-Ellison syndrome, the injection of secretin (1 U/kg) increases serum gastrin levels by more than 50%, or 120 pg/mL or greater in those with fasting gastrin levels less than 10-fold above normal. Imaging techniques, such as computed tomography (CT), magnetic resonance imaging, isotope scanning, endoscopic ultrasonography, videocapsule endoscopy, and balloon-assisted enteroscopy, may be used to detect the primary tumor, which is often located in either the pancreas or the proximal small bowel. In some patients, Zollinger-Ellison syndrome occurs as part of the multiple endocrine neoplasia syndrome (Chapter 231), particularly in association with hyperparathyroidism. Other hypergastrinemic hyperacidity syndromes are the retained gastric antrum syndrome (see later) and antral G-cell hyperfunction. In the latter, fasting serum gastrin levels are only modestly increased and do not rise after the injection of secretin, but they respond in an exaggerated way to meals, thereby leading to hyperacidity. When the condition occurs in an *H. pylori*–positive patient, bacterial eradication therapy may be curative. However, some patients with G-cell hyperfunction are *H. pylori* negative.

Ischemia

Stenosis or occlusion of the celiac trunk or the superior mesenteric artery (Chapter 143) also can lead to ulceration in the mucosa of the proximal digestive tract (Fig. 139-4). These ulcers typically occur in elderly patients who have known severe atherosclerosis or risk factors for it, but they can also occur in younger subjects with mesenteric obstruction due to other causes. Ischemic ulcers tend to heal slowly and to recur. Pallor of the mucosa, consistent with decreased mucosal blood flow, may be noted at endoscopy. Upper mesenteric ischemia is often associated with upper abdominal pain, which can be elicited by a meal or by physical activity. These symptoms may cause patients to decrease their food intake, leading to weight loss before their clinical presentation. The prevalence of upper mesenteric ischemia with secondary ulcer disease is unknown, in part owing to its variable presentation, often with a history of gradual symptoms; the lack of standardized and reliable diagnostic tests; and clinicians' unfamiliarity with the condition. Diagnostic evaluation includes a duplex ultrasound scan for vascular flow and conventional or CT angiography of the affected arteries. Validated functional tests for gastroduodenal mucosal perfusion are not widely available, but a technique for directly measuring mucosal oxygen saturation during endoscopy is investigational.

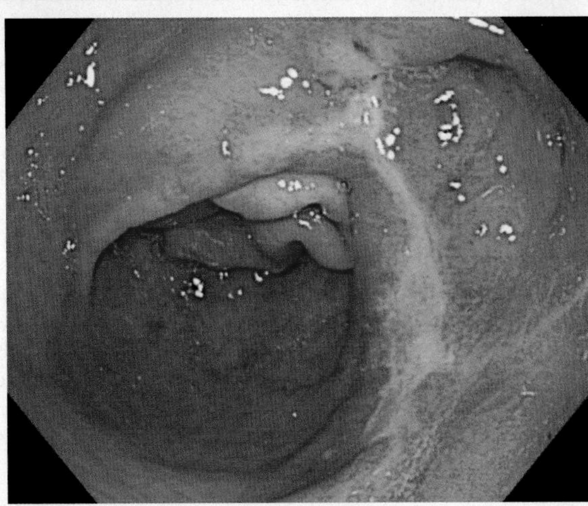

FIGURE 139-4. Endoscopic view of an irregular gastric ulcer at the posterior wall and smaller curvature in a patient with chronic mesenteric ischemia due to subtotal stenosis of the celiac trunk.

Stress Ulcers

Patients with severe medical conditions, such as major trauma, sepsis, extensive burns, head injury, or multiorgan failure, can develop stress ulcers in the stomach or duodenum. Major risk factors for stress ulceration in severely ill patients include mechanical ventilation, coagulopathy, and hypotension, but factors such as hepatic and renal failure and the use of ulcerogenic medications may contribute. Stress ulcers occur independently of *H. pylori* colonization. Ulcers associated with head injury are known as Cushing ulcers, and ulcers associated with extensive burns are known as Curling ulcers. Stress ulcers were once common in patients in intensive care units, but improvements in overall management, including respiratory and hemodynamic care, acid inhibition, and emphasis on adequate feeding, have reduced the incidence of these ulcers, which currently affect 1 to 2% of these patients. Stress ulcers may be asymptomatic, but they can also cause complications, especially bleeding.

Other Factors

Cameron Ulcer

Patients with large hiatal hernias (Chapter 138) may present with proximal gastric ulcers, termed *Cameron ulcers,* at the level of the hiatus, where the stomach is compressed. These ulcers are usually asymptomatic but may cause occult or overt bleeding. During upper gastrointestinal endoscopy, patients with large hiatal hernias and iron deficiency anemia should be carefully examined in normal and retroverted positions for the presence of Cameron ulcers.

Anastomotic or Marginal Ulceration

Patients who have undergone partial gastrectomy sometimes develop recurrent ulcers, often located at the anastomosis or within the jejunum immediately opposite the anastomosis. Ischemia and chronic inflammation in particular resulting from biliary reflux may cause such ulcers. If biopsies exclude cancer, treatment includes acid suppression and *H. pylori* eradication, if needed. Anastomotic ulcers after bariatric gastric surgery appear to be related to local ischemia. They have no clear correlation with *H. pylori,* and preoperative *H. pylori* eradication does not appear to reduce the incidence of such ulcers. Peptic ulcer disease can be associated also with the retained gastric antrum syndrome when the antrum is not completely excised from the detached duodenum during partial gastrectomy surgery. Because it then lacks exposure to acid and is thus not physiologically downregulated, it continues to secrete gastrin despite normal or even high acid levels. Marginal ulcers can also occur after bariatric Roux-en-Y gastric bypass surgery.

Other Microbial Organisms

Colonization with *Helicobacter heilmannii* (formerly known as *Gastrospirillum hominis*), which is probably a zoonotic organism, is associated with mild gastritis and sometimes with transient ulcer disease. Ulcer disease also may be infectious, resulting from secondary syphilis (Chapter 319), mycobacterial infection (Chapter 324), infection with herpes simplex virus type 1 (Chapter 374), varicella-zoster virus (Chapter 375), cytomegalovirus infection (Chapter 376), or Epstein-Barr virus (Chapter 377).

Alcohol

Short-term heavy alcohol use or long-term moderate to heavy alcohol use can lead to signs of acute and chronic gastritis. No evidence indicates that this type of gastritis is associated with a significant risk for peptic ulceration, although alcohol use increases the risk for bleeding in patients with peptic ulcer disease.

Hyperhistaminic Syndromes

Similar to the hypergastrinemic syndromes, persistent elevation of histamine can lead to hyperacidity as a result of the chronic stimulation of parietal cells. Elevated histamine levels are observed in two rare syndromes. *Systemic mastocytosis* (Chapter 255) is characterized by a proliferation of mast cells in the bone marrow, skin, liver, spleen, and gastrointestinal tract, often associated with both spontaneous and trigger-induced (e.g., alcohol) release of histamine and other vasoactive substances. Patients with systemic mastocytosis often have gastrointestinal symptoms, including pain, diarrhea, and blood loss. Ulceration results from chronic gastric acid hypersecretion. Clues to the diagnosis include symptoms of pruritus, urticaria, or rash. The bone marrow and affected organ mast cell infiltrates carry a specific *C-kit* mutation and express CD2 and CD25. Histamine hypersecretion leading to peptic ulcer disease also can occur in *chronic myelogenous leukemia* (Chapter 184) with basophilia.

Other Drugs

Oral bisphosphonates, used widely for osteoporosis (Chapter 243), may induce gastric erosions and ulcerations in an estimated 3 to 10% of treated patients. The risk for ulcer disease may be synergistically increased by NSAID use but is probably independent of *H. pylori* colonization. Although corticosteroid treatment can be complicated by peptic ulcer disease, the relative risk is only slightly increased, except in patients with serious comorbid diseases, using long-term or high-dose therapy, or with prior ulcers. Other patients who use corticosteroids are not at serious risk for ulcer disease and therefore do not require measures to prevent ulcers. Similarly, the use of aldosterone antagonists is also associated with an increased risk for peptic ulcer and ulcer bleeding, likely related to impaired mucosal healing.

Persons who use amphetamines and crack cocaine (Chapter 34) frequently develop ulcer disease, often with perforation, possibly as a result of vascular insufficiency. Chemotherapy, particularly when given selectively as a high-dose intra-arterial infusion in the celiac system, can be complicated by ulcer disease. Patients on anticoagulant therapy and those with other coagulopathies may rarely develop intramural hematoma of the gastrointestinal tract. Depending on the location, these hematomas may cause obstruction, but they can also leave large ulcers when they rupture into the lumen. Radiation therapy of the upper abdomen is sometimes complicated by chronic ischemic ulceration, especially as a late complication.

CLINICAL MANIFESTATIONS

The clinical manifestations of acid peptic disease (Table 139-2) do not always predict the various morphologic presentations found at endoscopy. Indeed, a silent ulcer may be recognized only when it presents abruptly with a complication, most commonly hemorrhage or perforation, or it may be discovered incidentally when a diagnostic test is performed for other reasons. Nevertheless, the typical presentation of acid peptic disease is recurrent episodes of pain. The pain is almost invariably located in the epigastrium and may radiate to the back or, less commonly, to the thorax or other regions of the abdomen (see Table 139-2). Some patients describe the pain as burning or piercing, whereas others describe it as an uncomfortable feeling of emptiness of the stomach, referred to as *painful hunger.* Indeed, the pain may improve with the ingestion of food, only to return in the postprandial period. The timing of the pain in relation to meals and to the soothing effects of food is nonspecific, however, and may also occur in patients with functional dyspepsia without ulcer. Nocturnal epigastric pain that awakens a patient several hours after a late meal is more likely to represent ulcer pain.

TABLE 139-2 KEY SYMPTOMS AND SIGNS OF PEPTIC ULCER

UNCOMPLICATED ULCER
No symptoms ("silent ulcer" in up to 40% of cases)
Epigastric pain
Pain may radiate to the back, thorax, other parts of abdomen (cephalad most likely, caudad least likely)
Pain may be nocturnal (most specific), "painful hunger" relieved by food, or continuous (least specific)
Nausea
Vomiting
Heartburn (mimics or associated with gastroesophageal reflex)
COMPLICATED ULCER
Severe abdominal pain
Shock
Abdominal board-like rigidity (and rebound and other signs of peritoneal irritation)
Free intraperitoneal air
Hemorrhage
Hematemesis and/or melena
Hemodynamic changes, anemia
Previous history of ulcer symptoms (80%)
Gastric outlet obstruction
Satiation, inability to ingest food, eructation
Nausea, vomiting (and related disturbances)
Weight loss

Aside from the pain during symptomatic episodes, patients may complain of retrosternal burning (heartburn) or acidic regurgitation into the throat, symptoms that reflect associated gastroesophageal reflux (Chapter 138), which is aggravated by hyperacidity or delayed gastric emptying. Nausea and vomiting may also occur but are nonspecific. The presence of significant diarrhea should raise the possibility of Zollinger-Ellison syndrome (Chapter 195), but diarrhea also may result from the intensive use of magnesium-containing antacids. In untreated patients, symptoms tend to be intermittent, with flares of daily pain lasting 2 to 8 weeks, separated by prolonged asymptomatic intervals. During periods of remission, patients may feel well and may be able to eat even heavy or spicy meals without apparent discomfort.

Physical Examination

The physical examination is usually unrevealing. If significant bleeding has occurred (Chapter 135), the patient may present with pallor and may be hypovolemic (Chapter 106). It is always useful to inquire about the characteristics of the stool because ulcer-related bleeding may manifest not only obviously in the form of hematemesis but also insidiously as melena (black feces). In the case of massive ulcer bleeding with the rapid bowel passage of blood, patients may also present with red rectal blood loss. When a patient has acute perforation, severe epigastric and abdominal pain usually develops, and the patient appears distressed. Characteristically, intense contracture of the abdominal muscles is apparent on palpation, together with rebound tenderness and other signs of peritoneal irritation. With large amounts of intra-abdominal air, percussion may reveal hypertympany over the liver.

DIAGNOSIS

In a patient who presents with symptoms consistent with ulcer disease, the diagnostic evaluation should proceed along two different but complementary paths: confirmation of the anatomic abnormality and investigation of its cause (Table 139-3). In most patients, it is advisable to follow both diagnostic paths simultaneously, but sometimes it is reasonable to skip the anatomic verification as a cost-saving strategy and proceed to management based on probable cause.

Anatomic Diagnosis

Upper gastrointestinal endoscopy (Chapter 134) is the primary investigative tool in patients suspected of having acid peptic disease. This technique can

TABLE 139-3 DIAGNOSTIC PATHS AND TOOLS IN ULCER DISEASE

PATH 1: MORPHOLOGIC DIAGNOSIS
Gastroduodenoscopy
Barium contrast (inferior alternative)
Endoscopic ultrasound (selected cases only)
Computed tomography (useful in selected cases)
PATH 2: ETIOLOGIC DIAGNOSIS
***Helicobacter pylori* Testing**
Histologic examination of gastric mucosa with appropriate stains
Stool antigen test
Carbon-13 urea breath test
Serum antibodies
Ulcer Associated with Nonsteroidal Anti-Inflammatory Drug Use
History of drug ingestion
Decreased platelet adherence
Molecular identification of drugs, pro-drugs, metabolites (complex, expensive)
Acid Hypersecretory Syndromes
Serum gastrin elevation
Gastrin provocative tests (intravenous secretin, meal)
Gastric analysis (acid titration)

detect erosive gastritis (see Fig. 139-1) or an ulcer in the gastric wall or duodenal bulb (see Fig. 139-2). Because of the high prevalence and the spontaneous improvement of dyspeptic symptoms, endoscopy generally should not be performed immediately; rather, its use should be restricted to patients with persistent or recurrent symptoms. However, immediate endoscopy is indicated in patients with alarm symptoms such as weight loss, dysphagia, anorexia, considerable vomiting, anemia, or signs of occult or overt bleeding.

Endoscopy, which is the gold standard for diagnosis, is both highly sensitive and highly specific for the detection of ulcer disease. The most common locations for a peptic ulcer are the stomach and duodenal bulb, but peptic ulcers sometimes occur in the esophagus, the small bowel, and a Meckel diverticulum lined with heterotopic gastric mucosa. Endoscopic ultrasound may detect an unsuspected submucosal component or enlarged lymph nodes, such as may occur in gastric neoplasia, especially lymphoma and linitis plastica (Chapter 192). Ulcers in the dorsal wall of the duodenal bulb, especially at the transition from the bulb to the postbulbar descending portion of the duodenum, are most difficult to visualize, and they sometimes require a side-viewing endoscope, particularly when endoscopic treatment is needed. Other regions where gastroduodenal ulcers can be easily missed are the cardia and the gastric angulus. Dieulafoy lesions may be difficult to diagnose because of their small mucosal defects and intermittent bleeding. Some patients require more than one endoscopy, preferably during acute bleeding, to localize the lesion. Endoscopy is also useful for ascertaining the presence of concomitant disorders, including esophagitis and duodenitis, or complications, such as bleeding or a visible vessel (see Fig. 139-2); obtaining biopsy specimens, such as for histologic examination and to assess for *H. pylori* (see Fig. 139-3); and performing therapeutic interventions.

In rare cases, such as stenosis that blocks the advancing endoscope, conventional barium contrast radiographs (Chapter 133) are indicated. Additional investigations by endosonography or CT are needed when underlying malignant disease is suspected. The endoscopist should obtain biopsy samples from all gastric ulcers, especially those with a suspicious appearance, to exclude potential malignant disease. Because duodenal ulcers are less likely to be malignant, biopsies are usually not required unless malignancy is specifically suspected.

Etiologic Diagnosis

Diagnosis must focus on establishing the cause of the ulcer. The first step is to determine whether *H. pylori* or NSAID use is present because these are the major risk factors for peptic ulcers and can be contributing factors in ulcers with other precipitating causes.

Testing for Helicobacter pylori

In populations with high *H. pylori* prevalence, nearly all patients with peptic ulcer disease are positive for *H. pylori*, so diagnostic testing has little value except when antimicrobial susceptibility testing is needed. The prevalence of *H. pylori* remains high in immigrants from developing countries, where most people become *H. pylori* positive in youth. In Western countries, approximately 50% of individuals who are older than 65 years are colonized with *H. pylori*, but the prevalence is less than 20% in those younger than 30 years. In these younger persons, the proportion of patients with ulcers who are *H. pylori* negative is higher than in older patients, making diagnostic testing for *H. pylori*, followed by targeted therapy in those who are positive for the bacterium, more attractive than empirical therapy.

The presence of *H. pylori* can be ascertained by four possible approaches. *Histologic examination* of gastric mucosal biopsies (either routine hematoxylin and eosin stain or a specific stain, such as Warthin-Starry stain), which is the standard procedure when diagnostic endoscopy is initially performed, is sensitive and specific for *H. pylori.* However, the accuracy of this technique may be affected by sampling error, improper orientation of the specimen, and recent therapy with proton pump inhibitors or antibiotics.

A second option is *serology*, which is a relatively simple, inexpensive test that has reduced predictive value in areas where the prevalence of *H. pylori* is low. Serology is not helpful to verify whether *H. pylori* has been eradicated with antibiotics because it may take more than 6 months or even 1 to 2 years for *H. pylori* antibodies to decrease to undetectable levels. None of the diagnostic tests that do not involve endoscopy can determine whether an ulcer is present.

A third option is a *stool H. pylori antigen test*, which is similar in accuracy to standardized serologic testing. Finally, the *carbon-13* or *carbon -14 urea breath test*, which relies on the detection of *H. pylori* urease activity, is a noninvasive and relatively simple test, but it is more expensive than stool or blood testing. Although the test usually becomes negative as soon as *H. pylori* treatment is begun, a minimum interval of 6 to 8 weeks after therapy has ended is recommended to reduce false-negative results.

Nonsteroidal Anti-inflammatory Drugs

NSAIDs are usually established as the putative cause of an ulcer based on information obtained from the patient. Assessment of NSAID use in an individual patient presenting with ulcer disease can be difficult both because NSAID use is common and often intermittent and because many different NSAIDs are widely available over the counter in most countries. NSAID use is usually evaluated by detailed medical history, focusing not only on current and recent drug use, and especially over-the-counter treatments but also on symptoms of pain, including musculoskeletal complaints. Further information from family members, family practitioners, and pharmacists is sometimes helpful. If surreptitious use of NSAIDs is suspected, direct serum and urine testing for aspirin and NSAID derivatives is feasible, or aspirin use can be assessed indirectly by a platelet adherence assay; however, these tests are not commonly used in clinical practice.

Hypersecretory Syndromes

Hypersecretory syndromes not related to *H. pylori* or NSAIDs are rare causes of ulcer disease and are diagnosed by special tests (see Table 139-3). Zollinger-Ellison syndrome should be strongly considered in patients with multiple ulcers, particularly in atypical locations such as distal to the duodenal bulb, and when diarrhea is present, because these finding are uncommon in *H. pylori*–related peptic ulcer disease. Hypergastrinemic syndromes (e.g., Zollinger-Ellison syndrome, antral G-cell hyperplasia) are best diagnosed by a determination of serum gastrin levels, both basal and after stimulation with intravenous secretin (gastrinoma detection) or a test meal (antral G-cell hyperplasia detection). When detected early, gastrinomas may be resectable (Chapter 195).

Gastric analysis, which is performed by placing a nasogastric tube to aspirate gastric juice and to quantify gastric acid output (both basal and after stimulation with subcutaneous pentagastrin), is indicated in only two rare circumstances: patients with elevated serum gastrin levels suggestive of Zollinger-Ellison syndrome or antral G-cell hyperplasia, but with equivocal responses to standard gastric provocative tests, and patients with indirect signs of gastric hypersecretion (e.g., enlarged folds and abundant clear fluid at endoscopy), normal gastrin levels, and negative provocative gastrin tests but who may still be hypersecretors, such as patients with recurrent ulcer disease despite a prior vagotomy with or without antrectomy. A basal acid output greater than 15 mEq/hour or greater than 5 mEq/hour in a postoperative patient is considered a positive test result.

The diagnosis of Zollinger-Ellison syndrome is best confirmed by gastric analysis showing a basal acid output greater than 15 mEq/hour in conjunction with a fasting serum gastrin level exceeding 1000 pg/mL in the presence of gastric pH less than 2. To skip the cumbersome gastric analysis, a gastric pH determination showing a fasting pH of 2 or less is adequate. For serum gastrin levels in the range 100 to 1000 pg/mL and intragastric pH greater than 2, an increase in the serum gastrin to more than 200 pg/mL after a secretin stimulation test is suggestive of the diagnosis. An elevated serum gastrin level alone is not sufficient to diagnose Zollinger-Ellison syndrome because serum gastrin levels tend to increase over time with atrophic gastritis and also can be markedly increased in patients receiving proton pump inhibitor therapy.

Other Causes

In patients in whom a gastroduodenal ulcer cannot be ascribed to colonization with *H. pylori*, use of NSAIDs, or a hypersecretory syndrome, the establishment of a definite etiologic diagnosis may require a more thorough evaluation, starting with a medical history that focuses on the use of other ulcerogenic agents and the presence of symptoms that could suggest an underlying systemic disease. The next step is to evaluate biopsy samples from ulcer borders and from the antrum, corpus, and duodenum. The ulcer specimens may reveal overt or suspicious signs of malignancy, in particular adenocarcinoma (Chapter 192) or lymphoma. In these cases, further diagnostic evaluation should include staging of the malignancy. Alternatively, the biopsies may provide evidence of other infectious conditions, specific types of gastritis, celiac disease, ischemia, amyloidosis, or a systemic inflammatory condition. These data can be combined with clues provided by the endoscopic evaluation, including the character and location of the ulcer, signs of ischemia, and signs of inflammation at other locations. Further evaluation should focus on the presence of systemic disorders and may include a chest radiograph, angiography, ileocolonoscopy, and abdominal CT.

Differential Diagnosis

The differential diagnosis of ulcer-like symptoms includes many disorders of the upper abdominal organs, including malignant diseases of the stomach (Chapter 192), duodenum (Chapter 193), pancreas (Chapter 194), or bile ducts (Chapter 196). The differential diagnosis of upper abdominal symptoms also includes liver and gallstone disease (Chapter 155), pancreatitis (Chapter 144), and motility disorders (Chapter 136). In many patients with upper abdominal dyspeptic complaints, no underlying cause can be identified. In this "nonulcer" or functional dyspepsia group, complaints characteristic of gastroesophageal reflux, ulcer symptoms, or dysmotility symptoms may be prominent. Some patients (generally 5%) benefit from eradication of *H. pylori*, with a slow decrease of dyspeptic complaints over 12 to 24 months, but functional dyspepsia is not a proven or widely accepted indication for treatment of *H. pylori*. If such treatment is considered, both the patient and the physician should be prepared for persistent symptoms despite eradication of *H. pylori* and potentially for the emergence of antimicrobial-resistant *H. pylori*, which may result in a spiral of multiple courses of therapy in an attempt to remove resistant organisms.

Diagnostic Scenarios: Acute or Initial Clinical Presentation

Younger (≤45 years old) patients without alarm symptoms or signs such as anemia, rapid weight loss, or other evidence of serious disease do not necessarily require endoscopy, and evidence indicates that malignant gastric disease is unlikely. When a physician is treating a patient who lives in an area of the world with a relatively high prevalence of *H. pylori* infection (>10% of the population is positive), a test-and-treat approach can begin with an *H. pylori* stool antigen determination, urea breath test, or *H. pylori* serologic examination. However, although commonly practiced, the test-and-treat approach has never been documented to improve outcomes, except in the setting of endoscopically confirmed peptic ulcer disease. If the *H. pylori* test is positive, the patient can be treated with the appropriate *H. pylori* eradication drugs (see later) and observed for 4 to 6 weeks. If a patient with dyspeptic symptoms is taking an NSAID, either orally or parenterally, the first therapeutic approach is to discontinue these drugs and to prescribe a proton pump inhibitor for 4 to 6 weeks. In patients who test negative for *H. pylori* and who are not taking NSAIDs or who do not improve after these drugs are discontinued, endoscopy is indicated to determine whether an ulcer is present.

Conversely, gastroenterologists more commonly proceed directly to endoscopy. If no abnormalities are apparent or the endoscopic study shows only "gastritis" without an overt ulcer, a biopsy should be obtained to ascertain by histologic examination or urease testing whether *H. pylori* is present. If *H. pylori* is found by endoscopic biopsy, eradication treatment may be pursued. However, the efficacy of *H. pylori* eradication for the relief of functional dyspeptic symptoms is only about 5 to 13% greater than with placebo,[A1][A2] and eradication therapy increases the risk for reflux-related symptoms (Chapter 138), especially in Asian patients.[5]

If endoscopic examination reveals an ulcer, its location determines the subsequent approach. An ulcer in the duodenal bulb has only a remote chance of representing a malignant lesion and need not routinely be examined by biopsy. By contrast, biopsy is mandatory for a gastric ulcerative lesion identified at endoscopy because malignant gastric disease may present with similar clinical manifestations and may resemble benign ulcer disease morphologically. Even if histologic assessment does not identify a malignant process, repeat endoscopy is recommended about 1 month after therapy to verify complete healing and for biopsy of the scar.

TREATMENT

Rx

Helicobacter pylori–Associated Ulcers

H. pylori–associated ulcers often heal spontaneously, but acid suppressive therapy accelerates healing and ameliorates symptoms. Four weeks of acid suppressive therapy heals 70 to 80% of ulcers, and this number increases to more than 90% after 8 weeks of therapy. If *H. pylori* colonization persists, however, ulcers recur in 50 to 90% of patients within 12 to 24 months; this rate can be reduced to 20 to 30% with maintenance acid suppression and to less than 5% with *H. pylori* eradication.[A3] Eradication treatment is therefore mandatory (Table 139-4). The success of eradication treatment strongly depends on therapy adherence and antimicrobial resistance. Resistance of *H. pylori* to metronidazole varies between 10 and 80% throughout the world. Clarithromycin resistance is increasing and ranges between 10 and 30% in many regions owing to the widespread use of macrolides to treat upper respiratory infections. Resistance to amoxicillin and tetracycline is rare and is not usually relevant in clinical practice. Because of this worldwide increase in prevalence of antimicrobial resistance, *H. pylori* eradication regimens continue to evolve.

The conventional regimen is "triple" therapy for 7 to 14 days.[6] Triple therapy combines a proton pump inhibitor with two antibiotics, usually combinations of amoxicillin, a nitroimidazole, and clarithromycin, the latter sometimes being replaced by levofloxacin.[A4] Triple treatment for 10 to 14 days has about a 4 to 8% advantage over 7-day therapy,[A5] which explains why 7-day therapy has become obsolete. Furthermore, double-dose proton pump inhibitor therapy (dose equivalent to omeprazole 40 mg twice daily) also increases eradication rates by approximately 10%. For patients in whom such therapy fails, a 10-day course of quadruple therapy is advised. This second-line regimen eradicates *H. pylori* in an additional 80% of patients.[7]

Because of the increased prevalence of antimicrobial resistance, triple therapies are increasingly being replaced by initial quadruple therapies.[8,9] Bismuth-based quadruple therapy consists of a proton pump inhibitor, a bismuth compound, and two antibiotics, usually tetracycline and a nitroimidazole (see Table 139-4). This regimen leads to eradication in 80 to 95% of patients. Non-bismuth-based quadruple therapies consist of a proton pump inhibitor plus three antibiotics, usually given for 10 days but often extended to 14 days (see Table 139-4). The three forms of non-bismuth-based quadruple therapy (sequential, hybrid, and concomitant therapy) differ in their antibiotic dosing schedule. Sequential therapy consists of a proton pump inhibitor with amoxicillin, usually given for 5 days, followed by a proton pump inhibitor with clarithromycin and a nitroimidazole for another 5 days. Ten-day sequential therapy is superior to 7- to 10-day triple therapy and equally effective as 14-day triple therapy.[A6] Hybrid therapy starts with the same 5-day combination of a proton pump inhibitor with amoxicillin and then continues the amoxicillin for the next 5 days together with clarithromycin and metronidazole. Concomitant therapy gives these same drugs all together for 10 to 14 days. Other combinations of antibiotics are occasionally used (see Table 139-4). Concomitant therapy is the most effective, in particular when given for 14 days with a proton pump inhibitor in a dose of 40 mg twice daily.[A7]

Continuation of acid suppressive therapy after antibiotic treatment is needed only when symptoms persist, or in cases of complicated ulcer disease until eradication of *H. pylori* has been confirmed. Ascertainment of therapeutic efficacy must be delayed at least 1 month after the end of treatment to prevent false-negative results related to the organism's temporary suppression but not eradication. When repeat endoscopy is needed (e.g., a gastric ulcer requires repeated histologic examination to exclude underlying malignancy), repeat screening for *H. pylori* can be performed using the gastric biopsy specimens for histologic examination, culture, or urease testing. If no clinical indication exists for repeat endoscopy, *H. pylori* status can be determined by a carbon-13 urea breath test, stool *H. pylori* antigen, or repeated serology. Serologic determination is based on a more than 40 to 50% decrease in immunoglobulin G antibody levels in the first 6 months after treatment compared with pretreatment levels in that patient; ideally, the (frozen) pretreatment and

TABLE 139-4 OVERVIEW OF ANTIBIOTICS USED FOR *HELICOBACTER PYLORI* ERADICATION

DRUG CLASS	DRUG	TRIPLE THERAPY* DOSE	BISMUTH-BASED QUADRUPLE THERAPY† DOSE	NON-BISMUTH-BASED QUADRUPLE THERAPY‡ DOSE
Acid suppression	Proton pump inhibitor	20-40 mg bid§	20-40 mg bid§	20-40 mg bid§
Standard antimicrobials	Bismuth compound‖		2 tablets bid	
	Amoxicillin	1 g bid	1 g bid	1 g bid
	Metronidazole¶	500 mg bid	500 mg tid	500 mg bid
	Clarithromycin	500 mg bid		500 mg bid
	Tetracycline		500 mg qid	
Salvage antimicrobials	Levofloxacin	500 mg bid	500 mg bid	500 mg bid
	Rifabutin	150 mg bid		
	Furazolidone	100 mg bid	100 mg bid	
	Doxycycline		100 mg bid	100 mg bid
	Nitazoxanide		500 mg bid	500 mg bid

*Triple therapy consists of a proton pump inhibitor or bismuth compound, together with two of the listed antibiotics, usually given for 7 to 14 days.
†Bismuth-based quadruple therapy consists of a proton pump inhibitor plus the combination of a bismuth compound and two antibiotics given for 7 to 14 days.
‡Non-bismuth-based quadruple therapy consists of a proton pump inhibitor, plus three antibiotics usually given for 10 days and sometimes extended to 14 days. The three forms of non-bismuth-based quadruple therapy differ in their antibiotic dosing schedules: (1) *sequential therapy* gives amoxicillin for the first half of the course, and then metronidazole and clarithromycin for the second half; (2) *hybrid therapy* starts with amoxicillin for the first half, and then continues the second half with amoxicillin, clarithromycin, and metronidazole; (3) *concomitant therapy* combines all three antibiotics throughout the 10- to 14-day therapy. Other combinations of antibiotics are occasionally used.
§Proton pump inhibitor dose equivalent to omeprazole 20 to 40 mg bid. (See Table 138-1 for doses of other proton pump inhibitors).
‖Bismuth subsalicylate or subcitrate.
¶An alternative is tinidazole 500 mg bid.

post-treatment specimens should be examined simultaneously by the same laboratory using the same assay.

After successful *H. pylori* eradication, the risk for recurrent infection in most populations is small. In a minority of patients, ulcers recur either owing to reinfection or in the presence of another ulcerogenic factor, particularly NSAID use.

Disease Related to Nonsteroidal Anti-inflammatory Drug Use

In patients who are diagnosed with acid peptic disease while they are taking NSAIDs or aspirin, the first step is to stop such therapy. Acid suppression with a proton pump inhibitor (in doses similar to those used for *H. pylori*) leads to healing of 85% of NSAID-induced gastric ulcers and more than 90% of duodenal ulcers within 8 weeks of therapy, whereas acid suppression with a histamine-2 (H_2)-receptor blocker, equivalent to ranitidine 300 mg twice daily (see Table 138-1), heals approximately 70% of ulcers within 8 weeks. The mucosal protective drug misoprostol (200 mg four times daily) has a similar effect to the H_2 blockers. Treatment must be continued for at least 8 weeks, and maintenance therapy is needed in patients who continue to take NSAIDs. Gastric ulcers, larger lesions, and recurrent lesions heal more slowly.

Ulcer occurrence during NSAID therapy suggests a causal relationship, but patients should also be tested for *H. pylori*. In patients who are *H. pylori* positive, eradication therapy should be considered because there are no clear clinical parameters distinguishing between these etiologic factors. In patients who continue to take NSAIDs, maintenance therapy with a proton pump inhibitor (see Table 138-1) is superior to *H. pylori* eradication for the prevention of recurrent ulcer,[A8] except in patients who use aspirin, for whom *H. pylori* eradication alone may be curative.

Idiopathic Ulcer Disease

Patients with idiopathic ulcer disease despite a thorough assessment for underlying causes are treated primarily with an acid suppressant, usually a proton pump inhibitor, because they are at considerable risk for recurrent ulcer disease. After the underlying cause is identified and adequately treated, acid suppressive therapy can be withdrawn if there are no additional risk factors for ulcer disease, such as NSAID therapy or *H. pylori* infection. If the cause of the idiopathic ulceration is not clarified and there is doubt about the adequacy of the diagnostic testing for *H. pylori*, empirical eradication therapy can be considered, especially when there is histologic evidence of chronic active gastritis without further explanation. If related to unidentified *H. pylori*, gastritis should slowly disappear after successful eradication therapy.

PREVENTION

Primary Prevention

A test-and-treat strategy for *H. pylori* colonization is sometimes considered for patients with dyspeptic symptoms, but there is no specific way to prevent *H. pylori*–associated ulcer disease. By contrast, primary prevention of NSAID-associated ulcer disease is widely advocated for patients at high risk because of a prior ulcer, severe concomitant disease, use of warfarin or high-dose corticosteroids, or older age (>65 years).[10] H_2 blockers (at a dose equivalent to ranitidine 300 mg twice daily; Table 138-1) partially prevent duodenal ulcer disease during NSAID therapy but have no effect on preventing gastric ulcers unless a higher dose (equivalent to famotidine 40 mg twice daily) is given. Proton pump inhibitors (at a dose equivalent to omeprazole 20 mg once daily; Table 138-1) and misoprostol (in doses varying between 400 and 800 mg/day) partially protect against both gastric and duodenal ulcers during NSAID use. Misoprostol and proton pump inhibitors are equally effective,[A9] but adherence with therapy is lower with misoprostol owing to its side effects. Patients should be advised of the importance of adherence because less than 80% adherence to gastroprotection is associated with a more than two-fold increased risk for ulcer disease compared with those who are fully adherent. During low-dose aspirin therapy, primary prevention of ulcers is advocated for the same risk groups, using a proton pump inhibitor[A8] or an H_2-receptor antagonist.[A10]

Secondary Prevention

Secondary prevention of *H. pylori*–associated ulcer disease is mandatory and consists of successful bacterial eradication. Testing to ascertain *H. pylori* status after eradication therapy is indicated in patients with prior complicated ulcer disease or with persistent or recurrent symptoms after therapy, as well as in patients who fail to complete the therapeutic course.

Secondary prevention of NSAID-related ulcer disease is preferentially achieved by the withdrawal of NSAIDs. In patients who must continue taking NSAIDs, a change to a selective COX2 inhibitor in combination with a proton pump inhibitor at a dose equivalent to esomeprazole 20 mg twice daily is advocated, especially for patients with complicated ulcer disease.[11] This combination is associated with a lower risk for secondary peptic ulcer complications than treatment with a COX2 inhibitor alone.

Secondary prevention of recurrent ulcers in patients who use aspirin may depend on *H. pylori* status. In *H. pylori*–positive patients, *H. pylori* eradication is as effective as a proton pump inhibitor for the prevention of recurrent ulcers. In *H. pylori*–negative patients, additional acid suppressive therapy at a dose equivalent to esomeprazole 20 mg twice daily should be prescribed.[A11] Secondary prevention of idiopathic ulcer disease consists primarily of maintenance therapy with a proton pump inhibitor and treatment of the underlying condition. When there is doubt about the accuracy of the diagnostic assessment for *H. pylori*, an empirical course of eradication treatment can be considered.

Complications

Hemorrhage

Hemorrhage (Chapter 135), which is the most common complication of peptic ulcer disease, occurs in about one in six patients with ulcers over the course of their ulcer activity. Ulcers caused by NSAIDs account for a larger proportion of these hemorrhages. Peptic ulcer is thus the most common cause of nonvariceal upper gastrointestinal bleeding, accounting for 40 to

TABLE 139-5 PARAMETERS OF THE ROCKALL, BLATCHFORD AND AIMS65 SCORING SYSTEMS FOR UPPER GASTROINTESTINAL BLEEDING*

SCORING CATEGORIES	SCORING PARAMETERS	*ROCKALL SYSTEM*[†]		*BLATCHFORD SYSTEM*[‡]		*AIMS65*[§]	
		Parameter	**Score**	**Parameter**	**Score**	**Parameter**	**Score**
Age	Age (yr)	60-79	1	N/A	—	>65	1
		≥80	2				
Clinical status	Systolic blood pressure	<100	2	100-109	1	≤90	1
				90-99	2		
				<90	3		
	Pulse	>100	1	>100	1	N/A	—
	Melena	N/A	—	Present	1	N/A	—
	Syncope	N/A	—	Present	1	N/A	—
	Altered mental status	N/A	—	N/A	—	Present	1
	Comorbidities	Any major comorbidity	2	Hepatic disease	2	N/A	—
		Renal or liver failure, or disseminated malignancy	3	Cardiac failure	2		
Laboratory parameters	Blood urea, mmol/L	N/A	—	6.5-7.9	2	N/A	—
				8.0-9.9	3		
				10-24.9	4		
				>25.0	6		
	Hemoglobin, g/L	N/A	—	Men; 120-130	1	N/A	—
				Women; 100-120	1		
				Men; 100-120	3		
				Men and women; <100	6		
	INR	N/A	—	N/A	—	>1.5	1
	Albumin	N/A	—	N/A	—	<3.0 g/dL	1
Endoscopy	Endoscopic diagnosis	No focus, or Mallory-Weiss tear	0	N/A	—	N/A	—
		Upper GI malignancy	2				
		All other diagnoses	1				
	Endoscopic SRH	None/dark spot only	0	N/A	—	N/A	—
		Blood/clot/vessel	2				

*The Blatchford (Stanley AJ, Ashley D, Dalton HR, et al. Outpatient management of patients with low-risk upper-gastrointestinal haemorrhage: multicentre validation and prospective evaluation. *Lancet.* 2009;373:42-47) and AIMS65 (Saltzman JR, Tabak YP, Hyett BH, et al. A simple risk score accurately predicts in-hospital mortality, length of stay, and cost in acute upper GI bleeding. *Gastrointest Endosc.* 2011;74:1215-1224) systems are pre-endoscopy scoring systems; the Rockall system (Rockall TA, Logan RF, Devlin HB, et al. Risk assessment after acute upper gastrointestinal haemorrhage. *Gut.* 1996;38:316-321) has a pre- and post-endoscopy component. The Blatchford system is a tool to select patients for early discharge and later endoscopy during office hours. The Rockall score can help to assess the risk for rebleeding and mortality. The AIMS65 predicts mortality.

[†]Scores before and after endoscopy. Low risk defined as scores of ≤2, high risk defined as scores ≥6.

[‡]Low risk defined as score of 0.

[§]Low risk defined as score of ≤1, high risk as score ≥2.

GI = gastrointestinal; INR = international normalized ratio; N/A = not applicable; PUD = peptic ulcer disease; SRH = stigmata of recent haemorrhage.

60% of cases in most populations. Bleeding is associated with a 5 to 15% risk for rebleeding and up to a 10% risk for mortality. Hemorrhage may occur along a continuum from a serious acute event associated with hemodynamic shock and high mortality to slow or intermittent blood loss leading to chronic anemia. Approximately 80% of patients with bleeding ulcers describe a prior history of symptomatic disease, and about 20 to 30% have suffered a previous hemorrhage. Assessment of the magnitude of bleeding is of paramount importance in determining the need for transfusion and subsequent management (Table 139-5). Initial hematocrit levels may be misleading and are likely to fall because of hemodilution. Rapid bleeding is usually apparent on the basis of clinical signs (pallor, systolic blood pressure ≤100 mm Hg, pulse ≥100/minute); immediate fluid resuscitation and transfusions are indicated to prevent circulatory collapse. Mortality is particularly related to complications of the bleed, such as aspiration, and exacerbation of underlying disease, such as pulmonary, cardiovascular, renal, and hepatic disease. On rare occasions, patients may actually bleed to death, especially when a larger artery is affected, such as when an ulcer in the posterior wall of the duodenal bulb perforates the gastroduodenal artery. The stopping of such bleeding is therefore a medical emergency.[12]

Initial treatment aims at hemodynamic stabilization. Endoscopy is the mainstay of therapy and should be performed emergently or within 24 hours of presentation in high-risk cases, especially patients who are hemodynamically unstable, require transfusion, or have more severe comorbidities. Endoscopy can be performed to ascertain the origin of the bleeding and, if necessary, provide therapy to stop the bleed and reduce the risk for rebleeding.

The appearance of the ulcer determines the need for endoscopic treatment and the risk for rebleeding (Table 139-6) and mortality. "Clean base" ulcers and those with flat and pigmented spots carry a low risk for rebleeding and do not require endoscopic treatment. In contrast, ulcers with active bleeding or stigmata of recent bleeding, in particular a visible vessel or adherent clot, require treatment to stop the bleed and reduce the otherwise high risk for recurrence.

TABLE 139-6 ENDOSCOPY RESULTS IN PATIENTS WITH BLEEDING ULCERS

ENDOSCOPY RESULT	ULCER CHARACTERISTICS*	RISK FOR RECURRENT BLEEDING (%)
Active bleeding	Arterial bleeding	80-90
	Oozing bleeding	10-30
Stigmata of recent bleeding	Nonbleeding visible vessel	50-60
	Adherent clot	25-35
	Flat pigmented spot	0-8
No signs of bleeding	Clean ulcer base	0-12

*The ulcer characteristics determine the risk for recurrent bleeding during follow-up.

Endoscopic therapy may lead to a three-fold reduction in episodes of recurrent bleeding and in the need for surgical intervention, as well as a 40% reduction in mortality. [A12] Treatment modalities include injection therapy with epinephrine or a sclerosant, thermocoagulation, and mechanical pressure by means of clips. Thermocoagulation can be performed by direct contact, such as with a heater probe, or by a noncontact method, such as argon plasma coagulation. The efficacy of these methods is generally comparable, except that epinephrine injection alone is inferior to the other modalities but can be useful when combined with any of the others. [A13] If an adherent clot is found, an attempt should be made to remove it by water flushing or snaring to allow an assessment of the underlying ulcer base and the treatment of any underlying visible vessels to reduce the risk for rebleeding.[A14]

The pre-endoscopy administration of intravenous proton pump inhibitor therapy (at a dose equivalent to a bolus of 80 mg esomeprazole, followed by a continuous infusion of 8 mg/hour until endoscopy) reduces bleeding and the need for emergent endoscopic treatment, but it has no effect on the need for transfusion or the occurrence of rebleeding or death.[A15] For patients with active bleeding or stigmata of recent bleeding, endoscopic treatment should be followed by an intravenous proton pump inhibitor given as a bolus at a dose equivalent to 80 mg esomeprazole over 30 minutes, followed by a continuous infusion at a dose equivalent to esomeprazole 8 mg/hour for 72 hours, to reduce rebleeding and the need for further intervention.[A16] Other therapies, including tranexamic acid, vasopressin, somatostatin, and octreotide, should be considered experimental (Chapter 135). Second-look endoscopy is not routinely indicated but can be considered in very high-risk cases, particularly when there is doubt about the adequacy of initial visualization or treatment.[13]

About 70 to 80% of rebleeds occur within the first 3 days and generally should be managed by repeat endoscopy. If endoscopy fails to stop the bleed or prevent further rebleeding, surgery and interventional radiology are equivalent options. Surgery includes stitching of the ulcer and occlusion of the feeding artery, usually the gastroduodenal artery. Interventional radiology uses angiography to insert a coil in the culprit vessel at the site of the bleed. Single-center observational experience suggests that each of these methods is equally effective in the hands of experienced clinicians, and the choice depends on local availability and expertise.

The risk for a fatal outcome of an upper gastrointestinal hemorrhage can be estimated based on five clinical and endoscopic parameters (see Table 139-5). In several studies, mortality in patients with a bleeding peptic ulcer was less than 2% among those with a score of 2 points or less, 10% in those with 3 to 5 points, and up to 46% in those with 6 points or more. Management of patients who recover after a peptic ulcer hemorrhage is similar to the treatment of patients with uncomplicated ulcers. Eradication of *H. pylori* provides excellent protection against both recurrence and rebleeding of *H. pylori*–related ulcers. NSAID-induced ulcers are preferentially managed by the withdrawal of NSAIDs or, if this is not feasible, by the combination of a COX2 inhibitor and a proton pump inhibitor at a dose equivalent to esomeprazole 20 mg twice daily. In patients with a history of ulcer bleeding and concomitant cardiovascular disease requiring antiplatelet therapy, the combination of low-dose aspirin and a proton pump inhibitor at a dose equivalent to esomeprazole 20 mg twice daily is associated with a lower risk for complicated ulcer than is clopidogrel monotherapy.[A17] If a patient who requires antiplatelet therapy presents with a bleeding ulcer, antiplatelet therapy should be continued or restarted as soon as possible if the risk for a cardiovascular event outweighs the risk for recurrent bleeding.[A18]

Perforation

Perforation may manifest as an acute event, whereby gastric contents spill into the peritoneal cavity, or more insidiously as the ulcer slowly penetrates into surrounding tissues. Acute free perforation typically causes abrupt and severe abdominal pain associated with abdominal muscular spasm that produces board-like rigidity of the abdomen and other manifestations of peritoneal irritation. Secondary hemodynamic shock is common. The clinical diagnosis can be confirmed in approximately 80% of patients by a plain chest radiograph with the patient standing (Fig. 139-5); a CT scan can be obtained if doubt persists. Leukocytosis and elevated C-reactive protein levels develop rapidly, and mild hyperamylasemia may occur. Treatment begins by correcting hemodynamic, fluid, and electrolyte imbalances. Nasogastric suction is helpful, and prophylactic antibiotics (e.g., amoxicillin-clavulanic acid 1 g every 8 hours intravenously) are usually administered. Unless a specific contraindication exists, emergency surgery is usually indicated, although more conservative approaches are sometimes appropriate. Given the success in achieving the long-term cure of ulcer disease through the eradication of *H. pylori* and the withdrawal of NSAIDs, suturing of the perforated ulcer may be adequate, permitting the patient to avoid a more radical vagotomy with or without gastric resection.

Intractability

Intractability is a term strictly applied to an ulcer that persists even after intensive and prolonged proton pump inhibitor therapy. Symptoms may or may not be present. These rare cases may result from poor compliance with recommended treatment, surreptitious use of ulcerogenic drugs, or other diseases (e.g., Crohn disease, ischemia, infection with bacteria other than *H. pylori*, viral infection). If these issues are recognized and these diagnoses are pursued, further complications and interventions such as surgical vagotomy and pyloroplasty can almost always be avoided.

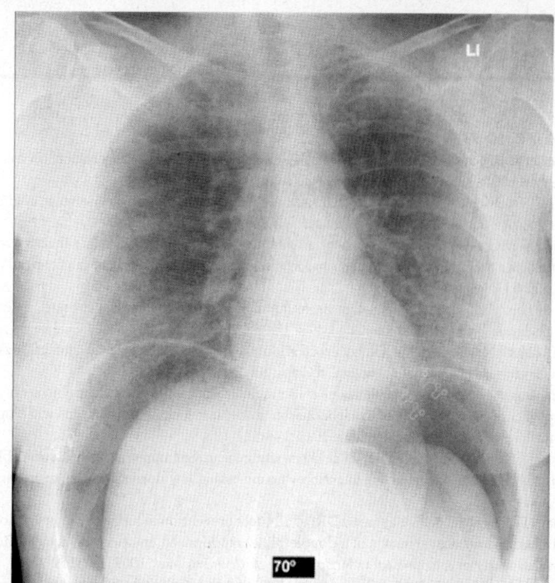

FIGURE 139-5. Plain chest radiograph in an upright patient with a perforated ulcer. The radiograph shows free air under the diaphragm.

Acid peptic disease related to alcohol or bisphosphonates should be addressed by discontinuing the precipitating agent. Treatment of Zollinger-Ellison syndrome requires high-dose proton pump inhibitors and/or surgery (Chapter 195). Those rare ulcers caused by Crohn disease (Chapter 141), vasculitis (Chapter 270), sarcoidosis (Chapter 95), polycythemia vera (Chapter 166), amyloidosis (Chapter 188), and other rare disorders should be addressed by treating the underlying condition. Stress ulcers and Cameron ulcers are treated by potent acid suppressive therapy (e.g., omeprazole 20 mg twice daily).

Stenosis

Gastric outlet obstruction is now a rare complication of ulcer disease because of the early detection and treatment of most ulcers. Most patients who develop clinically relevant gastric outlet obstruction have had an ulcer in the duodenal bulb and/or pyloric channel. Edema and inflammation play an important role, and occasionally a patient with active disease presents with symptoms of outlet obstruction as manifested by nausea, vomiting, and gastric stasis without a tight, chronic stenosis. Management therefore involves three key steps. The first is nasogastric tube aspiration and gastric lavage to clear the stomach of retained debris, followed by early endoscopy. This step facilitates an accurate diagnosis. Nasogastric suction may need to be maintained for several days if vomiting resumes when the tube is clamped. The second step consists of intense antisecretory therapy using intravenous proton pump inhibitors in a dose equivalent to a bolus of 80 mg esomeprazole over 30 minutes, followed by a continuous infusion of 8 mg/hour. Finally, the cause of the ulcer needs to be addressed, usually by eradicating *H. pylori* and withdrawing NSAIDs. If the initial treatment resolves the clinical situation and the patient can resume eating, it is often not necessary to undertake further treatment of the outlet stenosis; however, tight, fibrous scarring may require endoscopic balloon dilation or surgery.

PROGNOSIS

Most peptic ulcers heal spontaneously within weeks to months. However, if the underlying condition is not adequately treated, a large proportion of ulcers recur. Both initial and recurrent ulcers can give rise to complications. The four major complications are intractability, perforation, hemorrhage, and stenosis. Each distinct situation requires specific management approaches. Patients with complicated ulcer disease are at particular risk for recurrent complications and need careful assessment for secondary prevention. In patients who take long-term acid suppressive therapy with either H_2 antagonists or proton pump inhibitors, the risk for vitamin B_{12} deficiency (Chapters 164 and 218) is increased about two-fold.[14]

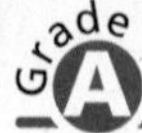

Grade A References

A1. Moayyedi P, Soo S, Deeks J, et al. Eradication of Helicobacter pylori for non-ulcer dyspepsia. *Cochrane Database Syst Rev*. 2006;2:CD002096.

A2. Mazzoleni LE, Sander GB, Francesconi CF, et al. Helicobacter pylori eradication in functional dyspepsia: HEROES trial. *Arch Intern Med*. 2011;171:1929-1936.

A3. Ford AC, Delaney BC, Forman D, et al. Eradication therapy for peptic ulcer disease in Helicobacter pylori positive patients. *Cochrane Database Syst Rev*. 2006;2:CD003840.

A4. Peedikayil MC, Alsohaibani FI, Alkhenizan AH. Levofloxacin-based first-line therapy versus standard first-line therapy for Helicobacter pylori eradication: meta-analysis of randomized controlled trials. *PLoS ONE*. 2014;9:e85620.

A5. Yuan Y, Ford AC, Khan KJ, et al. Optimum duration of regimens for Helicobacter pylori eradication. *Cochrane Database Syst Rev*. 2013;12:CD008337.

A6. Gatta L, Vakil N, Vaira D, et al. Global eradication rates for Helicobacter pylori infection: systematic review and meta-analysis of sequential therapy. *BMJ*. 2013;347:f4587.

A7. Molina-Infante J, Romano M, Fernandez-Bermejo M, et al. Optimized nonbismuth quadruple therapies cure most patients with Helicobacter pylori infection in populations with high rates of antibiotic resistance. *Gastroenterology*. 2013;145:121-128.

A8. Chan FK, Chung SC, Suen BY, et al. Preventing recurrent upper gastrointestinal bleeding in patients with Helicobacter pylori infection who are taking low-dose aspirin or naproxen. *N Engl J Med*. 2001;344:967-973.

A9. Graham DY, Agrawal NM, Campbell DR, et al. Ulcer prevention in long-term users of nonsteroidal anti-inflammatory drugs: results of a double-blind, randomized, multicenter, active- and placebo-controlled study of misoprostol vs lansoprazole. *Arch Intern Med*. 2002;162:169-175.

A10. Taha AS, McCloskey C, Prasad R, et al. Famotidine for the prevention of peptic ulcers and oesophagitis in patients taking low-dose aspirin (FAMOUS): a phase III, randomised, double-blind, placebo-controlled trial. *Lancet*. 2009;374:119-125.

A11. Chan FK, Wong VW, Suen BY, et al. Combination of a cyclo-oxygenase-2 inhibitor and a proton-pump inhibitor for prevention of recurrent ulcer bleeding in patients at very high risk: a double-blind, randomised trial. *Lancet*. 2007;369:1621-1626.

A12. Barkun AN, Martel M, Toubouti Y, et al. Endoscopic hemostasis in peptic ulcer bleeding for patients with high-risk lesions: a series of meta-analyses. *Gastrointest Endosc*. 2009;69:786-799.

A13. Laine L, McQuaid KR. Endoscopic therapy for bleeding ulcers: an evidence-based approach based on meta-analyses of randomized controlled trials. *Clin Gastroenterol Hepatol*. 2009;7:33-47.

A14. Kahi CJ, Jensen DM, Sung JJ, et al. Endoscopic therapy versus medical therapy for bleeding peptic ulcer with adherent clot: a meta-analysis. *Gastroenterology*. 2005;129:855-862.

A15. Sreedharan A, Martin J, Leontiadis GI, et al. Proton pump inhibitor treatment initiated prior to endoscopic diagnosis in upper gastrointestinal bleeding. *Cochrane Database Syst Rev*. 2010;7:CD005415.

A16. Sung JJ, Barkun A, Kuipers EJ, et al. Intravenous esomeprazole for prevention of recurrent peptic ulcer bleeding: a randomized trial. *Ann Intern Med*. 2009;150:455-464.

A17. Chan FK, Ching JY, Hung LC, et al. Clopidogrel versus aspirin and esomeprazole to prevent recurrent ulcer bleeding. *N Engl J Med*. 2005;352:238-244.

A18. Sung JJ, Lau JY, Ching JY, et al. Continuation of low-dose aspirin therapy in peptic ulcer bleeding: a randomized trial. *Ann Intern Med*. 2010;152:1-9.

GENERAL REFERENCES

For the General References and other additional features, please visit Expert Consult at https://expertconsult.inkling.com.

140

APPROACH TO THE PATIENT WITH DIARRHEA AND MALABSORPTION

CAROL E. SEMRAD

DEFINITIONS

Normal stool frequency ranges from three times per week to three times per day. As a symptom, diarrhea can be described as a decrease in stool consistency (increased fluidity), stools that cause urgency or abdominal discomfort, or an increase in the frequency of stool. Consistency is defined as the ratio of fecal water to the water-holding capacity of fecal insoluble solids, which are composed of bacterial mass and dietary fiber. Because it is difficult to measure stool consistency and because stool is predominantly (60 to 85%) water, stool weight becomes a reasonable surrogate of consistency.

As a sign, diarrhea is defined by the weight or volume of stool measured over a 24- to 72-hour period. Daily stool weights of children and adults are less than 200 g, and greater stool weights are an objective definition of diarrhea; however, this definition misses 20% of diarrheal symptoms in patients who have loose stools that are less than this daily weight.

Acute diarrheas persist for less than 2 to 3 weeks or, rarely, 6 to 8 weeks. The most common cause of acute diarrhea is infection. Chronic diarrheal conditions persist for at least 4 weeks and, more typically, 6 to 8 weeks or longer. The four mechanisms of diarrhea are osmotic, secretory, exudative, and altered motility. Because many diarrheal diseases are due to more than one of these mechanisms, it is clinically useful to categorize diarrhea as malabsorptive (fatty), watery, and inflammatory.

EPIDEMIOLOGY

Diarrhea is the second leading cause of mortality worldwide and is particularly problematic for elderly people and for children younger than 5 years of age in developing nations. Infectious diarrheal conditions cause approximately 750,000 worldwide childhood deaths annually, despite the improved use of oral rehydration solutions, zinc, and vitamin A supplements. Rotavirus infection (Chapter 380) is the most common cause of fatal childhood diarrhea, but the introduction of the oral monovalent rotavirus vaccine has significantly decreased its mortality rate in both developing and developed nations.

In the United States, norovirus has surpassed rotavirus as the leading cause of gastroenteritis requiring medical care.[1] Approximately 48 million Americans suffer from food-borne illness each year, including around 130,000 annual hospitalizations and 3000 deaths, most in elderly people. The major pathogens that cause diarrhea result in an estimated $14 to 16 billion in annual health care costs and days lost from work.

PATHOBIOLOGY

Fluid and Electrolyte Transport

Whether a hypotonic meal, such as a steak and water, or a hypertonic meal, such as milk and a doughnut, is consumed, the volume of the meal is augmented by gastric, pancreatic, biliary, and duodenal secretions. The permeable duodenum then renders the meal approximately isotonic with an electrolyte content similar to that of plasma by the time it reaches the proximal jejunum. As the intestinal slurry moves toward the colon, the Na^+ concentration in the luminal fluid remains constant, but Cl^- is reduced to 60 to 70 mmol/L, and bicarbonate (HCO_3^-) is increased to a similar concentration as the result of Cl^- and HCO_3^- transport mechanisms in the enterocyte and HCO_3^- secretion in the ileum (E-Fig. 140-1A and B). In the colon, K^{2+} is secreted, and the Na^+ transport mechanism of the colonocyte, together with the low epithelial permeability, extracts Na^+ and fluid from the stool. As a result, the Na^+ content of stool decreases to 30 to 40 mmol/L; K^{2+} increases from 5 to 10 mmol/L in the small bowel to 75 to 90 mmol/L; and poorly absorbed divalent cations, such as Mg^{2++} and Ca^{2++}, are concentrated in stool to values of 5 to 100 mmol/L. The anion concentrations in the colon change drastically because bacterial degradation of carbohydrate (i.e., unabsorbed starches, sugars, and fiber) creates short-chain fatty acids that attain concentrations of 80 to 180 mmol/L; at colonic pH, organic anions, such as acetate, propionate, and butyrate, are present. In the setting of carbohydrate malabsorption, the generation of high concentrations of these short-chain fatty acids may decrease stool pH to 4 or lower. The osmolality of the stool is approximately that of plasma (280 to 300 mOsm/kg H_2O) when it is passed.

At the cellular level, Na^{++} transport by the epithelium from lumen to blood (by Na^{++}-coupled sugar and amino acid transport in the small intestine, by Na^{++}/H^{++} exchange proteins in the small intestine and proximal colon, and by aldosterone-regulated $^{+}Na^{++}$ channels in the distal colon) creates a favorable osmotic gradient for absorption (see E-Fig. 140-1A and C). Chloride transport by the epithelium from blood to lumen (by cystic fibrosis transmembrane conductance regulator [CFTR] and the calcium-activated chloride channel in the small intestine and colon) creates an osmotic gradient for secretion (see E-Fig. 140-1B). Normally, the intestine is in a net absorptive state, regulated by extrinsic adrenergic nerves and proabsorptive neuropeptides and hormones (see E-Fig. 140-1D). Stimulation of secretion by neurotransmitters, hormones, and inflammatory mediators (Table 140-1) can offset this balance. A heterozygous missense mutation (c.2519G→T) in GUCY2C on chromosome 12 causes familial diarrhea by increasing GC-C signaling.

Diarrhea is due primarily to alterations of intestinal fluid and electrolyte transport and less to smooth muscle function. Each 24 hours, 8 to 10 L of fluid enters the duodenum. The diet supplies 2 L of this fluid; the remainder comes from salivary, gastric, hepatic, pancreatic, and intestinal secretions. The small intestine normally absorbs 8 to 9 L (80%) of this fluid and presents 1.5 L to the colon for absorption. Of the remaining fluid, the colon absorbs all but approximately 100 mL. Diarrhea can result from increased secretion by the small intestine or the colon if the maximal daily absorptive capacity of the colon (4 L) is exceeded. Alternatively, if the colon is diseased so that it cannot absorb even the 1.5 L normally presented to it by the small intestine, diarrhea results.

Watery diarrheas may be due to osmotic, secretory, or inflammatory mechanisms. With ingestion of a poorly absorbed (e.g., Mg^{2++}) or unabsorbable (polyethylene glycol, lactulose or, in lactase-deficient individuals, lactose) solute, the osmotic force of the solute pulls water and secondarily sodium and chloride ions into the intestinal lumen. A considerable proportion of the osmolality of stool results from the nonabsorbed solute. This gap between stool osmolality and the sum of the electrolytes in the stool causes osmotic diarrhea.

TABLE 140-1 STIMULI OF INTESTINAL SECRETION

AGENT	INTRACELLULAR MEDIATOR	RELATED DIARRHEAL ILLNESS
Cholera, *E. coli* heat labile toxin, *Salmonella, Yersinia*	cAMP	Travelers, endemic
E. coli heat stable toxin	cGMP	
Rotatoxin (NSP4)	?	Viral gastroenteritis
Serotonin, PAF	Ca	Inflammatory, allergic
PG, leukotrienes	cAMP, Ca	Invasive enteric bacteria* inflammatory bowel diseases
PG	cAMP	Villous adenoma
Histamine	Ca	Intestinal allergies, mastocytosis, scombroid poisoning
VIP	cAMP	VIPoma, ganglioneuromas
5-HT, substance P, bradykinin	Ca	Malignant carcinoid
Calcitonin	?	Medullary carcinoma thyroid
Acetylcholine	Ca	Insecticides, nerve gas poisoning, cholinergic drugs
Ricinoleic acid	cAMP, Ca	Laxative abuse†
Caffeine	cAMP	Coffee, sodas, tea

5-HT = 5-hydroxytryptamine; Ca = calcium; cAMP = cyclic adenosine monophosphate; cGMP = cyclic guanosine monophosphate; PAF = platelet-activating factor; PG = prostaglandin; VIP = vasoactive intestinal peptide.
**Shigella* sp, *Clostridium difficile*, enteroinvasive, *E. coli, Vibrio parahaemolyticus, Clostridium perfringens*.
†Also phenolphthalein, anthraquinone, bisacodyl, dioctyl sodium sulosuccinate, and senna.

Active chloride secretion or inhibited sodium absorption, which also creates an osmotic gradient favorable for the movement of fluids from blood to lumen, explains the pathophysiology of the secretory diarrheas. Agents that increase enterocyte cyclic adenosine monophosphate (cAMP) (e.g., cholera toxin, prostaglandins), cyclic guanosine monophosphate (cGMP) (e.g., *Escherichia coli* stable toxin), or intracellular ionized calcium (Ca^{2++}) (e.g., acetylcholine) (see Table 140-1) inhibit non-nutrient Na^{++} absorption and stimulate Cl^- secretion (see Table 140-1 and E-Fig. 140-1B and D).

Inflammatory diarrheas, which may be watery or bloody, are characterized by enterocyte damage, villus atrophy, and crypt hyperplasia. The damaged enterocyte membrane of the small intestine has decreased disaccharidase and peptide hydrolase activity, reduced or absent Na^{++}-coupled sugar or amino acid transport mechanisms, and reduced or absent sodium chloride absorptive transporters. Conversely, the hyperplastic crypt cells maintain their ability to secrete Cl^- (and perhaps HCO_3^-). If the inflammation is severe, immune-mediated vascular damage or ulceration allows blood, pus, and protein to leak (exudate) from capillaries and lymphatics and contribute to the diarrhea. Activation of lymphocytes, phagocytes, and fibroblasts releases various inflammatory mediators that induce intestinal chloride secretion (see E-Fig. 140-1D). Interleukin-1 (IL-1) and tumor necrosis factor, which also are released into the blood, cause fever, anorexia, and malaise.

ACUTE DIARRHEA

CLINICAL MANIFESTATIONS

Approximately 80% of acute diarrheas are due to infections with viruses, bacteria, and parasites. The remainder is due to medications that have an osmotic force, stimulate intestinal fluid secretion, damage the intestinal epithelium, or contain poorly or nonabsorbable sugars (e.g., sorbitol), or less commonly fecal impaction, pelvic inflammation (e.g., acute appendicitis [Chapter 142]), or intestinal ischemia (Chapter 143).

Food-Borne and Water-Borne Infectious Diarrhea

Most infectious diarrheas are acquired through fecal-oral transmission from water, food, or person-to-person contact (Table 140-2). Patients with infectious diarrhea often complain of nausea, vomiting, and abdominal cramps that are associated with watery, malabsorptive, or bloody diarrhea and fever (dysentery) (Chapters 302 through 312, 336, 337, 350 to 352, 356, 357, 379, and 380). As documented using polymerase chain reaction methods of diagnosis, most outbreaks of nonbacterial acute gastroenteritis in the United States and other countries are caused by noroviruses (Norwalk agent; Chapter 380). Rotavirus (Chapter 380) predominantly causes diarrhea in infants, usually in the winter months, but also may cause nonseasonal acute diarrhea in adults, particularly in elderly people. Mechanisms for diarrhea

TABLE 140-2 EPIDEMIOLOGY OF ACUTE INFECTIOUS DIARRHEA AND INFECTIOUS FOOD-BORNE ILLNESS

VEHICLE	CLASSIC PATHOGENS
Water (including foods washed in such water)	*Vibrio cholerae*, norovirus (Norwalk agent), *Giardia, Cryptosporidium*
Food	
Poultry	*Salmonella, Campylobacter, Shigella* sp
Beef, unpasteurized fruit juice	Enterohemorrhagic *Escherichia coli*
Pork	Tapeworm
Seafood and shellfish (including raw sushi and gefilte fish)	*V. cholerae, Vibrio parahaemolyticus*, and *Vibrio vulnificus; Salmonella* and *Shigella* sp; hepatitis A and B viruses; tapeworm; anisakiasis
Cheese, milk	*Listeria* sp
Eggs	*Salmonella* sp
Mayonnaise-containing foods and cream pies	Staphylococcal and clostridial food poisonings
Fried rice	*Bacillus cereus*
Fresh berries	*Cyclospora* sp
Canned vegetables or fruits	*Clostridium* sp
Sprouts	Enterohemorrhagic *E. coli, Salmonella* sp
Animal-to-person (pets and livestock) contact	*Salmonella, Campylobacter, Cryptosporidium*, enterohemorrhagic *E. coli*, and *Giardia* sp
Person-to-person (including sexual) contact	All enteric bacteria, viruses, and parasites
Daycare center	*Shigella, Campylobacter, Cryptosporidium*, and *Giardia* sp; viruses; *Clostridium difficile*
Hospitalization, antibiotics, or chemotherapy	*C. difficile*
Swimming pool	*Giardia* and *Cryptosporidium* sp
Foreign travel	*E. coli* of various types; *Salmonella, Shigella, Campylobacter, Giardia*, and *Cryptosporidium* sp; *Entamoeba histolytica*

Modified from Powell DW. Approach to the patient with diarrhea. In: Yamada T, Alpers DH, Owyang C, et al, eds. *Textbook of Gastroenterology*, 3rd ed. Philadelphia: Lippincott-Raven; 1999.

include decreased fluid absorption due to destruction of villus enterocytes and stimulation of fluid secretion by NSP4 rotatoxin and viral activation of the enteric nervous system. Ebola virus (*Filoviridae*) infects endothelial cells, macrophages, and dendritic cells. The mechanism for the massive watery diarrhea is not known (Chapter 381).

Food-borne bacterial diseases in the United States are primarily due to *Salmonella* (Chapter 308), *Campylobacter jejuni* (Chapter 303), and *E. coli* O157:H7 (Chapter 304), and less commonly *Shigella* (Chapter 309). The incidence of *Vibrio* infection is increasing owing to the consumption of raw shellfish. Outbreaks of *E. coli* O157:H7 have been associated with petting zoos, uncooked ground beef, and green leafy vegetables. These bacteria most often invade the distal small bowel and colon, where they multiply intracellularly and damage the epithelium. Diarrhea is due to the stimulation of intestinal secretion by inflammatory mediators, decreased absorption across the damaged epithelium, and exudation of protein into the lumen. *Shigella* species and enterohemorrhagic *E. coli* produce a similar toxin, the "Shiga toxin," which is cytotoxic to intestinal epithelial cells and causes inflammation, cell damage, and diarrhea with blood and pus.

Outbreaks of *Cryptosporidium* (Chapter 350) have been reported in water parks. This parasite causes diarrhea by adhering and fusing to the epithelial cell membrane in the small bowel, thereby causing cell damage. Organisms that are specific for seafood include *Vibrio parahaemolyticus* (Chapter 302), which causes either watery or bloody diarrhea, and *Vibrio vulnificus,* which causes watery diarrhea and, especially in patients with liver disease, a fatal septicemia. Ingestion of meat contaminated by anthrax (Chapter 294) causes fever, diffuse abdominal pain, and bloody stool or vomitus. Anthrax invades the intestinal mucosa; the organism, or anthrax toxin, causes inflammation, ulceration, and necrosis.

In addition to enteric infections, certain systemic infections (e.g., viral hepatitis [Chapter 148], listeriosis [Chapter 293], legionellosis [Chapter 314]), mycoplasma, and emerging infections (e.g., Hanta virus [Chapter 381], severe acute respiratory syndrome [SARS, Chapter 366], avian influenza [Chapter 364]) may cause or manifest with substantial diarrhea.

Environmental and Food Poisonings

Food poisoning refers to the accumulation of toxin in food owing to the growth of toxin-producing organisms, most commonly *Staphylococcus aureus* (Chapter 288), *Bacillus cereus, Clostridium perfringens* (Chapter 296), and *Clostridium botulinum* (Chapter 296). Diarrhea is usually of rapid onset, as early as 4 hours after ingestion, and is often associated with vomiting. Natural toxins also are responsible for mushroom (*Amanita*) poisoning (Chapter 110), which can also cause acute liver and kidney failure.

Environmental poisonings may be caused by heavy metals (arsenic from rat poison, gold, lead, mercury) that impair cell energy production. Arsenic (Chapter 22) also induces cardiovascular collapse at high doses. Insecticide (organophosphates and carbamates) poisoning occurs most commonly in field workers or from the ingestion of contaminated herbs or teas (Chapter 110); diarrhea, excessive saliva, and pulmonary secretions are caused by acetylcholine-stimulated chloride secretion in intestine and other epithelia. Patients often have associated vomiting and abdominal cramps.

Seafood is a common source of food poisoning, particularly fin fish and bivalve shellfish. Most of these toxins cause varying combinations of gastrointestinal (nausea, vomiting, diarrhea) and neurologic symptoms (tingling and burning around the mouth, facial flushing, sweating, headache, palpitations, and dizziness) within hours of seafood ingestion (Chapter 112). Similar symptoms are reported in patients with scombroid poisoning, which is caused by ingestion of decaying flesh of blood fish (tuna, mahi-mahi, marlin, or mackerel) that release large amounts of histamine (Chapter 112).

Marine dinoflagellates (algae) produce toxins that can cause paralytic shellfish poisoning, diarrhetic shellfish poisoning, and ciguatera (Chapter 112). Sporadic outbreaks of diarrhetic shellfish poisoning "red tides" occur when bivalve mollusks ingest dinoflagellates that produce saxitoxins (voltage-sensitive sodium-channel blocker) and okadaic acid (a lipid-soluble toxin that inhibits serine and threonine protein phosphatases 1 and 2A). Ingestion of contaminated mollusks by humans results in diarrhea and neurologic symptoms. Saxitoxins cause predominantly neurologic symptoms (paralytic, neurotoxic, or amnestic shellfish poisonings) and okadaic acid gastrointestinal symptoms (diarrhetic shellfish poisoning).

Food-chain passage of another dinoflagellate species (*Gambierdiscus toxicus*) to fin fish (mackerel, amberjack, snapper, grouper, or barracuda) results in the accumulation of ciguatoxin (Chapter 112) that causes a seafood poisoning called ciguatera. Ciguatoxin activates voltage-sensitive sodium channels and causes neurologic and gastrointestinal symptoms. Fish from the Albemarle-Pamlico estuary (eastern United States) ingest toxic dinoflagellates that cause *Pfiesteria piscicida* poisoning. The dinoflagellate toxins cause nausea, vomiting, abdominal pain, diarrhea, and neurologic symptoms such as fatigue, myalgias, pruritus, circumoral paresthesias, reversal of hot and cold sensation, psychiatric abnormalities, and memory loss. The neurologic symptoms may persist for months to years. Puffer fish poisoning by tetrodotoxin, a voltage-sensitive sodium-channel blocker produced by the fish, causes neurologic symptoms, respiratory paralysis, and death.

Traveler's Diarrhea

North American travelers to developing countries and travelers on airplanes and cruise ships are at high risk for acute infectious diarrhea. Common causes of traveler's diarrhea (Chapter 286) include enterotoxic or enteroaggregative *E. coli, Shigella,* giardiasis, and norovirus.[2,3] *E. coli* heat-stable toxin binds to guanylate cyclase in the enterocyte brush-border membrane, where it results in elevation of intracellular cGMP. *E. coli* heat-labile toxin, similar to cholera toxin, binds to the monosialoganglioside GM_1 in the brush-border membrane, thereby resulting in the activation of adenylate cyclase and the elevation of intracellular cAMP. cAMP and cGMP stimulate intestinal chloride secretion and inhibit the nutrient-independent absorption of sodium and chloride. Sodium-glucose absorption is not affected, hence the basis for oral rehydration therapy. Cholera toxin permanently binds to adenylate cyclase until the natural turnover of the intestinal epithelium in 5 to 7 days, thereby resulting in persistent secretion and severe diarrhea. DNA sequencing to detect genome sequences of *Vibrio* cholera isolates, suggest human introduction as the cause of recent outbreaks. Of the annual average of six cases of cholera reported in the United States, most are travel associated.

Antibiotic-Associated Diarrheas

Antibiotics are a common cause of hospital-acquired diarrheas that occur in approximately 20% of patients receiving broad-spectrum antibiotics; approximately 30% of these diarrheas are due to *Clostridium difficile* (Chapter 296). Strains that produce increased levels of toxins A and B and a binary toxin have emerged. These strains are associated with an increase in the incidence and severity of *C. difficile* infections, including fulminant *C. difficile* colitis that can lead to colectomy or even death. The A and B toxins produced by *C. difficile* can cause diarrhea. In animal models, IL-8, substance P, and leukotriene B_4 were found to mediate toxin A–stimulated intestinal fluid secretion. *C. difficile* can cause severe diarrhea, pseudomembranous colitis, or toxic megacolon.

Nosocomial Hospital Diarrhea

Diarrhea is the most common nosocomial illness among hospitalized patients and residents in long-term care facilities. Common causes include antibiotic-associated diarrhea, *C. difficile* infection, medications, fecal impaction, tube feeding, and underlying illness. Magnesium-containing laxatives, antacids, and lactulose cause osmotic diarrheas. Bisacodyl laxatives cause secretory diarrhea. Liquid formulations of medications cause diarrhea (elixir diarrhea) because of the high content of sorbitol or other nonabsorbable sugars (e.g., mannitol) used to sweeten the elixir; patients prescribed liquid medications through feeding tubes may receive more than 20 g of sorbitol daily. An important but poorly understood cause of diarrhea is enteral (tube) feeding (Chapter 216), particularly in critically ill patients, who often develop diarrhea. Dysmotility, increased intestinal permeability, and low sodium content in enteral formulas may be contributing factors.

Patients in mental health institutions and nursing homes have a high incidence of nosocomial infectious diarrhea (e.g., *C. difficile* and less commonly *Shigella, Salmonella,* hemorrhagic *E. coli, Giardia, Entamoeba histolytica*). Infectious diarrhea, 50% or more of which is caused by *C. difficile,* is also common in acute-care hospitals. Severe *C. difficile* infection has also been reported among peripartum women. If outside foods are not brought to hospitalized patients, the likelihood of a nosocomial infection caused by *Salmonella* or *Shigella* is extremely rare. Immunosuppressed patients are also susceptible to nosocomial viral infections (rotavirus, norovirus, adenovirus, and coxsackievirus).

Cancer Treatment and Medication-Related Diarrhea

Abdominal or whole body radiation virtually always causes an increased frequency of bowel movements that are often watery. Cancer chemotherapy with amsacrine, azacitidine, cytarabine, dactinomycin, daunorubicin, doxorubicin, floxuridine, 5-fluorouracil, 6-mercaptopurine, methotrexate, plicamycin, IL-2, and resveratrol may cause mild to moderate diarrhea. Irinotecan (CPT-11) or oxaliplatin and the combination of 5-fluorouracil plus leucovorin are frequent causes of severe watery diarrhea.

Olmesartan, an angiotensin II receptor antagonist (ARB), causes severe diarrhea as a result of a sprue-like enteropathy. Angiotensin-converting enzyme (ACE) inhibitors may cause abdominal pain and diarrhea resulting from visceral angioedema. Colchicine, neomycin, methotrexate, and *para*-aminosalicylic acid damage the enterocyte membrane. Cholestyramine, colestipol, and colesevelam bind bile salts and can result in malabsorptive diarrhea, especially in patients who have had an ileal resection. Gold therapy causes intestinal inflammation and diarrhea.

Daycare Diarrhea

More than 7 million children in the United States attend daycare, where diarrhea is extremely common, and secondary infection of family members occurs in 10 to 20% of cases. Most outbreaks of diarrhea are due to rotavirus or norovirus; less common causes are *Shigella* (Chapter 309), *Giardia* (Chapter 351), and *Cryptosporidium* (Chapter 350).

Runner's Diarrhea

Diarrhea occurs in 10 to 25% of individuals who exercise vigorously, especially women marathon runners and triathletes. Some athletes have associated abdominal cramps, urgency, nausea, or vomiting. The pathophysiology of runner's diarrhea is unknown. Release of intestinal secretogogues, especially prostaglandins, hormones, or ischemia, may be involved.

Diagnosis

Acute watery diarrhea may be due to infections, food toxins, or medications, or the acute diarrhea may signal the onset of a chronic disease (Fig. 140-1; see Tables 140-1 and 140-2) (Chapters 302 through 312, 336, 337, 351, 352, 356, 357, 379, and 380). The diagnostic approach in patients with fever and watery or bloody diarrhea should focus on stool cultures for *Campylobacter, Salmonella,* and *Shigella* sp. Routine stool culture is not indicated when diarrhea occurs after 3 to 5 days of hospitalization, except in patients with neutropenia, human immunodeficiency virus (HIV) infection, or signs of enteric infection. In patients with a history of recent antibiotic use, hospitalization, or peripartum, stools for *C. difficile* toxin should be obtained. Organisms that cause diarrhea but are not routinely tested by clinical microbiology laboratories include *Yersinia, Plesiomonas,* enterohemorrhagic *E. coli* serotype O157:H7, *Aeromonas, Cyclospora,* microsporidia, and noncholera *Vibrio.* Parasites such as *Giardia, Cryptosporidium,* and *Strongyloides* can be difficult to detect in stool but may be diagnosed by stool antigen testing or intestinal biopsy. Despite all testing techniques available, 20 to 40% of acute infectious diarrheas remain undiagnosed.

TREATMENT Rx

Goals for the treatment of diarrhea include fluid replacement, antidiarrheal agents, nutritional support, and antimicrobial therapy when indicated.[4] Because death in patients with acute diarrhea is caused by dehydration, the first task is to assess the degree of dehydration and to replace fluid and electrolyte deficits.

Fluid Replacement

Severely dehydrated patients should be treated with intravenous Ringer lactate or saline solution, with additional potassium and bicarbonate as needed. Oral rehydration solutions, which are used extensively to replace diarrheal fluid and electrolyte losses, are effective because they contain sodium, sugars, and, often, amino acids that use nutrient-dependent sodium uptake transporters. In alert patients with mild to moderate dehydration, oral rehydration solution is equally effective as intravenous hydration in repairing fluid and electrolyte losses. Oral rehydration solutions can be given to infants and children in volumes of 50 to 100 mL/kg over 4 to 6 hours; adults may need to drink 1000 mL/hour. Reduced-osmolarity solutions (Na^{++} 75 mmol/L, osmolarity 245 mmol/L versus Na^{++} 90 mmol/L, osmolarity 311 mmol/L in standard solutions) are better tolerated and effective in noncholera diarrhea but may cause hyponatremia in patients with high-volume diarrhea, particularly children.[5] Glucose-based solutions, although effective in rehydrating the patient, may worsen the diarrhea. In contrast to glucose-based solutions, polymeric rice-based solutions decrease diarrhea in cholera victims; rice is digested to many glucose monomers that aid in the absorption of intestinal secretions. These solutions may not decrease stool output in acute diarrhea, but they will effectively rehydrate the patient despite continued diarrhea. After rehydration has been accomplished, oral rehydration solutions are given at rates equaling stool loss plus insensible losses until the diarrhea ceases.

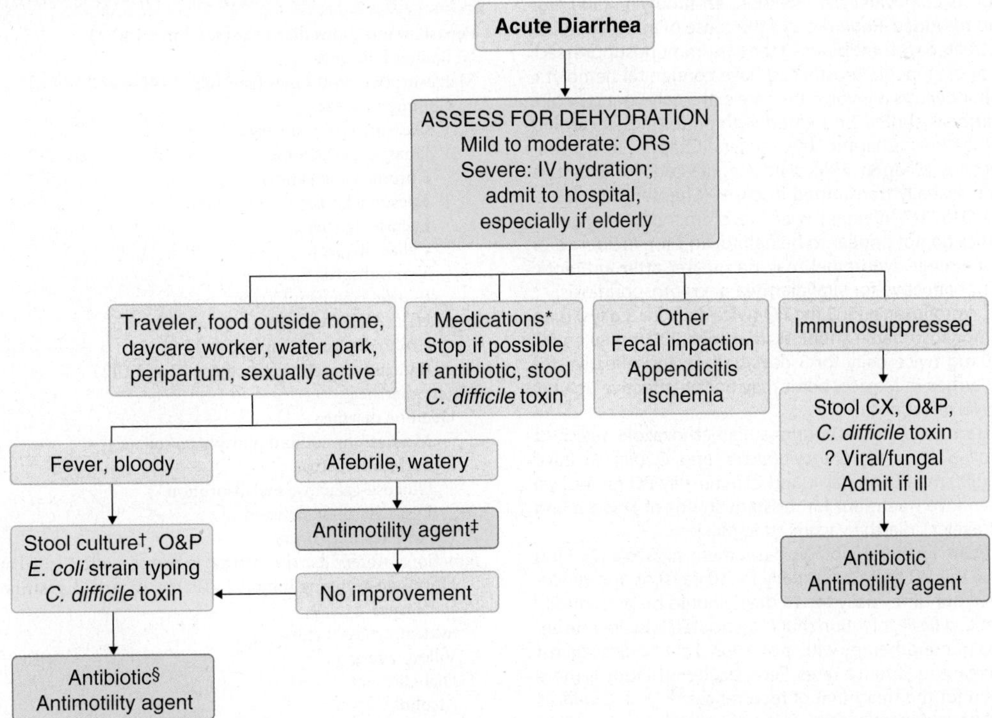

FIGURE 140-1. Approach to the diagnosis of acute diarrhea. *More than 700 medications cause diarrhea, including furosemide, caffeine, protease inhibitors, thyroid preparations, metformin, mycophenolate mofetil, sirolimus, cholinergic drugs, colchicine, theophylline, selective serotonin reuptake inhibitors, proton pump inhibitors, histamine-2 blockers, 5-ASA derivatives, angiotensin-converting enzyme inhibitors, bisacodyl, senna, aloe, anthraquinones, and magnesium- or phosphorus-containing medications. †Specifically request culture for *Yersinia, Plesiomonas,* enterohemorrhagic *Escherichia coli* serotype O157:H7, and *Aeromonas* if suspected. ‡If high suspicion for *Clostridium difficile* or invasive bacterial infection, wait for stool culture and toxin studies before starting. Racecadotril has antisecretory effects without paralyzing intestinal motility and can be used if available. §Not recommended for patients with bloody diarrhea due to *E. coli* O157:H7. CX = culture; IV therapy = intravenous rehydration; O&P = ova and parasites; ORS = oral rehydration solution.

Reducing Diarrhea

Bismuth subsalicylate (Pepto-Bismol, 525 mg orally [PO] every 30 minutes to 1 hour for five doses, may repeat on day 2) is safe and efficacious in bacterial infectious diarrheas. Opiates and anticholinergic drugs are not recommended for invasive bacterial infectious diarrheas because these drugs paralyze intestinal motility and predispose to increased colonization, invasion, and prolonged excretion of infectious organisms. The opiate loperamide is safe in acute or traveler's diarrhea, provided that it is not given to patients with dysentery (high fever, with blood or pus in the stool), and especially when administered concomitantly with effective antibiotics. A combination of loperamide (2 mg PO four times daily) plus simethicone (125 mg PO four times daily) may reduce the abdominal cramps and duration of traveler's diarrhea. Racecadotril (100 mg PO three times daily in adults, 1.5 mg/kg of body weight PO three times daily in children), an intestinal enkephalinase inhibitor that is antisecretory but does not paralyze intestinal motility, is effective in the treatment of acute diarrhea in children and adults. The diarrhea associated with enteral nutrition (Chapter 216) often can be managed with pectin (4 g/kg body weight daily) or, if there are no contraindications, with loperamide (2 mg PO four times daily for 3 to 7 days, maximal dose 16 mg daily), and diarrhea is not a reason to stop tube feeding unless stool volumes exceed 1 L/day.

Anxiolytics (e.g., diazepam 2 mg PO two to four times daily) and antiemetics (e.g., promethazine 12.5 to 25 mg PO once or twice daily) that decrease sensory perception may make symptoms more tolerable and are safe. Some foods or food-derived substances (green bananas, pectins [amylase-resistant starch], zinc) lessen the amount or duration of diarrhea in children. Unabsorbed amylase-resistant starches are metabolized in the colon to short-chain fatty acids that enhance fluid absorption. Zinc supplementation (20 mg of elemental zinc PO once daily) is effective in preventing recurrences of diarrhea in malnourished children; copper deficiency is a potential complication of prolonged zinc therapy.

Probiotics may be of benefit in children with acute diarrhea, predominantly that caused by rotavirus infection. *Lactobacillus* GG (10^{10} colony-forming units [CFU]/250 mL/day until diarrhea stops) added to an oral rehydration solution decreases the duration of diarrhea.

Antibiotics

While the clinician is awaiting stool culture results to guide specific therapy (Chapter 287), the fluoroquinolones (e.g., ciprofloxacin, 500 mg PO twice daily for 1 to 3 days, or levofloxacin, 500 mg PO daily for 1 to 3 days) are the treatment of choice when antibiotics are indicated (see Fig. 140-1). Trimethoprim-sulfamethoxazole (1 double-strength tablet PO twice daily for 5 days or 2 single-strength tablets PO twice a day for 5 days) is second-line therapy. If the symptom complex suggests *Campylobacter* infection, azithromycin (500 mg/day PO for 3 days) should be added. Regardless of the cause of infectious diarrhea, patients should be treated with antibiotics if they are immunosuppressed; have valvular, vascular, or orthopedic prostheses; have congenital hemolytic anemias (especially if salmonellosis is involved); or are extremely young or old.

Certain infectious diarrheas should be treated with antibiotics, including those associated with shigellosis (Chapter 309), cholera (Chapter 302), pseudomembranous enterocolitis (Chapter 296), parasitic infestations (Chapters 350 to 352 and 357), and sexually transmitted diseases (Chapter 285). Treatment of *E. coli* serotype O157:H7 infection is not recommended at present because current antibiotics do not appear to be helpful and the incidence of complications (hemolytic-uremic syndrome) may be greater after antibiotic therapy. Antibiotics are not effective for viral diarrhea or cryptosporidiosis.

For traveler's diarrhea, ciprofloxacin (500 mg PO twice daily for 3 days) is an effective treatment. The nonabsorbable antibiotic rifaximin (200 mg taken PO three times daily or 400 mg twice daily for 3 days) is safe and effective for treatment of traveler's diarrhea in Mexico, but it may not be effective against *Campylobacter* and *Shigella* infections.

Fluoroquinolone-resistant and trimethoprim-sulfamethoxazole–resistant strains of *Shigella, E. coli, Salmonella, Campylobacter,* and *C. difficile* have emerged. Azithromycin (500 mg PO on day 1 and 250 mg/day PO for 4 days) may be an effective alternative treatment for resistant strains of *Shigella* and *Campylobacter* and for traveler's diarrhea acquired in Mexico.

If *C. difficile* is suspected on an epidemiologic basis, metronidazole (250 mg PO four times daily or 500 mg PO three times daily for 10 days) or oral vancomycin (125 to 250 mg PO four times daily for 10 days) should be prescribed.[6] In patients with recurrent *C. difficile* infection that is associated with low serum antibody titers to toxin A, immunotherapy with monoclonal antibodies against toxin A and B[A1] may decrease recurrence rates. Fecal bacteriotherapy is more effective than vancomycin for the treatment of recurrences.[A2] Non–*C. difficile* antibiotic-induced diarrhea is generally mild and self-limited, and it usually clears spontaneously or in response to cholestyramine therapy (4 g PO four times daily for 2 weeks).

Treatment for chemotherapy-induced and radiation-induced mild to moderate diarrhea includes loperamide (2 mg PO four times daily) and nonsteroidal anti-inflammatory drugs (NSAIDs) (e.g., naproxen, 250 to 500 mg PO twice daily). Octreotide may be an effective treatment in those with severe diarrhea in doses up to 700 μg/day subcutaneously (SC).

PREVENTION

Rotavirus vaccination (Chapter 380) reduces the risk for infection and death and generally results in milder symptoms among those infected.[A3] Travelers to high-risk countries (Central America and parts of Latin America, Africa, Asia, the Middle East) should avoid ingestion of tap water and ice and of raw meat, raw seafood, and raw vegetables. An oral cholera vaccine against recombinant toxin B subunit and killed whole-cell (rBS-WC) is effective in preventing infection from the O1 El Tor strain and partially effective against enterotoxigenic *E. coli* strains.[A4] Cholera vaccination is recommended for relief workers and health professionals who work in endemic countries and for individuals who are immunocompromised or have chronic illnesses or hypochlorhydria. Rifaximin (200 to 600 mg/day PO for 2 weeks) and fluoroquinolones (e.g. norfloxacin 400/day PO for 2 weeks) are effective for reducing the risk for traveler's diarrhea in Mexico,[A5][A6] and the combination of rifaximin plus loperamide is better than either one alone.[A7] Bismuth subsalicylate (525 mg PO four times daily for up to 3 weeks) is also effective. Loperamide and NSAIDs are taken prophylactically by many runners who are susceptible to runner's diarrhea, but it is not clear whether they are effective. Oral probiotics (e.g., lactobacilli and bifidobacteria) are not effective for preventing antibiotic-associated acute diarrhea.[A8]

CHRONIC DIARRHEA

An estimated 5% of the U.S. population suffers from chronic diarrhea, and approximately 40% of these individuals are older than 60 years of age.[7] The causes of chronic diarrhea include persistent infectious or inflammatory diarrheas, malabsorptive syndromes, and watery diarrheas (Table 140-3).

CLINICAL MANIFESTATIONS

Patients with malabsorption (Table 140-4) can present with a variety of gastrointestinal or extraintestinal manifestations (Table 140-5). Significant malabsorption of fat and carbohydrate usually causes chronic diarrhea, abdominal cramps, gas, bloating, and weight loss. Steatorrhea (fat in the stool) manifests as oily, foul-smelling stools that are difficult to flush down the toilet. Stools may be large and bulky (e.g., pancreatic insufficiency) or watery (e.g.,

TABLE 140-3 CAUSES OF CHRONIC DIARRHEA

- Persistent infectious diarrheas (see Table 140-2)
  - Brainerd diarrhea
- Malabsorptive syndromes (see Tables 140-4 and 140-6)
  - Common causes
    - Gastric bypass surgery
    - Dumping syndrome
    - Chronic pancreatitis
    - Intestinal bacterial overgrowth
    - Lactase deficiency
    - Celiac disease
    - Tropical sprue
    - *Giardia lamblia* infection
    - HIV/AIDS-related
    - Crohn disease (Chapter 141)
    - Radiation enteritis (Chapters 20 and 142)
- Watery diarrhea
  - Osmotic diarrhea
    - Magnesium, sodium phosphate, sulfate
    - Sorbitol, fructose
    - Glucose-galactose malabsorption
    - Disaccharidase deficiencies
  - Rapid intestinal transit
- Functional watery diarrhea (irritable bowel syndrome; Chapter 137)
  - Hormone-secreting tumors (VIPoma, carcinoid, gastrinoma, medullary thyroid cancer)
  - Systemic mastocytosis
  - Villous adenoma
  - Diabetes
  - Alcohol
  - Factitious
- Idiopathic
- Inflammatory diarrheas
  - Inflammatory bowel disease (Chapter 141)
  - Eosinophilic gastroenteritis
  - Microscopic colitis (collagenous or lymphocytic)
  - Food allergy

AIDS = acquired immunodeficiency syndrome; HIV, human immunodeficiency virus; VIP = vasoactive intestinal peptide.

TABLE 140-4 CAUSES OF MALABSORPTION

MECHANISM OF MALABSORPTION	CONDITIONS
Impaired mixing	Partial/total gastrectomy Gastric bypass surgery
Impaired lipolysis	Chronic pancreatitis Pancreatic cancer Congenital pancreatic insufficiency Congenital colipase deficiency Gastrinoma
Impaired micelle formation	Severe chronic liver disease Cholestatic liver disease Bacterial overgrowth Crohn disease Ileal resection Gastrinoma
Impaired mucosal absorption	Lactase deficiency Congenital enterokinase deficiency Abetalipoproteinemia Giardiasis Celiac disease Tropical sprue Agammaglobulinemia Amyloidosis AIDS-related (infections, enteropathy) Radiation enteritis Graft-versus-host disease Whipple disease Eosinophilic gastroenteritis Megaloblastic gut Collagenous sprue Refractory celiac disease Lymphoma Bacterial overgrowth Autoimmune enteritis Short-bowel syndrome
Impaired nutrient delivery	Congenital lymphangiectasia Lymphoma Tuberculosis Constrictive pericarditis Severe congestive heart failure
Unknown	Hypoparathyroidism Adrenal insufficiency Hyperthyroidism Carcinoid syndrome

AIDS = acquired immunodeficiency syndrome.

TABLE 140-5 CLINICAL CONSEQUENCES OF MALABSORPTION OF NUTRIENTS, WATER, AND ELECTROLYTES

NUTRIENT MALABSORBED	CLINICAL MANIFESTATION
Protein	Wasting, edema
Carbohydrate and fat	Diarrhea, abdominal cramps and bloating, weight loss and growth retardation
Fluid and electrolytes	Diarrhea, dehydration
Iron	Anemia, cheilosis, angular stomatitis
Calcium and vitamin D	Bone pain, fractures, tetany
Magnesium	Paresthesias, tetany
Vitamin B_{12} and folate	Anemia, glossitis, cheilosis, paresthesias, ataxia (vitamin B_{12} only)
Vitamin E	Paresthesias, ataxia, retinopathy
Vitamin A	Night blindness, xerophthalmia, hyperkeratosis, diarrhea
Vitamin K	Ecchymoses
Riboflavin	Angular stomatitis, cheilosis
Zinc	Dermatitis, hypogeusia, diarrhea
Selenium	Cardiomyopathy
Essential fatty acids	Dermatitis
Copper	Anemia, mental deterioration, neuropathy

bacterial overgrowth, mucosal diseases). Individuals with malabsorption also can present with manifestations of vitamin and mineral deficiencies. Dyspnea can be caused by anemia from iron, copper, folate, or vitamin B_{12} deficiency. Manifestations of calcium, magnesium, or vitamin D malabsorption include paresthesias and tetany resulting from hypocalcemia or hypomagnesemia and bone pain from osteomalacia or osteoporosis-related fractures. Paresthesias and ataxia are manifestations of cobalamin and vitamin E deficiency. Alternatively, neuropathy may be due to malnutrition or copper deficiency. Dermatitis herpetiformis is a blistering, burning, itchy rash on the extensor surfaces and buttocks that is associated with celiac disease.

Inflammatory diarrheas may manifest with fever and abdominal pain or with edema to suggest chronic protein loss. Patients may have multiple, low-volume, bloody stools with tenesmus to suggest proctitis or have severe diarrhea as a result of graft-versus-host disease (GVHD) or celiac disease. Systemic manifestations of inflammatory bowel disease include polymigratory arthritis, sacroiliitis, erythema nodosum, pyoderma gangrenosum, leukocytoclastic angiitis, uveitis, and oral aphthous ulcers.

DIAGNOSIS OF CHRONIC DIARRHEA

A detailed history and physical examination lead to a diagnosis in 25 to 50% of patients with chronic diarrheas (see Table 140-1 and Fig. 140-2). The addition of stool culture and examination for ova and parasites, determination of stool fat, and flexible sigmoidoscopy or colonoscopy with biopsy raises the diagnostic rate to approximately 75%. The remaining 25% of patients with chronic diarrhea may need extensive testing and perhaps hospitalization to make a diagnosis.

A history of 10 to 20 daily bowel movements that do not respond to fasting suggests secretory diarrhea (Fig. 140-3). A history of peptic ulcer should suggest gastrinoma (Chapter 195) or systemic mastocytosis (Chapter 255). Physical examination is helpful only if the thyromegaly of medullary carcinoma (Chapter 246), the cutaneous flushing of the neuroendocrine tumors and systemic mastocytosis, the dermatographism of systemic mastocytosis, or the migratory necrolytic erythema of glucagonoma (Chapter 195) is evident. Autonomic dysfunction (e.g., postural hypotension, impotence, gustatory sweating) is almost invariably present in diabetic diarrhea.

Evaluation for malabsorption begins with a careful elicitation of bowel habits and a description of the stool, weight loss, travel, food or milk tolerance, underlying gastrointestinal, pancreatic, or liver diseases, abdominal surgery, radiation or chemotherapy treatments, family history, and drug and alcohol use.

Blood Tests

Blood measurements (see Fig. 140-2) of iron, folate, vitamin B_{12}, vitamin D, or prothrombin time (vitamin K) help evaluate malabsorption. Specific antibody tests should be sent when celiac disease is suspected (see later). Peripheral blood findings of leukocytosis, eosinophilia, elevated erythrocyte sedimentation rate, hypoalbuminemia, or low total serum protein suggests an inflammatory diarrhea, whose hallmark is the presence of blood, either gross or occult, and leukocytes in the stool. There are no bedside screening tests to establish the diagnosis in watery diarrheas.

Imaging

Malabsorption may be suggested if a flat plate radiograph of the abdomen shows pancreatic calcification (Chapter 133). Some diseases (e.g., previous gastric surgery, gastrocolic fistulas, blind loops from previous intestinal anastomoses, small intestine strictures, multiple jejunal diverticula, abnormal intestinal motility that could lead to bacterial overgrowth) may be shown by computed tomography (CT) or magnetic resonance imaging (MRI) of the abdomen after administration of oral contrast agents or by a traditional upper gastrointestinal radiographic series with small intestine follow-through. A small bowel barium study may show thickening of the intestinal folds (e.g., amyloidosis, lymphoma or Whipple disease), uniform or patchy abnormalities (e.g., lymphoma or lymphangiectasia), or flocculation of barium and ilealization of jejunum to suggest celiac disease. Routine contrast radiographs of the gastrointestinal tract usually are not helpful in the diagnosis of watery diarrheas, unless they show extensive small bowel resection, the presence of a tumor (carcinoid or villous adenoma), or a bowel filled with fluid (endocrine tumor). Abdominal contrast imaging, particularly CT or MR enterography that uses oral neutral contrast to enhance the bowel wall, may show diagnostic evidence of advanced inflammatory bowel disease or changes suggestive of eosinophilic gastroenteritis or radiation enterocolitis. Somatostatin receptor scintigraphy with indium-111–labeled octreotide can be useful in localizing gastrinomas, pancreatic endocrine tumors, and carcinoid tumors.

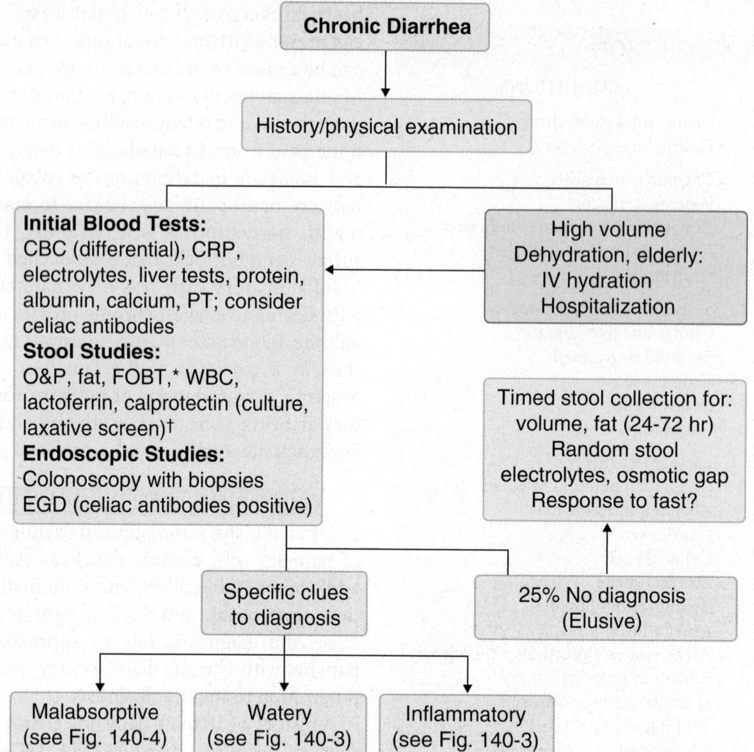

FIGURE 140-2. **Initial approach to chronic diarrhea. *Fecal occult blood testing (FOBT) is a sensitive test for underlying bowel inflammation. †Perform stool culture in those who are immunosuppressed; perform laxative screen if laxative abuse is suspected. CBC = complete blood count; CRP = C-reactive protein; EGD = esophagogastroduodenoscopy; IV = intravenous; O&P = ova and parasites; PT = prothrombin time; WBC = white blood cells.**

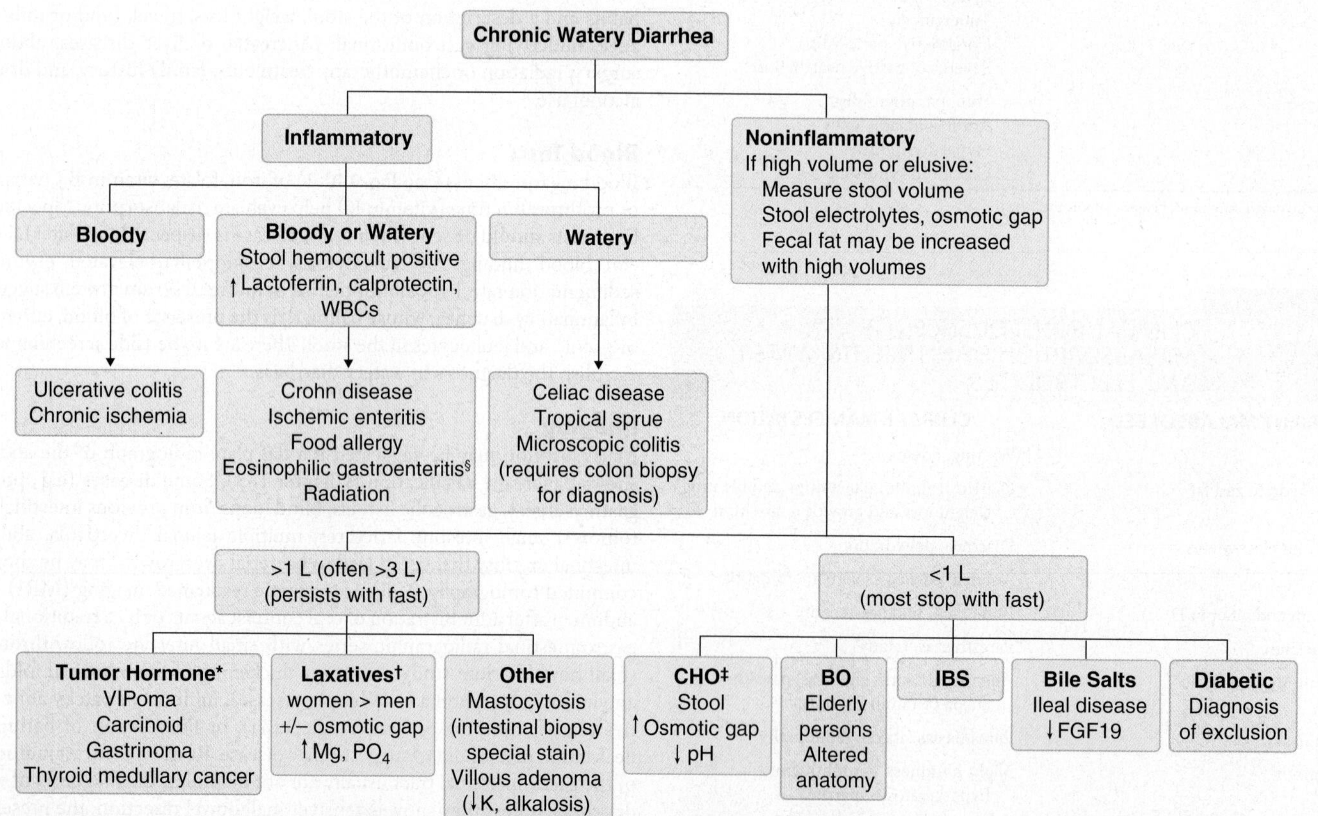

FIGURE 140-3. **Approach to the evaluation of watery diarrheas. Many diarrheas have more than one mechanism (i.e., osmotic, secretory, inflammatory). Other causes include medications, postsurgical (vagotomy, Nissan wrap, cholecystectomy), hyperthyroidism, and alcohol. *VIPoma: >3 L output daily "pancreatic cholera," elevated VIP level. Carcinoid: elevated urine 5-hydroxyindole acetic acid, positive OctreoScan. Gastrinoma (Zollinger-Ellison syndrome): elevated gastrin level, positive secretin stimulation test, diarrhea due to high volume of acid secretion. Thyroid medullary cancer: elevated calcitonin level. †May be high or low volume depending on dose ingested, may respond to fast. ‡Carbohydrate malabsorption (CHO) may be due to lactase deficiency, dietary fructose, sorbitol in diabetic candies or liquid medications. §Full-thickness biopsy may be needed for diagnosis. BO = bacterial overgrowth; FGF = fibroblast growth factor; IBS = irritable bowel syndrome; WBCs = white blood cells.**

Endoscopy and Biopsy

Upper endoscopy with distal duodenal biopsy should be undertaken if serologic tests for celiac disease are positive or diagnostic clues suggest small bowel mucosal malabsorption (Chapter 134). Small bowel biopsy is virtually always abnormal when the tTG immunoglobulin A (IgA) antibody level is very high (more than five-fold the normal range), and antiendomysial antibody (EMA) is positive. A biopsy may be avoided in this setting if gastrointestinal symptoms and the HLA risk alleles for celiac disease are present. Some patients may have patchy mucosal disease and require enteroscopy with jejunal biopsies for diagnosis. Wireless video capsule endoscopy (Chapter 134) and balloon-assisted enteroscopy are increasingly used to diagnose diseases that reside deep in the small bowel. Patients with severe watery or elusive diarrhea should have a colonoscopy to assess for villous adenomas, microscopic colitis, mastocytosis, or early inflammatory bowel disease. Colonoscopy also may show brown pigmentation suggestive of melanosis coli due to chronic use of anthracene laxatives. Terminal ileal biopsy may indicate infectious or inflammatory bowel disease.

Other Laboratory Tests

Malabsorption

If chronic diarrhea is the presenting symptom, a stool examination for ova and parasites and a stool antigen-capture enzyme-linked immunosorbent assay (ELISA) test for *Giardia* should be obtained. A stool test for fat on a high-fat diet (70 to 100 g/day) is the best available screening test for malabsorption (Table 140-6). If the fecal fat test result is negative, selective carbohydrate malabsorption or other causes of watery diarrhea should be considered. If the fecal fat test result is positive, further testing should be based on clinical suspicion for particular diseases. If pancreatic insufficiency is suspected, imaging studies of the pancreas should be performed. If bacterial overgrowth is suspected, culture of an intestinal aspirate or a breath test should be obtained. Small bowel contrast imaging is useful in detecting structural abnormalities that predispose to bacterial overgrowth (Table 140-7). If proximal mucosal damage is suspected, multiple small intestinal biopsy specimens should be obtained. If there are no clues, CT or MR enterography may help to detect middle and distal small bowel mucosal diseases. Some

TABLE 140-6 TESTS FOR THE EVALUATION OF MALABSORPTION*

TEST	COMMENTS
GENERAL TESTS OF ABSORPTION	
Quantitative stool fat test	Gold standard test of fat malabsorption, with which all other tests are compared. Requires ingestion of a high-fat diet (100 g) for 2 days before and during the collection. Stool is collected for 3 days. Normally, <7 g/24 hr is excreted on a high-fat diet. Borderline abnormalities of 8-14 g/24 hr may be seen in secretory or osmotic diarrheas that are not caused by malabsorption. There are false-negative findings if fat intake is inadequate. False-positive results can occur if the nonabsorbable fat olestra is ingested or mineral oil laxatives or rectal suppositories (e.g., cocoa butter) are given to the patient before stool collection.
Qualitative stool fat test	Sudan stain of a stool sample for fat. Many fat droplets per medium-power field (40×) constitute a positive test result. The nuclear magnetic resonance method determines the percentage of fat in the stool (normal, <20%). The test depends on an adequate fat intake (100 g/day). There is high sensitivity (90%) and specificity (90%) with fat malabsorption of >10 g/24 hr. Sensitivity drops with stool fat in the range of 6-10 g/24 hr.
Hydrogen breath test	Most useful in the diagnosis of lactase deficiency. An oral dose of lactose (1 g/kg body weight) is administered after measurement of basal breath H_2 levels. The sole source of H_2 in the mammal is bacterial fermentation; unabsorbed lactose makes its way to colonic bacteria, resulting in excess breath H_2. A *late peak* (within 3-6 hr) of > 20 ppm of exhaled H_2 after lactose ingestion suggests lactose malabsorption. Absorption of other carbohydrates (e.g., sucrose, glucose, fructose) also can be tested.
SPECIFIC TESTS FOR MALABSORPTION	
Tests for Pancreatic Function	
Secretin stimulation test	The gold standard test of pancreatic function. Requires duodenal test intubation with a double-lumen tube and collection of pancreatic juice in response to intravenous secretin. Allows measurement of bicarbonate (HCO_3^-) and pancreatic enzymes. A sensitive test of pancreatic function, but labor intensive and invasive.
Fecal elastase-1 test	Stool test for pancreatic function. Equal sensitivity to the secretin stimulation test for the diagnosis of moderate-to-severe pancreatic insufficiency. More specific than the fecal chymotrypsin test. Unreliable with mild insufficiency. False-positive results occur with increased stool volume and intestinal mucosal diseases.
Tests for Bacterial Overgrowth	
Quantitative culture of small intestinal aspirate	Gold standard test for bacterial overgrowth. Greater than 10^5 colony-forming units (CFU)/mL in the jejunum suggests bacterial overgrowth. Requires special anaerobic sample collection, rapid anaerobic and aerobic plating, and care to avoid oropharyngeal contamination. False-negative results occur with focal jejunal diverticula and when overgrowth is distal to the site aspirated.
Hydrogen breath test	The 50-g glucose breath test has a sensitivity of 90% for growth of 10^5 colonic-type bacteria in the small intestine. If bacterial overgrowth is present, increased H_2 is excreted in the breath. A hydrogen level (within 2 hr) of > 20 ppm suggests bacterial overgrowth. False-negative results occur with non–hydrogen-producing organisms. Concomitant measurement of breath methane improves test sensitivity.
Tests for Mucosal Disease	
Small bowel biopsy	Obtained for a specific diagnosis when there is a high index of suspicion for small intestinal disease. Several biopsy specimens (4-5) must be obtained to maximize the diagnostic yield. Distal duodenal biopsy specimens are usually adequate for diagnosis, but occasionally enteroscopy with jejunal biopsy specimens is necessary. Small intestinal biopsy provides a specific diagnosis in some diseases (e.g., intestinal infection, Whipple disease, abetalipoproteinemia, agammaglobulinemia, lymphangiectasia, lymphoma, amyloidosis). In other conditions, such as celiac disease and tropical sprue, the biopsy specimens show characteristic findings, but the diagnosis is made on improvement after treatment.
Tests of Ileal Function	
Schilling test	A test of vitamin B_{12} absorption (see Table 164-4 in Chapter 164).
^{75}SeHCAT test	This is a test of bile acid absorption. Seven days after ingestion of radiolabeled synthetic selenium–homocholic acid conjugated with taurine (^{75}SeHCAT), whole body retention is measured by a gamma-counting device. The result is expressed as a fraction of baseline ingestion. Retention values of <10% are abnormal and indicate bile acid malabsorption with a sensitivity of 80-90% and specificity of 70-100%. The radiation dose is equivalent to that of a plain chest x-ray. Liver disease and bacterial overgrowth may give false results. Not approved for use in the United States.

*Not all these tests are readily available. A strong suspicion for any disease may warrant foregoing an extensive work-up and obtaining the test with highest diagnostic yield. In some cases, empirical treatment, such as removing lactose from the diet of an otherwise healthy individual with lactose intolerance, is warranted without any testing.

TABLE 140-7 ABNORMALITIES CONDUCIVE TO BACTERIAL OVERGROWTH

STRUCTURAL
Afferent loop syndrome after gastrojejunostomy
Ileocecal valve resection
End-to-side intestinal anastomoses
Duodenal and jejunal diverticula
Strictures (Crohn disease, radiation enteritis)
Adhesions (postsurgical)
Gastrojejunocolic fistulas
MOTOR
Scleroderma
Diabetes mellitus
Idiopathic pseudo-obstruction
HYPOCHLORHYDRIA
Atrophic gastritis
Proton pump inhibitors
Acquired immunodeficiency syndrome
Acid-reducing surgery for peptic ulcer disease
MISCELLANEOUS
Immunodeficiency states
Pancreatitis
Cirrhosis
Chronic renal failure

individuals with celiac disease present with selective nutrient deficiencies without diarrhea. In these cases, tTG antibody tests and intestinal biopsy should be performed. In patients hospitalized for severe diarrhea or malnutrition, a more streamlined evaluation usually includes a stool for culture, ova and parasites, and fat; an abdominal imaging study; and a biopsy of the small intestine and colon.

Watery Diarrhea

Breath tests to measure the respiratory excretion of H_2 and methane after administration of carbohydrates can assess carbohydrate malabsorption or bacterial overgrowth (see Table 140-6).

The diagnosis of endocrine tumors, such as carcinoids, gastrinoma, VIPoma, medullary carcinoma of the thyroid, glucagonoma, somatostatinoma, and systemic mastocytosis, is made by showing elevated blood levels of serotonin, chromogranin A, or urinary 5-hydroxyindoleacetic acid and serum levels for gastrin, vasoactive intestinal peptide, calcitonin, glucagon, somatostatin, histamine, or prostaglandins (Chapter 195). Somatostatin receptor scintigraphy has proved to be sensitive and useful in the diagnosis and evaluation of Zollinger-Ellison syndrome (Chapter 195).

Inflammatory Diarrhea

Stool occult blood, white blood cells, or lactoferrin and calprotectin (components of leukocytes) are helpful tests for bowel inflammation. Video capsule endoscopy (Chapter 134) of the small bowel may detect ulcerations deep in the small bowel not reachable by standard upper or lower endoscopy and not detected with conventional barium contrast radiography. However, the risk for capsule retention in the small bowel is high in patients with Crohn disease or NSAID use, particularly when there is a history of obstructive symptoms. The most sensitive test for protein-losing enteropathy is measurement of intestinal protein loss by 24-hour stool excretion or clearance of α_1-antitrypsin.

Stool Examination in Elusive Diarrhea

An important adjunct to diagnosing the cause of diarrhea is to examine the stool. The greasy, bulky stool of steatorrhea and the bloody stool of gut inflammation are distinctive. Stool collections (see Table 140-6) can be analyzed for weight, volume, fat, electrolytes ($^+Na^{++}$, K^{++}, Cl^-), osmolality, pH, and a laxative screen (SO_4^{2-}, PO_4^{2-}, Mg^{2+}). Stool or urine can be analyzed for emetine (a component of ipecac), bisacodyl, castor oil, or anthraquinone.

Carbohydrate malabsorption lowers stool pH because of colonic fermentation of carbohydrate to short-chain fatty acids. Stool pH less than 5.3 usually means pure carbohydrate malabsorption, whereas in the generalized malabsorptive diseases, stool pH is greater than 5.6 and usually greater than 6.0.

The normal stool osmotic gap, which is the difference between stool osmolality (or 290 mOsm) and twice the stool Na^{++} and K^{++} concentrations, is 50 to 125. In secretory diarrheas, the colon's capacity for adjusting electrolyte concentrations is overwhelmed, the stool osmotic gap is less than 50, and stool electrolytes more nearly resemble plasma electrolytes ($^+Na^{++}$ concentrations are usually > 90 mmol/L, K^+ concentrations usually < 10 mmol/L), except for higher HCO_3^- concentrations (usually > 50 mmol/L). In osmotic diarrhea, the presence of uncharged solute or unmeasured cation in the colonic lumen draws in water, depresses stool Na^{++} (usually < 60 mmol/L) and K^+ concentrations, and results in a stool osmotic gap greater than 125. Stools with Na^{++} concentrations between 60 and 90 mmol/L and calculated osmotic gaps between 50 and 100 can result from either secretory or malabsorptive abnormalities. Patients with Mg^{2++}-induced diarrhea may be diagnosed by fecal Mg^{2+} values of more than 50 mmol/L. Sodium anion–induced diarrheas (Na_2SO_4, Na_2PO_4) mimic secretory diarrhea because the stool Na^{++} content is high (>90 mmol/L) and there is no osmotic gap; this diarrhea may be diagnosed by determining stool Cl^- concentration because these anions displace stool Cl^-, resulting in a depressed stool Cl^- value (usually < 20 mmol/L). A low stool osmolality suggests contamination of stool with urine or water in the case of factitious diarrhea.

SPECIFIC CAUSES OF CHRONIC DIARRHEA

Prolonged, Persistent Infectious Diarrheas

Prolonged infectious diarrheas (>2 weeks) may be due to persistent or recurrent infections. These diarrheas occur most commonly in children exposed to unsafe drinking water in developing countries, patients who have acquired immunodeficiency syndrome (AIDS) or are immunosuppressed for other reasons, and recent travelers. The most common causes in children in developing countries are enteropathogenic and enteroadherent *E. coli* infections (Chapter 304). Other common organisms include *Giardia* (Chapter 351), *Cryptosporidium* (Chapter 350), *Entamoeba* (Chapter 352), *Isospora* (Chapter 390), and microsporidia (Chapter 350). Recurrent or prolonged infectious diarrhea may lead to severe malnutrition and death (mortality rate, 50%). Treatment includes nutrition support with supplemental vitamin A (200,000 IU twice yearly) and zinc (20 mg elemental daily for 14 days). Severe disease may require total parenteral nutrition.

In patients with AIDS, protracted diarrhea may be caused by treatable agents such as *E. histolytica, Giardia,* or *Strongyloides* or by organisms such as *Cryptosporidium, Isospora belli,* and microsporidia that are difficult to treat or untreatable. The most effective treatment is retroviral therapy to improve the immune system (Chapter 388).

Up to 10% of travelers returning from developing countries have infectious diarrhea that persists for longer than 3 to 4 weeks. Stool should be examined for culture and for ova and parasites; in patients with a recent history of antibiotic use, stool also should be sent for *C. difficile* toxin. Any specific organisms that are identified should be treated. If treatment with trimethoprim-sulfamethoxazole or a fluoroquinolone has been unsuccessful, tetracycline (250 mg PO four times daily for 7 to 10 days) or metronidazole (250 mg PO three times daily for 7 to 10 days) can be tried. After documented infectious diarrhea, 25% of patients experience pain, bloating, urgency, a sense of incomplete evacuation, and loose stools for 6 months or longer; some of these patients have celiac disease, so screening (see later) is warranted in this setting. When no other cause is found, these patients are deemed to have postinfectious irritable bowel syndrome (Chapter 137).

Sporadic outbreaks of severe, prolonged diarrhea, often greater than 1 year in duration, occasionally have been reported. This form of prolonged diarrhea is called *Brainerd diarrhea.* The organism has yet to be identified. The diarrhea is difficult to treat; cholestyramine (4 g PO three times daily) may be helpful.

Malabsorptive Syndromes

Malabsorption is caused by many different diseases, drugs (e.g., the lipase inhibitor orlistat; Chapter 220), and nutritional products (the nonabsorbable fat olestra) that impair intraluminal digestion, mucosal absorption, or delivery of the nutrient to the systemic circulation (E-Fig. 140-2; see Table 140-4). Dietary fat is the nutrient most difficult to absorb. Fatty stools (steatorrhea) are the hallmark of malabsorption; a stool test for fat is the best screening test. Malabsorption does not always cause diarrhea. Clinical signs of vitamin or mineral deficiencies may occur in the absence of diarrhea. A careful history is crucial in guiding further testing to confirm the suspicion of malabsorption and to make a specific diagnosis (Fig. 140-4). The goals of treatment are to correct or treat the underlying disease and replenish losses of water, electrolytes, and nutrients.

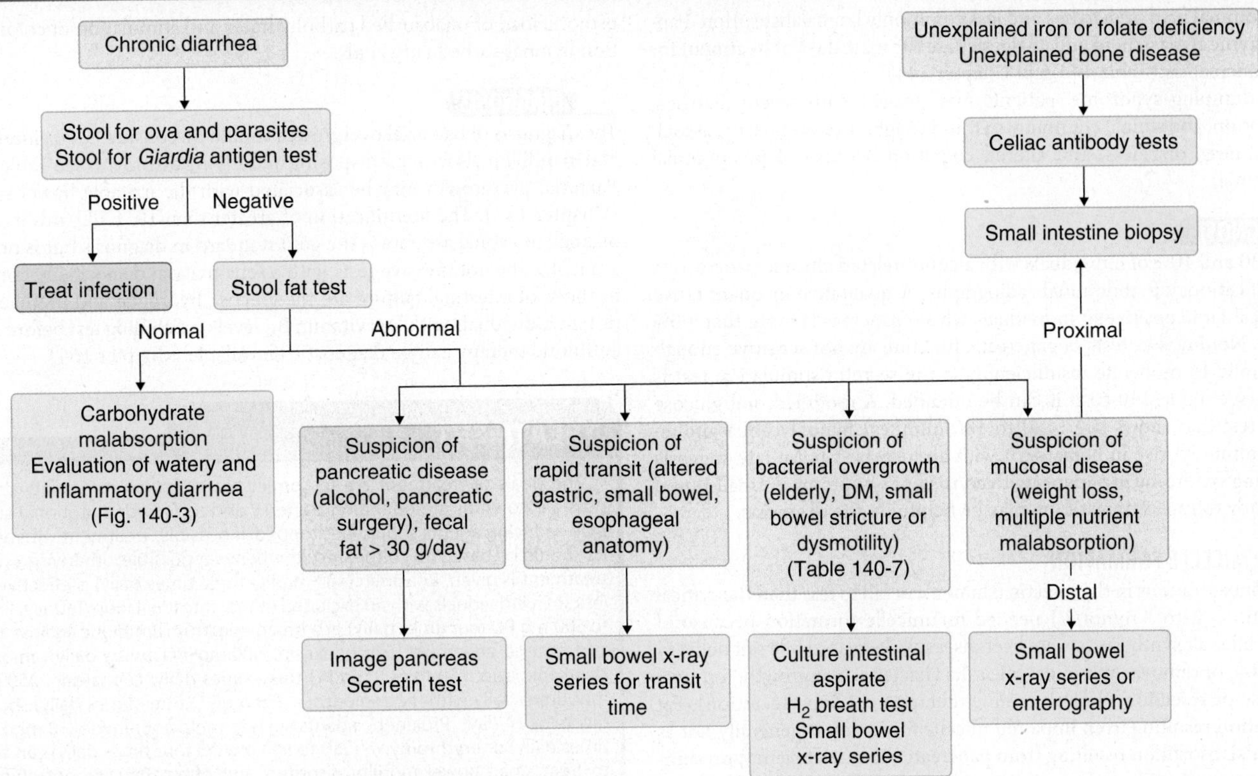

FIGURE 140-4. Approach to the diagnosis of malabsorption. DM = diabetes mellitus.

Conditions That Impair Intraluminal Digestion

Most digestion and absorption of nutrients occur in the small intestine (see E-Fig. 140-2). Carbohydrates and most dietary proteins are water soluble and readily digested by pancreatic enzymes. Pancreatic proteases (trypsinogen, chymotrypsinogen, procarboxypeptidases) are secreted from acinar cells in inactive forms. The cleavage of trypsinogen to trypsin by the duodenal brush-border peptidase enteropeptidase (enterokinase) allows trypsin to cleave the remaining trypsinogen and other proteases to their active form.

Most dietary lipids (long-chain triglycerides, cholesterol, and fat-soluble vitamins) are water insoluble and must undergo lipolysis and incorporation into mixed micelles before they can be absorbed across the intestinal mucosa. Pancreatic lipase, in the presence of its cofactor, colipase, cleaves long-chain triglycerides into fatty acids and monoglycerides. The products of lipolysis interact with bile salts and phospholipids to form mixed micelles, which also incorporate cholesterol and fat-soluble vitamins (D, A, K, and E) in their hydrophobic centers. Bicarbonate secreted from pancreatic duct cells is physiologically important to neutralize gastric acid because pancreatic enzyme activity and bile salt micelle formation are optimum at a luminal pH of 6 to 8.

IMPAIRED MIXING

Surgical alterations, such as partial gastrectomy with gastrojejunostomy (Billroth II anastomosis) or gastrointestinal bypass surgeries for obesity, result in the release of biliary and pancreatic secretions into the intestine at a site remote from the site of entry of gastric contents. This imbalance can result in impaired lipolysis and impaired micelle formation, with subsequent fat malabsorption. Bypass of the duodenum also impairs absorption of iron, folate, and calcium. Rapid transit through the jejunum contributes to the malabsorption of nutrients. Individuals with these conditions also have surgical anastomoses that predispose to bacterial overgrowth.

DUMPING SYNDROME

After esophageal (distal esophagectomy, myomectomy for achalasia), gastric (Nissan wrap, hiatal hernia repair, gastrojejunostomy), and bariatric (Roux-en-Y and duodenal switch gastric bypass) surgeries, the unregulated delivery of concentrated sugars and food into the duodenum and jejunum results in altered insulin regulation, maldigestion, osmotic movement of fluid into the intestinal lumen, and rapid transit such that intestinal contact time is insufficient for absorption of nutrients.

Treatment is with a diet that is low in concentrated sugars divided into six small meals. Administration of pectin (15 g with each meal) may slow gastric emptying. In patients who are refractory to dietary measures, a short-acting somatostatin analogue (e.g., octreotide, 25 to 200 μg SC three times daily) or the better tolerated intramuscular preparation (10 to 20 mg monthly) improves dumping symptoms. In patients with predominant reactive hypoglycemia 1 to 3 hours after a meal (late dumping), an α-glycosidase hydrolase inhibitor (e.g., acarbose, 50 to 100 mg PO three times daily) that blocks carbohydrate absorption in the small bowel may be beneficial. Continuous tube feeding is also effective.

IMPAIRED LIPOLYSIS

A deficiency in pancreatic lipase may be caused by the congenital absence of pancreatic lipase or by destruction of the pancreatic gland as a result of alcohol-related pancreatitis, cystic fibrosis, or pancreatic cancer. Pancreatic lipase also can be denatured by excess secretion of gastric acid (e.g., Zollinger-Ellison syndrome; Chapter 195). In such cases, lipase denaturation can be offset by treatment with a high-dose proton pump inhibitor (e.g., omeprazole 60 mg/day PO) to block acid secretion.

CHRONIC PANCREATITIS

Chronic pancreatitis (Chapter 144) is the most common cause of pancreatic insufficiency and impaired lipolysis. In the United States, chronic pancreatitis most commonly results from alcohol abuse; in contrast, tropical (nutritional) pancreatitis is most common worldwide. Malabsorption of fat does not occur until more than 90% of the pancreas is destroyed.

CLINICAL MANIFESTATIONS

Individuals with pancreatic causes of malabsorption typically present with bulky, fat-laden stools (usually > 30 g of fat daily), abdominal pain, and diabetes, although some present with diabetes in the absence of gastrointestinal symptoms. Stools usually are not watery because undigested triglycerides form large emulsion droplets with little osmotic force and, in contrast to fatty acids, do not stimulate water and electrolyte secretion in the colon. Deficiency of fat-soluble vitamins is seen only rarely, presumably because gastric and residual pancreatic lipase generates enough fatty acids for some micelle formation. In severe disease, subclinical protein malabsorption, manifested by the presence of undigested meat fibers in the stool, and subclinical carbohydrate malabsorption, manifested by gas-filled, floating stools, can occur. Weight loss, when it occurs, is most often caused by decreased oral intake to avoid abdominal pain or diarrhea and less commonly by malabsorption. Pancreatic enzyme replacement and analgesics are the mainstays of treatment for chronic pancreatitis (Table 144-5 in Chapter 144).

In the dumping syndrome, patients may present with severe diarrhea, malabsorption, abdominal cramping, gas, and weight loss. Some have associated sweatiness, dizziness, and altered cognition because of postprandial hypoglycemia.

DIAGNOSIS

Between 30 and 40% of individuals with alcohol-related chronic pancreatitis have calcifications on abdominal radiographs. A qualitative or quantitative test for fecal fat is positive in individuals whose pancreas is more than 90% destroyed. Noninvasive tests of pancreatic function are not sensitive enough to detect mild to moderate insufficiency, so the secretin stimulation test is preferred (see Table 140-6) if it can be obtained. A modified oral glucose tolerance test that shows late (120 to 180 minutes) hypoglycemia and an early (30 minutes) rise in hematocrit with an increased pulse rate suggests the dumping syndrome in patients with consistent symptoms. A small-bowel barium study to assess transit time may be helpful in the diagnosis.

IMPAIRED MICELLE FORMATION

Bile salt concentrations in the intestinal lumen can fall to less than the critical concentration (2 to 3 mmol/L) needed for micelle formation because of decreased bile salt synthesis (severe liver disease), decreased bile salt delivery (cholestasis), or removal of luminal bile salts (bacterial overgrowth, terminal ileal disease or resection, cholestyramine therapy, acid hypersecretion). Fat malabsorption resulting from impaired micelle formation is generally not as severe as malabsorption resulting from pancreatic lipase deficiency, presumably because fatty acids and monoglycerides can form lamellar structures, which to a certain extent can be absorbed. Malabsorption of fat-soluble vitamins (D, A, K, and E) may be marked, however, because micelle formation is required for their absorption.

Decreased Bile Salt Synthesis and Delivery

Malabsorption can occur in individuals with cholestatic liver disease or bile duct obstruction. The clinical consequences of malabsorption are seen most often in women with primary biliary cirrhosis because of the prolonged nature of the illness. Although these individuals can present with steatorrhea, osteoporosis or, less commonly, osteomalacia is the most common presentation. The cause of bone disease in these patients is poorly understood and often is not related to vitamin D deficiency. Bone disease is treated with calcium supplements (and vitamin D if a deficiency is documented), weight-bearing exercise, and a bisphosphonate (e.g., alendronate, 10 mg/day PO or 70 mg PO once weekly).

Intestinal Bacterial Overgrowth

In health, only small numbers of lactobacilli, enterococci, gram-positive aerobes, or facultative anaerobes can be cultured from the upper small bowel lumen. Motility and acid are the most important factors in keeping the number of bacteria in the upper small bowel low. Any condition that produces local stasis or recirculation of colonic luminal contents allows development of a predominantly "colonic" flora (coliforms and anaerobes, such as *Bacteroides* and *Clostridium*) in the small intestine (see Table 140-7). Anaerobic bacteria cause impaired micelle formation by releasing cholylamidases, which deconjugate bile salts. The unconjugated bile salts, with their higher pK_a, are more likely to be in the protonated form at the normal upper small intestinal pH of 6 to 7 and can be absorbed passively. As a result, the concentration of bile salts decreases in the intestinal lumen and can fall to less than the critical micellar concentration, causing malabsorption of fats and fat-soluble vitamins. Vitamin B_{12} deficiency and carbohydrate malabsorption also can occur with generalized bacterial overgrowth. Anaerobic bacteria ingest vitamin B_{12} and release proteases that degrade brush-border disaccharidases. Although anaerobic bacteria use vitamin B_{12}, they synthesize folate. Individuals with bacterial overgrowth usually have low serum vitamin B_{12} levels but normal or high folate levels; this helps distinguish bacterial overgrowth from tropical sprue, in which vitamin B_{12} and folate levels are usually low because of decreased mucosal uptake.

CLINICAL MANIFESTATIONS

Individuals with bacterial overgrowth can present with diarrhea, abdominal cramps, gas and bloating, weight loss, and signs and symptoms of vitamin B_{12} and fat-soluble vitamin deficiency. Watery diarrhea occurs because of the osmotic load of unabsorbed carbohydrates and stimulation of colonic secretion by unabsorbed fatty acids.

DIAGNOSIS

The diagnosis of bacterial overgrowth should be considered in elderly people and in individuals with predisposing underlying disorders (see Table 140-7).[8] Bacterial overgrowth may be associated with the irritable bowel syndrome (Chapter 137). The identification of greater than 10^5 CFU/mL in a culture of small intestinal aspirate is the gold standard in diagnosis but is not readily available. The noninvasive tests with a sensitivity and specificity comparable to those of intestinal culture are the glucose hydrogen and methane breath test; in individuals with low vitamin B_{12} levels, a Schilling test before and after antibiotic therapy can be diagnostic if available (Chapter 164).

TREATMENT

Rx

The goals of treatment are to correct the structural or motility defect, if possible; to eradicate offending bacteria; and to provide nutritional support. Acid-reducing agents should be stopped, if possible. Treatment with antibiotics should be based on culture results whenever possible; otherwise, empirical treatment is given. Rifaximin (400 mg PO three times daily) is effective,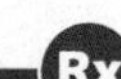 but less so in individuals with an excluded (blind) intestinal loop. Tetracycline (250 to 500 mg PO four times daily) or a broad-spectrum antibiotic against aerobes and enteric anaerobes (ciprofloxacin, 500 mg PO twice daily; amoxicillin-clavulanic acid, 250 to 500 mg PO three times daily; cephalexin, 250 mg PO four times daily with metronidazole, 250 mg PO three times daily) should be given for 14 days. Prokinetic agents such as metoclopramide (10 mg PO four times daily) or erythromycin (250 to 500 mg PO four times daily) can be tried to treat small bowel motility disorders, but often they are not efficacious. Octreotide (50 μg SC every day) may improve motility and reduce bacterial overgrowth in individuals with scleroderma. If the structural abnormality or motility disturbance cannot be corrected, the patient is at risk for malnutrition and deficiencies of vitamin B_{12} and fat-soluble vitamins. Cyclic treatment (1 to 3 weeks of every 4 to 6 weeks) with rotating antibiotics may be required in these patients to prevent recurrent bouts of bacterial overgrowth. If supplemental calories are needed, medium-chain triglycerides should be given because they do not depend on micelle formation for their absorption. Monthly treatment with vitamin B_{12} should be considered, along with supplemental vitamins D, A, K, and E and calcium.

ILEAL DISEASE

Disease of the terminal ileum is most commonly due to Crohn disease (Chapter 141), which also may lead to ileal resection, but it also can be caused by radiation enteritis, tropical sprue, tuberculosis, *Yersinia* infection, or idiopathic bile salt malabsorption. These diseases cause bile salt wasting in the colon.

The clinical consequences of bile salt malabsorption are related directly to the length of the diseased or resected terminal ileum. In an adult, if less than 100 cm of ileum is diseased or resected, watery diarrhea results because of stimulation of colonic fluid secretion by unabsorbed bile salts. Bile acid diarrhea responds to cholestyramine (2 to 4 g taken at breakfast, lunch, and dinner).[9] If more than 100 cm of ileum is diseased or resected, bile salt losses (>3 g/day) in the colon exceed the capacity for increased bile salt synthesis in the liver, the bile salt pool shrinks, and micelle formation is impaired. As a result, steatorrhea ensues, and fatty acid–induced intestinal secretion synergizes with the bile acid–induced secretion to cause diarrhea. Treatment is with a low-fat diet, vitamin B_{12} (300 to 1000 μg SC once every month or 2 mg/day PO), dietary supplements of calcium (500 mg PO two or three times daily, monitor 24-hour urine calcium for adequacy of dose), and a multiple vitamin and mineral supplement. An antimotility agent should be given for diarrhea. Bile salt binders may worsen diarrhea. Screening for fat-soluble vitamin deficiencies (vitamins A and E, 25-OH vitamin D, and prothrombin time) and bone disease (bone densitometry, serum calcium, intact parathyroid hormone, 24-hour urine for calcium) should be done.

Three long-term complications of chronic bile salt wasting and fat malabsorption are renal stones, bone disease (osteoporosis and osteomalacia), and gallstones. Oxalate renal stones occur as a consequence of excess free oxalate absorption in the colon. Free oxalate is generated when unabsorbed fatty acids bind luminal calcium, which is then unavailable for binding oxalate. Renal oxalate stones sometimes can be avoided with a low-fat, low-oxalate diet and calcium supplements. Bone disease is caused by impaired micelle formation with a resulting decrease in absorption of vitamin D; year-round sun exposure reduces this complication. Vitamin D (50,000 U PO one to three times per week) and calcium supplements (500 mg PO two to three times daily day) should be given to susceptible individuals, but vitamin D levels and serum and urinary calcium must be monitored for response to treatment because excess vitamin D can be toxic. The mechanism of gallstone formation in these individuals is unclear; pigmented gallstones are most common.

Conditions That Impair Mucosal Absorption

PATHOBIOLOGY

Nutrients are absorbed along the entire length of the small intestine, with the exception of iron and folate, which are absorbed in the duodenum and proximal jejunum, and bile salts and cobalamin, which are absorbed in the distal ileum. The efficiency of nutrient uptake at the mucosa is influenced by the number of villus absorptive cells, the presence of functional hydrolases and specific nutrient transport proteins on the brush-border membrane, and transit time. Transit time determines the contact time of luminal contents with the brush-border membrane and influences the efficiency of nutrient uptake across the mucosa.

Mucosal malabsorption can be caused by specific (usually congenital) brush-border enzyme or nutrient transporter deficiencies or by generalized diseases that damage the small intestinal mucosa or result in surgical resection or bypass of the small intestine. The nutrients malabsorbed in these general malabsorptive diseases depend on the site of intestinal injury (proximal, distal, or diffuse) and the severity of damage. The main mechanism of malabsorption in these conditions is a decrease in surface area available for absorption. Some conditions (infection, celiac disease, tropical sprue, food allergies, and GVHD) are characterized by intestinal inflammation and villus flattening; others are characterized by ulceration (ulcerative jejunitis, NSAIDs, Crohn disease), infiltration (amyloidosis), or ischemia (radiation enteritis, mesenteric ischemia).

Long-chain fatty acids are transported across the microvillus membrane of villus epithelial cells by the fatty acid transport protein FATP4. The bile salts from mixed micelles remain in the intestinal lumen and are absorbed in the distal ileum by sodium-dependent co-transport. Oligosaccharides and larger oligopeptides (products of pancreatic enzyme digestion), sucrose, and lactose are hydrolyzed further by enzymes present in the brush-border membrane of villus epithelial cells before they are absorbed. Although only sugar monomers (glucose, galactose, fructose) can be taken up at the apical epithelial cell membrane, dipeptides and tripeptides are readily taken into the cell.

Water-soluble vitamins are readily absorbed throughout the small intestine. Fat-soluble vitamins, minerals, and cobalamin are more difficult to absorb because of the requirement for micelle formation (vitamins D, A, K, and E), a divalent charge (magnesium, calcium, iron), or selected sites of uptake in the intestine (iron, cobalamin). Calcium is absorbed best in the proximal small intestine by a vitamin D–dependent calcium channel (TRPV6). Magnesium is absorbed in the small intestine by members of the transient receptor potential family (TRPM6 and TRPM7). Mutations in TRPM6 have been identified in the rare disorder hereditary hypomagnesemia. Ferrous iron is transported into intestinal epithelial cells by a proton-coupled metal-ion transporter (Nramp2) that has specificity for Fe^{2++} and other divalent cations (Zn^{2++}, Mn^{2++}, Co^{2++}, Cd^{2++}, Cu^{2++}, Ni^{2++}, and Pb^{2++}). The absorption of calcium and nonheme iron is enhanced by solubilization with hydrochloric acid. Intraluminal compounds such as oxalate, phytate, and long-chain fatty acids bind to calcium and magnesium, decreasing their absorption. Individuals with severe mucosal disease or short-bowel syndrome with high fecal fluid outputs lose magnesium and zinc from endogenous secretions.

Folates (Chapters 164 and 218) are both taken in the diet and produced by bacteria in the colon. Dietary folates are absorbed in the proximal small intestine through a reduced folate carrier (RFC1). Deficiency can be caused by poor intake or malabsorption secondary to intestinal disease or drugs. The cobalamins (Chapters 164 and 218) are abundant in foods containing animal proteins (e.g., meat, seafood, eggs, milk). Cobalamin (vitamin B_{12}) deficiency in industrialized countries is rarely due to poor dietary intake but rather reflects the inability to absorb cobalamin. This inability may be caused by a lack of intrinsic factor, consumption of cobalamin by overgrowth of anaerobic bacteria in the small bowel lumen, ileal disease or resection, or defective transcobalamin II. Large amounts of cobalamin are present in the liver (2 to 5 mg), and cobalamin is reabsorbed from bile through the enterohepatic circulation, thereby limiting daily losses to less than 1 μg. It usually takes 10 to 12 years for cobalamin deficiency to develop after it is eliminated from the diet, but deficiency can occur more rapidly (2 to 5 years) with malabsorptive syndromes. If lack of gastric acid causes food-cobalamin malabsorption, treatment with oral cyanocobalamin supplementation (Chapter 164) is curative.

LACTASE DEFICIENCY

EPIDEMIOLOGY

Acquired lactase deficiency is the most common cause of selective carbohydrate malabsorption. Most individuals, except those of northern European descent, begin to lose lactase activity by the age of 2 years. The prevalence of lactase deficiency is highest (85 to 100%) in persons of Asian, African, and Native-American descent.

PATHOBIOLOGY

The persistence or nonpersistence of lactase activity is associated with a single nucleotide polymorphism C/T_{-13910} that is found upstream of the lactase gene on chromosome 2q21-22. Hypolactasia is associated with the C/C_{-13910} genotype in diverse ethnic groups. The mechanism by which this variant downregulates the lactase gene is not known, but functional studies suggest genotype-dependent alterations in levels of messenger RNA.

Clinical Manifestations

Adults with lactase deficiency typically complain of gas, bloating, and diarrhea after the ingestion of milk or dairy products but do not lose weight. Unabsorbed lactose is osmotically active, drawing water followed by ions into the intestinal lumen. On reaching the colon, bacteria metabolize lactose to short-chain fatty acids, carbon dioxide, and hydrogen gas. Short-chain fatty acids are transported with sodium into colonic epithelial cells, facilitating the reabsorption of fluid in the colon. If the colonic capacity for the reabsorption of short-chain fatty acids is exceeded, an osmotic diarrhea results (see later discussion of carbohydrate malabsorption in watery diarrheas).

Diagnosis

The diagnosis of acquired lactase deficiency can be made by empirical treatment with a lactose-free diet, which results in resolution of symptoms; by the hydrogen breath test after oral administration of lactose; or by genetic testing.[10] Many intestinal diseases cause secondary reversible lactase deficiency, including viral gastroenteritis, celiac disease, giardiasis, and bacterial overgrowth.

CONGENITAL ENTEROPEPTIDASE (ENTEROKINASE) DEFICIENCY

Enteropeptidase is a brush-border protease that cleaves trypsinogen to trypsin, triggering the cascade of pancreatic protease activation in the intestinal lumen. The rare congenital deficiency of enteropeptidase results in inability to activate all pancreatic proteases and leads to severe protein malabsorption. It manifests in infancy as diarrhea, growth restriction, and hypoproteinemic edema.

ABETALIPOPROTEINEMIA

Formation and exocytosis of chylomicrons at the basolateral membrane of intestinal epithelial cells are necessary for the delivery of lipids to the systemic circulation. One of the proteins required for assembly and secretion of chylomicrons is the microsomal triglyceride transfer protein, which is mutated in individuals with abetalipoproteinemia. Children with this disorder have fat malabsorption and the consequences of vitamin E deficiency (retinopathy and spinocerebellar degeneration). Biochemical tests show low plasma levels of apoprotein B, triglyceride, and cholesterol. Membrane lipid abnormalities result in red blood cell acanthosis (burr cells). Intestinal biopsy is diagnostic; the tissue is characterized by engorgement of epithelial cells with lipid droplets. Calories are provided by treatment with a low-fat diet containing medium-chain triglycerides. Poor absorption of long-chain fatty acids sometimes can result in essential fatty acid deficiency. High doses of fat-soluble vitamins, especially vitamin E, often are needed. Mutations in the apolipoprotein B gene (hypobetalipoproteinemia) and intracellular retention of chylomicrons (Anderson disease) cause a similar although less severe clinical syndrome with rare fat malabsorption.

CELIAC DISEASE

DEFINITION AND EPIDEMIOLOGY

Celiac disease is an inflammatory condition of the small intestine precipitated by the ingestion of wheat, rye, and barley in individuals with certain genetic predispositions.[11] Screening studies for the antiendomysial (EMA) and anti–tissue transglutaminase (anti-tTG) antibodies that are associated with celiac disease suggest a prevalence in white populations of approximately 1%. High-risk groups for celiac disease include first-degree relatives and individuals with type 1 diabetes mellitus, autoimmune thyroid disease, primary biliary cirrhosis, Turner syndrome, or Down syndrome. Approximately 20% of patients diagnosed with irritable bowel syndrome or with microscopic (lymphocytic) colitis have celiac disease.

PATHOBIOLOGY

Environmental and genetic factors are important in the development of celiac disease. Approximately 15% of first-degree relatives of affected individuals are found to have celiac disease. Predisposition has been mapped to the human leukocyte antigen (HLA)-D region on chromosome 6. More than 90% of northern Europeans with celiac disease have the DQ2 heterodimer encoded by alleles DQA1*0501 and DQB1*0201, compared with 20 to 30% of controls. A smaller celiac group carries HLA DQ8. Many non-HLA alleles identified in genome-wide association studies account for a small portion of genetic risk. Most such genes are involved in adaptive and innate immune responses. Overlap variants have been identified in diabetes, rheumatoid arthritis, and Crohn disease.

The alcohol-soluble protein fraction of wheat gluten, the gliadins, and similar prolamins in rye and barley trigger intestinal inflammation in susceptible individuals. Oat grains, which have prolamins rich in glutamine but not proline, are rarely toxic. Gliadins and similar prolamins with high proline content are relatively resistant to digestion by human proteases. Many gliadin and prolamin peptides have been identified that stimulate HLA-DQ2 and DQ8 restricted intestinal T-cell clones from individuals with celiac disease. In blood lymphocyte comprehensive screen assays, three immunodominant prolamin peptides have been identified from wheat, barley, and rye in DQ2 celiac individuals; dominant peptides differ in those with DQ8. The DQ2 protein expressed on antigen-presenting cells has positively charged binding pockets; tTG (the autoantigen recognized by EMA) may enhance intestinal inflammation by deamidation of select glutamine residues in gliadin and similar prolamins to negatively charged glutamic acid. In the deamidated form, most gliadin peptides have a higher binding affinity for DQ2 and are more potent stimulants of gluten-sensitized T cells. Villous atrophy may be caused by inflammation that is triggered by γ-interferon released from DQ2- or DQ8-restricted CD4 T cells in the lamina propria. Alternatively, intraepithelial lymphocytes may directly kill intestinal epithelial cells under the influence of IL-15 released from stressed enterocytes.

CLINICAL MANIFESTATIONS

Celiac disease usually manifests early in life, at approximately 2 years of age (after wheat has been introduced into the diet), or later in the second to fourth decades of life, but it can occur at any age.[12] It may first manifest clinically after abdominal surgery or an episode of infectious diarrhea.

Breast-feeding and the time of introduction of wheat in the diet may lessen the risk or delay the onset of celiac disease in infants at risk. Adults with celiac disease in the United States often present with anemia or osteoporosis without diarrhea or other gastrointestinal symptoms. These individuals most likely have proximal disease that impairs iron, folate, and calcium absorption but an adequate surface area in the remaining intestine for absorption of other nutrients. Other extraintestinal manifestations of celiac disease include rash (dermatitis herpetiformis), neurologic disorders (peripheral neuropathy, ataxia, epilepsy), psychiatric disorders (depression, paranoia), reproductive disorders (infertility, spontaneous abortion), short stature, dental enamel hypoplasia, pancreatitis, chronic hepatitis, or cardiomyopathy.

Individuals with significant mucosal involvement present with watery diarrhea, weight loss or growth retardation, and the clinical manifestations of vitamin and mineral deficiencies. Cobalamin deficiency is more common (10% of patients) than previously thought and usually corrects itself on a gluten-free diet. Symptomatic individuals require supplementation of vitamin B_{12}. Diarrhea is caused by many mechanisms, including a decreased surface area for water and electrolyte absorption, the osmotic effect of unabsorbed luminal nutrients, an increased surface area for chloride secretion (crypt hyperplasia), and the stimulation of intestinal fluid secretion by inflammatory mediators and unabsorbed fatty acids. Some individuals have impaired pancreatic enzyme secretion caused by decreased mucosal cholecystokinin release or bacterial overgrowth that may contribute to diarrhea. Individuals with nonceliac gluten sensitivity have wheat-related intestinal and extraintestinal symptoms similar to those of celiac disease but lack intestinal inflammation or celiac serologic markers. Fermentable oligosaccharides, disaccharides, monosaccharides, and polyols (FODMAPs) or gluten may be the offending agent.

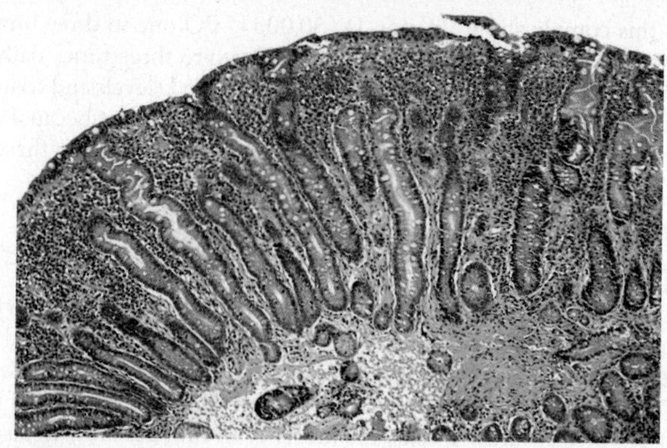

FIGURE 140-5. Intestinal biopsy appearance of flattened villi, hyperplastic crypts, and increased intraepithelial lymphocytes. (Courtesy John Hart, MD.)

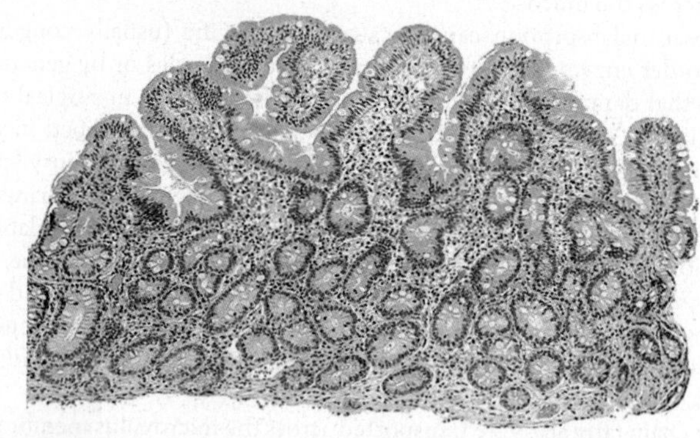

FIGURE 140-6. Regeneration of villi after initiation of a gluten-free diet. (Courtesy of John Hart, MD.)

DIAGNOSIS

Anti-tTG IgA antibody testing, when obtained with a serum IgA level, is a cost-effective strategy for screening high-risk groups; very high titers of the anti-tTG IgA and EMA antibodies are virtually diagnostic of celiac disease. EMA immunoglobulin A (IgA) antibodies, detected by indirect immunofluorescence, are highly sensitive (90%) and specific (95 to 99%) for active celiac disease in skilled laboratory testing. An enzyme-linked immunosorbent assay (ELISA) test to detect antibodies against tTG has equal sensitivity to the EMA test but is less specific. The anti-deamidated gliadin (a biotinylated synthetic γ-gliadin peptide with glutamic acid substituted for glutamine) IgA and IgG antibody immunofluorometric assay has a sensitivity and specificity that approaches that of anti-tTG IgA antibody.[13]

Patients with mild disease may have negative antibody studies. Anti-tTG, gliadin peptide, and EMA IgA antibodies tests are negative in individuals with selective IgA deficiency (present in up to 2.6% of individuals with celiac disease). In these patients, anti-tTG or gliadin peptide IgG antibodies may be helpful in diagnosis and monitoring. In equivocal cases (negative serologic findings and equivocal biopsy result or positive serologic findings and normal biopsy result), HLA genotyping is useful to exclude the diagnosis of celiac disease in persons who lack the DQ2 or DQ8 gene.

The diagnosis of celiac disease is confirmed by characteristic abnormalities seen on a small intestinal biopsy sample and improving when a gluten-free diet is instituted (Figs. 140-5 and 140-6). Biopsy is still required for diagnosis in most adults, who commonly present with atypical symptoms or are asymptomatic first-degree relatives detected by screening. In children, biopsy is not required if the patient has a greater than 5-fold increase in anti-tTG, a positive EMA serologic test, a DQ2 or DQ8 genotype, and typical gastrointestinal symptoms.[14] Mucosal flattening may be observed endoscopically as scalloped or reduced duodenal folds. Characteristic features found on intestinal biopsy include blunted or absent villi, crypt hyperplasia, increased intraepithelial lymphocytes, and infiltration of the lamina propria with plasma cells and lymphocytes. In some individuals, the only abnormal biopsy finding is increased intraepithelial lymphocytes. A hypoplastic mucosa indicates irreversible (end-stage) intestinal disease.

TABLE 140-8 VITAMIN AND MINERAL DOSES USED IN THE TREATMENT OF MALABSORPTION

VITAMIN	ORAL DOSE	PARENTERAL DOSE
Vitamin A*	Water-soluble A, 25,000 U/day†	
Vitamin E	Water-soluble E, 400-800 U/day†	
Vitamin D‡	25,000-50,000 U/day	
Vitamin K	5 mg/day	
Folic acid	1 mg/day	
Calcium§	1500-2000 mg elemental calcium/day Calcium citrate, 500 mg calcium/tablet† Calcium carbonate, 500 mg calcium/tablet†	
Magnesium	Liquid magnesium gluconate† 1-3 tbsp (12-36 mEq magnesium) in 1-2 L of ORS or sports drink sipped throughout the day Magnesium chloride hexahydrate† 100-600 mg elemental magnesium/day	2 mL of a 50% solution (8 mEq) both buttocks IM
Zinc	Zinc gluconate† 20-50 mg elemental zinc/day‖	
Iron	150-300 mg elemental iron/day Polysaccharide-iron complex† Iron sulfate or gluconate	Iron sucrose¶ Sodium ferric gluconate complex¶ Iron dextran (as calculated for anemia) (IV or IM¶; Chapter 159)
B-complex vitamins	1 megadose tablet/day	
Vitamin B_{12}	2 mg/day	1 mg IM or SC/mo**
Copper	copper sulfate 2-3 mg/day	1-2 mg IV/day

IM, intramuscularly; IV, intravenously; ORS = oral rehydration solution; SC = subcutaneously.
*Monitor serum vitamin A level to avoid toxicity, especially in patients with hypertriglyceridemia.
†Form best absorbed or with least side effects.
‡Monitor serum calcium and 25-OH vitamin D levels to avoid toxicity.
§Monitor 24-hr urine calcium to assess adequacy of dose.
‖If intestinal output is high, additional zinc should be given. Monitor for copper deficiency with high doses.
¶Parenteral therapy should be given in a supervised outpatient setting because of the risk for fatal reactions. Decreased risk for fatal reactions when compared with iron dextran.
**For vitamin B_{12} deficiency, 1 mg IM or SC twice per week for 4 wk, then once per month.

TREATMENT Rx

Treatment consists of a lifelong gluten-free diet,[15] and even asymptomatic EMA-positive patients benefit.A10 Wheat, rye, and barley grains should be excluded from the diet. Rice and corn grains are tolerated. Oats (if not contaminated by wheat grain) are tolerated by most. Early referral to a reputable celiac support group or website is often helpful in maintaining dietary compliance. Owing to secondary lactase deficiency, a lactose-free diet should be recommended until symptoms improve. Bone densitometry should be performed on all individuals with celiac disease because up to 70% have osteopenia or osteoporosis. Patients with diarrhea and weight loss should be screened for vitamin and mineral deficiencies. Documented deficiencies of vitamins and minerals should be replenished (Table 140-8), and women of childbearing age should take folic acid supplements. Bone mass often improves on a gluten-free diet alone. Patients with vitamin D or calcium deficiency should receive supplements (Chapter 218), with the dose monitored by 25-OH vitamin D levels and a 24-hour urine test for calcium.

PROGNOSIS

Of patients with celiac disease treated with a gluten-free diet, 90% experience symptomatic improvement within 2 weeks. The most common cause of a poor dietary response is continued ingestion of gluten. Other possibilities include a missed intestinal infection (see later), an alternative diagnosis (e.g., ARB use particularly in elderly patients with a sprue-like enteropathy but negative celiac serologic findings, agammaglobulinemia [diagnosed by hypogammaglobulinemia and lack of plasma cells on small bowel biopsy], autoimmune enteritis [diagnosed by a positive antienterocyte antibody and crypt apoptosis or loss of goblet cells on small bowel biopsy]), bacterial overgrowth, pancreatic insufficiency, microscopic colitis, or other food allergies (cow's milk, soy protein). Up to 40% of patients with celiac disease with symptomatic improvement have incomplete histologic recovery on a gluten-free diet; in such patients, a stricter diet may further improve symptoms and histology. In a small percentage of patients, symptoms and enteropathy do not improve despite a strict gluten-free diet. In such patients, repeat intestinal biopsy is indicated. Some patients will have collagen deposition beneath the surface epithelium (collagenous sprue) or a polyclonal population of intraepithelial lymphocytes (refractory celiac disease type I), Others will have ulcerative jejunitis or a monoclonal population of intraepithelial T cells with an aberrant phenotype or clonal T-cell receptor-γ gene rearrangements (refractory celiac disease type II), which are predictive of enteropathy-associated T-cell lymphoma (Chapter 185) that portends a poor prognosis. Video capsule endoscopy and device-assisted enteroscopy may be helpful in establishing these diagnoses. Patients with collagenous sprue, autoimmune enteritis, or refractory celiac disease type I often respond to prednisone (20 to 40 mg/day PO) or budesonide (9 mg PO daily).

Patients with celiac disease have a higher likelihood of having other autoimmune conditions, such as type 1 diabetes, thyroiditis, rheumatoid arthritis, inflammatory bowel disease, systemic lupus erythematosus, Sjögren syndrome, primary biliary cirrhosis, autoimmune hepatitis, vitiligo, and pancreatitis. Interestingly, approximately one third of patients with idiopathic sporadic ataxia have transglutaminase 6 antibodies, consistent with gluten-induced disease.

Individuals with celiac disease are at increased risk for B-cell lymphoma (Chapter 185),[16] gastrointestinal tract carcinomas (esophageal, small bowel, and colonic adenocarcinomas), and increased mortality; a strict gluten-free diet for life may lessen these risks. Intestinal T-cell lymphoma is rare and should be suspected in individuals who have abdominal pain, recurrence of symptoms after initial response to a gluten-free diet, or refractory celiac disease.

TROPICAL SPRUE

Tropical sprue is an inflammatory disease of the small intestine associated with the overgrowth of predominantly coliform bacteria. It occurs in residents or travelers to the tropics, especially India, Southeast Asia, Puerto Rico, and parts of the Caribbean. With the expansion of tourism and the global economy, this may be an under-recognized cause of enteropathy or mistaken for celiac disease.[17] Individuals classically present with diarrhea and megaloblastic anemia secondary to vitamin B_{12} and folate deficiency, but some have anemia only. Intestinal biopsy characteristically shows subtotal and patchy villous atrophy in the proximal and distal small intestine, which may be caused by the effect of bacterial toxins on gut structure or by the secondary effects of vitamin B_{12} deficiency on the gut (megaloblastic gut). Diagnosis is based on history, documentation of vitamin B_{12} or folate deficiency, and the presence of an abnormal small intestinal biopsy report. Treatment is a prolonged course of tetracycline (250 mg PO four times daily) or doxycycline (100 mg PO two times daily), folic acid (5 mg/day PO), and, with coexistent deficiency, vitamin B_{12} injections (1000 μg weekly) until symptoms resolve. Relapses or reinfection occurs in 20%, mainly in natives of the tropics.

GIARDIA LAMBLIA

Giardia lamblia (Chapter 351) infection, the most common protozoal infection in the United States, can cause malabsorption in individuals infected with many trophozoites, especially the immunocompromised or IgA-deficient hosts. Malabsorption occurs when many organisms cover the epithelium and cause mucosal inflammation, which results in villous flattening and a decrease in absorptive surface area. Stool for ova and parasites at this stage of infection is often negative because of the attachment of organisms in the proximal small intestine. Diagnosis can be made by a stool antigen-capture ELISA test but may require duodenal aspiration and biopsies.

HUMAN IMMUNODEFICIENCY VIRUS

Diarrhea, malabsorption, and wasting are common in individuals with AIDS but are seen less frequently with improved antiretroviral therapy (Chapter 390). In patients who are receiving highly active antiretroviral therapy, diarrhea is more likely to be due to protease inhibitors than to enteric infection.

Malabsorption is usually due to infection with cryptosporidia, *Mycobacterium avium-intracellulare* complex, *I. belli*, or microsporidia. An organism can be identified by stool examination or intestinal biopsy approximately 50% of the time. *AIDS enteropathy* (a term used if no organism is identified) also can cause malabsorption. Mechanisms of malabsorption and diarrhea include villous atrophy, increased intestinal permeability, rapid small bowel transit (in patients with protozoal infection), and ultrastructural damage of enterocytes (in AIDS enteropathy). Among individuals with AIDS and diarrhea, results of fecal fat absorption are frequently abnormal. Serum albumin, vitamin B_{12}, and zinc levels are often low. Vitamin B_{12} deficiency is caused mainly by ileal disease, but low intrinsic factor and decreased transcobalamin II may be contributing factors. Management of malabsorption should focus on restoring the immune system by treating the underlying HIV infection with antiviral therapy. If possible, the offending organism should be treated with antibiotics. If the organism cannot be eradicated, chronic diarrhea and malabsorption result; treatment in these cases consists of antimotility agents and a lactose-free, low-fat diet. Pancreatic enzyme replacement therapy can be tried in HIV-infected individuals who are taking highly active antiretroviral therapy or nucleoside analogues and who have fat malabsorption of obscure origin. If supplemental calories are needed, liquid oral supplements that are predigested and high in medium-chain triglycerides (semi-elemental) are tolerated best. Vitamin and mineral deficiencies should be screened for and treated.

WHIPPLE DISEASE

Whipple disease (Chapters 142 and 275), a rare cause of malabsorption, manifests with gastrointestinal complaints in association with systemic symptoms, such as fever, joint pain, or neurologic manifestations.[18] Approximately one third of patients have cardiac involvement, most commonly culture-negative endocarditis. Occasionally, individuals present with ocular or neurologic disease without gastrointestinal symptoms. Men are affected more commonly than women, particularly white men. The organism responsible for causing Whipple disease is a gram-positive actinomycete, *Tropheryma whippelii.* The epidemiology and pathogenesis of Whipple disease are poorly understood. The prevalence of the disease is higher in farmers than in other workers, which suggests that the organism lives in the soil. Using polymerase chain reaction, *T. whippelii* has been detected in sewage and in duodenal biopsy specimens, gastric juice, saliva, and stool of individuals without clinical disease. Whether the latter represents a carrier state or the presence of nonpathogenic organisms is not known. Immunologic defects, IL-16, and an association with the HLA-B27 gene may be disease factors. Small intestinal biopsy shows villous blunting and infiltration of the lamina propria with large macrophages that stain positive with the periodic acid–Schiff method and are filled with the organism. It is important to distinguish these macrophages from macrophages infected with *M. avium-intracellulare* complex, which stain positive on acid-fast staining and are found in individuals with AIDS. Treatment is with a prolonged course of broad-spectrum antibiotics (e.g., ceftriaxone, 2 g/day intravenously (IV) or meropenem 1 g IV three times daily; then trimethoprim 160 mg and sulfamethoxazole 800 mg PO two times daily for 1 year[A11] or trimethoprim 160 mg and sulfamethoxazole 800 mg PO two times daily for 1 year). Relapses occur, but initial treatment with parenteral ceftriaxone or meropenem appears to be associated with a low relapse rate.

GRAFT-VERSUS-HOST DISEASE

Diarrhea occurs frequently after allogeneic bone marrow or stem cell transplantation (Chapter 178). Immediately after transplantation, diarrhea is caused by the toxic effects of cytoreductive therapy on the intestinal epithelium. From 20 to 100 days after transplantation, diarrhea is usually due to GVHD or infection. Patients with GVHD present clinically with a skin rash, hepatic cholestasis, buccal mucositis, anorexia, nausea, vomiting, abdominal cramps, and diarrhea. The diagnosis of GVHD in the gastrointestinal tract can be made on biopsy of the stomach, small intestine, or colon. In mild cases, the mucosa appears normal on inspection at endoscopy, but apoptosis of gastric gland or crypt cells can be found on biopsy. In severe cases, denudation of the intestinal epithelium results in diarrhea and malabsorption and often requires parenteral nutritional support. Octreotide (50 to 250 μg SC three times daily) may be helpful in controlling voluminous diarrhea. Treatment of GVHD is with steroids and antithymocyte globulin combined with parenteral nutritional support until intestinal function returns.

SHORT-BOWEL SYNDROME

Malabsorption caused by small bowel resection or surgical bypass is called the short-bowel syndrome. The most common causes in the United States are massive resection of the jejunum, owing to strangulated bowel, volvulus, or ischemia (mesenteric or after intra-abdominal surgery), and jejunal exclusion, owing to gastric bypass surgery. Short-bowel syndrome resulting from Crohn disease and radiation enteritis now is less common because of improved medical and radiation therapies. The severity of malabsorption depends on the site and extent of resection; the capacity for hyperplasia,[19] dilation, and elongation; and the function of the residual bowel. Mechanisms of malabsorption after small bowel resection include a decreased absorptive surface area, decreased luminal bile salt concentration, rapid transit, and bacterial overgrowth. Limited jejunal resection usually is tolerated best because bile salt and vitamin B_{12} absorption remain normal. Ileal resection is less well tolerated because of the consequences of bile salt wasting and the limited capacity of the jejunum to undergo adaptive hyperplasia. Adaptive hyperplasia in residual small bowel after resection depends on nutrients, endogenous secretions (pancreatic and biliary juice), local factors (trefoil peptides, prostaglandins, polyamines), growth hormone, and growth factors (epidermal growth factor [EGF], insulin-like growth factor-1 [IGF1], transforming growth factor-α [TGFα], interleukin 11 [IL11]). The glucagon-like peptide 2 (GLP2) produced in L cells in the terminal ileum and colon is a potent stimulant of adaptive hyperplasia in the jejunum in response to a meal, Using intestinal stem cell technology, epithelial organoids have been successfully grown in culture systems.

When less than 100 cm of jejunum remains, the colon takes on an important role in caloric salvage and fluid reabsorption. Malabsorbed carbohydrates are digested by colonic bacteria to short-chain fatty acids, which are absorbed in the colon.

TREATMENT

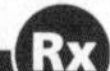

Parenteral nutrition may be avoided by a diet rich in complex carbohydrates, oral rehydration solutions, and acid-reducing and antimotility agents. In comparison, individuals with fewer than 100 cm of jejunum and no colon have high jejunostomy outputs and often require intravenous fluids or parenteral nutrition to survive. These individuals waste sodium, chloride, bicarbonate, magnesium, zinc, and water in their ostomy effluent. Dietary modifications should include a high-salt, nutrient-rich diet given in small meals. An oral rehydration solution with a sodium concentration greater than 90 mmol/L is absorbed best. Oral vitamin and mineral doses higher than the usual U.S. recommended daily allowances are required (Table 140-8). Vitamin B_{12} should be given parenterally (500 to 1000 μg SC every month). Magnesium deficiencies are often difficult to replenish with oral magnesium because of its osmotic effect in the intestinal lumen. A liquid magnesium preparation added to an oral rehydration solution and sipped throughout the day may minimize magnesium-induced fluid losses. Potent antimotility agents, such as tincture of opium (0.5 to 1 mL PO four times daily) or liquid morphine 20 mg/mL (1 mL PO four times daily), often are needed to slow transit and maximize contact time for nutrient absorption. High-volume jejunostomy outputs can be lessened by inhibiting endogenous secretions with a proton pump inhibitor (e.g., omeprazole, 40 mg PO one or two times daily, or lansoprazole, 30 mg PO one or two times daily) and, in severe cases, octreotide (100 to 250 μg SC three times daily; if effective, convert to an equivalent long-acting monthly dosage). The benefit of octreotide may be offset by its potential to inhibit intestinal adaptation and impair pancreatic enzyme secretion with doses greater than 300 μg/day.

In the most severe cases, supplemental calories must be provided by nocturnal tube feeding or parenteral nutrition. Treatment with growth hormone (0.1 mg/kg/day SC) with or without glutamine (30 g/day PO) for 4 weeks may reduce parenteral nutrition requirements in patients who have had massive intestinal resections. Teduglutide (0.05 mg/kg/day SC), a glucagon-like peptide-2 analogue that stimulates adaptive hyperplasia in remnant intestine after resection, reduces parenteral nutrition requirements.[20] Small bowel transplantation should be considered for individuals who require parenteral nutrition to survive and then develop progressive liver disease or venous access problems.[21]

PROGNOSIS

Long-term complications include bone disease, renal stones (oxalate stones if the colon is present, urate stones with a jejunostomy), gallstones, bacterial overgrowth, fat-soluble vitamin deficiencies, essential fatty acid deficiency, and D-lactic acidosis.

Conditions That Impair Nutrient Delivery to the Systemic Circulation

Insoluble lipids (present in chylomicrons) are exocytosed across the basolateral membrane of epithelial cells into the intestinal lymphatics. From there, they enter the mesenteric lymphatics and the general circulation through the thoracic duct. Sugar monomers, amino acids, and medium-chain fatty acids are transported across the basolateral membrane of intestinal epithelial cells into capillaries and into the portal circulation. Sugar monomers are transported across the basolateral membrane by the facilitative glucose transporter isoform (GLUT2) and amino acids by facilitative amino acid carriers (see E-Fig. 140-1C).

IMPAIRED LYMPHATIC DRAINAGE

Diseases that cause intestinal lymphatic obstruction, such as primary congenital lymphangiectasia (malunion of intestinal lymphatics), and diseases that result in secondary lymphangiectasia (lymphoma, tuberculosis, Kaposi sarcoma, retroperitoneal fibrosis, constrictive pericarditis, severe heart failure) result in fat malabsorption. The increased pressure in the intestinal lymphatics leads to leakage and sometimes rupture of lymph into the intestinal lumen, with the loss of lipids, γ-globulins, albumin, and lymphocytes. The diagnosis of lymphangiectasia can be made by intestinal biopsy, but the specific cause may be more difficult to identify. Individuals with lymphangiectasia malabsorb fat and fat-soluble vitamins and have protein loss into the intestinal lumen. The most common presentation is hypoproteinemic edema. Nutritional management includes a low-fat diet and supplementation with medium-chain triglycerides, which are absorbed directly into the portal circulation. Fat-soluble vitamins should be given if deficiencies develop.

WATERY DIARRHEA

Watery diarrhea may be due to osmotic, secretory, inflammatory, or often combined mechanisms (see Fig. 140-3).

Ingestion of Nonabsorbable or Poorly Absorbable Solutes

MAGNESIUM AND SODIUM PHOSPHATE AND SULFATE DIARRHEAS

Magnesium, phosphate, and sulfate are poorly absorbed minerals. Individuals who ingest significant amounts of magnesium-based antacids or high-potency multimineral and multivitamin supplements or those who surreptitiously ingest magnesium-containing laxatives or nonabsorbable anion laxatives, such as Na_2PO_4 (neutral phosphate) or Na_2SO_4 (Glauber or Carlsbad salt) may develop osmotically induced, watery diarrhea that may be high volume.

SORBITOL AND FRUCTOSE DIARRHEA

Dietetic food, chewing gum, candies, and medication elixirs that are sweetened with sorbitol, which is an unabsorbable carbohydrate, can cause diarrhea. Excessive consumption of pears, prunes, peaches, and apple juice, which also contain sorbitol and fructose, a poorly absorbable sugar, can result in diarrhea.[22] Most soft drinks are now sweetened with fructose-containing corn syrup and may be a cause of diarrhea when ingested in high concentrations.

Glucose-Galactose Malabsorption and Disaccharidase Deficiencies

Primary and secondary lactase deficiency is the most common cause of disaccharidase deficiency (see discussion of malabsorption). Congenital lactase deficiency causes diarrhea at birth with the first breast-feed. Congenital sucrose-isomaltose deficiency manifests in infancy when table sugar is introduced into the diet. Glucose-galactose malabsorption is due to mutations in the *SGLT1* gene and causes diarrhea at birth. The mechanism of diarrhea in these disorders is osmotic. Stools are acidic owing to conversion of unabsorbed sugars to short-chain fatty acids in the colon. Treatment is the substitution of fructose for other sugars in the diet. Patients who develop gas, bloating, or diarrhea after the ingestion of mushrooms may have a deficiency in the disaccharidase trehalase.

Rapid Intestinal Transit

A small amount of carbohydrate in the diet is unabsorbed by the normal small intestine. Diets that are high in carbohydrate and low in fat may allow rapid gastric emptying and rapid small intestinal motility, thereby leading to carbohydrate malabsorption and osmotic diarrhea. Rapid transit time also occurs in thyrotoxicosis (Chapter 226). Because of the production of H_2 and carbon dioxide gas by colonic bacteria, abdominal gas and cramping may be the predominant symptoms.

Bile Acid Malabsorption

Ileal malabsorption of bile salts results in the stimulation of colonic fluid secretion and watery diarrhea. Three types of bile acid malabsorption induce diarrhea. Type 1 results when severe disease (e.g., Crohn disease), resection, or bypass of the distal ileum allows bile salts to escape absorption (see earlier). Type 2 may be congenital, rarely, owing to a defect in the apical sodium bile acid transporter, or more commonly may be idiopathic. The idiopathic type has been associated with decreased levels of FGF19, an intestinal fibroblast growth factor that normally downregulates bile salt synthesis in the liver and increased levels of 7-α-hydroxy-4-cholesten-3-one (C4) (a marker of bile acid synthesis) in blood. The result is increased bile salt production that overwhelms reabsorption in the ileum. Type 3 is caused by various conditions, including prior cholecystectomy, celiac disease, pancreatic insufficiency, microscopic colitis, bacterial overgrowth, gastric surgery, or vagotomy. Postulated mechanisms include a bile salt storage problem, increased production, decreased recycling, or saturation of absorption.

TREATMENT Rx

Diarrhea due to types 1 and 2 often responds to cholestyramine (2 to 4 g PO two to four times daily) or the more potent and better tolerated bile salt binder, colesevelam (625-mg tablet PO two to six times daily). Fat-soluble vitamin deficiency is a potential risk with chronic use of bile salt binders. Although many patients with type 3 respond to cholestyramine or colesevelam, some do not. In these patients, motility-altering drugs such as opiates (e.g., loperamide, 2 to 4 mg PO two to four times daily) and anticholinergics (e.g., hyoscyamine sulfate, 0.125 to 0.250 mg PO two to four times daily) may be of benefit.

Functional Watery Diarrhea (Irritable Bowel Syndrome)

See Chapter 137.

TRUE SECRETORY DIARRHEAS

Endocrine diseases that can cause secretory diarrheas (see Fig. 140-3) include carcinoid tumors (Chapter 232), gastrinomas (Chapter 195), VIPomas of the pancreas (Chapter 195), and medullary carcinoma of the thyroid (Chapter 246). Diarrhea is also seen in 60 to 80% of patients with systemic mastocytosis (Chapter 255). Diarrhea resulting from gastrinoma is distinct in that it is caused by high volumes of hydrochloric acid secretion that overwhelm the reabsorptive capacity of the colon and by maldigestion of fat owing to pH inactivation of pancreatic lipase and precipitation of bile salts.

Villous Adenomas

Large (4 to 18 cm) villous adenomas (Chapter 193), particularly in the rectum or occasionally the sigmoid colon, may cause secretory diarrhea of 500 to 3000 mL/24 hours characterized by hypokalemia, chloride-rich stool, and metabolic alkalosis. Increased numbers of goblet cells and increased prostaglandin E_2 are responsible for the diarrhea. Chloride wasting in the stool and metabolic alkalosis are also found in congenital chloridorrhea, which is caused by a defect in the intestinal Cl^-/HCO_3^- transporter. The metabolic alkalosis distinguishes these two diarrheas from most other diarrheas that cause metabolic acidosis. A villous adenoma is usually diagnosed by colonoscopy. The prostaglandin antagonist indomethacin (25 to 100 mg/day PO) reduces the diarrhea in some patients; resection is curative.

Diabetes Mellitus–Related Diarrhea

Constipation is more common than diarrhea in patients with diabetes. High-volume, watery diarrhea, often with nocturnal incontinence, occurs in 20% of patients with poorly controlled type 1 diabetes. These patients usually have concomitant neuropathy, nephropathy, and retinopathy. The diarrhea may be due to several causes, including celiac disease, anal incontinence, bacterial overgrowth related to dysmotility, medications (metformin, acarbose), and autonomic neuropathy. If no specific cause is found, clonidine (initial dose 0.1 mg PO twice daily and titrated slowly to a maximal dose of 0.5 to 0.6 mg PO twice daily) may be helpful. Patients with neuropathy frequently have impaired anal sphincter function, and high-dose loperamide (4 mg PO four times daily) may improve the incontinence.

Alcoholic Diarrhea

Diarrhea related to alcohol ingestion (Chapter 33) may be due to rapid intestinal transit, decreased bile and pancreatic secretion, nutritional deficiencies such as folate or vitamin B_{12}, or alcohol-related enteric neuropathy. Diarrhea may be acute with binge drinking, or it may be chronic and watery and persist for days or weeks. The diarrhea slowly resolves with abstinence from alcohol, proper nutrition, and the repletion of vitamin deficiencies.

Factitious Diarrhea

Approximately 30% of patients referred to tertiary centers have chronic diarrhea from laxative abuse. The diarrhea is usually severe and watery, often with nocturnal symptoms. Some patients may have abdominal pain, weight loss, nausea, vomiting, hypokalemic myopathy, and acidosis. Stool volumes range from 300 to 3000 mL per day depending on the dose of laxative ingested. In the United States, bisacodyl is the most common cause. Other culprits include anthraquinone (senna, cascara, aloe, rhubarb) or osmotic laxatives (neutral phosphate, Epsom salts, and magnesium citrate). Some patients abuse other agents that cause diarrhea, such as the diuretics furosemide and ethacrynic acid.

More than 90% of laxative abusers are women who have underlying eating disorders such as anorexia nervosa or bulimia (Chapter 219) or middle-aged women who have complicated medical histories and who often work in health care. In patients with unexplained diarrhea, laxative screening of stool and urine (see later) should be performed to exclude this syndrome before an extensive medical evaluation is performed for other causes of chronic diarrhea.

Chronic Idiopathic Secretory Diarrhea

In a small subset of patients with secretory diarrhea, no cause is found despite an extensive evaluation. These cases are labeled as chronic idiopathic secretory diarrhea. In most patients, the diarrhea resolves within 6 to 24 months, which suggests a possible postinfectious or Brainerd diarrhea. If no diagnosis is found after thorough testing and a search for surreptitious laxative abuse, a therapeutic trial with bile salt–binding drugs (e.g., cholestyramine, 4 g PO before meals three times daily, or the more potent colesevelam, 625-mg tablet two to six times daily) or opiates (e.g., loperamide, 2 mg PO four times daily, maximal dose 16 mg daily) is warranted.

INFLAMMATORY DIARRHEAS

Diarrhea resulting from inflammation is characterized by watery or bloody stools, fecal leukocytes, and loss of protein in the stool (see Fig. 140-3).

Inflammatory Bowel Disease

See Chapter 141.

Eosinophilic Gastroenteritis

Eosinophilic gastroenteritis is an increasingly recognized condition of unknown etiology characterized by infiltration of eosinophils in the mucosa, muscle, or serosal layers of the gastrointestinal tract.[23] Approximately 50% of patients have atopic histories. Infestation with nematodes (Chapter 357) must be excluded before this diagnosis is made. Diarrhea occurs in 30 to 60% of patients with mucosal disease. Patients with involvement of the muscle layer often present with abdominal pain, nausea, and vomiting indicative of gastric outlet or intestinal obstruction. Peripheral eosinophilia is present in most patients. The disease may involve the entire gastrointestinal tract from esophagus to anus, or it may be isolated to a segment. With diffuse involvement, patients may have steatorrhea, protein-losing enteropathy, and blood loss.

Microscopic (Collagenous and Lymphocytic) Colitis

These two conditions, collectively known as *microscopic colitis,* may or may not be the same disease or variants of the same disease.[24] Lymphocytic colitis is equally prevalent in men and women, whereas collagenous colitis occurs 10 times more often in middle-aged or elderly women. These conditions may be associated with autoimmune disease or with NSAID use. There is an increased prevalence (15%) of microscopic colitis among individuals with celiac disease. These diseases may be categorized as either inflammatory or secretory diarrheas. An epidemiologic relationship to medications such as NSAIDs, H_2-receptor blockers, proton pump inhibitors, selective serotonin reuptake inhibitors, and smoking has been reported, and increased luminal prostaglandin levels may cause the diarrhea. Enteric infections, food hypersensitivity, or intraluminal bile has been proposed as a trigger for prostaglandin release from lymphocytes.

Antidiarrheal agents such as loperamide (2 mg PO four times daily) are the mainstay of therapy, and the disease usually has a benign and self-limiting course.[25] Budesonide (9 mg PO daily) is the most effective therapy.A12 In patients who do not tolerate or respond to it, alternatives include bismuth subsalicylate therapy (8 chewable 262-mg tablets PO daily) and 5-aminosalicylates (e.g., mesalamine, 400 to 800 mg PO three times daily). Patients with refractory disease may require corticosteroids (e.g., prednisone, 40 mg/day PO), a trial of azathioprine or anti–TNF-α antibodies, or, as a last resort, fecal stream diversion surgery.

Food Allergy

Food allergies or sensitivities, especially to cow's milk and soy protein, are a well-established cause of enterocolitis in children, with an estimated frequency of 5%. Symptoms of abdominal cramps, diarrhea, and sometimes vomiting occur shortly after ingestion of the allergen (Chapter 253). The role of food allergy in causing diarrhea in adults is less clear owing to the lack of a reliable diagnostic test. Allergy testing correlates poorly with intestinal allergy. The most common food allergens are milk, soy, eggs, seafood, nuts, and wheat. Sequential elimination diets can be diagnostic and therapeutic.

RADIATION ENTERITIS

Patients who receive pelvic radiation for malignancies of the female urogenital tract or the male prostate may develop chronic radiation enterocolitis 6 to 24 months after total doses of radiation greater than 40 to 60 Gy (Chapters 20 and 142), but symptoms can develop as late as 20 years after treatment. Early abnormalities include an increase in inflammatory mediators, an increase in cholinergic stimulation of intestinal tissue, and endothelial cell apoptosis that precedes epithelial cell apoptosis. The last finding suggests that vascular injury is the primary event. Diarrhea may be caused by bile acid malabsorption if the ileum is damaged, by bacterial overgrowth if radiation causes small intestinal strictures or bypass, or by radiation-induced chronic inflammation of the small intestine and colon. Rapid transit also may contribute to malabsorption and diarrhea.

TREATMENT Rx

Treatment is often unsatisfactory. Anti-inflammatory drugs (sulfasalazine, corticosteroids) and antibiotics have been tried with little success. Cholestyramine (4 g PO three times daily) and NSAIDs (e.g., naproxen, 250 to 500 mg PO twice daily) may help, as may opiates (loperamide, 2 mg PO four times daily, or loperamide-*N*-oxide, 3 mg PO two times daily).

PROTEIN-LOSING GASTROENTEROPATHY

Severe protein loss through the gastrointestinal tract can be caused by mucosal diseases such as lymphangiectasia, lymphatic obstruction, bacterial or parasitic infection, gastritis (Chapter 139), gastric cancer, collagenous colitis, inflammatory bowel disease (Chapter 141), celiac disease, sarcoidosis (Chapter 95), lymphoma (Chapter 185), tuberculosis (Chapter 324), Ménétrier disease (Chapter 192), eosinophilic gastroenteritis, and food allergies. A variety of extraintestinal diseases, including systemic lupus erythematosus (Chapter 266), heart failure (Chapter 58), and constrictive pericarditis (Chapter 77), also can be causative. Patients with systemic lupus erythematosus (Chapter 266) may present with protein-losing enteropathy as the only manifestation of their disease. Treatment focuses on the underlying disease.

MISCELLANEOUS DISEASES

Although acute mesenteric arterial or venous thrombosis manifests as an acute bloody diarrhea, chronic mesenteric vascular ischemia (Chapter 143) may manifest as watery diarrhea. Gastrointestinal tuberculosis (Chapter 324) and histoplasmosis (Chapter 332) manifest as diarrhea that may be either bloody or watery, as do certain immunologic diseases, such as Behçet syndrome or Churg-Strauss syndrome. All of these diseases may be misdiagnosed as inflammatory bowel disease (Chapter 141). Neutropenic enterocolitis, an ileocolitis that occurs in patients with neutropenia and leukemia, sometimes is caused by *C. difficile* infection.

TREATMENT OF CHRONIC DIARRHEA Rx

Antidiarrheal Therapy

Antidiarrheal agents are of two types: those used for mild to moderate diarrheas and those used for severe secretory diarrheas. A major shortcoming of opiates, the most commonly prescribed antidiarrheal agents, is that they have no antisecretory effect. Rather, they act by decreasing intestinal motility, thereby allowing longer contact time with the mucosa for improved fluid absorption. The exception is racecadotril, an enkephalinase inhibitor, that blocks intestinal fluid secretion without affecting motility.

Bulk-forming agents (psyllium, 7 g in 8 oz water PO up to five times daily] and methylcellulose [3 to 6 tablets twice daily with 300 mL of water]) act by binding water and increasing the consistency of stool. Pectin has been shown to have proabsorptive activity. These agents may be useful in patients with fecal incontinence. Bismuth subsalicylates (524 mg PO every hour up to eight doses daily) have mild antisecretory and antimotility effects and are effective and safe in mild diarrheas.

The opiates may be symptomatically useful in mild to moderate diarrheas. Paregoric, deodorized tincture of opium, codeine, and diphenoxylate with atropine largely have been supplanted by loperamide. Loperamide does not pass the blood-brain barrier and has a high first-pass metabolism in the liver; it has a high therapeutic-to-toxic ratio and is essentially devoid of addiction potential. It is safe in adults, even in total doses of 24 mg/day. The usual dose is 2 to 4 mg two to four times daily. Opiates may be harmful in patients with severe diarrheas because large volumes of fluid may pool in the intestinal lumen (third space), and stool output is no longer a reliable gauge for replacing fluid losses. The antimotility effects are a problem in infectious diarrheas because stasis may enhance bacterial invasion and delay clearance of microorganisms from the bowel. Opiates and anticholinergics also are dangerous in severe inflammatory bowel disease or severe *C. difficile* infection, where they may precipitate megacolon.

Antidiarrhea agents that are used for the treatment of severe secretory and inflammatory diarrheas generally have profiles with more serious side effects. The somatostatin analogue octreotide (initial dose, 100 to 600 µg SC in two to four divided doses daily; maximal dose, 1500 µg daily) lessens diarrhea in the carcinoid syndrome and in neuroendocrine tumors because it inhibits hormone secretion by the tumor. It is also effective in the treatment of dumping syndrome and chemotherapy-related diarrheas. Long-acting subcutaneous octreotide preparations (20 to 30 mg intramuscularly intragluteally every month) are now available for once-a-month dosing. Octreotide can suppress pancreatic enzyme secretion and make diarrhea worse; it also may be of only limited usefulness in short-bowel syndrome and AIDS diarrhea. Agents such as phenothiazine and calcium-channel blockers have mild antisecretory effects, but side effects limit their use. Clonidine (initial dose, 0.1 mg PO twice daily, titrated slowly to a maximal dose of 0.5 to 0.6 mg twice daily) is most useful in opiate withdrawal diarrhea and is sometimes useful in diabetic diarrhea; postural hypotension may limit its use, particularly in patients with diabetes. Alosetron (0.5 mg PO twice daily for 4 weeks, maximal dose 1 mg PO twice daily) may be justified for severe diarrhea-predominant irritable bowel syndrome; associations with ischemic colitis and severe constipation have limited its use. Indomethacin (250 to 500 mg PO twice daily), a cyclooxygenase blocker that inhibits prostaglandin production, is useful in the treatment of diarrheas caused by acute radiation, AIDS, or villous adenomas of the rectum or colon; occasionally, it may be useful in neuroendocrine tumors and food allergy. For eosinophilic gastroenteritis, corticosteroids (prednisone, 20 to 40 mg/day PO for 7 to 10 days) are the mainstay of therapy, but disodium cromoglycate (200 mg PO four times daily) also may be useful; food elimination diets are not usually effective. Treatment of inflammatory bowel disease is described in Chapter 141.

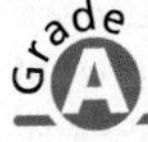

Grade A References

A1. Lowy I, Molrine DC, Leav BA, et al. Treatment with monoclonal antibodies against *Clostridium difficile* toxins. *N Engl J Med*. 2010;362:197-205.

A2. van Nood E, Vrieze A, Nieuwdorp M, et al. Duodenal infusion of donor feces for recurrent *Clostridium difficile*. *N Engl J Med*. 2013;368:407-415.

A3. Richardson V, Hernandez-Pichardo J, Quintanar-Solares M, et al. Effect of rotavirus vaccination on death from childhood diarrhea in Mexico. *N Engl J Med*. 2010;362:299-305.

A4. Sur D, Lopez AL, Kanungo S, et al. Efficacy and safety of a modified killed-whole-cell oral cholera vaccine in India: an interim analysis of a cluster-randomised, double-blind, placebo-controlled trial. *Lancet*. 2009;374:1694-1702.

A5. Hu Y, Ren J, Zhan M, et al. Efficacy of rifaximin in prevention of travelers' diarrhea: a meta-analysis of randomized, double-blind, placebo-controlled trials. *J Travel Med*. 2012;19:352-356.

A6. Alajbegovic S, Sanders JW, Atherly DE, et al. Effectiveness of rifaximin and fluoroquinolones in preventing travelers' diarrhea (TD): a systematic review and meta-analysis. *Syst Rev*. 2012;1:39.

A7. DuPont HL, Jiang ZD, Okhuysen PC, et al. A randomized, double-blind, placebo-controlled trial of rifaximin to prevent travelers' diarrhea. *Ann Intern Med*. 2005;142:805-812.

A8. Allen SJ, Wareham K, Wang D, et al. Lactobacilli and bifidobacteria in the prevention of antibiotic-associated diarrhoea and *Clostridium difficile* diarrhoea in older inpatients (PLACIDE): a randomised, double-blind, placebo-controlled, multicentre trial. *Lancet*. 2013;382:1249-1257.

A9. Lauritano EC, Gabrielli M, Scarpellini E, et al. Antibiotic therapy in small intestinal bacterial overgrowth: rifaximin versus metronidazole. *Eur Rev Med Pharmacol Sci*. 2009;13:111-116.

A10. Kurppa K, Paavola A, Collin P, et al. Benefits of a gluten-free diet for asymptomatic patients with serologic markers of celiac disease. *Gastroenterology*. 2014;147:610-617.

A11. Feurle GE, Junga NS, Marth T. Efficacy of ceftriaxone or meropenem as initial therapies in Whipple's disease. *Gastroenterology*. 2010;138:478-486.

A12. Miehlke S, Madisch A, Kupcinskas L, et al. Budesonide is more effective than mesalamine or placebo in short-term treatment of collagenous colitis. *Gastroenterology*. 2014;146:1222-1230.

GENERAL REFERENCES

For the General References and other additional features, please visit Expert Consult at https://expertconsult.inkling.com.

141

INFLAMMATORY BOWEL DISEASE

GARY R. LICHTENSTEIN

DEFINITION

Inflammatory bowel disease refers to two chronic idiopathic inflammatory disorders, ulcerative colitis and Crohn disease. Characteristic clinical, endoscopic, and histologic features are critical for the diagnosis of these disorders, but no single individual finding is absolutely diagnostic for one disease or the other. Ulceration from Crohn disease may be transmural and may occur anywhere in the gastrointestinal tract, most commonly in the distal ileum and proximal colon. The hallmark of ulcerative colitis is continuous ulceration starting in the rectum and limited to the colon. Approximately 10% of patients with inflammatory bowel disease have indeterminate colitis, a term used when Crohn colitis cannot be distinguished from ulcerative colitis.

EPIDEMIOLOGY

Inflammatory bowel disease occurs worldwide, but the highest incidence is found in North America, the United Kingdom, and northern Europe. Data suggest an increasing incidence and prevalence over time and in different regions around the world, although ulcerative colitis remains slightly more prevalent than Crohn disease.[1] The incidence of ulcerative colitis in North America is estimated to be 19.3 per 100,000 person years and 24.3 per 100,000 person years in Europe, with a prevalence of approximately 250 per 100,000 persons in North America and 500 per 100,000 persons in Europe. The incidence of Crohn disease in North America is estimated to be 20.2 per 100,000 person years and 12.7 per 100,000 person years in Europe, with a prevalence of approximately 320 per 100,000 in North America and in Europe.

Crohn disease and ulcerative colitis may occur at any age, but both have their peak incidence in the second to fourth decade, with a second peak in the seventh decade. The female-to-male ratio for both ulcerative colitis and Crohn disease suggests no gender preference.

Crohn disease and ulcerative colitis are polygenic disorders, for which family history is a risk factor. Crohn disease and ulcerative colitis occur in all ethnic and socioeconomic groups, but their incidence is highest in white Caucasians and Jewish people of Eastern European (Ashkenazi) descent. In North America and the United Kingdom, however, the incidence of Crohn disease in African Americans and African Caribbeans appears to be approaching that of whites. Studies of migrants from underdeveloped countries in South Asia to the United Kingdom suggest an increased prevalence of inflammatory bowel disease in subsequent generations, presumably as a result of environmental influences.

Cigarette smoking is associated with a worse prognosis in patients with Crohn disease but an improved course in ulcerative colitis. Nonsteroidal anti-inflammatory drugs (NSAIDs) appear to be associated with new onset of inflammatory bowel disease and with exacerbations of disease. Appendectomy has been suggested as protective against the development of ulcerative colitis. Diet does not clearly affect the course of inflammatory bowel disease.

PATHOBIOLOGY

Although the trigger for inflammatory bowel disease is not known, three major pathways likely activate the disease: a genetic predisposition, immune dysregulation, and an environmental antigen. A possible explanation is that the inability of the innate immune system to clear microbial antigens, combined with increased intestinal epithelial permeability to antigens, eventually leads to an overactive adaptive immune response.

Genetics

Of patients with inflammatory bowel disease, 5 to 20% have another family member with inflammatory bowel disease. First-degree relatives have a 10- to 15-fold increased risk for developing inflammatory bowel disease. The concordance rate of developing Crohn disease in identical twins, siblings, and first-degree relatives is 50%, 0 to 3%, and 5 to 10%, respectively. Ulcerative colitis follows similar genetic patterns but with slightly lower risk rates. Twenty percent of patients with a positive family history of inflammatory bowel disease will have discordant disease type: one family member with Crohn disease and another with ulcerative colitis.

More than 163 gene susceptibility loci have been linked to inflammatory bowel disease, with at least 30 specific for Crohn disease and more than 20 specific for ulcerative colitis. Some of these genes also may correlate with the severity of disease. The first gene discovered to be associated with Crohn disease was *NOD2/CARD15*, which is located on chromosome 16 (16q12) and expressed in intestinal epithelial Paneth cells, macrophages, and dendritic cells. This gene is involved in the expression of an intracellular receptor that senses muramyl dipeptide, a peptidoglycan component of gram-positive bacteria. Activation of *NOD2* leads to activation of nuclear factor κ-B (NF-κB), which mediates transcription of numerous proinflammatory cytokines. A mutation in the leucine-rich domain of the NOD2 protein, which interacts with bacterial lipopolysaccharide, leads to failure in activation of NF-κB and is associated with the development of Crohn disease.

The *ATG16L1* gene on chromosome 2 and the *IRGM* gene on chromosome 5 also have been associated with increased susceptibility to Crohn disease. Both are members of a family of genes involved in autophagy, an autonomous process that involves the maintenance of cellular homeostasis and organelle turnover, as well as the processing of intracellular pathogens, the subsequent presentation of antigens, and the regulation of cell signaling. Toll-like receptor-4 gene polymorphisms are associated with both Crohn disease and ulcerative colitis. Polymorphisms of the interleukin-23 (IL-23) receptor gene are associated with ulcerative colitis and a varied risk for Crohn disease. Human leukocyte antigen (HLA) class II polymorphisms, especially in HLA-DR molecules, may confer increased risk for ulcerative colitis and possibly Crohn as well. The *OCTN1* gene, located on chromosome 5q31, and the *DLG5* gene, located on chromosome 10, have been found to be associated with Crohn disease. *DLG5*, which encodes a scaffolding protein that is important for maintaining epithelial integrity in various organs, may interact with the *NOD2/CARD15* gene to increase susceptibility to Crohn disease. *OCTN1* encodes for an ion channel and also increases the risk for Crohn disease; mutations in this gene may disrupt ion channels through altered function of cation transporters and cell-to-cell signaling in the intestinal epithelium.

Inflammatory bowel disease also has been associated with Turner syndrome (Chapter 233), glycogen storage type Ib (Chapter 207), and the Hermansky-Pudlak syndrome (triad of albinism, platelet aggregation defect, and accumulation of ceroid-like pigment in tissue; and Chapter 173). Inflammatory bowel disease is associated with various diseases that have known genetic predisposition, including ankylosing spondylitis (Chapter 265), psoriasis (Chapter 438), atopy (Chapter 249), eczema (Chapter 438), celiac sprue (Chapter 140), cystic fibrosis (Chapter 89), primary sclerosing cholangitis (Chapter 155), multiple sclerosis (Chapter 411), autoimmune thyroid disease (Chapter 226), autoimmune hemolytic anemia (Chapter 160), primary biliary cirrhosis (Chapter 155), myasthenia gravis (Chapter 422), and Cogan syndrome (Chapter 270).

PATHOPHYSIOLOGY

Microbes likely play a part in the development of inflammatory bowel disease. In several animal models of colitis, colitis does not develop in a sterile environment but can be induced after the introduction of commensal bacteria. Diverting the fecal stream away from active mucosal inflammation, such as in an ileostomy, also helps alleviate inflammation in Crohn disease. Crohn disease and ulcerative colitis preferentially occur in the terminal ileum and colon, which contain the highest concentration of bacteria, on the order of approximately 10^{12} organisms per gram of luminal contents. Antibiotics, particularly antibiotics with broad-spectrum anaerobic coverage, are helpful in the treatment of Crohn disease. More recently, several genetic polymorphisms associated with sensing the intestinal microbial environment and triggering an immune response have been linked to inflammatory bowel disease.

Both Crohn disease and ulcerative colitis are products of a dysregulated innate immune system that triggers T cells and a humoral response. T_H17 cells, which are activated in Crohn disease and ulcerative colitis, are stimulated by IL-23, which is produced by antigen-presenting cells.

Pathology

Crohn Disease

As a result of a dysregulated immune system, patients with Crohn disease develop aphthous ulcers, which are superficial mucosal ulcers. As the disease progresses, the ulceration becomes deeper, transmural, and discrete; it may form a serpiginous pattern and may occur anywhere from the esophagus to the anus in a noncontinuous pattern. The most common location for ulceration is the ileocecal region. In some patients, chronic disease leads to the formation of fibrotic strictures, and approximately 30% of patients may develop fistulas.

In early Crohn disease, the histopathologic findings are characterized by an acute inflammatory infiltrate in the lamina propria, with cryptitis, and crypt abscesses. Later in the disease process, the crypt architecture becomes distorted, with a lymphocytic infiltrate and a resulting branching and shortening of the crypts. Noncaseating granulomas, which are present in up to 15% of endoscopic biopsy specimens and as many as 70% of surgical specimens, are not unique to Crohn disease but help confirm the diagnosis when other classic features are present.

Surgical specimens also may show transmural intestinal wall inflammation and fat creeping on the serosal surface.

Ulcerative Colitis

In mild ulcerative colitis, the mucosa is granular, hyperemic, and edematous in appearance. As the disease becomes more severe, the mucosa ulcerates, and the ulcers may extend into the lamina propria. Ulcerative colitis starts in the rectum and may extend proximally in a continuous pattern, but it affects only the colon. Pseudopolyps may form owing to epithelial regeneration after recurrent acute attacks. With chronic disease, the colonic mucosa may lose the normal fold pattern, the colon may shorten, and the colon may appear narrowed.

In early ulcerative colitis, the histopathologic findings are characterized by epithelial necrosis, an acute inflammatory infiltrate in the lamina propria, cryptitis, and crypt abscesses. In chronic disease, a predominant lymphocytic infiltrate and distortion of crypt architecture are seen.

CLINICAL MANIFESTATIONS

Symptoms of inflammatory bowel disease are varied and may be a consequence of the location of the disease, the duration of disease, and any anatomic complications of the disease, such as strictures and fistulas in Crohn disease (Table 141-1).

Symptoms

Crohn Disease

The terminal ileum is affected in about 70% of patients with Crohn disease. Primary ileal disease occurs in 30% of patients, whereas ileocolonic disease occurs in 40%. Symptoms may include abdominal pain, typically in the right lower quadrant, diarrhea, hematochezia, and fatigue. With more severe disease, fever and weight loss may be present. Some patients may present with obstructive symptoms, such as abdominal pain, abdominal distention, and nausea.

Only approximately 5% of patients develop Crohn disease in the upper gastrointestinal tract, and esophageal Crohn disease occurs in less than 2% of patients. Subjects with upper gastrointestinal Crohn disease may present with dysphagia, odynophagia, chest pain, or heartburn. Gastroduodenal disease occurs in 0.5 to 4% of patients and commonly occurs along with distal disease. Symptoms may include upper abdominal pain. Isolated jejunal disease is rare; if the jejunum is involved, there is also distal small bowel

TABLE 141-1 CLINICAL CHARACTERISTICS OF CROHN DISEASE AND ULCERATIVE COLITIS

CHARACTERISTICs	CROHN DISEASE	ULCERATIVE COLITIS
Peak age of onset (years of age)	15-30, 2nd peak in the 7th decade	20-40, 2nd smaller peak beyond the 7th decade
Sex distribution (F/M)	1.2/1	1/1
Potential sites of gastrointestinal involvement	Esophagus to anus	colon
Skipped areas of involvement	+	–
Transmural inflammation	+	–
Type of ulceration	Usually discrete	Continuous
Fistula	+	–
Stricture	–	–
Perianal disease (fissure, skin tags)	+	–

involvement. Up to 30% of patients have perianal disease (Chapter 145) that may include the development of fistulas, abscesses, fissures, and skin tags. Symptoms of perianal disease include pain and discharge. Fever may be present if there is an abscess.

Fistulas, which are internal tracts that can occur anywhere in the gastrointestinal tract and connect to various sites, occur in 20 to 40% of Crohn patients. Penetrating Crohn disease also may cause intra-abdominal and perianal abscesses owing to a fistula with a blind end or intestinal perforation. External fistulas, which present with symptoms of fluid discharge from the cutaneous opening, can be enterocutaneous or perianal. Internal fistulas can be enteroenteric, rectovaginal, or enterocolonic. Patients may present with persistent abdominal pain and fever with an abscess in this location.

Ulcerative Colitis

As with Crohn disease, symptoms and signs of ulcerative colitis depend on the extent and severity of disease. At the time of diagnosis, 14 to 37% of patients have pancolitis, 36 to 41% have disease extending beyond the rectum, and 44 to 49% have proctosigmoiditis. Symptoms include hematochezia, diarrhea, tenesmus, production of excessive mucus, urgency to defecate, and abdominal pain. In the setting of proctitis or proctosigmoiditis, patients may have constipation with difficulty defecating. With more extensive and severe colonic involvement, patients also may have weight loss and fever. They also may have nausea and vomiting because of abdominal pain, fatigue because of anemia, and peripheral edema because of hypoalbuminemia.

Physical Examination

Signs on physical examination are representative of the type of disease as well as its location and severity. Oral ulcers may be present in Crohn disease. The location of abdominal tenderness usually reflects the location of intestinal involvement. In Crohn disease, abdominal tenderness is classically in the right lower quadrant and may include fullness or a mass depending on the severity of inflammation. Peritoneal signs may occur when penetrating Crohn disease causes intestinal perforation. Rectal examination may reveal skin tags, hemorrhoids, fissure, and fistulae.

Extraintestinal Manifestations

Arthropathy, the most common extraintestinal manifestation (Table 141-2), affects up to 10 to 20% of subjects.[2] Peripheral arthralgias, arthritis, ankylosing spondylitis (Chapter 265), and sacroiliitis may exacerbate with gastrointestinal symptoms. Dermatologic disorders, such as erythema nodosum (10 to 15%; see Fig. 440-24) and pyoderma gangrenosum (1 to 2%; Chapter 261), develop in up to 15% of patients. Eye disorders, especially uveitis and episcleritis (Chapter 423), may occur in 5 to 15%. Patients with inflammatory bowel disease also have up to a 10% risk for renal calculi, especially calcium oxalate stones (Chapter 126), in the setting of fat malabsorption with Crohn disease in the small bowel. Uric acid stones can occur in the setting of severe volume depletion. Patients with inflammatory bowel disease, especially patients with ulcerative colitis, are at increased risk for primary sclerosing cholangitis—2 to 7.5% of patients develop this disorder, and 70-80% of patients with this disorder have inflammatory bowel disease (Chapter 155).

Extraintestinal Complications

Patients with inflammatory bowel disease are susceptible to extraintestinal complications from the disease itself or medications used to treat disease. These complications include osteoporosis, osteomalacia, arthritic complications, thromboembolic events, pulmonary disease, and renal, dermatologic, and neurologic complications. Osteoporosis occurs in approximately 15% of patients, and steroid therapy (Chapter 35) is the major risk factor; avascular necrosis of the hip and septic arthritis are unusual complications of steroids or other immunosuppressive therapies. Cheilitis may be a result of iron deficiency anemia (Chapter 159). Patients with inflammatory bowel disease are at an increased risk for thromboembolic disease, especially in the setting of active intestinal disease, even when compared with other autoimmune diseases such as rheumatoid arthritis and celiac disease. Secondary amyloidosis with renal involvement can be a consequence of chronic inflammation. Asthma is the most common pulmonary disorder observed in association with Crohn disease. Patients also are at risk for multiple sclerosis (Chapter 411) and for peripheral neuropathy (Chapter 420) from vitamin B_{12} deficiency, which may occur as a result of poor absorption owing to active small bowel disease or surgical resection.

DIAGNOSIS

When diarrhea (Chapter 140) is the predominant symptom, the initial evaluation should include a thorough medical history, testing for infectious colitis (Chapter 140), and screening for endocrine-metabolic disorders such as hyperthyroidism (Chapter 226) and hypocalcemia (Chapter 245). Infections with organisms such as *Shigella* (Chapter 309), *Amoeba* (Chapter 352), *Giardia* (Chapter 351), *Escherichia coli* O157:H7 (Chapter 304), and *Campylobacter* (Chapter 303) can be accompanied by bloody diarrhea, abdominal cramps, and an endoscopic mucosal appearance identical to that of ulcerative colitis. Stool studies are needed to diagnose or exclude these infections. If hematochezia and abdominal pain are the predominant symptoms, the differential diagnosis is broad (Table 141-3).

TABLE 141-2 EXTRAINTESTINAL COMPLICATIONS OF INFLAMMATORY BOWEL DISEASE

COMPLICATIONS	CROHN DISEASE	ULCERATIVE COLITIS
Ocular disorders (uveitis, episcleritis)	+	+
Arthropathy	+	+
Oral ulcers	+	–
Skin disorders (pyoderma gangrenosum, erythema nodosum)	+	+
Nephrolithiasis	+	+
Primary sclerosing cholangitis	+	+
Bone disorders (osteoporosis, osteomalacia)	+	–
Thromboembolic disease	+	+
B_{12} deficiency	+	–

TABLE 141-3 DIFFERENTIAL DIAGNOSIS OF ILEITIS AND COLITIS

INFECTIONS	**MEDICATIONS/TOXINS**
BACTERIAL	NONSTEROIDAL ANTI-INFLAMMATORY DRUGS
Aeromonas	PANCREATIC ENZYME SUPPLEMENTS—FIBROSING COLOPATHY
Campylobacter jejuni	PHOSPHOSODA BOWEL PREPARATIONS
Chlamydia (proctitis)	RADIATION
Clostridium difficile	**INFLAMMATORY**
Mycobacterium tuberculosis	APPENDICITIS
Salmonella	DIVERTICULAR DISEASE
Shigella	EOSINOPHILIC GASTROENTERITIS
Enterohemorrhagic *Escherichia coli*	NONGRANULOMATOUS ULCERATIVE JEJUNOILEITIS (CELIAC DISEASE)
Yersinia	**NEOPLASIA**
VIRAL	CARCINOID
Cytomegalovirus	CARCINOMA PRIMARY OR METASTATIC
Herpes simplex virus (proctitis)	LYMPHOMA
Human immunodeficiency virus	MYCOSIS FUNGOIDES
FUNGAL	MALIGNANT HISTIOCYTOSIS
Histoplasma capsulatum	**MISCELLANEOUS**
PARASITIC	AMYLOIDOSIS
Entamoeba histolytica	SARCOIDOSIS
Helminths	ENDOMETRIOSIS
VASCULAR	TUBO-OVARIAN ABSCESSES
COLLAGEN VASCULAR DISEASE	
Behçet disease	
Churg-Strauss syndrome	
Henoch-Schönlein purpura	
Systemic lupus erythematosus	
Polyarteritis nodosa	
ISCHEMIA	

Modified from Aberra FN, Lichtenstein GR. Crohn disease. In Talley NJ, Kane SV, Wallace MD, eds. *Practical Gastroenterology and Hepatology: Small and Large Intestine.* Wiley-Blackwell, 2010:225-235.

Diagnostic Evaluation

Endoscopic Evaluation

In a patient with symptoms suggestive of inflammatory bowel disease and no evidence for an infection to explain the symptoms, endoscopic evaluation is essential. Colonoscopy is the initial endoscopic test for patients who present with lower gastrointestinal symptoms such as diarrhea and hematochezia, except in the presence of acute severe peritoneal symptoms. Colonoscopy to the terminal ileum is important if there is a potential diagnosis of inflammatory bowel disease. Small bowel imaging (such as small bowel follow-through or computed tomography [CT] enterography) also may be needed to determine whether there is small bowel disease or to determine the distribution of disease. Capsule endoscopy is useful if all other endoscopic and radiologic testing is nondiagnostic, but Crohn disease of the small bowel is still suspected. Findings on capsule endoscopy should be followed by endoscopy to obtain biopsies. Capsule endoscopy should not be performed if Crohn disease is complicated by a known small bowel stricture.

Crohn Disease

Early endoscopic findings in Crohn disease include superficial small mucosal ulcers, also called aphthous ulcers. As the severity of Crohn disease progresses, the ulcerations become deeper and may become round, linear, or serpiginous. Intersecting longitudinal and transverse ulcers cause a cobblestone mucosal appearance, with "stone" areas representing normal mucosa (Fig. 141-1). Areas of ulceration, which are typically interspersed with normal "skip" areas, may occur anywhere from the esophagus to anus but are most common in the ileocecal region. Isolated colonic disease occurs in 25% of patients, and 60% will have rectal involvement, thereby making it at times difficult to differentiate from ulcerative colitis.

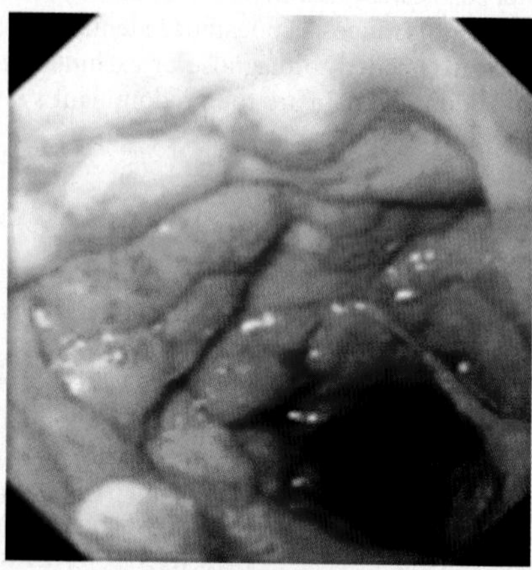

FIGURE 141-1. Endoscopic appearance of Crohn disease with cobblestoning.

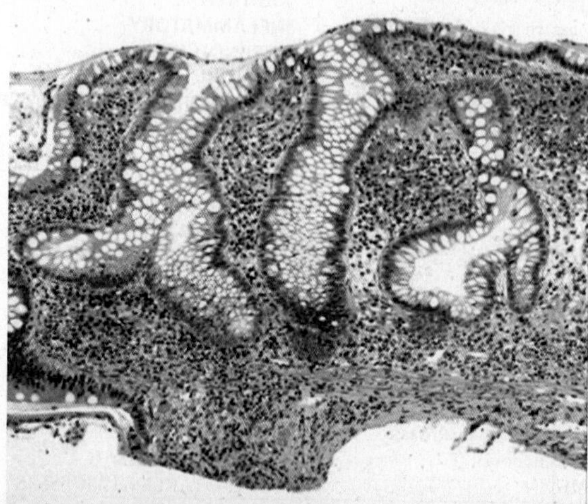

FIGURE 141-2. In ulcerative colitis, histopathology from colonic biopsies reveals features of crypt distortion and lymphocytic infiltration in the mucosa. (Modified from AGA Institute GastroSlides 2010.)

The diagnosis of inflammatory bowel disease is contingent upon accurate histopathologic results, so biopsy of the affected area(s) is key. Findings of an inflammatory infiltrate in the lamina propria and distortion of the crypt architecture support the diagnosis (Fig. 141-2). The diagnosis of Crohn disease may be made by histopathologic examination alone if noncaseating granulomas are seen, but granulomas are rarely found on endoscopic biopsies. The diagnosis of Crohn disease is usually based on a combination of information gleaned from histopathologic findings, colonoscopy, and small bowel imaging. A skip pattern of ulceration, ulceration in the small bowel or upper gastrointestinal tract, or the presence of fistulas support the diagnosis of Crohn disease. Colonic and small bowel ulceration occur in several other disorders, including infections that may not be detected by routine stool studies (such as enterohemorrhagic *E. coli*), vascular disorders, immune-related enterocolitis, neoplasia, diverticulitis, radiation, and medications such as NSAIDs (Table 141-3).

Ulcerative Colitis

The diagnosis of ulcerative colitis is based on endoscopic findings and histopathology. Early in the disease process, patients develop diffuse mucosal erythema with loss of the normal mucosal vascular pattern. In mild disease, the mucosa may have a granular and edematous appearance. As the disease becomes more severe, the mucosa becomes more friable, bleeds easily when the mucosa is touched, and may eventually ulcerate (Fig. 141-3). Endoscopic findings, which start in the rectum and may extend proximally in a continuous pattern, affect only the colon. The term "backwash ileitis" describes a spillover effect from ulcerative colitis and should not be construed as actual involvement of the terminal ileum by ulcerative colitis. Pseudopolyps may form owing to epithelial regeneration after recurrent attacks in patients with long-standing disease. With chronic disease, the colonic mucosa may lose its normal fold pattern, and the colon may shorten and appear narrowed. A new endoscopic index based on the observed vascular pattern, bleeding, and ulceration shows promise for grading the severity of ulcerative colitis and assessing its response to treatment.[3]

Features such as crypt distortion, continuous mucosal inflammation starting from the rectum, absence of granulomas, and absence of small bowel disease are consistent with ulcerative colitis. Early in the disease process, chronic inflammatory findings, such as crypt distortion, may not be present, and the diagnosis may be more difficult to confirm.

Radiology

Radiologic imaging is vital and almost always should be obtained when inflammatory bowel disease, particularly Crohn disease, is suspected. Barium studies such as an upper gastrointestinal series, small bowel follow-through, and barium enema are usually necessary to diagnose fistulas and strictures in Crohn disease. If Crohn disease is suspected by colonoscopic examination, a small bowel follow-through is generally obtained to assess the extent, severity, and type of disease (strictures and fistulas) in the small intestine. CT enterography and magnetic resonance imaging (MRI) enterography are alternatives to a small bowel follow-through. CT enterography may be preferred for the detection of abdominal abscesses, whereas MRI may be preferred for the detection of perineal abscesses and strictures.

Laboratory Findings

Anemia may result from chronic disease, blood loss, or nutritional deficiencies of iron, folate, or vitamin B_{12}. A modestly elevated leukocyte count is

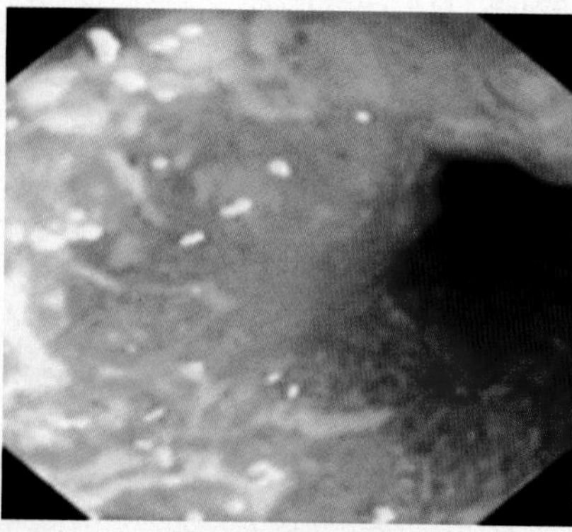

FIGURE 141-3. Endoscopic appearance of ulcerative colitis.

indicative of active disease, but a marked elevation suggests an abscess or another suppurative complication. The erythrocyte sedimentation rate and C-reactive protein are nonspecific serum inflammatory markers that are commonly used to monitor the activity of disease. Hypoalbuminemia is an indication of malnutrition and is common with active disease. Ileal disease or resection of more than 100 cm of distal ileum results in a diminished serum vitamin B_{12} level because of malabsorption.

Serologic Markers

Serologic markers are supportive but may not be used independently to diagnose inflammatory bowel disease. Anti–*Saccharomyces cerevisiae* antibodies (ASCA), which are antibodies to yeast, are present in 40 to 70% of patients with Crohn disease and in less than 15% of patients with ulcerative colitis. The combination of elevated ASCA immunoglobulin A (IgA) and IgG titers is highly specific for Crohn disease, ranging from 89 to 100%. Perinuclear antineutrophil cytoplasmic antibodies (pANCA) are present in 20% of Crohn patients, primarily in colon-predominant disease, and in 55% of patients with ulcerative colitis. ASCA-positive and pANCA-negative disease are associated with a sensitivity of 55% and specificity of 93% for Crohn disease. The antimicrobial antibodies anti-I2 (Crohn disease–related protein from *Pseudomonas fluorescens*), anti-Cbir1 (flagellin-like antigen), and anti-OmpC (*E. coli* outer membrane porin C) are also associated with Crohn disease.

TREATMENT

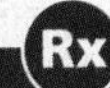

The aim of medical therapy is to reduce inflammation and subsequently induce and maintain clinical remission. Medications used to treat inflammatory bowel disease include the categories of 5-aminosalicylate (5-ASA), antibiotics, corticosteroids, immunomodulators, and biologics (infliximab, adalimumab, certolizumab pegol, golimumab, vedolizumab, and natalizumab (Table 141-4).[4] The specific medical therapy selected is based on the location, extent (nonpenetrating and nonstricturing, stricturing, and penetrating and fistulizing disease), and severity of disease (Fig. 141-4; see Fig. 141-3). Supportive medical therapy, such as antidiarrheal and antispasmodic medications, also may be used.

Categories of Medical Therapy

5-Aminosalicylate

5-ASA, which acts as a topical anti-inflammatory within the lumen of the intestine, is used to treat mild to moderate ulcerative colitis and as maintenance therapy for patients in remission.[A1] Sulfasalazine is the combination of a sulfapyridine with 5-ASA; 5-ASA is responsible for the anti-inflammatory property of this drug, whereas sulfapyridine is the carrier that allows 5-ASA to be delivered into the colon. Other oral formulations of 5-ASA allow it to be delivered to the intestine by different mechanisms. Mesalamine is released in the intestine based on a pH delivery model, whereas sulfasalazine, olsalazine, and balsalazide are released in the intestine by bacterial cleavage of a covalent bond between 5-ASA and a prodrug. For rectal and sigmoid disease, 5-ASA suppository and enema preparations are also effective for induction and maintenance of remission in patients with ulcerative colitis.[A2][A3] Adverse events associated with 5-ASAs are rare and may include nausea, dyspepsia, hair loss, headache, worsening diarrhea, and hypersensitivity reactions.

Corticosteroids

Corticosteroids are primarily used to treat flares of ulcerative colitis and Crohn disease. Oral formulations may be used for mild to moderate disease, whereas systemic corticosteroids are used for moderate to severe disease.

TABLE 141-4 MEDICAL THERAPIES FOR INFLAMMATORY BOWEL DISEASE

DRUG	DOSE	RELEASE SITE
5-AMINOSALICYLATES		
Sulfasalazine (Azulfidine)	2-6 g/day	Colon
Mesalamine (Asacol, Lialda, Apriso)	2.4-4.8 g/day	Distal ileum, colon
Olsalazine (Dipentum)	1-3 g/day	Colon
Balsalazide (Colazal)	6.25 g/day	Colon
Mesalamine (Pentasa)	2-4 g/day	Duodenum, jejunum, ileum, colon
Mesalamine (Rowasa), enema, suppository	4 g/day (enema) 1 g/day (suppository)	Rectum/sigmoid Rectum
Mesalamine (Canasa), suppository	1 g/day (suppository)	Rectum
CORTICOSTEROIDS		
Budesonide (Entocort EC)	Induction: 9 mg PO daily Maintenance: 6 mg PO daily	Small intestine
Budesonide (MMX, UCERIS)	Induction 9 mg PO daily	Colon
Prednisone	0.25-0.75 mg/kg PO daily	Systemic
Methylprednisolone	40-60 mg IV daily	Systemic
IMMUNOMODULATORS		
6-Mercaptopurine	1.5 mg/kg/day	Systemic
Azathioprine	2.5 mg/kg/day	Systemic
Methotrexate	Induction: 25 mg SC weekly × 4 mo. Maintenance: 15-25 mg SC weekly	Systemic
Cyclosporine	2-4 mg/kg/day IV	Systemic
BIOLOGICS		
Infliximab	Induction: 5 mg/kg IV weeks 0, 2, 6 Maintenance: 5-10 mg/kg IV every 8 weeks	Systemic
Adalimumab	Induction: 160 mg SC week 0, 80 mg week 2 Maintenance: 40 mg SC every other week	Systemic
Golimumab	Induction: 200 mg SC week 0 and 100 mg week 2 Maintenance: 100 mg SC every 4 weeks	Systemic
Certolizumab pegol	Induction: 400 mg SC weeks 0, 2, 4 Maintenance: 400 mg SC every 4 weeks	Systemic
Natalizumab	300 mg IV every 4 weeks	Systemic
Vedolizumab	Induction: 300 mg IV at 0, 2, and 6 weeks Maintenance: 300 mg IV every 8 weeks	Systemic

IV = intravenously; PO = orally; SC = subcutaneously.

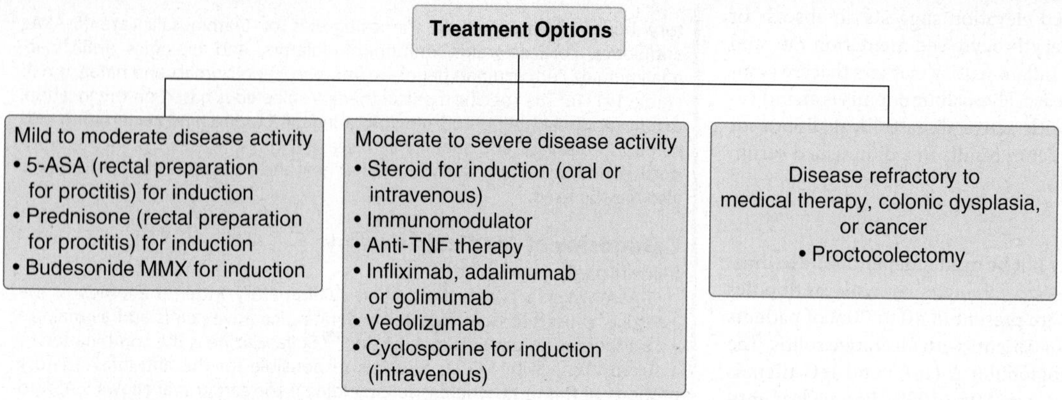

Treatment Options

Mild to moderate disease activity	Moderate to severe disease activity	Disease refractory to medical therapy, colonic dysplasia, or cancer
• 5-ASA (rectal preparation for proctitis) for induction • Prednisone (rectal preparation for proctitis) for induction • Budesonide MMX for induction	• Steroid for induction (oral or intravenous) • Immunomodulator • Anti-TNF therapy • Infliximab, adalimumab or golimumab • Vedolizumab • Cyclosporine for induction (intravenous)	• Proctocolectomy

FIGURE 141-4. Ulcerative colitis treatment algorithm.

Enteric-coated budesonide, a pH-dependent ileal release formulation, is an oral corticosteroid with high topical activity and low systemic bioavailability (10%). Enteric-coated budesonide is indicated for treatment of active mild to moderate ileocecal Crohn disease. Budesonide MMX is a budesonide formulation that is released in the colon and is available for treatment of mild to moderately active ulcerative colitis. Oral corticosteroids such as prednisone and methylprednisolone are used for moderate to severe disease, starting at doses ranging from 40 to 60 mg/day. Intravenous methylprednisolone is used for severe disease, with dosing ranging from 40 to 60 mg/day. Maintenance with systemic corticosteroids is not recommended because of their substantial side effects (Chapter 35).

Immunomodulatory therapy

In patients who remain symptomatic despite 5-ASA therapy or who have moderate to severe Crohn disease or ulcerative colitis, the thiopurine analogues (6-mercaptopurine and azathioprine) may be used.[A4] Methotrexate also may be used for moderate to severe Crohn disease.[A5] Azathioprine, the prodrug of 6-mercaptopurine, typically is prescribed at a dose of 2 to 3 mg/kg/day; the equivalent dose of 6-mercaptopurine is 1.5 mg/kg/day. A disadvantage of the thiopurine analogues is the slow clinical response that may not be evident for as long as 12 weeks. Their side effects include allergic reactions, pancreatitis, myelosuppression, nausea, infections, hepatotoxicity, and malignancy, especially lymphoma.[5] The white blood cell count and liver chemistries must be monitored routinely. Methotrexate, which is a folic acid antagonist, is given as 25 mg intramuscularly (IM) or subcutaneously (SC) once per week for 16 weeks for active Crohn disease and, 15 mg to 25 mg IM or SC once per week for maintaining remission.

Antibiotics

The exact mechanism for the beneficial effect of broad-spectrum antibiotics in the treatment of inflammatory bowel disease is not known. Potential mechanisms include eliminating bacterial overgrowth, eradicating a bacterially mediated antigenic trigger, and potential immunosuppressive properties (e.g., metronidazole). The primary role of antibiotics is in Crohn disease, where metronidazole (10 to 20 mg/kg/day for 4 to 8 weeks), ciprofloxacin (500 mg orally (PO) twice daily for 4 to 8 weeks), or both are primary inductive therapies for perianal fistulae and fissures.[A6] Metronidazole also may be a helpful adjunctive treatment for colonic Crohn disease and to prevent postoperative recurrence in Crohn disease as well. In addition, a novel enteric form of rifaximin may be of benefit for mild to moderate Crohn disease.

Biologicals

Anti–Tumor Necrosis Factor-α Agents

Monoclonal antibody therapy directed against tumor necrosis factor-α (anti–TNF-α) include infliximab, which is a chimeric mouse-human IgG1 monoclonal antibody that is approved to treat moderate to severe Crohn disease, fistulizing Crohn disease, and moderate to severe ulcerative colitis that has failed to respond to conventional therapy. Adalimumab (Humira) and certolizumab pegol (Cimzia) have been approved to treat moderate to severe Crohn disease that has failed to respond to conventional therapy, and adalimumab (Humira) and golimumab (Simponi) have been approved to treat moderate to severe ulcerative colitis that has failed to respond to conventional therapy. Adalimumab and golimumab are fully human IgG1 antibodies that are self-administered subcutaneously. Certolizumab pegol, which is a chimeric pegylated Fab fragment to TNF-α, also is administered subcutaneously. Before anti-TNF therapy is considered, risk versus benefit needs to be assessed in each individual patient, given the potential risk for infection and malignancy.[6]

Antiadhesion Molecules

Natalizumab, a humanized IgG4 monoclonal antibody, binds to the α_4 subunit of $\alpha_4\beta_1$ and $\alpha_4\beta_7$ integrins expressed on all leukocytes except neutrophils. Natalizumab inhibits the interactions between α_4 integrins on the surface of leukocytes and adhesion molecules on vascular endothelial cells in the gastrointestinal tract, thereby preventing adhesion and recruitment of leukocytes. Natalizumab is approved for the treatment of moderate to severe Crohn disease that is refractory to other therapies, but there are strict guidelines for prescribing natalizumab because of its associated risk for progressive multifocal leukoencephalopathy (Chapter 370).

Another small adhesion molecule, vedolizumab, is approved for patients with moderate to severe ulcerative colitis and adult patients with moderate to severe Crohn disease when one or more standard therapies (corticosteroids, immunomodulators, or TNF blocker medications) have not provided an adequate response. Because this agent is gut-selective and is not associated with impairment of central nervous system immunosurveillance, the risk for progressive multifocal leukoencephalopathy appears to be very low in this molecule.

Crohn Disease Medical Therapy

Mild to Moderate Crohn Disease

Sulfasalazine (3 to 6 g/day), is superior to placebo for treating active ileocolonic and colonic Crohn disease, with response rates ranging from 45 to 55% for mild to moderate disease, but is not clearly effective for small bowel disease alone (Fig. 141-5).[7] Mesalamine may provide a modest benefit compared with placebo for mild to moderate disease. However, the 5-ASAs are not effective for maintaining remission in Crohn disease. In a phase 2 randomized trial of patients with moderately active Crohn disease (800 mg of extended intestinal release rifaximin twice daily for 12 weeks) induced remission in 63% of patients compared with 43% of controls, with few adverse events. For mild to moderate Crohn disease involving the distal small intestine or proximal colon budesonide (9 mg/day) provides approximately a 70% response rate after 8 weeks and is significantly more effective than mesalamine (4 g/day) for distal ileal and right colonic disease.[A7] As a maintenance agent at 3 or 6 mg, the effects of budesonide wane and disappear within 1 year.

Upper gastrointestinal Crohn disease (jejunal, duodenal, gastric, and esophageal) is uncommon, and few clinical trials are available to assess therapies for this location. Because local therapies such as 5-ASAs and budesonide are not released in these locations, systemic immunosuppressants (azathioprine, mercaptopurine, infliximab, adalimumab, and certolizumab pegol) are the mainstays of therapy.

Moderate to Severe Crohn Disease

Patients with moderate to severe disease are initially treated with systemic corticosteroids, but corticosteroids should not be used as maintenance therapy. Options to induce a remission or maintain a steroid-induced remission include 6-mercaptopurine, azathioprine, methotrexate, infliximab, adalimumab, and certolizumab. Infliximab (5 mg/kg at 0, 2, and 6 weeks and then every 8 weeks) alone or infliximab plus azathioprine (2.5 mg/kg/day) is more effective than azathioprine alone,[A8] and initial combined therapy (corticosteroids, daily azathioprine, and infliximab) is preferable to reserving it only for patients who do not respond to corticosteroids plus azathioprine or who have aggressive disease.[8] Infliximab therapy also can decrease the need for hospitalization and surgery.[A9]

Of patients with Crohn disease who are treated for at least 1 year with infliximab and an antimetabolite agent, approximately 50% will experience a relapse within 1 year after discontinuation of infliximab. Patients who do not respond to conventional therapy, including an anti-TNF agent, may be considered for natalizumab.

For severe Crohn disease, patients should be hospitalized, given nothing by mouth, rehydrated with intravenous fluids, and administered parenteral corticosteroids. Patients who respond to parenteral corticosteroids should be switched to high-dose oral corticosteroids (prednisone, 40 to 60 mg/day), with the dose of prednisone gradually reduced. Patients who have severe Crohn disease and who do not respond to parenteral corticosteroids within a week should be considered for either infliximab or surgery.[9] A course of total parenteral nutrition (Chapter 217) may be useful as adjunctive therapy.

Fistulizing Crohn Disease

Fistulas (Chapter 145) occur in one third of patients with Crohn disease, and perianal fistulas represent the most common location. Asymptomatic internal fistulas rarely require therapy. A concomitant abscess, which may occur in the

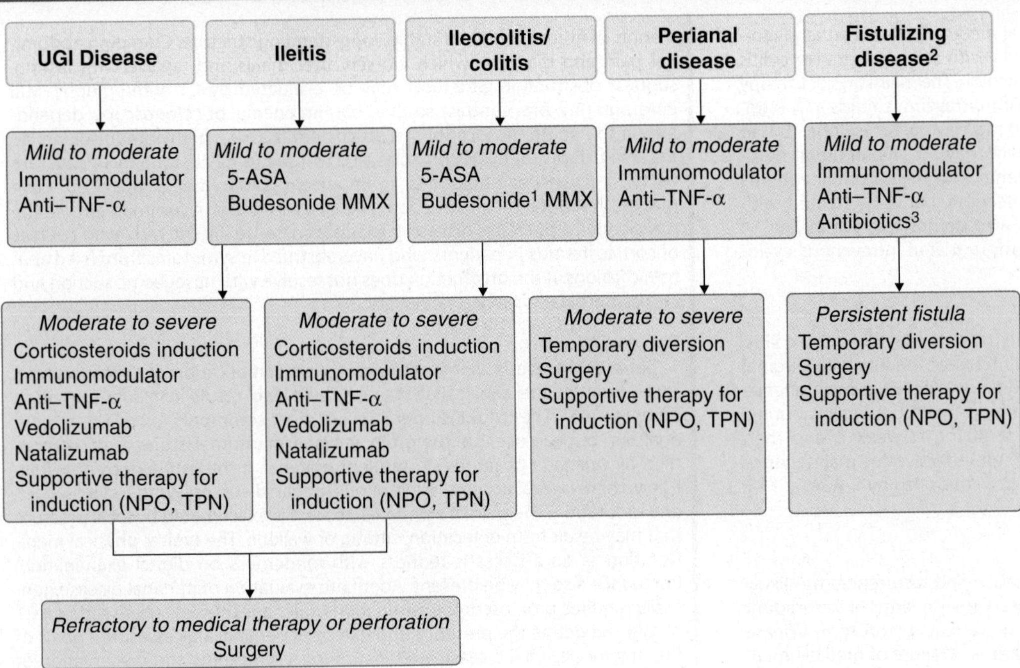

FIGURE 141-5. **Crohn disease treatment algorithm.** NPO = nothing by mouth; TNF-α = tumor necrosis factor-α; TPN = total parenteral nutrition; UGI = upper gastrointestinal.

setting of a fistula, must be excluded before initiating immunosuppressive therapy. Surgery may be required. Medical treatment depends on the location and associated complications.

High-output enterocutaneous fistulas in the setting of proximal small bowel involvement can lead to outputs of more than 500 mL/day and can cause severe volume depletion. Initial management requires volume repletion. In the postoperative setting, a fistulous opening is usually in the area of a wound, and it is imperative to protect the healing skin from infection caused by the drainage from either an ostomy bag or a catheter used for a high-output fistula. High-output fistulas will rarely close spontaneously and typically will require surgical closure. Low-output fistulas may be treated initially with azathioprine (or 6-mercaptopurine), methotrexate, or anti–TNF-α therapy (infliximab, adalimumab, or certolizumab).

Perianal fistulas are classified into simple and complex (Chapter 145). A simple fistula is located below the dentate line (i.e., most of the anal sphincter) and has one track. A complex fistula passes through the intersphincteric (high location), transsphincteric, or suprasphincteric region and may have multiple tracks. Simple fistulas respond well to medical therapy, initially with metronidazole (10 to 20 mg/kg/day PO for 4 to 8 weeks) and ciprofloxacin (500 mg PO twice daily for 4 to 8 weeks) for the fistula and treatment of concurrent mucosal disease. Treatment with immunomodulators or anti–TNF-α agents is also beneficial. Patients with fistulas without rectal mucosal Crohn disease may respond well to fistulotomy, whereas patients with mucosal involvement may benefit from seton placement rather than fistulotomy. Complex fistulas usually require a combination of surgical and medical therapy. In the setting of intractable disease, colonic or ileal diversion may allow for rectal and perianal healing; in severe cases, proctocolectomy may be necessary.

For Crohn disease–related rectovaginal fistulas, medical therapy with antimetabolite therapy or anti–TNF-α agents is usually considered before surgery. Surgical therapy such as fistulotomy and mucosal flap may be considered.

Enterovesicular or colovesicular fistulas may be treated with antimetabolite therapy or anti–TNF-α agents, or both, but recurrent urinary tract infection is an indication for surgery. Surgery usually involves resection of involved bowel and closure of the bladder defect.

Asymptomatic internal fistulas such as enteroenteric fistulas, do not require surgical intervention, but treatment with an immunomodulator may be considered. Internal fistulas, such as cologastric and coloduodenal, may cause substantial symptoms because of bypass of part of the intestine. If medical management fails or if an abscess forms, surgery is recommended.

Medical Management of Ulcerative Colitis

The anatomic distribution of ulcerative colitis guides therapy. Options include suppositories, retention enemas, topical foam, oral therapy, and parenteral therapy. Suppositories are effective to treat proctitis in the distal 20 cm of the colon. Topical foam and enemas are effective for distal and left-sided colitis. Oral therapy and parenteral therapy are effective for all locations of disease.

Proctitis

For active ulcerative proctitis, topical 5-ASA (enema and suppository) in combination with oral treatment is superior to oral treatment alone.[10] Topical 5-ASA is superior to topical corticosteroids for treatment of active ulcerative proctitis, rectal 5-ASA therapy produces a faster response when given with oral 5-ASA. Corticosteroid enemas, suppositories, or foam also can be used if 5-ASA fails. 5-ASA or corticosteroid retention enemas can be used for active disease up to the splenic flexure (i.e., the rectum, sigmoid colon, and descending colon). Another approach to proctitis or distal colitis is an oral aminosalicylate, although a response may not be evident for 3 to 4 weeks. Additionally, once-a-day extended-release budesonide (budesonide MMX) is effective for mild to moderately active ulcerative proctosigmoiditis, with fewer steroid-related side effects than conventional corticosteroids.[A10]

Extensive Colitis

In patients with ulcerative colitis of mild to moderate activity and extension of disease proximal to the splenic flexure, the initial drug of choice is an oral 5-ASA; efficacy increases with increasing doses. Even with more extensive disease, supplementation of oral 5-ASA with 5-ASA enemas or suppositories may help reduce the symptoms of urgency that result from rectal involvement, and budesonide MMX provides incremental benefit. In patients with more than five or six bowel movements per day, in patients in whom a more rapid response is desired, or in patients who have not responded to 3 to 4 weeks of 5-ASA, the treatment of choice is oral prednisone. Patients with severe diarrhea, systemic symptoms, or significant amounts of blood in their stool should be started on 40 mg/day; most patients respond to oral corticosteroids within a few days. After the symptoms are controlled, prednisone can be tapered gradually by 5 mg every 1 to 2 weeks. Patients who respond to oral prednisone and can be fully withdrawn from it should be maintained on 5-ASA.

If patients with severe ulcerative colitis do not begin to respond to corticosteroids at the equivalent dose of methylprednisolone 60 mg IV within 5 days or do not completely respond within 7 to 10 days, options include colectomy, infliximab, or cyclosporine. In a phase 2 trial, tofacitinib (an oral inhibitor of Janus kinases at doses ranging from 0.5 mg to 15 mg twice daily for 8 weeks) improved symptoms in patients with moderate to severe active ulcerative colitis. For patients whose disease flares whenever the corticosteroids are withdrawn or their corticosteroid dose is lowered, the continuation of high-dose corticosteroid therapy is the most common management error. In patients whose disease flares when their steroid dose is reduced, a trial of an immunomodulator (azathioprine or 6-mercaptopurine), infliximab, adalimumab, golimumab, or vedolizumab should be attempted. If the patient requires a substantial dose (>15 mg/day of prednisone) for more than 6 months, a trial of an immunomodulator, infliximab, adalimumab, golimumab, or vedolizumab should be considered for maintenance of remission,[A11] and attempts should be made to reduce the steroid dose.

The most common indication for hospitalization in patients with ulcerative colitis is intractable diarrhea, although blood loss is also common. Patients with severely active ulcerative colitis should be evaluated for toxic megacolon by abdominal radiography or CT. Antidiarrheal medications and anticholinergic medications are contraindicated in patients with severe ulcerative colitis because of the risk for precipitating toxic megacolon. The mainstays of therapy for severe ulcerative colitis are rehydration with intravenous fluids and intravenous corticosteroids (hydrocortisone, 300 mg/day; prednisolone, 60 to 80 mg/day; or methylprednisolone, 40 to 60 mg/day). Total parenteral nutrition (Chapter 217) may be necessary in patients with malnutrition. Patients with peritoneal signs or signs of systemic infection should be treated with parenteral antibiotics (Chapter 142). Patients who do not improve in 7 to 10 days should be considered for either colectomy, a trial of intravenous cyclosporine, or a trial of infliximab.

Maintenance Therapy

Aminosalicylates reduce recurrent disease in patients with ulcerative colitis, and essentially all patients should receive maintenance therapy with original or newer 5-ASA preparations. Corticosteroids are not effective as maintenance therapy and should not be used in this way. Azathioprine,[A12] 6-mercaptopurine, infliximab,[A13] adalimumab (160 mg at week 0, 80 mg at week 2, and then 40 mg every other week), and golimumab[A14] are effective for maintenance therapy in patients whose ulcerative colitis is not controlled by 5-ASA.

Surgical Therapy

Crohn Disease

Surgical resection does not cure Crohn disease and recurrences are likely after resection, so the approach should be conservative in terms of the amount of bowel resected. Nevertheless, nearly 50% of patients with Crohn disease undergo surgery within 10 years of their diagnosis.[11] Failure of medical management is a common cause for resection in patients with Crohn disease, but complications (e.g., obstruction, fistula, and abscess) are often the indications for resection. For Crohn disease of the small bowel, the most common surgical procedure is segmental resection for obstruction or fistula; the incidence of a recurrence severe enough to require repeat surgery after ileal or ileocolic resection is approximately 25% after 10 years and 35% after 15 years. For patients with extensive colonic disease that includes the rectum, the procedure of choice is total proctocolectomy with a Brooke (end) ileostomy. Total colectomy with ileal pouch anal anastomosis is not appropriate in Crohn colitis because recurrence of Crohn disease in the ileal segment of the new pouch would require a repeat operation and loss of a long segment of ileum.

Ulcerative Colitis

For ulcerative colitis, colectomy is a curative procedure. Approximately 40% of patients with extensive ulcerative colitis eventually undergo colectomy, usually because their disease has not responded adequately to medical therapy. Emergency colectomy may be required in patients with toxic megacolon or a severe fulminant attack without toxic megacolon. The standard operation for ulcerative colitis is proctocolectomy and a Brooke ileostomy. The most popular alternative operation is total proctocolectomy with an ileal pouch anal anastomosis. In this procedure, a pouch is constructed from the terminal 30 cm of ileum and the distal end of the pouch is pulled through the anal canal. Ileoanal anastomosis is sometimes complicated by inflammation in the ileal pouch (termed *pouchitis*), which can be treated with antibiotics (typically, metronidazole, 500 mg three times daily or 20 mg/kg/day, or ciprofloxacin, 500 mg twice daily for 2 weeks). The decision for or against colectomy and among types of surgery is influenced by the patient's age, social circumstances, and duration of disease, and this decision requires expert consultation. When other indications are equivocal, the risk for malignancy (see later) may be an indication for colectomy.

Complications

Crohn Disease

Abscesses

Abscesses, which are common complications in Crohn disease, result from extension of a mucosal fissure or ulcer through the intestinal wall and into extraintestinal tissue. Leakage of intestinal contents through a fissure into the peritoneal cavity results in an abscess. Abscesses occur in 15 to 20% of patients with Crohn disease, especially in the terminal ileum. The typical clinical manifestation of an intra-abdominal abscess is fever, abdominal pain, abdominal tenderness, and leukocytosis. A CT scan is the preferred modality to diagnose intra-abdominal abscess. Broad-spectrum antibiotic therapy, including anaerobic coverage, is indicated. Percutaneous drainage of abscesses in patients with Crohn disease may improve the clinical picture but does not provide adequate therapy because of persistent communication between the abscess cavity and the intestinal lumen. Resection of the involved intestine is usually required for definitive therapy.

Obstruction

Obstruction is a common complication of Crohn disease, particularly in the small intestine, and is a leading indication for surgery. In Crohn disease, small bowel obstruction may be caused by mucosal thickening from acute inflammation, by muscular hyperplasia and scarring as a result of previous inflammation, or by adhesions. Obstruction also may occur because of impaction of a bolus of fibrous food in a stable, long-standing stricture. Cramping abdominal pain and diarrhea, which worsen after meals and resolve with fasting, suggest obstruction. Strictures may be evaluated by CT enterography, MRI enterography, oral contrast studies, barium enema, or colonoscopy, depending on the anatomic location.[12] Corticosteroids (e.g., methylprednisolone, 40 to 60 mg/day IV, or hydrocortisone, 200 to 300 mg/day IV for 5 to 14 days) are useful if acute inflammation is an important component of the obstructive process, but not if the obstruction is caused by fibrosis. A common error in the management of Crohn disease is inappropriate treatment with long courses of corticosteroids in patients who have obstructive symptoms from fixed anatomic lesions. If the obstruction does not resolve with nasogastric suction and corticosteroids, surgery is necessary.

Perianal Disease

Perianal disease is a potentially disabling complication of Crohn disease. Ulcerations in the anal canal may coalesce and result in fistula formation (Chapter 145). The fistulous openings are most commonly found in the perianal skin but can occur in the groin, vulva, or scrotum. Fistulas are accompanied by drainage of serous or purulent material. If the fistula does not drain freely, there is local accumulation of pus (perianal abscess) with redness, pain, and induration. The pain of a perianal abscess is exacerbated by local pressure that may result from defecation, sitting, or walking. The typical physical manifestation of an abscess is redness with tenderness on digital examination; fluctuance also may be present. Adequate evaluation of perianal disease generally requires proctoscopic examination under anesthesia. Cross-sectional CT or MRI can define the presence and extent of perianal abscesses. The goals of therapy for perianal disease are relief of local symptoms and preservation of the sphincter. Limited disease can be approached with sitz baths and metronidazole, but most cases also require adequate external drainage. Azathioprine, infliximab, adalimumab, or certolizumab pegol may be useful in healing perianal disease, but the disease may reactivate when the drug is stopped. Persistent severe perianal Crohn disease can result in destruction of the anal sphincter and subsequent fecal incontinence.

Ulcerative Colitis

One of the most significant complications of ulcerative colitis is toxic megacolon, which is dilation of the colon to a diameter greater than 6 cm associated with worsening of the patient's clinical condition and the development of fever, tachycardia, and leukocytosis. Physical examination may reveal postural hypotension, abdominal tenderness over the distribution of the colon, and absent or hypoactive bowel sounds. Agents that reduce gastrointestinal motility, such as antispasmodics and antidiarrheal agents, are likely to initiate or exacerbate toxic megacolon. Medical therapy is designed to reduce the likelihood of perforation and return the colon to normal motor activity as rapidly as possible. The patient is given nothing by mouth, and nasogastric suction is begun. Intravenous fluids should be administered to replete water and electrolyte abnormalities, broad-spectrum antibiotics (e.g., ampicillin-sulbactam, given as 1 g ampicillin plus 0.5 g sulbactam, 1.5 to 3 g every 6 hours for 5 to 14 days; levofloxacin, 500 mg/day IV, plus metronidazole, 500 mg IV or PO twice daily; cefazolin, 500 mg IV three times daily, plus metronidazole, 500 mg IV or PO twice daily; or trimethoprim-sulfamethoxazole, 8 to 10 mg/kg/day IV or PO in two to four divided doses, plus metronidazole, 500 mg IV or PO twice daily for approximately 7 days or until symptomatic improvement) are given in anticipation of possible peritonitis as a result of perforation, and parenteral corticosteroids are administered at a dose equivalent to more than 40 to 60 mg of prednisone per day. Signs of improvement include a decrease in abdominal girth and the return of bowel sounds. Deterioration is marked by the development of rebound tenderness, increasing abdominal girth, and cardiovascular collapse. If the patient does not begin to show signs of clinical improvement during the first 24 to 48 hours of medical therapy, the risk for perforation increases markedly, and surgical intervention colectomy is indicated.

Follow-Up

Colon Cancer, Dysplasia, and Colonoscopic Surveillance

The risk for colorectal cancer is increased beginning after 8 years of disease and continues to increase in subsequent years.[13] The incidence of colorectal adenocarcinoma is 60% higher in persons with inflammatory bowel disease than in the general population and has been stable over time. Patients with extensive ulcerative colitis have a markedly increased risk for colon cancer, patients with left-sided disease have an intermediate risk, and patients with long-standing ulcerative colitis are at risk for colorectal cancer even if their symptoms have been relatively mild or even quiescent for 10 to 15 years.

Colon cancers are commonly submucosal and may be missed at colonoscopy. Colon cancer in patients with ulcerative colitis is most commonly associated with dysplastic changes in the mucosa, often at multiple sites in the colon. Although recent data have demonstrated that most dysplasia is visible, not all dysplasia can be identified by visual inspection, so microscopic examination of biopsy specimens is required.

Current practice guidelines recommend colonoscopy with random biopsies in patients with long-standing ulcerative colitis beginning 8 years after the onset of disease and repeated every 1 to 2 years. If the specimens show dysplasia, colectomy is recommended.

The risk for colon cancer in patients with Crohn colitis is similar to the risk in patients with a similar extent of ulcerative colitis. Surveillance colonoscopy is also recommended in patients with Crohn colitis.

Pregnancy

Fertility in women with inflammatory bowel disease usually is normal or only minimally impaired, and the incidence of prematurity, stillbirth, and developmental defects in the offspring of women with inflammatory bowel disease, except fetal complications may be somewhat more likely when the mother's disease is clinically active, regardless of drug therapy. Previous proctocolectomy or the presence of an ileostomy is not an impediment to successful completion of a pregnancy, but women who have had ileal pouch anal anastomosis surgery with a total proctocolectomy have markedly reduced fertility.

If a woman's disease is inactive at the time of conception, it is likely that it will remain inactive during the course of the pregnancy. Ulcerative colitis that is active at the time of conception tends to worsen. In patients with active Crohn disease at the time of conception, the degree of activity remains the same in two thirds of women; of the other one third, some improve clinically and others deteriorate.

Sulfasalazine does not harm the fetus, but pregnant women have an increased requirement for folic acid and sulfasalazine interferes with folate absorption by competitively inhibiting the jejunal enzyme folate conjugase. Therefore, women who are taking sulfasalazine and who are pregnant or considering pregnancy should receive folate supplementation (1 mg twice daily) to ensure that the fetus receives adequate amounts for normal development. The use of corticosteroids by pregnant women with inflammatory bowel disease is associated with an increased rate of premature rupture of the membranes and a higher rate of cleft lip. In general, it appears that the risk to the pregnancy of treatment with sulfasalazine or corticosteroids is less than the risk in allowing disease activity to go untreated.

Most of the data on the teratogenicity of azathioprine and 6-mercaptopurine in pregnancy are derived from the transplant literature and involve higher doses than are commonly used for inflammatory bowel disease. Reported fetal effects in the transplant population include congenital malformations, immunosuppression, prematurity, and growth retardation. The risks of these medications in the inflammatory bowel disease population are not completely known, given that only small a number of such patients have been formally studied.

Although the IgGl Fc antibody components of infliximab, adalimumab, and golimumab cross the placenta, these agents are considered to be safe during pregnancy. Certolizumab's Fc component is IgG4 and does not cross the placenta to the same extent. However, the risks of these various agents are not completely known, because only a relatively small number of patients have been formally studied.

PROGNOSIS

Ulcerative Colitis

Recurrent flares and remissions characterize typical ulcerative colitis. A rapidly progressive initial attack results in serious complications in approximately 10% of patients. Complete recovery after a single attack may occur in another 10% of patients. Some patients may actually have had an acute undetected infection rather than true ulcerative colitis. The probability that a patient with clinically inactive disease will remain in remission the following year is 80 to 90%. By comparison, patients with clinically active disease have a 70% probability of relapse during the following year.

Patients who present with ulcerative proctitis have the best overall prognosis, and only approximately 5% of patients with proctitis will require colectomy over a lifetime. Severe complications are very uncommon, but the disease will spread more proximally in the colon in up to 50% of patients. Ulcerative colitis–related mortality has decreased substantially since the introduction of corticosteroids, and recent studies suggest that long-term survival rates for patients with ulcerative colitis are similar to those of the general population.

Crohn Disease

The manifestations of Crohn disease wax and wane. A patient with clinically active Crohn disease has a 70 to 80% chance of having active disease in the subsequent year, whereas 80% of patients in remission will remain so over the following year. Over the course of a 4-year period, approximately 25% of patients will have persistently active disease after diagnosis, 25% will remain in remission, and 50% will have a fluctuating course with years of remission and years with clinically active disease. Approximately 75 to 80% of all patients with luminal and fistulizing Crohn disease will require surgical intervention for their disease, with approximately 50% of them requiring surgery within 6 months of diagnosis. The rate for a second surgery for luminal Crohn disease ranges from 25 to 38% within 5 years, and 40 to 70% will need reoperation by 15 years.

Patients with Crohn disease have an increased mortality rate, approximately 1.3 to 1.5 times higher than the general population, unrelated to whether they have small intestine or large intestine involvement, or both. This excess mortality, which is most notable in the first few years after diagnosis, is most commonly related to complications of Crohn disease (e.g., colorectal cancer, shock, volume depletion, protein-calorie malnutrition, and anemia). Whether aggressive use of immunomodulators and biologic therapy will alter the natural course of disease is unknown.

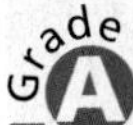

Grade A References

A1. Feagan BG, Macdonald JK. Oral 5-aminosalicylic acid for maintenance of remission in ulcerative colitis. *Cochrane Database Syst Rev*. 2012;10:CD000544.

A2. Marshall JK, Thabane M, Steinhart AH, et al. Rectal 5-aminosalicylic acid for maintenance of remission in ulcerative colitis. *Cochrane Database Syst Rev*. 2012;11:CD004118.

A3. Marshall JK, Thabane M, Steinhart AH, et al. Rectal 5-aminosalicylic acid for induction of remission in ulcerative colitis. *Cochrane Database Syst Rev*. 2010;1:CD004115.

A4. Chande N, Tsoulis DJ, MacDonald JK. Azathioprine or 6-mercaptopurine for induction of remission in Crohn's disease. *Cochrane Database Syst Rev*. 2013;4:CD000545.

A5. McDonald JW, Wang Y, Tsoulis DJ, et al. Methotrexate for induction of remission in refractory Crohn's disease. *Cochrane Database Syst Rev*. 2014;8:CD003459.

A6. Khan KJ, Ullman TA, Ford AC, et al. Antibiotic therapy in inflammatory bowel disease: a systematic review and meta-analysis. *Am J Gastroenterol*. 2011;106:661-673.

A7. Ford AC, Bernstein CN, Khan KJ, et al. Glucocorticosteroid therapy in inflammatory bowel disease: systematic review and meta-analysis. *Am J Gastroenterol*. 2011;106:590-599.

A8. Colombel JF, Sandborn WJ, Reinisch W, et al. Infliximab, azathioprine, or combination therapy for Crohn's disease. *N Engl J Med*. 2010;362:1383-1395.

A9. Costa J, Magro F, Caldeira D, et al. Infliximab reduces hospitalizations and surgery interventions in patients with inflammatory bowel disease: a systematic review and meta-analysis. *Inflamm Bowel Dis*. 2013;19:2098-2110.

A10. Travis SP, Danese S, Kupcinskas L, et al. Once-daily budesonide MMX in active, mild-to-moderate ulcerative colitis: results from the randomised CORE II study. *Gut*. 2014;63:433-441.

A11. Danese S, Fiorino G, Peyrin-Biroulet L, et al. Biological agents for moderately to severely active ulcerative colitis: a systematic review and network meta-analysis. *Ann Intern Med*. 2014;160:704-711.

A12. Timmer A, McDonald JW, Tsoulis DJ, et al. Azathioprine and 6-mercaptopurine for maintenance of remission in ulcerative colitis. *Cochrane Database Syst Rev*. 2012;9:CD000478.

A13. Reinisch W, Sandborn WJ, Rutgeerts P, et al. Long-term infliximab maintenance therapy for ulcerative colitis: the ACT-1 and -2 extension studies. *Inflamm Bowel Dis*. 2012;18:201-211.

A14. Sandborn WJ, Feagan BG, Marano C, et al. Subcutaneous golimumab maintains clinical response in patients with moderate-to-severe ulcerative colitis. *Gastroenterology*. 2014;146:96-109.

GENERAL REFERENCES

For the General References and other additional features, please visit Expert Consult at https://expertconsult.inkling.com.

142

INFLAMMATORY AND ANATOMIC DISEASES OF THE INTESTINE, PERITONEUM, MESENTERY, AND OMENTUM

JOHN F. KUEMMERLE

CONGENITAL STRUCTURAL ABNORMALITIES

Meckel Diverticulum

A Meckel diverticulum, which is the most common congenital anomaly of the gastrointestinal (GI) tract, is present in 2% to 3% of the population and is more common in men.[1] Meckel diverticulum occurs when the omphalomesenteric or vitelline duct connecting the fetal yolk sac to the primordial gut fails to close during development. Located on the antimesenteric border, the Meckel diverticulum is commonly found within about 100 cm of the ileocecal valve and typically is 1 to 10 cm in size. Heterotopic tissue is found in about 50% of Meckel diverticula, most commonly gastric or pancreatic tissue.[2] The presence of heterotopic tissue correlates with the development of symptomatic complications, with a lifetime risk of about 6%.

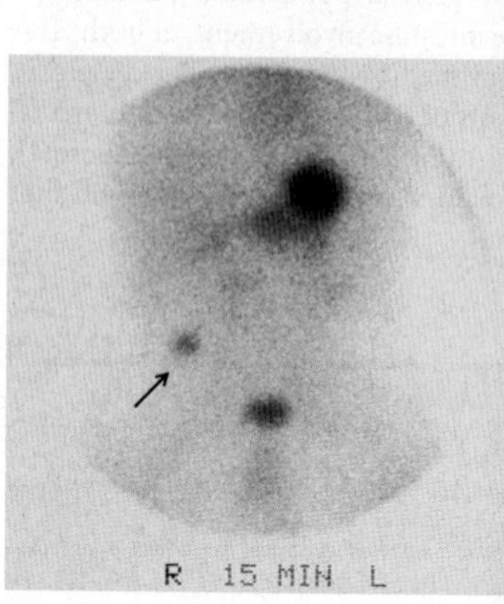

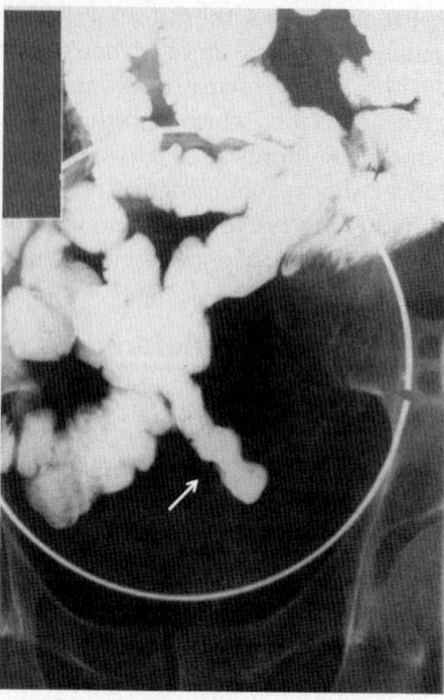

FIGURE 142-1. Meckel diverticulum. Nuclear medicine imaging with ^{99m}Tn pertechnetate scan shows tracer uptake in a Meckel diverticulum (*arrow* in left panel) and in the stomach and bladder. Barium radiography in the same patient also shows the Meckel diverticulum (*arrow* in right panel).

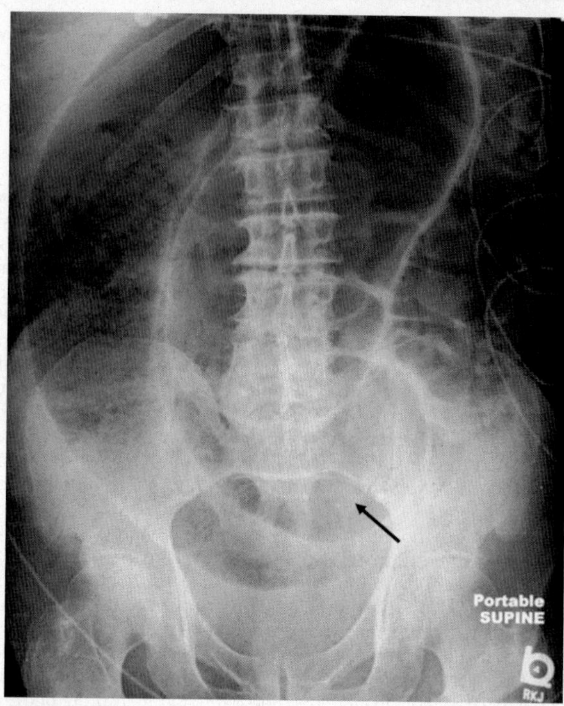

FIGURE 142-2. Sigmoid volvulus. Plain abdominal radiograph shows the presence of a sigmoid volvulus *(arrow)*.

CLINICAL MANIFESTATIONS

The complications from a Meckel diverticulum include bleeding, obstruction, diverticulitis, and perforation. Bleeding can occur when the production of acid from heterotopic gastric mucosa causes ileal ulcerations. Obstruction can result from volvulus around the diverticulum, intussusception of the diverticulum into the intestine, or herniation of the diverticulum and adjacent intestine. Inguinal, femoral, and umbilical hernias all can occur. Repeated and chronic inflammation at the neck of the diverticulum and nearby ileum also can lead to intestinal fibrosis and bowel obstruction. The most common complications are intestinal bleeding in children and obstruction in adults.

DIAGNOSIS

The diagnosis of a Meckel diverticulum can be challenging. Radionuclide imaging with sodium pertechnetate (^{99m}Tn) can be used in cases of bleeding because both normal and heterotopic gastric mucosa take up the tracer (Fig. 142-1). This test has high sensitivity and specificity in children but higher rates of false-positive and false-negative tests in adults. Crohn disease (Chapter 141) and other ileal inflammatory diseases can yield false-positive results. Radiographic imaging with a barium small bowel follow-through typically is not helpful because the diverticulum does not fill with barium contrast. Angiography can visualize the vestigial vitelline artery that arises from the superior mesenteric artery or a superior mesenteric artery branch that directly feeds the diverticulum or adjacent ileum. Both small bowel capsule endoscopy (Chapter 134) and double-balloon enteroscopy can identify a Meckel diverticulum during the evaluation of obscure bleeding.

TREATMENT AND PROGNOSIS Rx

The management of bleeding, obstruction, or perforation that occurs in association with a Meckel diverticulum is open or laparoscopic surgical resection of the diverticulum and possibly of adjacent ulcerated and bleeding ileum.[3] The surgical resection of a Meckel diverticulum incidentally identified at the time of surgery for another condition is controversial given the low lifetime risk of complications but can be considered in young men, patients with large diverticula, or patients with suspected heterotopic tissue. After identification and treatment, the prognosis is excellent because the Meckel diverticulum is removed, and the risk of complications is eliminated.

Intestinal Atresia and Stenosis, Malrotation, Gastroschisis, and Omphalocele

The congenital disorders of intestinal atresia and stenosis, malrotation, gastroschisis, and omphalocele disorders usually present early in infancy and childhood, but sometimes the diagnosis of stenosis or malrotation may be made in adulthood. With the exception of pyloric stenosis, significant long-term morbidity and mortality are associated with these anomalies even after surgical correction. Patients with malrotation or gastroschisis typically present with complications of their surgery, including adhesions, bowel obstruction, or abdominal wall hernias. Patients with intestinal atresia and resulting short gut syndrome also have significant morbidity and mortality related to intestinal failure.

ACQUIRED STRUCTURAL DISORDERS

Volvulus

Intestinal volvulus, which is pathologic twisting of the intestine around the mesentery, can result in obstruction of the proximal bowel. Mesenteric involvement may lead to vascular compromise, bowel necrosis with resulting perforation, and peritonitis. The most susceptible regions for volvulus are the sigmoid colon, cecum, and occasionally the transverse colon with an estimated annual incidence of two to six cases per 100,000.[4] Elderly persons, especially individuals who are institutionalized, are at the highest risk. Small bowel volvulus is uncommonly observed in U.S. adults but can result from preexisting anomalies such as malrotation or congenital bands of Ladd.

CLINICAL MANIFESTATIONS

Volvulus can present with symptoms and signs of acute bowel obstruction (Chapter 132), including pain that may be out of proportion to physical findings. Nausea and vomiting are usually present. The presentation can also be more insidious or intermittent with constipation, laxative use, and a previously recognized dilated colon. Physical findings include abdominal distention, tympanic percussion, rebound, guarding, and rigidity. Escalating pain and tenderness can indicate colonic ischemia and perforation.

DIAGNOSIS

The diagnosis of colonic volvulus can be made using abdominal radiographs, which demonstrate a distended colon, loss of haustrations, and a typical "bent inner tube" sign with the apex in the right upper quadrant of the abdomen (Fig. 142-2). In cases of a cecal volvulus, the dilated cecum is observed in the epigastrium or in the left upper quadrant. A water-soluble contrast enhanced radiograph can identify the point of obstruction due to volvulus.

TREATMENT AND PROGNOSIS

Rx

Patients with colonic volvulus should have nothing per oral cavity (NPO) with nasogastric (NG) tube decompression and receive appropriate fluid volume resuscitation. In the absence of complete obstruction or signs of ischemia or perforation, patients with a sigmoid volvulus can undergo emergent colonoscopy and attempted reduction, which is successful in up to 75% of cases.[5] Surgical intervention is indicated for volvulus involving the cecum, transverse colon, or small intestine, as well as after colonoscopic reduction of a sigmoid volvulus because of the risk of recurrence. The mortality rate is about 9% for sigmoid volvulus, 7% for cecal volvulus, and about 17% for combined sigmoid and cecal volvulus or transverse colon volvulus.[6]

Intussusception

Intestinal intussusception occurs when a segment of bowel invaginates into the adjacent distal intestine and results in bowel obstruction and ischemia. Intussusception usually involves just the small intestine, but it can also present as small intestinal intussusception into the colon. Although intussusception is a common cause of small bowel obstruction in pediatric patients, especially after rotavirus vaccination (Chapter 380), it is rare in adults and accounts for only about 5% of small bowel obstruction. The cause of intussusception is infrequently identified in children, but a cause can be identified in about 90% of adult cases.[7] Typical precipitating causes in adults include inflammatory bowel disease (Chapter 141), postoperative adhesions, Meckel diverticula, feeding tubes, and small intestinal polyps and tumors (including leiomyomas, neurofibromas, and lymphomas).

CLINICAL MANIFESTATIONS

Most patients present with symptoms of partial bowel obstruction, including pain, nausea, and vomiting, and some patients have diarrhea with occult or overt bleeding. The clinical picture can be confusing when the patient has intermittent symptoms from a spontaneously resolved event. A mass may be palpable on examination. Passage of "currant jelly" stools is characteristic of intussusception, especially in children.

DIAGNOSIS

The diagnosis of intussusception is usually made using computed tomography (CT), which reveals a characteristic alternating high- and low-attenuation target-like or sausage-shaped lesion that represents the invaginated intestinal segments. However, because of the confusing presentation of intussusception in adults, a combination of plain radiographs, upper GI series, and barium enema frequently is required for an adequate evaluation.

TREATMENT AND PROGNOSIS

Colonic intussusceptions are treated surgically in adults because of the high likelihood that a colonic malignancy is the causative lesion.[8] For small intestinal intussusception, pneumatic reduction is successful in children and has been tried in adults in whom no other significant causative lesion is present. However, adults with small intestinal intussusception frequently have an underlying pathological cause, so their treatment consists primarily of surgical intervention and bowel resection, which not only resolves the obstruction but also provides a diagnosis of the causative lesion. If the predisposing cause can be diagnosed and corrected, the prognosis is good, and recurrence rates are low. If the underlying cause is not fully correctable such as with neurofibromatosis (Chapter 417) or adhesions, intussusceptions may recur.

Hernias

Anatomically, hernias comprise a herniated viscus, the hernial sac (internal wall of the hernia lined by peritoneum), and the hernial ring. Whereas an external hernia occurs when the viscus lies outside the abdomen, an internal hernia occurs when the viscus lies in an abnormal location within the abdominal cavity. Secondary hernias can occur at previous sites of incision or injury. Incisional, inguinal, and umbilical hernias comprise 90% of all hernias.[9] Hernias are common and occur in about 5% of the population within their lifetimes. For inguinal hernias alone, the lifetime cumulative incidence is estimated to be 43% in men and 6% in women.[10] By comparison, femoral, umbilical, and incisional hernias occur twice as often in women.

CLINICAL MANIFESTATIONS, DIAGNOSIS, AND TREATMENT OF SPECIFIC HERNIAS

Rx

Epigastric hernias occur at sites of congenital weakness in the midline between the xiphoid and umbilicus along the linea alba. Small epigastric hernias may be asymptomatic or difficult to identify. Larger epigastric hernias can present as nodules, sometimes with tenderness. Multiple hernias may be present. They can be repaired surgically if symptomatic or if complications are present.

Umbilical hernias occur in association with obesity, in multiparous women, and in patients with ascites. They present as a protuberant mass palpable at the umbilicus. Incarceration of small bowel or omentum is common, and strangulation occurs in about one third of umbilical hernias. Umbilical hernias can be repaired surgically if they are symptomatic or associated with complications, but ascites should be controlled for the hernia repair to succeed.

Groin hernias present with bulging in this region, particularly with Valsalva maneuvers. Whereas direct inguinal hernias occur at the site of weakness at the base of the Hesselbach triangle, indirect inguinal hernias occur lateral to the Hesselbach triangle. Both direct and indirect inguinal hernias are above the inguinal ligament. Femoral hernias occur below the inguinal ligament in the femoral canal. Pain is typically mild, but more severe pain or colicky abdominal pain suggests incarceration or strangulation. Palpation can reveal the presence of a groin hernia that increases in size with standing or increased intra-abdominal pressure, such as a Valsalva maneuver, but palpation may be difficult in obese patients. In unclear cases, CT imaging can be helpful. The differential diagnosis of an inguinal bulge also includes adenopathy, lipoma or other tumors, testicular torsion of an undescended testicle, and abscess. Femoral hernias should be repaired when first diagnosed because of their risk for strangulation, but watchful waiting is an acceptable option for men with minimally symptomatic inguinal hernias.[A1] The treatment of symptomatic groin hernias is surgical, now usually by open mesh-based techniques or laparoscopic repair, which appear to provide equivalent results.[A2] Because the presence of strangulation can reliably be made only at surgery, more severe symptoms warrant early surgical intervention.

Pelvic hernias occur through a weakened pelvic floor and are sixfold more common in women, especially with advancing age. The most common form is an obturator hernia, but less common forms include a sciatic hernia through the sciatic foramen or perineal hernias through the pelvic floor musculature. Most obturator hernias present with acute bowel obstruction. A tender mass may be palpable near the obturator canal on rectal or vaginal examination. Inner thigh pain on internal rotation of the hip may be present in 50% of patients. Diagnosis can be aided using CT imaging. The treatment is surgical.

Incisional hernias can develop after 1% to 4% of laparotomy incisions. Incisional hernias may cause chronic abdominal discomfort, especially with maneuvers that increase intra-abdominal pressure. Repair is usually performed with prosthetic mesh.

More rare hernias include lumbar hernias (which are more common in men and after surgery for trauma), Spigelian hernias occurring through the linea semilunaris in elderly patients, and internal hernias that occur when an intraperitoneal organ protrudes into a separate compartment within the abdomen. Some hernias occur in surgically created defects or because of congenital defects (e.g., paraduodenal, pericecal, or foramen of Winslow). Up to 15% of internal hernias occur through mesenteric or omental defects. Most patients present with intermittent symptoms of pain and bowel obstruction or strangulation. Radiologic studies can be of variable assistance. The differential diagnosis should include volvulus, adhesions, and tumors. Surgery is needed to reduce the herniated viscus and close any defect.

INFLAMMATION OF THE INTESTINE AND COLON

Appendicitis

Appendicitis is the most common intra-abdominal pathology that requires emergency surgery. The lifetime prevalence of appendicitis is 8.7% in men and 6.9% in woman. Lifetime rates of appendectomy are higher, 12% in men and 23% in women, because the diagnosis may be difficult to confirm noninvasively and because of the practice of operating on patients in whom the condition is highly suspected.

About one third of patients have luminal obstruction of the vermiform appendix, most commonly caused by an appendicolith but also occasionally by lymphoid hyperplasia or tumors, including carcinoid tumors (Chapter 232). Gangrenous appendicitis is almost always associated with luminal obstruction.

TABLE 142-1 DIFFERENTIAL DIAGNOSIS OF ACUTE APPENDICITIS

SURGICAL CAUSES

Intestinal obstruction
Intussusception
Acute cholecystitis
Mesenteric adenitis (especially from adenoviral infection; Chapter 365)
Meckel diverticulitis
Right-sided colonic diverticulitis

UROLOGIC CAUSES

Right nephrolithiasis
Right pyelonephritis

GYNECOLOGIC CAUSES

Ectopic or tubal pregnancy
Ruptured or torsed ovarian cyst
Right-sided salpingitis or tubo-ovarian abscess

MEDICAL CAUSES

Yersinia (Chapter 312) or *Campylobacter* (Chapter 303) enterocolitis
Crohn ileitis
Pneumonia
Diabetic ketoacidosis
Herpetic neuralgia (especially right 10th and 11th nerves)
Porphyria
Tuberculous colitis

TABLE 142-2 SCORING SYSTEM FOR ACUTE APPENDICITIS*

	VARIABLE	VALUE
Symptoms	Migration of pain to the right iliac fossa	1
	Anorexia	1
	Nausea or vomiting	1
Signs	Tenderness in right lower quadrant	2
	Rebound of pain	1
	Elevation of temperature (≥37.3°C)	1
Laboratory	Leukocytosis (WBC count >10,000/μL)	2
	Shift to the left (>75% neutrophils)	1
Total score		10

*An aggregate score of 5 or 6 is compatible with the diagnosis of acute appendicitis. A score of 7 or 8 indicates a probable appendicitis, and a score of 9 or 10 indicates a very probable acute appendicitis.
WBC = white blood cell.
Adapted from Alvarado, A. A practical score for the early diagnosis of acute appendicitis. *Ann Emerg Med.* 1986;15:557-564.

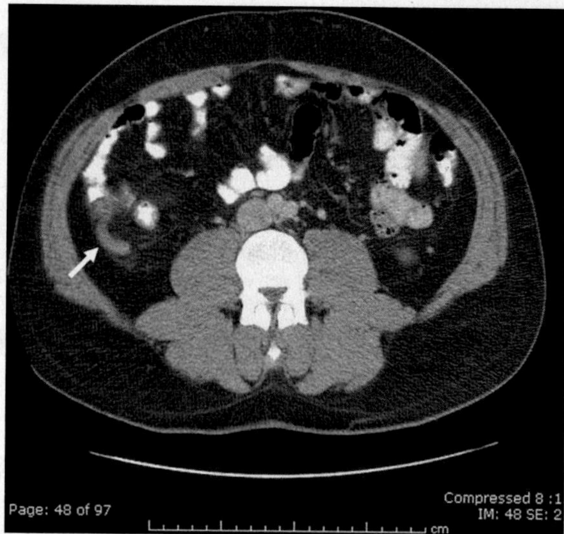

FIGURE 142-3. Appendicitis. A computed tomography scan shows an inflamed appendix with a diameter greater than 1 cm *(arrow)* consistent with acute, uncomplicated appendicitis. (Courtesy of Charlene Prather, MD.)

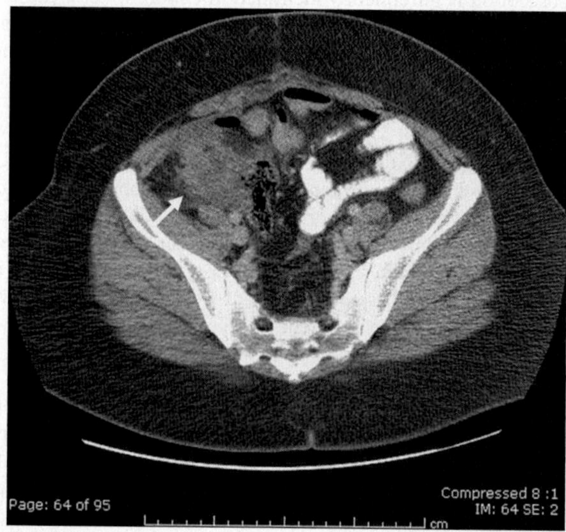

FIGURE 142-4. Appendicitis. A computed tomography scan shows appendicitis complicated by perforation with abscess formation *(arrow)*. (Courtesy of Charlene Prather, MD.)

CLINICAL MANIFESTATIONS AND DIAGNOSIS

The differential diagnosis of appendicitis is extensive (Table 142-1).[11] Current guidelines for diagnosis include characteristic history and physical findings of abdominal pain; localized tenderness; or other signs of acute appendicitis, including increased right lower quadrant pain with cough, pain with flexion and internal rotation of the hip, pain with passive extension of the right hip, and increased right lower quadrant pain during palpation of the left lower quadrant. Laboratory evidence of inflammation include leukocytosis, greater than10,000/μL but usually less than 18,000/μL unless perforation has occurred, with left shift, and elevated markers (Table 142-2) such as the C-reactive protein or procalcitonin level. However, none of these tests are accurate enough to make or exclude the diagnosis of appendicitis.[12] The preferred diagnostic test is multidetector CT (Fig. 142-3), which has a sensitivity and specificity of at least 94%[A3] and perhaps higher, and can also detect perforation (Fig. 142-4). Ultrasonography is less sensitive and specific, 83% and 93%, respectively, but is useful when CT is contraindicated, such as in pregnant women or a suspected ectopic pregnancy.

TREATMENT AND PROGNOSIS

When acute appendicitis is suspected, emergent surgical consultation and appendectomy are indicated. Laparoscopic appendectomy is increasingly used in preference to open appendectomy because of lower rates of postoperative complications and a more rapid return to normal eating and activity.[A4] Preoperative antibiotics (e.g., cefotetan, 2 g intravenously, or cefoxitin, 2 g intravenously followed by three postoperative doses or ticarcillin–clavulanic acid) reduce infectious complications in otherwise uncomplicated appendicitis. Because perforation of the appendix increases the risk of mortality from 0.0002% to 3% and increases the morbidity rate from 3% to 47%, the traditional approach is that a negative laparotomy is an acceptable trade-off to missing true appendicitis. A nonoperative approach using antibiotics to treat uncomplicated appendicitis can reduce routine surgical morbidity but at the expense of about a 2% risk of rupture and 1% risk of gangrenous appendicitis.[A5] For a perforated appendix with abscess formation, immediate appendectomy yields similar results to a strategy of percutaneous ultrasound- or CT-guided drainage, intravenous (IV) antibiotics, and laparoscopic appendectomy about 10 weeks later.[A6] In the setting of perforation, once-daily dosing with ceftriaxone and metronidazole for 7 to 10 days is as good as triple-dose therapy.[A7]

Complications develop in more than 15% of patients, with an overall mortality rate of about 3% in patients with perforated appendicitis. Complications are uncommon in surgically treated nonperforated appendicitis. Patients who have appendectomies for suspected but not confirmed appendicitis have a prognosis that depends on whether they had an underlying disease, such as Crohn (Chapter 141) or carcinoid (Chapter 232).

Diverticulitis of the Colon

Colonic diverticula are technically pseudodiverticula. They form when the colonic mucosa and submucosa herniate through the muscularis propria of

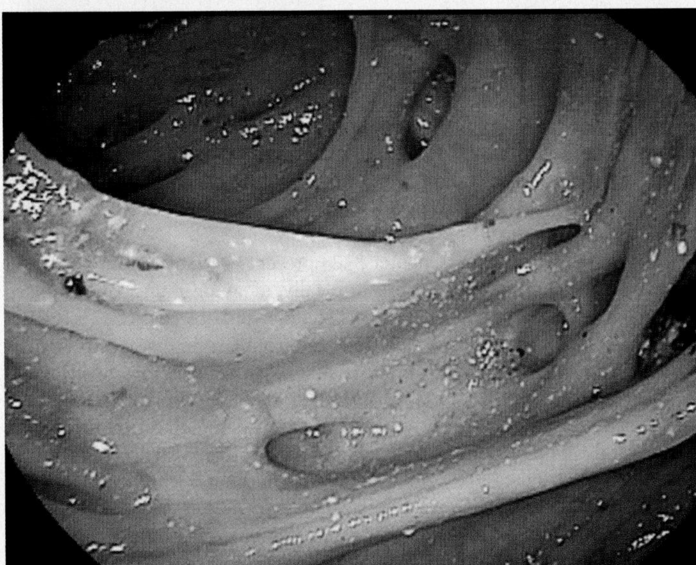

FIGURE 142-5. Sigmoid diverticulosis. The colonoscopic appearance of sigmoid diverticulosis coli.

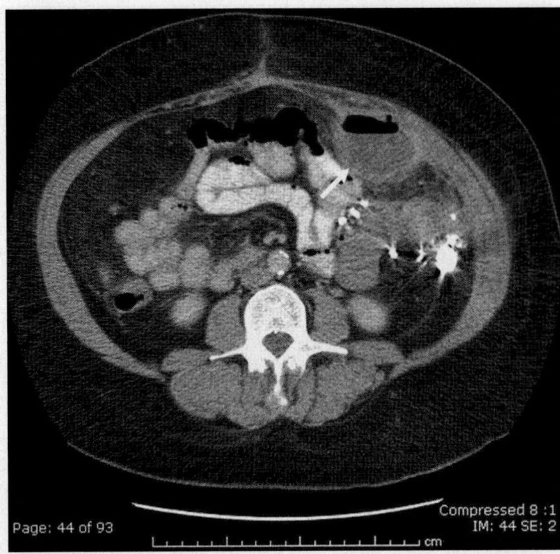

FIGURE 142-6. Diverticulitis. A computed tomography scan shows acute diverticulitis with perforation. An abscess *(arrow)* is seen presenting as an air-filled collection. (Courtesy of Charlene Prather, MD.)

the colon. A spectrum of problems can result from diverticulosis, including diverticulitis, which is an infected diverticulum, or diverticular bleeding, which is manifested as acute lower GI bleeding (Chapter 135). Diverticular disease (Fig. 142-5 and E-Fig. 142-E1) affects about 10% of middle-aged adults and increases in prevalence up to about 80% in elderly adults.

Colonic diverticula form at the site where the nutrient artery, the vasa recta, penetrates the muscularis propria. Diverticulosis in Western populations is most common in the left colon and has been thought to be associated with the low-fiber content of the typical Western diet, although recent epidemiologic studies cast doubt on this hypothesis. Diverticulosis can occur anywhere in the colon, however, and it is more commonly observed in the right colon in Asian populations.

The lifetime risk of diverticulitis is up to 25%.[13] Diverticulitis is thought to occur when impacted material in the diverticulum compresses the blood supply, thereby resulting in a microperforation. Diverticulitis can be complicated further by free perforation, abscess, or fistula formation.

CLINICAL MANIFESTATIONS

The majority of patients with colonic diverticulosis are asymptomatic. Patients with diverticulitis commonly present with localized pain, fever, and anorexia. The pain may radiate to the back, flank, or suprapubic region. Nausea and vomiting, constipation or diarrhea, or urinary symptoms may be variably present. Physical examination typically reveals left lower quadrant tenderness, sometimes with localized guarding or a palpable mass. Rebound tenderness or peritoneal signs should suggest the presence of free perforation. Visible diverticular bleeding is rare in the setting of acute diverticulitis. Leukocytosis is present. When the acutely inflamed diverticulum is adjacent to the bladder, sterile pyuria may be found.

DIAGNOSIS

The diagnosis of acute diverticulitis can be confirmed in the appropriate setting by leukocytosis and an ultrasound examination or a CT scan showing diverticulosis coli with localized inflammation of the colonic wall and pericolic fat at the site of acute diverticulitis. A CT scan also can demonstrate free perforation, abscess, or fistula formation (Fig. 142-6). Because of the increased risk of perforation, invasive testing such as barium enema or colonoscopy is contraindicated when a diagnosis of acute diverticulitis is being entertained. The differential diagnosis of acute diverticulitis includes inflammatory bowel disease (Chapter 141), gastroenteritis, appendicitis, and colon cancer (Chapter 193) with perforation.

TREATMENT

Rx

Uncomplicated acute diverticulitis can be treated with antibiotics. A 7- to 10-day course of oral antibiotics (e.g., ciprofloxacin 750 mg twice daily and metronidazole 500 mg four times daily), perhaps after a single IV dose of antibiotics, is as effective and safe as hospitalization for IV antibiotics.[A8] Patients who can tolerate clear liquids can be treated in the outpatient setting with gradual advancement of their diet. Patients who are unable to tolerate eating should be admitted to the hospital for IV fluids and antibiotics (e.g., levofloxacin 750 mg daily and metronidazole 500 mg every 6 hours or piperacillin–tazobactam 3.375 g every 6 hours).

Although the risks associated with one episode of uncomplicated diverticulitis are low, with a mortality rate that is less than 1%, complicated diverticulitis, defined as diverticulitis with abscess, fistula formation, free perforation, or obstruction, is associated with increased inpatient morbidity in up to 25% of cases and has a mortality rate as high as 5%. Furthermore, these risks increase with a second episode of complicated diverticulitis. Elective segmental colectomy typically has been recommended to patients after 2 to 3 episodes of complicated diverticulitis and in young patients even after a first episode. However, recent evidence suggests that the risk of complicated diverticulitis after recovery from uncomplicated diverticulitis is only about 5% and is lower not higher after subsequent episodes of uncomplicated diverticulitis. As a result, prophylactic surgery is not indicated in patients whose diverticulitis is uncomplicated and can be medically treated.[14] Patients with diverticulitis with abscess formation require percutaneous CT-guided drainage and subsequent surgery, usually laparoscopic, typically after 6 weeks. Acute diverticulitis can be complicated by colitis or late stricture formation. About 40% of patients with complicated diverticulitis have significant morbidity, and their mortality rate is about 6%, but it is only about 2% in patients without perforation. There is no convincing evidence that a high-fiber diet prevents recurrent diverticular disease[15] or that nuts or any particular foods should be favored or avoided.

Other Intestinal Inflammatory Conditions

SMALL INTESTINAL ULCERS

Most primary idiopathic ulcers are found in the mid- to distal ileum, where they can be solitary or multiple. A careful history is necessary to exclude other precipitating causes of small intestinal ulcers, including drug exposure and other systemic diseases (Table 142-3). Pathologically, these ulcers can be differentiated from Crohn disease or chronic ulcerative jejunoileitis by the absence of granulomas. Barium contrast studies including enteroclysis can make the diagnosis, and CT or magnetic resonance enterography can also be helpful. In the absence of bowel obstruction, wireless capsule endoscopy is often the preferred test. Therapy with anti-inflammatory or immunosuppressive medications has not proven helpful. Therapy is typically directed to complications, including perforation and obstruction, with segmental surgical resection. However, the risk of ulcer recurrence is high.

Drug-induced ulcerations are common and can result from nonsteroidal anti-inflammatory drugs (NSAIDs), potassium chloride preparations, vasoactive medications, antimetabolites, and cocaine. Wireless capsule endoscopy can make the diagnosis (Fig. 142-7). NSAID-induced injury is similar to Crohn disease, with transmural injury and the risk of stricture formation. Treatment is aimed at avoiding the offending agent, if possible. Unlike for

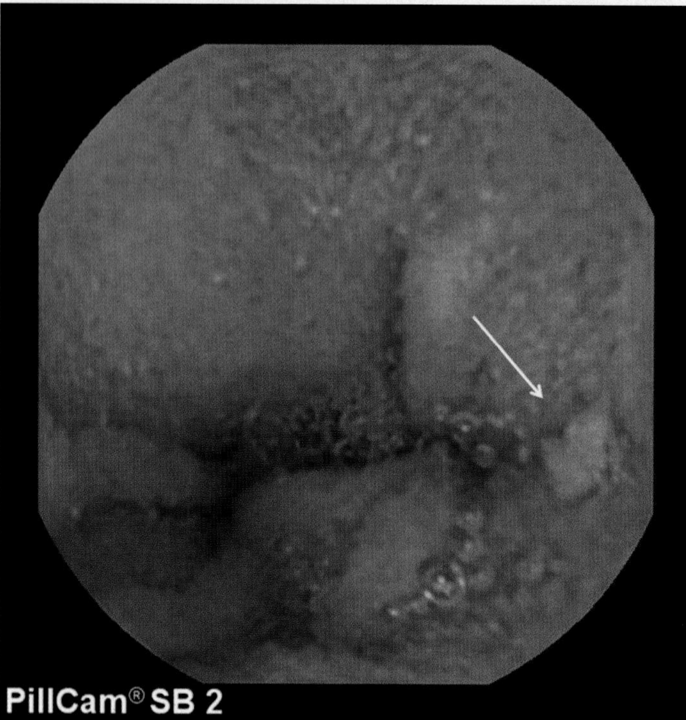

FIGURE 142-7. Nonsteroidal anti-inflammatory drug (NSAID)—induced enteropathy. The wireless capsule endoscopy appearance of a jejunal ulceration *(arrow)* caused by NSAID use.

TABLE 142-3 CAUSES OF SMALL INTESTINAL ULCERS

CATEGORY	CAUSES
Acidic	Meckel diverticulum, Zollinger-Ellison syndrome
Drug-induced	Potassium chloride, NSAID, antimetabolite
Idiopathic	Primary ulcer, Behcet disease
Infectious	Tuberculosis, typhoid, *Yersinia* infection, *Strongyloides* superinfection
Inflammatory	Crohn disease, SLE, chronic jejunoileitis
Metabolic	Uremia
Neoplastic	Malignant histiocytosis, lymphoma, adenocarcinoma
Radiation	Radiation enteritis
Vascular	Mesenteric vascular insufficiency, vasculitis, arteritis

NSAID = nonsteroidal anti-inflammatory drug; SLE = systemic lupus erythematosus.

gastric ulceration, data are conflicting as to whether the concomitant use of a proton pump inhibitor mitigates or exacerbates the condition.[16]

A variety of systemic conditions also can manifest with small intestinal ulcerations. Patients with Crohn disease (Chapter 141) can cause ulcers of any portion of the GI tract. Systemic lupus erythematosus (Chapter 266), rheumatoid arthritis (Chapter 264), scleroderma (Chapter 267), polyarteritis nodosa (Chapter 270), and Henoch-Schönlein purpura (Chapter 270) can present with small intestinal ulcerations that are thought to be secondary to microthrombosis and vasculitis. Mesenteric vasculitis presents as nausea, vomiting, fever, and GI bleeding.

Behçet disease (Chapter 270) is a systemic process that causes intestinal ulcers, typically in the ileocecal region, in fewer than 1% of cases. Although symptoms are similar to those of Crohn disease, pathologically Behçet disease-related ulcers are deep and do not have surrounding inflammation or granulomas. The optimal treatment of this disease has yet to be delineated. Patients frequently are treated with immunomodulators (Chapter 270), and surgery is reserved for ulcer-related complications.

Sarcoidosis (Chapter 95) uncommonly involves the intestine. Its presentation is similar to Crohn disease, with small and large intestinal ulceration and noncaseating granulomas. Patients commonly have nausea, vomiting, diarrhea, abdominal pain, and protein-losing enteropathy. Treatment is targeted to controlling the systemic disease.

Mycobacterium tuberculosis (Chapter 324) typically involves the distal ileum and cecum. A waxing and waning course can mimic the symptoms and location commonly seen in Crohn disease. The diagnosis is suspected based on a history of exposure, particularly in endemic regions, and confirmed by colonoscopy with biopsy, stains, and culture. Treatment is as for disseminated tuberculosis (Chapter 324).

Histoplasma capsulatum (Chapter 332) presents with ulcerations and polypoid masses that mimic tumors, typically in an immunocompromised patient. Patients present with diarrhea, bleeding, and obstruction. The granulomas seen on biopsy must be differentiated from Crohn disease, tuberculosis, and sarcoidosis. Treatment involves managing the systemic infection.

Neutropenic enterocolitis, or typhlitis (E-Fig. 142-E2), is an inflammation of the intestine or colon, usually during the neutropenic phase 10 to 14 days after high-dose induction chemotherapy.[17] It involves right lower quadrant abdominal pain, distention, and diarrhea, sometimes with bleeding. These findings in of themselves are nonspecific and are similar to *Clostridium difficile*–associated colitis (Chapter 296), ischemic colitis (Chapter 143), or pseudo-obstruction (Chapter 136). Diagnosis is based on typical CT scan findings of thickened bowel wall; bowel distention, especially of the cecum; and associated inflammatory changes. Treatment is conservative, with bowel rest and decompression when bowel dilation is present, and broad-spectrum antibiotics. Leukocyte-stimulating agents are often used to reverse the neutropenia (Chapter 167). Treatment of bleeding is supportive with transfusions and correction of any coagulopathy. Surgery is indicated in the setting of intractable bleeding or perforation. The symptoms resolve rapidly with resolution of neutropenia.

VISCERAL ANGIOEDEMA

Visceral angioedema can be idiopathic, or it can be a complication of hereditary and acquired C1 esterase inhibitor deficiency (Chapter 252), hypocomplementemia, drugs (especially angiotensin-converting enzyme inhibitors), or foods. Patients with GI angioedema commonly present with abdominal pain and distention, nausea, vomiting, and diarrhea. Some patients also have evidence of mucous membrane swelling, hives, wheezing, or dyspnea. On CT scan, thickened, fluid-filled loops of small bowel and ascites may also be seen. Symptoms commonly occur episodically, persist for 1 to 3 days and may recur periodically. The diagnosis is established by discontinuing the implicated drug or food, low serum levels of C4, low C1 esterase quantitative levels, or reduced C1 esterase functional activity. C1 esterase inhibitor deficiency can be treated successfully with C1 inhibitor therapy (Chapter 252).

RADIATION ENTERITIS

Radiation injury (Chapters 20 and 140) can occur in the small or large intestine as a result of therapy for gynecologic, urologic, rectal, or retroperitoneal tumors. Acute injury, which can occur during the course of treatment, is associated with nausea, diarrhea, and abdominal or rectal discomfort. The risk is related to radiation dose. Chronic injury typically presents 6 months to 2 years after treatment and presents with progressive bowel obstruction owing to continued inflammation and fibrosis.[18] Patients with radiation proctitis present with rectal pain, bleeding, and occasionally diarrhea.

Acute radiation injury is usually self-limited to the period of treatment, but up to 5% of patients can progress to chronic radiation injury to the small intestine, and up to 15% of patients experience chronic radiation proctitis. Radiation enteritis and stricture formation can be seen on barium radiographs or CT scans. The characteristic neovascularization pattern of telangiectasias from radiation proctitis is seen on endoscopy.

One third to half of patients develop bleeding, which can be minor and intermittent or more substantial. Whereas patients who do not require transfusion have a 70% chance of remission, patients with chronic radiation enteritis who need transfusion have a low rate of remission (20%) and have subsequent high morbidity and even mortality rates. Less invasive treatment options include sucralfate enemas. Several small studies suggest a benefit from endoscopic argon plasma coagulation.

An algorithmic approach emphasizing specific approaches, as outlined earlier, to each specific symptom, can improve outcome compared with routine clinical care.[A9] Surgery, which can be required in up to one third of patients with strictures or bleeding, is associated with a high complication rate and should be avoided if possible.[19]

PERITONEAL DISORDERS

Peritonitis

Peritonitis, which is a local or generalized inflammation that involves the visceral and parietal peritoneum, can occur as a primary or secondary process. Primary peritonitis in adults is the spontaneous infection of ascites in a patient with cirrhosis (Chapter 153) in the absence of an overt intra-abdominal source. The use of acid-suppressive therapy appears to increase the risk of developing spontaneous bacterial peritonitis threefold in hospitalized patients with cirrhosis.

Secondary peritonitis develops when disease or injury to the intestine results in bacterial contamination from a perforated viscus (e.g., peptic ulcer disease, appendicitis, diverticulitis, penetrating trauma, or iatrogenic), from iatrogenic causes (e.g., peritoneal dialysis [Chapter 131] or surgical contamination), from granulomatous disease (e.g., tuberculosis or fungal infections), or from chemical or aseptic exposures (e.g., bile, urine, or radiographic barium).[20]

CLINICAL MANIFESTATIONS AND DIAGNOSIS

Abdominal pain is the hallmark of peritonitis. It can be sudden in onset in the setting of a perforated viscus or more insidious in nature in the setting of granulomatous or chemical causes. Patients with peritonitis typically lie supine with flexed knees and exhibit shallow breathing. Physical examination reveals a distended abdomen with tenderness to palpation, localized or generalized guarding, and rigidity. Associated symptoms include fever, nausea, vomiting, and leukocytosis with a left shift. Some patients with bacterial peritonitis rapidly develop septic shock (Chapter 108).

Granulomatous peritonitis has a more insidious presentation, and 70% of patients have symptoms for 4 months before diagnosis. Systemic symptoms include fever, malaise, anorexia, and weight loss. The abdomen is diffusely tender. Leukocytosis can be absent.

Patients with tuberculous peritonitis often have a positive skin test result or infiltrates on their chest radiograph. The peritoneal fluid typically has a high protein level (<3 g/dL), a low glucose (<30 mg/dL), and elevated leukocytes (<250 cells/μL); fluid stains and cultures are unhelpful, but polymerase chain reaction–based tests can be diagnostic. The laparoscopic appearance of tuberculous peritonitis is characteristic, with fibrous masses from the parietal peritoneum and granulomas.

Plain abdominal radiographs may show evidence of paralytic ileus, and free air under the diaphragm on upright views confirms the presence of a perforated viscus. CT scan is more sensitive, 70% to 100%, than plain radiographs for detecting free air and may also demonstrate the underlying cause (Fig. 142-8).

In young patients, appendicitis and a perforated duodenal ulcer (Chapter 139) are common causes. In older patients, perforated diverticula and cancer (Chapter 193) are more common. In young women, tubal pregnancy and a ruptured tubo-ovarian abscess must be considered (Chapters 285 and 299).

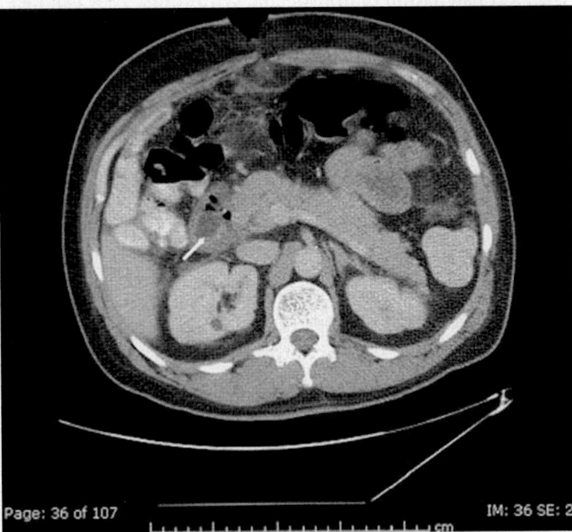

FIGURE 142-8. Peritonitis. A computed tomography scan in a patient with peritonitis showing a thickened duodenal wall from a perforated duodenal ulcer found at the time of surgical exploration. (Courtesy of Charlene Prather, MD.)

Secondary peritonitis is usually caused by a mixed flora of bacteria, including *Escherichia coli, Streptococcus faecalis, Pseudomonas aeruginosa, Klebsiella mirabilis, Bacteroides fragilis, Clostridium* spp., and anaerobic streptococci.

TREATMENT AND PROGNOSIS (Rx)

Treatment of acute suppurative peritonitis relies on prompt adequate resuscitation with IV fluids and broad-spectrum IV antibiotics. Treatment regimens include: piperacillin–tazobactam, 3.375 g every 6 hours; ampicillin–sulbactam, 3.0 g every 6 hours; ciprofloxacin, 400 mg every 12 hours, and metronidazole, 1 g every 12 hours; levofloxacin, 750 mg every 24 hours; cefepime, 2 g every 12 hours, and metronidazole, 1 g every 12 hours; or imipenem–cilastatin sodium, 500 mg every 6 hours. Early diagnosis and surgical intervention for acute peritonitis from perforated viscus is critical. The mainstay of treatment for tuberculous peritonitis is at least 6 months of a multidrug regimen (Chapter 324).

Chemical aseptic peritonitis can be complicated by secondary bacterial infection. Treatment is similar to that of acute suppurative peritonitis, with intervention to control the source of peritoneal contamination.

The outcome of peritonitis depends on its cause as well as the rapidity of treatment. The mortality rate can be as low as 15% in patients who have correctable causes, such as a perforated appendix, and who do not develop multiorgan failure before treatment but as high as 50% for postoperative infective peritonitis.

PERITONITIS AS A COMPLICATION OF CHRONIC AMBULATORY PERITONEAL DIALYSIS

The most common complication of chronic ambulatory peritoneal dialysis is infectious peritonitis from bacterial contamination (Chapter 131), which commonly results from poor technique.[21] In contrast to polymicrobial acute suppurative peritonitis, peritonitis complicating chronic ambulatory peritoneal dialysis is typically monomicrobial with gram-positive cocci in the majority of cases and gram-negative species in the remainder of cases. Fungal peritonitis is rare. Symptoms can be milder than in other forms of peritonitis, with patients often presenting with diffuse abdominal pain, low-grade fever, and leukocytosis. The exchange fluid is characteristically turbid and may be the only sign of infection. The diagnosis is based on these physical findings, turbid dialysate with less than 100 leukocytes/μL, and a positive dialysate culture that determines the microbe involved. Treatment is with intraperitoneal antibiotics. The dialysis catheter should be removed in the setting of an inadequate response to therapy, fungal or tuberculous peritonitis or concomitant skin infection.

ADHESIONS

Peritoneal adhesions, which are the most commonly observed cause of bowel obstruction,[22] can occur at any time after a laparotomy. Patients who have had intra-abdominal infection, ischemia, and peritonitis are at increased risk. Patients present with complete or incomplete bowel obstruction, which is usually manifested as colicky abdominal pain, nausea, and vomiting (including feculent vomiting), abdominal distention, and an absence of flatus or stooling. Bowel obstruction can be diagnosed on plain radiographs or CT scan from the presence of dilated bowel and air-fluid levels, with decompressed bowel distal to the site of obstruction (Fig. 142-9). Treatment of bowel obstructions is with NG tube decompression and fluid resuscitation. A nonoperative approach can be attempted in cases of partial bowel obstruction or in patients who have had numerous prior laparotomies, which make surgical exploration more complicated. However, urgent laparotomy for lysis of adhesions must be performed before bowel ischemia develops. In patients with chronic abdominal pain, surgical exploration for the intent of lysing adhesions without clear evidence of obstructing adhesions should be avoided. Patients who develop postoperative adhesions can progress to bowel obstruction and develop recurrent adhesions despite surgical lysis of the adhesions. Data suggest that oxidized regenerated cellulose and hyaluronate carboxymethylcellulose adhesion barriers can safely reduce clinically relevant consequences of adhesions.A10

PERITONEAL CARCINOMATOSIS AND MALIGNANT ASCITES

Peritoneal carcinomatosis results when malignancy spreads throughout the peritoneal cavity and eventually encases the viscera. The cause can be primary tumors of the peritoneal cavity (e.g., mesothelioma and sarcoma), dissemination of an intra-abdominal malignancy (e.g., gastric, colon, pancreatic,

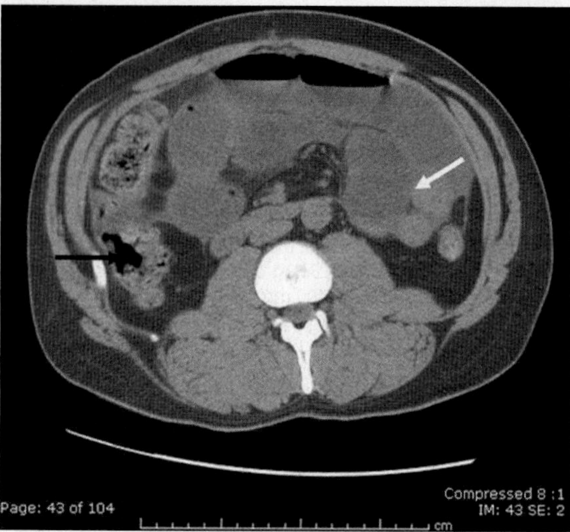

FIGURE 142-9. Small bowel obstruction. A computed tomography scan shows dilated, fluid-filled small bowel *(white arrow)* and a nondilated colon *(black arrow)* in a patient with a small bowel obstructions from adhesions in the midileum found at the time of surgical exploration. (Courtesy of Charlene Prather, MD.)

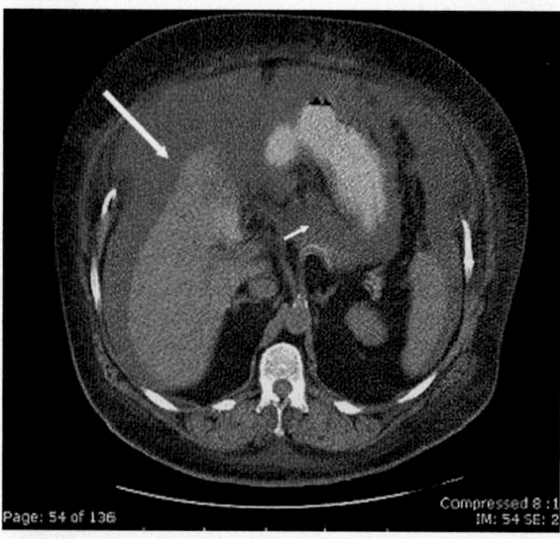

FIGURE 142-10. Malignant ascites. A computed tomography scan shows ascites *(large arrow)* in a patient with gastric cancer *(small arrow)*. (Courtesy of Charlene Prather, MD.)

ovarian, or neuroendocrine tumors), lymphomas, metastatic spread from extra-abdominal malignancy (e.g., breast, lung, or melanoma), and pseudomyxoma peritonei (a rare condition with gelatinous peritoneal implants from mucinous neoplasms of the appendix or ovary).

CLINICAL MANIFESTATIONS AND DIAGNOSIS

The presentation of peritoneal carcinomatosis is nonspecific, with complaints of abdominal pain, anorexia, nausea, vomiting, malaise, and weight loss. Ascites is the most common physical finding. Malignant ascites is rare, accounting for less than 10% of cases of ascites.

Although ultrasound examination may document ascites, CT is preferred to identify carcinomatosis and the origin of the underlying cause (Fig. 142-10). Diagnostic paracentesis can be performed to obtain cell count and differential, culture, and cytologic examination. A serum to ascites albumen ratio of less than 1.1 mg/dL suggests malignant ascites, but the differential diagnosis also includes pancreatic ascites (Chapter 144), nephrotic syndrome (Chapter 121), and peritoneal tuberculosis. Laparoscopy can disclose the typical tumor implant stubbing the peritoneum. Biopsy and appropriate stains can verify the presence of mesothelioma (Chapters 99 and 191) by detecting hyaluronic acid on Alcian stain in a specimen that has a negative carcinoembryonic antigen stain and no mucin on a periodic acid-Schiff stain. By contrast, carcinomas have no hyaluronic acid but show mucin and have a positive carcinoembryonic antigen stain.

TABLE 142-4 MESENTERIC DISEASES

PRIMARY INFLAMMATORY DISEASE
Panniculitis
Retractile mesenteritis
CYSTS
Developmental
Traumatic
Neoplastic
Infectious
TUMORS
Benign tumors
Lipoma
Leiomyoma
Hemangioma
Malignant tumors
Liposarcoma
Leiomyosarcoma
Rhabdomyosarcoma
Metastatic tumor
Mesenteric fibromatosis

TREATMENT AND PROGNOSIS

Rx

Treatment is typically palliative owing to the late presentation of disease. Malignant ascites responds poorly to diuretic therapies, and repeated therapeutic paracentesis may be needed. Recent data suggest some benefit from cytoreductive surgery and hyperthermic intraperitoneal chemotherapy.[23]

DISEASES OF THE MESENTERY AND OMENTUM

The differential diagnosis of mesenteric and omental disorders include a variety of rare disorders, including inflammation, cysts, and tumors that can be benign or malignant (Table 142-4).

Mesenteric panniculitis presents in middle or later age with a slight male predilection. Symptoms typically include nonspecific abdominal pain, weight loss, nausea, vomiting, and low-grade fever, but patients occasionally can present with an acute abdomen. A palpable mass is felt in the majority of patients. The diagnosis can be confirmed by CT scan. Lesions should be biopsied to exclude malignancy but generally are not amenable to complete resection. Significant improvement in the symptoms of this generally self-limited process has been reported with progesterone, corticosteroids, azathioprine, or cyclophosphamide, but evidence to recommend their general use is lacking.

Mesenteric and omental cysts and solid tumors are rare disorders. Patients present with a constellation of nonspecific symptoms. They can be identified with CT scan. Surgical resection will provide the definitive diagnosis and determine whether a benign or malignant condition is present.

Mesenteric fibromatosis (desmoid tumors) is a rare noninflammatory condition that may be associated with familial adenomatosis coli (Chapter 193) and Gardner syndrome (Chapter 193). Fibromatoses are locally aggressive tumors that may present as stable or rapidly growing intraabdominal masses. They have a high rate of recurrence after incomplete surgical resection, in patients with multicentric disease, or if precipitated by surgical trauma itself.

Grade A References

A1. Fitzgibbons RJ Jr, Giobbie-Hurder A, Gibbs JO, et al. Watchful waiting vs repair of inguinal hernia in minimally symptomatic men: a randomized clinical trial. *JAMA*. 2006;295:285-292.

A2. Karthikesalingam A, Markar SR, Holt PJ, et al. Meta-analysis of randomized controlled trials comparing laparoscopic with open mesh repair of recurrent inguinal hernia. *Br J Surg*. 2010;97:4-11.

A3. Kim K, Kim YH, Kim SY, et al. Low-dose abdominal CT for evaluating suspected appendicitis. *N Engl J Med*. 2012;366:1596-1605.

A4. Ohtani H, Tamamori Y, Arimoto Y, et al. Meta-analysis of the results of randomized controlled trials that compared laparoscopic and open surgery for acute appendicitis. *J Gastrointest Surg*. 2012;16:1929-1939.

A5. Varadhan KK, Neal KR, Lobo DN. Safety and efficacy of antibiotics compared with appendicectomy for treatment of uncomplicated acute appendicitis: meta-analysis of randomised controlled trials. *BMJ*. 2012;344:e2156.

A6. St Peter SD, Aguayo P, Fraser JD, et al. Initial laparoscopic appendectomy versus initial nonoperative management and interval appendectomy for perforated appendicitis with abscess: a prospective, randomized trial. *J Pediatr Surg*. 2010;45:236-240.

A7. St Peter SD, Tsao K, Spilde TL, et al. Single daily dosing ceftriaxone and metronidazole vs standard triple antibiotic regimen for perforated appendicitis in children: a prospective randomized trial. *J Pediatr Surg*. 2008;43:981-985.

A8. Biondo S, Golda T, Kreisler E, et al. Outpatient versus hospitalization management for uncomplicated diverticulitis: a prospective, multicenter randomized clinical trial (DIVER Trial). *Ann Surg*. 2014;259:38-44.

A9. Andreyev HJ, Benton BE, Lalji A, et al. Algorithm-based management of patients with gastrointestinal symptoms in patients after pelvic radiation treatment (ORBIT): a randomised controlled trial. *Lancet*. 2013;382:2084-2092.

A10. ten Broek RP, Stommel MW, Strik C, et al. Benefits and harms of adhesion barriers for abdominal surgery: a systematic review and meta-analysis. *Lancet*. 2014;383:48-59.

GENERAL REFERENCES

For the General References and other additional features, please visit Expert Consult at https://expertconsult.inkling.com.

143 VASCULAR DISEASES OF THE GASTROINTESTINAL TRACT

STEPHEN CRANE HAUSER

INTESTINAL ISCHEMIA

Intestinal ischemia can occur as a result of a variety of conditions that decrease intestinal blood flow. Both diminished arterial blood flow to the gut and compromised venous circulation from the intestine can cause intestinal or mesenteric ischemia. Several conditions, such as adhesions and malignancy (Chapter 193), may predispose to mesenteric ischemia by secondarily diminishing blood flow through extrinsic compression of otherwise normal intestinal arteries or veins (Table 143-1). These disorders and esophageal varices (Chapters 135 and 153) are discussed elsewhere.

TABLE 143-1 CONDITIONS PREDISPOSING TO SECONDARY MESENTERIC ISCHEMIA

Adhesions
Herniation
Volvulus
Intussusception
Mesenteric fibrosis
Retroperitoneal fibrosis
Carcinoid syndrome
Malignancy (peritoneal, mesenteric, colonic)
Neurofibromatosis
Amyloidosis
Trauma

EPIDEMIOLOGY

Intestinal ischemia is responsible for about one per 1000 hospital admissions. When considering the diagnosis of intestinal ischemia, it is important to distinguish *primary* (occlusive or non-occlusive) from *secondary* (extrinsic to the blood vessel) mesenteric ischemia, *acute* manifestations from *chronic*, *arterial* versus *venous*, and *small bowel* versus *colonic* ischemia. Risk factors for intestinal ischemia include older age (all of the disorders discussed) and conditions that predispose to arterial embolism (e.g., cardiac arrhythmias, cardioversion, heart failure, cardiomegaly, dyskinesia, valvular heart disease, recent myocardial infarction, cardiac catheterization, intracardiac thrombus, atheromatous cholesterol embolism), occlusion of arteries (atherosclerosis, fibromuscular dysplasia, abdominal aortic aneurysm, trauma, vasculitis), low-flow states (sepsis, dialysis, reduced cardiac output, vasoconstrictive drugs), and pathologic thromboses (largely venous; hypercoagulable and hyperviscosity states, portal hypertension, trauma, malignancy, inflammation).

PATHOBIOLOGY

Arterial or venous disease of the esophagus, stomach, duodenum, and rectum is very unusual for anatomic reasons. The esophagus receives its main blood supply segmentally through multiple small vessels from the aorta, right intercostal artery, bronchial arteries, inferior thyroid artery, left gastric artery, short gastric artery, and left phrenic artery. Likewise, the stomach, duodenum, and rectum have numerous arterial inputs with rich collateralization. Patients who have undergone extensive surgical resection of the esophagus, stomach, or duodenum are at increased risk for ischemia. Vasculitic disorders, which can involve small or large arteries or veins, may affect the esophagus, stomach, duodenum, or rectum.

The arterial supply of blood to the small and large intestine is from the *celiac artery, superior mesenteric artery* (SMA), and *inferior mesenteric artery* (IMA). Collateral vessels, which vary from person to person, may include the meandering mesenteric artery or arc of Riolan at the base of the mesentery (connecting the SMA and IMA), the marginal artery of Drummond along the mesenteric border (connecting the SMA and IMA), the pancreaticoduodenal arcade (connecting the celiac artery and SMA), the arc of Barkow (connecting the celiac artery and SMA), and the arc of Buhler (connecting the celiac artery and SMA). These collaterals can rapidly enlarge in response to localized mesenteric ischemia. During states of low arterial flow, such as in patients with low systemic arterial blood pressure, "watershed" areas such as the splenic flexure, which is the farthest away from arterial flow, are more likely to be involved. By contrast, when a major arterial vessel such as the IMA is suddenly occluded, the splenic flexure is less likely to be involved because of collaterals from the SMA circulation.

Intestinal blood flow, which accounts for approximately 10% of the cardiac output, increases to as much as 25% of the cardiac output after eating a meal. Blood flow to the intestine is regulated by the sympathetic nervous system and a variety of systemic (angiotensin II, vasopressin) and local (prostaglandins, leukotrienes) humoral factors.

Mesenteric ischemia can occur as a result of decreased *arterial* blood flow, which can be *occlusive* (arterial embolus, arterial thrombus, and vasculitis) or *nonocclusive* (low-flow states). *Venous* obstruction (thrombosis, vasculitis) can also result in mesenteric ischemia.

Whatever the cause of mesenteric ischemia, the gut is able to adapt to as much as a 75% reduction in normal blood flow for as long as 12 hours. Increased flow through available and newly opened collateral vessels and increased oxygen extraction help compensate. However, with a more prolonged and more severe reduction in blood flow, generalized mesenteric arterial vasoconstriction often develops and can become irreversible, even with correction of the original underlying condition (i.e., relief of focal arterial obstruction or resolution of a low-flow state). Hypoxia and reperfusion injury by oxygen radicals, reduced endothelial synthesis of nitric oxide, and an enhanced cellular inflammatory response cause microvascular and end-organ damage. Initially, the end-organ damage is primarily mucosal, but damage can rapidly progress to transmural necrosis (gangrene). Some ischemic segments of bowel will heal with fibrosis (strictures).

CLINICAL MANIFESTATIONS

Symptoms of small intestinal ischemia at initial evaluation may be acute (sudden, lasting hours),[1] subacute (days), or chronic (intermittent, occurring over a period of weeks to months).[2] With acute and many subacute manifestations, abdominal pain is often the cardinal symptom. Usually the pain is severe, persistent and periumbilical or poorly localized. Initially, the pain is typically more severe than the findings on abdominal palpation (i.e., pain out of proportion to tenderness). With or without pain, other initial features may include fever, altered mental status, abdominal distention, difficulty eating, nausea, vomiting, and diarrhea. With small bowel ischemia, overt gastrointestinal (GI) bleeding (Chapter 135) is a late and ominous finding that often suggests small bowel infarction.

Findings on physical examination can include hypotension, tachycardia, abdominal distention, initially increased and later decreased bowel sounds, and nonspecific diffuse abdominal tenderness, often mild at first. Over time, peritoneal signs with localized to generalized abdominal tenderness, rebound, and rigidity may become manifest. Occult GI bleeding can be an early finding.

DIAGNOSIS

As the diagnostic evaluation commences, appropriate attention must be directed concurrently to emergent therapy, including fluid resuscitation, antibiotics, and invasive procedures (Fig. 143-1).

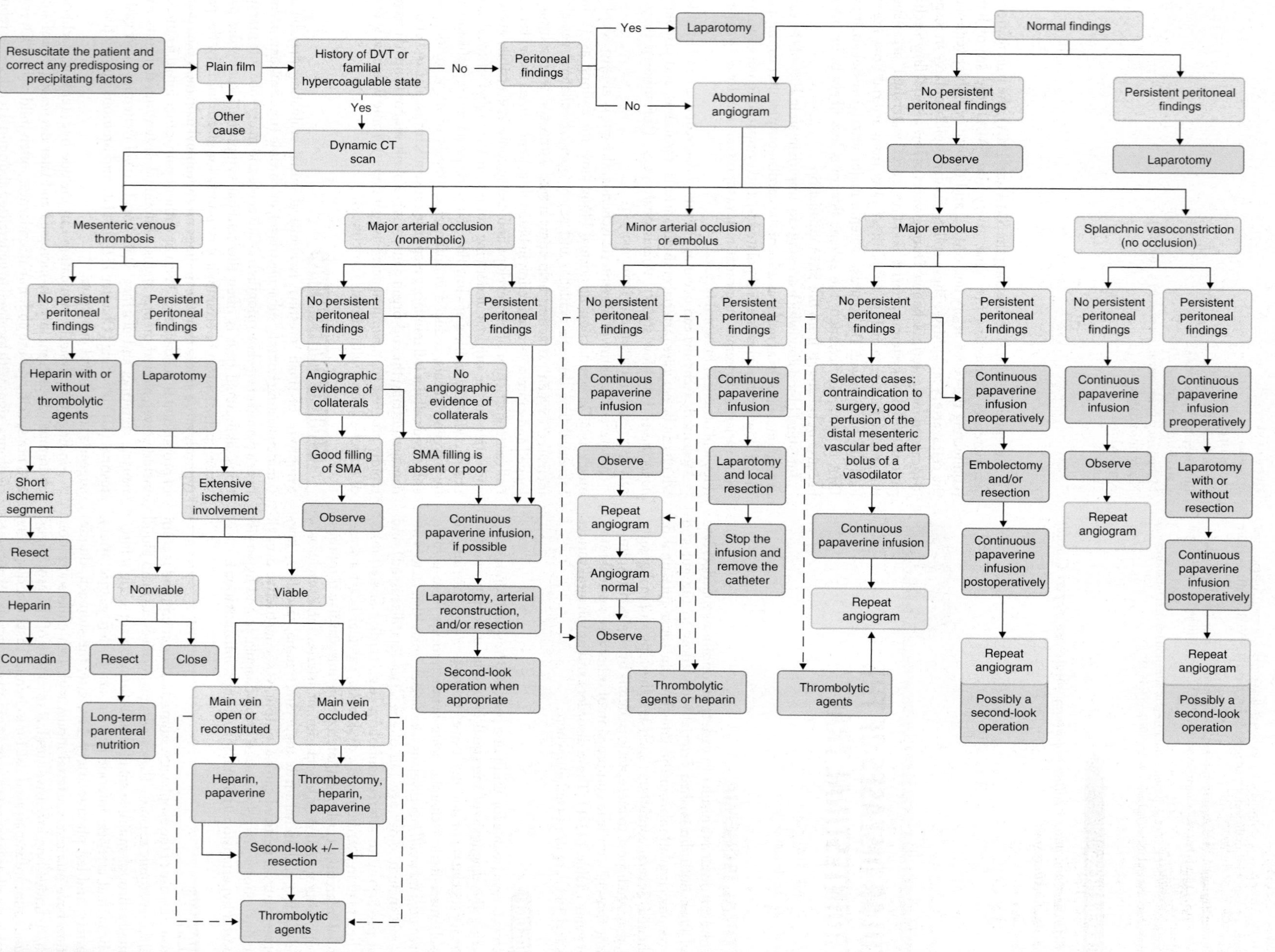

FIGURE 143-1. **Algorithm for managing patients with suspected acute mesenteric ischemia: diagnosis and management.** *Solid lines* indicate an accepted management plan; *dashed lines* indicate an alternative management plan. CT = computed tomography; DVT = deep vein thrombosis; SMA = superior mesenteric artery. (From American Gastroenterological Association Medical Position Statement: guidelines on intestinal ischemia. *Gastroenterology*. 2000;118:951-953 [corrected algorithm in *Gastroenterology*. 2000;119:281].)

Initial Diagnostic Evaluation

The initial laboratory findings in patients with an acute onset of small bowel ischemia can be entirely normal. Nonspecific abnormalities such as leukocytosis with a predominance of neutrophils and hemoconcentration may be observed. Elevated serum levels of amylase, lactate, aminotransferases, lactate dehydrogenase, creatine kinase, and phosphate often portend more advanced (necrotic) small bowel ischemia, but these findings lack sensitivity as well as specificity.

Noninvasive Imaging

The presence or absence of radiographic features suggestive of ischemia in patients with acute-onset mesenteric ischemia varies and depends on the duration and extent of ischemia. Plain abdominal radiographs are useful in helping exclude secondary causes of mesenteric ischemia, as well as other causes of acute abdominal pain, nausea, vomiting, or distention, such as obstruction and perforation. Radiographic findings such as "thumbprinting" (caused by submucosal hemorrhage), an ileus pattern, or formless loops of small bowel, or with more advanced disease, pneumatosis intestinalis or portal venous gas (often a sign of transmural necrosis or gangrene) occasionally may be observed. Contrast-enhanced abdominal-pelvic computed tomography (CT) is also helpful to exclude alternative diagnoses. CT may demonstrate entirely normal findings in acute mesenteric ischemia, or findings such as segmental bowel wall thickening, submucosal hemorrhage, mesenteric stranding, mesenteric venous thrombosis, pneumatosis, and portal venous gas may be present (Fig. 143-2). Multidetector CT angiography (CTA) has a greater sensitivity and specificity (each up to 95%) than traditional CT (≈65%) and is the preferred imaging study to diagnose acute small bowel mesenteric ischemia. Magnetic resonance angiography (MRA) is less sensitive for more peripheral emboli. Subacute manifestations of bowel ischemia may be due to a wide variety of causes, including mesenteric venous thrombosis, which is best diagnosed by CT scan. However, the time needed to obtain a CT scan should not delay resuscitation or arteriography in very ill patients with suspected acute-onset ischemia.

TREATMENT Rx

Acutely ill patients require prompt, definitive diagnosis and treatment,[3] which often requires selective mesenteric angiography (Fig. 143-3). Options for arterial reconstruction in appropriately selected patients include open surgery or endovascular treatment.[4] If transmural intestinal necrosis (gangrene) is suspected from peritoneal signs, pneumatosis, or portal venous gas on imaging procedures, emergency laparotomy is indicated. The presence of predisposing conditions (e.g., arrhythmias, systemic hypotension) and their extraintestinal manifestations (e.g., heart failure, sepsis, respiratory insufficiency, acute renal failure, anemia) dictate the initial therapy,, which includes volume replacement, optimization of cardiac output, management of respiratory function, avoidance of splanchnic vasoconstrictors such as digoxin, and administration of broad-spectrum antibiotics (e.g., meropenem, imipenem-cilastatin, metronidazole and a third-generation cephalosporin, ciprofloxacin and metronidazole, or piperacillin) until symptoms resolve to cover aerobic gram-negative and anaerobic organisms and to prevent sepsis secondary to translocation of bacteria across ischemic gut mucosa.

PROGNOSIS

Acute primary arterial mesenteric ischemia involving the small bowel is an urgent condition, which, if unidentified or untreated, can result in death within hours. Mortality rates may be as high as 70% but are much lower with early diagnosis and prompt therapy. Overall, patients with colonic ischemia have a much better prognosis than do those with small bowel ischemia. Patients with mesenteric venous thrombosis also have a much better prognosis than do those with acute primary arterial mesenteric ischemia of the small intestine.

Specific Ischemic Bowel Syndromes

SUPERIOR MESENTERIC EMBOLISM

Embolization to the intestine through the SMA (*SMA embolus*) accounts for 5% of peripheral emboli and nearly 50% of cases of primary noncolonic mesenteric ischemia. Emboli originate most commonly from the heart, with

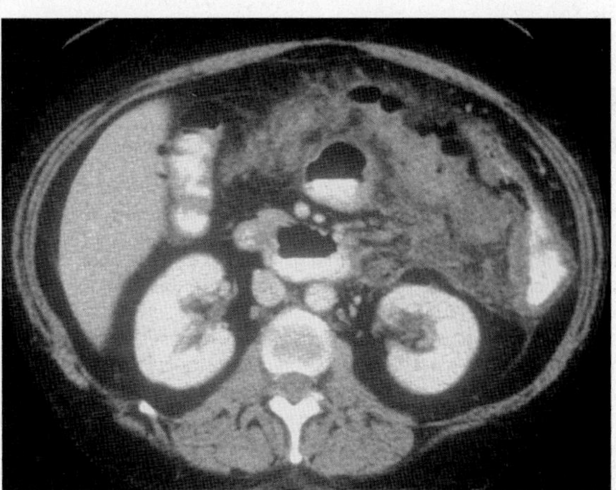

FIGURE 143-2. Computed tomography of the abdomen in a patient with ischemic colitis as a result of superior mesenteric vein thrombosis. A segmental area of the transverse colon demonstrates a thick wall, as well as considerable fluid and soft tissue stranding in the adjacent mesentery. (From Johnson CL, Schmit GD, eds. *Mayo Clinic Gastrointestinal Imaging Review*. Boca Raton, FL: Mayo Clinic Scientific Press, Taylor and Francis Group; 2005. By permission of the Mayo Foundation for Medical Education and Research. All rights reserved).

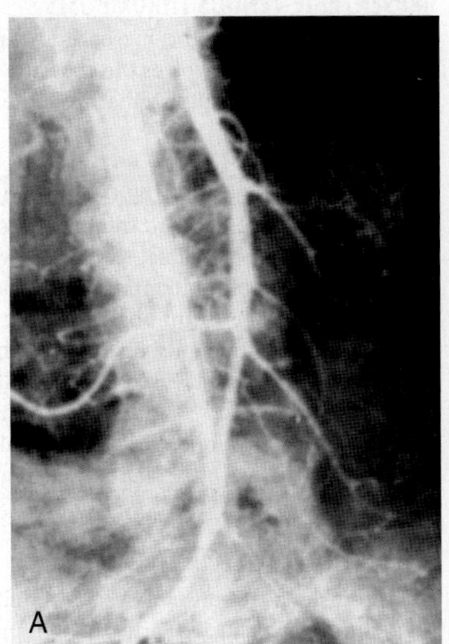

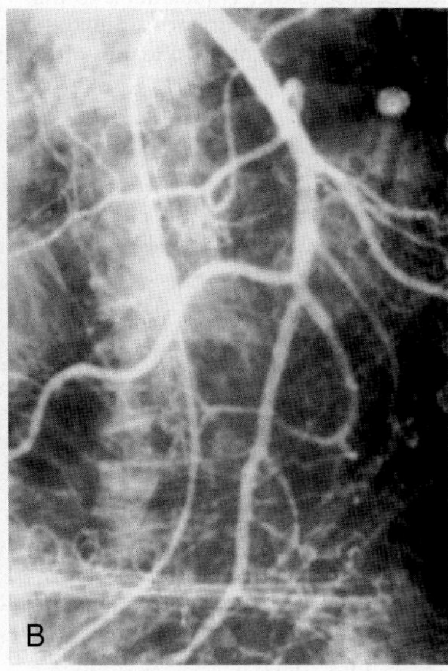

FIGURE 143-3. Selected films from superior mesenteric angiography. A, Diffuse vasoconstriction characteristic of nonocclusive mesenteric ischemia. B, Intra-arterial infusion of papaverine (30-60 mg/hr) resulted in vasodilation.

TABLE 143-2 CONDITIONS ASSOCIATED WITH EMBOLIZATION TO THE GASTROINTESTINAL TRACT

Cardiac arrhythmias
Valvular heart disease
Heart failure
Myocardial infarction
Intracardiac thrombus
Cardiac catheterization
Cardioversion
Atherosclerosis of the aorta

an aortic origin being less common (Table 143-2), and tend to obstruct beyond the origin of the SMA.

CLINICAL MANIFESTATIONS AND DIAGNOSIS

Patients who are evaluated early in the course of their illness may have entirely normal CT scans, or the CT findings may be consistent with mesenteric ischemia without features that would suggest alternative diagnoses (e.g., perforation, obstruction). Multidetector CTA is much more likely than standard CT to diagnose embolic disease reliably in the mesenteric arterial vasculature. Selective mesenteric angiography offers the possibility of therapy as well as diagnosis.

TREATMENT Rx

Select patients with acute onset of a partial or small SMA branch occlusion may be candidates for thrombolytic therapy (e.g., streptokinase, urokinase, tissue plasminogen activator) infused through an arterial catheter directly into the vicinity of the embolus; this therapy can lyse the embolus and resolve symptoms such as abdominal pain. Because segmental arterial embolic occlusion of a small portion of the SMA vascular bed results in widespread splanchnic visceral arterial vasoconstriction, which may persist even after the original inciting event (i.e., an embolus) is rectified, infusion of a vasodilator such as papaverine (often given as a 60-mg bolus followed by a continuous infusion of 30 to 60 mg/hr for 12-48 hours) through an arterial catheter reverses this reflex vasoconstriction and improves the outcome, including mortality rates. The same scenario occurs with other arterial occlusive lesions (SMA thrombi), arterial nonocclusive disease (nonocclusive mesenteric ischemia), and disorders associated with mesenteric venous occlusion.

Patients evaluated in the course of their acute embolic illness with peritoneal signs require laparotomy, with or without resection and with or without embolectomy, which is usually performed during surgical exploration. A "second-look" operation 24 hours after embolectomy to make sure that all necrotic tissue has been resected may be necessary.

Any patient in whom SMA embolization is diagnosed requires preoperative systemic anticoagulation (e.g., intravenous heparin) to prevent propagation of clot around the embolus and to guard against further embolization to the intestine or other organs (i.e., brain, coronary arteries, kidneys, extremities). Anticoagulation is usually discontinued before surgery and is often resumed 24 to 48 hours postoperatively, depending on the operative findings. Mortality can be as high as 70%.

SUPERIOR MESENTERIC THROMBOSIS

Thrombosis of the SMA (*SMA thrombus*) accounts for nearly 15% of cases of primary noncolonic mesenteric ischemia. Risk factors include older age, atherosclerosis (e.g., hypertension, diabetes mellitus, hyperlipidemia, smoking history), low-flow states, hypercoagulable states, and less often vasculitis and aortic or mesenteric aneurysms.

CLINICAL MANIFESTATIONS AND DIAGNOSIS

Nearly one-third of these patients have a history of symptomatic chronic mesenteric ischemia (see later) antedating their acute manifestation of SMA thrombosis. Proximal mesenteric arterial occlusions are well recognized by multidetector CTA, MRA, and Doppler ultrasonography, but similar abnormalities are common in asymptomatic elderly persons. Similar to acute SMA embolism, the diagnosis is confirmed by selective mesenteric angiography, with intra-arterial infusion of a vasodilator used to reverse reflex-generalized vasoconstriction.

TREATMENT Rx

Although thrombolytic therapy has been helpful in a limited number of case reports, surgical thrombectomy or bypass grafting, with or without bowel resection, is the most common therapeutic approach. Because many thrombi occur near the SMA origin, angioplasty may be therapeutic in very select cases, but the risk for reocclusion is high. Similar to acute SMA embolism, anticoagulation (intravenous heparin) is important preoperatively and at some point postoperatively in the acute state, as is administration of broad-spectrum antibiotics (see Small Intestinal Ischemia).

ACUTE NONOCCLUSIVE, NONCOLONIC PRIMARY ARTERIAL ISCHEMIA

Nonocclusive mesenteric ischemia, which accounts for about 20% of primary noncolonic mesenteric ischemia cases, is caused by low arterial blood flow to the intestine. Risk factors include advanced age, decreased systolic blood pressure (e.g., cardiac arrhythmia, heart failure, myocardial infarction, shock, sepsis, burns, pancreatitis, hemorrhage, multiple organ failure, dialysis, perioperative states), vasospasm (e.g., digoxin, vasopressin, amphetamines, cocaine), and atherosclerotic disease.

CLINICAL MANIFESTATIONS AND DIAGNOSIS

The clinical findings are generally indistinguishable from those of embolic or thrombotic vascular disease except that symptoms may be less acute. As a result, patients initially may be seen without acute abdominal pain but rather with more nonspecific symptoms such as distention, nausea, emesis, diarrhea, fever, altered mental status, and borderline or low systolic blood pressure. Selective mesenteric angiography establishes the diagnosis (lack of embolus or thrombus, alternating areas of vessel spasm and dilation, vascular pruning and spasm).

TREATMENT Rx

The best specific treatment is prolonged intra-arterial instillation of a vasodilator (e.g., papaverine, often given as a 60-mg bolus followed by a continuous infusion of 30-60 mg/hr) to reverse the vasospasm. Avoidance of vasospastic medications and optimization of cardiac output, blood volume, and blood pressure are crucial. Anticoagulation is generally not necessary, but broad-spectrum antibiotics (similar to those recommended earlier) should be administered to cover aerobic gram-negative and anaerobic organisms. Although many of these patients have serious conditions that predispose them to low-flow states and their ultimate prognosis depends on the outcomes of these serious conditions, the diagnosis and treatment of acute nonocclusive mesenteric ischemia with therapeutic angiography can be life saving.

MESENTERIC VENOUS THROMBOSIS

Occlusive disease of the mesenteric venous circulation *(mesenteric venous thrombosis)* usually involves the superior mesenteric vein (SMV) and may be accompanied by symptoms that are acute (hours to days) or subacute (weeks to months) in onset.[5]

EPIDEMIOLOGY AND PATHOBIOLOGY

Thrombosis of the SMV accounts for about 10% of cases of primary noncolonic mesenteric ischemia. Colonic involvement with ischemic colitis is much less common. In contrast to arterial occlusive disease, risk factors for and causes of SMV thrombosis are more numerous and diverse. Individuals with a personal or family history of a hypercoagulable state or deep vein thrombosis are at increased risk for SMV thrombosis. Hypercoagulable states, hyperviscosity syndromes, portal hypertension, intra-abdominal infections (e.g., pyelophlebitis, diverticulitis, appendicitis) or inflammation (e.g., Crohn disease, pancreatitis), malignancy, vasculitis, and trauma may all cause thrombosis of the SMV (Table 143-3).

CLINICAL MANIFESTATIONS

Symptoms in acute-onset cases are similar to those observed in acute occlusive and nonocclusive arterial mesenteric ischemia—abdominal pain, anorexia, nausea, vomiting, abdominal fullness, diarrhea, and constipation—but tend to persist over a longer time period. Some patients may have bacteremia, especially infection with *Bacteroides* spp. GI hemorrhage, if present, is

TABLE 143-3 RISK FACTORS FOR MESENTERIC VENOUS THROMBOSIS

HYPERCOAGULABLE AND HYPERVISCOSITY STATES
Protein S deficiency
Protein C deficiency
Antithrombin III deficiency
Factor V Leiden mutation
Hyperfibrinogenemia
Antiphospholipid syndrome
Primary myeloproliferative neoplasm
Sickle cell disease
Estrogen or progesterone
INTRA-ABDOMINAL INFECTIONS AND INFLAMMATION
Appendicitis
Diverticulitis
Crohn disease
Abscess
Pancreatitis
Cholecystitis
Pyelophlebitis
Neonatal omphalitis
PORTAL HYPERTENSION
Variceal sclerotherapy
MALIGNANCY
TRAUMA
VASCULITIS

often indicative of infarction. However, many patients with SMV thrombosis experience more vague symptomatic abdominal pain, nausea, distention, or diarrhea over a period of weeks to months (subacute).

DIAGNOSIS

Abdominal-pelvic contrast-enhanced CT, which is the preferred diagnostic test, usually (>90% sensitivity) demonstrates SMV thrombosis with or without portal vein or splenic vein thrombosis. By definition, chronic mesenteric venous thrombosis is asymptomatic and usually detected as an incidental CT finding in patients with portal hypertension, pancreatitis (acute or chronic), or malignancy. The presence of abundant collateral vessels suggests chronic or sometimes subacute mesenteric venous obstruction.

Small bowel radiography may demonstrate segmental bowel wall thickening and separation of bowel loops. Selective mesenteric angiography is not generally necessary.

TREATMENT Rx

Therapy for acute-onset cases may include laparotomy with or without bowel resection when infarction is suspected, fluid resuscitation, broad-spectrum antibiotics (similar to those recommended earlier to cover aerobic gram-negative and anaerobic organisms), avoidance of vasoconstrictors, and anticoagulation (e.g., intravenous heparin) in the absence of GI bleeding. Selected patients may be candidates for thrombolytic therapy (e.g., streptokinase, urokinase, tissue plasminogen activator) followed by anticoagulation. Underlying conditions such as hypercoagulable states, portal hypertension, intra-abdominal infections, intra-abdominal inflammation, and malignancy require concomitant diagnosis and therapy. The indications for anticoagulation in the chronic setting are uncertain, and it is generally avoided in patients who have portal hypertension but do not have symptoms related to their mesenteric venous thrombosis.

CHRONIC MESENTERIC ISCHEMIA

Chronic atherosclerotic stenosis of the visceral arteries is the cause of most cases of chronic mesenteric ischemia, sometimes called *intestinal angina.*

EPIDEMIOLOGY AND PATHOBIOLOGY

Risk factors for chronic mesenteric ischemia are principally older age and the same risk factors for atherosclerosis. Some patients may develop chronic mesenteric ischemia after their malignancy is treated with radiotherapy, chemotherapy, or both. Rarely, vasculitis or an aortic aneurysm can be manifested as chronic mesenteric ischemia. Atherosclerotic stenoses usually involve the origins of two or all of the three major visceral arteries supplying the intestine. However, many age-matched patients also harbor atherosclerotic lesions and do not have symptoms of chronic mesenteric ischemia.

CLINICAL MANIFESTATIONS

Patients typically complain of episodic ischemic abdominal pain. The pain is usually upper or midabdominal, typically begins 15 to 30 minutes after a meal, lasts 1 to 3 hours, and progresses in severity over time, as well as occurs after smaller meals and more frequently after meals. Patients may lose weight as a result of fear of eating (sitophobia). Nausea, vomiting, bloating, diarrhea, and constipation can also occur. Malabsorption with steatorrhea; otherwise unexplained gastroduodenal ulcerations; and small bowel biopsy findings of villous atrophy, nonspecific surface cell flattening, and chronic inflammation may be seen in some patients. More than half of patients have a bruit on abdominal examination. In some patients with episodic symptoms, acute thrombotic mesenteric ischemia develops suddenly.

DIAGNOSIS AND TREATMENT Rx

Atherosclerotic lesions usually can be identified by Doppler ultrasonography because they are proximal in these vessels and demonstrate increased flow velocity through areas of marked stenosis. Multidetector CTA and MRA are also useful to screen for arterial stenoses consistent with chronic mesenteric ischemia in symptomatic patients, but neither technique is adequately sensitive to exclude the diagnosis of chronic mesenteric ischemia when the pretest probability is high. Thus, selective mesenteric angiography is important to ensure that the anatomic findings are consistent with the diagnosis. Patients must be evaluated thoroughly to exclude other causes of abdominal pain (i.e., gastric cancer, gastroparesis, gastric volvulus, partial small bowel obstruction, small bowel bacterial overgrowth states, pancreatic cancer, biliary disease, paraesophageal hernias). For symptomatic patients with appropriate findings on angiography and no other causes of symptoms, surgical reconstruction provides better long-term outcomes than angioplasty and stenting in patients who are not at too high risk for surgery.[6]

ISCHEMIC COLITIS

EPIDEMIOLOGY AND PATHOBIOLOGY

Ischemic colitis, which is the single most common cause of mesenteric ischemia, accounts for nearly 50% of all cases and for almost one in 2000 hospital admissions. Many cases are acute and self-limited and occur in persons older than 60 years without any apparent cause; these cases are probably attributable to transient nonocclusive hypoperfusion involving a segment of the colon. It is controversial whether subtle hypercoagulable states contribute to the pathogenesis of idiopathic cases. Atherosclerotic or thrombotic occlusion of the IMA or its branches and low-flow states are recognizable causes of ischemic colitis. Less common causes include hypercoagulable states (especially in younger persons); iatrogenic ligation of the IMA (e.g., with aortic surgery); embolism; vasculitis; and any cause of colonic obstruction, including malignancy, stricture, and fecalith, that can produce localized compression of the vasculature with an upstream segment of ischemia. Other unusual associations include long-distance running (dehydration, mechanical trauma to the vasculature, generally involving the cecum), pit viper bite, scuba diving, and intra-abdominal infections or inflammatory disease. A variety of medications, illicit drugs, and chemicals also can result in a chemical picture identical or similar to ischemic colitis (Table 143-4), sometimes probably secondary to vasoconstriction that can affect other parts of the GI tract, liver, and other organ systems (e.g., cocaine, amphetamines, pseudoephedrine), sometimes caused by constipation (e.g., alosetron), sometimes caused by a hypercoagulable effect (e.g., estrogens), and sometimes as a result of a chemical effect (e.g., sodium polystyrene with sorbitol enemas).

CLINICAL MANIFESTATIONS

The clinical presentation of ischemic colitis is acute and, in most patients, includes abdominal pain (mostly left lower quadrant), often with urgency, diarrhea, and passage of bright red blood per rectum.[7] Anorexia, nausea, vomiting, abdominal distention, and passage of maroon material per rectum may also occur. Although the blood loss is not usually enough to require transfusion, some patients may be orthostatic because of loss of blood and fluid. Fever, tachycardia, abdominal tenderness over the affected portion of the colon, and distention may be found on physical examination.

TABLE 143-4 MEDICATIONS AND DRUGS ASSOCIATED WITH ISCHEMIC COLITIS

Digitalis
Vasopressin
Pseudoephedrine
Amphetamines
Cocaine
Ergot
Sumatriptan
Gold
Danazol
Estrogens
Progestins
Alosetron
Psychotropics
Nonsteroidal anti-inflammatory drugs
Various enemas
Tegaserod
Interferon/ribavirin

DIAGNOSIS

Laboratory findings range from normal to nonspecific findings such as leukocytosis and hemoconcentration to those observed in persons with bowel necrosis (see earlier). Evaluation of patients younger than 50 years should include tests for thrombophilic disorders (Chapter 176).

Plain radiographs of the abdomen may reveal "thumbprinting" or may be normal. Similar to small bowel ischemia, CT scanning can be useful to help exclude other disorders, especially in more symptomatic and ill patients; the findings may be consistent with segmental colonic edema and inflammation, with or without adjacent pericolonic inflammatory stranding. These radiographic features are consistent with ischemic colitis in an appropriate clinical setting but are nonspecific and may be seen in patients with other disorders such as acute diverticulitis (Chapter 142), infectious colitis (Chapter 140), and inflammatory bowel disease (Chapter 141). The diagnosis is best made by colonoscopy, which should provide endoscopic and histologic findings consistent with acute ischemic colitis: segmental patchy ulceration, edema, erythema, single stripe sign, and submucosal bluish purple hemorrhagic nodules (Fig. 143-4).

Typically, visceral angiography is not required because most patients with ischemic colitis have self-limited involvement of the left colon or distal transverse colon–splenic flexure with sparing of the rectum, and findings on urgent angiography in these patients are usually normal. However, about 10% of patients with acute ischemic colitis have predominantly right-sided involvement of the cecum, ascending colon, hepatic flexure, and proximal transverse colon. Because the arterial supply to the right colon is through the ileocolic branch of the SMA, there may be concomitant distal ileal ischemia, often owing to low-flow states (especially hemodialysis patients) or embolization. These patients have more pain, less bleeding, and a much worse outcome and are at risk for small bowel necrosis.

Differential Diagnosis

Gastrointestinal infections, such as with *Escherichia coli* O157:H7, *Clostridium difficile, Klebsiella oxytoca*, and cytomegalovirus (CMV), can mimic ischemic colitis clinically and even histologically. Acute-onset inflammatory bowel disease involving the colon can also be difficult to distinguish from ischemic colitis. However, patients with subacute or chronic pain, diarrhea, obstructive symptoms, weight loss, or bleeding may be thought to have complicated diverticular disease, Crohn disease, or malignancy with stricture, and chronic ischemic stricture of the colon may not be correctly diagnosed until after surgery is performed.

Stool culture can exclude infection, especially with *E. coli* O157:H7, *C. difficile,* and parasites. In immunocompromised patients, colonic biopsy can be performed to diagnose CMV infection.

TREATMENT Rx

Patients with right-sided ischemic colitis require multidetector CTA or visceral angiography not only for diagnosis but also for intra-arterial administration of vasodilators (e.g., papaverine as a 60-mg intravenous bolus followed by an infusion of 30 to 60 mg/hr). Some patients may require urgent surgery.

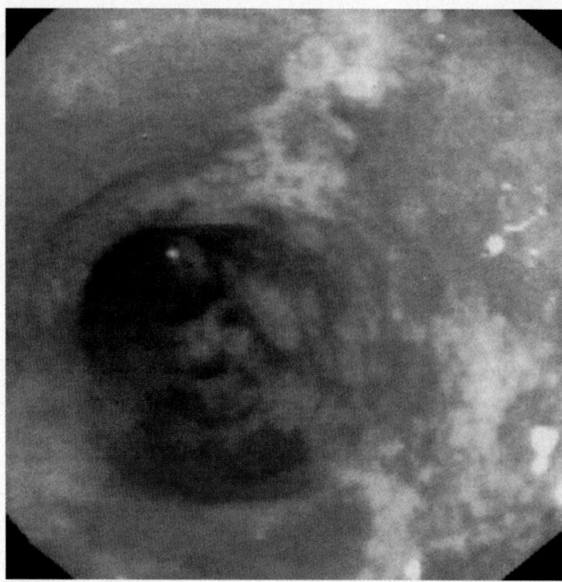

FIGURE 143-4. Endoscopy of the splenic flexure of the colon in a patient with ischemic colitis. Note the shallow, irregular, exudative ulceration with interspersed erythema. (From Emory TS, Carpenter HA, Gostout CJ, et al, eds. *Atlas of Gastrointestinal Endoscopy and Endoscopic Biopsies*. Washington, DC: Armed Forces Institute of Pathology, American Registry of Pathology; 2000.)

The clinical course in patients with right-sided ischemic colitis may be subacute, with a mortality rate as high as 50% or greater.

By contrast, left-sided acute ischemic colitis, which accounts for most cases, tends to resolve within hours to a few days with supportive therapy, including volume replacement, correction of any low-flow state; broad-spectrum antibiotics (similar to those recommended earlier for patients with small bowel ischemia); avoidance of vasoconstrictive medications; and rarely, blood transfusion; surgery is required only in patients with signs and symptoms of transmural necrosis, perforation, or massive bleeding. Occasional patients with acute-onset left-sided ischemic colitis have persistent or recurrent symptoms of pain, diarrhea, bleeding, sepsis, or stricture formation that develop over a period of weeks to months and may require segmental surgical resection.

PROGNOSIS

As many as 10% to 20% of patients may require urgent surgery. Nonocclusive ischemic colitis, acute renal failure, extent of bowel ischemia, serum lactate, and duration of catecholamine therapy predict survival.

VASCULITIS

Many vasculitic syndromes can involve the GI tract. Usually, but not always, other organ systems are also involved.

Large and Medium Vessel Vasculitis

Takayasu arteritis (Chapters 78 and 270) and *giant cell arteritis* (Chapter 271), which affect large to medium-sized muscular arteries, rarely involve the GI tract. Takayasu arteritis has been associated rarely with inflammatory bowel disease.

Medium to Small Vessel Vasculitis

Polyarteritis nodosa (Chapter 270) is characterized by segmental microaneurysms typically involving small- and medium-sized arteries. The small bowel is involved more commonly than the large bowel. Many patients will have abdominal pain, fever, hypertension, and multiple organ involvement. GI bleeding or perforation will develop in some patients. The gallbladder, spleen, pancreas, and liver may also be involved. About one-third of patients with polyarteritis nodosa are infected with hepatitis B virus.

Both *granulomatosis* with *polyangiitis* (Chapter 270) and *Churg-Strauss syndrome* (Chapter 270) affect small- and medium-sized arteries. Although GI involvement is not common in Wegener granulomatosis with granulomatous inflammation, in up to one third of patients with Churg-Strauss syndrome, abdominal pain or GI bleeding may develop as a result of ischemia. Mesenteric venous involvement can also occur with Churg-Strauss syndrome.

Thromboangiitis obliterans (Buerger disease; Chapter 80) involves small- and medium-sized arteries and can cause multiple distal occlusions of the mesenteric arterial circulation. Patients with *Behçet disease* (Chapter 270) often have lymphocytic inflammation of small- and medium-sized arteries, as well as veins. Similar to Crohn disease, the ileocecal region is frequently involved with ulceration. Abdominal pain, diarrhea, GI bleeding, and perforation may occur.

Degos disease, also known as malignant atrophic papulosis, is a rare condition characterized by vasculitis of small- and medium-sized arteries. Multiple organ systems can be affected, and GI perforation owing to mesenteric ischemia represents a major cause of mortality.

Small Vessel Vasculitis

Small vessel involvement with immunoglobulin A immune complex deposition in blood vessel walls is typical in *Henoch-Schönlein purpura* (Chapter 270). These patients usually have palpable purpura, arthritis, nephritis, and abdominal pain, as well as GI bleeding. *Hypersensitivity vasculitis* (Chapter 270), which affects small arterioles, venules, and capillaries, is related to a variety of drugs, infections, and chemicals; on occasion there may be GI involvement. *Cryoglobulinemia* (Chapter 187) with immune complex involvement of small blood vessels can sometimes involve the GI tract. These patients are often infected with hepatitis C virus.

HEMORRHAGIC VASCULAR DISORDERS

Angiodysplasia

DEFINITION AND EPIDEMIOLOGY

Angiodysplasia or vascular ectasia is a thin-walled, dilated, punctate red vascular structure in the mucosa or submucosa of the bowel; it typically involves adjacent venules, capillaries, and arterioles.[8] Angiodysplasia is found in the colon, especially the right colon, in up to 1% of persons and is found also in the stomach and small bowel but rarely in the esophagus. Angiodysplastic lesions may be single or multiple, and they increase in frequency with age. Some data suggest associations with chronic renal failure (Chapter 130), von Willebrand disease (Chapter 173), and aortic stenosis (Chapter 75); whether correction of these associated disorders diminishes future GI hemorrhage (Chapter 135) from angiodysplasia is uncertain.

CLINICAL MANIFESTATIONS

Clinically, these lesions can produce painless bleeding, which may be occult and manifest only by guaiac-positive stools or iron deficiency anemia, or the bleeding may be overt, with hematochezia, maroon stools, melena, and hematemesis.

DIAGNOSIS

Endoscopic procedures most often make the diagnosis of bleeding secondary to angiodysplasia (Fig. 143-5). In some patients, endoscopic procedures may need to be repeated, especially in volume-depleted patients and after the administration of narcotics. Small bowel angiodysplasia, beyond the reach of both a colonoscope from below and an extended-length endoscope from above, may be the cause of major bleeding (Chapter 135) and require video capsule endoscopy (Chapter 134) or small bowel balloon-assisted enteroscopy for diagnosis and treatment.

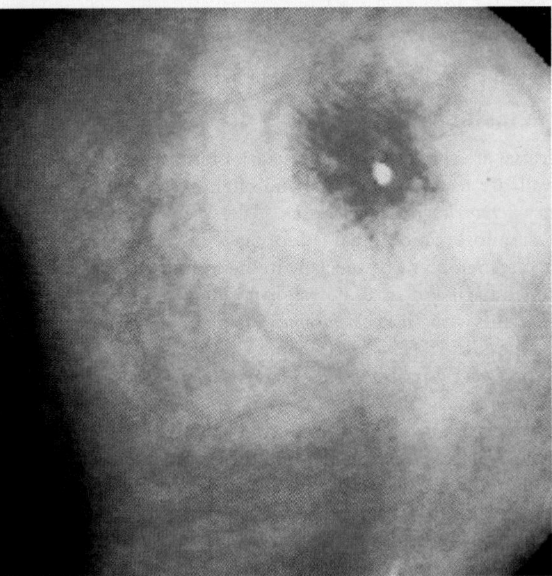

FIGURE 143-5. Endoscopy of the sigmoid colon in a patient with angiectasia. The lesion is discrete and contains a tight, radiating cluster of ectatic mucosal vessels. (From Emory TS, Carpenter HA, Gostout CJ, et al, eds. *Atlas of Gastrointestinal Endoscopy and Endoscopic Biopsies*. Washington, DC: Armed Forces Institute of Pathology, American Registry of Pathology; 2000.)

TREATMENT Rx

Electrocoagulation laser therapy or argon plasma coagulation can be accomplished during endoscopy. When very active bleeding makes urgent colonoscopy technically difficult, visceral angiography can be diagnostic and permit embolization of bleeding lesions or intra-arterial infusion of a vasoconstrictor. Rarely, bowel resection is required.

PROGNOSIS

More than 90% of GI angiodysplasias never bleed. When angiodsyplasias are found incidentally in patients who have no history of past or concurrent bleeding, they typically should not be treated.

Dieulafoy Lesion

Dieulafoy lesion is an unusually large submucosal artery typically found in the proximal portion of the stomach within 6 cm of the gastroesophageal junction. Similar lesions may also occur in the rectum; colon; small bowel; and far less often, the esophagus. Dieulafoy lesion is manifested clinically as sudden, massive bleeding, which may be recurrent.

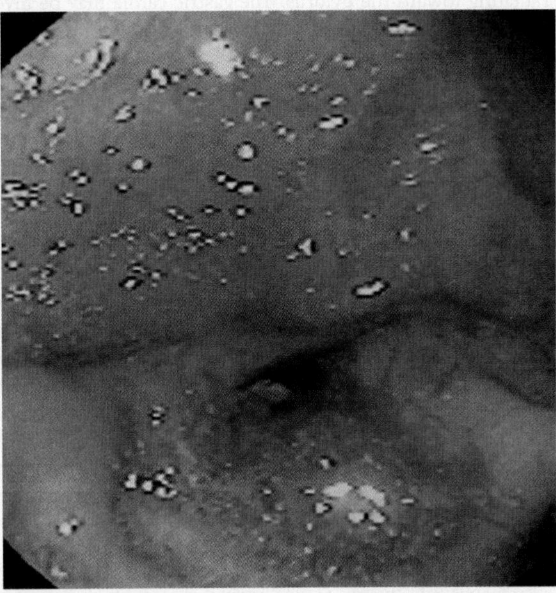

FIGURE 143-6. Endoscopy of the stomach in a patient with Dieulafoy lesion. Note the visible vessel manifested as a pale protuberance surrounded by a clot with adjacent normal-appearing mucosa. (From Emory TS, Carpenter HA, Gostout CJ, et al, eds. *Atlas of Gastrointestinal Endoscopy and Endoscopic Biopsies*. Washington, DC: Armed Forces Institute of Pathology, American Registry of Pathology; 2000.)

DIAGNOSIS AND TREATMENT Rx

Urgent endoscopy is required to identify what is usually a very small vascular protuberance (Fig. 143-6) but can rapidly become inapparent when the acute bleeding stops. Ulceration is not seen, and repeat endoscopic procedures during active bleeding may be required to make the diagnosis. Sometimes the diagnosis requires angiography during a bleeding episode. Endoscopic injection and electrocoagulation therapy are generally effective, but endoscopic band therapy and hemoclips may also be used, and surgery is sometimes required.

PROGNOSIS

Endoscopic therapy is successful long term in nearly 90% of patients.

Other Ectasias

Telangiectases are similar to angiodysplasias but occur in all the layers of the bowel wall, are usually congenital and often occur in other organ systems. *Hereditary hemorrhagic telangiectasia* (Osler-Weber-Rendu disease; Chapter 173) is an autosomal dominant disorder with telangiectases involving the lips; mucous membranes, especially in the mouth and nose; GI tract, especially the stomach and small bowel; liver; lung; retina; and central nervous system. Patients with *Turner syndrome* (Chapter 235) or *scleroderma* (Chapter 267), and the *CREST syndrome* (Chapter 267) (calcinosis, Raynaud phenomenon, esophageal dysmotility, sclerodactyly, telangiectasia) may also have GI tract telangiectases.

Vascular ectasias involving venules and capillaries can also be seen in the small bowel *(congestive enteropathy)*; in the colon *(congestive colopathy)*; and more commonly, in the stomach *(congestive gastropathy)* in patients with portal hypertension (Chapter 153). In contrast to angiodysplasias, these lesions tend to be more diffuse, appear as multiple, fine punctate red spots or as a mosaic pattern similar to the gastritis of *Helicobacter pylori* and are more often found in the proximal than the distal part of the stomach. Therapies that decrease portal hypertension can reduce or eliminate these lesions and bleeding from them.

Gastric antral vascular ectasia (GAVE), or watermelon stomach, also involves venules and capillaries with thrombosis as well as ectasia. Erythematous streaks similar to the stripes on a watermelon are typically seen in the antrum radiating toward the pylorus. The gastric cardia may be involved as well. Patients usually have occult bleeding and less often melena. GAVE is associated with connective tissue diseases (e.g., systemic lupus erythematosus [Chapter 266], mixed connective tissue disease [Chapter 267], scleroderma [Chapter 267]), pernicious anemia (Chapter 164), and portal hypertension (Chapter 153). However, unlike congestive gastropathy, treatment of portal hypertension does not eliminate GAVE or bleeding from it. Argon plasma coagulation is the usual therapy if iron replacement alone is not effective. Antrectomy is rarely needed.

Neoplastic Vascular Lesions

Hemangiomas are uncommon, usually benign vascular tumors that can be found throughout the GI tract, often in the rectum or colon. They may be single or multiple, bluish purple, and sessile or polypoid. In some persons, these lesions are multiple and associated with skin lesions, such as the *blue rubber bleb nevus syndrome* with purple-blue cutaneous hemangiomas or the *Klippel-Trenaunay* syndrome with port-wine-colored cutaneous hemangiomas, hemihypertrophy, and varicose veins. Rare vascular malignant neoplasms of the GI tract include *angiosarcomas* and *hemangioendotheliomas*.

Miscellaneous Vascular Disorders

Aortoenteric fistulas, which most commonly occur after surgery for an aortic aneurysm (Chapter 78), may be related to infection of the graft and can result in torrential GI bleeding. Many of these fistulas communicate with the duodenum. Evaluation of bleeding in persons who have previously undergone abdominal aortic surgery should include urgent extended-length upper endoscopy to document a fistula or diagnose another definitive source of the bleeding. Angiography and radiographic tests (CT, magnetic resonance imaging [MRI]) are helpful only if the findings are abnormal (i.e., there is evidence of a fistula) because of their poor sensitivity for the presence of aortoenteric fistulas. If no clear alternative source for the bleeding can readily be found, explorative surgery is indicated. *Atrioesophageal fistulas* can occur as a consequence of thermal damage within the heart or esophagus, such as after radiofrequency ablation procedures for atrial fibrillation or for Barrett esophagus.

Celiac artery compression syndrome (median arcuate ligament syndrome) is a very rare pseudo-ischemic syndrome. Patients are often young and healthy and have postprandial upper abdominal pain, most likely caused by extrinsic compression of the celiac axis by the median arcuate ligament of the diaphragm. Sitophobia can result in considerable weight loss, and there may be a loud systolic bruit in the epigastric region on physical examination. Visceral angiography supports the diagnosis, but bruits and celiac axis compression may occur without symptoms. Surgical therapy is indicated after other possible causes of the patient's symptoms have been excluded.

Patients with *Ehlers-Danlos syndrome type IV* (Chapter 260) can develop small bowel ischemia and perforation as well as arterial rupture. Similar vascular catastrophes with GI or intraperitoneal hemorrhage can occur in patients with *pseudoxanthoma elasticum type I* (Chapter 260) or with *visceral artery aneurysms* (secondary to atherosclerosis, fibrodysplasia, portal hypertension, pregnancy, pancreatitis, vasculitis, or trauma).

HEPATIC AND SPLENIC VASCULAR DISEASE

Budd-Chiari Syndrome

Budd-Chiari syndrome can occur as a result of any process that interferes with the normal flow of blood out of the liver, including constrictive pericarditis (Chapter 77) and veno-occlusive disease (Chapter 150). Hepatic vein thrombosis, which is the main cause of Budd-Chiari syndrome, may involve one, two, or all three of the major hepatic veins, with or without partial or complete occlusion of the inferior vena cava. Often, Budd-Chiari syndrome is caused by a hypercoagulable state (Chapter 176), such as a chronic myeloproliferative disorder (e.g., polycythemia vera [Chapter 166], essential thrombocythemia [Chapter 166], myeloid metaplasia [Chapter 166]), paroxysmal nocturnal hemoglobinuria, or other hypercoagulable conditions (Chapter 176), such as factor V (Leiden) gene mutation, antiphospholipid antibody syndrome, protein C deficiency, protein S deficiency, or antithrombin III deficiency. A high percentage of these patients harbor *JAK2* V617F mutations. Nearly 50% of patients with Budd-Chiari syndrome have more than one risk factor. Malignancies (direct compression or invasion of hepatic veins, hypercoagulable state), infections (liver abscess), pregnancy, inflammatory disorders (e.g., Behçet syndrome, inflammatory bowel disease, connective tissue disease, sarcoidosis), and membranous obstruction (webs) of the inferior vena cava are also associated with Budd-Chiari syndrome.

CLINICAL MANIFESTATIONS

The syndrome is usually subacute or chronic, occurs over a period of weeks to months, and is characterized by the insidious onset of upper abdominal pain, hepatomegaly, and ascites. Fulminant and acute presentations, including encephalopathy, jaundice, ascites, and liver failure, are rare.

DIAGNOSIS

Liver function testing usually reveals normal or mild to moderate nonspecific elevations in serum aspartate and alanine aminotransferase levels. *JAK2* mutation analysis should be part of the initial evaluation. Doppler ultrasonography of the liver is the initial diagnostic test of choice, but the absence of hepatic venous flow or venous thrombosis (or both) is also readily apparent with contrast-enhanced CT scanning or MRA. Hepatic venography can confirm the diagnosis (Fig. 143-7) and, with imaging of the inferior vena cava, as well as selective venous pressure measurements, can help guide therapy.

TREATMENT Rx

Therapy includes diagnosis and treatment of underlying conditions, anticoagulation (intravenous heparin; see Table 81-4 in Chapter 81) to prevent the propagation of thrombi, and treatment of ascites (e.g., diuretics; Chapter 153). To decompress the congested liver, most patients require interventional radiologic procedures, such as angioplasty, stenting, or transjugular intrahepatic portosystemic shunts, to restore hepatic venous flow.[9,10] Surgical procedures such as surgical shunts to drain the portal or mesenteric venous system into the inferior vena cava can also decompress the liver. Liver transplantation (Chapter 154) should be considered for patients with fulminant liver failure, cirrhosis, or both. Most patients with Budd-Chiari syndrome require lifelong warfarin anticoagulation (Chapter 38) even after liver transplantation. Selective JAK2 inhibitors (Chapter 166) are being tested in preclinical and clinical studies.

PROGNOSIS

Overall, the 5-year survival rate of patients with the Budd-Chiari syndrome is more than 80%. Indices such as levels of serum albumin and bilirubin, the international normalized ratio, ascites, and encephalopathy, and the Child-Pugh score (see Table 153-2 in Chapter 153) can be useful in determining the prognosis. About 50% of patients will have at least one episode of major bleeding, half of which are related to invasive therapy.

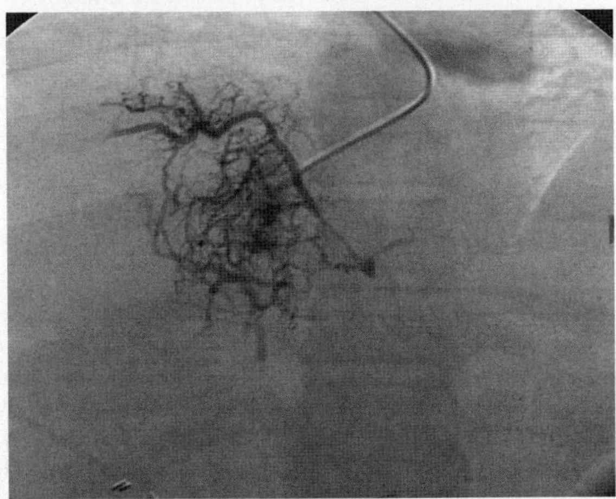

FIGURE 143-7. **Budd-Chiari syndrome. A hepatic vein contrast study depicts the "spider web" pattern of venovenous collaterals attempting to bypass a thrombosed hepatic vein. (Courtesy of Patrick Kamath.)**

Portal Vein Thrombosis

In adults, cirrhosis, hypercoagulable states, intra-abdominal malignancy, inflammatory disorders (e.g., pancreatitis, Crohn disease), and medical procedures (e.g., splenectomy, cholecystectomy, gastrectomy, liver transplantation, transjugular intrahepatic portosystemic shunt) are most often the cause of acute portal vein thrombosis. Similar to Budd-Chiari syndrome, a substantial number of these patients harbor *JAK2* V617F mutations.

CLINICAL MANIFESTATIONS AND DIAGNOSIS

Clinical manifestations include portal hypertension with variceal bleeding and ascites. Abdominal pain and diarrhea may indicate extension of the thrombus into the SMV with intestinal ischemia. The diagnosis of acute portal vein thrombosis is confirmed by Doppler ultrasound, multidetector CTA, or MRA. CT imaging may reveal multiple small liver abscesses.

TREATMENT

Rx

Anticoagulation (see Table 81-4 in Chapter 81) therapy for at least 3 months is recommended for patients with acute portal vein thrombosis and should be continued long term in those persons with permanent thrombotic risk factors not otherwise correctable, as well as in patients with extension of thrombus into the mesenteric veins.[11]

High fever, chills, a tender liver, and sepsis suggest pylephlebitis, which usually requires treatment with parenteral antibiotics such as piperacillin–tazobactam, ticarcillin–clavulanate, carbapenem, or a third-generation cephalosporin plus metronidazole for at least 6 weeks. Blood cultures can help to guide the choice and course of antibiotics, which should be administered intravenously for at least 2 weeks.

Treatment is less clear in cirrhotic patients with acute or chronic portal vein thrombosis. Endoscopy for the diagnosis and treatment of varices (Chapter 134), with or without pharmacologic treatment of the portal hypertension (e.g., β-blockade with propranolol; Chapter 153), is often beneficial, and surgical shunts are rarely necessary. Antibiotics, such as those recommended previously for pylephlebitis, should be administered in patients with any sign of infection.

Chronic portal vein thrombosis is defined as an obstructed portal vein replaced by collateral veins. Doppler ultrasonography, multidetector CTA, or MRA will confirm the diagnosis. Patients may be asymptomatic but often have hypersplenism and portal hypertension (e.g., subclinical encephalopathy, rare ascites). Some patients may develop jaundice owing to biliary cholangiopathy and will require endoscopic placement of biliary stents. Endoscopic screening and treatment of varices (Chapter 134), with or without pharmacologic treatment of portal hypertension (Chapter 153), is recommended. After treatment of the varices, long-term anticoagulation therapy (Chapter 81) should be considered in noncirrhotic patients whose permanent thrombotic risk factors are not otherwise correctable unless there is a contraindication.

PROGNOSIS

Mortality rates after treatment of acute portal vein thrombosis are less than 10%, and the prognosis for patients with chronic portal vein thrombosis over 5 years is similar.

Splenic Vein Thrombosis

Splenic vein thrombosis is usually secondary to malignancy (e.g., pancreatic cancer), pancreatitis, or trauma. In many of these patients, isolated gastric varices develop and are difficult to treat by therapeutic endoscopy. Liver function and portal pressure are normal. Most patients with splenic vein thrombosis have splenomegaly (Chapter 168). Doppler ultrasonography, MRI, and CT assist in making the diagnosis. Patients with symptomatic isolated splenic vein thrombosis (e.g., gastric variceal bleeding, hypersplenism) are best treated by splenectomy.

Hepatic and Splenic Arterial Disease

Hepatic arterial disease may be nonocclusive or occlusive. Nonocclusive disease, termed *ischemic hepatitis,* occurs when arterial blood flow to the liver is insufficient, usually because of cardiogenic hypotension, volume depletion, or sepsis. Typically, serum aminotransferase rises acutely to levels greater than 1000 U/L. With restoration of adequate hepatic arterial blood flow, serum aminotransferase levels eventually fall back to their baseline by about 40% to 60% per day. Hepatic artery thrombosis is extremely rare except in post–liver transplantation (Chapter 154) patients, in whom it may be manifested as mild abnormalities in liver function test results, bile duct injury (e.g., biliary stricture, cholangitis, liver abscess), or liver failure. Doppler ultrasonography and angiography confirm the diagnosis, and these patients often require biliary stents, drainage of abscesses, surgical reconstruction of the hepatic artery, or retransplantation of the liver.

The splenic artery or hepatic artery may be predisposed to the development of aneurysmal dilation, usually secondary to atherosclerosis, trauma, portal hypertension, pancreatitis, pregnancy, infection, or vasculitis. Common clinical manifestations include abdominal pain and intra-abdominal hemorrhage. Hemobilia may occur with hepatic artery aneurysms. Angiography is usually required to make the diagnosis. Symptomatic as well as sizable (variably defined, usually 1 cm or greater for a hepatic aneurysm and 2 cm or greater for a splenic artery aneurysm) aneurysms require surgery. Splenic artery aneurysms discovered during pregnancy are more likely to bleed and should be treated, usually by interventional radiology.

Fistulas from the hepatic artery to the portal vein can occur as a result of trauma, malignancy, or the inherited disorder hereditary hemorrhagic telangiectasia. The resultant portal hypertension may cause abdominal pain, ascites, and GI bleeding, and involvement of the hepatic artery may result in biliary strictures and hepatobiliary infection. Radiographic embolization of these fistulas, surgery, or liver transplantation may be required.

GENERAL REFERENCES

For the General References and other additional features, please visit Expert Consult at https://expertconsult.inkling.com.

144

PANCREATITIS

CHRIS E. FORSMARK

ACUTE PANCREATITIS

DEFINITION

Acute pancreatitis, which is a discrete episode of cellular injury and inflammation in the pancreas, is triggered by the release of activated digestive enzymes into the pancreas and peripancreatic tissues. Acute pancreatitis usually presents with symptoms of abdominal pain, nausea, and vomiting accompanied by an elevation in serum levels of amylase, lipase, or both and by radiographic evidence of pancreatic inflammation, edema, or necrosis. Although pancreatic morphology and function may recover after such an episode, complete recovery is unlikely if the initial damage is substantial, particularly if the original episode is associated with significant pancreatic necrosis. With repeated episodes, there can be a shift from acute inflammation, necrosis, and apoptosis to a milieu of chronic inflammation, the activation of pancreatic stellate cells, continued tissue destruction, and ultimately the fibrosis characteristic of chronic pancreatitis. About 25% of patients with acute pancreatitis will have recurrence, and about 10% will develop chronic pancreatitis.[1]

EPIDEMIOLOGY

Acute pancreatitis, which is the most common cause of hospitalization for a gastrointestinal condition in the United States,[2] accounts for approximately 275,000 hospitalizations yearly. This rate of hospital admissions has doubled over the past 2 decades. The incidence of acute pancreatitis ranges from 13 to 45 per 100,000 population. The total cost of caring for these patients is substantial, with estimates of $6 billion annually. The incidence of acute pancreatitis is increasing in the United States and in many other countries, perhaps because of heightened clinical suspicion for the diagnosis, the more widespread use of serum-based and radiologic testing, and an increasing incidence of gallstones in the midst of the obesity epidemic.

The risk of acute pancreatitis increases fourfold between ages 25 and 75 years. The risk is two- to threefold higher among the black population in the United States compared with whites. Increased abdominal adiposity but not body mass index increases the risk of acute pancreatitis approximately twofold.

PATHOBIOLOGY

The mechanisms that lead to acute pancreatitis include exposures to potential disease triggers and genetic polymorphisms that predispose to acute pancreatitis. Acute pancreatitis is characterized by premature activation of pancreatic digestive enzymes within the pancreas. In many models of pancreatitis, abnormal calcium signaling and the activation of specific protein kinases lead to the generation of inflammatory mediators, the activation of enzymes within the acinar cell, misdirected exocytosis, and ultimately the cellular injury and death that characterize acute pancreatitis.[3] The activation of trypsinogen to trypsin may be a critical initial step, with trypsin having the capacity to activate other proteases within the gland. These activated enzymes produce cellular injury and death. Necrosis may involve not only the pancreas but also surrounding fat and structures, leading to fluid extravasation into the retroperitoneal spaces ("third-space" losses). Although some degree of microscopic necrosis may be present in most cases of acute pancreatitis, more substantial necrosis (visible on an enhanced contrast computed tomography [CT] scan) is termed *acute necrotizing pancreatitis* and is distinguished from the milder *acute interstitial pancreatitis*, in which necrosis is not visible on a CT scan.

In addition to local damage within and around the pancreas, acute pancreatitis may be associated with distant organ system failure. The release of inflammatory cytokines and activated digestive enzymes into the systemic circulation can produce a systemic inflammatory response syndrome (SIRS; Chapters 106 and 108) and associated organ system failure. The most common manifestations of this process in severe acute pancreatitis include hypotension, renal failure, and respiratory failure. Gallstones and alcohol account for about 70% to 80% of all cases of acute pancreatitis, and the cause remains unknown in about 10% of cases (Table 144-1).

TABLE 144-1 CAUSES OF ACUTE PANCREATITIS

ETIOLOGY	EXAMPLES	COMMENTS
Gallstones	Gallstones Microlithiasis	Best detected by EUS
Drugs and toxins	Ethyl and methyl alcohol Tobacco	
	Azathioprine, 6-mercaptopurine, pentamidine, didanosine, sulfonamides, thiazides, aminosalicylates, valproic acid, and others	Usually idiosyncratic
	Scorpion venom Insecticides	Caused by hyperstimulation of pancreatic secretion
Metabolic	Hypertriglyceridemia	Usually requires triglyceride level >1000 mg/dL
	Hypercalcemia	
Trauma	Post-ERCP	Risk varies with indication and may be reduced by rectal NSAIDs and pancreatic duct stents
	Blunt or penetrating trauma Postoperative	
Obstruction of the pancreatic duct	Benign pancreatic duct stricture Benign ampullary stricture (e.g., celiac disease, diverticulum) Ampullary adenoma or adenocarcinoma Pancreatic ductal adenocarcinoma Intraductal papillary mucinous neoplasm	
	Pancreas divisum	Controversial
	Sphincter of Oddi dysfunction	
Infections	Cytomegalovirus, mumps, rubella, Coxsackie B *Candida*, histoplasmosis Ascaris	
Genetics	*PRSS1* mutations	Mutation sufficient to cause disease
	CFTR mutation *SPINK1* mutation Others (chymotrypsin C, calcium sensing receptor, claudin-2, others)	Mutations or polymorphisms predispose to pancreatitis
Autoimmune pancreatitis	Type 1 Type 2	Elevations in serum levels of IgG4 may be seen in Type 1
Idiopathic pancreatitis		

ERCP = endoscopic retrograde cholangiopancreatography; EUS = endoscopic ultrasonography; NSAID = nonsteroidal anti-inflammatory drug.

Gallstones and Obstruction

Passage of a gallstone through the ampulla of Vater, with transient obstruction of the pancreatic duct, is the initiating event for gallstone pancreatitis. Only about 5% of all patients with gallstones develop pancreatitis, and patients with smaller gallstones (≤5 mm), which can pass the cystic duct and reach the ampulla, are at highest risk. Microlithiasis describes very tiny gallstones that are not easily visible on standard transabdominal ultrasonography but may cause gallstone pancreatitis.

In addition to gallstones and microlithiasis, pancreatic duct obstruction owing to pancreatic ductal adenocarcinoma (Chapter 194), ampullary adenoma or carcinoma, or intraductal papillary mucinous neoplasm can cause acute pancreatitis. Benign strictures of the ampulla may cause acute pancreatitis, owing to duodenal diseases such as celiac disease and periampullary diverticula. Sphincter of Oddi dysfunction, defined by high pressures of the pancreatic sphincter, and pancreas divisum, in which the larger dorsal pancreas drains through the smaller minor papilla, are controversial causes of acute pancreatitis because patients with them often have coexistent underlying genetic mutations that contribute to this disease.

Alcohol

Long-standing use of substantial alcohol (Chapter 33), usually more than 5 years of intake averaging more than 5 to 8 drinks daily, is required before pancreatitis develops. Even then, the absolute risk of pancreatitis is only 2% to 5%, thereby emphasizing important cofactors such as a high-fat diet, genetic variability, and smoking. Interestingly, binge drinking does not appear to be a risk factor for pancreatitis, and many patients develop their first episode of pancreatitis several days after stopping drinking. The mechanism by which alcohol causes pancreatic injury is uncertain but likely involves a mixture of direct toxicity, oxidative stress, and alterations in pancreatic enzyme secretion.

Drugs, Toxins, and Metabolic Factors

Serum triglyceride levels greater than 500 mg/dL and usually greater than 1000 mg/dL can cause acute pancreatitis (Chapter 206). The mechanism is not known. Pancreatitis also can be precipitated by the administration of estrogens, which can exacerbate underlying hypertriglycideremia. Hypercalcemia is an exceedingly rare cause of acute pancreatitis. Drug-induced pancreatitis is rare and is generally an idiosyncratic event. Implicated drugs include 6-mercaptopurine and azathioprine (up to a 4% attack rate), didanosine, pentamidine, valproic acid, furosemide, sulfonamides, and aminosalicylates. Toxins that may cause acute pancreatitis include methyl alcohol (Chapter 110), organophosphate insecticides, and venom from certain scorpions (Chapter 359).

Trauma

Iatrogenic trauma to the pancreas and pancreatic duct during performance of an endoscopic retrograde cholangiopancreatography (ERCP; Chapter 134) is a common cause of pancreatitis. The risk of acute pancreatitis ranges from less than 5% for patients with simple common bile duct stones or malignancy to as high as 20% for patients with suspected sphincter of Oddi dysfunction.[4] Penetrating trauma and blunt trauma, ranging from a contusion to the gland to a severe crush injury and even transection of the gland, can also cause acute pancreatitis. Ischemic injury to the gland can occur after surgical procedures, especially in patients who undergo cardiopulmonary bypass.

Infections

Ascaris lumbricoides (Chapter 357) may cause pancreatitis by obstructing the pancreatic duct as the worms migrate through the ampulla. A number of viruses may infect the pancreatic acinar cells directly, including cytomegalovirus (Chapter 376), Coxsackie B virus (Chapter 379), Echovirus (Chapter 379), and mumps virus (Chapter 369). Fungal infections of the pancreas are exceedingly rare but may be seen in the setting of immunosuppression.

Genetic and Autoimmune Causes

Mutations in several genes predispose to the development of acute and chronic pancreatitis.[5] Most patients with these mutations will not develop pancreatitis, but those who do often develop relapsing acute pancreatitis and ultimately chronic pancreatitis.

Gain-of-function mutations in the cationic trypsinogen gene (*PRSS1*) predispose to hereditary pancreatitis with such a high penetrance that nearly all affected individuals will ultimately develop chronic pancreatitis (see later) and have a more than 35-fold lifetime risk of developing pancreatic ductal adenocarcinoma (Chapter 194) by age 70 years. Mutations in the cystic fibrosis conductance regulator (*CFTR*; Chapter 89), serine protease inhibitor Kazal type 1 (*SPINK1*), chymotrypsin C (*CTC*), calcium-sensing receptor gene, and claudin-2 genes predispose to both relapsing acute and chronic pancreatitis. With the exception of *PRSS1*, these mutations are best viewed as cofactors that interact with other risk factors and disease modifiers to cause pancreatitis.

Two forms of autoimmune pancreatitis, classically presenting as chronic pancreatitis (see later), have been identified.[6] Type 1 is a systemic disease that affects the salivary glands, retroperitoneum, biliary ducts, kidneys, and other organs and rarely presents as acute pancreatitis. Type 2 only affects the pancreas and may occasionally present as unexplained acute pancreatitis.

CLINICAL MANIFESTATIONS

Abdominal pain, nausea, and vomiting are the hallmark symptoms of acute pancreatitis. The abdominal pain is usually in the epigastric region and often radiates to the back. The pain is steady, reaches its maximum intensity over 30 to 60 minutes, and persists for days. These characteristic symptoms may be masked in patients who present with delirium, multiple organ system failure, or coma.

The physical examination usually reveals tachycardia, and more severe cases often present with or develop hypotension, tachypnea, and fever. Confusion, delirium, and even coma may occur. The abdomen is often distended with diminished bowel sounds. Tenderness to palpation of the abdomen, which may be epigastric or more diffuse, is typical, and rebound and guarding are observed in more severe cases. Dullness to percussion in the lower lung fields may be noted owing to a pleural effusion. Rare physical findings include ecchymoses of the flank (Grey Turner sign) or umbilicus (Cullen sign), which occur when fluid and blood track into these spaces from the retroperitoneum. Jaundice may be present if there is biliary obstruction by a stone.

The presence of dyspnea, tachypnea, oxygen desaturation, hypotension, or tachycardia portends a worse prognosis. Severe acute pancreatitis is defined by the presence of organ system failure (usually cardiovascular, renal, or pulmonary) or by the presence of pancreatic complications such as pancreatic and peripancreatic necrosis (Table 144-2).[7]

TABLE 144-2 COMPLICATIONS OF ACUTE PANCREATITIS

COMPLICATION	EXAMPLES
Systemic complications	Hypotension and shock Adult respiratory distress syndrome Acute renal failure Disseminated intravascular coagulation Hypocalcemia Hypertriglyceridemia Hyperglycemia Encephalopathy and coma
Gastrointestinal bleeding	Stress ulceration Pseudoaneurysm

Local complications	Acute peripancreatic fluid collection
	Pseudocyst
	Pancreatic necrosis (infected or sterile)
	  Acute necrotic collection
	  Walled-off pancreatic necrosis
	Duodenal or biliary obstruction

DIAGNOSIS

The diagnosis of acute pancreatitis requires the presence of two of three primary features: abdominal pain, elevations in serum amylase or lipase levels, and imaging studies consistent with acute pancreatitis. Accurate diagnosis also requires that other conditions that can mimic acute pancreatitis, such as intestinal infarction or small bowel obstruction, be excluded. It is equally important to define the most likely cause and the severity of pancreatitis because both strongly influence management.

Laboratory Tests

Amylase and Lipase

Nearly all patients with acute pancreatitis have an elevation in serum levels of amylase or lipase within a few hours after the onset of symptoms. Elevation more than three times the upper limit of normal is the recommended cutoff for diagnosing acute pancreatitis. Lipase remains elevated longer than amylase. Amylase and lipase levels may be normal in rare patients with acute pancreatitis, particularly if the measurement is delayed for several days after the onset of symptoms. In addition, marked hypertriglyceridemia can interfere with the accurate measurement of amylase and lipase. Both enzymes are cleared by the kidney, and renal failure can raise the level of these enzymes up to five times the upper limit of normal in the absence of pancreatitis. Both amylase and lipase can be elevated in a variety of other conditions, some of which may mimic acute pancreatitis. These include intestinal ischemia and infarction (Chapter 143), bowel obstruction (Chapter 142), cholecystitis (Chapter 155), and choledocholithiasis (Chapter 155). In addition, amylase may be elevated from ectopic pregnancy, acute salpingitis, and a variety of extraabdominal conditions such as parotitis (Chapter 369), lung cancer (Chapter 191), head trauma (Chapter 399), and others. In some patients, only amylase or lipase levels may be elevated. Given its improved specificity, equal cost, and equal sensitivity, lipase is preferred over amylase as a single diagnostic test.[8] Frequent serial measurements of amylase or lipase levels in patients with acute pancreatitis are not helpful in clinical decision making.

Other Laboratory Tests

In addition to amylase and lipase levels, all patients should have blood testing for renal function, liver chemistries, electrolyte concentrations, and levels of calcium and triglycerides. In severe pancreatitis, leukocytosis, hemoconcentration, and azotemia may be seen. Hyperglycemia, hypocalcemia, and mild hypertriglyceridemia can develop in more severe cases. Liver chemistries may be elevated in patients with gallstone pancreatitis. Elevations in alanine aminotransferase levels more than three times the upper limit of normal are most suggestive of gallstones as the cause of pancreatitis, although any significant elevation in liver chemistries should raise the possibility of gallstones (Chapter 155).

Imaging Studies

Imaging studies are used not only in establishing the diagnosis but also in determining the etiology and prognosis. In most patients, ultrasonography,

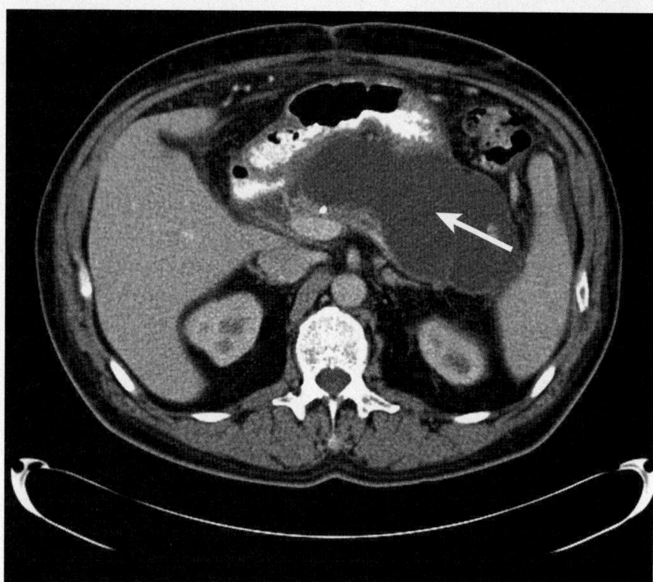

FIGURE 144-1. A computed tomography scan demonstrating a large area of pancreas that does not enhance with intravenous contrast *(arrow)*, consistent with pancreatic necrosis.

CT, or magnetic resonance imaging (MRI) are used in a complementary fashion.[9]

Abdominal ultrasonography can confirm the presence of acute pancreatitis by documenting pancreatic enlargement, edema, or associated peripancreatic fluid collections. Visualization of the pancreas may be inadequate owing to body habitus or overlying intestinal gas. Ultrasonography is accurate in identifying a ductal gallstone as the definitive cause of acute pancreatitis. Alternatively, gallstones in the gallbladder or a dilated common bile duct strongly suggests gallstones as the cause of acute pancreatitis.

Computed tomography is more accurate than ultrasonography for confirming the diagnosis of acute pancreatitis and for documenting the presence of pancreatic necrosis and peripancreatic fluid collections. CT is also particularly helpful in excluding some of the intraabdominal conditions that can mimic acute pancreatitis. However, CT is less accurate than ultrasonography in identifying gallstones. On contrast-enhanced CT, the pancreatic parenchyma that opacifies with intravenous contrast is considered still viable, but the parenchyma that does not opacify is necrotic (Fig. 144-1). The amount of pancreatic necrosis has some prognostic importance, but the degree of necrosis cannot be accurately identified on CT until 3 or more days after the onset of the disease. CT scans are not routinely required in patients with acute pancreatitis but should be performed in patients with a first attack, with severe disease, with disease that is slow to improve, or when the diagnosis is not clear.[10]

Magnetic resonance imaging is equivalent to CT in its ability to document the presence of acute pancreatitis, identify the presence of necrosis, and document nonpancreatic diseases that could mimic acute pancreatitis. In addition, *magnetic resonance cholangiopancreatography (MRCP)* is much better than CT in identifying the presence of gallstones and in assessing abnormalities of the pancreatic duct, such as pancreas divisum or a disrupted pancreatic duct. MRI is more difficult than CT to perform in critically ill patients.

Endoscopic procedures, including ERCP and endoscopic ultrasonography, are important in both diagnosis and therapy of acute pancreatitis. Endoscopic ultrasonography, which is primarily used to establish the cause when the initial evaluation is unrevealing, is particularly accurate in identifying underlying malignancy, premalignant lesions such as ampullary adenoma, and small gallstones or microlithiasis. ERCP is never used as a diagnostic test but may be used to evaluate rare causes of pancreatitis, such as pancreas divisum or sphincter of Oddi dysfunction, in patients with unexplained relapsing pancreatitis.

Determining Etiology

To identify the cause of acute pancreatitis, the history should focus on alcohol and tobacco use, previous biliary colic, drug history, family history, and recent trauma. Alcohol use may need to be corroborated with family members. All patients should undergo transabdominal ultrasonography, with CT or MR considered for patients who have a first attack or a severe attack, who fail to rapidly improve, or who do not have a clear diagnosis. Gallstones should be suspected if stones are seen on ultrasonography, CT, or MRI or if liver chemistries are abnormal, particularly if liver chemistries improve or normalize over a few days. If these initial studies are unrevealing, endoscopic ultrasonography is usually performed to assess for small gallstones, microlithiasis, or underlying malignancy, particularly in patients older than age 40 years. More specialized investigations such as ERCP, sphincter of Oddi manometry, or genetic testing are usually reserved for patients seen in referral centers after multiple attacks of pancreatitis.

On initial evaluation, about 25% of patients do not have an identified cause, but surreptitious alcohol use and microlithiasis are probably the most common underlying causes in these patients. After a detailed evaluation, approximately 10% of patients are ultimately diagnosed with idiopathic pancreatitis.

Determining and Predicting Severity

Severe pancreatitis is defined as organ system failure that persists for more than 48 hours or by local pancreatic and peripancreatic complications such as necrosis, acute fluid collections, or pseudocysts. Moderately severe pancreatitis is characterized by transient organ failure for less than 48 hours, by a local complication, or by a systemic complication owing to worsening of an underlying comorbid disease. Mild acute pancreatitis implies the absence of these features.

Organ failure can be single or multiple, early or late in onset, and progressive and persistent or transient. Patients may exhibit altered mental status, hypoxia, tachypnea, massive third space fluid loss, and intravascular volume depletion. In severe acute pancreatitis, renal failure, pulmonary failure, and circulatory failure most commonly occur as part of the SIRS response. Multiple organ system failure, particularly if it persists beyond 48 hours after admission, is associated with prolonged hospitalization, intensive care unit (ICU) admission, need for surgery, and death.

Local pancreatic and peripancreatic complications help define the severity of acute pancreatitis. The degree of pancreatic necrosis, which is defined on contrast-enhanced CT as areas of pancreas that do not enhance with intravenous contrast infusion, correlates with a worse outcome, particularly if infection develops in the devitalized necrotic tissue. Fluid collections may also accumulate around the pancreas in various retroperitoneal and peritoneal spaces. Much of this inflammatory fluid usually resolves, but some may form into a more circumscribed *pseudocyst* over several weeks. However, some fluid collections seen on contrast-enhanced CT may initially be termed *pseudocysts* when in reality they contain solid necrotic material as well as fluid and actually represent *walled-off pancreatic necrosis* that will require a different therapeutic approach than simple pseudocysts.

TREATMENT Rx

General Supportive Care

The majority of patients will recover within several days, but it is usually not possible to identify these patients accurately at the time of admission. Patients initially should not be given any oral food or fluids. In patients with more severe pancreatitis, admission to an ICU is appropriate.[11] Pain control usually requires parenteral narcotics (e.g., hydromorphone 1-2 mg every 4-6 hours initially or via patient controlled analgesia). Antiemetic agents (Table 132-5) are often required. Early and aggressive hydration (e.g., ≥250 cc/hr or even more) in the first 12 to 24 hours may be necessary to normalize the blood urea nitrogen (BUN), hematocrit, and vital signs and to generate adequate urine output.[12] Lactated Ringer solution may be preferred over normal saline.[A1] Care must be taken to ensure patients receive sufficient volume but not enough to cause fluid overload or the development of an abdominal compartment syndrome.

Patients can begin to be fed, beginning with a low-fat solid diet, when bowel sounds have returned and nausea has resolved, without necessarily waiting until all abdominal pain has resolved.[A2] Early nasoenteric feeding is no better than an oral diet started 72 hours after admission, with enteral feeding reserved for those who cannot tolerate oral feeding.[A3] Enteral nutrition with an elemental or semi-elemental formula is associated with fewer complications and less cost compared with total parenteral nutrition.

Treatment of Complications

Most patients who develop acute gallstone pancreatitis have already passed the offending gallstone into the duodenum, but those with a persistent or multiple stones are at higher risk of developing cholangitis and possibly more severe pancreatitis. Early ERCP is recommended in patients with gallstone pancreatitis and concomitant cholangitis (fever, jaundice, right upper quadrant pain) and in patients who have strong evidence of a persistent bile duct stone at 48 hours after admission based on a visible persistent stone on an imaging study, jaundice, a persistently dilated bile duct, or worsening liver chemistries. By comparison, early ERCP is not recommended for patients with severe pancreatitis, as evidenced by early and progressive organ system failure, but without cholangitis or suspicion of a persistent bile duct stone.[A4] When unsure, endoscopic ultrasonography or MRCP can help identify persistent bile duct stones before consideration of ERCP.

The systemic complications that develop in patients with severe acute pancreatitis are similar to those commonly encountered in other ICU patients, as well as specific metabolic issues that occur in the setting of severe pancreatitis. Hyperglycemia, which develops particularly if parenteral nutrition is used, contributes to higher rates of infections. Hypocalcemia is common in severe pancreatitis, but ionized calcium levels are usually normal and treatment is not needed in the absence of signs of hypocalcemia (Chvostek's sign or Trousseau sign; Chapter 245). Hypertriglyceridemia is usually mild, but even levels greater than 1000 mg/dL usually drop promptly when the patients do not eat. However, occasional patients with sustained severe hypertriglyceridemia may require plasmapheresis.

Acute peripancreatic fluid collections are common in acute pancreatitis, and most fluid collections will resolve spontaneously. Some, however, will mature into an encapsulated, fluid-filled pseudocyst outside of the confines of the pancreas. A pseudocyst also does not require therapy unless it causes abdominal pain or obstruction of a hollow viscus or it is associated with infection or bleeding; in these situations, endoscopic therapy is preferred.[A5] Arterial bleeding from a pseudoaneurysm caused by a pseudocyst may be massive and require an emergent CT scan for diagnosis followed by embolization.

In addition, patients with necrotizing pancreatitis may develop infected pancreatic necrosis. Infection of preexisting necrosis typically occurs 2 to 3 weeks into the illness and is heralded by fever, leukocytosis, and worsening abdominal pain. The responsible organisms are usually gram-negative rods and other intestinal flora, but *Staphylococcus aureus* is an important agent as well. If infected necrosis is suspected, a contrast-enhanced CT scan should be obtained to identify the extent of necrosis and assess for indirect evidence of infected necrosis (i.e., gas in the necrotic collection). A CT-directed fine-needle aspiration of the necrotic area for culture and Gram stain can allow antibiotic therapy to be tailored; otherwise, broad-spectrum empiric antibiotics should counter possible infective agents (Table 108-2). Prophylactic antibiotics to prevent infection in patients with preexisting sterile pancreatic necrosis is not recommended, although many patients with severe or necrotizing pancreatitis may ultimately receive antibiotics for treatment of various hospital-acquired infections. Ideally, conservative therapy is continued for at least 4 weeks to allow the infected necrotic material to demarcate, begin to liquefy, and become encapsulated so it can be more easily drained. Percutaneous, endoscopic, or minimally invasive surgical draining procedures are as effective and safer than early open surgical debridement,[A6] which is reserved for very rare patients with progressive clinical deterioration.

Any hospital-acquired infection (Chapter 282) dramatically worsens prognosis. Common infections include urinary tract infections (Chapter 284), pulmonary infections (Chapter 97), line infections, and *Clostridium difficile* (Chapter 296).

Prevention

The use of a rectal nonsteroidal anti-inflammatory drug suppository (e.g., indomethacin 100 mg or diclofenac 100 mg) placed either just before or just after ERCP reduces the risk of post-ERCP pancreatitis by about 50%.[A7] Placement of a temporary pancreatic duct stent provides equivalent protection. By comparison, preventing recurrent acute pancreatitis is more challenging. Abstinence from alcohol (Chapter 33) and tobacco (Chapter 32), which can be achieved in many patients, can reduce recurrent attacks[A8] and should be strongly encouraged. Cholecystectomy (Chapter 155) prevents subsequent attacks of gallstone pancreatitis and should be undertaken within a few weeks of discharge, at the latest. In patients who are not surgical candidates, endoscopic sphincterotomy provides reasonable protection from subsequent attacks. Control of serum lipids (Chapter 206) prevents subsequent attacks of hyperlipidemic pancreatitis. Therapy of lesions that obstruct the pancreatic duct such as strictures, ampullary adenomas, and possibly sphincter of Oddi dysfunction and pancreas divisum may also prevent recurrences.

PROGNOSIS

The case-fatality rate for acute pancreatitis has decreased over time and now averages approximately 1% to 2%. More than 80% of all patients with acute pancreatitis recover promptly and are discharged within a few days. In patients with severe acute pancreatitis, however, the mortality rate is between 10% and 20%. The mortality rate may even approach 30% in patients with more severe and numerous comorbid conditions and in patients who develop pancreatic necrosis, particularly infected necrosis, or organ system failure.

A number of scoring systems and other methods have been developed in an attempt to help guide clinicians predict prognosis, but none has been documented to be superior to experienced clinical judgment. The Ranson criteria, which are of historical interest only, have been replaced by APACHE (Acute Physiology and Chronic Health Evaluation) II and by more simplified systems using multiple-factor scoring. Practice guidelines suggest a cutoff of greater than 8 APACHE II points as the definition of severe disease, but this cutoff has a high false positive rate. An elevated BUN or hematocrit that does not return to normal with fluid therapy is associated with increased mortality rates. A C-reactive protein level greater than 150 mg/L at 48 hours is as accurate as many multifactorial scoring systems at predicting poor outcome. The BISAP score (BUN >25 mg/dL, impaired mental status, SIRS, age >60 years, and pleural effusion) has a possible score of 0 to 5, depending on the number of criteria present. Mortality ranges from less than 1% for a BISAP score of 0 or 1 up to 27% for a BISAP score of 5. For patients with alcoholic pancreatitis, the risk of progression to chronic pancreatitis is about 14% in patients who stop drinking and smoking after the first episode of acute pancreatitis but greater than 40% in those who do not change these behaviors.

CHRONIC PANCREATITIS

DEFINITION

Chronic pancreatitis, which is a syndrome with multiple predisposing risk factors, culminates in a final common pathway of irreversible and permanent pancreatic damage characterized by chronic inflammation, destruction of normal cellular (acinar) structures, and fibrosis. Chronic pancreatitis usually evolves after episodes of acute pancreatitis, some of which may have been subclinical, but the transition between acute and chronic pancreatitis may be difficult to identify.

EPIDEMIOLOGY

The prevalence of symptomatic chronic pancreatitis in Western countries is about 50 per 100,000 population, with an estimated incidence of five to 12 cases per 100,000. In the United States, chronic pancreatitis accounts for about 125,000 outpatient visits and 25,000 hospitalizations yearly. Interestingly, the prevalence of histologic evidence of chronic pancreatitis in autopsy studies approaches 5%. Many people apparently develop chronic damage to the pancreas as a consequence of normal aging, other diseases, or exposure to toxins (e.g., social consumption of alcohol) but do not develop any symptoms or signs of chronic pancreatitis during life.

PATHOBIOLOGY

Multiple episodes of acute inflammation, whether clinical or subclinical, eventually change the inflammatory milieu of the pancreas, with a shift to chronic inflammation, cellular loss, and the activation of pancreatic stellate cells with production of fibrosis. This process becomes self-sustaining and produces the characteristic histologic features in which a chronic fibrosis gradually replaces the acute inflammation.

The pathophysiology of pain, the most common symptom of chronic pancreatitis, is complex, involving both local pancreatic nociception as well as central nervous system responses. Chronic pancreatitis associated pain produces visceral, spinal cord, and central hyperalgesia, and the pain may become self-perpetuating even if therapy on the pancreas is successful.

Alcohol and Tobacco

Alcohol causes about 40% of all cases of chronic pancreatitis in the United States and other developed countries.[13] As with acute pancreatitis, which clinically or occasionally subclinically will precede chronic pancreatitis, substantial and prolonged ingestion of alcohol is usually required, on the order of 5 to 8 drinks daily over more than 5 years. The risk of chronic pancreatitis is only 2% to 5% in patients who consume this much alcohol, pointing to important cofactors such as host genetics and cigarette smoking. There is also evidence that tobacco alone can cause chronic pancreatitis, and smoking alone may be responsible for up to 25% of cases. The combination of alcohol and tobacco is synergistic in causing chronic pancreatitis.

Genetics

Hereditary pancreatitis is an autosomal dominant disease characterized by early onset of acute and chronic pancreatitis, the development of exocrine and endocrine pancreatic insufficiency, and a very high risk of pancreatic ductal adenocarcinoma (Chapter 194). Mutations in the trypsinogen (*PRSS1*) gene appear to cause a gain in function in which the mutant trypsinogen, once activated to trypsin, is difficult to inactivate. This trypsin, if present in an amount that overwhelms normal protective mechanisms, can activate other pancreatic enzymes and lead to pancreatic damage and eventually to chronic pancreatitis. One of the protective mechanisms is a trypsin inhibitor called SPINK1. Loss of function mutations in *SPINK1* mutations may predispose to chronic pancreatitis, but unlike PRSS1 mutations, are not sufficient alone to cause chronic pancreatitis. Major mutations in the cystic fibrosis conductance regulator (CFTR) lead to cystic fibrosis (Chapter 89), which may be associated with chronic pancreatitis and pancreatic atrophy. Some mutations in CFTR predispose to chronic pancreatitis without causing the sinopulmonary features of cystic fibrosis. Combined mutations of SPINK1 and CFTR may place patients at particularly high risk for chronic pancreatitis. Other mutations and polymorphisms associated with chronic pancreatitis include chymotrypsin C and the calcium-sensing receptor gene. Polymorphisms of claudin 2, an X-linked gene, work synergistically with alcohol and may partially explain the increased risk of alcoholic chronic pancreatitis in men.

Other Causes

Autoimmune pancreatitis most often presents as a mass-like lesion with obstructive jaundice, mimicking cancer. It may also present as chronic pancreatitis and rarely as acute pancreatitis. Type 1 autoimmune pancreatitis, which usually occurs in the fifth or sixth decade of life, is characterized by focal or diffuse swelling of the pancreas, elevations in serum IgG4, and involvement of other organs. Biliary strictures, salivary gland inflammation, retroperitoneal fibrosis, and renal lesions are commonly seen. Histology shows infiltration of these organs by chronic inflammatory cells and especially by plasma cells bearing IgG4 on their surfaces. The target of the autoimmune process is not known. Type 2 autoimmune pancreatitis is limited to the pancreas and occurs in a broader age group, including children.

Tropical pancreatitis is seen primarily in southern India. Characteristic features include childhood onset, exocrine insufficiency, diffuse pancreatic calcifications, and inevitable diabetes. There is a strong genetic component (SPINK1 and others), but cofactors such as malnutrition and dietary toxins have been suggested. In southern India, this disease is becoming rarer and is being replaced by alcohol and tobacco as the most common cause of chronic pancreatitis.

Recurrent or severe acute pancreatitis, particularly a severe acute attack that causes substantial pancreatic necrosis, can destroy enough of the gland to produce exocrine and endocrine insufficiency. In addition, diseases that cause repeated attacks of pancreatitis can lead to chronic pancreatitis. One example is *hypertriglyceridemia*, which causes acute pancreatitis but commonly leads to chronic pancreatitis.

CLINICAL MANIFESTATIONS

The most common symptom of chronic pancreatitis is pain. The pain may be episodic or constant and is generally felt in the epigastrium with radiation to the back. If pain is episodic, the patient may be labeled as having acute pancreatitis or an acute flare of chronic pancreatitis. When pain is severe, nausea and vomiting may occur. Pain may worsen, improve, or remain stable over time. Pain is the symptom that is most responsible for medical care and the symptom that most detracts from quality of life. A small percentage of patients do not have pain and instead present with exocrine (steatorrhea, weight loss) or endocrine (diabetes) pancreatic insufficiency.

Most patients present initially with an episode of acute pancreatitis but then develop evidence of chronic pancreatitis; others have obvious chronic pancreatitis at their first presentation. The disease tends to be progressive over time even if the original cause (e.g., alcohol) is removed.

DIAGNOSIS

The diagnosis may be suspected based on the clinical features but must be confirmed by tests that identify either structural damage to the pancreas or derangements in pancreatic function (Table 144-3). Chronic pancreatitis is a slowly progressive disease, and visible damage to the gland (e.g., on a CT scan) and functional failure (e.g., steatorrhea or diabetes) may not be apparent for years. All diagnostic tests are most accurate when the disease is far advanced, and all are far less accurate in the early stages of disease. Early diagnosis, when pain may be severe but imaging study results are normal or equivocal, is difficult.

No clear cause is found in a significant number of patients with chronic pancreatitis. In modern studies from referral centers, almost half of women and about 25% of men are labeled as having *idiopathic chronic pancreatitis.* Some have underlying genetic mutations that put them at particular risk, but gene testing may not be feasible or possible. Even if genetic testing is performed, many commercially available screens (e.g., for CFTR) only test a small percentage of all known mutations, and management will not necessarily be affected. Genetic testing for *PRSS1* is recommended if the family history is suggestive of an autosomal dominant disorder. Others may be surreptitiously using alcohol or may be smokers.

Tests of Pancreatic Structure

Plain abdominal radiographs may demonstrate diffuse or focal pancreatic calcification in patients with advanced chronic pancreatitis. Although specific for chronic pancreatitis, these findings are quite insensitive.

Abdominal ultrasonography is of limited accuracy owing to its inability to visualize the entire pancreas. A dilated pancreatic duct, pancreatic calcifications, gland atrophy, or changes in echotexture are seen in about 60% of patients.

Computed tomography is the most widely used diagnostic test for chronic pancreatitis. High-quality images can be obtained of the pancreas and pancreatic duct. Characteristic findings include a dilated pancreatic duct, ductal or parenchymal calcifications, and atrophy (Fig. 144-2). These structural changes take years to develop, so CT is not as accurate in early or less advanced chronic pancreatitis. Similar to CT, MRI allows detailed images of the pancreas, and the addition of MRCP allows even better assessment of pancreatic duct morphology. At some centers, secretin is administered at the time of MRCP to allow better visualization of the pancreatic duct.

Endoscopic retrograde cholangiopancreatography provides the most detailed images of the pancreatic duct. Changes in the duct include dilation,

TABLE 144-3 DIAGNOSTIC TESTS FOR CHRONIC PANCREATITIS

STRUCTURAL	FUNCTIONAL
Biopsy	Hormonal (secretin) test
Endoscopic ultrasonography	Using an oroduodenal tube
Endoscopic retrograde cholangiopancreatography	Using an endoscope
Magnetic resonance imaging with magnetic resonance cholangiopancreatography	Fecal elastase
Computed tomography	Serum trypsin
Ultrasonography	Fecal fat
Plain radiography	Blood glucose

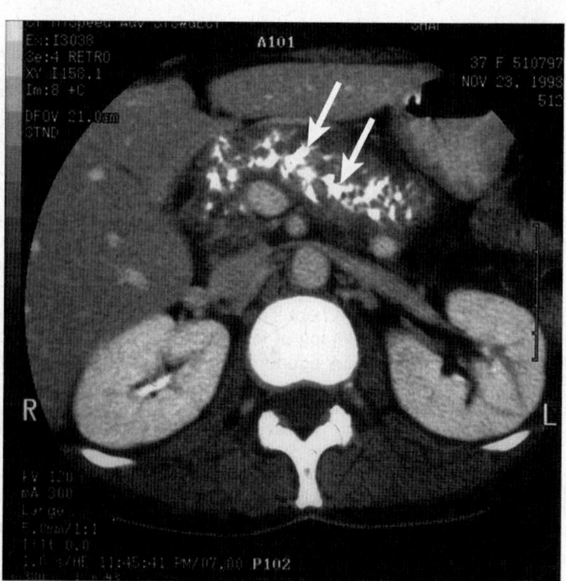

FIGURE 144-2. A computed tomography scan demonstrating diffuse pancreatic calcification in a patient with long-standing chronic pancreatitis *(arrows)*.

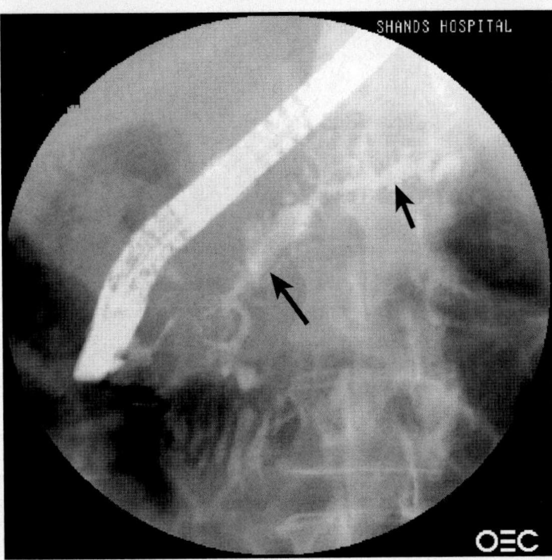

FIGURE 144-3. Endoscopic retrograde cholangiopancreatography demonstrating a very irregular pancreatic duct with areas of dilation and structuring in a patient with chronic pancreatitis *(arrows)*.

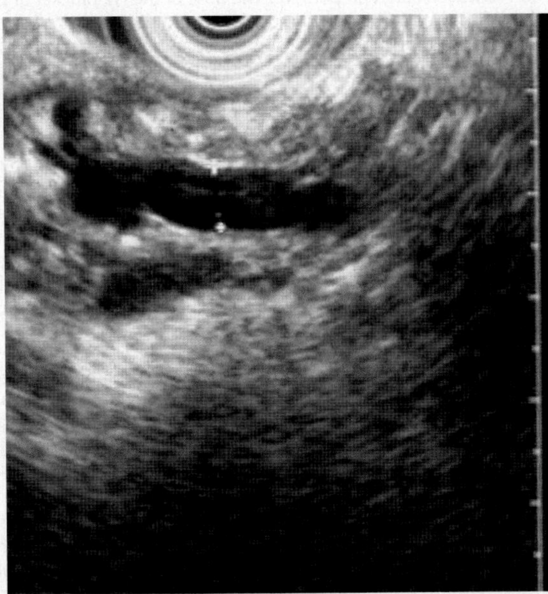

FIGURE 144-4. Endoscopic ultrasonography in a patient with chronic pancreatitis, demonstrating a dilated pancreatic duct (*marks* on margin of main duct).

irregularity, ductal stones, and strictures (Fig. 144-3). These findings are not completely specific for chronic pancreatitis and can be seen in other situations, including pancreatic cancer, after a pancreatic duct stent, and in very elderly individuals. Because of its risk, ERCP should be undertaken only when therapy involving the pancreatic duct is appropriate. Endoscopic ultrasonography allows very detailed images of pancreatic parenchyma and duct (Fig. 144-4) without the risk of ERCP. Normal endoscopic ultrasound results exclude chronic pancreatitis, but very abnormal endoscopic ultrasound results are highly consistent with chronic pancreatitis. However, many endoscopic ultrasound studies show intermediate findings, which are not specific for chronic pancreatitis.

Tests of Pancreatic Function

Serum trypsinogen is abnormally low in patients with far advanced chronic pancreatitis. Levels below 20 ng/mL are seen in patients with chronic pancreatitis that is sufficient to cause functional failure (e.g., steatorrhea). Serum levels of amylase and lipase are of little diagnostic utility for chronic pancreatitis. Serum glucose is elevated in those with endocrine insufficiency.

Quantification of fat in stool during a 72-hour collection while on a high-fat diet can be used to document steatorrhea but is rarely performed. Qualitative analysis of fat with Sudan staining of a stool specimen has poor sensitivity and specificity. Fecal levels of pancreatic elastase are diminished in patients with advanced chronic pancreatitis and steatorrhea. Fecal elastase below 100 mcg/g stool is consistent with advanced chronic pancreatitis. The test can be performed while patients are taking pancreatic enzyme therapy.

One pancreatic function test involves passing an oroduodenal tube and administering a supraphysiologic dose of secretin. Pancreatic secretions are collected over the course of 1 hour and analyzed for their bicarbonate concentration. A normal study is defined by a peak bicarbonate concentration of greater than 80 mEq/L. This test result becomes abnormal earlier in the disease process than any other test but is not widely available. An alternative, using endoscopy instead of a tube, is slightly less sensitive.

Diagnostic Approach

As the disease advances, typically over years, the structural and functional damage accumulate to the point that essentially all diagnostic test results are positive. In most patients, the diagnosis can be or will have been established by routine tests such as CT or MRI. Endoscopic ultrasonography and ERCP are rarely needed for diagnostic purposes in patients with longstanding chronic pancreatitis. The diagnostic challenge lies with patients who present with a severe pain syndrome suggestive of chronic pancreatitis but who have normal CT or MRI results. In these patients, endoscopic ultrasonography is the best choice unless the patient can have access to a secretin-based pancreatic function test. ERCP should not be used for purely diagnostic purposes because of the risk of complications, especially post-ERCP pancreatitis.

TREATMENT Rx

Abdominal Pain

Pseudocysts, obstruction of a surrounding hollow organ (e.g., duodenum or bile duct), and superimposed carcinoma cause chronic pain. A good-quality CT or MRI is usually sufficient to exclude these possibilities and to help choose appropriate therapy. Patients who have a dilated (generally >5 mm) pancreatic duct are candidates for endoscopic and surgical decompression therapy to relieve pain. Patients without ductal dilation are generally not appropriate for endoscopic and surgical therapy and must rely instead on medical therapy (Table 144-4).

Medical therapy starts with vigorous and structured attempts to assist patients in stopping alcohol and tobacco, if applicable. Most patients require analgesics. It is appropriate to start with the less potent agents first (e.g., tramadol, 50 mg four times daily), although many patients require more potent agents (Table 30-4) and may benefit from an adjunctive agent (e.g., gabapentin, pregabalin, selective serotonin-reuptake inhibitors, or tricyclic antidepressants; see Table 30-3 in Chapter 30) to potentiate the narcotic effect.[A9] Antioxidants (mixtures of selenium, vitamins E and C, β-carotene, and methionine) have been studied in two large randomized trials, with mixed results. Pancreatic enzyme therapy (see later) may have some beneficial effect on pain.[14]

Endoscopic retrograde cholangiopancreatography can be used to dilate ductal strictures and place stents. Ductal stones, if they are not too large and are not impacted, may also be removed. Lithotripsy of larger stones is usually required to reduce the stone to manageable fragments. This approach is technically successful in more than 80% of carefully selected patients, with pain relief in 70% to 80% of patients. Unfortunately, only a subset of patients with chronic pancreatitis has ductal anatomy that is amenable to this type of therapy.

Endoscopic ultrasound-guided celiac plexus block, which uses a local anesthetic and a steroid, or neurolysis, which uses absolute alcohol, can reduce the pain of chronic pancreatitis for weeks to months. However, the durability of those approaches has not been demonstrated, so they should be viewed as temporizing measures at best.

Surgery to decompress the pancreatic duct can provide more effective and durable long-term outcomes than endoscopic therapy for chronic pancreatitis.[A10][A11] The most commonly performed procedure involves a longitudinal incision of the pancreatic duct from the body of the pancreas to as close to the duodenum as possible, and this "filleted" duct is overlaid with a defunctionalized Roux limb. At the time of surgery, ductal strictures can be incised and ductal stones can be removed. The procedure is relatively simple in those with a dilated pancreatic duct (>5 mm) and preserves maximal pancreatic parenchyma. Pain relief in the short term is good (>80%), with about 50% obtaining long-term relief of pain. Alternative surgical procedures for pain include partial pancreatic resection, typically the head of the gland. More ambitious procedures, including pancreaticoduodenectomy and total pancreatectomy, usually coupled with autotransplantation of harvested islet cells, are performed as a last resort at a small number of specialized centers.

TABLE 144-4 TREATMENT FOR PAIN ASSOCIATED WITH CHRONIC PANCREATITIS

TREATMENT	EXAMPLES
Medical therapy	Alcohol and tobacco cessation Analgesics and adjunctive agents Antioxidants Non–enteric-coated enzymes
Neurolysis	Celiac plexus block or neurolysis EUS guided CT guided
Endoscopic therapy	Stent Stone removal, lithotripsy
Surgical therapy	Pancreaticojejunostomy (modified Puestow operation) Partial pancreatic resection (Whipple operation, duodenum preserving pancreatic head resection, others) Total pancreatectomy with islet cell autotransplantation

CT = computed tomography; EUS = endoscopic ultrasonography.

TABLE 144-5 ENZYME THERAPY FOR EXOCRINE PANCREATIC INSUFFICIENCY*

PRODUCT	AVAILABLE STRENGTHS	COMMENTS
	USP lipase units/capsule or tablet	
Zenpep	3000; 5000; 10,000; 15,000; 20,000; 25,000	Enteric-coated capsule
Creon	3000; 6000; 12,000; 24,000; 36,000	Enteric-coated capsule
Pancreaze	4200; 10,500; 16,800; 21,000	Enteric-coated capsule
Ultresa	13,800; 20,700; 23,000	Enteric-coated capsule
Pertzye	8000; 16,000	Enteric-coated capsule with bicarbonate
Viokace	10,440; 20,880	Non–enteric-coated tablet

*For the treatment of pain, non–enteric-coated preparations are used. For exocrine insufficiency, cotreatment with acid-reducing medications is necessary when using non–enteric-coated preparations.

Exocrine Insufficiency

Steatorrhea and maldigestion do not occur until approximately 90% of pancreatic enzyme secretion is lost usually after at least 5 to 10 years of chronic pancreatitis. Patients may note weight loss and oily stools but often do not complain of diarrhea. Patients with chronic pancreatitis and exocrine insufficiency maldigest fat, protein, and carbohydrates, but fat maldigestion is most severe. In addition to weight loss, malabsorption of fat-soluble vitamins, particularly vitamin D, is common. A formal 72-stool fat analysis, which is the most accurate method to document steatorrhea and to gauge effectiveness of therapy, is rarely done. Instead, the clinical features and a fecal elastase less than 100 mcg/g stool, coupled with an appropriate response to enzyme replacement therapy, is the best substitute for 72-hour fecal fat testing.

Pancreatic enzymes (Table 144-5) include both enteric-coated (capsules) and non-enteric-coated (tablets) preparations. Non–enteric-coated preparations are the agents of choice if the goal is to treat pain. They can also be used to treat exocrine insufficiency, although the enteric-coated preparations are used more frequently for this indication. No generic products are currently available. The goal of enzyme therapy, which is to administer at least 10% of normal pancreatic output with each meal, translates to approximately 90,000 USP units of lipase with each meal. Because most patients are still producing some digestive enzymes and have a compensatory increase in gastric lipase, it may not be necessary to prescribe the full dosage of 90,000 USP units with each meal. An initial starting dosage of 50,000 to 70,000 units of lipase per meal, with subsequent assessment of the clinical response, is reasonable.

If non–enteric-coated preparations are used, then cotreatment with an H2-blocker or proton pump inhibitor (Table 138-1) is required to prevent acid denaturation of enzymes, a critical point of emphasis. Enzymes should be administered during and immediately after the meal. Supplementation with vitamin D and calcium is appropriate because osteoporosis and osteopenia are very common. Supplementation with other fat- and water-soluble vitamins may also be needed.

Successful enzyme replacement therapy is generally defined as weight gain, absence of visible oil in the stool, and normalization of fat-soluble vitamin levels. Failure of enzyme therapy is most often caused by an inadequate dose. Increasing the dose up to the full 90,000 USP units with meals and encouraging compliance is appropriate as a first step. In patients using a non–enteric-coated preparation, the dose of the H2-blocker or proton pump inhibitor can be increased to reduce the acid destruction of enzymes. Some patients may not respond because a second disease, such as small intestinal bacterial overgrowth (Chapter 140), is contributing to the malabsorption.

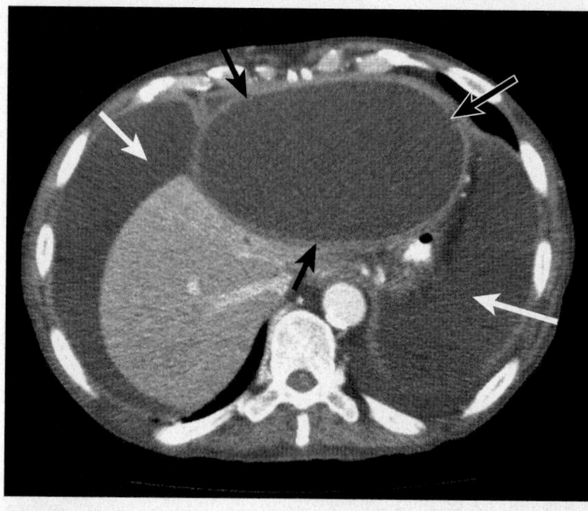

FIGURE 144-5. On computed tomography, a large pseudocyst is seen *(black arrows)*. In addition, ascites surrounding the liver *(white arrow)* is caused by a leak from the pseudocyst (pancreatic ascites).

Endocrine Insufficiency

Diabetes mellitus (Chapter 229) is a very late complication of chronic pancreatitis. Some patients will develop type 2 diabetes, some develop type 3C diabetes in which there is a loss of both insulin and glucagon secretion.[15] In such patients, overly aggressive therapy may lead to hypoglycemia, which cannot be reversed by the usual natural glucagon surge. Treatment-induced hypoglycemia can be fatal in these patients, especially if they are also malnourished. As a result, treatment should avoid exceedingly tight glucose control.

Complications

Pseudocysts, when they are discovered in patients with chronic pancreatitis, are generally mature and have a visible capsule surrounding them. As in acute pancreatitis, pseudocysts in chronic pancreatitis do not require therapy if they are not producing symptoms and are not rapidly enlarging. By comparison, symptomatic pseudocysts require drainage by endoscopic, percutaneous, or surgical procedure.

Pseudocysts may leak into the peritoneal compartment (pancreatic ascites) or track into the chest (pancreatic pleural effusion). Patients usually present with abdominal distention or dyspnea, respectively, rather than abdominal pain. Amylase level in the fluid is usually greater than 4000 U/L. Endoscopic therapy with stent placement across the connection between pseudocyst and pancreatic duct is highly effective in this situation (Fig. 144-5).

Cystic neoplasms require resection. Features that suggest a cystic neoplasm include a cyst with a thick wall or nodules in the wall, a cyst with multiple internal septations, or a cyst occurring in a patient who does not have a history of pancreatitis.

Chronic pancreatitis is also a strong risk factor for pancreatic ductal adenocarcinoma (Chapter 194), with a lifetime risk of about 4% to 5%. The risk is much higher in patients with hereditary pancreatitis and in patients who smoke. Equally important, it may be very difficult to distinguish cancer from benign disease, particularly in those with autoimmune pancreatitis.

PREVENTION

There is not currently any reliable method to prevent chronic pancreatitis, although patients who have fewer episodes of acute pancreatitis are less likely to develop chronic pancreatitis. Patients at risk for chronic pancreatitis and patients with recurrent episodes of acute pancreatitis should avoid alcohol and tobacco. Patients with autoimmune pancreatitis should be treated with steroids (see earlier) to reduce the risk of progression.

PROGNOSIS

The prognosis of chronic pancreatitis is heavily influenced by its cause, as well as by concurrent smoking and ongoing alcohol use. With prolonged follow-up of 10 to 20 years, the majority of patients will develop exocrine or endocrine insufficiency. The survival rate of patients with chronic pancreatitis is lower than in age-matched control participants. Death is usually not attributable to pancreatitis itself but rather to malignancy, postoperative complications, and complications of tobacco and alcohol.[16] Overall, the 10-year survival rate approximates 70% and the 20-year survival rate is 45%. Patients who are older, smoke, or have alcohol as the cause are at highest risk of mortality.

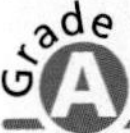

Grade A References

A1. Wu BU, Hwang JQ, Gardner TH, et al. Lactated Ringer's solution reduces systemic inflammation compared with saline in patients with acute pancreatitis. *Clin Gastroenterol Hepatol*. 2011;9: 710-717.

A2. Larino-Noia J, Lindkvist B, Iglesias-Garcia J, et al. Early and/or immediately full caloric diet versus standard refeeding in mild acute pancreatitis: a randomized open-label trial. *Pancreatology*. 2014;14:167-173.

A3. Bakker OJ, van Brunschot S, van Santvoort HC, et al. Early versus on-demand nasoenteric tube feeding in acute pancreatitis. *N Engl J Med*. 2014;371:1983-1993.

A4. Petrov MS, van Santvoort HC, Besselink MG, et al. Early endoscopic retrograde cholangiopancreatography versus conservative management in acute biliary pancreatitis without cholangitis: a meta-analysis of randomized trials. *Ann Surg*. 2008;247:250-257.

A5. Varadarajulu S, Bang JY, Sutton BS, et al. Equal efficacy of endoscopic and surgical cystogastrostomy for pancreatic pseudocyst drainage in a randomized trial. *Gastroenterology*. 2013;145: 583-590.

A6. Bakker OJ, van Santvoort HC, van Brunschot S, et al. Endoscopic transgastric vs surgical necrosectomy for infected necrotizing pancreatitis: a randomized trial. *JAMA*. 2012;307:1053-1061.

A7. Sethi S, Sethi N, Wadhwa V, et al. A meta-analysis on the role of rectal diclofenac and indomethacin in the prevention of post-endoscopic retrograde cholangiopancreatography pancreatitis. *Pancreas*. 2014;43:190-197.

A8. Nordback I, Pelli H, Lappalainen-Lehto R, et al. The recurrence of acute alcohol-associated pancreatitis can be reduced: a randomized controlled trial. *Gastroenterology*. 2009;136:848-855.

A9. Olesen SS, Bouwense SA, Wilder-Smith OH, et al. Pregabalin reduces pain in patients with chronic pancreatitis in a randomized, controlled trial. *Gastroenterology*. 2011;141:536-543.

A10. Dite P, Ruzicka M, Zboril V, et al. A prospective, randomized trial comparing endoscopic and surgical therapy for chronic pancreatitis. *Endoscopy*. 2003;35:553-558.

A11. Cahen DL, Gouma DJ, Laramee P, et al. Long-term outcomes of endoscopic vs surgical drainage of the pancreatic duct in patients with chronic pancreatitis. *Gastroenterology*. 2011;141: 1690-1695.

GENERAL REFERENCES

For the General References and other additional features, please visit Expert Consult at https://expertconsult.inkling.com.

145

DISEASES OF THE RECTUM AND ANUS

ROBERT D. MADOFF

ANATOMY

The Rectum

The rectum and anal canal make up the final portion of the hindgut. Several definitions exist to delineate the boundaries of each. In general, the rectum begins at the level of the sacral promontory, where the taeniae coli splay to form a continuous longitudinal muscle layer and extends 12 to 18 cm distally. The peritoneum covers the upper two thirds of the rectum anteriorly and is more limited laterally. The rectum and its mesentery are surrounded by endopelvic fascia, and this anatomic package contains the relevant lymphovascular structures that should be removed intact in rectal cancer surgery. The rectum has two or three curves within its lumen created by submucosal folds called the valves of Houston. The second valve is often used as a rough guideline for the intraperitoneal cavity anteriorly.

Blood supply to the rectum originates from the inferior mesenteric artery and internal iliac arteries. The inferior mesenteric artery terminates as the superior rectal (hemorrhoidal) artery, which supplies the rectum and the upper third of the anal canal. Additionally, internal iliac arteries give off the middle rectal (hemorrhoidal) arteries and the inferior rectal (hemorrhoidal) arteries (inferior via the internal pudendal artery) to supply the distal rectum and anal canal. The majority of the rectum drains into the superior hemorrhoidal venous plexus and then to the inferior mesenteric vein and portal and hepatic system. By contrast, the caudal rectum and the anal canal drain into the systemic venous circulation through the inferior and middle rectal veins into the internal iliac veins and inferior vena cava. As a general rule, the lymphatic drainage of the rectum follows the arterial supply via the inferior mesenteric and internal iliac lymph nodes. Innervation to the rectum involves both the sympathetic and parasympathetic plexus. Whereas the sympathetic nerves arise from the first three lumbar segments of the spinal cord, the parasympathetic nerve supply originates from the caudal three sacral nerve roots.

The Anal Canal

The anal canal, which begins at the level of the *levator ani* muscle and extends to the anal verge opening, is about 2.5 to 5 cm in length and is surrounded by the internal and external anal sphincter muscles. The anorectal junction, which can be easily appreciated on digital rectal examination, is the point where the rectum angulates posteriorly from the axis of the anal canal. The internal anal sphincter, which is responsible for about 70% of the resting anal tone, is an extension of the inner circular smooth muscle layer of the rectum. The external sphincter muscle comprises skeletal muscle and is under voluntary control.

The dentate (pectinate) line lies about 2 cm proximal to the anal verge (opening). Hemorrhoids are classified as proximal or distal to the dentate line.

The mucosal lining changes histologically along the course of the anal canal. Superiorly, the anal canal consists of columnar epithelium that mirrors the rectum. Approximately 1 to 2 cm above the level of the dentate line is a transitional zone, where columnar, cuboidal, transitional, and squamous epithelia cells are found. This admixture of cells constitutes the derivation of the term "basaloid" because it relates to the anal canal cancers and marks the proximal boundary for anal cancer surveillance. Distal to this line, the squamous epithelium extends to the anal verge and perianal skin, eventually adding glandular and hair follicles that resemble skin elsewhere on the body. Infected anal glands are a frequent cause of perianal abscess and fistula. Lymphatic drainage below the dentate line drains to the inguinal nodes. The external anal sphincter is innervated by fibers from S4 and the internal pudendal nerve. Somatic sensation of the anal canal comes from the inferior rectal nerve via the pudendal nerve. This somatic sensation ceases 1 to 2 cm above the dentate line, which explains why hemorrhoid ligation can be performed without anesthesia.

SPECIFIC ANORECTAL CONDITIONS

Hemorrhoids

EPIDEMIOLOGY AND PATHOBIOLOGY

An estimated 10 million or more individuals in the United States experience symptoms related to hemorrhoids each year, and these individuals generate more than 1 million annual office visits. The overall prevalence of symptomatic hemorrhoids is estimated to be approximately 5%, but many anorectal complaints attributed to "hemorrhoids" are caused by other conditions, so the true incidence and prevalence of hemorrhoids are unknown.[1]

Despite the commonly held notion that hemorrhoids are always abnormal, they actually are normal structures, identifiable even in fetuses. Hemorrhoids are vascular cushions that consist of connective tissue, smooth muscle, and both arterioles and veins. Functionally, they may aid with overall continence by serving as a malleable gasket to optimize the seal of the anal canal.

Hemorrhoids are *not* rectal varices, which are a distinct entity caused by portal hypertension. *Hemorrhoidal disease* is a more appropriate term to describe the pathologic state that generates symptoms. The arteriolar component explains why hemorrhoidal bleeding is typically bright red in color and can be copious in quantity. Causative factors that can provoke hemorrhoidal symptoms include constipation, diarrhea, older age, pregnancy, and prolonged straining at stool. Repeated stretching of the anal canal also may damage the supporting tissue and result in downward displacement of the vascular cushions. Although none of these precipitating factors has been established rigorously, each can cause either increased abdominal pressure or obstruction of venous return, thereby leading to engorgement and enlargement of the vascular cushions.

CLINICAL MANIFESTATIONS AND DIAGNOSIS

The most common symptom of internal hemorrhoids is bright red bleeding. This bleeding is typically painless and is most often seen on the toilet tissue or in the toilet bowel. The quantity of blood is variable, but some patients complain of blood dripping or squirting into the toilet bowl. Passage of dark blood or blood mixed in the stool suggests a more proximal source. Internal

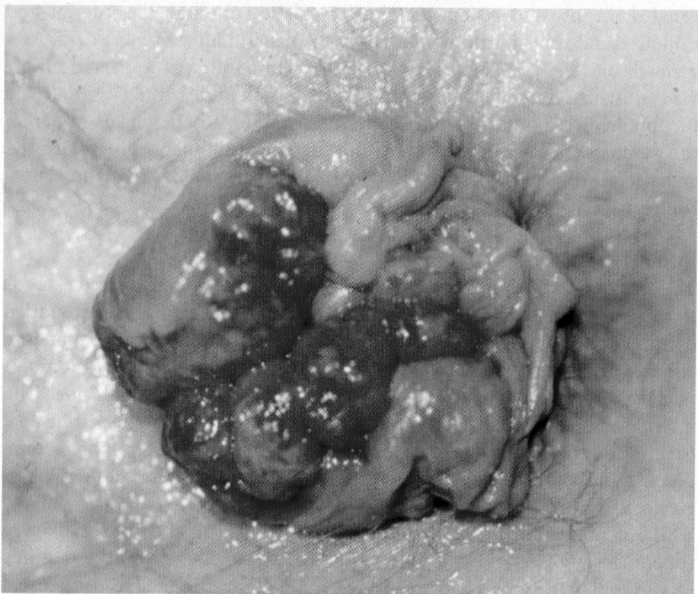

FIGURE 145-1. Grade 4 nonreducible internal and external hemorrhoids.

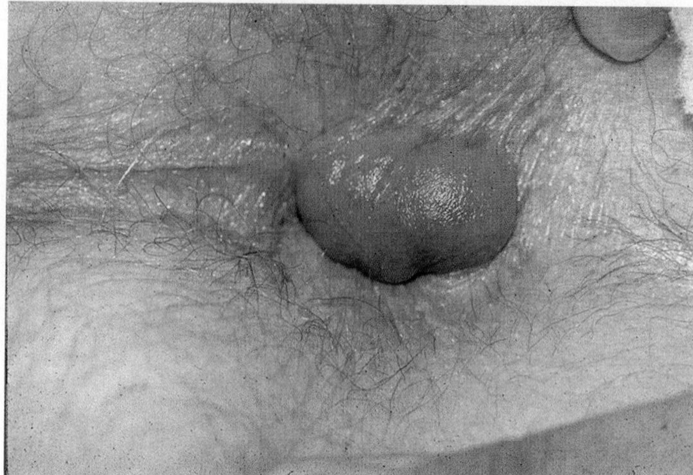

FIGURE 145-2. Thrombosed external hemorrhoid.

hemorrhoids are classified based on the symptoms they cause. As internal hemorrhoids enlarge, they become associated with redundant rectal mucosa that protrudes from the anus with defecation. Grade 1 hemorrhoids bleed but do not prolapse. Early protrusion reduces spontaneously (grade 2); more advanced protrusion requires digital reduction (grade 3) and, at its most advanced, becomes irreducible (grade 4) (Fig. 145-1). Internal hemorrhoids are insensate and are not itchy themselves, but they can cause itching owing to associated perianal soiling or mucus deposition caused by mucosal prolapse. Additionally, patients may complain of mucus discharge, extra tissue at the verge (i.e., mucosal prolapse), or a sensation of incomplete evacuation.

Individuals with anorectal symptoms frequently present complaining of "hemorrhoids" or are even referred from other physicians with a diagnosis of hemorrhoids. Although hemorrhoids may be present, they are often not the source of the underlying complaint. Therefore, it is always incorrect—and sometimes dangerous—for the physician to apply this diagnosis without completing an adequate evaluation. Fortunately, the initial evaluation is simple, and the correct diagnosis is often suspected based on history alone and confirmed by a limited visual and endoscopic examination. Internal hemorrhoids are best visualized with a slotted anoscope. Rectal bleeding should never be attributed to hemorrhoids alone, even if hemorrhoids are visible; at a minimum, flexible sigmoidoscopy is required to exclude more proximal pathology. For more concerning symptoms or high-risk patients (e.g., personal or family history of colorectal cancer, persistent bleeding despite therapy, unscreened individuals older than age 50 years), a full evaluation of the large intestine should be performed by colonoscopy.

External hemorrhoids are usually asymptomatic and should be differentiated from perianal skin tags, which occasionally cause difficulties with hygiene. External hemorrhoids become symptomatic when they thrombose to cause acute-onset pain and swelling (Fig. 145-2). Thrombosed external hemorrhoids are diagnosed by simple inspection. Occasional patients who present with extensive, circumferential thrombosis require urgent surgical consultation.

TREATMENT Rx

Grade 1 hemorrhoids often respond to dietary manipulation alone, including increased dietary fiber, addition of a fiber supplement, and increased water intake (Table 145-1). The goal, which may not be readily achievable, is approximately 25 to 30 g of fiber and 8 glasses of water daily. More advanced hemorrhoids require specific therapy, which is almost always office based. The most popular and simplest technique is rubber band ligation, whereby a tiny rubber band (internal diameter ≈1 mm) is placed around a quantity of redundant rectal mucosa and prolapsing hemorrhoid well above the dentate line.[A1] The banded tissue sloughs in 7 to 14 days, an event sometimes heralded by rectal bleeding. Banding can be repeated at 3- to 4-week intervals until bleeding and protrusion are controlled. Bands placed too close to the dentate line cause immediate severe pain and must be removed promptly. Patients who are at high risk of bleeding because of intrinsic coagulopathies or treatment with anticoagulant agents should not undergo rubber band ligation owing to the increased risk of postprocedure bleeding. Alternative therapies for moderate internal hemorrhoids include injection sclerotherapy and infrared coagulation, both of which are office-based procedures.

Operative hemorrhoidectomy is needed in only a minority of patients with advanced disease. Indications for hemorrhoidectomy include irreducible prolapse, a substantial external component, and failure of more conservative therapies. The most common approach is an excisional hemorrhoidectomy, which is generally performed on an outpatient basis. A more recent approach is the stapled hemorrhoidopexy, which entails resecting a ring of rectal mucosa proximal to the internal hemorrhoids using a circular stapling device. This technique is associated with less postoperative pain and a shorter period of disability, but its drawbacks include a higher recurrence rate than conventional surgery as well as a small but worrisome risk of significant complications, such as chronic pain, rectovaginal fistula, and staple line bleeding. Another alternative approach is Doppler-guided hemorrhoidal artery ligation, after which recurrence rates are 5% to 15%.[A2]

Thrombosed external hemorrhoids are usually treated by excision in the office under local anesthesia. However, because the pain associated with thrombosis generally abates within 7 to 10 days, patients who present with resolving symptoms are often best managed conservatively with standard doses of over-the-counter analgesics, Sitz baths, and 25 g/day of fiber supplementation.

TABLE 145-1 INTERNAL HEMORRHOIDS: GRADING AND MANAGEMENT

GRADE	SYMPTOMS AND SIGNS	MANAGEMENT
1	Bleeding No prolapse	Dietary modifications* Rubber band ligation Infrared coagulation Injection sclerotherapy
2	Prolapse with spontaneous reduction Bleeding, seepage	Rubber band ligation Infrared coagulation Dietary modifications Injection sclerotherapy Doppler hemorrhoidal artery ligation
3	Prolapse requiring digital reduction Bleeding, seepage	Surgical hemorrhoidectomy Surgical hemorrhoidopexy Rubber band ligation Dietary modifications Doppler hemorrhoidal artery ligation
4	Prolapsed, cannot be reduced Strangulated	Surgical hemorrhoidectomy Urgent hemorrhoidectomy

*Dietary modifications include increasing the consumption of fiber, bran, or psyllium and water. Dietary modifications are always appropriate for the management of hemorrhoids and to prevent recurrence after banding or surgery (or both).

Perianal Abscess

EPIDEMIOLOGY AND PATHOBIOLOGY

Several superficial and deep spaces around the rectum and anal canal normally contain loose areolar tissue but serve as potential sites for perianal infections. Perianal abscess is a common condition, but its incidence is not well documented. Approximately 80% of perianal abscesses are caused by infection of the anal glands that track toward the skin, but other causes include simple skin infections, trauma, inflammatory bowel disease, anorectal surgery, malignancy, and immunosuppression.[2]

CLINICAL MANIFESTATIONS AND DIAGNOSIS

Patients most commonly present with complaints of perianal pain and swelling. In most cases, a local area of erythema, tenderness, and fluctuance can be appreciated on physical examination. However, these findings are often absent in an intersphincteric abscess, which is a small abscess in the plane between the internal and external sphincter muscles, as well as in supralevator and deep ischiorectal abscesses. These abscesses should be suspected based on a history of increasing pain and fever, as well as the physical finding of focal perianal tenderness.

As with all acutely painful anal conditions, digital examination should generally be avoided. Likewise, office instrumentation with an anoscope or proctoscope is contraindicated because these examinations cause substantial pain and yield little if any diagnostic information. When the cause of the acute pain cannot be determined in the office, prompt examination under anesthesia should be performed. Adjunctive computed tomographic (CT) scanning, magnetic resonance imaging (MRI), or endorectal ultrasound can provide valuable information in occult, recurrent or complex disease.

TREATMENT Rx

Treatment for perianal abscess is prompt incision and drainage,[A3] which usually can be performed in the office. Large or deep (e.g., postanal or horseshoe) abscesses are best evaluated in the operating room with proper sedation. Antibiotics do not adequately penetrate abscess cavities, and extension of a local infection can lead to sepsis and complex long-term problems. Therefore, antibiotic therapy is inadequate and should never be given in an attempt to avoid or delay incision and drainage. Antibiotics generally are not indicated after incision and drainage, but exceptions include immunocompromised patients (those with poorly controlled HIV, transplant recipients, patients undergoing chemotherapy, patients with diabetes), patients with extensive cellulitis or severe systemic symptoms, and patients at high risk for endovascular infection (e.g., patients with cardiac shunts or prosthetic valves). In patients who fail to improve after incision and drainage, prompt surgical reevaluation is usually warranted because the problem is likely to be a residual abscess that requires further drainage.[3]

Anal Fistula

EPIDEMIOLOGY

An anal fistula, which represents the chronic form of a perianal abscess, usually manifests as one or more chronic tracts from the anal canal to the perianal skin. The incidence of anal fistula is about 8.6 per 100,000. Fistulae are two to three times more common in men than in women.

PATHOBIOLOGY

After a perianal abscess is drained, there is about a 30% to 50% chance that the internal opening—the site at the dentate line where the infected gland originated—will remain patent, thereby leaving a source for recurrent infection. Multiple or atypical anal fistulae should raise always the diagnostic suspicion of Crohn disease, which is isolated to the perianal area in approximately 10% of cases.

Anal fistulae are characterized by their relationship to the sphincter complex. The simplest and most common (≈70%) fistula is intersphincteric—located in the plane between the internal and external sphincter muscles. Transsphincteric fistulas (about 20%-25%), which traverse both the internal and external sphincter muscles, are classified either as low fistulae, which traverse only the distal external sphincter, or high fistulae, which traverse the more proximal portions of the external sphincter. Suprasphincteric fistulae originate at the dentate line and loop over the entire sphincter complex. Extrasphincteric fistulae have internal openings remote from the dentate line; most originate from a pelvic abscess caused by a ruptured appendix (Chapter 142), diverticulitis (Chapter 142), or Crohn disease (Chapter 141). A horseshoe fistula is one with external openings on both sides of the midsagittal plane; these most commonly have a single internal opening in the posterior midline.

CLINICAL MANIFESTATIONS AND DIAGNOSIS

Anal fistulae sometimes present as recurrent abscesses in the same location as the original one or as persistent purulent drainage from an abscess site that has failed to heal completely. Patients may often think the area has healed for several weeks or longer before experiencing the same feeling of a "boil" forming in the identical area, spontaneously rupturing, and relieving their symptoms.

The diagnosis of an anal fistula is established by history and by visualization of an external opening in the perianal skin. A fibrous fistula track can sometimes be palpated along the course of the fistula from the skin toward the anal canal. An internal opening is occasionally visible on anoscopy, but it is not necessary to identify one to make a presumptive diagnosis.

TREATMENT Rx

Treatment of anal fistulae is surgical. Most fistulae are cured by being laid open to eliminate the original source of infection at the internal opening. The fistula track heals by secondary intention. However, this approach divides sphincter muscle and puts the patient at risk for impaired fecal continence in proportion to the quantity of muscle involved. In general, intersphincteric and low transsphincteric fistulae can be safely laid open if the patient has normal baseline continence and no underlying predisposing factors for diarrhea (e.g., colitis) or recurrent fistulas (e.g., Crohn disease). Because the anterior sphincter mechanism is relatively short and subject to injury after vaginal delivery, fistulotomy for anterior fistulae in women must be undertaken only after careful consideration.

When a high fistula is identified, the first step is often placement of a seton, a suture, or other material (now commonly a Silastic vessel loop) that is passed though the fistula tract, out the anus, and secured to itself. The seton guarantees that the external fistula opening will not heal over, so a recurrent abscess is much less likely to supervene. After being left in for several weeks, the tract has often scarred around the seton and become fibrotic; treatment options to eliminate the internal opening include endorectal advancement flap repair and ligation of the intersphincteric fistula tract. Because Crohn disease-associated fistulae tend to be multiple and recurrent, fistulotomy is avoided, except for the most superficial fistulae. In general, patients with Crohn disease are best served by placement of long-term draining setons and medical therapy for their underlying disease (Fig. 145-3).

Anal Fissure

EPIDEMIOLOGY

Anal fissures can occur at any age but most frequently affect young adults. Men and women are equally affected.

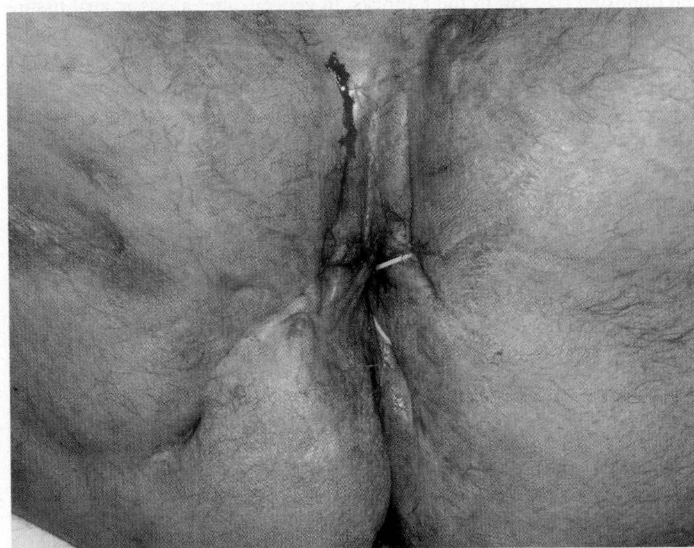

FIGURE 145-3. **Crohn disease fistulae.** Silastic setons in place with several additional draining tracts and evidence of prior surgery.

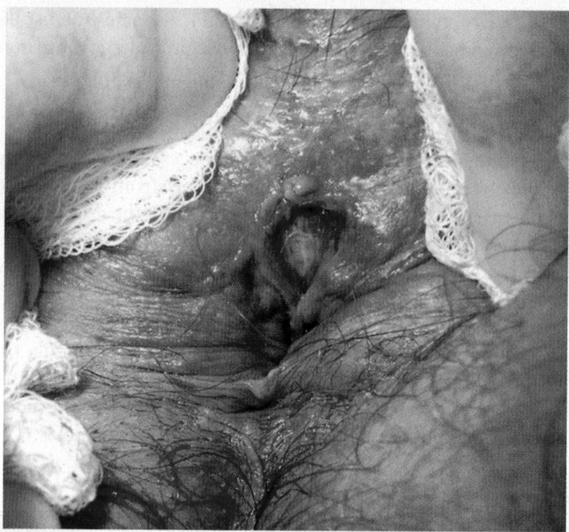

FIGURE 145-4. Anal fissure. This longitudinal tear occurs just inside the anal margin.

PATHOBIOLOGY

An anal fissure is a longitudinal tear in the anoderm that occurs just inside the anal margin (Fig. 145-4). The underlying pathophysiology of anal fissures is hypertonia of the internal anal sphincter. Typical anal fissures occur at the midline; most commonly, they occur posteriorly, but about 15% are found anteriorly or both anteriorly and posteriorly. "Off-the-midline" fissures may represent a routine fissure, but they generally require examination under anesthesia with culture, biopsy, and pathological evaluation to exclude causes such as anal cancer, Crohn disease, syphilis, HIV, leukemia, or tuberculosis.

CLINICAL MANIFESTATIONS AND DIAGNOSIS

Patients with anal fissures generally present with pain after a bout of constipation or a period of excessive diarrhea. After subsequent bowel movements, patients describe severe anal pain that may persist for hours or even continue until exacerbation by the next bowel movement. There is sometimes an association with minor bright red bleeding, most commonly seen in small quantities that streak the stool or the toilet tissue. Whereas an acute anal fissure appears as a superficial split in the perianal skin and anoderm, chronic anal fissures, defined by their presence for at least 6 to 8 weeks, are associated with a "sentinel" skin tag (so called because its presence should suggest the presence of an underlying fissure) and a hypertrophied anal papilla located just proximal to the fissure at the dentate line. Well-established fissures may have fibrotic margins and visible internal anal sphincter fibers at their base.

Most fissures can be readily observed on physical examination by applying opposing traction to the buttocks. In general, after a classic anal fissure is identified, no further examination is performed at that time. Digital and endoscopic examination typically should be delayed until the patient has healed to avoid causing pain. However, patients should be advised that they will require subsequent flexible sigmoidoscopy to exclude proximal pathology.

TREATMENT Rx

All therapies are directed at the underlying hypertonia of the internal anal sphincter. Approximately 40% of fissures heal with fiber supplementation and increased fluid intake alone, including the great majority of acute fissures. Patients are also advised to take warm Sitz baths for symptomatic relief, especially after bowel movements.

Two pharmacologic approaches can augment diet and Sitz baths: topical sphincter relaxants and botulinum toxin injection. Topical nitroglycerine ointment (0.2%-0.8%) or diltiazem gel (2%) applied to the anal orifice two to four times daily reduces sphincter tone and often leads to healing. Both drugs have similar efficacy, but nitroglycerine has the significant disadvantage of causing headaches, lightheadedness, or syncope owing to systemic vasodilation in approximately 25% of patients. Unfortunately, these nonsurgical approaches are only marginally better than placebo for healing chronic fissures, and recurrent fissures occur in approximately 50% of patients.[A4]

For patients who fail medical therapy or who are simply too miserable subjectively to pursue it, lateral internal sphincterotomy is an appropriate and generally safe approach that is easily performed under monitored local anesthesia in an outpatient setting.[A5] Recovery is rapid, and fissure healing is expected in more than 90% of cases. Sphincterotomy as first-line therapy provides higher healing rates, fewer relapses, and fewer side effects than topical nitroglycerine, with fewer symptoms, greater satisfaction, and no difference in continence at long-term follow-up.[A6] However, a small percentage of patients who undergo sphincterotomy develop minor seepage or actual incontinence, so sphincterotomy should be avoided in individuals who have underlying impaired continence, known sphincter injuries, or diarrheal disorders. When such patients have refractory fissures, a trial of botulinum toxin injection is often a good alternative.

Pruritus Ani

EPIDEMIOLOGY

The reported incidence of pruritus ani ranges from 1% to 5% in the general population, although is likely much higher. Men are more commonly affected than women (4 : 1), and this condition is most common in the fourth through the sixth decades of life. Primary or idiopathic pruritus is responsible for 50% to 90% of all cases of pruritus ani.

CLINICAL MANIFESTATIONS AND DIAGNOSIS

Pruritus ani, or perianal itching, is a very common symptom but is not a disease. The most common cause is likely inadequate perianal hygiene, often exacerbated by scratching, which leads to excoriation of the skin and further inflammation. Secondary causes include dermatologic, infectious, systemic, and lower gastrointestinal disease, as well as local irritants. Some of these sources include prolapsing hemorrhoids, anal fistulas, anal incontinence, as well as specific dermatologic conditions such as contact dermatitis, psoriasis, lichen sclerosis, squamous intraepithelial neoplasia (Bowen disease), and perianal Paget disease (intraepidermal adenocarcinoma).

The diagnosis is typically based on a history of intractable itching despite trials of several over-the-counter medications and physical examination to exclude an obvious inciting source.[4] The severity of the condition can be classified as stage 0—normal skin; stage 1—red and inflamed skin; stage 2—lichenified skin; or stage 3—lichenified skin as well as coarse ridges and often ulcerations.

TREATMENT Rx

A therapeutic trial of symptomatic empiric management is effective in more than 90% of patients. Options include improved hygiene, avoidance of potential contact allergens (e.g., soaps and over the counter topical treatments), and use of either talc to absorb excess moisture or a barrier cream such as zinc oxide. Mechanical scratching will perpetuate the cycle of inflammation and must be strictly avoided. Some patients benefit from the avoidance of certain foods, including caffeinated beverages, alcohol, milk, chocolate, and tomatoes. Mild topical steroids such as 1% hydrocortisone are sometimes helpful, but stronger steroid preparations are frequently counterproductive and should be avoided when they are not indicated for a specific dermatologic diagnosis. The placement of a small fluff of absorbent cotton at the anal verge can help to wick away moisture and collect any drainage before it can be in prolonged contact with the skin. Other adjuncts include drying the perianal skin with a hairdryer after bathing and replacing toilet paper with nondetergent, nondeodorant, nonalcohol hypoallergenic wipes. Skin biopsies and dermatologic consultation should be obtained when a primary dermatologic condition is suspected or when the perianal irritation fails to heal with conservative therapy.

Fecal Incontinence

EPIDEMIOLOGY AND PATHOBIOLOGY

Involuntary loss of stool or flatus is a relatively common problem that, when severe, can be socially isolating and debilitating. About 2% of individuals in the United States report incontinence symptoms, but the prevalence is substantially higher in patients visiting primary care providers and gastroenterologists.[5] Almost half of U.S. nursing home patients suffer from fecal incontinence. Factors such as embarrassment, denial, and the degree of symptoms hinder a determination of true prevalence. Patients presenting with fecal incontinence often have concomitant urinary incontinence

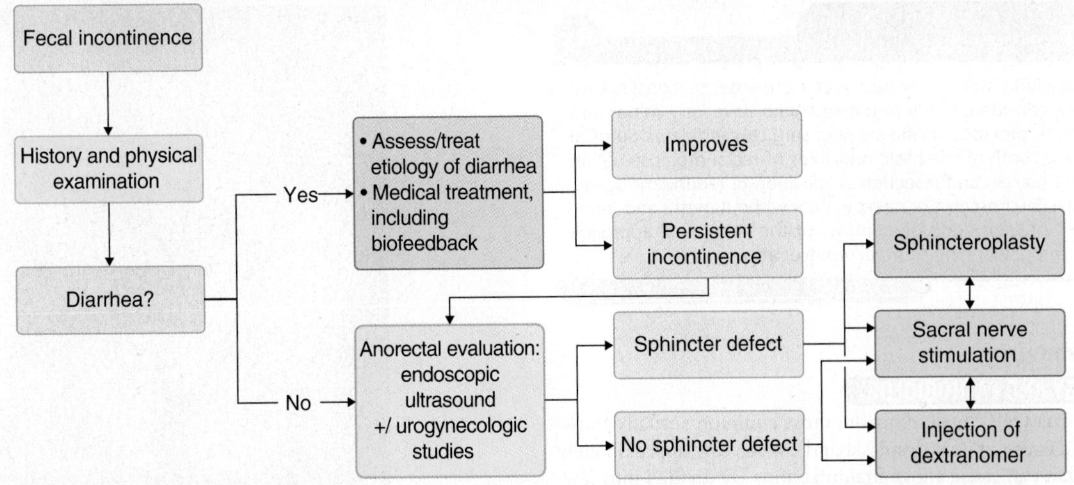

FIGURE 145-5. **Algorithm for fecal incontinence.** (Adapted from Madoff RD, Parker SC, Varma MG, Lowry AC. Fecal incontinence in adults. *Lancet*. 2004;364:621-632)

(Chapter 26), and up to 25% of women with fecal incontinence have at least one associated pelvic floor disorder.

Normal continence involves the coordinated interaction between multiple different neuronal pathways and the pelvic and perineal structures. In addition, several factors, including bowel motility, stool consistency, evacuation efficiency, mental status, and sphincter integrity, all play roles in normal regulation. Sphincter disruption related to vaginal delivery is a common cause that often affects young women; many incontinent women who present later in life have an underlying sphincter injury for which they can no longer compensate. Other causes of incontinence include fecal impaction, surgical or traumatic sphincter injury, rectal prolapse, neurologic disorders (e.g., diabetic neuropathy, stroke, multiple sclerosis, brain or spinal cord injury), chronic diarrheal states, dementia, impaired mobility, and poor access to toilet facilities.

CLINICAL MANIFESTATIONS AND DIAGNOSIS

Because incontinence is a symptom and not a disease, the diagnosis is based on history alone. Specific evaluation of the incontinent patient can include anal manometry, anal ultrasonography, pudendal nerve testing, and defecography. Anal endoscopic ultrasonography, which is generally the most helpful test, accurately depicts sphincter anatomy and reliably identifies sphincter defects. Some patients with fecal incontinence may have concomitant disorders such as impaired evacuation, pelvic prolapse, or urinary incontinence, urogynecologic evaluation should be performed when appropriate.

TREATMENT Rx

Mild incontinence is often treated successfully with dietary management, addition of a fiber supplement, and use of an antimotility agent such as loperamide 2 to 4 mg up to four times daily. Biofeedback is sometimes successful.A7

For individuals with sphincter disruption, surgical repair usually leads to substantial improvement (Fig. 145-5). Another alternative is sacral nerve stimulation, which is highly effective for fecal incontinence,A8 with about 40% of patients regaining continence and another 45% noting improvement at 36-months. A less invasive option that stimulates the posterior tibial nerve has shown encouraging early results.

For patients without a sphincter defect, sacral nerve stimulation is one option, but another option is transanal submucosal injection of dextranomer in stabilized hyaluronic acid.[6] These injections add bulk to the perianal tissues, thereby allowing the perianal tissues to coapt together. After two treatments of four injections at each, fecal incontinence decreases by about 50%, but many patients require repeat injections.[7] This treatment should not be used in patients who are immunosuppressed or who have had prior radiation therapy, rectal prolapse, or inflammatory bowel disease.

For patients with severe refractory incontinence, creation of a colostomy should be strongly considered. Initial reluctance notwithstanding, most patients regain control of their bowel function and report a substantially improved quality of life.

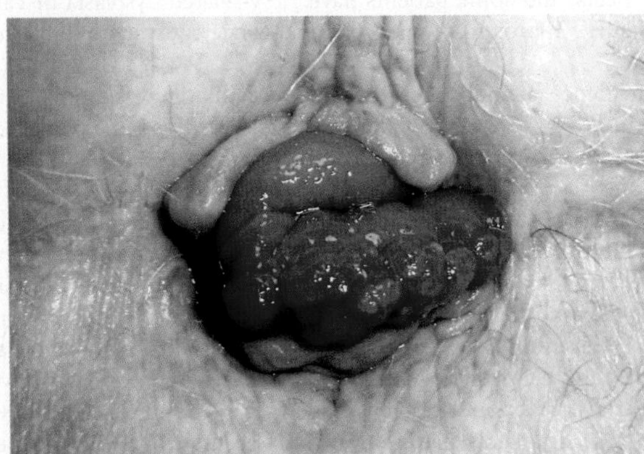

FIGURE 145-6. **Rectal mucosal prolapse. The main clinical manifestation of rectal prolapse is the protruding rectal mass.**

Rectal Prolapse

EPIDEMIOLOGY AND PATHOBIOLOGY

Rectal prolapse is a full-thickness protrusion of the rectum beyond the anal sphincter. It occurs in about 1% of adults older than age 65 years, and about 90% of cases are in women. Prolapse is caused by an internal rectal intussusception that eventually becomes more severe and protrudes externally. Risk factors include multiparity, a history of pelvic surgery, higher body mass index, chronic diarrhea or constipation, connective tissue disorders, and neurologic diseases. Uncorrected prolapse frequently leads to fecal incontinence by mechanically stretching the sphincter complex and causing a stretch injury to the pudendal nerves.

CLINICAL MANIFESTATIONS AND DIAGNOSIS

The main clinical manifestation of rectal prolapse is the protruding rectal mass (Fig. 145-6).[8] The protrusion most commonly occurs with bowel movements, but with time, it may occur with coughing or sneezing, and eventually it can occur spontaneously. Approximately 75% of patients have at least minor complaints of fecal incontinence, and complaints of "constipation," which are often caused by unsuccessful attempts to evacuate the intussuscepting rectum, occur in 15% to 65%. Other associated symptoms include chronic mucus discharge, pelvic discomfort, and minor bleeding. Patients can rarely present with an incarcerated or strangulated prolapse that mandates urgent intervention.

The diagnosis of rectal prolapse is confirmed on physical examination. Full-thickness prolapse, which is characterized by concentric mucosal folds, must be differentiated from circumferential mucosal prolapse, which is characterized by radial folds. The prolapse is often best demonstrated by having the patient strain on a commode. Ancillary studies do not routinely alter management, but colonoscopy may help exclude other pathology. Defecography is most helpful to diagnose internal rectal intussusception and associated pelvic floor abnormalities, such as rectocele and enterocele.

TREATMENT Rx

Nonoperative measures will not correct rectal prolapse, so conservative measures should be considered only in patients who have very minor and minimally symptomatic prolapse or who are poor surgical candidates. Surgical techniques use one or both of the basic principles of rectal prolapse repair: rectal fixation to the sacrum and resection or plication of redundant bowel. Both transabdominal (laparoscopic or open, with or without mesh) and transperineal approaches provide good outcomes, but the abdominal approach may be associated with lower long-term recurrence rates.

Human Papillomavirus

EPIDEMIOLOGY AND PATHOBIOLOGY

Human papillomavirus (HPV), which is the most common sexually transmitted infection, is a cause of anal dysplasia and cancer. The approximately 40 HPV subtypes that can cause anogenital infections are divided into low-risk types (e.g., types 6 and 11) that cause anal warts (condyloma acuminata) and high-risk types (e.g., types 16, 18, and 33) that can cause anal dysplasia and cancer. HPV infection is associated with cervical, vulvar, vaginal, and penile cancers, and some patients have HPV-related dysplasia or cancer in multiple sites. Approximately 90% of anal cancers are attributable to HPV infection.

The incidence of anal cancer has been steadily increasing, from 0.6 per 100,000 in 1973 to 1.0 per 100,000 in 2001. Over this same period of time, the female-to-male ratio decreased from 1.6 to 1 to 1.2 to 1. In the United States alone, an estimated 5000 or more individuals will develop anal cancer annually, and more than 700 will die from it. These epidemiologic trends have been attributed to a particularly rapid increase in anal cancers among men who have sex with men, especially men infected with HIV. Anal HPV, including the high-risk serotypes, is highly prevalent in at-risk populations (sex workers, intravenous drug users, transplant recipients, men who have sex with men, and HIV-positive men and women). Furthermore, anal dysplasia is common in at-risk populations, as evidenced by the 40% to 60% prevalence rate of high-grade anal dysplasia among HIV-positive men who have sex with men seen in specialty clinics in New York and San Francisco. Other associated risk factors for both dysplasia and anal cancer include a history of other HPV-related genital dysplasia or malignancy (cervical, vaginal or vulvar), prior sexually acquired diseases, anoreceptive intercourse, multiple sexual partners, and cigarette smoking.

ANAL WARTS

CLINICAL MANIFESTATION AND DIAGNOSIS

Anal warts can occur in the perianal skin and within the anal canal. The lesions are raised, epithelialized (when external), and narrow based. They can appear as scattered individual warts or as a confluent mass (Fig. 145-7).

TREATMENT Rx

External warts can be treated with topical podophyllin or imiquimod, but extensive warts usually require surgical excision or fulguration. Untreated warts can rarely progress to form Bushke-Löwenstein tumors—giant, locally invasive condyloma acuminata that frequently contain in situ or invasive cancer. Anal warts, especially in high-risk patients, have a high risk of recurrence and often require multiple treatments for eradication.

ANAL CANCER

CLINICAL MANIFESTATIONS AND DIAGNOSIS

The most common symptoms of anal cancer are bleeding, pain, and a palpable mass. The cancer may be seen externally as an ulcerated mass or may be palpated within the anal canal. Anal dysplastic lesions may appear as anal warts or as flat, pigmented lesions, or they may be invisible to the naked eye. They are best visualized using anal microscopy after topical application of 3% to 5% acetic acid (see later). Biopsy is necessary to make the diagnosis.

Thorough palpation of the inguinal lymph nodes is important to detect the presence of any clinically relevant adenopathy, but proper staging for anal canal malignancies requires a chest, abdominal, and pelvic CT scan. The size of the primary lesion should be measured, sometimes complemented by lower endoscopic ultrasonography or MRI to assess the size and depth of the lesion, as well as whether the sphincter is involved.[9]

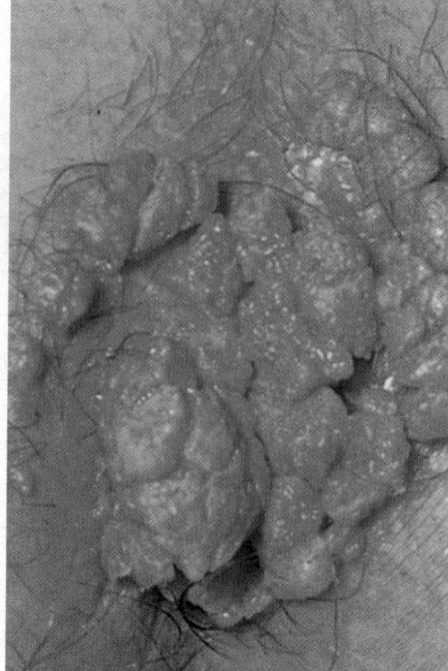

FIGURE 145-7. **Anal condyloma. These can occur as individual warts or as a confluent mass.**

The terminology of anal cancer is complex, but the great majority of tumors (including epidermoid, cloacogenic, and basaloid carcinomas) are variants of squamous cell carcinoma. The terminology of preinvasive squamous anal lesions is even more confusing because several terms exist for histologically identical pathology. The terms *anal dysplasia, anal intraepithelial neoplasia* (AIN), and *squamous intraepithelial lesion* (SIL) are used interchangeably. SILs are divided into low-grade and high-grade groups; AIN is similarly divided into AIN 1, 2, and 3, with AIN 2 and 3 being classified as high-grade lesions. Squamous cell carcinoma in situ corresponds to high-grade SIL and AIN 3; these terms are preferable to *Bowen disease*, which has historically been applied to this lesion. Other significant but less common anal cancers include adenocarcinoma, melanoma, and Paget disease.

Squamous cell carcinoma of the anus is divided into two groups based on tumor location: cancers of the anal margin (extending from the anal orifice for a distance up to 5 cm) and cancers of the anal canal. Tumors visible externally, but extending into the anal canal, are considered anal canal lesions.

TREATMENT Rx

Management of patients with anal dysplasia is controversial. Many authorities advocate a screening and treatment approach based on that used for cervical cancer, another HPV-associated disease. High-risk individuals are screened with anal Papanicolaou smears, and high-definition anal microscopy (analogous to colposcopy of the cervix) is performed when abnormal cytology is detected. Using this technique, dysplastic lesions can be identified and focally ablated or treated with topical imiquimod or 5-fluorouracil. Reported complete response rates vary significantly (≈30%-80%), and side effects (pain, irritation, and ulceration) may require withdrawal of therapy.[10] More extensive dysplasia requires microscopy-directed targeted ablation in the operating room.

Chemoradiotherapy is now standard first-line treatment for squamous cell cancer of the anal canal. Current radiation protocols most frequently use 45-Gy external beam radiation therapy in 25 fractions, with a boost to the primary tumor and involved inguinal nodes to a total dose of 54 to 59 Gy. Standard chemotherapy uses 5-fluorouracil (1000 mg/m^2 per 24 hours continuous infusion for 96 hours, starting on days 1 and 29) in combination with mitomycin C (most commonly 10 mg/m^2 intravenous bolus on days 1 and 29). Abdominoperineal resection with permanent colostomy is reserved for tumors that fail to respond to chemoradiation and those that recur. Similarly, groin dissection is performed only when involved inguinal nodes fail chemoradiation.

Early squamous cell cancers of the anal margin can be locally excised if a satisfactory margin can be obtained without injuring the anal sphincter and if there is no evidence of nodal spread. More advanced anal margin tumors are treated with chemoradiotherapy as described for anal canal tumors. Combined chemoradiation therapy is the primary treatment for most squamous cell carcinomas of the anal canal.

PREVENTION

In a randomized trial, use of an HPV vaccine reduced anal intraepithelial neoplasm by about 50% in men who have sex with men.[A9] Vaccination is warranted in all such individuals.

Other Sexually Transmitted Anorectal Diseases

A number of sexually transmitted diseases (Chapter 285) of the anorectum occur most frequently in individuals who practice anoreceptive intercourse. Common causative agents include *Treponema pallidum* (Chapter 319), *Neisseria gonorrhoeae* (Chapter 299), *Chlamydia trachomatis* (Chapter 318), herpes simplex (Chapter 374), and HIV (Chapter 384). Other sexually transmitted pathogens are *Shigella* (Chapter 309), *Campylobacter jejuni* (Chapter 303), *Haemophilus ducreyi* (Chapter 301), *Calymmatobacterium granulomatis* (Chapter 316), *Entamoeba histolytica* (Chapter 352), *Giardia lamblia* (Chapter 351), and *Isospora belli* (Chapter 353).

The widely variable presentations range from asymptomatic to anal pain, pruritus, discharge, fever, cramps, and bloody diarrhea. Clinical suspicion followed by appropriate and specific testing is necessary to make the correct diagnosis, and clinicians should consider the possibility of simultaneous infections. Treatment addresses the specific infection.

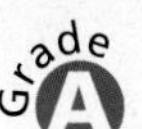

Grade A References

A1. Shanmugam V, Thaha MA, Rabindranath KS, et al. Rubber band ligation versus excisional haemorrhoidectomy for haemorrhoids. *Cochrane Database Syst Rev*. 2005;3:CD005034.

A2. Elmer SE, Nygren JO, Lenander CE. A randomized trial of transanal hemorrhoidal dearterialization with anopexy compared with open hemorrhoidectomy in the treatment of hemorrhoids. *Dis Colon Rectum*. 2013;56:484-490.

A3. Malik AI, Nelson RL, Tou S. Incision and drainage of perianal abscess with or without treatment of anal fistula. *Cochrane Database Syst Rev*. 2010;7:CD006827.

A4. Nelson RL, Thomas K, Morgan J, et al. Non surgical therapy for anal fissure. *Cochrane Database Syst Rev*. 2012;2:CD003431.

A5. Nelson RL, Chattopadhyay A, Brooks W, et al. Operative procedures for fissure in ano. *Cochrane Database Syst Rev*. 2011;11:CD002199.

A6. Brown CJ, Dubreuil D, Santoro L, et al. Lateral internal sphincterotomy is superior to topical nitroglycerin for healing chronic anal fissure and does not compromise long-term fecal continence: six-year follow-up of a multicenter, randomized, controlled trial. *Dis Colon Rectum*. 2007;50:442-448.

A7. Norton C, Cody JD. Biofeedback and/or sphincter exercises for the treatment of faecal incontinence in adults. *Cochrane Database Syst Rev*. 2012;7:CD002111.

A8. Ratto C, Litta F, Parello A, et al. Sacral nerve stimulation in faecal incontinence associated with an anal sphincter lesion: a systematic review. *Colorectal Dis*. 2012;14:e297-e304.

A9. Palefsky JM, Giuliano AR, Goldstone S, et al. HPV vaccine against anal HPV infection and anal intraepithelial neoplasia. *N Engl J Med*. 2011;365:1576-1585.

GENERAL REFERENCES

For the General References and other additional features, please visit Expert Consult at https://expertconsult.inkling.com.

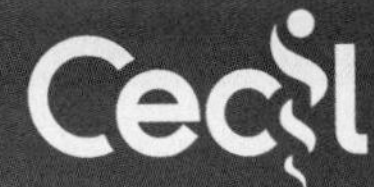

XIII

DISEASES OF THE LIVER, GALLBLADDER, AND BILE DUCTS

146

APPROACH TO THE PATIENT WITH LIVER DISEASE

PAUL MARTIN

The liver serves multiple key functions, including metabolism of the products of ingested food, production of amino acids to form proteins, detoxification of ingested drugs, conversion of nitrogenous substances from the gut into urea, formation of clotting factors, metabolism of bilirubin, processing of lipids absorbed from the intestine, and excretion of its products as bile. The liver also stores glycogen, which is a source of glucose, and helps contain infections by removing bacteria from the blood stream. These diverse functions reflect the activities of hepatocytes, bile duct cells called cholangiocytes, Kupffer cells, endothelial cells, and portal fibroblasts.

The liver has a dual blood supply: 70% delivered by the portal vein, which drains the intestine, and the remainder by the hepatic artery. After arrival in the liver, nutrient-rich portal blood passes along the hepatic sinusoids in close contact with lining hepatocytes before draining into the hepatic vein. The hepatocytes detoxify, metabolize, and synthesize the products of digestion. Bilirubin, which is produced by breakdown of red cells and other hemoproteins by reticuloendothelial cells predominantly in the liver and spleen, is transported to the hepatocytes, bound to albumin, and solubilized by them for biliary excretion.

Liver disease causes loss of hepatocellular activity, with diminished detoxification, excretory, and synthetic functions. Hepatocyte dysfunction results in impaired production of clotting factors, albumin, and other proteins, as well as reduced endogenous formation of lipids. Hepatocyte injury from a variety of causes, including viruses, alcohol, autoimmune disorders, and drug hepatotoxicity, is accompanied by leakage of cellular enzymes into the systemic circulation (Chapter 147). Coagulopathy, decreased serum albumin, and hyperbilirubinemia are observed in more profound hepatocellular injury. Portal hypertension occurs because of disruption of the low-pressure intrahepatic blood flow from the portal to the systemic venous circulation owing to hepatic fibrosis. Consequences of portal hypertension include accumulation of abdominal ascites and the development of portal-systemic venous collaterals with portal-systemic shunting, thereby resulting in the formation of varices and hepatic encephalopathy. Vascular disorders, including portal vein thrombosis, can result in portal hypertension in the absence of parenchymal liver disease.

The diversity of the liver's functions, its complicated blood supply, and its intimate relationship with the biliary tree contribute to the divergent manifestations of liver diseases. The initial complaint often reflects whether the cause is diffuse, such as acute viral hepatitis with widespread hepatocyte injury that manifests as malaise or fatigue, or whether the cause is discrete, such as when biliary obstruction from a gallstone in the common bile duct manifests with severe abdominal pain. Patients may present with multiple complaints, such as nausea and anorexia owing to hepatocellular disease accompanied by right upper quadrant discomfort due to stretching of the hepatic capsule by parenchymal cell edema and inflammation. Patients with more advanced liver disease, such as decompensated cirrhosis (Chapter 153), may have marked hepatocellular dysfunction with jaundice and coagulopathy in addition to portal hypertension with ascites and bleeding esophageal varices. Many patients who present with hepatic symptoms or signs may have extrahepatic disease; for example, a tender, enlarged liver may be caused by a systemic disorder, such as heart failure with hepatic congestion, rather than a primary hepatic disorder. In patients with cirrhosis, the initial presentation of previously unrecognized liver disease may be a major complication such as variceal hemorrhage, which in turn can precipitate hepatic encephalopathy and other features of frank hepatic decompensation.

HISTORY

Patients with liver disorders come to medical attention for a variety of reasons, ranging from the incidental discovery of abnormal liver chemistries to decompensated cirrhosis. Many complaints related to liver disease, such as fatigue, are nonspecific; unless liver disease is considered in the differential diagnosis, recognition of the hepatic origin of these complaints may be delayed.

In clinical practice, a frequent manifestation of asymptomatic liver disease is discovery of abnormal liver biochemistries during a life insurance application, annual physical examination, or attempt to donate blood.[1] It is important to inquire about occasions when liver biochemistries may have been obtained, to determine whether hepatic dysfunction is long-standing or more recent. In a patient with hepatic dysfunction, inquiry should be made about the presence of malaise, anorexia, fatigue, and weight change. Jaundice (Chapter 147) is a dramatic manifestation of possible liver disease. A patient may first notice lighter-colored stools or dark urine rather than scleral icterus. The absence of these latter changes suggests that unconjugated hyperbilirubinemia is due to hemolysis rather than intrinsic liver disease. Not infrequently, a patient may be unaware of jaundice until it is noted by others.

Abdominal pain (Chapter 132) related to liver disease can have a variety of causes. Symptomatic gallstones (Chapter 155) can manifest with the abrupt onset of severe epigastric or right upper quadrant discomfort, often after a large meal and frequently associated with nausea and vomiting. The pain is often steady rather than colicky and can radiate widely, including to the chest and back. A patient may not be able to achieve a position that lessens the pain, which may last several hours. More persistent pain, particularly if associated with weight loss and jaundice, raises concern about malignant bile duct obstruction. Pain is also common in parenchymal liver disease in the absence of biliary tract disease. Many patients with chronic hepatocellular disorders, such as chronic hepatitis C (Chapter 149) or nonalcoholic fatty liver disease (Chapter 152), complain of vague right upper quadrant discomfort that has no particular relieving or aggravating factors. Abdominal pain, which can be severe, is also frequent in acute viral hepatitis (Chapter 148), as well as with the hepatic congestion that results from back pressure in heart failure or hepatic vein occlusion, as in Budd-Chiari syndrome (Chapter 143).

Fatigue, anorexia, and malaise can be present in both acute and chronic liver disease. In acute liver disorders such as acute viral hepatitis (Chapter 148), drug-induced liver disease (Chapter 150), or an acute manifestation of autoimmune hepatitis (Chapter 149), patients may report profound fatigue, nausea, and malaise with decreased appetite and substantial associated weight loss. Distaste for cigarettes is said to be characteristic of acute viral hepatitis. Fatigue is also prominent in chronic liver disease such as chronic hepatitis C (Chapter 149). Pruritus is a prominent feature of cholestatic disorders, such as primary biliary cirrhosis, sclerosing cholangitis, or cholestatic drug reactions, particularly when patients are frankly icteric; however, pruritus also occurs in chronic parenchymal liver disease, most notably chronic hepatitis C, and in acute viral hepatitis. Easy bruisability in those with liver disease reflects coagulopathy and thrombocytopenia.

Fever in a patient with hepatic dysfunction is experienced in the prodrome of acute hepatitis A, as well as in alcoholic hepatitis and drug-induced liver disease. In a patient with suspected biliary obstruction, fever suggests complicating bacterial cholangitis or acute cholecystitis. Ascites is most frequently a manifestation of cirrhosis and portal hypertension in a patient with liver disease. Patients note increasing abdominal girth, which may be preceded by ankle edema. Weight gain owing to fluid retention may be masked by concomitant loss of muscle mass. The onset of ascites in the absence of a history of liver disease suggests a vascular event, such as hepatic vein occlusion (Chapter 143), or a nonhepatic cause of ascites, such as nephrotic syndrome or heart failure. Accumulation of ascites in a patient with liver disease may be subtle, with a slowly increasing waist circumference, or it may be more rapid, such as in a cirrhotic patient who receives fluid resuscitation after gastrointestinal bleeding. Although ascites in a patient with liver disease implies the presence of cirrhosis, ascites also can complicate severe acute liver disease, including alcoholic hepatitis and viral hepatitis, in which it suggests a poor prognosis.

Hepatic encephalopathy (Chapter 153), which is a neuropsychiatric disorder in patients with liver disease, can range from subtle cognitive impairment to deep coma. Early symptoms include a disturbed sleep pattern with nocturnal insomnia and daytime somnolence. More advanced encephalopathy can result in impairment of memory, confusion, and difficulty completing routine tasks. However, new-onset confusion or coma in a patient with liver disease should not be presumed to reflect hepatic encephalopathy unless other explanations, such as sedative overdose or subdural hematoma, have been excluded. Important precipitants of hepatic encephalopathy in a cirrhotic patient include gastrointestinal bleeding, bacterial infection (e.g., spontaneous bacterial peritonitis), electrolyte imbalance, and renal insufficiency, all of which need to be excluded during the initial clinical evaluation. In a patient with acute liver failure, coma as a consequence of cerebral edema may be impossible to distinguish from advanced hepatic encephalopathy unless the increased intracranial pressure results in papilledema.

Gastrointestinal hemorrhage resulting from bleeding varices is usually profuse and often abrupt in onset. It classically manifests with hematemesis or melena (Chapter 135), and coexisting postural hypotension and presyncope can reflect profound blood loss. The increased protein load in the gut can precipitate hepatic encephalopathy. Nonvariceal causes of gastrointestinal bleeding in a patient with liver disease include portal gastropathy (Chapter 135).

RISK FACTORS FOR LIVER DISEASE

An important aspect of the history is identification of possible risk factors for liver disease. The history should include directed questioning about alcohol consumption, including frequency and pattern (Chapter 33). The age of initial alcohol use and whether consumption has increased with age should be ascertained. Family members also should be asked about their perception of the patient's alcohol use and whether it has resulted in difficulties in personal relationships or work performance. Other clues to alcohol abuse are a history of convictions for driving under the influence of alcohol, motor vehicle accidents, and physical symptoms of alcohol dependence (Chapter 33). More circumspect questioning may be required to elicit a history of recreational drug use, especially given societal disapproval of this activity. Not infrequently, a patient with suspected viral hepatitis admits to smoking marijuana or snorting cocaine but does not acknowledge intravenous drug use. With the increasing frequency of nonalcoholic fatty liver disease as a cause of hepatic dysfunction (Chapter 152), comorbid conditions such as diabetes mellitus, hyperlipidemia, or weight gain should be noted.[2]

Medication use, whether prescription or over the counter, must be assessed because drug-induced liver disease is an important cause of apparently cryptogenic hepatic dysfunction and is not limited to therapeutic drugs (Chapter 150). Increasingly, herbal and "natural" products (Chapter 39) are ingested for a variety of maladies, and patients may fail to disclose their use because they do not perceive these agents to have side effects or may sense that the physician does not endorse their use.[3] As with alcohol, it is important to quantify the amount of medication ingested and over what period. The social history should include details about recent travel and contact with individuals with viral hepatitis through intimate, household, or occupational contact. It is also important to ask about vigorous physical activity that can result in elevated aminotransferase levels of nonhepatic origin.

ASSESSING DURATION OF LIVER DISEASE

The differential diagnosis in a patient with liver disease is determined to a large extent by manifesting symptoms, such jaundice or ascites. In many patients, however, the timing of more subtle findings such as elevated aminotransferases is difficult to determine. Prior blood test results should be retrieved to determine whether hepatic dysfunction is long-standing or more recent. Hepatic dysfunction of less than 6 months' duration is regarded as acute and is frequently self-limited, whereas abnormalities that persist for more than 6 months are unlikely to resolve spontaneously. If the patient has had a cholecystectomy, it is important to determine the indication. Incidental gallstones are sometimes assumed to be the cause of abnormal liver chemistries in a patient with parenchymal liver disease and can lead to an unnecessary operation. Thrombocytopenia owing to portal hypertension in a patient with unrecognized cirrhosis may have been investigated in the past without a firm conclusion being reached.

REVIEW OF OTHER ORGAN SYSTEMS

While focusing on liver-related symptoms, it is important not to overlook other diagnostic clues, associated disorders, and complications. Sicca symptoms, including dry eyes and mouth, are common in primary biliary cirrhosis (Chapter 155); florid features of scleroderma and CREST syndrome (Chapter 267) are other associations. Dyspnea in a patient with hepatic dysfunction may reflect cardiac failure with hepatic congestion (Chapter 58). Other explanations include hepatopulmonary syndrome (Chapter 153), with the characteristic complaint of platypnea–dyspnea (often with chest tightness) that is worse in the upright position owing to aggravation of the ventilation-perfusion mismatch because of intrapulmonary shunting. A hydrothorax in decompensated cirrhosis can cause dyspnea, as can emphysema in patients with liver disease caused by α_1-antitrypsin deficiency. A history of premature menopause is common in middle-aged women with cirrhosis, as is decreased libido and sexual potency in cirrhotic men. Arthralgias are often reported in viral hepatitis, and hemochromatosis (Chapter 212) may manifest with involvement of the proximal interphalangeal joints or chondrocalcinosis of the knees; increased skin pigmentation and diabetes mellitus are other features of this disorder. Accelerated osteopenia occurs in many liver diseases, including primary cirrhosis, primary sclerosing cholangitis, and alcoholic cirrhosis; osteopenia may be aggravated by corticosteroid use in autoimmune chronic active hepatitis. Alcoholic peripheral neuropathy (Chapter 416) can manifest with pain and paresthesia. Tremor and inattentiveness in a younger patient with hepatic dysfunction suggests Wilson disease (Chapter 211). Diarrhea and rectal bleeding in a patient with cholestatic liver disease suggests associated inflammatory bowel disease (Chapter 141).

FAMILY HISTORY

The family history should inquire not only about relatives with liver disease but also associated extrahepatic conditions. Hereditary hepatic conditions (see later), such as Wilson disease and hemochromatosis, may occur in several members of a sibship. In α_1-antitrypsin deficiency, some family members may experience predominantly emphysema rather than cirrhosis. Similarly, renal failure in a family member of a patient with hepatic cysts suggests adult polycystic disease (Chapter 127). A family history of inflammatory bowel disease may be a clue to primary sclerosing cholangitis in a patient with cholestatic liver chemistries. The history in patients with suspected alcoholic liver disease may reveal other family members with alcoholism.

PHYSICAL EXAMINATION

General Condition

In a patient with suspected liver disease, it is crucial to resist the temptation to palpate the abdomen immediately, thus potentially ignoring other important diagnostic clues. Apart from seeking icterus, the initial observation should note whether muscle wasting, cutaneous stigmata of liver disease, abdominal distention, and peripheral edema are present. The vital signs may reflect the hyperdynamic circulation characteristic of cirrhosis, with a resting tachycardia, wide pulse pressure, and low blood pressure resulting from peripheral vasodilation. Fetor hepaticus, which is described as a musty smell, may be detected when a cirrhotic patient exhales and must be distinguished from more frequent halitosis caused by poor dental hygiene.

Mucocutaneous Findings

Icterus (Fig. 146-1) is best confirmed by examination of the sclera or, if necessary, under the tongue, where elastin tissue retains bilirubin. Grayish skin discoloration in hemochromatosis may be most evident in the skin folds in the groin or axilla. Acanthosis nigricans can be observed in nonalcoholic fatty liver disease (Chapter 152). A Kayser-Fleischer ring (see Fig. 211-2), caused by the deposition of copper in Descemet membrane, is a brownish circle around the periphery of the iris and may require slit lamp examination to detect; it always should be sought in a patient with suspected Wilson disease (Chapter 211). Poor dentition is characteristic in alcoholic or drug-abusing individuals, and excessive dental caries may result from decreased saliva production in sicca syndrome. Parotid gland swelling is occasionally observed in alcoholic patients. Central cyanosis and clubbing are found in the hepatopulmonary syndrome. Temporal muscle wasting and "paper money" facial skin,

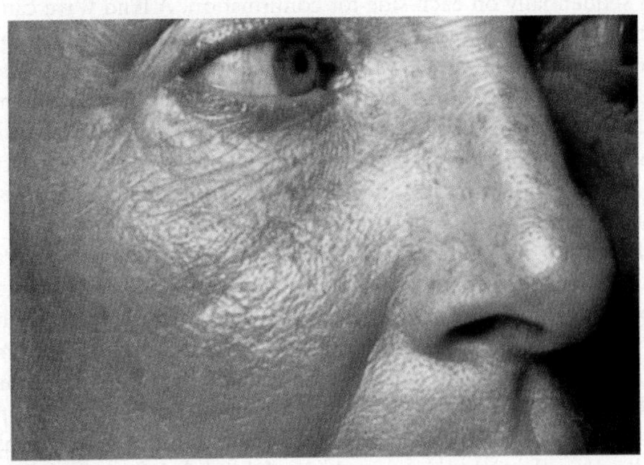

FIGURE 146-1. Scleral icterus.

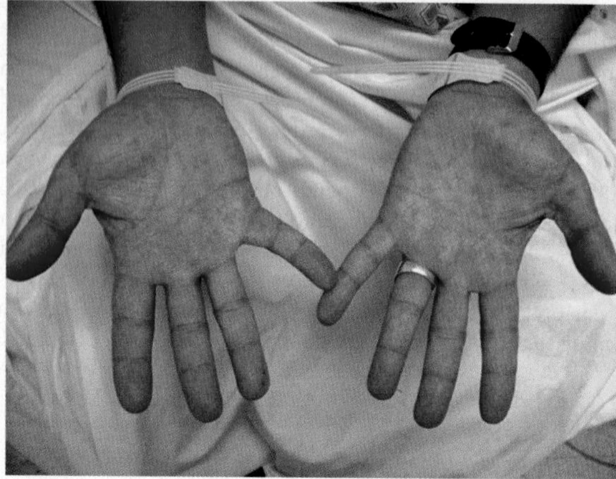

FIGURE 146-2. Palmar erythema.

owing to atrophy with telangiectasia, are signs of advanced liver disease. Xanthelasma from lipid deposits may be observed on the eyelids and skin around the orbits in patients with cholestatic liver disease. Spider nevi on the face and thorax are not pathognomonic of liver disease, especially in women, but they are suggestive if more than a few are present. Palmar erythema (Fig. 146-2) may be normal in women but suggests liver disease in men. Dupuytren contracture (see Fig. 152-1), the retraction of the palmar fascia with subsequent contracture of the palms and fingers can be a sign of alcoholic liver disease, although it is also described in patients with epilepsy or diabetes mellitus, as well as in individuals who have work-related contractures. Petechiae and ecchymoses reflect impaired production of clotting factors and hypersplenism in advanced liver disease. Patches of white discoloration on the nails may be present in advanced liver disease. Scratch marks from pruritus may be observed on the trunk and extremities of patients with cholestatic liver disease. Sparing of the center of the back can lead to a less pigmented butterfly-shaped area because patients cannot reach that area with their fingernails.

Examination of the Abdomen

Abdominal distention with ascites and dilation of collateral veins owing to portal hypertension represent florid signs of advanced liver disease. Caput medusae (Fig. 146-3) in the periumbilical area implies recanalization of the umbilical vein with portal hypertension.

Abdominal percussion may confirm the presence of ascites (Fig. 146-4). Shifting dullness results from movement of ascites to the most dependent portion of the abdomen. The subject should be examined in the supine position, with percussion of the abdomen from the midline toward the right or left flank. A change from a tympanic sound to a dull sound signifies a change from air to fluid, and the location of that change identifies the surface of the fluid pool. Next, the examiner should percuss below the point at which dullness is elicited and ask the subject to turn toward the examiner. With the subject on his or her side, the examiner percusses again at the same point where tympany converted to dullness. If that spot is now tympanic, shifting dullness has been detected as a result of movement of the air-fluid boundary; this finding supports the presence of ascites. This maneuver should be performed sequentially on each side for confirmation. A fluid wave can be felt by placing the medial border of one hand on the abdomen and tapping the right or left lateral abdominal walls; the resulting wave is felt by the first hand. Scrotal edema and abdominal wall hernias are often present in patients with long-standing ascites. Abdominal tenderness in a patient with ascites suggests peritonitis (e.g., spontaneous bacterial peritonitis or the result of a perforated viscus). However, it is important to note that abdominal tenderness is frequently absent in spontaneous bacterial peritonitis.

The liver is dull to percussion. Percussion of the right upper quadrant can determine the liver span, normally 6 to 12 cm in the midclavicular line. The liver span may be diminished in a patient with cirrhosis, whereas hepatomegaly (Fig. 146-5) is detected in hepatic congestion resulting from heart failure, nonalcoholic fatty liver disease, and cholestatic forms of cirrhosis. The liver is best examined with the patient in the supine position, arms parallel to the side of the body, and knees bent to relax the abdominal muscles. Palpation should begin in the right lower quadrant of the abdomen and move upward toward the rib cage so that the liver edge is felt on the way up. A normal liver

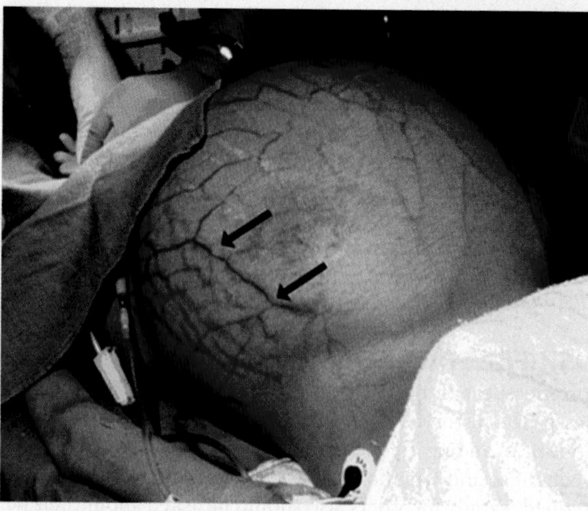

FIGURE 146-3. Caput medusae. Photograph shows caput medusae accentuated by a large amount of ascites in a patient being prepared for liver transplantation. An extensive plexus of veins is seen emanating from the umbilical region and radiating across the anterior abdominal wall. Note the large vein coursing inferiorly along the right flank (*arrows*). This is the superficial epigastric vein, which drains into the external iliac vein. (From Henseler KP, Pozniak MA, Le FT, et al. Three-dimensional CT angiography of spontaneous portosystemic shunts. *Radiographics.* 2001;21:691-704.)

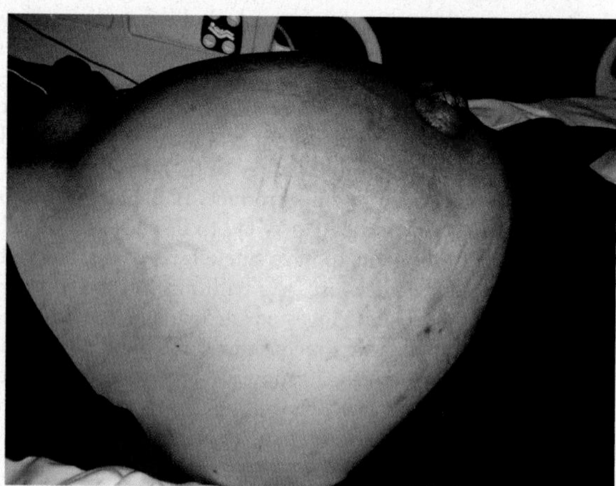

FIGURE 146-4. Ascites.

edge is smooth and sometimes slightly tender when palpated. In general, a liver edge that is felt up to 2 cm below the right costal margin is considered normal, but a normal-sized liver can be displaced downward by other abnormalities, such as emphysema. In thin subjects, the liver edge may be felt on deep inspiration, even if it is normal in size.

The liver can feel hard and irregular, as in cirrhosis, or slightly tender, enlarged, and smooth, as in acute viral hepatitis, alcoholic hepatitis, or hepatic congestion owing to congestive heart failure. The liver can extend across the midline, and the left lobe can be felt in the epigastrium. When the location of the edge of the liver is unclear, the scratch test may be helpful. The bell of the stethoscope is placed on the right upper quadrant over the rib cage while scratching the surface of the abdominal wall from the mid-abdomen toward the liver; the sound of the scratch is amplified in an area under which the liver lies.[4] In the presence of ascites, the liver edge may be detected by exerting quick pressure with the fingertips below the rib cage.

A palpable gallbladder suggests obstruction of the biliary system, whereas tenderness elicited by palpation during inspiration (the Murphy sign) suggests acute cholecystitis. Marked hepatic tenderness with hepatomegaly is observed in patients with a hepatic abscess (Chapter 151).

Splenomegaly (Chapter 168) is suggested by dullness to percussion between the 9th and 11th ribs in the left midaxillary line. A palpable spleen tip implies portal hypertension in a patient with chronic liver disease, although an enlarged spleen also can be detected in acute viral hepatitis and infiltrative disorders that involve both the liver and the spleen (see Table 168-7). Rectal examination is obligatory if gastrointestinal bleeding is suspected because of melena, anemia, or unexplained hepatic encephalopathy.

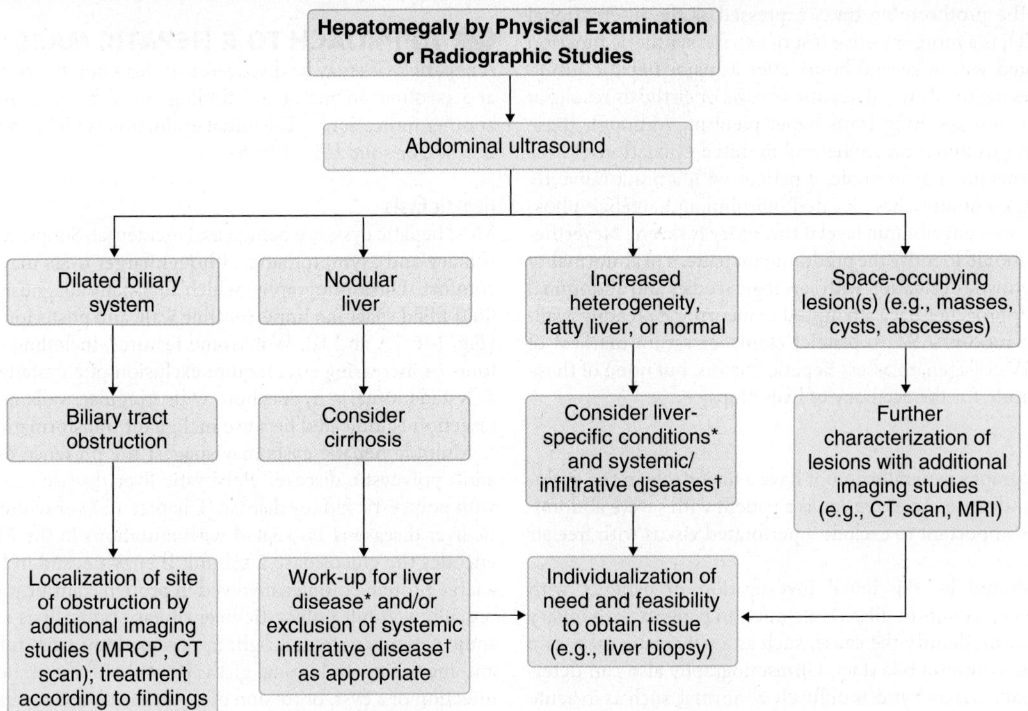

FIGURE 146-5. **Diagnostic approach to hepatomegaly. *Conditions to be excluded include viral hepatitis; alcohol- and drug-induced liver disease; steatohepatitis; autoimmune liver diseases; and metabolic disorders, including hemochromatosis, Wilson disease, and α_1-antitrypsin deficiency. †Systemic and infiltrative diseases include amyloidosis, lymphoma, sarcoidosis, and infectious processes such as disseminated tuberculosis and fungemia. CT = computed tomography; MRCP = magnetic resonance cholangiopancreatography; MRI = magnetic resonance imaging.**

TABLE 146-1 APPROACH TO COMMON HEPATIC COMPLAINTS

PRESENTATION	COMMON SYMPTOMS	COMMON PHYSICAL SIGNS	DIAGNOSTIC STUDIES	COMMON DIAGNOSES
Ascites	Abdominal distention and pain, ankle edema	Flank dullness Shifting dullness Fluid wave	Ultrasound with Doppler Diagnostic paracentesis Urinalysis	Cirrhosis Budd-Chiari syndrome Heart failure Nephrotic syndrome
Hepatic encephalopathy	Sleep disorientation, confusion, coma	Asterixis Altered mentation Fetor hepaticus	Serum ammonia Blood cultures Stool Hemoccult Serum creatinine and electrolytes	Decompensated cirrhosis Acute liver failure Other metabolic encephalopathies (renal, respiratory)
Hepatic mass	None or abdominal pain	Hepatic bruit or rub	α-Fetoprotein Ultrasound CT scan MRI Biopsy	Benign lesions: Hemangioma, adenoma, focal nodular hyperplasia Malignant lesions: Hepatocellular carcinoma, cholangiocarcinoma, metastases
Abdominal pain	Nausea, vomiting, fever	Right upper quadrant tenderness Palpable gallbladder Murphy sign	Ultrasound HIDA scan Paracentesis for ascites if present	Biliary colic Acute cholecystitis Hepatic congestion Hepatic metastases

CT = computed tomography; HIDA = hepatobiliary iminodiacetic acid; MRI = magnetic resonance imaging.

Complete Physical Examination

The presence of rales and elevation of the jugular venous pressure suggest heart failure or pericardial disease as a cause of hepatic congestion. Loss of secondary sexual characteristics in liver disease is reflected by a loss of axillary and pubic hair, as well as feminization of body habitus in a male patient. Testicular atrophy also may be present. Peripheral edema is common in decompensated cirrhosis and may occur before ascites is obvious.

Neuropsychiatric alterations can include subtle changes in personality or more overt hepatic encephalopathy. Constructional apraxia (e.g., inability to draw a five-pointed star or to write legibly) in a fully conscious patient is a typical finding in hepatic encephalopathy. Asterixis, which is characterized by a series of extensor and flexor wrist movements,[5] can be elicited by having the patient extend the arms, with dorsiflexion of the wrists, while separating the fingers for at least 15 seconds. Tremors (Chapter 410) are nonspecific but are also common in advanced cirrhosis.

DIAGNOSTIC STUDIES (TABLE 146-1)

Laboratory Studies

The initial evaluation of liver disease involves a battery of blood tests, which can assess hepatic necroinflammation (serum aminotransferases), cholestatic biliary tract dysfunction (alkaline phosphatase, γ-glutamyl transpeptidase), excretory function (bilirubin), and synthetic function (coagulation factors, albumin) (Chapter 147). In hepatocellular dysfunction caused by viral hepatitis (Chapter 148), aminotransferase levels are elevated, with the serum alanine aminotransferase (ALT) level higher than the aspartate aminotransferase (AST) level. In alcoholic hepatitis (Chapter 152), AST elevation exceeds that of ALT. In patients with biliary obstruction or cholestatic liver diseases (Chapter 155), such as primary biliary cirrhosis or a cholestatic drug reaction, bilirubin and generally alkaline phosphatase levels are elevated. Impairment of synthetic function leads to a decreased serum albumin level over days to weeks. The prothrombin time, expressed as the international normalized ratio (INR), is a more sensitive test of hepatic synthetic function and becomes prolonged within several hours after a major hepatic insult. Portal hypertension owing to advanced hepatic fibrosis or cirrhosis results in a decreased platelet count resulting from hypersplenism. Although these general patterns of liver dysfunction are helpful in initial evaluation of liver disease, they are nonspecific. For example, a patient with a predominantly hepatocellular process commonly has elevated bilirubin and alkaline phosphatase levels and a low serum albumin level if the injury is severe. Nevertheless, these blood tests should identify the predominant pattern of abnormality and direct further diagnostic evaluation with serologic studies and abdominal imaging. A variety of approaches have attempted to incorporate readily available tests, such as the ratio of AST to platelet count, or serum markers of fibrosis, such as type IV collagen, to assess hepatic fibrosis, but none of these alternatives can substitute for the accuracy of liver biopsy.

Abdominal Imaging

Plain abdominal radiographs generally do not have a major role in the evaluation of suspected liver disease. An exception is a patient with severe abdominal pain, in whom it is important to exclude a perforated viscus with free air under the diaphragm.

Ultrasonography should be the initial investigation in patients with obstructive jaundice. It can confirm dilated bile ducts in patients with biliary obstruction and often can identify the cause, such as a pancreatic mass or a gallstone lodged in the common bile duct. Ultrasonography also can determine whether the hepatic parenchyma is diffusely abnormal, such as in acute viral hepatitis; it can identify bright hepatic echo texture in nonalcoholic fatty liver disease or a coarsened echo texture in cirrhosis. In addition to confirming the presence of ascites, ultrasonography can identify other signs of portal hypertension, such as splenomegaly or intra-abdominal varices. A Doppler flow study can evaluate blood flow through the portal and hepatic vessels. An ultrasound study can identify hepatic masses and distinguish a cystic mass from a solid lesion (see later). Computed tomography (CT) and magnetic resonance imaging (MRI) add greater detail to the assessment of the hepatic vasculature, hepatic masses, and hepatic vascular structures. MRI can obtain a detailed cholangiogram, thereby avoiding a more invasive endoscopic retrograde cholangiopancreatography in many patients with suspected bile duct obstruction or disease (Chapters 133 and 134). Liver elastrography assesses hepatic fibrosis by measuring liver stiffness by propagation of waves in liver tissue. Generally liver stiffness correlates with fibrosis. *Fibroscan,* which uses high-frequency shear waves, can predict the amount of fibrosis in most patients, but it is less accurate in patients with a high body mass index or extensive steatosis.[6]

Liver Biopsy

Liver biopsy remains the definitive test to assess the severity of hepatic inflammation and fibrosis extent in diffuse hepatocellular disease. In addition, it can confirm certain diagnoses suspected by noninvasive testing, such as autoimmune hepatitis, or it can suggest other diagnoses, such as drug hepatotoxicity. However, because of its potential complications, such as intra-abdominal bleeding, biopsy is recommended only when less invasive testing does not yield a definitive diagnosis or prognosis or when additional information, such as quantitative determination of hepatic copper in Wilson disease or hepatic iron in hemochromatosis, is necessary for definitive diagnosis (see later).

Transjugular pressure measurements are indicated in patients with atypical presentations of portal hypertension (e.g., when it is unclear whether liver disease is the cause) or to titrate medications to reduce portal pressure. A catheter is advanced under fluoroscopy into the hepatic vein, and the free hepatic venous pressure is measured. The catheter is then advanced further until it becomes "wedged" in a small hepatic vein venule. A small balloon occludes the venule, and the wedged hepatic vein pressure, which reflects hepatic sinusoidal pressure, is obtained. The portal pressure gradient, which is derived by subtracting the free pressure measurement from the wedged pressure measurement, is normally less than 5 mm Hg. Varices form at a gradient greater than 10 mm Hg, whereas ascites and variceal hemorrhage occur only when the gradient greater than 12 mm Hg. A transjugular approach also increases the safety of liver biopsy in the presence of ascites, coagulopathy, or thrombocytopenia when standard percutaneous liver biopsy is hazardous. Endoscopy is indicated to screen for varices in any patient suspected of having cirrhosis to determine the need for prophylaxis against hemorrhage.

APPROACH TO A HEPATIC MASS

A hepatic mass may be discovered under a number of different circumstances and is often an incidental finding on abdominal imaging performed for another indication.[7,8] The initial evaluation is directed as to whether the mass is cystic or solid (Fig. 146-6).

Hepatic Cysts

Most hepatic cysts are benign and incidental. Simple hepatic cysts are usually solitary and asymptomatic, although larger cysts may cause abdominal discomfort. Ultrasonography, which is usually diagnostic, shows an anechoic fluid-filled space, an imperceptible wall, and posterior acoustic enhancement (Fig. 146-7A and B). Worrisome features, including the presence of symptoms or increasing size, require exclusion of a cystadenoma. On ultrasound a cystadenoma is hypoechoic with irregular walls and septations. Hepatic resection is indicated because malignant transformation can occur.

Multiple hepatic cysts may suggest the presence of autosomal dominant adult polycystic disease.[9] Polycystic liver disease can occur in conjunction with polycystic kidney disease (Chapter 127) or without it. Isolated polycystic liver disease is associated with mutations in the *PRCKSCH* gene, which encodes the glucosidase 2 subunit β enzyme, and in Sec63, which is part of a large protein complex involved in protein translocation in the endoplasmic reticulum. Adult polycystic liver disease typically is symptomatic, although some patients note dull right upper quadrant pain, fullness, sense of a mass, and increasing abdominal girth. Rupture of a cyst, hemorrhage into a cyst, infection of a cyst, or torsion of a cyst may cause severe pain. Physical examination may include hepatomegaly, cachexia due to weight loss, and ascites. As cysts increase in number and size with age, they may become palpable. On ultrasound, multiple fluid-filled cysts are present without internal echoes unless bleeding or infection has occurred. Interventions indicated for symptoms include aspiration or resection. Polycystic liver disease usually does not result in clinical hepatic impairment, and prognosis depends on the severity of any concurrent polycystic renal disease. In some cases, however, large, symptomatic, or bleeding cysts may raise the consideration of liver transplantation, often with combined kidney transplantation (Chapter 131) for associated renal cysts and failure.

Caroli disease, which is a rare congenital abnormality with cystic dilatation of the intrahepatic biliary tree, can be associated with cholangitis and biliary stones. Many patients ultimately develop cholangiocarcinoma (Chapter 155). Magnetic resonance cholangiopancreatography demonstrates intrahepatic dilatations with normal ducts in between and a normal common bile duct. Endoscopic treatment is indicated for cholangitis, although resection or liver transplantation may ultimately be required.

Solid Hepatic Mass

Most solid hepatic masses are asymptomatic, but some patients may have vague right upper quadrant discomfort. The abrupt onset of more severe pain suggests a complication, such as hemorrhage or rupture. The approach to a solid hepatic mass (Fig. 146-8) is influenced by the presence or absence of underlying chronic liver disease, such as chronic viral hepatitis, as well whether an extraheptic malignancy with possible hepatic metastases is a concern. If chronic liver disease is present, a solid mass must be assumed to represent primary hepatocellular carcinoma (Chapter 196) until proved otherwise. By comparison, a solid lesion in the absence of underlying liver disease is more likely to be benign and incidental. Benign hepatic adenomas are commonly discovered in young to middle-aged women and are not associated with hepatic dysfunction. With modern contrast studies, it is usually possible to make a confident radiologic diagnosis about the nature of a solid hepatic mass. Important examples include the initial peripheral filling and retention of contrast dye by a hemangioma (see Fig. 146-8A, B, and C), the rapid arterial filling of a hepatocellular carcinoma with subsequent "washout" of contrast during the portal venous phase (see Fig. 196-5), or the central scar typical of focal nodular hyperplasia (see Fig. 146-8D), although biopsy is indicated if it is not possible to exclude malignancy.

Hepatic hemangiomas are the most common benign solid hepatic mass. On ultrasound, the lesion is hyperechoic. It has a typical hypervascular appearance on contrast CT or MRI. Generally, no intervention is required unless there is a clear association with abdominal symptoms, increasing size, or a complication such as rupture.

Hepatic adenomas (Chapter 196) are benign epithelial hepatic tumors associated with use of oral contraceptives with a higher estrogen content. On ultrasound, adenomas are hyperechoic, reflective of their fat content,

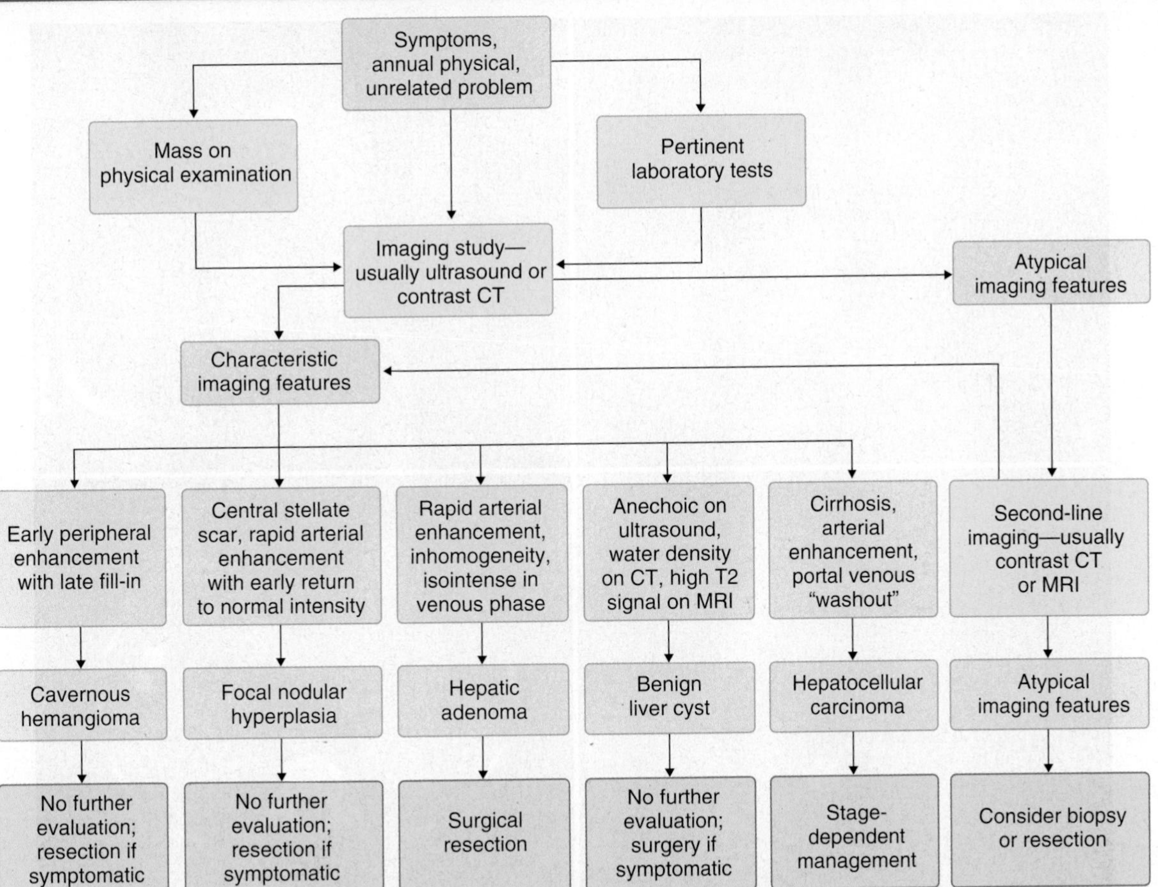

FIGURE 146-6. Approach to evaluating the patient with a mass lesion in the liver. Flow chart showing an algorithm for evaluating and managing common liver mass lesions. CT = computed tomography; MRI = magnetic resonance imaging. (From Roberts LR. Liver and biliary tract tumors. In: Goldman L, Schafer AI, eds. *Goldman's Cecil Medicine*, 24th ed. Philadelphia: Saunders; 2012.)

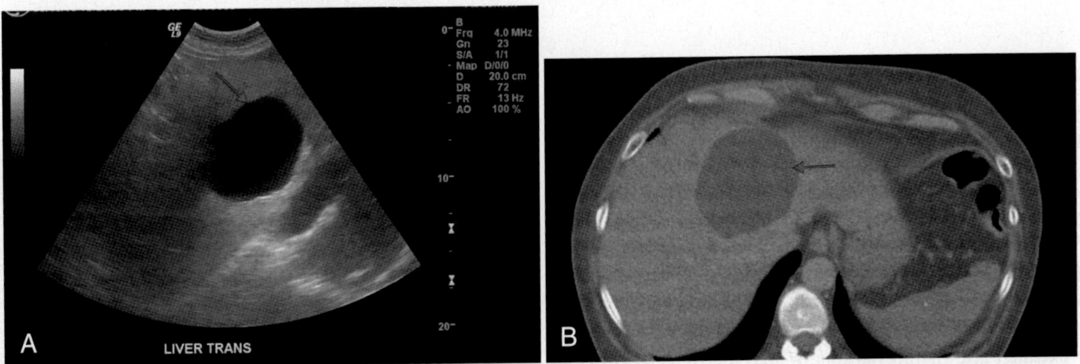

FIGURE 146-7. Simple hepatic cyst. A, Ultrasound demonstrates clear contents and an imperceptible wall (*arrow*). B, On a computed tomographic scan, a simple hepatic cyst is characterized by the lack of septation and an imperceptible wall (*arrow*). (Courtesy Dr. B. Madrazo.)

but become anechoic if hemorrhage has occurred. Contrast CT and MRI show arterial enhancement and varying signal intensity reflecting steatosis and hemorrhage if present. Biopsy may be needed for diagnosis. Potential complications of adenomas, especially if greater than 5 cm, include spontaneous hemorrhage and rupture, as well as rare malignant transformation. Discontinuation of oral contraceptives may lead to a decrease in size. Prophylactic hepatic resection is indicated for adenomas greater than 5 cm.

Focal nodular hyperplasia, which is a benign lesion characterized by a central scar and is thought to represent a hyperplastic response due to a vascular malformation. Identification of the scar by ultrasound, CT, or MRI is diagnostic (see Fig. 146-8D). Observation in the absence of symptoms is advised.

Nodular regenerative hyperplasia is characterized by multiple regenerative 1- to 3-mm nodules clustered around portal triads. It is associated with a variety of systemic disorders, predominantly autoimmune, including rheumatoid arthritis, systemic lupus erythematosus, and polymyalgia rheumatica, neoplastic such as myeloproliferative syndromes, and medications including thiopurines. Symptoms, if present, reflect associated portal hypertension. Diagnosis is by biopsy, which shows hypertrophied hepatocytes clustered around the center of the nodules with peripheral atrophy. Management is directed to the associated portal hypertension (Chapter 153).

Hepatocellular carcinoma (Chapter 196) is a frequent complication of cirrhosis of any cause as well as chronic hepatitis B infection even in the absence of cirrhosis. Patients usually will have evidence of cirrhosis with hepatic dysfunction. Because surveillance for hepatocellular carcinoma is now recommended in individuals at risk, this tumor is increasingly identified when asymptomatic and potentially curable.[10] On ultrasound, hepatocellular carcinoma appears solid. Owing to its predominantly arterial blood supply compared with that of normal hepatic parenchyma, intravenous contrast is

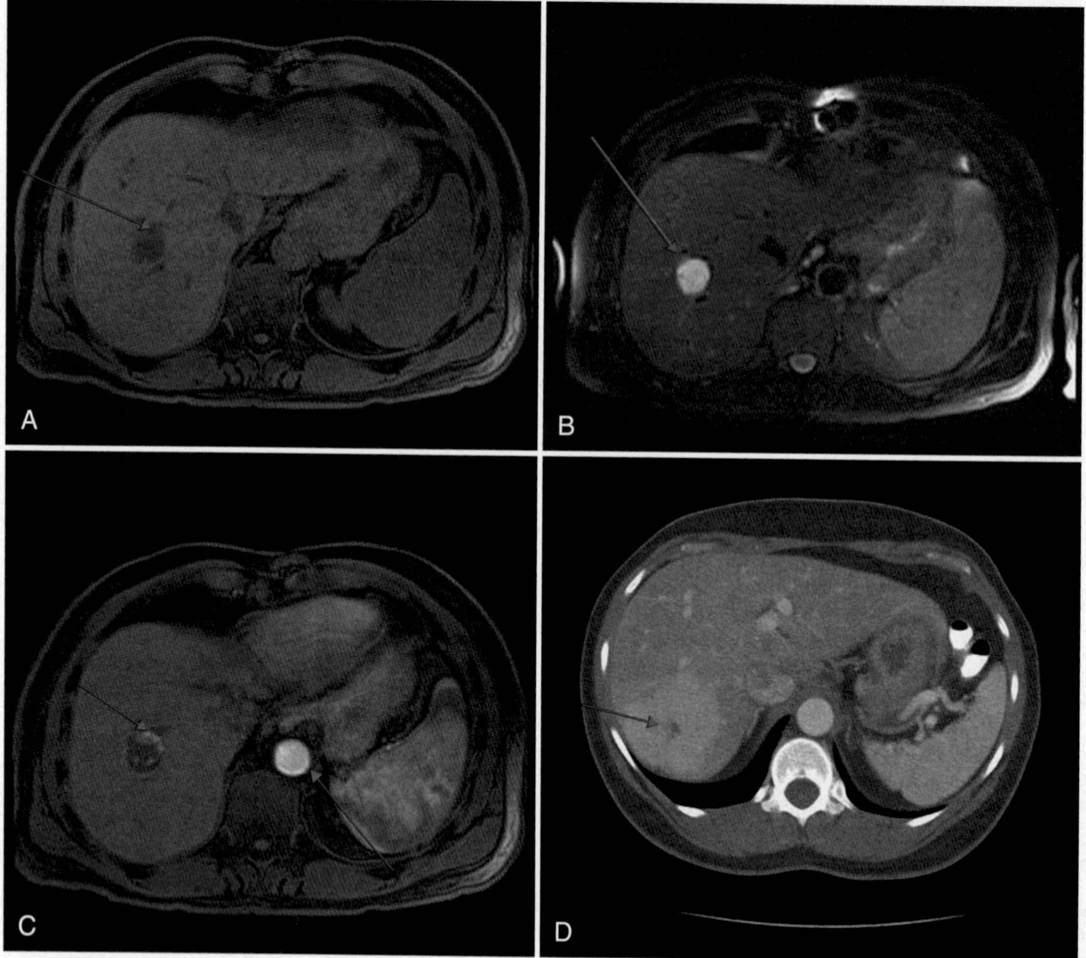

FIGURE 146-8. **Solid hepatic mass. A,** Hemangioma seen as a solid mass (*arrow*) on the T1 phase of a magnetic resonance (MR) imaging scan. **B,** Hemangioma on MR T2 image is characterized by a high signal density (*arrow*). **C,** A hemangioma fills slowly (*arrow*) from the periphery after intravenous contrast is administered (*arrow*). **D,** Focal nodular hyperplasia is characterized by a central scar (*arrow*) in the late venous phase of a contrast computed tomographic scan. (Courtesy Dr. B. Madrazo.)

rapidly taken up by a hepatic cellular carcinoma and then "washes out" on CT scan or MR imaging (see Fig. 196-5). Serum α-fetoprotein is elevated in approximately 60% of cases. Therapeutic options depend on the tumor's size and severity of associated liver disease.

APPROACH TO THE PATIENT WITH INHERITED LIVER DISEASE

The major inherited liver diseases in adults are hemochromatosis, Wilson disease, cystic fibrosis, and α_1-antitrypsin deficiency. These disorders may be suspected by their extrahepatic manifestations or may be detected during evaluation of unexplained hepatic dysfunction.

Hereditary hemochromatosis (Chapter 212), which is the most common inherited liver disorder, is most frequently due to mutations in the *HFE* gene (located on chromosome 6p22.2), typically at C282Y and H63D. Approximately 1 in 250 individuals of Northern European descent are homozygous for C282Y, the major *HFE* mutation, although only a minority develop phenotypic manifestations.[11] Liver blood test abnormalities, if present, are nonspecific. Definitive diagnosis is confirmed by detection of C282Y homozygote or compound heterozygote (C282Y/H63D). MRI or CT scan can confirm excessive hepatic iron. Liver biopsy is unnecessary for diagnosis but is advised for a serum ferritin greater than 1000 μg/L because the patient is likely to be cirrhotic. Iron accumulates in hepatocytes but not Kupffer cells in a periportal to pericentral gradient (Fig. 146-9). By comparison, secondary iron overload accumulates in Kupffer cells in conditions such as ineffective erythropoiesis. Quantitative iron measurement in liver tissue, calculated as the μmol of iron/g dry weight liver/age, can confirm the diagnosis. Treatment of hemochromatosis is by phlebotomy (Chapter 212).

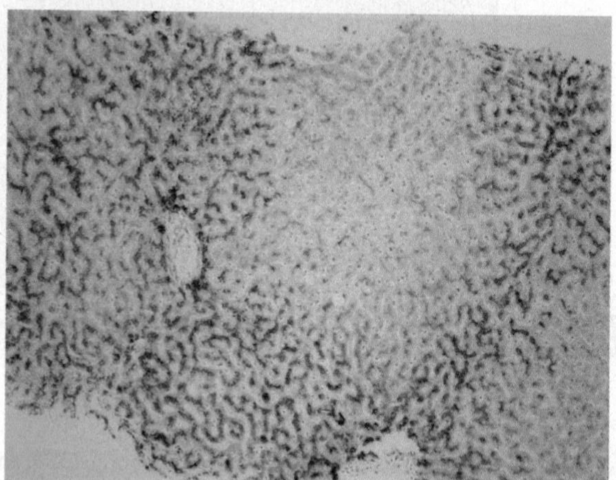

FIGURE 146-9. **Liver biopsy in hemochromatosis (Perls Prussian blue stain for iron).** Iron deposition is found in a periportal distribution, predominantly in parenchymal cells (hepatocytes). (From Bacon BR. Inherited and metabolic disorders of the liver. In: Goldman L, Schafer AI, eds. *Goldman's Cecil Medicine*, 24th ed. Philadelphia: Saunders; 2012.

α_1-Antitrypsin deficiency, which results from inherited mutations in this serine protease inhibitor, prevents its export from hepatocytes, where its accumulation causes liver inflammation, fibrosis, and cirrhosis. Deficiency of circulating α_1-antitrypsin results in panlobular emphysema (Chapter 88) even in nonsmokers. The disease is most frequent in persons of European ancestry. Inheritance is autosomal recessive with codominant inheritance because each allele provides 50% of circulating α_1-antitrypsin. A large number of alleles have been identified in the proteinase inhibitor (Pi) gene,

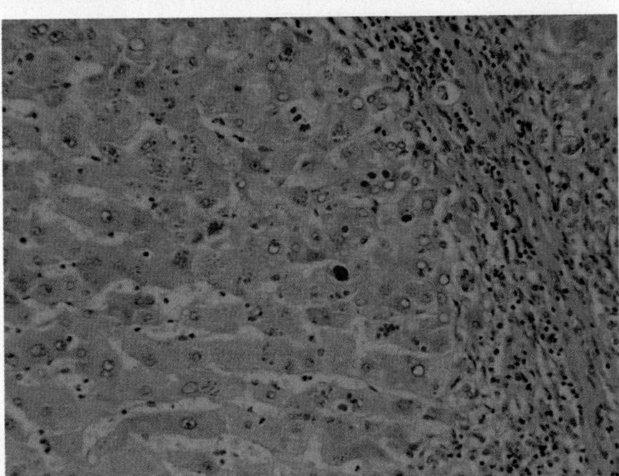

FIGURE 146-10. Liver biopsy in α_1-antitrypsin deficiency. On a periodic acid–Schiff, diastase-resistant stain, α_1-antitrypsin globules, with a characteristic magenta color, are found at the periphery of the lobule. (From Bacon BR. Inherited and metabolic disorders of the liver. In: Goldman L, Schafer AI, eds. *Goldman's Cecil Medicine*, 24th ed. Philadelphia: Saunders; 2012.)

with MM associated with normal circulating α_1-antitrypsin levels and the most common abnormal alleles, S and Z, associated with reduced levels. PiZZ homozygotes, who have the most severe α_1-antitrypsin deficiency, have only 15% of normal circulating levels and are prone to liver and lung disease. Liver disease has a bimodal distribution, with neonatal hepatitis and cholestatic jaundice manifesting in early life and cirrhosis in adulthood. Only approximately one third of adults with the PiZZ phenotype develop cirrhosis, thereby implying that other cofactors are involved in disease progression.[12] Other phenotypes with α_1-antitrypsin deficiency (e.g., PiMZ or PiSZ) increase the risk for liver disease, whereas null variants have lung but not liver disease. The condition may be suspected by a low α_1-1 globulin level on a routine protein electrophoresis, and the diagnosis can be confirmed by demonstration of a low serum α_1-antitrypsin level followed by Pi testing to determine the phenotype. Liver function tests are generally nonspecific, although the albumin level can be low and the INR prolonged if cirrhosis is present. Liver biopsy, which shows the extent of fibrosis, is characterized by periodic acid–Schiff (PAS)-positive, diastase-resistant globules in the periphery of the lobule (Fig. 146-10). No specific therapy is available for the liver disease, although weekly intravenous α_1-antitrypsin protein concentrate infusions, which are approved by the U.S. Food and Drug Administration, might prevent progression of lung disease by restoring serum and alveolar α_1-antitrypsin levels.

Wilson disease (Chapter 211) is excessive copper accumulation in liver and extrahepatic tissues owing to an inherited disorder in copper transport from hepatocytes to bile.[13] Hepatic manifestations include chronic hepatitis and cirrhosis, most typically appearing by the fourth decade of life, although they can manifest later. A characteristic finding in a fulminant manifestation of Wilson disease is hemolysis with an abnormally low alkaline phosphatase level, jaundice, and coagulopathy. More typically, patients have elevated aminotransferase levels without hemolysis at presentation. Diagnosis usually is based on an elevated 24-hour urinary copper level and low serum ceruloplasmin levels, but in unclear cases the quantification of increased hepatic copper content by biopsy is definitive. Copper chelation prevents disease progression.

Cystic fibrosis (Chapter 89) is usually dominated by pulmonary complications, but liver disease is an important cause of morbidity and mortality in adults.[14] In patients with elevated alkaline phosphatase and bilirubin levels, biliary cirrhosis (Chapter 155) can develop owing to abnormal bile viscosity. Ursodeoxycholic acid may improve biochemical test results but has no clear benefit on outcome. Liver transplantation (Chapter 154) may be necessary for decompensated cirrhosis.

GENERAL REFERENCES

For the General References and other additional features, please visit Expert Consult at https://expertconsult.inkling.com.

147

APPROACH TO THE PATIENT WITH JAUNDICE OR ABNORMAL LIVER TESTS

PAUL D. BERK AND KEVIN M. KORENBLAT

JAUNDICE AND HYPERBILIRUBINEMIA

DEFINITION

Jaundice, from the French *jaune* ("yellow"), is the yellow-orange discoloration of the skin, conjunctivae, and mucous membranes that results from an elevated plasma bilirubin level. Mild hyperbilirubinemia may be clinically undetectable, but jaundice becomes evident at plasma bilirubin greater than 3 to 4 mg/dL, depending on the patient's normal skin pigmentation, the conditions of observation, and the bilirubin fraction that is elevated. Hyperbilirubinemia may result from hepatocellular dysfunction (pure hyperbilirubinemia) or from either increased bilirubin production or inherited or acquired defects in specific aspects of hepatic bilirubin disposition.

PATHOBIOLOGY

Bilirubin Metabolism

Bilirubin Production

Bilirubin is the degradation product of the heme moiety of hemoproteins, a class of proteins involved in the transport or metabolism of oxygen (Fig. 147-1). Normal adults produce approximately 4 mg of bilirubin per kilogram of body weight per day. Between 70 and 90% of bilirubin is derived from the hemoglobin of erythrocytes, which are sequestered and destroyed by the mononuclear phagocytic cells of the reticuloendothelial system, principally in the spleen, liver, and bone marrow. The remainder results primarily from the turnover of nonhemoglobin hemoproteins such as myoglobin, the P-450 cytochromes, catalase, and peroxidase, principally in the liver; a minor fraction reflects ineffective erythropoiesis, which is the premature destruction of newly formed erythrocytes within the bone marrow. Although bilirubin production occurs principally in the liver, bilirubin has proved to have antioxidant properties, and recent studies suggest that a limited, regulated production of bilirubin from heme may occur in many cell types and contribute to regulating the intracellular antioxidant environment.[1]

The two-step conversion of heme to bilirubin begins with the opening of the heme molecule at its α bridge carbon by the microsomal enzyme *heme oxygenase,* a process that results in the formation of equimolar quantities of carbon monoxide and the green tetrapyrrole biliverdin. This nontoxic, water-soluble pigment is the main excretory product of heme in birds, reptiles, and amphibians. However, biliverdin cannot cross the placenta. Accordingly, its reduction to bilirubin in mammals by a second enzyme, *biliverdin reductase,* allows its transplacental removal from the fetus into the maternal circulation. The unconjugated bilirubin produced in the periphery is transported to the liver in plasma. Because of its insolubility in aqueous media, it is kept in solution by tight but reversible binding to albumin. A number of compounds, including sulfonamides, furosemide, and radiographic contrast agents, can competitively displace bilirubin from its binding sites on albumin, a phenomenon that is of little clinical significance except in neonates, in whom the resulting increased concentration of unbound bilirubin raises the risk for kernicterus.

Disposition of Bilirubin by the Liver

Excretion of bilirubin from the body is a major function of the liver (see Fig. 147-1), where the specialized microanatomy enhances the extraction of tightly protein-bound compounds from the circulation. Hepatic translocation of bilirubin from blood to bile involves four distinct steps: (1) uptake of unconjugated bilirubin, principally by an incompletely characterized facilitated transport process and to a lesser extent by diffusion; (2) intracellular binding, mainly to various cytosolic proteins of the glutathione-*S*-transferase family; (3) conversion of unconjugated bilirubin to bilirubin monoglucuronides and diglucuronides by a specific uridine 5′-diphosphoglucuronosyltransferase (UDP-glucuronosyltransferase) isoform designated UGT1A1, encoded by the *UGT1* gene complex; and (4) transfer of bilirubin monoglucuronides and diglucuronides into bile by a canalicular membrane

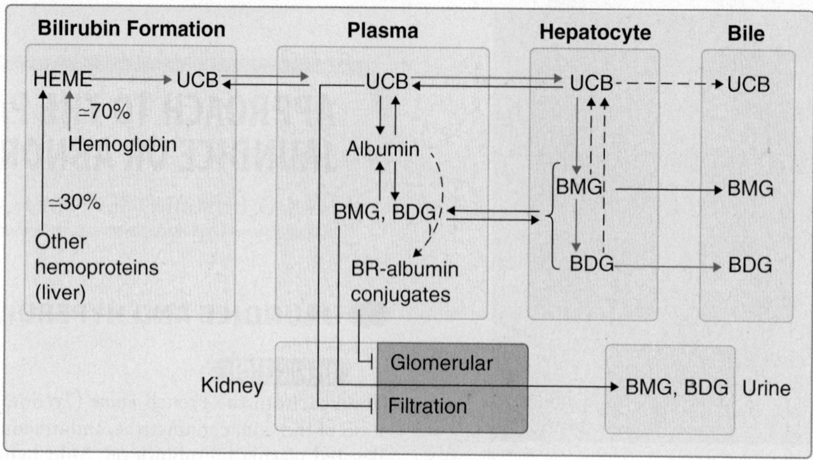

FIGURE 147-1. **Overview of bilirubin metabolism.** Unconjugated bilirubin (UCB) formed from the breakdown of heme from hemoglobin and other hemoproteins is transported in plasma reversibly bound to albumin and is converted in the liver to bilirubin monoglucuronide (BMG) and diglucuronide (BDG), the latter being the predominant form secreted in bile. BMG and BDG together normally account for less than 5% of normal serum bilirubin. In patients with hepatobiliary disease, BMG and BDG accumulate in plasma and appear in urine. Bilirubin glucuronides in plasma also react nonenzymatically with albumin and possibly other serum proteins to form protein conjugates, which do not appear in urine and have a plasma half-life similar to that of albumin. BR = bilirubin.

adenosine triphosphate (ATP)-dependent transporter designated multidrug resistance–associated protein 2 (MRP2) or canalicular multispecific organic anion transporter (cMOAT). MRP2/cMOAT is encoded by the gene *ABCC2,* a member of ATP-binding cassette (ABC) transporter superfamily of genes. ABC genes transport molecules across intracellular and extracellular membranes. The superfamily is divided into seven subfamilies. MRP2/cMOAT belongs to the MRP family, whose substrates include drug conjugates and unmodified anticancer drugs, which are pumped out of cells.

Conjugation of unconjugated bilirubin to bilirubin monoglucuronides and diglucuronides is a critical process that greatly increases the aqueous solubility of bilirubin, thereby enhancing its elimination from the body while simultaneously reducing its ability to diffuse across biologic membranes, including the blood-brain barrier. In newborn infants, a decreased capacity to conjugate bilirubin leads to unconjugated hyperbilirubinemia (physiologic jaundice of the newborn). If severe, this hyperbilirubinemia may lead to irreversible central nervous system toxicity. Phototherapy by exposure to blue light converts bilirubin to water-soluble photoisomers that are readily excreted in bile, thereby protecting the central nervous system from bilirubin toxicity. Gilbert syndrome and Crigler-Najjar syndrome types 1 and 2, which result from genetic defects in bilirubin conjugation, are characterized by unconjugated hyperbilirubinemia; by contrast, Dubin-Johnson syndrome, which results from inheritable defects in MRP2/cMOAT (see later), is characterized by conjugated or mixed hyperbilirubinemia. The recent discovery of the causative mutations in Rotor syndrome, which is also characterized by conjugated or mixed hyperbilirubinemia, has led to the finding of an additional step in bilirubin transport, characterized by the export of intracellular bilirubin conjugates across the sinusoidal membrane and their subsequent reuptake by transporters in downstream hepatocytes. The process, which is also involved in the disposition of drug metabolites, is believed to prevent the local saturation of upstream hepatocytes with bilirubin and drug conjugates.[2]

Enterohepatic Circulation and Excretion of Bilirubin

Normal human bile contains an average of less than 5% unconjugated bilirubin, 7% bilirubin monoconjugates, and 90% bilirubin diconjugates. Following canalicular secretion, conjugated bilirubin passes down the gastrointestinal tract without reabsorption by either the gallbladder or intestinal mucosa. Although some bilirubin reaches the feces, most is converted to urobilinogen and to related compounds by bacteria within the ileum and colon, where the urobilinogen is reabsorbed, returns to the liver through the portal circulation, and is re-excreted into bile in a process of enterohepatic recirculation. Any urobilinogen not taken up by the liver reaches the systemic circulation, from which it is cleared by the kidneys. Normal urine urobilinogen excretion is 4 mg/day or less. With hemolysis, which increases the load of bilirubin entering the gut and therefore the amount of urobilinogen formed and reabsorbed, or with liver disease, which decreases its hepatic extraction, plasma urobilinogen levels rise and more urobilinogen is excreted in the urine. Severe cholestasis, bile duct obstruction, or antibiotics that reduce or eliminate the bacterial conversion of bilirubin to urobilinogen markedly decrease the formation and urinary excretion of urobilinogen.

Unconjugated bilirubin ordinarily does not reach the gut except in neonates or, by ill-defined alternative pathways, in the presence of severe unconjugated hyperbilirubinemia (e.g., Crigler-Najjar type 1). In these circumstances, unconjugated bilirubin is reabsorbed from the gut, thereby amplifying the hyperbilirubinemia.

Measurement of Bilirubin in Plasma

The total plasma bilirubin concentration in normal adults is less than 1 to 1.5 mg/dL, depending on the measurement method. Modern analytic techniques show that normal plasma contains principally unconjugated bilirubin, with only a trace of conjugated bilirubin. Clinical laboratories typically quantify plasma bilirubin by a reaction in which bilirubin is cleaved by a diazo reagent, such as diazotized sulfanilic acid, to azodipyrroles that are readily quantitated spectrophotometrically. Bilirubin conjugates react rapidly ("prompt" or "direct"-reacting bilirubin). Unconjugated bilirubin reacts slowly because the site of attack by the diazo reagent is protected by internal hydrogen bonding. Accordingly, accurate measurement of the total plasma bilirubin concentration requires addition of an accelerator, such as ethanol or urea, to disrupt this internal hydrogen bonding and to ensure complete reaction of any unconjugated bilirubin.

The "indirect"-reacting bilirubin is calculated by subtracting the direct-reacting bilirubin from the total. Although physicians traditionally equate the direct-reacting fraction of bilirubin in plasma with conjugated bilirubin and the indirect fraction with unconjugated bilirubin, this approach is, at best, a rough approximation. The unqualified interpretation of direct and indirect fractions as reflecting conjugated and unconjugated bilirubin, respectively, may lead to diagnostic errors, particularly in the diagnosis of hereditary hyperbilirubinemias. In common practice, 10 to 20% of the bilirubin in normal plasma gives a prompt (direct) diazo reaction even though more than 95% of total bilirubin in normal plasma is unconjugated. Thus, at virtually any total bilirubin concentration, a direct-reacting fraction of less than 15% of the total bilirubin can be considered as essentially all unconjugated. When the direct-reacting fraction is greater than 15%, a simple dipstick test for bilirubinuria may clarify the situation. Unconjugated bilirubin is not excreted in urine regardless of the height of its plasma concentration because its binding to albumin is too tight for effective glomerular filtration and it is not secreted by the tubules. The canalicular transport mechanism for excretion of bilirubin conjugates is especially sensitive to injury. Accordingly, in parenchymal liver disease or mechanical bile duct obstruction, bilirubin conjugates within the hepatocyte or biliary tract may reflux into the blood stream, resulting in a mixed or, less often, a purely conjugated hyperbilirubinemia. Conjugated bilirubin, which is normally loosely bound to albumin, is readily filtered at the glomerulus; even modest degrees of conjugated hyperbilirubinemia result in bilirubinuria, which is *always* a pathologic finding. With prolonged conjugated hyperbilirubinemia, some of the conjugated bilirubin binds *covalently* to albumin and produces what is designated the δ-bilirubin fraction. Although δ-bilirubin gives a direct diazo reaction, it is not filterable by the glomerulus and does not appear in the urine; it disappears slowly from the plasma, with the 14- to 21-day half-life of the albumin to which it is bound. δ-Bilirubin can account for the slow rate at which conjugated (direct) hyperbilirubinemia sometimes resolves as hepatitis improves or biliary obstruction is relieved. Although δ-bilirubin is not easily measured, its presence can be inferred when an elevated direct-reacting bilirubin persists after bilirubinuria resolves.

Transcutaneous bilirubinometry is an alternative method for measuring bilirubin in infants with neonatal jaundice. The method is based on the measurement of the light reflected from the percutaneous transmission of visible light and is conceptually analogous to pulse oximetry.[3]

Bilirubin Kinetics

The plasma unconjugated bilirubin concentration ([UCB]) is determined by a balance between the bilirubin production rate (BRP) and hepatic bilirubin clearance (C_{BR}) according to the relationship:

$$[UCB] \approx BRP/C_{BR}$$

C_{BR} is analogous to the creatinine clearance test of kidney function; it is a measure of the rate at which bilirubin is extracted from plasma, and it is a true quantitative test of liver function. Whereas BRP and C_{BR} are not easily quantified clinically, investigative measurements have yielded useful pathophysiologic insights. This equation indicates that [UCB] is directly proportional with increases in BRP and inversely proportional with CBR, thereby providing a basis for classifying unconjugated hyperbilirubinemias according to their pathogenesis.

Increased Bilirubin Production

An increased production of bilirubin and a resulting unconjugated hyperbilirubinemia can be caused by hemolysis, an accelerated destruction of transfused erythrocytes, resorption of hematomas, or ineffective erythropoiesis owing to lead poisoning, megaloblastic anemias related to deficiency of either folic acid or vitamin B_{12}, sideroblastic anemia, congenital erythropoietic porphyria, or myeloproliferative or myelodysplastic diseases. In these settings, other liver tests are typically normal and the hyperbilirubinemia is modest, rarely exceeding 4 mg/dL; higher values imply concomitant hepatic dysfunction. However, after brisk blood transfusion or resorption of massive hematomas caused by trauma, the increased bilirubin load may be transiently sufficient to lead to frank jaundice. The causes of hemolysis are numerous (Chapters 160 to 163). Besides specific blood disorders, mild hemolysis accompanies many acquired diseases. In the setting of systemic disease, which may include a degree of hepatic dysfunction, hemolysis may produce a component of conjugated hyperbilirubinemia in addition to an elevated unconjugated bilirubin concentration. Prolonged hemolysis may lead to the formation of bilirubin gallstones, which may cause biliary tract disease (Chapter 155).

Decreased Hepatic Bilirubin Clearance

Decreased Bilirubin Uptake

Kinetic studies suggest that hepatocellular bilirubin uptake involves both facilitated and diffusive components. Several drugs (e.g., rifampin, novobiocin, and various cholecystographic contrast agents) competitively inhibit the hepatocellular uptake of bilirubin, thereby suggesting the existence of a component of facilitated uptake. Decreased hepatic bilirubin uptake is also believed to contribute to the unconjugated hyperbilirubinemia of Gilbert syndrome, although the principal molecular basis for that syndrome is a reduction in bilirubin conjugation. The identity of the bilirubin transporter remains controversial.

Impaired Bilirubin Conjugation

The most frequent cause of decreased bilirubin clearance is a decrease in bilirubin conjugating activity. Bilirubin conjugation with glucuronic acid is catalyzed principally by a specific UDP-glucuronosyltransferase, which is designated UGT1A1 and encoded by the *UGT1* gene complex. The *UGT1A1* gene is assembled by alternative splicing of a bilirubin-specific variant of exon 1, designated exon A_1, with four common exons (exons 2 to 5) that encode the shared carboxyl terminal end of all *UGT1*-encoded proteins. Its promoter region normally contains an $A(TA)_6TAA$ TATA box–like construct.

APPROACH TO THE PATIENT WITH HYPERBILIRUBINEMIA

Hyperbilirubinemia and jaundice (see Fig. 146-1) may result from isolated disorders of bilirubin metabolism, liver disease, or obstruction of the biliary tract. Jaundice represents the most visible sign of hepatobiliary disease of many causes (Table 147-1).

Genetic Disorders of Bilirubin Conjugation

The hereditary hyperbilirubinemias (Table 147-2) are a group of five syndromes in which hyperbilirubinemia occurs as an isolated biochemical abnormality, without evidence of either hepatocellular necrosis or cholestasis.[4]

CRIGLER-NAJJAR AND GILBERT SYNDROMES

Crigler-Najjar syndrome types 1 and 2 and Gilbert syndrome are hereditary forms of unconjugated hyperbilirubinemia that have been known for more than two decades to result principally from mutations in *UGT1A1*. In Crigler-Najjar type 1, essentially no functional enzyme activity is present, whereas patients with Crigler-Najjar type 2 have up to 10% of normal and patients with Gilbert syndrome have 10 to 33% of normal activity, leading to bilirubin concentrations of 18 to 45, 6 to 25, and 1.5 to 4 mg/dL, respectively (see Table 147-2). Because total UGT1A1 enzymatic activity must be reduced to less than 50% of normal to produce unconjugated hyperbilirubinemia, phenotypic expression of mutations in this enzyme requires either homozygosity or double heterozygosity, and each of these disorders is inherited as an autosomal recessive trait. Patients with Crigler-Najjar types 1 and 2 are either homozygotes or double heterozygotes for structural mutations within the coding region. In Western countries, patients with Gilbert syndrome are typically homozygous for an $A(TA)_7TAA$ promoter mutation; this polymorphism is designated *UGT1A1*28*. Structural mutations in exon 1 of UGT1A1 causing modest reductions in UGT1A1 enzymatic activity have been reported in some Japanese patients with Gilbert syndrome. To date, 130 different mutations in *UGT1A1* associated with hereditary hyperbilirubinemia have been identified, including 59 linked to Crigler-Najjar type 1 and 48 to Crigler-Najjar type 2.[5] Recent studies have identified mutations of multiple additional regions of *UGT1A* and also of the solute carrier protein SCLO1B1, both of which participate to varying degrees in the defective glucuronidation capacity of these three syndromes.[6] The resulting complex genotypes may pose a risk not only for hyperbilirubinemia but also for susceptibility to glucuronidation-associated drug toxicity and, perhaps, for subtle diverse benefits as well.[7]

Crigler-Najjar Syndrome Type 1

Crigler-Najjar type 1 is characterized by striking unconjugated hyperbilirubinemia that appears in the neonatal period, persists for life, and is unresponsive to phenobarbital. The majority of patients (type 1A) exhibit defects in the glucuronide conjugation of a spectrum of substrates in addition to bilirubin as the result of mutations in one of the common exons (2 to 5) of the *UGT1* complex. In a smaller subset (type 1B), a mutation in the bilirubin-specific exon A1 limits the defect to bilirubin conjugation. Fifty-nine structurally diverse *UGT1A1* mutations can cause Crigler-Najjar type 1; their common feature is they all encode proteins with absent or, at most, traces of enzymatic activity. Before the availability of phototherapy, most patients with Crigler-Najjar type 1 died of bilirubin encephalopathy (kernicterus) in infancy or early childhood.[8] Optimal treatment for a neurologically intact patient includes (1) approximately 12 hours/day of phototherapy from birth throughout childhood, perhaps supplemented by exchange transfusion in the neonatal period; (2) use of tin-protoporphyrin to blunt transient episodes of increased hyperbilirubinemia; and (3) early liver transplantation, before the onset of brain damage.[9] Plasmapheresis has been used to temporarily control abrupt increases in bilirubin[10] and transplantation with isolated allogeneic hepatocytes has been evaluated as an experimental therapeutic approach.

Crigler-Najjar Syndrome Type 2

Bilirubin concentrations are typically lower in Crigler-Najjar type 2, and plasma bilirubin levels can be reduced to 3 to 5 mg/dL by phenobarbital. At least 48 different mutations of *UGT1A1* have been associated with Crigler-Najjar type 2; all encode a bilirubin-UDP-glucuronosyltransferase with markedly reduced but detectable enzymatic activity. Although uncommon in Crigler-Najjar type 2, kernicterus has occurred at all ages, typically associated with factors that temporarily raise the plasma bilirubin concentration above baseline (e.g., fasting, intercurrent illness). For this reason, phenobarbital therapy is often recommended; a single bedtime dose usually maintains clinically safe plasma bilirubin concentrations.

Gilbert Syndrome

Gilbert syndrome is the most common form of the hereditary hyperbilirubinemias, with a genotypic prevalence of approximately 12% and a

TABLE 147-1 DIFFERENTIAL DIAGNOSIS OF HYPERBILIRUBINEMIA AND JAUNDICE

ISOLATED DISORDERS OF BILIRUBIN METABOLISM

Unconjugated Hyperbilirubinemia
- Increased bilirubin production
  - *Examples:* Hemolysis, ineffective erythropoiesis, blood transfusion, resorption of hematomas
- Decreased hepatocellular uptake
  - *Examples:* Drugs (e.g., rifampin)
- Decreased conjugation
  - *Examples:* Gilbert and Crigler-Najjar syndromes, physiologic jaundice of the newborn, breast milk jaundice, HIV protease inhibitors

Conjugated or Mixed Hyperbilirubinemia
- Decreased canalicular transport: Dubin-Johnson syndrome
- Decreased reuptake of bilirubin conjugates: Rotor syndrome

LIVER DISEASE

Acute or Chronic Hepatocellular Dysfunction
- Acute or subacute hepatocellular injury
  - *Examples:* Viral hepatitis A, B, C, E; hepatotoxins (e.g., ethanol, acetaminophen, mushroom *[Amanita phalloides]* poisoning); drugs (e.g., isoniazid, α-methyldopa), metabolic diseases (e.g., Wilson disease, Reye syndrome); pregnancy-related (e.g., acute fatty liver of pregnancy, HELLP); hepatic ischemia (e.g., hypotension, postoperative, hepatic artery thrombosis)
- Chronic hepatocellular disease
  - *Examples:* Hepatitis B, B + D, C, and E; hepatotoxins (e.g., vinyl chloride, vitamin A), nonalcoholic and alcoholic fatty liver disease; autoimmune hepatitis; metabolic disease (Wilson disease, hemochromatosis, α_1-antitrypsin deficiency)

Hepatic Disorders with Prominent Cholestasis
- Familial cholestatic disorders
- Single gene disorders
  - *Examples:* Benign recurrent intrahepatic cholestasis types 1-3; progressive familial intrahepatic cholestasis types 1-3
- Familial cholestatic disorders of unknown pathogenesis
  - *Examples:* Aagenaes syndrome, Navajo neurohepatopathy, North American Indian cholestasis
- Diffuse infiltrative disorders
  - *Examples:* Granulomatous diseases (e.g., mycobacterial and fungal infections, sarcoidosis, lymphoma, drugs), amyloidosis, infiltrative malignancies
- Inflammation of intrahepatic bile ductules and/or portal tracts
  - *Examples:* Primary biliary cirrhosis, liver allograft rejection, graft-versus-host disease, drugs (e.g., chlorpromazine, erythromycin)
- Miscellaneous conditions
  - *Examples:* Uncommon presentations of viral or alcoholic hepatitis, intrahepatic cholestasis of pregnancy, contraceptive jaundice, estrogens, anabolic steroids, postoperative cholestasis, cholestasis of sepsis, total parenteral nutrition, bacterial infections, drugs

OBSTRUCTION OF THE BILE DUCTS

Choledocholithiasis
- *Examples:* Cholesterol gallstones, pigment gallstones

Diseases of the Bile Ducts
- Inflammation, infection
  - *Examples:* Primary sclerosing cholangitis, AIDS cholangiopathy, hepatic arterial chemotherapy, postsurgical strictures
- Neoplasms (e.g., cholangiocarcinoma)

Extrinsic Compression of the Biliary Tree
- Neoplasms
  - *Examples:* Pancreatic carcinoma, metastatic lymphadenopathy, hepatoma
- Pancreatitis with or without pseudocyst formation
- Vascular enlargement (e.g., aneurysm, cavernous transformation of portal vein)

AIDS = acquired immunodeficiency syndrome; HELLP = hemolysis, elevated liver enzymes, and low platelets; HIV = human immunodeficiency syndrome.

phenotypic prevalence of approximately 7% in whites. Its high prevalence may explain the frequency of mild unconjugated hyperbilirubinemia in liver transplant recipients. Plasma bilirubin concentrations are most often less than 3 mg/dL, although both higher and lower values are frequent, with increases of two-fold to three-fold commonly occurring with fasting and intercurrent illness. The phenotypic distinction between mild Gilbert syndrome and a normal state is often blurred. Phenobarbital's ability to induce hepatic enzyme activity normalizes both the bilirubin concentration and C_{BR}. Oxidative drug metabolism and the disposition of many, but not all, xenobiotics that are metabolized by glucuronidation appear to be normal in Gilbert syndrome. A critical exception is the antitumor agent irinotecan (CPT-11), whose active metabolite (SN-38) is glucuronidated specifically by UGT1A1. In patients with Gilbert syndrome, CPT-11 can cause intractable diarrhea, myelosuppression, and other serious toxicities. Significant adverse events have not been described when individuals with Gilbert syndrome are prescribed many other agents that are metabolized by glucuronidation. Although Gilbert syndrome has no association with disease, occasional reports have demonstrated an association of the *UGT1A1*28* allele with decreased risk for cardiovascular and specific neoplastic diseases, an association that has been attributed to the vasodilatory and antioxidant effects of bilirubin and heme oxygenase.

UNCONJUGATED HYPERBILIRUBIN IN THE NEWBORN PERIOD

Most neonates develop mild unconjugated hyperbilirubinemia between days 2 and 5 after birth because of hepatic immaturity and low UGT1A1 levels. Peak bilirubin levels are typically less than 5 to 10 mg/dL, and levels return to normal within 2 weeks as mechanisms fostering bilirubin disposition mature. Prematurity, with hemolysis, is associated with higher bilirubin levels that may require phototherapy. The progestational steroid 3α,20β-pregnanediol and certain fatty acids that are found in breast milk (but not serum) of some mothers inhibit bilirubin conjugation and can cause excessive neonatal hyperbilirubinemia *(breast milk jaundice).* By comparison, a UGT1A1 inhibitor, which is found in maternal serum, causes *transient familial neonatal hyperbilirubinemia* (Lucey-Driscoll syndrome).

CONJUGATED OR MIXED HYPERBILIRUBINEMIA

Two phenotypically similar but mechanistically distinct inherited disorders, Dubin-Johnson syndrome and Rotor syndrome, are characterized by conjugated or mixed hyperbilirubinemia with normal values for other standard liver tests (see Table 147-2). Dubin-Johnson syndrome results from any of several mutations in the gene encoding the ATP-dependent canalicular organic anion transporter MPR2/cMOAT (see Fig. 147-1). Individuals with Rotor syndrome exhibit the simultaneous disruption of two genes that code for the organic anion transporting polypeptides OATP1B1 and OATP1B3, which mediate the reuptake by downstream hepatocytes of conjugated bilirubin secreted into the sinusoid via the sinusoidal efflux transporter ABCC3 in more upstream hepatocytes.[11] Despite the conjugated hyperbilirubinemia, patients with Rotor syndrome are not cholestatic and can be distinguished noninvasively both from normal subjects and persons with Dubin-Johnson syndrome by their two-fold to five-fold increase in total copropophryin

TABLE 147-2 PRINCIPAL FEATURES OF THE HEREDITARY DISORDERS OF BILIRUBIN METABOLISM

FEATURE	CRIGLER-NAJJAR SYNDROME *Type I*	CRIGLER-NAJJAR SYNDROME *Type II*	GILBERT SYNDROME	DUBIN-JOHNSON SYNDROME	ROTOR SYNDROME
Incidence	Very rare	Uncommon	Up to 12% of population	Uncommon	Rare
Total serum bilirubin (mg/dL)	18-45 (usually >20), unconjugated	6-25 (usually ≤20), unconjugated	Typically ≤4 in absence of fasting or overt hemolysis; mostly unconjugated	Typically 2-5, less often ≤25; approximately 60% direct reacting	Usually 3-7, occasionally ≤20; approximately 60% direct reacting
Defect(s) in bilirubin metabolism*	Bilirubin UGT1A1 conjugating activity markedly reduced: trace to absent	Bilirubin UGT1A1 conjugating activity reduced: ≤10% of normal.	Complex haplotype Bilirubin UGT1A1 conjugating activity typically reduced to 10-33% of normal; reduced bilirubin uptake in some cases; mild hemolysis in up to 50% of patients	Impaired canalicular secretion of conjugated bilirubin owing to MRP2/cMOAT mutation	Impaired hepatic secretion or storage of conjugated bilirubin owing to impaired reuptake of bilirubin conjugates resulting from simultaneous OATP1B1 and OATP1B3 mutations.
Routine liver tests	Normal	Normal	Normal	Normal	Normal
Serum bile acids	Normal	Normal	Normal	Usually normal	Normal
Plasma sulfobromophthalein removal (% retention of 5 mg/kg dose at 45 min)†	Normal	Normal	Usually normal (<5%); mild 45-min (<15%) retention in some patients	Slow initial decline in plasma concentration (retention ≤20% at 45 min) with secondary rise at 90-120 min	Very slow initial decline in plasma concentration (45-min retention = 30-45%) without secondary rise
Oral cholecystography	Normal	Normal	Normal	Faint or non-visualization of gallbladder	Usually normal
Pharmacologic responses/special features	No response to phenobarbital	Phenobarbital reduces bilirubin by ≤75%	Phenobarbital reduces bilirubin, often to normal	Increased bilirubin concentration with estrogens; diagnostic urine coproporphyrin isomer pattern (total is normal, with isomer I increased to ≥80% of total)	Characteristic urine coproporphyrin excretion pattern (total is increased ≤2.5-fold in ~65% of cases but isomer I always <80% of total)
Major clinical features	Kernicterus in infancy if untreated; may occur later despite therapy	Rare late-onset kernicterus with fasting	None	Occasional hepatosplenomegaly	None
Hepatic morphology/histology	Normal	Normal	Normal; occasionally increased lipofucin pigment	Liver grossly black; coarse, dark centrilobular pigment	Normal
Bile bilirubin fractions‡	>90% unconjugated	Largest fraction (mean 57%) monoconjugates	Mainly diconjugates but monoconjugates are increased (mean 23%)	Mixed conjugates, reported increase in diconjugates	Increased conjugates
Inheritance (all autosomal)	Recessive	Recessive	Promoter mutation is recessive; missense mutation often dominant	Recessive; rare kindred appears dominant	Recessive
Diagnosis	Clinical and laboratory findings, lack of response to phenobarbital	Clinical and laboratory findings, response to phenobarbital	Clinical and laboratory findings; promoter genotyping; liver biopsy rarely necessary	Clinical and laboratory findings; liver biopsy unnecessary if coproporphyrin studies available; BSP disappearance	Clinical and laboratory findings; urine coproporphyrin analysis; BSP disappearance
Treatment	Phototherapy or tin protoporphyrin as short-term therapy; liver transplantation definitive	Consider phenobarbital if baseline bilirubin ≥8 mg/dL	None necessary	Avoid estrogens; no other therapy necessary	No treatment necessary

*UGT1A1 = bilirubin specific isoform of the UGT1 family of uridine diphosphate glucuronosyltransferases.
†Sulfobromophthalein (BSP) studies: Previously used to help distinguish Dubin-Johnson and Rotor syndromes if coproporphyrin isomer studies not available. However, BSP is no longer approved for clinical use in the United States.
‡Bilirubin in normal bile: <5% unconjugated bilirubin, with an average of 7% bilirubin monoconjugates and 90% bilirubin diconjugates.

excretion into the urine (see Table 147-2). Both syndromes carry a benign prognosis without specific therapy.

LIVER AND BILIARY TRACT DISEASE

Jaundice is a common sign of generalized hepatobiliary dysfunction, both acute and chronic. Icteric hepatobiliary disease is readily distinguished from the isolated disorders of bilirubin metabolism because the increase in plasma bilirubin concentration occurs in association with other markers of hepatobiliary disease (Fig. 147-2). Liver diseases can be categorized as those in which the primary injury results from inflammation and hepatocellular necrosis, inhibition of bile flow (cholestasis), or a combination of the two. The cholestatic disorders can be further subdivided into those resulting from mechanical obstruction of the bile duct flow and those from intrahepatic cholestasis, from a multitude of conditions that include several familial cholestatic syndromes; infiltrative disorders (Chapters 149 to 153), particularly those involving the intrahepatic biliary tree; certain other inflammatory or neoplastic conditions; and drug reactions (see Table 147-1 and Chapters 149 to 153).

Familial Cholestasis Syndromes

Bile secretion, which is essential both for the elimination of metabolic wastes and for the solubilization and subsequent absorption of specific nutrients, is a complex, energy-dependent process in which three ABC transporters (ATP8B1, ABCB11, and ABCB4) play critical roles. ATP8B1, also known as

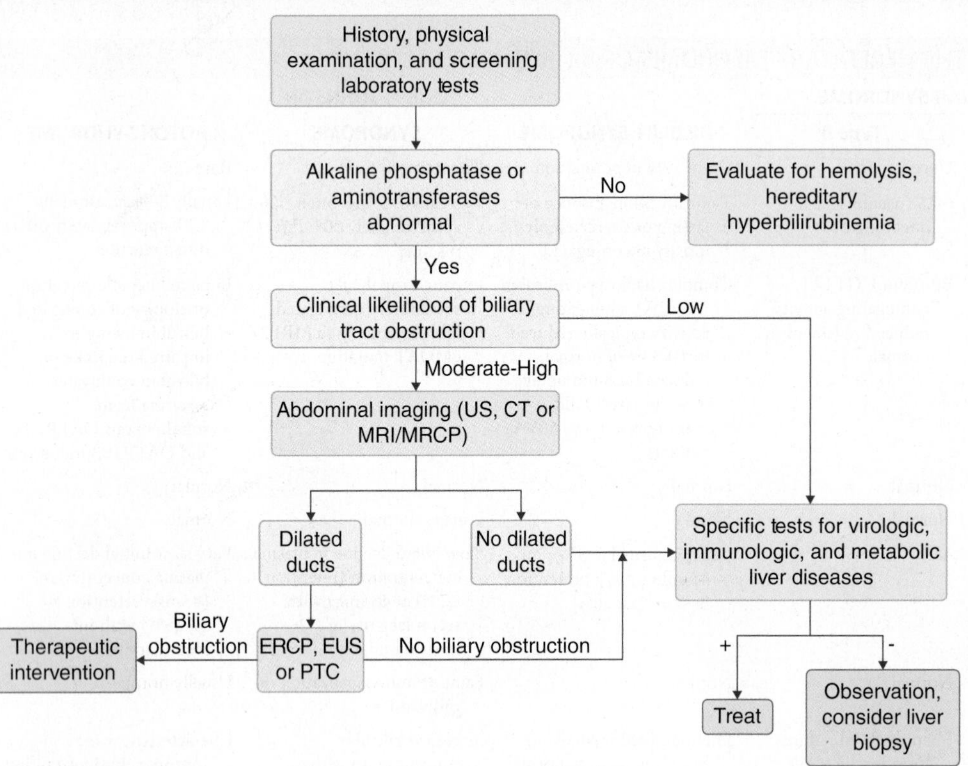

FIGURE 147-2. **Diagnostic algorithm for the evaluation of hyperbilirubinemia and other liver test abnormalities and signs and symptoms suggestive of liver disease.** CT = computed tomography; ERCP = endoscopic retrograde cholangiopancreatography; EUS = endoscopic ultrasound; MRCP = magnetic resonance cholangiopancreatography; MRI = magnetic resonance imaging; PTC = percutaneous transhepatic cholangiogram; US = ultrasound. (Modified from Lidofsky SD, Scharschmidt BF. Jaundice. In: Feldman M, Scharschmidt BF, Sleisenger MH, eds. *Gastrointestinal and Liver Disease.* 6th ed. Philadelphia: WB Saunders; 1998:227.)

familial intrahepatic cholestasis 1 (FIC1), is a phosphatidylserine flippase that translocates phosphatidylserine from the outer (canalicular) to the inner (cytoplasmic) leaflet of the canalicular plasma membrane; ABCB11, also known as the bile salt export pump (BSEP) or the sister of P glycoprotein (SPGP), translocates bile salts from the interior of the hepatocyte across the canalicular membrane into the bile. ABCB4 (multidrug resistance-associated protein 3 [MDR3]) is a phosphatidylcholine (lecithin) floppase translocating phosphatidylcholine outward from the cytoplasmic to the canalicular leaflet of the canalicular membrane.[12] A major function of ATP8B1 and ABCB4 is to maintain an appropriate physicochemical state of the canalicular membrane by regulating the balance of appropriate membrane phospholipids. Three different forms of severe pediatric cholestatic liver disease (designated progressive familial intrahepatic cholestasis types 1, 2, and 3) result from severe, homozygous mutations in these transporters. Less severe, nonprogressive cholestatic liver diseases (designated benign recurrent intrahepatic cholestasis [BRIC] types 1, 2, and 3) result from less severe mutations in these same genes.

Progressive familial intrahepatic cholestasis describes three phenotypically related syndromes of cholestasis during infancy and end-stage liver disease during childhood. All three disorders are inherited in an autosomal recessive pattern. In types 1 and 2, γ-glutamyl transpeptidase (GGT) levels are low despite elevations in alkaline phosphatase; by comparison, elevations in both GGT and alkaline phosphatase occur in type 3. In contrast to the selective bilirubin transport defect in Dubin-Johnson syndrome, the conjugated hyperbilirubinemia in these syndromes is caused by generalized bile secretory failure. Type 1 is the result of mutations in the *FIC1* gene that is also the cause of BRIC type 1. Types 2 and 3 are the result of mutations in genes *ABCB11* and *ABCB4,* respectively. *ABCB11* encodes a bile salt export pump, and *ABCB4* encodes the multidrug resistance protein 3 (MDR3), a protein responsible for the translocation of phosphatidylcholine.

Benign recurrent intrahepatic cholestasis is a rare, autosomal recessive disorder characterized by recurrent attacks of malaise, pruritus, and jaundice beginning in childhood or adulthood and varying in duration from weeks to months. Intervals between attacks may vary from months to years. This benign disorder does not progress to chronic liver disease or cirrhosis, and there is complete resolution between episodes. Treatment during the cholestatic episodes is symptomatic. Type 1 results from a mutation in the gene *familial intrahepatic cholestasis 1 (FIC1),* which is more severely mutated in progressive FIC1. It encodes the translocase protein ATP8B1 that transports aminophospholipids from the outer to the inner leaflet of various cell membranes. Phenotypically similar benign recurrent intrahepatic cholestasis type 2 and type 3 variants result from mutations in *ABCB11* and *ABCB4,* respectively.

Acquired Conjugation Defects

A modest reduction in bilirubin conjugating capacity occurs in advanced hepatitis or cirrhosis (Chapters 149 and 153). However, in these settings, conjugation is better preserved than other aspects of bilirubin disposition, such as canalicular excretion. Pharmacologic and metabolic perturbations may lead to acquired reductions in bilirubin conjugation. Unconjugated hyperbilirubinemia related to selective inhibition of UGT1A1 occurs with several human immunodeficiency virus (HIV) protease inhibitors (e.g., indinavir, atazanavir). Various other drugs (e.g., pregnanediol and the antibiotics novobiocin, chloramphenicol, gentamycin) also may cause unconjugated hyperbilirubinemia by inhibiting UGT1A1. In all settings in which UGT1A1 inhibitors cause unconjugated hyperbilirubinemia, the degree of hyperbilirubinemia is greater in patients with underlying Gilbert syndrome.

Jaundice in Pregnancy

Jaundice in pregnancy (Chapter 239) includes any liver disease that occurs during pregnancy. Conditions unique to pregnancy include a generally modest and self-limited elevation of the aminotransferase and bilirubin levels during the first trimester, often in patients with hyperemesis gravidarum. Intrahepatic cholestasis of pregnancy, which occurs during the second and third trimesters, is associated with intrauterine demise and resolves spontaneously after delivery. Mutations in genes encoding biliary transporters, especially *ABCB4,* have been reported in some but not all cases. Acute fatty liver or the HELLP (*h*emolysis, *el*evated *l*iver enzymes, and *l*ow *p*latelets) syndrome occurs in association with preeclampsia in the third trimester (Chapters 172 and 239). Acute fatty liver may resemble fulminant hepatic failure, with early delivery a prerequisite to maternal recovery.

Postoperative Jaundice

This multifactorial syndrome can be caused by increased bilirubin production (e.g., breakdown of transfused erythrocytes, resorption of hematomas), decreased hepatic bilirubin clearance (e.g., bacteremia, endotoxemia, parenteral nutrition, perioperative hypoxia), or both. Hyperbilirubinemia, which is the main biochemical feature, is often accompanied by a several-fold increase in alkaline phosphatase, GGT, or both levels. Aminotransferases are, at most, minimally elevated, and synthetic function is typically normal. The differential diagnosis includes biliary obstruction (Chapter 155) or hepatocellular injury related to shock, anesthetic injury (Chapter 150), or viral hepatitis (Chapter 148). Postoperative jaundice per se is not a threat to the patient, and it usually resolves in parallel with the patient's overall condition.

DIAGNOSIS

Accurate diagnosis and the distinction between acute and chronic disease often depend on appropriate selection and interpretation of a spectrum of laboratory and imaging studies. Tests used in initial evaluation of liver disease fall into two categories: tests that indicate injury, such as release of intracellular enzymes, and tests that measure, or at least reflect, actual function. Tests that reflect injury do not measure liver function and should not be called liver function tests. Liver tests must be chosen with care and interpreted within the overall clinical context. In specific situations, serial determinations are often helpful to assess the course of disease or the effects of therapy

Serum Enzyme Tests

The levels of hepatic enzymes found in plasma are a measure of hepatocyte turnover or injury. Enzymes released during normal hepatocyte turnover are believed to be the basis for normal circulating levels. Cell injury and cell death activate phospholipases that create holes in the plasma membrane, thereby increasing the release of intracellular contents.

Aminotransferases

The aminotransferases (formerly called transaminases) catalyze transfer of the α-amino group of aspartate (aspartate aminotransferase [AST]) or alanine (alanine aminotransferase [ALT]) to the α-keto group of α-ketoglutarate, with pyridoxal phosphate (vitamin B_6) as a cofactor. Laboratory methods that assay aminotransferase activity require supplementation with vitamin B_6 to avoid falsely decreased activity in subjects who are vitamin B_6 deficient.

Normal serum levels, which are established locally from samples obtained from normal populations, may vary appreciably in different populations but are typically 40 IU/L or less (see Appendix). Values can exceed 1000 IU/L in acute hepatocyte injury, for example, from viral infection (Chapter 148) or toxins (Chapter 150). ALT is a purely cytosolic enzyme. Distinct isoforms of AST are present in cytosol and mitochondria, and AST is also found on the plasma membrane. Expression of the mitochondrial isoform and its physiologic export from the hepatocyte are upregulated by ethanol. Circulating levels of AST and ALT are elevated in most hepatic diseases, and the degree of aminotransferase activity found in plasma roughly reflects the current activity of the disease process. There are, however, critical exceptions. In even the most severe cases of alcoholic hepatitis, aminotransferase levels greater than 200 to 300 IU/L are uncommon (Chapter 152). In nonalcoholic fatty liver disease, normal values for ALT may be found in an appreciable fraction of patients with active nonalcoholic steatohepatitis, fibrosis, or even cirrhosis. By contrast, aminotransferase activities of 1000 IU/L or greater are often present in even mild acute viral hepatitis (Chapter 148) or shortly after acute biliary obstruction, for example, during passage of a gallstone (Chapter 155). Conversely, aminotransferase levels may decline during the course of massive hepatic necrosis because liver injury is so extensive that little enzyme activity remains (Chapter 154). In rare circumstances, antibodies to AST result in an antibody-enzyme complex called a macroenzyme that has a delayed clearance from the circulation.

Aminotransferase levels are useful in several distinct ways. First, they provide a relatively specific screening test for hepatobiliary disease. Although AST levels may be increased with disease of other organs (notably myocardial and skeletal muscle), values 10 times the upper limit of normal or greater almost invariably indicate hepatobiliary pathology. Moreover, in the total clinical context, the source of increased aminotransferase activity is usually obvious. Aminotransferase levels are also used to monitor the activity of an acute or chronic parenchymal liver disease and its response to therapy. However, levels in a given patient may correlate poorly with the severity of the disease as assessed by liver biopsy, particularly in chronic hepatitis C (Chapter 149) and nonalcoholic fatty liver (Chapter 152).[13] Aminotransferases are also often normal despite advanced cirrhosis (Chapter 153), in which they are of limited prognostic value. Finally, aminotransferase levels may provide diagnostic clues. AST levels 15 or more times normal are unusual in chronic bile duct obstruction without cholangitis, and AST levels 6 or more times normal are uncommon in alcoholic liver disease in the absence of other causes. In most liver diseases, the ratio of AST to ALT is usually 1 or less; however, ratios are typically 2 or higher in alcoholic fatty liver and alcoholic hepatitis (Chapter 152), reflecting increased synthesis and secretion of mitochondrial AST into plasma and selective loss of ALT activity because of the pyridoxine deficiency commonly seen in alcoholism. An elevated AST/ALT ratio also occurs in fulminant hepatitis related to Wilson disease (Chapters 146 and 211).

Alkaline Phosphatase

Alkaline phosphatases are widely distributed enzymes (e.g., liver, bile ducts, intestine, bone, kidney, placenta, and leukocytes) that catalyze the release of orthophosphate from ester substrates at an alkaline pH. The normal activity level in adult serum is highly dependent on the measurement method, age, and sex. Two widely used current methods have upper limits of normal in adults of 85 and 110 IU/L (see Appendix). Higher levels are normal in children and in pregnancy. Results must always be compared with the appropriate normal range. In bone, alkaline phosphatase participates in the deposition of hydroxyapatite in osteoid. In other sites, including the liver, its phosphatase activity may facilitate movement of molecules across cell membranes. Serum alkaline phosphatase activity principally reflects the contribution of hepatic and bone isoforms; the intestinal form may account for 20 to 60% of the total after a fatty meal. There is a substantial placental contribution to the alkaline phosphatase level late in pregnancy; the Regan isozyme, a variant that appears identical to the placental form, is associated with hepatocellular cancer (Chapter 196), lung cancer (Chapter 191), and other tumors.

Elevations in the serum alkaline phosphatase activity in cholestatic hepatobiliary disease result from two distinct mechanisms: increased synthesis and secretion of the enzyme and solubilization from the apical (canalicular) surface of hepatocytes and the luminal surface of biliary epithelial cells by the increased local concentrations of bile acids that occur with cholestasis. Serum alkaline phosphatase activity also may be increased in bone disorders (e.g., Paget disease [Chapter 247], osteomalacia [Chapter 244], bone metastases [Chapter 202]), during rapid bone growth in children, in the later stages of pregnancy, with chronic renal failure (Chapter 130), and, occasionally, in the presence of malignancy not involving bones or liver. The source is often obvious, but when it is not, fractionation techniques can distinguish hepatobiliary alkaline phosphatase from other forms. A simpler alternative is to measure serum levels of GGT or 5′-nucleotidase (5′-NT), which tend to parallel levels of alkaline phosphatase in hepatobiliary disease but are usually not increased in bone disease. With a serum half-life of approximately 1 week, serum alkaline phosphatase levels may remain elevated for days to weeks after resolution of biliary obstruction. This delay may be especially misleading when it is accompanied by prolonged direct-reacting hyperbilirubinemia owing to delayed clearance of δ-bilirubin.

Modest increases in serum alkaline phosphatase activity (<3 times normal) occur in many hepatic parenchymal disorders, including hepatitis and cirrhosis. In the absence of bone disease, larger increases (3 to 10 times normal) usually indicate obstruction of bile flow. Although the highest levels usually reflect obstruction of the common bile duct, elevations also can occur with obstruction of intrahepatic bile ducts from infiltrative conditions that arise from granulomatous processes (sarcoidosis [Chapter 95], *Mycobacterium avium-intracellulare* infection [Chapter 325], mycobacteria tuberculosis [Chapter 324]), malignancy (lymphoma, cholangiocarcinoma, or metastatic cancer), or amyloidosis (Chapter 188).

Other Hepatic Enzymes

5′-NT is a plasma membrane enzyme that cleaves orthophosphate from the 5′ position on the pentose sugar of adenosine or inosine phosphate. Leucine aminopeptidase (LAP) is a ubiquitous cellular peptidase. The serum levels of both usually increase in cholestasis. Accordingly, their major use is to confirm whether an elevated serum alkaline phosphatase is of hepatobiliary origin. Both enzymes may be increased in the latter stages of a healthy pregnancy.

GGT is present in many tissues. Its serum activity increases in hepatobiliary disease but also after myocardial infarction; in neuromuscular diseases, pancreatic disease (even in the absence of biliary obstruction), pulmonary disease, and diabetes; and during the ingestion of ethanol and other inducers of microsomal enzymes. Nevertheless, because serum GGT levels are usually normal in bone disease, the enzyme may be helpful in confirming the hepatic origin of alkaline phosphatase. Measurement of GGT has been proposed as a sensitive screening test for hepatobiliary disease and for monitoring abstinence from ethanol. Because of its low specificity, many persons who test positive have no identifiable liver disease on further study. GGT offers no clear advantage over LAP or 5′-NT for identifying the source of increased serum alkaline phosphatase activity except in pregnancy. Serum GGT levels may be normal despite elevated hepatobiliary alkaline phosphatase levels in certain rare disorders, including benign recurrent intrahepatic cholestasis and progressive familial intrahepatic cholestasis types 1 and 2 (see earlier and Chapter 155).

Lactate dehydrogenase levels are often elevated in hepatic ischemia and other conditions that result in hepatic necrosis; otherwise the enzyme is too ubiquitous in other body tissues to be diagnostically useful.

Tests Based on Clearance of Metabolites and Drugs

A major function of the liver is to remove various metabolites and toxins from the blood (Chapter 150). In liver disease, clearance of such molecules may be impaired because of loss of parenchymal cells, diminished bile secretion, biliary obstruction, decreased cellular uptake or metabolism, or reduced or heterogeneous hepatic blood flow. When a metabolite is produced at a relatively constant rate (e.g., bilirubin), its serum level can be a sensitive indicator of liver function. The removal rate from plasma of certain exogenous drugs and dyes can be similarly interpreted. However, plasma removal rates of sulfobromophthalein (BSP) and indocyanine green, once widely used as tests of liver function, have essentially been abandoned.

Bilirubin

The differential diagnosis of hyperbilirubinemia (see earlier) includes generalized liver disease, inherited disorders of bilirubin metabolism (e.g., Gilbert, Crigler-Najjar, Dubin-Johnson, and Rotor syndromes) and nonhepatic conditions (e.g., hemolysis). Higher bilirubin levels correlate with a poorer prognosis in most forms of chronic liver disease.

Ammonia

Ammonia, a byproduct of amino acid metabolism, is removed from blood by the liver, converted to urea in the Krebs-Henseleit cycle, and excreted by the kidneys (Chapter 115). In the setting of portosystemic shunting or severe hepatic dysfunction (e.g., fulminant hepatic failure), ammonia levels rise. Measurements of blood ammonia are principally used to confirm a diagnosis of hepatic encephalopathy or response to treatment of the encephalopathy. However, serum ammonia levels do not strongly correlate with the severity of hepatic encephalopathy (Chapter 153). Correlations may be somewhat better if the measurement is made rapidly on an iced arterial blood sample. Elevated ammonia levels also occur when ammonia production is increased by intestinal flora (e.g., after a high-protein meal or gastrointestinal bleeding), by the kidney (in response to metabolic alkalosis or hypokalemia), or in rare genetic diseases that affect the pathway of urea synthesis (Chapter 205).

Drug Clearance

The rate of hepatic clearance of compounds such as lidocaine and aminopyrine from the circulation can be measured chemically or with radiolabeled tracers. Although such tests can quantify hepatic function, they are rarely used in clinical practice.

Tests Reflecting Hepatic Synthetic Function

Coagulation Tests

See also Chapters 38 and 171.

Prothrombin Time

The prothrombin time (PT) reflects the plasma concentrations of both extrinsic and common pathway factors, that is, factors VII, X, and V, prothrombin, and fibrinogen. A prolonged PT most often results from vitamin K deficiency, liver disease, or both. Vitamin K, a fat-soluble vitamin, is found in many foods and is also synthesized by gut bacteria (Chapter 174). Vitamin K deficiency can be caused by poor dietary intake and malabsorptive states, including the fat malabsorption that results from cholestasis, and it also occurs with antibiotic suppression of gut flora, particularly in patients who receive inadequate vitamin K replacement.

The half-lives of clotting factors are typically less than 1 day. Factor VII, which has the shortest half-life, is usually the earliest and most severely depressed during periods of defective hepatic synthesis. Because the PT is dependent on the level of factor VII, it responds rapidly with changes in hepatic synthetic function; it is useful for following the course of acute liver diseases, in which a significant or growing prolongation of the PT may indicate a poor prognosis (Chapter 148). An abnormal PT that is due solely to vitamin K deficiency usually becomes normal within 24 to 48 hours after parenteral repletion. However, if decreased synthesis of clotting factors reflects hepatocyte dysfunction, there may be little or no response to vitamin K.

Although the prolongation of PT with liver disease is generally accepted as indicative of defective clotting factor synthesis, the synthesis of both procoagulant and anticoagulant proteins is disturbed in liver disease.[14] The physiologic consequences of this rebalancing of coagulation may preserve the coagulation response. Prolongation of the PT may also reflect disseminated intravascular coagulation (Chapter 175), which should always be considered in the context of both acute liver failure and end-stage chronic liver disease.

Partial Thromboplastin Time

This test reflects both the intrinsic and common pathway factors, that is, all of the classical clotting factors except factor VII, and is, therefore, complementary to the PT. It is especially useful in detecting circulating anticoagulants (Chapter 175) but adds little to the PT in evaluating hepatic synthetic function.

Albumin

Albumin is produced solely by the liver. Its plasma concentration reflects a balance between its synthetic rate of approximately 100 to 200 mg/kg/day and its plasma half-life of approximately 21 days. The synthetic rate is affected by the patient's nutritional state, thyroid and glucocorticoid hormone levels, plasma colloid osmotic pressure, exposure to hepatotoxins (e.g., alcohol), and presence of systemic disorders, liver disease, or both. Many conditions increase albumin losses and shorten its plasma half-life, including nephrotic syndrome (Chapter 121), protein-losing enteropathy (Chapter 140), severe burns (Chapter 111), exfoliative dermatitis, and major gastrointestinal bleeding (Chapter 135). In cirrhosis with ascites (Chapters 153 and 154), hypoalbuminemia indicates diminished synthesis or redistribution into ascitic fluid. Thus, a reduced serum albumin concentration can be considered an indicator of decreased hepatic synthetic function only when these factors are not involved.

Hematologic Tests in Liver Disease

In moderate to severe acute liver diseases, varying degrees of cytopenias can be seen with all three cell lineages. The most common finding is thrombocytopenia from hypersplenism, which can be a surrogate marker of portal hypertension. Anemia may reflect low-grade hemolysis or marrow depression. Bone marrow suppression may be caused by ethanol or drugs, and aplastic anemia is an uncommon but well-recognized complication of acute viral hepatitis (Chapters 148 and 165). Zieve syndrome (hemolytic anemia and hypertriglyceridemia) is a rare but well-characterized complication of severe alcoholic liver disease (Chapters 152 and 153). Modest leukopenia, often with atypical lymphocytes, also may be present. Chronic liver disease, especially if cholestatic, may be accompanied by target cells in the peripheral blood smear. Target cells are erythrocytes with an expanded cell membrane that reflects abnormalities in serum lipids. Spur cells (acanthocytes), most often found in advanced alcoholic cirrhosis, reflect a still greater increase in membrane cholesterol.

Tests for Specific Liver Diseases

Patients who present with a picture of acute or chronic parenchymal liver disease are most likely to fall into one of three categories: viral or toxic hepatitis, including alcoholic liver disease; autoimmune liver disease; or an inherited or acquired metabolic disorder (Chapter 146). Specific tests for viral antigens, nucleic acids, and antibodies are available for the conventional hepatitis viruses, including A, B, C, D (delta), and E, chronic forms of which are being increasingly seen in immunosuppressed patients (Chapters 148 and 149), as well as Epstein-Barr virus (Chapter 377), cytomegalovirus (Chapter 376), and herpesviruses (Chapters 374 and 375), which are well-established but less common causes of liver disease. The major autoimmune diseases of the liver include primary biliary cirrhosis (Chapter 155), autoimmune hepatitis (Chapter 149), primary sclerosing cholangitis (Chapter 155), and various overlap syndromes. The starting point for establishing a specific diagnosis within this category is the search for specific autoantibodies in serum, including antimitochondrial antibodies against epitopes of the pyruvate dehydrogenase complex, which are virtually diagnostic of primary biliary cirrhosis (Chapter 155), and antinuclear, anti–smooth muscle, and anti–liver/kidney microsomal antibodies, which suggest a diagnosis of one of the subtypes of autoimmune hepatitis (Chapter 149). The most prevalent of the hereditary metabolic disorders affecting the liver include hemochromatosis, α_1-antitrypsin deficiency, and Wilson disease (Chapter 211). Nonalcoholic fatty liver disease is the most frequent acquired metabolic liver disease. The disorder is not associated with any known serologic markers, although nonspecific elevations in antinuclear antibody may be present (Chapter 152).

Liver Biopsy

Liver biopsy can be of great help in the diagnosis of diffuse or localized parenchymal diseases, including chronic hepatitis, cirrhosis, and primary or metastatic malignancy in the liver. The value of liver biopsy in acute hepatitis or acute cholestatic jaundice may be primarily prognostic because the histologic changes in these settings may be nonspecific. However, drug-induced liver injury due to certain specific agents (Chapter 150) may display diagnostic features. Liver biopsy for assessment of diffuse disease can be performed percutaneously after localization of the liver by physical examination or ultrasonographic visualization. When specific lesions, such as tumors, must be sampled, the biopsy can be guided by ultrasonographic or radiographic imaging or performed under direct visualization during laparoscopy. Relative or absolute contraindications include coagulopathy, high-grade biliary obstruction, biliary sepsis, ascites, and right pleural disease. Although liver biopsy remains the standard for assessment of hepatic histology in diffuse disease (Chapter 146), the procedure's invasiveness and concern for sampling error have generated interest in noninvasive measures of hepatic fibrosis. These noninvasive studies fall into two categories. One category uses magnetic resonance imaging or ultrasound to measure liver stiffness as a surrogate for fibrosis. The second category comprises panels of biomarkers accessible by blood testing to predict the severity of necroinflammation and fibrosis. These serologic panels typically include standard laboratory measures of hepatic injury (GGT, total bilirubin) and other serum markers (e.g. haptoglobin, hyaluronic acid, apolipoprotein A1). However, the ability of currently available noninvasive markers to assess the extent of hepatic fibrosis reliably across the clinically relevant histologic spectrum, especially in an individual patient, remains to be established.[15]

APPROACH TO THE PATIENT WITH JAUNDICE OR ABNORMAL LIVER TESTS

History, Physical Examination, and Initial Laboratory Studies

Patients with liver disease may present with jaundice or with other signs or symptoms, or the disease may be detected in the asymptomatic patient by the finding of abnormal liver tests during a routine evaluation. Regardless of how the patient comes to medical attention, the diagnostic approach (see Fig. 147-2) begins with a careful history and physical examination (Chapter 146) and screening laboratory studies (complete blood cell count, measurement of plasma bilirubin concentration, assay of ALT, AST, and alkaline phosphatase levels, and PT) to formulate an initial differential diagnosis.[16] The ability to distinguish expeditiously between liver disease and extrahepatic biliary tract obstruction is the major goal of the initial evaluation, in part because the latter may call for prompt surgical intervention. Appropriate selection of second-level laboratory tests and imaging studies leads to a definitive diagnosis in most patients. Care in selecting tests, particularly imaging studies, can both maximize the likelihood of making a correct diagnosis and protect the patient from unnecessary discomfort, risk, and expense.

If the patient is asymptomatic and hepatic tests other than bilirubin are normal, hemolysis or an isolated disorder of bilirubin metabolism should be considered. If signs, symptoms, or laboratory abnormalities indicate hepatobiliary disease, certain patterns of findings help to distinguish intrinsic liver disease from biliary obstruction (Table 147-3). Pain in the right upper quadrant accompanied by a predominant increase in serum alkaline phosphatase activity suggests biliary obstruction (Chapter 155), as does a history of biliary surgery, right upper quadrant scars, or an abdominal mass. Fever and rigors, indicative of cholangitis, strengthen this conclusion. The incidences of gallstone disease and malignant neoplasm increase with age, although risk factors such as obesity or recent extensive diet-induced weight loss increase the risk for gallstones. Other risk factors (e.g., hepatitis exposure, transfusions, intravenous drug use, alcohol use, certain medications, obesity, and family history of genetic diseases) and a predominant elevation in serum aminotransferase levels favor a diagnosis of parenchymal liver disease. Physical evidence of cirrhosis (e.g., spider angiomas, gynecomastia, ascites, splenomegaly) supports the diagnosis of chronic parenchymal disease.

Despite the general validity of these patterns, many exceptions exist. In particular, parenchymal disorders with prominent cholestasis may mimic biliary obstruction. Both alkaline phosphatase and GGT are usually elevated in patients with cholestasis; the combination of an elevated alkaline phosphatase and normal GGT suggests that the alkaline phosphatase is from bone. Conversely, an isolated elevation of GGT may result from certain drugs (e.g., diphenylhydantoin) or alcohol consumption even in the absence of liver disease. Because of the risk for life-threatening infection in the setting of unrelieved biliary tract obstruction, this possibility must always be considered and excluded if an alternative diagnosis is not definitely established.

TABLE 147-3 OBSTRUCTIVE JAUNDICE VERSUS CHOLESTATIC LIVER DISEASE

FEATURE	SUGGESTS OBSTRUCTIVE JAUNDICE	SUGGESTS PARENCHYMAL LIVER DISEASE
History	Abdominal pain Fever, rigors Prior biliary surgery Acholic stools	Anorexia, malaise, myalgias, suggestive of viral prodrome Known infectious exposure Use of injection drugs or intranasal cocaine Exposure to known hepatotoxin Family history of jaundice
Physical examination	High fever Abdominal tenderness Palpable abdominal mass Abdominal scar	Ascites Other stigmata of liver disease (e.g., prominent abdominal veins, gynecomastia, spider angiomata, asterixis, encephalopathy, Kayser-Fleischer rings)
Laboratory studies	Predominant elevation of serum bilirubin and alkaline phosphatase Prothrombin time that is normal or normalizes with vitamin K administration Elevated serum amylase	Predominant elevation of serum aminotransferases Prolonged prothrombin time that does not correct with vitamin K administration Blood tests indicative of specific liver disease

Imaging Studies

If extrahepatic obstruction is suspected, its site and nature can now be determined in virtually all patients (see Fig. 147-2). A reasonable initial step is the use of a noninvasive imaging study (Chapter 133) such as ultrasonography or magnetic resonance cholangiopancreatography to determine whether the intrahepatic, extrahepatic biliary system, or both are dilated, implying mechanical obstruction. Because of its lesser expense, portability, and convenience, ultrasound is often the procedure of choice, especially if gallstones are suspected. Magnetic resonance cholangiopancreatography may provide more precise resolution, including stricturing of intrahepatic ducts characteristic of primary sclerosing cholangitis. However, each of these techniques can fail to identify dilated ducts, particularly in patients with cirrhosis. Conversely, a modest degree of ductal dilatation is common in a patient with a previous cholecystectomy and does not necessarily signify current obstruction. If dilated ducts are found, the biliary tree should be examined by endoscopic retrograde cholangiopancreatography (ERCP) or percutaneous transhepatic cholangiography (PTC) (Chapter 134). ERCP involves positioning an endoscope in the duodenum, inserting a catheter through the ampulla of Vater, and injecting contrast medium into the distal common bile duct, pancreatic duct, or both. PTC involves percutaneous passage of a needle through the hepatic parenchyma into a peripheral bile duct, followed by injection of contrast medium into the biliary tree through the peripheral duct. The choice of procedure is based on the suspected site of obstruction (proximal vs. distal); the presence of coagulopathy; a history of abdominal surgery that might complicate PTC or ERCP; the likely need for a therapeutic procedure (e.g., stent placement or endoscopic sphincterotomy); and the skills of available staff. Endoscopic ultrasound (EUS) is a complementary approach that permits internal ultrasonographic analysis of the pancreas, extrahepatic bile ducts, and regional lymph nodes and blood vessels. EUS combined with fine needle aspiration permits tissue sampling of abnormalities in areas such as the bile ducts and pancreas that typically have been difficult to sample percutaneously.

Selection of Imaging Tests

Liver ultrasound is an ideal screening test to evaluate the liver architecture, assess for surface nodularity and parenchymal mass lesions, and exclude biliary obstruction. Ultrasound is relatively inexpensive in comparison to other imaging modalities, is widely available, and avoids ionizing radiation. The identification of mass lesions on ultrasound will commonly prompt further cross-sectional imaging with either computed tomography or magnetic resonance imaging. If there is evidence of biliary obstruction on imaging or, if obstruction is still considered likely despite imaging findings, direct

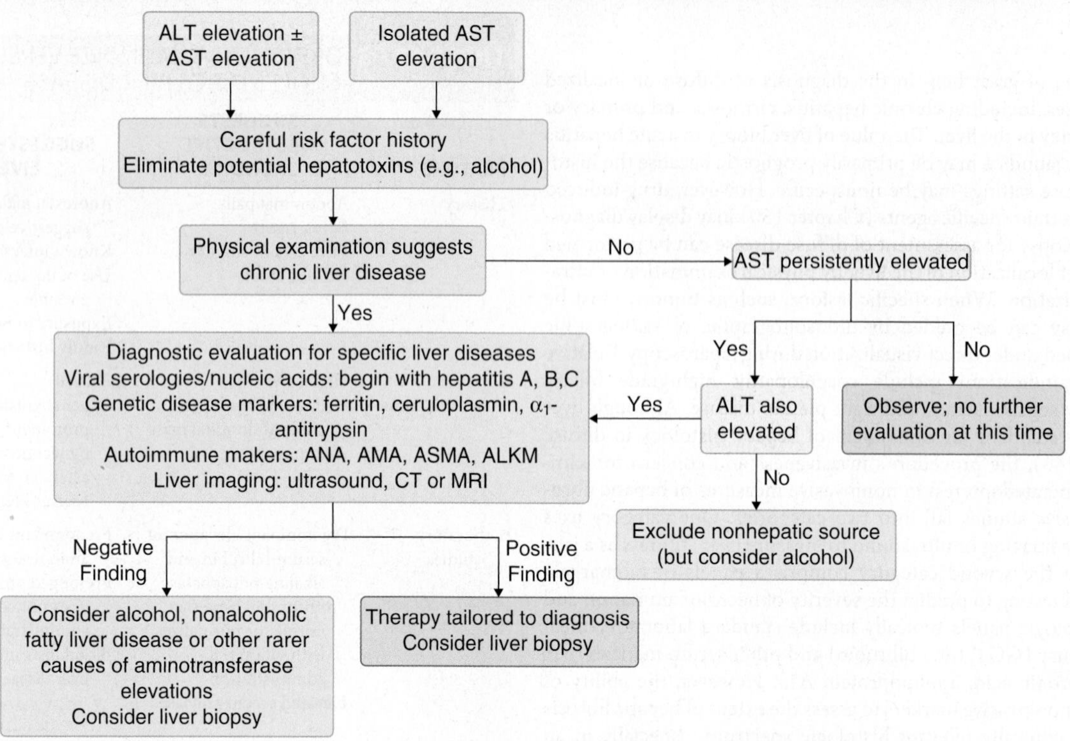

FIGURE 147-3. Approach to the evaluation of isolated elevated levels of serum alanine aminotransferase (*ALT*), aspartate aminotransferase (*AST*), or both in the asymptomatic patient. ANA = antinuclear antibody; AMA = antimitochondrial antibody; ASMA = anti–smooth muscle antibody; ALKM = anti–liver/kidney microsomal antibody; CT = computed tomography; MRI = magnetic resonance imaging.

cholangiography by ERCP or PTC, which offer therapeutic as well as diagnostic capabilities, may be an appropriate choice. If obstruction is considered possible but not highly likely, noninvasive imaging with MRCP is a reasonable study. Individual radiology suites have different levels of expertise for these procedures, and the local radiology staff may be quite helpful in recommending the best procedure for a given patient.

The apparently healthy patient with an isolated abnormality of the aminotransferase or alkaline phosphatase levels requires careful evaluation to identify any underlying disease while avoiding unneeded testing. Often, no significant disease is found despite extensive evaluation. Common causes of abnormal enzyme tests include alcohol consumption, hepatitis C infection, nonalcoholic fatty liver disease, bone disease, and muscle injury.

Asymptomatic Aminotransferase Elevation

Epidemiologic data suggest that up to 25% of asymptomatic adult Americans have a mild to moderate elevation of aminotransferase levels. The incidental discovery of such abnormalities is currently the most frequent means by which liver disease is first recognized. Whereas up to one third of such patients have no elevation on subsequent testing, many others prove to have steatohepatitis (Chapter 152) or chronic hepatitis C (Chapter 149). Further evaluation is generally indicated only in patients with persistent abnormalities (Fig. 147-3). Initial screening should include a careful history of exposure to hepatotoxins (alcohol, prescription drugs, over-the-counter medications, herbs, chemicals, and occupational exposures). If the abnormal test was an AST, a hepatic origin for the enzyme elevation should be confirmed with an ALT determination. If the ALT is normal, a muscle source is likely or the elevation may reflect the presence of a macroenzyme. If the ALT level is abnormal, the patient should be screened serologically for hepatitis B, C, and (at least in immunosuppressed patients) E; markers of autoimmune liver disease; and serologic markers of inherited metabolic disorders (Chapter 146). AST abnormalities caused by alcohol-induced injury should become normal with several weeks of abstinence. If the abnormalities persist for 6 to 12 months without an apparent cause, liver biopsy should be considered.

Asymptomatic Alkaline Phosphatase Elevation

Many patients with isolated elevation of the alkaline phosphatase level have nonhepatic causes, such as pregnancy or bone disease. The origin of an elevated alkaline phosphatase should be confirmed with a fasting sample because intestinal alkaline phosphatase may be elevated after a meal (Fig. 147-4).

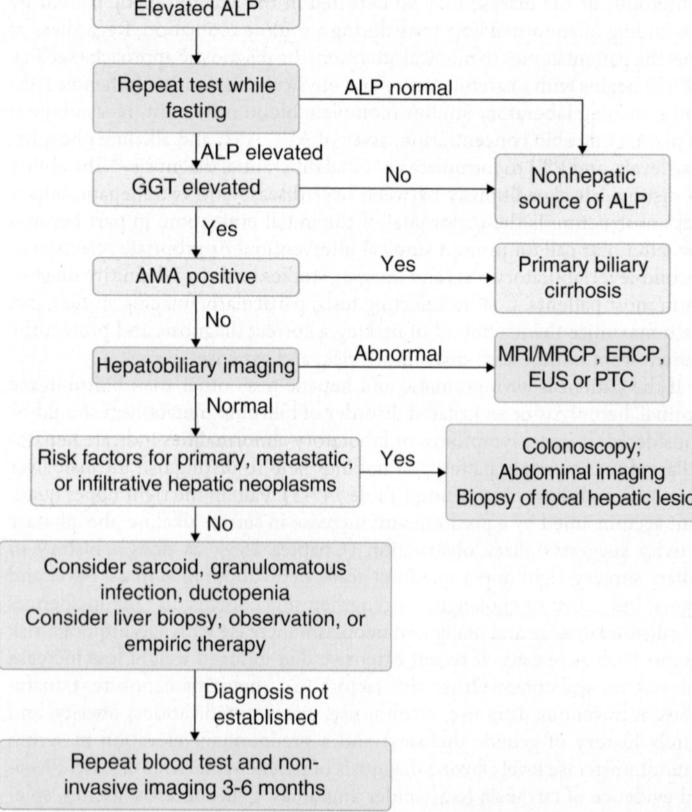

FIGURE 147-4. Approach to the asymptomatic patient with isolated elevated levels of serum alkaline phosphatase (*ALP*). In cases with a high index of suspicion of biliary tract disease (e.g., sclerosing cholangitis), cholangiography may be warranted even in the face of normal ultrasound imaging. AMA = antimitochondrial antibody; CT = computed tomography; ERCP = endoscopic retrograde cholangiopancreatography; EUS = endoscopic ultrasound; GGT = γ-glutamyl transpeptidase; MRCP = magnetic resonance cholangiopancreatography; MRI = magnetic resonance imaging; PTC = percutaneous transhepatic cholangiogram; US = ultrasonography.

A hepatic source is highly likely if the serum GGT is also abnormal. Serologic studies should include an antimitochondrial antibody test; a positive result suggests primary biliary cirrhosis (Chapter 155). A careful history identifies patients at risk for intrahepatic cholestasis related to drugs or toxins. Essentially all other patients with persistently abnormal alkaline phosphatase should receive a hepatobiliary sonogram or other noninvasive imaging test. Demonstration of dilated intrahepatic or extrahepatic bile ducts should prompt direct visualization of the biliary tract by ERCP or PTC (Chapters 134 and 155). Evidence of an intrahepatic mass should prompt thorough evaluation for possible malignancy (Chapters 155 and 196). Because colon cancer often metastasizes to liver, colonoscopy may be useful in appropriate cases (Chapter 193). Infiltrative diseases, including amyloidosis and granulomatous hepatitis (Chapter 151), should be considered. In the absence of evidence of biliary obstruction or a cause identifiable by noninvasive means, liver biopsy should be strongly considered to complete the evaluation of cholestatic liver test abnormalities.

GENERAL REFERENCES

For the General References and other additional features, please visit Expert Consult at https://expertconsult.inkling.com.

148

ACUTE VIRAL HEPATITIS

JEAN-MICHEL PAWLOTSKY

Infection with a hepatotropic virus causes an acute episode of liver inflammation, referred to as *acute hepatitis,* which can lead to either spontaneous clearance of the infectious agent or its persistence, which in turn leads to chronic infection for a subset of these viruses. Five hepatitis viruses are responsible for the vast majority of acute hepatitis cases (Table 148-1): hepatitis A virus (HAV); hepatitis B virus (HBV); hepatitis C virus (HCV); hepatitis D, or delta, virus (HDV), which is a defective viroid using the hepatitis B surface antigen (HBsAg) as its envelope; and hepatitis E virus (HEV).[1] Other viruses may cause acute inflammatory liver disease, including members of the Herpesviridae family such as human cytomegalovirus, Epstein-Barr virus, or herpes simplex virus. It is unclear to what extent other viruses, such as parvovirus B19 or human herpesvirus 6, can also cause acute hepatitis. Patients who present with an acute viral hepatitis syndrome but negative virologic tests are referred to as having non-A-to-E hepatitis, perhaps attributable to hepatotropic viruses that have yet to be identified. The worldwide incidence of acute viral hepatitis is decreasing because of global improvement in hygiene and the development and use of efficient vaccines against HAV and HBV, and perhaps in the future, HEV.

TABLE 148-1 VIRUSES RESPONSIBLE FOR ACUTE VIRAL HEPATITIS AND LIKELIHOOD OF CHRONIC EVOLUTION

VIRUS	EVOLUTION TO CHRONIC VIRAL HEPATITIS
Hepatitis A	Never
Hepatitis B	>90% (perinatal acquisition) to < 1% (adult infection)
Hepatitis C	50-80%
Hepatitis D or delta	2% (coinfection) to 90% (superinfection)
Hepatitis E	Occasionally in immunosuppressed patients
Other viruses Human cytomegalovirus Epstein-Barr Herpes simplex Human herpesvirus 6 Parvovirus B_{19}	May establish chronic infection, not associated with chronic hepatitis

GENERAL FEATURES OF ACUTE VIRAL HEPATITIS

PATHOBIOLOGY

Acute viral hepatitis is characterized by acute necroinflammation of the liver. Because none of the hepatotropic viruses is cytopathic, liver injury is mediated by a strong cytotoxic T cell–mediated reaction against infected hepatocytes that express viral antigens at their surface. Proinflammatory cytokines, natural killer cells, and antibody-dependent cellular cytotoxicity also appear to play a role in liver necroinflammation. Successful immune elimination may lead to viral clearance, which may or may not be associated with lifelong immunity, depending on the infecting agent. The immune reaction is sometimes so potent that the patient develops subfulminant or even fulminant hepatitis that requires liver transplantation (Chapter 154). In some patients—the proportion varies, according to the virus responsible for acute hepatitis—the immune response fails and chronic infection is established (Chapter 149).

CLINICAL MANIFESTATIONS

After infection, there is an incubation period of a few days to a few weeks, depending on the causative agent (Fig. 148-1). This incubation period is generally characterized by nonspecific symptoms, including fatigue, nausea, loss of appetite, flulike symptoms, and/or right upper quadrant pain (Table 148-2). The incubation period is often characterized by leukopenia and relative lymphocytosis. Immune-mediated symptoms, including rash, hives, arthralgias, angioneurotic edema, and fever, are observed in 10 to 20% of patients during the preicteric phase.

During the acute stage of the disease, symptoms may vary widely, from asymptomatic to subicteric, icteric or severe, and fulminant. The icteric form, which is not frequent, is characterized by fatigue, anorexia, nausea, dysgeusia, jaundice, dark urine, light-colored stool, and weight loss. Physical examination reveals jaundice and hepatic tenderness. Hepatomegaly and splenomegaly may be present. On laboratory testing, acute viral hepatitis is characterized by elevated total and direct serum bilirubin levels and aminotransferase levels that are often greater than 10 times the upper limit of normal. Cholestatic acute hepatitis is associated frequently with prolonged and fluctuating jaundice and pruritus. After 1 to 3 weeks, on average, both clinical and laboratory signs progressively improve and return to normal. Some patients, however, may experience a relapse before definitive resolution.

Signs of hepatic failure (Chapter 154), including changes in personality, aggressive behavior, sleeping disorders, and hepatic encephalopathy

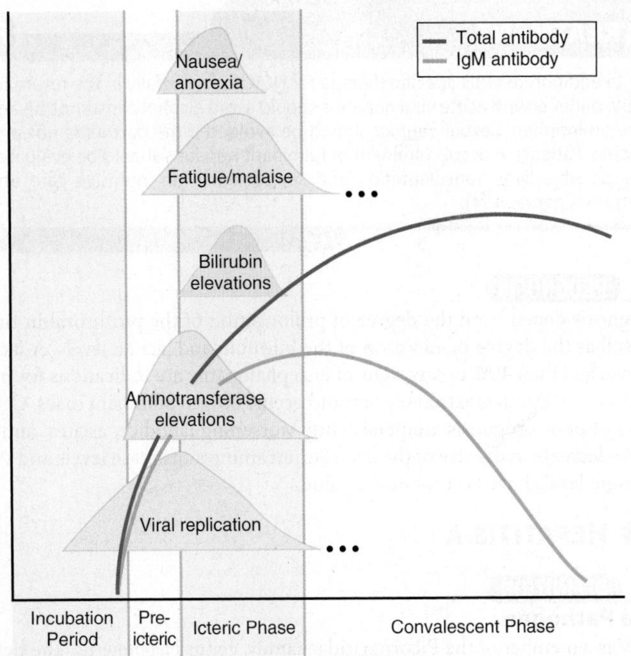

FIGURE 148-1. Typical course of acute viral hepatitis. IgM = immunoglobulin M.

TABLE 148-2 CLINICAL MANIFESTATIONS OF VIRAL HEPATITIS

PHASES OF INFECTION	DURATION*	MANIFESTATIONS*
Incubation	2-20 wk	Virus detectable in blood Aminotransferase and bilirubin levels normal No antibody detectable
Preicteric	3-10 days	Nonspecific symptoms: fatigue, anorexia, nausea, vague right upper quadrant pain Viral titers peak Aminotransferase levels begin to rise Serum sickness–like reaction (≈10-20% of cases) with rash, hives, arthralgias, fever
Icteric	1-3 wk	Jaundice appears; dark urine and light stools seen Nonspecific symptoms worsen Weight loss, dysgeusia, pruritus may occur Hepatosplenomegaly may develop Aminotransferase levels typically >10 times normal Antibodies appear Viral titers decline Rare extrahepatic manifestations (aseptic meningitis, encephalitis, seizures, ascending flaccid paralysis, nephrotic syndrome, seronegative arthritis)
Recovery	Up to 6 mo	Symptoms resolve gradually Antibody levels rise Aminotransferase and bilirubin levels normalize
Chronic	After 6 mo	See Chapter 149

*Varies by virus.

TABLE 148-3 LABORATORY TESTING FOR SUSPECTED ACUTE VIRAL HEPATITIS

GENERAL EVALUATION
Alanine aminotransferase
Aspartate aminotransferase
Alkaline phosphatase
International normalized ratio (INR)
FIRST-LINE DIAGNOSTIC TESTS
Anti-HAV IgM
HBsAg, anti-HBc IgM
Anti-HCV antibodies
HCV RNA
SECOND-LINE DIAGNOSTIC TESTS
Anti-HAV IgM present: none
HBsAg present: HBeAg, anti-HBe antibodies, HBV DNA, HDV antigen, anti-HDV antibodies
HCV RNA present with or without anti-HCV antibodies: none
No virologic marker: See Fig. 147-3

HAV = hepatitis A virus; HBc = hepatitis B core; HBeAg = hepatitis B e antigen; HBsAg = hepatitis B surface antigen; HBV = hepatitis B virus; HCV = hepatitis C virus; HDV = hepatitis D virus; IgM = immunoglobulin M.

characterize fulminant forms of acute viral hepatitis. Coma can supervene rapidly, and widespread hemorrhage may develop.

DIAGNOSIS

The diagnosis of acute hepatitis is suspected based on elevated serum aminotransferase levels, which are generally more than 10 times the upper limit of normal (Table 148-3). Total and direct bilirubin levels are elevated if the acute hepatitis is subicteric or icteric. Alkaline phosphatase levels may be elevated in cases of cholestatic hepatitis.

Serologic and eventually molecular testing identifies the causal agent. Liver biopsy or a noninvasive assessment of liver inflammation and fibrosis are generally not required. All cases of acute hepatitis should be reported to the local, state, or national health department as soon as possible after diagnosis.

TREATMENT

In addition to virus-specific therapy for HCV and hopefully in the future for HBV, patients with acute viral hepatitis should avoid alcohol consumption and acetaminophen. Sexual contact should be avoided if the partner is not protected. Patients with subfulminant or fulminant hepatitis should be evaluated for possible liver transplantation and supported in an intensive care unit setting (Chapter 154).

PROGNOSIS

Prognosis depends on the degree of prolongation of the prothrombin time, as well as the degree of elevation of the bilirubin and lactate levels. A factor V level less than 40% or any signs of encephalopathy are indications for hospitalization. Death is extremely rare and occurs only in fulminant cases. Other signs of poor prognosis are persistently worsening jaundice, ascites, and an acute decrease in the size of the liver. Serum aminotransferase levels and viral genome levels have no prognostic value.

HEPATITIS A

DEFINITION

The Pathogen

HAV is a member of the Picornaviridae family, genus *Hepatovirus*. The hepatitis A viral particle is a 27-nm nonenveloped icosahedral nucleocapsid that expresses the hepatitis A antigen and contains a positive-stranded RNA genome approximately 7.5 kb long. At least four different HAV genotypes have been described in humans (genotypes I, II, III, and VII), with genotype I predominating worldwide. Other genotypes have been isolated in nonhuman primates. It is currently unclear to what extent different genotypes are associated with distinct clinical courses of infection.

EPIDEMIOLOGY

HAV infection has a worldwide distribution, and infections can be sporadic or occur in epidemic outbreaks. The incidence of acute cases and the seroprevalence vary according to the hygiene, sanitation, housing, and socioeconomic standards of the region, with seroprevalences as low as approximately 13% in Sweden but up to 100% in many developing countries. In developing countries, infection generally occurs at a young age and most of the population has been exposed and is protected after age 10 years. In developed countries, however, infection can occur at any age, and the prevalence of exposed, immune subjects slowly increases with age. In the United States, according to the Centers for Disease Control and Prevention, the incidence of acute hepatitis A declined from 12.0 cases per 100,000 individuals in 1995 to 0.5 cases per 100,000 individuals by 2012.

HAV is generally transmitted via the oral-fecal route, most often directly from person to person or through the ingestion of fecally contaminated food or water. Transmission by blood transfusion has been reported, and isolated cases of apparent perinatal transmission have been described. High-risk groups for acute hepatitis A include travelers to developing countries, children in daycare centers and their parents, men who have sex with men, injection drug users, hemophiliacs who receive plasma products, and persons in institutions.

PATHOBIOLOGY

The genome serves as a messenger RNA and contains a single open reading frame that encodes both structural and nonstructural viral proteins. After attachment to a specific receptor at the surface of hepatocytes, the virus penetrates into cells and is uncoated. Subsequent events occurring exclusively in the cytoplasm include translation of the single open reading frame into a polyprotein that is later processed to generate the mature viral proteins; replication in a membrane-bound replication complex that generates new viral genomes, which are subsequently used for viral protein production and viral particle assembly; and packaging of newly formed genomes into new particles that are exported out of the cells. The virus is secreted into bile and, to a lesser extent, serum.

CLINICAL MANIFESTATIONS

Typically, the incubation period is 15 to 45 days (see Table 148-2). In most cases, acute infection takes a mild and often unrecognized course. The incidence of symptomatic, icteric cases increases with the age at infection. Acute hepatitis A in adults may require hospitalization in up to 13% of cases[2]; prolonged courses of 6 to 9 months have been reported in 10% of adult patients with a diagnosis of acute hepatitis A. Hepatitis A is the most common cause of relapsing cholestatic hepatitis.

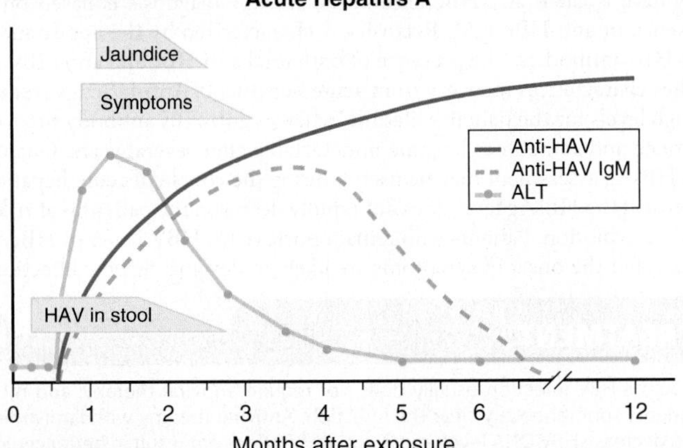

FIGURE 148-2. Serologic course of acute hepatitis A. ALT = alanine aminotransferase; HAV = hepatitis A virus; IgM = immunoglobulin M.

DIAGNOSIS

The diagnosis of acute hepatitis A is based on the detection of anti-HAV immunoglobulin M (IgM) in serum by enzyme immunoassay. IgM serum levels peak during the second month of infection (Fig. 148-2). HAV RNA can be transiently detected in stool and other body fluids by polymerase chain reaction (PCR) 3 to 10 days before the onset of illness and for 1 to 2 weeks thereafter; however, HAV RNA testing is generally not necessary. When the infection resolves, anti-HAV IgM disappears after 4 to 12 months, but anti-HAV IgG persists for life and confers definitive and durable protection against infection.

TREATMENT Rx

Because HAV infection is self-limited, no specific antiviral treatment is required. In severe cases, patients may need to be hospitalized. If liver function is deteriorating, patients may need to be assessed for liver transplantation, which is the only therapeutic option for acute liver failure (Chapter 154).

PREVENTION

HAV vaccines (Chapter 18) consist of inactivated hepatitis A antigen purified from cell culture. Two doses of the vaccine are recommended at a 6- to 18-month interval. All vaccines are highly immunogenic, and virtually all healthy persons who are vaccinated develop protective anti-HAV antibodies. Patients with chronic liver disease also respond to vaccination but may display lower anti-HAV titers. An accelerated vaccine schedule, with vaccination on days 0, 7, and 21, is also effective and may be recommended for those planning to travel to endemic areas. HAV vaccines are well tolerated, and no serious adverse events have been linked with their administration; they can be safely administered with other vaccines or immunoglobulins without compromising the development of protective antibodies. A combination HAV and HBV vaccine is also available. Seroconversion rates are lower in patients with human immunodeficiency virus (HIV) infection and in other immunocompromised individuals.

HAV vaccination is recommended for nonimmune individuals who plan to travel to endemic countries, medical health professionals, men who have sex with men, persons who are in contact with hepatitis A patients, and individuals with chronic liver diseases. A childhood vaccination program leads to a significant decline in HAV infection, justifying its use as part of control efforts in endemic countries. Serologic testing for anti-HAV IgG can be performed before vaccination in adults born in endemic countries and in individuals older than 50 years born in industrialized areas; persons with detectable IgG are protected and should not be vaccinated. For post-exposure prophylaxis, both HAV vaccination and immunoglobulin are effective. Immunoglobulin confers a slightly lower rate of protection than vaccine, and HAV vaccine and immunoglobulin should be used together in this setting.

Long-term follow-up studies after complete HAV vaccination show that anti-HAV titers sharply decline during the first year after vaccination but remain detectable in almost all individuals for at least 10 years. Protective anti-HAV antibody titers persist for at least 27 years after the successful vaccination of children and young adults.

PROGNOSIS

Acute hepatitis A infection generally resolves without complications in 3 to 4 weeks and never evolves to chronic infection. Prolonged elevation of serum aminotransferase levels has been reported. Relapses a few weeks after the acute case also have been observed. Prolonged courses may occur in children and immunosuppressed individuals.

Cholestatic hepatitis A is unusual and has a good prognosis, with full recovery within a few weeks. Fulminant hepatitis A is rare, occurring in less than 0.1% of cases, but its incidence and mortality increase with the patient's age at acquisition. In the United States, 4% of all cases of fulminant hepatitis are caused by HAV infection. Overall, mortality of acute hepatitis A is 1.8% in patients older than 50 years. In patients with chronic hepatitis B, superinfection with HAV is associated with a 6- to 23-fold higher morbidity and mortality.

ACUTE HEPATITIS B

DEFINITION

The Pathogen

HBV is a member of the Hepadnaviridae family, genus *Hepadnavirus*. The infectious virion, the Dane particle, is 42 to 47 nm in diameter. It possesses an envelope and a capsid or core that contains the partially double-stranded, circular DNA genome. The HBV genome is the smallest known human virus genome, with approximately 3000 nucleotides.

EPIDEMIOLOGY

Two billion individuals worldwide have been in contact with HBV, and more than 350 million individuals have chronic infection. In the United States, approximately 0.5% of the population is chronically infected. HBV virions are produced and circulate in very high amounts in HBV-infected individuals, who are highly contagious. Four principal routes of transmission are responsible for acute HBV infections: (1) sexual transmission, which is the principal route in industrialized areas; (2) perinatal mother-to-infant transmission, which is associated with a very high (>90%) rate of chronic infection and is the principal cause of HBV transmission in Asia; (3) horizontal transmission through nonsexual interindividual contact, which is frequent at a young age in Africa and is associated with evolution to chronicity in approximately 15% of cases; and (4) percutaneous transmission by blood and blood products, unsafe medical or surgical materials, or injection drug use.

In industrialized countries, groups at high risk for HBV infection include individuals born in areas where HBV is endemic, including immigrants and adopted children; individuals who were not vaccinated as infants and whose parents were born in regions where HBV is endemic; household and sexual contacts of HBsAg-positive individuals; persons who have ever injected drugs; persons with multiple sexual partners or a history of sexually transmitted disease; men who have sex with men; inmates of correctional facilities; patients infected with HCV or HIV; patients undergoing renal dialysis; recipients of blood or blood products before 1987; and health care workers.

PATHOBIOLOGY

The HBV genome contains at least four overlapping open reading frames that encode a number of structural and nonstructural viral proteins. The pre-S/S gene encodes the three surface proteins—small (S), middle (M), and large (L)—that express HBsAg. The pre-C/C gene encodes the core protein that expresses the hepatitis B core (HBc) antigen and the hepatitis B e (HBe) protein, a nonstructural protein that plays a role in immune tolerance to HBV replication. The P gene encodes the HBV polymerase, whose two motifs—a reverse transcriptase motif and an RNAse H motif—code for two enzymes involved in HBV replication. Finally, the X gene encodes the X protein, which is a transactivator involved in HBV replication that bears oncogenic properties. The blood of infected patients contains not only infectious viruses but also a large excess of empty, noninfectious HBV envelopes.

The complex HBV life cycle involves multiple steps: fixation to an as yet unidentified receptor complex at the surface of hepatocytes; internalization; fusion and release of the nucleocapsid containing the HBV DNA genome and the associated HBV polymerase molecule in the cell cytoplasm; transport into the nucleus, where decapsidation occurs and the DNA genome molecule is released; transformation of the viral genome by the viral polymerase into a covalently closed circular DNA, which is the episomal form responsible for persistence of the HBV genome in the nucleus of infected hepatocytes; generation of messenger RNAs and viral protein synthesis; generation of a pregenomic RNA, which serves as a template for reverse transcription that generates the long DNA strand; degradation of the pregenomic RNA by the RNAse H activity of the viral polymerase; DNA-dependent DNA polymerase activity of the reverse transcriptase motif, which synthesizes the short complementary DNA strand in newly formed nucleocapsids; and, finally, budding into the endoplasmic reticulum, maturation, and export of newly formed virions.

Nine HBV genotypes (A through I), which differ by approximately 8% of their genomic nucleotide sequence, have different geographic distributions and may be associated with different clinical outcomes. Genotype A predominates in Northern and Western Europe, whereas genotype D is the most frequent genotype in the Mediterranean area and in Eastern Europe. In non-Asian populations in the United States, genotype A predominates in men who have sex with men, whereas genotype D is the most frequent in intravenous drug users. In Asia and in Asian immigrants living in industrialized countries, genotypes B and C predominate. Genotype C has been associated with a higher incidence of severe liver disease and hepatocellular carcinoma compared with genotype B in Asia, perhaps because this genotype spread earlier than the others.

CLINICAL MANIFESTATIONS

Typically, the incubation period is 30 to 150 days. Jaundice has been reported in up to one third of adult patients with acute hepatitis B, but most cases are unrecognized.[3] Among symptomatic patients (see Table 148-2), the manifestations are similar to those of other causes of acute viral hepatitis.

DIAGNOSIS

Four markers should be sought for the diagnosis of acute hepatitis B: HBsAg, total anti-HBc antibodies, anti-HBc IgM, and anti-HBs antibodies (Table 148-4). Acute hepatitis B is characterized by the simultaneous presence of both HBsAg and anti-HBc IgM (Fig. 148-3). Total anti-HBc antibodies are also present, whereas anti-HBs antibodies are not. During the convalescence phase, patients lose HBsAg before the appearance of anti-HBs antibodies; they have isolated anti-HBc antibodies, and the diagnosis is based on the presence of anti-HBc IgM. Recovery is characterized by the appearance of anti-HBs antibodies. The presence of both total anti-HBc and anti-HBs antibodies characterizes recovery from acute hepatitis B. Anti-HBc IgG remains at high levels for the patient's lifetime, whereas anti-HBs antibody titers may fluctuate and sometimes become undetectable after several years. Quantitative HBsAg assessment may be useful during the course of acute hepatitis B because if the HBsAg level does not rapidly decrease, the patient is at risk for chronic evolution. Patients who remain positive for HBV DNA or HBeAg 6 weeks after the onset of symptoms are likely to develop chronic infection.

TABLE 148-4 SEROLOGIC PROFILES OBSERVED IN DIFFERENT PHASES OF ACUTE, SELF-RESOLVING HEPATITIS B

PHASE OF INFECTION	HBsAg	ANTI-HBc IgM	TOTAL ANTI-HBc ANTIBODIES	ANTI-HBs ANTIBODIES
Incubation	+	+/−	+/−	−
Acute hepatitis	+	+	+	−
Convalescence	−	+	+	−
Recovery	−	−	+	+

HBc = hepatitis B core; HBs = hepatitis B surface; HBsAg = hepatitis B surface antigen; IgM = immunoglobulin M.

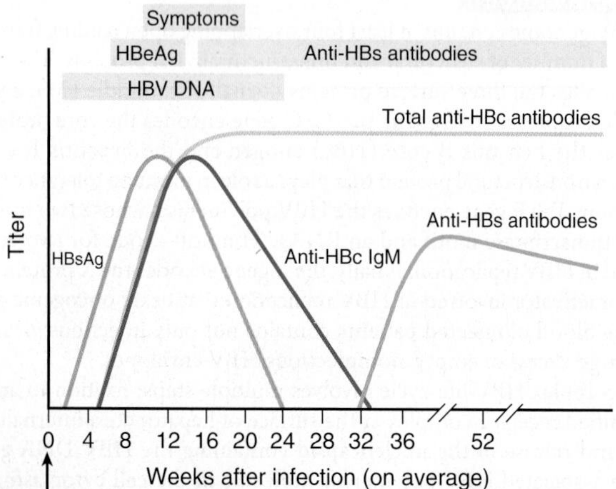

FIGURE 148-3. Kinetics of hepatitis B virus (HBV) markers during acute self-resolving hepatitis B. The *arrow* indicates infection. HBc = hepatitis B core; HBeAg = hepatitis B e antigen; HBs = hepatitis B surface; HBsAg = hepatitis B surface antigen; IgM = immunoglobulin M.

TREATMENT (Rx)

Acute HBV infection usually does not require antiviral therapy, and most patients spontaneously clear the infection. Antiviral therapy with lamivudine can decrease HBV DNA levels more rapidly but does not result in better clinical or biochemical improvement and may be associated with lower levels of protective anti-HBs at 1 year.[A2] In a small randomized trial of patients with severe but nonfulminant acute hepatitis B, lamivudine (100 mg daily) led to more rapid viral clearance but no difference in clinical outcomes.[A3] Nevertheless, nonrandomized data suggest that early antiviral therapy is safe and may reduce the need for liver transplantation in patients with fulminant hepatitis B. Although most of the experience has been with lamivudine (100 mg daily), more potent drugs with no risk for HBV resistance selection, such as tenofovir 300 mg daily or entecavir 0.5 mg daily, are recommended in this setting.[4]

PREVENTION

Because not everyone has been vaccinated, individuals who are aware that they are infected with HBV should take steps to avoid transmitting the infection to others. This is accomplished by ensuring that their sexual contacts and household members are vaccinated; using barrier protection during sexual intercourse; not sharing instruments such as toothbrushes, razors, and combs; cleaning blood spills with detergent or bleach; and not donating blood, organs, or sperm.

Prevention of HBV infection is based on vaccination. Universal infant vaccination programs have been initiated in many countries. High-risk individuals (e.g., health care workers, dialysis patients, family members and sexual partners of HBV carriers, pregnant women, and men who have sex with men) should be screened for HBV infection by HBsAg and anti-HBs antibody testing, and seronegative persons should be vaccinated.[5]

Vaccination consists of the administration of recombinant HBsAg in three injections at 0, 1, and 6 months in adults. A lower dose is given at the same time points in newborns, children, and adolescents. Adults on dialysis require four injections at months 0, 1, 2, and 6. HBV vaccination elicits a potent neutralizing response, characterized by the presence of anti-HBs antibodies at high titers. A titer greater than 10 U/L is considered protective. The seroconversion rate is higher than 90% in healthy individuals. HBV vaccines are well tolerated. Injection site reactions within 1 to 3 days, as well as mild general reactions, are common and transient. Postvaccination testing for anti-HBs antibodies to document seroconversion is not routinely recommended. However, persons who remain at risk for HBV infection, such as infants of HBsAg-positive mothers, health care workers, dialysis patients, and sexual partners of HBV carriers, should be tested to determine their response to vaccination.

Of vaccinated persons, 3 to 10% respond poorly or do not respond, especially smokers, obese patients, and elderly individuals. Nonresponders should receive another full course of vaccination, often with an increased dose. Other options include intradermal application and the coadministration of adjuvants and cytokines. One third to two thirds of vaccinated individuals lose their anti-HBs antibodies after 10 to 15 years. It is unclear whether these persons are still protected. Thus, persons at risk should receive booster immunization if anti-HBs antibodies have been lost.

When nonimmune persons or vaccinated individuals with an anti-HBs titer below 10 IU/L have contact with HBV-contaminated materials (e.g., needles) or have sexual intercourse with an HBV-infected person, active-passive immunization (i.e., infusion of hepatitis B immunoglobulin) plus active immunization (vaccination) is recommended within 48 hours after exposure. Vaccination alone is sufficient in persons with anti-HBs antibody titers between 10 and 100 IU/L, and no action is required if the anti-HBs titer is above 100 IU/L.

Infants born to HBsAg-positive mothers must receive hepatitis B immunoglobulin and be vaccinated within 12 hours of birth; this regimen reduces the rate of vertical HBV transmission from 95% to less than 5%. Mothers with

HBV DNA levels above 5×10^7 IU/mL should also be treated during pregnancy with a potent nucleoside/nucleotide analogue with no teratogenic risk; the safest and most potent drug in this setting is tenofovir. Cesarean section is not needed if active-passive immunization is to be performed. Mothers of vaccinated infants can breast-feed, unless oral antiviral medications are present in the breast milk.

PROGNOSIS

Fulminant hepatitis is more frequent in acute HBV infection than in other types of acute viral hepatitis, with an incidence of approximately 0.1%. Factors associated with adverse outcomes of acute hepatitis B include advanced age, female sex, and perhaps some strains of virus. Whether infection with a precore mutant strain is associated with more severe or fulminant disease is still debated.

Among patients infected at birth, the rate of spontaneous recovery after an acute HBV infection is less than 5%, whereas adult infections spontaneously resolve in 95 to 99% of cases. Spontaneous resolution confers lifelong immunity, which is usually characterized by the presence of anti-HBs antibodies. Anti-HBs antibodies may become undetectable several years after resolution, but patients rapidly produce protective antibodies if they are re-exposed to HBV.

ACUTE HEPATITIS C

DEFINITION

The Pathogen

HCV is a member of the Flaviviridae family, genus *Hepacivirus*. The genome is a single-stranded, positive, linear RNA molecule whose 5′ end contains an internal ribosome entry site involved in polyprotein translation; the genome also includes one single open reading frame and a short 3′ noncoding region involved in replication. The genome is contained in a protein capsid or core, which itself is surrounded by a lipid bilayer envelope into which two inserted viral glycoproteins mediate attachment of the viral particle to receptor molecules at the surface of target cells.

EPIDEMIOLOGY

HCV is present in all continents, and an estimated 170 million individuals are chronically infected. In industrialized countries, the incidence of HCV infection has declined considerably owing to blood screening and measures to prevent viral infections in intravenous drug users. However, approximately 17,000 new cases of acute hepatitis C still occur annually in the United States according to the Centers for Disease Control and Prevention. In France, approximately 2500 new infections occur each year. HCV incidence and prevalence are higher in developing areas of the world, where the main route of HCV infection is unsafe medical or surgical procedures; only approximately 50% of blood products are screened for anti-HCV antibodies in these countries, and approximately 40% of all injections are given with reused equipment. Egypt's estimated 9% prevalence is the highest worldwide, owing to unsafe injection campaigns for the treatment of schistosomiasis. Although the incidence of acute hepatitis C has declined in Egypt during the past 15 years, up to 10% of cases of acute hepatitis are still caused by HCV.

HCV is transmitted almost exclusively by infected blood. Preventive screening with highly sensitive enzyme immunoassays and, more recently, nucleic acid testing has virtually eliminated the risk for post-transfusional HCV infection (theoretical risk: 1 in 2 million donations in the United States, 1 in 8 million donations in France). As a result, the principal route for HCV transmission in industrialized countries is now intravenous drug use, which is responsible for 60 to 80% of new cases. The incidence of HCV infection in this high-risk group is as high as 39 per 100 person years. In this context, imprisonment is an important risk factor for acquiring HCV infection in industrialized countries.

Nosocomial transmission through the use of improperly decontaminated materials or the contaminated hands or gloves of health care workers is responsible for a substantial number of new infections worldwide. HCV also can be transmitted by tattooing, piercing, or acupuncture if standard precautions are not implemented. Although HCV can be acquired after accidental needlestick exposure, the risk for infection is low (<1%), and health care workers have only a slightly higher prevalence of HCV than the general population. HCV can be transmitted to household members who share instruments such as scissors, razors, and combs. Sexual transmission is unusual, but outbreaks of acute hepatitis have been reported in HIV-positive communities of men who have sex with men. The risk for mother-to-infant transmission of HCV is less than 5% and is generally related to exposure to the mother's blood in the perinatal period. Cesarean sections are not recommended, and breast-feeding is not contraindicated. The risk for perinatal transmission is higher when the mother is coinfected with HIV. Other factors possibly associated with high transmission rates include the level of HCV viremia and maternal intravenous drug abuse. In 10 to 30% of cases, no apparent risk factor for HCV infection is identifiable, suggesting other potential sources of community-acquired hepatitis C.

PATHOBIOLOGY

Entry of HCV into cells is followed by fusion. Decapsidation of viral nucleocapsids liberates free genomic RNAs into the cell cytoplasm, where they serve, together with newly synthesized RNAs, as messenger RNAs for synthesis of the HCV polyprotein. The post-translational processing of the HCV polyprotein results in the generation of at least 10 proteins, including 3 structural proteins (the core protein and the two envelope glycoproteins) and 7 nonstructural proteins. HCV replication takes place in the replication complex that associates viral proteins, cellular components, and nascent RNA strands. It is catalyzed by the RNA-dependent RNA polymerase. Viral particle formation is initiated by the interaction of the core protein with genomic RNA. Newly produced virus particles leave the host cell via constitutive secretory pathways.

Phylogenetic analyses of HCV strains isolated in various regions of the world have identified seven main HCV genotypes, designated 1 through 7. These HCV types comprise a large number of subtypes, identified by lowercase letters (1a, 1b, etc.). The genotypes' nucleotide sequences differ by 31 to 34%, and their amino acid sequences differ by approximately 30%; in contrast, the subtypes' nucleotide sequences differ by between 20 and 23%, with marked differences in particular genomic regions. The high prevalence and diversity of HCV genotype 3 and 6 strains in Asia and of genotype 1, 2, 4 and 5 strains in Africa suggest that these types and subtypes emerged and diversified in these regions. In industrialized countries, a small number of HCV genotypes, including 1a, 1b, 2a, 2b, 2c, 3a, and 4a, have been introduced and spread rapidly among exposed populations. Subtypes 1a and 1b predominate all over the world. The most common genotypes in the United States are 1a and 1b (~75%), 2a and 2b (~15%), and 3a (~7%). Genotype 3a is more prevalent in Western Europe, where it accounts for up to 35% of cases, especially among intravenous drug users. Genotype 4 is highly prevalent in the Middle East and Africa. Its incidence and prevalence are increasing in intravenous drug users in industrialized countries. Genotype 5 is rare outside South Africa, and genotype 6 is rare outside Southeast Asia. Infections with different genotypes do not differ in terms of the clinical manifestations, progression, or disease severity (although this is debated), but the HCV genotype is an important determinant of the response to interferon-α–based therapies.

CLINICAL MANIFESTATIONS

HCV RNA becomes detectable in the serum 3 to 7 days after exposure. HCV RNA levels rise rapidly during the first weeks, followed by serum aminotransferase levels 2 to 8 weeks after exposure. Anti-HCV antibodies arise late in the course of acute hepatitis C and may not be present at the onset of symptoms and serum aminotransferase elevation.

After an incubation period that ranges from 15 to 120 days, acute hepatitis C usually remains asymptomatic and is undiagnosed.[6] Nonspecific symptoms such as fatigue, low-grade fever, myalgias, nausea, vomiting, or itching may be present. Jaundice occurs in only 20 to 30% of patients, usually 2 to 12 weeks after infection. Serum aminotransferase levels commonly exceed 10 times the upper limit of normal in the acute stage, even in the absence of symptoms. Fulminant hepatitis C has been reported but appears to be exceptional in the absence of another chronic underlying liver disease.

DIAGNOSIS

When acute hepatitis C is suspected, patients should be tested for both anti-HCV antibodies by enzyme immunoassay and HCV RNA with a sensitive molecular biology technique (i.e., an HCV RNA assay with a lower limit of detection of ≤ 50 IU/mL). Four marker profiles can be observed, based on the presence or absence of either marker (Table 148-5). The presence of HCV RNA in the absence of anti-HCV antibodies is strongly indicative of acute HCV infection, which will be confirmed by seroconversion (i.e., the appearance of anti-HCV antibodies) a few days to weeks later. Acutely infected patients can have both HCV RNA and anti-HCV antibodies at the time of diagnosis; in this case, it is difficult to distinguish acute hepatitis C from an acute exacerbation of chronic hepatitis C or acute hepatitis of another cause in a patient with chronic hepatitis C.

TABLE 148-5 PATTERNS OF HEPATITIS C VIRUS (HCV) MARKERS AND THEIR SIGNIFICANCE DURING ACUTE HEPATITIS C

ANTI-HCV ANTIBODIES	HCV RNA	DIAGNOSIS
−	−	Not acute hepatitis C
−	+	Acute hepatitis C
+	−	Probably not acute hepatitis C (retest in a few weeks)
+	+	Difficult to differentiate acute from chronic hepatitis C

HCV = hepatitis C virus.

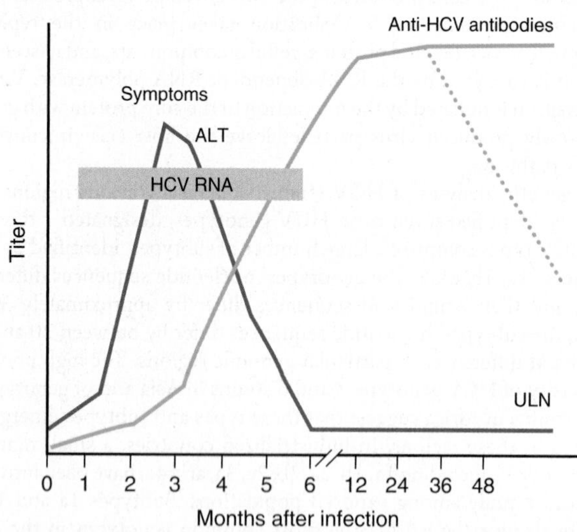

FIGURE 148-4. Kinetics of hepatitis C virus (HCV) markers during acute self-resolving hepatitis C. ALT = alanine aminotransferase; ULN = upper limit of normal.

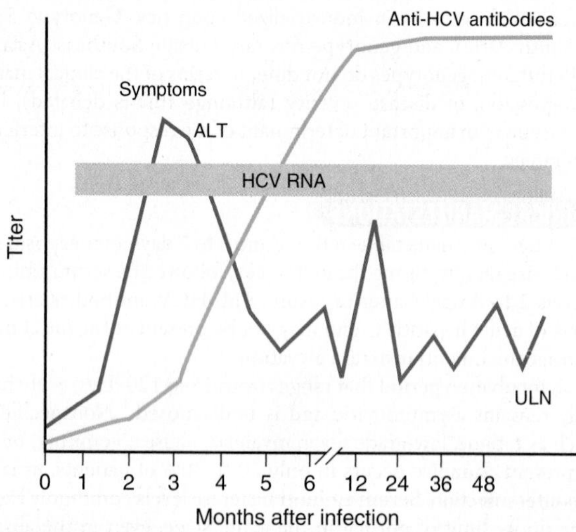

FIGURE 148-5. Kinetics of hepatitis C virus (HCV) markers during acute hepatitis C that evolves toward chronic infection. ALT = alanine aminotransferase; ULN = upper limit of normal.

Acute hepatitis C is very unlikely if both anti-HCV antibodies and HCV RNA are absent or if anti-HCV antibodies are present without HCV RNA (Fig. 148-4). Patients in the latter group should be retested in a few weeks, however, because HCV RNA may be temporarily undetectable owing to transient, partial control of viral replication before the infection becomes chronic (Fig. 148-5). Apart from such cases, the presence of anti-HCV antibodies in the absence of HCV RNA is generally seen in patients who have recovered from a past HCV infection. Nevertheless, this pattern cannot be differentiated from a false-positive enzyme immunoassay result, the exact prevalence of which is unknown.

TREATMENT Rx

Treatment of acute hepatitis C should be considered not only because it prevents chronic HCV infection, which can lead to serious clinical sequelae, but also because HCV viremia, which is associated with a risk for transmitting HCV to other persons, may have social, legal, and economic consequences, especially for infected health care workers. Classically, treatment of acute hepatitis C is based on the use of pegylated interferon-α2a or interferon-α2b at doses of 180 µg/week or 1.5 µg/kg/week, respectively.[A4] Treatment is usually administered for 24 weeks, but 12 weeks is probably sufficient in most patients, especially patients with baseline parameters that predict a rapid viral clearance, such as symptomatic disease, high alanine aminotransferase levels, and low HCV RNA levels.[A5] Ribavirin should be added in patients who have a delayed or slow HCV RNA decrease with treatment, genotype 1 infection, low or normal baseline alanine aminotransferase levels, or a combination of these. With this treatment, 70% to more than 90% of patients have sustained viral clearance. Although delaying treatment can avoid the side effects of treatment in the 20 to 50% of patients who will spontaneously clear the virus, immediate treatment provides higher rates of viral clearance, mostly because asymptomatic patients tend to be less adherent with the close following needed to monitor patients for the institution of appropriately timed delayed therapy.[A6]

If treatment fails to clear the virus, patients can be re-treated with a combination of pegylated interferon-α2a (180 µg/week) or interferon-α2b (1.5 µg/kg/week) and ribavirin (0.8 g/day) for 48 weeks. No randomized data are available for new anti-HCV drugs. However, given its efficacy in patients with chronic hepatitis C, the oral combination of sofosbuvir 400 mg daily and ribavirin (1 or 1.2 g/day according to body weight less or more than 75 kg) for 24 weeks can be used to treat acute hepatitis C. More data will be generated soon with other antiviral drug combinations without ribavirin.

After accidental needlestick exposure, neither immunoglobulin nor preemptive therapy is recommended. Patients should be monitored with HCV RNA and aminotransferase level testing at baseline, week 2, and 4 and 6 months after exposure. Patients who have documented infection should be treated as described earlier.

PREVENTION

Prevention of HCV transmission is based on standard precautions such as screening of blood and blood products, application of standard medical and surgical hygiene procedures, and safe use of syringes and materials for drug preparation in drug users. Needle exchange programs and education regarding the risks of drug use (including intranasal cocaine) and the risk for transmission from shared injection equipment are important.

No prophylactic vaccine is or will soon be available against HCV.

PROGNOSIS

Approximately 50 to 80% of patients are unable to clear HCV spontaneously and develop chronic infection.[7] Spontaneous recovery is more frequent if infection is acquired at birth (~50%) and if acute hepatitis is symptomatic. It is unclear whether the genotype influences recovery rates. Other factors associated with better rates of spontaneous recovery include female sex, early decline of HCV RNA levels, and high aminotransferase or bilirubin levels. Patients who spontaneously recover may retain detectable anti-HCV antibodies for years to decades, but they are not protected against HCV reinfection.

ACUTE HEPATITIS D OR DELTA

DEFINITION

The Pathogen

HDV, which is a satellite of HBV, can be transmitted only to patients who are acutely or chronically infected with HBV. Its single, negative-strand, circular RNA genome of approximately 1700 nucleotides folds in native conditions into a nearly complementary rodlike structure that contains a ribozyme. The HDV genome encodes one single structural protein, the hepatitis D (HD) protein, which expresses HDAg. The 36-nm infectious HDV virion comprises the HD protein and the genome, both enclosed within an HBsAg coat derived from empty HBV envelopes.

EPIDEMIOLOGY

Five percent of chronic HBV carriers, or 15 million to 20 million individuals worldwide, are also infected with HDV. The prevalence of HDV infection in

HBV-infected patients varies according to the geographic area because it is transmitted primarily through parenteral exposure. As a result, its prevalence is relatively higher in HBsAg-positive intravenous drug users in Western countries, where approximately 8 to 12% of HBsAg-positive patients are infected with HDV. By comparison, the prevalence of HDV has decreased substantially in southern Europe, probably owing to universal HBV vaccination programs, improvement in hygiene and living conditions, and implementation of standard precautions to prevent HIV infection. The incidence of HDV is increasing in Russia, Eastern Europe, Japan, and India.

PATHOBIOLOGY

HDV uses host RNA polymerase II for its replication, following the rolling circle model. Within cells, HDV RNA is associated with multiple copies of the HD protein to form a ribonucleoprotein complex. This complex is exported by the HBV envelope, which contains the three HBV envelope proteins, into the Golgi apparatus before being secreted.

HDV has at least eight genotypes, which differ from one another by at least 15% of their nucleotide sequences. Genotype I is the most prevalent HDV worldwide. Additional genotypes have recently been identified in Africa.

CLINICAL MANIFESTATIONS

HDV can be acquired at the same time as HBV (coinfection) or by a chronic HBsAg carrier (superinfection).[8] Coinfection is characterized by one or two episodes of acute hepatitis, depending on the respective amounts of HBV and HDV present in the inoculum; acute hepatitis can range from mild to fulminant. In contrast, when chronic HBV carriers are superinfected by HDV, acute hepatitis D is generally severe, often fulminant, and generally becomes chronic.

DIAGNOSIS

Three markers of HDV infection are total anti-HD antibodies, anti-HD IgM, and HDV RNA; the latter can be detected and quantified by real-time PCR. All HBsAg-positive patients should be tested.

In patients with an HBV-HDV coinfection, HDV RNA is only transiently present and is often missed. Anti-HBc IgM indicates concomitant acute HBV infection.

In HDV superinfection of a chronic HBsAg carrier, no anti-HBc IgM is present. HDV RNA is found in serum or plasma before and during the acute episode, whereas both total anti-HD antibodies and anti-HD IgM are present during the acute phase. Both serologic markers remain at high levels if the disease becomes chronic.

TREATMENT Rx

No treatments are of proven benefit for acute hepatitis D.[9]

PREVENTION

The most effective means of preventing HDV infection is HBV vaccination, because individuals who are protected against HBV cannot be infected with HDV. In chronic HBsAg carriers, standard hygiene and behavioral precautions should be practiced to avoid superinfection with HDV.

PROGNOSIS

In patients who are acutely coinfected with HBV and HDV, only approximately 2% become chronic HDV carriers. In contrast, when HDV infection is acquired by chronic HBV carriers, approximately 90% also become chronic carriers of HDV.

ACUTE HEPATITIS E

DEFINITION

The Pathogen

HEV is a member of the genus *Hepevirus* in the Hepeviridae family. HEV is a small, nonenveloped virus. Its genome is a positive sense, single-stranded RNA molecule. Five HEV genotypes have been described: genotypes 1 and 2 appear to be strictly human, whereas genotypes 3 and 4 appear to be of swine origin but can also infect humans.

PATHOBIOLOGY AND EPIDEMIOLOGY

HEV transmission is principally oral-fecal. HEV is endemic in most developing areas of the world, where acute infections are sporadic or occur during large epidemics related to the contamination of drinking water. Genotype 1 has been found principally in Asia and North Africa, whereas genotype 2 has been isolated in cases from Central America and Western Africa. No animal reservoir is known for these genotypes, and transmission appears to be linked to the contamination of food or drinking water. In industrialized countries, HEV genotypes 1 and 2 are not present. HEV genotypes 3 and 4 are endemic in swine, and zoonotic transmission appears to be the main route of transmission in Europe, the United States, and Asia. Diagnosed cases of acute hepatitis E have increased constantly in Western Europe and North America in recent years, and high HEV seroprevalences have been described in special at-risk populations, such as butchers or farmers. Transmission may be favored by the consumption of uncooked meat and direct contact with infected animals. It is now thought to be the most common cause of acute viral hepatitis worldwide.[10]

CLINICAL MANIFESTATIONS

The incubation period is 3 to 8 weeks. HEV infection causes only mild, nonspecific symptoms in the majority of cases, especially if the infection is acquired early in life. Immunocompetent individuals clear the virus spontaneously.[11] The peak of viremia occurs early during infection, whereas the peak of aminotransferase activity is reached approximately 6 weeks after infection. Severe disease is more frequent in pregnant women and in patients with underlying chronic liver disease, who may rarely progress to fulminant hepatic failure. In one European report, 5% of patients with Guillain-Barré syndrome (Chapter 420) had a preceding acute hepatitis E infection.[12]

DIAGNOSIS

Patients with otherwise unexplained acute hepatitis should be tested for hepatitis E. Diagnosis of acute hepatitis E is based on the detection of anti-HEV IgM antibodies, which appear within 6 weeks and persist for 3 to 12 months. Unfortunately, current assays lack sensitivity and specificity, and none are yet approved by the U.S. Food and Drug Administration. HEV RNA also can be detected in feces, serum, or plasma, where its presence is transient. Anti-HEV IgG generally persists for life after acute infection.

TREATMENT Rx

Treatment of acute hepatitis E is not recommended because the vast majority of patients recover spontaneously.[13] Severe and fulminant cases should be referred to specialized units, where ribavirin monotherapy can be successful.

PREVENTION

Improved public hygiene is the best defense against hepatitis E in developing countries. Travelers to areas of the world where HEV is endemic, particularly pregnant women, should be cautioned about drinking the water and eating uncooked food. An efficient prophylactic vaccine based on recombinant HEV proteins was 100% effective in a phase 3 trial[A7] and a hepatitis E vaccine is approved in China. However, the duration of protection is unclear, so the vaccine's efficacy in preventing the spread of HEV has yet to be determined.

PROGNOSIS

Acute cases can be severe in elderly patients, and fulminant cases are frequent among pregnant women who are infected during large-scale waterborne epidemics. Overall case fatality rates range from zero to 10%, and less than 1% of fatal cases of acute hepatitis in the United States are attributed to hepatitis E. HEV genotypes 3 and 4 are less virulent than genotypes 1 and 2. Sporadic cases in industrialized areas are generally benign. HEV does not commonly evolve into chronic infection, but immunosuppressed patients and HIV-positive individuals can become chronic carriers.

OTHER TYPES OF ACUTE VIRAL HEPATITIS

Infection by members of the Herpesviridae family, such as cytomegalovirus (Chapter 376), Epstein-Barr virus (Chapter 377), and herpes simplex virus

(Chapter 374), should be considered in the differential diagnosis of unclear episodes of elevated liver enzymes in the absence of markers of acute hepatitis virus infection, especially in immunocompromised individuals. For instance, cytomegalovirus infection can be associated with graft loss after liver transplantation (Chapter 154). Parvovirus B19 (Chapter 371) may persist in the liver and worsen liver disease in patients with chronic hepatitis B and perhaps in patients with chronic HCV infection. Human herpesvirus 6 variant A has been linked with syncytial giant-cell hepatitis.

Non-A-to-E Hepatitis

Rare patients develop acute hepatitis of presumed viral cause but have no markers of known hepatitis viruses. Some of these cases may be due to variants of known hepatitis viruses, in particular HBV, that are not detected by the usual serologic and molecular methods. However, the existence of other, unknown hepatotropic viruses cannot be excluded.

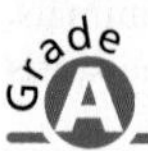

Grade A References

A1. Victor JC, Monto AS, Surdina TY, et al. Hepatitis A vaccine versus immune globulin for postexposure prophylaxis. *N Engl J Med*. 2007;357:1685-1694.
A2. Kumar M, Satapathy S, Monga R, et al. A randomized controlled trial of lamivudine to treat acute hepatitis B. *Hepatology*. 2007;45:97-101.
A3. Wiegand J, Wedemeyer H, Franke A, et al. Treatment of severe, nonfulminant acute hepatitis B with lamivudine vs placebo: a prospective randomized double-blinded multicentre trial. *J Viral Hepat*. 2014;21:744-750.
A4. Jeckel E, Cornberg M, Wedemeyer H, et al. Treatment of acute hepatitis C with interferon alfa-2b. *N Engl J Med*. 2001;345:1452-1457.
A5. Santantonio T, Fasano M, Sagnelli E, et al. Acute hepatitis C: a 24 week-course of peg-interferon alpha-2b versus a 12 week-course of peg-interferon alpha-2b alone or with ribavirin. *Hepatology*. 2014;59:2101-2109.
A6. Deterding K, Gruner N, Buggisch P, et al. Delayed versus immediate treatment for patients with acute hepatitis C: a randomised controlled non-inferiority trial. *Lancet Infect Dis*. 2013;13:497-506.
A7. Zhu FC, Zhang J, Zhang XF, et al. Efficacy and safety of a recombinant hepatitis E vaccine in healthy adults: a large-scale, randomised, double-blind placebo-controlled, phase 3 trial. *Lancet*. 2010;376:895-902.

GENERAL REFERENCES

For the General References and other additional features, please visit Expert Consult at https://expertconsult.inkling.com.

149

CHRONIC VIRAL AND AUTOIMMUNE HEPATITIS

JEAN-MICHEL PAWLOTSKY

DEFINITION

Chronic hepatitis is defined by chronic necroinflammation of the liver and may be due to various causes, including hepatotropic viruses, autoimmunity, alcohol (Chapter 152), and metabolic disorders (Chapter 146). Chronic infection by hepatitis viruses is by far the main cause of chronic hepatitis worldwide, with more than 500 million individuals chronically infected with hepatitis B virus (HBV) or hepatitis C virus (HCV). Chronic viral hepatitis B and C are the leading cause of cirrhosis (Chapter 153) and hepatocellular carcinoma (Chapter 196) worldwide and account for more than 1 million deaths per year. Chronic HBV infection can be associated with infection by hepatitis D virus (HDV). Hepatitis A virus does not cause chronic hepatitis. Hepatitis E virus (HEV) generally does not cause chronic hepatitis, except in immunosuppressed patients.

CLINICAL MANIFESTATIONS

The clinical symptoms of chronic viral and autoimmune hepatitis are typically nonspecific, and many patients have no symptoms. Fatigue, sleep disorders, and right upper quadrant pain may be present. Often the diagnosis is made when liver test abnormalities are identified by blood testing during a routine health evaluation or assessment for an unrelated problem or at the time of voluntary blood donation. More advanced symptoms include poor appetite, nausea, weight loss, muscle weakness, itching, dark urine, and jaundice. Patients can progress to full-blown cirrhosis (Chapter 153), with its typical clinical manifestations. If cirrhosis is present, weakness, weight loss, abdominal swelling, edema, bruisability, gastrointestinal bleeding, and hepatic encephalopathy with mental confusion may arise. Other findings may include spider angiomas, palmar erythema (see Fig. 146-2), ascites (see Fig. 146-4), edema, and skin excoriations.

TABLE 149-1 DIAGNOSIS OF CHRONIC HEPATITIS

DIAGNOSIS	SCREENING TESTS	CONFIRMATORY TESTS
Chronic hepatitis B	HBsAg	HBV DNA, HBeAg
Chronic hepatitis C	Anti-HCV antibodies	HCV RNA
Chronic hepatitis D	Anti-HDV antibodies	HDV RNA
Autoimmune hepatitis	ANA (anti-LKM1)	Exclusion of other causes and patterns of clinical disease
Drug-induced liver disease	History	Rechallenge, if necessary, if considered safe
Wilson disease	Ceruloplasmin	Urine copper concentration
Cryptogenic hepatitis	Exclusion of other causes	

ANA = antinuclear antibody; anti-LKM1 = anti–liver-kidney microsomal 1 antibody; HBeAg = hepatitis B e antigen; HBsAg = hepatitis B surface antigen; HBV = hepatitis B virus; HCV = hepatitis C virus; HDV = hepatitis D virus.

DIAGNOSIS

Levels of alanine aminotransferase (ALT) and aspartate aminotransferase (AST) are usually two to five times the upper limit of normal. The ALT level is generally higher than the AST level, but both can be normal in mild or inactive disease or 10 to 25 times the upper limit of normal during acute exacerbations. Biologic tests can establish the specific diagnosis (Table 149-1).

Alkaline phosphatase and γ-glutamyl transpeptidase levels are usually minimally elevated unless cirrhosis is present. Serum bilirubin and albumin levels and the prothrombin time are normal unless the disease is severe or advanced. Serum immunoglobulin levels are mildly elevated or normal in chronic viral hepatitis but may be very elevated in autoimmune hepatitis. Results that suggest the presence of advanced fibrosis are a platelet count below 160,000, AST levels higher than ALT levels, elevation in serum bilirubin, decrease in serum albumin, prolongation of the prothrombin time, elevation in α-fetoprotein levels, and presence of rheumatoid factor or high globulin levels.

Liver ultrasound can determine the texture and size of the liver and spleen, exclude hepatic masses, and assess the gallbladder, intrahepatic bile ducts, and portal venous flow. Computed tomography and magnetic resonance imaging of the liver are helpful if a mass or other abnormality is found by ultrasound. Hepatic transient elastography or acoustic radiation force impulse imaging can assess liver stiffness as a surrogate marker of fibrosis.

Liver biopsy is usually critical for diagnosis and to determine the severity of disease. Hepatocellular necrosis is typically eosinophilic degeneration or ballooning degeneration throughout the parenchyma, greater in the periportal area, spotty, or piecemeal. Fibrosis also typically begins in the periportal regions and can link adjacent portal areas or portal and central areas (bridging fibrosis), distort the hepatic architecture, and lead to cirrhosis and portal hypertension. The histologic grade of chronic hepatitis can be determined by combining scores for periportal necrosis and inflammation, lobular necrosis and inflammation, and portal inflammation. Recently, ultrasound-based methods or serologic markers have proved accurate for the assessment of mild disease and cirrhosis, but they are less accurate for identifying moderate to severe inflammation, except in patients with chronic hepatitis C. Patients with suspected chronic viral or autoimmune hepatitis should be evaluated carefully for fatty liver, alcohol-induced (Chapter 152) or drug-induced (Chapter 150) liver disease, and metabolic liver diseases (Chapter 146), each of which can coexist with hepatitis. Liver biopsy can exclude other diagnoses that mimic chronic hepatitis, including fatty liver, alcoholic liver disease, steatohepatitis (Chapter 152), drug-induced liver disease (Chapter 150), sclerosing cholangitis (Chapter 155), iron overload (Chapter 212), and veno-occlusive disease (Chapter 143).

TREATMENT AND PROGNOSIS

Rx

Chronic HBV infection is not curable, but it usually can be controlled by appropriate antiviral drugs. HCV infection is curable, and more than 80% of patients who have access to new therapies are cured. Autoimmune hepatitis responds to immunosuppression with corticosteroids and azathioprine.

CHRONIC HEPATITIS B

EPIDEMIOLOGY

More than 240 million individuals, or approximately 4% of the world's population, are chronic HBV carriers. Two billion individuals, or one human being in three, have been in contact with the virus. In North America, Western and Northern Europe, and Australia, less than 2% of the population is chronic hepatitis B surface antigen (HBsAg) carriers. In the United States, the prevalence is approximately 0.4%; that is, approximately 1.25 million Americans are infected. In Eastern Europe, South America, the Mediterranean basin, and the Indian subcontinent, the prevalence of chronic HBsAg carriage is between 2 and 8%. Highly endemic areas, with a rate of chronic HBsAg carriage exceeding 8%, include China, Southeast Asia, sub-Saharan Africa, and the native populations of the Far North of America.

HBV is the main cause of primary liver cancer (hepatocellular carcinoma, Chapter 196) worldwide, with approximately 350,000 new cases attributable to HBV every year. Hepatocellular carcinoma is more likely in the presence of underlying cirrhosis, but HBV has oncogenic properties of its own, and hepatocellular carcinoma can occur in noncirrhotic HBV patients.

PATHOBIOLOGY

HBV is not a cytopathic virus. Rather, liver injury in chronic hepatitis B is a consequence of the local immune response at the immune elimination phase. In particular, liver injury is related to cytotoxic T cells that recognize and kill infected hepatocytes that express HBV antigens at their surface and to the local production of cytokines. Chronic inflammation triggers fibrogenesis through the activation of hepatic stellate cells. The hepatitis B X protein may also directly activate fibrogenesis. As a result, many patients with chronic hepatitis B have progressive fibrosis, which may evolve into cirrhosis.

The rate of chronicity after an acute HBV infection is more than 95% among patients infected at birth. This risk diminishes as the age at acquisition increases, and it is less than 5% in those infected as adults. Chronic HBV infection is defined by HBsAg carriage that persists for more than 6 months after the acute episode. Chronic HBsAg carriage typically evolves through three phases: immune tolerant, immune elimination, and inactive.

The immune tolerant phase is generally short if the infection occurred during adulthood, but it persists for years to decades in patients infected at birth or during early childhood. At the immune tolerant stage, the immune response of the host "tolerates" HBV infection and does not cause liver inflammation or hepatocyte destruction. The immune tolerant phase is characterized by the presence of hepatitis B e antigen (HBeAg), very high levels of HBV DNA in blood, normal serum or plasma aminotransferase levels, and no or minimal inflammatory activity on liver biopsy.

The immune elimination phase is characterized by an active immune response that causes necroinflammatory lesions and triggers hepatic fibrogenesis and progressive fibrosis. ALT and AST levels are increased, but HBV DNA levels are lower than during the immune tolerant phase and frequently fluctuate. The immune elimination phase has a variable duration, ranging from a few weeks to several decades. HBeAg, when present, defines HBeAg-positive chronic hepatitis B; HBeAg can be cleared and replaced by anti-HBe antibodies, defined as HBe seroconversion; or HBeAg can be absent while anti-HBe antibodies are present and define HBeAg-negative chronic hepatitis B. Patients with HBeAg-positive chronic hepatitis B are infected with a wild-type virus and are able to secrete the HBe protein. Patients with HBeAg-negative chronic hepatitis B are infected with so-called precore mutant viruses, which cannot produce the HBe protein because they have a stop codon in the pre-C gene, and/or with core promoter mutant viruses, which produce considerably lower amounts of HBe protein. Because of the prevalence of the HBV genotype D in Euro-Mediterranean and African countries, HBeAg-negative/anti-HBe-positive chronic hepatitis B is seven to nine times more frequent than HBeAg-positive disease in those locations.

The inactive HBsAg carriage phase is the result of successful immune elimination leading to HBe seroconversion. ALT and AST levels are normal, HBV DNA is undetectable or at very low levels, and patients without preexisting cirrhosis have normal liver histology.

CLINICAL MANIFESTATIONS

Chronic hepatitis B is usually asymptomatic. The most common symptom is fatigue, but sleep disorders, difficulty concentrating, and upper right quadrant pain are often observed. Chronic hepatitis B is characterized biologically by elevated aminotransferase levels, and ALT levels can fluctuate substantially during the immune elimination phase. Moderate cholestasis, with mildly elevated alkaline phosphatase and γ-glutamyl transpeptidase levels, also can be present, especially in patients with cirrhosis.

HBeAg-negative chronic hepatitis B is generally more severe than the HBeAg-positive variety. The incidence of spontaneous HBe seroconversion among HBeAg-positive patients is 8 to 12% per year when they are in the immune elimination phase; HBe seroconversion often follows a transient ALT flare. Some of these patients evolve toward inactive HBsAg carriage, whereas others switch into an HBeAg-negative form of chronic hepatitis B, with elevated ALT levels and an HBV DNA level greater than 2000 IU/mL.

The annual incidence of cirrhosis varies from 2 to 10% in patients with chronic HBV infection, with a cumulative incidence of approximately 20% at 5 years. The risk for cirrhosis is two- to four-fold higher in HBeAg-negative patients compared with HBeAg-positive ones, probably because they are older and have more severe disease at the time of diagnosis. The annual incidence of hepatocellular carcinoma in patients with chronic hepatitis B varies from 1% in patients without cirrhosis to 2 to 8% in cirrhotic patients, with the higher rates occurring in older patients. Patients with cirrhosis (Chapter 153), hepatocellular carcinoma (Chapter 196), or both have the typical signs associated with these conditions. Rarely, chronic HBV infection is associated with extrahepatic manifestations, including glomerulonephritis (Chapter 121), most often in children, and polyarteritis nodosa (Chapter 270), mostly in adults.

DIAGNOSIS

Serologic markers used to diagnose chronic hepatitis B (Table 149-2) include HBsAg, anti-HBs antibodies, total anti–hepatitis B core (HBc) antibodies and anti-HBc immunoglobulin M (IgM), HBeAg, and anti-HBe antibodies. Molecular markers include HBV DNA and HBV resistance substitutions; real-time polymerase chain reaction (PCR)–based assays are the best way to detect and quantify HBV DNA.

Chronic HBV infection is defined by the persistence of HBsAg in the serum for more than 6 months after the acute episode. The majority of subjects with isolated anti-HBc antibodies are not viremic. However, some individuals who test positive for anti-HBc antibodies, but not for HBsAg or anti-HBs antibodies, may be viremic; in these cases, the virus's amino acid substitutions in the HBsAg sequence make HBsAg undetectable with current enzyme immunoassays. Other individuals may have such low-level HBV replication in their livers that HBV DNA is not detectable in blood ("occult" hepatitis B). Screening is recommended only in high-risk individuals.[1]

Serum or plasma ALT and HBV DNA levels are important markers of severity and prognosis. For both HBV and HCV, the assessment of severity, including the grade of necroinflammation and the stage of fibrosis, is based on the liver biopsy (Fig. 149-1). Noninvasive assessment using serologic markers, transient elastography, or acoustic radiation force impulse imaging can discriminate cirrhosis from mild hepatitis and fibrosis; although they are not accurate enough for intermediate stages, these methods will likely replace liver biopsy in the pretreatment assessment of the severity of chronic hepatitis B in many patients in the future.

PREVENTION AND TREATMENT

Rx

Patients with chronic hepatitis B should be vaccinated against hepatitis A virus, abstain from alcohol, and avoid immunosuppressive therapies unless absolutely necessary. HBV-infected patients who require corticosteroids, rituximab, or other chemotherapy for other conditions should receive entecavir 0.5 mg/day or tenofovir 300 mg/day during therapy and for 12 months after its cessation as prophylaxis against reactivation of hepatitis B.[A1]

The goals of therapy are to suppress HBV replication, reduce the histologic activity of chronic hepatitis, and lessen the risk for cirrhosis and hepatocellular carcinoma. HBV infection cannot be completely eradicated because of the

TABLE 149-2 VIROLOGIC MARKER PROFILES IN PATIENTS WITH CHRONIC HEPATITIS B VIRUS INFECTION

	HBsAg	ANTI-HBs Ab	HBeAg	ANTI-HBe Ab	Anti-HBc Ab IgM	Anti-HBc Ab TOTAL	HBV DNA
Chronic hepatitis							
HBeAg-positive	+	−	+	−	−*	+	$>2 \times 10^4$ IU/mL
HBeAg-negative	+	−	−	+	−*	+	$>2 \times 10^3$ IU/mL
Inactive carrier	+	−	−	+	−	+	$<2 \times 10^3$ IU/mL
Reactivation	+	−	+/−	+/−	+/−	+	$>2 \times 10^3$ IU/mL

*Anti-HBc IgM can be detected at low titers.
Ab = antibodies; Ag = antigen; HBc = hepatitis B core; HBe = hepatitis B e; HBs = hepatitis B surface; HBV = hepatitis B virus; IgM = immunoglobulin M.

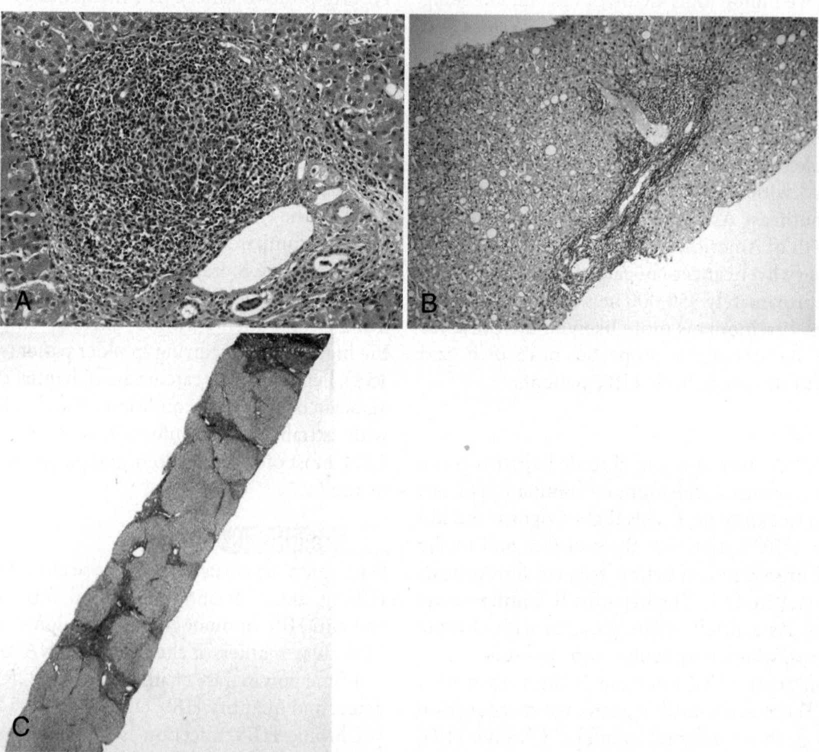

FIGURE 149-1. **Liver biopsies in patients with chronic hepatitis C. A, Lymphoid nodule with germinal center; minimal interface hepatitis (hematein-eosin, magnification 200×). B, Mild fibrosis, Metavir score F1 (picrosirius-hemalun, magnification 100×). C, Extensive fibrosis, Metavir score F3 (picrosirius-hemalun, magnification 20×). (Courtesy Prof. Elie-Serge Zafrani, Department of Pathology, Henri Mondor Hospital, Créteil, France.)**

persistence of covalently closed circular DNA in the nucleus of infected hepatocytes. As a result, therapy attempts to reduce HBV DNA levels as much as possible—ideally, below the limit of detection of real-time PCR assays (10 to 15 IU/mL)—to ensure a degree of viral suppression that will lead to biochemical remission, histologic improvement, and prevention of complications.

Two different types of drugs for the treatment of chronic hepatitis B are pegylated interferon-α (IFN-α) and nucleoside/nucleotide analogues. Pegylated IFN-α2a, administered subcutaneously at a dose of 180 μg/week for 48 weeks, improves various markers of HBV infection in both HBeAg-positive (Table 149-3) and HBeAg-negative (Table 149-4) patients.[A2] Pegylated IFN-α2b (1.5 μg/kg) is very similar to IFN-α2a and is used by many liver experts, although it is not currently approved for HBV. The most frequent side effects of IFN-α are flulike symptoms after the injections, fatigue, anorexia, weight loss, and alopecia. The most concerning side effects are neutropenia, thrombocytopenia, anxiety, irritability, depression, and suicidal ideation.

Nucleoside analogues (lamivudine, telbivudine, and entecavir) require triple phosphorylation to be active, whereas nucleotide analogues (adefovir and tenofovir) need only two phosphorylations to be active. These drugs are given orally (PO) once daily at the following dosages: 100 mg for lamivudine, 600 mg for telbivudine, 0.5 mg for entecavir, 10 mg for adefovir (administered as the pro-drug adefovir dipivoxil), and 300 mg for tenofovir (administered as the pro-drug tenofovir disoproxil fumarate). All have short-term benefits on various markers of HBV infection in HBeAg-positive (see Table 149-3) and HBeAg-negative (see Table 149-4) patients. Entecavir and tenofovir are two of the most potent inhibitors of HBV replication,[A3][A4] and they are the least likely to select for resistant HBV variants. These drugs are generally well tolerated. However, adefovir is nephrotoxic at doses higher than those used for HBV therapy; renal impairment and decreases in mineral bone density are rarely seen with tenofovir; myopathy is a rare complication of telbivudine, and peripheral neuropathy has been observed when telbivudine is combined with pegylated IFN-α.

Patients should be considered for treatment when their HBV DNA levels are greater than 2000 IU/mL and/or their serum ALT levels are abnormal if the liver biopsy shows moderate to severe active necroinflammation, fibrosis, or both. Indications for treatment must also take into account the patient's age and health status and the availability of antiviral agents in individual countries. Patients in the immune tolerant phase and those with mild hepatitis on liver biopsy (or noninvasive markers) should not be treated, but follow-up ALT levels and HBV DNA assays are mandatory. Patients with compensated cirrhosis and detectable HBV DNA may be considered for treatment even if their ALT levels are normal, their HBV DNA levels are below 2000 IU/mL, or both. Patients with decompensated cirrhosis require urgent antiviral treatment.

Two treatment strategies can be considered: a 48-week course of pegylated IFN-α or long-term oral treatment with nucleoside/nucleotide analogues. Whether their combined use improves the rate of sustained virologic response after treatment is currently under study. Pegylated IFN-α can provide a sustained virologic response, defined as a sustained HBe seroconversion (clearance of HBeAg, which is replaced by anti-HBe antibodies) and an HBV DNA level that remains below 2000 IU/mL after a 48-week course of treatment; an ALT flare can be observed at the time of HBeAg loss in patients in whom treatment is successful. Pegylated IFN-α treatment should be reserved for patients with the best chance of a sustained virologic response off

TABLE 149-3 SHORT-TERM (1-YEAR) RESPONSES TO APPROVED ANTIVIRAL THERAPIES AMONG TREATMENT-NAÏVE PATIENTS WITH HBeAg-POSITIVE CHRONIC HEPATITIS B

	PLACEBO/CONTROL GROUPS	PEGYLATED IFN-α2A (48 WK)	LAMIVUDINE (48-52 WK)	TELBIVUDINE (52 WK)	ENTECAVIR (48 WK)	ADEFOVIR (48 WK)	TENOFOVIR (48 WK)
Loss of serum HBV DNA (%)*	0-17	25	40-44	60	67	21	76
HBeAg loss (%)	6-12	30/34†	17-32	26	22	24	NA
HBe seroconversion (%)	4-6	27/32†	16-21	22	21	12	21
HBsAg loss (%)	0-1	3	1	0	2	0	3
ALT normalization (%)	7-24	39	41-75	77	68	48	68
Histologic improvement (%)	NA	38‡	49-56	65	72	53	74
Durability of response (%)§	NA	NA	50-80	≈80	69	≈90	NA

Modified from Lok AS, McMahon BJ. American Association for the Study of Liver Diseases practice guidelines: chronic hepatitis B—update 2009, http://www.aasld.org.
*HBV DNA levels were assessed with various molecular assays, with different lower limits of detection.
†Responses at week 48/week 72 (24 wk after stopping treatment).
‡Post-treatment biopsies at week 72 (24 wk after stopping treatment).
§No or short duration of consolidation treatment for lamivudine and entecavir; most patients had consolidation treatment for adefovir and telbivudine.
Ag = antigen; ALT = alanine aminotransferase; HBe = hepatitis B e; HBs = hepatitis B surface; HBV = hepatitis B virus; IFN = interferon; NA = not available.

TABLE 149-4 SHORT-TERM (1-YEAR) RESPONSES TO APPROVED ANTIVIRAL THERAPIES AMONG TREATMENT-NAÏVE PATIENTS WITH HBeAg-NEGATIVE CHRONIC HEPATITIS B

	PLACEBO/CONTROL GROUPS	PEGYLATED IFN-α2A (48 WK)	LAMIVUDINE (48-52 WK)	TELBIVUDINE (52 WK)	ENTECAVIR (48 WK)	ADEFOVIR (48 WK)	TENOFOVIR (48 WK)
Loss of serum HBV DNA (%)*	0-20	63	60-73	88	90	51	93
ALT normalization (%)	10-29	38	60-79	74	78	72	76
Histologic improvement (%)	33	48	60-66	67	70	64	72
Durability of response (%)	NA	≈20	≈10	NA	3	≈5	NA

*HBV DNA levels were assessed with various molecular assays, with different lower limits of detection.
ALT = alanine aminotransferase; HBeAg = hepatitis B e antigen; HBV = hepatitis B virus; IFN = interferon; NA = not available.
Modified from Lok AS, McMahon BJ. American Association for the Study of Liver Diseases practice guidelines: chronic hepatitis B—update 2009, http://www.aasld.org.

treatment—HBeAg-positive patients with high baseline ALT levels (more than three times the upper limit of normal) and HBV DNA levels below 2.10^6 IU/mL. Pegylated IFN-α therapy is contraindicated in patients with advanced cirrhosis and in immunosuppressed patients. Patients infected with HBV genotypes A and B generally respond better to IFN-α therapy than do patients infected with genotypes C and D, but the predictive value of the HBV genotype for an individual patient is weak. Patients who fail to achieve a sustained virologic response after a single course of pegylated IFN-α are candidates for nucleoside/nucleotide analogue therapy.

Long-term treatment with nucleoside/nucleotide analogues is indicated in the majority of patients with chronic hepatitis B. Tenofovir or entecavir, which are the most potent drugs with an optimal resistance profile, are recommended as first-line monotherapies. HBV DNA should be suppressed to undetectable levels (<10 to 15 IU/mL) with a sensitive real-time PCR-based assay. If the HBV DNA level is reduced but still detectable in a compliant patient, the other agent may be added; however, the long-term safety of combined tenofovir and entecavir is unknown. When HBeAg-positive patients seroconvert to negative or HBeAg-negative patients lose their HBsAg, treatment should be continued for an additional 6 to 12 months at least. In all other cases, treatment should be continued for life and adherence is particularly important.

Virologic breakthroughs—defined by a subsequent increase of the HBV DNA level of 1 log or more above the nadir level—in adherent patients are due to HBV resistance to the administered antiviral drug or drugs. HBV DNA levels most often increase back to baseline levels, and the virologic breakthrough is generally followed a few weeks later by a biochemical breakthrough in which a previously normal ALT level rises above normal. The cumulative rates of resistance in newly treated patients are 70% at 5 years for lamivudine, 17% at 2 years for telbivudine, 1.2% at 6 years for entecavir, 29% at 5 years for adefovir, and 0% at 6 years for tenofovir. These figures illustrate the high genetic barrier against resistance of entecavir and tenofovir. In a patient who develops resistance to any of the available nucleoside/nucleotide analogues, adding a second drug without cross-resistance or switching to tenofovir are the only efficient strategies, although the long-term safety of some of these combinations is not known. In patients with lamivudine, telbivudine, or entecavir resistance, treatment should be switched to tenofovir or tenofovir should be added. Patients who have resistance to adefovir should be switched to tenofovir and eventually also given lamivudine, telbivudine, or entecavir. In patients with tenofovir resistance (never reported thus far), any of these three drugs should be added. The combination of tenofovir and emtricitabine, a nucleoside analogue similar to lamivudine, in a single tablet (approved for HIV but not for HBV therapy) is also a valid option in cases of resistance to any of these drugs.

In patients with cirrhosis, nucleoside/nucleotide analogue therapy is the only option because pegylated IFN-α is contraindicated if cirrhosis is decompensated. Because resistance in this population can be life-threatening, some experts recommend de novo treatment with two potent drugs without cross-resistance. In those with decompensated disease, efficient antiviral treatment most often stabilizes the patient's condition and can also delay or obviate the need for liver transplantation. If transplantation is needed, post-transplant administration of anti-HBV immunoglobulins in combination with a potent nucleoside/nucleotide analogue prevents recurrent HBV in the vast majority of cases. With the advent of potent drugs with a high barrier to resistance, such as tenofovir or entecavir, the utility of immune globulins is debated.

PROGNOSIS

Every year, approximately 0.5% of inactive HBsAg carriers spontaneously lose HBsAg, and most of them acquire anti-HBs antibodies. Reactivations are possible in inactive HBV carriers, especially if they become immunosuppressed, such as when they are treated for other conditions with corticosteroids, rituximab, or other chemotherapeutic agents. HBV reactivations often evolve into a subfulminant or fulminant form.

The risk of cirrhosis (Chapter 153) in chronic hepatitis B is 2 to 10% per year, and it is significantly associated with a higher HBV DNA level, older age, alcohol consumption, coinfection with other hepatotropic viruses, and coinfection with human immunodeficiency virus (HIV). The cumulative incidence of liver decompensation is about 15 to 20% at 5 years in patients with compensated cirrhosis. The complications of cirrhosis, including hepatocellular carcinoma, are among the main causes of mortality in HBV-infected patients, and the annual incidence of death is about 3 to 4%.

The likelihood of developing hepatocellular carcinoma (Chapter 196) is approximately 1% per year in patients without cirrhosis and 2 to 8% per year in those with cirrhosis, and it is significantly associated with a higher HBV DNA level, male sex, old age, reversion from anti-HBe–positive to HBeAg-positive, and coinfection with other hepatotropic viruses. HBV carriers at risk for hepatocellular carcinoma should be screened every 6 to 12 months, with an ultrasound examination and an α-fetoprotein level.

CHRONIC HEPATITIS C

EPIDEMIOLOGY

HCV, which is present on all continents, is estimated to cause chronic infection in approximately 185 million individuals, or approximately 3% of the world's population. The prevalence of chronic HCV infection, which varies geographically, is estimated to be about 1.3% in the United States (affecting 2.7 million individuals),[2] 3.5% in Asia, 1.9% in the Americas overall, 5.2% in Africa, 1.7% in Europe, and 1.8% in Oceania. The highest prevalence is in Egypt (9% overall, but up to 40% in certain rural areas), where infection was initially spread by intramuscular injections for schistosomiasis during treatment campaigns several decades ago. By 2007, hepatitis C virus superseded HIV as a cause of death in the United States.

PATHOBIOLOGY

Acute HCV infection evolves into chronic infection in 50 to 80% of cases. Even patients who spontaneously recover and maintain detectable anti-HCV antibodies are not protected against reinfection. Persistence of infection is related to a qualitatively and quantitatively altered CD4+ T-helper cell and cytotoxic T lymphocyte response that fails to eradicate infection. The plasticity of the viral genomes is responsible for the coexistence of closely related but genetically different viral populations in equilibrium in the patient's replicative environment. This genetic diversity allows continuously generated variant viral populations to be selected by timely changes in the replicative environment.

Chronic HCV infection is responsible for necroinflammatory lesions of varying severity, sometimes associated with steatosis, which is the accumulation of triglycerides in hepatocytes. HCV is not a cytopathic virus. Liver injury in chronic hepatitis C is related to the action of immune effectors that recognize and kill infected hepatocytes that express HCV antigens at their surface. Chronic inflammation triggers fibrogenesis through the activation of hepatic stellate cells. Fibrosis progresses at nonlinear rates that are generally faster in older patients, in males, and in the presence of chronic alcohol intake, viral coinfections, or immunosuppression. The severity of chronic hepatitis is independent of the HCV RNA level and of the HCV genotype. This chronic inflammation and progression of fibrosis predispose patients to cirrhosis (Chapter 153) and hepatocellular carcinoma (Chapter 196).

CLINICAL MANIFESTATIONS

Acute hepatitis C (Chapter 148) is most often asymptomatic and therefore undiagnosed. The most common symptom associated with chronic HCV infection is fatigue, but it may remain inapparent for years. ALT levels are usually moderately elevated and fluctuate, but they can remain normal for weeks to months despite active hepatitis on liver biopsy. Moderate cholestasis can be present in patients with cirrhosis. Patients with cirrhosis (Chapter 153), hepatocellular carcinoma (Chapter 196), or both have the typical signs associated with these conditions.

HCV is the main cause of type II and type III mixed cryoglobulinemia (Chapter 187). Low levels of circulating cryoglobulins, which contain HCV RNA, anti-HCV antibodies, rheumatoid factor, and low levels of complement, can be found in 50 to 70% of cases, whereas elevated rheumatoid factor (Chapter 264) is found in 70% of cases. Fewer than 1% of HCV-infected patients develop symptoms of cryoglobulinemic vasculitis (Chapter 270), including fatigue, myalgias, arthralgias, rash (purpura, hives, leukocytoclastic vasculitis), neuropathy, and membranoproliferative glomerulonephritis. Cryoglobulinemia can be severe and lead to end-stage renal disease or severe neuropathies, and long-term cryoglobulinemia has been linked to non–Hodgkin B-cell lymphomas (Chapter 185).

Low titers of antinuclear and anti–smooth muscle antibodies can be found in HCV-infected patients, but they do not have any clinical significance. HCV has been reported to trigger the symptoms of porphyria cutanea tarda (Chapter 210), and an association with lichen planus (Chapter 438) has been suggested.

DIAGNOSIS

Chronic HCV infection is defined by the persistence of HCV RNA for more than 6 months. In patients with clinical, biologic, or both signs of chronic liver disease, chronic hepatitis C is diagnosed by the simultaneous presence of anti-HCV antibodies and HCV RNA. Detectable HCV replication in the absence of anti-HCV antibodies is observed almost exclusively in patients who are profoundly immunosuppressed, on hemodialysis, or agammaglobulinemic. In the United States, screening for HCV is recommended in high-risk individuals, and one-time screening is recommended in all persons born between 1945 and 1965 (Chapter 15).[3] The level of HCV replication does not correlate with the severity of liver disease or with the risk for progression to cirrhosis or hepatocellular carcinoma.

The HCV genotype, which has important therapeutic implications, should be determined. Anti-HCV IgM, which is found in approximately 50% of patients with chronic hepatitis, is of no significance. Laboratory testing often reveals high levels of monoclonal rheumatoid factor and cryoglobulins.

TREATMENT

Rx

Chronic HCV infection is curable. The goal of therapy is to achieve a sustained virologic response, defined by undetectable HCV RNA at 12 to 24 weeks after the end of therapy using a sensitive HCV RNA assay with a lower limit of detection of 10 to 20 IU/mL.[4]

The decision to treat chronic hepatitis C depends on a precise assessment of the severity of liver disease, the presence of absolute or relative contraindications to therapy, and the patient's willingness to be treated. Treatment typically requires a liver biopsy, but serologic markers of liver fibrosis, fibrogenesis, or both and transient elastography or acoustic radiation force impulse imaging have been validated in large series of patients with chronic hepatitis C. In patients with no indication for therapy or with contraindications to therapy, repeated assessments of aminotransferase levels are recommended on a yearly basis. Assessment of liver inflammation and fibrosis by liver biopsy or noninvasive serologic or ultrasound-based testing is indicated for patients with persistently or intermittently elevated aminotransferase levels.

Treatment strategies for chronic hepatitis C are evolving rapidly. Options vary in different countries based on the availability of newer medications.[5,6]

Historic Standard Therapy

For more than 15 years, the standard treatment for chronic hepatitis C has been the combination of ribavirin (0.8 to 1.4 g/day PO) with either pegylated IFN-α2a (180 μg subcutaneously [SC] once weekly) or pegylated IFN-α2b (1.5 μg/kg SC once weekly). This therapy yields sustained virologic response rates of the order of 50% in patients infected with HCV genotype 1 and 75-80% in those infected with HCV genotypes 2 or 3. Two inhibitors of the HCV protease, telaprevir (750 mg every 8 hours or 1250 mg every 12 hours PO) and boceprevir (800 mg every 8 hours PO), have been approved for use in combination with pegylated IFN-α and ribavirin exclusively in patients infected with HCV genotype 1, in whom this regimen yields sustained virologic response rates of the order of 65 to 75%. These regimens remain the only available treatments in many areas of the world where new therapies are not yet available.

The most common side effects of IFN-α are influenza-like symptoms (which can be prevented by acetaminophen), neutropenia, thrombocytopenia, irritability, difficulty concentrating, memory disturbances, thyroiditis, hair loss, sleep disorders, and weight loss. The principal side effect of ribavirin is hemolytic anemia. As a result of these side effects, dose modification is frequently required during therapy. Ribavirin should be decreased in 200-mg increments in patients with severe anemia. For IFN-induced side effects, the pegylated IFN-α dose should be decreased stepwise, from 180 to 135 to 90 μg/week for pegylated IFN-α2a, and from 1.5 to 1 to 0.5 μg/kg/week for pegylated IFN-α2b. In more than 50% of cases, telaprevir administration is associated with rash, which can be severe in approximately 5% of cases and can rarely manifest as *drug reaction with eosinophilia and systemic symptoms* (DRESS) syndrome or Stevens-Johnson syndrome. Boceprevir induces dysgeusia. Both telaprevir and boceprevir aggravate ribavirin-induced anemia.

The main contraindications to therapy with pegylated IFN-α and ribavirin are decompensated liver disease, renal failure, severe immunosuppression, solid organ transplantation, cytopenias, severe psychiatric disease, and active substance abuse. Ribavirin is also contraindicated in patients with anemia, significant coronary or cerebrovascular disease, or renal insufficiency. Because ribavirin is teratogenic, it is essential that adequate contraception be practiced during therapy and for at least 6 months thereafter in both men and women.

Newly Available Regimens

New treatment regimens (Chapter 360), which provide a sustained virologic response for 80 to 95% of patients, have changed the approach to hepatitis C in countries in which they are available.[7] Simeprevir (150 mg/day PO), which is an inhibitor of the HCV protease, has antiviral activity against genotypes 1 and 4 and a low barrier to resistance. Sofosbuvir (400 mg/day PO), which is a nucleotide analogue inhibitor of the HCV RNA-dependent RNA polymerase, is active against all HCV genotypes with a high barrier to resistance. Both drugs are well tolerated. Adverse reactions in patients receiving simeprevir are rash (including photosensitivity), pruritus, and nausea, as well as mild, transient hyperbilirubinemia not accompanied by changes in other liver parameters. The only side effects reported with sofosbuvir are headache and fatigue.

In patients for whom therapy is deemed appropriate, treatment is guided by the patient's HCV genotype and eligibility for pegylated IFN-α administration. Patients infected with HCV genotype 1 should be treated with one of five regimens: daily sofosbuvir plus weight-based ribavirin plus weekly pegylated IFN-α for 12 weeks; daily sofosbuvir plus daily simeprevir with or without weight-based ribavirin for 12 weeks; daily simeprevir plus weight-based ribavirin plus weekly pegylated IFN-α for 12 weeks followed by 12 weeks of pegylated IFN-α and ribavirin in treatment-naïve patients and for 36 weeks in treatment-experienced patients[A5,A6]; the combination of sofosbuvir with the NS5A inhibitor ledipasvir in one single pill with or without weight-based ribavirin for 12 weeks; or the combination of ritonavir-boosted paritaprevir, ombitasvir, and dasabuvir with or without weight-based ribavirin for 12 or 24 weeks.[A7] The combination of simeprevir, pegylated IFN-α, and ribavirin should not be used in patients who are infected with HCV subtype 1a with a detectable Q80K substitution in the HCV protease sequence before therapy and who should benefit from the other options.

Patients infected with HCV genotype 2 must be treated with daily sofosbuvir plus ribavirin for 12 weeks (eventually combined with pegylated IFN-α if the patient has failed prior therapy).[A5,A6,A8] Patients infected with HCV genotype 3 should be treated with either of two regimens: daily sofosbuvir plus weight-based ribavirin for 24 weeks or daily sofosbuvir plus weight-based ribavirin plus pegylated IFN-α for 12 weeks.

Patients infected with HCV genotype 4 should be treated with one of three regimens: daily sofosbuvir plus weight-based ribavirin plus weekly pegylated IFN-α for 12 weeks; daily sofosbuvir plus daily simeprevir with or without weight-based ribavirin for 12 weeks; or daily simeprevir plus weight-based ribavirin plus weekly pegylated IFN-α for 12 weeks followed by 12 weeks of pegylated IFN-α and ribavirin in treatment-naïve patients and 36 weeks in treatment-experienced patients. Patients infected with HCV genotypes 5 or 6 should be treated with daily sofosbuvir plus weight-based ribavirin plus weekly pegylated IFN-α for 12 weeks.[6]

Emerging Regimens

Numerous new anti-HCV drugs are in clinical development. They include protease inhibitors, nucleoside/nucleotide analogues, and non-nucleoside inhibitors of the HCV RNA-dependent RNA polymerase, inhibitors of the nonstructural 5A protein of HCV, and cyclophilin A inhibitors. Oral regimens with sustained virologic response rates greater than 90% are rapidly replacing IFN-based therapies.[6-8] Treatment regimens likely to become available soon include the combination of sofosbuvir with the NS5A inhibitor daclatasvir; and the triple combination of the protease inhibitor paritaprevir boosted by ritonavir, the NS5A inhibitor ombitasvir, and the non-nucleoside inhibitor of the HCV polymerase dasabuvir, with or without ribavirin.[A9-A16]

End-Stage Disease

In patients with end-stage liver disease, liver transplantation (Chapter 154) is the only option. However, in the absence of treatment, the graft becomes infected in 100% of patients who are viremic at the time of transplantation. Treatment with daily sofosbuvir and ribavirin until liver transplantation (up to 48 weeks) efficiently prevents graft infection when HCV RNA has been undetectable for at least 30 days before transplantation.

PROGNOSIS

Spontaneous HCV clearance in patients with chronic hepatitis C is exceptional. The HCV RNA level has no prognostic value in chronic hepatitis C. An estimated 20% of patients with chronic hepatitis C develop cirrhosis (Chapter 153) after an average of 20 years of progression in the absence of therapy. Cirrhosis remains compensated for many years in the vast majority of patients, but decompensation occurs at an annual rate of 2 to 5% in cirrhotic patients. After a first decompensation, the mortality rate related to portal hypertension, hepatocellular insufficiency, and hepatocellular carcinoma is 10% per year, with a 50% survival rate at 5 years. The risk for death increases with advancing age, male gender, and the severity of cirrhosis.

Hepatocellular carcinoma (Chapter 196) is rare in patients with chronic hepatitis C without cirrhosis. In patients with cirrhosis, the incidence of hepatocellular carcinoma is 2 to 4% per year, most often in patients with compensated cirrhosis. HCV has become the most common cause of hepatocellular carcinoma in most industrialized countries. However, hepatocellular carcinoma is less likely to develop in patients who have a sustained virologic response to treatment,[9] so this risk will hopefully decline now that better treatments are available.

Long-term follow-up shows that HCV does not recur in greater than 99% of patients who achieve a sustained virologic response, even in those who are immunosuppressed or receive chemotherapy. However, the liver disease may continue to evolve even after the infection has been eradicated. In addition, patients with chronic hepatitis C should abstain from alcohol and, unless there are other contraindications, should be vaccinated for hepatitis A and B (Chapter 18).

CHRONIC HEPATITIS D

EPIDEMIOLOGY

HDV infection occurs only in HBsAg carriers. Only approximately 2% of patients acutely coinfected with HDV and HBV develop chronic hepatitis D. In chronic HBV carriers superinfected by HDV, however, 90% of patients become chronic HDV carriers.

CLINICAL MANIFESTATIONS

Chronic hepatitis D is generally severe, with more than 80% of patients developing cirrhosis. Compared with patients who have chronic hepatitis B alone, patients with chronic infection with both HBV and HDV are three times as likely to develop hepatocellular carcinoma and twice as likely to die.

DIAGNOSIS

Markers of HDV infection should be sought at least once in every chronic HBsAg carrier. Both total anti-HD antibodies and anti-HD IgM remain at high levels in chronic HDV infection, and HDV RNA is present. Although all chronic HDV carriers also are chronic HBsAg carriers, chronic HDV carriers generally have low or undetectable HBV DNA levels because HDV inhibits HBV replication.

TREATMENT (Rx)

High doses (9 million units three times/week for 1 year) of standard, nonpegylated IFN-α result in sustained normalization of ALT levels 24 weeks after the end of therapy in approximately 50% of cases, sometimes for as long as 20 years. Some patients clear HDV RNA and, eventually, HBsAg.

Pegylated IFN-α2b, 1.5 μg/kg once weekly for 12 months, provides a sustained virologic response in 20 to 40% of cases.[A17] Although there is no clear consensus, most experts now recommend 1 year of pegylated IFN-α as first-line treatment of chronic HDV infection.

PREVENTION

Chronic HDV infection is best prevented by preventing primary HBV infection, because individuals who are protected against HBV cannot be infected with HDV. In chronic HBsAg carriers, standard hygiene and behavioral precautions should be practiced to avoid superinfection with HDV. Once acute HDV infection occurs, no secondary prevention strategy is successful.

CHRONIC HEPATITIS E

HEV infection is usually an acute self-limiting disease, but in developed countries it causes chronic infection with rapidly progressive cirrhosis in organ transplant recipients, patients with hematologic malignancies that require chemotherapy, and immunosuppressed HIV-infected individuals, either from a latent virus reactivated by immunosuppression or from a virus transmitted at the time of transplantation. Almost all cases of chronic infection have been in immunosuppressed patients.[10,11]

CLINICAL MANIFESTATIONS AND DIAGNOSIS

Chronic hepatitis E occurs after transplantation. Diagnosis is based on the detection of anti-HEV IgM antibodies. HEV RNA also can be detected in blood or feces, where its presence is transient. Solid organ transplant recipients with chronic hepatitis E harbor repeatedly positive anti-HEV antibodies and HEV RNA in blood.

TREATMENT AND PREVENTION (Rx)

There is no validated treatment of chronic HEV infection. Ribavirin (600 mg/day),[12] pegylated IFN, or a combination of the two has been used in small case series. Reducing the level of immunosuppression can result in viral clearance in approximately one third of patients. Whether candidates for transplantation or immunosuppressive therapies should be vaccinated to prevent chronic HEV infection remains to be determined.

AUTOIMMUNE HEPATITIS

Autoimmune hepatitis is a chronic inflammatory liver disorder characterized by the presence of autoantibodies in serum, high levels of serum immunoglobulins, and a frequent association with other autoimmune diseases.[13]

EPIDEMIOLOGY AND PATHOBIOLOGY

Autoimmune hepatitis typically manifests between the ages of 15 and 25 years or between the ages of 45 and 60 years, and it is more common in women. The incidence rate is approximately 1.7 per 100,000 population per year.[14] Along with primary biliary cirrhosis (Chapter 155) and primary sclerosing cholangitis (Chapter 155), autoimmune hepatitis is one of the three major autoimmune liver diseases.

Autoimmune hepatitis is believed to be caused by autoimmune reactions against normal hepatocytes in genetically predisposed persons or persons exposed to unidentified triggers of an autoimmune process against liver antigens. Associations are seen with the human leukocyte antigen (HLA) class I B8 and class II DR3 and DR52a loci. In Asians, autoimmune hepatitis is associated with HLA DR4.

CLINICAL MANIFESTATIONS AND DIAGNOSIS

Autoimmune hepatitis tends to be more severe at its onset than chronic hepatitis B or C, and it progresses to end-stage liver disease if not treated with immunosuppression. Although it is occasionally detected by elevated serum aminotransferase levels on a routine health evaluation, most patients present with fatigue and jaundice. Elevations of bilirubin or alkaline phosphatase indicate more severe or advanced disease. Patients typically have marked elevations in serum γ-globulin, specifically immunoglobulin G, as well as autoantibodies directed at non–organ-specific cellular constituents.

Type 1 (classic) autoimmune hepatitis is characterized by the presence of titers of 1 : 80 or higher (>1 : 20 in children) of antinuclear, anti–smooth muscle, antiactin, and anti-asialoglycoprotein receptor antibodies. Type 2 autoimmune hepatitis is characterized by similar elevations of anti–liver-kidney microsomal 1 antibodies and anti–liver cytosol 1 antibodies, without antinuclear or anti–smooth muscle antibodies. Liver biopsy shows features that are typical of all chronic types of hepatitis, except plasma cell infiltrates.

TREATMENT

Rx

The clinical symptoms and liver test abnormalities of autoimmune hepatitis generally respond promptly to prednisone, usually at a dose of 20 to 30 mg/day, with a decrease in serum aminotransferase levels to the normal or near-normal range within 1 to 3 months; higher doses may be required in patients with more severe disease. Lack of a biochemical or clinical response should lead to reevaluation of the diagnosis. Azathioprine 50 to 100 mg can be combined with prednisone or added later to reduce long-term steroid side effects. Maintenance doses, which are typically required indefinitely, are often 5 to 10 mg/day of prednisone combined with 50 to 150 mg/day of azathioprine. Sometimes patients can be maintained on azathioprine (2 mg/kg/day) alone. After 3 years or more of remission, therapy can be carefully withdrawn, but severe and even fatal flares can occur weeks to months later.

PROGNOSIS

The prognosis is generally related to the histologic stage of the disease. Patients who initially respond to therapy may do well for many years. Patients who progress to end-stage liver disease require liver transplantation (Chapter 154).[15]

CRYPTOGENIC CHRONIC LIVER DISEASE

Cryptogenic chronic liver disease refers to chronic hepatitis or cirrhosis of unknown cause after excluding hepatitis B, C, D, and E; autoimmune hepatitis; steatohepatitis (Chapter 152); alcoholic liver disease (Chapter 152); drug-induced hepatitis (Chapter 150); and inherited and metabolic liver diseases (Chapter 146). Tests to exclude these conditions include serum levels of α_1-antitrypsin, iron, and ceruloplasmin and, if necessary, urine and liver copper concentrations. In its later stages, nonalcoholic steatohepatitis may be associated with little or no fat.

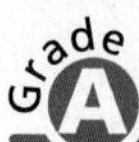

Grade A References

A1. Loomba R, Rowley A, Wesley R, et al. Systematic review: the effect of preventive lamivudine or hepatitis B reactivation during chemotherapy. *Ann Intern Med.* 2008;148:519-528.

A2. Lau GK, Piravisuth T, Luo KX, et al. Peginterferon alfa-2a, lamivudine and the combination for HBeAg-positive chronic hepatitis B. *N Engl J Med.* 2005;352:2682-2695.

A3. Chang TT, Gish RG, de Man R, et al. A comparison of entecavir and lamivudine for HBeAg-positive chronic hepatitis B. *N Engl J Med.* 2006;354:1001-1010.

A4. Marcellin P, Gane E, Buti M, et al. Regression of cirrhosis during treatment with tenofovir disoproxil fumarate for chronic hepatitis B: a 5-year open-label follow-up study. *Lancet.* 2013;381:468-475.

A5. Lawitz E, Mangia A, Wyles D, et al. Sofosbuvir for previously untreated chronic hepatitis C infection. *N Engl J Med.* 2013;368:1878-1887.

A6. Jacobson IM, Gordon SC, Kowdley KV, et al. Sofosbuvir for hepatitis C genotype 2 or 3 in patients without treatment options. *N Engl J Med.* 2013;368:1867-1877.

A7. Kowdley KV, Gordon SC, Reddy KR, et al. Ledipasvir and sofosbuvir for 8 or 12 weeks for chronic HCV without cirrhosis. *N Engl J Med.* 2014;370:1879-1888.

A8. Zeuzem S, Dusheiko GM, Salupere R, et al. Sofosbuvir and ribavirin in HCV genotypes 2 and 3. *N Engl J Med.* 2014;370:1993-2001.

A9. Sulkowski MS, Gardiner DF, Rodriguez-Torres M, et al. Daclatasvir plus sofosbuvir for previously treated or untreated chronic HCV infection. *N Engl J Med.* 2014;370:211-221.

A10. Kowdley KV, Lawitz E, Poordad F, et al. Phase 2b trial of interferon-free therapy for hepatitis C virus genotype 1. *N Engl J Med.* 2014;370:222-232.

A11. Afdhal N, Zeuzem S, Kwo P, et al. Ledipasvir and sofosbuvir for untreated HCV genotype 1 infection. *N Engl J Med.* 2014;370:1889-1898.

A12. Afdhal N, Reddy KR, Nelson DR, et al. Ledipasvir and sofosbuvir for previously treated HCV genotype 1 infection. *N Engl J Med.* 2014;370:1483-1493.

A13. Feld JJ, Kowdley KV, Coakley E, et al. Treatment of HCV with ABT-450/r-ombitasvir and dasabuvir with ribavirin. *N Engl J Med.* 2014;370:1594-1603.

A14. Zeuzem S, Jacobson IM, Baykal T, et al. Retreatment of HCV with ABT-450/r-ombitasvir and dasabuvir with ribavirin. *N Engl J Med.* 2014;370:1604-1614.

A15. Poordad F, Hezode C, Trinh R, et al. ABT-450/r-ombitasvir and dasabuvir with ribavirin for hepatitis C with cirrhosis. *N Engl J Med.* 2014;370:1973-1982.

A16. Ferenci P, Bernstein D, Lalezari J, et al. ABT-450/r-ombitasvir and dasabuvir with or without ribavirin for HCV. *N Engl J Med.* 2014;370:1983-1992.

A17. Wedemeyer H, Yurdaydin C, Dalekos GN, et al. Peginterferon plus adefovir versus either drug alone for hepatitis delta. *N Engl J Med.* 2011;364:322-331.

GENERAL REFERENCES

For the General References and other additional features, please visit Expert Consult at https://expertconsult.inkling.com.

150

TOXIN- AND DRUG-INDUCED LIVER DISEASE

WILLIAM M. LEE

DEFINITION

Toxin-induced and drug-induced hepatotoxicity, defined as any degree of liver injury caused by a drug or a toxic substance, is a frequent cause of acute liver injury and accounts for more than 50% of all cases of acute liver failure with hepatic encephalopathy in the United States. Hepatotoxicity has been described with many drugs, although the number of cases is low, given the number of prescriptions written.[1]

EPIDEMIOLOGY

Few data are available on the epidemiology of toxin-induced and drug-induced liver disease. The precise number of drug-induced liver injuries in the United States is unknown, but European data on adverse drug reactions indicate approximately 20 cases of drug-induced liver disease per 1 million people per year.[2] In developing parts of the world, drug-induced liver disease is much less common and is related to fewer drugs. It is estimated that less than 10% of actual cases are reported, so the true incidence of toxin-induced and drug-induced liver disease may be difficult to determine except in relatively closed populations.

PATHOBIOLOGY

The liver is central to the metabolism of exogenous substances. Most drugs and xenobiotics cross the intestinal brush border because they are lipophilic.

Biotransformation is the process by which lipophilic therapeutic agents are rendered more hydrophilic by the liver, resulting in drug excretion in urine or bile. In most instances, biotransformation changes a nonpolar to a polar compound through several steps. Foremost are oxidative pathways (e.g., hydroxylation) mediated by the cytochromes (CYPs) P-450 (Chapter 29). The next step is typically esterification to form sulfates and glucuronides, a process that results in the addition of highly polar groups to the hydroxyl group. These two enzymatic steps are referred to as *phase I* (CYP oxidation) and *phase II* (esterification). Other important metabolic pathways involve glutathione-*S*-transferase, acetylating enzymes and alcohol dehydrogenase, but the principal metabolic pathways for most pharmacologic agents involve CYPs and subsequent esterification.

Pathogenesis

The exact details of the pathogenesis of liver injury are unclear for most drugs.[3] A single drug may cause toxic effects in several ways. One overarching approach suggests that high-energy unstable metabolites of the parent drug, the result of CYP activation, bind to cell proteins or DNA and disrupt cell function. Perhaps the best example is acetaminophen. Although used universally for non-narcotic pain relief, acetaminophen, when taken in large quantities, causes profound centrilobular necrosis. The metabolic pathway of acetaminophen involves phase I and phase II reactions, glutathione detoxification, and the formation of reactive intermediates (E-Fig. 150-1). The presence of alcohol, which competes for CYP P-450 2E1, not only inhibits the formation of *N*-aminoparaquinoneamine (NAPQI) but also induces the enzyme so that its half-life is slowed and more enzyme is present. After the cessation of alcohol ingestion, NAPQI formation is enhanced by the presence of the induced enzyme and the lack of competition from alcohol. Toxicity is a dynamic process and may be most pronounced in the 24 hours after the cessation of alcohol. Glucuronidation and sulfation occur as the initial detoxifying step because the parent compound contains a hydroxyl group. Glucuronidation and sulfation capacity greatly exceeds daily needs, so even patients with very advanced liver disease continue to have adequate glucuronidation capacity, which explains why no obvious enhancement of toxicity is observed when cirrhotic patients take acetaminophen.

TABLE 150-1 FACTORS THAT MAY INFLUENCE THE METABOLIC FATE OF DRUGS

AGE
The elderly seem to be affected more often; adults are more susceptible than children to some drugs (acetaminophen, halothane, isoniazid) and less susceptible to others (aspirin, valproic acid)
ALCOHOL: ACUTE AND CHRONIC INGESTION
Induction of CYP2E1 affects drugs metabolized by this pathway, including acetaminophen and isoniazid
GENDER
Females are affected more often, but the reason is unknown
PREGNANCY
Effects of drugs in pregnancy have been poorly studied
PREEXISTING LIVER DISEASE
Hepatic disease may *protect* against idiosyncratic reactions and may *enhance* the toxicity of dose-dependent hepatotoxins (e.g., acetaminophen)
RENAL DISEASE
Slowed disappearance of the parent compound yields higher concentrations and affects P-450 (e.g., enhancement of tetracycline toxicity in renal disease)
CERTAIN FOODS
Grapefruit has an unknown substance that interferes with the metabolism of some drugs
CONCOMITANT DRUGS
Drug-drug interactions are common causes of adverse effects (e.g., valproate and chlorpromazine together lead to enhanced cholestasis)
GENETIC FACTORS
Enzyme polymorphisms (e.g., enhanced phenytoin liver disease in patients with defective epoxide hydrolase activity), HLA phenotypes (e.g., nitrofurantoin susceptibility)

Genetics

Enzyme Polymorphism

Although acetaminophen is a dose-related toxin, the rarity of idiosyncratic drug toxicity (1 in 10,000 patients) suggests the importance of environmental and host factors (Table 150-1). Genetically variant CYP isoenzymes may partially explain the observed individual variation in response to drugs. An example is debrisoquine, an antihypertensive drug marketed in Europe that is hydroxylated by CYP2D6, an isoform that is totally absent in 5% of normal individuals. Lack of CYP2D6 greatly prolongs the half-life of the parent compound in affected individuals. Another example is the phenomenon of fast versus slow acetylation, which affects different ethnic groups and has been implicated in the differential metabolism of isoniazid. Most of the known genetic variants that occur relatively frequently, however, cannot explain the formation of a toxic intermediate in only a rare individual.

Most drugs are small organic compounds, unlikely to evoke an immune response. Although some toxic drug reactions are associated with an obvious allergic response, most are not. Nevertheless, immune mechanisms not associated with systemic allergic immunoglobulin E (IgE) reactions or skin hypersensitivity might be involved. Studies suggest that the products of CYP P-450 metabolism, the highly reactive intermediates formed within the microsomes, covalently bind to the enzyme itself to form a drug-hapten adduct that disables the enzyme and injures the cell. Haptenization then evokes an immune response directed against the newly formed antigen or neoantigen. P-450s have been shown to traffic to the plasma membrane, thereby allowing the drug–P-450 adduct to become the target of a subsequent cytolytic attack. It is unclear whether the targets are these adducts or the smaller peptides processed and presented by the major histocompatibility complex class I and class II schemes. The association among neoantigens, autoantibodies, and hepatotoxic drugs implicates an immunologic mechanism, as does latency, which is the delay between the first ingestion and evidence of toxicity.[4]

Regardless of whether an individual drug causes significant cell necrosis, the drug–P-450 adducts can evoke an immune response. Any subsequent drug–P-450 adduct present on the hepatocyte surface would evoke a further response. Responses may be antibody mediated or occur as a result of direct cytolytic attack by primed T cells. Specific genetically determined components of the immune response may be important. A specific human leukocyte antigen (HLA) haplotype has been associated with hepatitis induced by amoxicillin-clavulanate and other polymorphisms encoding for increased susceptibility have been identified. However, it is unlikely that a single polymorphism will be found for most hepatocellular reactions, even when the phenotype of injury is well-characterized, such as for isoniazid. For every patient with a severe injury caused by drugs, there are often many more individuals with asymptomatic aminotransferase elevations that subsided despite continuing the drug—sometimes referred to as an *adaptive response.*

Other Mechanisms

In drug-induced cholestasis, disruption of specific transport channels in hepatocytes or cholangiocytes may be the key event. Estrogen or androgenic steroids may cause multiple canalicular membrane transport changes that affect, among others, the canalicular bile salt pump. For a few drugs, a specific uncoupling of mitochondrial respiration may lead to microvesicular steatosis and lactic acidosis.

Hepatotoxic Agents

Although there are a few dose-related toxins, most drugs involved in liver disease cause idiosyncratic, unpredictable toxicity.[5] The use of herbal and dietary supplements and the toxicity resulting from them appears to be increasing in the United States. Most common are body building supplements containing androgenic steroids that lead to severe cholestasis; weight loss products may cause hepatocellular injury of varying severity, including occasional fatalities.[6]

Intrinsic (Dose-Dependent) Agents

Acetaminophen (see later) and a few other agents seem to have a clear dose-response effect, although idiosyncrasy usually plays a role as well (Table 150-2). Some toxins, such as α-amanitine produced by *Amanita* mushrooms, cause dose-related injury. *Amanita* poisoning may occur after ingestion of the mushrooms *Amanita phalloides* (death cap) or *Amanita virosa* (deadly agaric). The dose-dependent toxic effect on the liver is attributed to amatoxin, an ingredient of the mushrooms that enhances the toxic effect by its enterohepatic recirculation characteristics; the toxic effect is exerted on each cycle of the recirculation through the liver.

TABLE 150-2 DRUGS AND TOXINS IN WHICH A DOSE-RESPONSE EFFECT IS OBSERVED

DRUG OR TOXIN	RESPONSE
Acetaminophen	Total dose, single vs. multiple time points
Amiodarone	Total dose over time
Bromfenac	Toxicity occurs only after extended use
Cocaine	Dose-related vascular collapse
Cyclophosphamide	Dose related, worse with previous ALT elevations
Cyclosporine	Cholestasis with toxic blood levels, CYP3A phenotype
Methotrexate	Aminotransferase, fibrosis; single dose/total dose
Niacin	Large doses cause vascular collapse
Oral contraceptives	Prolonged use causes hepatic adenomas
Tetracycline	Total dose, renal dysfunction
Toxins (yellow phosphorus, carbon tetrachloride, *Amanita* toxin, bacterial toxins)	Total dose

ALT = alanine aminotransferase.

TABLE 150-3 TYPES OF TOXIN AND DRUG REACTIONS

REACTION TYPE	IMPLICATED DRUGS OR TOXINS
Autoimmune (attack on cell surface markers)	Lovastatin, methyldopa, nitrofurantoin
Cholestatic (attack on bile ducts)	Anabolic steroids, carbamazepine, chlorpromazine, estrogen, erythromycin
Fibrosis (activation of stellate cells leads to fibrosis)	Methotrexate, vitamin A excess
Granulomatous (macrophage stimulation)	Allopurinol, diltiazem, nitrofurantoin, quinidine, sulfa drugs
Hepatocellular (damage to smooth endoplasmic reticulum and immune cell surface)	Acetaminophen, *Amanita* poisoning, diclofenac, isoniazid, lovastatin, nefazodone, trazodone, venlafaxine
Immunoallergic (cytotoxic cell attack on surface determinants)	Halothane, phenytoin, sulfamethoxazole
Mixed (see earlier)	Amoxicillin-clavulanate, carbamazepine, cyclosporine, herbs, methimazole
Oncogenic (hepatic adenoma formation)	Oral contraceptives, androgenic agents
Steatohepatitis (mitochondrial dysfunction: β-oxidation and respiratory chain)	Amiodarone, perhexiline maleate, tamoxifen
Vascular collapse (ischemic damage)	Cocaine, ecstasy, nicotinic acid
Veno-occlusive disease (endotheliitis of sinusoidal endothelial cells)	Busulfan, cytoxan

Idiosyncratic Reactions

Drug reactions occur in 1 in 1000 to 1 in 200,000 patients. Characteristics of these idiosyncratic reactions include their infrequent occurrence, varying time intervals between the initial exposure and the reaction, and varying severity of reactions in affected individuals. There are also similarities such as "class effects" (similar drugs exhibit similar features; Table 150-3), a consistent pattern for each drug, and the fact that rechallenge with a responsible agent usually leads to a more severe reaction with a shorter latency than seen after the initial exposure.

Antibiotics, anticonvulsants, and nonsteroidal anti-inflammatory drugs are associated more frequently with drug-induced liver disease, whereas hormones, antihypertensive drugs, digoxin, and antiarrhythmic drugs are implicated rarely. In some cases, idiosyncratic reactions are so infrequent that a drug continues to be used if its effectiveness or uniqueness makes the risk acceptable. An example is isoniazid, which is among the few drugs implicated in drug-induced liver injury in developing countries. In individuals receiving isoniazid as a single agent for tuberculosis prophylaxis, increased aminotransferase levels may develop in 15 to 20%, but severe hepatic necrosis develops in only 0.1 to 1% (Chapter 324)—a rate that is high in comparison to idiosyncratic drug reactions, yet low enough for isoniazid, because of its effectiveness, to remain a key drug. Drugs that require relatively high dosing, more than 100 mg/day, and that have high lipophilicity are associated with most liver injury, not those at lower dose levels.[7]

CLINICAL MANIFESTATIONS

Patients may have few or nonspecific complaints despite very elevated aminotransferase levels. Clinical features include nausea, fatigue, occasional right upper quadrant pain, and nonspecific symptoms similar to those seen in other forms of acute hepatitis (Chapter 148). Fever or pharyngitis (typically seen in phenytoin reactions) may be present. No specific physical findings to raise suspicion of drug toxicity are noted, except possibly a rash. Any patient in whom jaundice develops is at risk for having a severe or fatal outcome, and patients who continue taking the drug despite jaundice are at highest risk.

DIAGNOSIS

Abnormal aminotransferase levels with the use of a new drug should raise the suspicion for a drug-induced reaction and prompt immediate discontinuation of the drug rather than awaiting diagnostic tests to confirm or exclude the diagnosis. Immediate discontinuation of medication at the first sign of liver disease can prevent most fatal liver injuries.

Evaluation of a patient with a suspected drug reaction is directed toward establishing the timeline for all drugs or herbs the patient may have taken. Responsible drugs have usually been started between 5 and 90 days before the onset of symptoms. Evidence of viral hepatitis (Chapters 148), gallstones (Chapter 155), alcoholic liver disease (Chapter 152), pregnancy (Chapter 239), severe right heart failure (Chapter 58), or a period of hypotension (Chapter 106) points to these specific causes. Less commonly, cytomegalovirus (Chapter 376), Epstein-Barr virus (Chapter 377), or herpesviruses (Chapters 374 and 375) can cause hepatic injury, primarily in immunosuppressed individuals. If all these causes can be excluded, the temporal relationship fits, and the patient begins to improve after withdrawal of the drug, the diagnosis is more secure. Liver biopsy is of limited value because the histologic picture in most cases of drug-induced liver injury is no different from that of viral hepatitis (Chapter 148). Nevertheless, an occasional liver biopsy specimen in an enigmatic case might reveal eosinophils or granulomas, consistent with a drug reaction.

Types of Drug Reactions

Although most liver injury involves direct hepatocyte necrosis or apoptosis (hepatocellular injury), some drugs injure primarily the bile ducts or canaliculi and cause cholestasis without significant damage to hepatocytes. Other drugs affect sinusoidal cells or present a particular pattern of liver injury affecting multiple cell types (mixed type). Another approach to drug reactions emphasizes the histologic changes involved and the cell type (see Table 150-3 and E-Fig. 150-2).

Hepatocellular Reactions

Hepatocellular reactions are the most common type of drug-induced liver disease and account for 90% of cases (Table 150-4). They are characterized by a pattern of serum liver test results that reflect hepatocellular injury. Usually, improvement is quick after discontinuation of the drug (1 to 2 months), and fulminant, acute liver failure with hepatic encephalopathy develops in only a few patients.

Histologic findings include necrosis and cellular infiltration. The necrosis may be zonal (e.g., induced by acetaminophen or carbon tetrachloride) or diffuse (e.g., induced by halothane), and the inflammatory response consists of lymphocytes or eosinophils. Massive necrosis may cause acute liver failure and death.

Acetaminophen toxicity is the most common form of acute liver failure in the United States and is the best understood example of direct hepatocyte toxicity. The incidence of acetaminophen poisoning varies widely throughout the world, but it is becoming more frequent and widespread. Liver injury occurs predictably after an intentional suicidal overdose (Chapter 110); it also occurs when acetaminophen is used in excessive doses or sometimes even in therapeutic doses for pain relief. Enhanced toxicity occurs when patients are fasting or are chronic alcohol users because of enzyme induction and depletion of glutathione by alcohol and fasting; by comparison, acute alcohol intake may protect against acetaminophen toxicity during the period of alcohol ingestion. Thereafter, a rebound increase in available CYP2E1 results in increased toxicity in the 12 hours after ingestion because of enzyme

TABLE 150-4 SCORING SYSTEM TO ASSESS CAUSALITY OF HEPATOCELLULAR REACTIONS

FACTOR	SCORE*
TEMPORAL RELATIONSHIP OF START OF DRUG TO START OF ILLNESS	
Initial treatment: 5-90 days; subsequent treatment course: 1-15 days	+2
Initial treatment: <5 or >90 days; subsequent treatment course: >15 days	+1
From cessation of drug: ≤15 days†	+1
COURSE	
ALT decreases ≥ 50% from peak within 8 days	+3
ALT decreases ≥ 50% from peak within 30 days	+2
If the drug is continued, inconclusive	0
RISK FACTORS	
Alcohol‡	+1
No alcohol‡	0
Age ≥ 55 yr	+1
Age < 55 yr	0
CONCOMITANT DRUG	
Concomitant drug with suggestive time of onset	−1
Concomitant drug known to be a hepatotoxin with suggestive time of onset	−2
Concomitant drug with further evidence of involvement (rechallenge)	−3
NUMBER OF NONDRUG CAUSES	
Hepatitis A, B, or C; biliary obstruction; alcoholism (AST ≥ 2 × ALT); recent hypotension; and CMV, EBV, and HSV infection all excluded	+2
4-5 causes excluded	+1
<4 causes excluded	−2
Nondrug cause highly probable	−3
PREVIOUS INFORMATION ON HEPATOTOXICITY OF DRUG IN QUESTION	
Package insert mentions	+2
Published case reports but not on package label	+1
Reaction unknown	0
RECHALLENGE	
Positive (ALT doubles with drug alone)§	+2
Compatible (ALT doubles, compounding features)§	+1
Negative (increase in ALT but ≤ 2 × ULN)§	−2
Not done	0

Modified from Danan G, Benichou C. Causality assessment of adverse reactions to drugs. I. A novel method based on the conclusions of international consensus meetings: application to drug-induced liver injuries. *J Clin Epidemiol.* 1993;46:1323-1330; and Benichou C, Danan G, Flahault A. Causality assessment of adverse reactions to drugs. II. An original model for validation of drug causality assessment methods: case reports with positive rechallenge. *J Clin Epidemiol.* 1993;46:1331-1336.
*Causality is highly probable (score >8), probable (score 6-8), possible (score 3-5), unlikely (score 1-2), or excluded (score ≤0).
†For cholestatic reactions, ≤ 30 days.
‡For cholestatic reactions, alcohol, or pregnancy.
§For cholestatic reactions, substitute alkaline phosphatase (or total bilirubin) for ALT.
ALT = alanine aminotransferase; AST = aspartate aminotransferase; CMV = cytomegalovirus; EBV = Epstein-Barr virus; HSV = herpes simplex virus; ULN = upper limit of normal.

induction (see E-Fig. 150-1). Patients with an unintentional acetaminophen overdose may fare worse than suicidal patients because the former seek treatment later in their course, even though suicidal patients take larger doses. The better outcome after an acute overdose may be explained by earlier medical attention and the use of *N*-acetylcysteine, an effective antidote. Nevertheless, one fifth of suicide attempts using acetaminophen are associated with severe liver injury and the potential for a fatal outcome.

The extremely elevated aminotransferase values (often > 6000 IU/L, and sometimes as high as 30,000 IU/L) observed in suicidal and unintentional acetaminophen ingestion help distinguish these cases from viral hepatitis or other drug injury. This signature of hyperacute injury (high aminotransferase levels, low bilirubin levels) are almost pathognomonic of acetaminophen injury, which can go unrecognized if a careful history is not elicited.[8] The availability of an antidote makes this diagnosis especially important. The antidote *N*-acetylcysteine (Chapter 110) may be given by nasogastric tube on admission and for the next 72 hours to provide glutathione substrate. The standard treatment is intravenous *N*-acetylcysteine beginning at a dose of 140 mg/kg in 300 mL of 5% dextrose given over 1 hour, followed by a dose of 70 mg/kg in 5% dextrose given over a 1-hour period every 4 hours for 48 hours. A loading dose of 140 mg/kg PO can be given, followed by 70 mg/kg every 4 hours for 17 doses (72 hours). Expected survival rates are greater than 80%, although liver transplantation is occasionally required.

Cholestatic Reactions

Cholestatic reactions have been described for many drugs. Cholestasis is best defined as failure of bile to reach the duodenum, and common symptoms are jaundice and pruritus. *Pure cholestasis,* with no signs of hepatocellular necrosis, is seen almost exclusively in patients taking oral contraceptives, anabolic steroids, or sex hormone antagonists such as tamoxifen. Acute *cholestatic hepatitis* is characterized histologically by cholestasis (dilated canaliculi, brown granules in the cytoplasm of hepatocytes), some degree of liver cell necrosis and bile duct injury, and inflammatory infiltration by polymorphonuclear leukocytes. Drugs that cause this type of reaction include carbamazepine, trimethoprim-sulfamethoxazole, captopril, and body building dietary supplements containing androgenic compounds

Generally, drug-induced cholestasis takes longer to resolve than drug-induced hepatotoxicity. In some cases, segments of the intrahepatic biliary tree may be destroyed progressively, the so-called vanishing bile duct syndrome that occurs after a protracted course (>6 months) of drug-induced cholestasis. The result is a state of chronic cholestasis that resembles primary biliary cirrhosis (Chapter 155). Approximately 30 drugs have been implicated in the vanishing bile duct syndrome, including levofloxacin and, occasionally, other antibiotics. A sclerosing cholangitis–like syndrome with jaundice caused by intrahepatic and extrahepatic strictures in the bile ducts is sometimes observed in patients receiving intra-arterial floxuridine chemotherapy for hepatic metastases of colorectal cancer.

Immunoallergic Reactions

Drugs also may be associated with definite allergic reactions. A combined toxic-immunologic mechanism is involved in liver injury caused by halothane, a fluorinated hydrocarbon anesthetic that causes severe, often fatal liver injury after multiple exposures (Chapter 432). Other fluorinated hydrocarbons, including isoflurane and desflurane, occasionally result in the same response. Although halothane has never been withdrawn, its use has been limited by the advent of safer agents. Hypersensitivity reactions, such as fever, eosinophilia, and rash, are common. Halothane may induce fever, eosinophilia, and antimitochondrial antibodies. Direct cytotoxicity and immune-mediated toxicity are observed, consistent with the clinical observation that severe halothane toxicity occurs with repeated exposure. Although evidence of injury can usually be identified within 1 week of the first exposure, the interval to toxicity is shortened and the damage is more severe with each successive exposure, as befits an immune reaction.

Phenytoin (Chapter 403) induces the simultaneous onset of fever, rash, lymphadenopathy, and eosinophilia. The mechanisms responsible for the combined allergic and hepatotoxic reaction are unknown, but the slow resolution of the illness suggests that the allergen remains on the surface of the hepatocyte for weeks or months. A concurrent mononucleosis-like picture is frequently confused with a viral illness or streptococcal pharyngitis. If phenytoin is not discontinued promptly despite signs of hepatitis, a severe Stevens-Johnson drug eruption (Chapters 439 and 440) and prolonged fever may result. As with any therapeutic agent, rapid recognition of the presence of a toxic drug reaction and immediate discontinuation of the compound are key to limiting hepatic damage. Systemic features of an allergic reaction may not be obvious, even when eosinophilia or granulomas are present on liver biopsy.

Steatohepatitis

Fatty liver disease (Chapter 152) related to the metabolic syndrome is increasingly evident in the United States and elsewhere. Differentiating this underlying condition from de novo fatty liver caused by a drug reaction can be difficult. In addition, certain agents such as statins may be associated with aminotransferase elevations independent of fatty liver disease. As a general rule, statins very rarely cause significant liver injury and should not be withheld from patients with hypercholesterolemia, even when fatty liver is present (Chapter 206). Steatosis in the liver (Chapter 152) can be present in a microvesicular or macrovesicular pattern. Macrovesicular steatosis, the most common form, is characterized histologically by a single vacuole of fat filling up the hepatocyte and displacing the nucleus to the cell's periphery. Macrovesicular steatosis is typically caused by alcohol, diabetes, or obesity. Sometimes drugs such as corticosteroids or methotrexate may cause these hepatic changes. Amiodarone (Chapters 64 and 65) has been associated with a picture resembling alcoholic hepatitis, occasionally with progression to cirrhosis. The pathophysiology involves accumulation of phospholipids in the liver, eyes, thyroid, and skin. Treatment is primarily withdrawal of the drug and observation, although the half-life of amiodarone is prolonged. Tamoxifen, which has been used in long-term regimens for the prevention of recurrent breast cancer (Chapter 198), has also been associated with steatohepatitis evolving to cirrhosis.

In microvesicular steatosis, hepatocytes contain numerous small fat vesicles that do not displace the nucleus. Valproic acid, an anticonvulsant (Chapter 403), causes hepatotoxicity, either as a result of microvesicular fat deposition, resembling Reye syndrome, or in a more chronic, indolent fashion associated with macrovesicular fat accumulation. Toxicity is more severe and frequent in children. These lesions are associated with disruption of mitochondrial DNA, resulting in anaerobic metabolism that leads to lactic acidosis in the most severe cases. Macrovesicular and microvesicular lesions may be observed concomitantly in some patients, and microvesicular lesions are more often associated with a poor prognosis. Hepatocellular necrosis also may be present. Acute fatty liver of pregnancy (Chapters 147 and 239) and Reye syndrome are two examples of severe liver diseases caused by microvesicular steatosis.

Drugs involved in microvesicular steatosis include valproate, tetracycline, and fialuridine. Aspirin use in children has been associated with Reye syndrome, but the incidence of Reye syndrome has decreased dramatically since warnings were issued concerning aspirin use in children.

Effects of Sex Steroids

Anabolic steroids, such as methyltestosterone, may cause cholestasis. Androgens or estrogens may cause peliosis hepatis and benign or malignant tumors. Oral contraceptives (Chapter 238) may cause cholestasis, hepatic adenomas, or Budd-Chiari syndrome (hepatic vein thrombosis). Antiandrogens used to treat prostate cancer (Chapter 201), such as flutamide and nilutamide, and antipituitary drugs, such as cyproterone acetate, also have been associated with severe hepatocellular injury.

Other Drug Reactions

Other less severe drug reactions involving the liver include granulomatous reactions, fibrosis, ischemic injury, and chronic autoimmune liver injury (see Table 150-3). The type of reaction observed can be helpful in determining the probable agent because most drugs have a specific injury profile.

A pattern of veno-occlusive disease with obliteration of small intrahepatic veins, sinusoidal congestion, and necrosis is observed frequently in bone marrow transplant patients (Chapter 178) who receive chemotherapy with cyclophosphamide (Cytoxan) or busulfan. Symptoms, including rapidly accumulating ascites, painful hepatomegaly, and jaundice, develop soon after the chemotherapeutic regimen has begun. Oxiplatin can cause portal venular injury that leads to nodular regenerative hyperplasia and life-long portal hypertension. Rarely, herbal medicines (Chapter 39) such as pyrrolizidine alkaloids (*Crotalaria* and *Senecio* found in Jamaican bush tea) may cause veno-occlusive disease.

Toxins are associated with direct injury to hepatocytes in a dose-dependent fashion. Organic solvents such as carbon tetrachloride and trichloroethylene (Chapter 110) cause centrilobular injury. Yellow phosphorus, found in firecrackers and rat poisons, is a rare cause of liver injury from either accidental or intentional exposure. Symptoms of poisoning are similar to those of any other type of hepatitis.

Mushroom poisoning (Chapter 110), which follows the ingestion of *A. phalloides* and related species, typically occurs in amateur mushroom fanciers in a dose-related fashion. The associated muscarinic effects, including severe diarrhea, vomiting, and profuse sweating, predominate in the first hours after ingestion. Hepatic failure follows if antidotes (see later) are not given. The overall prognosis for spontaneous recovery is poor; liver transplantation may be life-saving.

Differential Diagnosis

The differential diagnosis of toxin-induced and drug-induced liver injury includes almost the entire spectrum of liver diseases. Some cases previously ascribed to drugs may now be linked to previously unsuspected hepatitis E (Chapters 148 and 149).[9] Because the clinical picture of drug-induced liver injury ranges from pure hepatocellular to pure cholestatic variants, a high index of suspicion must be maintained, even when toxin-induced or drug-induced liver injury is not obvious initially.

For dose-dependent hepatotoxins, the diagnosis may be easier to establish than for idiosyncratic drug reactions. Serum levels of acetaminophen, a thorough history, and characteristic biochemical abnormalities (high aminotransferase levels) usually reveal an acetaminophen overdose, whereas a diagnosis of *Amanita* poisoning depends on the history, symptoms of gastroenteritis (muscarinic reaction), and positive mushroom identification.

For idiosyncratic drug reactions, the diagnosis is sometimes more difficult to establish. A standardized reporting form called the Roussel-Uclaf Causality Assessment Method (RUCAM) (see Table 150-4), developed by an international panel, provides a worthwhile scoring system. These guidelines outline the steps an experienced clinician might use to assess the likelihood of a drug reaction. Causality assessment factors typically include the temporal relationship, course after cessation of the drug, risk factors, concomitant drugs, a search for nondrug causes (viral hepatitis), previous information concerning the drug, and response to rechallenge, which is typically not required. Recently, the Drug-Induced Liver Injury Network has used an expert opinion system that is helpful in defining phenotypes but is not readily applicable for day-to-day use.

TREATMENT Rx

Prompt discontinuation of a suspected drug is mandatory. Available antidotes should be used for acetaminophen (*N*-acetylcysteine) and *Amanita* poisoning (penicillin 300,000 to 1 million U/kg/day intravenously (IV) and thioctic acid 5 to 100 mg every 6 hours IV have been recommended, but there are no controlled trials). General supportive therapy ranges from intravenous fluid replacement to intensive monitoring and treatment of patients with hepatic encephalopathy secondary to acute liver failure (Chapter 153). *N*-Acetylcysteine is the standard antidote for acetaminophen overdose, but it may improve outcomes in some cases of acute liver failure not associated with acetaminophen, such as severe alcoholic hepatitis.[10] Almost 10% of patients die or require liver transplantation within six months after serious drug-induced liver injury and about another 20% have persistent evidence of liver injury.[11] Liver transplantation (Chapter 154) is performed in more than 50% of patients with idiosyncratic drug-induced acute liver failure because the survival rate in this setting without transplantation is less than 20%.

FUTURE DIRECTIONS

Research in pharmacogenomics may allow the patient's own genetic information to guide individualized drug therapy and monitoring of idiosyncratic drug reactions. The genetic information would probably concentrate initially on enzymes with variant alleles associated with poor metabolism, such as CYP1A2 or CYP2C19 for isoniazid, CYP2C9 for piroxicam, or CYP2D6 for nortriptyline. Better postmarketing surveillance of all drugs to identify those with previously unappreciated hepatotoxicity should be a high priority.

PREVENTION

It is reasonable to consider a drug reaction whenever an episode of apparent hepatitis is unexplained, particularly if a new agent has been introduced in the previous 3 months. It is prudent to defer embracing new drugs during their first year of introduction, particularly if they show no unique advantages over accepted formulations. Physicians must strive to instill in their patients a healthy level of alertness with regard to drug-induced liver injury, particularly for agents with known hepatotoxicity. Monitoring of aminotransferase levels on a monthly basis is suggested for known hepatotoxins such as isoniazid or diclofenac, but it is unlikely to be cost-effective when adverse reactions occur less frequently, such as in only 1 in 50,000 patients. Because many drug reactions develop within days, monitoring provides no guarantee. Most fatal drug reactions could have been prevented if the offending agent were withdrawn immediately, at the first sign of illness.

GENERAL REFERENCES

For the General References and other additional features, please visit Expert Consult at https://expertconsult.inkling.com.

151

BACTERIAL, PARASITIC, FUNGAL, AND GRANULOMATOUS LIVER DISEASES

K. RAJENDER REDDY

INFECTIONS OF THE LIVER

Infections of the liver can be due to a variety of pathogens, including bacteria, fungi, amebae, protozoa, helminths, spirochetes, and rickettsiae. The manifestations of these infections are protean; some are generic to all infections, whereas others are specific to particular infections. The epidemiology can vary and depend on the geographic region of the world. In endemic areas, *Entamoeba histolytica* is a key consideration in the differential diagnosis of a liver abscess (Table 151-1).

Bacterial Infections

PYOGENIC LIVER ABSCESS

DEFINITION

Pyogenic liver abscess is a focal collection of purulent bacterial material and necroinflammatory debris. It can be solitary or multiple and can be caused by one or more aerobic and anaerobic bacteria (Fig. 151-1).

EPIDEMIOLOGY

Pyogenic liver abscess has an estimated global incidence of approximately 1.1 to 2.3 per 100,000 person-years, whereas in the United States, the incidence is approximately 3.6 per 100,000 and has been rising.[1] Biliary obstruction, caused by either a malignant or benign disease, accounts for 50 to 60% of pyogenic liver abscesses, whereas portal pyemia, due to appendicitis or other intra-abdominal infections, accounts for about 20% of cases. Recently, a number of studies from Asia, where *Klebsiella pneumoniae* is the primary etiologic source of pyogenic liver abscess, have proposed a correlation with underlying colorectal neoplasms,[2] some of which were evident at the time of diagnosis but also with a 5- to 8-fold higher risk of newly diagnosed colorectal cancers in the 3 years after diagnosis.[3] However, it is yet to be determined whether these findings can be extrapolated to other regions of the world.

PATHOBIOLOGY

Bacteria can enter the liver through the portal system from infections in areas drained by the mesenteric system into the portal system, such as appendicitis (Chapter 142). Other mechanisms for pyogenic liver abscess include bacterial cholangitis due to benign or malignant obstruction and infection of the liver from a systemic bacteremia, such as an infection of the oral cavity. Pyogenic liver abscess can also be caused by blunt or penetrating trauma, including such unusual causes as the ingestion of a toothpick or fish bone that can cause an intestinal perforation, fistula to the liver, and subsequent abscess formation. Liver abscesses can occur in a transplanted graft owing to vascular compromise caused by hepatic artery thrombosis and ischemic bile duct strictures.

Multiple organisms can cause pyogenic liver abscess. The most common organism, *Klebsiella pneumoniae*,[4] often is associated with biliary tract

TABLE 151-1 FEATURES OF BACTERIAL AND AMEBIC ABSCESSES

	DEMOGRAPHICS	RISK FACTORS	SYMPTOMS	LABORATORY FINDINGS	RADIOGRAPHIC FEATURES	DIAGNOSIS	TREATMENT
Bacterial liver abscess	50-70 years old Male = female	Recent bacterial infection, biliary obstruction, diabetes mellitus	Fevers, chills, malaise, anorexia, diarrhea, cough, pleuritic chest pain, RUQ pain	Leukocytosis, anemia, elevated alkaline phosphatase and bilirubin, low albumin, positive blood cultures (50%)	Multifocal (50%), usually right lobe, irregular margins	Aspirate (70-80% positive)	Percutaneous drainage and antibiotics
Amebic liver abscess	18-50 years old Male > female	Alcohol intake, HLA-DR3, oral and anal sex, contaminated enema apparatus, travel to or living in an endemic area	Fever, RUQ pain, hepatic tenderness, anorexia, weight loss, uncommon to have colitis	Leukocytosis, no eosinophilia, mild anemia, elevated alkaline phosphatase, elevated ESR, positive serology	Single abscess (80%), usually right lobe, wall enhancement seen on CT scan with IV contrast	Aspirate (trophozoites rarely seen) can rule out superimposed bacterial infection, positive serology and risk factors	Metronidazole and iodoquinol

RUQ = right upper quadrant; ESR = erythrocyte sedimentation rate; CT = computed tomography; IV = intravenous.

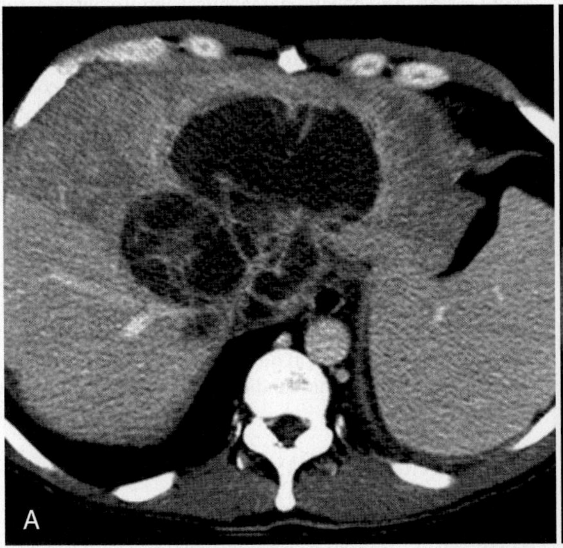

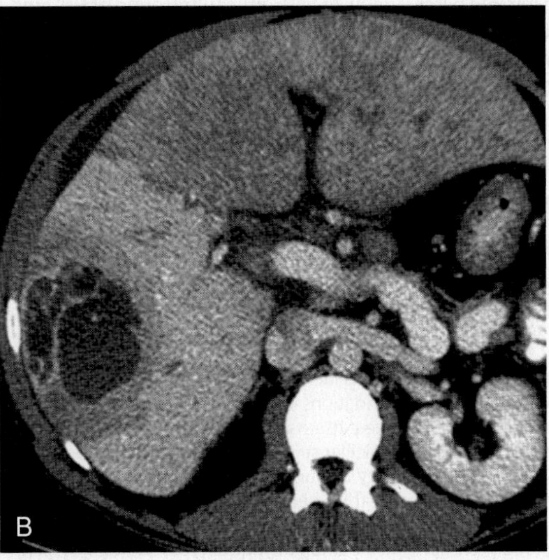

FIGURE 151-1. A and B, Computed tomographic scans of pyogenic liver abscess lesions. (Courtesy Dr. Chalermrat Bunchorntavakul, Bangkok, Thailand.)

disease. Other aerobes include *Escherichia coli*, group D streptococci, β-hemolytic streptococci, and *Staphylococcus aureus*. Anaerobic infection is often seen with colonic disease. Less common causes of liver abscesses include *Actinomyces*, *Nocardia asteroides*, *Yersinia pseudotuberculosis* and *Yersinia enterocolitica*, *Listeria monocytogenes*, *Campylobacter jejuni*, *Legionella pneumophila*, *Mycobacterium tuberculosis*, *Salmonella typhi* or *Salmonella paratyphi*, *Candida albicans*, and *Bartonella henselae*. Most often, the organism recovered from an abscess cavity is single, but multiple organisms can be isolated in as many as a third of patients. Bacteria may not be isolated from the abscess because of prior antibiotic therapy or the failure to perform proper anaerobic cultures.

CLINICAL MANIFESTATIONS

The signs and symptoms associated with a liver abscess typically include fever, right upper quadrant abdominal pain, chills, nausea, vomiting, weight loss, and jaundice. The presentation can be acute or indolent. An associated bacteremia is seen in approximately 50% of the patients, but frank sepsis is rare. About 10% of patients develop metastatic infection to other sites.[5]

DIAGNOSIS

Appropriate diagnosis requires a high degree of clinical suspicion, and diagnosis is sometimes delayed. Usually, however, the diagnosis is made promptly with the wide availability of the various radiologic modalities. The two common types of liver abscesses are pyogenic and amebic abscesses, and it is important to make a distinction because the prognosis and management differ. Amebic abscesses can become secondarily infected with other bacteria.

The diagnosis of an abscess is based on a constellation of clinical, bacteriologic, and radiologic features. Ultrasonography and computed tomography (CT) scanning are the most common radiologic modalities to diagnose an abscess cavity reliably, either as single or multiple lesions (see Fig. 151-1). CT is the preferred diagnostic indicator of an abscess, with sensitivity of more than 90%. Any concurrent biliary obstruction also can be diagnosed by these imaging modalities. Approximately 50% of patients have multiple abscesses. On CT, the lesion is seen as a fluid collection with irregular borders and wall edema. One drawback to this imaging modality is that no specific features differentiate a pyogenic abscess from other infectious causes (i.e., amebic or fungal). Another drawback is that a very early stage abscess may not be well formed and may have characteristics more suggestive of a solid mass. It is critical to distinguish an abscess from a tumor (Chapter 196) or a simple cyst, a process that can be complicated on noninvasive imaging by various events, such as bleeding into a cyst, calcification, necrosis, or bleeding into a tumor. A finding of smaller (<2 cm) peripheral lesions that surround a central abscess (the cluster sign) can help exclude a hepatic neoplasm. Calcification suggests bleeding into a tumor, but it also can be seen in the wall of an echinococcal cyst. Nonspecific radiologic features, including elevation of the right hemidiaphragm, right lower lung lobe atelectasis, and right pleural effusion, are seen in up to 30% of patients with pyogenic liver abscesses. Magnetic resonance imaging and tagged white blood cell scans add little to the diagnosis of a liver abscess.

Microbial cultures are essential. In addition to blood cultures, the abscess cavity should be aspirated percutaneously, with either ultrasound or CT guidance, and the aspirate should be cultured for aerobic and anaerobic organisms as well as for amebae if there is any suspicion of an amebic abscess. Blood cultures are positive in only approximately 50% of cases. In approximately 15 to 20% of cases, multiple organisms are identified in the abscess cavity, but 20 to 50% of cases may have negative cultures despite appropriate culture techniques.[6]

TREATMENT Rx

Immediate broad-spectrum antibiotic coverage and the prompt identification and treatment of the source of the infection are essential for successful outcomes. Any underlying biliary source must be resolved, and any biliary obstruction must be relieved.

As soon as the causative bacterium is identified, the antibiotic regimen can be tailored appropriately. Recommendations should be guided by the culture and by prevailing bacterial resistance patterns. Monotherapy with a β-lactam or β-lactamase inhibitor such as ampicillin-sulbactam (3 g IV every 6 hours) or piperacillin-tazobactam (4.5 g IV every 6 hours) or ticarcillin-clavulanate (3.1 g IV every 4 hours) can be used, or a third-generation cephalosporin such as ceftriaxone (1 g IV daily) *plus* metronidazole (500 mg IV every 8 hours) can be considered. Other regimens for consideration include a fluoroquinolone (such as ciprofloxacin 400 mg IV every 12 hours or levofloxacin 500 or 750 mg IV daily) *plus* metronidazole (500 mg IV every 8 hours) and monotherapy with a carbapenem such as imipenem-cilastatin (500 mg IV every 6 hours), meropenem (1 g IV every 8 hours), or ertapenem (1 g IV daily).

The duration of therapy is partly based on the response to therapy. An average of 4 to 6 weeks of antibiotic therapy is reasonable, and the last 2 to 4 weeks of the antibiotic regimen can be administered orally. Abscesses that are difficult to drain or slow to demonstrate radiographic resolution require longer courses of therapy. Importantly, radiologic abnormalities resolve more slowly than clinical and biochemical features do, so the latter should be used as an indicator for tailoring of the therapeutic regimen.

Antibiotics alone can sometimes successfully resolve small, multiple pyogenic abscesses, but most patients will require drainage of the abscesses. The standard approach is placement of a drain for about 7 days. Alternatively, needle aspiration, repeated as needed when the abscess is large enough to be drained percutaneously, provides equivalent results.[A1] [A2] Surgical drainage seldom is the first option except in patients who also have a surgically correctable precipitating lesion, such as appendicitis or biliary obstruction.[7] More often, biliary obstruction is treated with endoscopic retrograde cholangiopancreatography or transhepatic cholangiography with accompanying biliary drainage. For pyogenic abscesses in transplanted livers, management and proper biliary drainage may be difficult to achieve because of the diffuse nature of the biliary strictures.

PROGNOSIS

Abscesses smaller than10 cm can take up to 16 weeks to resolve, whereas abscesses larger than10 cm may take, on average, an additional 6 weeks to resolve. Mortality from pyogenic liver abscess is associated with older age and with comorbidities such as cirrhosis, diabetes, chronic renal failure, and malignant disease. Jaundice is an ominous sign. In developed countries, the mortality rate ranges from 2 to 12%.[8]

NON-ABSCESS HEPATIC BACTERIAL INFECTIONS

Bacterial infections of the liver can also cause more diffuse infections without frank abscess formation. Implicated organisms include *Listeria monocytogenes* (Chapter 293), *Yersinia enterocolitica* (Chapter 312), *Salmonella typhi* and *Salmonella paratyphi* (Chapter 308), *Legionella* (Chapter 314), *Ehrlichia* (Chapter 327), and gonococci (Chapter 299). There are no specific features associated with these infections, and these organisms do not necessarily cause abscesses. Patients with chronic liver disease are especially at risk for *Listeria* infection. Patients with active enteric *Yersinia* infection can have secondary liver involvement with or without liver abscesses. Disseminated gonococcal infections (Chapter 299) can cause a perihepatitis (Fitz-Hugh–Curtis syndrome), which can be manifested with right upper quadrant pain and tenderness.

Systemic bacteremia can cause a variety of hepatobiliary abnormalities, which may range from elevated aminotransferase and alkaline phosphatase levels (Chapter 147) to the cholestasis of sepsis with the development of jaundice. Several organisms can disrupt normal liver function after entering the blood stream, the most common of which are *E. coli*, *Klebsiella* spp, *Streptococcus pneumoniae*, and *Staphylococcus aureus*. Typically, in patients suffering from jaundice, sources of bacteremia include pneumonia, urinary tract infection, and soft tissue infection, although organisms may originate from a range of other sites. The hepatic biochemical abnormalities associated with bacteremia may be related to factors such as hemodynamic instability and liver hypoperfusion as well as to the infection. Associated renal failure, a blood transfusion–derived bilirubin load, and drugs may complicate the picture. The course of cholestasis may be prolonged for several days to a few weeks, but it typically resolves with resolution of the systemic infection. There is no specific treatment for the cholestasis related to a systemic infection, but it is important to rule out drug-induced cholestasis that may evolve as a consequence of one or more of the antibiotics.

Fungal Diseases of the Liver

Except for hepatosplenic candidiasis, clinically significant fungal diseases of the liver are unusual. Typically, other fungal infections will also be manifested as liver granulomas but will not show the high, swinging pyrexia that is characteristic of hepatosplenic candidiasis. Tissue cultures are required to confirm a diagnosis.

HEPATOSPLENIC CANDIDIASIS

EPIDEMIOLOGY AND PATHOBIOLOGY

Hepatosplenic candidiasis typically is caused by *Candida albicans*, but other species, including *C. tropicalis*, *C. parapsilosis*, *C. glabrata*, and *C. krusei*, have occasionally been reported. It occurs as part of disseminated candidiasis

(Chapter 338), almost exclusively in patients with acute leukemia but rarely in patients with lymphoma, aplastic anemia, and sarcoma. With the current widespread use of prophylactic antifungal agents early in the course of disease in patients with acute leukemia, hepatosplenic candidiasis develops in only 1 to 2% of patients, more commonly with acute lymphoblastic leukemia than with acute myeloid leukemia. Hepatosplenic candidiasis presumably results from translocation of *Candida* species from the gastrointestinal tract into the blood stream as a result of prolonged neutropenia and a breach in mucosal integrity.

CLINICAL MANIFESTATIONS AND DIAGNOSIS

Hepatosplenic candidiasis is manifested with persistent and high spiking fevers in a patient who was previously neutropenic and has now returned to a normal neutrophil count. Right upper quadrant pain, nausea, vomiting, and anorexia may accompany fever.

Patients typically have elevated levels of alkaline phosphatase and, less frequently, of aminotransferases, bilirubin, and leukocytes. CT, which is the imaging modality of choice, classically shows multiple lucencies representing microabscesses in the liver, spleen, and kidneys. If the CT scan is nondiagnostic but clinical suspicion remains high, magnetic resonance imaging should be performed. A definitive diagnosis is usually made on a liver biopsy specimen that shows multiple granulomas and may show yeast and hyphal forms with special stains. However, biopsy often will not show evidence of infection, especially in cases in which antifungal therapy has been used. Although biopsy is the only means to establish a definitive diagnosis, it often is not required because the clinical, laboratory, and radiographic manifestations of the disease are almost always sufficient to establish a specific diagnosis.

TREATMENT AND PROGNOSIS Rx

The mainstay of therapy is antifungal therapy. In clinically stable patients, oral fluconazole (400 mg, orally daily) can be used. In acutely ill patients, a lipid formulation of amphotericin B (3 to 5 mg/kg IV daily) is recommended. If the lipid formulation of amphotericin B is not used, other options are caspofungin (loading dose of 70 mg, then 50 mg IV daily), anidulafungin (loading dose of 200 mg, then 100 mg IV daily), and micafungin (100 mg IV daily). After 1 to 2 weeks, oral fluconazole at 400 mg daily should be started. Treatment should continue until the lesions resolve on follow-up CT scans, typically within 6 months of treatment. Patients receiving chemotherapy or stem cell transplants are at a higher risk for development of hepatosplenic candidiasis; if these treatments are indicated in patients who have a history of hepatosplenic candidiasis, fluconazole (400 mg orally, daily) should be used prophylactically to prevent relapse.

PROGNOSIS

With prolonged treatment with antifungal agents, there has been good success at treating hepatosplenic candidiasis.

OTHER FUNGAL DISEASES

Several additional fungal infections affect the liver, although rarely. *Coccidioides immitis* (Chapter 333) is often asymptomatic but may lead to fungal hepatitis characterized by increased alkaline phosphatase and the development of hepatic granulomas. Hepatic *Cryptococcus neoformans* (Chapter 336) infection is rare but has a higher prevalence in patients with AIDS, in whom it typically causes hepatomegaly. In the non–HIV-infected patient, disseminated cryptococcosis less frequently can result in focal granulomatous hepatitis, which may clinically mimic viral hepatitis, or can be manifested as obstructive jaundice secondary to sclerosing cholangitis. *Histoplasma capsulatum* (Chapter 332) infects individuals who inhale the fungus, but most cases are subclinical. In symptomatic hepatic histoplasmosis, two thirds of patients will present with hepatomegaly, with some showing splenic enlargement as well. On histologic examination, histoplasmosis can cause multiple granulomas diffusely distributed throughout the liver, although a more common finding is portal lymphohistiocytic infiltrate. *Paracoccidioides brasiliensis* (Chapter 335) most commonly infects adult men, and autopsy series have shown hepatic involvement in up to 50% of patients who die of this infection. Some individuals may present with hepatomegaly or jaundice, although jaundice is found in less than 6% of patients. Aminotransferase levels are often elevated in the early stages of the disease; changes in alkaline phosphatase or bilirubin levels tend to occur in the later stages. Biopsy may reveal lesions ranging from small granulomas to diffuse infiltration of yeast forms and fibrosis, often with bile duct involvement. In all of these examples, fungal cultures are necessary to establish a definitive diagnosis.

Parasitic, Protozoal, and Helminthic Infections of the Liver

AMEBIC LIVER ABSCESS

EPIDEMIOLOGY

Entamoeba histolytica (Chapter 352) is found throughout the world where the barriers between human feces and food and water are inadequate. After malaria, it is the second leading cause of death from parasitic diseases worldwide, accounting for an estimated 40,000 to 100,000 deaths annually. In the United States, most cases of amebiasis arise in immigrants from endemic areas and people living in states that border Mexico. Travelers to endemic areas are also at risk; ingestion of amebic cysts and colonization of the gastrointestinal tract can occur years before the development of a liver abscess. Amebic liver abscesses mainly affect men between the ages of 18 and 50 years but are also more common in postmenopausal women, thereby suggesting a hormonal protective effect. Other risk factors include alcohol intake, HLA-DR3, oral and anal sex, and contaminated enema apparatuses.[9]

PATHOBIOLOGY

E. histolytica has a simple life cycle consisting of the cyst (infectious form) and trophozoite (the motile stage associated with disease); it infects only humans and some nonhuman primates. Cysts are ingested and mature into trophozoites in the intestinal lumen. The development of amebic colitis is not essential for liver abscess formation. *E. histolytica* trophozoites penetrate through the mucosa and submucosal tissues and enter the portal circulation. *E. histolytica* blocks intrahepatic portal venules. When the trophozoites reach the liver, they create their unique abscesses, which are well-circumscribed regions of dead hepatocytes, liquefied cells, and cellular debris that are surrounded by a rim of connective tissue, a few inflammatory cells, and amebic trophozoites. The adjacent liver parenchyma is unaffected. Given the small numbers of amebae relative to the size of the abscess, it is suggested that *E. histolytica* can cause hepatocyte death without direct contact.

CLINICAL MANIFESTATIONS

Patients can present with amebic liver abscesses months to years after traveling to an endemic area, so a detailed travel history is essential for the diagnosis.[10] The disease should be suspected in patients with an appropriate travel history, fever, right upper quadrant pain, and substantial hepatic tenderness.[11] Jaundice is extremely uncommon. Symptoms are usually acute (<10 days in duration) but can be chronic, with anorexia and weight loss. Patients with acute disease tend to have multifocal disease, whereas patients with a more indolent course tend to have a solitary lesion. Laboratory data tend to demonstrate a leukocytosis without eosinophilia, mild anemia, elevated alkaline phosphatase level, and high erythrocyte sedimentation rate.

DIAGNOSIS

Although some individuals with amebic liver abscesses have concurrent amebic colitis, the majority of patients have no bowel symptoms; hence, the results of stool microscopy for *E. histolytica* trophozoites and cysts are usually negative. The diagnosis relies on identification of space-occupying lesions in the liver and a positive amebic serology. Both ultrasound and CT scan are sensitive (Fig. 151-2), but neither provides absolute specificity for amebic liver abscesses. Serologic testing of the blood is highly sensitive (>94%) and specific (>95%). False-negative test results can be obtained within the first 7 to 10 days of infection, but results on repeated testing will usually be positive. Polymerase chain reaction testing of the abscess aspirate has proved valuable for making the diagnosis in returning travelers. Aspiration of the lesion may be necessary to exclude a primary or secondary bacterial infection.

TREATMENT AND PROGNOSIS Rx

Metronidazole (500 to 750 mg orally three times daily or a loading dose of 15 mg/kg followed by 7.5 mg/kg every 6 hours intravenously) will usually provide evidence of clinical improvement within 72 to 96 hours but should be continued for 5 to 10 days. Nitroimidazole tinidazole at 2 g daily for 5 days is also effective. Drainage is not necessary, except in patients who have abscesses larger than 10 cm or do not respond within 5 days.[12] The abscess usually will shrink by about 50% within a week, but the mean time to complete radiologic resolution is 3 to 9 months. Repeated imaging in a clinically improving patient may lead to unwarranted concern and unnecessary treatment.[A3]

Treatment must also address the removal of all of the cysts from the intestinal lumen in patients with evidence of intraluminal infection (Chapter 352). A recommended treatment is diiodohydroxyquinoline (650 mg orally three times a day for 20 days) to prevent continued colonization and possible recurrence of the liver abscess. With prompt diagnosis and adequate medical treatment, the mortality rate from amebic abscess is 1 to 3%.

OTHER PROTOZOAN LIVER DISEASES

In addition to *Entamoeba histolytica*, other protozoan diseases that affect the liver include *Cryptosporidium*, *Toxoplasma gondii*, *Leishmania*, *Plasmodium*, and *Babesia microti* (Table 151-2).

HELMINTH INFECTIONS

Echinococcosis and Hydatid Cyst Disease

EPIDEMIOLOGY AND PATHOBIOLOGY

Human cystic echinococcosis is a zoonosis caused by the larval cestode *Echinococcus granulosus*. It is often referred to as hydatid cyst disease because of the watery cysts that characterize the infection.

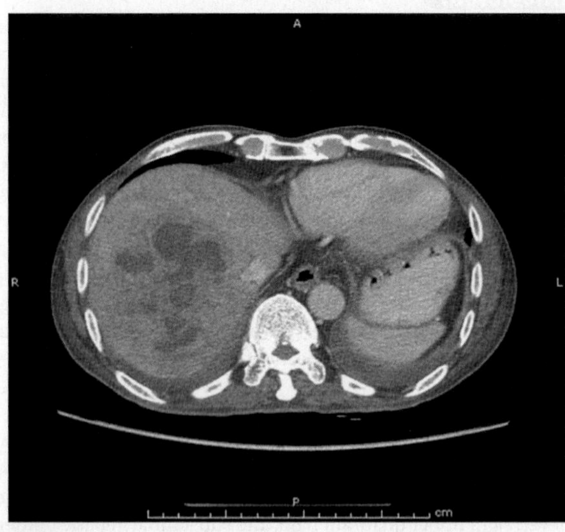

FIGURE 151-2. **Computed tomographic scan of an amebic liver abscess. (Courtesy Dr. Chalermrat Bunchorntavakul, Bangkok, Thailand.)**

The disease remains endemic in sheep-raising areas of the world, including Africa, the Mediterranean region of Europe, the Middle East, Asia, South America, Australia, and New Zealand. Dogs are the definitive hosts for *E. granulosus*, and sheep are the major intermediate hosts, although yaks, goats, and camels are other relevant intermediate hosts. Humans are only accidental hosts when they ingest food or water that is fecally contaminated with eggs. Human contact with sheepdogs that are in frequent contact with livestock is a major risk for infection.

The disease cycle begins when an adult tapeworm infects the intestinal tract of the definitive host (dogs usually). The adult tapeworm then produces eggs, which are expelled in the host's feces. Intermediate hosts become infected through the ingestion of parasitic eggs in fecally contaminated food. Inside the intermediate host, the eggs hatch and release tiny hooked embryos (called oncospheres), which travel in the blood stream and eventually lodge in the liver, lungs, or kidneys, where they develop into hydatid cysts. Inside these cysts grow thousands of tapeworm larvae, the next stage in the life cycle of the parasite.

CLINICAL MANIFESTATIONS

The initial infection is asymptomatic, but an enlarging hydatid liver cyst can cause abdominal pain, nausea, hepatomegaly, or a palpable mass.[13] Patients may describe symptoms of mild upper right quadrant pain, urticarial rash, and episodes of pruritus. If the cyst ruptures, serious complications can develop. Cysts that perforate into the peritoneum can lead to the development of extrahepatic cysts and may induce an allergic reaction leading to an increase of eosinophils in the blood, pruritic urticaria, and systemic anaphylaxis. In most cases, however, cysts rupture into bile ducts, which can result in cholestatic jaundice, cholangitis, or biliary pain.

DIAGNOSIS

On ultrasound or CT scans (Fig. 151-3), the hydatid cysts are often large with a flaky appearance that is referred to as hydatid sand. CT imaging also may show multiple daughter cysts or a fluid density cyst with peripheral focal areas of calcification. Fluid is of variable density, depending on the amount of proteinaceous debris.

Hydatid cysts of the liver can be diagnosed by a serologic assay, the Weinberg reaction, but it can be falsely negative in up to 38% of cases. An enzyme-linked immunosorbent assay may be more sensitive. Eosinophilia is not a feature unless the cyst ruptures; in fact, there are usually no changes in blood chemistries.

TABLE 151-2 PARASITIC INFECTIONS INVOLVING THE LIVER

	CHARACTERISTICS	ENDEMIC AREAS	RISK FACTORS	MAJOR HEPATIC MANIFESTATIONS
MAJOR PROTOZOA				
Entamoeba histolytica	Ingested cysts develop into invasive trophozoites that colonize the colon and occasionally spread to the liver by the portal blood	Mexico, regions of Central and South America, India, and regions of Africa	Male gender, alcohol intake, HLA-DR3, oral and anal sex, and contaminated enema apparatuses	Amebic liver abscesses develop as a tissue response to trophozoite invasion with acute and chronic manifestations (see text)
OTHER PROTOZOA				
Cryptosporidium sp and microsporidia	Ingested cysts develop into trophozoites in intestinal mucosa	Worldwide distribution	AIDS	Biliary tract infection with obstruction and cholangitis
Toxoplasma gondii	Ingestion of oocysts in contaminated soil or water or in infected meat; systemic spread of tachyzoites in the circulation	Worldwide distribution	Consumption of undercooked meat, contact with soil, and travel outside the United States, Europe, or Canada	Immunocompetent: asymptomatic or hepatomegaly and mild LFT elevations Immunocompromised: occasional overt hepatitis
Leishmania sp	Sand fly bite transmits promastigotes; proliferation in the reticuloendothelial system	Worldwide distribution	Children younger than 10 years and immunocompromised adults Contact with sand flies	Hepatosplenomegaly months to years after infection
Plasmodium sp	Mosquito (*Anopheles*) bite transmits sporozoites	Multiple regions throughout the world	Exposure to anopheline mosquito bites	Proliferation in hepatocytes causes hepatomegaly, enzyme elevations, and jaundice
Babesia microti	Tick bite transmits the agent, which parasitizes erythrocytes	Europe	Asplenia is a risk for fatal hepatic failure, especially bovine babesiosis	Mild liver enzyme elevations

TREATMENT AND PROGNOSIS

Drug therapy includes albendazole 400 mg twice a day for three- to six-month cycles, but treatment with albendazole alone is not effective, so drainage is essential to the effective treatment of hydatid cysts. In a randomized trial, percutaneous drainage consisting of puncture, aspiration, injection, and reaspiration of scolicidal solutions resulted in a rate of cyst disappearance similar to that of open surgical drainage, but with fewer side effects, provided patients received preprocedure and postprocedure albendazole therapy.[A4] Chlorhexidine, hydrogen peroxide, 80% alcohol, and 0.5% cetrimide are preferred scolicidal agents rather than hypertonic saline or formalin. If the cyst communicates with the biliary tree, however, injection of scolicidal agents carries an almost universal risk of secondary sclerosing cholangitis, and so it is contraindicated. In such cases, the cyst must be treated surgically, by either cystectomy or hepatic resection.

The prognosis is generally good, with complete cure expected after successful percutaneous or surgical treatment. However, spillage occurs in 2 to 25% of cases, depending on the location of the cyst and the surgeon's experience; the operative mortality rate varies from 0.5 to 4% for the same reasons.

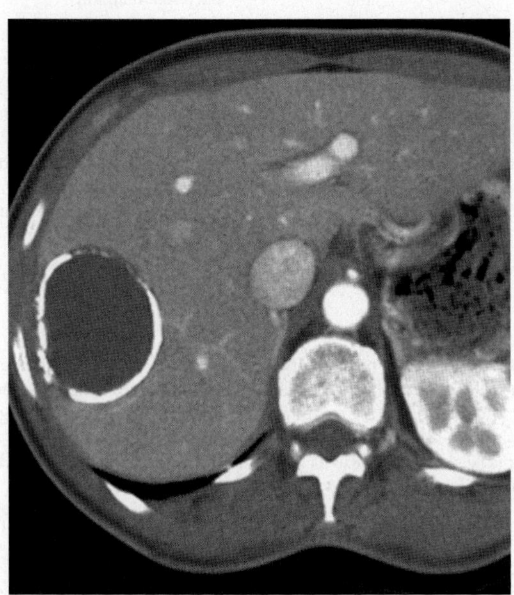

FIGURE 151-3. Computed tomographic scan of a hepatic echinococcal cyst.

Schistosomiasis

EPIDEMIOLOGY AND PATHOBIOLOGY

Schistosomiasis is an infection of trematodes. *Schistosoma* (Chapter 355) causes periportal fibrosis and liver cirrhosis by deposition of eggs in the small portal venules. *S. mansoni* and *S. japonicum* lead to liver disease. Infection with *S. mansoni* is found in parts of South America, Africa, and the Middle East. Infection with *S. japonicum* is found in the Far East, mostly China and the Philippines. Although primary infection does not occur in the United States, 5% of the world's population (200 million people) may be infected, thereby making it a major international health concern and highly prevalent in immigrants.

Humans become infected after contact with water that contains the infective stage (cercaria) of schistosomes. After penetration of the skin, the larvae migrate to the lungs and then to the venules of the mesentery, urinary bladder, or ureters. They release eggs in the venules of the mesentery, and the eggs enter the liver through the portal vein, where they become lodged in the terminal branches of the portal venules. The lodged eggs cause a granulomatous inflammation, and the lesions heal by periportal fibrosis. *S. japonicum* is more virulent than *S. mansoni* because its infections produce 10 times more eggs.

CLINICAL MANIFESTATIONS

Initial infection is manifested as itching that is caused by skin penetration by larvae.[14] Several weeks later, patients may complain of fever, diarrhea, chills, headaches, or hives. At this time, patients will have eosinophilia. During the next 5 to 15 years, periportal liver fibrosis develops and leads to presinusoidal portal hypertension, splenomegaly (Chapter 168), and gastroesophageal varices (Chapter 138). With *S. japonicum*, however, the progression can be much more rapid, with little interval between the acute and chronic disease. Hepatic function is generally well preserved, and patients usually present with hematemesis from ruptured gastroesophageal varices.

SYMPTOMS AND SIGNS	LABORATORY FINDINGS	RADIOGRAPHIC FEATURES	DIAGNOSIS	TREATMENT
Fever, RUQ pain, and substantial hepatic tenderness	Leukocytosis without eosinophilia, mild anemia, elevated serum AP, and high ESR	US, CT, and MRI can detect abscess but cannot always differentiate amebic from pyogenic. On CT or MRI, amebic abscess sometimes appears "cold" with bright rim.	Imaging, serology, stool antigen test (microscopic evaluation of stool has a poor yield)	Metronidazole, 500-750 mg PO tid × 5-10 days, or tinidazole, 2 g daily × 3 days Iodoquinol, 650 mg tid × 20 days, also needed to eradicate intestinal colonization
See Chapter 350	See Chapter 350	See Chapter 350	See Chapter 350	See Chapter 350
See Chapter 349	See Chapter 349	See Chapter 349	See Chapter 349	See Chapter 349
See Chapter 348	See Chapter 348	See Chapter 348	See Chapter 348	See Chapter 348
See Chapter 345	See Chapter 345	See Chapter 345	See Chapter 345	See Chapter 345
See Chapter 353	See Chapter 353	See Chapter 353	See Chapter 353	See Chapter 353

TABLE 151-2 PARASITIC INFECTIONS INVOLVING THE LIVER—cont'd

	CHARACTERISTICS	ENDEMIC AREAS	RISK FACTORS	MAJOR HEPATIC MANIFESTATIONS
MAJOR HELMINTHS				
Schistosoma sp	Cercaria in fresh water penetrate the skin, travel by the circulation to portal vein radicals	*S. mansoni* found in South America, Africa, and Middle East *S. japonicum* found in Far East (mostly China and Philippines)	Contact with fresh water containing cercaria of schistosomes	Progressive presinusoidal blood flow obstruction, periportal fibrosis, portal hypertension, varices, ascites, splenomegaly
Echinococcus granulosus	Eggs of small (3-7 mm) tapeworms in stool of canid hosts; ingested eggs produce larval oncospheres that migrate to the liver and form cysts in sheep, humans, and other intermediate hosts	Worldwide distribution, found especially in sheep-raising areas (Africa, the Mediterranean region of Europe, the Middle East, Asia, South America, Australia, and New Zealand)	Ingestion of food or water fecally contaminated with eggs and human contact with sheepdogs	Initial infection asymptomatic Liver cysts increase in diameter by 1-5 cm yearly and cause variable abdominal pain, hepatomegaly, and variable eosinophilia Occasional cyst rupture, secondary bacterial infection
Echinococcus multilocularis	Eggs of small tapeworms in stool of foxes; ingested eggs produce oncospheres in the liver of rodents, humans, and other intermediate hosts	Endemic in Northern Hemisphere	Human exposure increasing with growing fox populations	Metacestodes colonize the liver as a tumor-like mass of small vesicles
Fasciola sp	Leaf-shaped flukes up to 13 × 30 mm derived from ingested cysts; the fluke excysts in the duodenum, migrates directly across the bowel wall into the peritoneal cavity, and burrows directly into the liver (or occasionally out to the skin)	Worldwide distribution	Consumption of freshwater or aquatic plants contaminated by colonized livestock	Adult flukes live in the common and hepatic bile ducts, causing obstruction that leads to thickening of the ducts, dilation, and fibrosis of the proximal biliary tree
Opisthorchis sp and *Clonorchis sinensis*	Flukes of 8-25 mm derived from ingested cysts; the fluke excysts in the duodenum and migrates into the bile ducts	*Opisthorchis* sp: Southeast Asia, central and eastern Europe (particularly Siberia) *C. sinensis*: China, Japan, Vietnam, Korea	Consumption of raw, pickled, dried, smoked, or salted freshwater fish or crayfish originating from East Asia or, in the case of *Opisthorchis felineus*, Russia and eastern Europe	Acute: typically asymptomatic Chronic: abdominal pain, fever, anorexia, tender hepatomegaly, sometimes eosinophilia Late sequelae: intermittent biliary obstruction, cholelithiasis, cholecystitis, cholangitis, secondary bacterial abscesses, cholangiocarcinoma
Toxocara sp	Nematode infection disseminates to cause visceral larva migrans after ingestion of soil contaminated with dog or cat feces	Highest prevalence in southeastern United States	Consumption of food contaminated with soil containing eggs; distributed throughout the United States	Often an asymptomatic cause of eosinophilia (exclude *Trichinella*, *Strongyloides*, filaria, hookworm, schistosomiasis) Hepatomegaly is common, but nonhepatic manifestations dominate the clinical picture
OTHER HELMINTHS				
Ascaris lumbricoides	Ingested eggs develop into larvae that migrate to the lungs and are coughed and swallowed; develop into roundworms 15-30 mm long in the small intestine	Global distribution with higher prevalence in Africa, South America, India, and the Far East; 20% of the world's population is colonized	Consumption of fecally contaminated food or water, particularly in young children	Colonization is typically asymptomatic with eosinophilia Biliary migration of worms can cause symptomatic biliary obstruction, cholangitis, cholecystitis, and secondary bacterial liver abscess
Capillaria hepatica	Ingested eggs develop into larvae in the intestinal mucosa; larvae migrate to the liver by portal blood flow and develop into short-lived roundworms	Human infection is rare	Consumption of food contaminated with rodent feces	Fever, eosinophilia, and hepatomegaly; subsequent foci of liver fibrosis, granulomas, and calcification in involved areas
Strongyloides stercoralis	Ingested eggs develop into 1.5- to 2.5-mm nematodes that invade the hepatic vasculature, lymphatics, and biliary tract	Tropical and subtropical areas including southeast United States and southern and eastern Europe	Consumption of food contaminated with soil containing eggs, infection with HTLV-1, and immunocompromised individuals	Hepatic disease in the setting of immunosuppression: jaundice, abdominal pain; eosinophilia is uncommon

RUQ = right upper quadrant; AP = alkaline phosphatase; ESR = erythrocyte sedimentation rate; US = ultrasonography; CT = computed tomography; MRI = magnetic resonance imaging; ELISA = enzyme-linked immunosorbent assay; ERCP = endoscopic retrograde cholangiopancreatography; HTLV = human T-cell lymphotrophic virus.

Modified from Neuschwander-Tetri BA. Bacterial, parasitic, fungal, and granulomatous liver disease. In: Goldman L, Ausiello D, eds. *Cecil Textbook of Medicine.* 23rd ed. Philadelphia: WB Saunders; 2007.

SYMPTOMS AND SIGNS	LABORATORY FINDINGS	RADIOGRAPHIC FEATURES	DIAGNOSIS	TREATMENT
Initial infection presents as itching; later presentations include fever, diarrhea, chills, headaches, or hives Hematemesis from ruptured gastroesophageal varices	Eosinophilia and splenomegaly Seroconversion occurs within 4-6 weeks	Extensive calcification with typical "turtle-back" appearance along portal tracts	Rectal biopsy, liver biopsy, microscopic examination of stool	Praziquantel (single dose 40 mg/kg) with a second dose 6-12 weeks later if necessary
Enlarged hydatid cyst can cause abdominal pain, nausea, hepatomegaly, or a palpable mass Mild RUQ pain, urticaria, and episodes of pruritus	Positive Weinberg reaction (false-negative reaction in 38% of cases) or ELISA analysis Eosinophilia seen in ruptured cysts	On US or CT, cysts appear flaky, sometimes showing daughter cysts or peripheral focal calcification; fluid is of variable density	Imaging, Weinberg reaction, or ELISA	Albendazole (400 mg) 2× daily for 3-6 monthly cycles with 10- to 14-day intervals Drainage of the cyst is essential Surgical resection if the cyst communicates with the biliary tree
See Chapter 354	See Chapter 354	See Chapter 354	See Chapter 354	See Chapter 354
Acute: fever, abdominal pain, eosinophilia Chronic: symptomatic biliary obstruction, variable eosinophilia	Serologic tests include hemagglutination, complement fixation, ELISA, and counterimmunoelectrophoresis Anemia, leukocytosis, eosinophilia, elevated AP, and hypergammaglobulinemia are often seen	CT is most useful: liver shows hypodense nodules or tortuous tracks; thickening of the liver capsule, subcapsular hematoma, and parenchymal calcification may also be seen	Serology, stool examination	Triclabendazole, 10 mg/kg once or twice
Chronic infection presents as dyspepsia, abdominal pain, diarrhea, nausea, vomiting, anorexia, weight loss, fevers, hepatomegaly, and urticaria Acute presentation includes serum sickness, intrahepatic pigment stones, and facial edema Other rare complications are cholangitis, pancreatitis, and obstructive jaundice	Anemia, leukocytosis, eosinophilia, elevated AP, and hypergammaglobulinemia	US may detect flukes in biliary tree CT shows small hypodense nodules	Serology and stool examination	Praziquantel, 25 mg/kg q8h × 3 doses
See Chapter 358	See Chapter 358	See Chapter 358	See Chapter 358	See Chapter 358
Sensitized patients during pulmonary phase present with asthma-like symptoms, hemoptysis, chest pain, and cyanosis Urticaria and other allergic reactions sometimes seen Patients in intestinal phase show cognitive and nutritional impairment with abdominal pain, hepatomegaly, cholangitis, and obstructive jaundice	Leukocytosis with eosinophilia Hyperbilirubinemia occasionally seen	Movement of the worms within the biliary tree can sometimes be observed A "bull's-eye" appearance can be seen on cross-sectional imaging	Stool examination, imaging, and ERCP	Albendazole, 400 mg once
Persistent fever, eosinophilia, and hepatomegaly most common Splenomegaly, anorexia, nausea, vomiting, night sweats, and altered bowel habits also seen	Anemia, eosinophilia, moderately elevated liver enzymes, increased ESR, and hypergammaglobulinemia	US shows nonspecific hyperechoic areas in the portal spaces	Stool and liver biopsy	Mebendazole, 200 mg bid × 20 days
Recurrent urticaria, abdominal pain, diarrhea, and cough; mild jaundice and hepatomegaly in the absence of splenomegaly	Eosinophilia and hypoalbuminemia Patients may have elevated liver enzymes	Imaging studies not used in diagnosis	Serology and stool examination	Ivermectin, 200 μg/kg/day × 2 days, or albendazole, 400 mg/day × 7 days

DIAGNOSIS

Schistosomal eggs typically have lateral or terminal spines and are easy to detect on microscopic examination of feces or on a rectal biopsy specimen. Seroconversion occurs within 4 to 8 weeks of infection but cannot distinguish active infection from a history of exposure. Newer, more sensitive and specific molecular and immunodiagnostic techniques (including polymerase chain reaction–enzyme-linked immunosorbent assay systems) for detection of schistosome DNA in feces or serum and plasma have the potential to diagnose schistosomiasis in all stages of clinical disease, not only when the adult worms are producing eggs.[15] Imaging may show extensive calcification with the typical "turtle-back" appearance along the portal tracts reflecting the clustered, calcified eggs along the portal triads. Liver biopsy may demonstrate an egg of *S. mansoni* along with intense granulomatous change in the portal tract (Fig. 151-4).

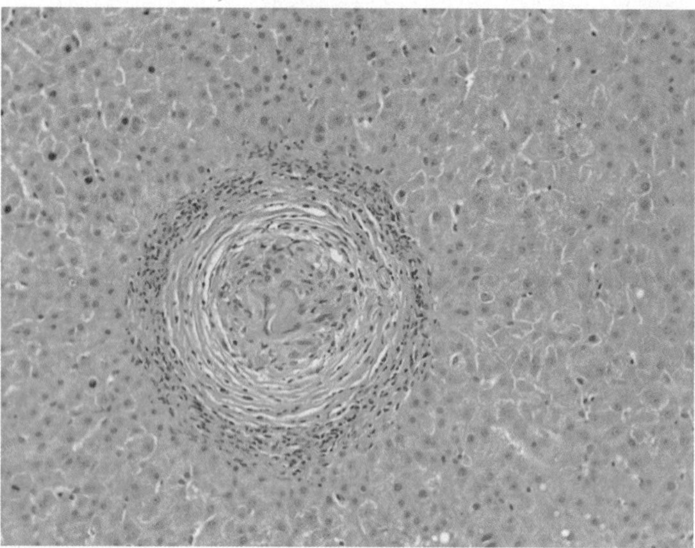

FIGURE 151-4. Liver biopsy specimen demonstrating an egg of *Schistosoma mansoni* and intense granulomatous change in the portal tract. (Courtesy Alberto Q. Farias, MD, São Paulo, Brazil.)

TREATMENT AND PROGNOSIS

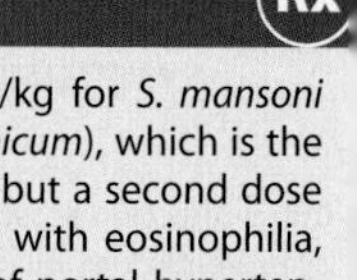

Praziquantel (a single or two divided doses of 40 mg/kg for *S. mansoni* infections, and two divided doses of 60 mg/kg for *S. japonicum*), which is the preferred treatment, A5 is effective in 70 to 100% of cases, but a second dose can be given 6 to 12 weeks later, particularly in patients with eosinophilia, high antibody titers, or persistent symptoms. Treatment of portal hypertension (Chapter 153) may be necessary. The mortality is 0.05% with heavy *S. mansoni* infection and 1.8% for severe *S. japonicum* infection. Bleeding from esophageal varices is the most serious complication. Chronic infection can lead to hepatocellular carcinoma.

GRANULOMATOUS DISEASES OF THE LIVER

Granulomas, which are found in up to 15% of liver biopsy specimens, can be an incidental finding or may represent a wide array of liver diseases (Table 151-3). A granuloma is an accumulation of epithelioid cells, including transformed macrophages, mononuclear cells, and other inflammatory cells. Granulomas may have associated necrosis (caseating), as in tuberculosis (Chapter 324), or may be non-necrotizing (noncaseating), as in sarcoidosis (Chapter 95). In addition, fibrin-ring granulomas are characterized by a vacuole encircled by a ring of fibrinoid necrosis and surrounded by lymphocytes and histiocytes, as seen in Q fever (Chapter 327).

An incidental granuloma requires minimal further evaluation. Tuberculosis should be excluded (Chapter 324). Sarcoidosis should also be considered as it is the most common cause of granulomas in the United States. An antimitochondrial antibody should be ordered to rule out primary biliary cirrhosis. The use of potentially causative drugs should be stopped (see Table 151-3).

Sarcoidosis

Sarcoidosis (Chapter 95), which is the most frequently identified cause of hepatic granuloma in the United States, affects all racial and ethnic groups and occurs at all ages. In patients with sarcoidosis, the liver is the third most commonly involved organ, after the lymph nodes and lungs; about 50 to 80% of patients with sarcoidosis will have granulomas in their livers. The classic granuloma is found mainly in the portal triads, with a cluster of large epithelioid cells and often with multinucleated giant cells.

CLINICAL MANIFESTATIONS AND DIAGNOSIS

Hepatic involvement of sarcoidosis is often subclinical, and only a minority of patients will present with pruritus, fever, abdominal pain, hepatomegaly,

TABLE 151-3 CAUSES OF GRANULOMATOUS LIVER DISEASE

DIAGNOSIS	SPECIAL AND UNIQUE FEATURES
Sarcoidosis	Evidence of pulmonary sarcoidosis, granulomas found on biopsy of other organs, elevated ACE level
Bacterial infections	
Mycobacterium tuberculosis	Caseating granulomas on biopsy, positive PPD response or interferon-gamma release assay, active pulmonary tuberculosis
Other mycobacteria (*M. avium-intracellulare, M. leprae, M. mucogenicum, M. bovis*)	HIV, exposure history
Other bacteria (brucellosis, listeriosis, melioidosis, tularemia, yersiniosis, bartonellosis, Q fever, syphilis, psittacosis)	Fever, exposure history
Viral infections (cytomegalovirus, Epstein-Barr virus, hepatitis C, hepatitis B, hepatitis A)	Serology for acute or recent exposure
Fungal infections (histoplasmosis, coccidioidomycosis, blastomycosis, nocardiosis, candidiasis)	Fever, immunocompromised
Parasitic infections (schistosomiasis, *Ascaris lumbricoides*, toxoplasmosis, visceral leishmaniasis)	Travel to endemic regions, positive serologic testing
Primary biliary cirrhosis	Female sex, positive AMA, elevated IgM
Malignant diseases (Hodgkin disease, non-Hodgkin lymphoma, renal cell carcinoma)	Evidence of malignant disease in kidney or bone marrow
Drug reactions (allopurinol, chlorpropamide, phenylbutazone, sulfonamides, carbamazepine, glyburide, quinidine, quinine, diltiazem, hydralazine, rosiglitazone, phenytoin, methyldopa, procainamide, amoxicillin–clavulanic acid, mebendazole, mesalamine, acetaminophen, pyrazinamide, halothane, isoniazid, norfloxacin)	Exposure history
Toxins (beryllium, copper sulfate, Thorotrast)	Previous exposure history
Miscellaneous (talc, Crohn disease, granulomatosis with polyangiitis, post–jejunoileal bypass, mineral oil lipogranulomas, hepatic allograft rejection, chronic granulomatous disease)	History of IV drug use, history of liver transplantation, diarrhea

ACE = angiotensin-converting enzyme; PPD = purified protein derivative; HIV = human immunodeficiency virus; AMA = antimitochondrial antibody; IV = intravenous.

cholestatic jaundice, or portal hypertension. In some patients, the granulomatous injury and destruction of the interlobular bile ducts eventually cause ductopenia and a histologic picture similar to primary biliary cirrhosis (Chapter 155). In other patients, damage to the large bile ducts may lead to a syndrome that mimics primary sclerosing cholangitis (Chapter 155). Other patients may present with focal liver lesions suggestive of malignant neoplasm.

Patients typically have markedly elevated serum alkaline phosphatase levels. Angiotensin-converting enzyme levels also are characteristically elevated but may not be helpful in differentiating sarcoidosis from other chronic liver diseases, such as primary biliary cirrhosis, in which it also may be elevated. The presence of noncaseating granulomas in a patient with clinically suspected sarcoidosis generally establishes the diagnosis. However, granulomas do not correlate with liver function test results or duration of disease.

TREATMENT AND PROGNOSIS

Rx

In general, hepatic sarcoidosis does not need to be treated except in patients with other indications for treatment (Chapter 95). Corticosteroids improve liver function test results but do not alleviate portal hypertension, and serial biopsies often show little improvement. Sarcoidosis that leads to portal hypertension and fibrosis may ultimately require liver transplantation (Chapter 154), although sarcoidosis may recur in the new organ.

Other Granulomatous Liver Diseases

In addition to sarcoidosis, another major cause of granulomatous liver disease is tuberculosis (Chapter 324). Military tuberculosis, caused by *Mycobacterium tuberculosis,* commonly results in hepatic granulomas, and patients present with hepatomegaly, abnormal liver function test results, or both. A biopsy revealing caseating granulomas along with a positive PPD (purified protein derivative) response and active pulmonary tuberculosis can help in establishing a diagnosis. Other mycobacteria are also known to cause granulomatous liver disease, including *M. avium-intracellulare, M. genavense,* and *M. scrofulaceum* (Chapter 325).

Other causes of granulomatous liver disease include zoonotic infections such as cat-scratch disease (Chapter 315), Q fever (Chapter 327), and brucellosis (Chapter 310). Cat-scratch disease, which primarily affects children, is caused by *Bartonella henselae,* with cats serving as the main reservoir for the organism. Patients typically present with lymphadenopathy associated with persistent pyrexia of unknown origin, abdominal pain, and weight loss. *B. henselae* can be identified by a Warthin-Starry stain, or an imaging study may demonstrate scattered defects in the liver. Q fever is caused by the intracellular gram-negative rickettsial organism *Coxiella burnetii.* Most infections are asymptomatic but may have self-limited influenza-like symptoms, pneumonia, and hepatitis. A liver biopsy specimen may demonstrate fibrin-ring granulomas (doughnut shaped) in the background of nonspecific reactive hepatitis and steatosis. Brucellosis, which is not common in the United States, is caused by at least four species of *Brucella*: *B. abortus, B. suis, B. melitensis,* and *B. canis.* The disease is manifested as recurrent high fevers, drenching sweats, malaise, arthralgia, fatigue, abdominal pain, anorexia, and headaches. Patients often have hepatomegaly and elevated serum levels of aminotransferases and alkaline phosphatase. The granulomas formed by this infection are typically smaller than those caused by sarcoidosis or tuberculosis, and a definitive diagnosis can be established through serologic testing.

It is important to keep in mind that hepatic granulomas are formed naturally as a consequence of the immune response, so they may be seen in infections with hepatic involvement. Many of the diseases noted can be manifested as granulomatous liver disease (see Table 151-3): listeriosis, yersiniosis, candidiasis, histoplasmosis, coccidioidomycosis, and schistosomiasis. Viral infections (e.g., cytomegalovirus, hepatitis A, hepatitis B, and hepatitis C), primary biliary cirrhosis, malignant diseases, and certain drug reactions have been etiologically linked to granulomatous liver disease. Table 151-3 categorically lists the major causes of hepatic granulomas and the means by which a differential diagnosis can be established.

Grade A References

A1. Singh O, Gupta S, Moses S, et al. Comparative study of catheter drainage and needle aspiration in management of large liver abscesses. *Indian J Gastroenterol.* 2009;28:88-92.

A2. Yu SC, Ho SS, Lau WY, et al. Treatment of pyogenic liver abscess: prospective randomized comparison of catheter drainage and needle aspiration. *Hepatology.* 2004;39:932-938.

A3. Chavez-Tapia NC, Hernandez-Calleros J, Tellez-Avila FI, et al. Image-guided percutaneous procedure plus metronidazole versus metronidazole alone for uncomplicated amoebic liver abscess. *Cochrane Database Syst Rev.* 2009;1:CD004886.

A4. Nasseri-Moghaddam S, Abrishami A, Taefi A, et al. Percutaneous needle aspiration, injection, and re-aspiration with or without benzimidazole coverage for uncomplicated hepatic hydatid cysts. *Cochrane Database Syst Rev.* 2011;1:CD003623.

A5. Danso-Appiah A, Olliaro PL, Donegan S, et al. Drugs for treating *Schistosoma mansoni* infection. *Cochrane Database Syst Rev.* 2013;2:CD000528.

GENERAL REFERENCES

For the General References and other additional features, please visit Expert Consult at https://expertconsult.inkling.com.

152

ALCOHOLIC AND NONALCOHOLIC STEATOHEPATITIS

NAGA P. CHALASANI

Alcoholic liver disease and nonalcoholic fatty liver disease (NAFLD), which represent two of the most common forms of liver disease, can lead to cirrhosis, liver failure, and death. Although these two conditions have different risk factors and natural histories, in both conditions (Table 152-1) the hepatocytes are characterized by macrovesicular steatosis, which is the accumulation of triglycerides as one large cytoplasmic globule that displaces the nucleus. In microvesicular steatosis, cytoplasmic accumulation of fat occurs as multiple small globules with a central nucleus.

ALCOHOLIC LIVER DISEASE

DEFINITION

Excessive alcohol consumption (Chapter 33) causes alcoholic liver disease and can significantly worsen other liver disorders, such as viral hepatitis (Chapter 149) and hemochromatosis (Chapter 212). Although most individuals who consume alcohol do not consume it excessively and do not develop any physical or social consequences, some alcoholics consume sufficient alcohol and, presumably because of other predisposing factors, develop alcoholic liver disease. Alcoholic liver disease is a spectrum of chronic liver diseases ranging from alcoholic fatty liver to alcoholic hepatitis and cirrhosis.

Alcoholic fatty liver disease will develop in nearly 90% of individuals who consume alcohol heavily (on average, >6 drinks per day), but only some individuals develop the more severe conditions of alcoholic hepatitis and alcoholic cirrhosis. Genetic predisposition is likely to play a role in the pathogenesis of acute alcoholic hepatitis and alcoholic cirrhosis, but these genetic factors have not been well defined.[1] Nearly 50% of the patients with alcoholic

TABLE 152-1 COMMON CAUSES OF MACROVESICULAR AND MICROVESICULAR STEATOSIS

MACROVESICULAR STEATOSIS	MICROVESICULAR STEATOSIS
Obesity, type 2 diabetes, metabolic syndrome, and dyslipidemia (nonalcoholic fatty liver disease)	Reye syndrome
Excessive alcohol consumption	Medications (valproate, antiretroviral medicines, intravenous tetracycline)
Hepatitis C (genotype 3)	Heat stroke
Wilson disease	Acute fatty liver of pregnancy
Lipodystrophy starvation	HELLP syndrome
Jejunoileal bypass	Inborn errors of metabolism (lecithin–cholesterol acyltransferase deficiency, cholesterol ester storage disease, Wolman disease)
Parenteral nutrition	
Medications (amiodarone, methotrexate, tamoxifen, corticosteroids, antipsychotics)	

HELLP = hemolysis, elevated liver enzymes, and low platelets.

hepatitis have preexisting cirrhosis (Chapter 153), and individuals who do not yet have cirrhosis are at high risk for its development, especially if they continue to consume alcohol.

EPIDEMIOLOGY

The true prevalence of alcoholic liver disease is not known, but nearly 1% of North American adults are believed to have alcoholic liver disease. Even this figure is considered an underestimation because milder forms of alcoholic liver disease are asymptomatic and often unrecognized. It has been estimated that alcoholic liver disease accounts for 40% of deaths from cirrhosis and 28% of all deaths from liver disease. It is the second most common indication for liver transplantation in the United States once abstinence from alcohol has been established.

PATHOBIOLOGY

The mechanisms underlying alcoholic liver injury can be broadly categorized into those caused by the effects of alcohol directly on hepatocytes and those caused by the effects mediated by Kupffer cells.[2] The hepatocyte mechanisms include the altered redox state induced by alcohol and aldehyde dehydrogenase reactions; the oxidative stress and lipid peroxidation caused by the induction of CYP2E1 enzymes and the mitochondrial electron transfer system; and the effects of alcohol on the nuclear transcription factors AMP kinase and SREBP-1c, protein adduct formation, and altered methionine and folate metabolism with resulting endoplasmic reticulum stress. Chronic alcohol consumption increases gut permeability, and the resulting portal endotoxemia activates Kupffer cells. Activated Kupffer cells release a number of proinflammatory mediators. These include tumor necrosis factor-α (TNF-α); transforming growth factor-β1; interleukins 1, 6, 8, and 10; and platelet-derived growth factor. TNF-α has plethora of biologic effects and causes hepatocyte apoptosis, whereas transforming growth factor-β1 and platelet-derived growth factor play important roles in stellate cell activation, collagen production, and hepatic fibrosis.

Among the known risk factors for development of alcoholic liver disease (Table 152-2), the amount of alcohol consumed is the single most important. For unclear reasons, only 30 to 35% of individuals with heavy and long-term drinking develop alcoholic hepatitis, and less than 20% develop cirrhosis. Women are at higher risk; for example, the risk of alcoholic cirrhosis increases after 10 years of alcohol consumption at quantities of more than 60 to 80 g/day in men, whereas in women, it can develop at quantities of only more than 20 g/day. Moreover, the peak incidence of alcoholic liver disease in women is approximately a decade earlier than in men. The type of alcoholic beverage consumed may not be as critical, but "spirits" and beer may be more hepatotoxic than wine. African American and Hispanic ethnic groups may be predisposed to more significant alcoholic liver injury. Both obesity and protein-calorie malnutrition, in which micronutrients and antioxidant capacity are diminished, also are important predispositions.

Polymorphisms in genes associated with alcohol metabolism (alcohol and aldehyde dehydrogenases and cytochrome P-450 enzymes) and dysregulated cytokine production (e.g., TNF-α) may also influence genetic susceptibility. In patients with other forms of chronic liver disease (e.g., viral hepatitis B or C), concomitant alcohol consumption significantly aggravates liver injury.

CLINICAL MANIFESTATIONS

Patients with alcoholic liver disease may have signs and symptoms from underlying alcoholism as well as those caused by liver disease. Stigmata of chronic alcoholism include palmar erythema (see Fig. 146-2), spider nevi, bilateral gynecomastia, testicular atrophy, bilateral parotid enlargement, and Dupuytren contractures (Fig. 152-1). The clinical features of liver disease will depend on the stage of alcoholic liver disease, that is, whether a patient has alcoholic fatty liver or more advanced liver disease, such as alcoholic hepatitis and cirrhosis.

Patients with alcoholic fatty liver disease are generally asymptomatic, but some patients may have anorexia, fatigue, right upper quadrant discomfort, and tender hepatomegaly. These patients may also have biochemical evidence of alcoholism and alcoholic liver disease with macrocytosis as well as elevated levels of aspartate aminotransferase (AST) and γ-glutamyl transpeptidase. Patients with alcoholic fatty liver typically do not have jaundice, ascites, or splenomegaly.

Patients with alcoholic hepatitis may have a more dramatic presentation with severe malaise, fatigue, anorexia, fever, evidence of protein-calorie malnutrition, and features of decompensated liver disease, including jaundice, coagulopathy, ascites, and encephalopathy. However, these classic features of acute alcoholic hepatitis are not universally present. Physical examination invariably shows at least some features of chronic alcoholism, and jaundice (see Fig. 146-1), ascites (see Fig. 146-4), and splenomegaly are common. The laboratory examination findings are typically abnormal. Common hematologic abnormalities include leukocytosis with neutrophil predominance, macrocytic anemia (Chapter 164), thrombocytopenia (Chapter 172), and prolonged prothrombin time. Liver biochemistries (Chapter 147) are abnormal with an elevated AST and ratio of AST to alanine aminotransferase (ALT), alkaline phosphatase, γ-glutamyl transpeptidase, and total bilirubin but decreased levels of serum albumin. The AST rarely exceeds 300 IU/L. Serum electrolyte abnormalities including hypokalemia (Chapter 117), hypomagnesemia (Chapter 119), hypocalcemia (Chapter 245), and hypophosphatemia (Chapter 119) are frequent. Patients with alcoholic cirrhosis have the same clinical features that are common to other types of cirrhosis (Chapter 153) but also with striking features of underlying chronic alcoholism.

DIAGNOSIS

The diagnosis of alcoholic liver disease strongly depends on the history of excessive alcohol consumption and the presence of liver disease. Although laboratory abnormalities are not specific for alcoholic liver disease, they can be suggestive in the context of excessive alcohol consumption. An AST/ALT ratio of more than 2 is typical in alcoholic liver disease, and ALT values greater than 150 to 200 IU/L are very rare in alcoholic liver disease. Serology testing for coexisting chronic viral hepatitis (Chapter 149) is critical. Diagnostic dilemmas arise when a patient denies excessive alcohol consumption in the face of clinical features that are suggestive of alcoholic liver disease. Interviewing family members about specific alcohol consumption may be helpful in the accurate ascertainment of alcohol consumption. Elevated blood levels of carbohydrate-deficient transferrin, which is a form of transferrin with fewer than the four sialic acid chains present in normal transferrin, can identify recent heavy alcohol consumption. Hepatic imaging by ultrasound, computed tomography, or magnetic resonance imaging will show changes consistent with hepatic steatosis or more advanced forms of liver disease, such as cirrhosis and portal hypertension. Imaging is also important to exclude other forms of liver disease, including malignant disease and

TABLE 152-2 RISK FACTORS FOR ALCOHOLIC LIVER DISEASE AND NONALCOHOLIC FATTY LIVER DISEASE (NAFLD)

ALCOHOLIC LIVER DISEASE	NAFLD
MAJOR	**MAJOR**
Amount and duration of alcohol consumption	Obesity
Female gender	Type 2 diabetes
Genetic factors	Dyslipidemia
Protein-calorie malnutrition	Metabolic syndrome
MINOR	**MINOR**
Type of beverage	Polycystic ovary syndrome
Binge drinking	Hypothyroidism
Obesity	Obstructive sleep apnea
African American and Hispanic ethnicity	Hypopituitarism
	Hypogonadism

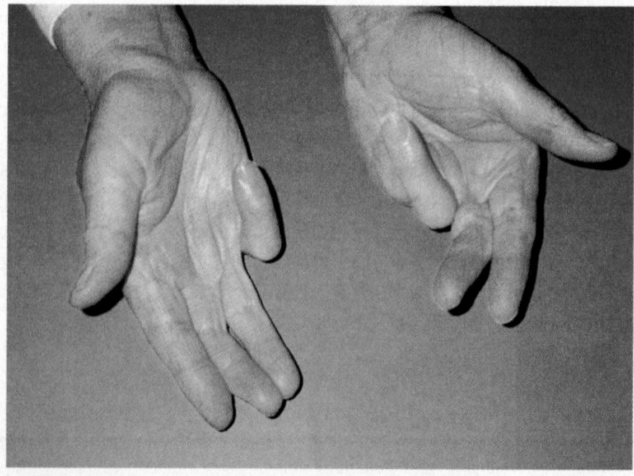

FIGURE 152-1. Dupuytren contracture. (From Gudmundsson KG, Jonsson T, Arngrimsson R. Guillaume Dupuytren and finger contractures. *Lancet*. 2003;362:165-168.)

biliary obstruction. Imaging findings specific for alcoholic liver disease include an enlarged caudate lobe, greater visualization of the right posterior hepatic notch, and focal fat sparing or geographic fat distribution.

Because specific treatment for alcoholic hepatitis may be harmful in patients with other liver diseases, it is important to exclude other predominant or coexisting liver diseases, including chronic viral hepatitis (Chapter 149) and drug-induced liver injury, especially from acetaminophen (Chapter 150), by history, blood tests, and biopsy if needed. Hyperferritinemia generally reflects an acute phase reactant, rather than an iron overload disorder, so it usually will return to normal when the acute liver injury resolves.

Liver biopsy is the key to precisely characterizing the nature of alcoholic liver disease and determining whether a patient has fatty liver or more advanced alcoholic hepatitis. Histologic features of alcoholic fatty liver include macrovesicular steatosis that is predominantly centrilobular (zone 3) in nature. In alcoholic hepatitis, the biopsy is more striking and reveals macrovesicular steatosis, lobular neutrophilic infiltration, Mallory hyaline, balloon degeneration of the hepatocytes, and perivenular fibrosis. In general, patients with alcoholic hepatitis also have histologic evidence of chronic liver injury in the form of more advanced fibrosis (periportal or bridging fibrosis or cirrhosis).

TREATMENT

Rx

Total abstinence, which is the most important treatment measure, is mandatory for the improvement of the clinical and histologic features of alcoholic liver disease. Its benefits are unequivocal, even in patients with severe decompensation. However, long-term abstinence is difficult to achieve, so a multidisciplinary approach with counseling and medications that promote abstinence should be considered. Disulfiram is not commonly used because of its poor tolerability and hepatotoxicity. Opioid antagonists, such as naltrexone (50 mg/day for up to 6 months or even longer), nalmefene (20 mg/day as maintenance), and acamprosate (333-mg tablets, 2 tablets three times each day for 1 year), can help promote abstinence when they are used as part of a multidisciplinary approach (Chapter 33).

Alcoholic fatty liver disease requires no specific treatment other than abstinence. Patients with alcoholic hepatitis, however, have increased short- and long-term mortality and should be considered for therapeutic interventions in addition to mandatory abstinence.[3] If a patient's liver biopsy findings are consistent with alcoholic hepatitis and there is no evidence of other inflammatory liver diseases, such as hepatitis C (Chapter 149), prednisolone (40 mg/day for 4 weeks) should be given to carefully selected patients with severe alcoholic hepatitis who have a score higher than 32 on Maddrey's discriminant function (4.6 × [patient's prothrombin time − control prothrombin time] + total bilirubin level) and encephalopathy but do not have gastrointestinal bleeding or systemic infection.[A1] Studies have suggested that a Model for End-Stage Liver Disease (MELD) score (see Table 153-2) higher than 21 can substitute for Maddrey's score to guide the use of prednisolone. Adding intravenous *N*-acetylcysteine (on day 1 at a dose of 150, 50, and 100 mg per kilogram of body weight in 250, 500, and 1000 mL of 5% glucose solution during a period of 30 minutes, 4 hours, and 16 hours, respectively; and on days 2 through 5, 100 mg per kilogram per day in 1000 mL of 5% glucose solution) to prednisolone appears to be superior to prednisolone alone in terms of a significantly lower mortality at 1 month (8% vs. 24%) and a somewhat but not significantly lower mortality at 6 months (22% vs. 34%; $P = .06$).[A2] Although randomized trials also have shown a benefit of pentoxifylline (400 mg three times daily for 28 days) for severe alcoholic hepatitis,[A3] prednisolone is more effective than pentoxifylline[A4] and the combination of pentoxifylline with prednisolone is no better than prednisolone alone.[A5]

The anti–TNF-α agents infliximab and etanercept are not effective and have significant side effects. All patients with alcoholic hepatitis and alcoholic cirrhosis should be assessed and treated for protein-calorie malnutrition and micronutrient deficiency. Hospitalized patients with severe decompensation should be considered for enteral nutrition (Chapter 216).

Complications such as ascites, spontaneous bacterial peritonitis, encephalopathy, variceal bleeding, hepatorenal syndrome, osteoporosis, and hepatopulmonary syndrome may occur in patients with decompensated alcoholic cirrhosis and must be managed carefully (Chapter 153). Liver transplantation is a reasonable option in patients with decompensated alcoholic cirrhosis, and observational data suggest that early liver transplantation can improve survival in patients with severe, medically refractory alcoholic hepatitis.[4] In general, however, 6 months of abstinence and strong social support are required for eligibility (Chapter 154). Patients with alcoholic cirrhosis are at risk for hepatocellular carcinoma (Chapter 196) and should be screened with semiannual liver imaging and serum α-fetoprotein levels. They are also at risk for extrahepatic malignant disease, notably head and neck, lung, and esophageal cancer. For Dupuytren contracture, injection of collagenase clostridium histolyticum can reduce the severity and improve the range of motion significantly.[A6]

PROGNOSIS

Alcoholic fatty liver is generally reversible with total abstinence for a few months. Alcoholic hepatitis carries high mortality, with nearly 40% of patients dying within 6 months after its presentation. Predictors of poor outcome include the severity of disease as quantified by approaches such as the MELD score[5] (Chapters 153 and 154) and the severity of fibrosis and the neutrophilic infiltration on liver biopsy.[6]

NONALCOHOLIC FATTY LIVER DISEASE

DEFINITIONS

On histologic examination, NAFLD resembles alcoholic liver disease, but it occurs in individuals without significant alcohol consumption. Average alcohol consumption of more than two drinks per day in men and more than one drink per day in women generally is not consistent with a diagnosis of NAFLD. In addition, the definition of NAFLD excludes patients with a history of exposure to steatogenic medications, such as amiodarone, methotrexate, and tamoxifen.

NAFLD encompasses a spectrum of abnormal liver histologic features, ranging from simple steatosis to nonalcoholic steatohepatitis (NASH) and cirrhosis. In simple steatosis, liver histology reveals macrovesicular steatosis without ballooning degeneration of hepatocytes or liver fibrosis. NASH, which is a more advanced form of NAFLD, is histologically characterized by macrovesicular steatosis, ballooning degeneration of the hepatocytes, and sinusoidal fibrosis.

EPIDEMIOLOGY

NAFLD is one of the most common causes of elevated liver enzymes and chronic liver disease in the Western world. Its incidence in adults and children is rising rapidly because of the ongoing epidemics of obesity (Chapter 220), type 2 diabetes mellitus (Chapter 229), and metabolic syndrome. Its prevalence is high in certain populations of patients; for example, nearly 80% of type 2 diabetic patients and 90% of morbidly obese individuals have imaging evidence of NAFLD. Nearly one third of adults in westernized countries are estimated to have NAFLD, and about 5% of adults may have NASH.[7] These percentages compare reasonably well with other data suggesting that the prevalence of cirrhosis from NAFLD is about 2%. Hispanics and whites are at higher risk for NAFLD, whereas its prevalence is intriguingly low in African Americans.

PATHOBIOLOGY

The major risk factors for NAFLD include obesity, type 2 diabetes mellitus (Chapter 229), metabolic syndrome, and dyslipidemia (see Table 152-2). Other comorbidities associated with NAFLD include polycystic ovary syndrome (Chapter 235), hypothyroidism (Chapter 226), hypopituitarism (Chapter 224), hypogonadism (Chapter 234), and sleep apnea (Chapter 100).

Two fundamental defects in NAFLD are insulin resistance/hyperinsulinemia and excessive levels of nonesterified fatty acids within the hepatocytes. An excessive influx of nonesterified fatty acids into the hepatocytes results in macrovesicular steatosis, which is predominantly centrilobular in location.

In addition, patients with NAFLD have increased de novo intrahepatic lipogenesis. Although patients with NAFLD robustly esterify free fatty acids into neutral triglycerides, free fatty acids within the hepatocytes are considered the primary mediators of cell injury (lipotoxicity). In the background of hepatic steatosis, factors that promote cell injury, inflammation, and fibrosis include oxidative stress, endoplasmic reticulum stress, apoptosis, adipocytokines, and stellate cell activation. The sources of oxidative stress include mitochondria and microsomes. Adipocytokines that play an important role in the pathogenesis of NAFLD include adiponectin and TNF-α. It is unclear why some patients with NAFLD exhibit NASH, whereas other patients with a comparable risk factor profile have only simple steatosis. There is a consistent and significant relationship of *PNPLA3* genetic polymorphisms with the severity of steatosis and other histologic features of NAFLD. However, the genetic factors that play a role in NASH and NAFLD have not been fully elucidated.

CLINICAL MANIFESTATIONS

NAFLD is often asymptomatic but may rarely cause fatigue and right upper quadrant pain. Physical examination may reveal hepatomegaly, palmar erythema (see Fig. 146-2), and spider nevi. If liver disease is advanced,

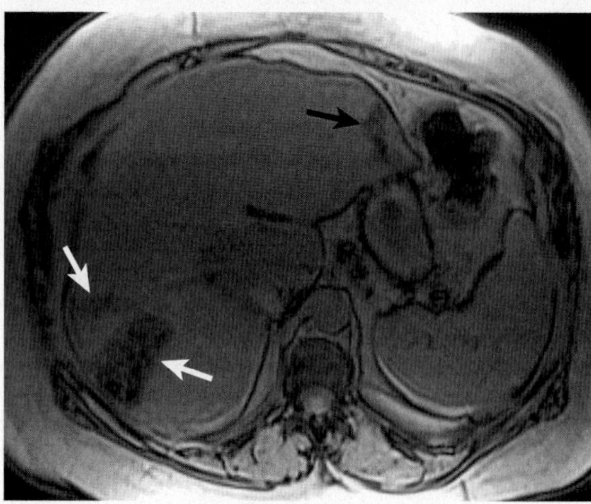

FIGURE 152-2. Magnetic resonance image of chronic liver disease due to nonalcoholic fatty liver disease. Out-of-phase T1-weighted images show focal fat infiltration of varying shapes in right lobe (*white arrows*) and left lobe (*black arrow*). (Courtesy Professor Kumar Sandrasegaran, Indiana University School of Medicine, Indianapolis, Ind.)

the features of liver failure, such as ascites, encephalopathy, and abdominal collateral vessels, are present. Simple steatosis is benign with a minimal risk of cirrhosis, whereas NASH is progressive and can lead to cirrhosis (Chapter 153) and liver failure (Chapter 154). In up to 20% of patients with NASH, liver histologic features will worsen and cirrhosis will develop during a 10- to 15-year period. Severe obesity, advancing age, and diabetes are believed to be risk factors for disease progression. Disease progression during the early phase can be identified only with a repeated liver biopsy, but in later stages, the signs and symptoms of portal hypertension (e.g., abdominal collateral vessels and low platelet count) indicate the development of cirrhosis. Patients with NASH-induced cirrhosis are at risk for development of hepatocellular carcinoma (Chapter 196). Patients with NAFLD have several metabolic risks that predispose them to atherosclerosis, and coronary artery disease is the single most common cause of death in patients with NAFLD.

DIAGNOSIS

NAFLD is generally suspected when aminotransferase levels are asymptomatically elevated in an individual with metabolic risk factors (obesity, diabetes, or the metabolic syndrome) or when liver imaging (ultrasound, computed tomography, or magnetic resonance imaging) obtained for another reason shows fatty infiltration (Fig. 152-2). The diagnosis of NAFLD requires that there is no history of previous or ongoing significant alcohol consumption, no exposure to steatogenic medications, and no evidence of other causes of liver disease, such as viral hepatitis B or C.[8] Elevated levels of aminotransferases, although common, are not required for the diagnosis of NAFLD. In contrast to alcoholic liver disease, ALT levels are higher than AST levels, but they rarely exceed 250 IU/L. In general, AST and ALT levels do not have diagnostic or prognostic significance. Mild hyperferritinemia is common and should not be confused with hereditary hemochromatosis (Chapter 212). Similarly, low-grade autoantibody (antinuclear antibody, anti–smooth muscle antibody) positivity is not uncommon and should not be confused with autoimmune liver disease (Chapter 149). Because steatosis is common in patients with Wilson disease (Chapter 211), serum ceruloplasmin levels should be obtained as part of the diagnostic evaluation.

Fatty liver on ultrasonography has a positive predictive value of only 77% and a negative predictive value of only 67% compared with liver biopsy. Abdominal magnetic resonance imaging is more accurate, but its high cost limits its usefulness in routine practice. Because neither of these imaging tests can differentiate simple steatosis from NASH or identify cirrhosis until hepatic fibrosis has caused nodular liver or overt portal hypertension, liver biopsy is required to establish the presence of NASH or cirrhosis. Common indications for a percutaneous liver biopsy in patients with NAFLD include persistently high aminotransferase levels, inability to exclude a competing or a coexisting cause (e.g., iron overload or autoimmune liver disease), and clinical suspicion of NASH and advanced fibrosis. In patients with NASH, liver histology shows steatosis, inflammation, ballooning, and fibrosis (Fig. 152-3). However, liver histology alone cannot reliably distinguish NASH from alcoholic hepatitis because these two entities have remarkably similar microscopic features.

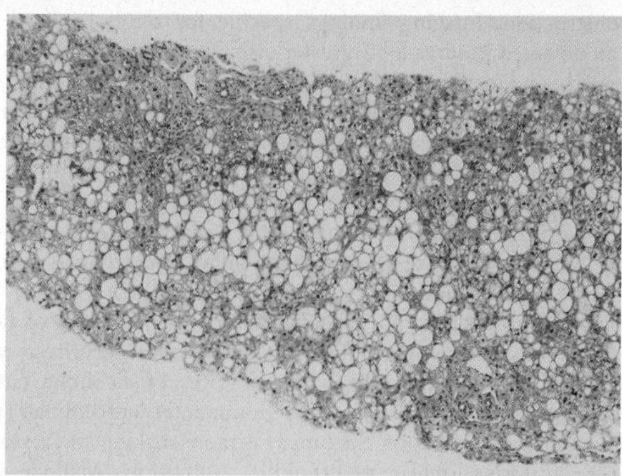

FIGURE 152-3. Liver biopsy specimen showing nonalcoholic steatohepatitis, with increased fat and with early cirrhosis. (Courtesy the NASH Clinical Research Network.)

TREATMENT Rx

Lifestyle modification with dietary restriction and regular exercise is the first choice of treatment for NAFLD.[A7] Weight reduction and increased physical activity consistently reduce liver fat, improve glucose control and insulin sensitivity, and may improve histopathologic features.[9] It is generally recommended that patients with NAFLD lose 10% of their body weight in a gradual fashion, but this goal is difficult to achieve. If resources are available, a multidisciplinary approach with behavioral therapy, dietary advice, and monitoring by a professional nutritionist and an exercise expert is more successful than a prescriptive approach.[10]

Statins (e.g., atorvastatin 20 mg daily) with or without vitamins C and E can improve liver test results and reduce subsequent NAFLD.[A8,A9] In one large trial, 800 IU of vitamin E administered daily for 2 years significantly improved liver histologic findings in adults,[A10] but other trials did not show such convincing benefits in children.[A11] Thiazolidinedione insulin sensitizers (pioglitazone and rosiglitazone) improve steatosis, inflammation, and ballooning, and perhaps fibrosis, but with the side effect of an average gain of nearly 10 pounds.[A12] Unfortunately, the weight gain that is common with thiazolidinediones may offset the histologic benefits that they offer. Treatment with pentoxifylline (400 mg three times daily) can also improve liver enzymes and liver histologic findings in individuals with NASH.[A13]

Patients with NAFLD often have dyslipidemia that puts them at excessive risk for coronary artery disease; their dyslipidemia (Chapter 206) should be treated aggressively with statins and other lipid-lowering agents, which can be safely administered to patients with NAFLD and NASH. In morbidly obese individuals with NASH and other significant metabolic comorbidities, foregut bariatric surgery can lead to significant improvement in hepatic histologic features, but the physician must exclude the presence of portal hypertension before offering this type of surgery.[11] Carefully selected patients with decompensated cirrhosis due to NASH can be treated with liver transplantation (Chapter 154), but recurrence during the post-transplantation period is common.

PREVENTION

The measures to prevent NAFLD include maintaining optimal body weight, exercising regularly, and treating any associated metabolic comorbidities such as diabetes and dyslipidemia. Avoidance of saturated fat, high fructose intake, and alcohol consumption may reduce the development of NAFLD.

PROGNOSIS

Steatosis alone is generally benign, whereas steatohepatitis is often progressive. One third of NAFLD patients may have remission within 7 years, mostly depending on modest weight reduction. Otherwise, however, data are sparse regarding the risk and risk factors for the progression of NAFLD and NASH to cirrhosis and liver failure.

Because NAFLD often coexists with one or more components of the metabolic syndrome, its presence reflects guarded long-term overall prognosis. The long-term complications in patients with simple steatosis generally result from cardiovascular disease and atherosclerosis, not from liver failure.

Patients with NASH also are at risk for liver failure and liver cancer (Chapter 196), in addition to their significantly increased risk of cardiovascular disease. For example, among patients with NASH on their initial biopsy, one third or more develop progressive fibrosis during a mean follow-up interval of about 5 years. Older age, diabetes, and ballooning and fibrosis on liver biopsy are important predictors of progression.

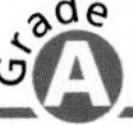

Grade A References

A1. Mathurin P, O'Grady J, Carithers RL, et al. Corticosteroids improve short-term survival in patients with severe alcoholic hepatitis: meta-analysis of individual patient data. *Gut.* 2011;60:255-260.
A2. Nguyen-Khac E, Thevenot T, Piquet MA, et al. Glucocorticoids plus *N*-acetylcysteine in severe alcoholic hepatitis. *N Engl J Med.* 2011;365:1781-1789.
A3. Parker R, Armstrong MJ, Corbett C, et al. Systematic review: pentoxifylline for the treatment of severe alcoholic hepatitis. *Aliment Pharmacol Ther.* 2013;37:845-854.
A4. Park SH, Kim DJ, Kim YS, et al. Pentoxifylline vs. corticosteroid to treat severe alcoholic hepatitis: a randomised, non-inferiority, open trial. *J Hepatol.* 2014;61:792-798.
A5. Mathurin P, Louvet A, Duhamel A, et al. Prednisolone with vs without pentoxifylline and survival of patients with severe alcoholic hepatitis: a randomized clinical trial. *JAMA.* 2013;310:1033-1041.
A6. Hurst LC, Badalamente MA, Hentz VR, et al. Injectable collagenase clostridium histolyticum for Dupuytren's contracture. *N Engl J Med.* 2009;361:968-979.
A7. Promrat K, Kleiner DE, Niemeier HM, et al. Randomized controlled trial testing the effects of weight loss on nonalcoholic steatohepatitis (NASH). *Hepatology.* 2010;51:121-129.
A8. Athyros VG, Tziomalos K, Gossios TD, et al. Safety and efficacy of long-term statin treatment for cardiovascular events in patients with coronary heart disease and abnormal liver tests in the Greek Atorvastatin and Coronary Heart Disease Evaluation (GREACE) study: a post-hoc analysis. *Lancet.* 2010;376:1916-1922.
A9. Foster T, Budoff MJ, Saab S, et al. Atorvastatin and antioxidants for the treatment of nonalcoholic fatty liver disease: the St. Francis Heart Study randomized clinical trial. *Am J Gastroenterol.* 2011;106:71-77.
A10. Sanyal AJ, Chalasani N, Kowdley KV, et al. Pioglitazone, vitamin E, or placebo for nonalcoholic steatohepatitis. *N Engl J Med.* 2010;362:1675-1685.
A11. Lavine JE, Schwimmer JB, Van Natta ML, et al. Effect of vitamin E or metformin for treatment of nonalcoholic fatty liver disease in children and adolescents: the TONIC randomized controlled trial. *JAMA.* 2011;305:1659-1668.
A12. Boettcher E, Csako G, Pucino F, et al. Meta-analysis: pioglitazone improves liver histology and fibrosis in patients with non-alcoholic steatohepatitis. *Aliment Pharmacol Ther.* 2012;35:66-75.
A13. Zein CO, Yerian LM, Gogate P, et al. Pentoxifylline improves nonalcoholic steatohepatitis: a randomized placebo-controlled trial. *Hepatology.* 2011;54:1610-1619.

GENERAL REFERENCES

For the General References and other additional features, please visit Expert Consult at https://expertconsult.inkling.com.

153

CIRRHOSIS AND ITS SEQUELAE

GUADALUPE GARCIA-TSAO

DEFINITION

Cirrhosis, which can be the final stage of any chronic liver disease, is a diffuse process characterized by fibrosis and conversion of normal architecture to structurally abnormal nodules (Fig. 153-1). These "regenerative" nodules lack normal lobular organization and are surrounded by fibrous tissue. The process involves the whole liver and generally is considered irreversible. Although cirrhosis is histologically an "all-or-nothing" diagnosis, clinically it can be classified by its status as compensated or decompensated. Decompensated cirrhosis is defined by the presence of ascites, variceal bleeding, encephalopathy, or jaundice, which are complications that result from the main consequences of cirrhosis: portal hypertension and liver insufficiency.

EPIDEMIOLOGY

Because many patients with cirrhosis are asymptomatic until decompensation occurs, it is difficult to assess the real prevalence and incidence of cirrhosis in the general population. The prevalence of chronic liver disease or cirrhosis worldwide is estimated to be 100 (range, 25 to 400) per 100,000 subjects, but it varies widely by country and by geographic region.

Cirrhosis is an important cause of morbidity and mortality worldwide and in the United States. According to the World Health Organization, about 800,000 people die of cirrhosis annually. In the United States, cirrhosis accounts for about 32,000 deaths each year, or a death rate of 10.3 per 100,000, thereby making it the 12th leading cause of death overall. Importantly, chronic liver disease and cirrhosis are the sixth leading cause of death in the United States in individuals between 25 and 44 years of age and fifth in individuals between 45 and 64 years of age. As chronic liver disease affects people in their most productive years of life, it has a significant impact on the economy as a result of premature death, illness, and disability.

Any chronic liver disease can lead to cirrhosis (Table 153-1). Chronic viral hepatitis C and alcoholic liver disease are the most common causes of cirrhosis, followed by nonalcoholic fatty liver disease (in particular, nonalcoholic steatohepatitis) and chronic hepatitis B (Chapters 149 and 152). However, other causes of cirrhosis include cholestatic and autoimmune liver diseases, such as primary biliary cirrhosis, primary sclerosing cholangitis (Chapter 155), and autoimmune hepatitis (Chapter 149), and metabolic diseases, such as hemochromatosis, Wilson disease, and α_1-antitrypsin deficiency (Chapter 146). When all potential causes have been investigated and excluded, cirrhosis is considered "cryptogenic." Many cases of cryptogenic cirrhosis are now thought to be due to nonalcoholic fatty liver disease (Chapter 152).

Although the entity termed primary biliary cirrhosis assumes the presence of cirrhosis, this term is actually misleading. Primary biliary cirrhosis (Chapter 155) is an immune-mediated cholestatic chronic liver disease that is characterized by progressive destruction of intrahepatic bile ducts and progresses over time from an initial stage in which fibrosis is minimal (stage 1) to a final stage in which there is well-established cirrhosis (stage 4).

PATHOBIOLOGY

Liver Fibrosis and Cirrhosis

The key pathogenic feature underlying liver fibrosis and cirrhosis is activation of hepatic stellate cells. Hepatic stellate cells, which are known as *Ito cells* or *perisinusoidal cells*, are located in the space of Disse between hepatocytes and sinusoidal endothelial cells. Normally, hepatic stellate cells are quiescent and serve as the main storage site for retinoids (vitamin A). In response to injury, hepatic stellate cells become activated, as a result of which they lose their vitamin A deposits, proliferate, develop a prominent rough endoplasmic reticulum, and secrete extracellular matrix (collagen types I and III, sulfated proteoglycans, and glycoproteins). In addition, they become contractile hepatic myofibroblasts.[1]

Unlike other capillaries, normal hepatic sinusoids lack a basement membrane. The sinusoidal endothelial cells themselves contain large fenestrae (100 to 200 nm in diameter) that permit the passage of large molecules with molecular masses up to 250,000 daltons. Collagen deposition in the space of Disse, as occurs in cirrhosis, leads to defenestration of the sinusoidal endothelial cells ("capillarization" of the sinusoids), thereby altering exchange between plasma and hepatocytes and resulting in a decreased sinusoidal diameter that is further exacerbated by the contraction of stellate cells.

Complications of Cirrhosis

The two main consequences of cirrhosis are portal hypertension, with the accompanying hyperdynamic circulatory state, and liver insufficiency (Fig. 153-2). The development of varices and ascites is a direct consequence of portal hypertension and the hyperdynamic circulatory state, whereas jaundice occurs as a result of an inability of the liver to excrete bilirubin (i.e., liver insufficiency). Encephalopathy is the result of both portal hypertension and liver insufficiency. Ascites, in turn, can become complicated by infection, which is called *spontaneous bacterial peritonitis*, and by functional renal failure, which is called *hepatorenal syndrome.*

Portal Hypertension and the Hyperdynamic Circulatory State

In cirrhosis, portal hypertension results from both an increase in resistance to portal flow and an increase in portal venous inflow. The initial mechanism is increased sinusoidal vascular resistance (Fig. 153-3) secondary to (1) deposition of fibrous tissue and subsequent compression by regenerative nodules (fixed component), which could theoretically be amenable to antifibrotic agents and could be ameliorated by resolving the underlying etiologic process, and (2) active vasoconstriction (functional component), which is amenable to the action of vasodilators such as nitroprusside and is caused by a deficiency in intrahepatic nitric oxide (NO) as well as enhanced activity of vasoconstrictors.

Early in the portal hypertensive process, the spleen grows and sequesters platelets and other formed blood cells, thereby leading to hypersplenism. In addition, vessels that normally drain into the portal system, such as the coronary vein, reverse their flow and shunt blood away from the portal system to the systemic circulation. These portosystemic collaterals are insufficient to decompress the portal venous system and offer additional resistance to portal

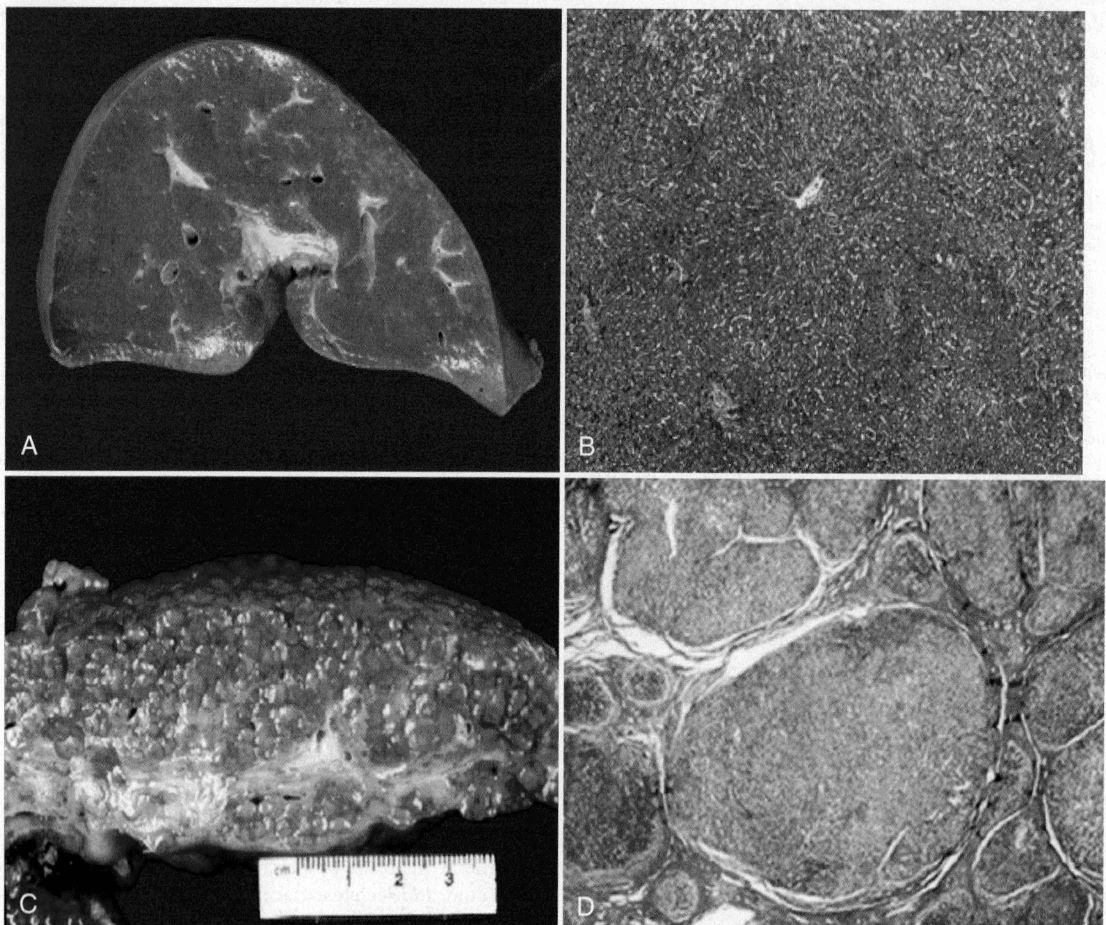

FIGURE 153-1. Gross and microscopic images of a normal and cirrhotic liver. **A**, Gross image of a normal liver with a smooth surface and homogeneous texture. **B**, On microscopic examination, liver sinusoids are organized, and vascular structures are normally distributed. **C**, Gross image of a cirrhotic liver. The liver has an orange-tawny color with an irregular surface and a nodular texture. **D**, On microscopic examination, the architecture is disorganized, and there are regenerative nodules surrounded by fibrous tissue.

TABLE 153-1 CAUSES OF CIRRHOSIS

MAIN FACTORS CAUSING CIRRHOSIS

Chronic hepatitis C
Alcoholic liver disease
Nonalcoholic fatty liver disease
Chronic hepatitis B

OTHER CAUSES OF CIRRHOSIS (<2% OF ALL CASES)

Cholestatic and autoimmune liver diseases
- Primary biliary cirrhosis
- Primary sclerosing cholangitis
- Autoimmune hepatitis

Intrahepatic or extrahepatic biliary obstruction
- Mechanical obstruction
- Biliary atresia
- Cystic fibrosis

Metabolic disorders
- Hemochromatosis
- Wilson disease
- α_1-Antitrypsin deficiency
- Glycogen storage diseases
- Abetalipoproteinemia
- Porphyria

Hepatic venous outflow obstruction
- Budd-Chiari syndrome
- Veno-occlusive disease
- Right-sided heart failure

Drugs and toxins
Intestinal bypass
Indian childhood cirrhosis

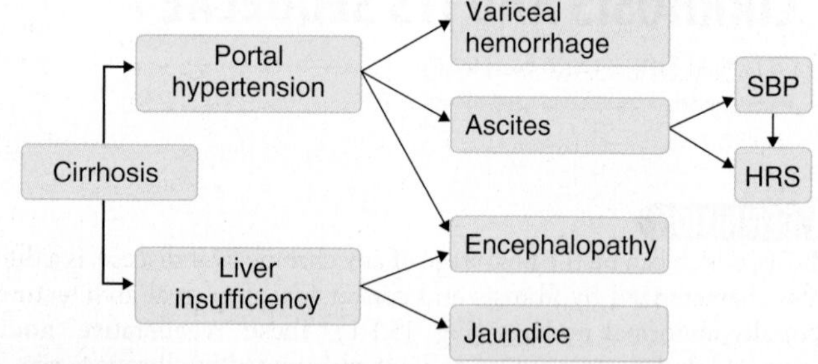

FIGURE 153-2. Complications of cirrhosis result from portal hypertension or liver insufficiency. Varices and variceal hemorrhage are a direct consequence of portal hypertension. Ascites results from sinusoidal portal hypertension and can be complicated by infection (spontaneous bacterial peritonitis [SBP]) or renal dysfunction (hepatorenal syndrome [HRS]). Hepatic encephalopathy results from portosystemic shunting (i.e., portal hypertension) and liver insufficiency. Jaundice results solely from liver insufficiency.

flow. As collaterals develop, an increase in portal blood inflow, which results from splanchnic vasodilation, maintains the portal hypertensive state. Splanchnic arteriolar vasodilation is, in turn, secondary to increased production of NO. Thus, the paradox in portal hypertension is that a deficiency of NO in the intrahepatic vasculature leads to vasoconstriction and increased resistance, whereas overproduction of NO in the extrahepatic circulation leads to vasodilation and increased portal flow.

In addition to splanchnic vasodilation, there is systemic vasodilation, which by causing a decreased *effective* arterial blood volume leads to activation of neurohumoral systems (renin-angiotensin-aldosterone system),

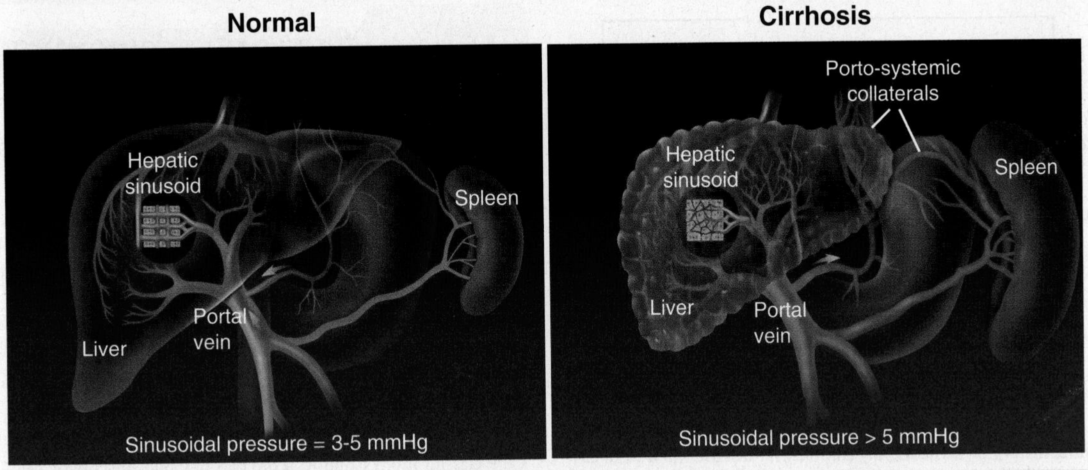

Normal

Hepatic sinusoid

Spleen

Portal vein

Liver

Sinusoidal pressure = 3-5 mmHg

Cirrhosis

Porto-systemic collaterals

Hepatic sinusoid

Spleen

Liver

Portal vein

Sinusoidal pressure > 5 mmHg

FIGURE 153-3. Hepatic sinusoidal pressure is increased in cirrhosis. In the normal liver (*left*), the intrahepatic vasculature is compliant, and the hepatic venous pressure gradient, which is a measure of sinusoidal pressure, is 5 mm Hg or lower. In the cirrhotic liver (*right*), the sinusoidal architecture is distorted by regenerative nodules and fibrosis that lead to increased intrahepatic resistance, portal hypertension, splenomegaly, and portosystemic collaterals; the hepatic venous pressure gradient is above 5 mm Hg. Complications of cirrhosis develop when the gradient increases above 10 to 12 mm Hg.

retention of sodium, expansion of plasma volume, and development of a hyperdynamic circulatory state. This hyperdynamic circulatory state maintains portal hypertension, thereby leading to the formation and growth of varices, and plays an important role in the development of all other complications of cirrhosis.

Varices and Variceal Hemorrhage

The complication of cirrhosis that results most directly from portal hypertension is the development of portal-systemic collaterals, the most relevant of which are those that form through dilation of the coronary and gastric veins and constitute gastroesophageal varices. The initial formation of esophageal collaterals depends on a threshold portal pressure, clinically established by a hepatic venous pressure gradient of 10 to 12 mm Hg, below which varices do not develop.

Development of a hyperdynamic circulatory state leads to further dilation and growth of varices and eventually to their rupture and variceal hemorrhage, one of the most dreaded complications of portal hypertension. Tension in a varix determines variceal rupture and is directly proportional to variceal diameter and intravariceal pressure and inversely proportional to variceal wall thickness.

Ascites and Hepatorenal Syndrome

Ascites, which is the accumulation of intraperitoneal fluid, in cirrhosis is secondary to sinusoidal hypertension and retention of sodium. Cirrhosis leads to sinusoidal hypertension by blocking hepatic venous outflow both anatomically by fibrosis and regenerative nodules and functionally by increased postsinusoidal vascular tone. Similar to the formation of esophageal varices, a threshold hepatic venous pressure gradient of 12 mm Hg is needed for the formation of ascites. In addition, retention of sodium replenishes the intravascular volume and allows the continuous formation of ascites. Retention of sodium results from vasodilation that is mostly due to an increase in NO production because NO inhibition in experimental animals increases urinary sodium excretion, lowers plasma aldosterone levels, and reduces ascites. With progression of cirrhosis and portal hypertension, vasodilation is more pronounced, thereby leading to further activation of the renin-angiotensin-aldosterone and sympathetic nervous systems and resulting in further sodium retention (refractory ascites), water retention (hyponatremia), and renal vasoconstriction (hepatorenal syndrome).

Spontaneous Bacterial Peritonitis

Spontaneous bacterial peritonitis, an infection of ascitic fluid, occurs in the absence of perforation of a hollow viscus or an intra-abdominal inflammatory focus, such as an abscess, acute pancreatitis, or cholecystitis. Bacterial translocation, or the migration of bacteria from the intestinal lumen to mesenteric lymph nodes and other extraintestinal sites, is the main mechanism implicated in spontaneous bacterial peritonitis. Impaired local and systemic immune defenses are a major element in promoting bacterial translocation and, together with shunting of blood away from the hepatic Kupffer cells through portosystemic collaterals, allow a transient bacteremia to become more prolonged, thereby colonizing ascitic fluid. Spontaneous bacterial peritonitis occurs in patients with reduced ascites defense mechanisms, such as a low complement level in ascitic fluid. Another factor that promotes bacterial translocation in cirrhosis is bacterial overgrowth attributed to a decrease in small bowel motility and intestinal transit time. Infections, particularly from gram-negative bacteria, can precipitate renal dysfunction through worsening of the hyperdynamic circulatory state.

Encephalopathy

Hepatic encephalopathy is brain dysfunction caused by liver insufficiency, portosystemic shunting, or both.[2,3] Ammonia, a toxin normally removed by the liver, plays a key role in its pathogenesis. In cirrhosis, ammonia accumulates in the systemic circulation because of shunting of blood through portosystemic collaterals and decreased liver metabolism (i.e., liver insufficiency). The presence of large amounts of ammonia in the brain damages supporting brain cells or astrocytes and leads to structural changes characteristic of hepatic encephalopathy (Alzheimer type II astrocytosis). Ammonia results in upregulation of astrocytic peripheral-type benzodiazepine receptors, the most potent stimulants of neurosteroid production. Neurosteroids are the major modulators of γ-aminobutyric acid, which results in cortical depression and hepatic encephalopathy. Other toxins, such as manganese, also accumulate in the brain, particularly the globus pallidus, where they lead to impaired motor function. Other yet-to-be-elucidated toxins may also be involved in the pathogenesis of encephalopathy.

Jaundice

Jaundice (Chapter 147) in cirrhosis is a reflection of the inability of the liver to excrete bilirubin and is therefore the result of liver insufficiency. However, in cholestatic diseases leading to cirrhosis (e.g., primary biliary cirrhosis, primary sclerosing cholangitis, vanishing bile duct syndrome), jaundice is more likely due to biliary damage than to liver insufficiency. Other indicators of liver insufficiency, such as the presence of encephalopathy or prolongation of the international normalized ratio, help determine the most likely contributor to hyperbilirubinemia (Chapter 147).

Cardiopulmonary Complications

The hyperdynamic circulatory state eventually results in high-output heart failure with decreased peripheral utilization of oxygen, a complication that has been referred to as *cirrhotic cardiomyopathy*. Vasodilation at the level of the pulmonary circulation leads to arterial hypoxemia, the hallmark of hepatopulmonary syndrome. Normal pulmonary capillaries are 8 μm in diameter, and red blood cells (slightly less than 8 μm) pass through them one cell at a time, thereby facilitating oxygenation. In *hepatopulmonary syndrome*, the pulmonary capillaries are dilated up to 500 μm, so passage of red cells through the pulmonary capillaries may be many cells thick. As a result, a large number of red cells are not oxygenated, which causes the equivalent of a right-to-left shunt.

Conversely, *portopulmonary hypertension* occurs when the pulmonary bed is exposed to vasoconstrictive substances that may be produced in the splanchnic circulation and bypass metabolism by the liver; the initial result

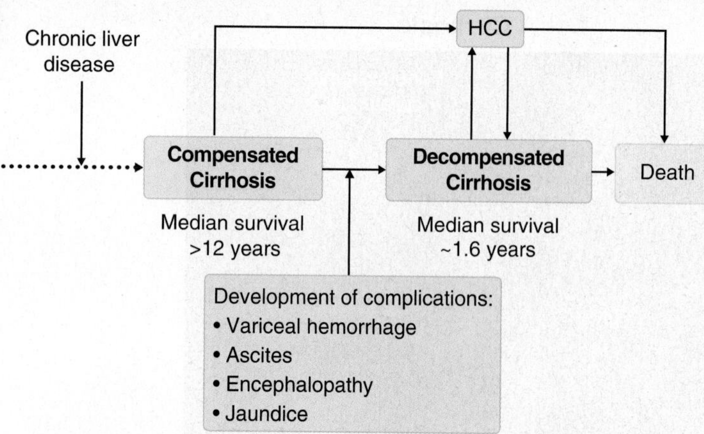

FIGURE 153-4. Natural history of cirrhosis. Any chronic liver disease will lead to cirrhosis. Initially, cirrhosis will be compensated (median survival, >12 years), but once complications (ascites, variceal hemorrhage, encephalopathy, jaundice) develop, it becomes decompensated (median survival, 1.6 years). Hepatocellular carcinoma (HCC) can develop at any stage and precipitate decompensation and death.

is reversible pulmonary hypertension. However, because these factors result in endothelial proliferation, vasoconstriction, in situ thrombosis, and obliteration of vessels, irreversible pulmonary hypertension ensues.

CLINICAL MANIFESTATIONS

The clinical manifestations of cirrhosis range widely, depending on the stage of cirrhosis, from an asymptomatic patient with no signs of chronic liver disease to a patient who is confused and jaundiced with severe muscle wasting and ascites. The natural history of cirrhosis is characterized by an initial phase, termed *compensated* cirrhosis, followed by a rapidly progressive phase marked by the development of complications of portal hypertension or liver dysfunction (or both), termed *decompensated* cirrhosis (Fig. 153-4).[4] In the compensated phase, liver synthetic function is mostly normal, and portal pressure, although increased, is below the threshold level required for the development of varices or ascites. As the disease progresses, portal pressure increases and liver function worsens, thereby resulting in the development of ascites, portal hypertensive gastrointestinal bleeding, encephalopathy, and jaundice. The development of any of these clinically detectable complications marks the transition from a compensated to a decompensated phase. Progression to death may be accelerated by the development of other complications, such as recurrent gastrointestinal bleeding, renal impairment (refractory ascites, hepatorenal syndrome), hepatopulmonary syndrome, and sepsis (spontaneous bacterial peritonitis). The development of hepatocellular carcinoma (Chapter 196) may accelerate the course of the disease at any stage (see Fig. 153-4). Transition from a compensated to a decompensated stage occurs at a rate of approximately 5 to 7% per year. The median time to decompensation, or the time at which half the patients with compensated cirrhosis will become decompensated, is about 6 years.

Compensated Cirrhosis

In this stage, cirrhosis is mostly asymptomatic and is diagnosed either during the evaluation of chronic liver disease or fortuitously during routine physical examination, biochemical testing, imaging for other reasons, endoscopy showing gastroesophageal varices, or abdominal surgery in which a nodular liver is detected. Nonspecific fatigue, decreased libido, or sleep disturbances may be the only complaints. About 40% of patients with compensated cirrhosis have esophageal varices. Nonbleeding gastroesophageal varices are asymptomatic, and their presence (without bleeding) does not denote decompensation.

Decompensated Cirrhosis

At this stage, there are signs of decompensation: ascites, variceal hemorrhage, jaundice, hepatic encephalopathy, or any combination of these findings. Ascites, which is the most frequent sign of decompensation, is present in 80% of patients with decompensated cirrhosis.

Variceal Hemorrhage

Gastroesophageal varices are present in approximately 50% of patients with newly diagnosed cirrhosis. The prevalence of varices correlates with the severity of liver disease and ranges from 40% in Child A cirrhotic patients (Table 153-2) to 85% in Child C cirrhotic patients.

TABLE 153-2 THE TWO MOST COMMONLY USED SCORING SYSTEMS IN CIRRHOSIS

1. CHILD-TURCOTTE-PUGH (CTP) SCORE (RANGE, 5-15)

	POINTS ASCRIBED		
Parameters	**1**	**2**	**3**
Ascites	None	Grade 1-2 (or easy to treat)	Grade 3-4 (or refractory)
Hepatic encephalopathy	None	Grade 1-2 (or induced by a precipitant)	Grade 3-4 (or spontaneous)
Bilirubin (mg/dL)	<2	2-3	>3
Albumin (g/dL)	>3.5	2.8-3.5	<2.8
Prothrombin time (seconds > control) or INR	<4 <1.7	4-6 1.7-2.3	>6 >2.3

CTP classification: Child A: score of 5-6; Child B: score of 7-9; Child C: score of 10-15

2. MODEL OF END-STAGE LIVER DISEASE (MELD) SCORE (RANGE, 6-40)

[0.957 × LN (creatinine in mg/dL) + 0.378 × LN (bilirubin in mg/dL) + 1.12 × LN (INR) + 0.643] × 10

INR = international normalized ratio; LN = natural logarithm.

Both the development of varices and the growth of small varices occur at a rate of 7 to 8% per year. The incidence of a first variceal hemorrhage in patients with small varices is about 5% per year, whereas medium and large varices bleed at a rate of approximately 15% per year. Large varices, severe liver disease, and red wale markings on varices are independent predictors of variceal hemorrhage. Bleeding from gastroesophageal varices can be manifested as overt hematemesis, melena, or both (Chapter 135).

Ascites and Hyponatremia

Ascites is the most common cause of decompensation in cirrhosis and occurs at a rate of 7 to 10% per year. The most frequent symptoms associated with ascites are increased abdominal girth, which is often described by the patient as tightness of the belt or garments around the waist, and recent weight gain. When it is present in small to moderate amounts, ascites can be identified on examination by bulging flanks, flank dullness, and shifting dullness (Chapter 146).

Hyponatremia, which is defined as a serum sodium concentration below 130 mEq/L (Chapter 116), is present in about 25% of patients with cirrhosis and ascites. However, patients with cirrhosis do not usually have significant neurologic manifestations or hyponatremia, presumably because it typically develops gradually. Nevertheless, hyponatremia is a marker of the severity of cirrhosis and is associated with poorer quality of life and the development of hepatic encephalopathy.[5]

Hepatorenal syndrome is a type of prerenal kidney injury that occurs in patients with cirrhosis and ascites.[6] It represents the extreme of the spectrum of abnormalities that lead to cirrhotic ascites and is the result of maximal peripheral vasodilation as well as maximal activation of hormones that cause the retention of sodium and water and intense vasoconstriction of the renal arteries. Hepatorenal syndrome is divided into two types based on clinical characteristics and prognosis. Type 1 hepatorenal syndrome is rapidly progressive *acute* kidney injury in which the rise in serum creatinine concentration occurs within a 2-week period. Type 2 hepatorenal syndrome is more slowly progressive and associated with ascites that is refractory to diuretics. Patients with hepatorenal syndrome usually have tense ascites that responds poorly to diuretics, but no specific symptoms or signs typify this entity.

Spontaneous Bacterial Peritonitis

About one third of cirrhotic patients are admitted for bacterial infection or acquire a bacterial infection during hospitalization, the most common being spontaneous bacterial peritonitis. The two most important predictors of the development of bacterial infection are the severity of liver disease and admission for gastrointestinal hemorrhage. The most frequent clinical manifestations of spontaneous bacterial peritonitis are fever, jaundice, and abdominal pain. On physical examination, there is typically abdominal tenderness, with or without rebound tenderness, or ileus (or both). However, up to one third of patients with spontaneous bacterial peritonitis initially may have no abdominal symptoms or symptoms of infection[7] and may present instead with encephalopathy, acute kidney injury, or evidence of shock.

Hepatic Encephalopathy

Hepatic encephalopathy, which is the neuropsychiatric manifestation of cirrhosis, occurs at a rate of approximately 2 to 3% per year. Hepatic encephalopathy associated with cirrhosis is of gradual onset and rarely fatal. It is manifested as a wide spectrum of neurologic and psychiatric abnormalities ranging from subclinical alterations to coma. Clinically, it is characterized by alterations in consciousness and behavior ranging from inversion of the sleep-wake pattern and forgetfulness (grade 1); to confusion, bizarre behavior, and disorientation (grade 2); to lethargy and profound disorientation (grade 3); to coma (grade 4). On physical examination, early stages may demonstrate only a distal tremor, but the hallmark of overt hepatic encephalopathy is the presence of asterixis (Chapter 154). In addition, patients with hepatic encephalopathy may have sweet-smelling breath, a characteristic termed *fetor hepaticus.*

Pulmonary Complications

Hepatopulmonary syndrome is associated with exertional dyspnea, which can lead to extreme debilitation. Clubbing of the fingers, cyanosis, and vascular spiders may be seen on physical examination. Hepatopulmonary syndrome is present in approximately 5 to 10% of patients awaiting liver transplantation.

Portopulmonary hypertension is manifested as exertional dyspnea, syncope, and chest pain. On examination, an accentuated second sound and right ventricular heave are prominent (Chapter 68).

DIAGNOSIS

The diagnosis of cirrhosis should be considered in any patient with chronic liver disease.[8] In asymptomatic patients with *compensated cirrhosis,* typical signs of cirrhosis may not be present, and the physical examination and laboratory test findings may be entirely normal. The diagnosis may often require histologic confirmation by liver biopsy, which is the "gold standard" for the diagnosis of cirrhosis. However, liver biopsy is an invasive procedure subject to sampling error, and the presence of cirrhosis can often be confirmed noninvasively by a combination of serum biomarkers, imaging techniques, and measurements of liver stiffness.

Physical Examination

On physical examination, stigmata of cirrhosis consist of muscle atrophy, mainly involving the bitemporal muscle regions and the thenar and hypothenar eminences; spider angiomas, mostly on the trunk, face, and upper limbs; and palmar erythema involving the thenar and the hypothenar eminences and the tips of the fingers. Although muscle atrophy is a marker of liver insufficiency, spider angiomas and palmar erythema are markers of vasodilation and a hyperdynamic circulation. Men may have hair loss on the chest and abdomen, gynecomastia, and testicular atrophy. Petechiae and ecchymoses may be present as a result of thrombocytopenia or a prolonged prothrombin time. Dupuytren contracture, which is a thickening of the palmar fascia, occurs mostly in alcoholic cirrhosis. A pathognomonic feature of cirrhosis is the finding on abdominal examination of a small right liver lobe, with a span of less than 7 cm on percussion, and a palpable left lobe that is nodular with increased consistency. Splenomegaly may also be present and is indicative of portal hypertension. Collateral circulation on the abdominal wall (caput medusae) may also develop as a consequence of portal hypertension. Absence of any of these physical findings does not exclude cirrhosis.

Laboratory Tests

Laboratory test results suggestive of cirrhosis include even subtle abnormalities in serum levels of albumin or bilirubin or elevation of the international normalized ratio. The most sensitive and specific laboratory finding suggestive of cirrhosis in the setting of chronic liver disease is a low platelet count (<150,000/μL), which occurs as a result of portal hypertension and hypersplenism. Other serum markers that are often abnormal include levels of aspartate aminotransferase, γ-glutamyl transpeptidase, hyaluronic acid, α_2-macroglobulin, haptoglobin, tissue metalloproteinase inhibitor 1, and apolipoprotein A. Combinations of these tests have been used to predict the presence of cirrhosis, but they are not as accurate as imaging studies.[9]

Imaging Studies

Confirmatory imaging tests include computed tomography, ultrasound, and magnetic resonance imaging. Findings consistent with cirrhosis include a nodular contour of the liver, a small liver with or without hypertrophy of the left or caudate lobe, splenomegaly, and, in particular, identification of intra-abdominal collateral vessels indicative of portal hypertension (Fig. 153-5). With increasing fibrosis, the liver becomes stiff, and this stiffness can be measured by ultrasound (transient elastography, acoustic radiation force impulse imaging) or magnetic resonance imaging. Measurement of liver stiffness, a new noninvasive technique, appears to be useful in the diagnosis of cirrhosis and in excluding its presence.[10] These tests are becoming more widely available, and typical findings on any of these imaging studies, together with a compatible clinical picture, are indicative of the presence of cirrhosis. A liver biopsy then would not be required unless the degree of inflammation or other features require investigation.

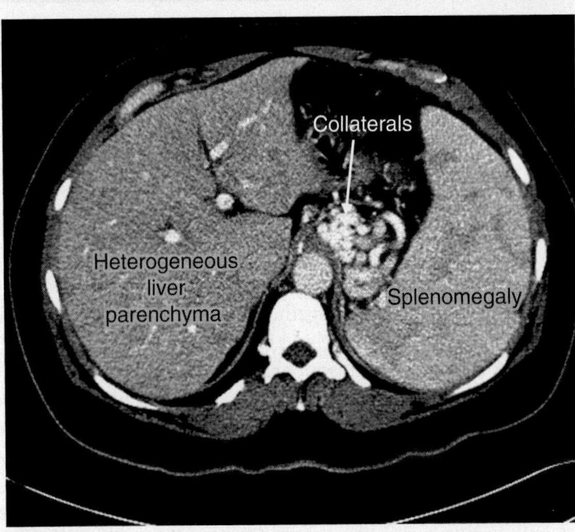

FIGURE 153-5. Computed tomography in a patient with compensated cirrhosis. The liver parenchyma is heterogeneous, there is splenomegaly, and, importantly, there are portosystemic collaterals.

In *decompensated cirrhosis,* detection of ascites, variceal bleeding, or encephalopathy in the setting of chronic liver disease essentially establishes the diagnosis of cirrhosis, so a liver biopsy is not necessary to establish the diagnosis. Patients with decompensated cirrhosis often exhibit malnutrition, more severe muscle wasting, more numerous vascular spiders, and hypotension and tachycardia as a result of the hyperdynamic circulatory state.

Portal Pressure Measurements

Direct measurements of portal pressure involve catheterization of the portal vein, are cumbersome, and may be associated with complications. Hepatic vein catheterization with measurement of wedged and free pressure is the simplest, safest, most reproducible, and most widely used method to indirectly measure portal pressure. Portal pressure measurements are expressed as the hepatic venous pressure gradient: the gradient between wedged hepatic venous pressure, which is a measure of sinusoidal pressure, and free hepatic or inferior vena cava pressure, which is used as an internal zero reference point. In a patient with clinical evidence of portal hypertension (e.g., varices), the hepatic venous pressure gradient is useful in the differential diagnosis of the cause of portal hypertension: it will be normal (3 to 5 mm Hg) in prehepatic causes of portal hypertension, such as portal vein thrombosis (Chapter 143), and in intrahepatic but presinusoidal causes, such as schistosomiasis (Chapter 355); but it will be abnormal (≥6 mm Hg) in sinusoidal causes of portal hypertension, such as cirrhosis, and in postsinusoidal causes, such as veno-occlusive disease. In patients with viral or alcoholic cirrhosis, a hepatic venous pressure gradient of 10 mm Hg or greater ("clinically significant" portal hypertension) predicts the development of complications of portal hypertension, and its reduction with pharmacologic therapy predicts a favorable outcome in patients with cirrhosis. In patients with variceal hemorrhage, a hepatic venous pressure gradient of more than 20 mm Hg predicts recurrent variceal hemorrhage and may portend death.

Complications of Cirrhosis

Varices and Variceal Hemorrhage

Upper gastrointestinal endoscopy (Chapter 134) remains the main method for diagnosis of varices and variceal hemorrhage. Varices are classified as small (straight, minimally elevated veins above the esophageal mucosal surface), medium (tortuous veins occupying less than one third of the esophageal lumen), or large (occupying more than one third of the esophageal lumen). The diagnosis of variceal hemorrhage is made when diagnostic esophagogastroduodenoscopy shows one of the following: active bleeding from a varix, a "white nipple" overlying a varix, clots overlying a varix, or varices with no other potential source of bleeding.

Ascites

The most common cause of ascites is cirrhosis, which accounts for 80% of cases. Peritoneal malignant disease (e.g., peritoneal metastases from gastrointestinal tumors or ovarian cancer), heart failure (Chapter 58), and peritoneal tuberculosis (Chapter 324) together account for another 15% of cases. The initial, most cost-effective, and least invasive method to confirm the presence of ascites is abdominal ultrasonography.

Diagnostic paracentesis is a safe procedure that should be performed in every patient with new-onset ascites, even in those with coagulopathy. Ultrasound guidance should be used in patients in whom percussion cannot locate the ascites or in whom a first paracentesis attempt does not yield fluid. The fluid in a patient with new-onset ascites should always be evaluated for albumin (with simultaneous estimation of serum albumin), total protein, and polymorphonuclear (PMN) blood cell count, and bacteriologic cultures and cytology should be performed. The PMN cell count and bacteriologic culture are useful to exclude infection (either spontaneous or secondary bacterial peritonitis), and cytologic evaluation is needed if peritoneal carcinomatosis is suspected. Depending on the clinical setting, additional tests can be performed on the fluid: glucose and lactate dehydrogenase levels (if secondary bacterial peritonitis is suspected), smear and culture for acid-fast bacilli (if peritoneal tuberculosis is suspected), and amylase level (if pancreatic ascites is suspected).

The serum-ascites albumin gradient and ascites protein levels are useful in the differential diagnosis of ascites (Table 153-3). The serum-ascites albumin gradient correlates with sinusoidal pressure and will therefore be elevated (>1.1 g/dL) in patients in whom the source of ascites is the hepatic sinusoid (e.g., cirrhosis or cardiac ascites). Protein levels in ascitic fluid are an indirect marker of the integrity of the hepatic sinusoids: normal sinusoids are permeable structures that "leak" protein, whereas sinusoids in cirrhosis are "capillarized" and do not leak as much protein. The three main causes of ascites—cirrhosis, peritoneal malignant disease or tuberculosis, and heart failure—can easily be distinguished by combining the results of both the serum-ascites albumin gradient and ascites total protein content. Cirrhotic ascites typically has a high serum-ascites albumin gradient and low protein, cardiac ascites has a high serum-ascites albumin gradient and high protein, and ascites secondary to peritoneal malignant disease typically has a low serum-ascites albumin gradient and high protein. A high serum B-type natriuretic peptide has a high diagnostic accuracy in the diagnosis of ascites due to heart failure.

Hepatorenal Syndrome

Hepatorenal syndrome, which is a diagnosis of exclusion, should be diagnosed only after diuretics have been discontinued, any condition that leads to worsening of the hemodynamic status of the cirrhotic patient has been excluded or treated, and intravascular volume has been expanded with albumin. Ascites unresponsive to diuretics is universal, and dilutional hyponatremia is almost always present. The differential diagnosis includes conditions that worsen vasodilation, such as sepsis, the use of vasodilators, and large-volume paracentesis not accompanied by albumin infusion; conditions that decrease effective arterial blood volume, such as gastrointestinal hemorrhage, overdiuresis, or diarrhea (often induced by overdoses of lactulose); conditions that induce renal vasoconstriction, such as nonsteroidal anti-inflammatory drugs; and nephrotoxic insults, such as from aminoglycosides.

TABLE 153-3 USING THE SERUM-ASCITES ALBUMIN GRADIENT AND THE ASCITES TOTAL PROTEIN LEVEL TO DIAGNOSE THE CAUSE OF ASCITES

CONDITION	SERUM-ASCITES ALBUMIN GRADIENT*	ASCITES TOTAL PROTEIN LEVEL†
Cirrhosis	High	Low
Malignant ascites	Low	High
Cardiac ascites	High	High

*High is more than 1.1 g/dL; low is less than 1.1 g/dL.
†High is more than 2.5 g/dL; low is less than 2.5 g/dL.

Spontaneous Bacterial Peritonitis

A high index of suspicion and early diagnosis are key in the management of spontaneous bacterial peritonitis. Diagnostic paracentesis should be performed in any patient with symptoms or signs of spontaneous bacterial peritonitis, including unexplained encephalopathy and renal dysfunction. Because spontaneous bacterial peritonitis is often asymptomatic and frequently community acquired, diagnostic paracentesis should be performed when any cirrhotic patient is admitted to the hospital, regardless of the cause for admission.

The diagnosis of spontaneous bacterial peritonitis is established by an ascitic fluid PMN count greater than 250/μL. Bacteria can be isolated from ascitic fluid in only 40 to 50% of cases, even with sensitive methods such as inoculation directly into a blood culture bottle. Spontaneous bacterial peritonitis is mostly a monobacterial infection, usually with gram-negative enteric organisms. However, the widespread use of antibiotic prophylaxis in cirrhosis has led to an increased prevalence of infections with multidrug-resistant organisms. Anaerobes and fungi very rarely cause spontaneous bacterial peritonitis; their presence, as well as a polymicrobial infection, should raise suspicion of secondary bacterial peritonitis.

Hepatic Encephalopathy

The diagnosis of overt hepatic encephalopathy is mainly clinical and based on a history and physical examination that shows alterations in consciousness and behavior as well as the presence of asterixis. Ammonia levels are unreliable, and there is poor correlation between the grade of hepatic encephalopathy and ammonia blood levels. High levels (>150 μmol/L) are, however, indicative of hepatic encephalopathy and can be useful in the evaluation of a patient with neurocognitive disturbances of unknown origin. Psychometric tests and an electroencephalogram, which typically shows generalized slow waves and the presence of triphasic waves, are commonly used in research but are not generally used for clinical diagnosis. Minimal or subclinical hepatic encephalopathy, which is present in up to 80% of patients with cirrhosis, is diagnosed solely on the basis of abnormal results of psychometric and neuropsychological tests of attention (e.g., number connection test, digit symbol test) and psychomotor function (e.g., grooved pegboard). Screening of cirrhotic patients for minimal hepatic encephalopathy is not widely recommended because diagnostic tests are not standardized and the benefits of treatment are uncertain.

Hepatopulmonary Syndrome and Portopulmonary Hypertension

The diagnostic criteria for hepatopulmonary syndrome are arterial hypoxemia with a PaO_2 of less than 80 mm Hg or an alveolar arterial oxygen gradient of greater than 15 mm Hg, along with evidence of pulmonary vascular shunting on contrast echocardiography (Chapter 55) or a ^{99m}Tc-labeled macroaggregated albumin scan demonstrating abnormal shunting of radioactivity to the brain.[11] Portopulmonary hypertension is diagnosed by the presence of mean pulmonary arterial pressure higher than 25 mm Hg on right-sided heart catheterization, provided pulmonary capillary wedge pressure is less than 15 mm Hg.

TREATMENT

Rx

Treatment of cirrhosis should ideally be aimed at interruption or reversal of fibrosis. Although antifibrotic drugs have not been shown to reverse fibrosis consistently or to improve outcomes in cirrhotic patients, eradication of the hepatitis C or the hepatitis B virus has been associated with reversal of fibrosis.[A1] Treatment of compensated cirrhosis is currently directed at preventing the development of decompensation by (1) treating the underlying liver disease (e.g., antiviral therapy for hepatitis C or B) to reduce fibrosis and to prevent decompensation; (2) avoiding factors that could worsen liver disease, such as alcohol, hepatotoxic drugs, and superimposed viral infections; and (3) screening for varices (to prevent variceal hemorrhage) and for hepatocellular carcinoma (to treat it at an early stage) (Fig. 153-6). Treatment of decompensated cirrhosis focuses on specific decompensating events and the option of liver transplantation. Increasingly, data reveal that different therapies for the same complication may be applicable to patients with different risk profiles, mainly based on severity of the disease (see Table 153-2).

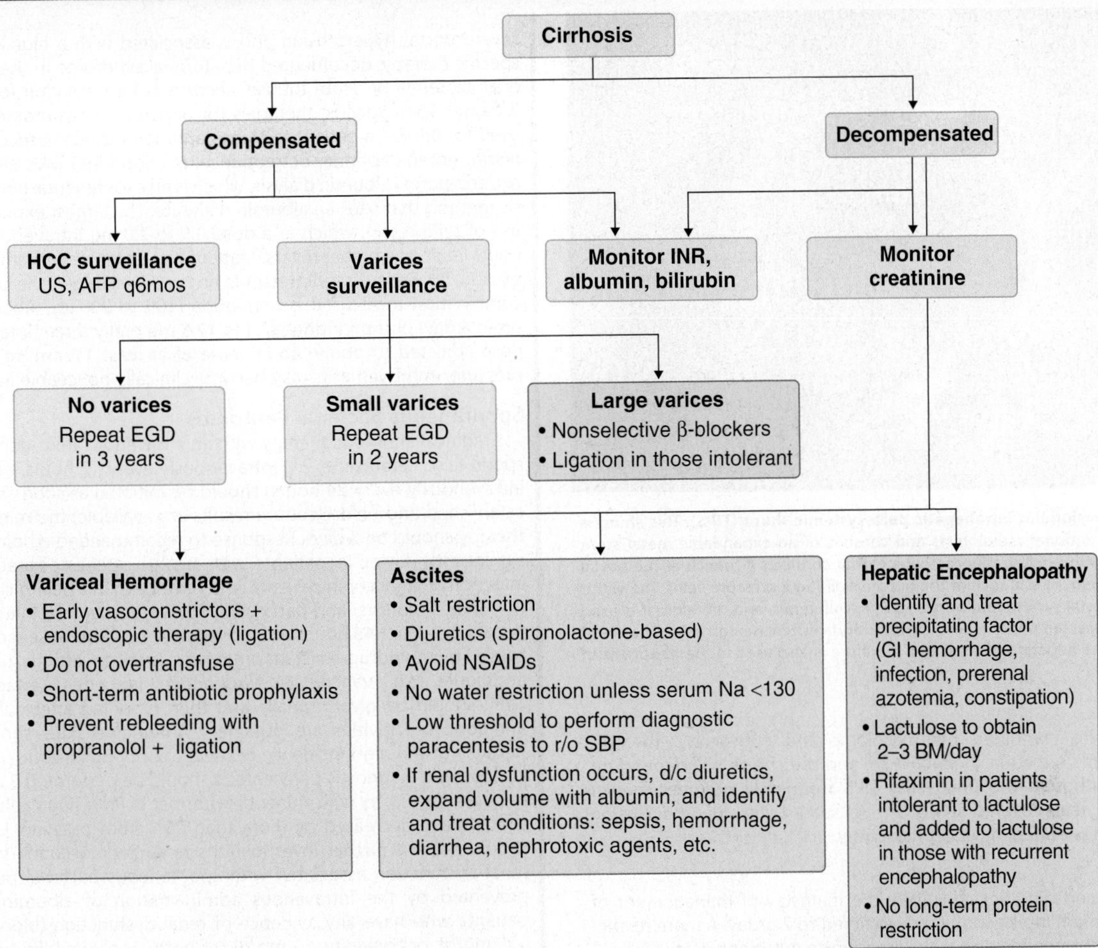

FIGURE 153-6. **Summary of the management of compensated and decompensated cirrhosis.** AFP = α-fetoprotein; BM = bowel movement; d/c = discontinue; EGD = esophagogastroduodenoscopy; GI = gastrointestinal; HCC = hepatocellular carcinoma; INR = international normalized ratio; Na = sodium; NSAIDs = nonsteroidal anti-inflammatory drugs; r/o = rule out; SBP = spontaneous bacterial peritonitis; US = ultrasound.

Varices and Variceal Bleeding

Reducing portal pressure decreases the risk for the development of varices and variceal hemorrhage as well as the risk for ascites and death. Nonselective β-adrenergic blockers (propranolol, nadolol) reduce portal pressure by producing splanchnic vasoconstriction and decreasing portal venous inflow. In patients with cirrhosis and medium or large varices that have never bled, nonselective β-blockers significantly reduce the risk for first variceal hemorrhage. Treatment options have included propranolol (initiated at a dose of 20 mg orally twice a day) and nadolol (initiated at a dose of 20 mg orally every day), with the dose titrated to produce a resting heart rate of about 50 to 55 beats per minute.[12] β-Adrenergic blockers also reduce portal pressure and lower the risk for development of ascites. Endoscopic variceal ligation (see Fig. 134-3), a therapy that aims to obliterate varices by placing rubber rings on variceal columns, is at least as useful as traditional nonselective β-blockers to prevent a first variceal hemorrhage.[A2] Ligation has no effect on portal pressure and can lead to hemorrhage from ligation-induced ulcers. Carvedilol (a nonselective β-blocker with vasodilating properties at a dose of 12.5 mg/day) has been shown to be superior to ligation[A3] and to lower portal pressure in patients who do not respond to propranolol[A4]; however, its use in patients with ascites may not be advisable because of its vasodilating effect. A rational approach is to start therapy with propranolol or nadolol and to use ligation in patients who cannot tolerate or have contraindications to β-blockers. In the compensated patient, carvedilol could be used in patients who cannot tolerate propranolol or nadolol.

In patients with no varices, nonselective β-blockers do not prevent the development of varices and are associated with more side effects. In patients with small varices, data are insufficient to recommend therapy with nonselective β-blockers. Endoscopy should be repeated every 2 to 3 years in patients with no varices, every 1 to 2 years in patients with small varices, and sooner in patients with decompensated disease so that effective therapy can be instituted before the varices grow in size and bleed.[13]

Patients with cirrhosis and variceal hemorrhage require resuscitation in an intensive care unit. However, overtransfusion should be avoided because it can precipitate rebleeding.[A5] Hemoglobin values should be maintained at about 8 g/dL. Prophylactic antibiotics should be used in this setting not only to prevent bacterial infections but also to decrease rebleeding and death.[A6] The recommended antibiotic is oral norfloxacin at a dose of 400 mg twice daily for 5 to 7 days, although intravenous ceftriaxone at a dose of 1 g/day for 5 to 7 days is preferable in patients with advanced liver disease (malnutrition, ascites, encephalopathy, and jaundice) or in those already receiving norfloxacin prophylaxis.[A7]

The most effective specific therapy for the control of active variceal hemorrhage is the combination of a vasoconstrictor with endoscopic therapy. Safe vasoconstrictors include terlipressin, somatostatin, and the somatostatin analogues octreotide and vapreotide[A8]; they can be initiated at admission to the hospital and continued for 2 to 5 days. The vasoconstrictor currently available in the United States is octreotide, which is used as a 50-μg intravenous bolus followed by an infusion at 50 μg/hour. The transjugular intrahepatic portosystemic shunt (TIPS) is generally recommended for patients who fail to respond to standard therapy (Fig. 153-7). In patients at high risk of failure, Child C (score 10-13) patients and Child B patients who have actively bleeding varices at endoscopy, preemptive TIPS placement (24 to 48 hours after admission) is associated with a reduced failure rate and a significant improvement in survival.[A9] Therefore, preemptive "early" TIPS should be considered in this high-risk subpopulation of patients with variceal hemorrhage. Even though patients with cirrhosis and coagulopathy (prolonged international normalized ratio or decreased platelet count) have a higher risk of not responding to hemostasis for variceal hemorrhage or bleeding from procedures (ligation, paracentesis, TIPS, surgery), neither recombinant factor VII nor eltrombopag has proved beneficial in randomized trials, and neither is recommended.

After control of hemorrhage, the 1-year recurrence of hemorrhage without treatment is high at about 60%. Therefore, therapy to prevent rebleeding should be instituted before the patient is discharged. The recommended therapy is combination of nonselective β-blockers (propranolol or nadolol), with or without isosorbide mononitrate, and endoscopic variceal ligation.[A10] The dose of β-blockers should be the maximal dose tolerated, and endoscopic variceal ligation should be repeated every 2 to 4 weeks until the varices are obliterated. Patients who had TIPS placed during the episode of acute variceal hemorrhage do not require β-blockers or ligation but do require periodic Doppler examination of the shunt to assess its patency.

Shunt therapy, either surgical or through radiologic placement of a TIPS, should be used in patients whose variceal bleeding has persisted

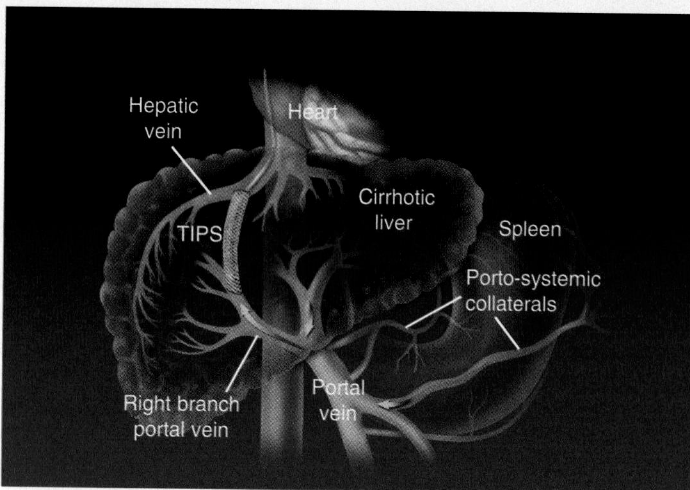

FIGURE 153-7. Transjugular intrahepatic portosystemic shunt (TIPS). This shunt is performed by interventional radiologists and consists of an expandable metal stent (most often coated with polytetrafluoroethylene) that connects a branch of the portal vein (high-pressure vein) to a branch of the hepatic vein (low-pressure vein). The shunt decompresses the portal system and portosystemic collaterals, and therefore it is used in the treatment of selected patients with cirrhosis and variceal hemorrhage. The shunt also decompresses the hepatic sinusoids and therefore is also used in the treatment of refractory ascites.

or recurred despite combined pharmacologic and endoscopic therapy. Both types of shunts are equally effective,A11 and the choice will depend on local expertise. Although the uncovered TIPS frequently occludes, newer polytetrafluoroethylene-covered stents are associated with lower occlusion rates and lower rates of hepatic encephalopathy.

Ascites

Salt restriction and diuretics constitute the mainstay of management of ascites. Dietary sodium intake should be restricted to 2 g/day. A more restrictive diet is not recommended and may compromise nutritional status.

Spironolactone, which is more effective than loop diuretics, should be started at a dose of 100 mg/day (once a day in the morning). The dose should be adjusted every 3 to 4 days to a maximal effective dose of 400 mg/day. Furosemide, at an escalated dose from 40 to 160 mg/day, can be started concurrently with spironolactone if ascites is tense or added subsequently if weight loss is inadequate or if hyperkalemia develops with spironolactone alone. The goal is weight loss of 1 kg in the first week and 2 kg/week subsequently. However, diuretics should be reduced if the rate of weight loss is more than 0.5 kg/day in patients without peripheral edema or more than 1 kg/day in patients with peripheral edema. Side effects of diuretic therapy include hypovolemic hyponatremia, hyperkalemia, renal dysfunction, encephalopathy, and, with spironolactone, painful gynecomastia.

In the 10 to 20% of patients with ascites who are refractory to diuretics, large-volume paracentesis, aimed at removal of all or most of the fluid, plus albumin at a dose of 6 to 8 g intravenously per liter of ascites removed, particularly when more than 5 L is removed at once, is a reasonable approach. The frequency of large-volume paracentesis is dictated by the rapidity at which the ascites reaccumulates. TIPS with uncovered stents is more effective than large-volume paracentesis plus albumin in preventing recurrent ascites but is associated with a higher rate of encephalopathy.A12 In patients requiring frequent large-volume paracentesis (more than twice per month), a polytetrafluoroethylene-covered TIPS should be considered. A peritoneovenous shunt, with use of a subcutaneously placed silicone tube that transfers ascites from the peritoneal cavity to the systemic circulation, can be used in patients who are not candidates for TIPS or liver transplantation. Automated flow pumps to move ascitic fluid to the bladder are under investigation.

Hyponatremia

Fluid restriction to 1.5 liters daily is recommended for severe hyponatremia (serum sodium concentration <130 mEq/L), but adherence with this recommendation is poor. Although V2-receptor antagonists such as tolvaptan are effective at increasing free water excretion and raising the serum sodium level in hyponatremic cirrhotic patients,A13 they have no overall effect on survival and are not approved for this use because of their hepatotoxicity. Because hyponatremia is a marker of neurologic dysfunction and increased mortality, short-term use of tolvaptan (15 mg/day, increased to 30 to 60 mg/day if needed) may be indicated only as a bridge to liver transplantation in patients in whom transplantation is imminent (Chapter 154).

Hepatorenal Syndrome

Because hepatorenal syndrome is a functional kidney injury that results from hemodynamic abnormalities secondary to end-stage liver disease and severe portal hypertension and is associated with a high mortality despite specific therapy, documented hepatorenal syndrome in the absence of prerenal azotemia or acute tubular necrosis is an indication for transplantation (Chapter 154). Specific therapies for hepatorenal syndrome that have been used to "bridge" a patient to transplantation include vasoconstrictors (terlipressin, norepinephrine, octreotide plus midodrine) plus albumin, TIPS, and extracorporeal albumin dialysis, which is an experimental hemofiltration dialysis method that uses an albumin dialysate. The largest experience is with the use of terlipressin, which at a dose 0.5 to 2.0 mg intravenously every 4 to 6 hours leads to a higher reversal rate of hepatorenal syndrome compared with placebo.A14 Because terlipressin is not yet available in the United States, the combination most used is octreotide (100 to 200 μg subcutaneously three times a day) plus midodrine (7.5 to 12.5 mg orally three times a day), with the dose adjusted to obtain an increase of at least 15 mm Hg in mean arterial pressure. Improvements may become clinically noticeable at day 7.

Spontaneous Bacterial Peritonitis

Empirical antibiotic therapy with an intravenous third-generation cephalosporin (e.g., cefotaxime, 2 g intravenously every 12 hours, or ceftriaxone, 2 g intravenously every 24 hours) should be initiated as soon as the diagnosis is established and before culture results are available; the minimal duration of therapy should be 5 days. Response to recommended empirical antibiotics is significantly lower in patients with health care–associated infections (i.e., infections that occur in patients who have been in a health care facility within the prior 3 months) and particularly low in nosocomial infections (i.e., infections that occur >48 hours after hospitalization)[14] because more infections are caused by multidrug-resistant organisms. In these settings, broader spectrum antibiotics (e.g., vancomycin-tazobactam, imipenem, ertapenem [Chapter 108]) should be given initially and then modified after culture results and antibiotic sensitivities are obtained. Aminoglycosides should be avoided because of the high incidence of renal toxicity in cirrhotic patients.

Repeated diagnostic paracentesis should be performed 2 days after antibiotics are started, by which time the number of PMN neutrophils in ascitic fluid should have decreased by more than 25% from baseline. Lack of response should prompt further investigations to exclude secondary peritonitis. The renal dysfunction associated with spontaneous bacterial peritonitis can be prevented by the intravenous administration of albumin, particularly in patients who have any evidence of renal dysfunction (blood urea nitrogen >30 mg/dL or creatinine >1 mg/dL, or both) or serum bilirubin concentration higher than 4 mg/dL at the time of diagnosis. Albumin has been used at a dose of 1.5 g per kilogram of body weight at diagnosis, repeated on the third day at an intravenous dose of 1 g per kilogram of body weight. However, this dosing is empirical and should not exceed 100 g per dose.

The administration of nonabsorbable (or poorly absorbable) antibiotics can prevent the development of spontaneous bacterial peritonitis and other infections in cirrhosis by selectively eliminating gram-negative organisms in the gut. However, the widespread use of prophylactic norfloxacin is associated with a higher rate of infections by antibiotic-resistant organisms. Long-term antibiotic prophylaxis with oral norfloxacin at a dose of 400 mg/day may be justified only in two groups: patients who have recovered from a previous episode of spontaneous bacterial peritonitis and patients who have an ascites protein level of less than 1 g/L with advanced liver and circulatory dysfunction as evidenced by the presence of jaundice, hyponatremia, or renal dysfunction.

Hepatic Encephalopathy

Treatment of overt hepatic encephalopathy starts by exclusion of alternative causes of altered mental status. Once the diagnosis of hepatic encephalopathy has been made, treatment involves identifying and treating the precipitating factor and reducing the ammonia level.[15] Precipitating factors include infections, overdiuresis, gastrointestinal bleeding, high oral protein load, and constipation. Narcotics and sedatives contribute to hepatic encephalopathy by directly depressing brain function. TIPS is a common precipitant of hepatic encephalopathy, and shunt reduction or occlusion may be required. Among agents aimed at decreasing ammonia production in the gut, lactulose (15 to 30 mL orally twice daily adjusted to obtain two or three soft bowel movements per day) has been the first choice for the treatment of episodic overt encephalopathy. Polyethylene glycol 3350-electrolyte solution (4 L orally or by nasogastric tube over 4 hours), however, may lead to a more rapid clinical response.A15 Other agents include orally administered nonabsorbable antibiotics, such as rifaximin (550 mg two times per day), neomycin (500 mg to 1 g three times per day), and metronidazole (250 mg two to four times per day). Drugs that may increase ammonia fixation in the liver, such as L-ornithine-L-aspartate, benzoate, and glycerol phenylbutyrate, are being studied.

Once an episode of overt encephalopathy has resolved, secondary prophylaxis with lactulose is recommended. If a precipitating factor has been identified and is well controlled or when liver function or nutritional status has improved, prophylactic therapy may be discontinued. In patients with recurrent encephalopathy, rifaximin together with lactulose is useful in preventing further recurrence.A16 Switching dietary protein from an animal source to a vegetable source may be beneficial in recurrent or persistent encephalopathy, but protein restriction is not necessary and should not be used long term.[16]

Pulmonary Complications

Hepatopulmonary syndrome rarely resolves spontaneously, and medical therapy is disappointing. TIPS is not generally recommended. The only viable treatment is liver transplantation (Chapter 154).

By comparison, liver transplantation is indicated only in a subset of patients with portopulmonary hypertension. In fact, a mean pulmonary arterial pressure higher than 45 mm Hg is an absolute contraindication to liver transplantation. The use of vasodilators should be considered in these patients (Chapter 68).

Surgical Therapy

Liver Transplantation

Orthotopic liver transplantation (Chapter 154), which is the definitive therapy for cirrhosis, is indicated when the risk for dying of liver disease is greater than the risk for dying of transplantation, as determined by a Child-Pugh score of 7 or higher (see Table 153-2) or a Model for End-Stage Liver Disease (MELD) score of 15 or higher. MELD (see Table 153-2), which is a mathematical model that estimates the risk for 3-month mortality, is used to determine the priority for liver transplantation (see E-Table 154-1). The number of available deceased donor organs is lower than the number of patients awaiting liver transplantation; as a result, 15 to 20% of patients awaiting liver transplantation in the United States die before an organ becomes available.

PRIMARY PREVENTION

Treatment of the underlying liver disease, before the development of cirrhosis, is a primary prevention strategy. Because the major causes of cirrhosis are related to lifestyle choices such as injection drug use (Chapter 34), alcohol consumption (Chapter 33), obesity, and unprotected sex, primary prevention programs that focus on encouraging alcohol abstinence, reducing high-risk behavior for hepatitis virus infection, weight reduction, and vaccination for hepatitis B are even better prevention strategies.

PROGNOSIS

The outcome of cirrhosis depends on the patient's stage. Patients with compensated cirrhosis die of liver disease only after transition to a decompensated stage. The 10-year survival rate of patients who remain in a compensated stage is approximately 90%, whereas their likelihood of decompensation is 50% at 10 years. Inception cohort studies of patients with compensated cirrhosis show a median survival of all patients, including those in whom decompensation develops over time, of about 10 years, whereas the median survival after decompensation is about 2 years. Survival is even lower in patients with refractory ascites, hyponatremia, or recurrent variceal hemorrhage and is lowest in patients who are hospitalized with an acute decompensating event, in whom 28-day mortality is about 30% and correlates with the number of organ failures present.[17] Hepatocellular carcinoma develops at a fairly constant rate of 3% per year and is associated with a worse outcome at whatever stage it develops.

Predictors of survival are different in compensated and decompensated patients. Parameters of portal hypertension (varices, splenomegaly, platelet count, γ-globulin) assume greater importance in compensated patients, whereas renal dysfunction, hemorrhage, and hepatocellular carcinoma are important predictive factors in patients with decompensated cirrhosis. In clinical practice, the Child-Pugh score is applicable to all cirrhotic patients, and the MELD score is used in decompensated patients to determine priority for liver transplantation.

Grade A References

A1. Marcellin P, Gane E, Buti M, et al. Regression of cirrhosis during treatment with tenofovir disoproxil fumarate for chronic hepatitis B: a 5-year open-label follow-up study. *Lancet*. 2013;381:468-475.

A2. Gluud LL, Krag A. Banding ligation versus beta-blockers for primary prevention in oesophageal varices in adults. *Cochrane Database Syst Rev*. 2012;8:CD004544.

A3. Tripathi D, Ferguson JW, Kochar N, et al. Randomized controlled trial of carvedilol versus variceal band ligation for the prevention of the first variceal bleed. *Hepatology*. 2009;50:825-833.

A4. Sinagra E, Perricone G, D'Amico M, et al. Systematic review with meta-analysis: the haemodynamic effects of carvedilol compared with propranolol for portal hypertension in cirrhosis. *Aliment Pharmacol Ther*. 2014;39:557-568.

A5. Villanueva C, Colomo A, Bosch A, et al. Transfusion strategies for acute upper gastrointestinal bleeding. *N Engl J Med*. 2013;368:11-21.

A6. Chavez-Tapia NC, Barrientos-Gutierrez T, Tellez-Avila F, et al. Meta-analysis: antibiotic prophylaxis for cirrhotic patients with upper gastrointestinal bleeding—an updated Cochrane review. *Aliment Pharmacol Ther*. 2011;34:509-518.

A7. Fernandez J, Ruiz del Arbol L, Gomez C, et al. Norfloxacin vs ceftriaxone in the prophylaxis of infections in patients with advanced cirrhosis and hemorrhage. *Gastroenterology*. 2006;131:1049-1056.

A8. Wells M, Chande N, Adams P, et al. Meta-analysis: vasoactive medications for the management of acute variceal bleeds. *Aliment Pharmacol Ther*. 2012;35:1267-1278.

A9. Garcia-Pagan JC, Caca K, Bureau C, et al. Early use of TIPS in patients with cirrhosis and variceal bleeding. *N Engl J Med*. 2010;362:2370-2379.

A10. Thiele M, Krag A, Rohde U, et al. Meta-analysis: banding ligation and medical interventions for the prevention of rebleeding from oesophageal varices. *Aliment Pharmacol Ther*. 2012;35:1155-1165.

A11. Henderson JM, Boyer TD, Kutner MH, et al. Distal splenorenal shunt versus transjugular intrahepatic portal systematic shunt for variceal bleeding: a randomized trial. *Gastroenterology*. 2006;130:1643-1651.

A12. Chen RP, Zhu Ge XJ, Huang ZM, et al. Prophylactic use of transjugular intrahepatic portosystemic shunt aids in the treatment of refractory ascites: metaregression and trial sequential meta-analysis. *J Clin Gastroenterol*. 2014;48:290-299.

A13. Dahl E, Gluud LL, Kimer N, et al. Meta-analysis: the safety and efficacy of vaptans (tolvaptan, satavaptan and lixivaptan) in cirrhosis with ascites or hyponatraemia. *Aliment Pharmacol Ther*. 2012;36:619-626.

A14. Gluud LL, Christensen K, Christensen E, et al. Systematic review of randomized trials on vasoconstrictor drugs for hepatorenal syndrome. *Hepatology*. 2010;51:576-584.

A15. Rahimi RS, Singal AG, Cuthbert JA, et al. Lactulose vs polyethylene glycol 3350-electrolyte solution for treatment of overt hepatic encephalopathy: the HELP randomized clinical trial. *JAMA Intern Med*. 2014;174:1727-1733.

A16. Bass NM, Mullen KD, Sanyal A, et al. Rifaximin treatment in hepatic encephalopathy. *N Engl J Med*. 2010;362:1071-1081.

GENERAL REFERENCES

For the General References and other additional features, please visit Expert Consult at https://expertconsult.inkling.com.

154

HEPATIC FAILURE AND LIVER TRANSPLANTATION

GREGORY T. EVERSON

In the United States, 130 programs perform about 6000 transplants per year, and about 17,000 patients are on waiting lists because recipients needing liver transplantation exceed the donor liver supply. The mortality rate while waiting on a list is 116 deaths per 1000 patient-years.

Since 1982, patient survival after liver transplantation has steadily increased by 20 to 30%, whether it is measured at 3 months, 1 year, 5 years, or 10 years, largely because of improvements within the first year after transplantation (Fig. 154-1). The positive shift in survival during the first 3 months after transplantation is related to improvements in surgical techniques and immediate postoperative care. By comparison, lack of further improvement beyond 3 months is because of long-term complications, such as recurrent hepatitis C (Chapter 149), recurrent autoimmune disease (Chapters 149 and 155), chronic allograft rejection, renal dysfunction (Chapter 130), hypertension (Chapter 67), and diabetes mellitus (Chapter 229). Further improvement in long-term survival after liver transplantation will require better management of these chronic complications.

GENERAL SELECTION CRITERIA

By far, the most common indication for liver transplantation is noncholestatic cirrhosis (Table 154-1). Livers may be donated from deceased donors (94%) or living donors (6%). Regardless of the type of transplantation, three fundamental questions must be addressed at the time of evaluation.[1]

1. Is liver transplantation indicated? The patient should have liver failure, complications of liver disease, or a metabolic condition that is best treated by liver transplantation and for which there are no alternative treatments.
2. Are there contraindications to transplantation (Table 154-2)? Comorbid conditions that could severely compromise graft or patient outcome must be identified.
3. Will the patient be able to tolerate and comply with immunosuppression and post-transplantation management? Inability to comply with the rigors of post-transplantation care and management could lead to graft loss and recipient death.

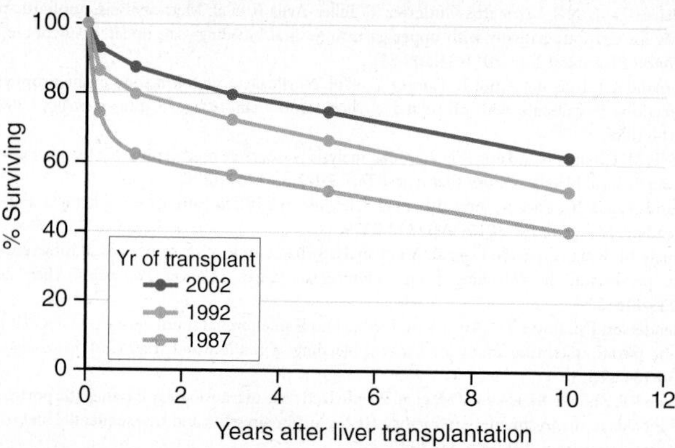

FIGURE 154-1. Survival of patients for three different years of transplantation, 1987, 1992, and 2002, by years after transplantation. The curves diverge early within the first year and then are nearly parallel, thereby suggesting that most of the improvement in survival is attributed to improvements in surgical techniques, intensive care unit management, and early post-transplantation care. Annual mortality rates between years 1 and 10 were 2.4% for the 1987 cohort, 3.1% for the 1992 cohort, and 2.8% for the 2002 cohort. (From Organ Procurement and Transplantation Network and Scientific Registry of Transplant Recipients. *OPTN/SRTR 2011 Annual Data Report*. Rockville, MD: Department of Health and Human Services, Health Resources and Services Administration, Healthcare Systems Bureau, Division of Transplantation; 2012).

TABLE 154-2 CONTRAINDICATIONS TO LIVER TRANSPLANTATION

Active substance abuse and inability to comply with rehabilitation
Inadequate social support, extreme psychosocial dysfunction, active psychosis, or other underlying psychosocial disease that makes it impossible for the patient to comply with peri-transplantation care and postoperative management
Unstable, active cardiopulmonary disease
- Symptomatic ischemic coronary disease not amenable to revascularization
- Severe pulmonary hypertension (mean PAP >45 mm Hg despite pharmacologic interventions)

Active, incurable extrahepatic malignant disease
- Metastatic nonhepatic malignant disease
- Hepatoma with macrovascular invasion, extrahepatic metastases, or exceeding Milan or UCSF criteria and not able to be downstaged
- Cholangiocarcinoma with percutaneous transperitoneal biopsy (likely seeding from the biopsy), tumor diameter >3 cm, or extrahepatic spread

Active, uncontrolled, and untreatable sepsis or other serious infectious disease
Active HIV infection with AIDS-defining illness, high-titer HIV RNA, very low CD4 count, or unresponsive to HAART
Anatomic anomaly or extensive vascular thromboses precluding hepatic transplantation

PAP = pulmonary artery pressure; UCSF = University of California, San Francisco; HIV = human immunodeficiency virus; AIDS = acquired immunodeficiency syndrome; HAART = highly active antiretroviral therapy.

TABLE 154-1 INDICATIONS FOR LIVER TRANSPLANTATION

CATEGORY	PERCENTAGE OF LISTED PATIENTS (TOTAL N = 15,748)	
Cirrhosis, non-cholestatic		72%
Hepatitis C	(27%)	
Alcoholic	(18%)	
Hepatitis C plus alcohol	(5%)	
Nonalcoholic steatohepatitis	(9%)	
Cryptogenic	(5%)	
Autoimmune	(4%)	
Hepatitis B	(3%)	
Other	(1%)	
Cholestatic liver disease		9%
Primary sclerosing cholangitis	(5%)	
Primary biliary cirrhosis	(3%)	
Other	(1%)	
Malignant neoplasms (primarily hepatocellular carcinoma)		7%
Acute liver failure		2%
Metabolic diseases		2%
Biliary atresia		1%
Other (e.g., Budd-Chiari syndrome) or unknown		8%

Based on Organ Procurement and Transplantation Network data as of May 30, 2014. http://optn.transplant.hrsa.gov/latestData/rptData.asp.

Medical Assessment

Certain components of the medical evaluation apply to all potential recipients. Viral serologies characterize the status of ongoing infection, prior exposure, or vaccination related to the hepatitis viruses (Chapters 148 and 149), Epstein-Barr virus (Chapter 377), cytomegalovirus (Chapter 376), and human immunodeficiency virus (HIV; Chapter 388). Colonoscopy is recommended for all patients older than 50 years to exclude colon cancer or polyps (Chapter 193) and in all patients with primary sclerosing cholangitis (Chapter 155) to detect inflammatory bowel disease (Chapter 141). Cardiopulmonary assessment (Chapters 51, 71, and 85) is performed in patients older than 50 years and in any patient with risk factors for coronary artery disease, such as hypertension, hypercholesterolemia, a significant family history, cigarette smoking, or diabetes. Cardiac catheterization (Chapter 57) is performed in patients with positive cardiac stress test results to confirm and to delineate the extent of coronary disease. Ultrasonography, computed tomography, and magnetic resonance imaging are useful to examine the biliary tract (Chapter 146), to exclude hepatocellular cancer (Chapter 196) or cholangiocarcinoma (Chapter 196), and to determine the patency of major vascular structures, such as the hepatic artery, celiac axis, splenic artery, portal vein, and superior mesenteric vein (Chapter 143).

The primary principle for consideration of liver transplantation is that a patient's predicted survival with transplantation must exceed expected survival without transplantation. For deceased donor liver transplantation, this principle is fulfilled by a Model for End-Stage Liver Disease (MELD) score of approximately 12 to 15 (see Table 153-2). In addition, certain complications of cirrhosis (Chapter 153), such as ascites, spontaneous bacterial peritonitis, encephalopathy, uncontrolled variceal hemorrhage, nutritional wasting, failure to thrive, and development of hepatoma (Chapter 196), shorten survival. Immediate evaluation and listing for transplantation are indicated for any patient with a MELD score of 15 or more or any of these complications.

Other complications that are not considered life-threatening may also be indications for consideration of liver transplantation. Examples include metabolic bone disease resulting in osteopenia and bone fractures (Chapters 243 and 244), inadequate nutrition, muscle wasting, severe fatigue, poor concentrating ability, and intractable pruritus.

Because the supply of donor livers is limited, transplant centers must select patients who have the greatest chance for a successful outcome. Elderly, obese, and deconditioned patients as well as patients with underlying vascular disease or long-standing diabetes mellitus are poor candidates for liver transplantation.

Surgical Assessment

The three phases of surgery are native liver dissection, the anhepatic phase, and revascularization of the graft. Native liver dissection, which is characterized by meticulous dissection and prompt control of bleeding vessels, can be complicated by morbid obesity, significant portal hypertension, portal thromboses, prior portosystemic shunt surgery, or prior abdominal surgery. The length of this phase is usually 1 to 2 hours, with blood losses ranging from 0 to 5 units of blood.

During the anhepatic phase, which usually lasts 1.5 to 3 hours and is associated with blood loss ranging from 0 to 5 units of blood, the vascular supply of the liver is completely interrupted, and the native liver is excised. Toward the end of the anhepatic phase, vessels are anastomosed, with the donor hepatic veins typically grafted to the recipient vena cava with only one caval anastomosis. Recipients with severe coagulopathy, cachexia, and nutritional deficiencies may be prone to excessive bleeding and metabolic complications.

When the venous clamps are removed, patients are at risk for primary fibrinolysis or consumptive coagulopathy. The arterial anastomosis is typically performed after unclamping to shorten the warm ischemia period.

Psychosocial Assessment

A patient referred for liver transplantation may have a history of alcohol, drug, or substance abuse. Psychosocial evaluation is important to help determine the risk of recidivism after transplantation. Today, nearly all transplant centers require a minimum 6-month period of documented abstinence and enrollment in education or rehabilitation programs. Social workers and psychiatrists may require the patient to undergo alcohol or drug treatment, counseling, and unannounced random screens for alcohol and drugs. Other key aspects of the psychosocial assessment include (1) evaluating the patient for any underlying psychiatric illness (Chapter 397), its severity, and how it should be managed; (2) defining and establishing social and psychological support for the potential recipient, including family, friends, and significant others; and (3) in living donor liver transplantation, evaluating the potential living donors.

Assigning Priority: Model for End-Stage Liver Disease

The prioritization of U.S. liver transplantation candidates and the allocation of deceased donor livers are based on the MELD score (see Table 153-2), which ranges from 6 (best prognosis) to 40 (worst prognosis). The 3-month mortality rate increases from 10% with a MELD score of 20 to 60% at a MELD score of 35, and essentially to 100% with a MELD score above 40. A patient's survival is not improved by deceased donor liver transplantation if the MELD score is below about 15. As a result, deceased donor livers must be made available more broadly if no local patient has a MELD score of 15 or higher and must be made available to local or regional patients with scores of 35 or higher. Patients with acute liver failure or post-transplantation patients with graft failure due to hepatic artery thrombosis have a MELD score of 40 and top priority status. This allocation system (E-Table 154-1) has improved transplantation rates and has not altered waiting list or post-transplantation mortality.

In patients with cirrhosis (Chapter 153), hyponatremia (Chapter 116) is associated with hepatorenal syndrome, ascites, and death from liver disease. Hyponatremia is an independent predictor of mortality up to a MELD score of 30. As a result, the MELD score is now adjusted for serum sodium concentration in allocating deceased donor livers.

The most common exception to liver allocation by MELD score is for hepatocellular carcinoma (Chapter 196) with a tumor diameter of more than 2 cm. Other exceptions can include patients with the hepatorenal syndrome (Chapter 153), the portopulmonary syndrome (Chapter 153), cholangiocarcinoma (Chapter 155), cystic fibrosis (Chapters 89 and 146), familial amyloid polyneuropathy (Chapter 188), and primary hyperoxaluria (Chapter 205) (E-Table 154-2).

DISEASE-SPECIFIC INDICATIONS FOR TRANSPLANTATION

Acute Liver Failure

Acute liver failure is defined as hepatic injury of fewer than 26 weeks in duration, an international normalized ratio of 1.5 or greater, and altered mental status in the absence of chronic liver disease except for Wilson disease (Chapter 211), vertically acquired hepatitis B, or autoimmune hepatitis (Chapter 149).[2] The main causes of acute liver failure in the United States are acetaminophen toxicity (Chapter 110), drug-induced liver injury (Chapter 150), viral hepatitis (Chapters 148 and 149), autoimmune hepatitis (Chapter 149), Wilson disease, mushroom poisoning (Chapters 110 and 150), acute hepatic ischemia (Chapter 143), Budd-Chiari syndrome, acute fatty liver of pregnancy (sometimes associated with the HELLP syndrome—hemolysis, elevated liver enzymes, low platelets; Chapters 160 and 239), and malignant infiltration of the liver (Chapter 196).

TREATMENT Rx

Patients with acute liver failure criteria should be transferred to the intensive care unit for enhanced monitoring, and a liver transplant center should be contacted for potential transfer of the patient. Specific treatments include *N*-acetylcysteine for acetaminophen hepatotoxicity (Chapters 110 and 150), *N*-acetylcysteine plus either silibinin or penicillin G for mushroom poisoning (Chapters 110 and 150), *N*-acetylcysteine and removal of the offending drug for drug-induced liver injury (Chapter 150), nucleos(t)ide analogues for hepatitis B (Chapters 148 and 149), acyclovir for herpes or varicella-zoster hepatitis (Chapters 374 and 375), dialysis and copper chelation for Wilson disease (Chapter 211), corticosteroids for autoimmune hepatitis (Chapter 149), delivery of the infant for acute fatty liver of pregnancy, and transjugular intrahepatic portosystemic shunting for the Budd-Chiari syndrome (Chapter 143). In addition, all causes of acute liver failure can cause a range of systemic complications.

A key issue in the general management of patients with acute liver failure is monitoring and treatment of encephalopathy. Progressive encephalopathy in acute liver failure is characteristically associated with cerebral edema and an elevated intracranial pressure (ICP). Elevated ICP is rare in patients with grade I (mild confusion) or grade II (agitated state) encephalopathy but occurs in 25 to 35% of patients with grade III encephalopathy (stuporous) and 65 to 75% of patients with grade IV (coma, but responsive to deep pain) encephalopathy. Irreversible brain injury is likely when the ICP is above 50 mm Hg and the cerebral perfusion pressure (mean arterial pressure minus ICP) is below 40 mm Hg for more than 2 hours. Liver transplantation may be contraindicated under these circumstances.

Because ammonia may play a role in the pathogenesis of cerebral edema, lactulose (20 g every 4 to 6 hours), rifaximin (550 mg twice daily), or both are recommended, especially for lower grades of encephalopathy. Patients with grade III/IV encephalopathy require intubation, mechanical ventilation, elevation of the head of the bed, sedation (e.g., propofol, initial dose of 0.005 mg/kg/minute IV, maintenance dose of 0.005 to 0.05 mg/kg/minute IV, which can be increased in increments of 0.005 mg/kg/minute every 5 minutes), and paralysis (cisatracurium, initial dose of 0.1 to 0.2 mg/kg IV, maintenance dose of 1 to 3 μg/kg/minute IV). Seizures (Chapter 403) should be treated with phenytoin (initial dose of 15 mg/kg IV, maintenance dose of 3 mg/kg every 12 hours IV), propofol (1 mg/kg IV loading dose, 3 to 7 mg/kg/hour IV maintenance), pentobarbital (13 mg/kg IV loading dose, 2 to 3 mg/kg/hour IV maintenance), or midazolam (0.2 mg/kg IV loading dose, 0.1 to 0.25 mg/kg/hour IV maintenance). Levetiracetam (500 [up to 1500] mg every 12 hours IV) may be used if renal function is preserved. Placement of an intracranial transducer for monitoring of ICP is desirable, but severe underlying coagulopathy may prohibit its placement. Elevated ICP may require treatment with mannitol (0.5 to 1.0 mg/kg every 4 to 6 hours IV), hypertonic saline (boluses every 2 to 4 hours of either 30 mL of 23.4% saline or 2 mL/kg of 7.5% saline), hyperventilation (target pH 7.45), pentobarbital (dose described before), and hypothermia (32° C to 34° C). The goal for these interventions is to maintain ICP below 20 mm Hg. Corticosteroids do not improve cerebral edema or lower ICP in acute liver failure,[3] and their use is not recommended.

Patients with acute liver failure are at increased risk for bacterial and fungal infections. Common infections include line sepsis, pneumonia (Chapter 97), and urinary tract infections (Chapter 284). Prolonged ventilation, dialysis, invasive procedures, and use of multiple antibiotics increase the risk for fungal infection (Chapter 282). Surveillance cultures of blood, urine, and sputum and periodic chest radiography are required every 2 days. Prophylactic antibiotic or antifungal therapy is not currently recommended.

In addition to an elevated international normalized ratio, many patients develop thrombocytopenia because of consumptive coagulopathy (Chapter 175). However, prophylactic use of transfusion of clotting factors or platelets should be restricted to the treatment of hemorrhage or in preparation for invasive procedures.

Patients with acute liver failure have a low systemic vascular resistance and a low mean arterial pressure. In patients with elevated ICP, the decrease in mean arterial pressure may further compromise cerebral perfusion pressure and blood flow. A goal of vasopressor therapy is to maintain cerebral perfusion pressure from 60 to 80 mm Hg. Treatment of hypotension to maintain a mean arterial pressure above 75 mm Hg may include dextrose-containing crystalloid, albumin, norepinephrine, and vasopressin (Chapter 106). Careful monitoring of volume status is critical, and care should be taken to avoid volume overload, which may worsen cerebral edema.

Acute renal failure (Chapter 120) is common in patients with acute liver failure, particularly when it is caused by acetaminophen, mushroom poisoning, or Wilson disease. Renal replacement therapy, when required, should be administered as continuous venovenous dialysis (Chapter 131). Intermittent modes of hemodialysis should be avoided because of their adverse hemodynamic effects.

In acute liver failure, hypoglycemia is a common complication that should be avoided and managed by continuous glucose infusions. Supplementation with phosphate, magnesium, and potassium (Chapter 117) may be required. Enteral feedings (Chapter 216) should be initiated early, and parenteral nutrition (Chapter 217) should be started if enteral feedings are contraindicated.

Selecting for Liver Transplantation

Clinical variables associated with reduced likelihood for spontaneous recovery include severe encephalopathy, advanced age, certain causes (hepatitis B, drug-induced hepatitis, sporadic non-A/non-B/non-C hepatitis, Wilson disease), long duration of jaundice, massive necrosis on liver biopsy, and markedly diminished liver volume on radiologic imaging. Transplant-free survival in patients with acute liver failure is approximately 50% for acetaminophen toxicity, hepatitis A, shock liver, and acute fatty liver of pregnancy/HELLP but less than 25% for all other causes.[4] Indications for listing for transplantation are based on the severity of disease but vary somewhat among countries (Table 154-3).[5]

TABLE 154-3 CRITERIA FOR SELECTION OF PATIENTS WITH ACUTE LIVER FAILURE FOR LIVER TRANSPLANTATION

KING'S COLLEGE, LONDON, UNITED KINGDOM
Acetaminophen toxicity
Acidosis (pH <7.3), or
INR >6.5 plus creatinine >3.4 mg/dL
Other causes of acute liver failure
INR >6.5, or
Any three of the following:
Age <10 years or >40 years
Non-A, non-B hepatitis or drug-induced disease
Duration of jaundice before encephalopathy >7 days
INR >3.5
Bilirubin >17.5 mg/dL
HÔPITAL PAUL-BROUSSE, VILLEJUIF, FRANCE
For all causes of acute liver failure:
Hepatic encephalopathy, and
Factor V <20% of normal in patient younger than 30 years or
Factor V <30% of normal in patient 30 years of age or older

INR = international normalized ratio.

Transplantation for acute liver failure accounts for less than 5% of all liver transplants. About 45% of patients with acute liver failure are listed for transplantation; about 10% die on the waiting list, about 5% improve without transplantation, and about 30% undergo liver transplantation. Overall 1- and 5-year survival rates after liver transplantation are 79% and 71%, respectively, but post-transplantation survival is better for patients with acute acetaminophen overdose and worse for patients with severe encephalopathy before transplantation. Living donor and auxiliary liver transplantation may be considered, but their use is controversial.

Chronic Liver Failure

Cirrhosis (Chapter 153) due to the hepatitis C virus (Chapter 149) is the most common indication for liver transplantation in the United States. Hepatitis C universally recurs in the liver allograft of recipients who are viremic at the time of liver transplantation and is associated with early graft loss and death of the patient. Pretransplantation treatment (Chapter 149) with an interferon-free, pangenotypic regimen of sofosbuvir (400 mg daily) plus weight-based ribavirin (1.0 to 1.2 g/day) for 48 weeks eliminates detectable hepatitis C virus RNA in nearly all patients within 4 weeks, and patients with undetectable hepatitis C virus RNA for 30 days or more before transplantation have only about a 4% risk of becoming viremic after transplantation.[6] A similar regimen given for 24 weeks after transplantation can achieve a sustained virologic response in about 70% of recipients with hepatitis C virus genotype I infection.[7] The combination of ledipasvir, sofosbuvir, and ribavirin yields sustained virologic response rates of approximately 90% in patients with decompensated cirrhosis and in transplant recipients with recurrent hepatitis C and advanced fibrosis or cirrhosis.

Alcoholic cirrhosis (Chapter 152) is a major albeit controversial indication for liver transplantation because many patients who totally abstain from alcohol may recover to the point that transplantation is no longer indicated.[8] Candidates for transplantation must typically adhere to at least 6 months of rehabilitation and document abstinence from alcohol by testing of urine or blood. Risk factors for noncompliance and return to alcohol use include polysubstance abuse, poor social support, joblessness, and underlying psychiatric illness. However, properly selected and compliant patients have excellent post-transplantation outcomes, even though 8 to 33% return to some degree of drinking. The 1-, 3-, and 5-year patient survival rates range from 81 to 92%, 78 to 86%, and 73 to 86%, respectively.

Transplantation for alcoholic hepatitis is even more controversial. One nonrandomized study from seven French liver transplant units suggested that carefully selected patients with severe alcoholic hepatitis could substantially benefit from liver transplantation, with a 2-year survival of 77% with transplantation compared with 23% without it.[9] It is not known whether this experience can be duplicated in other centers or countries, and alcoholic hepatitis currently is considered a relative contraindication to liver transplantation in most U.S. centers.

Patients with hepatocellular carcinoma (Chapter 196) are candidates for liver transplantation unless they have large tumors, multicentric tumors, macrovascular invasion, or extrahepatic spread. The Milan criteria recommend transplantation for a single hepatocellular carcinoma less than 5 cm in diameter or up to three hepatocellular carcinomas with no single lesion more than 3 cm in diameter. The post-transplantation survival of patients satisfying these Milan criteria is similar to that of patients transplanted for other indications. The University of California, San Francisco (UCSF) criteria recommend transplantation for a single tumor less than 6.5 cm in diameter or up to five tumors with total cumulative diameter of less than 8.5 cm. Patients who are "downstaged" by transarterial chemoembolization or other locoregional treatments from UCSF to Milan criteria have a post-transplantation outcome similar to that of patients who initially met Milan criteria.

The rare fibrolamellar variant of hepatocellular carcinoma constitutes only 0.85% of all cases of primary liver cancer. Compared with patients with typical hepatocellular carcinoma, patients with fibrolamellar carcinoma are younger (mean age, 39 years vs. 65 years) and more likely to be female (52% vs. 26%) and white (85% vs. 57%). Fibrolamellar carcinoma is characterized by broad bands of fibrosis, no association with cirrhosis, slow growth, and easier resection. Although post-transplantation recurrence rates of fibrolamellar carcinoma are similar to those for standard hepatocellular carcinoma, 5-year survival is higher in patients with fibrolamellar carcinoma.

Cholangiocarcinoma (Chapter 196), in the absence of underlying liver or biliary disease, typically is manifested in elderly patients with significant comorbidities and is not an indication for liver transplantation. By contrast, cholangiocarcinoma arising in younger patients with underlying biliary disease, such as primary sclerosing cholangitis (Chapter 155), may be considered for transplantation if staging is negative for vascular, lymphatic, or neural invasion. The 2- and 5-year post-transplantation survivals of patients with cholangiocarcinoma limited to the perihilar region of the liver and treated with adjuvant chemoradiation are 78% and 65%, respectively.[10] Factors associated with early recurrence and diminished survival are tumor diameter of more than 3 cm, performance of a percutaneous transperitoneal biopsy of the tumor, metastatic disease at time of surgery, and history of a prior malignant neoplasm.

Rare Primary Hepatic Malignant Neoplasms

Other primary hepatic malignant neoplasms—epithelioid hemangioendotheliomas, hemangiosarcomas, and hepatoblastomas—represent less than 10% of all tumors undergoing transplantation. Epithelioid hemangioendothelioma is generally thought to be indolent in nature, and reported post-transplantation survivals have been favorable. By contrast, hemangiosarcoma universally recurs, so transplantation is contraindicated.

In patients with liver metastases from primary endocrine tumors, such as carcinoid tumor (Chapter 232), gastrinoma, insulinoma, glucagonoma, and VIPoma (Chapters 195 and 230), liver transplantation is best restricted to those with metastases that are confined to the liver and are unresponsive to chemotherapy, local ablative therapies, surgical resection, and hormonal therapy.[11] Even in highly selected patients, tumor recurrence is the rule, with a 5-year post-transplantation patient survival of 52% but a disease-free 5-year survival of only 30%.

With the advent of effective antiviral regimens,[A1] the post-transplantation outcomes for patients transplanted for hepatitis B (Chapter 149) are now among the best for any indication,[12] with a 3-year survival of 87%. In the United States, potential recipients are treated before transplantation with either tenofovir or entecavir monotherapy, which is continued indefinitely in the post-transplantation period.

Nonalcoholic steatohepatitis (Chapter 152) has become an increasing indication for liver transplantation.[13] The likelihood of 1-, 3-, and 5-year survival is similar to that of other recipients because their higher risk for post-transplantation cardiovascular death is offset by a lower risk of graft failure.

For primary biliary cirrhosis (Chapter 153), the mean survival for patients with a serum bilirubin level above 10 mg/dL is only 1.4 years. By comparison, actuarial survival for patients undergoing liver transplantation is 83%, 78%, and 67% at 1 year, 5 years, and 10 years, respectively.[14] Although primary biliary cirrhosis may recur in the allograft, recurrence rarely leads to graft failure, retransplantation, or the patient's death.

Among patients with primary sclerosing cholangitis (Chapter 155), the 1-, 2-, 5-, and 10-year actuarial survival rates after liver transplantation are 94%, 92%, 86%, and 70%, respectively. Primary sclerosing cholangitis recurs after transplantation at a rate of approximately 4% per year, and recurrent primary sclerosing cholangitis occasionally may progress and require retransplantation.

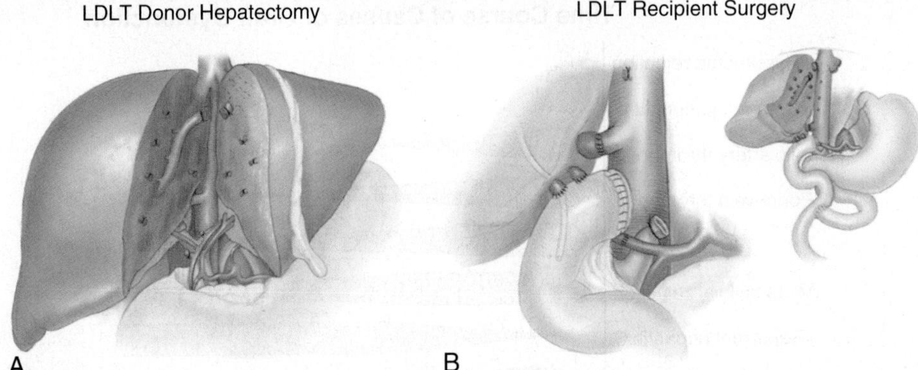

FIGURE 154-2. Living related donor hepatectomy (A) and orthotopic implantation of the right lobe graft (B). LDLT = living donor liver transplantation.

Up to 30% of patients with primary sclerosing cholangitis will develop cholangiocarcinoma, which diffusely infiltrates bile ducts, liver parenchyma, neural elements, lymphatic vessels, and surrounding tissues. Cholangiocarcinoma complicating primary sclerosing cholangitis, either before or after transplantation, reduces survival,[15] although the outcome is excellent if the cholangiocarcinoma is detected during surveillance imaging, treated with adjuvant chemoradiation, and then removed with the explant during transplantation.

In patients with autoimmune hepatitis (Chapter 149), 1-year patient survival rates after liver transplantation range from 83 to 92%, with an estimated 10-year survival of 75%. Recurrence is observed in 17% of patients after 4.6 ± 1 years, and an occasional patient with recurrent autoimmune hepatitis will require retransplantation.

For hemochromatosis (Chapter 212), liver transplantation now yields 1-, 3-, and 5-year survival rates similar to the survivals of all other transplant recipients. Patients with hemochromatosis who are considered for liver transplantation should undergo screening for hepatocellular carcinoma and also have a complete cardiologic evaluation. It is uncertain whether pretransplantation phlebotomy improves survival.

Patients with either the ZZ (n = 50) or SZ (n = 23) α_1-antitrypsin deficiency (Chapter 146) have excellent outcomes after liver transplantation.[16] Pulmonary evaluation is critical because one third of adults transplanted for α_1-antitrypsin deficiency will have significant underlying obstructive respiratory disease, which typically stabilizes and then improves after liver transplantation but sometimes may progress despite it.

In patients with polycystic liver disease, liver transplantation is rarely indicated but is highly successful in relieving symptoms of abdominal fullness, early satiety, and related complaints. The post-transplantation outcome is better for patients with isolated polycystic liver disease compared with polycystic liver in the setting of polycystic kidney disease (Chapter 127),[17] thereby highlighting the higher morbidity and mortality associated with cystic renal disease.

In patients with primary hyperoxaluria,[18] which is inherited as an autosomal dominant trait, liver transplantation is required to remove the source for the overproduction of oxalate and to halt the progression of renal disease. For patients with familial amyloid polyneuropathy, which is an inherited and fatal systemic amyloidosis that is caused by a point mutation in the transthyretin gene, liver transplantation halts the production of the amyloidogenic variant transthyretin, halts the progression of the disease, and significantly improves survival.[19]

An increasing number of HIV-infected patients are being considered for liver transplantation, primarily because of coinfection with hepatitis C virus.[20] Selection criteria include the absence of AIDS or AIDS-defining illness, adequate CD4 counts, low HIV levels, and lack of resistance to highly active antiretroviral therapies. The overall patient survival at 3 years after transplantation is 60% for HIV/hepatitis C virus coinfection, compared with 79% for hepatitis C virus monoinfection.

RISK FACTORS FOR POOR OUTCOME AFTER LIVER TRANSPLANTATION

Patients older than 60 years have about a 10% lower survival because of infection, cardiac complications, neurologic disease, and malignant disease. Survival is also lower in patients with ischemic heart disease, diabetes, persistent smoking, or chronic obstructive pulmonary disease, although patients who undergo liver transplantation for α_1-antitrypsin deficiency may show improvement in their pulmonary function test results.

LIVING DONOR LIVER TRANSPLANTATION IN ADULTS

Living donor liver transplantation is an option to expedite transplantation for adult patients with end-stage liver disease. Living donor liver transplantation already is the most common form of liver transplantation in Asia, where cultural barriers have limited liver donation from deceased donors, but it represents only 5% of all adult liver transplants in the United States. In adults, either the left or right lobe may be used, but most U.S. experts prefer the right hepatic lobe. In this procedure, the entire native liver of the recipient is removed and replaced with the right lobe of the liver from a living donor (Fig. 154-2).

The major clinical advantage of living donor liver transplantation is a reduction in recipient mortality, largely related to a reduction in pretransplantation mortality among patients who otherwise would languish on a waiting list. By comparison, both short-term and long-term survival after transplantation is nearly identical with living donor liver transplantation and deceased donor liver transplantation.[21]

The major disadvantage of living donor liver transplantation is donor safety. Most donors undergo successful right hepatectomy uneventfully, but significant complications, such as bile leakage and infection, occur in 10 to 20% of patients, and the death rate among living donors is 0.2%.[22] In the majority of donors, the quality of life returns to baseline by 6 months, although mild abdominal complaints and pain are common. More than 90% of donor-recipient pairs report that they have returned to their original predonation relationships at 1 year.

RECIPIENT OUTCOMES AFTER LIVER TRANSPLANTATION

Recipients of either deceased donor liver transplantation or living donor liver transplantation may encounter a number of complications that occur at different times after transplantation (Fig. 154-3).[23] Graft injury within the first 3 days is most often due to either primary nonfunction or hepatic artery thrombosis. Less common causes of graft dysfunction during this period include hyperacute rejection, portal vein thrombosis, and obstruction of the inferior vena cava. Between 3 and 14 days, graft dysfunction is most commonly related to acute cellular rejection, recurrent hepatitis C infection, hepatic artery thrombosis, or biliary leak or cholangitis. Infrequent causes of dysfunction during this period are portal vein thrombosis, drug hepatotoxicity, and functional cholestasis. From 14 days to 3 months, the most common causes of graft dysfunction include allograft rejection, recurrent hepatitis C infection, biliary complications, cytomegalovirus hepatitis, and drug hepatotoxicity. Vascular thromboses rarely are manifested after the first 3 months, and hepatitis B recurrence (in untreated patients) is typically delayed beyond 1 month.

The most severe form of early graft dysfunction is primary nonfunction, which is characterized by acute liver failure (encephalopathy, ascites, coagulopathy, unstable hemodynamics), elevated liver enzymes, and development of multiorgan failure (renal failure and pulmonary complications). Primary nonfunction is encountered in only 1% of recipients after living donor liver transplantation, because the graft is implanted quickly after it has been removed from the donor, but in 7 to 8.5% of recipients after deceased donor liver transplantation. Anywhere from 20 to 45% of recipients experience

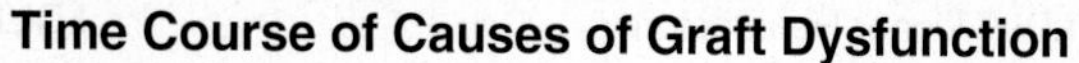

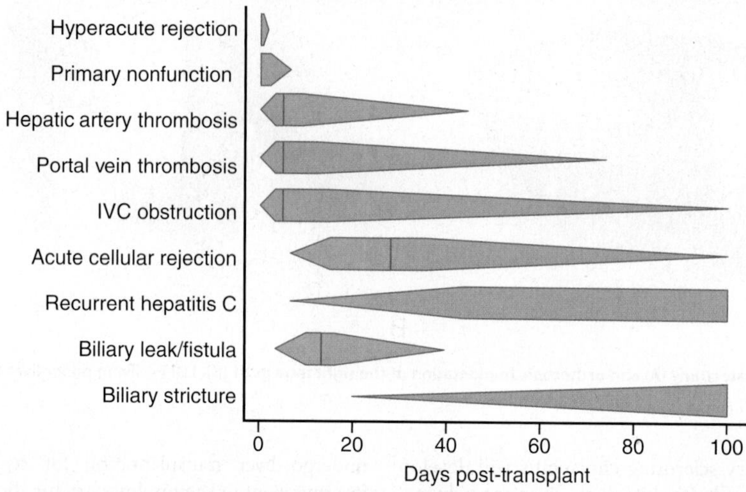

FIGURE 154-3. **The time course of graft dysfunction varies by etiology. Hyperacute rejection is rare (ABO incompatibility) but occurs within the first few hours to days. Primary nonfunction, vascular thrombosis, and biliary leaks are early events, and acute rejection episodes begin after the first 7 days. Recurrent hepatitis C may begin early but typically is manifested after the first 2 or 3 weeks after transplantation. Biliary strictures evolve more slowly and tend to be later events. IVC = inferior vena cava.**

Acute Allograft Rejection

Bile Duct Injury

Endothelialitis

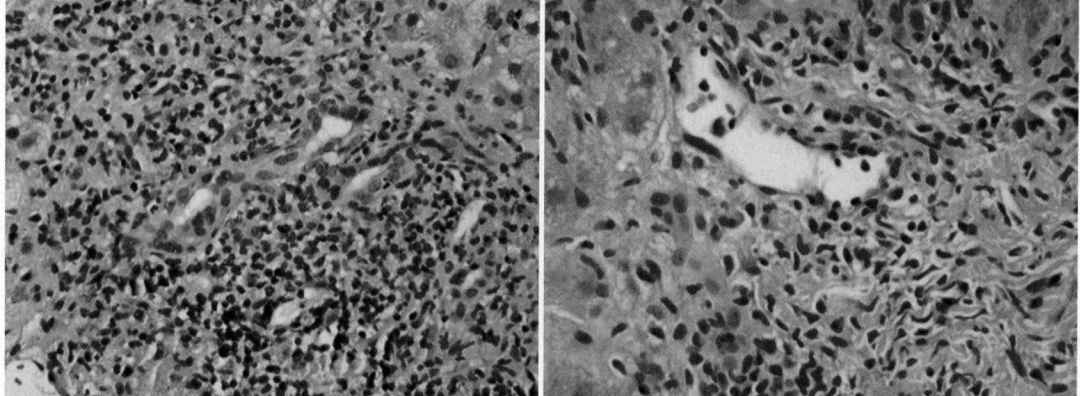

FIGURE 154-4. **Liver histology of acute allograft rejection (hematoxylin and eosin stain). The immune inflammatory response is centered around the portal triad, and the typical features include a mixed cellular infiltrate (eosinophils, neutrophils, plasma cells, lymphocytes), lymphocytic cholangitis, and endothelialitis.**

postoperative bleeding, including 5 to 15% who will need reoperation for bleeding. Hemorrhage is second only to infection as a cause of death.

Hepatic artery thrombosis, which complicates 3 to 10% of adult liver transplants, is one of the leading causes of graft failure in the immediate postoperative period. It is manifested as fever, bacteremia from a biliary source, and sudden elevations in liver enzymes. The preferred initial investigation of the hepatic artery is Doppler ultrasonography, followed by angiography if positive. In general, emergent revascularization is required for graft survival.

Portal Vein Thrombosis

Portal venous thrombosis, which is less common than hepatic arterial thrombosis, is manifested as hepatic failure and portal hypertension. Portal hypertension may be treated by radiologic thrombectomy, lytic therapy, stenting of underlying portal vein stenosis, or decompressive shunt surgery, but patients with significant hepatic dysfunction should be considered for revascularization or retransplantation.

Hepatic venous outflow obstruction may be manifested clinically by hepatic dysfunction, coagulopathy, and jaundice or even by hepatomegaly and ascites. Chronic outflow obstruction with preservation of graft function may be managed conservatively with diuretic therapy, radiologic evaluation of venous anastomoses, and angioplasty or stenting of outflow stenosis, but acute outflow obstruction can be a graft- and life-threatening condition that may require emergent revision of the outflow anastomosis.

Biliary tract complications, leaks, and strictures occur after approximately 5 to 30% of all liver transplants, usually within the first 3 months. Biliary scintigraphy can be diagnostic for large bile leaks, but cholangiography may be required for small, contained leaks. Anastomotic biliary strictures are focal and localized to the choledochocholedochostomy or choledochoenterostomy, whereas ischemic strictures are multiple and diffuse. Patients may present with jaundice, cholangitis, or asymptomatic elevations in liver test results. Choledocholithiasis may complicate strictures. Cholangiography is the "gold standard" for the diagnosis of biliary strictures as well as for their management with dilation and stenting. Surgical revision is reserved for patients in whom these procedures are unsuccessful, but diffuse ischemia strictures may necessitate retransplantation.

Rejection, which occurs in about 15 to 30% of liver transplants, usually is initially seen as an acute rejection within the first 30 days. Any acute rejection occurring beyond 30 days should raise the suspicion of subtherapeutic levels of immunosuppressive medications, drug interactions affecting immunosuppressant levels, or noncompliance of the patient with the medical regimen. Most patients are asymptomatic, although fever, malaise, abdominal pain, and worsening of portal hypertension with associated clinical manifestations can occur. Liver biopsy is essential for diagnosis. The classic findings are a mixed inflammatory infiltrate of lymphocytes, plasma cells, eosinophils, and neutrophils and nonsuppurative destructive cholangitis and endothelialitis (Fig. 154-4). Treatment consists of pulse doses of methylprednisolone (1 g IV daily for 1 to 3 days) and a taper of oral prednisone. Patients who fail to respond to corticosteroid treatment may be rescued by anti–T-cell therapy, such as thymoglobulin. In some cases in which the acute rejection may be mediated by B cells, plasmapheresis and anti–B-cell treatment (e.g., rituximab, 100 to 375 mg/m^2 weekly for two or three doses) may be required. Graft loss due to acute rejection is rare.

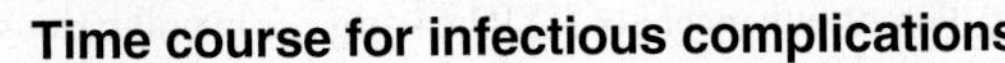

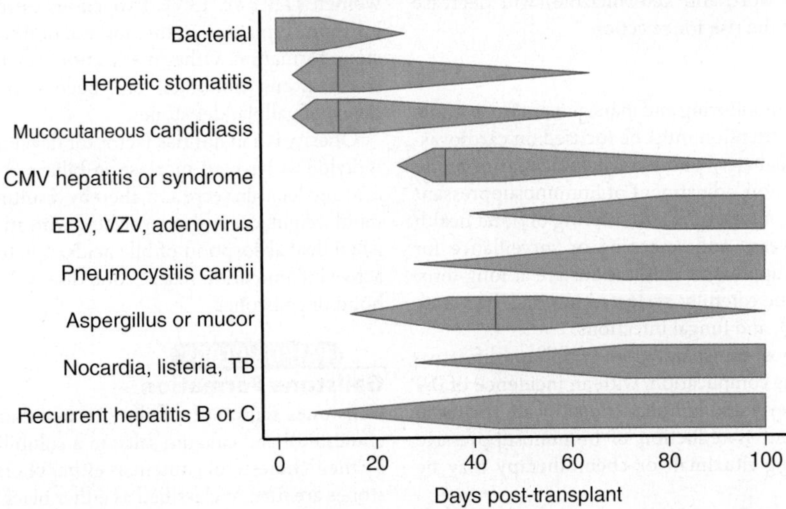

FIGURE 154-5. **The time course of infectious complications varies by type of infection. Bacterial and mucocutaneous viral or candidal infections occur early, and most of the others occur after the first 2 or 3 weeks after transplantation. CMV = cytomegalovirus; EBV = Epstein-Barr virus; VZV = varicella-zoster virus; TB = tuberculosis.**

Chronic allograft rejection occurs in 2 to 3% of liver transplants. Patients may be asymptomatic early in the course or present with jaundice or pruritus later in the course. Laboratory test results reveal elevated cholestatic liver enzymes, such as alkaline phosphatase or γ-glutamyltransferase, and bilirubin. Liver biopsy reveals paucity of inflammation, portal fibrosis, and loss of intralobular and interlobular bile ducts. Chronic rejection is poorly responsive to immunosuppressive therapy and often progresses to graft loss, need for retransplantation, and ultimately death.

Infections

Most infectious complications of liver transplantation occur within the first 3 months of transplantation (Fig. 154-5).[24] Bacterial and mucocutaneous herpetic (Chapter 374) or candidal (Chapter 338) infections dominate the immediate post-transplantation period. Other viral infections (such as cytomegalovirus [Chapter 376], Epstein-Barr virus [Chapter 377], varicella-zoster [Chapter 375], and adenovirus [Chapter 365]), *Pneumocystis jiroveci* infection (Chapter 341), or fungal infections tend to occur or to activate after the first 30 days. Hepatitis C replication begins immediately after transplantation in patients who are viremic at the time of transplantation, and recurrent hepatitis can occur as early as 7 days but more typically occurs after 30 days. Current strategies with nucleos(t)ides and hepatitis B immune globulin (Chapters 148 and 149) have essentially eliminated recurrent hepatitis B.

Approximately 80 to 90% of adults undergoing liver transplantation have serologic evidence of prior exposure to cytomegalovirus. Recipients who have positive cytomegalovirus serology or who receive a liver from a cytomegalovirus-positive donor are at risk for either cytomegalovirus syndrome (influenza-like illness) or cytomegalovirus hepatitis. Cytomegalovirus hepatitis requires liver biopsy for diagnosis (E-Fig. 154-1). The greatest risk is in a cytomegalovirus-negative recipient who receives a liver from a cytomegalovirus-positive donor (~60% risk for cytomegalovirus disease). Prophylaxis with oral valganciclovir (900 mg orally daily) during the first 90 days after transplantation effectively reduces risk for cytomegalovirus disease.

Immunosuppressive Medications

Immunosuppressive medications are managed by experts at the patient's liver transplant center. The primary care provider, however, should be aware of the typical maintenance immunosuppressive drugs, how they are monitored, and some of the common toxicities (Table 154-4). The backbone of most maintenance immunosuppressive regimens is an inhibitor of either calcineurin (cyclosporine and tacrolimus) or mTOR (sirolimus and everolimus). These immunosuppressants are metabolized through the hepatic enzyme CYP3A4, which is a pathway for the metabolism of about 60% of commonly prescribed medications. Coadministration of potent inhibitors of CYP3A4 (e.g., ritonavir, erythromycin, telaprevir, and boceprevir) with cyclosporine, tacrolimus, sirolimus, or everolimus will increase the plasma concentrations of the latter

TABLE 154-4 IMMUNOSUPPRESSIVE MEDICATIONS: MONITORING AND ADVERSE SIDE EFFECTS

TYPE	DOSE	MONITORING	ADVERSE EFFECTS
Cyclosporine[a]	100-200 mg bid	Blood level[b]	Nephrotoxicity[c] Neurotoxicity[d] Hypertension
Tacrolimus[e]	1-2 mg bid	Blood level[b]	Nephrotoxicity Neurotoxicity Diabetes mellitus[f]
Prednisone	5-20 mg qd	Clinical	Hypertension Diabetes mellitus[f] Neurotoxicity Fluid retention
Azathioprine	50-200 mg qd	CBC	Neutropenia Thrombocytopenia Anemia
Mycophenolate[g]	500-1500 mg bid	CBC	Neutropenia Dose-related increase in risk of HSV, CMV[h] Gastrointestinal symptoms
Sirolimus[i]	1-3 mg qd	Blood level	Neutropenia Thrombocytopenia Hyperlipidemia Vascular thrombosis
Everolimus[i]	1-2 mg bid	Blood level	Neutropenia Thrombocytopenia Hyperlipidemia

[a]Several different forms of cyclosporine are available. Additional adverse effects of long-term use of cyclosporine include hirsutism, gingival hyperplasia, and dyslipidemia.
[b]Dosages of cyclosporine and tacrolimus are adjusted primarily from trough plasma levels. There are different methods for measuring cyclosporine and tacrolimus levels. The therapeutic range will differ by the method used and whether whole blood or plasma is assayed.
[c]Nephrotoxicity is related to doses and plasma concentrations of cyclosporine or tacrolimus.
[d]Neurotoxicity includes paresthesias, neuropathy, and seizures. Neurotoxicity may be more common with tacrolimus than with cyclosporine.
[e]Several different forms of tacrolimus are available. Additional adverse effects of long-term use of tacrolimus include hirsutism, gingival hyperplasia, and dyslipidemia.
[f]Diabetes mellitus incidence is reduced by steroid withdrawal. Monotherapy with tacrolimus is more often associated with diabetes than is monotherapy with cyclosporine.
[g]Mycophenolate mofetil and mycophenolic acid are inhibitors of inosine 5′-monophosphate dehydrogenase and used as steroid-sparing or calcineurin inhibitor–sparing agents.
[h]Risk of CMV infection under mycophenolate immunosuppression is dose related, with greatest risk at doses of 3 g/day or more.
[i]Sirolimus and everolimus are inhibitors of mTOR, the mammalian target of rapamycin.
CBC = complete blood count; HSV = herpes simplex virus; CMV = cytomegalovirus.

drugs and increase the risk for toxicity. Potent enhancers of CYP3A4 (e.g., rifampin, phenobarbital, St. John's wort, and ketoconazole) will decrease plasma concentrations and increase the risk for rejection.

General Management Issues

The liver recipient requires ongoing monitoring and management to promote overall health and wellness. Special attention must be focused on cardiovascular risk factors (hypertension, diabetes, obesity, dyslipidemia, cigarette smoking), monitoring of renal function, adjustment of immunosuppressant medications, attention to drug-drug interactions, monitoring of bone health with bone densitometry every 2 years, and screening or surveillance for cancer. Patients receiving immunosuppressive medications are at long-term risk for infection, and fever should be carefully evaluated for viral, bacterial, atypical bacterial (e.g., tuberculosis), and fungal infections.

Epstein-Barr virus–associated post-transplantation lymphoproliferative disease is an uncommon but serious complication, with an incidence of 0.9 to 2.9% (Chapters 185 and 377). Fever and lymphadenopathy are the usual presenting findings. Initial treatment is reduction of immunosuppressive drugs, but other therapies including rituximab or chemotherapy may be required (Chapter 185).

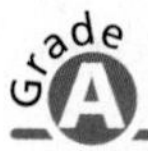

Grade A Reference

A1. Teperman LW, Poordad F, Bzowej N, et al. Randomized trial of emtricitabine/tenofovir disoproxil fumarate after hepatitis B immunoglobulin withdrawal after liver transplantation. *Liver Transpl.* 2013;19:594-601.

GENERAL REFERENCES

For the General References and other additional features, please visit Expert Consult at https://expertconsult.inkling.com.

155

DISEASES OF THE GALLBLADDER AND BILE DUCTS

EVAN L. FOGEL AND STUART SHERMAN

GALLBLADDER

Gallstones

EPIDEMIOLOGY

Gallstone disease is one of the most common and costly digestive diseases, with an estimated annual direct cost of $15 billion in the United States. Newly diagnosed gallstone disease occurs in more than one million people annually in the United States, and more than 750,000 cholecystectomies are now performed annually. The prevalence of gallstones is about 10 to 15% in American and European adults, with women affected about twice as often as men. Cholesterol gallstones are uncommon in individuals younger than 20 years, but a sharp increase is noted with each decade up to approximately the age of 70 years, particularly in women. About 20% of women and 10% of men have gallstones by 60 years of age. Together, approximately 12% of Americans or 36 million men and women harbor gallstones.

In the United States, the prevalence of stones is highest in Mexican American women (26%), followed by white women (17%) and African American women (14%). The prevalence of gallstones is extremely high in Native Americans, especially in women. In Chileans and Bolivians of Indian ancestry, gallstones are also common, and gallstone-associated cancer is the most common gastrointestinal cancer in these countries.

Environmental factors and genetic predisposition are likely to play an interactive role for gallstone formation. Pregnancy may contribute to the predominance of cholesterol stones in younger women as it is associated with progesterone-induced impaired gallbladder emptying and estrogen-mediated increased cholesterol saturation of bile. The prevalence of gallbladder stones in nulliparous women is approximately one tenth of that noted in multiparous women (1.3% vs. 13%). Exogenous estrogen administration in the form of hormone replacement therapy and oral contraceptives is also associated with stone formation. Other medications, including somatostatin analogues, ceftriaxone, and clofibrate, have been associated also with an increased incidence of gallbladder stones.

Obesity is a major risk factor for development of cholesterol stones. Obese individuals have an increase in biliary cholesterol secretion relative to bile acid and lecithin secretion, thereby resulting in bile supersaturation. However, rapid weight loss is also associated with an increased risk of gallstones. Diminished ileal absorption of bile acids, due to surgical resection or bypass or to active inflammation (e.g., Crohn disease), may also lead to an increased likelihood of gallstones.

PATHOBIOLOGY

Gallstone Formation

Gallstones represent a failure to maintain certain biliary solutes, primarily cholesterol and calcium salts, in a solubilized state. Gallstones are classified by their cholesterol content as either cholesterol or pigment stones. Pigment stones are further classified as either black or brown. Most cholesterol stones contain calcium salts in their core, and pure cholesterol gallstones are uncommon (10%). In most American populations, 70 to 80% of gallstones are cholesterol, and black pigment stones account for most of the remaining 20 to 30%.

In normal bile, cholesterol is soluble in the form of mixed micelles with optimal concentration of bile salts and phospholipids. With disproportionate concentrations, bile becomes supersaturated, and the excess cholesterol precipitates as monohydrate crystals. These crystals become embedded in gallbladder mucin gel with bilirubinate to form biliary sludge, which may eventually aggregate into a gallbladder stone.

Black pigment stones make up a small proportion of gallstones. These stones consist of polymerized calcium bilirubinate, precipitated as a result of exceeding the solubility of calcium and unconjugated bilirubin. In addition to increasing age, the formation of black pigment stones is more common in individuals who have conditions that create an excessive amount of unconjugated bilirubin (e.g., chronic hemolysis in hemoglobinopathies, cirrhosis, ineffective erythropoiesis), who are being fed by total parenteral nutrition (Chapter 217), or who have ileal diseases. Black pigment stones are typically tarry, are usually not associated with infected bile, and are located almost exclusively in the gallbladder.

By contrast, brown pigment stones are coarse in texture and are primarily formed in the bile duct as a result of bacterial infection that releases β-glucuronidase to hydrolyze glucuronic acid from bilirubin. Phospholipid hydrolysis also increases, thereby leading to precipitation of calcium, bilirubin, and free fatty acids and also resulting in the formation of brown pigment stones. Brown pigment stones account for 30 to 90% of gallstones in Asian populations, may also occur throughout the entire biliary tree, and are frequently associated with pyogenic cholangiohepatitis.

Gallbladder contractility is impaired in some patients with gallstones. Although gallbladder dysfunction can be the consequence of gallstone disease or of excessive cholesterol infiltration into the gallbladder's smooth muscle, evidence suggests that gallbladder stasis itself can lead to gallbladder stone formation. A normal gallbladder ejects 10 to 20% of its contents into the duodenum in response to enteric nervous stimulation. The presence of postprandial intestinal fat further increases gallbladder contractility, which is mediated by the enteric nervous system and cholecystokinin. Gallbladder stasis is frequently evident in patients with risk factors for forming gallstones, including obesity, pregnancy, rapid weight loss, and prolonged fasting (Table 155-1). Furthermore, gallbladder dysmotility is an independent risk factor for recurrent gallstones in patients who have been treated with extracorporeal shock wave lithotripsy.

Acute Calculous Cholecystitis

The most common complication of gallstone disease is acute cholecystitis, which occurs in 15 to 20% of symptomatic patients. Acute cholecystitis results when a stone becomes lodged at the gallbladder–cystic duct junction, where it impairs gallbladder outflow and drainage. The extent of inflammation and the progression of acute cholecystitis are related to the duration and degree of obstruction. In the most severe cases, this process can lead to ischemia and necrosis of the gallbladder wall. More often, the stone spontaneously dislodges, and the inflammation gradually resolves. Acute cholecystitis is primarily an inflammatory rather than an infectious process, but about 50%

TABLE 155-1 RISK FACTORS ASSOCIATED WITH GALLSTONE FORMATION

NONMODIFIABLE FACTORS	MODIFIABLE FACTORS
Increasing age Female gender Ethnicity Genetics, family history	Pregnancy and parity Obesity Low-fiber, high-calorie diet Prolonged fasting Medications: clofibrate, estrogens, octreotide Low-level physical activity Rapid weight loss Hypertriglyceridemia, low high-density lipoprotein Metabolic syndrome Gallbladder stasis Terminal ileal disease or resection Total parenteral nutrition, fasting state

of patients with acute cholecystitis have secondary bacteriobilia, most commonly with *Escherichia coli.*

CLINICAL MANIFESTATIONS

The clinical spectrum of cholelithiasis ranges from the asymptomatic state to fatal complications. Among patients with asymptomatic gallstones, approximate annual risks are 1% for biliary pain, 0.3% for acute cholecystitis, 0.2% for symptomatic choledocholithiasis, and 0.04 to 1.5% for gallstone pancreatitis. However, these low individual percentages represent a huge population-wide number of symptomatic patients, given the frequency of gallstones. Overall, about 1 to 2% of asymptomatic individuals with gallstones develop serious symptoms or complications each year related to their gallstones.

The majority of gallstones are asymptomatic and are discovered on imaging studies performed for other indications. In such individuals, the gallbladder fills and empties normally, and the gallstones remain in the gallbladder and do not obstruct the cystic duct. Over time, however, asymptomatic gallstones can become symptomatic and be manifested as biliary colic due to impaction of a gallstone at the neck of the gallbladder or cystic duct. Although the pain is commonly termed biliary colic, the majority of patients actually note constant pain due to obstruction of the cystic duct and a progressive increase in gallbladder wall tension, rather than the paroxysmal pain of typical colic. The pain usually is located in the right upper quadrant or epigastrium and frequently radiates to the back and right scapula. Although biliary colic classically occurs after fatty meals, an association with meals is present in only 50% of patients, and the pain often develops more than 1 hour after eating. The duration of pain is typically 1 to 5 hours, but it may persist up to 24 hours. Pain persisting beyond 24 hours suggests that acute inflammation or cholecystitis is present. Episodes of biliary colic are usually less frequent than one episode per week. Other symptoms, such as nausea and vomiting, accompany each episode in 60 to 70% of cases. Bloating and belching are also present in 50% of patients. Fever and jaundice occur much less frequently with simple biliary colic. Although some patients with gallstones have continuous pain, predominantly in the back or the left upper quadrant, rather than episodic pain, alternative causes should be considered in such patients.

Acute Calculous Cholecystitis

Patients with acute cholecystitis typically present with right upper quadrant pain similar to biliary colic. In acute cholecystitis, however, the pain is usually unremitting, may last several days, and is often associated with nausea, emesis, anorexia, and fever. On physical examination, patients usually have a low-grade fever, with localized right upper quadrant tenderness and guarding. The presence of Murphy sign, an inspiratory arrest during deep palpation of the right upper quadrant, is the classic physical finding of acute cholecystitis. A palpable right upper quadrant mass is appreciated in one third of patients and usually represents omentum that has migrated to the area around the gallbladder in response to the inflammation. Mild jaundice (bilirubin level < 6 mg/dL) may be present. Significant jaundice is rare with acute cholecystitis but when present suggests the presence of common bile duct stones, cholangitis, or obstruction of the common hepatic duct by severe pericholecystic inflammation because of the impaction of a large stone in Hartmann pouch, which mechanically obstructs the bile duct. High fever suggests ascending cholangitis, often with bacterial infection (Fig. 155-1). Acute cholecystitis may coexist with choledocholithiasis or its complications of acute cholangitis and gallstone pancreatitis.

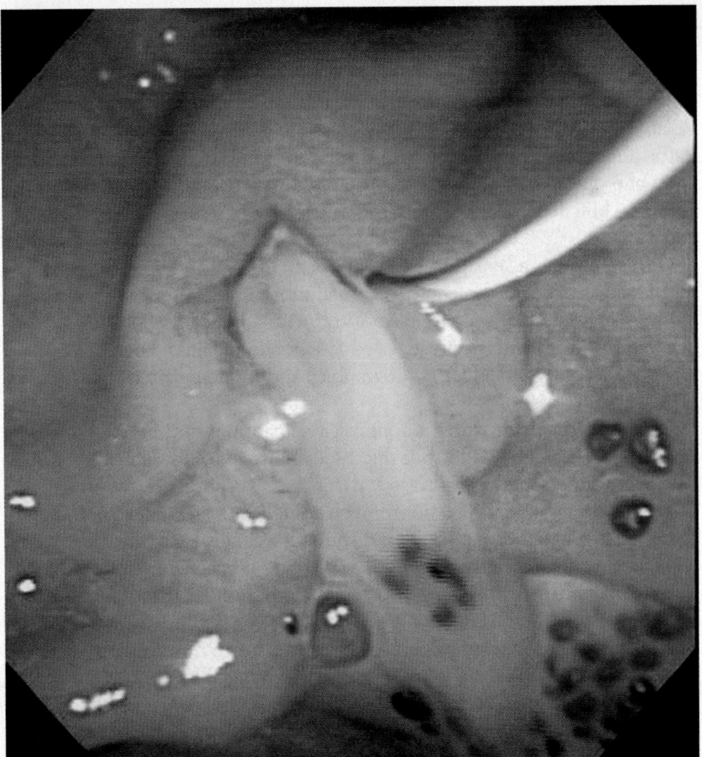

FIGURE 155-1. Endoscopic image of pus exiting the biliary orifice in this patient who presented with ascending cholangitis secondary to choledocholithiasis (note several small stones in duodenum).

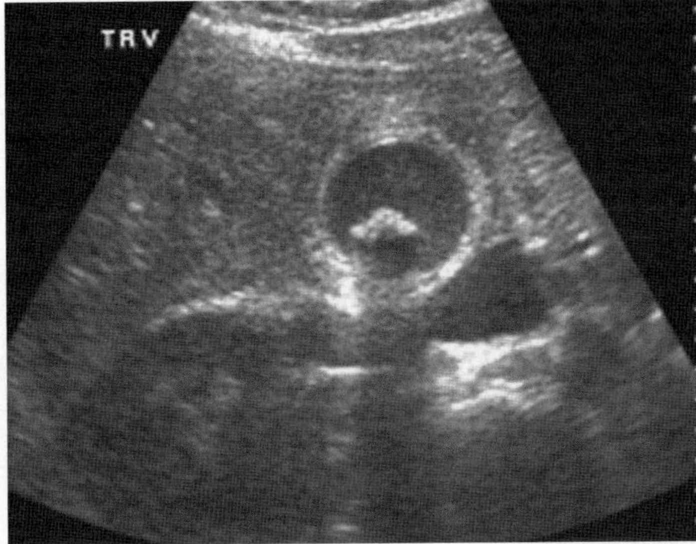

FIGURE 155-2. Ultrasound showing a gallstone. (From Afdhal N. Diseases of the gallbladder and bile ducts. In: Goldman L, Schafer A, eds. *Goldman's Cecil Medicine.* 24th ed. Philadelphia: Elsevier Saunders; 2012:1017.)

DIAGNOSIS

Transabdominal ultrasound is the radiologic procedure of choice to identify gallstones (Fig. 155-2).[1] Because the ultrasound waves cannot penetrate the stones, acoustic shadowing is seen posterior to the stones, thereby facilitating diagnosis. Free-floating gallbladder stones will also move to a dependent position when the patient is repositioned during scanning. If both of these features are present, the positive predictive value of ultrasound approaches 100%. Nonshadowing echoes alone, however, may be caused by gallbladder polyps. Gallstones may be missed because of a lack of contrasting bile around the stones, as may occur with an impacted cystic duct stone or when the gallbladder is filled with stones. Small gallstones may not cast an acoustic shadow. An ileus with increased abdominal gas, as can occur with acute cholecystitis or pancreatitis (Chapter 144), may limit visualization of the gallbladder. Overall, the false-negative rate of ultrasound for detection of gallstones is less than 5% but may increase to 15% with acute cholecystitis. Ultrasound may also demonstrate dilation of the intrahepatic and extrahepatic bile ducts. Dilated ducts may signify obstruction due to stones in the common bile duct, distal strictures, or malignant obstruction (Chapters 194 and 196).

Ultrasound has a sensitivity and specificity of 85% and 95%, respectively, for diagnosis of acute cholecystitis. In addition to the presence of gallstones, findings suggestive of acute cholecystitis include thickening of the gallbladder wall (>4 mm) and the presence of pericholecystic fluid. Focal tenderness directly over the gallbladder (sonographic Murphy sign) also is suggestive of acute cholecystitis.

Cholescintigraphy provides a noninvasive, anatomic, and functional evaluation of the liver, gallbladder, bile duct, and duodenum, although it has generally been superseded by ultrasound for this purpose, except in certain situations, such as identification of a suspected bile leak after cholecystectomy or a functional gallbladder disorder (see later). In this procedure, technetium Tc 99m–labeled iminodiacetic acid derivatives are injected intravenously, taken up by the liver, and excreted into the bile. These hepatobiliary iminodiacetic acid (HIDA) scans provide functional information about the liver's ability to excrete radiolabeled substances into a nonobstructed biliary tree. The tracer should be taken up by the liver, gallbladder, common bile duct, and duodenum within 1 hour. Nonvisualization of the gallbladder 1 hour after the injection of the radioisotope with filling of the bile duct and duodenum indicates an obstructed cystic duct and in the acute clinical setting is highly sensitive (95%) and specific (95%) for acute cholecystitis, although false-positive results are often seen in the setting of gallbladder stasis (e.g., critically ill patients, total parenteral nutrition). Slow uptake of the tracer by the liver suggests hepatic parenchymal disease. Filling of the gallbladder and bile duct with delayed or absent filling of the intestine may suggest an obstruction at the level of the major papilla.

Abdominal computed tomography (CT) is less sensitive than ultrasound for diagnosis of gallstones and is primarily indicated for the diagnosis of complications of gallstone disease, such as acute cholecystitis, choledocholithiasis, pancreatitis, and gallbladder cancer. By comparison, *plain abdominal radiographs* are of little value in the evaluation of gallbladder disease because only 15% of gallstones contain sufficient calcium to appear radiopaque. Plain films can be useful, however, for diagnosis of other causes of acute abdominal pain (e.g., perforated viscus, bowel obstruction). Rarely, abdominal films may show a calcified gallbladder wall (Fig. 155-3) in chronic cholecystitis or findings such as pneumobilia or gallstone-associated ileus in acute cholecystitis.

A CT scan also is frequently performed to evaluate an acutely ill patient with abdominal pain. The CT scan can detect gallstones, gallbladder wall thickening, pericholecystic fluid and edema, and air in the gallbladder or gallbladder wall (emphysematous cholecystitis), but it is generally less sensitive than ultrasonography for finding these conditions.

Magnetic resonance imaging is highly sensitive for diagnosis of both gallstones and common duct stones, but stones smaller than 3 mm may be missed. Endoscopic ultrasound provides excellent imaging of the gallbladder and biliary tree but is rarely the primary imaging modality for detection of a gallbladder stone. Endoscopic collection of bile for crystal analysis may serve as a surrogate for microlithiasis not seen on transabdominal ultrasound.

With cholecystitis, laboratory evaluation can show a mild leukocytosis, with a white blood cell count of 12,000 to 15,000 cells/μL. However, many patients have a normal white blood cell count. Leukocytosis greater than 20,000 cells/μL should suggest further complications of cholecystitis, such as gangrene, perforation, or cholangitis. Mild elevations in serum bilirubin, alkaline phosphatase, aminotransferase, and amylase levels may also be seen with acute cholecystitis.

TREATMENT

Rx

Silent Gallstones

The longer that stones remain silent, the less likely they are to cause symptoms. Furthermore, almost all patients will develop symptomatic disease before developing one of the serious complications of gallstones. Therefore, prophylactic cholecystectomy is not generally indicated in patients with asymptomatic gallstones.

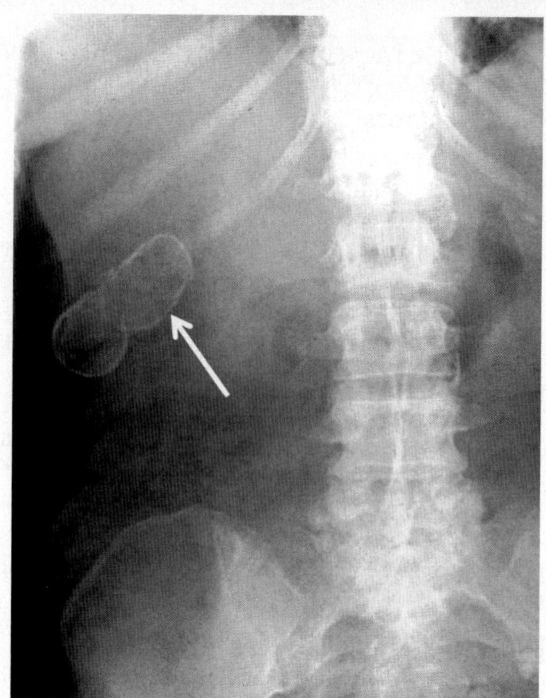

FIGURE 155-3. Plain abdominal radiograph illustrating a porcelain gallbladder. Note the calcified gallbladder wall.

In select groups of patients, however, prophylactic cholecystectomy should be considered, even when gallbladder stones are absent. A porcelain gallbladder with a calcified gallbladder wall is associated with a 5% or higher risk of malignant transformation, high enough to justify cholecystectomy. Patients with a long common channel between the bile and pancreatic ducts (i.e., anomalous pancreaticobiliary duct junction; see later) also are at significant risk for gallbladder cancer and should undergo prophylactic cholecystectomy. Acute cholecystitis is a potentially life-threatening condition in immunosuppressed patients, so prophylactic cholecystectomy is generally recommended before or at the time of major organ transplantation. Data also support cholecystectomy in patients undergoing bariatric weight loss surgery even in the absence of gallstones because of their nearly 30% risk for developing gallstones and requiring cholecystectomy during rapid weight loss in the first year after surgery. Prophylactic cholecystectomy adds minimal morbidity and mortality risks to most bariatric operations and is clearly indicated in patients with gallstones. Some patients with silent gallbladder stones may also benefit from prophylactic cholecystectomy. In patients with sickle cell disease (Chapter 163), for example, cholecystitis can precipitate a crisis with substantial operative risks. Large gallstones (>3 cm) are more frequently associated with acute cholecystitis and gallbladder carcinoma, so prophylactic cholecystectomy may also be indicated in these patients.

Symptomatic Gallstones

The operative management of gallstones has been the standard of care for more than a century. Early surgery within 24 hours is generally preferred for patients with biliary colic,[A1] and day surgery is as safe and effective as an overnight stay.[A2] More than 90% of these cholecystectomies are performed laparoscopically, with about 3% of elective procedures converted to an open procedure in the operating room. Contraindications to laparoscopic surgery include significant bleeding and Child's class C cirrhosis (Chapter 153). Some patients with severe chronic obstructive pulmonary disease or heart failure may not tolerate the pneumoperitoneum required for laparoscopic surgery, and the prior upper abdominal surgery may increase the difficulty of or preclude laparoscopic cholecystectomy. Serious complications of laparoscopic cholecystectomy are rare, with a reported incidence of 0.6 to 1.5% for any bile duct leaks and 0.3 to 0.6% for a major bile duct injury. Although these risks are higher than for open surgery, the overall mortality rate (<0.3%) is lower for laparoscopic surgery, and the postoperative recovery is much easier.

Nonsurgical options for the treatment of gallstone disease are rarely used today because of their limited efficacy and the widespread application of laparoscopic cholecystectomy. Oral dissolution therapy (e.g., ursodeoxycholic acid, 15 mg/kg/day) may be considered in symptomatic but not in asymptomatic patients who have cholesterol gallstones in a functioning gallbladder, but it completely dissolves stones in only 40% of patients, and stones recur in up to 50% of patients within 5 years after therapy is stopped. Lifelong therapy, therefore, may be necessary. The direct infusion of organic solvents (methyl *tert*-butyl ether, continuously infused and aspirated manually four to six times per minute, for an average of 5 hours/day, for 1 to 3 days) into the gallbladder also is efficacious only for cholesterol gallstones, and the recurrence rate is similar to that of oral dissolution therapy. Extracorporeal shock wave lithotripsy can be considered for a single stone of any type (i.e., cholesterol or calcium bilirubinate) 0.5 to 2 cm in diameter, but only a small percentage of symptomatic patients fit these criteria. As a result, this therapy is limited to a very select group of patients.

Acute Calculous Cholecystitis

After medical stabilization of the patient with intravenous fluids as needed, broad-spectrum antibiotics (e.g., piperacillin-tazobactam, 3.375 g every 6 hours; or ceftriaxone, 1 to 2 g once daily, plus metronidazole, 500 mg every 6 hours; or levofloxacin, 500 mg once daily, plus metronidazole), and parenteral analgesics as necessary (see Table 30-5), the treatment of choice for acute cholecystitis is cholecystectomy. When antibiotic therapy is initiated, the duration is tailored to clinical improvement. Laparoscopic cholecystectomy significantly reduces morbidity, length of hospital stay, and time to return to work, favoring patients compared with open surgery. However, the conversion rate to an open procedure is up to 25% compared with about 3% for elective laparoscopic surgery.

Prospective randomized trials have shown that early laparoscopic cholecystectomy (within 3 days of symptom onset) can be accomplished with a morbidity and mortality rate similar to that of delayed cholecystectomy,[A3] with no differences in the conversion rate to open cholecystectomy. Length of hospital stay, and therefore costs, are significantly reduced in patients undergoing early surgery. Because about 20% of patients fail to stabilize with initial medical therapy and require operation during the initial admission or before the end of the planned cooling-off period, the current recommendation is to proceed with early laparoscopic cholecystectomy for acute cholecystitis unless there are contraindications to it. If the bilirubin level is <4 mg/dL and the patient has no evidence of cholangitis, common duct exploration is probably not required.[A4]

In high-risk patients whose medical conditions preclude cholecystectomy, a percutaneous cholecystostomy can allow prompt gallbladder drainage. If such drainage and appropriate antibiotics do not lead to clear improvement within 24 hours, however, laparotomy is indicated because failure to improve after percutaneous drainage is usually caused by gangrene of the gallbladder or perforation. If cholecystostomy is successful and the acute episode resolves, the patient can electively undergo either cholecystectomy or percutaneous stone extraction and removal of the cholecystostomy tube. Alternatively, an endoscopic retrograde cholangiopancreatography (ERCP)–guided stent can be placed to drain the gallbladder if the cystic duct is patent.

PREVENTION

Moderate physical activity and dietary management (high fiber intake, avoidance of saturated fatty acids) may lower the risk of gallstone disease. Daily administration of cholecystokinin (3.5 μg) in patients receiving prolonged total parenteral nutrition may prevent formation of gallbladder sludge. Oral ursodeoxycholic acid (15 mg/kg/day) has been clearly demonstrated to be beneficial in prevention of gallstone disease during rapid weight loss[A5] and in patients who need long-term somatostatin therapy. For secondary prevention (i.e., in patients with gallstones already present), there are insufficient data to support the use of any medical therapy.

Complications of Acute Calculous Cholecystitis

Several complications of acute cholecystitis include empyema of the gallbladder, emphysematous cholecystitis, and gangrene leading to gallbladder perforation. Each of these complications can be associated with significant morbidity and mortality and therefore requires prompt surgical intervention. In 1 to 2% of patients with acute cholecystitis, the gallbladder will perforate into an adjacent hollow viscus, thereby creating a cholecystenteric fistula; the duodenum (79%) and the hepatic flexure of the colon (17%) are the most common sites. The episode of acute cholecystitis generally resolves as the gallbladder spontaneously decompresses after the fistula forms. If a large gallstone passes from the gallbladder into the small intestine, a mechanical bowel obstruction, termed gallstone ileus, may result. Gallstone ileus occurs in 10 to 15% of patients with a cholecystenteric fistula. Patients with gallstone ileus present with signs and symptoms of intestinal obstruction—nausea, vomiting, and abdominal pain. Abdominal films will demonstrate small bowel distention and air-fluid levels and may give additional clues to the source of the obstruction (pneumobilia or a calcified gallstone distant from the gallbladder). The initial management of gallstone ileus includes relieving the obstruction. Most frequently, this goal can be achieved by removing the gallstone through an enterotomy, although endoscopic retrieval of the offending stone can be done, depending on where the stone is located.

Acute Acalculous Cholecystitis

Acute acalculous cholecystitis, which accounts for 5 to 10% of all cases of acute cholecystitis, usually occurs in critically ill patients after trauma, burns, long-term parenteral nutrition, and major nonbiliary operations (e.g., abdominal aneurysm repair, cardiopulmonary bypass). The cause of acute acalculous cholecystitis remains unclear, although gallbladder stasis with increased bacterial colonization and ischemia have been implicated.

The symptoms and signs of acute acalculous cholecystitis are similar to those of acute calculous cholecystitis, with right upper quadrant pain and tenderness, fever, and leukocytosis. The disease often has a more fulminant course than acute calculous cholecystitis and more frequently progresses to gangrene, empyema, or perforation. Except for the absence of gallstones, ultrasound and CT findings are similar to those of calculous cholecystitis, including gallbladder wall thickening and pericholecystic fluid. On cholescintigraphy, the gallbladder does not fill; however, the false-positive rate (absent gallbladder filling without acute acalculous cholecystitis) may be as high as 40%.

Emergency cholecystectomy is recommended if the diagnosis is established or even if clinical suspicion is high because the risk of gangrene, perforation, or empyema exceeds 50%. Cholecystectomy rather than cholecystostomy is usually required, but percutaneous cholecystostomy or endoscopic gallbladder stenting is recommended in patients unable to undergo surgery. The mortality rate for acute acalculous cholecystitis can be as high as 40%, mostly because of the concomitant illnesses in patients who develop this disease.

Functional Gallbladder Disorder

Some patients present with typical symptoms of biliary colic but do not have any evidence of gallstones on ultrasound examination. If further investigations such as liver chemistries, amylase and lipase levels, CT scan, and even upper gastrointestinal endoscopy are unremarkable, the diagnosis of a functional gallbladder disorder should be considered.[2] The pathobiology is poorly understood, but one possibility is that the obesity epidemic has increased the population-wide accumulation of fat in the gallbladder wall—cholecystosteatosis—thereby decreasing the gallbladder's ability to empty. Some patients may have intermittent gallbladder outlet obstruction due to cystic duct spasm, poor coordination between the contraction of the gallbladder and the sphincter of Oddi, or dysmotility of the gallbladder. In a cholecystokinin-stimulated ^{99m}Tc-HIDA scan, cholecystokinin is infused intravenously after the gallbladder has filled with the ^{99m}Tc-labeled radionuclide, and a gallbladder ejection fraction is calculated 20 minutes later. An ejection fraction of less than 35% at 20 minutes is considered abnormal, and most of these patients have histopathologic evidence of chronic cholecystitis, although a low gallbladder ejection fraction is not specific for a functional gallbladder disorder (Table 155-2). The efficacy of laparoscopic cholecystectomy is controversial in this setting, but the Society of American Gastrointestinal and Endoscopic Surgeons recommends it. The percentage of patients undergoing cholecystectomy for functional gallbladder disorder in the United States during the past 15 years has increased from less than 5% to more than 20% of patients having the gallbladder removed.

Tumors of the Gallbladder

Benign

Cholesterol polyps are not true neoplasms but rather are cholesterol-filled projections of gallbladder mucosa that protrude into the lumen. These polyps account for approximately 50% of all polypoid gallbladder lesions, are usually

TABLE 155-2 SETTINGS IN WHICH A LOW GALLBLADDER EJECTION FRACTION MAY BE IDENTIFIED

Functional gallbladder disorder (chronic acalculous cholecystitis)
Cystic duct obstruction
Sphincter of Oddi dysfunction
Asymptomatic, healthy individuals
Diabetes
Pregnancy
Cirrhosis
Obesity
Celiac disease
Medications (narcotic analgesics, calcium-channel antagonists, oral contraceptive agents, benzodiazepines, histamine H_2-receptor antagonists)

smaller than 1 cm, are typically found incidentally on imaging studies as nonmobile filling defects, are usually asymptomatic unless associated with gallstones, and do not have malignant potential.

Adenomyosis consists of a hypertrophic gallbladder muscle layer with mucosal diverticula called Rokitansky-Aschoff sinuses. This condition may affect the gallbladder locally, particularly in the fundus, where it appears as a hemispheric lesion with a central dimple; segmentally, as an annular stricture; or diffusely, when it involves the entire gallbladder wall. The cause is not entirely clear but may be secondary to a gallbladder motility disorder. Isolated adenomyosis can cause biliary-type symptoms and can progress to gallbladder cancer, so prophylactic cholecystectomy is recommended.

Gallbladder adenomas are benign epithelial tumors with malignant potential. Adenomas usually are manifested as solitary, nonmobile filling defects on ultrasound. Polyps smaller than 0.5 cm, regardless of total polyp number, can be observed with serial imaging studies every 3 to 6 months. Larger polyps, however, may harbor a carcinoma in situ, and cholecystectomy is recommended for polyps larger than 1 cm and for any patients with biliary symptoms.

Malignant

Gallbladder cancer is the most common biliary tract malignant neoplasm and fifth most common gastrointestinal cancer overall, with approximately 7000 new cases diagnosed annually in the United States (2.5 cases/100,000 population). The usual age at onset is the sixth or seventh decade, with a female-to-male ratio of 3:1. Gallbladder cancer is more common in Native Americans, Mexicans, Alaskans, and American Hispanics as well as in residents of Israel, Chile, and northern Japan.

Perhaps because of chronic inflammation, gallbladder cancer is strongly associated with gallstones, which are identified in more than 90% of patients with gallbladder carcinoma. Conversely, only 1% of patients with gallstones develop gallbladder carcinoma. Choledochal cysts are associated with an increased risk of malignant neoplasms throughout the biliary tree, including the gallbladder, perhaps because of increased stasis, chronic inflammation, and infection. In patients with choledochal cysts, excision of extrahepatic cysts is recommended to avoid biliary tract cancer. By comparison, biliary sphincterotomy alone may be adequate for a type III extrahepatic cyst.

About 90% of gallbladder cancers are adenocarcinomas (90% scirrhous, 5% papillary, 5% colloid). The remaining tumors are anaplastic or squamous cell cancers. Gallbladder cancers spread by local extension and direct invasion of adjacent structures, including the common hepatic duct, liver, duodenum, and colon. Lymphatic drainage is to adjacent lymph nodes, and disseminated disease is to the liver and the peritoneal surface.

Most patients (80%) present with abdominal pain of less than 1 month in duration, which may be difficult to distinguish from symptoms of biliary colic or acute cholecystitis. Nausea and vomiting (50%) and weight loss (40%) are often present, and jaundice (30%) is a poor prognostic sign that typically signifies porta hepatis involvement with tumor. Up to 20% of gallbladder cancers are found at cholecystectomy performed for gallstones, whereas incidental cancers are found at 1% of cholecystectomies.

Diagnosis may be difficult preoperatively because laboratory test results may be normal or nonspecific even when advanced disease is manifested by hypoalbuminemia and anemia. There is no reliable tumor marker. Liver test results are abnormal when the tumor or periportal lymphadenopathy is associated with biliary obstruction. Ultrasonography has a sensitivity of 75 to 80% for detection of gallbladder cancer, with findings ranging from a complex luminal mass to gallbladder wall thickening, polypoid mass, or gallstones. CT or magnetic resonance cross-sectional imaging can assess the extent of disease, including regional and distant metastases. Endoscopic ultrasound may aid in determining the extent of local invasion and nodal involvement, but it rarely is necessary in the preoperative evaluation. ERCP is indicated only in patients who have clinical evidence of biliary obstruction and are being considered for stent placement to palliate their jaundice.

PREVENTION AND TREATMENT Rx

Patients with gallstones larger than 3 cm have a 10-fold increased risk for development of gallbladder cancer, so prophylactic cholecystectomy should be considered even in an asymptomatic patient. A porcelain gallbladder, with diffuse calcification of the gallbladder wall, is an indication for cholecystectomy in the asymptomatic patient because of the increased risk of cancer. Cholecystectomy also is indicated for any gallbladder polyp larger than 1 cm, in patients with choledochal cysts other than type III, in anomalous pancreaticobiliary union, and in adenomyosis of the gallbladder.

The resectability rates for gallbladder cancer range from 15 to 30%. When the tumor does not extend beyond the muscle layer of the gallbladder wall (T_1), simple cholecystectomy alone may be curative, with a 5-year survival rate approaching 100%. Tumors that extend through the gallbladder wall (stage II/III) require a more extensive resection (cholecystectomy, partial hepatectomy, lymph node dissection). Stage II tumors (no invasion beyond the gallbladder serosa) may have up to a 60 to 80% 5-year survival rate, whereas stage III tumors have a 25% 5-year survival rate. Median survival with unresectable (stage IV) disease is only 2 to 3 months. Radiation therapy has not been shown to be effective, whereas chemotherapy regimens in unresectable disease (typically similar to regimens for pancreatic cancer [Chapter 194]) are associated with response rates of approximately 20%. Because of the late presentation of this disease and spread of tumor at diagnosis, the overall 5-year survival is less than 10%.

BILE DUCTS

Bile Duct Stones

PATHOBIOLOGY

Bile duct stones, or choledocholithiasis, can be classified as either primary or secondary. Primary duct stones develop de novo within the bile ducts, whereas secondary stones develop in the gallbladder and subsequently pass into the bile duct. In the Western world, more than 85% of all bile duct stones are secondary. Primary duct stones typically occur in conditions associated with bile stasis (e.g., benign biliary strictures, sclerosing cholangitis, choledochal cysts, periampullary diverticula), which promotes bacterial overgrowth with subsequent bilirubin deconjugation and the breakdown of biliary lipids, thereby resulting in the formation of brown pigment stones.

CLINICAL MANIFESTATIONS

Bile duct stones are discovered incidentally in 5 to 12% of patients during the evaluation of gallbladder stones and suspected cholecystitis. It is difficult to determine whether the existing bile duct stones are asymptomatic in patients who present with biliary pain alone because pain can originate from either the gallbladder stones or bile duct stones. More than 50% of patients with retained bile duct stones experience recurrent symptoms during a follow-up period of 6 months to 13 years, and 25% of cases develop serious complications.

Common clinical symptoms and signs of bile duct stones include epigastric or right upper quadrant pain, fever, and jaundice (referred to as Charcot triad). Pain can be mild or severe, and severe episodes must be differentiated from other potentially life-threatening events. Occasional patients may present with painless jaundice and weight loss mimicking pancreaticobiliary malignant disease (Chapter 194).

DIAGNOSIS

Patients with cholangitis, with or without associated pancreatitis (Chapter 144), typically have elevated serum aminotransferase levels. The serum bilirubin level usually is less than 15 mg/dL with choledocholithiasis because most bile duct stones cause intermittent, incomplete biliary obstruction. In unusual cases, the serum aminotransferase levels can be profoundly elevated (up to 2000 IU/L), mimicking acute viral hepatitis.

Although ultrasound is the most common initial test for patients with suspected gallbladder stones, it has a low sensitivity rate (25 to 60%) for detection of bile duct stones, in part because the bile duct may not be dilated in acute obstruction. CT scan may demonstrate calcified bile duct stones (Fig. 155-4), but its sensitivity for this purpose is generally little better. CT is useful, however, for identifying other potential causes of biliary obstruction (e.g., mass lesion) and local complications, such as a liver abscess (Chapter 151). Magnetic resonance cholangiopancreatography (MRCP) and endoscopic ultrasound can detect bile duct stones with an accuracy comparable to that of ERCP (Fig. 155-5). Because of potential procedure-related risks, ERCP is now reserved for patients with confirmed or a high suspicion of biliary disease who are likely to require therapeutic intervention.

TREATMENT Rx

Given the potential serious complications of bile duct stones (i.e., cholangitis, pancreatitis), specific therapy is generally required regardless of symptoms.

About 85 to 90% of bile duct stones can be removed at ERCP by standard balloon dilation and basket extraction after biliary endoscopic sphincterotomy, with a complication rate, including pancreatitis, bleeding, cholangitis, cholecystitis, and perforation, of less than 10%. Endoscopic biliary orifice dilation without sphincterotomy may reduce some acute complications but increases the risk of pancreatitis and may lead to more subsequent procedures.

The 10 to 15% of bile duct stones that cannot be removed by standard ERCP are generally larger than 1.5 cm, impacted, or located above a stricture. Alternative therapies include the use of large-diameter dilation balloons (12 to 18 mm) and fragmentation by mechanical or electrohydraulic lithotripsy. Whenever stones cannot be completely removed endoscopically, biliary stents should be placed to ensure adequate biliary drainage and to prevent recurrent symptoms while awaiting further therapy. Long-term biliary stenting can also be used in patients with severe comorbid medical conditions that preclude surgery or repeated endoscopic interventions.

Ideally, patients with concomitant gallbladder and bile duct stones would be best treated with a single laparoscopic cholecystectomy and bile duct exploration, which is preferable to ERCP followed by cholecystectomy.[A6] However, only a minority of surgeons can successfully perform laparoscopic bile duct exploration, so open common bile duct exploration is generally performed if endoscopic and laparoscopic approaches are unsuccessful.

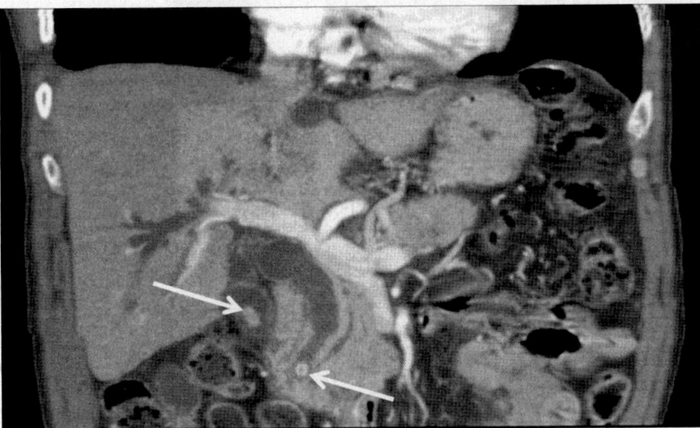

FIGURE 155-4. Computed tomography scan demonstrating calcified gallstones and a distal bile duct stone.

Complications of Bile Duct Stones

Cholangitis is a potentially life-threatening disease that results from bacterial infection of obstructed bile. Systemic toxicity occurs when intraductal pressure is sufficiently elevated to cause reflux of bacteria or endotoxin into the blood. About 80 to 90% of acute cholangitis is caused by choledocholithiasis, with the remaining cases caused by a benign biliary stricture (e.g., primary sclerosing cholangitis, chronic pancreatitis, postoperative bile duct injury, or narrowing at an anastomosis) or by malignant biliary obstruction, typically after previous endoscopic instrumentation and stent placement. In certain parts of the world, parasitic biliary obstruction (e.g., *Ascaris*; Chapter 357) may be manifested with cholangitis. The most common bacteria are gram-negative bacilli and *Streptococcus* spp, but *Enterococcus* spp are frequently seen in patients with occluded biliary stents. Prompt antibiotic therapy (e.g., intravenous ceftriaxone, 1 to 2 g once daily; ampicillin-sulbactam, 1.5 to 3 g every 6 hours; piperacillin-tazobactam, 3.375 g every 6 hours; ciprofloxacin, 400 mg twice daily; or levofloxacin, 500 mg orally once daily) is critical and usually can permit conservative management with endoscopic biliary decompression within 24 to 48 hours.[A7] However, urgent decompression is indicated if improvement is not seen within a few hours. The advantages of ERCP are that it can delineate the cause of obstruction, obtain bile for culture, and rapidly decompress the biliary tree definitively by removing the stone or temporarily by placing a stent without removing the stone. Routine stenting is not indicated after successful stone removal,[A8] unless the adequacy of biliary drainage is uncertain.

Acute gallstone pancreatitis accounts for up to 50% of cases of acute pancreatitis in Western countries (Chapter 144). Most patients quickly respond to conservative therapy, but some develop severe pancreatitis. Although early ERCP with biliary sphincterotomy and stone removal (Fig. 155-6) would appear

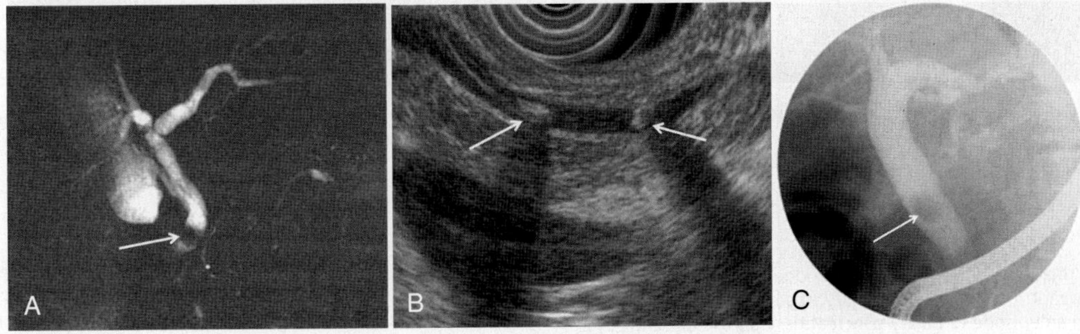

FIGURE 155-5. Common bile duct stones seen at magnetic resonance cholangiopancreatography (A), endoscopic ultrasound (B), and endoscopic retrograde cholangiopancreatography (C).

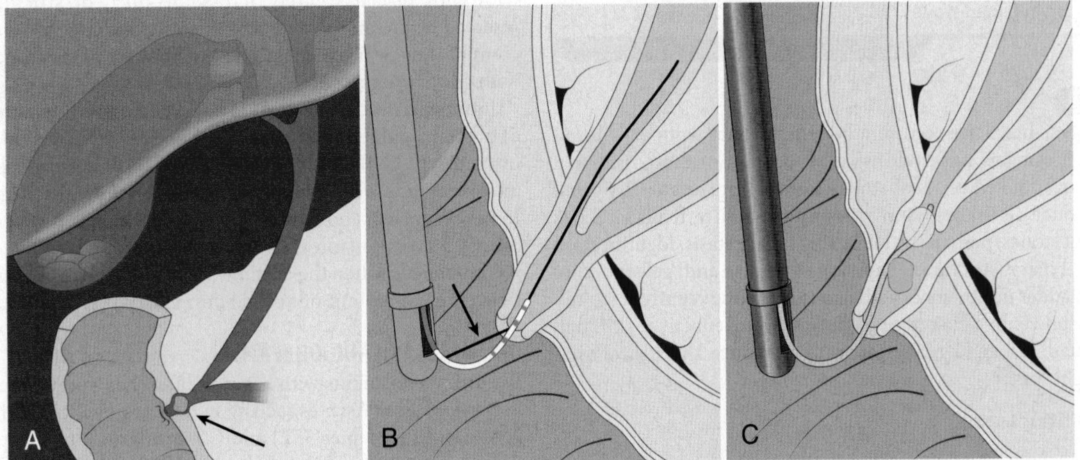

FIGURE 155-6. A, A stone that is impacted in the distal bile duct is causing biliary pancreatitis, with gallbladder stones also seen. B, Performance of biliary sphincterotomy. C, Subsequent stone removal by balloon sweep.

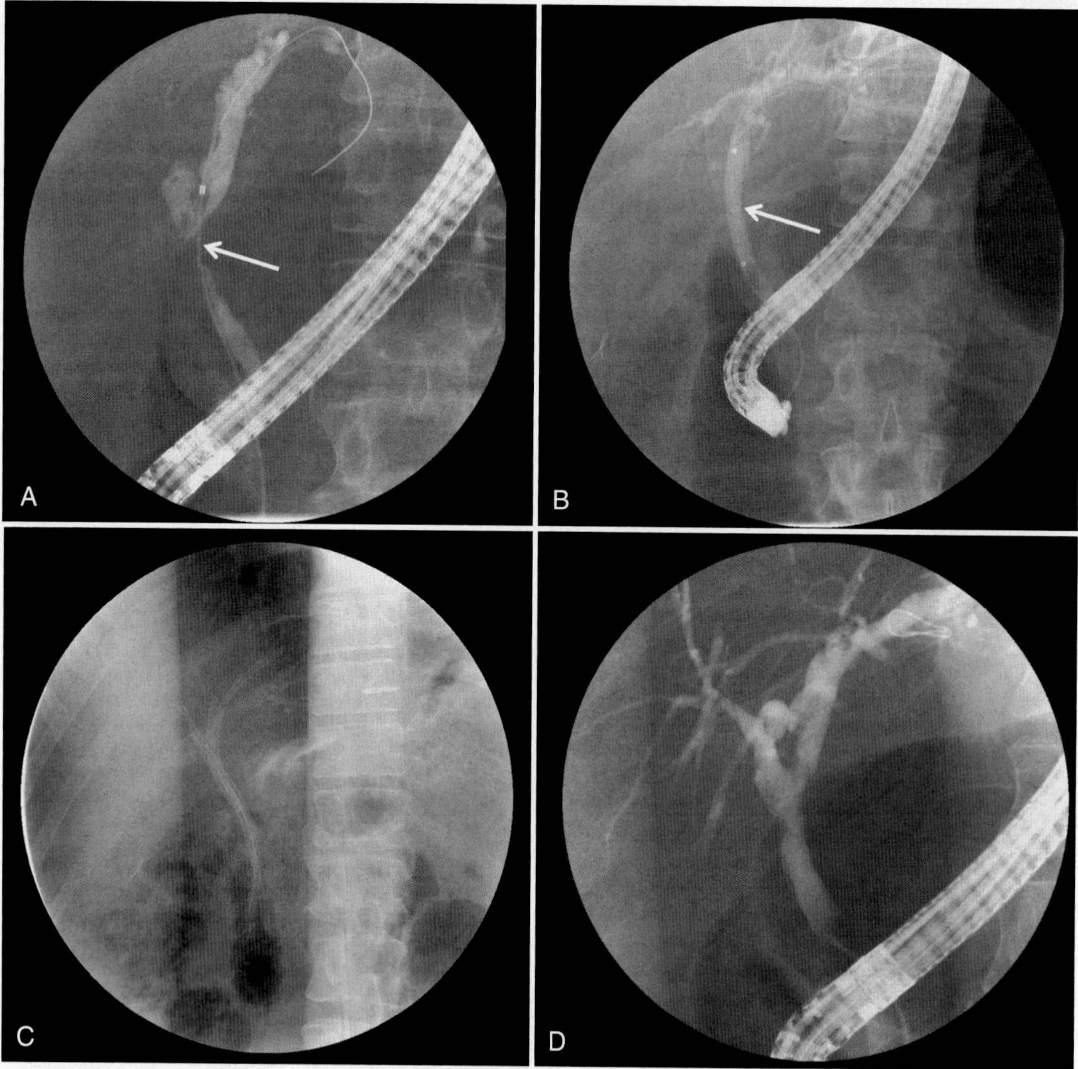

FIGURE 155-7. **Endoscopic retrograde cholangiopancreatography images obtained from a patient who presented with painless jaundice 8 months after cholecystectomy. A, Benign common hepatic duct stricture. B, Balloon dilation of the stricture. C, Multiple stents placed. D, Resolution of stricture after a 1-year stenting interval.**

to be an attractive therapeutic option, early ERCP does not reduce mortality or complications except in patients with biliary obstruction or cholangitis.[3] After recovery from an episode of biliary pancreatitis, laparoscopic cholecystectomy with intraoperative cholangiography is recommended to prevent further episodes, preferably during the same hospital admission.[A9] If a common bile duct stone is found at intraoperative cholangiography, laparoscopic or open common bile duct exploration and stone removal can be accomplished with high success rates in experienced hands, or postoperative ERCP can remove any retained stones.

PREVENTION

Up to 25% of patients may have recurrent bile duct stones, with or without a gallbladder, but it remains uncertain what proportion of these recurrent stones are in fact overlooked residual stones from a prior event. A dilated extrahepatic bile duct (≥13 mm) and periampullary diverticula are risk factors for recurrent stones, perhaps by increasing biliary stasis. Identification and treatment of biliary strictures, papillary stenosis, and gallstones in patients with gallbladder in situ are essential for preventing recurrent stones. Unfortunately, no preventive therapy has been proved effective, although ursodeoxycholic acid (15 mg/kg/day) appears to reduce the risk of gallstones during weight loss.[A4]

Benign Biliary Strictures

Postoperative extrahepatic bile duct strictures occur after 0.25 to 1% of cholecystectomies. Most such lesions are manifested as abnormal liver test results, obstructive jaundice, and cholangitis within 2 to 3 months postoperatively, although the presentation can be delayed. The cholangiogram commonly shows a short, smooth narrowing near the cystic duct stump with proximal duct dilation (Fig. 155-7). Strictures typically must be redilated, and stents are exchanged at 3- to 4-month intervals for 8 to 12 months until the stricture is nearly as open as the downstream bile duct. About 80% of patients will have a good result,[4] although some patients will ultimately require a bilioenteric bypass. Strictures more than 2 cm in length, strictures with clips placed securely across the duct, or strictures associated with resected segments of duct require surgical intervention. Biliary strictures complicating liver transplantation (Chapter 154) are usually treated similarly with good results.

Intrapancreatic common bile duct strictures, which may occur in 3 to 46% of patients with chronic pancreatitis, can lead to secondary biliary cirrhosis or recurrent cholangitis. With the complication of cholangitis or jaundice, intervention is clearly indicated, typically with ERCP and stent placement. In the absence of cholangitis or jaundice, either surgical repair or endoscopic biliary decompression with multiple plastic stents (Fig. 155-8) is generally recommended when the alkaline phosphatase level is consistently more than twice the upper limit of normal during a 6-month period of observation.

ORIENTAL CHOLANGIOHEPATITIS

Recurrent cholangitis with hepatolithiasis has a prevalence of more than 10% in parts of East Asia, especially in Taiwan, owing to infection with *Ascaris lumbricoides* (Chapter 357) and *Clonorchis sinensis* (Chapter 356). This condition results in local strictures and dilation of the intrahepatic biliary tree. Biliary stasis and subsequent bacterial infection cause brown stones to form. Most patients have recurrent cholangitis, but cholangiocarcinoma can also

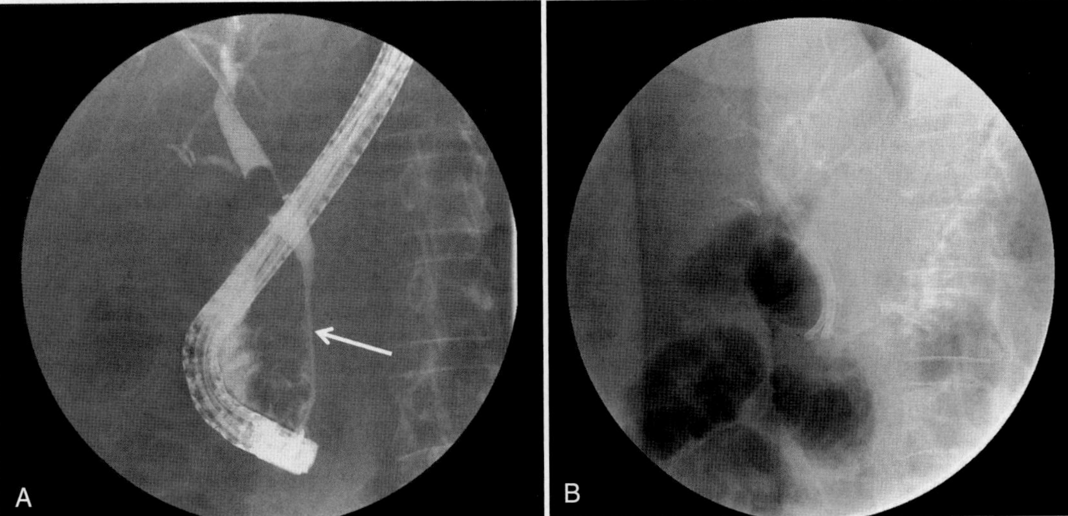

FIGURE 155-8. Endoscopic retrograde cholangiopancreatography images obtained from a patient with a history of alcohol abuse who presented with pruritus and was found to have markedly elevated alkaline phosphatase. A, A smooth distal bile duct stricture is seen *(arrow)*. B, Four stents have been placed through the stricture.

ensue. Ultrasound or CT can establish the diagnosis. Treatment includes intravenous fluids and antibiotics. Endoscopic stone removal is usually the preferred treatment, but localized surgical resection targeted to the cultured organisms may be necessary.

PRIMARY SCLEROSING CHOLANGITIS

DEFINITION

Primary sclerosing cholangitis is a chronic cholestatic disease characterized by fibrosing inflammation of segments of the intrahepatic and extrahepatic bile ducts.[5] It results in progressive narrowing of the duct lumen and ultimately may be manifested with recurrent episodes of ascending cholangitis or, alternatively, may progress to secondary biliary cirrhosis and its associated complications. Cholangiocarcinoma (Chapter 196) is a dreaded complication with a reported incidence of 25 to 40% at autopsy or liver transplantation.

EPIDEMIOLOGY

The true prevalence of primary sclerosing cholangitis is unknown, but current estimates are 0.2 to 8.5 per 100,000 in the U.S. population. Its prevalence is much higher in populations in which inflammatory bowel disease (Chapter 141) is more common. Affected men outnumber women in a 2 : 1 ratio, with the mean age at diagnosis of 32 to 40 years. However, primary sclerosing cholangitis has been reported in infants, children, and the elderly.

PATHOBIOLOGY

The cause of primary sclerosing cholangitis and the mechanisms responsible for its progression are unknown.[6] However, autoimmune and genetic causes are supported by its frequent association with inflammatory bowel disease and the increased prevalence of the HLA B8, DR3 haplotype. About two thirds of patients with primary sclerosing cholangitis have ulcerative colitis or Crohn colitis, and it is rarely associated with Crohn disease that is limited to the small bowel. However, only 1 to 13% of patients with colitis are diagnosed with primary sclerosing cholangitis during their lifetime. First-degree relatives of patients with primary sclerosing cholangitis have a 9- to 39-fold increased risk for development of the disease.

On pathologic examination, involved segments of bile ducts in strictured areas show diffuse thickening with a mononuclear inflammatory cell infiltrate. The most characteristic biopsy features are bile duct proliferation, periductal fibrosis, periductal inflammation, and loss of bile ducts. Obliterative cholangitis with a chronic inflammatory cell infiltrate and periductular "onion ring" fibrosis is strongly associated with primary sclerosing cholangitis but is infrequently observed in biopsy specimens. Given the patchy nature of the disease and possible lack of significant intrahepatic involvement, however, the histologic appearance of primary sclerosing cholangitis is variable and may resemble extrahepatic biliary obstruction, chronic active hepatitis, or, rarely, primary biliary cirrhosis.

CLINICAL MANIFESTATIONS

Most patients with primary sclerosing cholangitis are asymptomatic at presentation and are identified after investigation of an elevated alkaline phosphatase level (Chapter 147). Overall, about 90% of patients have an elevated alkaline phosphatase level, with or without mildly elevated serum aminotransferase levels. Fatigue, anorexia, malaise, and weight loss are common but may erroneously be attributed to a patient's inflammatory bowel disease. Patients may exhibit signs or symptoms of cholestatic liver disease, including pruritus, upper abdominal pain, and fever. The serum bilirubin concentration is elevated in only about 40% of patients at presentation. Some patients have anemia, hypoalbuminemia, or hypergammaglobulinemia, and a prolonged international normalized ratio suggests biliary obstruction or synthetic dysfunction. Nearly 90% of patients will have a positive perinuclear antineutrophilic cytoplasmic antibody, but this antibody is also nonspecific and may be found in both ulcerative colitis (Chapter 141) and autoimmune hepatitis (Chapter 149). Antinuclear or anti–smooth muscle antibodies are found in 25% of patients but are not specific, and a positive antimitochondrial antibody suggests primary biliary cirrhosis as the diagnosis.

DIAGNOSIS

Cholangiography is necessary to establish the diagnosis of primary sclerosing cholangitis (Fig. 155-9).[7] MRCP generally is the test of choice,[8] but ERCP may be indicated if MRCP is inconclusive, particularly when the disease is confined to small intrahepatic ducts. The role of biopsy remains uncertain owing to the segmental nature of the disease and the overlap of the histologic features with other disease states. Diffuse multifocal strictures are usually short, with intervening normal or dilated segments that give a beaded appearance. Other frequent findings on cholangiography include pseudodiverticula, mural irregularities, and biliary stones and sludge. Secondary causes of sclerosing cholangitis include obstruction (postoperative, autoimmune cholangiopathy, choledocholithiasis, and recurrent pyogenic cholangitis), ischemic (hepatic artery instillation of the chemotherapeutic agent 5-fluorouracil, radiation, and paroxysmal nocturnal hemoglobinuria), and neoplastic (cholangiocarcinoma, hepatocellular carcinoma, lymphoma, and metastasis).

TREATMENT Rx

The chronic cholestasis of primary sclerosing cholangitis can be treated with cholestyramine (4 to 8 g/day), ursodeoxycholic acid (15 mg/kg/day), rifampicin (300 to 600 mg/day), or phenobarbital (30 to 120 mg/day) with modest success. Fat-soluble vitamin deficiencies (Chapter 218) must be corrected. The prevalence of osteoporosis (Chapter 243) in primary sclerosing cholangitis is between 4 and 10%, so bone densitometry should be performed at diagnosis and every 2 to 3 years thereafter. Supplementation with oral vitamin D and calcium seems prudent, even in the absence of symptomatic deficiency. Treatment with bisphosphonates (Chapter 243) is reserved for

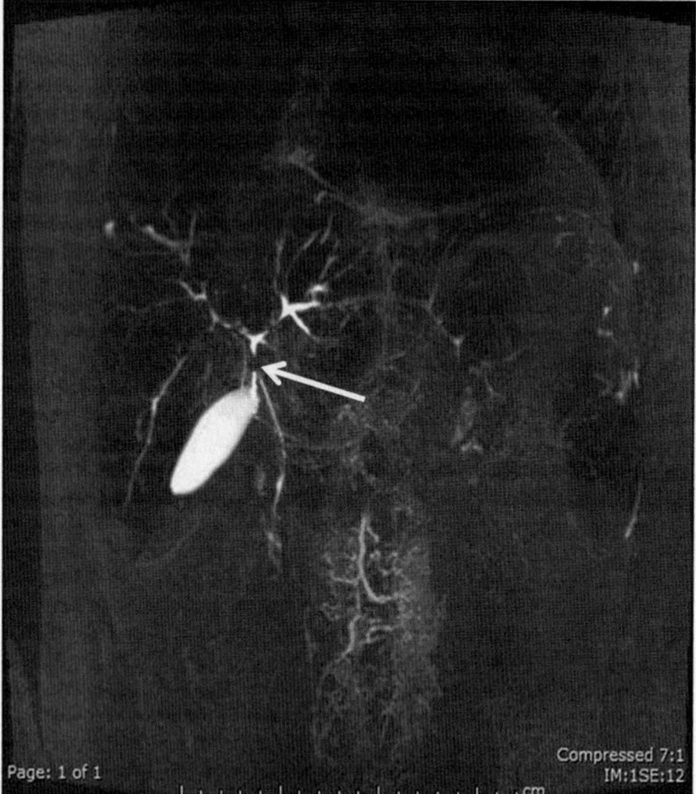

FIGURE 155-9. **Magnetic resonance cholangiopancreatography demonstrating the typical cholangiographic features of primary sclerosing cholangitis. Note the narrowed segment of the common bile duct *(arrow)* as well as the diffuse strictures and dilated segments of several intrahepatic bile ducts, giving the classic "beaded" appearance.**

patients with confirmed osteoporosis. Unfortunately, no medical treatment slows disease progression[A10]; ursodeoxycholic acid, D-penicillamine, corticosteroids, cyclosporine, methotrexate, and colchicine have all been shown to be ineffective for improving survival or delaying the time to liver transplantation. Whether repeated endoscopic treatment to maintain bile duct patency can improve outcomes is unknown.

Liver transplantation (Chapter 154) is the only potentially curative therapy. The 1-year and 5-year survival rates typically are in the 90% and 80% range, respectively. Primary sclerosing cholangitis may recur in the transplanted organ in 15 to 20% of patients.

PROGNOSIS

The natural history of primary sclerosing cholangitis is variable and incompletely understood. Asymptomatic patients have a much better prognosis than symptomatic patients, with 10-year actuarial survival rates of 80% and 50%, respectively. In symptomatic patients, the median time of survival until death or liver transplantation is 9 years, compared with 12 to 18 years for all patients with primary sclerosing cholangitis, regardless of symptoms. An elevated serum bilirubin level and hepatomegaly appear to correlate with a poor prognosis, whereas cholangiographic appearance, the presence or absence of inflammatory bowel disease, and the patient's age do not. Cholangiocarcinoma (Chapter 196) is a dreaded complication of primary sclerosing cholangitis, and the risk appears to be greatest in patients with long-standing ulcerative colitis and cirrhosis.

Choledochal Cysts and Anomalous Pancreaticobiliary Duct Junction

Choledochal cysts are uncommon anomalies of the biliary tree that are manifested as cystic dilation of the intrahepatic or extrahepatic ducts (or both). The incidence is 1 in 100,000 to 150,000 births in Western populations and 1 in 1000 in Asian populations. There is a 3 : 1 to 4 : 1 female-to-male preponderance. These cysts (E-Fig. 155-1) usually involve only the extrahepatic biliary tree, but they can present as extrapancreatic bile duct diverticula, involve only the intraduodenal part of the common bile duct, or present as multiple intrahepatic and extrahepatic cysts (Table 155-3). An anomalous pancreaticobiliary duct junction (E-Fig. 155-2) is frequently associated with choledochal cysts but may be found in isolation, especially in Asian populations.

TABLE 155-3 CLASSIFICATION OF CHOLEDOCHAL CYSTS

TYPES	DESCRIPTION	PROPORTION OF CHOLEDOCHAL CYSTS
I	Segmental or diffuse fusiform dilation of the bile duct	50-80%
II	Choledochal diverticulum	2%
III	Dilation of the intraduodenal portion of the bile duct	1.4-5%
IVa	Multiple intrahepatic and extrahepatic cysts	15-35%
IVb	Multiple extrahepatic cysts	
V (Caroli disease)	Single or multiple dilations of the intrahepatic ducts	20%

Patients with choledochoceles commonly have biliary colic, cholangitis, jaundice, or unexplained pancreatitis. Bile reflux may also result in acute pancreatitis or predispose to biliary cancers.

Cholangiography, preferably by ERCP, is the diagnostic "gold standard," although MRCP can also delineate the anatomy noninvasively. Because of the increased risk for development of biliary tract cancers, cyst resection (including cholecystectomy) is the generally recommended treatment, although it does not eliminate the risk entirely.[9]

Biliary Fistula

A biliary fistula represents an injury to the bile duct, most commonly seen as a complication of cholecystectomy, common bile duct exploration, or inadvertent operative injury of the bile duct or as a consequence of a local infection. Rarely, biliary fistulas result from long-standing untreated biliary tract disease. With more widespread use of laparoscopic cholecystectomy, the incidence of bile duct injury, including biliary fistula, has increased.

Postoperative bile duct leaks are usually manifested within a week after surgery, with patients presenting with abdominal pain (90%), tenderness (80%), fever (75%), nausea and vomiting (50%), and jaundice (40%). Clinically detectable ascites is rare. Biochemical testing is usually nonspecific, with variable elevations in serum liver test values and the white blood cell count.

Patients with suspected biliary fistulas often undergo abdominal ultrasonography or CT to look for evidence of a biloma as well as a hepatobiliary scan to diagnose the leak. However, ERCP is the most sensitive test to detect a biliary fistula. Treatment options for biliary leaks include percutaneously or endoscopically placed biliary drains or stents and surgical drainage and repair of the leak.

Vanishing Bile Duct Syndromes

The vanishing bile duct syndrome is characterized by a paucity of intrahepatic bile ducts, an elevated alkaline phosphatase level, and cholestasis. Causes include primary biliary cirrhosis, primary sclerosing cholangitis, autoimmune hepatitis (Chapter 149), graft-versus-host disease, chronic liver transplant rejection (Chapter 154), ischemia, intrahepatic chemotherapy, drug toxicity (e.g., ampicillin, amoxicillin, flucloxacillin, erythromycin, tetracycline, doxycycline, cotrimoxazole), human immunodeficiency virus (HIV) infection (Chapter 390), sarcoidosis (Chapter 95), and histiocytosis. Ursodeoxycholic acid (15 mg/kg) can increase bile flow, but the condition inexorably progresses to biliary cirrhosis, which ultimately requires liver transplantation.

PRIMARY BILIARY CIRRHOSIS

Primary biliary cirrhosis is an obliterative autoimmune cholangiopathy that involves the small and medium-sized bile ducts and that slowly progresses during a decade or so. As the ducts are obliterated, patients develop cholestasis, fibrosis, and, ultimately, liver failure.[10]

EPIDEMIOLOGY

About 95% of patients with primary biliary cirrhosis are women, and the peak age at onset is between 20 and 60 years. The incidence of the disease may be increasing. In the United States, the estimated annual incidence is about 4.5 per 100,000 per year for women and 0.7 for men. Because of the limited life expectancy of affected patients, the age- and gender-adjusted prevalence of primary biliary cirrhosis is about 65 per 100,000 in women and about 12 per 100,000 in men.

PATHOBIOLOGY

Although the mechanism of progressive destruction of the small interlobular ducts is unknown, primary biliary cirrhosis is considered to be an autoimmune disorder. Genome-wide studies show an association with HLA, interleukin-12A, and interleukin-12RB2 variants, suggesting that interleukin-12 signaling might be important. The disease progresses slowly and can eventually lead to biliary cirrhosis, portal hypertension, and liver failure. The classic histologic finding is noncaseating granulomas and paucity of bile ducts in the portal tracts.

CLINICAL MANIFESTATIONS

The most common symptoms are fatigue (50%), which can be debilitating and is unrelated to the degree of underlying liver disease, and pruritus (30%), but about 50% of patients are asymptomatic at the time of diagnosis. Many patients are initially seen by dermatologists for pruritus, which may be first noticed in pregnancy but persists after delivery.

Autoimmune syndromes associated with primary biliary cirrhosis include autoimmune thyroid dysfunction (Chapter 226), Sjögren syndrome (Chapter 268), Raynaud phenomenon (Chapter 267), and celiac disease (Chapter 140). Vitamin D malabsorption can also lead to metabolic bone disease (Chapters 243 and 244).

DIAGNOSIS

The first clue to primary biliary cirrhosis is an elevated serum alkaline phosphatase level, which should be confirmed by an elevated γ-glutamyl transpeptidase level (Chapter 147). The antimitochondrial antibody level has a sensitivity and specificity of more than 95% when the titer is higher than 1:40, and it may be positive even before there is any clinical or biochemical evidence of the disease. By comparison, the bilirubin level often is not elevated until later in the course of the disease, with most of the elevation typically due to an elevation in conjugated bilirubin. Total immunoglobulins are generally normal, but IgM levels can be elevated.

An ultrasound examination of the biliary tree is critical to confirm the absence of extrahepatic disease. A liver biopsy is occasionally needed to confirm the diagnosis, particularly in antimitochondrial antibody–negative patients, and to stage the disease.

TREATMENT Rx

Ursodeoxycholic acid therapy (12 to 15 mg/kg) improves serum bilirubin, alkaline phosphatase, and cholesterol levels and has a variable effect on pruritus. Unfortunately, it does not relieve fatigue, reduce mortality, or delay the need for liver transplantation.A11 Bezafibrate therapy also generally improves liver chemistry test results but not pruritus, liver-related mortality, or overall mortality.A12

There is no definite benefit from steroids, colchicine, azathioprine, or methotrexate. Bisphosphonates (Chapter 243) are commonly prescribed for the accompanying metabolic bone disease, but their benefit is uncertain.A13 Liver transplantation (Chapter 154) is indicated for refractory disease. The post-transplantation prognosis is excellent, with 2-year and 5-year survival rates of 80% and 70%, respectively. However, studies suggest an 8 to 40% recurrence in the transplanted liver.

PROGNOSIS

Up to two thirds of asymptomatic patients become symptomatic within 2 to 4 years. Significant bridging fibrosis or cirrhosis on biopsy carries a worse prognosis. Prognosis is also influenced by the serum bilirubin and albumin levels, the international normalized ratio, older age, and the presence of peripheral edema. Liver failure develops in about 25% of patients within 10 years after diagnosis, and median survival after diagnosis is 12 to 15 years.

Bile Duct Tumors

BENIGN

Benign bile duct tumors are exceedingly rare compared with malignant tumors and are much less common than benign gallbladder tumors. They can be divided into three histologic types (papillomas, adenomas, cystadenomas), may be solitary or multiple, and often are found incidentally during the evaluation of bile duct dilation or intraductal filling defects. Patients may be asymptomatic or have symptoms of biliary obstruction. Treatment typically consists of surgical bile duct resection with hepaticojejunostomy reconstruction. Even benign tumors tend to recur after excision, and some undergo malignant change.

CHOLANGIOCARCINOMA

Cholangiocarcinoma is discussed in Chapter 196.

Ampullary Tumors

Benign ampullary lesions seen on endoscopic or radiologic studies include heterotopic gastric mucosa, a lipoma, or an impacted common bile duct stone. Primary tumors of the ampulla of Vater can be premalignant or malignant, but the overwhelming majority (>95%) are either adenomas or adenocarcinomas. The prevalence of ampullary adenomas has been estimated to be 0.04 to 0.12% in autopsy series, but the prevalence is higher in patients with hereditary polyposis syndromes (Chapter 193), in which ampullary adenomas occur in up to 80% of individuals and progress to malignancy in 4%.

Malignant ampullary lesions are most commonly adenocarcinomas, although metastatic breast cancer, renal cell cancers, and melanomas also have been identified. Carcinoid tumors (Chapter 232) and other neuroendocrine tumors are rare. Ampullary adenomas probably follow an adenoma to carcinoma sequence similar to colorectal adenocarcinoma (Chapter 193), with a 25 to 85% risk of transformation to carcinoma.

Patients with ampullary lesions may present with biliary colic, obstructive jaundice, pancreatitis, or nonspecific upper abdominal pain, with or without fluctuating serum liver test results, malaise, and anorexia. However, ampullary lesions are often found incidentally on cross-sectional imaging or during upper endoscopy performed for a different indication.[11]

For ampullary adenomas, options include observation with surveillance biopsies and attempts to resect the lesion completely through endoscopy or surgery. Surveillance of an ampullary adenoma in the setting of familial adenomatous polyposis is reasonable if the lesion is small (<1 cm) and asymptomatic, but resection is preferred if advanced histology (e.g., villous features, dysplasia) is identified. Surgical resection has been the standard for ampullary tumors. Treatment modalities include pancreatoduodenectomy, which has a high rate of morbid and even fatal complications, and transduodenal excision, which is associated with high recurrence rates. The 5-year survival rates after pancreaticoduodenectomy range from 64 to 80% for patients with node-negative disease and from 17 to 50% for node-positive disease. Limited data exist regarding adjuvant therapy, the benefits of which are uncertain. A common practice is to treat these patients in a manner similar to patients with resected pancreatic adenocarcinomas (Chapter 194). Patients who present with unresectable disease tend to receive combination gemcitabine (1000 mg/m^2) plus cisplatin (25 mg/m^2) chemotherapy, each administered on days 1 and 8, every 3 weeks for eight cycles.A14 Palliative biliary stenting can be performed in individuals who have a short life expectancy.

In patients with small, localized, and clearly benign ampullary adenomas, endoscopic resection represents an alternative to surgical therapy in appropriately selected patients (E-Fig. 155-3). Whether endoscopic resection is effective for larger or higher risk adenomas is uncertain. Furthermore, recurrence rates after endoscopic papillectomy approach 20%, thereby emphasizing the need for careful follow-up endoscopic surveillance.

Sphincter of Oddi Dysfunction

Sphincter of Oddi dysfunction is a benign, noncalculous obstruction to flow of bile or pancreatic juice through the pancreaticobiliary junction. It may be manifested clinically by pain, pancreatitis (Chapter 144), abnormal liver test results, or abnormal pancreatic enzymes. Post-cholecystectomy pain resembling the patient's preoperative biliary colic occurs in at least 10 to 20% of patients.

Evaluation of patients with suspected sphincter of Oddi dysfunction includes standard serum liver chemistries, serum amylase and lipase levels, and an abdominal ultrasound examination or CT scan. The specimens for serum enzyme studies should be drawn during bouts of pain, if possible. Mild elevations (less than two times the upper limits of normal) are frequent in sphincter of Oddi dysfunction, whereas greater abnormalities are more suggestive of stones, tumors, and parenchymal liver disease. The findings on CT and abdominal ultrasound studies are usually normal, but abnormal liver or pancreatic enyzmes or a dilated bile duct or pancreatic duct may occasionally be found. ERCP and sphincter of Oddi manometry may be considered in patients who have objective evidence of pancreatic or biliary disease (abnormal liver or pancreatic enzymes or a dilated bile or pancreatic duct) or clinically significant or disabling symptoms and in whom definitive sphincter ablation is planned if abnormal sphincter function is found. In patients without objective evidence of pancreatic or biliary disease, ERCP and manometry are no longer recommended.[A15]

Medical therapy with nonspecific antispasmodics (e.g., dicyclomine, 10 to 20 mg every 6 hours; hyoscyamine, 0.375 mg every 12 hours) or smooth muscle relaxants (e.g., nifedipine, 60 mg daily) for a 1-month trial should be considered in patients with pancreaticobiliary-type pain (with or without abnormal liver enzyme, amylase, or lipase levels) or a dilated bile or pancreatic duct. If patients do not respond satisfactorily, ERCP and endoscopic sphincterotomy can improve pain in 55 to 95% of patients with abnormal findings on laboratory testing or abdominal imaging. Alternatively, only about 25% of patients without objective evidence of pancreatic or biliary disease improve after sphincterotomy.

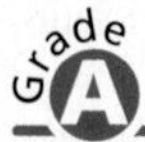

Grade A References

A1. Gurusamy KS, Koti R, Fusai G, et al. Early versus delayed laparoscopic cholecystectomy for uncomplicated biliary colic. *Cochrane Database Syst Rev*. 2013;6:CD007196.
A2. Vaughan J, Gurusamy KS, Davidson BR. Day-surgery versus overnight stay surgery for laparoscopic cholecystectomy. *Cochrane Database Syst Rev*. 2013;7:CD006798.
A3. Gurusamy KS, Davidson C, Gluud C, et al. Early versus delayed laparoscopic cholecystectomy for people with acute cholecystitis. *Cochrane Database Syst Rev*. 2013;6:CD005440.
A4. Iranmanesh P, Frossard JL, Mugnier-Konrad B, et al. Initial cholecystectomy vs sequential common duct endoscopic assessment and subsequent cholecystectomy for suspected gallstone migration: a randomized clinical trial. *JAMA*. 2014;312:137-144.
A5. Stokes CS, Gluud LL, Casper M, et al. Ursodeoxycholic acid and diets higher in fat prevent gallbladder stones during weight loss: a meta-analysis of randomized controlled trials. *Clin Gastroenterol Hepatol*. 2014;12:1090-1100.
A6. Ding G, Cai W, Qin M. Single-stage vs. two-stage management for concomitant gallstones and common bile duct stones: a prospective randomized trial with long-term follow-up. *J Gastrointest Surg*. 2014;18:947-951.
A7. Teoh AY, Cheung FK, Hu B, et al. Randomized trial of endoscopic sphincterotomy with balloon dilation versus endoscopic sphincterotomy alone for removal of bile duct stones. *Gastroenterology*. 2013;144:341-345.
A8. Zhang RL, Zhao H, Dai YM, et al. Endoscopic nasobiliary drainage with sphincterotomy in acute obstructive cholangitis: a prospective randomized controlled trial. *J Dig Dis*. 2014;15:78-84.
A9. Gurusamy KS, Nagendran M, Davidson BR. Early versus delayed laparoscopic cholecystectomy for acute gallstone pancreatitis. *Cochrane Database Syst Rev*. 2013;9:CD010326.
A10. Lindor KD, Kowdley KV, Luketic VA, et al. High-dose ursodeoxycholic acid for the treatment of primary sclerosing cholangitis. *Hepatology*. 2009;50:808-814.
A11. Rudic JS, Poropat G, Krstic MN, et al. Ursodeoxycholic acid for primary biliary cirrhosis. *Cochrane Database Syst Rev*. 2012;12:CD000551.
A12. Rudic JS, Poropat G, Krstic MN, et al. Bezafibrate for primary biliary cirrhosis. *Cochrane Database Syst Rev*. 2012;1:CD009145.
A13. Rudic JS, Giljaca V, Krstic MN, et al. Bisphosphonates for osteoporosis in primary biliary cirrhosis. *Cochrane Database Syst Rev*. 2011;12:CD009144.
A14. Valle J, Wasan H, Palmer DH, et al. Cisplatin plus gemcitabine versus gemcitabine for biliary tract cancer. *N Eng J Med*. 2010;362:1273-1281.
A15. Cotton PB, Durkalski V, Romagnuolo J, et al. Effect of endoscopic sphincterotomy for suspected sphincter of Oddi dysfunction on pain-related disability following cholecystectomy: the EPISOD randomized clinical trial. *JAMA*. 2014;311:2101-2109.

GENERAL REFERENCES

For the General References and other additional features, please visit Expert Consult at https://expertconsult.inkling.com.

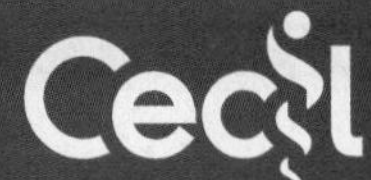

XIV

HEMATOLOGIC DISEASES

156

HEMATOPOIESIS AND HEMATOPOIETIC GROWTH FACTORS

KENNETH KAUSHANSKY

Hematopoiesis is the process by which bone marrow stem cells develop into all of the cell types present in the blood (erythrocytes, neutrophils, eosinophils, basophils, monocytes, platelets, T lymphocytes, B lymphocytes, natural killer cells) (Fig. 156-1). The regulation of the numbers of each cell type is carefully controlled by paracrine and endocrine hematopoietic growth factors, which exert antiapoptotic, proliferative, and differentiative effects on hematopoietic stem, progenitor, and maturing blood cells. Many of these glycoproteins are produced by recombinant DNA technology and have been among the most successful therapeutics in modern medicine.

HEMATOPOIETIC STEM AND PROGENITOR CELLS

Hematopoietic stem cells comprise one in 10^5 to 10^6 marrow cells and are not morphologically distinguishable from other progenitors or small lymphocytes but can be purified to homogeneity using physical characteristics and combinations of monoclonal antibodies (including $CD34^+$) to cell surface proteins.[1] The two critical characteristics of a hematopoietic stem cell are its ability to differentiate into all blood cell types and to self-renew. The decision to self-renew or differentiate is a stochastic process, at the stem cell stage and at the subsequent multipotent or unipotent stages of differentiation, that can be influenced by a number of cell extrinsic (growth factors and stromal proteins) and cell intrinsic (transcription factors) molecules. Hematopoietic stems cells reside in specialized microenvironments (niches) within the bone marrow. The complex and diverse stromal cell populations that comprise the stem cell niche provide signals that support critical stem cell properties such as maintenance, self-renewal capacity, and long-term multilineage repopulation ability.[2]

HEMATOPOIETIC CELL EXPANSION: HEMATOPOIETIC GROWTH FACTORS

A large number of transcription factors regulate stem cell number and differentiation state. Several molecular switches have been identified that determine hematopoietic cell fate.

Equally important to hematopoiesis is a group of hematopoietic growth factors that share structural homology and bind to nonredundant type I transmembrane proteins belonging to the cytokine receptor family. Many of these proteins are the physiological regulators of a specific lineage of blood cells (e.g., erythropoietin, granulocyte colony-stimulating factor, thrombopoietin); others appear to represent redundant hematopoietic growth-promoting activities of molecules essential for other biologic functions (e.g., interleukin-3 [IL-3], interleukin-11 [IL-11], granulocyte-macrophage colony-stimulating factor).

Erythropoietin is produced predominantly by the kidneys and to a lesser extent in the liver and acts on marrow erythroid progenitors to enhance their survival, proliferation, and differentiation. Levels of erythropoietin are inversely related to hemoglobin concentrations in the blood, as reflected in renal oxygen tension. In the presence of tissue (renal) hypoxia, the transcription factor hypoxia-induced factor (HIF) 1α is stabilized against proteasome-mediated destruction and drives erythropoietin transcription by binding to a critical hypoxia responsive element located in the 3′ untranslated region of the gene. Genetic elimination of erythropoietin or its receptor results in embryonic lethality, establishing that although other cytokines can influence erythropoiesis, red blood cell production is absolutely dependent on the hormone.

Granulocyte colony-stimulating factor stimulates the production of neutrophils from their marrow progenitors (Fig. 156-2). Levels of the hormone are also inversely related to neutrophil numbers but are regulated primarily by inflammatory stimuli, including tumor necrosis factor-α (TNF-α) and IL-1α acting on endothelial cells, fibroblasts, and macrophages. Similar to the action of erythropoietin on erythroid progenitors, granulocyte colony-stimulating factor acts to enhance the survival, proliferation, and differentiation of neutrophil progenitors. In addition, the cytokine acts to functionally activate the mature cells it helps to produce. Genetic elimination of granulocyte colony-stimulating factor or its receptor in mice reduces neutrophil levels to 25% of normal, the only hormone known to exert this great an impact on granulopoiesis.

Thrombopoietin, the primary regulator of platelet production, is produced in the liver and kidney and by marrow stromal cells and is regulated by both platelet receptor–mediated uptake and destruction and by transcriptional feedback inhibition of the thrombopoietin gene in marrow stromal cells by platelet granule proteins.[3] The plasma levels of free thrombopoietin are normally inversely related to bone marrow megakaryocyte (MK) and platelet mass. In a hypoproliferative thrombocytopenia, therefore, the resultant increase in plasma free thrombopoietin that is not bound to its MK and platelet receptors will drive a compensatory increase in thrombopoiesis. Similar to granulocyte colony-stimulating factor, thrombopoietin stimulates the survival, proliferation, and differentiation of its corresponding lineage, MKs and their precursors, and primes mature platelets to respond to platelet activation agonists. Genetic elimination of thrombopoietin or its receptor in mice or congenital nonsense or missense mutations in the gene for the thrombopoietin receptor in humans result in platelet levels approximately 10% of normal. Elimination of the thrombopoietin receptor in children leads to aplastic anemia by 1 to 2 years of age.

Other cytokine–receptor systems related to erythropoietin, granulocyte colony-stimulating factor, and thrombopoietin essential for one or more aspects of hematopoiesis include IL-7, critical for all types of lymphocyte production; IL-5, the primary regulator of eosinophil production; IL-4, responsible for immunoglobulin class switching in B lymphocytes; IL-15, essential for normal natural killer cell differentiation; and IL-2, a lymphocyte activation cytokine. They display modest effects on blood cell growth, but their genetic elimination fails to affect basal or stimulated production of those cells.

A second class of cytokines and receptors that influences hematopoiesis is exemplified by the c-kit receptor, a member of the receptor tyrosine kinase family of surface proteins, and its cognate ligand, stem cell factor (also termed steel factor or kit-ligand). Although the c-kit receptor is structurally distinct from members of the hematopoietic cytokine receptor family, possessing an intrinsic tyrosine kinase motif in its cytoplasmic domain, stem cell factor is structurally related to the cytokines that bind to members of the hematopoietic growth factor family. Genetic deletion of stem cell factor or the c-kit receptor results in the near complete elimination of hematopoietic stem cells, erythroid precursors and basophils, and mast cells. Two other hematopoietic members of this family of cytokines and receptors are Flt3 ligand and its receptor Flt-3 and monocyte colony-stimulating factor and its receptor, c-Fms. Similar to stem cell factor, both Flt3 ligand and monocyte colony-stimulating factor play nonredundant roles in hematopoiesis, inducing the formation of dendritic cells and monocytes, respectively.

The molecular mechanisms by which the hematopoietic growth factors affect blood cell survival, proliferation, and differentiation are becoming increasingly well understood. Binding of cognate ligand to each of the hematopoietic cytokine receptors results in activation of one or more tyrosine kinases, either tethered cytoplasmic kinases of the Janus (JAK) family for the hematopoietic cytokine receptor family or the intrinsic kinase of the cytokines that use the receptor tyrosine kinase class of receptors (stem cell factor, Flt3 ligand, and monocyte colony-stimulating factor). After activation, these kinases phosphorylate tyrosine residues within the cytoplasmic domains of each receptor, providing docking sites for cytoplasmic signaling intermediates possessing Src homology (SH)2 domains. Among the best characterized SH2 domain containing proteins that bind to hematopoietic receptors are nascent transcription factors, such as the signal transducers and activators of transcription (STAT) proteins; adapter proteins, including Grb2, Gab1, tensin2, and SHC; phosphatases, for example, SHP1 and SHP2; and the regulatory subunit (p85) of phosphoinositol-3-kinase (PI3K). When bound to one or more of the newly induced phosphotyrosine residues of the cytokine receptor or receptor tyrosine kinase, these secondary molecules are phosphorylated, either by JAK or other kinases, making them competent to bind additional molecules (e.g., the adapters that ultimately activate Ras, and p85 PI3K that binds its kinase [p110] subunit) or are activated as transcription factors (e.g., STATs). The downstream effector molecules then activated include a number kinases, transporter molecules, and transcription factors, ultimately leading to hematopoietic cell survival, proliferation, and differentiation.

CLINICAL USES OF HEMATOPOIETIC CELLS AND GROWTH FACTORS

The clinical development of erythropoietin, granulocyte colony-stimulating factor, and thrombopoietin mimetics represent some of the very best

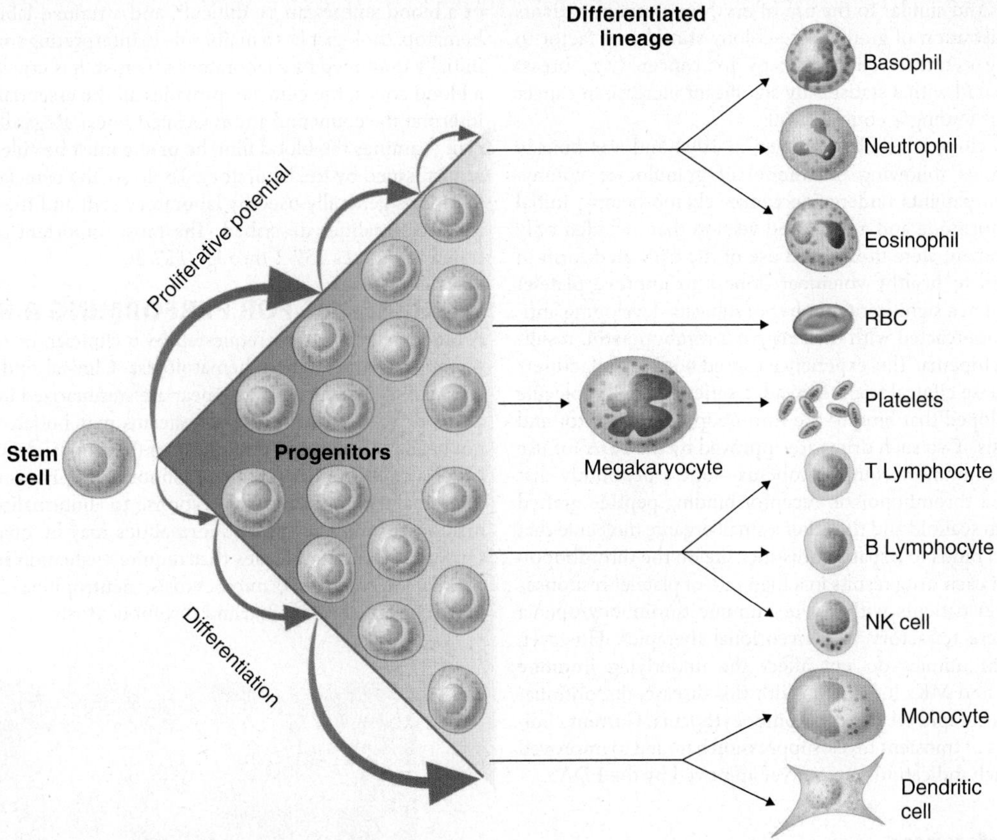

FIGURE 156-1. Hierarchical model of lymphohematopoiesis. NK = natural killer; RBC = red blood cell.

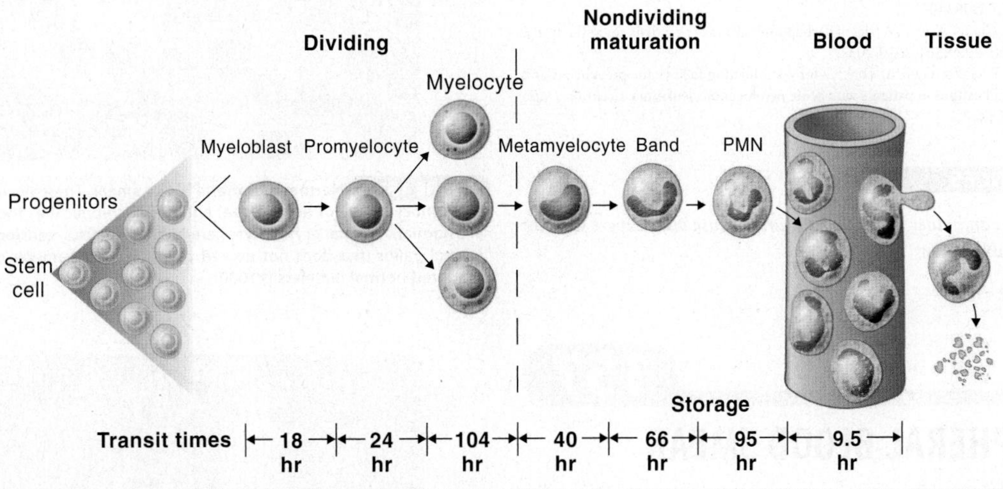

FIGURE 156-2. Neutrophil production system. PMN = polymorphonuclear leukocyte.

examples of harnessing recombinant DNA technology for therapeutic benefit. Patients with renal failure, widespread inflammation, or bone marrow replacement and those undergoing chemotherapy for cancer all experience variable degrees of anemia that are often very debilitating. Administration of erythropoietic stimulating agents almost invariably results in a rapid reticulocyte response and correction of the anemia. Most patients undergo an enhanced sense of well being as the blood hemoglobin concentration rises to 10 g/dL. Clinical trials have demonstrated the efficacy of these agents in patients with renal failure and with cancer, although recent analyses call into question the safety of these agents in some settings.[A1][A2] For example, patients receiving higher levels of the drug for anemia secondary to kidney failure progressed to requiring dialysis more frequently and experienced increased cardiovascular events, such as myocardial infarction and stroke, than patients on low levels of the hormone sufficient to maintain their blood Hgb at 10 g/dL or lower.[A3] And patients receiving erythropoietin for cancer also experienced increased relapses of their tumors than individuals not receiving the hormone. The only patients who regularly demonstrate a poor response are individuals with severe inflammation (Chapter 158). Overall, erythropoietic stimulating agents are safe and effective drugs for patients with anemia caused by a wide range of conditions, but their use and dose must be carefully considered.

Many patients undergoing cytotoxic therapy for cancer experience severe neutropenia and are thus at substantial risk for life-threatening infection. Clinical trials of recombinant granulocyte colony-stimulating factor in patients undergoing aggressive chemotherapy for leukemia and solid tumors resulted in the Food and Drug Administration (FDA) approval of the drug for use in patients undergoing chemotherapy of intensity sufficient to produce severe neutropenia (Chapter 167). The use of the drug is associated with the more rapid return of neutrophils to safe levels if administered soon after the inciting chemotherapy is completed but not at the nadir of neutrophil production and results in lower risk of severe infections. However, the use of granulocyte colony-stimulating factor has not enhanced survival in patients with any tumor type.[A4] And similar to the use of erythropoietin in patients with cancer, the administration of granulocyte colony-stimulating factor to some patients receiving cytotoxic chemotherapy for cancer, (e.g., breast cancer) has been associated with a statistically significant increase in cancer recurrence, although this finding is controversial.

Thrombopoietin was cloned and characterized in 1994 and was quickly advanced to clinical trials following the model of granulocyte colony-stimulating factor use in patients undergoing cancer chemotherapy. Initial results with the intact hormone and a truncated version that included only the receptor-binding domain were mixed, and use of the truncated form of the drug, administration to healthy volunteer donors to improve platelet apheresis yields, resulted in a significant number of subjects developing anti-drug antibodies that cross-reacted with their native thrombopoietin, resulting in severe thrombocytopenia. This experience caused both manufacturers of thrombopoietin to cease clinical trials. Instead, a series of small molecule mimics have been developed that bind to the thrombopoietin receptor and stimulate thrombopoiesis. Two such drugs are approved by the FDA for use in patients with severe immune thrombocytopenia—one a peptibody that contains four copies of a thrombopoietin receptor binding peptide grafted onto an immunoglobulin scaffold and the other a small organic molecule that is orally bioavailable and binds to a spatially distinct site on the thrombopoietin receptor. The use of each drug results in a high rate of platelet responses into the normal range in patients with severe immune thrombocytopenia (Chapter 172) who were refractory to conventional therapies. However, because thrombopoietin mimics do not affect the underlying immune destruction of platelets and MKs in patients with this disease, discontinuation of each drug results in rapid relapse of thrombocytopenia. Current clinical trials in other settings of transient myelosuppression have led to improved platelet recovery, but such indications are not yet approved by the FDA.

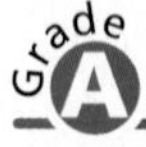

Grade A References

A1. Palmer SC, Saglimbene V, Craig JC, et al. Darbepoetin for the anaemia of chronic kidney disease. *Cochrane Database Syst Rev.* 2014;3:CD009297.

A2. Tonia T, Mettler A, Robert N, et al. Erythropoietin or darbepoetin for patients with cancer. *Cochrane Database Syst Rev.* 2012;12:CD003407.

A3. Pfeffer MA, Burdmann EA, Chen CY, et al. A trial of darbepoetin alfa in type 2 diabetes and chronic kidney disease. *N Engl J Med.* 2009;361:2019-2032.

A4. Gurion R, Belnik-Plitman Y, Gafter-Gvili A, et al. Colony-stimulating factors for prevention and treatment of infectious complications in patients with acute myelogenous leukemia. *Cochrane Database Syst Rev.* 2012;6:CD008238.

GENERAL REFERENCES

For the General References and other additional features, please visit Expert Consult at https://expertconsult.inkling.com.

157 THE PERIPHERAL BLOOD SMEAR

BARBARA J. BAIN

With the development of sophisticated automated instruments to count and characterize blood cells, Romanowsky (Wright-Giemsa or May-Grünwald-Giemsa)–stained peripheral blood smears are now performed on only a minority of blood specimens received in a hematology laboratory. Nevertheless, the blood smear remains important for a number of reasons: it can (1) verify the result of an automated instrument, (2) provide an immediate specific diagnosis, or (3) indicate a narrow range of diagnostic possibilities, permitting a focused rather than indiscriminate investigation.[1-3] A blood film can provide a rapid diagnosis in cases in which speed is crucial, such as in acute promyelocytic leukemia, thrombotic thrombocytopenic purpura, Burkitt lymphoma, and certain infections.[4,5] Sometimes a smear provides unexpected information that is of value in patient management.

Usually, blood smears are initially interpreted by a laboratory scientist. In some countries, it is customary for clinicians to examine the blood smears of their own patients because the clinician has the final responsibility for integrating all information and making a diagnosis. However, the interpretation of a blood smear can be difficult, and a trained laboratory hematologist or hematopathologist has a major role in interpreting smears that may have been initially examined by a laboratory scientist. It is crucial that, when requesting a blood count, the clinician provides all the essential information needed to interpret the count and any associated smear. Regardless of whether the clinician examines the blood film, he or she must be able to interpret the written report issued by the laboratory. To do so, the clinician must be familiar with the terms generally used by laboratory staff and the possible significance of the abnormalities described. The most important of these terms are illustrated in Figures 157-1 through 157-20.

REASONS FOR PERFORMING A BLOOD SMEAR

A blood smear may be requested by a clinician or initiated by a laboratory scientist or a laboratory hematologist. Clinical findings that should lead a clinician to request a blood smear are summarized in Table 157-1.

Laboratory scientists and physicians may initiate a blood smear that has not been requested by the clinician if the clinical details indicate the possibility of a significant hematologic abnormality. However, they are also likely to evaluate a blood smear in response to abnormalities revealed by an automated instrument. These abnormalities may be quantitative or qualitative. Quantitative abnormalities that require evaluation include anemia, polycythemia, macrocytosis, microcytosis, neutrophilia, lymphocytosis, eosinophilia, thrombocytopenia, and thrombocytosis.

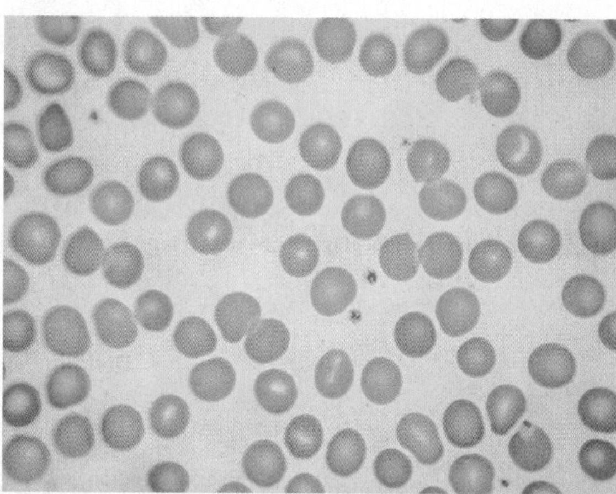

FIGURE 157-1. Normal peripheral blood smear. These normal red cells are described as *normocytic* (i.e., of normal size) and *normochromic* (i.e., their staining characteristics are normal). Normal erythrocytes are biconcave discs, causing them to have an area of central pallor that does not exceed one third the diameter of the cell. There are also scattered normal platelets (×1000).

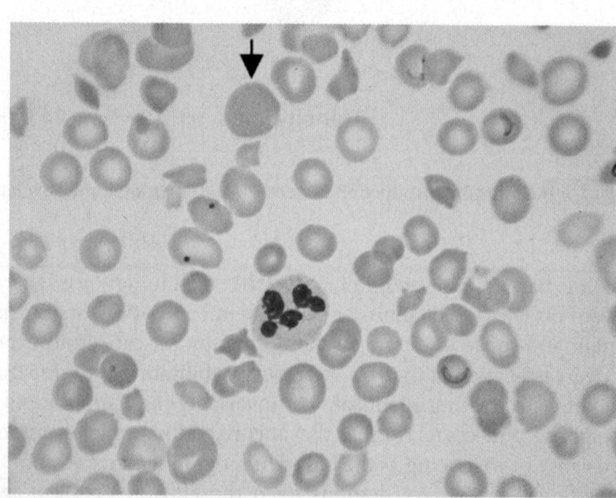

FIGURE 157-2. Smear showing multiple abnormalities. There is *anisocytosis,* defined as an increased variation in cell size; *poikilocytosis,* defined as an increased variation in cell shape; and *polychromasia,* defined as the presence of erythrocytes with a blue tinge to their cytoplasm—indicating a young cell recently released from the bone marrow in which the polychromasia is due to the presence of RNA. *Polychromatic cells* are erythrocytes with a blue tinge; because polychromatic cells are larger than normal mature erythrocytes, they are known as *polychromatic macrocytes (arrow).* The film also shows two cells containing bluish purple *Howell-Jolly bodies;* these inclusions are nuclear remnants (×1000).

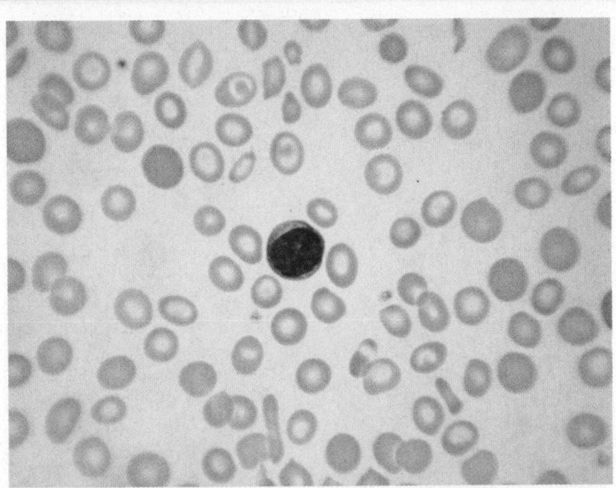

FIGURE 157-3. Microcytic red cells from a case of thalassemia minor. In a blood smear, a *microcyte* can be defined as a cell with a diameter less than that of the nucleus of a normal small lymphocyte. There are also some cells showing *hypochromia*, an area of central pallor that is larger than one third of the diameter of the red cell. In addition, there are two *target cells*, with a hemoglobinized area in the center of the area of pallor (×1000).

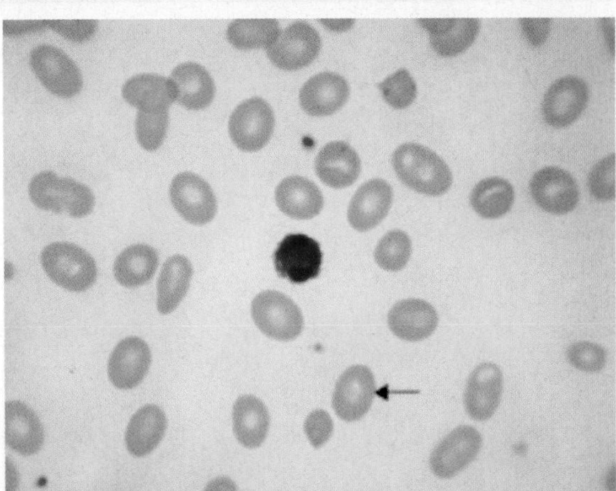

FIGURE 157-4. Macrocytic anemia. A *macrocyte* is recognized on a blood film as a cell with a diameter that is considerably greater than that of the nucleus of a small lymphocyte. In addition, this smear shows *oval macrocytes* (also known as *macro-ovalocytes*), defined as cells that are larger than normal and oval in shape *(arrow)*. They are of considerable diagnostic importance, being characteristic of megaloblastic anemia; they can also be seen in dyserythropoiesis (×1000).

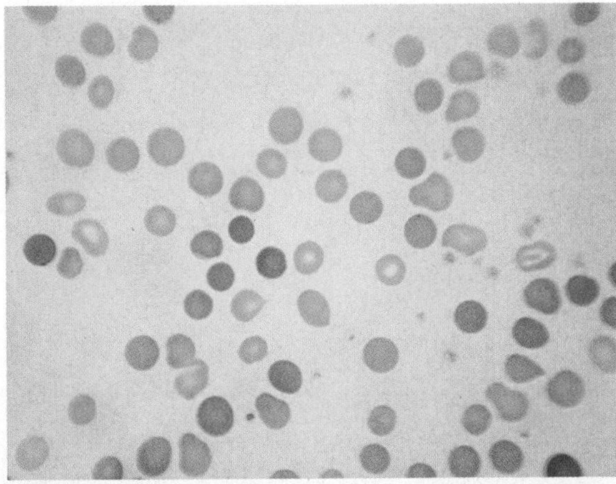

FIGURE 157-5. Hereditary spherocytosis. A *spherocyte* is a red cell that lacks central pallor because of its spherical shape. In hereditary spherocytosis, there are usually cells in which the central pallor is reduced rather than absent, and they are intermediate in shape between a spherocyte and a *discocyte,* which is an erythrocyte with the normal shape of a biconcave disc (×1000).

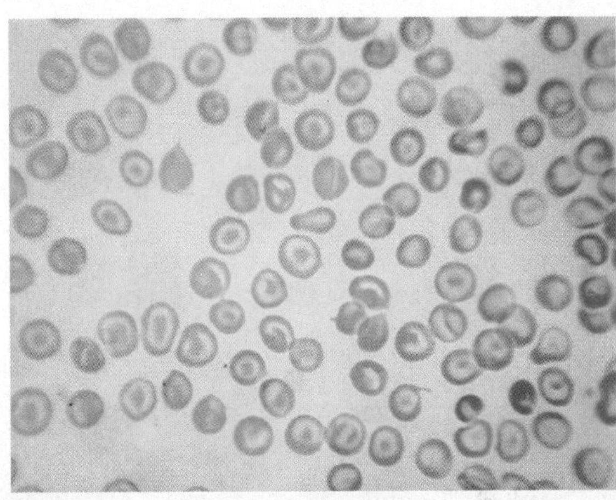

FIGURE 157-6. Target cells. A *target cell* is an erythrocyte with a hemoglobinized area in the middle of the normal area of central pallor (×1000).

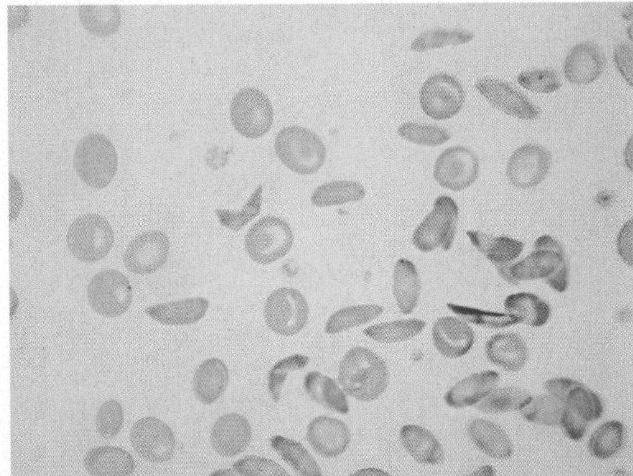

FIGURE 157-7. Sickle cells. A *sickle cell* is a cell with a sickle or crescent shape resulting from the polymerization of hemoglobin S. These cells are seen not only in sickle cell anemia (homozygosity for hemoglobin S) but also in compound heterozygous states such as sickle cell/hemoglobin C disease and sickle cell/β-thalassemia, which also lead to sickle cell disease. This smear also shows target cells and boat-shaped cells with a lesser degree of polymerization of hemoglobin S than in a classic sickle cell (×1000).

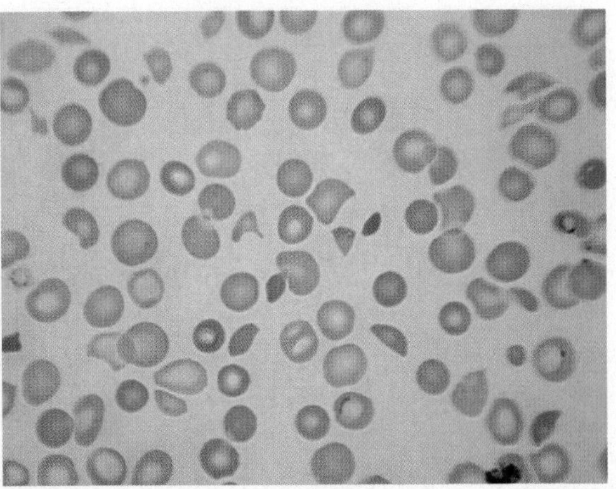

FIGURE 157-8. Red cell fragmentation. *Red cell fragments* or *schistocytes* are defined as fragments of erythrocytes. In addition to small angular fragments, there may be *microspherocytes,* cells of reduced size and spherical in form (also known as *spheroschistocytes*), and *keratocytes,* cells with two horn-like projections. Keratocytes can result from removal of a Heinz body, as well as from red cell fragmentation. Some schistocytes are referred to as *helmet cells* because of their typical shape. Schistocytes are seen in microangiopathic hemolytic anemias and in mechanical hemolysis (×1000).

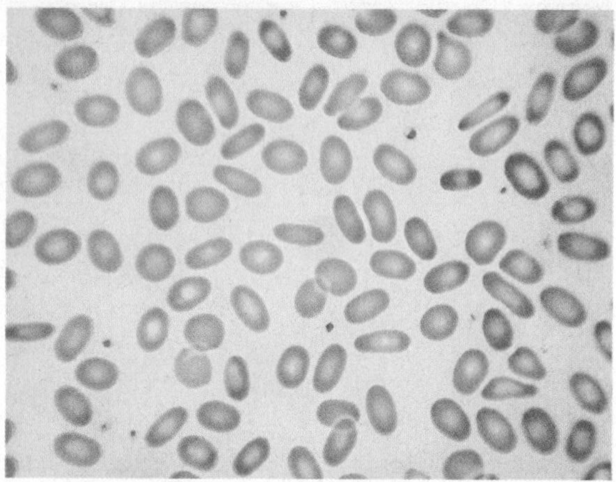

FIGURE 157-9. Hereditary elliptocytosis. An *elliptocyte* is an elliptical red cell. When seen in the numbers present in this smear, they are indicative of hereditary elliptocytosis; smaller numbers are seen in other conditions such as iron deficiency anemia, in which they are sometimes referred to as *pencil cells* (×1000).

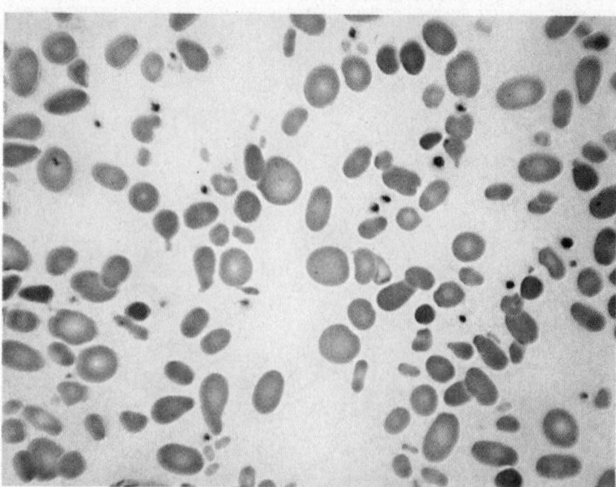

FIGURE 157-10. Hereditary pyropoikilocytosis. This smear shows striking poikilocytosis, including elliptocytes, microspherocytes and other fragments, and teardrop cells. This congenital condition, which is related to hereditary elliptocytosis, usually results from the inheritance of two different mutated genes from the two parents and is characterized by a severe hemolytic anemia (×1000).

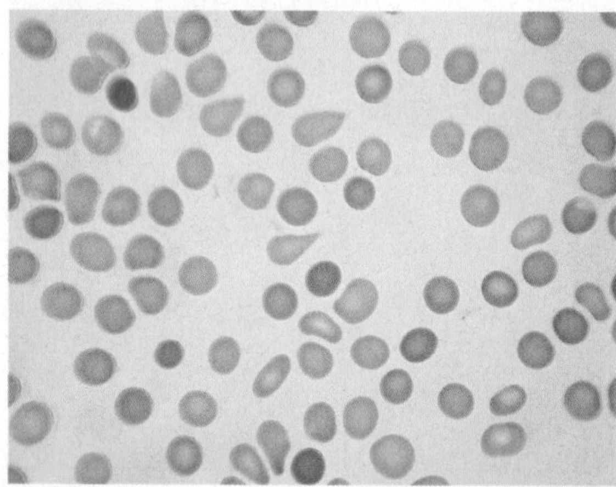

FIGURE 157-11. Teardrop poikilocytes. *Teardrop poikilocytes,* or *dacrocytes,* are teardrop-shaped red cells; they are characteristic of primary myelofibrosis but are also seen in megaloblastic anemia (×1000).

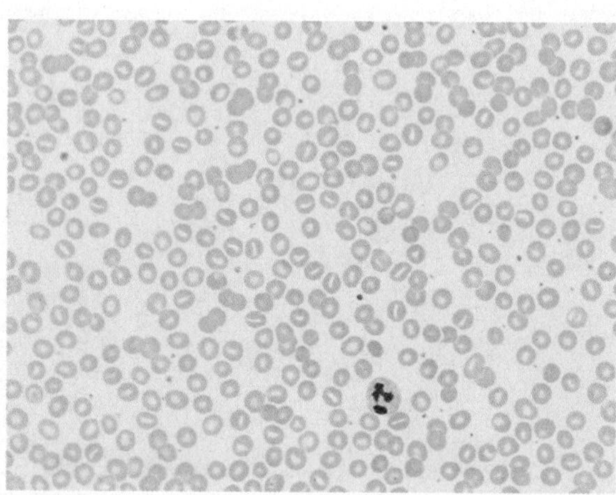

FIGURE 157-12. Stomatocytosis. A *stomatocyte* is a cell that appears to have a central mouth-shaped or slit-like stoma. Among the less common causes is hereditary stomatocytosis. Alcohol and hydroxycarbamide therapy are more common causes (×400).

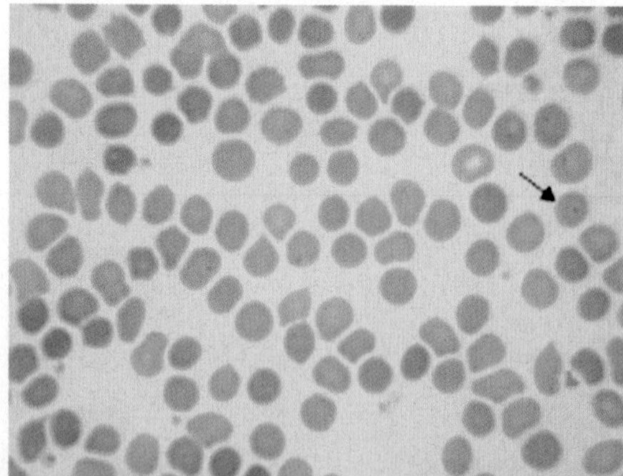

FIGURE 157-13. Numerous Pappenheimer bodies. A *Pappenheimer body* is an iron-containing red cell inclusion *(arrow)*. It is smaller and more angular than a Howell-Jolly body and stains navy blue rather than purple. Pappenheimer bodies are seen following splenectomy and in sideroblastic anemias (×1000).

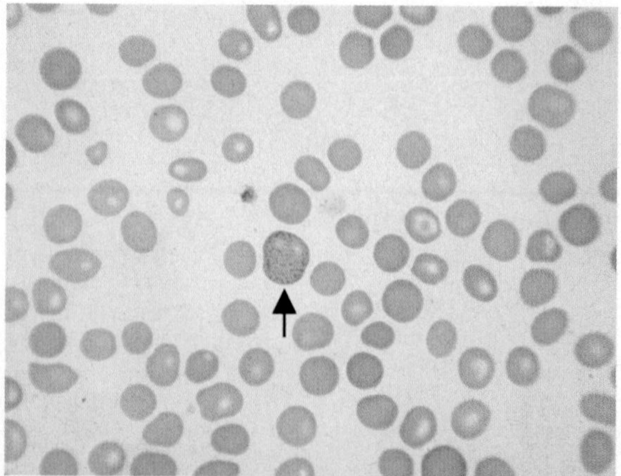

FIGURE 157-14. Basophilic stippling. *Basophilic stippling* means that there are fine (as in this case) or coarse purplish blue dots dispersed through the red cell *(arrow)*. They are a very nonspecific feature occurring in thalassemia trait, lead poisoning, pyrimidine 5′-nucleotidase deficiency, and dyserythropoiesis in general (×1000).

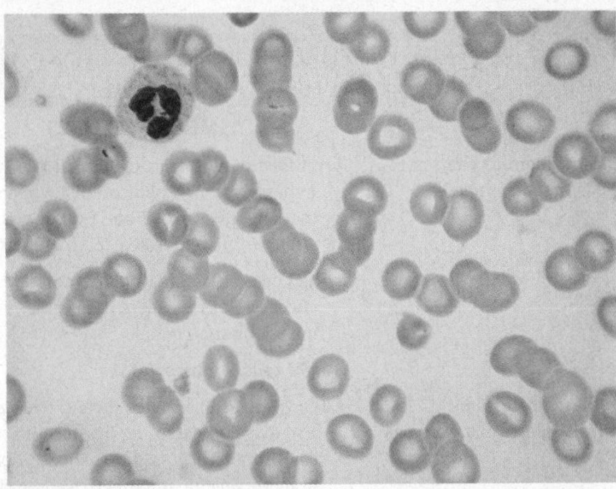

FIGURE 157-15. **Rouleaux formation.** *Rouleaux* are stacks of red cells, often compared to stacks of coins. They result from an increase of high-molecular-weight globulins in the plasma, either as a reactive change or as a result of secretion of a paraprotein in a plasma cell neoplasm (×1000).

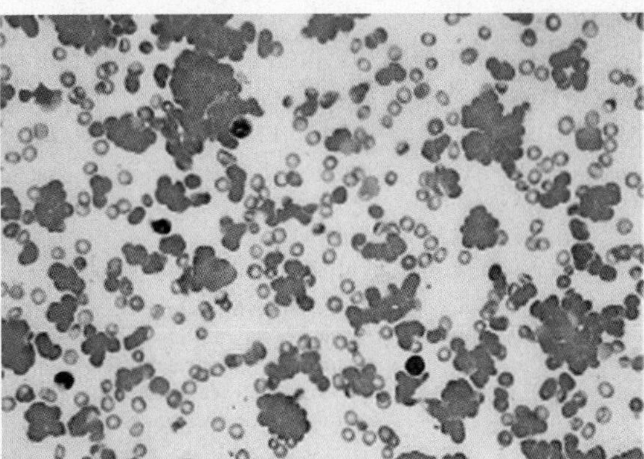

FIGURE 157-16. **Red cell agglutination.** *Red cell agglutinates* are irregular aggregates of red cells, as seen in *Mycoplasma pneumoniae* infection. They are also seen in other infections, such as infectious mononucleosis, and in chronic cold hemagglutinin disease (×100). (Courtesy of Jean Schafer.)

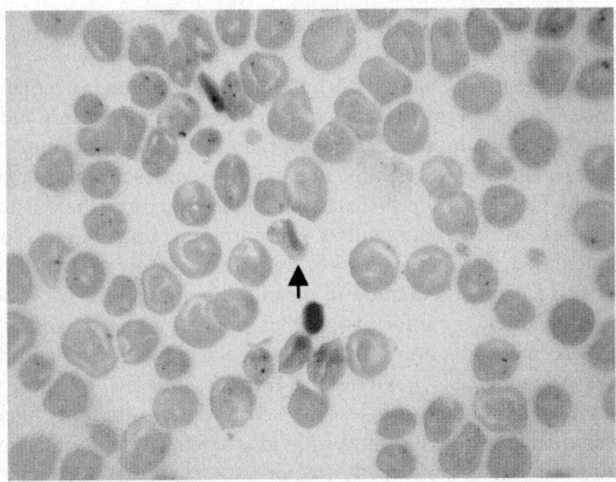

FIGURE 157-17. **Homozygous hemoglobin C.** Three *hemoglobin C crystals* are present, one indicated by an *arrow*. Hemoglobin C crystals are usually six-sided, with a long axis having parallel edges (×1000).

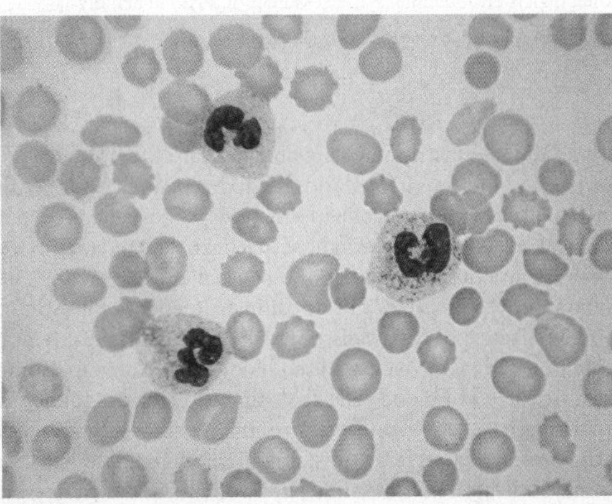

FIGURE 157-18. **Toxic granulation.** *Toxic granulation* refers to heavy staining of azurophilic granules of neutrophils. When accompanied by neutrophil vacuolation, it is often indicative of infection, but it can also result from inflammation, tissue damage, and normal pregnancy (×1000).

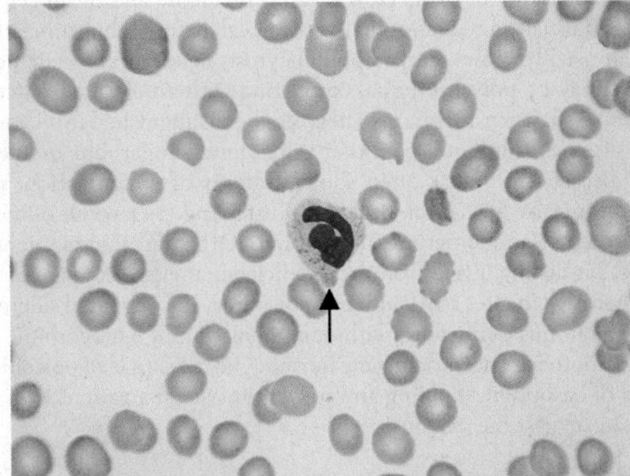

FIGURE 157-19. **Döhle body.** A *Döhle body (arrow)* is a pale blue-gray amorphous inclusion near the cell membrane of a neutrophil. Döhle bodies can result from infection and inflammation. Similar but different inclusions (larger and more angular) are seen in the May-Hegglin anomaly (×1000).

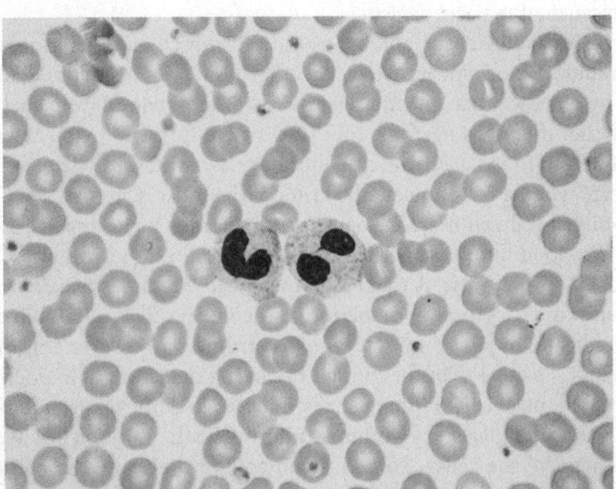

FIGURE 157-20. **Pelger-Huët anomaly.** A *Pelger-Huët anomaly* is a cytologic abnormality of neutrophils in which there is hypolobulation of nuclei and increased chromatin clumping. Nuclei may have a shape resembling a peanut or a pince-nez, as in the examples shown. The Pelger-Huët anomaly is inherited, but similar Pelger neutrophils are seen in myelodysplastic syndromes, in which the neutrophils may also be hypogranular (×1000). They can also be seen as an acquired reversible phenomenon in response to specific drugs, including tacrolimus and mycophenolate mofetil.

TABLE 157-1 CLINICAL FEATURES SUGGESTING THE NEED FOR A BLOOD SMEAR

CLINICAL FEATURE	REASON TO PERFORM A BLOOD SMEAR
Lymphadenopathy or splenomegaly	May be indicative of infectious mononucleosis or another reactive condition, or of leukemia or lymphoma
Clinically evident anemia	Helps in the differential diagnosis
Bruising or bleeding tendency, including unexplained retinal hemorrhages	May confirm thrombocytopenia or show morphologically abnormal platelets (which may have defective function); sometimes shows acute leukemia or other condition causing bone marrow failure
Acute renal failure	Hemolytic-uremic syndrome and thrombotic thrombocytopenic purpura should be confirmed or excluded
Jaundice and hypertension in a pregnant woman	May show schistocytes, supporting a diagnosis of HELLP syndrome
Bone pain	May indicate multiple myeloma, bone marrow infiltration, or sickle cell disease
Unexplained chest or abdominal pain or acute splenic enlargement in a child	Possible sickle cell disease
Unexplained hyperbilirubinemia	Assessment of possible hemolysis

HELLP = hemolysis, elevated liver enzymes, low platelets.

TABLE 157-2 USEFUL FEATURES FOR DETERMINING THE CAUSE OF MACROCYTIC ANEMIA

CAUSE	SMEAR FEATURES
Megaloblastic anemia (vitamin B_{12} or folic acid deficiency)	Oval macrocytes, teardrop poikilocytes, hypersegmented neutrophils; when severe, marked anisocytosis and poikilocytosis, which may include red cell fragments
Ethanol excess	Target cells and stomatocytes; anisocytosis and poikilocytosis less than in megaloblastic anemia
Liver disease	Target cells, stomatocytes
Myelodysplastic syndromes, including sideroblastic anemias	Other dysplastic features such as hypogranular and hypolobulated neutrophils; if erythropoiesis is sideroblastic, a population of hypochromic microcytic cells and Pappenheimer bodies
Chronic hemolytic anemia	Polychromasia; characteristic poikilocytes sometimes present (e.g., irregularly contracted cells if there is an unstable hemoglobin)

Modern automated instruments are able to "flag" the presence of qualitative abnormalities that require a blood film to be examined for confirmation of the abnormality or for further elucidation. "Flags" are generated in response to the electrical impedance or the light scattering characteristics of individual cells. Some instruments are dependent on cytochemical reactions of cells or on the cells' ability to polarize light. Most instruments can indicate the possibility of the presence of blast cells, reactive or other atypical lymphocytes, granulocyte precursors, or nucleated red blood cells. Some instruments can enumerate nucleated red blood cells. Instruments using a cytochemical reaction for peroxidase to help identify neutrophils, eosinophils, and monocytes may flag the appearance of large, unstained (i.e., peroxidase-negative) cells; such cells may indicate a harmless inherited peroxidase deficiency, but sometimes such cells are lymphoma cells, reactive lymphocytes, or leukemic blast cells. Instruments often flag the possibility of an erroneous platelet count, such as when there is an overlap in size between platelets and red cells or when light-scattering characteristics suggest the presence of platelet aggregates (a potential cause of pseudothrombocytopenia). A reported increase in basophil count should generally also be regarded as a flag because it often represents a pseudobasophilia, resulting from the presence of leukemia or lymphoma cells. Some instruments alert the instrument operator to the possible presence of malaria parasites.

International consensus guidelines indicate which automated instrument results require blood smear review. Whether a review is needed is determined in part by whether that specimen is the first one obtained from that patient and whether there has been a significant change from a previously validated result (referred to as a *delta check*). Laboratory computers can be programmed to indicate when a result meets the criteria for smear review.

Automated red cell measurements can, to some extent, replace examination of the blood film.[6] An increased red cell distribution width indicates the presence of anisocytosis. A decreased mean cell volume is usually a reliable indicator of microcytosis. A reduction in the mean cell hemoglobin concentration indicates hypochromia (for most instruments, however, this measurement is less sensitive than the human eye in the detection of hypochromia). An increased mean cell volume usually indicates macrocytosis, but examination of a smear is necessary both to confirm that the result is not artifactual and to elucidate the cause. Some instruments can measure the hemoglobin concentration in individual cells and thus flag the presence of hyperdense cells; however, a blood film is still necessary to distinguish spherocytes from irregularly contracted cells, sickle cells, and other cells that have an increased hemoglobin concentration. Most instruments produce a histogram of the size distribution of red cells, and some do the same for the distribution of hemoglobin concentration; either of these graphic representations may show dimorphic red cells (i.e., two populations of cells).

THE BLOOD SMEAR IN THE DIFFERENTIAL DIAGNOSIS OF ANEMIA

Microcytic Anemias

In microcytic anemias (Chapter 159), the automated count is of considerable importance and may permit a distinction between iron deficiency and thalassemia heterozygosity. In iron deficiency, there is initially a normocytic normochromic anemia; only when the deficiency becomes more severe is there microcytosis. Conversely, in β-thalassemia heterozygosity, there is usually a normal or near-normal hemoglobin concentration, but the red blood cell count is increased, and there is marked microcytosis (low mean cell volume) together with a parallel reduction in mean cell hemoglobin. The blood film provides supplementary information that can favor one diagnosis or the other. Iron deficiency is more likely to be associated with hypochromia and elliptocytes ("pencil cells"), whereas in β-thalassemia heterozygosity, there is microcytosis, hypochromia is less marked, and there are more likely to be target cells and basophilic stippling. Individuals with α-thalassemia involving the deletion of two α genes (–α/–α) or (– –/α α) have red cell indices similar to those of β-thalassemia heterozygosity; in this case, the blood film usually does not provide any additional diagnostically useful information, although individuals with nondeletional α-thalassemia due to hemoglobin Constant Spring have prominent basophilic stippling. When there is deletion of a single α gene, the blood count is either less abnormal or normal, and the blood smear does not provide any extra diagnostically useful information. The blood smear is, however, a useful supplement to the blood count in suggesting a diagnosis of hemoglobin H disease (Chapter 162). The count shows anemia, marked microcytosis (low mean cell volume and mean cell hemoglobin), and usually a reduction in the mean cell hemoglobin concentration. The smear usually shows marked poikilocytosis in addition to microcytosis, and there may be polychromasia, correlating with an elevated reticulocyte count. Iron deficiency anemia also needs to be distinguished from anemia of chronic disease. The blood counts may be quite similar, but in anemia of chronic disease, the smear often shows features of inflammation, such as increased rouleaux formation, background staining (as a result of increased plasma proteins), and sometimes neutrophilia. Other rare microcytic anemias that must be distinguished from iron deficiency include congenital sideroblastic anemia (Chapter 159) and lead poisoning. In congenital sideroblastic anemia, the film is dimorphic, with one population of hypochromic microcytes and another of normochromic normocytic cells. In lead poisoning, the presence of basophilic stippling and polychromasia in a patient with microcytosis can suggest the diagnosis.

Macrocytic Anemias

A blood film can be important in distinguishing true macrocytosis from factitious macrocytosis as a result of the presence of red cell agglutinates (see Fig. 157-16). Diagnostic features that can suggest the cause of macrocytosis are shown in Table 157-2.

A smear is particularly important in evaluating the possibility of a megaloblastic anemia (Chapter 164) (Figs. 157-4 and 157-21). Sometimes assays of

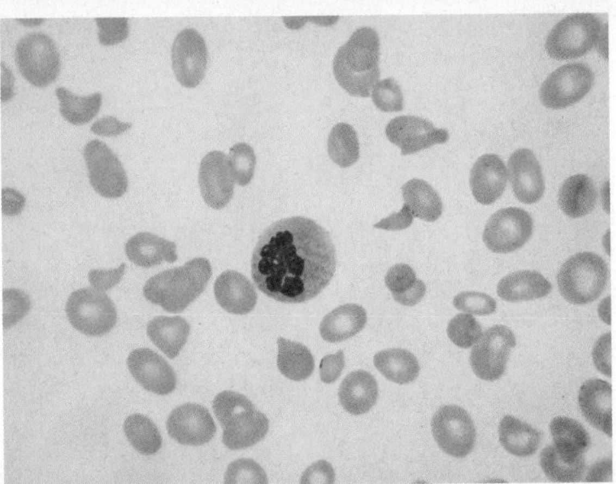

FIGURE 157-21. Hypersegmented neutrophils. A *hypersegmented neutrophil* is a neutrophil with more than five nuclear segments or lobes, as in this example from a patient with megaloblastic anemia. Neutrophil hypersegmentation is also said to be present if there are increased numbers of neutrophils with five lobes or if the median lobe count is increased (×1000).

TABLE 157-3 BLOOD SMEAR FEATURES SUGGESTING A SPECIFIC CAUSE OF INHERITED OR ACQUIRED HEMOLYTIC ANEMIA

BLOOD SMEAR FEATURES	CONDITIONS SUGGESTED
Spherocytes	Hereditary spherocytosis, autoimmune hemolytic anemia, alloimmune hemolytic anemia (e.g., hemolytic disease of the newborn, delayed hemolytic transfusion reaction), drug-induced immune hemolytic anemia, *Clostridium perfringens* sepsis
Elliptocytes	Hereditary elliptocytosis
Oval macrocytes plus stomatocytes	South-East Asian ovalocytosis
Irregularly contracted cells	Glucose-6-phosphate dehydrogenase deficiency, oxidant damage from chemicals or drugs in individuals with normal red cell enzymes (e.g., dapsone administration), liver failure due to Wilson disease (release of copper from liver), unstable hemoglobin, hemoglobin C homozygosity
Sickle cells and boat-shaped cells	Sickle cell disease (e.g., sickle cell anemia or compound heterozygous states such as S/C, S/D-Punjab, S/O-Arab, S/β-thalassemia)
Target cells	Hemoglobin C homozygosity, other hemoglobinopathies, hereditary xerocytosis
Stomatocytes	Hereditary stomatocytosis
Acanthocytes	Liver failure (spur cell hemolytic anemia)
Basophilic stippling	Lead poisoning, pyrimidine 5′-nucleotidase deficiency
Red cell fragments (schistocytes)	Microangiopathic hemolytic anemia (including hemolytic-uremic syndrome, thrombotic thrombocytopenic purpura, HELLP syndrome, and sometimes hemolysis associated with disseminated intravascular coagulation), mechanical hemolytic anemia (e.g., defective cardiac prosthetic valve, march hemoglobinuria)

HELLP = hemolysis, elevated liver enzymes, low platelets.

vitamin B_{12} and folate are normal despite a deficiency, and only the blood film features suggest the true diagnosis and indicate the need for further investigation.

Normocytic Normochromic Anemia

A blood smear is only occasionally useful in determining the cause of a normocytic normochromic anemia. Signs of inflammation may be present in anemia of chronic disease. Increased rouleaux formation and background staining can also indicate multiple myeloma. Polychromasia suggests the possibility of young red cells as a result of recent blood loss or hemolysis. Small numbers of acanthocytes may indicate hypothyroidism or anorexia nervosa. Dysplastic features, such as hypogranular or pseudo-Pelger neutrophils, suggest a myelodysplastic syndrome.

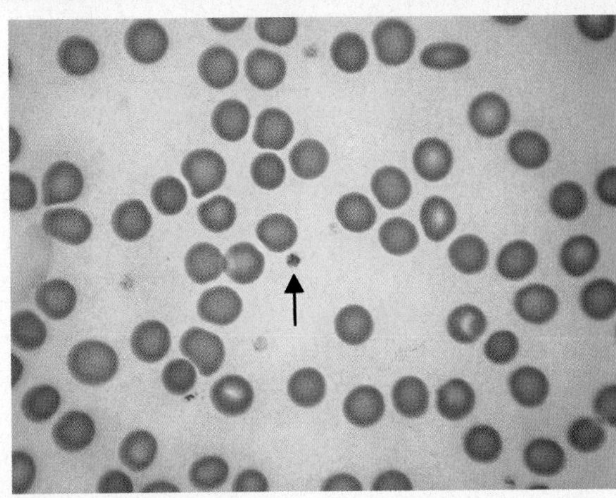

FIGURE 157-22. Normal-sized platelet *(arrow)*. Platelets have central granules, although this is not apparent in this photomicrograph (×1000).

Hemolytic Anemias

The possibility of hemolysis is suggested by the presence of polychromasia and macrocytosis. Specific causes of hemolysis are suggested by the presence of various poikilocytes, as shown in Table 157-3.

The distinction between spherocytes and irregularly contracted cells is important; both are dense cells with absent central pallor, but the differential diagnosis is quite different. Recognition of the features of oxidant damage is important in diagnosing glucose-6-phosphate dehydrogenase (G6PD) deficiency because sometimes an assay for G6PD performed during an acute hemolytic episode is normal (Chapter 161). In addition to irregularly contracted cells, there may be ghost cells, hemi-ghost cells ("blister cells"), and even Heinz bodies protruding from the red cells and confirmed on a Heinz body preparation. The observation of these features is an indication to repeat the assay when the acute hemolytic episode is over.

ASSESSMENT OF THROMBOCYTOPENIA, THROMBOCYTOSIS, AND PLATELET MORPHOLOGY

A blood smear is essential to validate the cell count whenever an automated count shows thrombocytopenia (e.g., a count $<60 \times 10^9$/L) (Chapter 172). This should be done quickly before patient management is altered, such as by postponing surgery or initiating further diagnostic workup. A platelet transfusion should never be given for an unexpected thrombocytopenia without microscopic confirmation of the count. A factitiously low platelet count is often the result of in vitro platelet aggregation (Chapter 171) and is occasionally the result of platelet satellitism, possibly also with platelet phagocytosis. To detect aggregates reliably, the edges and the tail of the smear should be examined. The presence of fibrin strands also suggests the activation of coagulation and an erroneous platelet count.

If a low platelet count is confirmed, the film may give clues to the cause (Chapter 172). Giant platelets (Figs. 157-22 and 157-23) occur in a number of inherited thrombocytopenias, including Bernard-Soulier syndrome and MYH9-related disorders (the May-Hegglin anomaly and related conditions). Small platelets are less common but are a feature of Wiskott-Aldrich syndrome and familial platelet disorder with propensity to myeloid malignancy. Agranular platelets occur in the gray platelet syndrome[7] and platelets with a reduced number of larger than normal granules are seen in Jacobsen/Paris-Trousseau syndrome. The presence of May-Hegglin inclusions (Döhle-like bodies; see Fig. 157-19) in neutrophils indicates that the cause of the thrombocytopenia is a mutation in *MYH9*. In acquired thrombocytopenias, increased platelet turnover is often accompanied by the presence of large platelets, whereas bone marrow failure is associated with platelets of normal size. It is important to look for red cell fragments to confirm or exclude a diagnosis of thrombotic thrombocytopenic purpura and atypical hemolytic-uremic syndrome in any patient with the apparent recent onset of

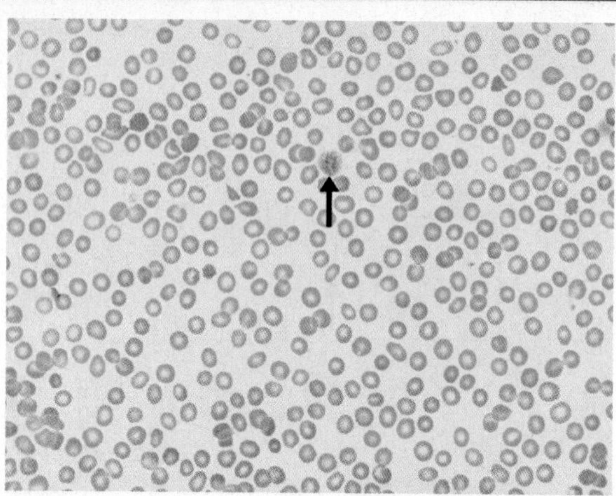

FIGURE 157-23. **Giant platelet *(arrow)*. Giant platelets are as large as or larger than normal red cells. Giant platelets can indicate increased platelet turnover or an inherited or acquired defect in thrombopoiesis (×1000).**

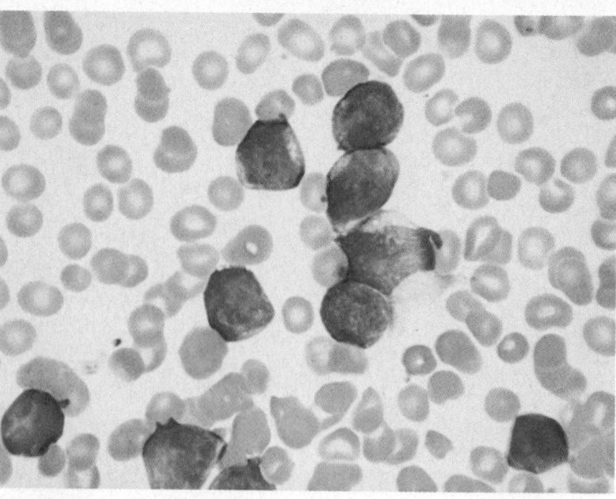

FIGURE 157-24. **Acute lymphoblastic leukemia. Numerous agranular blast cells with a high nuclear-to-cytoplasmic ratio are present. Platelets are decreased in number (×1000).**

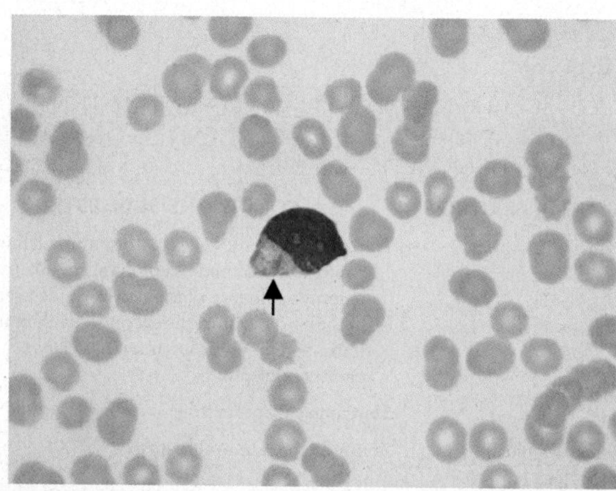

FIGURE 157-25. **Auer rod. An Auer rod *(arrow)* is a rod-shaped inclusion in the cytoplasm of cells of myeloid lineage formed by the crystallization of azurophilic granule constituents. Auer rods are seen only in acute myeloid leukemia and high-grade myelodysplastic syndromes. They are usually seen in blast cells but are occasionally found in maturing cells (×1000).**

thrombocytopenia; because platelet transfusions are usually contraindicated in these conditions, the smear should be examined before platelet transfusion is contemplated. The smear of any patient with the apparent recent onset of severe thrombocytopenia should be examined carefully for evidence of acute promyelocytic leukemia; the leukemic cells may be infrequent in the circulating blood. Hemorrhagic manifestations and a low platelet count can also be indicative of meningococcal septicemia; in some patients, organisms are seen in the blood smear and the diagnosis is confirmed; in other patients, only marked toxic changes in neutrophils are detected.

Thrombocytosis should also be confirmed on a smear. Factitiously elevated counts may be the result of the presence of red cell fragments (in microangiopathic or mechanical hemolytic anemia, burns, or accidental in vitro heating of the blood sample), white cell fragments (in acute leukemia and, less often, in lymphoma), cryoglobulin precipitates, or microorganisms (particularly *Candida* species). If the count is confirmed, the blood smear may be useful to indicate a likely cause (e.g., features of hyposplenism or the presence of basophilia in a myeloproliferative disorder).

It is sometimes necessary to examine a smear to confirm that an apparently normal platelet count is valid. This should always be done in patients with acute leukemia and an elevated white cell count; the presence of white cell fragments of a similar size to platelets can suggest that the platelet count is at a safe level when it is in fact dangerously low. Counting the ratio of platelets to other particles of similar size permits the count to be corrected. Any unexpectedly normal count should be confirmed; for example, the sudden rise of the automated platelet count in a patient being treated for a hematologic neoplasm may be the result of fungi that have colonized an indwelling intravenous line and are being shed into the blood stream.

LEUKOCYTOSIS AND LEUKOPENIA

The finding of leukocytosis is not necessarily an indication for a blood smear (Chapter 170). For example, this finding would be expected in a patient with infection or following surgery or trauma, in which case smear confirmation is not required. However, unexpected leukocytosis requires a smear. Artifactual elevation is unusual but can occur as a result of cryoglobulinemia, hyperlipidemia, or the presence of *Candida* species. Distinguishing reactive changes from leukemia on the basis of morphology is usually straightforward for myelocytosis but more difficult for lymphocytosis.[8] In reactive leukocytosis, there is usually toxic granulation, and Döhle bodies may be present (see Figs. 157-18 and 157-19). Vacuolation is particularly characteristic of bacterial infection, and there may be some degranulation of neutrophils. The hematologist should be aware of the changes induced by granulocyte colony-stimulating factor so that they are not confused with a response to infection; this cytokine can cause toxic granulation, Döhle bodies, vacuolation, and the presence of macropolycytes (giant neutrophils) and circulating neutrophil precursors. The changes typical of leukemia are discussed later.

Leukopenia (Chapter 167) usually requires a film for confirmation and elucidation. The exception is when it is expected in a given clinical context, such as when a patient has had recent chemotherapy. Rarely, an apparent leukopenia is artifactual, owing to the aggregation of neutrophils mediated by an autoantibody or resulting from infection-induced changes in adhesion molecules of the leukocyte surface membrane.

With some automated instruments, it is necessary to confirm that neutropenia is real. If the automated count is based on peroxidase cytochemistry, the presence of an inherited deficiency will lead to an apparent neutropenia associated with an increase of large, unstained (i.e., peroxidase-negative) cells. The scatter plot is characteristic, but because the same features could be due to acute leukemia with neutropenia and circulating blast cells, a smear is needed for confirmation.

LEUKEMIAS AND LYMPHOMAS

The blood smear is critical in the diagnosis of leukemias and lymphomas. The lymphoblasts of acute lymphoblastic leukemia are usually medium-sized agranular cells with relatively scanty cytoplasm (Fig. 157-24), whereas in acute myeloid leukemia, blast cells are generally larger, with more plentiful cytoplasm that may contain granules or Auer rods (Fig. 157-25). Myeloid blast cells vary in appearance according to whether they are myeloblasts or monoblasts. Myeloblasts are usually medium sized and may have plentiful granules, scanty granules, or no visible granules; they may contain Auer rods. Monoblasts are much larger cells with plentiful cytoplasm containing few granules and, very rarely, Auer rods. Megakaryoblasts are present in some patients and are sometimes cytologically distinctive because of their tendency to form cytoplasmic blebs or develop platelet-type granules.

Chronic myelogenous leukemia has a very characteristic blood smear (Fig. 157-26) in which the most numerous cells are myelocytes and mature neutrophils. Eosinophils and basophils are also present. Dysplastic features are generally absent. In atypical Philadelphia chromosome–negative chronic myeloid leukemia, monocytosis is more frequent and dysplastic features are present. Chronic myelomonocytic leukemia is characterized by increased

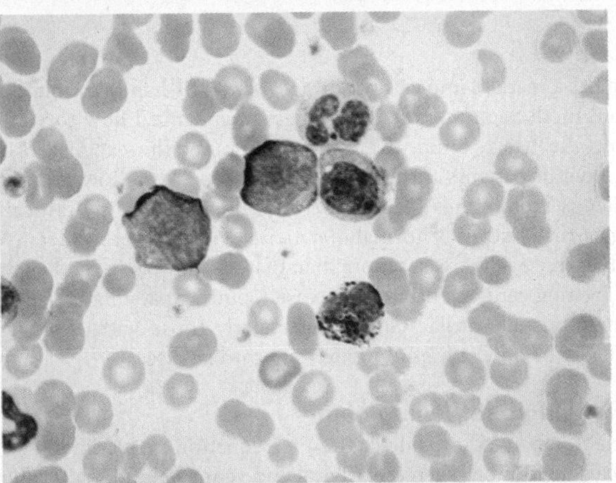

FIGURE 157-26. **Chronic myelogenous leukemia.** In this view there are myeloblasts, a myelocyte, a basophil, and a segmented neutrophil (×1000).

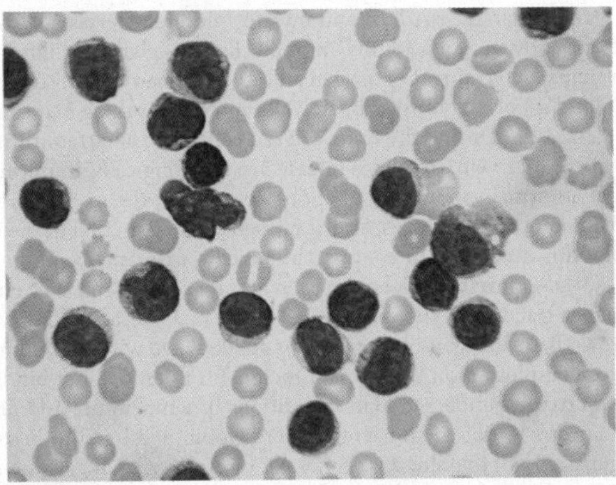

FIGURE 157-27. **Chronic lymphocytic leukemia.** There are large numbers of rather monotonous, mature small lymphocytes with chromatin clumping. Smear cells, reflecting the mechanical fragility of the cells, are characteristic but are not seen in this photomicrograph (×1000).

monocytes, some of them immature, with inconspicuous dysplastic features and infrequent granulocyte precursors.

Chronic lymphocytic leukemia also has a very characteristic blood film, with an increase of small, mature lymphocytes of rather uniform appearance. The chromatin is often irregularly clumped, creating a mosaic effect (Fig. 157-27). Smear cells are almost always increased in number but are not pathognomonic.

Lymphoma in leukemic phase often has cytologic features that aid in the diagnosis. Follicular lymphoma, Burkitt lymphoma, and splenic marginal zone lymphoma can all be distinctive.

THE INCIDENTAL DETECTION OF CLINICALLY SIGNIFICANT ABNORMALITIES

Sometimes the examination of a blood film reveals unexpected but clinically significant information. Examples are given in Table 157-4. Detection of microorganisms is particularly likely in patients with acquired immunodeficiency syndrome (AIDS), hyposplenic patients,[9] and patients with overwhelming sepsis, but sometimes they are detected in immunologically normal patients with only trivial symptoms. It should be noted that microorganisms in blood smears sometimes represent contaminants, particularly if specimens have been obtained by skin prick or from the umbilical cord and if there has been a delay in making the film.

CONCLUSION

Despite major advances in other diagnostic methods, the blood smear remains very useful in hematologic diagnosis. Sometimes it is critical either because it yields a diagnosis very quickly or because it provides information that is not available in any other way.

TABLE 157-4 INCIDENTAL BUT CLINICALLY RELEVANT BLOOD SMEAR OBSERVATIONS

OBSERVATION	POSSIBLE SIGNIFICANCE
Acanthocytes	Abetalipoproteinemia, neuroacanthocytosis (includes choreoacanthocytosis, McLeod phenotype, Huntington-like disease 2 and pantothenate-kinase associated neurodegeneration)
Howell-Jolly bodies, target cells, and acanthocytes	Hyposplenism (congenital, previous splenectomy, celiac disease, amyloidosis)
Cryoglobulin	Hepatitis C, multiple myeloma, Waldenström macroglobulinemia
Vacuolated lymphocytes	Inherited metabolic disorders
Parasites (e.g., malaria parasites, *Babesia*, microfilaria, trypanosomes, *Leishmania*)	Parasitic infection
Fungi (*Candida* spp, *Histoplasma capsulatum*, *Penicillium marneffei*, *Cryptococcus neoformans*, *Malassezia furfur*)	Disseminated fungal infection or, in the case of *Candida*, colonization of an indwelling intravenous line
Bacteria (e.g., pneumococcus, meningococcus, *Capnocytophaga canimorsus*, *Borrelia*, *Ehrlichia*, *Anaplasma*, *Yersinia pestis*)	Bacterial infection
Leukoerythroblastic blood film	Bone marrow infiltration (e.g., metastatic malignancy)

GENERAL REFERENCES

For the General References and other additional features, please visit Expert Consult at https://expertconsult.inkling.com.

158

APPROACH TO THE ANEMIAS

H. FRANKLIN BUNN

Anemia is defined as a significant reduction in the mass of circulating red blood cells. As a result, the oxygen binding capacity of the blood is diminished. Because blood volume is normally maintained at a nearly constant level, anemic patients have a decrease in the concentration of red cells or hemoglobin in peripheral blood. As shown in Table 158-1, hemoglobin and hematocrit levels vary with the age of the individual and, in adults, with gender. The values in women of childbearing age are 10% lower than those in men. At altitude, higher values are found, roughly in proportion to the elevation above sea level. Anemic patients' values are more than 1 standard deviation below the mean values for their gender. However, because of the wide range in normal hemoglobin and hematocrit levels, it is often difficult to document mild anemia. Anemia affects one fourth of the world's population, with a higher prevalence in low socioeconomic groups.[1]

Sometimes the diagnosis of anemia is confounded by a concomitant change in the plasma volume. For example, if a patient with a low red cell mass sustains a loss of plasma volume from dehydration, diarrhea, vomiting, or severe burns, the blood hemoglobin and hematocrit levels will be increased and may even be in the normal range. Another important example, discussed in detail later in this chapter, is acute hemorrhage, in which the loss of both red blood cells and plasma results in a false elevation of hemoglobin and hematocrit. In contrast, hemoglobin and hematocrit values may be falsely low in patients with an expanded plasma volume, such as in pregnancy or congestive heart failure.

PATHOBIOLOGY

Impact of Anemia on Oxygen Transport

In any organ or region of the body, the transport of oxygen is a product of three independent variables expressed in the Fick equation (Fig. 158-1). The middle variable—the oxygen carrying capacity of the blood—is, by definition, low in anemic patients. The two other variables in the Fick equation undergo compensatory changes that, as explained later, greatly enhance oxygen transport.[2]

TABLE 158-1 NORMAL VALUES FOR RED BLOOD CELL MEASUREMENTS

MEASUREMENT	UNIT	NORMAL RANGE (APPROXIMATE)*
Hemoglobin	g/dL	Males: 13.5-17.5 Females: 12-16
Hematocrit	%	Males: 40-52 Females: 36-48
Red blood cell (RBC) count	$\times 10^6/\mu L$ of blood	Males: 4.5-6.0 Females: 4.0-5.4
Mean cell volume (MCV)	fL	81-99
Mean cell hemoglobin (MCH)	pg	30-34
Mean cell hemoglobin concentration (MCHC)	g/dL	30-36
RBC size distribution width		
RDW-CV†	%	12-15
RDW-SD†	fL	37-47
Reticulocyte count (absolute number)	No./μL of blood	20,000-100,000
Reticulocyte percentage	% of RBCs	0.5-1.5

*Actual normal ranges for many of these values may vary slightly, depending on factors such as the location and type of laboratory instruments used, altitude above sea level, and patient age.
†Depending on analyzer instrument used, the RDW (red cell distribution width) can be reported as coefficient of variation (CV) and/or standard deviation (SD), RDW-CV and/or RDW-SD, respectively.

O_2 Delivery	= Blood Flow	×	Hb Concentration	× (Asat − Vsat)
In anemia:	↑Cardiac output Altered flow distribution		↑↑Plasma Erythropoietin	↑RBC 2,3-DPG ↓RBC O_2 affinity

FIGURE 158-1. The Fick equation expresses the three independent variables that determine the transport of oxygen to a given organ or tissue. The impact of anemia on each of these variables is shown beneath the equation. Asat = oxygen saturation of arterial blood (oxyhemoglobin/oxyhemoglobin + deoxyhemoglobin); 2,3-DPG = 2,3-diphosphoglycerate (2,3-bisphosphoglycerate); Hb = hemoglobin; RBC = red blood cell; Vsat = oxygen saturation of venous blood.

Blood Flow

Anemia has a marked impact on blood flow, the left-hand variable in the Fick equation. In all anemic individuals, there is enhanced flow to vital organs, including the heart, brain, liver, and kidneys, at the expense of nonvital organs. Anemic patients are pale because blood is diverted away from the skin and mucous membranes to preserve oxygen supply to the critical organs. Resting cardiac output is normal in patients with mild or moderate anemia, but with exercise, it increases more than that of a normal individual. In severe anemia, resting cardiac output is increased, putting patients at risk for developing high-output cardiac failure, particularly those with coronary artery insufficiency or other types of preexisting cardiac disease.

Oxygen Binding to Hemoglobin

The variable on the right side of the Fick equation is the difference in fractional oxygenation between the arterial and venous blood. This difference in oxygen saturation is determined by the hemoglobin oxygen-binding curve. A comparison between a normal individual and an anemic patient is shown in Figure 158-2. As shown in part A, the curve is shifted to the right in an anemic patient. At any given oxygen tension (Po_2), the oxygen saturation of hemoglobin is lower. Thus, red cells of anemic patients have decreased oxygen affinity. This change is due entirely to elevated levels of red cell 2,3-diphosphoglycerate (2,3-DPG) in red cells. This glycolytic intermediate is the principal determinant of oxygen affinity in human red cells. The Po_2 in arterial blood is normally approximately 95 mm Hg, resulting in nearly 100% oxygen saturation. During the transit of red cells from an artery through its capillary bed to its vein, oxygen is released to respiring cells. In normal individuals, at a normal venous Po_2 of about 40 mm Hg, the oxygen saturation is approximately 80%. Thus, as shown in Figure 158-2A, 20% of the oxygen in the blood is unloaded. In contrast, in patients with anemia and elevated red cell 2,3-DPG levels, the lower oxygen affinity of their red cells enables a much higher fraction of the oxygen (as much as 35%) to be unloaded. In Figure 158-2B, the oxygen-binding curves are depicted with the volume fraction of oxygen plotted on the *y*-axis. One gram of hemoglobin binds up to 1.34 mL of oxygen under standard conditions of temperature and pressure. Thus, in a normal individual having a hemoglobin of 15 g/dL, the oxygen-carrying capacity of the blood is 15 × 1.34, or 20 mL O_2/dL. As mentioned earlier, 20% of this oxygen will be unloaded, that is, 4 mL O_2/100 mL blood during arterial-venous transit. In contrast, an anemic patient with a hemoglobin of 7.5 g/dL has an oxygen-binding capacity that is half normal, or 10 mL O_2/dL. If this patient had red cells with normal oxygen affinity, 20%, or only 2 mL of oxygen, would be unloaded per 100 mL of blood. However, because the patient's red cells have a lower affinity for oxygen, 3.5 mL is unloaded, nearly as much as normal. Thus, the decrease in oxygen affinity is an important mechanism by which anemic patients compensate for the deficit in red cell mass.

Methemoglobinemia

In order for hemoglobin to reversibly bind oxygen, the iron atom in the heme must be in the reduced (Fe^{2+}) valence state. As red cells circulate, the heme iron slowly auto-oxidizes to Fe^{3+}, forming methemoglobin, which is incapable

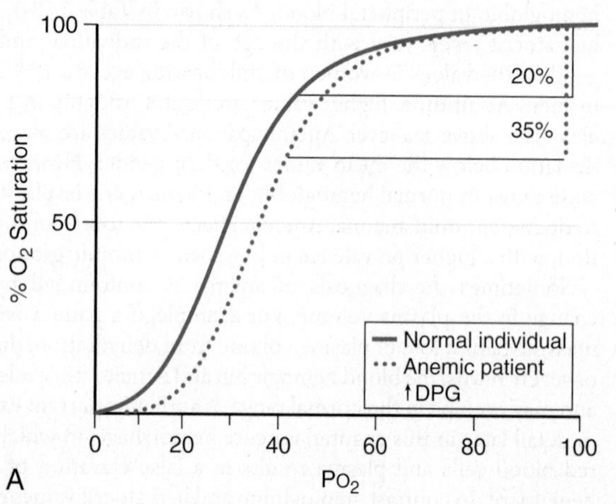

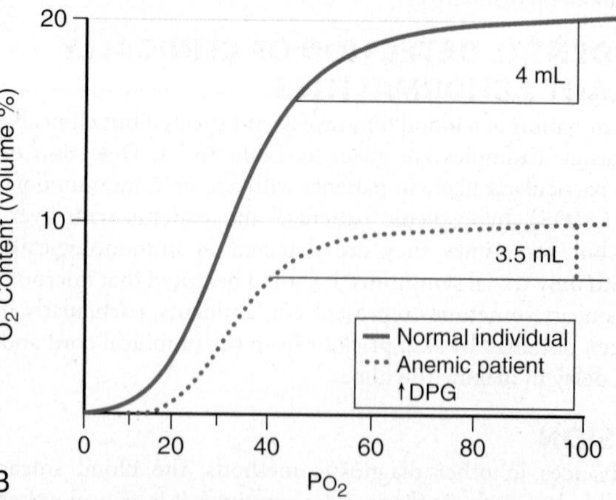

FIGURE 158-2. Oxygen-binding curves for hemoglobin of a normal individual and a patient with anemia. A, Conventional plot of percent of oxygen (O_2) saturation versus oxygen tension (Po_2). B, The *y*-axis shows the volume of oxygen in milliliters per 100 mL of blood. DPG = diphosphoglycerate.

of binding oxygen. Normal red cells are endowed with a very efficient enzymatic pathway composed of cytochrome b_5, cytochrome b_5 reductase, and NADH that rapidly reduces the iron in methemoglobin back to its functional Fe^{2+} form. Thus, normal red cells contain less than 0.5% methemoglobin. However, either an inherited deficiency in cytochrome b_5 reductase or exposure to an oxidant drug or toxin can result in methemoglobinemia.[3] Laboratory samples of blood containing methemoglobin are dark brown, whereas patients with greater than 10% methemoglobinemia have cyanosis, a blue discoloration of the skin indistinguishable from that commonly seen in patients having normal hemoglobin but low oxygen saturation owing to pulmonary or cardiac disease. In many hospitals and large clinical laboratories, the instrument that measures oxygen saturation in blood samples also provides an accurate determination of methemoglobin.

Patients with congenital methemoglobinemia inherit an autosomal recessive deficiency in cytochrome b_5 reductase. Heterozygote relatives have low or undetectable methemoglobin levels, whereas affected individuals (homozygotes and compound heterozygotes) generally have 10 to 35% methemoglobin. These individuals are usually asymptomatic because the methemoglobin is distributed primarily in the older population of red cells. Nevertheless, many affected individuals have cosmetic concerns. Treatment with oral ascorbic acid or riboflavin is effective in lowering the level of methemoglobin below the threshold of detectable cyanosis.

A variety of drugs can cause methemoglobinemia, including acetaminophen (Tylenol), dapsone, nitroprusside, amyl nitrate, procaine congeners used for local anesthesia[4], and recreational drugs (volatile nitrites called "poppers" and cocaine). It is not clear why only a very small fraction of those using these drugs develop this complication, but some affected individuals have been shown to be heterozygous for cytochrome b_5 reductase deficiency. When these drugs are taken in prescribed doses, methemoglobinemia seldom reaches levels high enough to cause clinical concern.

In contrast, individuals exposed to industrial toxins such as nitrite, nitrate, or aniline may develop life-threatening levels of methemoglobin. The threshold at which symptoms occur is highly variable. Acute induction of 20% methemoglobin may cause fatigue; at 30%, individuals often develop tachycardia. When methemoglobin exceeds 50%, patients experience weakness, breathlessness, and confusion. At 70 to 80%, coma and death may occur. The toxicity of methemoglobinemia is not just because of the inability of oxidized hemes to bind oxygen; the remaining functional (Fe^{2+}) hemes in the hemoglobin tetramer have increased oxygen affinity and therefore, as suggested in Figure 158-2, are much less effective in releasing oxygen to tissues. Patients with toxic methemoglobinemia can be effectively treated with intravenous infusion of methylene blue (1 to 2 mg/kg).

Regulation of Erythropoiesis by Erythropoietin

Anemia also affects the middle component of the Fick equation (see Fig. 158-1). As mentioned earlier, hemoglobin levels are, by definition, low in anemic patients. The resultant decrease in the oxygen-carrying capacity of the blood causes cellular hypoxia. In all cells of the body, a molecular sensor detects even modest degrees of low oxygen tension and induces a hypoxia-inducible transcription factor called HIF. HIF upregulates expression of the hormone erythropoietin in the kidney and, to a lesser extent, in the liver. Erythropoietin (Chapter 156) binds to a specific receptor abundantly expressed on erythroid progenitor cells in the bone marrow and salvages these cells from apoptosis, thereby enhancing red blood cell production. Normal individuals maintain nearly constant levels of circulating red cells by finely tuned regulation of erythropoietin production. In anemic patients, the hypoxic signal in the kidneys and, to a lesser extent, in the liver results in a robust induction of erythropoietin expression. As the hematocrit falls, the plasma erythropoietin level rises markedly; in severely anemic patients, it may be 1000-fold higher than normal (Fig. 158-3). In patients with anemia due to impaired red cell production, the erythroid progenitors are unresponsive to such high levels of plasma erythropoietin. In contrast, in patients whose anemia is due to hemolysis or blood loss, elevated erythropoietin levels maximize red cell production.

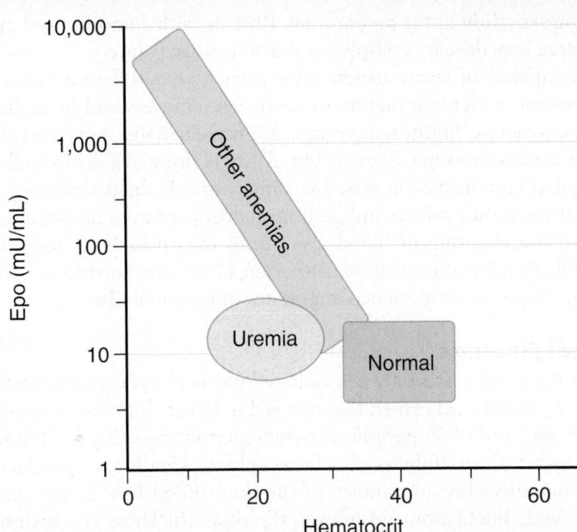

FIGURE 158-3. **Plasma erythropoietin (Epo) levels in patients with different degrees of anemia. The subset of anemia patients with chronic renal disease (labeled "Uremia") have much lower plasma erythropoietin levels than those with other types of anemia. Values for normal individuals are also shown.**

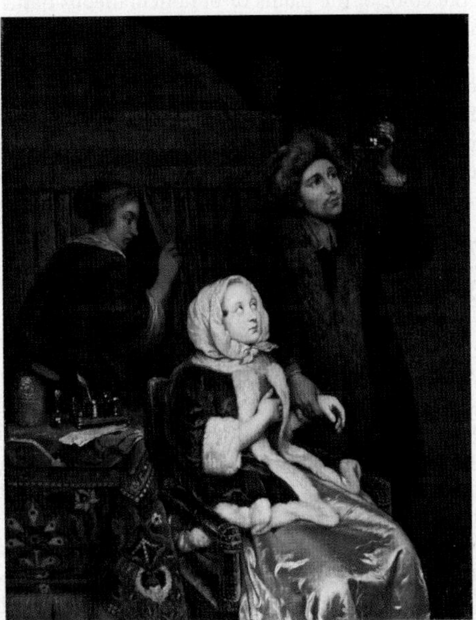

FIGURE 158-4. **"The Sick Lady," a 17th-century painting attributed to Caspar Netscher, from the Royal Collection, Buckingham Palace.**

CLINICAL MANIFESTATIONS

Figure 158-4 is a 17th-century painting of a pale young woman clutching her chest, apparently complaining of palpitations. Her physician is feeling her pulse, documenting her rapid, forceful heartbeat. These signs and symptoms, common in patients with very low hemoglobin levels, can be readily explained by the cardiovascular adjustments discussed in the preceding section. These clinical findings pertain to anemia per se, irrespective of cause, and are dependent on its severity and chronicity. The history and physical examination may reveal additional findings peculiar to specific causes of anemia or to other comorbid conditions. The degree to which symptoms occur in an anemic patient depends on several contributing factors. If the anemia has developed rapidly, there may not have been adequate time for compensatory adjustments to take place, and the patient may have more marked symptoms than if an anemia of equivalent severity had developed insidiously. Furthermore, the patient's complaints may depend on the presence of local vascular disease. For example, symptoms owing to ischemia in patients with angina pectoris, intermittent claudication, or transient cerebral episodes may be triggered by the development of anemia.

Symptoms

Many individuals with mild anemia have no complaints and are unaware that they have "tired blood." Others may complain of fatigue as well as dyspnea and palpitations, particularly following exercise. Patients with severe anemia are often symptomatic at rest and are unable to tolerate significant exertion. If the hemoglobin concentration falls below 7.5 g/dL, resting cardiac output is likely to rise, with an increase in both stroke volume and heart rate. The patient may be aware of this hyperdynamic state and complain of a rapid, pounding sensation in the precordium. Patients with compromised myocardial reserve may develop complaints due to cardiac failure.

The symptoms of severe anemia often extend beyond the cardiac or circulatory system. Patients sometimes experience dizziness and headache and, less often, syncope, tinnitus, or vertigo. Many are irritable and have difficulty sleeping or concentrating. Because blood flow is shunted away from the skin, patients may complain of increased sensitivity to cold. In like manner, gastrointestinal symptoms such as indigestion, anorexia, or even nausea are attributable to the shunting of blood away from the splanchnic bed. Females commonly develop abnormal menstruation, either amenorrhea or increased bleeding. Males may experience impotence or loss of libido.

Physical Findings

Pallor is the most commonly encountered physical finding in patients with anemia. As mentioned earlier, this sign is due to the shunting of blood away from the skin and other peripheral tissues, permitting enhanced blood flow to vital organs. The usefulness of pallor as a physical finding is limited by other factors that affect the appearance of the skin. Blood flow to the skin may undergo wide fluctuations. Moreover, the skin's thickness and texture vary widely among individuals. Those with a fair complexion may appear pale even though they are not anemic, whereas pallor is difficult to detect in deeply pigmented individuals. The amount of melanin in the epidermis is an important determinant of skin color. Pallor may be difficult to detect in patients who have increased melanin pigmentation due to Addison disease or hemochromatosis. Nevertheless, even in blacks, the presence of anemia may be suspected by the color of the palms or of noncutaneous tissues such as oral mucous membranes, nail beds, and palpebral conjunctivas. When the creases of the palm are as pale as the surrounding skin, the patient usually has a hemoglobin of less than 7 g/dL.

In addition to tachycardia, wide pulse pressure, and hyperdynamic precordium, a systolic ejection murmur is often heard over the precordium, particularly at the pulmonic area. In addition, a venous hum may be detected over the neck vessels. These findings disappear when the anemia is corrected.

DIAGNOSIS

Laboratory Evaluation of the Patient with Anemia

In the clinical assessment of the anemic patient, it is important to proceed in a systematic way so that the diagnosis can be established with a minimum of laboratory tests and procedures. A thorough history and careful physical examination are critical in the initial evaluation of the anemic patient. For example, a family history that reveals a dominant inheritance pattern would reinforce the tentative diagnosis of hereditary spherocytosis. The presence of fever, a new heart murmur, and splenomegaly is an anemic patient suggests subacute bacterial endocarditis.

In evaluating the anemic patient, the clinician must first ask whether the anemia is caused by decreased production of red cells or by loss of blood cells as a result of hemorrhage or hemolysis (Table 158-2). Blood loss may be either the sole cause of the anemia or a significant contributor. Therefore, examination of the stool for occult blood is an indispensable part of the evaluation of all anemic patients.

The laboratory work-up of anemia includes a complete blood count, red cell indices, reticulocyte count, and microscopic examination of the blood smear. In addition, in many cases a bone marrow examination is a critical component of the initial laboratory assessment.

TABLE 158-2 INITIAL ASSESSMENT OF ANEMIA

Decreased red cell production
Usually acquired
Onset is insidious
Reticulocyte count is inappropriately low
Red cell indices (MCV, MCHC) are informative
Bone marrow examination is often required for diagnosis
Increased red cell destruction (hemolysis)
Often inherited
Onset may be abrupt or insidious
Reticulocyte count is increased
Red cell morphology on peripheral blood smear is usually informative
Bone marrow examination is usually not indicated
Blood loss—must be ruled out in any patient with anemia

MCHC = mean cell hemoglobin concentration; MCV = mean cell volume.

Complete Blood Count

Most hospitals and clinical laboratories use equipment that provides high-throughput analyses of red cell, platelet, and white cell counts and white cell differential, along with measurements of cell size. The mean red cell volume (MCV) is normally 81 to 99 fL. These instruments also provide accurate determinations of hemoglobin concentration. The hematocrit, or fraction of packed red cells over total blood volume, is determined indirectly from the red cell count and the MCV. The mean concentration of hemoglobin within the red cell population (MCHC) is the quotient of hemoglobin divided by hematocrit. The MCV is particularly useful in classifying the anemias caused by decreased red cell production. Microcytic anemias have low MCV values and often low MCHC. Microscopic examination reveals small and often pale red cells. The MCV in the macrocytic anemias is increased, and large, oval cells (macro-ovalocytes) are seen. In contrast to the anemias of underproduction, the hemolytic anemias are either normocytic or slightly macrocytic owing to the preponderance of young red cells that are relatively large. Severe forms of thalassemia (Chapter 162) are an exception; there, microcytic red cells may be accompanied by brisk hemolysis.

Reticulocyte Count

This simple and cost-effective test is extremely useful for distinguishing anemias secondary to decreased red cell production from those caused by hemolysis. With the application of an appropriate supravital stain, the 1- to 2-day-old red cells in the peripheral blood reveal a network of purple strands, which are aggregates of ribosomes. The reticulocyte count in normal individuals is about 1%, consistent with a red cell lifespan of approximately 120 days. An elevated reticulocyte count reflects the release of an increased number of young cells from the bone marrow. The rate of red cell production can be assessed more quantitatively by determining the absolute reticulocyte count, the product of the percentage of reticulocytes and the red cell count. Thus, normal blood contains about 50,000 reticulocytes/mm^3. In interpreting this test, one should consider the distribution of reticulocytes between the bone marrow and the peripheral blood. When erythropoiesis is robust, marrow reticulocytes enter the circulation prematurely. These "shift reticulocytes" appear larger than average on a routine (Wright-stained) blood smear and have a lavender hue, called polychromatophilia. Because the circulation of shift reticulocytes in the peripheral blood is prolonged, the reticulocyte count should be divided by two. This correction should always be made if normoblasts are encountered in the peripheral blood because this finding indicates the premature release of newborn red cells into the circulation.

A failure to produce red cells is reflected in an inappropriately low reticulocyte count. In contrast, a significant elevation of reticulocytes is suggestive of hemolysis. Exceptions include the following:

- The brisk reticulocyte response seen in patients with hemorrhage
- Reticulocytosis encountered in patients recovering from impaired erythropoiesis (e.g., an individual with pernicious anemia who received an injection of cobalamin 1 week earlier)
- Mild to moderate elevations in reticulocytes (3 to 7%) encountered in myelophthisic anemia (Chapter 157), in which the orderly release of cells is affected by alterations of the marrow stroma owing to tumor, fibrosis, or granuloma

These exceptions are generally appreciated in the initial evaluation of the patient.

A number of ancillary laboratory tests described later under Hemolytic Anemias are useful in determining both the cause and extent of hemolysis.

Examination of the Blood Smear

In the evaluation of any patient with unexplained anemia, the physician should take the time to examine a well-stained peripheral blood film (Chapter 157). Many subtleties escape the attention of the technologist, whose primary aim is to confirm or refine the white cell differential count provided by automated cell counters. The clinician approaches the specimen with a prepared mind and can scrutinize it for specific abnormalities. Examination of the blood film can confirm the size and color of red cells estimated by red blood cell indices. In contrast to the mean statistical values provided by automated cell counters, microscopic examination can reveal variations in red cell size (anisocytosis) or shape (poikilocytosis), abnormalities that are helpful in diagnosing specific anemias. Examination of the blood smear is particularly important in a patient with hemolysis. Many types of hemolytic anemia have characteristic abnormalities in red cell morphology. The presence of abnormal white cells may be the first clue to a lymphoproliferative or primary bone marrow disorder.

Bone Marrow Examination

A microscopic examination of the bone marrow (aspirate with or without a core biopsy) is often useful and may be critical in the work-up of any *unexplained* anemia. Study of the bone marrow is informative in the diagnosis of anemias of underproduction, particularly those accompanied by abnormalities in white cells and/or platelets, suggesting disordered hematopoiesis. The more severe the anemia, the more likely it is that the procedure will be informative. An assessment of the quantity and quality of red cell precursors may identify a defect in cell production due to either hypoplasia or ineffective erythropoiesis. A marrow biopsy is required for estimating overall cellularity. The ratio of myeloid (M) to erythroid (E) precursors is normally about 2 : 1, but it may be artifactually increased by the inclusion of circulating leukocytes. The ratio is increased in patients with infection, a leukemoid reaction, or neoplastic proliferation of myeloid cells. Rarely, a high M/E ratio is due to selective aplasia of the red cell precursors. A decreased M/E ratio indicates erythroid hyperplasia. Erythroid maturation is normal in hemolysis and hemorrhage, but it is disordered when erythropoiesis is ineffective, such as in megaloblastic and sideroblastic anemias and in β-thalassemia major or intermedia. The bone marrow examination is also important in demonstrating the presence of cellular infiltrates such as those found in leukemia, lymphoma, or multiple myeloma. The demonstration of tumor, fibrosis, or granuloma usually requires a bone marrow biopsy, which provides information not available from bone marrow aspiration. A portion of the marrow specimen should be stained with Prussian blue. In addition to providing an assessment of iron stores, this iron stain is required for the identification of erythroid sideroblasts.

ANEMIA DUE TO BLOOD LOSS

The clinical presentation of anemia resulting from blood loss varies considerably, depending on the site, severity, and rapidity of the hemorrhage. At opposite extremes are acute fulminant bleeding producing hypovolemic shock and chronic occult blood loss leading to iron deficiency anemia.

Acute Blood Loss

Patients who have had a sudden hemorrhage present with clinical findings secondary to hypovolemia and hypoxia. Symptoms and signs depend on the severity of the process. The patient may experience weakness, fatigue, lightheadedness, or stupor and may appear pale, diaphoretic, and irritable. The vital signs reflect cardiovascular compensation for the acute blood loss. The degree of hypotension and tachycardia depends on the extent of the hemorrhage. Elicitation of postural signs is useful in the initial evaluation of a patient with acute blood loss. When a patient is lifted from a supine to a sitting position, an increase in the pulse of 25% or more or a fall in the systolic blood pressure of 20 mm Hg or more signifies significant hypovolemia (blood loss >1000 mL). Acute blood loss in excess of 1500 mL usually leads to cardiovascular collapse.

Following acute hemorrhage, the red cell mass and plasma volume are contracted in parallel; accordingly, there is often not a significant decrease in the hemoglobin or hematocrit level initially. This stress induces a moderate leukocytosis and a "shift to the left" in the white cell differential count. In both acute and chronic blood loss, the platelet count is often increased, particularly if the patient is already iron deficient. During the first few days after acute blood loss, there is usually an increase in reticulocytes. Severe hypoxia may trigger the release of nucleated red cells from the bone marrow into the peripheral blood. Because young red cells are larger than old ones, the MCV generally rises slightly. If significant blood loss continues, reticulocytosis will persist until iron stores have been exhausted. Internal bleeding is often accompanied by an increase in unconjugated bilirubin, reflecting an increase in the catabolism of heme from extravasated red cells. Patients with acute gastrointestinal blood loss sometimes have an elevation of blood urea nitrogen owing to impaired renal blood flow and perhaps to the absorption of digested blood protein.

These patients must be assessed promptly, and treatment must be initiated without delay. Patients with severe acute blood loss require transfusion of packed red cells, with central monitoring of the appropriate amount of volume replacement. The site or sites of bleeding should be emergently identified and controlled. In addition, an emergency coagulation profile should be obtained. The approach to the patient with shock is discussed in detail in Chapter 106.

Chronic Blood Loss

Chronic blood loss is usually due to lesions in the gastrointestinal tract or the uterus. Testing of stool specimens for occult blood is an essential but frequently overlooked part of the evaluation of anemia. It is sometimes necessary to examine serial specimens over a prolonged period because gastrointestinal bleeding may be intermittent. The hematologic manifestations of chronic blood loss are those of iron deficiency anemia, discussed in detail in Chapter 159.

ANEMIAS DUE TO DECREASED RED CELL PRODUCTION

As shown in Table 158-3, anemias caused by the underproduction of red cells can be conveniently classified according to red cell size: microcytic, macrocytic, and normocytic.

Microcytic Anemias

The presence of small red cells (MCV <77 fL) indicates a defect in the production of hemoglobin.[5] As shown in Figure 158-5, hemoglobin is composed of globin subunits into which heme is inserted. Heme is produced by the insertion of an iron atom into porphyrin (protoporphyrin IX). A defect in any of these three key components can cause microcytic anemia. Most individuals with microcytosis have either iron deficiency anemia (Chapter 159) or thalassemia (Chapter 162). A congenital or, more often, acquired impairment in porphyrin synthesis can lead to a buildup of excess iron in erythroid cells, resulting in the morphologic entity of ringed sideroblasts, which are identified in red cell precursors in the bone marrow (Chapter 159). Most patients with acquired sideroblastic anemia actually have a normal or somewhat elevated MCV but a broad distribution of red cell size, including a population of microcytes (because of this ambiguity, sideroblastic anemia appears in parentheses in Table 158-3). Iron deficiency anemia, the thalassemias, and sideroblastic anemia all involve some degree of ineffective erythropoiesis.

The anemias of chronic inflammation and malignancy, described in detail later, may be slightly microcytic owing to a defect in the availability of iron. However, these disorders are more often normocytic. Measurement of serum

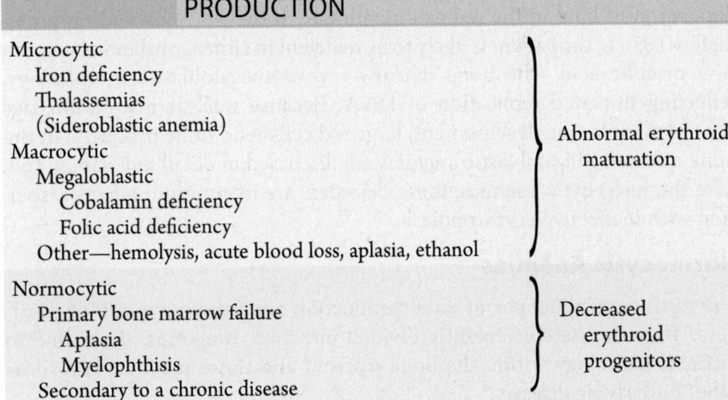

TABLE 158-3 ANEMIAS DUE TO DECREASED RED CELL PRODUCTION

Anemia	Mechanism
Microcytic	Abnormal erythroid maturation
Iron deficiency	
Thalassemias	
(Sideroblastic anemia)	
Macrocytic	
Megaloblastic	
Cobalamin deficiency	
Folic acid deficiency	
Other—hemolysis, acute blood loss, aplasia, ethanol	
Normocytic	Decreased erythroid progenitors
Primary bone marrow failure	
Aplasia	
Myelophthisis	
Secondary to a chronic disease	

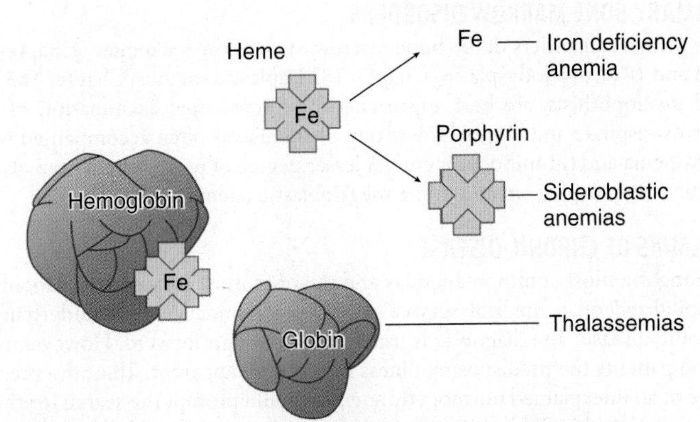

FIGURE 158-5. Components of hemoglobin that are deficient in the microcytic anemias.

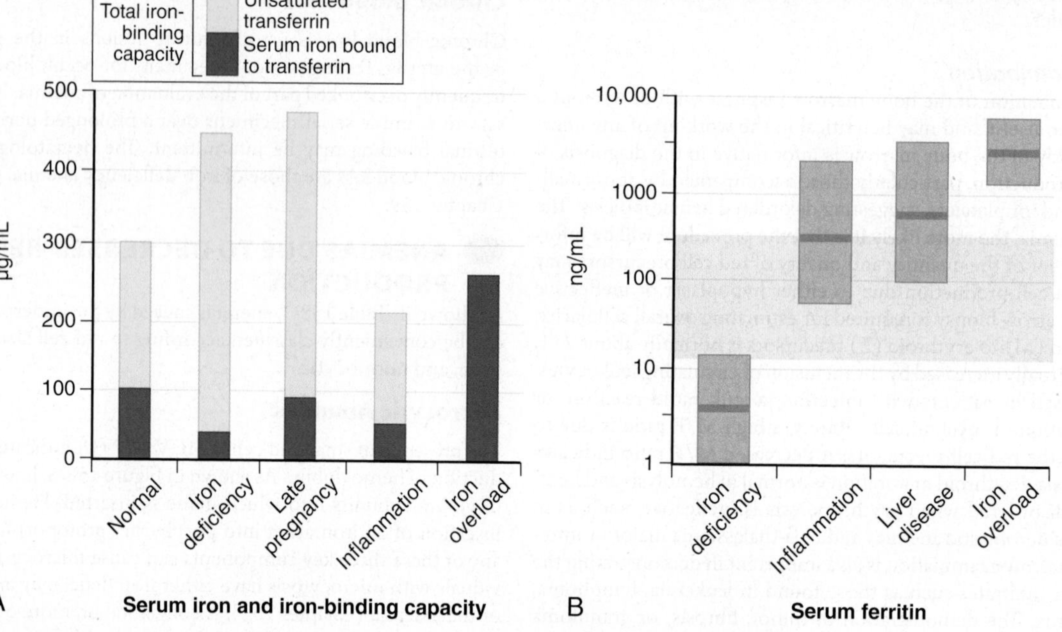

FIGURE 158-6. A, Serum iron and transferrin saturation in different conditions. B, Serum ferritin in different conditions. Note that the *y*-axis in panel B is on a log scale. The normal range (10 to 200 ng/mL) is shown by the beige shaded area.

iron and iron-binding capacity (Fig. 158-6A) and serum ferritin (Fig. 158-6B) particularly useful in distinguishing between iron deficiency and the anemia of chronic inflammation.

Macrocytic Anemias

A modest increase in red cell size is encountered in a variety of conditions, including liver disease, hypothyroidism, acute blood loss, hemolytic anemia, aplastic anemia, and alcoholism. Macrocytosis is so commonly seen in alcoholism that the MCV has been used as a clinical screen for abstinence from alcohol. Even in nonalcoholics, alcohol use can elevate the MCV. The macrocytes in liver disease and hypothyroidism may be related to an increased deposition of lipid in the red cell membrane. If the MCV exceeds approximately 105 fL, the patient is likely to be deficient in either cobalamin (vitamin B_{12}) or folic acid. The bone marrow reveals megaloblastic morphology, reflecting impaired replication of DNA. Because nuclear maturation lags behind cytoplasmic development, large red cells tend to be produced in the bone marrow. Megaloblastic anemias are discussed in detail in Chapter 164. Like the microcytic anemias, these disorders are maturation defects associated with ineffective erythropoiesis.

Normocytic Anemias

The normocytic anemias of underproduction are a diverse group of disorders. They can be conveniently divided into two categories: those due to intrinsic pathology within the bone marrow, and those secondary to some other underlying disease.

PRIMARY BONE MARROW DISORDERS

The primary disorders of the bone marrow, such as the leukemias (Chapters 183 and 184), myelodysplasia (Chapter 182), aplastic anemia (Chapter 165), and myelophthisis, are best approached by microscopic examination of a marrow aspirate and biopsy. This group of anemias is often accompanied by leukopenia and thrombocytopenia. A lesser degree of pancytopenia can also occur in hypersplenism and in the megaloblastic anemias.

ANEMIAS OF CHRONIC DISEASE

Among the most common anemias and the ones most prevalent in patients hospitalized on a medical service are those secondary to an underlying chronic disease. The diagnosis is usually quite straightforward. However, in some patients the predisposing illness may not be apparent. Thus, the presence of an unexplained normocytic anemia should prompt the search for the disorders listed in Table 158-4. Even if the presence of an underlying illness is established, the physician should investigate whether other factors such as blood loss or a nutritional deficiency are also contributing to the patient's

TABLE 158-4 ANEMIAS SECONDARY TO CHRONIC DISEASE

Inflammation
Chronic infections
Cancer
Connective tissue disorders
Renal insufficiency
Endocrine disorders
Hypothyroidism
Hypoadrenalism
Hypopituitarism
Hypogonadism—males
Liver disease
Aging

anemia. Generally, the anemias due to chronic inflammation, an endocrinopathy, or liver disease are of only moderate severity. In contrast, the anemia of uremia is often severe.

ANEMIA OF CHRONIC INFLAMMATION

If a systemic inflammatory disorder persists for more than a few weeks, it is nearly always accompanied by anemia. As shown in Table 158-4, the most common causes of chronic inflammation are infection, tumor, or a connective tissue disorder. Many chronic infections can be responsible, including tuberculosis, lung abscess, subacute bacterial endocarditis, pyelonephritis, and osteomyelitis. The pathogenesis is more complex in some types of chronic infections. For example, in AIDS (Chapter 393), the human immunodeficiency virus can directly attack hematopoietic cells and suppress erythropoiesis. In malaria and babesiosis, the parasite enters circulating red cells and triggers their destruction.

There is considerable variability in tumors' ability to evoke an inflammatory response. Many tumors express inflammatory cytokines as part of their profile of abnormal gene expression. In some cases, impaired supply of oxygen or nutrients to the interior of the tumor mass can lead to necrosis and an inflammatory response. Red cell production may be further compromised by encroachment of the bone marrow with leukemia, lymphoma, or metastatic tumor.

Anemia is also a feature of a broad range of inflammatory conditions that are not associated with either infection or cancer. In some of these disorders, the autoimmune attack on the patient's cells and tissues is met with a robust inflammatory response. Rheumatoid arthritis (Chapter 264) is the most commonly encountered connective tissue disorder and gives rise to the prototypical anemia of chronic inflammation. Even more intense inflammation and, accordingly, more severe anemia are seen in polymyalgia rheumatica and temporal arteritis (Chapter 271). In patients with systemic lupus erythematosus (Chapter 266), the anemia of chronic inflammation is often compounded by either immune hemolysis (Chapter 160) or renal insufficiency (discussed later).

PATHOBIOLOGY

Recently, the mechanism underlying the anemia of chronic inflammation has been elucidated by the discovery that plasma hepcidin levels are markedly increased as a result of induction by inflammatory cytokines. As shown in Figure 158-7, hepcidin blocks both iron absorption from the gut and the exit of iron from macrophages, thus explaining both reduced levels of serum iron and increased iron stores.

DIAGNOSIS

The anemia of chronic inflammation is associated with disordered iron homeostasis. Increased storage of iron in macrophages within the bone marrow, liver, and spleen results in elevated levels of serum ferritin (Fig. 158-6B). However, because of a block in the transfer of this excess iron into the plasma, serum iron is low (see Fig. 158-6A). The level of total transferrin in the serum is also low for unclear reasons. With the recent development of a reliable assay for hepcidin, elevated serum levels of this "master regulator" of iron homeostasis should become useful in the diagnosis of the anemia of chronic inflammation. Because of the impairment in iron availability, erythropoiesis is somewhat "iron deficient." The amount of cytoplasmic iron is decreased in erythroid precursors in the bone marrow, and the red cells that enter the circulation are slightly microcytic. This suppression of red cell production is earmarked by a low reticulocyte index. Because this block in iron utilization is subtle, the degree of anemia is seldom severe in patients with inflammatory disorders. If the hemoglobin is less than 8 g/dL, it is necessary to look for additional contributors such as hemolysis or bleeding.

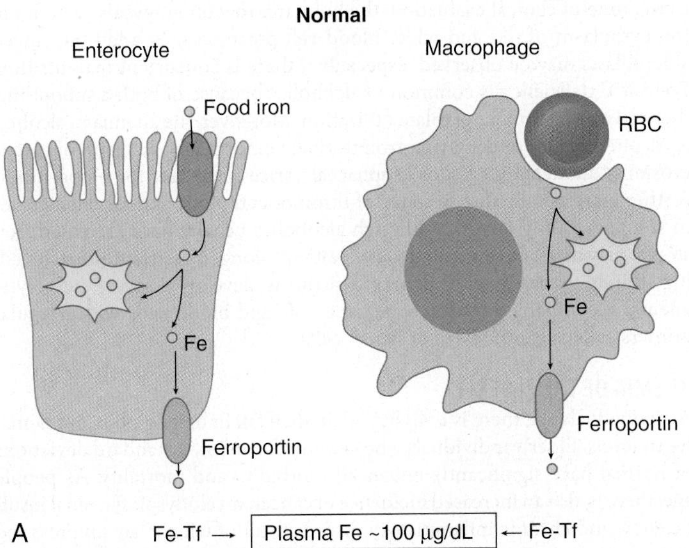

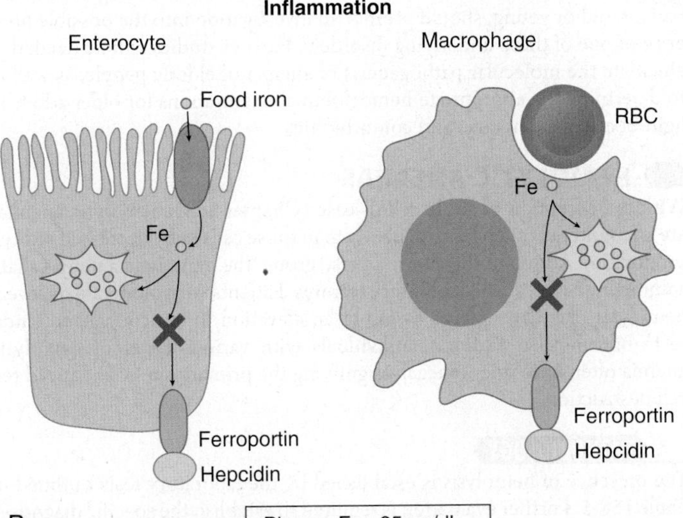

FIGURE 158-7. Pathogenesis of the block in iron availability in the anemia of chronic inflammation. The primary sources of iron in the plasma are from the breakdown of senescent red blood cells (RBCs) within macrophages and from duodenal absorption. **A,** In the presence of physiologically low levels of hepcidin in the plasma, there is efficient release of iron from the duodenal enterocyte and from macrophages through ferroportin. **B,** In patients with inflammation, the induction of plasma hepcidin by interleukin-6 and other cytokines results in the inactivation of ferroportin and the loss of iron egress from the duodenal enterocyte and from the macrophage.

TREATMENT Rx

Because the anemia of chronic inflammation is not severe, patients seldom require red cell transfusions. Some patients may benefit from recombinant erythropoietin therapy. However, the anemia is not fully corrected unless the underlying disease is effectively treated.

ANEMIA OF RENAL INSUFFICIENCY

A normocytic anemia almost always accompanies uremia (Chapter 130). Although the hemoglobin level is highly variable, the severity of the anemia is roughly proportional to the degree of impaired renal function. The cause of the kidney failure usually has little bearing on the extent of anemia. However, for any level of serum creatinine, patients with polycystic disease tend to be less anemic than those with other types of renal disease. In contrast to the anemias associated with other chronic disorders, the anemia of uremia can be very severe, with hemoglobin levels as low as 4 g/dL.

Examination of the bone marrow seldom reveals any abnormalities. Red cell morphology is usually normal. In a minority of patients, the peripheral blood smear reveals so-called burr cells characterized by an evenly scalloped border. Neither the degree of anemia nor the red blood cell lifespan is influenced by the presence of burr cells. In most patients, the corrected reticulocyte count is low, and the red blood cell survival is only modestly decreased. Thus, the low red blood cell mass is due to decreased red blood cell production.

PATHOBIOLOGY

The primary basis for the anemia is the diseased kidneys' inability to secrete adequate amounts of erythropoietin. Plasma erythropoietin levels are lower than those of nonuremic patients with a comparable degree of anemia (see Fig. 158-3). Erythropoiesis is further impaired but not abolished in patients who have undergone bilateral nephrectomy. In addition, red blood cell production may be suppressed by the accumulation of substances that are normally cleared by the kidneys.

Other factors may aggravate the anemia of renal disease. Uremic patients have a propensity to hemorrhage, owing to a qualitative defect in platelet function. As in other patients, chronic gastrointestinal blood loss leads to iron deficiency. Folic acid deficiency may also occur, owing to the poor nutrition of many patients or to the loss of this vitamin during dialysis. Patients whose renal failure is due to thrombotic thrombocytopenic purpura or hemolytic-uremic syndrome (Chapter 172) have a severe form of microangiopathic hemolytic anemia, with characteristic abnormalities of red blood cell morphology (Chapter 157).

TREATMENT Rx

Treatment of the anemia of uremia first focuses on reversing the renal failure. A prompt and dramatic correction of the anemia follows successful renal transplantation. Occasionally, polycythemia may be encountered after renal engraftment and may be a harbinger of impending rejection.

In patients who are not candidates for renal transplantation, the treatment of anemia of uremia has been revolutionized by the administration of recombinant human erythropoietin (rHuEPO). The rapid and complete responses that occur underscore the importance of erythropoietin in the pathogenesis of anemia. Figure 158-8 shows the hematologic response of one of the first patients treated with rHuEPO. Within a few days of initiating rHuEPO therapy, the hematocrit approached normal, necessitating a reduction in dose. Before rHuEPO treatment, this patient was overloaded with iron, as documented by increased serum ferritin and nearly full saturation of serum transferrin. As the

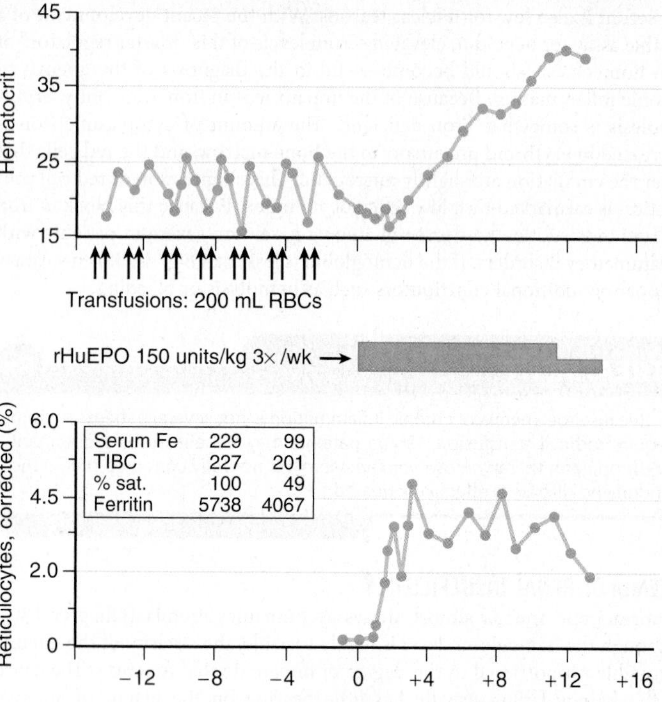

FIGURE 158-8. Response of a uremic patient to recombinant human erythropoietin (rHuEPO) therapy. Before therapy, the patient was severely anemic and transfusion dependent. Treatment with rHuEPO resulted in a reticulocytosis, followed by a progressive increase in hemoglobin. The dose of rHuEPO had to be lowered to prevent the hemoglobin from rising too high. Before rHuEPO therapy, the patient was severely iron overloaded. The marked increase in red cell mass following therapy was accompanied by a significant reduction in iron stores. RBC = red blood cell; TIBC = total iron-binding capacity. (From Eschbach JW, Egrie JC, Downing MR, et al. Correction of the anemia of end-stage renal disease with recombinant human erythropoietin: results of a combined phase I and II clinical trial. *N Engl J Med.* 1987;316:73-78.)

red cell mass increased rapidly following treatment, the robust utilization of iron stores resulted in a decline in serum ferritin and transferrin saturation. In contrast to this patient with iron overload, many uremic patients on dialysis therapy have normal or low iron stores before rHuEPO therapy and need the concomitant administration of iron to maximize the erythropoietic response. (See Erythropoietin Therapy in section on Approach to the Treatment of Anemia.)

ANEMIA OF ENDOCRINE HYPOFUNCTION

The in vitro proliferation of erythroid cells is stimulated by a number of hormones, including thyroxine, glucocorticoids, testosterone, and growth hormone. Therefore, it is not surprising that a mild to moderate normocytic anemia generally accompanies endocrine deficiency states, including hypothyroidism, Addison disease, hypogonadism, and panhypopituitarism.

In the anemia of hypothyroidism, erythropoiesis is suppressed, and the red blood cell lifespan is normal. A minority of patients have macrocytic red blood cells, sometimes owing to cobalamin deficiency. Patients with hypothyroidism have an increased incidence of pernicious anemia. Some patients, particularly females with menorrhagia, develop iron deficiency and a microcytic anemia. The anemia of hypothyroidism may be masked because of a reduction in plasma volume. Because the signs and symptoms of hypothyroidism are sometimes elusive (Chapter 226), this diagnosis should be considered in any patient with unexplained anemia.

The anemia of adrenal insufficiency, including Addison disease, may also be masked by a decrease in plasma volume. Untreated patients have an average hemoglobin level of about 13 g/dL. Upon hormone replacement, the plasma volume is rapidly reconstituted, and the hemoglobin level falls to 80% of its pretreatment value. With continued therapy, the red blood cell mass returns to normal.

Testosterone influences erythropoiesis in a physiologic manner. In males, the mean hemoglobin level increases from 13 to 15 g/dL during the transition from puberty to adulthood. Eunuchoid males usually have a mild anemia (hemoglobin ≈ 13 g/dL). Pituitary dysfunction or ablation is also associated with a mild anemia.

The anemias secondary to endocrine failure are all readily corrected when adequate hormone replacement is given.

ANEMIA OF CHRONIC LIVER DISEASE

Chronic liver disease, regardless of cause (Chapter 146), is usually accompanied by mild or moderate anemia that is normocytic or slightly macrocytic. An increased plasma volume may artificially lower the hematocrit, making the anemia seem worse than it is. Red cell morphology is normal, except for the presence of target cells (see Fig. 157-6) and occasional stomatocytes that have a slitlike rather than a circular area of central pallor. These morphologic features reflect an increased red cell membrane surface area due to increased deposits of cholesterol and phospholipid. The bone marrow is usually normal. Erythropoiesis fails to compensate for a modest shortening of the red cell lifespan. The mechanism underlying the anemia of chronic liver disease is not understood. The anemia is usually corrected if the patient regains normal hepatic function.

In patients with alcoholic liver disease (Chapters 152 and 153), the situation is much more complex. Many factors can contribute to the development of anemia. Alcohol in high doses suppresses not only erythropoiesis but also neutrophil and platelet production. In alcoholics who continue to drink up to the time of clinical evaluation, the bone marrow often reveals vacuoles in the cytoplasm of red and white blood cell precursors. In addition, ringed sideroblasts may be observed, especially if there is concurrent malnutrition. Folic acid deficiency is common in alcoholics because of both a suboptimal diet and an impairment of folate utilization. Moreover, the anemia in alcoholics is often compounded by gastrointestinal hemorrhage as a result of gastric erosions, duodenal ulcers, or esophageal varices. The risk for blood loss is further increased by the presence of thrombocytopenia and/or deficiencies in soluble clotting factors. Although alcoholics usually have increased iron stores, they may become iron deficient after prolonged gastrointestinal bleeding. Rarely, patients with alcoholic cirrhosis develop a severe hemolytic anemia accompanied by the appearance of rigid blood cells with irregular borders called acanthocytes or "spur" cells.

ANEMIA OF THE ELDERLY

As individuals age there is a slight and gradual fall in hemoglobin and hematocrit levels. Elderly individuals whose values fall below 2 standard deviations of normal have significantly enhanced morbidity and mortality. As people age, there is also an increased incidence of cancer, myelodysplasia, renal insufficiency, and chronic inflammatory disorders, all of which can suppress red cell production. Because of the high likelihood of comorbid conditions among the elderly,[6] it is not possible to affirm with any certainty whether aging per se is a cause of anemia. Nevertheless, a fall in hemoglobin in any patient, old or young, should prompt an investigation into the possible presence of one of these underlying disorders. Further studies will be needed to elucidate the molecular pathogenesis of anemia of elderly people, as well as to determine the appropriate hemoglobin concentrations for older adults in light of age, gender, race, and comorbidities.

HEMOLYTIC ANEMIAS

With the exception of sickle cell disease (Chapter 163), hemolytic anemias are encountered much less frequently than those caused by decreased red cell production. Although they are a diverse group, the hemolytic anemias share a number of clinical and laboratory features. Patients with moderate or severe hemolysis may have icterus owing to an elevation in nonconjugated (indirect) bilirubin. In addition, individuals with various types of hemolytic anemia often have splenomegaly, signifying the primary site of enhanced red cell destruction.

PATHOBIOLOGY

The presence of hemolysis is established by the laboratory tests outlined in Table 158-5. Further evaluation is required to establish the specific diagnosis. The clinician saves both time and money by using the available tests in a rational and orderly manner. Diagnosis of hemolytic anemias is greatly facilitated by the use of a logical and pathophysiologically based classification scheme. Table 158-6 groups these disorders going from the outside of the red cell into the cytoplasm, as well as by whether the defect is inherited or acquired. Hemolytic anemias due to environmental factors such as immune destruction or traumatic rupture (Chapter 160) are acquired. Abnormalities of red cell membrane proteins can also cause hemolysis. Mutations in

TABLE 158-5 LABORATORY FEATURES COMMON TO HEMOLYTIC ANEMIAS

Peripheral blood
- Increased reticulocyte count
- Polychromasia

Bone marrow—erythroid hyperplasia

Serum
- Increased nonconjugated (indirect) bilirubin
- Elevated lactate dehydrogenase (isoenzymes 1, 2, and 3)
- Decreased or absent haptoglobin
- Plasma hemoglobin
  - Extravascular hemolysis: moderately increased
  - Intravascular hemolysis: markedly increased

Urine
- Hemoglobinuria — In intravascular hemolysis
- Hemosiderin in urine sediment — In intravascular hemolysis

TABLE 158-6 CLASSIFICATION OF THE HEMOLYTIC ANEMIAS*

Classification	
Environmental factors	Acquired
Antibody: immunohemolytic anemias	Acquired
Mechanical trauma: TTP, HUS, heart valve	Acquired
Toxins, infectious agents: malaria, etc.	Acquired
Membrane defects	
Paroxysmal nocturnal hemoglobinuria	Acquired
Spur cell anemia	Acquired
Hereditary spherocytosis, etc.	Congenital
Defects of cell interior	Congenital
Hemoglobinopathies: sickle cell, thalassemia	Congenital
Enzymopathies: G6PD deficiency, etc.	Congenital

*A more detailed differential diagnosis of the hemolytic anemias is presented in Table 160-1 in Chapter 160.
G6PD = glucose-6-phosphate dehydrogenase; HUS = hemolytic-uremic syndrome; TTP = thrombotic thrombocytopenic purpura.

proteins of the red cell cytoskeleton may cause hemolysis of varying severity. The most commonly encountered is hereditary spherocytosis (Chapter 161). Acquired red cell membrane defects are rare. Paroxysmal nocturnal hemoglobinuria is discussed in Chapter 160, and spur cell anemia was mentioned earlier in the section on anemias secondary to chronic liver disease. The proteins in the cytosol of the red cell include hemoglobin and enzymes. Mutations in these proteins can result in inherited hemolytic anemias. Sickle cell disease (Chapter 163) and the thalassemias (Chapter 162) are the most commonly encountered hemoglobinopathies. Homozygous SS disease and the compound heterozygous states SC disease and S/β-thalassemia are pure hemolytic anemias. In contrast, anemia in the clinically significant forms of β-thalassemia is primarily due to ineffective erythropoiesis. By far the most common red cell enzyme defect is glucose-6-phosphate dehydrogenase deficiency (Chapter 161).

DIAGNOSIS

A number of laboratory tests are used to establish the presence of accelerated breakdown of red cells (see Table 158-5). As mentioned in the section Laboratory Evaluation of the Patient with Anemia, the reticulocyte count is the simplest and most cost-effective way to distinguish between hemolytic anemias and those due to decreased red cell production. In this test, a supervital stain or a probe for RNA reveals strands of polyribosomes that are present for only 24 to 48 hours after red cells exit the bone marrow. On a routine Wright or Romanowsky stain, these cells often appear relatively large, with a blue-gray hue (so-called polychromasia). The reticulocyte count is nearly always elevated in patients with hemolysis (unless there is concomitant marrow suppression, such as by folic acid or iron deficiency). This test is a reliable index of red cell production. Thus, in patients with hemolytic anemia, the bone marrow nearly always exhibits erythroid hyperplasia. Because this result is predictable, a bone marrow examination is seldom helpful in patients with hemolytic anemia, unless there is suspicion that the hemolysis is due to an underlying lymphoma.

A number of serum and urine tests are available to confirm the presence of hemolysis and assess its magnitude. As mentioned earlier, serum nonconjugated bilirubin is elevated in proportion to the severity of the hemolysis. Lactate dehydrogenase (LDH) isoforms type 1 through 3 are released from red cells during hemolysis, resulting in increased serum LDH. Most kinds of hemolytic anemia are extravascular, with red cell destruction mediated by macrophages in the spleen, liver, and bone marrow. In these patients, a relatively small amount of hemoglobin is released from engulfed red cells into the plasma, where it binds specifically to haptoglobin. The hemoglobin-haptoglobin complex is rapidly cleared from the circulation. Measurement of serum haptoglobin is a useful test of hemolysis. Most patients with clinically significant hemolysis have very low or absent levels. Less often, patients have intravascular hemolysis with much higher levels of free hemoglobin in the plasma, sufficient to traverse renal glomeruli and exceed the tubular reabsorption capacity. These patients have red or brown urine that, after centrifugation, tests positive with a "dipstick" that detects heme protein. Hemoglobinuria can be readily distinguished from myoglobinuria. In the former, both the plasma and the urine are pigmented. In the latter, the plasma remains colorless because the smaller myoglobin molecule rapidly traverses the glomeruli. Hemoglobinuria is often transient. For a week or so after the episode has abated, the urine sediment will contain hemosiderin, which can be readily detected with the Prussian blue iron stain.

After these general laboratory tests confirm the presence of hemolysis, an array of specific tests is available to establish the specific cause (Chapters 160 through 163).

APPROACH TO THE TREATMENT OF ANEMIA

As in other disorders, the effective treatment of anemia is based on a thorough diagnostic evaluation. Hematinics such as iron, cobalamin, or folic acid should not be administered unless a specific deficiency has been demonstrated or is anticipated. Although indiscriminate treatment with cobalamin is not harmful per se, it lulls both the patient and the physician into a false sense of security in the absence of a firm diagnosis. In contrast, the inappropriate use of iron preparations over a prolonged period can be directly harmful, leading to a state of iron overload in some incorrectly diagnosed patients.

Many kinds of anemias can be corrected if a precipitating cause can be uncovered and reversed. If a drug or toxin is responsible, its withdrawal may allow full recovery. Correction of anemia secondary to a chronic disease usually depends on whether the underlying condition can be reversed. One of the most dramatic dividends of successful renal transplantation is the rapid correction of the anemia of uremia.

Erythropoietin Therapy

The administration of erythropoiesis-stimulating agents (ESA) (epoetin alfa and darbepoetin alfa) is remarkably effective in certain circumstances. In addition to those with the anemia of chronic renal failure, selected patients with other types of anemia may benefit from ESAs. Treatment can lower transfusion requirements in patients with cancer or HIV infection in whom anemia has been aggravated by chemotherapy. In comparison with patients with renal failure, higher doses are required for those with cancer or AIDS to achieve the same increase in red cell mass. Treatment with ESAs has also been effective in some patients with primary bone marrow disorders, particularly myelodysplasia (Chapter 182). Transfusion requirements in surgical patients, both perioperatively and postoperatively, may be reduced by prior short-term administration of ESAs. Treatment may also benefit rare patients who are unable to receive blood transfusions because of either antigen incompatibility or religious convictions.

A note of caution has emerged from a number of large studies suggesting that high doses of ESAs that drive the hemoglobin level above 12 g/dL are associated with a slight but significant increase in the risk for thrombosis and cardiovascular mortality. Systematic reviews and meta-analyses of treatment with ESAs in patients with chronic kidney disease that target higher hemoglobin levels increase the risk for vascular access thrombosis and cardiovascular complications (Chapters 130 and 131),[A1][A2] and likewise for thromboembolic events in patients with cancer.[A3]

Primary bone marrow disorders pose a formidable therapeutic challenge. Aplastic anemia (Chapter 165) can be cured by both immunosuppressive therapy and stem cell transplantation. Long-lasting remissions can be achieved in an increasing fraction of patients with acute leukemias by chemotherapy, often coupled with stem cell transplantation (Chapter 178). Other primary bone marrow disorders that are unresponsive to these interventions are treated with supportive measures such as transfusions of red cells and platelets.

Red Cell Transfusion

The decision whether to transfuse an anemic patient is often challenging. The risks and complications of the administration of blood products are discussed in Chapter 177. Patients with chronic or long-standing anemia are able to compensate in several ways, discussed earlier in this chapter. A considerable reduction in red cell mass can be surprisingly well tolerated, especially if the patient is young or sedentary. Transfusion is seldom indicated in a patient with chronic anemia whose hemoglobin is 9 g/dL or greater. Those who are expected to respond to the administration of a specific agent such as iron, folic acid, or vitamin B_{12} can usually be spared transfusions.

Current evidence does not support the benefit of liberal transfusions in patients with asymptomatic anemia and heart disease. Indeed the American College of Physicians Guidelines on Treatment for Anemia in Patients with Heart Disease warns against both red cell transfusion and the use of ESAs in patients with cardiovascular disease who have mild to moderate anemia.[7] However, if the anemia is severe and accompanied by myocardial or cerebral ischemia or by congestive heart failure, prompt but slow administration of packed red cells is indicated. Whole blood should be given only if the patient is hypovolemic.

Splenectomy

Splenectomy is indicated in the treatment of certain hemolytic anemias. The efficacy of splenectomy correlates with the degree to which the abnormal or defective red cells are destroyed or sequestered in the spleen. Splenectomy is curative in nearly all patients with hereditary spherocytosis (Chapter 161). The operation may be also beneficial in selected patients with immunohemolytic anemia, congestive splenomegaly, spur cell anemia, and certain hemoglobinopathies and enzymopathies. The operative morbidity and mortality from elective splenectomy are very low. The procedure can often be done by laparoscopy. Occasional patients develop postoperative left subphrenic abscess. Following splenectomy, young children are at risk for developing overwhelming septicemia. This complication can be partially prevented by vaccination against pneumococcus and meningococcus. Post-splenectomy sepsis occurs rarely in adults. The risk for sepsis can be circumvented by partial splenectomy. Thrombocytosis generally develops promptly following splenectomy. However, in most cases it is transient. In patients with continued hemolysis or with a myeloproliferative disorder (Chapter 166), the thrombocytosis usually persists and may occasionally be associated with thromboembolic complications.

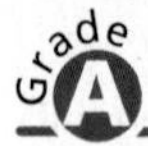

Grade A References

A1. Vinhas J, Barreto C, Assuncao J, et al. Treatment of anaemia with erythropoiesis-stimulating agents in patients with chronic kidney disease does not lower mortality and may increase cardiovascular risk: a meta-analysis. *Nephron Clin Pract*. 2012;121:c95-c101.

A2. Palmer SC, Navaneethan SD, Craig JC, et al. Meta-analysis: erythropoiesis-stimulating agents in patients with chronic kidney disease. *Ann Intern Med*. 2010;153:23-33.

A3. Tonia T, Mettler A, Robert N, et al. Erythropoietin or darbepoetin for patients with cancer. *Cochrane Database Syst Rev*. 2012;12:CD003407.

GENERAL REFERENCES

For the General References and other additional features, please visit Expert Consult at https://expertconsult.inkling.com.

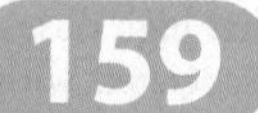

MICROCYTIC AND HYPOCHROMIC ANEMIAS

GORDON D. GINDER

The oxygen-carrying hemoglobin molecule executes the principal function of the mature erythrocyte. The hemoglobin content of erythrocytes is determined by the coordinated production of globin protein, the heme porphyrin ring, and the availability of iron. A deficiency in any of these three critical components of hemoglobin results in hypochromic and/or microcytic anemia (see Fig. 158-5).[1] Microcytic anemia is typically reported initially by automated red blood cell (RBC) indices. Hypochromic microcytic anemia can be confirmed on the peripheral blood smear (Fig. 159-1). Disorders of globin protein production typically produce microcytosis but not hypochromia and are discussed elsewhere (Chapter 162).

IRON DEFICIENCY ANEMIA

EPIDEMIOLOGY

Iron deficiency is by far the most common cause of anemia worldwide and is among the most frequently encountered medical problems seen by primary care physicians in the United States. More than 1.6 billion people, almost one fourth of the world's population, are anemic, and iron deficiency accounts for about half of the world's anemia burden.[2] It is estimated that between 2 and 5% of adolescent girls in the United States have iron deficiency sufficient to cause anemia. Elsewhere, the prevalence of iron deficiency–induced anemia is much higher, with estimates that up to 10% of the world population, or more than 500 million people, are affected. The prevalence rates are especially high in developing countries where dietary insufficiency and intestinal parasites are prevalent.

PATHOBIOLOGY

Most of the approximately 4 g of iron in the adult human body is incorporated into hemoglobin (approximately 2100 mg) in erythrocytes or myoglobin (approximately 300 mg) in muscle. The remainder is chiefly present as storage iron in the liver (1000 mg) and in the reticuloendothelial macrophages of the bone marrow and spleen (600 mg) (Fig. 159-2). Only a small

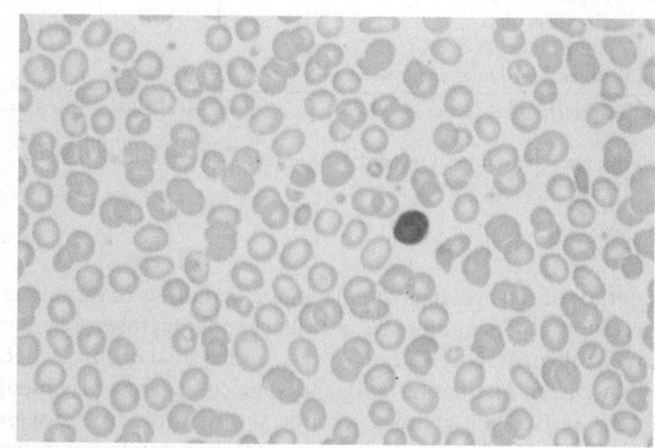

FIGURE 159-1. Iron deficiency anemia. Many of these red blood cells are microcytic (smaller than the nucleus of the normal lymphocyte near the center of the field) and hypochromic (with central areas of pallor that exceed half the diameter of the cells).

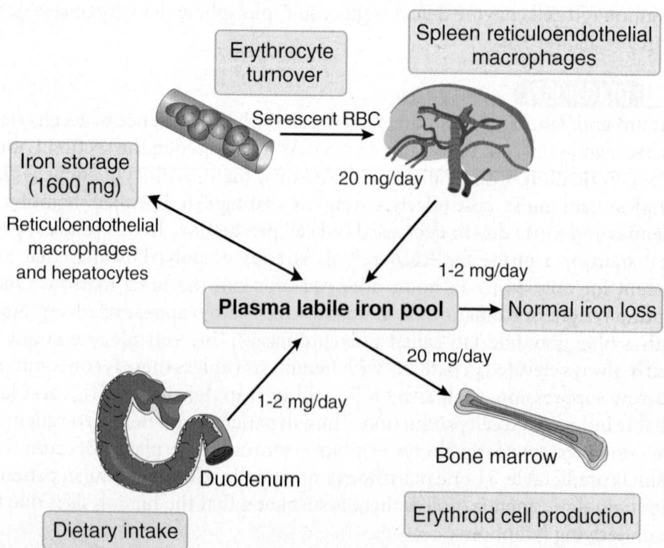

FIGURE 159-2. Iron homeostasis in normal humans. RBC = red blood cell.

amount of iron (3 to 7 mg) is freely circulating in plasma bound to transferrin, but this pool is kinetically very active, turning over every 3 to 4 hours. Because of the potent conservation mechanisms of iron recycling through the reticuloendothelial macrophage system, only an average of about 1 to 2 mg of iron is normally lost per day, largely through mucosal sloughing, desquamation, and, in females of reproductive age, menstruation.

The ability of iron to donate or accept electrons readily through conversion between the ferrous (Fe^{2+}) and ferric (Fe^{3+}) states makes it a critical component of the hemoglobin and myoglobin porphyrin rings that transport oxygen as well as cytochromes and various other vital enzymes. Free iron is extremely toxic owing to its capacity to catalyze the formation of free radicals, which lead to cellular damage. Therefore, the majority of body iron that is not stably incorporated into porphyrin rings is associated with proteins. Transferrin is the major protein associated with circulating plasma iron, and ferritin is the major protein associated with stored intracellular iron both in the cytoplasm and in mitochondria. Because the normal rate of iron loss is low, only about 1 to 2 mg/day of dietary iron is needed to maintain homeostasis. The average Western diet contains about 20 mg/day, and the efficiency of iron absorption in the duodenum is usually sufficient to maintain the amount of iron required for homeostatic balance.

Control of iron absorption by the duodenal crypt cells is critical because of the lack of any regulated physiologic mechanism for iron excretion. As a result, excessive iron intake can lead to deleterious iron overload, with concomitant organ damage (Chapter 212). Nonheme dietary iron is dissolved in part by the low pH of the stomach effluent. After reduction to the ferrous state by ferroreductase, iron is transferred across the apical crypt cell membrane by divalent metal transporter-1 (DMT-1). Several levels of regulation are involved in iron absorption by the intestine. One of these is modulated by dietary intake; thus, after a large influx of dietary iron, the duodenal absorptive capacity is diminished. A second regulatory mechanism modulates the iron absorption capacity based on total body iron stores. Finally, the so-called erythropoietic regulator modulates the capacity for enterocyte absorption based on the iron needed for erythropoiesis. A paradoxical increase in iron absorption through this mechanism occurs in certain types of anemia characterized by predominantly intramedullary destruction of erythroid cells (causing ineffective erythropoiesis): sideroblastic anemia, the thalassemias (Chapter 162), and congenital dyserythropoietic anemias.

Once inside the intestinal absorbing cell, iron is stored in complex with ferritin. Circulating plasma iron is complexed with the iron transport protein transferrin. The transferrin-iron complex is then taken up by erythroid precursors through the transferrin receptor. The high density of transferrin receptors on erythroid precursors ensures the preferential uptake of iron by these cells and explains why erythropoiesis proceeds normally until a critical deficiency of transferrin-bound iron, reflecting a depletion of total body iron, is present. The levels of transferrin, transferrin receptor, ferritin, and other proteins important in iron metabolism are regulated by the iron regulatory proteins IRP-1 and IRP-2.

Hepcidin, a 25-amino acid peptide, is the central regulator of iron homeostasis through its effects on intestinal absorption, macrophage recycling of iron from senescent RBCs, and iron mobilization from hepatic stores.[3] Thus, hepcidin affects all major sites of iron uptake and storage. Hepcidin is produced in the liver and acts as a negative regulator of iron absorption by the intestine and of iron release from storage in the macrophages and hepatocytes (see Fig. 158-7). It is believed that hepcidin binds to ferroportin, the major iron transporter in the membranes of the enterocyte, macrophage, and hepatocyte, causing the internalization and degradation of ferroportin. This process blocks the transport of iron across the membrane of the basolateral crypt cell, preventing its incorporation into transferrin-bound plasma iron. Likewise, loss of ferroportin function blocks the major export pathway of iron stores from macrophages and hepatocytes. Hepcidin production is upregulated by iron and downregulated by hypoxia, consistent with its homeostatic role. Because hepcidin is also upregulated by inflammatory cytokines, it is believed to play an important role in the paradoxical lack of transferrin-bound iron available for erythropoiesis in the face of adequate or even excess iron stores found in the anemia of chronic inflammation (see later and Chapter 158).

Blood Loss

Iron deficiency anemia results from an imbalance between available body iron for hemoglobin production and the minimal amount needed to sustain normal hemoglobin production during erythropoiesis (see Fig. 159-2). Because of the combined effectiveness of dietary absorption and retention of iron under normal circumstances, this mismatch is most often due to blood loss, with the gastrointestinal (GI) tract being the most common site (Chapter 135) in men and nonmenstruating women. In developed countries, the blood loss is usually secondary to benign or neoplastic lesions of the GI tract (Chapters 192 and 193) or chronic ingestion of drugs that cause GI mucosal damage (Chapter 139). The most common offending agents are alcohol and salicylates or other nonsteroidal anti-inflammatory agents. In developing countries, helminthic infections, including hookworm (Chapter 357) and schistosomiasis (Chapter 355), are among the most common causes of GI blood loss.

Genitourinary tract blood loss resulting in iron deficiency is most common in menstruating women. Less common are urinary tract malignancies (Chapter 197) and hemoglobinuria due to intravascular hemolysis (Chapter 160). Respiratory tract blood loss is far less common as a cause of iron deficiency.

Reproduction and Growth

In most cases, an increased iron requirement is due to blood loss; other causes include rapid growth in infancy and adolescence and pregnancy and lactation in adulthood. It is estimated that failure to satisfy the increased iron requirements during pregnancy with supplemental iron may result in a deficiency equivalent to a cumulative blood loss of up to 1500 mL.

Inadequate Iron Intake

The other major cause of iron deficiency is inadequate iron intake. Only diets that lack 1 to 2 mg/day fail to provide adequate iron. The average Western meal contains about 6 mg of iron, so dietary insufficiency is not a common cause of iron deficiency. Certain diets that lack iron or contain large quantities of phytates from cereals or tannate from tea, both of which inhibit intestinal iron absorption, may result in iron deficiency. Although iron is usually readily absorbed, primarily in the duodenum, pathologic states that can impair the process include generalized intestinal malabsorption (Chapter 140), atrophic gastritis (Chapter 139) with achlorhydria, and extensive gastric surgery. In contrast, chronic use of histamine-2 (H_2) receptor blockers or proton pump inhibitors does not appear to cause iron deficiency. In the United States, celiac disease (Chapter 140) is an increasingly common cause of iron deficiency, with resulting anemia.

CLINICAL MANIFESTATIONS

Because of compensatory physiologic mechanisms, patients with mild iron deficiency anemia may be asymptomatic. Iron deficiency in these patients may be recognized during the evaluation of an underlying disease process or as part of routine laboratory studies. The findings of microcytosis and hypochromia occur only after the hematocrit has fallen to approximately 30%, so neither finding may be present in early stages.

The anemia of iron deficiency, like other anemias, manifests with nonspecific symptoms such as weakness, pallor, dizziness, decreased exercise tolerance, or irritability. Because iron is a critical component of the porphyrin complex in muscle as well as many essential metabolic enzymes, its deficiency affects other organ systems besides the erythron, often resulting in a degree of fatigue, exercise intolerance, and weakness out of proportion to the hemoglobin level. Repletion of iron in iron-deficient individuals may improve cognitive and exercise performance. In addition, intravenous iron treatment in patients with heart failure and coexisting iron deficiency (to which heart failure patients are prone) can improve symptoms, functional capacity, and quality of life, irrespective of the presence or absence of anemia.[A1]

Rare patients, most frequently elderly women, may have dysphagia due to an esophageal stricture or web (Plummer-Vinson syndrome). A clinical manifestation unique to iron deficiency is pica, which is an unusual craving for certain non-nutritional substances. Pica may manifest as a craving for ice (pagophagia) or, less commonly, for clay (geophagia) or starch (amylophagia); pagophagia is believed to be the most specific for iron deficiency.

Physical findings that may be associated with the iron-deficient state include glossitis and angular stomatitis. Other less common but highly specific findings are spooning of the fingernails (koilonychia) and blue-tinged sclerae.

DIAGNOSIS

The diagnosis of iron deficiency anemia is made by laboratory testing. Because microcytic hypochromic RBCs are a sine qua non of this type of anemia, initial screening consists of a determination of hemoglobin levels, mean corpuscular volume, erythrocyte hemoglobin content, and reticulocyte

TABLE 159-1 LABORATORY FINDINGS FOR IRON STUDIES IN MICROCYTIC AND HYPOCHROMIC ANEMIAS

ANEMIA	SERUM IRON	TIBC	TRANSFERRIN SATURATION (%)	SERUM FERRITIN	SERUM TRANSFERRIN RECEPTOR	MARROW RE IRON	MARROW RINGED SIDEROBLASTS
Iron deficiency anemia	Low	High	0-15	Low (<30 μg/L)	High	Absent	Absent
Anemia of chronic disease	Low	Normal or low	5-15	Normal or high	Normal	Normal or high	Absent
Sideroblastic anemia	High	Normal	60-90	High	Normal or high	High	Present

RE = reticuloendothelial; TIBC = total iron-binding capacity.

count. In experienced hands, the peripheral blood smear (Chapter 157) is an excellent indicator of iron deficiency anemia. In iron deficiency anemia, most erythrocytes are smaller in diameter than the nucleus of a typical lymphocyte, and the area of central pallor is greater than 50% of the total diameter of the erythrocyte (see Fig. 159-1). Variability of erythrocyte size distinguishes iron deficiency anemia from other conditions that give rise to microcytosis; the calculated variability in RBC volume (the so-called RBC volume distribution width, or RDW) is elevated early in iron deficiency anemia.

The definitive diagnosis of iron deficiency anemia is made by tests that measure total body iron stores: the absence of iron stores that can be mobilized is unique to this microcytic hypochromic anemia. Transferrin and transferrin-bound iron levels may not be reliable indicators of iron deficiency because they are also abnormal in the anemia of chronic disease, despite adequate total body iron stores (see Fig. 158-6).

The serum ferritin level is the most reliable, noninvasive, and cost-effective indicator that is routinely available in most clinical laboratories (Table 159-1). In a large study of 259 anemic patients, a serum ferritin level less than 18 μg/L was diagnostic of iron deficiency with greater than 95% specificity and a 55% sensitivity. At a serum ferritin level of 45 μg/L, the sensitivity rose to approximately 70%, and a level higher than 100 μg/L in populations with a less than 40% prevalence of iron deficiency excluded a diagnosis of iron deficiency with more than 90% sensitivity. Although some recent studies have questioned the accuracy of the routine determination of stainable marrow iron, this test is still generally considered to be the "gold standard" for tests of iron deficiency. However, determination of total bone marrow iron stores is rarely necessary to diagnose iron deficiency anemia, except when there is some other complicating process.

One setting in which serum ferritin levels can be spuriously elevated is chronic inflammation or chronic disease. A meta-analysis involving 8796 subjects suggested that measurement of C-reactive protein (CRP) and α_1-acid glycoprotein (ACP) to assess for the level of inflammation can improve the accuracy of ferritin level as an indicator of iron deficiency.[4] The soluble serum transferrin receptor (sTfR) level is an excellent measure of total erythroid precursor mass. The sTfR is aberrantly elevated in the presence of iron deficiency, so it is considered a useful test for this condition. A number of studies have demonstrated the utility of the sTfR/ferritin ratio in distinguishing iron deficiency from the anemia of chronic disease. However, the lack of reliable standards and a meta-analysis of efficacy of the test indicating that additional data are needed to define the diagnostic accuracy of the sTfR[5] have prevented this assay from becoming routinely available in clinical practice.

TREATMENT

Rx

The treatment of iron deficiency anemia is replenishment of body iron stores. However, the underlying cause should always be investigated before treatment is begun because in many cases it is a correctable and potentially fatal GI lesion (Chapter 135).

Oral Administration

The preferred route of iron administration is oral. Oral iron is most readily absorbed in the absence of food, especially in the setting of decreased stomach acid production owing to atrophic gastritis, gastric surgery, or chronic suppression of gastric acid with an H_2 antagonist or proton pump inhibitor. The major obstacle to oral iron replacement is unacceptable side effects, chiefly epigastric discomfort or nausea; diarrhea or constipation also occurs in some patients. Reducing the dose often eliminates nausea and epigastric discomfort. Despite the development of a number of orally effective iron-containing compounds, the original salt, ferrous sulfate (325 mg three times daily), remains the most useful. Although some newer oral iron preparations, such as ferrous gluconate (300 mg two or three times daily) or ferrous fumarate (325 mg two or three times daily), may induce fewer GI side effects per milligram of iron, they are also less well absorbed, so there is no net advantage to these costlier formulations except for patients who cannot tolerate ferrous sulfate. Given both the low toxicity and the low cost of oral iron replacement, a therapeutic trial is an alternative means of confirming a diagnosis of iron deficiency anemia.

Parenteral Administration

In situations in which primary blood loss is uncontrollable, iron cannot be absorbed owing to severe malabsorption, or oral iron is not tolerated despite concerted efforts to minimize side effects, parenteral iron is an effective alternative treatment. Intramuscular dosing is limited to 100 mg/injection, so intravenous administration is recommended. Sodium ferric gluconate (given intravenously at a dose of 125 mg over 10 minutes) is the preferred form of parenteral iron owing to the low incidence of adverse reactions. A multi-institutional, double-blind, randomized, placebo-controlled trial of more than 2500 patients showed similar adverse events in patients receiving sodium ferric gluconate versus those receiving placebo, and only one life-threatening complication occurred; in comparison, there were 23 such events among 3768 patients treated with iron dextran in a historical control arm. One limitation of sodium ferric gluconate is that the maximum dose deliverable in a single injection is approximately 125 mg, and a total dose of 500 to 2000 mg is usually required for adequate repletion. Although large doses of iron dextran can be delivered in a single intravenous injection, this is currently reserved for situations in which rapid iron replacement is required because of the life-threatening anaphylactic and delayed adverse reactions that occur in 0.6 and 2.5% of cases, respectively. If iron dextran is to be given intravenously, premedication with diphenhydramine and a slow test-dose injection of 30 to 40 mg diluted in normal saline are recommended.

Newer iron preparations for intravenous use include ferric carboxymaltose, iron isomaltoside 1000, and ferumoxytol. These preparations allow the administration of much higher doses of intravenous iron in a shorter time and can be used safely to replenish iron stores, sometimes even in a single treatment session.

The response to iron repletion therapy is usually quite rapid, with elimination of symptoms within a few days. Increased reticulocytosis usually begins within 4 to 5 days, and the hemoglobin level often rises within 1 week and reaches a normal level after 6 weeks of therapy if adequate iron replacement is achieved. The goal of therapy, which is to reach a serum ferritin level of greater than 50 mg/L, usually takes 4 to 6 months. Therapy must be continued after adequate replacement is achieved if the underlying cause of iron deficiency is not reversible. Because of the avidity of transferrin receptor–rich erythroid precursors for transferrin-bound iron, the serum ferritin level usually does not rise until hemoglobin levels reach normal.

Failure to Respond to Iron Therapy

An incomplete or lack of response to oral iron therapy, as determined by failure to normalize the hemoglobin level, usually means either that iron replacement has not been adequate (most commonly due to noncompliance with oral iron because of its side effects) or that iron deficiency is not the primary cause of the anemia (e.g., coexisting anemia of chronic disease). Less common causes of failure to respond to oral iron include iron malabsorption (e.g., celiac disease, atrophic gastritis) or blood loss in excess of iron replacement. Refractoriness to oral iron due to celiac disease can be screened by testing for anti-tissue transglutaminase (TTG) antibodies; autoimmune atrophic gastritis by serum gastrin, parietal cell, or intrinsic factor antibodies; and *Helicobacter pylori* infection and gastritis by antibody screening or fecal antigen and urease breath test.

TMPRSS6, also called matriptase-2, is a type II transmembrane serine protease that suppresses hepcidin production. Several types of mutations in *TMPRSS6* that are either sporadic or familial (usually autosomal recessive) have recently been described as causes of iron-refractory iron deficiency anemia (IRIDA). Associated with inappropriately increased levels of urinary hepcidin, the defect causes impaired iron absorption and recycling, leading to IRIDA. Characteristically, these patients exhibit no hematologic improvement in response to oral iron intake and are only partially responsive to parenteral iron because of abnormal iron utilization.[6,7]

PROGNOSIS

In most cases, iron deficiency anemia can be corrected rapidly by either oral or parenteral replacement, but the long-term prognosis ultimately depends on the clinical course of the underlying cause. It is critical that the patient undergo a full evaluation to determine the underlying cause of the iron deficiency, especially because an occult gastrointestinal lesion, often malignant, may be present, particularly in patients older than 50 years (Chapters 192 and 193).

ANEMIA OF CHRONIC DISEASE AND INFLAMMATION

DEFINITION

Anemia of chronic disease (or *anemia of chronic inflammation*) refers to anemia that occurs in the setting of a chronic disease state, usually one associated with elevated levels of inflammatory cytokines. Although anemia of chronic inflammation usually manifests as a normochromic normocytic process (Chapter 158), between 20 and 50% of cases are associated with microcytic RBC indices. The anemia is usually mild to moderate, and it may not be symptomatic.

EPIDEMIOLOGY

Anemia of chronic inflammation is believed to be the second most common cause of anemia, after iron deficiency. It is the most common type of anemia encountered among hospitalized patients. The wide spectrum of underlying diseases includes acute and chronic infections, inflammatory and autoimmune diseases, cancers, and chronic kidney diseases.

PATHOBIOLOGY

There are three major mechanisms of anemia of chronic inflammation, and all are believed to result from the effects of abnormal levels of inflammatory cytokines. The first is dysregulated iron homeostasis, manifested by low serum iron (hypoferremia) in the presence of normal or elevated serum ferritin levels and abundant reticuloendothelial macrophage iron stores. The functional consequence is a limited availability of iron for erythroid progenitor cells and resultant restriction of erythropoiesis. Pro-inflammatory stimuli, including lipopolysaccharides, interferon-γ, and tumor necrosis factor-α (TNF-α), upregulate DMT-1, which increases iron uptake by the reticuloendothelial cells. At the same time, these stimuli cause the downregulation of ferroportin expression; ferroportin is the protein required for the release of ferrous iron from storage cells and for the transport of dietary iron from duodenal enterocytes into the circulation.

Because hepcidin is an iron-regulated, acute phase reactant peptide that blocks both iron uptake in the gut and iron release from hepatocytes and macrophage stores, its upregulation by lipopolysaccharides, interleukin (IL)-6, and possibly IL-1 (indirectly, through induction of IL-6) results in another mechanism of anemia. Also, patients with hepatic adenomas that secrete high levels of hepcidin have iron-refractory anemia in the presence of normal or elevated ferritin and macrophage iron stores, despite the absence of elevated inflammatory cytokine levels. Elevated urinary hepcidin concentrations correlate with ferritin levels in patients with anemia of inflammation, iron overload, and iron deficiency.[8] These relationships are depicted in Figure 158-7.

A third pathophysiologic feature of anemia of chronic inflammation is the inhibition of erythroid progenitor expansion. Interferon-γ is the most potent inhibitory factor of erythropoiesis, but similar inhibition is believed to be mediated by IL-1, TNF-α, and interferon-β. These mediators of inflammation act to increase erythroid progenitor apoptosis, downregulate erythropoietin receptors, and antagonize pro-hematopoietic factors. The action of erythropoietin appears to be directly antagonized by these pro-inflammatory cytokines, which would explain why responsiveness to erythropoietin seems to be inversely related to the severity of the underlying chronic inflammation and the levels of interferon-γ and TNF-α. Finally, increased erythrophagocytosis in the presence of inflammation results in a modest shortening of RBC half-life.

CLINICAL MANIFESTATIONS

The clinical manifestations in patients with anemia of chronic inflammation are usually dominated by the underlying disease process. The anemia in this condition is usually mild, with hemoglobin levels in the range of 8 to 10 g/dL. However, supervening blood loss, absolute iron deficiency, or other aggravating factors can produce life-threatening anemia. Even mild to moderate anemia contributes to the debilitating effects of the underlying disease, adversely affecting performance status and quality of life. Moreover, the presence of anemia is associated with a poorer overall prognosis in many of the underlying chronic diseases, although correction of anemia has not been directly demonstrated to improve survival.

DIAGNOSIS

The clinical diagnosis of anemia of chronic disease presenting with microcytic hypochromic RBC indices is one of exclusion, based on low serum iron in the presence of normal or increased total body iron stores (see Table 159-1). Serum ferritin is the best single laboratory marker for assessing iron storage, and it is almost invariably normal or elevated in anemia of chronic disease. If both the serum iron and the transferrin saturation are reduced, reflecting dysregulation of iron homeostasis, the diagnosis of anemia of chronic disease can be made in the appropriate clinical setting after the exclusion of other causes of anemia, such as coexistent blood loss, thalassemia (Chapter 162), and drug-induced suppression of erythropoiesis. In the presence of inflammation, however, up to 30% of patients with true iron deficiency have serum ferritin levels greater than 100 μg/L, potentially obscuring the diagnosis of iron deficiency. Assays for sTfR are useful to diagnose iron deficiency in the presence of the inflammation associated with anemia of chronic disease, but problems with standardization have limited this test's availability in clinical practice. Examination of the bone marrow for reticuloendothelial macrophage iron stores (hemosiderin) and erythroblasts containing iron granules (sideroblasts) can provide definitive evidence of absent iron stores in the setting of anemia of chronic inflammation. A low serum erythropoietin level is also useful in supporting a diagnosis of anemia of chronic inflammation, but only when the hemoglobin level is less than 10 g/dL.

TREATMENT Rx

Treatment of the Underlying Disease

The most effective treatment for anemia of chronic disease is successful treatment of the underlying inflammatory disease process, whether it is an acute or chronic infection, treatable cancer, renal failure, or rheumatoid arthritis. Even if definitive treatment is not possible, quality of life and perhaps prognosis can improve if symptomatic anemia is treated directly. Unfortunately, anemia of chronic inflammation remains undertreated, even in developed countries.

Blood Transfusion

Blood transfusion (Chapter 177) offers the immediate resolution of anemia, but it is indicated chiefly when the anemia is life threatening or seriously limits the patient's functioning. These situations almost always involve supervening blood loss or some other acute process that compounds the anemia of chronic disease. Transfusion is not recommended for the long-term treatment of mild or moderate anemia of chronic inflammation because of the secondary risks, which include transfusional iron overload, human leukocyte antigen (HLA) sensitization in the case of potential renal transplantation, and other side effects of transfusion.

Intravenous Iron and Erythropoietin Therapy

If iron replacement is needed for anemia of chronic inflammation, parenteral iron administration is usually required to replenish stores because of the block in intestinal absorption (see Parenteral Administration under Iron Deficiency Anemia). In hemodialysis patients receiving erythropoietin therapy, intravenous iron therapy improves anemia and increases both ferritin and transferrin saturation levels more than oral iron replacement; however, when intravenous iron replacement raises the transferrin saturation to greater than 20%, there appears to be an increased risk for developing bacteremia, underscoring the complex relationship between iron homeostasis and immunity.

Erythropoietin therapy is currently approved for use in patients with chronic kidney disease[9] or HIV infection, and in cancer patients who are undergoing myelosuppressive treatment. In patients with chronic kidney disease, the hemoglobin concentration goal should be 10-12 g/dL in chronic kidney disease[A2] (Chapter 130) and >9 g/dL but not >11 g/dL in end-stage renal disease patients on dialysis[A3][A4] (Chapter 131).

Patients with demonstrated iron deficiency should receive supplemental iron with intravenous iron gluconate (see the earlier discussion) while being treated with erythropoietin. There is increasing evidence that addition of iron in this setting reduces the need for higher dose erythropoietin with its attendant risks.

In patients undergoing chemotherapy for cancer whose hemoglobin is less than 10 g/dL, erythropoietin therapy improves quality of life and performance status[A5] but increases the risk of thromboembolic complications and death.[A6] Current recommendations are for cautious use during chemotherapy and against routine use in inpatients not receiving chemotherapy.

PROGNOSIS

The overall prognosis of anemia of chronic inflammation is determined almost exclusively by the course of the underlying disease. It is well established that the degree of anemia correlates well with the severity of the underlying disease process and therefore with levels of inflammatory cytokines. In the absence of a supervening process, anemia of chronic inflammation is not life threatening, and treatment of the anemia per se has not been proved to affect overall survival.

SIDEROBLASTIC ANEMIAS

DEFINITION

This heterogeneous group of anemias is distinguished by the characteristic finding of excessive mitochondrial iron in erythroblasts, as manifested by iron-laden, ringed sideroblasts in the bone marrow in the presence of moderate to severe anemia. These disorders result from mitochondrial defects either in the biosynthesis of the heme porphyrin ring or in the metabolism of iron. Both hereditary and acquired types of sideroblastic anemia have been described. Although often characterized by microcytic and sometimes hypochromic anemia, these disorders can manifest with normochromic normocytic RBCs; if the anemia is associated with myelodysplasia (Chapter 182), macrocytic RBC indices may be present.

EPIDEMIOLOGY

Although acquired sideroblastic anemias are relatively rare, they are much more prevalent than hereditary forms. The true incidence of acquired sideroblastic anemia is not well established, in part owing to the heterogeneity of causes and clinical presentations. Hereditary X-linked sideroblastic anemias usually manifest in childhood or early adulthood.

PATHOBIOLOGY

Genetics

The pathophysiologic mechanisms of hereditary sideroblastic anemias are much better understood than those of the more common idiopathic, acquired variety associated with myelodysplasia.[10,11] Two main forms of X-linked hereditary sideroblastic anemia have been characterized, and both result from defects in the heme synthesis pathway (Fig. 159-3). The first type is caused by mutations in the gene coding for erythroid-specific δ-aminolevulinic acid synthase, known as *ALAS-2*, on the X chromosome. These mutations may affect the affinity of the enzyme for pyridoxal phosphate or its structural stability, catalytic site, or susceptibility to mitochondrial proteases. In those cases in which the affinity of ALAS-2 for pyridoxal phosphate is altered, pyridoxine supplementation can ameliorate the associated anemia. The other major group of X-linked sideroblastic anemias results from defects in the adenosine triphosphate binding cassette (ABC) protein known as hABC7. The hABC7 protein is believed to be involved in iron-sulfur [FeS] cluster formation. Because [FeS] cluster–associated proteins include ferrochelatase and the cytosolic IRP-1, defects in hABC7 are believed to result in defective iron metabolism or inadequate incorporation of iron into the heme porphyrin ring by ferrochelatase. This type of X-linked sideroblastic anemia is associated with ataxia.

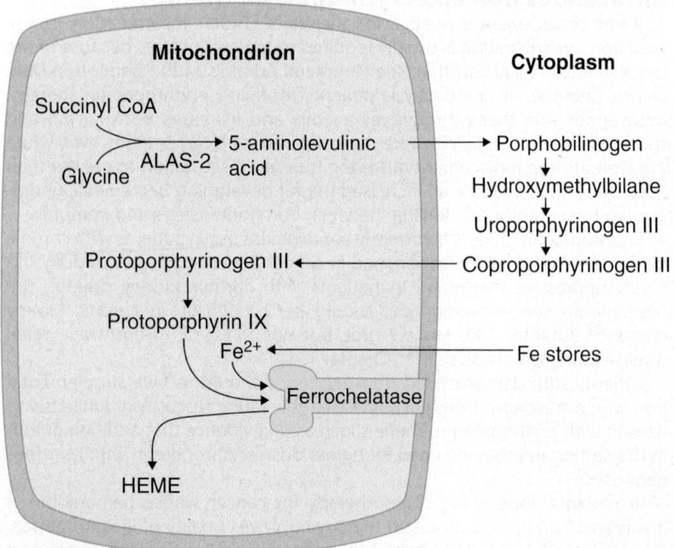

FIGURE 159-3. The heme synthesis pathway. ALAS-2 = δ-aminolevulinic acid synthase; CoA = coenzyme A.

In addition to the two X-linked causes, both autosomal dominant and recessive forms of hereditary sideroblastic anemia have been described. However, the exact mechanisms involved in these disorders are not known.

Other types of hereditary sideroblastic anemia are believed to result from mutations in the mitochondrial genome rather than in nuclear genes. The inheritance of these disorders is complex, owing to the exclusively maternal inheritance pattern of mitochondria; the ovum is the only source of embryonic mitochondria.

Exposure to Drugs or Toxins

The most common form of acquired sideroblastic anemia results from nutritional deficiency or exposure to exogenous drugs or toxins, especially alcohol. Although sideroblastic anemia is not a common finding in alcoholism, the high incidence of alcohol abuse in Western cultures accounts for its frequency as a cause. Alcohol directly inhibits erythropoiesis, but sideroblastic anemia is usually seen only in the setting of concurrent alcoholism and nutritional deficiencies. Other well-documented drug exposures associated with sideroblastic anemia include isoniazid, chloramphenicol, and cycloserine. Sideroblastic anemia has also been attributed to lead exposure (Chapter 22), but there are limited primary data to support this association. Deficiency of pyridoxine causes sideroblastic anemia in animals and may also occur in the setting of alcoholism in humans, although ethanol is believed to be an antagonist of the interaction of pyridoxal phosphate with 5-aminolevulinic acid as a cofactor in the first step of heme biosynthesis. Copper deficiency, though rare, has also been associated with sideroblastic anemia, usually in the setting of an overdose of bivalent cation chelators such as penicillamine or trientine, used to treat the copper overloading found in Wilson disease (Chapter 211).

Idiopathic Forms

The major cause of acquired sideroblastic anemia is idiopathic, in association with myelodysplastic syndromes (Chapter 182). Refractory anemia with ringed sideroblasts is characterized by abnormalities in all three hematopoietic cell lineages, in addition to the presence of ringed sideroblasts.[12]

A second form, known as pure sideroblastic anemia, is less frequently associated with cytogenetic abnormalities, is characterized by dysplasia only in erythroid progenitors, and lacks cytopenias other than anemia. The prognosis in this type of acquired idiopathic sideroblastic anemia is much better than that in refractory anemia with ringed sideroblasts, in part because of a very low incidence (about 10%) of evolution to acute leukemia.

Because of the important differences in prognosis, it is imperative to evaluate cytogenetics and marrow morphology at the time of diagnosis. Recent evidence suggests that mitochondrial DNA mutations and attendant mitochondrial cytopathies account for many, if not all, cases.

CLINICAL MANIFESTATIONS

Because of the heterogeneous nature of the sideroblastic anemias, many of the clinical manifestations vary according to the underlying pathophysiologic cause. The anemia is usually moderate to severe, with hemoglobin levels in the range of 4 to 10 g/dL. The peripheral blood smear frequently reveals hypochromia, often with basophilic stippling. Microcytosis is often seen in hereditary forms, but normochromic, normocytic, or even macrocytic RBCs may be seen, especially in the setting of myelodysplasia or in a rare X-linked hereditary form known as Pearson syndrome.

DIAGNOSIS

The most useful diagnostic laboratory test for sideroblastic anemia is bone marrow morphology with Prussian blue iron staining, which reveals abnormally large and numerous bluish green siderosomes within at least 15% of erythroblasts, giving the characteristic appearance of ringed sideroblasts (Fig. 159-4). These ringed sideroblasts distinguish this disorder from iron deficiency anemia and anemia of chronic inflammation. Bone marrow findings in idiopathic acquired sideroblastic anemias include dyspoietic features of erythroid and/or myeloid and megakaryotic cell lineages.

Iron studies usually reveal normal iron stores or evidence of iron overload, which is caused by the ineffective erythropoiesis found in sideroblastic anemia as well as by the transfusion therapy often required for its treatment. Iron deficiency can occur coincident with sideroblastic anemia, complicating

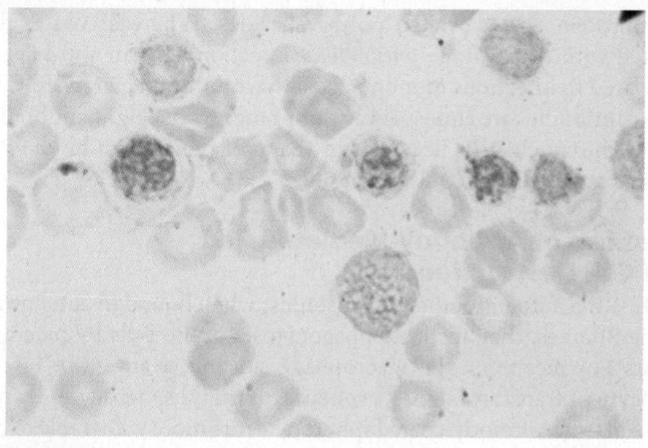

FIGURE 159-4. Sideroblastic anemia. Prussian blue iron stain of the bone marrow shows ringed sideroblasts, which are nucleated red blood cell precursors with perinuclear rings of iron-laden mitochondria.

the diagnosis owing to the lack of characteristic ringed sideroblasts, particularly in myelodysplastic syndromes in which thrombocytopenia leads to GI blood loss. If coexisting iron deficiency is suspected, a repeat bone marrow examination after iron repletion has failed to correct the anemia reveals the diagnostic ringed sideroblasts.

TREATMENT

Treatment of Underlying Disease

Most forms of sideroblastic anemia lack a specific therapy aimed at the underlying mechanism. Exceptions are those types caused by alcohol or drugs, for which removal of the offending agent usually results in resolution, or at least improvement, of the anemia. Abstinence from alcohol usually reverses the abnormalities in heme biosynthesis in 1 to 2 weeks, as evidenced by the disappearance of ringed sideroblasts in the marrow.

Pyridoxine markedly improves the relatively rare cases of nutritional deficiency, which are usually associated with alcoholism, and some forms of X-linked hereditary sideroblastic anemias in which the binding of pyridoxine by ALAS-2 is defective. Because of its low toxicity in moderate doses, a trial of pyridoxine, 100 to 200 mg/day orally for up to 3 months, is worthwhile in all patients. In responsive cases, reticulocytosis occurs within 2 to 3 weeks, and the hemoglobin level improves over several months. High-dose pyridoxine has been shown to overcome the defect in ALAS-2 activity in some patients with X-linked sideroblastic anemia, but prolonged high-dose therapy can be associated with peripheral neuropathy.

Transfusion

The mainstay of therapy for most severe sideroblastic anemias remains RBC transfusions. Because of the risks of long-term transfusion therapy, treatment should be aimed at achieving a normal performance status rather than a specific target hemoglobin level. Iron stores should be monitored regularly, and iron chelation therapy should be used in the setting of iron overload.

Erythropoietin

Therapy with erythropoietin, with or without granulocyte colony-stimulating factor (G-CSF), benefits a small percentage of patients with acquired sideroblastic anemia due to myelodysplasia. A meta-analysis of 17 studies in which 205 patients were treated with erythropoietin showed an overall response rate of only 16%. However, patients with a diagnosis other than refractory anemia with ringed sideroblasts who were not transfusion dependent had response rates greater than 50%, whereas none of the patients who had refractory anemia with ringed sideroblasts and a serum erythropoietin level greater than 200 U/L responded. Studies using a combination of erythropoietin and G-CSF showed somewhat higher response rates, although none of these studies was large or randomized. Allogeneic bone marrow transplantation (Chapter 178) benefits eligible patients whose myelodysplasia (Chapter 182) has a high risk for evolving into acute leukemia.

PROGNOSIS

As with the underlying pathophysiology, the prognosis in sideroblastic anemias is highly variable. Secondary acquired forms of the disease due to alcohol or toxins respond well to withdrawal of the offending agent, with rapid and often complete normalization of erythropoiesis. The pure sideroblastic anemia variant of myelodysplasia-associated sideroblastic anemia can usually be managed well for many years with transfusions and, if necessary, concordant iron chelation therapy. Other myelodysplasia-related sideroblastic anemias generally have a poor prognosis because of the frequent coexistence of pancytopenia and the relatively high incidence of progression to acute leukemia.

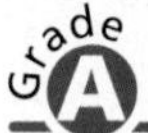

Grade A References

A1. Anker SD, Colet JC, Filippatos G, et al. Ferric carboxymaltose in patients with heart failure and iron deficiency. *N Engl J Med.* 2009;361:2436-2448.

A2. Pfeffer MA, Burdmann EA, Chen CY, et al. A trial of darbepoetin alfa in type 2 diabetes and chronic kidney disease. *N Engl J Med.* 2009;361:2019-2032.

A3. Drueke TB, Locatelli F, Clyne N, et al. Normalization of hemoglobin level in patients with chronic kidney disease and anemia. *N Engl J Med.* 2006;355:2071-2084.

A4. Singh AK, Szczech L, Tang KL, et al. Correction of anemia with epoetin alfa in chronic kidney disease. *N Engl J Med.* 2006;355:2085-2098.

A5. Ludwig H, Crawford J, Osterborg A, et al. Pooled analysis of individual patient-level data from all randomized, double-blind, placebo-controlled trials of darbepoetin alfa in the treatment of patients with chemotherapy-induced anemia. *J Clin Oncol.* 2009;27:2838-2847.

A6. Tonia T, Mettler A, Robert N, et al. Erythropoietin or darbepoetin for patients with cancer. *Cochrane Database Syst Rev.* 2012;12:CD003407.

GENERAL REFERENCES

For the General References and other additional features, please visit Expert Consult at https://expertconsult.inkling.com.

160

AUTOIMMUNE AND INTRAVASCULAR HEMOLYTIC ANEMIAS

MARC MICHEL

DEFINITION

Hemolytic anemia (HA) is defined as anemia caused by a shortened lifespan of mature red blood cells (RBCs) in the peripheral circulation. Hemolysis and accelerated destruction of RBCs can take place within the vasculature (i.e., intravascular hemolysis) or mainly in the liver and the spleen (i.e., extravascular hemolysis). HA can be the consequence of an intrinsic and often genetically determined defect of the RBC membrane (discussed in Chapter 161) or an RBC constituent (hemoglobin [Hb] structure [Chapters 162 and 163] or enzyme machinery [Chapter 161]), or HA can result from an extrinsic and usually acquired disorder of the RBC membrane (immune, infectious, toxic) (Table 160-1).

Autoimmune hemolytic anemia (AIHA) is an acquired autoimmune disease in which autoantibodies directed against autologous RBC membrane antigens lead to their accelerated destruction. The diagnosis of AIHA is thus based on the presence of a positive result on the direct antiglobulin test (DAT), also known as the direct Coombs test, and on the absence of any other hereditary of acquired cause of hemolysis. In AIHA, hemolysis is mainly extravascular, but some features of concomitant intravascular hemolysis may also be present at onset. Beyond AIHA, other causes of immune-mediated HAs that do not involve autoantibodies may occur, as with certain drug-induced HAs or in a posttransfusional hemolytic reaction because of the presence of alloantibodies or other more complex mechanisms (Chapter 177). *Paroxysmal nocturnal hemoglobinuria (PNH)* is a rare and potentially life-threatening acquired clonal blood disorder with protean manifestations in which RBC membranes are highly vulnerable to damage by activated complement. The resulting chronic intravascular hemolysis is the hallmark of the classical hemolytic form of the disease, and the release of free Hb contributes to most of its clinical manifestations.

AUTOIMMUNE HEMOLYTIC ANEMIA

EPIDEMIOLOGY

Autoimmune hemolytic anemia can affect both children (mainly before the age 5 years) and adults and is estimated to have an overall (not age-adjusted) annual incidence of approximately one to three per 100,000 individuals. Whereas boys tend to be more frequently affected than girls, the female-to-male sex ratio is 1.5 to 2 in adults. Among adults, most patients are older than 40 years of age, and the peak incidence occurs around the seventh decade of

TABLE 160-1 PRINCIPAL CAUSES OF HEMOLYTIC ANEMIAS

INTRACORPUSCULAR	EXTRACORPUSCULAR
DISORDERS OF THE RBC MEMBRANE	**IMMUNOLOGIC**
Inherited	• Autoimmune HA
• Hereditary spherocytosis	• Alloimmunization
• Elliptocytosis	• Drug-induced HA
• Hereditary stomatocytosis	**MECHANICAL**
Acquired	• Thrombotic thrombocytopenic purpura
• Paroxysmal nocturnal hemoglobinuria	• Hemolytic-uremic syndrome
HEMOGLOBINOPATHY	• Other microangiopathies
Qualitative defect in hemoglobin	• HELLP syndrome
• Sickle cell disease	• Prosthetic heart valve dysfunction
• Unstable hemoglobins	• Acanthocytosis
Quantitative defect in hemoglobin	**INFECTIOUS**
• β-Thalassemia	• Malaria
• α-Thalassemia	• Babesiosis; *Clostridium perfringens*; gram-positive bacteria
RBC ENZYME ABNORMALITY	**TOXIC**
• G6PD deficiency	• **Exogenous:** thermal burns; industrial copper, arsine, lead poisoning, spider bite, snake bite, mushroom ingestion.
• Pyruvate kinase deficiency	• **Endogenous:** Wilson disease
• Others: pyrimidine 5′ nucleotidase deficiency	• **Drug related**

HA = hemolytic anemia; HELLP = hemolysis, elevated liver function tests, low platelets; RBC = red blood cell.

life. This age distribution may be related to the increased frequency of underlying lymphoproliferative malignancies in elderly adults, resulting in an age-related increase in secondary AIHA caused by lymphoma. Most cases of AIHAs develop sporadically; familial cases are very uncommon. AIHA usually occurs as an isolated immune "cytopenia" but can sometimes be associated simultaneously or sequentially with immune thrombocytopenia (ITP) as *Evans syndrome* or autoimmune neutropenia. Among AIHAs, the so-called warm AIHA (wAIHA; see Diagnosis and Classification section) accounts for 70% to 80% of all cases in adults and almost 90% of the cases in children. Whereas *paroxysmal cold hemoglobinuria (PCH)* is a very uncommon AIHA subtype seen almost exclusively in children, *cold agglutinin disease (CAD)* occurs almost exclusively in adults older than 50 years of age. AIHA can be primary (or idiopathic), or it can occur in association with or disclose an underlying disease (secondary AIHA).

PATHOBIOLOGY

The pathogenesis of AIHA is a complex multistep process involving not only the autoantibodies but also various effectors of the immune system, including the complement system, macrophages, and B and T lymphocytes. Whereas the mechanisms leading to hemolysis have been partially elucidated (antibody-dependent, cell-mediated cytotoxicity, and complement-dependent cytotoxicity being primarily involved), the mechanisms leading to the breakdown of self-tolerance are far from fully understood.

Red Blood Cell Antibodies

IgG anti–RBC autoantibodies mediate the destruction of RBCs mainly by the process of extravascular hemolysis. In contrast, when lytic components of the complement system participate in the process, the destruction of RBCs usually occurs directly within the circulation (intravascular hemolysis). The participation of lytic complement components in IgG-mediated AIHA is rare.

In warm (or warm-reactive) AIHA, the autoantibody targeting RBCs is mainly of the IgG1 isotype. It is able to bind macrophages via its Fc-γ receptors, thereby causing extravascular hemolysis to take place mainly in the spleen. The autoantigens on RBC membranes targeted by the autoantibody are, in decreasing frequency, the following: (1) peptides from the Rhesus system (~one third of the cases); (2) band 3 protein; and (3) glycophorin A, an RBC membrane glycoprotein. In other cases, the antibodies have specificity for antigens in the Kell or Duffy blood group system (very rarely the ABO antigens), and in less than 10% of cases of wAIHA, no specificity can be found. Cold agglutinins are IgM antibodies that react with polysaccharides on the RBC surface, mainly with the I/i antigens or less commonly with the Pr glycoprotein and sialylated polysaccharides. Whereas cold agglutinins associated with *Mycoplasma pneumoniae* infection have an anti-I specificity, those related to infectious mononucleosis have anti-i specificity. In CAD, the cold autoantibodies are almost always anti-I monoclonal IgM antibodies with a VH4-34 heavy chain, a heavy-chain shape of the antigen-binding surface that favors attachment to polysaccharides.

Mechanism of Antibody-Mediated Red Blood Cell Destruction

IgG anti–RBC autoantibodies are opsonins; when bound to autoantigens on RBC membranes, they instigate phagocytosis of the cells by macrophages. Using its Fcγ receptors, the macrophage can ingest an entire IgG-coated erythrocyte or transform it into a spherocyte (microspherocyte) by nibbling away its surface. Antibody-coated spherocytes are more vulnerable to osmotic forces than normal, unsensitized RBCs and ultimately surrender to macrophages, especially in the splenic sinusoids, where blood flows sluggishly. The rate of hemolysis in AIHA depends on the amount of autoantibody on the RBC surface, the affinity and avidity of autoantibodies for the RBC autoantigen, and the number of macrophages in the environment of the antibody-coated erythrocyte. Populations of autoantibodies with high avidity cause a higher rate of RBC destruction than populations with low avidity. Free (monomeric) IgG competes with antibody-coated RBCs for interaction with the Fc receptors of macrophages, but the IgG normally present in plasma has only a minor influence on the hemolytic rate. The importance of the subclasses of IgG is unclear, but IgG3 antibodies seem more potent than IgG1 antibodies in promoting phagocytosis.

The basis of RBC destruction in CAD is the ability of IgM antibodies to fix complement, with each IgM molecule having two binding sites for C1q. When blood cools sufficiently in the extremities, it allows the cold agglutinins to bind RBC. The adherent IgM attracts C1q, which initiates the generation of C3b and C4b on the RBC's surface. On entering the warmer visceral circulation, the RBC releases the cold agglutinin, but the C3 fragments remain engaged to the CR1 of macrophages, thereby enabling phagocytosis of the RBC.

The efficiency of this process depends on the amount of cold agglutinin on the RBC surface and the thermal amplitude of the cold agglutinin. These factors account for the great variability of severity in CAD. The abnormal production of autoantibody directed toward RBC antigens could be the consequence of different and nonmutually exclusive mechanisms: an immune response toward some cryptic antigens or molecular mimicry with cross reactivity between external antigens and autoantigens. Polyclonal activation of both B and T cells is likely to play a role in wAIHA. A positive DAT result is more frequently observed in patients with chronic infections with hypergammaglobulinemia such as HIV (Chapter 393) or leishmaniasis (Chapter 348). In other noninfectious settings with hypergammaglobulinemia and immune dysregulation such as in the *autoimmune lymphoproliferative syndrome (ALPS)* or in *angioimmunoblastic T-cell lymphoma*, a significant proportion of patients have a positive DAT result with or without active hemolysis. Regarding T-cell activation, there is a disequilibrium of the CD4+ T helper 1(Th1)/Th2 balance in patients with active AIHA compared with healthy control participants, with an increase of Th2 cells subsets and an increased expression of both interleukin-4 (IL-4) and IL-10 and a reduced expression of interferon-γ and IL-12. This "Th2 pattern" promotes the induction and proliferation of autoreactive B cell clones. More recently, it has been shown that the production of the effector cytokine IL-17 is strongly associated with AIHA compared with healthy donors and correlates with the severity of the disease. This observation suggests some future therapeutic potential for the use of anti-IL17 monoclonal antibodies in AIHA.

The role of a regulatory T cells (Tregs) defect in the loss of tolerance in wAIHA has been mainly suggested through the study of animal models (e.g., New Zealand Black mice). In humans, few data on the potential role of Tregs in AIHA is available. Some Tregs specific for autoantigens from the Rhesus system are able to inhibit the Th1 effector immune response in vitro through an IL-10–dependent mechanism. Indirect evidence suggesting that a decrease in the number or function of Tregs is likely to play a role in AIHA in humans comes from the **immune dysregulation polyendocrinopathy enteropathy X-linked** (IPEX) syndrome (Chapter 250). IPEX syndrome is a rare inherited disease linked to the dysfunction of the transcription factor FOXP3, widely considered to be the master regulator of the regulatory T-cell lineage. Patients diagnosed with an IPEX syndrome have a high risk of developing a number of autoimmune manifestations (enteropathy; endocrinopathies, including diabetes), including in a lesser extent AIHA.

CLINICAL MANIFESTATIONS

Clinical symptoms of AIHA are those of anemia (unusual fatigue, exertional dyspnea, tachycardia) or those attributable to active hemolysis (jaundice with or without dark urine). Moreover, specifically in patients with high-affinity cold agglutinins, exposure to cold can precipitate episodes of acrocyanosis by inducing massive agglutination of RBCs in the capillary circulation of the hands, feet, or both. Mild splenomegaly may be present, especially in wAIHA; splenomegaly is uncommon in CAD unless there is an underlying B-cell lymphoma. AIHA is associated with an increased risk of venous thromboembolism.[3]

The usual clinical and biologic features of AIHA are shown in Table 160-2. Elevated serum levels of indirect bilirubin and lactate dehydrogenase (LDH) and a reduced serum haptoglobin concentration are the usual albeit nonspecific signs of HA. Laboratory signs of intravascular destruction of RBCs (hemoglobinemia, hemoglobinuria, and hemosiderinuria) are unusual in the setting of AIHA. After HA has been recognized, the diagnosis of AIHA is usually rather easy. It is based first on the identification of anti-RBC autoantibody by means of the DAT, also known as the Coombs test, and then on the exclusion of other causes of HA. To rule out other causes of hereditary or acquired hemolysis, ethnicity must be taken into account, and the history should also focus on previous personal episodes of unexplained anemia with or without jaundice and any familial history of HA or splenectomy. Moreover, a careful analysis of the peripheral blood smear is essential, keeping in mind that an increase in the number of spherocytes can be observed in approximately 30% to 40% of AIHAs.

DIAGNOSIS

The Direct Antiglobulin (Coombs) Test

The DAT that reveals antibody-coated RBCs is central to the diagnosis of autoimmune HA. The indirect antiglobulin (Coombs) test was devised to test for the presence of incomplete antibodies in the patient's serum, not on RBC surfaces. As presently used, the standard antiglobulin reagent contains antibodies against all four classes of IgG and components of complement (usually C3 and C4).

A positive DAT result requires cautious interpretation when there are no other features of AIHA. False-positive test results are not unusual. The reported incidence of positive DATs in normal blood donors and general populations of hospitalized patients varies widely, from one in 100 to one in 15,000. Differences in the technique used to perform the test account for this variation. The usual reason for a false-positive DAT result is nonspecific, low-avidity adherence of IgG to RBCs. In rare cases, however, the result is not a false-positive result but a harbinger of the development of AIHA. False-negative DAT results in true AIHA are very rare and are usually due to low-affinity autoantibodies that spontaneously elute from the RBC in vitro or to amounts of erythrocyte-coating antibodies that are below the limit of detection by the antiglobulin test. Before considering the diagnosis of DAT-negative AIHA[4] as a possibility, every other potential cause of HA has to be excluded. The distinction between a true-positive and a false-positive DAT result can be made by eluting the antibody from the RBCs and testing its ability to bind to normal RBCs. In a false-positive reaction, the eluted antibody does not bind to normal RBCs, but binding does occur in a true-positive test.

Classification of Aiha: Warm versus Cold Autoimmune Hemolytic Anemia (see Table 160-2)

After the diagnosis of AIHA is made, the classification of the AIHA type is essential.

According to the DAT pattern and the optimal temperature at which the autoantibody reacts with human RBCs, AIHAs are typically subdivided in four major subtypes: (1) wAIHA, (2) cold AIHA (including the chronic CAD), (3) mixed-type AIHA, and (4) the exceptional PCH. The great majority of cold-reactive autoantibody are so-called "cold agglutinins," cold hemolysins being indeed much less common. A small proportion (~5%) of patients may exhibit both cold-reactive and warm-reactive autoantibodies defining mixed AIHA. The distinction between cold and wAIHA is very important because the mechanisms of RBC injury, the primary site of hemolysis, and especially the therapeutic approaches are significantly different. Table 160-2 summarizes the main features of the different types of AIHA.

In wAIHAs, which represent 70 to 80% of all AIHAs in adults, the DAT pattern is either solely IgG positive or IgG and C3 positive, autoantibodies are of IgG isotype (mainly IgG_1), and they bind and react optimally with RBCs at a temperature of 37° C (range, 35 to 40° C). In wAIHA, the hemolysis is mainly extravascular and occurs predominantly in the spleen. On the other hand, in AIHAs caused by cold autoantibodies, which account for 15% to 20% of AIHAs, the usual DAT pattern is IgG negative and C3 positive, and circulating cold agglutinins are detectable in the serum at a significant titer (i.e., >1/64). Cold autoantibodies that are also cold agglutinins are almost exclusively of IgM isotype. However, the RBC antigen-reactive IgM immunoglobulins themselves that are able to activate the classical complement pathway on RBC membranes in vivo are seldom found fixed on the RBCs membrane on laboratory testing because they are rapidly eluted ex vivo. Cold antibodies typically react with RBCs at temperatures below 30° C (optimum, 4° C) and lead to various degree of extravascular hemolysis, predominantly in the liver. In rare cases of AIHAs (~10%) known as mixed-type AIHAs, autoantibodies (mostly of IgM isotype) can react with RBCs within a wide

TABLE 160-2 MAIN CHARACTERISTICS OF VARIOUS TYPES OF AIHA

AIHA TYPE	EPIDEMIOLOGY/ TYPE OF HEMOLYSIS	SECONDARY FORMS	AUTOANTIBODY ISOTYPE	OPTIMAL TEMPERATURE	DAT PATTERN	ELUATE	AUTOANTIBODY SPECIFICITY (TARGETED RBC ANTIGENS)
Warm AIHA	~70%-80% of all AIHA; adults > children (mean age, 3 yr); EV hemolysis; subacute onset (rarely abrupt with associated IV hemolysis)	~50% of cases (see Table 160-3)	IgG ≫ IgA, IgM	37° C	IgG ± C3d	IgG	Antigens of the Rh system, band 3, glycophorin, A
Cold agglutinin syndrome	~20%-30% of all AIHA cases in adults; age >50 yr; EV hemolysis	CAD associated with monoclonal IgM κ gammopathy in 90% of cases ± features of definite clonal B-cell lymphoproliferative disorder	IgM ⋙ IgA or IgG; cold agglutinin titer >1/500	4° C	C3	Negative	I antigen > i ≫ Pr
Cold transient AIHA	Children, young adults; IV hemolysis	Infections (*Mycoplasma pneumoniae*, EBV, other viruses)	Polyclonal IgM; cold agglutinin titer ≥1/64	4° C	C3	Negative	I > i antigens
Paroxysmal cold hemoglobinuria	Children (rare); exceptional in adults; acute IV hemolysis	Infections (*M. pneumoniae*, virus)	IgG (Donath-Landsteiner hemolysin)	>30° C	C3	Negative	P + c antigens (biphasic hemolysins)
Mixed-type AIHA	Adult; mainly EV hemolysis	Mainly B-cell lymphoma	IgG, IgM	Wide range (4°-37° C)	IgG ± C3	IgG	Polyreactivity

AIHA = autoimmune hemolytic anemia; CAD = cold agglutinin disease; DAT = direct antiglobulin test; EBV = Epstein-Barr virus; EV = extravascular, Ig = immunoglobulin; IV = intravascular range of temperatures (thermal amplitude from 4° to 37° C). Last, PCH is a very uncommon AIHA subtype that is seen almost exclusively in children. It is caused by an IgG hemolysin that reacts with autologous RBCs only at low temperatures (2° to 10° C) and can be detected only by means of the Donath Landsteiner test, a test available only in few referral laboratories. Besides these four distinct subtypes of AIHAs, drug-induced HAs must be regarded as a distinct entity.

In addition to the distinction between warm and cold AIHA, which is an essential step in diagnosis because it does influence the therapeutic strategy, AIHAs are also classified as (1) primary (or idiopathic) or (2) secondary, depending on the presence or absence of an underlying disease or condition promoting immune dysregulation. On average, 50% to 60% of wAIHAs are secondary (see Table 160-3 for associated conditions); therefore, a minimal workup must be performed at time of diagnosis in every patient to search for an underlying disease or condition (Table 160-4). It is important to emphasize that a presumably primary form of wAIHA can precede by many years the occurrence of a non-Hodgkin lymphoma, and therefore patients with wAIHA must be followed even after a remission of AIHA has been obtained.

Regarding AIHAs due to cold autoantibodies, in children and young adults they are mainly secondary to either bacterial (*M. pneumoniae* infection) or viral (Epstein-Barr virus [EBV] or cytomegalovirus) infection. In adults older than 50 years of age, although rare, chronic CAD is by far the most common cause of AIHA caused by cold autoantibodies.[5] Although chronic CAD in an older adult has long been considered as a primary (i.e., idiopathic) form of AIHA, it is now recognized that in about 90% of cases, it is associated with a monoclonal IgM κ and with other features of a clonal B-cell lymphoproliferative disorder in approximately 75% of cases. Thus, chronic CAD should be viewed more as a true lymphoproliferative disease characterized by clonal expansion of B cells with most often features of lymphoplasmacytic lymphoma in the bone marrow. HA is seldom very severe in the setting of chronic CAD, and it is classically exacerbated by exposure to cold or infections.

TABLE 160-3 MAIN DISORDERS OR CONDITIONS ASSOCIATED WITH SECONDARY WARM-REACTIVE AUTOIMMUNE HEMOLYTIC ANEMIAS

Hematologic disorders and lymphoproliferative diseases
- Chronic lymphocytic leukemia,* acute lymphoblastic leukemia,† LGL leukemia
- B-cell lymphoma,* Hodgkin lymphoma
- Angioimmunoblastic T-cell lymphoma
- Castleman disease
- Myelodysplasias, myelofibrosis

Solid tumors
- Thymoma
- Ovarian dermoid cyst
- Carcinomas

Autoimmune and inflammatory diseases
- Systemic lupus erythematosus, antiphospholipid syndrome
- Rheumatoid arthritis
- Inflammatory bowel disease
- Pernicious anemia, thyroiditis
- Myasthenia gravis
- Autoimmune hepatitis, giant cell hepatitis*
- Sarcoidosis
- Eosinophilic fasciitis

Infections
- Viruses: EBV,* hepatitis C, CMV
- Bacteria: tuberculosis, brucellosis, syphilis

Drugs

Primary immunodeficiencies
- Common variable immunodeficiency
- Hyper-IgM syndrome,† ALPS†
- IPEX syndrome,† APECED syndrome†

Others
- Pregnancy
- After allogeneic bone marrow transplantation or liver or small bowel transplant*
- Rosai-Dorfman disease

*Diseases that can also be associated with cold autoimmune hemolytic anemia and cold agglutinins.
†Seen almost exclusively in childhood.
ALPS = autoimmune lymphoproliferative syndrome; APECED = autoimmune polyendocrinopathy with candidiasis and ectodermal dystrophy; CMV = cytomegalovirus; EBV = Epstein-Barr virus; IPEX = immune dysregulation, polyendocrinopathy, enteropathy X-linked.
LGL = large granular lymphocytes.

TREATMENT Rx

The management of AIHA is, regardless the subtype, mainly empirical or based on retrospective uncontrolled studies. Very few prospective studies have been reported (mainly in CAD), and only two randomized controlled studies have been performed in wAIHA to date.

Supportive Care and Transfusion

Regardless the type of AIHA, folic acid supplementation (5-10 mg/day) is warranted in patients with active AIHA to prevent further depletion of folate stores (caused by increased erythropoiesis), which may be misinterpreted as a treatment failure. RBC transfusions are also indicated in patients with disabling symptoms of anemia or a poor underlying cardiovascular condition (i.e., coronary artery disease or heart failure). Although younger patients may tolerate a stable Hb level as low as 6 g/dL, in patients with comorbidities, maintaining an Hb level of at least 8 g/dL is usually recommended. It is important for the managing physician to understand that no patient with symptomatic AIHA should be denied blood transfusions because of an "incompatible crossmatch." The blood bank should be informed of the patient's status. Indeed, the patient's positive DAT result almost always interferes with compatibility testing, so the role of the blood bank is to provide packed RBCs that are the "least incompatible" ones in regard to the specificity of the patient's autoantibody. It is possible that DNA-based methods might become clinically feasible to replace hemagglutination assays in these situations in the future.[6] Close communication and cooperation between the clinician and the specialist in transfusion medicine is therefore essential for reducing the risks associated with transfusion in patients with AIHA. Because transfused RBCs can be destroyed by the patient's autoantibodies, rapid transfusion of large volumes of RBCs must be avoided because they can have serious consequences. This risk is increased if the patient also has alloantibodies induced by previous transfusions or pregnancy. Packed RBCs units should therefore not be administered at a rate that exceeds 1 mL/kg/hour. There is no strong evidence supporting the efficacy of plasma exchange in enhancing the response to blood transfusions.

Although this is not supported by strong evidence-based data, in cold AIHA, it is usually recommended to transfuse prewarmed (at a temperature close to 37° C) packed RBCs by means of a specific warming device to minimize the risk of hemolysis.

Treatment of Acute Cold Autoimmune Hemolytic Anemias

In cases of transient cold AIHAs induced by an infection, the onset is usually abrupt, and the degree of anemia may be profound and sometimes life threatening, requiring transfusions of prewarmed packed RBCs, which must not be postponed. Besides supportive care, the use of antibiotics is justified in case of pneumonia caused by infection with *M. pneumoniae*. A short course of corticosteroids can sometimes be considered in case of severe cold AIHA secondary to a viral infection (EBV) to reduce the duration of anemia, but this approach is not evidence based and not uniformly recommended.

Treatment of Chronic Cold Agglutinin Disease

The treatment of CAD has long been only supportive and symptomatic. Avoidance of cold is still the mainstay in the management of CAD, especially to avoid cold-induced circulatory symptoms, but this measure is often not sufficient to avoid episodes of hemolysis. With cold exposure, in cases of infections and acute phase reactions, the level of both C_3 and C_4 increase because of enhanced production, resulting in exacerbation of complement-dependent

TABLE 160-4 RECOMMENDED WORKUP IN WARM-REACTIVE AUTOIMMUNE HEMOLYTIC ANEMIA

1. Antinuclear antibodies (± anti-DNA Abs if ANA positive)
2. Anticardiolipin antibodies and lupus anticoagulant*
3. Serum protein electrophoresis and immunoelectrophoresis
4. Immunophenotyping of peripheral lymphocytes
5. CT scan of the thorax, abdomen, and pelvis (in the absence of obvious SLE or APS)
6. Bone marrow biopsy: recommended only in the presence of hypogammaglobulinemia, or monoclonal gammopathy, or abnormal lymphadenopathy on the CT scan

*Especially in case of previous episode of venous and/or arterial thrombosis or in case of recurrent miscarriage in women, and systematically before splenectomy.
Abs = antibodies; ANA = antinuclear antibodies; APS = antiphospholipid syndrome;
CT = computed tomography; SLE = systemic lupus erythematosus.

cytotoxicity caused by autoantibody directed toward autologous RBCs, leading to increased hemolysis as well as agglutination. Consequently, prompt treatment of febrile infections or illnesses as well as prevention of infection by means of influenza with or without pneumococcal vaccines is strongly recommended in patients with CAD. In case of exacerbation of hemolysis and severe anemia, transfusion of prewarmed packed RBCs must be considered because patients with CAD are often elderly with comorbid conditions. Whereas CAD is usually considered a rather indolent and slowly progressive lymphoproliferative disease with a relatively good prognosis, transfusion dependency may be observed in some patients with recurrent episodes of active hemolysis.

In patients with CAD who have active hemolysis and need to be treated, a number of single-agent therapies have shown little or no efficacy, and their use should therefore be avoided because they all have a significant toxicity. These include corticosteroids, alkylating agents, interferon-α, immunosuppressives, and cladribine. Oral cyclophosphamide and chlorambucil have shown favorable responses in a minority of patients with CAD. Because hemolysis takes place mainly in the liver in CAD, splenectomy should be avoided in these individuals because it is notoriously ineffective. In transfusion-dependent patients with normal or slightly elevated reticulocyte counts, the transient use of an erythropoiesis-stimulating agent off label may be useful as a transfusion-sparing strategy. Plasma exchanges can be temporarily helpful in cases of severe hemolysis or in preparation for surgery requiring cold exposure, such as lung–heart surgery. For patients with active or relapsing symptomatic episodes of HA, rituximab given either alone or in combination with fludarabine can be an option, especially in patients with an underlying B-cell lymphoma. An algorithm for the management of cold AIHAs is proposed in Figure 160-1. Last, because the hemolytic activity of cold agglutinins is complement dependent, the efficacy of eculizumab, an anti C5 humanized monoclonal antibody licensed in PNH (see later section Paroxysmal Nocturnal Hemoglobinuria), seems theoretically promising. Because only very few case reports have shown the efficacy of eculizumab, this approach should be only considered as a last-resort option in case of life-threatening exacerbation of HA not controlled by RBC transfusions.

Treatment of Primary Warm Autoimmune Hemolytic Anemias

First-line Treatment: Corticosteroids

Primary wAIHAs usually have a chronic course and, except for the very few patients who are unusual for having a mild compensated hemolysis with a normal or almost normal Hb level, treatment is needed in the large majority of the cases to improve RBC survival and significantly and durably increase the Hb level (Fig. 160-2). Corticosteroids are the cornerstone of therapy in wAIHAs, and they must be given as first-line treatment. As noted later under the discussion of rituximab, a recently reported randomized trial showed that rituximab and prednisolone combined, compared with prednisolone alone, increased the rate and duration of response as first-line treatment of warm antibody-reactive AIHA.[A1] Intravenous immunoglobulin (IgIV) has only little efficacy in wAIHAs, and because of their cost, they should be considered (at a total dose of 2 g/kg over 2 days) only in patients with severe, transfusion-dependent AIHA and in the absence of response to corticosteroids. The corticosteroid regimen is usually based on oral prednisone or prednisolone at the initial daily dose of 1 to 2 mg/kg. By analogy with other autoimmune diseases, the use of intravenous methylprednisolone at a dose of 250 to 1000 mg/day for 1 to 3 days may be considered in patients with profound anemia, although no clinical trials supporting their higher efficacy are available. The starting dose of oral prednisone is usually maintained for 3 to 4 weeks and then tapered progressively in case of at least partial initial response. There is no agreement on the total duration of treatment, but because the likelihood of early relapse is high when the treatment is prematurely stopped, corticosteroids should be maintained for at least 3 months after a complete response (defined by an increase of the Hb level back to normal and no active hemolysis) is achieved. Except for children, the use of alternate-day prednisone before stopping the treatment is not recommended. The effect of corticosteroids can take few days to 2 weeks, and one or several blood transfusions may be necessary at AIHA onset, especially in case of severe anemia in young children or elderly adults for maintaining a "safe" Hb level. After 2 to 3 weeks of treatment with corticosteroids, a clinically significant response is observed in 80% to 85% of the cases. Except for the few patients who are truly refractory to corticosteroids, the major issue that clinicians have to deal with when treating patients with wAIHA is that approximately 50% to 60% of them turn out to be dependant to corticosteroids. Thus, flares of relapses or wAIHA may occur either within weeks after withdrawal of corticosteroids or even while on treatment when the dose of daily prednisone is decreased below a threshold, which is usually between 10 to 15 mg, a dose that is associated with several adverse events in the long term. Overall, only one third of the patients can be considered to be in complete remission off treatment 1 year after disease onset.

Second-line Treatment

Danazol

In patients dependent on corticosteroids, the use of danazol, an attenuated androgen analog, at 400 to 800 mg/day can be helpful as a corticosteroid-sparing strategy in adults requiring a dose of daily prednisone greater than 15 mg to maintain a remission. However, because of its common masculinizing side effects, its use is usually rather limited in females, and its potential liver toxicity makes its long-term use also problematic in men.

Rituximab

The efficacy of rituximab, the well-known chimeric monoclonal antibody that targets CD20 antigen on B lymphocytes, was first shown in refractory wAIHA in children with a response rate reaching up to 100% in some studies. In adults, rituximab has also shown (both through retrospective but also a few prospective studies, including a randomized controlled trial) to be highly effective in primary wAIHAs, with an 80% to almost 100% response rate at 1 year. Rituximab can be effective in patients who have failed to respond to splenectomy (see later discussion),[7] and, conversely, patients who do not respond to rituximab are able to achieve a response after splenectomy. The

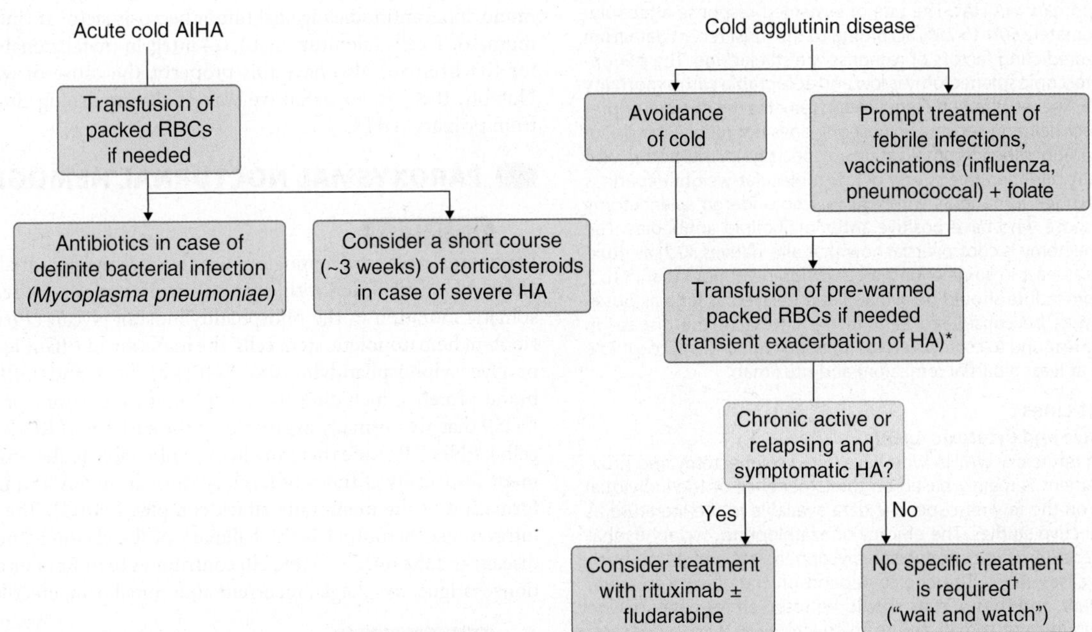

FIGURE 160-1. **Proposed algorithm for the management of cold-reactive autoimmune hemolytic anemias (AIHAs). HA = hemolytic anemia; RBC = red blood cell. *The short-term use of an erythropoiesis stimulating agent can be considered off-label; †Unless the underlying B cell-clonal lymphoproliferative disorder requires any specific management.**

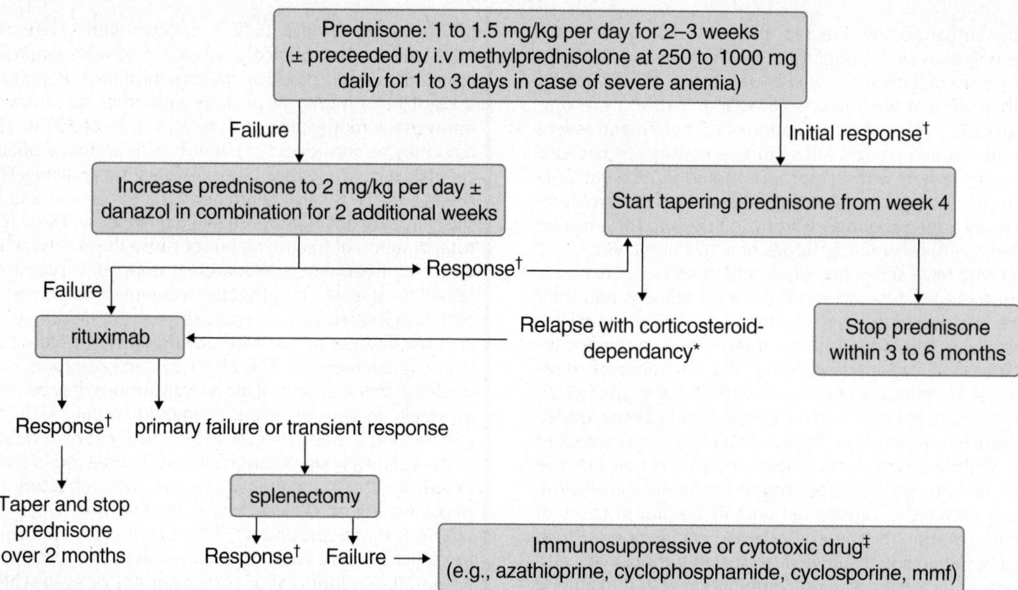

FIGURE 160-2. **Proposed algorithm for the treatment of primary warm-reactive autoimmune hemolytic anemia (AIHA) in adults. IV = intravenous; mmf = mycophenolate mofetil. *Dose of prednisone ≥10 mg/day needed to maintain at least a partial response (i.e., Hb level >10g/dL with at least a 2 g increase from baseline without recent transfusion). †Partial response defined as a hemoglobilin level >10g/dL with at least a 2 g increase from baseline and complete response defined as a normal hemoglobin level withouth hemolysis. ‡In alphabetical order (no evidence for preferring any one of these drugs).**

usual dose of rituximab is 375 mg/m² by intravenous infusion once a week for 4 weeks, but other regimens can be used. The safety profile is usually acceptable, although late-onset neutropenia and opportunistic infections, such as *Pneumocystis jiroveci* pneumonia, may rarely occur. Therefore, the systematic use of primary antibiotic prophylaxis should be considered in patients with AIHA treated with rituximab. Taken together the data from the literature clearly support, whenever possible, the use of rituximab (off-label use) in patients with chronic active or relapsing wAIHA who need to pursue a daily dose of prednisone (or prednisolone) of 15 mg or greater to maintain at least a partial remission. If rituximab is administered before splenectomy, vaccination against *Streptococcus pneumoniae* with or without *Haemophilus influenzae* type B or *Neisseria meningitides* must be systematically administered whenever possible 2 weeks before rituximab because splenectomy may be required thereafter.

Splenectomy

Splenectomy has long been the main and preferred second-line option for the treatment of primary wAIHAs. The rate of sustained response after splenectomy is approximately 60% to 70% according to the most recent data from the literature, but predicting factors of response are still lacking. The perioperative risk of laparoscopic splenectomy is low and acceptable with a mortality rate of less than 1%. The most feared complication remains the rare but unpredictable risk of overwhelming sepsis. Laparoscopy does not reduce the risk of postoperative thromboembolic complications, especially in the portal vein system. A systematic perioperative course of low-molecular-weight heparin is therefore recommended in patients with wAIHA who undergo splenectomy and especially in those who have positive antiphospholipid antibodies. The best time for splenectomy is controversial now that alternatives such as rituximab are available at least in some countries. In children younger than 5 to 7 years of age, this procedure should be avoided and delayed as long as possible. In adults, it must be considered early in the course of the disease in patients who fail to respond to corticosteroids (or need high and unacceptable doses to maintain at least a partial remission) and rituximab.

Other Treatment Lines

Immunosuppressive and Cytotoxic Agents

In patients with refractory wAIHA who have failed splenectomy and rituximab, the management is mainly based on the experience of the individual hematologist and on the few retrospective data available in the literature as opposed to prospective studies. The efficacy of azathioprine, cyclophosphamide, and to a lesser extent cyclosporine and mycophenolate mofetil has been reported in small cases series. The choice depend on the efficacy-to-safety ratio for each patient, and these drugs should be reserved for patients who have failed to respond to rituximab and to splenectomy or who, because of comorbidities, are not suitable candidates for splenectomy.

DRUG-INDUCED IMMUNE HEMOLYTIC ANEMIA

There are several mechanisms by which a drug can induce HA, and true drug-induced AIHAs are rare.[8] Many drugs or drug metabolites have the potential to elicit antidrug antibodies. Drugs that form covalent bonds with proteins in the RBC membrane can bind antidrug antibodies to the RBC surface, causing a positive DAT result and, in some cases, initiating antibody-mediated destruction of RBCs. Other drugs, such as the cephalosporins, can bind to RBC membranes and take up IgG nonspecifically from plasma. In these cases, there is no antidrug antibody. The diagnosis of drug-induced immune-mediated HA should be considered if the patient has a history of taking a suspected medication, there is acute complement-mediated hemolysis, only complement components are detectable on the RBC surface, or the patient's serum reacts with RBCs in the presence of the suspected drug. Some drugs can induce true autoantibodies against RBCs. Fludarabine, a purine nucleoside analogue used in the treatment of chronic lymphocytic leukemia, and monoclonal antibodies against tumor necrosis factor-α (infliximab and adalimumab), T cells (alemtuzumab), α4 integrin (natalizumab), and IL-2 receptor (daclizumab) also have this property, the cause of which is unknown. Notably, there is no definitive way of distinguishing drug-induced AIHA from primary AIHA.

PAROXYSMAL NOCTURNAL HEMOGLOBINURIA

DEFINITION

Paroxysmal nocturnal hemoglobinuria is a rare and potentially life-threatening clonal blood disorder with protean manifestations caused by an acquired somatic mutation in the phosphatidylinositol glycan *(PIG)-A* gene. In pluripotent hematopoietic stem cells, the mutation in *PIG-A* leads to a deficiency of glycosylphosphatidylinositol (GPI)-anchors and GPI-anchored membrane proteins, including the complement regulatory proteins CD55 and CD59 that are normally expressed on the surfaces of RBCs (and other blood cells). PNH RBCs are therefore highly vulnerable to the activation of complement (especially at times of fever, acidosis or hypoxia) and the unregulated formation of the membrane attack complex (MAC). The resulting chronic intravascular hemolysis is the hallmark of the classic hemolytic form of the disease and the release of free Hb contributes to most of its clinical manifestations (fatigue, dysphagia, recurrent abdominal pain, erectile dysfunction).

EPIDEMIOLOGY

Paroxysmal nocturnal hemoglobinuria can present at any age but most commonly between 10 and 50 years. The mean age at diagnosis is about 34 years (median age is about 40 years), and the female-to-male ratio is close to 1. The median survival time after diagnosis is approximately 20 years. It is a rare disorder with an estimated prevalence in the population of one in 10^5 to one in 10^6. A family history of PNH is unusual.

PATHOBIOLOGY

Genetics

Paroxysmal nocturnal hemoglobinuria is caused by a somatic mutation that causes a defect in the RBC membrane.[9] The disease begins in a single hematopoietic stem cell in which the *PIGA* gene on the short arm of the active X chromosome acquires a somatic mutation. The *PIGA* gene encodes PIG-A, an enzyme that is essential for the synthesis of glycosylphosphatidylinositol (GPI). The lipid GPI forms a peptide link with the C-terminal amino acid of numerous proteins, normally anchoring them to the RBC membrane. The somatic mutation in a hematopoietic stem cell affects *PIG-A* in blood cells of all lineages. Almost 150 different mutations of *PIG-A* have been identified. Most of them inactivate *PIG-A* and cause total loss of the GPI anchor in the descendants of the affected hematopoietic stem cell. RBCs with complete deficiency of GPI are termed *PNH III erythrocytes*, and those with partial deficiency are called *PNH II erythrocytes*. The coexistence of PNH III and PNH II RBCs in the same patient indicates the presence of two mutant clones. A small number of hematopoietic stem cells in normal people bear the *PIG-A* mutation; they have no proliferative advantage and persist in small numbers. In normal blood, the frequency of PIG-A–deficient cells is about one in 50,000 RBCs. In contrast to those with PNH, however, the deficient cells in normal subjects arise from committed hematopoietic cells. The presence of PIG-A–deficient cells in normal subjects suggests that PNH involves not only the *PIG-A* mutation but also a second step, perhaps another mutation, that allows competitive expansion of the mutated clone.

Functional Consequences of Deficiency of GPI

The membrane inhibitor of reactive hemolysis (CD59, or protectin) and CD55, an inhibitor of C3 convertase, are two of the many proteins that GPI anchors to the RBC under normal circumstances. They prevent polymerization of C9, the final step in assembly of the MAC that begins with cleavage of C5 to C5b. Deficiencies of CD59 and CD55 on PNH RBC membranes thereby allow unimpeded assembly of the MAC on the erythrocyte surface (and the surfaces of other blood cells derived from the mutated hematopoietic stem cell clone), thereby initiating intravascular hemolysis. A variety of nonspecific factors, such as a reduction in the pH of blood, can activate complement. The morning hemoglobinuria of PNH is probably the result of subtle acidification of blood during sleep.

CLINICAL MANIFESTATIONS

Classically, a patient with PNH arises in the morning and passes dark urine. The typical but actually rarely described paroxysms of hemoglobinuria occur on a background of chronic, low-grade intravascular hemolysis that causes constant hemosiderinuria in PNH. About one third of cases evolve into aplastic anemia (Chapter 165). Transformation to acute myelogenous leukemia is a rare event. Abdominal pain, dysphagia, and erectile dysfunction are additional clinical features. The basis of these symptoms is probably the scavenging by free plasma Hb of nitric oxide, a vasodilatory regulator of vasomotor and smooth muscle tone. In about one third of cases, venous thrombosis occurs in unusual sites and can cause Budd-Chiari syndrome by obstructing the hepatic veins, portal vein thrombosis or less frequently cerebral vein thrombosis (Chapter 143). Splenomegaly is uncommon; hepatomegaly and ascites suggest the complication of hepatic vein thrombosis and the resultant portal hypertension. Hemosiderinuria is the result of chronic intravascular hemolysis. Subtle or overt signs of bone marrow damage (coexisting leukopenia and thrombocytopenia) are frequent. The extent of RBC destruction in PNH depends on the number of PNH (versus normal) RBCs in blood, the level of GPI on the RBC membrane (PNH III cells are devoid of GPI), and the degree of activation of complement at the cell surfaces. The anemia is often aggravated by iron deficiency caused by chronic urinary iron loss in the form of hemosiderinuria. Long-term, repeated episodes of hemoglobinuria may lead to iron deficiency. Therefore, a DAT-negative HA associated with iron deficiency should raise suspicion of PNH. The basis of the tendency to develop venous thrombosis[10] is unclear. Hypercoagulability caused by the release of prothrombotic materials from RBC and platelet membranes (the latter being also abnormal in PNH) and impaired fibrinolysis has been implicated. Nitric oxide scavenging by free plasma Hb may also cause vasoconstriction and endothelial cell dysfunction, leading to the activation and aggregation of platelets.

DIAGNOSIS

Often, the clinical picture is virtually diagnostic. The diagnosis can be established by demonstrating, by flow cytometry, a deficiency of CD59 on erythrocytes. Another reagent with utility in flow cytometry is Aerolysin, a bacterial protein that binds to the GPI anchor. The fluorescinated Aerolysin variant (FLAER) is also a very good and reliable reagent to study GPI-linked antigens on leukocytes, helpful for diagnosing PNH. Flow cytometry can also measure the proportions of PNH III and PNH II RBCs in blood, providing information about the severity of the disease. The usual cut-off being the presence more than 5% GPI-AP–deficient polymorphonuclear cells in the peripheral blood, the clone size is usually correlated with the degree of intravascular hemolysis.

TREATMENT Rx

Eculizumab, a humanized monoclonal antibody against C5 that is essential for formation of the MAC, can reduce the signs of intravascular hemolysis, the requirement for transfusions, and the tendency to thrombosis. In a randomized trial,[A2] [A3] the dose of the antibody was 600 mg every week for 4 weeks followed 1 week later by a 900-mg dose and then by 900 mg every other week for a total treatment period of 52 weeks. A thrombotic event is a strong indication for eculizumab treatment. A molecular basis for poor response to eculizumab was recently elucidated in a small population of Japanese patients who were found to have a missense mutation in the gene encoding C5 that made the complement factor incapable of binding to eculizumab and being blocked by it.[11] Peptide inhibitors of C3 activation have been shown to prevent hemolysis and C3 opsonization of PNH RBCs and are potential therapeutic candidates.[12]

Warfarin can also be used in patients with a history of a thrombosis. Oral iron can correct the iron deficiency; treatment with iron does not exacerbate the hemolysis. Transfusions are helpful in supportive care. Aplastic anemia (Chapter 165) has been treated successfully with immunosuppressive agents (antithymocyte globulin, usually at a dose of 1.5 mg/kg/day for 7-14 days) with or without cyclosporine (3-5 mg/kg for at least 3 months). Allogeneic bone marrow transplantation (Chapter 178) is risky but can be curative.

OTHER EXTRACORPUSCULAR HEMOLYTIC ANEMIAS

Hemolytic Transfusion Reactions

The cause of hemolytic transfusion reactions (Chapter 177) is intravascular lysis of the donor's RBCs by antibodies (alloantibodies or isoantibodies) in the recipient that bind to one or more blood group antigens on the transfused cells. The recipient's isoantibodies can be natural anti-A or anti-B antibodies, or they can be induced by previous transfusions or pregnancy. Whether IgM or IgG, the isoantibodies trigger the assembly of lytic complement components on the surface of the donor's RBC. The rapid formation of large amounts of C3a and C5a fragments causes hypotension and bronchial and smooth muscle spasm. Renal failure is a consequence of severe, prolonged hypotension; the main renal lesion is renal cortical ischemia secondary to shunting of blood away from the kidneys. Hb itself is not nephrotoxic. The signs and symptoms of a hemolytic transfusion reaction are nonspecific and include fever, back pain, urticaria, dyspnea, hypotension, and evidence of disseminated intravascular coagulation. These nonspecific signs appear and worsen during administration of the transfusion. Immediate steps must be taken to stop the transfusion, submit the transfused blood and a sample of the patient's blood to the blood bank, and order tests of plasma and urine for free Hb. Management is further discussed in Chapter 177.

Other Causes of Intravascular Hemolysis

Conditions in which vascular abnormalities, toxins, infections, or drugs damage RBCs and cause them to lose pieces of membrane and ultimately fragment into Hb-containing bits should be considered in the differential diagnosis of intravascular hemolysis (see Table 160-3). Most of these conditions are readily apparent from the history and physical examination. Treatment focuses on the underlying cause of the hemolysis.

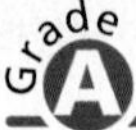

Grade A References

A1. Birgens H, Frederiksen H, Hasselbalch HC, et al. A phase III randomized trial comparing glucocorticoid monotherapy versus glucocorticoid and rituximab in patients with autoimmune haemolytic anaemia. *Br J Haematol.* 2013;163:393-399.

A2. Hillmen P, Young NS, Schubert J, et al. The complement inhibitor eculizumab in paroxysmal nocturnal hemoglobinuria. *N Engl J Med.* 2006;355:1233-1243.

A3. Brodsky RA, Young NS, Antonioli E, et al. Multicenter phase 3 study of the complement inhibitor eculizumab for the treatment of patients with paroxysmal nocturnal hemoglobinuria. *Blood.* 2008;111:1840-1847.

GENERAL REFERENCES

For the General References and other additional features, please visit Expert Consult at https://expertconsult.inkling.com.

161

HEMOLYTIC ANEMIAS: RED BLOOD CELL MEMBRANE AND METABOLIC DEFECTS

PATRICK G. GALLAGHER

The mature erythrocyte differs from all other cells in the body. Lacking a nucleus, DNA, RNA, and ribosomes, it cannot synthesize RNA, DNA, or protein. It does not divide, it has no mitochondria, it cannot perform the Krebs cycle, and it lacks an electron transport system for oxidative phosphorylation. After enucleation, the reticulocyte, the precursor of the mature erythrocyte, leaves the marrow and enters the circulation equipped with a full complement of enzymes, transporters, signaling molecules, and all other proteins necessary to perform the essential functions of the red blood cell (RBC) during its lifespan.

The erythrocyte membrane accounts for only about 1% of the total weight of an RBC, yet it plays a critical role in the maintenance of normal RBC homeostasis through a number of mechanisms. These include retention of vital compounds and removal of metabolic waste, regulation of erythrocyte metabolism and pH, and import of iron required for hemoglobin (Hb) synthesis during erythropoiesis. The membrane maintains a slippery exterior so that erythrocytes do not aggregate or adhere to endothelial cells. The membrane skeleton, a network of proteins on the inner surface of the RBC, provides the strength and flexibility needed to maintain the normal shape and deformability of the erythrocyte.

The principal functions of erythrocyte metabolism in the mature erythrocyte include maintenance of adequate supplies of adenosine triphosphate (ATP), production of reducing substances to act as antioxidants, and control of oxygen affinity of Hb by production of adequate amounts of 2,3-diphosphoglycerate (2,3-DPG). Because the mature erythrocyte has lost its ability to perform oxidative phosphorylation, its energy is supplied by anaerobic glycolysis though the Embden-Meyerhof pathway, by oxidative glycolysis through the hexose monophosphate (HMP) shunt, and through nucleotide salvage pathways.

THE ERYTHROCYTE MEMBRANE

Composed of a lipid bilayer and an underlying cortical membrane skeleton (Fig. 161-1), the membrane provides the erythrocyte the deformability and stability required to withstand its travels through the circulation. In one circulatory cycle throughout the body, an erythrocyte is subjected to high sheer stress in the arterial system, dramatic size and shape changes in the microcirculation with capillary diameters as small as 7.5 μm and marked fluctuations in tonicity, pH, and Po_2.

Membrane Lipids

Red blood cell membrane lipids are asymmetrically distributed across the bilayer membrane, reflecting a steady state involving a constant exchange of phospholipids between the two bilayer hemileaflets. Glycolipids and cholesterol are intercalated between the phospholipids in the bilayer with their long axes perpendicular to the bilayer plane. Glycolipids, located in the external half of the bilayer with their carbohydrate moieties extending into the aqueous phase, carry several important RBC antigens and serve other important functions. Phospholipids are asymmetrically organized, with the choline phospholipids, phosphatidylcholine and sphingomyelin, primarily in the outer half of the bilayer, and the amino phospholipids, phosphatidylethanolamine and phosphatidylserine (PS), in the inner half of the bilayer. In pathologic states, such as thalassemia, sickle cell disease, and diabetes, loss of phospholipid asymmetry with externalization of PS leads to activation of blood clotting through conversion of prothrombin to thrombin and facilitates macrophage attachment to erythrocytes, marking them for destruction. Mature erythrocytes are unable to synthesize fatty acids, phospholipids, or cholesterol de novo and depend on lipid exchange and fatty acid acylation as mechanisms for phospholipid repair and renewal.

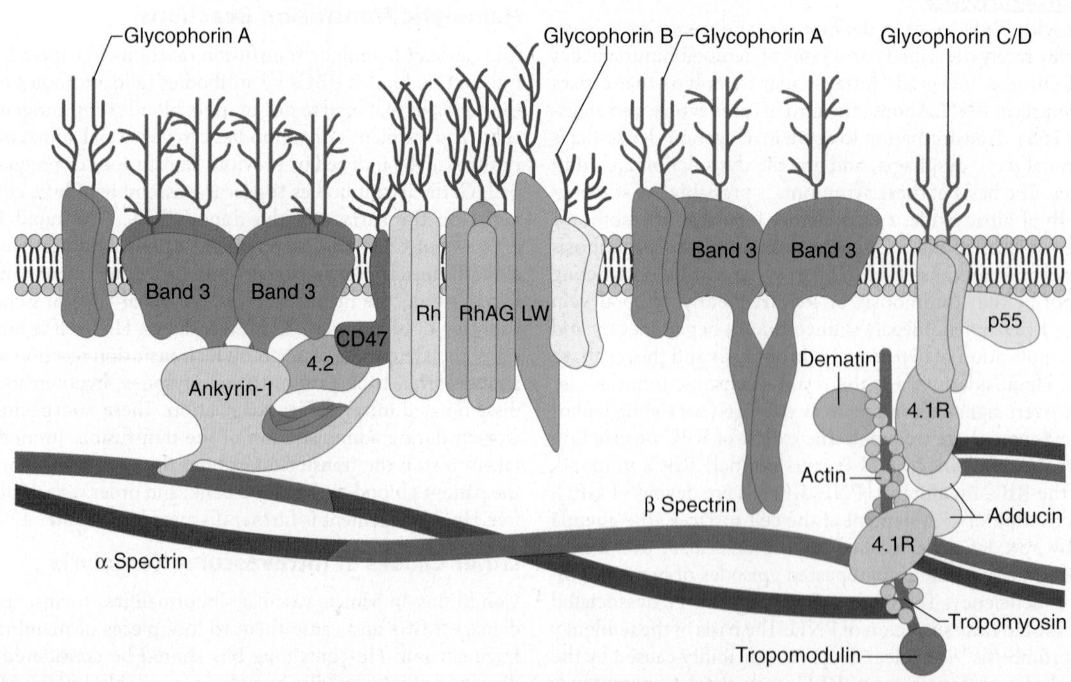

FIGURE 161-1. The erythrocyte membrane. A model of the major proteins of the erythrocyte membrane is shown: α and β spectrin, ankyrin, band 3 (the anion exchanger), 4.1 (protein 4.1) and 4.2 (protein 4.2), actin, and glycophorin. (From Perrotta S, Gallagher PG, Mohandas N. Hereditary spherocytosis. *Lancet.* 2008;372:1411-1426.)

Membrane Proteins

Membrane proteins are classified as *integral*, penetrating or crossing the lipid bilayer and interacting with the hydrophobic lipid core, or *peripheral*, interacting with integral proteins or lipids at the membrane surface but not penetrating into the bilayer core. Integral membrane proteins include the glycophorins, the Rh proteins, Kell and Duffy antigens, and transport proteins such as band 3 (AE1, anion exchanger 1, SLC4A1), Na^+,K^+-ATPase, Ca^{2+}-ATPase, and Mg^{2+}-ATPase. Numerous membrane receptors and antigens are present on integral membrane proteins. Peripheral membrane proteins are on the cytoplasmic membrane face and include enzymes such as glyceraldehyde-3-phosphate dehydrogenase and the structural proteins of the spectrin-actin–based membrane skeleton.

Integral Membrane Proteins

Band 3, the major integral protein of the RBC, has two primary functions, ion transport and maintenance of protein–protein interactions. Band 3 mediates chloride–bicarbonate exchange and provides a binding site for glycolytic enzymes, Hb, and the skeletal proteins ankyrin, protein 4.1, and protein 4.2. A single *N*-glycan chain attached to an Asn in the membrane spanning domain of band 3 is composed of *N*-acetyl-D-lactosamine units arranged in an unbranched, linear fashion in fetal erythrocytes (i antigen) and in a branched fashion in adult cells (I antigen).

The glycophorins are the next most abundant family of integral membrane proteins. They provide most of the negative surface charge required by RBCs to avoid sticking to each other and to the vascular wall. They are involved in transmembrane signaling and carry receptors for *Plasmodium falciparum*, a number of viruses and bacteria, and several blood group antigens.

Peripheral Membrane Proteins

Spectrin is the major component of the membrane skeleton. It is composed of two subunits, α and β spectrin, that are structurally related but functionally distinct. Spectrin is highly flexible and assumes a variety of conformations, an unusual property that may be critical for normal membrane pliancy. The spectrin-based membrane skeleton is linked to the plasma membrane through the actin–protein 4.1 junctional complex; through spectrin–ankyrin interactions; and through binding of a multiprotein complex containing Rh proteins, Rh-associated glycoproteins, CD47, LW, glycophorin B, and protein 4.2 to ankyrin. Protein 4.1, a protein necessary for normal membrane stability, interacts with spectrin, actin, and other proteins of the RBC membrane. Ankyrin serves as the primary linkage protein for the high-affinity binding of spectrin to the inner membrane through interactions with the cytoplasmic domain of band 3. Protein 4.2 is a peripheral membrane protein that helps link the skeleton to the lipid bilayer through interactions with ankyrin and band 3.

Erythrocyte membrane disorders result from alterations in the quantity or quality (or both) of individual proteins and their dynamic interactions with each other. Disruption of the vertical protein–protein interactions of the membrane, that is, the spectrin-ankyrin–band 3 linkage or the band 3–protein 4.2 interaction, leads to uncoupling of the membrane skeleton from the lipid bilayer. This leads to membrane instability with loss of lipids and some integral membrane proteins, resulting in loss of membrane surface area and the phenotype of spherocytosis. Disruption of the horizontal interactions of membrane skeleton proteins, including perturbation of spectrin self-association or junctional complex protein–protein interactions, leads to membrane instability, altered membrane deformability and mechanical properties, and the phenotype of elliptocytosis.

DISORDERS OF THE ERYTHROCYTE MEMBRANE

Hemolytic anemias caused by defects in the erythrocyte membrane comprise an important group of hereditary anemias. Hereditary spherocytosis (HS), hereditary elliptocytosis (HE), and hereditary pyropoikilocytosis (HPP) are the most common disorders among this group.[1] Detailed clinical studies carried out years ago have now been complemented by biochemical and genetic studies, providing both a better understanding of the pathogenesis of these disorders and a better understanding of the normal biology of the erythrocyte membrane.

Hereditary Spherocytosis

DEFINITION

Hereditary spherocytosis is a group of disorders characterized by spherical erythrocytes on the peripheral blood smear. Clinical, laboratory, and genetic heterogeneity characterize this group of disorders.

EPIDEMIOLOGY

Hereditary spherocytosis affects approximately one in 2000 to 3000 individuals of northern European ancestry. Found worldwide, it is much more common in whites than individuals of African ancestry.

PATHOBIOLOGY

The primary defect in HS is the loss of erythrocyte membrane surface area caused by defects in erythrocyte membrane proteins, including α spectrin, β spectrin, ankyrin, band 3, and protein 4.2. Qualitative or quantitative defects of one or more of these membrane proteins lead to membrane instability, which, in turn, leads to membrane loss. In approximately two thirds of HS patients, inheritance is autosomal dominant. In the remaining patients, inheritance is nondominant owing to a de novo mutation or autosomal recessive inheritance. Cases with autosomal recessive inheritance are caused by defects in either α spectrin or protein 4.2. Rare cases of homozygous HS have been reported, resulting in fetal death or severe hemolytic anemia. In most cases, HS mutations are "private," that is, each individual has a unique mutation, implying that there is no selective advantage to HS.

The spleen plays a critical, albeit secondary, role in the pathophysiology of HS. Splenic destruction of poorly deformable spherocytes is the primary cause of hemolysis experienced by HS patients. Abnormal erythrocytes are trapped in the splenic microcirculation and ingested by phagocytes. Moreover, the splenic environment is hostile to erythrocytes, with low pH, low glucose, and low ATP concentrations and high local concentrations of toxic free radicals produced by adjacent phagocytes, all contributing to membrane damage.

CLINICAL MANIFESTATIONS

The clinical manifestations of the spherocytosis syndromes vary widely.[2] The classic triad of HS is anemia, jaundice, and splenomegaly. Rarely, patients may have severe hemolytic anemia presenting in utero or shortly after birth and continuing through the first year of life. These patients may require multiple blood transfusions, and in some cases, splenectomy in the first year of life. Many patients with HS escape detection throughout childhood. In these patients, the diagnosis of HS may not be made until they are being evaluated for unrelated disorders later in life or when complications related to anemia or chronic hemolysis occur. Although the lifespan of an erythrocyte in these patients may be shortened to only 20 to 30 days, they adequately compensate for their hemolysis with increased bone marrow erythropoiesis.

Chronic hemolysis leads to the formation of bilirubinate gallstones, the most frequently reported complication in patients with HS. Although gallstones have been observed in early childhood, most appear in adolescents and young adults. Routine interval ultrasonography to detect gallstones should be performed even if patients are asymptomatic.

Other complications of HS include aplastic, hemolytic, and megaloblastic crises. Aplastic crises occur after virally induced bone marrow suppression and present with anemia, jaundice, fever, and vomiting. The most common etiologic agent in these cases is parvovirus B19 (Chapter 371). Hemolytic crises, usually associated with viral illnesses and occurring before 6 years of age, are generally mild and present with jaundice, increased spleen size, and a decrease in hematocrit. Megaloblastic crises occur in HS patients with increased folate demands, such as the pregnant patient, growing children, or patients recovering from an aplastic crisis.

Uncommon manifestations of HS include skin ulceration, gout, chronic leg dermatitis, cardiomyopathy, spinal cord dysfunction, movement disorders, and extramedullary erythropoiesis. In patients with untreated severe HS, poor growth and findings attributable to extramedullary hematopoiesis, such as hand and skull deformities, may be found.

DIAGNOSIS

Patients with HS may present at any age, usually with anemia, hyperbilirubinemia, or an abnormal blood smear. In evaluating a patient with suspected HS, particular attention should be paid to the family history, including questions about anemia, jaundice, gallstones, and splenectomy. The initial laboratory investigation should include a complete blood count with a peripheral smear, reticulocyte count, direct antiglobulin test (Coombs test), and serum bilirubin. When the peripheral smear or family history is suggestive of HS, an incubated osmotic fragility test or flow cytometric analysis of eosin-5-maleimide–labeled erythrocytes (EMA binding) (discussed later) should be obtained. Rarely, additional, specialized testing is required to confirm the diagnosis.

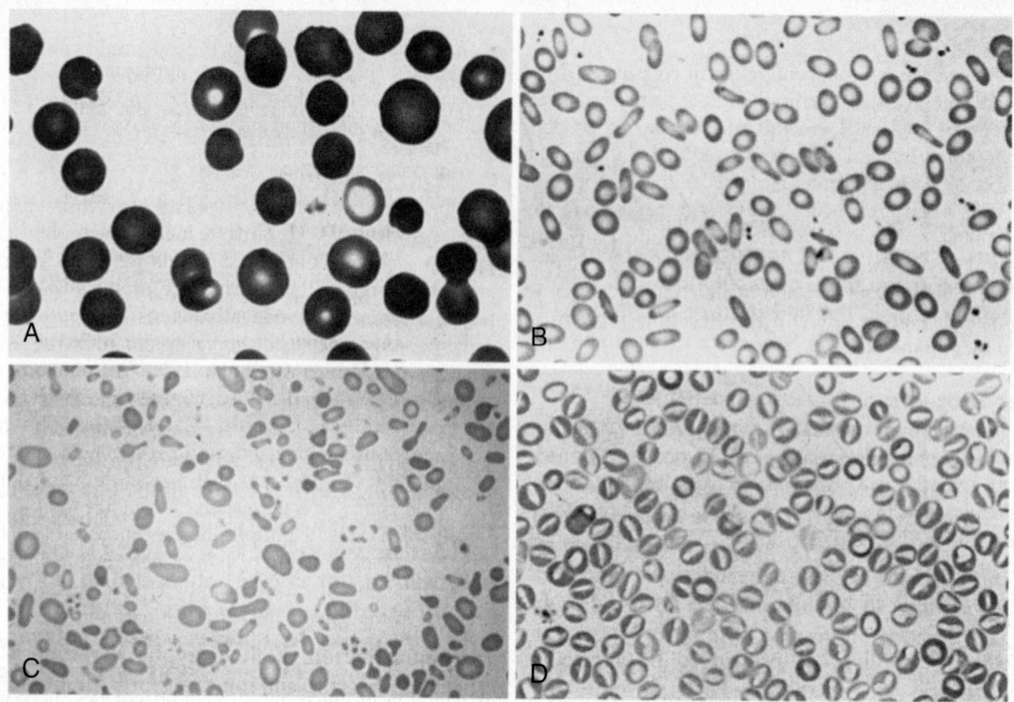

FIGURE 161-2. Peripheral blood smears in disorders of erythrocyte shape. A, Hereditary spherocytosis. Characteristic spherocytes lacking central pallor are seen. B, Hereditary elliptocytosis. Smooth, cigar-shaped elliptocytes are seen. C, Hereditary pyropoikilocytosis. Pronounced microcytosis, poikilocytosis, fragmentation of erythrocytes, and elliptocytes are seen. D, Hereditary stomatocytosis.

Overall, laboratory findings in HS are heterogeneous. Erythrocyte morphology is distinctive but not diagnostic (Fig. 161-2, *A*). Typical HS patients have blood smears with easily identifiable spherocytes lacking central pallor. Some patients present with only a few spherocytes on peripheral smear, but others present with numerous small, dense spherocytes and bizarre erythrocyte morphology. Specific morphologic findings have been identified in patients with certain membrane protein defects such as pincered erythrocytes (band 3) or spherocytic acanthocytes (β spectrin). When examining a smear in a case of suspected spherocytosis, it is important to have a high-quality smear with the erythrocytes well separated and some cells with central pallor in the field of examination because spherocytes are a common artifact on peripheral blood smears. The presence of spherocytosis on peripheral blood smear is not diagnostic of HS. Other disorders with spherocytes on peripheral blood smear are listed in Table 161-1.

The mean corpuscular hemoglobin concentration (MCHC) is increased (between 34.5 and 38) owing to relative cellular dehydration.[3] The mean corpuscular volume (MCV) is usually normal or slightly decreased.[4] Many cell counters provide a histogram of MCHCs claimed to be accurate enough to identify nearly all patients with HS.

In a normal erythrocyte, a redundancy of cell membrane gives the cell its characteristic discoid shape and provides it abundant surface area. In spherocytes, there is a decrease in surface area relative to cell volume, resulting in their abnormal shape. This change is reflected in the increased osmotic fragility found in these cells. Osmotic fragility is tested by adding increasingly hypotonic concentrations of saline to RBCs. Normal erythrocytes are able to increase their volume by swelling, but spherocytes, which are already at maximal volume for surface area, burst at higher saline concentrations than normal. Approximately one fourth of HS individuals will have a normal osmotic fragility on freshly drawn RBCs, with the osmotic fragility curve approximating the number of spherocytes seen on peripheral smear. However, after incubation at 37° C for 24 hours, HS RBCs lose membrane surface area more readily than normal because their membranes have become leaky and unstable. Thus, incubation accentuates the defect in HS erythrocytes and brings out the defect on osmotic fragility, making incubated osmotic fragility the standard test in diagnosing HS (Fig. 161-3, *bottom panel*). When the spleen is present, a subpopulation of very fragile erythrocytes that have been conditioned by the spleen form the tail of the osmotic fragility curve. This tail disappears after splenectomy. The osmotic fragility test suffers from poor sensitivity, with as many as 20% of mild cases of HS missed after incubation. It is unreliable in patients who have small numbers of spherocytes and in

TABLE 161-1 DISORDERS WITH SPHEROCYTES ON PERIPHERAL BLOOD FILM

Hereditary spherocytosis
Autoimmune hemolytic anemia
Thermal injuries
Microangiopathic and macroangiopathic hemolytic anemias
Hepatic disease
Clostridial septicemia
Transfusion reactions with hemolysis
Poisoning with certain snake, spider, and *Hymenoptera* venoms
Severe hypophosphatemia
Heinz body anemias
ABO incompatibility (neonates)

patients who have been recently transfused. It is abnormal in other conditions in which spherocytes are present.

Eosin-5-maleimide binding is a flow cytometry–based test used in the diagnosis of HS.[5] EMA is a fluorescent dye that binds to band 3 and Rh-related proteins in the erythrocyte membrane. In HS, the mean fluorescence of EMA-stained erythrocytes is lower compared with control because of the reduction of band 3 and related proteins, typically decreased to approximately 65% of normal (Fig. 161-3, *top panel*). Although primary defects of band 3 protein are seen in only about 25% of HS patients, decreased fluorescence intensity is also observed in the erythrocyte membranes of HS patients with defects in other membrane proteins such as ankyrin and spectrin. This is thought to be attributable to transmission of long-range effects of mutant protein defects across the membrane lattice, ultimately influencing the amount of EMA binding to band 3. EMA binding has good sensitivity and specificity and is simple and rapidly performed.

Specialized testing is available for studying difficult cases or cases in which additional information is desired. Useful tests for these purposes include structural and functional studies of erythrocyte membrane proteins, such as protein quantitation, limited tryptic digestion of spectrin, spectrin, and ion transport. Membrane frigidity and fragility may be examined using an ektacytometer. Complementary DNA and genomic DNA analyses are available when a molecular diagnosis is desired.

Other laboratory manifestations in HS are manifestations of ongoing hemolysis. Increased serum bilirubin, increased lactate dehydrogenase,

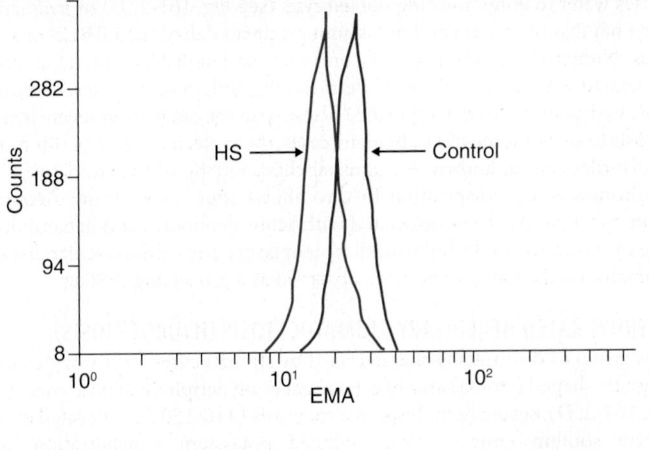

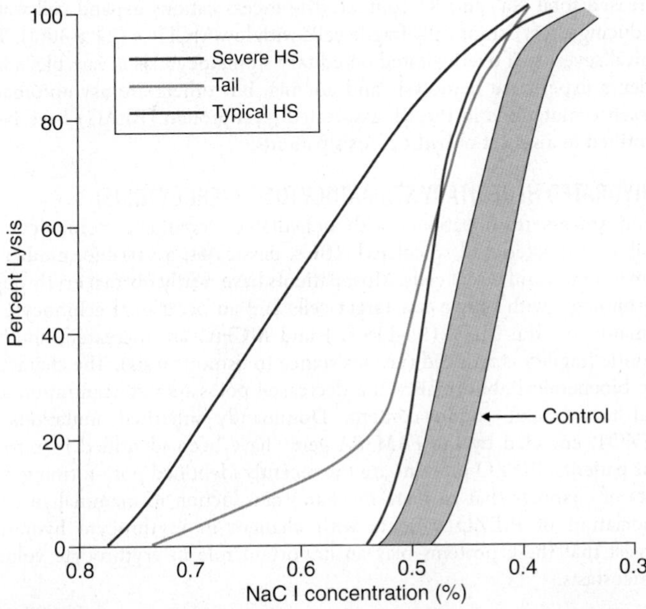

FIGURE 161-3. **Testing in hereditary spherocytosis.** *Top panel,* Eosin-5-maleimide (EMA) binding. Histogram of fluorescence of EMA-labeled erythrocytes from a normal control and a patient with typical hereditary spherocytosis. Decreased fluorescence in observed from HS erythrocytes. *Bottom panel,* Osmotic fragility curves in hereditary spherocytosis. The *shaded region* is the normal range. Results representative of both typical, and severe spherocytosis are shown. A tail, representing fragile erythrocytes conditioned by the spleen, is common in spherocytosis patients prior to splenectomy. (From Gallagher PG. Abnormalities of the erythrocyte membrane. *Pediatr Clin North Am* 2013;60:1349-1352.)

increased urinary and fecal urobilinogen, and decreased serum haptoglobin reflect increased erythrocyte destruction.

After diagnosing a patient with HS, family members should be examined for the presence of HS. This can be of great epidemiologic importance, particularly for very old and very young patients. Prenatal diagnosis of HS has been made in a few cases, but this is rarely necessary.

TREATMENT AND PROGNOSIS Rx

Splenic sequestration and destruction is the primary determinant of erythrocyte survival in HS patients. Splenectomy cures or alleviates anemia in most patients, reducing or eliminating the need for transfusions. The risk for cholelithiasis is also decreased to nearly background levels. After splenectomy, spherocytes remain in the peripheral blood, but their lifespan becomes near normal.

In the past, splenectomy was routinely performed in all HS patients. However, the risk of overwhelming postsplenectomy infection; the emergence of penicillin-resistant pneumococci; and the growing recognition of the increased risk of postsplenectomy cardiovascular disease, particularly thrombosis and pulmonary hypertension, have led to reevaluation of the role of splenectomy in the treatment of HS. In addition, with growing globalization, the important role of the spleen in protection of individuals living in or traveling to geographic regions where parasitic diseases such as malaria or babesiosis occur has reemerged. When splenectomy is considered, health care providers, the patient, and family members must review and weigh the benefits of splenectomy against the immediate and long-term risks of the procedure. Considering the risks and benefits, a reasonable approach is to splenectomize all patients with severe spherocytosis and all patients who have significant signs or symptoms of anemia, including growth failure, skeletal changes, leg ulcers, and extramedullary hematopoietic tumors. Other candidates for splenectomy are older HS patients who have vascular compromise of vital organs. Whether patients with moderate HS and compensated, asymptomatic anemia should undergo splenectomy is controversial.[6]

When splenectomy is indicated, laparoscopic splenectomy has become the method of choice. This technique results in less postoperative discomfort, a quicker return to preoperative diet and activities, shorter hospitalization, decreased costs, and smaller scars. Even massive spleens can be removed laparoscopically because the spleen is placed in a large bag, diced intraoperatively, and eliminated through suction catheters. Partial splenectomy, initially advocated for infants and young children with significant anemia associated with erythrocyte membrane disorders to allow for palliation of hemolysis and anemia while maintaining some residual splenic immune function, is now being suggested by some for most HS patients. Updated UK guidelines,[7] which reflect changes in current opinion about surgical management, include (1) preference for a laparoscopic approach, (2) performance of splenectomy ideally after the age of 6 years, (3) no indication for extended thrombosis prophylaxis after splenectomy for HS, and (4) avoidance of splenectomy in patients with some forms of hereditary stomatocytosis because of an increased risk of venous thromboembolism.

Before splenectomy, patients should be immunized with vaccines against pneumococcus, *Haemophilus influenzae* type B, and meningococcus. Postsplenectomy care includes counseling of patients or parents to seek prompt medical care in case of febrile illness. Use of routine antibiotics after splenectomy for prevention of pneumococcal sepsis is controversial. Data are lacking to indicate or refute their prescription. Before splenectomy and, in severe cases, after splenectomy, HS patients should take folic acid (1 mg/day orally) to prevent folate deficiency.

Hereditary Elliptocytosis and Related Disorders

DEFINITION

Hereditary elliptocytosis is characterized by the presence of elliptical or oval cigar-shaped erythrocytes on peripheral blood smears of affected individuals (see Fig. 161-2, *B*).

EPIDEMIOLOGY

Hereditary elliptocytosis has been estimated to occur in approximately one in 2000 to 4000 individuals. The true incidence of HE is unknown because its clinical severity is heterogeneous, and many patients are asymptomatic. It is common in African Americans and people of Mediterranean ancestry, presumably because elliptocytes confer some resistance to malaria. In parts of Africa, the incidence of HE approaches one in 100.

PATHOBIOLOGY

The principal defect in HE is mechanical weakness or fragility of the erythrocyte membrane skeleton. Qualitative and quantitative defects in a number of RBC membrane proteins have been described in HE, including α spectrin, β spectrin, protein 4.1, and glycophorin C. Most defects occur in spectrin, the principal structural protein of the erythrocyte membrane skeleton. αβ Spectrin heterodimers self-associate into tetramers and higher order oligomers that are critical for erythrocyte membrane stability as well as erythrocyte shape and function. Most spectrin defects in HE impair the ability of spectrin dimers to self-associate into tetramers and oligomers, thereby disrupting the membrane skeleton. Structural and functional defects of protein 4.1 appear to disrupt the spectrin–actin contact in the membrane skeleton. Glycophorin C variants are also deficient in protein 4.1. The precise pathobiology of how elliptocytes are formed in these syndromes is unclear.

Genetically, HE is heterogeneous with multiple genetic loci. A wide variety of mutations have been described in the α spectrin, β spectrin, protein 4.1, and glycophorin C genes, including point mutations, gene deletions and insertions, and messenger RNA processing defects. Several mutations have been identified in a number of individuals of the same genetic background, suggesting a "founder effect" for these mutants, which supports the hypothesis that there has been genetic selection for elliptocytosis because these RBCs confer some resistance to malaria. Most cases of HE are inherited in an autosomal dominant pattern, with rare cases of de novo mutations.

CLINICAL MANIFESTATIONS

The clinical presentation of HE is heterogeneous, ranging from asymptomatic carriers to patients with severe, life-threatening anemia. Most patients with HE are asymptomatic and are diagnosed incidentally during testing for unrelated conditions. Asymptomatic carriers have been identified who possess the same molecular defect as an affected HE relative but who have normal peripheral blood smears. The erythrocyte lifespan, normal in most patients, is decreased in only about 10% of patients. This subset of HE patients with decreased erythrocyte lifespan experience hemolysis, anemia, splenomegaly, and intermittent jaundice. Many of these patients have parents with typical HE and thus are homozygotes or compound heterozygotes for defects inherited from each of the parents. Symptoms may vary among members of the same family, indeed, they may vary in the same individual at different times.

Hereditary Pyropoikilocytosis

Hereditary pyropoikilocytosis is a rare cause of anemia with distinctive erythrocyte morphology on peripheral blood smear (see Fig. 161-2, *C*) and has a picture similar to that seen in patients with severe burns. Patients typically present in infancy with severe anemia and peripheral blood smear findings of elliptocytosis, poikilocytosis, pyknocytosis, and fragmentation. Microspherocytosis is common, and the MCV is usually very low (50-70 fL). Most patients are of African ancestry, and at least one third of HPP patients have a parent or sibling with typical HE. Patients with HPP tend to experience severe hemolysis and anemia in infancy that gradually improves, evolving toward typical HE later in life.

DIAGNOSIS

Cigar-shaped elliptocytes on peripheral blood smear are the hallmark of HE (see Fig. 161-2, *B*). These normochromic, normocytic elliptocytes vary in number from a few to 100%, with the likelihood of hemolysis not correlating with the number of elliptocytes present. Ovalocytes, spherocytes, stomatocytes, and fragmented cells may also be seen. In some cases, pyknocytes may be prominent. Elliptocytes may be seen in association with other disorders, including megaloblastic anemias, hypochromic microcytic anemias (iron deficiency anemia and thalassemia), myelodysplastic syndromes, and myelofibrosis; however, elliptocytes generally make up less fewer one third of RBCs in these conditions. History and additional laboratory testing usually clarify the diagnosis of these disorders. In typical cases, the incubated osmotic fragility is normal, but in severe HE and HPP, incubated osmotic fragility is increased, and EMA binding is decreased.

Other laboratory findings in HE are similar to those found in other hemolytic anemias and are nonspecific markers of increased erythrocyte production and destruction. The reticulocyte count generally is less than 5% but may be higher when hemolysis is severe.

Similar to HS, specialized laboratory procedures are available to study the erythrocyte membranes of HE and HPP patients. These studies are not routinely required to make the diagnosis of HE or HPP, but they may be helpful in studying problematic cases and in elucidating the underlying molecular defects.

TREATMENT

Therapy is rarely needed in patients with HE. In rare cases, occasional RBCs transfusions may be required. In cases of severe HE and HPP, splenectomy has been palliative because the spleen is the site of erythrocyte sequestration and destruction. Many practitioners think that the same indications for splenectomy in HS should be applied to patients with symptomatic HE or HPP. Postsplenectomy patients with HE or HPP experience increased hematocrits, decreased reticulocyte counts, and improvement in clinical symptoms.

Patients should be followed for signs of decompensation during acute illnesses. Interval ultrasonography to detect gallstones should be performed. In patients with significant hemolysis, folate should be administered daily.

Hereditary Stomatocytosis Syndromes

Red blood cell hydration is primarily determined by the intracellular concentration of monovalent cations. A net increase in sodium and potassium ions causes water to enter, forming *stomatocytes* (see Fig. 161-2, *D*) or *hydrocytes*, but a net loss of sodium and potassium produces dehydrated RBCs, or *xerocytes*. Numerous descriptions of congenital or familial hemolytic anemias associated with abnormal cation permeability and, in some cases, disturbed RBC hydration have been reported.[8] These span the range from severe hydrocytosis to severe xerocytosis. In many cases, the molecular bases of this group of disorders are unknown. An unusual characteristic of the stomatocytosis syndromes is a predisposition to thrombosis after splenectomy. Acquired stomatocytosis has been associated with acute alcoholism and hepatobiliary disease, vinca alkaloid administration, neoplasms, and cardiovascular disease. Stomatocytosis is also sometimes observed as a processing artifact.

OVERHYDRATED HEREDITARY STOMATOCYTOSIS (HYDROCYTOSIS)

This group of disorders is characterized by stomatocytes, erythrocytes with a mouth-shaped (stoma) area of central pallor on peripheral blood smear (see Fig. 161-2, *D*), severe hemolysis, macrocytosis (110-150 fL), elevated erythrocyte sodium concentration, reduced potassium concentration, and increased total Na^+ and K^+ content. The excess cations expand cell water, producing large, osmotically fragile cells with low MCHCs (24%-30%). The clinical severity of overhydrated hereditary stomatocytosis is variable; some patients experience hemolysis and anemia, but others are asymptomatic. Missense mutations in the Rh-associated glycoprotein (RhAG) have been identified in a subset of hydrocytosis patients.

DEHYDRATED HEREDITARY STOMATOCYTOSIS (XEROCYTOSIS)

Blood smears from patients with dehydrated hereditary stomatocytosis exhibit contracted and spiculated RBCs, dessicytes, a variable number of stomatocytes, and target cells. Most patients have nearly normal erythrocyte morphology, with only a few target cells and an occasional echinocyte or stomatocyte. The MCV (95-115 fL) and MCHC are increased, and the osmotic fragility is reduced (i.e., resistance to osmotic lysis). The characteristic biochemical abnormality is a decreased potassium concentration and total monovalent cation content. Dominantly inherited mutations in PIEZO1, encoded by the *FAM38A* gene, have been identified in xerocytosis patients. PIEZO proteins are the recently identified pore-forming subunits of channels that mediate mechanotransduction in mammalian cells. Association of PIEZO variants with changes in erythrocyte hydration suggest that these proteins play an important role in erythrocyte volume homeostasis.

INTERMEDIATE SYNDROMES AND HEREDITARY STOMATOCYTOSIS VARIANTS

Hydrocytosis and xerocytosis represent the extremes of a spectrum of RBC permeability defects. A number of families with features of both conditions have been reported. Some patients with severe permeability defects have little or no hemolysis. The proportion of stomatocytes and the degree of sodium influx do not correlate with each other, and neither correlates with the amount of hemolysis or anemia.

ERYTHROCYTE METABOLISM

The primary functions of the erythrocyte, gas transport and exchange, are maintained without a net change in energy state. However, several critical functions of the erythrocyte depend on the production and expenditure of energy. As erythrocytes age, glucose utilization and ATP levels fall, leading to decreased membrane deformability and, ultimately, a shortened lifespan. Lower potassium levels, higher sodium levels, and decreased membrane lipids are also seen in ATP-deficient, aging erythrocytes.

Erythrocytes do not undergo oxidative phosphorylation and do not store glycogen; thus, they must constantly catabolize glucose from the blood stream through the Embden-Meyerhof pathway and the HMP shunt as a source of energy (Fig. 161-4). Erythrocytes incorporate glucose from the plasma through facilitated transfer, with erythrocyte glucose levels rapidly equilibrating with changes in blood glucose levels. Glucose is the preferred carbohydrate of the RBC, but fructose and mannose are metabolized almost as readily. Inside the erythrocyte, glucose is converted to glucose-6-phosphate or to fructose by sorbitol. Glucose-6-phosphate follows one of three pathways: (1) most (~90%) enters the Embden-Meyerhof pathway, where it is converted into lactate, pyruvate, and ATP; (2) some (~5%-10%) enters the HMP shunt to produce reduced intermediates and ribulose 5-phosphate, the latter of which eventually enters the Embden-Meyerhof pathway; and (3) a tiny fraction (<1%) is converted to glucose-1-phosphate and then to glycogen.

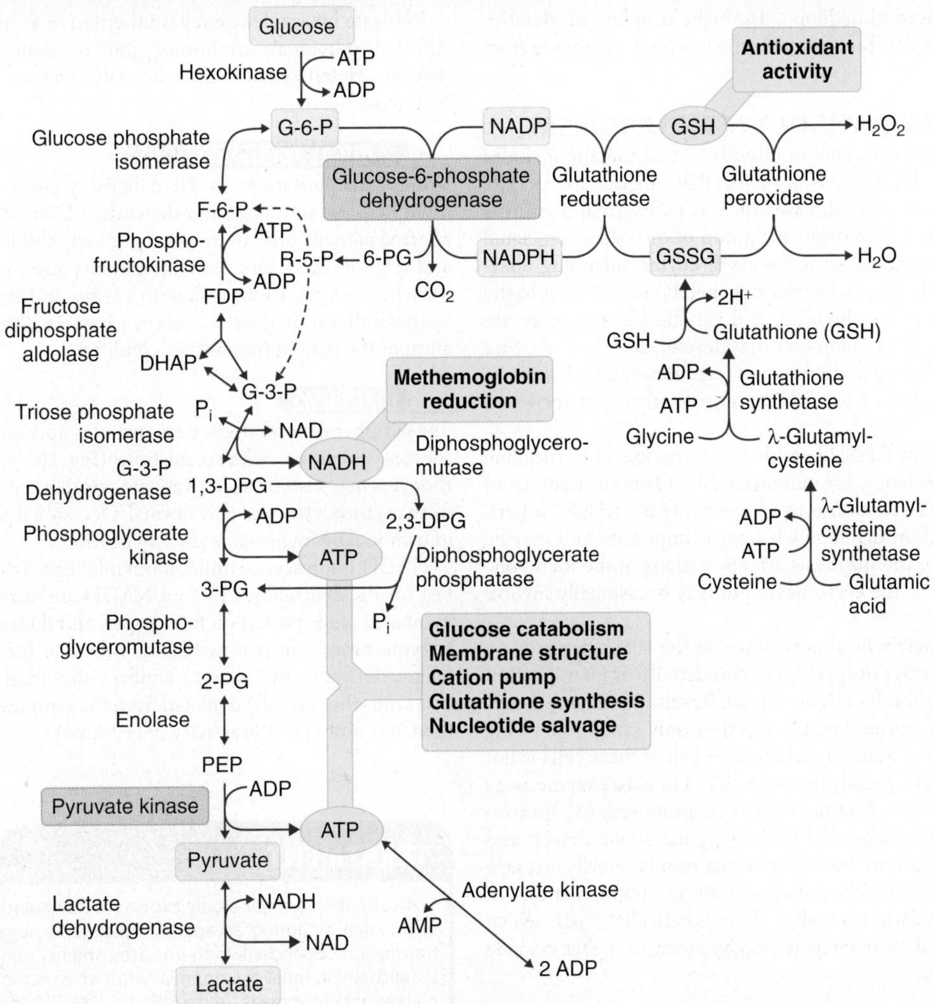

FIGURE 161-4. **Pathways of energy metabolism in the erythrocyte. Glucose-6-phosphate may be degraded anaerobically to lactate through the Embden-Meyerhof pathway or oxidatively through the hexose monophosphate shunt. Pentose phosphates (R-5-P) can reenter anaerobic glycolysis as fructose-6-phosphate (F-6-P) and glyceraldehyde-3-phosphate (G-3-P) after conversion by enzymes of the terminal pentose phosphate pathway or as a product of adenosine or inosine degradation. 2,3-Diphosphoglycerate (2,3-DPG) may be generated instead of adenosine triphosphate (ATP) through diversion of triose through the Rapoport-Luebering shunt. Glutathione may be synthesized directly from constituent amino acids; its cycling from oxidized (GSSG) to reduced forms (GSH) depends on reduced pyridine cofactor (NADPH) generation. ADP = adenosine diphosphate; DHAP = dihydroxy-acetone phosphate; FDP = fructose-1,6-diphosphate; NAD = nicotinamide adenine dinucleotide; NADP = nicotinamide adenine dinucleotide phosphate; NADPH = nicotinamide adenine dinucleotide phosphate, reduced form; PEP = polyestradiol phosphate.**

Embden-Meyerhof Pathway

The Embden-Meyerhof pathway of glycolysis is the primary source of ATP, 2,3-DPG and nicotinamide adenine dinucleotide, reduced form (NADH) in erythrocytes (see Fig. 161-4). Most of the energy generated by erythrocytes is through the Embden-Meyerhof pathway followed by storage as high-energy phosphates such as ATP or as reducing energy in the form of glutathione or pyridine nucleotides (NADH and nicotinamide adenine dinucleotide phosphate, reduced form [NADPH]). This pathway metabolizes about 90% of erythrocyte glucose with the catabolism of 1 mole of glucose yielding 2 moles of ATP and 2 moles of lactate. Two moles of ATP per mole of metabolized glucose seems insignificant compared with the Krebs cycle of intermediary metabolism, in which 1 mole of glucose metabolized produces 38 moles of ATP. However, this ATP production is adequate to renew 150% to 200% of the total RBC ATP every hour.

The Embden-Meyerhof pathway is also the primary source of NADH, a necessary cofactor for NADH methemoglobin reductase, which maintains heme iron in the reduced state. Without this reaction, heme iron would be oxidized to methemoglobin, which is not a functional oxygen transporter.

Finally, the Rapoport-Luebering shunt of the Embden-Meyerhof pathway (see Fig. 161-4) produces 2,3-DPG, a compound found in high concentrations in erythrocytes but in low concentrations in other cells. After it is formed, under physiologic conditions of pH and solute concentrations, 2,3-DPG binds reversibly to tetramers of deoxyhemoglobin with greater affinity than it does to oxyhemoglobin. By binding to deoxyhemoglobin, it allosterically upregulates the release of the remaining oxygen bound to the Hb, enhancing the ability of erythrocytes to release oxygen near tissues that need it most.

Hexose Monophosphate Shunt (Pentose Phosphate Pathway)

In the HMP shunt (see Fig. 161-4), glucose-6-phosphate undergoes oxidation followed by a series of reactions to yield fructose-6-phosphate and glyceraldehyde-3-phosphate, intermediates in the glycolytic pathway. The HMP shunt is the primary source of erythrocyte NADPH, with 2 moles of NADPH produced for each mole of glucose metabolized. NADPH is required for the reduction of oxidized glutathione and some protein sulfhydryl groups.

Mature erythrocytes synthesize large amounts of reduced glutathione (GSH). GSH protects erythrocytes from oxidants, including hydrogen peroxide (H_2O_2), superoxide anions (O_2^-), and hydroxyl radicals (OH), which are produced as byproducts of the oxidation of heme by oxygen. Oxidants are also produced by activated phagocytes (e.g., during infection) and by erythrocytes after exposure to certain agents. When oxidants accumulate, they damage cellular proteins and lipids. Detoxification of H_2O_2 is significantly enhanced by glutathione peroxidase. GSH is converted to oxidized glutathione (GSSG) and to mixed disulfides with protein thiols. GSH levels are restored by glutathione reductase. In this process, NADPH is oxidized to nicotinamide adenine dinucleotide phosphate (NADP), which stimulates the HMP shunt to regenerate NADPH.[9] After oxidant stress, hypoxia, or acidosis, erythrocytes can increase the amount of glucose metabolized through the HMP shunt up to 10- to 20-fold to generate increased amounts of reduced glutathione. The tight coupling of glutathione metabolism with the HMP shunt protects the mature erythrocyte from oxidative stress.

DISORDERS OF ERYTHROCYTE METABOLISM

Congenital nonspherocytic hemolytic anemia (CNSHA) traditionally includes erythrocyte disorders not due to defects of the RBC membrane or Hb, immune-mediated disease, or other diseases such as paroxysmal nocturnal hemoglobinuria. CNSHA is a heterogeneous group of disorders associated with various metabolic abnormalities of the erythrocytes, including enzymopathies of glucose, glutathione, and nucleotide metabolism. Similar to the membrane disorders, clinical, biochemical, and genetic heterogeneity are typical within the enzymopathies. Hemolysis may develop as a result of either enzyme or antioxidant deficiency or dysfunction (e.g., abnormal substrate or cofactor binding), altered activation or inhibition characteristics, or decreased stability or specific activity.

Peripheral blood smears in CNSHA, with the exception of pyrimidine 5′-nucleotidase (P5N) deficiency, are unremarkable. Osmotic fragility of fresh erythrocytes is normal. Response to splenectomy is variable. Inheritance is heterogeneous. A thorough family history is important and may be of assistance in determining the diagnosis. Manifestations of the metabolic defect are usually confined to the erythrocyte but may occasionally involve nonerythroid cells.

Definitive diagnosis of metabolic abnormalities of the RBCs depends on qualitative or quantitative assays of specific enzyme activity or identification of the specific genetic mutation by DNA analysis. Results of enzyme assays should be interpreted with caution because (1) they only sample surviving RBCs in the peripheral blood, and the metabolic milieu of these cells is not necessarily comparable to cells already hemolyzed; (2) in vitro enzyme assay conditions may not accurately reflect the in vivo environment; (3) transfusions before the assay may obscure the underlying metabolic defect, and (4) leukocyte contamination may lead to spurious results. Finally, average enzyme activity may not accurately reflect activity in subpopulations of erythrocytes. This is particularly true when there is reticulocytosis, which may yield artificially elevated mean enzyme activity owing to higher enzyme levels found in reticulocytes.

Disorders of the Embden-Meyerhof Pathway

Defects of the Embden-Meyerhof pathway are inherited in an autosomal recessive fashion, and usually hemolysis is seen only in homozygotes or compound heterozygotes.[10] Heterozygotes, whose erythrocytes contain less than normal amounts of mutant enzyme, are clinically normal.

An exception is phosphoglycerate kinase deficiency, an X-linked disorder with hemolysis found only in males. In this group of disorders, hemolysis is chronic, is not typically influenced by drugs or other inciting agents, and is attributed to insufficient levels of erythrocyte ATP. Splenomegaly from trapping of mutant erythrocytes is common. The hostile splenic environment contributes to the shortened erythrocyte lifespan. When performing specific diagnostic enzyme assays, measurement of glycolytic intermediates may assist in diagnosis because concentrations of intermediates are increased upstream of a defect and decreased downstream of a defect.

PYRUVATE KINASE DEFICIENCY

Pyruvate kinase (PK) deficiency accounts for approximately 90% of inherited defects of the Embden-Meyerhof pathway and is the second most common inherited erythrocyte enzymopathy associated with anemia after glucose-6-phosphate dehydrogenase (G6PD) deficiency (see later). PK deficiency is found worldwide, but it is most common in individuals of northern European descent.

PATHOBIOLOGY

Pyruvate kinase catalyzes the conversion of phosphoenolpyruvate (PEP) to pyruvate, generating ATP. Deficient or defective PK leads to decreased levels of erythrocyte ATP, disturbing many cellular processes such as signaling and maintenance of water and ion content, leading to energy failure and dehydration. Upstream catabolites accumulate in the erythrocyte, including 2,3-DPG, which shifts the oxygen dissociation curve to the right, enhancing tissue oxygenation and ameliorating some of the physiologic effects of anemia. Early PK-deficient reticulocytes retain the ability to use oxidative phosphorylation to produce ATP, bypassing their defect. This ability is lost as reticulocytes mature and is markedly dampened in the hypoxic environment of the spleen.

Pyruvate kinase deficiency is inherited in an autosomal recessive manner. Affected individuals are homozygous or compound heterozygotes for PK defects. Heterozygotes are clinically normal or exhibit very minimal hemolysis.

CLINICAL MANIFESTATIONS

Clinical manifestations in PK deficiency are heterogeneous, ranging from asymptomatic to transfusion-dependent hemolytic anemia.[11] More severely affected patients present in infancy or early childhood with anemia, jaundice, and splenomegaly. Occasionally, patients may escape detection until later in life when complications related to anemia and chronic hemolysis occur such as cholelithiasis or aplastic crisis or when the diagnosis is made during evaluation of the patient for another condition.

DIAGNOSIS

The peripheral blood smear demonstrates normocytic, normochromic erythrocytes, sometimes with spiculations (Fig. 161-5, *A*). Poikilocytes and acanthocytes may also be seen. Reticulocytosis is common. Osmotic fragility of fresh erythrocytes is usually normal. Occasional patients exhibit a population of osmotically fragile cells after incubation.

NADH fluorescence under ultraviolet light is a commonly used screening test for PK deficiency. PEP and NADH are mixed with the patient's blood, incubated, and spotted on filter paper, and fluorescence is measured. Direct enzyme assay, which uses PEP as substrate for PK, can be performed on leukocyte-free hemolysate to confirm abnormal fluorescence tests. Leukocytes must be carefully depleted from the samples because they contain more than 300 times the PK activity of erythrocytes.

TREATMENT Rx

Most patients require only expectant management, with only rare transfusions, such as during an aplastic episode. In severe cases, patients may be transfusion dependent. In these cases, splenectomy typically lessens hemolysis and ameliorates the anemia. After splenectomy, some patients develop marked reticulocytosis, up to 50% to 70%. This paradoxical reticulocytosis is attributed to increased reticulocyte survival after removal of the hostile splenic environment.

OTHER DISORDERS OF THE EMBDEN-MEYERHOF PATHWAY

Other abnormalities of the Embden-Meyerhof pathway have been described. Hexokinase deficiency is quite uncommon, with great phenotypic variability in reported cases. Severely affected patients have had anemia beginning in infancy and may require blood transfusions. Glucose phosphate isomerase (GPI) deficiency is the third most common hemolytic enzymopathy. GPI deficiency usually presents in infancy or early childhood with moderate to severe hemolytic anemia. Rare cases of GPI deficiency may also be complicated by neurologic symptomatology. Phosphofructokinase deficiency may involve erythrocytes, muscle, or both. The presentation is usually in adolescence with exertional myopathy (Chapter 207). Hemolytic anemia has been described in isolated cases of 2,3-bisphosphoglycerate mutase deficiency and phosphoglycerate kinase deficiency.

Disorders of Nucleotide Metabolism

Mature erythrocytes lack the ability to synthesize purine and pyrimidine nucleotides de novo. However, they are able to form some nucleotides through salvage pathways.

PYRIMIDINE 5′-NUCLEOTIDASE DEFICIENCY

Pyrimidine 5′-nucleotidase degrades the pyrimidine nucleotides of RNA to cytidine and uridine, which can diffuse out of the cell. When P5N is deficient, nondiffusible, partially degraded RNAs accumulate, leading to the marked basophilic stippling characteristic of P5N-deficient erythrocytes (see Fig. 161-5, *B*). These accumulated pyrimidine nucleotides inhibit the transport of GSSG (oxidized glutathione) out of RBCs, leading to high levels of erythrocyte glutathione. Clinically, the patient has mild to moderate hemolytic anemia and splenomegaly. The cause of the hemolysis remains cryptic. Typically, splenectomy does not ameliorate the hemolysis and anemia.

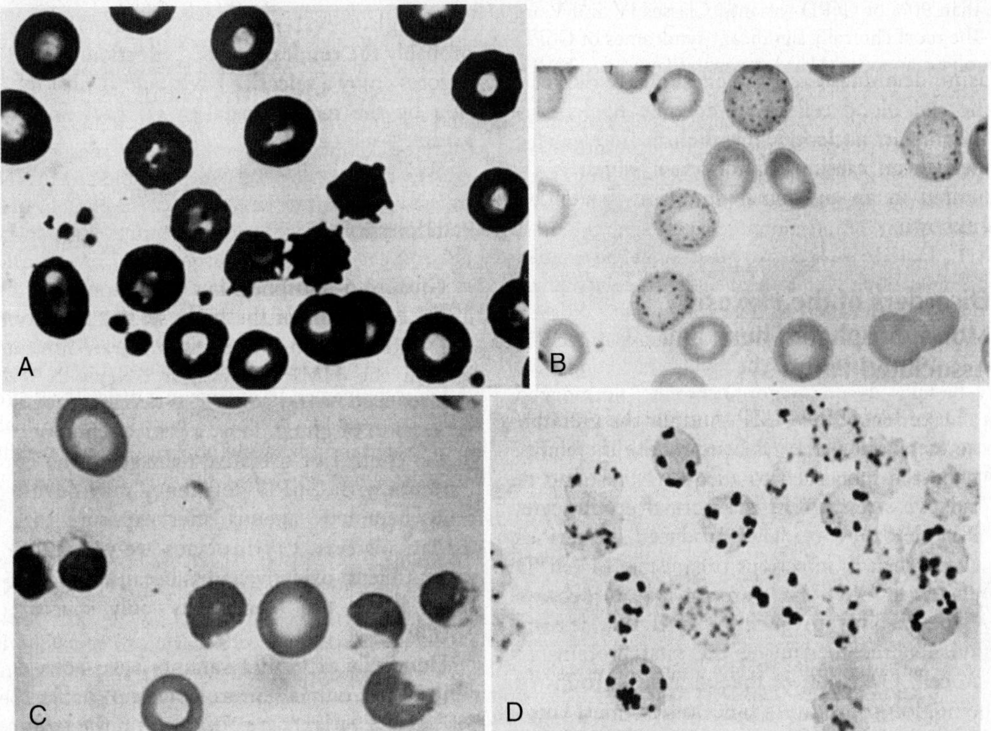

FIGURE 161-5. Peripheral blood smears in erythrocyte enzymopathies. A, Pyruvate kinase deficiency. B, Pyrimidine 5′-nucleotidase deficiency; C, Glucose-6-phosphate dehydrogenase (G6PD) deficiency. D, Heinz bodies in G6PD deficiency. (B from Paglia DE. Disorders of erythrocyte glycolysis and nucleotide metabolism. In: Handin RI, Lux SE, Stossel TP, eds. *Blood: Principles and Practice of Hematology*. Philadelphia: JB Lippincott; 1995:1877-1896.)

Disorders of the Hexose Monophosphate Shunt (Pentose Phosphate Pathway) and Associated Pathways

Disorders of the HMP shunt or of the glutathione metabolic pathways (see Fig. 161-4) compromise the ability of the RBC to respond adequately to oxidative stress. In normal erythrocytes, GSH detoxifies oxidants produced by various agents and infection. In G6PD-deficient erythrocytes, because of the inability to generate NADPH, GSH levels are inadequate, leaving the cell susceptible to oxidant stress. Oxidation of Hb sulfhydryl groups leads to the production of methemoglobin and intracellular Hb precipitates called *Heinz bodies*. Heinz bodies (see Fig. 161-5, *D*), usually visualized on peripheral blood smears with supravital stains such as methyl violet, attach to and damage the erythrocyte membrane. They induce clustering of immunoglobulins and band 3 protein, marking the erythrocyte for opsonization by phagocytes and eventual removal from the circulation. Heinz bodies are "pitted" from circulating cells by the spleen and are commonly seen on smears of patients after splenectomy. "Bite cells," erythrocytes with localized invaginations, possibly at the site of Heinz body injury or removal, are seen during acute hemolytic episodes. In addition to damage from Heinz body formation, GSH-deficient erythrocytes undergo peroxidation of membrane phospholipids and oxidative cross-linking of spectrin, decreasing membrane deformability and further promoting splenic trapping.

GLUCOSE-6-PHOSPHATE DEHYDROGENASE DEFICIENCY

G6PD deficiency is the most common inherited disorder of erythrocyte metabolism, affecting more than 400 million people worldwide.[12] The high prevalence of G6PD deficiency is thought to be attributable to genetic selection because G6PD-deficient erythrocytes have a selective advantage against invasion by the malaria parasite *Plasmodium falciparum*.

EPIDEMIOLOGY AND PATHOBIOLOGY

G6PD is the initial and rate-limiting step in the HMP shunt (see Fig. 161-4), which converts NADP into NADPH. NADPH is required for the generation of glutathione, a critical constituent in the prevention of oxidative damage to the cell. G6PD-deficient patients may develop acute hemolytic anemia after exposure to oxidative stress. Although G6PD is a ubiquitous enzyme, erythroid cells are particularly susceptible to oxidative stress because the HMP shunt is their only source of NADPH.

Hundreds of G6PD variants have been described, but only a few are common. Variants are classified on the basis of biochemical characteristics; electrophoretic mobility; ability to use substrate analogue, Km for NADP and G6PD; pH activity profile; and thermal stability. The normal enzyme, Gd^{B}, is present in 99% of white Americans and 70% of African Americans. A normal variant, Gd^{A+}, found in 20% of African Americans, has a faster electrophoretic mobility than Gd^{B}. Gd^{A-}, the most common variant associated with hemolysis, is found in about 10% of African Americans and in many Africans. Gd^{A-} has decreased catalytic ability compared with Gd^{A+}. Gd^{Med}, the second most common variant associated with hemolysis, is common in the Mediterranean area, in India, and in Southeast Asia, with a prevalence of up to 5% to 50%. Gd^{Med} exhibits markedly decreased catalytic activity. Gd^{Canton}, a variant common in Asian populations, produces a clinical syndrome similar to Gd^{A-}.[13,14]

Gd^{B} activity decreases as normal cells age, with a half-life of approximately 60 days. Despite very low levels of or no active G6PD, older erythrocytes maintain the ability to produce NADPH and maintain a GSH response to oxidative stress. The Gd^{A-} variant has a half-life of only 13 days, so young cells have a normal amount of enzyme activity, but older RBCs are grossly deficient. Because of this heterogeneity in G6PD levels, individuals with the Gd^{A-} variant experience only limited hemolysis after oxidant exposure.

More than 100 mutations in the *G6PD* gene, localized to Xq28, have been described. Most mutations are amino acid substitutions that influence enzyme kinetics, stability, or both, with a few rare deletions and splicing mutations described. Because it is X-linked, G6PD deficiency primarily affects males. Males have only one G6PD allele and express only one G6PD type. Females can express one or two G6PD types. The Lyon hypothesis specifies that only one X chromosome is active in any given cell; thus, any given cell in a heterozygous female is either normal or deficient. In females who are heterozygous for G6PD deficiency, average G6PD activity may be normal or mildly, moderately, or severely reduced, depending on the degree of lyonization. G6PD-deficient erythrocytes in heterozygous females are susceptible to the same oxidant stress as G6PD-deficient cells in males, but, typically, the overall degree of hemolysis is less because there is a smaller population of vulnerable cells.

CLINICAL MANIFESTATIONS

G6PD deficiency is divided into five classes based on clinical severity and degree of enzyme deficiency. Class I is characterized by CNSHA without precipitating cause and severe G6PD deficiency. Class II is characterized by intermittent hemolysis and severe G6PD deficiency. Class III is characterized by hemolysis after oxidant stress and mild G6PD deficiency. Class II and III together represent more than 90% of G6PD variants. Classes IV and V are clinically asymptomatic. The most clinically significant syndromes of G6PD deficiency are acute hemolytic anemia (AHA); neonatal jaundice (NNJ); and rarely, CNSHA.

Acute hemolytic anemia is the most dramatic clinical presentation of G6PD deficiency with acute intravascular hemolysis after exposure to an oxidative stress.[15] Oxidative stresses include ingestion of certain drugs such as primaquine or sulfa-containing compounds, exposure to naphthalene (mothballs), ingestion of fava beans, or infection, the latter being the most common cause of hemolysis. Table 161-2 lists drugs that should be avoided in G6PD-deficient patients. Presenting symptoms include irritability, fever, nausea, abdominal pain, and diarrhea within 48 hours of oxidant exposure. Hemoglobinuria, jaundice, and anemia ensue. The spleen and liver may be enlarged and tender. Cases with severe anemia may precipitate congestive heart failure. Laboratory findings include a normochromic, normocytic anemia with anisocytosis and reticulocytosis. Poikilocytes and bite cells may be seen. Heinz bodies, a classic finding in G6PD deficiency, may be seen but are an inconsistent finding because these damaged cells are rapidly cleared from the circulation in the spleen. Additional laboratory findings may include hemoglobinuria and the presence of free Hb in the blood.

Another clinically significant syndrome of G6PD deficiency is NNJ. Jaundice is seldom present at birth, with the peak incidence of onset between days 2 and 3 of life. The severity of hyperbilirubinemia is variable. It may be severe, resulting in kernicterus or even death. In most cases, however, hyperbilirubinemia is adequately treated with phototherapy. In NNJ, it is important to note that the anemia is very rarely severe. The etiology of NNJ remains controversial. NNJ is increased in G6PD-deficient infants who also carry a polymorphism of the uridine diphosphoglucuronyl transferase (*UDPGT1*) gene associated with Gilbert syndrome.

Chronic nonspherocytic hemolytic anemia is associated with uncommon variants of G6PD deficiency, usually mutant enzymes unable to maintain basal NADPH production. Presentation may be in the neonatal period when NNJ is accompanied by anemia in a male. The degree of chronic anemia in CNSHA caused by G6PD deficiency has been variable. Some patients have compensated hemolysis, but others require intermittent transfusions. Transfusion dependence occurs in the most severe cases.

TABLE 161-2 AGENTS TO BE AVOIDED BY GLUCOSE-6-PHOSPHATE DEHYDROGENASE–DEFICIENT PATIENTS*

ANTIMALARIALS

Primaquine (people with the African A$^-$ variant may take it at reduced dosage, under surveillance)
Pamaquine
Chloroquine (may be used under surveillance when required for prophylaxis or treatment of malaria)

SULFONAMIDES AND SULFONES

Sulfanilamide
Sulfapyridine
Sulfadimidine
Sulfacetamide (Albucid)
Acetyl sulfisoxazole (Gantrisin)
Salicylazosulfapyridine (Salazopyrin)
Dapsone
Sulfoxone
Glucosulfone sodium (Promin)
Sulfamethoxazole-trimethoprim (Septrin)

OTHER ANTIBACTERIAL COMPOUNDS

Nitrofurans—nitrofurantoin, furazolidone, nitrofurazone
[Nalidixic acid]
Chloramphenicol
p-Aminosalicylic acid

ANALGESICS

Acetylsalicylic acid (aspirin): moderate doses can be used
Acetophenetidin (Phenacetin)
Safe alternative: Paracetamol

ANTHELMINTICS

β-Naphthol
Stibophen
Niridazole

MISCELLANEOUS

Vitamin K analogues (1 mg of menaphthone can be given to babies)
Naphthalene (moth balls)
Probenecid
Dimercaprol (BAL)
Methylene blue
Arsine†
Phenylhydrazine†
Acetylphenylhydrazine†
Toluidine blue
Mepacrine

*Drugs in bold print should be avoided by people with all forms of glucose-6-phosphate dehydrogenase (G6PD) deficiency. Drugs in normal print should be avoided, in addition, by G6PD-deficient people of Mediterranean, Middle Eastern, and Asian origin. Items in normal print and within square brackets apply only to people with the African A$^-$ variant.
†These drugs or chemicals may cause hemolysis in normal people if given in large doses. Many other drugs may produce hemolysis in certain individuals.

DIAGNOSIS

The G6PD reaction (glucose-6-phosphate + $NADP^+$ → 6-phosphogluconolactone + NADPH + H^+) reduces $NADP^+$ to NADPH. Formation of NADPH and NADH can be observed directly because they fluoresce in the visible spectrum when illuminated with long-wave ultraviolet light. Based on this observation, several simple screening tests performed using inexpensive long-wave ultraviolet light have been devised. These tests are semiquantitative, categorizing a sample as normal or deficient. They are unreliable after an acute hemolytic episode and do not typically detect female heterozygotes. Positive screening test results should be confirmed by spectrophotometric assay or DNA studies.

Definitive assay of the enzyme depends on direct spectrophotometric measurement of NADPH production. Although more sensitive than screening tests, this still requires 20% to 30% G6PD-deficient cells to obtain an abnormal result. Sensitivity can be increased by comparing the level of G6PD deficiency with levels of other age-dependent erythrocyte enzymes, especially when testing is temporally in close proximity to an acute hemolytic episode. The cyanide-ascorbate test measures the ability of erythrocytes to prevent the oxidation of Hb by ascorbate. Using intact erythrocytes, as few as 10% to 15% deficient cells can be detected, making this test useful for detecting female heterozygotes and males after a hemolytic episode. This test also detects other perturbations of the HMP shunt or glutathione metabolism.

TREATMENT Rx

The best treatment for an individual with AHA is careful prescription of medications and avoidance of inciting agents (see Table 161-2). Outside of acute hemolytic episodes, these patients do not require any special therapy. AHA episodes are managed with particular attention to hematologic, cardiopulmonary, and renal complications of hemolysis. Management of NNJ does not differ from that recommended for other causes of neonatal hyperbilirubinemia. In CNSHA, management is expectant. Exposure to oxidant stresses should be avoided. Blood transfusions may be necessary during acute hemolytic episodes. In severe cases of CNSHA, splenectomy may ameliorate the anemia.

Disorders of Glutathione Metabolism

Defects of glutathione metabolism may be associated with hemolysis. Erythrocytes from patients lacking glutathione synthetase or γ-glutamylcysteine synthetase, enzymes involved in glutathione synthesis, have very low levels of GSH. Clinically, these disorders resemble G6PD deficiency. There is mild to moderate chronic hemolytic anemia with increased susceptibility to oxidant stress.

GENERAL REFERENCES

For the General References and other additional features, please visit Expert Consult at https://expertconsult.inkling.com.

162

THE THALASSEMIAS

MARIA DOMENICA CAPPELLINI

DEFINITION

The thalassemias, or more comprehensively the thalassemia syndromes, are a heterogeneous group of inherited hemolytic anemias characterized by deficient or absent production of one of the globin chains of hemoglobin. This leads to imbalanced globin chain synthesis that is the hallmark of all the thalassemia syndromes.

EPIDEMIOLOGY

Taken together, the thalassemias are the most common single-gene disorder in the world population, with estimated carrier numbers of more than 270 million, and more than 300,000 children are born each year with one of the thalassemia syndromes or one of the structural hemoglobin variants. The extremely high frequency of the hemoglobin disorders compared with other monogenic diseases reflects natural selection mediated by the relative resistance of carriers against *Plasmodium falciparum* malaria. Other factors that may be involved include the widespread practice of consanguineous marriage, increased maternal age in the poorer countries, and gene drift and founder effects. For these reasons, the thalassemias are most frequent in southeastern and southern Asia, in the Middle East, in the Mediterranean countries, and in northern and central Africa. However, as the result of mass migrations of African populations from high-prevalence areas, thalassemias are now encountered worldwide.

PATHOBIOLOGY

Normal adult red cells contain 97% adult hemoglobin (HbA: $\alpha_2\beta_2$), with approximately 2.5% of the minor component HbA_2 ($\alpha_2\delta_2$) and a small amount of fetal hemoglobin (HbF: $\alpha_2\gamma_2$). Because the stable tetramer $\alpha_2\beta_2$ is the major component of hemoglobin after birth, there are two main forms of thalassemia: α-thalassemias and β-thalassemias. Because β-chain synthesis is fully activated only after birth, it follows that the β-thalassemias are not expressed as a disease in intrauterine life; they are manifested as γ-chain synthesis declines during the first year of life. In contrast, because α chains are shared by both fetal and adult hemoglobin, α-thalassemias are manifested in both fetal and adult life.

As knowledge about their genetic basis and pathophysiologic mechanisms has evolved, the thalassemia syndromes can now be classified at genetic and clinical levels (Table 162-1).[1]

TABLE 162-1 GENETIC AND CLINICAL CLASSIFICATIONS OF THE THALASSEMIAS

	GENETIC		CLINICAL
α-Thalassemias	α^0		α-Minor
	α^+		HbH disease
		Deletion (−α)	Hydrops fetalis
		Nondeletion (α^T)	
β-Thalassemias	β^0		β-Minor
	β^+		Thalassemia intermedia
		Variant with high HbA_2	Thalassemia major
		Normal HbA_2	
		Silent	
		Dominant	
		Unlinked to β-gene cluster	
δβ-Thalassemia	$(\delta\beta)^0$		δβ-Minor
	$(\delta\beta)^+$		Thalassemia intermedia
	$(^A\gamma\delta\beta)^0$		
HPFH	Deletion		Silent increase HbF
	Nondeletion		
	Unlinked to β-gene cluster		

HbA = adult hemoglobin; HbF = fetal hemoglobin; HbH = hemoglobin H; HPFH = hereditary persistence of fetal hemoglobin.

Genetics

Six different types of globin chains (α,β,γ,δ,ε,ζ) are found in normal human hemoglobin at different stages of development. In the very early embryo, hemoglobin synthesis is restricted to the yolk sac and the production of hemoglobins Gower 1 ($\zeta_2\varepsilon_2$), Gower 2 ($\alpha_2\varepsilon_2$), and Portland ($\zeta_2\gamma_2$). Subsequently, at about 8 weeks of gestation, the fetal liver takes over, synthesizing predominantly HbF ($\alpha_2\gamma_2$) and a small amount (<10%) of HbA. Between about 18 weeks and birth, the liver is progressively replaced by bone marrow as the major site of red cell production; this is accompanied in the later stages of gestation by a reciprocal switch in production of HbF and HbA, which continues until, by the end of the first year, HbF production has dropped to less than 2%. The globin genes are encoded in separate gene clusters. The α cluster (ζ,α_2,α_1) lies at the telomere of chromosome 16; the β cluster ($\varepsilon,{}^G\gamma$ and ${}^A\gamma,\delta,\beta$) lies at chromosome 11p15.5. In both clusters, the genes are aligned 5′ to 3′ in the order in which they are expressed during development. Both sets of genes are under the regulation of enhancer-like elements (hypersensitive site [HS]−40 for α cluster and locus control region for β cluster) that lie some distance away at the 5′ end of the cluster. Deletion of these enhancer elements results in inactivation of any related globin gene. There are two α genes/alleles ($\alpha_2$and α_1) that differ by a few nucleotides in intron 2 and the 3′ untranslated region but produce identical protein products. The output of the α_2 gene exceeds that of the α_1 gene by two- to three-fold. The α cluster also contains pseudo-ζ and pseudo-α genes that are not translated into protein products. The region around a DNase1 hypersensitive site at 40 kilobases (kb) upstream of the ζ-globin gene (HS-40) is the major regulator of α-globin gene expression. The β cluster contains a single pseudo-β gene; the βcluster enhancer consists of five elements marked by erythroid-specific DNase1 hypersensitive sites lying 6 to 20 kb upstream of the ε-globin gene, each of which contains several binding sites for erythroid-specific and other transcription factors. All together, these elements are known as the locus control region, and each element contributes to the overall locus control region activity. In addition, there is an erythroid-specific hypersensitive site approximately 20 kb downstream of the β-globin gene; when the cluster is activated, the upstream and downstream hypersensitive sites are brought into proximity with the gene promoters to activate their transcription.

The individual globin genes share many general features; they consist of three coding sequence exons separated by two introns in identical position but of variable length for a total length of approximately 1500 nucleotides. This structure has been highly conserved throughout evolution. The upstream regions flanking the first exon contain a number of sequence motifs that are necessary for specifying correct transcriptional initiation. A TATA box is found at 30 base pairs upstream of the initiation site together with one or more CCAAT sites at 70 base pairs upstream. The gene promoters also contain a CACCC or CCGCCC box that binds erythroid Krüppel-like factor (EKLF) 1, and some have binding sites for erythroid transcription factor GATA-1. In model systems, mutations introduced into such sequences lead to reduction in the level of transcription.[2]

All the thalassemias have a similar pattern of inheritance; in most cases, the gene defects are transmitted in a mendelian autosomal fashion. Thus, the severe, symptomatic varieties usually result from the interaction of more than one genetic determinant. The inheritance of α-thalassemia is more complicated because it involves the products of the linked pairs of α genes (αα) (see Clinical Manifestations).

Molecular Basis of Thalassemias

The α- and β-thalassemias are divided into disorders in which no chains are produced from the affected chromosomes (α^0 and β^0) and those in which the output of the chains is reduced (α^+ and β^+). For the α-thalassemias, the most common molecular defects are deletions of one or both α genes, which are designated −α and − −, respectively. The single α gene is believed to have arisen by crossover between two misaligned α genes on the homologous chromosome that can give rise to chromosomes with either single (−α) or triplicated (ααα) α-globin genes. Depending on the point of crossover, deletions may remove between 2.5 and 5.3 kb of sequence, with the loss of 3.7 ($-\alpha^{3.7}$) or 4.2 ($-\alpha^{4.2}$) kb being the most prevalent. Full duplication of the α-globin gene locus, including the upstream regulatory element, has also been reported in subjects of different ancestry, suggesting that this type of homologous genetic recombination occurs relatively frequently in globin loci. To date, more than 20 different deletions that involve both α genes, resulting from illegitimate or nonhomologous recombination, have been reported. The lengths of deletion vary from 5.2 to more than 40 kb; the most common are those from Southeast Asia, the Mediterranean, and the Philippines, designated $--^{SEA}$, $--^{MED}$, and $--^{FIL}$, respectively. Nondeletion types of α-thalassemia (α^{α}) are much less common than the deletion forms; in most cases, they result from single oligonucleotide mutations at regions of the α gene sequence that are critical for normal expression. Because expression of the α_2 gene is two to three times greater than that of the α_1 gene, it is not surprising that most of the nondeletion mutants predominantly affect expression of the α_2 gene. The mutations may affect the initiation codon or splicing signals, cause frame shifts, or introduce premature stop codons. At least five single-nucleotide variants affect the natural termination codon (TAA) of the α_2-globin gene. Among these, hemoglobin Constant Spring ($\alpha^{cs}\alpha$) is the most common and extensively studied. Finally, there are several α-globin variants that are so unstable that they undergo rapid, postsynthetic degradation. In such situations, β chains remain in excess within the red cell, and the patient carriers of these α-chain variants, by definition, have α-thalassemia. To date, 17 unstable α variants have been shown to produce the phenotype of α-thalassemia to a greater or lesser extent.[3]

Like the α-thalassemias, the β-thalassemias are classified as β^0 (in which no β-globin is produced) and β^+ (in which some β-globin is produced but less than normal). In some cases, the defects in β-chain production are so mild that they are designated β^{++}. So far, more than 200 different thalassemic mutations of the β-globin gene have been reported; most are point mutations within the gene or its immediate flanking sequence. A few β-thalassemia mutations that segregate independently of the β-globin gene cluster have been described, presumably involving *trans*-acting regulatory factors. The distribution of alleles is highly variable from one population to another, but within each population, there are only a few alleles that are common. The nondeletion forms of β-thalassemia account for most β-thalassemia alleles. An updated list of these mutations is accessible at the Globin Gene Server website (*http://globin.cse.psu.edu*). They include transcriptional mutations, RNA processing mutations, and mutations affecting translation.

Simple deletions of the β-globin gene are rare, ranging in size from 290 base pairs to more than 60 kb. The 619–base pair deletion at the 3′ end of the β gene is relatively common among Sind and Punjabi populations in India and Pakistan. The remaining deletions are restricted to single families, are necessarily β^0-thalassemias, and interestingly are associated with unusually high levels of HbA_2 in heterozygotes. Large deletions that affect the entire β-globin gene cluster $(\varepsilon\gamma\gamma\delta\beta)^0$are rare and restricted to single families. Finally, some highly unstable β-chain variants may be manifested as a dominant form of β-thalassemia.[4]

The δβ-thalassemias and hereditary persistence of fetal hemoglobin (HPFH) are the result of deletions affecting various parts of the β-globin locus. These deletions are partially compensated by an increased expression of the γ genes that raises the level of HbF. The length of deletion accounts for different forms of δβ-thalassemia, including both ${}^G\gamma$ and ${}^A\gamma$ genes or only ${}^A\gamma$, and varies from 9 to 100 kb. Hemoglobin Lepore is a hybrid of δ and β chains resulting from a crossover between the two misaligned genes; this hemoglobin is synthesized inefficiently and gives rise to a form of δβ-thalassemia. Deletions of δ and β genes are also the molecular basis for many forms of HPFH that, however, usually have higher levels of compensatory HbF production than the δβ-thalassemias. Other HPFHs are due to point mutations in the promoter region upstream from the transcription start site in either the ${}^G\gamma$ or ${}^A\gamma$ genes that alter the binding of one or more transcription factors; they are known as nondeletion HPFHs. Genetic studies have identified three major quantitative trait loci that account for 20 to 50% of the common variation in HbF levels in patients with β-thalassemia and sickle cell disease as well as in healthy adults.

CLINICAL MANIFESTATIONS

The clinical manifestations (phenotype expression) of thalassemia syndromes are extremely variable and depend on the degree of globin chain imbalance.

α-Thalassemias

As previously mentioned, there are two major classes of α-thalassemias: α^0, in which both α genes are inactivated (– –/); and α^+, in which only one of the pair is defective because of α gene deletion or mutation (–α or $\alpha\alpha^T$).[5] The clinical spectrum of α-thalassemias correlates well with the number of the affected α genes, that is, from normal to the loss of all four genes. The inheritance of a normal allele (αα) with one of the α^+ or α^0 alleles most frequently results in α-thalassemia minor (– –/αα; –α/αα; $-\alpha^T/\alpha\alpha$; $\alpha^T\alpha$ /–α;–α/–α). In general, carriers of such genotypes have lower levels of total hemoglobin, mean corpuscular volume, and mean cell hemoglobin but higher red blood cell count than normal. The greatest differences are seen in mean cell hemoglobin, which is usually less than 26 pg. The peripheral blood smear is variable, showing various degrees of hypochromia with some target cells and occasional poikilocytes (Chapter 157). In carriers of α^0-thalassemia (– –/αα), it is possible to generate a few red cell HbH inclusions (β_4). The carriers of nondeletional forms ($\alpha\alpha^T/\alpha\alpha$) show slightly more marked hematologic changes than those for deletional forms. The hemoglobin constitution of adult carriers of α^+- or α^0-thalassemia is indistinguishable from normal but has slightly lower levels of HbA_2. Traces of hemoglobin Bart (γ_4) in the neonatal period are detectable in a large proportion of neonates with α-thalassemia, and they decline during the first 6 months after birth. The α-thalassemias are common in areas where β-thalassemias are also found at a high frequency. Thus, the coinheritance of α- and β-thalassemia trait may occur and even ameliorate the hematologic parameters. In some cases, for genetic counseling in families in which α- and β-thalassemias are present, genotype determination is essential. The unstable mutant Hb^{CT} causes a severe reduction in α_2-globin expression from the affected chromosome; therefore, the carriers and particularly the homozygotes have a more severe phenotype than α-thalassemia minor but not as severe as most cases of HbH disease.

HbH disease most frequently results from the interaction of α^+- and α^0-thalassemia, and not surprisingly most patients originate from the populations of southeastern Asia, the Mediterranean, and the Middle East. HbH disease is a diagnosis attributed to subjects older than 6 months having a sufficient globin imbalance to produce detectable levels of HbH (>1 to 2%) in their peripheral blood together with inclusion bodies (β_4 tetramers) in their red cells. The clinical phenotypes encompass a wide spectrum from mild clinical manifestations to thalassemia intermedia and are included in the so-called non–transfusion-dependent thalassemias.[6] The predominant features of HbH disease are a hypochromic, microcytic anemia with jaundice and hepatosplenomegaly. Because the main mechanism of the anemia is hemolysis rather than dyserythropoiesis, only a few patients have clinical evidence of an expanded erythron. The most common complication of HbH disease is the development of hypersplenism due to severe splenomegaly. Other complications include gallstones, leg ulcers, increased risk of infection, folic acid deficiency, and increased risk of venous thrombosis mainly after splenectomy. Hemoglobin levels range in different series from 3 to 12 g/dL, with fluctuations that may occur after exposure to an oxidant drug, infection, or transient aplasia possibly due to intercurrent viral infection. Rarely, patients with HbH disease require regular blood transfusions. The anemia is associated with reticulocytosis and typical thalassemic changes of the red cell indices. The relative amount of HbH varies from 1 to 40%. The values of HbA_2 are always reduced. The peripheral blood film shows hypochromia with variable anisopoikilocytosis, target cells, and basophilic stippling. The characteristic feature of HbH disease is that it is always possible to generate multiple inclusions in the red cells after incubation with brilliant cresyl blue. The bone marrow shows marked erythroid hyperplasia.[7]

The most severe form of α-thalassemia is hydrops fetalis, in which all four α-globin genes are deleted (genotype – –/– –). It is incompatible with life. In fact, because α-globin chains are absent during gestation, hemoglobin Bart (γ_4) becomes the dominant hemoglobin. Because of its high oxygen affinity, hemoglobin Bart is unable to deliver oxygen to tissues, and the intrauterine consequences are progressive severe anemia, severe ineffective erythropoiesis with marked extramedullary erythropoiesis, massive organomegaly, heart failure, severe hypoalbuminemia, and edema. Infants with hydrops fetalis syndrome die either in utero (30 to 40 weeks of gestation) or soon after birth. The hemoglobin levels range from 3 to 20 g/dL; the peripheral blood film is characterized by marked anisopoikilocytosis, large hypochromic macrocytes, and many nucleated red cells. The hemoglobin consists almost entirely of hemoglobin Bart (80 to 90%), with some remaining HbH and Portland. Mothers of these infants often have a history of previous neonatal deaths. Without medical care, women carrying these fetuses may have delivery and postpartum complications (e.g., retained placenta, eclampsia, sepsis) (Chapter 239).

There are several reports describing α-thalassemia in association with mental retardation (so-called ATR-16 syndrome). These conditions are mainly due to large deletions (one or two megabases) of the tip of chromosome 16 including the α-globin gene cluster. However, several cases have no deletions or other apparent abnormalities of the α-globin gene cluster. It has been shown that these patients with a peculiar phenotype characterized by severe mental retardation, dysmorphic facies, genital abnormalities, and α-thalassemia have a disorder that maps to the X chromosome (ATR-X syndrome).

β–Thalassemias

The β-thalassemias include a considerably heterogeneous group of disorders of hemoglobin synthesis, all of which are characterized by a reduced output of the β chains of adult hemoglobin.[8] The clinical classification includes thalassemia major (TM, transfusion dependent), thalassemia intermedia (TI, of intermediate severity, non–transfusion dependent), and thalassemia minor (asymptomatic) (Fig. 162-1 and Table 162-1). The severity of the clinical manifestations correlates well with the degree of imbalance of globin chains; depending on the β-globin gene defects and their interaction, the production of β-globin chains is quantitatively reduced to different degrees, whereas the synthesis of α-globin continues as normal, resulting in accumulation of excess unmatched α-globin chains in the erythroid precursors. The free α-globin chains are not able to form stable tetramers; they therefore precipitate in the erythroid precursors, forming inclusion bodies that damage the red cell membrane, thereby causing premature destruction of erythroid precursors in the bone marrow (ineffective erythropoiesis). Ineffective erythropoiesis leads to a sequence of events responsible for bone marrow expansion, anemia, hemolysis, splenomegaly, and increased iron absorption. Any factor that reduces the degree of chain imbalance and the magnitude of α-chain excess, such as coinheritance of α-thalassemia or an innate ability to increase fetal hemoglobin, will ameliorate the clinical expression of the disease (Fig. 162-2).

The major forms of β-thalassemia (still sometimes called Cooley anemia) are disorders in which life can be sustained only by regular blood transfusions. This condition usually results from the homozygous state or from the compound heterozygous state for severe β-gene mutations ($β^0$). The typical forms of TM become manifested during the first year of life, during which γ chains are switched off but not replaced by β-chain synthesis. These infants, left untreated, are incapable of maintaining a hemoglobin level above 5 g/dL and show marked bone deformities and growth retardation. They develop the "thalassemic" facies due to frontal bossing of the skull and protrusion of the jaws and cheekbones. The magnitude of the increase in erythropoiesis may result in extramedullary masses arising usually from the sternum and ribs. Progressive hepatosplenomegaly is a constant finding leading to pancytopenia. The early childhood of the untreated or inadequately treated TM patients is interspersed with various complications including recurrent infections, spontaneous fractures, gallstones, and leg ulcers. The mortality rate in such patients was formerly high around puberty. Fortunately, this is no longer the case in children with well-treated TM. TM children well transfused to maintain a hemoglobin level above 9 g/dL have relatively normal growth and development, and their future course depends on whether they have received adequate iron chelation (see Treatment). Many children who are adequately transfused and are fully compliant with iron chelation therapy develop normally, enter puberty, and become sexually mature. At present, we are dealing with an adult population of TM patients who may suffer from the side effects of long-term treatment, namely, transfusion-associated infections (particularly hepatitis B and C and, in some populations, HIV infection) and organ damage (liver, heart, endocrine glands) due to unsatisfactory long-term iron chelation. The main causes of death in adult TM patients still remain cardiac complications, although liver cirrhosis is also increasing because of the prolongation of life.[9]

Heart failure in these patients is multifactorial, involving chronic anemia, remaining iron overload, myocarditis, pericarditis, and probably other

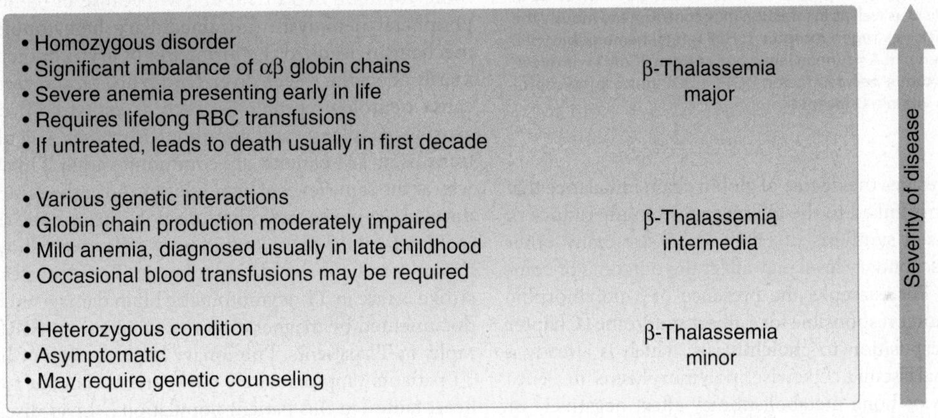

	Severity of disease
• Homozygous disorder • Significant imbalance of αβ globin chains • Severe anemia presenting early in life • Requires lifelong RBC transfusions • If untreated, leads to death usually in first decade	β-Thalassemia major
• Various genetic interactions • Globin chain production moderately impaired • Mild anemia, diagnosed usually in late childhood • Occasional blood transfusions may be required	β-Thalassemia intermedia
• Heterozygous condition • Asymptomatic • May require genetic counseling	β-Thalassemia minor

A

	Thalassemia major more likely	Thalassemia intermedia more likely
Clinical		
Presentation (years)	<2	>2
Hb levels (g/dL)	<7	7-10
Liver/spleen enlargement	Severe	Moderate to severe
Hematologic		
HbF (%)	>50	10-50 (may be up to 100%)
HbA_2 (%)	>3.5	<4-4.5
Genetic		
Parents	Both carriers of high HbA_2 β-thalassemia	One or both carriers: high HbF β-thalassemia, borderline HbA_2
Molecular		
Type of β-chain mutation	Severe	Mild/silent
Coinheritance of α-thalassemia	No/rare	Yes
Hereditary persistence of fetal hemoglobin	No	Yes
δβ-thalassemia	No	Yes
Gγ Xmnl polymorphism	No	Yes

B

FIGURE 162-1. **A, Clinical classification of β-thalassemias, from β-thalassemia minor to β-thalassemia major, according to the disease severity. β-Thalassemia minor subjects are asymptomatic, whereas at the severe extreme, β-thalassemia major patients are transfusion dependent. In between is a wide spectrum of clinical phenotypes labeled thalassemia intermedia because of different genetic interactions characterized by moderate to severe transfusion-independent anemia. B, Tentative criteria to differentiate thalassemia major from thalassemia intermedia at presentation. HbA = adult hemoglobin; HbF = fetal hemoglobin; RBC = red blood cell.**

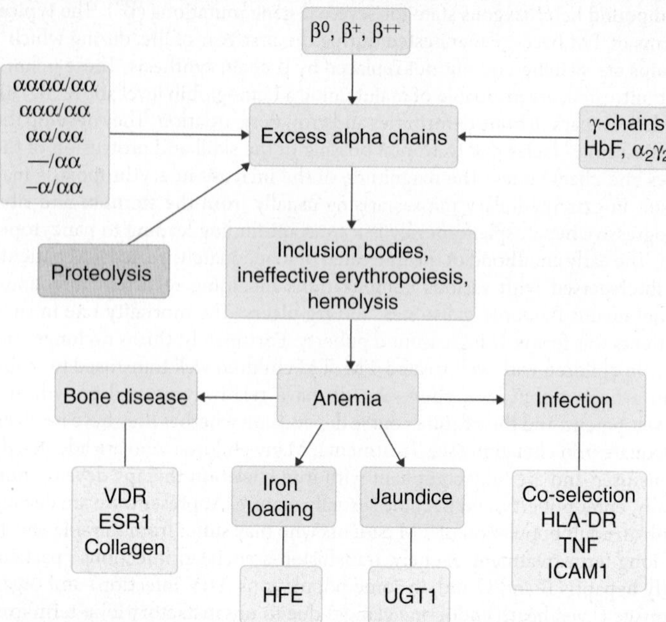

FIGURE 162-2. **Pathophysiology of β-thalassemias and modifiers of globin chain imbalance.** The severity of ineffective erythropoiesis is dependent on the degree of excess free α chains that result primarily from three different mechanisms: (1) inheritance of severe, mild, or silent β-chain mutations; (2) coinheritance of determinants associated with increased γ-chain production; and (3) coinheritance of α-thalassemia. A phenotype of thalassemia intermedia may result from the increased production of α-globin chains by a triplicated (ααα) or quadruplicated (αααα) α genotype associated with β heterozygosity. Inheritance of polymorphisms or mutations of genes involved in bone, iron, and bilirubin metabolism as well as in infection may contribute to modify the clinical course of the disease. ESR1 = estrogen receptor 1; HbF = fetal hemoglobin; HFE = hereditary hemochromatosis gene; HLA = human leukocyte antigen; ICAM1 = intercellular adhesion molecule 1; TNF = tumor necrosis factor; UGT1 = UDP-glucose:glycoprotein glucosyltransferase 1; VDR = vitamin D receptor.

mechanisms. Furthermore, besides the degree of globin chain imbalance that is dependent on genetic factors linked to the globin genes (coinheritance of α-thalassemia, innate increased synthesis of HbF), there are many other genetic modifiers that at the secondary level may affect the outcome of complications in different ways. For example, the presence of a polymorphic variant in the UGT1A1 promoter responsible for Gilbert syndrome (Chapter 147) may increase the predisposition to cholelithiasis, which is already a common complication in thalassemia. Likewise, polymorphisms in genes involved in iron homeostasis or bone metabolism may affect negatively or positively the degree of iron overload or the osteopenia and osteoporosis, respectively (see Fig. 162-2). Environmental factors, including social conditions, nutrition, and the availability of medical care, have also been implicated in the variable severity of TM clinical manifestations.

TI belongs to the non–transfusion-dependent group of thalassemia disorders; it is a clinical term used to describe patients with anemia and splenomegaly but without the full spectrum of clinical severity found in TM.[10] The clinical phenotypes of TI lie between those of thalassemia minor and major, encompassing a wide clinical spectrum. Mildly affected patients are almost completely asymptomatic until adult life, experiencing only mild anemia and spontaneously maintaining hemoglobin levels between 7 and 10 g/dL. Patients with more severe TI generally present between the ages of 2 and 6 years, and although they are able to survive without regular transfusion therapy, growth and development can be retarded. Most TI patients are homozygotes or compound heterozygotes for mild to moderate β-gene mutations ($\beta^+/\beta^+;\beta^0/\beta^+$); less commonly, only a single β-globin gene is affected. Because the clinical severity of the disease is dictated by the different extent of globin chain imbalance, at least three different mechanisms may promote the mild clinical characteristics of TI compared with TM: inheritance of mild or silent β-gene mutations; coinheritance of determinants associated with increased γ-chain production, which contributes to neutralizing the large proportion of unbound α chains; and coinheritance of α-thalassemia, which reduces the synthesis of α chains, thereby reducing the α/non-α chain imbalance.

Three main factors are responsible for the clinical sequelae in TI patients: rate of ineffective erythropoiesis, chronic anemia, and iron overload. The ineffective erythropoiesis primarily depends on the underlying molecular defects as already mentioned and is due to precipitation of free α chains in erythroid precursors in the bone marrow, causing membrane damage and premature cell death in the marrow. The degree of ineffective erythropoiesis is the primary determinant of the anemia of TI; peripheral hemolysis of mature, circulating red cells and an overall reduction in hemoglobin synthesis are secondary. Hemolysis and damaged red cells that expose negatively charged membrane phosphatidyl-serine residues have been linked to the development of the hypercoagulable state and increased risk of pulmonary hypertension in the TI patient population.[11]

Chronic anemia and chronic ineffective erythropoiesis lead to an inappropriate increase in gastrointestinal iron absorption, resulting in iron overload. In contrast, in TM, iron loading mainly results from transfusional iron infusion. It has been shown that chronic anemia and ineffective erythropoiesis, which are characteristic of TI, are associated with reduced expression of hepcidin, a hepatic peptide that plays a central role in iron homeostasis (Chapter 212). Moreover, the growth and differentiation factor 15 (GDF15) secreted by erythroid precursors and overexpressed in the presence of ineffective erythropoiesis may suppress hepcidin synthesis. More recently a molecule named erythroferrone, secreted by erythroblasts, has been identified and may also play a role in hepcidin regulation in TI. Taken together, ineffective erythropoiesis (leading to increased GDF15) and chronic anemia/hypoxia result in hepcidin suppression, increased dietary iron absorption from the gut, and increased release of recycled iron from the reticuloendothelial system, leading to an iron overload situation similar to that observed in patients with hereditary hemochromatosis syndromes (which are characterized by impaired hepcidin production)[12] (Chapter 212).

As a consequence of these pathophysiologic processes, several complications have been identified as unique in TI patients compared with TM patients, especially in splenectomized naïve patients. Cholelithiasis is much more common in TI than in TM because of ineffective erythropoiesis and peripheral hemolysis. Extramedullary hematopoiesis, as a compensatory mechanism, leads to the formation of erythropoietic tissue masses that primarily affect the spleen, liver, lymph nodes, and vertebrae. These masses may cause neurologic problems, such as spinal cord compression (sometimes causing paraplegia) and intrathoracic masses. Leg ulcers that are rare in well-transfused TM patients are common in adult TI patients; it remains unclear why at the same level of hemoglobin and at the same HbF level some patients develop leg ulcers and others do not. Thrombotic risk is definitely increased in TI patients. Several studies have collectively shown that the incidence of thromboembolic events is higher in TI splenectomized patients. Although stroke is rare in TI, asymptomatic brain damage including ischemia has been documented by magnetic resonance imaging (MRI) and computed tomography in TI patients. Pulmonary hypertension (Chapter 68) is prevalent in TI patients (approximately 60%) and is thought to be the primary cause of heart failure in this patient population.[13] Liver disease due to viral infection is less frequent than in TM; however, abnormal liver enzymes are frequently observed in TI patients, primarily because of hepatocyte damage resulting from iron overload. In some of the oldest patients with TI (>40 years), hepatocellular carcinoma (Chapter 196) due to long-term untreated iron accumulation has been detected with resultant cirrhosis in the liver as found in hereditary hemochromatosis (Chapter 212).[14]

Hypogonadism, hypothyroidism, and diabetes mellitus are rare. Although patients with TI generally experience puberty late, they have normal sexual development and are usually fertile. Women with TI may have spontaneous successful pregnancies, although complications during pregnancy may occur.[15]

Thalassemia minor is the heterozygous state of β-thalassemia. Subjects with thalassemia minor are "carriers" of a single β-globin gene defect, and they are usually asymptomatic except for a mild anemia of pregnancy. The carriers are usually identified as part of a family study, incidentally during an intercurrent illness, or as part of a population survey. The anemia is mild, microcytic and hypochromic, and associated with an elevated level of HbA_2. The blood smear shows characteristic microcytosis and hypochromia, with some variation in size and shape of the red cells. The presence of target cells is variable. The hematologic features are remarkably similar among different ethnic group. Carriers of β-thalassemia with normal HbA_2 have been observed in settings in which an individual with mild TI was found to have one parent with typical β-thalassemia minor with elevated HbA_2, whereas the other showed either minimal or no hematologic abnormalities and normal HbA_2. Subjects with normal HbA_2 are usually carriers of silent β^{++} mutations (β^{++}). Coincidental iron deficiency can lower elevated HbA_2 levels to the normal range.

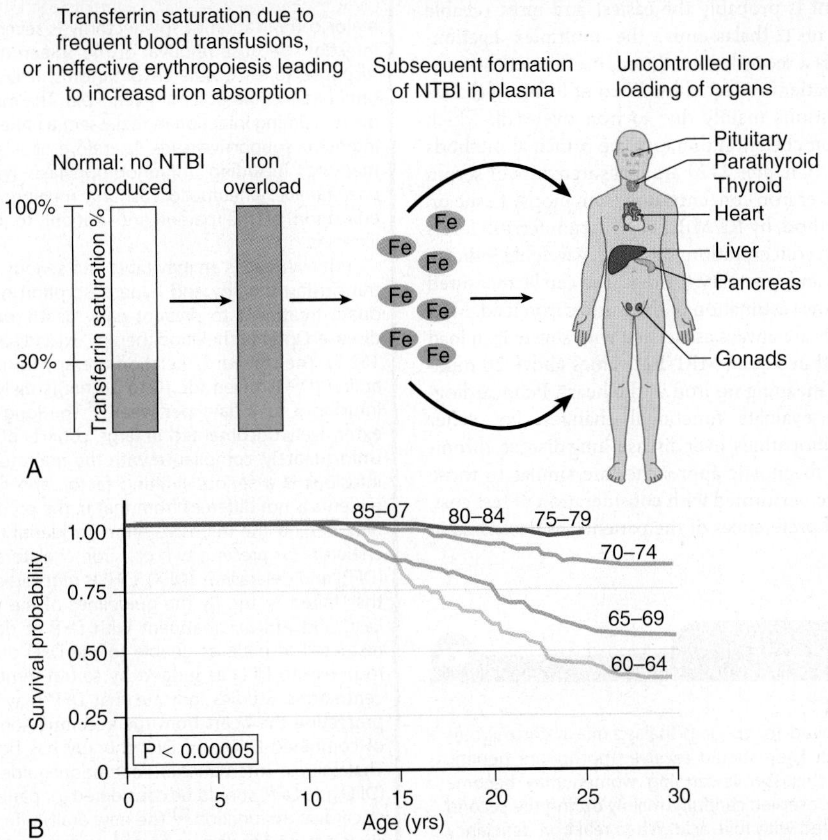

FIGURE 162-3. A, Transfusion iron overload and specific organ loading. B, Survival of Italian thalassemia major patients by cohort of birth. NTBI = non–transferrin-bound iron.

δβ-Thalassemia and Hereditary Persistence of Fetal Hemoglobin

The clinical manifestations of $(\delta\beta)^0$-thalassemias are similar to those of TI, whereas the heterozygotes are distinguished from β-thalassemia heterozygotes by normal levels of HbA_2 together with an increased HbF level of 5 to 20%. Homozygotes for Hb_{Lepore} may have phenotypes similar to either TM or TI. Subjects affected by deletion or nondeletion forms of HPFH are usually asymptomatic.

Any of the β-thalassemia defects may be coinherited with β-chain variants (HbS, HbC, HbE) and cause a clinically relevant β-thalassemia phenotype of different severity. These variants further illustrate that β-thalassemia syndromes have a wide clinical spectrum and that specific therapeutic approaches may completely change the clinical course and the natural history of these disorders (Fig 162-3).

Hemoglobin E and Hemoglobin E Thalassemias

Hemoglobin E (HbE) is caused by a substitution of glutamic acid by lysine at codon 26 of the β-globin gene. It is an common mutation, especially in the Indian subcontinent and Southeast Asia and among people who have emigrated from those regions. The frequency of HbE approaches 60% in many regions of Thailand, Laos, and Cambodia. HbE results in reduced synthesis of the β-E chain and therefore has the phenotype of a mild form of β-thalassemia. HbE trait has little clinical significance; it may be associated with slight microcytosis without anemia, but it could be mistaken for iron deficiency without appropriate laboratory testing. Homozygous HbEE individuals have mild anemia and microcytosis, occasional splenomegaly, and peripheral blood smears showing red cell changes similar to those seen in thalassemia traits, including target cells.

HbE interacts with different forms of α-thalassemia to produce a wide variety of clinical disorders. Its coinheritance with β-thalassemia, a condition called HbE/β-thalassemia, is the most common severe form of β-thalassemia in Asia and globally represents about 50% of the clinically severe β-thalassemias.[16]

DIAGNOSIS

The diagnosis of thalassemia may be required in a patient with an appropriate, suggestive clinical picture or for the identification of a heterozygote subject as part of a family study or population screening program. The general approach is common to any form of thalassemia, regardless of presentation. The primary evaluation is based on hematologic changes; the red cell indices by electronic cell counter and the red cell morphology examined on a well-stained blood film are sufficient to direct further investigations. Individuals with mean corpuscular volume below 80 fL and mean corpuscular hemoglobin below 27 pg with normal iron parameters need to be further investigated. The red blood cell number is usually higher than normal. In the presence of anemia with thalassemic red cell changes, the next step is the evaluation of hemoglobin fractions (HbA, HbA_2, HbF, or hemoglobin variants) by electrophoresis on cellulose acetate at alkaline pH or, even better, by high-performance liquid chromatography that enables the precise measurement of HbA_2, HbF, and HbA and the provisional identification of a large number of hemoglobin variants, including HbE. An HbA_2 level above 3.5% associated with hypochromic microcytic red cells is diagnostic of β-thalassemia minor. HbA_2 values between 3.2 and 3.5% (borderline) should be interpreted with care because they could be due to interaction of more than one thalassemic defect (α and β), a silent β mutation, or concomitant iron deficiency. If iron deficiency is present, it should be corrected and the HbA_2 estimation repeated. The majority of individuals with thalassemic red cell indices with normal or low HbA_2 and normal HbF will be α^0-thalassemia carriers or α^+-thalassemia homozygotes. Carriers of α^0-thalassemia may have a few red cells with HbH inclusions. Microcytosis with low or normal HbA_2 levels with elevated HbF (2 to 20%) indicates heterozygosity for δβ-thalassemia. Patients with HPFH usually have normal red blood cell indices but increased levels of HbF with different intercellular distribution (homogeneous or pancellular with the exception of heterocellular HPFH) compared with δβ-thalassemia (uneven or heterocellular).

A radioactive method for measuring the α/β-globin synthesis ratio was introduced in the mid to late 1960s, and it was largely directed at prenatal diagnosis in the pre-DNA era. Although it gives a quantitative assessment of globin production, today its use is limited to difficult cases because of interaction of different globin chain defects. The definitive diagnosis of the thalassemia syndromes involves the identification of the underlying mutations through DNA analysis. There are several methods available for the diagnosis of any particular mutation, such as polymerase chain reaction (PCR) restriction enzyme analysis, PCR allele-specific oligonucleotides, gap PCR, and direct sequencing that at present is probably the easiest and most reliable method. For deletion forms of α-thalassemia, the multiplex ligation-dependent probe amplification is a recently introduced, useful method.

During their clinical course, patients affected by different forms of thalassemia develop several complications mainly due to iron overload, which requires monitoring to direct iron chelation therapy. The principal methods of determining body iron levels (Chapter 212) are measurements of serum ferritin level and assessment of liver iron concentration from biopsy tissue or, as an alternative noninvasive method, by R2 MRI. High serum ferritin levels (>2500 μg/L) and high liver iron concentration (>15 g/dry weight) indicate high risk of significant morbidity and mortality. Cardiac iron can be measured by a T2* MRI procedure that allows estimation of the cardiac iron load. MRI T2* values below 10 milliseconds are always associated with severe iron load and high risk of heart failure within 1 year. MRI T2* values above 20 milliseconds are considered normal, meaning no iron in the heart. Echocardiography may also be useful to evaluate functional changes. For other complications, including endocrinopathies, liver disease, lung disease, thrombophilia, and bone disease, the diagnostic approaches are similar to those used in clinical practice; these are performed with consideration of test cost, performance characteristics, and preferences of the patients, as described in the corresponding chapters.

TREATMENT Rx

Conventional Treatment

No specific treatment is required for α- or β-thalassemia heterozygotes (carriers, thalassemia minor), but they should receive appropriate genetic counseling. During pregnancy, thalassemia-carrying women may become more anemic, so they should be observed carefully, mainly during the second and third trimesters, and supported with folic acid. When real iron deficiency is associated with thalassemia traits, iron supplementation should be provided, monitoring transferrin saturation and ferritin. A few cases of in utero blood transfusions have been reported with hemoglobin Bart hydrops fetalis syndrome; most of the infants have been delivered prematurely by cesarean section, subsequent development has been abnormal, and survivors required regular blood transfusions after birth. HbH patients in general have high hemoglobin levels (8 to 9 g/dL) and do not need regular blood transfusion. Supplementation with folic acid (2 to 5 mg/day) is generally recommended, especially in pediatric patients. The major complications in HbH disease are hemolytic crises that may occur during or after acute infections; in such cases, immediate intervention, including blood transfusions and treatment for infections, should be promptly administered.

The clinical management of TM and TI remains the major issue. The quality and duration of life of TM and TI patients have been transformed in this century, with life expectancy increasing well into the third and fourth decades. Nevertheless, prolongation of life is accompanied by several complications, partly due to the underlying disorder and partly as a consequence of the treatment with blood transfusions and iron overload. Moreover, we are starting to deal with aging-related complications in the context of a multiorgan disease that requires management by a team of clinicians who have specific knowledge of thalassemias in adults, working together with different specialists and well-trained nurses. The conventional treatment of TM patients includes regular transfusion therapy and iron chelation. The definition of the optimal transfusion and iron chelation regimen has been the most important advance in the management of TM patients, with the primary objective being to control the ineffective erythropoiesis, its consequences, and the body iron burden. The optimal transfusion regimen involves regular blood transfusions, usually administered every 2 to 5 weeks, to maintain the pretransfusion hemoglobin levels above 9 to 10.5 g/dL. The decision to initiate lifelong transfusion therapy should be based on a definitive diagnosis of severe thalassemia, taking into account the molecular defects, the severity of anemia on repeated measurement, the level of ineffective erythropoiesis, and the clinical criteria (such as failure to thrive or bone changes). It is advisable that TM patients receive leukoreduced packed red cells to minimize transfusion reactions and pathogen transmission. Adverse reactions to red blood cell transfusions may occur during or after transfusion and can be hemolytic and nonhemolytic. Transfusion-related acute lung injury is rare but severe and must be immediately managed (Chapter 177).

Many patients with TM require splenectomy because of hypersplenism. However, optimal clinical management may delay or even obviate the need for splenectomy that was common in the past. Splenectomy should be considered for patients whose annual blood consumption increases progressively and is responsible for significant increases in iron stores despite good chelation therapy or in the presence of symptoms due to spleen enlargement. Clinical problems related to leukopenia or thrombocytopenia due to hypersplenism could also be the reasons for considering splenectomy.[17] The major complication of splenectomy is severe and sometimes overwhelming infection. Because removal of the spleen may reduce the primary immune response to encapsulated organisms, it is advisable to delay splenectomy until patients are at least 5 years old. The mortality rate for postsplenectomy overwhelming infection in thalassemia patients is approximately 50% despite intensive supportive care. Therefore, it is mandatory to adopt preventive measures including immunoprophylaxis (vaccination against *Streptococcus pneumoniae*, pneumococcus, and meningococcus), chemoprophylaxis, and education of the parent and patient to recognize and to report febrile illnesses.

Iron overload is an inevitable and serious complication of long-term blood transfusion therapy and hyperabsorption of dietary iron that requires adequate treatment to prevent early death, mainly from iron-induced cardiac disease. Optimal chelation therapy extends complication-free survival (see Fig. 162-3). The standard chelation therapy for more than 40 years was deferoxamine (DFO), given for 10 to 24 hours daily as a continuous subcutaneous infusion 5 to 7 days per week.[A1] The long-term efficacy of DFO has been extensively documented in large cohorts of patients in Italy and elsewhere. Unfortunately, compliance with the rigorous regimen of daily subcutaneous infusions is a serious limiting factor, and life expectancy in noncompliant patients is not different from that in the pre-DFO era. This has been the rationale behind the intensive effort to identify alternative, orally effective iron chelators. At present, two oral iron chelators are on the market: deferiprone (DFP) and deferasirox (DFX). DFP is registered in Europe and more recently in the United States. By the guidelines of the EMEA countries (Europe, Middle East, and Africa), treatment with DFP at doses of 75 to 100 mg/kg/day is restricted to patients unable to use DFO or patients with an unsatisfactory response to DFO as judged by serum ferritin levels and by liver iron concentrations. Studies indicate that DFP may be more effective than DFO in protecting the heart from the accumulation of iron.[A2][A3] A potential benefit of combined DFO and DFP therapy has been observed, and according to Thalassemia International Federation guidelines, a combination treatment (DFO and DFP) should be considered for patients with high levels of heart iron or cardiac dysfunction.[A4] The new orally effective iron chelator DFX has been shown to be effective and safe in removing excess iron from different organs, including the heart.[A5] DFX is now available in most countries throughout the world as first-line treatment. Its use has clearly demonstrated that iron chelation is not a standard treatment, but it should be individualized according to age, history of compliance with previous chelation, and other factors. Monitoring and adjustment of iron chelation by repeated measurements of ferritin, calculation of iron intake by transfusions, and, whenever possible, measurement of cardiac and liver iron at least once by MRI are mandatory.

The management of TI patients is more complicated because of the wide heterogeneity of TI phenotypes. A number of options are currently adopted for treatment of TI patients, including transfusion therapy, splenectomy, modulation of HbF production, and hematopoietic stem cell transplantation (HSCT). However, increasing evidence is documenting the benefit of transfusion therapy in decreasing the incidence of complications. Thus, although the common practice has been to initiate transfusion when complications ensue, it may be worthwhile to start transfusion therapy earlier as a preventive approach, which will also help alleviate the increased risk of alloimmunization with delayed initiation of transfusion. The initiation of iron chelation therapy in patients with TI depends not only on the amount of excess iron but also on the rate of iron accumulation, the duration of exposure to excess iron, and various other factors in individual patients.[18]

Bone Marrow Transplantation and Experimental Therapies

Allogeneic HSCT (Chapter 178) in thalassemia syndromes has been increasingly successful during the last 2 decades, mainly in β-thalassemia major.[19] Predictors of poor transplant outcome are hepatomegaly, history of irregular chelation, and hepatic fibrosis. Patients are categorized into three risk classes. Class 1 patients have none of these adverse risk factors, class 2 patients have one or two adverse risk factors, and class 3 patients have all three. In the most recent update of the Pesaro group's experience, the probability of thalassemia-free survival for patients younger than 17 years at the time of HSCT receiving the allograft from an HLA-identical relative was 87% and 85%, respectively, in patients belonging to class 1 and class 2 and much lower in young patients in class 3. The progressive adjustment of conditioning regimens in class 3 patients and in adults (>17 years) has significantly reduced the incidence of transplant-related mortality in patients in class 3. Only 25 to 30% of patients with diseases potentially curable by HSCT have a suitable HLA-compatible sibling. Bone marrow transplantation from unrelated donors increases significantly the incidence of acute and chronic graft-versus-host disease, particularly in thalassemia. A study from the Eurocord cooperative group reported the outcome of 33 patients with thalassemia belonging to class 1 and class 2 (Pesaro classification) who received cord blood hematopoietic stem cells from an HLA-identical sibling; no patient died of transplant-related complications, suggesting that related cord blood HSCT is a safe procedure for thalassemia patients.[20]

An alternative treatment of β-thalassemia consists of the pharmacologic stimulation of HbF synthesis. In humans, hemoglobin switch from HbF to HbA occurs in the period around birth as a result of γ- to β-globin gene switching. A number of pharmacologic agents able to reactivate HbF synthesis have been identified, including hypomethylating agents, histone deacetylase inhibitors, and hydroxyurea. Whereas the effect of these pharmacologic treatments (particularly hydroxyurea) in sickle cell disease is clear (Chapter 163), their benefit on the clinical course of β-thalassemia is presently limited. The discrepancy between these two conditions in the response to HbF inducers may be mainly related to the higher level of HbF required in β-thalassemia to achieve clinical results compared with those observed in sickle cell disease. The limited clinical response to γ-globin inducers observed in the majority of β-thalassemic patients may be also a reflection of the unfavorable effects of these agents on the other globin genes (i.e., increased α-globin synthesis). A new molecule, sotatercept (ACE-011), an activin-type IIA receptor fusion protein, has recently been shown to increase the release of mature erythrocytes into the circulation by acting mainly on late-stage erythropoiesis. Clinical data in healthy volunteers have shown that treatment with sotatercept results in increased red blood cell parameters. A phase IIa, multicenter, open-label, dose-finding study to determine a safe and active dose level of sotatercept in adult patients with β-thalassemia intermedia is ongoing.

Gene therapy (Chapter 44) is an attractive approach for thalassemia syndromes; however, this strategy poses major challenges in terms of controlling transgene expression, which should be erythroid specific and sustained over time. Treatment of β-thalassemia, sickle cell disease, and other disorders through lentivirus-mediated gene transfer has been reported in murine and primate models, but until now few patients have been treated.

UNSTABLE HEMOGLOBINOPATHIES

More than 80 rare mutant hemoglobins have been reported to cause hemolytic anemia by either amino acid replacements or deletions that significantly lower solubility. These mutant hemoglobins form intracellular precipitates that can be detected as so-called Heinz bodies when the blood smear is exposed to a supravital stain. Structural abnormalities include mutations that weaken the linkage between heme and globin, disrupt secondary (α-helical) structure, or introduce a charged or polar side group into the hydrophobic interior of the globin subunit.

This disorder, sometimes called congenital Heinz body hemolytic anemia, is inherited in an autosomal dominant manner. Severely affected individuals have jaundice, splenomegaly, and, on occasion, dark brown urine due to the release of heme and aberrant conversion to dipyroles. The instability of a few of these globin mutants is so extreme that they cannot be detected by routine laboratory methods. This results in a thalassemia phenotype with microcytosis and ineffective erythropoiesis. Like individuals with glucose-6-phosphate dehydrogenase deficiency (Chapter 161), those with unstable hemoglobin mutants often lack clinical symptoms and signs of hemolysis until they develop an infection or are exposed to an oxidant drug.

The diagnosis can be established by a combination of a positive Heinz body preparation and either abnormal hemoglobin electrophoresis or demonstration of a precipitate after exposure of a hemolysate to heat or isopropanol. Some clinics have access to a reference laboratory that can identify the specific mutation by α- and β-globin DNA sequencing.

Most individuals with this disorder do not require treatment; some are symptomatic from severe anemia. Splenectomy generally results in a significant increase in red cell mass. However, the fraction of Heinz body–positive red cells increases markedly after splenectomy, and these patients are now at significant risk for development of pulmonary hypertension and cor pulmonale.

Grade A References

A1. Fisher SA, Brunskill SJ, Doree C, et al. Desferrioxamine mesylate for managing transfusional iron overload in people with transfusion-dependent thalassaemia. *Cochrane Database Syst Rev.* 2013;8:CD004450.

A2. Pennell DJ, Berdoukas V, Karagiorga M, et al. Randomized controlled trial of deferiprone or deferoxamine in beta-thalassemia major patients with asymptomatic myocardial siderosis. *Blood.* 2006;107:3738-3744.

A3. Fisher SA, Brunskill SJ, Doree C, et al. Oral deferiprone for iron chelation in people with thalassaemia. *Cochrane Database Syst Rev.* 2013;8:CD004839.

A4. Tanner MA, Galanello R, Dessi C, et al. A randomized placebo-controlled, double-blind trial of the effect of combined therapy with deferoxamine and deferiprone on myocardial iron in thalassemia major using cardiovascular magnetic resonance. *Circulation.* 2007;115:1876-1884.

A5. Taher AT, Porter J, Viprakasit V, et al. Deferasirox reduces iron overload significantly in nontransfusion-dependent thalassemia: 1-year results from a prospective, randomized, double-blind, placebo-controlled study. *Blood.* 2012;120:970-977.

GENERAL REFERENCES

For the General References and other additional features, please visit Expert Consult at https://expertconsult.inkling.com.

163

SICKLE CELL DISEASE AND OTHER HEMOGLOBINOPATHIES

MARTIN H. STEINBERG

SICKLE CELL DISEASE

DEFINITION

Sickle cell disease, caused by a mutation in the β-globin gene (*HBB*), consists of a group of chronic hemolytic anemias, all characterized by vaso-occlusive events, hemolytic anemia, vasculopathy, widespread acute and chronic organ damage, and premature mortality.

EPIDEMIOLOGY

The prevalences of the various forms of sickle cell disease and of the sickle cell trait (HbAS), which is not truly a form of sickle cell disease,[1] vary in the United States and worldwide (Table 163-1 and Fig. 163-1). The sickle hemoglobin mutation became prominent in equatorial Africa, the Middle East, and India several thousand years ago, when deforestation, the rise of agriculture, and stagnant pooling of water permitted *Plasmodium falciparum* infection to become endemic. Individuals with HbAS were more likely to survive to reproductive age and had a selective advantage where falciparum malaria was present. Slave trading and war spread this mutation from Africa and other sites of origin to the Americas, throughout the Mediterranean basin, and eastward to the Indian subcontinent. In some sites in Africa, half the population has HbAS. The partial protection provided from severe malaria by HbAS, HbC, HbE, α-thalassemia, and β-thalassemia along with other red blood cell traits is the source of the selective pressure maintaining the high prevalence of these carrier states.

PATHOBIOLOGY

Globin, the protein portion of hemoglobin, harbors the iron-containing porphyrin heme ring and permits the molecule to operate efficiently in oxygen transport and its other physiologic functions (Fig. 163-2). Mutations can alter the primary amino acid sequence of the globin polypeptide, sometimes resulting in clinically significant diseases called hemoglobinopathies, of which sickle cell disease is an example. Sickle hemoglobin (HbS: $\alpha_2\beta_2^S$) is caused by an adenine (A) to thymidine (T) substitution (GAG → GTG) in codon 6 of the β-globin gene (*HBB*), resulting in replacement of the normal glutamic acid residue by a valine (Glu6Val) (Fig. 163-3). HbS polymerizes when it is deoxygenated, a property only of hemoglobin variants that have the *HBB* Glu6Val substitution. Critical amounts of HbS polymer within sickle erythrocytes cause cellular injury and lead to the phenotype of sickle cell disease, which is recognized by hemolytic anemia and vaso-occlusion. Other hemoglobin variants, such as HbE and HbC, are also common. More than 1000 hemoglobin mutations are known, and they can occasionally affect the stability and function of hemoglobin and cause hemolytic anemia (Chapter 158), disordered oxygen transport Chapter 166), or methemoglobinemia (Chapter 158). However, most globin mutations are clinically insignificant. Thalassemias (Chapter 162) are also caused by mutations in globin genes, but these mutations affect globin gene expression, reducing or preventing the synthesis of globin, although the structure of any globin produced is usually normal.

Sickle cell anemia (homozygosity for HbS) is noteworthy for its clinical heterogeneity. Any patient can have almost all known disease complications; some have almost none but die suddenly; some skip one or more

TABLE 163-1 GENETIC AND LABORATORY FEATURES OF COMMON SICKLE HEMOGLOBINOPATHIES*

GENOTYPE	GENETICS	PREVALENCE AMONG AFRICAN AMERICANS†	HEMATOCRIT (%)	MCV (fL)	HbS (%)	HbA_2 (%)	HbF (%)	SEVERITY‡
Sickle cell anemia (HbSS)	Homozygous HbS	1:600	18-28	85-95	>85	2-3	2-15	4
HbSS-α-thalassemia	Homozygous HbS α^+-thalassemia	30% of HbSS patients	25-33	70-85	>85	4-6	2-15	4
HbSC disease (HbSC)	Compound heterozygous HbS, HbC	1:800	28-40	70-85	50	2-3	1-8	2
HbS-β^0-thalassemia (HbS-β^0-Thal)	Compound heterozygous HbS, β^0-thalassemia	1:1600	20-30	65-75	>85	4-6	5-15	4
HbS-β^+-thalassemia (HbS-β^+-Thal)	Compound heterozygous HbS, β^+-thalassemia	1:1600	30-40	60-70	70-95	4-6	2-10	1-3
HbSE disease (HbSE)	Compound heterozygous HbS, HbE	Rare§	30-45	70-80	60	2-3	1	1-2
HbS-HPFH	Compound heterozygous HbS and gene deletion HPFH	Rare	38-45	70-80	70	2	20-30	0
Sickle cell trait (HbAS)¶	Heterozygous HbS	1:12	38-50	80-90	35-40	2-3	<1	0
Normal (HbAA)	Homozygous HbA	—	38-50	80-90	0	2-3	<1	—

Hb = hemoglobin; HPFH = hereditary persistence of HbF; MCV = mean corpuscular volume.

*Many other abnormal globin genes can be found as compound heterozygotes with the HbS gene. The most common of these are α-thalassemia, HbD, HbO (Arabia), HbG (Philadelphia), HPFH, Hb Hope, and Hb Lepore. Average ranges of laboratory values are shown, but these can vary according to the patient's age.

†These figures differ by the prevalence of the involved genes in the population studied. In West and Central Africa, where the disease is most common, approximately 2% of all newborns have sickle cell disease. The prevalence of the HbC trait in African Americans is 3%, and that of the β-thalassemia trait is 1%. About 30% of African Americans carry an α-thalassemia gene, which can alter the phenotype of sickle cell disease by causing microcytosis, reduced cell density, and less hemolysis.

‡Severity of disease compared with sickle cell anemia, clinically the most severe genotype. This is a qualitative ranking of the clinical severity of each genotype; within each genotype, there is great clinical heterogeneity.

§Although this combination is still a rare genotype, the rising Asian population in the United States (HbE is a Southeastern Asian gene) will make it more frequent with time. With few cases reported compared with the other genotypes, the phenotype of HbSE disease is not totally defined. It may resemble HbS-β^+-thalassemia with symptoms appearing mainly in adults.

¶Sickle cell trait should not be classified as a form of sickle cell disease. About 8% of African Americans are carriers of HbS. Carriers are hematologically normal with a normal life expectancy. The few abnormalities traceable to the presence of HbS besides the renal lesions (see Table 163-3) include a four-fold increased risk of pulmonary embolism, an increased risk of splenic infarction at high altitude, and a higher risk of dying during the course of exertional heat illness.

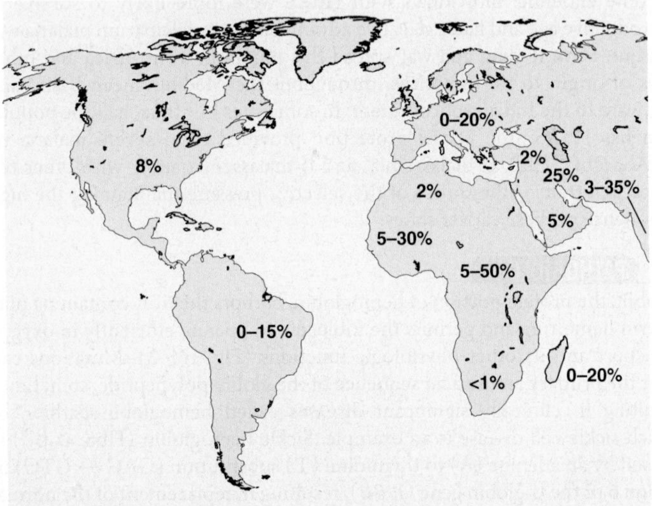

FIGURE 163-1. Worldwide prevalence of the sickle cell trait. Shown are the percentages of individuals with sickle cell trait in regions of the world where the hemoglobin S (HbS) gene is often present. In each geographic area, the prevalence of sickle cell trait can vary markedly according to racial or ethnic group, by historical migration patterns, and even from village to village. Not shown is the high concentration of the HbS gene in areas of Europe such as London, Manchester, and Paris, where migrants from Africa or Afro-Caribbean populations have settled.

complications of the disease but suffer intensely from others. Thus, this prototypical single-gene, mendelian disorder has exceptional phenotypic variability. Understanding of the pathobiology of the disease suggests many loci where the disease phenotype can be influenced by modifying genes. These genes affect the pathogenesis of sickle cell anemia by modulating fetal hemoglobin (HbF) concentration and mean corpuscular HbS concentration, and polymorphisms have also been noted in some genes that affect inflammation, oxidant injury, nitric oxide (NO) biology, vasoregulation, cell-cell interaction, blood coagulation, and hemostasis.[2]

HbF concentrations vary among patients with sickle cell anemia and among the erythrocytes of each individual.[3,4] Because HbF reduces HbS concentration and also directly inhibits HbS polymerization, its concentration within each cell and its distribution among all cells influence cellular heterogeneity. The sickle mutation is found on several different haplotypes of the β-globin gene cluster, reflecting different origins of the mutation in Africa and the Middle East; these haplotypes are associated with different HbF levels. The Senegal haplotype is associated with higher HbF levels than other African haplotypes are. The Arab-Indian haplotype, reflective of the HbS mutation that originates outside Africa, is associated with average HbF levels two to five times greater than in African haplotypes. Generally speaking, patients with higher HbF are more likely to have a less severe clinical course. Conversely, the Bantu haplotype, with lower HbF levels, may be associated with more disease complications. Nevertheless, there is great phenotypic heterogeneity within a particular haplotype group.

In sickle cell disease, erythrocytes are heterogeneous as a result of the highly variable cellular distribution and concentration of HbF and the varying increments of membrane damage. Cation homeostasis is impaired in some sickle cells.[5] A reduced capacity of sickle cells to maintain normal potassium gradients is mediated by activation of the Gardos, K^+/Cl^-, and other cotransport channels. As a result, sickle erythrocytes vary in their density and deformability. Irreversibly sickled cells (Fig. 163-4) always appear deformed because of permanent membrane damage, even though they may not contain HbS polymer. In some dense cells, the mean corpuscular hemoglobin concentration reaches 50 g/dL (normal, 27 to 38 g/dL), and deoxyHbS polymerization is exquisitely sensitive to the mean corpuscular hemoglobin concentration. Individuals with the highest numbers of irreversibly sickled cells and dense cells have the most hemolysis and anemia but not necessarily the highest incidence of acute vaso-occlusive events like painful episodes.

Hemolysis is mainly extravascular because of erythrophagocytosis by macrophages that recognize the damaged sickle erythrocyte. A variable amount of hemolysis is intravascular, and this liberates excessive amounts of hemoglobin into the circulation, thereby depleting haptoglobin and scavenging NO. This process promotes a vasoconstrictive, proinflammatory phenotype (Fig. 163-3). Certain complications of sickle disease, such as pulmonary

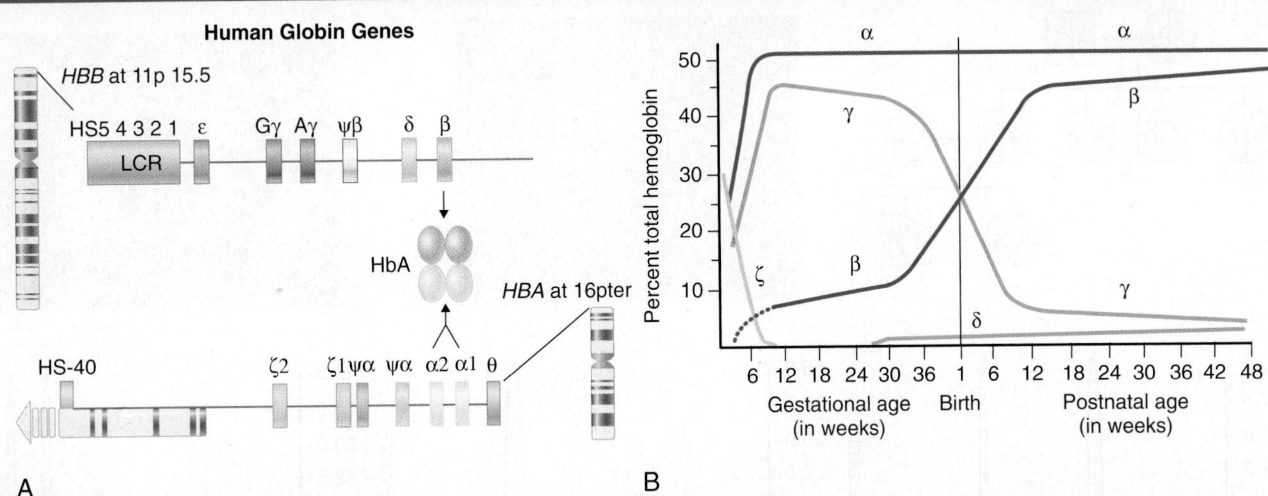

FIGURE 163-2. Human globin genes. A, The β-like globin gene cluster on chromosome 11 (*top*) and the α-like globin gene cluster (*bottom*) are shown. Two β-globin chains and two α-globin chains combine to form the normal hemoglobin A (HbA) tetramer, represented between the globin genes. Each globin chain contains one heme group, and oxygen transport takes place sequentially at the four iron-containing heme groups. Fetal hemoglobin (HbF) is composed of two α-globin and two γ-globin chains; the minor hemoglobin of adults, HbA_2, contains two α-globin and two δ-globin chains. Normally present at a level of only 2 to 3%, HbA_2 concentration is increased to 4 to 6% in most carriers of β-thalassemia. The ζ (*HBZ*) and ε (*HBE1*) genes are normally expressed only in the embryo. The 5′ ψα gene has been found to be expressed at a very low level and is now called the μ-globin gene (*HBM*). The θ-globin gene (*HBQ1*) is also expressed at low levels. Neither the θ nor the μ gene has been found in a functional hemoglobin. Any of the globin chains participating in hemoglobin formation may have a mutation altering its amino acid sequence. HbS, HbE, and HbC mutations affect the β-globin gene (*HBB*). Other mutations can affect the α-globin (*HBA1, HBA2*), γ-globin (*HBG1, HBG2*), and δ-globin (*HBD*) genes. LCR = locus control region. **B,** Expression of globin genes during development. The α chains are expressed throughout gestation and adult life, the fetal γ-globin chains are expressed predominantly in utero, and the β-globin and δ-globin genes are expressed mainly postnatally. This switching of gene expression patterns accounts for the different hemoglobins present in the embryo, fetus, and adult. It also accounts for the observation that disorders of α-globin can affect both fetus and adult, whereas β-globin chain diseases usually are not clinically apparent in the first months of life, when HbF levels are still high.

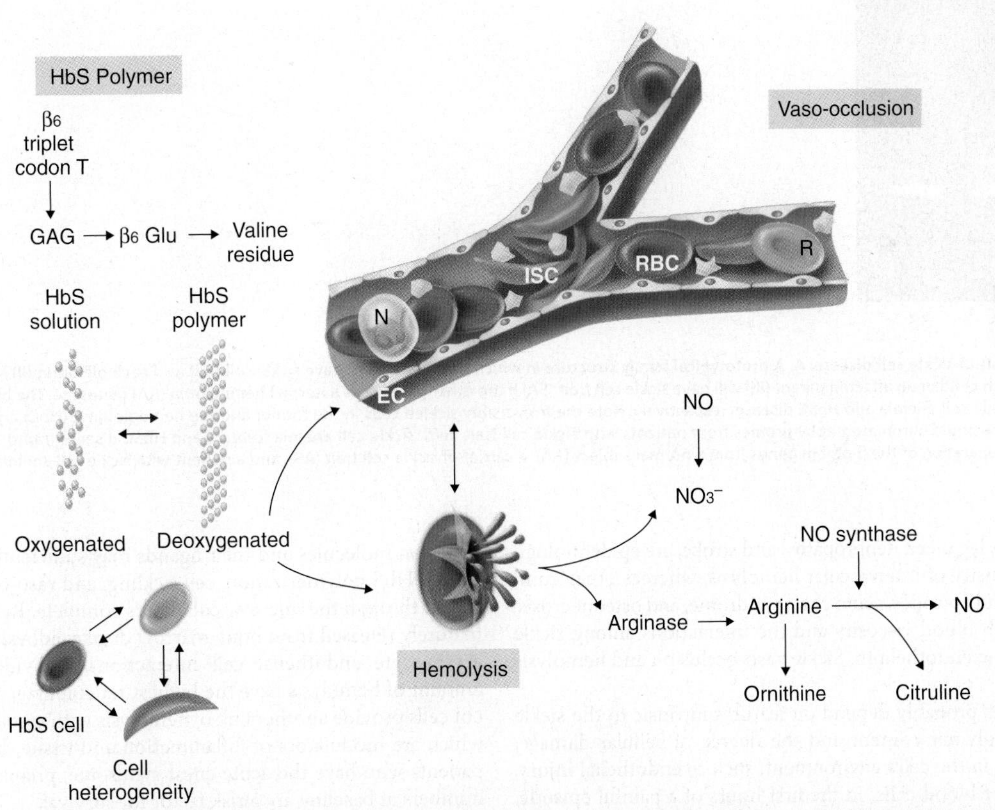

FIGURE 163-3. Pathophysiology of sickle cell disease. An adenine (A) to thymidine (T) transversion (A6T) at codon 6 in the β-hemoglobin gene on chromosome 11 (*HBB*) leads to the substitution of a glutamic acid codon by a valine codon. β^6 valine allows the hemoglobin S (HbS) molecule ($\alpha_2\beta_2^S$) to polymerize when it is deoxygenated. DeoxyHbS polymer injures the erythrocyte and leads to a heterogeneous population of sickle cells with damaged membrane cytoskeleton, reduced cation and water content, and altered distribution of membrane lipids. In the vasculature, sickle cells interact with endothelium and other blood cells to cause vaso-occlusion. Some damaged erythrocytes hemolyze intravascularly, thereby releasing heme into the plasma to scavenge nitric oxide (NO) and to reduce hemoglobin to methemoglobin and nitrate. NO, by binding soluble guanylate cyclase, converts cyclic guanosine triphosphate to guanosine monophosphate, thereby relaxing vascular smooth muscle and causing vasodilation. A state of reduced endothelial NO bioavailability in sickle cell disease impairs the homeostatic vascular functions of NO, such as inhibition of platelet activation and aggregation and transcriptional repression of genes transcribing cell adhesion molecules. Hemoglobin, heme, and heme iron catalyze the production of oxygen radicals and protein nitration, potentially further limiting NO bioavailability and activating endothelium. Lysed erythrocytes also liberate arginase, which destroys L-arginine, the substrate for NO production, providing another mechanism for endothelial NO deficiency. The normal balance of vasoconstriction versus vasodilation is therefore skewed toward vasoconstriction as well as endothelial activation and proliferation. EC = epithelial cell; ISC = irreversibly sickled cell; N = neutrophil; R = reticulocyte; RBC = red blood cell.

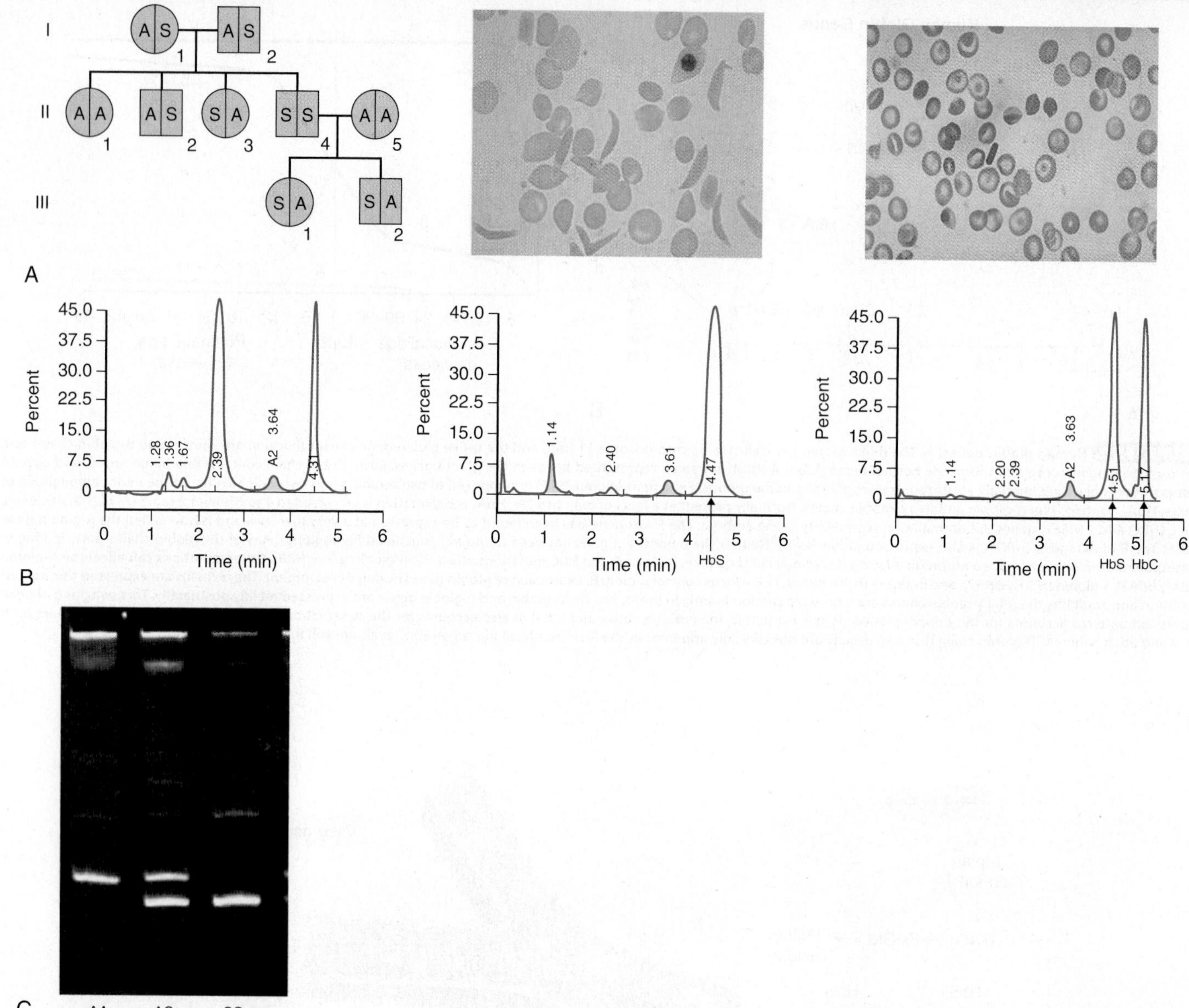

FIGURE 163-4. Diagnosis of sickle cell disease. A, A prototypical family structure in which both parents (I) have sickle cell trait and each offspring (II) has a 25% chance of having sickle cell anemia (SS). Each child of an affected parent (III) will have sickle cell trait (SA) if the other parent has a normal hemoglobin (AA) genotype. The blood films (*center and right*) are from patients with sickle cell anemia and HbSC disease, respectively. Note the irreversibly sickled cells in the former and the hemoglobin C (HbC) crystal and target cells in the latter. B, High-performance liquid chromatography profiles from patients with sickle cell trait (*left*), sickle cell anemia (*center*), and HbSC disease (*right*). C, Amplification refractory mutation system–based separation of the β-globin genes from a normal subject (AA), a carrier of sickle cell trait (AS), and a patient with sickle cell anemia (SS).

hypertension, priapism, leg ulcer, nephropathy, and stroke, are epidemiologically linked to the intensity of intravascular hemolysis, whereas other complications, such as painful episodes, acute chest syndrome, and osteonecrosis, are associated with high blood viscosity and the interactions among sickle cells, leukocytes, and the endothelium. Sickle vaso-occlusion and hemolysis are inextricably linked.

Vaso-occlusive events probably depend on features intrinsic to the sickle erythrocyte, such as polymer content and the degree of cellular damage, interacting with factors in the cell's environment, such as endothelial injury, vascular tone, and other blood cells. In the first hours of a painful episode, the number of dense erythrocytes falls; it rises again as pain resolves. These observations suggest the possibility that more deformable, more adherent cells might initiate vaso-occlusion, whereas dense cells become sequestered or destroyed in the microvasculature. Endothelial cells are responsive to many biologic modifiers that can be generated during sickle vaso-occlusive episodes and inflammation. Their activation and damage may be provoked by adherent sickle cells and shear stresses that cause release of oxidant radicals, expression of endothelin, and disturbed NO balance. Cellular damage enables adhesive interactions among sickle cells, endothelial cells, and leukocytes. Reperfusion injury can also induce endothelial activation and inflammation. The association of sickle and endothelial cells by a variety of adhesion molecules and their ligands may sufficiently delay cellular passage so that HbS polymerization, cell sickling, and vaso-occlusion happen before transit through the microvasculature is complete. Reticulocytes that are prematurely released from bone marrow display adhesive ligands that facilitate erythrocyte–endothelial cell interactions. Individuals with the greatest amount of hemolysis have the highest reticulocyte counts, and these adherent cells provide another link of hemolysis with vaso-occlusion. Neutrophils, which are modulators of inflammation and tissue damage, are increased in patients who have the acute chest syndrome, priapism, or stroke, and their numbers at baseline are a risk factor for survival.

CLINICAL MANIFESTATIONS

Sickle cell disease is a phenotype that results from different genotypes. Most patients have sickle cell anemia, HbSC disease, or HbS-β-thalassemia (see Table 163-1). Although the complications of disease are found in all genotypes, genotypes with higher cellular concentration of HbS are clinically more severe. Within milliseconds to seconds after HbS deoxygenation, depending on the intracellular concentration of HbS, HbS polymer appears in the sickle erythrocyte. In HbAS, each cell contains only 30 to 40% HbS, so polymer is not found under most conditions (see Fig. 163-4). Therefore, carriers have only subtle abnormalities and a normal life expectancy.

TABLE 163-2 FEATURES OF SICKLE CELL ANEMIA

Painful episodes: associated with higher hemoglobin and beneficially affected by high HbF
Acute chest syndrome: associated with higher hemoglobin and beneficially affected by high HbF
Stroke: associated with lower hemoglobin and little affected by HbF
Osteonecrosis: associated with higher hemoglobin and beneficially affected by high HbF
Priapism: associated with lower hemoglobin and little affected by HbF
Proliferative retinopathy: associated with higher hemoglobin and HbSC disease
Splenic infarction and sequestration more common in HbSC disease
Leg ulcers: associated with lower hemoglobin and beneficially affected by high HbF
Gallstones
Aplastic crisis due to B19 parvovirus
Osteopenia: bone marrow hyperplasia
Nutritional deficiencies: folic acid, zinc, calories
Pneumococcal disease and sepsis
Placental insufficiency

The features of sickle cell anemia change as life advances (Table 163-2). The switch from HbF to HbS underlies the clinical shift in life's first decade. This time is typified by acute problems: high risks of severe life-threatening infection, acute chest syndrome, splenic sequestration, and stroke. Chronic organ damage (renal failure, pulmonary hypertension, and late effects of previous cerebrovascular disease) becomes paramount in adults.

Most patients with sickle cell anemia have moderate anemia with a hematocrit between 25 and 30%. Some patients appear to have more severe hemolysis, with hematocrits less than 20%, marked reticulocytosis, and extreme elevation of serum lactate dehydrogenase. Patients with the most profound hemolysis appear more likely to have stroke, pulmonary hypertension, priapism, and leg ulcers (Fig. 163-5). Many patients with HbSC disease, especially adult men, have almost normal hematocrits and may have a higher incidence of sickle retinopathy, perhaps owing to their increased blood viscosity. Symptoms of anemia, such as weakness and dyspnea, are not the hallmarks of sickle cell disease, yet hemoglobin concentration can be a prognostic indicator for certain complications (see Table 163-2). A consequence of hemolysis is increased turnover of bile pigments, regulated in part by promoter polymorphisms in the uridine diphosphate glucuronosyltransferase 1A (*UGT1A*) gene, which is also associated with unconjugated hyperbilirubinemia and Gilbert syndrome (Chapter 147). As a result, more than half of all adults have cholelithiasis (Chapter 155). Hemolytic anemia places patients at risk for acute development of severe anemia when erythropoiesis is temporarily interrupted by parvovirus B19 infection (Chapter 371), which is the predominant cause of the aplastic crisis. Aplastic crisis is typified by a plummeting hematocrit, reticulocytopenia, and a bone marrow without erythroid precursors. It is a transient process, most common in children, and often requires blood transfusion to maintain circulatory competence until a spontaneous recovery follows. Rarely, if a patient's diet is inadequate, hemolysis-induced accelerated turnover of erythrocytes causes folic acid deficiency and megaloblastic anemia (Chapter 164).

Much of the epidemiologic data on the rate of complications in sickle cell disease discussed here antedates the widespread use of hydroxyurea in adults and its increasing use in very young children who have not yet developed complications of this disease. This, plus the use of chronic transfusions for prevention of stroke in many children, will change the phenotype of disease as these individuals advance to adulthood.

Ages 20 to 40 Years

Although any complication can occur at any age, certain events tend to predominate in different age groups. In the absence of hydroxyurea treatment or chronic transfusion, life's first decades are characterized by acute painful episodes, acute chest syndrome, and stroke. Delayed growth and sexual development, more severe in patients with sickle cell anemia than in those with HbSC disease, become major issues of concern to the adolescent, but sexual maturation is eventually achieved.

Psychosocial problems are common in adolescents with sickle cell disease. Difficulties with medical staff often begin in adolescence and frequently center on issues of pain management and inpatient stay.

The Painful Episode

Pain, presumed to be initiated by sickle vaso-occlusion, often starts in young children as the hand-foot syndrome or dactylitis: painful swelling of the hands and feet caused by inflammation of the metacarpal and metatarsal periosteum. Acute painful episodes are the most commonly encountered vaso-occlusive events in patients of all ages, but what triggers an acute painful episode is usually unknown. Commonly, painful episodes begin with little warning; some patients, however, may sense one in the offing. These episodes, which last hours to many days, can wax and wane in intensity and migrate from site to site. No useful laboratory test can tell whether a vaso-occlusive pain episode is occurring, and the history remains the best clue. Sickle cell pain is described as worse than postoperative or traumatic pain. Some women describe the pain of childbirth as paling in comparison with the pain experienced during painful episodes. These agonizing attacks of acute pain must be separated from chronic pain perhaps caused by osteoporosis of the spine, pain associated with osteonecrosis of the hips and shoulders, neuropathic pain, opioid-induced hyperalgesia, and the milder aches, pains, and soreness that are frequently present between severe episodes.

Almost all patients have acute painful episodes, but they vary greatly in number, severity, and frequency. Painful episodes are often stereotypical, affecting individuals in the same manner from episode to episode. Patients usually know whether the pain they are experiencing is different from their typical painful episode, and the wise physician should heed a patient's advice about the need for hospitalization or the likelihood that the pain has an alternative explanation.

In studies antedating the widespread use of hydroxyurea (see later), about 40% of patients did not have pain requiring a hospital visit in a given year, whereas 3% had more than six painful episodes per year. Having more than three pain episodes requiring hospitalization per year was associated with increased mortality among patients 20 years and older. Studies based on pain diaries suggest that pain is present on about half of all days and that most episodes are managed at home and not in a medical setting, so hospital visits underestimate the frequency of pain.

Most studies show that HbF levels are inversely related to the frequency of painful episodes. Concurrent α-thalassemia may increase the pain rate because it is associated with increased hematocrit. The day-to-day management of sickle cell disease often equates with the management of acute and chronic pain.

The pain accompanying acute chest syndrome, acute cholecystitis, splenic sequestration crisis, splenic infarction, or right upper quadrant syndrome may sometimes be mistaken for an uncomplicated pain episode. Acute painful episodes often precede the acute chest syndrome by 24 to 72 hours, and pain episodes occasionally end with multiorgan failure. Unexplained death can occur during acute painful episodes, perhaps as a result of an arrhythmia secondary to unrecognizable myocardial damage or perhaps as a sequela of pulmonary hypertension. Currently, it is not possible to foretell whether a "usual" pain episode will have an unexpected mortal outcome or presage acute chest syndrome, but the presence of atypically severe pain or an uncommonly high leukocyte count, low hematocrit, and thrombocytopenia should be cause for extra scrutiny.

Cerebrovascular Disease

A major complication of sickle cell anemia in early life is cerebrovascular disease that includes silent cerebral infarction and stroke caused by stenosis and occlusion of large vessels (Chapter 407).[6] Sickle erythrocytes and anemia-related high blood flow velocity lead to vascular damage. Hemorrhagic stroke in adults is a result of rupture of aneurysms or moyamoya disease, a proliferation of small vessels secondary to stenotic lesions (Chapter 407), and is associated with a mortality rate of more than 20%. Stroke is most common in HbS homozygotes, with much lower rates among those with HbSC disease or HbS-β^+-thalassemia. In the pre-hydroxyurea and pre-transcranial Doppler screening era, the incidence of stroke in sickle cell anemia was approximately 0.5 event per 100 patient-years until the age of 40 years, and the risk of having a first stroke was 11% by age 20 years, 15% by age 30 years, and 24% by age 45 years. These statistics have changed as a result of the use of transfusion to reduce the occurrence of stroke in children found to be at high risk by transcranial Doppler screening. Severe anemia, acute chest syndrome, and elevated systolic blood pressure are associated with ischemic strokes, whereas an elevated leukocyte count is a risk factor for hemorrhagic stroke. Concurrent α-thalassemia may protect patients with sickle cell anemia from stroke, perhaps because these patients have less hemolysis and a higher hematocrit. Subclinical neurologic events and silent cerebral infarction are even more common than stroke and are associated with decreased intellect and an increased likelihood of overt stroke. Neurologically

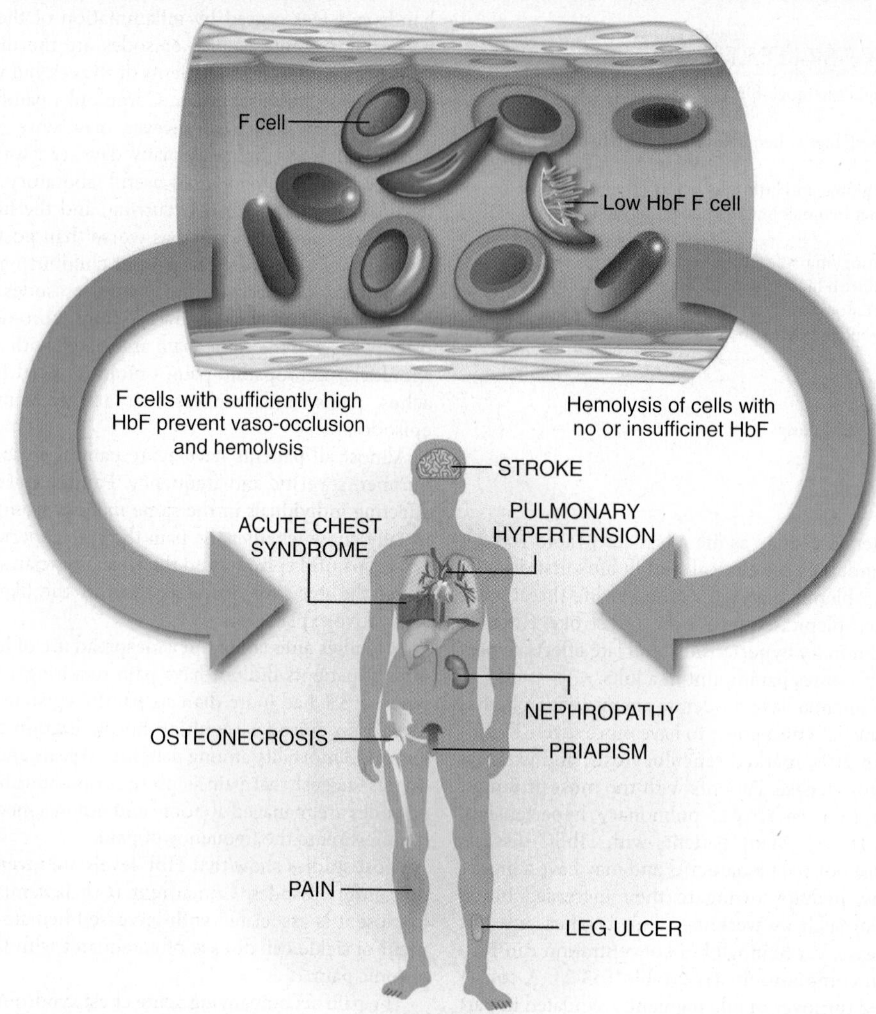

FIGURE 163-5. F cells and the subphenotypes of sickle cell anemia. The amount of HbF/F cell and the distribution of F cells vary among patients. In the example shown, some F cells have sufficiently high HbF concentration (bright red and magenta F cells), and their HbS will not polymerize or contains little polymer at physiologically relevant oxygen saturations. In some F cells (darker and brownish red), HbS polymerization will occur at venous oxygen saturations. Other cells with little or no HbF will have HbS polymers and sickle at high oxygen saturation; some of these cells will hemolyze intravascularly. Such cells, by releasing their hemoglobin intravascularly, can provoke certain subphenotypes of sickle cell disease. HbF = fetal hemoglobin.

intact adults without a stroke history have poorer cognitive performance than that of healthy controls.[7]

Acute Chest Syndrome

Acute chest syndrome, characterized by fever, chest pain, wheezing, cough, hypoxia, and a new lung infiltrate, is a sometimes lethal complication that affects more than half of all patients with sickle cell anemia.[8] It is the second most common reason for hospitalization and is a frequent cause of death in adults. The syndrome is more frequent in children, in whom its course is often mild, than in adults, in whom it tends to be more severe.

Commonly, acute chest syndrome develops after several days in individuals hospitalized for an acute painful episode (see earlier discussion). Acute chest syndrome also often occurs postoperatively, even when patients are properly prepared with blood transfusion. Other causes include rib infarction with atelectasis and regional hypoxia; fat emboli from the bone marrow (Chapter 98); infection with chlamydia, parvovirus B19, or other viral agents; microvascular or large-vessel in situ thrombosis; thromboembolic disease[9]; and vascular injury and inflammation. Fat embolism can be identified by finding lipid within pulmonary macrophages obtained by bronchopulmonary lavage, but this nonstandardized test is not recommended.

In most cases of acute chest syndrome, a cause cannot be found early enough to guide treatment.

Acute Anemia

Acute anemia can result from sequestration of blood in the spleen or liver; an aplastic crisis caused by parvovirus B19 infection (Chapter 371); or a severe vaso-occlusive event, such as acute chest syndrome or multiorgan failure. Transfusion may be needed. Megaloblastic arrest of erythropoiesis is uncommon if the diet is adequate in folic acid.

Infection

Because patients with sickle cell anemia are functionally asplenic early in life and hyposplenic later, they have increased susceptibility to infection with encapsulated bacteria. Persistent splenomegaly but not normal splenic function is common in patients with sickle cell disease in Africa, related to endemic malaria, and in Saudi Arabia, where half of the sickle cell disease population has α-thalassemia. Splenomegaly and splenic function often persist in patients with HbSC disease—hence the reduced incidence of infection but increased risk of splenic sequestration and infarction in adults. Prevention of mortality from pneumococcal infection is the basis for screening of newborns for sickle cell disease and the use of prophylactic oral penicillin in affected individuals. Pneumococcal vaccines (Chapter 18) are also recommended.

Pregnancy

There is no absolute contraindication to pregnancy for patients with sickle cell anemia, and fertility is probably normal. All approved methods of contraception can be used satisfactorily.

These are "high-risk" pregnancies, and close cooperation between the hematologist and obstetrician generally achieves good results; but the rates of pyelonephritis, pregnancy-induced hypertension (Chapter 239), and cesarean section are increased, and babies are more likely to have low birthweight. Limited data suggest that with good prenatal care, transfusions do not improve the outcome.

Osteonecrosis and Bone Diseases

Osteonecrosis of the hip and shoulder joints (Chapter 248) affects about half of all patients with sickle cell anemia or HbSC disease. Its onset is insidious but progressive, and most patients with early-stage disease progress to collapse of the femoral head within 2 years. Osteonecrosis of the hip usually is manifested with pain in and around the affected joint or at times with spasm of the surrounding muscles. Patients with higher hematocrits and with sickle cell anemia–α-thalassemia have the highest prevalence of osteonecrosis. Osteonecrosis can be detected very early by magnetic resonance imaging, but only more advanced disease is visible on plain radiographs.

Osteomyelitis (Chapter 272) is often difficult to distinguish from bone infarction. Osteomyelitis is usually caused by staphylococcal infection, but salmonella infection is a particular cause of sickle cell osteomyelitis.

Leg Ulcers

About 5 to 10% of patients with sickle cell anemia older than 10 years develop leg ulcers, but leg ulcers are rare in HbSC disease, in HbS-β^+-thalassemia, in Saudi Arabs with sickle cell disease, and in children before the age of 10 years. In the tropics, leg ulcers are more common. Small and superficial leg ulcers heal spontaneously with rest and careful local hygiene. Control of local inflammation and infection remains the mainstay of treatment. Dressing the ulcer with an Unna boot protects the involved area and is a reasonable method of conservative management. Deep, large, painful ulcers may require large doses of narcotic analgesics, prolonged bedrest, and even surgery.

Priapism

Priapism, a prolonged undesirable painful erection, may be seen in 40% of men with sickle cell anemia. Priapism in sickle cell anemia is usually bicorporal, with only the corpora cavernosa affected. Venous outflow is obstructed rather than arterial flow increased. In bicorporal priapism, the glans remains soft, and urination is normal. Recurrent, self-limited attacks of priapism can last for several hours with tolerable discomfort. These episodes have been termed stuttering priapism and usually have a nocturnal onset. Erectile function is usually preserved between attacks. Major episodes of priapism often but not always follow a history of stuttering attacks, last for days, and can be excruciatingly painful; they often end in impotency. Affected patients have a higher incidence of stroke, pulmonary hypertension, renal failure, leg ulcers, and premature death than individuals without priapism do, perhaps reflecting the severity of vasculopathy.

Digestive Diseases

Sickle hepatopathy, hepatic crisis, and right upper quadrant syndrome are terms applied to sickle cell–associated liver disease.[10] Liver disease may be related to intrahepatic and extrahepatic cholestasis, viral hepatitis (Chapter 148), cirrhosis, hypoxia, infarction, erythrocyte sequestration, iron overload (Chapter 212), or drug reactions (Chapter 150). Bilirubin levels can top 60 mg/dL, and such high levels are a poor prognostic sign portending liver failure. Differentiation among these potential causes can be difficult. Increased bilirubin levels (Chapter 147) are often a manifestation of hemolytic anemia and are related to polymorphisms of the UGT1A1 promoter.

Gallstones

Cholelithiasis (Chapter 155), a consequence of the accelerated bile pigment turnover typical of hemolytic anemia, can appear in the first decade of life, and more than half of all adults are affected. Depending on the degree of calcification, pigmented gallstones may be either radiopaque or radiolucent. Ultrasonography is the preferred means of detection, and laparoscopic cholecystectomy is the preferred method of dealing with symptomatic stones. Documented episodes of acute cholecystitis and typical obstructive jaundice are much less frequent than the presence of stones. If stones are asymptomatic or symptoms and laboratory findings suggesting cholecystitis are equivocal, careful observation may be the best course.

Beyond the Fifth Decade

Pulmonary Hypertension

Echocardiographic studies show that 30 to 43% of adults with sickle cell anemia have a tricuspid regurgitant jet velocity of more than 2.5 m/second (Chapter 55), and 5 to 10% of patients will have cardiac catheterization–documented pulmonary hypertension (Chapter 68). Both elevated tricuspid regurgitant jet velocity and true pulmonary hypertension are associated with a six- to ten-fold increased risk in mortality.[11] Increased tricuspid regurgitant jet velocity and the coexistence of relative systemic hypertension, renal disease, and intimal and smooth muscle proliferative changes in conduit vessels suggest the presence of a more widespread vasculopathy, which may be responsible for the observed mortality risk. Sickle cell anemia patients with pulmonary arterial hypertension have milder hemodynamics and symptoms compared with patients with idiopathic pulmonary arterial hypertension, particularly early in the course of disease, yet their survival is similar.

TABLE 163-3 RENAL ABNORMALITIES IN SICKLE CELL DISEASE*

Distal nephron
Impaired urine concentrating ability (hyposthenuria)
Impaired urine acidification—incomplete renal tubular acidosis
Impaired K^+ excretion
Hematuria
Papillary necrosis
Proximal tubule
Increased phosphate reabsorption
Increased β_2-microglobulin reabsorption
Increased uric acid secretion
Increased creatinine secretion
Hemodynamic changes
Increased glomerular filtration rate
Increased renal plasma flow
Decreased filtration fraction
Glomerular abnormalities
Proteinuria
Nephrotic syndrome with focal glomerular sclerosis
Chronic renal failure

*In carriers of sickle cell trait, because of its hypertonicity and oxygen content, HbS can polymerize in the renal medulla and lead to hyposthenuria, possibly an increased risk of urinary tract infection during pregnancy, papillary necrosis, and hematuria. A rare tumor, medullary carcinoma, arises from distal nephrons and is associated with sickle cell trait.

Nephropathy

Hyposthenuria is present in almost all patients with sickle cell anemia and even in most people with HbAS (Table 163-3). Clinically, the loss of urine concentrating ability is not important unless access to fluid is restricted. Isosthenuria, distal renal tubular acidosis, and impaired potassium excretion are signs of medullary dysfunction.

Glomerular hyperfiltration, increased creatinine secretion, and a very low serum creatinine concentration are characteristic of young patients with sickle cell anemia, so renal dysfunction can be present even with normal serum creatinine values. Glomerulopathy begins very early in life, but an increasing prevalence of renal failure is a hallmark of an aging population of sickle cell anemia patients. About 4% of patients with sickle cell anemia and 2% of those with HbSC develop renal failure, at median ages of 23 and 50 years, respectively. Among sickle cell anemia patients, 60% of those older than 40 years have proteinuria and 30% have renal insufficiency. Nephrotic syndrome is found in 40% of adults with creatinine levels above 1.5 mg/dL. Survival time for patients with sickle cell anemia after the diagnosis of sickle renal failure is 4 years, even with dialysis.

Eye Disease

Proliferative sickle retinopathy is present in less than 20% of patients with sickle cell anemia but in more than 40% of those with HbSC disease by the third decade of life. Vitreal hemorrhage and retinal detachment can occasionally lead to visual loss, but proliferative lesions may regress spontaneously. Screening for proliferative retinopathy by fluorescence angiography is recommended in patients with HbSC disease to guide possible laser photocoagulation.

Cardiovascular Complications

Cardiac complications of sickle cell disease are complex and can be manifested as both right and left ventricular systolic and diastolic dysfunction, elevated cardiac output, cardiomegaly, and myocardial ischemia. Progressive heart damage may result from iron overload in heavily transfused and poorly chelated patients, although this seems far less common than in β-thalassemia.

The heart is usually enlarged, with a hyperactive precordium and systolic ejection murmurs. Myocardial infarction is rare and when present suggests small-vessel disease.

Patients with sickle cell anemia usually have blood pressures that are in the normal range yet inappropriately high compared with controls who have similar levels of anemia. "Relative" hypertension in sickle cell anemia may reflect endothelial cell damage and increased NO scavenging by plasma hemoglobin. Survival is decreased, and the risk of stroke is increased as blood pressure rises. Treatment goals of 120/80 mm Hg or lower are generally the same as for other patients (Chapter 67).

DIAGNOSIS

Normocytic, microcytic, or macrocytic hemolytic anemia with reticulocytosis, increased levels of lactate dehydrogenase and aspartate aminotransferase, and a compatible clinical history should suggest the presence of sickle cell disease. Nevertheless, because of the multiple genotypes and considerable clinical heterogeneity of each genotype, milder cases may not be diagnosed for many years.

The Blood

In sickle cell anemia, the erythrocytes are normocytic or macrocytic, depending on the reticulocyte count. Microcytosis in a suspected case of sickle cell disease can be seen early in life, when iron deficiency has developed, or when β-thalassemia or α-thalassemia coexists with HbS. Sickled cells are usually present in the peripheral blood smear in sickle cell anemia and in HbS-β^0-thalassemia (see Fig. 163-4A) but are less common in other forms of sickle cell disease. In HbSC disease, target cells are prominent, and HbC crystallizes in some cells (see Fig. 163-4A). Irreversibly sickled cell numbers remain relatively constant over time, and their presence has no value for establishing whether a patient is experiencing a vaso-occlusive episode.

Hemoglobin Composition of the Blood

After 1 year of age, hemoglobin fractions are sufficiently stable to be relied on for diagnosis, but the high HbF concentrations of early infancy often make the results of hemoglobin analysis at that time difficult to interpret. In patients with sickle cell anemia, except in infancy, HbS almost always forms more than 80% of the hemolysate. HbS is best detected by high-performance liquid chromatography, which is also the method of choice for quantitation of the hemoglobin fractions in newborns and adults (see Fig. 163-4B). High-performance liquid chromatography provides excellent resolution of hemoglobin fractions, gives quantitative results, and is automated. HbF levels in adults average about 6% but can vary between 1 and 20%. DNA-based methods of detecting HbS are specific but usually are not needed for uncomplicated cases. Nevertheless, they are necessary for antenatal diagnosis and, sometimes, for genetic counseling (see Fig. 163-4C).

Family Studies

Hemoglobinopathies are inherited as codominant traits (see Fig. 163-2), implying that both normal and mutant alleles are expressed and are easily detectable. However, the sickle cell phenotype (see Table 163-1) is present only in homozygotes for HbS and in compound heterozygotes like HbSC disease. Family studies (see Fig. 163-4) can suggest a patient's hemoglobin genotype.

PREVENTION AND TREATMENT Rx

Primary Prevention

In populations with a high prevalence of the HbS gene, heterozygote detection is simple, but there is little proven benefit of a broad screening effort to detect carriers. A preferred approach consists of educational programs about sickle cell disease and HbAS, followed by counseling for couples who are planning families. These couples are offered the choice of testing, after which the risks of having affected fetuses can be discussed and the availability of antenatal diagnosis presented.

General Measures

Sickle cell disease is a chronic disorder for which good nutrition and timely immunizations are critical. Work should be encouraged.

Children beyond the age of 5 years do not routinely need continued antibiotic prophylaxis. Neonatal screening to detect newborns with sickle cell disease allows early administration of prophylactic penicillin and antipneumococcal immunization. These measures reduce the incidence of and mortality from pneumococcal bacteremia in children younger than 5 years who have sickle cell anemia.

Because of increased rates of red blood cell production and inadequate nutrition, folic acid, 1 mg daily, is generally recommended but may not be necessary with a good dietary intake. There is no evidence that high concentrations of inhaled oxygen are of preventive value.

The transition from pediatric to adult care is a time of heightened vulnerability, and this period should be managed jointly by pediatric and adult providers in a structured program.

Hydroxyurea

Hydroxyurea, the sole drug approved by the U.S. Food and Drug Administration for treatment of sickle cell anemia, increases HbF in most patients. In a multicenter trial in adults with sickle cell anemia, hydroxyurea reduced the incidence of pain and acute chest syndrome by almost 50%, with little risk during more than 17.5 years of observation.[A1] In follow-up studies, cumulative mortality was reduced almost 40%, and the favorable result was related to the ability of the drug to increase HbF and to reduce painful episodes and the acute chest syndrome.[A2] Children have a more robust HbF response to hydroxyurea than adults do, and a study in children with a mean age of 13 months showed clinical results similar to those of the adult multicenter trial, whereas hemoglobin concentration and HbF levels were higher than those of placebo-treated controls.[A3] Cancer and leukemia have been reported in adults with sickle cell disease treated with hydroxyurea, but whether the incidence is higher than in the general population is not known. Hydroxyurea should be used in nearly all adults and children with sickle cell anemia and HbS-β^0-thalassemia (Table 163-4).[12] However, not all patients who might benefit from this treatment receive it. A controlled clinical trial of hydroxyurea in HbSC disease has not been done.

Treatment of Common Complications

Painful Episodes

A decision as to whether hospitalization is needed can be made after an assessment of the duration and severity of the pain and the response to treatment. Associated factors, such as excessive tachycardia, hypotension, body temperature higher than 38.3°C (101°F), marked leukocytosis, fall in the hematocrit and platelet count, hypoxia, or new infiltrate on chest radiography, should prompt admission. On physical examination, there is sometimes localized swelling and pain over an involved bone. Low-grade fever and a mild increase in leukocytosis above baseline can accompany uncomplicated painful episodes, but higher temperature elevations may point to infection or extensive tissue damage.

The cornerstones of pain management (Chapter 30) are fluid replacement and opioid analgesics. Because almost every patient is hyposthenuric, urinary output in patients with sickle cell anemia may exceed 2 L/day, making them susceptible to dehydration. Pain is often accompanied by reduced fluid intake and increased water losses, so increased fluid intake is essential. Administration of 5% dextrose in water or 0.25 to 0.5 normal saline should be used for

TABLE 163-4 HYDROXYUREA TREATMENT IN SICKLE CELL ANEMIA*

BASELINE EVALUATION
Blood counts, RBC indices, HbF level, serum chemistries, pregnancy test, willingness to adhere to all recommendations for treatment, not receiving chronic RBC transfusions
INITIATION OF TREATMENT
Hydroxyurea 10-15 mg/kg/day or, for adults, 500 mg every morning for 6-8 wk
CONTINUATION OF TREATMENT
If counts are acceptable by CBC every 2 wk (granulocytes, ≥2000/mm³; platelets, ≥80,000/mm³), escalate dose in increments of 200 to 500 mg every 6-8 wk. When a stable nontoxic dose of hydroxyurea is reached, CBC may be done at 4- to 8-wk intervals. Most good responses require 1000 to 2000 mg/day, and a final dose of 30 mg/kg/day should be the maximum.
GOALS OF TREATMENT
Less pain, increase in HbF (usually measured every 6-8 wk) or MCV, increased hematocrit if severely anemic, acceptable toxicity Failure of HbF to increase may be due to biologic inability to respond to treatment or, more often, to poor compliance with treatment. If compliance is documented, the dose can be increased cautiously to 2000-2500 mg/day (maximum dose, 30 mg/kg).

CBC = complete blood count; HbF = fetal hemoglobin; MCV = mean corpuscular volume; RBC = red blood cell.

*Special caution should be exercised in patients with compromised renal or hepatic function and in those who are habituated to narcotics. Contraception should be practiced by both men and women. Without chronic RBC transfusions or an intercurrent illness suppressing erythropoiesis, a trial period of 6 to 12 months is probably adequate.

initial fluid replacement. Although needs vary, hydration and serum electrolyte values should be monitored closely to avoid iatrogenic heart failure or electrolyte imbalance. The daily fluid intake should be approximately 3 to 5 L for adults and 100 to 150 mL/kg for children. Oxygen should be reserved for patients who are hypoxic or have acute respiratory distress. Infection should always be considered and treated early if it is present. Treatment with intravenous magnesium sulfate in addition to standard therapy for vaso-occlusive episodes in children aged 4 to 18 years has been found to have no effect on hospital length of stay, pain scores, or cumulative analgesia.[A4]

Analgesic management presupposes that other treatments, such as hydration, oxygen, and antimicrobial agents, are used if needed. The key to successful pain management is individualized treatment and dosing, taking into account prior pain management and prior use of opioids. Patient-controlled analgesia and a scheduled regimen of drug dosing are preferable, and analgesics on an as-needed basis should be avoided. Frequent reassessment of the effects of treatment is paramount so that opioid doses can be titrated for pain relief and tapered when relief is obtained. Morphine and hydromorphone are the principal opioids used; meperidine should be avoided because its metabolites (e.g., normeperidine) can cause central nervous system excitation. Pain management (Chapter 30) is complicated by the influence of learned pain behavior, pain memories, and pain therapy–induced pain. Management proves extremely difficult in perhaps 10% of all patients, and enormous doses of opioids are often required for relief. High opioid doses are associated with allodynia (pain produced by a non-noxious stimulus to the skin), opioid-induced hyperalgesia, and neuropathic pain.

Stroke

For new strokes due to cerebral infarction, after initial stabilization and transfusion, chronic red blood cell transfusion reduces the chance of recurrence. Long-term management of hemorrhagic stroke is unclear, and whether transfusion reduces its recurrence is unknown. Increased intracranial flow velocity, measurable by transcranial Doppler flow measurement only in children, increases the risk of stroke, but its sensitivity is only 10%, with a far from perfect specificity. Children found to be at risk for stroke by transcranial Doppler flow velocities should be started on chronic transfusions, but it is unclear whether or when such transfusions may be discontinued.

Acute Chest Syndrome

Routine treatments for acute chest syndrome initially include bronchodilators (e.g., albuterol nebulizer, 0.25 mL in 2.5 mL normal saline, or albuterol metered-dose inhaler during the acute episode), incentive spirometry, empirical antimicrobial agents in febrile patients as used for community-acquired pneumonia (e.g., ceftriaxone or azithromycin or levofloxacin for 5 to 7 days [Chapter 97]), and supplemental oxygen when hypoxia is noted by continuous or frequent monitoring of blood oxygen saturation. Opioids are often needed, but their dose should be titrated carefully to avoid respiratory depression and worsening of hypoxia.

Blood transfusion is the cornerstone of treatment when a patient becomes hypoxic, develops respiratory distress, has a clinically significant fall in the hematocrit and platelet count or increase in leukocyte count, or shows any sign of multiorgan failure, such as impaired mentation, rhabdomyolysis, renal failure, or liver failure. Both simple transfusion and exchange transfusions appear to reverse many adverse findings of the acute chest syndrome, but controlled studies have never tested the superiority of either method. Although the death rate in acute chest syndrome is less than 10%, a few patients have a rapidly deteriorating course with sudden development of the acute respiratory distress syndrome (Chapter 104), as manifested by increased oxygen requirements, extensive pulmonary opacification, and multiorgan failure. Excessive hydration, fat emboli, and widespread vaso-occlusion are potential contributing causes. Successful management of severe acute chest syndrome and acute respiratory distress syndrome requires close coordination among physicians and nurses. Some patients have repeated episodes of severe acute chest syndrome, and chronic transfusion can reduce the recurrence rate. Hydroxyurea also reduces the rate of acute chest syndrome by about 50%.

Osteonecrosis and Bone Disease

Treatment with reduced weight bearing, nonsteroidal anti-inflammatory drugs, and physical therapy is the mainstay of conservative management but does not retard progression of osteonecrosis and bone disease. Total hip arthroplasty can be successful, but about one third of prostheses fail within 4 to 5 years.

Diffuse osteoporosis (Chapter 243) is usually present, and osteomalacia (Chapter 244) due to vitamin D deficiency is common in both children and adults. If vitamin D deficiency is present, treatment with calcium (1000 mg PO daily) and vitamin D (50,000 IU PO every week for 2 months, then 50,000 IU PO every other week) is reasonable.

Priapism

Conservative treatment of priapism includes analgesics and hydration. No evidence supports the use of transfusion. Aspiration and irrigation of the corporeal bodies should be performed if more than 4 hours have elapsed from the onset of erection if the episode differs from prior episodes of stuttering priapism. Operative treatment, which should be considered after 24 to 48 hours of priapism, includes the creation of shunts between the corpora cavernosa and corpus spongiosum. Oral α-adrenergic agonists, such as etilefrine and pseudoephedrine, and phosphodiesterase-5 inhibitors, like sildenafil and tadalafil, have been used successfully to prevent severe acute attacks but are not useful for treating acute major priapism once it has occurred.[13]

Pulmonary Hypertension

Pulmonary arterial hypertension can be determined definitively only by right-sided heart catheterization, although echocardiography or measurement of blood N-terminal pro-brain natriuretic peptide levels can suggest its existence. As these patients are often asymptomatic early in the course of their disease, a consensus group convened by the American Thoracic Society recommended echocardiography for risk stratification in sickle cell disease adults every 1 to 3 years.[14]

Management of patients with few symptoms and minimally elevated tricuspid regurgitant jet velocity is not informed by clinical trials. For symptomatic individuals, optimization of hydroxyurea, transfusions, anticoagulation, bosentan, and epoprostenol have all been used. A controlled trial of sildenafil based on tricuspid regurgitant jet velocity and low exercise capacity was stopped early because of increased hospitalization for pain[A5] (Table 163-5).

Renal Disease

In a small randomized trial, 6 months' treatment with 25 mg/day of captopril caused a 37% reduction in microalbuminuria, compared with a 17% increase in placebo-treated patients; such treatment would be reasonable in patients with known microalbuminuria, but whether screening for this or long-term treatment is worthwhile is unknown.[A6] Nonsteroidal anti-inflammatory drugs reduce the glomerular filtration rate in sickle cell anemia and should be avoided in older individuals with creatinine levels of 1.2 mg/dL or higher. Dialysis and renal transplantation are used in end-stage sickle cell nephropathy, but with outcomes less favorable than in other types of renal failure.

Surgery and Anesthesia

Blood transfusion should be given before all surgeries requiring general anesthesia and selected other surgeries. Simple transfusion to a hematocrit of about 30% before surgery is as effective as exchange transfusion in preventing postoperative complications and causes fewer transfusion-related complications.[A7] In some low-risk surgeries, preoperative transfusion might not be necessary.

Implantable infusion ports and catheters have higher risks of complications in sickle cell anemia, including thrombosis of large veins and bacteremia. Low-dose warfarin may retard thrombosis of these devices.

Red Blood Cell Transfusion and Iron Chelation Therapy

Acute transfusions of packed red blood cells can be life-saving, and chronic transfusions reduce the incidence of stroke[A8] and severity of most complications of sickle cell disease. However, repeated transfusions produce iron overload, alloimmunization, loss of venous access, and viral infection. Whether exchange transfusion is preferable to simple transfusion in the acute chest syndrome or other acute complications has not been tested in clinical trials. For severe symptomatic anemia and stroke prophylaxis, simple transfusions are preferred. The customary level of chronic stable anemia alone is seldom

TABLE 163-5 PULMONARY COMPLICATIONS OF SICKLE CELL DISEASE

ACUTE CHEST SYNDROME
Diagnosis: chest pain, fever, cough, wheezing, new infiltrate on chest radiograph, hypoxemia
Management: simple or exchange transfusions, pain relief, oxygen if hypoxemic, bronchodilators, incentive spirometry, antibiotics (broad coverage)
PULMONARY HYPERTENSION
Screening evaluation: echocardiography with tricuspid regurgitant jet velocity ≥ 2.5 m/sec; elevated N-terminal pro-brain natriuretic peptide (≥160 pg/mL); reduced 6-minute walk distance (≤350 m)
Definitive diagnosis: screen by echocardiography beginning at age 18 yr; repeat echocardiography periodically according to symptoms or every 1 to 3 years. If tricuspid regurgitant jet velocity > 3.0 m/sec, refer for right-sided heart catheterization that provides a definitive diagnosis.
Management: Consider anticoagulation, treatment of iron overload and nocturnal hypoxemia. Optimize hydroxyurea, consider chronic transfusions and pulmonary vasodilator therapy.
ASTHMA
ABNORMAL PULMONARY FUNCTION

an indication for transfusion. With aging and the onset of renal failure, anemia worsens and can become symptomatic. Transfusion may become necessary, although judicious use of erythropoietin (e.g., darbepoetin, 0.45 μg/kg every 2 weeks, increased as needed) can often restore the hematocrit to prerenal failure levels only and should not be targeted at even higher levels because of the potential adverse effects of hyperviscosity.

It is advised that patients undergo erythrocyte phenotyping to determine their red blood cell antigens before embarking on a chronic transfusion program. Otherwise, alloimmunization occurs in about one fourth of frequently transfused patients. In the presence of multiple alloantibodies, it may be difficult to find compatible blood.[15]

With repeated transfusion, iron overload inevitably develops and can result in heart and liver failure and many other complications (Chapter 212). Serum ferritin is an inaccurate means of estimating tissue iron burden. For deciding when to begin iron chelation and for observing the effects of chelation, magnetic resonance imaging is now the standard, leaving little indication for liver biopsy to measure iron concentration.

Chelation of excessive iron can be achieved with deferasirox (20 mg/kg orally daily).[A9] Increases in serum creatinine concentration and proteinuria occur in about 40% of patients. Desferrioxamine is a parenteral chelator and is usually started at a dose of 25 to 30 mg/kg given subcutaneously five times per week as 8- to 12-hour continuous infusions (Chapter 212). Side effects include gastrointestinal and skin reactions, ototoxicity, retinal toxicity, bone and growth abnormalities, and *Yersinia* infection resulting from the sudden mobilization of iron. Another oral chelator, deferiprone, is less potent than deferasirox or desferrioxamine but is especially useful when magnetic resonance imaging shows high levels of cardiac iron. Side effects requiring discontinuation of deferiprone, seen in 5 to 10% of patients, include agranulocytosis, neutropenia, arthropathy, and gastrointestinal symptoms.[16]

Stem Cell Transplantation

Successful stem cell transplantation (Chapter 178) can cure sickle cell anemia, but only about 10% of patients have suitable donors. Myeloablative stem cell transplantation carries a 5 to 10% mortality rate and is poorly tolerated in adults. A nonmyeloablative regimen that uses total body irradiation and treatment with alemtuzumab and sirolimus has led to stable mixed chimerism in about 50% of adults transplanted with an HLA-identical family donor, with no graft-versus-host disease observed.[17] In another small study, similar results were observed for HLA-haploidentical transplants, thereby expanding the numbers of patients who could be offered this treatment.[18]

Future Directions

Experimental treatments to induce higher levels of HbF (thereby reducing HbS polymer), to decrease the adherence of sickle erythrocytes to endothelium, and to modulate the oxygen affinity of hemoglobin in the sickle cell are undergoing clinical trials. Where malaria is endemic, antimalaria prophylaxis reduces episodes of malaria and increases mean hemoglobin levels. Gene therapy, tried in a few patients with β-thalassemia syndromes with some early success, has not yet been reported in sickle cell disease, but trials should soon begin.

PROGNOSIS

Average life expectancy for patients with sickle cell anemia in the United States was reported to be between 50 and 60 years, but these figures do not reflect better supportive care or widespread use of hydroxyurea; patients with HbSC disease typically live 60 to 70 years. Patients with HbS-β^0-thalassemia are likely to have a life expectancy similar to that of those with sickle cell anemia, and the lifespan for patients with the HbS-β^+-thalassemia may resemble that of patients with HbSC disease. Death is often caused by pulmonary disease and infection, and another 20% of deaths are related to organ failure. However, death in adults often is unexpected, happening in the midst of an acute event such as an acute painful episode and occurring within the first 24 hours of hospitalization. In areas of the developing world without access to modern medical care, death in childhood is still common.

OTHER HEMOGLOBINOPATHIES

Hemoglobinopathies other than those associated with HbS, HbE (Chapter 162), and HbC rarely cause clinically recognizable disorders. HbC (*HBB* Glu6Lys) and HbE (*HBB* Glu26Lys) are common β-globin variants. HbC is present in about 2% of African Americans, and HbE is seen in Southeast Asia, where, in some areas, the gene frequency may reach 50%. HbE is a β-hemoglobin variant that is produced at a slightly reduced rate and hence has the phenotype of a mild form of β-thalassemia.[19] Heterozygotes with HbC or HbE are asymptomatic, although the blood of HbC trait carriers contains target cells, and HbE carriers may have mild anemia and microcytosis. Even homozygotes for HbC and HbE have virtually no clinical disease, only mild hematologic abnormalities such as microcytosis, target cells, and mild anemia. Screening testing can be done by high performance liquid chromatography.

Compound heterozygotes for HbE and β-thalassemia usually have the phenotype of transfusion-dependent β-thalassemia, although genotype-phenotype correlations are difficult to make because of the likelihood that other genes affect the expression of disease. Because of immigration from Southeast Asia, HbSE disease is increasingly common in North America and Europe. It resembles HbS-β^+-thalassemia.

Rare hemoglobinopathies may change the affinity of hemoglobin for oxygen, render it susceptible to oxidation, or cause molecular instability. Amino acid substitutions involving heme-binding residues may lead to irreversible iron oxidation, methemoglobinemia, and cyanosis (Chapter 158). Patients with these conditions have congenital pseudocyanosis but are usually asymptomatic and need no treatment.

Substitutions at contacts between globin subunits may alter the affinity of hemoglobin for oxygen. When hemoglobin-oxygen affinity is increased, less oxygen is available in tissues, erythropoietin production is enhanced, and erythrocytosis results (Chapter 166). No treatment is usually required because the erythrocytosis is mild. Hemoglobin-oxygen affinity may also be reduced by some mutations, resulting in anemia or cyanosis. Hemoglobin instability, produced by several molecular mechanisms (including introduction of proline residues into the α-helix, substitutions near the heme ring, and deletion or addition of amino acids), often causes loss of heme from the molecule and hemolytic anemia. Hemoglobin Köln is the most common example of this class of hemoglobinopathy, but more than 200 unstable variants have been described. Oxidant drugs sometimes provoke increased hemolysis. Splenectomy is sometimes an effective treatment when the anemia is severe.

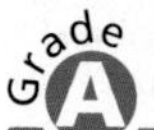

Grade A References

A1. Charache S, Terrin ML, Moore RD, et al. Effect of hydroxyurea on the frequency of painful crises in sickle cell anemia. *N Engl J Med.* 1995;332:1317-1322.

A2. Steinberg MH, Barton F, Castro O, et al. Effect of hydroxyurea on mortality and morbidity in adult sickle cell anemia: risks and benefits up to 9 years of treatment. *JAMA.* 2003;289:1645-1651.

A3. Wang WC, Ware RE, Miller ST, et al. Hydroxycarbamide in very young children with sickle-cell anaemia: a multicentre, randomised, controlled trial (BABY HUG). *Lancet.* 2011;377:1663-1672.

A4. Goldman RD, Mounstephen W, Kirby-Allen M, et al. Intravenous magnesium sulfate for vaso-occlusive episodes in sickle cell disease. *Pediatrics.* 2013;132:e1634-e1641.

A5. Machado RF, Barst RJ, Yovetich NA, et al. Hospitalization for pain in patients with sickle cell disease treated with sildenafil for elevated TRV and low exercise capacity. *Blood.* 2011;118:855-864.

A6. Sasongko TH, Nagalla S, Ballas SK. Angiotensin-converting enzyme (ACE) inhibitors for proteinuria and microalbuminuria in people with sickle cell disease. *Cochrane Database Syst Rev.* 2013;3:CD009191.

A7. Howard J, Malfroy M, Llewelyn C, et al. The Transfusion Alternatives Preoperatively in Sickle Cell Disease (TAPS) study: a randomised, controlled, multicentre clinical trial. *Lancet.* 2013;381:930-938.

A8. DeBaun MR, Gordon M, McKinstry RC, et al. Controlled trial of transfusions for silent cerebral infarcts in sickle cell anemia. *N Engl J Med.* 2014;371:699-710.

A9. Meerpohl JJ, Schell LK, Rucker G, et al. Deferasirox for managing transfusional iron overload in people with sickle cell disease. *Cochrane Database Syst Rev.* 2014;5:CD007477.

GENERAL REFERENCES

For the General References and other additional features, please visit Expert Consult at https://expertconsult.inkling.com.

164 MEGALOBLASTIC ANEMIAS

AŚOK C. ANTONY

DEFINITION

Megaloblastic anemias, a group of disorders characterized by a distinct morphologic pattern in hematopoietic cells, are commonly due to a deficiency of vitamin B_{12} (cobalamin) or folate. These anemias are globally prevalent and carry a significant burden of morbidity. Folate and cobalamin are both required to sustain one-carbon metabolism, which involves the transfer of one-carbon groups such as methyl-, formyl-, methylene-, methenyl-, and formimino- in enzyme reactions essential for pyrimidine and purine biosynthesis, including the synthesis of three of the four nucleotides of DNA. Thus, a deficiency in cobalamin or folate results in the common biochemical feature of a defect in DNA synthesis along with lesser alterations in RNA and protein synthesis, leading to a state of unbalanced cell growth and impaired cell division. The majority of megaloblastic cells have DNA values between 2 and 4 N because of delayed cell division. This is morphologically expressed as larger-than-normal "immature" nuclei with finely particulate chromatin, whereas the relatively unimpaired RNA and protein synthesis results in large cells with greater "mature" cytoplasm and cell volume. The microscopic appearance of this nuclear-cytoplasmic asynchrony (or dissociation) is morphologically described as *megaloblastic*. Megaloblastic hematopoiesis commonly is manifested with anemia, the most easily recognized clinical manifestation of a global defect in DNA synthesis affecting all rapidly proliferating cells. Precise identification of the deficient vitamin and the cause of the deficiency (Table 164-1) dictates the dose and duration of replacement therapy.

EPIDEMIOLOGY

Cobalamin

Nutrition

Cobalamin is a red, water-soluble vitamin with a complex structure that generally resembles the heme molecule but with cobalt replacing iron in the center of the pyrrole ring. The recommended daily allowance of cobalamin is 2.4 μg for men and nonpregnant women, 2.6 μg for pregnant women, 2.8 μg for lactating women, and between 1.5 and 2 μg for children 9 to 18 years old. Cobalamin is produced in nature only by microorganisms, and humans receive cobalamin solely from the diet. Meat from parenchymal organs is richest in cobalamin (>10 μg/100 g wet weight); fish and animal muscle, milk products, and egg yolks have 1 to 10 μg/100 g wet weight. An average nonvegetarian Western diet with abundant meat, milk, and other dairy products and eggs contains 5 to 7 μg/day of cobalamin, which is adequate to sustain normal cobalamin equilibrium. Herbivores can receive minuscule amounts of cobalamin from nitrogen-fixing soil bacteria (genus *Rhizobium*) present in the roots and nodules of legumes; from fresh produce contaminated by tiny insects or cobalamin-rich manure; from dried seaweed varieties (nori, chlorella, and spirulina); and from tempeh (fermented soybean cake). However, these are not reliable sources of cobalamin. For vegetarians, the consumption of eggs, milk, and dairy products generally provides less than 0.5 μg/day of cobalamin and cannot sustain cobalamin balance.[1] Near-vegetarians who infrequently consume animal-source foods (often because of poverty) also have a cobalamin status that is only marginally better than that of lacto-ovovegetarians and are also at risk for cobalamin deficiency.

Cobalamin is stored exceptionally well in tissues. Of the total body content of 2 to 5 mg in adults, half is in the liver. With a daily loss of 1 μg, dietary

TABLE 164-1 ETIOPATHOPHYSIOLOGIC CLASSIFICATION OF COBALAMIN AND FOLATE DEFICIENCIES

COBALAMIN DEFICIENCY
Nutritional cobalamin deficiency (insufficient cobalamin intake): vegetarians, poverty-imposed near-vegetarians, breast-fed infants of mothers with pernicious anemia
Abnormal intragastric events (inadequate proteolysis of food cobalamin): atrophic gastritis, hypochlorhydria, proton pump inhibitors, H_2-blockers
Loss/atrophy of gastric oxyntic mucosa (deficient intrinsic factor molecules): total or partial gastrectomy, adult and juvenile pernicious anemia, caustic destruction (lye)
Abnormal events in the small bowel lumen
Inadequate pancreatic protease (R-factor-bound cobalamin not degraded, cobalamin not transferred to intrinsic factor)
Insufficient pancreatic protease: pancreatic insufficiency
Inactivation of pancreatic protease: Zollinger-Ellison syndrome
Usurping of luminal cobalamin (inadequate binding of cobalamin to intrinsic factor)
By bacteria: stasis syndromes (blind loops, pouches of diverticulosis, strictures, fistulas, anastomosis), impaired bowel motility (scleroderma), hypogammaglobulinemia
By *Diphyllobothrium latum* (fish tapeworm)
Disorders of ileal mucosa/intrinsic factor–cobalamin receptors (intrinsic factor–cobalamin not bound to intrinsic factor–cobalamin receptors [also known as cubam receptors])
Diminished or absent cubam receptors: ileal bypass, resection, fistula
Abnormal mucosal architecture or function: tropical/nontropical sprue, Crohn disease, tuberculous ileitis, amyloidosis
Cubam receptor defects: Imerslund-Gräsbeck syndrome, hereditary megaloblastic anemia
Drug effects: metformin, cholestyramine, colchicine, neomycin
Disorders of plasma cobalamin transport (TCII-cobalamin not delivered to TCII receptors): congenital TCII deficiency, defective binding of TCII-cobalamin to TCII receptors (rare)
Metabolic disorders (cobalamin not used by cells)
Inborn enzyme errors (rare)
Acquired disorders (cobalamin functionally inactivated by irreversible oxidation): nitrous oxide inhalation
FOLATE DEFICIENCY
Nutritional causes
Decreased dietary intake: poverty and famine, institutionalization (psychiatric facilities, nursing homes), chronic debilitating disease, prolonged feeding of infants with goat's milk, special slimming diets or fad foods (folate-rich foods not consumed), cultural or ethnic cooking techniques (food folate destroyed)
Decreased dietary intake and increased requirements
Physiologic: pregnancy and lactation, prematurity, hyperemesis gravidarum, infancy
Pathologic
Intrinsic hematologic diseases involving hemolysis with compensatory erythropoiesis, abnormal hematopoiesis, or bone marrow infiltration by malignant disease
Dermatologic disease: psoriasis
Folate malabsorption
With normal intestinal mucosa
Drugs: pyrimethamine, proton pump inhibitors (by inhibition of proton-coupled folate transporters); anticonvulsants (reduced absorption and induction of microsomal liver enzymes)
Hereditary folate malabsorption (mutations in proton-coupled folate transporters) (rare)
With mucosal abnormalities: tropical and nontropical sprue, regional enteritis
Defective CSF folate transport: cerebral folate deficiency (mutation or autoantibodies to folate receptors) (rare)
Inadequate cellular utilization
Folate antagonists (methotrexate)
Hereditary enzyme deficiencies involving folate
Drugs (multiple effects on folate metabolism): alcohol, sulfasalazine, triamterene, pyrimethamine, trimethoprim-sulfamethoxazole, phenytoin, barbiturates
MISCELLANEOUS MEGALOBLASTIC ANEMIAS NOT CAUSED BY COBALAMIN OR FOLATE DEFICIENCY
Congenital disorders of DNA synthesis
Orotic aciduria
Lesch-Nyhan syndrome
Congenital dyserythropoietic anemia
Acquired disorders of DNA synthesis
Deficiency: thiamine-responsive megaloblastic anemia (thiamine transporter 1 mutation)
Erythroleukemia; refractory sideroblastic anemias (pyridoxine responsive?)

CSF = cerebrospinal fluid; TCII = transcobalamin II.

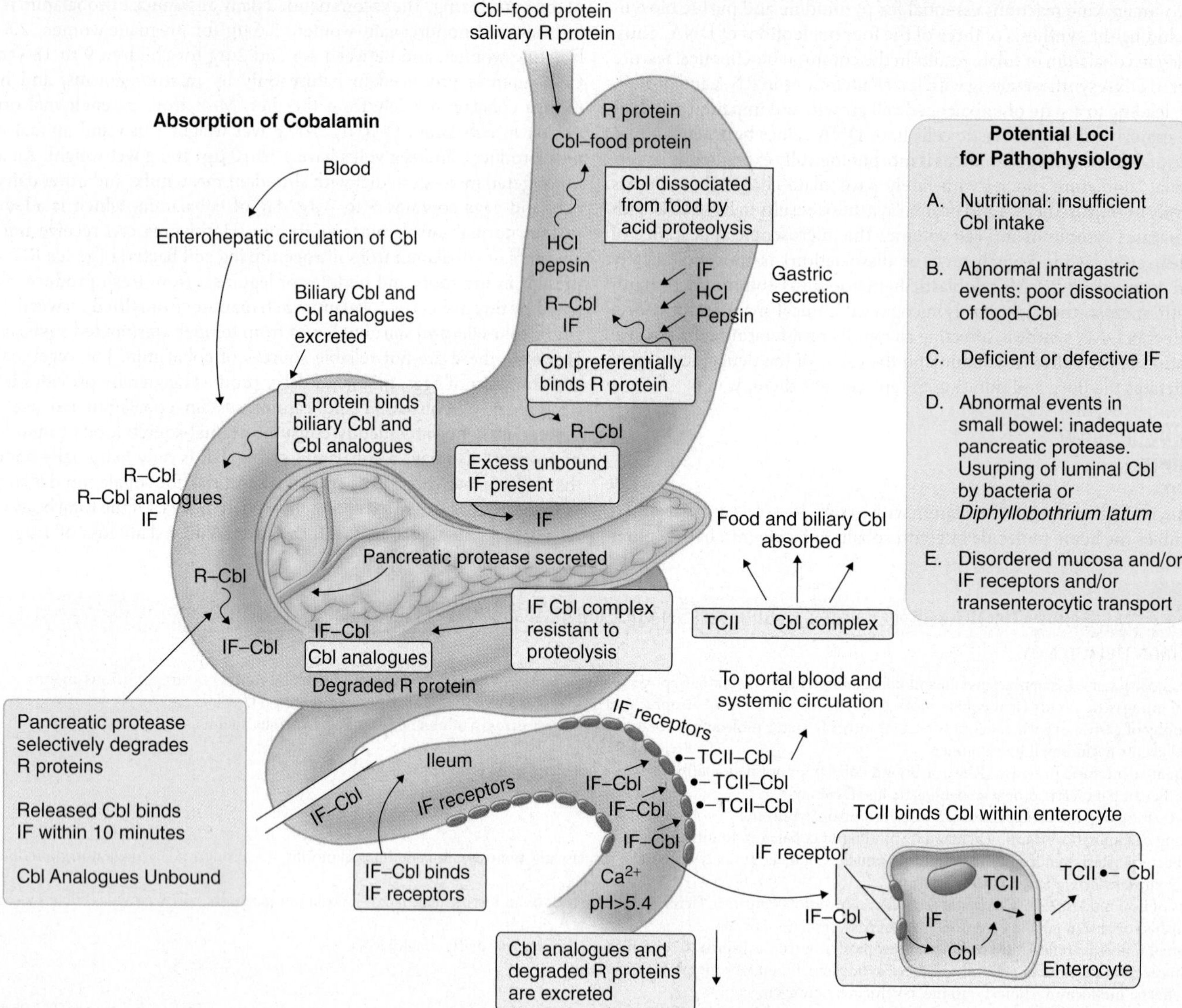

FIGURE 164-1. Components and mechanism of cobalamin absorption, with an indication of the locus for malabsorption. Cbl = cobalamin; IF = intrinsic factor; TCII = transcobalamin II. (From Antony AC. Megaloblastic anemias. In: Hoffman R, Benz EJ Jr, Silberstein LE, et al, eds. Hematology: Basic Principles and Practice. 6th ed. Philadelphia: Elsevier Saunders; 2013:473-504.)

cobalamin deficiency can take 5 to 10 years to become apparent. However, it takes about 3 to 4 years to deplete cobalamin stores if dietary cobalamin is abruptly malabsorbed (e.g., ileal resection), thereby interfering with an efficient enterohepatic circulation, which accounts for the turnover of 5 to 10 µg of cobalamin per day and reabsorption of 75% of cobalamin secreted into bile. Although cobalamin resists high-temperature cooking, it is unstable to light and can be converted to inactive analogues.

Folates

Nutrition

Folates are synthesized by microorganisms and plants. Rich food sources include green leafy vegetables (spinach, lettuce, broccoli), beans, fruit (bananas, melons, lemons), yeast, mushrooms, and animal protein (muscle, liver, kidney). The recommended daily allowance of folate is 400 µg for adult men and nonpregnant women, 600 µg for pregnant women, 500 µg for lactating women, and 300 to 400 µg for children 9 to 18 years of age. A balanced Western diet can prevent folate deficiency, but the net dietary intake of folate in many developing countries is more often grossly insufficient to sustain folate balance. Folates are susceptible to breakdown during prolonged cooking (boiling for more than 15 minutes), which can destroy 50 to 95% of folate.

PATHOBIOLOGY

Cobalamin

Normal Physiology

There are specialized protein chaperones that sequentially bind, sequester, and thereby protect cobalamin through its long odyssey—from the moment it is dissociated from food in the stomach to its final destination within cells as a cofactor for crucial enzyme reactions.

Absorption and Transport

Cobalamin in food is usually in coenzyme form (as deoxyadenosylcobalamin and methylcobalamin) and bound to proteins (Fig. 164-1). In the stomach, peptic digestion at low pH is a prerequisite for the release of cobalamin from food protein. Once it is released, cobalamin preferentially binds a high-affinity cobalamin-binding protein called R protein, which is secreted in salivary and gastric juice. These cobalamin–R protein complexes, along with unbound intrinsic factor, which is secreted by gastric parietal cells, pass into the duodenum, where pancreatic proteases degrade R proteins. This allows transfer of cobalamin to intrinsic factor.

The stable intrinsic factor–cobalamin complexes then pass through the jejunum to the ileum, where they specifically bind to intrinsic factor–cobalamin receptors (also called cubam receptors—a complex of two proteins, cubilin and amnionless) on the microvilli of ileal mucosal cells. Within enterocytes, cobalamin is transferred to transcobalamin II; this complex is then released into the circulation, from which it efficiently binds to high-affinity transcobalamin II receptors on cell surfaces. When cobalamin status is compromised, this is the fraction that is primarily reduced. There is, however, another protein, transcobalamin I, that binds the bulk (approximately 75%) of serum cobalamin but does not deliver it to cells, so it functions much like a storage protein for the cobalamin in blood. Because the cobalamin from this compartment of transcobalamin I–bound cobalamin—which is relatively invariant in serum—is also measured in serum cobalamin assays, this accounts for the relative insensitivity of this test, which aims to discover if there is a reduction in the functionally relevant transcobalamin II–bound cobalamin.[1,2] A third minor protein, transcobalamin III, binds a wide spectrum of cobalamin analogues that are rapidly cleared by the liver into bile for efficient fecal excretion.

Cellular Processing

More than 95% of intracellular cobalamin is bound to two intracellular enzymes: methylmalonyl coenzyme A (CoA) mutase and methionine synthase. In mitochondria, deoxyadenosylcobalamin is a coenzyme for methylmalonyl-CoA mutase, which converts methylmalonyl-CoA to succinyl-CoA so that it can be easily metabolized. In the cytoplasm, methylcobalamin is a coenzyme for methionine synthase, which catalyzes the transfer of methyl groups from methylcobalamin to homocysteine to form methionine. The methyl group of 5-methyltetrahydrofolate (methyl-THF) is donated to regenerate methylcobalamin, thereby forming the THF that is essential to sustain one-carbon metabolism. The methionine so formed can be adenylated to *S*-adenosylmethionine, which donates its methyl group in a critical series of biologic methylation reactions involving more than 80 proteins, phospholipids, neurotransmitters, RNA, and DNA. The close functional interrelationship between cobalamin and folate within cells (involving the common enzyme methionine synthase, the single enzymatic reaction of which is a metabolic step for which both cobalamin and folate are essential) explains why cobalamin deficiency leads to a functional folate deficiency and is also the basis for similar clinical (hematologic) manifestations involving perturbed DNA.

Pathogenesis of Cobalamin Deficiency

Nutritional Cobalamin Deficiency

Severe cobalamin deficiency in the West is likely to be pernicious anemia.[2] However, vegetarianism and poverty-imposed near-vegetarianism are more common causes worldwide in all age groups. Up to three quarters of the population in resource-limited countries (particularly women and children), who subsist on a monotonous diet low in animal-source foods, have subtle evidence of cobalamin deficiency; many also have folate and iron deficiency.[3] Low maternal cobalamin status compromises the amount of cobalamin delivered to the fetus; moreover, low cobalamin content of breast milk predisposes one third of their infants to cobalamin deficiency, thereby establishing a vicious intergenerational circle of cobalamin (and multiple nutrient) deficiency. As large swaths of the populations are exposed to war or famine, those teetering on the brink of cobalamin (and folate) deficiency will eventually come to light clinically.

Inadequate Dissociation of Cobalamin from Food Protein

In affluent countries, failure to fully release food cobalamin because of chronic gastric atrophy and achlorhydria is common among one third to one half of elderly individuals with low cobalamin status. This is estimated to be 10-fold more common than pernicious anemia.

Absent Secretion of Acid and Intrinsic Factor

Total gastrectomy invariably leads to cobalamin deficiency in 2 to 10 years, thus warranting prophylactic cobalamin (and iron) replacement. After partial gastrectomy or bariatric gastric bypass surgery (Chapter 220) and in those receiving long-term H_2-blockers or proton pump inhibitors, multifactorial cobalamin deficiency may result from decreased secretion of intrinsic factor, hypochlorhydria, or intestinal bacterial overgrowth of cobalamin-consuming organisms.

In pernicious anemia, autoimmune gastritis involving destruction of the gastric parietal cell mass leads to atrophy of the fundus and body of the stomach, absence of intrinsic factor and hydrochloric acid, and eventually severe cobalamin malabsorption and deficiency. Pernicious anemia is found in persons of all ages, races, and ethnic origins; however, the precise global incidence is not known because population-based studies, which rely on finding diagnostic serum anti–intrinsic factor antibodies (found in serum of 60% and gastric juice of 75%), will miss a substantial number of patients. Nevertheless, with this approach, nearly 2% of free-living individuals older than 60 years in southern California had undiagnosed pernicious anemia, with minimal clinical manifestations of cobalamin deficiency; significantly, in this cohort, 4% of white and African American women had pernicious anemia. About 30% of patients have a positive family history, and there is an association with other autoimmune diseases (e.g., polyglandular autoimmune syndrome, Graves disease, Hashimoto thyroiditis, vitiligo, Addison disease, idiopathic hypoparathyroidism, myasthenia gravis, and type 1 diabetes).

Abnormal Events Precluding Absorption of Cobalamin

Although pancreatic insufficiency (Chapter 140) can preclude transfer of R protein–bound cobalamin to intrinsic factor, with the early use of pancreatic protease replacement, cobalamin deficiency is uncommon. Endogenous pancreatic protease can, however, be inactivated by massive gastric hypersecretion arising from a gastrinoma in Zollinger-Ellison syndrome (Chapter 195). Further, if the pH of the luminal contents in the ileum is less than 5.4, the binding of the intrinsic factor–cobalamin complex to cubam receptors will be precluded.

Bacterial overgrowth in the small bowel (arising from stasis, impaired motility, and hypogammaglobulinemia; Chapter 142) favors colonization by bacteria, which can usurp free cobalamin before it can bind to intrinsic factor. This can be reversed by a short course of antibiotics. Individuals heavily infested with the fish tapeworm *Diphyllobothrium latum* (acquired by consuming raw or partially cooked freshwater fish) can become cobalamin deficient when these long (10 m) adult worms in the jejunum avidly usurp cobalamin. After expulsion of worms (with an oral dose of praziquantel 10 to 20 mg/kg), cobalamin replenishment is curative.

Disorders of the Intrinsic Factor Receptors or Mucosa

Because the distal ileum has the greatest density of cubam receptors, the removal, bypass, or dysfunction of only 1 to 2 feet of terminal ileum will result in cobalamin malabsorption. Among drugs (see Table 164-1), metformin, when it is used in full doses for type 2 diabetes, is notorious for inducing cobalamin malabsorption and low cobalamin levels after 5 years or more.[4] Although it is preventable by calcium (1.2 g/day), many with metformin-induced low cobalamin levels will progress to cobalamin deficiency, warranting cobalamin replacement and prophylaxis.

Acquired Cobalamin Deficiency

Nitrous oxide (N_2O) irreversibly inactivates cobalamin and results in a state of functional intracellular cobalamin deficiency, which can be bypassed by the administration of 5-formyl-THF (leucovorin). N_2O exposure can induce megaloblastosis in those with marginal or low cobalamin stores, but chronic intermittent (surreptitious, accidental, or occupational) exposure more frequently leads to neuromyelopathic manifestations. Capsules used for making whipped cream are a cheap and easy source of N_2O, allowing for abuse in the community.

Folates

Normal Physiology

Specialized mechanisms also exist to ensure the digestion, absorption, and uptake of folates into cells—and across both the placenta to the fetus and the choroid plexus into the nervous system—to support intracellular enzymes that are critical for synthesis of DNA.

Absorption and Transport

In general, only half the folate in food, which is mainly in polyglutamylated form, is nutritionally available (bioavailable), whereas 85% of folic acid added to food or ingested as a supplement is bioavailable. The small intestine can absorb folic acid unchanged, but food folate polyglutamates must be hydrolyzed to monoglutamate by folate polyglutamate hydrolase at the brush border before transport into enterocytes, so food preparation (dicing, purée-ing) can facilitate absorption. A jejunal luminal surface proton-coupled folate transporter, which has a low pH optimum, facilitates the efficient transport of folate into enterocytes, where it is reduced to THF and methylated before release by a cellular exporter protein into plasma as methyl-THF.[5] The serum folate level is maintained by dietary folate intake and an efficient enterohepatic circulation. From plasma, there is a rapid uptake of folates into tissues by cell membrane–associated folate receptors, which bind physiologically relevant methyl-THF, folic acid, and some newer antifolates with high affinity at concentrations found in serum. After folate receptor–mediated endocytosis, a proton-coupled folate transporter then helps export folate from acidified endosomes into the cytoplasm of cells. The sequentially coordinated function of folate receptors and proton-coupled folate transporters of the choroid plexus is also required to maintain the ratio of cerebrospinal fluid (CSF) folate to blood folate of up to 3 : 1. After glomerular filtration, folate receptors on the brush border membranes of proximal renal tubular cells bind luminal folate and transport it back into blood. Cells have an exquisite molecular mechanism for sensing and responding to folate deficiency by upregulating folate receptors to restore folate homeostasis. Reduced-folate carriers are also folate transporters that primarily mediate the uptake of pharmacologic folates (methotrexate and folinic acid) into cells. Passive diffusion also operates to transport folate across biologic membranes at supraphysiologic folate concentrations.

Intracellular Metabolism and Cobalamin-Folate Interactions

After cellular uptake, methyl-THF must first be converted to THF by methionine synthase. Only then can the THF be polyglutamylated by folate polyglutamate synthase, which allows it to be retained intracellularly to play a central role in one-carbon metabolism. THF can be converted to 10-formyl-THF (for de novo biosynthesis of purines) and to methylene-THF.

The central role of methylene-THF is that it can be used either in the thymidylate cycle via thymidylate synthase for the synthesis of thymidine and DNA or in the methylation cycle via methionine synthase (but only after its conversion to methyl-THF by methylene-THF reductase). Inactivation of methionine synthase during cobalamin deficiency results in accumulation of the substrate methyl-THF, which cannot be polyglutamylated and thus leaks out of the cell, resulting in an intracellular THF deficiency and compromised one-carbon metabolism (E-Table 164-1).

Pathogenesis of Folate Deficiency

Folate deficiency can arise from decreased supply (reduced intake, absorption, transport, or utilization) or increased requirements (from metabolic consumption, destruction, or excretion). One individual may have multiple causes of folate deficiency, but specific tests to define each mechanism are not available clinically. Nutritional folate insufficiency is the most common cause of folate deficiency worldwide in all age groups, with women and children in resource-limited (developing) countries at highest risk. Indeed, more than 90% of pregnant women in resource-limited countries consume less than the estimated average requirement of folate, cobalamin, and iron. Although fortification of food with folate has dramatically reduced the prevalence of folate deficiency in the United States, it can still be found among some chronic alcoholics and the elderly, infirm, or socially isolated individuals who consume imbalanced diets.

Nutritional Causes (Decreased Intake or Increased Requirements)

With an abrupt reduction in folate consumption, body stores of folate are adequate for approximately 4 months. However, these stores are depleted faster in individuals in chronically negative folate balance who often have multiple nutritional deficiencies (and diseases) that tip them into frank folate deficiency. A seasonal reduction in folate-rich foods, poverty, cultural or ethnic diets that are intrinsically low in folates, cooking techniques that destroy folate, and anorexia that accompanies chronic illnesses are among the many reasons for folate deficiency.

Patients with intrinsic hematologic diseases involving increased cell proliferation or with increased compensatory erythropoiesis in response to chronic peripheral red blood cell destruction have increased requirements for folate. Indeed, folate deficiency in the face of chronic hemolysis can lead to an acute reticulocytopenic (aplastic) crisis, an unexpected increase in transfusion requirements, or a fall in platelets. Exfoliative skin diseases (Chapter 436) also cause folate deficiency when there is an increased demand from excess loss of skin cells.

Pregnancy and Infancy

Poor folate intake during pregnancy is a common cause of megaloblastic anemia in developing countries because pregnancy and lactation require additional folate for growth of the fetus and maternal tissues. Physiologic transplacental folate transport by folate receptors relies on the continued intake of adequate dietary folate by the mother; if it is compromised by poor nutrition or increased needs (short intervals between pregnancies, twin pregnancies), poor pregnancy outcomes will result. This can be manifested by premature, low-birthweight infants and other midline developmental abnormalities in the fetus ranging from neural tube defects (such as anencephaly, encephalocele, meningocele, and spina bifida) to neurocristopathies (such as ventricular septal defects, cleft lip, and cleft palate). Periconceptional folate supplementation studies suggest that mothers who fail to consume sufficient folate during pregnancy have children who exhibit subtle changes that are manifested in early childhood; these include behavioral abnormalities (hyperactive/inattentive with peer problems, emotionally reactive, aggressive, anxious/depressed symptoms, and somatic complaints or withdrawn[6] and autistic disorder[7]) as well as cognitive dysfunction,[8] poor academic performance, and delayed language acquisition.

Cerebral folate deficiency can be caused either by a congenital mutation in folate receptors or by autoantibodies to folate receptors, which perturbs folate transport into the CSF, leading to severe developmental regression in early childhood associated with movement disturbances, epilepsy, and leukodystrophy. Blocking autoantibodies to folate receptors, which develop against consumed bovine milk folate-binding proteins that share epitopes with human folate receptors, can also be found in two autism spectrum disorders: Rett syndrome and infantile low-functioning autism with neurologic abnormalities. When it is diagnosed early, cerebral folate deficiency responds to high doses of folinic acid, which normalizes CSF folates and induces a partial to complete recovery in 12 months. When it is induced by autoantibodies, a bovine milk–free diet will also help decrease the autoantibody titer.

Hereditary folate malabsorption, which is due to a mutation in the proton-coupled folate transporter, results in compromised intestinal folate absorption and folate transfer into the CSF. Patients present with folate deficiency anemia, hypoimmunoglobulinemia with recurrent infections, chronic diarrhea, neurologic abnormalities (seizures or mental retardation), and low to undetectable CSF folate levels. High parenteral doses of folinic acid can ensure passive diffusion into the CSF and lead to significant clinical improvement in these children.

Tropical and Nontropical (Celiac) Sprue

With the development of intestinal mucosal abnormalities, patients are at increased risk for folate malabsorption. In tropical sprue (Chapter 140), a dramatic response to a 4- to 6-month course of oral folic acid (5 mg/day) plus tetracycline (250 mg four times a day) can effect a cure in 60% or more of patients. When it is prolonged (>3 years), malabsorption of cobalamin can develop together with iron deficiency (Chapter 159), pellagra, and beriberi (Chapter 218).

Drugs

Excess alcohol consumption at the expense of a balanced diet is a common cause of folate deficiency in the United States. Inhibition of dihydrofolate reductase by trimethoprim and pyrimethamine or methotrexate can be acutely reversed by folinic acid. Pyrimethamine and proton pump inhibitors inhibit the proton-coupled folate transporter, whereas anticonvulsants can reduce folate absorption and induce microsomal liver enzymes. Antineoplastics and antiretroviral antinucleosides can also induce megaloblastosis by perturbing DNA synthesis.

CLINICAL MANIFESTATIONS

The finding of macrocytosis (increased mean corpuscular volume [MCV]) on a routine complete blood count may be the first clinical manifestation. In other patients, the findings may be dominated by the condition causing the deficiency of cobalamin or folate, such as malabsorption, alcoholism, or malnutrition (see Table 164-1).

The clinical manifestations of folate deficiency may include hematologic (pancytopenia with megaloblastic bone marrow), cardiopulmonary (secondary to anemia), gastrointestinal (megaloblastosis with or without malabsorption), dermatologic (hyperpigmentation of the skin, premature graying), infertility (sterility), and psychiatric (primarily a flat affect) symptoms. If such patients have additional neurologic findings, either associated cobalamin deficiency or other diseases that predispose to folate deficiency must be considered, such as alcoholism with thiamine deficiency, which may result in peripheral neuropathy (dry beriberi) with Wernicke-Korsakoff syndrome, with or without heart failure from cardiovascular disease (wet beriberi) (Chapters 218 and 416). Because megaloblastosis due to either folate or cobalamin deficiency results in functional folate deficiency, the hematologic manifestations of both deficiencies, including pancytopenia with megaloblastic bone marrow, are indistinguishable. However, only cobalamin deficiency results in a patchy but widespread demyelinating process, which is expressed clinically as cerebral abnormalities and subacute combined degeneration of the spinal cord (Chapter 416). Either hematologic or neurologic manifestations may dominate the clinical picture.

Chronic hyperhomocysteinemia (Chapter 209) is a risk factor for several diseases (Table 164-2), many of which are benefited by folate supplementation or homocysteine-lowering therapy with combined folic acid, cobalamin, and pyridoxine. Thus, by inference, patients can present with any of these conditions arising from long-standing hyperhomocysteinemia or poor folate status.

DIAGNOSIS

Diagnostic Approach to the Patient

The general approach to a patient with megaloblastic anemia is first to recognize that megaloblastic anemia is present; then to distinguish whether folate, cobalamin, or combined folate and cobalamin deficiencies have led to the anemia; and finally to diagnose the underlying disease and mechanism causing the deficiency[9] (see Table 164-1).

TABLE 164-2 EFFECTS OF HOMOCYSTEINE-LOWERING THERAPY ON NONHEMATOPOIETIC SYSTEMS

FOLIC ACID, COBALAMIN, AND PYRIDOXINE SUPPLEMENTATION
Reduction in hip fracture[A1]
Reduction in progression of carotid intima-media thickness (a surrogate marker of early subclinical arteriosclerosis)[A2]
Reduction in age-related macular degeneration[A3]
Reduction in rate of brain atrophy[A4]
Reduction in rate of cognitive decline (folate plus cobalamin only)[A5]
FOLIC ACID SUPPLEMENTATION
Reduction in stroke[A6]
Reduction in age-related (sensorineural) hearing loss[A7]
Reduction in phenytoin-induced gingival hyperplasia[A8]
FOLIC ACID FORTIFICATION OF FOOD (POPULATION-BASED STUDIES)
Reduction in neural tube defects (anencephaly, spina bifida, encephalocele, meningocele, iniencephaly)
Reduction in cleft lip with or without cleft palate
Reduction in severe congenital heart disease (endocardial cushion defects, conotruncal defects)
Reduction in congenital pyloric stenosis, stenosis of the pelvic-ureteric junction, limb reduction defects, omphalocele
Reduction in stroke mortality
Decreased risk of preterm births, low-birthweight and small-for-gestational-age babies
No evidence of increase in cancer[A9]
DELETERIOUS EFFECT OF HOMOCYSTEINE-LOWERING THERAPY
Diabetic nephropathy[A10]

Although deficiencies of cobalamin and folate are only two of the many causes of macrocytosis (Fig. 164-2), they become increasingly more likely as the MCV increases. Because perturbed DNA synthesis from any cause (including folate and cobalamin deficiency) results in megaloblastosis of bone marrow precursor cells, the red cells released into the circulation have an MCV that is often greater than 110 fL; on the peripheral blood smear, these large cells appear oval (macro-ovalocytes). Compared with mature red cells, which normally have a central area of pallor that occupies about one third of the cell diameter, the central pallor of macro-ovalocytes is significantly reduced. By contrast, thin macrocytes, which contain an increased cell surface without a proportionate increase in volume, have a much larger area of central pallor (more than one-third the cell diameter). When reticulocytes, which are normally 20% larger than mature red cells, are prematurely released from the bone marrow during the stress of acute blood loss or hemolysis, these so-called shift reticulocytes are even larger. Therefore, assessment of the corrected reticulocyte count is a good starting point to distinguish whether the macrocytic anemia is due to increased reticulocytosis (see Fig. 164-2); if reticulocytopenia is evident, data from the history, physical findings, and peripheral smear showing either thin macrocytes or macro-ovalocytes will help narrow the differential diagnosis. The frequency with which a high MCV is found depends on the patient population studied. In U.S. hospitals, up to two thirds of cases of macrocytosis (MCV ≥100) can be due to chemotherapy or antiretroviral therapy, alcoholism, or liver disease. In resource-limited regions, insufficient intake of cobalamin, folate, and iron can result in a dimorphic anemia (with a large red cell distribution width from a mix of macro-ovalocytic and microcytic cells).

History and Physical Examination

The underlying condition predisposing to folate deficiency usually began within the previous 6 months and often dominates the overall clinical picture. By contrast, cobalamin deficiency takes several years to be manifested clinically. Therefore, the underlying condition is more chronic and symptoms develop more insidiously; defining the cause is a clinical challenge that necessitates a detailed history, physical findings, and the judicious use of laboratory studies.

The dietary history may be revealing (food faddism, vegetarianism), whereas the medical or family history may uncover gluten sensitivity, autoimmune diseases, epilepsy treated with an anticonvulsant, use of offending

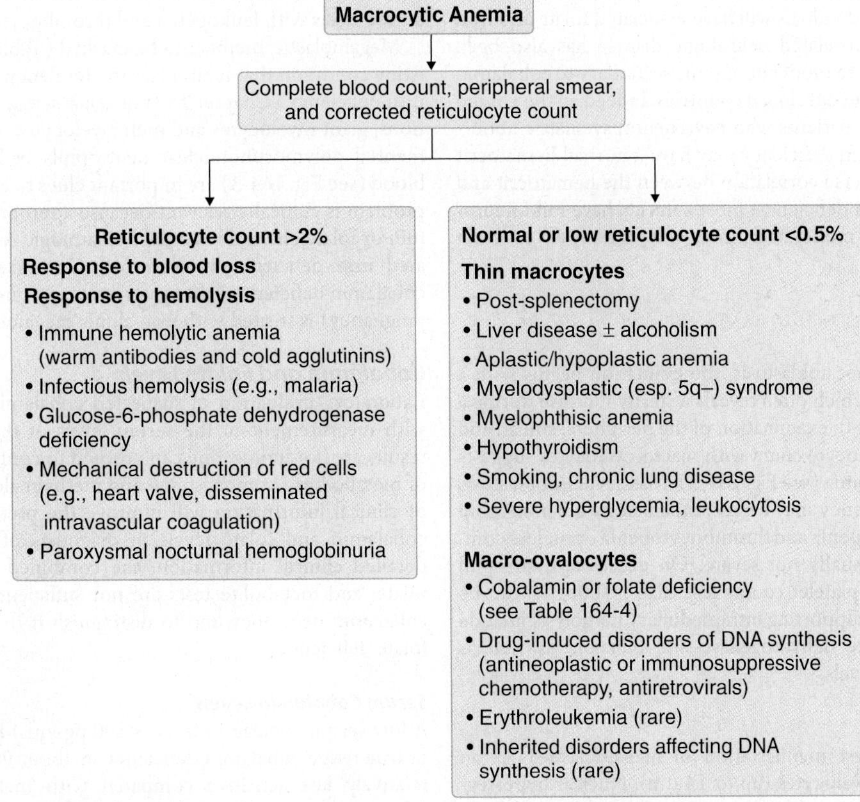

FIGURE 164-2. Algorithm for the evaluation of patients with macrocytosis.

drugs, hemolytic anemia, past surgery (e.g., gastrectomy, fistula, bowel resection), inhalation of N_2O, or travel history predictive for tropical sprue.

Physical examination of cobalamin-deficient vegetarians or those with pernicious anemia may reveal well-nourished individuals. By contrast, patients with folate deficiency are poorly nourished and may have other stigmata of multiple deficiencies from malabsorption (Chapter 140). Associated deficiency of iron and vitamins A, D, and K or protein-calorie malnutrition, or both, may give rise to angular cheilosis, bleeding mucous membranes, dermatitis, osteomalacia, and chronic infections. Varying degrees of pallor with lemon-tint icterus (a combination of pallor and icterus best observed in fair-skinned individuals) are common features of megaloblastosis. The skin may reveal either a diffuse brownish pigmentation or abnormal blotchy tanning. Premature graying is observed in both light- and dark-haired individuals. Examination of the mouth may reveal glossitis, with a smooth (depapillated), beefy-red tongue with occasional ulceration of the lateral surface. Thyromegaly may be observed with pernicious anemia and associated autoimmune thyroid disease. Heart failure from severe anemia may be accompanied by mild splenomegaly reflecting extramedullary hematopoiesis.

In prolonged cobalamin deficiency, neurologic examination reveals evidence of involvement of the posterior columns as well as of the pyramidal, spinocerebellar, and spinothalamic tracts. Posterior column dysfunction results in loss of position sense in the index toes (before great toe involvement) (Chapter 416) and loss of the ability to discern vibration of a high-pitched (256 cycles/second) tuning fork. Diminished vibratory sensation and proprioception of the lower extremities are the most common early objective signs. Neuropathic involvement of the legs precedes that of the arms. Upper motor neuron signs may be modulated by the subsequent involvement of peripheral nerves. A Romberg sign and a Lhermitte sign may be elicited. Loss of sphincter and bowel control or involvement of cranial nerves, such as optic neuritis, may be accompanied by other dysfunction of the cerebral cortex, including dementia, psychoses, and disturbances of mood. Cognitive impairment is not uncommon among vegetarians with cobalamin deficiency; a study reported that half had impaired recall and serial sevens, and one quarter had impaired naming. Objective findings of abnormal evoked potential (by the auditory oddball paradigm with P300 latency) are seen in half of these patients. The coexistence of folate deficiency with neurologic disease should prompt investigations to exclude cobalamin and other nutrient deficiencies arising from dietary insufficiency or malabsorption.

Nutritional cobalamin deficiency in resource-limited countries can be manifested as florid pancytopenia, mild hepatosplenomegaly, fever, and thrombocytopenia, with the neuropsychiatric syndrome developing as a later manifestation. Many of these individuals will have associated folate and iron deficiency. However, cobalamin-related neurologic disease has also been found in patients with only mild to moderate anemia secondary to cobalamin deficiency in both developing and developed countries. Indeed, in the United States, between 25 and 50% of patients who have neuropsychiatric abnormalities attributable to cobalamin deficiency may have a normal hematocrit and MCV. There is often an inverse correlation between the hematocrit and neurologic disease in cobalamin deficiency; most subjects have mild neurologic deficits, and 25% have only moderate deficits, with paresthesias or ataxia as the initial symptoms.

Laboratory Tests

Megaloblastosis

To establish the diagnosis of megaloblastosis, the evaluation begins with a complete blood count, MCV (which often reveals a steady increase during a period of several months or years), examination of the peripheral smear, and reticulocyte count; a low reticulocyte count with macro-ovalocytes suggests an underlying megaloblastic anemia (see Fig. 164-2). Classic megaloblastosis from cobalamin or folate deficiency may be accompanied by a hemoglobin level of less than 5 g/dL. Neutropenia and thrombocytopenia occur less commonly than anemia and are usually not severe. On occasion, neutrophil counts less than 1000/μL and platelet counts less than 50,000/μL can be seen. Additional abnormalities supporting intramedullary hemolysis include elevated levels of serum lactate dehydrogenase and bilirubin as well as decreased serum haptoglobin levels.

Peripheral Smear

In peripheral blood, the earliest manifestation of megaloblastosis is an increase in MCV with macro-ovalocytes (up to 14 μm). Nuclear hypersegmentation of neutrophils, diagnosed if more than 5% of polymorphonuclear leukocytes have five lobes or if 1% have six lobes on the smear (Fig. 164-3),

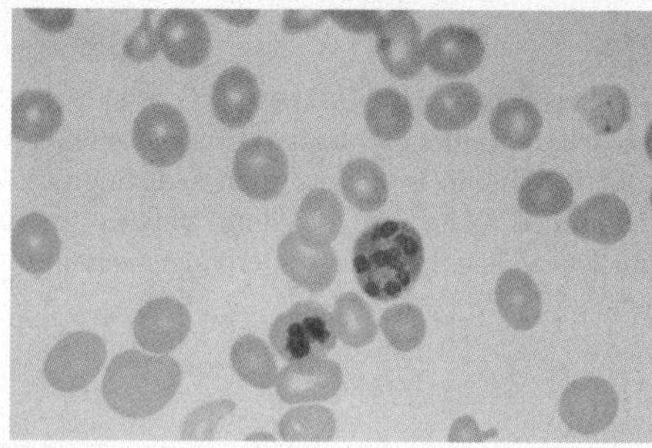

FIGURE 164-3. **Megaloblastic anemia. The peripheral blood has oval macrocytes (large red blood cells) and marked neutrophil hypersegmentation.**

TABLE 164-3 COMMON CONDITIONS PREDISPOSING TO MASKED MEGALOBLASTOSIS

Inadequate dietary intake of cobalamin, folate, and iron
Vegetarianism
Near-vegetarianism (in resource-limited settings)
Cobalamin *plus* iron deficiency
Post-gastrectomy
Pernicious anemia
Celiac disease (late manifestation)
Folate *plus* iron deficiency
Celiac disease (early manifestation)
Pregnancy in a woman not taking iron and folate supplements
Alcoholism with liver disease and gastrointestinal bleeding
Miscellaneous common clinical combinations
Rheumatoid arthritis with NSAIDs and gastrointestinal bleeding with methotrexate
Thalassemia with folate or cobalamin deficiency
Any patient with cancer receiving chemotherapy with chronic bleeding or iron deficiency
Antiretroviral therapy plus iron deficiency/thalassemia

NSAIDs = nonsteroidal anti-inflammatory drugs.

strongly suggests megaloblastosis, especially in association with macro-ovalocytosis. However, neutrophil hypersegmentation is not sensitive for the diagnosis of mild cobalamin deficiency, and macrocytosis is absent in nearly 50% of cases. There may be associated teardrop-shaped erythrocytes and anisocytosis with leukopenia and thrombocytopenia.

Megaloblastic anemia can be masked (Table 164-3) when there is a coexisting condition that neutralizes the tendency to generate large cells, such as iron deficiency (Chapter 159) or thalassemia (Chapter 162). In these situations, giant myelocytes and metamyelocytes in bone marrow and hypersegmented polymorphonuclear neutrophils in bone marrow and peripheral blood (see Fig. 164-3) are important clues to a masked megaloblastosis. This problem is clinically relevant because appropriate replacement with cobalamin or folate elicits a maximal hematologic response only when any associated iron deficiency is corrected. Conversely, if a combined iron and cobalamin deficiency (after gastrectomy) or iron and folate deficiency (with pregnancy) is treated with iron alone, megaloblastosis will be unmasked.

Cobalamin and Folate Levels

Laboratory evaluation of suspected cobalamin or folate deficiency begins with measurement of the serum levels of these vitamins. If any of these results are borderline, one can proceed to confirmatory tests by serum levels of metabolites (homocysteine and methylmalonic acid) (Table 164-4). Use of clinical information will improve the pretest probability of low serum cobalamin and folate levels in diagnosis of deficiency. Indeed, without detailed clinical information, the combined results of serum cobalamin, folate, and metabolite tests are not sufficiently unambiguous to diagnose cobalamin deficiency and to distinguish it from combined cobalamin plus folate deficiency.

Serum Cobalamin Levels

A low serum cobalamin level (<200 pg/mL) is a valuable clinical indicator of true tissue cobalamin deficiency in about 90% of patients. It is, however, relatively less sensitive compared with metabolite levels. Even among 173 unambiguously cobalamin-deficient patients, about 5% had normal cobalamin levels. Serum cobalamin is less than 300 pg/mL in 99% of patients

TABLE 164-4 STEPWISE APPROACH TO THE DIAGNOSIS OF COBALAMIN AND FOLATE DEFICIENCY

MEGALOBLASTIC ANEMIA OR NEUROLOGIC-PSYCHIATRIC MANIFESTATIONS CONSISTENT WITH COBALAMIN DEFICIENCY *PLUS* TEST RESULTS OF SERUM COBALAMIN AND SERUM FOLATE

Cobalamin* (pg/mL)	Folate† (ng/mL)	Provisional Diagnosis	Proceed with Metabolites?‡
>300	>4	Cobalamin or folate deficiency unlikely	No
<200	>4	Consistent with cobalamin deficiency	No
200-300	>4	Rule out cobalamin deficiency	Yes
>300	<2	Consistent with folate deficiency	No
<200	<2	Consistent with combined cobalamin plus folate deficiency or with isolated folate deficiency	Yes
>300	2-4	Consistent with folate deficiency or with anemia unrelated to vitamin deficiency	Yes

TEST RESULTS OF METABOLITES: SERUM METHYLMALONIC ACID AND TOTAL HOMOCYSTEINE

Methylmalonic Acid (normal = 70-270 nM)	Total Homocysteine (normal = 5-14 μM)	Diagnosis
Increased	Increased	Cobalamin deficiency confirmed; folate deficiency still possible (i.e., combined cobalamin plus folate deficiency possible)
Normal	Increased	Folate deficiency likely; <5% may have cobalamin deficiency
Normal	Normal	Cobalamin and folate deficiencies excluded

*Serum cobalamin levels: abnormally low, <200 pg/mL; clinically relevant low-normal range, 200-300 pg/mL. Methylmalonic acid is usually above 1000 nM in clinical cobalamin deficiency
†Serum folate levels: abnormally low, <2 ng/mL; clinically relevant low-normal range, 2-4 ng/mL. Homocysteine is usually above 25 μM in clinical folate deficiency. See E-Table 164-1 for additional limitations in the clinical interpretation of serum folate concentrations.
‡Any frozen-over sample from the serum folate or cobalamin determination can be subjected to metabolite tests.

with clinical hematologic or neurologic manifestations of cobalamin deficiency, whereas a cobalamin level above 300 pg/mL suggests folate deficiency or another cause of macrocytosis or neurologic disease. There have recently been several reports of patients who have had florid clinical evidence of cobalamin deficiency but whose serum cobalamin levels (by competitive binding luminescence assays) were either normal or in the high-normal range[10]; this is apparently due to the interference with the test by high titers of anti–intrinsic factor antibodies associated with pernicious anemia, a serious instance of a false-negative test result. This will lead to clinical manifestations if it is uncorrected. Therefore, if the clinical scenario is strongly suggestive of cobalamin deficiency but the test result is normal, the patient deserves a therapeutic trial with cobalamin. Confirmation of cobalamin deficiency with metabolites and detection of anti–intrinsic factor antibodies can allow retrospective diagnosis of pernicious anemia. Individuals with neuropsychiatric disorders attributed to cobalamin deficiency may not have anemia and only minimally depressed cobalamin levels. The serum cobalamin concentration can be falsely low in the absence of true cobalamin deficiency in patients with folate deficiency (one third of patients), pregnancy, multiple myeloma, transcobalamin I deficiency, and megadose vitamin C therapy.

An increase in cobalamin levels may be an unexpected finding in patients tested for cobalamin deficiency, for example, with high transcobalamin I and II levels (in myeloproliferative neoplasms, hepatic tumors, or active liver disease) and when transcobalamin II–producing macrophages are activated (in autoimmune diseases, monoblastic leukemias, and lymphomas). Approximately 10% of the U.S. population, especially the elderly, probably have metabolic evidence of true cobalamin deficiency.

Serum Folate Levels

In combination with a clinical picture of megaloblastic anemia and measurement of serum cobalamin, the serum folate level is the cheapest and best initial test for diagnosis of folate deficiency. Although red blood cell folate levels by earlier microbiologic assays correlated well with hepatic folate stores, the current assays for red blood cell folates are unreliable for routine clinical use.

The serum folate level is highly sensitive to the intake of a single folate-rich meal. Nutritional folate deficiency first leads to a decline in the serum folate level below normal (<2 ng/mL) in about 3 weeks; thus, it is a sensitive indicator of negative folate balance. Isolated reduction of serum folate in the absence of megaloblastosis (i.e., a false-positive result) occurs in one third of hospitalized patients with anorexia and acute alcohol consumption, in normal pregnancy, and in those using anticonvulsants. Because these groups are also at high risk for folate deficiency, additional testing with metabolites or an empirical therapeutic trial is indicated. Both cobalamin deficiency and malaria, which are common in resource-limited countries, can falsely elevate serum folate levels and mask the diagnosis of folate deficiency. In this scenario, the dietary history of folate intake is a better predictor of folate deficiency (see later).

Metabolite Levels: Homocysteine and Methylmalonic Acid

The serum methylmalonic acid (MMA) and homocysteine levels are highly sensitive tests, both of which rise in proportion to the severity of cobalamin deficiency; by contrast, the serum homocysteine level alone rises with folate deficiency (see Table 164-4). Therefore, an increase in both metabolites cannot differentiate between isolated cobalamin deficiency and combined cobalamin plus folate deficiency. These are too expensive to use as initial screening tests. Serum MMA levels are elevated in more than 95% of patients with clinically confirmed cobalamin deficiency (with median values of 3500 nM). Serum homocysteine concentrations are elevated in both cobalamin deficiency (median values of 70 μM) and folate deficiency (median values of 50 μM). Both homocysteine and MMA rise with dehydration or renal failure. Propionic acid, derived from anaerobic fecal bacterial metabolism, can raise MMA, which can be lowered by a course of metronidazole. The abnormally high metabolites return to normal in a week with the appropriate (deficient) vitamin replacement.

Clinicians can use serum MMA and homocysteine to assist in the diagnosis of patients with the following: borderline cobalamin and folate levels (see Table 164-4); existing conditions known to perturb folate and cobalamin tests, leading to difficulties in interpreting the results; low levels of both cobalamin and folate, in which case a high MMA level is useful to confirm cobalamin deficiency (rather than attributing the condition to folate deficiency alone); and low serum cobalamin levels when there is an alternative explanation for the syndrome that led to the test (e.g., a diabetic or alcoholic patient with peripheral neuropathy, or an alcoholic patient with a high MCV and low cobalamin level without anemia).

Bone Marrow Examination

In a plausible clinical setting for a patient with severe hematologic disease, the identification of nucleated red cells with megaloblastic features in the peripheral smear and classic macro-ovalocytes and hypersegmented polymorphonuclear neutrophils—which reflects the morphology in the bone marrow—can help clinch the diagnosis of megaloblastosis. If they are not found, a bone marrow aspirate can be invaluable in making a rapid diagnosis of megaloblastosis in a patient with severe anemia lacking classic findings. In the outpatient setting, when there is less urgency and anemia is only mild to moderate in a patient with a suggestive peripheral smear or when the clinical presentation is primarily neuropsychiatric, a good case can be made to initiate the sequence of diagnostic tests without bone marrow aspiration and to proceed with the measurement of serum levels of vitamins or metabolites (see Table 164-4 and Fig. 164-2).

On the bone marrow aspirate (Fig. 164-4), which is better than biopsy for observing megaloblastosis, the cells are actually proliferating very slowly despite what looks like exuberant cell proliferation with numerous mitotic figures. In early cobalamin or folate deficiency, normoblasts may dominate the marrow, with only a few megaloblasts seen, but the full spectrum of megaloblastic hematopoiesis is observed in severe deficiency and is accompanied by varying degrees of pancytopenia. In contrast to the normally dense chromatin of comparable normoblasts, megaloblastic erythroid precursors have an open, finely stippled, reticular, sieve-like pattern. The orthochromatic megaloblast, with its hemoglobinized cytoplasm, continues to retain its large, sieve-like immature nucleus, in sharp contrast to the clumped chromatin of orthochromatic normoblasts. Up to 90% of megaloblastic cells die in the bone marrow, with remnants of apoptotic cells giving an impression of myelodysplastic syndrome. These are scavenged by macrophages in a process

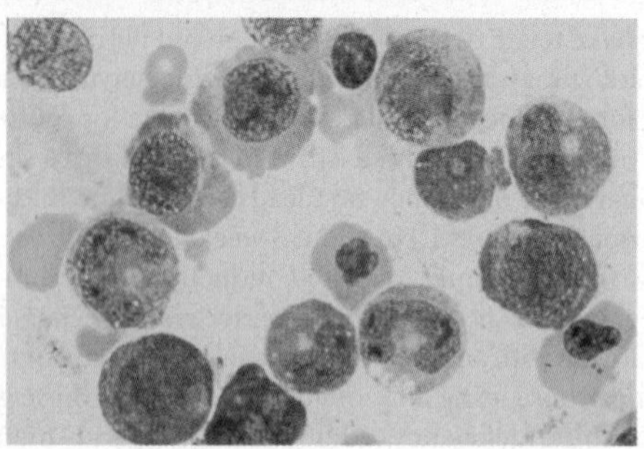

FIGURE 164-4. **Megaloblastic anemia. A bone marrow aspirate shows red blood cell precursors that are giant megaloblasts with nuclear-cytoplasmic dissociation (nuclear maturation lagging behind cytoplasmic maturation). Megaloblastic changes in the leukocyte series are shown by the "giant metamyelocyte."**

called ineffective erythropoiesis or intramedullary hemolysis. There is an increase in white blood cell production, with megaloblastic leukocytes also having a sieve-like chromatin. Giant (20 to 30 μm) metamyelocytes and "band" forms are pathognomonic for megaloblastosis. Hypersegmented polymorphonuclear leukocytes will be seen in the marrow and peripheral blood. Megakaryocytes may be normal or increased in number and can exhibit complex hypersegmentation, with liberation of fragments of cytoplasm and giant platelets into the circulation. The net output of platelets is decreased in severe megaloblastosis.

Determining the Cause of the Vitamin Deficiency

By the time that megaloblastic anemia is established, the cause of folate deficiency is usually clear from the history, physical examination, and clinical setting. With rare exceptions, adults with cobalamin deficiency have either cobalamin malabsorption or dietary cobalamin insufficiency. Whereas dietary cobalamin insufficiency is diagnosed by a dietary history and is easily prevented by small doses of prophylactic daily oral cobalamin, all other causes of cobalamin malabsorption respond to either parenteral cobalamin (warranting multiple loading doses followed by monthly maintenance) or daily high doses of oral cobalamin (1 to 2 mg/day). This raises a fundamental question: Why do we need to pursue the cause of cobalamin malabsorption? One practical reason is to determine the need for additional diagnostic tests (e.g., intestinal biopsy, examination of stool for malabsorption or *D. latum* infestation) to institute specific therapy (e.g., gluten-free diet, folate, antibiotics, anthelmintics). This evaluation, in turn, dictates whether cobalamin replacement should be lifelong.

The Schilling test, which was discontinued in 2003, provided such leads on the locus and mechanism of cobalamin malabsorption. Nowadays, without this test, the low sensitivity of serum anti–intrinsic factor antibodies allows only 60% of patients with pernicious anemia to be confidently identified through this measurement. Even poorer performance characteristics have rendered serum antiparietal cell antibodies diagnostically unhelpful. Although increased fasting levels of gastrin and low levels of pepsinogen I (a combination that suggests oxyntic gastric mucosal damage, like atrophy and hypochlorhydria) lack specificity, their sensitivity for detection of pernicious anemia is 90 to 92%. Therefore, some hematologists combine the specific but insensitive serum anti–intrinsic factor antibody test with the sensitive but nonspecific serum gastrin or pepsinogen I abnormalities to rule out pernicious anemia in patients with cobalamin deficiency in view of the loss of availability of the Schilling test.[11]

Because most of the conditions predisposing to cobalamin deficiency (see Table 164-1) should be clinically evident by the time that cobalamin deficiency is apparent, it is possible to identify several conditions through a detailed dietary history or past medical history. Such an exercise can point to esophagogastroduodenal disease, pancreatic insufficiency, impaired bowel motility, or other autoimmune diseases. The physical examination can also provide additional clues and suggest focused testing for rarer conditions (stool for ova; serum anti–tissue transglutaminase antibodies, lipase, or gastrin; intestinal biopsy; or radiographic contrast studies for stasis, strictures, or fistulas). Thus, by this classical medicine approach, it should be possible to identify the basis for cobalamin malabsorption and the duration of therapy in most instances (even without the Schilling test). For the younger patient with megaloblastic anemia, distinguishing juvenile pernicious anemia from congenital intrinsic factor deficiency warrants measurement of gastric juice for intrinsic factor and achlorhydria, and Imerslund-Gräsbeck syndrome requires DNA to detect mutations in cubam receptor (amnionless, cubilin) genes (see Table 164-1).

TABLE 164-5 CAUSES OF MEGALOBLASTIC ANEMIA NOT RESPONDING TO THERAPY WITH COBALAMIN OR FOLATE

Wrong diagnosis
Combined folate and cobalamin deficiencies being treated with only one vitamin
Associated iron deficiency
Associated hemoglobinopathy (e.g., sickle cell disease, thalassemia)
Associated anemia of chronic disease
Associated hypothyroidism

The utility of measurement of blood levels of holotranscobalamin (cobalamin-bound transcobalamin II) to evaluate cobalamin deficiency requires further clinical validation.

TREATMENT Rx

If a severely anemic patient is decompensated or decompensation is imminent, after blood is drawn for diagnostic studies, the patient is transfused slowly with initially only 1 U of packed red cells under diuretic coverage, and both cobalamin and folate are immediately started at full doses (parenteral cobalamin 1 mg/day plus folic acid 1 mg/day), even before the type of vitamin deficiency has been established. If the patient is only moderately symptomatic, transfusions should be avoided because a dramatic improvement in well-being is likely to occur within 2 to 3 days of starting full-dose vitamin replacement, even before hematologic improvement. If the patient is well compensated or in the ambulatory setting, diagnostic testing should proceed in an orderly sequence (see Fig. 164-2 and Table 164-4) before therapy is initiated.

Drug Dosage

Established Cobalamin Deficiency

For patients with severe cobalamin deficiency from any cause, an aggressive scheme to replace cobalamin rapidly is 1 mg/day of intramuscular or subcutaneous cyanocobalamin (week 1), 1 mg twice weekly (week 2), 1 mg/week for 4 weeks, and then 1 mg/month for life. For mild cobalamin deficiency, one can employ oral cobalamin 2 mg/day for 3 months, which exploits passive intestinal diffusion, through which 1 to 2% of the oral dose is absorbed. Once stores are fully replenished, those with cobalamin malabsorption can either continue with monthly maintenance or be switched to daily oral cobalamin 2 mg/day. For nutritional cobalamin deficiency, lifelong daily oral cobalamin (5 to 10 μg), with either tablets or equivalent cobalamin-fortified foods, should be instituted, but only after cobalamin stores are replenished. It is worth reminding patients that food intake reduces absorption of oral cobalamin by 50%.

In cobalamin deficiency associated with either pernicious anemia or food cobalamin malabsorption, the malabsorption of iron (due to achlorhydria) requires oral iron coadministered with organic acids (e.g., ascorbic acid) or total-dose parenteral iron replacement (e.g., low-molecular-weight iron dextran) (Chapter 159) to elicit a complete hematologic response.

An incomplete response must trigger a search for additional conditions (Table 164-5).

Subclinical Cobalamin Deficiency

The entity of subclinical cobalamin deficiency is encountered when an apparently asymptomatic patient has serum cobalamin values that either hover or fluctuate just above or just below normal cutoff values for many months and sometimes even inexplicably return to the normal range. This can sometimes be due to a deficiency of transcobalamin I, which binds the bulk of serum cobalamin but is of little clinical significance. Some experts proceed to obtain metabolite studies and then ignore cobalamin values if the MMA level is normal. Others periodically observe these patients and treat with cobalamin only when patients exhibit symptoms or signs of frank cobalamin deficiency. Yet others err on the side of caution, preferring to preemptively replenish depleted cobalamin stores and thereby circumvent any potential for the patient to develop impaired cognitive function, which can be detected only by specialized neurophysiologic testing, or even frank cerebral atrophy, which has been documented by magnetic resonance imaging.[A4] Accordingly, they empirically treat those with borderline cobalamin levels for 6 months with oral cobalamin (1 to 2 mg/day) and reassess serum cobalamin levels to ensure that values have returned to a mid to upper end of the normal range. This approach warrants repeated testing of cobalamin levels 6 to 12 months later to evaluate whether there has been an interim fall in cobalamin levels. At that time, options of either instituting cobalamin for the long term or alternating treatment for the first 6 months with no treatment for the next 6 months can be discussed with the patient.

Established Folate Deficiency

Oral folate (folic acid) at doses of 1 mg/day results in adequate absorption despite intestinal malabsorption of physiologic food folate. Therapy should be continued until complete hematologic recovery is documented; the subsequent duration of therapy is dictated by the cause. Folinic acid bypasses any block in one-carbon metabolism induced by methotrexate, trimethoprim-sulfamethoxazole, or N_2O.

Prophylaxis with Cobalamin or Folate

Several conditions are prevented by specific treatment designed either to lower homocysteine or to improve folate status (E-Table 164-2; see also Table 164-2). As one example, in elderly subjects with mild cognitive impairment, homocysteine lowering by a cocktail that included cobalamin and folate during 2 years did slow the rate of brain atrophy by almost 30%.[A4] For vegetarians, cobalamin-fortified foods (soy or rice beverages, fortified cereals, nutritional yeast) or oral cobalamin tablets 5 to 10 µg/day should suffice. For those with malabsorption of cobalamin from any other mechanism (see Table 164-1), cobalamin replacement is achieved with 1- to 2-mg tablets taken orally each day.

Periconceptional folate supplementation for all normal women (400 µg/day of folic acid) and for women who have previously delivered a baby with a neural tube defect (4 mg/day of folic acid) is now standard and prevents nearly three quarters of neural tube defects. Women of childbearing age who are taking anticonvulsant medications (phenytoin, phenobarbital, carbamazepine) are also at increased risk for delivering babies with neural tube defects and should routinely take 1 mg of folic acid daily. Moreover, administration of folic acid before initiation of phenytoin can eliminate the risk of gingival hyperplasia.[A8] Folate supplementation throughout pregnancy also helps prevent premature delivery of low-birthweight infants and is recommended for premature infants and lactating mothers. Folic acid supplements (1 mg/day orally) are taken by patients with hemolysis or myeloproliferative diseases and also to reduce the toxicity of methotrexate in patients with rheumatoid arthritis and psoriasis. Those individuals in whom cobalamin deficiency develops while they are receiving long-term folate replacement will present with a pure neurologic syndrome and not necessarily anemia.

The mandatory fortification of food (flour, enriched pasta, cornmeal, cereal foods) with 140 and 150 µg of folic acid per 100 g in the United States and Canada, respectively, has led to several beneficial effects (see Table 164-2). Indeed, 94% of U.S. adults who do not consume supplements or consume less than 400 µg/day of folic acid from supplements do not exceed the upper intake limit for folic acid (>1 mg/day), which has potential to mask cobalamin deficiency. Studies that have investigated adverse effects of fortification on development or progression of cancer have not identified that this is an issue.[A9] Moreover, folate deficiency–related anemia has nearly been eliminated in older U.S. adults after folate fortification.[12]

Prophylaxis in Resource-Limited Settings

Children of mothers from resource-limited countries with nutritional folate and cobalamin deficiency are at risk for cognitive dysfunction as toddlers and as young children[13]; hence, they deserve early prophylaxis with both folate and cobalamin. The serious and chronic problem of iron, folate, and cobalamin deficiency, especially among women in North India, which is due to poor dietary intake, and the high incidence of neural tube defects[14] warrant improving their nutrition through the use of iron, folate, and vitamin B_{12} supplements. Moreover, all pregnant women living in resource-limited malarious areas are at risk for iron, folate, and vitamin B_{12} deficiency[15] and malaria, so they should routinely be given intermittent preventive treatment according to the latest guidelines; currently, it is sulfadoxine-pyrimethamine (Chapter 345) together with insecticide-treated bed nets, plus 1 mg folic acid, prophylactic vitamin B_{12} (~10 to 25 µg), and replacement doses of oral iron. Likewise, women requiring antimalarial treatment should also be given iron, folate, and vitamin B_{12} to enable optimal hematopoiesis. Finally, although *Plasmodium falciparum* possesses two folate transporter proteins, in vitro as well as clinical studies using low-dose folic acid (1 mg/day) in 467 pregnant women with malaria have demonstrated benefit; by contrast, high-dose folic acid (5 mg/day) can "feed the parasite" and is contraindicated. Finally, optimizing the nutrition of the approximately 500 million adolescent girls before they become pregnant is a priority because maternal death is one of the most common causes of death for teenage girls between 15 and 19 years of age.

PROGNOSIS

The general response to cobalamin replacement is a dramatic improvement in well-being, with alertness, a good appetite, and resolution of a sore tongue. Megaloblastic hematopoiesis reverts to normal within 12 hours and resolves by 48 hours; the only persistent findings may be giant metamyelocytes in the bone marrow and hypersegmented neutrophils in the blood for up to 14 days. The reticulocyte count peaks by days 5 to 8, followed by a rise in the red cell count, hemoglobin level, and hematocrit. By the end of the first week, the white blood cell count rises, sometimes with a transient left shift, as does the platelet count; all three cell counts should normalize in 2 months.

With cobalamin replacement, the degree of reversal of neurologic damage is generally inversely related to the extent of disease and the duration of signs and symptoms. Most neurologic abnormalities improve in up to 90% of patients with documented subacute combined degeneration, and most signs and symptoms of less than 3 months' duration are reversible. With signs and symptoms of longer duration, there is invariably some residual neurologic dysfunction. The maximal response often takes up to 6 months, but recovery beyond 12 months is unusual.

Incorrect treatment of cobalamin deficiency with folate does not improve the neuropsychiatric abnormalities, which will continue to progress; hematologic improvements often occur, however. Alternatively, there may be associated iron deficiency or hypothyroidism that needs specific replacement or another hemoglobinopathy (e.g., sickle cell disease, thalassemia) that limits the normalization of hemoglobin values (see Tables 164-3 and 164-5).

In patients with pernicious anemia, subsequent iron deficiency anemia (Chapter 159), osteoporosis (Chapter 243) with fractures of the proximal end of the femur and vertebrae, gastrinoma and gastric cancer (Chapter 192), and cancer of the buccal cavity and pharynx can develop. Some experts recommend periodic upper endoscopic surveillance.

CLINICAL PRACTICE IN RESOURCE-LIMITED SETTINGS

Masking of Folate Deficiency with Associated Cobalamin Deficiency or Malaria

In resource-limited settings where vegetarianism or poverty-imposed near-vegetarianism is common, nutritional cobalamin as well as folate deficiency and hemolysis accompanying malaria often coexist. In such settings, the serum folate level is artificially raised in cobalamin deficiency and returns to baseline only after cobalamin replacement; likewise, the serum folate level is increased during hemolysis, which releases the extant 30-fold higher erythrocyte folate concentration into plasma. In this setting, measurement of the serum folate concentration will reveal normal to high values, predictably underestimate the tissue folate status, and completely miss the diagnosis of mild to moderate folate deficiency (see E-Table 164-1). By contrast, the dietary history or more formal assessment with a variety of methods (such as 24-hour recall, estimated/weighed record, or locally validated food frequency questionnaires), which are established methods to evaluate the quality and quantity of nutrients consumed, can predict the dietary folate and cobalamin intake of a population and identify those at risk for nutritional insufficiency.[15] Indeed, knowledge of dietary folate and cobalamin intake trumps the results of conventional blood tests for folate deficiency, which are seriously flawed in this clinical setting. In summary, all individuals at risk for nutritional anemia due to deficiency of iron, folate, and cobalamin (both adults and children) should be given prophylactic oral cobalamin, folate, and iron replacement; and in malarious zones, these should be combined with antimalarial drugs and insecticide-treated bed nets.

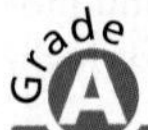

Grade A References

A1. Yang J, Hu X, Zhang Q, et al. Homocysteine level and risk of hip fracture: a meta-analysis and systematic review. *Bone*. 2012;51:376-382.

A2. Qin X, Xu M, Zhang Y, et al. Effect of folic acid supplementation on the progression of carotid intima-media thickness: a meta-analysis of randomized controlled trials. *Atherosclerosis*. 2012;222:307-313.

A3. Christen WG, Glynn RJ, Chew EY, et al. Folic acid, pyridoxine, and cyanocobalamin combination treatment and age-related macular degeneration in women: the Women's Antioxidant and Folic Acid Cardiovascular Study. *Arch Intern Med*. 2009;169:335-341.

A4. Smith AD, Smith SM, de Jager CA, et al. Homocysteine-lowering by B vitamins slows the rate of accelerated brain atrophy in mild cognitive impairment: a randomized controlled trial. *PLoS ONE*. 2010;5:e12244.

A5. Walker JG, Batterham PJ, Mackinnon AJ, et al. Oral folic acid and vitamin B-12 supplementation to prevent cognitive decline in community-dwelling older adults with depressive symptoms—the Beyond Ageing Project: a randomized controlled trial. *Am J Clin Nutr*. 2012;95:194-203.

A6. Wang X, Qin X, Demirtas H, et al. Efficacy of folic acid supplementation in stroke prevention: a meta-analysis. *Lancet*. 2007;369:1876-1882.

A7. Durga J, Verhoef P, Anteunis LJ, et al. Effects of folic acid supplementation on hearing in older adults: a randomized, controlled trial. *Ann Intern Med*. 2007;146:1-9.

A8. Arya R, Gulati S, Kabra M, et al. Folic acid supplementation prevents phenytoin-induced gingival overgrowth in children. *Neurology*. 2011;76:1338-1343.

A9. Vollset SE, Clarke R, Lewington S, et al. Effects of folic acid supplementation on overall and site-specific cancer incidence during the randomised trials: meta-analyses of data on 50,000 individuals. *Lancet*. 2013;381:1029-1036.

A10. House AA, Eliasziw M, Cattran DC, et al. Effect of B-vitamin therapy on progression of diabetic nephropathy: a randomized controlled trial. *JAMA*. 2010;303:1603-1609.

GENERAL REFERENCES

For the General References and other additional features, please visit Expert Consult at https://expertconsult.inkling.com.

165

APLASTIC ANEMIA AND RELATED BONE MARROW FAILURE STATES

GROVER C. BAGBY

DEFINITION

Aplastic anemia is a life-threatening syndrome characterized by failure of the bone marrow to produce peripheral blood cells and their progenitors. Diverse diseases and environmental factors can cause this syndrome, but its hallmark is bone marrow hypocellularity and hypoplasia of the erythroid, myeloid, and megakaryocyte lines (Fig. 165-1).

EPIDEMIOLOGY

The annual incidence is 2 per 1 million persons in Europe and North America and 4 to 7 per 1 million persons in Asia. No age group is exempt, and although the syndrome occurs most often in young adults, the age distribution of newly diagnosed patients is bimodal, with peaks at 15 to 25 years and at 60 to 65 years.

PATHOBIOLOGY

Pathology

Peripheral blood pancytopenia is universally present in patients with aplastic anemia, but because other disorders can cause pancytopenia, bone marrow biopsy is required to establish the diagnosis. The diagnosis will be clear-cut if the biopsy specimen is of sufficient size and has been obtained from an anatomic site that has never been exposed to extensive trauma or irradiation. As shown in Figure 165-1B, some residual lymphoid cell populations can be found in marrow specimens. Although these lymphoid cells may be of pathophysiologic importance, it is the absence of *nonlymphoid* hematopoietic cells that is important in establishing the diagnosis of this syndrome. However, if the hematopoietic marrow has been suppressed (or "replaced") by the infiltration of neoplastic cells or fibroblasts, the diagnosis of aplastic anemia cannot be made. Therefore, the diagnosis requires not only a dearth of hematopoietic cells in the marrow but also an "empty" bone marrow.

Some bone marrow failure syndromes affect only one lineage. In those cases, only the marrow precursors of that lineage are missing. In patients with agranulocytosis, for example, there are rare neutrophils and neutrophil precursors present, and the ratio of erythroid to myeloid cells is very high. Likewise, in patients with the disorder known as pure red cell aplasia, few erythroid cells are detectable in the marrow, but the other lineages are well represented and functional. These two disorders are examples of bone marrow failure syndromes but are not examples of aplastic anemia, which involves global suppression of all hematopoietic lineages.

Pathophysiology

Marrow aplasia in a few patients (10 to 15%) can be attributed to an inherited bone marrow failure syndrome,[1] but most cases are acquired. In all cases, it is clear that the causative factors, genetic or environmental, injure pluripotent hematopoietic stem cells. This is in contrast to the case of the lineage-restricted disorders, wherein the causative agents and factors suppress the growth and development of unipotent progenitor cells committed to that particular lineage. Radiation, viral diseases, cytotoxic drugs, and chemicals are known causes of aplastic anemia, but the most common form of acquired aplastic anemia is immunologically mediated, and evidence is emerging that some marrow failure states attributed to viral infection or to idiosyncratic drug reactions may also result from immune suppression of hematopoiesis. The pathogenesis of the major causes of aplastic anemia and related bone marrow failure states is outlined in Table 165-1.

Pathogenesis

Autoimmune Aplastic Anemia

Acquired Aplastic Anemia

In patients with the most common form of acquired aplastic anemia, autologous T lymphocytes suppress the replicative activity and induce the death of hematopoietic stem and progenitor cells. Evidence supporting this model is found in studies demonstrating the following: removal of T lymphocytes from cultured bone marrow cells enhances hematopoiesis in vitro; patients with aplastic anemia can be effectively treated with immunosuppressive therapy alone[2]; oligoclonal T cells in the marrow and blood of aplastic anemia

TABLE 165-1 MAJOR CAUSES OF APLASTIC ANEMIA AND RELATED BONE MARROW FAILURE STATES

- Autoimmune aplastic anemia
  - Acquired
  - Drug induced
  - Infections
    - Hepatitis
    - Epstein-Barr virus
- Autoimmune-mediated failure of single hematopoietic lineages
  - Agranulocytosis
  - Pure red cell aplasia
- Direct stem cell toxicity
  - Radiation
  - Chemicals
  - Drugs
- Other aplastic states
  - Pregnancy
  - Paroxysmal nocturnal hemoglobinuria
  - Inherited bone marrow failure syndromes

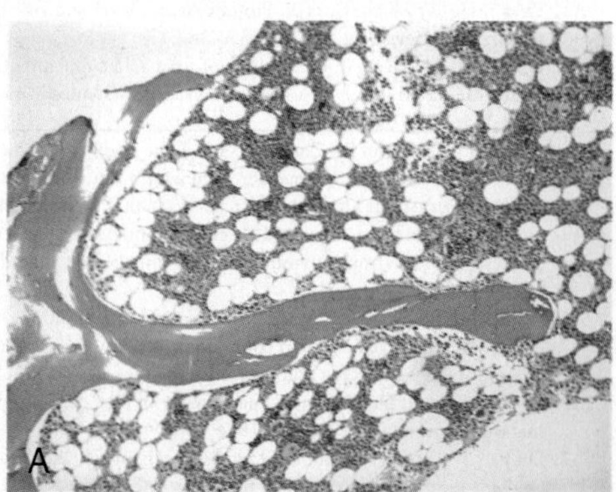

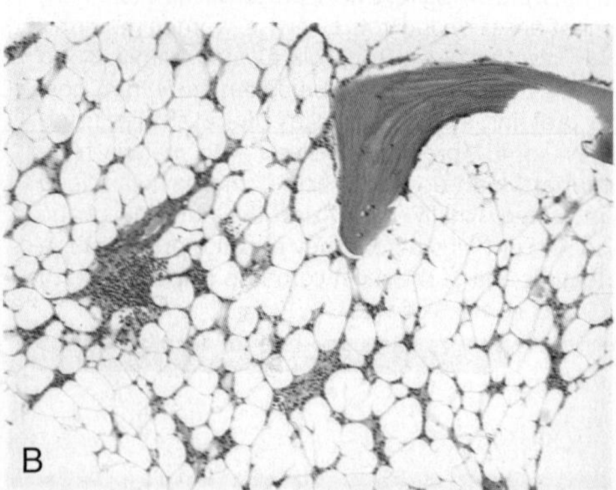

FIGURE 165-1. Two bone marrow biopsy samples from different patients. A, This specimen, from a normal individual, shows an abundance of hematopoietic cells, including myeloid and erythroid precursors and normal-appearing megakaryocytes. **B,** A specimen from a patient with severe aplastic anemia shows few detectable hematopoietic cells, and those that can be seen (one small nest) are largely lymphocytes. Lymphoid cells are often detectable and probably play an important pathophysiologic role in many cases of acquired idiopathic aplastic anemia, a disorder that is most often immunologically mediated. (Courtesy Dr. Ken Gatter, Oregon Health and Science University.)

patients contain high intracellular levels of the myelosuppressive cytokines interferon-γ and tumor necrosis factor-α; the interferon-γ/tumor necrosis factor-α–positive T-cell populations are suppressed in patients who respond to immunosuppressive therapy but are not suppressed in patients who do not respond; and the syndrome can be modeled in mice by infusing alloreactive lymphocytes that induce marrow failure. The mechanisms by which such autoinhibitory T-cell clones arise are unclear, but a loss of function in the regulatory T-cell population may play a role.[3]

Drug Induced

Although a wide variety of drugs have been associated with aplastic anemia, the association is loose. Much of the evidence is circumstantial, and apart from drugs that are known to be directly toxic to the marrow (e.g., chemotherapeutic agents; Table 165-2), the cases are not related to total dose of the suspect agent. These "idiosyncratic" reactions are likely to be autoimmune. Some agents, chloramphenicol being the classic example, are capable of inducing both types of injury. High doses can lead to myelosuppression in all treated patients (which abates after discontinuation of the drug), but even low doses can cause rare idiosyncratic aplastic responses as well (which do not remit after discontinuation of the agent). Drugs that have been repeatedly associated with aplastic anemia are listed in Table 165-2.

Infections

HEPATITIS. About 2 to 5% of patients with severe aplastic anemia have had viral hepatitis (Chapters 148 and 149). Some cases were associated with hepatitis A or B, but most patients with the hepatitis-aplasia syndrome have had hepatitis of unclear type (non-A, -B, -C, -E, or -G). Most patients with this syndrome are younger than 20 years. The natural course is rapid, with a 1-year mortality rate of more than 90%. The immune system is probably involved in the pathophysiologic mechanism of this syndrome because T-cell clonotypes are shared among patients with this type of aplasia[4] and immunosuppressive therapy has been reported to induce meaningful remissions.

EPSTEIN-BARR VIRUS. In rare patients with aplastic anemia, evidence of active Epstein-Barr virus (EBV) infection has been discovered (Chapter 377). Because the virus does not infect progenitor cells or stem cells, it is most likely that EBV induces an aberrant immune response that generates either immunoglobulin- or T-lymphocyte–mediated hematopoietic suppression. Because only a minority of EBV-infected aplastic patients describe a history of typical infectious mononucleosis, it is equally likely that the aplastic state came first and that EBV infection or reactivation was a second event.

TABLE 165-2 DRUGS AND TOXINS ASSOCIATED WITH APLASTIC ANEMIA

DOSE DEPENDENT

Antineoplastic Agents

Antimetabolites: fluorouracil, mercaptopurine, 6-thioguanine, methotrexate, cytosine arabinoside, gemcitabine, fludarabine, cladribine, pentostatin, hydroxyurea

Alkylating and cross-linking agents: busulfan, cyclophosphamide, chlorambucil, nitrogen mustard, melphalan, cisplatin, carboplatin, ifosfamide, nitrosoureas (BCNU and CCNU), mitomycin C

Cytotoxic antibiotics: daunorubicin, doxorubicin, mitoxantrone

Plant alkaloids: vinblastine, paclitaxel

Topoisomerase inhibitors: etoposide

Antimicrobial Agents

Chloramphenicol, dapsone, fluorocytosine

Anti-inflammatory and Antirheumatic Agents

Colchicine

Insecticides

Chlordane, chlorophenothane (DDT), lindane, parathion

Other Chemicals

Benzene

Benzene-containing chemicals: kerosene, chlorophenols, carbon tetrachloride

DOSE INDEPENDENT

Idiosyncratic, likely immune mediated

(*Note:* Most agents on this list should be considered to be possibly associated with aplastic anemia.)

Antimicrobial Agents

Chloramphenicol, dapsone, sulfonamides, tetracycline, methicillin, amphotericin, quinacrine, chloroquine, pyrimethamine

Anticonvulsants

Hydantoins, carbamazepine, phenacemide, primidone, ethosuximide

Anti-inflammatory Agents

Phenylbutazone, indomethacin, ibuprofen, oxyphenbutazone, sulindac, naproxen

Antiarrhythmic Drugs

Quinidine, tocainide, procainamide

Metals

Gold, arsenic, mercury, bismuth

Antihistamines

Cimetidine, ranitidine, chlorpheniramine, pyrilamine, tripelennamine

Diuretics

Acetazolamide, furosemide, chlorothiazide, methazolamide

Hypoglycemic Agents

Chlorpropamide, tolbutamide

Antithyroid Drugs

Propylthiouracil, potassium perchlorate, methylthiouracil, methimazole, carbimazole

Antihypertensive Agents

Methyldopa, enalapril, captopril

Sedatives

Chlordiazepoxide, chlorpromazine, meprobamate, prochlorperazine

Autoimmune-Mediated Failure of Single Hematopoietic Lineages

Agranulocytosis

Agranulocytosis is characterized by severe neutropenia and suppression of granulopoiesis (also see Chapter 167). This disorder can be an idiosyncratic reaction to certain drugs and most likely involves immune suppression of granulopoietic progenitor cells. The disease almost always abates when the offending drug is discontinued. Agranulocytosis also occurs in patients with established autoimmune diseases, including systemic lupus erythematosus, Sjögren syndrome, and rheumatoid arthritis. In some cases, the disorder is caused by myelosuppressive antibodies; in others, it is caused by T lymphocytes that suppress granulopoiesis. Immunosuppressive therapy is often effective in such patients and should be used in patients whose agranulocytosis is severe and associated with recurrent infections.

Pure Red Cell Aplasia

Severe normochromic, normocytic anemia (Chapter 158) with a marked decrease in reticulocyte number is sometimes associated with selective hypoplasia of the erythroid marrow without loss of megakaryocytes and myeloid precursor cells. In immunocompromised hosts and patients with chronic hemolytic diseases, this disorder, known as pure red cell aplasia, can be caused by parvovirus B19 infection (Chapter 371), an agent that infects erythroid precursor cells and likely generates an erythroid suppressive immune response. This disease can also be mediated by T lymphocytes or natural killer cells that suppress cells of the erythroid lineage and in more uncommon cases by antibody-dependent suppression of erythropoiesis. Pure red cell aplasia can also develop as a complication of thymoma (Chapter 99) and in these circumstances is likewise caused by oligoclonal T-cell expansion that specifically suppresses erythroid progenitor cells. This disorder can also be associated with drug exposure (e.g., isoniazid, chlorpropamide, and phenytoin), lymphoid neoplasms (chronic lymphocytic leukemia; Chapter 184), and myelodysplasia (Chapter 182). Rarely, adults with Diamond-Blackfan anemia present with isolated erythroid suppression, but the degree to which the erythroid marrow is suppressed in such patients rarely matches the profound suppression seen in acquired cases of immune-mediated pure red cell aplasia.

Direct Stem Cell Toxicity

Radiation

The severity of myelosuppression induced by radiation and the degree to which the marrow can recover from that injury depend on the radiation dose, the timing of exposure, and the fraction of hematopoietic tissues exposed. Low-dose total body radiation causes transient marrow suppression. High doses of total body radiation (700 to 1000 cGy) induce severe injury to the stem cell pool with persistent and life-threatening marrow failure. In the past, direct radiation injury to hematopoietic stem cells was the accepted explanation for stem cell injury, but recent evidence indicates that injury to other tissues (especially the gut) results in the release of endogenous factors that themselves suppress hematopoiesis.[5] When limited bone marrow sites are irradiated to very high doses (4000 cGy or more), the relatively radioresistant bone marrow stromal cells are eradicated, and thereafter that marrow space can never fully support hematopoietic activity.

Chemicals

Benzene suppresses the bone marrow in a dose-dependent manner, and chronic exposure to it has been linked with aplastic anemia and myeloid leukemogenesis. Benzene and many of its catabolites are directly toxic to stem cells, damage DNA, suppress the supportive function of the bone marrow microenvironment, and accentuate the responsiveness of hematopoietic progenitor cells to intramedullary apoptotic cues that arise during the inflammatory response. Kerosene, carbon tetrachloride, and chlorophenols contain benzene, as do many other like products used for paint stripping, refinishing, and degreasing (see Table 165-2).

Drugs

Many agents in use for the treatment of malignant diseases are predictably myelosuppressive and can induce aplastic anemia because they are directly toxic to stem and progenitor cells in the marrow (see Table 165-2). These myelosuppressive responses are completely predictable and dose dependent. In practical terms, unless the patient receives a drug overdose or has an undiagnosed genetic disorder that predisposes the patient to respond to the agent in an exaggerated way (e.g., Fanconi anemia [FA]), most patients treated for neoplastic diseases develop reversible bone marrow aplasia or hypoplasia and recover bone marrow function within a matter of days.

Other Aplastic States

Pregnancy

Aplastic anemia can be diagnosed in pregnancy. In addition, some patients with aplastic anemia have become pregnant after the diagnosis. The prognosis in both instances is poor, and most fatal outcomes are due to bleeding complications. Some women who have been fortunate enough to recover bone marrow function post partum develop aplastic anemia with a subsequent pregnancy. The pathogenesis and causal relationship between pregnancy and aplastic anemia remain unknown but may reflect a high level of immunologic activation during pregnancy.

Paroxysmal Nocturnal Hemoglobinuria

Paroxysmal nocturnal hemoglobinuria (PNH) is an acquired disorder that results from the expansion of a clone of hematopoietic stem cells whose progeny are incapable of anchoring essential proteins to their membranes (Chapter 160).[6] The defect is caused by an inactivating somatic mutation of *PIGA*, an X-linked gene that encodes a protein essential for synthesis of the membrane anchor glycosyl phosphatidylinositol (GPI). Some of the GPI-anchored proteins (e.g., CD55 and CD59) are important in normal red cells to protect them from activated complement. Consequently, the loss of CD55 and CD59 results in chronic intravascular hemolysis. Two less clearly defined features of PNH are high relative risks of thromboembolism (Chapter 176) and aplastic anemia. The emergence of "PNH clones" is not uncommon in patients with acquired aplastic anemia, and experimental evidence supports the idea that the evolution of *PIGA*-deficient stem cells is an adaptive response to the immune attack. How the *PIGA*-deficient cells fend off cytotoxic T cells is less clear, but it is likely that their pool expands because they accomplish that task somehow. The most reasonable model is one in which, in the setting of an immune attack, *PIGA*-deficient stem cells are more fit than normal stem cells, but the complement-sensitive red cells to which they give rise as a result of this "tradeoff" have an unusually short lifespan.

Inherited Bone Marrow Failure Syndromes

Some inherited bone marrow failure syndromes can be manifested in adolescence and adulthood. They include dyskeratosis congenita, FA, and Diamond-Blackfan anemia. The molecular pathogenesis of the bone marrow failure seen in these diseases is under active investigation.[7] Although the genetic basis of these disorders has been well defined in the past decade, the canonical functions of the proteins encoded by these genes is distinct (Table 165-3) for each disease. For example, in dyskeratosis, the mutations occur in genes that encode proteins and RNAs involved in telomere maintenance. In FA, the mutations involve proteins involved in the DNA damage response, and in Diamond-Blackfan anemia, inactivating mutations involve ribosomal proteins known to be involved in ribosome biogenesis.[8] Whether loss of these canonical functions is linked with the pathogenesis of marrow failure is

TABLE 165-3 DISTINGUISHING CLINICAL FEATURES OF THE INHERITED BONE MARROW FAILURE SYNDROMES THAT MAY BE INITIALLY DIAGNOSED IN ADULTHOOD

DISTINGUISHING FEATURES	DISEASES: FANCONI ANEMIA	DISEASES: DYSKERATOSIS CONGENITA	DISEASES: DIAMOND-BLACKFAN ANEMIA
History	Skeletal and renal malformations, low birthweight, pancytopenia, family member with bone marrow failure, myelodysplasia, acute myelogenous leukemia, or squamous cell carcinoma at an early age Family member with Fanconi anemia	Intrauterine growth retardation, developmental delay, and short stature Family history of myelodysplasia, acute myelogenous leukemia, marrow failure, abnormal fingernails or toenails, leukoplakia, head and neck cancer, or pulmonary fibrosis	Low birthweight, arm and thumb deformities at birth
Physical findings	Thumb and radial malformations, hyperpigmented skin lesions (cafe au lait spots), short stature, myelodysplasia, acute myelogenous leukemia, squamous cell carcinoma at young age, renal and cardiac malformations, microcephaly, hypogonadism	Lacy reticular pigmentation of skin, dystrophic fingernails and toenails, premature graying of hair, hair loss, short stature, oral leukoplakia, squamous cell cancer of head and neck, pulmonary fibrosis, osteopenia, hypogonadism	Triphalangeal thumbs, short stature, arm anomalies
Genes inactivated	*FANCA, FANCB, FANCC, FANCD1* (also known as *BRCA2*), *FANCD2, FANCE, FANCF, FANCG* (also known as *BRCA2, FANCD2, FANCE, FANCF XRCC9*), *FANCI, FANCJ* (also known as *BRCA2, FANCD2, FANCE, FANCF BACH1,* and *BRIP1*), *FANCL* (also known as *PHF9* and *POG*), *FANCM* (also known as *Hef*), *FANCN* (also known as *PALB2*), *FANCO* (also known as *RAD51C*), and *FANCP* (also known as *BRCA2, FANCD2, FANCE, FANCF SLX4*) These genes encode proteins known to protect the genome from excessive damage induced by chemical cross-linking agents. These genes account for most cases of Fanconi anemia.	*DKC1, TERC, TERT, TINF2, NOLA2* (also known as *NHP2*) and *NOLA3* (also known as *NOP10*), and *WRAP53* These genes encode proteins known to participate in maintenance of telomeres. They account for only half of dyskeratosis cases, so there are additional genes to be discovered.	*RPS7, RPS10, RPS17, RPS19, RPS24, RPS26, RPL5, RPL11, RPL26,* and *RPL35A* These genes encode ribosomal proteins. They account for only half of cases, so there are additional genes to be discovered.
Screening and diagnostic tests	1. Chromosomal breakage test on skin fibroblasts or peripheral blood lymphocytes (in response to mitomycin C or diepoxybutane) 2. Complementation analysis (flow cytometric analysis of G_2 arrest in melphalan-exposed cells after transduction with retroviral vectors expressing normal Fanconi anemia genes) 3. Gene sequencing	1. Quantitative analysis of telomere length (flow-FISH) in lymphocytes 2. Gene sequencing	*Note:* Isolated erythroid failure is more common than full-blown aplastic anemia. 1. There are no screening tests, although serum ADA is often elevated. 2. Gene sequencing

ADA = adenosine deaminase; FISH = fluorescent in situ hybridization.

unclear. In fact, studies on hematopoietic cells have revealed noncanonical functions of some of these proteins. Some of the FA proteins, for example, participate directly or indirectly in stem cell survival signaling pathways. Interestingly, some of the pathways disrupted in mutant cells result in hyperactivation of precisely those same cytokine signaling pathways involved in the pathogenesis of acquired autoimmune aplastic anemia.[9]

Genetics

The genetic basis of inherited bone marrow failure syndromes is being rapidly solved. Some of these syndromes (e.g., Shwachman-Diamond syndrome, amegakaryocytic thrombocytopenia, and severe congenital neutropenia) are almost always diagnosed in early life. However, some may be first diagnosed in adulthood (e.g., dyskeratosis congenita, FA, and Diamond-Blackfan anemia). It is critically important to consider these three disorders early in the evaluation of adults with aplastic anemia because the treatment of such patients with conventional stem cell transplantation regimens is associated with high mortality rates (especially in dyskeratosis congenita and FA). Furthermore, current immunosuppressive therapy, an important therapeutic option in patients with acquired aplastic anemia, plays no role in these diseases. The clinical and laboratory manifestations of these three diseases and the findings that should prompt genetic testing in such patients are reviewed in Table 165-3. Whereas the stem cell defects can be identified during fetal development, adults who present with these diseases were not born with aplastic anemia. Instead, aplasia develops over time and can give rise to symptoms in adulthood. Prospective studies of children and adults who present with bone marrow failure have indicated that nearly 10% will have previously unsuspected FA. Diagnostic consideration of a hereditary form of aplastic anemia should not be limited to children.

CLINICAL MANIFESTATIONS

The natural course of aplastic anemia is influenced by its severity. Patients with hypoplastic bone marrows have severe aplastic anemia if they meet two of the following laboratory criteria: absolute neutrophil count of less than 0.5 $\times 10^9$/L; platelet count of less than 20 $\times 10^9$/L; or reticulocyte count of less than 20 $\times 10^9$/L. Patients who do not have severe aplastic anemia often progress to severe aplasia, but the pace is slow (about 40% will have progressed in 5 years). Severe aplastic anemia is a life-threatening condition that, untreated, is associated with a mortality rate of 80% in the 24 months after diagnosis. Treatment of any cohort of patients with severe aplastic anemia will prolong life, and many patients, particularly those who have received stem cell transplants, will be cured.

History

Symptoms of this syndrome, cause notwithstanding, are almost always reflective of low blood counts. The most common presenting symptoms are those associated with thrombocytopenia and anemia. Low platelet counts are associated with bleeding, often epistaxis and bleeding gums, bruising with minor or no trauma, and menorrhagia. Anemia accounts for the nearly universal symptoms of fatigue and dyspnea on mild exertion. Some aplastic patients may present with intercurrent bacterial or fungal infection (because of severe neutropenia), but these cases are less common. Family histories that include any of the features listed in Table 165-3 should raise suspicion of an inherited bone marrow failure syndrome.

Physical Examination

Pallor and tachycardia at rest are common signs of anemia but can be absent or unnoticeable in younger patients and in patients whose aplasia is of recent onset. Hemorrhagic manifestations classic for thrombocytopenia are often found: petechiae (cutaneous or palatal), ecchymoses, and epistaxis. The most common form of aplastic anemia, autoimmune, is rarely associated with lymphadenopathy or hepatosplenomegaly, and when such findings are present, alternative diagnoses should be considered and painstakingly ruled out. Likewise, concerns of an inherited bone marrow failure disease should be triggered by the following: short stature; endocrinopathies; osteopenia; findings of developmental anomalies of the skin, nails, hands, or arms; and malformations of the heart, liver, or genitourinary tract (see Table 165-3).

Initial Laboratory Findings

Pancytopenia (anemia, leukopenia, and thrombocytopenia) is a universal presenting finding. The morphology of neutrophils, platelets, and red cells on peripheral blood smear is usually normal unless there is concurrent iron deficiency due to bleeding.

DIAGNOSIS

The evaluation of pancytopenic patients first requires examination of the peripheral blood smear. If there are morphologic or clinical signs of vitamin B_{12} or folic acid deficiency (e.g., hypersegmented neutrophils and oval macrocytes), those disorders should be ruled out because a bone marrow aspiration and biopsy would not be required in those conditions. In severe aplastic anemia, the peripheral blood smear will not show nucleated red blood cells or other signs that the marrow might be infiltrated with abnormal cells. All patients in whom vitamin B_{12} and folate deficiency have been ruled out (Chapter 164) require a bone marrow aspiration and biopsy. Obtaining both types of samples is important. The biopsy best assesses overall bone marrow cellularity and provides the most sensitive evidence for some infiltrative processes. The aspirated sample can be examined microscopically for the presence of abnormal cells but also provides cells for cytogenetic analyses (which can provide evidence supporting hypoplastic myelodysplasia and acute leukemia). Rarely in the early stages of aplasia, the biopsy finding can be somewhat cellular. A repeated biopsy in 1 to 2 weeks might be required to establish the diagnosis clearly. As summarized in Figure 165-2, once the diagnosis of aplastic anemia has been made, a series of additional tests must be obtained. In light of the life-threatening nature of this disease, the tests must be obtained simultaneously, but they serve three distinct purposes.

Ruling Out Aplastic Anemia Variants That Must Be Treated Differently

The best therapeutic option for many different aplastic states is often matched sibling donor stem cell transplantation, but there are some aplastic states that are managed differently. For example, a child with an inherited marrow failure syndrome might have a human leukocyte antigen (HLA)–identical sibling who also has the same genetic defect. If such a diagnosis has been overlooked in the recipient and donor, the recipient will most likely die because the donor cells are unfit for transplantation and the conditioning regimen will be too toxic. For example, patients with FA are highly intolerant of radiation and cross-linking agents used in conventional conditioning regimens, and patients with dyskeratosis suffer excessive post-transplantation morbidity and mortality. Patients with dyskeratosis congenita and children with the Shwachman-Diamond syndrome are also intolerant of conventional transplantation regimens and often suffer severe pulmonary and hepatic toxicity. Although patients with Diamond-Blackfan anemia are more tolerant of standard conditioning regimens, they are more apt to respond to glucocorticosteroid therapy, and if they are transplanted with stem cells from an undiagnosed affected sibling, they too will do poorly. Finally, patients with PNH should be identified with flow cytometric quantification of CD55- and CD59-deficient hematopoietic cells because more than half of patients with severe aplastic anemia will have PNH clones, and on treatment with immunosuppressive therapy, the PNH clone often expands, resulting in hemolysis and thrombosis.

Tests Helpful in Supportive Care

At some point during the course of the disease, red cell and platelet transfusions will be necessary. Irradiated and filtered blood products are used to prevent transfusion-associated graft-versus-host disease (GVHD), to reduce alloimmunization, and to reduce the complication of cytomegalovirus (CMV) infection. ABO and HLA typing are required. Infections can be of bacterial, viral, or fungal origin and must be quickly diagnosed and treated not only because the patients are often neutropenic but also because, once definitive therapy begins, the patient will be immunosuppressed. In the acutely infected, severely neutropenic patient, once culture and biopsy specimens are obtained, empirical antibiotic therapy should be given without waiting for the culture results. Post-transplantation CMV infection is best avoided in CMV-seronegative recipients by use of CMV-negative blood products (Chapter 177).

Evaluating the Patient as a Candidate for Stem Cell Transplantation

Timing of treatment depends on the severity of the aplastic anemia and the age of the patient (Table 165-4). Patients with mild marrow hypoplasia and mild bone marrow suppression can be observed closely to determine what the pace of hypoplasia might be. In patients up to 40 years of age with either severe acquired aplastic anemia or transfusion dependence, steps should be taken to evaluate them promptly for stem cell transplantation therapy by

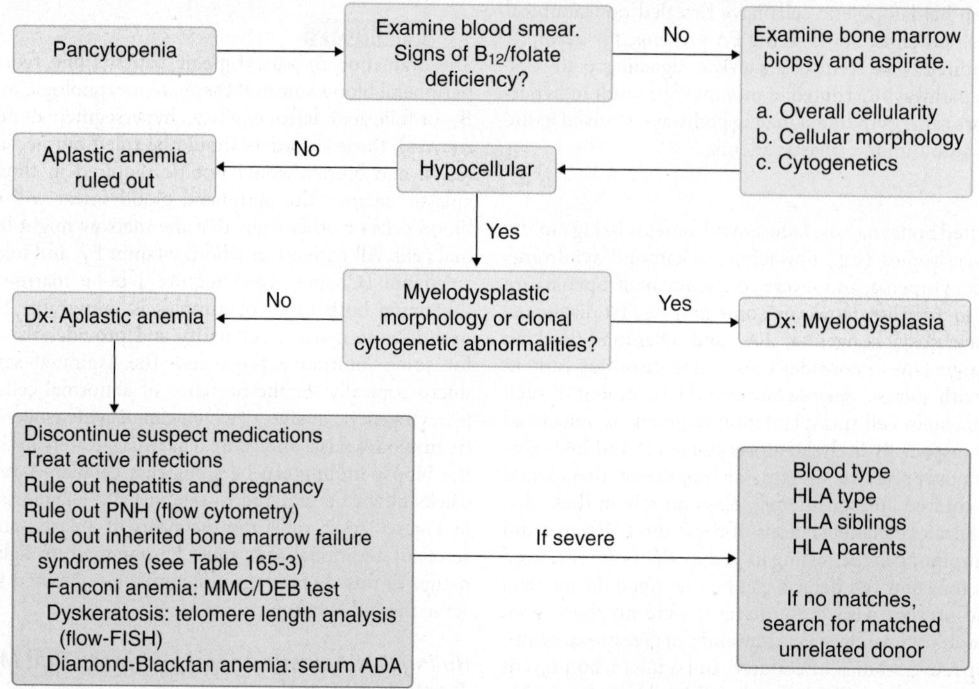

FIGURE 165-2. Diagnostic management of patients with aplastic anemia. Patients who present with pancytopenia will require bone marrow biopsy and aspiration unless there are signs of vitamin B_{12} or folate deficiency. If the bone marrow is as cellular as that shown in Figure 165-1A, the diagnosis of aplastic anemia has been effectively ruled out because the diagnosis requires bone marrow hypocellularity (see Fig. 165-1B). In all patients, regardless of severity, suspect medications should be discontinued, active infections should be treated without delay, and paroxysmal nocturnal hemoglobinuria (PNH) should be excluded, as should pregnancy and hepatitis. Microscopic evidence in the bone marrow sample of myelodysplastic changes and evidence of a clonal chromosomal abnormality indicate that the patient has "hypoplastic" myelodysplasia and should be treated accordingly. For patients with positive family histories or any one of the findings listed in Table 165-3 and for all patients younger than 40 years, inherited marrow failure syndromes should be ruled out with screening tests. Patients with severe aplastic anemia are those who have at least two of the following: absolute neutrophil count of less than 0.5×10^9/L, platelet count of less than 20×10^9/L, or reticulocyte count of less than 20×10^9/L. These patients must be treated with definitive therapy and should be evaluated for stem cell transplantation with human leukocyte antigen (HLA) typing (patient and family members) and, if necessary, a search for matched unrelated donors. ADA = adenosine deaminase; DEB = diepoxybutane; FISH = fluorescent in situ hybridization; MMC = mitomycin C.

TABLE 165-4 TREATMENT RECOMMENDATIONS FOR PATIENTS WITH SEVERE ACQUIRED IDIOPATHIC APLASTIC ANEMIA*

	AGE < 20 YEARS		AGE 20-40 YEARS		AGE > 40 YEARS	
HLA-identical sibling?	Yes	No	Yes	No	Yes	No
First-line treatment	MSBMT	IST	MSBMT	IST	IST	IST
Second-line treatment	IST or second MSBMT	IST or MUDT or CBT	IST	IST, eltrombopag, or MUDT	MSBMT	IST For failures, consider eltrombopag, clinical trials, or MUDT

*This general set of recommendations cannot be applied to patients with inherited bone marrow failure syndromes because they do not respond to immunosuppressive therapy.
CBT = umbilical cord blood transplantation; HLA = human leukocyte antigen; IST = immunosuppressive therapy; MSBMT = matched sibling bone marrow transplant; MUDT = matched unrelated donor transplant.
Modified from Bacigalupo A, Passweg J. Diagnosis and treatment of acquired aplastic anemia. *Hematol Oncol Clin North Am.* 2009;23:159-170.

seeking HLA-identical siblings and, in appropriate cases, searching for matched unrelated donors.

Differential Diagnosis

Most classic aplastic anemia patients have immunologically mediated disease. Notwithstanding strong evidence in support of this mechanism from some research laboratories during the past 30 years, there exists no validated screening tool or certified test that can either rule in or rule out immune-mediated disease, a fact complicated by the evidence that some cases of drug- and virus-induced disease are also immunologically mediated. Therefore, idiopathic autoimmune aplastic anemia remains a diagnosis of exclusion. For this reason, the obligation of the diagnostician is to consider disease induced by chemical or viral agents and radiation and disease associated with pregnancy. It is also most important to rule out PNH and inherited bone marrow failure syndromes (see Fig. 165-2).

Cytotoxic Drugs, Chemicals, and Radiation

A fastidiously obtained medication history is important. Any drug with the potential of inducing aplastic anemia should be discontinued. It is equally important to ask patients about alternative therapies that they might not consider to be "medicines." Some herbal remedies are known to contain molecules (e.g., phenylbutazone) not listed on the label but that are associated with aplasia (see Table 165-2). A history of exposure to radiation or to chemicals with myelosuppressive capacities (see Table 165-2) should likewise be obtained. Tests for benzene metabolites detect only acute exposure and are not reliable indicators of cumulative exposure in individual patients. Although it is intuitively obvious and prudent to discontinue the use of agents that might have inflicted severe stem cell injury, by the time the injury has progressed to the point of severe aplastic anemia, most of these patients are in need of the same types of therapy prescribed for patients with autoimmune aplastic anemia.

Idiosyncratic Drug Responses

If a medication history uncovers an exposure to an agent known to be associated with idiosyncratic (not related to dose) responses, the agent must likewise be discontinued. Because it is likely that these responses are immunologically mediated, the patient should be treated no differently from patients with severe idiopathic aplastic anemia, and the patient should be evaluated as a stem cell transplantation candidate. If, during the diagnostic evaluation of the patient and potential donors, there are signs that the marrow is recovering on its own, a more conservative approach can be taken.

Paroxysmal Nocturnal Hemoglobinuria

PNH can be ruled out by screening for CD55 and CD59 on the surface of granulocytes, monocytes, and red cells by flow cytometry. The proper diagnosis of PNH requires the absence of these or other GPI-anchored proteins on at least two hematopoietic cell types. Other characteristic features of this syndrome can be a high low-density lipoprotein level, high indirect bilirubin, low haptoglobin, and a positive urine hemosiderin test result.

Fanconi Anemia

FA should be considered in any adult of any age with a family history of aplastic anemia, acute myelogenous leukemia or myelodysplasia, or squamous cell carcinoma at an unusually young age. This disease should also be considered in any patient with any physical finding listed in Table 165-3 or in patients with a family member who has any of these findings. Unfortunately, some patients with FA meet none of these criteria, so some hematologists, including this author, advocate testing for FA in all patients with aplastic anemia younger than 40 years. This disease can be ruled out by obtaining a chromosomal breakage test (see Table 165-3). Here, either lymphocytes or skin fibroblasts are exposed to cross-linking agents (e.g., mitomycin C or diepoxybutane) for a period of 2 to 3 days, after which metaphase chromosomes are examined for chromosomal breaks and quadriradial forms (four-armed interchromosomal structures). If the clinical context is suggestive (see Table 165-3) but results of the lymphocyte chromosomal breakage test are negative or equivocal, testing of skin fibroblasts is required to rule out the diagnosis. Once the diagnosis is made, history, physical examination, blood counts, and chromosomal breakage tests should be performed on all immediate family members.

There are at least 15 different FA genes (see Table 165-3), and sequencing of them all with cells from every patient is not practical at this time. Fortunately, the involved gene can be first identified by a variety of more affordable complementation analyses. In this type of test, normal FA genes are introduced into primary cells of the patient in vitro, and the one gene that corrects the defect (i.e., reduces hypersensitivity to cross-linking agents [melphalan, mitomycin C, or diepoxybutane]) represents the gene of interest. That gene can then be fully sequenced to identify the precise mutation, information that will be of value to family members. In rare instances, it can also aid in applying preimplantation genetic diagnosis and in vitro fertilization, a process that has successfully resulted in unaffected offspring and ideal cord blood stem cell donors for transplantation of an affected sibling.

Dyskeratosis Congenita

Dyskeratosis congenita should be considered in any aplastic adult of any age with a family member who has had aplastic anemia. It should likewise be considered if either the patient or a family member has had acute myelogenous leukemia, myelodysplasia, nail dystrophy, lacy skin pigmentation, pulmonary fibrosis, oral leukoplakia, squamous cell carcinoma at an unusually young age, or any other physical finding listed in Table 165-3. This disease can be frequently ruled out by quantifying the length of telomeres in circulating white cells by a flow cytometric method. Because some of the physical findings overlap, FA should be ruled out in all patients being evaluated for dyskeratosis congenita. The dyskeratosis test quantifies telomere length with fluorescence in situ hybridization. Lymphocytes from dyskeratosis patients have extremely short telomeres (i.e., at or less than the first percentile). If two or three leukocyte types from a given patient are above the first percentile, the diagnosis of dyskeratosis is unlikely. If telomeres are in the diagnostic range, genetic testing is warranted. It is not yet known whether this test will become a "gold standard" test as reliable as the chromosomal breakage test is for FA because some investigators report that very short telomeres can be found in patients who have other causes of bone marrow failure. Unlike the genetic strategy employed with FA (at least today), complementation analyses are not routinely performed in dyskeratosis. The molecular diagnosis is based on gene sequencing. Once the diagnosis is made and even before the establishment of a molecular genetic diagnosis (see Table 165-3), all immediate family members of the patient should be seen individually, their history taken, and their physical examination performed along with peripheral blood counts and telomere length analysis.

Diamond-Blackfan Anemia

Diamond-Blackfan anemia is an inherited bone marrow failure syndrome that more often exhibits selective erythroid failure and is therefore an unusual cause of full-blown severe aplastic anemia. Although some patients can present in adulthood, most are discovered within the first year of life and present with anemia but less commonly neutropenia and thrombocytopenia. Phenotypic abnormalities like short stature and skeletal defects are the exception in this disease. Caused by mutations in one of at least 10 ribosomal proteins, there are no simple screening tests as reliable as those used for FA and dyskeratosis congenita. However, in patients with unexplained erythroid failure, the finding of an elevated adenosine deaminase level in the serum, although unexplained, is strongly suggestive of this disease, and genetic diagnosis should be considered. Because no validated screening test exists yet, there are no reliable or standardized complementation tests, and genetic diagnosis requires the application of gene sequencing methods (see Table 165-3).

Other Diagnostic Considerations

Aplastic anemia has been reported in recipients of organ allografts, in which mismatched T cells (either from the donated graft or from blood products that had not been irradiated) induce severe aplasia; in patients with myelodysplasia (Chapter 182); in patients with congenital and acquired immunodeficiency states (Chapter 250); and in patients with established autoimmune diseases including systemic lupus erythematosus (Chapter 266) and eosinophilic fasciitis[10] (Chapter 440), a disease characterized by painful swelling of the skin and subcutaneous tissue.

TREATMENT Rx

For patients with milder forms of aplastic anemia, aggressive therapy may not be indicated. A passive approach is more problematic in patients with FA and dyskeratosis congenita because transplantation early in life is better tolerated, immunosuppressive therapy is ineffective, and stem cell transplantation provides the only hope for cure of bone marrow failure. If there is evidence of an underlying autoimmune-mediated disease (e.g., isolated granulopoietic or erythroid failure in patients with rheumatic diseases or thymoma), immunosuppressive therapy alone is often highly effective. In fact, for severe aplastic anemia, immunosuppressive therapy either alone or associated with stem cell transplantation is required. Hematopoietic growth factors alone have been disappointingly ineffective until recently in studies using eltrombopag, a small-molecule agonist of the thrombopoietin receptor (Chapter 172). In a phase II study (starting with 50 mg daily and increasing as needed to a maximum of 150 mg daily, for a total of 12 weeks), this agent induced responses in at least one cell lineage in 44% of patients with refractory severe aplastic anemia,[11] and some responders have done well for two or more years.[12] Because of the theoretical potential for this agent to enhance clonal evolution, its role in the treatment of patients remains to be elucidated, and there are ongoing clinical trials being conducted to that end. Eltrombopag also can restore trilineage hematopoiesis in a subset of patients who are refractory to immunosuppressive therapy.

Hematopoietic Stem Cell Transplantation: Matched Sibling Donor

For patients with severe aplastic anemia, stem cell transplantation offers the advantages of immunosuppression, an infusion of new "healthy" stem cells, and the expectation that the lymphoid cells that suppressed the marrow in the first place will be replaced by more normal cells that have no myelosuppressive capacity. This expectation is supported by large retrospective studies suggesting that stem cell transplantation is superior to immunosuppressive therapy alone for the treatment of severe aplastic anemia, especially in patients younger than 40 years. In the past, this approach was relevant to a minority of patients because only 25 to 30% will have an HLA-matched sibling, but substantial improvements in outcomes for recipients of matched unrelated stem cell transplants have made such stem cell sources reasonable to consider, particularly in patients who have failed to respond to immunosuppressive therapy.[13] No perfectly designed study comparing "front-end" immunosuppressive therapy with stem cell transplantation has been conducted, so patients need to be clearly informed about the risks and benefits of each approach. For patients considering transplantation as a first-line therapy, the unique risks of early treatment-related mortality and later risk of GVHD should be reviewed (Chapter 178). Patients considering immunosuppressive therapy without transplant should be aware of the risks of recurrence and late life-threatening clonal evolution to myelodysplasia or acute leukemia.

Unless the donor is a twin (in which case, peripheral blood–derived stem cells may be preferable[14]), stem cells derived from the bone marrow, not the peripheral blood, should be the source of donor cells.[15] Studies testing the comparative effectiveness of peripheral blood as a source of stem cells have reported that the peripheral blood source is associated with excess mortality stemming from an increased incidence of chronic GVHD. The recipient (in whom congenital marrow failure syndromes have been ruled out) initially receives high-dose cyclophosphamide with either horse antithymocyte

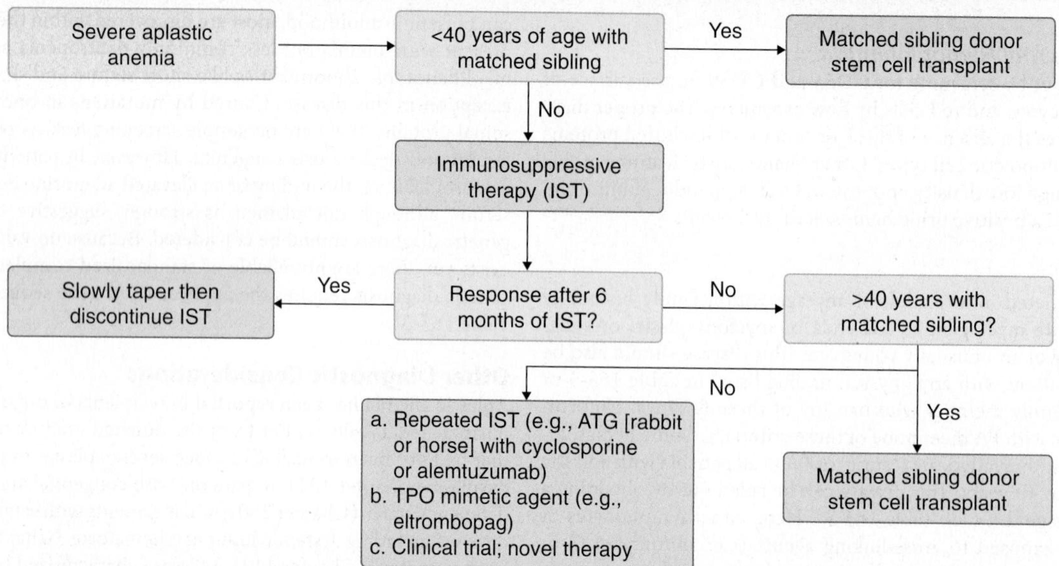

FIGURE 165-3. A therapeutic approach to management of severe aplastic anemia. There are no published results that clarify whether first-line therapy with immunosuppressive therapy (IST) alone is inferior to stem cell transplantation for patients with aplastic anemia. One accepted approach[18] takes into account the high incidence of complications in older patients receiving transplants and suggests matched sibling donor stem cell transplants for any patient younger than 40 years. The remainder receive IST. Because remissions can occur late, 6 months of therapy is required. If there is no response in a patient older than 40 years who also has a matched sibling, stem cell transplantation can be considered at that time. For those without a matched donor, reasonable alternatives are repeated IST, eltrombopag, and enrollment in a clinical trial of novel therapy. A similar approach focusing on the patient's age as a key element in the decision tree is outlined in Table 165-4. ATG = antithymocyte globulin; TPO = thrombopoietin.

globulin (ATG) or alemtuzumab[16,17] as the preparative regimen. Immunosuppressive therapy begins 2 to 4 days before infusion of stem cells. Common post-transplantation immunosuppression combines cyclosporine and methotrexate. The complication of graft failure with this approach is infrequently seen (<5%), grades II to IV acute GVHD is seen in 30 to 50% of recipients, 25% have chronic GVHD, and short-term (2-year) survival after transplantation is nearly 90%. Ten-year survival rates are highly age dependent: 83%, 73%, and 68% for recipients in the first, second, and third decades of life, respectively. In patients 40 years of age or older, the 10-year survival rate is only 51%. Treatment choices adjusted for age of the patient are presented in Table 165-4.

Hematopoietic Stem Cell Transplantation: Matched Unrelated Donor

The use of bone marrow from an HLA-matched unrelated donor should be considered for patients who have no HLA-identical siblings, have failed to respond to immunosuppressive therapy, and are refractory to transfused platelets. As it is with matched related donors, the use of peripheral blood–derived stem cells is associated with higher mortality than is seen with marrow-derived stem cells. Results have not been as favorable as those associated with the use of marrow from HLA-identical siblings, but this strategy has improved in the past decade in part because of more accurate selection of HLA-matched donors and in part because of adjustments made with pretransplantation conditioning regimens. In fact, in some pediatric populations, some centers are now reporting identical outcomes in children transplanted with marrow cells from HLA-matched related and matched unrelated donors. Conditioning regimens that exclude ATG are associated with inferior outcomes, and less toxic conditioning regimens appear to have improved survival (65% for patients older than 16 years and 75% for those 16 years of age or younger). The improvements have been encouraging enough to recommend strongly that unrelated donor searches be initiated at the time of diagnosis for any patient younger than 30 years. Adults older than 30 years should be considered candidates for alternative donor stem cell transplantation if two attempts at immunosuppressive therapy have failed because newer fludarabine-based conditioning regimens have improved outcomes of matched unrelated donor transplants substantially.

Immunosuppressive Therapy

Treatment with ATG alone prolongs survival compared with supportive care alone, and for patients with mild aplastic anemia (not severe), either no treatment or ATG alone is sufficient. In patients with severe aplastic anemia, however, the combination of ATG and cyclosporine is superior to treatment with ATG alone.[A1] The combination reduces mortality and induces more rapid and higher overall response rates than does ATG as a single agent. Doses vary from center to center, but ATG is given at doses of 12 to 40 mg/kg/day for 4 to 5 days, and cyclosporine doses of 5 to 10 mg/kg/day (targeting blood levels of 150 to 250 ng/mL) are prescribed for 6 months, after which cyclosporine is slowly tapered during a period of 1 year or more. The median time to response is 120 days. Complete responses are defined as the resolution of pancytopenia and the development of normal blood counts. Relapses are uncommon in complete responders (10%). Partial responders are those whose counts do not normalize but who no longer require transfusion support. Forty percent to 60% of these patients will relapse in 5 years, but most will respond to a repeated course of immunosuppressive therapy. Some will require chronic immunosuppressive therapy with cyclosporine to remain transfusion independent. Those with unresponsive relapses have a poor prognosis. The humanized anti-CD52 monoclonal antibody alemtuzumab is also effective in severe acquired aplastic anemia, although best results are obtained in the relapsed and refractory settings. Its activity has been attributed to its lymphocytotoxic properties. In a conditioning regimen in transplantation trials, it has reduced the incidence of chronic GVHD, so its use is increasing in practice both for immunosuppressive therapy alone and for stem cell transplantation.

All age groups can benefit from immunosuppressive therapy. Long-term survival rates do vary with the age of the treated population. In patients younger than 20 years, 10-year survival rates are 80%, but these rates progressively decline to 25% in patients older than 70 years. However, when adjusted for the survival of an age-matched population by the standardized mortality ratio, the corrected risk for death is highest in young patients and declines as age increases. Advanced age is not a contraindication to the prescription of immunosuppressive therapy.

There are some caveats of importance related to the use of immunosuppressive therapy in aplastic anemia patients. First, patients may experience allergic reactions during infusions of ATG. This should not necessarily dissuade one from continuing this agent. Slowing the infusion after premedication with glucocorticosteroids and antihistamines often solves this problem. Fever and rigor can be signs of cytokine release from damaged cells in the T-cell pool, so they likewise should not be used as a reason to stop treatment. Second, if a responsive patient later relapses, a second course of ATG is frequently effective and can be used, although alemtuzumab is effective in relapsing patients as well. Third, it seems clear that a long interval between diagnosis of aplastic anemia and the initiation of immunosuppressive therapy is a negative predictor of response. Treatment should begin as soon as possible, certainly within 3 weeks of initial diagnosis. Fourth, the inclusion of hematopoietic growth factors during immunosuppressive therapy provides no benefit.

An approach to the management of severe aplastic anemia is shown in Figure 165-3, which complements Table 165-4.

Diamond-Blackfan Anemia

Although the mechanism by which glucocorticosteroids induce remissions in patients with Diamond-Blackfan anemia is unknown, nearly 80% of patients initially respond. Prednisone treatment is started at 2 mg/kg/day and is tapered after the hemoglobin increases to 10 g/dL. Most patients require a low every-other-day dose, but 15% remain in remission off steroids altogether. In those cases, survival to 40 years of age is nearly universal. Of patients who require ongoing steroid support, 75% reach the age of 40 years. Only half of the patients with steroid-resistant severe anemia survive to the age of 40 years. Pure red cell aplasia may respond to a synthetic erythropoietin receptor agonist.

Supportive Care

Platelet Transfusions

In the absence of bleeding or infection, platelet transfusions are commonly administered only when the platelet count declines to 10,000/mL or less (Chapters 172 and 177), but in the presence of active infection or bleeding, transfusion thresholds are often set at 20,000/mL or higher. If bleeding and infection coexist, it is prudent to rule out disseminated intravascular coagulation because fresh-frozen plasma or cryoprecipitate may be required along with platelet transfusions. Drugs (e.g., aspirin) that inhibit platelet function should be avoided, as should activities that might result in trauma. Menstrual activity should be suppressed with oral contraceptives or other agents.

Red Cell Transfusions

Filtered packed red blood cells should be provided to meet the needs of the patient's daily activities. Because there is substantial interindividual variation and because comorbidities influence exercise tolerance, there can be no firmly established hemoglobin target number for everyone. As a general rule, however, the number is higher in elderly patients than in young patients. Children with hemoglobin levels as low as 6 g/dL can compensate reasonably. Adults with underlying cardiopulmonary disease may have symptomatic anemia at 8 g/dL. If chronic transfusion therapy is required, the development of iron overload may require chelation therapy.

Management of Infections

The major infectious challenges result from the immunosuppression used (either as primary therapy or as a component of a stem cell transplantation regimen) more than from the neutropenia. For that reason, antibacterial, antiviral, and antifungal prophylaxis is routinely used in transplant recipients. In many centers, patients treated with immunosuppressive therapy alone are treated similarly for a 2- to 3-month period after ATG administration. Importantly, the onset of fever requires prompt clinical evaluation and antibiotic therapy as described in Chapter 281.

PREVENTION

Apart from public health measures controlling exposures to benzene, aromatic hydrocarbons, and radiation, little can be done to prevent acquired aplastic anemia. In the inherited bone marrow failure syndromes, prevention is achievable. Once the proband is identified, other affected family members, carriers, and siblings with no mutant allele can be identified, and genetic results can be applied in family planning even to the extent of preimplantation genetic diagnosis followed by in vitro fertilization. Because all somatic cells of children and adults with FA are hypersensitive to alkylating agents and oxidative stress, they must not receive standard doses of radiation or alkylating agents either for transplant conditioning or for treatment of squamous cell carcinoma.

Clonal evolution (e.g., to myelodysplasia and acute leukemia) occurs in 10 to 20% of patients with acquired aplastic anemia and up to 40% of children and adults with dyskeratosis congenita and FA. This complication likely evolves through a process of clonal selection and adaptation and for that reason is seen less commonly in patients completely responsive to treatment than in those with less than complete responses (who therefore have ongoing suppression of hematopoiesis). This suggests that more effective strategies of immunosuppressive therapy may better control ongoing marrow damage and decrease the incidence of clonal evolution.

PROGNOSIS

Acquired Idiopathic Aplastic Anemia

The severity of aplastic anemia and age are key determinants of long-term survival. Both these factors influence the choice of therapy (see Table 165-4). Early intervention is associated with a better prognosis, which should dictate the pace of diagnostic evaluation. Matched sibling donor transplants are associated with higher response rates, lower relapse rates, long-term survival rates approximating 80%, and lower incidence of clonal evolution. Immunosuppressive therapy is associated with long-term (10-year) survival rates of 70 to 75% in responders. Infection represents the most common cause of death in patients of any age treated with either immunosuppression alone or stem cell transplantation. Somatic mutations can identify patients with markedly increased risks of progressing to a myelodysplastic syndrome.[19]

Inherited Bone Marrow Failure Syndromes

Patients with dyskeratosis congenita and FA will not respond to immunosuppressive therapy. Stem cell transplantation with nonmyeloablative approaches has the potential of curing the marrow failure component of these diseases but does nothing to reduce the other common life-threatening complication of squamous cell carcinoma. There are good theoretical reasons for anticipating that successful transplantation will reduce the likelihood of clonal evolution to myelodysplasia and acute leukemia. Unfortunately, the decision to transplant is influenced by other key factors, as described earlier. In light of these complexities, no clear-cut when-to-transplant rule can be applied to all patients with these diseases, but it is generally accepted that transplantation early in childhood is associated with fewer short- and long-term complications. Taking these difficult issues into account, all patients should be evaluated early in an experienced transplantation center, and family members should be screened by hematologists, geneticists, and genetic counselors with use of specialty laboratories.

In patients with dyskeratosis, small case series report good outcomes after fludarabine-containing nonmyeloablative conditioning regimens, but studies of sufficient size are not available to permit concrete recommendations except that patients should be referred to an experienced center in light of the other organ systems at risk (e.g., lung). In patients with FA, with proper conditioning regimens, matched sibling donor transplant recipients have expected 3-year survival rates of about 85%, and matched unrelated recipients (when fludarabine-containing nonmyeloablative approaches are used) have 3-year survival rates of 50%. In patients with Diamond-Blackfan anemia, sibling donor transplant recipients have 3-year survival rates of about 80%, but disease-free survival rates after matched unrelated donor transplants have been poor (20 to 30%).

Future Treatments

For patients with acquired aplastic anemia, studies designed to selectively target the T-cell clones responsible for hematopoietic suppression may provide more effective and less toxic strategies for immunosuppressive therapy. For all patients with aplastic anemia, further improvements in matched unrelated transplantation should make this modality more widely available for patients who are not now considered optimal candidates. GVHD control will continue to improve. For children with nonsevere aplastic anemia, the 10-year progression-free survival rate is only about 25%, suggesting that prospective trials of early intervention are warranted. For patients with inherited bone marrow failure syndromes, the genes for which have been largely identified, the possibility of stem cell gene therapy holds enormous theoretical promise and has been nicely validated in murine models of the disease.

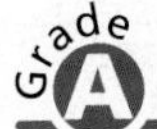

Grade A Reference

A1. Gafter-Gvili A, Ram R, Gurion R, et al. ATG plus cyclosporine reduces all-cause mortality in patients with severe aplastic anemia: systematic review and meta-analysis. *Acta Haematol.* 2008; 120:237-243.

GENERAL REFERENCES

For the General References and other additional features, please visit Expert Consult at https://expertconsult.inkling.com.

166

POLYCYTHEMIA VERA, ESSENTIAL THROMBOCYTHEMIA, AND PRIMARY MYELOFIBROSIS

AYALEW TEFFERI

DEFINITION

Polycythemia vera (PV), essential thrombocythemia (ET), and primary myelofibrosis (PMF) belong to the category of myeloproliferative neoplasms (MPNs), under the 2008 World Health Organization (WHO) classification system for hematologic malignancies (Table 166-1). These disorders represent stem cell–derived clonal myeloproliferation with a propensity to evolve into acute myeloid leukemia (AML), also called blast-phase MPN. PV, ET, and PMF, together with chronic myelogenous leukemia (CML), used to be

TABLE 166-1 WORLD HEALTH ORGANIZATION CLASSIFICATION OF MYELOID MALIGNANCIES

1. Acute myeloid leukemia (AML) and related precursor neoplasms* (Chapter 183)
2. Myeloproliferative neoplasms (MPN)
   2.1. Classic MPN
      2.1.1. Chronic myelogenous leukemia, *BCR-ABL1* positive (CML)
      2.1.2. Polycythemia vera (PV)
      2.1.3. Primary myelofibrosis (PMF)
      2.1.4. Essential thrombocythemia (ET)
   2.2. Nonclassic MPN
      2.2.1. Chronic neutrophilic leukemia (CNL)
      2.2.2. Chronic eosinophilic leukemia, not otherwise specified (CEL-NOS)
      2.2.3. Mastocytosis
      2.2.4. Myeloproliferative neoplasm, unclassifiable (MPN-U)
3. Myelodysplastic syndromes (MDS) (Chapter 182)
   3.1. Refractory cytopenia† with unilineage dysplasia (RCUD)
      3.1.1. Refractory anemia (ring sideroblasts <15% of erythroid precursors)
      3.1.2. Refractory neutropenia
      3.1.3. Refractory thrombocytopenia
   3.2. Refractory anemia with ring sideroblasts (RARS; dysplasia limited to erythroid lineage and ring sideroblasts ≥15% of bone marrow erythroid precursors)
   3.3. Refractory cytopenia with multilineage dysplasia (RCMD; ring sideroblast count does not matter)
   3.4. Refractory anemia with excess blasts (RAEB)
      3.4.1. RAEB-1 (2%-4% circulating or 5%-9% marrow blasts)
      3.4.2. RAEB-2 (5%-19% circulating or 10%-19% marrow blasts or Auer rods present)
   3.5. MDS associated with isolated del(5q)
   3.6. MDS, unclassifiable
4. MDS/MPN
   4.1. Chronic myelomonocytic leukemia (CMML)
   4.2. Atypical chronic myeloid leukemia, *BCR-ABL1* negative
   4.3. Juvenile myelomonocytic leukemia (JMML)
   4.4. MDS/MPN, unclassifiable
      4.4.1. Provisional entity: refractory anemia with ring sideroblasts associated with marked thrombocytosis (RARS-T)
5. Myeloid and lymphoid neoplasms with eosinophilia and abnormalities of *PDGFRA*,‡ *PDGFRB*,‡ or *FGFR1*‡ (Chapter 170)
   5.1. Myeloid and lymphoid neoplasms with *PDGFRA* rearrangement
   5.2. Myeloid neoplasms with *PDGFRB* rearrangement
   5.3. Myeloid and lymphoid neoplasms with *FGFR1* abnormalities

*Acute myeloid leukemia–related precursor neoplasms include "therapy-related myelodysplastic syndrome" and "myeloid sarcoma."
†Either mono- or bicytopenia: hemoglobin level <10 g/dL, absolute neutrophil count $<1.8 \times 10^9$/L, or platelet count $<100 \times 10^9$/L. However, higher blood counts do not exclude the diagnosis in the presence of unequivocal histologic or cytogenetic evidence for myelodysplastic syndrome.
‡Genetic rearrangements involving platelet-derived growth factor receptor α/β (*PDGFRA/PDGFRB*) or fibroblast growth factor receptor 1 (*FGFR1*).

referred to as "myeloproliferative disorders." Because CML is invariably linked to the Philadelphia translocation (i.e., *BCR-ABL1*), the other three are operationally labeled "*BCR-ABL1*–negative MPN."

EPIDEMIOLOGY

According to a recent systematic review, reported annual incidence rates ranged from 0.01 to 2.61, 0.21 to 2.27, and 0.22 to 0.99 per 100,000 for PV, ET, and PMF, respectively.[1] The combined annual incidence rates for PV, ET, and PMF are 0.84, 1.03, and 0.47 per 100,000, respectively. Population-based studies suggest a median age at diagnosis of approximately 71 years when all three MPN variants are considered together and a male-to-female ratio of approximately 50%. Other studies indicate a lower age distribution for ET and a slight male preponderance for PMF. Family studies suggest a five- to sevenfold increased risk of MPN among first-degree relatives of patients with *BCR-ABL1*–negative MPN and the possibility of a hereditary component to disease susceptibility was further elaborated by *JAK2* haplotype studies. PMF has been associated with exposure to ionizing radiation (e.g., in Hiroshima survivors), heavy exposure to petroleum derivatives, and thorium dioxide (Thorotrast) contrast medium, but in the vast majority of cases, there is no such exposure history.

PATHOBIOLOGY

These diseases are clonal in nature, deriving from a genetically transformed hematopoietic, bone marrow stem cell that results in clonal myeloproliferation. In 2005, a *JAK2* gain-of-function mutation (*JAK2*V617F) was reported

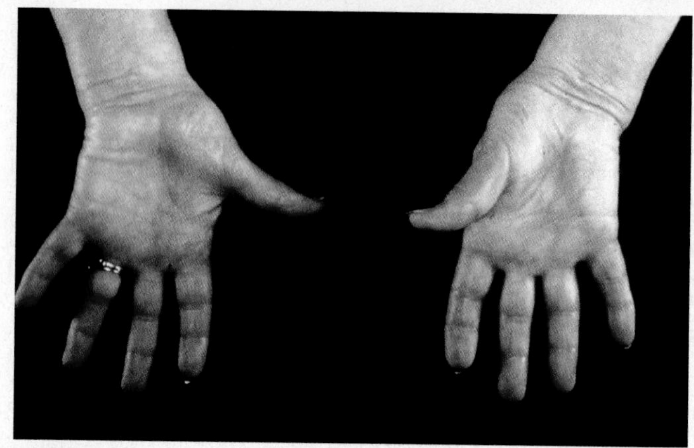

FIGURE 166-1. Erythromelalgia: painful red discoloration of the hands or, more commonly, the toes.

in *BCR-ABL1*–negative MPN. Subsequent studies using sensitive assays have revealed the presence of this mutation in approximately 95% of patients with PV and 60% of those with ET or PMF. Most of the remaining 5% of patients with PV carry another *JAK2* mutation (*JAK2* exon 12). In other words, virtually all patients with PV carry a *JAK2* mutation. Approximately 5% to 10% of *JAK2*V617F-negative patients with ET or PMF carry a *MPL*W515 mutation, which is equally JAK-STAT relevant (Table 166-2). In 2013, calreticulin (*CALR*) mutations were discovered in the majority of patients with ET or PMF who do not express *JAK2* or *MPL* mutations.[2] *CALR* mutations are relatively specific to ET and PMF and display mutational frequencies of approximately 20% and 25%, respectively. Additional mutations seen in MPN are listed in Table 166-2. Most of these latter mutations originate at the progenitor cell level, but they do not necessarily represent the primary clonogenic event, are not mutually exclusive, or follow a predictable hierarchy.

The above-listed molecular alterations in *BCR-ABL1*–negative MPN induce biologic changes that are demonstrated in animal models or ex vivo. For example, *JAK2* or *MPL* mutations induce PV-, ET-, or PMF-like disease in mice by experimental manipulation of mutant allele burden. These mutations are also believed to contribute to the growth factor independence or hypersensitivity of erythroid or megakaryocyte colony-forming progenitor cells. Bone marrow fibrosis, osteosclerosis, and angiogenesis in PMF are currently believed to be reactive and cytokine mediated.

CLINICAL MANIFESTATIONS

Essential Thrombocythemia

At presentation, microvascular and vasomotor symptoms are found in 25% to 50% of ET patients. Major thrombosis is seen in 11% to 25% of patients at diagnosis and 10% to 22% during follow-up, and major hemorrhage is observed in 2% to 5% at diagnosis and 1% to 7% during follow-up. Vasomotor disturbances (e.g., headaches, lightheadedness, visual symptoms such as blurring and scotomata, palpitations, chest pain, erythromelalgia, and distal paresthesias) are not infrequent in ET and might be the result of abnormal platelet–endothelium interactions. Erythromelalgia (Fig. 166-1) is the most dramatic vasomotor symptom, characterized by erythema, warmth, and pain in the distal extremities; this symptom is rare but not entirely specific for ET. Life-threatening complications of ET include large-vessel thrombosis (both arterial and venous), hemorrhage, and transformation of the disease into either a fibrotic phase resembling PMF or AML. Venous thrombosis in ET occurs both in sites common to other thrombotic diatheses (e.g., pulmonary embolism and lower extremity deep vein thrombosis and pulmonary embolism) but also in more unusual sites (e.g., cerebral sinus thrombosis, retinal vein thrombosis, and hepatic and portal vein thrombosis).

Major hemorrhage in ET is most common in the gastrointestinal (GI) tract and may be precipitated by aspirin (ASA) or nonsteroidal antiinflammatory drug (NSAID) use. Hemorrhage also occurs in the central nervous system (CNS) and the retina, but such events are, fortunately, uncommon. Paradoxically, patients with extreme thrombocytosis may be at special risk for bleeding, in part related to the development of an acquired von Willebrand syndrome that is thought to be related to platelet adsorption of large multimers of von Willebrand protein (Chapter 173). Fibrotic and leukemic transformations of ET are rare events (<5% of patients) during the first 10 years after diagnosis, but the risk increases with time.

TABLE 166-2 SOMATIC MUTATIONS IN *BCR-ABL1*–NEGATIVE MYELOPROLIFERATIVE NEOPLASMS (MPN), INCLUDING POLYCYTHEMIA VERA (PV), ESSENTIAL THROMBOCYTHEMIA (ET), AND PRIMARY MYELOFIBROSIS (PMF). MUTATIONAL FREQUENCIES IN BLAST PHASE (BP) DISEASE ARE ALSO PROVIDED*

MUTATIONS	CHROMOSOME LOCATION	MUTATIONAL FREQUENCY	PATHOGENETIC RELEVANCE
JAK2 (Janus kinase 2): *V617F*	9p24	PV: ~96% ET:~55% PMF: ~65%	Contributes to abnormal myeloproliferation and progenitor cell growth factor hypersensitivity
JAK2 exon 12 mutation	9p24	PV: ~3%	Contributes to primarily erythroid myeloproliferation
CALR (Calreticulin): exon 9 deletions and insertions	19p13.2	PMF: ~25% ET: ~20% PV: 0%	Wild-type *CALR* is a multifunctional Ca^{2+} binding protein chaperone mostly localized in the endoplasmic reticulum
MPL (myeloproliferative leukemia virus oncogene): MPN-associated *MPL* mutations involve exon 10	1p34	ET:~3% PMF: ~10%	Contributes to primarily megakaryocytic myeloproliferation
LNK (as in links), or *SH2B3* (a membrane-bound adaptor protein): MPN-associated mutations are monoallelic and involve exon 2	12q24.12	PV: rare ET: rare PMF: rare BP-MPN: ~10%	Wild-type *LNK* is a negative regulator of JAK2 signaling.
TET2 (TET oncogene family member 2): mutations involve several exons	4q24	PV: ~16% ET: ~5% PMF: ~17% BP-MPN: ~17%	TET proteins catalyze conversion of 5mC to 5hmC, which favors demethylated DNA. Both TET1 and TET2 display this catalytic activity. *IDH* and *TET2* mutations might share a common pathogenetic effect.
ASXL1 (additional sex combs-like 1): exon 12 mutations	20q11.1	ET: ~3% PMF: ~13% BP-MPN: ~18%	Wild-type *ASXL1* is needed for normal hematopoiesis and might be involved in coactivation of transcription factors and transcriptional repression.
IDH1/IDH2 (isocitrate dehydrogenase): exon 4 mutations	2q33.3/15q26.1	PV: ~2% ET: ~1% PMF: ~4% BP-MPN: ~20%	*IDH* mutations induce loss of activity for the conversion of isocitrate to 2-KG and gain of function in the conversion of 2-KG to 2-HG. 2-HG might be the mediator of impaired TET2 function in cells with mutant *IDH* expression.
EZH2 (enhancer of zeste homolog 2): mutations involve several exons	7q36.1	PV: ~3% PMF: ~7% MDS: ~6%	Wild-type *EZH2* is part of a histone methyltransferase (polycomb repressive complex 2 associated with H3 Lys-27 trimethylation). MPN-associated *EZH2* mutations might have a tumor suppressor activity, which contrasts with the gain-of-function activity for lymphoma-associated *EZH2* mutations.
DNMT3A (DNA cytosine methyltransferase 3a): most frequent mutations affect amino acid R882	2p23	PV: ~7% PMF: ~7% BP-MPN: ~14%	DNA methyl transferases are essential In establishing and maintaining DNA methylation patterns in mammals
CBL (Casitas B-lineage lymphoma proto-oncogene): exon 8/9 mutations	11q23.3	PV: rare ET:rare MF: ~6%	CBL is an E3 ubiquitin ligase that marks mutant kinases for degradation. Transforming activity requires loss of this function.
IKZF1 (IKAROS family zinc finger 1): mostly deletions including intragenic	7p12	CP-MPN: rare BP-MPN: ~19%	IKZF1 is a transcription regulator and putative tumor suppressor
TP53 (tumor protein p53): exons 4 through 9	17p13.1	PMF: ~4% BP-MPN ~27%	A tumor suppressor protein that targets genes that regulate cell cycle arrest, apoptosis, and DNA repair
SF3B1 (splicing factor 3B subunit 1): mostly exons 14 and 15	2q33.1	PMF: ~7%	SF3B1 is a component of the RNA spliceosome. *SF3B1* mutations are closely associated with ring sideroblasts.
SRSF2 (serine/arginine-rich splicing factor 2): exon 2	17q25.1	PMF: ~17%	SRSF2 is a component of the RNA spliceosome, whose dysfunction promotes defects in alternative splicing.
U2AF1 (U2 small nuclear RNA auxiliary factor 1)	21q22.3	PMF: ~16%	U2AF1 is a subunit of the U2 small nuclear ribonucleoprotein auxiliary factor involved in pre-mRNA processing

*See text for references.

BP-MPN = blast phase MPN; CP-MPN= chronic phase MPN; ET = essential thrombocythemia; 5hmC = 5-hydroxymethylcytosine; 5mC = 5-methylcytosine; MF includes both PMF and post-ET/PV myelofibrosis; MPN = myeloproliferative neoplasms; PMF = primary myelofibrosis; PV = polycythemia vera; 2-KG = 2-ketoglutarate; 2-HG = 2-hydroxyglutarate.

Polycythemia Vera

Table 166-3 lists the typical clinical and laboratory features of PV. Increased red blood cell (RBC) mass in PV might result in blood hyperviscosity, which leads to a plethora of symptoms and signs. Headaches are frequent, but blurry vision, altered hearing, mucous membrane bleeding, shortness of breath, and malaise are also observed. At least two thirds of PV patients have splenomegaly. Thrombosis occurs, most commonly arterial thrombosis, in about 40% of patients. As in ET, venous thrombosis can occur in unusual sites, such as mesenteric, portal, or hepatic veins (the latter also being called Budd-Chiari syndrome). Bleeding, especially from the GI tract, is seen in PV but less often than thrombosis. Pruritus is common in PV and may be provoked by warm water ("aquagenic"). Erythromelalgia (described earlier under ET) might also trouble some patients with PV, as do other vasomotor symptoms, such as paresthesias and headaches.

TABLE 166-3 CLINICAL AND LABORATORY FEATURES OF POLYCYTHEMIA VERA

Persistent leukocytosis
Persistent thrombocytosis
Microcytosis secondary to iron deficiency
Increased red blood cell mass
JAK2 mutations
Increased leukocyte alkaline phosphatase
Splenomegaly
Generalized pruritus (usually after bathing)
Arterial and venous thrombosis, including unusual thrombosis (e.g., Budd-Chiari syndrome)
Erythromelalgia (acral dysesthesia and erythema; see Fig. 166-1)

Primary Myelofibrosis

Most patients with PMF present with anemia and marked splenomegaly. The anemia of PMF is multifactorial. Contributing factors include ineffective hematopoiesis and hypersplenism. Spleen and liver enlargement in PMF is secondary to extramedullary hematopoiesis (EMH) and may be associated with hypercatabolic symptoms, including profound fatigue, weight loss, night sweats, and low-grade fever. Patients also experience peripheral edema; diarrhea; early satiety; and, occasionally, complications of portal hypertension, including variceal bleeding and ascites.

Splenomegaly in PMF may be complicated by splenic infarction manifested by left upper quadrant abdominal pain and referred left shoulder pain. CT imaging in such cases can be unremarkable or may show wedge-shaped or rounded low-attenuation lesions in the spleen. EMH occurs in a great diversity of sites throughout the body. Common sites besides the spleen and liver include lymph nodes, skin, pleura, peritoneum, lung, and paraspinal and epidural spaces. The latter may result in spinal cord or nerve root compression, which is a medical emergency requiring corticosteroids to reduce edema and immediate radiotherapy. Other clinical features of PMF include diffuse and sometimes regional bone and joint pain.

DIAGNOSIS

At present, the 2008 WHO criteria are used for the diagnosis of ET, PV, and PMF (Table 166-4). These criteria are based on morphology and cytogenetic and molecular studies (Fig. 166-2). Almost all patients with PV carry a *JAK2* mutation (*JAK2*V617F or *JAK2* exon 12 mutations). *JAK2*V617F is, however, not specific to PV and is also found in ET (~60% of cases), PMF (~60% of cases), and other myeloid neoplasms (usually <5% of cases). *JAK2* exon 12 mutations are relatively specific to *JAK2*V617F-negative PV and occur in approximately 3% of all patients with PV. *JAK2* exon 12 mutation-positive PV patients are characterized by predominantly erythroid myelopoiesis, subnormal serum erythropoietin (Epo) levels, and younger age at diagnosis. Taken together, the presence of a *JAK2* mutation excludes secondary myeloproliferation (e.g., secondary polycythemia or reactive thrombocytosis; see later discussion), and its absence makes a diagnosis of PV very unlikely. Among the 30% to 40% of ET or PMF patients who do not harbor *JAK2* mutations, the majority (60% to 70%) carry *CALR* mutations, and 5% to 10% carry *MPL* mutations. In other words, 80% to 90% of patients with ET or PMF carry one of the three MPN-specific mutations: *JAK2, CALR,* or *MPL*.

As outlined in Figure 166-2, the diagnostic work-up for suspected MPN, including PV, ET, and PMF, should start with peripheral blood mutation screening for *JAK2*V617F.[3] The presence of the mutation confirms the presence of an underlying MPN, but it is not specific to any one of the three MPN variants. In the absence of *JAK2*V617F, the next step is to screen for *JAK2* exon 12 mutation for PV and *CALR* mutations for ET and PMF (see Fig. 166-2). *MPL* mutations are studied only when both *JAK2* and *CALR* mutations are absent in suspected cases of ET or PMF. Bone marrow examination is recommended to confirm the diagnosis in triple-negative cases (i.e., wild type for *JAK2, CALR,* and *MPL*) and to distinguish between ET and prefibrotic PMF. Clinically, patients with ET and PV present with thrombocytosis and erythrocytosis, respectively. Patients with PMF usually present with peripheral blood leukoerythroblastosis (i.e., presence of nucleated RBCs, metamyelocytes, or myelocytes [Fig. 166-3] and bone marrow fibrosis with morphologically atypical megakaryocytes [Fig. 166-4]). Bone marrow morphology can also help distinguish clonal from reactive myeloproliferation (Fig. 166-5).

Table 166-5 includes a comprehensive list of causes of erythrocytosis,[4] including congenital and secondary polycythemia. The diagnostic approach to congenital polycythemia should start with measurement of serum Epo level. The presence of a subnormal serum Epo level, in the absence of PV, suggests the presence of a germline mutation of the erythropoietin receptor. If the serum Epo level is normal or elevated, the next step is to measure the p50 (the oxygen tension at which hemoglobin is 50% saturated). Decreased p50 suggests the presence of either high oxygen-affinity hemoglobinopathy or 2,3-bisphosphoglycerate (2,3-BPG) deficiency. If the p50 is normal, then the possibility of *VHL* mutations (usually associated with increased serum Epo level) should be considered first because they constitute the most frequent mutations in congenital polycythemia. Gene expression studies can identify two different phenotypic expressions of polycythemia vera in terms of disease duration, hemoglobin level, splenomegaly, and the risk of thromboembolism.[5]

Table 166-6 outlines the different causes of thrombocytosis, and Figure 166-5 provides an algorithmic approach to its diagnosis. Figure 166-6 illustrates the value of peripheral blood smear examination in the differential diagnosis of thrombocytosis. Other causes of bone marrow fibrosis are outlined in Table 166-7. The diagnosis of post-PV or post-ET myelofibrosis requires full documentation of a previous morphologic diagnosis of PV or ET, respectively.

TABLE 166-4 THE 2008 WORLD HEALTH ORGANIZATION DIAGNOSTIC CRITERIA FOR POLYCYTHEMIA VERA, ESSENTIAL THROMBOCYTHEMIA, AND PRIMARY MYELOFIBROSIS

CRITERIA	POLYCYTHEMIA VERA*	ESSENTIAL THROMBOCYTHEMIA*	PRIMARY MYELOFIBROSIS*
Major criteria	1. Hb >18.5 g/dL (men); >16.5 g/dL (women) *or* Hb/Hct >99th percentile of reference range *or* Hb >17 g/dL (men) or>15 g/dL (women) if associated with a sustained increase of ≥2 g/dL from baseline, not otherwise explained *or* Elevated RBC mass >25% above mean normal predicted value	1. Platelet count ≥450 × 10^9/L	1. Megakaryocyte proliferation and atypia[†] accompanied by either reticulin or collagen fibrosis *or* In the absence of fibrosis, megakaryocyte changes accompanied by increased marrow cellularity and granulocytic proliferation
	2. Presence of *JAK2*V617F or similar mutation	2. Megakaryocyte proliferation with large and mature morphology; no or little granulocyte or erythroid proliferation	2. Not meeting WHO criteria for CML, PV, MDS, or other myeloid neoplasm
		3. Not meeting WHO criteria for CML, PV, PMF, MDS, or other myeloid neoplasm	3. Demonstration of *JAK2*V617F or other clonal marker *or* No evidence of reactive marrow fibrosis
		4. Demonstration of *JAK2*V617F or other clonal marker *or* No evidence of reactive thrombocytosis	
Minor criteria	1. BM trilineage myeloproliferation 2. Subnormal serum Epo level 3. EEC growth		1. Leukoerythroblastosis 2. Increased serum LDH 3. Anemia 4. Palpable splenomegaly

*Diagnosis of polycythemia vera (PV) requires meeting either both major criteria and one minor criterion or the first major criterion and two minor criteria. Diagnosis of essential thrombocythemia requires meeting all four major criteria. Diagnosis of primary myelofibrosis (PMF) requires meeting all three major criteria and two minor criteria.

[†]Small to large megakaryocytes with an aberrant nuclear-to-cytoplasmic ratio and hyperchromatic and irregularly folded nuclei and dense clustering.

CML = chronic myelogenous leukemia; EEC = endogenous erythroid colony; Epo = erythropoietin; Hct = hematocrit; Hb = hemoglobin; LDH = lactate dehydrogenase; MDS = myelodysplastic syndrome; RBC = red blood cell; WHO =World Health Organization.

With permission from Patnaik MM, Tefferi A. The complete evaluation of erythrocytosis: congenital and acquired. *Leukemia*. 2009;23:834-844.

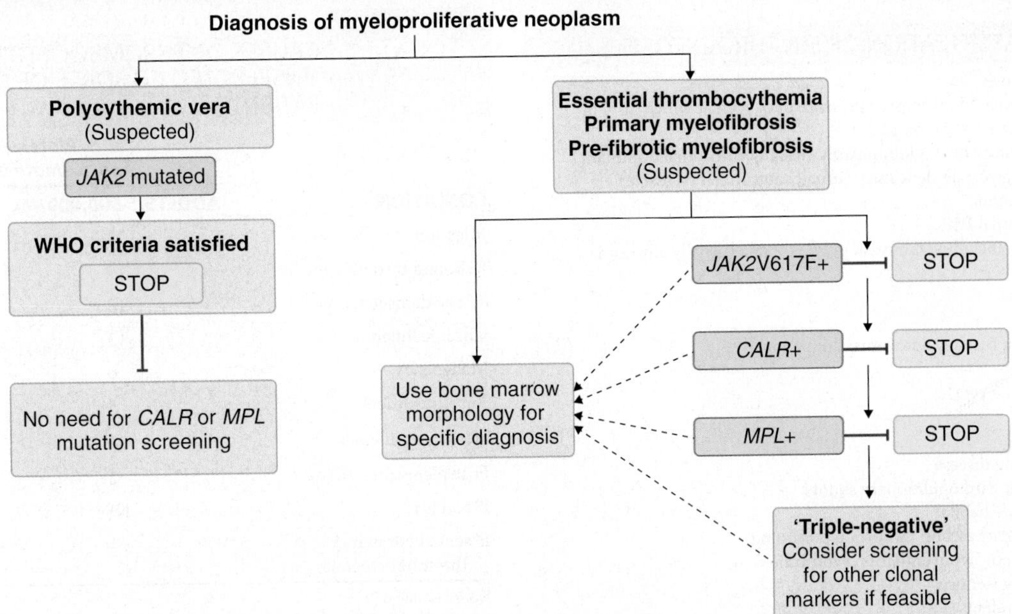

FIGURE 166-2. A diagnostic algorithm for polycythemia vera (PV), essential thrombocythemia (ET), primary myelofibrosis (PMF), and chronic myelogenous leukemia (CML) (With permission from Tefferi A, Pardanani A. Genetics: CALR mutations and a new diagnostic algorithm for MPN. *Nat Rev Clin Oncol.* 2014;11:125-126.)

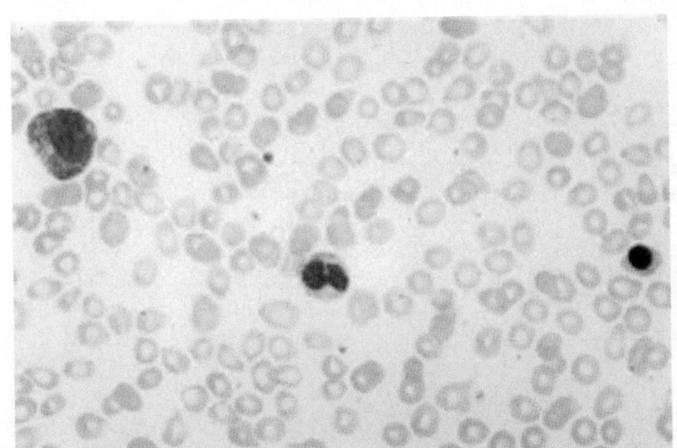

FIGURE 166-3. Myeloproliferative neoplasm. A peripheral blood smear from a patient with agnogenic myeloid metaplasia shows a leukoerythroblastic picture. The characteristic findings are teardrop-shaped red blood cells (dacryocytes), nucleated red blood cells (erythroblasts), and immature granulocyte precursors.

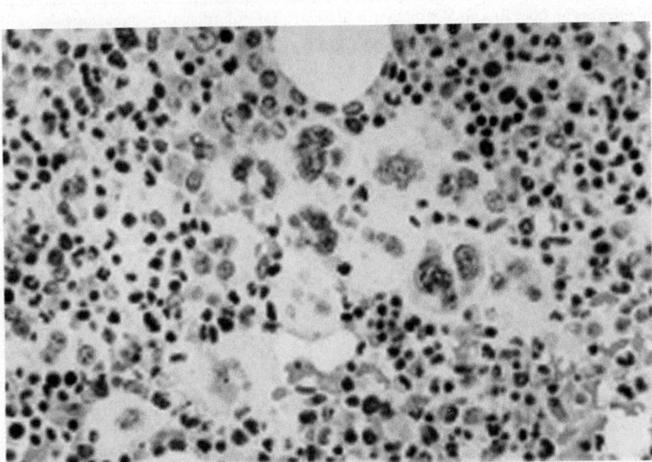

FIGURE 166-5. Myeloproliferative neoplasm. Bone marrow shows megakaryocytic clusters seen in essential thrombocythemia and other conditions associated with clonal thrombocytosis. These are not typically found in the bone marrow of individuals with other (secondary or reactive) types of thrombocytosis.

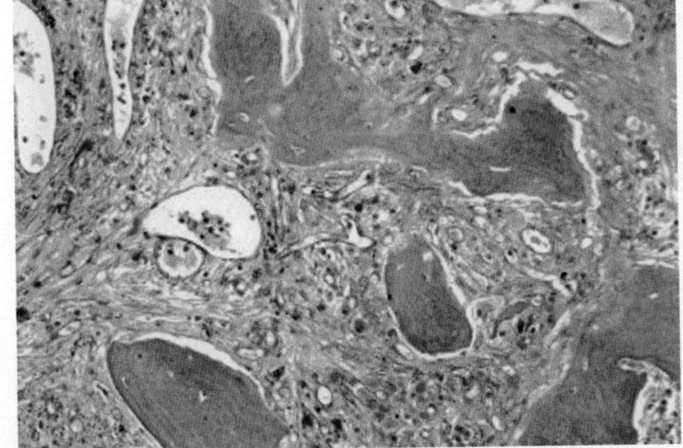

FIGURE 166-4. A bone marrow biopsy specimen from a patient with primary myelofibrosis shows reticulin fibrosis, osteosclerosis, and intrasinusoidal hematopoiesis.

TREATMENT

Rx

Essential Thrombocythemia and Polycythemia Vera

Drug therapy in ET or PV has not been shown to either improve survival or prevent disease transformation into post-ET or post-PV MF or blast-phase MPN. Instead, the main objective of specific therapy in ET or PV is either to prevent thrombosis in high-risk patients (i.e., age 60 years or older or presence of thrombosis history) or alleviate non–life-threatening symptoms, including microvascular disturbances (e.g., headaches, acral paresthesia, erythromelalgia), pruritus, or symptomatic splenomegaly. Microvascular symptoms are usually effectively treated with low-dose aspirin (81 mg/day). The cause of MPN-associated pruritus is poorly understood, but its dramatic response to JAK inhibitor therapy (see later discussion) suggests a causal relationship to cytokines that use JAK-STAT signaling. Other therapies for MPN-associated pruritus include antihistamines, selective serotonin reuptake inhibitors, interferon- (INF-α), and phototherapy. Symptomatic splenomegaly is usually managed by treatment with hydroxyurea (starting dose, 500 mg orally twice a day).

Observation alone is acceptable in asymptomatic young ET patients without a history of thrombosis[6]; the presence of microvascular symptoms,

TABLE 166-5 CLASSIFICATION OF ERYTHROCYTOSIS

1. Congenital erythrocytosis
   a. Associated with reduced P50 (partial pressure of oxygen at which 50% of hemoglobin is saturated with oxygen)
      i. High oxygen affinity hemoglobinopathy (usually autosomal dominant)
      ii. 2,3-Bisphosphoglycerate deficiency (usually autosomal recessive)
      iii. Methemoglobinemia
   b. Associated with normal P50
      i. *VHL* mutations, including Chuvash polycythemia (usually autosomal recessive)
      ii. *PHD2* mutations
      iii. *HIF2-α* mutations
      iv. *EPOR* mutations (usually autosomal dominant)
2. Acquired erythrocytosis
   a. Clonal (polycythemia vera)
   b. Secondary
      i. Hypoxia driven
         (1) Chronic lung disease
         (2) Right-to-left cardiopulmonary shunts
         (3) High-altitude habitat
         (4) Tobacco use or carbon monoxide poisoning
         (5) Sleep apnea or hypoventilation syndrome
         (6) Renal artery stenosis
      ii. Hypoxia independent
         (1) Use of androgen preparations or erythropoietin injection
         (2) After renal transplant
         (3) Cerebellar hemangioblastoma or meningioma
         (4) Pheochromocytoma, uterine leiomyoma, renal cysts, or parathyroid adenoma
         (5) Hepatocellular carcinoma or renal cell carcinoma

With permission from Patnaik MM, Tefferi A. The complete evaluation of erythrocytosis: congenital and acquired. *Leukemia.* 2009;23:834-844.

TABLE 166-6 CAUSES OF THROMBOCYTOSIS IN UNSELECTED COHORTS OF CONSECUTIVE PATIENTS

	Platelet Count (Approximate % of Patients)	
CONDITION	**ADULTS, >500,000/ML**	**>1 MILLION/ML**
Infection	22	31
Rebound thrombocytosis	19	3
Tissue damage (surgery)	18	14
Chronic inflammation	13	9
Malignancy	6	14
Renal disorders	5	<1
Hemolytic anemia	4	<1
Postsplenectomy status	2	19
Blood loss	NS	6
Essential (primary) thrombocythemia	3	14

NS = not stated.
From Tefferi A, Gilliland DG. Classification of chronic myeloid disorders: from Dameshek towards a semi-molecular system. *Best Pract Res Clin Haematol.* 2006;19:365-385.

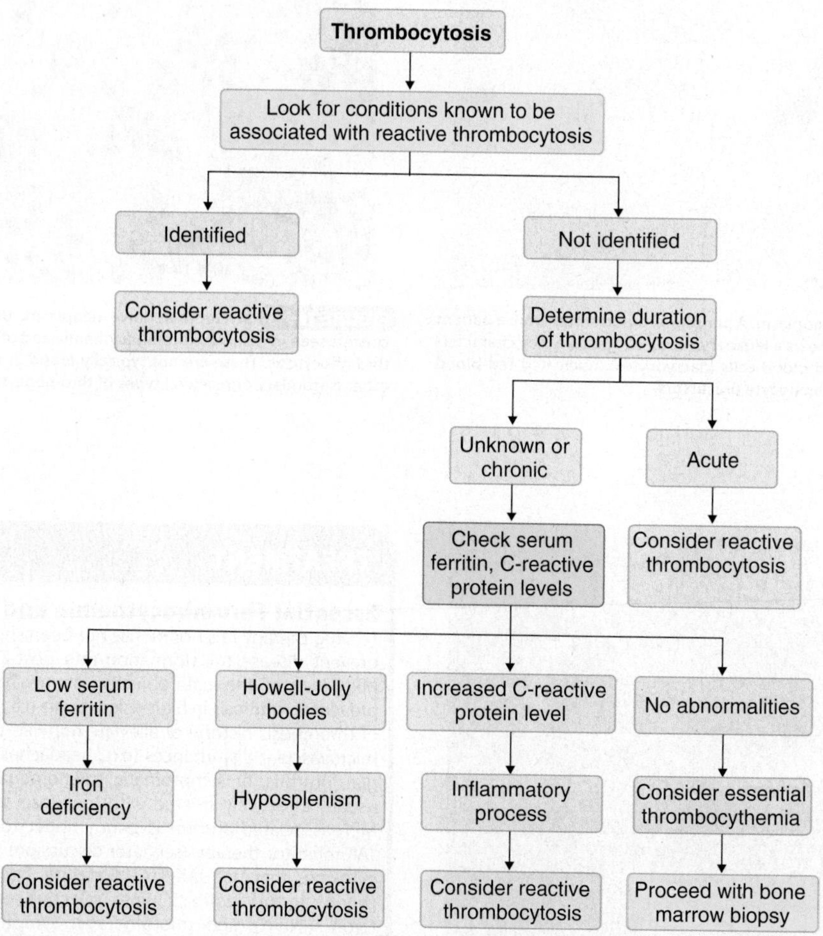

FIGURE 166-6. Diagnostic evaluation of thrombocytosis in routine clinical practice.

cardiovascular risk factors, or the *JAK2*V617F mutation justifies the use of once-daily aspirin therapy. Cytoreductive therapy for the prevention of thrombosis is indicated only in the presence of high-risk disease (Table 166-8). Randomized studies have demonstrated the value of low-dose aspirin (40-100 mg/day) in PV[A1] and hydroxyurea (starting dose, 500 mg orally twice a day)[A2] or anagrelide (starting at 1 mg daily)[A3] in high-risk patients with ET. Based on noncontrolled but prospective evidence, most experts agree that low-dose aspirin therapy (81 mg/day) should also be considered for ET and hydroxyurea therapy for high-risk PV (see Table 166-8). In addition, treatment with phlebotomy is required for all patients with PV, and the target hematocrit count in aspirin-treated patients should be less than 45% based on the most recent information from a controlled study.[A4]

In high-risk patients with ET in whom cytoreductive therapy is indicated, a platelet target of less than 400×10^9/L is reasonable and supported by data from retrospective studies. Hydroxyurea remains the first drug of choice for both high-risk ET and PV. High-risk PV or ET patients who are either intolerant or resistant to hydroxyurea are effectively managed by INF-α or busulfan.

Enthusiasm for the use of recombinant IFN in the MPNs was dampened by drug toxicity that often led to its discontinuation. The addition of a polyethylene glycol (PEG) moiety to IFN-α results in a longer half-life, allowing less frequent administration, more drug stability, less immunogenicity, and less toxicity, leading to the increased use of PEG-IFN-α instead of recombinant IFN.

Among the two second-line drugs, this author prefers the use of INF-α for patients younger than age 65 years and busulfan in the older age group. Because the long-term health effects of INF-α and impact on survival and disease complications are unknown, a controlled study is needed before INF-α is recommended for first-line therapy in either PV or ET. Busulfan is started at 4 mg/day orally and withheld in the presence of platelets below 100×10^9/L or white blood cell count below 3×10^9/L, and the dose is reduced to 2 mg/day if the corresponding levels are less than 150×10^9/L and less than 5×10^9/L.

There is unsubstantiated fear among primary caregivers regarding drug leukemogenicity with use of hydroxyurea or busulfan; there are no controlled studies in either PV or ET that shows this to be the case. A recent large retrospective study in PV, involving more than 1500 patients showed no evidence for leukemogenicity attached to either hydroxyurea or busulfan. Pregnancy in ET is associated with increased risk (~35% vs. approximately 15% in the control population) of first trimester spontaneous abortion. There is no association between the increased risk of spontaneous abortion and the degree of thrombocytosis. Low-risk pregnant patients with ET or PV are managed the same way as their nonpregnant counterparts, and the use of low-dose aspirin has been associated with a decreased prevalence of first trimester miscarriages in retrospective studies. High-risk pregnant women with ET (i.e., women with previous thrombosis) require cytoreductive therapy just like other high-risk patients. In such patients, there is anecdotal evidence on the safety of using IFN-α.

Major bleeding occurs in fewer than 10% of ET patients. Extreme thrombocytosis (i.e., platelet count >1 million/μL) appears to be a risk factor for

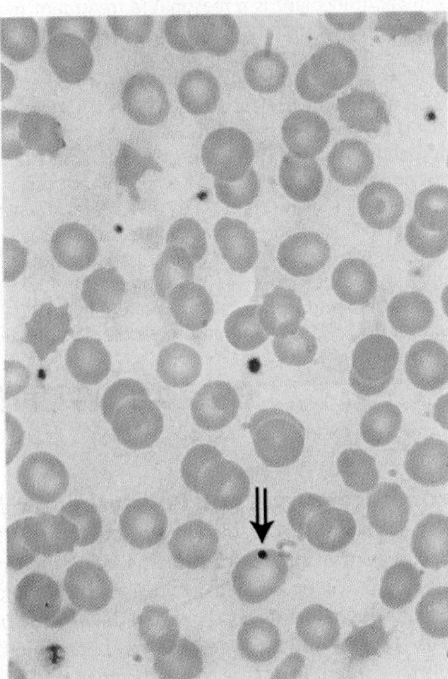

FIGURE 166-7. Peripheral blood smear showing Howell-Jolly bodies *(arrow)* in red blood cells, a finding typical of surgical or functional hyposplenism.

TABLE 166-7 CAUSES OF BONE MARROW FIBROSIS

MYELOID DISORDERS
Primary myelofibrosis
Metastatic cancer
Chronic myeloid leukemia
Myelodysplastic syndrome
Atypical myeloid disorder
Acute megakaryocytic leukemia
Other acute myeloid leukemias
Gray platelet syndrome
LYMPHOID DISORDERS
Hairy cell leukemia
Multiple myeloma
Lymphoma
NONHEMATOLOGIC DISORDERS
Connective tissue disorder
Infections (tuberculosis, kala-azar)
Vitamin D deficiency rickets
Renal osteodystrophy

TABLE 166-8 RISK STRATIFICATION AND RISK-ADAPTED THERAPY IN ESSENTIAL THROMBOCYTHEMIA, POLYCYTHEMIA VERA, AND PRIMARY MYELOFIBROSIS

RISK GROUPS: PV AND ET	MANAGEMENT: ET	MANAGEMENT: PV	MANAGEMENT: PMF	IPSS RISK GROUPS: PMF
Low risk (age <60 yr *and* no thrombosis history)	Low-dose aspirin	Low-dose aspirin + phlebotomy[§]	Observation	Low-risk (no risk factors[¶])
Low risk with extreme thrombocytosis*	Low-dose aspirin[†]	Low-dose aspirin[†] + phlebotomy	Conventional management[‖]	Intermediate-1 risk (one risk factor[¶])
High-risk (age ≥60 yr *or* thrombosis history)	Low-dose aspirin + hydroxyurea[‡]	Low-dose aspirin + phlebotomy + hydroxyurea[‡]	Allo-SCT if age <65 yr or experimental therapy	Intermediate-1 risk with transfusions or unfavorable karyotype
			Allo-SCT if age <65 years or experimental therapy	Intermediate-2 risk (2 risk factors[¶])
			Allo-SCT if age <65 yr or experimental therapy	High-risk (≥3 risk factors[¶])

*Extreme thrombocytosis is defined as a platelet count of $>1000 \times 10^9$/L.
†Clinically significant acquired von Willebrand syndrome (ristocetin co-factor activity <30%) should be excluded before the use of aspirin in patients with extreme thrombocytosis because of bleeding risk.
‡In hydroxyurea-intolerant or -resistant patients, interferon-α (age < 60 years) or busulfan or pipobroman (age older than 60 years) might be used.
§In the presence of aspirin therapy, the hematocrit target can range between 38% and 50% and is set at a level that maintains best performance status.
‖Androgen preparations or thalidomide with prednisone for anemia; hydroxyurea for symptomatic splenomegaly.
¶The International Prognostic Scoring System (IPSS) uses five risk factors for inferior survival: age older than 65 years, hemoglobin <10 g/dL, leukocyte count $>25 \times 10^9$/L, circulating blasts ≥1%, and presence of constitutional symptoms.
Allo-SCT = allogeneic stem cell transplantation; ET = essential thrombocythemia; PMF = primary myelofibrosis; PV = polycythemia vera.

bleeding, in part because of the acquired von Willebrand disease syndrome. Measuring ristocetin cofactor activity in patients with extreme thrombocytosis and holding the use of aspirin therapy if the value is less than 30% have been recommended.

Primary Myelofibrosis

Conventional therapy for PMF is largely palliative and has not been shown to improve survival. Anemia and symptomatic splenomegaly are the main indications for treatment in PMF. Conventional drugs used for the treatment of PMF-associated anemia include androgen preparations (e.g., oral fluoxymesterone 10 mg two times a day), danazol (400-600 mg/day orally), prednisone (30-40 mg/day), and erythropoiesis-stimulating agents (ESAs).[7] The use of ESAs may exacerbate PMF-associated splenomegaly, and it is ineffective in transfusion-dependent patients. Prostate cancer screening in men is necessary when considering treatment with androgen preparations. Response rates to prednisone, androgen preparations, or danazol are in the vicinity of 20% and response durations average about one to two years.

Recent studies have shown the value of thalidomide and thalidomide-like drugs such as lenalidomide in the treatment of anemia in PMF. Thalidomide as a single agent (50-200 mg/day orally) is not as effective as the drug combined with prednisone (30 mg/day) where reported response rates range from 20% to 62% for anemia, 25% to 80% for thrombocytopenia, and 7% to 30% for splenomegaly. Response rates with lenalidomide are somewhat similar, but the drug works best in the presence of del(5q) cytogenetic abnormality (see Chapter 182 on myelodysplastic syndrome.) The occurrence of peripheral neuropathy with thalidomide and severe pancytopenia with lenalidomide therapy has limited their use in most patients with the disease.

The drug of choice for symptomatic splenomegaly in PMF is hydroxyurea (starting dose, 500 mg orally twice a day). Hydroxyurea-refractory cases have been often managed by splenectomy in the past since the value of other conventional drugs in this regard has been limited (see section below on experimental drug therapy). Indications for splenectomy in PMF have included mechanical discomfort, symptomatic portal hypertension (i.e., associated with ascites or variceal bleeding), and frequent RBC transfusions. The perioperative mortality rate of splenectomy in PMF is between 5% and 10%. Postsplenectomy complications occur in approximately 50% of the patients and include bleeding, thrombosis, hepatomegaly, extreme thrombocytosis, leukocytosis, and an increase in circulating blasts. Prophylactic therapy with hydroxyurea has been advised to prevent postsplenectomy thrombocytosis. Transjugular intrahepatic portosystemic shunt might be considered to alleviate symptoms of portal hypertension.

Extramedullary hematopoiesis is the main cause of hepatosplenomegaly in PMF and post-PV or post-ET MF. Nonhepatosplenic EMH also occurs in PMF and might involve the vertebral column (spinal cord compression) lymph nodes, lung (pulmonary hypertension), pleura (effusion), small bowel, peritoneum (ascites), urogenital tract, skin, or heart. Diagnosis is usually tissue based, but imaging studies are sometimes used; MF-associated pulmonary hypertension can be confirmed by a technetium-99m sulphur colloid scintigraphy, which shows diffuse pulmonary uptake.

Radiotherapy has been a treatment option in both hepatosplenic and nonhepatosplenic EMH. Splenic irradiation (100-500 cGy in 5-10 fractions) induces transient reduction in spleen size but might be associated with life-threatening pancytopenia. More recent studies suggest the relative safety and value of lower dose treatment (100 cGy total dose in four daily fractions of 25 cGy). Radiation therapy works best for nonhepatosplenic EMH. Single-fraction (100-400 cGy) involved field therapy has also been shown to benefit patients with MF-associated pulmonary hypertension or extremity pain.

Quality of life–relevant symptoms in MF include profound fatigue, night sweats, weight loss, pruritus, bone pain, and nonproductive cough. Conventional drug therapy is inadequate in the management of these symptoms. Recent studies of JAK inhibitor therapy in PMF or post-PV, or post-ET MF suggest major benefit in terms of constitutional symptoms and cachexia.

Experimental Drug Therapy in Myeloproliferative Neoplasms

JAK-inhibiting ATP mimetics currently represent the most popular investigational drug therapy in MF.[8] Ruxolitinib is now approved by the Food and Drug Administration for use in MF, and momelotinib is currently being compared with ruxolitinib in a randomized phase 3 study. Ruxolitinib is a JAK1/JAK2 inhibitor. Two randomized studies comparing ruxolitinib with either placebo or best supportive care have now been published. In the COMFORT-1 trial that compared the drug with placebo, A5 the spleen size reduction response rate was approximately 42% for ruxolitinib versus less than 1% for placebo. In addition, about 46% of patients experienced substantial improvement in their constitutional symptoms, such as night sweats, pruritus, and fatigue. However, the use of the drug versus placebo was associated with anemia (31% vs. 13.9%) and thrombocytopenia (34.2% vs. 9.3%). The COMFORT-2 trial compared ruxolitinib with "best available therapy." A6 The spleen size reduction response was 28.5% with ruxolitinib versus 0% otherwise, and the use of the drug was associated with thrombocytopenia (44.5% vs. 9.6%), anemia (40.4% vs. 12.3%), and diarrhea (24.0% vs. 11.0%). The long-term outcome of ruxolitinib is associated with high treatment discontinuation rate and the occurrence of severe withdrawal symptoms during ruxolitinib treatment discontinuation ("ruxolitinib withdrawal syndrome"), characterized by acute relapse of disease symptoms, accelerated splenomegaly, worsening of cytopenias, and occasional hemodynamic decompensation. The 3-year follow-up information on COMFORT-2 suggested a 55% drug discontinuation rate and a slight but significant improvement in survival without any evidence of drug effect on *JAK2*V617F allele burden or bone marrow fibrosis. A7 Furthermore, reports have now associated ruxolitinib therapy with serious opportunistic infections.

Momelotinib (MMB, GS-0387, CYT387) is a JAK1 and JAK2 inhibitor. Among the first 60 patients treated in a phase 1 and 2 study,[9] Dose-limiting toxicities included grade 3 headache and hyperlipasemia (elevated lipase). Anemia and spleen responses were 59% and 48%, respectively. Most patients experienced constitutional symptoms improvement. The drug is currently undergoing phase 3 study and being compared with ruxolitinib.There is clearly a need to evaluate more drugs before making any conclusions regarding the value of anti-JAK2 therapy in MF or related MPN. It is also becoming evident that some of the salutary effects of these drugs might be the result of a potent anticytokine activity.

Allogeneic Stem Cell Transplantation

Allogenic stem cell transplant is a reasonable treatment modality in PMF, especially in the presence of high-risk disease.[10] However, there is a nontrivial risk of treatment-associated mortality and morbidity. In one study, for example, 5-year disease-free survival and treatment-related mortality rates were 33% and 35% for matched related and 27% and 50% for unrelated transplants, respectively. The respective chronic graft-versus-host disease and relapse rates for matched related transplants were 40% and 32%, respectively. Outcome did not appear to be favorably affected by reduced intensity conditioning (RIC). In another RIC transplant study, the 5-year disease-free survival rate was estimated at 51%, chronic graft-versus-host disease at 49%, and relapse at 29%. Splenectomy before transplant might not affect outcome. There is currently much interest in evaluating the use of JAK inhibitors before transplant with favorable and unfavorable experiences reported by different investigators, warranting the need for more studies before recommending such a strategy.

PROGNOSIS

Essential Thrombocythemia and Polycythemia Vera

Neither ET nor PV is currently a curable disease, and current therapy has not been shown to prolong survival. In a study of 1545 patients with PV, survival was adversely affected by older age, leukocytosis, abnormal karyotype, and venous thrombosis.[11] The first three also predicted leukemic transformation, which was 2.3% at 10 years and 5.5% at 15 years. Leukemic transformation was associated with treatment exposure to pipobroman or P32/chlorambucil but not to hydroxyurea or busulfan.

In WHO-defined ET, an international study identified age 60 years or older, thrombosis history, cardiovascular risk factors (CVR), leukocyte count greater than 11 × 10(9)/L, and the presence of *JAK2*V617F as independent predictors of arterial thrombosis and male gender as a predictor of venous thrombosis.[12] In a subsequent prognostic model,[13] thrombosis risk was lowest in the absence of these risk factors and intermediate or high otherwise. In ET, *CALR* mutations have been correlated with male sex, younger age, lower leukocyte count, lower hemoglobin level, higher platelet count, and longer thrombosis-free survival time.[14] Fibrotic or leukemic transformation in ET or PV is relatively infrequent (a combined rate of <10% in the first 15 years of disease).

Current risk stratification in PV and ET is designed to estimate the risk of thrombosis (see Table 166-8). Age 60 years or older and history of thrombosis are the two key risk factors used to classify patients with PV or ET into low- (no risk factors) and high- (one or two risk factors) risk groups. In addition, because of the potential risk for bleeding, low-risk patients with extreme thrombocytosis (platelet count $>1000 \times 10^9$/L) are considered separately. With the recent discovery of *CALR* mutations and their association with lower risk of thrombosis, the thrombogenic effect of *JAK2*V617F is increasingly being realized. Accordingly, more recent studies have identified the presence of *JAK2*V617F or cardiovascular risk factors as additional risk factors for thrombosis in ET.

Primary Myelofibrosis

The most robust prognostic model for PMF is the Dynamic International Prognostic Scoring System (DIPSS)-plus, which relies on eight adverse parameters: age older than 65 years, hemoglobin less than 10 g/dL, leukocyte count greater than 25×10^9/L, circulating blasts 1% or greater, constitutional symptoms, unfavorable karyotype, RBC transfusion need, and platelet count less than 100×10^9/L. The four DIPSS-plus risk categories based on these risk factors are low (no risk factors), intermediate-1 (one risk factor), intermediate-2 (two or three risk factors), and high (four or more risk factors), with respective median survival periods of 15.4, 6.5, 2.9, and 1.3 years. More recently, *ASXL1* mutations have been identified as a DIPSS-plus independent risk factor. Furthermore, *CALR* mutations in PMF were associated with younger age; higher platelet count; and lower incidences of anemia, leukocytosis, and spliceosome mutations and longer overall survival time. The best survival in PMK was found in the presence of *CALR* and absence of *ASXL1* mutation (i.e., $CALR^{+}ASXL1^{-}$) and worst survival in patients with $CALR^{-}ASXL1^{+}$ mutational status.[15]

CONCLUDING COMMENTS

Despite the seminal discoveries of *JAK2, MPL,* and *CALR* mutations, the pathogenesis of *BCR-ABL1*–negative MPN remains complex and poorly understood. It is becoming increasingly evident that *JAK2* is not the whole story with these diseases, and we should therefore curb our expectations from anti-JAK2 treatment strategies and instead pay attention to additional pathogenetic insight from correlative laboratory studies. In the end, one must recognize the relatively indolent natural history of ET and PV and avoid unnecessary treatment, especially in low-risk patients. There is currently an unmet need for treatment in PMF, and this is where the real challenge is and where progress is needed. It is hoped that that next-generation sequencing will help identify additional new mutations and prognostically relevant molecular signatures in MPN.

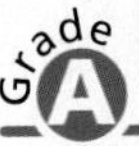

Grade A References

A1. Squizzato A, Romualdi E, Passamonti F, et al. Antiplatelet drugs for polycythaemia vera and essential thrombocythaemia. *Cochrane Database Syst Rev.* 2013;4:CD006503.

A2. Harrison CN, Campbell PJ, Buck G, et al. Hydroxyurea compared with anagrelide in high-risk essential thrombocythemia. *N Engl J Med.* 2005;353:33-45.

A3. Gisslinger H, Gotic M, Holowiecki J, et al. Anagrelide compared with hydroxyurea in WHO-classified essential thrombocythemia: the ANAHYDRET Study, a randomized controlled trial. *Blood.* 2013;121:1720-1728.

A4. Marchioli R, Finazzi G, Specchia G, et al. Cardiovascular events and intensity of treatment in polycythemia vera. *N Engl J Med.* 2013;368:22-33.

A5. Verstovsek S, Mesa RA, Gotlib J, et al. A double-blind, placebo-controlled trial of ruxolitinib for myelofibrosis. *N Engl J Med.* 2012;366:799-807.

A6. Harrison C, Kiladjian JJ, Al-Ali HK, et al. JAK inhibition with ruxolitinib versus best available therapy for myelofibrosis. *N Engl J Med.* 2012;366:787-798.

A7. Cervantes F, Vannucchi AM, Kiladjian JJ, et al. Three-year efficacy, safety, and survival findings from COMFORT-II, a phase 3 study comparing ruxolitinib with best available therapy for myelofibrosis. *Blood.* 2013;122:4047-4053.

GENERAL REFERENCES

For the General References and other additional features, please visit Expert Consult at https://expertconsult.inkling.com.

167

LEUKOCYTOSIS AND LEUKOPENIA

NANCY BERLINER

The normal peripheral white blood cell count (WBC) ranges between 4500/μL and 10,000/μL, with a mean of 7500/μL, and is composed of neutrophils, lymphocytes, monocytes, basophils, and eosinophils. Because neutrophils usually represent about 60% of the peripheral WBC, derangement in the WBC usually reflects elevation or reduction in the absolute neutrophil count. Leukocytosis, an elevated WBC, and leukopenia, a depressed WBC, may be secondary to an underlying disease or exposure, or they may be manifestations of a primary hematologic disorder. This chapter outlines both the primary and secondary causes of leukocytosis and leukopenia, focusing particularly on neutrophilia and neutropenia.

NORMAL NEUTROPHIL DYNAMICS

Neutrophils arise from multipotent progenitor cells in the bone marrow that also give rise to erythrocytes, megakaryocytes, eosinophils, basophils, and monocytes. Neutrophil precursors in the marrow mature over 6 to 10 days to form a storage pool of mature neutrophils (Fig. 167-1). Together the marrow populations make up about 95% of the body's total granulocyte mass (20% neutrophil precursors, 75% mature bands and neutrophils). The circulating neutrophil pool thus represents only the remaining approximately 5% of the body's total neutrophils, just over half of which at any given time are adherent to the vascular endothelium and the spleen, a phenomenon termed *margination*. These marginated neutrophils are poised for immediate release into the circulation during times of stress. The remaining neutrophils circulate freely in the blood. The lifespan of neutrophils in the peripheral blood was thought to be very short, only 6 to 12 hours; however, newer in vivo studies suggest that they circulate for up to 3 to 4 days.[1] They subsequently migrate into tissues, where they can survive for 1 to 4 days. Changes in neutrophil number reflect these dynamics. Neutrophilia can occur as the result of increased marrow production, increased release of neutrophils from the storage pool, or mobilization of neutrophils from the marginated pool. Neutropenia, on the other hand, may be due to decreased marrow production, increased margination with or without sequestration by the spleen, or increased destruction of peripheral cells.

NEUTROPHILIA

Most cases of neutrophilia are reactive or secondary to an underlying inflammatory process. This includes neutrophilia due to infection, chronic inflammation, stress, drugs, nonhematologic malignancy, marrow stimulation (as in hemolysis or idiopathic thrombocytopenic purpura), or splenectomy. Primary causes of neutrophilia may be congenital, including hereditary neutrophilia, Down syndrome, and leukocyte adhesion deficiency (LAD), or acquired as in the case of chronic myelogenous leukemia and other myeloproliferative neoplasms (Table 167-1).

TABLE 167-1 DIFFERENTIAL DIAGNOSIS OF NEUTROPHILIA

- Primary hematologic etiologies
  - Congenital neutrophilia
    - Hereditary neutrophilia
    - Chronic idiopathic neutrophilia
    - Down syndrome
    - Leukocyte adhesion deficiency (LAD)
      - LAD-1
      - LAD-2
  - Acquired hematologic neoplasms
    - Myeloproliferative neoplasm
      - Chronic myelogenous leukemia
      - Polycythemia vera
- Secondary to other disease entities
  - Infection
    - Acute via release from marginated and storage pools
    - Chronic via increased myelopoiesis (e.g., tuberculosis, fungal infection, chronic abscess, other chronic infections)
  - Chronic inflammation
    - Rheumatic disease: juvenile rheumatoid arthritis, rheumatoid arthritis, Still disease, and others
    - Inflammatory bowel disease
    - Granulomatous disease
    - Chronic hepatitis
  - Cigarette smoking
  - Stress
  - Drug induced
    - Corticosteroids
    - β-Agonists
    - Lithium
    - Recombinant cytokine administration
  - Nonhematologic malignancy
    - Cytokine-secreting tumors (lung, tongue, kidney, urothelial tumors)
    - Marrow metastasis (myelophthisis)
  - Marrow stimulation
    - Hemolytic anemia, immune thrombocytopenia
    - Recovery from marrow suppression
    - Recombinant cytokine administration
  - Post-splenectomy

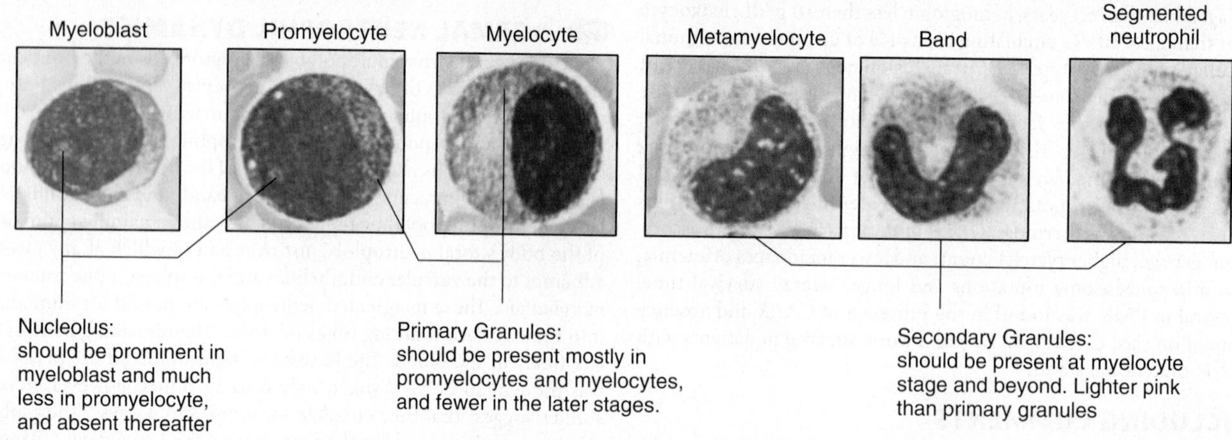
Myeloblast
Promyelocyte
Myelocyte
Metamyelocyte
Band
Segmented neutrophil
Nucleolus: should be prominent in myeloblast and much less in promyelocyte, and absent thereafter
Primary Granules: should be present mostly in promyelocytes and myelocytes, and fewer in the later stages.
Secondary Granules: should be present at myelocyte stage and beyond. Lighter pink than primary granules

FIGURE 167-1. **Myeloid maturation in the bone marrow. Nucleoli are prominent in myeloblasts, much less frequent in promyelocytes, and absent in more mature forms. Primary granules are present in the cytoplasm of promyelocytes and myelocytes, and secondary granules predominate beyond the myelocyte stage.**

ETIOLOGY

Secondary Causes of Neutrophilia

Infection

Many acute bacterial infections can present with a modest leukocytosis with a "left shift," referring to the circulation of more immature myeloid cells. This left shift most commonly is restricted to release of an increased number of band forms; however, in severe stress, one may see circulating metamyelocytes and even earlier cells (see Fig. 167-1) in the peripheral blood. Leukocytosis occurs within minutes to hours of infection owing to release of neutrophils from both the marrow and marginated pools. Examination of these neutrophils on peripheral smear may reveal evidence of toxic granulation (see Fig. 157-18), Döhle bodies (see Fig. 157-19), and cytoplasmic vacuoles. Certain infections (e.g., *Clostridium difficile* or tuberculosis in particular) are known to cause elevations in the WBC to greater than 30,000/μL in about one fourth of infected patients and may result in a *leukemoid reaction,* defined as a WBC of greater than 50,000/μL with a pronounced left shift (Fig. 167-2).

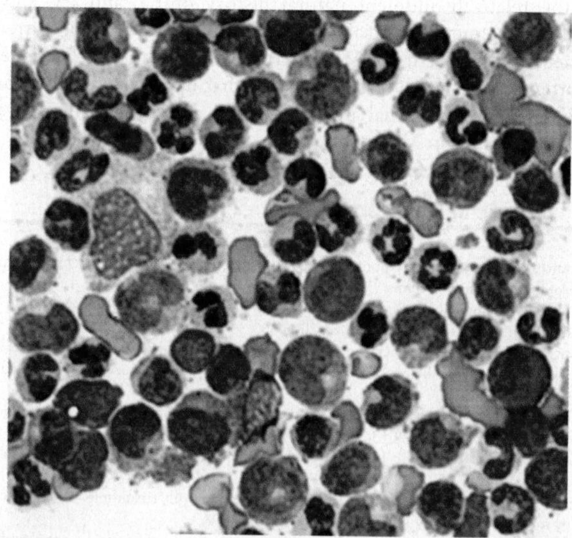

FIGURE 167-2. **Peripheral blood from a patient with leukemoid reaction. From this smear, it would be impossible to distinguish this from chronic phase chronic myelogenous leukemia (Chapter 184). Distinction would depend on determination of presence or absence of *BCR-ABL* fusion.**

Chronic Inflammation

Leukocytosis due to chronic inflammation results from increased leukocyte (specifically neutrophil and monocyte) production as opposed to altered neutrophil distribution. Mature neutrophil pools become depleted with ongoing inflammation, and the myeloid compartment of the marrow expands to increase neutrophil production. Myriad cytokines, including tumor necrosis factor-α (TNF-α), granulocyte colony-stimulating factor (G-CSF), granulocyte-macrophage colony-stimulating factor (GM-CSF), macrophage inflammatory protein-1 (MIP-1), interleukin-1 (IL-1), IL-6, and IL-8, have been implicated in this marrow stimulation (Chapter 156). Chronic inflammatory conditions that are particularly associated with leukocytosis and neutrophilia include juvenile rheumatoid arthritis, rheumatoid arthritis, Still disease, Crohn disease, ulcerative colitis, granulomatous infection, and chronic hepatitis. The WBC and neutrophil elevation in these cases is typically more modest than that seen in acute infection or inflammation.

Cigarette Smoking

Cigarette smoking can cause a leukocytosis and neutrophilia in about 25 to 50% of chronic smokers that can persist for even up to 5 years after quitting smoking. The mechanism by which this occurs is unknown, although there is recent evidence that cigarette smoke slows neutrophil apoptosis.[2]

Stress

Within minutes of exercise, surgery, or stress, one can see an elevation in circulating neutrophils. This is presumed to be due to the effects of catecholamines on marginated neutrophils, with release of neutrophils into the circulation. Some cases of stress-induced neutrophilia can be prevented by pretreatment with β-adrenergic antagonists (e.g., propranolol), supporting the role of catecholamines in the process. Exercise-induced neutrophilia, however, is not blocked by propranolol, suggesting that it may instead be due to flow and mechanical perturbation of neutrophils in the lungs. An elevated WBC has also been noted in the setting of acute myocardial infarction, but whether this is a risk factor for cardiac ischemia or a result of inflammation is unclear.

Drug Induced

Probably the most well-known and widely used drugs associated with leukocytosis are corticosteroids. Other drugs that are associated with elevations in the neutrophil count include β-agonists and lithium. Lithium causes neutrophilia by increasing the production of endogenous colony-stimulating factors (CSFs). G-CSF or GM-CSF treatment likewise may result in neutrophilia, and although this is the desired effect, the neutrophilia can be quite pronounced if not appropriately monitored.

Nonhematologic Malignancy

Leukocytosis can be seen in a number of nonhematologic malignancies. Some tumors (lung, tongue, kidney, bladder) are thought to secrete G-CSF as an ectopic hematopoietic growth factor. Other tumors (lung, stomach, breast), when metastasized to the bone and bone marrow, can cause a *leukoerythroblastic reaction,* characterized by left-shifted leukocytosis, thrombocytosis, and red cell abnormalities including nucleated and teardrop-shaped red blood cells (Fig. 167-3). The presence of nonhematopoietic entities invading the bone marrow (metastatic cancer, fibrosis, granulomatous disease) is termed *myelophthisis.*

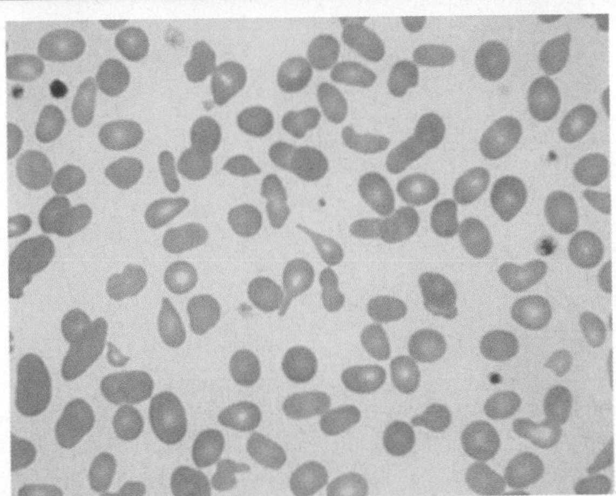

FIGURE 167-3. Myelophthisic changes in erythrocyte morphology. Note prominent teardrop forms. (From Rose M, Berliner N. Disorders of red blood cells. In: Andreoli TE, Benjamin IJ, Griggs RC, et al, eds. *Andreoli and Carpenter's Cecil Essentials of Medicine*, 8th ed. Philadelphia: Saunders; 2010:522, Fig. 49-2.)

Marrow Stimulation

Peripheral destruction of red cells and platelets, as seen with hemolytic anemia and idiopathic thrombocytopenic purpura, can result in stimulation of the bone marrow and a "spillover" leukocytosis. Recovery of cell counts following marrow suppression, as in the case of chemotherapy, can result in a rebound leukocytosis that may last several weeks.

Primary Causes of Neutrophilia

Hereditary Neutrophilia

Hereditary neutrophilia is an autosomal dominant genetic disease that is characterized by an elevated WBC in the 20,000 to 100,000/μL range with splenomegaly and widened diploe of the skull. The neutrophils in this disorder appear to function normally, and patients have no increased risk for bacterial infection or other sequelae. Hereditary neutrophilia caused by an autosomal-dominant *GCSF3* gene mutation has been reported, causing constitutive activation of the G-CSF receptor.

Chronic Idiopathic Neutrophilia

Chronic idiopathic neutrophilia is a condition marked by leukocytosis in the 11,000 to 40,000/μL range with a normal bone marrow biopsy. In one series with a 20-year follow-up, patients with this condition had no medical sequelae from this elevated WBC.

Pelger-Huët Anomaly

Patients with the Pelger-Huët anomaly (PHA) are often misdiagnosed as having a left-shifted WBC because many of their mature neutrophils are misinterpreted as band forms. Although these patients do not actually have leukocytosis, the anomaly often raises suspicion for an acute infection or inflammatory process because of this apparent left shift. PHA is due to a mutation in the lamin B receptor gene and manifests with mature neutrophils and condensed, clumped chromatin within a bilobed nucleus (see Fig. 157-20). These neutrophils, however, function normally. A number of drugs can reversibly induce pseudo-PHA, including colchicine, sulfonamides, ibuprofen, taxoids, and valproate. Pseudo-PHA is also seen in some patients with myelodysplasia (Chapter 182). Vitamin B_{12} or folate deficiency can cause increased nuclear lobation of neutrophils in patients with PHA, perhaps leading to a missed diagnosis. With correction of the vitamin deficiency, however, the aberrant neutrophil nuclear morphology returns.

Down Syndrome

Up to 10% of patients with Down syndrome develop transient myeloproliferative disorder (TMD) related to peripheral blood leukocytosis with blasts in association with an accumulation of megakaryoblasts in the blood, liver, and marrow. Similar reactions have also been reported in patients with trisomy 21 mosaicism who are phenotypically normal. TMD resolves spontaneously in most patients but can progress to acute megakaryoblastic leukemia (AMKL) in 23 to 30% of affected patients. This disorder is attributable to acquisition of mutations in the *GATA1* gene, which encodes a key transcription factor for hematopoietic regulation, leading to loss of normal GATA-1 expression and expression of a truncated GATA-1 protein. Evidence supports that these mutations are acquired during fetal life, and patients present in early infancy with TMD. The pathogenesis of progression to AMKL presumably requires additional genetic events and sequential epigenetic changes, and is the focus of intense study.[3,4]

Leukocyte Adhesion Deficiency

Patients with leukocyte adhesion deficiency (LAD) (see also Chapter 169) have persistent leukocytosis, defects in stimulus-dependent activation of neutrophils, recurrent infections, and delayed separation of the umbilical cord. LAD is an abnormality of leukocyte adhesion reflecting the loss of surface adhesion molecules. LAD-1 is due to absence or marked reduction in the common β chain of β2 integrins, resulting in loss of expression of leukocyte function–associated antigen 1 (LFA-1), the C3bi receptor, and GP150;95. This results in a failure to ingest and kill microbes opsonized by C3bi. In LAD-2, neutrophils lack sialyl Lewis X, the ligand for L-selectin expressed on endothelial cells. Neutrophils appear morphologically normal but are defective in chemotaxis, adherence, and phagocytosis.[5]

Familial Cold Urticaria

Familial cold urticaria is marked by episodic fevers, leukocytosis, urticaria, rash, conjunctivitis, and muscle and skin tenderness with cold exposure. The rash is composed of infiltrating neutrophils. The syndrome appears to be related to decreased levels of C1-esterase inhibitor and is associated with mutations in the *CIAS1* gene on chromosome 1q.

Chronic Myelogenous Leukemia and Other Myeloproliferative Disorders

Chronic myelogenous leukemia (CML), chronic neutrophilic leukemia (CNL), and the other myeloproliferative neoplasms (namely polycythemia vera [PV] and essential thrombocythemia [ET]) are discussed in detail in Chapters 184 and 166. They are the principal acquired primary hematologic disorders associated with neutrophilia. They are marked by clonal expansion of myeloid precursors and increased release of both immature and mature myeloid cells into the peripheral blood. CML on presentation often has to be distinguished from a leukemoid reaction. In contrast to a leukemoid reaction, CML is characterized by the presence of abnormalities of other blood cell lines ("panmyelosis") and by the presence of specific abnormalities. Therefore, the peripheral blood smear in CML (but not leukemoid reaction) demonstrates increased numbers in all cells of the neutrophilic series, classically with a greater proportion of myelocytes to metamyelocytes, and may display concomitant basophilia, eosinophilia, anemia, and thrombocytosis. CNL, a rare myeloproliferative neoplasm, is characterized by hepato/splenomegaly and leukocytosis of at least 25,000/μL, with more than 80% of leukocytes being segmented neutrophil/band forms and less than 10% being immature granulocytes, in contrast to CML.[6] CML is characterized by the diagnostic presence of the Philadelphia chromosome [t(9;22)], which can be identified in the peripheral blood by the detection of the *BCR-ABL* translocation by fluorescence in situ hybridization (FISH) or reverse transcription–polymerase chain reaction (RT-PCR). At least 50% of patients with CNL, in contrast, harbor mutations in the receptor for CSF-3 (*CSF3R; GCSFR*).[6] PV and ET, on the other hand, are notable for also having a marked increase in red cell mass and a marked thrombocytosis, respectively, which is often accompanied by leukocytosis.

The leukocyte alkaline phosphatase (LAP) score was historically used in the laboratory evaluation of granulocytosis as a diagnostic marker for myeloproliferative neoplasm. The LAP score is very low (usually 0) in the setting of CML and elevated in PV. The LAP score has a very wide normal range and in practical terms was only definitively helpful in the setting of CML because "high" LAP scores can also be seen in infectious and inflammatory settings. With the availability of direct molecular genetic diagnosis of CML by assay for the *BCR-ABL* fusion gene, it can no longer be recommended as a diagnostic test.

Post-splenectomy

Patients develop leukocytosis following splenectomy, and this may be longstanding, reflecting the loss of a major site of neutrophil margination. This is of no clinical importance, except insofar as it leads to unnecessary evaluation for other pathology.

CLINICAL MANIFESTATIONS AND DIAGNOSIS

As outlined previously, acquired leukocytosis is most commonly the result of acute or chronic infection or inflammation. When it occurs in the absence of

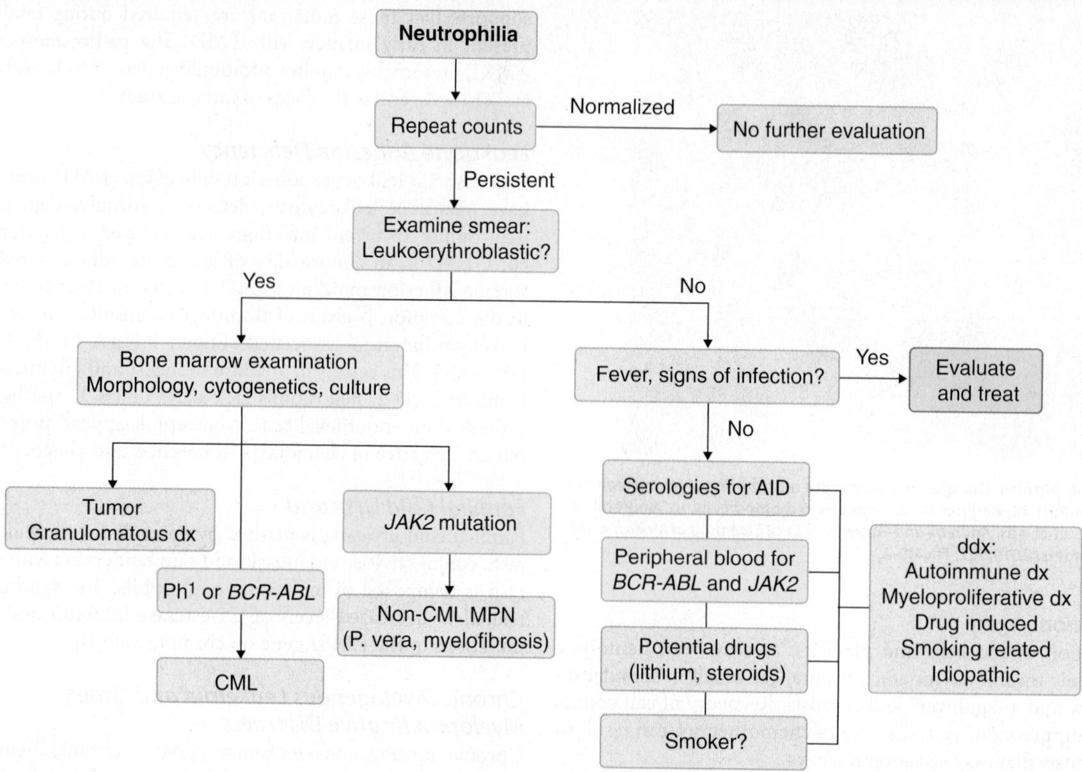

FIGURE 167-4. **Diagnostic approach to neutrophilia.** AID = autoimmune disease; CML = chronic myelogenous leukemia; ddx = differential diagnosis; dx = disease; MPN = myeloproliferative neoplasm; Ph[1] = Philadelphia chromosome; PV = P. vera, ET = essential thrombocytopenia.

fever, aberrations in acute phase reactants, effusions and edema, or other signs and symptoms of inflammation, it still may be secondary to drugs or an underlying nonhematologic malignancy. As such, it should be seen as the sign of a healthy hematopoietic system responding to an outside stress. Bone marrow evaluation is therefore rarely indicated. However, persistence of leukocytosis in the absence of signs and symptoms of inflammation or infection, nonhematologic malignancy, and offending drugs should prompt an evaluation for a primary myeloproliferative disease or clonal hematologic neoplasm, particularly when there is evidence of a leukoerythroblastic reaction. CML and other myeloproliferative neoplasms can be ruled out by molecular diagnosis on the peripheral blood, as described previously and in Chapter 166. In this setting, bone marrow examination is indicated to evaluate for marrow infiltration by infection, tumor, or fibrosis and should include cultures for tuberculosis and fungal infection as well as cytogenetics and flow cytometry (Fig. 167-4).

Leukocytosis Due to Expansion of Other Cell Lines

Monocytosis and lymphocytosis can also lead to elevations of the WBC. Monocytosis is defined by an absolute monocyte count of greater than 500/μL and usually occurs in the setting of chronic inflammation resulting from infections like tuberculosis, syphilis, or subacute bacterial endocarditis, autoimmune or granulomatous disease, and sarcoidosis. It can also be seen in malignancies, such as preleukemic states, nonlymphocytic leukemia including acute myelomonocytic and monocytic leukemia, histiocytosis, Hodgkin disease, non-Hodgkin lymphoma, and various carcinomas. Finally, it can be seen in the setting of chronic neutropenia, after splenectomy, and in the setting of recovery from marrow suppression (Table 167-2).

Lymphocytosis is defined by an absolute lymphocyte count of more than 5000/μL. The most common causes of an elevated lymphocyte count are viral infections such as Epstein-Barr virus and the hepatitis viruses. Although most bacterial infections cause neutrophilia, pertussis and cat-scratch disease due to *Bartonella henselae* can cause an impressive lymphocytosis. Other infections that may cause a secondary lymphocytosis include toxoplasmosis and babesiosis. Hypersensitivity reactions due to drugs or serum sickness may also be associated with lymphocytosis. Primary disorders that cause a lymphocytosis include chronic lymphocytic leukemia (CLL) and monoclonal B-cell lymphocytosis (Table 167-3; see also Table 184-2 and Chapter 184).

Eosinophilia is defined by an absolute eosinophil count of more than 400/μL. Eosinophils proliferate under the influence of IL-5 and play a role in phagocytosis and modulating toxicity due to mast cell degranulation in hypersensitivity reactions. Eosinophilia is therefore most often seen in the setting of drug reactions, allergy, atopy, and asthma. A variety of infections, particularly parasitic infections and, to a lesser degree, fungal infections, can be associated with an increased number of circulating eosinophils. Eosinophilia can also be the result of autoimmune and inflammatory conditions, as in Churg-Strauss vasculitis. Atheroembolic disease and adrenal insufficiency may also cause eosinophilia. A number of cancers have been associated with polytypic expansion of eosinophils, including lymphomas and solid tumors. There are also a number of clonal disorders of eosinophils that occur in the setting of some leukemias. Finally, there is a heterogeneous group of disorders termed *hypereosinophilic syndromes*. A *FIP1L1-PDGFRA* fusion gene has confirmed that some of these are primary clonal disorders of eosinophils; the clonality of other hypereosinophilic syndromes can be difficult to establish (see Table 170-1).

TABLE 167-2 DIFFERENTIAL DIAGNOSIS OF MONOCYTOSIS

Infection
Granulomatous disease (tuberculosis, fungal disease)
Endocarditis
Syphilis
Autoimmune diseases
Lupus, rheumatoid arthritis
Giant cell arteritis
Vasculitis
Inflammatory bowel disease
Sarcoid
Malignancy
Primary hematologic malignancy
Chronic myelomonocytic leukemia
Acute myelomonocytic leukemia
Lymphoma
Solid tumors
Neutropenia
Associated with chronic neutropenia
Recovery form marrow suppression
Post-splenectomy

TABLE 167-3 DIFFERENTIAL DIAGNOSIS OF LYMPHOCYTOSIS

Infection
- Viral infection
  - Epstein-Barr virus
  - Cytomegalovirus
  - Hepatitis
- Bacterial infection
  - Pertussis
  - Bartonella
  - Tuberculosis
  - Syphilis
  - Rickettsia
  - Babesia

Hypersensitivity reactions
- Serum sickness
- Drug hypersensitivity

Primary hematologic disease
- Chronic lymphocytic leukemia
- Monoclonal B-cell lymphocytosis
- Non-Hodgkin lymphoma

NEUTROPENIA

The risk for infection in the setting of neutropenia is highly dependent on the size of the neutrophil storage pool. Although neutropenia is defined by an absolute neutrophil count of less than 1500/μL, patients with neutrophil counts below this number may have different risks and rates of infection depending on the cause of neutropenia. For instance, patients who are neutropenic owing to chemotherapy, marrow failure, or marrow exhaustion experience infection at much higher rates than those with chronic neutropenic syndromes and immune-mediated neutropenia. Neutropenia may be congenital or acquired. The following sections first discuss congenital neutropenic disorders, the study of which has provided critical insights into normal myelopoiesis, and then the secondary causes of neutropenia (Table 167-4).

ETIOLOGY

Primary Causes of Neutropenia

Ethnic and Benign Familial (Constitutional) Neutropenia

The normal range of the neutrophil count is genetically determined and can be variable. A number of racial and ethnic groups have been observed to have a relatively large proportion of members who are neutropenic by comparison to the published normal range, usually based on young, largely white individuals. This is termed *constitutional neutropenia* and is seen among a variety of ethnic groups, including African Americans, Yemenite Jews, Falasha Jews, and African Bedouins. Single-nucleotide polymorphisms in the gene for the Duffy antigen receptor for chemokine *(DARC)* have been shown to associate with race and are a postulated candidate to explain racial and ethnic differences in neutrophil counts.[7] There is also an autosomal dominantly inherited condition called *benign familial neutropenia* that is characterized by neutrophil counts in the 800 to 1400/μL range. Neither ethnic nor benign familial neutropenia has been shown to be associated with *any* increased risk for infection.

Severe Congenital Neutropenia

First described by Rolf Kostmann in 1956, severe congenital neutropenia (SCN) is a disorder of severe neutropenia with neutrophil counts of less than 500/μL, presenting in the neonatal period with recurrent bacterial infections. These infections can occur as early as the first months of life and often include omphalitis and perirectal abscesses. There is often an increase in other myeloid cell lines, including monocytes and eosinophils. Bone marrow biopsy in SCN patients reveals a "maturation arrest" with an absence of mature neutrophil elements. SCN can follow autosomal dominant and recessive and X-linked patterns of inheritance and has been shown to be associated with mutations in a variety of genes, as summarized in Table 167-5.

Neutrophil elastase (ELA2, now ELANE) is a serine protease that is synthesized at high levels in the promyelocyte stage of neutrophil maturation and is packaged in primary granules. It was originally hypothesized that mutations in ELANE led to its defective cellular trafficking and cytoplasmic accumulation, subsequently triggering neutrophil apoptosis. Newer evidence, however, supports a mechanism by which accumulation of the mutant

TABLE 167-4 DIFFERENTIAL DIAGNOSIS OF NEUTROPENIA

Congenital neutropenia
- Ethnic and benign familial (constitutional) neutropenia
- Severe congenital neutropenia
  - Autosomal dominant (*ELANE* mutation)
  - Autosomal recessive (Kostmann syndrome; *HAX2* mutation)
  - X-linked (*WASP* mutation)
  - Other rare defects (*G-CSFR* mutation, unknown)
- Cyclic neutropenia
- Shwachman-Diamond syndrome
- Fanconi anemia
- Dyskeratosis congenita
- Glycogen storage disease type Ib
- Myelokathexis
- Chédiak-Higashi syndrome
- Griscelli syndrome type II
- Hermansky-Pudlak syndrome II
- Barth syndrome

Acquired neutropenia
- Infection
- Postinfection
- Drug induced
- Immune neutropenia
  - Primary immune neutropenia
  - Secondary to autoimmune disease
    - Rheumatoid arthritis
      - Felty syndrome
      - Large granular lymphocyte disease
    - Systemic lupus erythematosus
    - Wegener granulomatosis
    - Hyperthyroidism
  - Pure white cell aplasia associated with thymoma
  - Large granular lymphocyte disease
- Primary bone marrow failure
  - Aplastic anemia
  - Myelodysplastic syndrome
  - Acute leukemia
- Margination and hypersplenism
- Vitamin and mineral deficiencies (including B_{12}, folate, copper)
- Chronic idiopathic neutropenia in adults (CINA)

ELANE = neutrophil elastase; G-CSFR: granulocyte colony-stimulating factor receptor; WASP = Wiskott-Aldrich syndrome protein.

TABLE 167-5 CONGENITAL NEUTROPENIA SYNDROMES

SYNDROME	INHERITANCE PATTERN	GENE
SCN	Autosomal dominant	*ELANE* (~60%)
	Autosomal recessive	*HAX1* (~5%)
	X-linked	*WASP* (~5%)
	X-linked	*TAZ* (rare)
	Autosomal recessive	*G6PC3* (~2%)
	Autosomal dominant	*Gfi1* (rare)
	Autosomal dominant	*G-CSFR* (rare)
CYCLIC NEUTROPENIA	Autosomal dominant	*ELANE*
OTHER CONGENITAL SYNDROMES		
Shwachman-Diamond syndrome	X-Linked	*SBDS*
Fanconi anemia	Autosomal recessive	*FANCA-FANCO*
Dyskeratosis congenita	Variable	Telomerase and related genes
Glycogen storage disease type 1b	Autosomal recessive	*G-6-PT*
Myelokathexis	Autosomal dominant	*CXCR4*
Chédiak-Higashi syndrome	Autosomal recessive	*LYST*
Griscelli syndrome type 2	Autosomal recessive	*RAB27A*
Hermansky-Pudlak syndrome type 2	Autosomal recessive	*AP3B1*

ELANE = neutrophil elastase; G6PC3 = glucose-6-phosphatase catalytic subunit 3; G-6-PT = glucose-6-phosphatase translocase; G-CSFR = granulocyte colony-stimulating factor receptor; LYST = lysosomal trafficking regulatory gene; SBDS = Shwachman-Bodian-Diamond syndrome; SCN = severe congenital neutropenia; WASP = Wiskott-Aldrich syndrome protein.

neutrophil elastase in the endoplasmic reticulum activates the unfolded protein response, leading to apoptosis. SCN due to these mutations is inherited in an autosomal dominant fashion. Hax-1 is a mitochondrial protein with weak homology to bcl-2, and its absence results in mitochondrial-dependent apoptosis. It is the mutated protein implicated in the original autosomal recessive cases of SCN described by Kostmann. Although all SCN cases were originally referred to as *Kostmann syndrome*, that term is now reserved for this subgroup of autosomal recessive SCN. Wiskott-Aldrich syndrome protein (WASP) regulates actin polymerization in hematopoietic cells, and deficiency in this protein results in the Wiskott-Aldrich syndrome, characterized by small platelets in low number, sinopulmonary infections, and eczema. Another phenotype of mutated WASP, however, is X-linked thrombocytopenia and neutropenia. Mutations in the glucose-6-phosphatase catalytic subunit 3 (*G6PC3*) are the most recently discovered cause of a subset of SCN patients; homozygous loss of this metabolic enzyme also appears to lead to activation of the unfolded protein response and increased apoptosis of neutrophil precursors.[8]

SCN was formerly a disease of infancy and early childhood because few, if any, patients survived to adulthood. However, the advent of the availability of recombinant G-CSF and the observation that G-CSF is able to raise neutrophil counts and prevent infection in most patients have allowed these children to survive. Some patients require very high doses of G-CSF, but responses are seen in 80 to 90% of individuals. Increased survival led to the emerging realization that SCN predisposes to the development of myelodysplasia and acute leukemia (MDS/AML), with the development of MDS/AML at a rate of approximately 2% per year, and a cumulative risk of about 30% over 10 years.[9] Patients refractory to, or requiring very high doses of, G-CSF appear to have a higher risk for leukemic transformation. As discussed later, development of MDS/AML is often associated with the acquisition of a mutation in the gene encoding for the G-CSF receptor. Considerable controversy exists concerning the potential contribution of G-CSF administration to the risk for malignant transformation in children with SCN who receive lifelong treatment with G-CSF (see later under Treatment).

Two classes of G-CSF receptor mutations have been associated with SCN and either hyper-responsiveness or hyporesponsiveness of the receptor. Initial studies aimed at demonstrating that SCN was caused by mutation of the G-CSF or G-CSF receptor gene did not implicate such mutations in the pathogenesis of a significant number of patients with SCN. However, a small number of patients have been shown to have mutations in the G-CSF receptor gene that block ligand binding and produce a G-CSF-resistant form of SCN. More important, however, the studies identified an acquired missense mutation that introduces a stop codon and leads to the deletion of the distal intracellular domain of the receptor known to be responsible for differentiation signaling. This has been hypothesized to cause proliferation of hematopoietic progenitors at the expense of maturation and to be associated with hypersensitivity to G-CSF, suggesting that this mutation may play an important role in the development of MDS/AML in the setting of SCN. However, whether this mutation is in fact of pathogenetic importance to the development of MDS/AML and whether G-CSF influences the risk for developing the mutation and influencing leukemic transformation remain subjects of significant controversy.

Cyclic Neutropenia

Cyclic neutropenia is defined as periods of neutropenia (≤200/μL) lasting 3 to 5 days and occurring at approximately 21-day intervals. These periods of neutropenia may be marked by recurrent fevers, mouth sores, and infections of the skin, upper respiratory tract, and ears. The disorder can be dominantly inherited or sporadic. Congenital cyclic neutropenia has also been shown to be associated with mutations in the gene for neutrophil elastase in virtually all cases tested to date.[10] The diagnosis formerly required demonstration of transient neutropenia through frequent blood counts over a course of 6 weeks but now can be established by sequencing of the neutrophil elastase gene. It is successfully treated with G-CSF and is not associated with an increased risk for leukemic transformation. Rare cases of cyclic neutropenia acquired in adulthood have been associated with systemic diseases such as large granular lymphocytosis or T-cell lymphoma.

Other Congenital Syndromes with Associated Neutropenia

A number of other congenital syndromes are associated with neutropenia as one of the constellation of disease-associated abnormalities. These include Shwachman-Diamond syndrome, Fanconi anemia, dyskeratosis congenita, glycogen storage disease Ib, myelokathexis, Chédiak-Higashi syndrome, Griscelli syndrome II, and Hermansky-Pudlak syndrome II.[11]

Shwachman-Diamond syndrome usually begins as an isolated neutropenia but progresses to marrow failure and is also associated with pancreatic dysfunction and skeletal abnormalities. The responsible gene, the Shwachman-Bodian-Diamond syndrome gene (*SBDS*), is involved in the regulation of ribosomal RNA. These patients carry an increased risk for leukemic transformation.

Fanconi anemia is due to mutations in genes involved in DNA repair, and as such, it takes more time for marrow failure to develop in these patients (median age, 7 years). Patients with Fanconi anemia often have, in addition to marrow failure, short stature with upper limb anomalies and hyperpigmented cafe au lait spots, although about one third have no physical abnormalities. Screening is done by chromosomal fragility testing following exposure to diepoxybutane or mitomycin C as well as direct assessment for known Fanconi gene mutations. Stem cell transplantation is curative but carries a high risk for morbidity and mortality owing to the toxicity of preparative regimens.[12]

Dyskeratosis congenita (DKC) is a syndrome of nail dystrophy, leukoplakia, and skin pigmentation abnormalities with associated neutropenia or aplastic anemia, or both. It can be inherited in an autosomal dominant or recessive or X-linked fashion and has been shown to be associated with mutations in several genes that are implicated in telomere maintenance. It typically does not present until the second decade of life. Recent studies have demonstrated that DKC is one of several diseases associated with telomere abnormalities, with wide-ranging manifestations including pulmonary fibrosis and hepatic cirrhosis as well as bone marrow failure.

Glycogen storage disease Ib is inherited in an autosomal recessive fashion and characterized by intermittent neutropenia due to defects in the neutrophil respiratory burst with subsequent apoptosis of circulating neutrophils. Hepatomegaly and metabolic crises are also the hallmarks of this disease and are due to mutations in the gene for the glucose-6-phosphatase translocase enzyme.

The neutropenia of *myelokathexis* is due to retention of mature neutrophils in the bone marrow despite a low peripheral neutrophil count. During infection, however, patients with myelokathexis typically have a sudden rise in their neutrophil count, which makes their clinical course relatively more benign. There is an association between this condition and hypogammaglobulinemia and warts, the WHIM syndrome (*w*arts, *h*ypogammaglobulinemia, *i*mmunodeficiency, and *m*yelokathexis). It has been shown to be caused by heterozygous mutations in the gene encoding chemokine receptor CXCR4.

Chédiak-Higashi syndrome, Griscelli syndrome II, and *Hermansky-Pudlak syndrome II* are all syndromes of albinism and neutropenia due to defects in vesicular trafficking. Chédiak-Higashi syndrome is due to mutations in a lysosomal trafficking regulatory gene (*LYST*) and is characterized by oculocutaneous albinism, bleeding, progressive neurologic disease, and increased susceptibility to hemophagocytic syndrome. Patients with Griscelli syndrome II also have an increased susceptibility to hemophagocytic syndrome as well as albinism and periodic neutropenia; Griscelli syndrome II is caused by mutations in the gene encoding the small guanosine triphosphatase RAB27A, which is involved in the release of myeloperoxidase from the primary granules of neutrophils. Hermansky-Pudlak syndrome II is due to mutations in the *AP3B1* gene, which encodes a part of a protein transport complex that is involved in vesicular trafficking in many cell types and appears to be involved in the trafficking of neutrophil elastase. It is also marked by albinism, platelet abnormalities, and pulmonary fibrosis.

Barth syndrome is an X-linked autosomal recessive disorder characterized by neutropenia, cardiomyopathy, and growth retardation, with a high mortality rate through early childhood because of the heart disease. The causative mutation is in the *TAZ* gene, which encodes tafazzin protein that is critical to remodeling cardiolipin in the mitochondrial membrane.

Secondary Causes of Neutropenia

Infection-Related Neutropenia

Several viral infections have been shown to cause a transient neutropenia that typically resolves as the viremia abates. These include varicella, measles, rubella, hepatitis A and B, Epstein-Barr virus, influenza, parvovirus, and cytomegalovirus. The mechanisms are diverse and can involve redistribution, decreased production, and immune destruction of neutrophils. Human immunodeficiency virus and acquired immunodeficiency syndrome can likewise cause mulitfactorial leukopenia and neutropenia (Chapter 393). Patients often have splenomegaly with increased sequestration, but more commonly the neutropenia reflects immune-mediated destruction. A myriad of atypical infections like *Mycobacterium tuberculosis*, ehrlichiosis, rickettsia, tularemia, brucellosis, and some staphylococcal infections can cause a moderate neutropenia. Any infection leading to overwhelming sepsis can cause neutropenia, but this is usually through consumption of the marrow neutrophil reserve and is typically seen in newborns and elderly patients and not in individuals with an otherwise healthy and mature marrow. There is also increased margination of neutrophils during sepsis due to systemic activation of complement, exacerbating the neutropenia.

Drug-Induced Neutropenia and Neutropenia Due to Marrow Injury

Drug-induced neutropenia is the most common cause of neutropenia. Multiple drugs have been implicated in neutropenia and agranulocytosis, in both predictable and idiosyncratic patterns. Drug-induced neutropenias may reflect either suppression of marrow granulopoiesis or increased destruction or clearance of peripheral neutrophils. Many drugs cause direct dose-dependent marrow suppression, which is predictable and often mild. Others incite an idiosyncratic immune-mediated destruction that can present with profound agranulocytosis. The typical pattern of drug-induced neutropenia is a marked decline in the neutrophil count that occurs after about 1 to 2 weeks of exposure to the drug with a recovery that begins within days of stopping the drug. However, atypical cases can present long after drug initiation, and others may be associated with a longer interval before recovery of the neutrophil count (Fig. 167-5). Patients with drug-induced agranulocytosis may present with acute sepsis, and it is associated with a significant risk for acute mortality. Recovery is often preceded by the appearance of monocytes and immature neutrophil forms. The more hypercellular the marrow is at diagnosis, the earlier marrow recovery may occur. Some common drugs known to cause neutropenia, in addition to antineoplastic, antiviral, and immunosuppressive agents, include clozapine, the antithyroidal thioamides including carbimazole, methimazole and propylthiouracil, quinidine, procainamide, sulfasalazine, and Levamisole, which is widely used as a cocaine adulterant, causing cocaine-associated neutropenia. Neutrophil recovery is speeded by G-CSF, although there are no definitive data that this improves survival in this setting.

Radiation can also result in marrow injury leading to an acute or chronic marrow failure state; in high doses, it is also a risk factor for the development of myelodysplasia and leukemia. These malignant hematopoietic diseases can themselves cause marrow failure because the malignant cells proliferate within the marrow-occupying space and can cause marrow fibrosis, both of which lead to cytopenias. These diseases are discussed in greater detail in Chapters 182 and 183, respectively. Likewise, metastatic carcinoma to the bone can also cause marrow failure because the marrow becomes increasingly replaced by the metastatic cells.

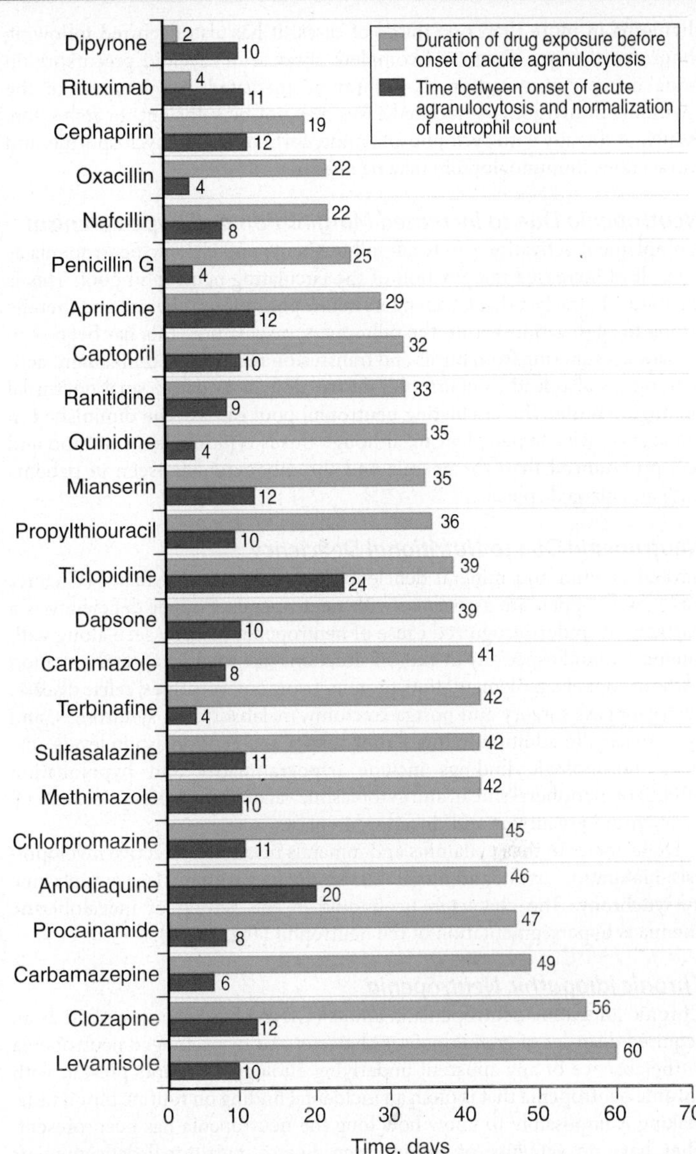

FIGURE 167-5. **Median duration of treatment and neutropenia. Only drugs with more than three definite or probable reports of the time between onset of acute agranulocytosis and normalization of neutrophil count and the duration of treatment before onset of acute agranulocytosis were considered. (From Andersohn F, Konzen C, Garbe E. Systematic review: agranulocytosis induced by nonchemotherapy drugs. *Ann Intern Med.* 2007;146: 657-665.)**

Immune Neutropenia

Infection and drugs cause immune-mediated neutrophil destruction. However, immune neutropenia can also occur as an isolated phenomenon (primary immune neutropenia) or as a manifestation of an underlying systemic autoimmune disease (secondary immune neutropenia). Primary autoimmune neutropenia is primarily a disease of children younger than 4 years; median age of onset is 6 to 12 months. Although infectious risk is increased, treatment is restricted to prophylactic antibiotics, with G-CSF reserved for acute infectious episodes. Ninety-five percent of patients undergo spontaneous remissions within 2 years. Nearly all of these patients have antineutrophil antibodies directed against antigens derived from the FcγIIIb receptor; these antibodies mediate neutrophil destruction by either sequestration in the spleen or complement-mediated neutrophil lysis.

Secondary autoimmune neutropenia is a disease of adults and can be seen in association with hyperthyroidism, Wegener granulomatosis, rheumatoid arthritis, and systemic lupus erythematosus (SLE). The role of antineutrophil antibodies in these patients is less clear. More than 50% of patients with SLE, for example, have antineutrophil antibodies, but many have normal neutrophil counts, and there is a poor correlation between the presence of the antibodies and neutrophil number.[13]

Felty syndrome and *large granular lymphocyte syndrome* deserve separate mention. Felty syndrome occurs in association with long-standing rheumatoid arthritis (RA) (Chapter 264) and is characterized by splenomegaly and profound neutropenia. Large granular lymphocyte syndrome often occurs in the setting of RA but can also occur as an isolated phenomenon. Both Felty syndrome and large granular lymphocyte syndrome are associated with a proliferation of large granular lymphocytes, with a characteristic surface phenotype ($CD3^+$, $CD8^+$, $CD16^+$, and $CD57^+$). In the setting of RA, these two syndromes were originally thought to be separate diseases, with Felty syndrome being polyclonal and large granular lymphocyte syndrome representing a monoclonal proliferation of larger granular lymphocytes. However, with increasing sensitivity of detection of monoclonal populations of lymphocytes, this distinction has become blurred. It has been observed that more than 90% of RA patients with either syndrome are human leukocyte antigen (HLA)-DR4-positive, leading to the postulate that the two entities represent the extremes of a single spectrum of disease. This HLA restriction is not found among non-RA patients with large granular lymphocytes. Both syndromes cause immune-mediated neutrophil destruction by a wide array of mechanisms, including antineutrophil antibodies and cell-mediated destruction. Some patients may also have G-CSF resistance mediated by inhibitory G-CSF antibodies.[14]

There are other rare forms of immune neutropenia. Isoimmune neonatal neutropenia is a moderate to severe neutropenia of the newborn due to transplacental passage of maternal immunoglobulin G antibodies against alleles inherited from the father, resulting in neutropenia in a manner similar to the development of anemia in Rh hemolytic disease. Pure white cell aplasia is a rare disease associated with severe pyogenic infections, and also with thymoma in more than two thirds of cases. It has also occurred following ibuprofen therapy. There is a complete absence of myeloid precursors on bone marrow examination. It is immune mediated, but removal of the thymoma in thymoma-associated cases may not be sufficient for remission. Adjuvant therapy with cyclophosphamide, corticosteroids, cyclosporine, and intravenous immunoglobulin may be needed.

Neutropenia Due to Increased Margination and Hypersplenism

Complement activation can result in both acute and chronic neutropenia as a result of increased margination of the circulating neutrophil pool. This is attributed to the fact that C5a renders neutrophils more adherent and thereby prone to aggregation within the pulmonary vasculature. This has been seen in patients suffering from burns and transfusion reactions. Complement activation may also lead to neutrophil destruction, as in paroxysmal nocturnal hemoglobinuria. The circulating neutrophil pool can also be diminished in association with hypersplenism, although this is typically less common and less pronounced than the anemia and thrombocytopenia seen in patients with an enlarged spleen.

Neutropenia Due to Nutritional Deficiency

Several vitamin and mineral deficiencies, particularly B_{12}, folate (Chapter 164), and copper, are associated with neutropenia. Copper deficiency is a particularly under-recognized cause of neutropenia (usually seen along with anemia), found especially in clinical situations like total parenteral nutrition without copper supplementation, protein-losing enteropathies, celiac disease, gastric bypass surgery and postgastrectomy, malabsorption syndromes, and zinc toxicity. In addition to low serum copper and ceruloplasmin levels, distinct morphologic findings include hypogranularity and hypolobation (PHA) on peripheral smear, and cytoplasmic vacuolization of myeloid as well as erythroid precursors and ringed sideroblasts.

Deficiencies in these vitamins and minerals result in ineffective myelopoiesis, maturation arrest, and megaloblastic changes with nuclear-cytoplasmic dyssynchrony. The characteristic finding in the setting of megaloblastic anemia is hypersegmentation of the neutrophil (Fig. 167-6).

Chronic Idiopathic Neutropenia

Chronic idiopathic neutropenia in adults (CINA) has been described as an acquired disorder of granulopoiesis characterized by prolonged neutropenia in the absence of any apparent underlying etiology.[15] Patients present with chronic neutropenia that is often an incidental finding on routine blood tests, making it impossible to know how long the neutropenia has been present. They have no evidence of autoimmune disease, nutritional deficiency, or myelodysplasia. The syndrome is heterogeneous, with a wide range of neutrophil counts. A group of patients with CINA from Greece were originally found to have increased production of transforming growth factor-β (TGF-β) and consequent suppression of granulopoiesis by the bone marrow. These patients tend to have very mild neutropenia, with an absolute neutrophil count (ANC) that is rarely less than 800. They may have an ethnic predisposition to neutropenia; indeed, the neutropenia has been demonstrated to be linked to a genetic polymorphism in the TGF-β locus. It seems likely, however, that these patients should be distinguished from other CINA patients, many of whom have an ANC below 200. The etiology of neutropenia in these patients is completely unknown. However, the natural history of CINA, even in the face of very low neutrophil counts, is generally benign. Most patients require no therapy, although those with very low counts must be treated with G-CSF when they develop fever in the setting of infections. Some patients with recurrent infections or troublesome aphthous ulcers require chronic G-CSF treatment. These patients typically respond to fairly low doses of G-CSF, and there is no reported increase in the development of MDS/AML.

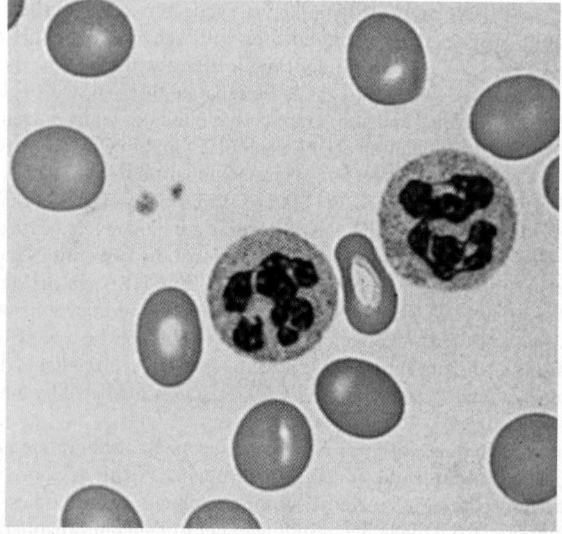

FIGURE 167-6. Peripheral blood with macrocytosis and hypersegmented neutrophils in megaloblastic anemia.

CLINICAL MANIFESTATIONS AND DIAGNOSIS

Neutropenia by itself is not associated with many clinical signs and symptoms other than those of the condition that may be causing it. It becomes clinically evident, however, when it results in infection. Although patients with an ANC below 1000/μL do have a slightly increased risk for infection, the risk is substantially increased once the neutrophil count falls below 500/μL. Given the lack of neutrophils, the signs and symptoms of infection may be attenuated; as such, pneumonia may be present with minimal infiltrate on chest radiograph, or a urinary tract infection may yield only a very mild pyuria. Given this, fever in any neutropenic patient must be considered an emergency with prompt acquisition of cultures and administration of empirical antibiotic therapy.

When fever, infection or sepsis, and neutropenia present concomitantly for the first time, it can be difficult to determine whether the neutropenia predated the infection or, conversely, if it is the result of the infection. Examination of the peripheral blood smear can be helpful in this regard because an elevation of band forms and evidence of toxic granulation suggest the latter.

Because drug-induced neutropenia is the most common cause of acquired neutropenia, a careful inventory of all drug and toxin exposures is warranted.[16] Likewise, there should be a careful evaluation for underlying malignant and inflammatory conditions as the precipitant of neutropenia. The time course of the neutropenia and infections can provide clues to the etiology of the neutropenia (acute versus chronic, persistent versus cyclic, neonatal versus childhood versus adult onset). Attention should be paid to the skin, bones, appendages, and nails because abnormalities in these may point toward one of the congenital neutropenia syndromes. Evaluation of the complete blood count, peripheral blood smear, and vitamin B_{12} and folate levels should also be performed.

When the neutropenia is not severe and is associated with anemia and thrombocytopenia, one should consider the possibility of hypersplenism. In many cases, the diagnosis can be made by the finding of palpable splenomegaly. However, especially in obese patients, abdominal imaging should be used to evaluate spleen size. Abdominal ultrasound allows the assessment of portal venous flow with Doppler studies. If splenic enlargement is confirmed, the etiology of the splenomegaly (Chapter 168) should be determined. It may reflect congestive splenomegaly secondary to portal hypertension (as a result of cirrhosis, fatty liver, or congestive heart failure, among others) or infiltrative splenomegaly due to a benign or malignant process. Felty syndrome should be considered in the setting of RA.

In patients with chronic neutropenia in the absence of a history of infection or drug or toxin exposure or an evident B_{12} or folate deficiency, bone marrow examination should be performed to rule out myelodysplasia, with assessment of morphology, flow cytometry for large granular lymphocyte syndrome, and cytogenetics. Once a normal marrow has been obtained, further bone marrow examination is not indicated in patients with CINA (Fig. 167-7).

TREATMENT AND MANAGEMENT Rx

The management of neutropenia is dependent on the etiology of the depressed neutrophil count as well as its severity and the presence or absence of fever or infection.[17] The approach to the patient with fever and neutropenia is discussed in more detail in Chapter 281. Neutropenia with fever is a clinical emergency because these patients are at risk for hemodynamic collapse and septic shock. Therefore, these patients should be evaluated thoroughly and cultured promptly, and antibiotics should be administered within 30 to 60 minutes of presentation before obtaining the results of the cultures. The timely empirical administration of a combination of antipseudomonal antibiotics in

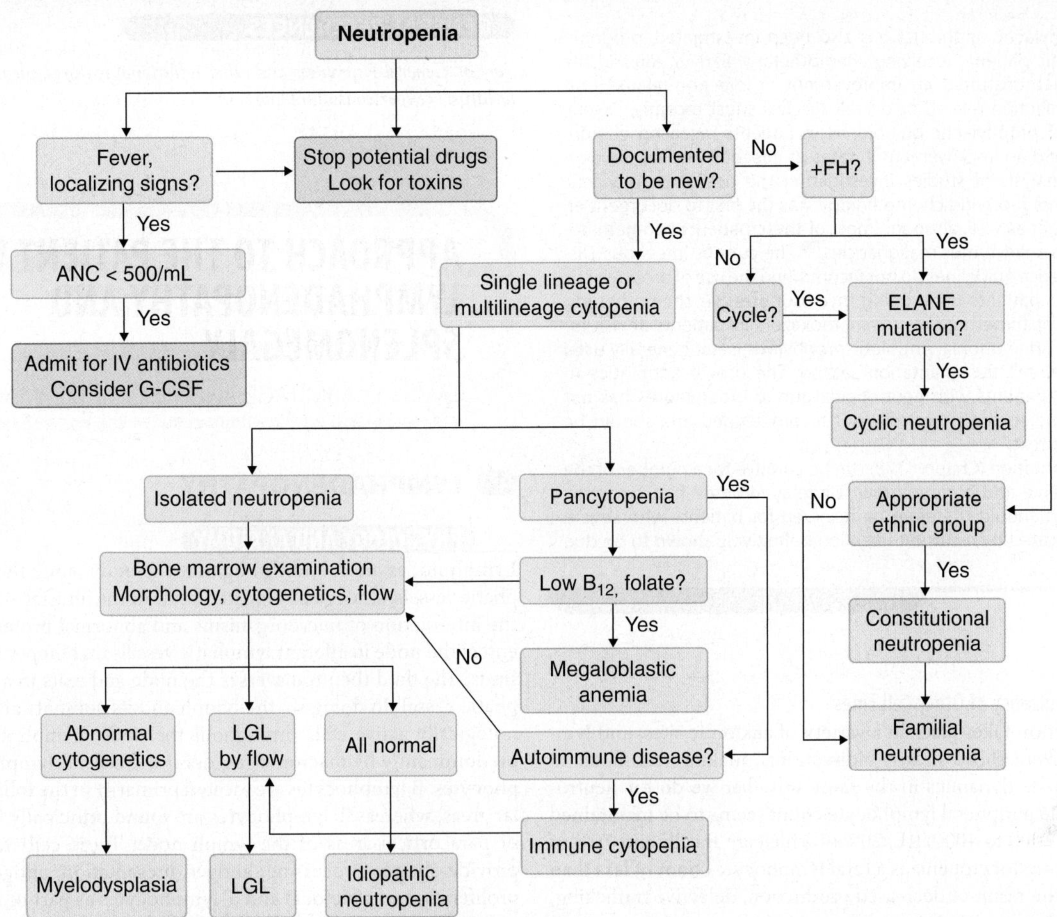

FIGURE 167-7. Diagnostic approach to neutropenia. ANC = absolute neutrophil count; ELANE = neutrophil elastase gene, FH = family history; G-CSF = granulocyte colony-stimulating factor; IV = intravenous; LGL = large granular lymphocyte syndrome.

patients with neutropenia at the onset of fever results in significant clinical benefit, with respect to both response and survival. With the advent of newer generation cephalosporins, studies have shown that monotherapy with a third- or fourth-generation cephalosporin at the onset of fever may be sufficient. A systematic review to assess the evidence for combination therapy versus monotherapy in cancer patients with febrile neutropenia in clinical trials has been recently updated.[A1] It concluded that randomized controlled trials have demonstrated the survival superiority of β-lactam monotherapy compared with β-lactam-aminoglycoside combination therapy.

The addition of a second antipseudomonal agent, vancomycin, or antifungal agent is warranted in patients considered at risk for resistant pseudomonal infection, resistant gram-positive infection, or fungal infections, respectively, or in the face of a failure to defervesce within 3 to 5 days of antibiotic administration. These considerations are discussed in more detail in Chapter 281.

How to manage the uninfected and afebrile neutropenic patient is more nuanced and dependent on the etiology of the neutropenia. Patients with immune-mediated neutropenia are typically treated with immunosuppressive therapy, including steroids, antithymocyte globulin, or cyclosporine, or a combination of these, aimed primarily at treatment of the underlying autoimmune disease. Patients usually respond to G-CSF, although in the setting of RA, this may induce a flare of joint symptoms. Patients with large granular lymphocyte syndrome often respond to therapy with low-dose methotrexate (10 mg/m^2 orally once a week), cyclosporine (100 to 600 mg or 2 to 10 mg/kg orally daily), or low-dose cyclophosphamide (50 to 100 mg orally daily).[18]

Patients with congenital neutropenia, including idiopathic, severe congenital, or cyclic neutropenia, are usually successfully managed with G-CSF for years. Before the use of G-CSF, the mean age of death for patients with severe congenital neutropenia was 2 to 3 years. Since the advent of G-CSF, however, life expectancy has been extended by decades into adulthood. Therapy is daily and chronic, given by subcutaneous injection, with doses varying by the type of neutropenia and the individual responsiveness to therapy. It is usually well tolerated, although accelerated bone loss has been observed. Growth and development do not appear to be affected. Patients with SCN typically require the highest doses, whereas those with idiopathic neutropenia require the lowest, and patients with cyclic neutropenia fall somewhere in between. An increased rate of MDS/AML has been reported with the use of G-CSF in patients with SCN, but this has occurred coincidentally with improved survival. The increased incidence of MDS/AML may then be due to the fact that patients are living longer with a disease whose natural history includes a risk for developing MDS or AML. Certainly, the observation that acquired mutations in the G-CSF receptor are present in 65 to 80% of patients with SCN who develop MDS or AML suggests a potential mutagenic pathway toward leukemogenesis, but whether this is enhanced or accelerated by the administration of G-CSF has yet to be determined. Patients with idiopathic and cyclic neutropenia do not develop MDS or AML, despite therapy with G-CSF. However, recent evidence suggests that the risk for MDS/AML in SCN patients is much higher in those requiring high doses of G-CSF (>10 μg/kg/day), and patients with idiopathic and cyclic neutropenia are usually responsive to much lower G-CSF doses.

In patients with CINA, G-CSF should be reserved for acute febrile episodes unless the patient has recurrent infections. Patients with CINA treated with G-CSF may experience significant side effects, including fever, gastrointestinal symptoms, and splenomegaly. Consequently, in patients with CINA requiring chronic G-CSF administration, the cytokine should be administered at the lowest dose necessary to prevent infections; it is usually sufficient to treat to maintain the ANC in the range of 300 to 500.

For patients with an inflammatory, infectious, or drug-induced neutropenia, the recommendation is to treat the underlying condition or stop the offending agent. This, however, is not always immediately possible, as in the cases of HIV-infected patients with opportunistic infections or on antiretroviral therapy, solid organ and bone marrow transplant recipients on immunosuppression and antiviral prophylaxis and treatment, and cancer patients undergoing chemotherapy. Prophylactic use of G-CSF in these patients has been shown to be effective in improving the ANC and decreasing rates of infection and febrile neutropenia, but has not been associated with a proven or consistent survival advantage.[A2] In light of these findings, many oncologic professional society guidelines recommend the use of prophylactic G-CSF in patients receiving chemotherapy who have a 20% or greater risk for developing febrile neutropenia based on age, comorbid illness, disease characteristics, and myelotoxicity of the chemotherapy regimen. In addition, it is recommended for use during hematopoietic stem cell transplantation, for patients receiving chemotherapy for non-Hodgkin lymphoma or dose-dense chemotherapy, and for patients with a history of febrile neutropenia receiving further chemotherapy.

The use of prophylactic antibiotics has also been investigated, predominantly in neutropenic patients receiving chemotherapy. Early studies in the 1980s and 1990s demonstrated an improvement in infection-related outcomes but not in infection-related or overall survival. Most recently, several randomized trials of prophylactic quinolones in patients receiving chemotherapy demonstrated an improvement in rates of infection and febrile neutropenia. A meta-analysis of studies investigating the use of prophylactic quinolones in patients receiving chemotherapy was the first to document an overall survival benefit as well, although most of these patients had hematologic as opposed to solid tumor malignancies.[A3] The current Infectious Diseases Society of America guidelines do not recommend the use of prophylactic antibiotics in cancer patients undergoing myelosuppressive chemotherapy, with the exception of trimethoprim-sulfamethoxazole in patients at risk for *Pneumocystis jirovecii* pneumonia. Antibiotic prophylaxis is not generally used outside of the stem cell transplantation setting. The use of antibiotics to prevent infection in patients with neutropenia due to other causes has not been extensively studied but is typically not recommended and should be based on clinical context.

Stem cell transplantation (Chapter 178) can be curative for a number of the congenital neutropenia and bone marrow failure syndromes. It is, however, not without risk and should therefore be reserved for patients with severe neutropenia complicated by recurrent infection definitively shown to be due to marrow failure.

Leukopenia Due to Deficiency of Other Cell Lines

Lymphocyte production takes place in a variety of anatomic sites, and lymphocyte trafficking from those sites is bidirectional, making it difficult to understand lymphocyte dynamics in the same way that we do for neutrophils. Despite this, the peripheral lymphocyte count seems to be maintained in a narrow range at 2000 to 4000/μL, 20% of which are B cells and 70% of which are T cells. Lymphocytopenia is a total lymphocyte count of less than 1500/μL. It can be the result of decreased production, defective trafficking, or increased loss or destruction. Decreased production can occur as a result of protein and calorie malnutrition; lymphocyte progenitor pool injury secondary to radiation, chemotherapy, or immunosuppressive agents; and congenital immunodeficiency states. Endogenous or exogenous glucocorticoid excess can cause lymphocytopenia by altering lymphocyte trafficking. This can also occur as the result of acute bacterial or fungal infections, certain viral infections, and granulomatous disease. Finally, many viruses can cause direct destruction of lymphocytes, as can antilymphocyte antibodies seen in patients with underlying autoimmune diseases. Lymphocytes can also be lost from intestinal lymphatics in cases of protein-losing enteropathy, primary disease of the gut or intestinal lymphatics, or gut edema secondary to severe heart failure. When lymphocytopenia is discovered, a comprehensive assessment of the immune system should be done, including lymphocyte subtyping, quantitative immunoglobulins, and skin testing to detect deficiencies of cell-mediated immunity. Treatment is typically aimed at the underlying disease, but intravenous immunoglobulin can be administered to patients who are hypogammaglobulinemic, and transplantation can be performed in patients with severe deficiencies of cell-mediated immunity due to impaired lymphocyte production and function.

Monocytopenia, eosinopenia, and basophilopenia can be seen in the setting of bone marrow failure syndromes or as a result of acute infection, malignancy, or severe injury. This is thought to be due to elevations in glucocorticoids, prostaglandins, and epinephrine. A rise in these humoral factors has the greatest impact on eosinophils such that a lack of eosinopenia in any of these settings should prompt suspicion for adrenal insufficiency, a primary myeloproliferative syndrome, parasitic infection, or primary hypereosinophilic syndrome. Monocytopenia is less frequently seen, probably owing to the diverse roles monocytes play in normal human physiology; prolonged and extreme monocytopenia may not be compatible with life.

Grade A References

A1. Paul M, Dickstein Y, Schlesinger A, et al. Beta-lactam versus beta-lactam-aminoglycoside combination therapy in cancer patients with neutropenia. *Cochrane Database Syst Rev*. 2013;6:CD003038.

A2. Cooper KL, Madan J, Whyte S, et al. Granulocyte colony-stimulating factors for febrile neutropenia prophylaxis following chemotherapy: systematic review and meta-analysis. *BMC Cancer*. 2011;11:404.

A3. Gafter-Gvili A, Fraser A, Paul M, et al. Meta-analysis: antibiotic prophylaxis reduces mortality in neutropenic patients. *Ann Intern Med*. 2005;142:979-995.

GENERAL REFERENCES

For the General References and other additional features, please visit Expert Consult at https://expertconsult.inkling.com.

168

APPROACH TO THE PATIENT WITH LYMPHADENOPATHY AND SPLENOMEGALY

JAMES O. ARMITAGE AND PHILIP J. BIERMAN

LYMPHADENOPATHY

PHYSIOLOGY AND ANATOMY

Lymph nodes are found throughout the body along the course of the lymphatic vessels, strategically located to allow the filtering of lymphatic fluid and the interdiction of microorganisms and abnormal proteins. Lymphatic fluid enters the node in afferent lymphatic vessels that empty into the subcapsular sinus. The fluid then transverses the node and exits in a single efferent lymphatic vessel. In doing so, the lymph and its contents are exposed to immunologically active cells throughout the node. Lymph nodes are populated predominantly by macrophages, dendritic cells, B lymphocytes, and T lymphocytes. B lymphocytes are located primarily in the follicles and perifollicular areas, whereas T lymphocytes are found principally in the interfollicular or paracortical areas of the lymph node. These cells function together to provide antigen processing, antigen presentation, antigen recognition, and proliferation of effector B and T lymphocytes as part of the normal immune response to microorganisms or foreign proteins.

Because the normal immune response leads to the proliferation and expansion of one or more cellular components of lymph nodes, it often results in significant lymph node enlargement. In young children, who are continuously being exposed to new antigens, palpable lymphadenopathy is the rule. In fact, the absence of palpable lymphadenopathy in them would be considered abnormal. In adults, lymph nodes larger than 1 to 2 cm in diameter are generally considered abnormal. However, lymph nodes 1 to 2 cm in diameter in the groin are sufficiently common to be considered normal.

Lymphoid proliferation is a normal response to exposure to foreign antigens. The location of the enlarged lymph nodes often reflects the site of invasion. For example, cervical lymphadenopathy would be typical in a patient with pharyngitis. Generalized immune proliferation and lymphadenopathy can occur with a systemic disorder of the immune system, disseminated infection, or disseminated neoplasia. Malignancies of the immune system might manifest as localized or disseminated lymphadenopathy.

DIAGNOSIS

Differential Diagnosis

The differential diagnosis of lymphadenopathy (Table 168-1) is vast, and the underlying causes are responsible for either proliferation of immunologically active cells or infiltration of the lymph node by foreign cells or substances. In practice, the cause of enlarged lymph nodes is often uncertain even in retrospect; in such cases, unrecognized infectious processes are generally blamed.

Infections by bacteria, mycobacteria, fungi, chlamydia, parasites, and viruses are the major causes of lymph node enlargement. Lymph nodes in the drainage area of essentially all pyogenic infections can enlarge. In certain infections, such as bubonic plague caused by *Yersinia pestis*, dramatic regional lymph node enlargement with fluctuant lymph nodes (i.e., buboes) can be a hallmark of the disease (Chapter 312). Other bacterial infections have lymph node enlargement as a prominent feature (e.g., cat-scratch disease; Chapter 315) and can mimic lymphoproliferative disorders. Mediastinal lymphadenopathy is seen in inhalational anthrax (Chapter 294). In some parts of the world, cervical lymphadenopathy is a sufficiently frequent manifestation of tuberculosis to lead to the institution of antituberculous therapy rather than biopsy. Disseminated lymphadenopathy can be seen in cases of infection by a variety of organisms such as *Toxoplasma*, Epstein-Barr virus (i.e., infectious mononucleosis), cytomegalovirus, and human immunodeficiency virus (HIV).

TABLE 168-1 CAUSES OF LYMPHADENOPATHY

Infection
- Bacterial (e.g., all pyogenic bacteria, cat-scratch disease, syphilis, tularemia)
- Mycobacterial (e.g., tuberculosis, leprosy)
- Fungal (e.g., histoplasmosis, coccidioidomycosis)
- Chlamydial (e.g., lymphogranuloma venereum)
- Parasitic (e.g., toxoplasmosis, trypanosomiasis, filariasis)
- Viral (e.g., Epstein-Barr virus, cytomegalovirus, rubella, hepatitis, HIV)

Benign disorders of the immune system (e.g., rheumatoid arthritis, systemic lupus erythematosus, serum sickness, drug reactions such as to phenytoin, Castleman disease, sinus histiocytosis with massive lymphadenopathy, Langerhans cell histiocytosis, Kawasaki syndrome, Kimura disease)

Malignant disorders of the immune system (e.g., chronic and acute myeloid and lymphoid leukemia, non-Hodgkin lymphoma, Hodgkin disease, angioimmunoblastic-like T-cell lymphoma, Waldenström macroglobulinemia, multiple myeloma with amyloidosis, malignant histiocytosis)

Other malignancies (e.g., breast carcinoma, lung carcinoma, melanoma, head and neck cancer, gastrointestinal malignancies, germ cell tumors, Kaposi sarcoma)

Storage diseases (e.g., Gaucher disease, Niemann-Pick disease)

Endocrinopathies (e.g., hyperthyroidism, adrenal insufficiency, thyroiditis)

Miscellaneous (e.g., sarcoidosis, amyloidosis, dermatopathic lymphadenitis, IgG4-related disease)

TABLE 168-2 MOST FREQUENT CAUSES OF LYMPHADENOPATHY IN ADULTS IN THE UNITED STATES

Unexplained

Infection
- In drainage area of infection (e.g., cervical adenopathy with pharyngitis)
- Disseminated (e.g., mononucleosis, HIV infection)

Immune disorders (e.g., rheumatoid arthritis)

Neoplasms
- Immune system malignancies (e.g., leukemias, lymphomas)
- Metastatic carcinoma or sarcoma

TABLE 168-3 FACTORS TO CONSIDER IN THE DIAGNOSIS OF LYMPHADENOPATHY

Associated systemic symptoms

Patient's age

History of infection, trauma, medications, travel experience, previous malignancy

Location: cervical, supraclavicular, epitrochlear, axillary, intrathoracic (hilar vs. mediastinal), intra-abdominal (retroperitoneal vs. mesenteric vs. other), iliac, inguinal, femoral

Localized vs. disseminated

Presence of tenderness or inflammation

Size

Consistency

A variety of nonmalignant disorders of the immune system can lead to localized or disseminated lymphadenopathy. Autoimmune diseases such as rheumatoid arthritis (Chapter 264) and systemic lupus erythematosus (Chapter 266) often have accompanying lymphadenopathy, which can pose a diagnostic challenge because of the increased incidence of lymphoma in patients with these disorders. In the lymphadenopathy that occurs as a reaction to drugs such as phenytoin, lymph node biopsy findings can sometimes be confused with lymphoma. Benign proliferative diseases of the immune system that can also be confused with lymphoma include Castleman disease (Chapters 185 and 393; angiofollicular lymph node hyperplasia), sinus histiocytosis with massive lymphadenopathy, and disorders seen more frequently in Asia, such as Kawasaki syndrome (Chapter 439) and Kimura disease.

All the cells in the immune system can become malignant. Several of these malignancies typically manifest as lymphadenopathy, and it can be seen in all of them. Lymphadenopathy as the initial manifestation is the rule for Hodgkin disease and non-Hodgkin lymphoma, and it is common in Waldenström macroglobulinemia and B-cell chronic lymphocytic leukemia; it is seen only occasionally in the myeloid leukemias (Chapters 183 through 186) and is rare in multiple myeloma. Malignancies of all organ systems can metastasize to the lymph nodes and cause lymphadenopathy, which is usually seen in the drainage area of the primary tumor—for example, axillary lymph nodes in patients with breast cancer, hilar and mediastinal lymph nodes in patients with lung cancer, and cervical lymph nodes in patients with head and neck cancer. However, widespread lymphadenopathy can also occur. Other disorders in which lymphadenopathy may be an initial finding include storage diseases such as Gaucher disease (Chapter 208), endocrinopathies such as hyperthyroidism (Chapter 226), sarcoidosis (Chapter 95), and dermatopathic lymphadenitis. Amyloidosis (Chapter 188) can cause lymphadenopathy in patients with multiple myeloma, hereditary amyloidosis, or amyloidosis associated with chronic inflammatory states.

Among patients with lymphadenopathy actually seen in practices in the United States, diagnoses are not determined in a high proportion (Table 168-2). In such cases, the lymphadenopathy is usually blamed on infection. When the lymphadenopathy is in the drainage site of a known infection (e.g., cervical lymphadenopathy in a patient with pharyngitis) or the patient has a known infection associated with lymphadenopathy (e.g., infectious mononucleosis; Chapter 377), this infectious assumption is usually correct. Alternatively, if a patient has an immunologic disorder that is known to cause lymphadenopathy, such as rheumatoid arthritis, this disorder is usually an acceptable explanation; however, progressive lymphadenopathy in such patients should trigger a biopsy because they are at increased risk for lymphoma. Localized, progressive lymphadenopathy, particularly when associated with fever, sweats, or weight loss, requires biopsy to exclude lymphoma.

Lymph Node Evaluation

Evaluation of a patient with lymphadenopathy includes a careful history, a thorough physical examination, laboratory tests, and sometimes imaging studies to determine the extent and character of the lymphadenopathy. The age of the patient and any associated systemic symptoms might be important clues (Table 168-3). Cervical lymphadenopathy in a child is much less worrisome than equally prominent lymphadenopathy in a 60-year-old adult. The occurrence of fever, sweats, or weight loss raises the possibility of a malignancy of the immune system. The explanation for the lymphadenopathy might become apparent with the identification of a site of infection, a particular medication, a travel history, or a previous malignancy.

Physical examination allows the identification of localized versus widespread lymphadenopathy. The particular sites of involvement can be important hints to the diagnosis because infection and carcinoma are likely to cause lymphadenopathy in the lymphatic drainage of the site of the disorder. In general, tender lymph nodes are more likely to be due to an infectious process, whereas painless adenopathy raises concern for malignancy. Lymph node consistency can also aid in the diagnosis: typically, lymph nodes containing metastatic carcinoma are rock hard, lymph nodes containing lymphoma are firm and rubbery, and lymph nodes enlarged in response to an infectious process are soft.

The larger the lymph node, the more likely it is that a serious underlying cause exists; lymph nodes greater than 3 to 4 cm in diameter in an adult are very worrisome. Physical examination to assess lymph node size is only marginally accurate and reproducible, although it is by far the most widely used method. More precise methods are available with various imaging techniques.

Imaging

Imaging studies, including routine radiographs, computed tomography (CT), ultrasonography, magnetic resonance imaging (MRI), and positron emission tomography (PET), can be used to assess the extent of lymphadenopathy in the chest and abdomen (Table 168-4). Chest radiographs are the most economical and easiest way to assess mediastinal and hilar lymphadenopathy but are not as accurate as CT of the chest. CT and ultrasonography are the most useful modalities for assessing abdominal and retroperitoneal lymphadenopathy. In most patients, CT is probably the most accurate approach, but ultrasonography has the advantage of being less expensive and not requiring radiation exposure. MRI and PET are not first-line studies for the assessment of lymphadenopathy. Although few randomized controlled trials have been published to date concerning the diagnostic accuracy of PET,[1] it is applied to the assessment of patients with lymphoma both at presentation and after treatment.[2] PET is usually positive in patients with Hodgkin disease and aggressive non-Hodgkin lymphomas and can be used to assess the presence of active lymphoma in patients with lymphadenopathy and a proven diagnosis; it is especially useful for re-evaluating patients after therapy because lymph nodes do not always regress to normal size after treatment, particularly those in the mediastinum and retroperitoneum, even though the malignancy has been eradicated.

TABLE 168-4 METHODS OF LYMPH NODE EVALUATION

Physical examination
Imaging
  Chest radiography
  Ultrasonography
  Computed tomography
  Magnetic resonance imaging
  Positron emission tomography
Sampling
  Needle aspiration
  Cutting needle biopsy
  Excisional biopsy

TABLE 168-5 APPROACH TO THE PATIENT WITH LYMPHADENOPATHY

Does the patient have a known illness that causes lymphadenopathy? Treat and monitor for resolution.
Is there an obvious infection to explain the lymphadenopathy (e.g., infectious mononucleosis)? Treat and monitor for resolution.
Are the nodes very large and/or very firm and thus suggestive of malignancy? Perform a biopsy.
Is the patient very concerned about malignancy and unable to be reassured that malignancy is unlikely? Perform a biopsy.
If none of the preceding is true, perform a complete blood cell count and, if unrevealing, monitor for a predetermined period (usually 2 to 8 weeks). If the nodes do not regress or if they increase in size, perform a biopsy.

TABLE 168-6 SOME DIAGNOSTIC CONSIDERATIONS FOR LOCALIZED LYMPHADENOPATHY

SITE	INFECTIONS	NEOPLASMS	OTHER
Cervical	Pharyngitis, other head and neck infections, mononucleosis, toxoplasmosis, TB	Head and neck cancers, thyroid cancer, lymphoma	
Supraclavicular		Intra-abdominal cancer (particularly left-sided nodes), lung cancer, lymphoma	
Axillary	Cat-scratch disease, distal infections, plague	Breast cancer, melanoma, lymphoma	Silicone implants
Mediastinal	TB, fungal infection, anthrax	Lymphoma, lung cancer, germ cell tumor	Sarcoidosis
Retroperitoneal	TB	Lymphoma, testicular cancer, kidney cancer, upper GI malignancy	Sarcoidosis
Mesenteric	Appendicitis, cholecystitis, diverticulitis, Whipple disease	Lymphoma, GI cancer	Inflammatory bowel disease, panniculitis
Inguinal	Distal or genital infection, plague, STDs	Lymphoma, melanoma, vulvar cancer	

GI = gastrointestinal; STD = sexually transmitted disease; TB = tuberculosis.

Interventional Evaluation

Lymph node aspiration or biopsy is often necessary for an accurate diagnosis of the cause of lymphadenopathy. Even then, morphologic findings alone may not be able to clearly distinguish between reactive changes in benign lymphadenopathies and neoplasm, particularly lymphoma; special studies on the specimens may be required to do so.[3] Fine-needle aspiration is currently popular and is an accurate means of diagnosing infection or carcinoma involving a lymph node. Although lymphomas can occasionally be diagnosed with this approach, it is inappropriate as an initial diagnostic maneuver for lymphoma. Cutting needle biopsy often provides sufficient material for an unequivocal diagnosis and subtyping of the lymphoma. However, excisional biopsy, which is most likely to provide the pathologist with adequate material to perform histologic, immunologic, and genetic studies, is also most likely to yield the correct diagnosis.

An Approach to the Patient with Lymphadenopathy

Patients with lymphadenopathy (Table 168-5) come to medical attention in several ways. Perhaps most common is a patient who feels a lymph node in the neck, axilla, or groin and seeks a physician's opinion. Lymphadenopathy might also be an unexpected finding on a routine physical examination or as part of an evaluation for another complaint. Finally, patients might be found to have unexpected lymphadenopathy on imaging studies of the chest or abdomen. When the nodes are multiple or larger than 2 to 3 cm, biopsy using mediastinoscopy, a paramediastinal incision, laparoscopy, or laparotomy is often required for diagnosis.

The approach to a patient complaining of newly discovered lymphadenopathy in the neck, axilla, or groin depends on the size, consistency, and number of enlarged lymph nodes and the patient's general health. In most cases, very large or very firm lymph nodes in the presence of systemic symptoms such as unexplained fever, sweats, or weight loss should lead to lymph node biopsy. Patients who have enlarged lymph nodes in the drainage area of a previously treated malignancy (e.g., neck nodes in a patient with a history of head and neck cancer) might be best approached by lymph node aspiration. Carcinoma can often be diagnosed in this manner, although it is a poor approach for the diagnosis of lymphoid malignancies. For cervical lymph nodes,[4] excisional biopsy should be delayed in a patient in whom head and neck cancer (Chapter 190) is a diagnostic consideration. These patients should initially undergo careful ear, nose, and throat examinations to avoid performing a biopsy that might complicate the patient's subsequent therapy. Some diagnostic possibilities for localized lymphadenopathy are presented in Table 168-6.

In the most common situation—that is, a lymph node is soft and is not larger than 2 to 3 cm and the patient has no obvious systemic illness—observation for a brief period is usually the best approach. Performance of a complete blood cell count and examination of a peripheral smear can be helpful in recognizing a systemic illness (e.g., infectious mononucleosis). These patients are often given antibiotics. If the lymph node does not regress over the course of a few weeks or if it gets bigger, a biopsy should be performed.

Part of the care of such patients involves the art of medicine and being responsive to the patient's particular needs. For example, biopsy might be performed more quickly in a patient who is very anxious about malignancy or who needs a definitive diagnosis expeditiously.

SPLENOMEGALY

DEFINITION

The spleen is the largest lymphatic organ in the body and is sometimes approached clinically as though it were a very large lymph node. Although it participates in the primary immune response to invading microorganisms and foreign proteins, the spleen has many other functions. It functions as a filter for the blood and is responsible for removing senescent red blood cells from the circulation, as well as blood cells and other cells coated with immunoglobulins. Blood enters the spleen, filters through the splenic cords, and is exposed to immunologically active cells in the spleen.

The splenic red pulp occupies more than half the volume of the spleen and is the site where senescent red cells are identified and destroyed and red blood cell inclusions are removed by a process known as *pitting*. In the absence of splenic function, basophilic inclusions known as *Howell-Jolly bodies* are seen in circulating red blood cells. The presence of Howell-Jolly bodies (Fig. 168-1) in peripheral blood indicates that the patient has undergone splenectomy or has a process that has rendered the spleen nonfunctional (e.g., sickle cell disease with repeated splenic infarcts, chronic graft-versus-host disease).

The white pulp of the spleen contains macrophages, B lymphocytes, and T lymphocytes; participates in the recognition of microorganisms and foreign proteins; and is involved in the primary immune response. Absence of this splenic function makes individuals particularly susceptible to certain

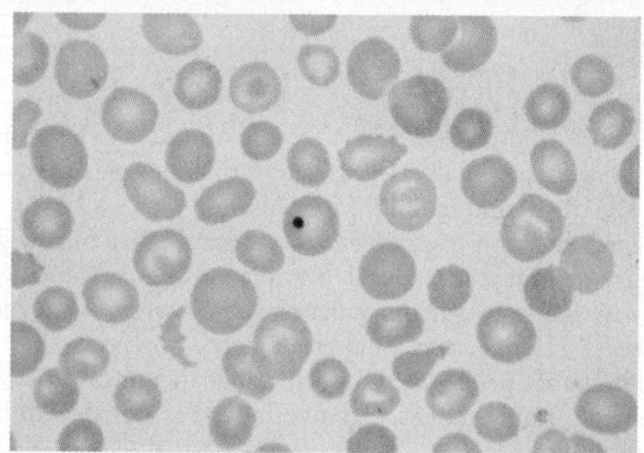

FIGURE 168-1. Howell-Jolly body in an erythrocyte. This is evidence of splenectomy or a nonfunctional spleen.

infections, including sepsis with encapsulated organisms such as *Streptococcus pneumoniae.* The risk for overwhelming sepsis is related to the age at the time of splenectomy or other cause of loss of splenic function. Children and young adults are at highest risk. If possible, all patients should undergo vaccination against *S. pneumoniae* and perhaps *Haemophilus influenzae* and *Neisseria meningitidis* before splenectomy. Some physicians have patients take oral penicillin (e.g., phenoxymethyl penicillin, 250 mg twice daily) indefinitely if splenectomy has been performed in childhood or adolescence.

PATHOBIOLOGY

As with lymphadenopathy, numerous conditions are associated with splenomegaly (Table 168-7). Certain bacterial infections such as endocarditis (Chapter 76), brucellosis (Chapter 310), and typhoid fever (Chapter 308) have splenomegaly as a frequent manifestation. Disseminated tuberculosis (Chapter 324) is often associated with splenomegaly, and splenomegaly can also be seen in cases of disseminated histoplasmosis (Chapter 332) and toxoplasmosis (Chapter 349). Splenomegaly is an almost constant accompaniment of malaria (Chapter 345). Rickettsial disorders such as Rocky Mountain spotted fever are frequently associated with splenomegaly. A wide variety of viral infections typically cause splenomegaly, including infectious mononucleosis associated with Epstein-Barr virus (Chapter 377) and viral hepatitis (Chapters 148 and 149). Splenomegaly can accompany HIV infection. Splenic abscesses, which are usually the result of hematogenous spread of pyogenic organisms, represent an unusual and difficult to diagnose cause of splenomegaly.

Splenomegaly is also seen in a variety of benign disorders of the immune system, including rheumatoid arthritis (Chapter 264); some of these patients have Felty syndrome and accompanying granulocytopenia. Splenomegaly can be detected in some patients with systemic lupus erythematosus (Chapter 266), certain drug reactions, and serum sickness.

Malignancies of the immune system and nonimmune organs can also lead to splenomegaly. Splenomegaly is usually seen in patients with chronic myeloid leukemia and is frequent in chronic lymphoid leukemia (Chapter 184). It can develop in patients with acute myeloid or lymphoid leukemia, non-Hodgkin lymphoma, Hodgkin disease, and Waldenström macroglobulinemia but is rare in multiple myeloma (Chapter 187). Isolated splenomegaly (i.e., without any enlarged lymph nodes) is characteristic of certain immune system malignancies, including hairy cell leukemia (Chapter 184), the prolymphocytic variant of chronic lymphocytic leukemia (Chapter 184), and splenic marginal zone lymphoma (Chapter 185). Metastasis of carcinomas and sarcomas to the spleen is unusual except for malignant melanoma; even with melanoma, however, palpable splenomegaly is an unusual finding.

Splenomegaly can develop as a result of increased pressure in the splenic circulation, especially in patients with portal hypertension caused by a variety of hepatic disorders, including alcoholic cirrhosis (Chapter 152). However, it also can be due to splenic or portal vein thrombosis. The first manifestation of an enlarged spleen in portal hypertension can be thrombocytopenia.

Hematologic disorders that can lead to palpable splenomegaly include autoimmune hemolytic anemia (Chapter 160), hereditary spherocytosis (Chapter 161), and a number of other anemias. The myeloproliferative neoplasms polycythemia vera (frequently), essential thrombocythemia (sometimes), and idiopathic myelofibrosis (usually) all can present with splenomegaly. In cases of idiopathic myelofibrosis, the spleen is frequently a site of extramedullary hematopoiesis (Chapter 166).

A variety of less common conditions can lead to splenomegaly. The storage disorder Gaucher disease (Chapter 208) usually manifests as splenomegaly.

TABLE 168-7 CAUSES OF SPLENOMEGALY

Infection
- Bacterial (e.g., endocarditis, brucellosis, syphilis, typhoid, pyogenic abscess)
- Mycobacterial (e.g., tuberculosis)
- Fungal (e.g., histoplasmosis, toxoplasmosis)
- Parasitic (e.g., malaria, leishmaniasis)
- Rickettsial (e.g., Rocky Mountain spotted fever)
- Viral (e.g., Epstein-Barr virus, cytomegalovirus, HIV, hepatitis)

Benign disorders of the immune system (e.g., rheumatoid arthritis with Felty syndrome, systemic lupus erythematosus, drug reactions such as to phenytoin, Langerhans cell histiocytosis, serum sickness)
Malignant disorders of the immune system (e.g., acute or chronic myeloid or lymphoid leukemia, non-Hodgkin lymphoma, Hodgkin disease, Waldenström macroglobulinemia, malignant histiocytosis)
Other malignancies (e.g., melanoma, sarcoma)
Congestive splenomegaly (e.g., portal hypertension secondary to liver disease, splenic or portal vein thrombosis)
Hematologic disorders (e.g., autoimmune hemolytic anemia, hereditary spherocytosis, thalassemia major, hemoglobinopathies, elliptocytosis, extramedullary hematopoiesis)
Storage diseases (e.g., Gaucher disease)
Endocrinopathies (e.g., hyperthyroidism)
Miscellaneous (e.g., sarcoidosis, amyloidosis, tropical splenomegaly, cysts)

TABLE 168-8 METHODS FOR EVALUATING THE SPLEEN

Physical examination
Imaging
- Ultrasonography
- Computed tomography
- Liver-spleen scanning
- Positron emission tomography

Biopsy
- Needle aspiration
- Splenectomy
  - Laparotomy (total or partial splenectomy)
  - Laparoscopy

Splenomegaly can be seen in endocrinopathies such as hyperthyroidism (Chapter 226). Sarcoidosis (Chapter 95) and amyloidosis (Chapter 188) can manifest as splenomegaly. *Tropical splenomegaly* is a term used to describe the palpable spleens found in patients who live in tropical areas, for which there may be numerous causes.

DIAGNOSIS

Evaluation of Spleen Size and Function

Physical Examination

The ability to perform an accurate physical examination and determine the presence of an enlarged spleen (Table 168-8) is an important skill, but it is not easily learned. Physical examination of the spleen can be performed with the patient supine or in the right lateral decubitus position. Inspection, percussion, auscultation, and palpation are all important parts of an accurate assessment. It is rare for a spleen to be so large that it is visible and can be seen to move with respiration. However, in patients with such a condition, it is possible to miss splenomegaly by failing to start palpation sufficiently low to find the edge. Occasionally, percussion of the left upper quadrant helps identify an area of dullness that moves with respiration and can lead to the identification of splenomegaly. Spleen size is generally recorded as the number of centimeters the spleen descends below the left costal margin in the midclavicular line on inspiration. Although auscultation is not usually a regular part of splenic examination, the existence of a splenic rub on inspiration can lead to the diagnosis of splenic infarction. The left kidney is sometimes confused with the spleen on physical examination, but its failure to move with respiration in the manner typical for the spleen usually allows its distinction.

Laboratory Evaluation

Laboratory studies are frequently valuable in assessing splenic function. In patients with an absent or nonfunctional spleen,[5,6] Howell-Jolly bodies will be seen in circulating red blood cells (see Fig. 168-1). Splenic hyperfunction (a condition often referred to as *hypersplenism*) is associated with cytopenias: the spleen is the normal reservoir for a significant proportion of platelets, and

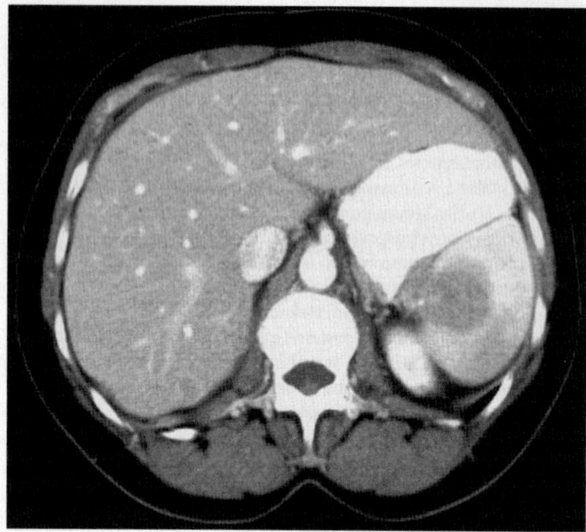

FIGURE 168-2. Enlarged spleen with metastatic adenocarcinoma.

this reservoir function can lead to thrombocytopenia in patients with splenomegaly. Patients with autoimmune hemolytic anemia usually have palpable splenomegaly, but patients with idiopathic (immune) thrombocytopenic purpura usually do not.

The spleen can be imaged with ultrasonography, CT,[7] traditional radionuclide scans, and PET (Fig. 168-2). Ultrasonography can provide an accurate determination of spleen size and is easy to repeat. CT frequently gives a better view of the consistency of the spleen and can identify splenic tumors or abscesses that would otherwise be missed. PET can aid in evaluating focal lesions in the spleen. The technetium-labeled liver-spleen scan can be important in identifying liver disease as the cause of splenomegaly; in patients with cryptogenic cirrhosis who are found to have thrombocytopenia, a technetium liver-spleen scan that shows higher activity in the spleen than in the liver might be the first hint of liver disease.

Because of the spleen's location and its propensity to bleed, needle aspiration or cutting needle biopsy of the spleen is rarely performed. In general, splenic "biopsy" involves splenectomy, which can be performed at the time of laparotomy or by laparoscopy. However, performing splenectomy laparoscopically usually leads to maceration of the organ and can reduce the diagnostic information. In very young children, in whom splenectomy leads to a high risk for serious infections such as pneumococcal septicemia, partial splenectomy can sometimes be performed. Patients who undergo splenectomy at the time of splenic trauma and rupture may have seeding of splenic cells to other sites in the abdomen (i.e., splenosis). Some patients have additional small or accessory spleens. Persistent, functional splenic tissue can be the explanation for recurrent immune thrombocytopenia after splenectomy and might be recognized by the absence of Howell-Jolly bodies in circulating red blood cells. Patients whose spleen has been removed often have thrombocytosis.

An Approach to the Patient with Splenomegaly

Patients with splenomegaly (Table 168-9) may come to medical attention for a variety of reasons. Patients may complain of left upper quadrant pain or fullness or early satiety. A splenic infarct, which typically manifests as left upper quadrant pain that sometimes radiates to the left shoulder, can be the first clue to the existence of an enlarged spleen. Rarely, splenomegaly initially manifests with the catastrophic symptoms of splenic rupture. Some patients are found to have splenomegaly as a result of evaluation for unexplained cytopenia. Splenomegaly can also be discovered incidentally on physical examination. In recent years, splenomegaly has frequently been discovered on imaging studies of the abdomen performed for other purposes.

The presence of a palpable spleen on physical examination is almost always abnormal. The one exception to this rule is a palpable spleen tip in a slender young woman. In general, the presence of a palpable spleen should be considered a serious finding, and an explanation should be sought. It is less clear whether the same rules apply to borderline splenomegaly discovered incidentally on routine imaging studies.

The approach to a patient with an enlarged spleen should focus initially on excluding a systemic illness that could explain the splenomegaly. Infectious mononucleosis, leukemia or lymphoma, rheumatoid arthritis, sarcoidosis, cirrhosis of the liver, malaria, and a host of other illnesses would be reasonable explanations for the splenomegaly. The systemic condition should be treated, and then the spleen should be re-evaluated. If the systemic illness can be treated successfully, the spleen should regress to normal size over time.

TABLE 168-9 APPROACH TO THE PATIENT WITH SPLENOMEGALY

Does the patient have a known illness that causes splenomegaly (e.g., infectious mononucleosis)? Treat and monitor for resolution.

Search for an occult infection (e.g., infectious endocarditis), hematologic disorder (e.g., hereditary spherocytosis), occult liver disease (e.g., cryptogenic cirrhosis), autoimmune disease (e.g., systemic lupus erythematosus), or storage disease (e.g., Gaucher disease). If found, manage appropriately.

If systemic symptoms are present and suggest malignancy, focal replacement of the spleen is seen on imaging studies, and no other site is available for biopsy, splenectomy is indicated.

If none of the above is true, monitor closely and repeat studies until the splenomegaly resolves or a diagnosis becomes apparent.

Patients with no obvious explanation for an enlarged spleen present a difficult diagnostic problem. Careful follow-up of these patients sometimes reveals occult liver disease or an autoimmune process that initially defied diagnosis. Concerns about malignancy, particularly in patients with systemic symptoms such as fever, sweats, or weight loss or in whom imaging studies show a focal abnormality, are sometimes indications for splenectomy. However, in the absence of such findings, it is generally preferable to monitor patients closely with repeated attempts to establish the diagnosis by approaches other than splenectomy. It is particularly important to avoid splenectomy in a patient with occult liver disease and portal hypertension.

Splenectomy was once performed routinely as part of the staging evaluation for Hodgkin disease or other lymphomas. Today, this procedure is rarely needed to choose the correct therapy, and it should be avoided. Splenectomy[8,9] can be an effective therapy for immune thrombocytopenic purpura (Chapter 172) and autoimmune hemolytic anemia (Chapter 160), and it is occasionally an appropriate therapy to relieve cytopenias in other conditions such as advanced myelofibrosis (Chapter 166). Radiofrequency ablation is an alternative to surgical removal.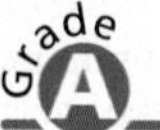 Splenectomized patients are at increased risk for infections, especially Gram-positive infections, and require careful follow-up[10,11] (Chapter 281).

Grade A Reference

A1. Feng K, Ma K, Liu Q, et al. Randomized clinical trial of splenic radiofrequency ablation versus splenectomy for severe hypersplenism. *Br J Surg.* 2011;98:354-361.

GENERAL REFERENCES

For the General References and other additional features, please visit Expert Consult at https://expertconsult.inkling.com.

169 DISORDERS OF PHAGOCYTE FUNCTION

MICHAEL GLOGAUER

Neutrophils and monocyte-macrophages are the key phagocytes of the innate immune system. Their principal innate immune role is to recognize and eliminate microorganisms that make their way past primary physical barriers, such as the epithelium and body secretions that protect the external and lining surfaces of the body. The neutrophil-pathogen interaction generates an army of antimicrobial mediators that results in efficient killing of pathogens.[1] Phagocytes identify foreign invaders through a series of pattern recognition receptors, most of which belong to the toll-like receptor family (Chapters 45 and 48). Whereas macrophages carry out sentinel duty looking for microbes in healthy tissue and act as a bridge between the innate and adaptive immune systems, neutrophils appear only in infected or damaged tissue after being recruited by inflammatory mediators released from activated macrophages and endothelial cells or by chemical signals released by invading microorganisms themselves (Table 169-1). After accumulation of these key immune cells at sites of infection, the microbes are eliminated through the process of phagocytosis, which is defined as the engulfment, internalization, and degradation of extracellular material.

NEUTROPHILS

Neutrophils develop in the bone marrow from myeloid precursors, migrate into the circulation, and, if required, make their way into infected or damaged tissue (Fig. 169-1). Their travels are essentially one-way trips because once they leave a compartment, they do not return. After release from the bone marrow compartment, a mature neutrophil has a blood half-life of 10 hours and may survive up to an additional 48 hours within infected or damaged tissue.

TABLE 169-1 PRIMARY IMMUNE ROLES OF MONOCYTE-MACROPHAGES AND NEUTROPHILS

MONONUCLEAR PHAGOCYTE FUNCTIONS
Elimination of invading pathogens
Elimination of cellular debris from sites of tissue damage and the blood stream
Wound healing and remodeling of normal tissue
Amplification of the innate immune response: release of immune regulators
Bridge to the adaptive immune system: presentation of antigens to lymphocytes
NEUTROPHIL FUNCTIONS
Elimination of invading pathogens

The Bone Marrow Compartment: The Site of Granulopoiesis

Neutrophils are the most abundant white blood cell and account for up to 70% of circulating leukocytes. Neutrophil numbers can increase rapidly by as much as 5- to 10-fold during periods of acute infection with a rate of continuous supply by the bone marrow of $5 \times 10^{10} - 10 \times 10^{10}$ neutrophils/day. Because these cells have a very short half-life in blood, the bone marrow compartment provides a steady supply of mature neutrophils with the capability to upregulate cell production rapidly during times of infection. Neutrophils originate in the bone marrow from a common population of hematopoietic stem cells through a 10- to 14-day process of proliferation, differentiation, and maturation (Chapter 156).

Steps in Granulopoiesis

The stages of neutrophil granulopoiesis in the bone marrow (Fig. 169-2) are identified by the major transitions from the pluripotent stem cell to the mature neutrophil. The *myeloblast* is the first recognizable progenitor cell committed to granulopoiesis. This proliferating cell is characterized by its large nucleus and agranular cytoplasm. The *promyelocyte* follows and displays the initial development of primary granules. *Myelocytes* occupy the next stage of neutrophil maturation and are characterized by development of the first specific or "secondary" (peroxidase-negative) granules. *Metamyelocytes,* which follow myelocytes, are incapable of further mitosis and are readily identifiable by their now numerous cytoplasmic granules. The functional maturation of metamyelocytes results in the development of *band* cells, which are usually slightly larger than mature neutrophils and have a horseshoe-shaped nucleus and a moderate to abundant supply of specific granules. Band cells can be found in the circulation during periods of acute infection. The final mature *neutrophil,* which is released into the circulation, has a diameter of approximately 10 µm with a characteristic nucleus that is segmented and multilobed and occupies about 20% of the cell's volume; the remaining

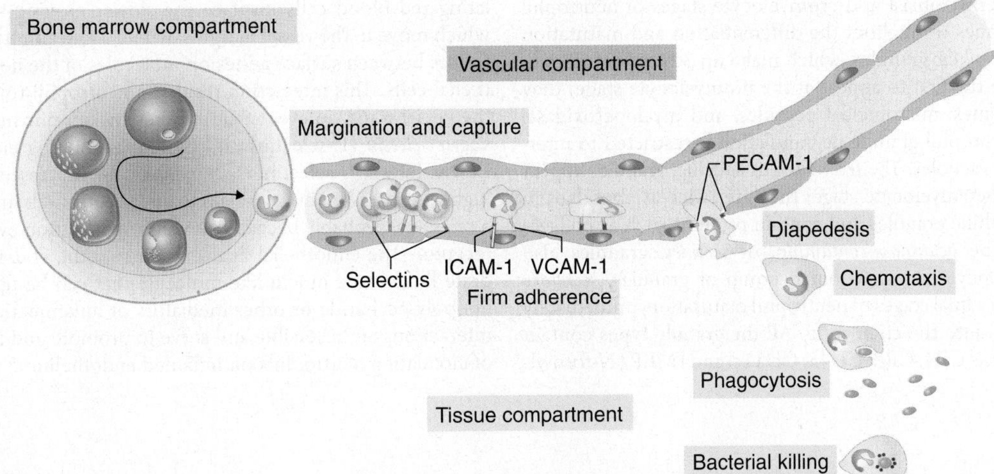

FIGURE 169-1. Life cycle of the neutrophil. The three major neutrophilic compartments (bone marrow, vascular, and tissue compartments) and the various steps involved in recruiting neutrophils to sites of infection are shown. ICAM = intercellular adhesion molecule; PECAM = platelet endothelial cell adhesion molecule; VCAM = vascular cell adhesion molecule.

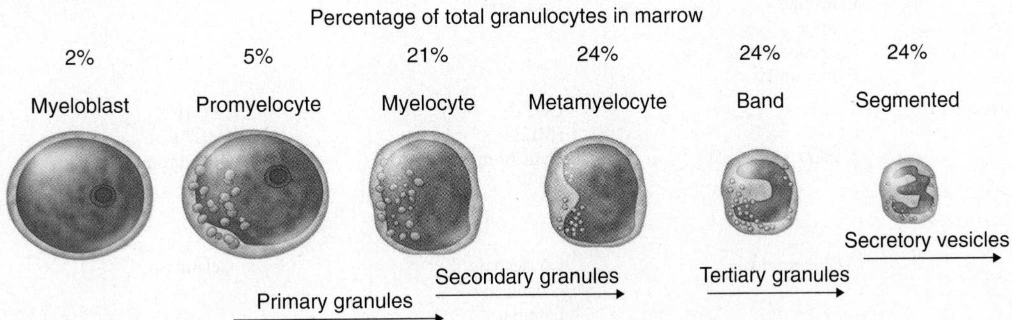

FIGURE 169-2. Cellular stages of granulopoiesis in bone marrow.

cytoplasm is taken up by granules. The distinctiveness of the granules reflects differences in content; as a result, granules formed at different stages carry specific types of matrix and membrane proteins.

Defects in granulopoiesis are manifested clinically as low circulating levels of neutrophils (neutropenia; Chapter 167). Verification of the stage at which neutrophil developmental arrest occurs can be determined by a bone marrow biopsy to assess the cellularity and characteristics of the neutrophil precursors present in the marrow space.

Regulation of Granulopoiesis

Granulopoiesis is driven by hematopoietic growth factors (Chapter 156). These factors, which are synthesized by a variety of cells, including fibroblasts and endothelial cells, are known to work together with other regulatory molecules, such as cytokines, to regulate hematopoiesis. Hematopoietic growth factors such as *interleukin-3* (IL-3), *granulocyte-macrophage colony-stimulating factor* (GM-CSF), and *granulocyte colony-stimulating factor* (G-CSF) bind to their target cells through specific receptors and are critical for the hematopoietic system to respond rapidly to infection or inflammation by dramatically increasing the production of leukocytes.

G-CSF is a potent cytokine that influences the proliferation, survival, maturation, and functional activation of cells from the neutrophil-granulocyte lineage. In normal individuals, circulating levels of G-CSF are very low (<100 pg/mL). However, in conditions of stress, G-CSF levels can rise to 20 times baseline levels, thereby resulting in a rapid increase in circulating neutrophils. G-CSF may regulate this increased granulopoiesis by increasing the mitotic pool at the promyelocyte and myelocyte stages and shortening neutrophil transit time in bone marrow.

Neutrophil Granules

One of the major mechanisms used by neutrophils to eliminate bacteria is a remarkable arsenal of antimicrobial proteins that are packed into cytoplasmic granules (Table 169-2). These antimicrobial proteins are securely contained within their respective granules and are released only when granules fuse with phagosomes or directly with the plasma membrane. Granulogenesis begins between the myeloblast and promyelocyte stages of neutrophil development and continues throughout the differentiation and maturation process of the cell. *Azurophilic* granules, which make up 30% of granules in a mature neutrophil, are the first to appear at the promyelocyte stage; they contain hydrolytic enzymes, microbicidal peptides, and myeloperoxidase. During phagocytosis, azurophil granule degranulation is restricted to internalization of phagocytic vacuoles. The *secondary,* or specific, granules appear later, beginning at the metamyelocyte stage; they are twice as abundant in the cytoplasm as azurophilic granules and contain proteins such as collagenase and lactoferrin. The *gelatinase-containing,* or *tertiary,* granules also appear at the metamyelocyte stage. A fourth group of granules, *secretory vesicles,* appears at the very final stages of neutrophil maturation, immediately before release of the cell into the circulation. All the granule types contain membrane proteins such as CR1, CR3, CD45, CD11c, and fMLP (*N*-formyl-methionyl-leucyl-phenylalanine) receptors, which are rapidly transported to the plasma membrane during activation to enhance neutrophil microbicidal activity.

A number of clinical conditions result from specific defects in granule development and formation. Initial assessment for granule defects can be made by microscopic evaluation of a peripheral blood smear (Chapter 157). Examples of obvious clinical diagnoses made with the peripheral smear include specific granule deficiency, which is characterized by bilobed nuclei in more than 80% of the neutrophils, and a significant decrease in cytoplasmic granularity. Abnormally large cytoplasmic granules are seen in individuals with Chédiak-Higashi syndrome.

The Vascular Compartment

Mature neutrophils are released from the postmitotic bone marrow compartment into the circulation, where they have an approximate lifespan of 8 to 12 hours and either circulate within the center of the blood vessel or attach to its endothelial lining, a process termed *margination.* Marginated neutrophils on the vessel walls are able to detach and reenter the circulation when required. For example, corticosteroids and epinephrine induce a rapid increase in circulating neutrophils by releasing neutrophils from the marginated pool. Neutrophils circulate until they are recruited to a site of infection. The initial phase of recruitment involves changes in the endothelial cell surface receptors lining the capillary beds closest to the site of infection or tissue damage. These critical changes in endothelial cells are mediated by immune regulators released by tissue macrophages, which initially detect the tissue damage or bacterial invasion. Emigration of circulating neutrophils from the vasculature to the site of infection or tissue damage requires three steps (see Fig. 169-1): capture and margination, firm adhesion to the endothelial wall, and diapedesis.

Margination and Capture

The marginated pool of neutrophils consists of neutrophils transiently retained against the walls of pulmonary capillaries and postcapillary venules. In the 20-μm diameter of a postcapillary venule, the smaller and faster circulating red blood cells displace the slower moving and larger neutrophils, which move to the vessel margins, where a low-affinity molecular interaction occurs between surface adhesion molecules of the neutrophil and the endothelial cells. This interaction results in neutrophil rolling and capture along the vessel walls, an event that requires the specific neutrophil receptors *leukocyte selectin* (L-selectin) and the corresponding endothelial ligand, sialyl Lewis (sLe). L-selectin is constitutively expressed in neutrophils, with highest expression in young circulating neutrophils and gradual decline with a cell's age, probably because previous margination events have depleted the receptor. The endothelial ligand for L-selectin, sLe, is a sialylated carbohydrate linked to a mucin-like molecule that can be upregulated by bacterial lipopolysaccharide or other mediators of inflammation. The selectin-ligand interactions are reversible and serve to promote and maintain accumulation of circulating neutrophils on inflamed endothelium.

TABLE 169-2 MEMBRANE AND MATRIX COMPONENTS OF NEUTROPHILIC GRANULES

COMPONENT	AZUROPHIL GRANULES (PRIMARY; PEROXIDASE POSITIVE)	SPECIFIC GRANULES (SECONDARY; PEROXIDASE NEGATIVE)	GELATINASE GRANULES (TERTIARY; PEROXIDASE NEGATIVE)	SECRETORY VESICLES
Antimicrobial proteins	Defensins Lysozyme Elastase Myeloperoxidase Cathepsin G	Lysozyme Lactoferrin	Lysozyme	
Membrane proteins and receptors	CD63 CD68 Alkaline phosphatase	CD11b fMLP-R Cytochrome b_{558} CR3	CD11b fMLP-R Cytochrome b_{558} CR3 CD45	CD11b fMLP-R Cytochrome b_{558} CR1 CD14 CD16
Matrix proteins	β-Glucuronidase	Collagenase Gelatinase Laminin	Gelatinase	Albumin

Modified from Edwards SW. *Biochemistry and Physiology of the Neutrophil.* Cambridge, UK: Cambridge University Press; 2005:55.

Adherence to the Endothelial Wall

Low-affinity, selectin-mediated transient interactions must be replaced by high-affinity, adhesive contacts between neutrophils and endothelial cells. During an acute inflammatory event, mediators derived from bacteria, damaged host cells, complement activation, or other immune cells are released from the site of infection and diffuse to the capillary beds, where they induce an immediate and transient vascular response that results in vascular leakage, which further encourages neutrophil margination. Endothelial cells adjacent to the site of inflammation, as well as the activated neutrophils that are bound to them, express integrin receptors that lead to high-affinity attachments between the neutrophils and endothelial cells. These high-affinity connections occur between neutrophil *β2 integrins* and their endothelial counterparts, the intercellular adhesion molecules (ICAMs). Integrins, which are a receptor family of heterodimeric transmembrane glycoproteins made up of an α- and β-subunit, are integral for cell adhesion. Neutrophil β2 integrins consist of three different α-subunits (CD11a, CD11b, and CD11c) that bind to a common β-subunit (CD18). The cytoplasmic tails of these transmembrane receptors possess phosphorylation sites for attachment of signal transduction and cytoskeletal proteins. The neutrophil integrins that mediate this adhesion step are *macrophage antigen-1* (Mac-1; CD11b/CD18) and *lymphocyte-associated function antigen-1* (LFA-1; CD11a/CD18). The receptors are stored in the neutrophil granule compartments to facilitate quick transfer to the plasma membrane during cell stimulation. The integrins bind to endothelial ICAM-1 and ICAM-2 and *vascular cell adhesion molecule-1* (VCAM-1), which are upregulated on the endothelial cell membranes when a cell is exposed to inflammatory cytokines. L-selectin receptors on neutrophils are concentrated on microvillus projections of the cell membrane, whereas the integrins are restricted to the body of the neutrophil. As a result, soon after initial contact during rolling interactions, the projections retract, thereby allowing integrins to interact with their ligands.

Diapedesis

Firm adherence through the L-selectin and integrin receptors facilitates transendothelial migration, or diapedesis, which marks the "point of no return" in the process of neutrophil recruitment to the site of injury. Unlike rolling and firm adhesion, which require heterophilic interactions between one class of molecules on the neutrophil and another class of molecules on the endothelial cell, diapedesis involves homophilic interactions between the same class of molecules on both cells—the *platelet-endothelial cell adhesion molecule-1* (PECAM-1 or CD31). PECAM-1 is expressed evenly on the surface of neutrophils and is concentrated at endothelial cell junctions. When they are firmly bound to the endothelial cell surface, neutrophils migrate between the closest tricellular endothelial cell junctions through interactions with PECAM-1 receptors. The neutrophil has now entered the tissue compartment, where it is primed for its final critical role in the elimination of microorganisms and cellular debris.

Laboratory Evaluation of Margination and Firm Adhesion

A defect in neutrophil margination or adhesion to the endothelial lining of the vascular compartment results in neutrophilia (elevated circulating neutrophil levels). This condition is usually associated with leukocyte adhesion deficiency (LAD), which is the result of a lack of CD11/CD18 receptor surface expression in peripheral blood neutrophils. If LAD is suspected, surface expression of these receptors can be measured with a flow cytometer and specific antibodies to CD11, CD18, or CD15 receptors.

The Tissue Compartment

Chemotaxis

Chemotaxis is the directed movement of cells up a chemical concentration gradient of a *chemoattractant.* Chemoattractants are soluble proteins or peptides, including bacterial products, complement factors, and chemokines produced by both inflammatory and noninflammatory cells, that are released from damaged or infected tissue. A concentration difference of 1% at the opposite ends of the neutrophil is sufficient to activate neutrophil chemotaxis. After a chemoattractant binds to its corresponding neutrophil membrane receptor, a series of cytoplasmic signaling pathways leads to activation of the neutrophil cytoskeleton. This activation results in the neutrophil assuming a polarized state characterized by an actin-rich leading lamella or pseudopod that drives cell motility.

Directional cell crawling, the intrinsic basis of chemotaxis, can be broken down into smaller processes, including extension of the cell membrane, adhesion to the tissue matrix, and contraction of the cell body in an organized and reversible manner. The actin-dependent protrusion of the leading edge, which is a sheetlike structure rich in actin filaments, is critical for normal neutrophil motility. The actin filaments within these lamellar regions are assembled into highly organized structures that push the membrane forward. These structures are formed by different collections of actin-binding proteins under the regulation of specific signal transduction cascades linking chemotactic receptors with cell movement. Defects in actin assembly also result in defects in chemotaxis and recurrent infections.

Actin Assembly Biology

Actin filaments are polar structures, with each end differing in its equilibrium-binding constant for actin monomers (Fig. 169-3). Filaments grow at the high-affinity or barbed end, whereas depolymerization occurs at the low-affinity or pointed end. This difference, generated by the ability of actin to bind and hydrolyze adenosine triphosphate, provides a physical polarity that regulatory proteins use to drive filament dynamics with high temporal and spatial precision. Three classes of proteins regulate the availability of high-affinity actin filament ends: filament-nucleating proteins (e.g., ARP2/3 de novo nucleation), filament-capping proteins (e.g., gelsolin), and filament-severing proteins (e.g., cofilin). Actin-nucleating factors bind actin monomers under conditions otherwise unfavorable for assembly and generate a new filament with a free high-affinity end available for assembly. Actin filament-capping proteins bind to the high-affinity filament end and regulate the addition of monomers by their presence or absence at the end of the filament. Actin-binding proteins are regulated by various second messengers,

Actin Assembly Regulation: Barbed End Regulation

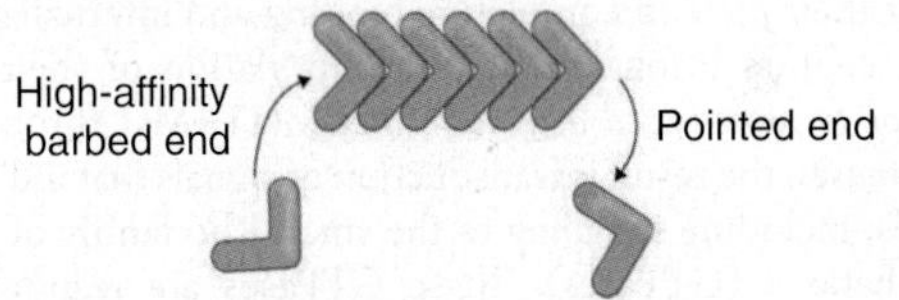

ARP 2/3 de novo nucleation

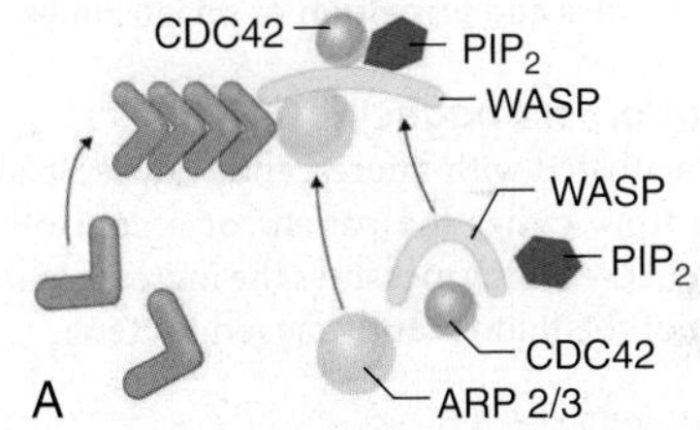

Capped barbed end

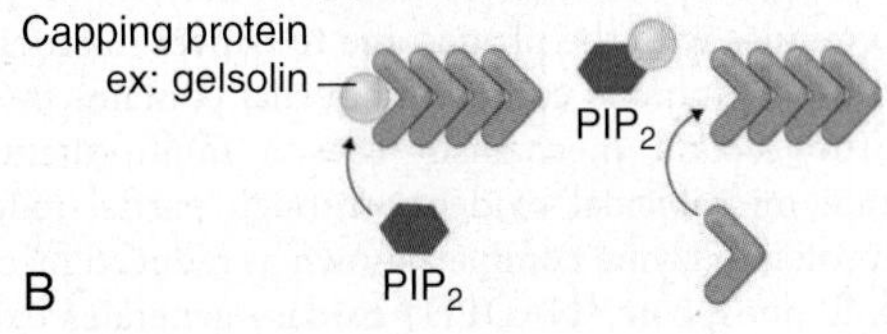

Cofilin-mediated severing

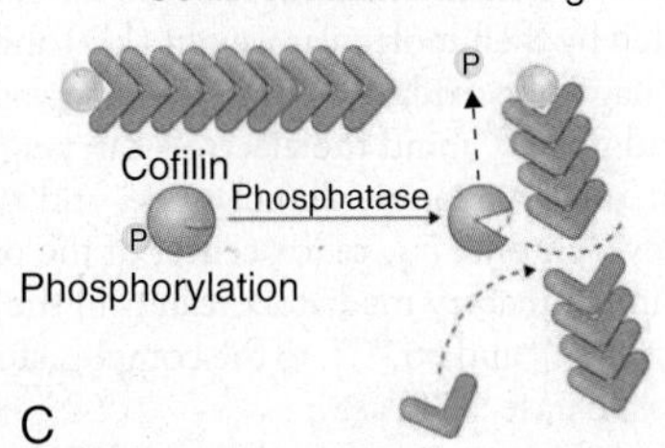

FIGURE 169-3. Regulation of actin assembly through the generation of free barbed ends by actin-binding proteins. A, The components below join together to form a nucleation complex (above). **B,** PIP_2 binds the capping protein, leading to its removal from the high-affinity end, allowing for addition and filament growth. **C,** A phosphatase removes the P from cofilin, thereby allowing it to sever the actin filament and leaving a free high-affinity end. PIP_2 = phosphatidylinositol 4,5-biphosphate; WASP = Wiskott-Aldrich syndrome protein.

including calcium. On stimulation, localized changes in the intracellular Ca^{2+} concentration lead to the rapid initiation of actin assembly and disassembly. The changes in actin filament length and the extent of cross-linkage between the filaments may account for the directional extension of actin-rich lamellae and contraction of the tail-like uropod at the other end of the cell. Movement in the neutrophil is therefore the result of lamellar protrusions resulting from the growth of actin filaments. Actin-rich lamellae will continue to be maintained as long as the neutrophil detects the chemoattractant gradient.

Laboratory Evaluation of Chemotaxis

A defect in neutrophil chemotaxis can be measured in the laboratory with a Boyden chamber, which uses a porous membrane to separate isolated neutrophils from a chemoattractant. A chemical gradient develops across the porous membrane and activates the neutrophils to crawl through the membrane toward the compartment containing the chemoattractant. Defects in chemotaxis can be determined by a lack of neutrophil transmigration through the membrane compared with control neutrophils from a healthy donor.

Phagocytosis

Phagocytosis is the process whereby neutrophils engulf and internalize invading pathogens into membrane compartments called *phagosomes.* Bacterial targets are "highlighted" or opsonized by antibodies (immunoglobulin G) or products from the classical complement pathway that coat the target and serve to mediate phagocytic adhesion. Neutrophilic phagocytosis involves two separate classes of receptors: *Fcγ receptors* (CD32 and CD16) for antibody-coated targets and *complement receptors* (CR1 and CR3) for complement-coated targets. CD32 and CR3 are functional receptors directly involved in neutrophilic phagocytosis, whereas CD16 and CR1 are coreceptors that assist their mate in completing binding and internalization. Activation of Fcγ receptors brings about phosphorylation of their cytoplasmic *immunoreceptor tyrosine-based activation motifs* (ITAMs) through activation of *Src family kinases;* the result is transduction of signals that induce extension of pseudopods, including signaling to the small Rho family of small guanosine triphosphatases (GTPases). These GTPases are responsible for the assembly of actin filaments, thereby leading to remodeling of the plasma membrane and the formation of actin-rich pseudopods, which are essential for the ingestion of particles and formation of phagosomes.

Laboratory Evaluation of Phagocytosis

Neutrophils can be incubated with fluorescently labeled bacteria after opsonization with serum from either the patient or a control. Phagocytosis is assessed by flow cytometry, which measures the increase in neutrophilic fluorescence after uptake of the fluorescently tagged bacteria.

Bacterial Killing

Phagocytes use two potent mechanisms for killing bacteria within the membrane-bound phagosome. The first involves fusion of the previously described storage granules with the phagosome to deliver microbicidal and lytic enzymes into the membrane compartment that contains the ingested microorganisms. The second mechanism uses a multiprotein enzyme complex to generate microbicidal oxidants through partial reduction of oxygen. The multiprotein enzyme complex known as reduced nicotinamide adenine dinucleotide phosphate (NADPH) oxidase generates oxidants by means of oxygen consumption, hence the term *respiratory burst.*

The NADPH enzyme system is made up of four essential polypeptide subunits that are denoted by their molecular weight (kD) and the superscript phox, which denotes phagocyte oxidase. Within the cytoplasmic membrane, the subunits $p22^{phox}$ and $gp91^{phox}$ bind the electron-carrying components of the oxidase (NADPH, a flavin adenine dinucleotide, and two nonidentical hemes) and form the cytochrome b_{558} redox center of the oxidase complex. Cellular activation by inflammatory mediators results in the addition of two cytosolic components, $p47^{phox}$ and $p67^{phox}$, to the complex along with the Rac small guanosine triphosphatase (GTPase).

The membrane-bound electron transport chain NADPH oxidase catalyzes the reduction of molecular oxygen to superoxide (O_2^-). The superoxide generated by this process is in turn catalytically converted to hydrogen peroxide and serves as a cosubstrate for myeloperoxidase to oxidize halides and to produce hypochlorous acid (HOCl), a very potent antimicrobial agent. These oxidants are able to kill bacteria within the phagosomes by oxidizing their cellular constituents.

Laboratory Evaluation of the Respiratory Burst and Bacterial Killing

Flow cytometry, a rapid and effective method for quantitatively assessing the respiratory burst, measures the fluorescence generated by cytoplasmic fluorescent probes such as dihydrorhodamine, which is converted to rhodamine by H_2O_2. The nitroblue tetrazolium (NBT) test is still used for rapid assessment of the respiratory burst when flow cytometry is not available.

Bacterial killing assays using a patient's neutrophils with either the patient's or control serum and bacteria such as *Staphylococcus aureus* or *Escherichia coli* are a definitive method to determine whether a given patient's neutrophils have an intracellular killing defect. Neutrophils from a healthy control subject phagocytose and kill approximately 95% of the bacteria within 2 hours. In assays in which an intracellular killing defect is present, neutrophils kill less than 10% of bacteria over a 2-hour period. It is necessary to confirm that there is no phagocytic defect before performing the bacterial killing assay to be sure that any defect in bacterial killing is not due to an internalization defect.

Neutrophil Extracellular Traps

Neutrophils use an extracellular process to contain and kill bacteria. Neutrophil extracellular traps (NETs) are formed by the release of chromatin and antimicrobial proteins from the neutrophil cytoplasm and granules. The chromatin forms a netlike meshwork that traps the bacteria and brings them in closer proximity to the antimicrobial elements adhered to the chromatin. Activation of NET formation requires simultaneous activation by at least two different receptors, and reactive oxygen species are essential to the process. IL-8 has been shown to be a potent activator of NET formation. The importance of NETs was highlighted by work showing that DNase expressing strains of group A streptococcus (GAS) and *Streptococcus pneumoniae* are more virulent than their non-DNase-expressing counterparts because of their ability to escape NETs.

CLINICAL MANIFESTATIONS

In addition to fever and recurrent infections, the most common findings in patients with phagocytic defects are oral infections resulting in gingival inflammation, periodontal bone loss, mobile or loose teeth, and premature loss of teeth (Table 169-3). An oral examination should be performed at the initial evaluation, followed by a full dental examination, depending on the findings. The history and laboratory tests can differentiate among the various clinical causes of disordered phagocytosis (Table 169-4).

DEFECTS IN LEUKOCYTE ADHESION

A defect in neutrophil adhesion to the endothelial lining leads to neutrophilia—an accumulation of neutrophils in the circulation, with very few neutrophils at sites of infection. Defects in neutrophil adhesion can be induced by drugs or due to a genetic defect. Drugs such as corticosteroids and epinephrine result in a transient leukocyte adhesive defect that results in an apparent dramatic increase in circulating neutrophils because of release of the marginated neutrophil pool. The major genetic disease that results in an adhesion deficiency is termed *leukocyte adhesion deficiency.*

Leukocyte Adhesion Deficiency

LAD-1

PATHOBIOLOGY

LAD-1 is an autosomal recessive inherited disorder in which patients have a mutation in the gene encoding CD18. The result is a deficiency of β2 integrin

TABLE 169-3 SYMPTOMS SUGGESTIVE OF A PHAGOCYTIC DISORDER

Recurrent infections that fail to resolve with conventional treatment
Recurrent infections of unusual severity
Recurrent infections in the lung, liver, or bone
Normally nonpathogenic bacteria or fungi identified in cultures from the infection sites
Aphthous ulcers
Severe periodontal diseases, including gingivitis
Lymphadenopathy or hepatosplenomegaly
Severe recurrent cutaneous infections with *Staphylococcus aureus*
Recurrent mycobacterial infections

receptors, which are required for neutrophil migration from the vasculature into the tissues, thereby impairing the binding of neutrophils to C3bi and endothelial ICAM-1 and ICAM-2. Indications of the disorder are high resting neutrophil counts accompanied by frequent dissemination, sepsis, and recurrent infections.[2]

CLINICAL MANIFESTATIONS AND DIAGNOSIS

Clinical manifestations in patients diagnosed with LAD-1 include delayed separation of the umbilical cord, bacterial and fungal infections, delayed wound healing, impaired pus formation, and severe destructive periodontitis with rapid tooth loss. Patients usually die during childhood. Flow cytometry is used to measure CD11/CD18 surface expression levels on neutrophils.

TREATMENT

Treatment is mainly supportive of early intervention for periodontal disease with prophylactic antibiotics in patients with recurrent infections. In severe cases, bone marrow transplantation is the treatment of choice.[3]

LAD-2 AND LAD-3

LAD-2, a variant of LAD-1, is associated with neutrophilia, the Bombay (hh) blood phenotype, dwarfism, and mental retardation. This disorder is due to a mutation in the guanosine diphosphate-fucose transporter gene, which

TABLE 169-4 DISORDERS OF PHAGOCYTIC FUNCTION

DISORDER	ETIOLOGY	IMPAIRED FUNCTION	CLINICAL CONSEQUENCE
DEGRANULATION ABNORMALITIES			
Chédiak-Higashi syndrome	Autosomal recessive; disordered coalescence of lysosomal granules Responsible gene found at 1q42-45. The encoded protein (LYST) has structural features homologous to a vacuolar sorting protein	Decreased neutrophilic chemotaxis, degranulation, and bactericidal activity; platelet storage pool defect; impaired NK function; failure to disperse melanosomes	Neutropenia, recurrent pyogenic infections, propensity for the development of marked hepatosplenomegaly in the accelerated phase, partial albinism
Specific granule deficiency	Autosomal recessive; abnormal regulation of various myeloid granule genes by a transacting factor	Impaired chemotaxis and bactericidal activity; bilobed nuclei in neutrophils; reduced content of neutrophil defensins, gelatinase, collagenase, vitamin B_{12}–binding protein, and lactoferrin	Recurrent infections, especially sinopulmonary and skin infections
ADHESION ABNORMALITIES			
Leukocyte adhesion deficiency type 1	Autosomal recessive; absence of CD11/CD18 surface adhesive glycoprotein (β2-integrins) on leukocyte membranes, most commonly arising from failure to express CD18 mRNA	Decreased binding of C3bi to neutrophils and impaired adhesion to ICAM-1 and ICAM-2	Neutrophilia, recurrent bacterial infection associated with lack of pus formation
Leukocyte adhesion deficiency type 2	Autosomal recessive; absence of neutrophil sialyl-Lewis^x	Decreased adhesion to activated endothelium expressing ELAM	Neutrophilia, recurrent bacterial infection without pus
Leukocyte adhesion deficiency type 3	Autosomal recessive; defects in activation of β1, β2, and β3 integrins	Severe leukocyte adhesion dysfunction; abnormal platelet aggregation	Neutrophilia, recurrent bacterial infection without pus, severe bleeding tendency
Neutrophil actin dysfunction	Altered polymerization of neutrophil cytoplasmic actin, perhaps arising from the presence of an inhibitor to F-actin formation	Impaired neutrophil adhesion, chemotaxis, and bacterial killing	Neutrophilia, recurrent bacterial infections without pus
DISORDERS OF CELL CHEMOTAXIS			
Hyperactive Chemotaxis			
Familial Mediterranean fever (FMF)	Autosomal recessive gene responsible for FMF on chromosome 16, which encodes for a protein called pyrin; pyrin may modify neutrophil activation	Excessive accumulation of neutrophils at inflamed sites	Recurrent fever, peritonitis, pleuritis, arthritis, amyloidosis
Depressed Chemotaxis			
Intrinsic defects of the neutrophil, e.g., leukocyte adhesion deficiency, Chédiak-Higashi syndrome, specific granule deficiency, neutrophil actin dysfunction, neonatal neutrophils	In the neonatal neutrophil, there is diminished ability to express β2 integrins and a qualitative impairment in β2 integrin function	Diminished chemotaxis	Propensity for the development of pyogenic infections
Direct inhibition of neutrophil mobility, e.g., drugs	Ethanol, glucocorticoids, cyclic AMP	Impaired locomotion and ingestion, impaired adherence	Possible causes of frequent infections; neutrophilia seen with epinephrine is the result of cyclic AMP release from the endothelium
Immune complexes	Bind to Fc receptors on neutrophils in patients with rheumatoid arthritis, systemic lupus erythematosus, and other inflammatory states	Impaired chemotaxis	Recurrent pyogenic infections
Hyperimmunoglobulin E syndrome	Disorders of cytokine signaling, most commonly due to autosomal dominant mutations in the *STAT3* gene	Impaired chemotaxis, impaired IgG opsonization of *Staphylococcus aureus*	Recurrent skin and sinopulmonary infections
DEFECTS OF MICROBICIDAL ACTIVITY			
Chronic granulomatous disease (CGD)	X-linked and autosomal recessive; failure to express functional gp91^{phox} (in the phagocyte membrane) and p22^{phox} (autosomal recessive). Other autosomal recessive forms of CGD arise from failure to express protein p47^{phox} or p67^{phox}	Failure to activate neutrophil respiratory burst leading to failure to kill catalase-positive microbes	Recurrent pyogenic infections with catalase-positive microorganisms
G6PD deficiency	Less than 5% of normal activity of G6PD	Failure to activate NADPH-dependent oxidase	Infections with catalase-positive microorganisms

TABLE 169-4 DISORDERS OF PHAGOCYTIC FUNCTION—cont'd

DISORDER	ETIOLOGY	IMPAIRED FUNCTION	CLINICAL CONSEQUENCE
Myeloperoxidase deficiency	Autosomal recessive; failure to process modified precursor protein arising from missense mutation	H_2O_2-dependent antimicrobial activity not potentiated by myeloperoxidase	None
Deficiencies of glutathione reductase and glutathione synthetase	Failure to detoxify H_2O_2	Excessive formation of H_2O_2	Minimal problems with recurrent pyogenic infections
IMPAIRED MACROPHAGE FUNCTION			
Defects in the interferon-γ–IL-12 axis	Interferon-γ receptor ligand-binding chain, interferon-γ receptor signaling chain, IL-12 receptor β_1 chain, IL-12 p40 deficiency; the interferon-γ receptor abnormalities may be autosomal dominant or recessive; the IL-12 receptor and IL-12 abnormalities are autosomal recessive	Impaired killing of microorganisms. Fatal BCG infection secondary either to an inability to produce IL-12 by dendritic cells and macrophages or to depressed bactericidal activity of macrophages lacking normal function of the interferon receptor	Infection with atypical mycobacteria, *Salmonella*, and *Listeria*
Hemophagocytic lymphohistiocystosis (HLH) and macrophage activation syndrome (MAS)	Primary inherited form with mutations in perforin gene and genes involved in exocytosis; secondary acquired forms associated with infections, malignancies, and (in MAS) rheumatologic disorders.	Hyperinflammatory state and hypercytokinemia; impairment of NK and cytotoxic T-cell function.	Fever, hepatosplenomegaly, pancytopenia, pulmonary and neurologic complications, increased serum ferritin and triglycerides

AMP = adenosine monophosphate; BCG = bacille Calmette-Guérin; ELAM = endothelial leukocyte adhesion molecule; G6PD = glucose-6-phosphate dehydrogenase; ICAM = intracellular adhesion molecule; IL-12 = interleukin-12; NADPH = nicotinamide adenine dinucleotide phosphate; NK = natural killer; phox = phagocyte oxidase.
Modified from Boxer LA. Quantitative abnormalities of granulocytes. In: Beutler E, Lichtman MA, Coller BS, et al, eds. *Williams Hematology*, 6th ed. New York: McGraw-Hill; 2001:836.

results in impaired expression of CD15s and other selectin ligands. Symptoms are similar to those of LAD-1, and the diagnosis is confirmed by flow cytometry for CD15s.

In the most recently described LAD-3,[4] there is a primary activation defect in all three β integrins (β1, β2, and β3), and mutations have been found in kindlin-3, which binds the cytoplasmic tail of integrin. Clinical manifestations include defects in platelet activation and severe bleeding tendency. Treatment includes blood transfusion during a bleeding episode.

DEFECTS IN NEUTROPHILIC CHEMOTAXIS

After phagocytes enter the tissue compartment from the vascular pool, they migrate up the concentration gradients of various chemoattractants to the site of focal infection. A number of chemotactic defects result in severe recurrent infections.

Hyperimmunoglobin E Syndrome

PATHOBIOLOGY

Hyperimmunoglobin E syndrome, or hyper-IgE syndrome, also referred to as Job syndrome, is a group of genetically diverse, multisystem disorders of cytokine signaling. The most common form of the syndrome involves dominant mutations in the gene for signal transducer and activator of transcription-3 (*STAT3*). Hyper-IgE syndrome is prevalent among white, Asian, and African populations, with equal frequency among males and females.[5]

CLINICAL MANIFESTATIONS AND DIAGNOSIS

The neutrophilic disorder is characterized by recurrent skin abscesses, pneumonia, and periodontal diseases. After birth, patients usually have moderate to severe dermatitis, eczematous skin eruptions, nonerythematous abscesses, pneumatoceles, and severe osteoporosis that can result in bone fractures. The organisms most commonly present at infected sites are *Staphylococcus aureus, Haemophilus influenzae, Escherichia coli,* and *Candida albicans.* Patients have elevated IgE levels (typically >1000 IU/mL) and eosinophilia. The defect in neutrophilic chemotaxis is less severe than that in Chédiak-Higashi syndrome (see later). Genetic testing of the *STAT3* gene, in conjunction with characteristic manifestations, such as immunologic and infectious complications and involvement of skeletal and connective tissue, is imperative to confirm diagnosis.[6] With implementation of prophylactic measures, accompanied by IgG infusion, good long-term prognosis can be seen.

TREATMENT Rx

Treatment includes prophylactic antibiotics, antifungal prophylaxis, IgG infusions, and aggressive treatment of infections.[7] In severe cases, hematopoietic stem cell transplantation may be considered.

Familial Mediterranean Fever

PATHOBIOLOGY

Familial Mediterranean fever, further discussed in Chapter 261, also known as recurrent polyserositis, is an autosomal recessive autoinflammatory disease that is widespread among people of Mediterranean descent, including Arabs, Armenians, and Sephardic Jews.[7] The genetic defect is a missense mutation in the *MEFV* gene, which encodes the protein pyrin. Pyrin is believed to be a transcription factor involved in downregulating inflammation, possibly through an effect on chemotaxis in neutrophils and monocytes. The *MEFV* mutation results in a hyperinflammatory response characterized by abundant neutrophilic infiltration into the peritoneal, pleural, and joint spaces.

CLINICAL MANIFESTATIONS AND DIAGNOSIS

The most common findings include acute, self-limited attacks of fever accompanied by pleuritis, peritonitis, arthritis, pericarditis, and erythematous skin lesions. Although first attacks may be observed during infancy, onset of clinical disease usually occurs in childhood or adolescence, with a relatively small number of adult-onset cases.

Leukocytosis has been observed during attacks, but the leukocyte count is normal between episodes. Genetic testing is available for the most common mutations. This disease can be fatal if renal failure develops as a result of amyloidosis (Chapter 188), which occurs in up to 25% of those affected.

TREATMENT Rx

The hyperinflammatory attacks can be reduced significantly and even the complications of amyloidosis can be prevented[8] with prophylactic colchicine, 0.6 mg orally two or three times daily, up to a maximum dose of 2.0 to 2.4 mg if needed and if tolerated.[A1] The prognosis is generally good for most affected individuals maintained with colchicine. Rilonacept, an IL-1 decoy receptor, has been found to reduce frequency of attacks and is a treatment option for patients with colchicine-resistant or -intolerant disease.[A2]

DISORDERS OF NEUTROPHILIC DEGRANULATION

Granules supply key membrane proteins, including receptors required for phagocytosis. Granule-related defects result in profound abnormalities in bacterial killing.

Chédiak-Higashi Syndrome

PATHOBIOLOGY

Chédiak-Higashi syndrome is a rare autosomal recessive disorder of the *LYST* gene, which encodes a protein responsible for lysosomal trafficking. Defective targeting of granules to the membrane results in large cytoplasmic granules that are unable to target to the plasma membrane in neutrophils, monocytes, and lymphocytes.

CLINICAL MANIFESTATIONS AND DIAGNOSIS

Symptoms are recurrent bacterial infections of the skin, mouth, and respiratory tract; partial albinism; peripheral neuropathy; and mild bleeding disorders as a result of a deficiency in serotonin- and adenosine phosphate–containing granules in platelets. Defects in myelopoiesis result in neutropenia. Death usually occurs by 7 years of age because of infection. Advanced disease is characterized by lymphocytic tissue infiltrates and pancytopenia.

Giant cytoplasmic granules are seen in the peripheral blood smear. Neutrophil function testing shows defects in chemotaxis and bacterial killing.

TREATMENT Rx

Prophylactic antibiotics should be used to prevent infections. Bone marrow transplantation from an HLA-matched donor may be successful if performed before the disease becomes advanced.

Specific Granule Deficiency

PATHOBIOLOGY

Specific granule deficiency (SGD) is an autosomal recessive disorder that manifests during infancy as the recurrent appearance of deep and superficial skin infections, respiratory infections, and abscesses. Azurophilic granules in neutrophils lack lactoferrin, defensins, gelatinase, collagenase, cytochrome *b*, and vitamin B_{12}-binding protein. Neutrophils are morphologically altered and have a bilobed rather than a trilobed nucleus.

CLINICAL MANIFESTATIONS AND DIAGNOSIS

This disorder is characterized by impaired neutrophil chemotaxis, reduced respiratory burst, and a defect in bacterial killing. Infections are commonly caused by *S. aureus*, *Pseudomonas aeruginosa*, and *C. albicans*. Flow cytometry is used to determine deficiency in lactoferrin and vitamin B_{12}-binding protein for diagnosis.

TREATMENT Rx

Treatment includes administration of parenteral antibiotics and drainage for infections. With aggressive treatment of infections, survival into adulthood is possible.

DISORDERS OF OXYGEN-DEPENDENT BACTERIAL KILLING

A genetic defect in any component of the respiratory burst results in delayed or ineffective bacterial killing.

Chronic Granulomatous Disease

PATHOBIOLOGY

Chronic granulomatous disease (CGD) is a genetic disease that occurs in about 1 in 200,000 live births. Neutrophils and macrophages cannot generate superoxide and are therefore unable to kill catalase-positive organisms. This condition results from mutations in one of the four structural genes of the NADPH oxidase complex. The most common genetic defect occurs in the 91-kD component of cytochrome b_{558}, which is coded on the X chromosome. The other mutations are autosomal recessive and have been detected in the 22-, 47-, and 67-kD structural proteins.

CLINICAL MANIFESTATIONS AND DIAGNOSIS

Children are prone to infections or granulomatous lesions in the lungs, skin, and liver. *S. aureus* is the most common organism, but other organisms include *Serratia marcescens*, *Burkholderia cepacia*, *Aspergillus* species, and *Nocardia* species. Staphylococcal liver abscesses are pathognomonic of CGD. Flow cytometry is used to measure the increase in fluorescence generated when dihydrorhodamine is converted to rhodamine by H_2O_2.

TREATMENT Rx

Abscesses can be removed by surgery. Trimethoprim-sulfamethoxazole prophylaxis (5 mg/kg/day divided into two equal doses) and antifungal prophylaxis with itraconazole (100 mg/day for <50 kg, 200 mg/day for >50 kg) have been shown to reduce the frequency of infections in these patients. Interferon-γ (50 μg/m^2 subcutaneously three times per week) prophylaxis is now considered "standard of care" in many centers. Bone marrow transplantation can also be considered for patients with refractory infections.[9] Gene therapy for CGD by gene-modified autologous hematopoietic stem cell transplantation has resulted in transient immune restoration but also genomic instability, monosomy 7, and clonal progression toward myelodysplasia. Future trials will be required to determine the role of gene therapy in clinical care.

Myeloperoxidase Deficiency

PATHOBIOLOGY

Myeloperoxidase (MPO) deficiency is a relatively common disorder (1 in 4000) in which the enzyme for conversion of neutrophilic hydrogen peroxide to HOCl is absent. This deficiency is not associated with increased susceptibility to infections, probably because of the accumulation of hydrogen peroxide, which is also bactericidal. Several genes have been reported to cause MPO deficiency, including *R569W*, *Y173C*, and *M251T*. The most common gene mutation related to MPO deficiency is the *R569W* gene, associated with the absence of MPO in neutrophils. Less frequently, patients with a mutation in *Y173C* gene have MPO that cannot fully mature. Differently, patients with a mutation in the *M251T* gene have fully mature MPO that are not functional.

CLINICAL MANIFESTATIONS AND DIAGNOSIS

MPO is usually asymptomatic, although patients with diabetes mellitus may occasionally experience candidal infections. The diagnosis is made by observation of a negative peroxidase stain of the peripheral blood smear.

TREATMENT Rx

Symptomatic patients may be treated with prophylactic antibiotics with routine control of blood glucose in those who have diabetes mellitus.

Glutathione Synthetase Deficiency

PATHOBIOLOGY

Glutathione synthetase (GSS) deficiency is a autosomal recessive disorder of glutathione metabolism with approximately 70 cases reported worldwide. Glutathione, which is a potent antioxidant found in granulocytes, is required for a normal respiratory burst and bacterial killing.

CLINICAL MANIFESTATIONS AND DIAGNOSIS

GSS deficiency can exist in mild, moderate, and severe forms. Patients with GSS deficiency typically have recurrent otitis and hemolytic anemia. Mildly affected patients typically present with hemolytic anemia; in the moderate form, metabolic acidosis occurs; and patients with the severe form in addition develop central nervous system impairment, such as seizures, mental retardation, and ataxia. The diagnosis is confirmed by verifying low or no glutathione synthetase in red blood cells, high levels of 5-oxoproline in the urine (up to 1 g/kg/day), and mutations in the glutathione synthetase *(GSS)* gene. Onset of symptoms ranges from birth to infancy and childhood.

TREATMENT

Treatment goals include supplementation with antioxidants, correction of acidosis with bicarbonate, and blood transfusion.

Severe Glucose-6-Phosphate Dehydrogenase Deficiency

PATHOBIOLOGY

Glucose-6-phosphate dehydrogenase (G6PD) deficiency is an X-linked disorder (>400,000 people) distributed throughout Africa, Asia, the Mediterranean, and the Middle East. The prevalence of G6PD deficiency is associated with the distribution of malaria and provides partial protection against malarial infection. White individuals with a severe reduction in G6PD activity are subject to recurrent infections, whereas Asians or blacks with similarly reduced G6PD levels are not. G6PD is crucial for regulating the availability of NADPH for the respiratory burst. Gene mutations associated with G6PD are located on the distal arm of the X chromosome and are frequently identified as missense mutations.

CLINICAL MANIFESTATIONS AND DIAGNOSIS

G6PD deficiency results in recurrent bacterial infections, hemolytic anemia (Chapter 161), and jaundice. The diagnosis can be made with flow cytometry to assess the respiratory burst and to demonstrate the absence of G6PD in all blood cells. The production of NADPH from NADP is detected thorough rapid fluorescent spot testing.

TREATMENT Rx

Treatment goals include abstaining from oxidative stressors and the consumption of fava beans. In severe cases of anemia, a blood transfusion is warranted.

MACROPHAGE-RELATED ABNORMALITIES

Accumulation of monocyte-macrophages at sites of infection occurs after the major influx of neutrophils. Macrophages have a critical role in antigen presentation to lymphocytes, thereby activating the adaptive arm of the immune system. A critical defect in macrophage signaling results in susceptibility to mycobacterial infection.

Interferon-γ Receptor-1 Defects

PATHOBIOLOGY

When macrophages phagocytose mycobacteria, they produce IL-12, which in turn stimulates T cells to produce interferon-γ (IFN-γ). IFN-γ is critical to the killing of mycobacteria and other intracellular bacteria. Patients with recurrent and severe mycobacterial infections who are not infected with human immunodeficiency virus should be assessed for abnormalities in pathways that lead to the generation and utilization of IFN-γ.

Patients with autosomal recessive mutations in the IFN-γ receptors typically have a complete loss of function of the IFN-γ receptors. Autosomal dominant mutations in the IFN-γ receptors result in normal ligand binding but defective intracellular signal transduction because of a cytoplasmically truncated form of the receptor.

CLINICAL MANIFESTATIONS AND DIAGNOSIS

Recessive mutations typically manifest as severe disseminated infections and poor formation of granulomas. Multifocal mycobacterial osteomyelitis is pathognomonic of an autosomal dominant mutation in the IFN-γ receptor. Flow cytometry confirms the absence of membrane expression of IFN-γ receptor-1 in the autosomal recessive form and up to 10-fold higher membrane expression levels of the cytoplasmically truncated receptor in the autosomal dominant form.

TREATMENT Rx

For patients with autosomal dominant mutations, subcutaneous IFN-γ is effective. For autosomal recessive patients completely lacking IFN-γ receptor function, hematopoietic stem cell transplantation should be considered. Long-term antibiotic prophylaxis against mycobacterial infections with azithromycin or clarithromycin is recommended.

Hemophagocytic Lymphohistiocytosis and Macrophage Activation Syndrome

PATHOBIOLOGY

Hemophagocytic lymphohistiocytosis (HLH), also known as *hemophagocytic syndrome*,[10] and the related *macrophage activation syndrome* are rare, often life-threatening syndromes of diverse etiologies. Their clinical manifestations reflect a state of extreme systemic inflammation and unregulated immune activation. These disorders have been traditionally classified as either (1) primary HLH that has an inherited basis and is seen in children,[11] or (2) secondary HLH that is seen in adults and is triggered by a variety of acquired disorders like infections, malignancies, and rheumatologic diseases. Macrophage activation syndrome has been considered to represent mainly the latter group, the rheumatologic forms of secondary HLH. However, the distinction between primary and secondary HLH is becoming increasingly blurred because genetic defects are also being discovered in adults with apparently acquired disease who have presentations of the syndrome that occur later in life. Genetic defects underlying HLH (and macrophage activation syndrome) generally cause impairment of natural killer (NK) cell and cytotoxic T-cell function. Mutations tend to occur in the perforin gene or in genes important for the exocytosis of cytotoxic granules.

CLINICAL MANIFESTATIONS AND DIAGNOSIS

The clinical manifestations of HLH result from its underlying hyperinflammatory state with hypercytokinemia. They include fever (often presenting as "fever of unknown etiology"), hepatosplenomegaly, various cutaneous manifestations, pulmonary involvement including acute respiratory failure with alveolar or interstitial infiltrates, various neurologic manifestations, bilineage or trilineage cytopenia, abnormal liver function tests, hypertriglyceridemia, and hypofibrinogenemia.

Conditions associated with secondary HLH include viral infections (herpes simplex virus, Epstein-Barr virus, cytomegalovirus, human immunodeficiency virus, parvovirus, influenza, and post vaccination); other infections (mycoplasma, bacterial, protozoal, fungal, and mycobacterial); malignancies (leukemia, Hodgkin and non-Hodgkin lymphoma, solid tumors like germ cell tumors); and immune deficiency states (including CGD and stem cell transplantation). Macrophage activation syndrome is now essentially considered to be HLH associated with rheumatic diseases, classically as a potentially lethal complication of systemic juvenile rheumatoid arthritis, but also with systemic lupus erythematosus, scleroderma, Sjögren syndrome, mixed connective tissue disorders, and Kawasaki disease.

A diagnostic hallmark of HLH, although sometimes not found early in the course of the disease, is histopathologic evidence of hemophagocytosis in the bone marrow.[12] Laboratory findings reflecting the hyperinflammatory state include extremely high serum levels of ferritin and soluble CD25 (i.e., the soluble IL-2 receptor, IL-2Rα).

TREATMENT Rx

A high index of suspicion is required to make an early diagnosis of HLH or macrophage activation syndrome so that treatment can be initiated promptly to attempt to prevent irreversible tissue damage. Most important is the identification and specific treatment of the underlying cause of the syndrome in any individual patient. Hematopoietic stem cell transplantation with reduced-intensity conditioning regimens is being increasingly considered when a genetic cause is identified. Combination therapy with (1) dexamethasone, etoposide with or without cyclosporine, or (2) corticosteroids, cyclosporine and antithymocyte globulin has been attempted, especially as a bridge to stem cell transplantation. Alemtuzumab, a monoclonal antibody to CD52-bearing lymphocytes, appears to be effective as a salvage agent for refractory HLH, leading to improvement and survival to transplantation in pediatric and adult patients.[13]

ASSESSING PHAGOCYTE FUNCTION: MAKING THE DIAGNOSIS

If a phagocyte functional disorder may be the underlying cause of recurrent infections in a patient, a complete blood count (CBC) and peripheral smear guide subsequent definitive testing (Fig. 169-4). Cultures from infected areas allow antimicrobial targeting and also provide critical diagnostic information. If the defect is a result of abnormal neutrophil development and maturation, the CBC will show neutropenia; a bone marrow biopsy might be required. Repeated CBC (twice per week for 6 weeks) is indicated if cyclic neutropenia is suspected because of a periodicity of the infections (Chapter 167).

If the CBC reveals neutrophilia, a defect in the recruitment of neutrophils into tissues is suggested. An assessment of the receptors required for transmigration by flow cytometry and specific antibodies to the surface receptors is indicated.

If circulating levels of phagocytes are normal yet the patient is experiencing recurrent infections, a phagocytic defect within the infected tissue is likely. Laboratory testing to evaluate chemotaxis, phagocytosis, and bacterial killing is indicated.

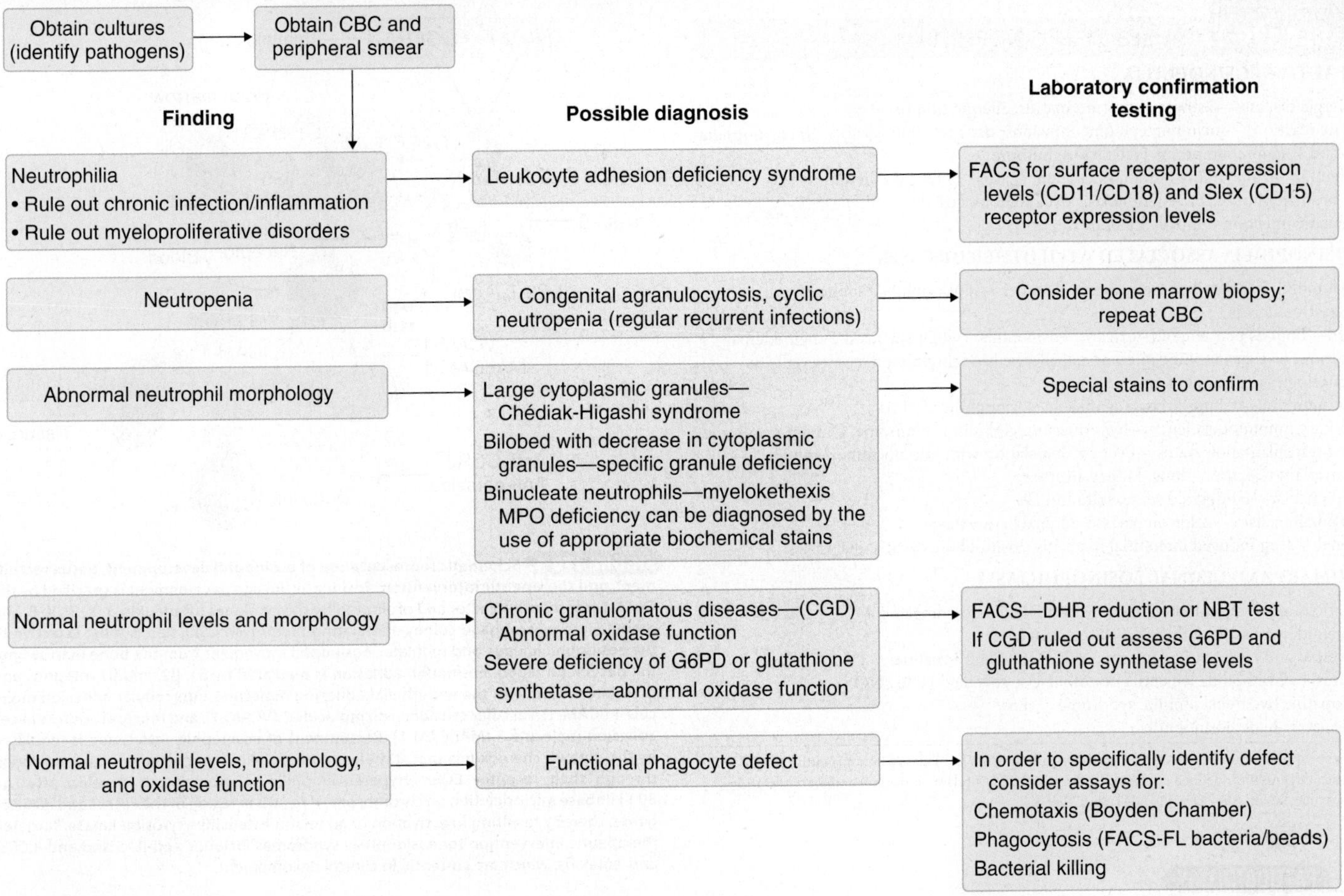

Obtain cultures (identify pathogens) → Obtain CBC and peripheral smear

Finding	Possible diagnosis	Laboratory confirmation testing
Neutrophilia • Rule out chronic infection/inflammation • Rule out myeloproliferative disorders	Leukocyte adhesion deficiency syndrome	FACS for surface receptor expression levels (CD11/CD18) and Slex (CD15) receptor expression levels
Neutropenia	Congenital agranulocytosis, cyclic neutropenia (regular recurrent infections)	Consider bone marrow biopsy; repeat CBC
Abnormal neutrophil morphology	Large cytoplasmic granules—Chédiak-Higashi syndrome Bilobed with decrease in cytoplasmic granules—specific granule deficiency Binucleate neutrophils—myelokethexis MPO deficiency can be diagnosed by the use of appropriate biochemical stains	Special stains to confirm
Normal neutrophil levels and morphology	Chronic granulomatous diseases—(CGD) Abnormal oxidase function Severe deficiency of G6PD or glutathione synthetase—abnormal oxidase function	FACS—DHR reduction or NBT test If CGD ruled out assess G6PD and gluthathione synthetase levels
Normal neutrophil levels, morphology, and oxidase function	Functional phagocyte defect	In order to specifically identify defect consider assays for: Chemotaxis (Boyden Chamber) Phagocytosis (FACS-FL bacteria/beads) Bacterial killing

FIGURE 169-4. **Approach to diagnosing a suspected phagocytic defect. CBC = complete blood count; DHR = dihydrorhodamine; FACS = flow cytometry; FL = fluorescent; G6PD = glucose-6-phosphate dehydrogenase; MPO = myeloperoxidase; NBT = nitroblue tetrazolium.**

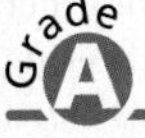

Grade A References

A1. Ozaltin F, Bilginer Y, Gulhan B, et al. Diagnostic validity of colchicine in patients with Familial Mediterranean fever. *Clin Rheumatol.* 2014;33:969-974.

A2. Hashkes PJ, Spalding SJ, Giannini EH, et al. Rilonacept for colchicine-resistant or -intolerant familial Mediterranean fever: a randomized trial. *Ann Intern Med.* 2012;157:533-541.

GENERAL REFERENCES

For the General References and other additional features, please visit Expert Consult at https://expertconsult.inkling.com.

170

EOSINOPHILIC SYNDROMES

MARC E. ROTHENBERG

DEFINITION

Eosinophilic syndromes are a heterogeneous group of disorders that involve eosinophilia, which is defined as the accumulation of eosinophils in peripheral blood and/or tissues. Circulating eosinophils normally account for only 1 to 3% of peripheral blood leukocytes, and the upper limit of the normal range is 350 cells/mm^3 of blood. Eosinophilia occurs in a variety of disorders (Table 170-1) and is usually arbitrarily classified according to the degree of blood eosinophilia: mild (351 to 1500 cells/mm^3), moderate (>1500 to 5000 cells/mm^3), or severe (>5000 cells/mm^3). Tissue eosinophilic disorders, such as eosinophil-associated gastrointestinal disorders and eosinophilic fasciitis, are not necessarily associated with blood eosinophilia, so their diagnosis is based on the microscopic identification of eosinophil-rich inflammatory infiltrates associated with tissue damage.

Historically, hypereosinophilic syndromes were generally classified as idiopathic and were defined by (1) the presence of eosinophilia (>1500 cells/mm^3 for at least 6 months) that remained unexplained despite a comprehensive evaluation for known causes of eosinophilia (such as drug reactions and infections) and (2) evidence of organ dysfunction directly attributable to the eosinophilia. Now, however, it is known that in some patients, an acquired genetic etiology is responsible. These include the (a) *FIP1L1*–platelet-derived growth factor receptor-α (*PDGFRA*) fusion gene associated with a microdeletion on 4q24; and (b) other abnormalities of 4q12 (*PDGFRA* fusion partners instead of *FIP1L1*), 5q31-33 (*PDGFRB*), 8p11-13 (*FGFR1*), 9p24 (*JAK2*), and 13q12 (*FLT3*). These are detected by conventional cytogenetics, fluorescent in situ hybridization (FISH), and reverse transcription–polymerase chain reaction (RT-PCR).[1] Identification of these diseases has important therapeutic implications because they can be treated with targeted agents like imatinib, a tyrosine kinase inhibitor.

EPIDEMIOLOGY

The most common cause of eosinophilia worldwide is helminth infections, which affect hundreds of millions of people. The most frequent cause in industrialized nations is atopic disease, which affects 10 to 30% of the population. Hypereosinophilic disorders such as *FIP1L1-PDGFRA*–associated disease and Churg-Strauss syndrome (Chapter 270) are very rare. For example, Churg-Strauss syndrome affects 4 to 6 cases per million per year, whereas true idiopathic hypereosinophilic syndromes may affect only 4000 to 5000 people worldwide. Other syndromes such as eosinophil-associated gastrointestinal disorders are more common, with a prevalence of approximately 1 in 2000 individuals.

TABLE 170-1 CAUSES OF EOSINOPHILIA

REACTIVE EOSINOPHILIA

Allergic diseases—asthma, atopic dermatitis, allergic rhinitis
Drug reactions—including cytokine infusions; drug reaction (rash) with eosinophilia and systemic symptoms (DRESS) syndrome
Infection—viral (human immunodeficiency virus) or fungal (allergic bronchopulmonary aspergillosis, coccidioidomycosis)
Parasitic infection—mostly helminths

EOSINOPHILIA ASSOCIATED WITH OTHER DISEASES

Eosinophil-associated gastrointestinal disorders—eosinophilic esophagitis, gastroenteritis
Skin—bullous pemphigoid, urticaria, eosinophilic cellulitis, episodic angioedema
Pulmonary—eosinophilic pneumonia, allergic bronchopulmonary aspergillosis
Neurologic—eosinophilic meningitis
Autoimmune—Churg-Strauss syndrome, eosinophilic fasciitis
Primary immunodeficiency—hyperimmunoglobulin E syndrome, Omenn syndrome
Post-transplantation status—liver (in association with immunosuppression)
Transplant rejection—lung, kidney, liver
Malignancy—Hodgkin disease, solid tumors
Hypoadrenalism—Addison disease, adrenal hemorrhage
Renal—drug-induced interstitial nephritis, eosinophilic cystitis, dialysis

PRIMARY AND CLONAL EOSINOPHILIAS*

Myeloid and lymphoid neoplasms with *PDGFRA* rearrangement
Myeloid neoplasms with *PDGFRB* rearrangement
Myeloid and lymphoid neoplasms with *FGFR1* abnormalities
Chronic eosinophilia leukemia not otherwise specified (CEL-NOS)
Idiopathic hypereosinophilic syndrome (HES)
Idiopathic hypereosinophilia

*These represent the revised World Health Organization (WHO) classification (Gottlib J. World Health Organization-defined eosinophilic disorders: 2011 update on diagnosis, risk stratification, and management. *Am J Hematol* 2011;86:677-688.)

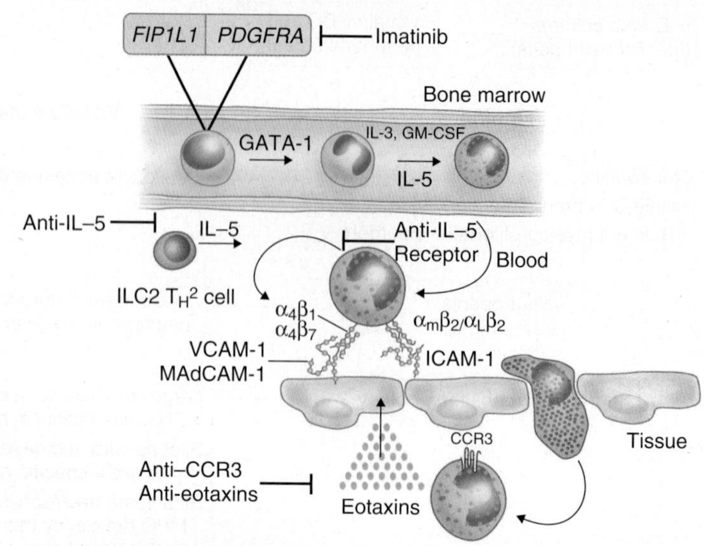

FIGURE 170-1. Schematic representation of eosinophil development, tissue recruitment, and therapeutic intervention. Eosinophil lineage development is specified by the GATA-1 transcription factor and promoted by the cytokines interleukin-3 (IL-3), IL-5, and granulocyte-macrophage colony-stimulating factor (GM-CSF). IL-5 is most selective to the eosinophil lineage and regulates eosinophil movement from the bone marrow into the peripheral blood. Eosinophil adhesion is mediated by β1, β2, and β7 integrins and their interaction with the endothelial adhesion molecules intercellular adhesion molecule 1 (ICAM-1), vascular cell adhesion molecule 1 (VCAM-1), and mucosal address in cell adhesion molecule 1 (MAdCAM-1). Recruitment of eosinophils into tissue is regulated by the eotaxin chemokines that stimulate eosinophilic chemoattraction and activation through their receptor CCR3. Hypereosinophilic syndromes can develop after an 800-kilobase microdeletion on chromosome 4 results in fusion of the *FIP1L1* and *PDGFRA* genes, thereby resulting in activation of an imatinib-sensitive tyrosine kinase. Targeted therapeutic intervention for eosinophilic syndromes includes anti-IL-5 and anti–CCR3/anti-eotaxins, which are currently in clinical development.

PATHOBIOLOGY

Eosinophils are multifunctional leukocytes that are produced in the bone marrow from pluripotential hematopoietic stem cells under regulation of the transcription factor GATA-1 and the cytokines interleukin-3 (IL-3), IL-5, and granulocyte-macrophage colony-stimulating factor (GM-CSF) (Fig. 170-1). They are capable of producing a wide variety of pro-inflammatory mediators and immunomodulatory molecules.[2] Eosinophils are under the regulation of helper type 2 T cells (T_H2) and type 2 innate lymphoid cells (ILC2) that secrete IL-4, IL-5, and IL-13. Notably, IL-5 is a cytokine that specifically regulates the selective differentiation of eosinophils, their release from bone marrow into the peripheral circulation, and their survival. IL-5 activity is counterbalanced by paired immunoglobulin-like receptors (PIR) expressed on eosinophils, which counterbalance cellular activation and inhibition. A humanized anti-IL–5 drug markedly lowers blood eosinophilia and reduces tissue eosinophilia more modestly. Recent preliminary studies in patients with severe asthma have shown that anti-IL–5 therapy improves asthma control, including exacerbations, and allows steroid reduction. Similarly, anti-IL–5 has a steroid-sparing effect in hypereosinophilic syndromes. Humanized anti-IL–5 therapy and cytotoxic anti-IL–5 receptor therapy are currently in clinical testing for a variety of indications, including eosinophilic esophagitis, asthma, and hypereosinophilic syndromes. IL-4 and IL-13 induce eosinophil recruitment and survival, expression of critical adhesion molecules on the endothelium that bind to the β1 and β2 integrins on eosinophils (such as intercellular adhesion molecule 1 [ICAM-1] and vascular cell adhesion molecule 1 [VCAM-1]), and eosinophil-active chemokines such as the eotaxins. The eotaxins are three structurally related eosinophil chemoattractant and activating proteins that signal exclusively through the eosinophil-selective receptor CCR3. In addition to regulating the baseline homing of eosinophils to the various tissues in which they normally predominantly reside under the regulation of ILC2, such as the gastrointestinal tract, the eotaxins are induced by T_H2-associated inflammatory triggers (e.g., IL-13) and thereby promote tissue accumulation of eosinophils. Humanized antibodies against the eotaxins and small-molecule inhibitors against CCR3 are promising new approaches for treating eosinophilic disorders that are in clinical development.

Eosinophil granules contain a crystalloid core composed of major basic protein (MBP-1 and MBP-2), as well as a matrix composed of eosinophil cationic protein (ECP), eosinophil-derived neurotoxin (EDN), and eosinophil peroxidase (EPO). MBP, EPO, and ECP have cytotoxic effects on a variety of tissues in concentrations similar to those found in biologic fluids from patients with eosinophilia. Additionally, ECP and EDN belong to the ribonuclease A superfamily and possess antiviral and ribonuclease activity. ECP can insert voltage-insensitive, ion-nonselective toxic pores into the membranes of target cells, and these pores may facilitate the entry of other toxic molecules. MBP directly increases smooth muscle reactivity by causing dysfunction of vagal muscarinic M_2 receptors, and this process has been postulated to contribute to the airway hyperresponsiveness associated with asthma. MBP also triggers degranulation of mast cells and basophils. Triggering of eosinophils by engagement of receptors for cytokines, immunoglobulins, and complement can lead to the generation of a wide range of inflammatory cytokines, including IL-1, IL-3, IL-4, IL-5, IL-13, GM-CSF, transforming growth factor α/β, tumor necrosis factor α, RANTES, macrophage inflammatory protein 1α (MIP-1α), and the eotaxins, thus indicating that eosinophils have the potential to modulate multiple aspects of the immune response. Additionally, eosinophils can directly activate T cells by antigen presentation and help polarize dendritic cells to promote a T_H2 phenotype.[3] Further eosinophil-mediated tissue damage is caused by toxic hydrogen peroxide and halide acids generated by EPO and by superoxide generated by the respiratory burst oxidase enzyme pathway in eosinophils. Eosinophils also generate large amounts of cysteinyl leukotriene C_4 (LTC_4), which is metabolized to LTD_4 and LTE_4. These three lipid mediators increase vascular permeability and mucus secretion and are potent stimulators of smooth muscle contraction. Finally, bipyramidal Charcot-Leyden crystals are derived from a nongranule lysophospholipase in eosinophils and are frequently found in sputum, feces, and tissues infiltrated by eosinophils.

CLINICAL MANIFESTATIONS

Hypereosinophilia is often recognized on a routine blood count in a patient who is asymptomatic or being evaluated for unrelated or nonspecific signs or symptoms. On other occasions, the possibility of eosinophilia may be specifically investigated in a patient with gastrointestinal or respiratory symptoms because helminthic disease or allergic causes are suspected. The clinical signs and symptoms of hypereosinophilic syndromes are heterogeneous because of the diversity of the causes and potential organ involvement. Common signs and symptoms include dermatitis, heart failure, neuropathy, and abdominal pain. One of the most serious complications of hypereosinophilia is cardiac disease secondary to endomyocardial thrombus formation and restrictive fibrosis (Chapter 60). Mitral and tricuspid valve regurgitation may result from progressive fibrotic damage to the chordae tendineae, and resultant heart failure can develop from valvular insufficiency and endomyocardial fibrosis. Cardiac involvement can occur in association with chronic eosinophilia from diverse causes, including parasitic infections. Hypereosinophilic syndromes can result in cerebral emboli from cardiac disease, diffuse encephalopathy, and peripheral neuropathy.

DIAGNOSIS

Differential Diagnosis

The differential diagnosis of eosinophilia includes reactive eosinophilia, eosinophilia associated with other primary disorders, and eosinophilia associated with clonal hematopoiesis (see Table 170-1). Evaluation of patients is based on their history and clinical characteristics (Fig. 170-2). The initial goal is to determine whether the eosinophilia is secondary to a reactive cause (i.e., in response to another primary trigger such as allergy, infection, solid tumor, vasculitis). If reactive causes are not identified, further evaluation should determine whether the eosinophilia is secondary to a clonal hematologic disorder. If no evidence of clonality is determined, the patient is considered to have an idiopathic hypereosinophilic syndrome. The diagnosis of idiopathic hypereosinophilic *syndrome* requires an absolute eosinophil count of greater than 1500 cells/mm^3 *and* evidence of organ involvement and dysfunction.[4] These diagnostic criteria have been challenged for reasons noted in the Treatment section. Eosinophilia of an as yet unknown etiology that does not meet these criteria should be called *idiopathic hypereosinophilia*.

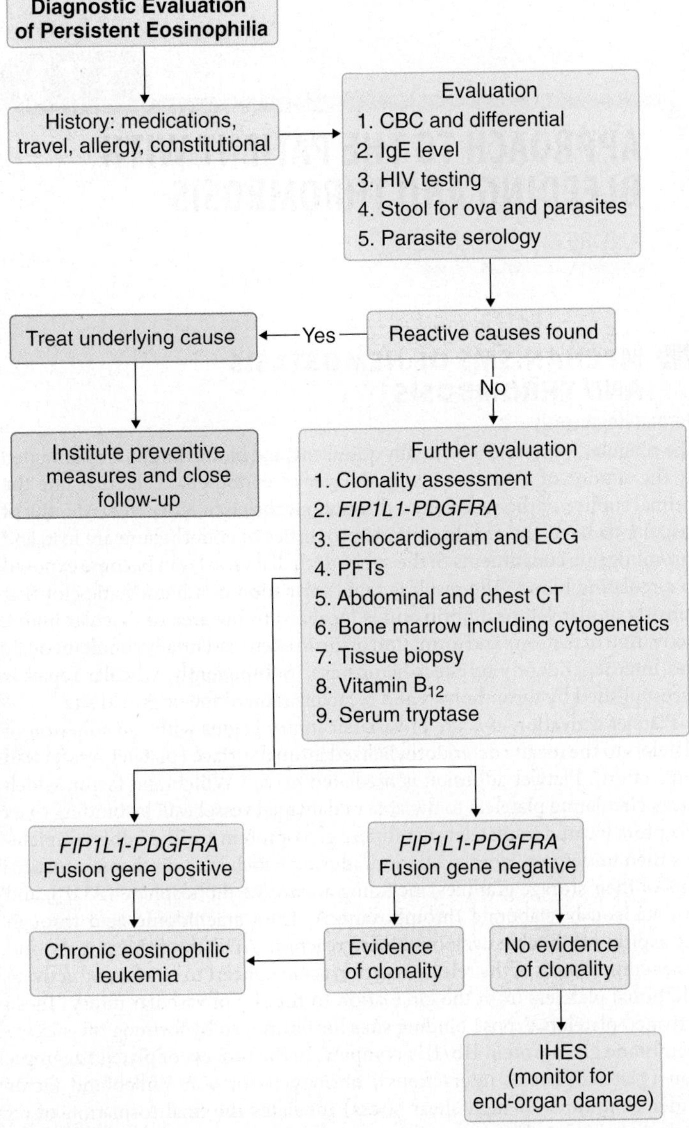

FIGURE 170-2. **Diagnostic evaluation of persistent eosinophilia.** CBC = complete blood count; CT = computed tomography; ECG = electrocardiogram; IgE = immunoglobulin E; IHES = idiopathic hypereosinophilic syndrome; HIV = human immunodeficiency virus; PDGFRA = platelet-derived growth factor receptor-α; PFTs = pulmonary function tests.

The differential diagnosis of eosinophilia requires a review of the patient's history, which may reveal wheezing (Chapter 87), rhinitis (Chapter 251), or eczema (indicating atopic causes); travel to areas where helminth infections (e.g., schistosomiasis [Chapter 355]) are endemic; the presence of a pet dog (indicating possible infection with *Toxocara canis* [Chapter 357]); symptoms of cancer; or drug ingestion (indicating a possible hypersensitivity reaction [Chapter 254]). Eosinophilia caused by drugs (Chapter 254) is usually benign but can sometimes be accompanied by tissue damage, as in hypersensitivity pneumonitis (Chapter 97) and in *DRESS syndrome* (drug reaction or rash with eosinophilia and systemic symptoms) (also see Chapter 440).[5] In most cases, the eosinophilia resolves when use of the drug ceases, but in some cases, such as eosinophilia-myalgia syndrome secondary to the ingestion of contaminated L-tryptophan, the disease can persist despite withdrawal of the drug.

The presence of abnormal morphologic features of eosinophils, an increase in immature and dysplastic cells in the bone marrow or blood, elevated levels of vitamin B_{12}, and splenomegaly raises suspicion of a clonal hypereosinophilic syndrome. In such cases, evidence of clonality (e.g., by analysis of X-chromosome inactivation patterns in female patients), an elevated level of mast cell tryptase (elevated in myelodysplastic variants of hypereosinophilic syndrome), the presence of aberrant lymphocyte phenotypes (elevated in lymphocytic variants of hypereosinophilic syndrome), abnormal cytogenetics, and the possible presence of specific fusion genes such as *FIP1L1-PDGFRA* should be investigated.

Other eosinophilic syndromes, such as Churg-Strauss syndrome, which is now referred to as eosinophilic granulomatosis with polyangiitis [EGPA] (Chapter 270), should be considered in patients with a history of worsening asthma, sinus disease, neuropathy, or blood eosinophilia and the presence of abnormal laboratory findings associated with inflammation and autoimmunity, such as an elevated erythrocyte sedimentation rate, C-reactive protein, and antineutrophil cytoplasmic antibodies.

An accumulation of eosinophils that is limited to specific organs is characteristic of particular diseases, such as eosinophilic cellulitis (Wells syndrome), eosinophilic esophagitis (Chapter 138), eosinophilic pneumonias (e.g., Löffler syndrome [Chapter 92]), and eosinophilic myositis (which now includes a genetic etiology caused by recessive mutations in calpain3 [*CAPN3*]).

Diagnostic Evaluation

Diagnostic studies that should be performed in patients with moderate to severe eosinophilia and considered in patients with persistent mild eosinophilia include morphologic examination of a blood smear, human immunodeficiency virus (HIV) screen, serial stool examinations for ova and parasites, parasite serology, and plasma immunoglobulin E (IgE) level.[6] Parasitic infections that cause eosinophilia are usually limited to helminthic parasites, with the exception of two enteric protozoans, *Isospora belli* (Chapter 353) and *Dientamoeba fragilis* (Chapter 353). *Strongyloides stercoralis* (Chapter 358) infection is important to diagnose because it can cause disseminated fatal disease in immunosuppressed patients; detection of such infection often requires serologic testing. Other infections to consider include trichinosis (Chapter 358), *T. canis* infection (Chapter 357), and HIV infection (Chapter 393).

Patients with sustained hypereosinophilia should be monitored closely for the subsequent development of cardiac disease. A pathologically similar disease, Löffler endomyocarditis (Chapter 60), has been noted in tropical regions, where antecedent parasite-elicited eosinophilia may be responsible for the cardiac damage. There should be a low threshold for a bone marrow analysis and testing for the presence of the *FIP1L1-PDGFRA* fusion gene in patients with hypereosinophilia. Testing for the presence of other activated tyrosine kinases (e.g., *PDGFRA* and *FGFR1*) should generally be reserved for individuals with bone marrow cytogenetic abnormalities.

TREATMENT

Rx

Reactive Hypereosinophilia and Hypereosinophilia Associated with Other Diseases

Treatment of reactive hypereosinophilia and hypereosinophilia associated with other diseases centers around identifying the cause and then treating the underlying disease process.[7,8] For example, reactive eosinophilia typically responds by removal of the inciting triggers (e.g., allergens, parasites, and medications). Eosinophilia associated with other disease processes typically improves after treatment of the underlying disease, such as dietary manipulation in patients with allergic eosinophilic gastroenteritis.

FIP1L1-PDGFRA–Positive Disease

As noted in the next section, other hypereosinophilic syndromes, treatment should be started as soon as possible to prevent potentially serious eosinophilia-mediated organ damage. Imatinib should be considered as first-line therapy in patients in whom the *FIP1L1-PDGFRA* fusion gene has been demonstrated and in selected patients with the characteristic clinical, laboratory, and molecular features of this myeloproliferative subtype of hypereosinophilic syndrome (e.g., male gender, tissue fibrosis, elevated serum vitamin B_{12} and tryptase levels). Clinical responses to imatinib in *FIP1L1-PDGFRA*–positive patients are rapid, with normalization of eosinophil counts generally occurring within 1 week of initiation of treatment and reversal of the signs and symptoms occurring within 1 month. Doses of imatinib as low as 100 mg daily appear to be effective in controlling symptoms and eosinophilia in most patients, but some recommend beginning imatinib treatment at 400 mg daily to achieve molecular remission and then decreasing the dose slowly while monitoring the patient closely for evidence of molecular relapse. In imatinib-resistant patients, sorafenib may be effective. The utility of imatinib therapy in hypereosinophilic patients without a demonstrable *FIP1L1-PDGFRA* mutation remains controversial, although some patients have responded. Nonmyeloablative allogeneic bone marrow transplantation (Chapter 178) has also been used successfully in several patients with hypereosinophilia.

Other Hypereosinophilic Syndromes

The current diagnostic criteria for hypereosinophilic syndromes that require at least 6 months of persistent eosinophilia of more than 1500 cells/mm^3 have been challenged because prompt diagnosis and treatment are required (before 6 months have passed) to prevent potentially serious end-organ damage. New diagnostic criteria have been proposed to address this limitation.[9]

Corticosteroids, which have been used for decades in the treatment of idiopathic hypereosinophilic syndromes, remain the first-line treatment for most patients, except those with *PDGFRA*-associated hypereosinophilia. The most appropriate initial corticosteroid dose and the duration of steroid therapy have not been subjected to randomized trials, but a general recommendation is to start with a moderate to high dose (≥40 mg prednisone equivalent) and taper very slowly while monitoring the eosinophil count closely. With this approach, most patients will respond initially, and some can be maintained on low doses of corticosteroids for prolonged periods.

Monoclonal anti-IL-5 antibody therapy (e.g., mepolizumab or reslizumab) for hypereosinophilia and eosinophil-associated asthma[A1][A2][A3] has a number of unique advantages related to the specificity of IL-5 for the eosinophil lineage. In patients treated with this agent, eosinophil counts are twice as likely to fall below 600/μL (95% vs. 45%, $P < .001$) with significantly lower prednisone doses.[A4] Of the cytotoxic therapies that have been used for steroid-refractory hypereosinophilia, hydroxyurea has been the most extensively studied at doses of 1 to 3 g/day. Vincristine at a dose of 1 to 2 mg intravenously can rapidly lower eosinophilia in patients with extremely high eosinophil counts (>100,000/mm^3) and may be useful for the treatment of children whose aggressive disease is unresponsive to other therapies. In patients who have corticosteroid-refractory hypereosinophilic syndromes or who develop intolerable side effects of steroid treatment, immunomodulatory agents that are sometimes helpful include interferon-α, cyclosporine, and alemtuzumab. Responses can often be achieved with relatively low doses of interferon-α (1 to 2 × 10^6 U/day) and may persist for prolonged periods. Because the effects of interferon-α on eosinophil numbers in peripheral blood may not become evident for several weeks, escalation to an effective dose may require several months. Rarely, patients have remained in remission for extended periods after cessation of interferon-α therapy, suggesting that interferon-α may be curative in a small subset of individuals. Low-dose (500 mg daily) hydroxyurea appears to act synergistically with interferon-α to lower the eosinophil count without increasing side effects.

PROGNOSIS

The prognosis of hypereosinophilic syndromes depends on the primary cause. Whereas *FIP1L1-PDGFRA*–positive disease and other forms of clonal disorders have a poor prognosis (25 to 50% 5-year mortality rate if responsiveness to therapeutic intervention is not achieved), the prognosis of hypereosinophilia from reactive and other causes is usually better and continues to improve.

A recent retrospective review of 247 cases of hypereosinophilic syndrome seen at the Mayo Clinic over a period of 19 years showed that only 23 patients died during this time, with the most common causes of death being cardiac dysfunction, infection, unrelated malignancy, and thromboembolic and vascular disease.[10] It was noted that targeted monitoring of at-risk end organs, combined with early treatment, may further improve survival and reduce morbidity.

FUTURE DIRECTIONS

Treatments on the horizon for hypereosinophilic disorders include targeted therapy against the eotaxin chemokines and their receptor CCR3, as well as anti-IL-5 and anti-IL-5 receptor–based antibody therapy.[11]

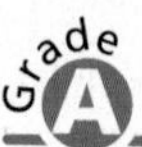

Grade A References

A1. Nair P, Pizzichini MM, Kjarsgaard M, et al. Mepolizumab for prednisone-dependent asthma with sputum eosinophilia. *N Engl J Med*. 2009;360:985-993.

A2. Haldar P, Brightling CE, Hargadon B, et al. Mepolizumab and exacerbations of refractory eosinophilic asthma. *N Engl J Med*. 2009;360:973-984.

A3. Castro M, Mathur S, Hargreave F, et al. Reslizumab for poorly controlled, eosinophilic asthma: a randomized, placebo-controlled study. *Am J Respir Crit Care Med*. 2011;184:1125-1132.

A4. Rothenberg ME, Klion AD, Roufosse FE, et al. Treatment of patients with the hypereosinophilic syndrome with mepolizumab. *N Engl J Med*. 2008;358:1215-1228.

GENERAL REFERENCES

For the General References and other additional features, please visit Expert Consult at https://expertconsult.inkling.com.

171 APPROACH TO THE PATIENT WITH BLEEDING AND THROMBOSIS

ANDREW I. SCHAFER

MECHANISMS OF HEMOSTASIS AND THROMBOSIS

Normal Hemostasis

The coagulation system is normally quiescent, and blood fluidity is maintained by the actions of a continuous monolayer of endothelial cells that line the intimal surface of the vasculature throughout the circulatory tree. At a site of vascular damage, the antithrombotic properties of endothelium are lost, and thrombogenic constituents of the subendothelial vessel wall become exposed to circulating blood. The result is rapid formation of a hemostatic clot that consists of platelets and fibrin and is localized to the area of vascular injury. Activation of platelets and formation of fibrin occur essentially simultaneously and interdependently to effect hemostasis. Subsequently, vascular repair is accomplished by thrombolysis and recanalization of the occluded site.[1]

Platelet activation at a site of vascular injury begins with the adhesion of platelets to the locally de-endothelialized intimal surface (platelet–vessel wall interaction). Platelet adhesion is mediated by von Willebrand factor, which sticks circulating platelets to the area of damaged vessel wall by binding to its receptors located in platelet membrane glycoprotein Ib. The adherent platelets then undergo a "release reaction," during which they discharge constituents of their storage granules, including adenosine diphosphate (ADP), and simultaneously elaborate thromboxane A_2 from arachidonic acid through the aspirin-inhibitable cyclooxygenase reaction. ADP, thromboxane A_2, and other components of the release reaction act in concert to recruit and activate additional platelets from the circulation to the site of vascular injury. These activated platelets expose binding sites for fibrinogen by forming the surface membrane glycoprotein IIb/IIIa complex. In the process of platelet aggregation (platelet-platelet interactions), fibrinogen (or von Willebrand factor under conditions of high shear stress) mediates the final formation of an occlusive platelet plug.

Fibrin, which anchors the hemostatic platelet plug, is formed from soluble plasma fibrinogen by the action of the potent protease enzyme thrombin (Fig. 171-1). The fibrin mesh is stabilized by covalent cross-linking mediated by factor XIII. Thrombin is formed from its inactive (zymogen) plasma

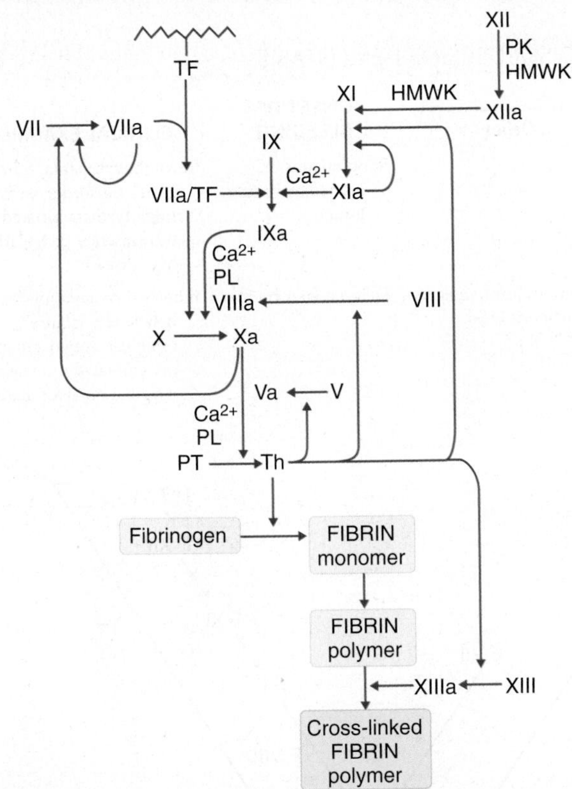

FIGURE 171-1. **Coagulation cascade. This scheme emphasizes an understanding of (1) the importance of the tissue factor pathway in initiating clotting in vivo, (2) the interactions among pathways, and (3) the pivotal role of thrombin in sustaining the cascade by feedback activation of coagulation factors. HMWK = high-molecular-weight kininogen; PK = prekallikrein; PL = phospholipid; PT = prothrombin; TF = tissue factor; Th = thrombin. (From Schafer AI. Coagulation cascade: an overview. In: Loscalzo J, Schafer AI, eds. *Thrombosis and Hemorrhage*. Cambridge, MA: Blackwell Scientific Publications; 1994:3-12.)**

precursor, prothrombin, by the action of activated factor X (Xa) and its cofactor, factor Va. This sequence of reactions has classically been referred to as the *common pathway* of coagulation. Factor X can be activated by either the *tissue factor (extrinsic) pathway* or the *contact activation (intrinsic) pathway* of coagulation. The tissue factor pathway is now considered to be the major physiologic initiator of coagulation activation. It is triggered by the formation of the complex of tissue factor, which is exposed on the surfaces of activated vascular and blood cells, with activated factor VII (VIIa). The contact activation pathway involves a series (or cascade) of zymogen-protease reactions that are initiated by factor XII, high-molecular-weight kininogen, and prekallikrein. Activated factor XII (XIIa) converts factor XI to XIa, which in turn activates factor IX to IXa. Factor IXa is the enzyme that converts factor X to Xa, a reaction that requires factor VIIIa as a cofactor.

Physiologic Antithrombotic Mechanisms

Intact, normal endothelium promotes blood fluidity by inhibiting platelet activation. It likewise plays a crucial role in preventing fibrin accumulation. Among the physiologic antithrombotic systems that produce this latter effect are (1) antithrombin III, (2) protein C and protein S, (3) tissue factor pathway inhibitor (TFPI), and (4) the fibrinolytic system. Antithrombin is the major protease inhibitor of the coagulation system[2]: it inactivates thrombin and other activated coagulation factors. Heparin functions as an anticoagulant by binding to antithrombin and greatly accelerating these reactions. Heparin and heparin sulfate proteoglycans are naturally present on endothelial cells, so antithrombin inactivation of thrombin and other coagulation proteases most likely occurs physiologically on vascular surfaces rather than in fluid plasma. Activated protein C, with its cofactor protein S, functions as a natural anticoagulant by destroying factors Va and VIIIa, two essential cofactors of the coagulation cascade. Thrombin itself is the activator of protein C, and this reaction occurs rapidly only on the surfaces of intact vascular endothelial cells, where thrombin binds to the glycosaminoglycan thrombomodulin. TFPI is a plasma protease inhibitor that specifically quenches tissue factor–induced coagulation. Finally, what little fibrin can be produced, despite these potent physiologic antithrombotic mechanisms, is digested rapidly by the endogenous fibrinolytic system. Fibrinolysis is mediated by the protease plasmin, which is generated from plasminogen in plasma by the action of endothelium-derived plasminogen activators.

EVALUATION OF THE PATIENT WITH A POSSIBLE BLEEDING DISORDER

History and Physical Examination

A thorough history is paramount in evaluating a patient for a possible systemic bleeding disorder. In addition to asking the patient about spontaneous bleeding episodes in the past, the responses to specific hemostatic challenges should be recorded. A bleeding tendency may be suspected if a patient previously experienced excessive hemorrhage after surgery or trauma, including common events such as circumcision, tonsillectomy, labor and delivery, menses, dental procedures, vaccinations, and injections. Conversely, a history of normal blood clotting after such specific challenges in the recent past is just as important to note. It may be a better test of the integrity of systemic hemostasis than any laboratory measurement can provide.

In a patient with a history of excessive or unexplained bleeding, the initial goal is to determine whether the cause is a systemic coagulopathy or localized anatomic or mechanical problem with a blood vessel. This situation is encountered most frequently in patients with excessive postoperative bleeding, which could be due to either local surgical trauma or a coagulation abnormality. A history of prior bleeding suggests a coagulopathy, as does the finding of bleeding from multiple sites. However, this is not always the case. Even diffuse bleeding may arise from anatomic rather than hemostatic abnormalities. An example of this is recurrent mucosal hemorrhage in patients with hereditary hemorrhagic telangiectasia (Chapter 173). Conversely, a single episode of bleeding from an isolated site may be the initial manifestation of a coagulopathy.

The history must include a survey of coexisting systemic diseases and drug ingestions that could affect hemostasis. Renal failure and the myeloproliferative disorders are associated with impaired platelet–vessel wall interactions and qualitative platelet abnormalities, connective tissue diseases and lymphomas are associated with thrombocytopenia, and liver disease causes a complex coagulopathy (Chapter 175). Ingestion of aspirin and other nonsteroidal anti-inflammatory drugs (NSAIDs) that cause nonselective inhibition of cyclooxygenase leads to platelet dysfunction; these drugs are often contained in over-the-counter preparations that patients may neglect to report without specific questioning. Other drugs, such as antibiotics, also may be associated with a bleeding tendency by causing abnormal platelet function or thrombocytopenia. Finally, it is important to elicit a family history of bleeding problems. Although a positive history provides an important clue to a possible inherited coagulopathy, a negative history does not exclude a familial cause; for example, 20% of patients with classic hemophilia have a completely negative family history of bleeding.

Mild bleeding events are commonly reported by patients with and without subsequently laboratory-documented bleeding disorders, sometimes making it difficult for hematologists to define a "significant bleeding history." Using a web-based questionnaire, 25% of subjects in a healthy population reported epistaxis, 18% easy bruising (more commonly in women), 18% prolonged bleeding after dental extraction, and 47% of women heavy menstrual bleeding.[3] More precise quantification of bleeding symptoms is being attempted by using "bleeding score" instruments such as the Vicenza bleeding score to help discriminate, in conjunction with laboratory testing, between healthy subjects and those with mild bleeding disorders.[4]

Patterns of clinical bleeding, as revealed by the history and physical examination, may be characteristic of certain types of coagulopathy (Table 171-1). In general, patients with thrombocytopenia or qualitative platelet or vascular disorders present with bleeding from superficial sites in the skin and mucous membranes. These may involve petechiae, which are pinpoint cutaneous hemorrhages that appear particularly over dependent extremities (characteristic of severe thrombocytopenia), ecchymoses (common bruises), purpura, gastrointestinal and genitourinary tract bleeding, epistaxis, and hemoptysis. In these types of disorders, bleeding tends to occur spontaneously or immediately after trauma. In contrast, patients with inherited or acquired coagulation factor deficiencies, such as hemophilia, or those on anticoagulant therapy tend to bleed from deeper tissue sites (e.g., hemarthroses, deep hematomas, retroperitoneal hemorrhage) and in a delayed manner after trauma.

Laboratory Testing

A few simple screening tests have traditionally been used in the initial evaluation of patients with a suspected coagulopathy: platelet count, bleeding

TABLE 171-1 CHARACTERISTIC PATTERNS OF BLEEDING IN SYSTEMIC DISORDERS OF HEMOSTASIS

TYPE OF DISORDER	SITES OF BLEEDING: General	Skin	Mucous Membranes	Other	ONSET OF BLEEDING	CLINICAL EXAMPLES
Platelet-vascular disorders	Superficial surfaces	Petechiae, ecchymoses	Common: oral, nasal, gastrointestinal, genitourinary	Rare	Spontaneous or immediately after trauma	Thrombocytopenia, functional platelet disorder, vascular fragility, disseminated intravascular coagulation, liver disease
Coagulation factor deficiency	Deep tissues	Hematomas	Rare	Common: joint, muscle, retroperitoneal	Delayed after trauma	Inherited coagulation factor deficiency, acquired inhibitor, anticoagulation, disseminated intravascular coagulation, liver disease

time, prothrombin time (PT) (also reported as the international normalized ratio, or INR), activated partial thromboplastin time (aPTT), and thrombin time (TT).[5] The North American Specialized Coagulation Laboratory Association (NASCOLA) has reported that most coagulation laboratories currently perform these tests, with the exception of the bleeding time, as their "bleeding disorder panels."

Thrombocytopenia, reported by electronic particle counting, should be verified by examination of the peripheral smear. Pseudothrombocytopenia, a laboratory artifact of ex vivo platelet clumping, may be caused by the ethylenediaminetetraacetic acid (EDTA) anticoagulant used in tubes for blood cell counts, by other anticoagulants, or by nonphysiologic cold agglutinins acting at room temperature. It should be suspected whenever a very low platelet count is unexpectedly reported in a patient who does not exhibit any clinical bleeding. Pseudothrombocytopenia is indicated by the finding of platelet clumps on the peripheral smear, and the diagnosis is supported by the finding of simultaneously normal platelet counts in blood samples obtained by finger stick, in tubes containing other anticoagulants, or in a tube maintained at 37° C before platelet counting. Examination of the blood smear can also reveal clues to the cause of real thrombocytopenia, such as fragmented red blood cells in thrombotic thrombocytopenic purpura.

The bleeding time was a widely used clinical screening test for disorders of platelet–vessel wall interactions. It measures the time to cessation of bleeding after a standardized incision over the volar aspect of the forearm. However, the test is prone to problems related to quality control, reproducibility, sensitivity, and specificity. Therefore, because von Willebrand disease is the most common genetic cause of abnormal platelet–vessel wall interactions, most experts now recommend replacing the bleeding time with specific tests for von Willebrand disease (VWD screen) in the initial evaluation of patients with a suspected coagulopathy (Chapter 173). As an additional replacement for the bleeding time, especially when a functional (qualitative) abnormality of platelets is suspected by characteristic mucocutaneous bleeding or bruising, a global assay of platelet function can be appended to the panel of screening tests. This is most commonly a platelet function analyzer (PFA) closure time. The PFA and other platelet function studies (see later) must be performed after discontinuation of drugs that interfere with platelet function (e.g., aspirin and other NSAIDs).

The PT measures the integrity of the extrinsic and common pathways of coagulation (factors VII, X, and V; prothrombin; and fibrinogen) (Fig. 171-2). The aPTT measures the integrity of the intrinsic and common pathways of coagulation (high-molecular-weight kininogen; prekallikrein; factors XII, XI, IX, VIII, X, and V; prothrombin; and fibrinogen). The sensitivity of the PT and aPTT in detecting coagulation factor deficiencies may vary with the reagents used to perform these tests, and each laboratory must determine its own reference standards. The TT is a screen for quantitative deficiencies and qualitative defects of plasma fibrinogen.

With a few notable exceptions, normal results for all these screening tests of hemostasis essentially exclude any clinically significant systemic coagulopathy. However, patients with factor XIII deficiency may have a serious bleeding diathesis but normal screening tests; specific tests for factor XIII deficiency should be performed if this disease is suspected (Chapter 174). The PT and aPTT detect only the more severe deficiencies of coagulation factors, usually at levels less than 30% of normal; specific factor levels should be determined if a mild coagulation factor deficiency is suspected. Rare disorders of fibrinolysis also may be associated with normal screening tests, necessitating more specialized tests when indicated (Chapter 174).

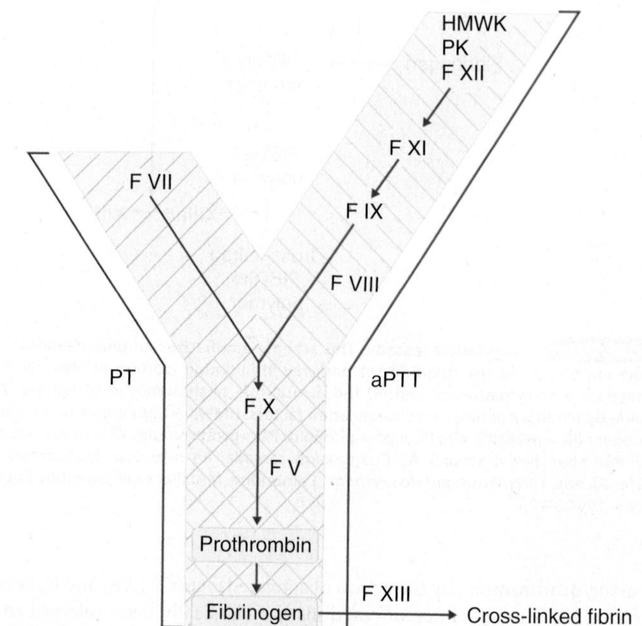

FIGURE 171-2. **Classic coagulation cascade. The prothrombin time (PT) measures the integrity of the extrinsic and common pathways, whereas the activated partial thromboplastin time (aPTT) measures the integrity of the intrinsic and common pathways. Factor (F) XIII deficiency is not detected by PT or aPTT. HMWK = high-molecular-weight kininogen; PK = prekallikrein.**

Abnormalities in these screening tests of hemostasis may be pursued by more specialized tests to establish a specific diagnosis (Fig. 171-3); other similar algorithms have been published.[6]

An abnormal VWD screen should be followed up with more specialized tests, including von Willebrand factor (VWF) multimer analysis, to identify the type of von Willebrand disease involved. Abnormalities in the PFA closure time should be followed by more specialized light transmission aggregometry (LTA) of platelets using a panel of agonists (ADP, epinephrine, collagen, arachidonic acid, ristocetin) that induce characteristic changes in light transmission (or optical density) in stirred suspensions of freshly isolated platelets in plasma (platelet-rich plasma, PRP). LTA is still considered the gold standard for platelet function testing[7] (see Fig. 171-3C and Chapter 173.)

The finding of a prolonged PT and/or aPTT indicates either a deficiency of one or more coagulation factors or the presence of an inhibitor (Fig. 171-4), usually an antibody, directed at one or more components of the coagulation system (see Fig. 171-3). These two possibilities can be distinguished by performing a simple inhibitor screen, which involves a 1 : 1 mix of the patient's plasma and normal plasma. The premise of the test is that even if the patient's plasma is completely deficient (0% level) in a certain factor, mixing it 1 : 1 with normal plasma (100% level) should bring the concentration of that factor to 50% in the mixture; this is sufficient to correct the prolonged PT or aPTT. If correction occurs with the inhibitor screen, individual coagulation factor levels should be assayed for a specific deficiency state. If the 1 : 1 mix fails to correct the prolonged PT and/or aPTT, an inhibitor is likely to be

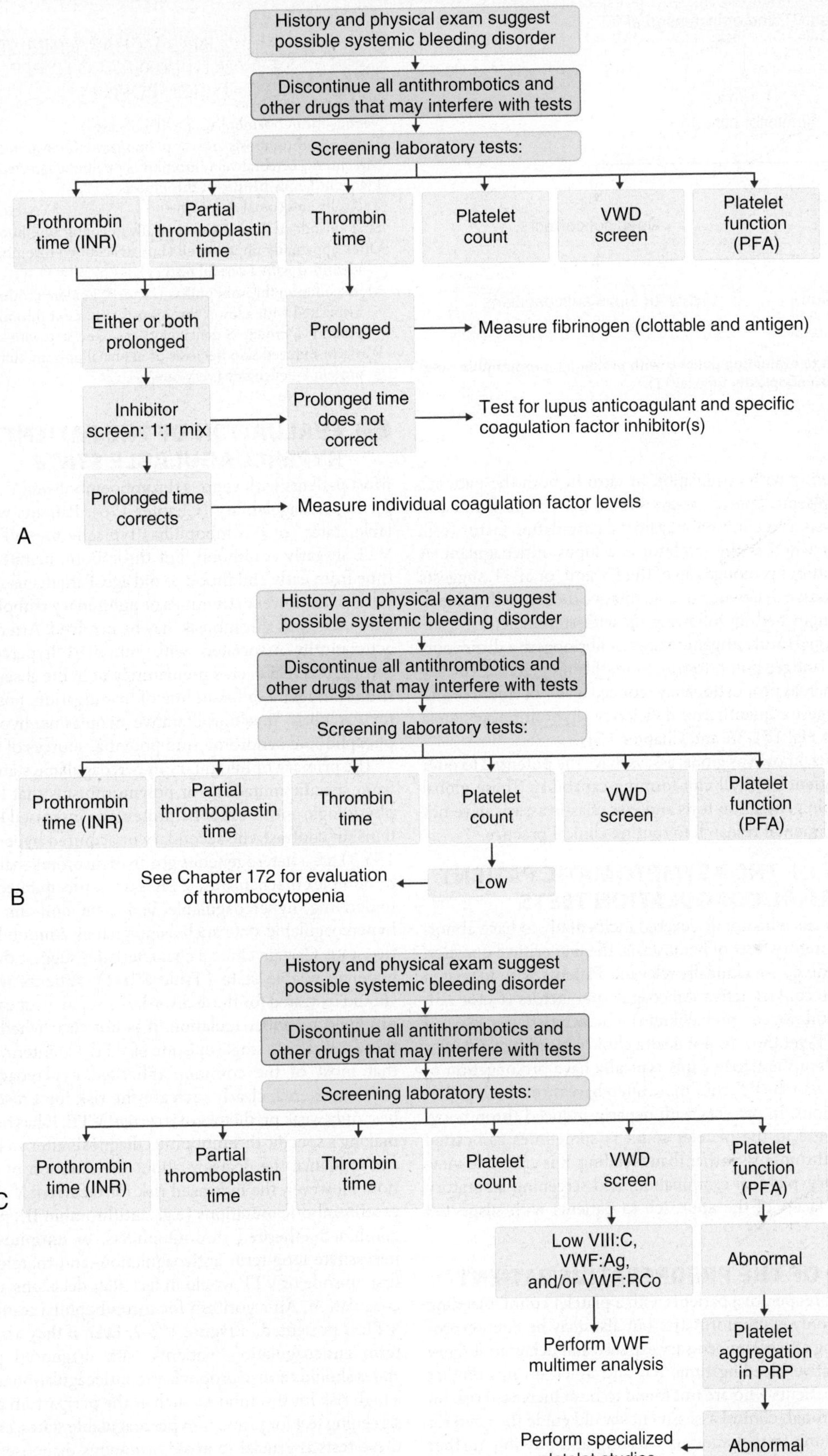

FIGURE 171-3. A to C, Algorithm for a clinical and laboratory approach to the diagnosis of a patient with a suspected systematic bleeding disorder (coagulopathy). The critical importance of a thorough personal and family history and physical examination is emphasized before initiating a laboratory work-up. INR = international normalized ratio; PFA = platelet function analyzer; VWF = von Willebrand factor; VIII:C = Factor VIII coagulant activity; VWF:Ag = von Willebrand factor antigen; VWF:RCo = von Willebrand factor: ristocetin cofactor activity; PRP = platelet-rich plasma.

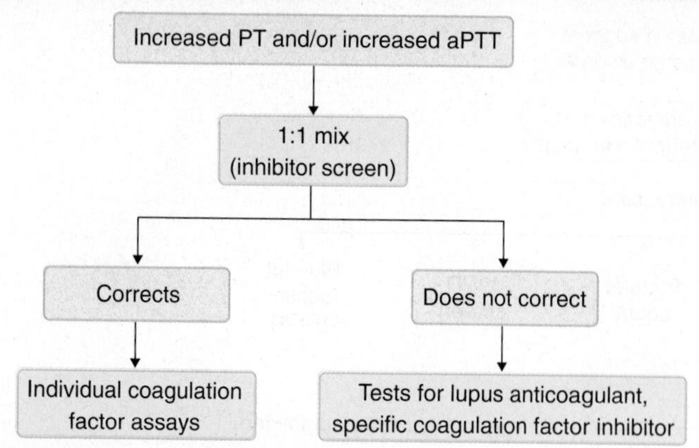

FIGURE 171-4. **Approach to evaluating patients with prolonged prothrombin time (PT) or activated partial thromboplastin time (aPTT).**

present, and it is interfering with coagulation in vitro in both the patient's plasma and the normal plasma. Specific assays should then be performed to determine whether there is a true inhibitor against a coagulation factor (e.g., factor VIII antibody) or whether the inhibitor is a lupus anticoagulant. A prolonged TT, with or without prolongation of the PT and/or aPTT, suggests the presence of a quantitative deficiency or a qualitative defect of fibrinogen. These can then be distinguished by following up with simultaneously performed clottable (functional) and antigenic assays of fibrinogen: a disproportionately low clottable fibrinogen points to a functional fibrinogen abnormality (dysfibrinogenemia), whereas proportionately reduced levels of clottable and antigenic fibrinogen suggest a quantitative deficiency (hypofibrinogenemia or afibrinogenemia) (see Fig. 171-3A and Chapter 174).

Newer coagulation tests, known as global assays, have the potential to offer fuller evaluation of a patient's overall clot-forming capability. These global assays, including thrombin generation tests and viscoelastic assays, have not yet advanced from experimental research to routine clinical practice.[8,9]

EVALUATION OF THE ASYMPTOMATIC PATIENT WITH ABNORMAL COAGULATION TESTS

In asymptomatic individuals who are discovered incidentally to have abnormalities in screening laboratory tests of hemostasis, the first critical question to ask is whether the findings are clinically relevant. Patients with inherited deficiencies of one of the contact activation coagulation factors (factor XII, high-molecular-weight kininogen, prekallikrein) characteristically have a markedly prolonged aPTT, yet they do not have a clinical bleeding tendency. Likewise, patients with lupus anticoagulants typically have prolongation of the aPTT and sometimes also the PT; they more often have thrombotic rather than bleeding complications. In patients with heparin-induced thrombocytopenia, a marked decrease in the platelet count is sometimes associated with arterial and venous thrombosis rather than bleeding. It is crucial to view the clinical setting, history, physical examination, and screening laboratory tests as complementary facets of the approach to patients with suspected coagulopathies.

EVALUATION OF THE PREOPERATIVE PATIENT

Routine screening of all preoperative patients with a platelet count, bleeding time, PT, and aPTT not only is uninformative but also may be counterproductive if follow-up testing causes unnecessary expense and delays in surgery (Chapter 431). Preoperative bleeding time, PT, and aPTT do not predict surgical bleeding risk in patients who are not found to be at increased risk on clinical grounds, so a thorough clinical assessment should guide the need for these preoperative screening tests. Laboratory testing and possibly further specialized tests of coagulation are indicated for patients whose bleeding histories are suspicious for a hemostatic abnormality. Preoperative screening tests of coagulation are probably warranted for patients who cannot cooperate with an adequate clinical assessment and for those who will be undergoing procedures in which even minimal postoperative hemorrhage could be hazardous. Recent guidelines for preinterventional and preoperative hemostatic evaluation have likewise concluded that bleeding risk requires a detailed personal and family history of hemorrhagic events and physical examination; but individuals with a negative history and without conditions that may interfere with systemic hemostasis should not undergo coagulation testing.[10]

TABLE 171-2 CLINICAL CHARACTERISTICS OF PATIENTS WITH INHERITED HYPERCOAGULABLE STATES (THROMBOPHILIA)

Venous thromboembolism (>90% of cases)
Deep vein thrombosis and/or pulmonary embolism most common
Mesenteric, cerebral vein thrombosis rare but characteristic
Frequent family history of thrombosis
Typically autosomal dominant
First episode of thrombosis typically in young adulthood (<40 years)
Often apparently unprovoked (but an acquired thrombosis trigger is frequently identified with a careful history)
More common thrombophilias (factor V Leiden, prothrombin 20210G→A) are associated with a lower thrombosis risk; rarer thrombophilias (antithrombin III, protein C, protein S deficiency) are associated with a higher thrombosis risk
Warfarin-induced skin necrosis or neonatal purpura fulminans with protein C or protein S deficiency (very rare)

EVALUATION OF THE PATIENT WITH A POSSIBLE HYPERCOAGULABLE STATE

Most patients with venous thromboembolism (VTE) have an inherited basis for hypercoagulability (Chapter 176). Patients with inherited hypercoagulable states (or thrombophilia) typically present with an initial episode of VTE in early adulthood, but thrombotic manifestations may begin at any time from early childhood to old age. Patients usually have deep vein thrombosis of the lower extremities or pulmonary embolism, but other uncommon sites of venous thrombosis may be involved. Arterial thrombosis is not characteristically associated with inherited hypercoagulable states. Arterial thrombosis that occurs prematurely or in the absence of apparent risk factors should trigger a different line of investigation, possibly including evaluation for vasculitis, myeloproliferative neoplasms, hyperhomocysteinemia, antiphospholipid syndrome, and potential sources of systemic embolization.

The primary or hereditary hypercoagulable states (see Table 176-1) result from specific mutations or polymorphisms that lead to decreased levels of physiologic antithrombotic proteins or increased levels of procoagulant proteins. In contrast, the secondary or acquired hypercoagulable states (see Fig. 176-3) are a heterogeneous group of disorders that predispose to thrombosis by complex mechanisms. VTE is often precipitated by the combination of an underlying hypercoagulable genotype and an acquired prothrombotic, hypercoagulable state such as pregnancy, immobilization, or the postoperative state. Certain clinical characteristics suggest the presence of an inherited hypercoagulable state (Table 171-2). Patients with recurrent thrombosis should be tested for these disorders and, in most cases, committed to lifelong prophylactic anticoagulation. It is not clear whether it is essential to order these tests after a single episode of VTE. Counterintuitively, it has been found that most of the common inherited hypercoagulable states—which, to varying extents, clearly increase the risk for a *first* episode of VTE—are at best only weak predictors of *recurrent* VTE. It has been argued, therefore, that making a specific thrombophilia diagnosis after an initial episode of VTE will not influence the decision about the duration of prophylactic anticoagulation. However, the increased risk for recurrent VTE with the more strongly prothrombotic mutations (e.g., antithrombin III, protein C or S deficiency), combined inherited thrombophilias, or antiphospholipid syndrome may necessitate long-term anticoagulation, and therefore their diagnosis after a first episode of VTE would in fact alter decisions about the duration of anticoagulation. An algorithm for thrombophilia testing after a first episode of VTE is presented in Figure 176-2. Even if they are not maintained on long-term anticoagulation, patients with diagnosed primary hypercoagulable states should receive prophylactic anticoagulation during situations that pose a high risk for thrombosis, such as the peripartum period. There is no simple screening test for primary hypercoagulable states, and the timing of obtaining these tests is crucial to avoid erroneous diagnoses. Acute thrombosis itself can cause transient decreases in the levels of antithrombin, protein C, and protein S. Heparin therapy can cause a decrease in plasma antithrombin activity. Warfarin therapy lowers the functional levels of protein C and protein S. Inherited deficiency states can be diagnosed spuriously under these conditions. Use of one of the newer anticoagulants can also interfere with laboratory tests, especially for lupus anticoagulant.

Patients who present with VTE have an increased risk for harboring an occult malignancy. This association is increased further in patients with recurrent and unprovoked thrombosis. There are conflicting opinions on whether an evaluation for occult malignancy in these patients must be exhaustive.

Most recommend that evaluation can be limited to a thorough history, physical examination, routine complete blood cell count and chemistries, test of fecal occult blood, urinalysis, mammogram (in women), and chest radiograph, with further testing guided by any abnormalities found in this initial evaluation. Others argue for routine computed tomography scanning of the chest, abdomen, and pelvis[11,12] (see algorithm in Fig. 176-3).

In addition to classic deep vein thrombosis and pulmonary embolism, certain characteristic types of thrombosis may provide important clues to the cause and trigger a more directed evaluation. Migratory, superficial thrombophlebitis (Trousseau syndrome) or nonbacterial thrombotic endocarditis strongly suggests the presence of an occult malignancy (Chapter 179). Hepatic vein thrombosis (Budd-Chiari syndrome; Chapter 143) or portal vein thrombosis may indicate a myeloproliferative neoplasm (Chapter 166) or paroxysmal nocturnal hemoglobinuria (Chapter 160). Extensive inferior vena cava thrombosis may occur with renal cell carcinoma (Chapter 197). Warfarin-induced skin necrosis strongly suggests underlying protein C or protein S deficiency. Recurrent, spontaneous miscarriages are characteristic of the antiphospholipid syndrome (Chapter 174), although they are also associated with other thrombophilias.

GENERAL REFERENCES

For the General References and other additional features, please visit Expert Consult at https://expertconsult.inkling.com.

172

THROMBOCYTOPENIA

CHARLES S. ABRAMS

Thrombocytopenia is defined as a platelet count of less than the normal range, typically below 140,000/μL. In the absence of qualitative platelet defects (Chapter 173), excessive bleeding does not occur in thrombocytopenic patients following trauma or surgery unless the platelet count is lower than 75,000/μL. In otherwise hemostatically normal patients, spontaneous hemorrhage typically does not occur with platelet counts above 30,000/μL. Patients with platelet counts of less than 5000/μL to 10,000/μL are at a high risk for spontaneous, life-threatening hemorrhage. However, there is no absolute threshold for spontaneous bleeding due to thrombocytopenia. Bleeding may occur at higher counts when fever, sepsis, severe anemia, and other hemostatic defects are present, or when platelet function is impaired by medication. Notably, a prolonged cutaneous bleeding time test (Chapter 171) does not accurately predict the risk for clinical bleeding. Therefore, it is critical that the physician consider the gamut of possibilities when diagnosing and managing a patient with a low platelet count.

Typically, the first step in diagnosing a patient with a low platelet count is to determine whether the thrombocytopenia is attributable to one of the three broad mechanisms for developing thrombocytopenia: (1) increased destruction of platelets, such as seen in immune-mediated causes; (2) decreased production of platelets, usually due to an underlying bone marrow disorder; or (3) sequestration of platelets within the spleen, as occurs in conditions that cause splenomegaly (hypersplenism).

Determining the cause of the patient's thrombocytopenia is essential to select the most appropriate therapy and to avoid unnecessary procedures. Because there is no easy test to differentiate among the three possibilities, clinical evaluation is critical. Therefore, a thorough history and physical examination, with attention to possible alternative explanations for thrombocytopenia, are mandatory. Particular attention should be paid to the duration of symptoms, which helps to determine whether the patient has acute or chronic thrombocytopenia. The clinician should also focus on the patient's recent exposure to new medications that might induce thrombocytopenia as a side effect.

Preliminary laboratory tests include a complete blood count (CBC) with a differential, along with an examination of the peripheral blood smear. Abnormalities in the number or morphology of the leukocytes or erythrocytes may indicate a systemic inflammatory disorder or a pathology within the bone marrow. Clumping of the platelets on the peripheral blood smear may indicate that the patient has pseudothrombocytopenia (Chapter 171). This anomaly is usually due to an antibody that binds to and thereby agglutinates platelets only in the presence of ethylenediaminetetraacetic acid (EDTA) or when the blood sample is allowed to cool to room temperature. Repeating the platelet count in a blood sample that has been anticoagulated with heparin and kept warm until it is analyzed can help exclude this spurious diagnosis. Any additional testing to determine the cause of thrombocytopenia is based solely on the available clinical information derived from the history and examination of the patient. For example, testing for human immunodeficiency virus (HIV) would be prudent in a patient with risk factors. A bone marrow aspirate and biopsy are typically not required for a patient with thrombocytopenia who has an otherwise normal CBC and peripheral blood smear. However, a bone marrow aspirate and biopsy should be considered in older patients and in patients for whom standard therapy has not been effective.

With the widespread use of the "routine CBC," asymptomatic individuals with incidentally discovered mild thrombocytopenia are being increasingly recognized. The clinical significance of mild thrombocytopenia (platelet counts between 100,000/μL and 150,000/μL) can be difficult to ascertain. Some of these individuals represent outliers of the normal distribution of platelet counts. However, others have thrombocytopenia that represents the early manifestation of an unrecognized disease. In the absence of other signs, many of these individuals are diagnosed with idiopathic (immune) thrombocytopenic purpura (ITP)—a disease that will be discussed later in this chapter. Studies of apparently healthy individuals who were incidentally discovered to have borderline thrombocytopenia have yielded some insight into their prognosis.[1] After a decade, approximately 10% will have developed ITP or another autoimmune disorder. However, approximately 90% of the subjects continued to manifest borderline thrombocytopenia without developing another disorder during this period of time. It can be concluded that most individuals with isolated and asymptomatic chronic mild thrombocytopenia simply represent the lower end of the normal platelet count distribution. Consequently, international consensus groups have set the threshold for the diagnosis of ITP at a platelet count of less than100,000/μL.

PATHOBIOLOGY

See Figure 172-1 for an approach to evaluating patients with chronic thrombocytopenia.

Increased Platelet Destruction

In the absence of splenomegaly, the presence of megakaryocytes in an otherwise normal bone marrow implies that thrombocytopenia is due to increased platelet destruction. An acute drop in a patient's platelet count also implies that a peripheral destructive process is the likely cause. For example, a patient who develops abrupt thrombocytopenia during hospitalization most likely has a low platelet count caused by an infection or by the introduction of a new medication. Both nonimmune and immune processes can lead to a shortened platelet lifespan. Nonimmune reasons for the accelerated destruction of platelets include sepsis, disseminated intravascular coagulation (DIC), thrombotic thrombocytopenic purpura (TTP), hemolytic-uremic syndrome (HUS), preeclampsia or eclampsia, cardiopulmonary bypass, and giant cavernous hemangioma. Thrombocytopenia that occurs in these circumstances usually resolves with treatment of the underlying disorder, and platelet transfusions are rarely necessary. Thrombocytopenia due to TTP, HUS, or heparin-induced thrombocytopenia (HIT) is more characteristically associated with microvascular occlusion or thrombosis than with bleeding (Table 172-1), so platelet transfusions are rarely necessary. In addition, reports have noted the clinical deterioration of patients with TTP or HIT following platelet transfusion, leading to the controversial suggestion that platelets should not be given to most patients with these disorders.

Immune-mediated platelet destruction can result from drugs, alloimmune sensitization, or autoimmunity. Medications should always be considered as a possible cause of acute thrombocytopenia. The list of potential offending agents is long, but drugs with strong evidence of antibody-mediated platelet destruction include quinine, quinidine, sulfonamides, and gold salts. In addition to stopping the offending medication, platelet transfusions might be required for severe thrombocytopenia.

Platelet Sequestration

Approximately 30% of the circulating platelet mass is normally sequestered within the spleen. Enlargement of the spleen due to portal hypertension or

Chronic thrombocytopenia

Platelet count less than 100,000/μL
- Exclude pseudothrombocytopenia on peripheral blood smear
- Abnormal blood smear or abnormality of WBC or RBC suggests bone marrow disorder
- Large spleen suggests hypersplenism
- Immune mediated; primary or secondary ITP; drug induced thrombocytopenia

Platelet count greater than 100,000/μL
- Exclude pseudothrombocytopenia on peripheral blood smear
- Follow CBC
  - Stable; continue to follow CBC
  - Platelet count less than 100,000 μL; see above algorithm

FIGURE 172-1. Systematic approach to the evaluation of chronic thrombocytopenia.

TABLE 172-1 DISORDERS THAT CAUSE BOTH THROMBOCYTOPENIA AND THROMBOSIS

Thrombotic thrombocytopenic purpura (TTP)
Hemolytic-uremic syndrome (HUS)
Heparin-induced thrombocytopenia (HIT)
Disseminated intravascular coagulation (DIC)
Paroxysmal nocturnal hemoglobinuria (PNH)
Vasculitis (such as systemic lupus erythematosus)
Antiphospholipid antibody syndrome (APS)

infiltration is accompanied by expansion of the splenic platelet pool. Because hypersplenism by itself rarely causes a platelet count of less than 40,000/μL to 50,000/μL, bleeding due to thrombocytopenia from hypersplenism alone is unusual. This in turn can result in moderate thrombocytopenia.

Decreased Platelet Production

Decreased platelet production occurs in primary diseases of the bone marrow, such as acute leukemia and aplastic anemia; myelophthisic processes in which bone marrow is affected by metastatic carcinoma, fibrosis, or other clonal hematopoietic disorders; following chemotherapy and/or radiation therapy; with ethanol toxicity; and during infections with viruses such as HIV, cytomegalovirus (CMV), Epstein-Barr virus (EBV), and varicella. Thrombocytopenia also occurs when normal megakaryocyte proliferation is impaired by myelodysplasia.

Thrombocytopenia due to decreased platelet production is often accompanied by abnormalities of both the white blood cells and red blood cells. This should be readily apparent by inspection of the CBC and review of the peripheral blood smear. When thrombocytopenia in this setting is accompanied by bleeding, the bleeding usually requires treatment by platelet transfusion. Additionally, when decreased platelet production cannot be readily reversed, prophylactic platelet transfusion to prevent bleeding is often considered. However, as will be discussed in the following section, prophylactic platelet transfusion is problematic because of the short lifespan of platelets and the potential to develop alloantibodies that will limit the effectiveness of future platelet transfusions.

PLATELET TRANSFUSIONS

Clinicians usually consider "wet" bleeding to be much more ominous than "dry" bleeding. Signs of wet bleeding include epistaxis, gingival bleeding, gastrointestinal bleeding, genitourinary bleeding, and bleeding around intravenous sites. Dry bleeding is defined as ecchymosis or petechiae (Fig. 172-2). Overt wet bleeding that is clearly due to thrombocytopenia is usually treated with platelet transfusion (Chapter 177). Prophylactic platelet transfusion for patients who are not bleeding is controversial. When making the decision whether to treat a nonbleeding patient with thrombocytopenia, the practitioner must consider the short lifespan of platelets (10 days), the 5-day shelf-life of stored platelets, and the potential for the patient to develop transfusion-induced platelet alloantibodies. In patients undergoing treatment for acute leukemia, recent clinical trials have supported the clinical practice of prophylactic platelet transfusions when the platelet count is below 5000/μL or 10,000/μL, rather than waiting until bleeding occurs in the severely thrombocytopenic patient.[A1] The indications for prophylactic platelet transfusions before interventional procedures is predominantly based on clinical experience and expert opinions, rather than on clinical trials. These recommendations are summarized in Table 172-2. Platelet transfusions should continue for several days following procedures where the risk for bleeding or the complications resulting from bleeding are high. For extremely high-risk procedures that involve the nervous and ocular systems, the prophylactic platelet transfusions should be continued for at least 7 to 10 days.

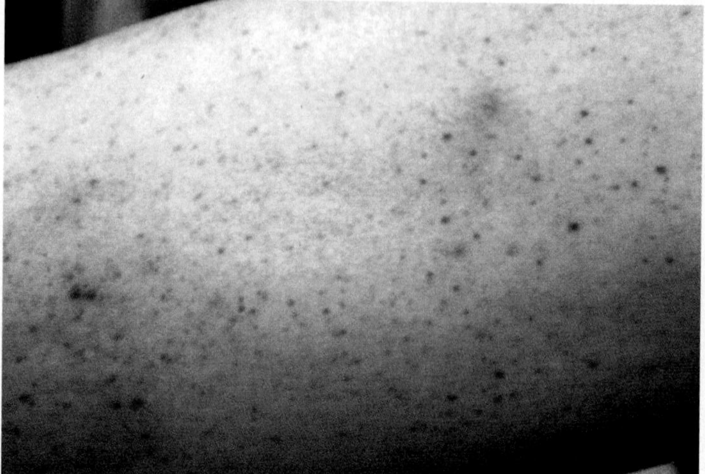

FIGURE 172-2. Petechiae. Multiple pinpoint, nonblanching, erythematous macules found predominantly on skin of dependent extremities in patients with severe thrombocytopenia.

TABLE 172-2 SUGGESTED MINIMUM PLATELET COUNTS BEFORE INVASIVE PROCEDURES

VERY-HIGH-RISK PROCEDURES—75,000/μL TO 100,000/μL
Neurosurgery
Ocular surgery (except cataract extraction)
Thyroid surgery
Prostatectomy
MODERATE-RISK PROCEDURES—50,000/μL
Liver Biopsy
Dental extraction
Most surgical procedures
LOW-RISK PROCEDURES—30,000/μL
Endoscopy
Bronchoscopy
Lumbar puncture (with scrupulous technique)
VERY-LOW-RISK PROCEDURES—NO PLATELET TRANSFUSIONS NECESSARY
Bone marrow biopsy
Cataract extraction

A donated unit of blood contains approximately 50 billion platelets. Infusing this number of platelets into a patient should increase his or her platelet count by 20,000/μL divided by the patient's body surface area in square meters. Therefore, transfusion into an average-sized patient should increase the recipient's platelet count by 10,000/μL to 12,000/μL. Bags of platelets used for transfusions are typically obtained by pooling platelets derived from four to eight blood donors. Therefore, a "unit" at one hospital may be derived from more donors than a "unit" obtained at another hospital.

Large quantities of platelets can be derived from a single donor by using apheresis technology (plateletpheresis) (Chapter 177). Because there is minimal loss of red blood cells with this technique, plateletpheresis allows one individual to donate very large numbers of platelets (equivalent to the number of platelets obtained from 6 to 10 units of donated blood). As discussed in the following section, the risk for platelet alloimmunization is partially dependent on the number of individuals donating platelets to a patient. Therefore, single-donor plateletpheresis can prevent or at least minimize alloimmunization.

Several trials have addressed how many platelets should be transfused into thrombocytopenic patients to maintain hemostasis and to minimize exposure to blood products (also see Chapter 177). The largest of these trials was the multicenter Platelet Dose (PLADO) Trial.[A2] In this study, patients with thrombocytopenia were randomized to receive transfusions of low-dose (110 billion/m^2), medium-dose (220 billion/m^2), or high-dose (440 billion/m^2) platelets while recovering from hematopoietic stem cell transplantation. Patients who received the low-dose therapy required more frequent platelet transfusions. However, overall they received fewer transfused platelets over the course of the study. Importantly, bleeding complications were identical with all platelet transfusion strategies. This study demonstrates that low doses of platelets (110 billion/m^2 of body surface area) are as safe as larger doses in patients with hypoproliferative thrombocytopenia who are receiving prophylactic platelet transfusion therapy.

Several complications of platelet transfusion therapy merit mention (also see Chapter 177). First, some patients can become alloimmunized against platelet antigens and can become refractory to future platelet transfusion therapy (discussed in detail later). Second, bacterial contamination of stored platelets is a much more common complication than the infectious risk associated with red blood cell transfusions. Unlike red blood cells, which are stored frozen after being harvested from donated blood, platelets are sensitive to cool temperatures and therefore need to be stored at room temperature. This method of storage results in more bacterial overgrowth in the transfusion bags. Transfusion-associated bacterial sepsis is one of the most frequently reported causes of transfusion-induced mortality in the United States, and platelet transfusions are the most common blood products associated with sepsis. It should also be noted that room temperature storage of platelets contributes to their short shelf life of approximately 5 to 7 days. Consequently, unlike the blood-derived products that can be frozen (such as red blood cells and plasma), there is a constant need for platelet donations year-round. In contrast to the risk for bacterial infection, the risk for viral infection from platelet transfusions is no higher than it is for red blood cell transfusions. From a single unit of platelets, the risk for being exposed to HIV is less than 1 in 2.5 million, the risk for exposure to hepatitis B virus is less than 1 in 750,000, and the risk for exposure to hepatitis C virus is less than 1 in 1 million.

Platelet transfusions have been considered contraindicated for thrombocytopenia caused by TTP or HIT. However, this recommendation is driven entirely by case reports of thrombotic events that have occurred soon after platelet transfusions have been given to such patients. This recommendation is not based on randomized trials designed to address this issue. Because thrombotic events are a known complication of both TTP and HIT, it is difficult to determine whether the thrombi that occurred in these patients were due to the platelet transfusions or merely to the intrinsic prothrombotic risk for TTP and HIT. In any case, there is usually no indication for platelet transfusions in patients with TTP and HIT because thrombosis is a much greater risk than hemorrhage in these disorders.

The Transfusion-Refractory Patient

Many patients do not have an optimal increase in their platelet count following transfusion. Although there are various definitions of platelet refractoriness, it is simplest to base this definition on the timing of platelet loss following transfusion. Patients who do not have the predicted rise in their platelet count (between 10,000/μL and 12,000/μL for every unit of donated platelets) should have their platelet count analyzed before their next platelet transfusion, 1 hour after that transfusion, and again 24 hours later. If their platelet count rises appropriately 1 hour after the transfusion but falls substantially 24 hours later, the patient has ongoing platelet consumption. This is often seen in patients with sepsis, DIC, or severe active hemorrhage, or as a result of the drug-mediated immune destruction of platelets. In these situations, the best therapy is to treat the underlying cause and to continue to support the patient with platelet transfusions as clinically indicated. Alternatively, some patients fail to have a significant increase in platelets even 1 hour after a transfusion. These patients may have (1) hypersplenism, (2) an autoantibody that eliminates not only endogenous platelets but also allogeneic platelets (as seen in patients with ITP), or (3) alloantibodies that react with antigens on the transfused platelets.

Alloantibodies develop in approximately 20% of patients who are repeatedly exposed to platelet transfusions, and these patients present some of the most challenging management issues in transfusion medicine (Chapter 177). The alloantibodies may be directed against human leukocyte antigen (HLA) class I antigens (HLA-A and HLA-B) or against platelet-specific antigens present on the surface of the platelets. Because it appears that HLA class II antigens present on the surface of leukocytes are essential for the development of antibodies directed against HLA class I antigens, efforts to remove the contamination of leukocytes in platelet transfusion preparations can minimize alloantibody formation. Therefore, filters that trap leukocytes during transfusions are useful to prevent patients from becoming refractory to future platelet transfusions. After a patient develops alloantibodies against transfused platelets, the clinician and the blood bank should attempt to identify whether the alloantibody is directed against an HLA class I antigen or against a platelet-specific antigen. If the alloantibody can be identified, platelets derived from donors matched for an HLA class I antigen or the platelet-specific antigen can be used. Corticosteroids, intravenous immunoglobulin, splenectomy, and recombinant factor VIIa are probably of no value in maintaining hemostasis in platelet-refractory patients. Antifibrinolytic agents (e.g., ε-aminocaproic acid) might be helpful for patients with bleeding that is predominantly in the oral cavity or in the genitourinary tract. However, antifibrinolytic agents are contraindicated in patients with DIC (Chapter 175) because these agents can precipitate thrombotic events.

SPECIFIC CAUSES OF THROMBOCYTOPENIA

Drug-Induced Thrombocytopenia

PATHOBIOLOGY

Drug-induced thrombocytopenia is one of the most frequent causes of cytopenias evaluated by physicians. The typical drug-induced thrombocytopenia is the result of an immune reaction elicited by either the drug or by one of its metabolites. Sometimes the drug is simply deposited on the platelet surface, and antidrug antibodies lead to accelerated platelet clearance, primarily in the spleen. More frequently, the drug binds to a protein on the platelet surface and induces a neoantigen that is ultimately recognized by the immune system.

In the absence of the drug or drug metabolites, this platelet neoantigen disappears, and the thrombocytopenia slowly resolves as new platelets are released from the bone marrow. This mechanism explains most drug-induced thrombocytopenias, but there are some exceptions. For example, chemotherapy and other bone marrow toxins can decrease platelet production and thereby induce thrombocytopenia by a mechanism independent of the immune system.

CLINICAL MANIFESTATIONS

Patients with drug-induced thrombocytopenia can have mild, moderate, or even severe forms. Almost all types of drug-induced thrombocytopenia predispose the patient to hemorrhagic but not thrombotic complications. The notable exception to this rule is heparin-induced thrombocytopenia (discussed separately in the next section). In acute or subacute cases of thrombocytopenia, it may be especially difficult to distinguish between drug-induced thrombocytopenia and the thrombocytopenia of an infection (viral or bacterial). In very ill patients, both possibilities must be considered in the management plan (see later section on Sepsis). Another difficult diagnostic dilemma is to discern drug-induced thrombocytopenia from ITP. For this distinction, the patient's medical history may be helpful. A gradually progressive thrombocytopenia is more consistent with ITP than with one induced by a medication. Conversely, the rapid onset of thrombocytopenia following the initiation of a new medication indicates that the drug is the most likely culprit. The time between the initiation of the offending drug and the development of thrombocytopenia has not been well documented for most medications. However, thrombocytopenia typically begins days to a few weeks after the administration of most medications with this type of toxicity. Presumably, this lag time represents the period required for the patient to develop an immune response against the drug-platelet complex. Medications that have been taken safely for years before the onset of thrombocytopenia are unlikely to be the offending agents. In addition to an assessment of the patient's prescribed medications, a careful and comprehensive evaluation of the patient's over-the-counter medications is necessary. Agents that contain quinine lead the list of often nonprescribed drugs that can induce life-threatening thrombocytopenia. Quinine is frequently contained in over-the-counter pills for leg cramps. Even the quinine in tonic water can induce severe thrombocytopenia ("gin and tonic purpura") when ingested by certain patients.

DIAGNOSIS

Some medications are much more likely to induce thrombocytopenia than others. Table 172-3 contains a partial list of drugs that frequently induce this type of toxicity. One particularly useful online database (www.ouhsc.edu/platelets/ditp.html) lists and periodically updates the level of evidence for specific drugs that may induce thrombocytopenia. With the exception of tests for HIT, laboratory tests for drug-induced thrombocytopenia do not have widespread applicability. Usually, drug-induced thrombocytopenia is proved only in retrospect, when the platelet count improves after the discontinuation of the suspected medication. Even then, the diagnosis is not conclusive unless thrombocytopenia recurs after rechallenging the patient with the offending drug (a practice that is almost never recommended).

TREATMENT Rx

The most efficacious method of treating drug-induced thrombocytopenia is to stop all suspected offending medications. Usually, no additional therapy is indicated. The thrombocytopenia typically begins to resolve without further intervention within days to a week of stopping the drug. The notable exceptions involve drugs with particularly long half-lives. Sulfonamides, quinine, and quinidine are particularly notorious for inducing severe or even life-threatening thrombocytopenia. In patients with profound thrombocytopenia (<10,000/µL to 15,000/µL) or at a high risk for bleeding, platelet transfusions are indicated. If ITP cannot be confidently excluded, and the thrombocytopenia is life threatening, specific treatment for ITP can also be initiated (see later in this chapter).

TABLE 172-3 DRUGS THAT ARE STRONGLY ASSOCIATED WITH THROMBOCYTOPENIA

ANTIBIOTICS AND ANTIVIRALS
Quinine, quinidine
Penicillin
Cephalosporin
Vancomycin
Trimethoprim-sulfamethoxazole
Sulfonamides, sulfonylureas
Linezolid
Valaciclovir
Ganciclovir
Indinavir
CARDIOVASCULAR MEDICATIONS
Abciximab
Tirofiban
Eptifibatide
Salicylates
Digoxin
Furosemide
MISCELLANEOUS
Cimetidine
Ranitidine
Famotidine
Valproate
Interferon

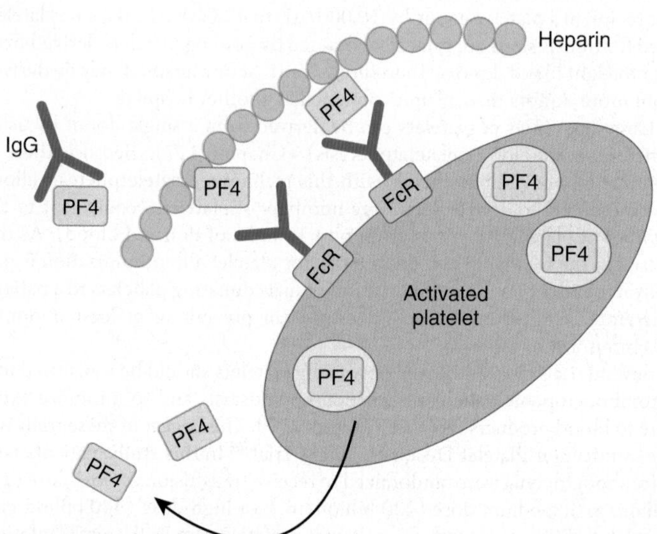

FIGURE 172-3. Pathophysiology of heparin-induced thrombocytopenia. Platelet factor 4 (PF4) is a protein that is stored in platelet granules and that is secreted from platelets upon their activation. Heparin can bind to PF4 and induce a conformational change within PF4 that in some patients produces an antibody-mediated immune response. Large complexes of immunoglobulin (Ig), heparin, and PF4 can accumulate on the platelet surface and stimulate the platelet when the Fc portion of the antibody interacts with the platelet's FcγRII receptor (FcR). Once activated, the platelets contribute to thrombosis. Additionally, the activated platelets secrete more PF4, which continues the process.

Heparin-Induced Thrombocytopenia

EPIDEMIOLOGY

A special case of drug-induced immune-mediated thrombocytopenia associated with arterial and venous thrombosis, rather than bleeding, is HIT.[2] It is seen in 2 to 5% of patients exposed to unfractionated heparin, and in 0.7% of patients given low-molecular-weight heparin. HIT almost never occurs in patients who are exposed only to fondaparinux.

PATHOBIOLOGY

To understand this disease, one must know that platelets can secrete a protein called platelet factor 4 (PF4) that can bind to heparin. HIT is caused by an antibody that binds to this PF4-heparin complex (Fig. 172-3). Large complexes of antibodies directed against heparin-bound PF4 accumulate on the surface of platelets. At times, these anti-PF4 immunoglobulins bind to the Fc receptor that is also present on the platelet surface, leading to activation of the platelet, release of more PF4, and a cycle of events that causes the stimulation of even more platelets. Ultimately, this also leads to the activation of the coagulation cascade. The activation of platelets and the clotting cascade leads to the formation of both thrombi and thrombocytopenia.

CLINICAL MANIFESTATIONS AND DIAGNOSIS

When thrombocytopenia is detected in a hospitalized patient, HIT must always be considered. Patients with this syndrome often have multiple potential causes of thrombocytopenia (such as other medications or infections). Therefore, it is important to exclude these other causes. Large retrospective studies of HIT have suggested that the onset of thrombocytopenia relative to the initiation of heparin therapy is useful in establishing or excluding this diagnosis. HIT typically occurs 4 to 14 days after patients are given heparin by any route (it even occurs after subcutaneous injections of "minidose" heparin or following extremely low doses by heparin flush). This lag time between heparin exposure and the appearance of HIT is due to the time it takes for the immune response to generate the requisite antibodies against the heparin-PF4 complex. Some patients who have been exposed to heparin within the past several months may already have preexisting antibodies against the heparin-PF4 complex in their circulation. Therefore, when these patients are re-exposed to heparin, they may develop an acute onset of HIT even within the first day of the reinitiation of heparin.

The unique timing of acute-onset HIT within hours of heparin re-exposure and the more typical development of HIT within 4 to 14 days of initial heparin exposure emphasize the importance of conducting a careful and critical history in establishing the diagnosis. HIT should be suspected in any patient who develops thrombocytopenia while on heparin therapy. It is important to note that the normal platelet count varies widely (140,000/μL to 450,000/μL), and some patients may have a substantial decrease in their platelet count but still remain within the normal range. Therefore, a greater than 50% decrease in the platelet count of a patient on heparin should raise the suspicion of this syndrome. HIT should also be suspected in any patient who develops a thrombotic event while on heparin therapy.

Although antibodies against the heparin-PF4 complex are almost always present in patients with HIT, these antibodies are also frequently present in heparin-treated patients who do not have this disorder (i.e., those patients with neither thrombocytopenia nor thrombosis). There are two general categories of laboratory assays for the diagnosis of HIT: functional assays and immunologic assays (Table 172-4). Functional assays analyze whether the combination of heparin and the patient's plasma can induce normal platelets to aggregate or to secrete serotonin; these assays have very high specificity but relatively low sensitivity. Immunologic assays test the patient's plasma for antibodies that bind to the heparin-PF4 complex; these assays have very high sensitivity but lack specificity. Consequently, a *negative immunologic assay* is useful in excluding this diagnosis, and a *positive functional assay* is useful in confirming the diagnosis of HIT. Several days may elapse before the test results are available. Therefore, in practice, these laboratory assays provide only confirmatory information. Urgent clinical decisions should *not* be deferred until such test results are available. The timing of the thrombocytopenia with respect to the heparin exposure and the degree of the platelet drop are the most important pieces of information needed by the physician when evaluating a patient suspected of having HIT.

Because platelets are consumed as they become activated, the clinical presentation of HIT is thrombocytopenia. However, it is unusual for the thrombocytopenia to actually cause bleeding in patients with HIT. Instead, HIT is a highly prothrombotic disorder. Both venous and arterial thromboses are common in HIT. Patients with HIT who do not have thrombosis on initial presentation still have a 20 to 30% chance of developing a thrombus within the next month. Nevertheless, the incidence of HIT-related clinical events is greatest immediately after diagnosis. More importantly, clinical studies report that the cessation of heparin alone frequently fails to prevent the development of new thrombotic events.

TABLE 172-4 LABORATORY ASSAYS FOR HEPARIN-INDUCED THROMBOCYTOPENIA

ASSAY	SENSITIVITY (%)	SPECIFICITY (%)	POSITIVE PREDICTIVE VALUE (%)	NEGATIVE PREDICTIVE VALUE (%)
Functional assay (e.g., serotonin release assay)	88	≈100	≈100	81
PF4/heparin enzyme immunoassay (ELISA)	95-98	86	93	95

ELISA = enzyme-linked immunosorbent assay; PF4 = platelet factor 4.

TREATMENT Rx

If a patient has HIT, all heparin should be stopped immediately. This includes subcutaneous injections of "minidose" heparin, heparin flushes of intravenous lines, and low-molecular-weight heparin; even heparin-coated intravenous catheters should be withdrawn. Alternative anticoagulation, such as a direct thrombin inhibitor like argatroban (Chapter 38), should be administered, at least until the platelet count normalizes. Although not as well studied, fondaparinux appears to be a viable alternative. In contrast, low-molecular-weight heparin should not be used because this drug can react with the pathologic HIT antibodies. Warfarin should also not be used initially in cases of acute HIT because of its delayed therapeutic effect and its association with venous limb gangrene. When the platelet count has returned to a normal level after an acute episode of HIT, however, warfarin can be slowly introduced at a dose of 5 mg or less daily and gradually increased to achieve an international normalized ratio (INR) of 2 to 3 for a duration of at least 4 to 6 weeks because HIT is a risk factor for subsequent venous thromboembolism.[3] Because patients rarely become profoundly thrombocytopenic as a result of HIT alone, platelet transfusions are typically not required. In fact, some reports suggest that platelet transfusions can actually precipitate thrombotic complications, although this premise remains controversial.

Sepsis

Along with the exposure to certain drugs, bacterial and viral infections are among the most common causes of acute thrombocytopenia in hospitalized patients. Acute thrombocytopenia can be caused by the deposition of antibody-antigen complexes on the platelet surface through an "innocent bystander" phenomenon. These antibody-coated platelets are then cleared from the circulatory system by Fc receptor–expressing macrophages in the spleen. Thrombocytopenia associated with infections can also be due to DIC. The treatment of sepsis-induced thrombocytopenia is directed at treating the underlying cause, along with the administration of platelet transfusions as clinically indicated.

Idiopathic (Immune) Thrombocytopenic Purpura

DEFINITION

ITP is an autoimmune disorder caused by circulating antiplatelet autoantibodies. An ITP-like picture can also be found in patients with autoimmune diseases, such as in systemic lupus erythematosus (Chapter 266); in low-grade lymphoproliferative disorders, such as chronic lymphocytic leukemia (Chapter 184); and in HIV infection (Chapter 393).

CLINICAL MANIFESTATIONS

ITP was originally thought to be a disease of young women. Although this description is appropriate for many individuals with this disorder, more recent data indicate that ITP can occur in patients of either sex and at any age. ITP is a chronic, recurring disorder in most adults with this disease. This is in stark contrast to pediatric patients, who usually suffer from acute ITP and rarely have the chronic variant of this disorder.

In contrast to patients with coagulation factor deficiencies who present with bleeding deep within their tissues, individuals with ITP (or other platelet disorders) typically have excessive mucocutaneous bleeding. Consequently, the clinician should inquire whether the patient has noticed epistaxis, gingival bleeding, easy bruising, hematuria, melena, or hematochezia. Female patients should also be asked about inappropriate or excessive vaginal bleeding. The physical examination should pay particular attention to signs of mucocutaneous bleeding. The patient should be thoroughly examined for petechiae (see Fig. 172-2) and ecchymosis as well as for evidence of hemorrhage within the conjunctiva, retina, and central nervous system.

DIAGNOSIS

In patients with ITP, the CBC is usually normal except for the thrombocytopenia, and their peripheral blood smear is remarkable only for a decreased number of platelets, some of which may be larger than normal. Splenomegaly is absent unless the ITP is due to an underlying disorder, such as lymphoma that is associated with splenomegaly. A bone marrow examination is usually not necessary in the absence of findings that suggest a different disease such as myelodysplasia.[4] If performed, the bone marrow aspirate and biopsy of ITP patients typically show normal or increased numbers of megakaryocytes. However, the rest of their bone marrow is otherwise normal. These bone marrow findings are similar to what is observed in the bone marrows of patients who have other forms of destructive thrombocytopenia. Antiplatelet antibody assays are insufficiently sensitive or specific to be clinically useful.

TREATMENT Rx

Because platelet production is assumed to be increased in patients with ITP as a result of the immune-mediated accelerated platelet destruction, traditional therapy has focused on moderating this immune response. For most of the latter half of the 20th century, splenectomy and corticosteroids were the sole therapies for ITP. Corticosteroids in the form of either prednisone (1 mg/kg orally daily) or high-dose dexamethasone (4-day pulses of 40 mg intravenously per day every 28 days for four to six cycles) are effective. Although corticosteroids remain first-line therapeutic modalities, immunomodulating agents, such as intravenous immunoglobulin (IVIg) and anti-D, as well as alternative immunosuppressives, have been introduced for the therapy of ITP. Alternatively, other immunosuppressives, such as cyclophosphamide, azathioprine, cyclosporine, mycophenolate mofetil, dapsone, interferon, and etanercept, might be useful.

For years, the basic mechanism of and rationale for ITP treatment revolved around altering the immune system by immunosuppressives, splenectomy, or immune modulators, such as IVIG or anti-D. A more recent addition to the ITP treatment regimen is rituximab, a "humanized" murine monoclonal antibody against CD20, which is a B-cell antigen. Although rituximab has not been approved by the U.S. Food and Drug Administration (FDA) for the treatment of ITP, it is currently widely used off label in patients who are unresponsive to splenectomy and corticosteroids. Response rates vary significantly between studies, ranging from 28% to 44% in larger trials. In a recent study of 133 newly diagnosed adult ITP patients with follow-up of up to 4 years, the combination of rituximab (375 mg/m^2 intravenously weekly for 4 weeks) plus dexamethasone (40 mg per day orally for 4 days) induced higher response rates and longer time to relapse, although also increased the incidence of grade 3 to 4 adverse events, than monotherapy with dexamethasone alone at the same doses.[A3]

Although most ITP patients have a compensatory increase in megakaryopoiesis in response to their rapid platelet destruction, plasma derived from some ITP patients was unexpectedly found to inhibit platelet production. This prompted a re-evaluation of whether impaired megakaryopoiesis contributes to the development of thrombocytopenia in this disease. Thrombopoietin (TPO) is a potent megakaryocyte colony-stimulating factor, and along with other cytokines, it increases the size and number of megakaryocytes (Chapter 156). TPO levels are not markedly elevated in ITP, suggesting that supplemental TPO could help to increase platelet production and correct the thrombocytopenia.

Early experiments demonstrated that recombinant as well as truncated forms of TPO significantly increased the platelet count in some refractory ITP patients. However, this also induced autoimmune autoantibodies against endogenous TPO, which resulted in profound and persistent thrombocytopenia. Therefore, both recombinant TPO and its truncated form were withdrawn from clinical trials. Subsequently, peptides were developed that bear no structural resemblance to TPO but still bind to and activate the TPO receptor; these agents are called *TPO receptor agonists*. Because these recombinant drugs bear little structural similarity to native TPO, they should not trigger autoimmune anti-TPO antibodies. The FDA has approved two of these drugs, and several more are being used in clinical trials. The first of these, called romiplostim (N-plate), is composed of several copies of a TPO receptor–binding peptide spliced into a recombinant antibody. This peptide agonist competes with TPO for binding to the TPO receptor and activates the receptor in an identical fashion as would endogenous TPO.[A4,A5] The second FDA-approved TPO receptor agonist is eltrombopag (Promacta). It is an oral drug that activates the TPO receptor by binding to the receptor's transmembrane region.[A4,A5]

Both subcutaneously administered romiplostim and orally administered eltrombopag are capable of increasing platelet counts in approximately 70% of patients with ITP. Remarkably, these drugs can also increase the platelet count in patients with ITP that is refractory to other treatment modalities, including splenectomy.[A4-A7] However, adverse events, including bone marrow fibrosis and thromboembolism, have been reported. It should be noted that the drugs' effects disappear soon after their discontinuation.

General Principles of ITP Therapy

Initial management of ITP is guided by both symptoms and platelet count.[4] Asymptomatic patients with platelet counts of greater than 30,000/μL can be followed without treatment. If the patient is bleeding and/or has a platelet count of less than 30,000/μL, treatment with prednisone is recommended (Table 172-5). Refractory patients may require splenectomy, other immunosuppressive medications, or one of the new thrombopoiesis-stimulating agents (Table 172-6). Splenectomy has a long history of success in this disorder, and durable complete response rates are approximately 66 to 70%. Approximately half of the remaining patients who do not have normal platelet counts following splenectomy achieve a partial response that is clinically meaningful. Unfortunately, 10 to 15% of patients derive no benefit from splenectomy, and there is no test to predict whether a particular patient will respond to this treatment.

ITP patients with severe thrombocytopenia (<5000/μL) and/or those who have internal bleeding should be promptly treated with high doses of pulse corticosteroids and IVIG. Platelet transfusions may be given concurrently with IVIG for critical bleeding. In Rh-positive patients who have not undergone a splenectomy, anti-D immune globulin may be substituted for IVIg. However, some patients develop autoimmune hemolysis from this treatment.

TABLE 172-5 THERAPY FOR THE INITIAL MANAGEMENT OF IDIOPATHIC THROMBOCYTOPENIC PURPURA

ORAL PREDNISONE

The effect is dose dependent—approximately 80% of patients respond to 1 mg/kg/day. Toxicity also increases with the dose and duration of treatment, and side effects include glucose intolerance, immunosuppression, osteoporosis, and cataracts. Relapse is typical once therapy is discontinued.

INTRAVENOUS IMMUNOGLOBULIN

The effect is more rapid than daily prednisone. Administered at a dose of 1 g/kg/day for 2 consecutive days or 0.4 g/kg/day for 5 consecutive days. The response rates are approximately 80%, and the effects typically last 2 to 4 weeks. Toxicity includes headache, allergic reactions, and rarely, thrombosis.

ANTI-D IMMUNOGLOBULIN

It is administered at a dose of 50 to 75 μg/kg IV. The response rates are dose dependent but can approach 75 to 80%. Hemolysis is a common toxicity but is usually mild. Rarely, hemolysis can be life threatening and can be associated with disseminated intravascular coagulation, renal failure, and end-organ infarction.

TABLE 172-6 THERAPY FOR THE MANAGEMENT OF REFRACTORY IDIOPATHIC THROMBOCYTOPENIC PURPURA

ORAL PREDNISONE

The effect is dose dependent and rapidly dissipates after discontinuation of the medication. Some patients can be maintained on a very low and tolerable daily dose (e.g., 5 mg). Long-term use is associated with infections, diabetes, osteoporosis, avascular necrosis, weight gain, and cataracts.

ORAL DEXAMETHASONE

This is administered at a dose of 40 mg/day for 4 consecutive days, repeated every 2 to 4 weeks for several months. Sustained response rates of 29 to 42% have been reported, although response rates are widely believed to be lower. Toxicity is similar to that of oral prednisone.

SPLENECTOMY

Durable (often lifelong), significant responses are seen in 65 to 70% of patients who undergo this procedure. More modest benefits are seen in another 10 to 15% of patients. There is no useful way to predict who will respond. Splenectomy is associated with surgical morbidity and some mortality (≈1-2%). Splenectomy produces lifelong immunosuppression to encapsulated and gram-positive organisms.

RITUXIMAB

This is given at a dose of 375 mg/m^2/wk IV for a total of 4 weeks. Significant responses are seen in 28 to 44% of patients, and these responses typically last for months. Toxicity includes reactivation of hepatitis B, immunosuppression, and rarely, progressive multifocal leukoencephalopathy.

THROMBOPOIETIN RECEPTOR AGONISTS

These are administered daily (eltrombopag) or weekly (romiplostim). An effect is typically seen in 2 to 3 weeks and disappears shortly after the discontinuation of the medication. Toxicity from long-term use is not well known but may include excessive thrombosis and bone marrow fibrosis.

Thrombotic Thrombocytopenic Purpura

DEFINITION

TTP is a consumptive thrombocytopenia associated with a mechanical hemolytic anemia.[5] The classic pentad of symptoms, which are thrombocytopenia, anemia, fever, neurologic problems, and renal abnormalities, are fully present in only a minority of patients. Many patients today have only hemolytic anemia and thrombocytopenia. The poor specificity of the clinical features of this disease and the nonspecific laboratory abnormalities makes TTP difficult to diagnose. Historically, patients with untreated TTP had a mortality rate of 90% within 3 months. With modern therapy, patients with TTP have a mortality rate of approximately 10 to 20%.

PATHOBIOLOGY

Some patients with recurrent TTP have very large multimers of von Willebrand factor (Chapter 173). Because larger multimers of von Willebrand factor are more efficient at binding and activating platelets than smaller multimers, it was speculated that TTP could be due to a deficiency of a protease that normally cleaves large multimers of von Willebrand factor into smaller, less sticky multimers. A genome-wide linkage analysis of patients with inherited and recurrent TTP (Upshaw-Schulman syndrome) demonstrated a deficiency of a metalloproteinase that has now been identified as ADAMTS13 (*a d*isintegrin-like *a*nd *m*etalloprotease with *t*hrombospondin type 1 motif, member *13*). Many patients with adult-onset TTP have an antibody against ADAMTS13 that thus causes an acquired deficiency of ADAMTS13. Inherited or acquired ADAMTS13 deficiency causes the accumulation of ultra-large multimers of von Willebrand factor in plasma, which leads to platelet activation and the microvascular thrombosis that is characteristic of this disease (Fig. 172-4). Because many patients can have a partial deficiency of ADAMTS13 without having TTP, clinical assays of ADAMTS13 enzymatic activity have not been useful in diagnosing TTP. Levels of ADAMTS13 below 5% of normal are hypothesized to be highly suggestive of TTP, but levels greater than this are not very helpful. This hypothesis still needs to be validated in large clinical trials. Consequently, analysis of ADAMTS13 enzymatic activity should not be used to diagnose TTP outside of a research setting at this time.

Some patients reportedly developed TTP soon after taking an antiplatelet drug of the thienopyridine class. Approximately 1 of 2000 patients taking ticlopidine will develop TTP. In several individuals with ticlopidine-induced TTP, an antibody against ADAMTS13 was identified. A few studies have also suggested that clopidogrel can induce TTP at an incidence as rare as 1 in 250,000. Because the incidence of TTP in the general population is approximately 1 in 100,000, it is difficult to determine whether there is a significant risk for TTP in patients who are prescribed clopidogrel. The thienopyridine-derivative prasugrel has also been implicated. It should be noted that some patients can also develop TTP after exposure to medications that directly injure the vascular endothelium (such as cyclosporin or tacrolimus). Most of these patients do not have TTP but have the related disorder HUS, discussed later in this chapter.

CLINICAL MANIFESTATIONS AND DIAGNOSIS

In TTP, patients can occasionally present with symptoms of excessive mucocutaneous bleeding, but they might present with signs of a thrombotic event (including phlebitis, myocardial infarction, or stroke). Many patients complain of abdominal pain, which is presumably due to intestinal ischemia. Signs of central nervous system disease, somnolence, and even coma can also be seen on presentation.

The two major hallmarks of TTP are microangiopathic hemolytic anemia and thrombocytopenia. Microangiopathic hemolytic anemia is a non-immune-mediated hemolytic anemia caused by red cell fragmentation. Patients with this disorder have typical laboratory findings of hemolytic anemia, including a decreasing hemoglobin concentration, a high lactate dehydrogenase (LDH) level, elevated indirect bilirubin, and an increased reticulocyte count. Examination of the peripheral blood smear (Chapter 157) shows torn red blood cells (schistocytes), and frequently also shows, early red blood cell precursor cells (nucleated red blood cells). The thrombocytopenia may be mild if the disease is diagnosed at an early stage, but advanced cases of TTP can have platelet counts of less than 10,000/μL. TTP should be considered in any patient who has evidence of hemolysis accompanied by thrombocytopenia.

Unlike most patients with typical thrombocytopenia, who tend to bleed excessively, patients with TTP have few hemorrhagic complications. Instead, they are markedly predisposed to thrombosis. In fact, a thrombotic complication in a thrombocytopenic patient is another clue that TTP might be the cause of the thrombocytopenia (see Table 172-1). Characteristically, the thrombotic occlusions are in the terminal arterioles and capillaries and are composed mainly of platelets within the damaged vascular lumen. In contrast to most blood clots, these occlusions contain very little fibrin and are referred to as *hyaline thrombi*. Before plasmapheresis was used in the treatment of this disease, TTP typically progressed and caused renal disease, neurologic symptoms, and fever. These symptoms are believed to be due to ischemia and infarction of the affected organs. Today, TTP is often diagnosed in its early stages, so patients may have only microangiopathic hemolytic anemia and thrombocytopenia.

TREATMENT Rx

The prompt initiation of plasma exchange (plasmapheresis with plasma replacement) reduces the mortality rate associated with TTP from 90% to approximately 15%. The mechanism of this benefit is not entirely known. A randomized trial demonstrated that plasma exchange is more beneficial than plasma infusion for the treatment of TTP. This implies that some of the benefit of plasmapheresis is attributable to the removal of a pathologic substance from the patient's plasma. Assuming that the pathogenesis of most acquired forms of TTP is the antibody-mediated inhibition of ADAMTS13, plasma exchange might have two benefits. First, it helps to remove the pathogenic antibody from the plasma. Second, the normal plasma infused into the patient during plasmapheresis repletes the deficiency of ADAMTS13. Both of these

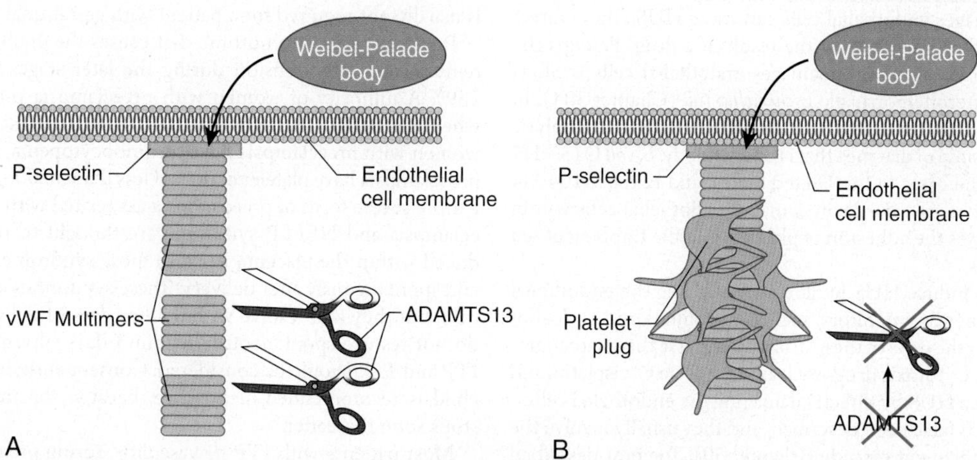

FIGURE 172-4. Pathophysiology of thrombotic thrombocytopenia purpura (TTP). A, Von Willebrand factor (vWF) is synthesized in endothelial cells and stored in Weibel-Palade bodies. The vWF is assembled into ultralarge multimers that are cleaved after they are released into the blood stream by the protease ADAMTS13. The resultant smaller multimers of vWF can bind to platelets to participate in normal hemostasis. B, Some patients with TTP have a deficiency of ADAMTS13. This results in the accumulation of ultralarge multimers of vWF within the circulation, which promotes the excessive adhesion of platelets. This produces large hyaline plugs of vWF and platelets that cause vascular occlusions.

benefits probably play a role in the efficacy of plasma exchange in the treatment of this disease.

Because patients with TTP can develop sudden thrombotic events (including stroke and myocardial infarction), and because patients can deteriorate quickly, it is prudent to initiate plasma exchange as rapidly as possible. Given the morbidity and mortality of untreated TTP, and given the relatively low risk of administering plasmapheresis, this therapy should be initiated even when the diagnosis is not certain. As discussed in the section on HUS (later in this chapter), plasmapheresis is not beneficial in children with Shiga toxin–induced microangiopathic hemolytic anemia or in patients who develop HUS following their exposure to endothelium-toxic drugs, such as chemotherapy.

Plasma exchange is administered to replace one entire plasma volume and is usually repeated once daily. An average-sized individual requires 20 to 30 units of fresh-frozen plasma for each plasmapheresis session. Therapy is usually administered daily, and patients are monitored for signs of improvement in their thrombocytopenia, hemolysis, neurologic symptoms, fever, and renal disease. Appropriate daily laboratory tests to monitor the patient are CBC, LDH, reticulocyte count, and creatinine. After the thrombocytopenia and hemolysis have been corrected for a few days, the daily plasmapheresis can either be discontinued or continued every other day for several more days. A typical duration of therapy is 1 to 2 weeks, although some patients require treatment far beyond this usual time course.

Approximately one third of patients relapse quickly after plasmapheresis is stopped. These patients require a reinitiation of plasma exchange and perhaps the addition of an immunosuppressive drug, such as a glucocorticoid. Some reports indicate that rituximab shows promise in reducing the incidence of relapse. However, given that this drug does not decrease antibody production for weeks to months after its administration, it is likely that if rituximab has any benefit in the treatment of TTP, it is probably only to minimize the incidence of late relapses.

Major complications of plasmapheresis do occur and are often attributable to the use of a central venous catheter. Hypotension, bacteremia, hemorrhage, and thrombosis are among the most common life-threatening complications of plasmapheresis therapy. Two specific complications deserve emphasis. First, patients taking an angiotensin-converting enzyme (ACE) inhibitor are susceptible to plasmapheresis-induced hypotension. This is due to these drugs' interference with bradykinin catabolism. Second, a patient who develops recurrent thrombocytopenia and a fever several days to a week into treatment may not be having an exacerbation of TTP but rather may be developing central line–induced sepsis. Therefore, a vigorous investigation for infection should be initiated in patients who appear to be relapsing early.

Hemolytic-Uremic Syndrome

DEFINITION

HUS is another cause of microangiopathic hemolytic anemia, and it may be difficult to distinguish from TTP. When acute renal failure is predominant, and there are no neurologic symptoms, many clinicians consider the syndrome to be HUS, not TTP.[6] In contrast to TTP, HUS is not caused by a deficiency of ADAMTS13. However, at this point, it is not clear whether ADAMTS13 levels will be clinically useful to distinguish between HUS and TTP. Because there is such overlap between the signs and symptoms of TTP and those of HUS, the distinction and diagnosis may be impossible to make in some cases.

PATHOBIOLOGY AND CLINICAL MANIFESTATIONS

A toxin that directly damages endothelial cells can cause HUS. These direct endothelial toxins are either infectious or the result of a drug. Perhaps the best-characterized infectious agent that damages endothelial cells is Shiga toxin, which produces enterohemorrhagic *Escherichia coli* (Chapter 304). In Shiga toxin–induced HUS, the renal disease and microangiopathic hemolytic anemia occur after an episode of diarrhea that is often bloody. *E. coli* O157:H7 is the cause of many of the cases in the United States, and *E. coli* O104:H4 causes some of the other cases.[7] The toxin damages endothelial cells within the glomeruli and promotes the adhesion of platelets and the trapping of red blood cells in the kidneys.

Several drugs can also induce HUS by directly damaging the endothelial cells. These include calcineurin inhibitors, such as tacrolimus and cyclosporine; sometimes, lowering the dose of these drugs can reverse the microangiopathic hemolytic anemia. Cytotoxic drugs such as mitomycin C, cisplatin, and bleomycin can also induce HUS by directly damaging the endothelial cells.

Inherited forms of HUS have been described, and they usually involve the dysregulation of the complement cascade (Chapter 50). The best-described genetic mutations cause the deficiency of factor H, which is a complement regulatory protease. HUS-inducing mutations in other components of complement regulation include those found in C3, CD46, and factor I.

TREATMENT AND PREVENTION (Rx)

Reducing the spread of Shiga toxin–producing *E. coli* is vital because antibiotics and antimotility drugs do not lower the risk for developing HUS symptoms. In contrast to TTP, there is little evidence that plasma exchange is beneficial. The clinical course and outcome of *E. coli* O104:H4–induced HUS are similar to infections with the more common O157:H7-induced HUS. Aggressive antibiotic therapy appears to be beneficial for reducing seizures and death. However, neither plasmapheresis nor glucocorticoids seem to be helpful. In a pilot study of 12 patients, *E. coli* O104:H4–associated HUS appeared to respond to immunoadsorption. The infusion of plasma or plasmapheresis is reportedly beneficial in the treatment of the atypical forms of HUS that are caused by the dysregulation of complement. Recent evidence suggests that some patients with atypical forms of HUS respond to eculizumab, an antibody that inhibits the terminal steps of the complement cascade.[8]

Disseminated Intravascular Coagulation

DIC is a pathologic condition that depletes components of the coagulation system, including platelets. Therefore, in contrast to TTP and HUS, the thrombocytopenia of DIC is associated with the consumption of coagulation factors and increased fibrinolysis. This often leads to prolongations of the prothrombin time (PT) and activated partial thromboplastin time (aPTT), as well as to increased levels of D-dimers. In its fully manifested state, DIC can be associated with arterial and venous thrombi, hemorrhage, microangiopathic hemolysis, thrombocytopenia, excessive fibrinolysis, and the deficiency of coagulation factors, such as fibrinogen. For a more complete review of DIC and related disorders, see Chapter 175.

Thrombocytopenia during Pregnancy

Thrombocytopenia occurs in approximately 10% of pregnant women. It may be due to a normal variant of pregnancy (gestational thrombocytopenia), a pregnancy-specific condition (preeclampsia and HELLP [*h*emolysis, *el*evated *l*iver enzymes, and *l*ow *p*latelets]) syndrome, or a condition exacerbated by pregnancy (ITP, vasculitis, TTP). A recent review estimated that thrombocytopenia occurs in approximately 7 to 10% of pregnancies, and about 75% of these cases are due to gestational thrombocytopenia, 15 to 20% are secondary to hypertensive disorders, 3 to 4% are due to an immune process, and the remaining 1 to 2% are rare constitutional thrombocytopenias, infections, and malignancies.[9] The prognosis and treatment vary tremendously based on the underlying cause.

Gestational thrombocytopenia (incidental thrombocytopenia of pregnancy) is a mild, asymptomatic thrombocytopenia that typically occurs late in pregnancy. There is no association with fetal thrombocytopenia, and this maternal thrombocytopenia resolves spontaneously after delivery. Other than thrombocytopenia during previous pregnancies, women with gestational thrombocytopenia have no prior history of a low platelet count. This lack of previous thrombocytopenia helps to distinguish gestational thrombocytopenia from ITP. Additionally, in contrast to other causes of maternal thrombocytopenia, gestational thrombocytopenia does not produce a platelet count lower than 70,000/μL. Consequently, deviation from standard obstetric care is usually not required for a patient with gestational thrombocytopenia.

Preeclampsia is a syndrome that causes the gradual development of proteinuria and hypertension during the later stages of pregnancy (Chapter 239). A minority of women with preeclampsia progress to have seizures; when this occurs, the syndrome is called *eclampsia*. Approximately 15% of women with preeclampsia have thrombocytopenia, and 5% of patients with preeclampsia have platelet counts of less than 50,000/μL. Some patients have a more severe form of preeclampsia associated with HELLP syndrome. Preeclampsia and HELLP syndrome are thought to result from a factor produced within the placenta because these syndromes usually resolve rapidly and spontaneously after delivery. These syndromes can also present postpartum, but they still resolve within a few days of delivery. If these syndromes do not resolve spontaneously within 3 days, alternative diagnoses, such as ITP and TTP, should be considered. Consequently, immediate delivery of the child is recommended, if possible, because the microangiopathic process stops soon thereafter.

Most patients with ITP or vasculitis during pregnancy have a history of thrombocytopenia before pregnancy. The antiplatelet IgG antibodies that cause this disease in the mother can cross the placenta and lead to thrombocytopenia in the fetus. However, the platelet count in the unborn child does not correlate well with the platelet count of the mother, and attempts to sample fetal blood to monitor platelet counts are associated with significant risk. Because most children born to women with ITP have a platelet count high enough for a successful delivery, the management of ITP focuses on keeping the maternal platelet count acceptable for the mother's safety. In the early stages of pregnancy, a platelet count of 30,000/μL to 50,000/μL is considered safe. In preparation for delivery, a platelet count of 50,000/μL to 80,000/μL is more desirable. This can be managed by the use of oral glucocorticoids, and if necessary, by the administration of IVIG. The safety of rituximab and thrombopoiesis-stimulating agents during pregnancy is not known. Splenectomy performed during the first trimester has a risk for inducing miscarriage, and this operation is technically difficult during the later stages of pregnancy because of uterine enlargement. There is no evidence that a cesarean section is safer than vaginal delivery.

The diagnosis of TTP during pregnancy can be difficult to make because many of the symptoms are identical to those of preeclampsia. If the symptoms develop during the early stages of pregnancy, when preeclampsia is unlikely, the diagnosis of TTP is more certain. The presence of hyperuricemia, hypoproteinemia, elevated liver transaminases, and direct bilirubin is more consistent with preeclampsia. The development of microangiopathic hemolytic anemia and thrombocytopenia in the peripartum period is presumed to be attributable to preeclampsia, and if it is safe to do so, immediate delivery of the fetus is desirable. Typically, the thrombocytopenia starts to resolve rapidly after delivery. If no improvement is seen by the third postpartum day, standard management for TTP, including plasma exchange, is recommended.

Post-transfusion Purpura and Neonatal Alloimmune Thrombocytopenia

Alloimmune thrombocytopenia is due to the sensitization to alloantigens, such as Pl^{A1} (HPA-1a). These alloimmune antibodies can cause thrombocytopenia approximately a week after a blood transfusion (post-transfusion purpura, or PTP).[10] A similar alloimmune antibody can cause thrombocytopenia in a fetus when it is produced by the mother (neonatal alloimmune thrombocytopenia, or NAIT). PTP causes profound thrombocytopenia 7 to 10 days after exposure to the small amount of platelets that contaminate most red blood cell transfusions. It can be treated with IVIG or by plasma exchange. NAIT can cause severe thrombocytopenia and bleeding in neonates, and it is treated with the transfusion of platelets derived from a Pl^{A1}-negative donor (most conveniently the newborn's mother), corticosteroids, and IVIg.

Vasculitis

Autoimmune diseases such as systemic lupus erythematosus, rheumatoid arthritis, and other forms of vasculitis can also cause thrombocytopenia. This can be due to an ITP-like process that occurs in patients with a propensity for the development of autoantibodies. The treatment for these patients is immunosuppression, similar to the treatment for other patients with ITP. Some patients with active vasculitis and endothelial inflammation consume circulating platelets by promoting their adhesion to the damaged vessel wall. This creates a clinical picture that is difficult to distinguish from that of TTP without a tissue diagnosis that documents vasculitis. Because of the difficulty of discerning TTP from a flare-up of vasculitis, these patients are often treated with both plasma exchange and immunosuppression.

Dilutional Thrombocytopenia

Thrombocytopenia does not typically occur after blood loss, possibly in part owing to the release of platelets from the splenic pool. Thrombocytopenia occasionally occurs after a massive hemorrhage. However, this is only when the hemorrhage is severe enough to necessitate the replacement of 1.5 to 2 times the total blood volume, which usually requires the transfusion of at least 15 to 20 units of packed red blood cells over a short period of time. Even in this circumstance, the thrombocytopenia is usually only mild to moderate. Therefore, the clinician should remain vigilant for another cause of the thrombocytopenia (such as DIC resulting from hemorrhage-induced hypotension and shock). When indicated, dilutional thrombocytopenia can be corrected with platelet transfusions.

Congenital Thrombocytopenias

Lifelong thrombocytopenia can be due to an inherited defect that affects platelet production or survival. These disorders can be autosomal dominant (May-Hegglin anomaly and Sebastian syndrome), autosomal recessive (Bernard-Soulier disease, Fanconi's anemia, gray platelet syndrome, and thrombocytopenia with absent radius syndrome), or X-linked (Wiskott-Aldrich syndrome). Many of these disorders are associated with other abnormalities in addition to thrombocytopenia. A congenital cause of thrombocytopenia should be suspected in a patient who has long-standing moderate thrombocytopenia that was presumed to be treatment-refractory ITP.

Grade A References

A1. Stanworth SJ, Estcourt LJ, Powter G, et al. A non-prophylaxis platelet transfusion strategy for hematologic cancers. *N Engl J Med.* 2013;368:1771-1780.

A2. Slichter SJ, Kaufman RM, Assmann SF, et al. Dose of prophylactic platelet transfusions and prevention of hemorrhage. *N Engl J Med.* 2010;362:600-613.

A3. Gudbrandsdottir S, Biryens HS, Fredericksen H, et al. Rituximab dexamethasone vs dexamethasone monotherapy in newly diagnosed patients with primary immune thrombocytopenia. *Blood.* 2013;121:1976-1981.

A4. Kuter DJ, Bussel JB, Lyons RM, et al. Efficacy of romiplostim in patients with chronic immune thrombocytopenic purpura: a double-blind randomised controlled trial. *Lancet.* 2008;37:395-403.

A5. George JN, Mathias SD, Go RS, et al. Improved quality of life for romiplostim-treated patients with chronic immune thrombocytopenic purpura: results from two randomized, placebo-controlled trials. *Br J Haematol.* 2009;144:409-415.

A6. Bussel JB, Provan D, Shamsi T, et al. Effect of eltrombopag on platelet counts and bleeding during treatment of chronic idiopathic thrombocytopenic purpura: a randomised, double-blind, placebo-controlled trial. *Lancet.* 2009;373:641-648.

A7. Cheng G, Saleh MN, Marcher C, et al. Eltrombopag for management of chronic immune thrombocytopenia (RAISE): a 6-month, randomised, phase 3 study. *Lancet.* 2011;377:393-402.

GENERAL REFERENCES

For the General References and other additional features, please visit Expert Consult at https://expertconsult.inkling.com.

173

VON WILLEBRAND DISEASE AND HEMORRHAGIC ABNORMALITIES OF PLATELET AND VASCULAR FUNCTION

WILLIAM L. NICHOLS

VON WILLEBRAND DISEASE

DEFINITION AND EPIDEMIOLOGY

Von Willebrand disease (VWD), a usually autosomal dominantly inherited condition affecting both males and females of all ethnicities, is the most common hereditary bleeding disorder worldwide, with prevalence estimates dependent on case definition. It may also occur less frequently as an acquired disorder (acquired von Willebrand syndrome [AVWS]). Von Willebrand factor (VWF) plasma levels are variably decreased (minimally to substantially) in at least 2.5% of humans, but approximately 0.1% (one in 1000) have definite VWD with medically significant bleeding symptoms related to low VWF, and approximately 0.01% (one in 10,000) have more severe forms of VWD that often result in referral to tertiary care centers, including hemophilia centers.[1-3]

PATHOBIOLOGY

Von Willebrand disease reflects deficiency or dysfunction of VWF, a multimeric plasma glycoprotein that mediates platelet adhesion and aggregation at sites of vascular injury (Chapter 171) and that also carries and stabilizes blood coagulation factor VIII (FVIII) in the circulation. The *VWF* gene is located on chromosome 12, with a partial pseudogene on chromosome 22 that potentially complicates DNA-based mutation detection (which remains primarily a research application, with evolving clinical diagnostic potential). The protein is synthesized by vascular endothelium as approximately 270-kD subunits (protomers) that are dimerized, processed and polymerized into very large (≤~20,000 kD) hemostatically active VWF multimers, and finally secreted into the blood. Vascular endothelial cells additionally provide a storage reservoir of multimerized VWF (in intracellular Weibel-Palade bodies) from which it can be released by stress or by drugs such as DDAVP (desmopressin). VWF is also synthesized and multimerized by bone marrow megakaryocytes and stored in circulating blood platelet α granules, from which it is secreted with platelet activation. Platelet-stored VWF represents about 10% of total blood VWF.

Multimerization of VWF is essential for its hemostatic activity that is mainly mediated by the higher-molecular-weight (larger) multimers. Circulating plasma VWF normally does not interact with platelets. However, when VWF binds to injured (deendothelialized) blood vessel walls, reflecting its collagen-binding activity, multimers can be stretched and unfolded by high intravascular shear forces, such as in the microvasculature, exposing and activating previously cryptic platelet-binding domains to promote platelet adhesion and aggregation to vessel-bound VWF. Simultaneously, activated (stretched) VWF multimers expose protomer cleavage sites for proteolysis by the circulating enzyme, ADAMTS13 (A Disintegrin And Metalloprotease domain with ThromboSpondin type 1 motifs, member 13), ultimately decreasing the size of VWF multimers and thereby downregulating VWF hemostatic function. Severe deficiency of ADAMTS13 is associated with the pathologic microangiopathy of thrombotic thrombocytopenic purpura (TTP) (Chapter 172), in which the microvascular thrombosis is mediated by ultralarge VWF multimers in the circulation.

Von Willebrand disease is classified into three major types that vary in severity and differ in clinical management, such that defining the VWD subtype is important. Type 1 VWD reflects partial quantitative deficiency of normally functioning VWF, of variable severity, and comprises 75% to 80% of individuals with symptomatic VWD. Type 2 VWD reflects qualitative VWF deficiency, with four subtypes (A, B, M, N), and comprises 20% to 25% of persons with VWD. Type 3 VWD reflects the virtual absence of VWF, with secondary near-absence of FVIII, and is rare (<1% of VWD). Inheritance of VWD is usually autosomal dominant, except that type 3 VWD is typically autosomal recessive in inheritance. Table 173-1 summarizes the classification of VWD subtypes and their basic pathophysiology.

The FVIII deficiency that often accompanies different types of VWD (see Table 173-1) is not genetically related to the disease; the gene that encodes FVIII is on the X chromosome, and its primary deficiency causes classic hemophilia (Chapter 174). FVIII deficiency in VWD is attributable to a primary deficiency or defect in the VWF molecule, which normally carries and stabilizes FVIII in the circulation. Therefore, FVIII is more rapidly cleared from the circulation, leading to its secondary deficiency in VWD.

TABLE 173-1 CLASSIFICATION OF VON WILLEBRAND DISEASE

TYPE	DESCRIPTION
1	Partial quantitative deficiency of VWF (~75%-80% of VWD)
2	Qualitative VWF defect (~20-25% of VWD)
2A	Caused by VWF mutations that decrease the proportion of large functional VWF multimers, leading to decreased VWF-dependent platelet adhesion and aggregation
2B	Caused by VWF mutations that increase platelet–VWF binding, resulting in depletion of large, functional VWF multimers. Circulating platelets are coated with mutant VWF, which may impair platelet adhesion and aggregation at sites of injury. Thrombocytopenia, persistent or intermittent, is observed in most cases. Distinguishing type 2B VWD may require RIPA to detect increased (abnormal) platelet aggregation response to low-dose ristocetin; the latter may also reflect platelet-type (pseudo) VWD caused by rare mutations in the platelet VWF receptor.
2M	Caused by VWF mutations that decrease VWF-dependent platelet adhesion and aggregation but do not deplete the large VWF multimers. Distinguishing between types 2A and 2M VWD requires VWF multimer gel electrophoretic analysis.
2N	Caused by VWF mutations that impair binding to FVIII, thereby shortening FVIII survival and lowering FVIII levels so that type 2N VWD can masquerade as an autosomal recessive form of hemophilia A. Discrimination from hemophilia A may require assays of VWF-FVIII binding.
3	Virtually complete VWF deficiency associated with markedly decreased FVIII (<1% of VWD)

FVIII = factor VIII coagulant activity; RIPA = ristocetin-induced platelet aggregation/aggregometry; VWD = von Willebrand disease; VWF = von Willebrand factor.
Adapted and modified from National Heart, Lung, and Blood Institute. *The Diagnosis, Evaluation, and Management of von Willebrand Disease.* Bethesda, MD: National Institutes of Health Publication 08-5832. December 2007 (released February 29, 2008), and Yawn BP, Nichols WL, Rick ME. Diagnosis and management of von Willebrand disease: guidelines for primary care. *Am Fam Physician.* 2009;80:1261-1268, 1269-1270.

CLINICAL MANIFESTATIONS

Individuals with VWD usually experience mucocutaneous bleeding symptoms such as easy bruising, prolonged or excessive bleeding from minor cuts or other injuries, nosebleeds or other mucosal bleeding such as gastrointestinal (GI) hemorrhage, or heavy menstrual bleeding in women, and they may be at increased risk for bleeding after surgery or invasive procedures, dental extractions, traumatic injury, or childbirth. Symptoms can range from relatively mild or infrequent bleeding in type 1 VWD to severe, life-threatening bleeding in type 3 VWD. As a group, women with VWD may be more affected by bleeding symptoms than men because of hemostatic challenges of menstruation and childbirth.

DIAGNOSIS

Clinical Assessment

The diagnosis of VWD (as in other bleeding disorders [Chapter 171]) begins with clinical assessment to evaluate for a personal and possible family history of abnormal bleeding, accompanied by focused physical examination to detect signs or symptoms of bleeding (e.g., petechiae, ecchymoses, hematomas, anemia), as well as findings that may suggest other causes of increased bleeding such as liver disease (e.g., hepatosplenomegaly, jaundice), joint or skin laxity (e.g., Ehlers-Danlos syndrome), telangiectasia (e.g., hereditary hemorrhagic telangiectasia [HHT]), or anatomic lesions on gynecologic examination. Because bleeding symptoms are common in apparently normal individuals, with a prevalence of certain symptoms as high as 25% to 50%, clinical assessment for VWD or other possible bleeding disorders can be challenging (Chapter 171).

The most important parts of the medical history include (1) family history of a known or suspected bleeding disorder; (2) review of personal surgical or other hemostatic challenges throughout life and recently, including dental extractions and traumatic injuries, and whether abnormal bleeding occurred and its severity; (3) mucocutaneous bleeding symptoms (e.g., bruising, nosebleeds, ecchymoses, GI bleeding, menorrhagia), including frequency, severity, and spontaneity of events; and (4) assessment for medical conditions that can increase the risk for bleeding, such as use of certain drugs that can impede normal hemostasis, including aspirin or other nonsteroidal antiinflammatory drugs (NSAIDs), clopidogrel, or warfarin or heparin or newer direct-acting oral anticoagulants; the presence of liver or kidney disease (e.g., cirrhosis, uremia); and a history of a low or high platelet count and blood or bone marrow disorders.[4]

Bleeding history scoring tools are being developed and applied for studying populations with VWD or other bleeding disorders but are not yet validated for routine clinical use.[5] However, in general, an increasing number of positive or abnormal clinical bleeding history items increases the likelihood that an individual has a bleeding disorder, including VWD, and may merit undergoing appropriate laboratory evaluation (Chapter 171).

Laboratory Evaluation

Because no simple, single laboratory test is available to screen for VWD, the initial laboratory evaluation requires measurements of plasma: (1) VWF antigen (VWF:Ag), (2) ristocetin cofactor activity (VWF:RCo), and (3) factor VIII coagulant activity (FVIII). All three tests are recommended for initial evaluation, and the results may not only establish the diagnosis but also suggest the type and severity of VWD if it is present.[6] These three tests are also used for monitoring therapy. Tests such as the bleeding time (BT) or platelet function analyzer (PFA-100, Siemens) assay lack sufficient sensitivity and specificity and are not recommended for routine screening.

If one or more of the three test results are abnormally low or if the ratio of VWF:RCo to VWF:Ag is below 0.5 to 0.7, additional laboratory evaluation may include selecting one or more of the following tests, based on the pattern of initial results together with clinical assessment and experience: (1) repeating the three initial VWD tests with timing and procedures optimized for conditions of the patient, the blood sample, and laboratory testing (see later discussion for additional information about these conditions); (2) VWF multimer analysis to help differentiate or exclude types 2A, 2B, or 2M VWD; (3) ristocetin-induced platelet aggregometry (RIPA), including low-dose ristocetin testing to evaluate for type 2B VWD or platelet-type (pseudo) VWD; (4) VWF-FVIII binding assay (or molecular DNA-based VWF testing) to evaluate for type 2N VWD; and (5) other tests such as VWF:CB (collagen-binding activity) or immunoassays reflecting VWF-platelet binding activity to supplement VWF:RCo testing. The latter tests (VWF:CB and VWF-platelet binding immunoassays) do not replace the VWF:RCo assay but can be useful as screening or supplementary tests.[7] Some of these tests

TABLE 173-2 PATTERNS OF LABORATORY TEST RESULTS FOR VON WILLEBRAND DISEASE DIAGNOSIS AND CLASSIFICATION*

CONDITION	VWF:RCo (IU/dL)	VWF:Ag (IU/dL)	FVIII (IU/dL)	VWF:RCo/VWF:Ag Ratio[¶]	RIPA	VWF MULTIMERS
Type 1 VWD	<30[†]	<30[†‡]	↓ or Normal	>0.5-0.7	Often normal	Normal
Type 2A VWD	<30[†]	<30-200[†‡]	↓ or Normal	<0.5-0.7	↓ or Normal	↓ HMW
Type 2B VWD	<30[†]	<30-200[†‡]	↓ or Normal	Usually <0.5-0.7	↑ (Low dose)	↓ HMW
Type 2M VWD	<30[†]	<30-200[†‡]†	↓ or Normal	<0.5-0.7	↓ or Normal	No ↓ HMW
Type 2N VWD	30-200	30-200	↓↓	>0.5-0.7	Normal	Normal
Type 3 VWD	<3	<3	↓↓↓ (1-9)	NA	Absent	NA
"Low VWF"[§]	30-50[§]	30-50[§]	Normal	>0.5-0.7	Normal	Normal
Normal	50-200	50-200	Normal	>0.5-0.7	Normal	Normal

*Values in the table represent prototypical cases without additional VWF (or other disease) abnormalities. Exceptions occur, and repeat testing and clinical experience may be necessary for clarification and interpretation of laboratory test results.

[†]VWF values <30 IU/dL (or %) are designated as the level for definite diagnosis of VWD (especially type 1 VWD) because (1) there is a high frequency of blood type O that is associated with "low VWF" levels but not necessarily VWD; (2) bleeding symptoms are reported by a significant proportion of individuals with no disease; and (3) no abnormality in the VWF gene has been identified in many individuals who have only mildly to moderately decreased VWF levels. VWF values of 30 to 50 IU/dL include both apparently normal persons and those with mild VWD.

[‡]VWF:Ag is <50 IU/dL in most persons with types 2A, 2B, or 2M VWD.

[§]Diagnosis of VWD is not precluded for persons with VWF:RCo of 30 to 50 IU/dL if there is supporting clinical or family evidence for VWD, nor is the use of agents to increase VWF levels precluded in those who have VWF:RCo of 30 to 50 IU/dL and who may be at risk for bleeding.

[¶]Until more laboratories clearly define a reference range, the VWF:RCo/VWF:Ag ratio of <0.5 to 0.7 is recommended to distinguish type 1 vs. type 2 VWD variants (A, B, or M).

FVIII = factor VIII coagulant activity; HMW = high-molecular-weight VWF multimers; IU/dL = international units per deciliter (e.g., 100 IU/dL = 100% of mean normal level); NA = not applicable; RIPA = ristocetin-induced platelet aggregation/aggregometry; VWD, von Willebrand disease; VWF = von Willebrand factor; VWF:Ag = von Willebrand factor antigen; VWF:RCo = von Willebrand factor ristocetin cofactor activity; ↓, ↓↓, ↓↓↓, ↑, refer to varying degrees of decrease, or an increase, of the test result compared to the laboratory reference range.

Adapted and modified from National Heart, Lung, and Blood Institute. *The Diagnosis, Evaluation, and Management of von Willebrand Disease.* Bethesda, MD: National Institutes of Health Publication 08-5832. December 2007 (released February 29, 2008), and Nichols WL, Rick ME, Ortel TL, et al. Clinical and laboratory diagnosis of von Willebrand disease: a synopsis of the 2008 NHLBI/NIH guidelines. *Am J Hematol.* 2009;84:366-370.

TABLE 173-3 VARIABLE CONDITIONS OF THE PATIENT, BLOOD SAMPLING, AND LABORATORY TESTING AFFECTING LABORATORY EVALUATION FOR VON WILLEBRAND DISEASE

Phlebotomy conditions: An atraumatic blood draw limits the exposure of tissue factor from the site and the activation of clotting factors, minimizing falsely high or low values. Lipemia should be avoided because it may interfere with photo-optical testing methods, especially some used for VWF:RCo assay.

Patient stress level: Undue stress, such as struggling or crying in children or anxiety in adults, may falsely elevate VWF and FVIII levels. Very recent exercise can also elevate VWF levels.

Additional conditions in the individual: The presence of an acute or chronic inflammatory illness may elevate VWF and FVIII levels, as may pregnancy or administration of estrogen or oral contraceptives. Individuals with blood group O have VWF levels approximately 25% lower than those of other ABO blood groups. African Americans have higher VWF levels than whites.

Sample processing: To prevent cryoprecipitation of VWF and other proteins, blood samples for VWF assays should be transported to the laboratory at room temperature. Plasma should be separated from blood cells promptly at room temperature, and the plasma should be centrifuged thoroughly to remove platelets. If plasma samples will be assayed within 2 hours, they should be kept at room temperature. Frozen plasma samples should be carefully thawed at 37° C and kept at room temperature for <2 hours before assay.

Sample storage: Plasma samples that will be stored or transported to a reference laboratory must be frozen promptly at or below −40° C and remain frozen until assayed. A control sample that is drawn, processed, stored, and transported under the same conditions as the tested person's sample may be helpful in indicating problems in the handling of important test samples. Activity of FVIII typically is 10% to 20% lower in frozen-thawed plasma than in fresh (nonfrozen) plasma and can be even lower if blood processing or storage conditions are suboptimal.

Laboratory testing: Calibrators for assays of VWF:Ag, VWF:RCo, and FVIII should be referenced to the WHO plasma standard. These three tests have relatively high coefficients of variation (CVs of 10%-30%), especially the VWF:RCo assay. The quality of laboratory testing also varies considerably among laboratories (high interlaboratory CV). Test results can be reported as international units per deciliter (IU/dL) rather than as a percentage (%) of mean normal, if WHO-linked calibrators are used. Referencing VWF testing results to the population reference range, rather than to ABO-stratified reference ranges, may be clinically useful.

CV = coefficient of variation; FVIII = coagulation factor VIII; VWF = Von Willebrand factor; VWF:Ag = VWF antigen; VWF:RCo = VWF ristocetin cofactor activity; WHO = World Health Organization.
Adapted and modified from National Heart, Lung, and Blood Institute. *The Diagnosis, Evaluation, and Management of von Willebrand Disease.* Bethesda, MD: National Institutes of Health Publication 08-5832. December 2007 (released February 29, 2008), and Nichols WL, Rick ME, Ortel TL, et al. Clinical and laboratory diagnosis of von Willebrand disease: a synopsis of the 2008 NHLBI/NIH guidelines. *Am J Hematol.* 2009;84:366-370.

have limited availability and are mainly performed in reference laboratories. Consultation with a hemostasis specialist can help guide test selection.

Multimer analysis visualizes the distribution of plasma VWF multimers, is technically complex, is qualitatively interpreted in conjunction with results of the initial three tests and available clinical information, and is used to help determine the VWD subtype. Therefore, VWF multimer analysis is not recommended for initial VWD screening and should only be performed if initial VWD testing identifies an abnormal result (e.g., abnormally low VWF:RCo or ratio of VWF:RCo to VWF:Ag) or clinical information suggests a high likelihood of abnormal VWF multimer analysis.

Table 173-2 provides prototypical laboratory values for VWD subtypes. Diagnosis, especially for individuals with mildly decreased VWF (30%-50% IU/dL), requires correlation of clinical assessment (personal and family history of bleeding) and results of laboratory testing, the latter preferably performed or repeated in the absence of conditions associated with elevation of baseline VWF and with careful attention to blood specimen collection, processing, transportation, and storage.

The laboratory evaluation of a person with possible VWD or AVWS is relatively complex, particularly because results of the laboratory tests can be influenced by certain conditions of the patient and by variables in the blood sample and laboratory testing methodology (Table 173-3). In interpreting test results, therefore, it is important to be aware of these variabilities and the status of the patient at the time of evaluation.

TREATMENT

Rx

Management of patients with VWD is focused on treatment or prevention of bleeding episodes. Three main approaches to treatment of VWD are used individually or in combination: (1) increasing plasma concentration of VWF and FVIII by releasing endogenous VWF stores through stimulation of endothelial cells with DDAVP (desmopressin: 1-desamino-8-D-arginine vasopressin); (2) replacing or supplementing VWF and FVIII by using human plasma-derived, viral-inactivated concentrates; and (3) promoting hemostasis using hemostatic agents that work by mechanisms other than increasing VWF and FVIII. Regular prophylaxis is seldom required, and treatment is given primarily before and after planned invasive procedures or in response to episodes of bleeding. Table 173-4 outlines usual durations of treatment for a variety of surgical and other invasive procedures.

TABLE 173-4 SUGGESTED DURATIONS OF VON WILLEBRAND FACTOR REPLACEMENT FOR DIFFERENT TYPES OF SURGICAL PROCEDURES

MAJOR SURGERY 7-14 DAYS*	MINOR SURGERY 1-5 DAYS*	OTHER PROCEDURES: IF UNCOMPLICATED, SINGLE VWF TREATMENT
Cardiothoracic	Biopsy: breast, cervical	Cardiac catheterization
Cesarean section	Complicated dental extractions	Cataract surgery
Craniotomy	Gingival surgery	Endoscopy (without biopsy)
Hysterectomy	Central line placement	Liver biopsy
Open cholecystectomy	Laparoscopic procedures	Lacerations
Prostatectomy		Simple dental extractions

*Individual cases may need longer or shorter duration depending on the severity of Von Willebrand disease and the type of procedure.
VWF = Von Willebrand factor.
Adapted and modified from National Heart, Lung, and Blood Institute. *The Diagnosis, Evaluation, and Management of von Willebrand Disease.* Bethesda, MD: National Institutes of Health Publication 08-5832. December 2007 (released February 29, 2008).

TABLE 173-5 INITIAL DOSING RECOMMENDATIONS FOR VON WILLEBRAND FACTOR CONCENTRATE REPLACEMENT FOR PREVENTION OR MANAGEMENT OF BLEEDING

MAJOR SURGERY/BLEEDING

Loading dose*: 40-60 U/kg
Maintenance dose†: 20-40 U/kg every 8 to 24 hours
Monitoring: VWF:RCo and FVIII trough and peak at least daily
Therapeutic goal: trough VWF:RCo and FVIII >50 IU/dL for 7-14 days
Safety parameter: do not exceed VWF:RCo >200 IU/dL or FVIII >250-300 IU/dL
May alternate with DDAVP for latter part of treatment

MINOR SURGERY/BLEEDING

Loading dose*: 30-60 U/kg
Maintenance dose†: 20-40 U/kg every 12 to 48 hours
Monitoring: VWF:RCo and FVIII trough and peak at least once
Therapeutic goal: trough VWF:RCo and FVIII >50 IU/dL for 3-5 days
Safety parameter: do not exceed VWF:RCo >200 IU/dL or FVIII >250-300 IU/dL
May alternate with DDAVP for latter part of treatment

*Loading dose is in VWF:RCo IU/dL.
†Dosing intervals reflect approximately 12-hour average half-lives of plasma VWF and FVIII without conditions resulting in shortened survival or enhanced clearance such as bleeding or surgery.
DDAVP = desmopressin: 1-desamino-8-D-arginine vasopressin; FVIII = factor VIII; VWF = Von Willebrand factor; VWF:RCo = VWF ristocetin cofactor activity.
Adapted and modified from National Heart, Lung, and Blood Institute. *The Diagnosis, Evaluation, and Management of von Willebrand Disease.* Bethesda, MD: National Institutes of Health Publication 08-5832. December 2007 (released February 29, 2008).

Desmopressin (DDAVP)

DDAVP is a synthetic derivative of the antidiuretic hormone and causes release of preformed VWF from endothelial cells. It is mainly used in type 1 VWD; is contraindicated for type 2B VWD (because it can cause thrombocytopenia); has limited efficacy for types 2A, 2M, or 2N VWD; and has no efficacy for type 3 VWD. DDAVP is generally administered for short time periods (48-72 hours) and usually not more frequently than at 24- to 48-hour intervals, owing to tachyphylaxis and side effects. If it is required for longer periods or more frequently, the patient should be monitored for fluid and electrolyte problems because DDAVP may cause symptomatic hyponatremia. DDAVP therapy is potentially mildly thrombogenic, especially for persons who are at increased risk for atherosclerotic cardiovascular disorders such as stroke or myocardial infarction.

The hemostatic dose of DDAVP is 0.3 μg/kg body weight infused intravenously over about 30 minutes or administered subcutaneously; however, a concentrated formulation for the latter is not available in the United States. For outpatients, DDAVP can also be administered nasally using a concentrated spray (Stimate, CSL Behring) that delivers 150 μg per nostril (300 μg total dose for persons ≥50 kg body weight). Peak increments of plasma VWF and FVIII occur about 1 to 2 hours after DDAVP, typically reaching two- to fourfold higher levels than at baseline, and decline toward baseline during the next 24 hours, reflecting VWF and FVIII plasma half-lives that are about 12 hours on average. However, plasma half-lives depend on the specific VWF subtype and phenotype and also vary considerably among individuals. Because of variability in response, before therapy with DDAVP, it is important to perform a treatment trial with pharmacokinetic monitoring of VWF and FVIII, measuring baseline (pre-DDAVP) and peak (~1 hour post-DDAVP) levels, supplemented with testing about 4 to 6 hours after DDAVP if a shortened survival of endogenous VWF is a consideration. A DDAVP treatment trial with extended monitoring can also help diagnose VWD variants with intrinsically heightened VWF clearance. Because of the problem of rapid tachyphylaxis, the trial of DDAVP should be performed at least 1 to 2 weeks before an elective procedure.

Factor Replacement Therapy

Alphanate SD/HT (Grifols), Humate-P (CSL Behring), and Wilate (Octapharma) are U.S. Food and Drug Administration–approved plasma-derived VWF concentrates for treatment of VWD by intravenous infusions. They also contain FVIII but differ in VWF/FVIII ratios and in content of large (high-molecular-weight) VWF multimers. Other VWF-containing concentrates include Koate-DVI (Talecris) and Wilfactin (LFB, France), which lacks FVIII (endogenous levels of which should rise secondarily within a few hours after infusion) and is not available in the United States. Cryoprecipitate is no longer recommended for VWF (or for FVIII) replacement, and its use should be limited to urgent situations when VWF concentrates are not available.

Table 173-5 outlines dosing and laboratory monitoring recommendations for treatment or prevention of bleeding in patients with VWD. Whenever possible, particularly for individuals with more severe forms of VWD, major surgeries or bleeding events should be managed in hospitals with appropriate laboratory capability and clinical staff, including a hematologist and a surgeon skilled in the management of bleeding disorders.

Other Hemostatic Agents

Treatment with combined oral contraceptive pills can ameliorate menorrhagia in women with VWD, mediated partly by hormonal effects on uterine tissues as well as by elevating blood levels of VWF and FVIII. Contraceptive hormonal skin patches have similar effects, and either type of therapy can also increase the risk for thromboembolic events. The levonorgestrel-releasing intrauterine device is an alternative to oral or skin-patch hormonal agents. For pregnancy and delivery in women with VWD, it is important to ensure that VWF and FVIII levels are normalized at the time of delivery, either spontaneously (which often occurs) or by therapy, including before administration of epidural anesthesia and postpartum.

ACQUIRED VON WILLEBRAND SYNDROME

Acquired von Willebrand syndrome refers to deficiencies or defects in VWF concentration, structure, or function that are not inherited but are consequences of other medical disorders. AVWS is less common than congenital (hereditary) VWD and is typically associated with several different mechanisms and medical conditions (Table 173-6).

Laboratory findings in AVWS are similar to those in congenital VWD (types 1, 2A, or 3). Although VWF:RCo values are typically decreased in AVWS (with variably decreased VWF:Ag or FVIII), sometimes only VWF multimer analysis is abnormal, with mild to moderate reduction or loss of the highest-molecular-weight (largest) multimers. This latter situation is more likely for AVWS associated with enhanced VWF proteolysis reflecting shear-induced conformational changes in VWF leading to increased proteolysis of VWF by ADAMTS13, such as with severe aortic valvular stenosis and other conditions causing abnormally high shear forces somewhere in the circulation (see Table 173-6).[8] Heyde's syndrome refers to AVWS caused by severe aortic stenosis and accompanied by GI bleeding from arteriovenous malformations (AVMs).

Acquired von Willebrand syndrome and disorders causing it should be considered in individuals found to have abnormal VWF test results and bleeding symptoms without a personal or family history consistent with hereditary VWD. Conversely, when bleeding occurs in association with one of the known causative conditions listed in Table 173-6, AVWS should be considered and initial VWD testing performed if indicated.

TREATMENT Rx

Treatment of AVWS should be focused first on elimination or amelioration of the associated causative disorder, if amenable to treatment (e.g., aortic valve replacement or repair for Heyde's syndrome). Survival of both endogenous

TABLE 173-6 CAUSES OF ACQUIRED VON WILLEBRAND SYNDROME

PATHOPHYSIOLOGIC CATEGORY*	DISEASE OR ASSOCIATION
Antibodies to VWF	Monoclonal gammopathies, lymphoproliferative disorders, or autoimmune diseases such as SLE
Shear-induced VWF conformational changes leading to increased proteolysis of VWF	Aortic valvular stenosis, VSD, hypertrophic obstructive cardiomyopathy, LVAD, or primary pulmonary hypertension
Markedly elevated blood platelet count	Essential thrombocythemia, polycythemia vera, myeloid metaplasia with myelofibrosis, or other myeloproliferative neoplasms
Removal of VWF from circulation by aberrant binding to tumor cells	Wilms' tumor and certain lymphoproliferative or plasma cell proliferative disorders
Decreased VWF synthesis	Hypothyroidism
Drugs associated with AVWS	Ciprofloxacin, valproic acid, hydroxyethyl starch, griseofulvin

*Pathophysiologic categories are listed in descending order of approximate prevalence.
AVWS = acquired von Willebrand syndrome; LVAD = left ventricular assist device; SLE = systemic lupus erythematosus; VWF, von Willebrand factor; VSD = ventricular septal defect.
Adapted and modified from Nichols WL, Rick ME, Ortel TL, et al. Clinical and laboratory diagnosis of von Willebrand disease: a synopsis of the 2008 NHLBI/NIH guidelines. *Am J Hematol.* 2009;84:366-370.

and infused VWF is often shortened in AVWS, and replacement therapy should be monitored with measurement of plasma VWF (VWF:RCo and VWF:Ag) and FVIII. For AVWS caused by monoclonal gammopathy of undetermined significance, intravenous immunoglobulin infusion may temporarily normalize plasma VWF and FVIII and stop abnormal bleeding by abrogating heightened VWF clearance. However, such treatment reflects an off-label product use.

BLEEDING CAUSED BY QUALITATIVE PLATELET DISORDERS

Hereditary Platelet Bleeding Disorders

Hereditary defects in platelet function can occur at all stages of the linked sequence of events involved in hemostatic platelet activation at sites of vascular injury, as described in Chapter 171: (1) platelet adhesion (Bernard-Soulier syndrome [BSS]), (2) platelet release reaction (storage pool disorders), and (3) platelet aggregation (Glanzmann thrombasthenia [GT]).[9,10] They lead to varying levels of severity of bleeding.

BERNARD-SOULIER SYNDROME AND GLANZMANN THROMBASTHENIA

These rare, autosomally recessive platelet hypofunctional disorders typically manifest moderately severe (minimally provoked or spontaneous) mucocutaneous bleeding symptoms during childhood and beyond as well as abnormal bleeding with hemostatic challenges such as surgery. BSS results from deficiency or dysfunction of the platelet membrane glycoprotein (GP) Ib-IX-V complex that is the principal receptor for binding VWF, mediating platelet adhesion to injured blood vessels. (In some ways, therefore, BSS is the platelet counterpart of VWD as an adhesion defect, the latter being caused by an abnormality in the plasma VWF rather than the platelets.) GT reflects deficiency or dysfunction of the platelet GPIIb-IIIa complex that is the principal receptor for binding plasma fibrinogen, mediating platelet aggregation. The platelet count and morphology are normal in GT, but BSS demonstrates moderate thrombocytopenia and enlarged (giant) platelets. BT or PFA-100 test results are typically markedly abnormal in both disorders but are nonspecific. Platelet aggregometry findings are usually diagnostic. BSS demonstrates an absence of aggregation response to ristocetin, but responses to other agonists are relatively normal. Conversely, GT demonstrates relatively normal response to ristocetin, contrasting with complete absence of aggregation response to other agonists, such as adenosine diphosphate, collagen, arachidonic acid, and epinephrine. Quantitative analysis of platelet membrane GPs by flow cytometry is evolving as a supplemental diagnostic tool for BSS and GT. Mutational DNA-based testing is primarily a research tool.

PLATELET STORAGE POOL DISORDERS

Platelet dense (δ) granule storage pool deficiency (DG-SPD) is more common than BSS and GT. Inheritance is typically autosomal recessive or occasionally dominant, with evolving understanding of different mutational causes. Bleeding symptoms are usually mild but may be clinically significant. Hermansky-Pudlak syndrome (HPS) is oculocutaneous albinism associated with platelet DG-SPD, with a propensity to develop pulmonary fibrosis or granulomatous colitis. DG-SPD can accompany some other hereditary disorders such as the X-linked Wiskott-Aldrich syndrome, in which it is associated with microthrombocytopenia, or Chédiak-Higashi syndrome with partial albinism and leukocyte inclusions. Isolated DG-SPD, including HPS, demonstrates normal platelet count and morphology by peripheral blood smear review. Results of BT, PFA-100, or platelet aggregometry testing may or may not be abnormal. Platelet content and secretion of adenosine triphosphate are decreased in DG-SPD, and platelet electron microscopy can diagnostically confirm absence or marked decrease of dense granules; however, these tests have limited availability.

Platelet α-granule deficiency manifests as the gray platelet syndrome, which is typically autosomal recessive in inheritance and may result in mild bleeding symptoms. Moderate thrombocytopenia is present, and peripheral blood smear review is usually diagnostic, demonstrating enlarged platelets that are "gray" (absence of granulomere staining, reflecting absence of α granules and their contents that include VWF). X chromosome–linked mutations of *GATA1*, the gene encoding a transcription factor essential for erythropoiesis and megakaryocytopoiesis, can cause a gray platelet syndrome–like disorder affecting males.

OTHER HEREDITARY PLATELET HYPOFUNCTIONAL DISORDERS

Hereditary platelet secretion disorders (defective release of α- and δ-granule contents without granule deficiency) comprise a variety of abnormalities affecting different platelet receptors or mechanisms of signal transduction and platelet activation, including defective platelet procoagulant activity, with or without thrombocytopenia or other syndromic features, and with variable bleeding propensity and symptoms. Some of these disorders are reviewed in Chapter 172.

TREATMENT Rx

For treating or preventing major bleeding events (e.g., certain surgical challenges), judicious use of platelet transfusion may be indicated for patients with more severe hereditary platelet bleeding disorders such as BSS and GT. To reduce the risk for platelet alloimmunization, single-donor apheresis platelet concentrates are preferred when available, and HLA-matched transfusions may sometimes be indicated. DDAVP administration has been reported to improve hemostasis in patients with DG-SPD, BSS, and some other hereditary platelet disorders. Treatment with recombinant activated coagulation factor VII (NovoSeven, NovoNordisk) has been reported as an alternative or salvage therapy for bleeding in GT and certain other platelet hypofunctional disorders. Antifibrinolytic therapy with epsilon-aminocaproic acid or tranexamic acid can be useful for dental extractions or for surgical procedures involving other tissues with high intrinsic fibrinolytic activity (e.g., nose, mouth and throat, extraocular tissues).[11]

Acquired Platelet Bleeding Disorders

DRUGS

Drugs are a relatively common cause of platelet hypofunction that can result in mild bleeding symptoms, particularly if other bleeding propensities are present, such as thrombocytopenia.[12] Aspirin, thienopyridines (e.g., clopidogrel, prasugrel, ticagrelor), dipyridamole, and inhibitors of platelet GPIIb/IIIa function are used therapeutically or prophylactically for atherosclerotic cardiovascular disorders such as coronary artery or cerebrovascular disease. In addition to aspirin, other NSAIDs can inhibit platelet arachidonic acid metabolism (Chapter 37) and contribute to bleeding. Other agents that may sometimes impair platelet function include certain selective serotonin reuptake inhibitors or antibiotics and some herbal or nutritional supplements. Laboratory testing for platelet hypofunction is not often indicated and may not yield diagnostic findings.

OTHER ACQUIRED PLATELET BLEEDING DISORDERS

Myelodysplastic and myeloproliferative disorders can sometimes manifest intrinsic platelet hypofunction disproportionate to thrombocytopenia or thrombocytosis when they are present. Cirrhosis or liver failure can cause platelet hypofunction as well as thrombocytopenia. Uremia may induce platelet hypofunction that can be ameliorated by dialysis and erythropoietin therapy. Antibodies causing autoimmune thrombocytopenia (Chapter 172) can sometimes cause acquired platelet hypofunction (e.g., acquired GT or BSS) in addition to the low platelet count.

TREATMENT

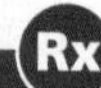

Review of patient medications and medical conditions and modifications of them when feasible and indicated can often suffice for recognition and management of acquired platelet hypofunctional disorders.

VASCULAR HEMORRHAGIC DISORDERS

Hereditary Vascular Hemorrhagic Disorders

Hereditary hemorrhagic telangiectasia, also called Osler-Weber-Rendu syndrome, is an autosomal dominant vascular disorder characterized by development of telangiectases and AVMs in the skin, mucous membranes, and certain viscera (especially the central nervous system, lung, and liver), with a propensity for severe recurring nosebleeds and GI bleeds resulting in chronic anemia and iron deficiency.[13] The diagnosis primarily relies on physical examination (Fig. 173-1). Several mutations in two genes have been described: endoglin in HHT type 1 and activin receptor-like kinase-1 (*ALK1*) in HHT type 2. These genes encode proteins that modulate transforming growth factor-β signaling in vascular endothelial cells, and mutations in them in HHT lead to the development of fragile telangiectatic vessels and AVMs. Molecular DNA-based testing has limited availability. Supportive treatment includes supplemental iron therapy for iron deficiency anemia. Among 24 patients with HHT, severe hepatic vascular malformations, and high cardiac output, bevacizumab (5 mg/kg every 14 days for a total of six injections) normalized the cardiac index in 20 of 24 patients (complete response in three; partial response in 17), with concomitant reductions in epistaxis and improvements in quality of life.[14] Tranexamic acid (1 gram three times daily) is effective for reducing recurrent epistaxis[A1], and intranasal administration is also being studied. In a small randomized trial, tamoxifen (20 mg per day for 6 months) also significantly reduced bleeding in patients with recurrent epistaxis.[A2]

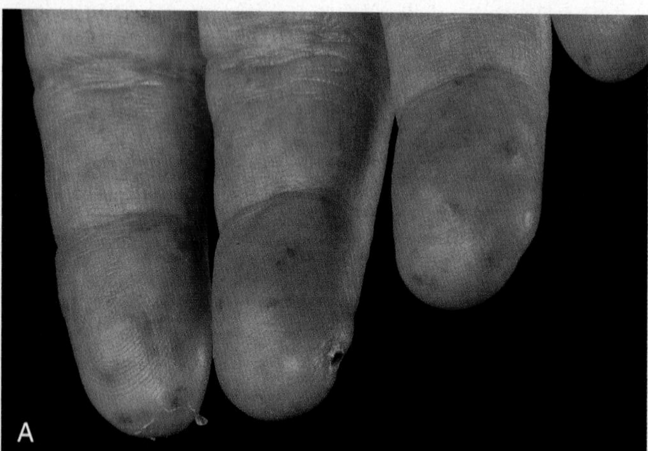

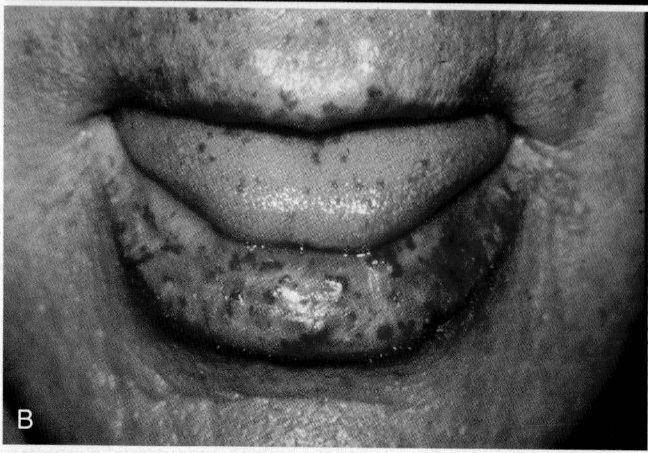

FIGURE 173-1. **Hereditary hemorrhagic telangiectasia (HHT).** Telangiectasias commonly occur on the fingers (A); face, lips, and tongue (B); and in other areas, including the nasal and gastrointestinal mucosa, and may develop in certain other internal organs. Skin or mucous membrane lesions typically blanch with pressure in contrast to petechiae, which do not. (A, Copyrighted and used with permission of the Mayo Foundation for Medical Education and Research, all rights reserved. B, Courtesy of Dr. Andrew Schafer.)

Ehlers-Danlos syndrome (Chapter 260) is caused by mutations in genes encoding fibrillar collagen or related genes and includes at least six subtypes that vary in clinical manifestations, severity, and prognosis.[15] Inheritance is primarily autosomal dominant. Principal manifestations of Ehlers-Danlos syndrome include skin or joint hyperextensibility, with an associated bleeding tendency including easy bruisability (purpura), surgical bleeding, poor wound healing, and menorrhagia in women. Diagnosis depends mainly on physical examination, supplemented with molecular DNA-based testing that currently has limited availability.

Acquired Vascular Hemorrhagic Disorders

Systemic amyloidosis, Waldenström macroglobulinemia, and cryoglobulinemia are dysproteinemic disorders reflecting monoclonal gammopathies or hyperglobulinemias (Chapters 187 and 188) that can manifest purpuric or other bleeding symptoms caused by either vascular deposition of immunoglobulin fragments (amyloidosis) or inhibition of platelet-vessel hemostatic functions by immunoglobulins.[16] Henoch-Schönlein purpura (Chapter 270) is primarily a transient disease of children that typically presents with a palpable purpuric rash of the lower extremities, arthralgias, abdominal pain and renal symptoms (hematuria, proteinuria) in some cases, manifestations of a systemic vasculitis characterized by deposition of immunoglobulin A–containing immune complexes in the skin, GI tract, and kidneys. Palpable purpura can also result from systemic sepsis or disseminated intravascular coagulation. Scurvy (Chapter 218) is caused by the effects of vitamin C deficiency on collagen structure and often presents with bruising or petechiae, including tiny perifollicular hemorrhages. Senile purpura or purpura simplex is thought to reflect partly the age-related changes of skin vascular structure and is typified by easy bruisability of the dorsa of the hands, forearms, and lower legs. Psychogenic purpuras are controversial entities that include Gardner-Diamond syndrome, which is characterized by recurring focal pain preceding development of ecchymoses, believed to reflect poorly understood psychosomatic mechanisms. It can be difficult to differentiate this rare syndrome from factitious or self-induced purpura and bleeding.

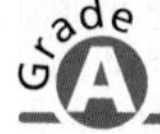

Grade A References

A1. Gaillard S, Dupuis-Girod S, Boutitie F, et al. Tranexamic acid for epistaxis in hereditary hemorrhagic telangiectasia patients: a European cross-over controlled trial in a rare disease. *J Thromb Haemost*. 2014;12:1494-1502.

A2. Yaniv E, Preis M, Hadar T, et al. Antiestrogen therapy for hereditary hemorrhagic telangiectasia: a double-blind placebo-controlled clinical trial. *Laryngoscope*. 2009;119:284-288.

GENERAL REFERENCES

For the General References and other additional features, please visit Expert Consult at https://expertconsult.inkling.com.

174 HEMORRHAGIC DISORDERS: COAGULATION FACTOR DEFICIENCIES

MARGARET V. RAGNI

COAGULATION DEFICIENCIES

Severe coagulation factor deficiencies, or coagulopathies, are typically characterized by spontaneous or traumatic bleeding, such as during surgery or trauma, and may result in life- or limb-threatening complications. By contrast, moderate and mild coagulopathies may remain clinically silent until they are detected coincidentally on routine laboratory screening tests (e.g., prothrombin time [PT], activated partial thromboplastin time [aPTT]) or when these tests are ordered to evaluate the cause of abnormal bleeding or bruising. Much of the morbidity of coagulopathies can be minimized or avoided altogether by prophylactic replacement of the deficient clotting factor proteins. In contrast to the lifelong clinical manifestations of hereditary or congenital coagulopathies, acquired coagulation deficiencies usually appear acutely in previously asymptomatic individuals; they may not be suspected and often remit spontaneously or after eradication of an inciting disease state or withdrawal of an offending medication. Acquired coagulation deficiencies may be associated with more severe bleeding than congenital deficiencies, in part because of the delay in diagnosis. In general, coagulation factor deficiencies may result from inadequate synthesis of coagulation factor proteins or from inhibition of activated clotting factor proteins by acquired antibodies or anticoagulant medications. Finally, qualitative defects of coagulation factors, either congenital or acquired, may also result in bleeding.

Hereditary Hemophilias

DEFINITION

The hemophilias include hemophilia A and hemophilia B, caused by deficiencies or defects in clotting factor VIII (antihemophilic factor) and factor IX (antihemophilic factor B, or Christmas factor), respectively. A deficiency of either of these intrinsic coagulation pathway proteins results in inadequate formation of thrombin at sites of vascular injury.

EPIDEMIOLOGY

Hemophilia A and B are sex-linked recessive disorders estimated to occur in 1 in 5000 and 1 in 30,000 male births, respectively. The higher incidence of hemophilia A may be due to the greater amount of DNA "at risk" for mutation in the factor VIII gene (186,000 base pairs) compared with the factor IX gene (34,000 base pairs). Hemophilia A and B are observed in all racial and ethnic groups, and in the United States, more than 20,000 individuals are affected. Although carrier testing, genetic counseling, and prenatal diagnosis are widely available in the United States through the network of federally funded hemophilia treatment centers (HTCs), fecundity rates remain high, and few confirmed carriers elect to terminate their pregnancies, even if an affected fetus is detected in utero. These decisions are likely influenced by the wide availability of safe and effective coagulation factor replacement concentrates and by the prospect of an eventual cure for the hemophilias through gene transfer. A substantial proportion (30%) of hemophilia cases arise as new, spontaneous mutations. Overall, the hemophilias are much more common than the autosomal recessive coagulation factor deficiencies (see later), which often affect progeny from consanguineous relationships and require the inheritance of two defective alleles for the bleeding manifestations to become evident.

PATHOBIOLOGY

Genetics

As with other sex-linked recessive diseases, the genes for factor VIII and factor IX are located on the long arm of the X chromosome. Males with a defective allele on their single X chromosome transmit this gene to all their daughters, who are obligate carriers, but to none of their sons. Because the offspring of female carriers inherit one affected X chromosome, half of their sons develop the coagulation disorder, and half of their daughters are obligate carriers. Female carriers may manifest bleeding symptoms, particularly postpartum bleeding, if the alleles on the X chromosome are unequally inactivated (lyonization); the defective hemophilic allele is expressed in preference to the normal allele, plasma factor VIII levels are below 50%, and phenotypic hemophilia results. Female hemophilia may arise as a result of mating between a hemophilic male and a female carrier (homozygous for the defective factor VIII or IX gene) or in carrier females who have the 45,XO karyotype (Turner syndrome) and are hemizygous for the defective hemophilia gene.

No single mutation is responsible for the hemophilias. Many missense and nonsense point mutations, deletions, and inversions have been described. Severe molecular defects predominate, with 40 to 50% of all cases of severe hemophilia A evolving from a unique inversion of intron 22 (the largest of the factor VIII introns). This inversion results from the recombination and translocation of DNA within intron 22 of the factor VIII gene, with areas of extragenic but homologous "nonfunctional" DNA located at a distance from intron 22. Other less common severe molecular defects include large gene deletions (5 to 10% of cases) and nonsense mutations (10 to 15% of cases). The encoded proteins resulting from these mutations are defective and do not express any factor VIII activity. Mild or moderate hemophilia A is commonly associated with point mutations and deletions. In contrast, factor IX mutations are more diverse, and severe hemophilia B is more likely caused by large deletions. Mutated clotting factor genes responsible for the hemophilias may also encode for the production of defective nonfunctional proteins that circulate in the plasma and are detected at normal quantitative levels by immunoassays but not by functional assays. A listing of the mutations that cause the hemophilias can be accessed through the Human Gene Mutation Database (www.hgmd.org).

CLINICAL MANIFESTATIONS

Hemophilia A and hemophilia B are said to be clinically indistinguishable, with clinical severity corresponding inversely to the circulating levels of plasma coagulant factor VIII or IX activity, respectively. However, several studies have found a higher bleeding frequency, greater factor use, and more frequent hospitalizations in hemophilia A, suggesting greater clinical severity than hemophilia B. Individuals with less than 1% of normal factor VIII or IX activity are classified as having "severe" disease, characterized by frequent spontaneous bleeding events in joints (hemarthrosis) and soft tissues and by profuse hemorrhage with trauma or surgery. Although spontaneous bleeding is uncommon in mild deficiencies (>5% normal activity), excess bleeding typically occurs with trauma or surgery. A moderate clinical course is associated with factor VIII or IX levels between 1 and 5%. Approximately 60% of all cases of hemophilia A are clinically severe, whereas only 20 to 45% of cases of hemophilia B are severe.

Severe hemophilia is typically suspected and diagnosed during infancy in the absence of a family history. Among newborns, intracranial hemorrhage is the leading cause of morbidity and mortality, with a cumulative incidence of 3.8%, according to data collected by the Centers for Disease Control and Prevention. Intracranial hemorrhage does not appear to be related to the mode of delivery, although half of such hemorrhages occur in the newborn period. Current guidelines suggest cesarean section delivery be considered for any known male infants with severe hemophilia A. Vacuum extraction may increase cephalohematoma formation and is discouraged. Circumcision within days after birth is accompanied by excessive bleeding in less than half of severely affected boys. The first spontaneous hemarthrosis in severely affected hemophiliacs usually occurs between 9 and 18 months of age, when ambulation begins; in moderately affected individuals, it generally does not occur until 2 to 5 years of age. The knees are the most prominent sites of spontaneous bleeds, followed by the elbows, ankles, shoulders, and hips; wrists are less commonly involved.

Acute hemarthroses (Fig. 174-1) originate from the subsynovial venous plexus underlying the joint capsule and produce a tingling or burning sensation, followed by the onset of intense pain and swelling. On physical examination, the joint is swollen, hot, and tender to palpation, with erythema of the overlying skin. Joint mobility is compromised by pain and stiffness, and the joint is usually maintained in a flexed position. Immediate or early replacement of the deficient clotting factor to normal hemostatic levels rapidly reverses the pain. Delayed treatment results in excess pain, morbidity, and joint damage. Optimal management includes *r*est, *i*ce, factor *c*oncentrate, and *e*levation (RICE). Swelling and joint immobility improve as the intra-articular hematoma resolves. Intra-articular needle aspiration of fresh blood is not recommended because of the risk for introducing infection. Short courses of oral corticosteroids may be helpful to reduce the acute joint symptoms in children but are rarely used in adults.

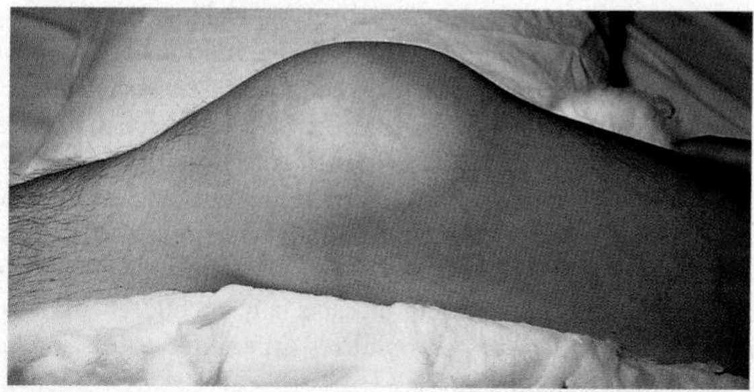

FIGURE 174-1. Acute hemarthrosis of the knee is a common complication of hemophilia. It may be confused with acute infection unless the patient's coagulation disorder is known because the knee is hot, red, swollen, and painful. (From Forbes CD, Jackson WF. *Color Atlas and Text of Clinical Medicine*, 3rd ed. London: Mosby; 2003.)

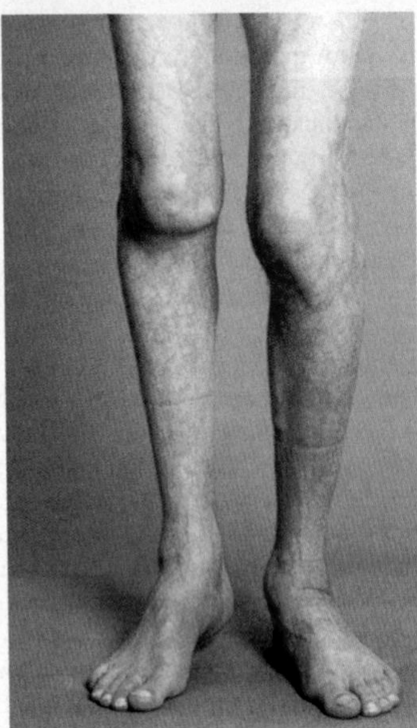

FIGURE 174-2. **Severe chronic arthritis in hemophilia. The knee is the most commonly affected joint. Both knees are severely deranged in this patient. Note that he is unable to stand with both feet flat on the floor. (From Forbes CD, Jackson WF. *Color Atlas and Text of Clinical Medicine*, 3rd ed. London: Mosby; 2003.)**

Recurrent or untreated bleeds result in chronic synovial hypertrophy and, eventually, damage to the underlying cartilage, with subsequent subchondral bone cyst formation, bony erosion, and flexion contractures. Abnormal mechanical forces from weight bearing can produce subluxation, misalignment, loss of mobility, and permanent deformities of the lower extremities (Fig. 174-2). These changes are accompanied by chronic pain, swelling, arthritis, and disability. Plain radiographs and clinical examination of chronic hemarthroses often underestimate the extent of bone and joint damage; serial magnetic resonance imaging is superior to radiography or computed tomography and is the most sensitive and specific means of detecting and monitoring early and progressive disease.

Intramuscular hematomas account for about 30% of hemophilia-related bleeding events and are rarely life threatening. They are usually precipitated by physical or iatrogenic trauma (e.g., after intramuscular injections) and may compromise sensory and motor function or arterial circulation if they entrap and compress vital structures in closed fascial compartments. The latter occurrence, termed *compartment syndrome*, presents with the rapid onset of swelling and severe pain in an extremity, unrelieved by factor infusion and standard analgesics. This is considered a medical emergency and may require fasciotomy to preserve tissue and provide pain relief. Retroperitoneal hematomas may be confused clinically with appendicitis or hip bleeds but should be suspected in a patient who is hunched over and unable to stand erect owing to the pain of muscle extension in the presence of hematoma. Unless these bleeding episodes are treated immediately and aggressively, permanent anatomic deformity, such as flexion contracture, nerve damage, or pseudotumor formation (expanding hematomas that erode and destroy adjacent skeletal structures), may occur. Bleeding from mucous membranes is very common and may be exaggerated by the degradation of fibrin clots by fibrinolytic enzymes contained in secretions. Bleeding involving the tongue or the retropharyngeal space may rapidly produce life-threatening compromise of the airway. Gastrointestinal hemorrhage typically originates from anatomic lesions proximal to the ligament of Treitz and may be exacerbated by esophageal varices secondary to cirrhosis and portal hypertension or by the use of nonsteroidal anti-inflammatory drugs (NSAIDs) for the treatment of hemarthroses. Spontaneous bleeding in the genitourinary tract secondary to hemophilia is a diagnosis of exclusion after ruling out renal stones and infection. Ureteral blood clots produce renal colic, which may be confused with nephrolithiasis and may be worsened by the use of antifibrinolytic agents. A short course of steroids may be helpful, especially in children, to hasten their resolution. Ninety percent of hemophiliacs experience at least one episode of gross hematuria or hemospermia.

Intracranial bleeds occur in 10% of patients, are usually induced by trauma, and may be fatal in 30% of cases. The risk for developing an intracranial hemorrhage is approximately 2% per year. Neuromuscular defects, seizure disorders, and intellectual deficits may ensue.

Individuals with hemophilia cared for at HTCs have lower mortality and reduced costs of care compared with those receiving treatment elsewhere. The chronic care model practiced at HTCs emphasizes prevention to reduce joint disease and complications, optimization of factor dosing, and counseling regarding safe sports and the avoidance of aspirin and other drugs that inhibit platelet function.

DIAGNOSIS

The diagnosis of hemophilia[1] is suspected on the basis of a family and personal bleeding history and laboratory detection of prolongation of the aPTT (with normal PT). It is confirmed by significantly reduced plasma factor VIII or IX activity. As noted in Chapter 171, the aPTT is not a sufficiently sensitive screening test to be prolonged in mild hemophiliacs, in whom the factor VIII level is sometimes greater than 30% of normal. Severe hemophilia is usually recognized in infancy, with circumcision bleeding; by contrast, moderate or mild disease is recognized later in life after trauma or surgery. Hemophilia can be distinguished from von Willebrand disease (VWD; Chapter 173) by normal ristocetin cofactor and von Willebrand factor (VWF) antigen levels. In type 2N VWD, factor VIII is significantly lower than ristocetin cofactor and VWF antigen levels because of reduced factor VIII binding; this variant of VWD may require genotyping to distinguish it from hemophilia A. Other congenital intrinsic factor deficiencies (e.g., factor XI and XII) can be determined by coagulation factor–specific assays. Vitamin K deficiency (see later and Chapter 175) can be detected by the associated PT prolongation; deficiencies of factors II, VII, IX, and X; and resolution of the coagulation defect with vitamin K. The presence of heparin can be confirmed by correction of the aPTT after running the sample over a heparin absorption column. Failure of the aPTT to correct in a 1 : 1 mix with normal plasma suggests the presence of an inhibitor; specific inhibitors are associated with a single decreased factor level (usually factor VIII; see Alloantibody Inhibitors to Factors VIII and IX under Treatment), whereas blocking inhibitors cause nonspecific factor level changes associated with a positive hexagonal lipid assay (see Antiphospholipid Syndrome and Lupus Anticoagulant later).

Although existing laboratory tests quantify the amount of factor in plasma, which is useful diagnostically and prognostically, these assays are limited in their ability to fully evaluate a patient's clot-forming capability. Newer, so-called global assays have the potential to more objectively measure the hemophilic phenotype as well as the response to treatment, especially in patients who develop inhibitors and in those for whom traditional coagulation tests cannot fully measure laboratory response to bypassing agents (see later); global assays such as thrombin-generation tests and viscoelastic assays await full validation in clinical practice.[2]

TREATMENT Rx

Treatment and prevention of acute bleeding events in hemophilia A and B are based on replacement of the missing or deficient clotting factor protein to restore adequate hemostasis (Table 174-1). The morbidity, mortality, and overall cost of care for individuals with hemophilia are reduced significantly if care is provided by comprehensive HTCs that have the multispecialty expertise and laboratory capabilities to coordinate and monitor specific patient needs.

The goal of replacement therapy (Table 174-1) is to achieve plasma factor VIII and IX activity levels of 25 to 30% for minor spontaneous or traumatic bleeds (e.g., hemarthroses, persistent hematuria), at least 50% clotting factor activity for the treatment or prevention of severe bleeds (e.g., major dental surgery, maintenance replacement therapy after major surgery or trauma), and 80 to 100% activity for any life-threatening or limb-threatening hemorrhagic event (e.g., major surgery, trauma). After major trauma or if visceral or intracranial bleeding is suspected, replacement therapy adequate to achieve 100% clotting factor activity should be administered *before* diagnostic procedures are initiated. To calculate the initial dose, plasma factor VIII activity generally increases about 2% (0.02 IU/mL) for each unit of factor VIII administered per kilogram of body weight, and factor IX activity increases about 1% (0.01 IU/mL) for each unit of factor IX administered per kilogram of body weight. Therefore, a 70-kg individual with severe hemophilia A or B (factor VIII or IX activity <1% of normal) who requires replacement to 100% activity for major surgery should initially receive 3500 IU of factor VIII or 7000 IU of factor IX concentrate. The circulating half-lives of factors VIII and IX require subsequent dosing at half the initial dose every 8 to 12 hours and every 18 to 24 hours, respectively. However, this empirical dosing (based on calculations) should be individualized according to the peak recovery increment within 10 to 15 minutes after bolus infusion, as well as trough activity levels. The frequency of repeat dosing is also determined by the rapidity of pain relief, recovery of joint function, and resolution of active bleeding. Replacement is usually maintained

TABLE 174-1 FDA-APPROVED COAGULATION PROTEINS AND REPLACEMENT THERAPIES AVAILABLE IN THE UNITED STATES

COAGULATION PROTEIN DEFICIENCY	INHERITANCE PATTERN	PREVALENCE	MINIMUM HEMOSTATIC LEVEL	REPLACEMENT SOURCES
Factor I (fibrinogen)			50-100 mg/dL	Cryoprecipitate, FFP, fibrinogen concentrate
Afibrinogenemia	Autosomal recessive	Rare (<300 families)		
Dysfibrinogenemia	Autosomal dominant or recessive	Rare (>300 variants)		
Factor II (prothrombin)	Autosomal dominant or recessive	1 in 2 million births	30% of normal	FFP, factor IX complex concentrates
Factor V (labile factor)	Autosomal recessive	1 in 1 million births	25% of normal	FFP
Factor VII	Autosomal recessive	1 in 500,000 births	25% of normal	Recombinant factor VIIa (15-20 µg/kg), FFP, factor IX complex concentrates
Factor VIII (antihemophilic factor)	X-linked recessive	1 in 5000 male births	80-100% for surgery/life-threatening bleeds, 50% for serious bleeds, 25-30% for minor bleeds	Factor VIII concentrates (recombinant preferred)
Von Willebrand disease (also see Chapter 173)			>50% VWF antigen and ristocetin cofactor activity	DDAVP for mild to moderate disease (except type 2B; variable response to 2A); cryoprecipitate and FFP (not preferred, except in emergencies); factor VIII/VWF concentrates, viral attenuated, intermediate purity (preferred for surgery, for disease unresponsive to DDAVP, and for type 3
Type 1 and 2 variants	Usually autosomal dominant	1% prevalence		
Type 3	Autosomal recessive	1 in 1 million births		
Factor IX (Christmas factor)	X-linked recessive	1 in 30,000 male births	25-50% of normal, depending on extent of bleeding, surgery	Factor IX concentrates (recombinant preferred); FFP not preferred except in dire emergencies
Factor X (Stuart-Prower factor)	Autosomal recessive	1 in 500,000 births	10-25% of normal	FFP or factor IX complex concentrates
Factor XI (hemophilia C)	Autosomal dominant; severe type is recessive	4% of Ashkenazi Jews; 1 in 1 million general population	20-40% of normal	FFP or factor XI concentrate
Factor XII (Hageman factor), prekallikrein, high-molecular-weight kininogen	Autosomal recessive	Not available	No treatment necessary	—
Factor XIII (fibrin stabilizing factor)	Autosomal recessive	1 in 3 million births	5% of normal	FFP, cryoprecipitate, or viral-attenuated factor XIII concentrate

DDAVP = desmopressin; FDA = U.S. Food and Drug Administration; FFP = fresh-frozen plasma; VWF = von Willebrand factor.

for 10 to 14 days after major surgery to allow proper wound healing. Bolus dosing typically results in wide fluctuations in clotting factor activity levels and requires frequent laboratory monitoring to avoid suboptimal troughs. A continuous infusion regimen, consisting of 1 to 2 IU of factor VIII or IX concentrate per kilogram per hour after a bolus dose, maintains a plateau level without the need for frequent laboratory testing. Continuous infusion also reduces total concentrate consumption by 30 to 75% in surgical settings. Ongoing and completed phase I/II/III clinical trials of long recombinant factors VIII and IX, pegylated or fused to albumin or to the Fc domain of immunoglobulin G1 (IgG1), indicate these proteins are safe, effective, and prolong half-life 1.5- to 2-fold for factor VIII and 2- to 4-fold for factor IX, suggesting they may allow simpler dosing schedules and fewer intravenous factor infusions. A completed phase III clinical trial of recombinant factor IX-Fc fusion protein (rFIXFc) in adults with severe hemophilia B has demonstrated safety, efficacy, and a 3-fold longer circulating half-life than recombinant factor IX, such that some patients were able to dose every 10 to 14 days.[3] Similarly, recombinant factor VIII-Fc (rFVIIIFc) is safe, effective, and has a 1.5-fold longer half-life than recombinant factor VIII, resulting in dosing every 3 to 5 days.

Because of the potential thrombogenicity associated with the repeated administration of prothrombin complex concentrates to replace factor IX deficiency, high-purity, plasma-derived, or genetically engineered factor IX concentrates, which lack activated vitamin K–dependent clotting factors, are preferred in hemophilia B.

Cryoprecipitate (a cold precipitate of fresh-frozen plasma [FFP] after thawing at 4°C) and FFP contain factor VIII, but only FFP contains factor IX. However, neither cryoprecipitate nor FFP is an optimal replacement product for either hemophilia A or hemophilia B because these agents may transmit blood-borne pathogens and require large-volume infusion. All clotting factor concentrates available in the United States (see Table 174-1), whether plasma derived or genetically engineered, are equally efficacious and are considered extremely safe; none has been implicated in the transmission of blood-borne viral pathogens or prions. The second- and third-generation recombinant factor VIII and IX concentrates are manufactured free of added human or animal proteins in the culture medium or in the final formulation, eliminating the theoretical risks for transmission of prions or murine viruses.

Hemarthroses

The moderate or severe pain that accompanies acute hemarthroses responds to immediate analgesic relief, temporary immobilization, restraint from weight bearing, and clotting factor replacement. Narcotic analgesics, such as codeine or synthetic derivatives of codeine, should be prescribed alone or combined with doses of acetaminophen that are low enough to avoid hepatic toxicity in patients with chronic hepatitis. Although these medications do not possess significant anti-inflammatory activity, they are preferable to NSAIDs or aspirin, which can exacerbate bleeding complications through their inhibition of platelet aggregation.

Strategies intended to prevent end-stage joint destruction should be initiated at an early age. Although prophylaxis beginning soon after the first bleed is the recommended approach (see later), most adults have not had the benefit of early prophylaxis and thus have advanced arthropathy with reduced motion, disability, and pain, for which surgery may be recommended. Synovectomy through open surgery or arthroscopy removes the inflamed tissue and should result in substantially decreased pain and less recurrent bleeding. Nonsurgical synovectomy (synoviorthosis), which involves the intra-articular administration of a radioisotope, is particularly useful for high-risk patients and for those with alloantibody inhibitors to factor VIII or IX (see later). The occurrence of leukemia in several hemophilic children undergoing radioisotopic synoviorthosis has raised concerns about potential leukemogenesis, especially given the low background rate of cancers in individuals with hemophilia. Neither synovectomy nor synoviorthosis reverses joint damage, but both procedures may delay its progression. Non-weight-bearing exercises, such as swimming and isometrics, are important to periarticular muscle development and maintenance of joint stability for ambulation. Intractable pain and severe joint destruction secondary to repeated hemorrhage require prosthetic replacement. Chronic ankle pain responds best to open surgical or arthroscopic fixation and fusion (arthrodesis).

The ultimate strategy to minimize or eliminate progressive joint destruction by recurrent hemarthroses is predicated on the concept of prophylaxis—the scheduled administration of clotting factor concentrates several times weekly (twice a week for factor IX, three times a week for factor VIII) at doses to maintain trough factor activity levels greater than 1 to 2% of normal. In a prospective, randomized clinical trial, the Joint Outcomes Trial, prophylaxis with factor VIII (25 IU/kg every other day) was superior to episodic therapy (on demand) in young children with severe hemophilia in reducing joint bleeding and joint damage as shown by magnetic resonance imaging and radiography.[A2] These findings were confirmed in older children in the ESPRIT trial,[A3] with the best outcomes when prophylaxis was initiated before 3 years of age. In several adult studies of two- or three-times-weekly prophylaxis at 20 to 80 IU/kg, there were significantly fewer joint bleeds and pain and better quality of life than in those on on-demand therapy.[A4] Although prophylaxis uses more factor product at greater expense, the benefits of long-term prophylaxis to promote joint health and avert disability have led to the recommendation that it be initiated in young children with severe disease at the time of the first bleed. Compliance with prophylaxis is not easy because it requires intravenous factor, which is invasive, burdensome, and in small children may require central venous access devices, which may be complicated by infection.

With the development of long-acting factor VIII and IX,[4] currently in clinical trials, infusion frequency and bleeds may decrease and access devices may be avoided entirely. Some unanswered questions include the minimal effective dose for prophylaxis in children, and the role of generic versus personal pharmacokinetic studies to optimize dosing. The risk for bleeding is thought to be related to the time spent at nadir factor levels less than 1% (0.01 IU/mL) between dosing. It is generally agreed that spontaneous bleeding may be averted by maintaining factor levels at 1% (0.01 U/mL) or greater.

Factor Concentrate–Transmitted Viral Infections

In contrast to other at-risk groups, individuals with hemophilia were exposed at a young age to transmissible agents through clotting factors. These include hepatitis C virus (HCV), leading to infection in 90% of those transfused from the late 1970s through the mid-1980s, and human immunodeficiency virus (HIV) infection in 80% of those transfused with factor VIII products and 50% of those transfused with factor IX products from 1978 through the mid-1980s. Overall, of those with HCV infection (Chapter 148), 40% have coinfection with HIV, and hepatitis C remains the leading cause of death in hemophilia. With the implementation of viral inactivation and recombinant technologies, viral transmission has been virtually eliminated in hemophiliacs born since the 1990s. Nevertheless, among those exposed to HCV, 25% have liver fibrosis, and those with HIV coinfection have a 1.4-fold greater fibrosis rate. Combined antiretroviral therapy (cART) has slowed the rate of HCV progression in coinfected patients to rates observed in HCV-monoinfected hemophilic men.

GB virus C (GBV-C), formerly known as hepatitis G virus, observed in 15 to 25% of hemophiliacs, is susceptible to current viral attenuation procedures. Hepatitis A and B vaccination have rendered viral infections with these agents rare in those with hemophilia, and although parvovirus B19 (Chapter 371) seroprevalence approaches 80% in older adult hemophiliacs exposed to plasma-derived products, the long-term clinical consequences remain unclear. Cadaver and living-donor liver transplantation (Chapter 154) has improved the survival of hemophilic men with chronic hepatitis-induced liver failure and has also resulted in the phenotypic cure of hemophilia, confirming that the liver is the predominant source of normal synthesis of factors VIII and IX. Liver transplantation is also performed successfully in HIV/HCV-coinfected patients on cART therapy, although HCV recurrence remains a universal problem.

Ancillary and Other Therapies

Ancillary treatment strategies for the hemophilias include antifibrinolytic agents, such as ε-aminocaproic acid (50 mg/kg 3 to 4 times daily) or tranexamic acid (3 or 4 g given orally daily in divided doses), to minimize mucous membrane bleeding, and the application of fibrin glue to bleeding sites. Desmopressin (DDAVP), which is also used in VWD (Chapter 173), can be administered by nasal insufflation 2 hours before a scheduled surgical procedure (one spray per nostril, to provide a total dose of 300 μg; or, in patients weighing less than 50 kg, 150 μg administered as a single spray); alternatively, DDAVP can be administered intravenously (dissolved in 50 mL normal saline) over 30 minutes at a dose of 0.3 μg/kg. DDAVP is useful in patients with mild hemophilia A because an adequate incremental rise in factor VIII activity can circumvent the use of clotting factor concentrates. Repeated administration of DDAVP (intravenously or by intranasal spray) may be complicated by facial flushing, tachyphylaxis, hyponatremic seizures (primarily in children), and, rarely, angina.

Alloantibody Inhibitors to Factors VIII and IX

Alloantibodies—that is, antibodies to "foreign" infused factor VIII or, less frequently, factor IX—are usually detected in childhood after a median of 9 to 12 days of exposure to clotting factor. These inhibitors occur preferentially in those with a family history of inhibitors; those with large, multidomain factor VIII and factor IX gene deletions; blacks; and Hispanics. Among blacks, gene sequence data suggest that mismatched factor VIII transfusions may account for the high inhibitor risk. Although hemophiliacs with major deletions of the factor VIII gene have a very high (up to 90%) prevalence of inhibitors, its prevalence in those with factor VIII gene missense mutations is low (<10%), as it is in those with intron 22 inversion (20%) even though the latter have severe hemophilia. Algorithms have been developed to stratify inhibitor risk for individuals and subpopulations. The incidence of factor VIII alloantibodies among hemophilia A patients is 15 to 25%, whereas the incidence of factor IX alloantibodies among hemophilia B patients is 1.5 to 3%. The latter is most common in Scandinavians and is also associated with anaphylaxis and nephrotic syndrome. Increasing evidence from the RODIN study suggests that although inhibitor risk appears to be unrelated to factor type (e.g., recombinant vs. plasma-derived), it is significantly associated with early high-intensity factor exposure (i.e., >3 to 5 days), especially in those with a family history or an at-risk mutation (e.g., a large deletion mutation).[5,6]

The development of an alloantibody inhibitor is suspected when replacement therapy is ineffective in controlling bleeding symptoms. These antibodies, typically of the IgG4 subclass, completely neutralize clotting factor activity and prevent or reduce any increment in factor VIII or IX levels following bolus infusions of concentrate. Characterized as time and temperature dependent, inhibitors are quantitated in Bethesda units (BU): by definition, 1 BU is the amount of inhibitor that neutralizes 50% of the specific clotting factor activity in normal plasma. "High responders," or patients with high-titer inhibitors (>5 BU), mount an anamnestic antibody response to factor VIII clotting factor protein, usually within 5 to 7 days after subsequent exposure, and are no longer responsive to infused factor VIII. By contrast, "low responders," or patients with low-titer inhibitors (≤5 BU), do not manifest anamnesis, and such low-titer inhibitors can easily be overwhelmed by large amounts of human factor VIII or factor IX concentrate and can be successfully treated with three to four times the usual factor dose.

Management of patients with high-titer inhibitors against factor VIII or IX is difficult, and no single approach is uniformly successful.[7] There are two components: first, assurance of hemostasis using "bypass therapy," and second, eradication of inhibitor formation. Hemostasis can be provided by "bypass" agents that are used to treat bleeding episodes (see Table 174-1); specifically, the activated prothrombin complex concentrate FEIBA VH (75 to 100 IU/kg initially, then 50 to 100 IU/kg every 6 to 8 hours) and recombinant factor VIIa (90 μ/kg every 2 to 3 hours) can be administered until bleeding is controlled. In studies of congenital hemophilia A patients with alloantibody inhibitors, one dose of FEIBA VH or two doses of recombinant factor VIIa controlled hemarthrosis episodes 81 and 79% of the time, respectively. The activated and unactivated prothrombin complex concentrates contain activated vitamin K–dependent clotting factors that "bypass" the intrinsic pathway (factor VIII or IX) inhibitor. As a result, repeated administration over a short time may be complicated by potential thrombogenicity: the aPTT and clotting factor assays are not helpful in monitoring hemostasis in these cases. In patients with high-titer inhibitors to factor VIII or IX, recombinant factor VIIa may achieve effective hemostasis, but its use is limited by the need for frequent intravenous dosing, usually every 2 hours to start. Although continuous dosing has been used in some patients, general experience dictates that for surgery or procedures in which significant bleeding is likely, bolus dosing is required to achieve optimal hemostasis—a so-called "thrombin burst." The product has also been effective in patients who experience anaphylactic reactions or nephrotic syndrome after exposure to factor IX–containing replacement products or fresh-frozen plasma (FFP). Several studies have shown that prophylactic treatment in adult inhibitor patients with either rFVIIa, 90 μg/kg daily or 270 μg/kg daily, or FEIBA, 85 IU/kg weekly, can significantly reduce bleeding rates compared with on-demand treatment.[A5]

Eradication of inhibitors is usually attempted with "immune tolerance induction" regimens,[8] which are generally effective if initiated within 12 months of the inhibitor's detection. Tolerance regimens consist of daily doses of factor concentrates to accomplish desensitization to infused factor, a process associated with a 68% success rate. In an international randomized trial of high-dose factor VIII (200 IU/kg daily) vs. low dose (50 IU/kg three times weekly) for immune tolerance induction (ITI) in young inhibitor patients, there was no difference in inhibitor eradication, but there was greater bleeding (mostly hematomas) in the low-dose arm.[A6] These findings suggest improved hemostasis may be possible in the high-dose arm, despite inhibitor detection. The authors also initiated ITI only after waiting for the inhibitor titer to drop below 10 BU because tolerance took longer to achieve the higher the inhibitor titer.[A6] After tolerance was achieved, prophylaxis with factor VIII or IX concentrate two or three times weekly (at 20 to 30 IU/kg) appears necessary to maintain tolerance. Individuals with inhibitors since childhood for whom immune tolerance was not possible before adulthood are unlikely to respond to ITI. Alternative single or combination immunosuppressive agents (e.g., rituximab, mycophenolate, or cyclosporine) may be used as alternative therapies but appear to be variably effective.[9]

PREVENTION

Carrier Detection and Prenatal Diagnosis

Carrier detection and prenatal diagnosis have become technically feasible, very sensitive, and widely available. Noninvasive prenatal diagnosis by use of microfluidic digital PCR of maternal plasma DNA is an emerging technique that is based on relative mutation dosage from a blood sample of a pregnant carrier with or without an affected fetus, which may detect hemophilia as early as the 11th week of gestation. The application of these diagnostic tools, however, is influenced by ethical, cultural, religious, economic, educational, and personal considerations. For instance, carrier detection is particularly useful in identifying women who may be at risk for hemorrhagic complications during the delivery process and male offspring who are particularly vulnerable to intracerebral bleeds at birth. Alternatively, these techniques can provide important information used to make difficult reproductive decisions. Genetic testing should be performed only following genetic counseling and with no patient coercion to accept such testing.

PROGNOSIS

The life expectancy of individuals with severe hemophilia is approaching that of the normal population. The age-matched death rate in hemophilia is 2.7-fold greater than that in the general population, although ischemic heart disease mortality is nearly 60% lower than in the general population. Life expectancy is related to the severity of hemophilia: the mortality rate of severely affected patients is 4- to 6-fold greater than that of patients with mild deficiency. Among those with alloantibody inhibitors, mortality rates are significantly higher than in noninhibitor patients. The three leading causes of death are hepatitis C, HIV/AIDS, and central nervous system bleeding. Hepatitis C, the leading cause of death, accounts for more than half of the deaths, whereas deaths from HIV have declined with the availability of cART therapy (Chapter 388). Among those with HIV/HCV coinfection, cART also slows the progression of HCV-related liver disease. Predictors of hepatitis C disease progression in hemophilia include alcohol use, the use of acetaminophen for pain relief of hemophilic arthropathy, hepatitis B surface antigenemia, and HIV coinfection. Bleeding also accounts for causes of death: the lifetime risk for intracranial hemorrhage is 2 to 8%, and although it is the leading cause of morbidity and mortality in the newborn period, prospective monitoring of central nervous system function continues to be a priority as the population ages. Finally, with the essential elimination of disease transmission through blood products in this population, the usual problems of aging are increasingly being recognized in those with hemophilia, including atherosclerosis, hypertension, hyperlipidemia, obesity, and diabetes. The impact of these conditions on the natural history of hemophilia, given the recognized lower mortality from ischemic heart disease, remains to be seen. More data are needed to help guide clinical management of these patients.

FUTURE DIRECTIONS

Gene Therapy for Hemophilia a and B

The hereditary hemophilias are model diseases for gene therapy because they are caused by specific, well-defined gene mutations; a small, incremental rise in clotting factor synthesis can lead to substantially improved treatment and quality of life; and inadvertent overexpression by successful gene transfer would not be detrimental. Successful gene transfer techniques have been developed to provide long-term therapeutic benefits in hemophilic mice and dog models, and early success is now being reported in humans. In one study of gene transfer using serotype-8 pseudotyped adeno-associated virus vector (AAV8) carrying a codon-optimized factor IX transgene, factor IX expression of 1 to 6% was achieved in hemophilia B patients, persisting up to the present, up to 2 years later.[10] An immune response to the AAV capsid, associated with increases in alanine transaminase (ALT) and aspartate transaminase (AST) in some of the subjects, resolved with a 4-week course of oral steroids, but approaches to avert this immune response are underway, including modification to neutralize excess AAV. Other approaches include design of less immunogenic vectors and use of innovative delivery systems, such as platelets. Novel therapeutic approaches to enhance clotting factor replacement therapy include RNAi silencing of antithrombin III, a thrombin inhibitor, to promote hemostasis through thrombin generation; oral delivery systems using bioencapsulated proteins; and molecular modifications to enhance the desirable properties of clotting factor.

Acquired Hemophilias

EPIDEMIOLOGY AND PATHOBIOLOGY

Autoantibody inhibitors occur spontaneously in individuals with previously normal hemostasis (nonhemophiliacs). In contrast to alloantibody inhibitors in hemophilic men, which are directed against foreign infused clotting factor, autoantibody inhibitors are directed against a "self" clotting factor, most commonly factor VIII. These autoantibodies typically arise in individuals with no past bleeding history; thus the diagnosis may be missed until a prolonged aPTT and aPTT mix tests are obtained (Chapter 171). Although half of those with autoantibody inhibitors have no obvious underlying cause, autoimmune diseases, lymphoproliferative disorders, idiosyncratic drug reactions, pregnancy, and advanced age are associated in the other half.[11]

CLINICAL MANIFESTATIONS AND DIAGNOSIS

Massive hemorrhagic events, even more severe than in hemophilia patients with alloantibodies, and more commonly in soft tissues, may occur in those with autoantibodies because of a delay in diagnosis and treatment. The laboratory expression of autoantibodies is similar to that of alloantibodies, except that clotting factor activity is not completely neutralized. Residual clotting factor activities between 3 and 20% of normal are frequently observed in patients with autoantibodies.

TREATMENT Rx

The same principles of replacement therapy for alloantibodies apply to these acquired autoantibody inhibitors.[12] There are two goals of treatment: (1) stop the bleeding and assure hemostasis, and (2) eradicate the inhibitor. For hemostasis, recombinant factor VIIa, activated prothrombin complex concentrate (aPCC), or factor VIII bypass activity is commonly used, in similar doses used to achieve hemostasis with alloantibody. Data from the EACH2 registry (European Acquired Haemophilia Registry) indicate that optimal bleeding control is with bypass treatment (rFVIIa or aPCC), which was effective in 93%, compared with FVIII or DDAVP, 68%. Thrombotic events were reported in only 3.6% for all of these hemostatic agents combined. Eradication of the inhibitor was significantly better in those treated with steroids and cyclophosphamide (80%), than those treated with steroids alone (58%); and the combination is more effective in autoantibody patients than in alloantibody patients; this includes corticosteroids (prednisone 1 mg/kg/day orally), cytotoxic agents (e.g., cyclophosphamide 150 mg/day orally or 500 to 750 mg/m^2 intravenous bolus every 3 to 4 weeks), or a combination, with dose titration based on inhibitor levels and complicating cytopenias. Rituximab (anti-CD20 antibody)-based regimens (375 mg/m^2 intravenously weekly for 4 weeks) are also effective in 61%. High-dose intravenous gamma globulin (IVIG)-based regimens may be effective in 45%. These agents are tapered and discontinued after the autoantibody has disappeared. The time to complete remission is about 5 weeks for steroids with or without cyclophosphamide, whereas rituximab-based regimens require twice as long to achieve remission.

PROGNOSIS

Several large series of patients with acquired hemophilia reveal a substantial mortality rate of 15 to 25%, which is considerably higher than that observed with alloantibody factor VIII inhibitors. A large meta-analysis found that overall survival in acquired hemophilia was influenced primarily by the achievement of a complete remission, age younger than 65 years at diagnosis, and related diseases (malignancy vs. postpartum vs. others). As many as 17% of the deaths were associated with sepsis, and 71% of those arose as a complication of cyclophosphamide-induced neutropenia. Hemorrhagic complications were the primary cause of death, but these could be reduced if the inhibitor could be eradicated.

Von Willebrand Disease

The most common congenital bleeding disorder is von Willebrand disease (VWD). This disorder is inherited in an autosomal dominant fashion and affects both sexes, with a prevalence of 1 to 3% and no ethnic predominance. Homozygous patients are rare and carry a recessive mutant gene. VWF, the protein that is decreased or defective in VWD, is a large, multimeric glycoprotein encoded by the *VWF* gene, located on chromosome 12. A personal history of mucocutaneous bleeding, a family history, and decreased functional VWF constitute a diagnostic triad. Treatment is accomplished with DDAVP or VWF concentrates. Detailed discussion of VWD is provided in Chapter 173.

Factor XI Deficiency

EPIDEMIOLOGY

Factor XI deficiency has a prevalence of 1 in 1 million in the general population and 1 in 500 births in Ashkenazi Jewish families.[13] Factor XI is the only component of the contact phase (factor XII, prekallikrein, and high-molecular-weight kininogen) of the intrinsic pathway of coagulation that is associated with excessive bleeding complications when a deficiency exists.

PATHOBIOLOGY

Factor XI deficiency is predominantly an autosomal recessive trait, although some mutations may have a dominant transmission pattern. The factor XI gene (*FXI*) is located on chromosome 4, and the protein circulates as a homodimer, with each FXI monomer composed of 4 apple domains encoded by exons 3 through 10 and a protease domain encoded by exons 11 through 15. The Glu117 stop mutation in *FXI* is the most common cause of factor XI deficiency; it is secondary to poor secretion or stability of the truncated protein or decreased levels of messenger RNA. To date, more than 170 mutations of *FXI* have been identified in factor XI–deficient patients (see www.factorxi.org), but close correlation between hemorrhagic phenotype and genotype is lacking. Most are missense or nonsense mutations and are located across all 4 apple domains and the serine protease region. In Ashkenazi Jewish individuals, factor XI deficiency is common, with a heterozygote frequency of 8 to 10%; two predominant gene mutations occur with equal frequency and are designated type II (a stop codon in exon 5) and type III (a single base defect in exon 9). The most severe clinical disease is observed in patients homozygous for type II, who usually have less than 1% factor XI activity. Homozygous type III individuals also manifest severe symptoms, but typically less severe than those of type II patients; they have slightly higher factor XI levels of about 10 to 20%. Compound heterozygotes, type II/III, make up the bulk of factor XI–deficient patients; they have clinically mild disease, with factor XI levels between 30 and 50%. In non-Jewish individuals, the mutations are more variable, although Cys128 stop has been described in several kindreds, and Cys38Arg has been found in several French Basque families. One third of those who develop inhibitors are homozygous for Glu117 stop, which results in an absent *FXI*. Genotypic identification of affected patients is determined by measuring factor XI levels rather than by defining the specific gene defect.

CLINICAL MANIFESTATIONS

The clinical bleeding tendency in factor XI deficiency is less severe than that observed in severe hemophilia A or B and, in contrast to the hemophilias, does not correlate with the severity of the deficiency. Most individuals with less than 20% of normal factor XI activity experience excessive bleeding after trauma or surgery; however, a few do not bleed. In contrast, bleeding has been observed in approximately 35 to 50% of mildly affected patients with factor XI levels between 20 and 50% of normal. Spontaneous hemorrhagic episodes, hemarthroses, and intramuscular and intracerebral bleeds are unusual; traumatic and surgical bleeds typically involve the mucous membranes. Patients undergoing tonsillectomy, prostatectomy, or dental extraction are at highest risk for bleeding unless replacement therapy is administered. Women may experience significant menorrhagia, and it has been recommended that women with menorrhagia be screened for both VWD and factor XI deficiency. Patients with mild factor XI deficiency and coincident mild VWD have an increased risk for bleeding.

DIAGNOSIS

Factor XI deficiency is diagnosed in the laboratory by a prolonged aPTT, normal PT, and decreased factor XI activity ascertained in a specific quantitative clotting assay (normal range, 60 to 130%).

TREATMENT Rx

Not all individuals with factor XI deficiency bleed, so it may be reasonable to monitor with no treatment, especially if there is no family history of bleeding. For surgical or other major bleeding, FFP 15 to 20 mL/kg may be given, although potential complications include fluid overload and infection risk, which can be reduced with the use of pathogen-inactivated FFP, if available. Use of factor XI concentrate, which is available in Europe but not the United States, may be complicated by thrombosis, which occurs in approximately 10% of patients, particularly in older individuals with preexisting cardiovascular disease or malignancy. Replacement dosing levels should not exceed 70% of factor XI activity. Repeat dosing with FFP or factor XI concentrate should take into consideration the long (60- to 80-hour) biologic half-life of factor XI in vivo.

The decision to treat heterozygotes with factor XI at levels greater than 20% is empirical and should be based on individual history of bleeding after trauma or surgery. There is no clear evidence of benefit with the use of DDAVP. Because hemorrhagic complications originate most commonly from mucous membrane surfaces, antifibrinolytic agents such as ε-aminocaproic acid or tranexamic acid are frequently helpful as adjunctive therapy. In women with menorrhagia or postpartum hemorrhage, testing for VWD is recommended because both diseases may be present.

Alloantibody inhibitors, which neutralize the hemostatic effects of exogenously administered factor XI replacement, can develop in patients with severe factor XI deficiency who have been exposed to plasma or factor XI concentrate. Recombinant factor VIIa can prevent bleeding during or after surgery in these patients.

Deficiencies of Contact Activation Factors

Although factor XI plays an important role in the activation of factor IX in the intrinsic pathway generation of thrombin, it is only one of the four components of the contact phase of coagulation. Deficiencies in any of the other three factors (factor XII, prekallikrein, and high-molecular-weight kininogen) produce in vitro laboratory abnormalities. Even among those with severe factor XII deficiency (<1% activity), there is no clinical bleeding; however, up to 8 to 10% with severe factor XII deficiency actually experience venous thromboembolic events, which are occasionally fatal. This finding has led to speculation that factor XII deficiency may lead to hypercoagulability through defective participation of the contact phase proteins in the activation of fibrinolysis.

DIAGNOSIS

Deficiencies of each of these factors prolong the aPTT, often markedly, which may normalize after prolonged incubation of the patient's plasma at 37° C with a negatively charged activator of the aPTT assay (i.e., kaolin or celite). Specific assays are also available to quantitate each of the contact factors.

TREATMENT Rx

Deficiencies of the contact activation factors, however severe they are and however prolonged the associated aPTT may be, do not cause clinical bleeding problems, even in response to surgery or trauma. Therefore, no therapy is indicated for factor XII deficiency, prekallikrein deficiency, or high-molecular-weight kininogen deficiency. Routine anticoagulation regimens are used to treat thrombogenic events.

Factor XIII (Fibrin-Stabilizing Factor) Deficiency

Factor XIII is a transglutaminase that is activated by thrombin and functions to cross-link fibrin to protect it from lysis by plasmin. It is also involved in wound healing and tissue repair and seems to be crucial for maintaining a viable pregnancy. Homozygous severe deficiency states are rare and are inherited in an autosomal recessive manner, with a prevalence of 1 per 3 million births. Consanguinity is common. Most patients are deficient in the A subunit (FXIII-A). Half of the molecular defects that account for A-subunit deficiency are missense mutations.

CLINICAL MANIFESTATIONS

Heterozygous carriers are usually asymptomatic, but homozygotes have lifelong bleeding that typically starts shortly after birth with persistent bleeding around the umbilical stump. Intracranial bleeding events, usually precipitated by minimal trauma, occur commonly enough in infants (25%) to justify the initiation of a primary prophylaxis regimen of replacement therapy. Delayed bleeding after surgery and trauma is the hallmark of the disease; however, easy bruising, poor wound healing with defective scar formation and dehiscence, and hemarthroses are characteristic. Spontaneous abortions are increased in severely affected women.

DIAGNOSIS

The diagnosis is usually suspected on clinical grounds, given that factor XIII deficiency is not detected by conventional screening coagulation assays (i.e., aPTT, PT). Most laboratories use a rapid screening assay that assesses the ability of a fibrin clot to remain intact with incubation in 5 mol/L of urea or 1% monochloroacetic acid. With factor XIII levels less than 1% of normal, the clot dissolves within 2 to 3 hours.

TREATMENT

Replacement therapy for prophylaxis or the treatment of acute bleeds in factor XIII deficiency can be accomplished by administering cryoprecipitate, FFP, or, preferably, plasma-derived factor XIII concentrate (Corifact, CSL Behring), which is pasteurized for viral safety. Normal hemostasis is achieved with a factor XIII level of only 5% of normal. The dose is 10 to 20 U/kg intravenously, and because it has a long half-life (10 days), prophylactic replacement can be given every 3 to 4 weeks. Acquired alloantibody inhibitors can develop in severely affected individuals. Autoantibodies also occur, usually in association with systemic lupus erythematosus. Preliminary data from an ongoing clinical trial of recombinant factor XIII indicates it is safe and effective in preventing bleeds in factor XIII–deficient patients.[14]

Dysfibrinogenemia and Afibrinogenemia

Approximately 300 abnormal fibrinogens have been described, but few cause hemostatic symptoms. Abnormal fibrinogens are rare autosomally inherited proteins. Quantitative fibrinogen deficiencies (afibrinogenemia and hypofibrinogenemia) may result from mutations affecting fibrinogen synthesis or processing, whereas qualitative defects (dysfibrinogenemia) are caused by mutations that lead to abnormal polymerization, defective cross-linking, or defective assembly of the fibrinolytic system.

CLINICAL MANIFESTATIONS

More than 50% of the dysfibrinogenemias are asymptomatic, 25% are associated with a mild hemorrhagic tendency (commonly caused by defective release of fibrinopeptide A), and 20% predispose individuals to thrombophilia (usually caused by impaired fibrinolysis) (Chapter 176). Concurrent bleeding and thrombosis also may occur. The prevalence of dysfibrinogenemia in patients with a history of thromboembolic episodes approaches 0.8%. A high prevalence of dysfibrinogenemia has been reported among patients with chronic thromboembolic pulmonary hypertension, implicating changes in the molecular structure of fibrin in the development of this disorder (Chapter 68). Women experience a high incidence of pregnancy-related complications, such as spontaneous abortion and postpartum thromboembolic events. Thrombin times and reptilase times (plasma-based clotting times with the substitution of reptilase snake venom for thrombin) are not helpful in predicting whether an abnormal fibrinogen will be prothrombotic, prohemorrhagic, or asymptomatic. However, clinical history, fibrinopeptide release studies, and fibrin polymerization studies may be useful. Clinically insignificant dysfibrinogenemias may be acquired in association with hepatocellular carcinoma (Chapter 196).

In contrast to the hepatic synthesis of a qualitatively abnormal protein in dysfibrinogenemia, congenital afibrinogenemia, an autosomal recessive disorder, represents the markedly deficient production of a normal protein. Severe life-threatening hemorrhagic complications can occur at any site, beginning at birth with umbilical bleeding. Intracranial hemorrhage is a frequent cause of death. Poor wound healing is characteristic. All coagulation-based assays that depend on the detection of a fibrin clot end point are markedly prolonged. Afibrinogenemia is usually detectable by specific functional or immunologic assays. Platelet dysfunction may accompany afibrinogenemia and exacerbate bleeding.

DIAGNOSIS

Abnormalities are usually detected incidentally when routine coagulation screening assays reveal decreased fibrinogen concentrations and prolonged thrombin clotting times. On further evaluation, discordance between functional and immunologic fibrinogen levels (>50 mg/dL more antigenic than functional) is observed; clotting times using snake venom (reptilase or ancrod) are variably prolonged.

TREATMENT

Deficiencies of fibrinogen can be corrected by the administration of FFP, cryoprecipitate, or a viral-attenuated (pasteurized), plasma-derived fibrinogen concentrate (Riastap, CSL Behring). The target replacement goal is a plasma level of 100 mg/dL, and given a circulating biologic half-life of at least 96 hours, treatment every 3 to 4 days is adequate. Primary prophylaxis regimens may be useful in afibrinogenemia, with on-demand or prophylactic replacement for trauma or surgery. Individuals with thrombophilic manifestations should receive anticoagulation long term, depending on risk-benefit assessment (Chapter 176). Riastap is not recommended for use in dysfibrinogenemia. Solvent/detergent plasma (Octaplas, Octapharma), a pooled human plasma that reduces allergic reactions and transfusion-related acute lung injury (TRALI), or psoralen-treated FFP (when licensed by the U.S. Food and Drug Administration [FDA]) may provide an alternative therapy.

Factor V Deficiency

Factor V is a component of the prothrombinase complex that assembles factors Va and Xa on the phospholipid membrane of the platelet for prothrombin (factor II) activation to thrombin (Chapter 171).

CONGENITAL FACTOR V DEFICIENCY

Deficiency of factor V is a rare, autosomal recessive disorder (1 in 1 million births). The factor V Leiden protein, which is responsible for resistance to activated protein C and thrombophilia, does not affect factor V coagulant activity (Chapter 176). The severity of plasma factor V deficiency correlates less well with the risk for clinical bleeding than does the factor V content in platelet α-granules (which cannot be measured in the clinical laboratory). This observation illustrates the critical role of the platelet in promoting adequate hemostasis at bleeding sites and explains why transfusions of normal platelets may be preferred over FFP for the treatment of hemorrhagic episodes secondary to congenital or acquired factor V deficiency. Hemostasis can be maintained without correcting plasma factor V activity (to >25% of normal).

COMBINED DEFICIENCIES OF FACTORS V AND VIII

Factors V and VIII are structurally homologous proteins, and combined deficiencies of these factors occur as an autosomal recessive disorder with a prevalence of 1 in 100,000 births among Jews of Sephardic origin. The severity of bleeding is determined by the levels of these factors, which usually range from 5 to 30% of normal. Replacement therapy should be aimed at normalizing both clotting protein activities.

ACQUIRED FACTOR V DEFICIENCY

Acquired factor V deficiency has been described in individuals exposed to bovine factor V, which contaminates the thrombin preparations used topically to control bleeding during cardiovascular surgery. This abnormality probably represents the development of anti–bovine factor V antibodies that cross-react with the human factor V protein. Profuse bleeding accompanies this complication.

Deficiencies of Vitamin K–Dependent Coagulation

DEFICIENCIES OF FACTORS II, VII, AND X

PATHOBIOLOGY AND CLINICAL MANIFESTATIONS

The coagulopathies of vitamin K deficiency and liver failure are discussed in Chapter 175. Congenital deficiencies of factors II (prothrombin), VII, and X are rare autosomally inherited disorders. Heterozygotes (with factor levels approximately 20% of normal) are typically asymptomatic except in the immediate newborn period, when physiologic vitamin K deficiency exacerbates the underlying clotting factor deficiency. Homozygotes with clotting factor levels less than 10% of normal manifest variable symptoms. As with other coagulopathies, these deficiencies are usually suspected after neonatal umbilical stump bleeding. Thereafter, unless replacement or prophylactic therapy is provided, these patients are subject to mucosal bleeding from epistaxis, menorrhagia, and dental extractions; hemarthroses and intramuscular hematomas; and bleeding after surgery or trauma.

Acquired factor VII deficiency has been associated with Dubin-Johnson and Gilbert syndromes (Chapter 147). Acquired factor IX deficiency has been associated with Gaucher disease because factor IX binds to glucocerebroside (Chapter 208). Acquired factor X deficiency and amyloidosis are discussed later.

DIAGNOSIS

In the coagulation laboratory, factor VII deficiency is associated with a prolonged PT and a normal aPTT. This pattern localizes the deficiency to the extrinsic pathway. In contrast, deficiencies of factors II (prothrombin) and X prolong both the PT and the aPTT, with the defects localized to the common pathway of coagulation. A Russell viper venom–based clotting assay can differentiate between these two deficiencies; as a direct activator of factor X, the assay is prolonged with factor X deficiency but not with factor II deficiency. Mixing patient plasma with normal plasma results in a correction of these assays, and specific clotting assays using plasma deficient in the coagulation protein to be studied can confirm the diagnosis.

TREATMENT Rx

Replacement therapy is indicated for acute symptomatic bleeds and for prophylaxis before surgery. In addition to FFP, which has the potential to transmit blood-borne viruses, factor IX complex concentrates can be administered to achieve hemostatic levels of any of these vitamin K–dependent factors (to >25 to 30% of normal).

Bleeding complications caused by acquired IgG autoantibodies directed against any coagulation factor protein can be reversed rapidly, albeit temporarily, by extracorporeal immunoadsorption over a Sepharose-bound polyclonal antihuman IgG or staphylococcal A column, with concomitant replacement therapy and initiation of immunosuppression. Recombinant factor VIIa is increasingly used for surgery in those with rare congenital coagulation deficiencies but typically at lower doses than with hemophilia inhibitors—generally 10 to 15 μg/kg/day or less, for up to several days.

FACTOR DEFICIENCY IN AMYLOIDOSIS

Severe acquired deficiency of factor X, often accompanied by deficiencies of other vitamin K–dependent factors, occasionally occurs in individuals with systemic amyloidosis (Chapter 188). Because amyloid fibrils in the reticuloendothelial system bind endogenous and exogenous sources of factor X, replacement therapy with FFP or factor IX complex concentrates, even in large quantities, may not be sufficient. Recombinant factor VIIa concentrate has been used to reverse acute bleeding. Splenectomy may ameliorate recurrent bleeding complications.

Other Acquired Coagulation Abnormalities

ANTIPHOSPHOLIPID SYNDROME AND LUPUS ANTICOAGULANT

EPIDEMIOLOGY

The antiphospholipid antibody syndrome (APS) is associated with recurrent thrombosis or recurrent pregnancy loss with autoantibodies directed against phospholipids. Antiphospholipid antibodies (APAs) may include lupus anticoagulant (LA), anticardiolipin antibody (CL), or anti-β2-glycoprotein-I (anti-β2-GPI). Thrombocytopenia is also a common finding in this prothrombotic disorder. Rarely, multiorgan failure may arise from widespread thrombosis, termed *catastrophic APS*.

PATHOBIOLOGY

Our understanding of the role of individual antibodies in diagnosing APS continues to be enhanced with clinical studies, which may also contribute to the development of better diagnostic assays.[15] It has been suggested that the prothrombotic effects of APAs may derive from their ability to complex with β2-GPI in vivo (thereby negating their modulatory phospholipid-binding function) or through APA inhibition of protein C activation, interference with antithrombin III activity, and/or disruption of the annexin V "shield," thereby preventing normal clot breakdown (fibrinolysis). Although complement and inflammation play a role in fetal loss in a murine model of APS, the pathogenic mechanism of APS-associated pregnancy loss remains unclear. Although non-β2-GPI antibodies detected by CL enzyme-linked immunosorbent assay (ELISA) may play a role in early obstetric APS, and anti-β2-GPI antibodies with LA activity play a role in late miscarriage, additional studies are needed to better classify, understand, and manage this syndrome.

CLINICAL MANIFESTATIONS

APAs prolong coagulation in in vitro assays but are not generally associated with clinical bleeding. Rarely, clinical bleeding may occur when APA interacts with factor II (prothrombin), producing an acquired prothrombin (factor II) deficiency associated with accelerated clearance of LA-prothrombin complexes from the circulation. Bleeding tendencies also may arise when LA targets platelet membranes and produces quantitative and/or qualitative platelet abnormalities. Other clinical findings in APS include livedo reticularis (Chapter 80), valvular heart lesions, and nephropathy. Clinically, although both arterial and venous thrombosis (Chapter 176) may occur in APS, the most relevant is venous thrombosis and stroke in young adults. A diagnostic work-up in those with arterial thrombosis should include transesophageal echocardiography to exclude a cardiac source for arterial clots. In obstetric patients, other causes of miscarriage should be excluded. A case-control study has indicated that a history of recurrent spontaneous abortion associated with antiphospholipid syndrome is a risk factor for subsequent venous thromboembolism in the long term.[16] Nonpregnant individuals with APS-associated thrombotic manifestations have a 50% risk for experiencing recurrent events over a 5-year period. Typically, recurrent thrombotic and vascular episodes occur in a pattern consistent with the initial finding (e.g., venous recurrence following an initial deep vein thrombosis).

DIAGNOSIS

By international consensus, a diagnosis of APS is based on both clinical and laboratory criteria.[17] Clinical criteria include (1) arterial, venous, or small vessel thrombosis in any tissue or organ and (2) pregnancy morbidity. The latter includes one or more pregnancy losses before 10 weeks' gestation; one or more pregnancy losses before 34 weeks due to eclampsia, preeclampsia, or placental insufficiency; or three or more spontaneous abortions before 10 weeks. APS may be suspected in the setting of recurrent spontaneous miscarriages or pregnancy-related thromboembolic events; with the detection of cerebral arterial thromboses in young adults; in those with systemic lupus erythematosus (20 to 40%; Chapter 266) or other autoimmune diseases or lymphoproliferative malignancies; in those receiving psychotropic medications (e.g., chlorpromazine); or when incidental coagulation assays reveal aPTT prolongation.

Laboratory criteria[18] include one or more high-titer APAs (LA, CL, anti-β2-GPI) on at least two occasions at least 12 weeks apart. APAs can be detected by three assays: the LA assay, the CL ELISA assay, and the β2-GPI ELISA assay. The LA assay includes a screening test, based on a prolonged phospholipid-dependent clotting time; a mixing test that distinguishes the inhibitor (fails to correct in a 1 : 1 mix) from a deficiency state (corrects in a 1 : 1 mix); and a confirmatory test based on platelet neutralization to demonstrate that the inhibitor is phospholipid dependent (clotting time corrects) or a modified aPTT reagent based on the binding of hexagonal phase phospholipids to LA. The CL ELISA measures antibodies in dilute sera that bind to CL-coated plates, including those that bind to CL alone or bind to bovine β2-GPI and both IgG and IgM, but it may miss CL bound to human β2-GPI. The β2-GPI ELISA detects antibodies that bind to β2-GPI–coated irradiated plates, but it has reduced specificity owing to binding by nonpathogenic antibodies. Positivity in multiple assays is strongly associated with thrombosis and miscarriage: the risk for first thrombosis among asymptomatic individuals positive for LA, CL, and β2-GPI antibodies, so-called triple-positive patients, is 5.3% per year. Of the three assays, the β2-GPI ELISA is most strongly associated with thrombosis and early recurrent miscarriage; the LA assay is associated with venous thrombosis, stroke, and late miscarriage. The greatest weight is given to a positive LA test. From a practical standpoint, testing for all three antibodies at diagnosis is recommended to guide follow-up because oral anticoagulants may interfere with the LA test.

TREATMENT Rx

Because of the high risk for recurrent thromboembolism, patients with APS should receive antithrombotic therapy. The approach is based on achieving a balance between thrombosis risk and bleeding complications, especially in those with thrombocytopenia. Because of the limited information from randomized clinical trials, the recommendations for APS are similar to those for patients without APS—that is, to use unfractionated heparin or low-molecular-weight heparin (LMWH), with a 4- to 5-day overlap with warfarin, for acute venous thromboembolism (VTE), followed by long-term warfarin to a target international normalized ratio (INR) of 2.0 to 3.0. This recommendation is based on a randomized trial indicating no difference in bleeding rates with high-intensity (INR >3.0) versus low-intensity (INR 2.0 to 3.0) anticoagulation. In individuals with thrombocytopenia, more frequent monitoring of the INR may be warranted to avoid bleeding complications. The duration of anticoagulation in those both with and without APS is based on a balance between VTE recurrence and bleeding.

For women with APS and pregnancy loss but no past thrombosis, the goal is to prevent recurrent pregnancy loss. Based on prospective studies indicating higher birth rates with aspirin plus heparin, recommendations include low-dose aspirin (81 mg) in combination with prophylactic heparin or LMWH in the antepartum period.

Among those with APS-associated thrombocytopenia and a platelet count below 20 to 30 × 10^9/L, in the setting of bleeding or when bleeding potential exceeds the risk for bleeding with VTE treatment, management is similar to that for idiopathic thrombocytopenic purpura (Chapter 172). This includes steroids, intravenous immunoglobulin, and immunosuppressive agents (e.g., cyclophosphamide, azathioprine, off-label rituximab). Case reports indicate that danazol, dapsone, aspirin, and chloroquine may be helpful adjuncts. In pregnant women with APS-associated thrombocytopenia, treatment is advised before epidural anesthesia or cesarean delivery. In the latter case, early delivery under cover of intravenous immunoglobulin is recommended.

Treatment of APS-associated bleeding is dependent on the site and severity of bleeding. For anticoagulation bleeding, the anticoagulant should be withheld and an antidote (e.g., protamine) given, if available. For thrombocytopenia bleeding, platelet transfusions should be given, along with red blood cell transfusions, if necessary. If both thrombosis and bleeding occur, treatment should be directed at the component that is most life threatening. In those with a high bleeding risk, anticoagulants should be withheld or given at a lower dosage; those with a high thrombotic risk, despite thrombocytopenia, should be anticoagulated and given agents to boost platelet count simultaneously. For those who receive prolonged heparin, supplemental calcium and vitamin D should be administered to minimize the risks for osteoporosis.

In the life-threatening multisystem complication of catastrophic antiphospholipid syndrome, which is characterized by histopathologic evidence of small vessel thrombosis and dysfunction of multiple organs (e.g., lung, brain, heart, kidneys, skin, and/or gastrointestinal tract) over a short period of time, maximal anticoagulation, plasma exchange, and immunosuppressive therapy have been used. A recent report showed that eculizumab, an inhibitor of terminal complement, was effective in a patient with recurrent catastrophic antiphospholipid syndrome.[19]

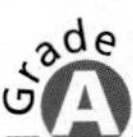

Grade A References

A1. Mahlangu J, Powell JS, Ragni MV, et al. Phase 3 study of recombinant factor VIII Fc fusion protein in severe hemophilia A. *Blood.* 2014;123:317-325.
A2. Manco-Johnson MJ, Abshire TC, Shapiro AD, et al. Prophylaxis versus episodic treatment to prevent joint disease in boys with severe hemophilia. *N Engl J Med.* 2007;357:535-544.
A3. Gringeri A, Lundin B, von Mackensen S, et al. A randomized clinical trial of prophylaxis in children with hemophilia A (the ESPRIT Study). *J Thromb Haemost.* 2011;9:700-710.
A4. Valentino LA, Mamonov V, Hellmann A, et al. A randomized comparison of two prophylaxis regimens and a paired comparison of on-demand and prophylaxis treatments in hemophilia A management. *J Thromb Haemost.* 2012;10:359-367.
A5. Leissinger C, Gringeri A, Antmen B, et al. Anti-inhibitor coagulant complex prophylaxis in hemophilia with inhibitors. *N Engl J Med.* 2011;365:1684-1692.
A6. Hay CRM, DiMichele DM. The principal results of the International Immune Tolerance Study: a randomized dose comparison. *Blood.* 2012;119:1335-1344.

GENERAL REFERENCES

For the General References and other additional features, please visit Expert Consult at https://expertconsult.inkling.com.

175

HEMORRHAGIC DISORDERS: DISSEMINATED INTRAVASCULAR COAGULATION, LIVER FAILURE, AND VITAMIN K DEFICIENCY

ANDREW I. SCHAFER

DISSEMINATED INTRAVASCULAR COAGULATION

DEFINITION

Disseminated intravascular coagulation (DIC), also referred to as consumptive coagulopathy or defibrination, is caused by a wide variety of serious disorders (Table 175-1). In most patients, the underlying process dominates the clinical picture, but in some cases (e.g., occult malignant neoplasm, envenomation), DIC may be the initial or predominant manifestation of the disorder. DIC never occurs in isolation, without an inciting cause.

TABLE 175-1 MAJOR CAUSES OF DISSEMINATED INTRAVASCULAR COAGULATION

INFECTIONS
Gram-negative bacterial sepsis
Other bacteria, fungi, viruses, Rocky Mountain spotted fever, malaria
IMMUNOLOGIC REACTIONS
Transfusion reactions (ABO incompatibility)
Transplant rejection
OBSTETRIC COMPLICATIONS
Amniotic fluid embolism
Retained dead fetus
Abruptio placentae
Toxemia, preeclampsia
Septic abortion
MALIGNANT NEOPLASMS
Pancreatic carcinoma
Adenocarcinomas
Acute promyelocytic leukemia
Other neoplasms
LIVER FAILURE
ACUTE PANCREATITIS
ENVENOMATION
RESPIRATORY DISTRESS SYNDROME
TRAUMA, SHOCK
Brain injury
Crush injury
Burns
Hypothermia or hyperthermia
Fat embolism
Hypoxia, ischemia
Surgery
VASCULAR DISORDERS
Giant hemangioma (Kasabach-Merritt syndrome)
Aortic aneurysm
Vascular tumors

PATHOBIOLOGY

DIC is pathophysiologically a thrombotic process. However, its clinical manifestation may be widespread hemorrhage in acute cases. The basic pathophysiologic mechanism (Fig. 175-1), regardless of cause, is entry into the circulation of procoagulant substances that trigger systemic activation of the coagulation system and platelets. This results in disseminated deposition of fibrin-platelet thrombi within the microvasculature.[1] In most cases, the procoagulant stimulus is tissue factor, a lipoprotein that is not normally exposed to blood. In DIC, tissue factor gains access to blood by tissue injury, its elaboration by malignant cells, or its expression on the surface of monocytes and endothelial cells by inflammatory mediators. Components of the inflammatory response and the coagulation system are reciprocally activated in some forms of DIC, such as sepsis. Tissue factor triggers generation of the coagulation protease thrombin, which induces fibrin formation and platelet activation. In some specific cases of DIC, procoagulants other than tissue factor (e.g., a cysteine protease or mucin in certain malignant neoplasms) and proteases other than thrombin (e.g., trypsin in pancreatitis, exogenous enzymes in envenomation) provide the procoagulant stimulus.

In acute, uncompensated DIC, coagulation factors are consumed at a rate in excess of the capacity of the liver to synthesize them, and platelets are consumed in excess of the capacity of bone marrow megakaryocytes to release them. The resulting laboratory manifestations under these circumstances are a prolonged prothrombin time (PT) and activated partial thromboplastin time (aPTT) and thrombocytopenia. Increased fibrin formation in DIC stimulates a heightened process of secondary fibrinolysis, in which plasminogen activators generate plasmin to digest fibrin (and fibrinogen) into fibrin(ogen) degradation products (FDPs). FDPs are potent circulating anticoagulants that further contribute to the bleeding manifestations of DIC. Intravascular fibrin deposition can cause fragmentation of red blood cells and lead to the appearance of schistocytes in blood smears; however, frank microangiopathic hemolytic anemia is unusual in DIC. Occlusive microvascular thrombosis in DIC can compromise the blood supply to some organs and

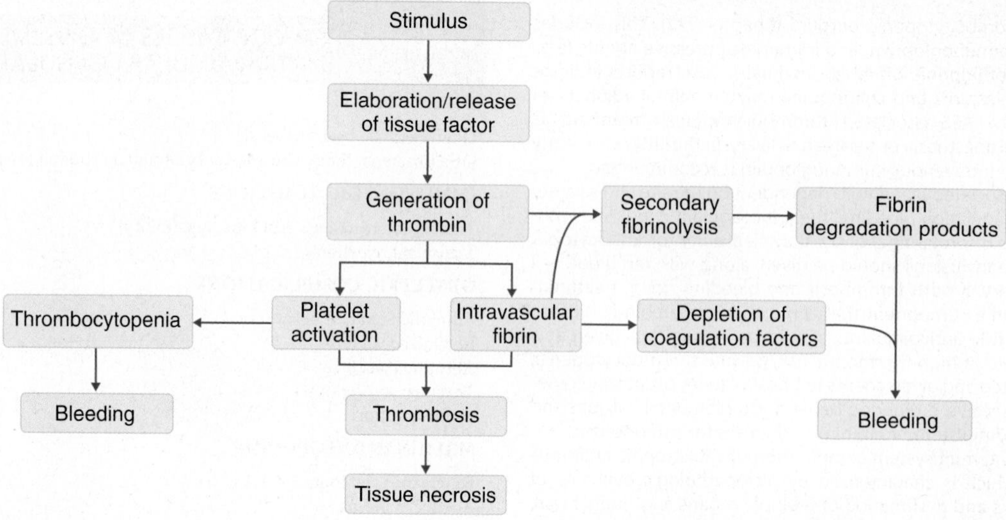

FIGURE 175-1. Pathophysiologic process of bleeding, thrombosis, and ischemic manifestations in patients with disseminated intravascular coagulation.

lead to multiorgan failure, particularly when it is accompanied by systemic hemodynamic and metabolic derangements.

Underlying Causes

DIC always has an underlying cause that generally must be identified and eliminated if the coagulopathy is to be managed successfully. The development of DIC in many of these disorders is associated with an unfavorable outcome. Infection is the most common cause of DIC. The syndrome is particularly associated with gram-negative or gram-positive sepsis (Chapter 108), although it can be triggered by a variety of other bacterial, fungal, viral, rickettsial, and protozoal microorganisms.

The placenta and uterine contents are rich sources of tissue factor and other procoagulants that are normally excluded from the maternal circulation; a spectrum of clinical manifestations of DIC may accompany obstetric complications when this barrier is breached, especially in the third trimester. These syndromes range from acute, fulminant, and often fatal DIC in amniotic fluid embolism to chronic or subacute DIC with a retained dead fetus. Other obstetric problems associated with DIC include abruptio placentae, toxemia, and septic abortion.

Chronic forms of DIC are caused by a variety of malignant neoplasms, particularly pancreatic cancer (Chapter 194) and mucin-secreting adenocarcinomas of the gastrointestinal tract (Chapter 193), in which thrombotic rather than bleeding manifestations predominate. Treatment with all-*trans*-retinoic acid has greatly reduced the incidence of severe DIC in patients with acute promyelocytic leukemia (Chapter 183). It is not known whether liver failure (see later) can cause DIC or whether its coexistence merely exacerbates intravascular coagulation because of impaired clearance of activated clotting factors, plasmin, and FDPs. Snake venom contains a variety of substances that can affect coagulation and endothelial permeability. Bites from rattlesnakes and other vipers can induce profound DIC by introduction of these exogenous toxins and release of endogenous tissue factor through tissue necrosis.

The likelihood and degree of DIC caused by trauma, surgery, and shock (Chapter 106) are related to the extent of tissue damage and the organs involved. The brain is a particularly rich source of tissue factor, so traumatic brain injury (Chapter 399) can precipitate acute DIC. Large aortic aneurysms (Chapter 78), giant hemangiomas, and other vascular malformations can cause subclinical or clinical DIC that is initiated locally within the abnormal vasculature but can "spill" into the systemic circulation.

CLINICAL MANIFESTATIONS

The clinical manifestations of DIC are determined by the nature, intensity, and duration of the underlying stimulus. The coexistence of liver disease exacerbates DIC of any cause. Low-grade DIC is often asymptomatic and diagnosed only by laboratory abnormalities. Thrombotic complications of DIC occur most often with chronic underlying diseases, as exemplified by Trousseau's syndrome in cancer (Chapter 176). DIC can be manifested as acrocyanosis and gangrene of the digits in critically ill, hemodynamically compromised patients receiving vasopressors. Hemorrhagic necrosis of the skin (Fig. 175-2) and purpura fulminans may also be manifestations of DIC.

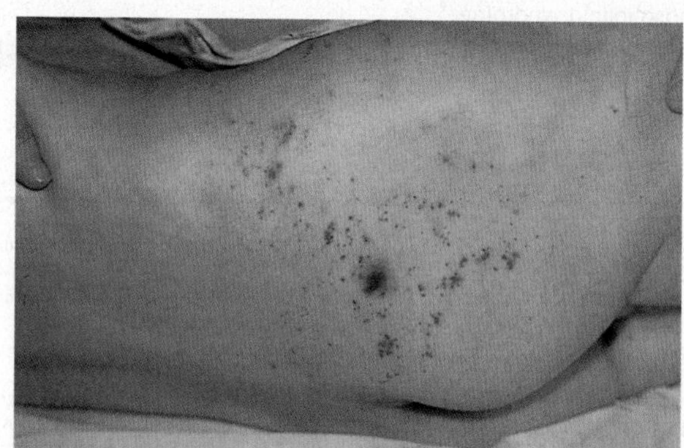

FIGURE 175-2. Disseminated intravascular coagulation resulting from staphylococcal septicemia. Note the characteristic skin hemorrhage ranging from small purpuric lesions to larger ecchymoses. (From Forbes CD, Jackson WF. Color Atlas and Text of Clinical Medicine. 3rd ed. London: Mosby; 2003.)

Bleeding is the most common clinical finding in acute, uncompensated DIC. Bleeding can be limited to sites of intervention or anatomic abnormalities, but it tends to be generalized in more severe cases, including widespread ecchymoses and diffuse oozing from mucosal surfaces and orifices.

DIAGNOSIS

The laboratory diagnosis of severe, acute DIC is not usually difficult. Consumption and inhibition of the function of clotting factors cause prolongation of the PT, aPTT, and thrombin time. Consumption of platelets causes thrombocytopenia. Secondary fibrinolysis generates increased titers of FDPs, which can be measured by latex agglutination or D-dimer assays. Some schistocytes may be seen in the peripheral blood smear, but this finding is neither sensitive nor specific for DIC. Chronic or compensated forms of DIC are more difficult to diagnose, with highly variable patterns of abnormalities in "DIC screen" coagulation tests.[2,3] Increased D-dimers and a prolonged PT are generally more sensitive measures than are abnormalities of the aPTT and platelet count. Overcompensated synthesis of consumed clotting factors and platelets in some chronic forms of DIC may actually cause shortening of the PT and aPTT or thrombocytosis (or both), even though elevated levels of D-dimers indicate secondary fibrinolysis in such cases.

The most difficult differential diagnosis of DIC occurs in patients who have coexisting liver disease. The coagulopathy of liver failure (see later section on liver failure) is often indistinguishable from that of DIC, partly because advanced hepatic dysfunction is in fact accompanied by a state of DIC. In liver failure, the combination of decreased synthesis of clotting factors, impaired clearance of activated clotting factors, secondary fibrinolysis, and thrombocytopenia from portal hypertension and hypersplenism may make the coagulopathy virtually impossible to differentiate from DIC. Thrombotic microangiopathies including thrombotic thrombocytopenic purpura and hemolytic-uremic syndrome, the syndrome of "hemolysis, elevated liver enzymes, and low platelet count" (HELLP) in obstetric patients,[4] and other forms of platelet consumption and thrombocytopenia (Chapter 172) are not accompanied by activation of clotting factors or secondary fibrinolysis; therefore, the PT, aPTT, thrombin time, and D-dimers are generally normal in these disorders. Schistocytes, often with frank hemolysis, are much more prominent in the peripheral smear in thrombotic thrombocytopenic purpura and hemolytic-uremic syndrome (Chapter 172) than in DIC.

Primary hyperfibrinolysis is disputed as a distinct entity.[5] Some patients with a serious clinical bleeding diathesis, however, have laboratory evidence of predominantly fibrinolysis, including high levels of FDPs (D-dimers) and severe hypofibrinogenemia, with relatively little consumption of coagulation factors and normal or nearly normal platelet counts. These unusual findings, which approximate the findings expected with fibrinolytic therapy, are encountered occasionally, particularly in patients with prostate cancer.

TREATMENT Rx

Successful treatment of DIC (Table 175-2) requires that the underlying cause be identified and eliminated. All other therapies, including hemodynamic support, replacement of coagulation factors and platelets, and pharmacologic inhibitors of coagulation and fibrinolysis, are just temporizing measures. Because of the difficulty of testing this complex syndrome with multiple causes by controlled, randomized clinical trials, current guidelines for treatment are generally not based on high-grade evidence.[6]

In many patients with asymptomatic, self-limited DIC who have only laboratory manifestations of the coagulopathy, no treatment may be necessary. In patients with DIC who are actively bleeding or who are at high risk for bleeding, the blood component treatments of choice are transfusions of platelets to improve the thrombocytopenia and fresh-frozen plasma to replace all consumed coagulation factors and to correct the prolonged PT and aPTT. Large volumes of plasma (e.g., >6 U/24 hours) may be required to ameliorate bleeding in severe cases. In some patients who have particularly profound hypofibrinogenemia, the additional transfusion of cryoprecipitate, a plasma concentrate that is enriched in fibrinogen, may be useful. The theoretical concern that these blood products could "fuel the fire" and exacerbate the DIC has not been supported by clinical experience.

The use of pharmacologic inhibitors of coagulation and fibrinolysis in DIC is controversial. Heparin is of theoretical benefit because it blocks thrombin activity and quenches intravascular coagulation and the resultant secondary fibrinolysis. In practice, heparin might exacerbate the bleeding tendency in acute DIC. Heparin is usually reserved for special forms of DIC, including those manifested by thrombosis or acrocyanosis and forms that accompany cancer, vascular malformations, retained dead fetus, and possibly acute promyelocytic leukemia, in which active bleeding is not present. In cases of DIC in which thrombosis or acral ischemia predominates, unfractionated heparin should be used by continuous infusion because of its short half-life and reversibility in the event of increased bleeding. Monitoring of the aPTT in the presence of DIC may be problematic, so heparin infusion in this setting should be followed mainly by clinical response and improvement in results of other tests of coagulation (e.g., thrombocytopenia). Antifibrinolytic agents, including ε-aminocaproic acid and tranexamic acid, are generally contraindicated in DIC. By blocking the secondary fibrinolytic response to DIC, these drugs cause unopposed fibrin deposition and may precipitate thrombosis. Antifibrinolytic agents may be effective in decreasing life-threatening bleeding in DIC, however, particularly in extreme cases in which aggressive blood component replacement fails to control the hemorrhage; in such situations, simultaneous infusion of low doses of heparin may reduce the risk for thrombosis. Bleeding and DIC laboratory parameters may also be improved with recombinant activated factor VII (rFVIIa) in patients whose bleeding is not controlled by standard measures.

Recombinant human activated protein C (rhAPC) was approved in 2001 for use in severe sepsis or septic shock, which is often accompanied by DIC. The mechanisms by which rhAPC is thought to modify disease course are through its actions on dysregulated coagulation and subsequent microvascular thrombosis as well as by its possible anti-inflammatory effects. However, subsequent trials failed to confirm the mortality reduction benefit of rhAPC in patients with septic shock or any of its prescribed subgroups[A1] or in groups that were less acutely ill, with lower risk of death from sepsis (Acute Physiology and Chronic Health Evaluation or APACHE II scores <25 or single-organ failure), and with extended infusions or in pediatric patients. Therefore, rhAPC was withdrawn by its manufacturer in 2011. Nevertheless, controversy has persisted with the subsequent publication of favorable meta-analyses and observational trials.[7] Although recombinant tissue factor pathway inhibitor, antithrombin III concentrates, and human soluble thrombomodulin may have some efficacy in improving laboratory parameters of DIC, the overall survival benefit with these agents in patients with DIC has not been demonstrated.

TABLE 175-2 TREATMENT OF DISSEMINATED INTRAVASCULAR COAGULATION

Identify and eliminate the underlying cause
No treatment if mild, asymptomatic, and self-limited
Hemodynamic support, as indicated, in severe cases
Blood component therapy
- *Indications:* active bleeding or high risk for bleeding
  - Fresh-frozen plasma
  - Platelets
  - In some cases, consider cryoprecipitate, antithrombin III

Drug therapy
- *Indications:* heparin for DIC manifested by thrombosis or acrocyanosis and without active bleeding; antifibrinolytic agents are generally contraindicated except with life-threatening bleeding and failure of blood component therapy

DIC = disseminated intravascular coagulation.

LIVER FAILURE

Bleeding complications in patients with advanced liver disease (Chapters 153 and 154) can be severe and even fatal and directly account for about 20% of the deaths associated with hepatic failure. The extent of the bleeding tendency depends on the severity and type of liver disease involved. About one third of deaths in patients undergoing liver transplantation are attributable to perioperative hemorrhage.

PATHOBIOLOGY

The pathophysiologic mechanism of bleeding in liver failure is complex and multifactorial.[8] Anatomic abnormalities resulting from portal hypertension are frequently the major cause of gastrointestinal bleeding in patients with liver disease. Upper gastrointestinal bleeding can be caused by esophageal varices or hemorrhagic gastritis (congestive gastropathy), whereas lower gastrointestinal bleeding, although seldom life-threatening, can be due to hemorrhoids.

The complexity of the systemic coagulopathy of liver failure is not surprising inasmuch as the liver is the principal organ site for the synthesis of coagulation and fibrinolytic factors as well as their protein inhibitors (Table 175-3). Therefore, the impaired hemostasis of liver failure is accompanied by opposing prothrombotic alterations. Hepatocytes produce all of the clotting factors except von Willebrand factor, and advanced parenchymal liver disease results in impaired synthesis of these proteins. Liver disease can also cause impairment in vitamin K–dependent γ-carboxylation of the procoagulant factors II, VII, IX, and X as well as the anticoagulant proteins C and S. Functional abnormalities of fibrinogen, termed dysfibrinogenemias, are frequently found in various forms of liver disease, particularly in hepatocellular carcinoma. Most forms of advanced liver disease are accompanied by some degree of DIC caused by impaired synthesis of inhibitors of blood coagulation and defective hepatocellular clearance of activated coagulation factors. DIC and bleeding risk are exacerbated by the enhanced fibrinolytic activity (hyperfibrinolysis) of liver disease caused by increased levels of tissue plasminogen activator accompanied by decreased synthesis of inhibitors of plasminogen activator and plasmin.

Quantitative and qualitative abnormalities of platelets also contribute to the bleeding diathesis of liver failure. Congestive splenomegaly secondary to portal hypertension causes increased pooling of platelets in the spleen (hypersplenism). The resultant thrombocytopenia, the degree of which generally correlates with spleen size, rarely causes a reduction in the platelet count to less than 30,000/mm^3. In alcoholic patients, suppression of bone marrow thrombopoiesis by the acute toxic effects of alcohol or folate deficiency may contribute to the thrombocytopenia. Qualitative platelet abnormalities have also been described in patients with liver disease.

Liver transplantation (Chapter 154) poses special problems to the coagulation system. During the anhepatic stage of surgery, which lasts about 2 hours, the complete cessation of synthesis of coagulation factors causes further prolongation of the PT and aPTT. Release of tissue plasminogen activator from the newly grafted liver leads to increased fibrinolysis and transient exacerbation of bleeding risk in the postoperative period.

CLINICAL MANIFESTATIONS

The most common hemorrhagic complication of liver disease is gastrointestinal bleeding, which is usually caused by anatomic abnormalities and exacerbated by the systemic coagulopathy of liver failure. Bleeding from other

TABLE 175-3 COAGULATION ABNORMALITIES IN LIVER DISEASE

ABNORMALITIES IN COAGULATION
Decreased synthesis of coagulation factors
Impaired vitamin K–dependent γ-carboxylation
Dysfibrinogenemia
Disseminated intravascular coagulation
Increased fibrinolytic activity
ABNORMALITIES IN PLATELETS
Thrombocytopenia (hypersplenism)
Abnormal platelet function

mucosal sites, extensive ecchymoses, or more serious hemorrhage into the retroperitoneum or central nervous system generally indicates more significant derangements of the coagulation system.

The severe coagulopathy in patients with liver disease makes liver biopsy a potentially hazardous procedure. The PT and platelet count may be the best guides to bleeding risk, but they too lack reliability as predictors of risk of bleeding with liver biopsy. In general, liver biopsy can be performed safely if the PT and aPTT do not exceed 1.5 times control values and the platelet count is higher than 50,000/mm^3. The American Association for the Study of Liver Diseases has concluded that the bleeding risk-benefit ratio of liver biopsy must be carefully considered on a case-by-case basis.[9]

DIAGNOSIS

Although the PT and aPTT are often prolonged in patients with advanced liver disease, the PT tends to be a more sensitive assay early in the course; a disproportionate prolongation of the aPTT should raise suspicion of a coexisting coagulation abnormality, such as a lupus anticoagulant or clotting factor inhibitor. A prolonged PT is also a useful prognostic indicator of poor outcome in patients with cirrhosis, acute acetaminophen hepatotoxicity, and acute viral hepatitis; in acute viral hepatitis, it is a better index of prognosis than are serum albumin and transaminases. A disproportionate prolongation of the thrombin time should suggest the presence of dysfibrinogenemia. Hypersplenism (Chapter 168), possibly associated with nutritional folate deficiency or the acute toxic effects of alcohol on bone marrow, often causes mild to moderate thrombocytopenia in patients with liver disease; however, consideration should be given to other coexisting causes of thrombocytopenia if the platelet count is significantly less than 30,000/mm^3.

The coagulopathy of liver failure is often indistinguishable from that of DIC, in part because some degree of DIC is in fact a necessary accompaniment of advanced liver disease. In general, patients with DIC have more marked decreases in levels of factor VIII and increases in D-dimer than do patients with liver failure. The simplistic notion that a prolonged PT (and sometimes also aPTT) as well as a thrombocytopenia creates a state of natural "auto-anticoagulation" in patients with liver failure ignores the complex pathophysiologic mechanism of the coagulopathy in this setting, which involves a delicate balance of not only antihemostatic abnormalities (leading to a bleeding tendency) but also prohemostatic abnormalities (leading to a simultaneous thrombotic tendency).[10] In fact, the risk of venous thromboembolism is two-fold higher in patients with liver failure than in controls, even in the presence of a prolonged international normalized ratio. The thrombotic risk is not just a localized one, involving portal vein and other abdominal venous thrombosis, but also a systemic one, involving lower extremity deep venous thrombosis and pulmonary embolism.

TREATMENT Rx

Therapy for the coagulopathy of liver disease may be directed at preventing the hemorrhagic complications of invasive procedures or treating active bleeding. The most effective treatment is blood component therapy with fresh-frozen plasma (which contains all the coagulation factors) and platelet transfusions (Chapter 177). Some patients require large volumes of fresh-frozen plasma (15 to 20 mL/kg) to lower the prolonged PT; rarely, plasmapheresis with plasma exchange is required to avoid fluid overload in these situations. Because of the short half-lives of some clotting factors, fresh-frozen plasma may have to be administered every 8 to 12 hours to maintain acceptable coagulation test parameters. In some patients, especially those with cholestasis, parenteral administration of vitamin K can at least partially reverse the coagulation abnormalities; however, in patients with advanced hepatocellular failure, vitamin K is largely ineffective. Prothrombin complex concentrates are relatively contraindicated in patients with liver failure, as in those with DIC, because of the risk of thrombotic complications. Because of immediate pooling of transfused platelets in the enlarged spleen of patients with hypersplenism, a higher than calculated dose of platelet concentrates is usually required to increase circulating platelet counts significantly. The oral thrombopoietin receptor agonist eltrombopag (25 to 100 mg daily) has been shown to increase platelet numbers in thrombocytopenic patients with hepatitis C virus infection complicated by advanced fibrosis and cirrhosis, allowing otherwise ineligible patients to use antiviral therapy, leading to increases in sustained virologic responses.[A2]

A Cochrane database meta-analysis of randomized clinical trials of recombinant human activated factor VII (rFVIIa) found no evidence to support or to reject its administration to patients with liver disease and upper gastrointestinal bleeding.[A3] Routine use of rFVIIa for the coagulopathy of liver disease cannot be recommended at this time. Desmopressin (DDAVP), which can shorten the bleeding time of patients with cirrhosis, may be considered as ancillary therapy in patients undergoing invasive procedures.

VITAMIN K DEFICIENCY

Vitamin K is required for γ-carboxylation of glutamic acid residues of the procoagulant factors II (prothrombin), VII, IX, and X and the anticoagulant factors protein C and protein S. This post-translational modification normally renders these proteins functionally active in coagulation. The PT is more sensitive than the aPTT in detecting vitamin K deficiency states because factor VII, the only vitamin K–dependent factor that is in the extrinsic pathway of coagulation, is the most labile of these proteins.

The two major sources of vitamin K are dietary intake and synthesis by the bacterial flora of the intestine. In the absence of malabsorption, nutritional deficiency alone rarely causes clinically significant vitamin K deficiency. The condition can arise, however, when eradication of gut flora is combined with inadequate dietary intake. This situation typically occurs in critically ill patients in intensive care units who have no oral intake and are receiving broad-spectrum antibiotics for prolonged periods. Vitamin K deficiency can also develop in patients receiving total parenteral nutrition unless the infusions are supplemented with vitamin K.

Vitamin K is absorbed predominantly in the ileum and requires the presence of bile salts. Clinically significant vitamin K deficiency occurs with malabsorption of fat-soluble vitamins secondary to obstructive jaundice (Chapter 155) or with malabsorption caused by intrinsic small bowel diseases, including celiac sprue, short-bowel syndrome, and inflammatory bowel disease (Chapters 140 and 141).

Warfarin (Chapter 38) acts as an anticoagulant by competitive antagonism of vitamin K. Rare cases of hereditary deficiency of the vitamin K–dependent coagulation factors may cause a lifelong bleeding tendency.

Correction of vitamin K deficiency, when it is clinically significant, can be achieved with oral supplementation, unless malabsorption is present, in which case parenteral vitamin K (10 mg subcutaneously daily) should be administered. Emergency treatment of bleeding caused by vitamin K deficiency is transfusion of fresh-frozen plasma.

Grade A References

A1. Ranieri VM, Thompson BT, Barie PS, et al. Drotrecogin alfa (activated) in adults with septic shock. *N Engl J Med.* 2012;366:2055-2064.

A2. Afdhal NH, Dusheiko GM, Giannini EG, et al. Eltrombopag increases platelet numbers in thrombocytopenic patients with HCV infection and cirrhosis, allowing for effective antiviral therapy. *Gastroenterology.* 2014;146:442-452.

A3. Martí-Carvajal AJ, Karakitsiou DE, Salanti G. Human recombinant activated factor VII for upper gastrointestinal bleeding in patient with liver disease. *Cochrane Database Syst Rev.* 2012;3:CD004887.

GENERAL REFERENCES

For the General References and other additional features, please visit Expert Consult at https://expertconsult.inkling.com.

176

THROMBOTIC DISORDERS: HYPERCOAGULABLE STATES

ANDREW I. SCHAFER

The hypercoagulable states, also referred to as thrombophilias, encompass a group of inherited or acquired conditions that are associated with an increased risk for thrombosis.

The primary hypercoagulable states are quantitative or qualitative abnormalities in specific coagulation proteins that induce a prothrombotic state. Most of these disorders involve inherited mutations and polymorphisms that lead to either a deficiency of a physiologic antithrombotic factor (typically associated with a loss-of-function mutation) or an increased level of a prothrombotic factor (typically associated with a gain-of-function mutation) (Table 176-1). Particularly when they are combined with other inherited prothrombotic mutations (multigene interactions), these primary hypercoagulable states are associated with a lifelong predisposition to thrombosis. The secondary hypercoagulable states, a diverse group of mostly acquired conditions, cause a thrombotic tendency by more complex, often multifactorial mechanisms. The trigger for a discrete, clinical thrombotic event is often the development of one of the acquired, secondary hypercoagulable states superimposed on an inherited state of hypercoagulability (Fig. 176-1).

PRIMARY HYPERCOAGULABLE STATES

Antithrombin III Deficiency

EPIDEMIOLOGY AND PATHOBIOLOGY

Inherited quantitative or qualitative deficiency of antithrombin III leads to increased fibrin accumulation and a lifelong propensity to thrombosis (Chapter 171). Antithrombin is the major physiologic inhibitor of thrombin and other activated coagulation factors; therefore, its deficiency leads to unregulated protease activity and fibrin formation.[1]

The frequency of asymptomatic heterozygous antithrombin deficiency in the general population may be 1 in 350. Most of these individuals have clinically silent mutations and never have thrombotic manifestations. The frequency of symptomatic antithrombin deficiency in the general population has been estimated to be between 1 in 2000 and 1 in 3000. Among all patients seen with venous thromboembolism (VTE), antithrombin deficiency is detected in only about 1 to 2%, but it is found in approximately 2.5% of selected patients with recurrent thrombosis or onset of thrombosis at a younger age (<45 years old).

Patients with type I antithrombin deficiency have proportionately reduced plasma levels of antigenic and functional antithrombin that result from a quantitative deficiency of the normal protein. Impaired synthesis, defective secretion, or instability of antithrombin in type I antithrombin-deficient individuals is caused by major gene deletions, single nucleotide changes, or short insertions or deletions in the antithrombin gene. Patients with type II antithrombin deficiency have normal or nearly normal plasma antigen accompanied by low activity levels, indicating a functionally defective molecule. Type II deficiency is usually caused by specific point mutations leading to single amino acid substitutions that produce a dysfunctional protein. More than 250 different mutations causing type I or type II antithrombin deficiency have been recognized to date.

The pattern of inheritance of antithrombin deficiency is autosomal dominant. Most affected individuals are heterozygotes whose antithrombin levels are typically about 40 to 60% of normal. These individuals may have the full clinical manifestations of lifelong hypercoagulability. Rare homozygous antithrombin-deficient patients generally have type II deficiency with reduced heparin affinity, a variant that is associated with a low risk for thrombosis in its heterozygous form; other forms of homozygous antithrombin deficiency are probably incompatible with life.

TABLE 176-1 PRIMARY HYPERCOAGULABLE STATES

DEFICIENCY OF ANTITHROMBOTIC FACTORS
Antithrombin (III) deficiency
Protein C deficiency
Protein S deficiency
INCREASED PROTHROMBOTIC FACTORS
Factor Va (activated protein C resistance; factor V Leiden)
Prothrombin (prothrombin G20210A mutation)
Factor IX Padua (factor IX R338L mutation)
Factors VII, XI, IX, VIII; von Willebrand factor; fibrinogen (epidemiologic data; molecular mechanisms unknown)

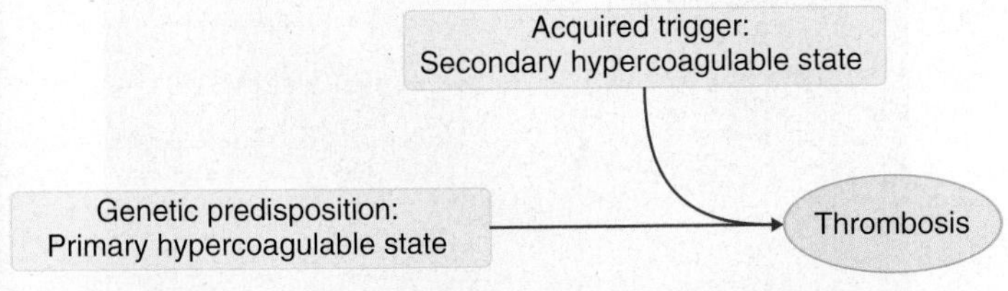

Acquired trigger: Secondary hypercoagulable state

Genetic predisposition: Primary hypercoagulable state

Thrombosis

FIGURE 176-1. **General scheme of thrombosis pathogenesis.** A clinical episode of thrombosis is triggered by an acquired trigger, often one of the secondary hypercoagulable states, superimposed on a genetic predisposition caused by a primary hypercoagulable state. The magnitude of the acquired trigger varies from major (e.g., knee or hip surgery) to minor (e.g., lengthy air travel) to subclinical (not overt and identifiable). Likewise, the magnitude of the lifelong genetic predisposition varies from major (e.g., heterozygous antithrombin III, protein C, or protein S deficiency; homozygous factor V Leiden or prothrombin gene mutation; or two or more primary hypercoagulable states) to minor (e.g., heterozygous factor V Leiden or prothrombin gene mutation).

Protein C Deficiency

Protein C deficiency leads to unregulated fibrin generation because of impaired inactivation of factors VIIIa and Va, two essential cofactors in the coagulation cascade.

EPIDEMIOLOGY

The prevalence of heterozygous protein C deficiency in the general population is about 1 per 200 to 500. Protein C deficiency is found in 2 to 5% of all patients with VTE.

PATHOBIOLOGY

As with antithrombin deficiency, two general forms of protein C deficiency are recognized: type I, in which quantitative deficiency of the protein is associated with a proportionate decrease in protein C antigen and activity; and type II, in which qualitative defects in protein C are associated with disproportionately reduced protein C activity relative to antigen. More than 270 mutations are known to cause protein C deficiency. In the more common type I deficiency, frameshift, nonsense, or missense mutations cause premature termination of synthesis or loss of protein C stability. In type II deficiency, different mutations can cause abnormalities in protein C activation or function. The mode of inheritance of protein C deficiency is autosomal dominant. As in antithrombin deficiency, most affected individuals are heterozygotes. Neonatal purpura fulminans, a very rare complication involving widespread and sometimes fatal thrombosis, occurs in homozygous protein C– or protein S–deficient individuals.

Protein S Deficiency

Protein S is the principal cofactor of activated protein C (APC), and its deficiency mimics that of protein C in causing loss of regulation of fibrin generation by impaired inactivation of factors VIIIa and Va. A population-based study showed that low levels of free protein S and total protein S could only marginally identify subjects at risk for venous thrombosis. Only when cutoff levels for free protein S were far below the normal range, or when unprovoked venous thrombosis was considered an outcome event, was even just a two-fold to five-fold increased risk found.[2]

EPIDEMIOLOGY

Protein S deficiency is estimated to occur in about 1 in 500 in the general population. Its frequency in all patients evaluated for VTE (1 to 3%) is comparable to that of protein C deficiency.

PATHOBIOLOGY

Protein S circulates in plasma partly in complex with C4b-binding protein; only free protein S, which normally constitutes about 35 to 40% of total protein S, can function as a cofactor of APC. As in antithrombin and protein

C deficiencies, quantitative (type I) and qualitative (type II) forms of inherited protein S deficiency are known. In addition, type III protein S deficiency is characterized by normal plasma levels of total protein S but low levels of free protein S.

More than 220 mutations of the protein S gene have been found to cause a deficiency state to date. Most involve frameshift, nonsense, or missense point mutations.

Activated Protein C Resistance (Factor V Leiden)

EPIDEMIOLOGY

The factor V Leiden mutation is remarkably frequent (3 to 8%) in healthy white populations of European ancestry but is far less prevalent in certain black and Asian populations. It causes APC resistance. In various studies, APC resistance was found in a wide range of frequencies (10 to 64%) in patients with VTE.

PATHOBIOLOGY

Almost all subjects with functional APC resistance have a single, specific point mutation in the gene for factor V, which is a critical target of the physiologic anticoagulant action of APC. In this mutation, termed factor V Leiden, guanine is replaced with adenine at nucleotide 1691 (G1691A), which leads to the amino acid substitution of Arg504 by Gln and renders factor Va incapable of being inactivated by APC. Heterozygosity for the autosomally transmitted factor V Leiden mutation increases the risk for thrombosis by a factor of 5 to 10, whereas homozygosity increases the risk by a factor of 50 to 100.

Prothrombin Gene Mutation (Prothrombin G20210A)

The substitution of G for A at nucleotide 20210 of the prothrombin gene has been associated with elevated plasma levels of prothrombin and an increased risk for venous thrombosis. The allele frequency for this gain-of-function mutation is 1 to 6% in white populations, but it is much less prevalent in other racial groups. The prothrombin G20210A mutation is found in 3 to 8% of all patients with VTE.

Other Primary Hypercoagulable States

The first X-linked thrombophilia was reported in a family with a gain-of-function mutation in the gene for coagulation factor IX (factor IX Padua). Juvenile thrombophilia in this family was associated with a five- to ten-fold increase in factor IX clotting activity (with normal quantitative protein levels). Hereditary thrombosis in a Japanese family was associated with a missense mutation in the prothrombin gene (prothrombin Yukuhashi) that causes impaired inhibition of its mutant thrombin product by antithrombin. Elevated levels of factor VIII coagulant activity are a significant risk factor for venous thrombosis and its recurrence, and family studies suggest that high factor VIII levels are often genetically determined.[3] Increased levels of factor VII, factor IX, factor XI, fibrinogen, von Willebrand factor, and thrombin-activatable fibrinolysis inhibitor as well as very low levels of tissue factor pathway inhibitor may also confer increased risk. Many other inherited abnormalities of specific physiologic antithrombotic systems may be associated with a thrombotic tendency. Most of these conditions are limited to case reports or family studies, their molecular genetic bases are less well defined, and their prevalence rates are unknown but are probably much lower than those of the disorders described earlier. The other primary hypercoagulable states include heparin cofactor II deficiency, dysfunctional thrombomodulin, and many fibrinolytic disorders that lead to impaired fibrin degradation, including hypoplasminogenemia, dysplasminogenemia, plasminogen activator deficiency, and certain dysfibrinogenemias that cause a thrombotic rather than a bleeding diathesis.

CLINICAL MANIFESTATIONS

The primary hypercoagulable states are associated with predominantly venous thromboembolic complications (see Table 171-2). Deep venous thrombosis (DVT) of the lower extremities and pulmonary embolism (PE) are the most frequent clinical manifestations. Venous thromboses occurring in more unusual sites include superficial thrombophlebitis and mesenteric and cerebral venous thrombosis (see Table 171-2). Arterial thrombosis involving the coronary, cerebrovascular, and peripheral circulations is not generally linked to any of the primary hypercoagulable states. However, venous thrombosis can result in arterial occlusion by paradoxical embolism across a patent foramen ovale. Also, epidemiologic studies have revealed increased overall risk of arterial thrombotic and atherosclerotic vascular disease in patients with a history of VTE and vice versa.[4] Recurrent pregnancy loss is probably increased in primary hypercoagulable states, but this association is not as strongly established as it is in antiphospholipid syndrome (see later under Secondary Hypercoagulable States).

The initial episode of VTE can occur at any age in patients with primary hypercoagulable states, but it typically takes place in early adulthood. Positive family histories of thrombosis can frequently be elicited. The risk for thrombosis varies among the individual primary hypercoagulable states and is highest in patients with deficiencies of antithrombotic factors (Table 176-2); it is markedly increased with the coexistence of multiple prothrombotic mutations. Patients with homozygous deficiency states tend to have more severe thrombotic complications. Warfarin-induced skin necrosis (Fig. 176-2) infrequently complicates the initiation of oral anticoagulant therapy in patients with heterozygous protein C or protein S deficiency. Because both these proteins depend on vitamin K for normal function, their plasma levels in patients with inherited deficiency states may drop to nearly zero within a few days of starting therapy with warfarin, a vitamin K antagonist, and lead to a transient prothrombotic imbalance and skin necrosis caused by dermal vascular thrombosis. Nevertheless, oral anticoagulation does provide effective long-term antithrombotic prophylaxis in these individuals.

In most patients with primary hypercoagulable states, discrete clinical thrombotic complications appear to be precipitated by acquired prothrombotic events (e.g., pregnancy, use of oral contraceptives, surgery, trauma, immobilization), many of which are the secondary hypercoagulable states discussed subsequently (see Fig. 176-1). For example, thrombosis complicates pregnancy, especially during the puerperium, in about 30 to 60% of women with antithrombin deficiency, 10 to 20% with protein C or protein S deficiency, and almost 30% with APC resistance (factor V Leiden) unless prophylactic anticoagulation is administered during this period.

TABLE 176-2 INHERITED HYPERCOAGULABLE STATES (THROMBOPHILIAS): EPIDEMIOLOGY AND RISK OF VENOUS THROMBOEMBOLISM (VTE)

	PREVALENCE (%)		RELATIVE RISK	
THROMBOPHILIA	***General Population****	***Unselected VTE***	***First VTE***	***Recurrent VTE***
Antithrombin deficiency	0.02-0.3	1-2	5-8	2.5
Protein C deficiency	0.2-0.5	2-5	5-8	2.5
Protein S deficiency	0.5	1-3	1.7-8	2.5
Factor V Leiden	3-8	10-65	5-10†	1.3
Factor II G20210A	1-6	3-8	1.5-3.8	1.4
Factor V Leiden and factor II G20210A	0.01	—	20-60	2.5

*Data refer to white populations. The prevalence of factor V Leiden and factor II G20210A is less than 0.1% in African, African American, and Asian populations.
†Relative risk of first VTE with homozygous factor V Leiden is up to 10-fold higher (50-100).Modified from Coppola A, Tufano A, Cerbone AM, et al. Inherited thrombophilia: implications for prevention and treatment of venous thromboembolism. *Semin Thromb Hemost.* 2009;35:683-694.

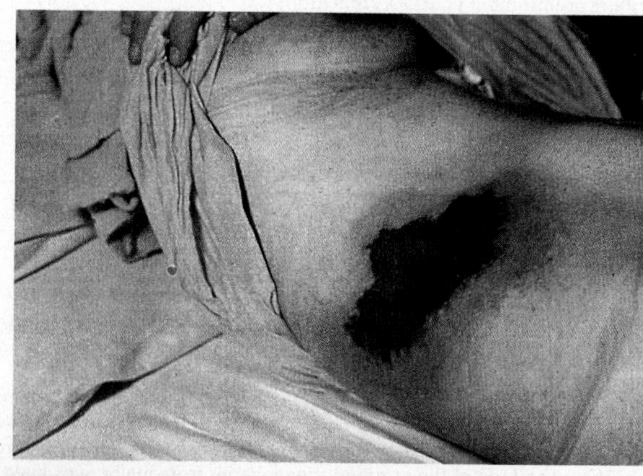

FIGURE 176-2. **Acute skin necrosis in a patient with protein C deficiency who was treated with heparin and warfarin for deep venous thrombosis that occurred after elective hip surgery.** Warfarin treatment was withdrawn and anticoagulation continued with heparin. Skin grafting of the affected area was required. (From Forbes CD, Jackson WF. Color Atlas and Text of Clinical Medicine. 3rd ed. London: Mosby; 2003.)

Although DVT and PE have been considered to simply reflect the clinical spectrum of manifestations of the same single entity (i.e., VTE), some distinct patterns for the two clinical events have become evident. When patients initially present with PE, regardless of cause, they are more likely to have PE again if VTE recurs, and likewise for DVT if VTE recurs.[5] In addition, certain hypercoagulable states have been noted to preferentially be manifested with either DVT or PE. Factor V Leiden poses a clearly higher risk for DVT than for PE (the so-called factor V Leiden paradox); conversely, individuals with underlying pulmonary disease (e.g., chronic obstructive pulmonary disease, pneumonia, or sickle cell disease) have a disproportionately higher likelihood of presenting with PE than with DVT as the primary manifestation of VTE.[6] The reasons that some individuals with VTE appear to be more embolism prone than others are not known.

DIAGNOSIS

Laboratory diagnosis (Chapter 171) of the primary hypercoagulable states requires testing for each of the disorders individually because no general screening test is currently available to determine whether a patient may have such a condition.[7] Factor V Leiden can be diagnosed by a DNA-based assay or by a functional test for APC resistance; the DNA-based assay is required to distinguish between heterozygous and homozygous states. DNA-based assay is required to identify the prothrombin G20210A mutation. In contrast, many different mutations have been found in the genes for antithrombin, protein C, and protein S, so DNA-based tests are not practical for the diagnosis of these inherited deficiency states. Therefore, they are detected by functional and immunologic tests. Because type II (qualitative) deficiencies of antithrombin, protein C, and protein S exhibit normal immunologic levels, functional assays for these proteins are better screening tests.

The diagnostic approach to a patient with a documented episode of VTE includes a thorough history, physical examination, and basic laboratory tests to search for possible precipitating conditions or triggers for the acute event and to rule out underlying acquired causes of hypercoagulability, including occult malignant disease, as discussed later in the section on secondary hypercoagulable states.

As noted in Chapter 171 (section under Evaluation of the Patient with a Possible Hypercoagulable State), the lack of evidence of clearly increased risk of thrombosis *recurrence* in patients with a history of VTE associated with most of the primary hypercoagulable states (thrombophilias) has made thrombophilia testing after a first episode debatable. This controversy is reflected by current practice guidelines.[8-11] An algorithm for thrombophilia testing is shown in Figure 176-3.

A reasonable diagnostic approach at this time is to screen at least all "strongly thrombophilic" patients after an initial episode of VTE: individuals with a documented event before 40 years of age, a positive family history, or unprovoked or recurrent VTE. Thrombophilia testing is not routinely recommended, however, indiscriminately in all patients after a first VTE episode or in those with overt provoking factors. Analysis of results from a randomized trial showed that recurrent VTE was not increased, at least during warfarin therapy, in the presence of factor V Leiden, prothrombin G20210A mutation, antithrombin deficiency, or elevated levels of factor VIII, factor XI, or homocysteine.[A1] However, there have been no controlled clinical trials to date that have assessed the benefit of testing for thrombophilia on the risk of recurrent VTE. Although indefinite anticoagulation is recommended for patients who have had two or more VTE events, regardless of whether a primary hypercoagulable state is found, testing of these individuals for thrombophilia is still useful to guide family screening strategies (see Fig. 176-3). Individuals with arterial thrombosis generally should not be tested for any of these disorders because primary hypercoagulable states (see Table 176-1) are not clearly associated with an increased risk for arterial thrombosis. In contrast, some of the secondary hypercoagulable states, including hyperhomocysteinemia and the antiphospholipid syndrome (see later), are associated with an increased risk for arterial as well as venous thrombosis.

In general, testing for primary hypercoagulable states is not recommended immediately after a major thrombotic event. Optimally, it should be performed in clinically stable patients at least 2 weeks after completion of oral anticoagulation following a thrombotic episode. This is because active thrombosis may transiently consume and deplete some of the antithrombotic proteins in plasma and lead to the erroneous diagnosis of inherited antithrombin, protein C, or protein S deficiency. In addition to acute thrombosis, pregnancy, estrogen use, liver disease, and disseminated intravascular coagulation may cause acquired deficiencies of antithrombin, protein C, or protein S. Anticoagulation may also interfere with some of the functional tests for

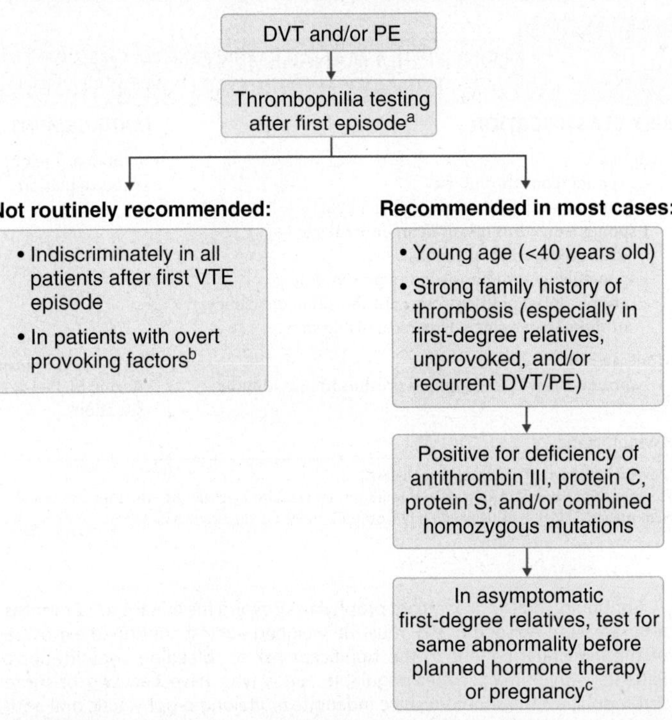

FIGURE 176-3. Algorithm for thrombophilia testing after a first episode of deep venous thrombosis (DVT) or pulmonary embolism (PE) and in asymptomatic, first-degree relatives. In the absence of strong evidence-based guidelines (see text), decisions about thrombophilia testing should be individualized, ranging from "not routinely recommended" to "recommended in most cases." VTE = venous thromboembolism. [a]Thrombophilia testing to include antithrombin III, protein C, protein S, factor V Leiden, prothrombin 20210A gene mutation, and lupus anticoagulant/antiphospholipid antibodies. [b]Provoking factors include active malignant disease, postoperative state, immobilization, trauma, active chronic inflammatory disease (e.g., extensive psoriasis), myeloproliferative neoplasm, pregnancy, oral contraceptives, and hormone replacement therapy. [c]In asymptomatic first-degree relatives of such individuals, avoidance is an alternative to testing.

primary hypercoagulable states. Heparin treatment can cause a decline in antithrombin levels to the deficiency range even in normal individuals. In contrast, warfarin can elevate antithrombin levels into the normal range in patients who do have an inherited deficiency state. Warfarin therapy, by its very mode of action, also predictably reduces the functional levels and, less prominently, the immunologic levels of protein C and protein S. This warfarin action thereby potentially leads to a misdiagnosis of inherited deficiency. When testing is indicated in patients in whom interruption of prophylactic oral anticoagulation is considered to be too risky, protein C and protein S levels can be determined after warfarin therapy has been discontinued under heparin coverage for at least 2 weeks.

As noted previously, functional assays are the best screening tests for antithrombin, protein C, and protein S deficiencies because they detect both quantitative and qualitative defects; antigenic (immunologic) assays detect only quantitative deficiencies of these proteins. Functional coagulation assays for protein C and protein S may yield spuriously low values, however, if APC resistance is present. APC resistance can be diagnosed by newer high-sensitivity and high-specificity coagulation assays or by DNA analysis of peripheral blood mononuclear cells for the factor V Leiden mutation.

TREATMENT Rx

The initial treatment of acute venous thrombosis or PE in patients with primary hypercoagulable states is not different from that in patients without genetic defects (Chapters 38 and 81). As in patients without known thrombophilia, thrombolytic therapy should be considered after massive venous thrombosis or PE. Acute management is initiated with at least 5 days of unfractionated or low-molecular-weight heparin or fondaparinux. Oral anticoagulation with warfarin can be started on the first day of parenteral anticoagulation use and continued for at least 6 months in patients with VTE in the absence of triggering factors (e.g., postoperative state), with regulation of the dose to maintain an international normalized ratio of the prothrombin time between 2.0 and 3.0.

TABLE 176-3 LONG-TERM MANAGEMENT OF PATIENTS WITH PRIMARY HYPERCOAGULABLE STATES*

RISK CLASSIFICATION	MANAGEMENT
High risk ≥2 spontaneous thromboses 1 spontaneous life-threatening thrombosis 1 spontaneous thrombosis at an unusual site (e.g., mesenteric, cerebral venous) 1 spontaneous thrombosis in the presence of antiphospholipid syndrome, antithrombin deficiency, or more than a single hypercoagulable state	Indefinite or lifelong anticoagulation
Moderate risk 1 thrombosis with an acquired prothrombotic stimulus	Vigorous prophylaxis during high-risk situations
Asymptomatic	

*Beyond initial period of thromboprophylaxis.
Modified from Bauer K. Approach to thrombosis. In: Loscalzo J, Schafer AI, eds. Thrombosis and Hemorrhage. 3rd ed. Philadelphia: Lippincott Williams & Wilkins; 2003:330-342.

Continuing oral anticoagulant prophylaxis beyond the initial 6 to 12 months after an acute episode of VTE must be weighed against continued exposure of the individual patient to the significant risk for bleeding complications. Patients with primary hypercoagulable states who have had two or more thrombotic events should receive indefinite or lifelong prophylactic oral anticoagulation (Chapter 38). Indefinite or lifelong anticoagulation is probably indicated for individuals with recurrent thrombosis even in the absence of identifiable primary hypercoagulable states.

The decision to continue prophylactic oral anticoagulation beyond the initial period after the first episode of thrombosis is more difficult (Table 176-3). After a single episode of thrombosis, patients with inherited hypercoagulable states should probably receive indefinite or lifelong anticoagulation if their initial episodes were life-threatening or occurred in unusual sites (e.g., mesenteric or cerebral venous thrombosis) or if they have more than one prothrombotic genetic abnormality. Some authorities also recommend indefinite or lifelong anticoagulation after an initial venous thromboembolic event in patients whose risk of recurrence likewise appears to be increased: those with isolated heterozygous deficiencies of antithrombin, protein C, or protein S and patients with homozygous factor V Leiden. In the absence of these characteristics, particularly if the initial episode was precipitated by a transient acquired prothrombotic situation (e.g., pregnancy, postoperative state, immobilization), it is reasonable at this time to discontinue warfarin therapy after 3 months and to administer subsequent prophylactic anticoagulation only during high-risk periods.

Asymptomatic individuals with known thrombophilia who have not had previous thrombotic complications do not require prophylactic anticoagulation except during periods of high risk for thrombosis. Because about half of the first-degree relatives of a patient with a primary hypercoagulable state should be affected, these individuals should be counseled about the implications of testing them and potentially making a diagnosis.

Management of pregnancy in women with primary hypercoagulable states requires special consideration because of the high risk for thrombosis, particularly during the puerperium.[12] Women with thrombophilia who have previously had thrombosis—and probably also asymptomatic women with thrombophilia—should receive prophylactic anticoagulation throughout pregnancy and for at least 6 weeks post partum, a particularly high-risk period. Coumarin derivatives cross the placenta and have the potential to cause both bleeding and teratogenic effects in the fetus; therefore, oral anticoagulants should not be used during pregnancy. Heparin does not cross the placenta and does not cause these fetal complications. Fixed-dose, low-molecular-weight heparin (instead of unfractionated heparin) is the anticoagulant of choice during pregnancy. Neither warfarin nor heparin induces an anticoagulant effect in a breast-fed infant when the drug is given to a nursing mother, so either can be given safely when indicated in the postpartum period.

Because warfarin-induced skin necrosis (see Fig. 176-2) is a rare problem, screening of all patients for inherited protein C or protein S deficiency, conditions that are known to predispose to this complication, is not indicated before starting warfarin therapy. Most cases can be avoided by not initiating warfarin therapy with high loading doses and by concomitant coverage with heparin. When the complication does occur, as manifested by painful red and subsequently dark, necrotic skin lesions (see Fig. 176-2) within a few days of starting warfarin, such therapy must be discontinued immediately, vitamin K administered, and heparin started (Chapter 38). The use of fresh-frozen plasma or purified protein C concentrate to normalize protein C levels rapidly can improve results. Despite this rare complication, warfarin is an effective, long-term prophylactic anticoagulant in patients with inherited protein C or protein S deficiency.

Antithrombin concentrate purified from normal human plasma or human recombinant antithrombin may be a useful adjunct to anticoagulation in "heparin-resistant" patients, who represent unusual cases of type II antithrombin deficiency, and in antithrombin-deficient patients with recurrent thrombosis despite adequate anticoagulation. Infusion of antithrombin concentrate can also be considered in some perioperative or obstetric settings in which anticoagulation poses an unacceptable bleeding risk.

SECONDARY HYPERCOAGULABLE STATES

DEFINITION

The secondary hypercoagulable states are diverse, mostly acquired disorders that predispose patients to thrombosis by complex, multifactorial pathophysiologic mechanisms. Many of these conditions also represent the acquired precipitating stimuli for clinical thrombotic events in individuals with a genetic predisposition (primary hypercoagulable states). Although each disorder causes thrombosis primarily through abnormalities in blood flow (rheology), the composition of blood (coagulation factors and platelet function), or the vessel wall, multiple overlapping mechanisms are operative in many of them.

Hyperhomocysteinemia

Hyperhomocysteinemia is an elevated blood level of homocysteine, a sulfhydryl amino acid derived from methionine by a transmethylation pathway (E-Fig. 176-1). Homocysteine is remethylated to methionine or catabolized to cystathionine. The major remethylation pathway requires folate and cobalamin (vitamin B_{12}) and involves the action of methylenetetrahydrofolate reductase (MTHFR); a minor remethylation pathway is mediated by betaine–homocysteine methyltransferase. Alternatively, homocysteine is converted to cystathionine in a trans-sulfuration pathway catalyzed by cystathionine β-synthase (CBS), with pyridoxine used as a cofactor.

Homozygous CBS deficiency states that lead to severe hyperhomocysteinemia (homocystinuria) (Chapter 209) cause premature arterial atherosclerotic disease and VTE as well as mental retardation, neurologic defects, lens ectopy, and skeletal abnormalities. By comparison, adults with heterozygous CBS deficiency, with resultant mild to moderate hyperhomocysteinemia, may have only venous or arterial thrombotic manifestations. Hyperhomocysteinemia resulting from inherited remethylation pathway defects usually involves reduced activity of MTHFR. In homozygous individuals with the autosomal recessive C677T mutation of the *MTHFR* gene, which occurs in 15% of certain populations, moderate hyperhomocysteinemia may occur and is correctable with folic acid, but it does not appear to be related to risk of venous thrombosis.[13] Acquired causes of hyperhomocysteinemia in adults most commonly involve nutritional deficiencies of the cofactors required for homocysteine metabolism, including pyridoxine, cobalamin, and folate.

Acquired and inherited hyperhomocysteinemia is a probable risk factor for both arterial and venous thrombosis. The mechanism of homocysteine-induced thrombosis and atherogenesis involves complex, probably multifactorial effects on the vessel wall. Homocysteine can cause vascular endothelial injury, conversion of the endothelial surface of blood vessels from an antithrombotic to a prothrombotic state, and smooth muscle cell proliferation. These toxic effects of homocysteine on the vessel wall may be mediated by oxidant stress.

Vitamin supplementation with folate, pyridoxine, and cobalamin can normalize elevated blood levels of homocysteine. However, several prospective clinical trials of homocysteine-lowering therapy have failed to show reduced rates of vascular events in patients with established vascular disease. It remains to be determined whether this disappointing lack of clinical benefit with homocysteine-lowering vitamin therapy indicates that homocysteine is not a direct atherogenic factor, or that vitamin therapy in this setting might have other, offsetting deleterious effects, or that possibly other mechanisms are operative.

Malignant Disease

Multiple abnormalities of hemostasis are involved in the hypercoagulable state in cancer patients, many of which initiate a systemic process of chronic disseminated intravascular coagulation (Chapter 175). The thrombotic tendency of patients with cancer may also be related to mechanical factors, such as immobility, indwelling central venous catheters, or a bulky tumor mass compressing vessels, and to comorbid conditions, such as sepsis, surgery, liver dysfunction secondary to metastases, and the prothrombotic effects of certain antineoplastic agents.

The incidence of thrombotic complications in cancer patients depends in part on the type of malignant disease. Hypercoagulability is most prominent in patients with pancreatic cancer (Chapter 194), adenocarcinoma of the gastrointestinal tract (Chapters 192 and 193), lung (Chapter 191), ovarian cancer (Chapter 199), and hematologic malignant neoplasms. The presence of underlying malignant disease compounds the independent risk for thrombosis in the postoperative state. There is a two-fold increase in risk of postoperative thrombosis (see later section, Postoperative State, Immobilization, and Trauma) in cancer patients compared with noncancer patients. Thrombosis most commonly occurs in patients with established or concurrently diagnosed malignant disease. In these patients, the risk of venous thrombosis has been found to be highest in the first few months after the diagnosis of malignant disease, then decreases progressively during the subsequent 15 years. The same large case-control study showed that the risk of venous thrombosis in cancer patients is approximately 12- to 17-fold increased in those who also have the factor V Leiden or the prothrombin G20210A mutation.

The increased risk of harboring an undiagnosed, usually occult malignant neoplasm in patients who present with VTE is now well established. The overall prevalence of undiagnosed cancer in patients with unprovoked VTE is approximately 6% at the time of thrombosis and 10% within the first year after thrombosis. Beyond thorough history, physical examination, and routine laboratory tests and radiography, the benefit of extensive evaluation for occult cancer including advanced imaging studies is not established, however.[14] An algorithm for evaluating a patient for occult malignant neoplasm after an episode of VTE is shown in Figure 176-4.

The most frequent thrombotic manifestations in patients with neoplasms are DVT and PE, but more unusual and distinctive thrombotic complications are also found. Trousseau's syndrome, characterized by migratory superficial thrombophlebitis of the upper or lower extremities, is strongly linked to cancer. Nonbacterial thrombotic endocarditis involves fibrin-platelet vegetations on heart valves, which produce clinical manifestations by systemic embolization (Chapter 60). Of patients with nonbacterial thrombotic endocarditis, 75% have underlying malignant neoplasms at autopsy. Trousseau's syndrome and nonbacterial thrombotic endocarditis are highly associated with adenocarcinomas. The occurrence of either syndrome in patients without known cancer demands a more vigorous search for occult malignant disease than in patients with DVT or PE. Thrombotic microangiopathy (Chapter 172), characterized by hemolysis with red blood cell fragmentation, thrombocytopenia, and microvascular thrombosis with involvement of target organs, occurs in about 5% of patients with metastatic carcinomas, most commonly those with gastric (Chapter 192), lung (Chapter 191), and breast (Chapter 198) primary sites.

Some antineoplastic agents themselves increase the risk of thrombosis in cancer patients. These include antiangiogenic agents (VTE with thalidomide and lenalidomide; arterial thrombosis with bevacizumab, sunitinib, sorafenib). In multiple myeloma (Chapter 187), the thrombotic risk of thalidomide is increased 10-fold when the drug is combined with high-dose dexamethasone and an anthracycline. Other thrombogenic chemotherapeutic agents include all-*trans*-retinoic acid and arsenic trioxide, particularly when used as induction chemotherapy for acute promyelocytic leukemia (Chapter 183); cisplatinum (causing both venous and arterial thrombosis); L-asparaginase (which can also cause bleeding); and methotrexate.[15]

TREATMENT Rx

Treatment of acute VTE in cancer patients should be initiated as in other patients, but subsequent prophylactic anticoagulation generally should be continued while active malignant disease is present.[16] In some patients, however, complete resolution of the VTE may allow treatment to be stopped safely.[A2] Anticoagulation can be difficult in many cancer patients; these patients may be resistant to warfarin prophylaxis. Anticoagulation can also be complicated by bleeding into tumors. Long-term treatment of cancer patients with low-molecular-weight heparin (LMWH) after VTE (Chapter 38) reduces recurrences and possibly decreases bleeding complications compared with treatment with warfarin. LMWH also reduces the risk of a first VTE in patients with cancer[A3] and is more effective than warfarin in doing so[A4], although it has not been shown to increase overall survival in this setting.[A5] Evidence-based practice guidelines have been published for the prevention and treatment of VTE in cancer patients.[A6]

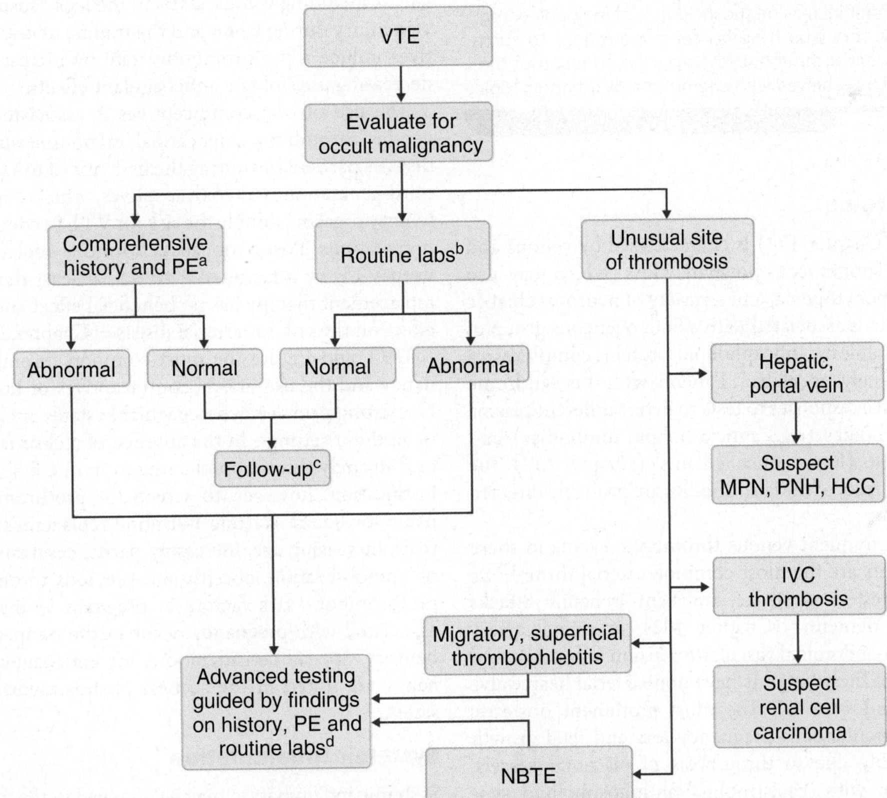

FIGURE 176-4. **Algorithm for evaluating a patient for occult malignant neoplasm after an unprovoked episode of deep venous thrombosis or pulmonary embolism or thrombosis at an unusual site. HCC = hepatocellular carcinoma; IVC = inferior vena cava; MPN = myeloproliferative neoplasm; NBTE = nonbacterial thrombotic endocarditis; PE = physical examination; PNH = paroxysmal nocturnal hemoglobinuria; VTE = venous thromboembolism. [a]Physical examination to include rectal (with stool sample for occult blood) and breast and pelvic examinations for women. [b]Routine laboratory evaluations to include chest radiography, complete blood count, basic chemistries, and calcium concentration. [c]Follow-up suggested at 6 to 12 months. [d]Advanced testing could include advanced imaging, endoscopies, cytologies, and the like.**

Myeloproliferative Neoplasms and Paroxysmal Nocturnal Hemoglobinuria

Thrombosis and, apparently paradoxically, bleeding are major causes of morbidity and mortality in patients with chronic myeloproliferative neoplasms (Chapter 166) and the related bone marrow stem cell disorder paroxysmal nocturnal hemoglobinuria (Chapter 160). In uncontrolled polycythemia vera (Chapter 166), increased whole blood viscosity contributes to the thrombotic tendency. Thrombocytosis, abnormal platelet function, and other less well understood factors are also probably involved in the hemostatic defect of the myeloproliferative neoplasms and paroxysmal nocturnal hemoglobinuria.

In addition to DVT and PE, some distinctive thrombotic manifestations are seen. Hepatic vein thrombosis (Budd-Chiari syndrome) and portal and other intra-abdominal venous thromboses (Chapter 143) are associated with myeloproliferative neoplasms and paroxysmal nocturnal hemoglobinuria (Chapter 160) and may be the initial manifestations of the disease. Myeloproliferative neoplasms, particularly polycythemia vera (Chapter 166) and essential thrombocythemia (Chapter 166), may cause erythromelalgia, a syndrome of microvascular thrombosis manifested by intense pain accompanied by warmth, duskiness, and mottled erythema, sometimes resembling livedo reticularis, in a patchy distribution in the extremities, most prominently in the feet; digital microvascular ischemia progressing to vascular insufficiency and gangrene may ensue (Chapter 80). A wide spectrum of neurologic manifestations may be caused by cerebrovascular ischemia, especially in patients with essential thrombocythemia.

TREATMENT Rx

Treatment of VTE in patients with the myeloproliferative neoplasms and paroxysmal nocturnal hemoglobinuria should be initiated as in patients without these hematologic disorders. In patients with thrombosis associated with polycythemia vera, the hematocrit should be maintained in the normal range with phlebotomies or chemotherapy, or with both (Chapter 166). Patients maintained at a hematocrit target of less than 45% have a significantly lower rate of cardiovascular death and major thrombosis than do those with hematocrit targets of 45 to 50%.[A7] Low-dose aspirin (100 mg daily) can prevent thrombotic complications without increasing the incidence of major bleeding in patients with polycythemia vera who have no contraindications to such treatment. In patients with essential thrombocythemia, cytoreduction of the elevated platelet count should be achieved with chemotherapy (Chapter 166).

Antiphospholipid Syndrome

Antiphospholipid syndrome (Chapter 174) is characterized by venous and arterial thrombosis, recurrent spontaneous pregnancy loss (which may also be due to thrombosis), thrombocytopenia, and a variety of neuropsychiatric manifestations.[17] The syndrome is associated with a heterogeneous group of autoantibodies that bind to anionic phospholipid-protein complexes, a protein cofactor of which is β_2-glycoprotein I. Patients with this syndrome have any combination of positive responses to tests to detect different plasma antiphospholipid-protein antibodies (e.g., anticardiolipin antibodies) and phospholipid-based clotting tests (lupus anticoagulants) (Chapter 257). The predominant prothrombotic effects of these antibodies are probably directed to the vessel wall.

DVT and PE are the most frequent venous thrombotic events in these patients. Cerebrovascular events are the most common arterial thrombotic complications and are manifested as stroke, transient ischemic attacks (Chapter 407), multi-infarct dementia (Chapter 402), or retinal artery occlusion. Peripheral and intra-abdominal vascular occlusion is encountered more rarely. About one third of these patients have nonbacterial heart valve vegetations (Libman-Sacks endocarditis). The most prominent obstetric complications are recurrent spontaneous pregnancy loss and fetal growth retardation, which are probably due to thrombosis of placental vessels. Patients are occasionally seen with "catastrophic" antiphospholipid syndrome involving a series of acute and sometimes fatal vascular occlusive events, or "thrombotic storm." Thrombotic complications are limited largely to patients with primary antiphospholipid syndrome and patients in whom the antibodies are associated with collagen vascular disease, not with drugs or infections.

TREATMENT AND PREVENTION Rx

Acute management of thrombosis in these patients is essentially the same as in other individuals. Monitoring of heparin anticoagulation is difficult in patients with a lupus anticoagulant because they already have a prolonged activated partial thromboplastin time at baseline; the use of low-molecular-weight heparin, which does not require monitoring, can circumvent this problem. Warfarin is effective in preventing recurrent thrombosis but usually requires prolonged or indefinite therapy with doses to achieve an international normalized ratio of 2.0 to 3.0. Whereas laboratory evidence of antiphospholipid antibodies in patients with a first episode of VTE is still usually considered an indication for indefinite anticoagulant therapy, a systematic review showed that the strength of this association is uncertain because of low-quality evidence supporting it.[18] No established treatment of women with antiphospholipid syndrome has been shown to prevent recurrent fetal loss. Treatment with prednisone and aspirin during pregnancy is not effective in promoting live birth and may increase the risk for prematurity.

Asymptomatic carriers of a "high-risk profile" of antiphospholipid antibodies (confirmed triple positive for anticardiolipin, lupus anticoagulant, and anti-β_2-glycoprotein I) are at considerable risk for a first thromboembolic event; some such individuals should even be considered for primary thromboprophylaxis.[19]

Pregnancy, Oral Contraceptives, and Hormone Replacement Therapy

Activation of the coagulation system is initiated locally in the maternal uteroplacental circulation, where the placenta is the source of increased thrombin generation. Platelet activation and increased platelet turnover also occur during normal pregnancy, and about 8% of healthy women have mild thrombocytopenia at term. Simultaneously, the fibrinolytic system is progressively blunted throughout pregnancy because of the action of placental plasminogen activator inhibitor type 2. The net effect of these coagulation changes is creation of a state of hypercoagulability that makes pregnant women vulnerable to thrombosis, particularly in the puerperium. These systemic alterations are compounded by prothrombotic mechanical and rheologic factors in pregnancy, including venous stasis in the legs caused by the gravid uterus, pelvic vein injury during labor, and the trauma of cesarean section. Oral contraceptives induce a prothrombotic state by increasing procoagulant effects and decreasing physiologic anticoagulant effects.

The use of oral contraceptives is associated with an increased risk for venous thrombosis, myocardial infarction, stroke, and peripheral arterial disease, particularly during the first year of use (Chapter 238). Unexpectedly, third-generation oral contraceptives, which contain less estrogen and a different progestin, double the risk for VTE in comparison to second-generation preparations. Postmenopausal hormone replacement increases the risk for deep VTE by a factor of 2 to 3.5, at least during the first year. Hormone replacement therapy has no beneficial effect and possibly even a detrimental effect on the risk for arterial disease (Chapter 240).

DVT and PE are the most common thrombotic complications of pregnancy and the use of oral contraceptives or hormone replacement therapy. Coexisting primary hypercoagulable states are an at least additive risk factor in all these settings. In the absence of a clear family history of clinical VTE or a strongly thrombophilic mutation in a first-degree relative, there is little justification, however, to screen for prothrombotic mutations with pregnancy or before starting hormone replacement therapy or oral contraceptives. Increasing age, increasing parity, cesarean delivery, prolonged bedrest or immobilization, obesity, and previous thromboembolism are additional prothrombotic risk factors in pregnant women. Most thrombotic events associated with pregnancy occur in the peripartum period, especially after delivery. Special considerations for anticoagulation in the setting of pregnancy are noted in the section on treatment of primary hypercoagulable states.

Systemic Inflammation

Systemic inflammation may be involved in the pathogenesis of VTE through vessel wall inflammation and damage as well as systemic hypercoagulability. Patients with autoimmune connective tissue diseases, particularly rheumatoid arthritis,[20] juvenile rheumatoid arthritis, and systemic lupus erythematosus, are at increased risk of VTE. Psoriasis, an immunoinflammatory disease that is associated with cardiovascular risk and atherothrombotic events, has also been shown in a cohort study to carry an increased risk of VTE; the risk was found to be highest in younger patients with severe psoriasis. Other skin diseases that are autoimmune in etiology were not associated with VTE risk in another population-based case-control study.

Postoperative State, Immobilization, and Trauma

Postoperative thrombosis (Chapter 433) is caused by a combination of local mechanical factors, including decreased venous blood flow in the lower extremities, and systemic changes in coagulation. The level of risk for postoperative thrombosis depends largely on the type of surgery performed. It is compounded by coexisting risk factors, such as an underlying inherited primary hypercoagulable state or malignant disease (see earlier sections), advanced age, and prolonged procedures. Postoperative DVT and PE, the most common thrombotic complications, are often asymptomatic and detectable only by noninvasive studies. The incidence of DVT after general surgical procedures is about 20 to 25%, with almost 2% of these patients having clinically significant PE. Without prophylaxis, the risk for DVT after hip surgery and knee reconstruction ranges from 45 to 70%, and clinically significant PE occurs in 20% of patients undergoing hip surgery. Although the process of thrombosis generally begins intraoperatively or within a few days of surgery, the risk for this complication can be protracted beyond the time of discharge from the hospital, particularly in hip replacement patients.

Patients who are bedridden or experiencing prolonged air travel are at increased risk for VTE. VTE is also one of the most common causes of morbidity and mortality in survivors of major trauma, and asymptomatic DVT of the lower extremities has been detected by venography in more than 50% of hospitalized trauma patients. The risk for venous thrombosis after trauma is increased by advanced age, need for surgery or transfusions, and presence of lower extremity fractures or spinal cord injury.

Mechanical methods of prophylaxis against VTE should be considered in high-risk postoperative patients and bedridden patients with medical conditions, either in combination with anticoagulant prophylaxis or instead of it in patients who have an unusually high risk for bleeding with anticoagulation. Such methods include graduated compression stockings, intermittent pneumatic compression devices, and venous foot pumps.

For long-distance travelers at increased risk of VTE, including those with previous VTE or hypercoagulable states, current recommendations include frequent ambulation, nonalcoholic hydration, calf muscle exercises, and the use of properly fitted, below-knee graduated compression stockings providing 15 to 30 mm Hg of pressure at the ankle during travel; compression stockings are not recommended for other long-distance travelers. The use of aspirin or anticoagulants to prevent VTE is not recommended for long-distance travelers at increased risk of VTE.[21]

Grade A References

A1. Kearon C, Julian JA, Kovacs MJ, et al. Influence of thrombophilia on risk of recurrent venous thromboembolism while on warfarin: results from a randomized trial. *Blood*. 2008;112:4432-4436.

A2. Napolitano M, Saccullo G, Malato A, et al. Optimal duration of low molecular weight heparin for the treatment of cancer-related deep vein thrombosis: The Cancer-DACUS Study. *J Clin Oncol*. 2014;32:3607-3612.

A3. Ben-Aharon I, Stemmer SM, Leibovici L, et al. Low molecular weight heparin (LMWH) for primary thrombo-prophylaxis in patients with solid malignancies—systematic review and meta-analysis. *Acta Oncol*. 2014;53:1230-1237.

A4. Di Nisio M, Porreca E, Otten HM, et al. Primary prophylaxis for venous thromboembolism in ambulatory cancer patients receiving chemotherapy. *Cochrane Database Syst Rev*. 2014;8:CD008500.

A5. Sanford D, Naidu A, Alizadeh N, et al. The effect of low molecular weight heparin on survival in cancer patients: an updated systematic review and meta-analysis of randomized trials. *J Thromb Haemost*. 2014;12:1076-1085.

A6. Farge D, Debourdeau P, Beckers M, et al. International clinical practice guidelines for the treatment and prophylaxis of venous thromboembolism in patients with cancer. *J Thromb Haemost*. 2013;11:56-70.

A7. Marchioli R, Finazzi G, Specchia G, et al. Cardiovascular events and intensity of treatment in polycythemia vera. *N Engl J Med*. 2013;368:22-33.

GENERAL REFERENCES

For the General References and other additional features, please visit Expert Consult at https://expertconsult.inkling.com.

177 TRANSFUSION MEDICINE

LAWRENCE T. GOODNOUGH

DEVELOPMENT OF TRANSFUSION MEDICINE

Concepts in blood transfusion and blood conservation include blood safety, blood inventory, and blood costs. The formation of clinical practice guidelines in patient blood management is based on effective blood utilization, new strategies in blood conservation, including pharmacologic alternatives to blood transfusion, and patients' informed consent for transfusion. The broad-based multidisciplinary constituency of transfusion medicine includes blood collection facilities, hospital-based transfusion services, research laboratories, and the commercial sector.

Patient-focused blood management is described in the Circular of Information[1] as "a professional judgment based on clinical evaluation that determines the selection of components, dosage, rate of administration...." Patient blood management therefore encompasses an evidence-based medical and surgical approach with preventive strategies that are emphasized to identify, evaluate, and manage anemia (e.g., pharmacologic therapy and reduced iatrogenic blood losses from diagnostic testing); to optimize hemostasis (e.g., pharmacologic therapy and point-of-care testing); and to establish decision thresholds (e.g., guidelines) for the appropriate administration of blood therapy.[2,3]

The medical director of the blood bank is responsible for issues related to blood inventory and safety, through the oversight of laboratory policies and procedures and quality management (Fig. 177-1). Management of the transfusion service includes coordinating blood transfusion and blood conservation activities and serving as a consultant to clinicians whose patients are undergoing massive transfusions, apheresis, or transplantation or who are having difficulty finding compatible blood products. Finally, the transfusion medicine specialist supervises quality assurance to satisfy regulatory and accreditation requirements.[4]

Blood Availability

Blood centers must be able to supply blood in response to acute crises. Sporadic shortages of blood and blood products (e.g., packed red cells, platelet products, albumin, intravenous immunoglobulin, and clotting factor concentrates) are potentially life threatening. Such shortages have been attributed to disruptions in production, increasingly strict criteria for accepting donors, product recalls, increased use (including off-label use), and stockpiling or other market issues.

In the United States, the Department of Health and Human Services monitors sentinel community blood services and hospital transfusion services to track blood collection and transfusion activity. Blood transfusion and collection activities peaked in 1986 and then declined until 1994. However, blood transfusion and collection subsequently increased 8.0% in 1997, 10.2% in 1999, and an estimated 4% to 5% annually thereafter.

Within the American Red Cross, which supplies about half of all blood products in the United States, a 3- to 4-day supply of red blood cell products is typical, but some independent centers have higher reserves. Use of frozen red cells as a hedge against inventory shortages has generally not been practical because the shelf life of thawed units is only 24 hours; however, an automated, functionally closed system for the glycerolization and deglycerolization processes allows a 2-week post-thaw shelf life. With such a system, many blood centers and transfusion services can expand their available red cell inventories as reserves. After disasters—human or natural—on-hand blood supplies are adequate in the short term and can be rapidly mobilized over great distances. Because of the need to maintain reserves, blood collection must routinely surpass the anticipated need for blood transfusion.[5]

Red Blood Cell Transfusion

Worldwide, more than 75 million units of whole blood are estimated to be donated every year, with yearly transfusion of 24 million blood units in the United States.

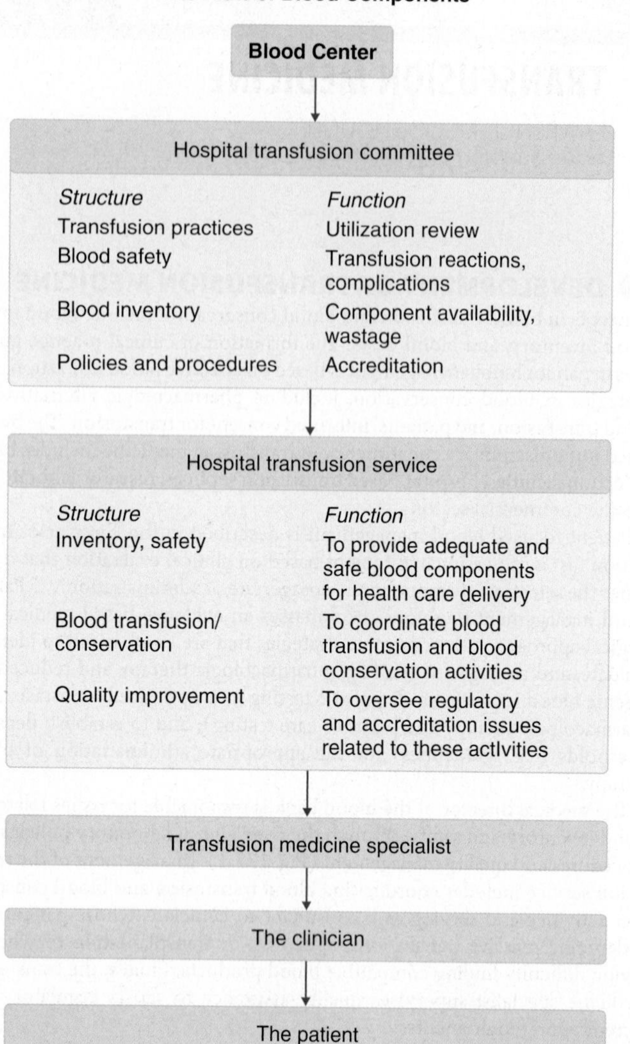

FIGURE 177-1. A hospital's transfusion committee and transfusion service can help treating physicians manage the availability, safety, and use of blood products. (From Goodnough LT. What is a transfusion medicine specialist? *Transfusion.* 1999;39: 1031-1033.)

Whole Blood

A unit of blood is collected as a donation of 450 mL ± 10% into a citrate anticoagulant that also contains phosphate and dextrose. The red cell and hemoglobin content is variable and dependent on the donor's hematocrit and the precise volume bled.

Whole blood is stored at 4 ± 2°C to diminish red cells' utilization of adenosine triphosphate and to preserve their viability, which should be at least 70% at the end of a shelf life of 35 days. After 10 days of storage, all predonation 2,3-diphosphoglycerate content in red cells is lost, but up to 50% is regenerated within 8 hours after transfusion.

In Western countries, whole blood is rarely used because within a few hours or days, some coagulation factors (especially factors V and VIII) and platelets decrease in quantity or lose viability. After a 7-day hold at 4°C, factor VIII levels fall to 0.32 ± 0.09 IU/mL, and factor V levels fall to 0.78 ± 0.15 IU/mL. At 4°C, platelets undergo a shape change from discoid to spherical that is irreversible after 8 hours, and their in vivo survival is reduced to 2 days.

Red Cell Components

Red cells are provided in various formats that differ with respect to the presence of additive solutions and the extent to which white cells are removed. Solutions that contain combinations of saline, adenine, phosphate, bicarbonate, glucose, and mannitol provide better red cell viability during storage and allow up to a 42-day shelf life. Red cells and red cells in additive solution can be used interchangeably, with the exception that red cells in additive solution are not recommended for exchange or massive transfusions in neonates.

Red cells should be refrigerated until the time of the transfusion because of the risk for bacterial proliferation within the pack at room temperature. Red cells that have been out of refrigeration for 30 minutes or longer cannot be returned to stock. A unit of red cells should be infused over a maximum period of 4 hours.

Irradiated Cellular Blood Components

Gamma-irradiated cellular blood components are used to prevent the occurrence of transfusion-associated graft-versus-host disease (see later).

Leukocyte-Reduced Blood Components

Blood components are depleted of leukocytes by means of filtration. A leukocyte-reduced component is defined as one with less than 5×10^6 residual white cells per liter, and 100% of tested units should meet this standard. Leukocyte removal should be performed while the cells are still intact by filtering the blood as soon as possible after collection.

Leukocyte reduction reduces the incidence of human leukocyte antigen (HLA) alloimmunization in multitransfused recipients, but immunization rates of 10 to 25% are still seen in women who have already been exposed to HLA alloantigens through previous pregnancy. Leukocyte reduction has less impact on refractoriness to random platelet donations because of the importance of nonimmune factors in the poor response to transfused platelets.

Leukocyte reduction also lowers the risk for nonhemolytic febrile reactions after the transfusion of red cells or platelets. Several studies suggest that leukocyte reduction has a beneficial impact on the rate of postoperative infection. The impact of leukocyte reduction on the incidence of transfusion-associated graft-versus-host disease is unknown.

Preventing Transmission of Cytomegalovirus

A small number of studies of prestorage leukocyte reduction have suggested its efficacy in preventing transfusion-transmitted cytomegalovirus (CMV) infection (Chapter 377), which occurs in 4% of cases, even with seronegative components. Prestorage leukocyte depletion reduces the infection rate to less than 1%, suggesting that this technology may be at least equivalent to serologic testing for CMV antibodies for the prevention of CMV transmission; however, CMV testing of leukocyte-reduced components continues to be performed by most transfusion services. Indications for CMV-seronegative components include transfusion in pregnancy, intrauterine transfusion, transfusions to neonates less than 37 weeks' gestation, transfusions to CMV-seronegative patients who are potential or actual recipients of allogeneic bone marrow or peripheral blood progenitor transplants when the donor is also CMV seronegative, and patients infected with human immunodeficiency virus (HIV).

Immunomodulatory Effects

Previous transfusion has an immunomodulatory benefit for the survival of renal allografts, even with the use of potent immunosuppressive drugs, although the exact mechanism of this benefit remains unknown. Retrospective studies suggest an adverse effect of transfusion on the rate of perioperative infections or recurrent cancers.

Typing and Crossmatching

Blood and blood components for transfusion must be compatible with the same blood type as the patient. Obtaining an accurate ABO/Rh grouping for a patient is the most significant serologic test performed before transfusion. When type-specific blood and components are unavailable or emergency circumstances do not allow their identification or use, type O-negative red cells should be used. Group O is the only choice for group O recipients and is the alternative choice for groups A, B, and AB.

Red cell antigens other than ABO and D are not routinely considered when selecting *donor* blood products for transfusion; the exception is when unexpected, clinically significant red cell antibodies are present in the patient, as determined by an antibody screen or previous identification. Red cell alloantibodies are produced by exposure to foreign red cell antigens through previous transfusion, pregnancy, or both. For an antibody to be considered clinically significant, it must be associated with a hemolytic transfusion reaction or decreased survival of transfused incompatible red cells. Most of the clinically significant antibodies are optimally reactive at 37°C or are detected by the antiglobulin test. If an antibody screen is negative in the *recipient,* the probability is greater than 99% that an ABO and Rh crossmatch will also be compatible. If no unexpected, clinically significant antibodies are detected and there is no record of their previous detection, only serologic testing for

ABO incompatibility is required (i.e., antiglobulin testing is not required when the crossmatch is performed).

Red Blood Cell Transfusion

If a transfusion is appropriate, a benefit should occur. In a large study of Jehovah's Witnesses (whose religious beliefs preclude the use of blood transfusion), the risk for death was higher in surgical patients with cardiovascular disease than in those without. A follow-up analysis of a subset of these patients reported that the odds of death in patients with a postoperative hemoglobin level less than 7 g/dL increased 2.5 times for each 1 gram decrease in the hemoglobin level; although no deaths occurred in 98 patients with postoperative levels of 7.1 to 8.0 g/dL, 34.4% of 32 patients with postoperative levels of 4.1 to 5.0 g/dL died. These data suggest that in surgery-induced anemia, survival is improved if blood transfusion is administered to maintain the hemoglobin concentration at greater than 7 g/dL. Data from randomized trials consistently support more restrictive policies for the transfusion of red blood cells[A1-A5] and platelets[A6-A9] (Table 177-1).

In a large, randomized trial of elderly patients undergoing repair of hip fracture, transfusion at a hemoglobin threshold of 10 g/dL was no better than transfusion for symptoms of anemia or at physician discretion for a hemoglobin level of less than 8 g/dL.[A4] In a multi-institutional study, 418 critical care patients received red cell transfusions when their hemoglobin levels dropped below 7 g/dL and had their levels maintained between 7 and 9 g/dL, whereas another 420 patients received transfusions when their hemoglobin levels dropped below 10 g/dL and had their levels maintained between 10 and 12 g/dL. Thirty-day mortality rates were not significantly different in the two groups, suggesting that a transfusion threshold as low as 7 g/dL may be as safe as a higher threshold of 10 g/dL in critically ill patients.[A2] A follow-up analysis found that the more restrictive strategy of red blood cell transfusion also appeared to be safe in most patients with cardiovascular disease.

A retrospective study analyzed the relationships among anemia, blood transfusion, and mortality in nearly 80,000 patients older than 65 years hospitalized for acute myocardial infarction. Anemia, defined as a hematocrit below 39%, was present on hospital admission in 44% of patients and was 33% or less in 10% of patients; blood transfusion in patients with hematocrit levels lower than 33% at admission was associated with a significantly lower 30-day mortality. On the basis of this study, transfusion to maintain hematocrit levels above 30% has been recommended in patients with acute myocardial infarction. In patients with heart failure, transfusion to maintain a hemoglobin level above 10 g/dL appears to improve outcomes. Among patients undergoing cardiac surgery, a restrictive perioperative transfusion strategy is as good as a more liberal strategy.[A3]

Clinical Practice Guidelines

The number of published clinical practice guidelines for red blood cell, platelet, and plasma transfusions attests to the increasing interest and importance of appropriate blood utilization by professional societies and health care institutions (Table 177-2). The guidelines acknowledge the necessity of considering patient covariables or other patient-specific criteria for making transfusion decisions. Among published guidelines, it is generally agreed that transfusion is not of benefit when the hemoglobin is greater than 10 g/dL but may be beneficial when the hemoglobin is less than 6 to 7 g/dL.[6] The selection of a discrete hemoglobin as a trigger for transfusion has been controversial. For example, the initial guidelines by the American Society of Anesthesiology (ASA) in 1996 identified a hemoglobin level of less than 6 g/dL as a transfusion trigger for acute blood loss, whereas the updated ASA guidelines in 2006 noted that "although multiple trials have evaluated transfusion thresholds on patient outcome, the literature is insufficient to define a transfusion trigger in surgical patients with substantial blood loss." Three guidelines have specified a hemoglobin threshold for patients with acute bleeding only, whereas the concept of an empirical hemoglobin concentration as a transfusion trigger has been refuted by a number of other published clinical practice guidelines. Arbitrary laboratory values are inadequate to define when red blood cell transfusions are appropriate, so that each patient must be evaluated individually and patient-specific anemia management strategies employed. Implementing real-time clinical decision support and best practice alerts into physician order entry for blood transfusions has resulted in improved blood utilization and improved patients outcomes.

Platelet Transfusion

The use of intensive chemotherapy regimens and bone marrow or stem cell transplantation has increased the demand for platelet products, particularly in patients with severe thrombocytopenia or bleeding complications. The use of apheresis platelet transfusions (i.e., a platelet unit collected from a dedicated donor through an apheresis procedure) has increased substantially, driven by the need for platelet inventories to support cardiac surgery, oncology, and stem cell transplantation programs. Emerging issues in platelet transfusion therapy include re-evaluation of the platelet threshold for prophylactic transfusion and modification of the dose of platelet transfusions. The problem

TABLE 177-1 KEY CLINICAL TRIALS IN RED BLOOD CELL AND PLATELET THERAPY

RED BLOOD CELL TRANSFUSION

CLINICAL SETTING	HEMOGLOBIN THRESHOLD (g/dL)	PATIENTS TRANSFUSED	DEVIATION FROM TRANSFUSION PROTOCOL	MEAN HEMOGLOBIN AT TRANSFUSION (g/dL)	PARTICIPATION OF ELIGIBLE PATIENTS	REFERENCE
Intensive care	7.0 vs. 10.0	67% 99%	1.4% 4.3%	8.5 ± 0.7* 10.7 ± 0.7*	41%	A2
Cardiothoracic surgery	8.0 vs. 10.0	47% 78%	1.6% 0%	9.1 (9.0-9.2) 10.5 (10.4-10.6)	75%	A3
Hip surgery	8.0 vs. 10.0	41% 97%	9.0% 5.6%	7.9 ± 0.6 9.2 ± 0.5	56%	A4
Acute upper GI bleeding	7.0 vs. 9.0	49% 86%	9% 3%	7.3 ± 1.4 8.0 ± 1.5	93%	A5

PLATELET TRANSFUSION

TYPE OF TRIAL	COMPARISONS	PATIENTS TRANSFUSED	PATIENTS TRANSFUSED OFF PROTOCOL	MEDIAN PLATELET COUNT AT TRANSFUSION ($\times 10^9$/L) (RANGE)	PATIENTS WITH GRADE 2 OR GREATER BLEEDING†	REFERENCE
Trigger for prophylactic platelet transfusion	Platelet count of 10×10^9/L vs. 20×10^9/L	135 120	5.4% 2.0%	9 (1-89) 14 (0-64)	21.5% 20%	A6
Platelet dose	Low vs. medium vs. high dose	417 423 432	21% 8% 14%	9 (7-16) 9 (7-19) 9 (7-12)	71% 69% 70%	A7
Prophylactic vs. therapeutic transfusion	Prophylactic vs. therapeutic	197 194	11% 22%	Not provided Not provided	19% 42%	A8
Prophylactic vs. therapeutic transfusion	Prophylactic vs. therapeutic	299 301	23% 14%	Not provided Not provided	43% 50%	A9

*Average daily hemoglobin.
†Different grading systems were used for documenting bleeding

TABLE 177-2 MEDICAL SOCIETY CLINICAL PRACTICE GUIDELINES

RED BLOOD CELL TRANSFUSION

YEAR	SOCIETY	RECOMMENDATIONS	REFERENCE
1988	NIH Consensus Conference	<7 g/dL (acute)	*JAMA* 1988;260:2700
1992	American Colleges of Physicians (ACP)	No number	*Ann Intern Med* 1992;116:393-402
1996/2006	American Society of Anesthesiologists (ASA)	<6 g/dL (acute) No number	*Anesthesia* 1996;84:732-747 *Anesthesia* 2006;105:198-208
1997/1998	Canadian Medical Association (CMA)	No number	*Can Med Assoc J* 1997;156:S1-24 *J Emerg Med* 1998;16:129-131
1998	College of American Pathologists (CAP)	6 g/dL (acute)	*Arch Pathol Lab Med* 1998;122:130-138
2001/2012	British Committee for Standards in Haematology	No number 7-8 g/dL*	*Br J Haematol* 2001;113:24-31 http://www.bcshguidelines.com/documents/BCSH_Blood_Admin_-_addendum_August_2012.pdf
2001	The NHMRC/Australasian Soc Blood Trans	7 g/dL	https://www.nhmrc.gov.au/guidelines-publications/cp78
2007/2011	Society of Thoracic Surgeons and Society of Cardiovascular Anesthesiologists	7 g/dL or 8 g/dL*	*Ann Thorac Surg* 2007;83:S27-86 *Ann Thorac Surg* 2011;91:944-982
2009	American College of Critical Care Medicine Society of Critical Care Medicine	7 g/dL 7 g/dL	*Crit Care Med* 2009;37:3124-157 *J Trauma* 2009;67:1439-1442
2011	Society for the Advancement of Blood Medicine	8 g/dL	*Trans Med Rev* 2011;25:232-246
2012	National Blood Authority, Australia	No number	http://www.nba.gov.au/guidelines/review.html
2012	American Association of Blood Banks	7-8 g/dL or 8 g/dL†	*Ann Intern Med* 2012;157:49-58
2012	Kidney Disease Improving Global Outcomes	No number	*Kidney Int* 2012;2:311-316
2012	National Cancer Center Network	7 g/dL	*JNCCN* 2012;10:628-653

PLATELET TRANSFUSION

YEAR	SOCIETY	RECOMMENDATIONS FOR TRIGGER FOR PROPHYLACTIC PLATELET TRANSFUSIONS‡	REFERENCE
1992	British Committee for Standards in Haematology	10×10^9/L	*Transfus Med* 1992;2:311-318
1994	College of American Pathologists	5×10^9/L	*JAMA* 1994;271:777-781
1998	Consensus Conference, Royal College of Physicians, Edinburgh	10×10^9/L	*Transfusion* 1998;38:796-797
2001	American Society of Clinical Oncology	10×10^9/L	*J Clin Oncol* 2001;19:1519-1538
2003	British Committee for Standards in Haematology	10×10^9/L	*Br J Haematol* 2003;122:10-23
2009	Italian Society of Transfusion Medicine and Immunohaematology	10×10^9/L	*Blood Transfus* 2009;7:132-150

PLASMA TRANSFUSION

YEAR	SOCIETY	PRINCIPAL INDICATIONS	REFERENCE
1984	Consensus Conference, National Institutes of Health	Replacement of clotting factor deficiencies Reversal of warfarin coagulopathy Massive blood transfusion Treatment of TTP Antithrombin III deficiency Immunodeficiencies	*JAMA* 1985;253:551-553
1992	British Committee for Standards in Haematology	1. Replacement of clotting factor deficiencies where factor concentrates are unavailable 2. Immediate reversal of warfarin effect 3. DIC 4. TTP	*Transfus Med* 1992;2:57-63
1994	College of American Pathologists	1. Coagulopathy (inherited or acquired) with bleeding or before an invasive procedure 2. Massive hemorrhage and transfusion 3. Reversal of warfarin coagulopathy 4. Antithrombin III deficiency 5. Immunodeficiencies 6. TTP	*JAMA* 1994;271:777-781
1997	Canadian Medical Association Expert Working Group	1. Acquired coagulation factor deficiencies (e.g., vitamin K deficiency, warfarin, liver disease) with bleeding or before an invasive procedure 2. Acute DIC 3. Massive hemorrhage and transfusion 4. TTP 5. Replacement of coagulation factor deficiencies where factor concentrates are unavailable	*Can Med Assoc J* 1997;156(11 Suppl):S1-S24

TABLE 177-2 MEDICAL SOCIETY CLINICAL PRACTICE GUIDELINES—cont'd

YEAR	SOCIETY	PRINCIPAL INDICATIONS	REFERENCE
2004	British Committee for Standards in Haematology	1. Replacement of coagulation factor deficiencies where factor concentrates are unavailable 2. DIC 3. TTP 4. Reversal of warfarin coagulopathy 5. Massive hemorrhage and blood transfusion	*Br J Haematol* 2004;126:11-28
2009	Italian Society of Transfusion Medicine and Immunohaematology	1. Correction of clotting factor deficiencies (factor concentrate unavailable) when the PT or aPTT is >1.5 (e.g., liver disease, warfarin coagulopathy, DIC, massive hemorrhage, and blood transfusion) 2. TTP 3. Reconstitution of whole blood for exchange transfusions 4. Hereditary angioedema where C1-esterase inhibitor is not available	*Blood Transfus* 2009;7:132-150
2010	American Association of Blood Banks[§]	1. Massive transfusion in trauma patients 2. Warfarin coagulopathy and intracranial hemorrhage	*Transfusion* 2010;50:1227-1239

*For patients with acute blood loss.
†For patients with symptoms of end-organ ischemia.
‡Consider higher threshold for patients with additional risk factors for bleeding.
§Only six questions relating to plasma use in specific scenarios were considered.
aPTT = activated partial thromboplastin time; DIC, disseminated intravascular coagulation; PT = prothrombin time; TTP = thrombotic thrombocytopenic purpura.
Modified from Goodnough LT, Levy JH, Murphy MF. Concepts of blood transfusion in adults. *Lancet.* 2013;381:1845-1854.

of platelet alloimmunization and the platelet transfusion–refractory patient is discussed in detail in Chapter 177.

Threshold for Platelet Transfusion

The appropriate threshold for prophylactic platelet transfusion depends on the clinical situation (Fig. 177-2). Prospective, randomized studies indicate that a platelet transfusion threshold of 10,000 cells/μL is as safe and effective as higher thresholds in patients undergoing chemotherapy or stem cell transplantation. A8-A10

For consumptive thrombocytopenias such as disseminated intravascular coagulation (Chapter 175), platelet therapy is supportive but not effective until the underlying cause is treated. Platelet transfusions are generally not indicated in patients with idiopathic thrombocytopenic purpura or the thrombotic microangiopathies, including thrombotic thrombocytopenic purpura and hemolytic-uremic syndrome (Chapter 172).

Platelet Dose

The AABB standards require that 75% of apheresis platelet products contain more than 3×10^{11} platelets; however, no consensus exists for a standardized platelet dose, and clinical trials have used a broad range of doses. In general, higher platelet doses result in greater incremental increases in the platelet count and prolonged time to the next transfusion; however, the estimated platelet half-life is similar, and there are no other differences in outcomes.

Low-dose platelet therapy (i.e., <1 platelet unit) may be more beneficial in thrombocytopenic patients who are receiving prophylactic platelet transfusions. The fixed platelet requirement for hemostasis is estimated at 7100/μL^3/day, and platelet needs above this threshold are mainly a result of platelet consumption. For patients who become thrombocytopenic as a result of myeloablative therapy, platelet survival decreases with increasing severity of thrombocytopenia. A trial of prophylactic platelet transfusions in patients with hypoproliferative thrombocytopenia found that low doses (1.1×10^{11} per square meter) of platelets led to a decreased number of transfusions but an increased number of platelets transfused (and donor exposures). A7 At doses between 1.1×10^{11} and 4.4×10^4 platelets per square meter, no effect on the incidence of bleeding was demonstrated.

Plasma Transfusion

Plasma therapy provides a source of clotting factors for patients with inherited or acquired coagulation disorders. Patients with inherited disorders such as hemophilia (Chapter 174) or von Willebrand disease (Chapter 173) are now treated primarily with clotting factor concentrates, which are blood derivatives from processed and treated commercial lots from pooled donors. For patients with acquired coagulopathies, there is little systematically derived, evidence-based guidance to inform plasma transfusion decisions. For patients with mild prolongation of coagulation assays such as prothrombin time and partial thromboplastin time (Chapter 171), plasma therapy has little or no value in prophylaxis for invasive procedures. Plasma therapy is indicated in patients undergoing massive hemorrhage (trauma, postpartum hemorrhage, or gastrointestinal bleeding) or for emergent reversal of warfarin-associated coagulopathy (Chapter 38), such as in patients with intracranial hemorrhage.[7] Recommended dosage in these settings is 15 to 30 mL/kg.

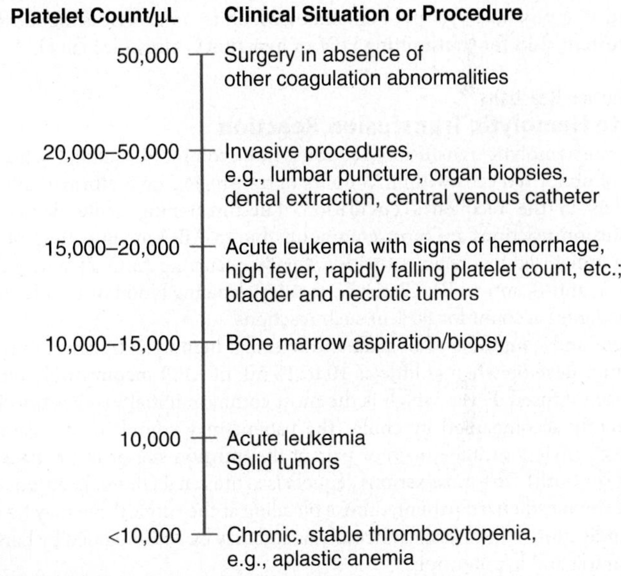

FIGURE 177-2. Threshold for providing platelet transfusions in thrombocytopenic patients.

BLOOD SAFETY

Adverse reactions associated with transfusion are listed in Table 177-3.

Errors in Transfusion Medicine

The mistransfusion rate (blood transfused to other than the intended recipient) is about 1 in 14,000 to 28,000 units. About two thirds of the errors occur in the clinical arena (patient misidentification and/or specimen mislabeling at the time of drawing blood for type and screen/crossmatch, incorrect identification of the recipient of the blood unit, and failure to recognize a transfusion reaction). Implementing a two-blood-specimen requirement to verify a patient's blood type before transfusion can minimize the issuing of mismatched blood products owing to wrong blood in the tube specimens. About

TABLE 177-3 TRANSFUSION-ASSOCIATED ADVERSE REACTIONS

ADVERSE REACTION	RISK PER UNIT INFUSED
Delayed serologic reactions	1 in 1600
Delayed hemolytic reactions	1 in 6700
Transfusion-related acute lung injury	1 in 8000
Graft-versus-host disease	Rare
Fluid overload	1 in 20
Febrile, nonhemolytic transfusion reactions	1 in 20-200
Allergic reactions	1 in 30-100
Anaphylactic reactions	1 in 150,000
Iron overload	After 80-100 U
Post-transfusion purpura	Rare
ABO-incompatible blood transfusions	1 in 30,000-60,000
Fatalities	1 in 600,000
Storage lesions	Unknown
Immunosuppressive effects	Unknown

Modified from Goodnough LT. Current issues in transfusion medicine. *Clin Adv Hematol Oncol.* 2005;3:614-616.

half of mistransfusions are ABO incompatible, and about 10% of these are fatal. The frequency of death as a result of ABO error can therefore be estimated at approximately 1 per 600,000 blood units, a risk that is higher than the current risks for transmitting HIV or hepatitis C virus (see later).

Transfusion Reactions

Acute Hemolytic Transfusion Reaction

An acute hemolytic transfusion reaction is most commonly defined as hemolysis of donor red cells within 25 hours of transfusion by preformed alloantibodies in the recipient's circulation. Life-threatening acute hemolytic transfusion reactions are most commonly due to ABO-incompatible blood being transfused to a recipient with naturally occurring ABO alloantibodies (anti-A, anti-B, anti-A, B). Clerical errors (mislabeling blood or misidentifying patients) account for 80% of such reactions.

Signs and symptoms of an acute intravascular hemolytic transfusion reaction may develop when as little as 10 to 15 mL of ABO-incompatible blood has been infused. Fever, which is the most common initial manifestation, is frequently accompanied by chills. The patient may complain of a general sense of anxiety or uneasiness or pain at the infusion site or in the back or chest (or both). The most serious sequela is acute renal failure. In an unconscious or anesthetized patient, diffuse bleeding at the surgical site may be the first indication of intravascular hemolysis and may be accompanied by hemoglobinuria and hypotension.

Treatment begins with immediate cessation of the transfusion. The risk for renal failure may be reduced by the administration of crystalloid fluids, including sodium bicarbonate (250 to 500 mg intravenously over a 1- to 4-hour period), to maintain urine pH at 7.0 and by diuresis with 20% mannitol (100 mL/m^2 in 30 to 60 minutes, followed by 30 mL/m^2/hour for 12 hours) or furosemide (40 to 120 mg intravenously).

Febrile Nonhemolytic Transfusion Reactions

Febrile nonhemolytic transfusion reactions are common and are estimated to occur in 0.5% of all red cell transfusions and up to 15% of platelet transfusions. A febrile transfusion reaction is defined as a rise in temperature greater than 1°C, which may be accompanied by chills, rigor, or both.

These reactions are thought to be due to a reaction of HLA or leukocyte-specific antigens on transfused lymphocytes, granulocytes, or platelets in the donor unit with antibodies in previously alloimmunized recipients. Multiply transfused individuals and multiparous women are most likely to experience this type of transfusion reaction. Febrile nonhemolytic transfusion reactions, especially those associated with platelet transfusions, may be caused by the infusion of biologic response modifiers, such as cytokines, that have accumulated in the platelet concentrate during storage.

Symptoms may occur during the transfusion or may not manifest until 1 to 2 hours after its completion. The diagnosis of a febrile nonhemolytic transfusion reaction is generally made by excluding other causes of fever (e.g., underlying patient condition, bacterial contamination of the unit, acute hemolytic transfusion reaction).

Febrile nonhemolytic transfusion reactions in susceptible populations can often be prevented by administering antipyretics before the transfusion of blood components. Prestorage leukocyte reduction is recommended to prevent reactions resulting from the accumulation of cytokines during storage.

Allergic Reactions

Allergic reactions can be mild, moderate, or life threatening and are associated with the amount of plasma transfused. From 1 to 5% of all blood transfusion recipients experience mild allergic reactions.

Anaphylactic transfusion reactions are sometimes associated with antibodies to immunoglobulin (Ig) A, which are common and have an incidence of approximately 1 in 700 individuals. However, the incidence of anaphylactic transfusion reactions is much lower—1 in 20,000 to 50,000.

Urticarial reactions are not well understood but are believed to be an interaction between antibodies in the recipient's plasma and plasma proteins in the donor blood. There is usually no specific identifiable antigen to which the patient is reacting. Symptoms are generally mild and include localized urticaria, erythema, and itching.

Anaphylactic or anaphylactoid reactions, which can occur after the transfusion of only a few milliliters of blood or plasma, include skin flushing, nausea, abdominal cramps, vomiting, diarrhea, laryngeal edema, hypotension, shock, cardiac arrhythmia, cardiac arrest, and loss of consciousness. Fever is notably absent. In some cases, there may be symptoms indicative of airway involvement, such as hoarseness, wheezing, dyspnea, and substernal pain. Management begins with discontinuation of the transfusion. Treatment is diphenhydramine (25 to 50 mg intravenously), but more severe episodes may require aggressive therapy (Chapters 252 and 253).

Patients who experience recurrent allergic or urticarial reactions can be treated with antihistamines and/or histamine-2 receptor antagonists (H_2 blockers) before transfusion. Washed red blood cells may be indicated for patients who experience repeated severe urticarial reactions. Severe allergic or urticarial reactions may require treatment with corticosteroids.[8]

Bacterial Contamination

Bacterial contamination may be introduced into a unit of blood through skin contaminants during venipuncture or from donors with asymptomatic bacteremia. Multiplication of bacteria can occur in blood and blood components stored at refrigerated temperatures but is more likely to occur in platelets stored at room temperature.

Bacterial contamination of red cells is most often due to *Yersinia enterocolitica,* followed by *Serratia liquefaciens,* whereas platelets are most often contaminated with *Staphylococcus* and Enterobacteriaceae. The incidence of bacterial contamination of red cells has been estimated to be 1 in 60,000, with an overall fatality rate of 1 in 1 million. The incidence of bacterial contamination of platelets was estimated to be 1 in 5000 before the initiation of bacterial detection systems in 2004, but it is now estimated to be 50% lower (1 in 10,000).

Recipients of units with low bacterial counts may have relatively mild symptoms such as fever and chills, but those receiving units with high bacterial counts may have severe or fatal reactions. Clinically, the patient may experience high fever, shock, hemoglobinuria, renal failure, and disseminated intravascular coagulation. The blood transfusion must be stopped immediately, the patient's blood and any untransfused blood must be cultured, and broad-spectrum antibiotics (Chapter 108) should be started.

Circulatory Overload

Acute pulmonary edema, caused by the circulatory system's inability to handle an increased fluid volume, can occur in any patient who is transfused too rapidly. Although the true frequency of this type of transfusion reaction is unknown, prospective surveillance studies estimate that 8% of patients have transfusion-associated circulatory overload (TACO). Susceptible populations are primarily very young patients, elderly patients, and patients with a small total blood volume or cardiopulmonary disease.[9,10] Treatment is the same as for heart failure (Chapter 59).

Delayed Reactions

A delayed hemolytic transfusion reaction generally occurs 3 to 7 days after transfusion of the implicated unit. Hemolysis is usually extravascular, and red cells are destroyed in the recipient's circulation by antibody produced as a result of an immune response to the transfusion. These reactions are most commonly due to an anamnestic response (secondary exposure to a red cell antigen) in a patient with a negative antibody screen despite a low level of antibody as a result of previous exposure to a foreign red cell antigen through either pregnancy or transfusion. Exposure to the same antigen a second time may cause IgG antibody to reappear within hours or days of the transfusion. This subsequent exposure to the antigen produces an anamnestic antibody response, resulting in increased production of IgG antibodies that are capable of reacting with any transfused cells present.

In most cases, anamnestic production of antibody does not result in acute hemolysis, but red cell destruction does occur between 3 days and 2 weeks after the transfusion. Patients are generally asymptomatic, and hemolysis may be noted only by a more rapid decline than usual in the patient's hemoglobin level or by an absence of the expected rise in hemoglobin. Fever, the most common initial symptom, is occasionally noted, along with jaundice; renal failure is rare. Prednisone (1 to 2 mg/kg/day) is indicated for more severe reactions.

Transfusion-Associated Graft-versus-Host Disease

Transfusion-associated graft-versus-host disease results from the transfusion of immunologically competent lymphocytes into an immunologically incompetent host. An individual's risk depends on whether the recipient is immunocompromised (and to what degree), the degree of HLA similarity between the transfusion donor and recipient, and the number of transfused T lymphocytes capable of multiplying and engrafting. The engrafted lymphocytes mount an immunologic response against the recipient's tissue, resulting in pancytopenia with bleeding and infectious complications. Symptoms usually appear within 12 days of transfusion. Transfusion-associated graft-versus-host disease is rare, but it is fatal in approximately 90% of affected patients.[11]

Transfusion-Related Acute Lung Injury

Transfusion-related acute lung injury (TRALI; Chapter 94) is an acute respiratory distress syndrome (Chapter 104) that occurs within 6 hours after transfusion and is characterized by dyspnea and hypoxia secondary to noncardiogenic pulmonary edema.[12,13] Although the actual incidence is almost certainly underreported, the estimated frequency is approximately 1 in 8000 transfusions. In a prospective nested case-control study, 16 of 668 (2.4%) of cardiac surgery patients developed TRALI, suggesting that the incidence of TRALI is particularly high in this population. In approximately 50% of cases, blood donor antibodies with HLA or neutrophil antigenic specificity can be shown to react with the recipient's leukocytes, leading to increased permeability of the pulmonary microcirculation.

Most recently, reactive lipid products from donor blood cell membranes that arise during the storage of blood products have been implicated in the pathophysiology of TRALI. Such substances are capable of neutrophil priming, with subsequent damage to the pulmonary-capillary endothelium of the recipient, particularly in patients who receive massive transfusions during cardiac surgery or for trauma or in patients receiving chemotherapy for malignancy. In each of these settings, the true incidence of TRALI may be underreported because the findings may be blamed on the underlying disease process or the surgical procedure. Similar to other causes of acute respiratory distress syndrome, therapy is supportive, and 90% of patients recover. Ongoing initiatives to reduce TRALI risks include recruiting male plasma donors or female donors with no prior history of pregnancy and screening female apheresis platelet donors for HLA antibodies and limiting donation to those who are HLA antibody negative.

Transmission of Blood Pathogens

Categories of transfusion-transmitted agents,[14] as well as those currently screened, are listed in Table 177-4. The implementation of nucleic acid testing of multiple minipools (donation samples, test well) from blood donations has markedly reduced the transmission of HIV and hepatitis C virus during the infectious window period. Current estimates of the risk per unit of blood are 1 in 1.4 million to 2.4 million for HIV and 1 in 872,000 to 1.7 million for hepatitis C virus (Fig 177-3). Restrictive transfusion strategies also reduce health care-associated infections. A11

Only 43% of the World Health Organization's 191 member states test blood for HIV, hepatitis C virus, and hepatitis B virus, so at least 13 million units of blood donated every year are not tested for these transmissible viruses. In the poorest countries, the cost of testing ($40 to $50 per blood

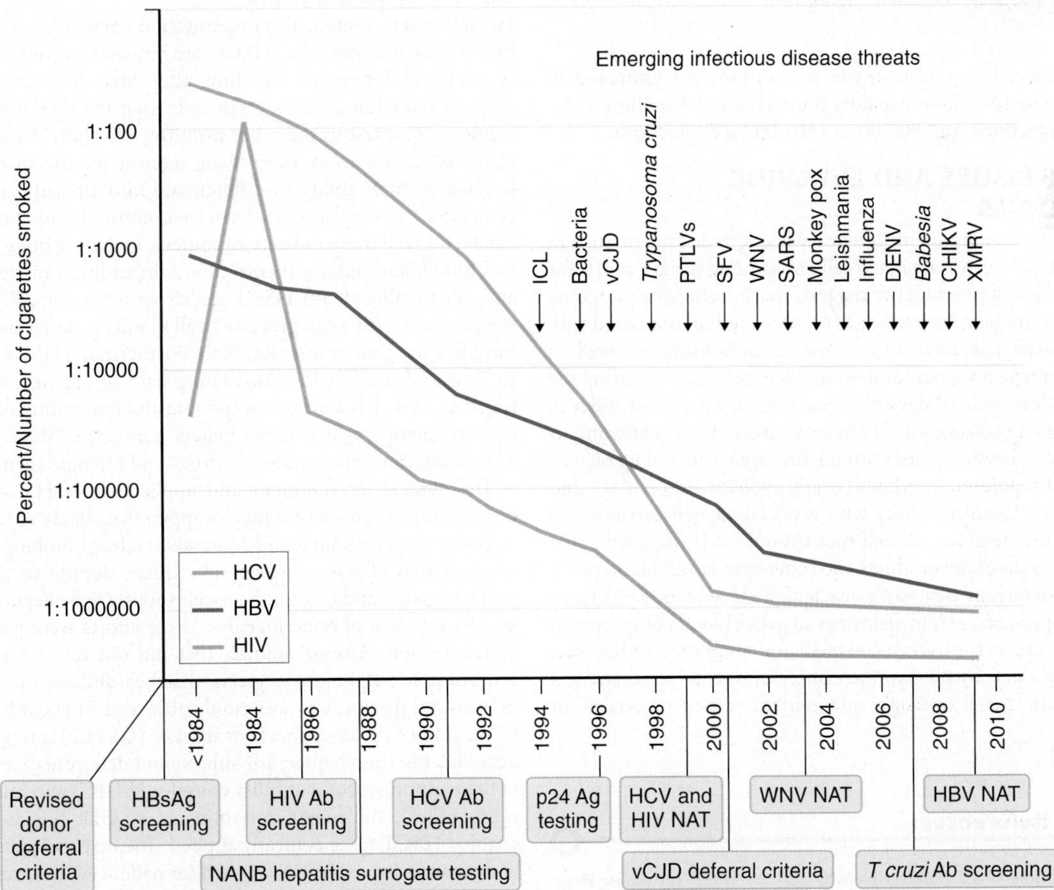

FIGURE 177-3. Risks for major transfusion-transmitted viruses (TTVs) linked to interventions, and accelerating rate of emerging infectious diseases (EIDs) of concern to blood safety. Evolution of the risks for transmission by blood transfusion of human immunodeficiency virus (HIV), hepatitis B virus (HBV), and hepatitis C virus (HCV). Major interventions to reduce risks are indicated below the time line on the *x*-axis. Emerging infectious disease threats over the past 20 years are indicated in the top right quadrant of the figure. Ab = antibody; Ag = antigen; CHIKV = Chikungunya virus; DENV = dengue virus; HBsAg = hepatitis B surface antigen; ICL = idiopathic CD4+ T lymphocytopenia; NANB = non-A, non-b hepatitis; NAT = nuclear acid testing; PTLV = primate T-lymphotopic virus; SARS = severe acute respiratory syndrome; SFV = simian foamy virus; vCJD = variant Creutzfeldt-Jakob disease; WNV = West Nile virus; XMRV = xenotropic murine leukemia virus–related virus.

TABLE 177-4 POTENTIAL RISKS OF BLOOD TRANSFUSION

1. Infectious agents
   - Transfusion-transmitted disease for which donors are tested*
     - Hepatitis B virus (HBV; 1970 [surface antigen]; 1986-1987 [core antibody]); 2009 [nucleic acid])
     - Human immunodeficiency virus (HIV; 1985 [antibody]; 1999 [nucleic acid])
     - Hepatitis C virus (HCV; 1986-1987 [alanine aminotransferase]; 1990 [antibody];1999 [nucleic acid])
     - Human T-cell lymphotropic virus (HTLV; 1988 [antibody])
     - West Nile virus (WNV; 2003 [nucleic acid])
     - Bacteria (in platelets only; 2004)
     - *Trypanosoma cruzi* (2007 [antibody])
     - Cytomegalovirus (CMV)
     - Syphilis
   - Transfusion-transmitted disease for which donors are not routinely tested
     - Hepatitis A virus (HAV)
     - Parvovirus B19
     - Dengue fever virus (DFV)
     - Malaria
     - *Babesia* sp
     - *Plasmodium* sp
     - *Leishmania* sp
     - *Brucella* sp
     - New variant Creutzfeldt-Jakob disease (nvCJD) prions
     - Unknown pathogens
2. Transfusion reactions
3. Alloimmunization
4. Medical errors (wrong blood to patient due to mislabeled specimen or patient misidentification)
5. Transfusion-associated acute lung injury (TRALI)
6. Transfusion-associated circulatory overload (TACO)
7. Iron overload
8. Immunomodulation
9. Storage lesions: age of blood

*The target of the screening assay (antibody, microbial antigen, or microbial nucleic acid) and the year of assay implementation are indicated in parentheses.From Goodnough LT. Blood management: transfusion comes of age. *Lancet.* 2013;381:1791-1792.

donation) is prohibitive. Every year, unsafe transfusions are estimated to account for 8 million to 16 million hepatitis B infections, 2.3 million to 4.7 million hepatitis C infections, and 80,000 to 160,000 HIV infections.

EMERGING ISSUES AND EVOLVING TECHNOLOGIES

Problems related to blood component storage have long been known, such as depletion of 2,3-diphosphoglycerate in red cell units during storage at 4°C for longer than 35 to 42 days. Some evidence suggests that in patients undergoing coronary artery bypass surgery, transfusion of older red cells is associated with a significantly increased risk for postoperative complications, as well as reduced survival. A prospective, randomized multicenter trial comparing the transfusion of blood less than 10 days old versus blood 21 days or older in adult patients undergoing coronary artery bypass surgery is currently underway in the United States. Erythropoiesis-stimulating agents, including recombinant human erythropoietin, modified erythropoietin molecules, and erythropoietin receptor agonists, along with artificial oxygen carriers, can potentially decrease the need for red cell transfusion.[15] It is important that oversight of these biotechnology products and other specialized blood products (e.g., solvent- or detergent-treated plasma, leukoreduced blood products, irradiated blood components, cytomegalovirus-negative blood components) be placed under the auspices the transfusion medicine committee. Otherwise, promotion of such products by the commercial sector directly to consumers undermines both institutional oversight and evidence-based rationales for their use.

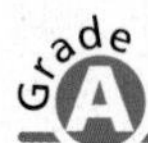

Grade A References

A1. Carson JL, Carless PA, Hebert PC. Transfusion thresholds and other strategies for guiding allogeneic red blood cell transfusion. *Cochrane Database Syst Rev.* 2012;4:CD002042.

A2. Hebert PC, Wells G, Blajchman MA, et al. A multicenter, randomized, controlled clinical trial of transfusion requirements in critical care. Transfusion Requirements in Critical Care Investigators, Canadian Critical Care Trials Group. *N Engl J Med.* 1999;340:409-417.

A3. Hajjar LA, Vincent JL, Galas FR, et al. Transfusion requirements after cardiac surgery: the TRACS randomized controlled trial. *JAMA.* 2010;304:1559-1567.

A4. Carson JL, Terrin ML, Noveck H, et al. Liberal or restrictive transfusion in high-risk patients after hip surgery. *N Engl J Med.* 2011;365:2453-2462.

A5. Villanueva C, Colomo A, Bosch A, et al. Transfusion strategies for acute upper gastrointestinal bleeding. *N Engl J Med.* 2013;368:11-21.

A6. Rebulla P, Finazzi G, Marangoni F, et al. The threshold for prophylactic platelet transfusions in adults with acute myeloid leukemia. Gruppo Italiano Malattie Ematologiche Maligne dell'Adulto. *N Engl J Med.* 1997;337:1870-1875.

A7. Slichter SJ, Kaufman RM, Assmann SF, et al. Dose of prophylactic platelet transfusions and prevention of hemorrhage. *N Engl J Med.* 2010;362:600-613.

A8. Wandt H, Schaefer-Eckart K, Wendelin K, et al. Therapeutic platelet transfusion versus routine prophylactic transfusion in patients with haematological malignancies: an open-label, multicentre, randomised study. *Lancet.* 2012;380:1309-1316.

A9. Stanworth SJ, Estcourt LJ, Powter G, et al. A no-prophylaxis platelet-transfusion strategy for hematologic cancers. *N Engl J Med.* 2013;368:1771-1780.

A10. Diedrich B, Remberger M, Shanwell A, et al. A prospective randomized trial of a prophylactic platelet transfusion trigger of 10 × 10(9) per L versus 30 × 10(9) per L in allogeneic hematopoietic progenitor cell transplant recipients. *Transfusion.* 2005;45:1064-1072.

A11. Rohde JM, Dimcheff DE, Blumberg N, et al. Health care-associated infection after red blood cell transfusion: a systematic review and meta-analysis. *JAMA.* 2014;311:1317-1326.

GENERAL REFERENCES

For the General References and other additional features, please visit Expert Consult at https://expertconsult.inkling.com.

178

HEMATOPOIETIC STEM CELL TRANSPLANTATION

ARMAND KEATING AND MICHAEL R. BISHOP

INTRODUCTION

Hematopoietic stem cell transplantation (HSCT) is a procedure by which hematopoietic stem cells (HSCs) are infused intravenously to restore hematopoiesis and immune function after high-dose chemotherapy with or without radiation therapy. Stem cells used for HSCT are of hematopoietic origin, in contrast to the more primitive pluripotent stem cells (embryonic stem cells), which are of growing interest for use in regenerative therapy because of their ability to differentiate into virtually any somatic cell. The term *HSCT* has replaced the term *bone marrow transplantation* because HSCs can be derived from a variety of sources, including bone marrow, the peripheral blood, and umbilical cord blood. In addition to treating blood cancers and other malignancies, HSCT can also provide clinically significant enzyme replacement. HSCs can give rise to all blood elements and may be genetically modified to enhance their function. Furthermore, HSCs may be manipulated ex vivo and used in the burgeoning field of regenerative medicine. Taken together, HSCT is a major component and foundation of the broader field of cellular therapy, which many believe forms the "third pillar" of medicine, complementing small molecule drugs and biologic agents.

The clinical development and application of HSCT originated in the observations of the severe myelosuppressive effects of radiation among survivors of the Hiroshima and Nagasaki nuclear bombings. There were intensive research efforts over the subsequent decade to develop methods to protect against and reverse the myelosuppressive effects of radiation, including the infusion of bone marrow. These efforts were primarily hindered by graft rejection. Among animals that did not reject their marrow grafts, a syndrome of weight loss, alopecia, diarrhea, and eventually death, referred to as "runting" disease, was commonly observed. This syndrome is now referred to clinically as graft-versus-host disease (GVHD) and is discussed in more detail later in this chapter. The subsequent determination and understanding of the major histocompatibility complex (MHC) and human leukocyte antigens (HLA), the major determinants of graft rejection, and of GVHD, enabled HSCT to be clinically applied. The first successful reports of clinical bone marrow transplantation, used for patients with severe combined immunodeficiency disorders, severe aplastic anemia, and advanced acute leukemias, occurred in the late 1960s and early 1970s. Subsequently in the 1980s, it was demonstrated that the administration of high-dose chemotherapy followed by HSCs obtained from the bone marrow or peripheral blood of the patients themselves improved outcomes and survival of patients with a variety of hematologic and solid tumors. HSCT is a standard treatment option for many malignancies, immunodeficiency states, metabolic disorders (e.g., Hurler syndrome), and defective hematopoietic states (e.g., severe aplastic anemia, thalassemia).

The three types of HSCT are allogeneic, autologous, and syngeneic. HSCs obtained from someone other than the patient are referred to as allogeneic, while HSCs obtained from the patient are referred to as autologous. In syngeneic HSCT, patients receive HSCs from an identical twin, a relatively rare event (<1%). The determination of the type of HSCT that a patient receives (i.e., allogeneic vs. syngeneic vs. autologous) is based on the disease to be treated, disease state (e.g., initial treatment vs. treatment of recurrent disease), the urgency to treat with HSCT, availability of a donor, and urgency in obtaining a donor.

As previously mentioned, HSCs may be obtained from the bone marrow, the peripheral blood, and umbilical cord blood. HSCs can be obtained directly from bone marrow by serial aspirations from the posterior iliac crests while the patient is under general anesthesia. Alternatively, HSCs can be obtained from peripheral blood after stimulation of the donor with hematopoietic growth factors such as granulocyte colony-stimulating factor (G-CSF) and plerixafor followed by leukapheresis. HSCs from bone marrow are used in both autologous and allogeneic HSCT, although less frequently than in the past. Peripheral blood HSCs are currently used in approximately 90% of autologous HSCT and in approximately 70% of allogeneic HSCT. The greater use of peripheral blood HSCs is related to their relative ease of procurement and moderate advantage in the rate of hematopoietic recovery after infusion compared with HSCs derived from bone marrow, but the outcomes of the two approaches are similar.[A1] The HSCs may be infused fresh or cryopreserved. Cryopreservation involves processing the cells in culture medium containing dimethyl sulfoxide (DMSO), placing them in specialized plastic bags, and then storing the cells indefinitely in the vapor phase of liquid nitrogen until needed. Cord blood HSCs are collected at the time of delivery, cryopreserved, and stored. For allogeneic donation, HSCs may also be infused on the day of collection. For autologous donation, HSCs are always cryopreserved.

ALLOGENEIC HEMATOPOIETIC STEM CELL TRANSPLANTATION

The distinctive characteristics of allogeneic HSCT are that the stem cell graft is free of contamination by malignant cells and contains lymphocytes, primarily T and natural killer (NK) cells that are capable of mediating an immunologic reaction against foreign antigens.[1] This latter characteristic can be a major advantage if the immunologic response is directed against malignant cells, referred to as the graft-versus-leukemia or graft-versus-tumor effect, which can potentially eradicate disease and reduce the chance of disease relapse. However, if the immunologic response is directed against antigens present on normal tissues, the graft-versus-host response, the destruction of normal organs can result and is described clinically as GVHD. The risk of both graft rejection (host-versus-graft reaction) and GVHD rises with the degree of HLA disparity between the donor and the recipient.

The graft-versus-leukemia effect first was recognized in animal models and subsequently was noted among patients undergoing allogeneic HSCT for acute and chronic leukemias. The clinical importance of the role that immunocompetent donor T cells play in mediating a graft-versus-leukemia effect was provided by initial observations of increased rates of relapse in patients who received allogeneic stem cell grafts from which T cells had been removed (T-cell depletion), an inverse correlation between relapse and severity of GVHD, and increased rates of relapse after syngeneic or autologous HSCT using the same myeloablative conditioning regimen. These data suggested that T cells within the allograft were involved directly in eradicating leukemia. Finally, the most compelling evidence for the importance of T cells mediating the graft-versus-leukemia effect arose from the clinical observation that infusion of allogeneic T cells alone, termed a donor lymphocyte infusion (DLI), at a time remote from the transplant conditioning regimen, successfully eradicated leukemia which had persisted or recurred after allogeneic HSCT. However, there is wide variability in the clinical effectiveness of the graft-versus-leukemia effect against different malignancies after allogeneic HSCT.

Sources of Donor Hematopoietic Stem Cells

As previously emphasized, HSCs are obtained from a donor other than the recipient or an identical twin in allogeneic HSCT. Because of the immunologic barriers that can result in graft rejection and GVHD, allogeneic HSCT requires that the donor and the recipient share key genes. The most important of these are HLA, which are derived from the MHC located on chromosome 6. The most important HLAs include HLA-DR, HLA-DP, and HLA-DQ loci. A single set of MHC alleles, described as a haplotype, is inherited from each parent, resulting in HLA pairs. A clinical "match" means that HLA in the donor match perfectly with those in the patient.

The choice of donor for an allogeneic HSCT takes into account several factors, including the patient's disease, disease state, and urgency in obtaining a donor. A fully HLA-matched sibling is the preferred donor source because of the sibling's availability and the observation that the risks of graft rejection and GVHD are lowest with these allogeneic HSCs. The probability of having a HLA match from a sibling is approximately 25% and increases with the number of siblings within a specific family. The probability can be estimated using the following formula: chance of having an HLA-matched sibling = 1 - $(0.75)^n$, where n is the number of potential sibling donors. There is approximately a 1% chance of a crossover event (i.e., genetic material switched between chromosomes during meiosis), primarily between the HLA-A and the HLA-B loci. The clinical outcomes for allogeneic HSCT using a sibling with a single HLA mismatch are similar to those with a fully HLA-matched sibling.

For patients who lack an HLA-identical sibling donor, the alternative sources for allogeneic HSCs include a fully HLA-matched volunteer unrelated donor, a fully or partially HLA-matched cord blood unit, or a partially HLA-matched first-degree family member. The genes encoding HLAs are numerous, and the odds that any two unrelated individuals are HLA identical for main loci are less than one in 10,000. More than 22 million volunteer donors are available worldwide; a donor can be found for about 50% of patients for whom a search is initiated. The probability of identifying a suitable volunteer is highly dependent upon race because of varying degrees of HLA diversity. For example, for persons of northern European extraction, the probability of a match can be as high as 90%. It usually takes about 2 to 4 months to locate an unrelated donor, which may be too long for some patients with rapidly progressive malignancies. When a suitable volunteer is not available or a donor is needed more urgently, HSCs from alternative donors can be considered, including partially HLA-matched ("haploidentical") relatives or umbilical cord blood. Haploidentical HSCs are readily available but have increased risks of graft rejection and GVHD. These risks can be reduced by T-cell depletion methods but lead to delayed immune reconstitution and competency posttransplant, leading to increased risks of infection and disease recurrence. Umbilical cord blood HSCs are taken at the time of delivery, stored in cord blood banks, and are readily available when needed.[2] Because of the unique immature biology of lymphocytes in umbilical cord blood, these transplants are associated with less GVHD; consequently, the HLA matching requirements are less strict, and two or three HLA mismatches may be acceptable. However, the small volume (50-150 mL) of cord blood that can be collected results in a limited number of HSCs, which often prohibits their use in adults because successful engraftment correlates with the number of HSCs per patient body weight. The limitation of cell dose can be overcome by the use of more than one cord blood unit. Cord blood HSCs are associated with delayed times to engraftment and immune reconstitution leading to an increased rate of infection. The other significant disadvantage is that after the cord blood unit is used, there is no possibility to obtain additional cells in the event of graft failure or if a DLI is required.

Conditioning and Preparation of Recipient

After an allogeneic stem cell source has been identified, the recipient patients then receive regimens with the intent of "conditioning" or "preparing" them for the infusion of HSCs (Fig. 178-1). These conditioning regimens are designed to be adequately immunosuppressive to overcome the host-versus-graft reaction and permit engraftment. They also are designed for tumor eradication in patients with an underlying malignancy. Most conditioning regimens use a combination of radiation and chemotherapy. Doses of total body and total lymphoid irradiation vary between 200 and 1440 cGy. The most commonly used chemotherapy agents in conditioning regimens are alkylating agents (e.g., cyclophosphamide). Conditioning regimens also may contain monoclonal antibodies that target T cells (e.g., alemtuzumab). The choice of a specific conditioning regimen depends on the disease that is being treated. The doses of chemotherapy and radiation used in these regimens are highly variable. When the doses result in a degree of myelosuppression and immunosuppression that is nearly universally fatal without the infusion of HSCs as a rescue product, they are referred to as "myeloablative." Allogeneic HSCT with myeloablative conditioning regimens has been performed successfully in patients older than 60 years of age; however, survival after these

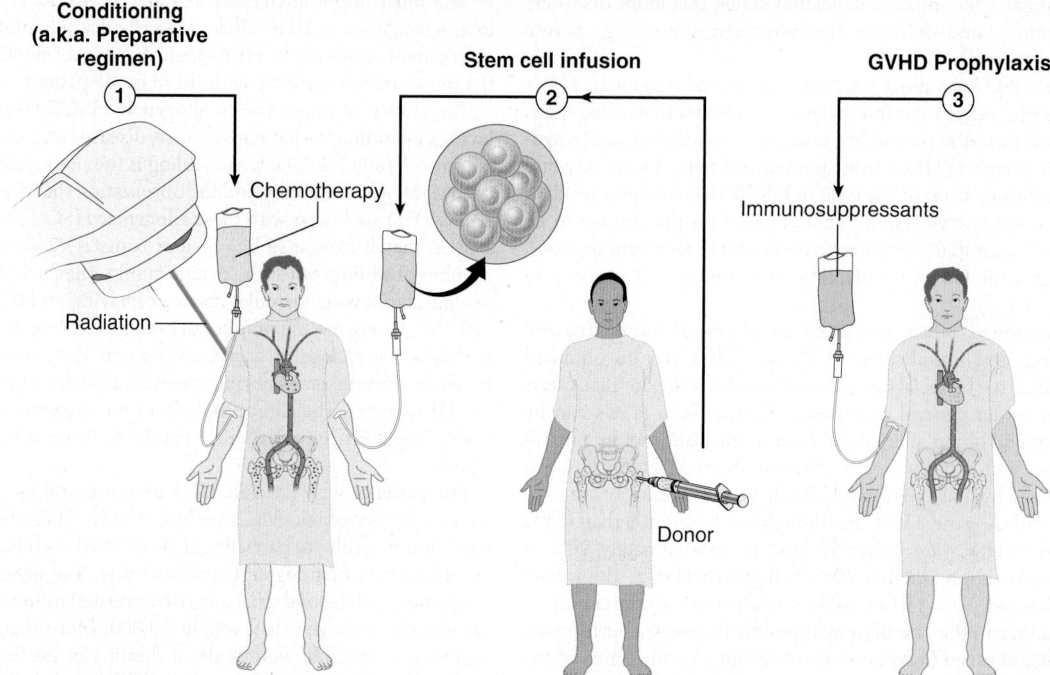

FIGURE 178-1. The process of allogeneic hematopoietic stem cell (HSC) transplantation. (1) The patient receives a conditioning regimen of chemotherapy or radiation therapy (or both) that is used to both eliminate the underlying malignancy and suppress the immune system to prevent rejection of the allogeneic HSCs. (2) Allogeneic HSCs are then collected directly from the bone marrow or from the blood of a related or unrelated stem cell donor and infused intravenously into the donor. (3) After the infusion of the HSCs, the patient receives immunosuppressant drugs to help prevent the development of graft-versus-host disease (GVHD).

transplants declines with increasing age, limiting the application of allogeneic transplantation to a minority of patients who potentially could benefit from this procedure. However, the demonstration that an immune-mediated graft-versus-leukemia effect plays a central role in the therapeutic efficacy of allogeneic HSCT led to the hypothesis that myeloablative conditioning regimens were not essential for tumor eradication. This idea subsequently led investigators to develop less intensive conditioning regimens, which were adequately immunosuppressive to permit the engraftment of donor HSCs but were associated with decreased toxicities compared with myeloablative regimens. These "nonmyeloablative" and "reduced-intensity" conditioning regimens increase the potential option of allogeneic HSCT for older patients and patients with preexisting comorbidities. However, the reduced doses in radiation and chemotherapy result in decreased antitumor activity and are associated with higher rates of disease recurrence after transplant.

Graft-Versus-Host Disease

After engraftment has occurred, patients are at risk for the development of GVHD, which represents the most important clinical challenge with allogeneic HSCT. GVHD is described as either acute, generally presenting within the first 100 days after transplant, or chronic, generally presenting after the first 100 days after transplant. However, clinical features of both acute and chronic GVHD may be observed at any time point after allogeneic HSCT. Current opinion holds that clinical manifestations rather than time after transplantation determine whether the clinical GVHD syndrome is considered acute or chronic. The broad category of acute GVHD includes "classic" acute GVHD, occurring within 100 days after transplantation or DLI and "persistent," "recurrent," or "late" acute GVHD, occurring beyond 100 days after transplantation or DLI. Risk factors for acute GVHD include HLA mismatch, a female donor (particularly a multiparous donor), more advanced age in the patient and the donor, and cytomegalovirus (CMV) seropositivity of the donor or patient, use of an unrelated donor or the use of a T cell–replete versus T cell–depleted graft.

Acute GVHD can often be diagnosed on the basis of clinical findings and is manifest by symptoms in several organ systems, but it primarily affects the skin, gastrointestinal tract, and liver. The skin manifestations range from a maculopapular rash to generalized erythroderma or desquamation. The severity of gastrointestinal GVHD is based on the quantity of diarrhea per day, and the severity of liver GVHD is scored on the basis of the bilirubin level. Organs may be involved in isolation or simultaneously. Histologic confirmation can be valuable in excluding other possibilities such as infection. Mild GVHD of the skin may demonstrate vacuolar degeneration and infiltration of the basal layer by lymphocytes. With more advanced disease, histologic findings of necrotic dyskeratotic cells with acantholysis may progress to frank epidermolysis. In the liver, early GVHD may be difficult to distinguish from hepatitis of other causes. A clinical grading system (Table 178-1) correlates with clinical outcome. Severity is described as grade I (mild) to grade IV (severe).

TABLE 178-1 CLASSIFICATION OF PATIENTS WITH ACUTE GRAFT-VERSUS-HOST DISEASE

	CLINICAL STAGING		
STAGE	**SKIN**	**LIVER**	**GUT**
+	Rash <25% BSA	Total bilirubin, 2-3 mg/dL	Diarrhea, 500-1000 mL/day
++	Rash 25%-50% BSA	Total bilirubin, 3-6 mg/dL	Diarrhea, 1000-1500 mL/day
+++	Generalized erythroderma	Total bilirubin, 6-15 mg/dL	Diarrhea >1500 mL/day
++++	Desquamation and bullae	Total bilirubin >15 mg/dL	Pain with or without ileus

	CLINICAL GRADING STAGE			
GRADE	**SKIN**	**LIVER**	**GUT**	**PS**
0 (none)	0	0	0	0
I	+ to ++	0	0	0
II	+ to +++	+	+	+
III	++ to +++	++ to +++	++ to +++	++
IV	++ to ++++	++ to ++++	++ to ++++	+++

BSA = body surface area; PS = performance status.

The best therapy for GVHD is prophylaxis.[3] The prophylactic use of a calcineurin inhibitor (e.g., cyclosporine, tacrolimus) in combination with methotrexate is effective in reducing the incidence of acute GVHD as well as improving the survival of transplant patients and is the most commonly used form of GVHD prophylaxis. Cyclosporine is a cyclic polypeptide that prevents T-cell activation by inhibiting interleukin-2 (IL-2) production and IL-2 receptor expression. Although effective as GVHD prophylaxis, cyclosporine imparts significant toxicities, including hypertension, nephrotoxicity, hypomagnesemia, a risk for seizures, hypertrichosis, gingival hyperplasia, tremors, and anorexia. Tacrolimus is a macrolide lactone that closely resembles cyclosporine in mechanism of action, spectrum of toxicities, and pharmacologic interactions. The combination of tacrolimus and methotrexate was demonstrated to be superior to cyclosporine and methotrexate in reducing grade II to IV acute GVHD when used as prophylaxis. For allogeneic HSCT, prophylactic immunosuppression is not lifelong; when immunologic tolerance is established, immunosuppressive agents can be slowly withdrawn and discontinued. The incidence of clinically significant GVHD (grades II-IV) in recipients of HLA-matched sibling grafts (T-cell replete) using tacrolimus and methotrexate for GVHD prophylaxis is approximately 30% to 40%. The incidence of grade II to IV GVHD in recipients of HLA-matched unrelated donor grafts is approximately 50% to 80%. Another strategy to prevent GVHD is to deplete the donor's T cells from the graft; the disadvantage of this approach is its association with increased rates of disease relapse and infection, and overall survival does not seem to be improved.

Moderate to severe GVHD (grades II-IV) requires treatment; the mainstay of therapy is corticosteroids. Methylprednisolone at a dose of 1 to 2 mg/kg/day achieves responses in 40% to 60% of patients. Higher doses of steroids are not of greater benefit. Steroid-refractory GVHD responds poorly to second line therapies such as antithymocyte globulin or various monoclonal antibodies (e.g., daclizumab, infliximab) and are associated with increased mortality rates. In general, whereas acute GVHD of the skin is most responsive to treatment, GVHD of the liver is least responsive. The fatality rate for acute GVHD may be as high as 50%.

Chronic GVHD occurs in 20% to 50% of long-term survivors. Chronic GVHD occurs most commonly between 100 days and 2 years from the transplant and has polymorphic features similar to a number of autoimmune diseases. Chronic GVHD is classified as either classic chronic GVHD, which consists only of manifestations that can be ascribed to chronic GVHD or acute and chronic GVDH overlap syndrome, in which features of both acute and chronic GVHD appear together. These distinctions are clinically relevant as "late-onset" acute GVHD and overlap syndrome subsets have been associated with poor survival rates in some studies. Chronic GVHD is most likely to develop in older patients who also had acute GVHD or received peripheral blood rather than bone marrow grafts. In 20% of cases, there is no history of prior acute GVHD. Adverse prognostic factors include thrombocytopenia, a progressive clinical presentation, extensive skin involvement, and an elevated bilirubin. Common manifestations include the sicca syndrome, lichen planus–like skin rash, scleroderma-like skin changes, esophageal and intestinal fibrosis, obstructive lung disease with or without pneumonitis, and elevated alkaline phosphatase with or without hyperbilirubinemia. Underlying immunologic deficiencies, including hypogammaglobulinemia, are common, placing patients at increased risk for infectious events.

Historically, chronic GVHD has been considered as limited or extensive. Whereas limited disease implies localized skin involvement with minimal or no liver involvement, extensive disease suggests generalized skin involvement with or without other organ involvement. This classification is relatively poorly reproducible and does not always provide useful prognostic information. A new chronic GVHD clinical staging system is now recommended for scoring of individual organs (scale, 0-3) that describes the severity for each affected organ or site at any given time and also measures functional impact. Treatment for chronic GVHD is guided by the extent of disease. Initiation of therapy before functional impairment is of critical importance. Treatments for chronic GVHD include corticosteroids, cyclosporine, thalidomide, ultraviolet light treatments, monoclonal antibodies, or other immunosuppressive agents. Alternative treatments include azathioprine, psoralen ultraviolet A, and extracorporeal photopheresis. Given that the most common cause of death in patients with chronic GVHD remains infection, all patients with GVHD should receive prophylactic antibiotics with or without intravenous immunoglobulin depending on levels.

SYNGENEIC HEMATOPOIETIC STEM CELL TRANSPLANTATION

Syngeneic HSCT uses stem cells from an identical twin. Because the HSCs are genetically identical with the recipient, the major advantage of a syngeneic HSCT is that it is not associated with GVHD or graft rejection, resulting in a relatively low risk of treatment-related morbidity and mortality. Another advantage of syngeneic HSCT, shared with allogeneic HSCT, is a lack of contamination of the graft by malignant cells. The major disadvantage of syngeneic HSCT is that it does not provide the graft-versus-leukemia effect associated with allogeneic HSCT. However, fewer than 1% of patients have an identical twin, and consequently, this is not an option for most patients.

AUTOLOGOUS HEMATOPOIETIC STEM CELL TRANSPLANTATION

The major rationale for autologous HSCT, using the patient's own HSCs, is that certain malignancies, such as leukemias and lymphomas, have a steep dose-response curve to chemotherapy and, to a relative degree, radiation.[4] However, the major limitation to the administration of higher doses of chemotherapy or radiation is the myelosuppressive effects of these therapies. Autologous HSCs (and for that matter, allogeneic and syngeneic HSCs) permit the administration of high-dose chemotherapy with or without radiation by restoring hematopoiesis. The major advantages of autologous HSCT compared with allogeneic HSCT are that (1) the patient can serve as his or her own donor, and (2) it may be performed in older patients with significantly lower morbidity and mortality because of the absence of GVHD as a major complication. However, autologous HSCT can be associated with more morbidity than conventional doses of chemotherapy. Although patients undergoing autologous transplantation have higher relapse rates than those undergoing allogeneic transplantation, the lower rate of other complications seems to translate into similar long-term outcomes.

INDICATIONS FOR TRANSPLANTATION

An estimated 60,000 HSC transplants are performed annually worldwide. They are used primarily for the treatment of hematologic malignancies, bone marrow failure states, and immune and enzyme deficiencies (Fig. 178-2).

Acute Myeloid Leukemia

Acute myeloid leukemia (AML) (Chapter 183) was one of the first malignancies in which all forms of HSCT were demonstrated to be effective. Allogeneic HSCT is capable of resulting in the long-term survival of 10% of patients with refractory AML. Long-term survival and an apparent cure rate of 20% to 40% have been achieved in patients treated in second or subsequent complete remission, and cure rates of 40% to 70% have been reported in patients given transplants in first complete remission.[5] Randomized controlled trials comparing autologous and allogeneic HSCT with conventional chemotherapy in patients with AML in first complete remission have demonstrated improved leukemia-free survival with both forms of HSCT. However, the data vary regarding an improvement in overall survival. Several meta-analyses demonstrate improved overall survival with allogeneic HSCT for AML in first complete remission, compared with nonallogeneic treatments in patients with intermediate- and high-risk cytogenetics but not for good-risk AML.[6] More recent studies indicate the importance of the presence of molecular mutations. For example, intermediate-risk AML with a normal karyotype represents a highly heterogeneous group with respect to prognosis based on molecular mutation status. Approximately one third of patients with normal karyotype AML harbor the *FLT3*-internal tandem mutation, which carries a poor prognosis, and may benefit from HLA-matched related HSCT transplantation, regardless of the presence of other mutations.

Acute Lymphocytic Leukemia

The results of conventional chemotherapy for acute lymphocytic leukemia (ALL) in children are excellent, except for ALL associated with the Philadelphia chromosome (Ph). In adults, however, although remission is frequently attained after intensive induction therapy, the probability of relapse is high is this disease, and some form of consolidation therapy is recommended, including allogeneic HSCT. Adverse prognostic factors include the presence of Ph, high white blood cell count, advancing age, and the presence of minimal residual disease. Studies suggest that HSCT improves overall survival compared with conventional chemotherapy alone, particularly for those who are Ph positive. The overall prognosis for both pediatric and adult patients with relapsed ALL is relatively poor, and the general treatment strategy is to obtain a second complete remission and then proceed to an allogeneic HSCT.

Myelodysplastic Syndrome

The only known curative treatment for myelodysplastic syndrome (MDS) (Chapter 182) is allogeneic HSCT. Unfortunately, the vast majority of patients are not considered candidates for this therapy for many reasons, including advanced age, comorbidities, donor availability, access to relatively

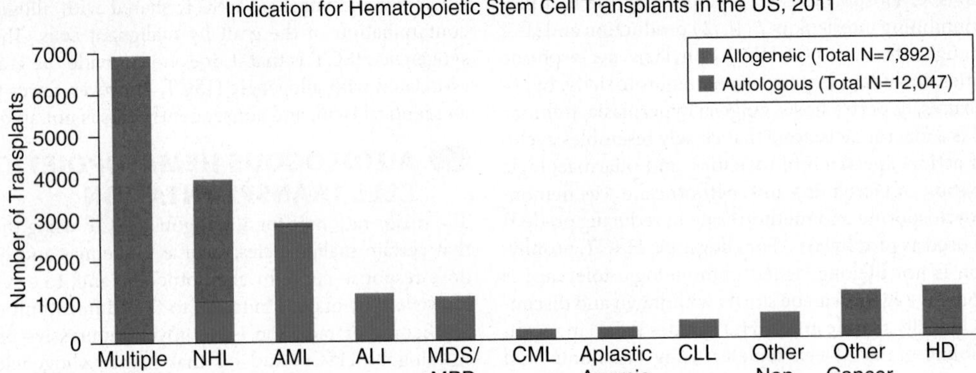

FIGURE 178-2. Indications for hematopoietic stem cell transplantation in the United States as Reported to the Center for International Blood & Marrow Research. AA = aplastic anemia; ALL = acute lymphocytic leukemia; AML = acute myeloid leukemia; CLL = chronic lymphocytic leukemia; HD = Hodgkin disease; MDS/MPD = myelodysplastic syndrome/myeloproliferative disorders; MM = multiple myeloma; NHL = non-Hodgkin lymphoma. (From Dunn, R. Current Uses and Outcomes of Hematopoietic Stem Cell Transplantation 2013: Summary Slides. Center for International Blood & Marrow Transplant Research. http://www.cibmtr.org/referencecenter/slidesreports/summaryslides/documents/2013 summary slides- final web version v2 4.14.2014.pptx)

well tolerated agents such as azacytidine or lenalidomide, and clinician or patient preferences. The best results have been obtained in relatively younger patients, who are earlier in their disease course and have not received any prior therapy. There is increasing evidence that reduced-intensity allogeneic HSCT may benefit even considerably older patients with MDS, and this is of importance given that the median age at diagnosis is in the seventh to eighth decades of life. The use of autologous HSCT for MDS remains investigational.

Chronic Myeloid Leukemia

Previously, allogeneic HSCT was the treatment of choice for chronic myeloid leukemia (CML) (Chapter 184); however, currently most CML patients are successfully treated with a tyrosine kinase inhibitor (TKI), such as imatinib. Consequently, in most cases, allogeneic HSCT is not performed in patients with CML in chronic phase, but it is reserved for patients in accelerated phase (AP) or blast crisis (BC) CML, those who are intolerant of or fail TKIs, and those with TKI-resistant mutations of *BCR-ABL*. Although the results of allogeneic HSCT in AP or BC CML are poor, results of posttransplant treatment with TKIs appear promising. In the TKI era, autologous stem cell collections, even in patients with hematopoiesis shown to be *BCR-ABL* negative by reverse transcription polymerase chain reaction, are rarely performed.

Myeloproliferative Neoplasms

Myeloproliferative neoplasms (Chapter 166), such as primary myelofibrosis, polycythemia vera, and essential thrombocythemia, usually are chronic in nature but can progress to a "spent" phase and develop myeloid metaplasia, which is characterized by bone marrow fibrosis and a generally poor prognosis with transformation into acute leukemia and a median survival time of less than 3 years. Conventional treatment options in this disease state are limited, and an accepted standard of care for myeloid metaplasia/myelofibrosis is allogeneic HSCT with increasing reports of the efficacy of nonmyeloablative allogeneic HSCT for these disorders in this older age population.

Non-Hodgkin Lymphoma

Although allogeneic, syngeneic, and autologous HSCT have all been reported to yield long-term, disease-free survival and an apparent cure for patients with advanced non-Hodgkin lymphomas (NHL) (Chapter 185), the current standard of care for patients with primary refractory or chemotherapy-sensitive relapsed NHL of specific histologies, including diffuse large B-cell lymphoma, remains autologous HSCT.

Autologous HSCT also has been used to treat patients with indolent follicular NHL resulting in disease-free survival rates as high as 60%. However, late relapses and the long overall survival period observed with conventional therapy make long-term follow-up necessary to document the efficacy of this approach. The demonstration of a potent graft-versus-leukemia effect against NHL is less clear. Consensus is currently lacking regarding the most appropriate role of HSCT (whether autologous or allogeneic) for patients with follicular lymphoma. Recent studies, however, suggest the potential value of nonmyeloablative allogeneic HSCT regimens in the context of clinical trials that incorporate rituximab or radioimmunoconjugates.

In the case of mantle cell lymphoma (MCL), further prospective trials are required, although autologous HSCT appears to improve progression-free and possibly overall survival in patients when used as part of front-line therapy. Patients with high-risk MCL are candidates for trials investigating the role of nonmyeloablative allogeneic HSCT.

Hodgkin Lymphoma

Based on a small prospective randomized trial conducted in the early 1990s, autologous HSCT has become the standard of care for patients with primary refractory and relapsed Hodgkin lymphoma (Chapter 186). The usual approach is to first treat these patients with second-line chemotherapy followed by the high-dose therapy and autologous HSCT. Allogeneic HSCT has had a limited role because of the efficacy of autologous HSCT and the significant treatment-related toxicities associated with myeloablative allogeneic HSCT. Data are accumulating on the efficacy of reduced-intensity allogeneic HSCT, especially in patients who relapse after autologous HSCT.

Multiple Myeloma

Although the advent of new agents, such as immunomodulatory derivatives and proteasome inhibitors, for the treatment of multiple myeloma (MM) (Chapter 187) is leading to a reappraisal of the role of autologous HSCT in the early treatment of the disease, current opinion indicates that standard of care remains induction therapy with novel agents followed by autologous HSCT.[7] Prospective comparisons of single versus tandem autologous transplants give conflicting results, although overall survival rates appear similar. Comparisons of tandem autologous versus autologous followed by allogeneic HSCT indicate improved complete remission rates and event-free survival but no increased overall survival and significantly worse nonrelapse mortality rates with the latter. Consensus appears to be to reserve a second transplant for patients who relapse after the first autologous HSCT, provided the duration of response was more than 1 year after the initial transplant.

Solid Tumors

High-dose chemotherapy plus transplantation has had success in the treatment of some chemotherapy-sensitive solid tumors, including germ cell tumors and childhood cancers such as neuroblastoma and Wilms tumor. In patients with germ cell tumors for whom platinum-based chemotherapy regimens fail to result in a cure, the use of high-dose chemotherapy and autologous HSCT has resulted in prolonged disease-free survival time, including patients with refractory disease. After initial promising results of autologous HSCT for advanced and metastatic breast cancer, several randomized trials failed to demonstrate an overall survival benefit, and the procedure is no longer performed for these indications.

Nonmalignant Conditions

Hematopoietic stem cell transplantation is also effective for treatment of nonmalignant disorders, including aplastic anemia, thalassemias, sickle cell disease[8], immunodeficiency disorders, and enzyme deficiency states. These latter indications are primarily for children and young adults. Allogeneic

HSCT can lead to long-term, disease-free survival times in more than 50% of patients with severe aplastic anemia (Chapter 165). When compared with standard immunosuppressive therapy, allogeneic transplantation is more likely to produce a complete and durable reversal of the hematologic abnormalities. Patients with aplastic anemia who are less heavily transfused have better outcomes with allogeneic transplantation. For patients with less severe aplastic anemia, patients older than 40 years, and those without a matched sibling donor, a trial of immunosuppression therapy is usually appropriate before consideration of allogeneic transplantation.

The hemoglobinopathies can be cured only by allogeneic HSCT, and the most extensive experience is with β-thalassemia (Chapter 162). Best results are obtained with HLA-identical sibling donor transplantations and in pediatric patients. Adults tend to have more advanced disease with greater iron overload and more organ dysfunction; hence, they have high treatment-related mortality rates. Studies with nonmyeloablative regimens are ongoing. There is considerably less experience with sickle cell disease (Chapter 163), partly because of reluctance to contemplate allogeneic HSCT in patients with an unpredictably variable clinical course.

Autologous HSCT has been investigated for almost 20 years for the treatment of severe autoimmune disease, including systemic lupus erythematosus, rheumatoid arthritis, scleroderma, and multiple sclerosis. Results have been promising in nonrandomized trials with approximately one third of patients exhibiting clinically significant responses, including medication-free remissions. The strategy has been to reconstitute the immune system without the presence of autoreactive T-cell clones. There has been a reluctance to consider allogeneic HSCT, with its attendant morbidity and mortality, because in general patients with autoimmune diseases have a low probability of death from their underlying disorder, but HSCT can confer a long-term survival benefit in patients with diffuse cutaneous systemic sclerosis.[A2]

COMPLICATIONS AFTER HEMATOPOIETIC STEM CELL TRANSPLANTATION

Early complications associated with all forms of HSCT include direct organ toxicities from the conditioning regimen (e.g., mucositis) and prolonged cytopenias (7-14 days) resulting in infections and bleeding. As described earlier in this chapter, allogeneic HSCT can be associated with acute and chronic GVHD. Long-term complications, particularly secondary malignancies, require that patients continue to be monitored for the remainder of their lives. Through improved supportive measures, there has been steady improvement in survival after HSCT over time.[9] A simple index, based on pretransplant comorbidities, has been developed that reliably predicts nonrelapse mortality and survival.[10] This comorbidity index is useful for patient counseling before HSCT. The late toxicities of HSCT must always be kept in mind when considering the option of HSCT for patients.

Graft Rejection

Graft rejection occurs when immunologically competent cells of host origin destroy the transplanted cells of donor origin. This complication occurs more commonly in patients who receive transplants from alternative or HLA-mismatched donors, in T cell–depleted transplants, and in patients with aplastic anemia. Graft rejection is rarely, if ever, observed in patients undergoing autologous or syngeneic HSCT.

Infections

Infections are a major cause of morbidity and mortality after all forms of HSCT, but especially after allogeneic transplantation because of prolonged use of immunosuppression for the prevention or treatment of GVHD. Bacterial infections are frequently related to central venous catheters. Prophylactic antibiotics significantly reduce the incidence of infection but not mortality.[A3] *Aspergillus* infections typically occur in patients receiving prolonged high-dose steroids for the treatment of GVHD.[11] Viral infections include reactivation of CMV, human herpes virus 6, and Epstein-Barr virus (EBV) infections. Brincidofovir, an investigational oral nucleotide analog, and letermovir, a novel antiviral agent, reduce CMV events in recipients of HSCT.[A4][A5] Post-HSCT patients are also susceptible to seasonal respiratory viruses. Revaccinations for common childhood infections are required after transplantation.

Cardiac Toxicity

Most transplant centers screen potential patients for underlying cardiac abnormalities that would place them at a potentially increased risk during the procedure. Despite this screening, however, a small number of patients experience cardiotoxicity, either acutely during the transplant or at a later time, manifest as a cardiac arrhythmia, congestive heart failure, or cardiac ischemia because of the large volumes of fluids administered during the procedure or from the added physiological stress. Complications associated with a pericardial effusion can be seen in some patients during or after transplant and are more common in patients with disease near that area and those receiving radiation therapy in that field. An idiosyncratic cardiomyopathy, associated with the administration of high doses of cyclophosphamide, has been documented in a small number of patients. Viral cardiomyopathies also can be seen.

Engraftment Syndrome

Engraftment syndrome occurs during neutrophil recovery after both autologous and allogeneic HSCT. It consists of a constellation of symptoms and signs that may include fever, erythrodermatous skin rash, and noncardiogenic pulmonary edema, and, in its most extreme forms, acute renal failure and diffuse alveolar hemorrhage. These clinical findings reflect the manifestations of increased capillary permeability and extensive endogenous cytokine. Corticosteroid therapy is often dramatically effective for engraftment syndrome, particularly for the treatment of the pulmonary manifestations.

Pulmonary Toxicities

Pulmonary toxicities are common during and after transplantation. Patients who receive certain chemotherapeutic agents, such as 1,3-bis (2-chloroethyl)-1-nitrosourea (BCNU; carmustine) have an increased incidence of chemotherapy-induced lung tissue damage after transplant, which usually can occur several weeks after transplantation and can be treated successfully with the prompt initiation of corticosteroid therapy. In addition to these complications, patients who are undergoing allogeneic HSCT are at increased risk for pneumonitis caused by CMV and fungal infections due to the patient's increased immunosuppression, and adult respiratory distress syndrome or interstitial pneumonia of unknown etiology. Chronic GVHD also can manifest as bronchiolitis obliterans in the lung.

Liver Toxicity

The most common liver complication associated with transplantation is veno-occlusive disease (VOD)/sinusoidal obstruction syndrome (SOS) of the liver. Symptoms associated with VOD/SOS include jaundice, tender hepatomegaly, ascites, and weight gain. Progressive hepatic failure and multiorgan system failure can develop in the most severe cases. Predisposing factors appear to be previous hepatic injury, use of estrogens, and high-dose intensity conditioning.

Renal Toxicity

Acute renal failure requiring dialysis during the transplant occurs infrequently, although patients with underlying renal dysfunction are at risk for this complication. An idiopathic or cyclosporine-induced hemolytic-uremic syndrome can be a serious complication after allogeneic HSCT and poses a high mortality risk or can result in end-stage renal disease. Recently, nephrotic syndrome and membranous nephropathy have been described in long-term survivors; these complications seem to be associated more commonly with chronic GVHD and nonmyeloablative conditioning.

Secondary Malignancies

One complication of the chemotherapy or radiation therapy (or both) used to treat malignancy is the development of a secondary malignancy. There have been several reports of the development of secondary AML or MDS after autologous transplantation. Some studies have suggested that total-body irradiation may increase the risk for these complications. After allogeneic transplantation, the overall incidence of secondary malignancies is 2.2% at 10 years and 6.7% at 15 years after transplantation. Within the first 1 to 2 years, the most common malignancies are EBV-related lymphoproliferative disorders; solid tumors are more likely to occur more than 3 years after transplantation. Risk factors include the use of antithymocyte globulin to treat GVHD, the use of a T cell–depleted allogeneic graft, HLA incompatibility, and perhaps total-body irradiation.

Infertility and Hypogonadism

Many of the preparative regimens used for transplant are associated with a high incidence of permanent sterility, particularly regimens containing total-body irradiation. However, successful pregnancies have occurred in some patients after other regimens, particularly in younger patients. Gynecomastia occasionally occurs in males. A reproductive endocrinologist should be consulted before transplantation in patients for whom future fertility is important.

Endocrine Dysfunction

Iatrogenic Cushing syndrome and diabetes can occur and are commonly caused by long-term steroid therapy for chronic GVHD. Particularly disabling are steroid-induced myopathy, avascular necrosis of the hip, and osteoporosis. Because many patients take steroids for many months, tapering can be associated with malaise, nausea, hypotension, and musculoskeletal pains. In these situations, slower tapering over several months or reintroduction of physiological replacement doses (e.g., 5 to 7.5 mg/day of prednisone) is appropriate. Hypothyroidism is typically related to the use of total-body irradiation or local irradiation of the head and neck for lymphoma or other cancers. Osteoporosis occurs in 50% to 60% of patients after HSCT. The major contributing causes include hypogonadism, secondary hyperparathyroidism caused by low serum calcium, and posttransplant steroid therapy. Bone mineral density should be evaluated before and after transplantation; osteopenia should be treated as appropriate with bisphosphonates, calcium, vitamin D, estrogen, and testosterone (Chapter 243).

CONCLUSION

There has been much progress in increasing the safety of HSCT and in expanding the application of this treatment to more patients. Areas currently under development that may further improve the use and efficacy of transplantation include continuous improvements in supportive care for transplant patients and the broadened use of alternative donors. Better treatments are necessary for the treatment of GVHD, and innovative studies are ongoing. Future progress depends on the ability to identify safer and better-targeted antitumor therapies that can be incorporated in transplantation regimens without increasing toxicity or attenuating graft-versus-tumor responses. However, novel cellular therapies, including genetic modification of lymphocytes to enhance cancer-killing activity, hold considerable promise.

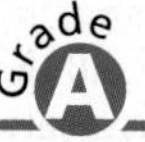

Grade A References

A1. Holtick U, Albrecht M, Chemnitz JM, et al. Bone marrow versus peripheral blood allogeneic haematopoietic stem cell transplantation for haematological malignancies in adults. *Cochrane Database Syst Rev.* 2014;4:CD010189.

A2. van Laar JM, Farge D, Sont JK, et al. Autologous hematopoietic stem cell transplantation vs intravenous pulse cyclophosphamide in diffuse cutaneous systemic sclerosis: a randomized clinical trial. *JAMA.* 2014;311:2490-2498.

A3. Kimura S, Akahoshi Y, Nakano H, et al. Antibiotic prophylaxis in hematopoietic stem cell transplantation. A meta-analysis of randomized controlled trials. *J Infect.* 2014;69:13-25.

A4. Marty FM, Winston DJ, Rowley SD, et al. CMX001 to prevent cytomegalovirus disease in hematopoietic-cell transplantation. *N Engl J Med.* 2013;369:1227-1236.

A5. Chemaly RF, Ullmann AJ, Stoelben S, et al. Letermovir for cytomegalovirus prophylaxis in hematopoietic-cell transplantation. *N Engl J Med.* 2014;370:1781-1789.

GENERAL REFERENCES

For the General References and other additional features, please visit Expert Consult at https://expertconsult.inkling.com.

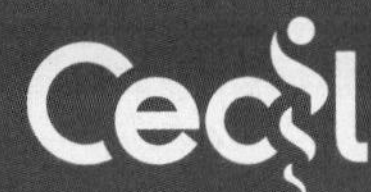

XV ONCOLOGY

179

APPROACH TO THE PATIENT WITH CANCER

JAMES H. DOROSHOW

INTRODUCTION TO THE CANCER PATIENT

Conveying or receiving an initial diagnosis of cancer, or the knowledge that cancer has recurred, are among the most difficult of human enterprises, and no amount of either specialized training or forewarning can adequately assuage the intensity of the emotions associated with these encounters. Patients often experience a storm of feelings that may limit useful discussion immediately following the receipt of a diagnosis of cancer. Unquestionably, it is difficult for even the most well-informed patient to process the complexities of his or her individual situation, including the range of additional diagnostic tests that may be required and the potentially vast array of treatment options and potential outcomes that lie ahead. And yet, at some point prior to the initiation of treatment, the physician and the patient must discuss the diagnosis, its implications, and therapeutic alternatives. Because of the wide range of potential prognoses (from curable disseminated testicular cancer to the limited lifespan of patients with locally advanced gastric or pancreatic cancer), it is often useful for family members or close friends to be present in the consulting room when detailed discussions of the complexities of either disease or therapy are conducted, both to provide emotional support and to be another "set of ears" during the visit. It is helpful to ask patients directly: "What do you understand about your diagnosis and treatment?" Family members or close associates of the patient may also be especially helpful in developing a written or digital record of the questions posed to and answered by health care providers; many patients find such a record to be especially helpful for later reference.

If the physician is not familiar with the latest treatment options, prompt referral to a specialist, whether a surgical oncologist, radiation oncologist, or medical oncologist, is imperative. The generalist should not be a therapeutic nihilist unless he or she is intimately involved in the field and is well versed in the potential risks and benefits of currently available therapies and clinical trials.

DIAGNOSIS

Diagnostic possibilities are protean for the wide range of human malignancies that may be discovered either in the presence of nonspecific but foreboding symptoms or signs (severe weight loss, hematuria, jaundice) or in asymptomatic individuals (e.g., during a routine physical examination). The importance of the medical history and physical examination, however, must be emphasized *whether or not* a pathologic diagnosis of cancer has already been confirmed. One of the most important considerations that underlies the approach to both the diagnostic work-up and choice of cancer treatment (surgical, radiation, or systemic therapy) is the patient's basic physiologic condition or "performance status" (Table 179-1). For example, a past medical history of prolonged tobacco smoking is not only relevant to a possible diagnosis of lung cancer but to the ability of a patient to tolerate potentially curable multimodality treatment. Underlying evidence of excessive alcohol consumption may play a role in both the tolerance for and metabolism of systemic chemotherapeutic agents. Family histories of cancer can provide prognostic indicators as well as suggest molecularly guided treatment approaches in, for example, women with possible *BRCA1*-related breast or ovarian cancer. It is also critical to assess the environment of care, including all of the patient's support systems, that may be sorely tested by the experience of a cancer diagnosis and the interventions that ensue therefrom. Finally, the physical examination will define the extent of certain sites of measurable malignancy—lymph node, splenic, or hepatic enlargement, for example—as well as the patient's muscle strength, the presence of possible malignant effusions, and potential central or peripheral neuropathies reflective of metastatic disease or paraneoplastic syndromes. But most importantly, it provides the treating physician with an initial sense of the patient's well-being, or lack thereof, prior to the initiation of therapy.

Diagnostic Procedures

A lesion that has been found on physical examination, or following radiographic studies prompted by abnormal laboratory results, will often undergo a percutaneous biopsy for pathologic evaluation. It is critical that the biopsy be representative of the entire tumor and be robust enough in size that appropriate investigations (e.g., special immunohistologic stains, flow cytometry, cytogenetics, hormone assays) can be performed before treatment is initiated. If there is a question whether the lesion is benign or malignant or about its proper classification, consideration should be given to additional biopsies, and consultation with a reference pathologist may be indicated. The recent emergence of a wide range of molecularly targeted systemic therapeutic agents active in solid tumors (see Table 179-4) has focused renewed attention on obtaining sufficient tissue from patients for performance of the essential molecular studies (DNA sequencing, RNA expression analyses, FISH [fluorescence in situ hybridization]) necessary to determine treatment choice. Although tumors removed by surgical resection are routinely of sufficient size to permit the full range of diagnostic examinations, active involvement of a skilled interventional radiologist or endoscopist is often required to produce both the size and number of tumor biopsies required for modern cancer therapeutic decision making. Finally, there is seldom a need for such rapid therapy that appropriate pretreatment evaluations cannot be performed. For some tumor sites such as the colon (Chapter 193), there is one predominant histology but critical molecular features of the tumor (presence or absence of a mutant *Ras* oncogene) that can define therapy; in others, such as the lung (Chapter 191), the distinction between small cell lung cancer and non–small cell lung cancer is critical for treatment. For breast cancer (Chapter 198), the treating physician is interested in a variety of factors, such as histology, tumor grade, the presence (and its degree) or absence of estrogen and progesterone receptor proteins, and the presence of HER2/neu overexpression. The rapidly increasing sophistication of molecular diagnostics has, furthermore, begun to improve the potential to localize cancers of unknown primary origin (Chapter 204).

Staging and Multidisciplinary Evaluation

After a tissue diagnosis has been established, staging follows to determine the extent of disease. The American Joint Committee on Cancer staging system is considered the standard in the United States and is based on the TNM (tumor, node, metastasis) system that is anatomically and pathologically based. The approach to staging from a clinical perspective depends on the type of cancer, but it commonly includes computed tomography (CT), magnetic resonance imaging (MRI), radionuclide scans, and, increasingly, positron emission tomography (PET). These studies are supplemented by routine hematologic and chemistry profiles, tumor markers (when appropriate), and in some cases, bone marrow aspiration and biopsy.

The goal of tumor staging is to define the extent of a patient's disease. Tumor stage provides critical prognostic information that will inform the therapeutic approach that is most appropriate. Accurate staging involves delineating the magnitude of the tumor determined by imaging procedures, as well as confirming the pathologic limits of disease spread from tissues removed at surgery. In essence, for most solid tumor patients, the tumor stage will establish whether the treatment will focus on a local (usually confined to an organ), regional, or disseminated pattern of malignancy and can determine whether the expected outcome of therapy is curative or palliative. On the other hand, hematopoietic malignancies are often disseminated at diagnosis and demand their own prognostic classifiers.

The focus of the staging work-up is to identify potential sites of metastases and to establish indicator lesions with which to monitor therapy. For most solid tumors, CT scans can accomplish both goals; however, in some circumstances, other imaging modalities are more appropriate for therapeutic monitoring (e.g., MRI when central nervous system [CNS] metastases are likely [small cell lung cancer], or combined PET/CT imaging to establish that a given lesion is likely to be malignant, or in diseases where early metabolic responses to treatment can be confirmed (such as for gastrointestinal stromal tumors). In patients with established advanced disease, indicator lesions for therapeutic monitoring should be carefully chosen prior to the initiation of treatment, be well documented in the medical record, and should be evaluated with the minimum frequency of imaging procedures required for accurate follow-up, consistent with evidence-based medical practice or the clinical protocol on which the patient is entered.

The consulting medical oncologist may often be advised by a local tumor board composed of other medical, surgical, and radiation oncologists,

TABLE 179-1 KARNOFSKY AND ZUBROD PERFORMANCE SCALES

KARNOFSKY PERFORMANCE STATUS SCALE

VALUE	LEVEL OF FUNCTIONAL CAPACITY
100	Normal, no complaints, no evidence of disease
90	Able to carry on normal activity, minor signs or symptoms of disease
80	Normal activity with effort, some signs or symptoms of disease
70	Cares for self, unable to carry on normal activity or to do active work
60	Requires occasional assistance but is able to care for most needs
50	Requires considerable assistance and frequent medical care
40	Disabled, requires special care and assistance
30	Severely disabled; hospitalization is indicated, although death is not imminent
20	Hospitalization is necessary; very sick, active supportive treatment necessary
10	Moribund; fatal processes progressing rapidly
0	Dead

EASTERN COOPERATIVE ONCOLOGY GROUP (ZUBROD) PERFORMANCE SCALE

PERFORMANCE STATUS	DEFINITION
0	Asymptomatic
1	Symptomatic; fully ambulatory
2	Symptomatic; in bed < 50% of day
3	Symptomatic; in bed > 50% of day
4	Bedridden

pathologists, radiologists, and members of the cancer care team (oncology nurses, social workers, and palliative care specialists). In such a multidisciplinary environment, the patient's overall prognosis can be reviewed and alternatives for care, including standard therapy, possible clinical trials, a second opinion, or no treatment, can be considered. The outcome of such an evaluation is usually viewed by patients and families as an important component in the coordinated development of an overall plan for either further diagnostic procedures or therapy. Finally, many oncologists actively participate in clinical trials that may make investigational drugs or other investigational procedures available for patients, or they may suggest referral to a tertiary cancer center where disease-specific clinical trials are available, as appropriate.

TREATMENT Rx

Therapeutic Plan

Intention of Treatment

Based on the multidisciplinary evaluation of an accurately staged patient, it should be possible to define whether the intent of treatment is curative or palliative. Whether or not this is done during a formal tumor board or multidisciplinary case conference, clarity must be reached regarding the specific choice of therapeutic options (and their potential risks and benefits, overall goals, and alternatives) when considered in the context of the wishes of the patient and family. This is particularly true when the side effects of treatment are substantial (such as for the multidisciplinary management of non–small cell lung cancer or esophageal cancer). For cancers amenable to surgery, resection is often an initial alternative if the patient is a suitable candidate for anesthesia (Chapter 432) and is otherwise in acceptable condition in terms of concomitant or comorbid illnesses. Determination of the patient's performance score (see Table 179-1) is a simple means of assessing functional status. If life expectancy is limited or if the patient is not a good candidate for surgery, more limited approaches to palliative radiation or systemic therapy may be appropriate. There are now substantial data suggesting that the extent of surgery required for an optimal long-term outcome may be reduced for certain solid tumors through the use of presurgical neoadjuvant chemotherapy, often as part of an "organ-sparing" approach. Concomitant and/or sequential multimodality treatments also have the potential to produce long-term disease-free remissions. When the best therapeutic outcomes require the combined skills of surgical, radiation, and medical oncologists, the need for coordination of care among a variety of specialists becomes paramount, and the use of predefined treatment regimens critical.

Therapeutic Paradigm and Therapeutic Index

The therapeutic paradigm in oncology, although still directed at improving the multidisciplinary care model, has begun to change from one focused on delivering treatments at the "maximally tolerated dose" for normal tissues, to therapy that is personalized based on both the molecular characteristics of the patient's tumor as well as any individual germline features that could modify treatment tolerance (Chapter 181). Based on the rapid expansion of our understanding of somatic mutations in human malignancies, and the ability to produce therapeutic molecules that can target specific deficiencies in tumoral DNA repair, growth factor signaling, or energy balance, for example, the currently developing approach to cancer therapeutics involves the employment of predictive molecular markers to guide all modalities of cancer care for the benefit of unique cancer patients. Hence, the focus of oncologists today is on the elaboration of treatments that can be administered with a high therapeutic index, defined as the comparison of the amount of treatment that is effective to the amount that causes toxicity; in this era of personalized cancer medicine, the goal of cancer therapy is to minimize normal tissue toxicity while preserving quality of life by advancing therapies or procedures that are targeted only to specific molecular dependencies in tumors.

Surgical Therapy

Surgery is used to biopsy a suspected lesion, remove the primary tumor, bypass obstructions, provide palliation, and prevent cancers in patients at very high risk because of genetic predispositions or chronic inflammatory states. Surgical staging also establishes the extent of disease. For example, patients with ovarian cancer (Chapter 199) benefit from surgical "debulking" to remove all visible disease, leaving minimal residual tumor, a process that may enhance the effectiveness of systemic treatment. Placement of a venous access device at the time of surgery, if considered proactively, may eliminate the need for a second surgical anesthesia.

Surgery remains the most common method to cure localized cancers such as breast cancer (Chapter 198), colorectal cancer (Chapter 193), and lung cancer (Chapter 191), but it is limited by the location of the tumor, its extension, and distant metastases. Even if a tumor cannot be removed, surgical biopsy provides confirmation of the diagnosis and additional tissue for molecular analysis. Occasionally, an obstructing lesion can be bypassed to provide palliation.

In specific circumstances when the primary tumor has been controlled, removal of a single metastasis (metastasectomy) can result in long-term survival; an example is resection of a solitary liver metastasis found at the time of colectomy for colorectal cancer. A variety of surgical techniques, such as radiofrequency ablation or cryoablation, can also be used to treat hepatic metastases in carefully selected patients. Adjuvant chemotherapy is often given after surgery in this situation to treat microscopic metastases.

The careful application of reconstructive surgery after a disfiguring procedure is critical to long-term physical and emotional well-being. Examples include postmastectomy breast reconstruction (Chapter 198) and plastic surgical procedures to correct deformities following head and neck surgery (Chapter 190).

Radiation Therapy

Ionizing radiation (Chapter 20) can be delivered using beams of high-energy rays, known as *teletherapy*, via a linear accelerator; by brachytherapy, through the application of sealed radioactive implants, seeds, wires, or plaques; and intravenously by using radioisotopes, either directly or attached to antibodies or other targeting molecules. Radiation interacts with water molecules to induce free radical species, including hydroxyl radicals, which damage DNA, proteins, and lipid membranes, leading to cell death. Like chemotherapy, radiation therapy is most effective against rapidly dividing cells that are well oxygenated.

The utility of radiation therapy is limited by the inapparent extension of disease outside a local treatment field, by the location of tumors next to normal structures that must be preserved, and by the presence of distant metastases. Normal tissue tolerance, which varies across different organs and tissues, often prevents the use of radiation doses that could uniformly eradicate cancers. Radiation therapy is also limited by tumor hypoxia: large, bulky tumors are frequently relatively radioresistant, whereas well-oxygenated tumors can be more effectively treated at lower doses. In addition to acute radiation-related toxicities (Chapter 20), late effects of radiation therapy include second malignancies, such as breast cancers that may occur decades after administering thoracic radiation fields during curative treatment for Hodgkin disease.

Radiation therapy can be used as primary treatment, as part of multimodality therapy, in the adjuvant setting, and for palliation. As a single modality, radiation therapy can be curative for early-stage malignancies such as laryngeal cancer (Chapter 190), cervical cancer (Chapter 199), and prostate cancer

(Chapter 201). Breast-conserving surgery (Chapter 198) requires the use of radiation to treat the remaining breast. Partial irradiation techniques using three-dimensional planning with external beam radiation have recently been developed and used in selected patients with appropriately placed and sized breast cancers. For localized prostate cancer (Chapter 201), implanted radioactive seeds of gold or palladium offer an alternative to surgery or external beam radiation therapy in certain patients.

Newer techniques, such as intensity-modulated radiation therapy (IMRT), permit more exact tailoring of the dose to the target, thereby reducing damage to the surrounding normal tissues. Stereotactic radiation therapy or gamma knife techniques allow the treatment of primary or metastatic brain tumors (Chapter 189) measuring up to 3 cm with enhanced accuracy, minimizing damage to normal brain. Particle-based treatment with protons has expanded in use, particularly for limited-stage prostate cancer, based on the potential to deliver higher radiation doses locally. However, there are no randomized studies demonstrating its superiority over other approaches using computational techniques to improve the specificity of radiation delivery (such as IMRT); it is also used for some uveal melanomas, base-of-skull tumors, and a few pediatric malignancies.

Low- to moderate-dose palliative radiation is used to ameliorate symptomatic cancer when cure is no longer the goal. For instance, radiation therapy can improve symptoms from brain metastases (Chapter 189), relieve pain from bone lesions, relieve some obstructing lesions, and sometimes improve hemoptysis caused by lung cancer (Chapter 191) or bleeding from a gynecologic malignancy (Chapter 199). Bone-seeking radioisotopes of samarium, strontium, or radium may relieve pain from bone metastases in prostate cancer (Chapter 201) or breast cancer (Chapter 198).

Systemic Therapy

Cancer Pharmacology

Principles

The fundamental goal of cancer pharmacology is the development of treatments that can be matched to the intrinsic sensitivity of specific tumors, and that can be delivered in concentrations that affect the molecular target of interest with an acceptable therapeutic index. Three properties of all cancer therapeutic agents underlie their clinical utility: (1) pharmacogenetics of the drug (how the germline or somatic expression of genes alters normal tissue toxicity or antitumor efficacy); (2) action of the drug (pharmacodynamics, or what the drug does to the tumor/body); and (3) delivery of the drug (pharmacokinetics, or what the body does to the drug).

Pharmacogenetics

Pharmacogenetics, the study of inherited interindividual differences in drug disposition and effects, is important in cancer therapy because genetic polymorphisms in drug-metabolizing enzymes may be responsible for variations in efficacy and toxicity observed with many chemotherapeutic agents. Drugs potentially affected by polymorphisms identified to date include the thiopurines, 5-fluorouracil, irinotecan, taxanes, and the platinum agents. In patients who are heterozygous or homozygous for deficiencies in metabolizing enzymes, toxicity can be dramatically enhanced. Testing for pharmacogenetic variations that predict for altered normal tissue tolerance is currently available for thiopurines and irinotecan.

Molecular Targeting and Pharmacodynamics

Molecular diagnostic testing to predict antitumor activity for hormonal and anti-HER2 therapeutics has been part of routine oncologic practice for the past two decades, but the recent past has witnessed a remarkable increase in the use of molecular diagnostic testing in cancer drug development and a consequent increase in the number of molecularly targeted anticancer agents that are prescribed only after demonstration of specific molecular abnormalities (predictive of response) in primary or metastatic tumor tissues.[1,2] Examples of such diagnostic/drug pairs include: EGFR mutations in lung adenocarcinomas and erlotinib; ALK tyrosine kinase translocations in lung adenocarcinomas and crizotinib; and $BRAF^{V600E}$ mutations in melanoma and vemurafenib. Recent advances in the process of cancer drug discovery, furthermore, have focused on demonstrating engagement of presumed molecular targets of drug action early in the development process (e.g., evidence of enzyme inhibition, protein dephosphorylation, or DNA damage) as the first step toward implementation of a predictive molecular test for the drug in clinical practice.

Pharmacokinetics and Drug Delivery

Dose selection in oncology is a critical issue primarily because anticancer agents have among the smallest therapeutic ratios in all of medicine. When tumors are responsive to treatment, higher doses may or may not be more effective but are likely to be more toxic to normal tissues. The clearance of a drug from both the systemic circulation and, potentially, from specific physiologic compartments (CNS, thoracic, or peritoneal effusions) is the most important determinant of the dose chosen for a particular patient. It is a composite of all the routes and mechanisms by which the drug can be eliminated from the body and thus determines dose and dose adjustments in the face of changes in drug metabolism, transport, or altered organ function. Although it is important to develop a clear understanding of drug half-lives to establish initial dosing schedules, drug clearance will be the actual determinant of the dose of drug that can be safely administered. Another aspect of drug delivery is the use of body surface area dosing versus flat dosing (using fixed amounts of a drug) in oncologic practice. Although dosing based on body surface area has a long history in oncology (unlike other areas of internal medicine), very little data support this approach; for most agents in common use, empirically determined pharmacokinetic variability from patient to patient is far greater than that which could reasonably be ameliorated by dosing based on weight or surface area.

Routes of Drug Dosing

Prior to the approval of imatinib (administered orally) for the treatment of chronic myelogenous leukemia in 2001, most anticancer agents were developed for parenteral use. However, although intravenous administration remains important, most new anticancer agents are developed for oral use; 7 of the 11 cancer drugs approved by the U.S. Food and Drug Administration (FDA) in 2012 are given by mouth. This change in the route of administration for new drugs brings to the forefront many drug delivery issues that had previously not been routinely considered in the oncology clinic, such as: treatment adherence (does the patient take his/her medication), variability in absorption due to food effects, emesis prior to drug absorption, first-pass metabolism in the liver or intestine, and difficulties in swallowing. For example, whether the orally administered anti-HER1/2 drug lapatinib is taken with food or on an empty stomach can alter its absorption by as much as 10-fold.

In addition to intravenous or oral dosing, anticancer drugs may be used: for intrathecal delivery (to overcome the blood-brain barrier) for the treatment or prevention of meningeal spread of leukemia; for intravesicle therapy of early-stage bladder cancer; for intra-arterial delivery of fluoropyrimidines or other agents to treat hepatic metastases from colon cancer or hepatocellular carcinoma; and for intraperitoneal administration of drugs such as platinum agents for ovarian cancer therapy, which provides a survival advantage for these agents compared with intravenous treatment. In almost all cases, administration of anticancer agents by other than the oral or intravenous routes requires intimate involvement of an oncologic specialist.

Clinical Trials

Clinical trials in oncology are defined by the steps in which new diagnostic approaches, therapeutic agents, or procedures are tested to determine whether they will become part of the standard care for cancer patients. During interventional (rather than observational) clinical trials, specific treatments or procedures are assigned to participants, and the effects of the interventions are measured. For trials of new oncologic drugs, the FDA recognizes several states in the drug development process. Exploratory studies of new drugs examined for the first time in humans (phase 0 trials) may be conducted in on a limited number of patients to define a drug's mechanism of action or biodistribution and to guide subsequent dosing in larger studies. Phase 1 trials define, using a variety of dose-escalation strategies, the maximum dose that can be safely administered to humans and the most appropriate schedule for drug administration, as well as the pharmacokinetic (and more recently pharmacodynamics) profile of the drug. Phase 2 trials often enroll 50 to 150 subjects and focus on testing the drug to determine its effectiveness and side-effect profile in a specific malignancy (or for a specific cancer-related molecular abnormality). If a drug demonstrates anticancer activity in a phase 2 study, phase 3 trials are performed to compare the usefulness of an investigational treatment to a control group receiving the standard of care; patients in most phase 3 studies are randomly assigned to the new or standard treatment to avoid a biased assessment of the results of the study. Finally, after approval of a new drug by the FDA, usually based on the results of phase 3 studies, phase 4 trials may be performed to collect safety information on larger patient populations to define the prevalence of side effects that may be rare but serious.

Drug Interactions

Many drug interactions affect the toxicity profile of anticancer agents, for the most part because concomitant administration of a second drug changes the clearance of the cancer therapeutic, potentially enhancing side effects if the clearance is decreased or diminishing efficacy because of reduced drug exposure. Most often these interactions occur because one drug affects the metabolism of the other by inhibiting or enhancing the activity of cytochrome P-450 isoforms (such as CYP3A) in the liver. This is particularly true for agents administered orally, such as imatinib, crizotinib, enzalutamide, pazopanib, and lapatinib. Concomitant drug-related as well as pharmacogenetic variations in proteins that affect the transport of anticancer agents across tumor and normal cell membranes, such as efflux pumps, also affect the sensitivity or resistance of many classes of cancer drugs. For example, certain drugs that are well-known inducers of hepatic metabolism (phenytoin and rifampin) also induce the expression of drug transport proteins.

Combination Therapy

Virtually all curative chemotherapy regimens developed for hematologic malignancies or solid tumors use combinations of active agents. Combination chemotherapy is usually superior to the use of single agents in adjuvant and neoadjuvant therapy as well. The improved results achieved by combination chemotherapy can be explained in several ways. Mechanisms of resistance to any particular single agent are almost always present in the tumor genome at diagnosis, even in clinically responsive tumors.[3,4] Tumors that are initially "sensitive" to systemic therapy rapidly acquire resistance to single agents, either as a result of selection of a preexisting clone of resistant tumor cells or because of a variety of potential acquired molecular changes (e.g., increased drug efflux, enhanced DNA repair, insensitivity to apoptosis) leading to clinical drug resistance. Combination therapy may address these phenomena by providing a broader range of mechanisms of drug action against initially resistant tumor cells, preventing or slowing the selection of resistant clones.

The development of combination systemic therapy regimens follows a set of principles (Table 179-2). For standard cytotoxic agents, each drug in the combination must be active against the tumor, and all drugs must be given at an optimal dose and on an appropriate schedule. The drugs should have different mechanisms of antitumor activity as well as different toxicity profiles, and the drugs should be given at consistent intervals for the shortest possible treatment time. The use of molecularly targeted agents in combination requires that each agent engages its specific target and that dual target inhibition produces a complementary enhancement of tumor growth inhibition. Toxicities of targeted agents should be moderate to allow prolonged administration and maximum target inhibition.

Therapeutic Settings

Systemic therapy is used in a variety of settings with or without and before, during, or after surgery and radiation therapy (Table 179-3). Considerable experimental evidence suggests that cancers are most sensitive to chemotherapy during early stages of growth because of higher growth fractions and shorter cell cycle times. Thus, a given dose of a cytotoxic drug may exert a greater therapeutic effect against a rapidly growing tumor than against a larger quiescent tumor.

Neoadjuvant therapy, also called primary or induction systemic therapy, is used before surgery or radiation therapy to decrease the size of locally advanced cancers, thereby permitting a more complete surgical resection or eradicating undetectable metastases. It also affords an opportunity to evaluate the effectiveness of treatment by histologic and molecular analysis of resected tissue. This approach is most often used for locally advanced breast cancer (Chapter 198).

TABLE 179-2 PRINCIPLES OF COMBINATION THERAPY

CYTOTOXIC AGENTS	MOLECULARLY TARGETED DRUGS
Drugs are each active against the tumor	Agent has therapeutic effect on molecular pathway in vivo
Drugs have different mechanisms of action	Agents have complementary effects on the same target or other targets in the same pathway or pathways that cross-talk to control tumor growth
Drugs have different clinical toxicities to allow full doses of each to be administered	Toxicities do not overlap with cytotoxics and are moderate to low to allow prolonged administration. Consider physiologic consequences of target engagement in relation to toxicity profile
Intermittent intensive therapy preferred to continuous treatment for cytoreduction and to reduce immunosuppression	Schedule chosen to maximize target inhibition

TABLE 179-3 COMMON EXAMPLES OF THERAPEUTIC SETTINGS

ADJUVANT THERAPY	NEOADJUVANT THERAPY	ORGAN-SPARING THERAPY	COMBINATION CHEMOTHERAPY
Stage I and II breast cancer	Stage III breast cancer	Anal cancer	Metastatic solid tumors*
Stage III colorectal cancer		Laryngeal cancer	Hematologic malignancies
Stage II lung cancer		Esophageal cancer	

*Usually palliative.

Organ-sparing therapy is another use of chemotherapy, radiation therapy, or both, to salvage organs that would have been surgically removed if cure were the intended result. This technique is often effective in patients with cancers of the larynx (Chapter 190), esophagus (Chapter 192), and anus (Chapter 193).

Adjuvant chemotherapy is used in patients whose primary tumor and all evidence of cancer (e.g., regional lymph nodes) have been surgically removed or treated definitively with radiation, but in whom the risk of recurrence is high because of involved lymph nodes or certain morphologic or biologic characteristics of the cancer. Common examples include cancers of the breast (Chapter 198) and colon (Chapter 193). The typical end points of chemotherapy, such as shrinkage of measurable tumor on serial radiographic studies, are not available in this situation; instead, relapse-free survival and overall survival are the principal measures of treatment effect. For an individual patient receiving adjuvant therapy, there is no way to determine whether such therapy is beneficial; hence, decisions are generally based on evidence from clinical trials.

Assessment of Response

Assessment of the response to therapy (usually performed using RECIST [Response Evaluation Criteria in Solid Tumors]) depends largely on tumor size, determined by either direct measurement or diagnostic imaging studies, using predefined categories. The categories of response are "complete response," with total absence of tumor and correction of tumor-associated changes measured twice at least 4 weeks apart; "partial response," defined as 30% or greater reduction in the sum of the longest diameters of up to 5 target lesions per organ confirmed by repeat measurement 4 weeks later; "progressive disease," characterized by either 20% or greater increase over the smallest sum of the longest diameters of target lesions or the development of new tumors; and "stable disease," defined as meeting criteria for neither partial response nor progressive disease. Leukemias are assessed by bone marrow biopsies and molecular diagnostic tests for residual disease, and multiple myeloma is typically assessed by the measurement of monoclonal proteins, peripheral blood counts, and percentages of malignant plasma cells in bone marrow samples, as well as imaging of bone lesions. Accurate assessment of response following systemic therapy is essential because of the tight relationship between the degree of response and the duration of disease control.

Classes of Therapeutic Agents

Cytotoxic Agents, Targeted Small Molecules, and Antibodies

The pharmacologic properties of the most commonly used cytotoxic and molecularly targeted chemotherapeutic agents approved by the FDA are described in Table 179-4, as well as their most common therapeutic indications. In all cases, current information from the manufacturer should be sought before therapy is initiated.

Administration of chemotherapy is best done by specifically trained individuals because of the dual acute risks of hypersensitivity reactions and extravasation. No doses or schedules are suggested in Table 179-4 because these agents are often used in combination, and the doses of each drug may need to be reduced when the compounds are combined. The treatment of special populations, including patients with significant obesity, during pregnancy, the elderly, and those with abnormal end-organ function, are addressed later in this chapter.

Unless otherwise specified, most cytotoxic chemotherapeutic agents are capable of producing some degree of nausea and vomiting, myelosuppression, alopecia, mucositis, and/or diarrhea after treatment; many agents are also teratogenic, mutagenic, and carcinogenic. Drugs used routinely to prevent agent-specific toxicities are also included in Table 179-4.

Over the past decade, several dozen small molecule anticancer agents with more precisely targeted mechanisms of action have become a standard part of oncologic practice (see Table 179-4). Although the molecular dependencies within tumor cells against which these drugs are targeted are broad in scope, including tyrosine kinase growth factors or their receptors, they are functionally much more specific than prior generations of systemic cancer therapies. This allows for a better appreciation of the clinical situations wherein certain drugs might be beneficial, as well as the possibility of developing agents for use in specific tumors based on their genetic susceptibilities. It is also noteworthy that the toxicity profiles of molecular targeted agents most often reflect alterations produced in biochemical pathways that control normal organ function, rather than a general pattern of toxicity consistent with injury to rapidly growing tissues, such as the bone marrow or gastrointestinal tract. Current research aims to clarify specific mutational profiles in the clinic that can be used to prospectively select patients for therapy (Chapter 181).

The development of monoclonal antibodies directed against antigens found on cancer cells represents an additional approach to molecular targeting of systemic therapy. Examples include cetuximab (targeting the epidermal growth factor receptor), rituximab (targeting the B-cell CD20 surface antigen), and trastuzumab (which blocks HER2). These monoclonal antibodies can be used alone, or labeled with a radioactive molecule, or conjugated to another

Text continued on p. 1218

TABLE 179-4 U.S. FDA-APPROVED DRUGS COMMONLY USED FOR THE SYSTEMIC TREATMENT OF CANCER

DRUG NAME	DRUG CLASS AND MECHANISM OF ACTION	PHARMACOKINETICS AND METABOLISM	TOXICITY	INDICATIONS
ALKYLATING AGENTS				
Bendamustine (Treanda)	Alkylating agent; bifunctional, with both alkylating and purine-like antimetabolite action	Biotransformation in liver; decrease dose for hematologic toxicity	Nausea, vomiting, and bone marrow suppression	CLL and B-cell non-Hodgkin lymphoma
Carboplatin (Paraplatin)	Platinum coordination compound; produces intrastrand and interstrand DNA cross-links leading to introduction of DNA breaks during replication	Rapidly cleared largely unchanged by kidney; patients with decreased CrCl experience greater thrombocytopenia	Thrombocytopenia; nephrotoxicity substantially less than cisplatin	Ovarian cancer, testicular cancer, lung cancer, head and neck cancer, breast cancer
Chlorambucil (Leukeran)	Bifunctional alkyl forms interstrand DNA cross-links with resultant inactivation of DNA; cell cycle nonspecific acting agent	Highly orally bioavailable; hepatic biotransformation	Dose-limiting myelosuppression; mucosal toxicity mild	CLL, Waldenström macroglobulinemia, non-Hodgkin lymphomas
Cisplatin (Platinol)	Platinum coordination compound; produces interstrand and intrastrand DNA cross-links leading to DNA breaks; cell cycle nonspecific	Rapid distribution and DNA binding to tissues; over 90% of drug is protein bound	Nephrotoxicity is dose-limiting; significant nausea and vomiting require expert management; ototoxicity; peripheral neuropathy; hypomagnesemia and potassium wasting	Testicular cancer, other germ cell tumors, ovarian cancer, bladder cancer, lung cancer, sarcomas, cervical cancer, endometrial cancer, gastric cancer, breast cancer, head and neck cancer
Cyclophosphamide (Cytoxan, Neosar)	Alkylating agent; cross links DNA, decreasing macromolecular synthesis; immunosuppressive	Hepatic biotransformation of parental pro-drug to alkylating species; metabolites excreted in urine	Bone marrow suppression moderate at standard doses; alopecia; hemorrhagic cystitis, SIADH, and pulmonary fibrosis infrequent	Breast cancer, Hodgkin and non-Hodgkin lymphomas, leukemias, neuroblastoma, retinoblastoma, other sarcomas, osteogenic sarcoma, Wilms tumor
Ifosfamide (Ifex)	Alkylating agent; alkylated metabolites interact with DNA; cell cycle nonspecific	Hepatic biotransformation; renal elimination	Myelosuppression; hemorrhagic cystitis (requires co-administration of the uroprotector mesna); nephrotoxicity; CNS toxicity (lethargy, stupor)	Germ cell tumors, sarcomas, non-Hodgkin lymphomas
Melphalan (Alkeran)	Alkylating agent; forms interstrand, intrastrand, or DNA protein cross-links; cell cycle nonspecific	Unpredictable absorption by GI tract; highly protein bound; hydrolyzed in plasma; partially eliminated by kidney	Myelosuppression; vomiting when used at high dose; associated with secondary leukemias when used chronically	Multiple myeloma, rhabdomyosarcoma, bone marrow ablation for stem cell transplantation
Oxaliplatin (Eloxatin)	Platinum coordination compound; produces interstrand DNA cross-links; not identical to other platins	Renal elimination following active metabolism; no excretion by liver and safe to use in face of liver dysfunction	Cumulative sensory neuropathy is dose-limiting and worse in the cold; fatigue and nausea common	Colorectal cancer
Temozolomide (Temodar)	Nonclassic alkylating agent that is affected by DNA methylation status	Oral bioavailability good; penetrates blood-brain barrier	Myelosuppression may be cumulative; treatable nausea; fatigue	Melanoma, brain tumors
ANTIMETABOLITES				
5-Azacitidine (Vidaza)	Antimetabolite; pyrimidine nucleoside analogue of cytidine; hypomethylates DNA, producing gene activation; directly incorporated into DNA, with cytotoxicity at higher doses	Hepatic metabolism; renal excretion	Dose-limiting myelosuppression; transient liver function abnormalities; nausea, vomiting, abdominal pain	Myelodysplastic syndrome
Capecitabine (Xeloda)	Pyrimidine antimetabolite; pro-drug form of 5-fluorouracil; inhibits DNA and RNA synthesis	Well absorbed after oral administration; metabolized to 5-fluorouracil in liver and in tumor	Myelosuppression, hand-foot syndrome, diarrhea, stomatitis, fatigue	Breast cancer, colorectal cancer
Cladribine (Leustatin), 2-chloro-2-deoxy-D-adenosine	Purine nucleoside antimetabolite; inhibits DNA synthesis and repair	Excreted primarily in urine as unchanged parent drug; excellent oral bioavailability	Bone marrow suppression, fever	Hairy cell leukemia, CLL, non-Hodgkin lymphoma
Clofarabine (Clofar)	Purine nucleoside antimetabolite; inhibits DNA synthesis and repair; activates apoptosis	Excreted in urine	Bone marrow suppression, hepatotoxicity, capillary leak syndrome	Relapsed acute lymphoblastic leukemia
Cytarabine* (Cytosar-U, Tarabine PFS)	Antimetabolite activated to cytarabine triphosphate in tissues; inhibits DNA synthesis; cell cycle specific, S phase	Deaminated in blood and tissues, with short terminal half-life	Bone marrow suppression, stomatitis, pancreatitis; with high doses, cerebral dysfunction, GI damage, hepatotoxicity, pulmonary edema, corneal damage, Ara-C syndrome	Acute myelocytic leukemia

Decitabine (Dacogen)	Antimetabolite that inhibits DNA methyltransferase, producing hypomethylation and gene activation	Deaminated in liver, blood, and GI tract; short half-life	Bone marrow suppression, nausea and vomiting, fatigue, abnormal liver function and blood sugar	Myelodysplastic syndrome
Fludarabine phosphate (Fludara)	Purine nucleotide antimetabolite; 2-fluoro-ara-ATP inhibits DNA synthesis by inhibition of ribonucleotide reductase and DNA polymerases	After IV dosing, 2-fluoro-ara-A widely taken up by tissues; drug and metabolites excreted by kidney	Neurotoxicity, including somnolence and demyelinating lesions, dose-limiting; myelosuppression (lymphopenia)	CLL; also used for low-grade non-Hodgkin lymphomas
Fluorouracil (5-FU, Adrucil)	Pyrimidine antimetabolite; inhibitor of thymidylate synthase; also alters RNA synthesis	Primarily metabolized by dyhydropyrimidine dehydrogenase in liver; remainder metabolized in tumor and other tissues to active species; renal excretion of remaining drug	Mucositis and diarrhea, myelosuppression; hand-foot syndrome when used as an IV infusion; rare cerebellar ataxia or cardiac ischemia	Colorectal cancer, other GI cancers, breast cancer, head and neck cancer
Gemcitabine (Gemzar)	Nucleoside analogue antimetabolite that inhibits ribonucleotide reductase and is incorporated into DNA following intracellular metabolism, leading to DNA synthesis inhibition	Metabolized by deamination in a variety of tissues and excreted both as parent drug and metabolites by the kidneys; elevated bilirubin requires dose reduction; increased creatinine enhances drug toxicity	Myelosuppression, nausea and vomiting, elevated transaminases, fever	Pancreatic cancer, breast cancer, non–small cell lung cancer, bladder cancer, ovarian cancer
Methotrexate (Folex, Mexate)	Folic acid analogue antimetabolite; inhibition of dihydrofolate reductase blocks nucleotide synthesis	Mainly renal excretion with minimal hepatic metabolism; strict attention to renal function required for dosing; third-space accumulation, including pleural effusions and ascites, with prolonged release and associated toxicity	Myelosuppression is dose-limiting; stomatitis and diarrhea common, especially if delayed excretion; renal toxicity can also be severe if drug elimination impaired	Acute leukemias, especially in children; non-Hodgkin lymphoma, breast cancer, head and neck cancer, sarcomas
Pemetrexed (Alimta)	Folic acid analogue antimetabolite; inhibits multiple enzymes in folate pathway, leading to altered DNA and RNA synthesis	Excreted as unchanged drug by kidney	Myelosuppression, nausea, diarrhea, rash, fatigue; must be given with folic acid and vitamin B_{12} to reduce toxicity	Mesothelioma, non–small cell lung cancer
Pralatrexate (Fotolyn)	Folic acid analogue antimetabolite	Renal excretion	Myelosuppression, mucositis, pyrexia; must be given with folic acid and vitamin B_{12} to reduce toxicity	Relapsed peripheral T-cell lymphoma
DIFFERENTIATING AGENTS				
All-*trans*-retinoic acid (ATRA)	Retinoid; induces cellular differentiation and/or apoptosis	Conjugated to glucuronic acid, with subsequent biliary excretion and enterohepatic circulation	Mucocutaneous, ocular, musculoskeletal, neurologic, hepatic toxicity; hyperlipidemia	Acute promyelocytic leukemia
Arsenic trioxide (Trisenox)	Arsenical differentiating agent	Hepatic metabolism; excreted in urine	Prolonged QT interval; acute promyelocytic leukemia differentiation syndrome (leukocytosis, fever, dyspnea, chest pain, hypoxia) that can be treated with corticosteroids; peripheral neuropathy	Acute promyelocytic leukemia
ENZYMES				
L-Asparaginase (Elspar)	Enzyme that hydrolyzes 1-asparagine to aspartic acid and ammonia, resulting in cellular deficiency of 1-asparagine, critical for tumor cells that lack asparagine synthetase; interferes with protein, DNA, and RNA synthesis	Metabolized in the vasculature by proteolysis	Hypersensitivity reactions; inhibitory effects on protein synthesis, with resultant decreases in hepatic synthesis of coagulation factors, pancreatitis, hyperglycemia, CNS depression, hepatotoxicity, transient renal dysfunction	Acute lymphoblastic leukemia
DNA-ACTIVE DRUGS WITH PLEIOTROPIC MECHANISMS OF ACTION				
Bleomycin (Blenoxane)	Antitumor antibiotic; produces free radical–related DNA strand breaks	Metabolized partially by intracellular aminopeptidases; renal excretion	Dose-related pulmonary fibrosis, fever, hypersensitivity reactions, skin toxicity, including Raynaud phenomenon	Testicular cancer and other germ cell tumors, Hodgkin and non- Hodgkin lymphomas; sclerosing agent for pleural effusions
Carmustine (BiCNU, BCNU)	Nitrosourea-class alkylating agent; alkylates DNA and may affect carbamoylation of amino acids	Taken up by CNS; metabolized in liver and excreted by kidney	Myelosuppression may be slow in onset and cumulative; severe nausea and vomiting, renal toxicity, interstitial lung disease	Glioblastoma
Daunorubicin (Cerubidine)	Anthracycline antibiotic; pleiotropic effects, including free radical formation, inhibition of topoisomerase II, altered mitochondrial metabolism, activation of pro-apoptotic signal transduction	Hepatic metabolism with biliary excretion; small amount of renal excretion leads to "orange-red" urine	Myelosuppression and mucositis are dose-limiting; alopecia, cumulative dose-related cardiotoxicity, extravasation injury	Acute myelocytic leukemia, acute lymphoblastic leukemia

TABLE 179-4 U.S. FDA-APPROVED DRUGS COMMONLY USED FOR THE SYSTEMIC TREATMENT OF CANCER—cont'd

DRUG NAME	DRUG CLASS AND MECHANISM OF ACTION	PHARMACOKINETICS AND METABOLISM	TOXICITY	INDICATIONS
Doxorubicin (Adriamycin, Rubex)	Anthracycline antibiotic; pleiotropic effects, including free radical formation, inhibition of topoisomerase II and DNA strand breaks, altered mitochondrial metabolism, activation of pro-apoptotic signal transduction	Hepatic metabolism to both active and inactive species, with 50% biliary excretion; "orange-red" urine	Myelosuppression and mucosal injury are dose-limiting; alopecia, cumulative dose-related cardiotoxicity (cardiomyopathy), nausea and vomiting, severe extravasation injury risk, secondary AML	Acute myelocytic leukemia, acute lymphoblastic leukemia, breast cancer, small cell lung cancer, Hodgkin and non-Hodgkin lymphomas, sarcomas, endometrial cancer, Wilms tumor, neuroblastoma
Doxorubicin liposomal (Doxil)	Anthracycline antibiotic with pleiotropic mechanisms of action	Liver	Myelosuppression, dose-related cardiotoxicity, extravasation injury, hand-foot syndrome	Ovarian cancer, breast cancer, Kaposi sarcoma
Epirubicin (Ellence)	Anthracycline antibiotic with pleiotropic mechanisms of action similar to others in class	Liver	Similar to doxorubicin; modestly less cardiotoxic; extravasation	Breast cancer adjuvant therapy
Etoposide (VP-16, VePesid)	Epipodophyllotoxin plant alkaloid; inhibits topoisomerase II, leading to decreased DNA synthesis	Extensively protein bound; hepatic metabolism; excreted as metabolites in bile and unchanged in urine	Dose-limiting myelosuppression, nausea and vomiting, stomatitis when used at high dose, secondary AML	Small cell lung cancer, germ cell tumors, lymphomas; high-dose therapy conditioning regimens
Idarubicin (Idamycin)	Anthracycline antibiotic with pleiotropic mechanisms of action similar to others in class	Hepatic metabolism with biliary excretion	Similar to doxorubicin; modestly less cardiotoxic; extravasation	Acute myelocytic leukemia
Irinotecan (Camptosar)	Semisynthetic camptothecin analogue that poisons DNA topoisomerase I, preventing religation of replication-related single-strand breaks	Partially inactivated in plasma; metabolized by esterases to active species SN-38, which is excreted into bile; patients with elevated bilirubin have increased toxicity	Myelosuppression; early and late diarrhea may be severe; flushing, alopecia	Colorectal cancer
Topotecan (Hycamtin)	Semisynthetic camptothecin analogue that inhibits DNA topoisomerase I, inhibiting transcription	Excreted primarily unchanged in urine	Severe myelosuppression is dose-limiting (both granulocytes and platelets); mild nausea, fatigue, diarrhea	Relapsed ovarian and small cell lung cancer
INHIBITORS OF MITOTIC FUNCTION				
Docetaxel (Taxotere)	Mitotic spindle poison that stabilizes tubulin polymers, leading to mitotic tumor cell death	Biliary excretion	Myelosuppression and alopecia, hypersensitivity reactions, fluid retention syndrome, peripheral sensorimotor neuropathy	Breast cancer, non–small cell lung cancer, ovarian cancer, gastric cancer, head and neck cancer
Eribulin mesylate (Halaven)	Semisynthetic natural product; microtubule inhibitor	Excreted primarily as unchanged parent compound in feces	Neutropenia, peripheral neuropathy, QT prolongation, fatigue, nausea	Metastatic breast cancer
Ixabepilone (Ixempra)	Microtubule inhibitor; analogue of epothilone B that binds to β-tubulin, suppressing function of microtubules and causing mitotic cell death	Metabolized by liver and excreted in feces; dose reduction required in face of liver dysfunction	Cumulative peripheral neuropathy, neutropenia, hypersensitivity reactions, fatigue, myalgias, stomatitis	Breast cancer
Paclitaxel (Taxol)	Taxane natural product; mitotic spindle poison that inhibits tubulin depolymerization	Hepatic metabolism, biliary excretion	Myelosuppression, mucositis, hypersensitivity reactions, cumulative peripheral neuromyopathy with arthralgias, cardiovascular toxicity with hypotension, arrhythmias	Non–small cell lung cancer, ovarian cancer, breast cancer, esophageal cancer, gastric cancer, head and neck cancer
Paclitaxel protein-bound particles (Abraxane)	Albumin nanoparticle-bound form of paclitaxel; same mechanism of action	Hepatic metabolism, biliary excretion	Hypersensitivity reactions, myelosuppression, neuropathy, arthralgias/myalgias, cardiotoxicity	Metastatic breast cancer, pancreatic cancer, non–small cell lung cancer
Vincristine (Oncovin)	Vinca alkaloid natural product; inhibits tubulin polymerization, arresting cells in metaphase	Hepatic metabolism, biliary excretion	Extravasation injury, dose-limiting peripheral neurotoxicity, constipation	Acute lymphocytic leukemia, neuroblastoma, Wilms tumor, Hodgkin and non-Hodgkin lymphomas, rhabdomyosarcoma
Vinorelbine (Navelbine)	Semisynthetic vinca alkaloid; inhibits tubulin polymerization during mitosis	Hepatic metabolism, biliary excretion	Myelosuppression, extravasation, milder neurotoxicity than other vincas	Non–small cell lung cancer, breast cancer

HORMONAL AGENTS				
Abiraterone acetate (Zytiga)	Inhibitor of androgen biosynthesis	Parent drug and metabolites excreted in stool; systemic clearance decreased in patients with liver dysfunction	Joint swelling, edema, hepatotoxicity	Castration-resistant metastatic prostate cancer
Anastrozole (Arimidex)	Nonsteroidal aromatase inhibitor; inhibits conversion of adrenal androgens to estrogens	Metabolized in liver, excreted into bile and urine	Hot flashes, headache, arthralgias	Adjuvant and metastatic breast cancer in postmenopausal women
Bicalutamide (Casodex)	Nonsteroidal antiandrogen that binds to prostatic androgen receptor	Hepatic metabolism	Worsening bone pain, hot flashes, gynecomastia	Prostate cancer (usually in conjunction with LHRH antagonist)
Degarelix (Firmagon)	GnRH receptor antagonist; binds to GnRH receptors in pituitary, decreasing gonadotropin release	Biliary excretion of parent and metabolites; lesser renal excretion of unchanged parent drug	Injection site reactions, hot flashes, weight gain, increased LFTs, QT prolongation	Prostate cancer
Enzalutamide (Xtandi)	Nonsteroidal antiandrogen; inhibits androgen receptor-mediated signal transduction	Hepatic metabolism, eliminated primarily in urine	Fatigue, arthralgias, dizziness, bone pain	Metastatic castration-resistant prostate cancer
Exemestane (Aromasin)	Steroidal aromatase inhibitor; binds and irreversibly inhibits aromatase, inhibits synthesis of estrogens by preventing conversion of adrenal androgens to estrogens	Metabolized in liver	Hot flashes, fatigue, arthralgias	Metastatic breast cancer in postmenopausal women
Flutamide (Eulexin)	Nonsteroidal antiandrogen; inhibition of nuclear binding of androgen in target tissues; its interference with testosterone at cellular level complements "medical castration" produced by LHRH analogues	Metabolized to active and inactive metabolites in liver	Worsening bone pain, hot flashes, gynecomastia, impotence	Prostate cancer (usually in conjunction with LHRH antagonist)
Fulvestrant (Faslodex)	Estrogen receptor antagonist; binds to estrogen receptor, causing degradation of estrogen receptor protein	Metabolized by liver, excreted in bile	Hot flashes, nausea, peripheral edema and weight gain, fatigue, arthralgias	Recurrent breast cancer in postmenopausal women
Goserelin (Zoladex)	Synthetic decapeptide analogue of LHRH; suppresses pituitary gonadotropins, with fall of serum testosterone into castrate range	Slowly released from depot injection site; not extensively metabolized; urinary excretion	Worsening bone pain, hot flashes, impotence, gynecomastia, breakthrough vaginal bleeding	Prostate cancer, breast cancer
Letrozole (Femara)	Nonsteroidal competitive inhibitor of aromatase; inhibits estrogen synthesis by blocking conversion of adrenal androgens to estrogens	Metabolized in liver, excreted by kidney	Hot flashes, fatigue, arthralgias	Adjuvant and metastatic breast cancer in postmenopausal women
Leuprolide (Lupron, Lupron Depot)	Synthetic LHRH analogue; suppresses secretion of GnRH, with resultant fall in testosterone secretion, producing "medical castration"	Metabolized to inactive peptide fragments; minor renal excretion	Increased bone pain, hot flashes, gynecomastia, lethargy, thromboembolic phenomena	Prostate cancer, breast cancer
Octreotide (Sandostatin)	Synthetic octapeptide analogue of somatostatin; suppresses secretion of serotonin and GI peptides; blocks carcinoid flush, decreases serum 5-HIAA, and controls other symptoms associated with carcinoid syndrome	Hepatic metabolism; renal excretion following hydrolysis in plasma	Hyper/hypoglycemia, hepatic dysfunction, diarrhea	Palliative treatment of carcinoid tumors and vasoactive intestinal peptide tumors (VIPomas)
Tamoxifen (Nolvadex)	Nonsteroidal antiestrogen; competes with estradiol for estrogen receptor protein; also has non–estrogen receptor–dependent effects on tumor cells	Metabolized in liver but not excreted in bile or urine	Hot flashes, nausea/vomiting, vaginal bleeding or discharge, endometrial hyperplasia, thrombophlebitis, hypercalcemia, visual disturbances	Adjuvant and metastatic estrogen receptor–positive breast cancer; also approved for chemoprevention of breast cancer in high-risk individuals

TABLE 179-4 U.S. FDA-APPROVED DRUGS COMMONLY USED FOR THE SYSTEMIC TREATMENT OF CANCER—cont'd

DRUG NAME	DRUG CLASS AND MECHANISM OF ACTION	PHARMACOKINETICS AND METABOLISM	TOXICITY	INDICATIONS
BIOLOGIC AND IMMUNOLOGIC MODIFIERS				
Aldesleukin (Human Recombinant IL-2, Proleukin)	Cytokine that supports T-cell proliferation, augments natural killer cell cytotoxicity, induces lymphokine-activated killer (LAK) cell development, and participates in activation of monocytes and B cells	Catabolized by proteolysis in many tissues; minimal renal or biliary excretion	Toxicities associated with continuous infusion (and to a lesser extent with bolus dosing) include: capillary leak syndrome, fever and chills, hypotension, edema, arrhythmias, nephrotoxicity, pulmonary edema, abnormal liver function, endocrinopathies, dermatologic complications, CNS toxicity, myelosuppression, sepsis	Renal cancer, melanoma
Erythropoietin (Aranesp, Epogen, Procrit)[†]	Hematopoietic growth factor; stimulates division and differentiation of committed erythroid progenitors in bone marrow	Proteolytically degraded in vasculature, with minimal excretion of intact peptide	Increased risk of thrombosis, stroke, myocardial infarction; headache, hypertension, and possible seizures; allergic reactions; can produce iron deficiency with prolonged use—concomitant iron dosing may enhance efficacy	Correction of anemia due to chronic renal failure or HIV-related infection, and symptomatic chemotherapy-induced anemia (however, risk of tumor progression limits use for patients being treated with chemotherapy for cure)
Filgrastim (G-CSF, Neupogen)	Hematopoietic growth factor; binds to specific cell surface receptors on progenitor cells to stimulate proliferation and differentiation of neutrophils	Elimination by proteolysis in vasculature and by the kidney	Pain at site of subcutaneous injection, allergic reactions, bone pain, low-grade fever, myalgia, arthralgia	Decreases incidence of infection after myelosuppressive chemotherapy; enhances myeloid engraftment after BMT; enhances peripheral progenitor cell yield prior to BMT
Interferon-α (Intron-A, Roferon)[‡]	Interferon antiviral immunostimulant with both antiproliferative and immunomodulatory properties	Catabolized in renal tubules	Fever and flulike symptoms, fatigue, myelosuppression, cardiotoxicity, depression, neurotoxicity	Hairy cell leukemia, Kaposi sarcoma
Ipilimumab (Yervoy)	CTLA-4-blocking monoclonal antibody that enhances the anticancer effect of activated T cells	No clear pharmacokinetic effects of altered renal or hepatic function	Fatigue, diarrhea and immune-mediated colitis, hepatitis, rash, pruritus, endocrinopathy	Metastatic melanoma
Sargramostim (GM-CSF, Leukine, Prokine)	Hematopoietic growth factor; binds to specific cell surface receptors to stimulate proliferation and differentiation of granulocytes and macrophages; not lineage specific	Metabolized in liver and kidney	Fever and capillary leak syndrome, pain at site of subcutaneous injection, allergic reactions, arthralgias, bone pain	Decreases incidence of infection after myelosuppressive chemotherapy; enhances myeloid engraftment after BMT; enhances peripheral progenitor cell yield
MOLECULARLY TARGETED AGENTS				
Aflibercept (Zaltrap)	VEGF inhibitor; decoy receptor that binds circulating VEGF thus inhibiting activation of VEGFR	Metabolized by proteolysis	Hemorrhage, GI fistulas and perforation, hypertension, altered wound healing, stomatitis, fatigue, myelosuppression	Colon cancer in combination with chemotherapy
Axitinib (Inlyta)	Multikinase inhibitor, including VEGFR1, 2, and 3; inhibits angiogenesis	Metabolized by hepatic P-450 enzymes; excreted in feces>urine; multiple interactions with CYP 3A4/5 inducers	Hypertension, hand-foot syndrome, fatigue, asthenia, stomatitis, hypothyroidism	Advanced renal cancer
Bevacizumab (Avastin)	Recombinant humanized monoclonal antibody against VEGF; inhibits angiogenesis by binding to VEGF, blocking receptor binding and subsequent stimulation of blood vessel growth	Prolonged (20-day) half-life after IV infusion	Fatigue, nausea, delayed wound healing, hypertension, proteinuria, thromboembolic phenomena and hemorrhage	Metastatic colorectal cancer, lung cancer, kidney cancer, breast cancer, ovarian cancer
Bortezomib (Velcade)	Reversible inhibitor of 26S proteasome; blocks breakdown of ubiquitinated intracellular proteins and disrupts ubiquitin-proteasome pathway	Undergoes oxidative metabolism (deboronation) as well as cytochrome P-450-dependent metabolism; dose reduction to 0.7 mg/m² required in face of moderate to severe liver dysfunction; adverse event profile unchanged in myeloma patients with CrCl < 50 mL/min	Myelosuppression, peripheral neuropathy, asthenia, diarrhea, hypotension	Multiple myeloma, non-Hodgkin lymphoma

Cetuximab (Erbitux)	Chimeric monoclonal antibody targeted against EGFR; blocks growth factor binding to EGFR, preventing cell signaling by tyrosine kinase phosphorylation	Half-life 5-7 days, with minimal renal or hepatic clearance	Hypersensitivity reactions (fever, dyspnea), acneiform rash, diarrhea, hypomagnesemia	Metastatic colorectal cancer (*K-Ras* wild-type); head and neck cancer in combination with radiation
Carbozantanib (Cometriq)	Multikinase inhibitor that targets RET, MET, VEGFR1-3, KIT, AXL, TIE-2, and FLT-3	Metabolized by hepatic CYP 3A4 and subject to interactions related to CYP3A4 substrates; excreted into urine and feces	Hypertension, GI perforation, diarrhea, stomatitis, hemorrhage, fatigue	Metastatic medullary thyroid cancer, prostate cancer, bone metastases
Crizotanib (Xalkori)	Tyrosine kinase inhibitor active against ALK, ROS, MET	Hepatic P-450-mediated metabolism; excreted in feces and urine	Hepatotoxicity, pneumonitis, QT prolongation, vision disturbance, nausea, fatigue	Non–small cell lung cancer positive for anaplastic lymphoma kinase (ALK) rearrangement
Dasatinib (Sprycel)	Multitargeted tyrosine kinase inhibitor; inhibits BCR-ABL, SRC, and multiple other kinases	Metabolized in liver by P-450 CYP3A4; multiple interactions with CYP3A4 inducers or inhibitors	Myelosuppression, fluid retention, diarrhea, rash, musculoskeletal pain	Resistant/refractory CML
Denosumab (Prolia)	IgG2 monoclonal antibody that targets RANKL, a ligand for the RANK receptor on osteoclasts, and decreases bone resorption	Prolonged elimination (>20 days) typical of monoclonal antibodies	Musculoskeletal and bone pain, arthralgias, abdominal pain, peripheral edema, hypersensitivity, hypocalcemia	Prevention of malignant bone fractures
Erlotinib (Tarceva)	Small molecule inhibitor of tyrosine kinase domain of EGFR	Hepatic metabolism with excretion in feces; CYP3A4 inducers and inhibitors may alter metabolism, and dose should be reduced by 50% in patients with hepatic dysfunction; renal dysfunction does not alter drug tolerability	Acneiform rash, fatigue, diarrhea, interstitial lung disease, weight gain, hepatic toxicity	Non–small cell lung cancer; pancreatic cancer in combination with gemcitabine
Everolimus (Affinitor)	mTOR inhibitor that inhibits signal transduction through PTEN/AKT pathway	Metabolized by CYP3A4 in liver	Pneumonitis, stomatitis, renal dysfunction, myelosuppression, hyperglycemia, altered lipids	Renal cell carcinoma; hormone receptor–positive breast cancer in combination with exemestane; neuroendocrine tumors
Ibrutinib (Imbruvica)	Oral inhibitor of Bruton tyrosine kinase; blocks signaling through the B-cell antigen receptor important for B-cell chemotaxis and adhesion	Metabolized in the liver by CYP3A (avoid use with strong CYP3A inhibitors such as ketoconazole or grapefruit); primarily eliminated unchanged in feces	Myelosuppression, renal dysfunction, bleeding	Mantle cell lymphoma
Imatinib (Gleevec)	Inhibits BCR-ABL tyrosine kinase	Hepatic metabolism, excreted in feces; inhibits CYP3A4 and CYP2D6; mild hepatic dysfunction requires dose reduction to 500 mg/day; mild to moderate renal dysfunction alters kinetics but does not affect drug tolerance	Myelosuppression, hypophosphatemia, fluid retention, nausea, fatigue, hemorrhage, myelosuppression, hepatotoxicity	CML; GIST
Lapatinib (Tykerb)	Inhibitor of both EGFR and HER2 tyrosine kinases	Metabolized by CYP3A4 in liver	Diarrhea, hand-foot syndrome, hepatotoxicity, decreased cardiac function	HER2-positive breast cancer in combination with capecitabine
Lenalidomide[§] (Revlimid)	Immunomodulatory and antiangiogenic agent, in part through downregulation of VEGF, TNF-α, and IL-6, and T-cell and NK cell activation	Renal excretion	Neutropenia, thrombocytopenia, diarrhea, pruritus, rash, fatigue, leg cramps	Myelodysplasia, multiple myeloma
Nilotinib (Tasigna)	Inhibits ATP site of BCR-ABL kinase	Metabolized in liver	Prolonged QT interval, rash, fatigue, myalgias, nausea, myelosuppression	Resistant/intolerant CML
Ofatumumab (Arzerra)	Monoclonal antibody against CD-20	Not known if dose requires modification for patients with renal impairment	Infusion reactions, tumor lysis syndrome, myelosuppression, hepatitis B reactivation, infection	Resistant CLL
Pazopanib (Votrient)	Inhibits multiple tyrosine kinases including VEGFR-1, VEGFR-2, PDGFR, FGF, Kit, Lck, and cFms	Hepatic P-450 metabolism; excreted in feces	Hepatotoxicity, QT prolongation, hypertension, fatigue, nausea, decreased cardiac function	Renal cell cancer, soft tissue sarcoma
Panitumumab (Vectibix)	Monoclonal antibody that binds EGFR, inhibiting ligand interaction	Prolonged (7-day) half-life	Acneiform rash (may be severe), diarrhea, infusion reaction, hypomagnesemia, pulmonary fibrosis	EGFR-expressing colorectal cancer

TABLE 179-4 U.S. FDA-APPROVED DRUGS COMMONLY USED FOR THE SYSTEMIC TREATMENT OF CANCER—cont'd

DRUG NAME	DRUG CLASS AND MECHANISM OF ACTION	PHARMACOKINETICS AND METABOLISM	TOXICITY	INDICATIONS
Pertuzumab (Perjeta)	Monoclonal antibody against HER2; blocks HER2-mediated signaling; associated with antibody-dependent cell-mediated cytotoxicity	Prolonged half-life	Decreased cardiac ejection fraction (particularly in patients previously exposed to anthracyclines), hypersensitivity reactions, nausea, diarrhea, rash	HER2-positive metastatic breast cancer in combination with trastuzumab and docetaxel for patients without prior anti-HER2 therapy
Ponatinib (Iclusig)	BCR-ABL kinase inhibitor; also inhibits BCR-ABL carrying the T315I resistance mutation; also inhibits other tyrosine kinases including VEGFR, FGFR, SRC, PDGFR, and FLT3	Hepatic metabolism with fecal excretion	Significant risk of arterial thrombosis, stroke, myocardial infarction; myelosuppression, hypertension, hepatotoxicity, fatigue, rash	Because of thrombotic risk, usage limited to patients with CML resistant to or intolerant of first- or second-line BCR-ABL inhibitors
Romidepsin (Istodax)	Histone deacetylase inhibitor; catalyzes removal of acetyl groups from lysines on histone proteins, enhancing transcription from less condensed chromatin	Metabolized by hepatic P-450 system	Nausea and vomiting, T-wave changes and QT prolongation on ECG, diarrhea, infections, hypomagnesemia, hypotension, myelosuppression, hypersensitivity reactions	Cutaneous T-cell lymphoma
Rituximab (Rituxan)	Chimeric antibody targeting B-cell CD20 surface antigen on lymphocytes	Proteolysis without substantial excretion	Hypersensitivity reactions, lymphopenia	Relapsed low-grade CD20-positive non-Hodgkin lymphomas
Rogorafenib (Stivarga)	Multikinase inhibitor; targets VEGFR2, TIE-2; inhibits angiogenesis	Hepatic metabolism with excretion into feces>urine	Hypertension, hepatotoxicity, fatigue, abdominal pain	Colorectal cancer, GIST
Ruxolitinib (Jakafi)	JAK1 and 2 kinase inhibitor; blocks JAK-dependent immune and hematopoietic signal transduction pathways	Hepatic metabolism with excretion into urine >feces	Myelosuppression, bruising, headache, weight gain, liver function abnormalities	Myelofibrosis
Sorafenib (Nexavar)	Multikinase inhibitor; inhibits RAF kinase, as well as VEGF and PDGF receptors; antiangiogenic	Metabolized in liver, excreted in feces; patients with severe liver or kidney dysfunction do not tolerate drug well	Rash, hand-foot syndrome, fatigue, diarrhea, hair loss, hypertension, arthralgias, myelosuppression, cardiac ischemia and QT prolongation	Renal cell carcinoma, hepatocellular carcinoma, thyroid cancer
Sunitinib maleate (Sutent)	Multitargeted tyrosine kinase inhibitor with activity against VEGFR1-3, FLT-3, PDGFR; antiangiogenic	Metabolized by P-450's in liver, with excretion in feces	Bleeding, decreased cardiac function, prolonged QT interval, hypertension, myelosuppression, nausea, rash, liver function abnormalities	Renal cell cancer, GIST, pancreatic neuroendocrine tumors
Temosirolimus (Torisel)	Inhibits mTOR kinase-dependent cell signaling	Metabolized in liver	Hypersensitivity reaction, bowel perforation, interstitial lung disease	Renal cell cancer
Thalidomide (Thalomid)	Immunomodulatory and antiangiogenic agent; inhibits TNF-α production; alters endothelial cell proliferation and cytokine production	Nonenzymatic hydrolysis; eliminated in urine	Teratogenicity, sedation, constipation, peripheral neuropathy, rash	Multiple myeloma
Trastuzumab (Herceptin)	Recombinant monoclonal antibody against HER2; downregulates expression of HER2 pathways; immune-mediated effects	Minimal renal or hepatic clearance	Hypersensitivity reactions, fever, and chills; nausea; enhances anthracycline cardiac toxicity	Metastatic or adjuvant HER2-expressing breast cancer or HER2-positive gastric cancer

Vemurafenib (Zelboraf)	Inhibits B-RAF kinase carrying V600E mutation	Metabolized by liver, excreted into feces	QT prolongation, liver function abnormalities, photosensitivity, alopecia, arthralgias, fever, rash, hyperkeratosis and skin papillomas	Malignant melanoma carrying B-RAF V600E mutation
Vismodegib (Erivedge)	Hedgehog pathway inhibitor; binds and inhibits Smoothened, a transmembrane G-protein receptor important for signal transduction in the hedgehog pathway	Hepatic metabolism, excretion in feces	Muscle spasms, fatigue, alopecia, weight loss, diarrhea	Advanced basal cell carcinoma
Vorinostat (Zolinza)	Histone deacetylase inhibitor; catalyzes removal of acetyl groups from lysines on histone proteins, enhancing transcription from less condensed chromatin	Metabolized in liver, eliminated in urine	Deep venous thrombosis, diarrhea, fatigue, alopecia, myelosuppression,	Cutaneous T-cell lymphoma
Zoledronic acid (Zometa)	Bisphosphonate inhibitor of osteoclastic bone resorption	Renal elimination	Bone pain, arthralgias and muscle pain, fever, fatigue, abnormal renal function, osteonecrosis of jaw, atypical subtrochanteric femoral fractures	Hypercalcemia of malignancy, multiple myeloma; prevention of bone fractures for patients with advanced breast and prostate cancer in concert with standard systemic therapy
DRUGS THAT AMELIORATE CHEMOTHERAPY SIDE EFFECTS				
Dexrazoxane (Zinecard)	Anthracycline protective agent that chelates iron and protects the heart by inhibiting formation of anthracycline-induced reactive oxygen species	Hepatic metabolism, excreted in urine	Myelosuppression, nausea and vomiting, stomatitis	Reduces cumulative cardiotoxicity when administered with anthracyclines; also ameliorates anthracycline-induced extravasation injury
Leucovorin (folinic acid, citrovorum factor, Wellcovorin)	Water-soluble folate vitamin; increases body and tumor pool of reduced folates; enhances 5-FU metabolite-mediated inhibition of thymidylate synthase	Renal excretion	Well tolerated by itself; occasional nausea	Prophylaxis and treatment of hematopoietic side effects of folic acid antagonists; enhanced efficacy of 5-FU for colon cancer and other GI malignancies
Mesna (Mesnex)	Synthetic sulfhydryl compound; metabolite, mesna disulfide, reacts chemically with urotoxic ifosfamide metabolites, resulting in their detoxification	Renal	Bad taste, diarrhea	Prophylaxis of cyclophosphamide/ifosfamide-induced hemorrhagic cystitis

*An intrathecal formulation, DepoCyt, is used for the treatment of carcinomatous meningitis.
†Dosing differs among agents.
‡Dosages differ among brands.
§An analogue of thalidomide, which is a severe human teratogen; restricted prescribing.
AML = acute myelogenous leukemia, ATP = adenosine triphosphate; bFGF, basic fibroblast growth factor; BMT = bone marrow transplantation; CrCe = creatine clearance, CHF = congestive heart failure; CLL = chronic lymphocytic leukemia; CML = chronic myelogenous leukemia; CNS = central nervous system; CSF = colony-stimulating factor; CTLA-4 = cytotoxic T-lymphocyte-associated protein 4; EGFR = epidermal growth factor receptor; ERBB2 = HER2/neu; FDA = U.S. Food and Drug Administration; FSH = follicle-stimulating hormone; G-CSF = granulocyte colony-stimulating factor; GM-CSF = granulocyte-macrophage colony-stimulating factor; GI = gastrointestinal; GIST = gastrointestinal stromal tumor; GnRH = gonadotropin-releasing hormone; 5-HIAA = 5-hydroxyindolacetic acid; HIV = human immunodeficiency virus; IL = interleukin; LFT = liver function test; LH = luteinizing hormone; LHRH = luteinizing hormone–releasing hormone; MAO = monoamine oxidase; mTOR = mammalian target of rapamycin; NSAID = nonsteroidal anti-inflammatory drug; PDGF = platelet-derived growth factor; SIADH = syndrome of inappropriate secretion of antidiuretic hormone; TKI = tyrosine kinase inhibitor; TNF = tumor necrosis factor; VEGF = vascular endothelial growth factor.

cytotoxin to enhance cell killing.[A2] Radioimmunoconjugate approaches have been most effective in the treatment of non-Hodgkin lymphoma (Chapter 185) and chronic lymphocytic leukemia (Chapter 184). The effectiveness of monoclonal antibodies in specific tumor types is not identical to small molecules developed against the same target, in part because of the induction of immunologically mediated mechanisms of tumor cell killing that are unique to antibodies.

Hormonal Therapies

Endocrine or hormonal therapy for cancer, the earliest form of systemic therapy, is almost entirely limited to breast cancer (Chapter 198) and prostate cancer (Chapter 201). Many premenopausal breast cancers are thought to be under the influence of estrogens, and hormonal deprivation (ablation) may produce long-term responses in properly selected patients (those with estrogen and/or progesterone receptor positivity who have predominantly soft tissue or bone disease). The antiestrogen tamoxifen is effective against breast cancer, and it may decrease the incidence of contralateral breast cancers in both premenopausal and postmenopausal women with breast cancer. It also has an estrogen-like activity that is responsible for an increased rate of endometrial cancers. Postmenopausal women who are candidates for hormonal therapy may also respond to tamoxifen; however, aromatase inhibitors (e.g., anastrozole, letrozole, exemestane), which decrease the conversion of metabolites in fat and muscle into estrogen, have been found to be more effective than tamoxifen as first-line therapy in both the adjuvant and metastatic settings.

Prostate cancer (Chapter 201) is usually androgen dependent, and androgen deprivation can produce meaningful responses. The recent introduction of more potent inhibitors of androgen biosynthesis (abiraterone) and androgen receptor-mediated signal transduction (enzalutamide)[A3] has further enhanced the range and effectiveness of androgen deprivation therapy for this disease.

The corticosteroids (Chapter 35), typically prednisone or dexamethasone, are widely used in the treatment of hematologic and oncologic cancers. In Hodgkin disease (Chapter 186), the non-Hodgkin lymphomas (Chapter 185), and multiple myeloma (Chapter 187), corticosteroids have antitumor activity. In solid tumor patients, they are used as antiemetics and for symptomatic relief of cerebral edema in cases of CNS metastases (Chapter 189), or as an adjunct to radiation therapy for spinal cord metastases.

Immunotherapy

Recently, several new approaches to improving cancer immunotherapy by blocking the negative effects on the immune system produced by tumors have yielded dramatic clinical benefits for patients with a variety of advanced cancers, including melanoma, kidney, and lung cancers. The survival of men and women with metastatic melanoma (Chapter 203) was significantly increased following treatment with an antibody (ipilumumab, anti-CTLA-4) that neutralizes proteins that protect tumor cells against destruction by the immune system.[A4] Additional antibodies that target other immunologic checkpoints (anti-PD-1 and anti-PD-L1) are in advanced stages of clinical investigation and are likely to provide substantive clinical benefits for patients with melanoma, renal cancer (Chapter 197), and non–small cell lung cancer.

Drugs for Prevention of Toxicity

In addition to the hematopoietic growth factors used to reduce the adverse effects of systemic cancer therapies on the bone marrow (discussed later under Management of Complications), there are drugs that have been developed to ameliorate important side effects of cytotoxic chemotherapy (see Table 179-4). These include dexrazoxane, an iron chelating agent that can prevent the cardiac toxicity of the anthracyclines (doxorubicin and daunorubicin); leucovorin, which can diminish the hematologic side effects of folic acid antagonists; and mesna, a thiol-containing compound that blocks damage to the bladder mucosa from metabolites of cyclophosphamide.

Bone Marrow or Hematopoietic Stem Cell Transplantation

Because the major dose-limiting toxicity of most chemotherapeutic agents is myelosuppression, approaches have been developed to harvest the pluripotent stem cells found in bone marrow, peripheral blood, or, less often, cord blood before marrow-damaging chemotherapy so that the stem cells can be reinfused later (Chapter 178). This technique is most effective for acute leukemias (Chapter 183), relapsed lymphomas (Chapter 185), and germ cell tumors (Chapter 200). The effectiveness of the approach is limited more by the inability to eradicate cancer cells than by the inability to achieve engraftment. Transplants may be syngeneic (from an identical twin), autologous (from oneself), allogeneic (from a matched donor such as a sibling or parent), or from a matched unrelated donor. Nonablative hematopoietic transplants that do not completely abolish myelopoiesis reduce toxicity and allow the treatment of older and medically infirm patients. Hematopoietic stem cell transplantation is discussed in detail in Chapter 178.

Special Treatment Populations

Obesity

Studies of practice patterns indicate that up to 40% of obese patients receive limited doses of chemotherapy that are not based on actual body weight. Concerns about toxicity or overdosing based on the use of actual body weight in obese patients with cancer are unfounded. The American Society of Clinical Oncology (ASCO) has published evidence-based practice guidelines that recommend that full cytotoxic chemotherapy doses be used to treat obese patients with cancer, especially when the goal of treatment is cure.[5]

Pregnancy

Cancer during pregnancy is not uncommon, with breast, cervical, ovarian, and thyroid cancers, melanoma, and hematologic malignancies being most common. This is an emotionally charged time, and clinical decision making is complicated by ethical, moral, cultural, and religious issues. If surgery can be safely accomplished, this may be the best course, even if it is only a temporizing measure. Radiation therapy carries the very real risk of radiation exposure to the fetus, and staging is almost always suboptimal and confined to ultrasound examinations. When the disease requires chemotherapy, changes in both the mother and fetus must be taken into account; for instance, there are major changes in drug clearance during pregnancy, along with gastrointestinal absorption and placental transfer, not to mention fetal pharmacokinetics and placental excretion. Many commonly used chemotherapeutic drugs are classified by the FDA as category D (positive human fetal risk, but the benefits in pregnant women may be acceptable despite the risk) or category X (studies in humans and animal have shown fetal malformations or there is evidence of fetal risk based on human evidence). If the mother's condition permits, it is advisable to defer chemotherapy (including anthracyclines and taxanes) during the first trimester and to treat life-threatening situations during the third trimester after extensive counseling with the parents.

Geriatrics

An increasing proportion of cancers occur in the older population. The physiologic changes that develop with age include: decreased excretion of drugs and metabolites from the kidneys, decreased volume of distribution of water-soluble drugs, and increased susceptibility to myelosuppression, cardiomyopathy, and neuropathy, related in part to comorbid conditions. As a general rule, the suitability of an older patient for therapy can be determined by a comprehensive geriatric assessment (CGA) that evaluates the patient's function, comorbidity, nutrition, medications, and resources. Geriatric assessment is discussed in detail in Chapter 24. By itself, age is not a barrier to surgery; rather, the patient's performance status and the CGA should determine the likelihood of a good recovery. Tolerance of radiation therapy seems to remain largely intact with increasing age. Chemotherapy decisions are also based on the performance status and CGA. Dosage adjustments are also made for individual glomerular filtration rates for patients aged 65 and older, where appropriate. The use of lower chemotherapy doses based on age alone is not advisable and may result in ineffective treatment.

Organ Dysfunction

Alterations in drug clearance play a critical role in the safe administration of anticancer agents. Over the past decade, pharmacokinetic studies have begun to detail the landscape of how specific levels of carefully defined renal or hepatic dysfunction alter the clearance and tolerance of many of the most commonly used drugs for the systemic treatment of cancer. For each new agent, prospective investigations are required to define usage parameters for each clinically defined level of organ dysfunction. It should be pointed out that alterations in pharmacokinetic parameters per se may occur with or without important changes in toxicity. Where evidence exists, applicable recommendations for chemotherapeutic drug use in the setting of renal or hepatic dysfunction are outlined in Table 179-4.

Management of Complications

Supportive Care

Nutritional Support

Nutrition is always a concern for patients newly diagnosed with cancer, even if they have not experienced weight loss. In fact, significant weight loss is an adverse prognostic factor for several cancers, especially lung cancer. Patients are often concerned about whether their diet contributed to development of the cancer and whether diet can influence the results of therapy. In most settings, neither of these scenarios is the case. Malnourished patients should be evaluated by a dietitian to determine whether they are ingesting sufficient calories and whether dietary supplements might be needed. Nutritional assessment is discussed in detail in Chapter 214. Some patients, such as those with head and neck cancers (Chapter 190) or esophageal cancers (Chapter 192), may require parenteral nutrition through a percutaneous gastrostomy tube. Total parenteral nutrition (Chapter 217) is rarely indicated. Larger-than-recommended doses of vitamins are also not helpful and may be toxic. It is important to determine whether over-the-counter and/or alternative medications (Chapter 39) are being contemplated or used by the patient because of the potential for drug interactions.

Psychosocial Support

Patients with a recent cancer diagnosis have increased risks of death from cardiovascular causes, especially during the first week after diagnosis. The need for continuing psychosocial support in the face of ongoing cancer treatment, and the associated anxiety, depression, and fear experienced by many patients, is substantive and may be beyond the ability of the immediate family to fulfill. In this setting, patients often benefit from participation in support groups or from direct one-on-one counseling, and from efforts to improve communication across all levels of care and support systems.

Hematopoietic Growth Factors

Growth factors, such as granulocyte colony-stimulating factor (G-CSF) and granulocyte-macrophage colony-stimulating factor (GM-CSF), speed recovery from white blood cell count depression, permitting chemotherapy to be given on schedule, without reducing the dosage in many cases (Chapter 156).[A5] However, such therapy does not decrease hospitalizations or improve survival. It is possible to determine which individuals are at greatest risk for febrile neutropenia (Chapter 167) and to treat them in advance, based on published guidelines.[6] Correction of anemia with erythropoiesis-stimulating agents (ESAs) (Epoetin alfa and Darbepoietin alfa), while possible, may be associated with complications of adverse cardiovascular events and even potentially tumor progression (Chapter 158).[7]

Prevention of Pathologic Bone Fractures

The bisphosphonates pamidronate and zoledronate are very effective not only for the treatment of tumor-induced hypercalcemia but also to reduce pathologic fractures in bones with metastatic lesions, particularly from breast cancer (Chapter 198), prostate cancer (Chapter 201), and myeloma (Chapter 187). They are also used to treat osteoporosis caused by chemotherapy-induced premature menopause in young women with breast cancer (Chapter 243). Denosumab is a human monoclonal antibody that binds to RANK ligand, a protein found on osteoclasts that is involved in bone breakdown. Some clinical trials have found denosumab to be superior to zoledronic acid for the prevention of skeletal-related events in cancer patients with bone metastases.[A6]

Symptom Management

Effective management of symptoms is critical to successful delivery of either curative or palliative treatment and maintenance of a patient's quality of life.

Nausea and Vomiting

Patients continue to fear chemotherapy because of the risk of nausea and vomiting. New antiemetics, used in combination, have made this side effect much less debilitating. Chemotherapeutic drugs can be ranked according to their probability of causing nausea and vomiting, with prophylactic treatment given accordingly. The availability of the serotonin 5-hydroxytryptamine type 3 (5-HT_3) receptor antagonists (dolasetron, granisetron, ondansetron) has dramatically improved our ability to completely control nausea and vomiting. More emetogenic regimens require combination therapy with a corticosteroid (usually dexamethasone), a 5-HT_3 antagonist, and a benzodiazepine (e.g., lorazepam) or the neurokinin-1 receptor antagonist, aprepitant.[A7] Aprepitant is particularly useful for the treatment/prevention of delayed nausea and vomiting. A double-blind randomized clinical trial of four combination regimens for controlling delayed nausea concluded that the addition of dexamethasone on days 2 and 3 was particularly effective.[A8]

Pain Control

Pain control[8] (Chapter 30) can be accomplished with a variety of analgesics, both non-narcotic and narcotic. Oncologists use a variety of scales for the evaluation of pain and start treatment with nonsteroidal anti-inflammatory drugs (NSAIDs) such as aspirin and acetaminophen, progress through ibuprofen and related drugs, and then through combinations of NSAIDs and narcotics to stronger narcotics. Newer narcotics are available in both short-duration and long-duration forms; some dermal patches last 72 hours, which is ideal for patients who have severe pain and are unable to take oral medications. Oral transmucosal fentanyl is more effective than standard-release morphine in this setting. Painful oral mucositis, a common complication of intensive therapy for hematologic malignancies, can be treated with local measures or with recombinant human keratinocyte growth factor. Oral anti-*Candida* drugs that are absorbed or partially absorbed from the gastrointestinal tract can help prevent pain from oral candidiasis. American Pain Society standards for pain management in cancer recommend both pharmacologic[9] and psychosocial[10] interventions as complementary approaches. A recently published meta-analysis of randomized controlled studies of various psychosocial interventions among adult cancer patients (e.g., relaxation training, cognitive behavioral therapy, and other education- and skills-based approaches) demonstrated medium-sized effects on both pain severity and interference with daily activities.

Malignant Effusions

Accumulations of fluid and malignant cells in the pleural, peritoneal, or pericardial spaces are common complications of epithelial and hematopoietic malignancies that frequently produce a significant array of symptoms, either at the time of diagnosis or accompanying tumor progression. Malignant pleural effusions (Chapter 99) are most commonly associated with cancers of the lung and breast or lymphomas, may be the result of lymphatic obstruction or direct invasion of pleural membranes, and can produce significant degrees of dyspnea, cough, or pain that require therapy. Diagnostic thoracentesis of sufficient volume (>60 mL), with cytologic analysis of the pleural effusion, has a reasonably high diagnostic yield for malignancy (60 to 90%). In patients with previously untreated lymphoma, breast cancer, or small cell lung cancer, objective response to the initiation of systemic chemotherapy may provide long-term symptomatic relief. However, in patients with recurrent lung or breast cancer, for example, pleural effusions that are confirmed to contain malignant cells may present difficult ongoing therapeutic challenges. For symptomatic patients, therapeutic thoracentesis, usually under ultrasound guidance, is required and may need to be repeated to reduce dyspnea. When frequent thoracenteses over short intervals are needed, a pleurodesis procedure is often performed, encompassing drainage of the pleural space with a chest thoracostomy and the instillation of a sclerosing compound (talc, doxycycline) that will initiate an inflammatory response of sufficient magnitude to obliterate the pleural space. Pleurodesis is at least temporarily successful in preventing fluid recurrence in most patients; when it is not, placement of an indwelling pleural catheter may provide long-term symptomatic relief of dyspnea.

Malignant ascites (peritoneal effusion) occurs most frequently in patients with intra-abdominal malignancies (gastric, ovarian, pancreatic, and primary peritoneal cancers) but can be observed as well in patients with advanced breast and lung cancers or lymphoma. Malignant ascites may be caused in part by increased permeability of the tumor vasculature that is a result of vascular endothelial growth factor overexpression, by inflammatory cytokine overproduction in the peritoneal space, or by lymphatic blockade secondary to carcinomatosis. Ultrasound-guided paracentesis provides relief of bloating, dyspnea, and the pain of abdominal distension, but will often need to be repeated, which carries the risk of dehydration, protein loss, electrolyte imbalance, bleeding, infection, and kidney dysfunction. A requirement for paracentesis at frequencies less than 1 week should prompt consideration of placement of a permanent catheter to allow self-drainage, although these devices carry a significant risk of infection.

Malignant pericardial effusions (Chapter 77) are most commonly related to direct extension or metastatic spread from lung or breast cancers, melanomas, and hematologic malignancies. As is the case for other malignant effusions, image-guided pericardiocentesis with cytologic examination of the fluid that has been evacuated will frequently provide diagnostic confirmation of malignancy; furthermore, even the removal of a relatively modest amount of fluid (<50 mL) may, at least partially, relieve the hemodynamic compromise produced by the effusion. The approach to a patient with malignant pericardial effusions is dictated by hemodynamic status (which can drive the choice between emergency pericardiocentesis or elective pericardiostomy) and by the predicted sensitivity of the inciting tumor to systemic therapy (untreated lymphoma versus chemotherapy-resistant lung cancer, for example).

ENDOCRINE MANIFESTATIONS OF CANCER

Clinical syndromes associated with ectopic hormone production may pose special diagnostic dilemmas, can produce a significant degree of morbidity or even death in cancer patients, and may be difficult to treat (Table 179-5). Management of these syndromes involves the simultaneous treatment of both the cancer and the syndrome caused by excessive hormone production. Many of the endocrine manifestations of cancer are caused by the production of small polypeptide hormones by tumors, some of which are derived from specific types of neuroendocrine cells. These cells are widely dispersed in a wide variety of organs, are often of neural crest origin, and can produce biogenic amines. The hormones produced from these tumors include adrenocorticotropic hormones (corticotropin, ACTH), calcitonin, vasoactive intestinal peptide, growth hormone–releasing hormone, corticotropin-releasing hormone (CRH), somatostatin, and other peptides. A second group of tumors, generally derived from squamous epithelium, produces parathyroid hormone–related proteins (PTHrP) and vasopressin.

Hypercalcemia of Malignancy

Humoral hypercalcemia is one of the most common endocrine syndromes related to an underlying malignancy. There are several different underlying mechanisms related to this pathophysiologic process, including ectopic production of PTHrP with activation of the PTH receptor to increase osteoclast

TABLE 179-5 SOME CLINICAL SYNDROMES OF ECTOPIC HORMONE PRODUCTION

Humoral hypercalcemia
- Parathyroid hormone–related protein
  - Squamous cell carcinoma
  - Breast cancer
  - Neuroendocrine tumors
  - Renal cell cancer
  - Melanoma
  - Prostate cancer
- Increased calcitriol
  - Lymphoma
  - Benign conditions: sarcoid, berylliosis, tuberculosis, fungal infections

Corticotropin
- Proopiomelanocortin
  - Small cell lung cancer
  - Pulmonary carcinoid
  - Medullary thyroid cancer
  - Islet cell tumor
  - Pheochromocytoma
  - Ganglioneuroma
- Corticotropin-releasing hormone
  - Medullary thyroid cancer
  - Paraganglioma
  - Prostate cancer
  - Islet cell tumors

Human chorionic gonadotropin
- Choriocarcinoma
- Testicular embryonal cell carcinoma
- Seminoma

Hypoglycemia
- Insulinoma
- Sarcomas or large retroperitoneal tumors

Inappropriate antidiuretic hormone secretion
- Small cell lung cancer
- Squamous cell head and neck cancer

Erythropoietin
- Renal cell cancer
- Hepatoma
- Pheochromocytoma
- Benign conditions: cerebellar hemangioblastoma, uterine fibroids

differentiation and bone resorption, with consequent hypercalcemia. Ectopic PTHrP (rather than PTH) production by several different types of cancer, most characteristically in squamous cell, breast, renal cell, and prostate cancer, as well as neuroendocrine tumors and melanoma (see Table 179-5), is one of the most common causes of hypercalcemia of malignancy.[11] Increased production of calcitriol, which increases calcium absorption with suppression of serum PTH levels, is another cause of malignant hypercalcemia that is most commonly observed in patients with lymphoma. Bone metastases, particularly in patients with breast cancer and myeloma, may produce hypercalcemia due to increased local production of PTHrP or other cytokines that increase bone resorption.

The treatment of malignant hypercalcemia is similar to that caused by hyperparathyroidism (Chapter 245) in that reversal of dehydration and the initiation of a saline diuresis should begin early; patients with a serum calcium in excess of 13 mg/dL should be treated with a bisphosphonate initially, with extended use of the bisphosphonate, as described earlier, for the prevention of bone fractures and recurrence of hypercalcemia (Chapter 245).

Other Ectopic Hormone Syndromes

Inappropriate secretion of ACTH is rare but resembles pituitary Cushing disease (Chapter 224); tumors that produce CRH include medullary thyroid cancer, prostate cancer, and islet cell neoplasms. Ectopic ACTH syndrome may become manifest as classic Cushing syndrome, with easy bruisability, centripetal obesity, muscle wasting, hypertension, diabetes, and metabolic alkalosis, although many patients with ectopic ACTH-producing cancers progress too quickly to develop prominent cushingoid manifestation clinically. Profound hypokalemia may predominate without all the classic features of Cushing syndrome in patients with small cell lung cancer.

Tumor-associated hypoglycemia, although uncommon, may be the result of: insulin overproduction by islet cell tumors; insufficient hepatic

TABLE 179-6 EVALUATION AND DIAGNOSIS OF PARANEOPLASTIC SYNDROMES

Characterize abnormality; obtain laboratory studies and biopsy as necessary.
Carefully elicit any additional symptoms and signs.
Eliminate common causes.
If there is no obvious etiology, consider a paraneoplastic syndrome.
If findings are consistent with a known syndrome, screen for underlying malignancy.
If signs and symptoms are consistent with a known paraneoplastic syndrome, undertake a search for an unknown primary cancer or recurrence or progression of a known primary tumor.
Screening should include a careful physical examination with breast, gynecologic, and prostate evaluations; basic hematology, chemistry, and urine studies; chest radiograph; and mammogram.
Computed tomography (CT) of the abdomen and pelvis or positron emission tomography (PET) scan is indicated if there are any suspicious symptoms, signs, or laboratory abnormalities.
Antibody testing for paraneoplastic neurologic syndromes and/or skin biopsy should be performed as indicated.
Consider treatment of cancer and/or appropriate palliative treatment, including immunosuppressive therapy for paraneoplastic symptoms when possible.

gluconeogenesis related to loss of functional hepatic mass by metastatic disease; and overexpression of insulin-like growth factor II, which can activate the insulin receptor in patients with large retroperitoneal sarcomas or hepatocellular carcinomas. In each of these cases, treatment with frequent small feedings can be prescribed; however, successful symptomatic management of hypoglycemia may be difficult without control of the primary tumor mass or metastases.

The clinical syndrome of inappropriate secretion of antidiuretic hormone is caused by ectopic production of vasopressin, primarily in patients with small cell lung cancer or squamous cancers of the head and neck, and occasionally in those with primary brain tumors. It is characterized by hyponatremia, hypo-osmolality, excessive urine sodium excretion, an inappropriately high urine osmolality for the low serum osmolality, and normal kidney, adrenal, and thyroid function (Chapter 116). Fluid (free water) restriction can provide adequate short-term management of symptomatic hyponatremia; however, treatment with demeclocycline, which blocks the effects of vasopressin on the kidney, provides more effective long-term therapy.

PARANEOPLASTIC SYNDROMES

The term *paraneoplasia*, which means "alongside cancer," has been commonly used to denote remote effects of cancer that cannot be attributed either to direct invasion or to distant metastases. These syndromes may be the first sign of a malignancy and affect up to 15% of patients with cancer (Table 179-6). However, if patients with cachexia are excluded, the incidence probably drops to only a few percent. Paraneoplastic syndromes may be the initial presenting sign or symptom of an underlying malignancy. Up to two thirds of paraneoplastic syndromes arise before an associated malignancy is diagnosed. In some cases, the paraneoplastic syndrome may be associated with relatively small tumors; recognition of these associations may lead to earlier diagnosis and possibly more effective therapy. Furthermore, one of the hallmarks in defining a paraneoplastic syndrome is that the course of the syndrome generally parallels the course of the tumor. Therefore, effective treatment of the underlying malignancy is often accompanied by improvement or resolution of the syndrome. Conversely, recurrence of the cancer may be heralded by the return of systemic symptoms. The numerous neurologic paraneoplastic syndromes[12] are reviewed in Chapter 411.

Dermatologic Paraneoplastic Syndromes

Associations between cutaneous syndromes and underlying malignancies may be difficult to confirm. Generally, the skin condition and cancer follow a parallel course, and the two diagnoses should be made at about the same time. Some skin lesions are almost always associated with malignancy. Others, however, are nonspecific and are most commonly seen with nonmalignant conditions, making it difficult or impossible to connect the skin disease with the underlying malignancy. In addition, biopsies of the skin lesion are usually nonspecific, showing features identical to those when the same lesion is seen without a malignant condition. The formation of tumor-related autoantibodies has rarely been associated with dermatologic paraneoplastic syndromes, although inflammatory cell infiltration may be seen.

Recognition of cutaneous manifestations of malignancy can be critical for the early diagnosis and successful treatment of cancer, but some syndromes are seen only with advanced, incurable disease. Cutaneous manifestations include direct involvement of the skin with tumor as well as the remote effects of cancer.[13,14] Both specific and nonspecific dermatologic adverse effects are also seen with cytotoxic chemotherapeutic agents, including alkylating agents, antimetabolites, anthracyclines, and antitumor antibiotics.

One of the best-known paraneoplastic syndromes is acanthosis nigricans, the pathogenesis of which is unclear. The tumor may produce factors that activate insulin-like growth factors or the insulin receptor in skin. Many tumors are known to produce transforming growth factor-α (TGF-α), which might activate epidermal growth factor receptors in skin, causing hyperpigmentation and thickening. The skin lesions arise as velvety, verrucous hyperpigmentation of the neck, axilla, groin, and mucosal membranes, including the lips, periocular area, and anus. Although acanthosis nigricans clearly occurs as a benign entity associated with obesity and endocrinopathy, its appearance in older adults, especially when it includes mucosal lesions, has been highly associated with malignancies of the gastrointestinal tract as well as other adenocarcinomas. The lesions often regress with successful treatment of the underlying tumor.

Rheumatologic Paraneoplastic Syndromes

In patients who have rheumatic disorders with atypical clinical presentation—particularly older patients, those with coexisting systemic symptoms, and patients who respond unexpectedly poorly to usual antirheumatic treatments—the possibility of an underlying occult malignancy should be considered.[15] Chemotherapeutic agents can also cause rheumatic adverse effects.[16]

One of the more common and specific rheumatologic paraneoplastic syndromes is hypertrophic osteoarthropathy, which arises as an oligoarthritis or polyarthritis of the distal joints, with clubbing, tender periostitis of the distal long bones, and noninflammatory synovial effusions (also see Chapter 275). Hypertrophic osteoarthropathy may affect up to 10% of patients with adenocarcinoma of the lung. It is also seen with a variety of other pulmonary malignancies, including lung metastases from other primary sites. The etiology is unknown. Laboratory studies often reveal an elevation in the erythrocyte sedimentation rate; bone radiographs show linear ossification of the distal long bones separated by a radiolucent zone from the underlying cortex (Fig. 179-1). Treatment is symptomatic with anti-inflammatory agents; successful treatment of the underlying tumor may also improve the signs and symptoms of this syndrome.

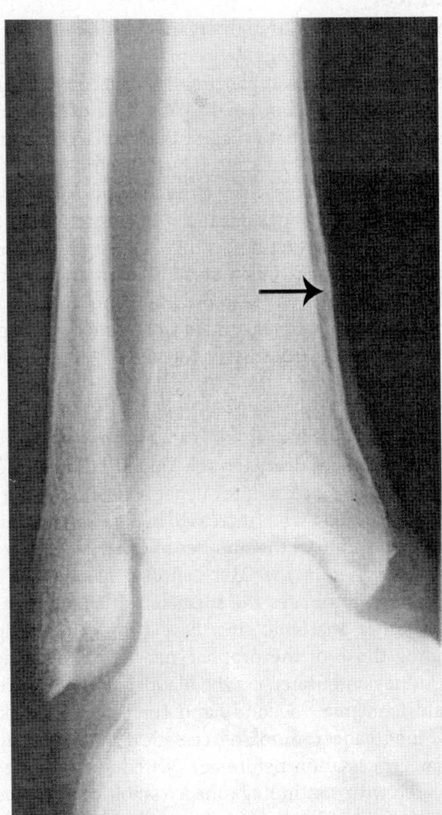

FIGURE 179-1. Hypertrophic pulmonary osteoarthropathy characterized by periosteal elevation of the tibia (*arrow*). (Courtesy Dr. Lynne S. Steinbach.)

Fever and Cachexia

Fever (Chapter 280), night sweats, and cachexia are nonspecific symptoms that, when seen in the absence of infection or a known disorder, suggest the diagnosis of an underlying malignancy. Cytokines clearly play a pathogenetic role in inducing both fever and cachexia. TNF-α, interleukins (particularly IL-1 and IL-6), and interferon-γ are produced directly by the tumor or by tumor-associated host inflammatory cells, such as macrophages, which results in a catabolic state. Cytokines may produce fever directly by acting at the level of the hypothalamic thermoregulatory center. In addition to the burden of tumor and the production of cytokines, cachexia may be caused or worsened by the side effects of cancer treatment, by intestinal blockage or malabsorption caused by tumor infiltration, and by depression.

Fever is generally cyclic and may be associated with drenching night sweats. Symptoms resolve with successful treatment of the underlying tumor, and return of fever usually heralds relapse. When treatment of the tumor is not possible or is ineffective, NSAIDs or steroids given around the clock significantly improve quality of life. Although cancer-related fever is most commonly seen in association with malignant lymphoproliferative disease (Chapters 185 and 186), renal cell carcinoma (Chapter 197), and leukemias (Chapters 183 and 184), it may also occur with other cancers, particularly in the face of extensive hepatic metastases.

Cachexia, or the cancer wasting syndrome, is probably the single most common paraneoplastic syndrome, eventually affecting up to 80% of patients with cancer. This syndrome is characterized by anorexia, muscle wasting, loss of subcutaneous fat, and fatigue. It appears to be caused by a combination of protein wasting, malabsorption, immune dysregulation, and increased glucose turnover in the setting of tumor-induced increases in energy expenditure. Successful treatment of the underlying tumor reverses the process; symptomatic treatment for patients with advanced disease is modestly successful at best. Megestrol acetate given in high concentrations in liquid form (400 to 800 mg/day) can improve appetite and result in weight gain, but at the cost of fluid retention.

SURVIVORSHIP AND FOLLOW-UP

Approximately 4% of the United States population (≈14 million people) is living with a history of cancer; about 60% of cancer survivors are age 65 or older.[17] Thus, there is a large and increasing number of individuals who are living longer during the period of cancer survivorship—from the end of active treatment to the point of recurrence or death from another condition. There has been a growing appreciation of the specific care needs of these patients, including: a defined program of surveillance to detect recurrence or second cancers and the late effects of cancer treatment; intervention to treat the consequences of the cancer and its treatment (such as lymphedema, fatigue, and psychosocial distress); prevention of new cancers through changes in diet, behavior, and physical activity; and the institution of a coordinated program of care for cancer survivors that may require a variety of specialty services. Long-term follow-up can be optimized by the provision of a survivorship care plan for patients that provides a comprehensive summary of all diagnostic and therapeutic procedures undergone, toxicities experienced, and therapeutic outcomes, as well as a specific program of individualized follow-up care. Although definitive follow-up regimens do not exist for most cancers, evidence-based templates for common malignancies have been developed by the American Society of Clinical Oncology and the National Comprehensive Cancer Network. Lastly, it must be remembered that issues of survivorship affect caregivers, who often experience a high degree of psychological distress, along with the patient, during and after the period of active treatment.

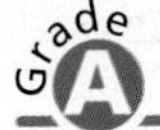

Grade A References

A1. Maemondo M, Inoue A, Kobayashi K, et al. Gefitinib or chemotherapy for non-small cell lung cancer with mutated EGFR. *N Engl J Med.* 2010;362:2380-2388.

A2. Verma S, Miles D, Gianni L, et al. Trastuzumab emtansine for HER2-positive advanced breast cancer. *N Engl J Med.* 2012;367:1783-1791.

A3. Scher HI, Fizazi K, Saad F, et al. Increased survival with enzalutamide in prostate cancer after chemotherapy. *N Engl J Med.* 2012;367:1187-1197.

A4. Hodi FS, O'Day SJ, McDermott DF, et al. Improved survival with ipilimumab in patients with metastatic melanoma. *N Engl J Med.* 2010;363:711-723.

A5. Mhaskar R, Clark OA, Lyman G, et al. Colony-stimulating factors for chemotherapy-induced febrile neutropenia. *Cochrane Database Syst Rev.* 2014;10:CD003039.

A6. Fizazi K, Carducci M, Smith M, et al. Denosumab versus zoledronic acid for treatment of bone metastases in men with castration-resistant prostate cancer: a randomized, double-blind study. *Lancet*. 2011;377:785-786.
A7. Basch E, Prestrud AA, Hesketh PJ, et al. Antiemetics: American Society of Clinical Oncology clinical practice guidelines update. *J Clin Oncol*. 2011;29:4189-4198.
A8. Roscoe JA, Heckler CE, Morrow GR, et al. Prevention of delayed nausea: a University of Rochester Cancer Center Community Clinical Oncology Program study of patients receiving chemotherapy. *J Clin Oncol*. 2012;30:3389-3395.

GENERAL REFERENCES

For the General References and other additional features, please visit Expert Consult at https://expertconsult.inkling.com.

180

EPIDEMIOLOGY OF CANCER

DAVID J. HUNTER

EPIDEMIOLOGY

Overview

The International Agency for Research on Cancer (IARC) estimates that over 14.1 million new incident cases of cancer (excluding non-melanoma skin cancer) occurred in 2012, of which over 8 million (57%) occurred in less developed regions (defined as Africa, Asia [excluding Japan], Latin America, and the Caribbean, plus Melanesia, Micronesia, and Polynesia in Oceania). Over 8.2 million deaths occurred, with over 5.3 million (65%) in less developed regions.[1] This is predicted to increase to 21.7 million incident cases and 13 million deaths by 2030 (Fig. 180-1), with the majority of this increase being due to the aging of populations, as well as increased total population.

The 10 most common cancers diagnosed worldwide in 2012 were lung (13%), breast (12%), colon/rectum (10%), prostate (8%), stomach (7%), liver (6%), cervix (4%), esophagus (3%), bladder (3%), and non-Hodgkin lymphoma (3%) (Fig. 180-2A), with 8 of these being among the 10 most common causes of cancer death: lung (19%), stomach (9%), liver (9%), colon/rectum (9%), breast (6%), esophagus (5%), prostate (4%), pancreas (4%), cervix (3%), and leukemia (3%) (Fig. 180-2B). These global estimates mask very large differences in regional incidence rates of specific cancers, with age-standardized incidence rates varying over five-fold between low- and high-incidence regions (Fig. 180-3); for some cancers there is a 20-fold difference between the lowest and highest incidence rates in individual countries. The burden of cancer on individual countries is a function of age-specific rates and population size. Thus, the country with the largest population in the world faces the largest number of cases of cancer, but the United States, with the world's third largest population, has the second largest number of cases of cancer, owing to high age-specific rates, and a high proportion of people in older age groups (Fig. 180-4).

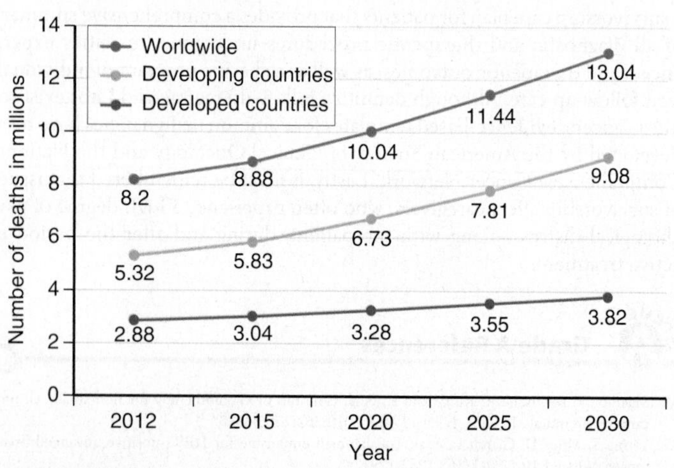

FIGURE 180-1. Projected Number of Cancer Deaths Worldwide, 2012-2030. (Data from Ferlay J, Soerjomataram I, Ervik M, et al. GLOBOCAN 2012 v1.0, Cancer Incidence and Mortality Worldwide: IARC CancerBase No. 11 [Internet]. Lyon, France: International Agency for Research on Cancer; 2013. Available from: http://globocan.iarc.fr. Accessed February 18, 2015.)

In the United States, the most common cancers predicted for 2014 for men are prostate, (27%), lung (14%), colorectal (8%), bladder (7%), melanoma (5%), renal (5%), non-Hodgkin lymphoma (4%), oropharyngeal (4%), leukemia (4%), and liver (3%), with 8 of these being among the 10 most common causes of cancer death: lung (28%), prostate (10%), colorectal (8%), pancreas (7%), liver (5%), leukemia (5%), esophagus (4%), bladder (4%), non-Hodgkin lymphoma (3%), and renal (3%), with the addition of pancreas (7%) and esophagus (4%). For women, these are breast cancer (20%), lung (13%), colorectal (8%), uterine (6%), thyroid (6%), non-Hodgkin lymphoma (4%), melanoma (4%), renal (3%), pancreas (3%), and leukemia (3%), with 7 of these being the among the top 10 causes of mortality: lung (26%), breast (15%), colon/rectum (9%), pancreas (7%), leukemia (4%), uterine (3%), and non-Hodgkin lymphoma (3%), with the addition of ovary (5%), liver (3%), and brain and other nervous system (2%).[2]

Demographic Factors

Age

The rates of most cancers increase with age, often in a log-linear (exponential) fashion; any population that experiences increases in life expectancy in the proportion of the population in older age groups will almost inevitably see an increase in the numbers of cases of cancer. Some cancers have different age-incidence curves, notably cancers that occur mostly in the first few years of life, such as retinoblastoma and neuroblastoma, or in young adulthood, such as testicular cancer. Hodgkin lymphoma has a bimodal age incidence curve with peaks in younger and older adults. Breast cancer rates increase with age in premenopausal women but plateau or increase more slowly postmenopausally.

Sex

Male breast cancer occurs at less than 1% of the rate of female breast cancer in most countries. For cancers that occur in both sexes, age-specific rates are often two- to three-fold higher in men than women; for smoking-related cancers, this is often due to higher prevalence and duration of smoking among men.

Causes of Cancer

People who migrate from low to high organ-specific cancer incidence countries tend to acquire the cancer incidence profile of their new country within one to three generations; for example, breast cancer risk among Asian American women with grandparents born in the United States is actually higher than for white U.S. women. These data suggest that the large international differences in cancer incidence rates are caused by environment and lifestyle differences between countries, rather than ethnic-specific differences in genetic susceptibility. Substantial changes in cancer incidence within countries over time, such as the rise in U.S. lung cancer incidence in the last 50 years (while stomach cancer incidence has fallen steadily) also suggest changes in the environmental determinants of these diseases. Thus, a high proportion of cancer cases are due to environment and lifestyle, and cancer epidemiologists have tried to establish these causative factors over the last 60 years.

Smoking

Smoking is the major modifiable cause of cancer in many countries, estimated to cause one third of cancer deaths in the United States and 21% of cancer deaths worldwide. While smoking prevalence has fallen in the United States over the past several decades, it has increased in many other countries, including the world's largest, China[3]; the number of cancer deaths from tobacco is likely to be much higher in the 21st century than in the 20th century. Although lung cancer dominates the spectrum of smoking-related cancers, cancers at many other anatomic sites have been convincingly related to smoking, including those of the oropharynx, larynx, esophagus, stomach, liver, pancreas, kidney and ureter, cervix, bladder, and colon/rectum, as well as acute myeloid leukemia.[4] Second-hand (or passive) smoking has been associated with lung cancer. Smoking cessation results in rapidly reduced rates of lung cancer; cessation before age 30 reduces lifetime risk by more than 90% compared with continuing tobacco smoking. However, the latency between smoking initiation and cancer occurrence is several decades, so the emergence of large numbers of smoking-related cancers occurs decades after smoking prevalence increases.

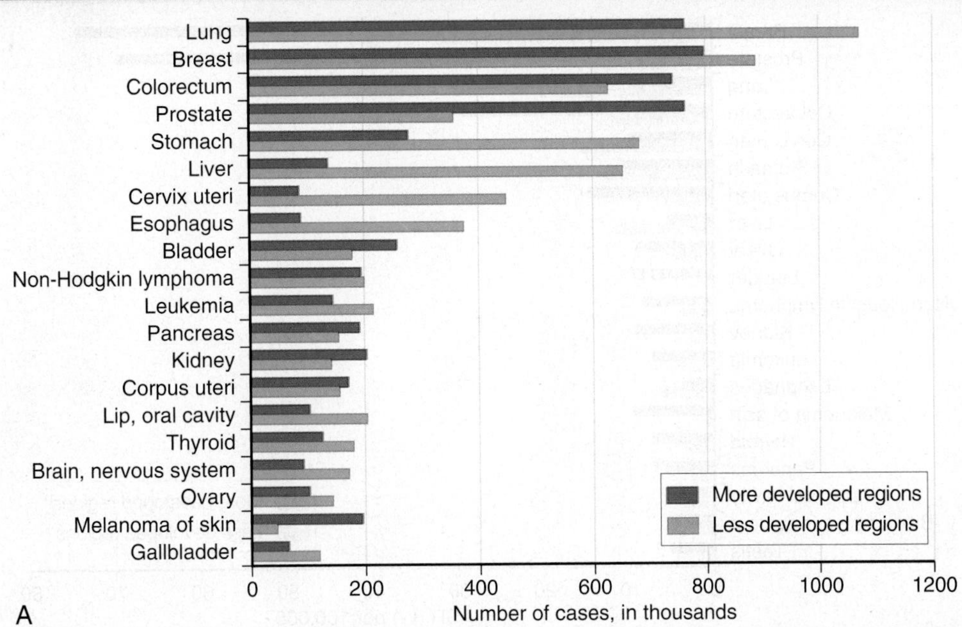

FIGURE 180-2A. **Global Annual Cancer Incidence, Both sexes, All ages.** (Data from Ferlay J, Soerjomataram I, Ervik M, Dikshit R, Eser S, Mathers C, Rebelo M, Parkin DM, Forman D, Bray, F. GLOBOCAN 2012 v1.0, Cancer Incidence and Mortality Worldwide: IARC CancerBase No. 11 [Internet]. Lyon, France: International Agency for Research on Cancer; 2013. Available from: http://globocan.iarc.fr. Accessed February 18, 2015.)

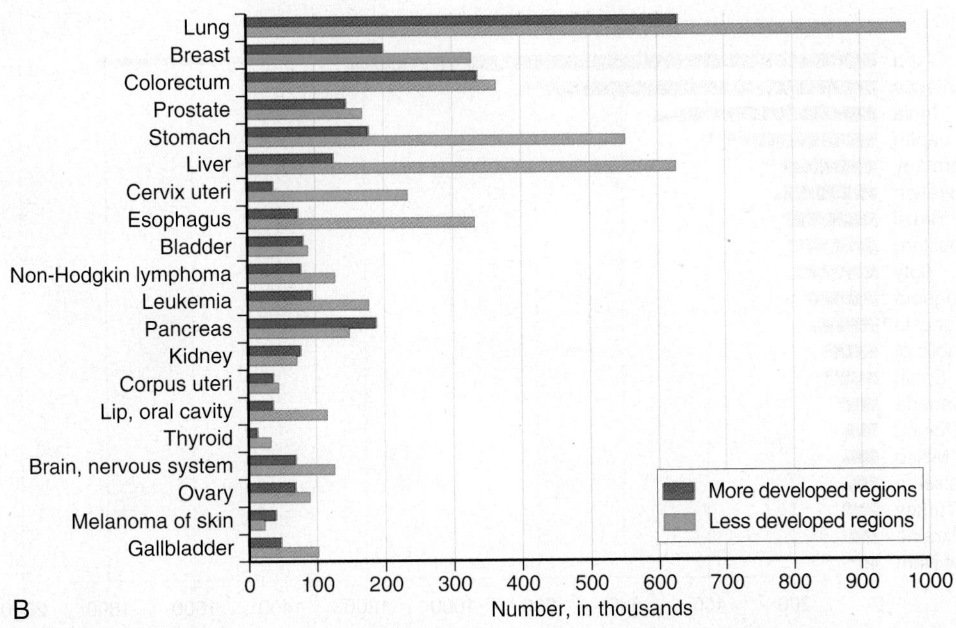

FIGURE 180-2B. **Global Annual Cancer Mortality, Both sexes, All ages.** (Data from Ferlay J, Soerjomataram I, Ervik M, Dikshit R, Eser S, Mathers C, Rebelo M, Parkin DM, Forman D, Bray, F. GLOBOCAN 2012 v1.0, Cancer Incidence and Mortality Worldwide: IARC CancerBase No. 11 [Internet]. Lyon, France: International Agency for Research on Cancer; 2013. Available from: http://globocan.iarc.fr. Accessed February 18, 2015.)

Infections

A substantial fraction of cancers, estimated to be about 16% globally, are caused by infectious agents, particularly in less developed countries (estimated to be ≈ 23%).[5] On the other hand, only 3% of cancers were estimated to be due to infections in the United Kingdom.[6] The major infectious agents are *Helicobacter pylori* (stomach cancer), human papillomavirus (HPV [cervical cancer]), and hepatitis B and C viruses (liver cancer).

Diet

Perhaps no field of epidemiology has been as complex and controversial as the relationship between diet and cancer. Authoritative sources have estimated that a large fraction of cancer incidence is associated with dietary factors; however, a definitive understanding of the mechanisms involved has been difficult, mainly because of difficulties in obtaining valid estimates of intake of specific foods and nutrients and dietary patterns. Foods or nutrients associated with one type of cancer may not be associated with other types of cancer; it is also difficult to distinguish between true etiologic differences between cancer at different sites and false-positive results for a specific cancer type. The World Cancer Research Fund has issued two large-scale summaries of the evidence, most recently in 2007,[7] and the critical recommendations on diet were to: (1) limit consumption of energy-dense foods (avoid sugary drinks); (2) eat mostly foods of plant origin; (3) limit intake of red meat, and avoid processed meat; and (4) limit consumption of salt, and avoid moldy cereals (grains) and legumes.

Part of the difficulty in making generalizations about the percent of cancer attributable to diet is the relationship between diet and body size, and whether to "count" this influence as a "dietary" or "anthropometric" factor. Well-nourished, more affluent societies tend to have taller and heavier populations, both factors positively related to risk of cancer at several sites.

Body Weight and Height

The role of overweight and obesity as risk factors for a wide variety of cancers has become more apparent in the last decade. Even this relationship can be

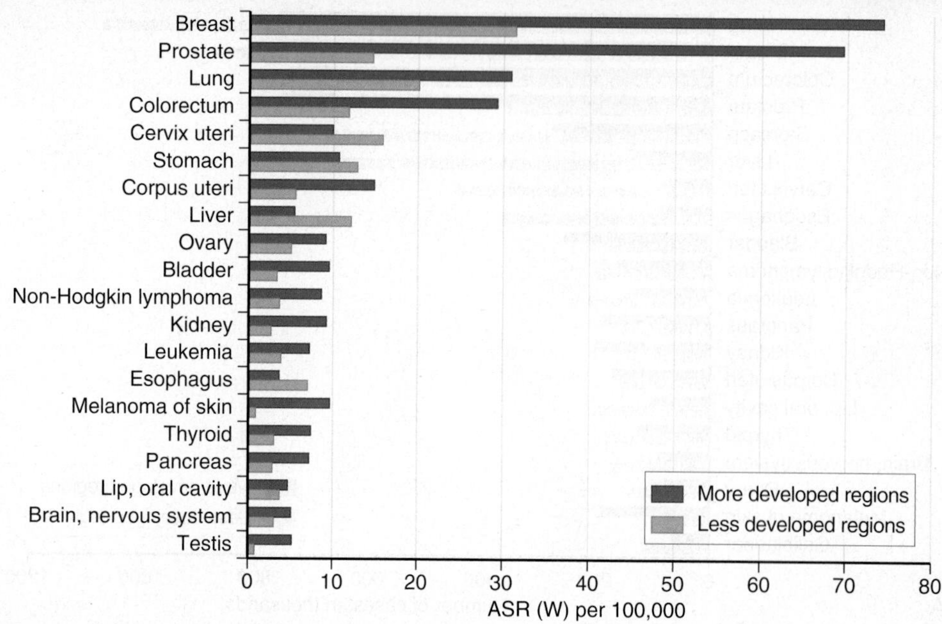

FIGURE 180-3. **Age-standardized Rate of Cancer Incidence, Both Sexes, All ages.** **(Data from Bray F, Ren JS, Masuyer E, Ferlay J. Estimates of global cancer prevalence for 27 sites in the adult population in 2008. Int J Cancer. 2013 Mar 1;132(5):1133-45. doi: 10.1002/ijc.27711. Epub 2012 Jul 26. Available from: http://globocan.iarc.fr. Accessed February 18, 2015.)**

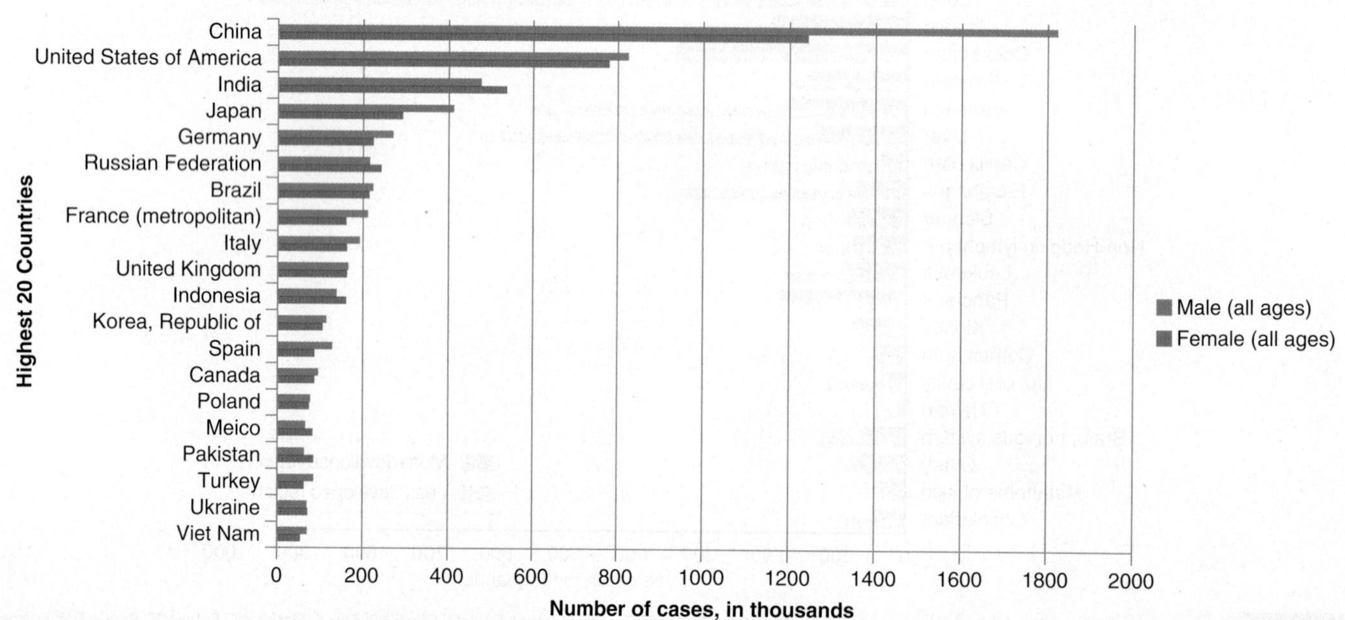

FIGURE 180-4. **Annual cancer incidence (excluding non-melanoma skin cancer) by number of cases, highest 20 countries.** **(Data from Ferlay J, Soerjomataram I, Ervik M, Dikshit R, Eser S, Mathers C, Rebelo M, Parkin DM, Forman D, Bray, F. GLOBOCAN 2012 v1.0, Cancer Incidence and Mortality Worldwide: IARC CancerBase No. 11 [Internet]. Lyon, France: International Agency for Research on Cancer; 2013. Available from: http://globocan.iarc.fr. Accessed February 18, 2015.)**

complex. For example, obesity is inversely related to the incidence of premenopausal breast cancer but positively related to postmenopausal breast cancer. Greater height is associated with modest increases in the risk of cancer at many sites. The secular trends of increasing height and weight in more affluent societies explain a substantial fraction of the increases in cancer rates over time.

Physical Inactivity

An independent role for physical activity in cancer causation is difficult to dissect from the fact that sedentary lifestyles are associated with overweight and obesity. Physical activity has occupational, recreational, and activities of daily living components and can be difficult to measure in epidemiologic studies. A majority of studies suggest that higher levels of physical activity are associated with lower colorectal cancer risk, independent of body weight, and many studies have also reported an inverse relationship with breast cancer. Whether or not this is due to uncontrolled confounding by body weight, a more active lifestyle is a key component of prevention of weight gain, and thus is recommended for prevention of at least these two types of cancer.

Alcohol

Consumption of alcohol is associated with cancer at several sites, notably cancers of the mouth, pharynx and larynx, esophagus, liver, breast, and rectum. Globally, about 5% of cancers were estimated to be due to alcohol, and for the United Kingdom the estimate is 4%. For breast cancer, the risk appears to increase linearly with increasing alcohol consumption, whereas for the aerodigestive cancers, such as esophageal cancer, the risk is most apparent for heavy drinking. Most authorities recommend no more than one alcoholic drink per day for women, and two for men.

Ionizing Radiation

Ionizing radiation is a clear cause of leukemia and thyroid cancer; however, minimization of exposure means that it is a relatively infrequent cause of cancer, estimated to account for about 2% of cancers in Western societies.

Ultraviolet Radiation

Ultraviolet radiation is the major cause of non-melanoma skin cancers and melanoma, and is estimated to account for 3 to 4% of cancers in the Western world. Avoidance of sunburns in early life may be particularly important for reducing the risk of melanoma.

Occupational Exposures

Starting with the work of Sir Perceval Potts on scrotal cancer in chimney sweeps, it has been appreciated that cancer at certain sites is more frequent in specific occupations. A wide variety of industrial chemicals, more common in certain occupations, are associated with risk of specific cancers. In advanced economies, efforts to minimize exposure usually ensure that risks are minimal, although it was estimated that almost 4% of cancers in the United Kingdom are still due to occupational exposures. In less developed economies, risks may be higher, owing to migration of "dirty" industries to less regulated environments, and a lower level of appreciation of the risks and need to protect workers from carcinogenic exposures.

Exogenous Hormones

Use of oral contraceptives increases the relative risk of breast cancer by about 30% while women are taking them; however, since most women taking oral contraceptives are in the 15- to 40-year age group, when breast cancer incidence rates are low, the absolute number of additional cases is small.[8] Ten or more years of use of oral contraceptives reduces ovarian cancer risk by more than 50%, as well as reducing risk of endometrial cancer.[9]

Use of postmenopausal hormones, particularly those combining estrogen and progestins, increases risk of breast cancer, although risk declines quickly after cessation[10] and decreases risk of colon cancer.[11] After the publication of the Women's Health Initiative findings of a positive association, use of postmenopausal hormones declined dramatically, and the incidence rate of breast cancer (mostly estrogen receptor positive) declined over the next few years, one of the few examples in which a rapid change in prevalence of a risk factor can be linked to a short-term change in cancer incidence.

Reproductive Factors

A variety of reproductive factors have been associated with risk of cancer in women. These include early age at menarche, late age at first birth, nulliparity or low parity, and late age at menopause, short duration of lactation (all increase risk of breast cancer), and nulliparity or low parity (increased risk of ovarian and endometrial cancer).

PREVENTION

Definitions of what risk factors are modifiable vary, but consensus estimates in the 1980s, 1990s, and the 2000s[12] agree that the majority of cancers are theoretically preventable by various combinations of risk factor reduction, and immunization against cancer-causing infectious agents.

Primary Prevention

Primary prevention refers to the strategy of reducing risk factor prevalence, and thus reducing the incidence of cancer. Reducing the prevalence of smoking and the use of other tobacco products is the single factor with the greatest potential for reducing cancer risk. Unfortunately, while per capita consumption of cigarettes has approximately halved in several high-income countries since the 1970s, global consumption is still increasing, fueled by younger age population structures in less developed countries, as well as the tobacco industry's marketing in countries where cigarette consumption was previously low.

Next to smoking, there is consensus that a diet that minimizes weight gain through the course of life is the next major potentially preventive factor. Although the precise content of the diet that is preventive remains unclear, consensus panels stress diets high in fruits and vegetables and low in meat and processed meat products. Minimal to moderate alcohol exposure reduces cancer risk.

Avoidance of sunburns and long periods of ultraviolet exposure will reduce risk of skin cancers. Hepatitis B and HPV vaccination are underused strategies globally; clinical interventions against *H. pylori* would probably reduce risk of stomach cancer, but this is unproven. Occupational health regulations and enforcement are needed to reduce risk of exposure to ionizing radiation and workplace carcinogens. Reduction in use of postmenopausal hormones has already been shown to reduce rates of estrogen-positive breast cancer. Reproductive factors such as age at menarche, parity, and age at first birth, although theoretically modifiable, are difficult to change (e.g., extreme physical activity delays menarche) or are socially determined in a way that tends to supersede concerns about future cancer risk.

Secondary Prevention

Secondary prevention aims to prevent cancer death in those diagnosed with cancer or a premalignant lesion, usually by treating at an early stage. The major success in cancer screening has been organized cervical cancer screening, which is responsible for dramatic reduction in cervical cancer deaths in countries such as the United States, where most cases occur in women with a history of suboptimal screening.[13] A decline in U.S. colorectal cancer incidence is at least partly due to screening for early cancers and premalignant colorectal adenomas, with fecal occult blood testing, sigmoidoscopy, and colonoscopy having different tradeoffs in terms of patient acceptance and test performance. The use of PSA screening for prostate cancer and mammography for breast cancer remains controversial. In both cases, there is plausibly a reduction in the death rate from each cancer in men or women screened, respectively. However, better appreciation of the harms of screening and "overdiagnosis" (i.e., detection and treatment of lesions that might never have come to clinical attention) has meant that recommendations have been changed in recent years. In the case of breast cancer, better treatment of the disease and better awareness by women of the need to seek early assessment of any lumps or changes in the breast may mean that the effectiveness of mammography in reducing death rates has changed over time.[14] A report for the U.S. Preventive Services Taskforce describes the evidence as "strong" that low-dose computed tomography screening reduces risk of lung cancer and lung cancer death, although the evidence is based on a single, large, good-quality study.[15]

Although many cancers can be cured if detected early enough, the sheer volume of cancers in less developed countries with limited infrastructure, plus the cost of frequent screening, means that organized screening activities will take time to develop. The exception may be cervical screening, for which HPV testing combined with gynecologic follow-up may provide a means of screening large numbers of women relatively rapidly, although this is by no means a trivial endeavor. Greater awareness of cancer symptoms and signs, combined with appropriate and prompt follow-up, will remain a mainstay of attempts to downstage cancers in less developed regions, and developing adequate diagnostic and treatment services may be required before instituting screening services.

TREATMENT Rx

Once cancer is diagnosed, appropriate treatment is not available to many in less developed countries, resulting in substantially higher case-fatality rates. Many of the most efficacious chemotherapy drugs are off-patent and relatively inexpensive; other modalities such as radiation can be offered at low cost per patient once a facility has been built and staff trained to use it. It is estimated that 80% of patients in the world have no access to opiates at the end of life,[16] a situation that could be remedied at low cost if international treaties that limit opiate export, as well as concerns about their abuse, could be addressed.

FUTURE DIRECTIONS

As for other non-communicable diseases, a broad range of actions need to be taken to prevent, detect, and treat cancers as incidence rates of many cancers increase and absolute rates increase faster because of the aging of populations around the world. Fortunately, several non-communicable diseases share similar risk factors,[17] particularly tobacco use and sedentary lifestyles/obesity; hence, efforts to limit the spread of these risk factors may be important in the control of cardiovascular disease, diabetes, and respiratory diseases, as well as cancer.[18] Access to even low-cost treatments requires major investments in health systems, but without these investments the human and economic costs of cancer will be greater still.

GENERAL REFERENCES

For the General References and other additional features, please visit Expert Consult at https://expertconsult.inkling.com.

181

CANCER BIOLOGY AND GENETICS

ADRIAN R. BLACK AND KENNETH H. COWAN

CANCER AS A GENETIC DISEASE

Cancer Development Is Driven by Random Mutations

Cancer develops from mutations in genes that regulate normal cellular processes; thus, cancer can be thought of as a genetic disease. Mutations that lead to cancer involve two types of genes: mutant genes that enhance the development of cancer are known as oncogenes, whereas genes that inhibit tumorigenesis are known as tumor suppressor genes. Alterations in the function of oncogenes and tumor suppressors allow cells to escape the normal controls that regulate tissue homeostasis, leading to the outgrowth of mutant cells and the subsequent development of cancer. Except in rare cases, such as seen with the *BCR-ABL* fusion gene in chronic myelogenous leukemia (CML), a single mutation is not sufficient to lead to cancer. Instead, cancer develops in a multistep process that requires accumulation of mutations that drive progression of normal tissues through benign precancerous lesions to aggressive malignant disease.[1]

The acquisition of these mutations is random, and tumor evolution follows a model of natural selection where mutations that bestow a growth and/or survival advantage allow for clonal expansion of the population of cells that carry the mutation. During this process, many mutations occur that are disadvantageous, and cells that carry these mutations die out. The timing of mutations is also a factor in the evolution of cancer. Some mutations that help drive cancer development are deleterious to normal cells but can provide a growth/survival advantage in cells in which other mutations have occurred. For example, activation of oncogenes in normal cells can lead to cell death through apoptosis (see later) or induce a permanent growth arrest known as senescence, and their oncogenic activity is only manifested if mutations that negate these effects have already occurred in the cell. The need for mutations to occur in the correct order represents an important brake on cancer progression. The sequential multistep nature of cancer is reflected in the preferential association of specific mutations with different stages of tumor progression, as has been elegantly demonstrated for the development of colon cancer (Fig. 181-1).[2]

Mutation Rate and Cancer Risk Factors

Because mutations occur randomly within the genome, it is impossible to predict who will get cancer or to know definitively why it developed in any particular patient. However, factors that increase the rate of mutation increase the risk of tumorigenesis. For example, exposure to environmental chemicals that damage DNA (mutagens) has long been recognized as a major risk for developing cancer, as exemplified by the association of exposure to tobacco smoke—which contains multiple mutagenic compounds—with lung, oral, and other cancers. Similarly, ionizing radiation, which causes DNA strand breaks and crosslinks, is also closely associated with cancer risk. This is seen in the high risk of leukemia in survivors of the nuclear bombs in Hiroshima and Nagasaki and in the association of exposure to ultraviolet radiation in sunlight and on tanning beds with melanoma and other skin cancers. Physiologically, increased cell proliferation also increases the risk of cancer because it enhances the rate at which mutations from DNA damage become fixed in the genome during replication, increases replication-associated mutations and chromosomal rearrangements, and accelerates expansion of the pool of

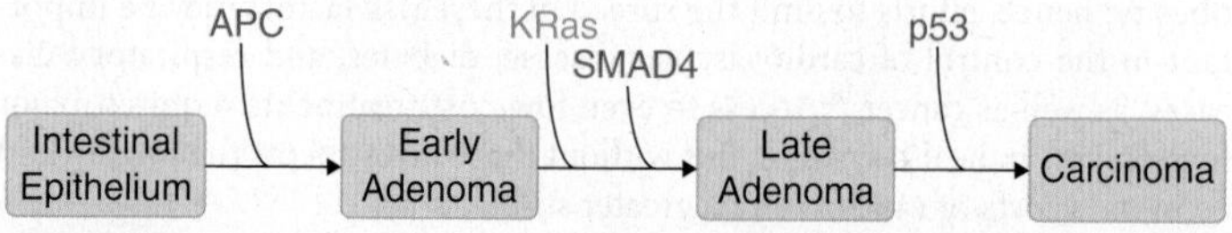

FIGURE 181-1. Genetic changes associated with different stages of colon cancer development. Scheme for accumulation of genetic changes in colon cancer in familial adenomatous polyposis patients, adapted from that originally proposed by Dr. Burt Vogelstein and colleagues at the Johns Hopkins University. Proto-oncogenes/oncogenes are indicated in green; tumor suppressor genes are indicated in red.

mutated cells. This effect is seen in the association of endometrial cancer with hormone replacement therapy, tamoxifen therapy, and obesity, which are all mitogenic in the endometrium owing to increases in estrogenic signaling.

Another major risk factor for cancer is chronic inflammation[3], such as that found in the increased risk of colon cancer for patients with inflammatory bowel disease and of stomach cancer for patients harboring *Helicobacter pylori* infections. Inflammatory cells increase the mutation rate by producing reactive oxygen species and other immune effectors that damage DNA, as well as through mitogenic cytokines that can directly increase tumor cell proliferation. Because mutations accumulate over time, increasing age itself is a major risk factor for most cancer types.

Genomic Instability and Cancer Development

Although the genome is continuously being damaged, cells have efficient mechanisms that keep the overall mutation rate low. Mechanisms for repair of replication errors and damaged nucleotides include mismatch repair, base-excision repair, and nucleotide-excision repair, whereas more severe damage and double strand breaks can be repaired by homologous recombination and non-homologous end joining. Mutations that disrupt these mechanisms dramatically increase the rate of mutation. Because cancer development requires ordered mutation of selected genes, efficient DNA repair means that the chances that appropriate mutation will accumulate in a cell to produce cancer within the lifetime of an individual are very low. Thus, it is not surprising that mutations that disrupt DNA repair are almost universally seen in cancer cells. Although these mutations do not directly provide an advantage to cells (and may even decrease survival), they dramatically increase the chance that cells will accumulate appropriate mutations for cancer development.

The contribution of DNA repair defects to cancer development[4] can be seen in the number of inherited cancer susceptibility syndromes that are due to mutations in DNA repair genes (Table 181-1). These mutations are also found in corresponding sporadic cancers. Mutations in mismatch repair genes (e.g., *MLH1*, *MSH2*) that cause the Lynch syndromes (also known as hereditary nonpolyposis colon cancer [HNPCC]) are commonly found in sporadic colon cancer. Mutations in *BRCA1* (involved in homologous recombination repair, non-homologous end joining, and nucleotide excision repair) or *BRCA2* (homologous recombination repair) that lead to familial breast and ovarian cancer are also common in sporadic disease.

DNA repair is essential for cell survival, and mutations in DNA repair genes can thus predispose to "synthetic lethality" in cancer cells. For example, inhibition of poly-ADP ribose polymerase (PARP) induces double strand breaks in cells with *BRCA1* or *BRCA2* mutations, but not in BRCA1/2 wild-type cells. The potential clinical relevance of this finding is supported by results from clinical trials.

Two Types of Cancer Genes

As mentioned, genes whose mutation contributes to the development of cancer are traditionally divided into two groups, oncogenes and tumor suppressor genes. The products of oncogenes, which are generally proteins referred to as oncoproteins, are positive drivers of cancer development. In contrast, tumor suppressor genes help to prevent the development of cancer in normal tissues and often counter the effects of oncogenes. Because mutations in oncogenes are activating, only one copy of the gene needs to be affected for the phenotype to be manifested; thus, oncogene mutations are dominant. The presence of two copies of tumor suppressor genes in the normal diploid genome means that both copies of these genes have to be inactivated to remove tumor suppressive activity. Thus, tumor suppressor mutations are recessive. This need for two "hits" for inactivation of tumor suppressors represents another brake on cancer development.

Familial Cancer Susceptibility Syndromes

Although most tumors are sporadic, there are a number of inherited syndromes that are associated with the risk of cancer. The vast majority of these syndromes are due to a germline mutation in one copy of a tumor suppressor gene (see Table 181-1). Because tumor suppressor genes are recessive, they remain phenotypically silent until the wild-type copy of the gene is mutated. However, the germline mutations provide the first "hit" for the loss of a tumor suppressor and vastly increase the risk of developing cancer. The dominant nature of mutations in oncogenes means that they are generally incompatible with normal development. Thus, although some familial syndromes are associated with oncogenes, these are relatively rare (see Table 181-1). Individuals with family histories of cancers that point to the possibility of an inherited disease should be offered genetic screening and counseling.

TABLE 181-1 HEREDITARY CANCER RISK SYNDROMES

SYNDROME	GENE	ASSOCIATED TUMORS
TUMOR SUPPRESSOR MUTATIONS		
Cowden	*PTEN*	Breast, thyroid, endometrial, colorectal, kidney, melanoma
Familial adenomatous polyposis	*APC*	Colorectal, stomach, intestinal, hepatoblastoma, thyroid, pancreatic, adrenal, bile duct, medulloblastoma
Familial gastric carcinoma	*CDH1* (E-Cadherin)	Stomach, breast
Familial malignant melanoma	*CDKN2* (p16^{INK4A} and p14^{ARF}), *CDK4*	Melanoma, pancreatic
Familial Wilms tumor	*WT1*	Wilms (kidney)
Hereditary retinoblastoma	*RB1* (pRB)	Retinoblastoma
Hereditary paraganglioma	*SDHA, SDHB, SDHC, SDHD* or *SDHAF2* (succinate dehydrogenase)	Paraganglioma, pheochromocytoma
Li-Fraumeni	*TP53* (p53)	Osteosarcoma, soft tissue sarcoma, leukemia, breast, brain, adrenal, melanoma, Wilms, stomach, colorectal, pancreatic, esophageal, lung, gonadal germ cells
Multiple endocrine neoplasia type 1	*MEN1*	Parathyroid, pituitary, islet cell, adrenal, carcinoid
Neurofibromatosis type 1	*NF1*	Neurofibroma, glioma, leukemia, breast, rhabdomyosarcoma, gastrointestinal stromal
Neurofibromatosis type 2	*NF2*	Neuromas, schwannomas, meningiomas, astrocytomas, gliomas
Peutz-Jeghers syndrome	*LKB1*	Colon, intestine, stomach, pancreas, cervix, ovary, testis, breast, thyroid
Von Hippel-Lindau	*VHL*	Kidney, adrenal, pheochromocytoma
DNA REPAIR GENE MUTATIONS		
Ataxia telangiectasia	*ATM*	Leukemia, lymphoma
Bloom	*BLM*	Leukemia, multiple solid tumors
Fanconi anemia	*FANCA, FANCC, FANCD2, FANCE, FANCF or FANCG*	Leukemia, multiple solid tumors
Hereditary breast and ovarian cancer	*BRCA1* or *BRCA2*	Breast, ovary, pancreatic, fallopian tube
Lynch (hereditary nonpolyposis colon cancer)	*MLH1, MSH2, MSH6 or PMS2*	Colorectal, endometrial, stomach, breast, ovarian, intestinal, pancreatic, prostate, urinary tract, liver, kidney
MYH-associated polyposis	*MUTYH*	Colorectal, intestinal
Xeroderma pigmentosum	*XPA, XPC, ERCC2, ERCC3, ERCC4, ERCC5*, or *DDB2*	Skin (basal cells, squamous), melanoma, tongue, eye
ONCOGENE MUTATIONS		
Costello	*HRAS*	Papilloma, rhabdomyosarcoma, neuroblastoma
Noonan	*PTPN11, SOS1, KRAS, NRAS, RAF1 or BRAF* (Ras-Erk pathway regulators)	Leukemia, rhabdomyosarcoma, neuroblastoma
Familial malignant melanoma	*CDK4*	Melanoma
Multiple endocrine neoplasia type 2	*RET*	Thyroid, parathyroid, pheochromocytoma

Oncogenes and Proto-oncogenes

Oncogenes are activated forms of normal cellular genes that are termed *proto-oncogenes*. The products of proto-oncogenes are involved in the regulation of multiple aspects of physiology, including proliferation, survival, and cell migration, and play an important role in development and tissue homeostasis. Mutations that activate oncogenes lead to loss of the normal control that governs the activity of proto-oncogenes and gives a growth or survival advantage to the cell. A single oncogene can affect multiple aspects of tumor progression and in rare cases may be all that is needed to support oncogenic transformation (e.g., the *BCR-ABL* oncogene in CML). In keeping with their diverse roles, proto-oncogenes perform diverse functions in the cell. They commonly function as signal transduction molecules, acting as extracellular ligands/growth factors (e.g., KGF, SIS, INT-2, WNT1), growth factor receptors (e.g., EGFR, HER2, FGFR), and signaling intermediates (e.g., the PI-3 kinase [PI-3K] catalytic subunit *PIK3CA*, PKCι, B-Raf, and the Ras proteins K-Ras, N-Ras, and H-Ras). They can also be involved in direct regulation of gene expression, acting as transcription factors (e.g., myc, fos, jun, myb), translation factors (e.g., eIF4E), or regulators of protein degradation (e.g., MDM2, Cbl). Other common roles are in promoting cell survival (e.g., Bcl2, MCL1) and cell cycle progression (e.g., cyclin D1, CDK4, cyclin E).

Oncogenes can be activated by multiple mechanisms, and a single oncogene can be activated by different mechanisms. Activation can result from mutations that lead to a qualitative change that affects the activity or regulation of the encoded oncoprotein, or by a quantitative effect that increases the levels of an oncoprotein in the cell (through increased gene expression or reduced protein turnover). Qualitative effects are generally due to point mutations that lead to loss of negative regulatory domains or, more commonly, to single amino acid changes that affect the activity or interactions of an oncoprotein. These mutations can (1) directly increase kinase activity (e.g., *B-Raf* mutations in melanoma and colon cancer, or *PIK3CA* mutations in colorectal, brain, and gastric cancers), (2) decrease negative regulation (e.g., C-terminal truncation of Src), (3) alter autoregulation (e.g., K-Ras, H-Ras, and N-Ras, seen in 50% of colon cancers), and (4) reduce protein degradation (e.g., phosphorylation site mutations of β-catenin, seen in colon cancer). These mutations often occur at a single site or limited region of the gene, so-called hot spots that localize to important functional regions of the protein encoded by the oncogene. For example, oncogenic mutations of *B-Raf* are commonly missense mutations of the valine residue in its activation loop (V600).

In addition to point mutations, gross chromosomal abnormalities can lead to activation of oncogenes. Increased gene copy number through gene amplification is a mechanism by which oncogenes become overexpressed. Gene amplification is extremely common in cancer and represents a major mechanism by which oncogenes are activated. Amplifications are detected histologically by karyotypic abnormalities such as double-minute chromosomes (DMs) and homogeneous staining regions (HSRs). Chromosomal translocations can also lead to overexpression of oncogenes by locating the gene next to a strong transcriptional element. For example, the t(8;14) translocation in Burkitt lymphoma transcriptionally activates the *MYC* oncogene by placing it in the immunoglobulin heavy chain locus. In many cases, translocations not only lead to increased expression of an oncoprotein but can also alter the protein itself. The t(7;9) translocation in T-cell acute lymphoblastic leukemia (ALL) places the *NOTCH1* gene (*TAN1*) next to the T-cell receptor promoter. However, the translocation is only partial and leads to overexpression of the transcriptionally active NOTCH1-IC fragment, and thus constitutively activates Notch signaling. Translocations can also lead to the production of fusion proteins that have distinct properties from the original proto-oncogene. For example, the t(9;22) translocation seen in CML fuses the B-cell receptor gene with *Abl* tyrosine kinase genes. The resultant BCR-ABL fusion protein is not only overexpressed and a constitutively active kinase, it is also aberrantly localized to the cytoplasm and thus phosphorylates different substrates from Abl. Although oncogenic chromosomal translocations are particularly prevalent in leukemias and lymphomas, they are also seen in solid tumors such as Ewing sarcoma, papillary thyroid cancer, and rhabdomyosarcoma (producing the *EWS-FLI*, *RET-PCP*, and *PAX3-FKHR* gene fusions, respectively).

Viral Infection and Cancer

Viral infection has been associated with up to 20% of cancers worldwide and is thus a major concern in oncology (Chapter 180). Known oncoviruses include: human papillomaviruses HPV-16 and HPV-18 (the main causative factors for cervical cancer), hepatitis B and hepatitis C viruses (linked to hepatocellular carcinoma), Epstein-Barr virus (linked to lymphomas and nasopharyngeal carcinoma), HTLV-I (linked to T-cell leukemia), Kaposi sarcoma herpesvirus (Kaposi sarcoma), and Merkel cell polyomavirus (Merkel cell carcinoma). Viral reproduction requires replication of viral DNA in the host cell. Oncoviruses achieve this by enlisting the host replicative machinery through expression of oncogenes (e.g., E6 and E7 of human papillomavirus and LMP1 and BARF1 of Epstein-Barr virus), which results in an increased risk of cancer in the infected tissue.

Tumor Suppressors

Whereas the term *oncogene* refers to a mutated version of a proto-oncogene, tumor suppressor genes are normal cellular genes whose inactivation contributes to the development of cancer. Although mutations of tumor suppressors are almost always recessive, occasionally mutation in a tumor suppressor gene can give rise to a "dominant negative" protein that can block the activity of the wild-type protein; such mutated forms of the tumor suppressor act as an oncogene (e.g., some c-cbl and p53 mutations).

As with proto-oncogenes, tumor suppressors are involved in multiple aspects of cellular physiology. They can be cell surface receptors and downstream mediators of growth inhibitory signaling [e.g., TGFβ receptor II (*TGFBR2*), SMAD4 (*DPC4*)], negative regulators of mitogenic signaling [e.g., APC, NF1, PTEN], negative regulators of the cell cycle [e.g., the retinoblastoma protein (pRB, *RB1*), $p16^{INK4a}$ (*CDKN2A*), p53 (*TP53*)], promoters of apoptosis (p53, *RASSF1A*), regulators of cell adhesion [e.g., E-cadherin (*CDH1*)], transcription factors [e.g., p53, pRB, Wilms tumor suppressor 1 (*WT1*)] or regulators of protein degradation (e.g., Von Hippel-Lindau protein (*VHL*)]. Genes involved in DNA damage repair and maintenance of genome stability are also considered tumor suppressors (see Table 181-1). As discussed earlier, although DNA repair defects do not directly contribute to the transformed phenotype, they greatly increase the chances that cancer will develop.

Inactivation of tumor suppressors can occur through point mutations in the gene. These can be missense mutations that lead to alterations in amino acid sequences (hot spots) that are critical for the activity of a tumor suppressive protein (e.g., Trp248 and His273 mutations in p53) or nonsense mutations that lead to a truncated protein (e.g., APC truncations in colon cancer). Tumor suppressor genes can also be inactivated by chromosomal deletion or rearrangement (e.g., inactivation of PML by the t[15;17] translocation in acute promyelocytic leukemia, which results in the RAR-PML fusion protein).

In addition to genetic changes, tumor suppressor genes can be inactivated epigenetically.[5] DNA methylation of the promoter region of genes, which results in transcriptional repression, is a normal regulatory mechanism that ensures correct gene expression and stable silencing during development. Aberrant promoter methylation of tumor suppressor genes is very common in cancer and represents a major mechanism by which these genes are inactivated. Reversal of this transcriptional repression allows for reexpression of the tumor promoters and forms the rationale for the use of drugs that inhibit DNA methylation, such as decitabine.

Once one copy of a tumor suppressor gene is disrupted, the most common mechanism for inactivation of the remaining wild-type copy is through loss of heterozygosity (LOH). LOH can occur when the wild-type gene is lost through deletion, chromosomal loss, or unequal recombination, which results in a single mutant copy remaining in the cell. Alternatively, copy neutral LOH can occur, in which the wild-type gene is replaced by the mutant gene through loss and reduplication or mitotic recombination.

miRNAs as Oncogenes and Tumor Suppressors

Although most of our knowledge of tumor suppressors and oncogenes is concentrated on genes that encode for protein, an important role for non-coding RNAs is rapidly emerging.[6] microRNAs (miRNAs) regulate the expression of other genes by binding to their mRNAs in a sequence specific manner and causing their degradation or inhibiting their translation. miRNAs that inhibit the expression of oncogenes act as tumor suppressors, whereas those that inhibit the expression of tumor suppressors have oncogenic properties and are known as oncomirs. Recent research is identifying miRNA profiles that are associated with particular cancer types, underlining the importance of these non-coding RNAs in tumor development.

Activities of Oncogenes and Tumor Suppressors Are Interrelated

Oncogenes and tumor suppressors are commonly part of signal transduction pathways (Fig. 181-2). A pathway that is activated in many cancers is the Ras/Raf/Erk signaling cascade. In addition to the Ras and Raf proteins (e.g., K-Ras, B-Raf), growth factor receptors that activate Ras (e.g., EGFR, HER2, PGDF, KIT) and downstream targets of the pathway (e.g., the transcription factors Fos and Jun) also act as oncoproteins to activate this pathway. In contrast, the NF1 tumor suppressor (see Table 181-1) negatively regulates the pathway by inactivating Ras. Another pathway that is activated in cancer is the PI-3K/AKT/mTOR pathway, in which growth factor receptors activate the Akt protein kinase through PI-3K-mediated phosphorylation of phosphatidylinositol (see Fig. 181-2). Although both PI-3K (PIK3A) and Akt can act as oncogenes in this pathway, the PTEN tumor suppressor negatively regulates the pathway by dephosphorylating phosphatidylinositol-(3,4,5) triphosphate. Thus, in addition to activation by direct mutation, proto-oncogenes can be activated indirectly through mutation of upstream oncogenes or tumor suppressors. Because only one oncogene or tumor suppressor needs to be mutated to activate a pathway, it is rare that two mutations are seen in the same pathway. An example can be seen in the APC/β-catenin pathway: although mutations in either APC or β-catenin are commonly found in colon cancer, mutation of these genes is mutually exclusive.

Signal transduction pathways in a cell do not act simply as linear pathways but participate in interlinked networks. Oncogenes and tumor suppressors

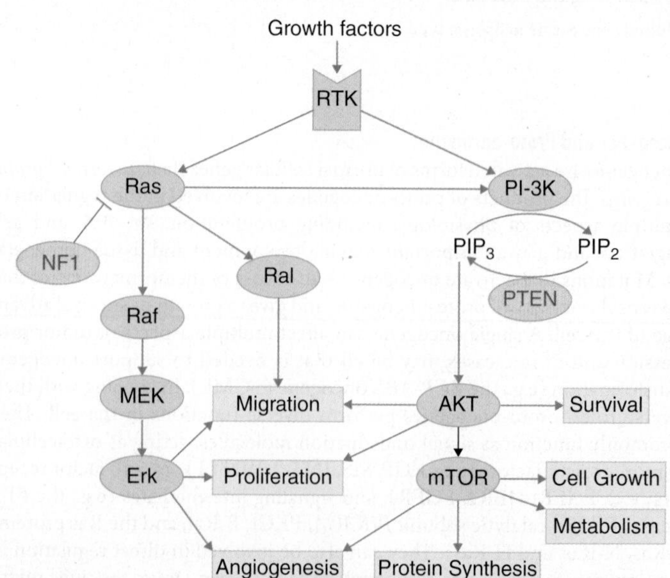

FIGURE 181-2. Ras/Erk and PI-3K/Akt pathways. Schematic diagram of the relationship between critical components of the Ras/Erk and PI-3K/Akt pathways are shown, along with downstream effects of pathway activation. Proto-oncogenes/oncogenes are indicated in green; tumor suppressors are indicated in red. Green arrows indicate activation, and the red T indicates inhibition. NOTE: mutations that affect oncogenes or tumor suppressors at any point along a signaling pathway can stimulate the pathway and have similar effects on downstream targets. RTK = receptor tyrosine kinase (e.g., EGFR, HER2, PDGFR). For details see section on "Activities of Oncogenes and Tumor Suppressors Are Interrelated"

are involved in this signaling crosstalk. For example, Ras activates both the Raf-Erk and the PI-3K/Akt pathways, and Ras-Erk signaling inactivates the *LKB1* tumor suppressor that is a negative regulator of AMPK signaling (see Table 181-1).

Oncogenes and Tumor Suppressors Are Not Restricted by Disease Site

Certain oncogenes and tumor suppressors are associated with particular cancer types, as can be seen in many familial syndromes. This often reflects the roles of particular signaling pathways in the normal tissue from which the cancer arises. For example, in keeping with the critical role of the Wnt/APC/β-catenin signaling pathway in regulating proliferation and stem cell maintenance in the normal intestinal epithelium, activation of this pathway through loss of *APC* or activation of β-catenin is found in the vast majority of colon cancers. Because the same signaling pathways can be important in multiple tissues, cancers in different disease sites can have mutations in the same oncogenes and tumor suppressors. For example, in addition to colon cancer, disruption of the Wnt/APC/β-catenin pathway is found in other cancer types including those arising in the pancreas, breast, and thyroid. This lack of disease site specificity for tumor suppressors can clearly be seen in the array of cancers that are associated with familial cancer susceptibility syndromes (see Table 181-1).

There are two pathways that appear to be of universal importance and are disrupted in most, if not all, cancers. These involve the tumor suppressor genes *RB1*, encoding the retinoblastoma protein (pRB), and *TP53*, encoding p53 (Fig. 181-3). pRB was the first tumor suppressor to be identified and is responsible for hereditary retinoblastoma. It is a central player in a pathway that senses the extracellular growth environment and controls whether or not a cell will proliferate. Disruption of this pathway in cancer cells thus divorces proliferation from the normal controls that maintain tissue homeostasis. pRB inhibits proliferation by repressing transcription of growth-related genes through binding to E2F transcription factors. The activity of pRB is regulated by cyclin-dependent kinases (cdks). When bound to cyclins, cdks phosphorylate pRB, and this blocks its ability to bind E2Fs and allows for transcription of E2F-regulated genes, many of which are proto-oncogenes. Expression of D-type cyclins (e.g., cyclin D1), regulatory molecules whose binding to cdks initiates the phosphorylation of pRB, is regulated by extracellular signaling and thus provides a link between cell proliferation and the extracellular growth environment. Activity of this pathway is negatively regulated by a number of cdk inhibitory proteins, including $p21^{CIP1}$, $p27^{KIP1}$, and $p16^{INK4A}$. Although mutations in pRB itself are relatively rare, mutations in multiple members of the pathway that mediate inactivation of pRB are a common feature of cancer (Table 181-2). In addition, oncogenes and tumor suppressors feed into this pathway through regulation of cyclins and cdk inhibitory protein.

p53 is the most commonly mutated tumor suppressor gene, with mutations seen in about 50% of all human cancers. Germline mutations in p53 are responsible for Li-Fraumeni syndrome (see Table 181-1). p53 is known as "the guardian of the genome" because it is a central player in the system that assesses DNA damage and the internal fitness of the cell to divide. DNA damage leads to transcriptional activation p53, which has two major effects dependent on the severity of the damage. If DNA damage is not too severe, p53 can induce cell cycle arrest by increasing expression of the cdk inhibitor $p21^{CIP1}$, which activates the pRB growth inhibitory pathway. This allows time for DNA to be repaired prior to the initiation of replication. With more severe DNA damage, p53 induces apoptosis through upregulation of proapoptotic proteins such as PUMA and Bax. In addition to p53 mutations, activation of oncogenes such as *MDM2* or loss of tumor suppressors like $p14^{ARF}$ can disrupt p53 activity in the cancer cell (see Fig. 181-3).

The importance of the p53 and the pRB-E2F pathway to cancer development can be seen in the targeting of these pathways by DNA tumor viruses. For example, the E6 and E7 oncogenes of human papillomavirus target p53 for degradation and prevent pRB binding to E2F, respectively.

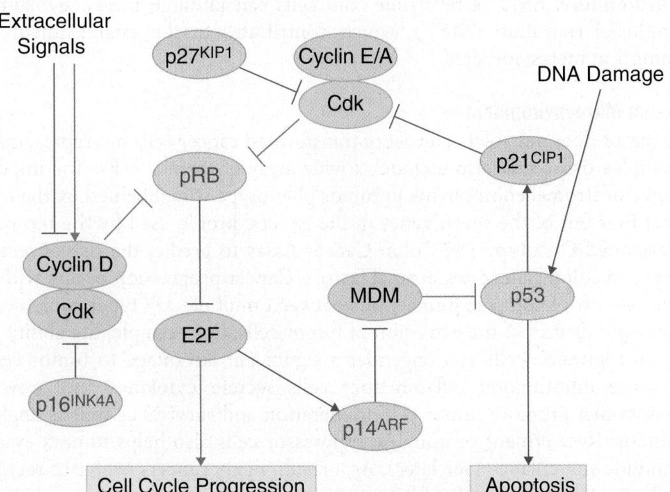

FIGURE 181-3. Interaction of the pRB/E2F and p53 pathways. Proto-oncogenes/oncogenes are indicated in green; tumor suppressors are indicated in red. Green and red connectors indicate growth/survival promoting and inhibitory effects, respectively. For details, see section on "Oncogenes and Tumors Are Not Restricted by Disease Site."

CRITICAL FEATURES OF THE CANCER PHENOTYPE

As cells accumulate oncogenic mutations, they progressively gain the ability to circumvent the normal mechanisms that control tissue homeostasis. Although diverse sets of mutations can lead to cancer, there are a set of general characteristics that must be acquired for tumors to develop. These phenotypic changes have been termed "hallmarks of cancer" and include the ability to sustain growth and resist growth inhibitory signals, resist apoptosis, stimulate angiogenesis, acquire replicative immortality, metastasize, deregulate cellular energetics, and avoid immune destruction (Table 181-3). These core characteristics, along with other factors that have a direct impact on cancer development and its clinical management, are discussed below.

Sustained Cell Proliferation

Normal tissue homeostasis is regulated by the balance between signals that promote proliferation and those that inhibit proliferation and induce differentiation. Multiple oncogenic mutations free cancer cells from this regulation by lessening their dependence on growth factors and weakening their sensitivity to negative signals. As noted earlier, direct disruption of cell

TABLE 181-2 pRB-E2F PATHWAY DISRUPTION IN CANCER

PROTEIN	GENE	COMMON CHANGES IN CANCER
pRB	*RB1* (tumor suppressor)	Mutation, deletion, methylation
p130	*RB2* (tumor suppressor)	Mutation
Cyclin D1	*CCND1* (oncogene)	Transcriptional activation, amplification, chromosome rearrangement
Cyclin E	*CCNE1* (oncogene)	Amplification
Cdk4	*CDK4* (oncogene)	Amplification, mutation
$p16^{INK4a}$	*CDKN2A* (tumor suppressor)	Deletion, methylation
$p27^{KIP1}$	*CDKN1B* (tumor suppressor)	Post-transcriptional downregulation

TABLE 181-3 THE HALLMARKS OF CANCER

- Sustaining proliferative signaling
- Evading growth suppressors
- Activating invasion and metastasis
- Enabling replicative immortality
- Inducing angiogenesis
- Resisting cell death
- Deregulating cellular energetics
- Avoiding immune destruction

The "hallmarks of cancer" comprise these biological capabilities acquired during the multistep development of human tumors. Underlying these hallmarks are "enabling characteristics," including genome instability and mutation and tumor-promoting inflammation. In addition to the cancer cells themselves, tumors recruit a repertoire of ostensibly normal cells that contribute to the acquisition of hallmark traits by creating a "tumor microenvironment."

Adapted from Hanahan D, Weinberg RA. Hallmarks of cancer: the next generation. *Cell.* 2011;144:646-674.

cycle regulation through the pRB-E2F pathway, and activation of growth promoting signaling pathways through oncogene activation and tumor suppressor inactivation, isolates cancer cells from the requirement for growth factors and the effects of negative growth signals. Similarly, loss of p53 contributes to continued proliferation in the presence of genetic damage that would normally cause growth arrest.

Replicative Immortality

Even in the presence of continuous positive growth signals, the majority of cells in normal tissues have a limited replicative potential. Once this limit is reached, cells either enter senescence or die through apoptosis (see later). Therefore, for a cancer to grow to a size where it becomes clinically relevant, this limit must be overcome. One of the major factors that limit replicative potential is the shortening of chromosomes during replication. Genetic material at the end of chromosomes is protected from this loss by repetitive DNA sequences known as telomeres. Telomeres also form specialized structures that protect chromosomes from cellular exonucleases and from fusion due to non-homologous end joining. Germline cells and some stem cells express an enzyme, telomerase, that is able to lengthen their telomeres following replication. However, for most cells in the body, replication leads to a progressive shortening of telomeres until they become unable to protect the chromosomes; the DNA ends are then recognized as DNA damage, and the cell becomes senescent or enters apoptosis. Tumor cells evade this fate by acquiring mechanisms to maintain telomere length above the critical minimum. This is mainly by reexpression of telomerase or, less commonly, through a recombination-based mechanism. Loss of telomeres can also contribute to genetic instability, because defects in the DNA damage response can allow continued replication in the presence of chromosomal fusions associated with telomere loss.

Apoptosis

Apoptosis is a physiologic mechanism of programmed cell death that involves a protease cascade, leading to activation of executioner caspases. It is induced by both external and internal signals and is integral to development and control of tissue damage. Many of the alterations that lead to cancer also trigger apoptosis, mainly through the intrinsic pathway. These include oncogene activation, uncontrolled E2F activity due to inactivation of the pRB pathway, and DNA damage. Thus, cancer progression requires mechanisms to overcome these apoptotic responses. A major mechanism of apoptosis that results from intrinsic cellular abnormalities involves the release of cytochrome c from mitochondria, which leads to activation of cytoplasmic caspases. The tumor suppressors Bax and Bim mediate the release of cytochrome c, whereas the oncogene *Bcl2* inhibits its release. Another mechanism by which apoptosis is reduced in cancer cells involves upregulation of inhibitors of apoptotic proteins (e.g., survivin, XIAP, cIAP) that can directly suppress caspase activity. Changes in the expression of survival proteins can result from mutation of oncogenes and tumor suppressors, or from oncogenic activation of prosurvival signaling pathways such as those involving Akt and the NF-κB transcription factors. As noted, loss of p53 activity is a major contributor to apoptosis resistance in cancer cells.

Although these changes help to reduce the effect of pro-apoptotic changes associated with tumor development, apoptosis is prevalent in many tumors, and cancer cells remain susceptible to apoptotic signals. This susceptibility forms much of the basis for the selectivity of cytotoxic chemotherapeutic agents, and changes affecting apoptosis represent a mechanism of drug resistance in cancer.

Stress Responses

The accumulation of genetic damage and mutations, along with the hostile environment in which tumors develop, places significant stress on cancer cells. Cells respond to stress by eliciting a stress response characterized by upregulation of chaperone proteins. Chaperones, such as the heat shock proteins hsp90 and hsp70, play a central role in regulation of protein folding and are expressed at low levels under normal conditions. Under stress, these proteins become limiting, and their upregulation protects cells from the deleterious effects of protein denaturation and reduces apoptosis. Cancer cells characteristically have a constitutive stress response and are dependent on elevated levels of chaperone proteins for survival. Notably, many oncogenes are highly dependent on chaperones for their activity, making these proteins potential targets for cancer therapy. While no antichaperone therapies have been approved to date, several—especially those targeting hsp90—have shown promise in clinical trials.

Angiogenesis

Without an ability to recruit new blood vessels through angiogenesis, tumors are reliant on diffusion of oxygen and nutrients from surrounding tissue and can only grow to a few millimeters in diameter. Angiogenesis is a normal physiologic response that is essential for normal development and wound healing but is dormant in most adult tissues. It is regulated by a balance of pro-angiogenic and anti-angiogenic signals; several factors switch this balance toward angiogenesis in cancers. Hypoxia, which develops in tumors as they outgrow the diffusion limit of oxygen, is a major physiologic inducer of angiogenesis. In addition, activation of oncogenic signaling and loss of tumor suppressors directly leads to secretion of angiogenic factors such as vascular endothelial growth factor (VEGF) and basic fibroblast growth factor (bFGF), and to downregulation of anti-angiogenic factors such as Tsp-1. Many tumors also recruit significant numbers of inflammatory cells that secrete pro-angiogenic factors. Angiogenesis in tumors differs from that in normal tissues; the tumor vasculature is not properly organized. Blood vessels in tumors are leaky to both water and macromolecules, which leads to an increase in intratumoral pressure. These vessels are also prone to collapse, leading to large areas of tumors that remain hypoxic. The properties of tumor vessels can present a problem for cancer therapy, particularly for those that require oxygen (e.g., ionizing radiation).

Angiogenesis is an attractive target for cancer treatment, and agents that target this process have entered the clinic. Bevacizumab, a monoclonal antibody that inhibits angiogenesis by binding VEGF-A, has been approved for treatment of refractory glioblastoma. Several approved multitargeted kinase inhibitors that block VEGF receptors, such as pazopanib, sorafenib, and sunitinib, may also partially act through effects on angiogenesis.

Invasion and Metastasis

For most solid tumors, the main clinical threat comes from their ability to metastasize. Metastasis is a complex multistep process that involves local invasion, intravasation, survival in the circulatory system, extravasation, and colonization. A key mechanism underlying this process is epithelial-to-mesenchymal transition (EMT), characterized by the loss of cell-cell junctions and polarity, together with the gain of mesenchymal markers such as vimentin. EMT, which is normally involved in developmental cell dispersal and tissue regeneration, is subverted in cancer cells, allowing them to gain enhanced migratory capacity, invasiveness, and increased resistance to apoptosis. EMT has also been linked to the acquisition of stem cell characteristics (see later) and may thus contribute to the population of the metastatic site. Multiple transcription factors, including Snail, Slug and Zeb1, as well as miRNAs, cooperate with oncogenic signaling changes to induce EMT in cancer cells. In addition to cell-inherent changes, environmental factors including hypoxia and tissue interactions modulate EMT.

A major change that drives EMT is downregulation of E-cadherin, a component of adherens junctions and a tumor suppressor in the Wnt/β-catenin pathway. In many cases, tumor cells only undergo partial EMT, with the degree of EMT varying both within a tumor and between different tumors. Furthermore, EMT is reversible, and cells can undergo mesenchymal-to-epithelial transition (MET), which contributes to the establishment of tumors at metastatic sites.

Tumor Microenvironment

A tumor does not solely consist of transformed cancer cells but represents a complex tissue that also includes a wide array of stromal cells. The importance of stromal components in tumor phenotype is highlighted by the fact that four out of the seven genes in the genetic profile used by the recently developed Oncotype DX Colon Cancer Assay to predict the risk of recurrence in colon cancer are stromal factors. Cancer progression occurs within the context of complex interactions between multiple cell types, which can be major drivers of the evolution of tumor cells. For example, the ability to recruit immune cells can engender a significant advantage to tumor cells because intratumoral inflammatory cells secrete cytokines and growth factors that promote tumor cell proliferation and survival as well as angiogenesis. Recruitment of immune suppressor cells also helps tumors evade immune surveillance (see later). As a result, many cancers evolve to recruit inflammatory cells, and infiltration by these cells is often seen in tumor biopsies.

Other cellular components of the stroma, such as fibroblasts, can also secrete growth factors that support survival and proliferation of cancer cells. Direct interaction of integrins on cancer cells with the extracellular matrix and other cells also enhances tumorigenesis by activation of focal adhesion kinase (FAK) and several oncogenic signaling pathways, including Mek/Erk and PI-3K/Akt signaling (see Fig. 181-2).

The Immune Response to Cancer

Accumulating evidence indicates that immune surveillance and removal of immunogenic transformed cells presents a physiologic barrier to cancer development. Cancer cells can evolve a number of mechanisms to evade the immune system. They can reduce immune recognition by downregulation of major histocompatibility complex (MHC) class I antigens or by expressing immune suppressive proteins such as PD-L1. Cancer cells also have direct effects on the immune system. They secrete factors such as TGF-β, VEGF, and IL-10 that reduce the immune response, potentiate immune checkpoints, and recruit T_{reg} cells and other immune suppressor cells. Exploitation of the immune response for cancer therapy is gaining momentum in the clinic.[7] A major strategy in immune therapy is to boost the antitumor response by targeting immune checkpoints. Ipilimumab, a humanized antibody approved for the treatment of melanoma, enhances T-cell activation through blockade of CTLA-4-mediated co-inhibition. Similar therapies targeting PD-1/PD-L1–mediated checkpoints have also recently demonstrated substantial clinical effectiveness. Cancer cells also express antigens that can be used in vaccine therapies. These include cancer-testis antigens that are normally only expressed on germline cells (e.g., NY-ESO-1) and tissue-specific antigens. Sipuleucel-T is a cancer vaccine against prostatic acid phosphatase (PAP); it is approved for metastatic hormone-refractory prostate cancer. Evidence indicates that immune responses may also play a role in the therapeutic effect of antibodies designed to target specific oncogenes (see following and Table 181-4).

Energy Metabolism

Cancer cells evolve changes in energy metabolism known as the Warburg effect. This is characterized by a vast increase in the uptake of glucose, which is preferentially channeled to glycolysis rather than aerobic respiration. Oncogenic alterations that underlie these changes in glucose uptake and metabolism include increased PI-3K/Akt/mTor signaling, as well as upregulation of c-Myc and hypoxia-inducible factor-1α (HIF-1α). A direct role for altered metabolism in carcinogenesis[8] is supported by mutations affecting succinate dehydrogenase in hereditary paraganglioma (see Table 181-1), succinate dehydrogenase or fumarate hydratase in some renal cell carcinomas, and isocitrate dehydrogenase-1 and -2 (*IDH1*, *IDH2*) in glioma. Although the exact advantage conferred by the Warburg effect remains to be established, a likely rationale is that increased glycolysis provides many of the intermediates required for macromolecular synthesis, and thus may be required to sustain tumor growth. In some cases, it may also reflect an adaptation to hypoxia in tumors. Altered energy metabolism has attracted attention as a potential biomarker and target for cancer therapy, with 2-deoxyglucose and inhibitors of 6-phosphofructo-2-kinase, and pyruvate kinase M2 already being tested in clinical trials. The increased glucose uptake in cancer cells also underlies the use of positron emission tomography for visualizing tumors in vivo.

Cancer Stem Cells

Normal proliferating tissues contain pluripotent self-renewing stem cells that have high proliferative potential and can differentiate into all of the cell types in the tissue. Stem cell division gives rise to daughter stem cells and to more differentiated, transit-amplifying progenitor cells. Transit amplifying cells then continue to divide and progressively differentiate to give rise to the full spectrum of a tissue's cellular components. Stem cells are rare within tissues and usually divide very slowly, with the bulk of the proliferation responsible for tissue renewal carried out by the transit-amplifying population. Stem cells can also be found in tissues that are traditionally considered to be nonproliferative, where they remain quiescent until required for tissue repair.

Increasing evidence indicates that cancer cells are not phenotypically identical cells but are organized similarly to proliferative tissues. Analysis of solid tumors and hematopoietic cancers has revealed the presence of populations of cells that have a high potential to regenerate cancers, whereas the bulk of cancer cells have a negligible regenerative potential. Moreover, these cells can regenerate tumors that recapitulate the heterogeneity of the original malignancy. Such cells are analogous to normal tissue stem cells with regard to their capacity for self-renewal and "tissue" regeneration, and are thus referred to as cancer stem cells. This analogy is strengthened by the fact that cancer stem cells express many of the markers that differentiate stem cells in the tissues from which the cancer arose. In addition to their ability for self-renewal, cancer stem cells differ from the bulk of cancer cells in that they are slowly dividing and relatively resistant to chemotherapy. Despite these differences, the precise relationship between the different populations of cancer cells remains to be established. For example, EMT can induce a cancer stem cell–like phenotype, opening the possibility that acquisition of "stemness" in cancer cells is a dynamic process, with cells able to enter and exit a stem cell state in response to microenvironmental cues or other stimuli.

Whatever the nature of cancer stem cells, the presence of a population of drug-resistant cells with self-renewing capacity has required a reevaluation of the criteria by which cancer treatments are assessed. Treatments that do not kill the cancer stem cell population are destined to result in relapse, no matter how efficiently they debulk the cancer. Future development of treatment regimens will have to consider efficacy against the minor population of cancer stem cells that may be difficult to detect after treatment.

Tumor Heterogeneity

In addition to the phenotypic heterogeneity associated with the presence of stem cells, cancers show considerable genetic and morphologic heterogeneity both within and between patients.[9] The genetic instability associated with cancer development, together with the stochastic nature of oncogenic mutations, supports genetic drift and the coevolution of cancer cells with different genetic lesions within a tumor. Morphologic heterogeneity within tumors is particularly noticeable in the stroma, which is affected not only by the ability of cancers to recruit different cell types but also by random factors such as tumor depth, variations in vascularization, and differences in the surrounding tissue. The resultant variation in microenvironment produces different evolutionary pressures that select for regional heterogeneity within the cancer cells of a tumor. Even in apparently homogeneous cancers that arise from clonal expansion of genetically identical cells, small variations in the microenvironment may allow for the survival of subpopulations of genetically distinct cells.

Heterogeneity across tumors has implications for therapy that are analogous to those seen with stem cells. Genetically distinct populations in different microenvironments would be expected to differ in their susceptibility to treatment. Thus, heterogeneous cancers are likely to have subpopulations of resistant cells that may evade therapy and lead to relapse. This is a particular concern for metastases, which are exposed to environmental pressures that are distinct from those of the original tumor.

EXPLOITATION OF TUMOR BIOLOGY FOR TARGETED THERAPIES

Targeted Therapies

Knowledge of the biology that underlies cancer development is being leveraged in the clinic,[10] with an increasing number of drugs that target molecular changes in cancer being evaluated in patients (Table 181-4). The promise of these therapies is that by targeting changes specific to cancer, highly effective treatments can be developed that do not have the side effects associated with traditional cytotoxic chemotherapy. The majority of agents in the clinic directly target oncogenic pathways, with most approved agents being either small molecules that target protein kinases or antibodies that disrupt signaling from cell surface receptors (see Table 181-4). Another strategy is to exploit the potential "synthetic lethality" that results from oncogenic changes, as seen with the susceptibility of cells with BRCA1 or BRCA2 mutations to inhibitors of PARP (see "Genome Instability and Cancer Development" section).

By their nature, targeted therapies are only effective in tumors with relevant mutations. Specific mutations may be common in tumors from a particular disease site, leading to targeted therapies being associated with specific cancer types (e.g., HER2 inhibitors and breast cancer, EGFR inhibitors in lung and colon cancer); however, only a subpopulation of tumors at a specific disease site will be susceptible to any given targeted therapy. For example, although breast cancers with overexpression of HER2 are responsive to trastuzumab (see Table 181-4), they represent only 20 to 25% of all breast cancers; furthermore, the majority of these HER2-expressing breast tumors do not respond to HER2 inhibitors. Tumors can also have mutations in downstream components of a signaling pathway that negate the action of a drug. For example, B-Raf is downstream of EGFR, and thus EGFR inhibitors are ineffective for tumors carrying mutations activating B-Raf, even if they overexpress EGFR. As a result, application of targeted therapies requires testing of tumors to determine if they have the correct genomic profile to respond to any given treatment. Optimal use of targeted agents requires that

TABLE 181-4 TARGETED CANCER THERAPIES

THERAPEUTIC AGENT	TYPE	TARGET	DISEASE	INDICATION	COMPANION TEST
Imatinib Dasatinib Nilotinib	Small molecule	BCR-ABL	CML, ALL	Philadelphia chromosome positive	Cytogenetic analysis, FISH, PCR
Ponatinib Bosutinib	Small molecule		CML and AML resistant to prior tyrosine kinase inhibitor therapy	Philadelphia chromosome positive	Cytogenetic analysis, FISH, RT-PCR
Imatinib	Small molecule	c-Kit	Gastrointestinal stromal tumors	CD117 (c-Kit) positive	Immunohistochemistry (c-Kit PharmDx)
Cetuximab Panitumumab	Monoclonal antibody	EGFR	Colorectal cancer, head and neck	*KRAS* wild-type in colon cancer	PCR (*therascreen* KRAS RGQ Kit)
Gefitinib Erlotinib	Small molecule	EGFR	NSCLC	Mutant EGFR	PCR (*therascreen* EGFR RGQ PCR Kit, cobas EGFR Mutation Test)
Tramatenib Dabrafenib Vemurafenib	Small molecule	B-Raf	Melanoma	V600 mutant BRAF	PCR (THxID, cobas 4800 BRAF V600 Mutation Test)
Trastuzumab	Monoclonal antibody	Her2	Breast, stomach, gastroesophageal	Her2 positive	Immunohistochemistry (PATHWAY, InSite, Bond Oracle, HercepTest), FISH (Inform, PathVysion, SPOT-Light, HER2 CISH PharmDx)
Lapatinib	Small molecule	Her2, EGFR	Breast	Her2 positive, trastuzumab resistant	
Everolimus	Small molecule	mTOR	Breast, pancreatic, renal cell, astrocytoma		
Bevacizumab	Monoclonal antibody	VEGF	NSCLC, metastatic colorectal, metastatic kidney, glioblastoma		
Ipilimumab	Monoclonal antibody	CTLA-4	Melanoma		

Companion tests in parentheses are U.S. Food and Drug Administration–stipulated tests for certain uses of the corresponding drug.
ALL = acute lymphoblastic leukemia; CML = chronic myelogenous leukemia; FISH = fluorescence in situ hybridization; NSCLC = non–small cell lung cancer; PCR = polymerase chain reaction.

the appropriate mutation or other molecular abnormality be present (see Table 181-4). Many new targeted drugs are being approved by the U.S. Food and Drug Administration, together with a companion diagnostic test for identification of relevant therapeutic targets.

Use of genetic testing and targeted therapies is blurring the classification of cancer based on disease site. The fact that similar genetic changes can occur in cancers from different organs means the same drug may be appropriately used to target the same molecular change in cancers originating from different histologies (see Table 181-4). This, together with the observation that only a subset of cancers respond to a targeted treatment, suggests that in the future the classification of tumors based on the genetic abnormalities they contain may be more relevant for the choice of therapy than the tissues from which they arise.

Efficacy and Resistance Associated with Targeted Therapies

When appropriate genetic changes are present, targeted therapies can be remarkably effective, particularly in homogeneous cancers that are driven by a single well-defined genetic lesion. This can be seen with Philadelphia chromosome–positive CML, which arises because of the aberrant tyrosine kinase activity of the *BCR-ABL* oncogene (Chapter 184). Imatinib, an inhibitor of Abl (along with PDGFRα and c-Kit) is highly effective in treating chronic-phase CML patients, turning it from a uniformly fatal disease to one with a 7-year survival of about 90%. It is important to note that despite its clinical efficacy, the majority of patients treated with imatinib harbor residual disease, and recurrence is observed when treatment is stopped. This is true for most targeted therapies which are labeled for continuous treatment until disease recurrence. Thus, even successful targeted therapies may not cure cancer but turn it into a chronic condition that requires ongoing treatment for continuing patient benefit.

Because of their specificity, most targeted therapies are particularly vulnerable to the development of resistance resulting from mutations that produce changes in the target protein. Mutations that affect drug binding or induce overexpression (such as amplification) can render a targeted therapy ineffective. The genetic instability present in tumors, along with the need for chronic treatment with these agents, exacerbates this problem. Resistance arising from mutation of the target can be overcome by use of agents that are insensitive to the mutation. For example, tyrosine kinase inhibitors such as dasatinib, nilotinib, or ponatinib can be effective against imatinib-resistant BCR-ABL. Where resistance is the result of mutations in another protein that reduces reliance on a particular target, the other proteins can be targeted if known. For example, the B-Raf inhibitor dabrafenib (see Table 181-4) is being tested in combination with EGFR inhibitors for treatment of tumors that are resistant to EGFR inhibitors owing to the V600-activating mutation of B-Raf (see Fig. 181-2).

Although targeted therapies have proven highly effective for homogeneous cancers, they have more limited efficacy in the majority of more heterogeneous tumors. This can be seen with CML, where imatinib has limited efficacy in patients experiencing blast crisis where additional molecular lesions have accumulated (Chapter 184). Targeted therapies are available that prolong survival of appropriately selected patients, but in most cases these treatments give rise to transient responses with rapid emergence of resistant disease. Treatment failure may arise from de novo mutations or from preexisting subpopulation(s) of resistant cells present in heterogeneous tumors. The rapid emergence of resistant tumors indicates that tumor heterogeneity is a particular concern. Use of combination therapies, where targeted agents are combined with either conventional chemotherapy or with other targeted therapies, is one strategy that can increase the efficacy of these agents (e.g., pertuzumab, a monoclonal antibody that targets HER2, has been approved for combined therapy with trastuzumab and docetaxel in breast cancer).

Side Effects of Targeted Therapies

Although targeted therapeutics may lack the systemic toxicity of traditional chemotherapy, they are not without side effects. With traditional chemotherapies, the therapeutic window is based on the increased susceptibility of cancer cells to their cytotoxic effects, and treatment is limited by their maximum tolerated dose (MTD). However, the concept of MTD is less appropriate for targeted therapies where side effects are a direct consequence of the intended action of the drug. Most oncogenes have normal cellular equivalents (proto-oncogenes) that regulate homeostasis in non-tumor tissues. Since proto-oncogenes can be inhibited by the targeted agents, disruption of normal tissue homeostasis may, in some cases, be an unavoidable consequence of targeted therapies. In many situations, such as the rash seen with EGFR inhibitors, side effects can provide an indication of whether the drug is altering its target. Severe side effects of targeted therapeutics, such as cardiac problems associated with HER2 inhibitors, are rare and generally reverse upon cessation of treatment.

Genetic Profiling and Personalized Medicine

Development of molecularly targeted cancer therapies opens the possibility that treatment could be tailored to the specific defect in the cancer of an individual patient. Such a personalized approach to cancer therapy has become feasible with recent technologic advances in DNA sequencing that allow mutational profiles of individual tumors to be determined over a short time interval. Technologies currently under development include array-based platforms for analysis of mutations in genes of interest, deep sequencing of known drivers of tumorigenesis (i.e., repeated reads of the sequence of interest), and whole genome or exome sequencing (Chapter 43). Each approach has its advantages and disadvantages. For example, deep sequencing can identify mutations in subpopulations of cells that may be missed by other methods, but this approach is more costly and time consuming. Approaches that rapidly test a limited number of genes, on the other hand, may miss changes that would be identified in whole genome/exome sequencing. Thus, the best strategy for personalized medicine remains to be determined. Because analysis is normally performed on biopsies of primary tumors, the problem of regional heterogeneity in tumors and potential genetic differences in metastases also needs to be addressed for successful implementation of more personalized treatments.

Genetic profiling of tumors can also be used to gain prognostic information. Our increasing knowledge of the biology and genetics of cancer has led to the development of mutation and expression signatures that are associated with various cancer phenotypes. As a result, several commercial tests that use the mutational status of a panel of genes to predict the risk of recurrence and/or aggressiveness for breast (e.g., MammaPrint, Oncotype DX), colon (e.g., Oncotype DX), and prostate (e.g., Prolaris, Oncotype DX) cancers are now available for use in the clinical setting.

GENERAL REFERENCES

For the General References and other additional features, please visit Expert Consult at https://expertconsult.inkling.com.

182

MYELODYSPLASTIC SYNDROMES

DAVID P. STEENSMA AND RICHARD M. STONE

DEFINITION

The myelodysplastic syndromes (MDS) are a heterogeneous group of bone marrow failure syndromes collectively characterized by ineffective hematopoiesis resulting in peripheral blood cytopenias, most commonly anemia. MDS have a tendency to evolve over time, and there is a risk of progression to acute myeloid leukemia (AML), which is arbitrarily defined by the World Health Organization (WHO) as the presence of 20% or more immature myeloid "blast" cells in the blood or bone marrow.

Although some investigators feel that MDS should not be considered a form of cancer because some cases remain stable for many years, and a few patients have a pathophysiology dominated by autoimmune suppression of hematopoietic progenitor cells and resembling aplastic anemia, MDS are classified as myeloid neoplasms by the WHO and other organizations. Many of the somatic gene mutations that are recurrent in MDS are also present in AML and other myeloid neoplasms, and there are typically one or just a few mutant clones in the bone marrow contributing to most of the marrow cellularity.[1]

The minimal diagnostic criteria for MDS as defined by the WHO include the presence of a meaningful and persistent cytopenia (i.e., hemoglobin <11 g/dL, absolute neutrophil count <1500/mm^3, or platelet count <100,000/mm^3) together with at least one of the following features: (1) greater than 5% blasts in the bone marrow, (2) an abnormal marrow karyotype with an acquired chromosome anomaly that is consistent with the diagnosis of MDS, (3) other evidence of clonal hematopoiesis besides marrow karyotype (e.g., abnormal result using a fluorescence in situ hybridization [FISH] panel of probes directed at common MDS-associated chromosomal abnormalities), or (4) greater than 10% cells in any given hematopoietic linage that appear dysplastic (i.e., morphologically abnormal, described further below) in a patient in whom other causes of dysplastic cell morphology such as nutritional deficiency have been ruled out. Patients sometimes have persistent cytopenias and do not quite meet these diagnostic criteria, yet no other diagnosis is apparent after detailed investigation. These disorders are sometimes termed *idiopathic cytopenias of undetermined significance* (ICUS), and such patients should be followed over time because they have a risk of developing overt MDS.[2]

EPIDEMIOLOGY

The incidence and prevalence of MDS have been difficult to estimate accurately, in part because of varying definitions and imprecise terminology historically, and also because until recently, MDS cases were not captured by most global cancer registries. The U.S. National Cancer Institute's Survey, Epidemiology, and End Results (SEER) data indicate that 10,000 to 12,000 new cases are diagnosed in the United States each year. However, analysis of insurance claims data, including Medicare claims, suggests that the actual incidence of MDS is much higher—at least 40,000 new U.S. cases per year, several times higher than the incidence of AML.[3] In addition, many geriatric patients who have cytopenias of uncertain etiology and may have MDS are incompletely evaluated (e.g., they do not undergo bone marrow aspiration) and never receive an MDS diagnosis.

The primary risk factor for development of MDS is aging, with disease a consequence of cumulative acquisition of somatic mutations in marrow stem cells. The rate at which MDS is diagnosed is slightly increased in workers in certain industries such as the petroleum industry and agricultural sector, probably owing to exposure to genotoxic hydrocarbons, accelerating acquisition of such mutations. There is a slight male predominance overall, perhaps representing patterns of occupational exposure. In Asia and Eastern Europe, MDS is typically diagnosed at younger ages than in the West; in the United States, the median age at which MDS is diagnosed is 71 years, whereas in China it is closer to 50 years.

Individuals who have been exposed to ionizing radiation or certain types of cytotoxic chemotherapy (e.g., alkylating agents such as chlorambucil or mephalan, or topoisomerase II inhibitors such as etoposide or doxorubicin) have an increased risk of developing MDS subsequently. The peak incidence of MDS diagnosis after alkylating agent or radiation exposure is 5 to 10 years later, whereas after a topoisomerase inhibitor exposure, it is 1 to 3 years. The risk never goes away entirely; even 50 years after the Hiroshima and Nagasaki atomic bomb events in Japan, radiation-exposed individuals continued to be diagnosed with MDS at a higher rate than the unexposed population. Patients with a chemotherapy or radiation exposure history are said to have therapy-related MDS (t-MDS) or "secondary" MDS.

Although familial MDS is rare, germline gene mutations in several genes, including *RUNX1* and *GATA2*, predispose to MDS.[4] *RUNX1* mutations are associated with a prodrome of thrombocytopenia that can be mistaken for immune thrombocytopenic purpura, whereas *GATA2* mutations are associated with a history of mycobacterial infections and monocytopenia.

PATHOBIOLOGY

MDS are clonal disorders, meaning that one or several stem or progenitor cells in the marrow that bear somatic gene mutations expand and proliferate at the expense of healthy stem cells and come to dominate the bone marrow. These clones can then acquire additional mutations that give rise to subclones that contribute to progression of disease. The process of somatic mutation acquisition can be accelerated through exposure to radiation or DNA-damaging chemicals, as noted earlier.

Marrow cellularity is usually normal or increased in MDS, but excessive apoptosis (i.e., programmed cell death) of hematopoietic cells within the bone marrow accounts for the peripheral blood cytopenias. Excessive apoptosis within the marrow characterizes earlier MDS, but as the disease progresses toward AML and one clone begins to dominate, intramedullary apoptosis may decrease. In addition, hematopoietic differentiation, which is disordered but still can proceed in earlier stages of the disease, may become completely impaired late in the disease, such that most developing hematopoietic cells are arrested at the myeloblast stage. If 20% or more of the cells in the marrow or blood are blast cells, this is considered AML; MDS by definition is associated with less than 20% blast cells.

Large gains and losses of chromosomal material within diseased cells, including monosomies, trisomies, and large chromosomal deletions, are detectable by routine metaphase karyotyping present in one half of patients with de novo MDS and more than 80% of patients with t-MDS.[5] Newer genetic techniques such as array-based comparative genomic hybridization may uncover cryptic chromosomal deletions in patients with MDS who have normal karyotype results.

More than 25 genes are now known to be recurrently mutated in MDS.[6,7] No one mutation dominates; MDS are associated with considerable genetic heterogeneity. These genes and the probable function of the proteins they encode are listed in Table 182-1. More than 90% of patients have at least one detectable clonal somatic mutation, and most patients with MDS have several such mutations detectable in their marrow cells. Mutations affecting epigenetic patterning (e.g., DNA methylation) and chromatin conformation (e.g., histone-DNA interactions) are common in MDS, and this may be why agents that affect DNA methylation, such as azacitidine and decitabine, are effective in some patients. In addition, mutations affecting pre-mRNA splicing are common, especially in patients with MDS subtype refractory anemia with ring sideroblasts, but the specific genes that are misspliced and give rise to an MDS phenotype are unclear.

A subset of patients with pathologic findings that resemble MDS will have autoimmune suppression of hematopoiesis, which may be driven by a clonal T-lymphocyte population.[8] Patients are more likely to have an immune component to their marrow failure if they are younger than 55 years and have a hypocellular marrow similar to that seen in aplastic anemia, a normal

TABLE 182-1 GENE MUTATIONS ASSOCIATED WITH MDS AND FUNCTIONAL CLASS OF THE ASSOCIATED PROTEIN

RECURRENTLY MUTATED GENES	MUTATION FREQUENCY IN MDS	ADDITIONAL NOTES
SPLICEOSOME COMPONENTS (ALTER PRE-mRNA SPLICING)		
SF3B1	20-25%	Strongly associated with presence of ring sideroblasts (60-80% of RARS cases), often co-occurs with *DNMT3A** mutations
*U2AF1**	5-10%	Often co-occurs with del(20q)
SRSF2	5-10%	More frequent in CMML (25-30%), often co-occurs with *RUNX1** or *ASXL1** mutations
ZRSR2	5-10%	
U2AF2, SFRA1, PRPF40B, SF1	<2% each	
EPIGENETIC PATTERN & CHROMATIN CONFORMATION MODIFIERS		
TET2	20%	More frequent in CMML (≈40%)
*DNMT3A**	10-15%	Associated with poor outcome after transplant
SETBP1	5-10%	More common in CMML; germline mutations cause Schinzel–Giedion syndrome
*ASXL1**	10-20%	More frequent in CMML (≈40%)
*EZH2**	6%	More frequent in CMML (≈12%)
KDM6A	<2%	Rare in MDS, more frequent in CMML
IDH1, IDH2	<2%	More frequent in AML than MDS
PHF6	<1%	
ATRX	Rare	Associated with acquired α-thalassemia (hemoglobin H inclusions in RBCs)
TRANSCRIPTION FACTORS		
*RUNX1**	10-15%	Germline mutations cause familial platelet disorder with propensity to AML (FPD-AML)
*ETV6**	<5%	Translocations common in AML; formerly known as *TEL*
MYBL2	<1%	
GATA2	Rare	Germline mutations cause familial MDS with monocytopenia
CEBPA	Rare	More frequently mutated in AML, germline mutations cause familial AML without preceding dysplasia
WT1	Rare	More frequently mutated in AML
GENOME STABILITY		
*TP53**	5-10%	Associated with very poor prognosis; associated with t-MDS and with complex karyotype
TYROSINE KINASE SIGNALING		As a group, these genes are more often mutated in myeloid malignancies with a proliferative component
*NRAS**, *KRAS, BRAF*	5-10% collectively	*NRAS* mutations more common in CMML and AML; first mutations described in MDS (1987)
JAK2	<5%	More frequent in RARS with thrombocytosis (RARS-T) (50%)
CBL, CBLB	<5%	More frequently mutated in CMML than MDS
FLT3, MPL, KIT	<1%	*MPL* mutated in (5%) of RARS-T, *FLT3* and *KIT* mutations are rare in MDS and much more common in AML
NF1	<1%	Germline mutations cause neurofibromatosis type 1
PTPN11	<1%	Rare in MDS, more frequent in JMML (30%)
OTHERS		
NPM1	<2%	Much more frequently mutated in AML
GNAS	<1%	
BCOR, BCORL1	<1%	
UMODL1	<1%	
ZSWIM4	<1%	
Cohesins (*RAD21, STAG1, STAG2, SMC3, SMC1A)*	Rare	

*Those mutations that appear to be independently associated with poor outcomes in MDS are denoted by an asterisk. (Bejar R. Clinical and genetic predictors of prognosis in myelodysplastic syndromes. *Haematologica* 2014;99:956-964.) AML = acute myelogenous leukemia; CMMS = chronic myelomonocytic leukemia; JMML = juvenile myelomonocytic leukemia; RARS = refractory anemia with ring sideroblasts; t-MDS = therapy-related MDS. Data based on Bejar R, Levine R, Ebert BL. *J Clin Oncol.* 2011;29:504-515, and others.

chromosome pattern or trisomy 8 rather than a more complex karyotype, a paroxysmal nocturnal hemoglobinuria cell population (Chapter 160) detectable by flow cytometry, and HLA-DR15 tissue type. Such patients may respond to immunosuppressive therapy with anti–T-cell therapies.

Most patients with MDS come to medical attention because they have anemia (which is present in 95% cases and is often macrocytic); one half of patients also have neutropenia, thrombocytopenia, or both at the time of diagnosis. The peripheral blood and bone marrow exhibit characteristic "dysplastic" cell morphologic abnormalities. In the peripheral blood, these include hypogranular neutrophils, hypolobated neutrophils such as the two-lobed pseudo-Pelger-Hüet cell, platelet size and granularity abnormalities, poorly hemoglobinized red cells, and circulating early myeloid cells such as small numbers of myeloblasts. Maturation abnormalities in the bone marrow include megaloblastoid erythroid maturation, multi-nucleated erythroid cells, ring sideroblasts (i.e., erythroid precursors with abnormal peri-nuclear iron-containing mitochondria visible with Perls' Prussian blue reaction), nuclear karyorrhexis, myeloid lineage abnormalities such as left-shifted myelopoiesis and the presence of hypogranular white cells, and megakaryocytic abnormalities such as micromegakaryocytes, very large hypernucleated megakaryocytes, or hypolobated megakaryocytes (Fig. 182-1). A mild increase in reticulin fibrosis is common in MDS, but severe reticulin fibrosis or collagen fibrosis are rare. Extramedullary hematopoiesis is uncommon in MDS, and the presence of splenomegaly or hepatomegaly should prompt consideration of another cause.

CLINICAL MANIFESTATIONS

The natural history of MDS is highly variable. Approximately half of patients will die of complications of the cytopenias, particularly infection due to both neutropenia and to functional neutrophil defects (i.e., impaired bactericidal activity due to hypogranularity). Among lethal infections in MDS, pneumonia and bacteremia due to gastrointestinal or urinary infections are the most common. Bleeding is the second leading common cause of death. In addition, anemia may exacerbate cardiovascular or cerebrovascular disease. Approximately 25% of patients will progress to AML, which is usually a fatal complication. Finally, because MDS is often diagnosed in elderly patients or in those with a history of cancer, unrelated causes are the chief contributor to death in at least one third of patients.

The clinical course in MDS is dominated by complications of the cytopenia, including mucosal bleeding, recurrent infections, and exertional dyspnea and fatigue. Fatigue correlates poorly with the degree of anemia and may be due in part to cytokine release by the abnormal clonal cells. Paraneoplastic manifestations including neutrophilic dermatosis (Sweet syndrome, Chapter 440), inflammatory arthritis, and other rheumatologic syndromes occur in 10 to 15% of patients. Repeated transfusions of red cells can lead to transfusional hemosiderosis and organ dysfunction, including hepatic and cardiac abnormalities. The frequency with which actual clinical complications of iron overload occur, as well as the importance of chelation therapy in MDS, are controversial topics.

DIAGNOSIS

The diagnosis of MDS is usually suspected when the patient is discovered to have cytopenias, especially macrocytic anemia in an older person that is not due to B_{12} or folate deficiency, medication effect (e.g., methotrexate or azathioprine), or alcohol abuse. The blood count abnormality may be an incidental finding, but most patients with MDS are symptomatic with fatigue, dyspnea, and other cytopenia-associated symptoms.

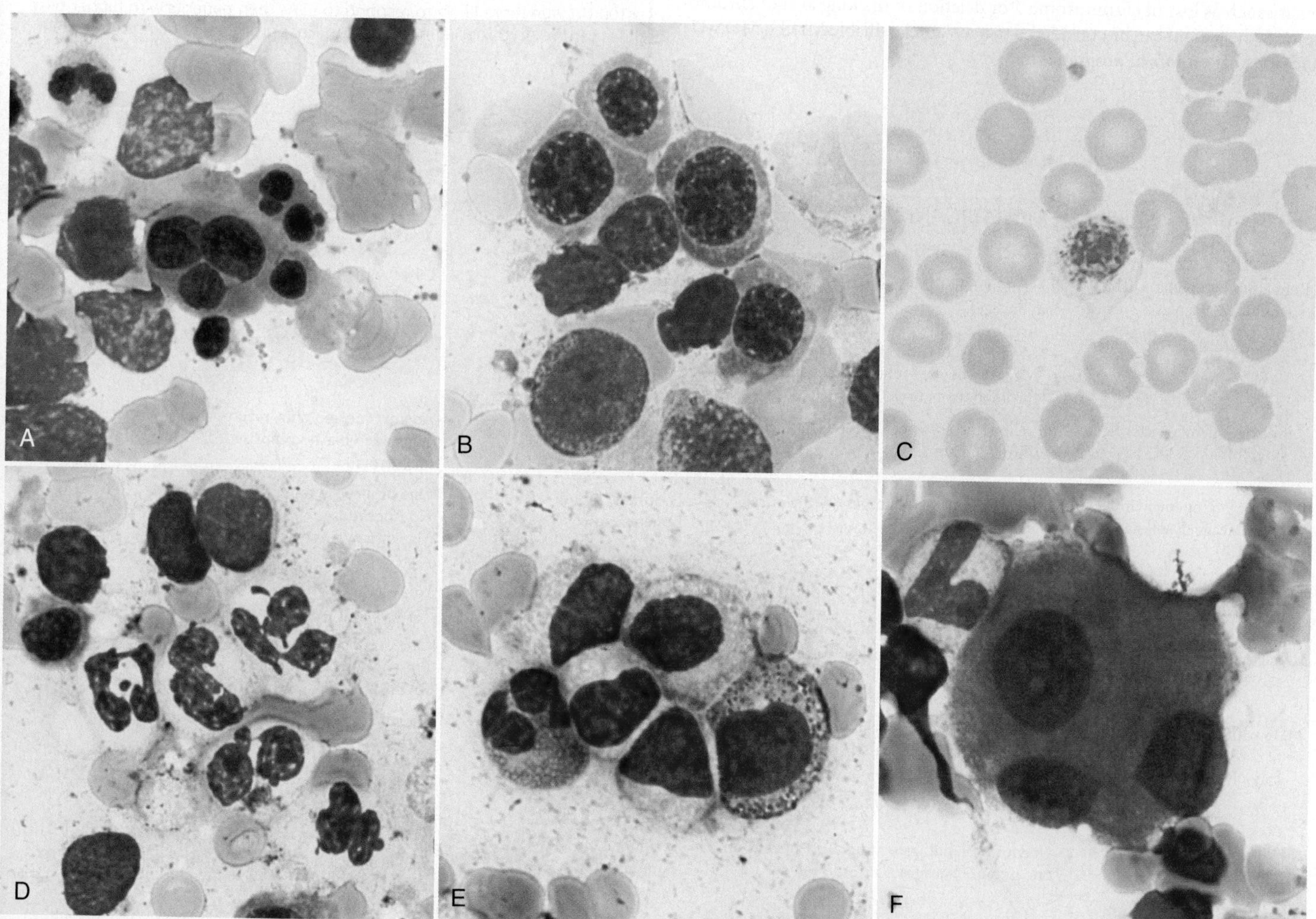

FIGURE 182-1. **Dysplastic cell morphologic abnormalities commonly observed in the peripheral blood or marrow of patients with myelodysplastic syndrome (MDS). A, Multi-nucleated erythroid precursor. B, Megaloblastoid maturation of erythroid precursors with "open" nuclear chromatin. C, Ring sideroblast (pathologic erythroid precursor). D, Hypogranular neutrophils. E, Pseudo-Pelger-Huët anomaly (hypolobated neutrophil). F, Abnormal nuclear lobation in a megakaryocyte—a "Pawn Ball" cell with three separated nuclei/nuclear lobes. *A, B, D,* and *F* are Wright-Giemsa–stained marrow aspirate; *C* is Perls' Prussian blue reaction of marrow aspirate; *E* is Wright-Giemsa–stained peripheral blood. (Figures courtesy Elizabeth A. Morgan, MD, PhD, Brigham & Women's Hospital.)**

A bone marrow aspirate is required to make the diagnosis, and bone marrow core (trephine) biopsy is also useful and can provide information about the marrow architecture and overall marrow cellularity.[9] Metaphase cytogenetics is essential, but FISH is only necessary if karyotyping fails because of an unsuccessful aspiration. FISH abnormalities are rarely detected in patients for whom at least 20 metaphases can be counted during karyotyping.

Not all that is dysplastic is MDS, and it is important to consider other potential causes for cytopenias and morphologic abnormalities. The differential diagnosis includes nonclonal disorders such as B_{12} or folate deficiency, copper deficiency, iron deficiency, HIV infection, medication exposure (especially cytotoxic chemotherapy agents), or an immune disorder such as T-cell large granular lymphocyte (T-LGL) leukemia. In patients with isolated sideroblastic anemia, it is important to rule out congenital sideroblastic anemias, including those due to germline mutations in *ALAS2*, which can present late in life.

In addition, MDS must be separated from aplastic anemia (Chapter 165), which can be oligoclonal but is not typically associated with Pelger-Hüet cells or other morphologic abnormalities, and the chromosome karyotype in aplastic anemia is usually normal. MDS can also be mistaken for AML or a myeloproliferative neoplasm (MPN) such as primary myelofibrosis. Cases in which MDS features, such as cytopenias, overlap with MPN features (Chapter 166), such as leukocytosis and splenomegaly, include chronic myelomonocytic leukemia (CMML). The WHO categorizes MDS/MPN overlap syndromes separately from MDS, and these cases have a unique mutational spectrum.

Several different MDS subtypes of varying risk of progression to leukemia are recognized by the WHO; these are listed in Table 182-2. If a patient has cytopenias but does not have characteristic MDS-associated morphologic abnormalities, yet has a typical MDS-associated marrow cytogenetic abnormality such as loss of chromosome 7 or deletion of the long arm of chromosome 5, the patient can be considered to have "unclassifiable MDS" (MDS-U) and does have a risk of progression.

TREATMENT Rx

Given the heterogeneity of MDS and the wide spectrum of functional status and comorbidities present in the typically older population with MDS, treatment must be individualized. Currently, lack of a specific well-characterized molecular target in most patients with MDS precludes a true biologically based approach to therapy. Algorithms for treatment (Fig. 182-2) are based primarily on the patient's prognosis, as discussed further below.

General Approach to the Patient

When choosing a potential therapy for a patient with MDS, clinicians should consider the patient's age, comorbidity and functional status, disease biology (currently based on assessment of bone marrow and peripheral blood findings plus cytogenetic analysis), and pace of evolution of the disease. Some patients with MDS have mild cytopenias and minimal or no symptoms, and they can reasonably be observed without therapy. For higher-risk patients (e.g., International Prognosis Scoring System [IPSS] intermediate 2 or high risk), immediate therapy is usually indicated because patients are usually severely cytopenic and have a life expectancy of less than 2 years. For lower-risk patients (IPSS low and intermediate 1 risk) a more cautious approach is appropriate. The only curative modality for MDS is allogeneic stem cell transplantation, so this option should be considered in developing a therapeutic plan if the patient is young enough and lacks other major medical problems.

Supportive Care

Hematopoietic Growth Factors and Other Approaches to Cytopenias

Because most patients with MDS are anemic, erythropoiesis-stimulating agents (ESA) including epoetin and darbepoetin are often used, even though these are not specifically U.S. Food and Drug Administration (FDA) approved for treatment of MDS. The benefits of ESAs are generally modest and of limited duration, and no prospective data confirm that they prolong survival. Patients with lower baseline serum erythropoietin levels (<500 U/L, and especially <100 U/L) are more likely to respond to ESAs than patients with higher baseline serum erythropoietin levels. An inappropriately low erythropoietin

TABLE 182-2 WORLD HEALTH ORGANIZATION (WHO) SUBTYPES OF MYELODYSPLASTIC SYNDROME

MDS SUBTYPE	DYSPLASIA	BLAST COUNT	OTHER FINDINGS
Refractory cytopenia with unilineage dysplasia (RCUD)	• Present in only 1 lineage (>10% of cells in that lineage): • Erythroid (subtype: refractory anemia) • Myeloid (subtype: refractory neutropenia) • Megakaryocytic (subtype: refractory thrombocytopenia)	• Peripheral blood: <1% • Bone marrow: <5%	• Cases with bilineage cytopenias may be included in this category, but marrow dysplasia must be limited to 1 lineage • Ring sideroblasts represent <15% of erythroid precursors
Refractory anemia with ring sideroblasts (RARS)	• Present in the erythroid lineage (>10% of erythroid precursors)	• Peripheral blood: none • Bone marrow: <5%	• Anemia (normocytic/macrocytic) • Ring sideroblasts comprise ≥ 15% of erythroid precursors
Refractory cytopenia with multilineage dysplasia (RCMD)	• Present in 2 or more lineages (>10% of cells in each affected lineage)	• Peripheral blood: <1% • Bone marrow: <5%	• One or more cytopenias • No Auer rods • May or may not have ≥ 15% ring sideroblasts
Refractory anemia with excess blasts-1 (RAEB-1)	• Present in 1 or more lineages (>10% of cells in each affected lineage)	• Peripheral blood: <5% • Bone marrow: 5-9%	• One or more cytopenias • No Auer rods • 2-4% blasts in the peripheral blood → RAEB-1
Refractory anemia with excess blasts-2 (RAEB-2)	• Present in 1 or more lineages (>10% of cells in each affected lineage)	• Peripheral blood: 5-19% • Bone marrow: 10-19%	• One or more cytopenias • Presence of Auer rods for any blast count <20% → RAEB-2
MDS with isolated deletion of chromosome 5q (5q− syndrome)	• Increased numbers of megakaryocytes, many small and with hypolobated/nonlobated nuclei • Dysplasia in other lineages less common	• Peripheral blood: no or rare blasts (<1%) • Bone marrow: <5%	• Anemia (often macrocytic) with or without other cytopenias/thrombocytosis • No Auer rods • Interstitial or terminal deletion of the long arm of chromosome 5
MDS, unclassifiable (MDS-U)	• Unequivocal, but present in <10% of cells of one or more lineages	• Peripheral blood: ≤1% • Bone marrow: <5%	• May progress to a specific MDS • Can also include cases otherwise classified as RCUD or RCMD but with 1% blasts in peripheral blood; RCUD but with pancytopenia • Cases with an MDS-associated chromosome abnormality (other than loss of Y chromosome or trisomy 8 or deletion of chromosome 20) but without dysplasia can be included in this category

Data based on Swerdlow SH, Campo E, Harris NL, et al, eds. *WHO Classification of Tumours of Haematopoietic and Lymphoid Tissues*. 4th ed. Lyon: IARC Press; 2008.

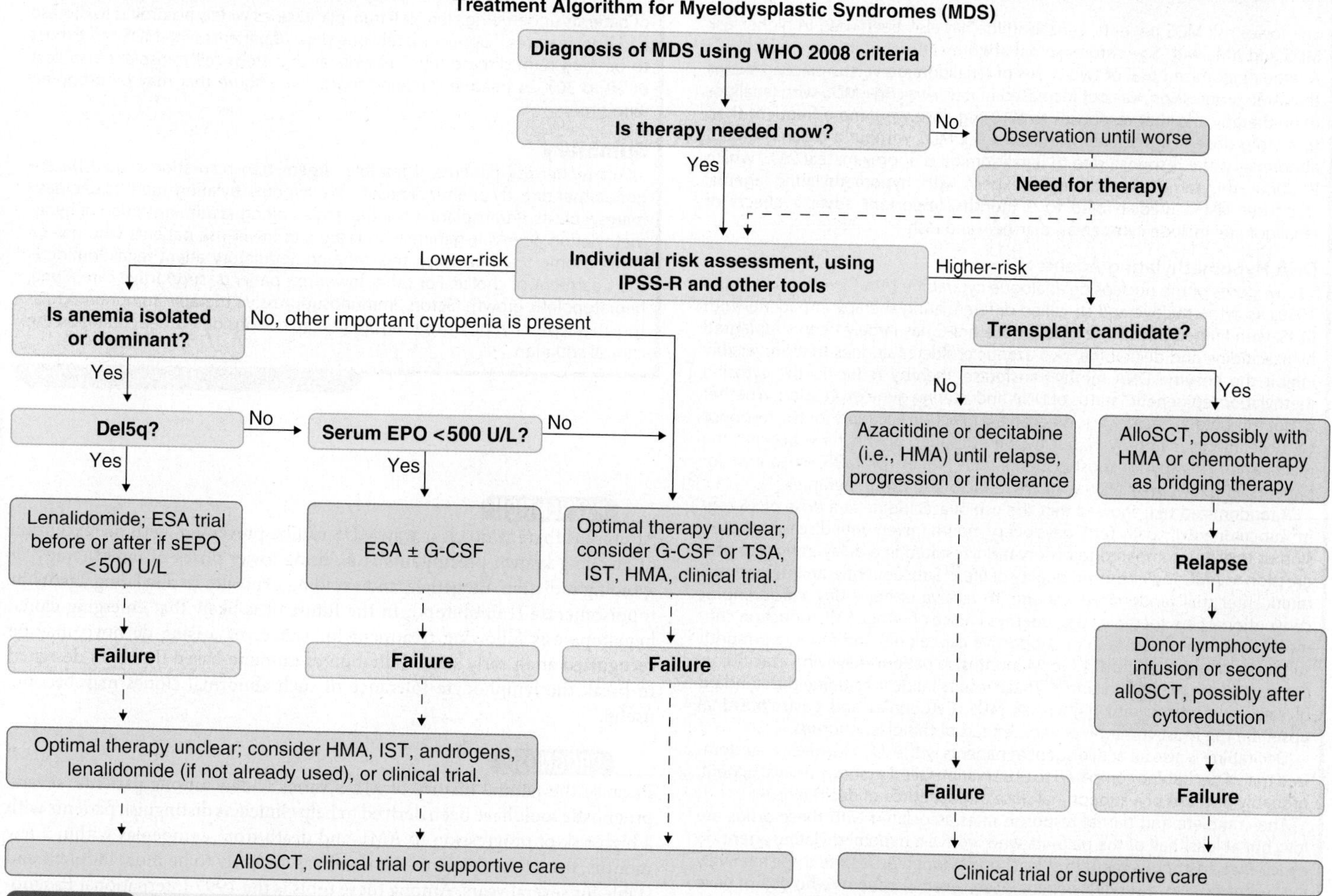

FIGURE 182-2. Suggested treatment algorithm for myelodysplastic syndrome (MDS). AlloSCT = allogeneic stem cell transplant; Del5q = deletion of long arm of chromosome 5 (5q−); EPO = erythropoietin; ESA = erythropoiesis-stimulating agent; G-CSF = granulocyte colony-stimulating factor; HMA = hypomethylating agent; IST = immunosuppressive therapy; sEPO = serum erythropoietin; TSA = thrombopoiesis-stimulating agent; WHO = World Health Organization.

response to a given degree of anemia is more likely in older patients because of the higher frequency of renal insufficiency. If no response is observed after 2 to 3 months of ESA therapy, the trial should be concluded. For patients with refractory anemia with ring sideroblasts (RARS), the addition of granulocyte colony-stimulating factor (G-CSF) to the ESA may potentiate the erythropoietic response.[10] A few patients will benefit from treatment with androgens, but the risk of prostate enlargement in men and other complications such as hepatotoxicity must be considered.

Although myeloid growth factors such as G-CSF can ameliorate the neutropenia often seen in MDS patients, such an approach (probably not leukemogenic, as was once feared) is not likely to reduce the risk of infections or provide other clinical benefit, probably because of the neutrophil dysfunction that may occur in addition to neutropenia. There is no clear role for prophylactic antibiotics.

The thrombopoiesis-stimulating agents romiplostim and eltrombopag have been approved to treat immune thrombocytopenic purpura. These agents have undergone limited study in MDS and are not FDA approved in MDS. They probably should not be used in higher-risk patients with excess blasts, because they could potentially promote leukemogenesis, but a therapeutic trial could be justified in a patient with lower-risk disease with severe thrombocytopenia or bleeding. Platelet transfusions (Chapters 172 and 177) should be used judiciously in MDS patients owing to the risk of alloimmunization, with prophylactic transfusion appropriate only in those with platelet counts less than 5000 to 10,000/mm^3. Patients with mucosal bleeding and refractory thrombocytopenia may benefit from treatment with antifibrinolytic agents such as aminocaproic acid.

Iron Chelation Therapy

The multiple red blood cell (RBC) transfusions needed by some patients with MDS may cause iron overload and tissue injury, but the frequency with which this complication occurs with clinical significance is unclear. Patients with higher serum ferritin levels fare less well than patients with lower values, both in the transplant and nontransplant settings. However, whether the ferritin is simply a marker of inflammation or more advanced disease, or whether the iron deposition in marrow, liver, heart, and pancreas directly results in this adverse outcome, remains uncertain. That uncertainty coupled with the rarity of reported deaths in MDS secondary to iron overload, as well as the toxicity of available chelators, makes the role of iron chelation therapy with agents such as deferasirox or deferoxamine in this disease quite controversial. Although it is reasonable to recommend a trial of iron chelation therapy in patients with lower-risk disease and high transfusional burdens (e.g., >20 to 40 RBC units transfused), there are no prospective data yet to suggest a clear-cut benefit in this setting. Retrospective data suggest that chelated patients live longer than nonchelated patients, but these studies are confounded by patient selection factors.[A1]

Disease-Modifying Therapy

Immunosuppressive Therapy

As described earlier, some patients with MDS display a pathophysiology that seems similar to aplastic anemia (Chapter 165), including T-lymphocyte–driven autoimmune attack against hematopoietic cells. Such patients may respond to anti–T-cell therapies, including antithymocyte globulin and calcineurin inhibitors such as cyclosporine or tacrolimus. However, although younger patients with normal karyotype, trisomy 8, paroxysmal nocturnal hemoglobinuria clones, or HLA-DR15 status seem to have a higher likelihood of benefitting, there are currently no good predictive strategies for selecting patients for immunosuppressive therapy.

Immunomodulatory Agents

Early reports showing improvements in anemia in some MDS patients during thalidomide therapy prompted a trial of the immunomodulatory lenalidomide in patients with lower-risk disease. An initial trial and a large phase II trial that followed clearly showed that patients with loss of chromosome 5q (5q−), either alone or in conjunction with other chromosomal abnormalities, had high response rates to lenalidomide, including a nearly 70% transfusion independence rate and better than 30% cytogenetic normalization rate, lasting a median of more than 2 years. Therefore, in the United States, lenalidomide has become the treatment of choice for such

5q− lower-risk MDS patients. Lenalidomide has also been used in higher-risk MDS and AML with 5q− chromosomal abnormalities, but it is less effective.[11] A large randomized trial of two doses of lenalidomide versus placebo shows that AML progression was not increased in lower-risk 5q− MDS with lenalidomide therapy and that responses to a 10-mg dose were more frequent than to a 5-mg dose.[A2] In patients with lower-risk MDS without a chromosome 5 abnormality, the response rate to lenalidomide is approximately 25%, which is about the same as one might expect with hypomethylating agents; responses last a median of 8 to 9 months. Important adverse effects of lenalidomide include cytopenias, diarrhea, and rash.

DNA Hypomethylating Agents

Low doses of the nucleoside analogue cytarabine (Ara-C) were used in the 1980s as cytoreductive and so-called differentiating therapy in patients with MDS, with limited effect. Use of low-dose Ara-C has largely been supplanted by azacitidine and decitabine, two azanucleoside analogues that irreversibly inhibit the enzyme DNA methyltransferase, thereby reducing the cytosine methylation "epigenetic" status of DNA and altering gene expression. Whether or not this putative epigenetic mechanism of action accounts for the response to these agents is unproven, but hypomethylating agents have become the mainstay of therapy for most patients with higher-risk MDS, as well as for patients with lower-risk MDS who are refractory to other therapies.

A randomized trial showed that the use of azacitidine at a dose of 75 mg/m^2 subcutaneously daily for 7 days every month (given until disease progression or toxicity), compared to observation, resulted in a delay in time to progression to AML and improved quality of life.[A3] Subsequently, an international multicenter trial randomized patients to receive either 7-day azacitidine or conventional care therapies (i.e., doctor's choice of either AML induction chemotherapy, low-dose Ara-C, or supportive care alone) and found a 9-month survival prolongation (from 15 to 24 months) in patients receiving azacitidine, compared with the control arm.[A4] These results made azacitidine the standard of care for patients with higher-risk MDS. Cytopenias and gastrointestinal upset are the most common adverse effects of this class of drugs.

Decitabine is also an active agent in patients with MDS. However, a randomized trial of decitabine compared to observation failed to show survival benefit, probably because of a suboptimal dose and schedule of decitabine.

The complete and partial response rates associated with these drugs are low, but at least half of the patients who receive a hypomethylating agent do experience an improvement in at least one cytopenia. Despite these relatively modest responses, a survival benefit is seen even in patients who do not have a complete response.[12] The major problem is that these agents are not curative, and once they fail, the patient's life expectancy is less than 6 months. There are numerous therapies in development that are being tested, but at present there is no standard of care for patients whose disease worsens while undergoing therapy with azacitidine or decitabine.

Stem Cell Transplantation

Because allogeneic stem cell transplantation (Chapter 178) is potentially curative, this modality should be considered in all patients with higher-risk MDS who are approximately 75 years old or younger and lack major comorbid conditions. Reduced-intensity conditioning stem cell transplantation is feasible in adults up to that age, whereas myelosuppressive stem cell transplants are generally reserved for those younger than approximately age 55. Studies considering both types of stem cell transplants suggest that patients with higher-risk disease should be referred immediately for stem cell transplantation if feasible.[13] The optimal conditioning regimen is unclear.

Relapses are common after stem cell transplantation. It is uncertain whether there is benefit from the administration of so-called bridging therapy with azacitidine or decitabine before a planned transplant in an effort to reduce the leukemic burden. Because most patients with MDS are older and uncommonly have a younger sibling who is a suitable stem cell donor, azacitidine or decitabine may be useful to stabilize a patient prior to transplant while an unrelated donor search is ongoing. Although the long-term outcome of patients undergoing stem cell transplant varies widely according to disease and host features,[14] approximately one third of patients with MDS can expect to be long-term disease-free survivors after a stem cell transplant at a cost of 20 to 30% in treatment-related mortality, a figure that may be dropping with time.

Summary

For higher-risk patients, if feasible, urgent transplantation should be the goal, either directly or after exposure to a hypomethylating agent to decrease marrow blasts. If transplant is not the goal, prolonged administration of hypomethylating agents is generally indicated. In lower-risk patients who have a chromosome 5 abnormality, the immunomodulatory agent lenalidomide is the treatment of choice. For other lower-risk patients, supportive care alone, hematopoietic growth factors, immunosuppressive therapy, immunomodulatory therapy, or hypomethylating agents can be considered, depending on the clinical situation.

PREVENTION

At present there is no clear way MDS can be prevented, with the exception of avoiding known precipitants (e.g., using lower doses of radiotherapy or avoiding radiation altogether, and avoiding exposure to alkylating agents or topoisomerase II inhibitors). In the future, it is likely that emerging clonal hematopoiesis following treatment for cancer or arising de novo may be recognized at an early stage. Initiation of immune-based therapies designed to break the lymphocyte tolerance of such abnormal clones may become useful.

PROGNOSIS

Because the natural history of MDS varies widely among patients, several prognostic tools have been derived to help clinicians distinguish patients with a high risk of progression to AML and death from cytopenias within a few months, from those patients whose disease is likely to be more indolent and stable for several years. Among these tools is the 1997 International Prognosis Scoring System (IPSS), which assessed patients' risk by scoring the number of cytopenias, the chromosome pattern (some anomalies are associated with a better prognosis than others), and the proportion of blast cells in the marrow. In 2012, a revised version of the IPSS (IPSS-R) was published; it included a broader range of cytogenetic abnormalities than the original IPSS and weighted abnormal cytogenetics more heavily.[15] The IPSS-R (Table 182-3) defines five different subgroups of MDS with varying risks of death and progression to AML.

Comorbid conditions also influence prognosis independently of the MDS. Other relevant factors that are not included in current prognostic models include serum ferritin and lactate dehydrogenase levels, aberrant expression of certain cell surface markers on myeloid cells detected by flow cytometry (e.g., CD5 or CD56 on myeloid cells), rarer cytogenetic abnormalities not included in the IPSS, and most importantly, the presence of certain molecular abnormalities.[16,17] Several molecular changes, including mutations in *EZH2*, *TP53*, *ASXL1*, *RUNX1*, and *ETV6* are associated with a poorer prognosis than would have been predicted by the IPSS; in patients with lower-risk disease, only *EZH2* retains independent prognostic value. Additionally, the presence of either a *TP53* or a *DNMT3A* mutation predicts for a worse outcome after stem cell transplant.

TABLE 182-3 2012 REVISED INTERNATIONAL PROGNOSTIC SCORING (IPSS-R) FOR MYELODYSPLASTIC SYNDROMES

RISK GROUP	INCLUDED KARYOTYPES	MEDIAN SURVIVAL, YEARS	25% OF PATIENTS TO AML, YEARS	PROPORTION OF PATIENTS IN THIS GROUP
Very good	del(11q), −Y	5.4	N/R	4%
Good	Normal, del(20q), del(5q) alone or with 1 other anomaly, del(12p)	4.8	9.4	72%
Intermediate	+8, del(7q), i(17q), +19, any other single or double abnormality not listed	2.7	2.5	13%
Poor	Abnormal 3q, −7, double abnormality include −7/del(7q), complex with 3 abnormalities	1.5	1.7	4%
Very poor	Complex, with >3 abnormalities	0.7	0.7	7%

TABLE 182-3 2012 REVISED INTERNATIONAL PROGNOSTIC SCORING (IPSS-R) FOR MYELODYSPLASTIC SYNDROMES—cont'd

PARAMETER	CATEGORIES AND ASSOCIATED SCORES				
Cytogenic risk group	Very good 0	Good 1	Intermediate 2	Poor 3	Very poor 4
Marrow blast proportion	≤2% 0	>2-<5% 1	5-10% 2	>10% 3	
Hemoglobin	≥10 g/dL 0	8-<10 g/dL 1	<8 g/dL 1.5		
Absolute neutrophil	$\geq 0.8 \times 10^9$/L 0	$<0.8 \times 10^9$/L 0.5			
Platelet count	$\geq 100 \times 10^9$/L 0	50 -100 $\times 10^9$L 0.5	$<50 \times 10^9$/L 1		

Possible range of summed scores: 0-10.

IPSS-R (see: http://www.mds-foundation.org/ipss-r-calculator/)

RISK GROUP	POINTS	% PATIENTS (*n* = 7012; AML DATA ON 6485)	MEDIAN SURVIVAL, YEARS	MEDIAN SURVIVAL FOR PATIENTS UNDER 60 YEARS	TIME UNTIL 25% OF PATIENTS DEVELOP AML, YEARS
Very low	0-1.5	19%	8.8	Not reached	Not reached
Low	2.0-3.0	38%	5.3	8.8	10.8
Intermediate	3.5-4.5	20%	3.0	5.2	3.2
High	5.0-6.0	13%	1.5	2.1	1.4
Very high	>6.0	10%	0.8	0.9	0.7

Top panel, Cytogenetic (chromosome) classification used in IPSS-R. *Middle panel,* Table for calculation of IPSS-R risk group. *Bottom panel,* Outcomes by risk group. Cytogenic (chromosome) classification used in IPSS-R.
Data from Steensma DP. The changing classification of myelodysplastic syndromes: what's in a name? *Hematology* 2009;2009:645-655.

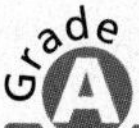

Grade A References

A1. Meerpohl JJ, Schell LK, Rücker G, et al. Deferasirox for managing iron overload in people with myelodysplastic syndrome. *Cochrane Database Syst Rev.* 2014;10:CD007461.

A2. Fenaux P, Giagounidis A, Selleslag D, et al. A randomized phase 3 study of lenalidomide versus placebo in RBC transfusion-dependent patients with low-/intermediate-1-risk myelodysplastic syndromes with del5q. *Blood.* 2011;118:3765-3776.

A3. Silverman LR, Demakos EP, Peterson BL, et al. Randomized controlled trial of azacitidine in patients with the myelodysplastic syndrome: a study of the cancer and leukemia group B. *J Clin Oncol.* 2002;20:2429-2440.

A4. Fenaux P, Mufti G, Hellstrom-Lindberg E, et al. Efficacy of azacitidine compared with that of conventional care regimens in the treatment of higher-risk myelodysplastic syndromes: a randomised, open-label, phase III study. *Lancet Oncol.* 2009;10:223-232.

GRADE REFERENCES

For the General References and other additional features, please visit Expert Consult at https://expertconsult.inkling.com.

183

THE ACUTE LEUKEMIAS

FREDERICK R. APPELBAUM

DEFINITION

Normal hematopoiesis (Chapter 156) requires tightly regulated proliferation and differentiation of pluripotent hematopoietic stem cells that become mature peripheral blood cells. Acute leukemia is the result of a malignant event or events occurring in an early hematopoietic precursor. Instead of proliferating and differentiating normally, the affected cell gives rise to progeny that fail to differentiate but continue to proliferate in an uncontrolled fashion. As a result, immature myeloid cells in acute myeloid leukemia (AML) or lymphoid cells in acute lymphoblastic leukemia (ALL)—often called blasts—rapidly accumulate and progressively replace the bone marrow, diminishing the production of normal red cells, white cells, and platelets. This loss of normal marrow function in turn gives rise to the common clinical complications of leukemia: anemia, infection, and bleeding. With time, the leukemic blasts pour out into the blood stream and eventually occupy the lymph nodes, spleen, and other vital organs. If untreated, acute leukemia is rapidly fatal; most patients die within several months after diagnosis. With appropriate therapy, however, the natural history of acute leukemia can be markedly altered, and many patients can be cured.

EPIDEMIOLOGY

Incidence

There were 14,590 new cases of AML and 6075 new cases of acute ALL in the United States in 2013, leading to 10,320 deaths from AML and 1430 deaths from ALL. The incidence of acute leukemia has remained relatively stable over the past 3 decades. Although acute leukemia accounts for only about 2% of cancer deaths, the impact of leukemia is heightened because of the young age of some patients. For example, with a maximum incidence between ages 2 and 10 years, ALL is the most common cancer in children younger than 15 years and accounts for one third of all childhood cancer deaths. The incidence of AML gradually increases with age, without an early peak. The median age at diagnosis of AML is about 60 years.

Determinants

In most cases, acute leukemia develops for no known reason, but sometimes a possible cause can be identified.

Genetic Predisposition

The concordance rate is virtually 100% in identical twins if one twin develops leukemia during the first year of life. Single germline mutations in *RUNX1*, *CEBPA*, and *GATA2* cause rare syndromes leading to acute leukemia without other manifestations. The incidence of acute leukemia is markedly increased in syndromes involving defective DNA repair, such as Fanconi's anemia and Bloom's syndrome, and in bone marrow failure syndromes associated with ribosomal abnormalities (Chapter 165), including Diamond-Blackfan syndrome, Shwachman-Diamond syndrome, and dyskeratosis congenita. Germline mutations in P53 (Li-Fraumeni syndrome) and abnormalities in chromosome number, as in Down and Klinefelter's syndromes, are also associated with an increased incidence of acute leukemia.

Radiation

Ionizing radiation (Chapter 20) is leukemogenic. The incidence of ALL, AML, and chronic myeloid leukemia (CML) is increased in patients given therapeutic radiation and among survivors of the atomic bomb blasts at Hiroshima and Nagasaki. The magnitude of the risk depends on the dose of radiation, its distribution in time, and the age of the individual. Greater risk results from higher doses of radiation delivered over shorter periods to younger patients. In areas of high natural background radiation (often from radon), chromosomal aberrations are reportedly more frequent, but an increase in acute leukemia has not been consistently found. Concern has been raised about the possible leukemogenic effects of extremely low-frequency nonionizing electromagnetic fields emitted by electrical installations. If such an effect exists at all, its magnitude is small.

Oncogenic Viruses

The search for a viral cause of leukemia has been pursued intensely, but only two clear associations have been found. Human T-cell lymphotropic virus type I (HTLV-I), an enveloped, single-stranded RNA virus, is considered the causative agent of adult T-cell leukemia (Chapter 378). This distinct form of leukemia is found within geographic clusters in southwestern Japan, the Caribbean basin, and Africa. Because HTLV-I seropositivity was found with increasing frequency among heavily transfused patients and intravenous drug users, screening of blood products for antibodies to HTLV-I is now routine practice in blood banks in the United States. Epstein-Barr virus (Chapter 377), the DNA herpes family virus that causes infectious mononucleosis, is associated with the endemic African form of Burkitt's lymphoma/leukemia (Chapter 185).

Chemicals and Drugs

Heavy occupational exposure to benzene and benzene-containing compounds such as kerosene and carbon tetrachloride may lead to marrow damage, which can take the form of aplastic anemia, myelodysplasia, or AML. A link between leukemia and tobacco use has been reported.

With the increasing use of chemotherapy and radiotherapy to treat other malignancies, as much as 10% of AMLs and a smaller percentage of ALLs are likely the consequence of prior therapy.[1] Prior exposure to alkylating agents such as melphalan and the nitrosoureas is associated with an increased risk for secondary AML, which often manifests initially as a myelodysplastic syndrome (Chapter 182), frequently with abnormalities of chromosomes 5, 7, and 8 but with no distinct morphologic features. These secondary AMLs typically develop 4 to 6 years after exposure to alkylating agents, and their incidence may be increased with greater intensity and duration of drug exposure. Secondary AML associated with exposure to topoisomerase II inhibitors, including the epipodophyllotoxins (teniposide or etoposide) and doxorubicin, tends to have a shorter latency period (1 to 2 years), lacks a myelodysplastic phase, has a monocytic morphology, and involves abnormalities of the long arm of chromosome 11 (band q23) or chromosome 21 (band q22). Recently, concern has been raised about an increased risk for second cancers including myeloid malignancies in patients receiving lenalidomide as maintenance therapy in multiple myeloma. Because patients frequently receive combination chemotherapy, it is often difficult to identify a single causative agent.

PATHOBIOLOGY

Clonality and Cell of Origin

The acute leukemias are clonal disorders, and all leukemic cells in a given patient are descended from a common progenitor. The clonal nature of acute leukemia suggests that there are leukemic stem cells capable of both self-renewal and proliferation. Leukemic stem cells in AML are rare among the leukemic mass, with a frequency of 0.2 to 10 per 10^6, and are within the primitive $CD34^{2+}$ $CD38^-$ fraction. Less is known about the ALL stem cell.

Classification

The World Health Organization (WHO) classification of acute leukemias is based on clinical, morphologic, immunophenotypic, cytogenetic, and molecular features (Table 183-1).

TABLE 183-1 WORLD HEALTH ORGANIZATION CLASSIFICATION OF ACUTE LEUKEMIAS

CLASSIFICATION SUBTYPES (2008)
Acute Myeloid Leukemia (AML) and Related Neoplasms
AML with recurrent genetic abnormalities
AML with t(8;21)(q22;q22); *RUNX1-RUNX1T1*
AML with inv(16)(p13.1q22) or t(16;16)(p13.1;q22); *CBFB-MYH11*
Acute promyelocytic leukemia (APL) with t(15;17)(q22;q12); *PML-RARA*
AML with t(9;11)(p22;q23); *MLLT3-MLL*
AML with t(6;9)(p23;q34); *DEK-NUP214*
AML with inv(3)(q21q26.2) or t(3;3)(q21;q26.2); *RPN1-EVI1*
AML (megakaryoblastic) with t(1;22)(p13;q13); *RBM15-MKL1*
Provisional entity: AML with mutated *NPM1*
Provisional entity: AML with mutated *CEBPA*
AML with myelodysplasia-related changes
Therapy-related myeloid neoplasms
AML, not otherwise specified
AML with minimal differentiation
AML without maturation
AML with maturation
Acute myelomonocytic leukemia
Acute monoblastic/monocytic leukemia
Acute erythroid leukemia
Pure erythroid leukemia
Erythroleukemia, erythroid/myeloid
Acute megakaryoblastic leukemia
Acute basophilic leukemia
Acute panmyelosis with myelofibrosis
Myeloid sarcoma
Myeloid proliferations related to Down syndrome
Transient abnormal myelopoiesis
Myeloid leukemia associated with Down syndrome
Blastic plasmacytoid dendritic cell neoplasm
B-Lymphoblastic Leukemia (ALL)/Lymphoma
B-lymphoblastic leukemia/lymphoma, not otherwise specified
B-lymphoblastic leukemia/lymphoma with recurrent genetic abnormalities
B-lymphoblastic leukemia/lymphoma with t(9;22)(q34;q11.2); *BCR-ABL1* (Philadelphia chromosome–positive ALL)
B-lymphoblastic leukemia/lymphoma with t(v;11q23); *MLL* rearranged
B-lymphoblastic leukemia/lymphoma with t(12;21)(p13;q22); *TEL-AML1* (*ETV6-RUNX1*)
B-lymphoblastic leukemia/lymphoma with hyperdiploidy
B-lymphoblastic leukemia/lymphoma with hypodiploidy
B-lymphoblastic leukemia/lymphoma with t(5;14)(q31;q32); *IL3-IGH*
B-lymphoblastic leukemia/lymphoma with t(1;19)(q23;p13.3); *TCF3-PBX1*
T-Lymphoblastic Leukemia (ALL)/Lymphoma

ALL = acute lymphoblastic leukemia.

Morphology

Leukemic cells in AML are typically 12 to 20 nm in diameter, with discrete nuclear chromatin, multiple nucleoli, and cytoplasm that usually contains azurophilic granules (Fig. 183-1). Auer rods, which are slender, fusiform cytoplasmic inclusions that stain red with Wright-Giemsa stain, are virtually pathognomonic of AML (Fig. 183-2). The French-American-British (FAB) morphologic system divides AML into eight subtypes: M0, M1, M2, and M3 reflect increasing degrees of differentiation of myeloid leukemic cells; M4 and M5 leukemias have features of the monocytic lineage; M6 has features of the erythroid cell lineage; and M7 is acute megakaryocytic leukemia. The WHO system also recognizes acute basophilic leukemia and acute leukemia with predominant myelofibrosis.

The leukemic cells in ALL tend to be smaller than AML blasts and relatively devoid of granules (see Fig. 183-1). ALL can be divided by FAB criteria into L1, L2, and L3 subgroups. L1 blasts are uniform in size, with homogeneous nuclear chromatin, indistinct nucleoli, and scanty cytoplasm with few, if any, granules. L2 blasts are larger and more variable in size and may have nucleoli. L3 blasts are distinct, with prominent nucleoli and deeply basophilic cytoplasm with vacuoles.

Immunophenotyping

Immunophenotyping by multiparameter flow cytometry is used to determine lineage involvement of newly diagnosed acute leukemias and to detect aberrant immunophenotypes, allowing the measurement of minimal residual disease after therapy. Most cases of AML express antigens seen on normal immature myeloid cells. The most immature forms of AML express CD34,

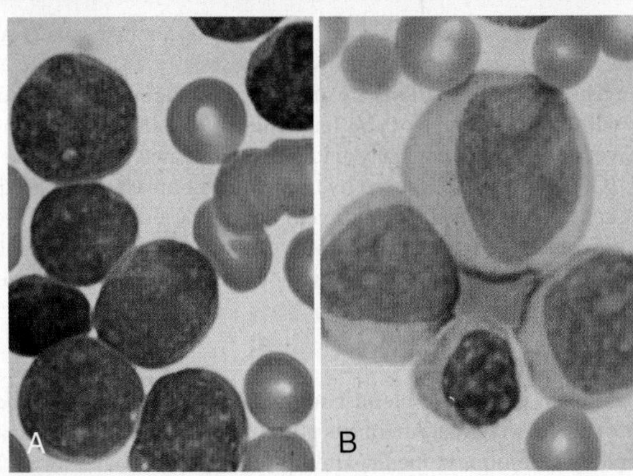

FIGURE 183-1. **Acute leukemia. A, Acute lymphoblastic leukemia (ALL). B, Acute myeloid leukemia (AML). Lymphoblasts in ALL are smaller, with a higher ratio of nuclear to cytoplasmic material and less distinct nucleoli than in the myeloblasts in AML. The nucleoli in the myeloblasts are clear and "punched out."**

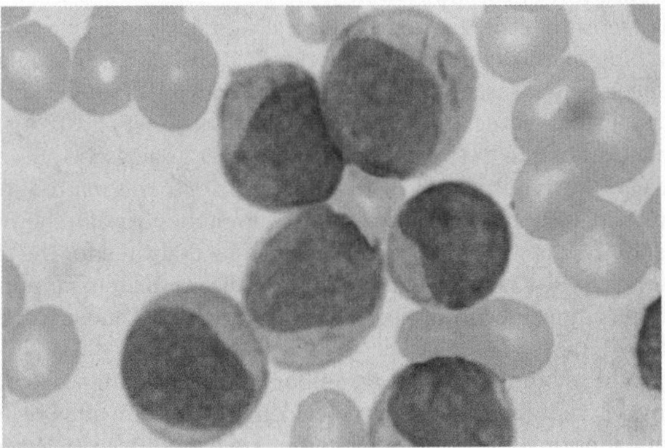

FIGURE 183-2. **Acute myeloid leukemia. The myeloblasts in the smear show Auer rods as cytoplasmic inclusions.**

CD117 and HLA-DR, whereas more differentiated forms express CD13 and CD33. CD14, CD15, and CD11b are expressed by AMLs with monocytic features, erythroid leukemias express CD36 and CD71, and megakaryocytic AMLs express CD41a and CD61. In 10 to 20% of patients, otherwise typical AML blasts also express antigens usually restricted to B- or T-cell lineage. Expression of a single lymphoid antigen by AML cells does not change either the natural history or the therapeutic response of these leukemias.

Approximately 75% of cases of ALL express B-lineage antigens and can be subdivided into four categories. The most immature group, pro-B ALL, expresses CD19 and/or CD 22 but not CD10 and represents about 10% of cases of ALL. Approximately 50 to 60% of cases of ALL express the early B-cell antigens CD19 and/or CD22 along with the common ALL antigen (CALLA, or CD10), a glycoprotein that is also found occasionally on normal early lymphocytes. CALLA-positive ALL is thought to represent an early pre-B-cell differentiation state. Approximately 10% of cases of ALL have intracytoplasmic immunoglobulin and are termed pre-B-cell ALL. Mature B-cell ALL is signified by the presence of surface immunoglobulin and accounts for less than 5% of cases of ALL. In general, the best therapeutic outcomes among B-cell ALL types are with early pre-B-cell (CALLA positive) ALL. The 25% of cases of ALL that express T-lineage antigens can be separated into three groups: (1) early T-precursor ALL expressing CD7 but not CD1a or CD3, (2) thymic T-ALL expressing CD1a but not surface CD3, and (3) mature T-ALL expressing surface CD3. The prognosis for thymic T-cell ALL is superior to that of the other forms of T-ALL. In about 25% of patients with ALL, the leukemic cells may also express a myeloid antigen, but with current therapies, this does not affect outcome.

Acute leukemias of ambiguous lineage are rare cases with no evidence of lineage differentiation (i.e., acute undifferentiated leukemia [AUL]) or those with blasts that express definitive markers of more than one lineage (i.e., mixed phenotype acute leukemia [MPAL]). MPAL can contain either distinct blast populations of different lineages (bilineal) or a single population expressing features of both lineages (biphenotypic). In general, the prognosis of patients with AUL or MPAL is poor when treated with standard chemotherapy.[2]

Cytogenetics and Molecular Biology

In most cases of acute leukemia, an abnormality in chromosome number or structure is found. These abnormalities are clonal, involving all the malignant cells in a given patient; they are acquired and are not found in the normal cells of the patient; and they are referred to as "nonrandom" because specific abnormalities are found in multiple cases and are associated with distinct morphologic or clinical subtypes of the disease. These abnormalities may be simply the gain or loss of whole chromosomes, but more often they include chromosomal translocations, deletions, or inversions. When patients with acute leukemia and a chromosomal abnormality receive treatment and enter into complete remission, the chromosomal abnormality disappears; when relapse occurs, the abnormality reappears. In many cases, these abnormalities have provided clues into the pathobiology of acute leukemia.

The most common cytogenetic abnormalities seen in AML can be categorized according to their underlying biology and prognostic significance.[3] The translocation t(8;21) and the inversion inv(16) result in abnormalities of a transcription factor made up of core binding factor-α (CBF-α) and CBF-β. The t(8;21) results in the fusion of CBF-α on chromosome 21 with the *MTG8* gene on chromosome 8, whereas inv(16) results in the fusion of CBF-β on the q arm of chromosome 16 with the *MYH11* gene on the p arm. Both of these "core binding factor" AMLs are characterized by a high complete response rate and relatively favorable long-term survival. An additional translocation with a favorable prognosis, t(15;17), involves two genes, *PML* and *RAR-α* (a gene encoding the α-retinoic acid receptor), and is invariably associated with acute promyelocytic leukemia (APL), the M3 subtype of AML. Translocations involving the *MLL* gene, located at chromosome band 11q23, are seen in 5-7% of AMLs. *MLL* is perhaps the most promiscuous oncogene partner in oncology, with more than 30 fusion partners identified. The prognosis of MLL-associated AML depends on the fusion partner, with t(9;11) and t(11;19) predicting an intermediate prognosis and all others considered unfavorable. Trisomy 8 is among the most common nonrandom cytogenetic abnormalities seen in AML; it accounts for 9% of cases and carries an intermediate prognosis. Trisomies of chromosome 21, chromosome 11, and other chromosomes are sometimes seen as well. Deletions of part or all of chromosome 5 or 7 each account for 6 to 8% of cases of AML. These abnormalities are seen with greater frequency in older patients and in patients with AML secondary to myelodysplasia or prior exposure to alkylating agents, and are associated with an unfavorable prognosis. The presence of multiple (more than three) cytogenetic abnormalities in individual cases of AML defines "complex cytogenetics" and also is associated with an unfavorable prognosis.

The identification of recurrent chromosomal abnormalities in acute leukemia, including translocations, inversions, and gene duplications, led to the identification and cloning of the involved genes. More recently, directed and genome-wide assays have provided a better understanding of the genomic landscape of AML.[4] AML cells appear to carry, on average, a total of approximately 13 mutations per cell, far less than found in epithelial cancers. Of these, on average 5 mutations are in genes recurrently mutated in AML (so called driver mutations), with the remainder being considered as passenger mutations. Among the recurrently mutated driver mutations, several are of significant prognostic importance and thus are part of the standard evaluation of AML. *CEBPA*, a gene encoding a leucine zipper transcription factor involved in myeloid differentiation, is mutated in 4 to 15% of cases of AML and is associated with a more favorable prognosis. *NPM1* encodes a nucleolar phosphoprotein with multiple functions. Mutations in *NPM1* are found in approximately 30% of AML cases and are also associated with a more favorable prognosis. *FLT3* is a receptor tyrosine kinase and is mutated in 30 to 35% of AML patients, one fourth of the time as a point mutation and three fourths of the time as an internal tandem duplication. Mutations in *FLT3* are associated with a poorer clinical outcome. Other driver mutations recurrently mutated in AML include *DNMT3A, IDH 1* and 2, *NRAS* and *KRAS, RUNX1, TET2,* and *TP53*. Although assays of the mutational status of these genes has not yet become standard, increasing numbers of studies are suggesting their possible utility both for prognosis and for treatment selection.[5]

Whole-genome sequencing of paired samples of skin and bone marrow in individuals who transform from myelodysplastic syndromes to secondary

AML shows that the genetic evolution of secondary AML is a dynamic process shaped by multiple cycles of mutation acquisition and clonal selection. The preexisting myelodysplastic syndrome–founding clone persists with transformation to AML. With the acquisition of each new set of mutations, all the preexisting mutations are carried forward, resulting in daughter subclones that contain increasing numbers of mutation during evolution.[6]

The most common cytogenetic abnormality seen in adults with ALL is the Philadelphia (Ph) chromosome, or t(9;22).[7] This translocation results in fusion of the *BCR* gene on chromosome 22 to the *ABL* tyrosine kinase gene on chromosome 9. This results in the constitutive activation of *ABL*, but the precise mechanism by which this activity leads to leukemia is unclear. The *BCR-ABL* fusion is associated with both ALL and CML (Chapter 184), with a difference in the breakpoint of *BCR* distinguishing the two. A slightly smaller 190-kD fusion protein is usually found in ALL, whereas a larger 210-kD protein is characteristic of CML. The frequency of t(9;22) in ALL increases with age: it is found in approximately 5% of childhood cases and 25% of adults. Before the development of specific tyrosine kinase inhibitors, ALL with t(9;22) had a poor prognosis; newer regimens combining tyrosine kinase inhibitors with chemotherapy are providing improved outcomes. The most common translocation seen in childhood ALL is t(12;21), which involves the genes *TEL* and *AML1*. Like the AML-associated t(8;21) and inv(16), t(12;21) is thought to result in abnormal DNA transcription by interfering with the normal function of CBF. Although t(12;21) is difficult to diagnose by routine cytogenetics, by molecular studies it has been shown to account for 25% of childhood ALL and 4% of adult ALL and has a favorable prognosis. Partial deletions in 9p, seen in 5 to 7% of adults with ALL, are also associated with a favorable outcome. Other abnormalities sometimes seen in B-cell ALL include t(8;14) and t(8;22), which result in translocation of the *MYC* gene on chromosome 8 and immunoglobulin enhancer response genes on chromosomes 14 or 22; they are associated with a poor therapeutic outcome. T-cell ALLs are frequently associated with abnormalities of chromosome 7 or 14 at the sites of T-cell receptor enhancer genes on these chromosomes. The leukemia cells in about 20% of patients with ALL have a propensity to gain chromosomes, sometimes reaching an average of 50 to 60 chromosomes per cell. Patients with such hyperdiploid leukemias tend to respond well to chemotherapy.

As in AML, directed and genome-wide evaluation of cases of ALL have revealed recurrent mutations in addition to those already identified through cytogenetics.[8] Among the most common are mutations in *PAX5* and *IKZF1* seen in 30 and 25% of cases of B-cell ALL respectively, and mutations in *NOTCH1* seen in 35% of cases of T-cell ALL.

CLINICAL MANIFESTATIONS

The signs and symptoms of acute leukemia are usually rapid in onset, developing over a few weeks to a few months at most; they result from decreased normal marrow function and invasion of normal organs by leukemic blasts. Anemia is present at diagnosis in most patients and causes fatigue, pallor, headache, and, in predisposed patients, angina or heart failure. Thrombocytopenia is usually present, and approximately one third of patients have clinically evident bleeding at diagnosis, usually in the form of petechiae, ecchymoses, bleeding gums, epistaxis, or hemorrhage. Most patients with acute leukemia are significantly granulocytopenic at diagnosis. As a result, approximately one third of patients with AML and slightly fewer patients with ALL have significant or life-threatening infections when initially seen, most of which are bacterial in origin.

In addition to suppressing normal marrow function, leukemic cells can infiltrate normal organs. In general, ALL tends to infiltrate normal organs more often than AML does. Enlargement of lymph nodes, liver, and spleen is common at diagnosis. Bone pain, thought to result from leukemic infiltration of the periosteum or expansion of the medullary cavity, is a common complaint, particularly in children with ALL. Leukemic cells sometimes infiltrate the skin and result in a raised, nonpruritic rash, a condition termed *leukemia cutis*. Leukemic cells may infiltrate the leptomeninges and cause leukemic meningitis, typically manifested by headache and nausea. As the disease progresses, central nervous system (CNS) palsies and seizures may develop. Although less than 5% of patients with ALL have CNS involvement at diagnosis, the CNS is a frequent site of relapse; therefore, CNS prophylaxis is an essential component of ALL therapy. Because the incidence of CNS disease is low in AML, there is no proven benefit to CNS surveillance or prophylaxis. Testicular involvement is seen in ALL, and the testicles are a frequent site of relapse. In AML, collections of leukemic blast cells, often referred to as *chloromas* or *myeloblastomas*, can occur in virtually any soft tissue and appear as rubbery, fast-growing masses.

Certain clinical manifestations are unique to specific subtypes of leukemia. Patients with acute promyelocytic leukemia (APL) of the M3 type commonly have subclinical or clinically evident disseminated intravascular coagulation (DIC; Chapter 175) caused by tissue thromboplastins released by the leukemic cells. Acute monocytic or myelomonocytic leukemias are the forms of AML most likely to have extramedullary involvement. M6 leukemia often has a long prodromal phase. Patients with T-cell ALL frequently have mediastinal masses.

DIAGNOSIS

Abnormalities in peripheral blood counts are usually the initial laboratory evidence of acute leukemia. Anemia is present in most patients. Most are also at least mildly thrombocytopenic, and up to one fourth have severe thrombocytopenia (platelets <20,000/μL). Although most patients are granulocytopenic at diagnosis, the total peripheral white cell count is more variable; approximately 25% of patients have very high white cell counts (>50,000/μL), approximately 50% have white cell counts between 5000 and 50,000/μL, and about 25% have low white cell counts (<5000/μL). In most cases, blasts are present in the peripheral blood, although in some patients the percentage of blasts is quite low or absent.

The diagnosis of acute leukemia is typically established by marrow aspiration and biopsy, usually from the posterior iliac crest. Marrow aspirates and biopsy specimens are usually hypercellular and contain 20 to 100% blast cells, which largely replace the normal marrow (see Figs. 183-1 and 183-2). Occasionally, in addition to the blast cell infiltrate, other findings are present, such as marrow fibrosis (especially with M7 AML) or bone marrow necrosis. Marrow samples should also be evaluated by immunophenotyping and cytogenetics. If AML is suspected, samples should be evaluated for the presence of mutations in *FLT3*, *NPM1*, and *CEBPA*. A diagnostic lumbar puncture is generally recommended in suspected cases of ALL, but not in asymptomatic cases of AML.

The prothrombin and partial thromboplastin times are sometimes elevated. In APL, reduced fibrinogen and evidence of DIC are often seen. Other laboratory abnormalities frequently present are hyperuricemia, especially in ALL, and increased serum lactate dehydrogenase. In cases of high cell turnover and cell death (e.g., L3 ALL), evidence of *tumor lysis syndrome* may be noted at diagnosis, including hypocalcemia, hyperkalemia, hyperphosphatemia, hyperuricemia, and renal insufficiency. This syndrome, which is more commonly seen shortly after therapy is begun, can be rapidly fatal if untreated.

Differential Diagnosis

The diagnosis of acute leukemia is usually straightforward but can occasionally be difficult. Both leukemia and aplastic anemia (Chapter 165) can manifest with peripheral pancytopenia, but the finding of a hypoplastic marrow without blasts usually distinguishes aplastic anemia. An occasional patient has hypocellular marrow and a clonal cytogenetic abnormality, which establishes the diagnosis of myelodysplasia (Chapter 182) or hypocellular leukemia. A number of processes other than leukemia can lead to the appearance of immature cells in the peripheral blood. Although other small round cell neoplasms can infiltrate the marrow and mimic leukemia, immunologic markers are effective in differentiating the two. Leukemoid reactions to infections such as tuberculosis can result in the outpouring of large numbers of young myeloid cells, but the proportion of blasts in marrow or peripheral blood almost never reaches 20% in a *leukemoid reaction* (Chapter 167). Infectious mononucleosis (Chapter 377) and other viral illnesses can sometimes resemble ALL, particularly if large numbers of atypical lymphocytes are present in the peripheral blood and the disease is accompanied by immune thrombocytopenia or hemolytic anemia.

TREATMENT Rx

With the development of effective programs of combination chemotherapy and advances in hematopoietic cell transplantation, many patients with acute leukemia can be cured. These therapeutic measures are complex and are best carried out at centers with appropriate support services and experience in treating leukemia. Because leukemia is a rapidly progressive disease, specific antileukemic therapy should be started as soon after diagnosis as possible, usually within 72 hours. The goal of initial chemotherapy is to induce a complete remission (CR) with restoration of normal marrow function. In general, induction chemotherapy is intensive and is accompanied by significant toxicities. Therefore, patients should be stabilized to the extent possible before specific antileukemic therapy is begun.

Preparing the Patient for Therapy

Severe bleeding usually results from thrombocytopenia, which can be reversed with platelet transfusions (Chapter 177). Once thrombocytopenic bleeding is stopped, continued prophylactic transfusions of platelets is warranted to maintain the platelet count higher than 10,000/μL. Occasionally, patients also have evidence of DIC, usually associated with the diagnosis of M3 AML. If M3 AML is suspected as the cause, all-*trans*-retinoic acid (ATRA) should be started without waiting for molecular confirmation of the diagnosis; the drug can be discontinued if the diagnosis is not M3 AML. If active bleeding is due to DIC (Chapter 175), low doses of heparin (50 U/kg) given intravenously every 6 hours can be of benefit. Platelets and fresh-frozen plasma (or cryoprecipitate) should be transfused to maintain the platelet count higher than 50,000/μL and the fibrinogen level greater than 100 mg/dL until the DIC abates. Whether heparin should be given prophylactically to patients with laboratory evidence of DIC but no active bleeding is an often debated but unsettled question.

Blood cultures should be obtained in patients with fever and granulocytopenia; while awaiting culture results, infection should be assumed and broad-spectrum antibiotics begun empirically (Chapters 167 and 281). It is preferable to bring an infection under control before starting initial chemotherapy if the patient has an adequate granulocyte count. However, patients often have infection but essentially no granulocytes; in this situation, delaying chemotherapy is unlikely to be beneficial.

Patients with very high blast counts may develop symptoms attributable to the effect of masses of these immature cells on blood flow (leukostasis). Although randomized trials are lacking, many experts suggest immediate leukapheresis and administration of hydroxyurea (3 g/m²/day orally for 2 or 3 days) in an effort to rapidly lower counts in asymptomatic patients with AML presenting with while blood cell counts greater than 100,000/μL and for ALL patients presenting with counts greater than 300,000/μL.[9] The most often affected organs are the CNS and lungs. If CNS symptoms occur, immediate whole-brain irradiation (600 cGy in one dose) should be added. If pulmonary symptoms occur, high-dose corticosteroids are often used.

Before treatment, management in all patients should be aimed at preventing the tumor lysis syndrome. Patients should be hydrated and given allopurinol 100 to 200 mg orally or intravenously three times a day before chemotherapy is initiated. Allopurinol prevents the conversion of xanthine and hypoxanthine to uric acid, but does not affect already formed uric acid. Patients presenting with very high white cell counts may have uremia and anuria secondary to greatly increased serum uric acid levels and intratubular crystallization, even before starting therapy. These patients should be treated with rasburicase 0.20 mg/kg/day for up to 5 days intravenously, given over 30 minutes. Rasburicase promotes the catabolism of already formed uric acid to allantoin. Urinary alkalinization, a past standard, is no longer recommended because, although it increases uric acid solubility, it also increases the possibility of xanthine and calcium phosphate precipitation in the kidney.

The diagnosis of leukemia usually comes as a profound psychological shock to the patient and family. Therefore, in addition to stabilizing the patient hematologically and metabolically, it is worthwhile to have at least one formal conference in which the patient and family are advised about the meaning of the diagnosis of leukemia and the consequences of therapy before treatment is initiated.

Treatment of Acute Lymphoblastic Leukemia

After the patient's condition has been stabilized, antileukemic therapy should be started as soon as possible.[10] Treatment of newly diagnosed ALL can be divided into three phases: remission induction, postremission therapy, and CNS prophylaxis.

Remission Induction

The initial goal of treatment is to induce CR, defined as the reduction of leukemic blasts to undetectable levels and the restoration of normal marrow function. A number of different chemotherapeutic combinations can be used to induce remission; all include vincristine and prednisone, and most add L-asparaginase and daunorubicin, administered over a period of 3 to 4 weeks. With such regimens, CR is achieved in 90% of children and 80 to 90% of adults (Table 183-2). Because vincristine, prednisone, and L-asparaginase are relatively nontoxic to normal marrow precursors, the disease often enters CR after a relatively brief period of myelosuppression. Failure to achieve CR is usually due to either the leukemic cells' resistance to the drugs or progressive infection. These two complications occur with approximately equal frequency.

Postremission Chemotherapy

If no further therapy is given after induction of CR, relapse occurs in almost all cases, usually within several months. Chemotherapy after CR can be given in a variety of combinations, dosages, and schedules. The term *consolidation chemotherapy* refers to short courses of further chemotherapy given at doses similar to those used for initial induction (requiring rehospitalization). Usually, different drugs are selected for consolidation chemotherapy than were used to induce the initial remission. In the case of ALL, such drugs include high-dose methotrexate, cyclophosphamide, and cytarabine, among others. Most regimens include six to eight courses of intensive consolidation therapy. Maintenance involves the administration of low-dose chemotherapy on a daily or weekly outpatient basis for long periods. The most commonly used maintenance regimen in ALL combines daily 6-mercaptopurine and weekly or biweekly methotrexate. The optimal duration of maintenance chemotherapy is unknown, but it is usually given for 2 to 3 years. Maintenance is most beneficial for patients with pro- and pre-B-cell ALL, less so for T-cell ALL, and of no apparent benefit for patients with mature B-cell ALL.

Central Nervous System Prophylaxis

Most chemotherapeutic agents that are given intravenously or orally do not penetrate the CNS well, and if no form of CNS prophylaxis is given, at least 35% of adults with ALL will develop CNS leukemia. With prophylaxis, relapse in the CNS as an isolated event occurs in less than 10% of patients. Systemic chemotherapy with high-dose methotrexate (e.g., 200 mg/m² intravenously over 2 hours, followed by 800 mg/m² over 22 hours) and cytarabine (e.g., 3 g/m² over 2 hours every 12 hours for four doses) can achieve therapeutic drug levels within the CNS. Alternatives are intrathecal methotrexate, intrathecal methotrexate combined with 2400 cGy radiation to the cranium, or 2400 cGy to the craniospinal axis.

Treatment of Burkitt-like ALL

Burkitt-like ALL (also called FAB L3 or mature B-cell ALL) is characterized by the presence of monoclonal surface immunoglobulin, cytogenetics showing t(8;14), and the constitutive expression of the *MYC* oncogene. Burkitt-like ALL, which accounts for 3 to 5% of adult cases of ALL, responds well to regimens that incorporate short, intensive courses of high-dose methotrexate (1.5 g/m² over 24 hours with leucovorin), cytarabine (3 g/m² over 2 hours every 12 hours for four doses), and cyclophosphamide (200 mg/m²/day for 5 days); this regimen yields high rates of complete response and cures in about 50% of

TABLE 183-2 COMMON REGIMENS FOR COMMON FORMS OF ACUTE LEUKEMIA

I. MANAGEMENT OF NEWLY DIAGNOSED ACUTE MYELOID LEUKEMIA

A. Induction—daunorubicin 60-90 mg/m²/day for 3 days (or idarubicin 10-12 mg/m²/day for 3 days) and cytarabine 200 mg/m²/day for 7 days
B. Postremission
  1. Favorable risk—cytarabine 3 g/m² over 3 hr q12h on days 1, 3, and 5 every month for 4 mo
  2. Intermediate risk—as for favorable risk; or, if HLA-matched related or unrelated donor exists, allogeneic hematopoietic cell transplantation
  3. Unfavorable risk—proceed to allogeneic transplantation if possible; if not, treat as for intermediate risk

II. MANAGEMENT OF NEWLY DIAGNOSED ACUTE PROMYELOCYTIC LEUKEMIA

A. Induction—ATRA 45 mg/m²/day until complete remission plus daunomycin 45-60 mg/m²/day for 3 days and cytarabine 200 mg/m²/day for 7 days
B. Consolidation #1—arsenic trioxide 0.15 mg/kg/day 5 days/wk for 5 wk; repeat course after 2-wk rest
   Consolidation #2—ATRA 45 mg/m²/day for 7 days and daunomycin 50 mg/m²/day for 3 days; repeat course 1 mo later
C. Maintenance—ATRA 45 mg/m²/day for 15 days every 3 mo plus 6-MP 100 mg/m²/day and MTX 10 mg/m²/wk for 2 yr

Or, if intermediate/good risk, consider:
  A. Induction: Arsenic trioxide 0.15 mg/kg/day plus ATRA 45 mg/m²/day until complete remission
  B. Consolidation: Arsenic trioxide 0.15 mg/kg/day 5 days/wk, 4 wk on, 4 wk off for 4 cycles
     ATRA 45mg/m²/day 2 wk on, 2 wk off for 7 cycles

III. MANAGEMENT OF NEWLY DIAGNOSED ADULT PH-NEGATIVE ACUTE LYMPHOID LEUKEMIA

A. Induction (and courses 3, 5, 7)—cyclophosphamide 300 mg/m² over 3 hr q12h for 6 doses on days 1, 2, 3; doxorubicin 50 mg/m² on day 4; vincristine 2 mg/day on days 4 and 11; and dexamethasone 40 mg/day on days 1-4 and days 11-14
B. Consolidation (courses 2, 4, 6, 8)—MTX 200 mg/m² over 2 hr, followed by 800 mg/m² over 22 hr on day 1; high-dose cytarabine 3 g/m² over 2 hr q12h for 4 doses on days 2 and 3
C. Four intrathecal treatments of MTX 12 mg alternating with cytarabine 100 mg are given during the first four courses of systemic therapy

ATRA = all-*trans*-retinoic acid; HLA = human leukocyte antigen; 6-MP = 6-mercaptopurine; MTX = methotrexate; Ph = Philadelphia chromosome [t(9;22)].

patients. Recent results suggest that the addition of rituximab may further improve outcomes.

Treatment of Philadelphia Chromosome–Positive ALL

Approximately 5% of pediatric cases and 25% of adult cases of ALL have cytogenetics showing t(9;22), the Ph chromosome. Historically, such patients had CR rates slightly lower than those seen in Ph-negative ALL and markedly reduced remission durations, averaging less than a year; few if any such patients were cured with conventional chemotherapy. Therefore, the general recommendation has been that such patients receive an allogeneic transplant during the first remission, if possible. With this approach, approximately 50% of patients can be cured. More recently, the addition of the tyrosine kinase inhibitor imatinib mesylate to conventional chemotherapeutic regimens has increased complete response rates, equaling those seen in Ph-negative ALL, but the impact of the addition of imatinib mesylate on the duration of remission is not yet known. Dasatinib, a second-generation BCR-ABL tyrosine kinase inhibitor, has demonstrated efficacy in relapsed/refractory adult Ph-positive ALL. Therapy with dasatinib and prednisone alone without chemotherapy appears sufficient to allow the majority of older patients with Ph-positive ALL to achieve an initial hematologic remission.[11]

Prognosis of ALL after Initial Chemotherapy

A number of factors are predictive of outcome in ALL, the most important of which are younger age, a lower white cell count at diagnosis, and favorable cytogenetics. With currently available treatment regimens, 80 to 85% of children and 35 to 40% of adults who initially achieve CR maintain that state for more than 5 years, and these patients are probably cured of their disease.

Treatment of Relapsed ALL

Most relapses occur within 2 years after diagnosis, and most occur in the marrow. Occasionally, relapse is initially found in an extramedullary site such as the CNS or testes. Extramedullary relapse is usually followed shortly by systemic (marrow) relapse and should be considered part of a systemic recurrence. With the use of chemotherapeutic regimens similar to those used for initial induction, 50 to 70% of patients achieve at least a short-lived second remission. A small percentage of patients for whom the initial remission was longer than 2 years may be cured with salvage chemotherapy. If the CNS or testes is the initial site of the relapse, specific therapy to that site is also required, along with systemic retreatment. Because the prognosis of relapsed leukemia treated with chemotherapy is so poor, hematopoietic stem cell transplantation is usually recommended in this setting. Newer agents active in recurrent ALL include nelarabine for T-cell ALL and the anti-CD19 targeted agent blinatumomab and the anti-CD22 immunoconjugate inotuzumab in B-cell ALL. Complete responses have also recently been reported in early trials using chimeric antigen receptor T cells targeting CD19.[12]

Hematopoietic Stem Cell Transplantation

The use of high-dose chemoradiotherapy followed by hematopoietic stem cell transplantation (Chapter 178) from an HLA-identical sibling can cure 20 to 40% of patients with ALL who fail to achieve an initial remission or who have a relapse after an initial CR; it can cure 50 to 60% of patients who undergo transplantation during a first remission. Although there is still considerable debate, several recent studies have reported improved survival for adults with high-risk or standard-risk ALL who receive a hematopoietic stem cell transplant during a first remission rather than being treated with standard chemotherapy.[A1,A2] The major limitations of transplantation are graft-versus-host disease, interstitial pneumonia, and recurrence of disease. If an HLA-identical sibling is not available, transplantation from a matched unrelated donor or transplantation of cord blood from a partially matched unrelated donor can be conducted, with results that approach those seen with matched related donors.

Treatment of Acute Myeloid Leukemia

Remission Induction

Treatment with a combination of an anthracycline and cytarabine (100 to 200 mg/m^2/day for 7 days) leads to CR in 60 to 80% of patients with AML. Prospective randomized trials have demonstrated that for patients aged 65 years or less idarubicin (10 to 12 mg/m^2/day for 3 days) or a higher dose of daunorubicin (60 to 90 mg/m^2/day for 3 days) is superior to the conventional daunorubicin dose of 45 mg/m^2/day for 3 days.[A3,A4] Profound myelosuppression always follows when these agents are used at doses capable of achieving CR. Failure to achieve CR is usually due to either drug resistance or fatal complications of myelosuppression. In a randomized study of adults with AML, five doses of intravenous gemtuzumab ozogamicin (3 mg/m^2 on days 1, 4, and 7 during induction and day 1 of each of the two consolidation chemotherapy courses) doubled the probability of event-free survival at 2 years.[A5]

Postremission Therapy

Intensive consolidation chemotherapy with repeated courses of daunorubicin and cytarabine at doses similar to those used for induction, high-dose cytarabine (1 to 3 g/m^2/day for 3 to 6 days), or other agents prolongs the average remission duration and improves the chances for long-term disease-free survival. The best results reported to date have generally been achieved with repeated cycles of high-dose cytarabine.[13] Unlike the situation with ALL, low-dose maintenance therapy is of limited benefit after intensive consolidation treatment. In AML, leukemic recurrence occurs less often in the CNS (approximately 10% of cases), most commonly in patients with the M4 or M5 variant. There is no evidence that CNS prophylaxis improves survival in AML.

Prognosis of AML after Initial Chemotherapy

Among patients in whom CR is achieved, 20 to 40% remain alive in continuous CR for more than 5 years, suggesting a probable cure. As with ALL, younger patients and those with a low white cell count at diagnosis have a more favorable outcome. The European LeukemiaNet recognizes four risk categories of AML based on cytogenetics and molecular testing.[14] The favorable group includes those with t(8;21) or inv(16) and those with normal cytogenetics but mutated *CEBPA* or mutated *NPM1* and wild-type *FLT3*. Intermediate I patients are those with normal cytogenetics but without mutations in *NPM1* and *CEBPA*, or with mutations in *FLT3*. Intermediate II includes those with t(9;11), t(11;19), or those with cytogenetics abnormalities not classified as favorable or unfavorable. Finally, the unfavorable group includes those with inv(3), t(6:9), −5 or del5, −7 or del7, and those with complex cytogenetics (Fig. 183-3). Patients with *DNMT3A* and *NPM1* mutations and those with *MLL* translocations appear to selectively benefit from higher dose induction.[15] Patients who have a preleukemic phase before their condition evolves into acute leukemia and those whose leukemia is secondary to prior exposure to chemotherapy have a poorer prognosis. Increased expression of the multidrug resistance gene 1 *(MDR1)* is also associated with a worse outcome.

Treatment of Recurrent AML

Patients whose AML recurs after initial chemotherapy can achieve a second remission in about 50% of cases after retreatment with daunorubicin-cytarabine or high-dose cytarabine. The likelihood of achieving a second

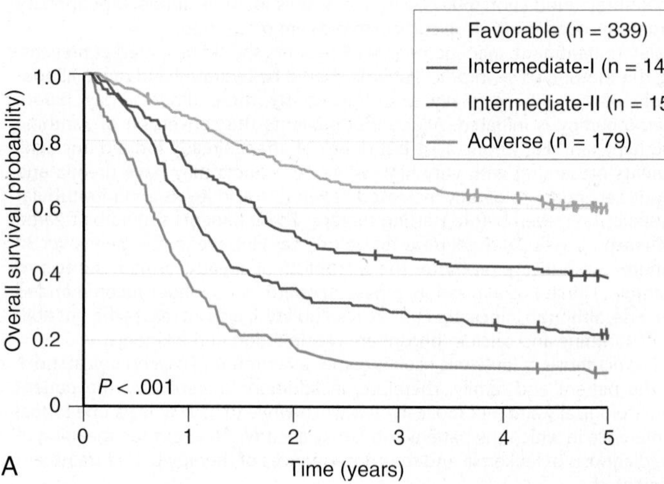

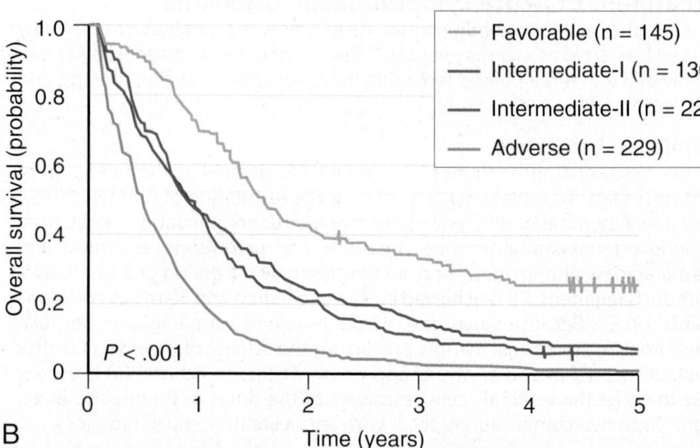

FIGURE 183-3. **Overall survival in acute myeloid leukemia according to European LeukemiaNet risk groups. A, Overall survival in patients younger than 60 years. B, Overall survival in patients 60 years and older. (From Mrózek K, et al. Prognostic significance of the European LeukemiaNet standardized system for reporting cytogenetic and molecular alterations in adults with acute myeloid leukemia. *J Clin Oncol.* 2012;30: 4515-4523).**

remission is predicted by the duration of the first remission: 70% in patients whose first remission persisted beyond 2 years, compared with less than 15% in those whose first remission lasted less than 6 months. Older patients may benefit from gemtuzumab ozogamicin (9 mg/m^2 intravenously on days 1 and 15), a form of antibody-targeted chemotherapy. Second remissions tend to be short-lived, however, and few patients in whom relapse occurs after first-line chemotherapy are cured by salvage chemotherapy.

Treatment of Acute Promyelocytic Leukemia

CR can be induced in at least 90% of patients with APL by using ATRA (45 mg/m^2/day orally until CR is achieved) in combination with an anthracycline.[16] Patients treated with ATRA usually have their coagulation disorders corrected within several days. A unique toxicity of ATRA in the treatment of APL is the development of hyperleukocytosis accompanied by respiratory distress and pulmonary infiltrates. The syndrome responds to temporary discontinuation of ATRA and the addition of corticosteroids. By combining ATRA with anthracyclines for induction and consolidation and then using ATRA as maintenance therapy, approximately 70% of patients can be cured. Arsenic trioxide (0.15 mg/kg/day intravenously until CR is achieved) is effective in patients with recurrent APL and appears to improve overall survival if used as part of consolidation therapy for patients in their first CR. The combination of ATRA plus arsenic trioxide without any chemotherapy has recently been shown to be as effective as the standard ATRA-chemotherapy combination for patients with low- or-intermediate risk APL (i.e., those who present with white blood cell counts <10,000/μL).[A6]

Hematopoietic Stem Cell Transplantation

For patients with AML in whom an initial remission cannot be achieved or for those who relapse after chemotherapy, hematopoietic stem cell transplantation (Chapter 178) from an HLA-identical sibling offers the best chance for cure. Fifteen percent of patients with end-stage disease can be saved by this treatment. If the procedure is applied earlier, the outcome is better: approximately 30% of patients who undergo hematopoietic stem cell transplantation at first relapse or second remission are cured, and 50 to 60% of patients are cured if hematopoietic stem cell transplantation is performed during the first remission. A large number of studies have prospectively compared the outcome of allogeneic hematopoietic stem cell transplantation with that of chemotherapy in patients with AML in first remission. The trends in all these studies have been toward higher treatment-related mortality but improved disease-free and overall survival time with allogeneic transplantation. Meta-analyses conclude that survival is improved with allogeneic transplantation from a matched sibling in first remission when compared with continued chemotherapy.[A7] This improvement is clearest in patients with unfavorable or intermediate-risk disease and is not seen in those in the favorable-risk category. The major limitations of allogeneic hematopoietic stem cell transplantation are lack of a matched sibling donor, graft-versus-host disease, interstitial pneumonia, and disease recurrence. Because transplant-related toxicities increase with patient age, some centers limit hematopoietic stem cell transplantation to those 65 years of age or younger. However, recent studies of reduced-intensity or nonmyeloablative allogeneic transplantation have shown encouraging results in patients with AML in remission at ages up to 75 years. Allogeneic transplantation using matched unrelated donors results in survival essentially equivalent to that seen using matched siblings, although there is a higher incidence of complications.[17] Autologous hematopoietic stem cell transplantation offers an alternative for patients without matched siblings to serve as donors. In randomized trials, the use of autologous transplantation after consolidation chemotherapy significantly prolonged the duration of disease-free survival for patients with AML in first remission but did not alter overall survival.[18]

Treatment of AML in Older Patients

The benefits of intensive consolidation chemotherapy in younger patients do not translate to patients older than 65 years, in part because older patients are less able to tolerate therapy, but also because AML in older patients is more often associated with unfavorable cytogenetics (particularly abnormalities of chromosomes 5 and 7) and more often overexpresses P-glycoprotein, resulting in the multidrug resistance phenotype. Accordingly, long-term survival rates of only 10 to 15% are seen with chemotherapy in patients older than 65 years. Otherwise healthy older patients can usually tolerate intensive chemotherapy and should be offered this treatment. However, intensive chemotherapy can cause more harm than good in older patients with poor performance status. In prospective randomized trials, low-dose cytarabine prolonged survival in older patients unfit for intensive therapy. Other alternative therapies for this group of patients include the demethylating agents azacitidine or decitabine or entry onto clinical trials.[19]

MANAGEMENT OF COMPLICATIONS

Treatment of acute leukemia, especially AML, is accompanied by a number of complications, the two most serious and frequent being infection and bleeding. During the granulocytopenic period that follows induction and consolidation chemotherapy, the risk for bacterial infection is high. A Cochrane review examined results of antibiotic prophylaxis compared with placebo in afebrile neutropenic patients. Antibiotic prophylaxis significantly decreased infection-related deaths, with the best results seen with quinolones.[A8] Despite prophylaxis, many patients are febrile while neutropenic, and patients can still develop important infections. The most common bacterial species vary somewhat from medical center to medical center, but *Staphylococcus* (primarily *S. epidermidis*) and *Enterococcus* species are the most frequent gram-positive organisms, whereas *Pseudomonas aeruginosa* and enteric organisms such as *Escherichia coli* and *Klebsiella* species are the most common gram-negative organisms isolated.

Even if no cause for fever is found, bacterial infection should be assumed, and, in general, all patients with fever and neutropenia should receive broad-spectrum antibiotics (Chapters 167 and 281). Monotherapy with an intravenous antipseudomonal agent, such as a carbapenem (e.g., imipenem-cilastatin), a cephalosporin (e.g., cefepime), or an antipseudomonal penicillin (e.g., piperacillin-tazobactam), is recommended as empirical therapy. Vancomycin should not be part of standard coverage in most patients but may be used in those with suspected catheter infections or severe mucositis and in patients with hemodynamic instability or altered mental status. Combination therapy with other gram-negative agents (e.g., aminoglycosides) may be needed. Once begun, antibiotics should be continued until patients recover their granulocyte counts, even if they become afebrile first. If documented bacteremia persists despite appropriate antibiotics, the physician should consider removal of indwelling catheters.

Invasive fungal infections are also common following chemotherapy for acute leukemia and are associated with significant morbidity and mortality. A review of randomized trials found a significant reduction in death from fungal infection in patients given antifungal prophylaxis. Posaconazole is considered by many to be more effective than fluconazole or itraconazole. In addition to being granulocytopenic, patients undergoing induction chemotherapy for leukemia have deficient cellular and humoral immunity, at least temporarily, and therefore are subject to infections common in other immunodeficiency states, including *Pneumocystis jirovecii* (formerly *Pneumocystis carinii*) infection and a variety of viral infections. *P. jirovecii* infection can be prevented by the prophylactic use of trimethoprim-sulfamethoxazole. In cytomegalovirus (CMV) -seronegative patients, CMV-seronegative or leukocyte-reduced blood products should be used to prevent primary infection (Chapter 376). Herpes simplex (Chapter 374) can often complicate existing mucositis and can be prevented with prophylactic acyclovir. Acyclovir is also useful for the prevention and treatment of herpes zoster (Chapter 375).

Myeloid growth factors (granulocyte or granulocyte-macrophage colony-stimulating factor; Chapter 156), if given shortly after the completion of chemotherapy, shorten the period of severe myelosuppression by, on average, 4 days. In most studies, this accelerated recovery has resulted in fewer days with fever and less use of antibiotics, but it has not improved the complete response rate or altered survival.

The platelet count that signals a need for platelet transfusion has been the subject of debate. Traditionally, platelet transfusions from random donors were used to maintain platelet counts greater than 20,000/μL, but more recently it has been demonstrated that lowering this threshold to 10,000/μL is safe in patients with no active bleeding. In contrast, a no-prophylaxis strategy results in more days with bleeding and a shorter time to first bleeding episode and therefore is not recommended.[A9] In 30 to 50% of cases, patients eventually become alloimmunized and require the use of HLA-matched platelets (Chapter 177). Transfusion-induced graft-versus-host disease (Chapter 177), manifesting as a rash, low-grade fever, elevated values in liver function tests, and decreasing blood counts, can be prevented by irradiating all blood products before transfusion.

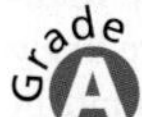

Grade A References

A1. Goldstone AH, Richards SM, Lazarus HM, et al. In adults with standard-risk acute lymphoblastic leukemia, the greatest benefit is achieved from a matched sibling allogeneic transplantation in first complete remission, and an autologous transplantation is less effective than conventional consolidation/maintenance chemotherapy in all patients: final results of the International ALL Trial (MRC UKALL XII/ECOG E2993). *Blood*. 2008;111:1827-1833.

A2. Ram R, Gafter-Gvili A, Vidal L, et al. Management of adult patients with acute lymphoblastic leukemia in first complete remission: systematic review and meta-analysis. *Cancer*. 2010;116:3447-3457.

A3. Fernandez HF, Sun Z, Yao X, et al. Anthracycline dose intensification in acute myeloid leukemia. *N Engl J Med*. 2009;361:1249-1259.

A4. Lowenberg B, Ossenkoppele GJ, van Putten W, et al. High-dose daunorubicin in older patients with acute myeloid leukemia. *N Engl J Med*. 2009;361:1235-1248.

A5. Castaigne S, Pautas C, Terré C, et al. Effect of gemtuzumab ozogamicin on survival of adult patients with de-novo acute myeloid leukaemia (ALFA-0701): a randomised, open-label, phase 3 study. *Lancet*. 2012;379:1508-1516.

A6. Lo-Coco F, Avvisati G, Vignetti M, et al. Retinoic acid and arsenic trioxide for acute promyelocytic leukemia. *N Engl J Med*. 2013;369:111-121.

A7. Koreth J, Schlenk R, Kopecky KJ, et al. Allogeneic stem cell transplantation for acute myeloid leukemia in first complete remission: a systematic review and meta-analysis of prospective clinical trials. *JAMA*. 2009;301:2349-2360.

A8. Gafter-Gvili A, Fraser A, Paul M, et al. Meta-analysis: antibiotic prophylaxis reduces mortality in neutropenic patients. *Ann Intern Med*. 2005;142:979-995.

A9. Stanworth SJ, Estcourt LJ, Powter G, et al. A no-prophylaxis platelet-transfusion strategy for hematologic cancers. *N Engl J Med*. 2013;368:1771-1780.

GENERAL REFERENCES

For the General References and other additional features, please visit Expert Consult at https://expertconsult.inkling.com.

184 THE CHRONIC LEUKEMIAS

SUSAN O'BRIEN AND ELIAS JABBOUR

CHRONIC MYELOGENOUS LEUKEMIA

DEFINITION

Chronic myelogenous leukemia (CML), also called chronic myeloid leukemia, is a clonal myeloproliferative neoplasm of the primitive hematopoietic stem cell that is characterized by overproduction of cells of the myeloid series, resulting in marked splenomegaly and leukocytosis. Basophilia and thrombocytosis are common. A characteristic cytogenetic abnormality, the Philadelphia (Ph) chromosome, which produces the fusion oncogene *BCR-ABL*, is present in the bone marrow cells in more than 90% of cases. Most patients (85 to 90%) present in the chronic phase. Eventually, if poorly controlled, CML evolves into the accelerated and blastic phases.

EPIDEMIOLOGY

CML constitutes one fifth of all cases of leukemia in the United States. It is diagnosed in 1 or 2 persons per 100,000 per year and has a slight male preponderance. This incidence of 4800 to 5000 cases annually has not changed significantly in the past few decades. The incidence of CML increases with age; the median age at diagnosis is 50 to 55 years. Ph-positive *BCR-ABL*-positive CML is uncommon in children and adolescents. No familial association of CML has been noted; for example, the risk is not increased in monozygotic twins or in relatives of patients with CML. Because of the availability of effective therapy, the annual mortality has been reduced from 15 to 20%, before 2000, to 1 to 2% currently.[1] Thus, the prevalence of CML is predicted to increase gradually, from 15,000 to 20,000 cases before 2000 up to 180,000 cases by 2030 in the United States.

Usually, no etiologic agent is incriminated in CML. Exposure to ionizing radiation (e.g., in survivors of the atomic bomb explosions in Japan in 1945, in those undergoing radiation treatment for ankylosing spondylitis or cervical cancer) increases the risk for CML; the peak incidence occurs 5 to 12 years after exposure and is dose related. No increase in the risk for CML has been demonstrated among individuals working in the nuclear industry. Radiologists working without adequate protection before 1940 were more likely to develop myeloid leukemia, but no such association has been found in recent studies. Benzene exposure increases the risk for acute myelogenous leukemia (AML) but not of CML. CML is not a frequent secondary leukemia after treatment of other cancers with radiation, alkylating agents, or both.

PATHOBIOLOGY

Molecular Pathogenesis

The Ph chromosome abnormality, present in more than 90% of patients with typical CML (Fig. 184-1), results from a balanced translocation of genetic material between the long arms of chromosomes 9 and 22: t(9;22)(q34;q11.2). The breakpoint at band q34 of chromosome 9 results in

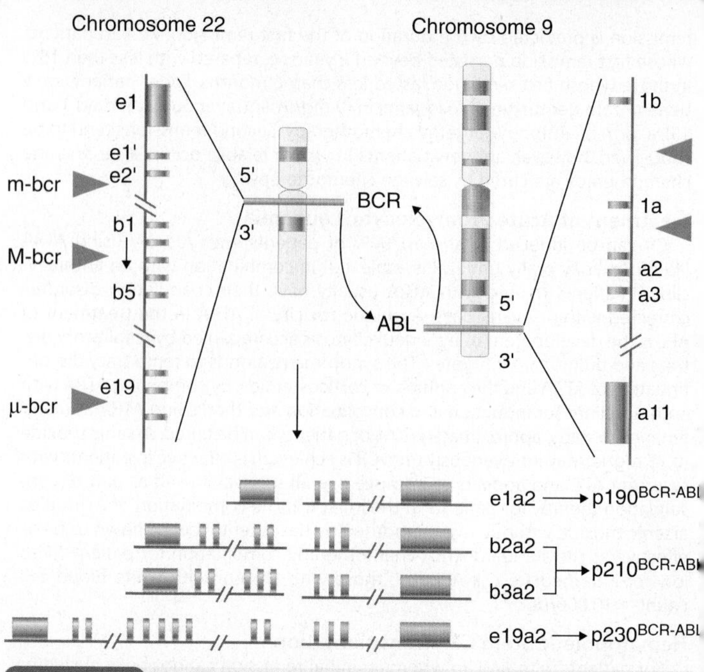

FIGURE 184-1. The Philadelphia chromosome. Originally described as a shortened long arm of chromosome 22, the Philadelphia chromosome (Ph) was later found to be the result of a balanced translocation of genetic material between the long arms of chromosomes 9 and 22: t(9;22)(q34;qll.2). This results in the juxtaposition of *ABL1* to *BCR*, producing a hybrid *BCR-ABL1* oncogene. Depending on the breakpoint on *BCR*, three oncoproteins may be produced: p210$^{BCR-ABL1}$, which is associated with 98% or more of the cases of Ph-positive chronic myelogenous leukemia (CML); p190$^{BCR-ABL1}$, which is associated with 60 to 80% of cases of Ph-positive acute lymphocytic leukemia (the other 20 to 40% of cases are p210$^{BCR-ABL1}$); and p230$^{BCR-ABL}$, which is associated with rare cases of Ph-positive CML.

translocation of the cellular oncogene *ABL1* (previously *c-ABL*) to a region on chromosome 22 coding for the major breakpoint cluster region (*BCR*). *ABL1* is a homologue of *v-ABL*, the Abelson virus that causes leukemia in mice. This translocation allows juxtaposition of a 5′ portion of a *BCR* and 3′ position of *ABL*; the two genetic sequences produce a new hybrid oncogene (*BCR-ABL1*), which codes for a novel BCR-ABLI oncoprotein with a molecular weight of 210 kD (p210$^{BCR-ABLI}$). The p210$^{BCR-ABLI}$ oncoprotein results in uncontrolled kinase activity of BCR-ABLI, which triggers the excessive proliferation and reduced apoptosis of CML cells, thereby giving CML cells a growth advantage over normal cells and suppressing normal hematopoiesis. Although in most cases 100% of the metaphases on cytogenetic analysis show *BCR-ABL1*, normal stem cells emerge on long-term bone marrow culture and after treatment with interferon-α (IFN-α), imatinib, and other BCR-ABLI-selective tyrosine kinase inhibitors (TKIs).

The constitutive activation of BCR-ABLI results in autophosphorylation and activation of multiple downstream pathways that affect gene transcription, apoptosis, cytoskeletal organization, cytoadhesions, and degradation of inhibitory proteins. The signal transduction pathways implicated involve RAS, mitogen-activated-protein (MAP) kinases, signal transducers and activators of transcription (STAT), phosphatidyl inositol 3-kinase (PI3K), MYC, and others. Many of these interactions are mediated through tyrosine phosphorylation and require binding of the BCR-ABLI to adapter proteins such as GRB-2, CRK, CRK-like protein (CRKL), and SCR homology-containing proteins (SHC). Although imatinib and new-generation TKIs (nilotinib, dasatinib, bosutinib, ponatinib) have been extremely successful at targeting BCR-ABLI, understanding of the pathophysiology of the downstream events of BCR-ABLI is important for the future development of agents that may target these events.

In Ph-positive acute lymphocytic leukemia (ALL), the breakpoint in *BCR* is proximal, in the minor *BCR*, resulting in a smaller *BCR* gene apposing *ABL1*; the resulting fusion gene, messenger RNA, and BCR-ABLI oncoprotein (p190$^{BCR-ABLI}$) are smaller. A third rare, "micro" *BCR* breakpoint distal to the major *BCR* produces a p230$^{BCR-ABLI}$ hybrid oncoprotein, which is associated with a more indolent CML course.

What induces this molecular rearrangement is unknown. Molecular techniques that amplify detection of *BCR-ABL1* have demonstrated its presence in the marrow cells of 25 to 30% of healthy volunteers and 5% of infants, but not in cord blood. Because clinical CML develops in only 1 to 2 of 100,000 individuals (i.e., 1 to 2 per 25,000 to 30,000 individuals who express *BCR-ABL* in their bone marrow), immune regulatory processes or additional molecular events presumably contribute to the development of CML.

BCR-ABL1 is found only in hematopoietic cells and has its origin close to the pluripotent stem cell. The Ph chromosome occurs in erythroid, myeloid, monocytic, and megakaryocytic cells; less commonly in B lymphocytes; rarely in T lymphocytes; and not at all in marrow fibroblasts. The fusion *BCR-ABL1* gene and the p210 protein can be found in cases of morphologically typical CML in which no cytogenetic abnormality occurs or in which changes other than the typical t(9;22) (q34;q11.2) are identified. These patients have a survival rate and a response to therapy similar to those of patients with Ph-positive CML. Patients with atypical CML (usually older and more frequently exhibiting anemia, thrombocytopenia, monocytosis, and dysplasia) who are Ph negative and *BCR-ABL1* negative have a worse prognosis than those who are either Ph positive or Ph negative and *BCR-ABL1* positive; they more closely resemble patients with myelodysplastic syndrome (Chapter 182). Thus, three groups of patients with CML can be identified: (1) those who are positive for Ph and *BCR-ABL1;* (2) those who are Ph negative but *BCR-ABL1* positive; and (3) those who are negative for Ph and *BCR-ABL1. PDGFB* (previously *SIS),* which codes for platelet-derived growth factor (PDGF) and is the homologue of the simian sarcoma virus, is also translocated from chromosome 22 to chromosome 9 in CML, but it is distant from the breakpoint and is not expressed.

The pathophysiologic mechanisms underlying CML resistance to TKIs is a fascinating topic that has now been replicated with other targeted therapies in other hematologic and solid tumors. Several mechanisms of resistance to TKIs have been identified; the most common are mutations in the BCR-ABLl kinase domain. More than 100 different mutations have been reported and can involve any of the important domains in the BCR-ABLl structure, including the P-loop (the area where adenosine triphosphate [ATP] binds), the activation loop, and the catalytic domain, as well as the amino acids where imatinib makes contact with BCR-ABLl. The different mutations have considerable variability with respect to resistance to imatinib and other TKIs. Some mutations are overcome by higher concentrations of imatinib than required to inhibit the wild-type form; others are completely insensitive to imatinib. Mutational analysis is useful in patients with imatinib resistance to identify those with the T3151 mutation, who do not respond to imatinib or the second-generation TKIs (dasatinib, nilotinib, bosutinib) but do respond to ponatinib therapy. Knowledge of the sensitivity of the different mutations, as determined by the IC_{50} for particular agents, can help select the TKIs.

CLINICAL MANIFESTATIONS

About 40 to 50% of patients diagnosed with CML do not have symptoms, and the disease is found on routine physical examinations or blood tests. In these patients, the white blood cell (WBC) count may be relatively low at diagnosis. The degree of leukocytosis correlates with tumor burden, as defined by spleen size.

The symptoms of CML, when present, are due to anemia and splenomegaly; they include fatigue, weight loss, malaise, easy satiety, and left upper quadrant fullness or pain. Rarely, bleeding or thrombosis occurs. Other rare presentations include gouty arthritis (from elevated uric acid levels), priapism (usually with marked leukocytosis or thrombocytosis), retinal hemorrhages, and upper gastrointestinal ulceration and bleeding (from elevated histamine levels due to basophilia). Headaches, bone pain, arthralgias, pain from splenic infarction, and fever are uncommon in the chronic phase but more frequent as CML progresses. Symptoms of leukostasis, such as dyspnea, drowsiness, loss of coordination, or confusion, which are due to leukocyte sludging in the pulmonary or cerebral vessels, are uncommon in the chronic phase despite WBC counts exceeding 50×10^9 cells/μL, but these symptoms appear more frequently in the accelerated or blastic phases of the disease.

Splenomegaly, the most consistent physical sign in CML, occurs in 30 to 50% of cases. Hepatomegaly is less common (10 to 20%) and usually minor. Lymphadenopathy is uncommon, as is infiltration of skin or other tissues. If present, these findings suggest Ph-negative CML or the accelerated or blastic phase of CML.

DIAGNOSIS

The diagnosis of typical CML is not difficult. Patients with untreated CML usually have leukocytosis ranging from 10 to 500×10^9/μL. The predominant cells are neutrophils, with a left shift extending to blast cells. Basophils and eosinophils are commonly increased. Monocytes may be slightly increased in some cases that overlap with chronic myelomonocytic leukemia (CMML; see later discussion). Thrombocytosis is common, whereas thrombocytopenia is rare and, if present, suggests a worse prognosis. A hemoglobin level of less than 11 g/dL is present in one third of patients. Some patients demonstrate a cyclic oscillation of the WBC count. The presence of unexplained myeloid leukocytosis (Fig. 184-2) with splenomegaly should lead to a bone marrow examination and cytogenetic and molecular analysis.

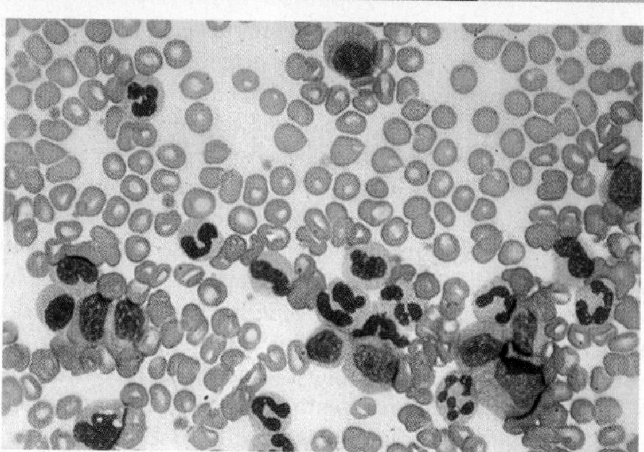

FIGURE 184-2. Chronic myelogenous leukemia, chronic phase. Peripheral smear shows leukocytosis, with representation by the entire spectrum of leukocyte differentiation, ranging from myeloblasts to mature neutrophils. (Courtesy Andrew Schafer, MD.)

Bone Marrow

The bone marrow is hypercellular, with marked myeloid hyperplasia and, at times, evidence of increased reticulin or collagen fibrosis. The myeloid-erythroid ratio is 15 : 1 to 20 : 1. About 15% of patients have 5% or more blast cells in the peripheral blood or bone marrow at diagnosis.

Cytogenetics

The presence of the t(9; 22) (q34; q11.2) abnormality establishes the diagnosis of CML. If the Ph chromosome is not found in a patient with suspected CML, molecular studies for the presence of the hybrid *BCR-ABL1* gene should be performed. About 25 to 30% of patients with a typical morphologic picture of CML who are Ph negative have the *BCR-ABL1* rearrangement. The Ph chromosome is usually present in 100% of metaphases, often as the sole abnormality. Between 10 and 15% of patients have additional chromosomal changes (loss of the Y chromosome, trisomy 8, an additional loss of material from 22q, or double Ph). Some patients have complex chromosomal changes involving chromosome 9 or chromosome 22 (Ph variants, three-way translocations).

Differential Diagnosis

CML must be differentiated from leukemoid reactions (Chapter 167), which usually produce WBC counts lower than 50×10^9/μL, and toxic granulocytic vacuolation, Döhle bodies in the granulocytes, absence of basophilia, and normal or increased leukocyte alkaline phosphatase (LAP) levels (which are typically low in CML). The clinical history and physical examination generally suggest the origin of the leukemoid reaction. Corticosteroids can rarely cause extreme neutrophilia with a left shift, but this abnormality is self-limited and of short duration.

CML may be more difficult to differentiate from other myeloproliferative or myelodysplastic syndromes (Chapters 166 and 182). Patients with myeloid metaplasia with or without myelofibrosis frequently have splenomegaly, neutrophilia, and thrombocytosis. Polycythemia vera with associated iron deficiency, which causes normal hemoglobin and hematocrit values, can manifest with leukocytosis and thrombocytosis. Such patients usually have a normal or increased LAP score, a WBC count less than 25×10^9/μL, and no Ph chromosome or *BCR-ABL1* rearrangement.

The greatest diagnostic difficulty lies with patients who have splenomegaly and leukocytosis but do not have the Ph chromosome. In some, the *BCR-ABL* hybrid gene can be demonstrated despite a normal or atypical cytogenetic pattern. Patients who are Ph negative and *BCR-ABLI* negative are considered to have Ph-negative CML or CMML (see later discussion). Isolated megakaryocytic hyperplasia can be seen in essential thrombocythemia (Chapter 166), with marked thrombocytosis and splenomegaly. Some patients who present with clinical characteristics of essential thrombocythemia (with marked thrombocytosis but without leukocytosis) have CML; cytogenetic and molecular studies showing the Ph chromosome, the *BCR-ABL1* rearrangement, or both lead to the appropriate diagnosis and treatment.

Rarely, patients have myeloid hyperplasia, which involves almost exclusively the neutrophil, eosinophil, or basophil cell lineage. These patients are described as having chronic neutrophilic, eosinophilic, or basophilic leukemia and do not have evidence of the Ph chromosome or the *BCR-ABL1* gene but may have other molecular abnormalities. Most patients with *chronic neutrophilic leukemia*, characterized clinically by sustained, mature neutrophilic leukocytosis, hepatosplenomegaly, and bone marrow granulocytic hyperplasia, have oncogenic mutations in the gene for colony-stimulated factor 3 receptor (*CSF3R*).[2] Patients with *chronic eosinophilic leukemia* (or clonal hypereosinophilic syndrome) (Chapter 170) have mutations in the genes for platelet-derived growth factor receptor-aα (*PDGFRA*) or *PDGFRB* or *FGFR1*; the prototypical abnormality is the *FIP1L1-PDGFRA* gene fusion.[3] Peripheral blood or bone marrow can be tested for these genetic markers by reverse transcription–polymerase chain reaction (RT-PCR) or interphase/metaphase fluorescent in situ hybridization (FISH), as can the *BCR-ABL1* rearrangement for CML.

Clinical Course

Evolution to Accelerated and Blastic Phases

More than 90% of patients present with CML in the benign or chronic phase. If symptomatic at presentation, it becomes asymptomatic once the disease is controlled. Death rarely occurs during the chronic phase of CML. When poorly controlled, CML evolves into an accelerated phase, usually defined by the presence of 15% or more blasts, 30% or more blasts plus promyelocytes, 20% or more basophils, thrombocytopenia (platelets $<100 \times 10^9/\mu L$) unrelated to therapy, or cytogenetic clonal evolution. The accelerated phase can be also characterized by worsening anemia; increasing splenomegaly or hepatomegaly; infiltration of nodes, skin, bones, or other tissues; and fever, malaise, and weight loss. In the accelerated phase, bone marrow studies may show dysplastic changes, increased percentages of blasts and basophils, myelofibrosis, and chromosomal abnormalities in addition to the Ph chromosome (clonal evolution). About 5 to 10% of patients present in the accelerated phase.

Before the era of imatinib therapy, the risk for developing accelerated or blastic phase CML was 10% per year in the first 2 years after diagnosis and 15 to 20% per year thereafter, unless therapies such as IFN-α or allogeneic hematopoietic stem cell transplantation (AHSCT) were used. With imatinib, the annual incidence of progression of CML from the chronic to the accelerated or blastic phase has been 2% in the first 10 years of observation (Fig. 184-3). Before imatinib therapy, the median survival of accelerated phase CML was 18 months or less, but survival has now increased to 4 years or more. In de novo accelerated phase CML, the estimated 8-year survival rate with TKI therapy is 75%.

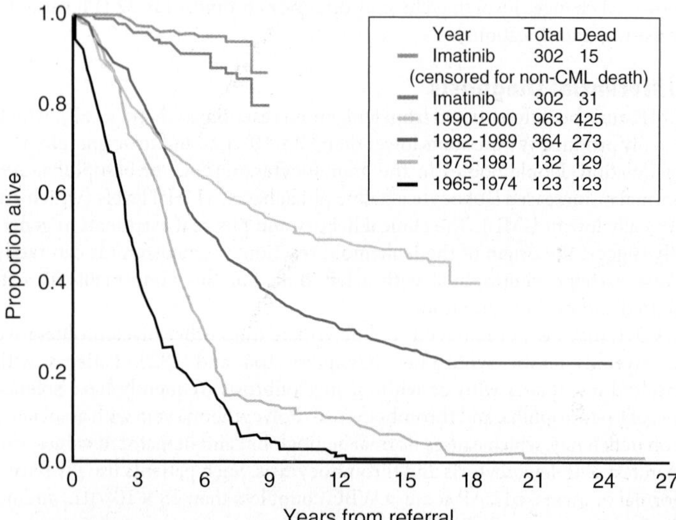

FIGURE 184-3. Survival of patients with Ph-positive chronic myelogenous leukemia (CML) in chronic phase CML. In single-institutional studies, industry-sponsored trials, and national reports where TKI therapy has full penetration, the estimated 8- to 10-year survival rates are high. The survival rates are lower where TKI treatment penetration is not optimal. A, From Bjorkholm M, Ohm L, Eloranta S, et al. Success story of targeted therapy in chronic myeloid leukemia: a population-based study of patients diagnosed in Sweden from 1973-2008. *J Clin Oncol.* 2011;29:2514-2520. B, From Chen Y, Wang H, Kantarjian H, et al. Trends in chronic myeloid leukemia incidence and survival in the United States from 1975-2009. *Leuk Lymphoma.* 2013;54:1411-1417.

The blastic phase of CML is diagnosed when 30% or more blast cells are present in the bone marrow and/or peripheral blood or when extramedullary blastic disease is present. Most patients develop features of the accelerated phase before progressing to the blastic phase, but 20% of patients evolve quickly into a blastic phase without warning. Most patients in the accelerated or blastic phase have additional chromosomal abnormalities (clonal evolution) such as duplication of the Ph chromosome, trisomy of chromosome 8, or development of an isochromosome 17. The extramedullary blastic phase of CML can occur in the spleen, lymph nodes, skin, meninges (especially in the lymphoid blastic phase), bones, and other sites; extramedullary transformation is usually followed shortly by evidence of marrow involvement. Blastic phase CML is associated with a very poor median survival time of 5 months. About 25% of patients develop a lymphoid blastic phase. Ph-negative and *BCR-ABL1*-negative CML often appear to overlap clinically with CMML in their behavior, progress, and response to therapy and seem to resemble the myelodysplastic syndromes (Chapter 182) more than Ph-positive CML. A male preponderance and older age are noted; splenomegaly is common (60 to 70%).

TREATMENT Rx

Today, there are five TKIs that have been approved for the treatment of CML. Imatinib mesylate was approved in 2001 by the U.S. Food and Drug Administration (FDA) for CML salvage and in 2002 for CML firstline therapy. Nilotinib, a more potent selective BCR-ABL1 TKI, was approved in 2007 for CML salvage and in 2010 for first-line CML therapy. Dasatinib, a dual BCR-ABL TKI, was approved for CML salvage therapy in 2006 and for first-line therapy in 2010. In 2012, two additional TKIs were approved for CML salvage: bosutinib, a dual SRC-ABL1 inhibitor, and ponatinib, a pan BCR-ABL1 kinase inhibitor with selective potency against the resistant T315I mutation. In 2012, omacetaxine mepesuccinate, a semisynthetic cephalotaxine that inhibits protein synthesis, was also approved for the treatment of CML following failure of two or more TKIs.

First-line therapy for CML today includes imatinib, nilotinib, or dasatinib.[4,5] Patients who demonstrate CML resistance or intolerance to treatment may be offered salvage TKI therapy with any of the other available TKIs. The choice of second-line therapy with a TKI versus allogeneic hematopoietic stem cell transplantation (AHSCT) depends on several factors: (1) the patient's age and general condition; (2) the availability of acceptable donors (related or matched unrelated); (3) whether a patient has intolerance or CML resistance to first-line TKI therapy; (4) the emerging mutation in the resistant CML clone; (5) whether there is additional clonal evolution at the time of relapse; (6) the response to second-line therapy with the new TKI; (7) the estimated safety and success of the AHSCT; and (8) additional comorbid conditions of the patients (e.g., diabetes, pulmonary conditions, cardiac status, prior history of pancreatitis or pulmonary hypertension) (Chapter 178).

Patients who present with or develop accelerated or blastic phase should receive second-line TKIs to reduce the disease burden and should be offered AHSCT as soon as possible (the exception possibly being de novo CML accelerated phase which may respond durably to first-line TKI therapy, particularly with achievement of a complete cytogenetic response). Patients who develop intolerance to first-line TKI in chronic phase could be offered second-line TKIs as durable therapy, particularly if they achieve complete cytogenetic response. Patients who develop resistance to a first-line TKI in chronic phase are offered a second-line TKI based on their mutation analysis. A T3151 mutation in the CML clone requires therapy with ponatinib and (as of today) early consideration of AHSCT until the results of ponatinib therapy mature. Mutations involving V299L, T315A, or F317LN/I/C are sensitive to nilotinib therapy. Mutations involving Y253H, E255KN, or F359N/C/I are sensitive to dasatinib and bosutinib therapy. Patients who harbor clonal evolution in the CML cells (additional chromosomal abnormalities in the Ph positive cells) or mutations at the time of second-line therapy, or those who do not achieve a complete cytogenetic response by 1 year of second-line TKI therapy, should be considered early for AHSCT. However, if there is no clonal evolution or mutations at the time of second-line therapy, and if the patient achieves complete cytogenetic response with second-line TKI therapy, responses are durable, and TKIs can be continued until evidence of cytogenetic relapse before AHSCT is considered as third-line therapy. Older patients (e.g., 65 to 70 years or older) may forgo a curative option of AHSCT in favor of several years of good disease control. In such patients, TKI therapy with or without additional (older) agents (hydroxyurea, cytarabine, decitabine, 6-mercaptopurine) may sustain less than a complete cytogenetic response (partial, minor) or a complete hematologic response for many years with a good quality of life, and without the risk for mortality or morbidities associated with AHSCT, particularly if the donor is not optimal (unrelated, mismatched). Treatment options and choice and timing of AHSCT in CML are detailed in Tables 184-1 and 184-2.

Recent trials with different TKIs have indicated that early and "deep" cytogenetic and molecular responses are predictive of improved progression-free and overall survival.[A1-A3][6]

Imatinib Mesylate

Since its discovery in 1999, imatinib mesylate has become standard therapy for CML. Imatinib is a 2-phenylaminopyrimidine derivative that binds to the canonical ATP lining the groove between the N and C lobes of the ABL1 kinase domain, thus blocking the phosphorylation of tyrosine residues on substrate protein. Blocking of ATP binding inactivates the ABLI kinase because it cannot transfer phosphate to its substrate. By inhibiting phosphorylation, imatinib prevents the activation of signal transduction pathways that induce the leukemic transformation processes that cause CML (Fig. 184-4). Imatinib inhibits several tyrosine kinases, including p210$^{BCR\text{-}ABLI}$, p190$^{BCR\text{-}ABLI}$, v-ABL, c-ABL, c-Kit, and PDGF receptor.

In a randomized trial of 1106 patients with newly diagnosed CML, imatinib 400 mg/day orally provided significantly higher rates of major cytogenetic response (87% vs. 35%) and complete cytogenetic response (76% vs. 14%), as well as lower rates of progression (8% vs. 26%) and transformation (3% vs. 9%) after 12 months of therapy, compared with the prior standard nontransplantation therapy (a combination of IFN-α and cytosine arabinoside).[A4] The longer term follow-up results continue to demonstrate excellent outcomes with imatinib therapy (Table 184-3; see Fig. 184-3); with a median follow-up of 8 years, the complete cytogenetic response rate (occurring at least once during therapy) is 83%, the estimated 8-year event-free survival rate is 81%, and the transformation-free survival rate 92%. The estimated 8-year survival rate is 85% (93% if only CML-related deaths are included). The annual rate of transformation was 1.5 to 2.8% in the first 3 years and decreased to less than 1% in the subsequent 5 years among patients who continued on imatinib therapy. Therapy with high-dose imatinib or with combinations of imatinib and other agents (e.g., peg-IFN-α2) did not show convincingly improved results compared with standard imatinib 400 mg daily.

Imatinib has a 5% or lower rate of serious side effects, which include nausea, vomiting, diarrhea, skin rash, muscle cramps, bone pain, periorbital or leg edema, weight gain, and rarely, hepatic, renal, or cardiopulmonary dysfunction; most of these are manageable with dose reduction or treatment interruption. Drug-related myelosuppression occurs in 10 to 20% of patients with newly diagnosed CML and is manageable with brief treatment interruptions, dose modifications, or both, or with the administration of growth factors (erythropoietin for anemia, granulocyte colony-stimulating factor for neutropenia). Imatinib and other TKIs may prolong the cardiac QTc interval; medications that contribute to QTc prolongation should be avoided. Hypophosphatemia associated with altered bone metabolism can occur, and the serum phosphate level should be monitored. Chromosomal abnormalities may appear in the Ph-negative diploid cells in 5 to 10% of responding patients, probably owing

TABLE 184-1 THERAPY OF CHRONIC MYELOID LEUKEMIA

First line	Imatinib 400 mg daily Nilotinib 300 mg twice daily Dasatinib 100 mg daily
Second/third line	Nilotinib, dasatinib, bosutinib, ponatinib Omacetaxine Allogeneic stem cell transplantation
Other	Decitabine, pegylated interferon Hydroxurea, cytarabine, decitabine Combinations of tyrosine kinase inhibitor–based regimens Investigational

TABLE 184-2 ROLE AND TIMING OF ALLOGENEIC STEM CELL TRANSPLANTATION IN CHRONIC MYELOID LEUKEMIA

CHRONIC MYELOID LEUKEMIA STATUS	TYROSINE KINASE INHIBITOR THERAPY	ALLOGENEIC STEM CELL TRANSPLANTATION
Accelerated or blastic phase	Interim therapy to minimal residual disease	As soon as possible
Imatinib failure in chronic phase with T3151 mutation	Ponatinib interim therapy to minimal residual disease	As soon as possible if no good response obtained
Imatinib failure in chronic phase; no clonal evolution, no mutations, good initial response	Long-term second-line tyrosine kinase inhibitors	Third-line post second tyrosine kinase inhibitors failure
Imatinib failure in chronic phase with clonal evolution or mutation or no cytogenetic response to second-line tyrosine kinase inhibitors	Interim therapy to minimal residual disease	Second line
Older (>65-70) post-imatinib failure in chronic phase	Long-term	May forgo allogeneic stem cell transplantation for many years of quality of life

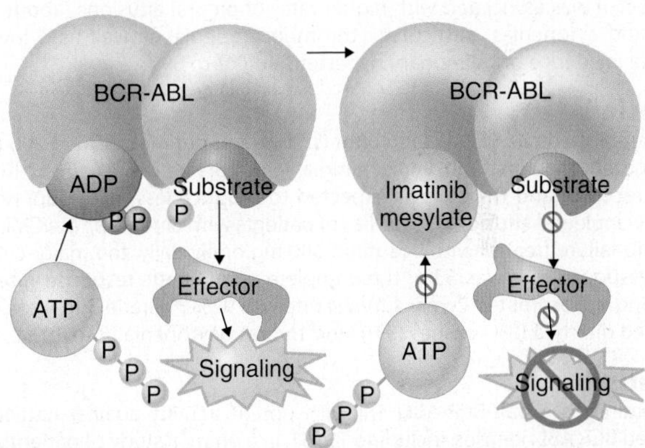

FIGURE 184-4. **Mechanism of action of imatinib. By occupying the adenosine triphosphate (ATP)-binding pocket of the ABL kinase domain, imatinib prevents substrate phosphorylation and downstream activation of signals, thus inhibiting the leukemogenic effects of BCR-ABL on cells in chronic myelogenous leukemia. ADP = adenosine diphosphate; P = phosphate group.**

TABLE 184-3 RESULTS OF TYROSINE KINASE INHIBITOR THERAPY IN CHRONIC PHASE CHRONIC MYELOGENOUS LEUKEMIA

THERAPY	LEUKEMIA STATUS	COMPLETE CYTOGENETIC RESPONSE (%) (AT INDICATED YEAR OF TREATMENT)	MAJOR/COMPLETE MOLECULAR RESPONSES (%) (AT INDICATED YEAR OF TREATMENT)	SURVIVAL (%) (AT INDICATED YEAR AFTER INITIATION OF TREATMENT)
Imatinib	First line	65 (5)	40/20 (5)	85 (8-10)
Nilotinib	First line	85-87 (4)	73-76/37-40 (4)	95-97 (4)
Dasatinib	First line	86 (2)	74/34 (4)	93 (4)
Dasatinib	Salvage	50 (5)	43 (6)	71 (6)
Nilotinib	Salvage	44 (4)	30-40 (4)	85 (3)
Ponatinib	Salvage	45-65 (2)	30-50 (2)	90 (2)
Bosutinib	Salvage	40 (2)	30 (2)	92 (2)
Omacetaxine	Salvage	10 (2)	—	85-90 (2)

to unmasking of a fragile stem cell prone to the development of CML or to chromosomal instability; such changes disappear spontaneously in 70% of cases and rarely evolve into a myelodysplastic syndrome or acute myeloid leukemia, probably as part of the natural course of CML.

Nilotinib

Nilotinib, a selective BCR-ABLI TKI 30 times more potent than imatinib, was initially approved for the treatment of CML after imatinib failure. In CML chronic phase after imatinib failure, nilotinib 400 mg orally twice daily was associated with complete cytogenetic response rates of 40 to 50%. The major molecular response rates, defined as BCR-ABL1 transcripts, 0.1% by International Scale [IS], are 30 to 40%, and the estimated 3-year survival rate is 80%. Subsequent studies compared nilotinib to imatinib in newly diagnosed patients with CML. In a three-arm randomized study,[A5] patients received imatinib 400 mg daily, nilotinib 400 mg twice a day, or nilotinib 300 mg twice daily. With a minimum follow-up of 4 years, the two arms of nilotinib demonstrate better early results compared with imatinib. There was no difference in the estimated 4-year survival rates (94%, 97%, 93%, respectively). Nilotinib therapy was associated with lower rates of fluid retention, diarrhea, headaches, muscle cramps, nausea and vomiting, and neutropenia. However, it was associated with higher rates of headache, rash, pruritus, and hyperglycemia, and with a low but notable incidence of pancreatitis (<2%), ischemic heart disease (4 to 5% vs. 1% with imatinib), and peripheral arterial occlusive disease (1.4 to 1.8% vs. 0%).

Dasatinib

Dasatinib, a dual SRC-ABL1 inhibitor, is 300 times more potent than imatinib. In chronic phase CML after imatinib failure, dasatinib therapy was associated with complete cytogenetic response rates of 45 to 60%, major molecular response rate of 43%, and estimated 6-year survival rate of 71%. A first-line study comparing dasatinib to imatinib (DASISION trial)[A6] randomized patients to receive either imatinib 400 mg daily or dasatinib 100 mg daily. With a minimum follow-up of 48 months, the incidence of complete cytogenetic response by 24 months was 86% with dasatinib and 82% with imatinib. The incidence of major molecular response was 74% vs. 60%. The rate of transformation to accelerated or blastic phase was 4.6% vs. 7%. The estimated 4-year progression-free survival rates were similar, 90%. The estimated 4-year survival rates were 93% and 92%, respectively. Dasatinib therapy was associated with lower rates of fluid retention, edema, myalgia, nausea, vomiting, and rashes. However, it was associated with higher rates of pleural effusions (about 10 to 15%) and cytopenias, particularly thrombocytopenia, as well as a low but notable incidence of pulmonary hypertension (<2 to 3%).

Bosutinib

Bosutinib, a dual SRC-ABLI inhibitor (similar to dasatinib), is 30 to 200 times more potent than imatinib. It has minimal inhibitory activity against c-Kit and PDGF receptor and therefore is expected to produce less myelosuppression and fewer pleural effusions. In studies of patients with chronic phase CML after imatinib failure treated with bosutinib 500 mg orally daily, the major cytogenetic response rate was 53%, the complete cytogenetic response rate was 41%, and the estimated 2-year survival rate was 92%.[A7] Grade 3 to 4 toxicities included diarrhea (8%), rashes (9%), and thrombocytopenia (5 to 10%).

Ponatinib

Ponatinib is a pan-BCR-ABLI TKI with potent activity against native and mutated BCR ABLI kinases, including T3151. In a phase II study of patients with chronic, accelerated, or blastic (CML) or Ph-positive acute lymphocytic leukemia, all of whom were resistant or intolerant to several TKIs, ponatinib showed high activity. In these chronic phase CML patients, the complete cytogenetic response rate was 44%, and the major molecular response rate was 30%. In the subset of patients with T3151 mutation, the major cytogenetic response rate was 70%, the complete cytogenetic response rate 66%, and the major molecular response rate 50%.[7] Significant side effects included pancreatitis (5 to 10%), thrombocytopenia (30%), and skin rash (30%). Because of the cumulative incidence of serious thrombotic events since the approval of ponatinib, the FDA has restricted its use to patients resistant to other TKIs. Additional clinical trials assessing the safety profile and different dose schedules of ponatinib are being considered.

Omacetaxine

Omacetaxine mepesuccinate, a semisynthetic analogue of homoharringtonine, is a first-in-class cephalotaxine that acts as a protein synthesis inhibitor that induces apoptosis in leukemic cells by reducing levels of multiple oncoproteins, including BCR-ABL1. Data pooled from two phase II trials of subcutaneous omacetaxine, 1.25 mg/m^2 twice daily for 2 weeks every 4 weeks until response, then for 1 week every 4 weeks, in patients with chronic phase CML after failure of two TKIs, a major cytogenetic response was reported in 20% and complete cytogenetic response in 10%.[8] Grade 3 to 4 side effects included cytopenias in 37 to 67% of patients, which were reversible. This led to FDA approval of omacetaxine for patients whose disease has progressed despite treatment with two TKIs.

Allogeneic Hematopoietic Stem Cell Transplantation

AHSCT (Chapter 178), a potentially curative therapy in selected patients with CML, is most effective during the chronic phase, when it is associated with a 20-year survival rate of 40 to 50%. Transplant-related mortality rates range from 5 to 50%, depending on the patient's age, whether the donor is related or unrelated, the degree of matching, and other, less important factors such as positivity for cytomegalovirus, preparative and post-transplantation regimen, and institutional expertise. Disease-free survival rates with related allogeneic stem cell transplantation are 40 to 80% in chronic phase, 15 to 40% in accelerated phase, and 5 to 20% in blastic phase. In chronic phase CML, patients younger than 30 to 40 years have disease-free survival rates of 60 to 80%, compared with only 30 to 40% for patients older than 50 years. A major limitation of allogeneic stem cell transplantation is the availability of related donors. Human leukocyte antigen (HLA)-compatible unrelated donors can be found for 50% of patients; the median time from initiation of the donor search to transplantation is 3 to 6 months.

Nonmyeloablative preparative regimens have expanded the indications for AHSCT to older patients and have reduced transplant-related mortality and complications (Chapter 178). Early results show acceptable degrees of engraftment, less mortality and organ damage, more persistent residual disease, and similar degrees of graft-versus-host disease. Patients whose CML recurs after AHSCT may respond to imatinib or new-generation TKIs, donor lymphocyte infusions, IFN-α, or a second AHSCT.

AHSCT can produce an estimated cure rate of 40% at 20 years. However, it is associated with a 1-year mortality rate of 5 to 40% and with morbidities such as cataracts, infertility, second cancers (5 to 10%), immune-mediated complications, and chronic graft-versus-host disease. Delaying AHSCT beyond 1 to 3 years after diagnosis may be associated with worse results and with occasional sudden blastic transformation, which may not be salvageable. The outcome of AHSCT may be even better after exposure to TKIs.

Choice of First-Line Chronic Myelogenous Leukemia Therapy

Currently, all three TKIs (imatinib, nilotinib, and dasatinib) are acceptable first-line therapies for CML. The choice of TKI may depend on patient and physician preferences and patient prior history and comorbidities (e.g., diabetes, pancreatitis, cardiopulmonary conditions, and pulmonary hypertension). Current oncology practice trends appear to increasingly favor nilotinib and dasatinib over imatinib as initial therapy because of their better early results, particularly the lower early incidence of CML transformation. However, the costs of TKIs may shift treatment paradigms in some emerging nations to using a particular TKI over others, or even to consider first-line AHSCT (total one-time procedure cost of \$30 to \$100,000) in situations in which patients or the national health care system cannot afford the burden of the TKI. Imatinib may become available in generic formulations in 2015. The price of generic imatinib is unknown but may be lower than that of other agents (\$2000 to \$10,000 per year). The choice of first-line TKI therapy may then depend on the differential pricing of generic imatinib versus dasatinib and imatinib and on the maturing long-term data (5 to 8 years) for survival, transformation-free survival, and event-free survival with the three TKIs. With an estimated 8-year survival rate of 93% with imatinib (considering only CML-related deaths) and the high efficacy of new-generation TKIs as salvage therapies, the survival benefit with dasatinib or nilotinib may or may not be apparent compared with imatinib first-line therapy, careful monitoring for cytogenetic relapse, and rapid institution of second-line TKI therapies at that time.

Treatment of Chronic Phase Chronic Myelogenous Leukemia after Failure of Therapy with Imatinib or Other TKIs

In several studies, the achievement of a complete cytogenetic response (Ph-positive metaphases 0%; BCR-ABLI transcripts 1%) at 12 months or later on TKI therapy was associated with significant survival benefit compared with achievement of lesser degrees of response. Therefore, achievement of complete cytogenetic response is now the primary end point of TKI therapy. The achievement of complete molecular response (nonmeasurable BCR-ABLI transcripts) offers the possibility of treatment discontinuation in the clinical trial setting. Lack of achievement of major molecular response or of complete molecular response should not be interpreted as a need to change TKI therapy or to consider AHSCT. Response assessments at earlier times on first-line TKI therapy (3 to 6 months) have shown better outcomes, with achievement of a major cytogenetic response by 3 to 6 months on imatinib therapy (Ph-positive metaphases 35%, or BCR-ABLI transcripts 10%). Although this is interpreted to mean that a change to a second TKI therapy may be considered if such an outcome is not obtained, no studies have shown that changing therapy from imatinib to second TKI for this indication has improved patient outcome. When nilotinib or dasatinib is used for first-line therapy, achievement of complete cytogenetic response by 3 to 6 months of TKI therapy has been associated with improved outcomes.

Currently, imatinib failure (requiring a change of therapy) should be strictly defined as failure to achieve a major cytogenetic response after 6 months of imatinib therapy and a complete cytogenetic response after 12 months or cytogenetic or hematologic relapse at any later time, on an optimal imatinib dose schedule (adjusting dose for significant side effects or for intolerance and checking for treatment compliance). With the use of second-generation TKIs in the first-line setting, failure of TKI therapy has been suggested to be lack of achievement of complete cytogenetic response or BCR-ABLl transcript levels of 1% by 3 to 6 months of therapy. Such patients (<10% of the denominator) have a worse event-free survival, although their survival at 3 to 5 years remains in the range of 90%, better or equivalent to what would be achievable with AHSCT. Thus, although the early surrogate response parameters at 3 to 6 months on first-line TKI therapy predict for differences in outcome, a change of therapy at that point in time has not been proved to improve longer term prognosis.

Patients with CML whose disease progresses on imatinib therapy may be treated with a newer generation TKI or with AHSCT, as discussed earlier. Patients with CML and failure on first-line dasatinib or nilotinib therapy may possibly be salvaged with ponatinib if the CML clones exhibit a T3151 mutation. If no such mutation is detected, they could be considered for other TKI therapies, AHSCT, treatment with omacetaxine, or combined-modality therapies including TKIs and older agents (hydroxyurea, cytarabine, decitabine). The choice of AHSCT as second-line versus later salvage therapy was discussed earlier.

Treatment of Accelerated and Blastic Phase Chronic Myelogenous Leukemia

Patients with accelerated or blastic phase CML may receive initial therapy with TKIs (newer generation TKIs like dasatinib or ponatinib are preferred over imatinib) to reduce the CML burden and may be considered for early AHSCT. Response rates with combinations of TKIs and chemotherapy are 40% in nonlymphoid blastic phase CML and 70 to 80% in lymphoid blastic phase CML. Median survival times are 6 to12 months and 12 to 24 months, respectively. The addition of TKIs to chemotherapy has improved the response rates and prolonged the median survival time in blastic phase CML.

At present, AHSCT is the only curative therapy for accelerated and blastic phase CML; overall cure rates are in the range of 15 to 40% and 5 to 20%, respectively. Patients with cytogenetic clonal evolution as the only accelerated phase criterion have a long-term event-free survival rate of about 60%. Otherwise, TKIs provide hematologic responses in 80% of patients and an estimated 4-year survival rate of 40 to 55% in accelerated phase CML, but only a 40% response rate and a median survival of 9 to 12 months in blastic phase CML. Patients in the accelerated or blastic phase should be encouraged to participate in investigational strategies to improve their prognosis. Patients with de novo CML accelerated phase have a better outcome with first-line TKI therapy than patients who evolve from chronic to accelerated phase. The estimated 6- to 8-year survival rates with TKI therapy in de novo accelerated phase CML are 60 to 80%. Such patients may continue on TKI therapy as their long-term treatment if they achieve a complete cytogenetic response on TKI therapy.

Special Therapeutic Considerations

Patients with severe leukocytosis and manifestations of leukostasis may benefit from initial leukapheresis. Severe thrombocytosis uncontrolled with anti-CML measures may respond to anagrelide, thiotepa, IFN-α, 6-mercaptopurine, 6-thioguanine, hydroxyurea, and platelet pheresis. CML during pregnancy may be controlled with pheresis in the first trimester and then with hydroxyurea until delivery. Use of IFN-α during pregnancy has been reported anecdotally to be safe. An analysis of 125 babies delivered to women with CML on imatinib therapy (who discontinued imatinib once the pregnancy was known) showed most babies to be healthy. However, the study demonstrated imatinib therapy to be associated with a syndrome of ocular, skeletal, and renal abnormalities in three babies delivered. Therefore, imatinib (and presumably other TKIs, although there is little experience with them) should be discontinued immediately once pregnancy is documented, but abortion is not recommended because fetal malformations are rare. Partners of men with CML on TKI therapy who become pregnant have delivered normal babies. Splenectomy can be useful as a palliative measure in patients with massive, painful splenomegaly, hypersplenism, or thrombocytopenia.

Monitoring Response to Therapy in Chronic Myelogenous Leukemia

With TKI therapy, complete cytogenetic response, major molecular response, and even complete molecular response have been achieved. These response rates improve with continued therapy and are higher with new-generation TKIs (dasatinib, nilotinib) compared with imatinib as first-line therapy (see Table 184-3). Techniques have been developed to measure these responses more accurately (rather than relying on only 20 metaphases by cytogenetic analysis), with less tedious and less painful procedures (peripheral blood rather than marrow studies), and at levels below the level of detection by routine cytogenetic evaluations. FISH studies with improved probes can measure 200 interphase cells using peripheral blood, and they have false-positive rates of less than 2 to 3%. Quantitative PCR tests usually measure the BCR-ABLl transcript levels (ratio of the abnormal message, BCR-ABLl, to a normal message, such as ABL1). BCR-ABLl transcript levels of 0.1% [IS], about a 3-log reduction of disease, have been associated with a very low risk for CML relapse on TKI therapy. This is referred to as a *major molecular response.* Undetectable BCR-ABL1 transcript levels, (usually <0.0032% [IS], or 4.5 log of reduction) are sometimes referred to as *complete molecular response.* The percentage of patients achieving complete molecular response is significantly higher with new-generation TKIs compared with imatinib.

In monitoring the response to TKI-based therapies, patients require a bone marrow analysis before treatment (to determine the percentages of blasts and basophils and clonal evolution) and FISH and quantitative PCR analyses. Quantitative PCR can be falsely negative at diagnosis in 5 to 8% of patients with unusual breakpoints and messages (e.g., b2a3 or b3a3) if proper procedures are not used. Thus, knowledge of the pretreatment BCR-ABL1 transcript levels avoids the false assumption of complete molecular response because of the false negativity. Bone marrow analysis may be useful at 6 and 12 months (to assess cytogenetic response and confirm complete cytogenetic response) and once every 1 to 3 years in patients with stable, durable complete cytogenetic responses (to look for chromosomal abnormalities in both Ph-positive and Phnegative cells). Monitoring in patients with confirmed durable complete cytogenetic responses can be continued with either FISH or quantitative PCR studies every 6 months (or more often, such as every 3 months, if there are concerns about significant and consistent increases in BCR-ABLl transcripts levels). Some CML experts have shifted from monitoring by marrow studies to monitoring by peripheral blood studies using molecular analysis, with or without FISH studies. Among patients achieving major molecular response, molecular analysis without FISH studies is sufficient.

Resistance to imatinib therapy (discussed earlier) requires a change of therapy to other TKIs, TKI combinations with chemotherapy, or consideration of AHSCT. It is important to emphasize that many patients with apparent CML resistance to a TKI therapy may be noncompliant with the treatment. This should be discussed clearly with patients when they exhibit signs of CML progression by either molecular or FISH studies. If they are noncompliant, they may continue on the same TKI treatment with emphasis on compliance and evaluated 3 to 6 months later, before CML resistance is declared.

Among patients in complete cytogenetic response on a particular TKI, failure to achieve a major molecular response does not, at present, indicate resistance to the particular TKI or a need to change therapy. Mutational studies are recommended in patients who develop cytogenetic or hematologic resistance or relapse on a particular TKI therapy, when considering changing therapy to another TKI. The detection rate of mutations in this situation is 30 to 50%. Mutational studies are not recommended in patients in complete cytogenetic response on a particular TKI because the detection rate of mutations are then very low (<3 to 5%).

FUTURE DIRECTIONS

In 2014, patients with CML have multiple treatment options, including several TKIs, omacetaxine (protein synthesis inhibition), and several older agents (hydroxurea, IFN-α, busulfan, 6-mercaptopurine, cytarabine, decitabine). Most patients with CML would be expected to live their normal functional life and to be functionally, although not molecularly, cured, as long as they continue therapy with TKI-based regimens, are compliant with the treatment, and are monitored closely for signs of resistance in order to change therapy in a timely manner and/or consider AHSCT before CML progression. Future directions will focus on the potential molecular cure of CML (i.e., achievement of a durable complete molecular response and its persistence after discontinuation of TKI therapy). This is not a trivial issue because, with effective TKI therapy and full treatment penetration worldwide (to 100% of all diagnosed patients and continuation of TKI therapy without interruptions), the prevalence of CML would increase annually and plateau in about 2030 to 2040 at a rate 35 times the incidence. This figure is estimated to be close to 160,000 patients with CML in the United States and about 3 million patients worldwide. This may represent a considerable burden on patients and the health care systems in relation to drug availability, compliance, potential development of long-term side effects, and costs. Therefore, it is critical to continue research into therapies that increase the rates of durable complete molecular responses. This may be achievable with the current more potent new-generation TKIs alone or in combination with other available (pegIFN-α, omacetaxine, decitabine) or investigational therapies (JAK2 inhibitors, hedgehog inhibitors, stem cell poisons, vaccines). Such strategies may improve the eradication of minimal residual disease, potentially obviating the need for indefinite therapy with TKIs. Further understanding of the pathophysiologic events downstream of BCR-ABLl may help in the development of new strategies to target them.

PROGNOSIS

Treatment of CML with imatinib and other TKIs has revolutionized the outcome of the disease. In patients with newly diagnosed CML, imatinib therapy is associated with an estimated 8- to 10-year survival rate of 85% (93% if non-CML deaths are censored). If this favorable trend continues with longer follow-up, the median survival time in CML may exceed 25 years. The annual mortality rate of CML with TKIs in the first decade of experience has been reduced from the historical rate of 10 to 20%, down to 2% (1% if only CML deaths are counted). Many well established poor prognostic factors in CML (e.g., older age, splenomegaly, presence of marrow fibrosis, deletion of 9q) have lost much of their prognostic importance since the advent of TKI therapy. With AHSCT, cures can be expected in 40 to 80% of patients with chronic phase CML, 15 to 40% of those with accelerated phase CML, and 5 to 20% of those with blastic phase CML.

CHRONIC MYELOMONOCYTIC LEUKEMIA AND ATYPICAL CHRONIC MYELOID LEUKEMIAS

DEFINITION AND EPIDEMIOLOGY

Although superficially resembling CML in its clinical and morphologic presentation, CMML should be considered a separate entity because of its particular clinical, therapeutic, and prognostic aspects. CMML is a hybrid entity manifesting as a proliferation of the myeloid monocytic series and dysplasia of the erythroid-megakaryocytic series. Patients with CMML are older (median age, 65 to 70 years) than most patients with CML.

PATHOBIOLOGY

The cytogenetic findings in patients with CMML are either normal or involve an additional chromosome 8 or findings other than the Ph chromosome. Patients with CMML have *RAS* mutations in 40 to 60% of cases.

CLINICAL MANIFESTATIONS AND DIAGNOSIS

Patients often present with symptoms related to anemia and thrombocytopenia (fatigue, bleeding). Other typical features include splenomegaly, leukocytosis, and monocytosis. Organ infiltration (lymph nodes, skin, liver) is less common. Basophilia and thrombocytosis are not presenting features. High-frequency mutations in the granulocyte colony-stimulating factor 3 receptor gene (*CSF3R*) in *chronic neutrophilic leukemia* (CNL) and in some patients with *atypical chronic myeloid leukemia* (aCML) have been identified. In addition, recurrent mutations in *SETBPl* (Set binding protein) have been identified in 25% of aCML patients.

TREATMENT AND PROGNOSIS Rx

AHSCT (Chapter 178), which is the only curative modality, should be considered first-line therapy in candidate patients. Other therapies include hydroxyurea to control leukocytosis, erythropoietin to improve anemia, azacitidine or decitabine (both approved by the FDA for the treatment of CMML), topotecan and cytarabine or other intensive anti-AML (Chapter 183) regimens for CMML transformation, splenectomy for symptomatic splenomegaly and/or hypersplenism, and investigational agents. Inhibition of Janus kinase 2 or SRC kinase signaling downstream of mutated CSF3R is being explored therapeutically.

Poor prognostic factors include the presence of anemia (hemoglobin <10 g/dL), thrombocytopenia, and more than 5% blasts. Median survival is 12 to 18 months.

HAIRY CELL LEUKEMIA

DEFINITION AND EPIDEMIOLOGY

Hairy cell leukemia (HCL) is an uncommon and indolent B-cell leukemia (1 to 2% of all leukemias). The median age at diagnosis is 50 years, and there is a 4 : 1 male preponderance.

PATHOBIOLOGY

The cell of origin of HCL is the B lymphocyte, as documented by the demonstration of heavy and light chain immunoglobulin gene rearrangements. In a series of 47 patients, all had a *BRAF V600E* activating mutation. Hairy cells express CD19, CD20, CD11C, CD103, FMC7, and CD22, but not CD21, CDS, CD10, or CD23. The cells demonstrate a κ or λ light chain phenotype. The cells also express CD25 (TAC), the low-affinity interleukin-2 (IL-2) receptor, and CD103, a unique hairy cell antigen. High levels of soluble IL-2 receptor (more than five times normal) are present in the sera of almost all patients with HCL, with extremely high levels noted in many cases. Immune dysfunction is wide ranging in HCL. Monocytopenia is universal; B and T lymphocytes are decreased in number; the CD4/CD8 (helper T/suppressor T) ratio is often inverted; and skin test reactivity to recall antigens is impaired, as is antibody-dependent cellular cytotoxicity. Humoral immunity is relatively preserved, with normal immunoglobulin levels. Marrow failure in HCL may be due in part to inhibitory factors (e.g., tumor necrosis factor) produced by the leukemic infiltrate; the pancytopenia is often more marked than would be anticipated from the degree of leukemic infiltration.

CLINICAL MANIFESTATIONS

Most patients present with pancytopenia and splenomegaly. Patients may also have fatigue, fever, weight loss, and infection secondary to granulocytopenia or monocytopenia. Leukocytosis is uncommon, and lymphadenopathy is rare. Anemia is present in up to 85% of patients, whereas leukopenia and thrombocytopenia are present in 60 to 75%. The cytopenias are caused by a combination of bone marrow failure due to leukemic infiltration and hypersplenism. Patients may experience repeated infections and, rarely, a systemic vasculitis resembling polyarteritis nodosa. Although bacterial infections occur, as would be expected with neutropenia, patients with HCL have a predilection to develop tuberculosis, atypical mycobacterial infections, and fungal infections, perhaps related to the severe monocytopenia that is characteristic of this disorder.

DIAGNOSIS

In conjunction with the clinical features, careful examination of the peripheral blood smear may demonstrate the occasional typical cells with cytoplasmic projections, giving rise to the name *haily cell leukemia* (Fig. 184-5). The hairy cells are 10 to 15 mm in diameter, with pale blue cytoplasm, a nucleus with a loose chromatin structure, and one or two indistinct nucleoli. Bone marrow aspiration is often inadequate owing to increased deposition of reticulum, collagen, and fibrin; bone marrow biopsy is usually necessary. Bone marrow involvement is interstitial or patchy, and the infiltrate is characterized by widely spaced nuclei due to the abundant cytoplasm, giving rise to the commonly described fried-egg appearance.

Hairy cells exhibit a strong acid phosphatase (isoenzyme 5) cytochemical reaction in 95% of cases, a reaction that is resistant to the inhibitory effect of tartaric acid (TRAP). Other lymphoproliferative diseases are rarely TRAP positive. Electron microscopy clearly demonstrates the microvillar projections. Often, ribosomal-lamellar complexes, which are characteristic but not diagnostic of HCL, can be identified. The peroxidase stain is negative, and lysozyme activity is absent in hairy cells, thereby differentiating these cells from monocytes.

Differential Diagnosis

The differential diagnosis must distinguish HCL from non-Hodgkin lymphoma (Chapter 185) or chronic lymphocytic leukemia (CLL) (see later), which can manifest with predominant splenomegaly and minimal lymphadenopathy. Some patients with a myelodysplastic syndrome (Chapter 182) or

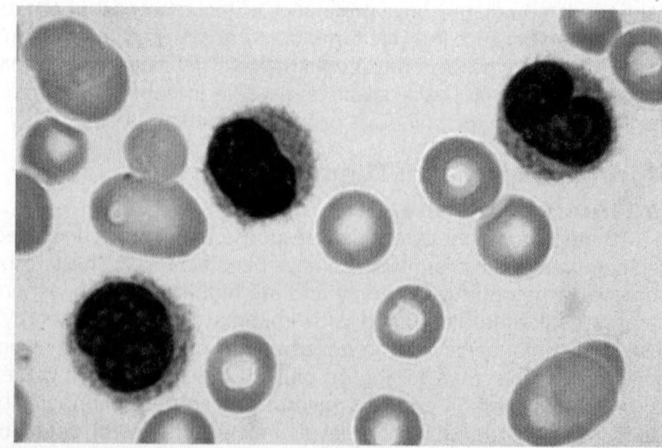

FIGURE 184-5. Hairy cell leukemia. Peripheral smear shows hairy cells with blue-gray cytoplasm; fine, hair-like projections (resembling ruffles); and oval or slightly indented nuclei with loose chromatin and indistinct nucleoli. (Courtesy Andrew Schafer, MD.)

chronic myeloproliferative neoplasm (Chapter 166) have splenomegaly nd pancytopenia with only a few atypical cells. Patients with other diseases, uch as systemic lupus erythematosus (Chapter 266) and other autoimmune liseases, B-cell and T-cell prolymphocytic leukemias (see later), infiltrative plenomegaly (Chapter 168), or tuberculosis (Chapter 324), may have splenomegaly and cytopenia, but these diagnoses can usually be made by history, physical examination, and appropriate blood and bone marrow tests. Splenomegaly, cytopenia, and nonaspirable marrow in a middle-aged man should create a high index of suspicion for HCL. Splenectomy or lymph node biopsy s sometimes necessary to establish the diagnosis in difficult cases. Cases of HCL variant manifest with higher WBC counts, are TRAP negative, have prominent nucleoli, and are only occasionally positive for antibodies against CD25. HCL variant does not respond as well to the agents that are usually effective in the management of typical HCL.

TREATMENT

Rx

A small proportion (<5%) of patients with HCL do not require therapy. These patients have mild cytopenias, are not transfusion dependent, have no history of infections, and have a low level of marrow infiltration by hairy cells. 2-Chlorodeoxyadenosine (cladribine), an adenosine analogue that *is* resistant to deamination by adenosine deaminase, produces complete remission in more than 80% of HCL patients after a single course of 0.1 mg/kg/day for 7 days given by continuous intravenous infusion, and it is now the recommended first-line therapy.[9] It can also be given at 0.14 mg/kg/day for 5 days as a short daily intravenous infusion. Remissions are durable, and patients who relapse can often attain a second remission after retreatment with cladribine. The drug is well tolerated, with a low infection rate. Despite long-lasting suppression of $CD4^+$ lymphocyte counts, there does not appear to be an increase in late opportunistic infections or second malignancies. Partial response to purine analogs is regarded as a poor prognostic factor, and a second course of purine analog therapy is recommended if patients do not enter complete remission, with the addition of rituximab to be considered. Rituximab in combination with a purine analogue is often used in the treatment of relapsed disease.

Deoxycoformycin (pentostatin; 4 mg/m^2 weekly or every 2 weeks for up to 6 months), an adenosine deaminase inhibitor, produces complete remission in 70 to 80% of patients. The response to treatment is rapid. Toxicity includes nausea and vomiting, infection, renal and hepatic dysfunction, conjunctivitis, and photosensitivity, albeit mild in most cases.

Human leukocyte interferon (HuIFN), or recombinant interferon-α (r-IFN-α), rapidly improves granulocyte, platelet, and hemoglobin levels (within 1 to 3 months); reduces spleen size; and decreases marrow infiltration. Peripheral blood cell counts return to normal in 80% of cases, but complete remission is uncommon. In addition, when treatment is discontinued, relapse occurs within 1 to 2 years. Rituximab, the monoclonal antibody targeting CD20, also produces responses; eight weekly infusions appear to be more effective than four. Two immunotoxins can produce responses in refractory patients. LMB2 is composed of the Fc portion of the anti-TAC antibody linked to a *Pseudomonas* exotoxin. Moxetumomab also contains a *Pseudomonas* exotoxin linked to an antibody targeting CD22. The B-RAF inhibitor, vemurafenib, has successfully been used to treat a patient with HCL, and a clinical trial in relapsed HCL is underway.[10] Splenectomy is recommended mainly for patients with splenic infarcts or massive splenomegaly.

PROGNOSIS

More than 85 to 90% of patients treated with cladribine or pentostatin are expected to be alive at 10 years.

CHRONIC LYMPHOCYTIC LEUKEMIA

DEFINITION

CLL is a neoplasm characterized by the accumulation of monoclonal lymphocytes of B-cell origin. The cells accumulate in the bone marrow, lymph nodes, liver, spleen, and occasionally other organs. After decades of chemotherapy-based treatment of CLL, recent progress has turned attention to mechanism-driven therapy with targeting of the B-cell receptor signaling pathway.[11]

EPIDEMIOLOGY

CLL is the most common leukemia (one third of all cases) in the Western world and is twice as common as CML. The disease occurs rarely in those younger than 30 years; most patients with CLL are older than 60 years. CLL increases in incidence exponentially with time; by age 80 years, the incidence rate is 20 cases per 100,000 persons per year. The male-to-female ratio is approximately 2 : 1. The incidence of CLL among Asians in Japan and China is only 10% of that in the United States and other Western countries. Intermediate incidence rates are seen in persons of Hispanic origin.

The cause of CLL is unknown. Ionizing radiation and viruses have not been associated with CLL, although hepatitis C infection has recently been associated with splenic lymphoma with villous lymphocytes (another indolent B-cell disorder). Familial clustering in CLL is more common than in other leukemias; first-degree relatives of patients have a two- to four-fold higher risk and develop CLL at a younger age compared with the general population. Farmers have a higher incidence of CLL than do those in other occupations, raising the possibility of an etiologic role for herbicides or pesticides. Agent Orange, the defoliating agent used in Vietnam, has been associated with the development of CLL.

PATHOBIOLOGY

Leukemia cells in CLL are homogeneous and have the appearance of normal mature lymphocytes. However, clonality can be documented by the presence of immunoglobulin gene rearrangements and the restriction to either κ or λ light chains on the cell surface. The cells express low-intensity monoclonal surface immunoglobulin (Smig; usually immunoglobulin [Ig] M ± IgD) and the pan-B-cell antigens CD19, CD20, CD23, and CD24 in almost all cases, as well as CD21 (which includes the receptor for the Epstein-Barr virus and the C3d component of complement) in more than 75% of cases. Almost all cells exhibit Ia antigen and receptors for the Fc fragment of IgG and spontaneously form rosettes with mouse erythrocytes. In addition to B cell antigens, CLL cells express CDS (Leu 1, Tl, and TlOl), a pan-T-cell antigen. Other T-cell antigens are absent. CD25 (TAC, IL-2 receptor) antigen is positive in about 25% of cases. T cells are increased in number at diagnosis, and the CD4/CD8 ratio is often inverted, owing to a relatively greater increase in $CD8^+$ cells. The CD4/CD8 ratio declines as the disease progresses and after therapy. The T cells have a blunted response to T-cell mitogens and decreased delayed hypersensitivity reactions to recall antigens. However, these T-cell functions are impaired by factors produced by the CLL cells because purified T cells have a normal response to T-cell mitogens.

GENETICS

Genes mutated in CLL include *TP53* (15% of patients), *SF3B1* (15%), *ATM* (9%), *MYD88* (10%), and *NOTCH1* (4%). Standard cytogenetic analysis identifies abnormalities in 40 to 50% of cases of CLL, but CLL cells have low mitotic activity. By FISH, the likelihood of detecting abnormalities increases to 80%. A 13q deletion is the most common abnormality; other abnormalities include llq deletion (15 to 20%), trisomy 12 (15 to 20%), and 17p deletion (5 to 10%). The 17p deletion increases in frequency as the disease progresses, recurs after therapy, and is associated with a very poor prognosis. The llq deletion also is associated with a poorer prognosis, whereas the 13q deletion, if present as the sole abnormality, is associated with a favorable prognosis.

CLINICAL MANIFESTATIONS

Most patients with CLL do not have symptoms, and the disease is diagnosed when absolute lymphocytosis is noted in the peripheral blood (Fig. 184-6)

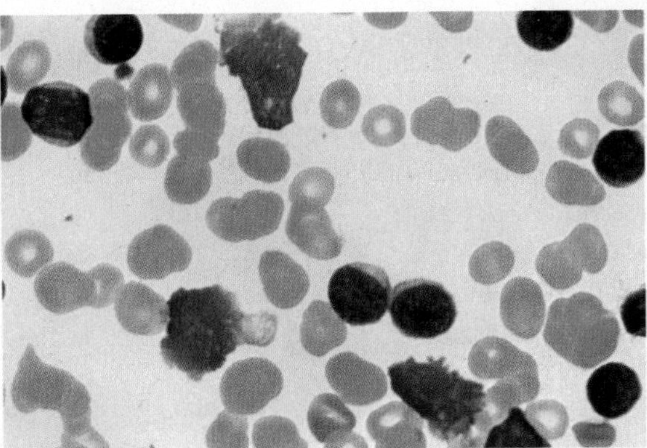

FIGURE 184-6. Chronic lymphocytic leukemia. Peripheral smear shows that the predominant leukocytes are "normal," mature-appearing lymphocytes, with occasional "smudge" cells. (Courtesy Andrew Schafer, MD.)

during evaluation for other illnesses or when the patient undergoes a routine physical examination. Symptoms such as fatigue, lethargy, loss of appetite, weight loss, and reduced exercise tolerance are nonspecific. Many patients have enlarged lymph nodes. B symptoms (fever, night sweats, weight loss) are rarely present initially, and their presence in later stages of the disease suggests transformation to large cell lymphoma (Richter transformation). The most common infections are sinopulmonary. As the disease progresses, the frequency of neutropenia, T-cell deficiency, and hypogammaglobulinemia increases, resulting in infections with gram-negative bacteria, fungi, and viruses such as herpes zoster and herpes simplex.

The major physical findings relate to infiltration of the reticuloendothelial system. Lymphadenopathy with discrete, soft, mobile lymph nodes is present in two thirds of patients at diagnosis. Later, as the lymph nodes enlarge, they can become matted. Enlargement of the liver or spleen is less common at diagnosis (approximately 10% and 40% of cases, respectively) but occurs more frequently with progression. Organ failure resulting from infiltration with CLL is uncommon. Infiltration of the central nervous system in CLL is rare, and central nervous system symptoms are more likely to be caused by opportunistic infections such as cryptococcosis or listeriosis.

DIAGNOSIS

CLL is characterized by absolute lymphocyte counts that typically range from 5000 to 600,000 × 10^9/μL in the peripheral blood. Even with markedly elevated WBC counts, hyperviscosity symptoms rarely occur, probably because of the small size and pliability of the cells. Anemia (hemoglobin <11 g/dL) is present in 15 to 20% of patients at diagnosis and thrombocytopenia (platelet count <100 × 10^9/μL) in 10%. However, bone marrow replacement and hypersplenism, which are seen with progressive disease, increase the frequency of anemia and thrombocytopenia. The anemia is usually normochromic and normocytic, and the reticulocyte count is normal unless the patient has autoimmune hemolytic anemia (Chapter 160), which usually results from the development of a warm-reacting IgG antibody. The diagnosis of autoimmune hemolytic anemia, which occurs in 10% of cases, is confirmed by a positive direct Coombs (DAT) test (80 to 90% of cases), reticulocytosis, a low serum haptoglobulin concentration, and an elevated unconjugated serum bilirubin level. In such patients, reactive erythroid hyperplasia as a response to the hemolysis may be masked in the bone marrow by the marked lymphocytic infiltration. Cold agglutinin hemolysis occurs rarely in CLL. Autoimmune thrombocytopenia (immune thrombocytopenic purpura; Chapter 172) can be diagnosed in 10 to 15% of cases. The antibodies causing red cell and platelet destruction are not produced by the CLL cells, and the mechanisms for the associated autoimmune diseases are not known. Pure red cell aplasia (Chapter 165) is an additional, underappreciated cause of anemia in CLL.

The lymphocytes in CLL are indistinguishable on light or electron microscopy from normal small B lymphocytes (see Fig. 184-6). On bone marrow aspiration, the proportion of lymphocytes is greater than 30% and may be up to 100%. Four patterns of lymphocyte infiltration on bone marrow biopsy occur: nodular (15%), interstitial (30%), mixed nodular and interstitial (30%), and diffuse (35%). Most early-stage cases have one of the first three patterns; diffuse histology is common in advanced-stage disease and becomes more prominent as the disease evolves. A diffuse histologic pattern confers a poor prognosis regardless of the stage of disease.

Differential Diagnosis

There are many diseases that can cause lymphocytosis, including pertussis (Chapter 313), cytomegalovirus (Chapter 370), Epstein-Barr virus mononucleosis (Chapter 377), tuberculosis (Chapter 324), toxoplasmosis (Chapter 349), chronic inflammatory disorders, and autoimmune syndromes. These diseases are seldom confused with B-cell CLL, largely because the lymphocytosis in these conditions is usually less than 15 × 10^9/μL and is not sustained. If doubt persists, immunophenotypic or molecular studies can distinguish the monoclonal lymphocytosis in CLL from the T-cell or polyclonal B-cell proliferation in the other disorders.

In individuals 62 to 80 years old, monoclonal CLL-phenotype B cells are found in about 5% of individuals with normal blood counts. In patients with greater than 4000 lymphocytes/mL, about 45% have CLL, about 40% have reactive lymphocytosis, and about 15% have monoclonal CLL-phenotype B cells that confer a 1.1% per year risk for developing CLL. The latter is a more recently recognized entity that has been termed *monoclonal B-cell lymphocytosis*. In patients ultimately diagnosed with CLL, B-cell clones were previously present in peripheral blood in 98% of patients, sometimes many years before diagnosis.

Other Chronic Lymphocytic Leukemias

The more difficult differential diagnosis is distinguishing CLL from other lymphoproliferative disorders such as prolymphocytic leukemia (PLL), splenic lymphoma with villous lymphocytes, HCL (see earlier section), the leukemic phase of mantle cell lymphoma, and Waldenström macroglobulinemia (Chapter 187). Although certain clinical features are more common in some of these disorders (e.g., marked splenomegaly with minimal or no lymphadenopathy in PLL, splenic lymphoma, and HCL vs. extensive lymphadenopathy with or without splenomegaly in CLL), none of these clinical features is specific. The differential diagnosis therefore depends largely on histopathologic and, more specifically, immunophenotypic features (Table 184-4).

Prolymphocytic Leukemia

PLL is an uncommon disease (incidence <5% that of CLL), and its characteristics of massive splenomegaly, minimal lymphadenopathy, and markedly elevated WBC count (often >100 × 10^9/μL), with 10 to 90% of the cells being prolymphocytes, distinguish this disease from typical B-cell CLL. Prolymphocytes are larger cells that have a distinct nucleolus and express FMC-7. The male-to-female ratio is 4 : 1, and the median age at diagnosis is 70 years. Survival is shorter than in CLL (median, 3 years), and response to therapies usually applied in CLL is poor. A serum paraprotein, typically IgG or IgA, is present in one third of cases. The immunoglobulin on the surface of the cells is occasionally IgG or IgA, not IgM ± IgD, as in CLL. Several karyotypic abnormalities have been reported in PLL, including t (11; 14) (q13; q32). Deletions of llq3, 23, and 17p are more common in B-cell PLL than in CLL. Abnormalities in the *TP53* oncogene are found in 75% of cases of B-cell PLL. One fifth of PLL cases express a T-cell phenotype.

Small Lymphocytic Lymphoma

Small lymphocytic lymphoma (SLL) shares histopathologic and immunophenotypic features with CLL, differing only in the lack of lymphocytosis in

TABLE 184-4 DIFFERENTIAL DIAGNOSIS OF INDOLENT LYMPHOPROLIFERATIVE DISORDERS

DISEASE	LYMPHADENOPATHY (%)	SPLENOMEGALY (%)	CELL OF ORIGIN (BIT)	POSITIVE MARKERS Smlg	CDS	CD19, CD20 (%)	Other
Chronic lymphocytic leukemia (CLL)	75	50	B (20 : 1)	Weak	>90%	90	Mouse red blood cell receptors
Prolymphocytic leukemia (PLL)	33	95	B (4 : 1)	Bright	T-cell PLL	75	FMC-7
Hairy cell leukemia	<10	80	B (T rare)	Bright	—	>90	CD25, CD11C, CD103
Lymphoma (leukemic phase)	90	90	B (T rare)	Bright	Some	>90	CD10
Splenic lymphoma with villous lymphocytes	10	80	B	Bright	20%	>90	FMC-7, CD22
Waldenström macroglobulinemia	33	33	All B	Weak	Some	Many	CD38, PCA-1
Large granular lymphocytosis	10	10	All T	Absent	-	-	CD2, CD3, CD8

CD2 = pan-T cell; CD3 = pan-mature T cell; CDS = pan-T cell, B-cell CLL; CD8 = T cell (suppressor cytotoxic); CD10 = early B cell; CD11C = hairy cell, activated T cell, NK cell; CD19 = early pan-B cell; CD20 = pan-B cell; CD25 = low-affinity interleukin-2 receptor; CD38 = activated B cell, thymocyte, plasma cell; FMC-7 = PLL, hairy cell leukemia; PCA-1 = plasma cell; Smlg = monoclonal surface immunoglobulin.

he peripheral blood. The bone marrow in SLL may or may not have more han 30% lymphocytes. LFA-1 adhesion protein is much more commonly expressed on SLL cells than on CLL cells. Other lymphomas, such as follicular and mantle cell lymphomas (Chapter 185), occasionally manifest a leukemic phase on initial presentation. Follicular lymphoma cells are often cleaved on light microscopy, have bright staining for Smlg, and are positive for FMC-7 and CD10. Lymph node biopsy should be performed to identify these cases with greater precision. The presence of lymphoma cells in the blood in follicular lymphoma is more common with advanced disease. Follicular lymphoma can usually be identified by the presence of the translocation t(14;18) and consequent *BCL2* rearrangement, both of which are rare in CLL. The WBC count in Waldenström macroglobulinemia (Chapter 187) is usually much lower than in CLL ($<10 \times 10^9/\mu L$), and many patients are leukopenic. The cells have a plasmacytoid appearance, CD38 and PCA-1 positivity, and more Smlg and cytoplasmic Ig. A serum monoclonal IgM peak is present in almost all cases of Waldenström macroglobulinemia but is uncommon in CLL.

T-Cell Leukemias

The predominant clinical manifestation of *Sézary syndrome* (a $CD4^+$ T-cell malignant disorder related to *mycosis fungoides*) is chronic exfoliative erythroderma with a low number of circulating monoclonal T cells. The clinical and laboratory differentiation from CLL is not difficult.

Other T-cell malignant disorders with peripheral blood involvement are *adult T-cell leukemia-lymphoma* and *large granular lymphocytosis*, also referred to as *large granular lymphoproliferative disorder*, T-cell lymphocytosis with neutropenia, or T-γ lymphocytosis syndrome. Adult T-cell leukemia-lymphoma is associated with a retrovirus (human T-lymphotropic virus I) and is common in Japan and the Caribbean. It frequently manifests with lytic bone lesions and hypercalcemia. In T-cell large granular lymphoproliferative disorders, the absolute lymphocyte count is usually low ($<5 \times 10^9/\mu L$). The disease is defined by clonal amplification of either $CD3^+$ cytotoxic T-lymphocytes or $CD3^-$ natural killer (NK) cells.[12] These patients often have splenomegaly, neutropenia, and rheumatoid arthritis–like symptoms. A subset, called NK-cell large granular lymphocytosis, has an NK-cell phenotype ($CD16^-$) and no molecular evidence of T-cell receptor rearrangement. The lymphocytes in large granular lymphoproliferative disorder have abundant cytoplasm with azurophilic granules. Most patients have a benign course, although repeated infections can occur.

Staging and Prognostic Factors

The natural history of CLL is heterogeneous, with survival times ranging from 2 to 20 years after diagnosis. Either of two validated clinical staging systems can be used. The Rai staging system (1975) defines five stages and is most frequently used in the United States, whereas the Binet system (1981) defines three stages and is most frequently used in Europe (Table 184-5). Patients with anemia and thrombocytopenia (Rai III and IV, Binet C) have the worst prognosis; patients with lymphocytosis alone (Rai 0, some Binet A patients) have an excellent prognosis. A group of patients with a lymphocyte count of less than $30 \times 10^9/\mu L$, hemoglobin greater than 13 g/dL, platelet count greater than $100 \times 10^9/\mu L$, fewer than three involved node areas, and lymphocyte doubling time greater than 12 months has been described as having "smoldering" CLL, with survival equal to that of an age- and sex-matched control population. Patients tend to progress through stages, with many patients developing more sites of involvement over time and eventually experience marrow failure; however, anemia and thrombocytopenia can develop abruptly, even without antibody-mediated destruction or markedly increased tumor burden.

Other adverse factors include a diffuse pattern of lymphocytic infiltration observed on bone marrow biopsy; molecular abnormalities, including deletion of llq or 17p; advanced age; male sex; elevated serum levels of thymidine kinase, β_2-microglobulin, and soluble CD23; rapid lymphocyte doubling time; an increased proportion of large or atypical lymphocytes in the peripheral blood; and lack of somatic mutation of the *VH* gene within the B-CLL cell or the presence of the ZAP-70 protein or CD38 on the CLL cell surface.

TREATMENT

Rx

The major therapeutic questions are when to treat and which therapeutic regimen to use. Recent progress has transformed the treatment of CLL, initially from chemotherapy to chemoimmunotherapy and now to mechanism-driven drugs that target the B-cell receptor signaling pathway.[13] Patients with CLL are usually older, and the prognosis of the disease is variable (with some early-stage cases being stable for 10 to 20 years). Treatment of early-stage CLL (Rai 0, Binet A) is delayed until the disease progresses. In randomized trials, early treatment with alkylating agents did not prolong survival and was associated with a heightened risk for developing second malignant tumors. Treatment of Rai stages III and IV (Binet stage C) is recommended at the time of diagnosis because of the morbidities associated with cytopenias and the poor survival time of these patients. Treatment of intermediate-stage disease (Rai I and II, Binet B) is recommended if symptomatic disease (fever, sweats, weight loss, severe fatigue) or massive lymphadenopathy, with or without hepatosplenomegaly, is present.

Medical Therapy

Chemotherapy

Fludarabine monophosphate (25 mg/m^2/day for 5 days every 4 weeks), an adenosine analogue, is approved by the FDA for treatment of relapsed CLL; it produces an overall response rate of 50 to 60%. The dose-limiting toxicity is myelosuppression. In a large randomized trial of initial therapy for CLL, fludarabine was compared with chlorambucil, the historical standard therapy; it resulted in higher overall and complete remission rates, longer duration of remission, and improved response rates on crossover. Ten-year follow-up showed a survival benefit in the fludarabine arm. Cladribine is used primarily in Europe, where it appears to have efficacy similar to fludarabine. Pentostatin has not been as widely studied in CLL as in HCL.

The combination of fludarabine and cyclophosphamide (FC) was a logical attempt to improve on the efficacy of fludarabine alone by combining it with the other most active agent in this disease, an alkylating agent. The FC combination has been compared with fludarabine alone in three randomized trials. All these trials consistently showed a higher complete response rate, higher overall response rate, and longer progression-free survival with the FC combination.

TABLE 184-5 RAI AND BINET STAGING SYSTEMS IN CHRONIC LYMPHOCYTIC LEUKEMIA

STAGE	LYMPHOCYTOSIS	LYMPHADENOPATHY	HEPATOMEGALY OR SPLENOMEGALY	HEMOGLOBIN (g/dL)	PLATELETS ×10^3/mL
RAI STAGING SYSTEM					
0	+	−	−	≥11	≥100
I	+	+	−	≥11	≥100
II	+	±	+	≥11	≥100
III	+	±	±	<11	≥100
IV	+	±	±	Any	<100
BINET STAGING SYSTEM					
A	+	±	± (<3 lymphatic groups* positive)	≥10	≥100
B	+	±	± (≥3 lymphatic groups* positive)	≥10	≥100
C	+	±	±	<10†	<100†

*The three lymphatic groups are (1) cervical, axillary, and inguinal nodes; (2) liver; and (3) spleen. Each group is considered one group whether unilateral or bilateral.
†The criterion is hemoglobin <10 g/dL and/or platelets <100×10^3/mL.

TABLE 184-6 DEFINITION OF REMISSION IN CHRONIC LYMPHOCYTIC LEUKEMIA: THE INTERNATIONAL WORKSHOP IN CHRONIC LYMPHOCYTIC LEUKEMIA–NATIONAL CANCER INSTITUTE WORKING GROUP CRITERIA

CRITERION	COMPLETE REMISSION	PARTIAL REMISSION
Physical examination		
Nodes	None ≥1.5 cm	≥50% decrease
Liver/spleen	Not palpable	≥50% decrease
Symptoms	None	N/A
Peripheral blood		
Neutrophils	≥1500 m/L	≥1500/mL or ≥50% increase from baseline
Platelets	>100,000/μL	>100,000/μL or ≥50% increase from baseline
Hemoglobin	>11 g/dL	11 g/dL or >50% increase from baseline
Lymphocytes	≤4000 /mL	>50% decrease
Bone marrow	<30%, no B-lymphoid nodules	50% reduction in infiltrate or B-lymphoid nodules

After therapy, many patients remain stable for months to years before progressive disease indicates the need for further treatment. The goal of treatment is to achieve complete response (Table 184-6).

Bendamustine is a potent alkylating agent that has some structural similarity to nucleoside analogues, but preclinical data suggest that it does not function as a nucleoside analogue. Bendamustine was recently approved by the FDA for the treatment of CLL based on a randomized trial comparing this agent to chlorambucil as initial therapy for patients with CLL.A8 Complete and overall response rates were higher with bendamustine, and progression-free survival was longer. The main side effect is myelosuppression.

Monoclonal Antibodies Alone and with Chemotherapy

Rituximab, a monoclonal antibody targeting the CD20 antigen, is associated with response rates of about 50% when given at the standard dose (375 mg/m^2/week for 4 weeks) as initial therapy for CLL and significantly lower rates when used in the salvage setting; complete responses are rare in either situation. The major benefit of this antibody appears to be its use in combination with chemotherapy. Fludarabine combined with rituximab produces better responses than those seen historically with fludarabine alone. In addition, progression-free and overall survival rates are better than those seen in the historical cohort. A three-drug regimen of fludarabine, cyclophosphamide, and rituximab (FCR) appears to produce the best and most durable complete remission rates when used as first-line therapy. A randomized trial compared the activity of FC to that of FCR. The complete response rate and the overall response rate were significantly higher with FCR, and progression-free and overall survival rates were significantly longer than with chemotherapy alone.A9 A trial of previously untreated CLL patients with coexisting conditions tested the efficacy of chlorambucil alone versus chlorambucil plus rituximab versus chlorambucil plus obinutuzumab, a glycoengineered anti-CD20 monoclonal antibody. Combining an anti-CD20 antibody with chemotherapy improved outcomes, and obinutuzumab was found to be superior to rituximab when each was combined with chlorambucil.A10

Alemtuzumab (Campath-IH; 30 mg intravenously three times a week for 4 to 12 weeks), a monoclonal antibody that binds to the CD52 antigen, was originally approved for the treatment of fludarabine-refractory CLL. One third of such patients can achieve remission. Recently, alemtuzumab was compared with chlorambucil as initial therapy for symptomatic patients with CLL. Alemtuzumab produced higher complete and overall response rates and longer progression-free survival. In the first-line treatment of high-risk CLL, the addition of subcutaneous alemtuzumab to oral FC chemotherapy (fludarabine plus cyclophosphamide) improved progression-free survival and overall survival (the latter only in patients younger than 75 years) compared with FC chemotherapy alone.A11 Alemtuzumab was withdrawn from the market in the United States and Europe in 2012 but is available free of charge from the company by compassionate request.

Ofatumumab is a humanized monoclonal antibody that binds to CD20, but to a different epitope than rituximab. This drug was recently approved by the FDA for the treatment of fludarabine- and alemtuzumab-refractory CLL. In the pivotal trial, the drug was given intravenously for 8 weeks and then monthly for 4 months.A12 The overall response rate in this highly refractory population was 58%; the median progression-free survival was 6 months, with a median overall survival of 13.7 months. As with other monoclonal antibodies, the predominant side effects are infusion reactions, which tend to be more common with the initial doses.

B-Cell Receptor Signaling Pathway Inhibitors

A new category of targeted agents, called B-cell receptor signaling pathway inhibitors, is providing significant increased efficacy in CLL. Several inhibitors are being tested, targeting different kinases in the B-cell receptor pathway. Recent data have demonstrated that B-cell receptor signaling inhibitors are very active, particularly for the treatment of relapsed CLL. Ibrutinib is a first-in-class, oral covalent inhibitor of Bruton tyrosine kinase, an essential enzyme in B-cell receptor signaling, homing, and adhesion. It has been granted accelerated approval by the FDA for use in CLL. A randomized trial compared the effect of ibrutinib with that of the anti-CD20 antibody ofatumumab, both used alone, in the treatment of patients with relapsed or refractory CLL or small lymphocytic lymphoma.A13 Ibrutinib significantly improved both progression-free and overall survival, compared with ofatumumab. Idelalisib is an inhibitor of phosphatidylinositol 3-kinase δ (PI3Kδ). Signaling through the B-cell receptor is mediated in part by activation of PI3Kδ. The δ isoform of PI3K is highly expressed in lymphoid cells, and it is the most critical isoform involved in the malignant phenotype of CLL. In a randomized, phase 3 study, patients with relapsed CLL who had clinically significant coexisting medical conditions that made them less able to undergo standard chemotherapy were randomized to receive eight intravenous infusions of rituximab plus either idelalisib 150 mg orally twice daily or placebo.A14 The combination of idelalisib and rituximab, compared with rituximab alone, significantly improved response rate, progression-free survival, and overall survival.

Chimeric Antigen Receptor–Directed T Cells

Chimeric antigen receptors (CARs) are fusion proteins that combine antigen moieties and costimulatory T-cell receptors to redirect T cells toward malignant cells. All CARs targeting CLL have thus far directed the T cells through recognition of CD19.[14] Complete remissions, including absence of residual disease by sensitive testing, has been produced in refractory patients. *Cytokine release syndrome*, which can be life-threatening, is the initial toxicity. (Cytokine release syndrome, a rare phenomenon, also occurs in graft-versus-host disease after transplantation, severe infections, hemophagocytic lymphohistiocytosis or macrophage activation syndrome, and monoclonal antibody therapy; cytokines trigger an acute systemic inflammatory response that leads to endothelial and organ damage, microvascular leakage, and heart failure.[15]) Late toxicity includes the need for immunoglobulin replacement due to simultaneous eradication of normal B cells. CARs targeting other antigens in CLL are being investigated.

Stem Cell Transplantation

Autologous stem cell transplantation has no proven benefit in terms of survival or longterm disease control in CLL. Data on allogeneic stem cell transplantation are limited to young patients with refractory disease, in whom a long-term control rate of 40 to 55% has been reported. Nonmyeloablative stem cell transplantation, which works mainly by its graft-versusleukemia effect, has been used in older patients with CLL with some success.

Radiation Therapy

In CLL, radiation therapy is used palliatively to shrink unsightly or painfully enlarged nodal masses or an enlarged spleen.

Autoimmune and Infectious Manifestations

Autoimmune hemolytic anemia and immune-mediated thrombocytopenia do not correlate closely with the activity of CLL. Prednisone (60 to 100 mg/day) is indicated as treatment for autoimmune hemolytic anemia (Chapter 160) and for some cases of immune-mediated thrombocytopenia (Chapter 172) in CLL. If there is no response in 3 to 4 weeks, the treatment has failed, and the dose should be tapered over 1 to 2 weeks. If a response is obtained, the dose is reduced by 25% each week over 4 weeks. Patients for whom corticosteroids fail often respond to low-dose oral cyclosporine 100 mg three times a day. Other therapeutic options include splenectomy, intravenous immunoglobulin, rituximab, and alemtuzumab. Intravenous immunoglobulin (400 mg/kg every 3 to 4 weeks) significantly decreases the incidence of infections in patients with recurrent infections and hypogammaglobulinemia. However, the cost of this therapy is substantial.

PROGNOSIS

Approximately one third of patients who present with early-stage CLL never require therapy and have the same survival as age-matched controls. Frequent characteristics of such patients include WBC less than 30×10^9/L, hemoglobin greater than 13 g/dL, nondiffuse pattern on bone marrow biopsy, and slow lymphocyte doubling time.

Factors associated with shorter time to treatment failure as well as either poorer response to at least chemotherapy-based regimes, or shorter remission durations, include an unmutated *IgVH* gene, presence of 17p or llq deletions, presence of ZAP70 and CD38, and mutations in *TP53, SF3Bl, ATM,* and *NOTCH*. A poor response to therapy is an adverse factor in all phases of the disease. As CLL progresses, the development of a prolymphocytic transformation (10% of cases) or transformation to large cell lymphoma (Richter transformation) portends a median survival time of less than 6 months. Other factors that may suggest transformation are the development of B symptoms (fevers, night sweats, weight loss), a markedly elevated lactate dehydrogenase level, or fluorodeoxyglucose-avid disease on positron emission tomography. A high incidence of second malignant tumors (10 to 20% of patients) either precedes or follows the diagnosis of CLL; the roles of therapy versus impaired immune surveillance as causative factors are unclear. Skin cancer, including melanoma, as well as colorectal and lung cancers particularly are common. CLL tends to develop in older people; in indolent cases, death occurs from other intercurrent illnesses seen in this age group. Almost all patients younger than 60 years and those with progressive disease die as a result of CLL, primarily from infections. Gram-positive organisms usually cause nonfatal infections early in CLL, but most deaths due to infection are associated with gram-negative bacterial or fungal infections. Infection with other opportunistic organisms, such as *Mycobacterium tuberculosis,* herpes virus, and *Pseudomonas jiroveci,* may also be fatal.

Grade A References

A1. Jabbour E, Kantarjian HM, Saglio G, et al. Early response with dasatinib or imatinib in chronic myeloid leukemia: a 3-year follow-up from a randomized phase 3 trial (DASISION). *Blood.* 2014;123:494-500.

A2. Hughes TP, Saglio G, Kantarjian H, et al. Early molecular response predicts outcomes in patients with chronic myeloid leukemia in chronic phase treated with frontline nilotinib or imatinib. *Blood.* 2014;12:1353-1360.

A3. Shah NP, Guilhot F, Cortes JE, et al. Long-term outcome with dasatinib after imatinib failure in chronic-phase chronic myeloid leukemia: follow-up of a phase 3 study. *Blood.* 2014;123: 2317-2324.

A4. Druker B, Guilhot F, O'Brien S, et al. Five-year follow-up of patients receiving imatinib for chronic myeloid leukemia. *N Engl J Med.* 2006;355:2408-2417.

A5. Larson RA, Hochhaus A, Hughes TP, et al. Nilotinib vs imatinib in patients with newly diagnosed Philadelphia chromosome-positive chronic myeloid leukemia in chronic phase: ENESTnd 3-year follow-up. *Leukemia.* 2012;26:2197-2203.

A6. Kantarjian HM, Shah NP, Cortes JE, et al. Dasatinib or imatinib in newly diagnosed chronic- phase chronic myeloid leukemia: 2-year follow-up from a randomized phase 3 trial (DASISION). *Blood.* 2012;119:1123-1129.

A7. Cortes JE, Kim DW, Kantarjian HM, et al. Bosutinib versus imatinib in newly diagnosed chronic-phase chronic myeloid leukemia: results from the BELA trial. *J Clin Oncol.* 2012;30:3486-3492.

A8. Knauf WU, Lissichkov T, Aldaoud A, et al. Phase III randomized study of bendamustine compared with chlorambucil in previously untreated patients with chronic lymphocytic leukemia. *J Clin Oncol.* 2009;27:4378-4384.

A9. Hallek M, Fischer K, Fingerle-Rowson G, et al. Addition of rituximab to fludarabine and cyclophosphamide in patients with chronic lymphocytic leukaemia: a randomised, open-label, phase 3 trial. *Lancet.* 2010;376:1164-1174.

A10. Goede V, Fischer K, Busch R, et al. Obinutuzumab plus chlorambucil in patients with CLL and coexisting conditions. *N Engl J Med.* 2014;370:1101-1110.

A11. Geisler CH, van T' Veer MB, Jurlander J, et al. Frontline alemtuzumab with fludarabine and cyclophosphamide prolongs progression-free survival in high-risk CLL. *Blood.* 2014;123:3255-3262.

A12. Wierda WG, Kipps TJ, Dürig J, et al. Chemoimmunotherapy with O-FC in previously untreated patients with chronic lymphocytic leukemia. *Blood.* 2011;117:6450-6458.

A13. Byrd JC, Brown JR, O'Brien S, et al. Ibrutinib versus ofatumumab in previously treated chronic lymphocytic leukemia. *N Engl J Med.* 2014;371:213-223.

A14. Furman RR, Sharman JP, Coutre SE, et al. Idelalisib and rituximab in relapsed chronic lymphocytic leukemia. *N Engl J Med.* 2014;370:997-1007.

GENERAL REFERENCES

For the General References and other additional features, please visit Expert Consult at https://expertconsult.inkling.com.

185

NON-HODGKIN LYMPHOMAS

PHILIP J. BIERMAN AND JAMES O. ARMITAGE

DEFINITION

Lymphomas are solid tumors of the immune system. Increasing knowledge of the biology of the immune system has led to a corresponding increase in the understanding of these malignancies. In addition to better systems of classification and clinical evaluation, this new knowledge has led to the development of new therapies. Beneficial treatment is available for essentially every patient with non-Hodgkin lymphoma. The overall survival of lymphoma patients has increased steadily over the past 30 years, and many patients can be cured.

EPIDEMIOLOGY

In the United States, approximately 70,000 new cases of non-Hodgkin lymphoma are diagnosed annually, and about 19,000 people are estimated to die each year of this disease. Non-Hodgkin lymphomas account for about 4% of new cancers in the United States and result in about 3% of cancer deaths. The U.S. lifetime risk for developing non-Hodgkin lymphoma is estimated to be 2.4% (1 in 42) for men and 1.90% (1 in 52) for women. In 2010 the U.S. age-adjusted incidence rate for non-Hodgkin lymphoma was about 26.82 per 100,000 for men and 17.39 per 100,000 for women.[1] The incidence rate increases dramatically with age and is higher in whites than in other ethnic groups.

Geographic differences in the incidence of non-Hodgkin lymphomas vary as much as five-fold. The highest rates are seen in the United States, Europe, and Australia, whereas lower rates are seen in Asia. Even more striking are geographic differences in the incidence of certain types of non-Hodgkin lymphoma, such as Burkitt lymphoma, follicular lymphoma, extranodal natural killer (NK)/T-cell nasal lymphoma, and adult T-cell leukemia/lymphoma (see later).

Between 1950 and the beginning of the 21st century, the incidence rate for non-Hodgkin lymphomas in the United States increased by about 3 to 4% yearly. Since then, the incidence rate for non-Hodgkin lymphoma has reached a plateau. Increases occurred among both men and women in all parts of the world. The increase in incidence was partially related to the aging population (Fig. 185-1) and to the acquired immunodeficiency syndrome (AIDS) epidemic (Chapter 393). Occupational and environmental exposures (e.g., agricultural chemicals) may also explain some of the increase. Finally, some of the increase may be explained by improvements in the ability of pathologists to diagnose lymphoma and by improvements in imaging techniques.

PATHOBIOLOGY

For most cases of non-Hodgkin lymphoma, the cause is unknown, although genetic, environmental, and infectious agents have been implicated (Table 185-1).[2-4]

Genetic Factors

Familial non-Hodgkin lymphoma clusters have been described, and there is a slightly higher risk for non-Hodgkin lymphoma among siblings and first-degree relatives of patients with lymphoma or other hematologic malignancies. There is increasing recognition that host genetics are involved in the development of lymphomas. The incidence of non-Hodgkin lymphoma has

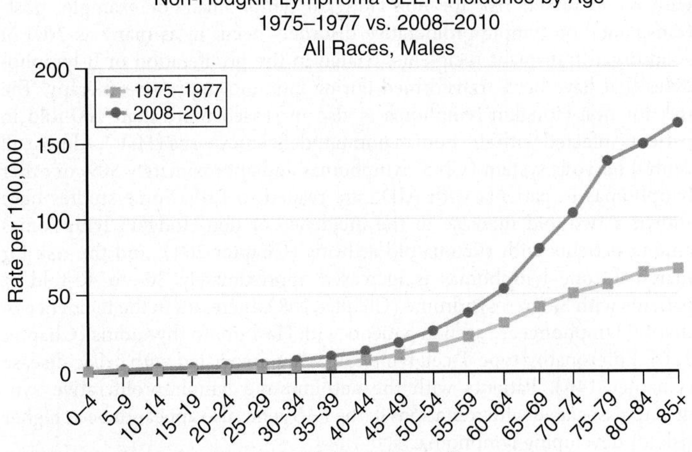

FIGURE 185-1. Non-Hodgkin lymphoma incidence by age in men, 1975-1977 versus 2008-2010. (From the Surveillance, Epidemiology, and End Results [SEER] Program of the National Cancer Institute, http://seer.cancer.gov/csr/1975_2010/.)

TABLE 185-1 FACTORS ASSOCIATED WITH THE DEVELOPMENT OF NON-HODGKIN LYMPHOMA

Inherited immune disorders
- Severe combined immunodeficiency disease
- Common variable immunodeficiency disease
- Wiskott-Aldrich syndrome
- Ataxia-telangiectasia
- X-linked lymphoproliferative disorder
- Autoimmune lymphoproliferative syndrome

Acquired immune disorders
- Solid organ transplantation
- Acquired immunodeficiency syndrome (AIDS)
- Methotrexate therapy for autoimmune disorders
- Rheumatoid arthritis and systemic lupus erythematosus
- Sjögren syndrome
- Hashimoto thyroiditis

Infectious agents
- Epstein-Barr virus
- Human T-lymphotropic virus type 1
- Human herpesvirus type 8
- Hepatitis C virus
- *Helicobacter pylori*
- *Borrelia burgdorferi*
- *Chlamydia psittaci*
- *Campylobacter jejuni*

Occupational and environmental exposure
- Herbicides
- Organic solvents
- Hair dyes
- Ultraviolet light
- Diet
- Smoking
- Drugs

been associated with polymorphisms in a variety of genes related to immunity, including chemokines, tumor necrosis factor, interleukin-10 (IL-10), and lymphotoxin-α. Polymorphisms in other genes related to the cell cycle and apoptosis have also been associated with an increased risk for developing lymphoma.

Immune System Abnormalities

Several inherited disorders increase the risk for developing non-Hodgkin lymphoma as much as 250-fold (see Table 185-1). In some of these conditions, the lymphoma may be related to Epstein-Barr virus (EBV; Chapter 377). For example, patients with X-linked lymphoproliferative disorder have mutations in the *SH2D1A* gene, which encodes proteins that regulate the host immune response against EBV-infected cells. Patients may develop fatal infectious mononucleosis or non-Hodgkin lymphoma after primary exposure to EBV. Acquired immunodeficiency states are also associated with an increased risk for non-Hodgkin lymphoma. For example, post-transplantation lymphoproliferative disorders occur in as many as 20% of solid organ transplant recipients, related to the proliferation of B lymphocytes that have been transformed during immunosuppressive therapy. The risk for non-Hodgkin lymphoma is also increased more than 100-fold in patients infected with the human immunodeficiency virus (HIV). Almost all central nervous system (CNS) lymphomas and approximately 50% of other lymphomas in patients with AIDS are related to EBV. Some studies have shown a two-fold increase in the incidence of non-Hodgkin lymphomas among patients with rheumatoid arthritis (Chapter 264), and the risk for marginal zone lymphomas is increased approximately 30- to 40-fold in patients with Sjögren syndrome (Chapter 268). Increases in the incidence of thyroid lymphoma are seen in patients with Hashimoto thyroiditis (Chapter 226). Enteropathy-type T-cell lymphomas are associated with celiac disease (Chapter 140). Patients with the autoimmune lymphoproliferative syndrome, associated with mutations in the *FAS* gene, also appear to be at higher risk for developing lymphoma.

Infectious Agents

EBV is associated with the majority of post-transplantation lymphoproliferative disorders and many AIDS-associated lymphomas. This viral genome is detectable in more than 95% of cases of endemic Burkitt lymphoma and in approximately 15 to 35% of cases of sporadic Burkitt lymphoma and AIDS-associated lymphomas. This virus is also associated with EBV-positive diffuse large B-cell lymphoma of elderly people, plasmablastic lymphoma, and extranodal NK/T-cell lymphoma.

The human T-lymphotropic virus type 1 (HTLV-1; Chapter 378) is detectable in virtually all cases of adult T-cell leukemia/lymphoma. The risk for lymphoma is approximately 3% in patients infected with HTLV-1. In endemic areas, up to 50% of all non-Hodgkin lymphomas may be related to HTLV-1.

Human herpesvirus-8 (HHV-8, Kaposi sarcoma–associated herpesvirus; Chapter 393), which is associated with expansion of the B-cell population, is also associated with primary effusion lymphoma (see later) in immunocompromised patients and with multicentric Castleman disease. Patients with primary effusion lymphoma are often coinfected with EBV.

Epidemiologic evidence has linked hepatitis C virus (Chapter 149) to lymphoplasmacytic lymphoma associated with type II cryoglobulinemia, nodal marginal zone lymphoma, and splenic marginal zone lymphoma. Chronic antigenic stimulation from this virus may lead to the emergence of malignant B-cell clones.

Helicobacter pylori is associated with gastric lymphoma (Chapter 192) of extranodal marginal zone/mucosa-associated lymphoid tissue (MALT). Colonized patients develop gastritis from chronic antigenic stimulation mediated by T cells, which respond to *H. pylori*–specific antigens and emergence of malignant B-cell clones. *Borrelia burgdorferi* (Chapter 321) has been associated with marginal zone B-cell lymphoma of the skin. Evidence also links *Chlamydia psittaci* (Chapter 318) with ocular adnexal lymphomas and *Campylobacter jejuni* with immunoproliferative small intestinal disease (Chapter 303).

Environmental and Occupational Exposure

Agricultural chemicals have been associated with an increased risk for developing non-Hodgkin lymphomas, and the strongest associations involve phenoxy herbicides such as 2,4-dichlorophenoxyacetic acid (2,4-D), which was also a component of Agent Orange (Chapter 19). An increased risk has also been associated with ionizing radiation (Chapter 20), organic solvents, hair dyes, and nitrates in drinking water, although contradictory results have been reported. Some studies have also linked non-Hodgkin lymphomas to high-fat diets and ultraviolet radiation (Chapter 180). The risk for non-Hodgkin lymphomas is increased approximately 20-fold after treatment for Hodgkin lymphoma (Chapter 186). Heavy smokers (Chapter 32) have an increased risk for developing follicular lymphoma. Low levels of vitamin D have been associated with increased risk for recurrent lymphoma, as well as poor outcome. Anti–tumor necrosis factor (anti-TNF) agents might be associated with an increased risk for developing lymphoma—particularly hepatosplenic T-cell lymphoma. There is also a reported association of breast implants with the development of anaplastic large cell lymphoma.

Pathology

Non-Hodgkin lymphomas are derived from cells of the immune system at varying stages of differentiation. In some cases, the cell of origin is directly linked to the morphology, immunophenotype, and clinical behavior of the lymphoma (Fig. 185-2 and Table 185-2).

The transformation of cells from the normal immune system into malignant lymphoma reflects the acquisition of specific genetic abnormalities. In many cases, cytogenetic studies can identify chromosomal translocations that underlie the development or progression of the lymphoma. In most cases of non-Hodgkin lymphoma, the activation of proto-oncogenes is the major abnormality, but occasionally chromosomal translocations can lead to fusion genes that code for chimeric proteins. In addition, some cases are associated with deletion of tumor suppressor genes. Specific genetic abnormalities are associated with some specific subtypes of non-Hodgkin lymphoma (Table 185-3). It is becoming clear that the tumor microenvironment from cells of the host immune system is important in tumor cell survival and response to therapy.[5,6]

Classification

Recognition of the Reed-Sternberg cell approximately 100 years ago made it possible to define Hodgkin lymphoma (Chapter 186) as a distinct entity, whereas other lymphomas were included under the heading "non-Hodgkin lymphomas." In the 1990s, a classification system incorporating morphologic, immunologic, genetic, and clinical information (the Revised

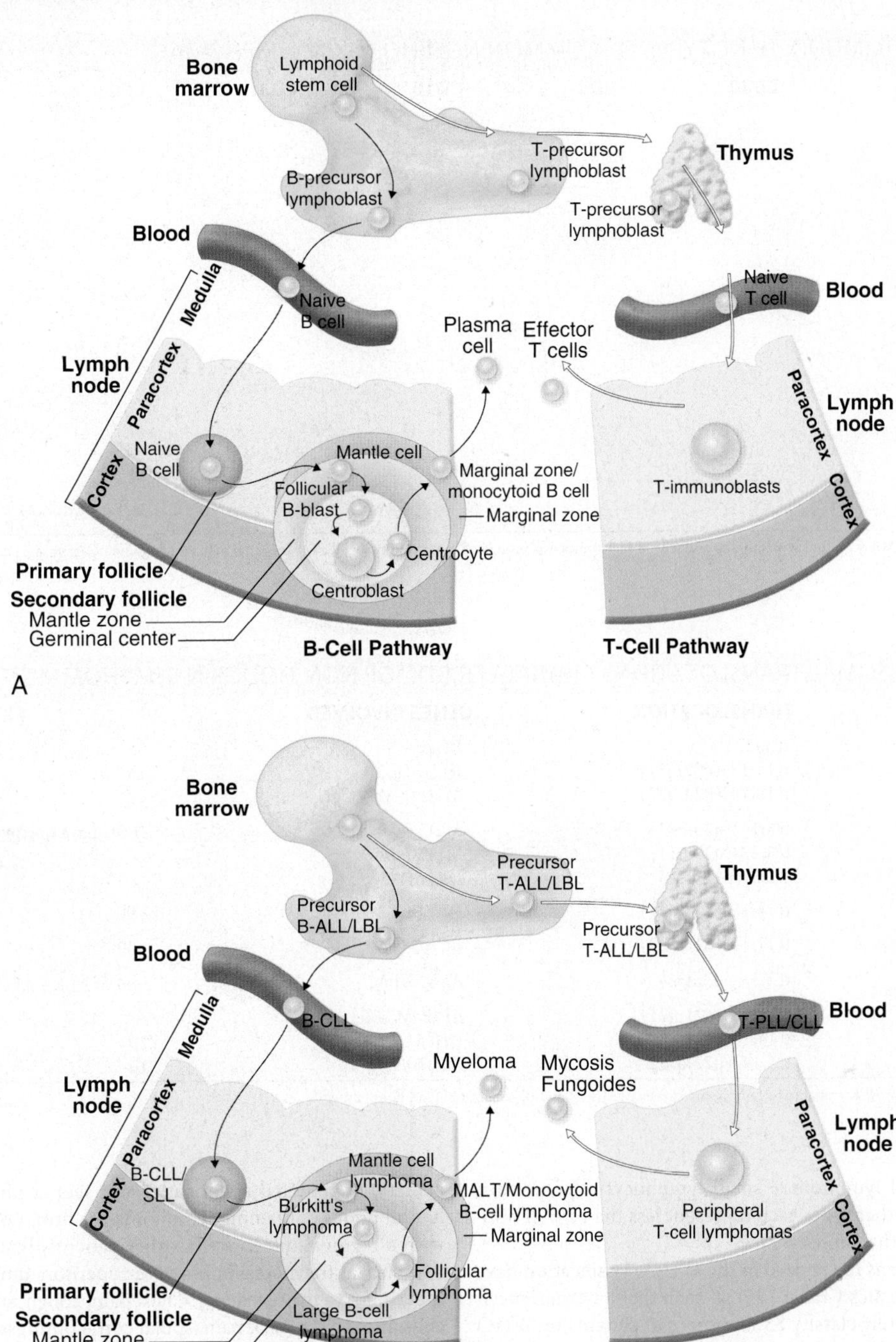

FIGURE 185-2. Postulated normal counterparts of currently recognized B- and T-cell malignancies. A, Schema of normal B- and T-cell differentiation. Bone marrow–derived lymphoid stem cells differentiate into committed B-cell precursors or into T-cell precursors that undergo further maturation in the thymus. These B- and T-cell precursors mature into naïve B or T cells that circulate to lymph nodes. After antigen exposure, normal B blasts proliferate and undergo further differentiation in the germinal center of the secondary follicle. The germinal center is surrounded by a mantle zone and a marginal zone. Antigen-specific B cells generated in the germinal center leave the follicle and reappear in the marginal zone. Thereafter, immunoglobulin-producing plasma cells accumulate in the lymph node medulla and subsequently exit to the periphery. Antigen-dependent T-cell proliferation occurs in the lymph node paracortex. After antigen exposure, mature T cells become immunoblasts and, subsequently, antigen-specific effector T cells that exit to the periphery. The postulated normal counterparts of many currently recognized T- and B-cell neoplasms are shown. **B,** T- and B-cell malignancies derived from the postulated normal counterparts shown in **A.** ALL = acute lymphoblastic leukemia; CLL = chronic lymphocytic leukemia; LBL = lymphoblastic lymphoma; MALT = mucosa-associated lymphoid tissue; PLL = prolymphocytic leukemia; SLL = small lymphocytic lymphoma.

European-American Lymphoma classification, or REAL) was developed to identify distinct clinicopathologic subgroups representing diseases that can be recognized by clinicians. This system was subsequently adopted as the World Health Organization (WHO) classification of lymphomas in 2008 (Table 185-4).[7]

The WHO classification divides lymphomas on the basis of B-cell or T/NK-cell origin and whether they are derived from primitive precursor cells or from more mature "peripheral" cells. Specific clinical and pathologic entities are recognized within each of these groupings. In the United States and Europe, 85 to 90% of non-Hodgkin lymphomas are B cell in origin.

The most frequent type is diffuse large B-cell lymphoma, which represents 31% of all non-Hodgkin lymphomas worldwide. The next most frequent type is follicular lymphoma, which represents 22% of cases. Follicular lymphoma is relatively more frequent in North America and Western Europe and less frequent in Asia. Less common types, each representing between 5 and 10% of all non-Hodgkin lymphomas, are extranodal marginal zone/MALT

TABLE 185-2 TYPICAL IMMUNOPHENOTYPES OF COMMON NON-HODGKIN LYMPHOMAS

LYMPHOMA	CD20	CD3	CD10	CD5	CD23	OTHER
Small lymphocytic	+	−	−	+	+	
Lymphoplasmacytic	+	−	−	−	−	Cytoplasmic Ig^+
Extranodal marginal zone MALT	+	−	−	−	−	
Nodal marginal zone	+	−	−	−	−	
Follicular	+	−	+	−		
Mantle cell	+	−	−	+	−	Cyclin $D1^+$
Diffuse large B cell	+	−				
Mediastinal large B cell	+	−				
Burkitt	+	−	+	−		TdT^-
Precursor T lymphoblastic	−	+/−				TdT^+, $CD1a^{+/-}$, $CD7^+$
Anaplastic large T cell	−	+/−				$CD30^+$, $CD15^-$, EMA^+, ALK^+
Peripheral T cell	−	+/−				Other pan-T variable

ALK = anaplastic lymphoma kinase; EMA = epithelial membrane antigen; MALT = mucosa-associated lymphoid tissue; TdT = terminal deoxynucleotidyl transferase.

TABLE 185-3 CHROMOSOMAL TRANSLOCATIONS CHARACTERISTIC OF NON-HODGKIN LYMPHOMA

LYMPHOMA SUBTYPE	TRANSLOCATION	GENES INVOLVED	FREQUENCY (%)
Diffuse large B cell	t(3q27) t(14;18)(q32;q21) t(18;14)(q24;q32)	*BCL6* *IgH, BCL2* *MYC (c-Myc), IgH*	35 15-20 <5
Burkitt	t(8;14)(q24;q32) t(8;22)(q24;q11) t(2;8)(p12;q24)	*MYC, IgH* *MYC, IgL* *IgK, MYC*	100% have one of these, most commonly t(8;14)
Follicular	t(14;18)(q32;q21)	*IgH, BCL2*	~90
Mantle cell	t(11;14)(q13;q32)	*BCL1, IgH*	>90
ALCL	t(2;5)(p23;q35)	*ALK, NPM*	>80 of ALK+ ALCLs
MALT	t(11;18)(q21;q21) t(14;18)(q21;q32) t(1;14)(p22;q32)	*API2, MALT1* *IgH, MALT1* *BCL10, IgH*	35 20 10

ALCL = anaplastic large cell lymphoma; ALK = anaplastic lymphoma kinase; MALT = mucosa-associated lymphoid tissue.

lymphomas, peripheral T-cell lymphomas, small lymphocytic lymphoma, and mantle cell lymphoma. Other types each represent less than 2% of non-Hodgkin lymphomas seen in the United States.

The non-Hodgkin lymphomas recognized in the WHO classification have clinically distinctive characteristics (Table 185-5), such that an experienced hematopathologist can accurately classify 85% or more of patients by WHO criteria when adequate material is available. Some diagnoses, such as follicular lymphoma, can be made with a high degree of accuracy without immunologic or genetic studies. The diagnosis of T-cell lymphomas cannot be made accurately without immunophenotyping. Cytogenetic studies and molecular genetic studies (fluorescent in situ hybridization, or FISH) can help resolve difficult differential diagnoses. For example, the presence of a t(8;14) translocation supports the diagnosis of Burkitt lymphoma, whereas a t(11;14) with cyclin D1 overexpression can confirm the diagnosis of mantle cell lymphoma (see Tables 185-2 and 185-3).

The use of DNA microarrays has allowed the identification of distinct subsets of patients with diffuse large B-cell lymphoma. Patients with histologically identical lymphomas can be divided into those with gene expression patterns resembling normal germinal center B cells (GCB), those whose tumors resemble activated post–germinal center B cells (ABC), or those with patterns resembling that seen in Hodgkin lymphoma. The last pattern is most frequently found in young women who present with large mediastinal masses. Use of immunohistochemistry to subdivide diffuse large B-cell lymphoma into GCB and ABC subtypes is widely used but does not correlate perfectly with DNA microarray results.

CLINICAL MANIFESTATIONS

The most common presentation of non-Hodgkin lymphoma is lymphadenopathy (Fig. 185-3; Chapter 168). In many cases, patients notice cervical, axillary, or inguinal adenopathy and seek a physician's advice. In general, lymph nodes containing lymphoma are firm, nontender, and not associated with a regional infection. In other patients, lymphadenopathy occurring in sites such as the mediastinum or retroperitoneum causes symptoms that bring the patient to the physician. Chest pain, cough, superior vena cava syndrome, abdominal pain, back pain, spinal cord compression, and symptoms of renal insufficiency associated with ureteral compression are characteristic.

Non-Hodgkin lymphomas are often associated with systemic symptoms that may lead to the diagnosis. The most obvious symptoms are fever, night sweats, and unexplained weight loss. Any of these symptoms without an obvious cause should lead a physician to consider the diagnosis of lymphoma. Other, less characteristic symptoms include fatigue, which is frequently present at the time of diagnosis if the patient is questioned carefully, and pruritus.

Non-Hodgkin lymphomas can involve essentially any organ in the body, and malfunction of that organ can cause symptoms that lead to the diagnosis. Examples include neurologic symptoms with primary brain lymphoma (Chapter 189), shortness of breath with MALT lymphomas in the lung, epigastric pain and vomiting with gastric MALT lymphomas or diffuse large B-cell lymphomas (Chapter 192), bowel obstruction with small bowel lymphomas (Chapter 193), testicular masses with diffuse large B-cell lymphoma (Chapter 200), and skin lesions with cutaneous lymphomas (Chapter 440). Many lymphomas involve the bone marrow and occasionally cause extensive myelophthisis (Chapter 165) and bone marrow failure. These patients may present with infections, bleeding, and anemia.

Non-Hodgkin lymphomas can also manifest with a variety of immunologic abnormalities. For example, autoimmune hemolytic anemia (Chapter 160) and immune thrombocytopenia (Chapter 172) can be the presenting manifestations of non-Hodgkin lymphoma, especially small lymphocytic

TABLE 185-4 WORLD HEALTH ORGANIZATION CLASSIFICATION OF NON-HODGKIN LYMPHOMA (2008)

PRECURSOR LYMPHOID NEOPLASMS

B-lymphoblastic leukemia/lymphoma
T-lymphoblastic leukemia/lymphoma

MATURE B-CELL NEOPLASMS

Chronic lymphocytic leukemia/small lymphocytic lymphoma
B-cell prolymphocytic leukemia
Splenic marginal zone lymphoma
Hairy cell leukemia
Splenic lymphoma/leukemia, unclassifiable
Lymphoplasmacytic lymphoma
Heavy chain diseases
Plasma cell neoplasms
Extranodal marginal zone lymphoma of mucosa-associated lymphoid tissue (MALT lymphoma)
Nodal marginal zone lymphoma
Follicular lymphoma
Primary cutaneous follicle center lymphoma
Mantle cell lymphoma
Diffuse large B-cell lymphoma, NOS (see Table 185-10 for variants and subtypes)
Burkitt lymphoma
B-cell lymphoma, unclassifiable, with features intermediate between diffuse large B-cell lymphoma and Burkitt lymphoma
B-cell lymphoma, unclassifiable, with features intermediate between diffuse large B-cell lymphoma and classical Hodgkin lymphoma

MATURE T- AND NK-CELL NEOPLASMS

Adult T-cell leukemia/lymphoma
Extranodal NK/T-cell lymphoma, nasal type
Enteropathy-associated T-cell lymphoma
Hepatosplenic T-cell lymphoma
Subcutaneous panniculitis-like T-cell lymphoma
Mycosis fungoides
Sézary syndrome
Primary cutaneous CD30$^+$ T-cell lymphoproliferative disorders
Peripheral T-cell lymphoma, NOS
Angioimmunoblastic T-cell lymphoma
Anaplastic large cell lymphoma, ALK positive
Anaplastic large cell lymphoma, ALK negative

ALK = anaplastic lymphoma kinase; MALT = mucosa-associated lymphoid tissue; NK = natural killer; NOS = not otherwise specified.

lymphoma/chronic lymphocytic leukemia as well as other subtypes, including diffuse large B-cell lymphoma. Peripheral neuropathies (Chapter 420), often associated with overproduction of a monoclonal protein, can be seen in a variety of subtypes but are most characteristic of lymphoplasmacytic lymphoma; sometimes they are also seen with POEMS syndrome (polyneuropathy, organomegaly, endocrinopathy, M protein, skin changes; Chapter 187). Paraneoplastic neurologic complications of non-Hodgkin lymphoma include demyelinating polyneuropathy, Guillain-Barré syndrome, autonomic dysfunction, and peripheral neuropathy. Paraneoplastic syndromes (Chapter 179) associated with non-Hodgkin lymphoma can affect the skin (e.g., pemphigus), kidney (e.g., glomerulonephritis), and miscellaneous organ systems (e.g., vasculitis, dermatomyositis, cholestatic jaundice).

The differential diagnosis in patients with non-Hodgkin lymphoma is broad. Any cause of lymphadenopathy or splenomegaly can potentially be confused with non-Hodgkin lymphoma (Chapter 168). However, this confusion is resolved by an appropriate biopsy. It is extremely important to recognize that the diagnosis of non-Hodgkin lymphoma must be considered in patients with compatible clinical presentations and then confirmed by an adequate biopsy read by an experienced hematopathologist. The diagnosis should never be inferred, and patients should not be treated until the diagnosis is confirmed by biopsy. This is also true for patients who achieve a

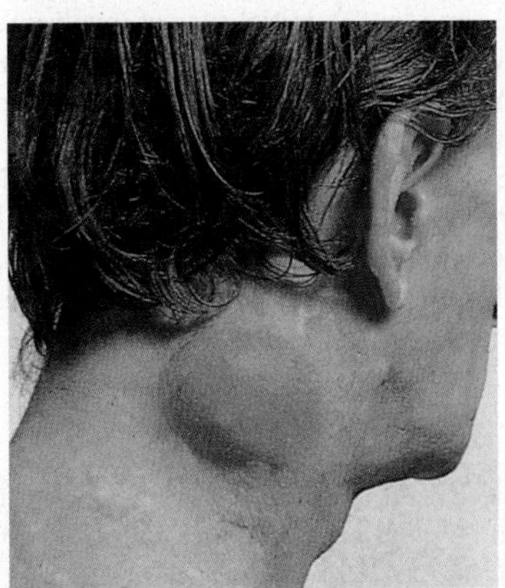

FIGURE 185-3. Non-Hodgkin lymphoma. Despite the redness of the skin over the enlarged lymph node in this patient, the lesion was completely painless. (From Forbes CD, Jackson WF. *Color Atlas and Text of Clinical Medicine*, 3rd ed. London: Mosby; 2003.)

TABLE 185-5 PRESENTING CLINICAL CHARACTERISTICS OF COMMON NON-HODGKIN LYMPHOMA SUBTYPES

TYPE OF LYMPHOMA	MEDIAN AGE (yr)	MALE (%)	STAGE (%) I	STAGE (%) IV	B SYMPTOMS (%)	BONE MARROW INVOLVED (%)
B-CELL LYMPHOMAS						
Small lymphocytic	65	53	4	83	33	72
Lymphoplasmacytic	63	53	7	73	13	73
Extranodal marginal zone MALT	60	48	39	31	19	14
Nodal marginal zone	58	42	13	40	37	32
Follicular	59	42	18	51	28	42
Mantle cell	63	74	13	71	28	64
Diffuse large B cell	64	55	25	33	33	16
Mediastinal large B cell	37	34	10	31	38	3
Burkitt	31	89	37	38	22	33
PRECURSOR B/T-CELL LYMPHOMAS						
Precursor T lymphoblastic	28	64	0	75	21	50
T-CELL LYMPHOMAS						
Anaplastic large T cell	34	69	19	39	53	13
Peripheral T cell	61	55	8	65	50	36

B symptoms = fevers, night sweats, and weight loss; MALT = mucosa-associated lymphoid tissue.
Adapted from Armitage JO, Weisenburger DD, for the Non-Hodgkin Lymphoma Classification Project. New approach to classifying non-Hodgkin lymphomas: clinical features of the major histologic subtypes. *J Clin Oncol.* 1998;16:2780-2795.

complete remission with initial therapy; they should not be treated for presumed relapse on the basis of symptoms or abnormal images without a biopsy.

DIAGNOSIS

Each new patient with a non-Hodgkin lymphoma should be thoroughly evaluated in a systematic manner (Table 185-6). Because subtle pathologic distinctions may alter therapy, the most important issue in managing non-Hodgkin lymphoma is to establish an accurate diagnosis. Core needle biopsies can occasionally be used for a primary diagnosis if the specimen is handled properly. Fine-needle aspirates should not be used to diagnose lymphoma, and they preclude an accurate diagnosis of the specific subtype of non-Hodgkin lymphoma. In most cases, an excisional biopsy is necessary (and is always preferred) for the initial diagnosis. Another biopsy should be performed if sufficient material is not obtained. Review by an experienced hematopathologist is essential.

Staging and Prognostic Systems

After diagnosis, a meticulous staging evaluation is necessary to estimate prognosis and determine therapy. Staging requires a careful history and physical examination; complete blood count; renal and hepatic function tests; serum lactate dehydrogenase (LDH) level; computed tomography (CT) of the chest, abdomen, and pelvis; and bone marrow biopsy. Positron emission tomography (PET) can identify initial sites of involvement and, after treatment, can distinguish persisting lymphoma from residual fibrosis in masses seen on CT. The most common staging system is the Ann Arbor classification, which separates patients into four stages based on anatomic sites of disease (Table 185-7). In addition, each stage is subdivided into A (no defined general symptoms) and B (unexplained weight loss >10% of body weight in the previous 6 months, unexplained temperature >38° C, or night sweats) categories. Known sites of disease can be reexamined later to evaluate the response to therapy.

Although a wide variety of patient factors (e.g., age, symptoms, LDH level) and tumor factors (e.g., bulk, gene expression pattern, proliferation rate) can affect treatment outcomes, two prognostic systems can help in choosing therapy and determining an accurate prognosis. The International Prognostic Index (IPI; Table 185-8) is the most widely used method to predict treatment outcome and survival. The IPI is based on five adverse factors (age >60 years, performance status ≤2, elevated serum LDH level, two or more extranodal sites of disease, Ann Arbor stage III or IV), which are summed to give the score. This index was developed for patients with diffuse aggressive lymphoma (predominantly diffuse large B-cell lymphoma), but it can be used to predict treatment outcome with any subtype. For young patients, an abbreviated index that uses only reduced performance status, elevated serum LDH level, and high stage can be applied. Because patients with follicular lymphoma rarely have a reduced performance status or a large number of extranodal sites, an alternative index termed the *Follicular Lymphoma International Prognostic Index* (FLIPI) was developed. It substitutes more than four nodal areas of involvement and a hemoglobin less than 12 g/dL as staging criteria and does a somewhat better job of predicting treatment outcome in follicular lymphoma.

Other prognostic indices have been developed for mantle cell lymphoma and the peripheral T-cell lymphomas.

TREATMENT Rx

Lymphomas may behave in an indolent or an aggressive manner. The behavior of many of these neoplasms is distinctive, but within each category, behavior is frequently influenced by disease site, tumor bulk, and performance status of the patient. Some lymphomas can be managed, at least initially, with observation, whereas other situations are medical emergencies, such as spinal cord compression (Chapter 189). It is important to consider three questions before starting therapy: (1) Does treatment have curative potential? (2) Can treatment prolong survival? (3) Will treatment alleviate symptoms?

SPECIFIC TYPES OF NON-HODGKIN LYMPHOMAS

Precursor T-Cell and B-Cell Lymphomas

These tumors are nodal or other solid tissue infiltrates of cells that are morphologically and immunophenotypically identical to the immature cells seen in B-cell or T-cell acute lymphoblastic leukemia (Chapter 183). Patients who have predominantly nodal disease with minimal or no involvement of the bone marrow are frequently classified as having *lymphoblastic lymphoma*, whereas those with more than 25% neoplastic cells in the marrow are classified as having *lymphoblastic leukemia*. These distinctions are arbitrary and reflect the stage of disease rather than different diagnoses. These neoplasms are more common in children than in adults.

B-cell precursor lymphomas frequently manifest as solid tumors with involvement of the skin and bones, whereas T-cell neoplasms typically

TABLE 185-6 TYPICAL EVALUATION OF A PATIENT NEWLY DIAGNOSED WITH NON-HODGKIN LYMPHOMA

1. Biopsy to establish diagnosis
2. Careful history and physical examination
3. Laboratory evaluation
   A. Complete blood count
   B. Chemistry screen, including lactate dehydrogenase
4. Imaging studies
   A. Computed tomography of chest, abdomen, and pelvis
   B. Positron emission tomography
5. Additional biopsies
   A. Bone marrow
   B. Any other suspicious site if results would change therapy

TABLE 185-7 STAGING OF NON-HODGKIN LYMPHOMA

STAGE	DESCRIPTION
I	Involvement of a single lymph node region (I) or a single extralymphatic organ or site (I_E)
II	Involvement of two or more lymph node regions on the same side of the diaphragm (II) or localized involvement of an extralymphatic organ or site and one or more lymph node regions on the same side of the diaphragm (II_E)
III	Involvement of lymph node regions on both sides of the diaphragm (III), which may also be accompanied by localized involvement of an extralymphatic organ or site (III_E) or by involvement of the spleen (III_S) or both (III_{SE})
IV	Diffuse or disseminated involvement of one or more extralymphatic organs or tissues with or without associated lymph node enlargement
Subtypes	
A	No B symptoms
B	B symptoms: unexplained weight loss ≥10% of body weight in prior 6 months, unexplained fever with temperature >38° C, or night sweats

Adapted from Carbone PP, Kaplan HS, Musshoff K, et al. Report of the Committee on Hodgkin Disease Staging Classification. *Cancer Res.* 1971;31:1860-1861.

TABLE 185-8 INTERNATIONAL PROGNOSTIC INDEX

CATEGORY	SCORE (NO. OF RISK FACTORS)
ALL PATIENTS*	
Low	0 or 1
Low intermediate	2
High intermediate	3
High	4 or 5
AGE-ADJUSTED INDEX, PATIENTS ≤60 YEARS†	
Low	0
Low intermediate	1
High intermediate	2
High	3

*Adverse factors for all patients: age >60 yr, ↑LDH, performance status 2-4, >1 extranodal site, Ann Arbor stage III or IV.
†Adverse factors for patients ≤60 yr: ↑LDH, performance status 2 –4, Ann Arbor stage III or IV.
LDH = lactate dehydrogenase.
Adapted from Shipp M, Harrington D, Anderson J, et al. A predictive model for aggressive non-Hodgkin lymphoma. *N Engl J Med.* 1993;329:987-994.

manifest as a mediastinal mass in a young male. Involvement of the CNS is common. Approximately 90% of patients who present with lymphoblastic lymphoma have a T-cell phenotype, whereas about 85% of patients who present with acute lymphoblastic leukemia have a B-cell phenotype. Adverse prognostic characteristics include CNS involvement, stage IV disease, and elevated LDH level.

TREATMENT Rx

Patients with either T-cell lymphoblastic lymphoma or precursor B-cell lymphoblastic lymphoma are typically treated with regimens modeled after those used for acute lymphoblastic leukemia (Chapter 183). These regimens frequently contain cytarabine and high-dose methotrexate, and they often include maintenance therapy. CNS prophylaxis with intrathecal chemotherapy, high-dose methotrexate, or cranial irradiation is often a component of these regimens.

Mature B-Cell Lymphomas

SMALL LYMPHOCYTIC LYMPHOMA AND CHRONIC LYMPHOCYTIC LEUKEMIA

Small lymphocytic lymphoma is defined as a lymph node or other tissue infiltrate that is morphologically and immunophenotypically identical to chronic lymphocytic leukemia (Chapter 184). Patients frequently are symptom free, and the diagnosis is often made when blood counts are performed for other reasons. Patients frequently have lymphadenopathy or splenomegaly. Fatigue is common. Hypogammaglobulinemia can occur and may lead to an increased susceptibility to infection.

A poor prognosis is associated with advanced stage and systemic symptoms, expression of high levels of CD38 and ZAP-70 on tumor cells, lack of rearranged immunoglobulin heavy chain genes, and genetic abnormalities such as del(17p) and del(11q). As many as 10% of patients exhibit transformation to diffuse large B-cell lymphoma (Richter syndrome), which is associated with a poor prognosis.

The median survival time is more than 10 years for patients without adverse characteristics, and these patients can often be managed initially with observation. Therapy is necessary for patients who have systemic symptoms, for those with rapidly progressive or symptomatic lymphadenopathy or splenomegaly, and for those who develop cytopenias.

TREATMENT 

Management must be individualized because therapy is unlikely to be curative, and patients are often elderly. A regimen consisting of fludarabine in combination with cyclophosphamide and rituximab (FCR) (Table 185-9) has a high complete remission rate and is frequently used in the United States for relatively young, fit patients.[A1] Fludarabine plus rituximab or the combination of chlorambucil and obinituzumab is used in elderly patients.[A2] Bendamustine plus rituximab (B-R) is an active combination. It is better tolerated but has a lower response rate than FCR.[A3] The immune modulator lenalidomide is also an active agent. The B-cell receptor pathway inhibitors ibrutinib and idelalisib are new highly active oral agents that may transform the management of this lymphoma.[8] Allogeneic hematopoietic stem cell transplantation may be curative, but few patients are candidates for this approach.

Patients may develop autoimmune thrombocytopenia (Chapter 172), autoimmune neutropenia (Chapter 167), and red blood cell aplasia (Chapter 165). These disorders may respond to treatment with corticosteroids, intravenous immune globulin, rituximab, or splenectomy, as used in patients without underlying lymphoma.

EXTRANODAL MARGINAL ZONE LYMPHOMA OF MUCOSA-ASSOCIATED LYMPHOID TISSUE (MALT LYMPHOMA)

MALT lymphomas are indolent tumors that originate in association with epithelial cells and are seen most commonly in the gastrointestinal tract, salivary glands, breast, thyroid, orbit, conjunctiva, skin, and lung. The majority of cases are stage I or II at diagnosis, although in some series as many as 30% disseminate to bone marrow or other sites. These lymphomas tend to remain localized for extended periods. Local treatment with surgery or radiation therapy cures a high proportion of localized neoplasms. Disseminated disease is treated similarly to follicular lymphoma (see later).

TABLE 185-9 COMBINATION CHEMOTHERAPY REGIMENS FOR NON-HODGKIN LYMPHOMA

REGIMEN	DOSE	DAYS OF ADMINISTRATION	FREQUENCY
R-CHOP			**EVERY 21 DAYS**
Cyclophosphamide	750 mg/m² IV	1	
Doxorubicin	50 mg/m² IV	1	
Vincristine	1.4 mg/m² IV*	1	
Prednisone, fixed dose	100 mg PO	1-5	
Rituximab	375 mg/m² IV	1	
R-EPOCH$			**EVERY 21 DAYS**
Etoposide	50 mg/m²/d IV¶	1-4	
Doxorubicin	10 mg/m²/d IV¶	1-4	
Vincristine	0.4 mg/m²/d IV¶	1-4	
Cyclophosphamide	750 mg/m² IV	5	
Prednisone	60 mg/m² bid PO	1-5	
Rituximab	375 mg/m² IV	1	
R-CVP			**EVERY 21 DAYS**
Cyclophosphamide	1000 mg/m² IV	1	
Vincristine	1.4 mg/m² IV*	1	
Prednisone, fixed dose	100 mg PO	1-5	
Rituximab	375 mg/m² IV	1	
FCR			**EVERY 28 DAYS**
Fludarabine	25 mg/m² IV	1-3	
Cyclophosphamide	250 mg/m² IV	1-3	
Rituximab	375 mg/m²	1	
B-R			**EVERY 28 DAYS**
Bendamustine	90 mg/m² IV	1-2	
Rituximab	375 mg/m² IV	1	

*Vincristine dose is often capped at 2 mg total.
$Doses are adjusted based on myelosuppression with previous cycle.
¶Continuous infusion.

Gastric MALT lymphomas are frequently associated with infection by *H. pylori*. About 75% of patients achieve remission after eradication of *H. pylori*, and more than 90% remain in remission for prolonged periods of time. Nonresponders are more likely to have submucosal invasion by endoscopic ultrasonography. Approximately 25% progress, of which about 25% develop diffuse large B-cell lymphoma. Response to antibiotic therapy is less likely if invasion is deeper, lymph node metastases are found, or the t(11;18) chromosomal translocation is present.

TREATMENT 

Patients may have tumors in more than one extranodal site, and these locations can sometimes be successfully treated with local therapy. Patients without symptoms can be monitored closely without therapy until symptoms progress. Patients with symptoms can be treated with rituximab, single-agent chemotherapy, or combinations.[A4] Gastric MALT lymphoma that does not respond to antibiotics can be treated with radiation, rituximab as a single agent (similar to its use in follicular lymphoma), or several traditional combination chemotherapy regimens (see Table 185-9).[9]

FOLLICULAR LYMPHOMA

Follicular lymphoma accounts for the majority of indolent or "low-grade" lymphomas in the United States. Follicular lymphoma is divided into three grades based on the proportion of large, transformed cells (centroblasts).

Patients with follicular lymphoma are frequently asymptomatic. The most common presenting complaint is painless lymphadenopathy. Some patients have cough or dyspnea related to pulmonary or mediastinal involvement or pleural effusions. Other patients have symptoms of abdominal pain or fullness related to subdiaphragmatic or splenic disease. A minority of patients have systemic symptoms of fevers, night sweats, or weight loss.

The clinical behavior and treatment of follicular lymphoma grades 1 and 2 are the same and are discussed in this section. Some grade 3 follicular lymphomas have a more aggressive clinical course and are treated similarly to diffuse large B-cell lymphoma (see later). This distinction between grade 3a (indolent behavior) and 3b (aggressive behavior) is based on the presence or absence of sheets of centroblasts, although this separation may not be reproducible among pathologists. Because of this, we favor treating all patients with grade 3 follicular lymphoma like diffuse large B-cell lymphoma.

TREATMENT Rx

Localized Disease

Approximately 5 to 15% of patients have localized disease (stage I or minimal stage II disease) at diagnosis. These lymphomas are usually treated with involved-field radiation, and most series report 10-year disease-free survival rates of approximately 50% and overall survival rates of 60 to 70%.[10] Some retrospective series have reported improved outcomes when chemotherapy plus rituximab is combined with radiation.[11]

Advanced Disease

Most patients with follicular lymphoma have extensive disease at diagnosis. The median survival time of these patients has improved after the addition of rituximab and is now 10 to 20 years. Spontaneous regression has been described. As many as 30 to 50% of patients experience transformation to a more aggressive histology—usually diffuse large B-cell lymphoma. Transformation is frequently associated with new systemic symptoms and rapidly progressive lymphadenopathy, an aggressive clinical course, and a poor prognosis.

Asymptomatic patients, especially elderly patients and those with other medical illnesses, are frequently managed with a "watch and wait" approach. Prospective trials have demonstrated that this approach does not influence overall survival, and patients can sometimes be observed for long periods before treatment is required. A5

Most patients with follicular lymphoma eventually require treatment because of systemic symptoms, symptomatic or progressive lymphadenopathy, splenomegaly, effusions, or cytopenias. In elderly patients, those who are poor candidates for intensive chemotherapy regimens, and those who want to avoid the side effects of chemotherapy, single-agent rituximab (375 mg/m^2 intravenously, given weekly for 4 consecutive weeks) yields an objective response rate of well over 50%. The median duration of response is approximately 1 to 2 years for patients who receive no additional therapy, but the response can be extended with ongoing administration of rituximab once every 2 or 3 months or by repeating the initial four doses every 6 months. When rituximab is combined with standard chemotherapy regimens (see Table 185-9), the response rate, duration of response, and survival are increased compared with the chemotherapy regimen alone. A6 A7 Maintenance rituximab is widely used and extends the duration of remission. A7 A8

Salvage Therapy

Most patients respond to initial chemotherapy. However, follicular lymphoma recurs in the majority of patients with advanced-stage disease. Patients who relapse usually respond to additional therapy, often with the same agents, although the duration of response becomes progressively shorter with repeated courses of therapy. Some patients respond to the radiolabeled antibodies tositumomab or ibritumomab. Radiation therapy may also be useful for patients with a localized site of symptomatic disease.

Prolonged remissions have been observed after autologous hematopoietic stem cell transplantation. Allogeneic hematopoietic stem cell transplantation may cure some patients with relapsed follicular lymphoma.

MANTLE CELL LYMPHOMA

Mantle cell lymphoma is a B-cell neoplasm composed of small lymphoid cells that may resemble small lymphocytic lymphoma or follicular lymphoma. It is most common in elderly patients and is usually at an advanced stage at the time of diagnosis. Males are more frequently affected, and extranodal disease, especially involvement of the bone marrow, Waldeyer's ring, and the gastrointestinal tract, is common. Mantle cell lymphoma is the most common cause of multiple lymphomatous polyposis, and many oncologists recommend that the gastrointestinal tract be evaluated with endoscopy during the initial evaluation.

Some patients present with involvement of the peripheral blood as well as the bone marrow, a clinical picture that resembles chronic lymphocytic leukemia (Chapter 184). The lymphocytes in both disorders are CD5$^+$, but the t(11;14) and overexpression of cyclin D1 seen in mantle cell lymphoma usually allow an accurate diagnosis.

The median survival of mantle cell lymphoma has significantly improved with new therapies. Occasional patients may have an indolent course without initial therapy—particularly those with a leukemic presentation. Patients have a poor outcome when treated with the same regimens used for diffuse large B-cell lymphoma. Regimens similar to those used for Burkitt lymphoma and lymphoblastic lymphoma are effective. The combination of bendamustine plus rituximab and regimens that incorporate high-dose cytarabine are efficacious. Maintenance rituximab seems to prolong remission duration. A9 Autologous hematopoietic stem cell transplantation for patients in their first remission is widely used.[12] Several new agents, including lenalidomide, bortezomib, and the Bruton tyrosine kinase inhibitor ibrutinib,[13] are very active and may become part of standard therapy. Allogeneic transplantation can be curative but is associated with considerable morbidity and mortality.

DIFFUSE LARGE B-CELL LYMPHOMA

These tumors are the most common type of non-Hodgkin lymphoma, but their morphology and genetic features are heterogeneous. Signs and symptoms are similar to those of other subtypes, although patients are more likely to have B symptoms or symptoms from the local tumor than are patients with follicular lymphoma.

The WHO classification of non-Hodgkin lymphomas has identified several variants and subtypes of diffuse large B-cell lymphoma (Table 185-10). Many of these are histologic or genetic subtypes or variants for which treatment is the same as the standard approach for diffuse large B-cell lymphoma. Other subtypes present unusual clinical syndromes or specific therapeutic problems.

TREATMENT Rx

Localized Disease

As many as 30% of patients with diffuse large B-cell lymphoma have stage I or minimal stage II disease. These patients are occasionally cured with radiation therapy alone, but initial treatment with chemotherapy is more effective. In the United States, most patients are treated with R-CHOP. Some patients can be treated with fewer courses of chemotherapy if radiotherapy is included. For patients with bulky disease, a complete course of chemotherapy is usually used. Some physicians advocate the use of PET scans to shorten the duration of therapy or eliminate the need for radiotherapy in complete responders.

TABLE 185-10 DIFFUSE LARGE B-CELL LYMPHOMA VARIANTS AND SUBTYPES

- Diffuse large B-cell lymphoma, not otherwise specified (NOS)
  - Common morphologic variants
    - Centroblastic
    - Immunoblastic
    - Anaplastic
  - Immunohistochemical subgroups
    - CD5$^+$ DLBCL
    - Germinal center B-cell like (GCB)
    - Non–germinal center B-cell like (non-GCB)
- Diffuse large B-cell lymphoma, subtypes
  - T-cell/histiocyte-rich large B-cell lymphoma
  - Primary DLBCL of the CNS
  - Primary cutaneous DLBCL, leg type
  - EBV-positive DLBCL of elderly people
- Other large B-cell lymphomas
  - Primary mediastinal (thymic) large B-cell lymphoma
  - Intravascular large B-cell lymphoma
  - DLBCL associated with chronic inflammation
  - Lymphomatoid granulomatosis
  - ALK-positive large B-cell lymphoma
  - Plasmablastic lymphoma
  - Large B-cell lymphoma arising in HHV-8-associated multicentric Castleman disease
  - Primary effusion lymphoma

ALK = anaplastic lymphoma kinase; CNS = central nervous system; DLBCL = diffuse large B-cell lymphoma; EBV = Epstein-Barr virus; HHV = human herpesvirus.

Advanced Disease

R-CHOP is the most widely used regimen for adults of all ages with advanced-stage diffuse large B-cell lymphoma. Among patients older than 60 years, 75% achieve a complete response, with a 10-year progression-free survival rate of 36.5% and a 10-year overall survival rate of 43.5%. In younger patients, the outcome is better.[A10] In younger patients, R-EPOCH and the intensive regimen R-ACVBP may yield superior results.[A11] Autologous transplantation in first remission may benefit very high-risk patients.[A12]

Salvage Therapy

A variety of chemotherapy regimens have been developed for patients who relapse after attaining a remission with initial chemotherapy. These regimens commonly contain agents such as cisplatin, cytarabine, etoposide, carboplatin, and ifosfamide. Response rates exceeding 50% can be observed with these combinations, although no more than 10% of patients achieve long-term disease-free survival. High-dose therapy followed by autologous hematopoietic stem cell transplantation has become accepted therapy for patients with relapsed diffuse large B-cell lymphoma. Approximately 20 to 50% of these patients attain long-term disease-free survival, depending on their response to conventional salvage chemotherapy.[A13] Several new drugs such as lenalidomide and ibrutinib seem to particularly benefit patients with ABC subtype.

Subtypes of Diffuse Large B-Cell Lymphoma

Primary mediastinal large B-cell lymphoma originates in the thymus and is most common in young women. This subtype shares genetic features with classic Hodgkin lymphoma. This entity is distinguished by the presence of a mediastinal mass, which usually causes symptoms of cough, chest pain, or superior vena cava syndrome. A very large mass (>10 cm) or the existence of a malignant pleural effusion is associated with a worse prognosis. Mediastinal large B-cell lymphoma is treated with the same chemotherapy regimens used for diffuse large B-cell lymphoma, followed, in some cases, by consolidative radiation therapy.[14] The prognosis is similar to that of other diffuse large B-cell lymphomas. Relapses often occur in extranodal sites such as the CNS, lungs, gastrointestinal tract, liver, ovaries, and kidneys.

Intravascular large B-cell lymphoma is an aggressive lymphoma caused by cells that infiltrate the lumens of small blood vessels. Widespread extranodal involvement is common. Focal neurologic deficits and mental status changes are frequent. Cases are often diagnosed at autopsy, although durable responses to combination chemotherapy have been described.

Primary effusion lymphoma is associated with HHV-8 and is seen in HIV-infected and other immunosuppressed patients. Effusions occur in serous body cavities. Peripheral lymphadenopathy is not seen. Prognosis is poor despite chemotherapy.

Plasmablastic lymphoma is most often seen in patients with HIV infection and frequently presents with involvement of the head and neck. This tumor does not express CD20 and thus does not benefit from treatment with rituximab.

Primary cutaneous diffuse large B-cell lymphoma of the leg (leg type) is one of two presentations of B-cell lymphoma in the skin. This tumor occurs mostly in older patients and follows an aggressive course. This neoplasm must be distinguished from primary cutaneous follicle center lymphoma, which might also be diagnosed as a cutaneous diffuse large B-cell lymphoma but follows an indolent course and requires only local therapy.

Double-hit and gray-zone lymphomas are newly described entities. Double-hit lymphomas have rearrangements of *Myc* in combination with *Bcl-2* and/or *Bcl-6*. They have a poor outcome when treated with standard chemotherapy regimens. Gray-zone lymphomas include those with features intermediate between diffuse large B-cell lymphoma and Burkitt lymphoma and those with features intermediate between mediastinal diffuse large B-cell lymphoma and classic Hodgkin lymphoma.[15]

BURKITT LYMPHOMA

Burkitt lymphoma is a highly aggressive B-cell lymphoma that is more common in children and immunosuppressed individuals than in healthy adults (see later). Widespread extranodal involvement is common. The endemic form of Burkitt lymphoma is seen most frequently in children who reside in equatorial Africa. Involvement of bones of the jaw is common in this form. The sporadic form of Burkitt lymphoma is seen most commonly in children in the United States. Males are more frequently affected. Both children and adults frequently have bulky abdominal disease, sometimes with involvement of the kidneys, ovaries, and breasts. Bone marrow involvement is seen in about one third of cases.

TREATMENT (Rx)

Tumors may progress extremely rapidly, so therapy should be started as soon as possible. Tumor lysis syndrome may occur because of the frequent presence of bulky disease, the high rate of tumor proliferation, and the extreme sensitivity of the tumor to chemotherapy. Patients are usually treated with specialized high-intensity regimens, including rituximab, of relatively short duration.[16] Treatment with the R-CHOP regimen used for diffuse large B-cell lymphoma has a poor outcome. CNS prophylaxis with intrathecal chemotherapy or high-dose methotrexate is required. Cure rates well in excess of 50% are typical with appropriate therapy. Excellent results have been described with R-EPOCH.

RARE TYPES OF B-CELL LYMPHOMA

Several rare types of lymphoma have distinct clinical features.

Lymphoplasmacytic lymphoma is an indolent lymphoma that frequently involves the bone marrow, peripheral blood, and spleen. Patients frequently have an immunoglobulin M (IgM) paraprotein (and therefore the disease could be called Waldenström macroglobulinemia) that may lead to symptoms of hyperviscosity, autoimmune phenomena, or neuropathies (Chapter 187). Plasmapheresis can reduce symptoms of hyperviscosity. Chemotherapy with alkylating agents, combination chemotherapy, or fludarabine all in combination with rituximab may be used.[A14] Newer agents such as bortezomib and ibrutinib are active.

Splenic marginal zone lymphoma is an indolent lymphoma that usually manifests with splenomegaly and lymphocytosis. A monoclonal gammopathy is frequently seen. Peripheral lymphadenopathy is unusual. Anemia and thrombocytopenia may respond to splenectomy. Chemotherapy with single agents or anthracycline-based combinations may be useful, and when the lymphoma is associated with hepatitis C, antiviral therapy may be effective. Responses to interferon have been described. This lymphoma appears to be particularly responsive to rituximab.

Nodal marginal zone B-cell lymphoma is an indolent disorder that is usually associated with generalized lymphadenopathy. The clinical course and prognosis are similar to those of follicular lymphoma, and it is usually treated in a similar manner.

Small intestinal immunoproliferative disease, a disorder seen most frequently in the Middle East, begins as a polyclonal process and can progress to a large B-cell lymphoma. The process is often associated with *C. jejuni* infection. Early in the disease, patients may respond to antibiotics, and frank lymphoma may respond to combination chemotherapy regimens.

Mature T-Cell Lymphomas (Peripheral T-Cell Lymphomas)

Peripheral (or mature) T-cell lymphomas are neoplasms of post-thymic T cells. These include relatively indolent disorders such as mycosis fungoides and $CD30^+$ cutaneous lymphoproliferative disorders, but most patients diagnosed with peripheral T-cell lymphoma have an aggressive neoplasm. Peripheral T-cell lymphomas represent only 10% of the non-Hodgkin lymphomas occurring in the United States. Unfortunately, the treatment for these lymphomas has not progressed as rapidly as the treatments for B-cell lymphomas.[17]

MYCOSIS FUNGOIDES

Mycosis fungoides (often referred to as *cutaneous T-cell lymphoma*) is an indolent malignancy that is most common in middle-aged and older adults.[18] The clinical course is usually a slow progression from isolated patches or plaques to thickened, more widespread plaques and then to multiple cutaneous tumors that may ulcerate (Chapter 440). A subset of patients presents with generalized erythroderma and circulating tumor cells, called *Sézary syndrome*. Lymph node and visceral involvement may occur late in the course of the disease.

TREATMENT

Cutaneous radiation therapy may be curative for patients with limited patch or plaque disease. Patients with early-stage disease (<10% body surface area) are frequently treated with skin-directed therapy that may include ultraviolet radiation, topical steroids, or topical nitrogen mustard.

Patients with more advanced disease frequently benefit from total skin electron beam therapy or extracorporeal photopheresis. Medical treatments include interferon-α, retinoids, monoclonal antibodies, histone deacetylase inhibitors (vorinostat, depsipeptide), the fusion toxin denileukin diftitox, and traditional cytotoxic chemotherapeutic agents.[A15] However, these treatments are usually only palliative. Results with autologous hematopoietic stem cell transplantation are usually poor, although allogeneic stem cell transplantation has yielded promising results in some cases.

ADULT T-CELL LYMPHOMA/LEUKEMIA

Adult T-cell lymphoma/leukemia, which is associated with HTLV-1 infection (Chapter 378), is most commonly seen in southern Japan and the Caribbean. Most infected patients are asymptomatic, and the lifetime risk for developing adult T-cell lymphoma/leukemia is approximately 3%.

Patients may have acute leukemia, aggressive lymphoma, or an indolent lymphoproliferative disease. Patients with aggressive disease present with generalized lymphadenopathy, hepatosplenomegaly, cutaneous infiltration, and hypercalcemia. Many patients have characteristic circulating tumor cells with a "flower" or "cloverleaf" nucleus.

TREATMENT Rx

Patients with indolent disease can sometimes be monitored without therapy. Aggressive disease is usually treated with combination chemotherapy, but there is no consensus on the best regimen.[A16] Historically, the 5-year survival rate has been less than 10%, although recent trials have reported better outcomes.

CD30$^+$ CUTANEOUS LYMPHOPROLIFERATIVE DISORDERS

These disorders represent a spectrum of diseases that may have an identical histologic appearance and overlapping clinical manifestations. Treatment decisions are often based on the clinical behavior of the lesions. These lymphomas express CD30 but do not express the anaplastic lymphoma kinase (ALK) protein (see later).

Lymphomatoid papulosis is a "histologically malignant" clonal disorder consisting of erythematous or skin-colored papules that frequently undergo spontaneous ulceration and necrosis over a period of weeks. The prognosis is excellent, although patients may eventually develop lymphoma.

Primary cutaneous anaplastic large cell lymphoma occurs most commonly in older men and also undergoes frequent spontaneous regression. The 5-year survival rate is greater than 90%. Treatment usually consists of local measures (surgery or radiation), although chemotherapy may be required.

PRIMARY SYSTEMIC ANAPLASTIC LARGE CELL LYMPHOMA

Anaplastic large cell lymphoma (ALCL) is an aggressive, CD30$^+$, T-cell non-Hodgkin lymphoma that is seen most frequently in young males. B-cell lymphomas with similar morphology can occur, but they have clinical features identical to other diffuse large B-cell lymphomas and are not considered part of this disease. A morphologically similar but biologically unrelated and clinically distinct neoplasm, primary cutaneous ALCL, occurs predominantly in older adults and represents part of the spectrum of cutaneous CD30$^+$ lymphoproliferative disorders (see earlier). Primary systemic ALCL frequently has a t(2;5) chromosomal translocation that leads to overexpression of ALK, a protein not normally detectable in lymphoid cells.

Patients usually have lymphadenopathy, and involvement of the skin, bone, and gastrointestinal tract may be observed.

A newly described entity of anaplastic large cell lymphoma of the breast is associated with breast implants. When localized, these patients may be cured with surgery including removal of the implant.

TREATMENT Rx

Patients are usually treated with chemotherapy regimens such as CHOP with or without the addition of etoposide.[19] Patients whose tumors express ALK have an excellent outcome, and 5-year survival rates of 70 to 90% have been observed. ALK-negative ALCL is more common in older patients and is associated with an inferior response rate and shorter survival time. Autologous hematopoietic stem cell transplantation may be curative for patients who relapse. The anti-CD30 antibody-drug conjugate brentuximab vedotin is highly active for patients with relapsed disease and may be incorporated into primary therapy. Patients whose lymphomas express ALK usually respond to the ALK inhibitor crizotinib.

PERIPHERAL T-CELL LYMPHOMAS, UNSPECIFIED

The largest group of patients with peripheral T-cell lymphomas is defined in the WHO classification as having "peripheral T-cell lymphoma, unspecified." These patients' signs and symptoms are similar to those of patients with aggressive B-cell lymphomas, although systemic symptoms (fevers, night sweats, and weight loss) and extranodal involvement are frequent. The diagnosis of peripheral T-cell lymphoma requires immunophenotyping to demonstrate the T-cell origin.

TREATMENT 

Patients are generally treated with the same regimens used for diffuse large B-cell lymphomas (e.g., CHOP with or without etoposide), often in combination with upfront autologous hematopoietic stem cell transplantation, although the outcome is substantially worse.[20] Patients who relapse after complete remission can sometimes be cured with hematopoietic stem cell transplantation.

UNUSUAL SUBTYPES OF T-CELL LYMPHOMA

Angioimmunoblastic T-cell lymphoma is associated with generalized lymphadenopathy, fever, weight loss, skin rash, and polyclonal hypergammaglobulinemia. Results of therapy are similar to those for peripheral T-cell lymphoma, unspecified.

Extranodal NK/T-cell lymphoma usually occurs in extranodal sites, especially the nose, palate, and nasopharynx. Involvement of the nose and face leads to the syndrome that was previously called lethal midline granuloma. This disorder is unusual in the United States, but it is frequent in Southeast Asia and Latin America. The prognosis is extremely poor, although patients with localized disease can sometimes be cured with aggressive combination radiation therapy and chemotherapy.

Hepatosplenic T-cell lymphoma is characterized by sinusoidal infiltration of the spleen, liver, and bone marrow, which leads to hepatosplenomegaly, systemic symptoms, and cytopenias. Lymphadenopathy is unusual. Patients are typically young males, and this disease can occur in allograft recipients and in the setting of immune dysfunction. The prognosis is poor, and remissions are rarely observed with chemotherapy.

Enteropathy-type T-cell lymphoma is usually seen in patients with gluten-sensitive enteropathy (Chapter 140). Patients typically present with abdominal pain and diarrhea and sometimes with bowel perforation. Treatment of celiac disease with a gluten-free diet may reduce the risk for lymphoma. The prognosis in these often undernourished patients is poor.

Subcutaneous panniculitis-like T-cell lymphoma manifests with multiple subcutaneous nodules and is often misdiagnosed as panniculitis. Patients with disseminated disease can have a syndrome consisting of fevers, weight loss, hepatosplenomegaly, pancytopenia, and phagocytosis of blood cells (hemophagocytic syndrome). Patients sometimes respond to combination chemotherapy regimens used for diffuse large B-cell lymphoma, interferon, and radiation therapy, but long-term disease-free survival is unusual.

SPECIAL CLINICAL SITUATIONS

The diagnosis and management of patients with the various types of non-Hodgkin lymphoma can be profoundly influenced by the site of origin of the lymphoma and by certain clinical characteristics of the patients. Examples of the latter include pregnant patients with lymphoma, elderly patients with lymphoma, and lymphoma in patients who are severely immunosuppressed.

Specific Primary Sites of Diffuse Large B-Cell Lymphoma

Approximately 30% of diffuse large B-cell lymphomas originate in extranodal sites. Presentation in certain extranodal sites is associated with unique clinical behaviors that may necessitate diagnostic studies or additional therapy beyond that used for patients with nodal presentations.

Patients with primary CNS lymphoma (Chapter 189) commonly have ocular involvement, and all patients with this diagnosis should have a slit lamp examination. Surgical resection of primary CNS lymphoma is usually not performed, and the primary role of surgery is for diagnosis. Primary lymphomas of the CNS are very sensitive to corticosteroids, but the best results have been observed with chemotherapy regimens that use high-dose methotrexate alone or in combination with other agents such as cytarabine and temozolomide. By comparison, conventional chemotherapy regimens, such as CHOP, are of little benefit. Whole brain irradiation is also effective therapy, although the incidence of leukoencephalopathy is extremely high, especially in elderly patients.[A17] Radiation therapy is frequently reserved for relapse rather than being used as adjunctive treatment with primary chemotherapy.

Treatment of primary testicular lymphoma, the most common testicular cancer in men older than 60 years (Chapter 200), usually consists of orchiectomy followed by combination chemotherapy. Relapse in the contralateral testicle is common, and most oncologists recommend adjuvant radiation to the scrotum. CNS involvement is common, and prophylactic intrathecal chemotherapy is usually recommended. Late relapses occur frequently.

Diffuse large B-cell lymphoma of the stomach and gastrointestinal tract is treated differently from gastric MALT lymphoma, even if there is a history of prior MALT lymphoma. Patients can be cured with surgery and adjunctive radiation or chemotherapy, although surgery is rarely performed for gastric lymphomas because of the morbidity associated with gastric resection. Patients should be treated with chemotherapy regimens used for other diffuse large B-cell lymphomas. Radiation therapy is sometimes used after chemotherapy, although the role of combined-modality treatment is not defined.

Lymphoma in AIDS and Post-transplantation Lymphoproliferative Disorders

Non-Hodgkin lymphoma is an AIDS-defining illness in HIV-infected individuals (Chapter 393), and the risk for developing a non-Hodgkin lymphoma is increased more than 150-fold after the diagnosis of another AIDS-defining illness. Most cases are diffuse large B-cell lymphomas or Burkitt lymphomas. AIDS-associated lymphomas behave aggressively and frequently involve the CNS and other unusual sites, such as the gastrointestinal tract, anus, rectum, skin, and soft tissue (Chapter 393). Factors associated with poor survival include low CD4 counts, poor performance status, older age, and advanced stage. The incidence of AIDS-associated non-Hodgkin lymphoma has declined, and the prognosis has improved considerably. Patients are generally treated in the same manner as non-immunocompromised patients, and the prognoses are similar. Intrathecal prophylaxis is generally recommended because of a higher risk for CNS involvement.

The risk for developing a non-Hodgkin lymphoma is also markedly increased in patients who have received a solid organ transplant. The histologic appearance of these lymphomas is variable, but they frequently resemble aggressive lymphomas in non-immunocompromised patients. Similar disorders can be seen in patients who are treated with methotrexate and other drugs for autoimmune disorders and in recipients of allogeneic hematopoietic stem cell transplants, especially if the transplants are T-cell depleted. These post-transplantation lymphoproliferative disorders, which may develop within weeks after surgery, are more common in patients who receive aggressive immunosuppression after transplantation. Involvement of extranodal sites is common, and lymphoma frequently involves the transplanted organ. Post-transplantation lymphoproliferative disorders may respond to reduction or withdrawal of immunosuppression. Some investigators have advocated the use of acyclovir or ganciclovir because these lymphomas are usually related to EBV, but this practice is controversial. High response rates are also seen with rituximab. Other patients require treatment with combination chemotherapy regimens.

Non-Hodgkin Lymphoma in Elderly Patients

More than 50% of patients who develop non-Hodgkin lymphomas are older than 60 years, and the prognosis is generally worse for elderly patients. These poorer outcomes are related to increased toxicity of drug therapy, lower remission rates, increased rates of relapse, and higher death rates from cardiovascular disease and causes other than the lymphoma itself. Older patients are more likely to have other adverse prognostic characteristics (see Table 185-8), which also contribute to poorer outcomes. The practice of arbitrary dose reductions based solely on age should be discouraged if patients have a good performance status and no comorbid illnesses.

Non-Hodgkin Lymphoma and Pregnancy

Non-Hodgkin lymphoma in pregnancy involves major clinical and ethical issues, and a multidisciplinary approach is needed (Chapter 239). Although chest radiographs are generally considered safe, ultrasound examination is usually used instead of CT for staging in the abdomen and pelvis.

Treatment can occasionally be delayed until after delivery; however, most women have a tumor that is potentially curable, and treatment delays may decrease the chance for cure. Other patients have conditions such as superior vena cava syndrome that require immediate treatment. After the first trimester, full-dose standard therapy such as R-CHOP-R may be used. Several studies indicate high probabilities of cure without significantly increased adverse long-term physical or intellectual deficits for the child. Although it is reasonable to offer therapeutic abortion for women in the first trimester, chemotherapy may also be successful in this situation. Regimens using methotrexate or abdominal radiation must be avoided.

DISEASES SOMETIMES CONFUSED WITH LYMPHOMA

A variety of conditions are associated with lymphadenopathy that can be confused with lymphoma.[21] The most common atypical lymphoid proliferations that can be confused with lymphoma are florid reactions to immune stimulation. Follicular hyperplasia with diffuse proliferation of B cells and T cells can be seen in a variety of autoimmune diseases (e.g., Sjögren syndrome, systemic lupus erythematosus, rheumatoid arthritis) and infectious processes (e.g., EBV, cytomegalovirus, cat-scratch disease) (Chapter 168). If the definitive diagnosis of lymphoma cannot be made even after immunologic and molecular studies, the patient should be closely observed. The clinical course or subsequent biopsies can usually resolve the confusion.

Castleman disease, or angiofollicular lymph node hyperplasia, usually appears with a hyaline vascular pattern of lymphoid proliferation, but a subset of patients has hyperplastic lymphoid follicles and sheets of plasma cells. Patients with Castleman disease often present with a localized lymphoid mass, but some patients have a systemic illness with fevers, night sweats, weight loss, and fatigue. Frequently, the systemic symptoms of Castleman disease are related to excessive production of IL-6. Castleman disease in HIV-infected patients is frequently associated with HHV-8. Patients with disseminated and plasma cell–rich forms of Castleman disease may occasionally progress to lymphoma. Patients with localized Castleman disease can be treated with surgical removal or radiation therapy. Patients with systemic disease may respond to treatment with high-dose corticosteroids. Patients with overexpression of IL-6 frequently benefit from treatment with an anti-IL-6 antibody. If other treatments fail, patients sometimes benefit from combination chemotherapy regimens, autologous or allogeneic hematopoietic stem cell transplantation, or both.

Sinus histiocytosis with massive lymphadenopathy, also known as *Rosai-Dorfman disease,* manifests as bulky lymphadenopathy in children and young adults. Extranodal sites such as the skin, upper airways, gastrointestinal tract, and CNS can be involved. The disease is usually self-limited, but it has been associated with autoimmune hemolytic anemia.

Kikuchi's disease (histiocytic necrotizing lymphadenitis) is a disease of unknown origin that most commonly affects young women. Symptoms most commonly consist of painless cervical lymphadenopathy that is often accompanied by fever, flu-like symptoms, and rash. Treatment is symptomatic, and manifestations usually resolve within weeks or months.

IgG4-related disease is a systemic immune-mediated fibrosing inflammatory disease in which various organs are infiltrated by IgG4-positive plasma cells. Patients often have accompanying asymptomatic lymphadenopathy that usually responds to corticosteroids.

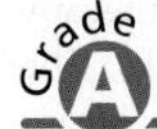

Grade A References

A1. Hallek M, Fischer K, Fingerle-Rowson G, et al. Addition of rituximab to fludarabine and cyclophosphamide in patients with chronic lymphocytic leukaemia: a randomized, open-label, phase 3 trial. *Lancet.* 2010;376:1164-1174.

A2. Goede V, Fischer K, Busch R, et al. Obinutuzumab plus chlorambucil in patients with CLL and coexisting conditions. *N Engl J Med.* 2014;370:1101-1110.

A3. Eichhorst B, Fink A-M, Busch R, et al. Chemoimmunotherapy with fludarabine (F), cyclophosphamide (C), and rituximab (R) (FCR) versus bendamustine and rituximab (BR) in previously untreated and physically fit patients (pts) with advanced chronic lymphocytic leukemia (CLL): results of a planned interim analysis of the CLL10 trial, an international, randomized study of the German CLL Study Group (GCLLSG). *Blood.* 2013;122(abstr. 526).

A4. Zucca E, Conconi A, Laszlo D, et al. Addition of rituximab to chlorambucil produces superior event-free survival in the treatment of patients with extranodal marginal-zone B-cell lymphoma: 5-year analysis of the IELSG-19 randomized study. *J Clin Oncol.* 2013;31:565-572.

A5. Ardeshna KM, Qian W, Smith P, et al. Rituximab versus a watch-and-wait approach in patients with advanced-stage, asymptomatic, non-bulky follicular lymphoma: an open-label randomised phase 3 trial. *Lancet Oncol.* 2014;15:424-435.

A6. Bachy E, Houot R, Morschhauser F, et al. Long-term follow up of the FL2000 study comparing CHVP-interferon to CHVP-interferon plus rituximab in follicular lymphoma. *Haematologica.* 2013;98:1107-1114.

A7. Rummel MJ, Niederle N, Maschmeyer G, et al. Bendamustine plus rituximab versus CHOP plus rituximab as first-line treatment for patients with indolent and mantle-cell lymphomas: an open-label, multicenter, randomized, phase 3 non-inferiority trial. *Lancet.* 2013;381:1203-1210.

A8. Salles G, Seymour JF, Offner F, et al. Rituximab maintenance for 2 years in patients with high tumour burden follicular lymphoma responding to rituximab plus chemotherapy (PRIMA): a phase 3, randomised controlled trial. *Lancet.* 2011;377:42-51.

A9. Kluin-Nelemans HC, Hoster E, Hermine O, et al. Treatment of older patients with mantle-cell lymphoma. *N Engl J Med.* 2012;367:520-531.

A10. Coiffier B, Thieblemont C, Van Den Neste E, et al. Long-term outcome of patients in the LNH-98.5 trial, the first randomized study comparing rituximab-CHOP to standard CHOP chemotherapy in DLBCL patients: a study by the Groupe d'Etudes des Lymphomes de l'Adulte. *Blood.* 2010;116:2040-2045.

A11. Récher C, Coiffier B, Haioun C, et al. Intensified chemotherapy with ACVBP plus rituximab versus standard CHOP plus rituximab for the treatment of diffuse large B-cell lymphoma (LNH03-2B): an open-label randomised phase 3 trial. *Lancet.* 2011;378:1858-1867.

A12. Stiff PJ, Unger JM, Cook JR, et al. Autologous transplantation as consolidation for aggressive non-Hodgkin's lymphoma. *N Engl J Med.* 2013;369:1681-1690.

A13. Gisselbrecht C, Glass B, Mounier M, et al. Salvage regimens with autologous transplantation for relapsed large B-cell lymphoma in the rituximab era. *J Clin Oncol.* 2010;28:4184-4190.

A14. Leblond V, Johnson S, Chevret S, et al. Results of a randomized trial of chlorambucil versus fludarabine for patients with untreated Waldenström macroglobulinemia, marginal zone lymphoma, or lymphoplasmacytic lymphoma. *J Clin Oncol.* 2012;31:301-307.

A15. Whittaker S, Ortiz P, Dummer R, et al. Efficacy and safety of bexarotene combined with psoralen-ultraviolet A (PUVA) compared with PUVA treatment alone in stage IB-IIA mycosis fungoides: final results from the EORTC Cutaneous Lymphoma Task Force phase III randomized clinical trial (NCT00056056). *Br J Dermatol.* 2012;167:678-687.

A16. Tsukasaki K, Utsunomiya A, Fukuda H, et al. VCAP-AMP-VECP compared with biweekly CHOP for adult T-cell leukemia-lymphoma: Japan Clinical Oncology Group study JCOG9801. *J Clin Oncol.* 2007;25:5458-5464.

A17. Thiel E, Korfel A, Martus P, et al. High-dose methotrexate with or without whole brain radiotherapy for primary CNS lymphoma (G-PCNSL-SG-1): a phase 3, randomized, non-inferiority trial. *Lancet Oncol.* 2010;11:1036-1047.

GENERAL REFERENCES

For the General References and other additional features, please visit Expert Consult at https://expertconsult.inkling.com.

186

HODGKIN LYMPHOMA

JOSEPH M. CONNORS

DEFINITION

Hodgkin lymphoma, formerly called Hodgkin disease, is one of the B-cell lymphomas. It consists of two major types: classic Hodgkin lymphoma, with a characteristic neoplastic cell, the Hodgkin-Reed-Sternberg cell; and the much less common (~5% of cases) nodular lymphocyte-predominant Hodgkin lymphoma, with a characteristic lymphocyte-predominant cell. Both types have a distinct natural history, and most important, an excellent response to treatment, with the large majority of patients being cured. Its management, which requires careful multidisciplinary cooperation, serves as a paradigm for the successful application of modern oncologic concepts. Highly effective multiagent chemotherapy is the cornerstone of treatment. Carefully selected patients may require the addition of radiation or, if the lymphoma recurs after primary treatment, high-dose chemoradiation therapy and autologous hematologic stem cell transplantation (HDC/HSCT). The major challenge to clinicians managing this neoplasm is to cure the disease while minimizing long-term toxicity.

EPIDEMIOLOGY

The incidence of Hodgkin lymphoma varies substantially around the world. The highest rates occur in the United States, Canada, Switzerland, and northern Europe. Intermediate rates are seen in southern and eastern Europe and low rates in eastern Asia. No clear explanation for this variation in incidence has been found. Postulated reasons include differences in the age at onset or genotype of any associated Epstein-Barr virus (EBV) infection; crowding during childhood as a result of lower socioeconomic status, predisposing to passage of an as yet undiscovered infectious vector; and intrinsic genetic differences in susceptibility.

Approximately 20,000 new cases are seen annually in North America and Europe. The age-adjusted incidence of Hodgkin lymphoma declined modestly over the 20 years before 1990 at a rate of approximately 0.9% per year but has leveled off since then and is now approximately 2.7 per 100,000. Age-adjusted annual mortality is 0.5 per 100,000. Hodgkin lymphoma occurs slightly more often in men and is seen more frequently in whites than African Americans and much less frequently in Asian populations. Much of the difference in incidence between whites and blacks in North America can be attributed to the higher incidence seen in higher socioeconomic classes. The cumulative lifetime risk for development of Hodgkin lymphoma is approximately 1 in 250 to 1 in 300 in North America.

The incidence of Hodgkin lymphoma is bimodal in distribution, rising from very low in childhood to an early peak in young adulthood (25 to 30 years) and a later peak in late adulthood (>50 years). In the Western world, only about 5% of cases occur in persons younger than 15 years and 5% in individuals older than 70 years. In contrast, the age distribution in the Indian subcontinent is strongly shifted into childhood.

PATHOBIOLOGY

The cause of Hodgkin lymphoma remains unclear. Hodgkin lymphoma is not associated with exposure to radiation, chemicals, biocidal agents, working in health care–related professions, or previous tonsillectomy. The leading suspect remains EBV, based on much suggestive evidence but no definitive proof.[1]

Epstein-Barr Virus

EBV is a large B-lymphocyte tropic herpesvirus (Chapter 377). Approximately 90% of the general population acquires infection with EBV by early adulthood. In the developing world, this infection usually occurs in childhood, but in developed countries, infection is often delayed into the teens, when it is associated with the syndrome of infectious mononucleosis in up to 30% of new cases. A history of infectious mononucleosis increases the likelihood for subsequent Hodgkin lymphoma three-fold. Antibodies to the viral capsid antigen reach higher levels in patients with Hodgkin lymphoma than in controls, and these higher levels appear several years before the neoplasm. In situ hybridization studies have demonstrated that the Hodgkin-Reed-Sternberg cells in approximately 50% of cases of Hodgkin lymphoma contain EBV-encoded small RNA (EBER), and in these cases, virtually all the Hodgkin-Reed-Sternberg cells are positive for the virus. The EBV genome is amplified 50-fold or more in Hodgkin-Reed-Sternberg cells and is monoclonal in an individual patient's Hodgkin-Reed-Sternberg cells. In some populations, virtually all cases of Hodgkin lymphoma occur in EBV-positive individuals, but up to 50% of patients in developed countries do not have EBV in their Hodgkin-Reed-Sternberg cells. Thus, although EBV may play an important role in the development of Hodgkin lymphoma, that role is neither straightforward nor universal.

Genetic Factors

Circumstantial evidence for a genetic contribution to the etiology of Hodgkin lymphoma comes from studies showing that Hodgkin lymphoma is almost 100-fold more likely to develop in the monozygotic twin of an affected individual than in a dizygotic twin. First-degree relatives of individuals with the disease have up to a five-fold increased risk for development of the lymphoma. Perhaps genetically predisposed individuals react differently to EBV, thereby increasing the chance that a lymphoid neoplasm will develop.

Polymerase chain reaction–based genotypic analysis has demonstrated the clonal derivation of Hodgkin-Reed-Sternberg cells, including identical *p53* mutations from multiple Hodgkin-Reed-Sternberg cells extracted from a single biopsy specimen, thereby unequivocally establishing clonality. The presence of clonal immunoglobulin gene rearrangements from multiple cells in the same biopsy specimen also confirms a B-cell origin. Only a few rare cases with a T-cell genotype have been reported, but these are exceptional. The presence of clonal somatic mutations provides proof of the germinal center origin of the neoplastic cells. Finally, identification of cells with identical immunoglobulin gene rearrangements both at diagnosis and at relapse verify that the B-cell clonality of the disease is preserved over time.

Despite their B-cell origin, the neoplastic cells of Hodgkin lymphoma are incapable of making intact antibodies, perhaps because they lack the ability to make the transcription factors necessary to activate the immunoglobulin promoter. B cells that are incapable of manufacturing antibody should undergo apoptosis, but the Hodgkin-Reed-Sternberg cells avoid self-destruction. The observation that the antiapoptotic nuclear transcription factor NFκB is constitutively activated in these cells may provide an explanation.

Classic cytogenetics has been unrevealing in Hodgkin lymphoma. Aneuploidy and hyperploidy consistent with the multinucleated nature of Hodgkin-Reed-Sternberg cells are frequent, but no consistent translocations have been detected. A germline *NPAT* mutation and multiple possible sites on chromosome 6 at 6p21.3[2,3] have been associated with an increased risk for Hodgkin lymphoma.

CLINICAL MANIFESTATIONS

Hodgkin lymphoma is usually manifested as lymphadenopathy (Chapter 168), typically in the cervical, axillary, or mediastinal areas, and only about 10% of patients present with nodal disease below the diaphragm. Although peripherally located nodes seldom reach large size, very large mediastinal masses or, less often, retroperitoneal masses can develop with only modest symptoms. Lymph node involvement in Hodgkin lymphoma is usually painless, but an occasional patient notes discomfort in involved nodal sites immediately after drinking alcohol.

Approximately 25% of patients with Hodgkin lymphoma have constitutional symptoms. The classic B symptoms, significant weight loss (>10% of baseline), night sweats, and persistent fever, usually signal widespread or locally extensive disease and imply a need for systemic treatment. Generalized pruritus, occasionally severe, can antedate the diagnosis of Hodgkin lymphoma by up to several years. Some patients have symptoms suggestive of a growing mass lesion, such as cough or stridor as a result of tracheobronchial compression from mediastinal disease or bone pain secondary to metastatic involvement. Because Hodgkin lymphoma can involve the bone marrow extensively, an occasional patient presents with symptomatic anemia or incidentally noted pancytopenia. Paraneoplastic neurologic or endocrine syndromes have been reported with Hodgkin lymphoma but are rare.

DIAGNOSIS

The diagnosis of classic Hodgkin lymphoma is based on recognition of Hodgkin-Reed-Sternberg cells (Fig. 186-1) or Hodgkin cells (or both) in an appropriate cellular background in tissue sections from a lymph node or extralymphatic organ, such as bone marrow, lung, or bone. Fine-needle aspiration biopsy is not adequate for the diagnosis of Hodgkin lymphoma. Open biopsy and standard histochemical staining are required to establish the diagnosis unequivocally and to determine the histologic subtype. Immunohistochemical studies can prove helpful in difficult cases or to distinguish special subtypes such as the lymphocyte-rich classic and nodular lymphocyte-predominant types. In classic Hodgkin lymphoma, scattered large Hodgkin-Reed-Sternberg cells either are multinucleated or have large polyploid nuclei. Variations include mononuclear cells that are similar to the usual polylobated or multinuclear cells but have only one large nucleus with a prominent nucleolus, as well as lacunar cells, which are Hodgkin-Reed-Sternberg variants with abundant cytoplasm that has retracted as an artifact of formalin fixation. The infrequent Hodgkin-Reed-Sternberg cells are usually present in a background mixture of polyclonal lymphocytes, eosinophils, neutrophils, plasma cells, fibroblasts, and histiocytes. A high number of associated macrophages have been demonstrated to be a strong predictor of treatment resistance. Occasionally, granulomas form with a prominent histiocytic component.

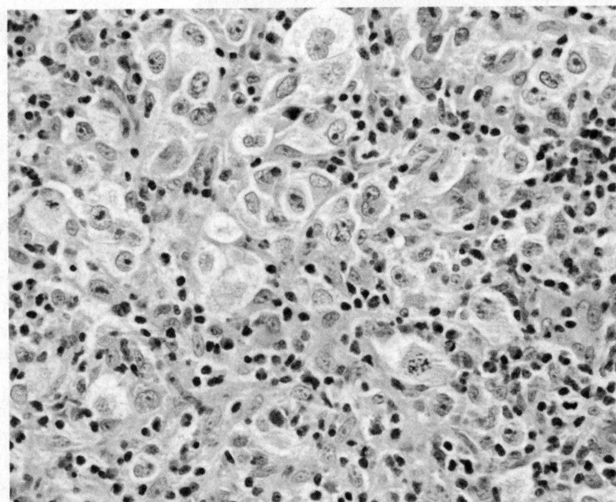

FIGURE 186-1. Nodular sclerosing Hodgkin lymphoma. This figure shows a typical case of classic nodular sclerosing Hodgkin lymphoma with many lacunar cells, occasional diagnostic Hodgkin-Reed-Sternberg cells, and the characteristic background of lymphocytes and eosinophils. (Photomicrograph courtesy of Randy D. Gascoyne, MD, British Columbia Cancer Agency.)

Hodgkin lymphoma can typically be classified into well-described subtypes (Table 186-1). Reproducibility of the distinctions among these subtypes has been confirmed in the current widely accepted World Health Organization classification of lymphoid neoplasms. With addition of the new category of lymphocyte-rich classic Hodgkin lymphoma, this newest classification scheme permits confident identification of nodular lymphocyte-predominant Hodgkin lymphoma as a separate entity. The most common subtype is nodular sclerosing, which has characteristic coarse bands of sclerosis surrounding nodules composed of typical Hodgkin-Reed-Sternberg cells in the usual background mixture of reactive and inflammatory cells.

The immunophenotype of the neoplastic cells in Hodgkin lymphoma can help identify the specific subtype. Typically, the Hodgkin-Reed-Sternberg cells stain positively for CD30 (80 to 100% of cases), CD15 (75 to 85% of cases), and B-cell-specific activating protein (BSAP), which is the product of the *PAX5* gene (>90% of cases). However, often only a minority of the malignant cells stain positively for the CD15 and BSAP markers. CD20, a generally reliable marker of B-cell lineage, is positive in about 40% of cases of classic Hodgkin lymphoma, but usually only in a minority of cells, and the staining can be weak. In contrast, nodular lymphocyte-predominant Hodgkin lymphoma almost always stains strongly positive for CD20 and for the specialized B-cell markers CD79a and CD45, but it is negative for CD30 and CD15. Anaplastic large cell lymphoma (Chapter 185) is positive for CD30 but reliably negative for CD15, CD20, and CD79a.

Differential Diagnosis

Depending on the site of occurrence and associated symptoms, the differential diagnosis of Hodgkin lymphoma includes non-Hodgkin lymphoma (Chapter 185), germ cell tumors (Chapter 200), thymoma (Chapter 422), sarcoidosis (Chapter 95), and tuberculosis (Chapter 324). However, the specific diagnosis is readily determined by obtaining an adequate biopsy specimen for review by an experienced hematopathologist. Proceeding to such a biopsy early in the assessment of patients with lymphadenopathy (Chapter 168), especially of the mediastinum, often saves time and spares the patient needless testing and delay in diagnosis.

With computed tomography (CT) and appropriate biopsy procedures to investigate enlarged central thoracic or intra-abdominal lymph nodes, the diagnosis of Hodgkin lymphoma seldom presents difficulty. The immunophenotype helps distinguish Hodgkin lymphoma from other diseases. For example, T-cell-rich B-cell lymphoma (Chapter 185) is distinguished from classic Hodgkin lymphoma by being CD30 and CD15 negative but positive for CD20 and CD45. However, T-cell-rich B-cell lymphoma (Chapter 185) can be very difficult to distinguish from nodular lymphocyte-predominant Hodgkin lymphoma because both are negative for CD30 and CD15 but positive for CD45. This distinction is best made by focusing on the histologic pattern of the neoplastic cells. In fact, the combination of appropriate immunohistopathologic evaluation by an expert hematopathologist and clinical assessment has virtually eliminated difficulties with the differential diagnosis. Problems mostly arise when inadequate or improperly processed material is all that is available for diagnosis.

TABLE 186-1 WORLD HEALTH ORGANIZATION CLASSIFICATION OF HODGKIN LYMPHOMA SUBTYPES

SUBTYPE NAME	FREQUENCY (%)*
Classic Hodgkin lymphoma	
Nodular sclerosis	70
Lymphocyte rich	3
Mixed cellularity	10
Lymphocyte depleted	1
Nodular lymphocyte-predominant Hodgkin lymphoma	7
Hodgkin lymphoma, not otherwise classifiable	9

*Frequency based on all new cases (N = 1043) seen in British Columbia since January 1998 when the category of lymphocyte-rich classic Hodgkin lymphoma became well established.

Staging

Physical Examination

Given its tendency to spread in an orderly fashion, usually from initially involved lymph nodes, the stage of Hodgkin lymphoma can be established by using readily available imaging and laboratory tests (Fig. 186-2 and Table 186-2). The evaluation should start with a careful history to search for the presence of localizing signs, such as bone pain, or the constitutional symptoms of fever, weight loss, or night sweats. The history may also reveal comorbid conditions that may affect the safe delivery of planned treatment. The physical examination may identify lymphadenopathy or organomegaly.

Laboratory Testing

Laboratory testing should include blood cell counts and the erythrocyte sedimentation rate, assessment of liver and renal function, serum albumin level, serum protein electrophoresis, and serologic testing for hepatitis B. Also, the patient should be tested for hepatitis C if liver enzyme abnormalities are detected and human immunodeficiency virus (HIV) antibody if the history indicates an increased risk or if the sites of extranodal disease are unusual. Bone marrow aspiration and biopsy are only useful for the minority of patients with constitutional (B) symptoms or those with lower than normal peripheral blood counts at diagnosis and may be rendered entirely unnecessary by fluorodeoxyglucose positron emission tomography if current studies are validated.[4]

TABLE 186-2 TESTS REQUIRED FOR STAGING OF HODGKIN LYMPHOMA

Complete history to search for B symptoms (fever, weight loss, night sweats) or other symptomatic problems suggesting more advanced disease
Physical examination for lymphadenopathy or organomegaly
Complete blood count
Serum creatinine, alkaline phosphatase, lactate dehydrogenase, bilirubin, and protein electrophoresis (including serum albumin level)
Chest radiograph, posteroanterior and lateral views
Computed tomography scan of the neck, thorax, abdomen, and pelvis
Fluorodeoxyglucose positron emission tomography with computed tomography (PET/CT)
Certain tests are required only for specific manifestations

MANIFESTATION/CONDITION	TEST
B symptoms or WBC count $<4.0 \times 10^9$/L, Hgb <120 g/L (women) or 130 g/L (men), or platelets $<125 \times 10^9$/L	Bone marrow biopsy and aspiration
Stage IA or IIA disease with upper cervical lymph node involvement (suprahyoid)	ENT examination

ENT = ear, nose, and throat; Hgb = hemoglobin; WBC = white blood cell.

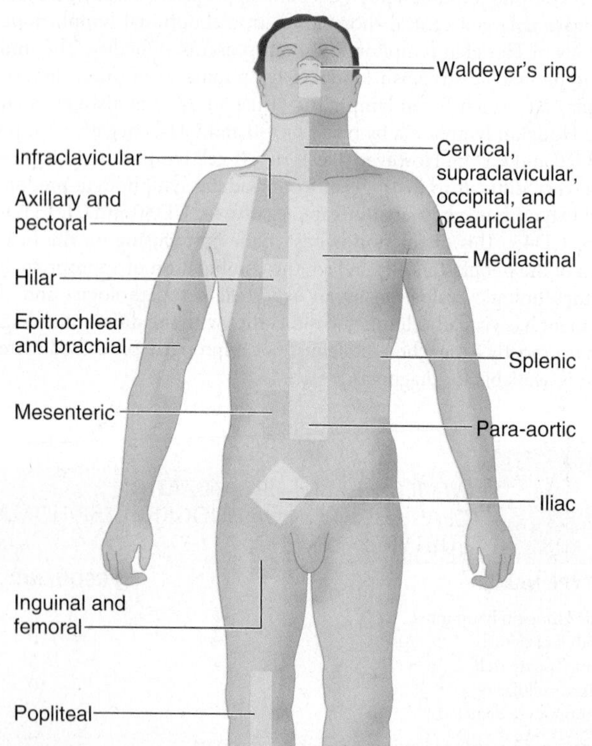

FIGURE 186-2. Anatomic definition of lymph node regions for staging of Hodgkin disease. (From Kaplan HS, Rosenberg SA. The treatment of Hodgkin disease. *Med Clin North Am.* 1966;50:1591-1610.)

Imaging

Imaging techniques to evaluate Hodgkin lymphoma continue to evolve (Fig 186-3). All patients should undergo contrast-enhanced CT scanning of the neck, thorax, abdomen, and pelvis with slices at intervals of 1 cm or less. Magnetic resonance imaging is occasionally useful when the extent of bone or soft tissue involvement must be determined precisely or for a patient with an absolute contraindication to the use of intravenous contrast agents.

Positron Emission Tomography

Fluorodeoxyglucose positron emission tomography (PET) is more sensitive and specific than CT or gallium scanning both for staging and for assessment of residual masses after treatment and is now considered mandatory for staging of Hodgkin lymphoma.[5] It may also be useful for the assessment of residual masses during or after planned treatment, allowing better selection of patients who should receive altered or additional therapy, especially radiotherapy.

Staging System

The Ann Arbor staging system with the Cotswold modification (Table 186-3) categorizes patients into four stages. The first three indicate the expanding extent of lymph node disease (see Fig. 186-2): stage I, a single nodal area; stage II, two or more nodal areas but still on one side of the diaphragm; and stage III, nodal disease on both sides of the diaphragm. The spleen and the lymphoid tissue of Waldeyer's ring each count as nodal sites in this system. Stage IV is reserved for extranodal disease, which for all practical purposes is disease in the bone marrow, lung, bone, or liver. Hodgkin lymphoma at any other extranodal site should prompt questioning of the diagnosis or a search for HIV infection.

Bulky disease is defined as the presence of any tumor mass with the largest diameter greater than 10 cm or a mediastinal mass with a transverse diameter exceeding one third of the largest transverse transthoracic diameter. With CT scanning, use of the mediastinal mass ratio is obsolete, and the term *bulky* is best assigned to tumors exceeding 10 cm in largest single diameter.

The E lesion designation identifies patients whose limited extranodal extension of Hodgkin lymphoma could be included in a reasonable involved field of irradiation. As part of staging, patients are further subdivided into those with or without fever, night sweats, or weight loss (B symptoms).

TREATMENT

Over the past 70 years, Hodgkin lymphoma has been transformed from a nearly uniformly fatal illness to one that is usually cured. This remarkable success has provided a paradigm on which much of modern oncologic treatment is based. The principles underlying combined-modality treatment and multiagent chemotherapy, the mainstays of today's successful treatment of many malignancies, were first demonstrated to be effective with Hodgkin lymphoma. The essential involvement of a multidisciplinary team, including pathologists, experts in diagnostic imaging, medical and radiation oncologists, nurses, and support staff, has served as a model for all cancer. The necessity to balance greater efficacy of initial treatment, which often requires an increase in intensity and therefore toxicity, against troublesome and occasionally fatal late complications has encouraged a long-term perspective and careful monitoring for late treatment-related side effects.

From a practical therapeutic viewpoint, patients with stage III or IV disease or bulky disease are defined as having advanced disease, whereas patients without these characteristics have limited-stage disease. In Europe, patients with limited disease are further subdivided into those with favorable and unfavorable outcomes. Cure rates exceed 90 to 95% for patients with nonbulky stage IA or IIA (limited) disease. However, for patients with advanced-stage disease, independent predictors of progression include gender, age, stage, hemoglobin level, white blood cell count, lymphocyte count, and serum albumin level (Table 186-4). Based on results obtained in the 1980s, the 80% of patients with fewer than four factors had a progression-free survival of 70%,

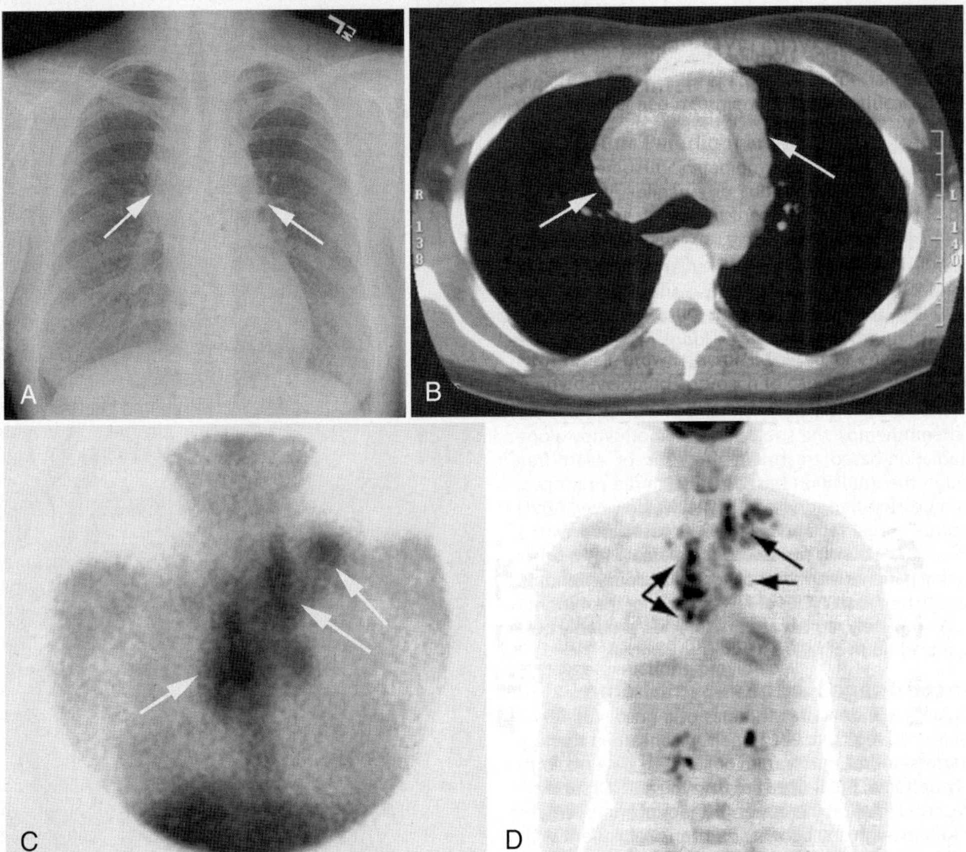

FIGURE 186-3. **Imaging of Hodgkin lymphoma.** Bulky Hodgkin disease as seen on chest radiograph (**A**), computed tomography (CT) of the chest (**B**), gallium scan (**C**), and positron emission tomography (PET) (**D**). The *arrows* indicate sites of disease. Note that the PET and CT scans provide more detailed information than the chest radiograph and gallium scan.

TABLE 186-3 MODIFIED ANN ARBOR STAGING SYSTEM FOR HODGKIN LYMPHOMA

STAGE	INVOLVEMENT
I	Single lymph node region (I) or one extralymphatic site (I_E)
II	Two or more lymph node regions, same side of the diaphragm (II), or local extralymphatic extension plus one or more lymph node regions, same side of the diaphragm (II_E)
III	Lymph node regions on both sides of the diaphragm (III); may be accompanied by local extralymphatic extension (III_E)
IV	Diffuse involvement of one or more extralymphatic organs or sites
A	No "B" symptoms
B	Presence of at least one of the following: Unexplained weight loss >10% of baseline during 6 mo before staging Recurrent unexplained fever >38° C Recurrent night sweats

TABLE 186-4 RATES OF PROGRESSION IN 5 YEARS IN PATIENTS WITH ADVANCED-STAGE HODGKIN LYMPHOMA

NO. OF FACTORS*	FREQUENCY (%)	PERCENTAGE WITH PROGRESSION-FREE SURVIVAL AT 5 YEARS
0-3	81	70
4-7	19	47

*Male sex, age older than 45 years, stage IV, hemoglobin level less than 10.5 g/dL, white blood cell count greater than 15,000/mL, lymphocyte count less than 600/mL or less than 8% of the white cell count, or serum albumin less than 4 g/dL.

but for the 20% who had four or more factors, the progression-free survival rate fell to less than 50%. However, with better attention to dose delivery, more current results indicate a spread of only 80% to 60% between these two groups.[6] A straightforward plan of treatment for the 90% of patients in whom Hodgkin lymphoma is diagnosed between the ages of 16 and 70 years can be based on clinical stage, the presence of B symptoms, and bulk of the largest tumor mass (Table 186-5).

TABLE 186-5 TREATMENT PLAN FOR HODGKIN LYMPHOMA BASED ON STAGE

STAGE	TREATMENT
IA or IIA, no bulky disease*	ABVD† × 4 if CR after 2 cycles, or ABVD × 2 + IRRT
IB, IIB, or any stage III or IV or bulky disease, any stage	ABVD† until 2 cycles past CR (minimum 6, maximum 8) or escalated BEACOPP†

*Bulky refers to disease with the largest diameter of any single mass equal to or greater than 10 cm.
†See text for drugs in each regimen. Optimal dosing must be individualized.
CR = complete response.

Treatment of Limited-Stage Hodgkin Lymphoma

More than 95% of the one third of patients with Hodgkin lymphoma initially found to have limited-stage disease can be cured regardless of the site of occurrence, the presence of disease above or below the diaphragm, or the histologic subtype. The challenge is to achieve this goal with the least toxicity and cost.

Two cycles of ABVD (Adriamycin [doxorubicin], bleomycin, vinblastine, and dacarbazine) chemotherapy followed by involved-field irradiation cures nearly 95% of patients with limited-stage disease, nearly completely eliminates the risk for infertility, premature menopause, and leukemia, and minimizes cardiopulmonary toxicity.[7] However, chemotherapy alone has been shown to be a viable alternative for patients with a good initial response to treatment and further reduces the risks of exposure to radiation.[A1] More intensified approaches have been tested for early-stage but unfavorable Hodgkin lymphoma with adverse prognostic factors such as bulky mediastinal mass, extranodal extension, elevated erythrocyte sedimentation rate (ESR), or three or more lymph node areas involved. In such patients, two cycles of BEACOPP (bleomycin, etoposide, Adriamycin, cyclophosphamide, vincristine, procarbazine, and prednisone), followed by two cycles of ABVD before involved-field radiotherapy, significantly improves tumor control compared with only four cycles of ABVD before involved-field radiotherapy, but long-term results do not differ.[8] The chemotherapy in the combined-modality treatment of limited-stage Hodgkin lymphoma eradicates subclinical disease and allows smaller fields of irradiation to be used. However, a substantial proportion of the excess, long-term mortality in patients with limited-stage Hodgkin lymphoma is due to cardiovascular disease and second neoplasms that are closely related to the use of irradiation.[9] In a randomized trial that compared four to six cycles of ABVD chemotherapy alone versus irradiation, either alone or augmented with two cycles of ABVD chemotherapy, the strategy of chemotherapy alone proved equivalent to irradiation-based treatment in terms of event-free and overall survival, although the irradiation-based approach did produce a modest improvement in progression-free survival. At 12 years, however, ABVD therapy alone without subtotal nodal radiation therapy is associated with a better overall survival (94% vs. 87%) owing to a lower rate of death from other causes. These data suggest that patients with limited-stage Hodgkin lymphoma can be successfully treated with four to six cycles of ABVD alone; for the minority whose lymphoma does not completely regress after two cycles, probably best assessed by PET scanning, the addition of radiation may be optimal.

Treatment of Advanced-Stage Hodgkin Lymphoma

In advanced-stage Hodgkin lymphoma (stages IIIA, IIIB, IVA, and IVB), ABVD has become the most widely used regimen. The addition of radiation therapy significantly improves progression-free survival at 10 years in patients with advanced-stage Hodgkin lymphoma, but it does not improve overall survival. The adverse long-term effects of radiation therapy and its lack of improvement in overall survival appear to outweigh any benefits for the usual patient with advanced-stage disease. A negative PET scan at the end of chemotherapy distinguishes between residual fibrosis and persistent lymphoma and identifies the three fourths of patients with a residual mass who do not require radiation therapy.[A2]

Recently devised regimens for patients with advanced Hodgkin lymphoma are the Stanford V regimen (doxorubicin, vinblastine, mechlorethamine, etoposide, vincristine, bleomycin, and prednisone) and escalated BEACOPP (bleomycin, etoposide, doxorubicin, cyclophosphamide vincristine, procarbazine, and prednisone) (see Table 186-5). As originally described, both include post-chemotherapy irradiation to sites of initial or residual tumor bulk (≥5 cm), but radiation does not appear to be routinely necessary after BEACOPP. Although initial results appeared quite promising, the Stanford V regimen is no more effective than standard ABVD.[A3] Assessing the role of escalated BEACOPP for advanced-stage Hodgkin lymphoma requires consideration of potential secondary treatments for those not cured by primary therapy. About 50% of patients who are not cured by primary chemotherapy can be effectively treated with HDC/HSCT (Chapter 178). Thus, although escalated BEACOPP offers better initial disease control, randomized trials have failed to demonstrate its superiority over ABVD for overall survival.[A4][A5]

Management of Refractory or Relapsed Hodgkin Lymphoma

HDC/HSCT has become the established treatment for most patients whose Hodgkin lymphoma persists or recurs despite primary chemotherapy. However, the treatment-related mortality, high levels of toxicity, and cost associated with HDC/HSCT demand that it be reserved for patients in whom it clearly increases the chance of cure over alternative treatments;[10] such patients include those whose disease progresses during or within 3 months of initial multiagent chemotherapy (refractory Hodgkin lymphoma) and those who relapse more than 3 months after multiagent chemotherapy (relapsed Hodgkin lymphoma). For relapsed lymphoma, controversy remains, however, for two special subgroups: patients who relapse solely in originally involved but unirradiated lymph nodes and without B symptoms or extranodal disease, who may obtain up to a 40 to 50% cure rate with wide-field irradiation, and patients who relapse without B symptoms more than 1 year after completion of primary chemotherapy, who may achieve up to a 30 to 40% cure rate with additional chemotherapy with or without irradiation. However, even these two subgroups may achieve up to an 80% 10-year disease-free survival rate after HDC/HSCT. Thus, data suggest that standard treatment for patients with progressive Hodgkin lymphoma after primary chemotherapy for advanced-stage disease should be HDC/HSCT regardless of the characteristics of the relapse.

Management of Complications

Follow-up and Late Complications of Treatment

Most adult patients with Hodgkin lymphoma are cured and experience minimal long-term toxicity from their treatment. However, the risk for certain predictable and rare and less predictable late effects warrants careful but not intrusive follow-up and selective intervention (Table 186-6). At the conclusion of treatment, a thorough reassessment of the initial sites of lymphoma should be completed to provide post-treatment baseline measurements. Patients should be seen by a specialist knowledgeable in the management of lymphoma, preferably about every 3 months for 2 years, then every 6 months for 3 years, then annually. Patients should be strongly encouraged to refrain from smoking, to perform careful breast and skin examinations on a regular basis, and to undergo regular immunizations for influenza annually, pneumococcus at diagnosis and 5 years after treatment, and diphtheria and tetanus every 10 years (Chapter 18). Patients who have received radiation to the head or neck area should follow a vigorous program of dental prophylaxis in anticipation of the deleterious effect of reduced saliva production and should have their thyroid-stimulating hormone (TSH) level checked annually in recognition of the 50% risk for eventual hypothyroidism.

TABLE 186-6 MONITORING AFTER SUCCESSFUL PRIMARY TREATMENT OF HODGKIN LYMPHOMA

RISK/PROBLEM	INCIDENCE/RESPONSE
Relapse	Ten to 30% of patients experience relapse. Careful attention should be directed to lymph node sites, especially if previously involved with disease and not treated with radiation. New persistent focal symptoms such as bone pain should be investigated with appropriate laboratory and imaging studies.
Dental caries	Neck or oropharyngeal irradiation may cause decreased salivation. Patients should have regular dental care and should make their dentist aware of the previous irradiation.
Hypothyroidism	After external beam thyroid irradiation at doses sufficient to cure Hodgkin lymphoma, at least 50% of patients eventually become hypothyroid. All patients who have been exposed to neck irradiation should have an annual TSH level determined. Patients whose TSH level becomes elevated should be treated with lifelong thyroxine replacement in doses sufficient to suppress TSH levels to low normal (Chapter 226).
Infertility	ABVD is not known to cause permanent gonadal toxicity, although temporary oligospermia or irregular menses may persist for 1 to 2 years after treatment. Direct or scatter radiation to gonadal tissue may cause infertility, amenorrhea, or premature menopause, but this adverse event seldom occurs with the current fields used for the treatment of Hodgkin lymphoma. In general, women who continue menstruating are fertile, but men require semen analysis to provide a specific answer.
Secondary neoplasms	Although uncommon, certain secondary neoplasms occur with increased frequency in patients who have been treated for Hodgkin lymphoma: acute myelogenous leukemia; thyroid, breast, lung, cervical, and upper gastrointestinal carcinoma; and melanoma. It is appropriate to "be vigilant" for these neoplasms for the remainder of the patient's life because they may have a lengthy induction period.

ABVD = doxorubicin (Adriamycin), bleomycin, vinblastine, and dacarbazine; TSH = thyroid-stimulating hormone.

Other potential long-term sequelae of Hodgkin lymphoma treatment[11] include second malignancies. Radiation therapy–related solid tumors, most commonly nonmelanoma skin cancers, lung, breast, and colorectal malignancies, have a median latency period of more than 14 years after treatment. Chemotherapy-related myelodysplasia and acute myelogenous leukemia are more likely to be caused by alkylating agents that are included in regimens like MOPP and BEACOPP compared with ABVD and have shorter latency periods (median of 3 years) after treatment.[11] Long-term (usually >10 years after treatment) cardiovascular complications are coronary artery disease (related to mediastinal irradiation) and cardiomyopathy (caused by the cardiotoxicity of cumulative doses of anthracycline chemotherapy). Chemotherapy, particularly alkylating agents in MOPP and BEACOPP but not ABVD regimens, can cause permanent infertility. Long-term survivors of childhood Hodgkin lymphoma (median age at diagnosis of 15 years) are at increased risk for neurocognitive impairment.[12]

Special Problems in the Management of Hodgkin Lymphoma

Hodgkin Lymphoma during Pregnancy

Between 0.5 and 1.0% of cases of Hodgkin lymphoma occur coincident with pregnancy (Chapter 239). When the lymphoma is discovered during pregnancy, it is almost always possible to keep it under control and allow the pregnancy to go to full term.

Standard staging tests (see Table 186-2) should be completed, except that imaging requiring radiation must be minimized. For example, abdominal ultrasonography can identify bulky retroperitoneal disease, and a single posteroanterior radiograph of the chest, with proper shielding, can identify bulky mediastinal disease.

Patients can often continue the pregnancy to term without any treatment of the lymphoma.[13] If symptomatic or progressive disease develops, systemic chemotherapy can be given in the second and third trimester with very low risk for injuring the fetus. An attractive alternative to multiagent chemotherapy is intermittent single-agent vinblastine, given in the lowest dose that can control symptoms until delivery, followed by a full course of six to eight cycles of multiagent chemotherapy after delivery.

Hodgkin Lymphoma and Acquired Immunodeficiency Syndrome

In patients with HIV infection, the incidence of Hodgkin lymphoma is increased as much as 5- to 10-fold, and the lymphoma manifests differently and pursues a more aggressive natural history (Chapter 393). Hodgkin lymphoma in HIV-positive individuals is almost always associated with EBV within Hodgkin-Reed-Sternberg cells. The histology is much more likely to be mixed cellularity or lymphocyte depleted. The disease most commonly develops in extranodal sites, especially the bone marrow. More than 80% of patients have advanced-stage disease, and most patients have B symptoms.

Patients are prone to opportunistic infections, and the interaction of chemotherapeutic agents with other medications may compromise the patient's ability to tolerate treatment. The best approach is a combination of highly active antiretroviral agents (Chapter 389), vigorous supportive care with antiherpetic and antifungal agents and neutrophil-stimulating growth factors, and standard multiagent chemotherapy. With appropriate supportive care, regimens such as ABVD can be delivered. However, more severe than normal toxicity must be anticipated, and although cure rates for the lymphoma are comparable to those seen in HIV-negative individuals, median overall survival is much shorter than that seen in the non-HIV-infected patients, typically 3 to 4 years.[14]

Hodgkin Lymphoma in the Elderly Population

Elderly patients with Hodgkin lymphoma have a worse outcome. For example, the 5-year overall survival rate falls from 80% in patients younger than 65 years to less than 50% in patients older than 65 years.[A4] Explanations include more advanced stage at diagnosis, comorbid diseases, delay in diagnosis, incomplete staging, inadequate adherence to treatment protocols, and failure to maintain full dose intensity.

Of note is that elderly patients achieve outcomes equivalent to those of younger patients when they receive similar doses of chemotherapy. The best approach for elderly patients is to attempt to treat them in a manner similar to younger patients, with vigorous supportive care and the addition of neutrophil growth factors if necessary to enable safe delivery of full doses. For patients with preexisting pulmonary or cardiac disease, it might be necessary to reduce or eliminate bleomycin or doxorubicin, respectively.

FUTURE DIRECTIONS

The ability to profile multigene expression patterns and identify genetic polymorphisms associated with specific malignancies may provide better insight into the molecular genesis of Hodgkin and other lymphomas.[15] Therapeutic agents more specifically targeted at the malignant Hodgkin-Reed-Sternberg cells, such as those coupling an antibody to the CD30 antigen with a cellular toxin, have proved remarkably effective and hold substantial promise to improve treatment outcome.[A5]

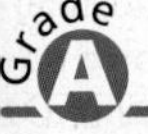

Grade A References

A1. Meyer RM, Gospodarowicz MK, Connors JM, et al. ABVD alone versus radiation-based therapy in limited-stage Hodgkin lymphoma. *N Engl J Med.* 2012;366:399-408.

A2. Engert A, Haverkamp H, Kobe C, et al. Reduced-intensity chemotherapy and PET-guided radiotherapy in patients with advanced stage Hodgkin lymphoma (HD15 trial): a randomised, open-label, phase 3 non-inferiority trial. *Lancet.* 2012;379:1791-1799.

A3. Gordon LI, Hong F, Fisher RI, et al. Randomized phase III trial of ABVD versus Stanford V with or without radiation therapy in locally extensive and advanced-stage Hodgkin lymphoma: an intergroup study coordinated by the Eastern Cooperative Oncology Group (E2496). *J Clin Oncol.* 2013;31:684-691.

A4. Mounier N, Brice P, Bologna S, et al. ABVD (8 cycles) versus BEACOPP (4 escalated cycles ≥ baseline): final results in stage III-IV low-risk Hodgkin lymphoma (IPS 0-2) of the LYSA H34 randomized trial. *Ann Oncol.* 2014;25:1622-1628.

A5. Viviani S, Zinzani PL, Rambaldi A, et al. ABVD versus BEACOPP for Hodgkin lymphoma when high-dose salvage is planned. *N Engl J Med.* 2011;365:203-212.

GENERAL REFERENCES

For the General References and other additional features, please visit Expert Consult at https://expertconsult.inkling.com.

187 PLASMA CELL DISORDERS

S. VINCENT RAJKUMAR

Plasma cell disorders are neoplastic or potentially neoplastic diseases associated with the clonal proliferation of immunoglobulin-secreting plasma cells (Table 187-1). They are characterized by the secretion of electrophoretically and immunologically homogeneous (monoclonal) proteins that represent intact or incomplete immunoglobulin molecules. Monoclonal proteins are commonly referred to as M proteins, myeloma proteins, or paraproteins.

Syndromes associated with plasma cell disorders and monoclonal proteins include premalignant disorders (monoclonal gammopathy of undetermined significance, smoldering multiple myeloma), malignant neoplasms (multiple myeloma, Waldenström macroglobulinemia), and disorders primarily related to the unique properties of the secreted monoclonal protein (cryoglobulinemia, immunoglobulin light chain [AL] amyloidosis, light chain deposition disease) (see Table 187-1).[1]

Serum Immunoglobulins

Intact immunoglobulins consist of two heavy (H) polypeptide chains of the same class and subclass and two light (L) polypeptide chains of the same type (Chapter 45). The heavy polypeptide chains are designated by Greek letters: γ in immunoglobulin G (IgG), α in immunoglobulin A (IgA), μ in immunoglobulin M (IgM), δ in immunoglobulin D (IgD), and ε in immunoglobulin E (IgE). The light chain types are kappa (κ) and lambda (λ). Both heavy chains and light chains have constant and variable regions with respect to the amino acid sequence. The class specificity of each immunoglobulin is defined by a series of antigenic determinants on the constant regions of the heavy chains (γ, α, μ, δ, and ε) and the two major classes of light chains (κ and λ). The amino acid sequence in the variable regions of the immunoglobulin molecule corresponds to the active antigen-combining site of the antibody.

In the majority of clonal plasma cell disorders, *intact* immunoglobulin molecules are secreted as monoclonal (M) proteins. In addition, there can also be abnormal secretion of excess monoclonal *free* light chains that are released without being bound to immunoglobulin heavy chains. In some patients, heavy chain expression is completely lost, and only monoclonal free light chains (commonly referred to as Bence Jones proteins) are secreted. Even less frequently, only heavy chains are secreted, resulting in heavy chain diseases (HCDs). Rare patients with multiple myeloma secrete no identifiable immunoglobulin (nonsecretory myeloma).

TABLE 187-1 PLASMA CELL PROLIFERATIVE DISORDERS

I. Premalignant monoclonal gammopathies
   A. Monoclonal gammopathy of undetermined significance (MGUS)
   B. MGUS in association with chronic lymphocytic leukemia and non-Hodgkin lymphoma
   C. Biclonal and triclonal gammopathies of undetermined significance
   D. Idiopathic Bence Jones proteinuria and light chain MGUS
   E. Smoldering multiple myeloma
II. Malignant monoclonal gammopathies
   A. Multiple myeloma and related malignant neoplasms (IgG, IgA, IgD, IgE, and free light chains)
      1. Symptomatic multiple myeloma
      2. Plasma cell leukemia
      3. Osteosclerotic myeloma (including POEMS syndrome)
      4. Solitary plasmacytoma of bone
      5. Solitary extramedullary plasmacytoma
   B. Waldenström macroglobulinemia (IgM)
III. Heavy chain diseases (HCDs)
   A. γ-HCD
   A. α-HCD
   A. μ-HCD
IV. Cryoglobulinemia (types I, II, and III)
V. Immunoglobulin light chain amyloidosis

Ig = immunoglobulin; POEMS = polyneuropathy, organomegaly, endocrinopathy, M protein, and skin changes.

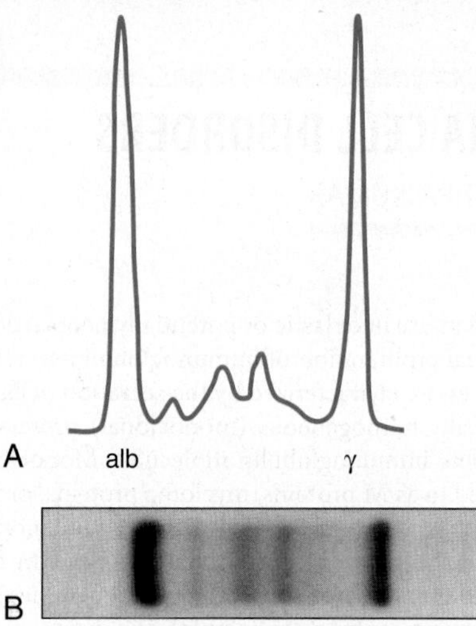

FIGURE 187-1. Serum protein electrophoresis showing a monoclonal (M) protein. **A, Monoclonal pattern of serum protein as traced by a densitometer after electrophoresis on agarose gel: tall, narrow-based peak of γ mobility. B, Monoclonal pattern from electrophoresis of serum on agarose gel (anode on the left): dense, localized band representing monoclonal protein of γ mobility. (From Kyle RA, Katzmann JA. Immunochemical characterization of immunoglobulins. In: Rose NR, Conway de Macario E, Folds JD, et al, eds. *Manual of Clinical Laboratory Immunology*. 5th ed. Washington, DC: ASM Press; 1997:156, with permission of the American Society for Microbiology.)**

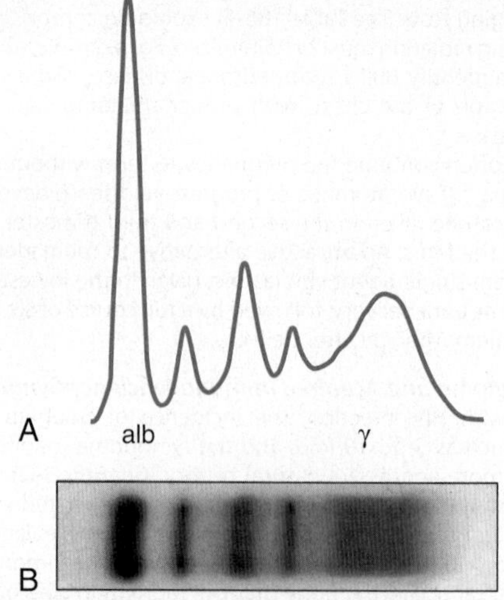

FIGURE 187-2. Serum protein electrophoresis showing increased polyclonal immunoglobulins. A, Polyclonal pattern from a densitometer tracing of agarose gel: broad-based peak of γ mobility. B, Polyclonal pattern from electrophoresis of agarose gel (anode on the left). The band at the right is broad and extends throughout the γ area. (From Kyle RA, Katzmann JA. Immunochemical characterization of immunoglobulins. In: Rose NR, Conway de Macario E, Folds JD, et al, eds. *Manual of Clinical Laboratory Immunology*. 5th ed. Washington, DC: ASM Press; 1997:156, with permission of the American Society for Microbiology.)

Identification of Monoclonal Proteins

Protein electrophoresis of the serum and urine detects M protein as a narrow peak (like a church spire) on the densitometer tracing or as a dense, discrete band on agarose gel (Fig. 187-1). Electrophoresis also permits quantitation of M proteins. Monoclonal light chains (Bence Jones proteinemia) are rarely seen on serum electrophoresis but are easily detected on urine electrophoresis. Urine electrophoresis requires a 24-hour urine collection.

Immunofixation of the serum and urine is performed when a peak or band is first seen on protein electrophoresis to identify the heavy and light chain types of the M protein. Immunofixation is also a more sensitive test than protein electrophoresis, and it should always be performed in conjunction with electrophoresis when multiple myeloma or related disorders are first suspected to detect small, unmeasurable M proteins that may be missed on electrophoresis. This is particularly important in oligosecretory myeloma, primary amyloidosis, and solitary plasmacytoma and after successful treatment of multiple myeloma or macroglobulinemia. In these instances, a small M protein can be concealed in the normal β or γ areas of the electrophoresis gel and may be overlooked.

Monoclonal proteins must be distinguished from an excess of polyclonal immunoglobulins (one or more heavy chain types and both κ and λ light chains, usually limited to the γ region), which produce a broad-based peak or broad band (Fig. 187-2). This finding is associated with chronic infectious or inflammatory states, including chronic liver disease.

Detection of Serum Free Light Chains

The serum free light chain assay measures the level of free κ and λ immunoglobulin light chains (i.e., light chains that are not bound to intact immunoglobulin). An abnormal κ/λ free light chain ratio (normal range, 0.26 to 1.65) indicates an excess of one light chain type versus the other and is interpreted as representing a monoclonal elevation of the corresponding light chain type. The serum free light chain assay is more sensitive than electrophoresis or immunofixation in detecting free monoclonal light chains and is useful in the diagnostic evaluation of plasma cell disorders and in risk stratification.

MONOCLONAL GAMMOPATHY OF UNDETERMINED SIGNIFICANCE

DEFINITION

Monoclonal gammopathy of undetermined significance (MGUS; formerly called benign monoclonal gammopathy) is a premalignant clonal plasma cell disorder characterized by the presence of a serum M protein in persons who lack evidence of multiple myeloma, macroglobulinemia, amyloidosis, or other related diseases. MGUS is defined by a serum M protein concentration lower than 3 g/dL; less than 10% clonal plasma cells in the bone marrow; and absence of lytic bone lesions, anemia, hypercalcemia, and renal insufficiency that can be attributed to a plasma cell disorder. The main clinical significance of MGUS is its lifelong risk of transformation to myeloma or related malignant disease at a fixed but unrelenting rate of 1% per year.

EPIDEMIOLOGY

More than 50% of patients in whom a serum M protein is detected have MGUS (Fig. 187-3). The prevalence of MGUS in the general population increases with age, from approximately 1% in persons 50 to 60 years old to more than 5% in those older than 70 years.[2] The age-adjusted prevalence is higher in men than in women and is twice as high in blacks compared with whites. There is an increased prevalence of MGUS as well as of multiple myeloma among blood relatives of individuals with monoclonal gammopathies.

PATHOBIOLOGY

MGUS represents a limited, nonmalignant expansion of monoclonal plasma cells. The etiology of MGUS is unknown, but age, male gender, family history, immunosuppression, and exposure to certain pesticides are known risk factors. It is hypothesized that infection, inflammation, or other antigenic stimuli, acting in concert with the development of cytogenetic abnormalities in the plasma cells, are the initiating pathogenetic events in most patients. Approximately 40% of MGUS is associated with plasma cell translocations involving the immunoglobulin heavy chain (IgH) locus on chromosome 14q32 (IgH-translocated MGUS), 40% with trisomies involving odd-numbered chromosomes (hyperdiploid MGUS), 15% with both trisomies and IgH translocations, and the remaining with other cytogenetic abnormalities. The primary IgH translocations seen in MGUS commonly involve one of five recurrent partner chromosome loci: 11q13 (*CCND1* [cyclin D1 gene]), 4p16.3 (*FGFR3* and *MMSET*), 6p21 (*CCND3* [cyclin D3 gene]), 16q23 (*c-maf*), and 20q11 (*mafB*).

CLINICAL MANIFESTATIONS

MGUS is asymptomatic and is usually diagnosed incidentally on laboratory testing. Patients with MGUS progress to multiple myeloma or related malignant disease at a rate of approximately 1% per year. The interval from the time of recognition of the M protein to the diagnosis of serious disease ranges from 1 to 32 years (median, 10.6 years), and the relative risk versus a control population is 25.0 for progression to multiple myeloma, 8.4 for primary amyloidosis, 46.0 for Waldenström macroglobulinemia, 2.4 for the development of other forms of non-Hodgkin lymphoma, and 8.5 for plasmacytoma.

DIAGNOSIS

MGUS is differentiated from multiple myeloma and smoldering multiple myeloma by the size of the M protein; the bone marrow plasma cell

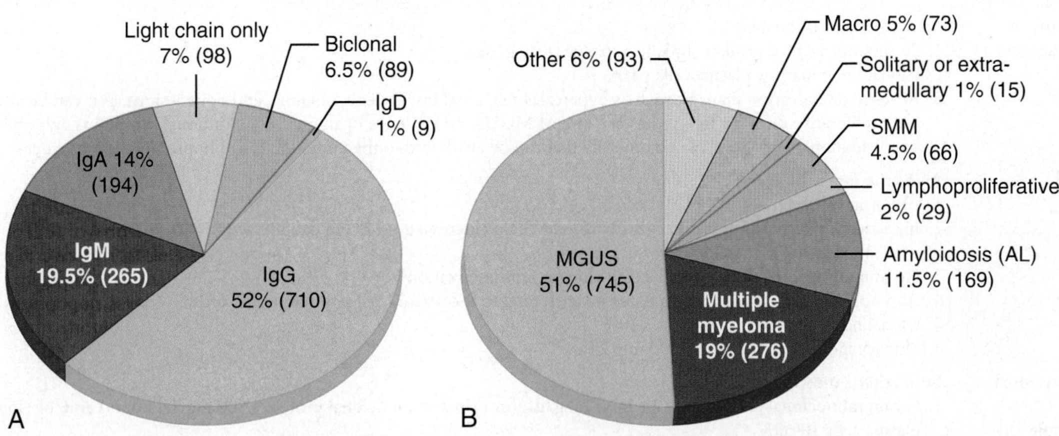

FIGURE 187-3. **Monoclonal gammopathy. A, Distribution of serum monoclonal proteins in patients seen at the Mayo Clinic. B, Diagnoses in cases of monoclonal gammopathy seen at the Mayo Clinic. Ig = immunoglobulin; Macro = Waldenström macroglobulinemia; MGUS = monoclonal gammopathy of undetermined significance; SMM = smoldering multiple myeloma.**

percentage; and the presence or absence of anemia, renal failure, hypercalcemia, or lytic bone lesions (Table 187-2). Because anemia and renal insufficiency are relatively common in the elderly population with MGUS, the causes of these conditions should be carefully investigated with adequate laboratory studies. For example, in a patient with anemia, tests to exclude iron, vitamin B_{12}, or folate deficiency must be performed. In certain instances, such as unexplained renal failure, a renal biopsy may be needed. Only patients with strong evidence of end-organ damage thought to be directly related to a plasma cell disorder can be considered to have myeloma or a related malignant disease.

Although a reduction in the levels of the immunoglobulin classes other than M protein (i.e., the normal polyclonal or background immunoglobulins) is more frequently seen in multiple myeloma or Waldenström macroglobulinemia, such reductions also occur in almost 40% of patients with MGUS.

Association of MGUS with Other Diseases

MGUS is associated with numerous diseases. However, because 3% of the general population older than 50 years has MGUS, it is often difficult to determine whether these reported associations are causal or coincidental. Some associations have been verified on the basis of epidemiologic studies; these include peripheral neuropathy (Chapter 420), proliferative glomerulonephritis, deep venous thrombosis (Chapter 81), osteoporosis (Chapter 243), and lymphoproliferative disorders (Chapter 185). A secondary form of MGUS also occurs with immunosuppression after organ transplantation (Chapter 49) and autologous or allogeneic stem cell transplantation (Chapter 178). M proteins also occur in the sera of some patients with chronic lymphocytic leukemia (Chapter 184) but have no recognizable effect on the clinical course.

Approximately 5% of patients with sensorimotor peripheral neuropathy of unknown cause (Chapter 420) have an associated monoclonal gammopathy (monoclonal gammopathy–associated neuropathy). In half of such patients, the M protein binds to myelin-associated glycoprotein. These patients have a slowly progressive sensory neuropathy more than motor neuropathy, beginning in the distal ends of the extremities and extending proximally. The clinical and electrodiagnostic manifestations of MGUS neuropathy resemble those of a chronic inflammatory demyelinating polyneuropathy. A causal relationship is usually assumed in younger patients and those without other conditions known to cause neuropathy in whom the neuropathy is severe and progressive. Therapeutic approaches include plasmapheresis and, occasionally, chemotherapy (similar to myeloma for IgG or IgA monoclonal proteins, and rituximab or rituximab-based regimens for IgM monoclonal proteins; see the later section on the treatment of multiple myeloma).

Monoclonal gammopathy is also thought to be the underlying cause of approximately 50% of idiopathic proliferative glomerulonephritis, including membranoproliferative glomerulonephritis and C3 glomerulopathy (Chapter 121). Certain skin disorders are also known to be associated with MGUS. Lichen myxedematosus (papular mucinosis, scleromyxedema) is associated with an IgG γ protein. Pyoderma gangrenosum (Chapter 440) and necrobiotic xanthogranuloma are other associated skin disorders.

PREVENTION AND TREATMENT Rx

No treatment is necessary for MGUS. Low-risk patients (Table 187-3) can be evaluated when symptoms suggestive of myeloma or related disorders occur. In all other patients with MGUS, the M protein level in serum and urine should be measured serially, together with periodic reevaluation of clinical and other laboratory findings, to determine whether multiple myeloma or another related disorder is present. In general, electrophoresis, complete blood count, and creatinine and calcium levels should be repeated at 6 months and, if stable, yearly thereafter.

PROGNOSIS

Differentiating a patient with MGUS in whom the disorder will remain stable for life from one in whom multiple myeloma, macroglobulinemia, or a related disorder will eventually develop is difficult when the M protein is first recognized. The size and type of the M protein at diagnosis of MGUS and an abnormal serum free light chain ratio are prognostic factors for progression (see Table 187-3). A study of 728 Swedish cases of MGUS observed for up to 30 years showed a cumulative risk of 15.4% for development of lymphoid disorder and a cumulative risk of 10.6% for progression to multiple myeloma (approximately 0.5% annual risk). Three factors were significantly associated with progression: (1) abnormal free light chain ratio (<0.26 or >1.65); (2) M-protein level of 1.5 g/dL and higher; and (3) reduction of one or two noninvolved immunoglobulin isotype levels (immunoparesis).[3] The first two of these confirm the factors considered by the Mayo Clinic group (see Table 187-3).

BICLONAL GAMMOPATHIES

Biclonal gammopathies occur in at least 5% of patients with clonal plasma cell disorders. A biclonal gammopathy of undetermined significance (analogous to MGUS) accounts for about two thirds of such patients. The remainder have multiple myeloma, macroglobulinemia, or other lymphoproliferative diseases. Rarely, triclonal gammopathies may occur.

LIGHT CHAIN MGUS AND IDIOPATHIC BENCE JONES PROTEINURIA

The diagnosis of typical MGUS requires expression of an intact heavy chain type. In some patients, a premalignant clonal plasma cell disorder characterized by the presence of monoclonal immunoglobulin light chains without expression of heavy chains can occur (light chain MGUS).[4] By definition, these patients should not have evidence of end-organ damage attributable to the light chain, and the clonal bone marrow plasma cell percentage should be

TABLE 187-2 CRITERIA FOR THE DIAGNOSIS OF PLASMA CELL DISORDERS

DISORDER	DISEASE DEFINITION
Monoclonal gammopathy of undetermined significance (MGUS)	All 3 criteria must be met: 1. Serum monoclonal protein (IgG, IgA, or IgM) <3 g/dL 2. Clonal bone marrow plasma cells <10% 3. Absence of end-organ damage, such as hypercalcemia, renal insufficiency, anemia, and bone lesions, that can be attributed to the plasma cell proliferative disorder (or, in the case of IgM MGUS, no evidence of anemia, constitutional symptoms, hyperviscosity, lymphadenopathy, or hepatosplenomegaly that can be attributed to the underlying lymphoproliferative disorder)
Light chain MGUS	All 6 criteria must be met: 1. Abnormal FLC ratio (<0.26 or >1.65) 2. Increased level of the appropriate involved light chain (increased κ FLC in patients with ratio >1.65 and increased λ FLC in patients with ratio <0.26) 3. No immunoglobulin heavy chain expression on immunofixation 4. Absence of end-organ damage that can be attributed to the plasma cell proliferative disorder 5. Clonal bone marrow plasma cells <10% 6. Urinary monoclonal protein <500 mg/24h
Smoldering multiple myeloma (also referred to as asymptomatic multiple myeloma)	Both criteria must be met: 1. Serum monoclonal protein (IgG or IgA) ≥3 g/dL (or urinary monoclonal protein ≥500 mg/24 hours) and/or clonal bone marrow plasma cells 10-60% 2. Absence of myeloma defining events or amyloidosis
Multiple myeloma	Both criteria must be met: 1. Clonal bone marrow plasma cells ≥10% or biopsy-proven bony or extramedullary plasmacytoma 2. Any one or more of the following myeloma defining events: • Evidence of end organ damage that can be attributed to the underlying plasma cell proliferative disorder, specifically: • Hypercalcemia: serum calcium >1 mg/dL (>0.25 mmol/L) higher than the upper limit of normal or >11 mg/dL (>2.75 mmol/L) • Renal insufficiency: creatinine clearance <40 mL per minute or serum creatinine >2 mg/dL (>177 µmol/L) • Anemia: hemoglobin value of >2 g/dL below the lower limit of normal, or a hemoglobin value <10 g/dL • Bone lesions: one or more osteolytic lesions on skeletal radiography, CT, or PET-CT • Any one or more of the following biomarkers of malignancy: • Clonal bone marrow plasma cell percentage ≥60% • Involved: uninvolved serum free light chain ratio ≥100 (involved free light chain level must be ≥100 mg/L) • >1 focal lesions on MRI studies (at least 1mm in size)
Waldenström macroglobulinemia	Both criteria must be met: 1. IgM monoclonal gammopathy (regardless of the size of the M protein) 2. >10% bone marrow lymphoplasmacytic infiltration (usually intertrabecular) by small lymphocytes that exhibit plasmacytoid or plasma cell differentiation and a typical immunophenotype (surface IgM$^+$, CD5$^{+/-}$, CD10$^-$, CD19$^+$, CD20$^+$, CD23$^-$) that satisfactorily excludes other lymphoproliferative disorders, including chronic lymphocytic leukemia and mantle cell lymphoma
Smoldering Waldenström macroglobulinemia (also referred to as indolent or asymptomatic Waldenström macroglobulinemia)	Both criteria must be met: 1. Serum IgM monoclonal protein ≥3 g/dL and/or bone marrow lymphoplasmacytic infiltration ≥10% 2. No evidence of end-organ damage, such as anemia, constitutional symptoms, hyperviscosity, lymphadenopathy, or hepatosplenomegaly, that can be attributed to a lymphoplasma cell proliferative disorder
Solitary plasmacytoma	All 4 criteria must be met: 1. Biopsy-proven solitary lesion of bone or soft tissue with evidence of clonal plasma cells 2. Normal bone marrow with no evidence of clonal plasma cells 3. Normal skeletal survey and either MRI of spine and pelvis or PET computed tomography (except for the primary solitary lesion) 4. Absence of end-organ damage, such as hypercalcemia, renal insufficiency, anemia, or bone lesions, that can be attributed to a plasma cell proliferative disorder
POEMS syndrome	All 4 criteria must be met: 1. Presence of a monoclonal plasma cell disorder (almost always λ type) 2. Peripheral neuropathy 3. Any one of the following 3 major features: sclerotic bone lesions, Castleman disease, elevated levels of vascular endothelial growth factor 4. Any one of the following 7 minor features: organomegaly, edema, endocrinopathy (excluding diabetes mellitus or hypothyroidism), typical skin changes, papilledema, thrombocytosis, polycythemia The features should have a temporal relationship to one another, with no other attributable cause

CT = computed tomography; FLC = free light chain; MRI = magnetic resonance imaging; PET = positron emission tomography.
Derived from Rajkumar SV, et al. International Myeloma Working Group updated Criteria for the diagnosis of multiple myeloma. *Lancet Oncology* 2014;15:e538-e548; and Kyle RA, Rajkumar SV. Criteria for diagnosis, staging, risk stratification and response assessment of multiple myeloma. *Leukemia*. 2009;23:3-9.

TABLE 187-3 RISK OF PROGRESSION OF MONOCLONAL GAMMOPATHY OF UNDETERMINED SIGNIFICANCE TO MYELOMA OR RELATED DISORDERS

RISK GROUP	RELATIVE RISK	CUMULATIVE ABSOLUTE RISK OF PROGRESSION AT 20 YEARS (%)*	CUMULATIVE ABSOLUTE RISK OF PROGRESSION AT 20 YEARS ACCOUNTING FOR DEATH AS A COMPETING RISK (%)†
Low risk: serum M protein <1.5 g/dL, IgG subtype, normal free light chain ratio (0.26-1.65)	1	5	2
Low-intermediate risk: any 1 factor abnormal	5.4	21	10
High-intermediate risk: any 2 factors abnormal	10.1	37	18
High risk: all 3 factors abnormal	20.8	58	27

*Estimates in this column represent the risk of progression assuming that patients do not die of other causes during this period.
†Estimates in this column represent the risk of progression calculated by use of a model that accounts for the fact that patients can die of unrelated causes during this time.
Ig = immunoglobulin.
Modified from Rajkumar SV, Kyle RA, Therneau TM, et al. Serum free light chain ratio is an independent risk factor for progression in monoclonal gammopathy of undetermined significance (MGUS). *Blood*. 2005;106:812-817. © The American Society of Hematology.
Also see reference 3.

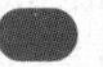

less than 10%. No therapy is indicated unless progression to malignancy occurs.

MULTIPLE MYELOMA

DEFINITION

Multiple myeloma is a malignant neoplasm of plasma cells characterized by bone marrow infiltration and extensive skeletal destruction resulting in anemia, bone pain, and fractures. Multiple myeloma (commonly referred to as myeloma) is defined by the presence of 10% or more clonal plasma cells on bone marrow examination or biopsy-proven plasmacytoma; and evidence of one or more myeloma defining events (see Table 187-2).[5] Patients with multiple myeloma must be differentiated from those with MGUS and smoldering multiple myeloma.

EPIDEMIOLOGY

Multiple myeloma accounts for 1% of all malignant disease and slightly more than 10% of hematologic malignant neoplasms in the United States. The annual incidence of multiple myeloma is 4 per 100,000. Its incidence in blacks is almost twice that in whites. Multiple myeloma is slightly more common in men than in women. The median age of patients at the time of diagnosis is about 65 years; only 2% of patients are younger than 40 years.

PATHOBIOLOGY

The cause of multiple myeloma is unclear. Exposure to radiation, benzene, and other organic solvents, herbicides, and insecticides may play a role. Multiple myeloma has been reported in familial clusters of two or more first-degree relatives and in identical twins.

Almost all cases of myeloma evolve from a premalignant MGUS phase, although the MGUS is clinically recognized before the diagnosis of myeloma in only a small minority of patients. The progression of MGUS to myeloma suggests a simple, random, two-hit genetic model of malignant transformation in which the risk of progression is fixed (approximately 1% per year) regardless of the duration of MGUS. Unfortunately, the precise mechanisms of progression are unknown, although several potentially pathogenetic abnormalities have been described in the clonal plasma cells. These include *RAS* and *p53* mutations, p16 methylation, *MYC* abnormalities, and secondary translocations. Changes in the bone marrow microenvironment may also play a role in the pathogenesis, including induction of angiogenesis and abnormal paracrine loops involving cytokines such as interleukin (IL)–6, which serves as a major growth factor for plasma cells.

The lytic bone lesions, osteopenia, hypercalcemia, and pathologic fractures in patients with myeloma are a result of abnormal osteoclast activity induced by the neoplastic plasma cells as well as inhibition of osteoblast differentiation. Osteoclasts are activated by stimulation of the transmembrane receptor RANK (receptor activator of nuclear factor κB), which belongs to the tumor necrosis factor receptor superfamily. The ligand for this receptor (RANKL) also has a decoy receptor, osteoprotegerin (OPG). In myeloma, there is an increase in RANKL expression by osteoblasts (and possibly plasma cells), accompanied by a reduction in the level of OPG. The resultant increase in the RANKL/OPG ratio causes osteoclast activation and increased bone resorption and turnover (Chapter 242). Other factors that may play a role in osteoclast activation include increased levels of macrophage inflammatory protein 1α, stromal cell–derived factor α, IL-3, IL-1β, and IL-6. In addition to these changes that promote osteoclast activation, there is simultaneous suppression of osteoblasts mediated by increased levels of IL-3, IL-7, and dickkopf 1 (DKK1). This combination leads to the pure osteolytic bone disease that is the hallmark of multiple myeloma.

Cytogenetic Abnormalities

As discussed earlier (see pathobiology of MGUS), primary translocations involving the IgH loci (chromosome 14q32) are seen in up to 40% of patients with multiple myeloma (IgH-translocated or nonhyperdiploid myeloma). Approximately 40% of patients do not have IgH translocations but have evidence of trisomies (hyperdiploid myeloma), 15% have both IgH translocations and trisomies, and 5% have other abnormalities. Although primary IgH translocations and trisomies originate at the MGUS stage, response to therapy and prognosis of myeloma are affected by the specific underlying abnormality (Table 187-4). Besides these cytogenetic abnormalities, other secondary cytogenetic abnormalities occur as late events during the course of symptomatic myeloma; these include activating mutations of N- and K-*RAS*, inactivating mutations of *p53*, and dysregulation of c-*MYC*. Complete or partial deletions of chromosome 13 are well described in myeloma and have prognostic value, but they also occur at the MGUS stage.

TABLE 187-4 STAGING AND PROGNOSTIC FACTORS IN MULTIPLE MYELOMA

STAGE/RISK FACTOR	MEDIAN SURVIVAL
INTERNATIONAL STAGING SYSTEM	
Stage I (serum β_2-microglobulin <3.5 mg/L and serum albumin ≥3.5 g/dL)	62 months
Stage II (neither stage I nor stage III)	44 months
Stage III (serum β_2-microglobulin ≥5.5 mg/L)	29 months
RISK STRATIFICATION*	
High-risk myeloma (any one of the following in the absence of trisomies): Translocations t(14;16), t(14;20) Deletion 17p	24-36 months
Intermediate-risk myeloma Translocation t4;14	Similar to standard-risk myeloma with bortezomib-based induction, transplantation, and maintenance
Standard-risk myeloma Translocations t(11;14), t(6;14) Trisomies	84-120 months
OTHER ADVERSE PROGNOSTIC FACTORS	
Elevated lactate dehydrogenase level	
Poor performance status	
Increased circulating plasma cells	
Plasmablastic morphology	
Increased plasma cell labeling index ≥1%	

*Typically detected in clonal plasma cells by fluorescence in situ hybridization of plasma cells.

TABLE 187-5 MAJOR CLINICAL MANIFESTATIONS OF MULTIPLE MYELOMA

CLINICAL FINDINGS	APPROXIMATE PERCENTAGE OF PATIENTS WITH ABNORMALITY AT DIAGNOSIS
Skeletal involvement: pain, reduced height, lytic bone lesions, pathologic fractures	80
Anemia (hemoglobin ≤12 g/dL): caused mainly by decreased erythropoiesis; produces weakness and fatigue	75
Renal insufficiency (serum creatinine ≥2 mg/dL): caused mainly by "myeloma kidney" from light chains or hypercalcemia, rarely from amyloidosis	20
Hypercalcemia (≥11 mg/dL)	15
Light chain amyloidosis	10
Evidence of monoclonal protein by immunofixation and serum free light chain assay	97
Evidence of clonal plasma cells ≥10% in bone marrow	96

CLINICAL MANIFESTATIONS

History

Bone pain, particularly in the back or chest and less often in the extremities, is present at the time of diagnosis in more than two thirds of patients (Table 187-5). The patient's height may be reduced by several inches because of vertebral collapse. Weakness and fatigue are common and are often associated with anemia. Fever is rare and, when present, is generally from an infection; in some patients, the infection itself is the initial feature. Other symptoms may result from renal insufficiency, hypercalcemia, nephrotic syndrome, radiculopathy, or amyloidosis (Chapter 188).

Physical Examination

Pallor is the most frequent physical finding. The liver is palpable in about 5% of patients and the spleen in 1%. Tenderness may be noted at sites of bone involvement. Radiculopathy may be caused by spinal compression fractures. On occasion, extramedullary plasmacytomas are palpable.

DIAGNOSIS

Laboratory Findings

A normocytic, normochromic anemia (Chapter 158) is present initially in approximately 75% of patients, but it eventually occurs in nearly every patient with multiple myeloma. Serum protein electrophoresis shows an M protein in 80% of patients. With serum immunofixation, an M protein can be detected in 93% of patients. When these serum studies are combined with urine electrophoresis plus immunofixation, an M protein can be detected in 97% of patients with myeloma. The serum free light chain assay is more convenient and can be used in place of urine studies in the diagnostic evaluation. The type of M protein is IgG in 52%, IgA in 21%, light chain only (Bence Jones proteinemia) in 16%, IgD in 2%, and biclonal gammopathy in 2%; the light chain type is κ in 65% of cases and λ in 35%. In 3% of patients, no secreted M protein can be identified; these patients are considered to have nonsecretory myeloma.

In the bone marrow, clonal plasma cells account for more than 10% of all nucleated cells in 96% of patients (Fig. 187-4). In 4% of patients, bone marrow examination shows less than 10% plasma cells, even though the patient otherwise meets the criteria for myeloma; because bone marrow involvement in myeloma may be focal rather than diffuse, repeated bone marrow examinations or biopsy of a discrete bone or extramedullary lesion may be required. In most cases, the plasma cells in myeloma are cytoplasmic Ig^+, $CD38^+$, $CD45^-$, $CD138^+$, $CD56^+$, and $CD19^+$; only a minority express CD10 and HLA-DR, and 20% express CD20. The clonality of the plasma cells is established by the κ/λ ratio, which is abnormal in myeloma (either >4 : 1, indicating a clonal κ population, or <1 : 2, indicating a clonal λ population). This is helpful for differentiation of monoclonal plasma cell proliferation in multiple myeloma from reactive plasmacytosis related to connective tissue disease, metastatic carcinoma, liver disease, and infection.

Radiologic Findings

Conventional radiographs reveal abnormalities consisting of punched-out lytic lesions (Fig. 187-5), osteoporosis, or fractures in nearly 80% of patients. The vertebrae, skull, thoracic cage, pelvis, and proximal ends of the humerus and femur are the most frequent sites of involvement. Technetium Tc99m bone scanning is inferior to conventional radiography and should not be used. Positron emission tomography (Fig. 187-6) and magnetic resonance imaging are increasingly used to evaluate patients in whom there is doubt about the magnitude of the disease burden, in those who have skeletal pain but no abnormality on radiographs, and for monitoring of the response to therapy.

Organ Involvement

Renal

At diagnosis, the serum creatinine value is increased initially in almost half of patients and is more than 2 mg/dL in 20%.

The two major causes of renal insufficiency are light chain cast nephropathy (*myeloma kidney*) and hypercalcemia. Light chain cast nephropathy is characterized by the presence of large, waxy, laminated casts in the distal and collecting tubules. The casts are composed mainly of precipitated monoclonal light chains. The extent of cast formation correlates directly with the amount of free urinary light chain and with the severity of renal insufficiency. Dehydration may precipitate acute renal failure.

Hypercalcemia (Chapter 245), which is present in 15 to 20% of patients initially, is a major and treatable cause of renal insufficiency. It results from destruction of bone. Hyperuricemia may contribute to renal failure. Besides light chain cast nephropathy and hypercalcemia, there are other mechanisms by which renal dysfunction can occur in myeloma. For example, light chain amyloidosis (Chapter 188) occurs in nearly 10% of patients and may produce nephrotic syndrome, renal insufficiency, or both. Acquired Fanconi syndrome (Chapter 122), characterized by proximal tubular dysfunction, results in glycosuria, phosphaturia, and aminoaciduria. Deposition of monoclonal light chains in the renal glomerulus (light chain deposition disease) may also produce renal insufficiency and nephrotic syndrome.

Neurologic

Radiculopathy (Chapter 400), the single most frequent neurologic complication, usually occurs in the thoracic or lumbosacral area and results from compression of the nerve by the vertebral lesion or by the collapsed bone itself. Compression of the spinal cord occurs in up to 10% of patients. Peripheral neuropathy (Chapter 420) is uncommon in multiple myeloma and, when present, is generally caused by amyloidosis. Rarely, myeloma cells diffusely infiltrate the meninges. Intracranial plasmacytomas almost always represent extensions of myelomatous lesions of the skull.

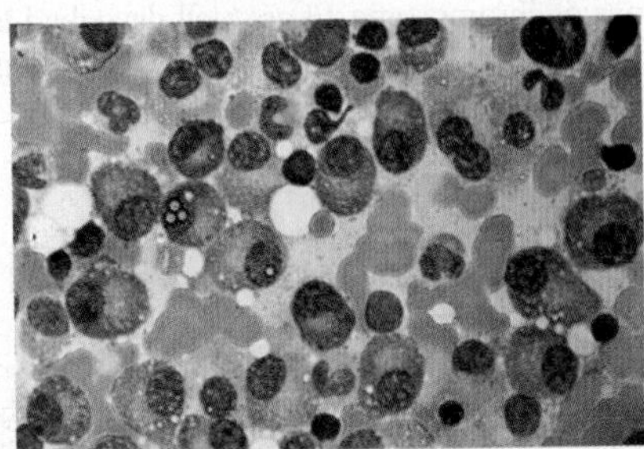

FIGURE 187-4. **Multiple myeloma. A bone marrow aspirate shows a predominance of plasma cells.**

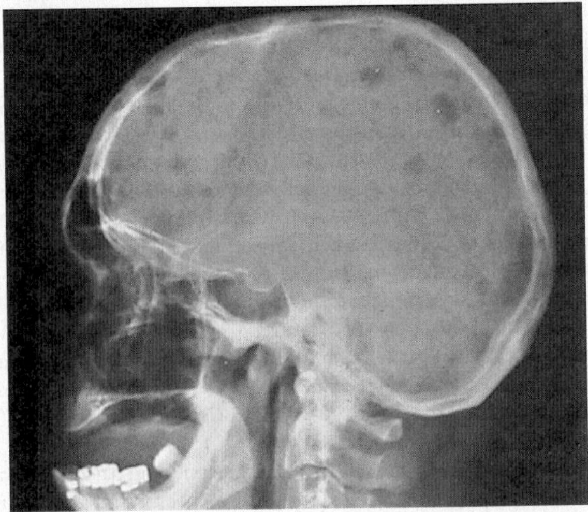

FIGURE 187-5. **Skull radiograph of a patient with multiple myeloma showing multiple lytic lesions.**

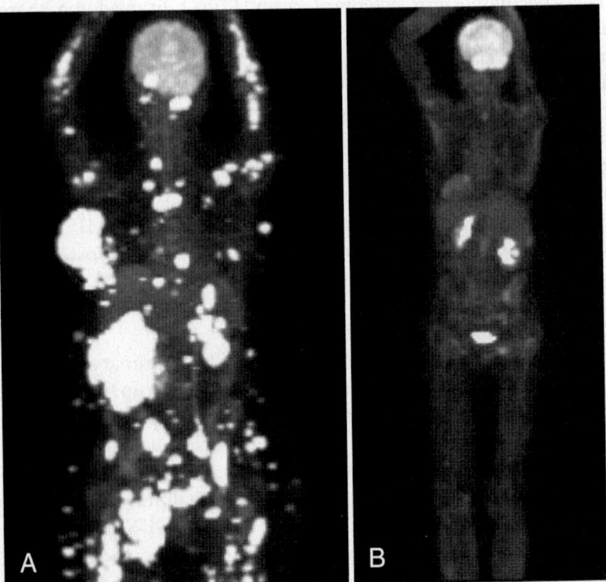

FIGURE 187-6. **Positron emission tomography in multiple myeloma. A, Extensive bone and extramedullary disease. B, Significant improvement after systemic chemotherapy for myeloma.**

Other Systemic Involvement

Hepatomegaly from plasma cell infiltration is uncommon. Plasmacytomas of the ribs are common and arise either as expanding bone lesions or as soft tissue masses. The incidence of infections is increased in patients with multiple myeloma. Historically, *Streptococcus pneumoniae* and *Staphylococcus aureus* have been the most frequent pathogens, but gram-negative organisms now account for more than half of all infections. The propensity for infection results from impairment of the antibody response, deficiency of normal immunoglobulins, and neutropenia. Bleeding from coating of the platelets by M protein may occur. Myeloma patients have an increased risk of deep venous thrombosis, particularly in relation to its therapy (see later).

PREVENTION AND TREATMENT Rx

Patients with MGUS or smoldering multiple myeloma should not be treated until evidence of multiple myeloma develops. The approach to treatment of multiple myeloma is illustrated in Figure 187-7.

Initial Therapy for Patients Who Are Candidates for Autologous Stem Cell Transplantation

In the approximately 50% of patients with newly diagnosed multiple myeloma who are considered candidates for autologous stem cell transplantation on the basis of good performance status, no or limited comorbid conditions, and younger physiologic age (<65 to 70 years), autologous peripheral blood stem cell transplantation (Chapter 178) with high-dose chemotherapy improves overall survival in comparison to conventional chemotherapy.[A1] Currently, it is not possible to eradicate myeloma cells completely with conditioning regimens, and reinfused autologous stem cells are usually contaminated by myeloma cells or their precursors. As a result, autologous transplantation is not curative, but it prolongs event-free and overall survival.

Initial therapy for stem cell transplant candidates typically consists of a non–melphalan-containing induction regimen for approximately 4 months followed by the stem cell collection. Most modern induction regimens have not been compared against each other in randomized trials, and the choice of regimen is dependent on availability and costs.[6] Common induction regimens include lenalidomide plus low-dose dexamethasone (Rd); bortezomib, thalidomide, plus dexamethasone (VTD); bortezomib, lenalidomide, plus dexamethasone (VRD); and bortezomib, cyclophosphamide, plus dexamethasone (VCD) (Table 187-6). VTD is associated with superior response rates and progression-free survival compared with thalidomide-dexamethasone (TD).[A2] In a randomized trial, lenalidomide plus low-dose dexamethasone (40 mg once a week) was associated with superior overall survival compared with lenalidomide and high-dose dexamethasone (40 mg on days 1 to 4, 9 to 12, and 17 to 20). As a result, high-dose pulse dexamethasone is no longer recommended in the context of initial therapy.[A3] Toxicities of lenalidomide include deep venous thrombosis, and all patients must be treated with prophylactic aspirin or an anticoagulant.

After induction therapy, peripheral blood stem cells adequate for one or two stem cell transplants are collected with the use of granulocyte colony-stimulating factor, with or without plerixafor or cyclophosphamide to aid in mobilization. Autologous stem cell transplantation (Chapter 178) is performed with melphalan 200 mg/m^2 as the conditioning regimen, followed by infusion of the peripheral blood stem cells. Patients who do not achieve a complete or very good partial response with the first autologous transplant can be considered for a second autologous transplant.[A4]

An alternative approach in patients with newly diagnosed disease is to cryopreserve stem cells for future use after initial therapy. Patients then continue initial therapy, such as lenalidomide plus low-dose dexamethasone, until progression or achievement of a plateau phase, with stem cell transplantation reserved for the first relapse. Data from randomized trials comparing early versus delayed transplantation indicate no significant difference in survival between the two strategies. The choice is based on the patient's preferences and other clinical conditions, but early transplantation is often preferred

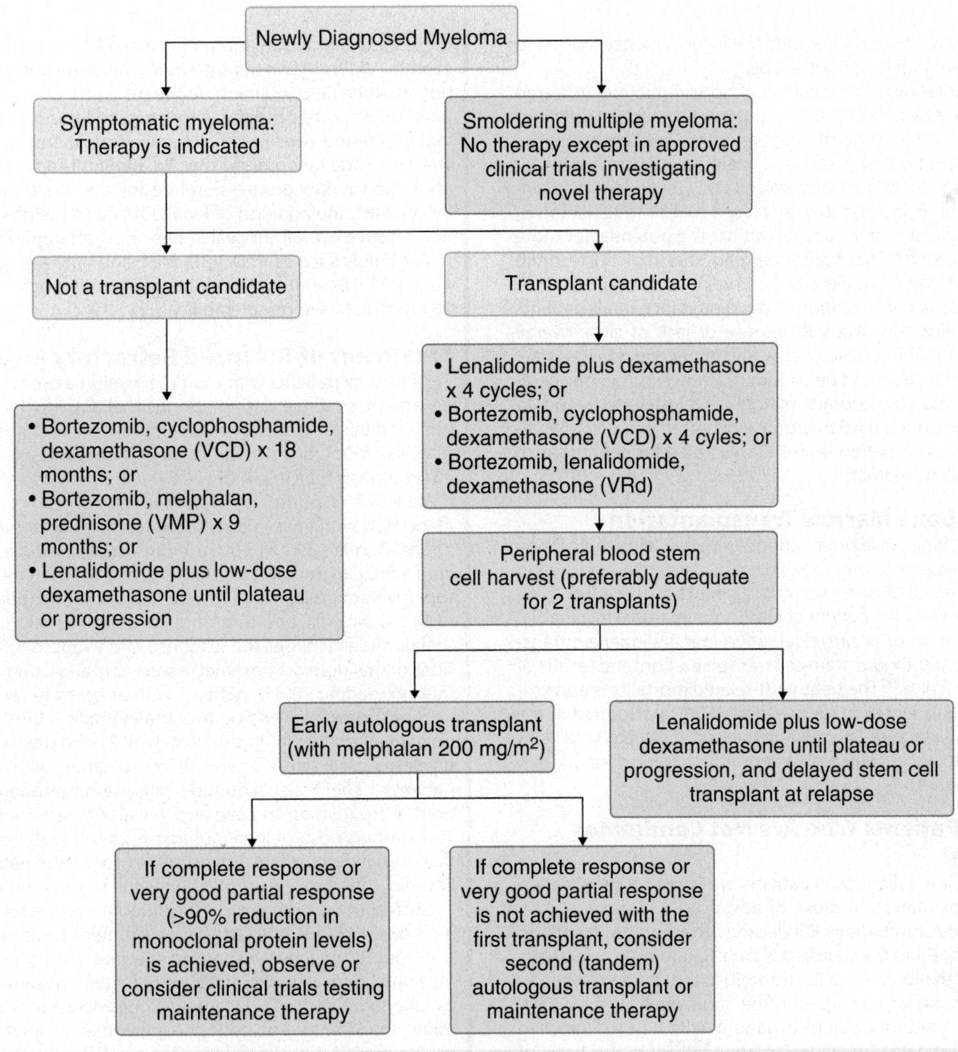

FIGURE 187-7. Therapeutic approach to newly diagnosed multiple myeloma.

TABLE 187-6 TREATMENT REGIMENS IN NEWLY DIAGNOSED MULTIPLE MYELOMA

REGIMEN	SUGGESTED STARTING DOSES*	OVERALL RESPONSE RATE (%)
REGIMENS FOR TRANSPLANT-ELIGIBLE AND TRANSPLANT-INELIGIBLE PATIENTS		
Lenalidomide-dexamethasone (Rd)	Lenalidomide, 25 mg orally, on days 1-21 every 28 days Dexamethasone, 40 mg orally, on days 1, 8, 15, 22 every 28 days Repeated every 4 weeks	70
Bortezomib-thalidomide-dexamethasone* (VTD)	Bortezomib, 1.3 mg/m^2 IV, on days 1, 8, 15, 22 Thalidomide, 100-200 mg orally, on days 1-21 Dexamethasone, 20 mg on day of/after bortezomib (or 40 mg on days 1, 8, 15, 22) Repeated every 4 weeks	95
Bortezomib-cyclophosphamide-dexamethasone* (VCD)	Cyclophosphamide, 300 mg/m^2 orally, on days 1, 8, 15 and 22 Bortezomib, 1.3 mg/m^2 IV, on days 1, 8, 15, 22 Dexamethasone, 40 mg orally, on days 1, 8, 15, 22 Repeated every 4 weeks	90
Bortezomib-lenalidomide-dexamethasone* (VRD)	Bortezomib, 1.3 mg/m^2 IV, on days 1, 8, 15 Lenalidomide, 25 mg orally, on days 1-14 Dexamethasone, 20 mg on day of and day after bortezomib (or 40 mg on days 1, 8, 15, 22) Repeated every 3 weeks	100
REGIMENS FOR TRANSPLANT-INELIGIBLE PATIENTS		
Melphalan-prednisone-thalidomide (MPT)	Melphalan, 0.25 mg/kg orally, on days 1-4 (use 0.20 mg/kg/day orally on days 1-4 in patients older than 75 years) Prednisone, 2 mg/kg orally, on days 1-4 Thalidomide, 100-200 mg orally, on days 1-28 (use 100-mg dose in patients >75 years) Repeated every 6 weeks	70
Bortezomib-melphalan-prednisone* (VMP)	Bortezomib, 1.3 mg/m^2 IV, on days 1, 8, 15, 22 Melphalan, 9 mg/m^2 orally, on days 1-4 Prednisone, 60 mg/m^2 orally, on days 1-4 Repeated every 35 days	70

*Doses of dexamethasone and bortezomib reduced from initial trial reports to once-weekly schedules.
Reproduced from Rajkumar SV. Treatment of multiple myeloma. *Nat Rev Clin Oncol.* 2011;8:479-491.

because its mortality is low (<1%), and it avoids the inconvenience, cost, and potential side effects of prolonged chemotherapy.

After stem cell transplantation, a short course of bortezomib administered as consolidation has been shown to improve response rates and progression-free survival.[A5] Similarly, studies suggest that long-term outcome may be improved by the administration of prolonged maintenance therapy after autologous stem cell transplantation. In randomized trials, lenalidomide maintenance (10 mg/day for the first 3 months, increased to 15 mg if tolerated) significantly prolongs progression-free survival but has the potential for more toxicity and second cancers.[A6,A7] There are emerging data that bortezomib maintenance administered every 2 weeks may also provide a similar benefit.[A8] At present, the routine use of consolidation and maintenance in all patients after transplantation remains controversial because of lack of clear overall survival benefit and concerns about toxicity, cost, and impact on quality of life. Consolidation and maintenance should be considered, however, in intermediate- and high-risk myeloma (bortezomib maintenance preferred) and in patients not achieving a very good partial response or better with transplantation (lenalidomide maintenance preferred) (see Table 187-4 for definitions of intermediate- and high-risk myeloma).

Role of Allogeneic Bone Marrow Transplantation

Most patients with multiple myeloma cannot undergo allogeneic bone marrow transplantation because of their age, lack of an HLA-matched sibling donor, or inadequate renal, pulmonary, or cardiac function (Chapter 178). There are no clear data showing the benefit of either conventional myeloablative allogeneic transplantation or nonmyeloablative (mini) allogeneic transplantation compared with autologous stem cell transplantation, and results of randomized trials are conflicting.[A9] The treatment-related mortality is approximately 20%. Allogeneic transplantation for myeloma is best performed in the context of clinical trials or as second-line salvage therapy in selected high-risk patients who are willing to accept the high treatment-related mortality rate associated with the procedure.

Initial Therapy for Patients Who Are Not Candidates for Transplantation

Approximately 50% of newly diagnosed patients are not considered candidates for stem cell transplantation because of advanced age, poor performance status, or associated comorbidities. For decades, the oral administration of melphalan and prednisone was the standard of care. Randomized trials have shown that the addition of thalidomide or bortezomib to the standard regimen of melphalan plus prednisone improves event-free and overall survival compared with melphalan plus prednisone alone in patients with newly diagnosed myeloma who are not candidates for transplantation.[A10,A11] On the basis of these data, melphalan and prednisone plus either thalidomide (MPT) or bortezomib (VMP) are two treatments for this population of patients. More recently, non–melphalan-containing regimens such as Rd, VRD, and VCD used in patients who are candidates for stem cell transplantation are being increasingly preferred over melphalan-based regimens in this group of patients as well. In a large randomized trial, Rd administered until progression was associated with superior progression-free and overall survival compared with MPT.[A12] By contrast, the addition of lenalidomide to melphalan and prednisone does not improve overall survival and is not recommended.[A13]

Regimens such as VCD, VRD, MPT, and VMP are typically given for approximately 12-18 months. Rd can be given until progression or for approximately 18 months, based on tolerability.

Treatment of Relapsed Refractory Myeloma

Almost all patients with multiple myeloma eventually relapse. Single-agent dexamethasone, alkylating agents, thalidomide, lenalidomide, and bortezomib, administered alone or in combination, are options for the treatment of relapsed refractory myeloma. Methylprednisolone, 2 g three times a week intravenously for a minimum of 4 weeks, then reduced to once or twice a week if there is a response, is helpful for patients with pancytopenia and may be associated with fewer side effects than with dexamethasone.

Thalidomide (50 to 200 mg/day orally) produces an objective response, with a median duration of about 1 year, in about a third of patients with refractory myeloma. Side effects are sedation, constipation, peripheral neuropathy, rash, bradycardia, and thrombotic events. The addition of dexamethasone to thalidomide increases the response rate to approximately 50%, and combinations of thalidomide, dexamethasone, and alkylating agents produce response rates exceeding 70% in patients with relapsed refractory disease.

Lenalidomide, an analogue of thalidomide, is better tolerated and produces objective benefits in approximately 40% of patients with relapsed refractory myeloma as a single agent; in combination with dexamethasone, 60% of patients benefit. Lenalidomide plus dexamethasone significantly prolongs time to progression and overall survival compared with dexamethasone alone. The starting dose of lenalidomide is 25 mg orally on days 1 to 21, every 28 days. Lenalidomide has significantly fewer nonhematologic toxicities than thalidomide does; myelosuppression is the most common adverse event.

Bortezomib, an inhibitor of the ubiquitin-proteasome pathway, acts through multiple mechanisms to arrest tumor growth, tumor spread, and angiogenesis. It produces objective responses in about a third of patients with refractory myeloma and is superior to single-agent dexamethasone. Bortezomib is usually combined with dexamethasone and other active agents (e.g., lenalidomide, thalidomide, or cyclophosphamide) to increase response rates. The usual dose is 1.3 mg/m^2 administered subcutaneously on days 1, 8, 15, and 22 every 28 days. The once-weekly subcutaneous dosing is associated with significantly lower neuropathy than the twice-weekly intravenous schedule. The most common adverse events are gastrointestinal side effects, fatigue, and neuropathy.

Options for the treatment of patients with myeloma refractory to lenalidomide and bortezomib include pomalidomide (an analogue of lenalidomide) and carfilzomib (a novel keto-epoxide tetrapeptide proteasome inhibitor).[7,8] Pomalidomide and carfilzomib have a response rate of approximately 25% in this population of patients and can be combined with other active agents to improve response rates. In a randomized trial, the addition of carfilzomib to lenalidomide and dexamethasone significantly improved progression-free survival.[A14]

Patients with relapsed refractory myeloma should also be considered for clinical trials. Promising investigational agents with single-agent activity include MLN 9708 (an oral proteasome inhibitor), marizomib (proteasome inhibitor), ARRY-520 (kinesin spindle protein inhibitor), monoclonal antibodies to CD38, and cyclin-dependent kinase inhibitors. Additional agents with potential activity in combination with standard anti-myeloma agents include panobinostat (histone deacetylase inhibitor) and elotuzumab (an anti–CS-1 antibody).

Role of Radiation Therapy

Palliative radiation in a dose of 20 to 30 Gy should be limited to patients who have multiple myeloma with disabling pain and a well-defined focal process that has not responded to chemotherapy and to patients with spinal cord compression from a plasmacytoma. Analgesics in combination with chemotherapy can usually control the pain (Chapter 30).

Management of Complications

Hypercalcemia

Hypercalcemia, present in 15 to 20% of patients at diagnosis, should be suspected in those with anorexia, nausea, vomiting, polyuria, polydipsia, constipation, weakness, confusion, or stupor. If hypercalcemia is untreated, renal insufficiency may develop. Hydration, preferably with isotonic saline plus prednisone (25 mg four times/day), usually relieves the hypercalcemia. Bisphosphonates, such as zoledronic acid or pamidronate, are recommended and will correct hypercalcemia in almost all patients (Chapter 243).

Renal Insufficiency

The most common cause of acute renal failure is light chain cast nephropathy in patients who have excess excretion of monoclonal protein in urine (myeloma kidney). Aggressive treatment of acute renal failure due to light chain cast nephropathy is critical for long-term overall survival. If the patient is not oliguric, intravenous fluids and furosemide are needed to maintain a high urine flow rate (100 mL/hour). If the underlying cause is thought to be light chain cast nephropathy on the basis of clinical findings (e.g., serum free light chains >150 mg/dL) or renal biopsy, plasmapheresis is recommended daily for 5 days to reduce the levels of circulating light chains. Hemodialysis is necessary for symptomatic azotemia. The mainstay of therapy is aggressive treatment of myeloma with a regimen such as bortezomib, thalidomide, and dexamethasone (VTD) or bortezomib, cyclophosphamide, and dexamethasone (VCD). Allopurinol is necessary if hyperuricemia is present.

Infection

Prompt, appropriate therapy for bacterial infections is necessary. Prophylactic antibiotics, such as trimethoprim-sulfamethoxazole, should be considered in patients taking high-dose corticosteroids. Acyclovir should be given as prophylaxis against herpes zoster in patients receiving bortezomib. Intravenously administered gamma globulin is reserved for patients with hypogammaglobulinemia and recurrent severe infections. Pneumococcal and influenza immunizations (Chapter 18) should be given to all patients.

Skeletal Lesions

Patients should be encouraged to be as active as possible but to avoid trauma. Pamidronate (90 mg infused intravenously during a 4-hour period every 4 weeks) or zoledronic acid (4 mg intravenously during at least 15 minutes every 4 weeks) reduces the incidence of bone pain, pathologic fractures, and spinal cord compression; such prophylaxis is now routinely recommended for all patients with myeloma bone disease and may improve overall survival.[A15] After 1 to 2 years, the dosing can be reduced to once every 3 months in patients who are stable to minimize the risk of osteonecrosis of the jaw, which is a complication of long-term bisphosphonate therapy.

Spinal cord compression from an extramedullary plasmacytoma (Chapter 400) should be suspected in patients who have severe back pain, weakness or paresthesias of the lower extremities, or bladder or bowel dysfunction. Initial treatment is with dexamethasone-based therapy or radiation therapy. If the neurologic deficit increases, surgical decompression is necessary.

Miscellaneous Complications

Symptomatic hyperviscosity (see later) is less common than in Waldenström macroglobulinemia. Anemia that persists despite adequate treatment of underlying myeloma often responds to erythropoietin.

PROGNOSIS

Multiple myeloma is considered incurable at present, but survival has improved significantly in recent years. The median survival is approximately 5 years, but it varies widely according to clinical stage and risk stratification factors (see Table 187-4).[9] In some patients, an acute or aggressive terminal phase is characterized by rapid tumor growth, pancytopenia, soft tissue subcutaneous masses, decreased M protein levels, and fever; survival in this subset is generally only a few months.

FUTURE DIRECTIONS

Future efforts must be directed toward identifying new active agents and developing effective combinations of active drugs. Studies are under way to improve the conditioning regimen used in autologous stem cell transplantation and to better integrate novel therapies with stem cell transplantation.

VARIANT FORMS OF MULTIPLE MYELOMA

Smoldering Multiple Myeloma

Smoldering (asymptomatic) multiple myeloma is defined by the presence of an M protein level higher than 3 g/dL in serum or 10 to 60% clonal plasma cells in bone marrow in the absence of myeloma defining events and amyloidosis.[10] Patients with smoldering multiple myeloma are biologically similar to those with MGUS but carry a much higher risk for progression to myeloma or related malignant disease: 10% per year for the first 5 years, 5% per year for the next 5 years, and 1 to 2% per year thereafter. As a result, patients must be observed more closely (every 3 to 4 months), but they should not be treated unless progression to symptomatic multiple myeloma occurs. A small randomized trial found improved survival with the use of Rd as preventive therapy in patients with high-risk smoldering multiple myeloma,[A16] but additional data are needed before this approach can be recommended as routine practice. However, patients with ultrahigh-risk features (such as serum free light chain ratio ≥100 or presence of one or more focal lesions on magnetic resonance imaging) are candidates for therapy similar to that for symptomatic myeloma because they are at imminent risk of progression.

Plasma Cell Leukemia

Patients with plasma cell leukemia have more than 20% plasma cells in the peripheral blood and an absolute plasma cell count of 2000/μL or higher.[11] Plasma cell leukemia is classified as primary when it is diagnosed in the leukemic phase (60%) or as secondary when there is leukemic transformation of a previously recognized multiple myeloma (40%). Patients with primary plasma cell leukemia are younger and have a greater incidence of hepatosplenomegaly and lymphadenopathy, higher platelet count, fewer bone lesions, smaller serum M protein component, and longer survival (median, 6.8 vs. 1.3 months) than do patients with secondary plasma cell leukemia. Treatment of plasma cell leukemia is unsatisfactory. An aggressive initial treatment regimen such as bortezomib, dexamethasone, thalidomide, cisplatin, doxorubicin, cyclophosphamide, and etoposide (VDT-PACE) for two cycles, followed by autologous stem cell transplantation and subsequent maintenance therapy with a bortezomib-based regimen, is a reasonable strategy if the patient's clinical condition permits such an approach. Secondary plasma cell leukemia rarely responds in a durable manner to chemotherapy because the patients have already received chemotherapy and are resistant.

Nonsecretory Myeloma

Patients with nonsecretory myeloma have no M protein in either serum or urine and account for only 3% of cases of myeloma. For the diagnosis to be made, the clonal nature of bone marrow plasma cells should be established by immunoperoxidase, immunofluorescence, or flow cytometric methods. Treatment and survival are similar to those of patients with typical myeloma. The serum free light chain assay is abnormal in more than 60% of patients and can be used to monitor the response to therapy.

Osteosclerotic Myeloma (POEMS Syndrome)

This syndrome is characterized by polyneuropathy, organomegaly, endocrinopathy, M protein, and skin changes (POEMS) (see Table 187-2). The major clinical features are a chronic inflammatory-demyelinating polyneuropathy with predominantly motor disability and sclerotic skeletal lesions. The bone marrow usually contains less than 5% plasma cells, and hypercalcemia and renal insufficiency rarely occur. Almost all patients have a λ-type

M protein. The diagnosis is confirmed by identification of monoclonal plasma cells obtained at biopsy of an osteosclerotic lesion.

If the lesions are in a limited area, radiation therapy substantially improves the neuropathy in more than 50% of patients. If the patient has widespread osteosclerotic lesions, treatment is with autologous stem cell transplantation or other systemic therapy similar to that used for myeloma.

Solitary Plasmacytoma (Solitary Myeloma) of Bone

The diagnosis of solitary bone plasmacytoma is based on histologic evidence of a solitary tumor consisting of monoclonal plasma cells identical to those in multiple myeloma. In addition, complete skeletal radiographs and magnetic resonance imaging of the spine and pelvis must show no other lesions of myeloma, and the bone marrow aspirate must contain no evidence of clonal plasma cells. An M protein may be present in serum or urine at diagnosis, but persistence of the M protein after radiation therapy is associated with an increased risk for progression to multiple myeloma. Treatment consists of radiation in the range of 40 to 50 Gy. Almost 50% of patients who have a solitary plasmacytoma are alive at 10 years, and disease-free survival rates at 10 years range from 15 to 25%. Progression to myeloma, when it occurs, usually takes place within 3 years, but patients must be monitored indefinitely. There is no convincing evidence that adjuvant chemotherapy decreases the rate of conversion to multiple myeloma.

Extramedullary Plasmacytoma

Extramedullary plasmacytomas outside the bone marrow are most commonly found in the upper respiratory tract (80% of cases), especially in the nasal cavity and sinuses, nasopharynx, and larynx. Extramedullary plasmacytomas may also occur in the gastrointestinal tract, central nervous system, urinary bladder, thyroid, breast, testes, parotid gland, or lymph nodes. Extramedullary plasmacytomas may be solitary, or they may occur in the context of existing myeloma. The diagnosis of solitary extramedullary plasmacytoma is based on detection of a plasma cell tumor in an extramedullary site, absence of clonal plasma cells on bone marrow examination, and absence of other bone or extramedullary lesions on radiographic studies. Treatment of solitary extramedullary plasmacytoma consists of either complete surgical resection or tumoricidal irradiation. The plasmacytoma may recur locally, metastasize to regional nodes, or, rarely, develop into multiple myeloma.

WALDENSTRÖM MACROGLOBULINEMIA (PRIMARY MACROGLOBULINEMIA)

DEFINITION

Waldenström macroglobulinemia is the result of the uncontrolled proliferation of lymphocytes and plasma cells in which an IgM M protein is produced.[12] The cause is unknown; familial clusters have been reported. The median age of patients at the time of diagnosis is about 65 years, and approximately 60% are male. The diagnostic criteria are IgM monoclonal gammopathy (regardless of the size of the M protein), 10% or greater bone marrow infiltration (usually intertrabecular) by clonal lymphocytes that exhibit plasmacytoid or plasma cell differentiation, and a typical immunophenotype (e.g., surface IgM^+, $CD5^{+/-}$, $CD10^-$, $CD19^+$, $CD20^+$, $CD23^-$) that would satisfactorily exclude other lymphoproliferative disorders, including chronic lymphocytic leukemia (Chapter 184) and mantle cell lymphoma (Chapter 185). A recurrent mutation of the *MYD88* gene (MYD88 L265P) has recently been shown to be present in most patients with Waldenström macroglobulinemia and is thought to be relatively specific for this disease.[13]

CLINICAL MANIFESTATIONS

Weakness, fatigue, and bleeding (especially oozing from the oronasal area) are common initial symptoms. Blurred or impaired vision, dyspnea, weight loss, neurologic symptoms, recurrent infections, and heart failure may occur. In contrast to multiple myeloma, lytic bone lesions, renal insufficiency, and amyloidosis are rare. Physical findings include pallor, hepatosplenomegaly, and lymphadenopathy. Retinal hemorrhages, exudates, and venous congestion with vascular segmentation ("sausage" formation) may occur. Sensorimotor peripheral neuropathy is common. Pulmonary involvement is manifested by diffuse pulmonary infiltrates and isolated masses.

Laboratory Evaluation

Almost all patients have moderate to severe normocytic, normochromic anemia. The serum electrophoretic pattern is characterized by a tall, narrow peak or dense band that is of the IgM type on immunofixation. Quantitative IgM levels are high. A monoclonal light chain is detected in the urine of 80% of patients, but the amount of urinary protein is generally modest.

The bone marrow aspirate is often hypocellular, but the biopsy specimen is hypercellular and extensively infiltrated with lymphoid cells and plasma cells. The number of mast cells is frequently increased. Rouleau formation is prominent (Chapter 157), and the sedimentation rate is markedly increased. About 10% of cases may have an associated type I cryoglobulinemia (see later).

DIAGNOSIS

Diagnosis requires the combination of typical symptoms and physical findings, the presence of an IgM M protein, and 10% or greater lymphoplasmacytic infiltration of the bone marrow. The lymphoplasmacytic cells express CD19, CD20, and CD22, whereas expression of CD5 and CD10 occurs in a minority. Asymptomatic patients with 10% or greater lymphoplasmacytic infiltration of the bone marrow are considered to have smoldering Waldenström macroglobulinemia. Multiple myeloma, chronic lymphocytic leukemia, and MGUS of the IgM type must be excluded.

Patients meeting the diagnostic criteria for Waldenström macroglobulinemia but who have less than 3 g/dL IgM protein at diagnosis have sometimes been classified as having lymphoplasmacytic lymphoma with an IgM M protein (Chapter 185). However, except for hyperviscosity, the clinical picture, therapy, and prognosis for these patients do not differ from those of patients with an IgM level of 3 g/dL or higher; thus, these patients are also considered to have Waldenström macroglobulinemia by the current definition.

PREVENTION AND TREATMENT Rx

Patients should not be treated unless they have anemia, constitutional symptoms (such as weakness, fatigue, night sweats, or weight loss), hyperviscosity, or significant hepatosplenomegaly or lymphadenopathy. Rituximab, a chimeric anti-CD20 monoclonal antibody (Chapter 36), produces a response in at least 50% of untreated patients. The most common regimen used as front-line therapy is the combination of rituximab with cyclophosphamide and dexamethasone (RCD).[14] This combination is highly active and also preserves the ability to mobilize stem cells for transplantation, if necessary. Alternatives include bendamustine plus rituximab (BR); rituximab, bortezomib plus dexamethasone; and cladribine with or without rituximab.[15]

In general, for minimally symptomatic patients, rituximab as a single agent is an excellent choice for initial therapy. For patients with more advanced symptoms, including severe anemia or hyperviscosity, combination approaches such as RCD or BR are preferred.

For relapse, the agents used as initial therapy can be given alone or in combination. Autologous stem cell transplantation can be considered for eligible patients with relapsed disease.

Spuriously low hemoglobin and hematocrit levels may occur because of the increased plasma volume from the large amount of intravascular M protein. Consequently, transfusions should not be given solely on the basis of the hemoglobin or hematocrit value. Symptomatic hyperviscosity should be treated by plasmapheresis. The median survival of patients with macroglobulinemia is 5 years.

HYPERVISCOSITY SYNDROME

Hyperviscosity syndrome occurs in patients with Waldenström macroglobulinemia who have high levels of serum IgM M protein (>5 g/dL) and occasionally in those with myeloma, especially of the IgA type. Hyperviscosity is disproportionately more common relative to the same serum concentration of IgM and IgA M proteins compared with IgG M proteins because of the inherent tendency of IgM and IgA molecules to polymerize. Typically, IgM forms pentamers, whereas IgA forms dimers or sometimes trimers, resulting in high-molecular-weight complexes. Chronic nasal bleeding and oozing from the gums are the most frequent symptoms of hyperviscosity, but postsurgical or gastrointestinal bleeding may also occur. Retinal hemorrhages are common, and venous congestion with sausage-like segmentation and papilledema may be seen (Fig. 187-8). The patient occasionally complains of blurring or loss of vision. Dizziness, headache, vertigo, nystagmus, decreased hearing, ataxia, paresthesias, diplopia, somnolence, and coma may occur. Hyperviscosity can precipitate or exacerbate heart failure. Most patients have symptoms when the relative viscosity is greater than 4 cP, but the relationship between serum viscosity and clinical manifestations is not precise. There have

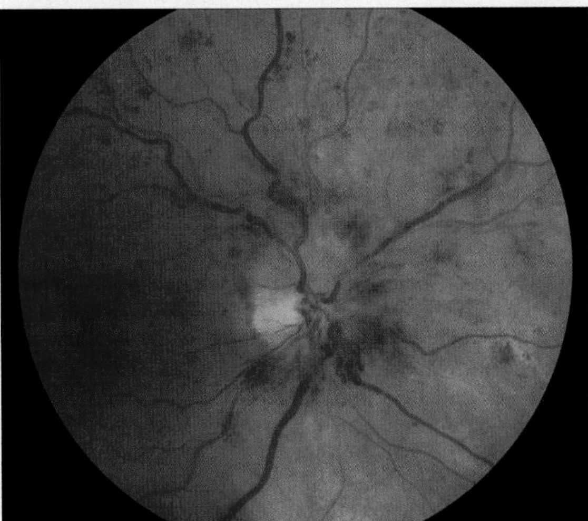

FIGURE 187-8. Hyperviscosity syndrome. Right eye retinal image in a patient with Waldenström macroglobulinemia and hyperviscosity syndrome showing sausaging (focal venular dilations), intraretinal hemorrhages, microaneurysms, and peripapillary cotton-wool spots and disc swelling (papilledema).

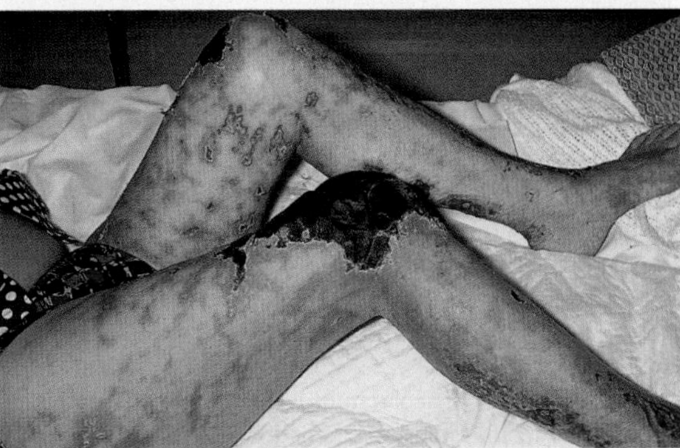

FIGURE 187-9. Skin infarction in cryoglobulinemia. The skin has a reticulated pattern as a result of leakage of red blood cells from damaged skin capillaries. Necrosis and ulceration have occurred in peripheral sites because of vessel blockage. This patient eventually required plastic surgery. (From Forbes CD, Jackson WF. *Color Atlas and Text of Clinical Medicine*. 3rd ed. London: Mosby; 2003.)

been no randomized trials on management of hyperviscosity syndrome. Patients with symptomatic hyperviscosity should be treated with plasmapheresis and with chemotherapy to treat the underlying malignant disease. Plasma exchange of 3 to 4 L with albumin should be performed daily until the patient is asymptomatic. Plasma exchange is rapidly effective (two or three exchanges) in the case of IgM M proteins, which are primarily distributed in the intravascular space; with IgG M proteins, in contrast, multiple attempts may be needed because a significant amount of IgG can exist in the extravascular space.

HEAVY CHAIN DISEASES

The HCDs are characterized by the presence of an M protein consisting of a portion of the immunoglobulin heavy chain in serum, urine, or both. These heavy chains are devoid of light chains and represent a lymphoplasma cell proliferative process. There are three major types: γ-HCD, α-HCD, and μ-HCD.

γ-HCD

Patients with γ-HCD often initially have a lymphoma-like illness, but the clinical findings are diverse and range from an aggressive lymphoproliferative process (Chapter 185) to an asymptomatic state. Hepatosplenomegaly and lymphadenopathy occur in about 60% of patients. Anemia is found in approximately 80% initially and in nearly all eventually. The electrophoretic pattern often shows a broad-based band more suggestive of a polyclonal increase than an M protein. The diagnosis depends on the identification of an isolated monoclonal γ heavy chain on serum immunofixation, without evidence of either monoclonal κ or λ light chain expression.

Treatment is indicated only for symptomatic patients and consists of chemotherapy with melphalan plus prednisone or regimens used to treat non-Hodgkin lymphoma (Chapter 185), such as cyclophosphamide, vincristine, and prednisone. The prognosis of γ-HCD is variable and ranges from a rapidly progressive downhill course of a few weeks' duration to the asymptomatic presence of a stable monoclonal heavy chain in serum or urine.

α-HCD

α-HCD is the most common form of HCD and occurs in patients from the Mediterranean region or the Middle East, generally in the second or third decade of life. About 60% are men. The gastrointestinal tract is most commonly involved, and severe malabsorption with diarrhea, steatorrhea, and weight loss is noted (Chapter 140). Plasma cell infiltration of the jejunal mucosa is the most frequent pathologic feature. Immunoproliferative small intestinal disease is restricted to patients with small intestinal lesions who have the pathologic features of α-HCD but do not synthesize α heavy chains.

The serum protein electrophoretic pattern is normal in half the cases; in the remainder, an unimpressive broad band may appear in the α_2 or β region. The diagnosis depends on identification of an isolated monoclonal α heavy chain on serum immunofixation, without evidence of either monoclonal κ or λ light chain expression. The amount of α heavy chain in urine is small.

In the absence of therapy, α-HCD is typically progressive and fatal. The usual treatment consists of antibiotics, such as tetracyclines, and the eradication of any concurrent parasitic infection. Patients who do not respond adequately to antibiotics are given chemotherapy similar to that used to treat non-Hodgkin lymphoma, for example, the cyclophosphamide, hydroxydaunomycin, vincristine (Oncovin), and prednisone (CHOP) regimen (Chapter 185).

μ-HCD

This disease is characterized by the demonstration of an isolated monoclonal μ chain fragment on serum immunofixation, without evidence of either monoclonal κ or λ light chain expression.

The serum protein electrophoretic pattern is usually normal, except for hypogammaglobulinemia. Bence Jones proteinuria has been found in two thirds of cases. Lymphocytes, plasma cells, and lymphoplasmacytoid cells are increased in the bone marrow. Vacuolization of the plasma cells is common and should suggest the possibility of HCD. The course of μ-HCD is variable, and survival ranges from a few months to many years. Treatment is with corticosteroids and alkylating agents.

CRYOGLOBULINEMIA

Cryoglobulins are plasma proteins that precipitate when cooled and dissolve when heated. They are designated idiopathic or essential when they are not associated with any recognizable disease. Cryoglobulins are classified into three types: type I (monoclonal), type II (mixed monoclonal plus polyclonal), and type III (polyclonal).

Type I Cryoglobulinemia

Type I (monoclonal) cryoglobulinemia is most commonly of the IgM or IgG class, but IgA and Bence Jones cryoglobulins have been reported. Most patients, even with large amounts of type I cryoglobulin, are completely asymptomatic from this source. Others with monoclonal cryoglobulins in the range of 1 to 2 g/dL may have evidence of vasculitis with pain, purpura, Raynaud phenomenon, cyanosis, and even ulceration and sloughing of skin and subcutaneous tissue (Fig. 187-9) on exposure to cold because their cryoglobulins precipitate at relatively high temperatures. Type I cryoglobulins are associated with macroglobulinemia, multiple myeloma, or MGUS. Therapy for patients with symptomatic type I cryoglobulinemia and significant symptoms is similar to that for Waldenström macroglobulinemia for the IgM type and multiple myeloma for the non-IgM type.

Type II Cryoglobulinemia

Type II (mixed) cryoglobulinemia typically consists of an immune complex of IgM M protein and polyclonal IgG, although monoclonal IgG or monoclonal IgA may also be seen with polyclonal IgM. Serum protein electrophoresis generally shows a normal pattern or a diffuse, polyclonal hypergammaglobulinemic pattern. The quantity of mixed cryoglobulin is usually less than 0.2 g/dL. Despite the monoclonal component, most patients do not have a clonal plasma cell disorder; rather, they have serologic evidence of infection with hepatitis C virus (Chapter 149). At present, hepatitis C is thought to be the cause of most cases of type II cryoglobulinemia.

Most clinical manifestations are related to the development of vasculitis and include palpable purpura, livedo reticularis, polyarthralgias, and neuropathy. Involvement of the joints is symmetrical, but joint deformities rarely develop. Raynaud phenomenon, necrosis of the skin, and neurologic involvement may be present. In almost 80% of renal biopsy specimens, glomerular damage can be identified. Nephrotic syndrome may result, but severe renal insufficiency is uncommon.

Early administration of corticosteroids is the most frequent therapy. Treatment should also target underlying hepatitis C infection with interferon alfa-2 or ribavirin (Chapter 149). Agents to treat the monoclonal component, such as cyclophosphamide, chlorambucil, azathioprine, or rituximab, are used if there is no response. Plasmapheresis (with a warmed circuit) is helpful in the acute management of symptoms by removal of circulating immune complexes.

Type III Cryoglobulinemia

Type III (polyclonal) cryoglobulinemia does not have a monoclonal component and is not associated with a clonal plasma cell proliferative disorder. Type III cryoglobulins are found in many patients with chronic infections or inflammatory diseases and are usually of no clinical significance unless they are associated with hepatitis C infection.

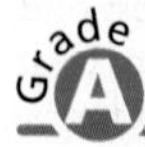

Grade A References

A1. Palumbo A, Cavallo F, Gay F, et al. Autologous transplantation and maintenance therapy in multiple myeloma. *N Engl J Med.* 2014;371:895-905.

A2. Cavo M, Tacchetti P, Patriarca F, et al. Bortezomib with thalidomide plus dexamethasone compared with thalidomide plus dexamethasone as induction therapy before, and consolidation therapy after, double autologous stem-cell transplantation in newly diagnosed multiple myeloma: a randomised phase 3 study. *Lancet.* 2010;376:2075-2085.

A3. Rajkumar SV, Jacobus S, Callander NS, et al. Lenalidomide plus high-dose dexamethasone versus lenalidomide plus low-dose dexamethasone as initial therapy for newly diagnosed multiple myeloma: an open-label randomised controlled trial. *Lancet Oncol.* 2010;11:29-37.

A4. Attal M, Harousseau JL, Facon T, et al. Single versus double autologous stem-cell transplantation for multiple myeloma. *N Engl J Med.* 2003;349:2495-2502.

A5. Cavo M, Pantani L, Petrucci MT, et al. Bortezomib-thalidomide-dexamethasone is superior to thalidomide-dexamethasone as consolidation therapy after autologous hematopoietic stem cell transplantation in patients with newly diagnosed multiple myeloma. *Blood.* 2012;120:9-19.

A6. Attal M, Lauwers-Cances V, Marit G, et al. Lenalidomide maintenance after stem-cell transplantation for multiple myeloma. *N Engl J Med.* 2012;366:1782-1791.

A7. McCarthy PL, Owzar K, Hofmeister CC, et al. Lenalidomide after stem-cell transplantation for multiple myeloma. *N Engl J Med.* 2012;366:1770-1781.

A8. Sonneveld P, Schmidt-Wolf IG, van der Holt B, et al. Bortezomib induction and maintenance treatment in patients with newly diagnosed multiple myeloma: results of the randomized phase III HOVON-65/GMMG-HD4 trial. *J Clin Oncol.* 2012;30:2946-2955.

A9. Krishnan A, Pasquini MC, Logan B, et al. Autologous haemopoietic stem-cell transplantation followed by allogeneic or autologous haemopoietic stem-cell transplantation in patients with multiple myeloma (BMT CTN 0102): a phase 3 biological assignment trial. *Lancet Oncol.* 2011;12:1195-1203.

A10. Hulin C, Facon T, Rodon P, et al. Efficacy of melphalan and prednisone plus thalidomide in patients older than 75 years with newly diagnosed multiple myeloma: IFM 01/01 Trial. *J Clin Oncol.* 2009;27:3664-3670.

A11. San Miguel JF, Schlag R, Khuageva NK, et al. Bortezomib plus melphalan and prednisone for initial treatment of multiple myeloma. *N Engl J Med.* 2008;359:906-917.

A12. Benboubker L, Dimopoulos MA, Dispenzieri A, et al. Lenalidomide and dexamethasone in transplant-ineligible patients with myeloma. *N Engl J Med.* 2014;371:906-917.

A13. Palumbo A, Hajek R, Delforge M, et al. Continuous lenalidomide treatment for newly diagnosed multiple myeloma. *N Engl J Med.* 2012;366:1759-1769.

A14. Stewart AK, Rajkumar SV, Dimopoulos MA, et al. Carfilzomib, lenalidomide, and dexamethasone for relapsed multiple myeloma. *N Engl J Med.* 2015;372:142-152.

A15. Morgan GJ, Davies FE, Gregory WM, et al. First-line treatment with zoledronic acid as compared with clodronic acid in multiple myeloma (MRC Myeloma IX): a randomised controlled trial. *Lancet.* 2010;376:1989-1999.

A16. Mateos M-V, Hernández M-T, Giraldo P, et al. Lenalidomide plus dexamethasone for high-risk smoldering multiple myeloma. *N Engl J Med.* 2013;369:438-447.

GENERAL REFERENCES

For the General References and other additional features, please visit Expert Consult at https://expertconsult.inkling.com.

188

AMYLOIDOSIS

MORIE A. GERTZ

DEFINITION

Immunoglobulin light chain amyloidosis is characterized by a clonal population of bone marrow plasma cells that produces a monoclonal light chain of the κ or λ type, as either an intact molecule or a fragment. The light chain protein, instead of conforming to the α-helical configuration of most proteins, misfolds and forms a β-pleated sheet.[1] This insoluble protein is deposited in tissues and interferes with organ function. The β-pleated sheet configuration is responsible for the tinctorial properties; when the protein is stained with Congo red and viewed under polarized light, apple-green birefringence is demonstrated and is required for the diagnosis. Systemic light chain amyloidosis (AL) must be distinguished from the much less common amyloidosis associated with chronic infection and inflammatory arthropathies (secondary amyloidosis or AA) or with inherited amyloid cardiomyopathies and neuropathies (familial amyloidosis or AF).

CLINICAL MANIFESTATIONS

Amyloidosis is particularly difficult to diagnose and is a challenge for internists. The presenting symptoms can be diverse and are mimicked by far more common disorders (Table 188-1). The signs include tongue enlargement with dental indentations (Fig. 188-1) and "pinch" or periorbital purpura (Fig. 188-2), a result of vascular fragility. The signs are specific but lack sensitivity in that they are present in no more than 20% of patients. No single imaging procedure or laboratory study is diagnostic for the disease. The clinician must therefore be aware of the possibility of amyloidosis, or it may be overlooked. The kidney is commonly involved in amyloidosis (50% of cases). The diagnosis should be suspected in any patient who presents with nondiabetic nephrotic-range proteinuria (Chapter 121).[2] One third of patients with amyloidosis have nephrotic syndrome that is manifested with dramatic increases in the blood cholesterol level (median, 270 mg/dL), and urinalysis for proteinuria should be done in patients with a sudden increase in the serum cholesterol level. A patient with nondiabetic proteinuria may receive an empirical course of corticosteroids for possible minimal-change glomerulopathy. This treatment delays the diagnosis of amyloidosis and allows other organs to become involved.[3] Ten percent of renal biopsy specimens from patients with nondiabetic nephrotic syndrome are subsequently shown to be involved by amyloidosis. The incidence of bleeding after percutaneous renal biopsy is not increased in patients with AL.

The heart is involved in approximately 50% of patients with amyloidosis, and the presentation is subtle because fatigue is often the only manifestation.[4] Because amyloid heart disease (Chapter 60) is a disorder of diastolic failure, the typical findings of cardiomyopathy (enlarged cardiac silhouette on chest radiography, depressed ejection fraction by echocardiography, and pulmonary vascular redistribution) are absent. The effect of amyloidosis on the heart is poor filling during diastole. Patients have low end-diastolic volume and, as a consequence, poor stroke volume, despite a completely

TABLE 188-1 SYMPTOMS, SIGNS, AND SYNDROME OF AMYLOIDOSIS

SYMPTOMS AND SIGNS
Common symptoms: fatigue, edema, dyspnea, anorexia, paresthesias
Rare symptoms: claudication, joint pain and stiffness, sicca syndrome
Common signs: periorbital purpura, glossomegaly, hepatomegaly
Rare signs: waxy infiltration of eyelids, shoulder pad sign
SYNDROMES
Nondiabetic nephrotic syndrome
Nonischemic cardiomyopathy with an echocardiogram showing "hypertrophy"
Hepatomegaly or increased alkaline phosphatase with no imaging abnormality
Peripheral neuropathy with monoclonal gammopathy of undetermined significance or chronic inflammatory demyelinating polyneuropathy with autonomic features
Atypical myeloma with monoclonal light chains and modest marrow plasmacytosis

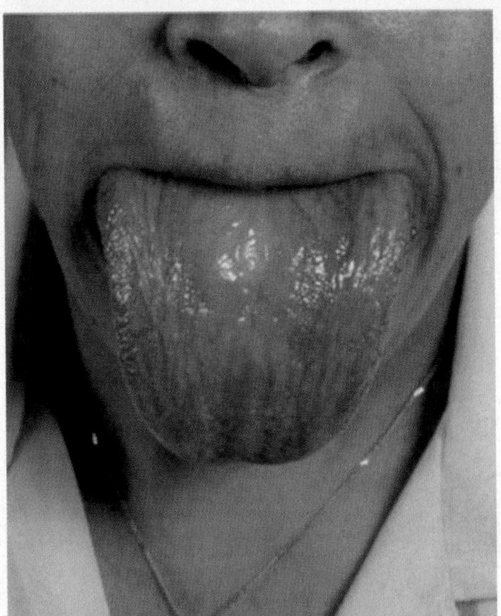

FIGURE 188-1. **Macroglossia (or glossomegaly) in a patient with amyloidosis.** (From Esplin BL, Gertz MA. Current trends in diagnosis and management of cardiac amyloidosis. *Curr Probl Cardiol.* 2013;38:53-96.)

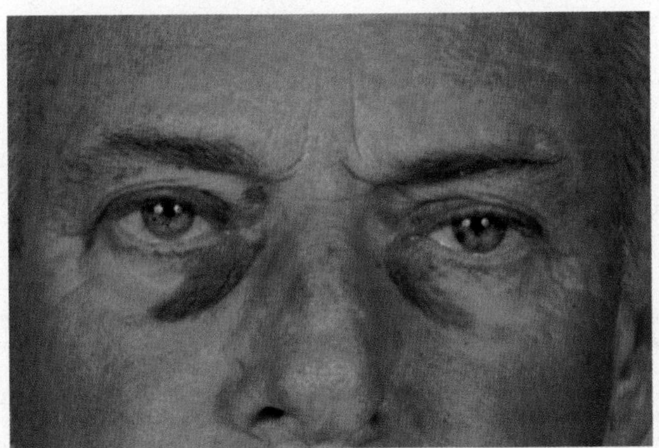

FIGURE 188-2. **Periorbital purpura in amyloidosis.** (From Kitchens CS. Purpura and other hematovascular disorders. In: Kitchens CS, Konkle BA, Kessler CM, eds. *Consultative Hemostasis and Thrombosis.* 3rd ed. Philadelphia: Elsevier; 2012.)

normal ejection fraction. Electrocardiography frequently shows a pseudoinfarct pattern, which can be interpreted as demonstrating silent ischemic infarction; this finding leads to coronary angiography, which is invariably negative (unless there is coincidental coronary artery disease). Echocardiography, which shows thickening of the heart walls due to amyloid infiltration, is frequently interpreted as showing left ventricular hypertrophy, and the cause of heart failure can be ascribed to silent hypertension or, alternatively, hypertrophic cardiomyopathy. Restrictive cardiomyopathy has been confused with pericardial disease, and patients have undergone unnecessary pericardiectomy, without clinical benefit. The classic granular sparkling appearance on the echocardiogram is not a useful diagnostic finding. Patients with amyloidosis rarely have symptoms of ischemic heart disease. Enhancement on magnetic resonance imaging with gadolinium is delayed in 69% of patients with cardiac amyloidosis. Myocardial enhancement is associated with increased ventricular mass and impaired left ventricular systolic function.

The liver is involved in 13% of patients. The typical presentation is hepatomegaly and an increased serum alkaline phosphatase value. Increased transaminase values and hyperbilirubinemia are late signs. Imaging is not helpful, and liver uptake is homogeneous. Many patients undergo evaluation for metastatic malignant disease. Liver biopsy is not associated with an increased rate of bleeding and is not contraindicated in the presence of hepatic amyloidosis. Rarely, patients present with spontaneous splenic rupture. Acquired deficiency of coagulation factor X (Chapter 174) is specific to AL and can be associated with clinically severe hemorrhage. Levels of coagulation factor X improve with effective therapy because the cause of low levels of circulating factor X is binding of factor X to the amyloid fibrils.

The peripheral neuropathy (Chapter 420) associated with amyloidosis begins in the lower extremities, is symmetrical, and is generally sensory or mixed sensorimotor. When a monoclonal protein is recognized, frequent diagnoses are chronic inflammatory demyelinating polyneuropathy and neuropathy associated with monoclonal gammopathy of undetermined significance because amyloidosis has not been considered in the differential diagnosis. Associated autonomic neuropathy occurs in approximately 4% of patients and can be characterized by orthostatic hypotension, which may be misattributed to cardiac failure. Autonomic dysmotility of the bowel is a common associated finding (Chapter 136). It can be upper intestinal, leading to pseudo-obstruction and recurrent emesis, or lower intestinal, characterized by alternating obstipation and fecal incontinence. Diarrhea caused by autonomic failure has been misdiagnosed as collagenous colitis when eosinophilic deposits are found in the bowel mucosa on hematoxylin-eosin staining in the absence of Congo red staining. Carpal tunnel syndrome (Chapter 420) occurs in approximately 13% of patients; it is not clinically distinguishable from the syndrome associated with repetitive stress injury but frequently fails to improve after surgical release. Rarely, interstitial lung disease, pseudoclaudication, periarticular deposits, and unexplained weight loss are presenting symptoms.

Systemic amyloidosis can be confused with early multiple myeloma (Chapter 187). Patients who present with vague symptoms of fatigue and edema are found to have a monoclonal protein in the urine, and a bone marrow biopsy specimen shows a clonal plasmacytosis with a median of 5% plasma cells in the bone marrow; however, a quarter of patients have more than 10% plasma cells in the bone marrow, a finding that qualifies as a diagnosis of multiple myeloma. These patients are often considered to have atypical multiple myeloma when the underlying amyloid syndrome is undetected. In these patients, a misdiagnosis of myeloma kidney or demyelinating neuropathy is made when an adequate diagnostic evaluation to exclude amyloidosis has not been performed.

DIAGNOSIS

Screening for Amyloidosis

In a patient with nondiabetic proteinuria, cardiomyopathy without ischemic risk factors, unexplained hepatomegaly, peripheral or autonomic neuropathy, or carpal tunnel syndrome, amyloidosis is not the most likely cause. The disorder occurs in only 8 per million persons per year, and routine biopsy is not appropriate whenever consistent symptoms are found. The classic physical finding of periorbital purpura occurs in only 10% of patients, is often limited to petechial eruptions over the eyelids, and is easily overlooked. Enlargement of the tongue occurs in 10 to 15% of patients; therefore, although it is specific, it is not sensitive for the diagnosis. Amyloidosis in patients with enlarged tongues may be unrecognized, or these patients may be evaluated for acromegaly or undergo unnecessary tongue biopsies because of the suspicion of squamous cell cancer. If biopsy is not an appropriate screening technique, what algorithm should be used to recognize AL?

By definition, amyloidosis is a plasma cell dyscrasia (Chapter 187); therefore, virtually all patients have a detectable immunoglobulin abnormality by immunofixation of the serum or urine, or they have abnormal results on a serum immunoglobulin free light chain assay. When a patient presents with a compatible clinical syndrome, these diagnostic studies should be completed before invasive diagnostic studies are performed (Fig. 188-3). Simple electrophoresis without immunofixation is inadequate because the monoclonal proteins are quantitatively very small in most patients and will not cause a detectable peak on serum protein electrophoresis. When these three diagnostic studies are used in combination, the sensitivity is 100%. If a monoclonal protein is detected, further investigations for amyloid should proceed, as described later. If a monoclonal protein is not found, three possibilities exist: (1) the patient does not have amyloidosis; (2) if the patient is known to have amyloidosis, it may be localized rather than systemic; or (3) if the patient is known to have systemic amyloidosis, it may be the senile systemic or familial type rather than the light chain type (see later section on other forms of amyloidosis).

Confirming the Diagnosis of Amyloidosis

In view of the grave prognosis associated with AL, the diagnosis must be confirmed by biopsy (with Congo red staining) in all cases.[5] Although it is reasonable to biopsy the kidney when proteinuria is the presenting symptom,

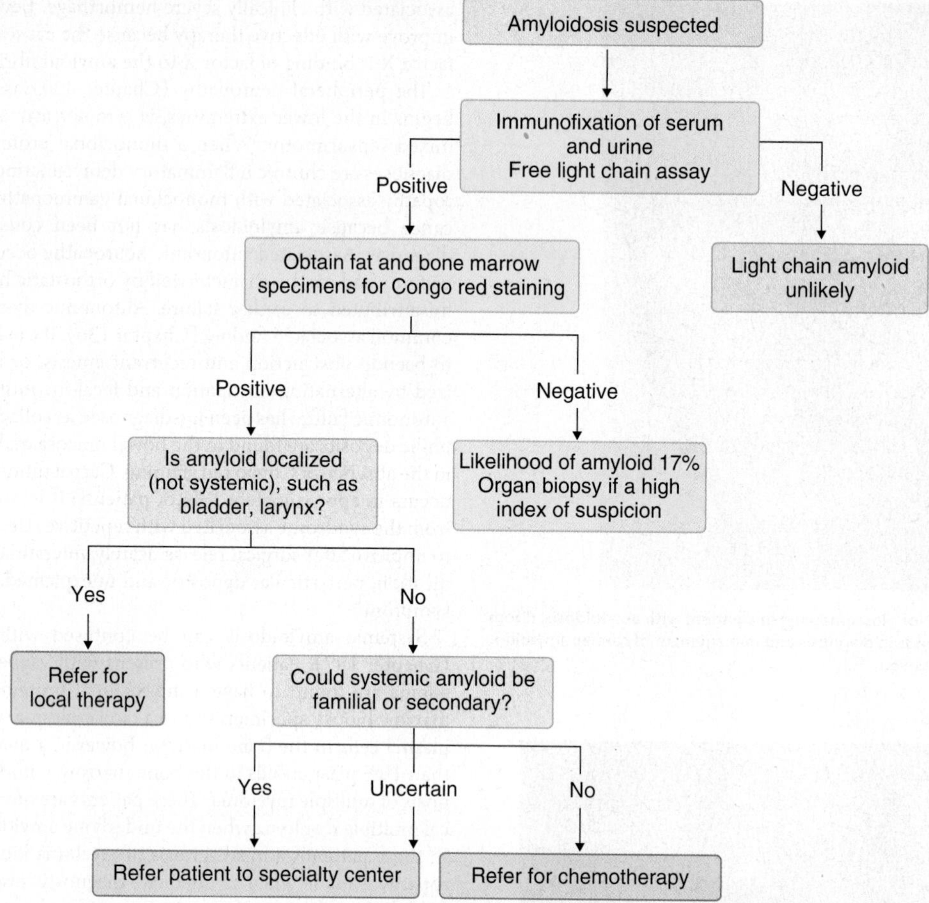

FIGURE 188-3. **Algorithm for the cost-effective pursuit of a diagnosis of systemic light chain amyloidosis.**

the heart when cardiomyopathy is recognized, the liver when there is hepatomegaly and increased alkaline phosphatase, or the nerve when there is a sensorimotor functional loss, these invasive and occasionally risky procedures are not required. Subcutaneous fat aspiration is an outpatient procedure that has a 24-hour turnaround time and recognizes amyloid deposits in 70% of patients. Bone marrow is a second convenient biopsy site, and this test is often required to exclude the possibility of associated multiple myeloma. Bone marrow biopsy is positive in 50% of patients. When both subcutaneous fat aspiration and bone marrow biopsy are done, amyloid is detected in 83% of patients. The remaining patients should have biopsy of the appropriate organ.

Once amyloid deposits are detected in tissues, further diagnostic evaluation is required. The presence of a monoclonal protein in the serum or urine and the presence of congophilic deposits in tissue do not verify that amyloidosis is light chain in origin. Further diagnostic studies are essential to classify the type of amyloid before therapy is initiated. Immunohistochemical studies on the tissue may be useful, but misfolding of the amyloid light chain often prevents epitopes from being recognized by commercial antisera; thus, false-negative results are common. Mass spectrometric analysis of the amyloid deposit can be done on paraffin-embedded tissue and validates the type of amyloid by direct amino acid sequencing, leaving no question about the origin of the amyloid protein as an immunoglobulin light chain. The incidence of monoclonal gammopathies in the elderly ranges from 3 to 5%. Therefore, that fraction of patients with senile systemic, localized, and familial amyloidosis (see section on other forms of amyloidosis) could be expected to have an associated monoclonal gammopathy, which would be misleading. Mass spectrometric analysis is feasible on subcutaneous fat tissue.

TREATMENT

Rx

Amyloidosis was previously thought to be untreatable and invariably fatal. With current therapy, response rates of about 70% regularly occur, and the median duration of survival is reportedly upward of 5 years.[6] Agents to reverse the misfolding of the protein and render it soluble would be ideal, but they are not available. The source of the immunoglobulin light chain is the clonal plasma cell population in the bone marrow. All known therapies are directed at destruction of the plasma cell clone.

The two treatment choices are generally traditional-dose chemotherapy and high-dose chemotherapy with autologous stem cell transplantation. Most patients are not candidates for high-dose therapy because of age, advanced cardiac dysfunction, or renal insufficiency. High-dose melphalan is a feasible approach in selected patients with cardiac AL and is associated with a high rate of hematologic and organ responses that lead to prolonged survival. Current therapies include combinations of melphalan, cyclophosphamide, dexamethasone, bortezomib, and lenalidomide. Treatment with a combination of bortezomib (1.5 mg/m^2 weekly or 1.3 mg/m^2 on days 1, 4, 8, and 11 every 28 days), cyclophosphamide (300 mg/m^2 orally weekly), and dexamethasone (40 mg weekly) has produced rapid and complete hematologic responses in the majority of patients with AL with few side effects.[7] Effective therapy has been associated with resolution of nephrotic syndrome, cardiac failure, and hepatomegaly. Imaging has shown amyloid deposits to regress after the suppression of light chain synthesis.

A systematic review and meta-analysis indicated that autologous hematopoietic stem cell transplantation does not appear to be superior to conventional chemotherapy in improving overall survival in patients with AL amyloidosis, although the quality of evidence was deemed low.[A1]

Assessing the Effect of Therapy

The serum immunoglobulin free light chain assay has been cited as a useful screening test for patients with a compatible clinical syndrome. This assay is also used to measure the therapeutic effect of intervention because the light chain level is quantifiable and reproducible. On the basis of current hematologic response criteria, successful therapy is characterized by a 50% reduction in the abnormal free light chain level.[8,9] Because the tissue toxicity associated with amyloid is related to the deposition of small amounts of light chain, it is unclear whether a successful outcome requires complete eradication of the light chain product. Studies have shown that patients achieving complete normalization of the free light chain have a better outcome, but it is uncertain whether patients who do not achieve this level of response should be subjected to more intensive treatment in an effort to remove this pathogenic amyloid serum precursor.

PROGNOSIS

The outcome of patients with AL depends on the extent of cardiac involvement (Chapter 60). With the advent of routine hemodialysis for this population, death due to renal failure is uncommon. The greater the involvement of the heart, the shorter a patient's survival. Echocardiography provides useful information about the ejection fraction, the thickness of the ventricular septum and left ventricular free wall, and the strain percentage (the rate at which wall shortening occurs). Doppler echocardiography allows quantitative measurements of diastolic function and reflects the slowing of blood flow into the ventricular chamber as the noncompliant left ventricle fills. This "stiffness," measured by the deceleration time, provides useful information and correlates well with survival.

Cardiac biomarkers are extremely sensitive measures of myocardial function, are reproducible, and can be used not only for prognosis but also to follow cardiac response after effective therapy. The serum troponin value is a powerful predictor of survival in patients with amyloidosis, and the N-terminal pro–brain natriuretic peptide value predicts survival after a diagnosis of amyloidosis. A staging system has been developed with these two cardiac biomarkers and the difference between involved and uninvolved free light chain levels to accurately predict survival.

OTHER FORMS OF AMYLOIDOSIS

Localized amyloidosis can be confused with systemic amyloidosis, but it has a much better prognosis. Localized AL amyloidosis represents a true plasma cell neoplasm and not a pseudotumor.[10] However, patients with localized amyloidosis generally do not require systemic therapy; management can be supportive or localized to the deposition. The location of the amyloid deposits can be a clue to the localized nature. Typical sites for localized amyloid deposition include the ureter, bladder, urethra, and prostate. Therapy entails cystoscopic resection or intravesical instillation of dimethyl sulfoxide. Most forms of cutaneous amyloidosis are localized, although nodular cutaneous amyloidosis has occurred in systemic AL. Tracheobronchial and laryngeal amyloidosis and nodular pulmonary amyloidosis are localized, are not associated with a plasma cell dyscrasia, and generally require only local therapy. Nodular pulmonary amyloidosis is often diagnosed after thoracotomy for a presumed malignant pulmonary nodule. Most cases of laryngeal amyloidosis are found when the patient presents to an otorhinolaryngologist with hoarseness and amyloid deposits are found on endoscopic biopsy. Patients with localized amyloidosis do not have a demonstrable monoclonal protein in the serum or urine and have a normal free light chain ratio. The localized amyloidosis found in Alzheimer disease is chemically unrelated to AL, and AL patients have no increased risk of dementia.

Senile systemic amyloidosis results from the deposition of a normal serum protein, transthyretin (TTR), in the myocardium. It has a much better prognosis than cardiac AL and generally necessitates endomyocardial biopsy for diagnosis; most patients are older than 70 years. When a monoclonal protein is present, it is incidental, and confirmation of type generally requires analysis of the amyloid-laden tissues. Therapy is supportive. The clinical presentation of senile systemic amyloidosis is not distinguishable from that of cardiac AL.

AF is uncommon in the United States and represents only 3% of cases of systemic amyloidosis. Patients present with the full clinical spectrum associated with amyloidosis, including cardiomyopathy, peripheral neuropathy, and proteinuria. Patients do not have a monoclonal protein because the deposited precursor is a mutant form of TTR, fibrinogen, lysozyme, or apolipoprotein A. Diflunisal (250 mg twice dail) can slow the rate of progression of the AF associated polyneuropathy.[A2] Selected patients with AF with polyneuropathy have benefited from liver transplantation because this disease is characterized by systemic accumulation of polymerized TTR in the peripheral nerves and systemic organs and liver transplantation stops the major production of amyloidogenic TTR.[11] In one hospital, the estimated probability of 10-year survival in patients with familial amyloid polyneuropathy was 100% after liver transplantation compared with 56% for the nontransplantation group, with the survival curves diverging at 6 years.[12]

One important form of AF in the United States is associated with an allele of the normal serum protein TTR in which isoleucine is substituted for valine at position 122 (TTR Val-122-Ile). The prevalence of this mutation in blacks in the United States is as high as 3.9%. Heterozygous inheritance of this mutant TTR is associated with late-onset cardiomyopathy in this population. Wall thickening is found on echocardiography. Heart failure is often mild at onset. The prognosis is far better than that of cardiac AL, and its recognition has important implications for genetic counseling.

SECONDARY AMYLOIDOSIS

Systemic AA is the rarest form in Western countries.[13] Previously, it was a consequence of uncontrolled sustained inflammation, usually infectious, and causes included tuberculosis and osteomyelitis. Cystic fibrosis, bronchiectasis, decubitus ulcers, and skin abscesses related to subcutaneous injection of illicit drugs are modern-day infectious causes. Today it occurs primarily in patients with difficult-to-control inflammatory syndromes, including Crohn's disease, juvenile arthritis, and ankylosing spondylitis. Organ damage results from the extracellular deposition of proteolytic fragments of the acute phase reactant serum amyloid A (SAA) as amyloid fibrils. However, because only a minority of patients with chronic inflammatory disorders actually develop this complication, disease-modifying factors must be also operative. The best characterized of these is the *SAA1* genotype. There has been a recent decline in numbers of patients presenting with AA amyloidosis due to rheumatic diseases, at least in part due to the use of disease-modifying antirheumatic therapy.[14]

The large majority of these patients present with proteinuria, nephrotic syndrome, or renal dysfunction. Diarrhea related to intestinal involvement (22%) and thyromegaly (9%) also occur.

Suppression of the inflammatory process results in regression of tissue amyloid deposits. Early diagnosis and rapid control of the underlying inflammatory disease are critical to prevent irreversible organ damage and to improve survival of patients with AA amyloidosis. Therefore, monitoring of patients with chronic, active inflammatory disease by serial testing of SAA, C-reactive protein, microalbuminemia, proteinuria, and other indicators of amyloid development, as well as possibly determination of the *SAA1* genotype, can guide approach to management. Anti– tumor necrosis factor-α agents have markedly reduced the incidence of AA from inflammatory arthritis. There are familial forms of AA associated with familial periodic fever syndromes, the most common being familial Mediterranean fever (Chapter 261) due to mutations in the tumor necrosis factor receptor. Interleukin-1 inhibitors (anakinra) have been used successfully in these inherited periodic fever syndromes.

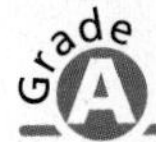

Grade A References

A1. Mhaskar R, Kumar A, Behera M, et al. Role of high-dose chemotherapy and autologous hematopoietic cell transplantation in primary systemic amyloidosis: a systematic review. *Biol Blood Marrow Transplant.* 2009;15:893-902.

A2. Berk J, Suhr O, Obici L, et al. Repurposing diflunisal for familial amyloid polyneuropathy: a randomized clinical trial. *JAMA.* 2013;310:2658-2667.

GENERAL REFERENCES

For the General References and other additional features, please visit Expert Consult at https://expertconsult.inkling.com.

189

TUMORS OF THE CENTRAL NERVOUS SYSTEM

LISA M. DEANGELIS

INTRACRANIAL TUMORS

General Approach to Brain Tumors

EPIDEMIOLOGY

About 23,000 new primary brain tumors and nervous system cancers are diagnosed annually in the United States, making central nervous system (CNS) tumors more than twice as common as Hodgkin disease and approximately one third as common as melanoma. There is no definitive evidence that any of them are linked to cell phone use. In contrast, intracranial metastases are five times more common than primary brain tumors. More than 120 types of primary brain tumors arise from the different cells that make up the CNS (Table 189-1). In addition to classifying tumors by their cell of origin, in clinical practice it is often useful to classify a tumor by its intracranial site as well, such as pineal region tumors or pituitary and suprasellar tumors.

TABLE 189-1 WORLD HEALTH ORGANIZATION CLASSIFICATION OF BRAIN TUMORS

TUMORS OF NEUROEPITHELIAL TISSUE
- Astrocytic tumors
  - Astrocytoma
  - Anaplastic (malignant) astrocytoma
  - Glioblastoma
  - Pilocytic astrocytoma
  - Pleomorphic xanthoastrocytoma
  - Subependymal giant cell astrocytoma
- Oligodendroglial tumors
  - Oligodendroglioma
  - Anaplastic (malignant) oligodendroglioma
- Ependymal tumors
  - Ependymoma
  - Anaplastic (malignant) ependymoma
  - Myxopapillary ependymoma (spinal tumor)
  - Subependymoma
- Mixed gliomas
  - Oligoastrocytoma
  - Anaplastic (malignant) oligoastrocytoma
- Choroid plexus
  - Choroid plexus papilloma
  - Choroid plexus carcinoma
- Neuronal and mixed neuronal—glial tumors
  - Gangliocytoma
  - Dysembryoplastic neuroepithelial tumor
  - Ganglioglioma
  - Anaplastic (malignant) ganglioglioma
  - Central neurocytoma
- Pineal parenchymal tumors
  - Pineocytoma
  - Pineoblastoma
- Embryonal tumors
  - Medulloblastoma
  - Primitive neuroectodermal tumor

TUMORS OF CRANIAL AND SPINAL NERVES
- Schwannoma
- Neurofibroma

TUMORS OF MENINGES
- Meningioma
- Hemangiopericytoma
- Hemangioblastoma

PRIMARY CENTRAL NERVOUS SYSTEM LYMPHOMAS

GERM CELL TUMORS
- Germinoma
- Embryonal carcinoma
- Yolk sac tumor (endodermal sinus tumor)
- Choriocarcinoma
- Teratoma
- Mixed germ cell tumors

CYSTS AND TUMOR-LIKE LESIONS
- Rathke cleft cyst
- Epidermoid cyst
- Dermoid cyst
- Colloid cyst of the third ventricle

TUMORS OF THE SELLAR REGION
- Pituitary adenoma
- Pituitary carcinoma
- Craniopharyngioma

METASTATIC TUMORS

Abridged and modified from World Health Organization classification.

PATHOBIOLOGY

In contrast to tumors arising elsewhere in the body, there is little distinction between benign and malignant tumors when they occur in the brain. The growth of brain tumors is restricted to the CNS; they rarely if ever metastasize to other organs. In the CNS, a malignant tumor is characterized by aggressive pathologic features, including local tissue invasion, neovascularity, regional necrosis, and cytologic atypia. These features confer a growth advantage to malignant cells and lead to rapid expansion and, frequently, to early regrowth after treatment. Tumors lacking these aggressive histologic features are preferably classified as low grade rather than benign. Many low-grade tumors continue to grow within the CNS, causing progressive neurologic disability and some may acquire a more malignant phenotype over time. The low-grade tumors that transform into high-grade neoplasms are primarily the intra-axial tumors that cannot be cured by resection because of their diffuse infiltration of brain. Almost all truly benign CNS tumors are extra-axial tumors, such as meningiomas and acoustic neuromas that can be cured with complete surgical resection.

CLINICAL MANIFESTATIONS

A patient with a brain tumor can present with one or both of two types of symptoms and signs. *Generalized symptoms,* which typically reflect the increased intracranial pressure (ICP) that often accompanies cerebral tumors, include headache, lethargy, personality change, nausea, and vomiting. *Lateralizing symptoms,* which reflect the specific location of the tumor include hemiparesis, hemisensory deficits, aphasia, visual field impairment, and seizures (Table 189-2).

Most patients have symptoms that progress during a week to a few months. A sudden intensification of symptoms may precipitate the patient's initial visit to the physician; however, a careful history usually reveals symptoms that predated the acute deterioration and slowly worsened over time. Two exceptions are the new appearance of a seizure in a previously asymptomatic individual (Chapter 403) and sudden hemorrhage into a tumor.

Symptoms of brain tumors can be produced by tumor invading brain parenchyma, tumor and edema compressing brain tissue, cerebrospinal fluid (CSF) obstruction caused directly by the tumor or by a shift of brain tissue, and herniation. Invasion and compression typically produce focal symptoms, many of which can be relieved if the compression is reduced. Obstruction of CSF flow and herniation are frequently a consequence of elevated ICP and typically produce generalized symptoms of headache, nausea, and vomiting, but they can also cause false localizing signs, such as an abducens nerve palsy as a result of diffuse increased ICP.

Headache (Chapter 398) is a presenting symptom of approximately 35% of brain tumors. It is more common in younger than in older patients and more common in patients who have rapidly growing tumors than in those whose tumors have evolved slowly (Fig. 189-1). Mental and cognitive abnormalities may be a reflection of local tumor (e.g., aphasia, alexia, agnosia) or of general impairment (e.g., lethargy, confusion, word finding difficulty, apathy). Seizures affect approximately one-third of patients with brain tumors, and they are especially common as the presenting and only symptom of a low-grade tumor. The seizures, which are focal because they originate at the site of the tumor, may remain restricted (e.g., focal motor seizures), or they may generalize secondarily, producing loss of consciousness, sometimes so quickly that the focal signature is missed by the patient or even an observant witness.

DIAGNOSIS

Imaging

Magnetic resonance imaging (MRI) is far superior to computed tomography (CT) and should be used in all cases of suspected intracranial tumor. MRI should be performed both without and with intravenous administration of gadolinium. A well performed MRI scan identifies any intracranial tumor, and a normal finding on MRI effectively excludes a neoplasm. The MRI of some extra-axial tumors (e.g., acoustic neuromas, meningiomas) is so characteristic that histologic confirmation is not required. A non–contrast-enhancing infiltrative lesion that is visible primarily on T2-weighted or fluid-attenuated inversion recovery images is most consistent with a low-grade glioma (Fig. 189-2), whereas a contrast-enhancing lesion with an area of central necrosis and surrounding edema is most likely to be a glioblastoma or possibly a brain metastasis. Although these diagnoses must be confirmed histologically, the preoperative diagnostic possibilities affect the surgical approach to the lesion.

Perfusion MRI after rapid infusion of gadolinium can measure the relative cerebral blood volume and neovascularity associated with a tumor; high perfusion is associated with higher grade of malignancy. This technique can help estimate the tumor grade preoperatively and guide the planning of treatment.

Magnetic resonance spectroscopy noninvasively assesses tissue composition. High-grade primary brain tumors are associated with a decrease in *N*-acetylaspartate and an increase in choline. More malignant tumors are

TABLE 189-2 FOCAL CLINICAL MANIFESTATIONS OF BRAIN TUMORS

Frontal lobe
Generalized seizures
Focal motor seizures (contralateral)
Expressive aphasia (dominant side)
Behavioral changes
Dementia
Gait disorders, incontinence
Hemiparesis (contralateral)
Basal ganglia
Hemiparesis (contralateral)
Movement disorders (rare)
Parietal lobe
Receptive aphasia (dominant side)
Spatial disorientation (nondominant side)
Cortical sensory dysfunction (contralateral)
Hemianopia (contralateral)
Agnosias
Occipital lobe
Hemianopia (contralateral)
Visual disturbances (unformed)
Temporal lobe
Complex partial (psychomotor) seizures
Generalized seizures
Behavioral changes
Olfactory and complex visual auras
Language disorder (dominant side)
Visual field defect
Corpus callosum
Dementia (anterior)
Memory loss (posterior)
Behavioral changes
Asymptomatic (middle)
Thalamus
Sensory loss (contralateral)
Behavioral changes
Language disorder (dominant side)
Midbrain/pineal
Paresis of vertical eye movement
Pupillary abnormalities
Precocious puberty (boys)
Sella/optic nerve/pituitary
Endocrinopathy
Bitemporal hemianopia
Monocular visual defects
Ophthalmoplegia (cavernous sinus)
Pons/medulla
Cranial nerve dysfunction
Ataxia, nystagmus
Weakness, sensory loss
Spasticity
Cerebellopontine angle
Deafness (ipsilateral)
Loss of facial sensation (ipsilateral)
Facial weakness (ipsilateral)
Ataxia
Cerebellum
Ataxia (ipsilateral)
Nystagmus

associated with a greater choline/*N*-acetylaspartate ratio and frequently contain areas with elevation of lactate and lipid.

Surgical resection is a major objective in the treatment of almost every kind of brain tumor, but resection must be balanced against possible damage to adjacent normal brain. The development of functional MRI (fMRI), which measures cerebral blood flow when areas of cortex are activated, has greatly enhanced the ability to localize critical neurologic functions and their relationship to the tumor preoperatively. When the fMRI is fused with the anatomic MRI, essential functions can be identified in relationship to the patient's tumor, and a safer and more complete resection may be planned.

On positron emission tomography (PET), high-grade tumors are usually hypermetabolic, whereas low-grade tumors are hypometabolic. New technologies using ^{11}C-methionine PET may differentiate low- from high-grade gliomas much more efficiently than deoxyglucose PET.

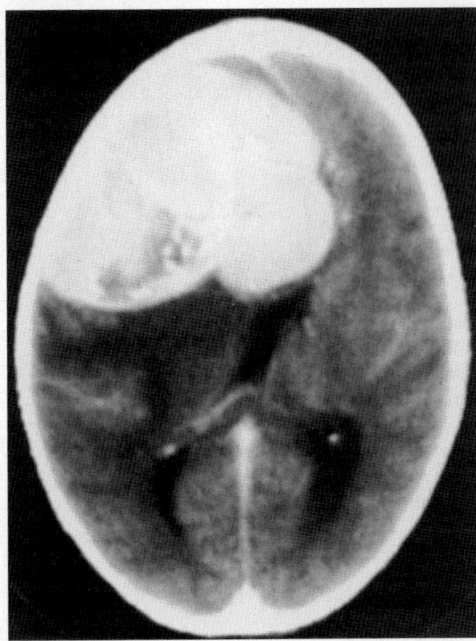

FIGURE 189-1. Meningioma. Computed tomography scan with contrast enhancement of a meningioma in a patient who presented with mild cognitive deficits, illustrative of the size that a slow-growing tumor can attain in the brain. The tumor was completely resected.

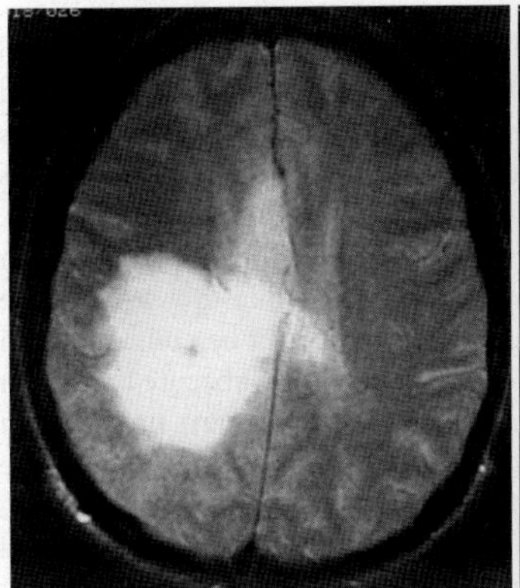

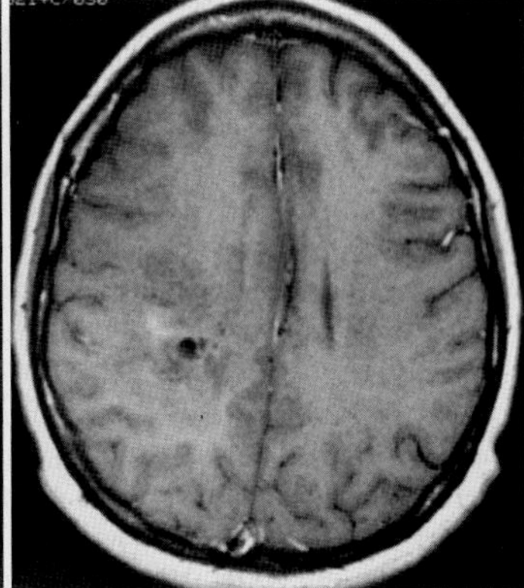

FIGURE 189-2. Glioma. Magnetic resonance imaging of a low-grade glioma. *Left*, T2-weighted image. *Right*, T1-weighted image, gadolinium contrast with minimum enhancement. The images are typical of this tumor, which is being detected with increasing frequency by magnetic resonance imaging in seizure patients. Many are invisible on computed tomography scans.

CT, without and with intravenous administration of contrast material, should be used only for patients who cannot undergo MRI. A CT scan, even with the administration of contrast material, may miss low-grade tumors and tumors in the posterior fossa.

Angiography no longer has a role in the diagnosis of intracranial tumors. However, angiographic embolization is occasionally useful preoperatively to reduce the vascularity of some meningiomas, thereby making a complete resection safer and more feasible.

Other Tests

Electroencephalography is rarely needed in the diagnosis or management of brain tumors. An electroencephalogram can occasionally be useful in a patient who has prolonged or unexplained stupor and in whom nonconvulsive status epilepticus is a consideration. Intraoperative monitoring is also used frequently to help guide resection of epileptogenic cortex adjacent to or within brain tumor tissue.

CSF analysis has little role in the diagnosis of most intracranial neoplasms. In primary CNS lymphoma (Chapter 185), the diagnosis may be established on CSF cytologic examination in about 15% of patients. The sensitivity of CSF cytology in the diagnosis of CNS lymphoma increases when it is combined with flow cytometry and is further enhanced by immunophenotypic and molecular genetic analyses of the CSF.[1] Rarely, a lumbar puncture is

TABLE 189-3 DIFFERENTIAL DIAGNOSIS OF INTRACRANIAL TUMORS

- Infection
  - Brain abscess
    - Bacterial
    - Fungal
    - Parasitic (e.g., cysticercosis)
  - Herpes encephalitis
- Vascular disease
  - Stroke
  - Intracranial hemorrhage
- Inflammatory conditions
  - Granuloma (sarcoid)
  - Multiple sclerosis: tumefactive single large lesion
- Vascular malformations
  - Cavernous angiomas
  - Venous angiomas
- Congenital abnormalities
  - Cortical dysplasia
  - Heterotopia

TABLE 189-4 TREATMENT OF BRAIN TUMORS

SYMPTOMATIC

- Glucocorticoids
- Antiepileptics
- Venous thromboembolism prophylaxis and treatment

DEFINITIVE

- Surgery
  - Goal is gross total excision
- Radiation therapy
  - Standard external beam
    - Fractionated
    - Usually focal
  - Stereotactic radiosurgery
- Chemotherapy
  - Limited by intrinsic drug resistance and blood-brain barrier

required to exclude inflammatory conditions or other processes that may be confused with a primary brain tumor. Lumbar puncture must be avoided in patients with cerebellar tumors because the release of pressure through the spinal needle may result in herniation of the cerebellar tonsils through the foramen magnum.

Differential Diagnosis

Patients who present with symptoms of raised ICP or the new onset of central neurologic symptoms, such as hemiparesis or seizure, should be evaluated rapidly. Prompt neuroimaging discloses a mass, and the radiographic features narrow the differential diagnosis (Table 189-3). Extra-axial tumors, such as a meningioma or acoustic neuroma, can be confused with a dural metastasis. Low-grade intra-axial tumors, which are nonenhancing on MRI, have been confused with infections such as herpes encephalitis when they involve the temporal lobe. Contrast-enhancing intra-axial tumors can be confused with a stroke, brain abscess, or focal plaque of demyelination. Subacute infarction can show brisk contrast enhancement, usually in a gyral pattern, unlike brain tumors in which enhancement is primarily in the white matter; however, the two are occasionally indistinguishable radiographically. Brain abscesses typically have a thinner enhancing wall than a malignant tumor and have restricted diffusion. Despite careful evaluation, patients thought to have a malignant glioma occasionally are found at surgery to have a brain abscess. A single large plaque of demyelination can also be confused radiographically with a brain tumor, and sometimes the diagnosis can be established only by biopsy.

When MRI suggests a primary brain tumor, there is no need for an extensive systemic search for a possible source of metastasis. Brain metastases are more common than primary brain tumors, but most occur in patients with known cancer, typically with active systemic disease. If an obvious systemic cancer is not revealed by a thorough physical examination, chest radiograph, routine blood tests, and urinalysis, the patient should proceed to craniotomy. Even if a brain metastasis is found at surgery, resection of a single brain metastasis is the appropriate treatment, and the pathologic examination of the lesion guides the subsequent search for the primary tumor.

TREATMENT (Rx)

The treatment for all brain tumors can be divided into two main categories: symptomatic and definitive (Table 189-4). Symptomatic treatment addresses the associated problems, such as cerebral edema, seizures, and thromboembolic disease, which can contribute substantially to clinical symptoms. Definitive treatment addresses the tumor itself.

Symptomatic Treatment

Symptomatic management includes the use of corticosteroids, anticonvulsants, and prophylaxis for deep venous thrombosis (Chapter 38). Corticosteroids decrease the vasogenic edema that surrounds primary and metastatic brain tumors. Blood vessels associated with tumor formation are leaky and do not share the normal morphologic and physiologic features that form the blood-brain barrier; corticosteroids effectively reconstitute the blood-brain barrier by decreasing the abnormal permeability of these neovessels. Clinical improvement may begin within minutes, and frequently patients are dramatically improved within 24 to 48 hours.

Dexamethasone is the most commonly used glucocorticoid because it has the least mineralocorticoid activity. The usual starting dose is 12 to 16 mg/day, but this can be adjusted to find the lowest possible dose that alleviates neurologic symptoms. After definitive treatment is instituted, many patients can be tapered off their corticosteroid completely. Chronic high-dose corticosteroid therapy is associated with substantial side effects (Chapter 35) and should be avoided if possible. Patients who will be taking glucocorticoids for 6 weeks or longer should receive prophylaxis against *Pneumocystis jiroveci* (formerly *Pneumocystis carinii*; Chapter 341).

Anticonvulsants are administered to any patient who has had a seizure, but prophylactic anticonvulsants should not be prescribed for patients who have never had a seizure, except in the immediate perioperative period.[A1] A taper should begin 2 to 3 weeks after craniotomy.

Venous thromboembolism, which occurs in about 25% of patients with brain tumors, can occur early in the illness or at any time during treatment. All patients undergoing neurosurgery should have pneumatic compression boots in the postoperative period to reduce the incidence of venous thromboembolism. Prophylactic anticoagulants have also been used successfully in the immediate postoperative period without increasing postoperative hemorrhage. Appropriately regulated anticoagulation (Chapter 38) is the optimal therapy for deep venous thrombosis and is not associated with an increased risk of intracerebral hemorrhage in patients with intracranial tumors. Inferior vena cava filters can be used for patients who have deep vein thrombi or pulmonary emboli and who cannot be fully anticoagulated.

Definitive Treatment

Surgery

Complete excision is the goal for a primary brain tumor. Surgical excision can often be accomplished for primary extra-axial tumors, such as meningiomas and acoustic neuromas, unless their intracranial location makes resection impossible. Tumors of the skull base are particularly difficult to remove, and partial resection for decompression is often performed to preserve neurologic function. The safe boundaries for resecting cortical lesions while preserving function can often be elucidated by preoperative fMRI and intraoperative cortical mapping. However, lesions involving critical structures, such as the brainstem or thalamus, cannot be excised safely.

Lesions that cannot be resected are still amenable to biopsy for diagnostic purposes. Stereotactic biopsy can reach lesions in almost any area of the brain with minimal morbidity. The risks of stereotactic biopsy include inadequate tissue sample to make a diagnosis; a tissue sample that does not accurately reflect the most malignant grade of the tumor; and a procedure-related complication, such as hemorrhage. Hemorrhage that causes neurologic impairment occurs in only 2% of stereotactic biopsies, typically in patients with glioblastoma.

Complete excision can cure an extra-axial primary brain tumor and is associated with prolonged survival and better neurologic outcome even in patients with primary intra-axial tumors. Gross total excision, as measured by postoperative neuroimaging, is associated with prolonged survival in patients with malignant gliomas and probably in those with low-grade gliomas as well. However, most low-grade gliomas are not amenable to gross total excision, and usually only partial excision is feasible. Macroscopic tumor can frequently be removed completely in patients with high-grade gliomas, but there is always remaining microscopic disease that infiltrates surrounding brain.

Some tumors, such as brainstem gliomas, are in such critical locations that biopsy is not attempted. Their characteristic radiographic appearance permits diagnosis and initiation of medical treatment.

Radiation Therapy

A course of external beam radiation therapy is delivered in small daily fractions to a total cumulative dose usually between 45 and 60 Gy. Dividing the treatment into small daily fractions permits sublethal repair in normal tissues and markedly reduces neurologic toxicity associated with cerebral irradiation. External beam irradiation, which is the most effective nonsurgical treatment of brain tumors, doubles median survival time of patients with malignant primary brain tumors or metastatic lesions. It can also be useful for recurrent meningiomas and acoustic neuromas. However, it only rarely cures any of these lesions, and most patients develop recurrent disease despite maximal radiation therapy.

Stereotactic radiosurgery has been developed to deliver high fractions of focused radiation therapy that spare normal surrounding tissue. The technique is limited to tumors that are 3 cm in diameter or smaller and is less useful for malignant gliomas because of their infiltrative nature.

The neurologic complications of radiation therapy, which are usually observed in patients months to years after completion of treatment, include radionecrosis, dementia, and leukoencephalopathy. The incidence is reported as less than 5%, and most patients die of their brain tumor before the delayed consequences of treatment can be observed. However, in long-term survivors (e.g., patients with low-grade glioma or children with medulloblastoma), the late consequences of radiation therapy are important. Dementia accompanying radiation-induced leukoencephalopathy can progress and result in severe neurologic impairment. Radionecrosis can mimic recurrent tumor with a large contrast-enhancing lesion on MRI. Corticosteroids can reduce the edema and sometimes are sufficient to treat small areas of radionecrosis. However, if the lesion is sufficiently large, resection may be required to decompress the mass and reduce the steroid requirements.

Chemotherapy

Chemotherapy for brain tumors has usually been disappointing because of the intrinsic resistance of these tumors to most conventional agents. Carboplatin and cisplatin are active agents against medulloblastoma, even when the tumor is disseminated in the CSF. Temozolomide (150 to 200 mg/m^2 for 5 days every 4 weeks) is active in all gliomas, and high-dose methotrexate (3 to 8 g/m^2 for 3 to 12 months) is effective for primary CNS lymphoma. For patients with glioblastoma, polymers impregnated with carmustine (BCNU) and placed in a resection cavity offer modest benefit compared with no chemotherapy, but they are associated with local tissue injury and edema.

Specific Types of Brain Tumors

PRIMARY EXTRA-AXIAL TUMORS

The most common primary extra-axial tumors are meningiomas, pituitary adenomas, and acoustic neuromas. These tumors arise within the intracranial cavity but are not tumors of brain tissue. Almost all are benign; because the brain is rarely invaded, complete excision often enables cure with full recovery of neurologic function. These tumors produce neurologic symptoms and signs by compressing the underlying brain; however, edema of the underlying brain is infrequent, so glucocorticoids have a limited role.

Meningiomas

EPIDEMIOLOGY

Meningiomas are usually benign. Between 5 and 10% of meningiomas are atypical or malignant variants with a more aggressive course.[2] Meningiomas are more common in women, may be multiple in about 10% of patients with sporadic meningioma, and are occasionally part of a familial syndrome. They occur with increased frequency in patients with neurofibromatosis type 2. *NF2* inactivation is seen in approximately 50% of sporadic tumors, and mutations in *AKT1*, *SMO*, and *TRAF7* have also been identified.

DIAGNOSIS

Meningiomas grow slowly and produce symptoms that are insidious in onset and typically slowly progressive. Tumors can reach a considerable size, but they grow so slowly that the brain accommodates to the progressive compression. Meningiomas typically occur in specific locations: over the convexity, along the falx and parasagittal area, in the olfactory groove, at the base of the skull near the sphenoid bone, in the cavernous sinus (Fig. 189-3), in the cerebellopontine angle, and in the foramen magnum. Cortical and parasagittal tumors typically are manifested with seizures or progressive hemiparesis. Tumors in the anterior cranial fossa can cause slowly progressive changes in personality and cognition. Meningiomas at the base of the skull are manifested with cranial neuropathies and gait difficulties when there is brainstem compression. Frequently, tumors are completely asymptomatic and are identified on neuroimaging done for another purpose, such as head trauma.

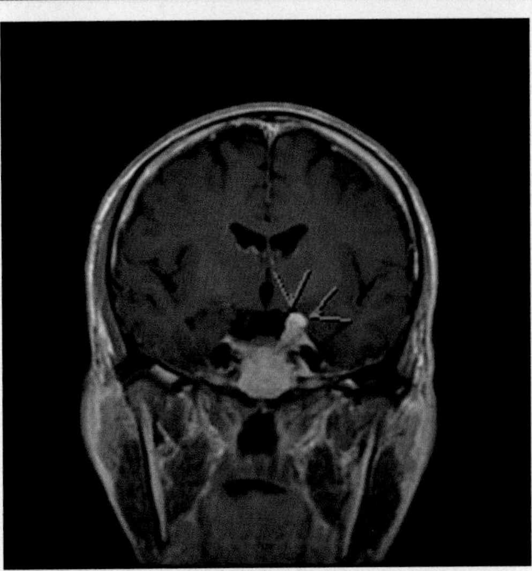

FIGURE 189-3. Skull base meningioma. A post-gadolinium coronal magnetic resonance image demonstrating a small left meningioma arising from the clinoid.

On MRI, meningiomas have a characteristic appearance consisting of a diffusely enhancing, dural-based lesion that is associated with a thin enhancing dural tail extending from the tumor. The radiographic features are often so characteristic that surgery is performed for therapeutic purposes only. The radiographic differential diagnosis includes the less common hemangiopericytoma and dural metastasis. Most meningiomas are not accompanied by significant edema, but marked edema is seen with high-grade malignant lesions or the secretory variant.

If small meningiomas are discovered in the absence of clinical symptoms or the symptoms are minor, lesions may be monitored with serial images because growth can be so slow.

TREATMENT Rx

If treatment is indicated, complete resection is often curative, but even completely resected benign tumors may recur (as many as 20% in some series), so radiologic follow-up is essential.[3] Tumors at the base of the skull often cannot be resected completely and tend to recur despite successive attempts at surgical resection. Stereotactic radiosurgery may be an alternative to surgery if the lesion is small or there is progressive or residual tumor. External beam radiation therapy may slow progression of recurrent lesions and is essential for the treatment of malignant meningiomas. No effective chemotherapy has yet been identified.[4]

Acoustic Neuromas

Acoustic neuromas (Chapter 428), better called vestibular schwannomas, are benign tumors that arise from the eighth cranial nerve. Acoustic neuromas are twice as common in women as in men; the peak age is between 40 and 60 years. Sporadic vestibular schwannomas are unilateral; bilateral acoustic neuromas are pathognomonic of neurofibromatosis type 2 (Chapter 417).

Acoustic neuromas usually arise from the vestibular portion of the nerve and typically are manifested with unilateral hearing loss, sometimes preceded or accompanied by tinnitus and a sensation of dizziness or unsteadiness but not true vertigo. The slow, progressive enlargement of the tumor produces ipsilateral facial numbness or weakness by compressing the fifth or seventh cranial nerve, respectively. Tumors originate within the internal auditory meatus but grow out of the acoustic canal and into the cerebellopontine angle, where they can compress the brainstem and cause ataxia and ipsilateral cerebellar signs. Cranial MRI with gadolinium delineates even small acoustic neuromas with ease (Fig. 189-4).

Treatment is often surgical; stereotactic radiosurgery may be an alternative for lesions smaller than 3 cm. It is preferable to treat the tumors when they are small to preserve facial nerve function and hearing.

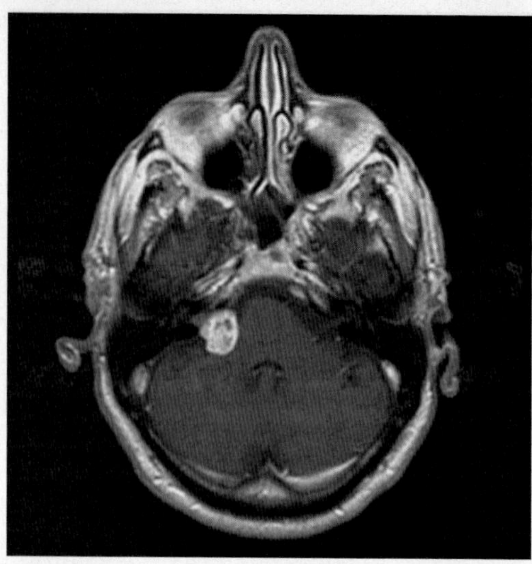

FIGURE 189-4. **Acoustic neuroma.** A post-gadolinium magnetic resonance image demonstrating a large right acoustic neuroma. The origin can be seen in the acoustic canal, but the tumor has grown into the cerebellopontine angle, where it is compressing the brainstem.

Pituitary Adenomas

Pituitary adenomas (Chapter 224) can be classified according to their size as microadenomas (<1 cm in diameter) or macroadenomas; by the presence or absence of endocrine function; and by the endocrinologic or neurologic syndromes caused by tumor compression. Microadenomas typically manifest with endocrine symptoms as described in Chapter 224. As pituitary tumors enlarge and become macroadenomas, they compress the surrounding neural structures, including the optic chiasm and optic nerves, typically causing bitemporal hemianopia and occasionally causing unilateral visual loss. Macroadenomas are frequently nonsecreting but destroy pituitary tissue, causing panhypopituitarism. Rarely, pituitary tumors manifest with the abrupt onset of headache, ophthalmoplegia, unilateral blindness, and even a depressed level of alertness or coma—a syndrome of *pituitary apoplexy* caused by hemorrhage or infarction.

Cranial MRI, particularly with coronal images and gadolinium administration, can completely outline the pituitary tumor and surrounding neural structures. All microadenomas and some macroadenomas can be treated with transsphenoidal pituitary surgery, which is associated with minimal morbidity. On occasion, residual or recurrent tumor necessitates radiation therapy. Some hormone-secreting tumors, particularly prolactinomas or growth hormone–secreting tumors, can be treated medically with cabergoline or somatostatin analogues such as octreotide, respectively (Chapter 224). These medications not only correct the hormonal excess but also shrink the tumor; they must be taken for life.

Other tumors in the pituitary and suprasellar region include craniopharyngiomas, suprasellar epidermoid cysts, Rathke cleft cysts, germinomas (discussed later), and lymphocytic hypophysitis, which is a benign inflammatory condition that usually is manifested with diabetes insipidus (Chapter 225). MRI frequently differentiates these conditions, which are usually suprasellar and erode into the pituitary fossa only secondarily. Some of these lesions also have characteristic radiographic features. These lesions are benign. Except for hypophysitis, which resolves completely with corticosteroid treatment (e.g., methylprednisolone 120 mg daily for 2 weeks and then tapered for 1 additional week), complete surgical excision is the curative therapy.

Other Extra-Axial Tumors

Pineal region tumors all have a characteristic clinical presentation that includes Parinaud syndrome, which consists of paresis of upward gaze, poor pupillary reaction to light with brisk reaction on accommodation, impairment of convergence, and convergence-retraction nystagmus. Some of these lesions may also cause hydrocephalus and symptoms of increased ICP. Pineal region tumors include pineal parenchymal tumors, such as pineocytomas and the more aggressive pineoblastomas, and germ cell tumors, including germinomas and nongerminomatous germ cell tumors. Germinomas can be completely cured with focal radiation therapy, whereas nongerminomatous germ cell tumors are more aggressive and frequently relapse despite chemotherapy plus cranial irradiation.

Chordomas are rare tumors of residual notochordal tissue. They usually occur at the base of the skull, are locally invasive, and are characterized by multiple recurrences despite surgery and radiation therapy. Chordomas are characterized by overexpression of the transcription factor brachyury. They also have activation of several receptor tyrosine kinases with overactivation of the downstream pathways, specifically the PI3K/AKT mTOR pathway. Inhibitors of the epidermal growth factor receptor and platelet-derived growth factor β have each been reported to produce responses and clinical benefit in patients with recurrent disease.[5] PI3K/AKT/mTOR inhibitors are under investigation.

Lipomas are benign tumors that can occur in midline structures, particularly near the corpus callosum. They can be cured by complete removal.

Arachnoid cysts are not tumors but can manifest with headache, seizures, or focal neurologic symptoms if they become large enough to compress underlying brain tissue. Many are completely asymptomatic and are found incidentally on neuroimaging. Only symptomatic cysts require removal.

PRIMARY INTRA-AXIAL TUMORS

Most primary intra-axial brain tumors are gliomas, including the astrocytomas, oligodendrogliomas, and ependymomas. Less common are medulloblastomas, other rare neuroectodermal tumors, and primary CNS lymphomas. All of these tumors have a tendency to invade brain tissue, and none can be completely excised surgically.

Glioma

DEFINITION

Astrocytomas, which are the most common glioma, are classified into one of four World Health Organization categories: grade I, the pilocytic astrocytoma; grade II, the fibrillary astrocytoma; grade III, the anaplastic astrocytoma; and grade IV, the glioblastoma. Pilocytic astrocytomas (grade I) are extremely low-grade focal tumors that are more common in children and may be associated with neurofibromatosis type 1; they are often cured by complete surgical excision. Fibrillary astrocytomas, anaplastic astrocytomas, and glioblastomas are diffuse tumors that infiltrate widely into brain; even grade II tumors progress over time, and most acquire the histologic features and growth patterns of grade III and IV tumors.

EPIDEMIOLOGY

Gliomas occur at any age, but the peak age is 20 to 30 years for an astrocytoma, 40 years for anaplastic astrocytoma, and 55 to 60 years for glioblastoma. Age is the single most important prognostic factor; younger patients live substantially longer than older patients. Histology is also critical; patients with glioblastoma do significantly worse than patients with lower-grade lesions. Performance status, duration of symptoms, and whether a complete resection has been achieved are also strong predictors of improved outcome and prolonged survival. For all grades of glioma, men are more frequently affected than women, and whites are significantly more frequently affected than blacks. Gliomas are typically single lesions, but multifocal disease is seen in approximately 5% of patients with high-grade tumors. A variant of gliomas, called gliomatosis cerebri, causes widespread infiltration of the entire brain; most patients have relatively low-grade pathologic findings on biopsy, but focal regions of high-grade transformation can exist.

PATHOBIOLOGY

At least 95% of gliomas are sporadic, and only 5% occur in patients with a family history of brain tumor. Furthermore, patients with a familial history of glioma usually do not fall into a well-recognized hereditary syndrome. However, neurofibromatosis 1 (von Recklinghausen disease; Chapter 417) is associated with an increased incidence of gliomas, particularly in the optic pathway, hypothalamus, and brainstem. Gliomas also occur with increased frequency in Turcot and Lynch syndrome, in which colorectal neoplasms are seen in association with a variety of CNS tumors. Somatic mutations of the isocitrate dehydrogenase 1 and 2 genes (*IDH1* and *IDH2*) have been identified in most low-grade gliomas and secondary glioblastomas; these patients have a better outcome than do those with wild-type *IDH* genes.[6] Molecular profiling has identified four subclasses of glioblastoma: (1) classical, defined by overactivation of the epidermal growth factor receptor pathway; (2) proneural, defined by *IDH* mutation and alterations of *PDGFRA* and expression of neural markers; (3) mesenchymal, defined by *NF1* loss and expression of mesenchymal markers; and (4) neural, characterized by expression of neuronal markers. These categories

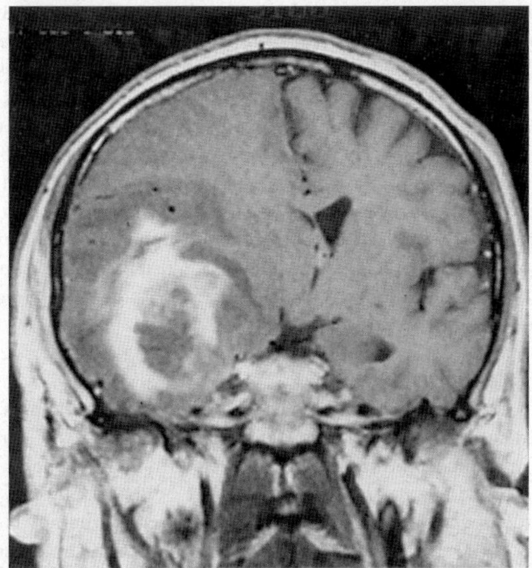

FIGURE 189-5. **Temporal lobe glioblastoma.** This T1-weighted gadolinium-enhanced magnetic resonance image shows a typical ring configuration of contrast material with central necrosis and marked mass effect.

define distinctly different pathways to histologically identical glioblastomas. The prognostic and therapeutic implications of these distinctions are under investigation.

CLINICAL MANIFESTATIONS AND DIAGNOSIS

Patients with gliomas often present with seizures, headache, and lateralizing signs such as hemiparesis, aphasia, or a visual field deficit.[7] On MRI, low-grade gliomas typically appear as diffuse, nonenhancing lesions with a propensity to occur in the frontal lobe and insular cortex. High-grade gliomas, which typically enhance with contrast material, occur in the cortical white matter and are accompanied by significant surrounding edema. Glioblastomas frequently have regions of central necrosis (Fig. 189-5), and hemorrhage can occur in 5 to 8% of patients.

TREATMENT Rx

For all gliomas, treatment frequently involves surgery, radiation therapy, and chemotherapy. The surgical goal of complete removal of all visible disease is often impossible. A prospective, randomized trial provided evidence for the use of intraoperative MRI guidance in optimizing the extent of resection of gliomas.[A2] The adequacy of resection is best assessed on a postoperative MRI study, without and with gadolinium, performed within 72 to 96 hours after surgery. Glioma resections with intraoperative stimulation mapping are associated with fewer severe neurologic deficits and more extensive resection. Surgical removal usually improves neurologic function and reduces dependency on corticosteroids.

Anaplastic Astrocytoma and Glioblastoma

All anaplastic astrocytomas and glioblastomas should be treated with postoperative radiation therapy to a dose of approximately 60 Gy. In a randomized trial of patients with glioblastoma, the alkylating agent temozolomide (75 mg/m^2 daily), administered concurrently with radiation therapy and followed by adjuvant temozolomide (150 to 200 mg/m^2 for 5 consecutive days every 4 weeks for six cycles), significantly improved survival (median, 14.6 months) compared with radiation therapy alone (median, 12.1 months; $P < .001$), and the 2-year survival rate more than doubled to 26.5%.[A3] Patients whose tumors contained a methylated promoter of the O^6-methylguanine-DNA methyltransferase (*MGMT*) DNA repair gene benefited most from the addition of temozolomide. On the basis of these data, combined treatment is the current standard of care for patients with glioblastoma. Chemotherapy is generally well tolerated and associated with minimal toxicity. Elderly patients often do poorly, but a randomized trial showed that radiation therapy (compared with supportive care only) results in a modest improvement in survival, without reducing quality of life or cognition, in elderly patients with glioblastoma.[A4] In the Nordic randomized phase III trial, standard radiation therapy was associated with poor outcomes in elderly patients with glioblastoma, especially those older than 70 years. Both temozolomide and hypofractionated radiation therapy should be considered as standard treatment options in elderly individuals with glioblastoma.[A5] The addition of bevacizumab (an anti-vascular endothelial growth factor molecule, initially at 10 mg/kg intravanously every 2 weeks) may further improve progression-free survival.[A6,A7] Recurrences can be treated with re-resection, additional chemotherapy or, occasionally, stereotactic radiosurgery or a combination of these. Despite aggressive treatment, disease recurs in almost all patients, and the median survival time is 15 months for glioblastoma. Patients with anaplastic gliomas (including anaplastic oligodendrogliomas) had an identical median survival of about 7 years whether the initial treatment was radiation therapy alone or chemotherapy alone.[A8] However, some young patients with anaplastic astrocytoma can survive much longer before the tumor recurs.

Optic and Brainstem Glioma

Optic gliomas, which can involve the optic nerve or optic chiasm, are usually associated with neurofibromatosis type 1. These gliomas are typically pilocytic tumors that can have an indolent course including rare spontaneous regression. They are often not amenable to surgical resection, and they can have a stuttering clinical course, with periods of visual loss punctuated by prolonged periods of visual stability. When necessary, radiation therapy or even chemotherapy may be useful, but often no treatment is required. Brainstem gliomas usually involve the pons, less often the medulla or midbrain. Brainstem gliomas are most commonly seen in children in the first decade of life but can be found even in elderly people; they can have a low-grade or high-grade histology, but outcome is primarily determined by the location of the tumor. In general, most brainstem gliomas have a dismal outcome with survival of 1 year or less, but relatively benign variants occasionally occur.

Low-Grade Astrocytoma

Low-grade astrocytomas have a variable course. In patients who present with isolated seizures that can be controlled easily with antiepileptics, treatment with radiation therapy or chemotherapy immediately after surgery may prolong progression-free but not overall survival, and such patients can be monitored until there is clinical or radiographic evidence of tumor progression. However, resection should be performed at diagnosis, if feasible.[8] Patients with progressive neurologic symptoms or cognitive impairment require immediate treatment after diagnosis, and focal radiation therapy to a total of about 54 Gy is the optimal choice. For low-grade gliomas, progression-free and overall survival appear to be better when chemotherapy is added to radiation therapy. An astrocytoma can progress as a low-grade tumor or transform to a higher-grade malignant neoplasm, a change that typically is associated with the appearance of contrast enhancement on MRI. Resection or a biopsy may be necessary in these patients, followed by radiation therapy if they have not received it previously; chemotherapy with temozolomide (150 to 200 mg/m^2 for 5 days every 4 weeks for anywhere from 6 to 24 cycles) is also used. Patients with an astrocytoma have a median survival of about 5 years, but the range is wide.

Oligodendroglioma

Oligodendrogliomas occur as low-grade tumors and, less commonly, as anaplastic lesions. Treatment of these tumors differs from that of their astrocytic counterparts because oligodendrogliomas are uniquely chemosensitive due to their characteristic loss of chromosomes 1p and 19q. As with the low-grade astrocytomas, treatment should be withheld in patients with low-grade oligodendrogliomas who have no symptoms other than well-controlled seizures. Patients with progressive neurologic symptoms or radiographic progression require treatment, and initial therapy is often chemotherapy, usually with single-agent temozolomide (150 to 200 mg/m^2 for 5 days every 4 weeks for 6 to 24 cycles) or the combination of procarbazine, lomustine, and vincristine (PCV). Radiation therapy is withheld until chemotherapy fails.

By comparison, all anaplastic oligodendrogliomas require immediate treatment. The standard approach includes focal radiation therapy. Adjuvant chemotherapy significantly prolongs disease-free and overall survival in patients with codeleted tumors but not in those with intact 1p and 19q chromosomes.[A9] However, there is a growing movement toward treatment of high-grade tumors with chemotherapy alone initially[9]; this can be considered only in neurologically healthy patients. Tumor progression should be treated with re-resection, radiation therapy if it has not been previously administered, and additional chemotherapy. Patients with low-grade oligodendrogliomas have a median survival time in excess of 15 years. Median survival is about 14 years for patients with a 1p/19q codeleted anaplastic oligodendroglioma compared with the median survival of about 3 years for patients with an intact 1p/19q.

Medulloblastoma

Medulloblastomas usually occur in the vermis of the cerebellum and principally affect children and young adults. Boys outnumber girls by about 2:1, and peak onset is 7 years of age; medulloblastoma in adulthood is rare and usually affects the cerebellar hemisphere.

Transcription profiles have identified four distinct subclasses that include: (1) the Wnt subtype driven by a stabilizing mutation in *CTNNB1* (β-catenin), which has an excellent prognosis; (2) the SHH subtype with mutations in *PTCH1, SMO, GLI2,* or *SUFU,* which has an intermediate prognosis; (3) group 3, which has an increased expression of *MYC* and has the worst prognosis; and (4) group 4, which is characterized by isochromosome 17q and marked male predominance. Medulloblastomas have a characteristic clinical presentation, with ataxia (due to cerebellar and brainstem involvement) and headache, nausea, and vomiting (due to increased ICP from obstructive hydrocephalus). Aggressive surgery with complete excision is strongly associated with improved outcome. Surgery is always followed by neuraxis radiation therapy. Chemotherapy with vincristine, etoposide, carboplatin, and cyclophosphamide significantly improves 5-year event-free survival from 60 to 74% but has not significantly prolonged overall survival, which is about 70 to 80% at 5 years when all patients are considered together. However, clinical high-risk patients do worse and standard-risk patients do better. It is unknown if molecular subclasses should supersede clinical stratification or dictate treatment selection. This vigorous therapy often results in delayed complications in survivors, including intellectual deficits, growth impairment, and endocrinologic dysfunction.[10] Late relapses as well as secondary neoplasms compromise long-term outcome.

Ganglioglioma

Gangliogliomas, as the name implies, possess both a glial component and a neoplastic neural component (ganglion cell). Some low-grade gangliogliomas are indolent and do not require additional treatment after surgical extirpation. Patients with anaplastic tumors may fare better than patients with malignant gliomas, but recurrence is the rule despite surgery and radiation therapy.

Primary Central Nervous System Lymphoma

Primary CNS lymphomas are associated with immunodeficiency states, particularly acquired immunodeficiency syndrome and organ transplantation, and are seen with increased frequency among the apparently immunocompetent population, in whom the median age at diagnosis is about 60 years. These tumors are usually diffuse large B-cell non-Hodgkin's lymphomas identical to systemic diffuse large B-cell lymphoma (Chapter 185). The tumor can involve the CSF, eye, and brain, where it is multifocal in about 40% of patients at presentation (Fig. 189-6). In contrast to all other brain tumors, surgical resection may not be associated with improved survival and can cause significant neurologic morbidity; therefore, biopsy is usually the preferred surgical approach. Chemotherapy is the primary treatment, and high-dose methotrexate (3 to 8 g/m^2 on alternate weeks for 3 to 12 months) is the most important chemotherapeutic agent. In most patients, radiation therapy is avoided because the necessary whole brain irradiation causes significant cognitive impairment when it is combined with chemotherapy and does not prolong survival.[A10] Corticosteroids (e.g., dexamethasone 8 to 16 mg/day), which are frequently used as part of the chemotherapeutic regimen, not only help manage the associated cerebral edema but also can cause tumor regression. With the use of multiagent chemotherapy, with or without cranial irradiation, median survival times is 3 to 5 years.

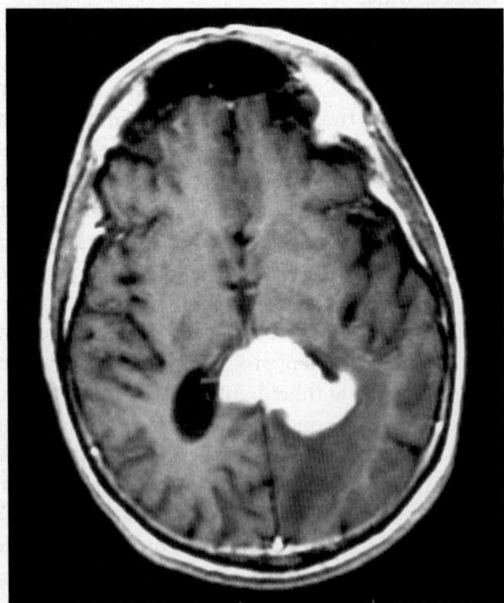

FIGURE 189-6. **Primary CNS lymphoma. A post-gadolinium magnetic resonance image demonstrating a diffusely enhancing splenial lesion. The periventricular location and absence of central necrosis are characteristic of primary CNS lymphoma.**

Other Intra-Axial Tumors

Rare, intra-axial cerebral tumors include the *ependymoma,* which is optimally treated with surgical excision followed by radiation therapy. *Choroid plexus papillomas* and *carcinomas* may be manifested with hydrocephalus or lateralizing signs. Resection may be sufficient for the benign papilloma, but carcinomas rapidly recur even when postoperative radiation therapy is also used. *Colloid cysts* of the third ventricle are benign tumors that can cause obstructive hydrocephalus; they may be treated with a third ventriculostomy or with resection by use of an intraventricular endoscope. *Hemangioblastomas* occur primarily in the cerebellum but can also occur in the spinal cord and the hemispheres. About 15% of patients with a hemangioblastoma have the autosomal dominant disorder von Hippel–Lindau disease (Chapter 417), which is characterized by hemangioblastomas in the CNS and retina, renal cell carcinoma, pheochromocytoma, endolymphatic sac tumors, and cysts in a variety of visceral organs. Hemangioblastomas are treated by surgical excision and require radiation therapy only for recurrence. Complete removal usually results in cure.

METASTATIC TUMOR

Brain Metastasis

DEFINITION AND EPIDEMIOLOGY

Every systemic cancer is capable of metastasizing to the brain. Melanoma (Chapter 203) has the greatest propensity to spread to the CNS, but the most common causes of CNS metastases are cancers of the breast (Chapter 198) and lung (Chapter 191), followed by cancers of the colon (Chapter 193) and kidney (Chapter 197). CNS metastases are being seen with greater frequency as patients with systemic cancers have prolonged survival with better treatments. In most patients with brain metastases, CNS disease develops late in the course of their illness, but a brain metastasis may be the initial presentation of a systemic cancer. In most of these patients, lung cancer is the primary site; in some, however, a primary site is never identified (Chapter 204).

CLINICAL MANIFESTATIONS AND DIAGNOSIS

Patients with brain metastases present with progressive neurologic symptoms and signs that typically include headache, seizures, and lateralizing signs. Metastases are best diagnosed by cranial MRI with gadolinium (Fig. 189-7). All lesions can be clearly seen by MRI, which is better than CT for visualizing the posterior fossa. Metastases, which are usually well-circumscribed lesions at the gray matter–white matter junction, are often associated with extensive edema. Hemorrhage into a metastasis occurs most frequently with metastases from melanoma, renal cancer, or thyroid cancer; however, because brain metastases from lung cancer are so common, they are the type most commonly associated with hemorrhage. Sometimes, hemorrhage into a brain metastasis is best visualized by noncontrast head CT.

TREATMENT Rx

Because brain metastases do not widely infiltrate into brain tissue and tend to have a pseudocapsule around them, they can be completely excised surgically. In randomized controlled studies, complete removal of a single brain metastasis substantially prolonged life and maintained neurologic function for a longer period. Postoperative whole brain radiation therapy significantly improves control of CNS disease after resection of a single brain metastasis, but it does not prolong survival because patients die of progressive systemic tumor. Consequently, the use of postoperative whole brain radiation therapy is frequently decided on an individual basis. If multiple lesions can be completely resected, these patients do as well as those with a single lesion that has been removed.

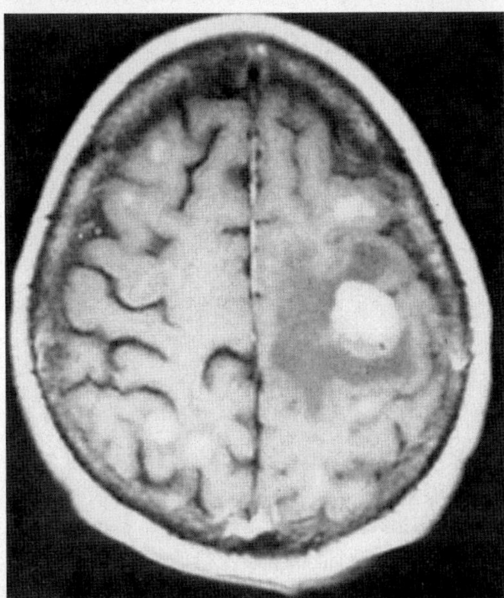

FIGURE 189-7. **Brain metastasis. Multiple metastases from breast carcinoma are seen on this T1-weighted gadolinium-enhanced magnetic resonance image. The multiple smaller tumors were not visible on computed tomography, even after a contrast agent was given.**

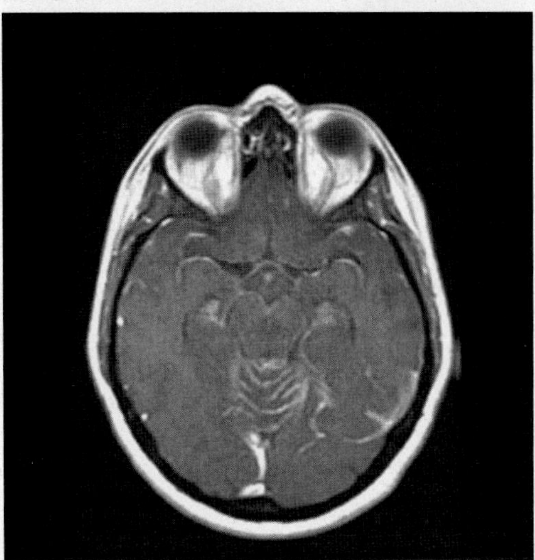

FIGURE 189-8. **Leptomeningeal metastases. A post-gadolinium cranial magnetic resonance image demonstrating enhancement of all sulci of the cerebellar vermis representing tumor cells in the subarachnoid space of this patient with breast cancer.**

Most patients with multiple brain metastases are best treated with a course of whole brain radiation therapy, most commonly 3 Gy in 10 fractions for a total of 30 Gy.[11] Some patients with single brain metastasis are also treated with whole brain irradiation if they are in poor general condition, have uncontrolled systemic disease, or are not good candidates for surgical treatment.

Stereotactic radiosurgery, with either a gamma knife that delivers gamma radiation from multiple cobalt sources or a linear accelerator that delivers x-rays to a highly focused area involving the tumor, has been effective for the treatment of one or a few brain metastases.[12] Most patients tolerate radiosurgery without difficulty, but the procedure is occasionally complicated by seizures or acute swelling that causes more neurologic dysfunction. Approximately 20 to 30% of patients develop radionecrosis, which may be indistinguishable clinically and on MRI from recurrent tumor. One advantage of stereotactic radiosurgery is that most of the normal brain is not exposed to the radiation.

Chemotherapy is used to treat brain metastases from only a few chemosensitive primary cancers, such as choriocarcinoma, small cell lung cancer, and, to a lesser extent, breast cancer. Because few patients have a significant response to chemotherapy, it is usually used as a last resort, although it has increasingly been employed in asymptomatic patients in whom brain metastases are identified at diagnosis on a screening MRI examination and who require chemotherapy for their systemic disease. The planned chemotherapy is often administered and the brain metastases will frequently respond in a fashion comparable to other systemic sites of disease. The choice of agents is based on the primary cancer type and the patient's prior drug exposures. Some targeted therapies have also been effective against brain metastases, such as in *BRAF* mutant melanoma, in which responses are seen after vemfurafenib.[13]

Leptomeningeal Metastasis

The brain is the most common intracranial site of metastases, but systemic cancer can spread to the dura and the leptomeninges as well. Dural metastases most commonly arise from breast (Chapter 198) or prostate (Chapter 201) cancer, frequently from a metastasis in the overlying calvaria, Metastasis to the leptomeninges often is manifested as multifocal neurologic symptoms and signs. These metastases involve the cranial nerves to cause diplopia or bulbar palsy (Fig. 189-8); the cervical and lumbar roots to cause limb pain or weakness; and the intracranial space to cause headache, nausea, vomiting, and elevated ICP. The diagnosis is established by the presence of tumor cells in the CSF, by cytologic examination or novel techniques to identify isolated cancer cells,[14] or by neuroimaging that definitively outlines tumor in the subarachnoid space (Fig. 189-9). Treatment frequently involves radiation therapy to symptomatic sites; intrathecal chemotherapy, usually through an intraventricular cannula (Ommaya reservoir); or systemic chemotherapy with agents or doses that penetrate into the CSF.

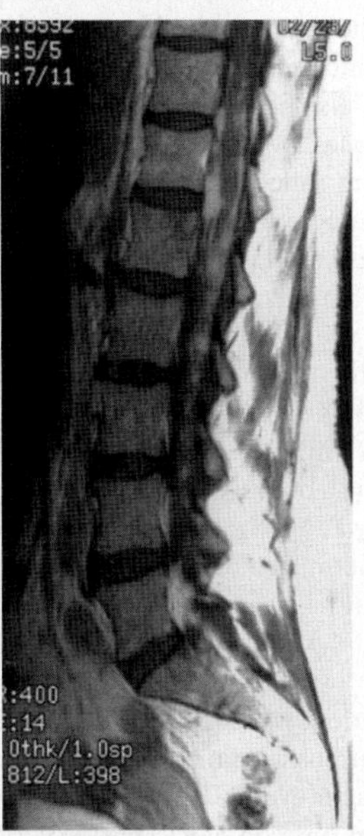

FIGURE 189-9. **Leptomeningeal metastases. Gadolinium-enhanced magnetic resonance imaging of the lumbosacral spine in a patient with leptomeningeal metastases from melanoma. Multiple enhancing nodules are seen on the cauda equina, and the conus medullaris and lower spinal cord are encased by tumor.**

SPINAL TUMORS

Tumors involving the spine can be classified according to the anatomic area they involve: extradural, intradural extramedullary, and intramedullary tumors (Table 189-5). Extradural tumors typically arise from the bone elements of the spine and cause neurologic symptoms and signs by spinal cord compression. Intradural but extramedullary tumors arise from the pachymeninges or nerve roots (meningiomas or schwannomas) and can cause either radicular symptoms or spinal cord compression. Intramedullary spinal cord tumors are rare; they arise from the spinal cord parenchyma and have a biology similar to that of brain tumors.

Extradural Tumors

EPIDEMIOLOGY AND CLINICAL MANIFESTATIONS

Most extradural tumors originate from a metastasis to the bone elements of the spine, typically the vertebral body and occasionally the vertebral lamina or spinous process. Less common are primary tumors of the spine, including chordoma, osteogenic sarcoma, plasmacytoma, and chondrosarcoma. Expansile growth of the bone tumor impinges on the spinal canal and, if untreated, compresses the spinal cord or the nerve roots as they exit the intervertebral foramina. Whereas most of these lesions arise from bone

TABLE 189-5 SPINAL TUMORS

Extradural
- Metastasis
- Primary bone tumors arising in the spine
  - Chordoma
  - Osteogenic sarcoma
  - Chondrosarcoma
  - Plasmacytoma

Intradural extramedullary
- Meningiomas
- Neurofibromas
- Schwannomas
- Lipomas
- Arachnoid cysts
- Epidermoid cysts
- Metastasis

Intramedullary
- Ependymoma
- Glioma
- Hemangioblastoma
- Lipoma
- Metastasis

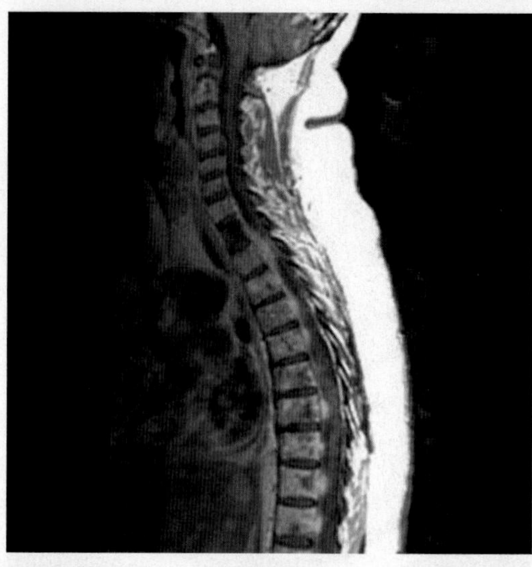

FIGURE 189-10. Multilevel epidural spinal cord compression. This patient with metastatic breast cancer has multiple areas of ventral epidural tumor seen throughout the thoracic spine on this post-gadolinium sagittal magnetic resonance image.

metastases, extradural tumors can also arise from paravertebral metastases that can grow through the intervertebral foramina and into the epidural space without affecting surrounding bone structures; very rarely, a direct metastasis to the epidural space is also seen. The most common primary cancers that cause extradural metastases are prostate cancer (Chapter 201), breast cancer (Chapter 198), and lung cancer (Chapter 191) as well as the lymphomas (Chapter 185). Hematologic malignant neoplasms may also be associated with paravertebral disease that grows through the intervertebral foramina.

Whether the mass is a primary bone tumor or a metastasis from a distant source, 98% of patients present with pain that is usually localized to the site of the tumor. Because there are more thoracic than cervical or lumbar vertebrae, the tumor and pain are likely to be in the middle or high back, a less common site for benign pain (Chapter 400). Motor impairment and sensory symptoms are present in about 50% of patients, whereas sphincter disturbances are found in only about 25% of patients. Back pain often precedes the development of any other neurologic symptom or sign, frequently by weeks and occasionally by months.

DIAGNOSIS

Severe back pain in a patient with cancer should be evaluated by MRI which does not require intravenous administration of contrast material. Plain films of the spine, bone scans, or even CT scans may show bone disease, but epidural tumor can be seen only on MRI (Fig. 189-10). Furthermore, MRI is the only technique that can reveal paravertebral or direct epidural metastasis. Patients who cannot have an MRI study should be imaged by CT with sagittal reconstruction images.

Differential Diagnosis

The differential diagnosis of extradural tumors includes epidural abscess (Chapter 413), acute or subacute epidural hematomas (Chapter 400), herniated intervertebral discs (Chapter 400), spondylosis (Chapter 400), epidural lipomatosis, and, rarely, extramedullary hematopoiesis. On occasion, a percutaneous needle biopsy or decompressive laminectomy is required to make a definitive diagnosis.

TREATMENT Rx

Epidural metastases require immediate treatment because patients can develop acute and unpredictable neurologic deterioration resulting in paraplegia. Patients should be started on high-dose corticosteroids (usually >20 mg IV dexamethasone), which rapidly relieve pain and may contribute to neurologic recovery. Surgery followed by postoperative radiation therapy is superior to radiation therapy alone in preserving the ability to walk and may prolong survival in a wide population of patients with metastatic spinal cord compression, but its advantage may be lost in patients 65 years of age and older.[A11] It is much easier to preserve neurologic function than to reverse impairment, so clinically silent areas of extradural tumor that are detected on MRI should be treated before neurologic compromise develops. Patients with epidural metastasis can have a good neurologic outcome if they are treated before the onset of severe neurologic compromise, but their overall survival is usually short because of the presence of widespread metastatic disease. Patients whose primary tumor arises in the spine, such as an osteogenic sarcoma (Chapter 202), should undergo definitive surgery; the need for postoperative radiation therapy is based on the tumor's histology.

Intradural Extramedullary Tumors

Meningiomas

Most intradural extramedullary tumors are benign. Meningiomas are benign, slow-growing tumors that occur primarily in middle-aged women and are predominantly located in the thoracic region. Back pain is a common symptom, but about 25% of patients have no pain and present with slowly progressive neurologic dysfunction, typically a gait disorder that has been progressing, frequently for years. Spinal MRI with gadolinium clearly delineates the lesion. Surgical resection is curative, and a complete resection can usually be accomplished easily.

Nerve Sheath Tumors

Nerve sheath tumors include schwannomas and neurofibromas. Both typically arise from the dorsal root, and the first symptom is often radicular pain that precedes symptoms of spinal cord compression by months or even years. Some patients with spinal neurofibroma or schwannoma have neurofibromatosis type 1 (Chapter 417), but most do not. The diagnosis is clearly established by gadolinium-enhanced MRI of the spine. The treatment is surgical, and complete removal results in cure.

Metastases

Metastasis to the spinal leptomeninges can be manifested as an intradural extramedullary lesion. A single large tumor nodule can cause focal symptoms and signs referable to that spinal level, but in most patients, multiple levels of the neuraxis are involved, causing multifocal neurologic symptoms and signs. Cervical and lumbosacral radicular pain as well as sensory and motor loss is seen in more than half of patients. The diagnosis is established by gadolinium-enhanced MRI showing multifocal nodules or sometimes a layer of cells coating the spinal cord or nerve roots (see Fig. 189-9). If imaging is negative, the diagnosis can be established by demonstrating tumor cells in the CSF. Treatment is complicated and frequently requires radiation therapy to symptomatic sites of disease, intrathecal chemotherapy best administered through an intraventricular cannula (Ommaya device), and occasionally systemic chemotherapy. Radiation therapy can ameliorate neurologic symptoms, particularly pain, but the disease often has a relentless progressive course, resulting in death in 3 to 6 months despite aggressive therapy. Because of the diffuse nature of the disease, surgery is not an option.

Intramedullary Tumors

Intramedullary spinal cord tumors are similar to neoplasms that arise in brain parenchyma. The most common spinal cord tumors are ependymomas and

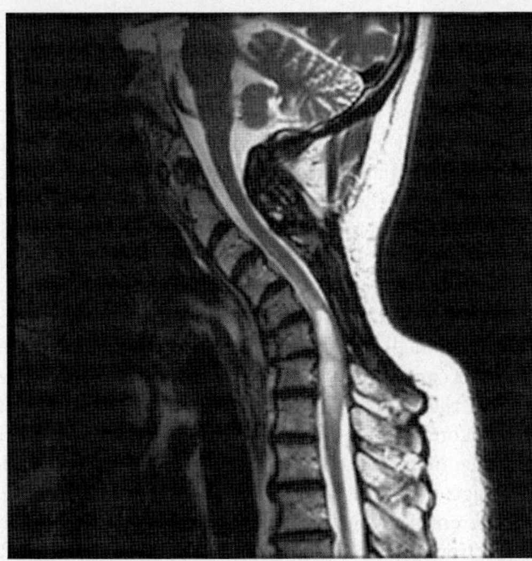

FIGURE 189-11. **Spinal cord astrocytoma.** T2-weighted sagittal magnetic resonance image demonstrating a lower cervical intramedullary low-grade astrocytoma; no enhancement was evident.

astrocytomas; hemangioblastomas (particularly in association with von Hippel–Lindau disease; Chapter 417), lipomas, and, rarely, intramedullary metastases are also seen.

CLINICAL MANIFESTATIONS AND DIAGNOSIS

All intramedullary tumors have a similar clinical presentation, and pain is a common initial symptom. Signs of spinal cord dysfunction subsequently ensue and reflect the location of the lesion. In addition, some intramedullary tumors are accompanied by a syrinx (Chapter 417), which can contribute to symptoms. The classic signs of intramedullary spinal cord lesions, such as dissociated sensory loss, sacral sparing, and early sphincter problems, are not sufficiently reliable to distinguish intramedullary from extramedullary lesions on the basis of clinical findings. The diagnosis is established by gadolinium-enhanced and T2-weighted MRI (Fig. 189-11).

TREATMENT Rx

Surgery is the first therapeutic intervention, both to obtain a definitive diagnosis and to resect the lesion. Complete resection of spinal cord tumors is possible, particularly in the case of ependymomas and hemangioblastomas. However, spinal cord tumors are rare, and only neurosurgeons experienced in removal of this type of lesion should perform the procedure. High-grade gliomas and residual ependymomas should be treated with postoperative radiation therapy.[15] Low-grade astrocytomas of the spinal cord can be treated with radiation therapy when the patient develops symptomatic neurologic impairment, but presymptomatic treatment does not prevent the development of impairment nor necessarily delay it. Intramedullary metastases do not require surgery because the diagnosis is usually straightforward; radiation therapy provides limited benefit because these patients typically have other CNS metastases.

Grade A References

A1. Mikkelsen T, Paleologos NA, Robinson PD, et al. The role of prophylactic anticonvulsants in the management of brain metastases: a systematic review and evidence-based clinical practice guideline. *J Neurooncol.* 2010;96:97-102.

A2. Senft C, Bink A, Franz K, et al. Intraoperative MRI guidance and extent of resection in glioma surgery: a randomised, controlled trial. *Lancet Oncol.* 2011;12:997-1003.

A3. Stupp R, Hegi ME, Mason WP, et al. Effects of radiotherapy with concomitant and adjuvant temozolomide versus radiotherapy alone on survival in glioblastoma in a randomised phase III study: 5-year analysis of the EORTC-NCIC trial. *Lancet Oncol.* 2009;10:459-466.

A4. Keime-Guibert F, Chinot O, Taillandier L, et al. Radiotherapy for glioblastoma in the elderly. *N Engl J Med.* 2007;356:1527-1535.

A5. Malmström A, Gronberg BH, Maroşi C, et al. Temozolomide versus standard 6-week radiotherapy versus hypofractionated radiotherapy in patients older than 60 years with glioblastoma: the Nordic randomized, phase 3 trial. *Lancet Oncol.* 2012;13:916-926.

A6. Chinot OL, Wick W, Mason W, et al. Bevacizumab plus radiotherapy-temozolomide for newly diagnosed glioblastoma. *N Engl J Med.* 2014;370:709-722.

A7. Gilbert MR, Dignam JJ, Armstrong TS, et al. A randomized trial of bevacizumab for newly diagnosed glioblastoma. *N Engl J Med.* 2014;370:699-708.

A8. Wick W, Hartmann C, Engel C, et al. NOA-04 randomized phase III trial of sequential radiochemotherapy of anaplastic glioma with procarbazine, lomustine, and vincristine or temozolomide. *J Clin Oncol.* 2009;27:5874-5880.

A9. Cairncross G, Wang M, Shaw E, et al. Phase III trial of chemoradiotherapy for anaplastic oligodendroglioma: long-term results of RTOG 9402. *J Clin Oncol.* 2013;31:337-343.

A10. Thiel E, Korfel A, Martus P, et al. High-dose methotrexate with or without whole brain radiotherapy for primary CNS lymphoma (G-PCNSL-SG-1): a phase 3, randomized, non-inferiority trial. *Lancet Oncol.* 2010;11:1036-1047.

A11. Chi JH, Gokaslan Z, McCormick P, et al. Selecting treatment for patients with malignant epidural spinal cord compression—does age matter? Results from a randomized clinical trial. *Spine.* 2009;34:431-435.

GENERAL REFERENCES

For the General References and other additional features, please visit Expert Consult at https://expertconsult.inkling.com.

190 HEAD AND NECK CANCER

MARSHALL R. POSNER

DEFINITION

The principal cancers of the head and neck include squamous cell cancers arising from the mucosal surfaces of the upper aerodigestive tract and a diverse group of salivary gland neoplasms. Unique cancers of the region include Epstein-Barr virus (EBV)–associated nasopharyngeal carcinoma, human papillomavirus (HPV)–associated oropharynx cancer (HPVOPC), thyroid malignant neoplasms (Chapter 226), esthesioneuroblastoma, and sinonasal undifferentiated carcinoma. A variety of other cancers arise from structures and tissues in the head and neck, including the more common skin cancers (Chapter 203), lymphomas (Chapters 185 and 186), and sarcomas (Chapter 202).

EPIDEMIOLOGY

Squamous cell carcinomas account for 95% of all malignant neoplasms of the head and neck, whereas salivary gland cancers represent nearly all of the remaining 5%. They represent 4% of all malignant neoplasms in the United States. Squamous cell cancers of the head and neck can be divided into two distinct groups based on pathogenesis, biology, and prognosis. Environmentally related cancers, caused principally by tobacco and alcohol, have been declining in incidence; however, they remain common. There has been an increasing incidence of HPV-related oropharynx cancer.[1] HPVOPC now represents about 75% of oropharynx cancers seen in the United States and Europe.[2] HPVOPC affects a younger population (50 to 60 years) than environmental cancers do (55 to 65 years). HPVOPC patients are also generally healthier and are not prone to comorbid illnesses and second cancers seen in environmentally related squamous cancers.

The mucosal surfaces of the head and neck are divided into six anatomic regions: the oral cavity, oropharynx, hypopharynx, larynx, nasopharynx, and paranasal sinuses. The site of anatomic origin for a squamous cell carcinoma of the head and neck has important albeit imperfectly defined implications for diagnosis, pathogenesis, spread, prognosis, and treatment. This is because of intrinsic differences in the biology of the mucosal cells and subsequent cancers at the sites of origin, carcinogenic viral tropisms, and differences in lymphatic drainage patterns and proximity to other structures in this compact region.

Oral Cavity

The oral cavity includes the floor of the mouth, anterior or oral aspect of the tongue, lips, buccal surfaces, hard palate, retromolar trigone, and gums. This region is easily appreciable by physical examination, and thus tumors in this area can frequently be detected early in their course. Tumors of the oral cavity, which are strongly related to the use of smokeless tobacco and other oral tobacco products (Chapter 32) and, in southern Asia, to betel nut and pan chewing, appear on the mid oral tongue and buccal and gingival surfaces in the sites where these products are held in contact with the mucosa for long periods. Anterior tongue cancers are more common in smokers. Lip cancers are particularly prevalent in transplant recipients and can be caused by DNA damage from solar ultraviolet light.

Oropharynx

The oropharynx consists of the tongue from the circumvallate papillae posteriorly to the epiglottis, the tonsils, the associated pharyngeal walls, and the soft palate. The oropharynx has become the most common location for head and neck tumors in the United States and is a common site of origin in Europe. This is due to a high rate of HPVOPC, which continues to increase in incidence.[3] HPVOPC is caused almost exclusively by HPV-16, a high-risk HPV type associated with cervical, anal, and vulvar cancers. Other high-risk HPV types account for 10 to 15% of new diagnoses. High-risk HPV types are transmitted in body fluids and infect squamous mucosal surfaces of the anogenital tract and the oropharynx. Whereas smoking does not increase the risk of HPVOPC, 50% of smokers with oropharynx cancer have HPV as a cause. Compared with environmental cancers, HPVOPC often presents with lower primary T stage (T1 and T2) and higher nodal stage (N2 and N3), and it is frequently a cause of cancer of unknown primary origin (Chapter 204) because of small and difficult-to-identify primary tumors.[4]

Hypopharynx

The hypopharynx comprises the piriform sinuses, the lateral and posterior pharyngeal walls, and the posterior surfaces of the larynx. These structures surround the larynx posteriorly and laterally. Tumors in this region can be difficult to detect because of the recesses and spaces surrounding the larynx. As a result, primary hypopharyngeal tumors may be asymptomatic and, like oropharyngeal tumors, may initially be recognized in an advanced state or diagnosed as an unknown primary (Chapter 204). These tumors are associated with tobacco (Chapter 32) and alcohol (Chapter 33) use.

Larynx

The larynx includes the vocal cords, the subglottis, and the supraglottic larynx as well as the thyroid, cricoid, and arytenoid cartilages. Tumors arising in the true vocal cords are frequently symptomatic early and rarely spread beyond the confines of the larynx, whereas subglottic and supraglottic cancers can be relatively asymptomatic and have a much higher and earlier risk of spread to the lymphatics and regional sites. Laryngeal cancers are strongly associated with smoking (Chapter 32).

Nasopharynx

The nasopharynx includes the mucosal surfaces and structures of the cavity behind the nasal passages. Nasopharyngeal cancers are common in the Pacific Rim, northern Africa, and the Middle East. In some areas of China and Southeast Asia, nasopharyngeal cancers occur with a frequency that rivals that of lung cancer. In North America, there are about 2000 cases each year, but numbers are increasing as high-risk ethnic populations settle in North America. Nasopharyngeal cancers are frequently associated with the presence of latent infection of the epithelial tumor cells by EBV, the etiologic agent of infectious mononucleosis (Chapter 377). Nasopharyngeal cancers are also associated with both environmental and genetic factors in susceptible populations that have migrated to North America and remain at high risk for this disease. Unlike other squamous cell carcinomas of the head and neck, nasopharyngeal cancers can occur at an early age, with a distinct peak in adolescence and young adulthood. Nasopharyngeal cancers are categorized into three histologic subtypes by the World Health Organization (WHO): the undifferentiated (WHO III) and nonkeratinizing forms (WHO II) are latently infected with EBV in 95% of cases and represent the majority of cases in North America and worldwide; the well-differentiated (WHO I) form is rarer and represents about 5% worldwide but about 15 to 25% of all nasopharyngeal cancers in North America, and it is usually associated with traditional risk factors such as smoking. Nasopharyngeal cancers have a high risk of early regional lymph node involvement, a prolonged natural history, and a very high risk of spread to distant sites.

Paranasal Sinuses

The paranasal sinuses comprise the maxillary, ethmoid, sphenoid, and frontal sinuses as well as the nasal cavity. These are relatively rare locations for tumors of the head and neck in North America, but there is an unexplained higher rate of malignant sinus disease among the Japanese. Squamous maxillary sinus cancers are more common in smokers. Up to 50% of cancers of the sinuses may be of salivary gland origin. Adenocarcinomas have often been related to exposure to dust from woodworking, tanning, or leather working (Chapter 19). On occasion, neuroendocrine tumors and the rare sinonasal undifferentiated carcinoma are found. Sinus cancers are frequently diagnosed late in their course at the time of symptomatic invasion of surrounding structures, including the orbit, nasal cavity, base of the skull, and cranial nerves.

Salivary Glands

Salivary glands occur in all the regions described as well as in the trachea and esophagus. Tumors can develop in all of the major and minor salivary glands with an incidence that is roughly proportional to the quantity of glandular tissue. The most common single site is the parotid. Although tumors can develop at any age, including childhood, the peak incidence is between 55 and 65 years of age. Salivary gland cancers have diverse histologic findings and manifest different behavior on the basis of their histologic classification. A substantial fraction of parotid salivary tumors can be benign. Risk factors for salivary gland cancers are poorly understood, but previous radiation therapy in adjacent areas increases the risk (Chapter 20).

PATHOBIOLOGY

Tobacco products and alcohol are major etiologic and risk factors for squamous cell carcinoma of the head and neck. Both show a clear dose response. Any irritating smoked product increases the risk for local cancer, but nicotine in tobacco as well as in other tobacco leaf components directly affects the oral mucosa and increases the risk for squamous cancer (Chapter 32). Alcohol is also a carcinogen, and alcohol consumption (Chapter 33) as well as its direct application in mouthwashes is associated with an increased risk. Moreover, alcohol affects local and systemic detoxification enzymes and may increase the carcinogenic potential of other environmental carcinogens. Other environmental risk factors include radiation exposure and solar radiation; welding, metal refining, diesel and wood stove exhaust, and asbestos exposure; chronic irritants; vitamin A deficiency; and immunosuppression.

Carcinogenic viruses are responsible for the increasing incidence of head and neck cancer in the United States and Europe. Pathogenic HPV subtypes, most frequently HPV-16, independently account for approximately 75% of oropharyngeal cancer cases. HPV is transmitted by epithelial contact and body fluids. There is increased risk of HPVOPC associated with increasing numbers of individual sexual partners, although the majority of HPVOPC patients do not have sexual activity above the average. HPV DNA can be found in the tumor cells, and the oncogenic viral proteins E6 and E7 are frequently expressed and are responsible and necessary for the growth and survival of the cancer cells by affecting critical signaling pathways. Men have a three-fold greater incidence of HPVOPC than women do, although the cause for this imbalance in incidence is not known. Of great importance, HPVOPC patients have a three-fold better prognosis than that of patients with environmentally related cancers. This is due to three factors: fewer comorbid illnesses in patients with HPVOPC; few second cancers caused by tobacco and alcohol; and increased sensitivity of HPVOPC tumors to treatments. The majority of nasopharyngeal cancer is caused by another more complex virus that infects keratinocytes, EBV (Chapter 377). The classic nasopharyngeal cancer, which is also called *lymphoepithelioma*, is associated with a brisk lymphoid infiltrate that can be confused with a lymphoma. Careful examination reveals the malignant epithelial cells, with EBV detectable in the tumor cells. EBV is also rarely associated with epithelial tumors of the oropharynx, tonsil, and salivary gland.

Several inherited diseases and genetic abnormalities are associated with the development of head and neck cancer.[5,6] Fanconi anemia (Chapter 165), a rare disorder of a family of related gene products, has been linked to the development of tongue cancer, as has Cowden syndrome (Chapter 181), which is associated with mutation of the *PTEN* gene. *NOTCH1* may function as a tumor suppressor gene rather than as an oncogene in head and neck squamous cell carcinoma. Finally, common inherited allelic variants of the alcohol dehydrogenase and P-450 genes may be associated with increased susceptibility to alcohol and other environmental carcinogens.

The development of environmentally related squamous cell carcinoma of the head and neck is a multistep process in which early genetic changes evolve into frank malignancy. In environmentally related cancers, an abnormal premalignant clone of mucosal cells may be localized to a single site within the head and neck, or clones may occur independently in many sites. The

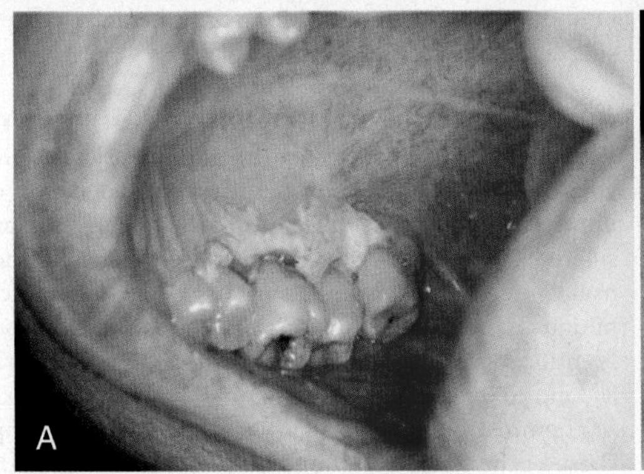

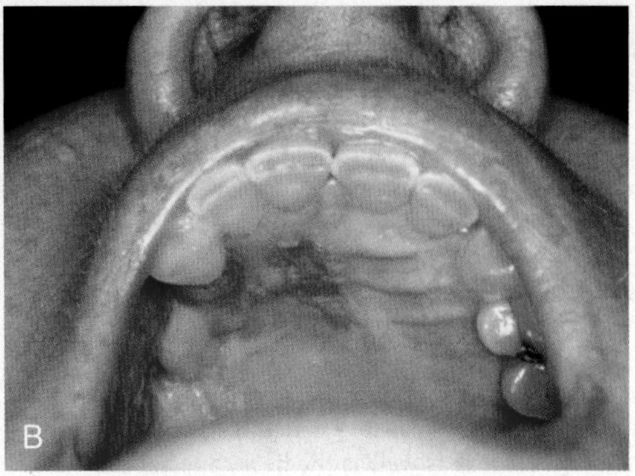

FIGURE 190-1. **High-risk early mouth lesions. A, Oral leukoplakia. B, Oral erythroplakia.**

pathogenesis of HPVOPC is less well understood. Second cancers are rare with HPVOPC in the short term, and long-term risk is unknown. In contrast, about 20% of patients with environmentally caused cancers will develop a second primary cancer, most commonly in the head and neck, lung, and esophagus; 5% of patients are initially seen with a synchronous second primary. In environmentally related cancers, the cell cycle is dysregulated by the early loss of p16, an inhibitor of cyclin D1, or by upregulation of cyclin D1; p53 is disabled through a number of mechanisms preventing programmed cell death; mitogenic signaling is enhanced by upregulation of epidermal growth factor (EGF) receptor function; cyclooxygenase 2 is overexpressed, thereby inhibiting apoptosis and promoting angiogenesis; and chromosomal instability with aneuploidy develops. Many of these early molecular and functional changes occur without obvious alteration in the physical appearance of the oral mucosa, although leukoplakia can occur. In HPVOPC, the RB and p53 pathways are inactivated by the HPV oncogenic proteins E6 and E7. As a result, the p16 protein is upregulated as a biomarker of HPV tumor origin. As a consequence of RB and p53 inactivation, these patients have dysregulation of cell growth and DNA damage control/programmed cell death, respectively. The differences between the genetic and molecular determinants of cancer in HPVOPC and environmentally related cancers can be differentially targeted for therapy.

In environmentally related cancers, high-risk early lesions can occasionally be identified as leukoplakia and erythroplakia. Leukoplakia (Fig. 190-1A) is diagnosed clinically as a white patch of mucosal tissue in the oral mucosa or larynx. It can unpredictably progress to cancer during a period of several years in approximately 30% of patients. Erythroplakia (Fig. 190-1B), a red hyperkeratotic change in the mucosa, is a more advanced premalignant lesion with an approximately 60% rate of progression to oral cancer. Surgical resection of leukoplakia or erythroplakia has no effect on the subsequent development of invasive cancer. There is no proven chemopreventive therapy for persons with oral premalignant lesions. Because continued smoking or alcohol consumption increases the risk for recurrence and second primaries dramatically, patients with prior environmentally related cancers should stop alcohol and tobacco use.

CLINICAL MANIFESTATIONS

The symptoms and clinical manifestations of tumors in the head and neck can vary broadly and are related to the structures at the site of the primary tumor as well as regional lymph node drainage. Small tumors of the oral cavity and larynx can be easily appreciated because of physical self-discovery or early compromise of the function of a critical structure. As a result of the propensity for squamous cell carcinoma of the head and neck to remain a local and regional disease, it is unusual for this cancer to be associated with abnormalities outside the head and neck. Salivary gland malignant neoplasms are less constrained and frequently spread distantly; however, because the primary tumors are also frequently accessible to direct physical examination and early discovery, it is still uncommon to identify these tumors as a result of metastatic spread outside the region.

Clinical manifestations of *tumors in the oral cavity* include a painless lump, a painful mass or ulcer, or simple thickening of the mucosa. Small lesions in the lateral aspect of the tongue and the floor of the mouth can cause pain referred to the mandible, gums, and ear because of the shared sensory nerves supplying these areas. Antibiotics can relieve symptoms and even reduce the size of a tumor or lymph nodes when superficial infection and inflammation are contributing to the pain; however, recurrent or continued pain in an adult should trigger early suspicion about more ominous disease. Speech may be affected late if the tumor causes restricted tongue motion or cranial nerve XII dysfunction. Gingival tumors can loosen teeth and invade the mandible along tooth sockets.

In true vocal cord cancer, hoarseness and other forms of voice change are common and expected early symptoms, but they may be later manifestations of *supraglottic and subglottic laryngeal tumors,* which become relatively large without affecting the voice. Tumors of the piriform sinus can affect the voice when they become large and impair the recurrent laryngeal nerve or are associated with deep local invasion; pain in the ear or pain on swallowing referred to the ear is also a common and important feature of these tumors. Adults with ear pain or persistent hoarseness should be referred to an otolaryngologist for evaluation. Because this posterior area is difficult to assess directly, primary tumors are frequently missed in routine office examinations. *Tumors of the supraglottic region, subglottic cancers, and cancers of the piriform sinus* can also be manifested as acute, emergency airway obstruction. Frequently, patients have a history of wheezing and mild upper airway distress in the period leading up to the emergency situation. On occasion, such findings are confused with adult-onset asthma.

A middle ear infection or effusion in an adult should also prompt an ear, nose, and throat evaluation. Nasopharyngeal cancer may be manifested as an ear infection in young adults. Hemoptysis or epistaxis may be the only clue to a nasopharyngeal cancer or a *paranasal sinus tumor*. Cranial nerve findings from deep invasion of the base of the skull are late events and include lateral gaze abnormalities, diplopia, facial pain, or facial nerve paralysis. *Sinus tumors* can also be associated with these later findings, although nasal stuffiness occurs frequently and can be confused with sinusitis. New and persistent symptoms of sinusitis or facial pain should raise suspicion of sinus cancer and prompt an evaluation.

Tumors in the tonsil or base of the tongue can cause local pain and referred ear pain; however, they are frequently asymptomatic and can attain a large size before becoming evident as a result of changes in speech ("hot potato voice"), a sense of globus, trismus, or restriction of tongue movement. Manifestation as a painless lump in the neck is increasingly common with the increased incidence of HPVOPC. Tumors of the tonsil or base of the tongue may also lose their mucosal component, not be seen or felt on direct inspection, and occur as a solid or cystic neck mass. Isolated neck masses can wax and wane with antibiotics. A mass, especially a cystic mass, in the neck in an adult is cancer and specifically HPVOPC until proved otherwise and should prompt an ear, nose, and throat evaluation and positron emission tomography (PET)/computed tomography (CT) imaging, fine-needle aspiration, and examination under anesthesia before excisional biopsy.

The staging of squamous cell carcinoma of the head and neck is based on the TNM (tumor, node, metastasis) staging system, and prognosis is related primarily to the N and T stages. The risk of the cancer's spreading to lymph nodes is directly related to the location of the primary and secondarily to the size of the primary. Tumors of the oropharynx have a high risk for nodal metastases, followed in risk by the supraglottic larynx and piriform sinus (hypopharynx), oral portion of the tongue, soft palate, oral cavity and floor of the mouth, and larynx. Nasopharyngeal cancer is often associated with extensive nodal spread, whereas paranasal sinus cancers rarely spread to the lymph nodes. The location of lymph node spread is determined in part by site. Nasopharyngeal cancer spreads to the posterior cervical lymph nodes as well as to the high cervical nodes. Oropharynx, larynx, and piriform sinus tumors spread to the high cervical nodes. Nodal metastases from these locations can be bilateral. Oral cavity tumors spread to the submental nodes and submandibular nodes. Spread tends to be orderly from the submandibular nodes to the midcervical nodes. Oral cavity cancers can have as high as a 20% risk of clinically unappreciated contralateral spread.

DIAGNOSIS

The relative accessibility of the head and neck to direct inspection makes physical examination critical for diagnosis and staging. Patients with localized symptoms or a sign such as an ulcer or a small mass should have a thorough head and neck office examination performed by their primary physician and by a specialist, including inspection of the visible structures and palpation of the base of the tongue and tonsil areas as well as the neck. Specialized office examination with fiberoptics should be included in the preliminary assessment. Regardless of whether cancer is suspected, excisional biopsies should be discouraged because margins are frequently violated and inadequate, thereby leading to larger re-excisions. A simple punch biopsy is sufficient for diagnosis, particularly in the oral portion of the tongue where tumors can spread readily through lymphatics.

When cancer is highly suspected and before definitive surgical intervention, PET/CT of the body and a high-resolution CT scan from the base of the skull to the clavicles, preferably with the spiral technique, are indicated. Magnetic resonance imaging (MRI) provides added information in evaluating soft tissue involvement, especially in the base of the tongue and the parapharyngeal spaces and for sinus tumors. MRI can distinguish between soft tissue masses and retained secretions, whereas PET/CT and high-resolution CT are more helpful in assessing nodal spread in the neck, and CT is effective in identifying extracapsular nodal extension and bone invasion, which are important prognostic and clinical findings. PET scanning provides an important adjunct to CT scanning and can identify occult disease. PET is particularly helpful when the patient has an "unknown primary tumor," before biopsy, to guide the evaluation and to reduce the risk of inadequate diagnostic and premature therapeutic procedures (Fig. 190-2).

When a biopsy indicates cancer or cancer is highly suspected, an examination under anesthesia with endoscopy can be performed to stage the primary tumor before definitive therapy is undertaken. This procedure, which may be part of definitive therapy, provides information about the extent of disease, the appropriateness of the planned definitive procedure, and the presence of second primaries. It is an absolute requirement before definitive therapy can be completed. Endoscopy and palpation under anesthesia can identify unexpected local spread or a synchronous second primary (found synchronously in about 5% of patients with environmentally related cancers), which can substantially alter the treatment plan.

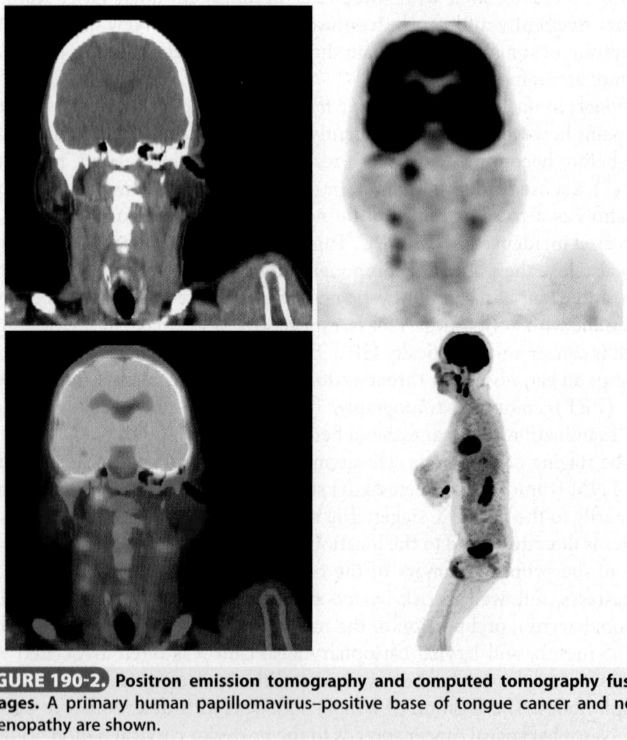

FIGURE 190-2. Positron emission tomography and computed tomography fused images. A primary human papillomavirus–positive base of tongue cancer and neck adenopathy are shown.

Approach to the Patient with an Unknown Primary Site

Patients frequently seek care from their primary physician because of an enlarged lymph node, a cystic mass, or a collection of lymph nodes in the upper part of the neck (Fig. 190-3). Such masses in an adult should be considered cancer until proved otherwise. Masses in the supraclavicular areas usually derive from primary tumors below the clavicles, and masses in the midneck and cervical regions are almost always from the head and neck. Identification of a primary site is critical to focus therapy, to reduce morbidity, and to determine prognosis.

The most common primary sites for painless lumps are the oropharynx (base of the tongue and tonsil) and piriform sinus. Oropharynx cancers are frequently due to HPV, and a positive HPV or EBV-encoded RNA (EBER) finding in the biopsy specimen or fine-needle aspirate is presumptive evidence of oropharynx or nasopharynx origin, respectively. Salivary gland cancers, lymphomas, melanomas, and skin cancers can also occur in this manner. Bilateral nodal disease or nodal disease with systemic symptoms may suggest lymphoma. By comparison, pain, warmth, and erythema may suggest an infectious etiology. Intraparotid nodes most likely represent metastases from skin malignant neoplasms. Physical examination should include a careful investigation for primary skin cancers. CT, PET, and MRI should be part of the initial evaluation. Fine-needle aspiration with HPV and EBER

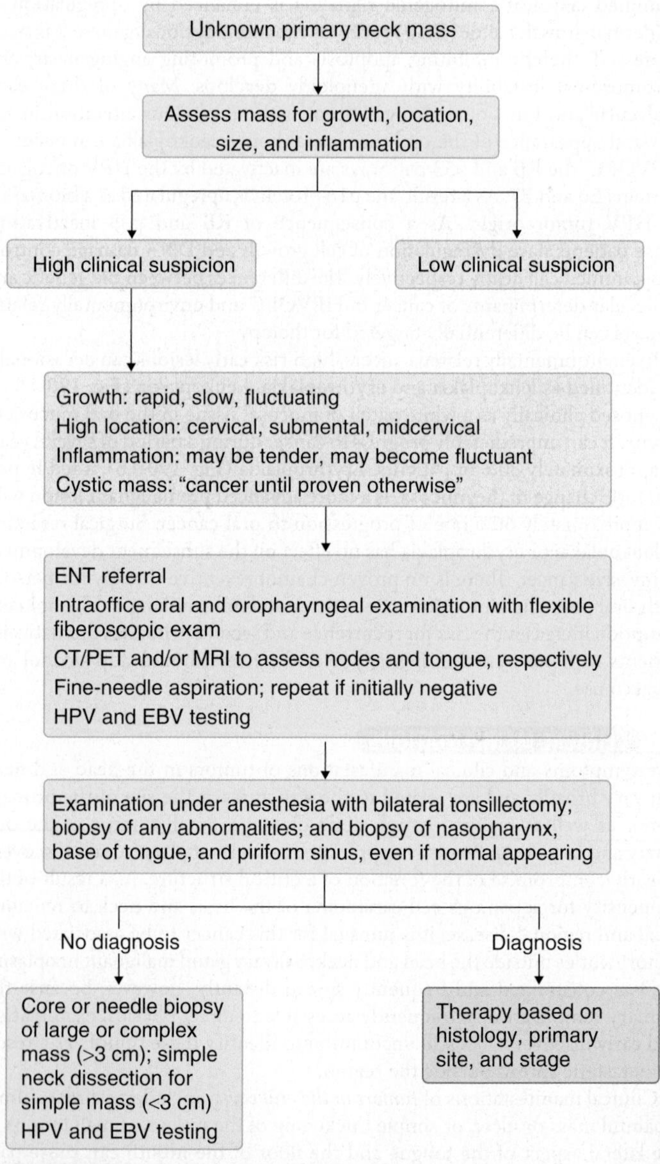

FIGURE 190-3. Evaluation of an unknown primary neck mass. CT = computed tomography; EBV = Epstein-Barr virus; ENT = ear, nose, and throat; HPV = human papillomavirus; MRI = magnetic resonance imaging; PET = positron emission tomography.

testing for squamous tumors should be performed. CT-guided biopsy may be indicated if the mass is difficult to approach. If squamous cells are identified, the tumor is most likely a squamous cell carcinoma of the head and neck. Next, endoscopy under anesthesia should be performed with bilateral tonsillectomy and directed biopsies of any abnormalities, areas of firmness, and the base of the tongue, nasopharynx, and ipsilateral piriform sinus, even if they appear normal. Core or excisional (single node <3 cm) biopsy of the lymph node should be performed if the pathologic findings are equivocal and a primary site is not confirmed. Neck dissection can be accomplished if a primary site is not identified and the patient has an N1 or small N2a/b manifestation. Some unknown primaries with squamous histology are never identified. Currently, HPV and EBV are the only molecular markers known to distinguish head and neck cancer from skin or salivary gland squamous cancer. EBV positivity indicates a nasopharyngeal cancer, and HPV an oropharyngeal primary. Although p16 immunohistochemistry is often used as a surrogate for HPV testing, it is not adequate for a final therapeutic decision to be made and may be positive in up to 20% of non-HPV cancers.

In contrast to squamous cell carcinoma of the head and neck, salivary gland cancers are heterogeneous in their natural history and treatment. The three most common histologic types are adenoid cystic carcinoma, mucoepidermoid cancer, and adenocarcinoma. Other histologic types include the aggressive salivary ductal cancer and squamous cell cancers, whereas less aggressive histologic varieties include adenocarcinoma ex pleomorphic adenoma and acinic cell carcinoma. Because adenoid cystic carcinoma travels along nerves and can spread hematogenously, careful assessment of the cranial nerves and the chest by CT is indicated before major surgery is undertaken. Patients should also be evaluated for bone and liver metastases. PET scan may not be positive in acinic cell carcinoma because of slow proliferation and metabolism in the malignant cells. Formal lymph node dissection is not indicated. Ethmoid and sphenoid sinus adenoid cystic carcinomas are locally and regionally aggressive and require specialized surgery and radiation therapy techniques for local and regional control. The behavior of mucoepidermoid carcinoma is determined by histology. Low- and intermediate-grade lesions rarely metastasize. Isolated high-grade tumors spread to local lymph nodes and by hematogenous routes and carry a high risk for the development of lung metastases. Local therapy should be directed at local and regional control with lymph node dissection. Radiation therapy is indicated for close microscopic margins or lymph node involvement. Adenocarcinoma, salivary ductal cancers, and squamous cell carcinoma are poor prognosis lesions with aggressive local and distant behavior. These tumors should be evaluated in the same fashion as aggressive mucoepidermoid carcinomas. Salivary ductal carcinomas may be positive for overexpression of EGFR2 or androgen receptor and should be tested for these markers to guide therapy with targeted agents. Acinic cell carcinoma and carcinoma ex pleomorphic adenoma are relatively rare. They have a propensity for local and regional recurrence if they are not removed in toto. Metastases are rare in acinic cell carcinoma and tend to be slow growing.

Other Tumors of the Head and Neck

Lymphomas in the head and neck frequently are manifested either as nodal disease in the neck or as tumor involving the lymphoid tissues of Waldeyer's ring (Chapters 185 and 186). A primary head and neck cancer may later develop in patients with lymphoma as a consequence of past exposure to tobacco, radiation therapy, or immunosuppression. The tonsil is a preferred site for mantle cell and undifferentiated lymphomas. Mucosa-associated lymphoid tissue lymphomas can affect the salivary glands.

In the context of an isolated neck mass, a systematic evaluation (see Fig. 190-3) should be undertaken, even in young adults without a smoking history. The sinonasal T-cell and natural killer cell lymphomas, also known as *lethal midline granulomas*, represent a unique family of lymphomas of the head and neck. These lymphomas are associated with EBV infection (Chapter 377). Solitary, extramedullary plasmacytoma can also occur in the nasopharynx or paranasal sinuses (Chapter 187).

Sarcomas that arise in the head and neck include osteogenic sarcomas (Chapter 202) and nerve sheath tumors. Paragangliomas, which are rare malignant tumors of the chief cells of nerve paraganglia, can be extensive, multicentric, and vascular. Rhabdomyosarcomas, which have a predilection for the orbit and sinuses, occur in younger persons; the prognosis tends to be better for tumors of the head and neck than for other locations. Olfactory neuroblastomas or esthesioneuroblastomas invade the nasal cavity and base of the skull.

Many skin tumors, including melanoma and squamous cell cancer, can be accompanied by adenopathy of the neck or parotid area (Chapter 203). An unusual skin appendage tumor, Merkel cell cancer, can be confused with other neuroendocrine epithelial tumors. Merkel cell tumors are associated with HIV infection and may, in up to 50% of cases, be caused by Merkel cell polyomavirus.

PREVENTION AND TREATMENT Rx

Selection of a treatment program for an individual patient is based on three factors: (1) the primary site and stage of the tumor; (2) the patient's comorbid conditions, including performance status and preferences; (3) and the biology of the tumor (Table 190-1). Early-stage lesions, T1N0 and T2N0, are defined by their size, and their prognosis is site specific. For example, early *larynx cancer* involving the true vocal cords has an excellent prognosis and can be treated by local excision. Voice-preserving larynx conservation surgery is effective for selected patients. Radiation therapy is equally effective for early cancer. When there is a risk of lymph node spread, radiation therapy must be given postoperatively, and the primary value of surgery is significantly diminished. Intensity-modulated radiation therapy allows radiation to be delivered in a more conformal manner to the tumor and areas at risk while sparing critical structures such as the spinal cord and noncritical but important structures such as the salivary glands and swallowing structures. Intensity-modulated radiation therapy is now a standard of care for almost all patients with head and neck cancer.[7]

Oral tongue, piriform sinus, and environmentally related oropharynx tumors have a poor prognosis and are difficult to stage accurately because of submucosal spread or lymphatic involvement. Stage I and stage II cancers are cured with local and regional surgery or radiation therapy in 70 to 90% of cases. Surgery may be preferred for oral cavity and anterior lesions. In surgically treated patients, those with a positive margin, two or more positive lymph nodes, or extracapsular spread have a significantly poorer survival rate (<30%) at 5 years. Perineural invasion and lymphovascular invasion may also be associated with a poor prognosis. Postoperative cisplatin-based chemoradiotherapy improves local and regional control as well as has a trend to increased survival, and it should be given to patients with a poor prognosis if their condition permits.[A1] At present, aside from HPV status and p16 immunohistochemistry, no molecular or immunohistochemical finding definitively adds to the information gleaned from pathology, staging, and performance status.[8]

TABLE 190-1 GENERAL APPROACH TO SQUAMOUS CELL HEAD AND NECK CANCER

STAGE	TNM	DISEASE-SPECIFIC SURVIVAL	TREATMENT APPROACH	SPECIAL CONDITIONS
I	T1N0	85-95%	Surgery or radiation therapy	Consider organ function and long-term toxicity
II	T2N0	75-90%	Surgery, radiation therapy, or chemoradiotherapy	Consider organ function Combined modality treatment for high-volume tumor Postoperative chemoradiotherapy for poor prognostic findings on pathologic staging
III	T3N0 T1-3N1	50-75%	Combined modality treatment	Primary chemoradiotherapy or TPF induction therapy or sequential therapy for organ function Postoperative chemoradiotherapy More aggressive approach (sequential therapy) for high-volume disease or hypopharynx tumors
IV	T1-3N2-3 T4N0-3 Any M1	20-60%	Combined modality treatment	Combined modality therapy Limited surgery Postoperative chemoradiotherapy Palliative therapy for M1 (curative therapy for isolated lung metastases)

When organ preservation and function are issues for stage III or stage IV cancers or when radiation therapy is required regardless of surgical outcome, primary chemoradiotherapy or sequential therapy should be considered.A2 A3 The curative treatment of intermediate (stage III, T1-3N1, T3N0) and locally advanced (stage IV, T1-3N2-3, T4) disease remains controversial. Long-term (3 years) survival rates in patients with stage III disease are generally between 50 and 75%, whereas only 15 to 50% of stage IV patients survive for 3 years. Intermediate-stage tumors are usually resectable, but organ preservation may be an important consideration. In many of these cases, a combined modality approach that includes chemotherapy and radiation therapy is the standard of care.A4

Patients with anterior lesions may do better with initial surgical treatment. The oral cavity is easy to access and is relatively forgiving for surgery and reconstruction; postoperative radiation therapy or chemoradiotherapy can be moderated in the absence of poor prognostic features. For intermediate and advanced tumors of the oral cavity, newer microvascular surgical techniques can substantially improve functional outcome and may help increase local-regional control. Radiation therapy or chemoradiotherapy remains a necessary adjunct to prevent recurrence. In contrast, tumors of oropharyngeal base of tongue or hypopharynx are almost always more extensive than is clinically appreciated, and functional outcome can be compromised by surgery followed by chemoradiotherapy. These may be more suited to a nonsurgical regional and systemic approach. In addition, patients with rapidly growing tumors are more suitable for a combined modality approach. Patients with extensive N2 or N3 nodal disease (stage IV) should be considered relatively unresectable because of a poor prognosis from regional recurrence and distant metastases. Certain locations, such as the nasopharynx and posterior pharynx, should also be considered for definitive radiation therapy, sequential therapy, or chemoradiotherapy.

Surgical therapy has changed radically in the last 5 years. Microvascular reconstructive techniques have improved outcomes in the oral cavity and have substantially reduced functional morbidity and permitted previously morbid resections to be accomplished with good functional outcomes. Transoral laser microdissection and transoral robotic surgery have created the opportunity to operate on previously "inoperable" tumors of the oropharynx and hypopharynx. Surgery with these technologies is performed without bystander tissue damage, which often leads to complications and required prolonged hospitalizations. These technologies are being integrated into combined modality approaches.

Radiation therapy has been proved by randomized trials to yield better local control and disease-free survival if it is given in twice-daily fractionated treatments rather than as daily therapy. However, the absolute benefit of hyperfractionated radiation therapy at 5 years is only 3 to 4%, and a twice-daily schedule is not advantageous with chemotherapy or better than chemotherapy and standard once-daily approaches. Studies strongly support the notion that altered fractionation radiation therapy with chemotherapy is substantially less efficacious or more toxic than standard fraction chemotherapy and that chemoradiotherapy with standard fractionation is more efficacious than altered fractionation alone. Proton beam radiation therapy has become available for tumors of the base of skull or those close to the eyes or the optic chiasm and is suitable in that context.

Induction chemotherapy is the delivery of chemotherapy before definitive local-regional treatment. Sequential therapy adds chemoradiotherapy (see later) to induction chemotherapy. Induction chemotherapy with docetaxel (75 mg/m^2), cisplatin (75 to 100 mg/m^2 by intravenous bolus), plus 5-fluorouracil (750 to 1000 mg/m^2/day for 4 to 5 days by intravenous infusion), repeated every 3 or 4 weeks (TPF), is an effective, standard regimen. For patients with advanced oropharynx, larynx, and hypopharynx tumors, sequential chemotherapy with chemoradiotherapy using concomitant carboplatin and once-daily radiation therapy improves survival and preserves function compared with radiation, surgery, or cisplatin and 5-fluorouracil chemotherapy (PF).

Chemoradiotherapy integrates chemotherapy and radiation therapy together and has led to significant improvements in overall survival in patients with advanced disease compared with radiation therapy alone. For example, patients with unresectable disease who received cisplatin (100 mg/m^2 by intravenous bolus) every 3 weeks during radiation therapy have significantly better survival than do those treated with radiation therapy alone. In a trial of patients with oropharyngeal carcinoma, those treated with carboplatin and 5-fluorouracil plus simultaneous radiation therapy had significantly better survival than did those treated by radiation therapy alone. Cetuximab plus radiation therapy has also proved effective in improving survival in patients with locally advanced head and neck cancer compared with radiation therapy alone in a single trial.A5 Compelling data for an improvement of cetuximab or equivalence with cisplatin-based chemoradiotherapy in either toxicity or survival has not been produced. Conventional chemoradiotherapy results in more favorable outcomes than chemotherapy with accelerated radiation therapy or very accelerated radiation therapy alone in patients with locally advanced head and neck carcinoma.

Patients with locally advanced or unresectable disease (or both) should receive chemotherapy and radiation therapy as part of a combined modality approach. Surgery may be integrated into this approach. Organ preservation should be offered to patients who can tolerate the treatment and participate in the post-treatment rehabilitation.

Treatment of *tumors of the paranasal sinuses* is a special case. They rarely metastasize, and treatment should focus on surgical resection with postoperative radiation therapy or chemoradiotherapy for resectable stage III and stage IV disease and on chemoradiotherapy for local and regional control of unresectable disease. Proton beam irradiation may be more suited for tumors in and around the base of the skull, optic chiasm, orbits, and brain.

Follow-up

Patients need lifelong follow-up. Surveillance examinations for second primaries and recurrences should be performed monthly to bimonthly in the first year and then less frequently over time. PET/CT scan can provide evidence of local-regional persistence approximately 12 to 16 weeks after completion of radiation therapy and can be used to guide early salvage surgery and neck management. Biannual PET/CT scan as postoperative surveillance can identify early metastases or recurrence and increase the rate and success of salvage surgery. Treatment failure after 5 years is uncommon, but second primaries and distant metastases may continue to be identified in environmentally related cancers and HPVOPC, respectively. It is important to counsel these patients to avoid tobacco products.

During radiation therapy and immediately after radiation therapy, patients benefit from pain medications, local anesthetics, mucolytics, and saline mouthwash. Patients must avoid alcohol-containing preparations or irritants. Long-acting agents such as fentanyl or time-release narcotics should be added when needed (Chapter 30). A percutaneous endoscopic gastrostomy feeding tube is often effective for maintaining weight, improving healing, and managing nutrition during radiation therapy. Because depression is a major problem, psychiatric support and antidepressants may be very helpful. Salivary function improves during more than 4 years after radiation therapy, but most improvement occurs in the first 2 years. Pilocarpine and cevimeline (Evoxac) are effective stimulants of salivary flow in about 20% of patients.

Long-term sequelae of radiation therapy include dependence on a feeding tube in patients treated with aggressive chemoradiotherapy or radiation therapy alone. Attention should be paid to preservation of swallowing function by means of training in speech and swallowing as well as by dilation in selected patients. Hypothyroidism occurs in up to 50% of patients and as early as 3 months after treatment. Patients should be monitored by determining serum thyroid-stimulating hormone levels at regular intervals and then treated as appropriate (Chapter 226). Dental failure is a common problem. Patients must be counseled to see their dentists regularly for cleanings and to obtain fluoride therapy daily for dental preservation. Patients are at substantial lifelong risk for complications from dental manipulations after radiation therapy. Bone necrosis is painful, can be confused with recurrent tumor, and requires vigorous antibiotic therapy, débridement, and possibly hyperbaric oxygen to promote healing. Late vascular compromise of the carotid artery should lead to routine carotid ultrasound beginning about 10 years after radiation therapy.

Patients with recurrent disease, a second primary, or metastatic disease must be evaluated for potential curability. Symptomatically, persistent pain may be the most important indicator of a recurrence, and repeated biopsy should be considered when a suspicious lesion is observed. If patients have a recurrence or second primary, curative treatment options are defined by their current stage, their previous therapy, and the interval from their original therapy. Patients who have previously been treated with surgery but not radiation therapy can undergo surgery and chemoradiotherapy as part of a curative treatment plan. Patients with a surgically treatable recurrence in an irradiated field should undergo surgery as appropriate. Surgical salvage may cure as many as 30% of patients with recurrent oral cavity, larynx, or hypopharyngeal tumors. The surgery must encompass the entire recurrence. A repeated course of radiation therapy or chemoradiotherapy is also acceptable in selected patients.

Patients who are incurable can be managed effectively with palliative therapy to improve quality of life and survival (e.g., tracheostomy for airway control, laryngectomy for pain and aspiration, percutaneous endoscopic gastrostomy tube for feeding). These maneuvers can improve comfort and care in appropriate patients.

Palliative chemotherapy can provide meaningful benefit to some patients. Response rates with single agents are generally poor, and combination therapy offers higher response rates (30 to 50%). The combination of a platinum (cisplatin or carboplatin) plus 5-fluorouracil with an anti-EGF receptor antibody, cetuximab, significantly improves survival, response rate, and progression-free survival compared with the same chemotherapy without cetuximab.

Salivary Gland Tumors

In contrast to squamous cell carcinoma of the head and neck, salivary gland cancers are heterogeneous in their natural history and treatment; however, the mainstays of therapy for these tumors are surgery and radiation therapy. Early symptoms of local-regional recurrence include cranial nerve dysfunction and progressive pain. A PET scan may be useful in distinguishing recurrence from the neuropathy that may result from radiation therapy.

There are no highly active agents or combinations for treatment of metastatic salivary gland tumors with the exception of anti-Her2 therapy for Her2-positive tumors. Local therapy can include surgical removal of isolated metastases, radio frequency ablation, and radiation therapy. Response rates are generally in the range of 20 to 35%, but prolonged responses are occasionally seen.

Future Directions

Antibodies that target newly identified molecular targets are being evaluated and may improve local and regional control as well as survival when they are delivered in combination with other therapies. Therapeutic vaccines may improve outcomes in EBV nasopharyngeal carcinoma and HPVOPC, and preventive vaccines in adolescents may prevent later malignant disease. New immune checkpoint blockade inhibitors appear to be showing promise in viral and environmentally caused head and neck cancers.

PROGNOSIS

The prognosis for patients with squamous cell carcinoma of the head and neck (see Table 190-1) is directly related to the presence of HPV, stage, and performance status. The risk for recurrence declines dramatically at 3 years after definitive treatment, and survival and possible cure can be defined after 5 years. HPV status[9] and then N (nodal) stage are the most important prognostic indicators of potential recurrence, with T (tumor) stage and smoking history being next.[10] Stage I patients (T1N0) have a 90% likelihood of tumor control, whereas stage II patients (T2N0) have greater than 70 to 85% tumor control. Tumor control in stage III patients (T1-2N1, T3N0-1) is site dependent, is HPV status and smoking history dependent, and varies from 35 to 95%. Patients with stage IVa and IVb environmentally related cancers (T1-3, N2-3, or T4NX) have a 20 to 50% tumor-specific 5-year survival rate compared with 60 to 90% 5-year survival for HPVOPC. Poor prognostic signs in advanced-stage (IVb) patients are related to N3 nodal disease, extracapsular extension, and invasion of basic structures (carotid artery encasement, base of the skull, pterygoid muscles). Patients with M1 disease are categorized as stage IVc. Patients with single lung metastases, whether as a second primary or as an isolated recurrence, can be cured. Cures with metastatic disease caused by HPVOPC may be seen after aggressive management. Patients with recurrent disease and no curative options have a median survival of 6 to 9 months.

Distant metastases occur in about 15 to 20% of patients, but this rate is increasing as better local and regional control prolongs survival in patients with locally advanced disease. Oropharyngeal, tonsil, and piriform sinus tumors have the highest risk for distant metastases. A single synchronous lung metastasis in a patient at initial evaluation or at follow-up can be cured in about 20% of cases.

Salivary gland cancers vary in behavior, depending on their histology. Adenocarcinoma, salivary ductal cancer, salivary squamous cell cancer, and high-grade mucoepidermoid cancer not only spread to lymph nodes but also spread rapidly hematogenously. The presence of lymph node metastases signals a high risk for distant metastases. Adenoid cystic carcinoma infrequently involves lymph nodes but spreads along nerves. Regional recurrences along cranial nerves are frequent and associated with "skip" lesions. Adenoid cystic carcinoma is also associated with the late development of lung metastases, but these patients can have a prolonged lifespan lasting more than 20 years. Low-grade mucoepidermoid cancer and acinic cell carcinoma have little risk of distant spread and are more notable for local recurrence if they are not completely removed.

Grade A References

A1. Cooper JS, Zhang Q, Pajak TF, et al. Long-term follow-up of the RTOG 9501/intergroup phase III trial: postoperative concurrent radiation therapy and chemotherapy in high-risk squamous cell carcinoma of the head and neck. *Int J Radiat Oncol Biol Phys.* 2012;84:1198-1205.

A2. Forastiere AA, Zhang Q, Weber RS, et al. Long-term results of RTOG 91-11: a comparison of three nonsurgical treatment strategies to preserve the larynx in patients with locally advanced larynx cancer. *J Clin Oncol.* 2013;31:845-852.

A3. Pointreau Y, Garaud P, Chapet S, et al. Randomized trial of induction chemotherapy with cisplatin and 5-fluorouracil with or without docetaxel for larynx preservation. *J Natl Cancer Inst.* 2009;101:498-506.

A4. Blanchard P, Bourhis J, Lacas B, et al. Taxane-cisplatin-fluorouracil as induction chemotherapy in locally advanced head and neck cancers: an individual patient data meta-analysis of the meta-analysis of chemotherapy in head and neck cancer group. *J Clin Oncol.* 2013;31:2854-2860.

A5. Bonner JA, Harari PM, Giralt J, et al. Radiotherapy plus cetuximab for locoregionally advanced head and neck cancer: 5-year survival data from a phase 3 randomised trial, and relation between cetuximab-induced rash and survival. *Lancet Oncol.* 2010;11:21-28.

GENERAL REFERENCES

For the General References and other additional features, please visit Expert Consult at https://expertconsult.inkling.com.

191

LUNG CANCER AND OTHER PULMONARY NEOPLASMS

FADLO R. KHURI

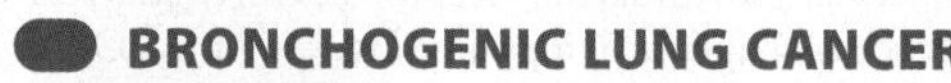

BRONCHOGENIC LUNG CANCER

DEFINITION

Lung cancer, or bronchogenic carcinoma, is a proliferative malignant neoplasm arising from the primary respiratory epithelium. Lung cancer is generally divided into two major histologic groups: *non–small cell lung cancer* (NSCLC), which accounts for approximately 85% of all lung cancers, and *small cell lung cancer* (SCLC). There are several other less common pulmonary neoplasms including carcinoid tumors, primary soft tissue sarcomas of the lung, pulmonary blastomas, and lymphoma.

EPIDEMIOLOGY

Lung cancer is by far the leading cause of cancer-related mortality globally, with an estimated 1.3 million new cases diagnosed worldwide each year, accounting for nearly 12% of all cancers and an estimated 1.1 million deaths each year. Among men, lung cancer is the most common malignant neoplasm (incidence rate of 35.5 per 100,000), whereas in women, lung cancer incidence (12.1 per 100,000) is next only to breast, cervix, and colon cancers. The incidence and mortality related to lung cancer in men have declined during the last two decades in Western countries but continue to increase in the developing world; in women, lung cancer deaths are increasing in most regions of the world. The most dramatic increases in lung cancer incidence and death globally are in China, which has experienced a 465% increase in lung cancer–related deaths during the past 30 years.

Risk Factors

Cigarette smoking is the most common risk factor for lung cancer, with roughly 85% of lung cancer patients having a tobacco-smoking history and approximately 50% being former smokers (defined as free from smoking for at least 12 months before diagnosis). The risk for development of lung cancer correlates with the number of cigarettes smoked per day and the cumulative duration of smoking time. Patients with a smoking history of at least 20 to 30 pack-years (defined as 1 pack per day of cigarettes for 20 to 30 years) are at substantially increased risk for development of lung cancer. Since the release of the first U.S. Surgeon General's Report on the Hazards of Smoking in 1964, the prevalence of cigarette smoking has declined considerably in the United States but continues to increase at an alarming rate in developing and third world countries. As a result, the number of cases of lung cancer diagnosed annually is likely to rise during the next few decades, and it is estimated that the majority of lung cancer cases will occur outside the United States and Europe by the year 2030. Smoking cessation is associated with a gradual reduction in risk for development of lung cancer, although it does not reach that of a never-smoker. Second-hand exposure to smoke is another risk factor that contributes to nearly 1% of all cases of lung cancer.

Because only about 11% of heavy smokers develop lung cancer, genetic susceptibility to lung cancer also appears to play a role. Patients with a family history of early lung cancer (before 60 years of age) have a two-fold higher risk for development of the disease. Women appear to be at a higher risk for development of lung cancer at the same smoking exposure level as that of men, but the reasons behind this remain unclear. In recent years, an increasing number of never-smokers have been diagnosed with lung cancer.

TABLE 191-1 HISTOLOGIC MARKERS IN NON–SMALL CELL LUNG CANCER

	PERCENTAGE IHC-POSITIVE CASES AMONG HISTOLOGIC CARCINOMA SUBTYPES			POSITIVE AND NEGATIVE PREDICTIVE VALUE OF ANTIBODY PANEL	
	Adenocarcinoma (n = 215)	*Squamous Cell Carcinoma (n = 123)*	*Large Cell Carcinoma (n = 22)*	*Adenocarcinoma*	*Squamous Cell Carcinoma*
p63	7.0	99.2	52		88.9, 99.5
Cytokeratin 5/6	9.8	99.2	68		84.9, 99.5
TTF-1	83.5	3.4	23	97.7, 76.9	
Cytokeratin 7	97.2	23.5	77	88.4, 93.6	
Mucin	43.4	13.4	0		

Modified from Sterlacci W, Savic S, Schmid T, et al. Tissue-sparing application of the newly proposed IASLC/ATS/ERS classification of adenocarcinoma of the lung shows practical diagnostic and prognostic impact. *Am J Clin Pathol.* 2012;137:946-956.
IHC = immunohistochemically; TTF-1 = thyroid transcription factor-1.

The etiology behind this is unclear at this time. These individuals are more likely to harbor certain genetic alterations in the tumor, such as mutations in the gene encoding epidermal growth factor receptor (EGFR) and rearrangement in the gene encoding anaplastic lymphoma kinase (ALK). Occupational exposure to asbestos leads to an estimated four-fold higher risk of lung cancer, with cigarette smoking having an additive effect on risk. There is a latency of several decades between asbestos exposure and the development of lung cancer, and risk is related to the duration of exposure as well as to the quantity and the type of asbestos fiber. The Environmental Protection Agency and the World Health Organization consider all forms of asbestos to be carcinogenic; accordingly, the use of asbestos is banned in nearly 50 countries.

Radon exposure has also been implicated in the development of 5 to 8% of lung cancer cases.[1] Household exposure to radon, which results from the radioactive decay of uranium, is high in certain geographic regions. The Environmental Protection Agency recommends that the household radon level be less than 4 picocuries/liter of air, and simple remedial methods are available to reduce radon exposures above this threshold. Exposure to ionizing radiation in the form of therapeutic radiation or frequent diagnostic radiographic tests is also associated with a higher risk for development of lung cancer, as to a lesser degree are exposures to metals such as arsenic, nickel, and chromium as well as to silica and general air pollution, including biomass fuels such as coal and wood smoke. A study estimated that human immunodeficiency virus is associated with an increased risk for development of lung cancer with a hazard ratio of 3.6.

PATHOBIOLOGY

Pathology

Lung cancer is broadly subdivided into NSCLC and SCLC on the basis of the distinct biologic behavior and response to chemotherapy of these two subsets. NSCLC comprises *adenocarcinoma*, *squamous cell carcinoma*, and *large cell carcinoma* subtypes. In the past several years, distinct differences between the various histologic subtypes that comprise NSCLC have been recognized, with an increasing emphasis placed on the identification of histologic subtype from diagnostic specimens.

Adenocarcinoma is now the most common histologic subtype of lung cancer; never-smokers who develop lung cancer most frequently have adenocarcinoma. It has gradually increased in incidence, surpassing squamous cell cancer during the past two decades, and now represents nearly 50% of all newly diagnosed cases of lung cancer in the United States. Adenocarcinoma has a higher predilection for distant metastasis compared with squamous cell histology. In 2011, a new classification system for lung adenocarcinoma was developed dividing adenocarcinomas into preinvasive, minimally invasive, and invasive types.[2] *Atypical adenomatous hyperplasia* refers to a localized proliferative lesion consisting of atypical type II pneumocytes or Clara cells and measuring less than 5 mm. *Adenocarcinoma in situ* refers to lesions smaller than 3 cm that lack any invasive characteristics. This entity was previously referred to as bronchioloalveolar carcinoma or noninvasive adenocarcinoma. Lesions 3 cm or smaller with a predominantly lepidic pattern and with invasion of less than 5 mm in greatest dimension are referred to as *minimally invasive adenocarcinoma*. Adenocarcinoma in situ and minimally invasive adenocarcinoma have a more than 95% 5-year survival rate when they are treated with surgical resection, making the establishment of a precise pathologic diagnosis of great significance. Invasive adenocarcinoma represents nearly 90% of all cases of adenocarcinoma. Based on the predominant characteristic features, it is categorized as lepidic, acinar, papillary, micropapillary, or solid predominant with mucin production.

Squamous cell lung cancer is decreasing in incidence in the United States, most likely because of the changing smoking habits of the population. Squamous tumors of the lung are generally centrally located and are almost always seen in patients with a significant smoking history. Squamous dysplasia and squamous cell carcinoma in situ are preinvasive lesions that can develop into invasive cancers.

In addition to morphologic features, immunohistochemical studies are important in establishing NSCLC histologic subtype. Adenocarcinoma specimens usually stain positive for cytokeratin 7 and thyroid transcription factor-1 (TTF-1) and are negative for cytokeratin 20. The majority of squamous cell tumors stain positive for p40 and p63, members of the p53 family of proteins, whereas adenocarcinomas occasionally stain positive for p63. On the basis of these findings, a panel of markers including TTF-1, p63, and p40 is frequently evaluated in diagnostic specimens of patients with lung cancer to accurately identify the histologic subtype (Table 191-1). Large cell carcinoma represents 3 to 4% of NSCLC and is characterized by a high mitotic rate, necrosis, and morphologic features of NSCLC. Large cell tumors stain positively for neuroendocrine markers such as chromogranin A and synaptophysin. Because this histologic subtype is often difficult to accurately diagnose owing to an abundance of necrotic tissue and a poor degree of differentiation, diagnosis requires an adequate tissue specimen. Large cell carcinoma is often associated with an aggressive clinical course and poor survival rates, even when it is found in the setting of early-stage disease. Large cell carcinoma is strongly associated with a history of prior smoking.

SCLC is diagnosed in approximately 13% of lung cancer cases in the United States, and its incidence has gradually declined during the past three decades. SCLC is strongly associated with smoking and is rare in never-smokers. Pathologic diagnosis can be challenging because of an abundance of necrotic tissue but is established by characteristic features, such as a high degree of mitosis and necrosis. Diagnostic work-up of SCLC includes immunostaining for TTF-1, chromogranin, synaptophysin, and CD56. Approximately 15% of SCLC specimens have mixed morphology with components of NSCLC.

Molecular Pathology

In recent years, a number of molecular abnormalities have been identified in lung cancer. Many of these represent novel targets for therapy, strengthening the rationale for obtaining adequate tumor tissue to conduct molecular studies as an essential component of the diagnostic work-up for lung cancer. With modern genomic techniques, a greater understanding of the molecular features that account for the long-recognized clinical heterogeneity of lung cancer is leading to individualized treatment approaches.[3]

Oncogenes

In lung adenocarcinoma, nearly two thirds of patients harbor an oncogenic mutation that can potentially be targeted with specific agents (Fig. 191-1A).[4] The most common are mutations involving *KRAS, EGFR, BRAF, HER2,* and *PIK3CA* and gene rearrangements involving *ALK, RET,* and *ROS1*. *KRAS* mutations are present in approximately 25% of lung adenocarcinoma patients and are usually associated with cigarette smoking. The most common sites of mutation in *KRAS* include codons 12, 13, and 61, resulting in amino acid substitutions, which cause impaired GTPase activity and constitutive

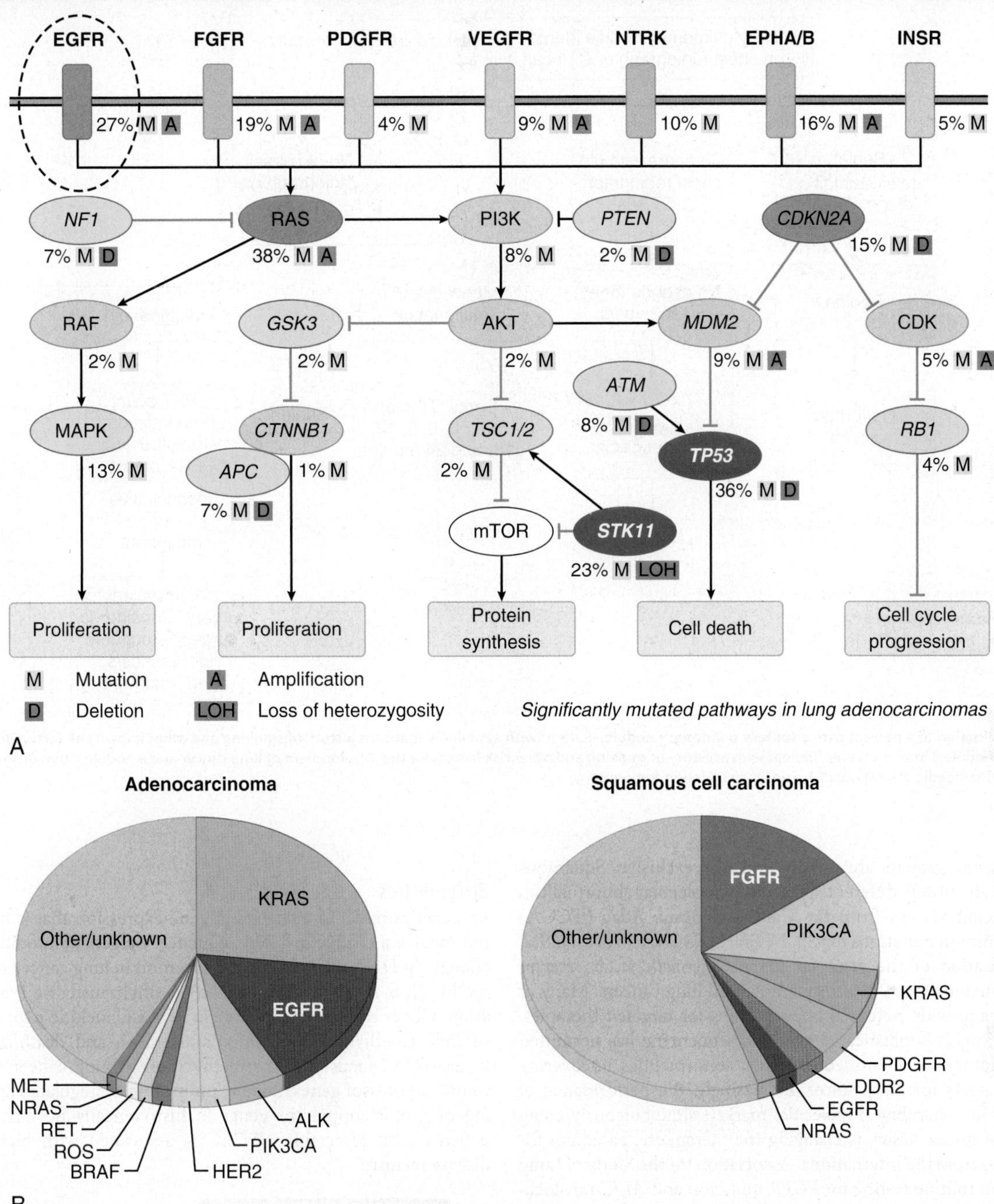

FIGURE 191-1. Altered signaling networks in lung cancer. A, Significantly mutated pathways in lung adenocarcinoma. (Modified from Ding L, Getz G, Wheeler DA, et al. Somatic mutations affect key pathways in lung adenocarcinoma. *Nature*. 2008;455:1069-1075.) B, Genetic profiles by histologic subtype. (From the Lung Cancer Mutation Consortium and modified from Sequist LV, Heist RS, Shaw AT, et al. Implementing multiplexed genotyping of non-small-cell lung cancers into routine clinical practice. *Ann Oncol*. 2011;22:2616-2624; Bergethon K, Shaw AT, Ou SH, et al. ROS1 rearrangements define a unique molecular class of lung cancers. *J Clin Oncol*. 2012;30:863-870; Weiss J, Sos ML, Seidel D, et al. Frequent and focal FGFR1 amplification associates with therapeutically tractable FGFR1 dependency in squamous cell lung cancer. *Sci Transl Med*. 2010;2:62ra93; Hammerman PS, Sos ML, Ramos AH, et al. Mutations in the DDR2 kinase gene identify a novel therapeutic target in squamous cell lung cancer. *Cancer Discov*. 2011;1:78-89.)

activation of RAS signaling. The prognostic value of *KRAS* mutation in patients with lung cancer is controversial.

Mutations in *EGFR* are observed in nearly 15% of white and almost 40% of Asian lung adenocarcinoma patients. Deletion mutations in exon 19 and a point mutation in exon 21 are located in the tyrosine kinase–binding domain of the receptor and result in constitutive activation of the signaling pathway, leading to proliferation, evasion of apoptosis, and enhanced angiogenesis. Patients with *EGFR*-activating mutations can derive robust and durable clinical benefit from treatment with EGFR tyrosine kinase inhibitors (TKIs). However, most of the benefit is limited in duration, and within 12 to 24 months, nearly 60% of these patients will develop a secondary mutation in exon 20 that confers resistance to EGFR TKI therapy. This mutation can also be found de novo in certain patients with lung adenocarcinoma along with an exon 19 or 21 mutation before exposure to EGFR TKI therapy. Another common mechanism of acquired resistance to EGFR TKI therapy is amplification of the growth factor receptor c-Met. In approximately 5% of patients with lung adenocarcinoma, gene rearrangement involving *ALK* is observed. Clinical features associated with the *ALK* gene rearrangement include never-smokers, adenocarcinoma histology, signet ring features on histopathologic evaluation, and younger age. The fusion gene results from inversion or translocation of portions of the *echinoderm microtubule-associated protein-like 4 (EML4)* with the *ALK* gene and leads to activation of downstream signals that can be inhibited by specific ALK kinase inhibitors. Crizotinib, an ALK inhibitor, induces objective tumor response in nearly two thirds of patients. *ALK* gene rearrangement is detected by fluorescent in situ hybridization, often in addition to immunohistochemistry. Other fusion abnormalities involving the *RET* and *ROS1* genes are each observed in 1% of lung adenocarcinoma specimens. It is noteworthy that *EGFR* and *KRAS* mutations

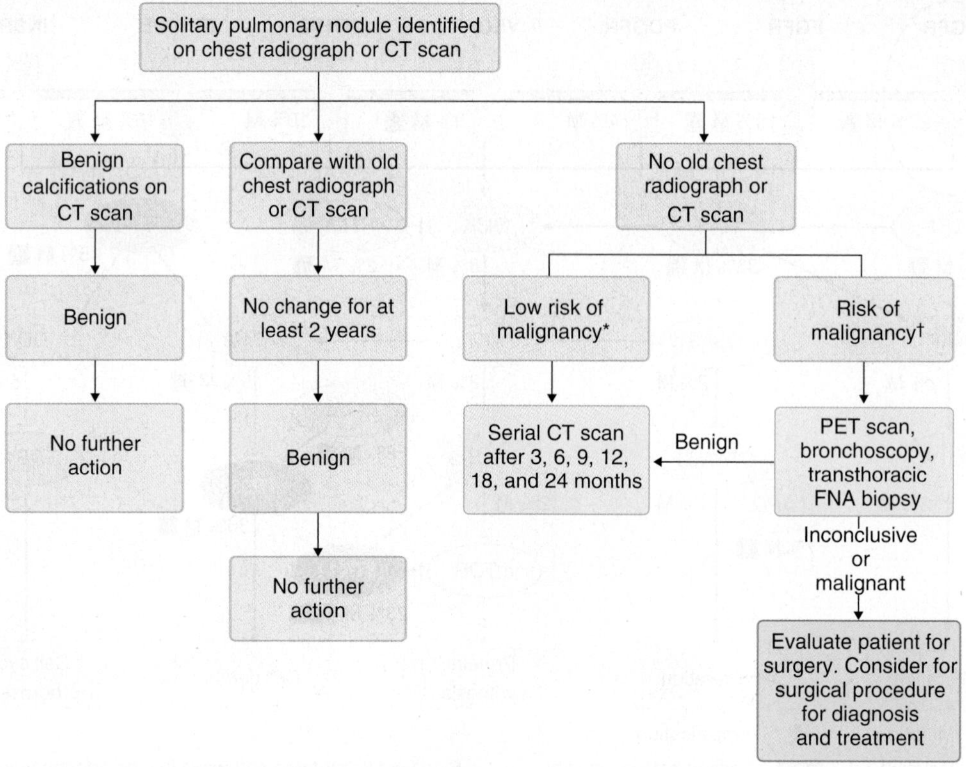

FIGURE 191-2. **Evaluation of a patient with a solitary pulmonary nodule.** *Patient with a minimal or absent history of smoking and other known risk factors for the development of lung cancer and a nodule 8 mm or smaller. †Patient with a history of smoking and other risk factors for the development of lung cancer and a nodule 8 mm or larger. CT = computed tomography; FNA = fine-needle aspiration; PET = positron emission tomography.

and *ALK* gene rearrangements are usually mutually exclusive. Squamous cell carcinoma has an entirely different spectrum of molecular abnormalities (Fig. 191-1B). Recent studies from the Cancer Genome Atlas (TCGA) project indicate common mutations in *p53, PTEN, PIK3CA, KEAP1, DDR2,* and *RB1*. Amplification of the gene for *fibroblast growth factor receptor* (FGFR) is also noted in 10 to 20% of squamous cell lung cancers. Many of these abnormalities provide potential opportunities for targeted therapies. The availability of highly sophisticated genomic sequencing has permitted the elucidation of hitherto unidentified molecular abnormalities, uncovering new therapeutic targets for lung cancer. Increasingly, the performance of "multiplex" testing for a number of molecular markers simultaneously, using limited amounts of tumor tissue, is changing the therapeutic paradigm for NSCLC. Guidelines from the International Association for the Study of Lung Cancer recommend routine testing for *EGFR* mutation and *ALK* translocation for all newly diagnosed patients with lung adenocarcinoma.[5] For patients with tumors of squamous cell histology, routine molecular testing is not yet recommended, although randomized clinical trials using this approach are in progress. In the absence of Food and Drug Administration–approved, molecularly directed therapies for squamous cancers, the use of standard chemotherapies is recommended for this disease at present.

Tumor Suppressor Genes

The function of multiple tumor suppressor genes is frequently lost in lung cancer, including *p53, Rb, LKB1,* and a number of genes found on the short arm of chromosome 3 (*3p*). *p53* mutation or loss correlates with cigarette smoking and has been detected in some preneoplastic lesions of the lung. Mutations of *p53* are common in both NSCLC (~50%) and SCLC (~80%). Mutations in *LKB1* are also common in NSCLC. The *STK11/LKB1* gene, which encodes a *serine/threonine kinase*, regulates cell polarity and functions as a tumor suppressor. One of the earliest genetic abnormalities in lung cancer occurs during the deletion of genetic material on chromosome 3p (p14-p23). The deletion occurs in approximately 50% of NSCLC and 90% of SCLC patients. The *FHIT* (fragile histidine triad) gene (3p14.2), which is abnormal in many lung cancers, may function as a tumor suppressor gene by limiting tumor growth and enhancing apoptosis. The Rb protein is not expressed in 90% of SCLC because of mutation or deletion. In NSCLC, Rb is normally expressed, but when Rb is phosphorylated, uncontrolled cell division can occur.

Epigenetics

Epigenetics refers to a change in gene expression that is heritable but does not involve a change in DNA sequence. Epigenetic modifications involving changes in DNA methylation are common in lung cancer and include hypomethylation, dysregulation of DNA methyltransferase I, and hypermethylation. Genes that are methylated in NSCLC include *p16, RARB, RASSF1A, MGMT* (methylguanine-methyltransferase), and death-associated protein kinase (DAP-kinase). Hypermethylation in lung cancer can often silence tumor suppressor genes, thereby promoting dysregulated cell growth. Silencing of tumor suppressor genes in histologically normal lymph nodes in patients with resectable NSCLC is associated with higher likelihood of disease relapse.

CLINICAL MANIFESTATIONS

Lung cancers grow from a single abnormal cell or small group of abnormal cells to develop into large macroscopic masses that may be several centimeters in diameter. Most lung cancers originate from the bronchial epithelium and are termed carcinomas. Primary noncarcinoma lung cancers are less common and include carcinoid, pulmonary blastomas (more common in younger patients), and sarcomas. Early lung cancers often are manifested as pulmonary nodules, defined as "a rounded opacity, well or poorly defined, measuring up to 3 cm in diameter" (see Fig. 191-2 for evaluation of a patient with a solitary pulmonary nodule). Abnormal lung tissues range in histologic grade from mildly atypical cells to aggressive cancers. Lesions such as atypical adenomatous hyperplasia are considered preinvasive lesions, with a continuum of cellular atypia through adenocarcinoma (Fig. 191-3).

Currently, only 15% of patients with lung cancer are asymptomatic when they are initially diagnosed. Diagnosis in these patients is often made incidentally on a chest radiograph obtained for other reasons (e.g., a preoperative study). The work-up for suspected lung cancers is dependent on the probability that the lesion in question is malignant or the stage of disease at presentation (see Fig. 191-2). Pulmonary nodules often are due to current or prior infection, although they may be the manifestation of early cancer. Results from the National Lung Screening Trial (NLST) showed that of all nodules detected, more than 95% were false positives and were noncancerous. However, most patients have symptoms and signs that are (1) caused by the pulmonary lesion itself—these include local tumor growth, invasion, and

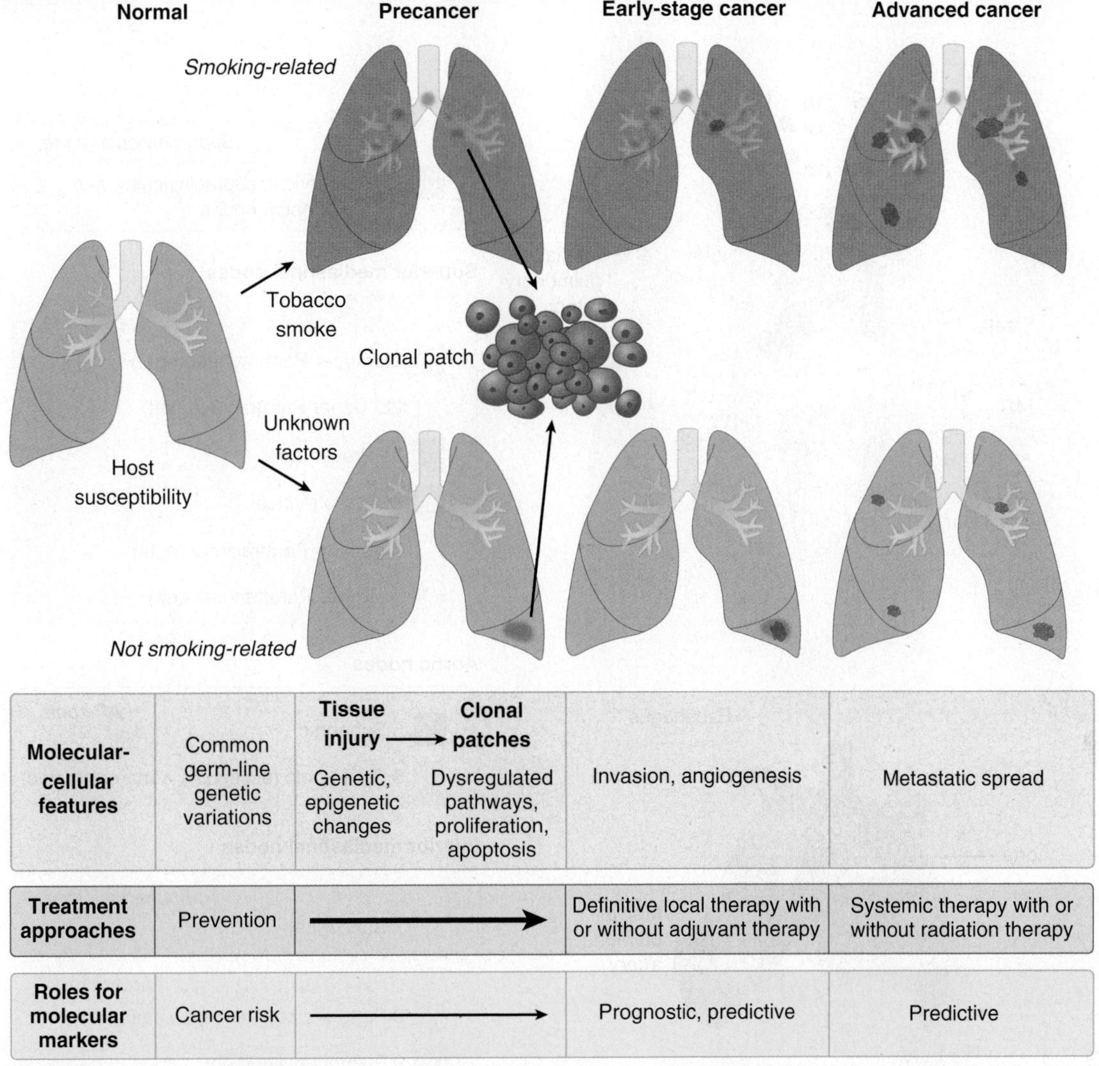

FIGURE 191-3. **Carcinogenesis of lung cancer.** (From Herbst RS, Heymach JV, Lippmann SM. Lung cancer. *N Engl J Med* 2008;359:1367-1380.)

bstruction; (2) intrathoracic-regional tumor spread to lymph nodes and djacent structures; (3) extrathoracic-distant spread of disease; or (4) para-eoplastic syndromes. Common presenting symptoms of lung cancer include ough, dyspnea, pain, hemoptysis, and weight loss; anorexia occurs in about 0% of patients, fatigue in one third of patients, and anemia and fever in 10 o 20% of patients. More than 80% of patients initially have three or more ymptoms or signs as a result of the lung cancer. Because the majority of atients with lung cancer have other tobacco-related cardiopulmonary dis-ases, such as emphysema/chronic obstructive pulmonary disease, ischemic eart disease, and others, these overlapping symptoms often result in a delay n diagnosis of the underlying malignant disease. Symptoms could also result rom local invasion or metastasis of the tumor, such as headache, bone pain, irway obstruction, cough, and hemoptysis. Paraneoplastic syndromes asso-iated with lung cancer include the syndrome of inappropriate antidiuretic ormone (Chapter 116), hypercalcemia (Chapter 245), pulmonary hyper-rophic osteoarthropathy (Chapter 275 and Fig. 275-1), Eaton-Lambert nyasthenic syndrome (Chapter 422), and Cushing's syndrome (Chapters 79 and 227). Hypercalcemia is common in squamous cell histology, whereas he syndrome of inappropriate antidiuretic hormone, Eaton-Lambert myas-henic syndrome, and Cushing's syndrome are most commonly associated vith SCLC.

DIAGNOSIS

Vith the advent of computed tomography (CT) screening, it is anticipated hat a greater subset of patients with lung cancer will be diagnosed before the nset of symptoms.[6] In patients with clinical or radiographic findings sugges-ive of lung cancer, CT scans of the chest and abdomen are indicated to etermine the location of the primary tumor, involvement of mediastinal ymph nodes (Fig. 191-4), and spread to other anatomic sites.

Diagnostic Procedures

Accurate diagnostic characterization of lung cancers is essential because the presence or absence of mediastinal nodal metastases is crucial in determining prognosis, assessing resectability, and selecting the appropriate treatment strategy for primary lung cancer. Enlarged lymph nodes identified by CT or positron emission tomography (PET) require histologic confirmation. It is debatable whether all patients require invasive mediastinal staging before surgical resection or other local treatment modality, such as stereotactic body radiation therapy (SBRT). Only 5 to 15% of patients with peripheral T1 tumors with a negative mediastinum by CT or PET have mediastinal nodal metastases.

Invasive Diagnostic Procedures

Important advances in surgical diagnosis have been established and refined in the last few years. Transbronchial needle aspiration (TBNA) allows staging of the mediastinum during diagnostic bronchoscopy. Sensitivity of TBNA is dependent on lymph node size, location, and needle size, being best suited for large, clinically positive lymph nodes. On-site cytopathologic analysis increases the likelihood of obtaining a malignant diagnosis. Linear array ultrasound technology combined with TBNA allows endobronchial ultrasound (EBUS) fine-needle aspiration (FNA) of mediastinal and hilar lymph node stations. EBUS-FNA is superior in performance to TBNA, with overall sensitivity approaching 90%. Among the diseases that are also associ-ated with enlarged and metabolically active mediastinal lymph nodes are sarcoidosis, tuberculosis, and multiple infectious causes, generally of a fungal, atypical, or viral nature (histoplasmosis, tuberculosis, and coccidioi-domycosis among the differential diagnoses), making it mandatory to obtain nodal tissue.

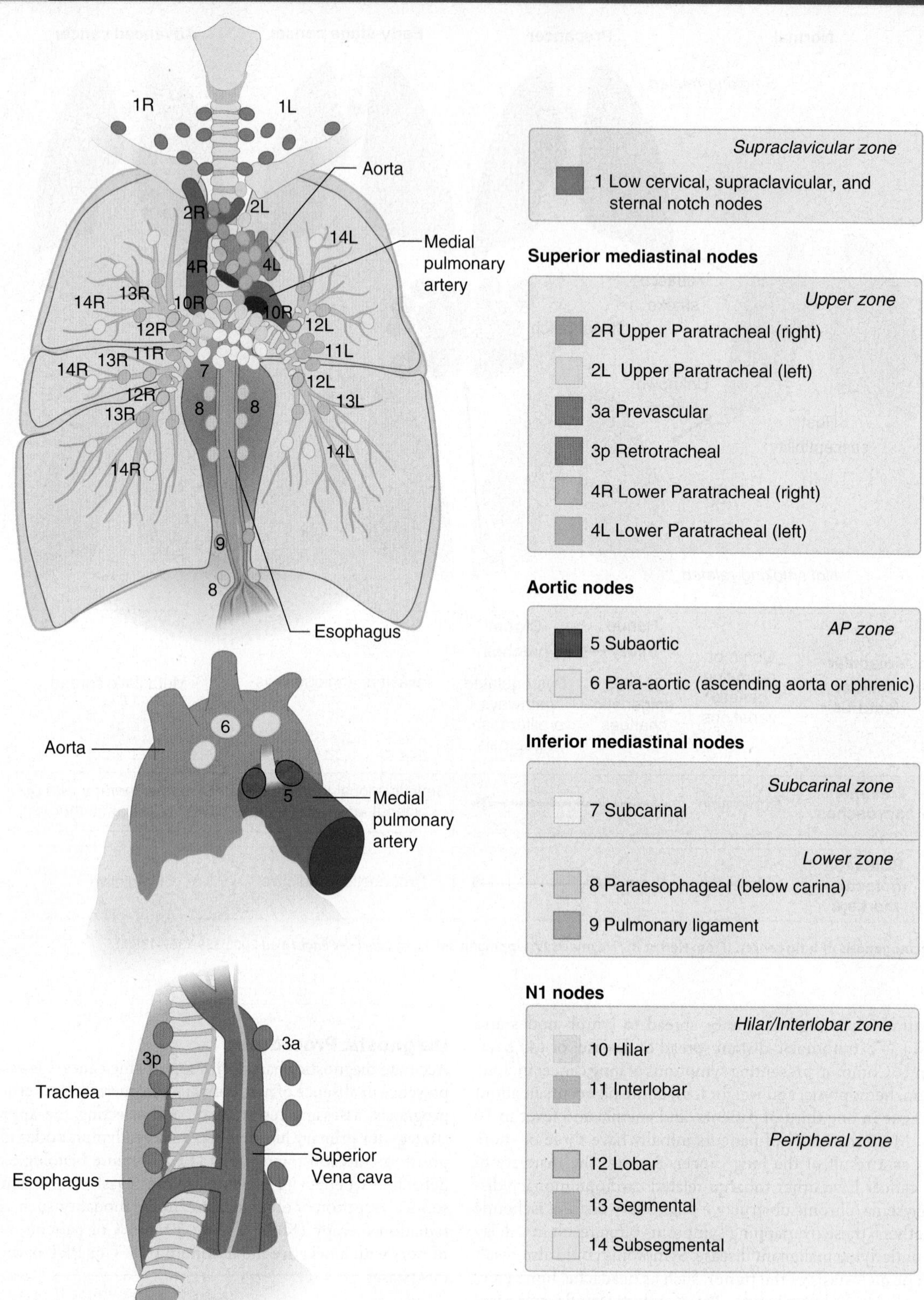

FIGURE 191-4. The International Association for the Study of Lung Cancer (IASLC) lymph node map. Included is the proposed grouping of lymph node stations into "zones" for the purposes of prognostic analyses. (From Rusch VW, Asamura H, Watanabe H. The IASCL lung cancer staging project. A proposal for a new international lymph node map in the forthcoming seventh edition of the TNM classification for lung cancer. *J Thorac Oncol.* 2009;4:568-577.)

Esophageal endoscopic ultrasonography (EUS), or EUS-FNA, allows sampling of inferior pulmonary ligament, periesophageal, and subcarinal lymph node stations (9, 8, and 7). Stations 2 and 4 are difficult to sample. The combination of EBUS-FNA and EUS-FNA can exceed 90% yield in obtaining a tissue diagnosis of lung cancer when it is present.

Mediastinoscopy involves surgical assessment of mediastinal lymph nodes for determination of tumor involvement. Cervical mediastinoscopy is the standard and allows sampling or removal of lymph node stations 2, 4, 7, and often 10. The complication rate is 2%, with few life-threatening complications. With video mediastinoscopy, sensitivity and specificity exceed 97%.

An anterior mediastinotomy (Chamberlain procedure) provides access to stations 5 and 6 (aortic and aortopulmonary window), generally not accessible with cervical mediastinoscopy. This is performed through an incision in the left second or third intercostal space or through excision of the second costal cartilage.

A biopsy is necessary to establish diagnosis and, in recent years, to conduct molecular studies that can further guide therapy. The most accessible site with the least invasive method is the preferred approach to obtaining diagnostic tissue. Whereas an FNA procedure is often adequate to establish diagnosis and can be accomplished by a transthoracic approach or by ronchoscopy, the yield is often inadequate to conduct molecular studies. herefore, a core needle biopsy to obtain sufficient tissue is recommended or patients with suspected lung cancer. For patients presenting with pleural r pericardial effusions, transthoracic aspiration of fluid is sufficient for diag-osis and staging. Cell blocks prepared from the fluid can be used to conduct nolecular studies, although the success rate depends on the number of viable ancer cells in the specimen. The diagnostic yield of pleural fluid in patients vith malignant effusion is approximately 50 to 70%. In instances in which epeated aspiration of pleural fluid is nondiagnostic, a video-assisted thora-oscopy procedure might be necessary to establish diagnosis. For patients vith localized lung tumors that are suggestive of cancer, it is reasonable to roceed with surgical resection without a diagnostic biopsy if all other poten-al causes are excluded.

With the recent use of molecularly targeted therapies, understanding of the nechanisms of resistance is an important determinant of subsequent thera-ies. Therefore, it is recommended to obtain additional tumor biopsy speci-nens at various time points during the course of treatment.

Diagnostic Imaging

n conjunction with standard thoracic imaging procedures, additional sites of isease may require evaluation based on presenting complaints. The most ommon sites of lung cancer metastasis include contralateral lung, liver, drenal gland, bones, and brain. Imaging of the brain is recommended to valuate for metastasis in patients with suggestive symptoms and signs or hose with lung adenocarcinoma larger than 3 cm and evidence of mediasti-al nodal involvement. Magnetic resonance imaging (MRI) and CT scan vith contrast enhancement are both acceptable modalities to evaluate for rain metastasis, although MRI is preferred for its superior sensitivity. Radio-uclide study of the bones is indicated in patients with bone pain or an nexplained elevation in serum alkaline phosphatase level.

PET using [^{18}F]fluorodeoxyglucose (FDG) is included as part of staging n patients with localized lung cancer; however, the use of FDG-PET scan o assess response to anticancer therapy and in surveillance after curative herapy is controversial at this time and is not recommended. MRI scan of he chest may be useful in determination of invasion of surrounding struc-ures, such as the brachial plexus, in patients with tumors involving the uperior sulcus of the lung, but its use in staging is generally restricted to reoperative settings.

Solitary Pulmonary Nodule

The management of pulmonary nodules differs by whether they are solid (soft issue attenuation) or subsolid (less than soft tissue attenuation without bscuring of the underlying lung architecture on CT). For larger nodules, CT haracteristics suggestive of malignancy include irregular margins, spicula-ion, invasion of adjacent structures, lymphadenopathy, and distant metasta-es. Asymptomatic single pulmonary nodules less than 3 cm in diameter, the solitary nodule," with normal surrounding lung architecture are found inci-lentally in up to 0.2% of chest radiographs; 10 to 70% are malignant. The otential for these lesions to be malignant increases with the patient's age, nodule size (< 4 mm vs. > 8 mm), growth rate, definite history of smoking, nd size changes compared with prior imaging studies. PET scans may be nelpful in defining abnormal mediastinal nodes in these patients. A pulmonary nodule that has not changed in size for more than 2 years is probably benign. For lesions larger than 8 mm, serial high-resolution CT scans are appropriate. Suspicious nodules should undergo definitive biopsy (see Fig. 191-2).

Staging

Stage is the most important determinant of prognosis in patients with lung ancer. The seventh edition of the *American Joint Committee on Cancer (AJCC) Cancer Staging Manual* is currently in use (Table 191-2). This staging system uses new T and M descriptors to determine lung cancer stage based on the TNM (tumor, node, and metastasis) profile of the patient. Individual T descriptors are defined on the basis of tumor size of less than 2, 2 to 3, 3 o 5, 5 to 7, and more than 7 cm. In the previous system, tumors were catego-ized on the basis of size of less than or more than 3 cm. Currently, satellite nodules in the same lobe as the primary tumor are categorized as T3 and nodules in another lobe of the ipsilateral lung as T4. Malignant pleural or pericardial effusion constitutes M1 disease. Presence of metastases within the horax constitutes M1a and extrathoracic disease is classified as M1b because patients with M1a disease have a slightly better prognosis than those with M1b. Nodal descriptors were not changed from the previous system.

The TNM staging system is also now recommended for SCLC, given its ability to ascertain prognosis in a more accurate manner. SCLC was previously classified as limited or extensive stage on the basis of the ability to administer radiation therapy to the tumor with a single port. Treatment guidelines for localized SCLC have not been affected.

TABLE 191-2 TREATMENT BY AMERICAN JOINT COMMITTEE ON CANCER (AJCC) STAGE

	T	N	M	MEDICALLY FIT	MEDICALLY UNFIT
Stage IA	1	0	0	Surgery	SBRT
Stage IB	2	0	0	Surgery plus adjuvant chemotherapy if T ≥4 cm	SBRT plus chemotherapy at progression
Stage IIA/B	1-2	1	0	Surgery plus adjuvant concurrent chemoradiation	Thoracic radiation plus chemotherapy
Stage IIIA	X-3 4	2 X	0 0		Concurrent or sequential chemoradiation
Stage IIIB	X-4	3	0	Concurrent chemoradiation	
Stage IVA	X	X	1a	Chemotherapy (if *EGFR* mutation, treat with EGFR TKI)	
Stage IVB	X	X	1b	Chemotherapy (if *EGFR* mutation, treat with EGFR TKI); radiation for palliation	

T = tumor; N = node; M = metastasis; SBRT = stereotactic body radiation therapy; EGFR = epidermal growth factor receptor; TKI = tyrosine kinase inhibitor. (From AJCC Cancer Staging Manual. 7th ed. New York: Springer-Verlag; 2018)

TREATMENT Rx

Non–Small Cell Lung Cancer

Surgery

Surgical management plays the major role in the treatment of patients with stage I, stage II, and selected stage III NSCLC. However, nearly 40% of patients with early-stage lung cancer are not candidates for surgery because of limiting comorbid conditions. The commonly used parameters for inoperability include pulmonary functions with baseline forced expiratory volume in the first second of expiration (FEV_1) of less than 40%, predicted postoperative FEV_1 of less than 30%, and severely limited diffusion capacity. Such patients are referred to as medically inoperable despite the presence of localized disease and may be candidates for SBRT, as discussed later.

The first step in managing localized lung cancer is to stage the mediastinal lymph nodes. For peripheral tumors that are not associated with mediastinal adenopathy and do not have FDG uptake in the nodes, many surgeons advo-cate proceeding with surgical resection and sampling mediastinal nodes intra-operatively. However, for patients with nodes that are positive on PET scan, sampling is strongly recommended before surgery. The false-positive rate for PET scan in the mediastinum for patients with localized lung cancer is approxi-mately 20%. The likelihood of nodal involvement in patients with negative PET scan is approximately 5 to 15%.

Lobectomy is the standard surgical procedure for patients with localized lung cancer who are medically fit.[7] If anatomic resection cannot be achieved with lobectomy, bilobectomy or pneumonectomy might be necessary. Sleeve resection refers to removal of the tumor along with the bronchus and anasto-mosis of the remaining ends of the bronchial tree. Surgical resection can be achieved by performing an open thoracotomy or by video-assisted thoracic surgery (VATS). VATS is gaining wider use because of lower morbidity, faster recovery from surgery, and better ability to administer postoperative systemic therapy. The ability to achieve an R0 resection is critical, and surgery should not be attempted if this is not deemed feasible during preoperative work-up. For patients with positive surgical margins, re-resection should be attempted whenever it is feasible. If not, postoperative radiation therapy should be administered. Robotic resection of lung cancers, including robotic lobectomy and pneumonectomy, has increased in use but is not as widely employed as VATS approaches.

Sublobar resections are not recommended because of the higher risk of local recurrence. An exception to this rule is for patients with peripheral tumors smaller than 2 cm, for which studies have demonstrated excellent outcomes. An ongoing study is comparing sublobar resection to standard lobectomy and will likely provide definitive answers to this important question.

A randomized comparison of mediastinal lymph node dissection to nodal sampling demonstrated comparable outcomes for patients with NSCLC. Another study compared sublobar resection followed by placement of ^{125}I brachytherapy to the tumor bed with surgery alone in patients who are not candidates for standard lobectomy. There was no difference in overall survival between the two groups, and therefore the brachytherapy approach is not recommended. Tumors involving the superior sulcus are managed with pre-operative chemoradiotherapy to enhance tumor resection and to gain local and distant tumor control. The decision to perform surgery for these anatomi-cally challenging tumors depends on the extent of local invasion, involvement of the brachial plexus, and mediastinal lymph node involvement.

The role of surgery in the management of stage III NSCLC with mediastinal nodal involvement continues to be controversial. Surgery alone is associated with a poor outcome. In a randomized study, patients with N2-positive disease who underwent chemoradiotherapy followed by surgery did not have improved survival compared with chemoradiotherapy alone and had an unacceptably high rate (almost 30%) of postoperative mortality. Therefore, trimodality therapy is not recommended for patients who require pneumonectomy. For patients with multistation N2 disease or bulky nodal disease, surgical resection is not recommended. Clearance of mediastinal nodes after induction therapy might be the most important predictor of benefit from surgical resection, which calls for restaging of the mediastinum after induction therapy if surgery is contemplated.

The role of surgery in patients with oligometastatic disease can be considered under certain situations. Surgical resection of both the primary and a solitary brain metastasis has resulted in 5-year survival rates of approximately 20%. There are also limited data with oligometastatic disease to the adrenal glands, but similar approaches with solitary metastasis at other distant sites are not recommended. This approach cannot be recommended for patients with mediastinal nodal involvement.

Radiation Therapy

Radiation therapy is an important part of multimodality therapy for NSCLC. It plays a major role in curative therapy for stage III disease and palliation of stage IV disease and has been successfully tested for patients with medically unresectable stage I disease. Significant improvements in the delivery of radiation therapy in the past two decades allow use of smaller radiation field size, reducing exposure of normal tissue to radiation and facilitating more effective treatment of tumor. Respiratory gating techniques allow the delivery of radiation therapy to the tumor regardless of the phase of respiration. SBRT involves the delivery of high-dose radiation to a limited tumor volume after stereotactic localization.

Stage I and Stage II NSCLC

SBRT[8] has emerged as an effective treatment option for patients with T1 and T2 tumors who are node negative but are medically inoperable because of comorbid illness. In one study, delivery of SBRT over three to five fractions resulted in nearly 90% local control rate, prompting studies of SBRT in medically fit patients and in combination with systemic therapy for early-stage NSCLC. SBRT has shown considerable efficacy for peripheral tumors; studies are ongoing to examine its use in centrally located tumors.

Radiation therapy is indicated for patients with positive surgical margins after surgery for early-stage NSCLC but not for those with negative surgical margins. A meta-analysis reported a detrimental effect for patients treated with postoperative radiation therapy, especially for those with N0 and N1 disease. Patients with involved mediastinal nodes (or N2 disease) demonstrated favorable survival with radiation therapy. This has also been observed in an analysis of the U.S. Surveillance, Epidemiology and End Results (SEER) database. A prospective study is under way in Europe to compare postoperative radiation therapy with observation in patients with surgically resected N2 disease.

Stage III NSCLC

Whereas surgery is appropriate for patients with T3N1 disease, administration of radiation therapy results in improved outcomes for patients with involvement of the mediastinal lymph nodes. A subset of N2-positive patients might benefit from multimodality therapy involving neoadjuvant chemoradiation followed by surgical resection, including stage IIIA patients with single-station or microscopic lymph node involvement and disease amenable to resection with lobectomy or bilobectomy. Preoperative radiation consists of 45 Gy once daily, and a dose of 60 Gy has been piloted with acceptable safety results.

For patients with stage III disease that is not appropriate for surgical resection, thoracic radiation therapy to a dose of 60 to 66 Gy in once-daily fractions with concurrent (rather than sequential) chemotherapy is the recommended treatment.[A1] This category includes patients with bulky mediastinal disease, involvement of contralateral or supraclavicular nodes (N3), and direct invasion of major structures such as the vertebrae, trachea, major blood vessel, or esophagus by the primary tumor (T4). A 5-year survival rate of 20 to 25% has been reported with combined chemoradiotherapy in this setting. The main adverse events include esophagitis and pneumonitis, the latter depending on the extent of normal lung tissue and the dose of radiation received by normal lung tissue. Radiation-related pneumonitis can occur immediately after radiation therapy or after 6 to 9 months.

Several efforts to improve on standard chemoradiotherapy have been undertaken in the past two decades. Hyperfractionated radiation therapy with administration of two or three fractions per day has demonstrated favorable results over once-daily fractionation, particularly in squamous cell carcinoma. However, logistical constraints have limited the adoption of this approach. Single-arm studies showed the use of higher doses of up to 74 Gy in once-daily fractions to be a promising approach. However, randomized studies have failed to show benefit to dose escalation to 70 Gy or higher in this population of patients. Therefore, 60 to 66 Gy remains the standard radiation dose for stage III NSCLC.

Stage IV NSCLC

In patients with advanced-stage NSCLC, radiation therapy can be effective for palliation of spinal cord compression, brain metastasis, airway obstruction, hemoptysis, and pain.

Spinal cord compression is an emergency situation, and neurosurgical evaluation should be initiated to assess whether surgery is advised, which can be the case when there is a large tumor burden and rapidly deteriorating motor and sensory function. Surgical decompression is used when neurologic compromise is early and the patient has well-controlled systemic disease and it is followed by radiation therapy. Spinal cord compression is usually managed with external beam radiation therapy to 30 Gy and corticosteroids. For brain metastases, resection of oligometastatic disease has been associated with better outcomes. Whole brain radiation therapy of 30 to 37.5 Gy given in 10 to 15 fractions can be administered when multiple metastases are present. Stereotactic radiosurgery can be used instead of whole brain radiation therapy for patients with low-volume brain metastasis limited to one to three lesions and brain lesions that progress after whole brain radiation therapy. Pain control in sites of bone metastasis or chest wall involvement can be achieved by a short course of radiation therapy. Palliative radiation therapy is also administered to 30 to 45 Gy during 2 to 3 weeks before the initiation of systemic therapy in patients with systemic disease who present with hemoptysis or postobstructive pneumonia.

Systemic Therapy

Systemic therapy refers to the use of cytotoxic or molecularly targeted agent therapy or both. Although it was initially developed for patients with advanced-stage lung cancer, the high propensity for metastasis of lung cancer cells has extended the use of systemic therapy to patients with earlier stages of the disease. A number of effective and well-tolerated cytotoxic agents have been developed during the past three decades that are used for the routine care of patients with lung cancer. In addition, many targeted agents are under clinical investigation; six are currently approved for use in NSCLC (Table 191-3): the EGFR TKIs erlotinib, gefitinib, and afatinib; the vascular endothelial growth factor (VEGF) monoclonal antibody bevacizumab; and crizotinib, an inhibitor of MET, ALK, and ROS1 tyrosine kinases.

Systemic Therapy in Early-Stage NSCLC

Even in the setting of optimal surgery, patients with early-stage NSCLC remain at high risk for disease recurrence or metastases due to the presence of micrometastasis, which can increasingly be quantified by the evaluation of circulating tumor cells or circulating tumor DNA. A consistent benefit of 5 to 15% in 5-year survival rate observed across multiple trials has resulted in the adoption of four cycles of adjuvant cisplatin-based two-drug combination regimens as the standard of care for stage II and stage IIIA NSCLC. In stage IA disease, however, the potential benefits of chemotherapy are largely outweighed by the risks, and there is an overall detrimental effect. For patients with stage IB disease, post hoc analyses have revealed that improvement in survival with adjuvant therapy was restricted to patients with tumors larger than 4 cm, but this observation has yet to be validated in prospective trials.

Whereas cisplatin-vinorelbine has been the most commonly used combination in clinical trials of adjuvant therapy, the use of newer, better tolerated agents effective in the treatment of advanced NSCLC, such as taxanes, gemcitabine, and pemetrexed, is increasing. It is hoped that the future use of adjuvant chemotherapy may be tailored to patients at high risk for recurrence, based on genomic or proteomic markers, with circulating tumor cells or circulating tumor DNA among the most promising tools at present.[9]

Locally Advanced NSCLC

For patients with stage III disease that is not amenable to surgical resection, concomitant administration of chemotherapy with radiation therapy has

TABLE 191-3 TARGETED AGENTS IN LUNG CANCER THERAPY

MOLECULAR TARGET	FDA-APPROVED AGENTS	INVESTIGATIONAL AGENT
EGFR	Erlotinib Gefitinib Afatinib	Dacomitinib Cetuximab
ALK translocation	Crizotinib Certinib	
ROS	Crizotinib	
VEGF	Bevacizumab	
B-Raf		Dabrafenib
HSP90		Ganetespib

FDA = Food and Drug Administration.

consistently demonstrated efficacy superior to that of sequential therapy. Both cisplatin- and carboplatin-based regimens are associated with meaningful survival results but have not been compared in this setting. The combination of cisplatin and etoposide allows administration of full systemic dose of chemotherapy with radiation therapy. The carboplatin and paclitaxel regimen involves administration of lower "radiosensitizing" doses of the two agents with radiation therapy followed by consolidation therapy with two cycles at regular doses. This approach has a favorable tolerability profile compared with cisplatin-based regimens. The use of induction or consolidation chemotherapy in other settings has not resulted in improved survival. With modern combined chemoradiotherapy, cure rates of nearly 20 to 25% are achieved in locally advanced NSCLC, with esophagitis and pneumonitis being the main toxicities.

Several systemic targeted agents, including cetuximab (a monoclonal antibody against EGFR), bevacizumab (a monoclonal antibody against VEGF), and ALK inhibitors, are under evaluation for the treatment of stage III disease. Ongoing studies continue to evaluate the role of EGFR TKIs in patients with activating *EGFR* mutations and locally advanced disease.

Advanced-Stage NSCLC

In patients with advanced-stage NSCLC, randomized trials have shown platinum-based systemic therapy to improve overall survival and quality of life compared with supportive care alone. Cisplatin treatment is associated with nausea, emesis, nephrotoxicity, and neurotoxicity, although the availability of highly effective antiemetic agents has greatly improved its tolerability. Carboplatin is a better tolerated alternative to cisplatin and is associated with ease of outpatient administration. The dose-limiting toxicity of carboplatin is thrombocytopenia. Two-drug combination regimens have proved superior to monotherapy with cisplatin alone or a nonplatinum compound, leading to the adoption of combination chemotherapy as the recommended treatment of advanced NSCLC.

A meta-analysis of randomized trials compared the efficacy of cisplatin to carboplatin in advanced-stage NSCLC and demonstrated comparable survival but a numerically higher incidence of treatment-related deaths with cisplatin-based regimens. Although cisplatin-based regimens have a narrow efficacy advantage, carboplatin-based regimens have found wider adoption because of their favorable therapeutic index.

A number of partner agents for platinum have demonstrated similar efficacy in advanced NSCLC in randomized trials, including etoposide, vinblastine, vindesine, vinorelbine, taxanes, gemcitabine, irinotecan, and pemetrexed. On the basis of several randomized studies, the choice of chemotherapy agent for frontline treatment is made on consideration of toxicity, preference of the patient, schedule, and cost. Recent trials involving superior supportive care have shown median survival for combinations of cisplatin with docetaxel, gemcitabine, or pemetrexed in the 10- to 11-month range. Combinations of three cytotoxic agents are not recommended because of a higher toxicity burden and lack of meaningful incremental benefit.

In randomized studies of patients with an activating *EGFR* mutation, treatment with gefitinib or erlotinib has been associated with improvements in progression-free survival and quality of life over platinum-based chemotherapy. This did not translate into a survival benefit because the majority of patients treated with chemotherapy were subsequently crossed over to receive an EGFR inhibitor on disease progression. The importance of molecular testing before initiation of EGFR inhibitor therapy in first-line treatment is highlighted by the inferior outcomes in wild-type patients treated with targeted therapy.[A2] Afatinib, an irreversible EGFR TKI, has recently demonstrated superiority over chemotherapy in patients with an activating *EGFR* mutation, leading to its approval in this setting.

Initial studies of the VEGF antibody bevacizumab for first-line therapy for advanced NSCLC were promising, although squamous histology was associated with a higher incidence of life-threatening hemoptysis. Further studies limited to patients with nonsquamous histology demonstrated a significant improvement in overall survival and progression-free survival with the addition of bevacizumab to carboplatin and paclitaxel chemotherapy, leading to the Food and Drug Administration approval of bevacizumab in this setting. Notable adverse events included bleeding, hypertension, proteinuria, and neutropenia.

The MET, ALK, and ROS1 TKI crizotinib demonstrated a response rate of nearly 60% and a clinical benefit rate of 90% in patients with ALK-positive advanced-stage NSCLC, with a median progression-free survival of 10 months.[A3] Accordingly, crizotinib is approved in this setting in the United States and Europe. The second-generation ALK inhibitor ceritinib also is useful and approved for the treatment of patients with ALK-positive metastatic NSCLC with disease progression or intolerance to crizotinib.[A4]

Role of Histology in Choice of Chemotherapy

Until recently, chemotherapy regimens were considered to be suitable for all histologic subtypes of NSCLC. This notion was dispelled in a randomized phase III study demonstrating superior survival for patients with nonsquamous advanced-stage NSCLC treated with cisplatin-pemetrexed and superior survival for patients with squamous histology receiving cisplatin-gemcitabine. Nanoparticle albumin-bound paclitaxel (nab-paclitaxel) is associated with a favorable response rate in patients with advanced NSCLC, which is restricted to patients with squamous histology. The biologic basis for the histologically specific therapeutic activity of these drugs is not presently known; however, the variable efficacy of pemetrexed and nab-paclitaxel based on histology should be considered when chemotherapy is selected for first-line treatment of advanced NSCLC.

Maintenance Therapy

In the first-line treatment of advanced-stage NSCLC, continuation of combination, multi–cytotoxic drug treatment beyond four to six cycles is associated with cumulative toxicities but no tangible benefit. Recently, single-agent maintenance therapy has proved to be useful in patients who have a demonstrated clinical benefit from four cycles of platinum-based combination chemotherapy. Current therapeutic strategies employ either a "switch maintenance" approach, which uses an alternative cytotoxic or targeted agent that has not been previously administered, or "continuation maintenance," which involves continuing the nonplatinum agent beyond four cycles.

Pemetrexed is the only cytotoxic agent that provides a survival advantage as maintenance therapy in advanced NSCLC. It has demonstrated similar benefit in both continuation and switch maintenance strategies in randomized trials for patients with advanced nonsquamous histology and has thus been approved for maintenance therapy in the United States and Europe. The EGFR TKI erlotinib also extends survival when it is used as maintenance therapy in patients who have experienced stable disease with a platinum-based combination for four cycles, with greater benefit in patients with an activating *EGFR* mutation. The use of bevacizumab maintenance has been adopted for patients who receive it as part of their initial treatment regimen because all pivotal randomized trials performed with bevacizumab used it as maintenance therapy after six cycles of combination treatment.

Docetaxel, pemetrexed, and erlotinib are also efficacious when they are used as salvage therapy for patients with advanced NSCLC who experience disease progression during or after platinum-based chemotherapy. Therefore, the relative merits of using the last two agents as maintenance therapy versus use after disease progression has become controversial. Careful discussion with patients with nonsquamous lung cancers who have responded to front-line chemotherapy regarding the value of maintenance therapy versus close observation is recommended.

Salvage Therapy

Virtually all patients with advanced NSCLC will eventually experience disease progression regardless of the extent of benefit from first-line chemotherapy. Salvage therapy for these patients provides a modest but real improvement in survival. Docetaxel, at a dose of 75 mg/m^2 every 3 weeks, was the first agent proven in this setting to improve survival compared with best supportive care or first-generation cytotoxic agents. Pemetrexed has efficacy as salvage therapy similar to that of docetaxel and a more favorable toxicity profile, but its use is restricted to patients with nonsquamous histology. Targeted therapy with erlotinib has also been demonstrated to enhance survival and progression-free survival in the salvage setting. Overall, the presently available salvage therapy options are associated with response rates of less than 10%, with a median progression-free survival of 3 months and overall survival of 8 months.

Crizotinib significantly improves progression-free survival and response rate compared with chemotherapy in the salvage setting for patients whose tumors exhibit an *ALK* rearrangement. The use of bevacizumab as salvage therapy for NSCLC is currently being examined in ongoing clinical trials. Combinations of cytotoxic or targeted agents for salvage therapy have not resulted in improved survival, and these are therefore not recommended.

Investigational Targeted Agents

The use of targeted therapies has gained considerable momentum in recent years, and many investigational targeted agents are in preclinical and clinical development. The irreversible EGFR inhibitor dacomitinib demonstrated a favorable efficacy profile compared with erlotinib in a randomized phase II study in an unselected population of patients and is presently being evaluated in phase III trials. Several new agents and combinations are under study for managing resistance to EGFR TKIs. Cetuximab, a monoclonal antibody against EGFR, produces a modest improvement in overall survival when it is combined with cisplatin and vinorelbine for first-line treatment of advanced NSCLC. The identification of predictive biomarkers to select patients is necessary for the use of this combination in routine care.

LDK378, a potent ALK inhibitor, produced a response rate of 60% in patients who developed disease progression during crizotinib therapy. Other novel ALK inhibitors are also under development for management of crizotinib resistance or as primary therapy. Heat shock protein 90 (HSP90) plays a critical chaperone function for ALK, and HSP90 inhibitors have recently been found to possess single-agent activity in this subgroup of patients.

Besides the VEGF monoclonal antibody bevacizumab, other strategies to inhibit angiogenesis, including small-molecule VEGF TKIs and vascular disrupting agents, have not been successful to date in advanced NSCLC. Efforts to identify biomarkers to predict benefit with bevacizumab and other antiangiogenic agents have also been unsuccessful and have consequently restricted optimal use of these agents.

Advances in genomic technology have made it possible to prospectively identify novel mutations that play a critical role in the growth of lung cancers. In adenocarcinoma, a fusion gene involving *ROS1*, observed in 1% of patients, also confers sensitivity to treatment with crizotinib. Another fusion involving the *RET* gene has been identified in 0.5 to 1% of patients. Patients with mutations in *BRAF* appear to respond to therapy with dabrafenib, a BRAF inhibitor. Recent DNA sequencing data from the Cancer Genome Atlas project in a cohort of patients with squamous cell lung carcinoma, together with the efforts of the Lung Cancer Mutation Consortium, have demonstrated several novel, potentially targetable mutations in this disease. Routine testing of tumor specimens of patients for molecular targets is increasingly seen as a strategy to personalize treatment options for lung cancer.

Management of Special Populations of Patients

Elderly patients represent a growing subset of lung cancer patients. In the United States, the median age at diagnosis of lung cancer is 70 years. Aging is associated with declines in physiologic and vital organ function that affect a patient's tolerance for systemic therapy, making current physical function and prospective quality of life considerations important factors in the choice of systemic treatment. Single-agent chemotherapy has a demonstrated survival benefit compared with supportive care in elderly patients; and for those with good performance status, platinum-based combinations are superior to single-agent therapy. The appropriate use of targeted agents may have clinical benefit in the elderly. The addition of bevacizumab to chemotherapy for non-squamous cancers in older patients is, however, associated with a narrow therapeutic index and is recommended only with great caution.

A substantial percentage of NSCLC patients present with reduced performance status, which limits their ability to tolerate combination chemotherapy. The median survival for advanced NSCLC patients with a performance status of 2 or worse (Eastern Cooperative Oncology Group scale) is dismal at less than 4 months; however, studies conducted exclusively in patients with a poor performance status indicate that chemotherapy may be beneficial for highly selected patients. It is important to consider the underlying cause of poor performance status in making treatment plans for this population of patients. For those with limiting comorbid conditions, a less aggressive approach with single-agent chemotherapy might be more appropriate. For those with a targetable mutation, appropriate targeted therapy can be administered regardless of the performance status in view of the greater potential for benefit.

Small Cell Lung Cancer

SCLC is characterized by enhanced initial sensitivity to systemic chemotherapy, although disease recurrence is common regardless of the extent of initial response. Approximately two thirds of patients present with extensive-stage SCLC, defined as the presence of metastatic disease outside the chest or large-volume thoracic disease that cannot be treated with radiation therapy. The median survival of untreated extensive-stage SCLC is less than 2 months, and the overall goal of treatment is palliation. The use of platinum-based chemotherapy results in response rates of 50 to 70% and median survival of 9 to 11 months. The regimen of four to six cycles of cisplatin and etoposide is considered the standard approach for the treatment of SCLC, extending to six cycles in responding patients, with no proven role for maintenance therapy. Carboplatin is considered an acceptable alternative in the treatment of extensive-stage disease. Despite the extent of initial response, disease recurrence develops in a median of 4 to 6 months. Disease that progresses during or within 90 days of administration of cisplatin-based chemotherapy is referred to as refractory relapse. Recurrence outside this time window represents a "sensitive" subgroup that might benefit from salvage treatment. Other approaches, such as high-dose chemotherapy, alternating chemotherapy regimens, dose-dense therapy, and three-drug combination regimens, have been unsuccessful in improving survival. In the Japanese population but not in Western patients, the regimen of cisplatin and irinotecan has demonstrated superior results over cisplatin and etoposide.

Salvage therapy has yielded only modest results in sensitive relapsed SCLC. Topotecan is the only agent to demonstrate clinical benefit in relapsed SCLC, with a response rate of 20% and a favorable symptom improvement profile but no improvement in overall survival in randomized studies. Several novel agents, including molecularly targeted agents against known targets, are presently being studied in efforts to improve the outcomes for patients with SCLC.

For patients with limited-stage SCLC, radiation therapy is used in combination with chemotherapy and can achieve cure for approximately 20 to 30% of patients. Earlier initiation of radiation therapy appears superior to a delayed approach and has been adopted as the standard in fit patients. A randomized study demonstrated superior survival of twice-daily radiation therapy fractions compared with the same dose given once daily along with concomitant chemotherapy, and this is being further evaluated in an ongoing trial.

Prophylactic cranial irradiation is associated with a modest improvement in 5-year survival for patients with limited-stage SCLC who achieve complete remission after combined modality therapy. This is due to the high risk of brain recurrence observed in patients with SCLC. Similarly, studies have demonstrated that prophylactic cranial irradiation results in modest improvement in overall survival and reduced risk of brain recurrence in patients with extensive-stage disease who achieve a favorable response to combination chemotherapy.

The role of surgery is limited to the less than 5% of SCLC patients presenting with peripheral lung lesions without mediastinal nodal involvement. In 10 to 15% of patients with SCLC, a mixed histology with NSCLC features is observed. These patients may demonstrate local progression after combined modality therapy resulting from the NSCLC component. Therefore, these individuals could be considered for surgical resection in selected situations.

Treatment advances in SCLC have, unfortunately, lagged behind those for NSCLC during the past two decades; consequently, survival outcomes for SCLC have not changed considerably. Concerted efforts to develop appropriate preclinical models to test new agents, genomic subcategorization of SCLC, and discovery of new systemic anticancer agents are necessary to improve outcomes for this aggressive disease.

SURVIVORSHIP AND SURVEILLANCE

As outcomes for lung cancer have improved in recent years, with a concomi tant increase in the number of survivors after surgery or chemoradiotherap an important part of lung cancer care has become defining the optimal survei lance, follow-up for second primary disease, and management of long-tern consequences of chemoradiotherapy. The importance of smoking cessatio cannot be overemphasized, given the high risk of enhanced complications o chemotherapy and the higher incidence of second primary tumors in lun cancer survivors. Patients should be provided with appropriate opportunitie to receive counseling and behavioral therapy and other treatment modalitie to assist their efforts to discontinue smoking (Chapter 32).

At present, there is no standard approach to optimal radiographic an clinical follow-up in patients who undergo surgical resection or chemoradio therapy. CT scans are commonly used for follow-up of these patients However, the relative merits of CT scan versus chest radiography, the fre quency of evaluation, and the role of FDG-PET scans are unclear and will b answered only by prospective clinical trials. For patients with advanced-stag disease, CT scans are used to assess response to therapy every two or thre cycles of treatment. In view of the proven role for salvage therapy, patient who are in follow-up after combination chemotherapy should be closel observed for development of new symptoms or clinical deterioration in addi tion to periodic radiographic studies.

Respiratory therapy should be offered and strongly recommended t patients with dyspnea after surgery or chemoradiotherapy. Because a hig proportion of these patients also have smoking-related pulmonary diseases referral to a pulmonologist should be considered in symptomatic patient Overall, a team approach that includes supportive care personnel, oncologi psychiatrists, nutritionists, oncologists, and appropriate additional specialist should be used to ensure the return of lung cancer survivors to normalcy t the fullest extent possible.

SUPPORTIVE CARE

Patients with lung cancer have a cure rate of only 16%, even in the mos advanced Western health systems, because the majority of patients presen with locally advanced or metastatic disease. Early discussion and institutio of palliative and supportive care are therefore critical for the patient to ensur maximal quality of life. Studies indicate that early integration of supportiv care helps maintain and improve quality of life, with one randomized tria finding that the addition of early palliative care to chemotherapy for patient with advanced disease can produce a meaningful impact on overall survival, a surprising but reaffirming finding.

EARLY DETECTION AND PREVENTION

Decades of research into the screening of high-risk individuals for earlie detection of lung cancer have recently met with success.[10] The NLST random ized more than 50,000 subjects between 55 and 74 years of age with a histor of cigarette smoking of at least 30 pack-years to screening with low-dose C scan or chest radiographs at baseline and 1 and 2 years after enrollment. Th rate of adherence to scans was more than 90% in both arms. Positive result were observed in nearly 25% and 7% of subjects with CT screening and ches radiograph, respectively. Among patients with a positive CT scan, 96.4% were deemed false positive after additional evaluation. Adverse event were uncommon. Screening with annual low-dose CT scans in high-ris ndividuals was associated with a reduction of 20% in lung cancer mortality and 6.7% in all-cause mortality. Nearly 80% of patients diagnosed with lung cancer with low-dose CT had stage I, II, or IIIA disease amenable to curative therapy.[A6] Subsequent analysis of the NLST data showed that screening with low-dose CT prevented the greatest number of deaths from lung cancer among participants who were at highest risk and prevented very few deaths among those at lowest risk.[A7] These results have led to the adoption of low-dose CT for early detection of lung cancer by major health organizations including the U.S. Preventive Services Task Force.[11,12] For lung nodules detected on low-dose CT screening, it has been shown that predictive tools based on patient and nodule characteristics can be used to accurately estimate the probability that they are malignant.[13]

Primary prevention of lung cancer focuses on ways to prevent individuals from smoking and promotion of smoking cessation, which remain the most effective means to prevent lung cancer. Smoking cessation efforts are often sporadic; but most studies indicate that patients who successfully quit smoking benefit from pharmacologic, psychological, and physician support.

Trials of supplemental β-carotene and vitamin E, stimulated by epidemiologic evidence of lower serum levels of these antioxidants in patients with lung cancer, not only have been unsuccessful but actually produced a higher risk of lung cancer in smokers. High concentrations of selenium in the blood are associated with a lower risk of lung cancer, but a phase III trial in patients with resected stage I lung cancer failed to show any benefit for selenium supplementation. These and other trials have indicated that lung cancer patients who continue to smoke have the highest incidence of recurrence and second primary tumor development.

OTHER PULMONARY NEOPLASMS

Malignant Mesothelioma

Malignant pleural mesotheliomas[14] are generally related to asbestos exposure, with a peak risk for development of the disease 30 to 35 years after the initial exposure. Additional possible risk factors include radiation and SV40 virus. Mesothelioma is generally diagnosed in the fifth to seventh decade of life (median age, 60 years), with a male-to-female preponderance of 5 : 1. Common symptoms include dyspnea (60%) and chest wall pain or discomfort (60%). Chest radiographs usually reveal the presence of a unilateral pleural effusion. Tumor progression and symptoms are generally the result of local progression, with symptomatic distant metastases a late occurrence. Cytologic evaluation of pleural fluid to establish diagnosis is difficult and often inaccurate. The diagnosis is generally made by a biopsy procedure under CT guidance or thoracoscopically, including VATS if necessary. Several staging systems have been proposed, but none has achieved complete acceptance. Treatment, depending on the extent of disease, includes surgery (thoracoscopy with sclerosis, pleurectomy, extrapleural pneumonectomy), radiation therapy, and, often, chemotherapy. These three modalities individually have not significantly improved survival rates, and chemotherapy or radiation therapy does not provide long-term palliation or relief of symptoms. Combination chemotherapy with pemetrexed and cisplatin is associated with symptomatic relief in patients with advanced, unresectable malignant mesothelioma and with a significant response rate in advanced disease. It is occasionally used as preoperative or induction chemotherapy before extrapleural pneumonectomy followed by radiation therapy. Multimodality and molecularly targeted agents are being evaluated. Mesothelioma unfortunately remains a nearly universally fatal illness, with a median survival of less than 12 months from the time of diagnosis.

Neuroendocrine and Other Lung Tumors

Neuroendocrine lung tumors are classified into four types: carcinoid tumors, atypical carcinoids, SCLC, and large cell neuroendocrine carcinomas. *Carcinoid tumors* (Chapter 232) are low-grade neuroendocrine tumors with a 10-year survival rate greater than 90%. Atypical carcinoid tumors are intermediate-grade tumors, significantly more aggressive than carcinoid, with 10-year survival of below 20%. *Large cell neuroendocrine carcinoma* is an aggressive neuroendocrine tumor that does not meet the criteria for carcinoid, atypical carcinoid, or SCLC. Considerable activity for everolimus and other inhibitors of the mammalian target of rapamycin (mTOR) has been demonstrated in low-grade carcinoid tumors.

Carcinoid tumors of the lung account for 1 to 2% of all lung neoplasms. These neuroendocrine tumors trace their origin to the Kulchitsky cell present in bronchial epithelium. Typical and atypical carcinoids differ in the number of mitoses (<2 per 10 high-power fields vs. 2 to 10 per 10 high-power fields, respectively), nuclear pleomorphism (absent vs. present), and regional lymph node metastases (5 to 15% vs. 20 to 28%). Distant metastases at initial evaluation are rare (<20%). Patients with typical carcinoid tumors usually live for many years, whereas patients with atypical carcinoid tumors have a 5-year mortality rate of 61 to 88%. Carcinoid tumors are not associated with cigarette smoking, are twice as common in women as in men, usually occur in patients younger than 40 years, and arise in the perihilar area of the lung. Treatment of bronchial carcinoid tumors is based on the stage of the disease. Mediastinal staging is usually followed by surgical resection. With mediastinal lymph node involvement, radiation therapy is recommended for typical carcinoid tumors if surgery cannot be performed. For atypical carcinoid or metastatic disease, chemotherapy (etoposide plus cisplatin every 3 weeks for four cycles) plus radiation therapy is commonly used, but there is no evidence for the benefit of one therapy over another.

Salivary gland carcinomas include mucoepidermoid carcinoma and adenoid cystic carcinoma, which represent approximately 0.2% of lung cancers. These slow-growing neoplasms arise from the bronchial glands and are usually treated with surgery.

Primary sarcomas of the lung are very rare and include malignant fibrous histiocytoma, fibrosarcoma, leiomyosarcoma, rhabdomyosarcoma, epithelioid hemangioendothelioma, angiosarcoma, and liposarcoma (Chapter 202). The primary treatment is surgery, but depending on the size and grade of the tumor and whether the margins are clear, radiation therapy or chemotherapy may also be given. Primary lymphomas of the lung are also very rare, accounting for approximately 0.3% of all primary lung cancers. The most common type is a low-grade small lymphocytic lymphoma, for which surgery and chemotherapy are the usual treatments (Chapter 185).

Grade A References

A1. Curran WJ Jr, Paulus R, Langer CJ, et al. Sequential vs. concurrent chemoradiation for stage III non–small cell lung cancer: randomized phase III trial RTOG 9410. *J Natl Cancer Inst.* 2011;103:1452-1460.

A2. Lee JK, Hahn S, Kim DW, et al. Epidermal growth factor receptor tyrosine kinase inhibitors vs conventional chemotherapy in non-small cell lung cancer harboring wild-type epidermal growth factor receptor: a meta-analysis. *JAMA.* 2014;311:1430-1437.

A3. Shaw AT, Kim DW, Nakagawa K, et al. Crizotinib versus chemotherapy in advanced ALK-positive lung cancer. *N Engl J Med.* 2013;368:2385-2394.

A4. Shaw AT, Kim DW, Mehra R, et al. Ceritinib in ALK-rearranged non-small-cell lung cancer. *N Engl J Med.* 2014;370:1189-1197.

A5. Temel JS, Greer JA, Muzikansky A, et al. Early palliative care for patients with metastatic non-small-cell lung cancer. *N Engl J Med.* 2010;363:733-742.

A6. National Lung Screening Trial Research Team, Aberle DR, Adams AM, Berg CD, et al. Reduced lung-cancer mortality with low-dose computed tomographic screening. *N Engl J Med.* 2011;365:395-409.

A7. Kovalchik SA, Tammemagi M, Berg CD, et al. Targeting of low-dose CT screening according to the risk of lung-cancer death. *N Engl J Med.* 2013;369:245-254.

GENERAL REFERENCES

For the General References and other additional features, please visit Expert Consult at https://expertconsult.inkling.com.

192 NEOPLASMS OF THE ESOPHAGUS AND STOMACH

ANIL K. RUSTGI

NEOPLASMS OF THE ESOPHAGUS

DEFINITION

The esophagus is a hollow tubular organ with primary physiologic functions related to contraction to permit propulsion of solid and liquid food contents into the stomach. The mucosa is a stratified squamous epithelium that covers the submucosa and muscle; the latter is skeletal muscle in the proximal esophagus and smooth muscle in the mid-distal esophagus. Cancers of the esophagus may be classified broadly into epithelial versus nonepithelial.

There are benign epithelial tumors referred to as squamous cell papillomas. Malignant epithelial tumors are classified into two main subtypes: esophageal squamous cell carcinoma and esophageal adenocarcinoma. Other, less common, esophageal epithelium-derived cancers include verrucous squamous cell carcinoma, adenosquamous carcinoma, adenoid cystic carcinoma, and mucoepidermoid carcinoma. Benign nonepithelial tumors include leiomyoma, granular cell tumors, fibrovascular polyp, hemangioma, lymphangioma, lipoma, and fibroma. Malignant nonepithelial tumors include leiomyosarcoma and other sarcomas, metastatic carcinoma (originating from breast, lung), and lymphoma.

Esophageal Squamous Cell Carcinoma

EPIDEMIOLOGY

Esophageal squamous cell carcinoma is the more common type of esophageal cancer worldwide and represents a leading cause of cancer-related mortality in men. Esophageal squamous cell carcinoma may have rates of up to 100 per 100,000 population in what is often termed the *Central Asian belt*, including regions around the Caspian Sea, Iran, India, and China; other areas of high incidence include some Mediterranean countries and South Africa. In the United States, esophageal squamous cell carcinoma is more common among African American males than white males, with risks of 15.1 per 100,000 compared with 2.9 per 100,000, respectively. Overall, although the U.S. incidence of esophageal squamous cell carcinoma is low in males or females younger than 50 years, it does increase with advancing age.

Risk Factors

Cancers in general are viewed in the context of hereditary or inherited forms versus sporadic or seemingly random diseases that are related to age, environmental exposures, and genetic alterations (Table 192-1). That being said, the hereditary basis for esophageal squamous cell carcinoma is exceedingly rare, consisting of a desquamating condition termed *tylosis palmaris et plantaris*. As implied, the desquamation most dramatically affects the hands and feet, but this extends to the esophagus as well. Another uncommon condition, Plummer-Vinson syndrome or Paterson-Brown Kelly syndrome, entails glossitis, cervical esophageal webs, and iron deficiency anemia. In both conditions, it is likely that chronic inflammation triggers the cascade of events that culminate in esophageal dysplasia and esophageal squamous cell carcinoma.

The preponderance of esophageal squamous cell carcinoma cases are attributable to cigarette smoking or alcohol, but especially so in combination, because there appear to be synergistic deleterious effects of various chemical carcinogens in both, including *N*-nitroso compounds, polycyclic aromatic hydrocarbons, and aromatic amines. The relative risk for esophageal squamous cell carcinoma is 6.2 in those who smoke more than 25 cigarettes on a daily basis. Cessation of cigarette smoking is helpful in attenuating risk after 10 years of abstinence. Cigarette smokers who partake in beer and whiskey have a 10- to 25-fold enhanced risk of developing esophageal squamous cell carcinoma. Indeed, it is the type of alcohol and the manner of distillation that are most critical. In endemic areas of the world, deficiencies of vitamins A, B_{12}, C, and E, folic acid, and certain minerals (zinc, selenium, molybdenum) are important risk factors. All these vitamins and minerals exert direct or indirect antioxidant effects, and their deficiencies impair epithelial and tissue homeostasis and regeneration.

Other risk factors for esophageal squamous cell carcinoma[1] include achalasia (Chapters 136 and 138), a disorder that involves aganglíosis of Auerbach's plexus, resulting in dysphagia, chest pain, and weight loss, among other symptoms. The emergence of esophageal squamous cell carcinoma may be observed 10 to 20 years after the identification of achalasia in patients. Because head and neck squamous cell carcinoma (HNSCC) (Chapter 190) shares many of the environmental and lifestyle risk factors with esophageal squamous cell carcinoma, particularly alcohol and tobacco smoking, HNSCC and esophageal squamous cell carcinoma may occur synchronously or metachronously. In different parts of the world, esophageal squamous cell carcinoma is also associated with chronic esophageal stricture due to lye ingestion, consumption of maté (a hot herb-based beverage), celiac sprue, human papillomavirus (HPV) infection (especially genotypes HPV-16, HPV-18, and HPV-33), and radiation injury.

TABLE 192-1 RISK FACTORS FOR ESOPHAGEAL CANCER

Esophageal squamous cell cancer
Tylosis palmaris et plantaris
Achalasia
Plummer-Vinson syndrome
Cigarette smoking
Alcohol
Chronic lye ingestion
Human papillomavirus infection
Radiation injury
Celiac sprue
Esophageal adenocarcinoma
Gastroesophageal acid reflux
Bile reflux
Obesity
Barrett esophagus

PATHOBIOLOGY

Esophageal squamous cell carcinoma involves the transition from normal squamous epithelium to squamous dysplasia to cancer. Esophageal squamous cell carcinoma initiation, progression, and metastasis are associated with a number of genetic alterations. Among these genetic alterations are overexpression of epidermal growth factor receptor *(EGFR)* and cyclin D1 oncogenes, and inactivation of *TP53*, *p16INK4A*, *E-cadherin*, and p120-catenin *(p120ctn)* tumor suppressor genes. The frequency of these changes varies greatly based upon various studies, but the oncogenic alterations generally appear early in dysplasia and early esophageal squamous cell carcinoma, whereas the inactivation of tumor suppressor genes appear as later events in established primary and metastatic esophageal squamous cell carcinoma. From a genomic viewpoint, the SOX-2 transcription factor, important in the pluripotent capacity of somatic cells, has been shown to be an important gene involved in esophageal squamous cell carcinoma pathogenesis and transformation by virtue of SOX-2 amplification. The ability to model esophageal squamous cell carcinoma in vitro and in vivo has witnessed great strides in recent years through the advent and characterization of three-dimensional organotypic culture models, xenograft transplantation mouse models, and genetically engineered mouse models. For example, conditional knockout of the *p120ctn* tumor suppressor gene in the esophagus of mice results in invasive esophageal squamous cell carcinoma.

CLINICAL MANIFESTATIONS

Symptoms and Signs

Although esophageal squamous dysplasia is typically not associated with symptoms, esophageal squamous cell carcinoma, which has a predilection for the proximal to midesophagus, may be associated with dysphagia, odynophagia, atypical or typical chest pain, gastrointestinal bleeding, nausea, vomiting, weight loss, and malnutrition. Esophageal squamous cell carcinoma may metastasize to local lymph nodes, lung, liver, and bone. Symptoms attributable to metastatic esophageal squamous cell carcinoma may involve bone-related pain, dyspnea, and evidence of jaundice and liver failure, depending upon the extent of metastatic disease.

Physical Examination

The patient should be evaluated for changes in hair, skin integrity, and nail beds as a reflection of malnutrition. Weight loss may result in general cachexia and muscle wasting. There may be lymphadenopathy in the anterior cervical and superclavicular regions. Hepatomegaly and complications of liver disease may be present with metastatic disease to the liver.

Laboratory Studies

There may be progressive iron deficiency anemia due to chronic indolent upper gastrointestinal bleeding. Additional abnormalities may be reflected in metabolic disturbances, such as metabolic alkalosis due to vomiting and hypernatremia due to dehydration. Liver enzyme abnormalities, both hepatocellular and cholestatic, may reflect metastasis to the liver. There are no specific markers for esophageal squamous cell carcinoma, but an elevated carcinoembryonic antigen (CEA) level may be used to aid in monitoring disease recurrence after therapy.

DIAGNOSIS

Barium swallow radiography is useful for the diagnosis of esophageal squamous cell carcinoma, with depiction of a filling defect due to the mucosal lesion or impaired transit of barium due to luminal growth (Chapter 138). However, definitive diagnosis involves direct visualization with upper endoscopy (Chapter 134); once the mass is visualized, biopsies are necessary for confirmation by histopathology and immunohistochemistry for

TABLE 192-2 TNM STAGING SYSTEM FOR CANCER OF THE ESOPHAGUS (AMERICAN JOINT COMMITTEE ON CANCER CRITERIA)

PRIMARY TUMOR (T)*	
TX	Primary tumor cannot be assessed
T0	No evidence of primary tumor
Tis	High-grade dysplasia†
T1	Tumor invades lamina propria, muscularis mucosae, or submucosa
T1a	Tumor invades lamina propria or muscularis mucosae
T1b	Tumor invades submucosa
T2	Tumor invades muscularis propria
T3	Tumor invades adventitia
T4	Tumor invades adjacent structures
T4a	Resectable tumor invading pleura, pericardium, or diaphragm
T4b	Unresectable tumor invading other adjacent structures, such as aorta, vertebral body, trachea, etc.

*(1) At least maximal dimension of the tumor must be recorded, and (2) multiple tumors require the T(m) suffix.
†High-grade dysplasia includes all noninvasive neoplastic epithelia that was formerly called carcinoma in situ.

LYMPH NODE (N)*	
NX	Regional lymph nodes cannot be assessed
N0	No regional lymph node metastasis
N1	Metastasis in 1-2 regional lymph nodes
N2	Metastasis in 3-6 regional lymph nodes
N3	Metastasis in 7 or more regional lymph nodes

*Number must be recorded for total number of regional nodes sampled and total number of reported nodes with metastasis.

DISTANT METASTASIS (M)	
MX	Metastasis cannot be assessed
M0	No distant metastasis
M1	Distant metastasis

From *AJCC Cancer Staging Manual*. 7th ed. New York: Springer-Verlag; 2010.

cytokeratins associated with proliferation and differentiation. Esophageal squamous cell carcinoma may involve local lymph nodes, which are best detected by endoscopic ultrasound (EUS); as needed, samples can then be analyzed by cytopathology following fine-needle aspiration (FNA). In high-volume centers in the United States, the cytopathologist will be in the procedure room with the gastroenterologist to provide an initial evaluation of the specimens obtained through FNA. Evaluation of metastatic disease involves chest and abdominal computed tomography (CT) scans. Bone scan might be useful in patients who are symptomatic with bone-related pain. Positron emission tomography (PET) has become increasingly used in some settings. In totality, these diagnostic modalities also allow for staging of esophageal squamous cell carcinoma (Table 192-2), which is important in guiding therapeutic options.[2]

TREATMENT Rx

Surgical Therapy

Surgery is the cornerstone of therapy for curative intent. Technical advances have led to improvements in both operative mortality and postoperative morbidity. The different surgical techniques include transthoracic, transhiatal, and radical en bloc resections. Depending upon the location of the esophageal squamous cell carcinoma, either total esophagectomy or subtotal esophagectomy is pursued. For the latter, jejunal or colonic interposition can be done. Although there is currently a lack of high-quality studies comparing minimally invasive esophagectomy (MIE) to conventional approaches, MIE can achieve equivalent or better perioperative mortality, morbidity, and oncologic outcomes compared to open surgery in selected patients.[3]

Medical Therapy

Depending upon the stage of disease, there is some variation in whether to proceed with preoperative (neoadjuvant) chemoradiation therapy (preferred for early stage) or postoperative (adjuvant) chemoradiation therapy.

A study in which patients were randomized to receive surgery alone or surgery plus postoperative chemotherapy with 5-fluorouracil and leucovorin and concurrent radiation therapy revealed that the median survival was 36 months for patients in the adjuvant arm compared with 26 months for those in the surgery-only arm. The 3-year overall survival rates were 50% (surgery plus adjuvant therapy) compared with 40% (surgery alone), respectively.

PROGNOSIS

The 5-year survival for treated esophageal squamous cell carcinoma is dependent upon stage and types of therapies used. For stages T1 and T2 without lymph node involvement, surgery alone may be curative in more than 60% of cases. The occurrence of major postoperative complications, which occur in about one third of patients, exerts a long-lasting negative effect on health-related quality of life in patients who survive for 5 years after esophagectomy for cancer. Dyspnea, fatigue, eating restriction, sleep difficulty, and gastroesophageal reflux progressively worsen more during follow-up in those who suffer such major postoperative complications compared with those without major surgical complications. For patients with metastatic disease, therapy is palliative, involving endoscopically placed expandable prosthetic stents to open the nearly obstructed lumen for passage of food contents, percutaneous endoscopic gastrotomy tubes for delivery of nutrition to the stomach distal to the mass lesion, total parenteral nutrition, pain control, and systemic chemotherapy.

Esophageal Adenocarcinoma

EPIDEMIOLOGY

Esophageal adenocarcinoma affects whites more than African Americans and males much more than females (3 : 1 to 5.5 : 1); it increases in incidence after the age of 40 years. The age-adjusted incidence annually is 1.3 per 100,000. In this chapter, esophageal adenocarcinoma is discussed as a separate entity from gastroesophageal (GE) adenocarcinomas (so-called GE junctional cancer) and gastric cardia adenocarcinomas, although there has been an increasing tendency to think of these in aggregate. The incidence of esophageal adenocarcinoma is increasing dramatically in developed countries, especially in the United States (by 4 to 10% annually) and Western/Northern Europe.

Etiology

Obesity (central) is an important risk factor for esophageal adenocarcinoma. This may be related to either mechanical factors that foster greater gastroesophageal reflux disease (GERD) or the release of proinflammatory cytokines and chemokines that track to the esophagus, or both. The major recognized precursor of esophageal adenocarcinoma is Barrett esophagus. Barrett esophagus is the replacement of the normal stratified squamous epithelium by an incomplete small intestinal epithelium (metaplasia) in the distal esophagus, projecting from the GE junction in a distal-proximal gradient. In turn, it has been demonstrated that Barrett esophagus is fostered by GERD but also by an admixture of bile acids in the acid refluxate. Patients with scleroderma (Chapter 267) may be at increased risk for Barrett esophagus. A small subset of Barrett esophagus patients may progress to esophageal adenocarcinoma through intermediate stages of low-grade and high-grade dysplasia. In Barrett esophagus, one case of esophageal adenocarcinoma is estimated to arise in 55 to 441 patient-years, which corresponds to an approximately 125-fold increased risk for esophageal adenocarcinoma compared with that in the general population.

PATHOBIOLOGY

Barrett esophagus involves transdifferentiation from normal esophageal epithelium to an epithelium of the small intestine with columnar enterocytes and secretory goblet cells, but without Paneth cells and enteroendocrine cells—hence the designation of incomplete intestinal metaplasia. By itself, the metaplasia of Barrett esophagus cannot become esophageal adenocarcinoma. However, if and when Barrett esophagus transitions to low-grade and high-grade dysplasia, there is the aforementioned risk for esophageal adenocarcinoma. Barrett esophagus is associated with abnormal DNA ploidy based on flow cytometry analysis, and certain genetic alterations in epidermal growth factor receptor signaling, *TP53*, and *p16INK4A*. Microsatellite instability may be noted as well. Whole genome approaches are revealing gains and losses of chromosomal regions that might lead to identification of known and previously unknown genes critical in the pathogenesis of esophageal adenocarcinoma.[4] Recent advances in genetically engineered mouse models have allowed the phenocopying of Barrett esophagus and esophageal adenocarcinoma through the direct targeting of interleukin (IL)-1β to the esophagus; and in another approach, through the global knockout of p63 (an important marker of stem cells and progenitor cells), Barrett esophagus is evident in the postnatal period.

CLINICAL MANIFESTATIONS

Symptoms and Signs

It is estimated that 5 to 15% of GERD patients may develop Barrett esophagus, but such population-based studies are difficult to pursue because vast millions of people are affected with GERD, and most GERD patients do not undergo upper endoscopy. Patients with Barrett esophagus may or may not have symptoms related to GERD. Chronic GERD with Barrett esophagus may be associated with distal esophageal strictures. With esophageal adenocarcinoma, patients may suffer from dysphagia, odynophagia, upper gastrointestinal bleeding, chest pain, nausea, vomiting, early satiety, weight loss, and malnutrition.

Physical Examination

Examination of the patient may reveal signs consistent with malnutrition and weight loss. Lymph adenopathy should be explored. There may be hepatomegaly. Paraneoplastic syndromes are unusual with esophageal adenocarcinoma (as well as with esophageal squamous cell carcinoma). Nevertheless, it is important to ensure that esophageal adenocarcinoma is not mistaken for a benign entity such as a primary esophageal motility disorder.

Laboratory Studies

Patients with esophageal adenocarcinoma may have iron deficiency anemia, metabolic derangements, and abnormal liver enzyme tests owing to metastatic disease. CEA may be elevated as a tumor serologic marker.

DIAGNOSIS

Barium swallow radiography may lead one to the suspicion of Barrett esophagus and can diagnose luminal mass lesions consistent with esophageal adenocarcinoma in the distal esophagus. However, the mainstay of diagnosis is upper endoscopy. At that time, a characteristic salmon-colored mucosa is visualized at the GE junction, with frondlike projections in a proximal direction. If the extent of Barrett esophagus is 3 cm or less, it is termed *short-segment Barrett esophagus*; if it is more than 3 cm, it is referred to as *long-segment Barrett esophagus*. This distinction is important in that the risk for esophageal adenocarcinoma in long-segment Barrett esophagus is greater than in short-segment Barrett esophagus. Noting that the normal esophageal mucosa is more pinkish-white in hue, one can visually distinguish the two different types of epithelia, with the caveat that the gastric cardia mucosa at the GE junction should not be mistaken for Barrett esophagus. Endoscopic mucosal biopsies from the Barrett esophagus region (with control biopsies from the normal esophagus and gastric cardia) are required for histopathologic diagnosis. Features of dysplasia are best appreciated in the absence of reflux-related esophagitis that can lead to nuclear architectural distortion; hence, suppression of acid production with proton pump inhibitor therapy for 6 to 8 weeks is needed, with a view to repeat biopsies.

If the patient has Barrett esophagus metaplasia, upper endoscopy should be repeated every 3 years. However, low-grade dysplasia (with confirmation by an expert pathologist) requires surveillance endoscopy every 6 to 12 months. High-grade dysplasia, if properly evaluated by the pathologist, may require reconfirmation, but then leads to either medical (radio frequency ablation [RFA], endoscopic mucosal resection) or surgical intervention because of the possibility of missed contiguous esophageal adenocarcinoma. EUS may be helpful in discriminating between high-grade dysplasia and esophageal intramucosal adenocarcinoma.

TREATMENT Rx

The principles are very similar to those applied to esophageal squamous cell carcinoma in terms of surgery. Preoperative chemoradiotherapy (carboplatin titrated to achieve an area under the curve of 2 mg/mL/min and paclitaxel 50 mg/m^2 for 5 weeks) and concurrent radiotherapy (at 41.4 Gy in 23 fractions, 5 days per week) significantly improves median survival from 24 months to 49 months among patients with potentially curable esophageal or esophagogastric-junction cancer.[A1] Overall prognosis for esophageal adenocarcinoma is not too dissimilar from that noted in esophageal squamous cell carcinoma. Major improvements in the treatment options for Barrett esophagus, the main precursor of esophageal adenocarcinoma, have witnessed dramatic growth (Chapter 138). RFA reduces progression of Barrett esophagus with low-grade dysplasia or possibly high-grade dysplasia to cancer.[A2] Endoscopic mucosal resection (EMR) is used for Barrett esophagus–related high-grade dysplasia or Barrett esophagus associated with intramucosal esophageal adenocarcinoma. For advanced, unresectable tumors, self-expanding stents, often with localized brachytherapy, can provide palliation.[5]

NEOPLASMS OF THE STOMACH

DEFINITION

Gastric neoplasms are predominantly malignant, and nearly 90 to 95% of these tumors are adenocarcinomas. Less frequently observed malignant diseases include lymphomas, especially non-Hodgkin's lymphoma, and sarcomas such as leiomyosarcoma. Benign gastric neoplasms include leiomyomas, carcinoid tumors, and lipomas.

Adenocarcinoma of the Stomach

EPIDEMIOLOGY

The great geographic variation in the incidence of gastric cancer worldwide indicates that environmental factors influence the pathogenesis of gastric carcinogenesis. Further support for this notion comes from observations that groups emigrating from high-risk to low-risk areas, such as Japanese individuals moving to Hawaii and Brazil, acquire the low risk of the area into which they emigrate, presumably because of adoption of the endogenous lifestyle and exposure to different environmental factors.

Gastric adenocarcinoma was the most frequently observed malignant disease in the world until the mid-1980s, and it remains extremely common among men in certain regions such as tropical South America, some parts of the Caribbean, and Eastern Europe. Regardless of gender, it remains one of the most common malignancies in Japan and China.

Whereas gastric cancer was the most common cancer in the United States in the 1930s, its annual incidence has steadily decreased. The annual incidence is now fewer than 10,000 new cases per year. However, although the incidence of gastric adenocarcinoma localized to the distal stomach has declined, the incidence of proximal gastric and GE junctional adenocarcinomas has been steadily increasing in the United States, a finding that perhaps reflects differences in pathogenic factors. Typically, gastric cancer occurs between the ages of 50 and 70 years and is uncommon before age 30. The rates are higher in men than in women by 2 : 1. Five-year survival is less than 20%.

Risk Factors

Risk factors for the development of gastric adenocarcinoma[6] can be divided into environmental and genetic factors as well as precursor conditions (Table 192-3). For example, *Helicobacter pylori* infection is significantly more common in patients with gastric cancer than in matched control groups. Epidemiologic studies of high-risk populations have also suggested that genotoxic agents such as *N*-nitroso compounds may play a role in gastric tumorigenesis. *N*-nitroso compounds can be formed in the human stomach by nitrosation of ingested nitrates, which are common constituents of the diet. High nitrate concentrations in soil and drinking water have been observed in areas with high death rates from gastric cancer. Atrophic gastritis (Chapter 139), with or without intestinal metaplasia, is observed in association with gastric cancer, especially in endemic areas. Pernicious anemia (Chapter 139) is associated with a several-fold increase in gastric cancer. Atrophic gastritis and gastric cancer have certain environmental risk factors in common. It is likely that atrophic gastritis and intestinal metaplasia represent intermediary steps to gastric cancer. The achlorhydria associated with gastritis related to *H. pylori* infection, pernicious anemia, or other causes favors the growth of bacteria capable of converting nitrates to nitrites. The nitrosamine *N*-methyl-*N*′-nitro-*N*-nitrosoguanidine causes a high rate of induction of adenocarcinoma in the glandular stomach of rats. At the same time, most patients with atrophic gastritis do not develop gastric cancer, a finding suggesting that neither atrophic gastritis nor achlorhydria alone is responsible.

Benign gastric ulcers do not appear to predispose patients to gastric cancer. However, patients who have a gastric remnant after subtotal gastrectomy for benign disorders have an increased relative risk for gastric cancer of 1.5 to 3.0 by 15 to 20 years after surgery.

TABLE 192-3 CONDITIONS PREDISPOSING TO OR ASSOCIATED WITH GASTRIC CANCER

ENVIRONMENTAL
Helicobacter pylori infection
Dietary: excess of salt (salted pickled foods), nitrates/nitrites, carbohydrates; deficiency of fresh fruit, vegetables, vitamins A and C, refrigeration
Low socioeconomic status
Cigarette smoking
GENETIC
Familial gastric cancer (rare)
Associated with hereditary nonpolyposis colorectal cancer
Blood group A
PREDISPOSING CONDITIONS
Chronic gastritis, especially atrophic gastritis with or without intestinal metaplasia
Pernicious anemia
Intestinal metaplasia
Gastric adenomatous polyps (>2 cm)
Postgastrectomy stumps
Gastric epithelial dysplasia
Ménétrier's disease (hypertrophic gastropathy)
Chronic peptic ulcer

PATHOBIOLOGY

Gastric adenocarcinomas can be divided into two types based on the Lauren classification: intestinal and diffuse. The intestinal type is typically in the distal stomach with ulcerations, is often preceded by premalignant lesions, and is declining in incidence in the United States. By contrast, the diffuse type involves widespread thickening of the stomach, especially in the cardia, and it often affects younger patients; this form may present as linitis plastica, a nondistensible stomach with the absence of folds and a narrowed lumen caused by infiltration of the stomach wall with tumor. Diffuse-type gastric cancers harbor mucin-producing cells. Other conditions may result in linitis plastica, such as lymphoma (Chapter 185), tuberculosis (Chapter 324), syphilis (Chapter 319), and amyloidosis (Chapter 188). The prognosis is generally worse in the diffuse type.

Key histopathologic features of gastric cancer include its degree of differentiation, invasion through the gastric wall, lymph node involvement, and the presence or absence of signet ring cells within the tumor itself. Other pathologic manifestations include a polypoid mass, which may be difficult to distinguish from a benign polyp. Early gastric cancer, a condition that is common in Japan and has a relatively favorable prognosis, consists of superficial lesions with or without lymph node involvement. Here, the Borrmann classification scheme is helpful: I, polypoid; II, fungating ulcer with sharp raised margins; III, ulcer with poorly defined infiltrative margins; and IV, infiltrative, mostly intramural lesion, not well demarcated.

The leading hypothesis explaining the way in which *H. pylori* predisposes to gastric cancer risk is the induction of an inflammatory response, in which IL-1β may be pivotal. Chronic *H. pylori* infection also leads to chronic atrophic gastritis with resulting achlorhydria, which in turn favors bacterial growth that can convert nitrates (dietary components) to nitrites. These nitrites, in combination with genetic factors, promote abnormal cellular proliferation, genetic mutations, and eventually cancer. In a mouse model of gastric cancer, *H. pylori* infection may play a role in the recruitment of bone marrow–derived stem cells that facilitate gastric carcinogenesis. Animal models can now recapitulate the cardinal features of gastric adenocarcinoma, either through the use of carcinogens or through genetic approaches.

Genetics

It is clear that genetic factors play a role in gastric cancer. For example, blood group A is associated with a higher incidence rate of gastric cancer, even in nonendemic areas. A three-fold increase in gastric cancer has been reported among first-degree relatives of patients with the disease. Furthermore, germline or inherited mutations in the genes for E-cadherin and α-catenin, albeit rare, have been described in diffuse hereditary gastric cancer, which is seen in young patients. In addition, in Lynch syndrome (Chapter 193), patients have associated extracolonic cancers, including gastric cancer. Patients with familial adenomatous polyposis (FAP) have an increased risk of distal (antral) gastric adenocarcinoma.

It now appears that several genetic mechanisms are important in gastric cancer: oncogene activation, tumor suppressor gene inactivation, and DNA microsatellite instability. For example, loss of heterozygosity of the *APC* (adenomatous polyposis coli) gene has been observed in gastric cancers. The p53 tumor suppressor gene product regulates the cell cycle at the G_1-S phase transition and probably also functions in DNA repair and apoptosis (programmed cell death). The *p53* gene is mutated not only in gastric cancer but also in gastric precancerous lesions, a finding suggesting that mutation of the *p53* gene is an early event in gastric carcinogenesis. Microsatellite DNA alterations or instability in dinucleotide repeats occur frequently in sporadic gastric carcinoma. Mutations in genes may accumulate as a result of DNA microsatellite instability.

CLINICAL MANIFESTATIONS

Symptoms and Signs

In its early stages, gastric cancer may often be asymptomatic or may produce only nonspecific symptoms that make early diagnosis difficult. Later symptoms include bloating, dysphagia, epigastric pain, or early satiety. Early satiety or vomiting may suggest partial gastric outlet obstruction, although gastric dysmotility may contribute to the vomiting in patients with nonobstructive cases. Epigastric pain reminiscent of that associated with peptic ulcer (Chapter 139) occurs in about one fourth of patients, but in most patients with gastric cancer, the pain is not relieved by food or antacids. Pain that radiates to the back may indicate that the tumor has penetrated the pancreas. When dysphagia is associated with gastric cancer, this symptom suggests a more proximal gastric tumor at the GE junction or in the fundus.

Signs of gastric cancer include bleeding, which can result in iron deficiency anemia that produces the symptoms of weakness, fatigue, and malaise, as well as (rarely) more serious cardiovascular and cerebrovascular consequences. Perforation related to gastric cancer is unusual. Gastric cancer metastatic to the liver can lead to right upper quadrant pain, jaundice, and fever. Lung metastases can cause cough, hiccups, and hemoptysis. Peritoneal carcinomatosis can lead to malignant ascites unresponsive to diuretics. Gastric cancer can also metastasize to bone.

Physical Examination

In the earliest stages of gastric cancer, the physical examination may be unremarkable. At later stages, patients become cachectic, and an epigastric mass may be palpated. If the tumor has metastasized to the liver, hepatomegaly with jaundice and ascites may be present. Portal or splenic vein invasion and thrombosis can cause splenomegaly. Lymph node involvement in the left supraclavicular area is termed *Virchow's node*, and periumbilical nodal involvement is called *Sister Mary Joseph's node*. The fecal occult blood test may be positive. Metastasis to the ovary is termed *Krukenberg's tumor*.

Paraneoplastic syndromes may precede or occur concurrently with gastric cancer. Examples include the following: Trousseau syndrome (Chapter 176), which is recurrent migratory superficial thrombophlebitis indicating a possible hypercoagulable state; acanthosis nigricans, which arises as raised and hyperpigmented skin lesions of flexor areas, neck, axilla, groin, and mucosal membranes; neuromyopathy with involvement of the sensory and motor pathways; and central nervous system syndromes with altered mental status and ataxia.

Laboratory Studies

Laboratory studies may reveal iron deficiency anemia. Microangiopathic hemolytic anemia has been reported. Abnormalities in liver tests generally indicate metastatic disease. Hypoalbuminemia is a marker of malnutrition. Protein-losing enteropathy is rare but can be seen in Ménétrier's disease, another predisposing condition. Serologic test results, such as those for CEA and CA72.4, may be abnormal. Although these tests are not recommended for initial diagnosis, they may be useful for monitoring disease after surgical resection.

DIAGNOSIS

The diagnostic accuracy of upper endoscopy with biopsy and cytologic examination approaches 95 to 99% for both types of gastric cancer.[7] Cancer may arise as a small mucosal ulceration, a polyp, or a mass (Fig. 192-1). In some patients, gastric ulceration may first be noted in an upper gastrointestinal barium contrast study. A benign gastric ulcer is associated with a smooth, regular base, whereas a malignant ulcer is associated with a surrounding mass, irregular folds, and an irregular base. Although these and other radiographic characteristics historically helped to predict benign versus malignant disease, upper gastrointestinal endoscopy with biopsy and cytologic examination is mandatory whenever a gastric ulcer is found in the radiologic study, even if the ulcer has benign characteristics.

Endoscopic ultrasonography (EUS) is very helpful in both diagnosis and staging of gastric cancer (Table 192-4). The extent of tumor, including gastric wall invasion and local lymph node involvement, can be assessed by EUS (Fig. 192-2), which provides information complementary to that obtained from CT scans. EUS can help guide aspiration biopsies of lymph nodes to determine their malignant features if any. CT of the chest, abdomen, and pelvis should be performed to document lymphadenopathy and extragastric organ (especially lung and liver) involvement. In some centers, staging of gastric cancer entails bone scans because of the proclivity of gastric cancer to metastasize to bone.

TREATMENT Rx

Surgical Therapy

The only chance for cure of gastric cancer remains surgical resection, which is possible in 25 to 30% of cases. If the tumor is confined to the distal stomach, subtotal gastrectomy is performed, with resection of lymph nodes in the porta hepatis and the pancreatic head. By contrast, tumors of the proximal stomach merit total gastrectomy to obtain an adequate margin and to remove lymph nodes; distal pancreatectomy and splenectomy are usually also performed as part of this procedure, which carries with it higher mortality and morbidity rates. The addition of para-aorta nodal dissection does not improve survival. Even if a curative procedure is not possible because of metastasis, limited gastric resection may be necessary for patients with excessive bleeding or obstruction. If cancer recurs in the gastric remnant, limited resection may again be necessary for palliation. Most recurrences in both types of gastric cancer are in the local or regional area of the original tumor.

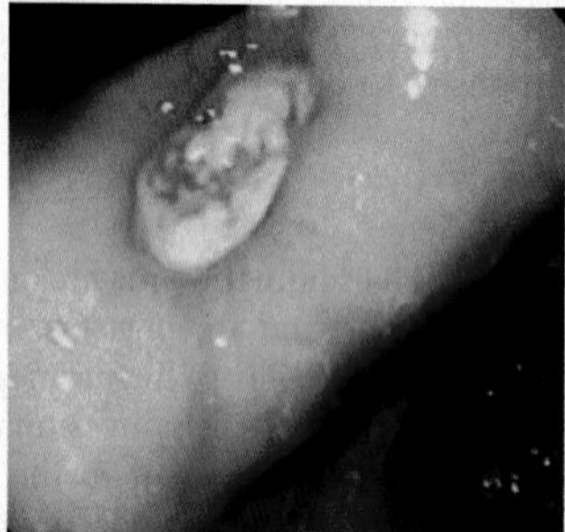
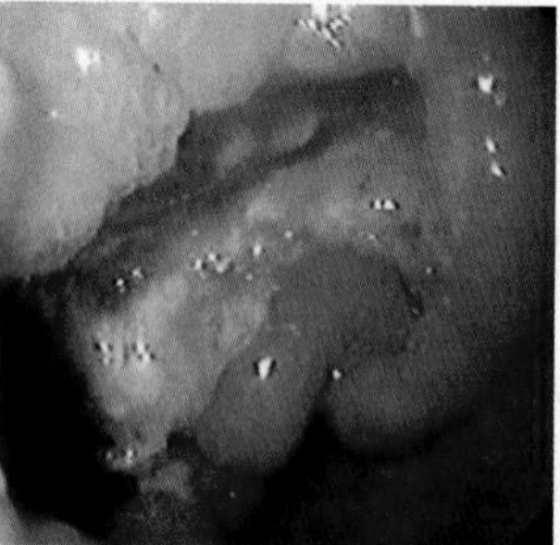

FIGURE 192-1. Benign (*left*) and malignant (*right*) gastric ulcer. Note the shaggy, thickened, and overhanging edges of the cancer. (Courtesy Pankaj Jay Pasricha, MD.)

TABLE 192-4 TNM STAGING OF STOMACH CANCER

PRIMARY TUMOR (T)	
TX	Primary tumor cannot be assessed
T0	No evidence of primary tumor
Tis	Carcinoma in situ: intraepithelial tumor without invasion of the lamina propria
T1	Tumor invades lamina propria, muscularis mucosa, or submucosa
T1a	Tumor invades lamina propria or muscularis mucosa
T1b	Tumor invades submucosa
T2	Tumor invades muscularis propria*
T3	Tumor penetrates subserosal connective tissue without invasion of visceral peritoneum or adjacent structures[†,‡]
T4	Tumor invades serosa (visceral peritoneum) or adjacent structures[†,‡]
T4a	Tumor invades serosa (visceral peritoneum)
T4b	Tumor invades adjacent structures
REGIONAL LYMPH NODES (N)	
NX	Regional lymph nodes(s) cannot be assessed
N0	No regional lymph nodes metastasis[§]
N1	Metastasis in 1-2 regional lymph nodes
N2	Metastasis in 3-6 regional lymph nodes
N3	Metastasis in 7 or more regional lymph nodes
N3a	Metastasis in 7-15 regional lymph nodes
N3b	Metastasis in 16 or more regional lymph nodes
DISTANT METASTASIS (M)	
M0	No distant metastasis
M1	Distant metastasis

**Note:* A tumor may penetrate the muscularis propria with extension into the gastrocolic or gastrohepatic ligaments, or into the greater or lesser omentum, without perforation of the visceral peritoneum covering these structures. In this case, the tumor is classified T3. If there is perforation of the visceral peritoneum covering the gastric ligaments or the omentum, the tumor should be classified T4.

†The adjacent structures of the stomach include the spleen, transverse colon, liver, diaphragm, pancreas, abdominal wall, adrenal gland, kidney, small intestine, and retroperitoneum.

‡Intramural extension to the duodenum or esophagus is classified by the depth of the greatest invasion in any of these sites, including the stomach.

§*Note:* A designation of pN0 should be used if all examined lymph nodes are negative, regardless of the total number removed and examined.

From *AJCC Cancer Staging Manual.* 7th ed. New York: Springer-Verlag, 2010.

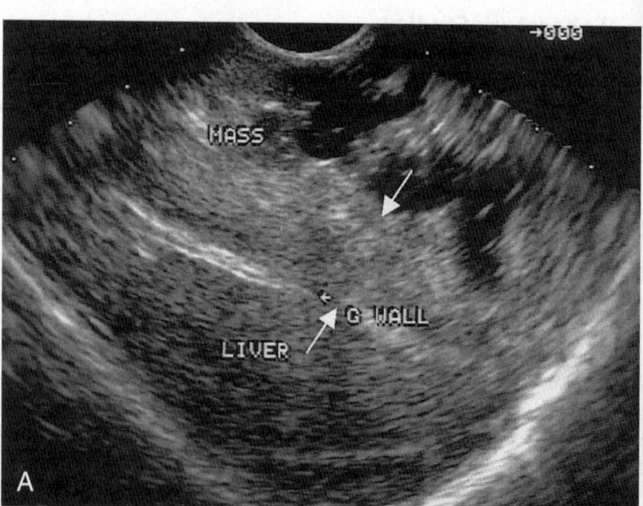

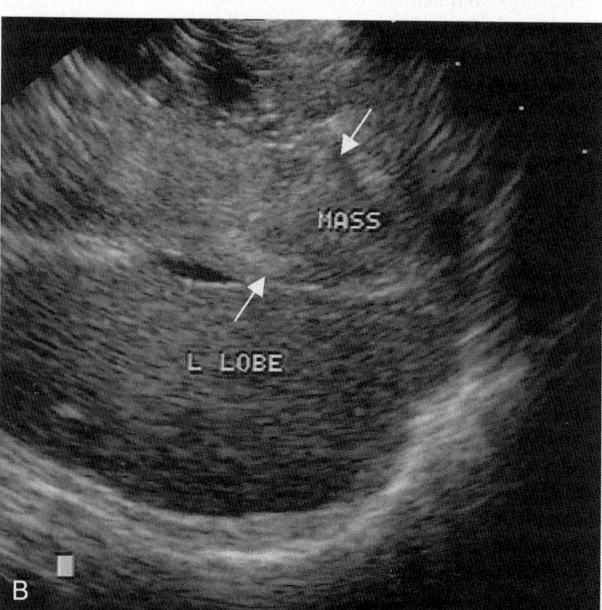

FIGURE 192-2. Gastric mass. Endoscopic ultrasonography depicting a large gastric mass that is compressing the liver and gallbladder wall (A) and, on a different view, the left lobe of the liver (B).

Medical Therapy

Gastric cancer is one of the few gastrointestinal cancers that is somewhat responsive to chemotherapy.[8] In patients with gastric cancer who undergo gastrectomy and extended lymph node dissection with curative intent, S-1 (an oral fluoropyrimidine, 80 mg daily for 4 weeks followed by 2 weeks off, repeated in 6-week cycles for 1 year starting within 6 weeks after surgery) significantly improves 3-year survival from 70 to 80%. Chemotherapy with the combination of epirubicin, cisplatin, and fluorouracil, given both preoperatively and postoperatively, significantly improves 5-year survival from 23 to 36% in patients with resectable GE cancer. Similarly, the combination of chemotherapy (fluorouracil and leucovorin) with radiation therapy has been shown to improve median survival from 27 to 36 months compared with surgery alone in patients with adenocarcinoma of the stomach or GE junction. With a more than 10-year median follow-up, overall survival and relapse-free survival demonstrate continued strong benefit from postoperative radiochemotherapy.[A3]

Single-agent chemotherapy treatment, which provides partial response rates of 20 to 30%, is reserved for patients with a poor performance status. Combination regimens that can yield partial response rates of 35 to 50% include the following: ECF, which is most popular in Europe (epirubicin, 50 mg/m^2 on day 1; cisplatin, 60 mg/m^2 on day 1; 5-fluorouracil, 200 mg/m^2/day as a continuous infusion through a central venous access device [CVAD] given throughout treatment, repeated every 21 days for a maximum of 8 cycles); CF (5-fluorouracil infusion, 1000 mg/m^2/day for 4 days; cisplatin, 75 to 100 mg/m^2 on day 1, every 4 weeks); or TCF (docetaxel [Taxotere], 75 mg/m^2 on day 1; cisplatin, 75 mg/m^2 on day 1; and 5-fluorouracil, 750 mg/m^2/day for 5 days, every 3 weeks), or capecitabine plus cisplatin. A randomized trial of triple chemotherapy for advanced esophagogastric cancer showed that oral capecitabine is at least as effective as infused fluorouracil, and that oxaliplatin (which does not require hydration) is at least as effective as cisplatin (which does require hydration) with respect to overall survival.[A4] Bevacizumab, a monoclonal antibody targeting vascular endothelial growth factor A (VEGF-A), administered at a dose of 7.5 mg/kg by intravenous infusion every 3 weeks, was found to increase progression-free survival and overall response rate when it was given along with capecitabine-cisplatin chemotherapy as first-line treatment of advanced gastric cancer.[A5] Ramucirumab (a VEGF receptor antagonist) given as 8 mg/kg intravenously every two weeks can improve median survival from 3.8 to 5.2 months in advanced gastric cancer.[A6] Trastuzumab (8 mg/kg intravenously once, then 6 mg/kg every 3 weeks) can increase survival of HER2-positive advanced gastric or GE junction cancer from 11.1 months to 13.8 months. Radiation therapy alone is ineffective and is generally employed only for palliative purposes in the setting of bleeding, obstruction, or pain. Gene therapy and immune-based therapy are currently only investigational in animal models.

General Methods

Implicit in the management of the patient with gastric cancer is meticulous attention to nutrition (jejunal enteral feedings or total parenteral nutrition), correction of metabolic abnormalities that arise from vomiting or diarrhea, and treatment of infection from aspiration or spontaneous bacterial peritonitis. *H. pylori* eradication treatment reduces the risk for metachronous gastric carcinoma by about two thirds. To maintain lumen patency, endoscopic laser treatment or prosthesis placement can be used in a palliative fashion.

PROGNOSIS

Approximately one third of patients who undergo a curative resection are alive after 5 years. In aggregate, the overall 5-year survival rate in patients with gastric cancer is less than 10%. Prognostic factors include anatomic location and nodal status. Distal gastric cancers without lymph node involvement have a better prognosis than proximal gastric cancers with or without lymph node involvement. Other prognostic factors include depth of penetration and tumor cell DNA aneuploidy. Linitis plastica and infiltrating lesions have a much worse prognosis than polypoid disease or exophytic masses. In the subset of mostly Japanese patients with early gastric cancer that is confined to the mucosa and submucosa, surgical resection may be curative and definitely improves the 5-year survival rate to more than 50%. In fact, when early gastric cancer is confined to the mucosa, endoscopic mucosal resection may be an alternative.

Lymphoma of the Stomach

EPIDEMIOLOGY

Gastric lymphoma represents about 5% of all malignant gastric tumors and is increasing in incidence. Most gastric lymphomas are non-Hodgkin's lymphomas (Chapter 185), and the stomach is the most common extranodal site for non-Hodgkin's lymphomas. Patients with gastric lymphoma are generally younger than those with gastric adenocarcinoma, but the male predominance remains.

CLINICAL MANIFESTATIONS

Patients commonly present with symptoms and signs similar to those of gastric adenocarcinoma. Lymphoma in the stomach can be a primary tumor, or it can be secondary to disseminated lymphoma.

B-cell lymphomas (Chapter 185) of the stomach are most commonly large cell with a high-grade type. Low-grade variants are noted in the setting of chronic gastritis and are termed *mucosa-associated lymphoid tissue* (MALT) lymphomas. MALT lesions are strongly associated with *H. pylori* infection.

DIAGNOSIS

Radiographically, gastric lymphomas usually arise as ulcers or exophytic masses; diffusely infiltrating lymphoma is more suggestive of secondary lymphoma. Thus, upper gastrointestinal barium studies usually show multiple nodules and ulcers for a primary gastric lymphoma and typically have the appearance of linitis plastica (see earlier) with secondary lymphoma. As with gastric adenocarcinoma, however, upper endoscopy with biopsy and cytologic examination are required for diagnosis and have an accuracy of nearly 90%. Apart from conventional histopathologic analysis, immunoperoxidase staining for lymphocyte markers is helpful in diagnosis. As with gastric adenocarcinoma, proper staging of gastric lymphoma involves EUS, chest and abdominal/pelvic CT scans, and bone marrow biopsy as needed.

TREATMENT Rx

Treatment of gastric diffuse large B-cell lymphoma is best pursued with combination chemotherapy with or without radiation therapy (Chapter 185). For MALT lesions, eradication of *H. pylori* infection with antibiotics should be attempted[9] (Chapter 139), but patients with refractory lesions that are confined to the stomach can sometimes be cured with chemoradiotherapy (Chapter 185).

Other Malignant Tumors of the Stomach

Leiomyosarcoma, which constitutes approximately 1% of all gastric cancers, usually occurs as an intramural mass with central ulceration. Symptoms may include bleeding accompanied by a palpable mass. Leiomyosarcomas are often relatively indolent; surgical resection yields a 5-year survival rate of about 50%. Metastasis can occur to lymph nodes and the liver. Other gastric sarcomas include liposarcomas, fibrosarcomas, myosarcomas, and neurogenic sarcomas.

Most gastrointestinal stromal tumors (GISTs)[10] have been associated with activating mutations in the C-*kit* gene; a subset of such tumors is associated with mutations in the platelet-derived growth factor receptor *(PDGFR)* gene. C-*kit* mutations are also found in chronic and acute myelogenous leukemia (Chapters 183 and 184), and approximately 50% of GISTs respond to imatinib mesylate, which should be continued for at least 3 years.[A7] If imatinib is not successful, sunitinib increases survival. If both fail, regorafenib, a multikinase inhibitor, can be tried.[11] Carcinoid tumors (Chapter 232) may begin in the stomach and are curable by removal if they have not yet spread to the liver.

Primary tumors can also spread to the stomach. In addition to lymphomas, other tumors found in the stomach include primary lung (Chapter 191) and breast (Chapter 198) cancers as well as malignant melanoma (Chapter 203).

Leiomyomas and Benign Tumors

Leiomyomas, which are smooth muscle tumors of benign origin, occur with equal frequency in men and women and are typically located in the middle and distal stomach. Leiomyomas can grow into the lumen, with secondary ulceration and consequent bleeding. Alternatively, they can expand to the serosa with extrinsic compression. Endoscopy may reveal a mass that has overlying mucosa or mucosa replaced by ulceration. On upper gastrointestinal series, leiomyomas are usually smooth with an intramural filling defect, with or without central ulceration. However, benign leiomyomas can be difficult to distinguish from their malignant counterparts radiographically or endoscopically; tissue diagnosis is imperative. Symptomatic leiomyomas should be removed, but those without associated symptoms do not require therapy.

Other benign gastric tumors include lipoma, neurofibroma, lymphangioma, ganglioneuroma, and hamartoma, the last associated with Peutz-Jeghers syndrome (Chapter 193) or juvenile polyposis (when restricted to the stomach).

Adenomas

Gastric adenomas and hyperplastic polyps are unusual but may be found in middle-aged and elderly patients. Polyps may be sessile or pedunculated. Although isolated gastric adenomatous polyps are generally asymptomatic, some patients may have dyspepsia, nausea, or bleeding. Gastric adenomas and hyperplastic polyps are smooth and regular on upper gastrointestinal series, but the diagnosis must be confirmed by upper endoscopy with biopsy. Pedunculated polyps that are larger than 2 cm or that have associated symptoms should be removed by endoscopic snare cautery polypectomy, whereas large sessile gastric adenomatous polyps may merit segmental surgical resection. If polyps progress to an intermediary stage of severe dysplasia or culminate in cancer, treatment is the same as for gastric adenocarcinoma.

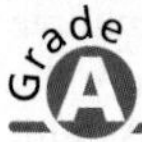

Grade A References

A1. van Hagen P, Hulshof MC, van Lanschot JJ, et al. Preoperative chemoradiotherapy for esophageal or junctional cancer. *N Engl J Med.* 2012;366:2074-2084.

A2. Phoa KN, van Vilsteren FG, Weusten BL, et al. Radiofrequency ablation vs endoscopic surveillance for patients with Barrett esophagus and low-grade dysplasia: a randomized clinical trial. *JAMA.* 2014;311:1209-1217.

A3. Smalley SR, Benedetti JK, Haller DG, et al. Updated analysis of SWOG-Directed Intergroup Study 0116: a phase III trial of adjuvant radiochemotherapy versus observation after curative gastric cancer resection. *J Clin Oncol.* 2012;30:2327-2333.

A4. Cunningham D, Starling N, Rao S, et al. Capecitabine and oxaliplatin for advanced esophagogastric cancer. *N Engl J Med.* 2008;358:36-46.

A5. Ohtsu A, Shah MA, Van Custem E, et al. Bevacizumab in combination with chemotherapy as first-line therapy in advanced gastric cancer: a randomized, double-blind, placebo-controlled phase III study. *J Clin Oncol.* 2011;29:3968-3976.

A6. Fuchs CS, Tomasek J, Yong CJ, et al. Ramucirumab monotherapy for previously treated advanced gastric or gastro-oesophageal junction adenocarcinoma (REGARD): an international, randomised, multicentre, placebo-controlled, phase 3 trial. *Lancet.* 2014;383:31-39.

A7. Joensuu H, Eriksson M, Sundby Hall K, et al. One vs three years of adjuvant imatinib for operable gastrointestinal stromal tumor: a randomized trial. *JAMA.* 2012;307:1265-1272.

GENERAL REFERENCES

For the General References and other additional features, please visit Expert Consult at https://expertconsult.inkling.com.

193

NEOPLASMS OF THE SMALL AND LARGE INTESTINE

CHARLES D. BLANKE AND DOUGLAS O. FAIGEL

NEOPLASMS OF THE SMALL INTESTINE

EPIDEMIOLOGY

The small intestine accounts for the majority of the length (≈75%) and absorptive surface (≈90%) of the gastrointestinal (GI) tract. Nonetheless, it is a rare site for the development of neoplastic disease, because only 1 to 2% of primary GI tumors originate in the duodenum, jejunum, or ileum. In fact, half of all small bowel neoplasms represent metastatic disease from other sites, particularly elsewhere in the GI tract. Although small bowel malignancies constitute less than 0.5% of all cancers, the incidence of small bowel tumors (especially carcinoids) has increased dramatically over the last several decades, which may possibly be a reflection of better diagnostic techniques. Overall, the mean age at diagnosis of a small bowel tumor is about 67 years (younger for those with sarcomas and lymphomas); neoplasms are more common in males, and they occur more frequently in African Americans than whites.

PATHOBIOLOGY

Adenocarcinomas, arising from mucosal glands, were formerly the most frequent primary small bowel tumor. They now constitute 25 to 33% of small bowel neoplasms, including benign growths, and 40% of all malignant tumors. Adenocarcinomas most commonly arise in the duodenum (65% of all small intestinal adenocarcinomas), even though the duodenum represents only a tiny fraction of the length of the small bowel. They occur less com monly in the jejunum and least commonly in the ileum. The majority are we or moderately differentiated.

Small bowel carcinoids, which derive from enterochromaffin cells in th crypts of Lieberkühn, are now the most common small bowel tumor accounting for up to 44% of malignancies. They tend to be quite well diffe entiated. In contrast to glandular tumors, small intestinal carcinoids tend t arise in the distal ileum, and up to 30% are multifocal. Other small bowe neuroendocrine tumors are occasionally seen, including biochemically activ neoplasms such as gastrinomas and somatostatinomas. Very rarely, high grade true small-cell carcinomas occur.

Malignant connective tissue tumors account for 10 to 17% of small bowe neoplasms. Gastrointestinal stromal tumors (GISTs), which derive from th interstitial cells of Cajal or a common precursor, account for approximatel 85% of these neoplasms (Fig. 193-1). GISTs, like adenocarcinomas, dispro portionately arise in the duodenum, and the small bowel itself is the secon most common primary site for these mesenchymal neoplasms (33% deriv from small bowel). Morphologically, GISTs often resemble leiomyosarcoma (Fig. 193-2), but they can be differentiated by the expression of the Ki protein (CD117). Other small bowel sarcomas, such as true leiomyosarco mas, are seen more rarely (Chapter 202).

Primary GI lymphomas are the most common extranodal lymphomatou variation, and the small intestine is the second most common GI site for suc tumors (Chapter 185). Lymphomas account for approximately 8% of sma bowel neoplasms. The ileum, rich in submucosal lymphoid follicles, is th most common small bowel site. Tumors may be low or higher grade and ca arise from precursor B or T lymphocytes. The overwhelming majority ar non-Hodgkin tumors (Fig. 193-3). Lymphomas involving the small bowe may also be a manifestation of true systemic disease.

Malignant melanoma (Chapter 203) can develop as a primary mucosa small bowel tumor, probably arising from schwannian neuroblasts associate with GI innervation. In addition, the small bowel is the most common G site for melanoma metastases.

Finally, a variety of common benign tumors may originate in the smal bowel, including adenomas, leiomyomas, and lipomas. Desmoids (most often seen in patients with familial adenomatous polyposis [FAP]), hamartomas, and hemangiomas are relatively rare. Benign growths are more common in the distal small intestine.

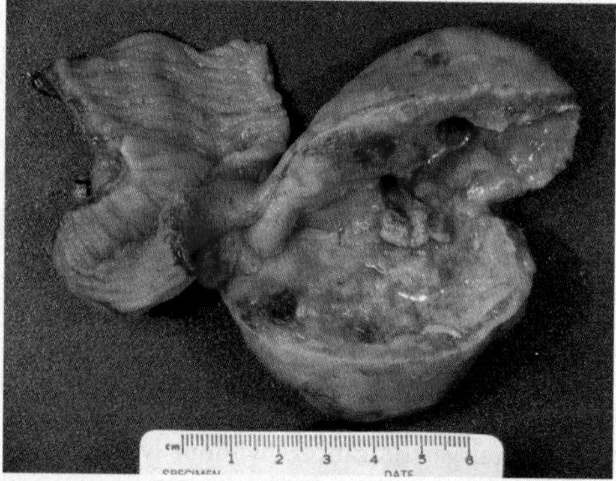

FIGURE 193-1. Small bowel gastrointestinal stromal tumor with ulceration.

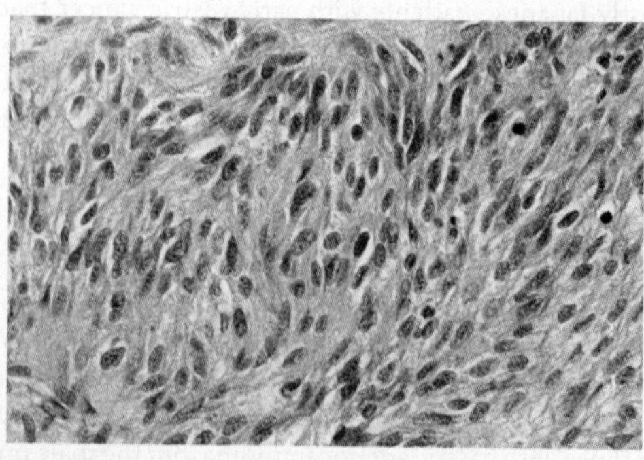

FIGURE 193-2. Histopathology of gastrointestinal stromal tumor.

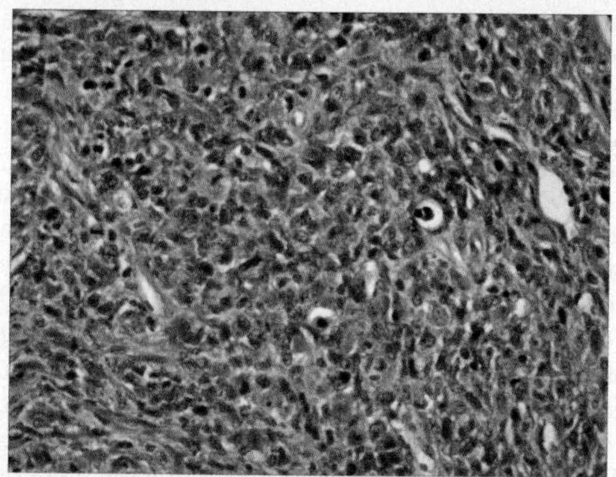

FIGURE 193-3. Histopathology of small bowel non-Hodgkin lymphoma. (Courtesy Dr. M.K. Washington.)

The small intestine can be involved with advanced cancers from other sites through direct invasion, extension of peritoneal metastases, or hematogenous spread. As noted, the small bowel is the most common GI site for melanoma metastases; involvement is also fairly common with ovarian, breast, lung, and other GI neoplasms.

Predisposing Conditions

Inflammatory bowel disease (Chapter 141) and some environmental factors (e.g., salt-cured foods, alcohol) predispose to small bowel adenocarcinomas. Data regarding tobacco exposure and obesity are conflicting. Additionally, many of the polyposis syndromes are associated with small bowel neoplasms. Most notably, FAP (see later) is associated with adenomas and carcinomas of the duodenum and jejunum, but especially in the ampullary and periampullary region. At least 90% of FAP patients develop duodenal adenomas, and up to 10% develop cancer. The risk of cancer is related to the number of polyps, their size and histologic type, and the presence of high-grade dysplasia. Patients with FAP should undergo regular screening for duodenal neoplasia with both forward- and side-viewing endoscopes beginning around the time of colectomy and repeated at 1- to 5-year intervals, depending on the presence and degree of duodenal polyposis. Patients with *MUTYH*-associated polyposis likewise develop duodenal neoplasia and should undergo screening. Patients with hereditary nonpolyposis colon cancer (HNPCC) are also at increased risk for small intestine adenocarcinoma, which may be the first manifestation of their disease. HNPCC-associated small bowel cancer may present at a young age (median, 39 years) and occurs with decreasing frequency from the duodenum to the ileum, with about 50% of occurrences in the duodenum. Screening may be considered beginning at age 30. Patients with sprue are at increased risk for small bowel lymphomas, and they have an almost 35-fold increased risk for developing adenocarcinomas.

CLINICAL MANIFESTATIONS

The most common presenting symptom of small bowel tumors is abdominal pain, especially for those that are true cancers. Weight loss, nausea, GI bleeding, and symptoms related to perforation are less common. Approximately 25% of patients have GI obstruction, and duodenal periampullary tumors can lead to obstructive jaundice. Most malignancies are symptomatic, whereas benign tumors may be asymptomatic in up to half of patients. Carcinoid tumors in the small bowel are often asymptomatic, although in the setting of advanced disease, they may secrete bioactive amines, leading to flushing, diarrhea, wheezing, and eventually symptoms of right heart failure (related to valvular fibrosis) (Chapter 232). This occurs more commonly with tumors originating in the jejunum and ileum. Benign tumors tend to be found incidentally, although intraluminal growth may eventually cause symptoms of obstruction, and some may grow large enough to ulcerate and bleed.

DIAGNOSIS

The physical examination in patients with small bowel tumors is often unremarkable, although a palpable mass and, in more advanced cases, ascites may be present. As discussed earlier, patients with periampullary neoplasms may be jaundiced and/or icteric. Obstructive signs such as hyperperistalsis may be present, and patients with lymphoma may also have splenomegaly or other signs of systemic involvement, such as lymphadenopathy. Laboratory findings may include iron deficiency anemia or increased hepatic enzymes (the latter is especially common in those with liver metastases or biliary obstruction). Serum levels of the carcinoembryonic antigen (CEA) tumor marker may be elevated in small bowel adenocarcinoma, especially in advanced cases, but it is neither sensitive nor specific enough for routine diagnostic use. Patients with neuroendocrine tumors may demonstrate elevated levels of serotonin, chromogranin A, tumor-specific bioactive amines (e.g., gastrin), or urinary 5-hydroxyindoleacetic acid. Variants of intestinal lymphomas may show heavy chain immunoglobulin A fragments in serum and urine.

Proper imaging is crucial for both diagnosis and staging of small bowel neoplasms, but no one method is clearly the best. Standard radiographic techniques of value include upper GI with small bowel follow-through (helpful in demonstrating both masses and potential mucosal defects), angiography (which may show a site of bleeding or tumor blush with specific neoplasms), and computed tomography (CT) or magnetic resonance imaging (MRI) enteroclysis (double-contrast studies are both sensitive and specific for small bowel masses). Transabdominal ultrasound and standard CT may indicate a primary mass as well as metastases; MRI appears to be superior to CT in detecting and characterizing liver metastases.

Primary neuroendocrine tumors and their metastases are often apparent on indium-111 octreotide scanning. A wide variety of histologies may have uptake on positron emission tomography (PET) scanning. PET does not yet have a well-defined role in the diagnosis of most small bowel malignancies, although PET scans are useful in those with GISTs, to monitor response to systemic therapy (see later). Plain films rarely are specific enough to lead to a diagnosis, but they may demonstrate intestinal obstruction.

Capsule endoscopy uses a wireless endoscopic device that allows minimally invasive imaging of the small intestine. The system consists of the capsule camera—a swallowable, self-contained, battery-operated device that transmits two images per second—a receiver worn on the patient's belt, and a computerized work station for downloading and viewing the images. The primary indications for capsule endoscopy are the evaluation of obscure GI bleeding and Crohn disease. Tumors are found in about 2 to 3% of patients undergoing capsule endoscopy for obscure GI bleeding, and they may be more common in younger patients. Tumors detected include lymphoma, adenocarcinoma, metastatic disease, carcinoid tumor, and GIST. Capsule endoscopy has also been used to assess the small intestines of patients with FAP and Peutz-Jeghers syndrome (PJS), although its clinical utility for routine screening of these patients has not been established.

Deep enteroscopy describes a group of related techniques to facilitate deep intubation of the small bowel with long endoscopes. The small bowel may be examined antegrade (through the mouth) or retrograde (through the colon), allowing the majority of the small bowel to be examined. Although more invasive than capsule endoscopy, deep enteroscopy has a similar diagnostic yield but allows for tissue sampling (biopsy) and therapy including polypectomy and control of bleeding.

Surveillance

Patients with FAP, *MUTYH* polyposis, PJS, and probably HNPCC require regular surveillance of the small intestine, with specific recommendations as noted earlier. Patients with sporadic small intestine adenomas and possibly carcinoid tumors should undergo colonoscopy because they are at increased risk for colonic neoplasia. No specific guidelines exist for following patients with resected small bowel adenocarcinomas.

Staging

The staging systems for small bowel tumors vary by histology. Adenocarcinomas and, more recently, neuroendocrine cancers and GISTs are staged using different classifications within the American Joint Committee on Cancer's TNM malignant tumors system. Intestinal non-Hodgkin lymphomas, whether primary or part of a systemic process, are staged in accordance with a modified Ann Arbor system originally used in Hodgkin disease (Chapter 185).

TREATMENT

Rx

In general, surgical excision is the treatment of choice for most localized small bowel tumors. The extent of excision necessary depends on the tumor's location and histology. Adenocarcinomas involving the first and second portions of the duodenum require pancreaticoduodenectomy, whereas those in the more distal small intestine may be treated with segmental or wide local resection, including regional lymph nodes. Low-grade neuroendocrine tumors should be managed with en bloc resection, again including regional nodes. GISTs, which very rarely spread to regional nodes, may be treated with excision without lymphadenectomy (except in cases with gross involvement of nodes). Primary surgery for lymphomas may be offered for low-stage malignancies and may also be required for complications of disease (e.g., intussusception). Local management of benign small bowel tumors varies from observation (incidentally discovered lipomas) to endoscopic polypectomy (small adenomas) to pancreaticoduodenectomy (periampullary villous adenomas) (Video 193-2).

The need for and types of adjuvant therapy vary as well. Fully resected benign tumors require no additional therapy. Adenocarcinomas are often treated according to the principles developed for colorectal cancer, with some experts advocating fluoropyrimidine-based systemic chemotherapy, at least for patients with nodal involvement. Older retrospective studies demonstrated no benefit from adjuvant systemic therapy, but its use has still increased almost three-fold over the last two decades. Chemoradiotherapy has occasionally been recommended for those with more locally advanced duodenal adenocarcinomas. So far, no randomized trials have proven either strategy offers any advantage. Fully excised well- to moderately differentiated neuroendocrine cancers do not require adjuvant therapy. Postoperative imatinib mesylate treatment clearly postpones the recurrence of high-risk GISTs (Grade A)[A1]; a survival benefit has been demonstrated for those with gastric and nongastric primaries. Questions remain regarding dose and ideal duration of therapy. There is no defined role for the postoperative treatment of other mesenchymal tumors. Lymphomas treated with excision alone have high rates of recurrence, and systemic chemotherapy is advocated for high-grade variants; some experts also recommend chemotherapy for low-grade subtypes.

Patients with advanced small bowel adenocarcinomas are often treated with systemic chemotherapy regimens known to be effective against cancers of similar histology originating in the colon. However, the data supporting any specific regimen are scant and are not derived from randomized trials. Approximately 90% of patients with incurable GISTs have durable disease control when treated with the tyrosine kinase inhibitor imatinib mesylate, and the median survival for patients with metastatic disease has recently improved from approximately 18 months to 5 years.

Patients with small bowel lymphomas may be treated with chemotherapy that is effective in similar tumors originating outside the GI tract.

PROGNOSIS

Patients with small bowel adenocarcinomas generally do worse than those with similarly staged colonic glandular tumors. Also, patients with duodenal primaries may have poorer outcomes than those with more distal small bowel cancers. In general, 5-year survival rates range from 4% for those with metastases to 80% for those with very early disease confined to the small bowel wall. Five-year survival in patients with small bowel carcinoids exceeds 50%. In the pre-imatinib era, patients with surgically resected small bowel GISTs had recurrence rates ranging to 90% or higher, depending on the tumor's size, precise location, and mitotic rates; those with more distal tumors had a worse prognosis than those with duodenal primaries. Patients with recurrences almost invariably died within 2 years because salvage surgery and systemic chemotherapy were ineffective. True life expectancy in the era of postoperative imatinib use is unknown, but the median survival of patients with advanced GISTs likely exceeds 5 years. Small intestinal lymphomas have 5-year survival rates surpassing 60%, although this is highly variable and depends on the histologic subtype.

NEOPLASMS OF THE LARGE INTESTINE

Colorectal cancer (CRC) is the third most common cancer in the United States. Disease that has spread beyond regional lymph nodes is, for the most part, incurable, and CRC in general remains the second leading cause of neoplastic death. The lifetime risk of developing CRC for the average individual is about 1 in 18 to 20.

EPIDEMIOLOGY

Almost three quarters of large bowel cancers arise proximally (i.e., are of colonic origin). Although CRC is primarily a disease of the elderly (median age ≈ 73 years), about 10% of cases occur in those aged 50 or younger. CRC incidence and mortality have decreased overall recently, although the incidence has been increasing in the young. Incidence rates for right-sided cancers have also been decreasing, possibly but not solely owing to effective distal large bowel screening with flexible sigmoidoscopy. CRC is slightly more common in men than in women and in African Americans than in whites. Men develop CRC an average of 5 to 10 years earlier than women; similarly, large bowel cancers seem to arise an average of 5 to 10 years earlier in African Americans than in whites. Significant geographic variation in incidence occurs, probably based more on environmental factors than on genetic ones, as suggested by migration studies.

PATHOBIOLOGY

Between 96 and 98% of CRCs are adenocarcinomas. Rarely seen histologies include neuroendocrine cancers, epidermoid carcinomas, lymphomas, and sarcomas (including GISTs). Composites, particularly adenocarcinomas with neuroendocrine differentiation, are frequently encountered.

Adenocarcinomas derive from colonic columnar glandular epithelium in the colorectal mucosal lining. They are equally common in males and females and are most frequently reported in the sigmoid colon. Adenocarcinomas most commonly present at a localized or regional (nodal) stage. About two thirds are of moderate grade. The majority are nonmucinous, although the mucinous phenotype constitutes up to one fifth of all CRCs. Another variant is the true signet ring carcinoma, identified by large quantities of single tumor cells with nuclear displacement by intracytoplasmic mucin. Data are controversial as to whether mucinous tumors have a worse prognosis, whereas signet ring histology is clearly associated with advanced disease and/or worse outcome.

Neuroendocrine cancers can have a variety of histologies ranging from bland, well-differentiated carcinoids to high-grade small-cell carcinomas. True carcinoids are the second most common histologic colorectal subtype. They are more common in nonwhites and make up the vast majority of non-adenocarcinoma epithelial cancers. Distal bowel carcinoids are hormonally inactive. Noncarcinoid neuroendocrine cancers tend to be high grade and commonly present with hepatic and other distant metastases.

Epidermoid carcinomas are rare overall but still account for up to one fourth of CRCs. Most are squamous cell subtypes. They are more common in women and Hispanic patients. Epidermoid carcinomas are located in the rectum more than 90% of the time, and they are usually moderately or poorly differentiated. Interestingly, they commonly present as localized cancers, regardless of their degree of differentiation.

Medullary carcinomas, which are more often right-sided and seen in older female patients, tend to have a lower incidence of lymph node involvement. The majority exhibit microsatellite instability, and they tend to have a relatively better prognosis.

Primary colorectal lymphomas are fairly rare, constituting 10 to 20% of all GI lymphomas but less than 1% of CRCs. They are much more common in males and in the elderly. The cecum is the most common site of origin. Tumors are usually of B-cell origin.

Sarcomas of the large bowel have no gender or racial predilections. More than 50% have been classified as leiomyosarcomas, and they are most commonly found in the rectum. Sarcomas are usually diagnosed at a localized stage, regardless of grade, although about 40% are actually poorly differentiated. Kaposi sarcomas and GISTs are other sarcoma histologies found in the large bowel; many of the distal tumors called "leiomyosarcomas" in older registries were likely true GISTs.

Predisposing Conditions

Predisposing conditions for colonic neoplasia include age (discussed previously), gender, race, inflammatory bowel disease, family history,[1] and defined inherited syndromes. Defined genetic cancer syndromes, however, account for only a small percentage of CRCs (see later). Patients with first-degree relatives who also have colon neoplasia (adenomas or carcinomas) are commonly seen. Individuals with a first-degree relative with CRC face a 2- to 3-fold increased risk for malignancy, and this risk rises to 5- or 6-fold if two first-degree relatives are affected. Patients whose relatives have adenomas face a 1.8-fold increased risk for CRC, and this rises to 2.6 if the relative is younger than 60 years.

Patients with ulcerative colitis and Crohn disease (Chapter 141) are at increased risk for CRC in proportion to the amount of bowel involved and the duration of illness.[2] For example, adenocarcinoma of the colon is 10 to 20 times more common in persons with ulcerative colitis than in the general population. Between 2 and 4% of all patients with long-term ulcerative colitis develop this malignancy, and the cumulative incidence over a 25-year period is approximately 12%. Overall, the incidence of colorectal adenocarcinoma is 60% higher in persons with inflammatory bowel disease than in the general population and has been stable over time. Patients with both ulcerative colitis and primary sclerosing cholangitis seem to be at even greater risk. For those with Crohn colitis, patients with extensive disease involving more than one third of the colon are at increased risk (six- to eight-fold), similar to those

TABLE 193-1 GENERAL FEATURES OF INHERITED COLORECTAL CANCER SYNDROMES

SYNDROME	POLYP HISTOLOGY	POLYP DISTRIBUTION	AGE OF ONSET	RISK OF COLON CANCER	GENETIC LESION	CLINICAL MANIFESTATIONS	ASSOCIATED LESIONS
Familial adenomatous polyposis	Adenoma	Large intestine, duodenum	16 yr (range, 8-34 yr)	100%	5q (*APC* gene)	Rectal bleeding, abdominal pain, bowel obstruction	Desmoids, CHRPE
Peutz-Jeghers syndrome	Hamartoma	Large and small intestine	First decade	Slightly above average	19p (*STK11*)	Possible rectal bleeding, abdominal pain, intussusception	Orocutaneous melanin pigment spots, other tumors
MUTYH-associated polyposis	Adenoma	Large intestine, duodenum	45-50 yr (range, 13-60 yr)	75% (range, 50-100%)	1p (*MUTYH* gene)	Rectal bleeding, abdominal pain, bowel obstruction	CHRPE, osteomas
Juvenile polyposis	Hamartoma (rarely adenoma)	Large and small intestine	First decade	≈9%	*PTEN, SMAD4, BMPR1*	Possible rectal bleeding, abdominal pain, intussusception	Pulmonary AVMs
Hereditary nonpolyposis colon cancer	Adenoma	Large intestine	40 yr (range, 18-65 yr)	30%	Mismatch repair genes*	Rectal bleeding, abdominal pain, bowel obstruction	Other tumors (e.g., ovary, uterus, pancreas, stomach)

*Including *hMSH2, hMSH3, hMSH6, hMLH1, hPMS1,* and *hPMS2.*
AVM = arteriovenous malformation; CHRPE = congenital hypertrophy of the retinal pigment epithelium.

with ulcerative colitis. Isolated proctitis is not a risk factor. Patients with ulcerative colitis or extensive Crohn disease should undergo screening colonoscopy every 1 to 2 years beginning 8 to 10 years after disease onset. At colonoscopy, a dye spray may be used to identify suspicious areas, and multiple biopsies (at least 32 for pan-colitis) are obtained with targeting of suspicious lesions. The purpose of this is to identify the presence of dysplasia. The presence of high-grade dysplasia, any dysplasia in a mass or lesion that cannot be excised endoscopically, or multifocal low-grade dysplasia should prompt colectomy.

Patients who have had ureterocolostomy and those with acromegaly are also at increased risk. Case-control studies suggest that obesity, low physical activity, smoking, excessive alcohol, high-fat diet, and lack of dietary fiber increase the CRC risk. Patients with *Streptococcus bovis* bacteremia or endocarditis have increased rates of CRC and should undergo colonoscopy.

Polyposis Syndromes

Several defined dominant and recessive genetic conditions have been identified that convey an increased risk of CRC (Table 193-1). These include FAP, HNPCC, *MUTYH*-associated polyposis, PJS, juvenile polyposis, *PTEN* hamartoma syndrome, and Cronkhite-Canada syndrome.

FAMILIAL ADENOMATOUS POLYPOSIS

FAP is an autosomal dominant condition characterized by the development of hundreds to thousands of adenomatous polyps and CRC by age 40 (Fig. 193-4). Estimates of disease prevalence are 1 in 8000 to 15,000 births.

PATHOBIOLOGY

FAP is inherited as an autosomal dominant disease with incomplete penetrance. It has been mapped to the adenomatous polyposis coli (*APC*) gene located on the long arm of chromosome 5 (5q21). *APC* is a tumor suppressor gene that is a critical regulator of intestinal epithelial cell growth. Inherited mutations generally result in a truncated gene product. Patients with the familial syndrome inherit one mutant copy of *APC*; when a loss-of-function mutation develops in the other *APC* allele, mucosal epithelial cell growth is no longer controlled normally, and polyps develop. Variable phenotypes can be partly attributed to differences in the location of the *APC* mutation, with attenuated FAP being seen in mutations at the 5′ and 3′ ends of the gene.

CLINICAL MANIFESTATIONS AND DIAGNOSIS

Adenomas begin to appear early in the second decade of life, and GI symptoms begin to appear in the third or fourth decade. Polyps are distributed relatively evenly throughout the colon, although a slight predominance has been noted in the distal colon. Almost all patients with FAP develop frank colorectal carcinoma by age 40 years if the condition is left untreated. Gastric polyps (mostly nonadenomatous) occur in 30 to 100% of patients, and duodenal adenomas are found in 45 to 90%. Periampullary duodenal cancer develops in approximately 10% of cases. Small bowel lesions that are distal to the duodenum rarely progress to malignancy. In attenuated FAP, fewer than 100

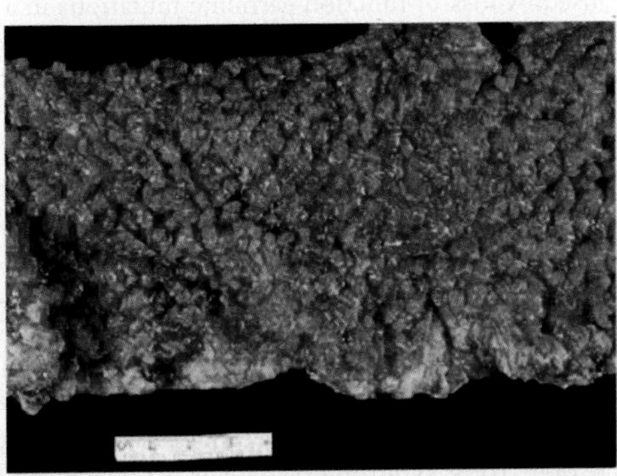

FIGURE 193-4. **Resected colon lined with hundreds of adenomatous polyps in a patient with familial adenomatous polyposis.**

colonic adenomas develop, there is a right colon predominance, and cancer develops approximately 10 years later. Genetic testing may identify the mutation in up to 85% of affected individuals and is useful for family screening.

TREATMENT Rx

The primary treatment option in FAP patients is total proctocolectomy with conventional ileostomy or ileoanal (pouch) anastomosis. Individuals with *APC* mutations and those with no identified mutation but clinical FAP in their families should be screened with annual sigmoidoscopy beginning at age 10 to 12 years. In families with known *APC* mutations, individuals who test negative do not require heightened surveillance but should undergo routine risk screening. FAP patients should be screened for duodenal polyposis with upper endoscopy beginning at age 20, with subsequent surveillance depending on polyp burden and histology. Cyclooxygenase-2 inhibition with sulindac or celecoxib may be considered in patients with small bowel adenomas or adenomas in the remnant rectum. Eicosapentaenoic acid supplementation has also been shown to decrease polyps in the remnant rectum.

GARDNER SYNDROME

Gardner syndrome is a phenotypic subtype of FAP that is also caused by mutations in the *APC* gene. It is distinguished by the presence of extraintestinal manifestations, including osteomas (particularly mandibular), soft tissue tumors (including lipomas, sebaceous cysts, and fibrosarcomas), supernumerary teeth, desmoid tumors, mesenteric fibromatosis, and congenital hypertrophy of the retinal pigment epithelium. The phenotypic differences between Gardner syndrome and FAP appear to result from variations in the location of the *APC* mutation, the presence of modifying genes, and environmental factors. Adenomatous polyps in Gardner syndrome have the same malignant potential as those found in FAP, and CRC screening and treatment recommendations are the same.

TURCOT SYNDROME

A hallmark of Turcot syndrome is the combination of colorectal polyposis and malignant diseases of the central nervous system. Mutations in the *APC* gene account for two thirds of cases, and the remaining one third result from mutations in the DNA mismatch repair genes that are also mutated in HNPCC. Central nervous system manifestations include medulloblastomas, glioblastomas, and ependymomas.

HEREDITARY NONPOLYPOSIS COLON CANCER

HNPCC, also known as Lynch syndrome, is the most common hereditary CRC syndrome and accounts for approximately 2% of all cases of CRC. It is an autosomal dominant trait and is highly penetrant. Clinically, HNPCC has been defined by the presence of all three of the following: (1) three or more relatives with histologically verified HNPCC-associated cancer (CRC or cancer of the endometrium, small bowel, ureter, or renal pelvis), one of whom is a first-degree relative of the other two, in the absence of FAP; (2) CRC involving at least two generations; and (3) one or more family members with cancer diagnosed before age 50.

PATHOBIOLOGY

HNPCC is caused by loss-of-function germline mutations in a set of genes involved in the repair of DNA base pair mismatches that occur during DNA replication (also known as the mutation mismatch repair system).

CLINICAL MANIFESTATIONS AND DIAGNOSIS

The median age for diagnosis of HNPCC is the mid-40s. Although several adenomas may be present, the diffuse polyposis characteristic of FAP is not found. Colonic neoplasia has a right-sided predominance (proximal to the splenic flexure). Although the cancers tend to be poorly differentiated, they generally have a better prognosis than similar sporadic CRCs. Synchronous and metachronous CRC is common. Patients with HNPCC are also at high risk for other malignant diseases, especially endometrial carcinoma, as well as cancers of the ovary, stomach, small bowel, hepatobiliary tract, ureter, and pancreas.[3] The Muir-Torre syndrome variant is associated with cutaneous lesions and visceral malignancies. Screening for HNPCC may begin with testing of the tumor for microsatellite instability, performing immunohistochemical staining for products of mismatch repair genes (including *hMSH2, hMSH6, hMLH1*, and *hPMS2*). A positive screen does not definitely indicate HNPCC, because up to 15% of sporadic tumors may have these features; this should be followed with germline testing.

TREATMENT Rx

Persons potentially affected with HNPCC should undergo a colonoscopy every 2 years beginning at age 21 and annually beginning at age 40. Patients with CRC or large adenomas should undergo subtotal colectomy. Women in HNPCC-affected families should have pelvic examinations every 1 to 3 years beginning at age 18; annual pelvic examinations, transvaginal ultrasonography, and endometrial biopsy have been recommended beginning at age 25. Prophylactic total abdominal hysterectomy with bilateral salpingo-oophorectomy may also be considered at the time of colectomy. Chemoprophylaxis with aspirin 600 mg daily may be considered; one randomized controlled trial did show benefit.[A2]

MUTYH-ASSOCIATED POLYPOSIS

MUTYH-associated polyposis is a recently described autosomal recessive syndrome caused by mutations in the *MUTYH* gene (also called *MYH* [mutY homologue]). It is characterized by colonic polyposis and a high rate of CRC. Approximately 0.4% to 0.7% of CRC patients are homozygous for *MUTYH* mutations.

PATHOBIOLOGY

MUTYH-associated polyposis is caused by a biallelic inherited defect in the *MUTYH* gene located on chromosome 1p. Inherited as an autosomal recessive trait, this leads to defects in base excision repair and acquired mutations of the *APC* gene and other genes, such as *KRAS*. This results in adenoma formation and the subsequent development of adenocarcinoma.

CLINICAL MANIFESTATIONS AND DIAGNOSIS

Phenotypically, affected patients are similar to those with attenuated FAP. Patients have five to hundreds of adenomas. Multiple hyperplastic polyps and serrated adenomas may also be seen. The onset is later than in classic FAP, with cancers more likely to be right sided and to occur at age 45 to 50. Associated extracolonic features include gastroduodenal polyps, duodenal carcinoma, breast and ovarian cancer in female carriers, bladder cancer, skin cancer, congenital hypertrophy of the retinal pigment epithelium, and osteoma. Monoallelic carriers do not appear to have an increased cancer risk.

The diagnosis is suggested by the presence of colonic polyposis in the absence of FAP, or when there appears to be recessive inheritance. In these cases, genetic testing for *MUTYH* gene mutations should be considered. Whether heterozygote carriers are at increased risk has not been established, but screening similar to that for individuals with first-degree relatives with CRC may be advisable (i.e., colonoscopy at age 40 and then every 5 years).

TREATMENT Rx

Patients with numerous polyps should undergo colectomy. Patients with mild disease and a relatively small number of polyps may be considered for colonoscopy with polypectomy and regular surveillance. Colonoscopy should be performed beginning at age 18 to 20 and repeated every 1 to 2 years. Regular endoscopic surveillance for duodenal polyps should also be performed beginning at age 25 to 30.

PEUTZ-JEGHERS SYNDROME

PJS is an intestinal hamartomatous polyposis of the upper and lower GI tract that is associated with characteristic mucocutaneous pigmentation. The average age at diagnosis is in the mid-20s. PHS predisposes to both intestinal and extraintestinal malignancies.

PATHOBIOLOGY

PJS is a rare autosomal dominant syndrome with high penetrance. The prevalence is between 1 in 8300 and 1 in 29,000. The gene responsible for the syndrome is the serine-threonine kinase *(STK11)* gene located on chromosome 19p; a mutation in *STK11* is found in approximately 60% of patients with this syndrome. The hamartomatous polyps in PJS are located predominantly in the small intestine (64 to 96%), stomach (24 to 49%), and colon (60%). Histologically, these polyps are benign; they are unique in that a layer of muscle that extends into the submucosa or muscularis propria may surround the glandular tissue. Adenomatous and hyperplastic polyps may also be found.

CLINICAL MANIFESTATIONS AND DIAGNOSIS

The most common symptoms are small bowel intussusception, obstruction, and GI bleeding that may require surgery and may be recurrent. PJS is associated with an increased risk of cancer, with an estimated 47% of patients developing a malignancy by age 65. The most common cancers are those of the small intestine, stomach, colon, pancreas, testes, breast, ovary, cervix, and uterus. More than 95% of patients have a characteristic pattern of melanin spots on the lips, buccal mucosa, and skin (Fig. 193-5). Because genetic testing is not widely available, first-degree relatives should be screened beginning at birth with an annual history, physical examination, and evaluation for melanotic spots, precocious puberty, and testicular tumors.

TREATMENT Rx

Standard medical care for patients with PJS involves an annual physical examination that includes evaluation of the breasts, abdomen, pelvis, and testes, as well as a complete blood cell count. Surveillance for cancer includes small bowel radiography every 2 years, esophagogastroduodenoscopy and colonoscopy every 2 years, and endoscopic ultrasound of the pancreas every 1 to 2 years. For women, annual Pap smear, transvaginal ultrasound, CA125, and mammography are recommended. Polyps larger than 1 cm should be removed endoscopically. Laparotomy and resection are recommended for recurrent or persistent small intestinal intussusception, obstruction, or intestinal bleeding.

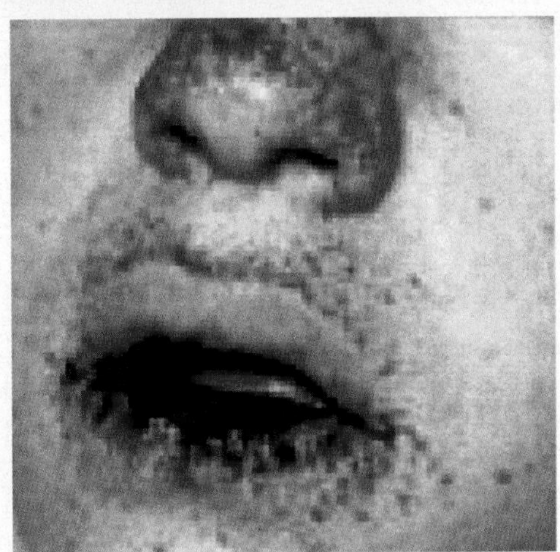

FIGURE 193-5. Mucosal pigmentation in a patient with Peutz-Jeghers syndrome.

JUVENILE POLYPOSIS

Familial juvenile (non-neoplastic, hamartomatous) polyposis is a rare (<1 in 100,000 births) syndrome characterized by 10 or more non-neoplastic hamartomatous polyps throughout the GI tract, or any number of polyps in a patient with a family history of juvenile polyposis. The syndrome is inherited in an autosomal dominant manner with high penetrance and is caused by mutations in the *SMAD4*, *PTEN*, or *BMPR1A* gene. The hamartomas are histologically distinct from the polyps seen in PJS. Patients generally present with rectal bleeding, anemia, abdominal pain, or intestinal obstruction in childhood or early adolescence. Extraintestinal symptoms include pulmonary arteriovenous malformations in some probands. The risk of malignancy in juvenile polyposis is reportedly as high as 20% and occurs in adulthood (median age, 37 years). Affected individuals should undergo regular colonoscopic surveillance. Patients with numerous, large, or high-grade dysplastic polyps may be considered for subtotal colectomy. Family members should be screened with colonoscopy every 3 to 5 years beginning at age 12 to 15 until age 40.

PTEN HAMARTOMA SYNDROME

PTEN hamartoma syndrome is a rare autosomal dominant syndrome consisting of multiple hamartomatous polyps of the skin and mucous membranes, including GI polyps, facial tricholemmomas, oral papillomas, and keratoses of the hands and feet. It was previously referred to as Cowden syndrome and Bannayan-Riley-Ruvalcaba syndrome. The causative genetic lesion has been mapped to the *PTEN* tumor suppressor gene. The rate of associated malignancy is high, particularly in the thyroid, breast, and reproductive organs. The polyps in *PTEN* hamartoma syndrome are benign. The incidence of CRC is approximately 10 times higher than in the general population.

CRONKHITE-CANADA SYNDROME

Cronkhite-Canada syndrome is a rare, sporadic, acquired condition characterized by multiple hamartomatous polyps throughout the GI tract, along with alopecia, dermal pigmentation, and atrophy of the nail beds. Symptoms include diarrhea, protein-losing enteropathy, GI bleeding, intussusception, and rectal prolapse. It carries a poor prognosis, with 5-year mortality rates as high as 55%. Patients are at risk for gastric and CRC, and endoscopic surveillance has been recommended.

MISCELLANEOUS GENETIC SYNDROMES

Recently, several new syndromes have been identified that predispose to CRC. In the serrated polyposis syndrome, affected individuals have multiple (≥5), large (at least 2 ≥ 10 mm), serrated adenomas, affected family members, and an increased CRC risk. Patients with defects in the epithelial cell adhesion molecule *(EPCAM)* gene have the phenotypic features of Lynch syndrome without mutations of the mismatch repair genes. Germline defects in the *POLE* and *POLD1* genes leads to DNA proofreading errors, polyposis, and/or CRC. The hereditary mixed polyposis syndrome is an autosomal dominant condition causing polyps of multiple and mixed morphologies and CRC; the causative genetic defect (a duplication spanning the 3′ end of the *SCG5* gene and a region upstream of the *GREM1* locus) has recently been discovered.

Polyps of the Colon

A polyp is defined as a grossly visible mass of epithelial cells that protrudes from the mucosal surface into the lumen of the intestine. A polyp may be sessile, flat, or pedunculated when it is attached by a stalk. Polyps are classified as either non-neoplastic or neoplastic (adenomatous). Polyps may rarely cause symptoms such as bleeding, prolapse, or obstruction. Neoplastic polyps have the potential to become malignant.

NON-NEOPLASTIC POLYPS

Non-neoplastic polyps account for approximately half of all mucosal polyps detected in the large bowel of average-risk individuals older than age 50 years. These polyps, which are also termed *nonadenomatous polyps*, can be subcategorized into hyperplastic, inflammatory, lymphoid, and juvenile polyps. Most non-neoplastic polyps are hyperplastic polyps that arise as a result of abnormal maturation of the mucosal epithelial cells; these polyps are usually small in diameter and are found predominantly in the distal sigmoid colon and rectum. Hyperplastic polyps are not malignant and are not thought to be associated with any measurable increase in malignant potential. Patients with inflammatory bowel disease may develop inflammatory pseudopolyps, which may require biopsy or removal to distinguish them from neoplastic polyps. Lymphoid polyps are regions of the mucosa that contain exaggerated intramucosal lymphoid tissue. Juvenile polyps usually develop in the rectum of children younger than 5 years and are termed *hamartomatous* because they are focal malformations that resemble tumors but are caused by abnormal development of the lamina propria; these polyps require no therapy unless they cause symptoms (e.g., obstruction, severe bleeding) or are part of a genetic syndrome.

ADENOMATOUS POLYPS

DEFINITION

Adenomatous polyps (or adenomas) are neoplastic polyps with malignant potential. They are benign glandular tumors that exhibit either low- or high-grade dysplasia under microscopy. Their anatomic distribution parallels that of colorectal adenocarcinoma. Adenomatous polyps manifest in a range of sizes and may be sessile, flat, or pedunculated in morphology. They are believed to be the precursor lesion to colorectal adenocarcinoma, a process that occurs along the adenoma-carcinoma sequence. Evidence supporting the adenoma-carcinoma sequence comes from several sources. Patients with genetic conditions that predispose to adenoma formation (e.g., FAP) develop cancer at high rates. Animal studies in which adenomas are induced by either carcinogens or genetic manipulation show carcinoma formation. Correlative evidence includes the observations that the epidemiology is similar for adenomas and carcinomas, that both lesions are more common in the same anatomic locations, and that adenomatous tissue can often be found in small adenocarcinomas. Intervention studies have shown that the removal of adenomatous polyps leads to a significant decrease in the risk for CRC.

EPIDEMIOLOGY

Adenomatous polyps are relatively common, particularly in elderly populations. Among healthy screening populations older than 50 years, adenomas are found in more than 15% of women and 25% of men. The prevalence of adenomas tends to be high in regions of the world where CRC is common. The importance of genetic risk factors is clear in the hereditary polyposis syndromes, and sporadic adenomas have a familial component; for example, individuals with a positive first-degree family history have a four-fold greater risk of developing adenomatous polyps. African Americans in the United States have an increased risk for developing adenomas and carcinomas relative to whites; the risk in Asian and Hispanic individuals is similar to that in whites.

PATHOBIOLOGY

The layer of epithelial cells lining the surface of the normal large bowel undergoes continuous self-renewal, with a turnover period of 3 to 8 days. Undifferentiated stem cells located at the base of invaginated crypts give rise to cells that migrate toward the lumen as they differentiate further into specialized enterocytes; these cells are subsequently removed by apoptosis, by extrusion, or by phagocytes underlying the epithelial layer. The development of adenomatous polyps is associated with a sequence-specific accumulation

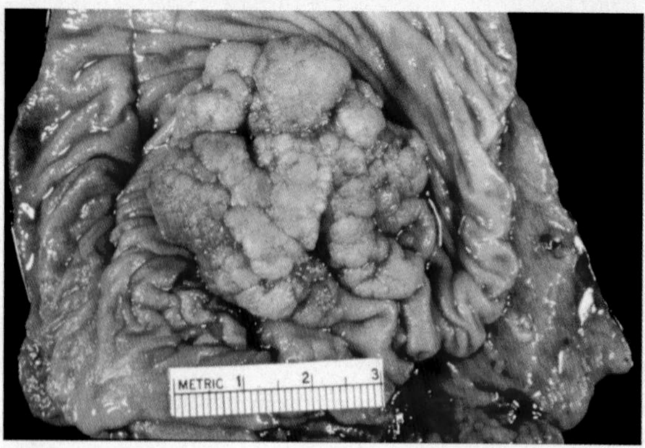

FIGURE 193-6. Villous adenoma. Large and sessile villous adenomas of the large bowel with finger-like projections into the gut lumen. (Courtesy Dr. M.K. Washington.)

of genetic lesions that cause an imbalance between epithelial cell proliferation and cell death. As a result, cells accumulate at the luminal surface, where they remain undifferentiated and continue to undergo cell division, eventually leading to the abnormal development of a mass of adenomatous tissue.

Adenomas are classified into three main histologic subtypes: tubular adenomas, villous adenomas (Fig. 193-6), and tubulovillous adenomas. Tubular adenomas account for 70 to 85% of all adenomas removed at colonoscopy. They are often small and pedunculated, and they consist of dysplastic tubular glands that divide and branch out from the mucosal surface; they rarely contain concomitant high-grade dysplasia or carcinoma. In contrast, villous adenomas (<5% of all adenomas) are generally large and sessile and are composed of strands of dysplastic epithelium that project, finger-like, into the lumen of the gut; they have a much higher prevalence of high-grade dysplasia or carcinoma. Tubulovillous adenomas (10 to 25% of all adenomas) have a mixture of tubular and villous architecture. Advanced adenomas are defined as those that measure 1 cm or greater or have any villous histology or high-grade dysplasia. Patients with advanced adenomas or multiple adenomas (three or more) are at much greater risk for synchronous (developing simultaneously) or metachronous (developing after a time interval) CRC.

CLINICAL MANIFESTATIONS

Patients with adenomatous polyps generally remain asymptomatic, but they may present with an asymptomatic positive stool occult blood test or with evident hematochezia. The lifetime incidence of additional adenomas in a patient with one known adenoma is 30 to 50%. Fewer than 5% of all adenomas eventually develop into carcinomas. Two critical factors that determine the likelihood of an adenoma developing into an invasive lesion are the size of the polyp and the grade of dysplasia. For polyps less than 1 cm, the risk for carcinoma is 1 to 3%; polyps between 1 and 2 cm have a 10% risk of becoming cancerous; and more than 40% of polyps greater than 2 cm progress to an invasive lesion. All adenomatous polyps contain some degree of dysplasia, but they can be further categorized as low- or high-grade to indicate the degree of dysplasia and the corresponding risk for invasive carcinoma. High-grade dysplasia is associated with a 27% rate of eventual transformation into carcinoma.

DIAGNOSIS

Adenomatous polyps in the colon and rectum can be diagnosed by endoscopy, barium radiography, or CT scanning (CT colography or virtual colonoscopy). Colonoscopy is the preferred method for diagnosing adenomas because of its high accuracy and the ability to immediately biopsy and resect most polyps. Barium enema, as assessed in the National Polyp Study, missed 52% of polyps measuring 1 cm or more. CT colography has good sensitivity for detecting large (>1 cm) polyps (>85%) and for detecting cancers (96%), but it is less sensitive and specific for smaller polyps. CT colography requires bowel preparation, exposes the patient to ionizing radiation, and cannot remove polyps. Colonoscopy may miss 6 to 12% of large (≥1 cm) polyps and 5% of cancers. Of note is that nonpolypoid (flat and depressed) colorectal neoplasms are found in about 9% of asymptomatic and symptomatic adults on colonoscopy and are more likely to contain a carcinoma than are polypoid lesions; these lesions may not be visible on barium radiography or CT.

Flexible sigmoidoscopy, which is often used to screen asymptomatic persons at average risk for colorectal adenocarcinoma, detects 50 to 60% of all polyps and cancers. Generally, patients who have polyps detected by barium radiography, CT colography, or flexible sigmoidoscopy should undergo colonoscopy to remove the lesion and search for additional polyps. In one study in which patients with polyps discovered by flexible sigmoidoscopy underwent subsequent colonoscopy, there was an 80% reduction in the incidence of CRC.

TABLE 193-2 COLONOSCOPY SURVEILLANCE INTERVALS

MOST ADVANCED FINDING	INTERVAL
No polyps or small (<10 mm) hyperplastic polyps	10 yr
1-2 adenomas, <1 cm	5-10 yr
3-10 adenomas or adenoma with villous features, ≥1 cm, or with high-grade dysplasia	3 yr
>10 adenomas	<3 yr
Sessile adenoma ≥ 2 cm, piecemeal excision	2-6 mo
Serrated lesions:	
<10 mm, no dysplasia	5 yr
≥10 mm or dysplasia	3 yr

SERRATED POLYPS

Sessile serrated adenomas/polyps (SSA/P) are a recently recognized neoplastic lesion with malignant potential. In the past, these have been confused with large, benign, hyperplastic polyps. SSA/P are characterized microscopically as having a disorganized and distorted crypt growth pattern. SSA/P are sessile or flat, may be difficult to distinguish on endoscopy and have a right colon predominance. The risk of progression to cancer is at least as high as for conventional adenomas. Pathogenesis is via hypermethylation of CpG islands ("CIMP-high") and *MLH1*, and have *BRAF* mutations, leading to polyps and tumors with microsatellite instability. Traditional serrated adenomas are a rare subtype that are histologically distinct from SSA/P and have a high prevalence of high-grade dysplasia and carcinoma in situ.

TREATMENT

Rx

The goal of treatment for neoplastic polyps is to remove or destroy the lesion during endoscopy. This recommendation is based on overwhelming evidence that endoscopic polypectomy reduces the subsequent incidence and mortality of CRC. Pedunculated adenomas are generally removed by snare polypectomy (Video 193-1), with subsequent submission of the tissue for pathologic analysis. Piecemeal snare resection may be required to remove sessile polyps. Surgical resection of a polyp is indicated when endoscopic resection of an advanced adenoma is not possible. The biopsied polyp must be evaluated histologically to determine the presence or absence of carcinoma; if a malignant lesion is found, its histologic grade, vascular and lymphatic involvement, and proximity to the margin of resection should be determined. Unfavorable histopathologic factors that should prompt surgical resection include poorly differentiated histology, vascular invasion, lymphatic invasion, and incomplete endoscopic resection. Malignant pedunculated polyps with cancer confined to the submucosa, with no evidence of unfavorable histologic features, can be definitively treated with endoscopic resection, without the need for surgical resection. Whether similar malignant sessile polyps can be managed nonoperatively is controversial. In these cases, the risk of surgery versus the risk of recurrence or lymphatic metastases needs to be balanced.

PROGNOSIS

Patients who have undergone resection of an adenomatous or sessile serrated polyp are at increased risk for the subsequent development of adenoma and colorectal adenocarcinoma. This risk is influenced by the size, histology, and number of adenomas, and the surveillance intervals differ (Table 193-2). Low-risk patients—those with only 1 or 2 small tubular adenomas—should undergo colonoscopy in 5 to 10 years. Patients with multiple (>2) adenomas, large (≥1 cm) adenomas, or adenomas with villous or high-grade histology should undergo colonoscopy in 3 years. Patients with numerous (>10) adenomas should undergo colonoscopy within 3 years. Patients who have had polypectomy of a large (≥2 cm) adenoma or an adenoma that had to be

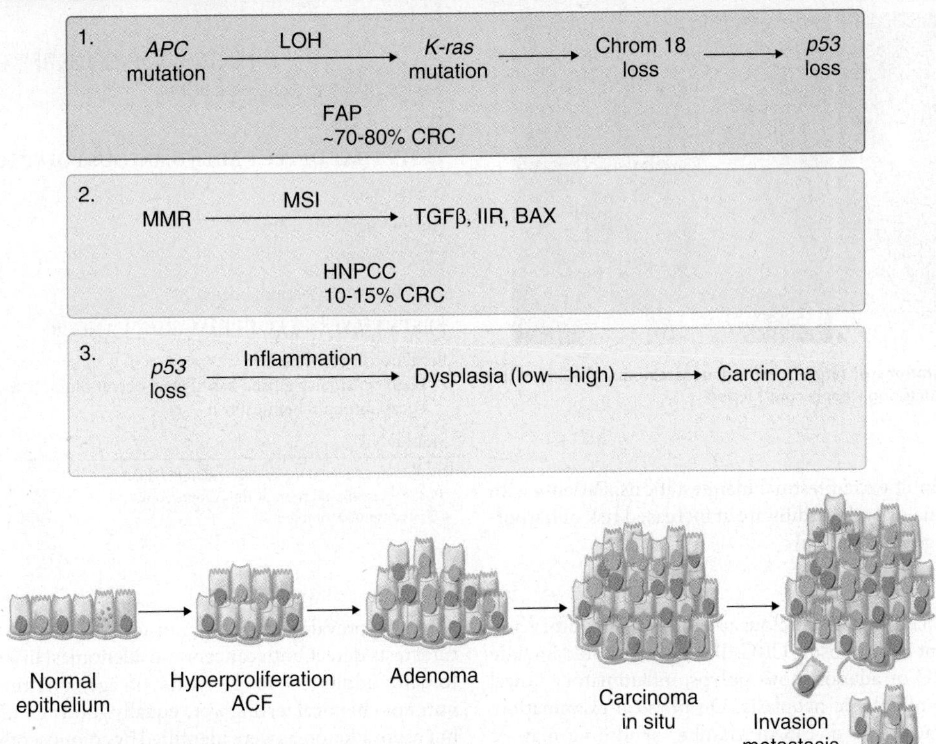

FIGURE 193-7. **The molecular basis of colorectal cancer. Sequence-specific genetic lesions result in the transition from normal large bowel mucosa to invasive carcinoma. ACF = aberrant crypt foci; BAX = apoptosis-related protein; CRC = colorectal cancer; HNPCC = hereditary nonpolyposis colorectal cancer; IIR = type II receptor; LOH = loss of heterozygosity; MMR = mutation mismatch repair; MSI = microsatellite instability; TGFβ = transforming growth factor-β.**

removed in pieces (piecemeal resection) should undergo colonoscopy within 6 months to evaluate the completeness of the resection. Patients with sessile serrated polyps smaller than 10 mm without dysplasia should undergo surveillance colonoscopy at 5 years. Patients with sessile serrated polyps 10 mm or larger, high-grade dysplasia, or a traditional serrated adenoma should undergo colonoscopy at 3 years (Video 193-3).

Adenocarcinoma of the Colon and Rectum

PATHOBIOLOGY

Colorectal cancer is caused by the accumulation of multiple genetic lesions over time. Except for hypermutated tumors, colon and rectal primaries have similar patterns of alterations. Both the tissue architecture and the cellular genotype change as the disease progresses (Fig. 193-7).[4] Three distinct molecular pathways have been recognized: chromosomal instability, microsatellite instability, and CpG island methylator phenotype (CIMP). These pathways are not mutually exclusive, and tumors may exhibit features of more than one.

The chromosomal instability pathway is the most common, accounting for up to 70% of sporadic CRC. The most common gene mutations are in the *APC* gene (a tumor suppressor gene) and *KRAS* (a proto-oncogene involved in the transduction of mitogenic signals across cell membranes). Germline mutations in *APC* are the cause of FAP. Chromosomal instability leads to aneuploidy (imbalance in chromosome number), genomic amplifications, and loss of heterozygosity where cells have only one allele of a gene owing to the loss of individual chromosomes during mitosis. Additional important affected genes include the mutated in colon cancer *(MCC)* gene (a tumor suppressor gene), *p53* (a regulator of the cell cycle), *VEGF, MYC, MET, LYN, PTEN,* and others. Many of the genetic changes affect the Wnt signaling pathway, which appears to be important for initiation and progression of CRC.

The microsatellite instability (MSI) pathway is caused by defects in DNA mismatch repair. Microsatellites are short, repeating nucleotide sequences that are prone to errors owing to their repetitive nature. MSI-high tumors have genetic defects in the mismatch repair genes, especially *MLH1, MSH2, MSH6,* and *PMS2*. Germline mutations in these genes are the cause of HNPCC (Lynch syndrome). Hypermethylation silencing of *MLH1* also results in MSI-high cancers. MSI-high tumors are more common in the right colon, in women, and have a lymphocytic infiltration and poor differentiation. They are associated with improved survival, despite being less responsive to some chemotherapeutic agents such as 5-fluorouracil.

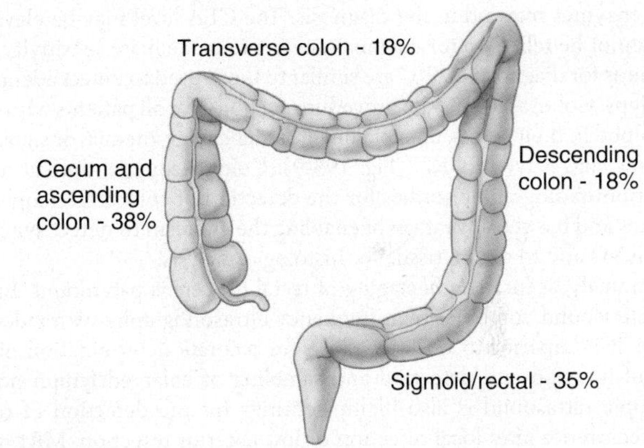

FIGURE 193-8. **Sites of development of large bowel adenocarcinoma.**

In the CIMP pathway, hypermethylation of DNA promoter regions leads to gene silencing, and silencing of tumor suppressor genes leads to carcinogenesis. In colorectal carcinogenesis, these include *APC, MCC, MLH1, MGMT,* and others. CIMP-high tumors are often poorly differentiated with mucinous or signet ring morphology, are MSI-high, and have *BRAF* mutations. The sessile serrated adenoma is likely the precursor lesion.

CLINICAL MANIFESTATIONS

The majority of patients with CRC present with symptoms; these may be emergent. Common symptoms related to primary disease include rectal bleeding with or without manifestations of anemia, abdominal pain, and change in bowel function. Patients with systemic disease may exhibit anorexia, weight loss, and symptoms related to hepatic dysfunction, such as jaundice, icterus, and ascites (the last may also be seen with peritoneal metastases). Symptoms vary depending on the primary site (Fig. 193-8). Proximal lesions are more likely to present with bleeding and associated symptoms; more distal disease has a higher risk of obstruction and perforation. Rectal cancers can also manifest with tenesmus and changes in stool caliber. They involve sacral nerve plexi, causing significant neuropathic pain. Patients with PJS or

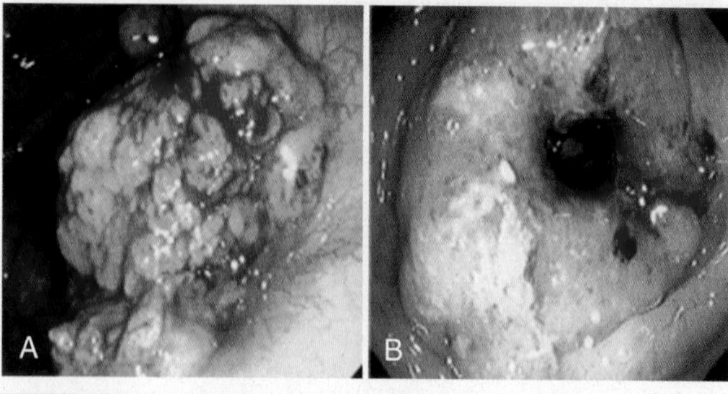

FIGURE 193-9. Two manifestations of large bowel adenocarcinoma. A, Exophytic growth within the lumen. B, Stricturing ("apple core") lesion.

TABLE 193-3 OPTIONS FOR COLORECTAL NEOPLASIA SCREENING*

TEST	INTERVAL
TESTS THAT DETECT ADENOMATOUS POLYPS OR CANCER	
Colonoscopy	Every 10 yr
Flexible sigmoidoscopy†	Every 5 yr
CT colography†	Every 5 yr
Double-contrast barium enema†	Every 5 yr
TESTS THAT DETECT PRIMARILY CANCER†	
Fecal occult blood tests	
High-sensitivity guaiac-based fecal occult blood test	Annually
Fecal immunochemical test	Annually
Stool DNA	Interval uncertain

*Beginning at age 50 for average-risk individuals.
†Positive test should prompt full colonoscopy.
CT = computed tomography.

Gardner syndrome may exhibit extraintestinal manifestations. Patients with *Streptococcus bovis* bacteremia or endocarditis are at increased risk of harboring CRC and should undergo colonoscopy.

DIAGNOSIS

The history, physical examination, and judicious use of both laboratory and radiologic tests are important in diagnosing CRC. The history should include the possibility of prior CRC or adenomatous polyps, inflammatory bowel disease, and family history of colonic neoplasia. On physical examination, extraintestinal lesions characteristic of PJS or Gardner syndrome may be noticed. Metastatic disease may be suggested by enlargement of left supraclavicular lymph nodes (Virchow's nodes) or the liver, or by the presence of an umbilical mass (Sister Mary Joseph's node) or ascites. The digital rectal examination may reveal a distal rectal cancer or spread of the tumor to the rectal shelf or pelvis (Blumer's shelf). The stool shows evidence of frank or occult blood in 40 to 80% of advanced cases. Iron deficiency anemia or an elevation in liver enzymes may aid in the diagnosis. The CEA level may be elevated, but it cannot be relied on for diagnosis, owing to inadequate sensitivity.

Methods for diagnosing CRC are similar to those used to detect adenomatous polyps. Colonoscopy is the procedure of choice for all patients who have occult blood in their stools, unexplained iron deficiency anemia, or signs and symptoms suggestive of CRC (Fig. 193-9). Colonoscopy is more accurate than barium radiographic studies for the detection of colorectal neoplasms of all sizes and has the advantage of enabling the clinician to detect synchronous cancers and to obtain tissue for histologic analysis.

Additionally, accurate *local* staging of rectal cancers is paramount. Endoscopic ultrasound combines high-frequency ultrasonography with videoendoscopy. It is superior to CT and allows an accurate determination of the degree of invasion and detection and sampling of enlarged lymph nodes. Endoscopic ultrasound is also highly sensitive for the detection of rectal cancer recurrence after local resection or low anterior resection. MRI using either endorectal or phased array coils can also provide accurate local staging of rectal cancer. Local staging of nonrectal large bowel cancer is generally not performed preoperatively, because this information is not used to guide therapy.

Many expert consensus guidelines now recommend CT scans of the abdomen and pelvis for CRC patients because advanced liver metastases would preclude resection of an asymptomatic primary. Chest imaging with plain films or CT is recommended as well. PET scans have specific uses in defined cases of CRC, such as precluding additional systemic disease before resection of a solitary metastatic site. They may also be used to further describe abnormalities seen on CT. However, there is no role for PET in the routine work-up. Plain abdominal films are mostly useful in diagnosing obstruction.

Screening

The purpose of screening is to reduce CRC-related mortality by removing the precursor adenomas and detecting prevalent cancers at earlier, more curable stages.[5] The long latency between adenoma development and subsequent cancer, on the order of 10 to 20 years, makes CRC a preventable disease through colonoscopy with polypectomy. It is an age-associated disease, and most patients should begin screening at age 50.[6] There is a range of options for average-risk individuals (Table 193-3). These can be divided into two categories: stool tests, which include tests for occult blood and abnormal DNA, and structural tests, which include colonoscopy, flexible sigmoidoscopy, CT colography, and double-contrast barium enema. Stool tests are best suited for detecting prevalent cancers (and some advanced adenomas), whereas structural tests detect both cancers and adenomas. In a randomized trial of asymptomatic adults 50 to 69 years of age, one-time colonoscopy and fecal immunochemical testing were equally good at finding prevalent colon cancer, but more adenomas were identified by colonoscopy.[A3] These tests may be used alone or in combination. Current multisociety guidelines recognize the multiple screening options but encourage the use of structural tests that have the ability to both detect and prevent CRC. For example, the American College of Physicians recommends that clinicians screen for CRC in average-risk adults starting at age 50, and in high-risk adults starting at age 40 (or 10 years younger than the age at which the youngest affected relative was diagnosed with CRC), using a stool-based test, flexible sigmoidoscopy, or optical colonoscopy in patients who are at average risk, but optical colonoscopy in patients who are at high risk. Clinicians should stop screening for CRC in adults older than 75 years or in adults with a life expectancy of less than 10 years.

Tests for fecal occult blood detect hemoglobin in the stool from bleeding tumors. These tests are either guaiac based or immunochemical based. The guaiac tests detect blood in stool through the pseudoperoxidase activity of heme or hemoglobin. The immunochemical tests react with human globin and are therefore more specific. Guaiac testing consists of collecting two samples from three consecutive stools. To improve test accuracy, individuals undergoing guaiac testing are instructed to avoid aspirin, nonsteroidal anti-inflammatory drugs (NSAIDs), vitamin C, red meat, poultry, fish, and some vegetables. Three large prospective randomized trials demonstrated that guaiac-based testing decreased CRC mortality by 15 to 33%, and this benefit appears to persist for 30 years.[7] One large U.S. study also showed a 20% decrease in CRC incidence, attributed to the relatively higher rates of colonoscopy in the study group. Guaiac-based tests have sensitivities for cancer from 35 to 80%. Immunochemical-based tests do not rely on a peroxidase reaction and therefore may have fewer false positives and false negatives. They are done essentially the same way as the traditional guaiac, but they do not require the dietary restrictions of guaiac-based tests and only one stool specimen is collected. The immunochemical tests have better adherence, find 2.5 times as many cancers and advanced adenomas as guaiac-based tests, and are now the preferred fecal occult blood test for screening. Fecal occult blood tests are repeated annually, and any positive test should prompt colonoscopy.

Stool DNA tests rely on the observation that both adenomas and carcinomas contain altered DNA, and this DNA is shed in the stool. Tests contain a multiple marker panel designed to detect exfoliated DNA markers. Collection kits are designed to facilitate stool collection (at least 30 g) and mailing. First-generation stool DNA tests had better sensitivity for CRC (52%) than a guaiac-based test (unrehydrated Hemoccult II; 13% sensitivity) but poor sensitivity for advanced adenomas (15%). Next-generation stool DNA testing with an updated marker panel can identify about 90% of patients with CRC and about 40% of patients with advanced adenomas, with an 87% specificity.[8] Stool DNA testing is more expensive than fecal occult blood testing, and the optimal screening interval has not been defined.

Flexible sigmoidoscopy is capable of examining the distal 60 cm of the colon, or roughly the splenic flexure to the rectum. It can be done with minimal bowel preparation, does not require sedation, and can be performed by primary care providers, nurses, or physician's assistants. Flexible sigmoidoscopy can detect distal cancers or polyps as well as colonoscopy can.[9] The detection of an adenoma should prompt referral for full colonoscopy, owing to the high prevalence of synchronous neoplasia in the unexamined proximal colon. In one randomized trial, a single flexible sigmoidoscopy performed once between ages 55 to 64 years reduced CRC incidence by 23% and mortality by 31%.[A4] In another randomized trial, screening with flexible sigmoidoscopy led to a significant 29% decrease in CRC incidence in both the distal and proximal colon, and a significant 50% decrease in mortality from cancers of the distal colon only.[A5] In a third trial, CRC incidence was reduced by 20% and death by 12%.[A6] Sigmoidoscopy should be repeated every 5 years and may be combined with yearly fecal occult blood testing.

Colonoscopy allows complete examination of the colon as well as adenoma removal, and thus cancer prevention. In the United States, it is generally done under sedation after an oral bowel preparation, and by physicians with specific training in colonoscopy and polypectomy. Large cohort studies have found an up to 1% cancer rate, 5 to 10% advanced adenoma rate (size > 10 mm, villous histology, or high-grade dysplasia), and at least 20% with 1 or more adenomas.[10] Major complication rates are less than 0.5%, with more than half due to polypectomy. There are no direct randomized studies assessing the efficacy of colonoscopy for screening, although there is a large amount of indirect evidence. Colonoscopy is generally used as the gold standard in assessing other screening methods. In a large randomized Minnesota study of fecal occult blood testing, a decrease in cancer incidence was observed that could be explained only by the use of colonoscopy and polypectomy at a higher rate in the screened population. Randomized and case-control studies of sigmoidoscopy demonstrate a CRC mortality benefit that should also apply to colonoscopy. The National Polyp Study, which followed patients after polypectomy, found that the incidence of CRC was reduced 76 to 90% compared to three reference populations. In another study of patients who had adenomas detected and removed by colonoscopy, the risk of death from CRC at 16 years was only 50% of what was expected in the general population,[11] with most of the reduced incidence found among patients who had low-risk adenomas removed.[12] The efficacy of colonoscopy is influenced by the quality of the exam, with the most important quality markers being the cecal intubation rate (indicating a complete exam) and the adenoma or polyp removal rate. Studies have demonstrated superior CRC prevention when the colonoscopy is performed by a physician with a high adenoma or polyp removal rate.[13] Physician experience and specialty are also important, with gastroenterologists preventing more CRC than other specialties.[14] If the initial screening colonoscopy is normal, further screening can be deferred for 10 years.[15]

Double-contrast barium enema evaluates the entire colon by coating the mucosal surface with high-density barium and insufflating with air via a rectal tube. Multiple radiographs are obtained while varying the patient's position under fluoroscopy. It requires a colon preparation and exposes the patient to a small amount of ionizing radiation. There are no studies of double-contrast barium enema as a screening test. It is 85 to 97% sensitive for colon cancer, but its sensitivity for detecting large adenomas is only 48 to 73%. It should be repeated every 5 years. The finding of a polyp larger than 5 mm should prompt colonoscopy.

CT colography (also known as virtual colonoscopy) uses multidetector CT technology to obtain two- and three-dimensional images of the entire colon. It requires an adequate colon preparation and gaseous distention of the bowel using a rectal tube. Tagging of residual stool with barium or iodinated contrast material is frequently used. CT scanning is performed with the patient in the supine and prone positions. No studies have been done to evaluate the efficacy of CT colography in decreasing CRC incidence or mortality. CT colography has been compared with standard colonoscopy for the detection of neoplasia in screening populations. The sensitivity of CT colography for large (≥10 mm) polyps is 85 to 92%, with a specificity of 83 to 86%. For polyps 5 mm or larger, CT colography is about 65% sensitive and 89% specific. Sensitivity for CRC (96%) is similar to that of colonoscopy. Laxative-free CT colography is accurate in detecting adenomas 10 mm or larger but less so for smaller lesions.[16] Although the optimal interval for testing has not been established, it is recommended that CT colography screening begin at age 50; if negative, it should be repeated at 5-year intervals. If a polyp larger than 5 mm is found, colonoscopy should be performed.

Staging

Accurate staging of CRC is of the utmost importance in determining both prognosis and the most relevant and effective therapy. The versions of the TNM classification system for large bowel cancers used by the American Joint Committee on Cancer and the International Union Against Cancer are identical (Table 193-4). Differing from many solid tumors (although not those of other GI origin, except for anal cancer), CRCs are not staged according to size. Stage I cancers penetrate into but not through the bowel wall (T1–2N0M0), whereas stage II cancers penetrate through the wall and can involve nearby organs without spreading to regional lymph nodes. About 40% of patients present with stage I or II disease in the United States. Stage III cancers involve regional lymph nodes and constitute about 40% of presenting cases. Stage IV colorectal tumors (distant metastasis or metastases) commonly involve liver, lung, distant nodes, and peritoneum, with about 20% of patients presenting with this stage. Rectal primaries, because of early access to the systemic circulation, may involve the lungs without liver metastases; this pattern of spread is distinctly unusual in proximal large bowel cancers.

TABLE 193-4 STAGING FOR COLORECTAL ADENOCARCINOMAS

STAGE	TUMOR	NODE	METASTASIS
0	Tis	N0	M0
I	T1, T2	N0	M0
IIA	T3	N0	M0
IIB	T4a	N0	M0
IIC	T4b	N0	M0
IIIA	T1, T2 T1	N1 N2a	M0 M0
IIIB	T3, T4a T2, T3 T1, T2	N1 N2a N2b	M0 M0 M0
IIIC	T4a T3, T4a T4b	N2a N2b N1, N2	M0 M0 M0
IVA	Any T	Any N	M1a
IVB	Any T	Any N	M1b

Tis = in situ; T1 = submucosa; T2 = muscularis propria; T3 = subserosa, pericolorectal tissues; T4a = visceral peritoneum; T4b = other structures.
N1a = 1 regional node; N1b = 2-3 regional nodes; N1c = satellite(s) without regional nodes; N2a = 4-6 regional nodes; N2b = ≥7 regional nodes.
M1a = 1 organ; M1b = >1 organ, peritoneum.

TREATMENT Rx

Chemoprevention

NSAIDs, including aspirin, are believed to reduce adenoma formation and inhibit colon cancer development by inhibiting cyclooxygenase and subsequent prostaglandin generation (Chapter 37). Prostaglandins (e.g., E_2) promote cell proliferation and tumor growth. The NSAIDs sulindac and celecoxib cause regression of existing adenomas and inhibit the formation of new adenomas in patients with FAP. Epidemiologic studies have shown decreased CRC rates in regular users of NSAIDs. Randomized trials of aspirin have shown 20 to 40% reductions in adenoma recurrence. A secondary analysis combining data from four European vascular event prevention trials reported up to a 70% reduction in the incidence of CRC when at least 75 mg of aspirin daily was continued for 5 or more years.[17] However, the 4 individual studies and two large American trials (Women's Health Trial, Physicians Health Study) did not find an aspirin benefit. Calcium supplementation (1200 mg/day) was shown to decrease the rate of metachronous adenomas by 20%. However, the large Women's Health Trial (36,000 participants) found that calcium (1000 mg) plus vitamin D (400 IU) had no effect in reducing CRC incidence. Currently, the routine use of aspirin and calcium for CRC prevention is not recommended, but it may be considered on an individual basis.

Dietary Prevention

Epidemiologic studies have reported correlations between CRC and obesity, smoking, inactivity, excessive alcohol use, and diets high in fat and low in fruits, vegetables, and fiber. These observations suggest that lifestyle modifications may decrease CRC risk. Unfortunately, three randomized intervention trials of modest dietary changes (10% less fat, 25 to 75% more fiber, 50% more fruits and vegetables) found no significant reductions in adenomas or CRC over 3 to 8 years of follow-up. Fish consumption is inversely associated with CRC incidence, and eicosapentaenoic acid supplementation decreases polyp burden in FAP.

Surgery

Resection is the primary treatment modality for patients with regionally confined CRC. Highly selected patients with metastatic disease may also undergo surgery with curative intent. The goal of curative surgery for colonic adenocarcinoma is margin-negative elimination of the tumor, plus en bloc removal of the primary feeding arterial vessel and corresponding lymphatics for that segment of bowel. A minimum of 12 lymph nodes should be retrieved for microscopic examination to assure staging accuracy. Synchronous colon cancers may be removed individually or with subtotal colectomy, and tumors adherent to adjacent structures should be resected en bloc. Prophylactic oophorectomy is no longer recommended, but women with one ovary grossly involved with cancer should undergo bilateral oophorectomy because of the relatively high risk of involvement of the other side. Laparoscopic resection is currently thought to be as effective as open resection and requires a modestly shorter recovery time. Very preliminary data suggest elderly patients undergoing a laparoscopic procedure have a lower chance of being discharged to a nursing home (as opposed to their own residences) than those treated with standard resection.

In general, surgical considerations for rectal primaries are similar. Total mesorectal excision (en bloc removal of the lymphovascular and fatty envelope surrounding the rectum) is recommended for distal cancers, whereas tumor-specific mesorectal excision (en bloc removal of the mesorectum 5 cm distal to the tumor) should suffice for upper rectal tumors. Local transanal excision is acceptable for selected low rectal cancers thought to have minimal risk of nodal involvement. Selection criteria include the following: T1 disease, size less than 3 cm, low grade (well differentiated), location within 8 cm of the anal verge, no lymphovascular invasion, and less than one third circumferential. The wide spectrum of symptoms that occur in most patients after resection and reconstruction of the rectum, ranging from increased bowel frequency to fecal incontinence or evacuatory dysfunction, has been termed *anterior resection syndrome*.

Resection of the primary formerly was recommended for patients presenting with synchronous CRC and unresectable metastases, regardless of whether the primary caused symptoms. This practice pattern obviously had the potential to delay systemic treatment in patients who were markedly more likely to die from their metastases before suffering significant complications from the intact large bowel tumor. Recent data suggest that stage IV patients with an asymptomatic primary tumor can safely begin systemic therapy without undergoing surgery, with only a small chance of developing serious complications requiring urgent operative interaction. Patients with rectal primaries may be at slightly higher risk for developing complications than those with tumors originating in the proximal large bowel.

Obstructing tumors that can be fully removed should be resected, with bowel anastomosis usually being acceptable in this setting. Proximal diversion alone, especially in the setting of very locally advanced unresectable cancer, may be necessary; if the primary tumor responds to the point where it can later be removed, resection followed by ostomy closure is reasonable. Endoscopic stenting may be useful to relieve acute obstruction. Perforated bowel is usually resected, with the choice of anastomosis, with or without diversion, depending on a number of factors, including degree of fecal contamination and general health of the patient.

Radiation Therapy

Radiation therapy may be used as curative or palliative treatment of large bowel cancers. In general, it is employed much more commonly in treating rectal versus colonic primaries. Single-institution trials have shown that irradiation improves local control following resection of high-risk proximal large bowel (colonic) cancers, but these findings were not confirmed in a randomized intergroup trial that closed early owing to slow accrual. Current recommendations for adjuvant radiation to the tumor bed following colon cancer resection include positive margins and localized perforation. Some authorities also advocate its use in colon cancers at particularly high risk of local recurrence (T4, T3N1-2 tumors in the ascending or descending colon), but that recommendation is not universally accepted. Irradiation may still play a role in treating colon cancer metastases to bone, brain, liver, and lung, as well as in cases of bleeding, obstruction, and locally advanced unresectable disease.

A major use for radiation in the definitive treatment of large bowel adenocarcinoma involves perioperative therapy for resectable rectal cancer. It is also commonly employed with chemotherapy for unresectable locally advanced invasive tumors, which occasionally may downsize and be surgically removed after therapy. As with colon primaries, irradiation may be used to palliate bleeding, obstruction, or selected metastases from rectal cancers.

Systemic and Combination Therapies

The backbone of CRC treatment in both the adjuvant and metastatic settings is a fluorinated pyrimidine. The most commonly used drug is 5-fluorouracil (5-FU), although oral prodrugs are increasingly being used. 5-FU targets the enzyme thymidylate synthase, inhibiting DNA synthesis and/or repair. It also may be incorporated into RNA, interfering with further processing. Although not particularly effective as a single agent (see later), 5-FU's efficacy can be enhanced by changing its means of administration (prolonging infusion) and by administering it with a variety of biochemical modulators, most commonly leucovorin. Other chemotherapeutic agents commonly used in treating advanced CRC include irinotecan, a topoisomerase I inhibitor, and oxaliplatin, a later-generation platin that forms bulky DNA adducts that inhibit replication. Recent effective biologics[18] include agents targeting vascular endothelial growth factor (bevacizumab) or circulating VEGF (aflibercept), the epidermal growth factor receptor (cetuximab, panitumumab), or a combination of the VEGF and various tyrosine kinase receptors (regorafenib).

Patients with resected stage I colon cancers have a high cure rate, and this cannot easily be improved on with systemic therapy. Stage II patients have a higher chance of relapse (event-free survival ≈ 76% at 3 years), and systemic therapy with 5-FU and leucovorin improved that figure by about 3% for an unselected group of node-negative patients. Patients harboring highly microsatellite-unstable tumors have a better prognosis in general but may actually have worse outcomes with 5-FU treatment, although that is controversial. Treatment of stage II patients remains controversial in general: some experts suggest that the proportional benefit of systemic therapy is as great as it is in stage III disease, while others point out the low absolute magnitude of benefit and do not advocate its use. Risk stratification using molecular markers has been attempted but has not been demonstrated to have predictive capabilities, with the exception of microsatellite instability and its described resistance to fluoropyrimidines. Some clinical categories of stage II disease are believed to be at particularly high risk for recurrence (e.g., obstruction). These patients usually receive postoperative chemotherapy, often with regimens commonly prescribed for patients with stage III cancer. Radiation has been tested in patients thought to be at higher-than-average risk of local relapse (T4 tumors), but its use is not standard. Other drugs useful in metastatic disease and resected node-positive patients (specifically oxaliplatin) are not routinely recommended nor used in those with stage II cancers.

Five-year disease-free survival for patients with stage III colon cancer ranges from 45 to 85%, depending on substage. Barring significant comorbidities or other confounding factors, all patients with node-positive disease receive adjuvant systemic therapy. Combinations of 5-FU and oxaliplatin (usually FOLFOX [fluorouracil, leucovorin, oxaliplatin]) clearly improve long-term survival rates[19] and represent standard care. Regimens containing irinotecan and biologics (bevacizumab, cetuximab) are highly effective in the treatment of advanced disease (see later), but oddly they do not clearly benefit patients when they are given in the postoperative setting. Patients who are not candidates for combination chemotherapy may be offered capecitabine, an oral prodrug activated to 5-FU in sequential enzymatic steps. Capecitabine has also been combined effectively and relatively safely with oxaliplatin for adjuvant use. An important outstanding question regarding adjuvant chemotherapy is whether a shorter duration (3 months vs. the standard 6) might be equally effective, as suggested in one small randomized trial.

Rectal Adenocarcinoma

Therapeutic considerations are slightly different for patients with primary rectal adenocarcinomas, owing to the difficulty of achieving negative circumferential (radial) margins. Specifically, the risk of local recurrence is much more significant. Adjuvant chemotherapy for rectal cancer is still controversial.[20] In general, rectal cancer patients undergoing standard resection for stage I tumors do not receive additional treatment. However, higher-risk patients (T2 disease, T1 with poorly differentiated histology, perineural or lymphovascular invasion, or close margins) treated with local excision should receive postoperative pelvic irradiation with or without 5-FU chemotherapy, or they should return to the operating room for total mesorectal excision. Irradiation is standard for those with stage II and III rectal adenocarcinomas to decrease local relapse rates, increase the chance of sphincter preservation (when used in selected preoperative settings for low-lying cancers), and possibly improve survival. The major considerations are timing (pre- or postoperative use), course (short or long), and whether to combine it with fluoropyrimidine-based chemotherapy. Short-course (5-day) preoperative irradiation without chemotherapy may be considered and used if tumor downsizing is not necessary. When short-course radiation is used, patients still require postoperative systemic therapy with either a fluoropyrimidine alone (stage II) or a fluoropyrimidine-oxaliplatin combination regimen (node-positive disease). Long-course irradiation (≈5.5 weeks) is particularly important when tumor response is necessary to make surgery easier or more feasible. It is usually combined with continuous-infusion 5-FU or capecitabine, and it can be given pre- or postoperatively (if the patient did not receive preoperative short-course radiation). Including oxaliplatin preoperatively does not improve results and is not recommended independent of a clinical trial, owing to its higher toxicity profile. Oxaliplatin may be used postoperatively if the pathology specimen demonstrates nodal involvement. With long-course irradiation, preoperative (compared with postoperative) treatment is less toxic and may offer improved local control. A7 However, it requires accurate preoperative staging (to avoid treating patients who might have stage I disease). Highly selected rectal cancer patients thought to be at low risk of local recurrence (T3N0 or T1-2N1) may receive total mesorectal excision plus best systemic therapy without irradiation, usually postoperatively.

Metastatic Colorectal Cancer

Metastatic disease is treated identically, regardless of the site of origin (colon vs. rectum). Patients with incurable metastatic CRC have a median survival of approximately 6 months with best supportive care alone; however, incremental gains made through the adoption of new systemic therapies have extended that time to nearly 2 years or more. For example, treatment with single-agent fluoropyrimidines leads to median survival in the 10- to 13-month range; adding one more effective chemotherapy drug (either irinotecan or oxaliplatin) affords survival of about 15 to 20 months, and adding both drugs to 5-FU has been reported to extend life to 23 months. Interestingly, long-term results seem to be similar regardless of which drug (oxaliplatin or irinotecan) is added to 5-FU first (although the toxicity pattern varies, depending on which drug is given), or even regardless of whether 5-FU is used first and combination chemotherapy is used subsequently, as long as patients are eventually exposed to all active agents.

Additional improvements have arisen through the development of drugs that are more convenient and/or less toxic than standard agents, although they may not be more effective. Capecitabine, an oral prodrug activated to 5-FU in three sequential enzymatic steps, can be substituted for that agent alone and in combination with oxaliplatin (although patients still need intravenous access for the latter drug).

Recent breakthroughs have mostly been related to use of biologic agents (Chapter 36). Drugs used successfully to date include several monoclonal antibodies and one oral tyrosine kinase inhibitor. Bevacizumab is a humanized monoclonal antibody directed against vascular endothelial growth factor, an important mediator of angiogenesis. Bevacizumab has little single-agent activity against CRC, but it improves the interval without progression when added to irinotecan- or oxaliplatin-containing chemotherapy. Bevacizumab with FOLFOX or FOLFIRI (fluorouracil, leucovorin, irinotecan) now represents first-line treatment for patients with advanced large bowel cancer in the United States,[A8] and many oncologists continue its use along with second-line fluoropyrimidine-based chemotherapy. Aflibercept, or VEGF trap, is a fusion protein with VEGF-binding portions from VEGFR and the Fc portion of IgG1. It prevents VEGF-A and B from binding to receptors. A second-line trial after oxaliplatin failure showed aflibercept with irinotecan- and fluoropyrimidine-based chemotherapy (FOLFIRI), improves survival over chemotherapy with placebo. It is unknown whether it is better to continue bevacizumab versus switching to aflibercept in the setting of second-line therapy.

The epidermal growth factor receptor (EGFR) is another important target in advanced CRC. Cetuximab and panitumumab are monoclonal antibodies (chimeric and human, respectively) directed against the EGFR. They have single-agent activity against CRCs, and both may be combined with irinotecan-based chemotherapy to improve progression-free survival. Panitumumab also improves progression-free survival front-line when combined with oxaliplatin-containing chemotherapy. Although both agents appear effective in front-line or later use, efficacy is restricted to patients whose tumors harbor wild-type *KRAS*.

Regorafenib is an oral inhibitor of angiogenic (VEGFR-1, -2, -3, and TIE-2), stromal (PDGFR-B, FGFR), and oncogenic (KIT, RET, BRAF) tyrosine kinases. It has activity in advanced CRC, improving progression-free and overall survival after failure of standard therapies.[A9]

Locally Directed Treatment of Metastatic Disease

Complete resection of hepatic or pulmonary metastases may result in long-term survival and is the standard of care for selected patients with CRC. The majority of data exist for hepatic metastasectomy. Actuarial 5-year survival rates have been in the 25 to 60% range. However, relapse after 5 years still occurs, suggesting that this percentage does not reflect the number actually *cured* with surgery. That figure, calculated from 10-year survival rates, is probably between 17 and 25%, which still compares quite favorably with the survival rate for patients with CRC metastatic to the liver who do not undergo surgery. The role of preoperative systemic therapy in potentially resectable patients remains controversial; if used, a fluoropyrimidine with either oxaliplatin or irinotecan +/− panitumumab (for wild-type *KRAS*) or irinotecan-based chemotherapy +/− cetuximab (for wild-type *KRAS*), or triple chemotherapy with a fluoropyrimidine, oxaliplatin, and irinotecan may be employed. In those undergoing metastasectomy, many experts advocate 6 months of postoperative fluoropyrimidine-based chemotherapy, often with oxaliplatin. Importantly, bevacizumab can impair wound healing, and most experts avoid its use in the immediate perioperative period.

Small liver metastases that are not resectable because of anatomic location or in a frail patient unable to undergo hepatic resection may be treated with radio frequency ablation, which uses alternating electric current to generate heat, destroying malignant cells through protein coagulation. Although it has never been directly compared with resection in a randomized trial, radio frequency ablation appears to offer inferior local control of disease. Some advocate the placement of a hepatic artery pump to infuse fluoropyrimidine-based chemotherapy to treat unresectable liver-predominant metastases. Other techniques useful in noncolorectal liver-based tumors (e.g., hepatocellular carcinoma), such as chemoembolization, have no proven role for large bowel liver metastases.

Surveillance

Surveillance should be undertaken in patients fit enough to undergo metastasectomy or systemic therapy for recurrent CRC. The American Society of Clinical Oncology recommends annual CT of the chest and abdomen for 3 years following resection of high-risk primary tumors, with pelvic CT added in cases of rectal origin. Colonoscopy should also be done at 3 years and then every 5 years, with flexible proctosigmoidoscopy offered to rectal cancer patients who have not received irradiation. Physical examinations should be performed every 3 to 6 months for 3 years, then biannually for at least 2 more years. CEA levels should be checked every 3 months for at least 3 years, although the benefits for improving outcome are uncertain.[A10]

PROGNOSIS

The prognosis for patients with CRC depends primarily on stage. Five-year survival for patients with proximal (colonic) adenocarcinomas ranges from a low of 6 to 8% for those with metastatic disease to approximately 95% for those with stage I resected tumors. Corresponding rates for rectal cancers are similar to slightly inferior overall, ranging from 4 to 72%. Besides TNM stage, additional factors that are prognostic for poorer outcomes in patients undergoing potentially curative resection include signet ring histologic subtype (see preceding discussion under Pathobiology), lymphovascular and perineural invasion, absence of host lymphoid response, presence of clinical obstruction preoperatively, high preoperative serum levels of the CEA tumor marker, positive margins, high tumor grade, and microsatellite-stable disease. Differing from many solid tumors originating outside the GI tract, CRCs do not have different prognoses based on size.

Genetic factors are important as well, even in the metastatic setting. Patients with tumors harboring *BRAF* mutations appear to have a worse outcome. *KRAS* mutations were formerly thought to be prognostic but now appear to be only predictive for lack of benefit from certain types of systemic therapy.

Colorectal cancer remains a significant problem despite the fact that most cases can be prevented. Large gains have been made in terms of overall survival, but the vast majority of patients with advanced disease still succumb to their malignancy. Minimal tailoring can currently be offered to patients (e.g., selecting a chemotherapeutic agent based on toxicity or not using an anti-EGFR antibody in those with *KRAS*-mutated tumors); the dream of truly individualized therapy remains elusive but is under active study.

Grade A References

A1. Joensuu H, Eriksson M, Hall KS, et al. One versus three years of adjuvant imatinib for operable gastrointestinal stromal tumor: a randomized trial. *JAMA*. 2012;307:1265-1272.

A2. Burn J, Gerdes AM, Macrae F, et al. Long-term effect of aspirin on cancer risk in carriers of hereditary colorectal cancer: an analysis from the CAPP2 randomised controlled trial. *Lancet*. 2011; 378:2081-2087.

A3. Quintero E, Castells A, Bujanda L, et al. Colonoscopy versus fecal immunochemical testing in colorectal-cancer screening. *N Engl J Med*. 2012;366:697-706.

A4. Atkin WS, Edwards R, Kralj-Hans I, et al. Once-only flexible sigmoidoscopy screening in prevention of colorectal cancer: a multicentre randomised controlled trial. *Lancet*. 2010;375:1624-1633.

A5. Schoen RE, Pinsky PF, Weissfeld JL, et al. Colorectal-cancer incidence and mortality with screening flexible sigmoidoscopy. *N Engl J Med*. 2012;366:2345-2357.

A6. Holme O, Loberg M, Kalager M, et al. Effect of flexible sigmoidoscopy screening on colorectal cancer incidence and mortality: a randomized clinical trial. *JAMA*. 2014;312:606-615.

A7. Sauer R, Liersch T, Merkel S, et al. Preoperative versus postoperative chemoradiotherapy for rectal cancer: results of the German CAO/ARO/AIO-94 randomized phase III trial after a median follow-up of 11 years. *J Clin Oncol*. 2012;30:1921-1933.

A8. Grothey A, Van Cutsem E, Sobrero A, et al. Regorafenib monotherapy for previously treated metastatic colorectal cancer (CORRECT): an international multicenter, randomized, placebo-controlled, phase 3 trial. *Lancet*. 2013;381:303-312.

A9. Loupakis F, Cremolini C, Masi G, et al. Initial therapy with FOLFOXIRI and bevacizumab for metastatic colorectal cancer. *N Engl J Med*. 2014;371:1609-1618.

A10. Primrose JN, Perera R, Gray A, et al. Effect of 3 to 5 years of scheduled CEA and CT follow-up to detect recurrence of colorectal cancer: the FACS randomized clinical trial. *JAMA*. 2014;311: 263-270.

GENERAL REFERENCES

For the General References and other additional features, please visit Expert Consult at https://expertconsult.inkling.com.

194

PANCREATIC CANCER

DANIEL LAHERU

DEFINITION

Pancreatic cancer usually refers to ductal adenocarcinomas of the pancreas, because more than 90% of pancreatic tumors arise from the ductal epithelium. Other major tumors of the pancreas include endocrine malignancies (Chapter 195), carcinoid tumors (Chapter 232), lymphomas (Chapter 185), and a variety of rare sarcomas.

EPIDEMIOLOGY

Pancreatic ductal adenocarcinoma (PDAC) has one of the highest incidence-to-mortality ratios of any disease. Although it represents the tenth leading cause of cancer in the United States, it is the fourth leading cause of cancer-related deaths,[1] because the vast majority of patients will die from their disease. Annually, approximately 40,000 individuals will die in the United States from PDAC or its complications. The incidence of pancreatic cancer is slowly increasing based on the changing demographics of the U.S. population. The risk of developing PDAC increases with age, with a mean age at onset of 71 years; the risk in men and women is equivalent. The average lifetime risk for developing PDAC is about 1 in 78 for both men and women. Globally, 70% of all pancreatic cancer cases occur in people living in advanced economies, with over 270,000 deaths per year worldwide. Some PDACs occur in association with other cancers or diseases, but most do not occur in association with a defined syndrome. The overwhelming majority of PDAC cases are sporadic—that is, occurring without a history of the disease in first-degree relatives. Smoking tobacco, as well as passive exposure to tobacco smoke in the environment, contributes significantly to the development of PDAC. Occupational hazards that have been associated with an enhanced risk of developing PDAC include exposure to chlorinated hydrocarbon solvents and heavy metals.

Approximately 10% of PDACs occur in families with a history of PDAC; in these patients, the risk of developing PDAC is increased seven-fold compared with the general population. Premalignant cystic lesions of the pancreas also occur in pancreatic cancer families. In addition to the recent discovery of the *PALB2* gene in 3% of these families, mutations in *ATM* or *BRCA2*, critical partners in the DNA damage repair pathway, as well as *p16*, have also been discovered.

Chronic pancreatic inflammation from alcohol misuse or genetic anomalies significantly enhances the risk of being diagnosed with PDAC. Although the association between chronic pancreatitis and the development of PDAC has been well known for decades, only recently have studies clarified how pro-inflammatory cytokines contribute to the progression from premalignant lesion to advanced tumor. In addition to chronic pancreatitis, the role of diabetes mellitus and obesity in the development of PDAC has been emphasized. Long-standing type 1 and type 2 diabetes mellitus may represent increased risk of PDAC, but the cause-and-effect relationship between pancreatic cancer and diabetes is complex. Recently, epidemiologic studies have focused on the development of PDAC in patients with type 3c diabetes (diabetes related to pancreatic disease, or pancreatogenic diabetes), a major subset of diabetes characterized by a severe deficiency of all glucoregulatory hormones (Chapter 229). Patients with type 3c diabetes appear to have the highest associated risk of developing PDAC, especially in the setting of coexisting chronic pancreatitis. Type 3c diabetes is also a consequence of PDAC in approximately 30% of patients. The increase in obesity in the U.S. population and the concomitant increase in associated diabetes mellitus are strongly associated with an enhanced lifetime risk of developing PDAC.

PATHOBIOLOGY

Understanding the molecular characteristics of cancers of the exocrine pancreas is critical for the development of targeted therapies. Pancreatic cancer is caused by inherited (germline) and acquired (somatic) mutations in cancer-causing genes. Several oncogenes and tumor suppressor genes have been demonstrated to be involved in the development of pancreatic cancer, both by contributing to the growth of the tumor itself as well as to the surrounding microenvironment. Oncogenes, typically inactive in normal cells, cause uncontrolled cell proliferation by inhibiting apoptosis and activating the cell cycle when mutations render them constitutively active. The *KRAS* oncogene, located on chromosome 12, is the most frequently mutated oncogene in pancreatic cancer in (>90% of tumors). It encodes a membrane-bound protein that has GTP-ase activity and is involved in signal transduction.[2] When activated by mutation, typically a point mutation in codon 12, the functions of *KRAS* are independent of growth factor control, leading to chronic activation of its downstream signaling partners, *PI3K*, *MAPK*, and *RAF*, causing inhibition of apoptosis and activation of the cell cycle, migration, angiogenesis, cytoskeletal remodeling, and unchecked proliferation. Tumor suppressor genes, when functioning normally, act in the opposite manner by enhancing apoptosis and inhibiting cell proliferation. The tumor suppressor *CDKN2A/TP16*, a cell cycle control gene, is commonly inactivated in pancreatic cancer, with 80 to 95% loss of activity leading to increased cell cycle progression. *TP53* is activated by DNA damage to stop cell cycle progression and repair damaged DNA or initiate apoptosis. Mutations in this tumor suppressor gene are commonly found in 50 to 75% of pancreatic tumors. Inactivation of *SMAD4* (DPC4), involved in regulating cell cycle progression through the transforming growth factor (TGF)-β pathway, is observed in over 50% of pancreatic cancers and is associated with worse prognosis and the development of metastases. Inactivation of *RB1* (in < 10% of pancreatic cancers) and *STK11* (responsible for Peutz-Jeghers syndrome) is also observed.

There are several major signaling pathways involved in pancreatic tumorigenesis. Hedgehog (Hh) signaling, critical in embryogenesis, regulates the cell cycle and apoptosis, aids in the formation of tumor stroma, and is often upregulated and abnormal in pancreatic cancers. The NOTCH pathway, also important in normal embryogenesis to prevent terminal differentiation of cells until appropriate, can be abnormally activated in pancreatic cancer, allowing cells to remain in an undifferentiated state that contributes to tumor growth. When the Wnt pathway is activated, β-catenin is stabilized and migrates into the nucleus, where it activates its target genes. The epidermal growth factor receptor (EGFR), TGF-β, and JAK/STAT pathways have also been found to be abnormal in pancreatic cancer cells, leading to the promotion of cell growth, proliferation, differentiation, and cell survival. Epigenetic modification, the process by which gene expression is altered by mechanisms other than changes in actual DNA sequence, also has a role in pancreatic cancer tumorigenesis. Telomere shortening and overexpression of microRNAs lead to chromosomal instability and dysregulation of gene expression, respectively, and are also observed.

In addition to cancer cells themselves, the tumor microenvironment is composed of stromal cells, inflammatory cells, and endothelial cells that all play a particularly important role in pancreatic cancer growth. Cancer cells secrete growth factors, including insulin-like growth factor (IGF)-1, fibroblast growth factor (FGF), TGF-β, vascular endothelial growth factor (VEGF), and platelet-derived growth factor (PDGF), that stimulate pancreatic stellate cells (also called myofibroblasts) to secrete excess amounts of extracellular matrix. The matrix and its stromal cells, in turn, secrete cytokines and growth factors that promote cancer cell growth, invasion, and dissemination and protect pancreatic cancer cells from apoptosis, as well as generating a desmoplastic reaction that interferes with the delivery of chemotherapy to the tumor site.[3] The local presence of TGF-β also leads to decreased helper T-cell activity, which suppresses the body's immune reaction against pancreatic cancer cells.

Precursor Lesions

A major advance in understanding the development of pancreatic cancer has been the appreciation that the majority of pancreatic adenocarcinomas progress sequentially from histologically normal ductal epithelium to low-grade pancreatic intraepithelial neoplasia (PanIN), to high-grade PanIN, to invasive carcinoma. This process is associated with the accumulation of specific gene alterations (Fig. 194-1).

CLINICAL MANIFESTATIONS

Symptoms of early PDAC are often subtle and include nonspecific gastrointestinal complaints (nausea, vague abdominal pain), fatigue, and weight loss of undetermined etiology.[4] Epigastric pain and obstructive jaundice often prompt the initial diagnostic work-up of the biliary tree, but are frequently late symptoms that are associated with advanced local or regionally disseminated disease. Because approximately 75% of pancreatic carcinomas are located in the head of the pancreas, it is not unexpected that clinical presentations are often related to compression or invasion of the biliary tree or pancreatic ducts. Deep or superficial venous thrombosis (Trousseau syndrome) is not infrequent, either early or late in the presentation of PDAC (Chapter 176). Observation of a palpably distended gallbladder (from obstruction of the distal common bile duct), or Courvoisier's sign, is uncommon.

The laboratory abnormalities that accompany PDAC at presentation include anemia and elevations of serum bilirubin, alkaline phosphatase, and aminotransferases. A majority of patients eventually develop signs of obstructive jaundice as well as hyperglycemia, reflective of associated diabetes mellitus. Unfortunately, pre-neoplastic cystic lesions of the pancreas often remain asymptomatic until discovered following acute symptoms (due to ductal obstruction) that precipitate an abdominal computed tomography (CT) scan. Early PanIN lesions are asymptomatic.

DIAGNOSIS

Differential Diagnosis

The differential diagnosis of PDAC includes conditions that can present as a solid pancreatic mass, including acute (or an exacerbation of chronic) pancreatitis, ampullary or distal cholangiocarcinomas with associated biliary obstruction and jaundice, and non-neoplastic cystic pancreatic neoplasms.

Cystic neoplasms of the pancreas are frequent, detectable in 2% of abdominal magnetic resonance imaging (MRI) examinations. Whereas serous cystadenomas are benign abnormalities that do not connect to pancreatic ducts and warrant surgery only if symptomatic, mucinous cystadenomas (MCN) are precursors of PDAC that often occur in the tail of the pancreas, more frequently in women in their 40s; they are overtly malignant in 15% of patients and require surgical resection. Intraductal papillary mucinous neoplasms (IPMN) of the pancreas occur in the head of the organ, are often polycystic, and contain malignant elements in 40% of patients; all patients with this lesion require surgery.

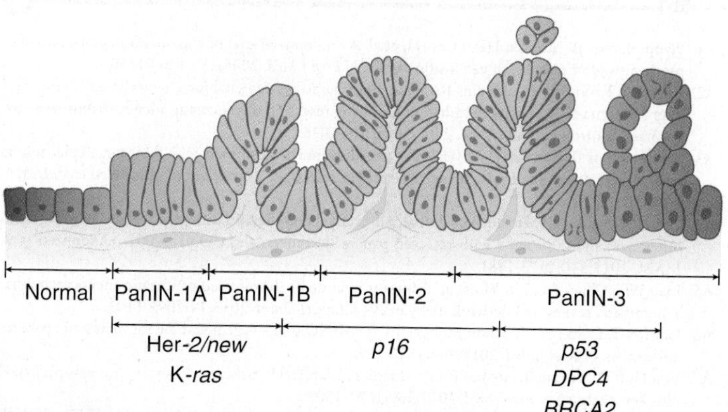

FIGURE 194-1. Genetic progression model of pancreatic adenocarcinoma. Molecular changes in the development of pancreatic ductal adenocarcinoma begin with early changes that include telomere shortening and development of mutations in *KRAS*; these are followed by loss of p16 function and expression of cyclin D1. Late changes include expression of p53 and loss of SMAD4/DPC4. PanIN = pancreatic intraepithelial neoplasia.

Imaging

CT scan with dynamic contrast and thin cuts through the pancreas is the imaging procedure of choice when PDAC is suspected. CT scans can provide information regarding the presence of metastatic disease, vascular invasion, and potential for resection. Endoscopic ultrasound (EUS) may provide additional information useful for preoperative assessment, including fine-needle aspiration biopsy under endoscopic guidance. It is important to point out that the typical desmoplastic reaction that can encase PDACs increases the possibility of false-negative biopsy findings. Patients with locally advanced or metastatic disease should have their diagnosis confirmed pathologically by fine-needle biopsy of the primary site or of a metastasis.

Biomarkers and Screening

A recent preliminary study identified two diagnostic panels based on microRNA expression in whole blood, with the potential to distinguish patients with pancreatic cancer from healthy controls.[5] However, so far, no serum- or tumor-based biomarkers or biomarker panels have been established that are both sensitive and specific enough for accurate early detection in clinical practice. CA19.9 is the most commonly used tumor biomarker for monitoring therapeutic progress in PDAC, but the lack of specificity of the assay is a concern, and CA19.9 therefore cannot be used for early detection. EUS is useful for the evaluation of cystic lesions and permits sampling of cystic fluid for genetic markers associated with the development of PDAC in cancer-prone families, as well as for cytologic studies.

TREATMENT

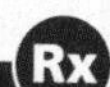

Resectable Pancreatic Cancer

Surgery offers the only chance to cure pancreatic cancer. Tumors are considered resectable if a clear fat plane is present around the celiac and superior mesenteric arteries, and if the mesenteric and portal veins are patent. Unfortunately, tumor will recur in the majority of patients who undergo resection. Adjuvant therapy is indicated to decrease the risk and delay the timing of locoregional and metastatic recurrence. It is typically started 1 to 2 months after surgery to allow the patient to recover from the complications associated with the underlying cancer as well as from surgery itself. Although no regimen has been proven substantially more effective than others, 6 months of adjuvant therapy with 5-fluorouracil (5-FU) or gemcitabine-based chemotherapy is an appropriate standard (Table 194-1). A meta-analysis has shown that chemotherapy with 5-FU or gemcitabine is the optimum adjuvant treatment for pancreatic adenocarcinoma and reduces mortality after surgery by about a third. Chemoradiation plus chemotherapy is less effective in prolonging survival and is more toxic than chemotherapy.[A5]

TABLE 194-1 SELECTED ADJUVANT STUDIES

STUDY	TREATMENT	1-YEAR SURVIVAL (%)	2-YEAR SURVIVAL (%)	5-YEAR SURVIVAL (%)	DISEASE-FREE SURVIVAL (MO)	MEDIAN SURVIVAL (MO)
ESPAC-1 (2004)[A1] N = 289	2 × 2 design: Observation v. Chemorad v. Chemo v. Chemorad plus chemo			11 v. 7 v. 29 v. 13	Chemorad, 10.7 v. no chemorad, 15.2 Chemo, 15.3 v. no chemo, 9.4	16.9 v. 13.9 v. 21.6 v. 19.9
RTOG-9704 (2008)[A2] N = 451	Gem/XRT v. 5-FU/XRT	69 v. 65	35 v. 39	20 v. 20	NR	20.5 v. 16.9
ESPAC-3 (2010)[A3] N = 1088	Gem v. 5-FU	70 v. 70	40 v. 40	NR	14.3 v. 14.1	23.6 v. 23
Johns Hopkins and Mayo Clinic Retrospective (2010)[6] N = 1272	Observation v. chemorad	58. v. 80	34.6 v. 44.7	16.1 v. 22.3		15.5 v. 21.1 ($P < .001$)
ACOSOG (2011)[7] N = 89	IFN-cisplatin-5-FU plus XRT	80	60	NR	14.1	25.4
CONKO-1 (2013)[A4] N = 354	Observe v. gem	72 v. 72	42 v. 47	11 v. 22	6.7 v. 13.4 ($P < .001$)	10.4 v. 21.7 ($P = .06$)

5-FU = 5-flourouracil; chemo = chemotherapy; chemorad = chemoradiation therapy; gem = gemcitabine; IFN = interferon; NR = not reported; XRT = radiation therapy.

TABLE 194-2 SELECTED METASTATIC PANCREATIC CANCER STUDIES

STUDY	CHEMOTHERAPY	RESPONSE RATE (% PARTIAL RESPONSE)	MEDIAN SURVIVAL (MO)	1-YEAR SURVIVAL (%)
Burris (1997)[A8] N = 126	5-FU v. gem	NR	4.4 v. 5.6 (P = .0025)	2 v. 18
Cunningham (2009)[A9] N = 533	Gem ± capecitabine	14 v. 7 (P = .008)	7.4 v. 6 (P < .05)	26 v. 19
Conroy (2011)[A6] N = 343	Gem v. FOLFIRINOX	9 v. 32	6.8 v. 11.1 (P < .0001)	17 v. 36
Van Hoff (2013)[A7] N = 861	Gem ± nab-paclitaxel	23 % v. 7%	8.5 v. 6.7 (P < .001)	35 v. 22 (P < .001)

5-FU = 5-fluorocil; FOLFIRINOX = combination chemotherapy with oxaliplatin, irinotecan, fluorouracil, and leucovorin; gem = gemcitabine; NR = rot reported.

Neoadjuvant (presurgical) therapy remains an option in the treatment of pancreatic cancer. It has the potential to downstage patients of borderline resectability who achieve a partial response with therapy, allowing them to undergo surgery with a higher likelihood of complete resection. In fact, 15 to 40% of patients who initially present with borderline or unresectable tumors may eventually be deemed appropriate to undergo surgery. In addition, neoadjuvant therapy spares some patients the risks and stress of a complex surgical procedure, because rapidly developing metastatic disease may be detected by routine restaging following the completion of neoadjuvant treatment. Unfortunately, chemotherapy-resistant cancer can be demonstrated in 15 to 35% of patients initially considered for surgery in this setting. The use of neoadjuvant treatment also guarantees that almost all patients will receive some form of chemotherapy and/or chemoradiation because they do not have any postoperative complications from which to recover. Studies show that 73 to 100% of patients are able to complete the majority of their neoadjuvant regimens. The chemoradiation component of neoadjuvant therapy also decreases local recurrence rates in patients who undergo surgery.

However, surgery is required for cure, and neoadjuvant therapy does delay potentially curable surgery. Although the same percentage of patients ultimately undergo surgery, there are no randomized trials favoring neoadjuvant over adjuvant treatment. Therefore, at this time neoadjuvant therapy is usually reserved for borderline resectable patients, whereas resectable patients are taken to surgery immediately, with adjuvant therapy administered following recovery. Patients treated with either adjuvant or neoadjuvant therapy have similar survival rates when resection can be completed successfully. Decisions regarding initial treatment should, if possible, be made in a multidisciplinary manner to achieve the most timely and coordinated therapy.

Metastatic Disease

For many years, 5-FU was the standard of care to treat advanced PDAC. In 1997, a phase III trial demonstrated a survival benefit for gemcitabine over bolus 5-FU, with a median survival of 5.65 months compared to 4.41 months, and 1-year survival of 18% versus 2%, favoring treatment with gemcitabine. Gemcitabine also had a superior clinical benefit response, described as improvement in pain, performance status, or weight in 24% of patients versus 5% in the 5-FU group; it is therefore appropriate treatment for patients with moderate performance status.

Gemcitabine has also been combined with targeted therapies; however, addition of the EGFR inhibitor erlotinib has been the only molecularly targeted agent shown to improve overall survival, albeit modestly. Newer combination regimens, both with improved efficacy based on phase III clinical trials for metastatic PDAC patients, include FOLFIRINOX (oxaliplatin, irinotecan, fluorouracil, and leucovorin)[A6] and the nab-paclitaxel and gemcitabine doublet[A7] (Table 194-2).

PROGNOSIS AND SUPPORTIVE CARE

The overall 5-year survival for all patients with pancreatic cancer is less than 5%. This is in part because there is no appropriate screening test for the general population, and presenting symptoms are vague. Once patients are diagnosed, only 15 to 20% present with resectable, and thus potentially curable, disease. In these patients, the somatostatin analogue pasireotide (900 mg subcutaneously twice daily for 7 days beginning in the morning of surgery) can reduce the risk of fistula leak with abscess by 50%.[A10] However, even in patients with early-stage disease, median survival is 20 to 24 months, with a 5-year survival of only 15 to 20% because the majority will eventually recur despite surgery and adjuvant or neoadjuvant therapy. Patients with locally advanced (≈25 to 30% at presentation) and metastatic disease (≈50 to 60% at presentation) have median survivals of 8 to 14 months and 4 to 6 months, respectively. Because many patients suffer from biliary obstruction, diarrhea, pain, and malnutrition, palliative care can provide great benefit. Surgery can also play an important palliative role; patients found to be unresectable may be improved symptomatically by a biliary or gastric bypass procedure, depending on the site of obstruction. Placement of both biliary and duodenal stents in the absence of a surgical approach may also improve pruritus, pain, or other complications of biliary tract obstruction. Palliative care for patients with PDAC necessitates scrupulous attention to pain management that often requires a multidisciplinary approach, as well as maintenance of hydration and adequate nutritional status.

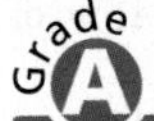

Grade A References

A1. Neoptolemos JP, Stocken DD, Friess H, et al. A randomized trial of chemoradiotherapy and chemotherapy after resetion of pancreatic cancer. *N Engl J Med*. 2004;350:1200-1210.
A2. Regine WF, Winter KA, Abrams RA, et al. Fluorouracil vs gemcitabine chemotherapy before and after fluorouracil-based chemoradiation following resection of pancreatic adenocarcinoma: a randomized controlled trial. *JAMA*. 2008;299:1019-1026.
A3. Neoptolemos JP, Stocken DD, Bassi C, et al. Adjuvant chemotherapy with fluorouracil plus folinic acid vs. gemcitabine following pancreatic cancer resection: a randomized controlled trial. *JAMA*. 2010;304:1073-1081.
A4. Oettle H, Neuhaus P, Hochhaus JT, et al. Adjuvant chemotherapy with gemcitabine and long-term outcomes among patients with resected pancreatic cancer: the CONKO-001 randomized trial. *JAMA*. 2013;310:1473-1481.
A5. Liao WC, Chien KL, Lin YL, et al. Adjuvant treatments for resected pancreatic adenocarcinoma: a systematic review and network meta-analysis. *Lancet Oncol*. 2013;14:1095-1103.
A6. Conroy T, Desseigne F, Ychou M, et al. FOLFIRINOX versus gemcitabine for metastatic pancreatic cancer. *N Engl J Med*. 2011;364:1817-1825.
A7. Von Hoff DD, Ervin T, Arena FP, et al. Increased survival in pancreatic cancer with nab-paclitaxel plus gemcitabine. *N Eng J Med*. 2013;369:1691-1703.
A8. Burris HA 3rd, Moore MJ, Andersen J, et al. Improvements in survival and clinical benefit with gemcitabine as first-line therapy for patients with advanced pancreas cancer: a randomized trial. *J Clin Oncol*. 1997;15:2403-2413.
A9. Cunningham D, Chau I, Stocken DD, et al. Phase III randomized comparison of gemcitabine plus capecitabine in patients with advanced pancreatic cancer. *J Clin Oncol*. 2009;27:5513-5518.
A10. Allen PJ, Gönen M, Brennan MF, et al. Pasireotide for postoperative pancreatic fistula. *N Engl J Med*. 2014;370:2014-2022.

GENERAL REFERENCES

For the General References and other additional features, please visit Expert Consult at https://expertconsult.inkling.com.

195

PANCREATIC NEUROENDOCRINE TUMORS

ROBERT T. JENSEN

DEFINITION

Pancreatic neuroendocrine tumors (pNETs) are also called islet cell tumors, but because the cell of origin of most of these tumors is unknown, the general term *pNET* is preferred. This term is also a misnomer, however, because pNETs can occur outside the pancreas. Eleven pNETs are well established (Table 195-1).[1] Other functional pNET syndromes have been rarely reported: pNETs secreting renin causing hypertension, pNETs secreting erythropoietin

TABLE 195-1 PANCREATIC NEUROENDOCRINE TUMORS

NAME OF TUMOR	NAME OF SYNDROME	MAIN SIGNS OR SYMPTOMS	LOCATION	MALIGNANCY (%)	HORMONE CAUSING SYNDROME
I. FUNCTIONAL pNET					
Gastrinoma	Zollinger-Ellison syndrome	Abdominal pain, diarrhea, esophageal symptoms	Pancreas—30% Duodenum—60% Other—10%	60-90	Gastrin
Insulinoma	Insulinoma	Hypoglycemic symptoms	Pancreas—100%	5-15	Insulin
Glucagonoma	Glucagonoma	Dermatitis, diabetes/glucose intolerance, weight loss	Pancreas—100%	60	Glucagon
VIPoma	Verner-Morrison, pancreatic cholera, WDHA	Severe watery diarrhea, hypokalemia	Pancreas—90% Other—10% (neural, adrenal, periganglionic tissue)	80	Vasoactive intestinal peptide (VIP)
Somatostatinoma	Somatostatinoma	Diabetes mellitus, cholelithiasis, diarrhea	Pancreas—56% Duodenum/jejunum—44%	60	Somatostatin
GRFoma	GRFoma	Acromegaly	Pancreas—30% Lung—54% Jejunum—7% Other—13% (adrenal, foregut, retroperitoneum)	30	Growth hormone–releasing factor (GRF)
ACTHoma	ACTHoma	Cushing's syndrome	Pancreas—4-16% of all ectopic Cushing's cases	>95	Adrenocorticotropic hormone (ACTH)
pNET causing carcinoid syndrome	pNET causing carcinoid syndrome	Diarrhea, flushing	Pancreas—<1% of all carcinoids	60-90	Serotonin, tachykinins
pNET causing hypercalcemia	pNET causing hypercalcemia	Signs/symptoms of hypercalcemia	Pancreas (rare cause of hypercalcemia)	>85	PTHrP, other unknown
CCKoma	CCKoma	Diarrhea, peptic ulcer, gallbladder disease,	Pancreas (1 case)	100	Cholecystokinin
II. NONFUNCTIONAL pNET					
Nonfunctioning PPoma	Nonfunctional PPoma	Weight loss, abdominal mass, hepatomegaly	Pancreas—100%	60-90	None: pancreatic polypeptide, chromogranin released, but no known symptoms due to hypersecretion

pNET = pancreatic endocrine tumor; PP = pancreatic polypeptide; PTHrP = parathormone-related peptide; WDHA = watery diarrhea, hypokalemia, and achlorhydria.

causing polycythemia, pNETs secreting luteinizing hormone that causes virilization, pNETs secreting insulin-like growth factor (IGF)-II or glucagon-like peptide (GLP)-1 causing hypoglycemia, and pNETs secreting enteroglucagon causing small intestinal hypertrophy1. In addition, pNETs synthesizing neurotensin, calcitonin, and ghrelin have been reported, but no distinct syndromes related to them have been generally accepted).

pNETs frequently are classified as functional or nonfunctional (see Table 195-1), depending on whether a clinical syndrome resulting from the autonomously released hormone is present).[2,3] Nonfunctional pNETs frequently release hormones and peptides (pancreatic polypeptide, neurotensin, α- and β-subunits of human chorionic gonadotropin, neuron-specific enolase, chromogranin A and breakdown products) that cause no distinct clinical syndromes.

EPIDEMIOLOGY

pNETs are uncommon, having a prevalence of less than 10 cases per 1 million population. Insulinomas, gastrinomas, and nonfunctional pNETs are the most common, with an incidence of 1 to 3 new cases per 1 million population.[4]

PATHOBIOLOGY

All pNETs share certain features. pNETs are classified as APUDomas (amine precursor uptake and decarboxylation), which share cytochemical features with carcinoid tumors, melanomas, and other endocrine tumors (pheochromocytomas, medullary thyroid cancer).[5] Except for insulinomas, these tumors are frequently malignant. All pNETs appear similar histologically, with few mitotic figures. Ultrastructurally, they have dense granules containing peptides, amines, and products of neuroendocrine differentiation (neuron-specific enolase, chromogranins, synaptophysin). The presence of chromogranin immunoreactivity in the tumor is now widely used to identify these tumors as endocrine tumors.

Molecular studies show that pNETs have a different pathogenesis than common gastrointestinal adenocarcinomas because they infrequently demonstrate mutations in common tumor suppressor genes (e.g., retinoblastoma gene, *p53*) or common oncogenes (*ras, c-Jun, c-Fos*).[6] Recent studies show important alterations are found in the *MEN1* gene, gene alterations affecting p53 and retinoblastoma activity, mutations in the DAXX-ATRX complex (important for transcription/chromatin remodeling), and the mTOR pathway.[7] Alterations in p16^{INK4a}, the *MEN1* gene, and the expression of growth factors, as well as chromosomal losses (1q, 3p, 3q, 6p, X) and gains (17p, 17q, 20q), have been associated with a worse prognosis in numerous studies.[8] A number of other factors have prognostic significance, the most important of which is the presence of liver metastases. Recently, classification systems including a TNM classification and a grading system (World Health Organization, ENETS [European Neuroendocrine Tumor Society], AJCC/UICC [American Joint Committee on Cancer/Union for International Cancer Control]) have been proposed for pNETs based on tumor size, presence of metastases, invasiveness, and proliferative indices; these classification systems have been recently shown to have prognostic value in a number of studies. Furthermore, they are important in choosing the proper treatment approach.[9]

Four autosomal dominant inherited disorders are associated with an increased occurrence of pNETs: multiple endocrine neoplasia type 1 (MEN 1; 80 to 100% develop pNETs), von Hippel-Lindau disease (VHL; 10 to 17% have pNETs), von Recklinghausen disease (neurofibromatosis [NF]-1; 12% develop duodenal somatostatinomas), and tuberous sclerosis (<1% develop pNETs).[10]

FUNCTIONAL PANCREATIC NEUROENDOCRINE TUMOR SYNDROMES

Zollinger-Ellison Syndrome (Gastrinomas)

DEFINITION AND EPIDEMIOLOGY

Zollinger-Ellison syndrome (ZES) is a clinical syndrome caused by a gastrin-releasing endocrine tumor usually located in the pancreas or duodenum and characterized by clinical symptoms and signs resulting from gastric acid hypersecretion (peptic ulcer disease, diarrhea, esophageal reflux disease).

ZES is diagnosed most frequently between the ages of 35 and 65 years and is slightly more common in men (60%).[11]

PATHOBIOLOGY

In recent surgical series, gastrinomas occur two to five times more frequently in the duodenum than in the pancreas. Duodenal gastrinomas are generally small (<1 cm), whereas pancreatic gastrinomas are generally larger. Occasionally ZES results from a gastrinoma in the splenic hilum, mesentery, stomach, or only in a lymph node or an ovary. Extrapancreatic gastrinomas producing ZES have been reported in the heart and as a result of small-cell lung cancer. As with other pNETs, malignancy can be reliably determined only by demonstrating the presence of metastatic disease, and no light microscopic or ultrastructural finding can clearly establish malignant behavior.

Gastrin stimulates parietal cells to secrete acid and also has a growth effect on cells of the gastric mucosa. Chronic hypergastrinemia thus leads to increased gastric mucosal thickness, prominent gastric folds, and increased numbers of parietal cells and gastric enterochromaffin-like cells. Patients with gastrinomas have increased basal and maximal acid outputs. *Helicobacter pylori* appears not to be important in the pathogenesis of the ulcer disease in ZES, in contrast to that of routine peptic ulcers (Chapter 139). Diarrhea is common because the large-volume gastric acid output leads to structural damage to the small intestine (inflammation, blunted villi, edema), interference with fat transport, inactivation of pancreatic lipase, and precipitation of bile acids. These same mechanisms, if prolonged, can lead to steatorrhea. If acid hypersecretion is controlled, the diarrhea will stop.

Twenty to 25% of ZES patients have MEN 1(MEN1/ZES) (Chapter 231). These patients have hyperplasia or tumors of multiple endocrine glands (parathyroid hyperplasia [>90%], pituitary tumors [60%], and pNETs [80 to 100%]). In 80 to 95% the gastrinomas are in the duodenum, frequently small (<0.5 cm), almost always multiple, and in 40 to 60% associated with lymph node metastases.

CLINICAL MANIFESTATIONS

Abdominal pain resulting from a peptic ulcer is the most common symptom (>80%). Most ulcers occur in the duodenum (>85%), but they occasionally occur in the postbulbar area, jejunum, or stomach, or in multiple locations. Initially, the pain is usually similar to that of patients with typical peptic ulcers (Chapter 139). With time, the symptoms become persistent and, in general, respond poorly to treatments aimed at eliminating *H. pylori* and to conventional doses of histamine-2 receptor antagonists, as well as to the now rarely used surgical treatments for ulcer disease. By comparison, conventional doses of proton pump inhibitors (PPIs) (e.g., omeprazole, lansoprazole, pantoprazole, esomeprazole, rabeprazole) can mask the symptoms of most patients with ZES and can also cause hypergastrinemia as seen in ZES. The widespread use of PPIs has delayed the diagnosis of ZES.[12]

Heartburn is also common (20%). Diarrhea (60 to 70%) occurs frequently and may be the first symptom (10 to 20%). In MEN1, ZES is the most common functional pNET syndrome (54%), although patients typically first develop renal stones related to hypercalcemia from hyperparathyroidism or have elevated prolactin levels resulting from pituitary tumors and only later develop ZES. However, studies show that 20 to 40% of patients with MEN1/ZES initially present with ZES symptoms.

In ZES patients, almost all the symptoms result from the effects of gastric acid hypersecretion, but late in the disease, patients can have tumor-related symptoms. Approximately one third of patients have metastatic liver disease at presentation, but less than 20% of other patients develop metastatic disease to the liver during a 10-year follow-up period.

Up to 5% of patients with ZES develop Cushing syndrome (Chapter 227) as a result of adrenocorticotropic hormone (ACTH) secretion by the gastrinoma. These patients usually have a metastatic gastrinoma in the liver, ZES without MEN 1, and a poor prognosis.

DIAGNOSIS

ZES should be suspected in any patient whose peptic ulcer disease is accompanied by diarrhea, is recurrent, does not heal with treatment, is not associated with *H. pylori* infection, is associated with a complication (bleeding, obstruction, esophageal stricture), is multiple or occurs in unusual locations, or is associated with a pancreatic tumor. ZES should also be suspected in patients with chronic secretory diarrhea (Chapter 140), peptic ulcer disease associated with large gastric folds, a family or personal history of renal stones or endocrinopathies, or the laboratory finding of hypercalcemia, hypergastrinemia, or gastric acid hypersecretion.

When suspected, the initial test is a fasting serum gastrin level, which is elevated in 99 to 100% of ZES patients. Recent studies report up to 60% of commercial gastrin assays are unreliable (over/underestimate true value), so a reliable assay should be used. Besides ZES, other causes of fasting hypergastrinemia include renal failure, *H. pylori* infections, and a physiologic response to achlorhydria or hypochlorhydria because of pernicious anemia, atrophic gastritis, or the use of PPIs. If the serum gastrin level is elevated, the fasting gastric pH should be determined. If the serum gastrin is more than 1000 pg/mL (normal, <100) and the gastric pH is less than 2.0, the patient almost certainly has ZES; approximately 40% of patients have this combination. If the gastrin is increased less than 10-fold and the gastric pH is higher than 2.0, basal acid output and a secretin test should be performed. Basal acid output is increased in patients with ZES, and more than 95% have a value greater than 15 mEq/hour if no previous gastric acid–reducing surgery has been performed. Because of their long duration of action, PPIs must be stopped for at least 1 week, if possible, to ensure that the cause of the hypergastrinemia is not the drug itself. Stopping a PPI in an undiagnosed ZES patient can lead to complications, so it needs to be done with care, and it is best to consult a group well versed in making the diagnosis.

Differential Diagnosis

A secretin test can exclude *H. pylori* infection, retained gastric antrum syndrome, antral G-cell hyperfunction or hyperplasia, chronic renal failure, and gastric outlet obstruction that may mimic ZES. Physiologically normal individuals show a less than 120 pg/mL increase in the gastrin level after intravenous secretin, whereas 94% of ZES patients with a fasting gastrin level that is elevated less than 10-fold above normal have a positive test. No false-positive results are reported except in patients with achlorhydria. In all patients with ZES, evaluation must exclude MEN 1 syndrome by searching for other endocrinopathies and assessing family history.

Imaging and Endoscopy

All patients should have imaging studies to localize the tumor. A cross-sectional imaging study such as triphasic computed tomography (CT) or magnetic resonance imaging (MRI) with contrast is usually the initial study because of their widespread availability.[13] Somatostatin receptor scintigraphy using single-photon emission CT (SPECT) after injection of indium-111–[diethylenetriamine pentaacetic acid-D-phenylalanine-1] octreotide is the most sensitive modality; it identifies 60% of primary gastrinomas and more than 90% of patients with metastatic liver disease, with a sensitivity equal to all conventional imaging studies (MRI, CT, ultrasound, angiography) combined.[14] For pancreatic gastrinomas, endoscopic ultrasound is particularly sensitive. Small duodenal gastrinomas (<1 cm) are frequently not detected by an imaging modality but can be found at surgery if routine duodenotomy is performed. Recent studies show that two new imaging techniques may be useful for small gastrinomas and other pNETs: the use of hybrid scanning with CT or MRI and somatostatin receptor scintigraphy (SRS) and the use of positron emission tomographic scanning, especially with gallium-68-labeled somatostatin analogues.

TREATMENT Rx

Medical Therapy

Patients need medical therapy directed at controlling the gastric acid hypersecretion and, if possible, surgical therapy to remove the gastrinoma. PPIs are now the drugs of choice. Because of their long duration of action, acid hypersecretion can be controlled in all patients with once- or twice-daily doses. The recommended starting dose for omeprazole is 60 mg once a day. In 30% of patients, higher doses are needed, particularly in patients with complicated disease (MEN 1), previous gastric surgery, or a history of severe esophageal reflux. With time the omeprazole dose can be reduced in most patients with uncomplicated disease to 20 to 40 mg/day. Patients must be treated indefinitely unless surgically cured. Long-term therapy is safe, and patients have been treated for up to 20 years with omeprazole without loss of efficacy, although reduced vitamin B_{12} levels may occur and require vitamin B_{12} supplementation (Chapter 164). Histamine-2 receptor antagonists are also effective, but frequent (every 4 to 6 hours) high doses are needed. Total gastrectomy, the historical treatment, is now performed only for patients who cannot or will not take oral antisecretory medications.[15] Selective vagotomy reduces acid secretion, but many patients continue to require a low dose of drug, and it is now rarely used. Parathyroidectomy should be performed in MEN 1 patients with hyperparathyroidism and ZES, because it reduces acid secretion and increases the sensitivity to antisecretory drugs.

Surgical Therapy

Surgical exploration for cure is recommended in all patients without unresectable liver metastases, MEN 1, or complicating medical conditions that limit life expectancy. Tumors are found by experienced endocrine surgeons in 95% of patients at surgery. Surgical resection decreases the metastatic rate, increases survival, and results in a 5-year cure rate of 30%. Patients with metastatic gastrinoma in the liver have a poor prognosis, with a 5-year survival rate of 30%.

Metastatic Disease

If the metastatic disease can be resected (>90%), surgery should be considered (5 to 15% of cases). If the metastatic disease is nonresectable and slowly increasing in size or is symptomatic, treatment with octreotide (100 to 450 μg two to three times daily) alone or in combination with interferon-α (1 to 5 million U, 3 to 7 days/week) is effective in inhibiting further tumor growth in 50 to 60% of patients. In a randomized multinational study, the somatostatin analog lanreotide was associated with significantly prolonged survival among patients with somatostatin-positive metastatic enteropancreatic neuroendocrine tumors of grade 1 or 2.[A1] If this treatment fails or if the tumor is rapidly growing, chemotherapeutic agents (streptozotocin, 5-fluorouracil, doxorubicin) or treatment with the mTOR inhibitor everolimus or the tyrosine kinase inhibitor sunitinib is recommended. Everolimus[A2] and sunitinib[A3] also have been shown in prospective randomized studies to more than double the progression-free survival time. For patients with extensive metastatic disease, somatostatin receptor–directed radiation therapy using analogues labeled with yttrium-90, lutetium-177, or indium-111 is increasingly used, but these therapies are still not approved.[16] Newer chemotherapy treatments using temozolomide show some promise in a small number of gastrinomas and other pNET patients. In advanced cases where metastases are confined to the liver, liver-directed therapies (embolization, chemoembolization, radioembolization) and local ablative methodologies such as radio frequency ablation, are increasingly used. Liver transplantation is occasionally performed in the rare patient with metastases limited to the liver.

PROGNOSIS

pproximately 25% of gastrinomas show aggressive growth. The most nportant prognostic predictor is the development of liver metastases. The resence of a large primary tumor, a pancreatic tumor, bone metastases, evelopment of ectopic Cushing syndrome, or a high fasting gastrin level is ssociated with aggressive growth.

lucagonomas

DEFINITION

lucagonomas are endocrine tumors of the pancreas that ectopically secrete lucagon, causing a specific syndrome (see Table 195-1).

PATHOBIOLOGY

lucagon hypersecretion explains the glucose intolerance. The exact origin f the rash is unclear; some studies report that prolonged glucagon infusions an cause the characteristic skin lesions. A role for possible zinc deficiency as been proposed because of the similarity of the rash to that seen with zinc eficiency (acrodermatitis enteropathica) and because the rash improves in ome patients who are given zinc. The hypoaminoacidemia is thought to be econdary to the effect of glucagon on amino acid metabolism by altering luconeogenesis. The wasting and weight loss are intrinsic parts of the glucaonoma syndrome, and recent studies suggest that a novel anorectic subtance distinct from glucagon is responsible.

CLINICAL MANIFESTATIONS

he cardinal clinical features are a distinct dermatitis (necrolytic migratory rythema, seen in 70 to 90%) (Fig. 195-1), diabetes mellitus and glucose ntolerance (40 to 90%), weight loss (70 to 96%), anemia (30 to 85%), ypoaminoacidemia (80 to 90%) with deficiencies of essential fatty acids, hromboembolism (10 to 25%), diarrhea (15 to 30%), and psychiatric disurbances (0 to 20%). The characteristic rash is usually found at intertrigiious and periorificial sites, especially in the groin and buttocks (see Fig. 95-1). It is initially erythematous, becomes raised, and develops central ullae whose tops detach, with the eroded areas becoming crusty. Healing ccurs with hyperpigmentation.

DIAGNOSIS

he diagnosis is established by demonstrating elevated plasma glucagon evels. Normal levels are 150 to 200 pg/mL; in patients with glucagonomas, evels usually (>90%) are higher than 1000 pg/mL. However, in some recent

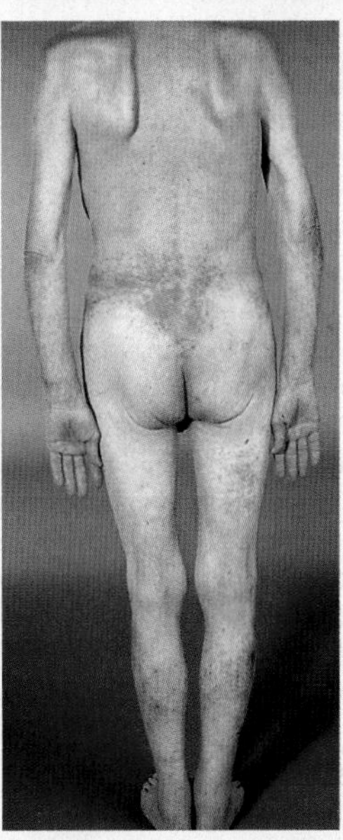

FIGURE 195-1. A patient with a glucagonoma with the characteristic rash (necrolytic migratory erythema). The rash is usually at intertriginous areas or periorificial sites and shows various stages of erythema, blistering, and crusting. (From Forbes CD, Jackson WF. *Color Atlas and Text of Clinical Medicine*. 3rd ed. London: Mosby; 2003.)

studies, up to 40% of patients had plasma glucagon values of 500 to 1000 pg/mL. Increased plasma glucagon levels also occur in renal insufficiency, acute pancreatitis, hypercorticism, hepatic diseases, celiac disease, severe stress and prolonged fasting, in patients treated with danazol, and in familial hyperglucagonemia. In these conditions, the level is usually less than 500 pg/mL except in patients with hepatic diseases or in those with familial hyperglucagonemia. Recently, two new glucagonoma-related syndromes have been described: Mahvash disease (characterized by mutations in the glucagon receptor, glucagon cell hyperplasia, hyperglucagonemia, but no symptoms of the glucagonoma syndrome) and glucagon cell adenomatosis (characterized by glucagon cell hyperplasia and occasional symptoms mimicking the glucagonoma syndrome).

Glucagonomas are generally large when discovered (mean, 5 to 10 cm), and they most frequently occur in the pancreatic tail (>50%). Liver metastases are commonly present at the time of diagnosis (45 to 80%).

TREATMENT

Subcutaneous administration of the synthetic long-acting somatostatin analogue octreotide (100 to 400 μg two to three times daily) controls the rash in 80% of patients and improves weight loss, diarrhea, and hypoaminoacidemia,[17] but it usually does not improve the diabetes mellitus. Increasingly, long-acting depot formulations of octreotide (octreotide-LAR) or lanreotide autogel are being given by monthly injection. Zinc supplementation and infusions of amino acids or fatty acids, or both, can diminish the severity of the rash. After tumor localization, surgical resection is preferred; even debulking of metastatic tumor may be of benefit. For advanced disease, treatment is similar to outlined for advanced nonresectable gastrinomas.

PROGNOSIS

The prognosis is now largely determined by the growth of the tumor per se, because the symptoms of glucagon excess can be largely controlled by somatostatin analogues. This is particularly true with glucagonomas; in many series, more than 50 to 80% are metastatic at presentation, and patients usually present late with large primary tumors. The mean 5-year survival rate is 50%; however, extended survivals (>15 years) are reported in some patients with treatment with somatostatin analogues and other tumor-directed therapies.

VIPomas

DEFINITION

The VIPoma syndrome, also called the Verner-Morrison syndrome, pancreatic cholera, and the WDHA syndrome (for watery diarrhea, hypokalemia, and achlorhydria), results from an endocrine tumor, usually in the pancreas, that ectopically secretes vasoactive intestinal polypeptide (VIP).

EPIDEMIOLOGY AND PATHOBIOLOGY

VIPomas in adults are found in the pancreas in 80 to 90% of cases; rare cases result from intestinal carcinoids, ganglioneuromas, ganglioneuroblastomas, and pheochromocytomas. In children younger than 10 years and rarely in adults (<5%), the VIPoma syndrome is caused by ganglioneuromas or ganglioneuroblastomas at extrapancreatic sites. VIPomas are usually large and solitary; 50 to 75% of these tumors occur in the pancreatic tail, and 40 to 70% have metastasized at diagnosis. VIPomas frequently secrete both VIP and peptide histidine methionine, but VIP is responsible for the symptoms. VIP is a potent stimulant of secretion in the small and large intestine, which causes the cardinal clinical features of the VIPoma syndrome. VIP also causes relaxation of gastrointestinal smooth muscle, and this may contribute to the dilated loops of bowel that are common in this syndrome, as well as a dilated atonic gallbladder that is sometimes seen. Hypochlorhydria is thought to result from the inhibitory effect of VIP on acid secretion, the flushing is related to the vasodilatory effects of VIP, and the hyperglycemia is caused by the glycogenolytic effect of VIP. The mechanism of the hypercalcemia remains unclear.

CLINICAL MANIFESTATIONS

The cardinal clinical feature is severe, large-volume, watery diarrhea (>1 L/day) (100%), which is secretory and occurs during fasting. Hypokalemia (67 to 100%) and dehydration (83%) commonly occur because of the volume of the diarrhea. Achlorhydria is occasionally noted, but hypochlorhydria is usually found (34 to 72% of cases). Flushing occurs in 20% of patients, hyperglycemia in 25 to 50%, and hypercalcemia in 41 to 50%. Steatorrhea is uncommon (16%) despite the volume of diarrhea.

DIAGNOSIS

The diarrhea of VIPomas characteristically persists during fasting and is large in volume (>3 L/day in 70 to 80%); the diagnosis is excluded when fasting stool volume is less than 700 mL/day. To differentiate VIPomas from other causes of large-volume fasting diarrhea, fasting plasma VIP levels should be determined. The normal value in most laboratories is less than 190 pg/mL, and elevated levels are present in 90 to 100% of patients in various series. The differential diagnosis of large-volume fasting diarrhea (>700 mL/day) includes ZES, diffuse islet cell hyperplasia, surreptitious use of laxatives, the pseudopancreatic cholera syndrome, and rarely, HIV infection (Chapter 390). Serum gastrin levels identify patients with ZES, and plasma VIP levels are normal in most patients who abuse laxatives, in 82% of patients with pancreatic islet cell hyperplasia, and in patients with HIV-induced secretory diarrhea.

TREATMENT Rx

The symptoms caused by the VIP are controlled initially in more than 85% of patients by daily doses of octreotide (50 to 400 μg once to three times daily) or by monthly injections of the depot form, octreotide-LAR or lanreotide autogel, but increased doses may be needed over time. Before the availability of octreotide, small numbers of patients were reported to respond to a variety of agents, including high-dose prednisone (60 to 100 mg/day; 40 to 50%), clonidine, lithium carbonate, indomethacin, loperamide, metoclopramide, and phenothiazines. After tumor localization studies, surgical resection should be attempted if it is possible to remove all visible tumor; however, more than 50% of patients have generalized liver metastases at diagnosis, so complete resection may not be possible. For patients with unresectable advanced disease, treatment is similar to outlined for advanced nonresectable gastrinomas.[18]

PROGNOSIS

The prognosis is now largely determined by the growth of the tumor per se, because the symptoms of VIP excess can be largely controlled by somatostatin analogues. This is particularly true in patients with VIPomas, because they frequently (>50%) present with advanced metastatic disease. The mean 5-year survival is 50 to 70%.

Somatostatinomas

Definition and Pathobiology

Somatostatinomas are endocrine tumors that occur in the pancreas or upper small intestine and ectopically secrete somatostatin. In the gastrointestinal tract, somatostatin inhibits basal and stimulated acid secretion, pancreatic secretion, intestinal absorption of amino acids, gallbladder contractility, and release of numerous hormones, including cholecystokinin and gastrin.

CLINICAL MANIFESTATIONS

Most reported somatostatinomas are diagnosed histologically as an endocrine tumor containing somatostatin-like immunoreactivity and are not associated with a distinct clinical syndrome (the somatostatinoma syndrome). The somatostatinoma syndrome includes diabetes mellitus, gallbladder disease, diarrhea, steatorrhea, and weight loss. Sixty percent of somatostatinomas occur in the pancreas, and 40% are found in the duodenum or jejunum. Pancreatic somatostatinomas occur in the pancreatic head in 60 to 80% of cases; 70 to 92% will have metastasized at diagnosis, and they are usually large (mean, 5 cm) and solitary. In contrast, duodenal somatostatinomas are smaller (mean, 2.4 cm), frequently associated with psammoma bodies on histologic examination (11%), and less frequently have metastases at diagnosis (30 to 40%).

The somatostatinoma syndrome occurs much more commonly (80 to 95% of all cases) in patients with pancreatic than duodenal or intestinal somatostatinomas. Duodenal somatostatinomas occur in up to 10% of patients with von Recklinghausen disease and are usually asymptomatic.

DIAGNOSIS

Somatostatinomas are usually found by accident, particularly during exploratory laparotomy for cholecystectomy, during endoscopy, or on imaging studies. The presence of psammoma bodies on histologic examination of a duodenal endocrine tumor or any duodenal lesions in patients with von Recklinghausen disease should raise the suspicion of a duodenal somatostatinoma. The diagnosis of the somatostatinoma syndrome requires the demonstration of increased concentrations of somatostatin-like immunoreactivity in the plasma and the resected tumor. However, other tumors outside the pancreas or intestine, such as small-cell lung cancer, medullary thyroid carcinoma, pheochromocytomas, and paragangliomas, may also have elevated concentrations of somatostatin-like immunoreactivity. Somatostatinomas can be imaged using somatostatin receptor scintigraphy or, if needed, other conventional imaging studies to assess the tumor's location.

TREATMENT Rx

Treatment with octreotide or lanreotide can improve symptoms. Surgery, if possible, should be performed. For patients with unresectable advanced disease, treatment is similar to outlined for advanced nonresectable gastrinomas.[19]

PROGNOSIS

Patients with intestinal somatostatinomas, which uncommonly cause the somatostatinoma syndrome and are less malignant, have an excellent prognosis (5-year survival rate, >80%), whereas those with pancreatic somatostatinomas, which frequently cause the somatostatinoma syndrome and present with metastatic disease (>70%), have a much reduced 5-year survival rate (<50%).

GRFomas

DEFINITION

GRFomas are endocrine tumors that frequently originate in the pancreas but also occur in other extrapancreatic locations and ectopically release growth hormone–releasing factor (GRF). The GRF causes acromegaly that is clinically indistinguishable from that caused by a pituitary adenoma.

PATHOBIOLOGY

GRFomas most commonly occur in the lung (54%). Most of the remainder occur in the gastrointestinal tract, including 30% in the pancreas. Pancreatic GRFomas are usually large (mean, 6 cm), 39% are metastatic at diagnosis, 40% occur in combination with ZES, and 33% are in patients with MEN 1.

DIAGNOSIS

GRFomas are an uncommon cause of acromegaly. These tumors occurred in none of 177 unselected patients with acromegaly in one study. However, any patient with acromegaly and abdominal complaints, with acromegaly but no pituitary tumor (Chapter 224), or with acromegaly and hyperprolactinemia (which occurs in 70% of GRFomas) should be suspected of having a GRFoma. The intra-abdominal features of GRFomas result from its metastases and are typical of any malignant pNET. The diagnosis is confirmed by performing a plasma assay for GRF and growth hormone.

TREATMENT

The effects of the GRF can be controlled with octreotide or lanreotide in more than 90% of patients. Treatment should be directed at the GRFoma per se, as described for the other more common pNETs. For patients with unresectable advanced disease, treatment is similar to that outlined for advanced nonresectable gastrinomas.

Nonfunctional Pancreatic Neuroendocrine Tumors

DEFINITION

Nonfunctional pNETs are endocrine tumors that originate in the pancreas and either secrete no peptides or secrete products that do not cause clinical symptoms.

PATHOBIOLOGY

Frequently secreted nonfunctional peptides include chromogranin A (100%), pancreatic polypeptide (60%), and the α-subunit (40%) and β-subunit of human chorionic gonadotropin. Immunocytochemically, even higher percentages contain these peptides as well as insulin (50%), glucagons (30%), and somatostatin (13%).

CLINICAL MANIFESTATIONS

Nonfunctional pNETs are frequently diagnosed only late in the course of disease after the patient presents with symptoms or signs of metastatic disease and a liver biopsy reveals metastatic pNET. Any symptoms or signs result from the tumor per se and include abdominal pain (36 to 56%), abdominal mass or hepatosplenomegaly (8 to 40%), weight loss or cachexia (8 to 46%), and jaundice (27 to 40%). In 20% of asymptomatic patients, tumors are found incidentally at surgery.

DIAGNOSIS

Any patients with a long survival (>5 years) after a diagnosis of metastatic pancreatic adenocarcinoma should be suspected of having a nonfunctional pNET. Most primary tumors are large (70% are > 5 cm), and 70% occur in the pancreatic head. Liver metastases are frequent (38 to 62%) at presentation. An elevated plasma chromogranin A or pancreatic polypeptide level or a positive somatostatin receptor scintigraphic scan is strong evidence that a pancreatic mass is a pNET. Malignancy correlates with vascular or perineural invasion, a proliferative index of more than 2%, a mitotic rate of 2 or higher, a size of at least 4 cm, capsular penetration, nuclear atypia, lack of progesterone receptors, and the presence of calcitonin immunoreactivity in the tumor.

TREATMENT

Tumor localization is needed in all patients. Survival is better in patients with smaller tumors, patients who are asymptomatic at presentation, patients with no metastases, and patients in whom surgical resection can be performed.

Surgical resection should be performed whenever possible. For patients with unresectable advanced disease, treatment is similar to that outlined for advanced nonresectable gastrinomas.

PROGNOSIS

The overall 5-year survival rate varies in different series from 30 to 70%, but it is heavily dependent on the extent of the disease at diagnosis, with survival rates of 96% in patients without metastases at presentation, decreasing to 30 to 50% for those with metastatic disease.[20]

ACTHomas and Other Uncommon Tumors

pNETs that ectopically secrete ACTH cause 4 to 16% of the cases of ectopic Cushing syndrome. Cushing syndrome (Chapter 227) occurs in 5% of all cases of ZES, but in patients with sporadic ZES it is a late feature, occurring with metastatic liver disease. Its development is associated with a poor prognosis, and the response to chemotherapy is generally poor; however, occasional patients benefit from the use of long-acting somatostatin analogues (octreotide, lanreotide).

Paraneoplastic hypercalcemia (Chapter 245) can result from a pNET that releases parathormone-related peptide or an unknown hypercalcemic substance. Tumors are generally large, with metastatic liver disease at diagnosis. Somatostatin analogues may help control the hypercalcemia, but surgery, chemotherapy, hepatic embolization, and chemoembolization are the mainstays of treatment.

pNETs causing the carcinoid syndrome (Chapter 232) are usually large, and 68 to 88% are malignant. Octreotide may control the symptoms. Surgery, chemotherapy, hepatic embolization, chemoembolization, or molecular targeted therapy (everolimus, sunitinib) may be helpful.

A single case of a pNET that secreted renin manifested with severe hypertension; the tumor was localized with somatostatin receptor scintigraphy, and the patient's symptoms improved significantly after tumor resection. A single case of an erythropoietin-secreting pNET resulting in polycythemia, and a single case of a pNET secreting IGF-II or GLP-1 causing hypoglycemia have been described.

Two symptomatic cases of pNETs that secreted luteinizing hormone have been described; virilization occurred in the female patient, whereas the male patient had increased acne and a rash. In both cases, the tumors were resectable, and symptoms improved postoperatively. A single case of a pNET secreting cholecystokinin (CCKoma) has been recently described, with the patients demonstrating peptic ulcer disease, gallbladder disease, diarrhea, and weight loss.[21] A case of a pNET secreting enteroglucagon causing small intestinal hypertrophy has also been described.

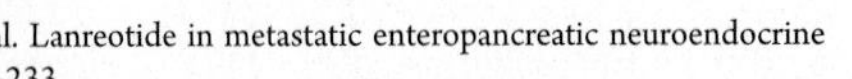

Grade A References

A1. Caplin ME, Pavel M, Cwikla JB, et al. Lanreotide in metastatic enteropancreatic neuroendocrine tumors. *N Engl J Med*. 2014;371:224-233.
A2. Yao JC, Shah MH, Ito T, et al. Everolimus for advanced pancreatic neuroendocrine tumors. *N Engl J Med*. 2011;364:514-523.
A3. Raymond E, Dahan L, Raoul JL, et al. Sunitinib malate for the treatment of pancreatic neuroendocrine tumors. *N Engl J Med*. 2011;364:501-513.

GENERAL REFERENCES

For the General References and other additional features, please visit Expert Consult at https://expertconsult.inkling.com.

196 LIVER AND BILIARY TRACT CANCERS

ROBIN K. KELLEY AND ALAN P. VENOOK

Malignancies arising from the liver parenchyma and biliary ductal epithelium are a heterogeneous group of cancers with generally poor prognosis, whose treatment is complicated by underlying liver injury, cirrhosis, or biliary obstruction in the majority of cases. These cancers collectively represent the third leading cause of cancer death worldwide and are rising in incidence, requiring clinician awareness of their presentation, evaluation, and treatment.

DEFINITION

Cancers arising from the liver and biliary tract include hepatocellular carcinoma, cholangiocarcinoma, and gallbladder adenocarcinoma, as well as other less common malignant histologies (Table 196-1, Fig. 196-1). Cholangiocarcinomas are further subclassified by their anatomic location along the biliary tract: intrahepatic (also known as peripheral) or extrahepatic, which includes hilar (also known as Klatskin tumors) and distal locations. The liver is a frequent site of metastasis from other primary cancers, requiring consideration of metastatic disease in the differential diagnosis of liver tumors. This chapter focuses on primary malignant tumors of the liver and biliary tract; metastatic disease to the liver is presented in other chapters, according to primary tumor of origin.

EPIDEMIOLOGY

Hepatocellular Carcinoma

Hepatocellular carcinoma is the most common primary tumor of the liver and the second leading cause of cancer death worldwide, accounting for approximately 782,000 new cases and 746,000 deaths worldwide each year based on estimates from 2012.[1] Over 80% of hepatocellular carcinoma cases

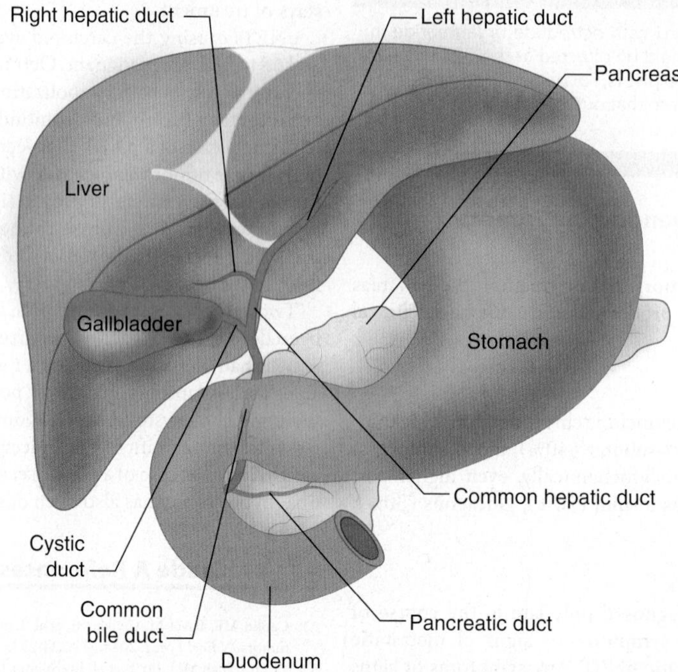

FIGURE 196-1. Anatomy of the liver and biliary tract. Hepatocellular carcinoma arises from liver parenchyma, and cholangiocarcinomas arise from the biliary ductal epitheliun within (intrahepatic or peripheral) or outside of (extrahepatic) the liver. Tumors arising from the confluence of the right and left bile duct at the hepatic hilum are called hilar cholan giocarcinoma or Klatskin tumors.

TABLE 196-1 PRIMARY MALIGNANT TUMORS OF THE LIVER AND BILIARY TRACT

TUMOR TYPE	APPROXIMATE ANNUAL INCIDENCE
Hepatocellular carcinoma	782,000 cases/yr worldwide*
Gallbladder carcinoma	145,000 cases/yr worldwide
Cholangiocarcinoma	9,810 cases/yr in United States†
Mixed hepatocellular-cholangiocarcinoma	Rare
Fibrolamellar hepatocellular carcinoma	Rare
Cystadenocarcinoma	Rare
Hepatic endothelioid hemangioendothelioma	Rare
Angiosarcoma and other sarcomas	Rare

*Includes cases of intrahepatic cholangiocarcinoma.
†Includes cases of gallbladder cancer and excludes cases of intrahepatic cholangiocarcinoma.

occur in developing countries (Fig. 196-2), which is attributed to an increased prevalence of hepatocellular carcinoma risk factors, particularly hepatitis B virus (HBV) and hepatitis C virus (HCV) (Chapters 148 and 149, Table 196-2). HBV and HCV together account for over 80% of all hepatocellular carcinoma cases worldwide.[2,3] HBV is endemic in regions including Asia and sub-Saharan Africa and is vertically transmitted from mother to fetus in utero. HCV, which may be acquired by intravenous drug abuse or from blood transfusion, is another important risk factor for hepatocellular carcinoma, leading to an estimated hepatocellular carcinoma incidence of 2 to 8% per year among patients with cirrhosis caused by HCV. Obesity, diabetes, and the metabolic syndrome are risk factors for nonalcoholic fatty liver disease, a condition of rising incidence, particularly in Western populations, which can lead to steatohepatitis, cirrhosis, and hepatocellular carcinoma. Nonalcoholic fatty liver disease, alcohol-related disorders, and HCV are leading causes of hepatocellular carcinoma in the United States. Other risk factors for hepatocellular carcinoma include hepatitis D virus (which requires coinfection with HBV for pathogenicity), hereditary hemochromatosis, α_1-antitrypsin deficiency, primary biliary cirrhosis, autoimmune hepatitis, male gender, and dietary exposure to fungal aflatoxins.

Biliary Tract Cancers

Although classified as a rare cancer, cholangiocarcinoma is the most commo primary biliary tract malignancy and the second most common primar cancer of the liver after hepatocellular carcinoma.[4] The incidence of intrahe patic cholangiocarcinoma appears to be increasing. Although most cases ar sporadic, there is an increased risk for cholangiocarcinoma with the followin conditions or exposures: primary sclerosing cholangitis, inflammatory bowe disease, viral hepatitis infection, congenital choledochal cysts or other struc tural abnormalities of the biliary tract, chronic pancreatitis, obesity, fluk infections and other causes of chronic cholangitis, bile duct adenomas, Caro disease, and diabetes mellitus.

Gallbladder adenocarcinomas are a rare tumor type in the United State but account for 145,000 cases and 109,000 deaths per year worldwide base on estimates from 2008. There is significant regional variation in incidence with higher incidence reported in India and areas of South America and Asi Risk factors for gallbladder adenocarcinoma include female gender, chroni cholelithiasis, chronic cholecystitis, a history of gallbladder polyps, an abnormalities of the common bile duct. Calcification of the gallbladde ("porcelain gallbladder") is often considered a risk factor, but it is only weakl associated with development of cancer.

Other Primary Liver Cancers

Other primary tumors of the liver are much less common, with poorly unde stood risk factors. Chronic inflammatory conditions, including viral hepatitis may be associated with the development of combined-histology liver tumor Exposure to polyvinyl chloride has been implicated in the development c hepatic angiosarcomas. The fibrolamellar variant of hepatocellular carcinom may occur more commonly in females. Hepatoblastoma tumors occur i infants and children, but almost never in adults.

PATHOBIOLOGY

Hepatocellular Carcinoma

Hepatocellular carcinoma is an epithelial neoplasm that arises fron malignant transformation of liver hepatocytes (Fig. 196-3A and B). Th pathogenesis of hepatocellular carcinoma is thought to be a multistep proces triggered by underlying liver injury (such as from viral hepatitis, alcohol, iro overload, or aflatoxin exposure) in the majority of cases. Subsequent inflam mation, necrosis, regeneration, cell turnover, and proliferation result in th progressive accumulation of genetic damage and somatic (acquired

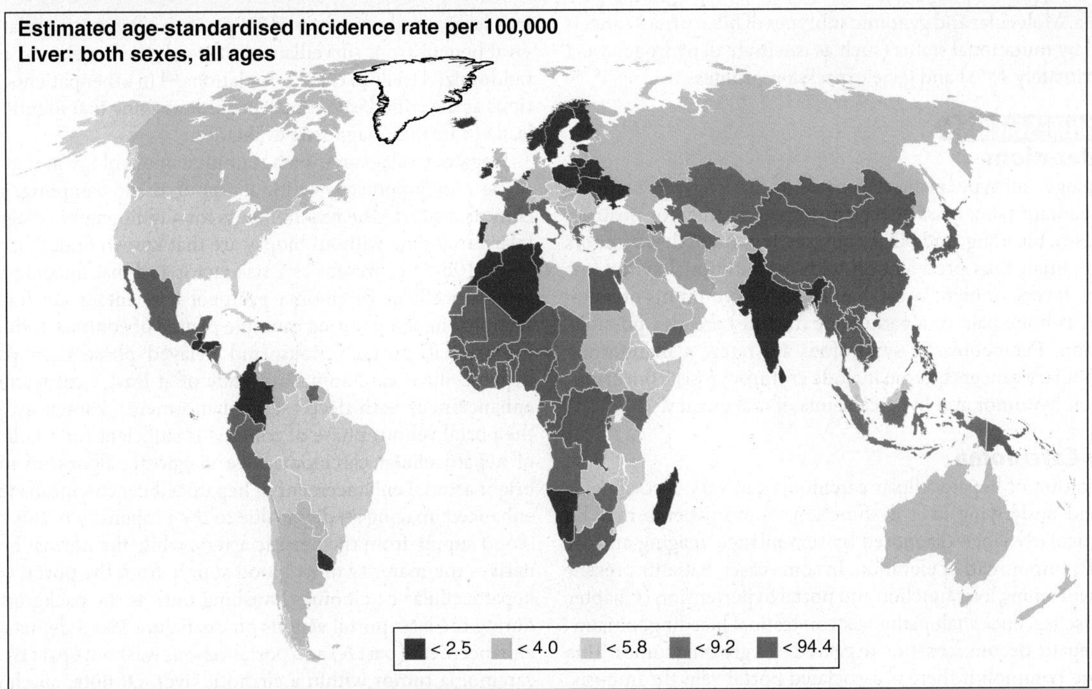

FIGURE 196-2. Global incidence of liver cancer. The incidence of liver cancer is highest in less developed regions, particularly Eastern and South-Eastern Asia and Middle and Western Africa.

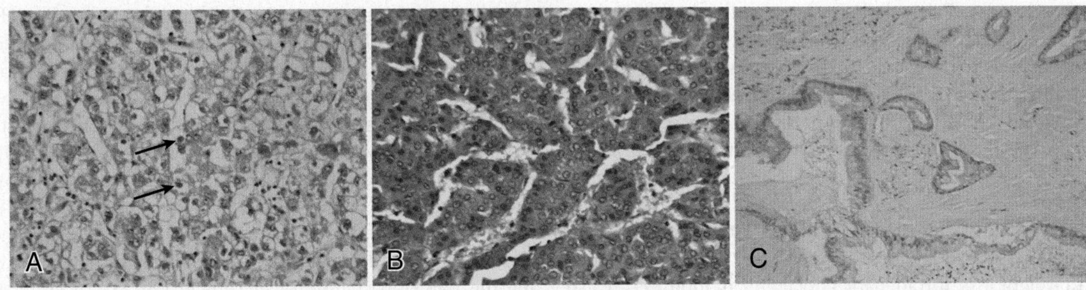

FIGURE 196-3. Histology of hepatocellular carcinoma and cholangiocarcinoma. A, Hepatocellular carcinoma (40×) with clear cell features and Mallory hyaline inclusions (*black arrow*). B, Hepatocellular carcinoma (40×) with trabecular pattern and small cell change. C, Hilar cholangiocarcinoma (20×) with dense fibrous stromal reaction. (Courtesy Dr. Linda Ferrell, Department of Pathology, University of California, San Francisco.)

TABLE 196-2 RISK FACTORS FOR HEPATOCELLULAR CARCINOMA

RISK FACTOR	INCIDENCE OF HEPATOCELLULAR CARCINOMA*
Asian male HBV carriers over age 40	0.4-0.6%/yr
Asian female HBV carriers over age 50	0.3-0.6%/yr
HBV carrier with family history of HCC	Higher incidence than without family history
African/North American Blacks with HBV	HCC occurs at younger age
HBV carriers with cirrhosis	3-8%/yr
HCV cirrhosis	3-5%/yr
Stage 4 primary biliary cirrhosis	3-5%/yr
Hereditary hemochromatosis with cirrhosis	Unknown
α_1-Antitrypsin deficiency with cirrhosis	Unknown
Other cause cirrhosis	Unknown

Modified from Bruix J, Sherman M. Management of hepatocellular carcinoma: an update. *Hepatology.* 2011;53:1020-1022.
*Data from Nordenstedt H, White DL, El-Serag HB. The changing pattern of epidemiology in hepatocellular carcinoma. *Digest Liver Dis.* 2010;42(Suppl 3):S206-S214.
HCC = hepatocellular carcinoma.

mutations.[5] Activation of oncogenes or inactivation of tumor suppressor genes, dysplasia, and subsequently carcinoma can arise. The most well-described mutations in hepatocellular carcinoma are point mutations or deletions resulting in inactivation of the tumor suppressor *TP53* in over 50% of cases and mutations in β-catenin *(CTNNB1)* in approximately 30% of cases. Alterations in Wnt, cell cycle, and chromatin-remodeling pathways have been described and may be associated with the etiology of underlying liver injury. In HBV-associated hepatocellular carcinoma, a unique mechanism of malignant transformation is direct viral DNA integration into the host genome, which appears to favor specific loci. A recurrent locus for HBV integration is the *TERT* gene which encodes telomerase reverse transcriptase. HBV integration can activate *TERT,* resulting in malignant transformation and immortalization in a subset of HBV-associated hepatocellular carcinomas.

Biliary Tract Cancers

Cholangiocarcinomas are a histologically diverse group of epithelial cancers that may arise from multiple different cell types within the liver, including biliary epithelial cells or hepatic progenitor cells, and are often surrounded by a dense stroma with cancer-associated fibroblasts (see Fig. 196-3C). Cholangiocarcinomas are associated with underlying inflammation and cholestasis, which activate growth factors and a proliferative response. Overexpression of Notch1 and AKT have been implicated in a process of hepatocyte conversion into cholangiocyte precursors of intrahepatic cholangiocarcinoma. Molecular and genomic subtypes of biliary tract cancers can also be defined by mutational status (such as isocitrate dehydrogenase-1 mutation in approximately 15%) and gene expression profiles.

CLINICAL MANIFESTATIONS

General Considerations

Regardless of histologic subtype, primary tumors of the liver can manifest with right upper quadrant pain, mass effect causing early satiety or obstructive symptoms, nausea, bleeding, and biliary obstruction. All of these tumors have metastatic potential; thus presentation with constitutional symptoms (such as weight loss, fevers, or night sweats) and signs or symptoms of metastatic disease (such as bone pain or a pathologic fracture) are also possible, though less common. Paraneoplastic syndromes are rarely a manifesting symptom in hepatobiliary cancers but can include erythrocytosis from erythropoietin production by tumor and hypercalcemia of malignancy.

Hepatocellular Carcinoma

The clinical presentation of hepatocellular carcinoma can vary according to extent of tumor and underlying liver dysfunction. Some patients may be asymptomatic, particularly when diagnosed by surveillance imaging and/or α-fetoprotein (AFP) tumor marker elevation. In some cases, patients present with symptoms of worsening liver function and portal hypertension (Chapter 153), such as new ascites, encephalopathy, gastrointestinal bleeding, or jaundice, as a result of hepatic decompensation triggered by a growing tumor. This presentation is more common if there is associated portal vein thrombosis. In other cases, there may be chronic progressive upper abdominal pain because of tumor involvement of the sensitive liver capsule, sudden onset acute pain from tumor bleeding or rupture, or a palpable mass leading to the diagnosis of hepatocellular carcinoma. Constitutional symptoms such as cachexia, fatigue, and weight loss may be present with advanced stages. On physical examination, patients with hepatocellular carcinoma may have an enlarged liver with tenderness. Particularly in large and rapidly growing tumors, a bruit may be auscultated over the liver surface. Ascites, jaundice, signs of portal hypertension such as caput medusae and splenomegaly, and asterixis may be variably present if there is associated decompensation in hepatic function (Chapter 153). The tumor marker AFP is elevated in approximately 70% of cases but is not diagnostic (see later discussion).

Biliary Tract Cancers

Extrahepatic cholangiocarcinomas most often manifest with signs and symptoms of biliary obstruction, such as jaundice, pruritus, pale stools, dark urine, anorexia, nausea, and weight loss. Intrahepatic cholangiocarcinomas can also cause obstruction, but generally only when there is extensive disease present. Less commonly, complications such as biliary fistulae and hemobilia can occur. Gallbladder cancers are often diagnosed incidentally during cholecystectomy, but in some cases can be associated with right upper quadrant pain, biliary colic, or a tender, palpable mass. Infections of the biliary tract can produce symptoms including right upper quadrant pain, fever, chills, nausea, vomiting, and jaundice. Cholangitis can result from biliary obstruction by tumors throughout the biliary tract and can lead to complications such as abscess, bacteremia, or sepsis syndrome.

Diagnosis and Staging

General Considerations

The approach to patients with the finding of a liver mass requires assessment of risk factors and extent of underlying liver disease, if present. The diagnostic evaluation, staging, and treatment options are guided by whether underlying liver disease is present as well as by its extent. The differential diagnosis for hepatocellular carcinoma and biliary tract cancers includes benign liver lesions (such as hemangiomas, adenomas, abscesses, and regenerative nodules), malignant tumors of other primary liver histologies, mixed-histology tumors, and metastatic disease. It is recommended that diagnostic evaluation and procedures in patients with hepatobiliary tumors be performed in expert centers because the unique interplay of underlying liver disease, disease-specific imaging findings and staging, and risks for biopsy.

Hepatocellular Carcinoma

In patients with known cirrhosis or other risk factors for hepatocellular carcinoma (see Table 196-2), a liver mass may be identified during a program of surveillance by imaging and/or elevated serum AFP level, in the absence of other signs or symptoms of cancer. A randomized, controlled trial of surveillance by ultrasound and AFP every 6 months compared to no surveillance in a large, predominantly HBV-positive Chinese population showed a su vival benefit from surveillance, although the benefit has not been proved randomized trials in other populations.[A1] In other patients, clinical manifest tions as described earlier may prompt imaging that identifies a liver mass an leads to further diagnostic evaluation.

Hepatocellular carcinoma is unique in oncology in that a diagnosis can b made radiographically without tumor tissue sampling, in the appropria clinical context. The requirements for a radiographic diagnosis of hepatoce lular carcinoma without biopsy are that known underlying liver disease (se Table 196-2) is present as a risk factor and that imaging is performed usir a hepatocellular carcinoma protocol that entails contrast-enhanced cros sectional imaging during multiple phases of contrast administration (inclu ing arterial, portal venous, and delayed phases). In patients at risk fo hepatocellular carcinoma, a nodule of at least 1 cm featuring arterial phas enhancement with decreased enhancement (known as "washout") durir the portal venous phase of contrast is sufficient for a radiographic diagnos of hepatocellular carcinoma (see diagnostic algorithm in Fig. 196-4). Th bright arterial enhancement of hepatocellular carcinoma lesions on contras enhanced imaging studies is due to the propensity of this tumor to parasitiz blood supply from the hepatic artery, while the normal hepatic parenchym derives the majority of its blood supply from the portal vein. This results i hepatocellular carcinomas "washing out" as the background liver brighter during the later portal venous phase. Figure 196-5 depicts the classic arteri enhancement (part A) and portal venous washout (part B) of a hepatocellul carcinoma tumor within a cirrhotic liver. Of note, an elevated AFP level not sufficiently sensitive or specific for diagnosis of hepatocellular carcinom in cirrhotic patients with a liver mass. A biopsy is warranted to confirm th diagnosis of hepatocellular carcinoma if either arterial enhancement or port venous washout is not present. In patients with small lesions who may b eligible for curative surgery or transplantation, consultation with a hepatol gist and/or experienced liver surgeon, should be obtained before performin percutaneous biopsy, because of risk for tumor seeding (Fig. 196-4).

Once a patient has been radiographically and/or pathologically diagnose with hepatocellular carcinoma, the staging for extent of disease require cross-sectional imaging of the chest, abdomen, and pelvis, AFP measur ment, and a bone scan, if symptoms or signs of bone metastases (such as bon pain or markedly elevated alkaline phosphatase value) are present. Th staging of hepatocellular carcinoma also requires a thorough assessment c underlying liver function, which affects prognosis and treatment option independent of tumor extent. Several hepatocellular cancer–specific, joir tumor staging and liver disease scoring systems have been developed, incluc ing the Barcelona Clinic Liver Cancer (BCLC) staging system, the Okud classification, and the Cancer of the Liver Italian Program (CLIP) scorin system, though there is no consensus regarding which is superior.[6]

Other Liver Tumors and Biliary Tract Cancers

For patients without known risk factors for hepatocellular carcinoma, or diagnostic enhancement features of hepatocellular carcinoma are not me pathologic confirmation by biopsy or cytologic examination is required fo diagnosis of liver tumors. As is the case with suspected hepatocellular carci nomas, however, there is concern for tumor seeding of the needle track b percutaneous or endoluminal biopsy. Referral to an expert center is recom mended to guide the diagnostic evaluation in potential surgical candidates.

Endoluminal approaches such as by endoscopic retrograde cholangiopan creaticogram (ERCP) cytologic brushing, or endoscopic ultrasound fin needle aspiration are preferred in patients with early stages of disease tha may be amenable to curative surgery or transplantation. Staging of biliar tract and other rarer types of liver cancer generally includes cross-section imaging of the chest, abdomen, and pelvis. A mass in the gallbladde fossa suggests primary gallbladder cancer. Unlike hepatocellular carcinom cholangiocarcinomas characteristically display progressive enhancemen during the portal venous phase of contrast imaging (Fig. 196-7). Biliar obstruction and ipsilateral hepatic lobe atrophy and contralateral hypertro phy may be present and can sometimes obscure identification of the actu tumor mass. For biliary tract cancers, CA-19-9 and carcinoembryonic antige (CEA) tumor markers may be elevated and can help to monitor respons to treatment, although levels can be confounded if biliary obstructio and hyperbilirubinemia are present. Upper and lower endoscopy are indi cated to exclude metastatic disease in patients diagnosed with intrahepati cholangiocarcinoma, which otherwise can be difficult to discriminate fron metastatic disease radiographically and histologically. Cholangiography (b ERCP or magnetic resonance cholangiogram) may be indicated for bot

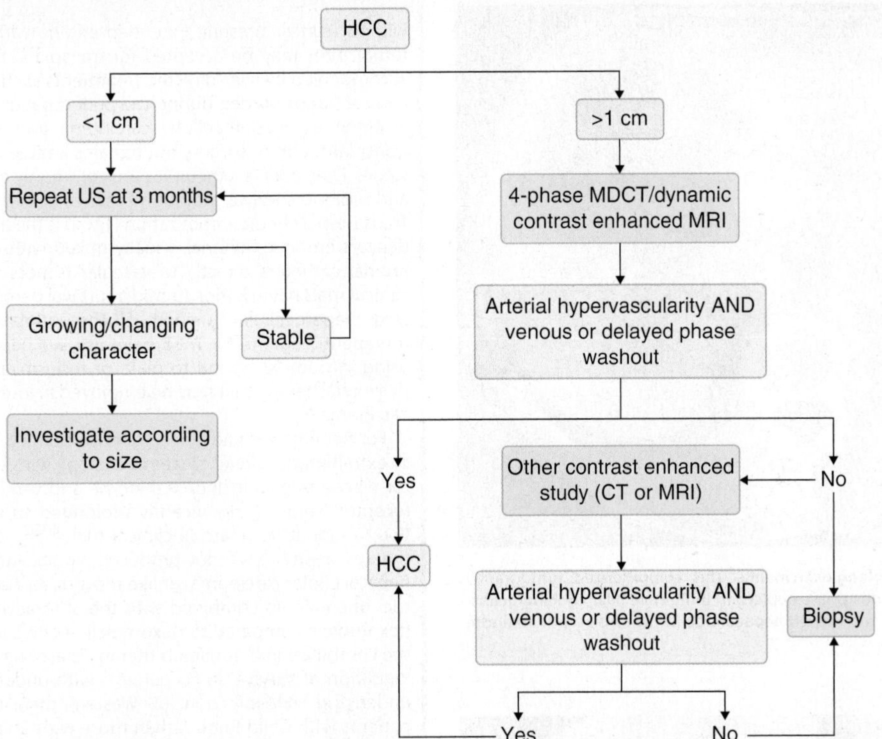

FIGURE 196-4. Hepatocellular carcinoma (*HCC*) diagnostic algorithm. American Association for the Study of Liver Diseases (AASLD) diagnostic algorithm for suspected hepatocellular carcinoma. CT = computed tomography; MDCT = multidetector CT; MRI = magnetic resonance imaging; US = ultrasound.

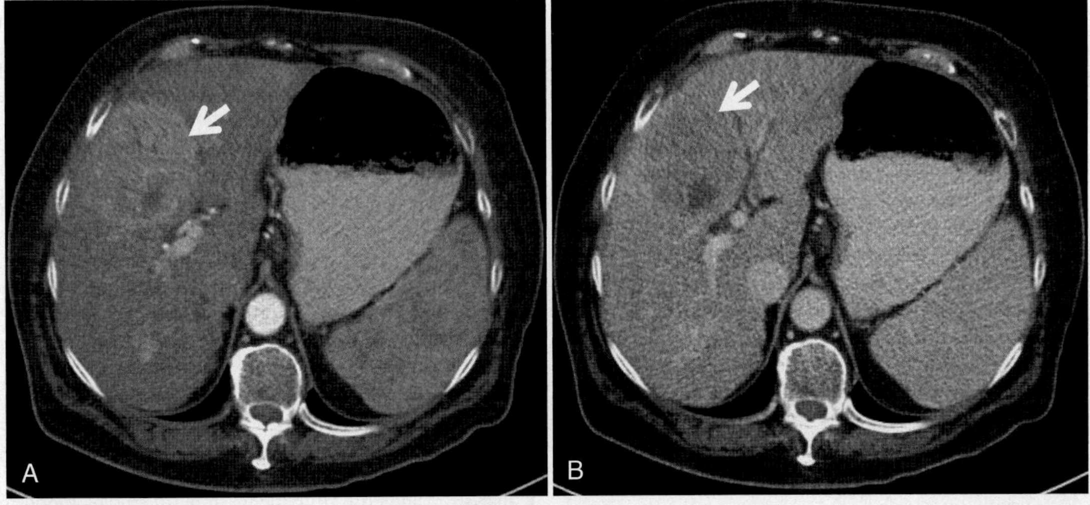

FIGURE 196-5. Imaging of hepatocellular carcinoma. In this contrast-enhanced computed tomography scan of the liver of a patient with hepatocellular carcinoma, a tumor in the right hepatic lobe demonstrates arterial phase enhancement (*white arrow,* panel A) followed by "wash-out" in the portal venous phase (white arrow, panel B).

diagnostic and therapeutic purposes (such as stent placement), particularly if biliary obstruction is present. A diagnostic laparoscopy to exclude peritoneal disease should be considered before undertaking a laparotomy for curative resection in patients with newly diagnosed gallbladder adenocarcinoma and cholangiocarcinoma, because of the propensity for radiographically occult peritoneal metastases, which would have an impact on surgical decision making. Staging of biliary tract cancers and other liver tumors follows the Tumor, Node, Metastasis (TNM) system of the American Joint Committee on Cancer.

TREATMENT Rx

General Considerations

The treatment of patients with hepatobiliary cancers requires management of underlying liver disease as well as the tumor itself. In patients with active HBV infection or prior exposure, close monitoring of liver function and viral load is advisable; antiviral therapy may be required to prevent reactivation, which can occur with immunosuppressive therapy (Chapter 35).[7] Management of liver tumors in patients with cirrhosis may necessitate treatment for complications of portal hypertension or liver dysfunction (Chapter 153). In patients with biliary tract cancers, biliary obstruction is a common complication that often requires endoscopic stent placement, percutaneous drainage, or antibiotic therapy if cholangitis develops. Chemotherapy and supportive care medications may need dose adjustments depending on the degree of liver dysfunction.

Hepatocellular Carcinoma

The treatment of early stages of hepatocellular carcinoma depends on the degree of liver dysfunction. In patients with preserved liver function and without significant portal hypertension, surgical resection can be curative and is better than catheter-based options.[A2] Among patients with increasing degrees of portal hypertension, however, surgical outcomes are significantly poorer than in patients without portal hypertension. For individuals with contraindications to surgery or inadequate projected future liver remnant

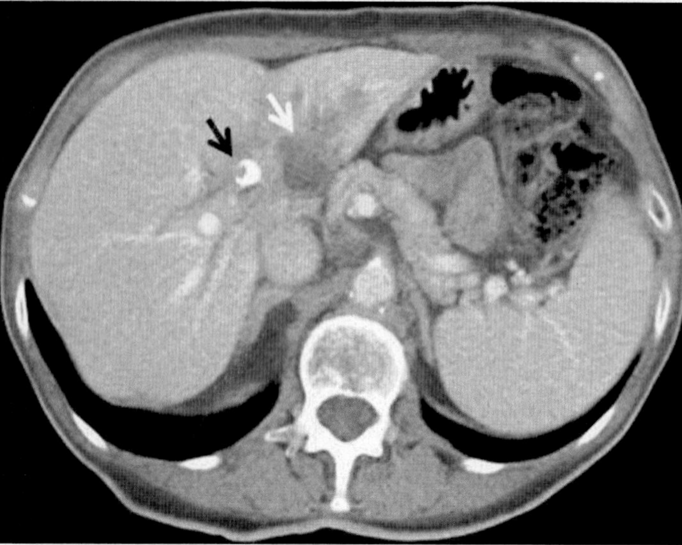

FIGURE 196-6. Imaging of cholangiocarcinoma. This computerized tomography image with contrast in portal venous phase depicts an infiltrative hilar cholangiocarcinoma (Klatskin tumor) extending into the left hepatic lobe (*white arrow*) with an endobiliary stent in place (*black arrow*).

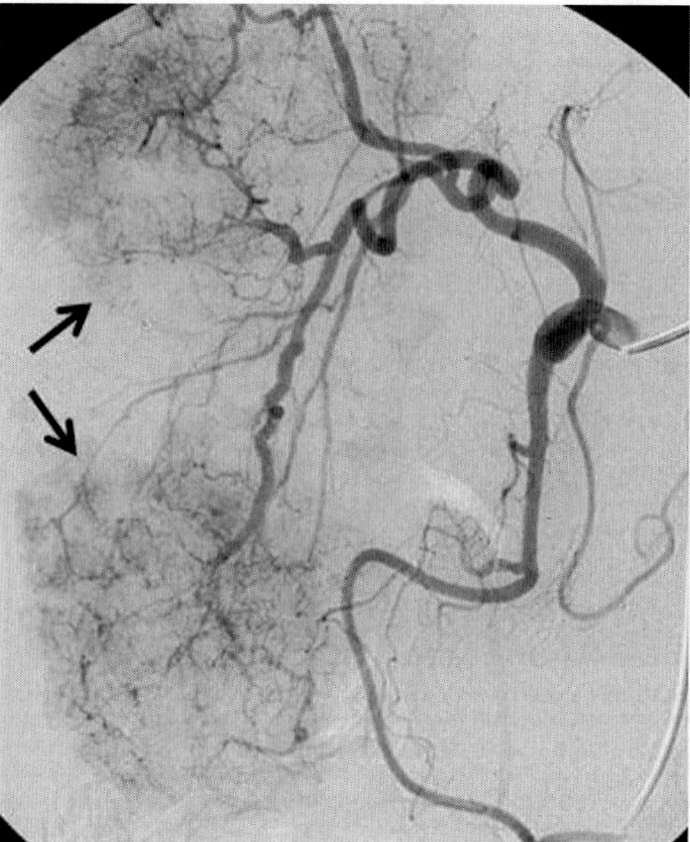

FIGURE 196-7. Trans-arterial chemoembolization (TACE) of hepatocellular carcinoma. This common hepatic artery angiogram from a 42-year-old woman with hepatitis B shows two distinct areas of "tumor blush" corresponding to underlying hepatocellular carcinoma lesions (*black arrows*) that were treated by TACE. (Courtesy Dr. Nicholas Fidelman, Department of Interventional Radiology, University of California, San Francisco.)

function, ablation of small tumors using probes that convey radiofrequency or microwaves, or by ethanol injection, can provide long-term control, and is sometimes curative.

For patients with early stages of hepatocellular carcinoma by the Milan Criteria (one lesion ≤ 5 cm or up to 3 lesions ≤ 3 cm each, without any evidence of vascular involvement or extrahepatic spread), orthotopic liver transplantation is an approved treatment with potential for long-term survival, achieving survival outcomes similar to patients undergoing transplantation for cirrhosis without cancer present. Extended criteria with parameters including larger tumor sizes may be accepted for transplantation at selected centers, often accompanied by liver-directed treatments such as embolization or ablation to control tumor burden during the period patients are waiting for transplant.[8]

When the hepatocellular carcinoma tumor burden exceeds criteria for transplantation or surgery but remains limited to the liver (BCLC intermediate stage), liver-directed therapies are commonly employed to delay progression and prolong survival, although these treatments are not likely to be curative. Transarterial chemoembolization (TACE) is the most common approach, which delivers embolic material, usually mixed with chemotherapeutic agents, via arterial catheters directly to vascular tumors within the liver. Randomized, clinical trials have demonstrated a survival benefit from TACE for intermediate-stage hepatocellular carcinoma.[A3] The optimal embolic material and chemotherapeutic agents for TACE have not yet been defined. Radioembolization using yttrium-90 bound to glass or resin microspheres is another arterially delivered therapy that may be employed in intermediate-stage hepatocellular carcinoma.[9]

For patients with advanced disease characterized by vascular involvement or extrahepatic spread, systemic therapy with sorafenib, a multikinase inhibitor whose targets include Raf kinase and vascular endothelial growth factor receptor isoforms, significantly prolonged survival compared to placebo in two randomized, phase III clinical trials.[A4][A5] Conventional cytotoxic chemotherapy agents have not produced significant improvements in survival in hepatocellular carcinoma, unlike most other cancers, although a randomized trial of sorafenib combined with the anthracycline chemotherapeutic agent doxorubicin compared to doxorubicin alone suggested improved survival for the combination.[10] Sorafenib therapy is associated with greater absolute prolongation of survival in (1) patients with underlying HCV than in those with underlying HBV infection, (2) Western than in Asian populations, and (3) patients with Child-Pugh A than those with Child-Pugh B or poorer liver function, underscoring the clinical and biologic heterogeneity of hepatocellular carcinoma. In a recently reported phase III trial, sorafenib was found to be superior to sunitinib in overall survival, and also less toxic, in patients with hepatocellular carcinoma.[A6]

Biliary Tract Cancers

Surgical resection is the definitive therapy for patients with localized biliary tract cancers,[11] including gallbladder cancer. For patients with distal cholangiocarcinoma, a Whipple pancreaticoduodenectomy may be required. Liver transplantation for early-stage hilar cholangiocarcinoma after neoadjuvant chemotherapy and/or chemoradiation may be an option at selected centers.[12] In gallbladder cancer, cholecystectomy with en bloc hepatic resection and porta hepatis lymphadenectomy is recommended for patients with a gallbladder mass identified preoperatively on imaging or intraoperatively. A staging laparoscopy may be performed in advance to exclude occult peritoneal carcinomatosis. For patients with early-stage gallbladder cancer diagnosed incidentally on review of surgical pathologic findings after a cholecystectomy performed for benign causes, patients with tumors invading no deeper than the lamina propria (T1a) and negative surgical margins may be treated with observation only. Those found to have invasion to the muscular layer (T1b) or beyond may require additional hepatic resection and lymphadenectomy but should be referred to a center with expertise in the management of biliary tract cancers for evaluation and treatment.[13]

After surgical resection for patients with cholangiocarcinoma and gallbladder cancers, adjuvant therapy with chemotherapy and/or radiation, is often employed in fit patients, although randomized data are lacking. A large meta-analysis including 6710 patients from 20 studies suggested higher survival rates with the use of adjuvant chemotherapy, chemoradiation, or radiation.[14] In contrast, however, a randomized phase III trial comparing adjuvant treatment with gemcitabine or fluorouracil plus folinic acid versus observation in patients with periampullary cancers did not show a benefit for adjuvant therapy in a subset analysis of patients enrolled with a diagnosis of biliary tract cancers, although interpretation was limited by small sample size.[A7]

In patients with advanced biliary tract cancers not amenable to resection, combination chemotherapy with gemcitabine plus cisplatin improved survival compared to gemcitabine alone in a randomized phase III trial.[A8]

END-OF-LIFE CARE

The majority of patients diagnosed with primary hepatobiliary cancers will succumb to their cancer or complications thereof within a relatively short period of time; therefore, palliative care and end-of-life care play an integral role in management. As with most advanced cancers, pain control, treatment of nausea and constipation, and family and social support are essential. Bone metastases may require palliative radiation or stabilization procedures Patients with advanced stages of hepatobiliary cancers, particularly hepatocellular carcinoma, are also at risk for developing complications of end-stage liver disease, such as intractable ascites, jaundice, pruritus, encephalopathy infections, and gastrointestinal bleeding (Chapter 135). Diuretic therapy, therapeutic paracentesis, and endoscopic management of gastrointestinal bleeding may be required. In biliary tract cancers, biliary obstruction and recurrent cholangitis also may require endoscopic or percutaneous biliary drainage and antibiotic therapy for palliation. Hospice referral may be appropriate when patients have progressed on standard anticancer therapies and/or are ineligible for further anticancer therapy because of extent of disease, liver dysfunction, poor performance status, or patient preferences.

In the United States, hepatocellular carcinoma is associated with a high incidence of health disparity, including immigrant status, racial or ethnic minority, and lower socioeconomic status. Providers must have an awareness of cross-cultural issues surrounding disclosure of diagnosis, pain control, use of alternative therapies, and end-of-life care. Pain management in patients with active substance abuse or a history of substance abuse (a risk factor for hepatocellular carcinoma) may be complicated by tolerance and/or dependency. In some cases, patients and caregivers may require providers' reassurance before using opiates or other analgesics for pain control because of concerns about addiction. Palliative care specialists and social workers provide important ancillary services in the end-of-life care for patients with hepatobiliary cancers.

PREVENTION

Screening and surveillance for hepatocellular carcinoma is associated with improved outcomes in selected populations, although a role for routine screening and surveillance has not been established across populations at risk and remains controversial. HBV vaccination programs have also been shown to reduce the incidence of hepatocellular carcinoma. Effective antiviral therapy for underlying HBV or HCV in patients with active viral hepatitis may be associated with a reduced risk for developing hepatocellular carcinoma.[15-17,A9] Prevention and treatment of alcohol-related disorders, obesity, and other conditions associated with nonalcoholic fatty liver disease are appropriate measures to mitigate hepatocellular carcinoma risk factors and minimize ongoing liver injury, although prospective evidence for cancer risk reduction is limited.

There is limited evidence to support preventive measures or screening for biliary tract cancers. For patients with primary sclerosing cholangitis at increased risk for cholangiocarcinoma, periodic screening by noninvasive imaging and serum CA-19-9 marker measurements may be considered, although with limited supporting data.

PROGNOSIS

The prognosis of patients with hepatocellular carcinoma and biliary tract cancers is generally poor. For patients with hepatocellular carcinoma or intrahepatic cholangiocarcinoma, the overall 5-year survival across stages is approximately 20%. Among the minority of patients with hepatocellular carcinoma or intrahepatic cholangiocarcinoma diagnosed with localized stages of disease, the 5-year relative survival rate approaches 30%, although this figure is substantially higher in patients with early stages of disease who undergo curative ablation, surgery, or transplantation, among whom 5-year cause-specific survival rates generally approximate or exceed 60%.[18,19] For patients diagnosed with advanced stages of hepatocellular carcinoma or cholangiocarcinoma, the 5-year survival rate declines to approximately 3%, and the median overall survival remains less than a year with or without treatment.

For patients with gallbladder adenocarcinoma, the 5-year overall survival is approximately 15% across stages, with high rates of metastatic recurrence even among those with resectable disease. The prognosis of patients with rarer types of primary liver cancers such as fibrolamellar hepatocellular carcinoma, hepatic endothelioid hemangioendothelioma, or hepatic angiosarcoma is extremely heterogeneous and generally based on limited data from retrospective case series.

Grade A References

A1. Zhang BH, Yang BH, Tang ZY, et al. Randomized controlled trial of screening for hepatocellular carcinoma. *J Cancer Res Clin Oncol.* 2004;130:417-422.

A2. Yin L, Li H, Li AJ, et al. Partial hepatectomy vs. transcatheter arterial chemoembolization for resectable multiple hepatocellular carcinoma beyond Milan Criteria: a RCT. *J Hepatol.* 2014;61:82-88.

A3. Liu Z, Gao F, Yang G, et al. Combination of radiofrequency ablation with transarterial chemoembolization for hepatocellular carcinoma: an up-to-date meta-analysis. *Tumour Biol.* 2014;35:7407-7413.

A4. Llovet JM, Ricci S, Mazzaferro V, et al. Sorafenib in advanced hepatocellular carcinoma. *N Engl J Med.* 2008;359:378-390.

A5. Cheng AL, Kang YK, Chen Z, et al. Efficacy and safety of sorafenib in patients in the Asia-Pacific region with advanced hepatocellular carcinoma: a phase III randomised, double-blind, placebo-controlled trial. *Lancet Oncol.* 2009;10:25-34.

A6. Cheng AL, Kang YK, Lin DY, et al. Sunitinib Versus Sorafenib in Advanced Hepatocellular Cancer: Results of a Randomized Phase III Trial. *J Clin Oncol.* 2013;31:4067-4075.

A7. Neoptolemos JP, Moore MJ, Cox TF, et al. Effect of adjuvant chemotherapy with fluorouracil plus folinic acid or gemcitabine vs observation on survival in patients with resected periampullary adenocarcinoma: the ESPAC-3 periampullary cancer randomized trial. *JAMA.* 2012;308:147-156.

A8. Valle J, Wasan H, Palmer DH, et al. Cisplatin plus gemcitabine versus gemcitabine for biliary tract cancer. *N Engl J Med.* 2010;362:1273-1281.

A9. Liaw YF, Sung JJ, Chow WC, et al. Lamivudine for patients with chronic hepatitis B and advanced liver disease. *N Engl J Med.* 2004;351:1521-1531.

GENERAL REFERENCES

For the General References and other additional features, please visit Expert Consult at https://expertconsult.inkling.com.

197 TUMORS OF THE KIDNEY, BLADDER, URETERS, AND RENAL PELVIS

DEAN F. BAJORIN

RENAL CELL CARCINOMA

DEFINITION

Cancers of the kidney are a heterogeneous group of neoplasms, the majority of which are of epithelial origin and malignant. Renal cell carcinoma, classically referred to as clear cell carcinoma or hypernephroma, is not a single malignancy. Rather, renal cell carcinoma comprises a group of distinguishable entities, each with a strong relationship between its morphologic and genetic features.[1] The World Health Organization recognizes these biologic and histologic differences in its classification system of kidney cancers (Table 197-1). The metastatic potential depends on the histologic subtype and ranges from the most virulent conventional clear cell carcinomas (65% of total tumors but accounting for 90% of the metastases), to the more indolent papillary and chromophobe carcinomas (25% of the total but only 10% of the metastases), and to the benign oncocytomas (10% of all tumors).

EPIDEMIOLOGY

There will be over 63,000 new cases of kidney and renal pelvis tumors in the United States in 2014, resulting in approximately 13,000 deaths.[2] These cancers represent the sixth most common form of cancer in men and the eighth most common in women. The increase in incidence of renal cell cancers may be in part related to early detection as a consequence of computed tomography (CT) and magnetic resonance imaging (MRI) of the abdomen for other medical conditions. The ratio of males to females is approximately 2 : 1 to 3 : 1, and the incidence is highest in African Americans

TABLE 197-1 CLASSIFICATION OF RENAL CELL NEOPLASMS

BENIGN	MALIGNANT
Oncocytoma	Clear cell (conventional) renal cell carcinoma
Papillary (chromophil) adenoma	Papillary (chromophil) renal cell carcinoma
Metanephric adenoma	Chromophobe renal cell carcinoma
Nephrogenic adenofibroma	Collecting duct carcinoma
	Medullary carcinoma
	Mixed tubular and spindle cell carcinoma
	Renal cell carcinoma, unclassified

Modified from Storkel S, Eble JN, Adlakha K, et al. Classification of renal cell carcinoma: Workgroup No. 1. Union Internationale Contre le Cancer (UICC) and the American Joint Committee on Cancer (AJCC). *Cancer.* 1997;80:987-989.

TABLE 197-2 HISTOLOGIC SUBTYPES, GENETICS, AND SYNDROMES

HISTOLOGIC SUBTYPE	PERCENT	MAJOR GENETIC/ MOLECULAR DEFECTS	OTHER GENETIC/MOLECULAR DEFECTS	ASSOCIATED SYNDROMES
Conventional clear cell	75	LOH 3p Mutation of 3p25 (VHL)	+5q, −8p, −9p, −14q *TP53* mutation, *c-erB-1* oncogene expression	Von Hippel-Lindau Hereditary RCC
Papillary 1	5	*C-Met* gene mutation 7q31	Trisomy 7, −4q, −6q, −9p, −13q, +12, +16, +20	Hereditary papillary renal cell carcinoma (HPRCC)
Papillary 2	10	Fumarate hydratase 1q42	−9p, −11q, −14q, −17p, −21q *PRCC-TFE3* gene fusion	Hereditary leiomyomatosis renal cell carcinoma (HLRCC)
Chromophobe	5	Birt-Hogg Dubé 17p11	−1p, −2p, −6p, −13q, −21q, −Y *TP53* mutation	Birt-Hogg Dubé
Oncocytoma	9.7	Birt-Hogg Dubé 17p11	−1, −Y, 11q Rearrangement	Familial oncocytoma Birt-Hogg Dubé
Collecting duct	0.4	−18, −Y	−1q, −6p, −8p, −11, −13q, −21q *c-erB-1* oncogene expression	Renal medullary carcinoma

Modified from Zambrano N, Histopathology and molecular genetics of renal tumors. *J Urol.* 1999;162:1246-1258.

and lowest in Asians and Pacific Islanders. The mean age at diagnosis is in the sixth to seventh decade of life. Aside from genetic predisposition, risk factors associated with renal cell carcinoma include cigarette smoking, obesity, hypertension, and the use of diuretics. Cigarette smoking has been associated with greater risk in both men and women. The risk may decrease after smoking cessation but requires about 20 years. Obese persons have an increased risk for renal cell carcinoma, and the risk rises with increasing body mass index. Although there is an elevated risk associated with diuretic use, this association is hard to distinguish from the increased risk associated with hypertension. Renal cell carcinoma is more prevalent in patients with preexisting renal conditions such as polycystic kidney disease, horseshoe kidney, and chronic renal failure requiring hemodialysis.

PATHOBIOLOGY

The classification system for renal cell carcinomas permits a better understanding of the cell of origin for the various subtypes and their chromosomal abnormalities (Table 197-2). The classic clear cell carcinoma constitutes approximately 65% of tumors and is believed to be derived from the proximal convoluted tubule. It is generally solitary and well circumscribed, with a golden yellow color resulting from the abundant cytoplasmic lipid. Higher grade tumors contain less lipid and glycogen. Approximately half of the tumors exhibit either a solid or acinar growth pattern characterized by solid sheets of tumor cells accompanied by a rich capillary vascular network. Papillary renal cell carcinomas comprise from 7 to 14% of primary epithelial renal neoplasms. The majority of patients present with unilateral tumors. Multifocality, either bilateral or multifocal lesions in the same kidney, is present in approximately 45% of cases. The majority of these tumors exhibit a broad morphologic spectrum, including papillary, papillary-trabecular, and papillary-solid areas; associated necrosis is a common finding. The classic papillary pattern is characterized by discrete papillary fronds lined by neoplastic epithelial cells and containing a central fibrovascular core, easily recognized on low magnification. These tumors are divided into type 1 and type 2 lesions, based on cytologic features and genetic differences. Chromophobe renal cancers account for 6 to 11% of renal epithelial tumors. Characteristically, these tumors are solitary and discrete but not encapsulated. The typical histologic findings consist of large round-to-polygonal cells with well-defined cell borders and pale basophilic cytoplasm admixed with a smaller population of polygonal cells with eosinophilic cytoplasm. These tumors may be quite large at diagnosis, with resectable tumors reported as big as 23 cm.

Clear cell carcinoma is characterized by the loss of genetic material from the short arm of chromosome 3 (3p) and mutations in the von Hippel-Lindau *(VHL)* gene. In patients with von Hippel-Lindau (VHL) disease, these losses and mutations occur in virtually all cases. The more common sporadic tumors also have somatic mutations and hypermethylation in the same region in approximately 75 to 80% of cases. Conventional clear cell tumors have a mutation in the VHL gene, which is inactivated by a point mutation or by epigenetic gene silencing by promoter methylation. The loss of *VHL*, responsible for ubiquination and degradation of hypoxia-inducible factor (HIF), leads to upregulation of HIF-responsive genes responsible for angiogenesis and cell growth. Two of these upregulated genes are platelet derived growth factor (PDGF) and vascular endothelial growth factor (VEGF), which are pro-angiogenic proteins thought to induce the neovascularity in both primary and metastatic clear cell cancers. Patients with VHL more commonly develop tumors at an earlier age and frequently have multiple tumors. Other tumors associated with the syndrome include central nervous system hemangioblastomas, pancreatic neuroendocrine tumors, pheochromocytomas, retinal angiomas, and epididymal cystadenomas. More recent molecular characterization of renal cell carcinoma shows alterations in genes responsible for maintenance of chromatin states such as *PBRM1*, the SWI/SNF chromatin remodeling complex including *ARID1A* and *SMARCA4*, and members of the PI3K/AKT pathway.[3]

The majority of sporadic papillary renal cell carcinomas are characterized by trisomy of chromosomes 7 and 17 and loss of chromosome Y. Chromophobe renal cell cancers have genetic loss on chromosomes 1 and Y, as well as combined chromosomal losses affecting chromosomes 1, 6, 10, 13, 17, and 21. Hereditary papillary renal cell cancer is a result of germline mutations and activation of the *MET* proto-oncogene, which is located on chromosome 7p. These cells have aberrant hepatocyte growth factor receptors that are unable to deactivate after binding by the growth factor. Somatic *MET* gene amplifications also have been observed in approximately 10% of sporadic papillary renal cancer. Hereditary leiomyomatosis renal cell carcinoma, characterized by alteration of the gene fumarate hydratase, is associated with uterine leiomyomas (more common) or leiomyosarcoma (rare), cutaneous nodules (leiomyomas), and type 2 papillary renal cell carcinoma, which is often solitary and frequently develops metastases. Birt-Hogg Dubé syndrome is a rare disorder predominantly associated with chromophobe renal cancers but in which clear cell and chromophobe/oncocytic tumors can develop. Birt-Hogg-Dubé syndrome is characterized by fibrofolliculomas, pulmonary cysts, pneumothorax, and bilateral renal tumors. The gene associated with Birt-Hogg Dubé syndrome has been mapped to 17p and expresses a novel protein, folliculin, whose function is not yet characterized.

CLINICAL MANIFESTATIONS

Although renal cell carcinoma has a high propensity for metastases and is associated with paraneoplastic syndromes, the majority of patients are asymptomatic at presentation. Historically, renal cell carcinoma was characterized by the presenting triad of hematuria, a palpable mass, and pain in as many as 10% of patients. However, there has been a stage migration resulting in the detection of tumors at earlier stages with the increased use of abdominal imaging for unrelated medical conditions in modern series. Up to 48% of tumors may be discovered in this manner, and less than 5% of patients have a palpable mass at presentation. The more common manifesting symptoms are anemia, weight loss, malaise, and anorexia (Table 197-3). Patients presenting with renal cell carcinoma frequently have associated paraneoplastic syndromes. Hypercalcemia has been observed in approximately 20% of patients and can be due to the secretion of parathyroid hormone, parathyroid hormone–like peptide, and interleukin-6 (IL-6), which have been shown to stimulate osteoclastic bone resorption. Other associated syndromes include hypertension, erythrocytosis (from ectopic erythropoietin production), and the rare Stauffer's syndrome, which is the presence of liver dysfunction without the presence of hepatic metastases; the hepatic dysfunction resolves after surgical resection of the tumor.

TABLE 197-3 PRESENTING SYMPTOMS AND SIGNS OF RENAL CELL CARCINOMA (BOTH LOCALIZED AND METASTATIC DISEASE)

SYMPTOMS AND SIGNS	PERCENT
Anemia	52
Hepatic dysfunction	32
Weight loss	23
Hypoalbuminemia	20
Malaise	19
Hypercalcemia	13
Anorexia	11
Thrombocytosis	9
Night sweats	8
Fever	8
Hypertension	3
Erythrocytosis	4
Chills	3

Modified from Kim HI, Belldegrun AS, Freitas DG, et al. Paraneoplastic signs and symptoms of renal cell carcinoma: implications for prognosis. *J Urol.* 2003;170:1742-1746.

DIAGNOSIS

The complete evaluation for patients with suspected renal cell carcinoma should include a complete blood count, a chemistry profile, a bone scan, and a CT scan of the chest, abdomen, and pelvis. CT is the most reliable method for detecting and staging of renal cell carcinoma. The "ideal" CT scan for renal masses can be divided into four phases, including the pre-contrast images, the arterial phase (~25 seconds after injection), the nephrographic phase (~90 seconds into the injection), and the excretory phase. The most important phases for imaging renal tumors are the pre-contrast and nephrographic images because renal lesions appear low in density in contrast to the uniformly enhanced renal parenchyma. The arterial phase is helpful for identifying renal arteries and small hypervascular masses. The excretory phase aids in assessing the collecting system and the renal pelvis. The CT scan is also helpful in detecting regional metastases, and three dimensional CT imaging is now possible in cases in which nephron-sparing surgery or partial nephrectomy is planned. The additional use of ultrasonography and MRI can help distinguish benign from malignant lesions of the kidney and in treatment planning. Ultrasound is used when distinguishing cysts from solid lesions. MRI has the advantage of imaging tumors in patients with poor renal function in whom intravenous contrast may be contraindicated. MRI is also helpful for delineating any thrombi that may be extending into the renal vein or inferior vena cava, and magnetic resonance angiography can be used to determine the number and location of renal arteries in patients who are candidates for partial nephrectomy. Once the evaluation is complete, the clinical stage is assessed using the (Tumor, Node, Metastasis (TNM) system (Table 197-4).

TABLE 197-4 TNM STAGING OF RENAL CELL CARCINOMA

TUMOR, NODES, AND METASTASES CLINICAL CLASSIFICATION	
Primary Tumor (T)	
TX	Primary tumor cannot be assessed
T0	No evidence of primary tumor
T1	Tumor 7 cm or less in greatest dimension, limited to the kidney
T1a	Tumor 4.0 cm or less in greatest dimension limited to kidney
T1b	Tumor more than 4 cm but not more than 7 cm in greatest dimension; limited to kidney
T2	Tumor more than 7 cm in greatest dimension, limited to kidney
T2a	Tumor more than 7 cm but less than or equal to 10 cm in greatest dimension, limited to the kidney
T2b	Tumor more than 10 cm, limited to the kidney
T3	Tumor extends into major veins or the perinephric tissues but into the ipsilateral adrenal gland and not beyond Gerota's fascia
T3a	Tumor grossly extends into renal vein(or its segmental (muscle containing) branches, or tumor invades perirenal and/or renal sinus fat but not beyond Gerota's fascia
T3b	Tumor grossly extends into the vena cava below the diaphragm
T3c	Tumor grossly extends into vena cava above diaphragm or invades the wall of the vena cava
T4	Tumor invades beyond Gerota's fascia (including contiguous extension into the ipsilateral adrenal gland)
N—Regional Lymph Nodes	
NX	Regional lymph nodes cannot be assessed
N0	No regional lymph node metastasis
N1	Metastasis in regional lymph node(s)
M—Distant Metastasis	
Mx	Distant metastasis cannot be assessed
M0	No distant metastasis
M1	Distant metastasis
STAGE GROUPING	
Stage I	T1 N0 M0
Stage II	T2 N0 M0
Stage III	T1 N1 M0
	T2 N1 M0
	T3a N0 or N1 M0
	T3b N0 or N1 M0
	T3c N0 or N1 M0
Stage IV	T4 N0 M0
	T4 N1 M0
	Any T Any N M1

From *AJCC Staging Manual*, 7th ed. New York: Springer-Verlag; 2010.

TREATMENT

Rx

Localized Disease

The historical standard of care for patients with a renal cell carcinoma is a radical nephrectomy. Kidney cancers routinely selected for radical nephrectomy include large and centrally localized tumors that have effectively replaced the majority of the normal renal parenchyma, tumors associated with regional adenopathy (of benign or malignant etiology), those with inferior vena cava or right atrial extension, and even those in which metastatic disease is evident. Nephrectomy can be performed through a flank, transperitoneal, or transthoracic incision. The ipsilateral adrenal gland is also removed, but a regional lymph node dissection is optional and controversial. The increasing percentage of small tumors has resulted in a corresponding decrease in patients undergoing radical nephrectomy with excellent long-term survival.[4] Both open and laparoscopic approaches can be used for partial nephrectomy to control disease and preserve renal function. Laparoscopic nephrectomy offers a minimally invasive alternative to the classic radical nephrectomy. Partial nephrectomy for tumors of 7 cm or less, whether performed by open or minimally invasive laparoscopic technique, accomplishes rates of local tumor control and survival similar to radical nephrectomy. Partial nephrectomy reduces the risk for renal insufficiency over time.[5] Management with a partial nephrectomy is further supported by the fact that approximately 35% of renal cortical tumors are the indolent papillary or chromophobe carcinomas.

Renal cell carcinomas are resistant to both radiation therapy and cytotoxic chemotherapy; hence, those modalities of treatment have no role in the adjuvant setting after nephrectomy. Immunotherapy agents and approved drugs targeting VEGF or mammalian target of rapamycin (mTOR), beneficial in metastatic disease, have not been shown to affect survival favorably after nephrectomy.

Metastatic Disease

Approximately 30% of patients with renal cell carcinoma present with metastatic disease, and an additional 20 to 30% of patients with surgically resected primary tumors will relapse with metastases. Complications of metastatic disease include pain from either an unresectable primary tumor or skeletal metastases. Radiation therapy is frequently used for palliation of bone metastases and for patients with multiple brain metastases. Palliative nephrectomy is sometimes used to provide symptomatic relief of pain. Surgical resection of the primary tumor is considered a mainstay of treatment even in the patient with metastatic disease and has been shown to extend survival in patients with metastatic disease. Surgical resection of metastatic sites of disease (metastasectomy) may also extend survival and even cure a subset of patients. The patients most likely to benefit from surgical resection of metastatic disease are those with a disease-free interval of greater than 1 year, those with a solitary site of metastasis, and those with lung metastases. Long-term survival has been observed when the solitary site of resection was the lung (up to 45%) and even the brain (up to 20%). Renal cell carcinoma is resistant to most conventional chemotherapy agents, with responses seen in less than 10% of patients.

Immunotherapy with either IL-2 or interferon-α (IFN-α) has been the historical standard treatment for patients with metastatic disease. High-dose intravenous IL-2, a potentially curative therapy, requires a dedicated inpatient setting because of its severe toxicities, including hypotension, pulmonary edema, renal failure, and central nervous system toxicity. However, most toxicities are reversible and complete or partial responses are seen in approximately 15 to 20% of patients; approximately 4% of patients achieve long-term, disease-free survival.[6] IFN-α therapy is less toxic than IL-2 and has an overall response rate of approximately 15%, but long-term survival is not observed. Reversible toxicities of IFN-α treatment include flulike symptoms, including fever, chills, myalgias, mild myelosuppression, and mild hepatic dysfunction.

Renal cell carcinoma has been an ideal candidate for the development of drugs targeting the downstream effects of *VHL* mutations.[7] Clinical trials have shown the benefit of tyrosine kinase inhibitors (TKIs), such as sunitinib,[A1] axitinib,[A2] pazopanib,[A3] and sorafenib,[A4] which block the actions of VEGF and PDGF; all are approved for the treatment of metastatic disease. Common side effects include fatigue, diarrhea, hypertension, and hand-foot syndrome, a condition in which blisters appear at areas of contact. The combination of IFN plus bevacizumab, an antibody that blocks the VEGF receptor, is superior to IFN alone and also has been approved for first-line treatment.[A5] Side effects include hypertension and an increased risk for bleeding. Two drugs targeting the mTOR pathway are also approved for the treatment of renal cell carcinoma both as first-line treatment and for patients whose disease has progressed despite TKI treatment. Temsirolimus, an intravenous mTOR inhibitor, improves survival of patients with untreated poor risk disease (those with more than three risk factors, see later).[A6] Everolimus, an oral mTOR inhibitor, improves the outcomes of patients who have been previously treated with sunitinib, sorafenib, or bevacizumab.[A7] Common side effects include fatigue, skin rash, and mouth sores.

PROGNOSIS

Progression-free survival and overall survival rates for resected nonmetastatic renal cortical tumors substantially differ according to multiple factors including age, size, grade and pathologic state (Figure 197-1, and also E-Figures 197-1, 197-2, and 197-3). The prognosis declines considerably for patients with more advanced disease, with long-term survival seen in only 20% of stage III patients and 5% or less in stage IV patients. Of the more commo histologic subtypes of renal cell carcinoma, the prognosis of clear cell carc noma is less favorable than that of papillary renal cell carcinoma; chromo phobe renal cell carcinoma is the most favorable. For patients with metastat disease, five clinical features associated with shorter survival are low perfo mance status, high lactate dehydrogenase, low hemoglobin, high calcium, an absence of prior nephrectomy. Three strata groups have been defined usin survival data from patients treated with immunotherapy: (1) favorable (zer risk factors) with a median survival of 20 months; (2) intermediate (1 or risk factors), with a median survival of 10 months; and (3) poor (three c more risk factors) with a median survival of 4 months. IL-2 immunotherap and surgical resection of solitary metastases can result in long-term surviv of a small percentage of patients with renal cell cancer. Drugs targeting VEG and the mTOR pathway are now the standard of care for patients with meta static disease.

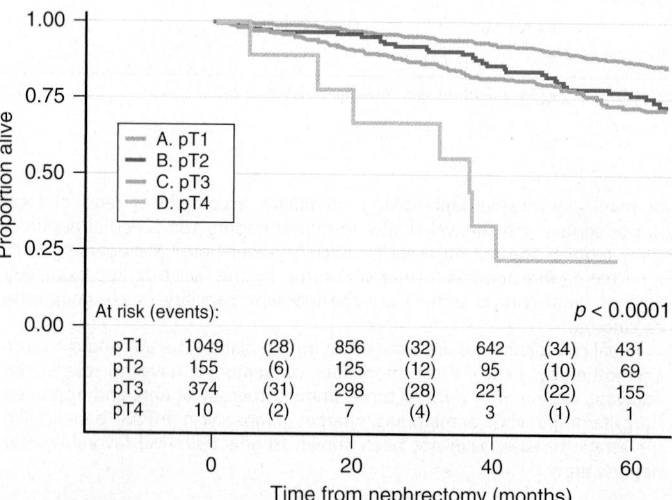

FIGURE 197-1. Overall survival after resection of localized kidney cancer according to pathologic tumor (pT) classification. Curve A indicates pT1 tumors; curve B, pT2 tumors; curve C, pT3 tumors, curve D, pT4 tumors. (The "pT" categories correspond to the "T" categories in the TNM staging categories shown in Table 197-4). (From Russo P, Jang TL, Pettus JA, et al. Survival rates after resection for localized kidneys cancer: 1989-2004. *Cancer*. 2008;113:84-96.)

BLADDER CANCER

DEFINITION

A spectrum of tumors arise from the urothelial lining of the bladder, rena pelvis, ureters, and urethra, of which transitional cell carcinoma is the mos common. The vast majority of tumors arise from the bladder, with a minorit arising from the upper tracts (renal pelvis and ureters) and even less fre quently from the proximal urethra. Although transitional cell cancers posses a variable natural history, they have a proclivity for multifocality, high recur rence rates, and progression to higher pathologic stages. These tumors ar generally grouped into the three broad categories of non–muscle invasive muscle-invasive, and metastatic disease, each of which differs in clinica behavior, prognosis, and primary management. For non–muscle invasiv tumors, the aim is to prevent recurrences and progression to a more advance stage. In muscle-invasive disease, the medical challenge is to integrate th modalities of surgery, chemotherapy, and/or radiation to optimize cure an minimize morbidity. For metastatic disease, chemotherapy is used to palliat the symptoms of most patients, but there is a subset of patients in whic combination chemotherapy may result in long-term cure. Long-term cure i directly related to stage and grade, ranging from 99% for low-grade Ta tumor to up to 15% for metastatic disease.

EPIDEMIOLOGY

An estimated 74,000 new cases of bladder cancer will be diagnosed in th United States in 2014, of which approximately 15,000 patients are expecte to succumb to their disease. The ratio of males to females is 3 : 1, similar i all racial groups; it is the fourth most common cancer in men. The 5-yea survival for all stages is 78%, resulting in a high prevalence (>500,000 peopl in the United States living with bladder cancer); it is twice as prevalent i whites as in African Americans and is less frequently observed in Asians. Th vast majority of patients (90%) are over 50 years of age at diagnosis, with a median age of 73 at diagnosis. There is a lifetime risk of 2.4% of men an women developing bladder cancer.

Carcinogens or their metabolites implicated in the carcinogenesis o bladder cancer are believed to be excreted in the urine, where they can act directly on the urothelial lining. The latency period from initial exposure to the development of cancer is almost 20 years, making it difficult to establish a definitive cause and effect relationship between a putative carcinogen and the development of disease. Cigarette smoking is the leading risk factor for bladder cancer, believed to contribute to half of the cancers in men and one quarter of the cancers in women. A longer duration of exposure is associated with a higher risk than a more intense exposure (in cigarettes/day) over a shorter time period. Overall, smokers have a two- to four-fold higher relative risk for bladder cancer than nonsmokers. Smoking is associated with cellular atypia of the urothelium; individuals who never smoked show atypia in only 4% of cases in contrast to a 50% incidence of atypia in smokers.

Polycyclic aromatic hydrocarbons such as 2-naphthylamine, 4-aminobiphenyl and benzidine, and benzene or exhausts from combustion gases are associated with an increased risk for bladder cancer. Occupations reported to be at higher risk include aluminum workers, dry cleaners, manufacturers of preservatives and polychlorinated biphenyls, and pesticide applicators. Arylamines, also implicated in carcinogenesis, are metabolically activated to electrophilic compounds by N-hydroxylation in the liver by cytochrome P-450 IA2 and detoxified by N-acetylation; studies suggest that individuals with a fast oxidizer and slow acetylator phenotype are at highest risk.

Occupations associated with a higher exposure to arylamines such as workers in the dye, rubber, or leather manufacturing industries are believed to be at higher risk for developing bladder cancer. *Schistosoma haematobium* infection enhances formation of carcinogenic N-nitroso compounds and results in an increased risk for both squamous and transitional cell carcinomas of the bladder. An association has been observed between squamous cell carcinoma (but not transitional cell tumors) and the presence of chronic urinary tract infections seen in paraplegics and patients with chronic bladder stones and indwelling Foley catheters. The chemotherapy agent cyclophosphamide can increase the risk for bladder cancer nine-fold when used chronically, and phenacetin-containing compounds have been implicated in the development of renal pelvis and ureteral tumors.

PATHOBIOLOGY

Urothelial tumors occur anywhere along the urinary tract, including the renal pelvis, ureters, bladder, and the urethra. Over 90% of tumors originate in the bladder, 8% in the renal pelvis, and the remaining 2% originate in the ureter and urethra. Transitional cell carcinomas comprise 90 to 95% of urothelial tumors; squamous cell (keratinizing) tumors (3%), adenocarcinomas (2%), and small cell tumors (1%) are the remainder. Mixed-histology tumors, consisting of predominantly transitional cell carcinoma with areas of squamous, adenocarcinomatous, or neuroendocrine elements are frequently observed. Squamous cell tumors are more frequent in the distal urethra, and adenocarcinomas occur in the embryonal remnant of the urachus on the dome of the bladder and in periurethral tissues. In endemic areas of *S. haematobium* infections (such as Egypt), 40% of tumors are squamous cell carcinomas. Rare tumors of the bladder include lymphoma, sarcoma, and melanoma.

The majority (70-80%) of newly detected bladder cancers are classified as non–muscle invasive tumors and include exophytic papillary tumors confined to the mucosa (Ta), tumors invading the lamina propria (T1), and carcinoma in situ (CIS). Non–muscle invasive bladder tumors are typically graded according to the World Health Organization/International Society of Urologic Pathology (WHO/ISUP) grading system as low-grade and high-grade. If the grading system is not specified, a numeric system can be used: well differentiated (G1), moderately differentiated (G2), poorly differentiated (G3), and undifferentiated (G4). Grading is more important for noninvasive Ta tumors because almost all invasive bladder tumors (T1 or greater) are high grade. Primary CIS, or Tis, without a concurrent Ta or T1 tumor, constitutes 1 to 2% of new bladder cancer cases. More frequently, Tis is found in the presence of multiple papillary tumors, either immediately adjacent to another lesion or involving remote mucosa in the bladder. Tis is, by definition, high-grade disease; it is regarded as a precursor to more invasive tumors because 60% of untreated tumors develop more invasive disease within 5 years. T1 tumors are an aggressive, invasive malignancy. Virtually all T1 tumors are high grade, and 50% have associated Tis. Disease in 50% of patients recurs by 1 year and in 90% within 5 years. A minority of primary tumors at diagnosis is found to invade the muscularis propria (T2), extend to perivesicular fat (T3), or extend into immediately adjacent organs (T4); all primary tumors stage T2 or higher are high grade.

The natural history of a urothelial tumor is to recur either at the same location or at a separate site in the urothelial tract and at the same or a more advanced stage. Several studies support the controversial concept that these recurrences are clonal in origin. The epidermal growth factor receptor (EGFR) is highly expressed (~80%) in bladder cancers; the Her2/Neu growth factor receptor is less frequently expressed (~50-70%). Studies suggest that higher expression of these receptors is associated with a more advanced and/or more aggressive phenotype of disease. Bladder cancer has a very high somatic mutation rate (7.7 per megabase) compared to that of other cancers, exceeded only by lung cancer and melanoma.[8] Epigenetic modifying genes *MLL2, ARID1A, KDM6A,* and *EP300* are significantly mutated in bladder cancer; approximately 75% have at least one inactivating mutation. Genes that regulate the cell cycle are also frequently mutated, including *TP53* in 49% and *RB1* in 13% of tumors. Amplifications of *ERBB2, MDM2,* and *EGFR* occur in a minority of tumors and represent potential therapeutic targets.

CLINICAL MANIFESTATIONS

Hematuria is the manifesting symptom in 80 to 90% of bladder cancer cases, but other patients may present with a urinary tract infection. Individuals over 40 years of age who develop hematuria should have an evaluation for the presence of urothelial cancer that includes urinary cytology, cystoscopy, and imaging of the urinary tract by either an ultrasound or CT scan. Screening of asymptomatic individuals for hematuria increases the probability of diagnosing bladder cancer at an earlier stage but does not improve survival; thus, it is not routinely recommended. Urinary frequency and nocturia may be present either as a consequence of irritative symptoms or a reduced bladder capacity. Pain, when present, typically reflects the location of the bladder tumor. Lower abdominal pain may occur as a result of a bladder mass, and rectal discomfort and perineal pain can result from tumors invading the prostate or pelvis. Tumors of the renal pelvis, ureter, or bladder in which the ureteral orifice is obstructed can cause hydronephrosis, reduced renal function, and flank pain. Patients with more advanced disease can present with anorexia, fatigue, weight loss, or pain from a metastatic bone lesion. The physical examination is frequently unremarkable in patients presenting with bladder tumors because the vast majority of patients have organ-confined tumors.

DIAGNOSIS

The mainstay of bladder cancer diagnosis and staging is the cystoscopic evaluation. The procedure includes examination under anesthesia to determine if a palpable mass (either mobile or not) is present. A nonmobile tumor mass is indicative of disease invading the pelvic sidewall that is unlikely to be resectable. Urine is obtained to evaluate for the presence of malignant cells. A cystoscope is inserted to visually inspect the bladder and detail the size, number, location, and growth pattern (papillary or solid) of all lesions. All visible disease undergoes transurethral resection of the bladder tumor to determine the histologic subtype and depth of invasion. Adequate evaluation, particularly in large tumors that may be invasive, requires that muscle is identified in the pathologic specimen. Repeat biopsy of the resected area is occasionally required to ensure that no muscle invasion is present, because invasion into muscle requires consideration of surgical removal of the bladder rather than endoscopic resection of the tumor. Biopsies from any areas of erythema are performed to assess for CIS. The urethra is inspected during withdrawal of the cystoscope, and biopsies are taken if clinically indicated. Patients with a positive cytologic findings but no apparent tumor within the bladder undergo selective retrograde catheterization of the ureters up to the renal pelvices to determine whether upper tract disease is present.

The decision whether to obtain images of the abdomen and pelvis is based on the cystoscopy results and the pathology of the tumor. Either a CT or magnetic resonance urogram can evaluate the upper urinary tracts, and a CT or MRI may distinguish whether a tumor extends to the perivesical fat (T3), prostate, or vagina (T4) and whether regional lymph nodes are involved (N+). In the case of larger, invasive tumors, the presence or absence of distal metastases can be documented with physical examination, CT of the abdomen and pelvis, a chest radiograph, and radionuclide bone scan.

All patients with carcinoma of the bladder or related sites are staged using the TNM system, advocated by the American Joint Committee on Cancer (AJCC) (Table 197-5). The TNM system categorizes the depth of invasion of the primary tumor, nodal metastases in the pelvis (or retroperitoneum for upper tract disease) on the basis of the number and size of regional nodal involvement, other nonregional lymph node sites, and any visceral sites of disease.

TREATMENT Rx

Non–Muscle Invasive Disease

The standard treatment for non–muscle invasive tumors is a complete endoscopic resection. The majority of patients develop new tumors, 30% of which progress to a higher stage, mandating vigilant surveillance at 3-month intervals with cystoscopy, urine cytology, and repeat transurethral resection when indicated. Additional treatment in the form of adjuvant intravesical therapy depends on the number of lesions, the size, the depth of invasion, and the number of prior tumors in that individual. Prophylactic or adjuvant intravesical therapy is typically instituted in the setting when a patient has shown either a repeated tendency to develop new lesions in the bladder or is at high risk for recurrence or progression de novo. Intravesical therapy is not warranted for the first Ta tumor that is low grade. Instances of high recurrence and progression warranting intravesical therapy include multifocal or large lesions, high-grade papillary lesions, T1 tumors, CIS, or a combination of these. It is never advised for muscle-invasive tumors because agents instilled in the bladder do not penetrate beyond a few layers of cells. After allowing sufficient time for healing after the endoscopic resection, intravesical therapy is most frequently initiated with the immunologic agent bacillus Calmette-Guérin (BCG) weekly for 6 weeks, followed by a prolonged maintenance

TABLE 197-5 TNM DEFINITIONS FOR CANCERS OF THE BLADDER, URETER AND RENAL PELVIS

PRIMARY TUMORS OF THE BLADDER (T)

TX	Primary tumor cannot be assessed
T0	No evidence of primary tumor
Ta	Noninvasive papillary carcinoma
Tis	Carcinoma in situ (i.e., flat tumor)
T1	Tumor invades subepithelial connective tissue
T2	Tumor invades musculearis propria
pT2a	Tumor invades non-muscle invasive muscularis propria (inner half)
pT2b	Tumor invades deep muscularis propria (outer half)
T3	Tumor invades perivesical tissue
pT3a	Microscopically
pT3b	Macroscopically (extravesical mass)
T4	Tumor invades any of the following: prostatic stroma, seminal vesicles, uterus, vagina, pelvic wall, abdominal wall
T4a	Tumor invades the prostatic stroma, uterus, vagina
T4b	Tumor invades the pelvic wall, abdominal wall

REGIONAL LYMPH NODES FOR UROTHELIAL TUMORS OF THE BLADDER (N)

NX	Regional lymph nodes cannot be assessed
N0	No lymph node metastasis
N1	Single regional lymph node metastasis in the true pelvis (hypogastric, obturator, external iliac, or presacral node)
N2	Multiple regional lymph node metastases in the true pelvis (hypogastric, obturator, external iliac, or presacral node)
N3	Lymph node metastasis to the common iliac lymph nodes

PRIMARY TUMORS OF THE URETER AND RENAL PELVIS (T)

TX	Primary tumor cannot be assessed
T0	No evidence of primary tumor
Ta	Papillary noninvasive carcinoma
Tis	Carcinoma *in situ*
T1	Tumor invades subepithelial connective tissue
T2	Tumor invades the muscularis
T3	(For renal pelvis only) Tumor invades beyond muscularis into peripelvic fat or the renal parenchyma
T3	(For ureter only) Tumor invades beyond muscularis into periureteric fat
T4	Tumor invades adjacent organs or through the kidney into perinephric fat

REGIONAL LYMPH NODES FOR UROTHELIAL TUMORS(N) OF URETER AND RENAL PELVIS

NX	Regional lymph nodes cannot be assessed
N0	No regional lymph node metastasis
N1	Metastasis in a single lymph node, ≤2 cm in greatest dimension
N2	Metastasis in a single lymph node, >2 cm but ≤5 cm in greatest dimension; or multiple lymph nodes, ≤5 cm in greatest dimension
N3	Metastasis in a lymph node, >5 cm in greatest dimension

DISTANT METASTASIS FOR ALL UROTHELIAL TUMORS (M)

MX	Distant metastasis cannot be assessed
M0	No distant metastasis
M1	Distant metastasis

AJCC STAGE GROUPINGS FOR BLADDER CANCER

0a	Ta, N0, M0
0is	Tis, N0, M0
I	T1, N0, M0
II	T2a, N0, M0
	T2b, N0, M0
III	T3a, N0, M0
	T3b, N0, M0
	T4a, N0, M0
IV	T4b, N0, M0
	Any T, N1-3, M0
	Any T, any N, M1

AJCC STAGE GROUPINGS FOR CANCER OF THE RENAL PELVIS AND URETER

0a	Ta, N0, M0
0is	Tis, N0, M0
I	T1, N0, M0
II	T2, N0, M0
III	T3, N0, M0
IV	T4, N0, M0
	Any T, N1, M0
	Any T, N2, M0
	Any T, N3, M0
	Any T, any N, M1

From *AJCC Staging Manual*, 7th ed. New York: Springer-Verlag; 2010.

schedule.[9] Occasionally, other chemotherapeutic agents or cytokines are used when BCG is contraindicated. Treatment outcome is assessed at the 3- and 6-month evaluations following treatment to determine whether the bladder has been rendered tumor-free. If disease persists, either a repeat course of BCG treatment or even an immediate cystectomy may be recommended. Bladder toxicity caused by urothelial irritation can occur and includes bladder irritability or spasms, hematuria, and pain on urination. A rare complication of BCG is development of a systemic tuberculosis infection requiring treatment with systemic antituberculosis agents (Chapter 324). BCG is highly effective in eradicating Tis, with 70% of patients disease-free at 1 year and 40% at 10 years. Selected tumors in the ureter or renal pelvis can be managed by ureteroscopic resection, in some cases by instillation of BCG through the renal pelvis, or nephroureterectomy. Tumors of the prostatic urethra are frequently managed by cystoprostatectomy, particularly if a complete resection cannot be accomplished.

Muscle-Invasive Tumors

For patients with tumors infiltrating the muscularis propria, the standard of care in the United States is a radical cystectomy and pelvic lymphadenectomy because of the high incidence of cancer extending into the perivesicular fat or into regional lymph nodes. A prostatectomy is also performed in men; in women, the urethra, uterus, fallopian tubes, ovaries, and anterior vaginal wall are removed. Urinary flow can be directed through either a conduit diversion or a continent reservoir. With a conduit diversion, urine is drained directly from the ureters to a loop of small bowel that is anastomosed to the skin surface with no internal reservoir. Urine is collected in an external appliance. Alternatively, a low-pressure continent reservoir can be created from a detubularized segment of bowel attached to the abdominal wall with a continent stoma that can be self-catheterized at regular intervals. Low-pressure reservoirs also can be anastomosed to the urethra, creating an internal orthotopic neobladder that permits the patient to void via the normal urethra. The standard pelvic lymphadenectomy includes the distal common iliac, external iliac, obturator, and hypogastric nodes; improved survival and decreased local recurrence are associated with an increased number of lymph nodes removed. Complications of cystectomy include recurrent urinary infections, hyperchloremic acidosis, oxalate stones, incontinence, and impotence. Perioperative chemotherapy in addition to surgery is a standard of care for patients with muscle-invasive bladder cancer.[10] Neoadjuvant chemotherapy before cystectomy for muscle-invasive bladder cancer increases survival.[A8] This survival benefit is achieved only with cisplatin-based combinations, which require that the patient has normal renal function and a good performance status. Some physicians prefer immediate cystectomy followed by adjuvant chemotherapy for tumors with a high risk for relapse. However, no evidence from prospective, randomized trials exists to support this approach in contrast to a proved survival benefit from neoadjuvant chemotherapy. Radical cystectomy is effective at providing long-term disease control in 75 to 80% of patients with organ-confined disease; approximately 50% of those with tumors extending into the perivesical tissues; and up to a third of patients with regional lymph node involvement. Metastatic disease in the pelvic lymph nodes despite a normal preoperative CT scan is very frequent. Bilateral pelvic lymph node dissection in addition to cystectomy improves survival.[11] Some patients prefer a nonsurgical, bladder-sparing approach using radiation treatment rather than a cystectomy. Radiation with chemotherapy sensitization is preferred over radiation alone because of better tumor control.[A9] The best candidates for this approach are patients with a solitary early-stage lesion and no evidence of hydronephrosis. This tri-modality treatment for bladder preservation first requires a successful, near-complete transurethral resection of tumor followed by concurrent chemotherapy and radiation. External beam treatments are typically delivered in five daily fractions per week, ranging from 2.0 to 2.5 Gy, to a total treatment dose of approximately 65 Gy. Toxicities include inflammation of the skin, impotence, fatigue, and irritative symptoms from the bladder and bowel; persistent proctitis is rare. In this approach, cystectomy is reserved for patients whose disease failed to achieve complete response. The 5-year disease-free survival with this approach is 50%, with the majority of patients retaining a normally functioning bladder.

Metastatic Disease

Patients with metastatic disease are treated predominantly with chemotherapy. Cisplatin-based chemotherapy is the standard of care, and the two most commonly used regimens are gemcitabine plus cisplatin (GC) and the four-drug regimen of methotrexate, vinblastine, doxorubicin, and cisplatin (MVAC); six cycles of therapy are given over a 6-month period. The most frequently observed toxicities include anemia, thrombocytopenia, neutropenic fever, mucositis, and fatigue. The GC regimen is better tolerated and has less severe toxicities than MVAC. The median survival of patients treated with both regimens is approximately 14 months, and the 5-year survival is 15% or less. Patients with a good performance status and whose metastatic disease is limited to the lymph nodes (i.e., no visceral metastases) have the highest likelihood of response, and a 20 to 33% chance of 5-year disease-free survival.[12] The addition of paclitaxel to the GC doublet has not improved survival for all patients with metastatic bladder cancer but can be integrated with post-chemotherapy surgery in patients with local-regional metastases resulting in long-term cure.[13] Based on the high vascularity of bladder cancer and prior studies suggesting the benefit of bevacizumab which blocks the effects of VEGF, a national intergroup randomized trial is comparing the GC doublet plus either bevacizumab or placebo.[14] Multiple medical conditions preclude the use of cisplatin-based chemotherapy.[15] Patients with impaired renal function are treated with carboplatin-based therapy rather than cisplatin because it is less toxic to the kidneys. Carboplatin plus gemcitabine is the standard of care in patients ineligible for cisplatin.[A10]

PROGNOSIS

Cancer of the urinary bladder is a common but heterogeneous disease. Non–muscle invasive TaG1 lesions, easily treated with endoscopic resection alone, almost never progress. At the other end of the spectrum of non–muscle invasive disease, aggressive transitional cell carcinoma in situ requires intravesical immunotherapy with BCG in addition to endoscopic resection. This intravesical treatment can substantially reduce recurrence and progression, with 5-year disease-free survival rates of 60%. Muscle-invasive disease is most frequently cured with an integrated approach of systemic chemotherapy for micrometastases followed by cystectomy and pelvic lymphadenectomy; cure rates for T2 tumors can be as high as 80% with this multimodality approach. Bladder-sparing approaches associated with an improved quality of life are possible using external beam radiation. Metastatic urinary bladder cancer is a fast-growing and often lethal malignancy; despite aggressive chemotherapy only a small proportion (~15%) of patients are disease-free at 5 years.

CANCERS OF THE RENAL PELVIS AND URETERS

Approximately 10% of transitional cell carcinomas occur in the ureters and the renal pelvis. These tumors can arise either de novo or in the setting of prior tumors; the risk for developing an upper tract tumor in patients with multifocal carcinoma in situ of the bladder approaches 25% by 10 years. These tumors are morphologically similar to the tumors in the bladder and behave in a similar manner. Hematuria is the most common manifesting symptom, although patients with large tumors and/or ureteral obstruction can present with flank pain. A CT scan or MRI is used to stage the extent of primary disease and detect regional metastases. Low-grade tumors can be treated endoscopically, but high-grade tumors are most commonly treated with a nephroureterectomy. In contrast to cystectomy, a regional lymphadenectomy is not routinely performed. In renal pelvis tumors, the ureter is removed in addition to a nephrectomy because of the high risk for multifocal tumors along the entire upper tract and the inability to monitor the ureteral stump with accuracy. Systemic chemotherapy is used for unresectable primary tumors, patients with regional adenopathy, or recurrent tumors. Upper tract transitional cell carcinomas are staged according to the TNM system (see Table 197-5). Treatment for advanced, nonsurgical disease is with chemotherapy; these urothelial tumors have the same sensitivity to chemotherapy as bladder cancer, with similar response rates and 5-year survival rates. Cisplatin-based chemotherapy is used in patients with normal renal function, and carboplatin-based chemotherapy is considered if there is renal insufficiency from obstruction, a prior nephroureterectomy, or medical comorbidity.

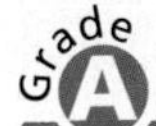

Grade A References

A1. Motzer RJ, Hutson TE, Tomczak P, et al. Sunitinib versus interferon alfa in metastatic renal-cell carcinoma. *N Engl J Med.* 2007;356:115-124.

A2. Rini BI, Escudier B, Tomczak P, et al. Comparative effectiveness of axitinib versus sorafenib in advanced renal cell carcinoma (AXIS): a randomized phase 3 trial. *Lancet.* 2011;378:1931-1939.

A3. Motzer RJ, Hutson TE, Cella D, et al. Pazopanib versus sunitinib in metastatic renal-cell carcinoma. *N Engl J Med.* 2013;369:722-731.

A4. Escudier B, Eisen T, Stadler WM, et al. Sorafenib for treatment of renal cell carcinoma: final efficacy and safety results of the phase III treatment approaches in renal cancer global evaluation trial. *J Clin Oncol.* 2009;27:3312-3318.

A5. Escudier B, Pluzanska A, Koralewski P, et al. AVOREN Trial investigators. Bevacizumab plus interferon alfa-2a for treatment of metastatic renal cell carcinoma: a randomised, double-blind phase III trial. *Lancet.* 2007;370:2103-2111.

A6. Hudes G, Carducci M, Tomczak P, et al. Global ARCC Trial. Temsirolimus, interferon alfa, or both for advanced renal-cell carcinoma. *N Engl J Med.* 2007;356:2271-2281.

A7. Motzer RJ, Escudier B, Oudard S, et al. RECORD-1 Study Group. Efficacy of everolimus in advanced renal cell carcinoma: a double-blind, randomised, placebo-controlled phase III trial. *Lancet.* 2008;372:449-456.

A8. International Collaboration of Trialists. International phase III trial assessing neoadjuvant cisplatin, methotrexate, and vinblastine chemotherapy for muscle-invasive bladder cancer: long-term results of the BA06 30894 trial. *J Clin Oncol.* 2011;29:2171-2177.

A9. James ND1, Hussain SA, Hall E, et al. Radiotherapy with or without chemotherapy in muscle-invasive bladder cancer. *N Engl J Med.* 2012;366:1477-1488.

A10. De Santis M, Bellmunt J, Mead G, et al. Randomized phase II/III trial assessing gemcitabine/carboplatin and methotrexate/carboplatin/vinblastine in patients with advanced urothelial cancer who are unfit for cisplatin-based chemotherapy: EORTC study 30986. *J Clin Oncol.* 2012;30:191-199.

GENERAL REFERENCES

For the General References and other additional features, please visit Expert Consult at https://expertconsult.inkling.com.

198

BREAST CANCER AND BENIGN BREAST DISORDERS

NANCY E. DAVIDSON

Invasive breast cancer, the most common nonskin cancer in women in the United States, will be diagnosed in approximately 232,000 women in 2014 and will result in approximately 40,000 deaths. Incidence and mortality from breast cancer appear to be dropping in the United States and parts of Western Europe. This decline is believed to reflect early detection by screening mammography and widespread use of adjuvant systemic therapy, as well as decreased use of hormone replacement therapy.

BREAST CANCER

EPIDEMIOLOGY AND PATHOBIOLOGY

Multiple risk factors for the development of breast cancer have been identified (Table 198-1). The principal risk factor is gender. Breast cancer is largely a disease of women, although it does occur in men at an incidence of approximately 1% that seen in women. A second critical risk factor is age. Approximately 75% of breast cancer cases in the United States are diagnosed in women older than 50 years of age.

Family history is a third critical risk factor. Approximately 20% of breast cancer occurs in women with a family history of breast cancer; increased risk

TABLE 198-1 RISK FACTORS FOR BREAST CANCER

RISK FACTOR	RELATIVE RISK
Any benign breast disease	1.5
Postmenopausal hormone replacement (estrogen with progestin)	1.5
Menarche at < 12 yr	1.1-1.9
Moderate alcohol intake (two to three drinks/day)	1.1-1.9
Menopause at > 55 yr	1.1-1.9
Increased bone density	1.1-1.9
Sedentary lifestyle and lack of exercise	1.1-1.9
Proliferative breast disease without atypia	2
Age at first birth > 30 yr or nulliparous	2-4
First-degree relative with breast cancer	2-4
Postmenopausal obesity	2-4
Upper socioeconomic class	2-4
Personal history of endometrial or ovarian cancer	2-4
Significant radiation to chest	2-4
Increased breast density on mammogram	2-4
Older age	>4
Personal history of breast cancer (in situ or invasive)	>4
Proliferative breast disease with atypia	>4
Two first-degree relatives with breast cancer	5
Atypical hyperplasia and first-degree relative with breast cancer	10

is associated with a diagnosis of breast cancer in first-degree relatives younger than 50 years. Of breast cancer cases, 5 to 8% occur in high-risk families. Several familial breast cancer syndromes with associated molecular abnormalities have been identified. Chief among them is the breast-ovarian cancer syndrome, which is linked to germline mutations in the breast cancer susceptibility genes, *BRCA1* and *BRCA2*. These mutations are inherited in an autosomal dominant fashion and can therefore be transmitted through the maternal or paternal line. Extensive studies suggest that a germline mutation in either of these genes is associated with a 50 to 85% lifetime risk for developing breast cancer. Testing for *BRCA1* and *BRCA2* mutations is now viewed as a standard option for women with clinical features suggestive of a hereditary breast cancer syndrome; these include multiple family members with early-onset breast or ovarian cancer, bilateral breast cancer, or Ashkenazi Jewish heritage. Careful counseling about the implications of a positive or negative test and about the limitations of testing is a prerequisite for testing.

Other hereditary cancer syndromes (Chapter 181) include germline loss-of-function mutations in *PALB2*,[1] the Li-Fraumeni syndrome (which is linked with germline mutations in the *p53* tumor suppressor gene), and Cowden syndrome (which is associated with inherited mutations in the *PTEN* gene). Finally, in addition to these high-penetrance genetic susceptibility syndromes, recent results from genome-wide association studies have identified a number of low-penetrance genetic associations, including single nucleotide polymorphisms in a variety of genes. If or how to incorporate these low-penetrance traits into clinical practice remains to be established. Whole-genome sequencing of breast cancers is exposing the scope of tumor diversity and helping to pinpoint avenues for precise diagnostics and targeted therapy.[2]

Reproductive risk factors include early menarche, late menopause, nulliparity, and late first pregnancy. In aggregate, these factors result in prolonged estrogen exposure of the breast. The emerging association between postmenopausal obesity and breast cancer likely reflects estrogen exposure as well. Certain types of breast pathology, including atypical hyperplasia and lobular carcinoma in situ, are also associated with increased risk. The possibility that increased breast density as assessed by mammography is a risk factor has also been raised. Finally, much interest has focused on the possibility that exogenous environmental factors predispose to breast cancer. Among the factors that appear to enhance breast cancer risk are ionizing radiation during adolescence, prolonged use of hormone replacement therapy, ongoing use of oral contraceptives, and alcohol consumption. Large studies have failed to show any convincing association between exposure to estrogenic pesticides or a high-fat diet and breast cancer.

CLINICAL MANIFESTATIONS

Breast cancer usually manifests as a mammographic abnormality or a physic change in the breast, including a mass or asymmetrical thickening, nippl discharge, or skin or nipple changes. Two unusual clinical manifestation include Paget disease of the nipple and inflammatory breast cancer. Th former is a form of adenocarcinoma involving the skin and ducts and i manifested as nipple excoriation. The latter is recognized as a constellation c redness, warmth, and edema that often reflects tumor cell infiltration c dermal lymphatics of the breast; it should not be mistaken for simpl mastitis.

Nipple discharge may be associated with breast malignancy. Althoug milky discharge is seldom associated with a malignant diagnosis, patient with a clear or bloody nipple discharge require breast examination and mam mography and often excisional biopsy of any suspicious area. Ductograph and sometimes ductoscopy may be used to identify the inciting lesion. bloody discharge is frequently caused by an intraductal papilloma.

Breast pain is common, especially as a premenstrual symptom in premeno pausal women. But it may also be associated with an underlying malignancy Patients with localized noncyclic breast pain should undergo breast examina tion and bilateral mammography. If these are normal, ultrasound or magneti resonance imaging (MRI) may be used to exclude the small possibility of malignancy.

DIAGNOSIS

Diagnostic evaluation is generally triggered by suspicious findings on screening mammogram or detection of a palpable breast abnormality by th patient or health care provider. For both clinically occult and clinically appar ent lesions, pathologic evaluation is mandatory to establish a diagnosis Today, fine-needle aspiration and core needle biopsy have replaced incisiona or excisional biopsy as the standard diagnostic measures. These procedures can be performed in the office in patients with suspicious palpable lesions For women with nonpalpable lesions, biopsy guided by mammography ultrasonography, or MRI is now standard. Stereotactic- or ultrasound-guided core needle biopsies are almost as accurate as, and associated with lowe complication rates than, open surgical biopsy. These technologies permit ar accurate diagnosis that can be followed by definitive treatment planning. It is axiomatic, however, that further evaluation must be undertaken for suspicious lesions that give an equivocal diagnosis after needle aspiration or core biopsy. Finally, bilateral breast imaging is always recommended to identify any unsuspected lesions in the contralateral breast that may also require evaluation.

Staging and Prognostic and Predictive Markers

Although staging originally reflected the clinical assessment of tumor size, nodal status, and evidence of metastatic disease, pathologic staging is the most accurate estimate of tumor involvement and prognosis. The staging system for breast cancer was revised in 2010 (Tables 198-2 and 198-3).

Most patients with breast cancer present with stage I or II disease in the absence of symptoms. In these patients, laboratory studies can be limited to blood counts, chemistry panel, and chest radiograph, and more extensive radiologic evaluation is not warranted because of low yield. In contrast, women with clinical evidence of stage III or IV disease should undergo more intensive evaluation of common sites for metastases, including lung, liver, and bone, through computed tomography and radionuclide scanning.

The two most important determinants of prognosis for early-stage breast cancer are pathologic lymph node status and tumor size. Other factors that contribute to prognosis are the expression of the estrogen receptor-α (ER), progesterone receptor (PR), and HER2 proteins; these are conventionally measured by immunohistochemistry (IHC), although in situ hybridization (ISH) for *HER2* gene amplification is also employed. Poor prognosis is associated with high lymph node burden, poor histologic grade, large tumor size, absence of ER and PR expression, and overexpression of HER2.

Recently, the focus has been on the development of predictive markers to guide selection of therapy. The three established predictive markers for breast cancer are ER, PR, and HER2, and these should be routinely evaluated in every invasive cancer. Many tumors that express ER or PR, or both, are responsive to endocrine therapy, whereas those that lack ER and PR expression seldom respond to such therapy. Overexpression of the HER2 protein by IHC or *HER2* gene amplification by ISH is associated with response to the HER2-targeted therapies. Evidence that links expression of ER, PR, or HER2 to chemotherapy efficacy is equivocal.

TABLE 198-2 AMERICAN JOINT COMMITTEE ON CANCER TUMOR, NODE, METATASIS STAGING SYSTEM FOR BREAST CANCER

TNM STAGING

PRIMARY TUMOR (T)

Definitions for classifying the primary tumor (T) are the same for clinical and pathologic classification. If the measurement is made by the physical examination, the examiner uses the major headings (T1, T2, or T3). If other measurements, such as mammographic or pathologic measurements, are used, the subsets of T1 can be used. Tumors should be measured to the nearest 0.1-cm increment.

TX	Primary tumor cannot be assessed
T0	No evidence of primary tumor
Tis	Carcinoma in situ
Tis (DCIS)	Ductal carcinoma in situ
Tis (LCIS)	Lobular carcinoma in situ
Tis (Paget)	Paget disease of the nipple with no tumor

Note: Paget disease associated with a tumor is classified according to the size of the tumor.

T1	Tumor 2 cm or less in greatest dimension
T1mic	Microinvasion 0.1 cm or less in greatest dimension
T1a	Tumor more than 0.1 cm but not more than 0.5 cm in greatest dimension
T1b	Tumor more than 0.5 cm but not more than 1 cm in greatest dimension
T1c	Tumor more than 1 cm but not more 2 cm in greatest dimension
T2	Tumor more than 2 cm but not more than 5 cm in greatest dimension
T3	Tumor more than 5 cm in greatest dimension
T4	Tumor of any size with direct extension to (a) chest wall or (b) skin, only as described below
T4a	Extension to chest wall, not including pectoralis muscle
T4b	Edema (including peau d'orange) or ulceration of the skin of the breast or satellite skin nodules confined to the same breast
T4c	Both T4a and T4b
T4d	Inflammatory carcinoma

REGIONAL LYMPH NODES (N)

Clinical

NX	Regional lymph nodes cannot be assessed (e.g., previously removed)
N0	No regional lymph node metastasis
N1	Metastasis to movable ipsilateral axillary lymph node(s)
N2	Metastases in ipsilateral axillary lymph nodes fixed to one another (matted) or in clinically detected ipsilateral internal mammary nodes in the absence of clinically evident axillary lymph node metastasis
N2a	Metastases in ipsilateral axillary lymph nodes fixed to one another (matted) or to other structures
N2b	Metastases only in clinically apparent ipsilateral internal mammary nodes and in the absence of clinically evident axillary lymph node metastasis
N3	Metastasis in ipsilateral infraclavicular lymph node(s), with or without axillary lymph node involvement, or in clinically apparent ipsilateral internal mammary lymph node(s) and in the presence of clinically evident axillary lymph node metastasis; or metastasis in ipsilateral supraclavicular lymph node(s), with or without axillary or internal mammary lymph node involvement
N3a	Metastasis in ipsilateral infraclavicular lymph node(s)
N3b	Metastasis in ipsilateral internal mammary lymph node(s) and axillary lymph node(s)
N3c	Metastasis in ipsilateral supraclavicular lymph node(s)

Pathologic (pN)

pNX	Regional lymph nodes cannot be assessed (e.g., previously removed or not removed for pathologic study)
pN0	No regional lymph node metastasis histologically
pN0(i–)	No regional lymph node metastasis histologically, negative IHC
pN0(i+)	Malignant cells in regional lymph node(s) 0.2 mm or less (detected by IHC including isolated tumor cell(s)
pN0(mol–)	No regional lymph node metastasis histologically, negative molecular findings (RT-PCR)
pN0(mol+)	No regional lymph node metastasis by IHC or histology, positive molecular findings (RT-PCR)
pN1	Metastasis in 1 to 3 axillary lymph nodes, or in internal mammary nodes with microscopic disease detected by sentinel lymph node dissection, but not clinically detected
pN1mi	Micrometastasis (greater than 0.2 mm and/or more than 200 cells, none greater than 2.0 mm)
pN1a	Metastasis in 1 to 3 axillary lymph nodes with a least 1 metastasis greater than 2 mm
pN1b	Metastasis in internal mammary nodes with micrometastases or macrometastases detected by sentinel lymph node dissection but not clinically detected
pN1c	Metastasis in 1 to 3 axillary lymph nodes and in internal mammary nodes with micrometastases or macrometastases detected by sentinel lymph node dissection, but not clinically detected
pN2	Metastasis in 4 to 9 axillary lymph nodes or in clinically detected internal mammary lymph nodes in the absence of axillary lymph node metastasis
pN2a	Metastasis in 4 to 9 axillary lymph nodes (at least 1 tumor deposit greater than 2.0 mm)
pN2b	Metastasis in clinically detected internal mammary lymph nodes in the absence of axillary lymph node metastasis
pN3	Metastasis in 10 or more axillary lymph nodes, or in infraclavicular lymph nodes, or in clinically detected ipsilateral internal mammary lymph nodes in the presence of 1 or more positive axillary lymph nodes; or in more than 3 axillary lymph nodes and in internal mammary lymph nodes with micrometastases or macrometastases detected by sentinel lymph node biopsy but not clinically detected; or in ipsilateral supraclavicular lymph nodes
pN3a	Metastasis in 10 or more axillary lymph nodes (at least 1 tumor deposit greater than 2.0 mm), or metastasis to the infraclavicular lymph nodes
pN3b	Metastasis in clinically detected ipsilateral internal mammary lymph nodes in the presence of 1 or more positive axillary lymph nodes; or in more than 3 axillary lymph nodes and in internal mammary lymph nodes with micrometastases or macrometases detected by sentinel lymph node dissection, but not clinically detected
pN3c	Metastasis in ipsilateral supraclavicular lymph nodes

DISTANT METASTASIS (M)

MX	Distant metastasis cannot be assessed
M0	No clinical or radiographic evidence of distant metastasis
cM0(+)	No clinical or radiographic evidence of distant metastases but deposits of molecularly or microscopically detected tumor cells in blood, bone marrow, or nonregional nodes without symptoms or signs of metastases
M1	Distant detectable metastases as determined by classic clinical and radiologic means and/or histologically proved greater than 0.2 mm

STAGE GROUPING

Stage 0	Tis	N0	M0
Stage IA	T1	N0	M0
Stage IB	T0 or T1	N1mi	M0
Stage IIA	T0	N1	M0
	T1	N1	M0
	T2	N0	M0
Stage IIB	T2	N1	M0
	T3	N0	M0
Stage IIIA	T0	N2	M0
	T1	N2	M0
	T2	N2	M0
	T3	N1	M0
	T3	N2	M0
Stage IIIB	T4	N0	M0
	T4	N1	M0
	T4	N2	M0
Stage IIIC	Any T	N3	M0
Stage IV	Any T	Any N	M1

Note: Stage designation may be changed if postsurgical imaging studies show distant metastases, provided that the studies are carried out within 4 months of diagnosis in the absence of disease progression and provided that the patient has not received neoadjuvant therapy.

IHC = immunohistochemistry; RT-PCR = reverse-transcriptase polymerase chain reaction; TNM = tumor, node, metastasis.

TABLE 198-3 TUMOR, NODE, METASTASIS (TNM) STAGE AND SURVIVAL

STAGE	TNM CATEGORY*	RECURRENCE FREE AT 10 YEARS (NO SYSTEMIC ADJUVANT THERAPY) (%)
0	TisN0M0	98
I	T1N0M0	80 (all stage I patients)
	T ≤ 1 cm	90%
	T > 1-2 cm	80-90
IIA	T0N1M0; T2N0M0	60-80
IIA	T1N1M0	50-60
IIB	T2 N1M0	5-10 worse than IIA and based on node status
IIB	T3N0M0	30-50
IIIA	T0 or T1 or T2N2M0; or T3N1 or N2M0	10-40
IIIB	T4N0 or N1 or N2M0	5-30
IIIC	Any T, N3M0	15-20
IV	Any T, any NM1	<5

*See Table 198-2 for TNM definitions.
TNM = tumor, node, metastasis.

TABLE 198-4 CARCINOMA IN SITU: DUCTAL VERSUS LOBULAR

FEATURE	LOBULAR CARCINOMA IN SITU	DUCTAL CARCINOMA IN SITU
Age	Younger	Older
Palpable mass	No	Uncommon
Mammographic appearance	Not detected on mammography	Microcalcifications, mass
Immunophenotype	E-cadherin negative	E-cadherin positive
Usual manifestation	Incidental finding on breast biopsy	Microcalcifications on mammography or breast mass
Bilateral involvement	Common	Uncertain
Risk and site of subsequent breast cancer	25% risk for invasive breast cancer in either breast over remaining lifespan	At site of initial lesion; 0.5% risk/yr of invasive breast cancer in opposite breast
Prevention	Consider tamoxifen or raloxifene or aromatase inhibitor	Consider tamoxifen or raloxifene if estrogen receptor positive
Treatment	Yearly mammography and breast examination	Lumpectomy ± radiation; mastectomy for large or multifocal lesions

Modern molecular techniques have provided further insight into molecular classification of breast cancer. Integrating data derived from analysis by genomic DNA copy number arrays, DNA methylation, exome sequencing, messenger RNA arrays, microRNA sequencing, and reverse-phase protein arrays, multiple genetically distinct types of breast cancer have been identified.[3,4] Transcriptional profiling has suggested that breast cancers can be divided into at least four molecular subsets: luminal A and B, HER2, and basal. The luminal subtypes frequently express ER, but luminal A appears to be associated with a better prognosis and higher likelihood of response to endocrine therapy than luminal B. The basal subtype is dominated by tumors that lack expression of ER, PR, and HER2—the so-called triple-negative breast cancer that lacks a readily identified molecular target. Multigene assays that evaluate these gene expression patterns are under investigation, and several multigene assays are available in clinical practice. One such assay, Oncotype Dx, may assist in the identification of women with early-stage steroid receptor–positive breast cancer who would benefit from the addition of chemotherapy to tamoxifen. A second assay, Mammaprint, may be useful to identify young women with breast cancer with poor prognosis. A number of other assays are under development, and both the Oncotype Dx and Mammaprint assays are the subject of large randomized trials to refine the conditions for their optimal use.

TREATMENT Rx

Local Treatment of Early-Stage Breast Cancer

In Situ Carcinoma

Thanks to heightened breast cancer awareness and use of screening mammography, in situ carcinomas now account for 20 to 25% of newly diagnosed cases of breast cancer (Table 198-4). Most of these are ductal carcinoma in situ (DCIS). These lesions are associated with approximately a 30% risk for subsequent invasive breast cancer in the same breast. The risk for metastatic breast cancer with a diagnosis of DCIS is extremely small. As a consequence, management decisions are centered on the involved breast, and axillary lymph node evaluation is not routinely performed. Total mastectomy, the traditional therapy, has a high likelihood of cure, but studies suggest that breast conservation is appropriate for many women with DCIS. The major contraindications include poor cosmesis, extensive disease, or patient preference. Several models have suggested that size and grade of lesion and surgical margin status are important determinants of local outcome. Excision to obtain tumor-free margins is critical. Careful mammographic examination of the specimen and postexcision mammography of the breast are crucial to confirm that the DCIS has been adequately excised. A large randomized trial showed that radiotherapy plus lumpectomy decreased the likelihood of in situ or invasive recurrence compared with lumpectomy alone. Other data sets suggest that some women with favorable histologic findings who are willing to undergo close surveillance are candidates for local excision alone. In addition, the use of tamoxifen for 5 years can reduce ipsilateral breast cancer recurrence and contralateral breast cancer diagnosis by approximately 50%.

Controversy continues over whether lobular carcinoma in situ (LCIS) is truly a malignant lesion. LCIS is usually an incidental finding on a breast biopsy done for other indications, and it appears to be associated with a 25% risk for development of invasive breast cancer in either breast. Women with LCIS are generally managed expectantly with regular breast examination and mammography. Bilateral total mastectomy is sometimes considered for women with LCIS who have other risk factors or extreme anxiety. Finally, these women are candidates for tamoxifen or raloxifene or an aromatase inhibitor as a risk-reduction strategy based on the results of several large breast cancer chemoprevention trials.

Invasive Breast Cancer

Surgery

Although radical mastectomy (removal of the breast, axillary contents, and underlying chest musculature) was the mainstay for breast cancer treatment for many years, it is seldom performed today. Multiple randomized trials have consistently shown that breast conservation therapy (BCT) with lumpectomy plus radiotherapy provides identical survival rates to modified radical mastectomy (removal of the breast and lymph nodes) for women with stages I and II breast cancer. Medical contraindications to BCT include multifocal disease, previous radiotherapy, ongoing pregnancy that precludes the timely use of radiotherapy, poor cosmesis, and patient preference. Although the number of patients who receive BCT has increased substantially, there are wide geographic differences within the United States. Patients who undergo mastectomy should be counseled about the availability of a number of autologous tissue and implant options for reconstruction, either at the time of surgery or any time thereafter.

Because the likelihood of distant micrometastatic spread is highly correlated with the number of pathologically involved axillary lymph nodes, axillary dissection has traditionally been used to provide prognostic information. A drive toward limiting axillary surgery to minimize the incidence of postoperative lymphedema (see later) has led to the development of sentinel node techniques. A radioactive tracer, blue dye, or both are injected into the area around the primary breast tumor. The injected substance tracks rapidly to the dominant axillary lymph node—the sentinel node—which can be located and removed by the surgeon. If the sentinel node is tumor free, the remaining nodes are likely to be tumor free as well and no further axillary surgery is required. Currently, women with palpable axillary nodes and those with more extensively involved sentinel nodes are counseled to undergo axillary dissection. For women with small tumors and a clinically negative axilla, large randomized trials of sentinel node management and traditional axillary dissection suggest similar outcomes.[A1] Data suggest that it may also be possible to omit further axillary surgery for patients with a low burden of disease in sentinel nodes.

Adjuvant Radiotherapy

Radiotherapy has been a cornerstone in breast conservation therapy because women who undergo lumpectomy alone have a breast cancer recurrence rate of up to 40%, whereas the rate of recurrence is less than 10% with whole-breast radiotherapy. As a result, radiotherapy to the conserved breast reduces the breast cancer death rate by approximately 15%.[A2] Attempts to identify women whose tumors are so favorable that radiotherapy can be withheld are ongoing. One large trial suggested that women older than 70 years with small ER-positive tumors who receive tamoxifen gain little with radiotherapy. Current research is also focused on the possibility that radiotherapy can be delivered safely and effectively to a smaller field (partial breast radiotherapy) or over a shorter period.

The role of postmastectomy radiotherapy continues to be a matter of debate. Based on the results of individual randomized trials and a meta-analysis suggesting a survival advantage, many radiation oncologists recommend postmastectomy radiation to women with more than three involved nodes and discuss its use for those with involvement of one to three nodes, in whom a smaller benefit is seen.[A3]

Adjuvant Systemic Therapy for Early-Stage Breast Cancer

Adjuvant systemic therapy is defined as the use of chemotherapy, endocrine therapy, or biologic therapy, or a combination of these, after definitive local therapy for early breast cancer. Its goal is to suppress or eradicate clinically occult micrometastases. Because current testing does not permit the definitive identification of the patient with micrometastases, recommendations for adjuvant systemic therapy are based on menopausal status, lymph node status, tumor size, and the extent of expression of the ER, PR, and HER2 proteins in breast cancer cells. The treatment algorithms that are currently used are the result of more than 50 years of clinical trials; the results of these trials have been compiled in sequential overview analyses that have evaluated the worldwide experience with use of endocrine therapy and chemotherapy.[A4][A5] These analyses have shown that adjuvant therapy results in a proportional reduction in risk for recurrence across all patients regardless of risk for recurrence; this implies that the absolute benefit of adjuvant systemic therapy is greatest for individuals with the greatest risk for recurrence. Tools to assist the clinician and patient to make decisions about the use of adjuvant therapy include guidelines based on evidence and expert consensus such as the National Comprehensive Care Network (NCCN) and St. Gallen conference guidelines, as well as web-based algorithms such as Adjuvant Online (Table 198-5).[5]

Adjuvant Endocrine Therapy

Tamoxifen (20 mg/day for 5 years) has been the most widely used endocrine therapy. It improves outcomes in women of all ages with ER- or PR-positive breast cancer. Its side-effect profile includes an increased risk for thromboembolic events and uterine cancer, especially in postmenopausal women, because of its estrogen agonist properties. Potential benefits include promotion of bone density and lowering of cholesterol. An active area of research is the effects on outcome of altered activity of the tamoxifen metabolizing enzyme, CYP2D6, by either coadministration of pharmacologic inhibitors or by single-nucleotide polymorphism variants in the *CYP2D6* gene.

In recent years, the role of estrogen deprivation has been the subject of intense scrutiny—ovarian suppression or ablation for premenopausal women and aromatase inhibition for postmenopausal women. Ovarian ablation through surgery or radiotherapy is the oldest form of systemic therapy for breast cancer. More recent work has focused on the use of luteinizing hormone–releasing hormone (LHRH) agonists as a means of effecting a temporary and reversible ovarian suppression. Two large meta-analyses sought to define the role of these approaches. A meta-analysis of trials addressing the efficacy of LHRH agonists in women with early-stage ER-positive breast cancer suggested the following: (1) monotherapy with LHRH agonist has significant activity; (2) the efficacy of LHRH monotherapy is similar to that of certain chemotherapy regimens; and (3) LHRH agonists appear to add benefit to adjuvant chemotherapy, especially in women younger than 40 years, who are less likely than older women to become postmenopausal as a consequence of adjuvant chemotherapy. Unfortunately, these trials did not routinely include tamoxifen because its value in premenopausal breast cancer was recognized only after accrual for these ovarian suppression studies was completed. In sum, however, it appears that ovarian ablation or suppression is a viable strategy for premenopausal women with steroid receptor–positive breast cancer.

In premenopausal women, the combination of LHRH agonist plus aromatase inhibitor may be better than LHRH agonist plus tamoxifen. For example, in a recent randomized trial of hormone-receptor-positive early breast cancer in premenopausal women, adjuvant treatment with the aromatase inhibitor exemestane plus ovarian suppression, as compared with tamoxifen plus ovarian suppression, significantly reduced recurrence.[A6]

In postmenopausal women, the primary source of estrogen is the conversion of androgens synthesized by the adrenal glands to estrogen through the activity of CYP19 or aromatase in peripheral tissues such as mammary and adipose tissues. The aromatase inhibitors (anastrozole, letrozole, and exemestane) specifically inhibit this conversion, leading to further estrogen deprivation in older women. Randomized trials have shown that efficacy of aromatase inhibitors is similar or superior to that of tamoxifen and that these drugs have an acceptable side-effect profile.[A7] Multiple trials have compared monotherapy with tamoxifen, aromatase inhibitor, or sequential therapy; in aggregate, they suggest that the use of an aromatase inhibitor at some point should be considered for most postmenopausal women with steroid receptor–positive

TABLE 198-5 ADJUVANT TREATMENT GUIDELINES FOR PATIENTS WITH EARLY-STAGE INVASIVE BREAST CANCER*

PATIENT GROUP*	TREATMENT
FAVORABLE HISTOLOGY (TUBULAR OR COLLOID)	
ER- and/or PR-Positive Breast Cancer	
<1 cm and pN0 or pN1mi	No adjuvant therapy
1-2.9 cm and pN0 or PN1mi	Consider adjuvant hormonal therapy†
≥3 cm or node-positive	Adjuvant hormonal therapy ± adjuvant chemotherapy†
ER- and PR-Negative Breast Cancer	
<1 cm and pN0	No adjuvant therapy
1-2.9 cm	Consider adjuvant chemotherapy
≥3 cm or node-positive	Adjuvant chemotherapy
HORMONE RECEPTOR–POSITIVE (ER- AND/OR PR-POSITIVE) BREAST CANCER	
Lymph Nodes Negative	
≤0.5 cm	Consider adjuvant hormonal therapy
0.6-1.0 cm well differentiated and no unfavorable features‡	Consider adjuvant hormonal therapy†
>1 cm	Adjuvant hormonal therapy ± adjuvant chemotherapy†
Lymph Nodes Positive	
	Adjuvant hormonal therapy + adjuvant chemotherapy
HORMONE RECEPTOR–NEGATIVE (ER- AND PR-NEGATIVE) BREAST CANCER	
≤0.5 cm and pN0	No adjuvant therapy
0.6-1.0 cm and pN0 or pNmi	Consider chemotherapy
>1 cm or lymph-node positive	Adjuvant chemotherapy
HER2 POSITIVE	
	Trastuzumab should be added to the suggested treatment above for all node-positive patients and considered for pN0 tumors that are > 5 mm

Modified from National Comprehensive Cancer Network Guidelines. Available at http://www.nccn.org.
*Data are insufficient to make chemotherapy recommendations for patients 70 years and older. Treatment should be individualized for these patients based on life expectancy and comorbidity.
†In ER-positive or PR-positive patients, decisions regarding the added value of chemotherapy in addition to hormonal therapy alone in N0 patients can be aided by the use of the Oncotype Dx assay to assess recurrence score.
‡Unfavorable characteristics include high-grade tumor, blood vessel or lymphatic invasion by tumor, and high tumor proliferation rate (high S phase by flow cytometry or high Ki-67 value by immunohistochemistry) or HER2-positive status or high recurrence score.
ER = estrogen receptor; PR = progesterone receptor.

invasive breast cancer.[6] Side effects include postmenopausal symptoms, osteoporosis and fractures, and arthralgias. Aromatase inhibitors are not useful for receptor-negative breast cancer, nor should they be used as monotherapy in premenopausal women. The simultaneous administration of tamoxifen plus aromatase inhibitor does not improve outcome over aromatase inhibitor alone.

Duration of endocrine therapy appears to be quite important. Direct evidence suggests that at least 5 years of adjuvant endocrine therapy is associated with better outcomes than shorter periods. Two large, recently reported trials suggest that 10 years of tamoxifen is better than 5 years.[A8] Optimal duration of aromatase inhibitor therapy is under study.

Adjuvant Anti-HER2 Therapy

Increased understanding of growth and death pathways of breast cancer led to the identification of critical nonendocrine pathways that are potential targets for therapy. The transmembrane HER2/neu protein is overexpressed in approximately 20% of breast cancers, generally because of gene amplification. The efficacy and safety of the monoclonal antibody trastuzumab in the treatment of women with HER2-overexpressing metastatic breast cancer laid the foundation for several adjuvant trials that in aggregate showed that the addition of 1 year of trastuzumab to chemotherapy reduced the risk for recurrence by approximately 50% in women with high-risk HER2-positive early breast cancer.[A9] Thus, use of trastuzumab is considered for many women with

HER2-positive tumors. More recent trials suggest that 1 year of therapy is better than 6 months and 2 years is no better than 1 year.[A10] Important questions remain regarding long-term risks and benefits, the use of trastuzumab in the absence of chemotherapy, and the role of other anti-HER2 agents such as lapatinib, pertuzumab, or trastuzumab, and emtansine in addition to or in place of trastuzumab.

Adjuvant Chemotherapy

Individual trials and the Early Breast Cancer Trialists Collaborative Group meta-analysis have shown the benefit of adjuvant chemotherapy. Benefit varies by age and nodal status such that, in the meta-analysis, the absolute benefit is greatest in women younger than 50 years, in whom 15-year breast cancer mortality decreased from 42% to 32%, whereas it decreased from 50% to 47% for women aged 50 to 69 years.

These trials established several principles that guide chemotherapy use. Combination therapy appears to be more effective than single-agent chemotherapy. Effective agents include anthracyclines, taxanes, antimetabolites, and cyclophosphamide. Randomized trials demonstrated that 3 to 6 months of therapy is preferred over longer durations. Dose reduction below the standard level is associated with inferior outcome, but dose escalation through the use of colony-stimulating factors or autologous stem cells support leads to excess toxicity without improved outcome. Regimens that use colony-stimulating factors to accelerate the schedule of chemotherapy administration have been more successful.

Increased use of adjuvant chemotherapy and longer survival led to concerns about toxicity. Acute side effects of therapy are nausea and vomiting, bone marrow suppression, and hair loss; all are reversible, and the first may be mitigated by the use of modern antiemetics. Careful use of colony-stimulating agents can minimize complications of neutropenia, but current evidence argues against the use of erythroid-stimulating agents for chemotherapy-induced anemia. Induction of menopause is a common concern for premenopausal women. Its likelihood is related to the type and duration of chemotherapy and the age of the patient; most women older than 40 years will suffer drug-induced menopause. Doxorubicin-related cardiomyopathy is noted in approximately 1% of women who received doxorubicin-containing adjuvant chemotherapy. Use of standard adjuvant chemotherapy regimens results in a very small increase in the incidence of acute leukemia, but there is no evidence of increased incidence of other second tumors. Effect of chemotherapy on cognitive function is an area of study.

Sequencing of Adjuvant Therapy

Women frequently receive several adjuvant interventions, including chemotherapy, radiotherapy, endocrine therapy, and/or anti-HER2 therapy. A logical question is how best to sequence these therapies.

Because a large randomized trial showed that concurrent chemotherapy plus tamoxifen led to worse outcome than chemotherapy followed by tamoxifen, most practitioners delay the administration of endocrine therapy until after completion of chemotherapy. Conversely, the benefit of trastuzumab appears to be greater when it is coadministered with taxane chemotherapy rather than following completion of taxane. A randomized trial showed no clear difference between the sequence of chemotherapy followed by radiotherapy compared with radiotherapy followed by chemotherapy.

A number of trials have tested the concept that administration of systemic therapy before primary surgery would improve outcome over the standard sequence of surgery followed by systemic therapy. Together they suggest that, compared with adjuvant therapy, preoperative (also termed *neoadjuvant*) systemic therapy improves the rate of breast conservation but does not enhance disease-free or overall survival. The possibility that preoperative therapy can provide an in vivo assessment of tumor response to therapy is suggested by the correlation between the finding of a pathologic complete response (absence of invasive cancer in the surgical specimen) and long-term disease-free survival in some studies.

Follow-Up of Early-Stage Breast Cancer Survivors

A critical question is how longitudinal medical follow-up should be conducted in women who have received appropriate local and systemic therapy for early breast cancer. Randomized trials have addressed the question of the value of serial laboratory and radiology testing, as well as the role of primary care versus oncology specialist follow-up. On the basis of these and other studies, the American Society of Clinical Oncology has published evidence-based guidelines for follow-up of asymptomatic survivors of early-stage breast cancer. These guidelines are summarized in Table 198-6.

TABLE 198-6 FOLLOW-UP GUIDELINES FOR PATIENTS WITH EARLY-STAGE BREAST CANCER: AMERICAN SOCIETY OF CLINICAL ONCOLOGY GUIDELINES

PROCEDURE OR TEST	FREQUENCY
History and physical examination* (eliciting of symptoms of breast cancer)	Every 3-6 mo for first 3 yr, every 6-12 mo for next yr, then yearly
MAMMOGRAPHY	
Mastectomy patients	Yearly
Lumpectomy patients	Yearly
Pelvic examination	Age appropriate
Breast self-examination	Monthly
Complete blood cell counts and chemistry studies	The literature does not support the use of these tests
Chest radiography, bone scans, PET scans, breast MRI, liver imaging, and tumor marker studies	Not recommended for routine follow-up in asymptomatic patients
Patient education regarding signs and symptoms of recurrence	Each visit

Modified from Khatcheressian JL, Hurley P, Bantug E, et al. Breast cancer follow-up and management after primary treatment: American Society of Clinical Oncology clinical practice guideline update. *J Clin Oncol.* 2013;31:961-965.

*Limited evaluation: assess for pain, dyspnea, weight loss, and other major changes in function. The limited examination should include an assessment of nodes, axillae, lumpectomy or mastectomy site, chest, and abdomen. Patients should be instructed regarding symptoms of recurrence.

MRI = magnetic resonance imaging; PET = positron emission tomography.

Stage III Breast Cancer

Locally advanced or inoperable stage III breast cancer accounts for approximately 10% of breast cancers. It is characterized by large primary tumor, fixed tumor or lymph nodes, or neoplastic invasion of the skin or chest wall. Inflammatory breast cancer falls into this category. It has a clinical presentation of breast swelling, warmth, and erythema and may or may not be associated with a mass. Because as many as one third of women with locally advanced breast cancer have distant metastases at the time of diagnosis, many oncologists perform an evaluation for distant disease even in asymptomatic patients. Diagnosis is usually established by fine-needle aspiration or core biopsy, and combined-modality therapy is used to maximize control of local disease and distant micrometastases. Several months of preoperative endocrine therapy or chemotherapy results in tumor regression in most patients, thereby allowing definitive breast surgery of some type to be performed. Postoperative radiotherapy is generally employed to enhance local control, and some studies suggest that administration of further chemotherapy, hormone therapy, anti-HER2 therapy, or a combination thereof (depending on the features of the cancer) is then desirable. Multimodality therapy results in a 5-year disease-free survival rate of approximately 50%.

Stage IV or Metastatic Breast Cancer

Although seldom curable, advanced breast cancer is a highly treatable illness. Palliation or prevention of symptoms without excess toxicity is the primary goal of treatment. The median survival after diagnosis of metastatic breast cancer is 2 to 3 years, although the range is great, and a small cadre of long-term survivors has been described. Several recent clinical trials have documented small improvements in survival with some of the newer therapies.

Most women with metastatic breast cancer present with symptoms or abnormalities on physical examination. Less than 10% of women present initially with metastatic disease; rather, advanced disease is normally diagnosed in women with a previous diagnosis of early breast cancer for which they received treatment. Common sites for metastases include bone, soft tissues, lung, liver, and brain. If metastatic disease is suspected, relevant hematologic, biochemical, and radiographic evaluation is indicated to assess location and severity of involvement. Because of the import of the diagnosis, pathologic confirmation is preferred. This permits verification of recurrent disease, exclusion of other diagnoses, and reassessment of biologic features such ER, PR, and HER2. Elevation of tumor markers (e.g., CA-27-29, carcinoembryonic antigen) or the presence of circulating tumor cells is not diagnostic of recurrent disease, although these markers may be useful adjuncts in the assessment of the effects of therapy.

The role of surgery in metastatic breast cancer is limited. It is useful in certain circumstances such as resection of a chest wall nodule or solitary brain metastasis or orthopedic stabilization to treat or prevent a long-bone fracture. Radiotherapy is a mainstay in the management of advanced disease. It may be used at any time during the patient's course to treat localized disease such as chest wall recurrence, brain metastases, or painful bony metastases. Systemic treatment is the primary mode for management of disseminated disease. Key principles for selection of therapy include maximal palliation of symptoms, minimization of treatment-related toxicity, and prevention of disease complications. An algorithm for treatment of stage IV breast cancer is shown in Figure 198-1.

Endocrine Therapy

Endocrine therapy is preferred as the first intervention for metastatic breast cancer whenever feasible because of its favorable therapeutic index. Factors that support the use of endocrine therapy include the expression of hormone

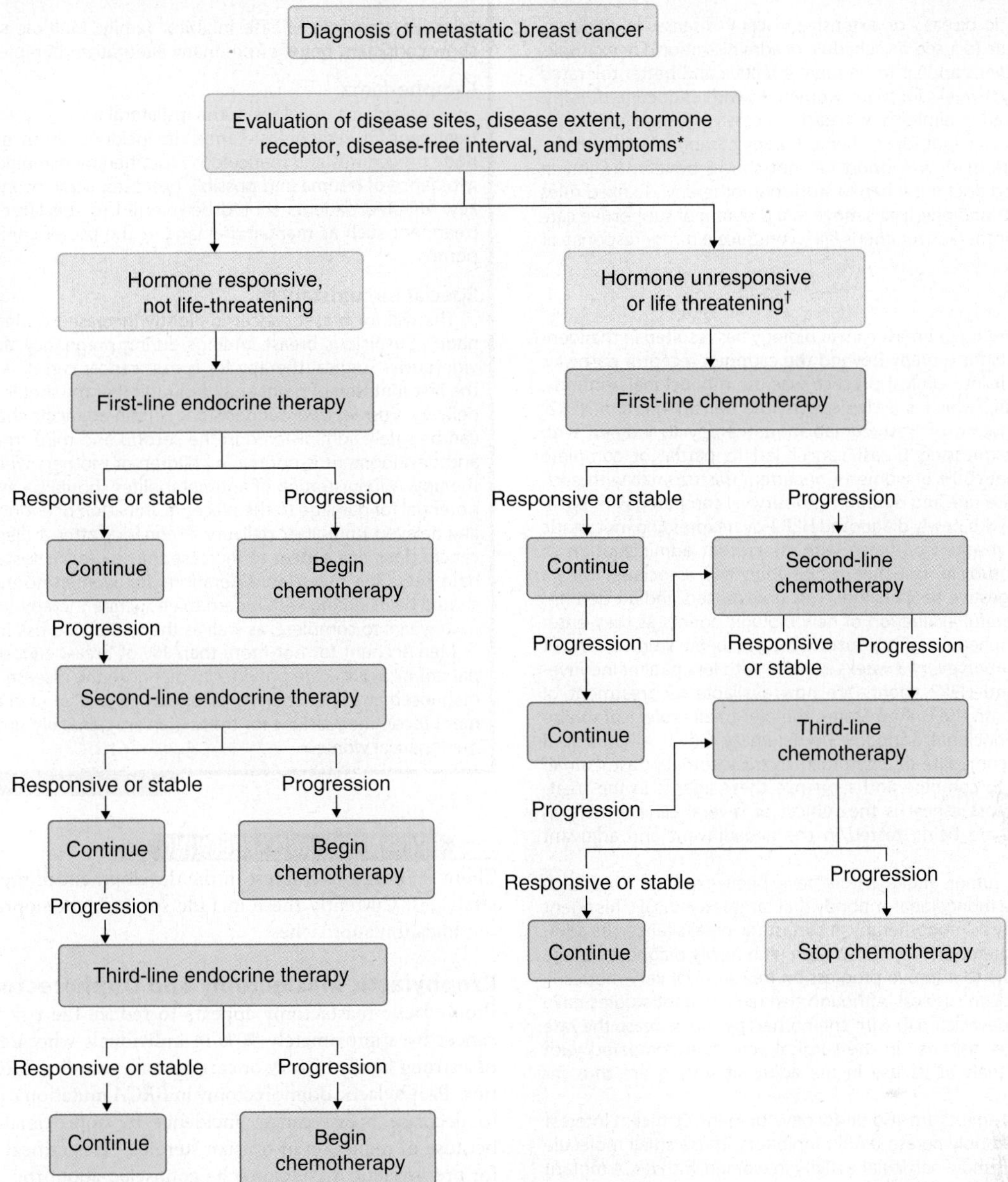

FIGURE 198-1. **An algorithm used for the systemic treatment of stage IV breast cancer. *Consider use of bisphosphonate or denosumab if bone involvement. †Consider integration of anti-HER2 therapy if tumor is HER2 overexpressing.**

receptors, a long disease-free interval, and absence of symptoms or visceral disease. More than half of the women who meet these criteria respond to an initial course of hormone therapy, with a median response duration of 9 to 12 months. Length of response is a good predictor for the likelihood of response to a second course of endocrine therapy when the first agent fails. A second course of endocrine therapy is less likely to be successful, and the duration of response is shorter; again, duration of response predicts for likelihood of success with third-line therapy. Successful application of this algorithm can result in good disease control with little toxicity for several years in some women.

A number of types of hormone therapy are now available. These include the selective estrogen receptor modulator (SERM) tamoxifen, the selective estrogen receptor–degrading agent fulvestrant, the aromatase inhibitors, and ovarian suppression by oophorectomy or LHRH agonists. Selection is usually made on the basis of efficacy, toxicity, and menopausal status. Serial administration of agents is the norm, although one study in estrogen receptor–positive postmenopausal metastatic breast cancer showed that the combination of the aromatase inhibitor anastrozole with fulvestrant was superior to anastrozole alone or sequential anastrozole and fulvestrant.[A11] Other combination therapies (with the possible exception of ovarian suppression plus tamoxifen) do not improve outcomes. Recent work has also demonstrated the value of everolimus but not temsirolimus combined with an aromatase inhibitor to improve progression-free survival compared with an aromatase inhibitor alone in patients with hormone receptor–positive advanced breast cancer previously treated with nonsteroidal aromatase inhibitors.[A12]

Several months of therapy are needed before the efficacy of a newly introduced endocrine therapy can be assessed. Patients and clinicians should be aware of the possibility of *treatment-related tumor flare*—a syndrome of worsening symptoms and increased circulating tumor markers—that can occur within the first few weeks of treatment. This response is usually of short duration and should not be confused with disease progression.

Chemotherapy

Most women with advanced breast cancer experience endocrine-unresponsive disease at some point and become candidates for palliative chemotherapy. Serial chemotherapy is the norm. Patients receive two to four cycles of therapy and then are evaluated for disease stabilization or improvement. Duration of therapy is variable for those who are responding to therapy. Several trials compared the approach of continuing therapy until time of disease progression with the approach of administering therapy, followed by a "drug holiday," with resumption of therapy at the time of disease progression. In sum, these studies suggest that survival is the same with these two approaches but that quality of life, as judged by the patients, is often better with continued therapy. Thus, decisions about continuation or cessation of a therapy are driven by perception of side effects and benefits by the patient and clinician.

Many active agents for breast cancer are now available. These include well-established drugs such as cyclophosphamide, doxorubicin, and methotrexate, as well as newer agents such as paclitaxel, docetaxel, vinorelbine, capecitabine, gemcitabine, carboplatin, ixabepilone, pegylated doxorubicin, and nano-albumin–bound paclitaxel. All these agents are active individually and in combination. There is considerable debate about the value of combination therapy compared with sequential single-agent therapy for metastatic breast cancer. Current guidelines suggest the use of serial monotherapy unless the patient has highly symptomatic disease or extensive visceral disease. In addition, much attention has been focused on schedule of administration. For example, weekly paclitaxel regimens appear to be more effective and better tolerated than regimens of every 3 weeks for many women. As with endocrine therapy, response rates and duration diminish with each successive change in therapy. As with early breast cancer, high-dose chemotherapy combined with autologous stem cell or bone marrow support has not shown benefit. A difficult question for patient and doctor is when to stop chemotherapy. No fixed rules exist, but many patients and physicians move to a program of supportive care if two successive chemotherapy regimens fail to produce a tumor response or disease stabilization.

Biologic Agents

Enhanced understanding of breast cancer biology has resulted in the identification of new targets for therapy beyond the estrogen receptor pathway. The first agent brought into clinical practice was the monoclonal antibody, trastuzumab (Herceptin), which is active against the transmembrane HER2/neu protein. Administration of trastuzumab monotherapy to women with metastatic HER2-overexpressing breast cancer led to partial or complete tumor regression in about 30% of women. Concurrent trastuzumab with paclitaxel increased response rate and duration and survival compared with paclitaxel alone for women with newly diagnosed HER2-overexpressing metastatic breast cancer. Similar results were seen with concurrent administration of trastuzumab and doxorubicin, but this combination was associated with a 20% incidence of congestive heart failure. This unexpected finding demonstrates the need for careful evaluation of new biologic agents as they enter the clinic. Dose and schedule of trastuzumab have been studied, and it appears that administration every 3 weeks is active with less patient inconvenience. Three other anti–HER2 agents are now available for treatment of advanced breast cancer in the United States, the oral small molecular inhibitor lapatinib; the monoclonal antibody pertuzumab, which inhibits HER dimerization; and the conjugate of a cytotoxic to trastuzumab, trastuzumab emtansine.[A13,A14] How to combine and sequence these agents in the treatment of metastatic breast cancer is the subject of several clinical trials; in addition these agents are being tested in the neoadjuvant and adjuvant settings.

Strategies to block tumor angiogenesis have been explored. One such agent is bevacizumab, a monoclonal antibody that targets the VEGF. This agent has only modest activity as monotherapy in metastatic breast cancer. Its addition to taxane-based chemotherapy for women with newly diagnosed stage IV breast cancer appears to improve progression-free survival very modestly without a major impact on survival. Although two neoadjvuant studies have suggested that use of bevacizumab with chemotherapy can increase the rate of pathologic complete response in the surgical specimen compared with chemotherapy alone, trials of its use in the adjuvant setting are thus far negative.

Many other targeted agents are also under development. Of recent interest are the poly-ADP-ribose polymerase (PARP) inhibitors. These small molecule inhibitors of DNA repair show particular activity in women with *BRCA* mutant breast cancer in early studies; more definitive testing is in progress.

Supportive Care

Bone Health

Because palliation of symptoms and prevention of complications of metastatic disease are the primary goals of treatment for advanced breast cancer, careful attention to supportive care is vital. Bone is the most common site of metastasis in breast cancer, and bone disease can be a source of significant morbidity. Several studies have shown that regular administration of a bisphosphonate such as zoledronate or pamidronate or the anti-RANKL monoclonal antibody denosumab, in addition to endocrine therapy or chemotherapy, can reduce pain and lower the incidence of skeletal complications of disease. Although such therapy is now the norm, several issues remain unaddressed, including the optimal treatment interval and duration of therapy in metastatic breast cancer.

Given the propensity of breast cancer therapy to spread to bone and to lead to estrogen deprivation and osteopenia or osteoporosis (Chapter 243), the use of bisphosphonates in the adjuvant setting is under evaluation. Although individual trials have not shown improved outcomes with the use of bisphosphonates in the adjuvant setting,[A15] a recently presented meta-analysis suggests that these agents may be useful in the setting of estrogen deprivation such as in postmenopausal patients.

Postmenopausal Symptoms

Postmenopausal symptoms as a consequence of therapy or natural aging are common in breast cancer survivors. In general, hormone replacement therapy should be avoided in women with a history of breast cancer. A short course of treatment can be considered in patients with early-stage breast cancer who have truly disabling symptoms. Topical estrogens are considered for women with vaginal dryness that does not respond to lubricants. Vasomotor symptoms may be reduced with the use of certain antidepressants of the selective serotonin release inhibitor family. Multiple studies have failed to show consistent benefit from many alternative therapies.

Lymphedema

Lymphedema develops in the ipsilateral arm in up to 15% of women after treatment for early breast cancer. Its incidence is lower with sentinel lymph node procedures and meticulous radiotherapy planning. Prevention includes avoidance of trauma and possibly exercises. Early recognition of symptoms is key. Affected patients should be referred to specialists for consideration of treatment such as manual drainage or the use of compression stockings or pumps.

Special Circumstances

The risk for breast cancer is slightly increased during and just after pregnancy. Suspicious breast findings during pregnancy should be investigated vigorously. Surgical therapy for breast cancer can be safely performed after the first trimester of pregnancy, but radiotherapy should be delayed until after delivery. Current data suggest that certain adjuvant chemotherapy regimens can be safely administered in the second and third trimesters of pregnancy, and development is normal in children of mothers who receive this chemotherapy. Administration of antimetabolites should be avoided because of the potential for damage to the placenta. Initiation of endocrine therapy is generally delayed until after delivery. Pregnancy after a diagnosis of early breast cancer does not appear to increase the risk for metastatic disease in limited data sets. The major considerations for women contemplating pregnancy should be its timing with regard to endocrine therapy, which may require 5 or more years to complete, as well as the underlying risk for disease recurrence.

Men account for not more than 1% of breast cancer cases. Failure of the patient or health care provider to diagnose the disease means that it may be diagnosed at a later stage. Most breast cancers in men express ER, and treatment recommendations for these men are generally similar to those for postmenopausal women.

PREVENTION AND SCREENING

There is enormous interest in the development of breast cancer prevention strategies. Currently these include surgical, chemopreventive, and lifestyle modification approaches.

Prophylactic Mastectomy and Oophorectomy

Prophylactic mastectomy appears to reduce the risk for developing breast cancer by approximately 90% in individuals who are at high risk because of a strong family history or carriage of a germline *BRCA1* or *BRCA2* mutation. Prophylactic oophorectomy in *BRCA* mutation carriers has been shown to decrease breast cancer incidence by approximately 50%, presumably because of reduction in ovarian steroids.[7] It is critical that women who opt for prophylactic mastectomy be counseled about the possibility that cancer may develop in remnants of breast tissue that remain after prophylactic mastectomy.

Chemoprevention

The observation that adjuvant endocrine therapy with the SERM tamoxifen also decreased contralateral breast cancer led to evaluation of tamoxifen as a chemopreventive for well women who are at high risk for breast cancer. Meta-analysis of four randomized trials of tamoxifen versus placebo for high-risk women confirmed a 38% reduction in invasive breast cancer with tamoxifen. The largest trial, NSABP P01, randomized 13,388 high-risk women to receive either tamoxifen or placebo for 5 years. Risk factors used to determine eligibility were age 60 years or older, a diagnosis of lobular carcinoma in situ, or age 35 to 59 years with a constellation of risk factors that, when combined, resulted in a 1.67% or greater risk for breast cancer within 5 years. This study showed a 50% decrease in the diagnosis of breast cancer across all age groups at a cost of increased risk for endometrial cancer and thromboembolic events in women older than 50 years. These data led to the approval of tamoxifen to reduce the incidence of breast cancer in women at high risk as defined by the eligibility criteria for this prevention trial.

Other SERMs have been studied as chemopreventive agents.[8,9] Two trials have documented the utility of raloxifene as a breast cancer risk-reduction strategy. In one trial, raloxifene administration reduced the incidence of breast cancer in postmenopausal women of average breast cancer risk and elevated cardiovascular risk. A second trial showed that raloxifene was less effective than tamoxifen in preventing invasive breast cancer in postmenopausal women at high risk for breast cancer.[A16] Raloxifene use was associated with fewer uterine cancers than tamoxifen but carries the same risk for thromboembolic events. It is approved by the FDA for risk reduction in high-risk postmenopausal women. Two large studies of an aromatase inhibitor (exemestane or anastrozole) show that either of these drugs lowers the incidence of breast cancer in moderate- to high-risk postmenopausal women by approximately 50%.[A17,A18] A vitamin A derivative, fenretinide, showed some impact as a chemopreventive agent for secondary prevention in premenopausal breast cancer survivors but has not found a place in routine practice. Finally, large epidemiologic studies have raised the possibility that aspirin or certain statins might also decrease breast cancer risk, but these agents have not been prospectively tested.

Lifestyle Modification

Prevention strategies that involve lifestyle alterations have been suggested. The Women's Health Initiative did not show a clear role for a low-fat diet as a means of breast cancer prevention. Regular exercise, especially during adolescence, may be associated with reduced breast cancer risk. By extrapolation from the epidemiologic studies mentioned previously, abstinence from alcohol might slightly reduce the risk for breast cancer.

Screening

Screening strategies for breast cancer have traditionally included the triad of breast self-examination (BSE), clinical breast examination (CBE) by a health care professional, and screening mammography in well women. Although widely promulgated as an important component of early detection, two large randomized trials of conventional BSE versus observation failed to show any clinical advantage with BSE. As a result, many experts now promote breast awareness rather than regular BSE. The independent value of CBEs has not been rigorously assessed. Rather, it has been studied in conjunction with screening mammography, in which case the two interventions appear to decrease mortality from breast cancer by 25 to 30% in women older than 50 years. Considerable controversy continues over the value of screening mammography in women 40 to 50 years of age and those over 70 years of age as well, as the optimal interval between mammograms for women aged 50 to 70 years. Currently, the American Cancer Society recommends annual screening mammography for women older than 40 years of age who are at standard risk for breast cancer. In contrast, the U.S. Preventive Services Task Force recommends that women between 40 and 50 years of age be counseled about the risks and benefits of screening mammography and that screening mammography can be used at 2-year intervals for women aged 50 to 75 years (Table 198-7). However, women aged 40 to 49 years with a two-fold increased risk for breast cancer have similar benefit-to-harm ratios for biennial screening mammography, as do average-risk women aged 50 to 74 years. A study of digital versus conventional film screen mammography failed to show an overall advantage for digital mammography but suggests that digital mammography may be more useful for women with dense breasts. The survival benefits of mammography come at the cost of false positive results that lead to anxiety and further evaluation. According to various estimates, more than half of the women screened by mammography have false-positive results over 10 years of screening, and 7 to 9% get recommendations for breast biopsy.[10] Other studies have estimated an overdiagnosis rate of 3.3% for invasive cancer and from 18 to 32% for carcinoma in situ.[11] In general, screening is unlikely to be worthwhile for women with a life expectancy of less than ten years.[12]

The knowledge that screening mammography fails to diagnose approximately 10 to 15% of breast cancers has led to the evaluation of other imaging modalities. Of these, MRI is the most mature.[13] MRI has been promoted as a useful screening tool for women at high risk by virtue of the *BRCA* mutation; indeed, the American Cancer Society has recommended consideration of screening MRI for women whose predicted risk for breast cancer exceeds 20%. MRI has been shown to detect breast cancer in the contralateral breast in 3% of women with a newly diagnosed breast cancer whose contralateral mammogram showed no abnormality. Use of MRI in the general population is limited by the fact that it is highly sensitive but lacks specificity. As a result, MRI has not translated into improved selection of surgical treatments or a reduction in the number of operations. Insufficient information exists about other breast imaging modalities such as ultrasound and radionuclide imaging to support their use in screening asymptomatic women.

TABLE 198-7 BREAST CANCER SCREENING

TEST	ACS	USPSTF
Mammography		
40-<49 yr	Annual	Insufficient evidence to support
>49 yr	Annual if healthy	Every 2 yr, 50-75 yr
Clinical breast examination	Every 3 yr, 20-39 yr Annually, ≥40 yr	Insufficient evidence to support
Breast self-examination	Optional	Not recommended

ACS = American Cancer Society; USPSTF = U.S. Preventive Services Task Force.

BENIGN BREAST LESIONS

Benign breast disease includes mastalgia (pain and tenderness), mastitis (including infectious and noninfectious inflammatory conditions), trauma, and benign tumors. In addition, mastalgia can be caused by extramammary conditions, such as myocardial ischemia, pneumonia, pleural irritation, esophageal spasm, costochondritis, rib fracture, and varicella-zoster virus (preceding the skin eruption). After these conditions have been ruled out, mastalgia is considered to be a benign condition that is self-limited. It can be cyclical or noncyclical in timing (where it is thought to be related to hormonal activity), and it may occur in postmenopausal women, even in the absence of hormone replacement therapy.

Mastitis is due to breast inflammation or infection, and it can occur in either nonlactating or lactating women. The typical presentation in nonlactating women is occurrence in their 40s with the acute onset of severe breast pain and tenderness followed by erythema and swelling that tends to be localized in the nipple-areolar area. The cause in most cases is considered to be rupture of dilated subareolar ducts that leads to an inflammatory response to leakage of intraductal contents into periductal tissue. Infection is difficult to rule out, and, in practice, patients are often treated with empirical antibiotics; if symptoms do not resolve within 7 to 10 days on antibiotics, ultrasound is required to rule out abscess. If the latter is found, incision and drainage are required. The most important differential diagnosis with mastitis is inflammatory carcinoma, as noted previously. Therefore, failure to improve with antibiotics or to find an abscess should lead to evaluation by a breast surgeon. Mastitis in lactating women is often due to infection caused by a break in the skin of the nipple or milk stasis. *Staphylococcus aureus, Staphylococcus albus,* and sometimes *Escherichia coli* or streptococci are the most common pathogens. Treatment requires antibiotics and milk removal.

Nonproliferative and Proliferative Benign Breast Lesions

Nonproliferative benign breast lesions include (1) inflammatory fat necrosis, which follows surgical or blunt trauma, and generally resolves spontaneously; (2) lymphocytic mastitis, which may be seen in diabetic patients; and (3) granulomatous mastitis, associated with foreign body reactions (e.g., silicone and paraffin for breast augmentation and reconstruction after cancer surgery), sarcoid, or certain infections. Other nonproliferative benign breast lesions appear as tumor-like processes, including (4) fibroadenoma, a very common (~25% of women), usually solitary, sharply demarcated, smooth lesion in younger age groups; (5) phyllodes tumor (previously known as cystosarcoma phyllodes); (6) intraductal papilloma, solitary lesions that may be accompanied by bloody nipple discharge; (7) fibrocystic breast disease, which is now more appropriately called *fibrocystic changes* because it is observed clinically in up to 50% and histologically in 90% of women, composed of varying amounts of fibrosis and cysts sometimes associated with calcifications and inflammation; and (8) simple or complex cysts, which should be aspirated with ultrasound guidance and, when the fluid is not clear, sent for cytologic analysis.

Proliferative benign breast lesions include ductal or lobular hyperplasia; atypical hyperplasias are associated with increased risk for breast cancer.

Breast Cancer Risk

The increasing use of mammography has increased the frequency of breast biopsies, which, in turn, has increased the finding of benign breast lesions, the most common findings on biopsy. The benign breast lesions listed in the previous section encompass the general histologic spectrum of (1) nonproliferative lesions, (2) proliferative lesions without atypia, and (3) atypical hyperplasia, listed in ascending order of risk for breast cancer. A large number of retrospective and prospective studies have shown an overall relative risk for breast cancer of 1.5 to 1.6 for women with biopsy-proved benign breast disease compared with women in the general population. A study of 9087 women with all types of benign histologic findings, followed for a median of 15 years at the Mayo Clinic, found that 707 of them developed breast cancers. Increased risk for cancer persisted for at least 25 years after the original biopsy. Of the three broad histologic categories, the relative risk for cancer development was 4.24 associated with atypia, 1.88 with proliferative changes without atypia, and 1.27 with nonproliferative lesions. It is not known whether the finding of a benign breast lesion with atypical histologic findings represents an actual precursor lesion for cancer or if it is only a marker for a general tendency to develop breast cancer. The observations that approximately half of breast cancers in these patients arise in the contralateral breast suggests the latter hypothesis.

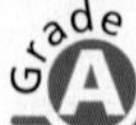

Grade A References

A1. Rao R, Euhus D, Mayo HG, et al. Axillary node interventions in breast cancer: a systematic review. *JAMA*. 2013;310:1385-1394.
A2. Early Breast Cancer Trialists' Collaborative Group (EBCTCG), et al. Effect of radiotherapy after breast-conserving surgery on 10-year recurrence and 15-year breast cancer death: meta-analysis of individual patient data for 10,801 women in 17 randomised trials. *Lancet*. 2011;378:1707-1716.
A3. McGale P, Taylor C, Correa C, et al. Effect of radiotherapy after mastectomy and axillary surgery on 10-year recurrence and 20-year breast cancer mortality: meta-analysis of individual patient data for 8135 women in 22 randomised trials. *Lancet*. 2014;383:2127-2135.
A4. Early Breast Cancer Trialists' Collaborative Group (EBCTCG). Comparisons between different polychemotherapy regimens for early breast cancer: meta-analyses of long-term outcome among 100,000 women in 123 randomised trials. *Lancet*. 2012;379:432-444.
A5. Early Breast Cancer Trialists' Collaborative Group (EBCTCG). Relevance of breast cancer hormone receptors and other factors to the efficacy of adjuvant tamosifen: patient-level meta-analysis of randomized trials. *Lancet*. 2011;378:771-784.
A6. Pagani O, Regan MM, Walley BA, et al. Adjuvant exemestane with ovarian suppression in premenopausal breast cancer. *N Engl J Med*. 2014;371:107-118.
A7. Dowsett M, Cuzick J, Ingle J, et al. Meta-analysis of breast cancer outcomes in adjuvant trials of aromatase inhibitors versus tamoxifen. *J Clin Oncol*. 2010;28:509-518.
A8. Davies C, Pan H, Godwin J, et al. Long-term effects of continuing adjuvant tamoxifen to 10 years versus stopping at 5 years after diagnosis of oesteroen receptor-positive breast cancer: ATLAS, a randomized trial. *Lancet*. 2013;381:805-816.
A9. Perez EA, Romond EH, Suman VJ, et al. Trastuzumab plus adjuvant chemotherapy for human epidermal growth factor receptor 2-positive breast cancer: planned joint analysis of overall survival from NSABP B-31 and NCCTG N9831. *J Clin Oncol*. 2014;32:3744-3752.
A10. Goldhirsch A, Gelber RD, Piccart-Gebhart MJ, et al. 2 years versus 1 year of adjuvant trastuzumab for HER2-positive breast cancer (HERA): an open-label, randomised controlled trial. *Lancet*. 2013;382:1021-1028.
A11. Mehta RS, Barlow WE, Albain KS, et al. Combination anastrozole and fulvestrant in metastatic breast cancer. *N Engl J Med*. 2012;367:435-444.
A12. Baselga J, Campone M, Piccart M, et al. Everolimus in postmenopausal hormone-receptor-positive advanced breast cancer. *N Engl J Med*. 2012;366:520-529.
A13. Baselga J, Cortés J, Kim SB, et al. Pertuzumab plus trastuzumab plus docetaxel for metastatic breast cancer. *N Engl J Med*. 2012;366:109-119.
A14. Verma S, Miles D, Gianni L, et al. Trastuzumab emtansine for HER2-positive advanced breast cancer. *N Engl J Med*. 2012;367:1783-1791.
A15. Coleman RE, Marshall H, Cameron D, et al. Breast-cancer adjuvant therapy with zoledronic acid. *N Engl J Med*. 2011;365:1396-1405.
A16. Vogel VG, Costantino JP, Wickerham DL, et al. Update of the National Surgical Adjuvant Breast and Bowel Project Study of Tamoxifen and Raloxifene (STAR) P-2 Trial: preventing breast cancer. *Cancer Prev Res*. 2010;3:696-706.
A17. Goss PE, Ingle JN, Alés-Martínez JE, et al. Exemestane for breast-cancer prevention in postmenopausal women. *N Engl J Med*. 2011;364:2381-2391.
A18. Cuzick J, Sestak I, Forbes JF, et al. Anastrozole for prevention of breast cancer in high-risk postmenopausal women (IBIS-II): an international, double-blind, randomised placebo-controlled trial. *Lancet*. 2014;383:1041-1048.

GENERAL REFERENCES

For the General References and other additional features, please visit Expert Consult at https://expertconsult.inkling.com.

199 GYNECOLOGIC CANCERS

DAVID SPRIGGS

GENERAL CONSIDERATIONS

The role of the internist or primary care practitioner in the care of women with gynecologic cancers has three important components: awareness and prompt diagnosis of gynecologic cancers, primary care of the patient with active cancer, and care and surveillance of cancer survivors. Diagnosis of these cancers relies on both the collection of appropriate clinical history and routine gynecologic examination. None of these malignancies are common, but in every case, early detection and treatment leads to superior outcomes. Both demographic trends and the increased effectiveness of cancer treatment will contribute to a growing population of cancer survivors receiving care in the non-oncologist's practice.

CERVICAL CANCER

EPIDEMIOLOGY

Cervical cancer is an important worldwide health problem, often affecting younger women in the prime of life. Newly diagnosed cervical cancer will affect over 500,000 women annually and will lead to over 250,000 deaths, making it the third most common cancer in women around the world. Because of the long natural history of premalignant and early cervical cancer, annual cytologic screening (Pap smear) has dramatically reduced the incidence of advanced cervical cancer in the developed world and areas with good medical infrastructure. Cervical cancer remains an important cause of cancer death in the developing world, often striking young women in their most productive years. It is primarily a disease afflicting patients of lower socioeconomic status whose access to advanced medical care is limited. The overall 5-year survival rate for cervical cancer is approximately 67% in the United States (~12,000 new cases and roughly 4000 deaths in 2014) but depends on the group prevalence of annual screening to detect early-stage disease.[1] Younger women and white women have better outcomes than older women and black and Hispanic women based on many factors, including early diagnosis of localized cancers. Other factors linked to higher incidence of cervical cancer include age of first intercourse, parity (more live births linked to higher risk), current cigarette smoking, and male human papillomavirus (HPV)-related factors. Regions with a higher frequency of penile cancer and lower rates of male circumcision have a higher incidence of cervical cancer diagnoses. High prevalence of other sexually transmitted diseases is also a known risk factor, including *Chlamydia trachomatis* and herpes simplex virus infections. Finally, host immunity appears to play a major role. Both human immunodeficiency virus (HIV) infection and immune suppression related to transplantation are associated with dramatic increases in the incidence of cervical cancer.

PATHOBIOLOGY

Infection with specific, carcinogenic strains of HPV has been established as the necessary causal event for nearly all cervical cancer.[2] This includes both the most common squamous cell cancers (85%) and the less common, more difficult to detect, adenocarcinomas. Not all HPV strains are linked to cervical cancer, and the most common cancer-related subtypes include 16, 18, 32, 33, 35, 45, 52, and 58. Although the prevalence of the genotype will show substantial regional variation, over 70% of all cervical cancers can be linked to HPV 16, 18, and 45. Many other HPV strains can cause infection but will not lead to cervical cancer. HPV infection tends to occur soon after sexual initiation, and in most women will be cleared by the immune system within 24 months. In some cases the HPV DNA is incorporated into the host DNA and can continue to produce viral proteins (persistence). Often the HPV DNA is silenced and will go through a period of latency but can be reactivated later. The HPV protein E7 mediates immortalization through abrogation of the G1/S transition through interaction with the Rb protein. Other targets of E7 include a variety of cyclin-dependent kinases and cyclins that are critical for cell cycle regulation. The E6 protein binds to p53 and promotes its degradation, leading to decreased capacity for DNA damage repair. E6 also upregulates the cellular telomerase complex and contributes to immortalization of HPV-infected epithelial cells. As a consequence of inactivation of Rb and p53, there is loss of cell cycle regulation and a variety of subsequent mutations appear to accumulate. Mutational load appears to play a dominant role in the eventual development and progression of cervical cancer.

SCREENING

HPV infection of cervical epithelial cells leads to a failure of cellular differentiation and to cytologic abnormalities of the cervical epithelium referred to as cervical intraepithelial neoplasia (CIN). Whereas early, or low-grade, CIN often resolves, higher grades of CIN (CIN 2/3) appear to be linked to viral integration into host DNA and a failure to clear the infection. Persistent CIN can be detected by Pap cytologic testing during its long preinvasive phase, and this fact has led to the success of screening strategies in developed countries. Current recommendations mandate initiation of cytologic (Pap) testing at age 21 and every 2 years until age 30, when women with persistently negative screening tests can be screened every 3 years until age 65.[3,4] For women in the 30- to 65-year age group, a combined screening strategy of cytologic and HPV testing is preferred. The combination of HPV testing and liquid-based cytology has a sensitivity of 96.7%; patients testing positive for HPV 16/18 should all be referred for colposcopy, regardless of their cytologic result. At age 65, women with multiple negative cytologic screening tests may discontinue screening. Any woman with a cytologic screen revealing CIN 2 or other abnormalities should be referred to a gynecologist for colposcopy and appropriate subsequent management. CIN 2/3 implies probable viral integration, so a woman with a history of CIN 2/3 should undergo more frequent and extended screening.

CLINICAL MANIFESTATIONS AND DIAGNOSIS

Early cervical cancer is generally asymptomatic, and thus detection is highly dependent on screening and routine gynecologic care. In advanced stages, patients may present with vaginal discharge or bleeding, pelvic pain, or abnormalities of bowel, bladder, or sexual function. The diagnosis of cervical cancer is usually based on positive cytologic status and direct inspection by vaginal speculum examination. Early cervical cancers are detected primarily by colposcopy and direct biopsy. The staging of cervical cancer is based on both expert clinical evaluation of resectability and imaging studies of both the pelvis and potential sites of distant metastases (lymph nodes, lungs, and abdominal sites).

TREATMENT

Rx

The primary treatment of localized cervical cancer is stage dependent. Staging of cervical cancer depends on the clinical evaluation of a skilled gynecologic oncologist; the International Federation of Gynecology and Obstetrics (FIGO) staging system is summarized in Table 199-1. In general, treatment of early-stage cervical cancer is exclusively surgical. The appropriate procedure will depend on patient age, comorbidities, stage, and tumor size. Radical hysterectomy with nodal dissection is the most common procedure, although younger patients with low risk for metastatic disease may undergo simple hysterectomy or even radical trachelectomy for highly selected patients who desire preservation of fertility. Patients with low-stage cervical cancer who have certain high-risk pathologic findings after surgery may benefit from radiation or chemotherapy.

There is some variability in treatment recommendations for patients with FIGO stage IB to IIA. Younger women with smaller tumors may be offered radical hysterectomy, whereas bulkier tumors and older patients may be better served by definitive chemoradiation. Patients with FIGO stage IIB to IV should all be treated with combinations of cisplatin and external beam radiation.[A1] It is important to note that the combination of cisplatin and external beam radiation can provide an opportunity for cure and long-term survival, even in stage IV cancer of the cervix.

Patients with recurrent cancer of the cervix or patients with distant metastases at diagnosis are very rarely curable. Death is usually related to local recurrence, but distant metastatic spread to the lung, peritoneum, or bone is also common in cervical cancer. Platinum-based chemotherapy remains the mainstay of palliative treatment. The addition of bevacizumab, a humanized anti-vascular endothelial growth factor (VEGF) monoclonal antibody, to combination chemotherapy in patients with recurrent, persistent, or metastatic cervical cancer has been associated with an improvement of 3.7 months in median overall survival.[A2] Recurrent or persistent tumors within the prior radiation field are particularly difficult to manage with chemotherapy. Local problems such as pain, bleeding, and fistulas between the bladder, vagina, and bowel are common in the advanced stages of this disease.

TABLE 199-1 APPROACH TO CERVIX CANCER BY STAGE*

STAGE	BRIEF DEFINITION	USUAL TREATMENT
0	Carcinoma in situ	Conization, hysterectomy
IA1	Microscopic stromal invasion < 3 mm	Conization, hysterectomy
IA2	Microscopic stromal invasion 3 to 5 mm	Radical hysterectomy
IB1	Visible lesion < 4 cm in greatest dimension	Radical hysterectomy
IB2	Visible lesion > 4 cm in greatest dimension	Chemoradiation
IIA	Tumor beyond the uterus, no parametrial involvement	Radical hysterectomy (selected)
IIB	Tumor beyond the uterus with parametrial extension	Chemoradiation
IIIA	Tumor involves lower third vagina but no pelvic wall extension	Chemoradiation
IIIB	Tumor extends to pelvic wall or hydronephrosis or regional lymph nodes	Chemoradiation
IVA	Involvement of mucosa of bowel or bladder	Chemo-radiation
IVB	Distant metastatic disease	Chemotherapy only

*Cervical cancer is staged clinically and not by either radiographic or pathologic findings. Chemoradiation generally includes weekly cisplatin treatment. Metastatic disease chemotherapy is generally based on cisplatin doublet treatment.

PROGNOSIS AND CARE OF SURVIVORS

Patients with a history of CIN 2/3 or other noninvasive disease require regular cytologic examinations, because the onset of cancer in patients with HPV 16/18 infection can occur years after primary infection. Early-stage cancer of the cervix is highly curable. Although perioperative complications can occur for any major operation, late complications of radical hysterectomy are not common but may include lymphedema and persistent bladder or rectal dysfunction. Patients with more advanced stage disease appropriately treated with chemoradiation combinations have long-term survival rates from 30 to over 80% percent, based on stage and underlying health. The late complications of chemoradiation are similar but probably more common, affecting 5 to 10% of survivors. Fistulas can occur between pelvic organs, including bladder, vagina, small bowel, and rectum. Other bladder problems may include urgency, incontinence, and chronic cystitis with loss of bladder capacity. Rectal problems include pain, diarrhea or constipation, urgency, and incontinence. Skeletal complications can include pelvic insufficiency fractures, associated with pain in as many as 10% of patients after radiation. Vaginal stenosis, dryness, and dyspareunia are common but usually can be managed with vaginal dilators and appropriate lubricants. Late complications of cisplatin-based chemotherapy include neuropathy, as well as renal insufficiency with chronic wasting of potassium and magnesium. Multimodality therapy regimens including radiation, surgery, and chemotherapy pose a higher risk for late complications and impaired patient quality of life decades after primary curative treatment.

PREVENTION

Our understanding of the pathobiology of HPV-derived cervical cancer supported the development of vaccines for the prevention of the most common oncogenic subtypes of HPV infection (Chapter 373). There are now licensed vaccines that immunize against HPV 16, 18, and selected other high-risk types. They are both safe and effective in substantially reducing the risk for cervical dysplasia and carcinoma.[A3][A4] HPV vaccines require administration before sexual activity and can be highly effective in reducing the risk for cervical cancer. Both the approval trials and subsequent follow-up trials reveal a high level of safety and durable type-specific immunity that seems to persist for more than 5 years after a series of three initial vaccinations.[A5] Additional HPV type coverage may eventually be available, but it is already clear from population-based studies that the vaccine can reduce the incidence of precursor lesions such as cervical dysplasia. Beyond immunization, prevention is absolutely linked to regular screening for early HPV-related lesions and appropriate management during the premalignant phase of the disease.

ENDOMETRIAL CANCER

EPIDEMIOLOGY

Endometrial cancer arises from the epithelium of the uterine lining, in distinction to uterine sarcomas that have their tissue of origin in the smooth muscle of the myometrium. Endometrial cancer is the most common gynecologic cancer in the United States, with over 52,000 new cases each year. Death from endometrial cancer occurs in approximately 8600 women each year. The risk factors for endometrial cancer include advancing age, estrogen exposure, obesity, and multiparity. As populations age across the world, the incidence of endometrial cancer is generally rising. The median age for the development of endometrial cancer is 60 years, and most endometrial cancers are diagnosed after age 50. Exposure to exogenous or endogenous estrogens appears to be a strong risk factor. Early menarche, late menopause, nulliparity, and unopposed estrogen in hormone replacement therapy are all implicated in higher endometrial cancer risk. Obesity is associated with higher levels circulating estrogens related to peripheral conversion of androstenedione to estrogen. Even the low rates of tamoxifen (a selective estrogen receptor modulator)-induced endometrial cancer are probably related to weak estrogenic effects on the endometrium.

PATHOBIOLOGY

Endometrial cancers can be divided into two large categories for understanding risk and biology. The more common tumors (type 1 cancers; 85%) are distinguished by endometrioid histology, a more differentiated grade, and a relationship to unopposed estrogen exposure. These type 1 malignancies tend to present as stage I or II cancers (confined to the uterus) and generally have a better prognosis than the type 2 cancers. They often retain expression of progesterone receptors.[5] On a molecular level, these tumors are more likely to be diploid, have wild-type *p53*, and be associated with loss of *PTEN* and microsatellite instability. In contrast, type 2 endometrial cancers are poorly differentiated, often have serous or clear cell histology, and often manifest at advanced stages with higher risk for dissemination. At the molecular level, type 2 endometrial cancers are aneuploid, carry mutations or loss of *p53* and lack *PTEN* deletion or other abnormalities of the PI3 kinase/AKT pathway.[6]

Most endometrial cancers are sporadic, but small percentages (3-5%) of type 1 cancers are associated with a cancer family history consistent with Lynch syndrome (hereditary nonpolyposis, colorectal cancer [HNPCC]). This familial cancer syndrome is associated with early-onset colon, ovary, renal, and endometrial cancers, related to germline mutations in one of the mismatch repair genes *MLH1, MSH2,* and *MSH6*. The development of endometrial cancer before 50 years of age with an appropriate family history or histologic appearance should prompt genetic testing of the patient, to guide both proband and family preventive management.

CLINICAL MANIFESTATIONS AND DIAGNOSIS

The 80% survivorship in endometrial cancer is predominantly related to the high likelihood of detection while the cancer is confined to the uterus. Abnormal uterine bleeding in postmenopausal women always should be regarded as suspicious. Abnormal vaginal discharge or nonspecific gastrointestinal symptoms also may be present at the time of diagnosis. It is important to recall that the routine Pap smear is not an appropriate diagnostic procedure to exclude endometrial cancer. The classic dilatation and curettage (D&C) has largely been replaced by an office endometrial biopsy. The D&C and hysteroscopy are now usually reserved for uterine bleeding problems that are difficult to diagnose. Common sites of spread for endometrial cancer at the time of diagnosis include pelvic or periaortic lymph nodes, ovary, and peritoneal implants. The recently revised FIGO staging system for endometrial cancer is shown in Table 199-2.

TABLE 199-2 APPROACH TO ENDOMETRIAL CANCER BY STAGE*

STAGE	BRIEF DEFINITION	USUAL TREATMENT
IA G1/2	Invasion to less than half the myometrial thickness	TAH and BSO, no XRT
IA G3	Invasion to less than half the myometrial thickness, poorly differentiated, serous cancer	TAH and BSO, consider chemotherapy, no XRT
IB G1/2	50% or more invasion of myometrial thickness	TAH and BSO, no XRT
IB G3	50% or more invasion of myometrial thickness, poorly differentiated	TAH and BSO, consider chemotherapy, no XRT
II	Uterine and cervical involvement	TAH and BSO, consider VBT
IIIA	Invades corpus serosa or adnexa	TAH and BSO, tumor-directed chemo-XRT and chemotherapy
IIIB	Vaginal or parametrial invasion	TAH and BSO, tumor-directed chemo-XRT and chemotherapy
IIIC1	Pelvic lymph node involvement	TAH and BSO, tumor-directed chemo-XRT and chemotherapy
IIIC2	Paraaortic lymph node involvement	TAH and BSO, tumor-directed chemo-XRT and chemotherapy
IVA	Invasion of bowel or bladder	TAH and BSO, tumor-directed chemo-XRT and chemotherapy
IVB	Distant metastatic disease	Chemotherapy only

*Endometrial cancer (FIGO 2009) staging is based on pathologic findings. Stages I and II endometrial cancer do not show a survival benefit from adjuvant radiation therapy. High-risk disease may benefit from adjuvant chemotherapy, but the studies are ongoing. For stage III and IV disease, complete debulking is preferred and platinum-based chemotherapy is generally needed. The use of volume-directed radiotherapy for gross residual disease is under investigation.
TAH and BSO = total abdominal hysterectomy and bilateral salpingo-oophorectomy ; XRT = radiation therapy; VBT = vaginal brachytherapy irradiation.

TREATMENT Rx

For the vast majority of patients with endometrial cancer, surgical resection represents the primary approach to management. In many cases, surgery resection (total hysterectomy with bilateral salpingo-oophorectomy, lymph node assessment) will be sufficient for both staging and treatment. Laparoscopic or robotic surgery has replaced open hysterectomy in many situations and appears to be a less morbid procedure.[A6] The role and extent of lymph node dissection and the use of sentinel node biopsy are areas of active surgical research. These advances continue to decrease the morbidity and length of hospitalization associated with primary surgical treatment. Following primary surgery, patients are staged by pathologic findings and stratified by risk factors to assign appropriate adjuvant therapy (see Table 199-2). Important risk factors for recurrence include stage (as determined by metastatic deposits, lymph node involvement, and depth of myometrial invasion), tumor histology, cytologic grade, and lymphovascular space involvement. General treatment approaches, by stage, are shown in Table 199-2. High-risk patients with stage 1 disease historically received adjunctive radiotherapy with significant reduction in local recurrence, but there is no evidence supporting a long-term survival impact of radiation.[A7-A9] In type 2 endometrial cancers of serous histology, patients with even the lowest stage disease are at risk for distant recurrence and adjuvant chemotherapy is increasingly used.

For patients with higher stage (Stage III or IV) disease, complete surgical resection of gross disease appears to be the important determinant of survival. Platinum-based chemotherapy has been increasingly identified as effective and has replaced whole-abdominal radiation therapy as the mainstay of adjuvant therapy. Combinations of carboplatin and paclitaxel are generally well tolerated and will reduce recurrence in both high-risk and advanced stage disease groups. Even patients with substantial residual disease after surgery can sometimes achieve long remissions following platinum-based treatment. As with most solid tumors, recurrent cancer is difficult to cure. An exception appears to be local recurrence in patients who did not receive prior radiation. In that select group, radiation therapy should be given with curative intent. Otherwise, metastatic endometrial cancer can be managed with other systemic chemotherapies; the patterns of drug sensitivities are similar to those seen in recurrent ovarian cancer. Common sites of metastatic disease include the peritoneal cavity, liver, bone, lung, and occasionally brain. The comorbidities commonly associated with age and obesity can play an important role in the treatment choice for endometrial cancer. For patients whose overall health precludes a surgical procedure, curative radiation therapy can be offered. Although the long-term complications of definitive radiation treatment can be significant, it may be the best choice for patients with a compromised performance status.

PREVENTION

For sporadic endometrial cancers, the best prevention strategy appears to be a high degree of suspicion in the context of postmenopausal bleeding. Because of its location, these tumors are rarely asymptomatic late in their natural history and surgical extirpation is usually curative. In families with HNPCC, a total hysterectomy with bilateral salpingo-oophorectomy should be strongly considered in confirmed carriers who have completed their childbearing.

PROGNOSIS

Stage I and II endometrial cancers have an excellent cancer-specific prognosis. The common comorbidities of obesity and age (diabetes, hypertension, cardiovascular disease) complicate their overall management, but most of these patients will survive their cancers without recurrent disease. A substantial minority of patients with more advanced disease can still be cured at the time of primary therapy with combinations of surgery, chemotherapy, and sometimes radiation. Patients with persistent or recurrent disease will generally succumb to their illness within a 2- to 3-year period.

Late complications of surgical resection tend to be quite limited; some mild lymphedema is the most common late toxicity. Pelvic radiation has more reported late complications, including bowel, bladder, and sexual dysfunction, but recent advances in computer-based treatment plans may provide a better long-term risk-to-benefit ratio. The long-term adverse effects of adjuvant chemotherapy are rare but can include neuropathy and occasional renal injury.

UTERINE SARCOMAS

Gynecologic sarcomas most often arise in the uterus. The two most common malignant histologic types are carcinosarcoma of the uterus and leiomyosarcoma. Carcinosarcoma of the uterus is generally sporadic and is managed with a combination of complete surgical resection and adjuvant combination chemotherapy. Like endometrial cancer, even advanced stage carcinosarcoma can be successfully treated by multimodality therapy, but recurrent disease is rapidly fatal. Leiomyosarcoma is a malignant smooth muscle tumor arising in the myometrium. Surgical resection is the mainstay of treatment, and the role of adjuvant chemotherapy or radiotherapy is unproved. Recurrent leiomyosarcoma can be treated with surgery (for localized disease) and chemotherapy.

CANCERS OF THE FALLOPIAN TUBE AND OVARY

EPIDEMIOLOGY

Ovarian cancer is a generic term for a family of diseases, including epithelial ovarian cancers, germ cell tumors of the ovary, and stromal cancers arising in the ovary. Cancer originating in the epithelium of the fallopian tube and ovarian surface is the fourth most common lethal cancer in American women. Approximately 22,000 new cases of ovarian cancers will be diagnosed each year, and because most are diagnosed at advanced stages, roughly 15,000 of these women will eventually die of their disease despite current therapy. Internationally, the incidence of ovarian cancer is highest in white women, and societies characterized by low parity, high-fat diets, and older populations. Ovarian cancer incidence is highest in North America and Europe, with lower incidence in Asia and Sub-Saharan Africa. In the United States, risk factors for ovarian cancer include family history of breast or ovarian cancer, early menarche, delayed menopause, and nulliparity, whereas oral contraceptives, aspirin, and breast-feeding are consistently shown to reduce risk. The median age of onset for ovarian cancer is approximately 60 years, although familial ovarian cancers occur roughly 10 years earlier than the sporadic form.

The indolent borderline tumors of the ovary (or tumors with low malignant potential) form a distinct group of epithelial ovarian cancers characterized by slow growth, rare metastatic spread, and a very different pattern of genetic alterations. These rare borderline tumors are primarily managed by surgical resection as necessary.

PATHOBIOLOGY

The histologic appearance (and accompanying genetic characteristics) allows epithelial ovarian cancers to be divided into serous, mucinous, clear cell, and endometrioid cancers. Although distinct on histologic and molecular grounds, the clinical management of these ovarian cancers has not yet diverged. High-grade serous ovarian cancer (HGSOC) comprises over 80% of the total number of patients and is the best characterized subset of ovarian tumors.[7]

At least 85% of ovarian cancers are sporadic and not associated with heritable abnormalities. However, approximately 10 to 15% of HGSOCs are linked to families carrying germline mutations that are inherited in an autosomal dominant fashion. The affected genes include *BRCA1* and *BRCA2*, which are critical cell cycle checkpoint regulators involved in the maintenance of DNA integrity, particularly in the homologous recombination pathway that is important for double-strand DNA repair. Certain ethnic populations founded from small ancestral populations such as the Ashkenazi Jews have a high frequency of mutations in these genes. In addition to these genes, other less common germline mutations in DNA repair–linked genes, including *CHEK2, ATM,* and *PALB2,* also can increase ovarian cancer risk. Affected members of these breast/ovarian cancer families have an increased risk for both early-onset breast and ovarian cancer and a high lifetime risk for these cancers. In sporadic ovarian cancers, these same genes may be lost through somatic mutation or gene silencing. It is now estimated that 50% or more of all ovarian cancers have a BRCA-like phenotype. Interestingly, *BRCA1/2* mutated ovarian cancer appears to have a superior survival compared to sporadic ovarian cancer.[8] Mutations in *BRCA1* or *BRCA2* confer a "collateral sensitivity" to cisplatin and other chemotherapy agents that induce double-stranded DNA damage. This collateral weakness has been targeted through the development of poly-ADP-ribose polymerase inhibitors.[A10] A smaller group of familial ovarian cancers is linked to families with Lynch syndrome (HNPCC) and impairment of DNA mismatch repair.

It is now accepted that most serous ovarian cancers arise through a well-defined series of mutations in the fallopian tube epithelium. Through sequential losses of the homologous DNA repair competence (via loss *of BRCA1, BRCA2, PALB2,* or other genes in the DNA repair pathway) and *p53* function, a defined sequence of events leads to serous carcinoma in situ and eventually carcinoma involving the ovary, lymph nodes, and peritoneal surfaces of the abdominal organs. The lifetime risk for women carrying an altered, high-risk allele for one of these genes may approach 70% or more, depending on environmental factors and modifying alleles when the second, nonpathogenic allele is lost.

CLINICAL MANIFESTATIONS

The diagnosis of ovarian cancer is complicated by the nonspecific nature of the initial symptoms.[9] Unfortunately, small adnexal masses are usually silent, but as a mass increases in size, symptoms include pelvic fullness, constipation, urinary frequency, and dyspareunia. In more advanced disease, the most common symptoms include fatigue, malaise, early satiety, bloating, and loss of appetite. Abdominal girth increase is often noted as malignant ascites accumulates.

DIAGNOSIS

Ultrasonography or computed tomography of the abdomen and pelvis will usually strongly support the diagnosis and lead to early surgical intervention. Although peritoneal fluid cytology can sometimes be diagnostic, percutaneous biopsy of adnexal masses should *not* be part of the initial workup, to avoid contamination of the peritoneal cavity by an otherwise confined tumor. CA-125 is a normal mucin antigen from MUC16 that is often found at abnormally high levels in the serum of patients with ovarian cancer (and sometimes in other cancers, including lung, pancreas, and uterus). However, serologic findings can be supportive but is not diagnostic in affirming or excluding the diagnosis of ovarian cancer because a variety of benign conditions also can elevate the CA-125 value.

TREATMENT Rx

The treatment of ovarian cancer begins at the time of exploratory laparotomy, and adequate primary surgery remains the most important determinant of ovarian cancer survival. The surgery should be performed by a trained gynecologic oncologist in a highly experienced center to achieve the best outcome. Adequate initial surgery should include a total abdominal hysterectomy with bilateral salpingo-oophorectomy, omentectomy, and lymph node dissection. The upper abdomen and diaphragm should be inspected and biopsy samples obtained. Every effort should be made to remove any visible cancer. If complete resection is not achievable, cytoreduction to tumor bulk less than 1 cm is still useful and will permit intraperitoneal chemotherapy. If a successful complete resection is not possible, neoadjuvant chemotherapy and deferred surgery is an acceptable choice, although the projected survival is inferior to complete primary resection.[A11]

At the completion of primary surgery, a stage is assigned to the patient's tumor, based on extent of involvement as shown in Table 199-3. Using a combination of residual tumor bulk, tumor histology, grade and stage, one of four treatment plans is chosen, as illustrated in Figure 199-1. For stage IA or IB, grade 1 or 2 tumors, observation alone is the most acceptable treatment because these patients have a tumor recurrence rate below 5%. For all stage IC cancers, all grade 3 tumors, and the rare stage IIA tumors, the recommendation should be for three to six cycles of platinum-based chemotherapy. For stage IIB to IIIC tumors, with residual disease less than 1 cm in greatest dimension, six cycles of platinum-based intraperitoneal treatment is preferred, and bulkier disease or stage IV disease should receive intravenous platinum-based therapy.[10][A12] These strategies are indicated in Table 199-3.

Following primary chemotherapy, reassessment of extent of residual disease by CA-125 and computed tomography is performed. For patients with persistent or resistant disease, other palliative chemotherapy can be offered but the outlook for such patients is quite poor. Patients in complete remission can be observed expectantly. Nearly all relapses will occur within a 3-year period, and regular quarterly follow-up is recommended in the United States. Over 75% of patients with advanced ovarian cancer will relapse in 12 to 30 months after diagnosis; although patients can be successfully treated for years, curative treatment is not yet available. Choice of chemotherapy at the time of recurrence depends on treatment-free interval, comorbidities, and residual toxicities. Active agents for retreatment include with carboplatin, gemcitabine, liposomal doxorubicin, pemetrexed, and bevacizumab.[11]

SCREENING AND PREVENTION

Although screening procedures have been aggressively sought for 25 years, there are no screening strategies that currently can be recommended, even for high-risk patients and definitely not for the general population of postmenopausal women. Combinations of serum CA-125 screening, transvaginal ultrasound testing, and panels of circulating serologic markers have all failed to achieve the requisite sensitivity and specificity in large-scale testing.[A13] Testing for germline and somatic mutations is increasingly important to

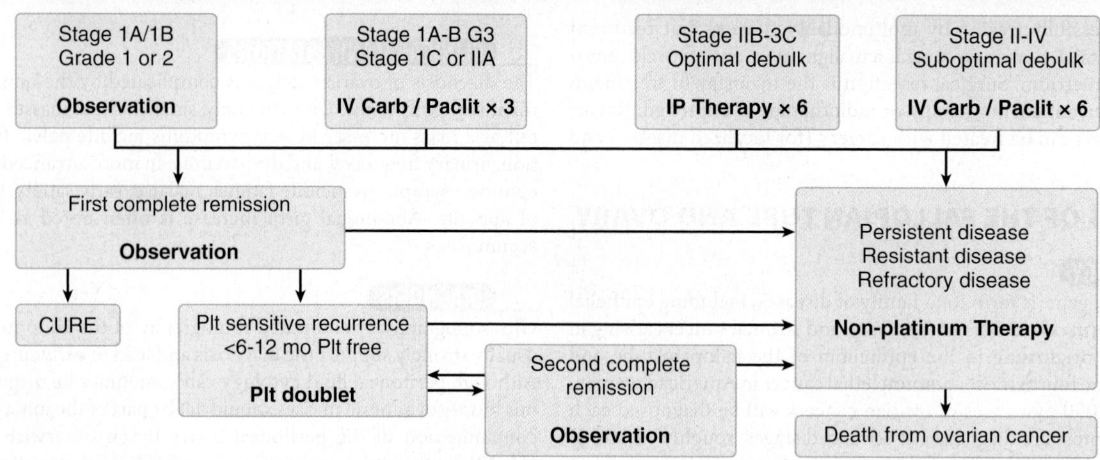

FIGURE 199-1. Ovarian cancer disease states model. The bulk of ovarian cancer management occurs after relapse. Primary therapy is allocated as indicated in the upper portion of the figure. The subsequent treatment depends on the elapsed time since the last exposure to a platinum complex drug. Patients with a platinum-free interval exceeding 6 to 12 months usually will receive a platinum-containing doublet and may attain a second (or greater) complete remision. Shorter intervals of platinum-free time will go on to nonplatinum single-agent treatment and have a median life expectancy of 1 to 2 years. Carb = carboplatin; Paclit = paclitexel; Plt = platinum.

TABLE 199-3 APPROACH TO OVARIAN CANCER BY STAGE*

FIGO STAGE	BRIEF DEFINITION	USUAL TREATMENT
IA G1/2	One ovary, no surface involvement	Staging laparotomy, observation only
IA G3	One ovary, no surface involvement; poorly differentiated	Staging laparotomy, chemotherapy for 3 cycles
IB G1/2	Both ovaries, no surface involvement	Staging laparotomy, observation only
IB G3	50% or more invasion of myometrial thickness, poorly differentiated	Staging laparotomy, chemotherapy for 3 cycles
IC	Surface involvement, positive cytology, or intraoperative spillage	Staging laparotomy, chemotherapy for 3 cycles
IIA	Extension to tubes or uterus	Staging laparotomy, chemotherapy for 3-6 cycles
IIB	Other pelvic organ extension	Staging laparotomy, chemotherapy for 3-6 cycles
IIC	Pelvic extension plus surface involvement, positive cytology, or intraoperative spillage	Staging laparotomy, chemotherapy with IP route preferred
IIIA	Microscopic tumor outside the true pelvis	Staging laparotomy, chemotherapy with IP route preferred
IIIB	Tumor < 2 cm in dimension outside the pelvis	Staging laparotomy, chemotherapy with IP route preferred
IIIC	Tumor > 2 cm outside the true pelvis or positive lymph nodes	Staging laparotomy, chemotherapy with IP route preferred
IV	Involvement of liver parenchyma, extension beyond the abdomen, cytology positive pleural effusion, inguinal lymph nodes	Chemotherapy

*Staging laparotomy includes total abdominal hysterectomy, bilateral salpingo-oophorectomy and omentectomy. A pelvic lymph node dissection and upper abdominal exploration is also required. In well-staged, early-stage disease (IA/IB), the need for chemotherapy is based primarily on histologic grade. In advanced disease, optimal debulking to < 1 cm residual disease permits the use of intraperitoneal treatment (IP). All primary therapy should include a platinum drug and a second, non–cross-reactive drug such as paclitaxel or liposomal doxorubicin.

predict the response to therapy and prognosis.[12] The routine genetic testing of women with newly diagnosed ovarian cancer is recommended, in the appropriate circumstance, to discover families bearing *BRCA1/2* mutations who will require further monitoring.

Prevention strategies for ovarian cancer remain limited. Oral contraceptive use for 5 years or more can reduce ovarian cancer incidence by approximately 50%.[13] For high-risk women with mutations in *BRCA1* or *BRCA2*, a prophylactic salpingo-oophorectomy by age 40 can reduce ovarian cancer risk by more than 90% and will also reduce breast cancer incidence. Low-dose aspirin use has also been associated with reduced ovarian cancer risk.[14]

PROGNOSIS AND SURVIVOR MANAGEMENT

Women who remain disease-free for 3 years are likely to be cured of their ovarian cancer. Among patients with recurrence, median survival seems highly dependent on their initial stage and success of their primary debulking surgery. Patients with optimally debulked stage IIIC disease have a median survival in excess of 5 years, whereas patients with stage IV and patients with suboptimal debulking surgery have median survivals of 30 to 48 months. The terminal phase of ovarian cancer is generally characterized by progressive inanition and eventual intestinal obstruction. Ovarian cancer survivors may have intestinal adhesions from surgery and chronic neuropathy or electrolyte wasting from primary chemotherapy. Those ovarian cancer survivors living with chronic ovarian cancer are often able to continue to have productive work and family lives for several years after the diagnosis of ovarian cancer.

VULVAR CANCER

Cancer of the vulva is a relatively rare gynecologic malignancy that represents less than 5% of gynecologic cancer and is primarily seen in postmenopausal women. Like cervical cancer, the etiology of vulvar cancer is prior infection with HPV. Patients with vulvar cancer complain of itching, pain, and local discomfort, often arising in the presence of atrophic changes of the vulvar epithelium. The treatment of vulvar cancer is surgical excision with good margins and possible dissection of one or both inguinal lymph node regions in advanced disease. Recurrent or unresectable vulvar cancer also can be treated with external beam radiation, often in combination with cisplatin in radiation sensitizing doses.

UTERINE FIBROIDS

Uterine fibroids are the most common female pelvic tumor, with a prevalence as high as 40% during the reproductive years and as high as 70 to 80% by age 50. Fibroids, which are almost always benign monoclonal tumors, arise from disordered smooth-muscle cells in the uterine myometrium. A variety of somatic mutations, especially of the *MED12* gene on the X chromosome, have been described. Fibroids depend on estrogen and progesterone and usually shrink after menopause.[15] In early pregnancy and the postpartum period, however, they can grow rapidly.

The majority of fibroids are asymptomatic, but they can cause pelvic pressure, pain, and heavy uterine bleeding. Diagnosis is typically made by physical examination and confirmed by ultrasound. Although fibroids are not premalignant tumors, a uterine sarcoma can have similar symptoms at presentation.

Noninvasive, hormonally based anti-progesterone therapies such as oral ulipristal acetate (5 or 10 mg per day for 13 weeks) can reduce the size of fibroids, decrease dysfunctional uterine bleeding and pain, and improve overall quality of life. A14 A15 For persistent symptoms, surgical removal of the fibroid or of the uterus itself can be performed during laparotomy or by laparoscopic surgery. Power morcellation, a process by which the uterus is divided into smaller fragments that can be removed in stages laparoscopically, is no longer routinely recommended because of the small but finite risk of disseminating pieces of potentially malignant tissue found in a small percentage of fibroid uteruses.[16] Robotically assisted and laparoscopic hysterectomy have similar morbidity profiles, but the use of robotic technology results in substantially higher costs. Other strategies for the treatment of symptomatic uterine fibroids include uterine artery embolization, transvaginal temporary uterine artery occlusion, and MRI-guided focused ultrasound.

OTHER GYNECOLOGIC CANCERS

Any structure of the müllerian tract can undergo malignant transformation. Other types of gynecologic cancer include germ cell tumors of the ovary (homologs of testicular cancer), stromal tumors of the ovary, and cancers of the vagina, vulva, and vulvar adnexa. These are all much less common than the tumors described earlier. Because of the rarity of these cancers, early referral to experts in gynecologic oncology is essential. Survivors of these rare forms of gynecologic cancer will share the residual side effects that affect survivors of cervical, endometrial, and ovarian cancers, such as potential alterations of bowel, bladder, and sexual function, as well as lymphedema and the consequences of early menopause.

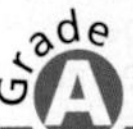

Grade A References

A1. DiSilvestro PA, Ali S, Craighead PS, et al. Phase III randomized trial of weekly cisplatin and irradiation versus cisplatin and tirapazamine and irradiation in stages IB2, IIA, IIB, IIIB, and IVA cervical carcinoma limited to the pelvis: a Gynecologic Oncology Group study. *J Clin Oncol.* 2014;32:458-464.

A2. Tewari KS, Sill MW, Long HJ 3rd, et al. Improved survival with bevacizumab in advanced cervical cancer. *N Engl J Med.* 2014;370:734-743.

A3. Munoz N, Manalastas R Jr, Pitisuttithum P, et al. Safety, immunogenicity, and efficacy of quadrivalent human papillomavirus (types 6, 11, 16, 18) recombinant vaccine in women aged 24-45 years: a randomised, double-blind trial. *Lancet.* 2009;373:1949-1957.

A4. Paavonen J, Naud P, Salmeron J, et al. Efficacy of human papillomavirus (HPV)-16/18 AS04-adjuvanted vaccine against cervical infection and precancer caused by oncogenic HPV types (PATRICIA): final analysis of a double-blind, randomised study in young women. *Lancet.* 2009; 374:301-314.

A5. Lu B, Kumar A, Castellsague X, et al. Efficacy and safety of prophylactic vaccines against cervical HPV infection and diseases among women: a systematic review & meta-analysis. *BMC Infect Dis.* 2011;11:13.

A6. Walker JL, Piedmonte MR, Spirtos NM, et al. Recurrence and survival after random assignment to laparoscopy versus laparotomy for comprehensive surgical staging of uterine cancer: Gynecologic Oncology Group LAP2 Study. *J Clin Oncol.* 2012;30:695-700.

A7. Kong A, Johnson N, Kitchener HC, et al. Adjuvant radiotherapy for stage I endometrial cancer: an updated Cochrane systematic review and meta-analysis. *J Natl Cancer Inst.* 2012;104:1625-1634.

A8. Nout RA, van de Poll-Franse LV, Lybeert ML, et al. et al. Long-term outcome and quality of life of patients with endometrial carcinoma treated with or without pelvic radiotherapy in the post operative radiation therapy in endometrial carcinoma 1 (PORTEC-1) trial. *J Clin Oncol.* 2011;29: 1692-1700.

A9. Nout RA, Putter H, Jurgenliemk-Schulz IM, et al. Five-year quality of life of endometrial cancer patients treated in the randomised Post Operative Radiation Therapy in Endometrial Cancer (PORTEC-2) trial and comparison with norm data. *Eur J Cancer.* 2012;48:1638-1648.

A10. Ledermann J, Harter P, Gourley C, et al. Olaparib maintenance therapy in platinum-sensitive relapsed ovarian cancer. *N Engl J Med.* 2012;366:1382-1392.

A11. Vergote I, Trope CG, Amant F, et al. Neoadjuvant chemotherapy or primary surgery in stage IIIC or IV ovarian cancer. *N Engl J Med.* 2010;363:943-953.

A12. Burger RA, Brady MF, Bookman MA, et al. Incorporation of bevacizumab in the primary treatment of ovarian cancer. *N Engl J Med.* 2011;365:2473-2483.

A13. Buys SS, Partridge E, Black A, et al. Effect of screening on ovarian cancer mortality: the Prostate, Lung, Colorectal and Ovarian (PLCO) Cancer Screening Randomized Controlled Trial. *JAMA.* 2011;305:2295-2303.

A14. Donnez J, Tatarchuk TF, Bouchard P, et al. Ulipristal acetate versus placebo for fibroid treatment before surgery. *N Engl J Med.* 2012;366:409-420.

A15. Donnez J, Tomaszewski J, Vazquez F, et al. Ulipristal acetate versus leuprolide acetate for uterine fibroids. *N Engl J Med.* 2012;366:421-432.

GENERAL REFERENCES

For the General References and other additional features, please visit Expert Consult at https://expertconsult.inkling.com.

200

TESTICULAR CANCER

LAWRENCE H. EINHORN

EPIDEMIOLOGY

Testicular tumors are relatively uncommon and account for only 1% of male malignancies in the United States. The incidence of testicular cancer is increasing globally, although mortality rates remain low.[1] The primary age group is 15 to 35 years for nonseminomatous tumors and a decade older for seminomas.

Male patients with a history of cryptorchidism have a 10- to 40-fold increased risk for the development of testicular cancer. The normally descended testis in these men is also at higher risk, suggesting a dysgenetic abnormality.

PATHOBIOLOGY

More than 95% of tumors of the testis originate from germ cells.[2] Germ cell tumors can be seminomas or nonseminomatous germ cell tumors. Seminomas are more likely to be confined to the testis (stage I) and small-volume metastases to the retroperitoneal lymph nodes are exquisitely sensitive to radiation therapy. Pure seminomas never have elevated serum α-fetoprotein (AFP) levels. Nonseminomatous germ cell tumors consist of embryonal cell carcinomas, choriocarcinomas, yolk sac tumors, or teratomas, alone or mixed with other elements. Teratomas do not secrete human chorionic gonadotropin (hCG) or AFP and do not usually metastasize; they grow by local extension and are completely resistant to radiation therapy and chemotherapy.

Most germ cell testicular cancers in adults are associated with the cytogenetic abnormality i12p—an isochromosome of the short arm of chromosome 12—which is a highly specific finding in germ cell tumors. Genome-wide associated studies (GWAS) have identified association with variants in several genes, most strongly with *KITLG*.[3] Sertoli cell tumors, Leydig cell tumors, and lymphomas are the most common non–germ cell tumors. In men older than 60 years, most tumors are non-Hodgkin lymphoma (Chapter 185), with a predilection for bilateral involvement.

CLINICAL MANIFESTATIONS

Most patients with testicular cancer are initially evaluated because of testicular pain or because of a mass in or enlargement of one testis. Others are asymptomatic, and the cancer is first detected during a routine physical examination. Less commonly, the diagnosis is made during an evaluation for infertility, in part because testicular cancer can cause oligospermia.

Metastatic spread is either lymphatic or hematogenous. Lymphatic metastases usually go initially to the ipsilateral retroperitoneal lymph nodes, where they may be associated with flank pain. Lymphatic metastases may continue in a superior direction to the posterior mediastinum and eventually to the left supraclavicular lymph nodes. A large retroperitoneal mass or a supraclavicular lymph node may be palpable on physical examination. Hematogenous spread usually occurs first to the pulmonary parenchyma bilaterally. Pulmonary symptoms such as chest pain, shortness of breath, dyspnea on exertion, coughing, or hemoptysis are seen only with extensive pulmonary metastases. Other sites of hematogenous spread include the liver, bone, or brain. Significant elevation of the serum hCG level may produce gynecomastia.

DIAGNOSIS

Patients with a palpable mass in the testis should be suspected of having testicular cancer, especially if there is a history of cryptorchidism. Other causes of testicular and scrotal abnormalities may be included in the differential diagnosis. Acute pain in the testis suggests torsion. Painful enlargement

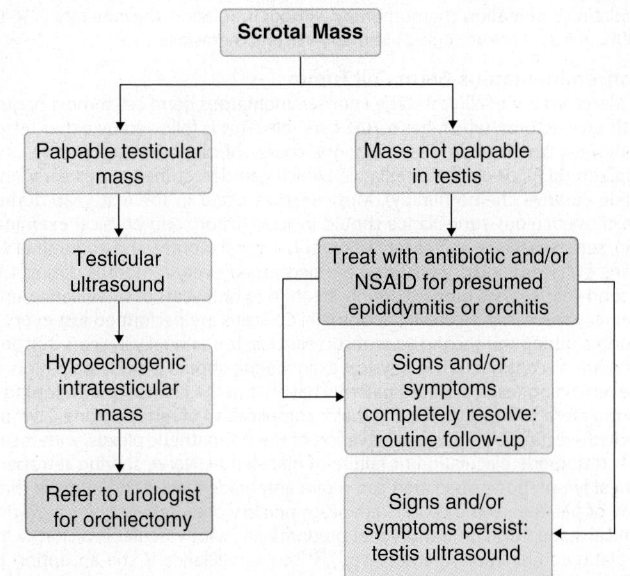

FIGURE 200-1. **Management of a scrotal mass. NSAID = nonsteroidal anti-inflammatory drug.**

may be due to a hydrocele, which may be caused by an underlying primary testicular malignancy. Pain and tenderness adjacent to the testis may be due to epididymitis or a varicocele. Tenderness of the testis itself on physical examination may reflect orchitis. However, an underlying neoplasm should always be considered.

Any testicular symptoms, including pain or a suspected mass, require evaluation. Testicular ultrasound is the test of choice in all suspicious cases. A hypoechogenic mass within the testis must be presumed to be testicular cancer and requires referral to a urologist (Fig. 200-1).

When orchiectomy reveals the diagnosis of testicular cancer, a staging evaluation is performed to determine the extent of disease and appropriate therapy. Clinical stage I disease is confined to the testis; stage II disease reflects spread to the retroperitoneal lymph nodes; and stage III is supradiaphragmatic disease, with either nodal metastases to the posterior mediastinum or supraclavicular region or hematogenous spread, especially to the lungs.

In addition to a full history and physical examination, serum hCG and AFP levels should be determined. Because the serum half-life is 1 day for hCG and 5 days for AFP, an AFP level of 1000 may take more than a month to normalize after orchiectomy, even if the tumor has been completely removed and there are no metastases. Imaging studies to define the extent of disease include abdominal and pelvic computed tomography (CT) and a chest radiograph. If the chest radiograph does not show pulmonary metastases, a chest CT scan should be performed. Bone scans and head CT scans can be reserved for patients with symptoms suggestive of osseous and central nervous system metastases, respectively.

TABLE 200-1 DEFINITION OF POOR RISK DISEASE (ALL NONSEMINOMATOUS GERM CELL TUMOR)

Presence of any of the following:
- Human chorionic gonadotropin (hCG) > 50,000 mIU/mL
- α-Fetoprotein (AFP) > 10,000 ng/mL
- Non-pulmonary visceral metastases (e.g., bone liver, brain)
- Primary mediastinal nonseminomatous germ cell tumor

PREVENTION AND TREATMENT Rx

A careful testicular examination is a mandatory part of the physical examination in men, especially young men (Chapter 15), and is the key means of detecting tumors at an early stage.[4] With the patient lying supine or standing up, the testis is gently palpated with the thumb and second and third fingers; the entire anterior, posterior, and lateral surfaces of the testis should be examined. Men ages 15 to 34 years should be taught to perform the examination on themselves.[5]

Local and Regional Disease

Seminomas

Approximately 70% of seminomas are initially diagnosed at clinical stage I.[6] Although the cure rate with orchiectomy alone is 85%, treatment also can include 2000 cGy para-aortic irradiation[A1] or adjuvant carboplatin.[A2] The preferred option, however, is surveillance, which avoids unnecessary therapy in 85% of patients as well as potential late consequences of therapy.[A3]

Twenty percent of patients with seminoma are initially found to have stage II disease (positive abdominal CT scan). For these patients, radiation therapy has a 90% cure rate; in patients who are not cured by radiation therapy, subsequent combination chemotherapy (cisplatin combined with etoposide, with or without bleomycin) is usually curative. If the transverse diameter of the tumor is greater than 3 cm, if there are multiple anatomic levels of nodal metastases, or if stage III disease is present, the preferred initial treatment is cisplatin combination chemotherapy without irradiation; the cure rate is 90 to 100% unless there are non-pulmonary visceral metastases.[7]

Nonseminomatous Germ Cell Tumors

Management of clinical stage I nonseminomatous germ cell tumors begins with orchiectomy, which has a 70% cure rate. This is followed by either retroperitoneal lymph node dissection; one course of bleomycin, etoposide, and cisplatin (BEP); or close surveillance (which can detect metastases early and guide curative chemotherapy). Most relapses occur in the first year, during which meticulous surveillance should include history and physical examination, serum markers, and chest radiograph every 2 months and abdominal CT scans every 4 months. All studies are performed every 4 months during the second year, every 6 months during the third to fifth years of surveillance, and annually thereafter. However, abdominal CT scans are performed just every 6 months during the second year of surveillance, but annually in years 3-5, and then are discontinued. The physical examination should include palpation of the remaining testis, because patients have a 1 to 2% chance of developing a contralateral primary tumor. The major complication of retroperitoneal lymph node dissection is inadvertent severing of the sympathetic plexus, with resultant retrograde ejaculation or failure of ejaculation. Nerve-sparing retroperitoneal lymph node dissection can retain antegrade ejaculation in more than 95% of patients. Some centers advocate primary chemotherapy for high-risk clinical stage I disease (embryonal predominant with vascular invasion) with cisplatin combination chemotherapy,[A4] but surveillance is still an option in these patients.

For clinical stage II disease with persistently elevated serum markers or a transverse tumor diameter greater than 3 cm, chemotherapy is preferred. Other patients with stage II disease are treated with retroperitoneal lymph node dissection, often followed by close surveillance (as described earlier, but without abdominal CT scans) or adjuvant chemotherapy. Testicular cancer has a higher cure rate with surgery alone, despite nodal metastases, than any other cancer.

Chemotherapy for Disseminated or Persistent Disease

The combination of bleomycin, etoposide, and cisplatin (BEP) repeated every 3 weeks for three or four courses cures 70% of patients with metastatic disease and is the standard chemotherapy for disseminated testicular cancer. Poor-risk disease (Table 200-1) has a 50 to 60% cure rate with standard three-drug therapy, intermediate-risk disease (hCG 5000 to 50,000 IU/mL or AFP 1000 to 10,000 ng/mL) has a 75% cure rate, and all other forms of metastatic disease (good risk) have a 90 to 100% cure rate. Approximately 60% of patients receiving chemotherapy have good-risk disease, and just three courses of BEP is an adequate duration of therapy.

In the 30% of metastatic germ cell tumors that are not cured by initial combination chemotherapy, the use of standard-dose salvage therapy (ifosfamide, cisplatin, and either vinblastine or paclitaxel)[8] or high-dose carboplatin and etoposide therapy, followed by peripheral blood stem cell transplantation, can cure 25 to 70% of refractory cases, depending on patient characteristics. Late relapse beyond 2 years from completion of chemotherapy occurs in 2 to 3% of patients with metastatic disease. This usually is manifested by a rise in serum AFP. Optimal approach is evaluation for site(s) of metastases and surgical resection if feasible.

PROGNOSIS

Sequelae in Long-Term Survivors

Testicular cancer is the most curable solid tumor, with a 10-year survival rate of more than 95%. However, the typically normal life expectancy of individuals with the disease who were treated at a young age has led to the emergence of significant morbidities.

Testicular cancer survivors, particularly those who were initially treated with a combination of chemotherapy and irradiation, are at increased risk for developing second malignancies. These may include a wide variety of solid tumors and hematologic malignancies. Etoposide and cisplatin are associated with cumulative dose-dependent development of myelodysplastic syndrome (Chapter 182) and secondary leukemia.[9] Patients are also at increased risk for developing metachronous contralateral testicular cancer.

Increased cardiovascular risk in long-term survivors manifests most prominently as hyperlipidemia (Chapter 206) and metabolic syndrome (Chapter 229). The risk for metabolic syndrome is especially increased in survivors with testosterone levels in the lowest quadrille.[10] The clinical significance of low-grade hypogonadism among testicular cancer survivors has not been well studied. Although 10-year paternity rate in testicular cancer survivors is reduced by 30% compared with that in the general population, the majority of individuals who attempt paternity after treatment will become biologic fathers without medical assistance. Other long-term complications in survivors may include peripheral neuropathy, ototoxicity, and chronic renal insufficiency.

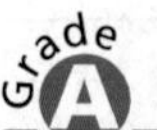

Grade A References

A1. Jones WG, Fossa SD, Mead GM, et al. Randomized trial of 30 versus 20 Gy in the adjuvant treatment of stage I testicular seminoma. *J Clin Oncol.* 2005;23:1200-1208.

A2. Oliver RTD, Mason MD, Mead GM, et al. Radiotherapy versus single-dose carboplatin in adjuvant treatment of stage I seminoma: a randomised trial. *Lancet.* 2005;366:293-300.

A3. Nichols C, Roth B, Albers P, et al. Active surveillance is the preferred approach to clinical stage I testicular cancer. *J Clin Oncol.* 2013;31:3490-3493.

A4. Alberts P, Siener R, Krege S, et al. Randomized phase III trial comparing retroperitoneal lymph node dissection with one course of bleomycin and etoposide plus cisplatin in the adjuvant treatment of clinical stage I non-seminomatous germ cell tumors. *J Clin Oncol.* 2008;26:2966-2972.

GENERAL REFERENCES

For the General References and other additional features, please visit Expert Consult at https://expertconsult.inkling.com.

201

PROSTATE CANCER

ERIC J. SMALL

DEFINITION

Prostate cancer is the most common noncutaneous malignant neoplasm in men in the United States, where it results in about 32,000 deaths each year, making it the second most common cause of cancer death in men. Prostate cancer is a single histologic disease with marked clinical heterogeneity ranging from indolent, clinically unimportant disease to a virulent, rapidly lethal phenotype.

EPIDEMIOLOGY

The incidence of clinically diagnosed prostate cancer reflects the effects of screening by the prostate-specific antigen (PSA) assay. Before PSA testing was available, about 19,000 new cases of prostate cancer were reported each year in the United States; this number reached 84,000 by 1993 and peaked at about 300,000 new cases in 1996. Since 1996, the reported annual incidence of prostate cancer in the United States has declined to about 190,000, a number that may more closely estimate the true incidence of clinically detectable disease. The death rate from prostate cancer has declined by about 1% per year since 1990. The age-specific decrease in the mortality rate has been greatest in men younger than 75 years. Men older than 75 years still account for two thirds of all prostate cancer deaths. Whether this decline is due to early detection (screening) or to improved therapy has not been established.

Risk factors for prostate cancer[1] include increasing age, family history, African American ethnicity, obesity, and dietary factors. Epidemiologic studies have suggested that nutritional factors such as reduced fat intake and increased soy protein may have a protective effect against the development of prostate cancer. The incidence of prostate cancer among African Americans is nearly twice that observed among white Americans. Prostate cancer is diagnosed in African Americans at a more advanced stage, and disease-specific survival is lower in African Americans. The relative contributions of biologic, genetic, and environmental differences, as well as differences in health care access, are not well established. Prior vasectomy and benign prostatic hypertrophy (BPH) (Chapter 129) do not increase the risk. Prostatic intraepithelial neoplasia, particularly when it is high grade, is recognized as a premalignant lesion, so its presence on biopsy increases the likelihood of subsequent malignancy.

PATHOBIOLOGY

Prostate cancer is more common among relatives of men with early-onset prostate cancer. However, although many genetic abnormalities with both loss and gain of function have been identified, none occur in more than 10% of patients with prostate cancer. For example, germline mutation (G84E) of $H0XB_{13}$, a homeobox transcription factor gene that is important in prostate development, has been associated with significantly increased risk of hereditary prostate cancer.[2] Consistent patterns of changes associated with an increased likelihood for the development of prostate cancer have not been identified.

Approximately half of prostate cancers demonstrate genetic rearrangements,[3,4] including fusion of promoters or enhancers of androgen-responsive genes such as *TMPRSS2* (transmembrane protease, serine 2) with oncogenic *ETS (E-26)* transcription factors such as *ERG (ETS-related gene)*. Gene fusions lead to overexpression of these oncogenic transcription factors.

Testosterone is required for maintenance of a normal, healthy prostatic epithelium, but it is also a prerequisite for the development of prostate cancer. Prostate cancers express robust levels of androgen receptor (AR), and signaling through the AR results in growth, progression, and invasion of prostate cancer. Inhibition of signaling, typically by the surgical or pharmacologic reduction of testosterone levels, results in prostate cancer apoptosis and involution. Ultimately, however, androgen-deprivation therapy (ADT) loses clinical efficacy. The biologic events surrounding the clinical development of "androgen-deprivation–resistant prostate cancer," also called castration-resistant prostate cancer (CRPC), are not well delineated, but amplification of the AR, which is a common event in these patients, presumably makes the cancer sensitive to minute levels of androgen or other ligands of the AR. Androgens produced through accessory pathways by the adrenal gland and upregulation of enzymatic regulators of androgen synthesis pathways within CRPC cells provide additional sources of ligand. The identification of AR splice variants that are constitutively active and ligand independent raises this as a potential mechanism by which true hormone resistance develops. The development of resistance to potent androgen signaling inhibition may be associated with the emergence of aggressive, lethal CRPC with neuroendocrine differentiation. Whether this reflects a process of transdifferentiation or clonal selection is not known.

CLINICAL MANIFESTATIONS

Most patients with early-stage, organ-confined disease are asymptomatic. Obstructive voiding symptoms (hesitancy, intermittent urinary stream, decreased force of stream) generally reflect locally advanced disease with growth into the urethra or bladder neck, although these symptoms can be indistinguishable from BPH (Chapter 129). Locally advanced tumors can also result in hematuria and hematospermia. Prostate cancer that has spread to the regional pelvic lymph nodes occasionally causes edema of the lower extremities or discomfort in the pelvic and perineal areas. Metastasis occurs most commonly to bone, where it is frequently asymptomatic, but it can also cause severe and unremitting pain. Bone metastasis can result in pathologic fractures or spinal cord compression. Although visceral metastases are rare as presenting features of prostate cancer, there is an increasing incidence of pulmonary, hepatic, pleural, peritoneal, and central nervous system metastases that appear to be treatment emergent.

DIAGNOSIS

More than 60% of patients with prostate cancer are asymptomatic, and the diagnosis is made solely because of an elevated screening PSA level. A palpable nodule on digital rectal examination (DRE), which is the next most common clinical presentation, generally prompts biopsy. Much less commonly, prostate cancer is diagnosed because of advanced disease that causes obstructive voiding symptoms, pelvic or perineal discomfort, lower extremity edema, or symptomatic bone lesions.

Although the DRE has a low sensitivity and specificity for the diagnosis of prostate cancer, biopsy of a nodule or area of induration reveals cancer 50% of the time, suggesting that prostate biopsy should be undertaken in all men with palpable nodules. The PSA level has a far better sensitivity but a low specificity because conditions such as BPH and prostatitis can cause false-positive PSA elevations (Chapter 129). By use of a PSA threshold of 4 ng/mL, 70% to 80% of tumors are detected. Far greater accuracy is achieved with age-specific PSA thresholds. Thus, for men age 40 to 49 years, a PSA greater than 2.5 is considered abnormal; for men 50 to 59 years, a PSA greater than 3.5 is abnormal; for men 60 to 69 years, a PSA greater than 4.5 should prompt further evaluation; and patients age 70 to 79 years should have a PSA of 6.5 or less. The positive predictive value for a single PSA level above 10 ng/mL is greater than 60% for cancer, but the positive predictive value for a PSA level between 4 and 10 ng/mL is only about 30%. Assays of the PSA fraction that circulates unbound (percentage of free PSA) may help distinguish prostate cancer from benign processes; in patients with PSA levels of 4 to 10 ng/mL, the percentage of free PSA appears to be an independent predictor of prostate cancer, and a cutoff value of free PSA less than 25% can detect 95% of cancers while avoiding 20% of unnecessary biopsies.

Transrectal ultrasonography with biopsies is indicated when the PSA level is elevated, when the percentage of free PSA is less than 25%, or when an abnormality is noted on DRE. Extended field specimens (preferably up to six biopsies on each side) are generally obtained. Seminal vesicles are sampled in high-risk patients. A bone scan is warranted only in patients with PSA levels above 10 ng/mL, and abdominal and pelvic computed tomography or magnetic resonance imaging is usually unrevealing in patients with PSA levels below 10 to 20 ng/mL.

The prognosis of patients with prostate cancer correlates with histologic grade and extent (stage) of disease. More than 95% of prostate cancers are adenocarcinomas, and multifocality is common. Although uncommon, a neuroendocrine variant is increasingly being identified, because of increased awareness but also as a manifestation of the development of resistance to potent androgen signaling inhibition. The histologic (Gleason) grade of adenocarcinomas range from 3 to 5. The Gleason score, which refers to the sum of the two most common histologic patterns seen on each tissue specimen, ranges from 6 (3 + 3) to 10 (5 + 5). In general, tumors are classified as well differentiated (Gleason score of 6), of intermediate differentiation (Gleason score of 7), or poorly differentiated (Gleason score of 8-10). Neuroendocrine differentiation is a histologic diagnosis that is confirmed by staining for chromogranin A or synaptophysin.

Clinical stage is defined by the extent of disease based on the physical examination, imaging studies, and pathology. Stage T1 is nonpalpable prostate cancer detected only on pathologic examination, noted either incidentally after transurethral resection for benign hypertrophy (T1a and T1b) or on a biopsy specimen obtained because of an elevated PSA level (T1c, the most common clinical stage at diagnosis). Stage T2 is a palpable tumor that appears to be confined to the prostate gland (T2a in one lobe or T2b in two lobes), and stage T3 is tumor with extension through the prostatic capsule (T3a if it is focal or T3b if seminal vesicles are involved). T4 tumors are those with invasion of adjacent structures, such as the bladder neck, external urinary sphincter, rectum, levator muscles, or pelvic sidewall. Nodal metastases can be microscopic and detectable only by biopsy or lymphadenectomy, or they can be visible on imaging studies. Distant metastases are predominantly to bone, but occasional visceral metastases occur.

PREVENTION

The precise role for screening remains controversial.[5-7] Currently, many organizations recommend screening with PSA, but the U.S. Preventive Services Task Force recommends against screening.[8] Of two large randomized screening trials using PSA levels, one reported a reduction in prostate cancer–specific mortality,[A1] but neither found an overall reduction in mortality rate.[A1,A2] Overall, PSA screening reduces prostate cancer death at 11 years by 21% (absolute reduction, 0.10 deaths per 1000 persons-years or 1.07 deaths per 1000 men) but not all-cause mortality.[A3] Although overall mortality from prostate cancer has fallen during the screening era, there is no direct evidence that there is a causal relationship.[A4] Screening of men at high risk for developing prostate cancer (family history and African Americans) has not been specifically tested. Randomized trials have shown that vitamins C and selenium are not effective in preventing prostate cancer,[9] and vitamin E supplementation increases prostate cancer by 17%.[10] The use of 5α-reductase inhibitors (both finasteride and dutasteride) unambiguously reduces the risk for development of prostate cancer.[A5,A6] However, this approach has not been widely adopted, primarily because of attendant side effects, most notably sexual dysfunction.

TREATMENT

Rx

Localized Prostate Cancer

Principles of Therapy

The principal therapeutic options for men with localized prostate cancer include (1) active surveillance[11]; (2) retropubic or perineal radical prostatectomy, with or without postoperative radiation therapy to the prostate margins and pelvis; (3) external-beam radiation therapy; and (4) brachytherapy (either permanent or temporary radioactive seed implants), with or without external-beam radiation therapy to the prostate margins and pelvis.

Treatment options require individualization, taking into account the patient's comorbidity, life expectancy, likelihood of cure, and personal preferences based on an understanding of the potential morbidity associated with each treatment. A multidisciplinary approach to integrate surgery, radiation therapy, and androgen deprivation is increasingly recommended. For higher risk patients with a greater likelihood of nodal micrometastases, androgen deprivation is often combined with radiation therapy encompassing both the prostate and the pelvis. In patients at extremely high risk of micrometastatic disease or with comorbidities, systemic therapy alone without concurrent local therapy may be appropriate.

Prostate-specific antigen screening has led to the early detection of a large number of nonpalpable tumors, for which conventional clinical means of staging are inadequate. Thus, less emphasis is being placed on clinical stage, and more emphasis is being placed on Gleason score, PSA values, and other predictors of outcome. Careful risk assessment is required to identify patients who are appropriate candidates for definitive local treatment.

Several studies have confirmed that serum PSA level, clinical stage, and biopsy Gleason score can be used to predict the final pathologic stage after prostatectomy and that these are independent predictors of clinical outcome. For example, in a radiation therapy series, clinical stage T3 or higher, PSA level above 10 ng/mL, and biopsy Gleason score of 7 or higher were risk factors for poor outcome (death or PSA elevation); the 5-year survival rate without PSA elevation was 85% for patients with none of these adverse features (good risk), 65% for patients with one adverse feature (intermediate risk), and 35% for patients with two or three adverse features (poor risk). Similar statistics are cited in radical prostatectomy series. The percentage of biopsy specimens that are positive and the rate of increase in the PSA value are each independent predictors of outcome after radical prostatectomy and can be used to counsel patients about their therapeutic options. A number of multivariable prognostic models have been developed and validated and have been used to develop simple nomograms or online risk calculators.

Low- to Intermediate-Risk Disease

In one randomized trial of patients younger than 75 years with clinical stage T1b, T1c, or T2 prostate cancer, radical prostatectomy compared with no therapy significantly reduced the relative risk of death caused by prostate cancer by about 40% (an 11% absolute risk reduction) and the overall mortality rate by a similar absolute amount at 18 years.[A7] Reductions in progressive disease and metastases were also significant. The adverse effects on quality of life differed between the two strategies—more sexual dysfunction and urinary leakage after radical prostatectomy and more urinary obstruction with active surveillance—but were of similar magnitude.[A8] Nerve-sparing radical prostatectomy was not routinely performed in this study, and many patients already had palpable disease, so the implications for less advanced disease with newer surgical techniques are not known. In another randomized trial of men with localized prostate cancer, radical prostatectomy did not significantly reduce all-cause or prostate-cancer mortality compared with observation through at least 12 years of follow-up, although patients with a PSA greater than 10 ng/mL and possibly patients with intermediate-risk or high-risk tumors may benefit.[A9]

Active surveillance is an increasingly important option for men with low-risk disease. Careful observation of PSA and serial biopsies identifies patients who will never need local therapy. In large active surveillance series, anywhere from 50% to 75% of patients never require local therapy.

Nerve-sparing procedures and careful dissection techniques have decreased the risk of postoperative urinary incontinence and impotence. Postoperative urinary incontinence is reported to occur in fewer than 10% of cases. Postoperative impotence depends on a variety of factors, including the patient's age, preoperative erectile function, extent of cancer, and whether a nerve-sparing procedure was performed. In general, impotence rates of 10% to 50% are cited. Robotic-assisted laparoscopic prostatectomies have gained popularity but have not been shown to result in better outcomes. After a radical prostatectomy, the PSA should become undetectable; a detectable PSA implies the presence of cancer cells, either locally or at a metastatic site. Immediate (adjuvant) postoperative radiation therapy improves biochemical progression-free survival and local control in patients with one or more pathologic risk factors (capsule penetration, positive surgical margins, invasion of a seminal vesicle) after radical prostatectomy.

Conventional external-beam radiation therapy is being replaced by three-dimensional conformal radiation therapy or intensity-modulated radiation therapy, which permits higher doses to the target tissue with less toxicity. Randomized trials suggest a benefit with higher doses of radiation. Brachytherapy, which is the placement of permanent or temporary radioactive seeds directly into the prostate, is adequate for intracapsular disease with no more than minimal transcapular extension; otherwise, it should be combined with external-beam radiation therapy.

High-Risk Disease

Patients with adverse risk features (Gleason score of 8 to 10, PSA >10, stage T3) are at high risk of nodal and micrometastatic disease and are generally treated with aggressive local therapy in combination with androgen deprivation, which is synergistic with radiation therapy.[A10,A11] Taken in the aggregate, trials suggest that 4 months of androgen deprivation with radiation therapy can improve local control and prolong progression-free survival in patients with intermediate-risk features, and long-term androgen deprivation (up to 3 years) prolongs local control, progression-free survival, and overall survival in patients with high-risk features compared with radiation therapy alone.[A12,A13] Patients with stage T3 disease and Gleason scores of 7 have intermediate outcomes, with 8-year survival rates of about 70%; patients with stage T3 disease and Gleason scores of 8 to 10 have 8-year survival rates after radiation therapy of about 50%. Compared with ADT alone, the addition of radiation therapy to ADT improved the overall survival rate at 7 years from 66% to 74% in patients with locally advanced prostate cancer.[A14] Several randomized controlled trials suggest that patients with high-risk disease who are treated surgically and have capsule penetration, positive margins, or seminal vesicle involvement should receive immediate adjuvant radiation therapy.

Recurrent Disease

Between 30% and 50% of men treated with radiation therapy or prostatectomy have evidence of disease recurrence, as defined by a climbing PSA level. PSA doubling time is predictive of survival, and a short PSA doubling time (<3-6 months) is associated with a higher likelihood of systemic disease. For selected patients with clear local recurrences, low PSA levels, and prolonged PSA doubling times, local salvage therapy (surgery for patients previously treated with radiation therapy, radiation therapy for patients previously treated with surgery, and androgen deprivation) can be considered. Although

ADT readily controls PSA levels, it is unknown whether it prolongs life in patients with PSA-only recurrent disease.

Advanced Disease

In patients whose radical prostatectomy surgery reveals microscopic involvement of lymph nodes, immediate androgen deprivation prolongs survival compared with deferment of androgen deprivation until osseous metastases are detected.[12] Similarly, patients who are at high risk of nodal invasion and who undergo external-beam radiation benefit from concurrent short-term hormonal therapy.[A15]

In patients with newly diagnosed metastatic prostate cancer, ADT is the mainstay of treatment and results in symptomatic improvement and disease regression in approximately 80% to 90% of patients. ADT can also be achieved by orchiectomy or by medical castration with a luteinizing hormone–releasing hormone (LHRH) agonist (leuprolide acetate, goserelin acetate). Intermittent ADT, typically consisting of 12 months of therapy followed by time off therapy before resuming ADT is an option in patients with nonmetastatic disease and is potentially useful in patients with metastatic prostate cancer.

Some LHRH agonists cause a transient worsening of signs and symptoms during the first week of therapy as a result of a surge in luteinizing hormone and testosterone, which peaks within 72 hours; an antiandrogen (flutamide, bicalutamide, or nilutamide) should be given with the first LHRH injection to prevent a tumor flare. Medical castration occurs within 4 weeks. The duration of hormone sensitivity is 5 to 10 years for node-positive or high-risk localized (or recurrent) prostate cancer, but it is closer to 24 months in patients with overt metastatic disease. The most common side effects of androgen ablation are loss of libido, impotence, hot flashes, weight gain, fatigue, anemia, and osteoporosis. Bisphosphonates and denosumab reduce bone mineral loss associated with androgen deprivation.

Castration-Resistant Prostate Cancer

Typically, the first manifestation of resistance to androgen deprivation is a climbing PSA level in the setting of anorchid levels of testosterone.[13] In about 15% of patients, discontinuation of antiandrogen therapy (flutamide, bicalutamide, nilutamide) while continuing treatment with LHRH agonists results in a PSA decline that can be associated with symptomatic improvement and can persist for 4 months or more. If antiandrogen withdrawal fails, treatment with secondary hormonal manipulations, such as ketoconazole or estrogens, is appropriate. Sipuleucel-T is an autologous dendritic cell product that has been shown to prolong life[A16] and is appropriate for patients with castration-resistant metastatic prostate cancer who do not have cancer-associated pain, visceral metastases, rapidly progressive disease, or the need for systemic steroids.

As noted earlier, AR amplification is a common event in castration-resistant prostate cancer. Consequently, novel agents that target the AR axis have demonstrated dramatic improvements in response proportion, progression-free survival, and overall survival. Agents that target either the ligand (e.g., the androgen biosynthesis inhibitor abiraterone acetate), as well as agents that target the receptor (e.g., enzalutamide, a direct AR antagonist) in this pathway have been shown to increase survival in metastatic castration-resistant prostate cancer patients, have been approved for use by the Food and Drug Administration, and have dramatically changed the therapeutic landscape.[A17-A20] The optimal sequencing or combination of these agents is under investigation, as is the treatment of metastatic castration-resistant prostate cancer resistant to these agents, including treatment-emergent neuroendocrine variants.

Radium 223 is an α-emitting agent that localizes to metastatic prostate cancer lesions in bone and has been shown to provide a survival advantage in patients with bone-predominant disease and no visceral metastases.[A21] The optimal sequencing and combination of this agent with others is under investigation.

Thereafter, treatment with chemotherapeutic regimens, such as docetaxel plus corticosteroids or mitoxantrone plus corticosteroids, may be effective. Randomized phase III trials have demonstrated a survival advantage of approximately 25% in patients receiving taxol-based therapy compared with mitoxantrone,[A22] and docetaxel-prednisone is now considered a standard therapeutic approach in patients with metastatic, androgen deprivation–resistant prostate cancer. After therapy with docetaxel, patients who remain candidates for further chemotherapy can be treated with cabazitaxel, an agent shown to prolong life in this group of patients. In general, serial PSA levels are the best (albeit imperfect) way to follow up with patients, and a decline of 30% to 50% is associated with improved survival. Zoledronic acid or denosumab is indicated in castration-resistant prostate cancer patients with bone metastases because each reduces the incidence of skeletal-related events.

Palliative Care

Many patients with advanced prostate cancer have bone pain or functional impairments that adversely affect quality of life, and the provision of appropriate palliative care is an integral component of their management. In addition to the usual analgesics, glucocorticoids serve as anti-inflammatory agents and can alleviate bone pain. For patients with widespread bone metastases and pain not easily controlled with analgesics or local irradiation, samarium-153 or radium-223 can be administered intravenously; they are selectively concentrated in bone metastases and are effective in alleviating pain in many patients.

The approach to the treatment of patients with prostate cancer is detailed in Table 201-1.

TABLE 201-1 APPROACH TO THE TREATMENT OF PROSTATE CANCER

EXTENT OF CANCER	THERAPEUTIC OPTIONS
Organ confined: low risk (usually T1 or T2, GS = 7, PSA <10 ng/mL)	Active surveillance Radical prostatectomy External-beam radiation therapy to prostate Brachytherapy
Organ confined: intermediate risk (usually T2, GS = 7, PSA = 10-20 ng/mL)	Active surveillance Radical prostatectomy External-beam radiation therapy to prostate, possibly to pelvis, with or without ADT Brachytherapy
Organ confined: high risk (usually T3, GS >7, PSA >20 ng/mL)	Radical prostatectomy (with adjuvant radiation therapy, if needed) External-beam radiation therapy to prostate and pelvis (usually with ADT) Brachytherapy plus radiation therapy (usually with ADT)
Climbing PSA level after local therapy	ADT: antiandrogen monotherapy or combined ADT Salvage radiation therapy (for patients with prior prostatectomy) Salvage radical prostatectomy (for patients with prior radiation therapy) Surveillance Investigational therapy
Node positive	ADT Pelvic or prostate radiation therapy + ADT Investigational therapy
Metastatic: untreated hormone-refractory prostate cancer	ADT Second-line hormones Sipuleucel-T immunotherapy Chemotherapy Investigational therapy

ADT = androgen-deprivation therapy; GS = Gleason score; PSA = prostate-specific antigen.

PROGNOSIS

In general, the 10-year PSA progression-free survival rate is 70% to 80% with well-differentiated tumors, whether treatment is with radiation therapy or surgery; 50% to 70% for intermediate risk tumors; and 30% for high risk tumors. For patients with a climbing PSA level after radical prostatectomy, time to detectable PSA, Gleason score at the time of prostatectomy, and PSA doubling time are important prognostic variables. The likelihood of bone metastases at 7 years ranges from 20% for good-prognosis patients to 80% for poor-prognosis patients. Patients require periodic surveillance and careful comprehensive medical care.[14]

For patients with microscopic nodal disease, the 10-year survival rate approaches 80% in men treated with androgen deprivation. The median survival period in men treated with androgen deprivation for established metastatic disease ranges from 2 to 6 years. The median survival period for men with metastatic castration-resistant prostate cancer approaches 3 years, a dramatic improvement from the survival reported even 5 years ago.

FUTURE DIRECTIONS

Molecular markers can not only identify patients at risk for the development of progressive disease but also act as therapeutic targets. In addition, the genomic characterization of prostate cancer subtypes will lead to risk-adapted therapy. Enhanced understanding of AR biology may permit the development of specific hormonal therapies and guide the more rational use of existing agents.

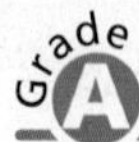

Grade A References

A1. Schröder FH, Hugosson J, Roobol MJ, et al. Screening and prostate-cancer mortality in a randomized European study. *N Engl J Med.* 2009;360:1320-1328.
A2. Andriole GL, Grubb RL 3rd, Buys SS, et al. Mortality results from a randomized prostate-cancer screening trial. *N Engl J Med.* 2009;360:1310-1319.
A3. Schröder FH, Hugosson J, Roobol MJ, et al. Prostate-cancer mortality at 11 years of follow-up. *N Engl J Med.* 2012;366:981-990.
A4. Ilic D, Neuberger MM, Djulbegovic M, et al. Screening for prostate cancer. *Cochrane Database Syst Rev.* 2013;1:CD004720.
A5. Andriole GL, Bostwick DG, Brawley OW, et al. Effect of dutasteride on the risk of prostate cancer. *N Engl J Med.* 2010;362:1192-1202.
A6. Thompson IM Jr, Goodman PJ, Tangen CM, et al. Long-term survival of participants in the prostate cancer prevention trial. *N Engl J Med.* 2013;369:603-610.
A7. Bill-Axelson A, Holmberg L, Garmo H, et al. Radical prostatectomy or watchful waiting in early prostate cancer. *N Engl J Med.* 2014;370:932-942.
A8. Steineck G, Helgesen F, Adolfsson J, et al. Quality of life after radical prostatectomy or watchful waiting. *N Engl J Med.* 2002;347:790-796.
A9. Wilt TJ, Brawer MK, Jones KM, et al. Radical prostatectomy versus observation for localized prostate cancer. *N Engl J Med.* 2012;367:203-213.
A10. D'Amico AV, Chen MH, Renshaw AA, et al. Androgen suppression and radiation vs radiation alone for prostate cancer: a randomized trial. *JAMA.* 2008;299:289-295.
A11. Jones CU, Hunt D, McGowan DG, et al. Radiotherapy and short-term androgen deprivation for localized prostate cancer. *N Engl J Med.* 2011;365:107-118.
A12. Bolla M, van Poppel H, Collette L, et al. Postoperative radiotherapy after radical prostatectomy: a randomized controlled trial (EORTC trial 22911). *Lancet.* 2005;366:572-578.
A13. Roach M 3rd, DeSilvio M, Lawton C, et al. Phase III trial comparing whole-pelvic versus prostate-only radiotherapy and neoadjuvant versus adjuvant combined androgen suppression: radiation Therapy Oncology Group 9413. *J Clin Oncol.* 2003;21:1904-1911.
A14. Warde P, Mason M, Ding K, et al. Combined androgen deprivation therapy and radiation therapy for locally advanced prostate cancer: a randomised, phase 3 trial. *Lancet.* 2011;378:2104-2111.
A15. Bria E, Cuppone F, Giannarelli D, et al. Does hormone treatment added to radiotherapy improve outcome in locally advanced prostate cancer?: meta-analysis of randomized trials. *Cancer.* 2009;115:3446-3456.
A16. Kantoff PW, Higano CS, Shore ND, et al. Sipuleucel-T immunotherapy for castration-resistant prostate cancer. *N Engl J Med.* 2010;363:411-422.
A17. de Bono JS, Logothetis CJ, Molina A, et al. Abiraterone and increased survival in metastatic prostate cancer. *N Engl J Med.* 2011;364:1995-2005.
A18. Ryan CJ, Smith MR, de Bono JS. Abiraterone in metastatic prostate cancer without previous chemotherapy. *N Engl J Med.* 2013;368:138-148.
A19. Scher HI, Fizazi K, Saad F, et al. Increased survival with enzalutamide in prostate cancer after chemotherapy. *N Engl J Med.* 2012;367:1187-1197.
A20. Beer TM, Armstrong AJ, Rathkopf DE, et al. Enzalutamide in metastatic prostate cancer before chemotherapy. *N Engl J Med.* 2014;371:424-433.
A21. Parker C, Nilsson S, Heinrich D, et al. Alpha emitter radium-223 and survival in metastatic prostate cancer. *N Engl J Med.* 2013;369:213-223.
A22. de Bono JS, Oudard S, Ozguroglu M, et al. Prednisone plus cabazitaxel or mitoxantrone for metastatic castration-resistant prostate cancer progressing after docetaxel treatment: a randomised open-label trial. *Lancet.* 2010;376:1147-1154.

GENERAL REFERENCES

For the General References and other additional features, please visit Expert Consult at https://expertconsult.inkling.com.

202

MALIGNANT TUMORS OF BONE, SARCOMAS, AND OTHER SOFT TISSUE NEOPLASMS

JAMES H. DOROSHOW

PRIMARY BONE TUMORS

DEFINITION

Primary bone tumors arise from cells that are normal components of bone tissues and that have the potential to metastasize. They are relatively uncommon malignancies (accounting for 0.2% of all neoplasms in the Surveillance, Epidemiology, and End Results [SEER] database, with 1.8 new cases per 100,000 population per year). Malignant bone tumors must be distinguished from a variety of more common benign bone lesions, such as osteochondromas and enchondromas.

CLINICAL MANIFESTATIONS AND DIAGNOSIS

Patients with primary malignant and benign bone tumors present with pain, swelling, and occasionally pathologic fracture of the involved bone. If radiologic studies suggest a malignant primary bone tumor (see characteristics of each subtype described later), an orthopedic oncologist should be consulted before carrying out a biopsy because improper biopsy technique may compromise subsequent surgical care, particularly limb-sparing surgery. Staging of patients with bone tumors generally requires computed tomography (CT) scans of the chest, abdomen, and pelvis to evaluate whether metastatic disease is present. Characterization of the primary bone tumor may benefit from magnetic resonance imaging (MRI) assessment of soft tissue extension or CT scan assessment of cortical bone involvement, or both.

MAJOR PRIMARY MALIGNANT BONE TUMORS

Myeloma, the most common primary bone malignancy, is covered in Chapter 187.

Osteosarcoma

Osteosarcoma is the most common malignant sarcoma of bone, representing about 35% of cases. It has a bimodal age distribution with the highest incidence in patients younger than 20 years of age, most likely related to the normal rapid bone growth that occurs during adolescence. In this age group most tumors arise in the metaphyseal areas of the long bones of the extremities, particularly around the knee. Males are affected more commonly than females at a ratio of 3 : 2. A second peak of incidence occurs in adults older than 60 years. The sites of origin in these older patients are somewhat more heterogeneous, with craniofacial and pelvic bones each accounting for 20% of tumors. Osteosarcomas are classified based on location, cell type, and tumor grade. All osteosarcomas contain varying amounts of osteoid, with most also containing some cartilage and fibrous tissue.[1,2] Radiographically, osteosarcomas usually present as mixed osteoblastic and osteolytic lesions, although pure forms of either appearance can occur. Periosteal elevation (Codman's triangle), cortical destruction, and tumor extension into soft tissue are common on plain radiographs or MRI.

The incidence of osteosarcoma is increased in families that carry germline deletions of retinoblastoma (*RB*), *TP53* (Li-Fraumeni), or *RecQ* DNA helicase (Rothman-Thompson, Werner, or Bloom syndrome) genes. Consistent with these observations, although most younger patients with osteosarcomas have no apparent predisposing factor or family history of bone tumors, alterations in the *TP53* and *RB* genes of such sporadic tumors occur in 40% and 60% of patients, respectively. In older patients, a variety of conditions may predispose to osteosarcoma, most convincingly antecedent Paget disease or prior radiation therapy.

TREATMENT Rx

Osteosarcoma is a highly proliferative neoplasm that metastasizes rapidly, most often by hematogenous spread; the most common site of metastasis is the lung. Despite aggressive surgical resection of the primary bone tumor, the incidence of recurrence with metastatic disease is high in the absence of systemic treatment, consistent with the concept that most patients present with clinically inapparent micrometastatic disease. The development of effective systemic chemotherapy with doxorubicin and cisplatin, with or without methotrexate, has had a profoundly positive effect on treatment outcome, with 5-year disease-free survival rates exceeding 65% in patients younger than 40 years with nonmetastatic extremity tumors.[A1] However, subsequent progress has been less striking.[3] Most patients are managed with initial neoadjuvant chemotherapy, delayed resection of the primary tumor, and then further postoperative chemotherapy. Serum alkaline phosphatase levels, often elevated in patients with osteosarcoma, can be used to monitor disease status.

Modern surgical techniques have allowed resection of most extremity osteosarcomas without amputation. Although resection of lung metastases can be curative in about 20% of selected patients, detection of radiographically-apparent metastatic disease at presentation significantly worsens prognosis. Long-term disease control in older adults with osteosarcoma is substantially lower than in younger patients, with a 5-year overall survival rate of 22% in one series of patients older than 65 years, most likely because of fundamental differences in the underlying molecular pathophysiology of tumors in older adults. Although osteosarcoma is generally considered to be relatively radiation resistant, radiation can play a palliative role in selected patients.

Chondrosarcoma

Chondrosarcoma is a malignant tumor characterized by hyaline cartilage differentiation; it is the second most common sarcoma of bone, representing 25% of bone sarcomas. The peak incidence is in the fifth to seventh decades of life. The most common primary sites are in the pelvis, proximal femur, and proximal humerus. Patients present with long-standing complaints of swelling, pain, or both. Radiographically, chondrosarcoma usually appears as a mixed lytic and sclerotic lesion.[4] MRI provides the optimal modality for determining the extent of marrow replacement by conventional intramedullary chondrosarcoma. Distinguishing low-grade chondrosarcomas from benign central enchondromas can be difficult; location in the axial skeleton and size larger than 5 cm favors malignancy.

Up to 15% of chondrosarcomas arise from preexisting peripheral osteochondromas and, similar to their benign counterparts, harbor mutations in the exostosin *(EXT)* gene. The remaining 85% of chondrosarcomas arise in a central location, some in preexisting enchondromas. Chondrosarcomas are divided into three grades, with higher grade tumors characterized by greater cellularity and cellular atypia. In one series, 61% of patients had grade 1 tumors; only 4% of such patients developed metastases. In contrast, 36% of patients had grade 2, and 3% grade 3 tumors; among this combined group, 29% developed metastases.

TREATMENT

Unlike osteosarcoma and Ewing sarcoma, chondrosarcomas generally grow slowly, metastasize less commonly, and have an excellent prognosis after adequate surgical resection. Although chondrosarcomas are considered relatively radiation resistant, radiation therapy may provide palliation for patients with large or recurrent, unresectable central chondrosarcomas.

Ewing Sarcoma

Ewing sarcoma and primitive neuroectodermal tumors (PNET) are a family of small round cell sarcomas that represent 16% of primary bone sarcomas. The molecular hallmark of Ewing sarcoma is the translocation between the Ewing sarcoma protein (EWS) and an ETS (E26 transformation-specific or E-twenty-six) family transcription factor. In 85% of cases, the t(11;22)(q24;q12) translocation between *EWSR1* and *FLI1* is detected, although other fusion genes have also been described.[5,6]

As with osteosarcoma, the peak incidence occurs during the second decade of life, but unlike osteosarcoma, the incidence of Ewing sarcoma is unimodal, being distinctly unusual in older adults and in nonwhites. Ewing sarcoma tends to arise in the diaphyseal region of long bones, in the pelvis, or in the ribs. Ewing tumors are characterized radiologically by a permeative or "moth-eaten" appearance of the affected bone, with a multilayered "onion-skin" periosteal reaction. MRI studies frequently document a significant soft tissue mass associated with the bone lesion. Unlike other sarcomas of bone, Ewing sarcoma may present with symptoms of an inflammatory systemic illness, with intermittent fevers, anemia, leukocytosis, and an increased sedimentation rate.

Eighty-five percent of Ewing's family sarcomas contain a t(11;22)(q24;q12) chromosomal translocation that juxtaposes the EWS gene on chromosome 22 with FLI1, an ETS family transcription factor. Another 15% contain a variant in which EWS is juxtaposed to ERG, another ETS family member on chromosome band 21q22. Because Ewing sarcoma resembles other small round cell tumors microscopically, reverse transcription–polymerase chain reaction and fluorescent in situ hybridization studies that document such translocations play a critical role in confirming the diagnosis. Ewing sarcoma/PNET cells characteristically express the CD99/MIC2 cell membrane glycoprotein.

TREATMENT

Patients with localized disease treated with multimodality therapy can achieve a 5-year event-free survival rate of 70%, but the 5-year overall survival rate of patients who present with overt bone or bone marrow metastatic disease at diagnosis is less than 20%.[5] The development of effective systemic chemotherapy regimens has substantially improved long-term control of Ewing sarcoma.[7] After completion of staging procedures, patients are treated with neoadjuvant chemotherapy. One highly active regimen alternates cycles of vincristine, doxorubicin, and cyclophosphamide with ifosfamide and etoposide. After 3 months of chemotherapy, the primary tumor is resected, radiated, or both, depending on the location and extent of the primary tumor. Chemotherapy is then resumed for a total of up to 1 year of treatment. Using such an approach, the mean 5-year event-free survival rate for patients who present with nonmetastatic disease is 73%.[A2][8] Insulin-like growth factor-1 receptor antagonists have demonstrated clinical activity in recent clinical trials for chemotherapy-refractory disease.

METASTATIC TUMORS TO BONE

Tumors metastatic to bone are important causes of cancer-related morbidity. Effective prevention and treatment of skeleton-related metastases are important parts of clinical care for many cancer patients. The most common tumors that metastasize to bone are breast cancer in women and prostate cancer in men followed by cancers of the lung, kidney, gastrointestinal tract, and thyroid.

Bone metastases typically present with localized or referred pain and less commonly as a new bone fracture. Plain radiographs may demonstrate blastic or lytic lesions. Although bone metastases from prostate cancer are often blastic and multiple myeloma usually lytic, most other tumors have a mixed appearance. In patients with one documented bone metastasis or in patients with widely metastatic disease and bone pain, a radiologic survey can identify bone metastases that may ultimately place the patient at risk for a pathologic fracture. Radionuclide bone scans are useful to delineate the extent of bone metastases and in following response to therapy. However, a negative study result must be interpreted cautiously because tumors that are potentially purely lytic (particularly multiple myeloma) may not be detectable by bone scan. In such tumors, a plain skeletal survey or CT or MRI scan is preferable. Routine screening for bone metastases is not indicated for cancer patients with no symptoms or signs of bone involvement.

TREATMENT Rx

In the absence of fracture or impending fracture, painful bone metastases are treated with external-beam radiation therapy. In patients with numerous bone metastases, systemic chemotherapy or endocrine therapy can play an important palliative role. Pathologic fractures or imminent fractures are generally managed by operative internal fixation.

PREVENTION

In patients with breast cancer, prostate cancer, and multiple myeloma, bisphosphonate therapy increases the time to a first skeletal event.[A3] Bisphosphonate therapy also appears to prolong survival in patients with metastatic breast cancer. The optimal schedule and duration of administration of bisphosphonates to maximize benefit and minimize potential complications remain to be established.

SARCOMAS AND OTHER CONNECTIVE TISSUE NEOPLASMS

DEFINITION

Sarcomas are tumors of mesenchymal origin that make up approximately 1% of human cancers.[9] They are a heterogeneous group of malignant neoplasms of connective tissues, including bone and soft tissue, comprising more than 50 histologic subtypes. Mesenchymal cells (derived from mesoderm), as well as neural crest cells (from ectoderm), give rise to connective tissues and provide critical functions such as support and nourishment to neural tissues. When growth, differentiation, or survival of these cells is aberrant, tumors arise, and this is the family of neoplasms to which sarcomas belong. Sarcomas include a vast array of tumor types related to muscle, stromal tissue, adipose tissue, blood and lymphatic vessels, nerves and nerve sheaths, cartilage, bone, and other fibrous tissues.

EPIDEMIOLOGY

Although very rare in adults, true sarcomas represent a disproportionately large number of cancers in the pediatric population (≈15% of pediatric cancers). The overall incidence of sarcomas of soft tissue and bone is approximately 15,000 cases per year in the United States. The prevalence of sarcomas significantly exceeds the incidence because sarcomas can be cured with expert multidisciplinary care. Hence, the initial evaluation and management of patients suspected of having sarcomas should be performed by an experienced team with relevant expertise and interdisciplinary capabilities (including expertise in sarcoma pathology, surgical specialization, and radiotherapeutic experience and judgment, as well as access to the latest systemic therapeutic agents).[10]

Certain patients are at high risk of developing sarcomas, most notably individuals in families with Li-Fraumeni syndrome and those with neurofibromatosis (at risk for malignant peripheral nerve sheath tumors and gastrointestinal stromal tumors [GISTs]) or familial polyposis (at risk for intra-abdominal desmoid tumors). Other risk factors include exposure to radiation (including radiation therapy for other cancers, such as patients with prior irradiated breast cancer or survivors of retinoblastoma). Chemical carcinogens can also increase the risk of sarcoma development, such as the increased incidence of sarcomas in Vietnam veterans exposed to Agent Orange or the greatly increased risk of hepatic angiosarcomas associated with occupational exposure to polyvinyl chloride. However, the vast majority of sarcomas appear to be sporadic, with no evident inciting risk factors.

PATHOBIOLOGY

Sarcomas and other connective tissue neoplasms are a heterogeneous mixture of diseases with a wide range of clinical behaviors and outcomes. Some soft tissue neoplasms, such as localized tenosynovial giant cell tumors, can be cured by expert resection, but more advanced tumors of this type (referred to as pigmented villonodular tenosynovitis) often lead to debilitating amputations or even death because of metastatic disease. Expert pathological review is necessary for the diagnosis of specific sarcoma subtypes; unfortunately, interobserver variability can impair even the most elegant diagnostic categories, such as those promulgated by the World Health Organization. Increasingly, knowledge of the molecular pathways that drive sarcomas has provided more objective diagnostic tools, including novel immunohistochemical staining patterns and genetic markers. In general, sarcomas may exhibit differentiation patterns consistent with defined connective tissues (e.g., well-differentiated liposarcoma may appear as only slightly bizarre fat cells under the microscope), or they may be unclassifiable. In any case, as diagnostic tools have evolved, it has become possible to place poorly differentiated tumors more accurately into certain histopathologic categories based on the expression of lineage-related proteins (e.g., smooth muscle actin expression may help categorize tumors as leiomyosarcomas) or on the basis of genomic markers (e.g., overexpression of chromosome 12 material or the *MDM2* gene locus is most consistent with a dedifferentiated liposarcoma). Recent studies have revealed that mesenchymal-to-epithelial transition (MET) may be operative in sarcomas, and MET may be an important basic biological and clinical process in tumors of mesenchymal original in general.[11]

CLINICAL MANIFESTATIONS AND DIAGNOSIS

Given the variety of sarcoma subtypes, it is understandable that the clinical course of these diseases can range from rapidly evolving and immediately life-threatening to indolent lesions that can take decades to evolve (e.g., atypical lipomatous tumors, also known as well-differentiated liposarcomas). Most patients with sarcomas present with a mass, often nontender, with a history of abnormal growth over time. For extremity tumors of soft tissues, it is important to note that many benign tumors (e.g., lipomas) cannot be easily distinguished from more worrisome neoplasms or even from frankly malignant sarcomas. Therefore, it is important to include sarcoma in the differential diagnosis of any mass.

The initial biopsy or surgical approach to a sarcomatous lesion is often the most important, and a poorly oriented biopsy or a suboptimal surgical procedure can make the difference between cure with full limb function and disease recurrence with the need for amputation or mutilating surgical re-resection. The National Comprehensive Cancer Network has developed expert consensus guidelines for clinical practice that emphasize the importance of expert management from the moment a suspected sarcoma presents. The initial diagnosis includes appropriate imaging studies of relevant anatomic areas, including plain radiographs, CT, or MRI to define the anatomic area of the mass and surrounding tissue, as well as systemic staging because sarcomas can spread in well-defined patterns to distal sites such as the lung or liver. The decision to proceed to diagnostic biopsy, with optimal orientation, is an important one, and for certain lesions, forgoing incisional biopsy and proceeding directly to expert surgical excision may be justified. The most important consideration is to make the correct diagnosis, and there must be sufficient amounts of properly prepared and expertly oriented tissues for optimal diagnostic analysis. In certain tumors with pathognomonic molecular markers (e.g., the translocation between chromosomes X and 18 that characterizes synovial sarcoma or the balanced translocation between chromosomes 12 and 16 that defines myxoid and round cell liposarcoma), molecular analyses such as fluorescence in situ hybridization may help mak the diagnosis. New molecular subtypes of sarcoma enter the pathology liter ture frequently; these new diagnostic categories may lead to the use of nove molecularly targeted therapies. Nowhere has this been more evident than i the rapid evolution of effective therapy against the major pathobiologic caus of GISTs (see below).

The diagnosis of a soft tissue sarcoma is made by evaluating biopsy materi in a clinical context, which includes understanding the tumor's anatomi location and imaging characteristics. Such contextual diagnostics are critic to understanding whether a lesion may represent a primary sarcoma c whether it may be the first presentation of metastases from an occult primar tumor located elsewhere. Given the broad spectrum of sarcomas, the diag nostic considerations are quite far reaching, especially because many benig pathophysiologic conditions can mimic sarcomas.

TREATMENT

The most important element of treatment is expert multidisciplinary care. The range of options is too broad to categorize simply, and the specific details of each patient's anatomy, comorbidities, functional status, and personal preferences must be taken into account when defining treatment options and management plans. Therefore, the care of virtually all sarcoma patients should be managed by an expert multidisciplinary team with expertise in advanced surgical or orthopedic oncology techniques, radiation therapy, reconstructive surgery, physical therapy and rehabilitation medicine, systemic therapies such as conventional cytotoxic chemotherapy, hormonal therapy, and modern molecularly targeted therapy with agents such as kinase inhibitors, and psychosocial support and specialized nursing care. Therefore, appropriate referral to obtain expert opinion and to define the diagnostic and treatment options for patients with suspected sarcomas is recommended.

For most localized masses for which sarcoma is in the differential diagnosis, the first step is to obtain the correct diagnosis in a manner that does not compromise patient outcome or function. The need for biopsy must be considered first because some small, localized sarcomas are best approached through definitive surgical excision following careful staging and expert review of imaging studies. For suspected sarcomas in deeper locations, such as within muscle compartments, or for large visceral lesions, biopsy may be necessary to ascertain that the process is in fact a sarcoma, as well as to fully characterize the histopathologic subtype. This may make the difference between initial management with chemotherapy, as might be appropriate for a highly chemosensitive disease, versus surgery, which might be appropriate for a less chemosensitive disease such as dedifferentiated liposarcoma. Expert opinion varies regarding the utility and timing of adjuncts to surgical resection, such as radiation therapy or systemic cytotoxic chemotherapy.

In general, expert surgical resection is the first-line of therapy for localized sarcomas. Preoperative systemic chemotherapy may be appropriate for some rhabdomyosarcomas. Many expert teams favor preoperative radiation therapy for certain sarcomas; irradiation of a large primary tumor can deliver smaller doses to surrounding normal tissues preoperatively compared with postoperatively, but this is a matter of personal preference. A randomized trial of preoperative versus postoperative radiation therapy for large sarcomas of the extremity was performed in Canada, and outcomes were similar, with subtle differences: patients who received preoperative radiation had a higher incidence of serious postoperative wound complications, but the long-term functional outcomes were slightly more favorable.

Many sarcoma centers disagree about the relative value of cytotoxic chemotherapy, although there is no doubt that chemotherapy has greatly improved disease control rates and cure rates of certain subtypes of aggressive sarcomas such as rhabdomyosarcoma. For other forms of sarcoma originating in bone (e.g., chondrosarcoma) or soft tissue (e.g., leiomyosarcoma, synovial sarcoma), there is no strong evidence that systemic chemotherapy increases cure rates or long-term clinical outcomes, although there may be some improvement in local disease control and recurrence-free survival. This has led to discordant expert opinion: many experts believe that the risks and toxicities of aggressive chemotherapy justify the benefit of longer disease-free survival, but others believe that such toxicities are not reasonable without a major improvement in overall survival. Limited series of postoperative adjuvant therapy are often contradictory owing to the relatively small patient groups under study, as well as divergent patient selection factors, such as the inclusion of those with a lower risk of recurrence or death from metastatic disease. Inclusion of a sizable percentage of sarcoma patients with low-risk disease no doubt dilutes the results of even a reasonably effective therapy and runs the risk of making the study result negative.

It is also critical to recognize that treatment may differ radically depending on the histologic diagnosis. The best example of this is GIST (also see Chapters 192 and 193), a form of sarcoma that, in more than 95% of cases, is driven by aberrant tyrosine kinase signaling.[12] Routine systemic chemotherapy is completely ineffectual against this disease; however, tyrosine kinase inhibitor therapy (e.g., with imatinib mesylate or sunitinib malate) produces dramatic tumor regressions and tumor control in more than 85% of patients. Fortunately, pathologists are increasingly able to recognize this disease histopathologically, and immunohistochemistry to detect CD117 (the Kit receptor tyrosine kinase) and DOG1 (a membrane antigen that is reasonably specific for GIST), as well as tumor genotyping via molecular genetics have significantly increased the accuracy of GIST diagnosis in the past decade. Imatinib has been approved by the Food and Drug Administration to decrease the risk of disease recurrence following resection of GISTs with significant potential for relapse. However, patients with a low risk of relapse have not derived substantive benefits from adjuvant imatinib because they have a very good chance of being cured by surgery alone.[A5] GIST is an excellent example of a sarcoma in which critical therapy decisions must be made in the context of the proper molecular diagnosis.[13]

For soft tissue sarcomas other than GIST, radiation therapy can play a meaningful role in preventing disease recurrence, especially for lesions that arise in the extremities. Radiation therapy can also provide significant palliation of unresectable disease, and it can be surprisingly effective in certain tumors such as desmoid tumor. However, radiation-associated sarcomas are increasingly common after therapeutic radiation therapy (e.g., in patients cured of breast cancer with radiation therapy), and an increasing incidence of poorly differentiated sarcomas or vascular sarcomas has been reported in patients after irradiation for other diseases.

As noted earlier, traditional cytotoxic chemotherapy is effective at increasing disease control and cure rates for certain sarcomas (especially those most prevalent in pediatric patients, such as rhabdomyosarcoma). It is less effective in improving long-term cure rates for patients with most other forms of soft tissue and bone sarcomas, such as liposarcoma, leiomyosarcoma, synovial sarcoma, and other subtypes. Nonetheless, appropriate use of chemotherapy can lead to objective responses in certain patients and can palliate those with metastatic disease with disease control and prolongation of progression-free survival. Targeted therapies hold potential promise for some sarcomas. For example, pazopanib, a multitargeted tyrosine kinase inhibitor at 800 mg once daily, improves the overall survival period from 10.7 to 12.5 months in patients who have metastatic nonadipocytic soft tissue sarcoma and who have had previous chemotherapy.[A6] Furthermore, a recent study demonstrated the first effective treatment for an uncommon, vasculogenic sarcoma of young adults, alveolar soft part sarcoma, with a multikinase inhibitor (cediranib) that primarily targets the vascular endothelial growth factor.

Sarcoma experts often disagree about the relative value and toxicity of combination chemotherapy as opposed to sequential single-agent chemotherapy. In patients with very aggressive and highly symptomatic sarcomas, clinicians may choose a combination chemotherapy regimen, even if there is a greater risk of toxicity, to ensure some measure of rapid disease control or even a greater chance of disease regression. In contrast, in patients with asymptomatic metastatic disease (e.g., a sarcoma patient with indolent pulmonary metastases and no symptoms), the optimal choice might be single-agent chemotherapy to avoid toxicity and to maximize the choice of subsequent chemotherapeutic agents after the benefit of the first agent is fully realized. There are no definitive data from properly powered randomized trials demonstrating that any chemotherapy for metastatic sarcoma of soft tissue (other than GIST) improves overall survival.[A7] All experts agree that owing to the complexity of the trials, the diseases, and the clinical settings, one must allow for variations in interpretations for individual patients. This explains the greatly discordant practice patterns observed across the country based on referrals, provider experience, and patient characteristics and preferences.

PROGNOSIS

Discussing prognosis for sarcomas overall is difficult because they represent such a variety of diseases with widely divergent natural histories. It is estimated that approximately 50% of patients with localized sarcomas can be cured, and the risk of recurrence is related to variables such as tumor grade (low-grade tumors have a lower risk of recurrence or metastasis compared with intermediate- or high-grade tumors), tumor size, and tumor location or depth. For patients with recurrent or metastatic sarcoma, outcome depends on many factors, including the time from initial diagnosis to the first appearance of metastatic disease; a longer disease-free interval is associated with longer survival, probably indicating a slower rate of tumor proliferation. Another factor that may determine outcome is the number of metastatic lesions; it is possible that oligoclonal metastases, with few lesions, can be surgically resected, which itself may be associated with improved survival.

Advances in targeted therapies have also affected survival, as documented by the dramatic improvements in survival and disease control for GIST and other kinase-driven sarcomas, such as dermatofibrosarcoma protuberans, giant cell tumor of bone, perivascular epithelioid cell–oma (PEComa), tenosynovial giant cell tumor, and alveolar soft part sarcoma. The natural history of these diseases will almost certainly be changed by a more mechanistic understanding of the underlying neoplasia-promoting signals that cause the transformation and maintenance of the sarcoma. Expert multidisciplinary management of sarcomas is critical to improving outcomes, and ongoing translational and therapeutic research will provide dividends far beyond the relatively low incidence and prevalence of these mesenchymal cell neoplastic disorders.

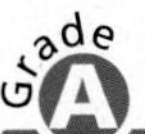

Grade A References

A1. Bernthal NM, Federman N, Eilber FR, et al. Long-term results (>25 years) of a randomized, prospective clinical trial evaluating chemotherapy in patients with high-grade, operable osteosarcoma. *Cancer*. 2012;118:5888-5893.

A2. Womer RB, West DC, Krailo MD, et al. Randomized controlled trial of interval-compressed chemotherapy for the treatment of localized Ewing sarcoma: a report from the Children's Oncology Group. *J Clin Oncol*. 2012;30:4148-4154.

A3. Barrett-Lee P, Casbard A, Abraham J, et al. Oral ibandronic acid versus intravenous zoledronic acid in treatment of bone metastases from breast cancer: a randomized, open-label, non-inferiority phase 3 trial. *Lancet Oncol*. 2014;15:114-122.

A4. Gastrointestinal Stromal Tumor Meta-Analysis Group (MetaGIST). Comparison of two doses of imatinib for the treatment of unresectable or metastatic gastrointestinal stromal tumors: a meta-analysis of 1640 patients. *J Clin Oncol*. 2010;28:1247-1253.

A5. DeMatteo RP, Ballman KV, Antonescu CR, et al. Placebo-controlled randomized trial of adjuvant imatinib mesylate following the resection of localized, primary gastrointestinal stromal tumor (GIST). *Lancet*. 2009;373:1097-1104.

A6. van der Graaf WT, Blay JY, Chawla SP, et al. Pazopanib for metastatic soft-tissue sarcoma (PALETTE): a randomised, double-blind, placebo-controlled phase 3 trial. *Lancet*. 2012;379:1879-1886.

A7. Sharma S, Takyar S, Manson SC, et al. Efficacy and safety of pharmacological interventions in second- or later-line treatment of patients with advanced soft tissue sarcoma: a systematic review. *BMC Cancer*. 2013;13:385.

GENERAL REFERENCES

For the General References and other additional features, please visit Expert Consult at https://expertconsult.inkling.com.

203 MELANOMA AND NONMELANOMA SKIN CANCERS

LYNN M. SCHUCHTER

MELANOMA

EPIDEMIOLOGY

Current estimates are that one of 37 men and one of 56 women will be diagnosed with melanoma during their lifetimes. Each year in the United States, approximately 76,690 new cases of invasive melanoma are detected, and 9480 patients die of melanoma. The explanation for the rising incidence is thought to be increasing sun exposure, especially early in life. Melanoma is the leading cause of death from cutaneous malignant disease, and it accounts for 1% to 2% of all cancer deaths in the United States. Melanoma affects all age groups; the median age at diagnosis is 50 years. Melanoma is largely a disease of whites, with a very low incidence in African Americans, Asians, and Hispanics.

PATHOBIOLOGY

Exposure to sunlight, especially ultraviolet (UV) radiation (Chapter 20), has been strongly implicated as a causative factor in the development of melanoma. Melanomas originate from melanocytes, which are located predominantly in the basal cell layer of the epidermis and use the enzyme tyrosinase to synthesize melanin pigment, which serves to protect against UV damage (Chapter 435). Worldwide, the incidence of melanoma in whites generally correlates inversely with latitude; that is, rates are generally higher closer to the equator and become progressively lower near the poles.

Risk Factors

Risk factors for melanoma include family history of melanoma, prior melanoma or nonmelanoma skin cancer, inherited genetic susceptibility, and sun

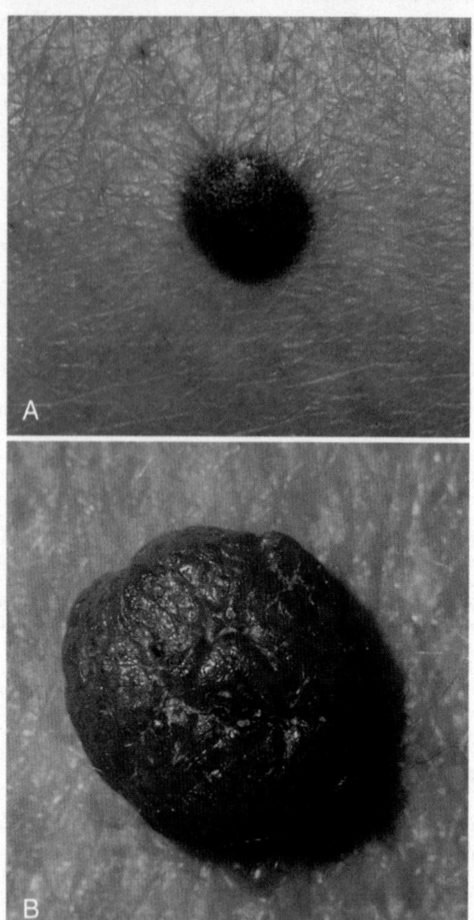

FIGURE 203-1. Nevi. A, Common benign nevus. B, Dermal nevus.

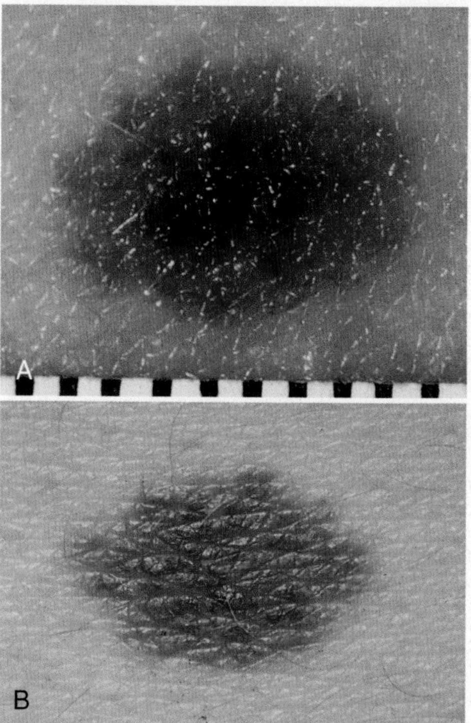

FIGURE 203-2. Dysplastic nevi. A and B, Examples of dysplastic nevi.

exposure. Artificial exposure to UV radiation by indoor tanning is likewise a risk factor for melanoma. Individuals with fair complexions, blond or red hair, blue eye color, and freckles, who have a tendency to burn rather than tan, have higher rates of melanoma. The pattern of sun exposure may also be important; intermittent intense exposure, rather than long-term exposure, may carry a higher risk of melanoma.

Individuals with an increased number of typical or benign moles, atypical moles, or dysplastic nevi (Figs. 203-1 and 203-2) also have an increased risk for melanoma. Atypical moles or dysplastic nevi are important precursor lesions of melanoma and serve as markers for increasing risk. For example, individuals with dysplastic nevi have a 6% lifetime chance of developing melanoma, and this risk increases to as high as 80% in individuals who have dysplastic nevi and a strong family history of melanoma.

Genetics

Approximately 10% of patients with melanoma have a family history of melanoma.[1] Several chromosomal loci determine susceptibility to melanoma, the most important of which is *p16/CDKN2A*, a gene located on chromosome 9p21. This gene is a member of a class of molecules that play a central role in cell cycle regulation. Of the members of melanoma-prone families, 25% to 40% have mutations in this gene. The risk of developing cutaneous melanoma in an individual who is a *CDKN2A* carrier is between 30% and 90% by age 80 years and varies by geographic location. Testing for mutations in the *p16/CDKN2A* locus is commercially available, but its clinical utility is unclear at this time. Genetic variability in melancortin-1 receptor (MC1R) plays a key role in pigmentation of skin and hair and more recently has been implicated in melanoma predisposition.

Somatic mutations in primary and metastatic melanoma primarily involve the mitogen activated protein kinase pathway. Activating mutations in *B-RAF* can be found in approximately 50% of melanomas, and 20% of melanomas are associated with a mutation in *N-RAS*. Recent studies have found that melanoma on mucous membranes, acral skin (soles, palms), and skin with chronic sun damage (i.e., lentigo maligna melanoma) have frequent mutations in *c-kit*. Thus, distinct patterns of genetic alterations are found in primary melanomas based on anatomic location and extent of sun exposure. Uveal melanoma is associated with mutations in *GNAQ/GNA11*. Monosomy of chromosome 3 and somatic mutations in the gene encoding BRCA-1 associated protein (BAP) on chromosome 3 have been associated with worse outcome and the development of metastatic melanoma. The discovery of somatic mutations in melanoma and associated aberrant signal transduction pathways has provided leads for the development of molecularly targeted therapy for patients with advanced melanoma.

CLINICAL MANIFESTATIONS

Early detection and recognition of melanoma are key to improving survival. The signs of early melanoma are based on the clinical appearance of the pigmented lesion and a change in the shape, color, or surface of an existing mole. Most patients report a preexisting mole at the site of the melanoma. Itching, burning, or pain in a pigmented lesion should increase suspicion, although melanomas often are not associated with local discomfort. Bleeding and ulceration are signs of a more advanced melanoma. Most melanomas are varying shades of brown, but they may be black, blue, or pink. The ABCDEs for the recognition of melanoma are asymmetry, border irregularity, color variation, diameter greater than 6 mm, and evolution or a change in a skin lesion. The "ugly duckling" sign is recognizing a pigmented lesion that looks different from other skin lesions and is therefore suspicious.

Cutaneous melanoma has been divided into four subtypes. Superficial spreading melanoma, which accounts for 70% of all melanomas, can be located on any anatomic site (Fig. 203-3). Lentigo maligna melanoma, which represents 4 to 10% of all melanomas, tends to occur more commonly in chronically sun-exposed skin in older patients, frequently on the head and neck (Fig. 203-4); clinically, it appears as a macular (flat) lesion, arising in a lentigo maligna. Nodular melanoma (Fig. 203-5) accounts for 15% to 30% of melanomas and manifests as a rapidly enlarging elevated or polypoid lesion, often blue or black. The ABCDE rule does not always apply as well to nodular melanomas. Acral lentiginous melanoma manifests as a darkly pigmented, flat to nodular lesion on the palm, on the sole, or subungually; sunlight is not thought to play a causative role in this form of melanoma. Histologic subtype does not directly correlate with clinical behavior. However, recent data suggest that histologic subtype may correlate with specific genetic abnormalities.

Ocular melanomas arise from the pigmented layer of the eye. Uveal melanoma is the most common intraocular malignancy of adults. Melanomas

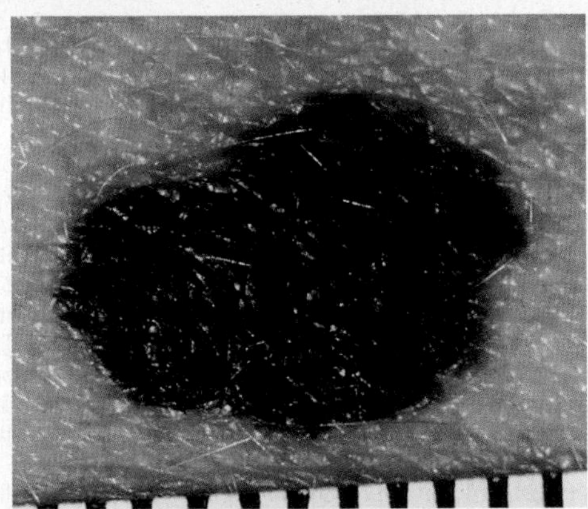

FIGURE 203-3. Superficial spreading melanoma.

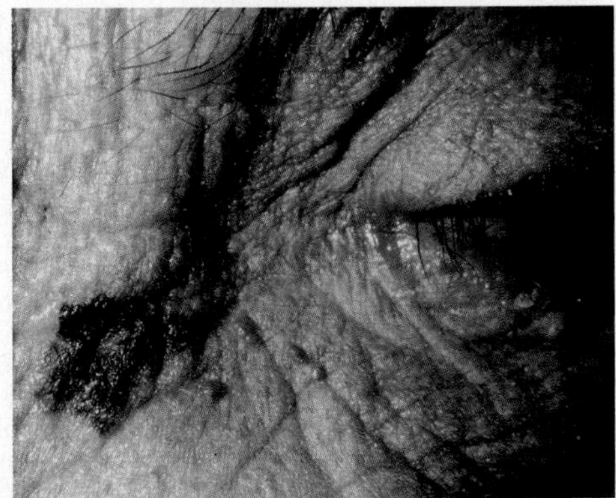

FIGURE 203-4. Lentigo maligna melanoma.

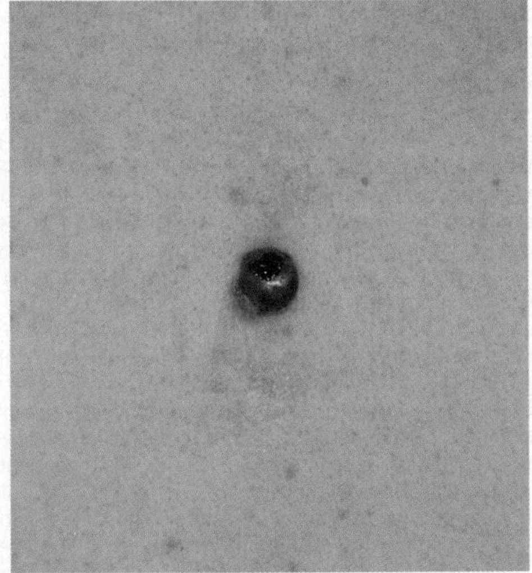

FIGURE 203-5. Nodular melanoma.

can also arise from noncutaneous sites, including mucosal epithelium in the gastrointestinal tract, anorectal area, genitourinary tract, and nasal and nasopharyngeal mucosa. Melanomas of the vulva and vagina are relatively rare. In general, mucosal melanomas are diagnosed at a more advanced stage of disease. The mainstay of treatment is surgical.

DIAGNOSIS

Any skin lesion suggestive of melanoma should be sampled using biopsy with complete excision, including a 1- to 2-mm margin of normal skin and some subcutaneous fat. An incisional biopsy may be necessary for lesions too large for complete excision. The role of sentinel lymph node biopsy (SLNB) is explained in detail in the Treatment section. Shallow shave biopsies, curettage, cryosurgery, laser, and electrodessication are contraindicated in lesions suggestive of melanoma. Other lesions that can be confused with melanoma include blue nevi, pigmented basal cell carcinoma (BCC), seborrheic keratosis, and hemangiomas (Table 203-1).

TABLE 203-1 CLINICAL FEATURES OF COMMON NEVI, DYSPLASTIC NEVI, AND MELANOMAS

DISEASE	CHARACTERISTICS
Common acquired nevi (moles)	These tend to be small, flat, and round; the border is regular, smooth, and well defined; the color is homogeneous, usually no more than two shades of brown; any site is affected; lesions are usually <6 mm.
Dysplastic nevi (atypical moles)	These occur predominantly on the trunk; they tend to be large, usually >5 mm, with a flat component; the border is characteristically fuzzy and ill defined. The shape can be round, oval, or misshapen. The color is usually brown but can be mottled with dark brown, pink, and tan. Some individuals have only one to five moles; others have more than 100.
Melanoma	The border is more irregular; lesions tend to be larger, often >6 mm; substantial heterogeneity of color is noted, ranging from tan-brown, dark brown, black, pink, red, gray, blue, or white.

Prognostic Factors

As with most malignancies, the outcome of melanoma depends on the stage and extent of disease at presentation. For localized melanoma, the most important prognostic factor is involvement of regional lymph nodes. The most important prognostic factor related to the primary tumor is the depth of invasion (Breslow's thickness) of the melanoma, which is measured in millimeters from the top of the epidermis to the underlying dermis. Increasing thickness is associated with an increased risk for recurrence, regional lymph node involvement, and death from melanoma. Whereas patients whose melanomas are smaller than 1 mm thick have about an 80% to 90% 10-year survival rate, patients whose melanomas are greater than 4 mm thick have only a 40% to 50% 10-year survival rate. Other poor prognostic factors related to the primary melanoma include the presence of ulceration, an increasing level of invasion (Clark's level), a high mitotic rate, and the presence of microscopic satellites. Regional lymph node involvement (stage III) has a major impact on survival, with 5-year survival rates ranging from 20% to 70%, depending on the number of involved lymph nodes. Melanomas that arise on the extremity tend to have a better prognosis, and women tend to do better than men.

Staging System for Melanoma

Staging and prognosis for melanoma are based on the TNM system, in which T refers to tumor, N to nodes, and M to metastasis, which was updated in 2009 (E-Table 203-1). Stages I and II indicate clinically localized primary melanoma, stage III indicates regional involvement (lymph nodes or in-transit metastases), and stage IV is metastatic disease beyond the regional lymph nodes (i.e., lung, liver, brain).

Patient Evaluation

The initial evaluation of a patient with melanoma includes a personal history, a family history, a total skin examination, and palpation of regional (draining) lymph nodes. The focus is to identify risk factors, signs or symptoms of metastases, dysplastic nevi, and additional melanomas. A chest radiograph and liver enzyme tests may be performed at the discretion of the physician. Most patients who present with melanoma do not have distant metastatic disease at presentation; therefore, extensive evaluations with computed tomography (CT) to search for distant metastases have an extremely low yield and are not indicated in asymptomatic patients. More extensive staging evaluation with CT or positron emission tomography (PET) can be considered in patients with high-risk disease (primary melanoma >4 mm thick or node-positive disease), in whom the risk of distant metastatic disease is higher.

TREATMENT

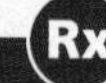

Primary Melanoma

After melanoma is diagnosed, the standard treatment is surgical excision. Several prospective randomized trials have been conducted to define the optimal surgery for primary melanoma. The extent of the surgery depends on the thickness of the primary melanoma. Large surgical excisions are no longer required, and most wide excisions can be performed with primary closure. For melanoma in situ, excision with a 0.5-cm border of clinically normal skin is sufficient. For melanomas less than 1 mm thick, a 1-cm margin is recommended. If the thickness is between 1 and 4 mm, a 1- to 2-cm margin is recommended.[A1] For melanomas thicker than 2 mm, 2-cm resection margin also is sufficient and safe. In cosmetically sensitive areas (face) or anatomically difficult areas (ear, hands), it may be difficult to achieve the desired margin, but at least a 1-cm margin should be obtained whenever possible.

Management of Regional Lymph Nodes

Clinically Normal Regional Lymph Nodes

In approximately 10% to 20% of patients who do not have clinically apparent lymph node involvement, lymph nodes contain occult micrometastases. The risk for occult lymph node involvement rises with increasing tumor thickness. Results from randomized trials fail to show a survival benefit from elective or prophylactic lymph node dissections in patients with clinically negative lymph nodes.

Sentinel lymph node biopsy is a technique that accurately evaluates whether microscopic melanoma cells involve regional lymph nodes. The technique relies on the concept that specific regions of the skin drain specifically to an initial lymph node within the regional nodal basin through an organized pathway of afferent lymphatic channels. This technique is performed by injecting the primary melanoma site with blue dye (isosulfan blue), radiolabeled colloid, or both. When both modalities are used in combination, a sentinel node can be identified in 98% of patients; biopsy of the node accurately determines whether melanoma cells have metastasized to that specific lymph node basin. The sentinel node technique also promotes a more comprehensive histologic examination of lymph nodes because limited amounts of pathologic material are submitted.

Sentinel lymph node biopsy allows earlier identification of metastases and is an important staging tool. The likelihood of detecting melanoma in SLNB increases with thickness of the primary lesion. SLNB is recommended to patients with melanoma 1 mm thick or thicker. The use of this technique for patients with thinner melanomas, that is, less than 1 mm thick can be considered if the primary has high risk features, is controversial. The SLNB is generally performed at the same time as the wide excision of the primary tumor. If the SLNB result is negative for melanoma, no further lymph node surgery is required. If melanoma is detected by the SLNB, complete lymph node dissection remains the standard of care. A recently reported randomized trial showed that the use of SLNB in patients with intermediate-thickness of thick primary melanomas provides accurate and important staging information; enhances regional disease control; and among patients with nodal metastases, improved melanoma-specific survival.[A2]

Clinically Apparent Regional Lymph Nodes

Surgical (therapeutic) lymphadenectomy is the preferred treatment of cytologically (fine-needle aspiration) positive or pathologically proven regional lymph node involvement with melanoma. The goal is to provide long-term, disease-free survival and reduce local morbidity of enlarged lymph nodes.

Adjuvant Therapy

Postsurgical adjuvant therapy can be considered for patients at high risk for recurrence (melanomas ≥4 mm thick or node-positive disease). These patients have at least a 25% to 75% chance of dying of melanoma. Adjuvant treatment options include interferon-α (IFN-α), enrollment in a clinical trial, or observation. High-dose IFN-α is the only U.S. Food and Drug Administration (FDA)—approved adjuvant therapy for patients with melanoma. Randomized clinical trials have shown that therapy with IFN-α can prolong disease-free survival but has not consistently demonstrated improvement in overall survival. The treatment is given for 1 year and is associated with considerable side effects, which require close monitoring. Intermediate and low doses of IFN-α as well as pegylated IFN-α have also been evaluated in a series of clinical trials. Pegylated IFN-α was recently approved by the FDA for treatment of patients with stage III melanoma. Numerous vaccine studies are ongoing but are considered experimental at present. Ipilimumab, a monoclonal antibody targeting CTLA-4, has been shown to prolong survival in patients with metastatic melanoma. Currently, ipilimumab is being studied in multiple phase III trials as an adjuvant therapy in patients with high risk melanoma.

Treatment and Course of Advanced Melanoma (Stage IV)

Melanoma can metastasize to virtually any organ, especially the lung, skin, liver, and brain. Until recently, the overall survival period for patients with metastatic melanoma has ranged from 5 to 11 months, with a median survival period of 9 months. However, new approaches with immunotherapy and molecularly targeted therapy based on somatic mutation profile have led to several recent FDA approvals of new agents that have redefined the standard of care for patients with metastatic melanoma.[2]

New immunotherapy approaches include ipilimumab, which blocks cytotoxic T-lymphocyte antigen 4 (CTLA-4).[3] Immunotherapy with ipilimumab has been shown to be better than dacarbazine alone (3-year survival rate, 21% vs. 12%) for previously untreated metastatic melanoma. Ipilimumab, 3 mg/kg intravenously every 3 weeks for a total of four doses, is FDA approved for patients with unresectable stage III or stage IV melanoma.[A3] Treatment with ipilimumab results in immune-mediated adverse reactions, including enterocolitis, hepatitis, dermatitis, and endocrinopathies such as hypopituitarism and hypothyroidism. Dose interruption of ipilimumab and corticosteroids are the main stays of treatment for this side effect mediated by T-cell activation and proliferation.

A second investigational approach to inhibit regulation of T-cell activation is to block the PD-1/PD-L1 (programmed cell death) pathway. Monoclonal antibodies targeting both PD-1 and PD-L1 are now in clinical trials. The first-in-class anti PD-1 antibody nivolumab, a fully human IgG4 monoclonal PD-1 antibody, has shown impressive clinical activity in patients with advanced melanoma.[A4] Another PD-1 inhibitor recently FDA approved is lambrolizumab, which also has significant clinical activity (response rate >40%) with fewer immune adverse events than traditionally seen with ipilimumab. Combining anti-CTLA-4 with anti-PD-1 immunotherapy has been encouraging in early non-randomized studies.[4]

The discovery of somatic genetic mutations in melanoma has provided leads for the development of molecularly targeted therapies. The MAP (mitogen-activated protein) kinase pathway, which is activated in most melanomas because of mutations in *BRAF*, *NRAS*, and *c-kit*, has been the focus of most clinical investigations of signal transduction (kinase) inhibitors. In patients with metastatic melanoma whose tumors harbor the *V600E BRAF* mutation, vemurafenib (960 mg orally twice daily),[A5] trametinib (2 mg orally twice daily), and dabrafenib (150 mg orally twice daily) each can increase 6-month survival rate significantly compared with dacarbazine. Squamous cell carcinoma (SCC) and keratoacanthomas develop in approximately 20% of patients with melanoma treated with vemurafenib because of paradoxical activation of MAPK signaling. Nevertheless, vemurafenib provides a median overall survival time of about 16 months in treated patients with *BRAF V600*–mutant metastatic melanoma. Recently, combination targeted therapy with dabrafenib (BRAF inhibitor) and trametinib (MEK inhibitor)[5] has been FDA approved based on results showing a 70% response rate and an acceptable safety profile. Combination therapy with several different regimens has now been shown to provide better progression free survival, better overall survival, and no increase in side effects in patients with metastatic melanoma.[A6][A7] Preliminary results also show that imatinib can induce regression in patients whose melanomas are driven by *KIT* mutations.

Surveillance and Follow-up

Patients should be educated on the clinical characteristics of melanoma, the importance of safe sun exposure strategies, and the performance of monthly self-examinations of the skin. Patients should be followed regularly for evidence of local or regional recurrence, distant metastatic disease, and a second primary melanoma. The intensity of the surveillance and the extent of the investigation are influenced by risk for recurrence with more frequent follow-up visits in patients who have thicker tumors or node-positive disease because these patients are at greater risk for recurrence.

For patients with low-risk melanoma (≤1 mm), visits are recommended every 6 months for 2 years and then annually. The surveillance guidelines for patients with high-risk melanoma include evaluation every 3 to 4 months for 2 years and then every 6 months for 3 years. After 5 years, patients are seen once a year. Patients are generally followed for 10 years. However, lifelong dermatologic examination is recommended, particularly for patients with dysplastic nevi or a family history of melanoma. In general, a history and physical examination are performed at each visit. Periodic chest radiographs, laboratory studies, and other imaging studies are performed at the discretion of the treating physician. The physical examination should include a thorough skin examination because at least 3% of patients develop an additional primary cutaneous melanoma within 3 years. Regional lymph nodes should be thoroughly examined, especially in patients without prior nodal surgery. For the remainder of the examination, one should keep in mind the frequency of metastases to lung, liver, and brain. Follow-up studies may include a complete blood cell count and chemistry studies, including liver enzyme tests. An elevated lactate dehydrogenase level suggests metastatic melanoma.

PREVENTION

The most important measures to prevent melanoma are to reduce excessiv[e] sun exposure, particularly to the midday sun, and to avoid sunburns. Sun[-]screen products with a sun protection factor (SPF) of 15 or greater an[d] protective clothing are recommended, and one randomized trial foun[d] that regular sunscreen use reduced incident melanoma by 50% and invasive melanoma by 75%.[6] Sunscreens block primarily UVB rays, which are considered to be the major causative agent of cutaneous cancers. Newer sunscreen products also block UVA rays, which may contribute to the risk of melanoma.

Screening for skin cancer, whether by self-examination or by a health care provider, is controversial (Chapter 15). Many public health experts do not recommend screening for adults in the general population, but some organizations do. On the basis of the type and number of nevi, family history of melanoma, prior melanoma, and history of severe sunburns, clinicians can identify patients who are at high risk for melanoma and who may benefit from screening programs. In several population studies, screening has detected melanomas at an earlier, curable stage. Physicians, other health care providers, and the public should be educated regarding the early signs of melanoma and the need for prompt biopsy of a suspicious pigmented lesion.

Patients with clinically atypical nevi (see Fig. 203-2), particularly if they have a family history of melanoma, require a regular dermatologic surveillance program. Regular skin examinations should be performed every 6 to 12 months, preferably assisted by the use of serial photography.

Recent studies have focused on the impact of vitamin D levels on the risk for melanoma, and results have been conflicting. The potential health benefits of vitamin D continue to be evaluated, both in terms of melanoma prevention and risk.

BASAL AND SQUAMOUS CELL SKIN CANCER

Nonmelanoma skin cancer (BCC and SCC) is the most common malignant disease in the United States.[7] Although national statistics are imprecise, an estimated 900,000 to 1,200,000 of nonmelanoma skin cancers are diagnosed annually in the United States. SCC accounts for 20%, and most of the remainder are BCC. SCC is associated with a higher absolute mortality rate; most of the 2300 annual deaths from nonmelanoma skin cancer in the United States arise from this tumor.

EPIDEMIOLOGY

Overall, skin cancer incidence rates are rising because of increased recreational sun exposure, longer life expectancy, and depletion of the ozone layer. More than 99% of nonmelanoma skin cancers occur in whites. These skin cancers are most commonly seen in elderly persons, especially those with fair skin and long-standing sun exposure. However, nonmelanoma skin cancers are increasingly being seen in people in their 30s and 40s. The lifetime risk of developing BCC is 30%.

PATHOBIOLOGY

Basal cell carcinoma arises from a pluripotential stem cell within the skin. Acquired mutations in the patched gene 1 (*PTCH1*), a tumor suppressor gene in the hedgehog signaling pathway, have been identified in cases of sporadic BCC. Sporadic BCC are also associated with mutations in the genes encoding p53 and ras.

Squamous cell carcinoma of the skin is a malignant disease of epidermal keratinocytes. Many such carcinomas are derived from actinic keratosis, a precursor that appears as a rough, scaly, often erythematous papule, which often is more apparent on palpation than on visual examination. Estimates of the likelihood of progression of actinic keratosis to SCC range from 0.025% to as high as 20%. Mutations in the gene encoding the p53 protein and in the *RAS* oncogene have been found in both actinic keratosis and SCCs. Mutations in *p16* have also been reported in SCCs.

Risk Factors

The most important risk factor is exposure to UV radiation from sunlight. The most clearly established association is with UVB radiation, but increasing evidence suggests that UVA is probably carcinogenic as well (Chapter 20). The timing and pattern of sun exposure are associated with different types of skin cancer. In general, SCC is associated with cumulative sun exposure and occurs most frequently in areas maximally exposed to the sun (e.g., the face, back of hands, and forearms). Intermittent, intense exposure to the sun, particularly in childhood, is associated with an increased risk for BCC. There is evidence for a dose-response relationship between artificial UV radiation exposure by use of tanning beds and the risk of skin cancers, especially BCC, and the association is stronger for individuals with a younger age at exposure.[8] Individuals who have fair skin, light-colored eyes, red hair, a tendency to burn rather than tan, and a history of severe sunburns are at increased risk for nonmelanoma skin cancers. Other risk factors, primarily for SCC, include chronic arsenic exposure, therapeutic radiation, chronic inflammatory skin conditions, psoralen plus UVA (PUVA) treatment for psoriasis and other diseases, and immunosuppression. Most cases in African American patients are associated with scarring or burns rather than UV exposure. Human papillomavirus infection (Chapter 373) has also been implicated in some SCCs, particularly in the autosomal dominant disorder epidermodysplasia verruciformis.

Basal cell carcinoma can be seen in association with several conditions, including the basal cell nevus syndrome (also called nevoid basal cell carcinoma syndrome or Gorlin syndrome), albinism, and xeroderma pigmentosum. The basal cell nevus syndrome is a rare autosomal dominant disorder caused by germline mutations in the patched gene (*PTCH*).

CLINICAL MANIFESTATIONS

Basal Cell Carcinoma

Approximately 90% of BCCs occur on sun-exposed areas such as the face, neck, ears, scalp, and arms. The nose is the most common site. Typical BCC appears as slowly growing, shiny, skin-colored to pink translucent papules with telangiectasia and a "pearly," rolled border (Fig. 203-6). As the tumor grows, the center may become ulcerated and bleed, although there is usually no associated pain or tenderness. BCC rarely metastasizes and is usually curable with a variety of treatments. Although the mortality rate is low, these cancers may result in significant morbidity owing to invasive local growth with potential disfigurement and destruction of skin, bone, and cartilage. Clinical trials with inhibitors of the hedgehog pathway for patients with advanced BCC have demonstrated very encouraging clinical activity.

Squamous Cell Carcinoma

This type of skin cancer usually appears on areas of skin that are heavily damaged by sun exposure. The most common sites include the head or neck, back, forearms, and dorsum of the hand. Clinically, SCC occurs as a discrete scaly erythematous papule on an indurated base that can develop on normal-appearing skin or on an actinic keratosis (Fig. 203-7). The lesion may grow

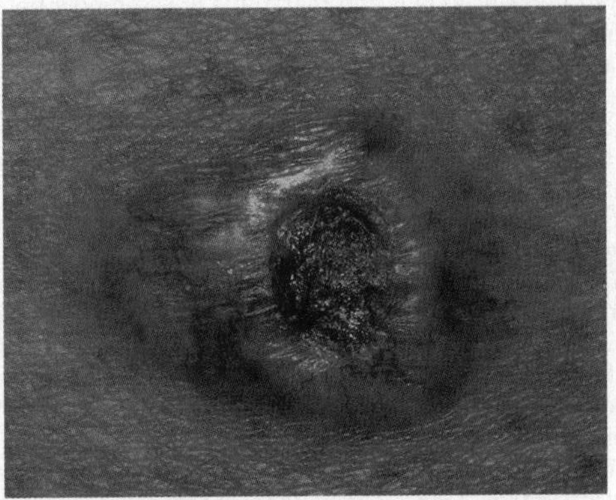

FIGURE 203-6. Basal cell carcinoma.

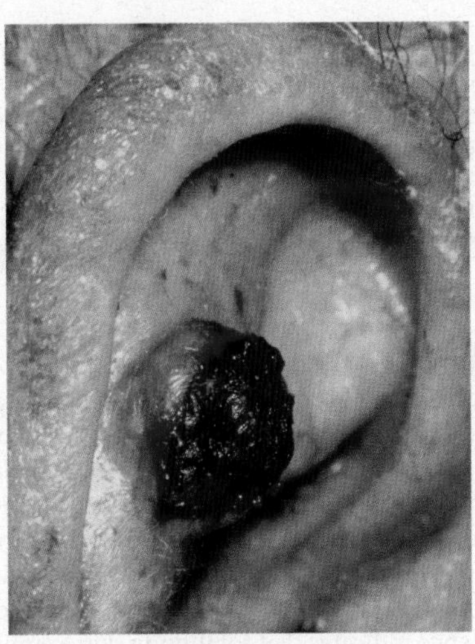

FIGURE 203-7. Squamous cell carcinoma of the skin.

over time and may become ulcerated, itchy, or painful and may bleed. Keratoacanthoma is a variant that is characterized by rapid growth and a crateriform appearance with a central plug. Bowen disease, or SCC in situ, manifests as an erythematous, scaly, sharply defined plaque.

Untreated SCC may cause significant local destruction. However, unlike BCC, SCC carries a 0.5% to 5% risk for metastasis. Higher risk lesions are those that are larger than 2 cm, are moderately or poorly differentiated, have perineural involvement, are located on the ear or the lip, arise in scars, or occur in immunosuppressed patients. Most metastases develop in regional lymph nodes, although metastases may also occur in lung, liver, brain, skin, or bone. For patients with lymph node metastases, the 5-year survival rate is less than 50%.

DIAGNOSIS

The diagnosis of BCC and SCC is frequently suspected by inspection alone, but histologic confirmation is usually indicated. Either a shave or a punch biopsy technique is acceptable (Chapter 436). Care should be taken to include the base of the lesion if a shave biopsy technique is used.

TREATMENT

Rx

Basal Cell Carcinoma

Basal cell carcinomas are classified as low or high risk based on their clinical features, location, and histology. Treatment options includes cryotherapy (liquid nitrogen), electrosurgery (i.e., curettage and electrodessication), topical treatment (i.e., 5-fluorouracil, photodynamic therapy, or imiquimod), surgical excision, Mohs' surgery, or radiation therapy. Mohs' microsurgery involves serial excisions of a skin cancer with subsequent microscopic examinations for residual tumor, providing histologic control of the surgical margins to achieve the lowest recurrence rate while maximally preserving uninvolving tissue.[9] The procedure should be considered when treating recurrent cases; microscopically aggressive forms, such as the morpheaform subtype; lesions greater than 2 cm in greatest diameter; and tumors of the ears, eyelids, nose, nasolabial folds, and lips. Cure rates for BCC range between 90% and 99%.

Treatment of advanced BCC and metastatic BCC can now be approached using targeted therapy. Vismodegib, an inhibitor of the hedgehog signaling pathway, has recently been FDA approved.[10] In a nonrandomized study, treatment with vismodegib provided objective tumor responses in 30% to 43% of patients and a complete response in 20% of patients with locally advanced or metastatic basal-cell carcinoma. Side effects associated with therapy include muscle spasms, taste abnormalities, diarrhea, and fatigue.

Squamous Cell Carcinoma

As with BCC, SCC can also be cured by traditional surgical excision or Mohs' surgery, cryotherapy, topical therapies, and radiation therapy. Topical 5-fluorouracil, photodynamic therapy, and imiquimod have roles in the management of in situ SCC. The optimal approach for a specific patient requires consideration of likelihood of the lesion recurring or metastatic potential, cosmetic factors, and the expertise of the treating physicians.

Mohs' micrographic surgery provides the lowest recurrence rate, with cure rates greater than 90%. Mohs' microsurgery is especially useful for recurrent tumors or lesions that have an increased risk of metastasis. Cetuximab, a monoclonal antibody that targets epidermal growth factor receptor (EGFR), has some antitumor activity in patients with advanced SCC of the skin.

Follow-up

Patients with BCC and SCC require ongoing follow-up to detect local recurrences and to recognize new skin cancers. The likelihood of developing a second BCC or SCC has been estimated to be 15% over 3 years. In addition, these patients have an increased risk of developing cutaneous melanoma. Patient education regarding modification of risk factors (i.e., sun exposure) is an important component of follow-up.

PREVENTION

Primary prevention strategies are aimed at reducing long-term sun exposure.[11] Public education and patient education should encourage the regular use of sunscreens with a SPF of 15 or greater, especially in childhood, and sun-protective clothing (e.g., a broad-brimmed hat). Avoidance of tanning parlors and minimizing of total sun exposure, especially to the midday sun, is recommended. The thinning of the ozone layer has been linked to increased UV radiation and increases in the incidence of nonmelanoma skin cancers. Currently, no evidence indicates that total-body skin examination is effective at reducing mortality or morbidity from nonmelanoma skin cancer.

Grade A References

A1. Gillgren P, Drzewiecki KT, Niin M, et al. 2-cm versus 4-cm surgical excision margins for prima cutaneous melanoma thicker than 2 mm: a randomised, multicentre trial. *Lancet.* 2011;37 1635-1642.

A2. Morton DL, Thompson JF, Cochran AJ, et al. Final trial report of sentinel-node biopsy versus nod observation in melanoma. *N Engl J Med.* 2014;370:599-609.

A3. Robert C, Thomas L, Bondarenko I, et al. Ipilimumab plus dacarbazine for previously untreate metastatic melanoma. *N Engl J Med.* 2011;364:2517-2526.

A4. Robert C, Long GV, Brady B, et al. Nivolumab in previously untreated melanoma without BRA mutation. *N Engl J Med.* 2015;372:320-330.

A5. Chapman PB, Hauschild A, Robert C, et al. Improved survival with vemurafenib in melanoma wi BRAF V600E mutation. *N Engl J Med.* 2011;364:2507-2516.

A6. Robert C, Karaszewska B, Schachter J, et al. Improved overall survival in melanoma with combin dabrafenib and trametinib. *N Engl J Med.* 2015;372:30-39.

A7. Larkin J, Ascierto PA, Dréno B, et al. Combined vemurafenib and cobimetinib in BRAF-mutate melanoma. *N Engl J Med.* 2014;371:1867-1876.

GENERAL REFERENCES

For the General References and other additional features, please visit Expert Consu at https://expertconsult.inkling.com.

204

CANCER OF UNKNOWN PRIMARY ORIGIN

JOHN D. HAINSWORTH AND F. ANTHONY GRECO

DEFINITION

The first signs or symptoms of cancer are frequently the result of metastase to visceral or nodal sites. In most such patients, the clinical diagnosis of meta static cancer is evident and is confirmed by biopsy of a metastatic lesion Subsequent clinical evaluation with a comprehensive history, physical exami nation, complete blood cell count, screening chemistries, chest and abdomi nal computed tomography (CT) scans, and directed radiologic studies base on specific symptoms or signs identifies the primary tumor site as well as th extent of metastatic disease. Patients who have no primary tumor locate after this clinical evaluation are defined as having *cancer of unknown primar origin*. Further clinical and pathologic evaluation identifies the primary sit in only a few patients, and approximately 80% never have a primary sit identified during their subsequent clinical course.

EPIDEMIOLOGY

In patients whose primary site of cancer remains undetectable, the primar site has presumably remained small or, less likely, regressed spontaneousl Before the routine use of CT or magnetic resonance imaging (MRI) fo diagnosis, large autopsy series identified primary sites (usually <2 cm i diameter) in 85% of patients with cancer of unknown primary origin, usuall in the pancreas, lung, and various other gastrointestinal (GI) sites. With th use of CT and MRI for diagnosis, however, primary sites are identified a autopsy in only 50% to 70% of patients.[1]

Approximately 4% of all patients with cancer have metastatic diseas without a known primary site; the annual incidence is approximately 80,00 cases in the United States. Cancer of unknown primary site occurs wit approximately equal frequency in men and women, and it increases in incidence with advancing age.

DIAGNOSIS

The initial clinical and pathologic evaluations should focus on identifying a primary site, when possible, and on identifying patients for whom specific treatment is indicated.

Biopsy and Pathologic Evaluation

The diagnosis of metastatic cancer should be confirmed by biopsy of the most accessible metastatic lesion. A fine-needle aspiration is usually sufficient to confirm the diagnosis of metastatic cancer but does not provide adequate material for optimum pathologic evaluation. Therefore, a larger biopsy (surgical or core needle) should be performed if technically feasible.

TABLE 204-1 RECOMMENDED EVALUATION AFTER INITIAL LIGHT MICROSCOPIC DIAGNOSIS

DIAGNOSIS	CLINICAL EVALUATION*	SPECIAL PATHOLOGIC STUDIES
Adenocarcinoma (or poorly differentiated adenocarcinoma)	PET CT of the chest and abdomen Men: serum PSA Women: mammography, breast MRI Colonoscopy (patients with colon cancer "profile") Additional directed radiologic or endoscopic studies to evaluate abnormal symptoms, signs, laboratory values	Men: PSA stain Women: estrogen and progesterone receptor stains (if clinical features suggest metastatic breast cancer) Molecular tumor profiling
Poorly differentiated carcinoma	PET CT of the chest and abdomen Serum hCG and AFP Additional directed radiologic or endoscopic studies to evaluate abnormal symptoms, signs, and laboratory values	Immunoperoxidase staining Molecular tumor profiling Electron microscopy (if other studies are indeterminate or conflicting)
SCC, cervical nodes	PET Direct laryngoscopy with visualization; biopsy of the nasopharynx, pharynx, hypopharynx, and larynx Fiberoptic bronchoscopy (if laryngoscopy results are negative)	—
SCC, inguinal nodes	PET Complete examination of perineal area (including pelvic examination) Anoscopy Cystoscopy	—

*In addition to a history, physical examination, complete blood cell counts, chemistry profile, and chest radiograph.
AFP = α-fetoprotein; CT = computed tomography; hCG = human chorionic gonadotropin; MRI = magnetic resonance imaging; PET = positron emission tomography; PSA = prostate-specific antigen; SCC = squamous cell carcinoma.

The initial light microscopic evaluation identifies adenocarcinoma in approximately 60% of patients with cancer of unknown primary site. Other diagnoses obtained by initial light microscopy include poorly differentiated carcinoma (25%), squamous carcinoma (10%), and poorly differentiated neoplasm (inability to distinguish among carcinoma, lymphoma, melanoma, and sarcoma; 5%).[3]

Additional pathologic evaluation is essential in all poorly differentiated tumors. Immunochemical (IHC) stains can usually identify the tumor lineage (e.g., carcinoma vs. lymphoma vs. sarcoma) when the histologic diagnosis is "poorly differentiated neoplasm." Because more than 50% of these patients have lymphoma, this distinction is important. When the histologic diagnosis is "poorly differentiated carcinoma," IHC staining sometimes identifies germ cell tumors or neuroendocrine carcinoma.

In patients with adenocarcinoma, it is seldom possible for the pathologist to determine a primary site by light microscopic examination of histology. IHC stains can narrow the diagnostic spectrum, particularly when interpreted in conjunction with clinical features. In several situations, IHC stains are quite specific, including prostate-specific antigen (PSA) for prostate cancer (Chapter 201), estrogen and progesterone receptors for breast cancer (Chapter 198), and leukocyte common antigen for non-Hodgkin lymphoma (Chapter 185). Other diagnoses suggested by immunoperoxidase staining include neuroendocrine carcinomas, melanomas (Chapter 203), and sarcomas (Chapter 202).

Occasionally, electron microscopy or analysis for tumor-specific chromosomal abnormalities (i12p in germ cell tumors, Chapter 200; t11:22 in Ewing tumor; immunoglobulin gene rearrangements in non-Hodgkin lymphoma, Chapter 185) are useful in the evaluation of poorly differentiated tumors if results of other pathologic studies are inconclusive.

Molecular tumor profiling is a new diagnostic method that is in the process of changing the management of patients with cancer of unknown primary origin. Gene expression profiles differ in various normal body tissues, and most cancers retain expression profiles specific to their tissue of origin. Molecular profiling assays can correctly predict the tissue of origin in 85% to 90% of metastatic cancers by detecting tissue-specific gene expression patterns.[4,5] Although the accuracy of the profiling predictions is more difficult to quantitate in patients with cancer of unknown primary origin (because most primaries never become manifest), current evidence indicates a similar high accuracy rate.[6,7] Therefore, molecular tumor profiling is a valuable addition to the pathologic evaluation, and is indicated when histologic examination and IHC do not identify a tissue of origin.

Search for the Primary Site

After completion of the brief, directed initial evaluation necessary to make the diagnosis of cancer of unknown primary origin (see the Definition section), further diagnostic studies should be limited (Table 204-1). The value of positron emission tomography (PET) in identifying a primary site is debated; in the only prospective study to date, PET results did not augment results of CT scanning.[8] Other routine radiologic and endoscopic evaluations of asymptomatic areas are rarely useful in identifying a primary site and therefore are not recommended. Levels of serum tumor markers, including carcinoembryonic antigen, CA-125, CA-19-9, and CA-15-3, are frequently increased in patients with carcinoma of unknown primary site; however, these elevations are nonspecific and should not be used to infer a primary site even though they can be useful in monitoring response to treatment.

Specific clinical presentations should trigger additional diagnostic evaluation. In all men with metastatic adenocarcinoma, serum PSA should be measured. Mammography and breast MRI should be considered in women with metastatic adenocarcinoma, particularly if clinical features are consistent with metastatic breast cancer (e.g., axillary node involvement, pleural effusion, lytic or blastic bone metastases). In patients younger than 50 years of age with poorly differentiated carcinoma, serum human chorionic gonadotropin and α-fetoprotein (AFP) levels should be measured to screen for germ cell tumors. Patients with metastatic squamous carcinoma involving cervical lymph nodes should have a thorough endoscopic evaluation of the head and neck, including visualization of the structures from the nasopharynx to the larynx and biopsy of any suspicious areas (Chapter 190). Fiberoptic bronchoscopy should also be considered in patients who have low cervical adenopathy and in whom no head or neck primary site is established by endoscopic examination. In patients with metastatic squamous carcinoma involving inguinal lymph nodes, all perineal structures should be carefully inspected, including by anoscopy, a urologic evaluation, and a pelvic examination in women.

TREATMENT Rx

Management of Specific Treatable Subsets

Because patients with cancer of unknown primary site have advanced disease, therapeutic nihilism has been common. However, several subsets of patients can benefit from specific treatment, and they can be identified on the basis of clinical and pathologic features (Table 204-2). These patients are important to recognize and treat appropriately because some individuals in each group have the potential for long-term survival.

Adenocarcinoma

Women with Axillary Lymph Node Metastases

Metastatic breast cancer should be suspected in women who have axillary lymph node involvement with adenocarcinoma, particularly when other metastatic sites are not evident. In these patients, pathologic evaluation of the

TABLE 204-2 SPECIFIC PATIENT SUBSETS AND RECOMMENDED TREATMENT

SUBSET-IDENTIFYING FEATURES		
HISTOLOGIC	**CLINICAL**	**TREATMENT RECOMMENDATIONS**
Adenocarcinoma	Women, isolated axillary adenopathy	Treat as stage II breast cancer
Adenocarcinoma, poorly differentiated carcinoma	Women, peritoneal carcinomatosis (Occasionally men?)	Treat as stage III ovarian cancer
Adenocarcinoma	Men, elevated PSA or blastic bone metastases	Treat as advanced prostate cancer
Adenocarcinoma, poorly differentiated carcinoma	Single metastatic lesion	Definitive local therapy (resection or radiation therapy [or both]) with or without chemotherapy
Adenocarcinoma	Colon cancer profile	Treat as metastatic colorectal cancer
Squamous	Cervical adenopathy	Treat as locally advanced head or neck cancer
Squamous	Inguinal adenopathy	Definitive local therapy (node dissection with or without radiation therapy) with or without chemotherapy
Poorly differentiated carcinoma	Young men with midline tumor or elevated hCG or AFP	Treat as extragonadal germ cell tumor
Neuroendocrine carcinoma, poorly differentiated	Diverse clinical presentations	Treat as advanced stage small cell lung cancer
Neuroendocrine carcinoma, well differentiated	Usually liver metastases	Treat as metastatic carcinoid tumor

AFP = α-fetoprotein; hCG = human chorionic gonadotropin; PSA = prostate-specific antigen.

initial lymph node biopsy should include staining for estrogen and progesterone receptors and for *HER-2* expression; elevated levels provide strong evidence for the diagnosis of breast cancer.

When no other metastases are identified, these women should be treated as if they had stage II breast cancer, which is potentially curable with appropriate therapy (Chapter 198). Modified radical mastectomy identifies a breast primary site in 44% to 82% of women even when the breast examination and mammographic findings are normal. Axillary lymph node dissection followed by radiation therapy to the breast appears to give results similar to those of mastectomy, although these two options for primary therapy have not been compared directly. Adjuvant systemic therapy should follow standard guidelines for the treatment of women with stage II breast cancer.

Women with Peritoneal Carcinomatosis

Adenocarcinoma involving the peritoneum in women usually originates from the ovary (Chapter 199), although carcinomas arising in the GI tract or breast can occasionally produce this syndrome. However, diffuse peritoneal carcinomatosis occasionally occurs in women who have histologically normal ovaries or who have had previous bilateral oophorectomy. The peritoneum is frequently the only site of tumor involvement, and serum CA-125 levels are usually elevated. When histologic features suggest ovarian cancer, this syndrome has been called *peritoneal papillary serous carcinoma* or *primary extraovarian serous carcinoma*.

Even when the histologic features are not typical, women with adenocarcinoma of unknown primary site involving the peritoneum often have cancers with biologic characteristics similar to those of ovarian cancer (Chapter 199). Treatment of these patients should follow guidelines for stage III ovarian cancer. When feasible, a full laparotomy with maximal surgical cytoreduction should be performed followed by combination chemotherapy with a taxane/platinum–containing regimen. Measurement of serial serum CA-125 levels provides an accurate assessment of the efficacy of treatment. A few of these patients may have complete responses and long-term survival, particularly when initial surgical cytoreduction leaves minimal residual disease. A similar syndrome of peritoneal carcinomatosis that is responsive to chemotherapy for ovarian cancer has rarely been reported in men.

Men with Skeletal Metastases or Elevated Serum Prostate-Specific Antigen Levels

Metastatic prostate cancer (Chapter 201) should be suspected in men with adenocarcinoma predominantly involving bone, particularly if the metastases are blastic. An elevated serum PSA level or tumor immunostaining for PSA confirms the diagnosis of prostate cancer. Occasionally, men with adenocarcinoma of unknown primary site and patterns of metastasis unusual for prostate cancer (e.g., lung metastases, mediastinal lymph node metastases) are found to have elevated serum PSA levels. These patients should be treated according to guidelines for advanced prostate cancer. Androgen ablation produces excellent responses and substantial palliation in most patients.

Single Metastatic Lesion

Occasionally, a single metastatic lesion containing adenocarcinoma or poorly differentiated carcinoma is identified, and a complete evaluation reveals no other evidence of disease. Such presentations can include a single lymph node or subcutaneous site or single lesions in various visceral sites, including bone, liver, lung, brain, and adrenal gland. The possibility of an unusual primary site mimicking a metastatic lesion should be considered (e.g., a subcutaneous nodule from a primary apocrine or sebaceous carcinoma rather than a metastasis), but this possibility can usually be excluded on the basis of clinical or pathologic features. PET is useful in excluding other metastatic lesions.

For patients with only a single identifiable lesion, definitive local therapy is recommended, guided by the site of tumor involvement. Such therapy may include surgical resection, radiation therapy, or a combination of these modalities. Although most of these patients eventually develop other metastatic sites, a significant disease-free interval is often experienced, and local treatment provides substantial palliation. The role of systemic chemotherapy in addition to definitive local therapy is not well defined; younger patients with poorly differentiated carcinoma or poorly differentiated adenocarcinoma are often treated with a short course of a taxane/platinum–based regimen.

Colon Cancer Profile

The accurate recognition of patients likely to respond to treatment for advanced colon cancer has become increasingly important because the efficacy of colon cancer treatment has improved substantially. In patients with cancer of unknown primary origin, a "colon cancer profile" includes (1) metastases predominantly in the liver, peritoneum, or both; (2) adenocarcinoma with histologic features typical of GI origin; and (3) typical immunohistochemical staining (CK20 positive, CK7 negative, and CDX-2 positive).[9] Patients with this profile should be treated according to guidelines for metastatic colorectal cancer (Chapter 193).

Squamous Cell Carcinoma

Cervical Adenopathy

Squamous cell carcinoma (SCC) of unknown primary site is relatively uncommon. Most patients with this syndrome have involvement of cervical lymph nodes, usually in the upper or midcervical area. Often, patients with this syndrome are middle aged or elderly and have a history of substantial tobacco or alcohol use or both. A primary site in the head and neck region should be suspected (Chapter 190); however, complete endoscopic evaluation fails to identify a primary site in approximately 15% of these patients. Even if other test results are negative, PET identifies a primary site in the head and neck region in approximately 25% of such patients and should be part of the initial evaluation.

Even when no primary site is identified, these patients should receive treatment with concurrent chemotherapy and radiation therapy,[10] as is currently recommended for locally advanced SCC arising in the head and neck. Combined modality therapy produces 5-year disease-free survival rates of 50% to 60%; multiple involved lymph nodes or nodes larger than 2 cm are adverse prognostic features (Chapter 190).

Inguinal Adenopathy

Occasionally, metastatic squamous cell cancer is found in inguinal lymph nodes. In most of these patients, a primary site can be located in the perineal or anorectal area. For the occasional patient in whom no primary site is identified, long-term survival can result from local therapy with inguinal lymph node dissection, with or without radiation therapy. Recently, combined-modality treatment with concurrent chemotherapy and radiation therapy has improved cure rates in patients with several SCCs arising in this region (e.g., cervix, anus, bladder). Although data are incomplete, a reasonable approach is the addition of chemotherapy with a platinum–5-fluorouracil regimen, as described for locally advanced carcinoma of the cervix.

Poorly Differentiated Carcinoma

Extragonadal Germ Cell Cancer Syndrome

Young men with clinical features of extragonadal germ cell tumors, including tumors in the mediastinum or retroperitoneum or those associated with elevated serum levels of human chorionic gonadotropin or AFP, should be treated according to guidelines for extragonadal germ cell tumors (Chapter 200). Some of these patients can be proven to have germ cell tumors by identifying an i12p chromosomal abnormality even when the diagnosis is not possible with other standard pathologic techniques. Approximately 30% to 40% of such patients achieve complete responses and long-term survival after chemotherapy with cisplatin, etoposide, and bleomycin as used for advanced germ cell tumors.

Anaplastic Lymphoma

An appropriate initial pathologic evaluation should identify most histologically atypical lymphomas. Occasionally, IHC staining for leukocyte common antigen is negative or cannot be adequately performed in patients with anaplastic lymphoma. The disease in some of these patients can be recognized using other IHC stains (e.g., Ki-1, CD-30), molecular genetic analysis (detection of immunoglobulin gene rearrangements), or molecular tumor profiling. All patients with lymphomas identified by special pathologic studies should be treated using standard guidelines for aggressive non-Hodgkin lymphoma (Chapter 185).

Neuroendocrine Carcinoma

In approximately 10% of poorly differentiated carcinomas, neuroendocrine features are identified by either IHC staining or electron microscopy. Treatment of these patients is discussed later (see Neuroendocrine Carcinoma).

Other Poorly Differentiated Carcinomas

In most patients with poorly differentiated carcinoma, there are no clinical or pathologic features that allow their assignment to any of the treatable subsets. These patients have a prognosis similar to patients with adenocarcinoma of unknown primary site, and treatment should follow similar guidelines.

Neuroendocrine Carcinoma

Poorly Differentiated Neuroendocrine Carcinoma or Small Cell Anaplastic Carcinoma

These high-grade neuroendocrine tumors are now reliably identified using widely available IHC stains. Although the origin of these tumors remains obscure, they are often highly sensitive to combination chemotherapy; platinum–etoposide chemotherapy as used in the treatment of small cell lung cancer, produces an overall response rate of approximately 60%, and 15% to 20% of patients have complete responses. In patients with locoregional disease, the addition of radiation therapy after chemotherapy is reasonable.

Low-Grade (Carcinoid-Type) Neuroendocrine Tumors

Occasionally, low-grade neuroendocrine tumors are found at a metastatic site. In almost all cases, the liver is the site of involvement, and the histologic features suggest a carcinoid (Chapter 232) or islet cell tumor of GI origin (Chapter 195). Various clinical syndromes caused by the secretion of vasoactive peptides (e.g., serotonin, vasoactive intestinal peptide, gastrin) have been described. Similar to other carcinoid tumors, these tumors often have indolent biologic characteristics, and patients can frequently survive for several years despite multiple liver metastases. Unlike poorly differentiated neuroendocrine tumors, these tumors are relatively resistant to chemotherapy, and intensive combination regimens should usually be avoided. Management of these patients should follow guidelines for metastatic carcinoid tumors (Chapter 232) and may include the use of somatostatin analogues, local ablative procedures (e.g., surgical resection, radiofrequency ablation, chemoembolization), targeted agents (e.g., sunitinib, everolimus), or fluorouracil-based chemotherapy regimens.

Empiric Chemotherapy

Approximately 70% to 80% of patients with adenocarcinoma or poorly differentiated carcinoma of unknown primary site do not fit into any of these defined clinical subsets. In these patients, treatment with empiric chemotherapy (usually taxane–platinum or gemcitabine–platinum combinations) has been of modest benefit, producing response rates of 30% to 45% and a median survival time of 9 to 11 months. However, empiric chemotherapy regimens, designed at a time when there was substantial overlap in the systemic therapy of different tumor types, are no longer able to provide adequate "coverage" as therapy for different cancers becomes more specific. At present, the standard of care is shifting from empiric chemotherapy to site-specific treatment, directed by the molecular tumor profiling prediction of the site of tumor origin.

Site-Specific Therapy Directed by Molecular Tumor Profiling

Molecular tumor profiling results in a prediction of the primary site in more than 90% of patients with cancer of unknown origin. Site-specific therapy has several potential advantages over empiric therapy, including the ability to appropriately incorporate tumor-specific targeted agents and to avoid unnecessary treatment in patients with unresponsive tumor types. In a group of 194 patients with cancer of unknown primary, assay-directed site-specific treatment produced a median survival period of 12.5 months.[11] Patients predicted to have more responsive tumor types (and therefore likely to derive the most benefit from site-specific treatment) had a median survival period of 13.4 months compared with 7.6 months for less treatment-responsive tumor types. In general, treatment responses and survival were consistent with the cancer type predicted; patients predicted to have breast or ovarian tumors had median survival periods of more than 24 months with site-specific treatment.[12] As additional treatment results become available, it is likely that molecular assay-directed, site-specific therapy will become the new treatment standard, with empiric chemotherapy reserved for patients whose tumors are unclassifiable by molecular profiling.

GENERAL REFERENCES

For the General References and other additional features, please visit Expert Consult at https://expertconsult.inkling.com.

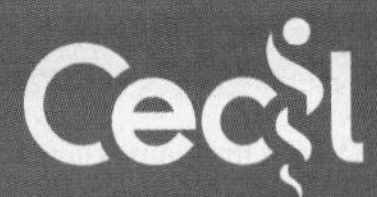

INDEX

Page numbers followed by "*f*" indicate figures, "*t*" indicate tables, and "*b*" indicate boxes.

D

E

Q

R

X

Y

Z

GUIDE TO THE APPROACH TO COMMON SYMPTOMS, SIGNS, AND LABORATORY ABNORMALITIES—cont'd

	CHAPTER	SPECIFIC TABLES OR FIGURES
Abdomen		
Hepatomegaly	146	Figure 146-5
Splenomegaly	168	Tables 168-7, 168-9
Acute abdomen	142, 143	Figure 143-1; Table 142-1
Abdominal swelling/ascites	142, 153	Table 153-3
Rectal bleeding/positive stool	135, 193	Figures 135-3, 135-4, 135-6; Table 135-4
Hemorrhoids	145	Table 145-1
Musculoskeletal/Extremities		
Arthritis	256	Figure 256-1
Edema	51	Figure 51-8
Cyanosis	51	
Clubbing	51	Figure 51-10
Neurologic		
Delirium	28	Figure 28-1; Tables 28-1, 28-2
Psychiatric disturbances	397	Tables 397-1 to 397-4, 397-6 to 397-8, 397-10, 397-11, 397-13, 397-14
Coma	404	Tables 404-1 to 404-4
Stroke	407, 408	Figure 407-1; Tables 407-2, 407-3, 407-5, 407-6, 408-5, 408-6
Movement disorders	409, 410	Tables 409-4, 410-1 to 410-8
Neuropathy	420	Figure 420-1; Tables 420-1 to 420-5, E-Table 420-1
Skin and Nails		
Suspicious mole	203	Table 203-1
Nail diseases	442	Table 442-4
COMMON LABORATORY ABNORMALITIES		
Hematology/Urinalysis		
Anemia	158	Tables 158-2 to 158-6
Polycythemia	166	Figure 166-2; Table 166-4
Leukocytosis	167	Figure 167-4; Table 167-1
Lymphocytosis	167	Table 167-3
Monocytosis	167	Table 167-2
Eosinophilia	170	Figure 170-2; Table 170-1
Neutropenia	167	Figure 167-7; Tables 167-4 and 167-5
With fever	281	Figure 281-1
Thrombocytosis	166	Figure 166-6; Table 166-6
Thrombocytopenia	172	Figure 172-1; Tables 172-1, 172-3
Prolonged PT or PTT	171	Figure 171-3
Urinalysis	114, 120	Tables 114-2, 120-6
Chemistries		
Abnormal liver enzymes	147	Figures 147-2 to 147-4
Elevated BUN/creatinine		
Acute	120	Figure 120-1; Tables 120-1 to 120-5
Chronic	130	Table 130-1
Hyperglycemia	229	Tables 229-1, 229-2
Hypoglycemia	230	Tables 230-1, 230-2
Electrolyte abnormalities	116, 117	Figure 116-4; Tables 116-6, 116-7, 117-2, 117-3
Acid-base disturbances	118	Figures 118-1, 118-2; Tables 118-1 to 118-6
Hypercalcemia	245	Figure 245-3; Tables 245-2 to 245-4
Hypocalcemia	245	Figure 245-4; Table 245-6
Hypo- and hyperphosphatemia	119	Tables 119-2, 119-3
Magnesium deficiency	119	Table 119-1
Elevated Pco_2	86	Figure 86-2
Chest Radiograph/ECG		
Solitary pulmonary nodule	191	Figure 191-2
Pleural effusion	99	Tables 99-4 to 99-6
ECG abnormalities	54	Tables 54-2 to 54-5

BUN = blood urea nitrogen; ECG = electrocardiogram; PT = prothrombin time; PTT = partial thromboplastin time.

GUIDE TO THE APPROACH TO COMMON SYMPTOMS, SIGNS, AND LABORATORY ABNORMALITIES

	CHAPTER	SPECIFIC TABLES OR FIGURES
SYMPTOMS		
Constitutional		
Fever	280	Tables 280-1 to 280-8
Fatigue	274	E-Table 274-1
Poor appetite	132	Table 132-1
Weight loss	132, 219	Figure 132-4; Tables 132-4, 219-1, 219-2
Obesity	220	Figure 220-1
Snoring, sleep disturbances	100, 405	Table 405-6
Head, Eyes, Ears, Nose, Throat		
Headache	398	Tables 398-1, 398-2
Visual loss, transient	423, 424	Tables 423-2, 424-1
Ear pain	426	Table 426-3
Hearing loss	428	Figure 428-1
Ringing in ears (tinnitus)	428	Figure 428-2
Vertigo	428	Figure 428-3
Nasal congestion, rhinitis, or sneezing	251, 426	Figure 251-1; Table 251-2
Loss of smell or taste	427	Table 427-1
Dry mouth	425	Table 425-7
Sore throat	429	Figure 429-2; Table 429-1
Hoarseness	429	
Cardiopulmonary		
Chest pain	51, 137	Tables 51-2, 137-5, 137-6
Bronchitis	96	
Shortness of breath	51, 83	Figure 83-3
Palpitations	51, 62	Figure 62-1; Tables 51-4, 62-5
Dizziness	51, 62, 428	Figure 62-1; Table 428-1
Syncope	62	Figure 62-1; Tables 62-1, 62-2, 62-4
Cardiac arrest	63	Figures 63-2, 63-3
Cough	83	Figure 83-1; Tables 83-2, 83-3
Hemoptysis	83	Tables 83-6, 83-7
Gastrointestinal		
Nausea and vomiting	132	Figure 132-5; Table 132-5
Dysphagia, odynophagia	132, 138	Table 132-1
Hematemesis	135, 153	Figure 135-3; Table 135-1
Heartburn/dyspepsia	132, 137, 138, 139	Figures 132-6, 138-2; Tables 137-3, 137-4, 139-1
Abdominal pain		Figures 132-1, 132-2; Tables 132-2, 132-3, 142-1
Acute	132, 142	Figure 132-3; Tables 132-2, 137-1
Chronic	132, 137	
Diarrhea	137, 140	Figures 137-1, 140-1 to 140-4
Melena, blood in stool	135	Figures 135-3, 135-4, 135-6; Table 135-4
Constipation	136, 137	Figures 136-3, 136-5, 137-1; Table 136-2
Fecal incontinence	145	Figure 145-5
Anal pain	145	
Genitourinary		
Dysuria	284, 285	Tables 284-3, 284-5, 285-2
Frequency	284	Table 284-3
Incontinence	26	Tables 26-1 to 26-3
Urinary obstruction	123	Tables 123-1 to 123-3
Renal colic	126	Figure 126-1
Vaginal discharge	285	
Menstrual irregularities	236	Figure 236-3; Tables 236-3, 236-4
Female infertility	236	Table 236-5
Hot flushes	240	Table 240-1
Erectile dysfunction	234	Figure 234-10
Male infertility	234	Figures 234-8, 234-9; Table 234-7
Scrotal mass	200	Figure 200-1
Genital ulcers or warts	285	Table 285-1